TEXTBOOK OF

CRITICAL CARE

Section Editors:

EDWARD ABRAHAM, MD
Section Head, Critical Care Medicine
Professor of Medicine, Division of Pulmonary Sciences and Critical Care Medicine
University of Colorado Health Sciences Center
Denver, Colorado

RINALDO BELLOMO, MB BS (HONS), MD, FRACP
Associate Professor of Medicine
University of Melbourne
Director of Intensive Care Research and Staff Specialist in Intensive Care
Austin and Repatriation Medical Centre
Heidelberg, Melbourne, Victoria, Australia

JEFFREY S. GROEGER, MD
Professor of Clinical Medicine
The Weill Medical College of Cornell University
Medical Director, Special Care Unit—Critical Care Medicine
Department of Anesthesiology and Critical Care Medicine
Memorial Sloan-Kettering Cancer Center
New York, New York

DANIEL A. HENRY, MD
Associate Professor
Department of Radiology
Medical College of Virginia School of Medicine
Virginia Commonwealth University
Medical College of Virginia Hospital
Richmond, Virginia

MICHAEL L. HESS, MD, FACC
Professor of Medicine
Chairman, Division of Cardiopulmonary Laboratories and Research
Medical College of Virginia School of Medicine
Virginia Commonwealth University
Richmond, Virginia

JOANN I. LAMB, MA, MSN, PA-C, FCCM
Physician Assistant
Lenox Hill Hospital
Clinical Instructor
Pace University–Lenox Hill Hospital Physician Assistant Program
New York, New York

PETER K. LINDEN, MD, DMD
Associate Professor, Departments of Anesthesiology/Critical Care Medicine and Medicine
University of Pittsburgh School of Medicine
Associate Director, Liver Intensive Care Unit
University of Pittsburgh Medical Center
Pittsburgh, Pennsylvania

MICHAEL R. PINSKY, MD, CM, FCCP, FCCM
Professor, Department of Anesthesiology/Critical Care Medicine
Director of Research, Division of Critical Care Medicine
University of Pittsburgh School of Medicine
Pittsburgh, Pennsylvania

KENNETH WAXMAN, MD, FACS
Director of Surgical Education
Santa Barbara Cottage Hospital
Santa Barbara, California

GARY P. ZALOGA, MD, FCCM
Director, Critical Care Medicine
Department of Medicine
Washington Hospital Center
Washington, DC

Managing Editor:

INGER GRENVIK
Pittsburgh, Pennsylvania

TEXTBOOK OF CRITICAL CARE

FOURTH EDITION

Senior Editor

AKE GRENVIK, MD, PhD, FCCM
Distinguished Service Professor of Critical Care Medicine
University of Pittsburgh School of Medicine
Director Emeritus, Multidisciplinary Critical Care Training Program
University of Pittsburgh Medical Center
Pittsburgh, Pennsylvania

Editors

STEPHEN M. AYRES, MD, FCCM
Professor of Medicine
Dean Emeritus, Medical College of Virginia School of Medicine
Director, International Health Programs
Virginia Commonwealth University
Richmond, Virginia

PETER R. HOLBROOK, MD, FCCM
Professor of Anesthesia and Pediatrics
George Washington University School of Medicine
Chief Medical Officer
Children's National Medical Center
Washington, DC

WILLIAM C. SHOEMAKER, MD, FCCM
Professor of Anesthesia and Surgery
University of Southern California School of Medicine
Los Angeles, California

W.B. SAUNDERS COMPANY
A Division of Harcourt Brace & Company
Philadelphia London Toronto Montreal Sydney Tokyo

W.B. SAUNDERS COMPANY
A Division of Harcourt Brace & Company

The Curtis Center
Independence Square West
Philadelphia, Pennsylvania 19106

Library of Congress Cataloging-in-Publication Data

Textbook of critical care / William C. Shoemaker . . . [et al.]; senior editor, Ake Grenvik; editors, Stephen M. Ayres, Peter R. Holbrook, William C. Shoemaker; section editors, Edward Abraham . . . [et al.].—4th ed.

p. cm.

Includes bibliographical references and index.

ISBN 0–7216–7246–9

1. Critical care medicine. I. Shoemaker, William C. II. Grenvik, Ake.
[DNLM: 1. Critical Care. 2. Intensive Care Units. WX 218 T355 2000]

RC86.7.T453 2000 616′.028—dc21

DNLM/DLC 98–28550

TEXTBOOK OF CRITICAL CARE ISBN 0-7216-7246-9

Printed in the United States of America.

Last digit is the print number: 9 8 7 6 5 4 3 2 1

This book is the product of more than 300 authors, all with excellent reputations for their devotion to outstanding, state-of-the-art management of critically ill patients during the worst phase of their disease when in need of intensive care. While we acknowledge the wisdom and foresight of the founders of the ***Society of Critical Care Medicine*** *and the important influence of the many leaders who have served as presidents of this Society, we realize that the true heroes are the patients themselves. Therefore, we wish to dedicate this new edition of our textbook to all current and future ICU patients.*

CONTRIBUTORS

KAREEM ABU-ELMAGD, MD, PhD
Associate Professor of Surgery and Advisor, Premedical Enrichment Program, University of Pittsburgh School of Medicine, Pittsburgh, Pennsylvania. Associate Professor of Surgery, Monsoura University, Monsoura, Egypt.
Intestinal and Multiple Organ Transplantation

AMAL M. ABU-GHOSH, MD
Fellow, Georgetown University Medical Center, Washington, D.C.
Hematopoietic Colony-Stimulating Factors

CHARLES G. ALEX, MD
Associate Professor of Medicine, Loyola University of Chicago Stritch School of Medicine, Maywood, Illinois. Director, Medical Intensive Care Units, Loyola University Medical Center; Foster G. McGaw Hospital, Maywood; Edward Hines, Jr. Veterans Administration Hospital, Hines, Illinois.
Assessment of Pulmonary Function in Critically Ill Patients

NICK G. ANAS, MD
Associate Clinical Professor, Department of Pediatrics, University of California, Los Angeles, UCLA School of Medicine, Los Angeles. Director, Pediatric Intensive Care, Children's Hospital of Orange County, Orange; Harbor-UCLA Medical Center, Torrance, California.
Drowning and Near-Drowning

HARRY L. ANDERSON III, MD
Assistant Professor of Surgery and Anesthesia, University of Pennsylvania School of Medicine. Attending Surgeon, Hospital of the University of Pennsylvania, Philadelphia, Pennsylvania.
Extracorporeal Life Support for Respiratory Failure and Multiple Organ Failure

DEREK C. ANGUS, MB, ChB, MPH
Associate Professor of Anesthesiology, Critical Care Medicine, and Medicine, University of Pittsburgh School of Medicine, Pittsburgh, Pennsylvania.
Appraising and Using Evidence in Critical Care

DONALD ARMSTRONG, MD
Professor of Medicine, Cornell University Medical College. Attending Physician, Memorial Sloan-Kettering Cancer Center, New York, New York.
Infections in Patients with Neoplastic Disease

JUAN A. ASENSIO, MD, FACS
Assistant Professor of Surgery, University of Southern California School of Medicine. Unit Chief, Trauma Surgery "A" Service, Department of Surgery, Division of Trauma Surgery and Critical Care, and Senior Attending Surgeon, Los Angeles County–University of Southern California Medical Center, Los Angeles, California.
Exsanguination; Penetrating Injuries of the Neck; Thoracic Injuries

STEPHEN M. AYRES, FCCM, MD
Professor of Medicine, Dean Emeritus, Medical College of Virginia School of Medicine, and Director, International Health Programs, Virginia Commonwealth University, Richmond, Virginia.
Introduction; Rapid Identification of Coronary Artery Insufficiency; Heat Stroke; The Ethics of Resource Allocation in the Intensive Care Unit

JUAN CARLOS AYUS, MD, FACP
Professor of Medicine, Baylor College of Medicine. Attending Physician, Methodist Hospital, Houston, Texas.
Sodium and Potassium Disorders

TIMOTHY J. BABINEAU, MD
Assistant Professor of Surgery, Harvard Medical School. Associate Program Director, General Surgery Residency, Beth Israel Deaconess Medical Center, Boston, Massachusetts.
Total Parenteral Nutrition for the Critically Ill Patient

EDWARD D. BALL, MD
Professor of Medicine, University of California School of Medicine. Director, Blood and Marrow Transplantation Program, and Co-Head, Conjoint Division of Hematology/Oncology and Bone Marrow Transplantation, University of California, San Diego, La Jolla, California.
Bone Marrow Transplantation

NILS U. BANG, MD, PhD
Professor, Pathology, Medicine, and Physiology, Indiana University School of Medicine. Director, Thrombosis and Hemostasis Services, Riley Hospital for Children, Indianapolis, Indiana.
Diagnosis and Management of Bleeding Disorders

CAROL A. BARCH, MN, CRNP, CNRN
Guest Instructor, University of Pittsburgh School of Nursing. Coordinator, Stroke Institute Program, University of Pittsburgh Medical Center, Pittsburgh, Pennsylvania.
Management of Acute Ischemic Stroke

RAFAEL BARRERA, MD
Instructor, The Weill Medical College of Cornell University and Memorial Hospital for Cancer and Allied Diseases, New York, New York.
Medical Complications in the Patient with Cancer

ROBERT H. BARTLETT, MD
Professor, General and Thoracic Surgery, University of Michigan Medical School. Attending Surgeon, University of Michigan Medical Center, Ann Arbor, Michigan.
Extracorporeal Life Support for Respiratory Failure and Multiple Organ Failure

THOMAS G. BAUMGARTNER, PharmD, MEd, FASHP, BCNSP
Clinical Professor, University of Florida at Gainesville, Colleges of Pharmacy, Medicine, Nursing, and Dentistry. Clinical Pharmacy Specialist, Shands Health Science Center, Gainesville, Florida.
Nutrition for the Critically Ill Geriatric Patient

DANIEL G. BAUSCH, MD, MPH
Research Assistant Professor, Department of Tropical Medicine, Tulane School of Public Health and Tropical Medicine; Assistant Professor, Department of Medicine, Section of Infectious Diseases, Tulane University School of Medicine, New Orleans, Louisiana.
Malaria and Other Tropical Infections in the Intensive Care Unit

ELIZABETH BEALE, MD
Research Associate, Department of Surgery, University of Southern California School of Medicine, Los Angeles, California.
Adrenal Insufficiency

RINALDO BELLOMO, MB BS (HONS), MD, FRACP
Associate Professor of Medicine, University of Melbourne. Director of Intensive Care Research and Staff Specialist in Intensive Care, Austin and Repatriation Medical Centre, Heidelberg, Melbourne, Victoria, Australia.
Prevention of Acute Renal Failure; Renal Replacement Therapy in the Intensive Care Unit; Acute Renal Failure in Infants and Children

MICHAEL K. BELZ, MD
Attending Physician, Tacoma General Hospital and St. Joseph Hospital, Tacoma, Washington.
Cardiac Pacemakers and Implantable Defibrillators in the Intensive Care Unit Setting

HOWARD BELZBERG, MD, FCCM, FCCP, FACP
Assistant Professor of Surgery, University of Southern California School of Medicine. Associate Director, Trauma/Critical Care, Los Angeles County–University of Southern California Medical Center, Los Angeles, California.
Adrenal Insufficiency; Critical Care Applications of Large Data Bases

GORDON R. BERNARD, MD
Professor of Medicine, Vanderbilt University School of Medicine, Nashville, Tennessee.
Management Controversies in Acute Respiratory Distress Syndrome

WALTER L. BIFFL, MD
Assistant Professor of Surgery, University of Colorado School of Medicine. Trauma Surgeon, Denver Health Medical Center, Denver, Colorado.
Role of the Gut in Multiple Organ Failure

CAROLE BIRDSALL, EdD, ANP, CCRN, FCCM
Associate Professor, Hunter College, City University of New York, New York, New York.
Complementary Modalities of Care: A Future That Is Here Now

GEORGE L. BLACKBURN, MD, PhD
Associate Professor of Surgery and S. Daniel Abraham Chair in Nutrition Medicine, Harvard Medical School. Director, Nutrition Support Service, Beth Israel Deaconess Medical Center, Boston, Massachusetts.
Total Parenteral Nutrition for the Critically Ill Patient

THOMAS P. BLECK, MD, FCCM
Louise Nerancy Professor of Neurology and Professor of Neurological Surgery and Internal Medicine, University of Virginia School of Medicine. Director, Neuroscience Intensive Care Unit, University of Virginia Health Sciences Center, Charlottesville, Virginia.
Seizures in Critically Ill Patients; Neuromuscular Disorders in Critical Care

ELANA J. BLOOM, MD
Clinical Assistant Professor, University of Pittsburgh Medical Center. Private Practice, Pittsburgh, Pennsylvania.
Bone Marrow Transplantation

RICHARD J. BOLD, MD
Assistant Professor, Department of Surgery, Division of Surgical Oncology, University of California, Davis, School of Medicine, Davis; University of California–Davis Cancer Center, Sacramento, California.
Cellular Signaling and Cell Death

CLARK ANDREW BONHAM, MD
Assistant Professor of Surgery, University of Pittsburgh School of Medicine, Pittsburgh, Pennsylvania.
Principles of Immunosuppression

LARRY BORTENSCHLAGER, MD
Attending Physician, Department of Critical Care Medicine, Methodist Hospital, Indianapolis, Indiana.
Obesity in the Critically Ill Patient

STEPHEN A. BOWLES, MD
Assistant Professor, Department of Anesthesiology/Critical Care Medicine, University of Pittsburgh School of Medicine. Staff, University of Pittsburgh Medical Center, Pittsburgh, Pennsylvania.
Pancreas Transplantation

PHILIP G. BOYSEN, MD
Professor of Anesthesiology and Medicine, and Chair, Department of Anesthesiology, University of North Carolina at Chapel Hill School of Medicine, Chapel Hill, North Carolina.
Pulmonary Aspiration

FRANCISCO BRACHO, MD
Fellow, Georgetown University Medical Center, Washington, D.C.
Hematopoietic Colony-Stimulating Factors

GORDON L. BRAY, MD
Medical Director, Baxter-Healthcare–Hyland, Immunology, Glendale, California.
Bleeding Disorders of Childhood

LAURENT J. BROCHARD, MD
Professor of Intensive Care Medicine, Université Paris XII, and Service de Réanimation Médicale, Hôpital Henri Mondor, Creteil, France.
Noninvasive Ventilation

BRIAN A. BROZNICK, CPTC
Executive Director/CEO, Center for Organ Recovery and Education, Pittsburgh, Pennsylvania.
History and Organization of Organ Transplantation

DEREK A. BRUCE, MB, ChB
Clinical Associate Professor of Neurosurgery, University of Texas Southwestern Medical Center at Dallas Southwestern Medical School. Attending Neurosurgeon, Children's Medical Center of Dallas and Medical City Dallas Hospital, Dallas, Texas.
Pediatric Neurosurgical Emergencies

SUSAN I. BRUNDAGE, MD, MPH
Trauma/Surgical Critical Care Fellow and Clinical Instructor, University of Washington School of Medicine; Harborview Medical Center, Seattle, Washington.
Trauma to the Pregnant Patient

TIMOTHY G. BUCHMAN, PhD, MD, FACS, FCCM
Professor of Surgery, Anesthesiology, and Medicine, Washington University School of Medicine. Director of Burn, Trauma, Surgical Critical Care, Barnes-Jewish Hospital, Saint Louis, Missouri.
Regulation of Gene Expression

JAVIER BUENO, MD
Visiting Instructor in Surgery, University of Pittsburgh School of Medicine, Pittsburgh, Pennsylvania.
Intestinal and Multiple Organ Transplantation

MITCHELL S. CAIRO, MD, FAAP
Professor of Pediatrics, Medicine, and Pathology, Georgetown University School of Medicine, Washington, D.C.
Hematopoietic Colony-Stimulating Factors

CARLOS CARAMELO, MD
Associate Professor Autonoma, University of Madrid. Attending Physician, Renal Laboratory, Fundacion Jimenez Diaz, Madrid, Spain.
Sodium and Potassium Disorders

JOSEPH A. CARCILLO, JR, MD
Assistant Professor, Department of Anesthesiology, Critical Care Medicine, and Pediatrics, University of Pittsburgh School of Medicine. Associate Director, Pediatric Intensive Care Unit, Children's Hospital of Pittsburgh, Pittsburgh, Pennsylvania.
Genetic Influences on Critical Illness

GRAZIANO C. CARLON, MD
Professor of Anesthesiology, The Weill Medical College of Cornell University. Member, Department of Anesthesiology and Critical Care Medicine, Memorial Hospital, New York, New York.
Intensive Care of the Cancer Patient

RICHARD W. CARLSON, MD, PhD, FCCM
Professor of Medicine, Mayo Medical School, Scottsdale; Professor of Clinical Medicine, University of Arizona College of Medicine, Tucson. Chair, Department of Medicine, Maricopa Medical Center, Phoenix, Arizona.
Injuries by Venomous and Poisonous Animals; Anaphylactic Reactions; Building Bedside Collaborative Practice

VIRGINIA R. CARLSON, MSN, MBA, RN, FCCM
Department Director, Intensive Care Unit, Dartmouth-Hitchcock Medical Center, Lebanon, New Hampshire.
Barriers to Effective Patient Care

DONNA A. CASTELLO, DO
Assistant Professor, Department of Anesthesiology, Albany Medical College. Attending Anesthesiologist, Albany Medical Center Hospital, Albany, New York.
Conventional Airway Access

SANTIAGO CHAHWAN, MD
International Research Fellow, Department of Surgery, Division of Trauma Surgery and Critical Care, University of Southern California–Los Angeles County Medical Center, Los Angeles, California.
Exsanguination; Thoracic Injuries

JEAN CHASTRE, MD
Professor of Medicine, Université Páris 7. Assistant Director, Intensive Care Unit, Hôpital Bichat, Paris, France.
Severe Community-Acquired Pneumonia; Nosocomial Pneumonia

LAKSHMIPATHI CHELLURI, MD, MPH
Associate Professor, Department of Anesthesiology/Critical Care Medicine, University of Pittsburgh School of Medicine. Attending Physician, University of Pittsburgh Medical Center, Pittsburgh, Pennsylvania.
Critical Care of Kidney Transplant Recipients

GLENN CHERTOW, MD, MPH
Assistant Professor of Medicine in Residence, University of California School of Medicine. Director, Clinical Services, Division of Nephrology, Moffitt-Long Hospitals and Mount Zion–University of California Medical Center, San Francisco, California.
Renal Replacement Therapy in the Intensive Care Unit

WALTER J. CHWALS, MD
Professor of Surgery and Pediatrics, and Chief, Section of Pediatric Surgery, University of Chicago Pritzker School of Medicine. Surgeon-in-Chief, University of Chicago Children's Hospital, Chicago, Illinois.
Pediatric Enteral and Parenteral Surgical Nutrition

JACQUELINE J. COALSON, PhD
Professor of Pathology, University of Texas Medical School at San Antonio, San Antonio, Texas.
Bacterial Pneumonia in Adult Respiratory Distress Syndrome; Pathology of Acute Lung Injury

TIMOTHY J. COLE, MD
Assistant Professor, Department of Radiology, Medical College of Virginia School of Medicine, Virginia Commonwealth University; Medical College of Virginia Hospitals, Richmond, Virginia.
Critical Care Imaging of the Chest

JAMES A. COOK, PhD
Professor of Physiology, Medical University of South Carolina College of Medicine, Charleston, South Carolina.
Prostaglandins, Thromboxanes, Leukotrienes, and Other Products of Arachidonic Acid

LYNN COPPAGE, MD
Assistant Professor, Department of Radiology, Medical University of South Carolina College of Medicine, Charleston, South Carolina.
Critical Care Imaging of the Chest

EDWARD E. CORNWELL III, MD
Associate Professor of Surgery, Johns Hopkins University School of Medicine. Chief of Trauma, Johns Hopkins Hospital, Baltimore, Maryland.
Abdominal Trauma

ROBERT J. CORRY, MD
Professor of Surgery, University of Pittsburgh School of Medicine. Director of Pancreas Transplantation, University of Pittsburgh Medical Center, Pittsburgh, Pennsylvania.
Pancreas Transplantation

PAUL J. CORSO, MD, FACS, FACC
Clinical Professor of Surgery, George Washington University School of Medicine and Health Sciences. Director, Section of Cardiac Surgery, Washington Hospital Center, Washington, D.C.
New Techniques in Management of the Cardiac Surgery Patient

JOHN A. DALLER, MD, PhD
Surgical Critical Care Fellow, Multidisciplinary Critical Care Training Program, University of Pittsburgh School of Medicine, Pittsburgh, Pennsylvania.
Alternative Organ Donor Categories

JOSEPH M. DARBY, MD
Associate Professor, Department of Anesthesiology/Critical Care Medicine and Department of Surgery, University of Pittsburgh School of Medicine. Medical Director, Trauma/Surgical Intensive Care Unit, Presbyterian University Hospital, Pittsburgh, Pennsylvania.
Brain Death—Definition, Determination, and Physiologic Effects on Donor Organs

LAKSHMANA DAS NARLA, MD
Associate Professor of Radiology and Pediatrics, Medical College of Virginia School of Medicine, Virginia Commonwealth University, Richmond, Virginia.
Chest Imaging in Pediatric Intensive Care

JAMES H. DAUBER, MD, FCCP
Professor of Medicine, University of Pittsburgh School of Medicine. Medical Director of Lung Transplantation, University of Pittsburgh Medical Center, Pittsburgh, Pennsylvania.
Critical Care Aspects of Lung Transplantation

ANDREW R. DAVIES, MBBS, FRACP
Intensivist, Alfred Hospital, Melbourne, Victoria, Australia.
Independent Lung Ventilation

JILL K. DAVIES, MD
Instructor, Department of Obstetrics and Gynecology, University of Colorado School of Medicine, Denver, Colorado.
Trauma to the Pregnant Patient

GUY DE L. DEAR, MB, FRCA
Assistant Professor of Anesthesiology, Duke University School of Medicine. Attending Anesthesiologist, Duke University Medical Center, Durham, North Carolina.
Hyperbaric Oxygen in Critical Care

GERMAN D. DEJOYA, MD
Senior Fellow, Critical Care Medicine, Multidisciplinary Critical Care Medicine Training Program, University of Pittsburgh School of Medicine, Pittsburgh, Pennsylvania.
Brain Death—Definition, Determination, and Physiologic Effects on Donor Organs

MARGARIDA DE MAGALHAES-SILVERMAN, MD
Associate Professor, Department of Medicine, Division of Hematology/Oncology, University of Iowa School of Medicine, Iowa City, Iowa.
Bone Marrow Transplantation

DEMETRIOS DEMETRIADES, MD, PhD, FACS
Professor of Surgery, University of Southern California School of Medicine. Attending Surgeon and Chief, Division of Trauma and Critical Care, Los Angeles County–University of Southern California Medical Center, Los Angeles, California.
Common Bedside Procedures in the Intensive Care Unit; Penetrating Injuries of the Neck

ANDRÉ DE TROYER, MD, PhD
Director, Laboratory of Cardiorespiratory Physiology, Brussels School of Medicine. Professor of Medicine, Chest Service, Erasme University Hospital, Brussels, Belgium.
Respiratory Muscle Function

MICHAEL A. DEVITA, MD
Assistant Professor, Department of Anesthesiology/Critical Care Medicine and Department of Internal Medicine, University of Pittsburgh School of Medicine. Assistant Medical Director, Institute for Quality and Medical Management, University of Pittsburgh Medical Center, Pittsburgh, Pennsylvania.
Forgoing Life-Sustaining Therapy in Intensive Care

JOHN W. DEVLIN, PharmD
Adjunct Assistant Professor of Pharmacy, College of Pharmacy and Allied Health Professions, Wayne State University. Clinical Pharmacy Specialist, Surgery/Critical Care, Detroit Receiving Hospital and University Health Center, Detroit, Michigan.
Alterations in Drug Disposition in the Elderly

DONALD J. DEYO, DVM
Assistant Professor of Anesthesiology and Coordinator of Large Animal Services, University of Texas Medical Branch, University of Texas Medical School at Galveston, Galveston, Texas.
Brain Function Monitoring

S. FORREST DODSON, MD
Assistant Professor of Surgery, University of Pittsburgh School of Medicine, Pittsburgh, Pennsylvania.
Future of Transplantation (Including Xenografting)

ALBERT D. DONNENBERG, PhD
Professor of Medicine and Interim Director, Blood and Marrow Transplant Program, University of Pittsburgh School of Medicine, Pittsburgh, Pennsylvania.
Bone Marrow Transplantation

JOHN J. DOWNES, MD
Emeritus Professor of Pediatrics and Anesthesiology, University of Pennsylvania School of Medicine. Director of Respiratory Rehabilitation Service, Division of Critical Care Medicine, Department of Anesthesiology and Critical Care Medicine, Children's Hospital of Philadelphia, Philadelphia, Pennsylvania.
Distal Airway Disorders in Infants and Children: Bronchiolitis and Asthma

ROBERT J. DOWNEY, MD
Assistant Attending Surgeon, Department of Anesthesiology and Critical Care Medicine, Memorial Sloan-Kettering Cancer Center, New York, New York.
Surgical Problems in the Critically Ill Oncologic Patient

HOWARD R. DOYLE, MD
Assistant Professor of Surgery and Medical Informatics, Department of Surgery, University of Pittsburgh School of Medicine, Pittsburgh, Pennsylvania.
Multiple Organ Procurement

JEFFREY M. DRAZEN, MD
Parker B. Francis Professor of Medicine, Harvard Medical School. Chief, Pulmonary and Critical Care Division, Department of Medicine, Brigham and Women's Hospital, Boston, Massachusetts.
Life-Threatening Asthma

CHRISTOPHER J. DUNATOV, MD
Fellow, Critical Care Medicine, Division of Pulmonary and Critical Care Medicine, University of Virginia Health System, Charlottesville, Virginia.
Seizures in Critically Ill Patients

THOMAS D. EAST, PhD
Associate Professor (Medical Informatics), Research Associate Professor (Bioengineering), and Associate Professor of Anesthesiology, University of Utah School of Medicine, Salt Lake City. Assistant Director, Medical Informatics, Central Urban Region–IHC, and Director, Medical Informatics, South Salt

Lake Valley-IHC and Cottonwood Hospital/Intermountain Health Care, Inc., Murray, Utah.
Computerized Management of Mechanical Ventilation

DAVID H. EBB, MD
Instructor in Pediatrics, Harvard Medical School. Assistant Pediatrician, Massachusetts General Hospital, Boston, Massachusetts.
Bleeding Disorders of Childhood

MICHAEL EDMOND, MD, MPH
Associate Professor of Internal Medicine, Divisions of Quality Health Care and Infectious Diseases, Medical College of Virginia School of Medicine, Virginia Commonwealth University. Hospital Epidemiologist, Medical College of Virginia Hospitals, Richmond, Virginia.
Antimicrobial Resistance and Other Epidemiologic Considerations in the Intensive Care Unit

M. FRANCESCA EGIDI, MD
Associate Professor of Internal Medicine, University of Tennessee, Memphis, College of Medicine; University of Tennessee Medical Center, Memphis, Tennessee.
Pancreas Transplantation

FREDERICK J. EHLERT, PhD
Professor, Department of Pharmacology, University of California, Irvine, College of Medicine, Irvine, California.
Receptor Physiology

MARTIN R. EICHELBERGER, MD
Professor of Surgery and Pediatrics, George Washington University School of Medicine and Health Sciences. Director, Trauma and Burn Services, Children's National Medical Center, Washington, D.C.
Intensive Care Management of the Injured Child

KENNETH A. ELLENBOGEN, MD
Professor of Medicine, Medical College of Virginia School of Medicine, Virginia Commonwealth University, Richmond, Virginia.
Cardiac Pacemakers and Implantable Defibrillators in the Intensive Care Unit Setting

JOSEPH ESPAT, MD
Surgical Oncology Fellow, Memorial Sloan-Kettering Cancer Center, New York, New York.
Surgical Problems in the Critically Ill Oncologic Patient

ANDRÉS ESTEBAN, MD, PhD
Director, Intensive Care Unit, Hospital Universitario dé Getafe, Madrid, Spain.
Nitric Oxide in Critical Illness

JEAN-YVES FAGON, MD, PhD
Professor of Medicine, Université Paris V. Director, Intensive Care Unit, Hŏpital Broussais, Paris, France.
Severe Community-Acquired Pneumonia; Nosocomial Pneumonia

PETER F. FEDULLO, MD
Professor of Medicine, University of California, San Diego, School of Medicine, La Jolla. Director, Medical Intensive Care Unit, UCSD Medical Center, San Diego, California.
Pulmonary Embolism and Deep Venous Thrombosis

I. ALAN FEIN, MD
Clinical Assistant Professor, University of Miami School of Nursing. Medical Director, Advanced Life Support Training Center, Baptist Health Systems. President, Critical Care Management Consultants, Miami, Florida.
Utilization and Allocation of Critical Care Resources

SANDRA L. FEIN, MA, RN
Educational Consultant, Miami, Florida.
Utilization and Allocation of Critical Care Resources

ALPHA A. FOWLER III, MD
Professor of Medicine, Department of Internal Medicine, Division of Pulmonary/Critical Care Medicine, Medical College of Virginia School of Medicine, Virginia Commonwealth University, Richmond, Virginia.
Structural Basis of Pulmonary Function

BRADLEY P. FUHRMAN, MD
Professor of Pediatrics and Anesthesiology, State University of New York at Buffalo School of Medicine and Biomedical Sciences. Chief, Pediatric Critical Care, Children's Hospital of Buffalo, Buffalo, New York.
Congestive Heart Failure in Infants and Children; Partial Liquid Ventilation

TISHA FUJII, DO
Fellow, Critical Care Medicine, St. Vincent Hospital and Medical Center, New York, New York.
Anaphylactic Reactions; Building Bedside Collaborative Practice

ANN S. FULCHER, MD
Assistant Professor, Medical College of Virginia School of Medicine, Virginia Commonwealth University. Director, Abdominal Magnetic Resonance, Medical College of Virginia Hospitals, Richmond, Virginia.
Computed Tomography and Magnetic Resonance Imaging of the Abdomen in the Critical Care Patient

WILLIAM J. FULKERSON, MD
Professor of Medicine, Department of Medicine, Division of Pulmonary and Critical Care Medicine, Duke University School of Medicine, Durham, North Carolina.
Fiberoptic Bronchoscopy in the Intensive Care Unit

JOHN J. FUNG, MD, PhD
Professor of Surgery, University of Pittsburgh School of Medicine. Chief, Division of Transplantation Surgery, Thomas E. Starzl Transplantation Institute, University of Pittsburgh Medical Center, Pittsburgh, Pennsylvania.
Principles of Immunosuppression; Intensive Care of Liver Transplant Recipients; Future of Transplantation (Including Xenografting)

TOMAS GANZ, PhD, MD
Professor of Medicine and Pathology, University of California, Los Angeles, UCLA School of Medicine, Los Angeles, California.
Macrophage Function

TODD W. B. GEHR, MD
Associate Professor of Medicine, Department of Internal Medicine, Division of Nephrology, Medical College of Virginia School of Medicine, Virginia Commonwealth University. Staff, Medical College of Virginia Hospitals, Richmond, Virginia.
Clinical Assessment of Renal Function; Adult Acute and Chronic Renal Failure

JEFFREY A. GELFAND, MD
Professor of Medicine and Dean for Research, Tufts University School of Medicine. Senior Vice President, Research and Technology, New England Medical Center, Boston, Massachusetts.
Cytokines in Disease

LARRY M. GENTILELLO, MD
Associate Professor of Surgery, University of Washington School of Medicine. Associate Director, Trauma Intensive Care Unit, Harborview Medical Center, Seattle, Washington.
Accidental Hypothermia

HUGO GOMEZ, MD
International Research Fellow, Department of Surgery, Division of Trauma Surgery and Critical Care, Los Angeles County–University of Southern California Medical Center, Los Angeles, California.
Exsanguination; Thoracic Injuries

EDGAR R. GONZALEZ, PharmD
Associate Professor of Emergency Medicine and Associate Professor of Pharmacy, Medical College of Virginia, Virginia Commonwealth University, Richmond, Virginia.
Inotropic Therapy and the Critically Ill Patient

JOSEPH A. GOVERT, MD
Assistant Professor, Department of Medicine, Division of Pulmonary and Critical Care Medicine, Duke University School of Medicine, Durham, North Carolina.
Fiberoptic Bronchoscopy in the Intensive Care Unit

GEORGE A. GREGORY, MD
Professor of Anesthesia and Pediatrics, University of California, San Francisco, School of Medicine, San Francisco, California.
Resuscitation of the Newborn

AKE GRENVIK, MD, PhD, FCCM
Distinguished Service Professor of Critical Care Medicine, University of Pittsburgh School of Medicine. Director Emeritus, Multidisciplinary Critical Care Training Program, University of Pittsburgh Medical Center, Pittsburgh, Pennsylvania.
Air Embolization; History and Organization of Organ Transplantation; Alternative Organ Donor Categories; Future of Transplantation (Including Xenografting); Forgoing Life-Sustaining Therapy in Intensive Care

JEFFREY S. GROEGER, MD
Professor of Clinical Medicine, The Weill Medical College of Cornell University. Medical Director, Special Care Unit—Critical Care Medicine, Department of Anesthesiology and Critical Care Medicine, Memorial Sloan-Kettering Cancer Center, New York, New York.
Medical Complications in the Patient with Cancer

JACQUARD GUENON, MS
Chief Technology Officer, Wired Ventures Ltd., San Francisco, California.
Critical Care Applications of Large Data Bases

DAVID W. HAAS, MD
Associate Professor of Medicine, Division of Infectious Diseases, Vanderbilt University School of Medicine. Director, Clinical Infectious Diseases Services, Vanderbilt University Medical Center, Nashville, Tennessee.
Central Nervous System Infections

ANGELA M. HADBAVNY, MS, PharmD
Adjunct Clinical Instructor, Duquesne University School of Pharmacy. Critical Care Clinical Pharmacy, Specialist and Clinical Research Study Coordinator, Department of Critical Care Medicine, St. Francis Medical Center, Pittsburgh, Pennsylvania.
Sedatives and Analgesics in Critical Care

PERRY V. HALUSHKA, PhD, MD
Professor of Pharmacology and Medicine, Medical University of South Carolina College of Medicine, Charleston, South Carolina.
Prostaglandins, Thromboxanes, Leukotrienes, and Other Products of Arachidonic Acid

DAVID HANPETER, MD
Assistant Unit Chief, Trauma Surgery "A" Service, Department of Surgery, Division of Trauma Surgery and Critical Care, Los Angeles County–University of Southern California Medical Center, Los Angeles, California.
Exsanguination; Thoracic Injuries

JOHN M. HARLAN, MD
Professor of Medicine and Head, Division of Hematology, University of Washington School of Medicine, Seattle, Washington.
Neutrophil-Endothelial Cell Interactions

MAURENE A. HARVEY, RN, MPH, CCRN, FCCM
Consultant, Critical Care, Inc., Pasadena, California.
Building Bedside Collaborative Practice

ANDREA HASTILLO, MD
Associate Professor of Medicine, Division of Cardiology, Medical College of Virginia School of Medicine, Virginia Commonwealth University, Richmond, Virginia.
Conduction Disturbances and Cardiac Arrhythmias in the Critically Ill

MARILYN T. HAUPT, MD
Professor of Medicine, Oregon Health Sciences University School of Medicine. Medical Director, Critical Care Services, Oregon Health Sciences University Hospitals and Clinics, Portland, Oregon.
Anaphylactic Reactions

DAVID HEIMBACH, MD
Professor of Surgery, University of Washington School of Medicine. Director, Burn Center, Harborview Medical Center, Seattle, Washington.
Accidental Hypothermia

ELIZABETH A. HENNEMAN, RN, PhD, CCRN
Assistant Clinical Faculty, University of California, Los Angeles, UCLA School of Nursing. Clinical Nurse Specialist, UCLA Medical Center, Los Angeles, California.
Preventing Complications in the Intensive Care Unit

DANIEL A. HENRY, MD
Associate Professor, Department of Radiology, Medical College of Virginia School of Medicine, Virginia Commonwealth University; Medical College of Virginia Hospital, Richmond, Virginia.
Critical Care Imaging of the Chest

LYNN J. HERNAN, MD
Assistant Professor of Pediatrics and Anesthesiology, State University of New York at Buffalo School of Medicine and Biomedical Sciences. Associate Director, Pediatric Intensive Care Unit, Children's Hospital of Buffalo, Buffalo, New York.
Congestive Heart Failure in Infants and Children; Partial Liquid Ventilation

CARL ANTHONY HESS, MD
Associate Clinical Professor, Department of Anesthesiology, University of California, Irvine, College of Medicine, Irvine. Director, Memorial Pain Associates; President, PRISM Pain Management; Staff Anesthesiologist, Anaheim Memorial Medical Center, Anaheim, California.
Acute Pain in the Intensive Care Unit

MICHAEL L. HESS, MD, FACC
Professor of Medicine and Chairman, Division of Cardiopulmonary Laboratories and Research, Medical College of Virginia School of Medicine, Virginia Commonwealth University, Richmond, Virginia.
Applied Cardiovascular Physiology in the Critically Ill; Contemporary Thrombolytic Therapy in Acute Myocardial Infarction; Interventional Therapies for Cardiogenic Shock; Inotropic Therapy and the Critically Ill Patient

THOMAS L. HIGGINS, MD, FACP, FCCM
Associate Professor of Medicine and Anesthesiology, Tufts University School of Medicine, Boston. Director, Adult Critical Care Service, Baystate Medical Center, Springfield, Massachusetts.
Severity of Illness Indices and Outcome Prediction: Development and Evaluation

MICHAEL H. HINES, MD
Assistant Professor, Cardiothoracic Surgery, and Director, Extracorporeal Membrane Oxygenation, Wake Forest University School of Medicine. Attending Surgeon, Wake Forest University Baptist Medical Center, Winston-Salem, North Carolina.
Use of Mechanical Circulatory Support Systems in Critically Ill Patients

ELIZABETH HINGSBERGEN, MD
Assistant Professor of Radiology and Pediatrics, Medical College of Virginia School of Medicine, Virginia Commonwealth University. Medical Staff, Children's Hospital, Richmond, Virginia.
Chest Imaging in Pediatric Intensive Care

MICHAEL J. HOCKSTEIN, MD, FCCP
Medical Director, Surgical Intensive Care Unit, Washington Hospital Center, Washington, D.C.
New Techniques in Management of the Cardiac Surgery Patient

STUART HOROWITZ, PhD
Director, Research and Technology, The Heart and Lung Institute, Jewish Hospital, Louisville, Kentucky.
Apoptosis in Critical Illness

JOHN W. HOYT, MD
Clinical Professor of Anesthesiology/Critical Care Medicine, University of Pittsburgh School of Medicine. Chairman, Department of Critical Care Medicine, St. Francis Medical Center, Pittsburgh, Pennsylvania.
Sedatives and Analgesics in Critical Care

F. IDA HSU, BA
Research Assistant, Memorial Sloan-Kettering Cancer Center, New York, New York.
Surgical Problems in the Critically Ill Oncologic Patient

RUSSELL D. HULL, MB BS, MSc
Professor of Medicine, University of Calgary Faculty of Medicine. Director, Thrombosis Research Unit, Foothills Hospital, Calgary, Alberta, Canada.
Treatment of Massive Pulmonary Embolism; Diagnosis and Treatment of Venous Thromboembolism

DAVID H. INGBAR, MD
Professor of Medicine and Pediatrics, Pulmonary, Allergy and Critical Care Division, University of Minnesota School of Medicine. Medical Director, Critical Care; Medical Director, Medical ICU; and Co-Medical Director, Respiratory Care, Fairview University Medical Center, Minneapolis, Minnesota.
Life-Threatening Hemoptysis

JULIE R. INGELFINGER, MD
Associate Professor of Pediatrics, Harvard Medical School. Chief, Pediatric Nephrology, Massachusetts General Hospital, Boston, Massachusetts.
Hypertensive Emergencies in Infants and Children

MICHAEL R. JACOBS, MB, BCh, PhD, MRCPath
Professor of Pathology, Case Western Reserve University School of Medicine. Director, Clinical Microbiology, University Hospitals of Cleveland, Cleveland, Ohio.
Laboratory Diagnosis of Infection

YVES JANIN, MD
Senior Fellow, Division of Cardiology, Medical College of Virginia School of Medicine, Virginia Commonwealth University, Richmond, Virginia.
Contemporary Thrombolytic Therapy in Acute Myocardial Infarction; Interventional Therapies for Cardiogenic Shock

RANDEEP S. JAWA, MD
Surgical Resident, Howard University College of Medicine, Washington, D.C.
Cellular Effectors of the Septic Process

KHURSHEED N. JEEJEEBHOY, MBBS, PhD, FRCPC
Professor of Medicine, Nutrition, and Physiology, University of Toronto Faculty of Medicine. Gastroenterologist, St. Michael's Hospital, Toronto, Ontario, Canada.
Micronutrient Deficiencies

DENNIS M. JENSEN, MD
Professor of Medicine, Division of Gastroenterology, Department of Medicine, University of California, Los Angeles, UCLA School of Medicine, Los Angeles, California.
Severe Gastrointestinal Hemorrhage

HOWARD JOLLES, MD
Senior Associate Consultant, Mayo Clinic Jacksonville, Jacksonville, Florida.
Critical Care Imaging of the Chest

VERN C. JUEL, MD
Assistant Professor of Neurology, University of Virginia School of Medicine, Charlottesville, Virginia.
Neuromuscular Disorders in Critical Care

GREGORY J. JURKOVICH, MD
Professor of Surgery, University of Washington School of Medicine. Chief of Trauma, Harborview Medical Center, Seattle, Washington.
Accidental Hypothermia; Trauma to the Pregnant Patient

ROBERT M. KACMAREK, PhD, RRT, FCCM
Associate Professor, Department of Anesthesia, Harvard Medical School. Director, Respiratory Care Services, Massachusetts General Hospital, Boston, Massachusetts.
Controlled Mechanical Ventilation

ALLEN B. KAISER, MD
Professor and Vice-Chairman of Clinical Affairs, Department of Medicine, Vanderbilt University School of Medicine; Vanderbilt University Medical Center, Nashville, Tennessee.
Central Nervous System Infections

GEORGE J. KALOYANIDES, MD, FACP
Professor, Department of Medicine, State University of New York at Stony Brook Health Sciences Center, School of Medicine, Stony Brook, New York.
Drug-Kidney Interactions

YOOGOO KANG, MD
Professor of Anesthesiology and Critical Care Medicine, University of Pittsburgh School of Medicine. Director, Hepatic Transplantation Anesthesiology and Critical Care Medicine, Department of Anesthesiology/Critical Care Medicine, University of Pittsburgh Medical Center, Pittsburgh, Pennsylvania.
Multiple Organ Procurement

BARBARA S. KANNEWURF, PharmD
Clinical Fellow, School of Pharmacy, Medical College of Virginia, Virginia Commonwealth University, Richmond, Virginia.
Inotropic Therapy and the Critically Ill Patient

JILL D. KAPLAN, MD
Assistant Professor of Neurology, University of California, San Francisco, School of Medicine. Attending Neurologist, Mt. Zion Hospital, San Francisco, California.
Postoperative Confusion

JOAN E. KAPUSNIK-UNER, PharmD
Associate Clinical Professor, University of California, San Francisco, School of Medicine, San Francisco. Senior Knowledge Engineer, First Data Bank, San Bruno, California.
Antimicrobial Therapy in the Critical Care Setting

ROBERT KATZ, MD
Associate Professor of Pediatrics, University of New Mexico School of Medicine. Director, Pediatric Intensive Care Unit, University of New Mexico Hospital, Albuquerque, New Mexico.
Acute Parenchymal Disease in Childhood

CLIFFORD J. KAVINSKY, MD, PhD
Assistant Professor of Medicine, Rush Medical College of Rush University. Assistant Director, Section of Cardiology, Rush-Presbyterian St. Luke's Medical Center, Chicago, Illinois.
Severe Heart Failure in Cardiomyopathy: Pathogenesis and Treatment

JEFFREY A. KAZZAZ, PhD
Assistant Professor, State University of New York at Stony Brook Health Sciences Center, School of Medicine, Stony Brook. Senior Staff Scientist, Cardiopulmonary Research Institute, Winthrop-University Hospital, Mineola, New York.
Apoptosis in Critical Illness

ROBERT J. KEENAN, MD, FRCSC
Professor of Surgery, University of Pittsburgh School of Medicine. Surgical Director of Lung Transplantation, University of Pittsburgh Medical Center, Pittsburgh, Pennsylvania.
Critical Care Aspects of Lung Transplantation

JOHN A. KELLUM, MD
Assistant Professor of Anesthesiology/Division of Critical Care Medicine and Medicine, University of Pittsburgh School of Medicine, Pittsburgh, Pennsylvania.
Diagnosis and Treatment of Acid-Base Disorders; Appraising and Using Evidence in Critical Care

JOHN M. KELLUM, MD, FACS
Professor, Department of Surgery, Medical College of Virginia School of Medicine, Virginia Commonwealth University, Richmond, Virginia.
Intra-abdominal Sepsis

AJAI KHANNA, MD, FRCS
Assistant Professor of Surgery, Department of Surgery, University of California, San Diego, School of Medicine, La Jolla. Attending Transplant Surgeon, UCSD Medical Center, Department of Surgery, San Diego, California.
Principles of Immunosuppression

NABIL E. KHOURY, MD
Clinical Assistant Professor, Department of Internal Medicine, Case Western Reserve University School of Medicine, Cleveland, Ohio. Division Head, Emergency Medicine, and Medical Director, Clinical Decision Unit, Henry Ford Medical Center, West Bloomfield, Michigan.
Clinical Decision Units and Acute Medical Emergencies

THOMAS KILLIP, MD
Professor of Medicine, Albert Einstein College of Medicine of Yeshiva University, Bronx, New York. Director, Heart Institute, Beth Israel Medical Center, New York, New York.
Treatment of Myocardial Infarction

IVAN KIROV, MD
Fellow, Children's Hospital of Orange County, Orange, California.
Hematopoietic Colony-Stimulating Factors

W. ANDREW KOFKE, MD, FCCM
Professor and Vice-Chairman, Department of Anesthesiology, West Virginia University School of Medicine, Morgantown, West Virginia.
Neuropathophysiology

MICHAEL C. KONTOS, MD
Assistant Professor, Department of Medicine, Division of Cardiology, Medical College of Virginia School of Medicine, Virginia Commonwealth University, Richmond, Virginia.
Echocardiography in Critical Care

ROBERT L. KORMOS, MD
Associate Professor of Surgery, University of Pittsburgh School of Medicine. Director, Artificial Heart Program, University of Pittsburgh Medical Center, Pittsburgh, Pennsylvania.
Multiple Organ Procurement

DAVID J. KRAMER, MD
Associate Professor of Anesthesiology/Critical Care Medicine, Medicine, and Surgery, University of Pittsburgh School of Medicine. Co-Director, Liver Transplant Intensive Care Unit Service, University of Pittsburgh Medical Center–Presbyterian University Hospital, Pittsburgh, Pennsylvania.
Intensive Care of Liver Transplant Recipients

JOHN W. KREIT, MD
Assistant Professor of Medicine, University of Pittsburgh School of Medicine. Director, Medical Intensive Care Unit, VA Medical Center, Pittsburgh, Pennsylvania.
Mechanics of the Respiratory System

FRED J. LAINE, MD
Associate Professor of Radiology and Otolaryngology, Medical College of Virginia School of Medicine, Virginia Commonwealth University, Richmond, Virginia.
Imaging of the Central Nervous System in the Critical Care Patient

LUIS LANDÍN, MD, PhD
Associate Professor, Department of Medicine, Universidad de Alcala de Henares. Attending Physician, Intensive Care Unit, Hospital Ramón y Cajal, Madrid, Spain.
Nitric Oxide in Critical Illness

EDWIN LEE, MD
Director of Endocrinology, Gessler Clinic, Winter Haven, Florida.
Neuroendocrine Immunology in the Critically Ill Patient

KEITH LEWIS, MD
Instructor, Department of Pediatrics, University of California, Los Angeles, UCLA School of Medicine, Los Angeles. Fellow, Pediatric Critical Care, Harbor-UCLA Medical Center, Torrance; Children's Hospital of Orange County, Orange; Charles R. Drew–Martin Luther King Medical Center, Los Angeles, California.
Drowning and Near-Drowning

YUCHI LI, PhD
Research Scientist, Cardiopulmonary Research Institute, Winthrop-University Hospital, Mineola, New York.
Apoptosis in Critical Illness

PETER K. LINDEN, MD, DMD
Associate Professor, Departments of Anesthesiology/Critical Care Medicine and Medicine, University of Pittsburgh School of Medicine. Associate Director, Liver Intensive Care Unit, University of Pittsburgh Medical Center, Pittsburgh, Pennsylvania.
Infections After Solid Organ Transplantation

DOUGLAS P. LOHMANN, ME
Coordinator of Circulatory Support, Wake Forest University Baptist Medical Center, Winston-Salem, North Carolina.
Use of Mechanical Circulatory Support Systems in Critically Ill Patients

JOSÉ A. LORENTE, MD, PhD
Attending Physician, Intensive Care Unit, Hospital Universitario dé Getafe, Madrid, Spain.
Nitric Oxide in Critical Illness

JOHN M. LUCE, MD
Professor of Medicine and Anesthesia, University of California, San Francisco, School of Medicine. Associate Director, Medical-Surgical Intensive Care Unit, San Francisco General Hospital, San Francisco, California.
Management of HIV and AIDS-Related Infection in the Intensive Care Unit

PHILIP D. LUMB, MB, BS, FCCM
Eric A. Walker Professor and Chairman, Department of Anesthesia, Pennsylvania State University College of Medicine. Director, Division of Anesthesia, South Central Operating Team, Penn State Geisinger Health System, Milton S. Hershey Medical Center, Hershey, Pennsylvania.
Conventional Airway Access

DREW A. MacGREGOR, MD
Assistant Professor of Anesthesiology (Critical Care) and Assistant Professor of Medicine (Pulmonary/Critical Care), Wake Forest University School of Medicine. Associate Medical Director, Adult Intensive Care Unit, Wake Forest University Baptist Medical Center, Winston-Salem, North Carolina.
Basic Pharmacologic Principles and Drug Monitoring

NEIL R. MacINTYRE, MD
Professor of Medicine, Duke University School of Medicine. Medical Director, Respiratory Care, Duke University Medical Center, Durham, North Carolina.
Patient-Ventilator Interactions; Weaning from Ventilatory Support in Hypoxemic Respiratory Failure

ROBERT C. MACKERSIE, MD, FACS
Professor of Surgery, University of California, San Francisco, School of Medicine. Director, Trauma Services, San Francisco General Hospital, San Francisco, California.
Transfusion Therapy

LUIS MALDONADO, MD
Assistant Professor, University of South Florida College of Medicine. Attending Staff, Tampa General Hospital, Tampa, Florida.
Proximal Airway Disorders in the Pediatric Patient

ROBERT J. MANGIALARDI, MD
Attending Physician, Centennial Medical Center, Nashville, Tennessee.
Management Controversies in Acute Respiratory Distress Syndrome

JOHN J. MARINI, MD
Professor of Medicine, University of Minnesota Medical School—Minneapolis. Chairman of Academic Medicine, and Director of Pulmonary and Critical Care Medicine, Regions Hospital, St. Paul, Minnesota.
Partial Ventilatory Assist; Initial Management of Acute Hypoxemia

IGNAZIO ROBERTO MARINO, MD, FACS
Associate Professor of Surgery, University of Pittsburgh School of Medicine. Associate Director, Transplant Division, Veterans Affairs Medical Center. Director, European Medical Division, University of Pittsburgh Medical Center, Pittsburgh, Pennsylvania.
Multiple Organ Procurement

LAWRENCE F. MARSHALL, MD
Professor and Head, Division of Neurosurgery, University of California, San Diego, School of Medicine, La Jolla. Chief, Neurosurgery, UCSD Medical Center, San Diego, California.
Management of Traumatic Brain Injury in the Intensive Care Unit

G. DANIEL MARTICH, MD
Assistant Professor of Anesthesiology and Critical Care Medicine, University of Pittsburgh School of Medicine. Co-Director, Cardiothoracic Intensive Care Unit, University of Pittsburgh Medical Center–Presbyterian Hospital; Medical Director, Critical Care Information Systems, University of Pittsburgh Medical Center, Pittsburgh, Pennsylvania.
Heart Transplantation

TOM A. MARTIN, PharmD, BCPS
Clinical Assistant Professor of Pharmacy, School of Pharmacy, University of North Carolina at Chapel Hill, Chapel Hill; Clinical Assistant Professor of Pharmacy Practice, School of Pharmacy, Campbell University, Buies Creek. Pharmaceutical Care Coordinator for Critical Care, Department of Pharmacy, Wake

Forest University Baptist Medical Center, Winston-Salem, North Carolina.
Basic Pharmacologic Principles and Drug Monitoring

GEORGE V. MAZARIEGOS, MD
Assistant Professor of Surgery, University of Pittsburgh School of Medicine. Co-Director, Liver Transplant Intensive Care Unit Service, Presbyterian University Hospital and Children's Hospital of Pittsburgh, Pittsburgh, Pennsylvania.
Intensive Care of Liver Transplant Recipients; Intestinal and Multiple Organ Transplantation

JERRY McCAULEY, MD
Associate Professor of Medicine and Surgery, University of Pittsburgh School of Medicine. Director of Transplantation Nephrology, University of Pittsburgh Medical Center, Pittsburgh, Pennsylvania.
Critical Care of Kidney Transplant Recipients

DAVID J. McCONKEY, PhD
Assistant Professor, Department of Cancer Biology, University of Texas Medical School at Houston; University of Texas M. D. Anderson Cancer Center, Houston, Texas.
Cellular Signaling and Cell Death

KRISTINE M. McCULLOCH, MD
Associate Professor, University of Illinois, College of Medicine. Attending Neonatologist, University of Illinois Hospital at Chicago Medical Center; Michael Reese Hospital and Medical Center; St. Elizabeth's Hospital, Chicago, Illinois.
Surfactant Physiology, Metabolism, Function, and Therapy

LISA McDUFFIE, MD
Research Fellow, Department of Surgery, Division of Trauma Surgery and Critical Care, Los Angeles County–University of Southern California Medical Center, Los Angeles, California.
Exsanguination

JEFFREY P. McGOVERN, MD
Assistant Clinical Professor of Medicine, Baylor College of Medicine, Houston, Texas.
Oxygenation Strategy

MAGED S. MIKHAIL, MD
Associate Professor of Anesthesiology and Surgery, University of Southern California School of Medicine, Los Angeles County–University of Southern California. Associate Director, Intensive Care Unit and Anesthesia, USC/Kenneth Norris Cancer Hospital, Los Angeles, California.
Hyperthermia; Anesthesia for High-Risk Patients

ADELAIDA M. MIRO, MD
Associate Professor of Anesthesiology/Critical Care Medicine, University of Pittsburgh School of Medicine, Pittsburgh, Pennsylvania.
Acute Respiratory Failure in Patients with Chronic Obstructive Pulmonary Disease

JEROME MODELL, MD
Associate Vice President for Health Affairs and Professor of Anesthesiology, University of Florida College of Medicine, Gainesville, Florida.
Pulmonary Aspiration

ERNESTO P. MOLMENTI, MD
Instructor, Department of Surgery, University of Pittsburgh School of Medicine, Pittsburgh, Pennsylvania.
Future of Transplantation (Including Xenografting)

RICHARD E. MOON, MD, CM, FACP, FCCP, FRCP(C)
Professor of Anesthesiology and Associate Professor of Pulmonary Medicine, Duke University School of Medicine. Medical Director, Hyperbaric Center, and Attending Anesthesiologist/Pulmonologist, Duke University Medical Center, Durham, North Carolina.
Hyperbaric Oxygen in Critical Care

ERNEST E. MOORE, MD
Professor and Vice-Chairman of Surgery, University of Colorado School of Medicine. Chief, Department of Surgery, Denver Health Medical Center, Denver, Colorado.
Role of the Gut in Multiple Organ Failure

MATTHEW L. MORONT, MD
Pediatric Trauma Fellow, The George Washington University School of Medicine and Health Sciences, and Children's National Medical Center, Washington, D.C.
Intensive Care Management of the Injured Child

GABRIELLE F. MORRIS, MD
Chief Resident, Neurosurgery, University of California, San Diego, Medical Center, San Diego, California.
Management of Traumatic Brain Injury in the Intensive Care Unit; Modern Management of Acute Spinal Cord Injury

WILLIAM J. MORRIS, MD
Pediatric Neurosurgeon, Mary Bridge Children's Hospital, Tacoma, Washington.
Pediatric Neurosurgical Emergencies

INGRID MROZ, MS, RN, CCRN, ARNP
Adjunct Assistant Professor, University of Vermont, Burlington, Vermont. Clinical Nurse Specialist, Intensive Care Unit, Dartmouth-Hitchcock Medical Center, Lebanon, New Hampshire.
Barriers to Effective Patient Care

JAMES A. MURRAY, MD
Assistant Professor of Surgery, University of Southern California, Los Angeles, California.
Abdominal Trauma

ANNE L. NACLERIO, MD
Clinical Instructor, Pediatrics, George Washington University School of Medicine and Health Sciences. Fellow, Critical Care Medicine, Children's National Medical Center, Washington, D.C.
Evaluating Pediatric Critical Care

JANICE M. NEWSOME, MD
Assistant Instructor, Department of Radiology, Medical College of Virginia School of Medicine, Virginia Commonwealth University, Richmond, Virginia.
Interventional Radiology for the Critically Ill Patient

RONALD LEE NICHOLS, MD, MS, FACS
Professor of Surgery, Tulane University School of Medicine, New Orleans, Louisiana.
Infections in the Surgical Critical Care Unit

J. V. NIXON, MD
Professor of Medicine, Medical College of Virginia School of Medicine, Virginia Commonwealth University. Director, Echocardiography Laboratories, Richmond, Virginia.
Echocardiography in Critical Care

SCOTT NORWOOD, MD, FACS, FCCM
Regional Director for Trauma Services, East Texas Medical Center, Tyler, Texas.
Catheter Colonization and Catheter-Related Bacteremia

RICHARD NOWAK, MD, MBA
Clinical Associate Professor, Department of Surgery, Division of Emergency Medical Services, University of Michigan Medical School, Ann Arbor. Vice-Chairman, Department of Emergency Medicine, Henry Ford Medical Center, Detroit, Michigan.
Clinical Decision Units and Acute Medical Emergencies

DAVID R. NUNLEY, MD, FCCP
National Research Service Award Fellow, University of Pittsburgh Medical Center, Pittsburgh, Pennsylvania.
Critical Care Aspects of Lung Transplantation

TIMOTHY E. OAKS, MD
Assistant Professor, Cardiothoracic Surgery, and Director, Thoracic Transplantation, Wake Forest University School of Medicine. Attending Surgeon, Wake Forest University Baptist Medical Center, Winston-Salem, North Carolina.
Use of Mechanical Circulatory Support Systems in Critically Ill Patients

K. PATRICK OBER, MD
Professor of Internal Medicine (Endocrinology and Metabolism), Wake Forest University School of Medicine, Winston-Salem, North Carolina.
Endocrine Emergencies

DANILA ODER, BA
Administrative Assistant, Department of Surgery, Los Angeles County–University of Southern California Medical Center, Los Angeles, California.
Critical Care Applications of Large Data Bases

WALTER J. O'DONNELL, MD
Associate Professor of Medicine, MCP Hahnemann School of Medicine, Philadelphia. Vice Chairman for Clinical Affairs, Department of Medicine, Allegheny General Hospital, Pittsburgh, Pennsylvania.
Life-Threatening Asthma

GARY J. ORDOG, MD, FAACT
Medical Director, Henry Mayo Newhall Memorial Hospital, Valencia, California; University of California, Los Angeles Medical Center, Los Angeles, California.
Medical Toxicology in Critical Care Medicine

SEBASTIAN ORDUNA, MD
International Research Fellow, Department of Surgery, Division of Trauma Surgery and Critical Care, Los Angeles County–University of Southern California Medical Center, Los Angeles, California.
Exsanguination; Thoracic Injuries

STEVEN L. OREBAUGH, MD
Assistant Professor of Anesthesiology and Assistant Clinical Professor of Emergency Medicine, University of Pittsburgh School of Medicine. Staff Anesthesiologist and Emergency Physician, University of Pittsburgh Medical Center–Southside, Pittsburgh, Pennsylvania.
Air Embolization

JOHN T. OWINGS, MD
Assistant Professor of Surgery, University of California, Davis, School of Medicine, Davis, California. Attending Physician, University of California, Davis Medical Center, Sacramento, California.
The Coagulopathy of Trauma

JOSEPH E. PARRILLO, MD
Professor of Medicine, Rush Medical College of Rush University. James B. Herrick Professor of Medicine; Chief, Section of Cardiology; and Chief, Section of Critical Care Medicine, Rush-Presbyterian St. Luke's Medical Center, Chicago, Illinois.
Severe Heart Failure in Cardiomyopathy: Pathogenesis and Treatment

CYRUS J. PARSA, MD
Resident, Department of Surgery, University of California–Davis–East Bay, Oakland, California.
Intravenous and Intra-arterial Access

M. H. PARSA, MD
Associate Clinical Professor of Surgery, College of Physicians and Surgeons, Columbia University. Director, Trauma Center, and Chief, Vascular Access and Hyperalimentation Service, Harlem Hospital Center, New York, New York.
Intravenous and Intra-arterial Access; Invasive and Noninvasive Monitoring

DAVID L. PATERSON, MBBS, FRACP
Chief, Infectious Disease Section, University of Pittsburgh Medical Center, European Medical Division, Pittsburgh, Pennsylvania.
Pneumonia in the Immunosuppressed Patient

D. GLENN PENNINGTON, MD
Howard Holt Bradshaw Professor of Surgery and Chairman, Department of Cardiothoracic Surgery, and Director, Division of Surgical Sciences, Wake Forest University School of Medicine. Attending Surgeon, Wake Forest University Baptist Medical Center, Winston-Salem, North Carolina.
Use of Mechanical Circulatory Support Systems in Critically Ill Patients

JAY I. PETERS, MD
Professor of Medicine, University of Texas Medical School of San Antonio. Director of Critical Care, University of Texas Health Science Center at San Antonio, San Antonio, Texas.
Bacterial Pneumonia in Adult Respiratory Distress Syndrome

STEVEN M. PINCUS, MD, PhD
Associate Professor, Department of Internal Medicine, Division of Hematology/Oncology, Saint Louis University School of Medicine. Attending Physician, Director, Blood and Marrow Transplant Program; and Director, Blood and Marrow Processing Laboratory, Saint Louis University Hospital, St. Louis, Missouri.
Bone Marrow Transplantation

MAURICIO PINEDA-ROMAN, MD
Attending Physician, Department of Medicine, Maricopa Medical Center, Phoenix, Arizona.
Injuries by Venomous and Poisonous Animals

GRAHAM F. PINEO, MD
Professor of Medicine, University of Calgary Faculty of Medicine. Director, Thrombosis Research Unit, Foothills Hospital, Calgary, Alberta, Canada.
Treatment of Massive Pulmonary Embolism; Diagnosis and Treatment of Venous Thromboembolism

SUSAN K. PINGLETON, MD
Professor of Medicine, University of Kansas School of Medicine. Director, Division of Pulmonary and Critical Care Medicine, University of Kansas Medical Center, Kansas City, Kansas.
Adjunctive Respiratory Therapy

MICHAEL R. PINSKY, MD, CM, FCCP, FCCM
Professor, Department of Anesthesiology/Critical Care Medicine, and Director of Research, Division of Critical Care Medicine, University of Pittsburgh School of Medicine. Staff, University of Pittsburgh Medical Center, Pittsburgh, Pennsylvania.
Heart-Lung Interactions

FRED PLUM, MD
Professor, Department of Neurology and Neuroscience, Cornell University Medical College. Senior Attending Neurologist, The New York Hospital, New York, New York.
Evaluation of Coma

MURRAY M. POLLACK, MD
Professor of Anesthesiology and Pediatrics, George Washington University School of Medicine and Health Sciences. Chairman, Department of Critical Care Medicine, Children's National Medical Center, Washington, D.C.
Evaluating Pediatric Critical Care

DAVID J. POWNER, MD, FCCM
Professor, Department of Anesthesiology/Critical Care Medicine and Department of Medicine, University of Pittsburgh School of Medicine. Director, Multidisciplinary Critical Care Training Program, University of Pittsburgh Medical Center, Pittsburgh, Pennsylvania.
Brain Death—Definition, Determination, and Physiologic Effects on Donor Organs; Alternative Organ Donor Categories

RICHARD C. PRIELIPP, MD
Associate Professor, Cardiac Anesthesiology, and Section Head, Critical Care, Wake Forest University School of Medicine, Winston-Salem, North Carolina.
Neuromuscular Blocking Drugs in Patients in the Intensive Care Unit

DONALD S. PROUGH, MD
Professor of Anesthesiology, Neurology, and Pathology and Rebecca Terry White Distinguished Chair of Anesthesiology, University of Texas Medical Branch, Galveston, Texas.
Brain Function Monitoring

GINA A. QUAID, MD
Post-doctoral Fellow, University of Cincinnati School of Medicine, Cincinnati, Ohio.
Cellular Effectors of the Septic Process

NAGARAJAN RAMAKRISHNAN, MBBS
Senior Research Fellow, Division of Critical Care Medicine, University of Pittsburgh School of Medicine, Pittsburgh, Pennsylvania.
Appraising and Using Evidence in Critical Care

RADHA RAMAMRUTHAM, MD
Senior Resident, Maricopa Medical Center, Phoenix, Arizona.
Injuries by Venomous and Poisonous Animals

ABDUL S. RAO, MD, DPhil
Director, Section of Cellular Transplantation, Thomas E. Starzl Transplantation Institute, University of Pittsburgh Medical Center, Pittsburgh, Pennsylvania
Future of Transplantation (Including Xenografting)

GARY E. RASKOB, MSc, PhD
Associate Professor, Department of Biostatistics and Epidemiology and Department of Medicine, University of Oklahoma College of Medicine, Oklahoma City, Oklahoma.
Diagnosis and Treatment of Venous Thromboembolism

ARLINE REINKING-HANF, RN, MS, CCRN, CEN, HNC
Nurse Massage Therapist, Complementary Medicine Services, New York Presbyterian Hospital; Massage Therapy Coordinator, Beth Israel Medical Center, New York, New York.
Complementary Modalities of Care: A Future That Is Here Now

JORGE REYES, MD
Associate Professor of Surgery, University of Pittsburgh School of Medicine. Director, Pediatric Transplant Surgery, Children's Hospital of Pittsburgh, Pittsburgh, Pennsylvania.
Intestinal and Multiple Organ Transplantation

TELFER B. REYNOLDS, MD
Clayton G. Loosli–Hastings Foundation Professor of Medicine, University of Southern California School of Medicine, Los Angeles, California.
Acute Hepatic Failure

PAMELA R. ROBERTS, MD
Assistant Professor of Anesthesia/Critical Care, Wake Forest University School of Medicine, Winston-Salem, North Carolina.
Calcium Magnesium, and Phosphorus Disorders

WILLIAM C. ROBERTS, MD
Medical Director, Baylor Cardiovascular Institute, Baylor University Medical Center, Dallas, Texas.
The Coronary Arteries in Unstable Angina Pectoris, Acute Myocardial Infarction, and Sudden Coronary Death

MARJORIE ROBINSON, PharmD
Assistant Clinical Professor, NOVA Southeastern University, Fort Lauderdale, Florida.
Antimicrobial Therapy in the Critical Care Setting

JOSEP ROCA
Associate Professor, University of Barcelona School of Medicine. Chief, Pulmonology, Hospital Clinic, Barcelona, Spain.
Principles of Gas Exchange

ROBERTO RODRIGUEZ-ROSIN
Professor of Medicine and Chairman, Department of Medicine, University of Barcelona School of Medicine. Head, Respiratory Medicine Service, Hospital Clinic, Barcelona, Spain.
Principles of Gas Exchange

STEPHANIE A. ROHOVSKY, MD
Clinical Fellow in Surgery, Harvard Medical School. Chief Resident, Surgery, Beth Israel Deaconess Medical Center, Boston, Massachusetts.
Total Parenteral Nutrition for the Critically Ill Patient

MARJORIE ROMKES, PhD
Assistant Professor, Department of Environmental and Occupational Health and the Center for Clinical Pharmacology, University of Pittsburgh, Pittsburgh, Pennsylvania.
Genetic Influences on Critical Illness

CLAUDIO RONCO, MD
Professor of Nephrology, Postgraduate School of Nephrology, University of Padua, Padua, Italy. Associate of Clinical Nephrology, Department of Nephrology, St. Bortolo Hospital, Vicenza, Italy.
Prevention of Acute Renal Failure; Renal Replacement Therapy in the Intensive Care Unit; Acute Renal Failure in Infants and Children

MASSIMO RONCONI, MD
Director of Neonatology, Division of Pediatrics and Neonatology, Department of Child Health, St. Bortolo Hospital, Vicenza, Italy.
Acute Renal Failure in Infants and Children

ALLAN H. ROPPER, MD
Chairman, Department of Neurology, Tufts University School of Medicine. Chief of Neurology, St. Elizabeth's Medical Center, Boston, Massachusetts.
Postoperative Confusion

ALAN J. ROSENBLOOM, MD
Assistant Professor, Department of Anesthesiology/Critical Care Medicine, University of Pittsburgh School of Medicine. Attending Physician, Liver Transplantation Intensive Care Units, Thomas E. Starzl Transplantation Institute, University of Pittsburgh Medical Center, and Presbyterian University Hospital, Pittsburgh, Pennsylvania.
Principles of Immunosuppression

BRADLEY ROTH, MD
Assistant Unit Chief, Trauma Surgery "A" Service, Department of Surgery, Division of Trauma Surgery and Critical Care, Los Angeles County-University of Southern California Medical Center, Los Angeles, California.
Thoracic Injuries

STEN RUBERTSSON, MD, PhD, EdICM
Assistant Professor, Department of Anesthesiology/Intensive Care, Uppsala University Hospital, Uppsala, Sweden.
Cardiopulmonary-Cerebral Resuscitation

LEWIS J. RUBIN, MD
Professor of Medicine and Physiology and Head, Division of Pulmonary and Critical Care Medicine, University of Maryland School of Medicine, Baltimore, Maryland.
Pulmonary Hypertension

WITOLD B. RYBKA, MD
Professor of Medicine, Pennsylvania State University College of Medicine. Head, Hematology/Oncology, Penn State Geisinger Cancer Center, Milton S. Hershey Medical Center, Hershey, Pennsylvania.
Bone Marrow Transplantation

PETER SAFAR, MD, Drhc, FCCM, FCCP
Professor, Department of Anesthesiology/Critical Care Medicine, University of Pittsburgh School of Medicine, and Safar Center for Resuscitation Research, Pittsburgh, Pennsylvania.
Cardiopulmonary-Cerebral Resuscitation

AMAR SAFDAR, MD
Fellow in Medicine, Cornell University Medical College. Fellow, Infectious Disease Service, Memorial Sloan-Kettering Cancer Center, New York, New York.
Infections in Patients with Neoplastic Disease

STEVEN A. SAHN, MD
Professor of Medicine and Director, Division of Pulmonary and Critical Care Medicine, Allergy and Clinical Immunology. Co-Director, Asthma and Allergy Center, Medical University of South Carolina School of Medicine, Charleston, South Carolina.
Pleural Disease in the Intensive Care Unit

R. MATTHEW SAILORS, ME
Research Assistant, Department of Medical Informatics, University of Utah School of Medicine, Salt Lake City. Informaticist/Programmer, Cottonwood Hospital/Intermountain Health Care, Inc., Murray, Utah.
Computerized Management of Mechanical Ventilation

ANGUS C. SAMPATH, DSc, MD
Clinical Professor Emeritus, Department of Pathology, College of Physicians and Surgeons, Columbia University. Director, Microbiology Laboratories, and Associate Director, Department of Pathology, Harlem Hospital Center, New York, New York.
Intravenous and Intra-arterial Access

MERLE A. SANDE, MD
Professor and Chairman, Department of Medicine, University of Utah School of Medicine, Salt Lake City, Utah.
Antimicrobial Therapy in the Critical Care Setting

CATHERINE S. H. SASSOON, MD
Associate Professor of Medicine, University of California, Irvine, College of Medicine, Irvine. Staff Physician, VA Medical Center, Long Beach, California.
Oxygenation Strategy

THOMAS J. SAVIDES, MD
Assistant Professor of Clinical Medicine, Division of Gastroenterology, University of California, San Diego, School of Medicine, La Jolla, California.
Severe Gastrointestinal Hemorrhage

GREGORY J. SCHEARS, MD
Assistant Professor of Anesthesiology and Pediatrics, University of Pennsylvania School of Medicine. Assistant Anesthesiologist and Pediatrician, Division of Critical Care Medicine, Department of Anesthesiology and Critical Care Medicine, Children's Hospital of Philadelphia, Philadelphia, Pennsylvania.
Distal Airway Disorders in Infants and Children: Bronchiolitis and Asthma

WILLIAM R. SCHILLER, MD, FACS
Clinical Professor of Surgery, University of Arizona College of Medicine, Tucson. Director, Burn and Trauma Center, Maricopa Medical Center, Phoenix, Arizona.
Burn Care and Inhalation Injury

ROBERT SCHLICHTIG, MD
Director, Intensive Care Unit, Noble Hospital, Westfield, Massachusetts.
Acid-Base Balance (Quantitation)

SIDNEY H. SCHNOLL, MD, PhD
Professor, Departments of Internal Medicine and Psychiatry, Medical College of Virginia School of Medicine, Virginia Commonwealth University. Chairman, Addiction Medicine, Medical College of Virginia Hospitals, Richmond, Virginia.
Drug Abuse, Overdose, and Withdrawal Symptoms

ANTON C. SCHOOLWERTH, MD, MSHA
Professor of Medicine and Chief, Nephrology Division, Department of Internal Medicine, Medical College of Virginia School of Medicine, Virginia Commonwealth University, Richmond, Virginia.
Clinical Assessment of Renal Function; Adult Acute and Chronic Renal Failure

ROBERT SELBY, MD
Associate Professor of Surgery, University of Southern California School of Medicine. Chief of Division of Hepato-Biliary and Pancreas Surgery and Liver Transplantation, Los Angeles County–University of Southern California Medical Center, Los Angeles, California.
Intestinal and Multiple Organ Transplantation

MICHAEL G. SENEFF, MD
Associate Professor of Anesthesiology and Medicine, George Washington University School of Medicine and Health Sciences. Director, Intensive Care Unit, George Washington University Medical Center, Washington, D.C.
Benchmarking and Clinical Reengineering in the Intensive Care Unit

CURTIS N. SESSLER, MD
Professor of Medicine, Pulmonary and Critical Care Medicine, Medical College of Virginia School of Medicine, Virginia Commonwealth University. Medical Director of Critical Care, Medical College of Virginia Hospitals, Richmond, Virginia.
Structural Basis of Pulmonary Function

LELAND SHAPIRO, MD, FACP
Assistant Professor of Medicine, University of Colorado School of Medicine, Denver, Colorado.
Cytokines in Disease

RON SHAPIRO, MD
University of Pittsburgh School of Medicine. Director of Renal Transplantation, Thomas E. Starzl Institute, University of Pittsburgh Medical Center, Pittsburgh, Pennsylvania.
Critical Care of Kidney Transplant Recipients

JERRY L. SHENEP, MD
Professor of Pediatrics, University of Tennessee, Memphis, College of Medicine. Associate Member, Department of Infectious Diseases, St. Jude Children's Research Hospital, Memphis, Tennessee.
Pathogenesis of Gram-Positive Bacterial Infection

RICHARD K. SHEPARD, MD
Assistant Professor, Department of Medicine, Division of Cardiology, Medical College of Virginia School of Medicine, Virginia Commonwealth University, Richmond, Virginia.
Conduction Disturbances and Cardiac Arrhythmias in the Critically Ill

WILLIAM C. SHOEMAKER, MD, FCCM
Professor of Anesthesia and Surgery, University of Southern California School of Medicine, Los Angeles, California.
Resuscitation Algorithms in Acute and Emergency Conditions; Invasive and Noninvasive Monitoring; Diagnosis and Treatment of Shock and Circulatory Dysfunction; Hemodynamic Evaluation and Management of Acute Illnesses in the Emergency Department; Pericardial Tamponade; Pathophysiology and Management of Acute Respiratory Distress Syndrome After Surgery, Trauma, and Other Acute Illnesses

WILLIAM S. SIBBALD, MD, FRCP(C)
Professor, Faculty of Medicine, University of Western Ontario. Coordinator, Critical Care Trauma Center, Victoria Hospital, London, Ontario, Canada.
Applied Cardiovascular Physiology in the Critically Ill

WILLIAM SILVESTER, MD
Senior Lecturer, University of Melbourne. Hospital Intensive Care Specialist, Intensive Care Unit, Austin and Repatriation Medical Centre, Heidelberg, Melbourne, Victoria, Australia.
Renal Replacement Therapy in the Intensive Care Unit

KEVIN P. SIMPSON, MD
Assistant Professor of Medicine and Assistant Chairman, Department of Medicine, Loyola University of Chicago Stritch School of Medicine, Maywood, Illinois.
Weaning from Respiratory Support in Airflow Obstructive States

NINA SINGH, MD
Associate Professor of Internal Medicine, University of Pittsburgh School of Medicine. Chief, Transplantation and Infectious Diseases, Veterans Affairs Medical Center, Pittsburgh, Pennsylvania.
Pneumonia in the Immunosuppressed Patient

ARTHUR S. SLUTSKY, MD
Professor of Medicine, Surgery, and Biomedical Engineering, University of Toronto Faculty of Medicine. Division Director, Respiratory Medicine, University of Toronto; Mount Sinai Hospital, Toronto, Ontario, Canada.
Constant Gas Flow and High-Frequency Ventilation

ROBERT C. SMALLRIDGE, MD, FACP
Professor of Medicine, Mayo Medical School, Rochester, Minnesota. Chair, Division of Endocrinology, Mayo Clinic Jacksonville, Jacksonville, Florida.
Thyroid Emergencies

HOWARD S. SMITH, MD
Assistant Professor, Department of Anesthesiology, Albany Medical College. Director, Pain Management Center, Albany Medical Center Hospital, Albany, New York.
Conventional Airway Access

JOSEPH S. SOLOMKIN, MD
Professor of Surgery, University of Cincinnati School of Medicine, Cincinnati, Ohio.
Cellular Effectors of the Septic Process

STEPHANIE E. SPOTTSWOOD, MD, MSPH
Assistant Professor, Medical College of Virginia School of Medicine, Virginia Commonwealth University, Richmond, Virginia.
Chest Imaging in Pediatric Intensive Care

THOMAS E. STARZL, MD, PhD
Distinguished Professor of Surgery, University of Pittsburgh School of Medicine. Director, Transplant Division, Veterans Affairs Medical Center, and Director, Thomas E. Starzl Transplantation Institute, University of Pittsburgh Medical Center, Pittsburgh, Pennsylvania.
Multiple Organ Procurement; Intestinal and Multiple Organ Transplantation; Future of Transplantation (Including Xenografting)

MICHAEL L. STEER, MD
Professor of Surgery, Harvard Medical School. Surgeon, Beth Israel Deaconess Medical Center, Boston, Massachusetts.
Acute Pancreatitis

STEVEN M. STEINBERG, MD, FACS
Professor of Surgery, Case Western Reserve University School of Medicine. Director, Department of Surgery, Mt. Sinai Medical Center, Cleveland, Ohio.
Infections in the Surgical Critical Care Unit

DAVID M. STEINHORN, MD
Associate Professor of Pediatrics, State University of New York at Buffalo. Associate Director of Pediatric Intensive Care Unit, Children's Hospital of Buffalo, Buffalo, New York.
Partial Liquid Ventilation

JEFFREY A. STERNBERG, MD
Clinical Fellow in Surgery, Harvard Medical School. Chief Resident in Surgery, Beth Israel Deaconess Medical Center, Boston, Massachusetts.
Total Parenteral Nutrition for the Critically Ill Patient

BRYANT W. STOLP, MD, PhD
Assistant Professor of Anesthesiology and Associate, Cell Biology, Duke University School of Medicine. Attending Anesthesiologist, Duke University Medical Center, Durham, North Carolina.
Hyperbaric Oxygen in Critical Care

SUSAN A. STUART, RN, BSN, MPM, CPTC
Assistant Executive Director, Center for Organ Recovery and Education, Pittsburgh, Pennsylvania.
History and Organization of Organ Transplantation

JOERG-PATRICK STÜBGEN, MD, FRCPC
Assistant Professor, Department of Neurology and Neuroscience, Cornell University Medical College. Assistant Attending Neurologist and Neurologist for Intensive Care Units, The New York Hospital and Hospital for Special Surgery, New York, New York.
Evaluation of Coma

MICHAEL J. SULLIVAN, MD
Assistant Professor of Anesthesia, University of Southern California, Los Angeles, California
Hemodynamic Evaluation and Management of Acute Illnesses in the Emergency Department

DALE SWIFT, MD
Assistant Clinical Professor of Neurosurgery, University of Texas Southwestern Medical School at Dallas. Attending Neurosurgeon, Children's Medical Center of Dallas and Medical City Dallas Hospital, Dallas, Texas.
Pediatric Neurosurgical Emergencies

KAREN N. SWISHER, MS, JD
Associate Professor, Health Law, and Associate Director, Williamson Institute for Health Studies, Medical College of Virginia School of Medicine, Virginia Commonwealth University, Richmond, Virginia.
Legal Issues in the Delivery of Critical Care Medicine; The Ethics of Resource Allocation in the Intensive Care Unit; Legal and Risk Management Issues Surrounding Managed Care

PETER N. SWISHER, MA, JD
Professor of Law, University of Richmond Law School, Richmond, Virginia.
Legal and Risk Management Issues Surrounding Managed Care

RICHARD A. SZUCS, MD
Assistant Professor, Medical College of Virginia School of Medicine, Virginia Commonwealth University, Richmond, Virginia.
Computed Tomography and Magnetic Resonance Imaging of the Abdomen in the Critical Care Patient

ROBERT W. TAYLOR, MD
Director, Critical Care Training Program, Saint Louis University School of Medicine; St. John's Mercy Medical Center, St. Louis, Missouri.
Pathophysiology of Acute Lung Injury

WILLIAM R. TAYLOR, MD
Assistant Clinical Professor of Surgery, Division of Neurosurgery, University of California, San Diego, School of Medicine, La Jolla. Staff, UCSD Medical Center, San Diego, California.
Management of Traumatic Brain Injury in the Intensive Care Unit; Modern Management of Acute Spinal Cord Injury

CHARLES TEO, MD
Associate Professor, Department of Neurosurgery, University of Arkansas for Medical Sciences. Chief, Division of Pediatric Neurosurgery, Arkansas Children's Hospital, Little Rock, Arkansas.
Pediatric Neurosurgical Emergencies

DURAIYAH THANGATHURAI, MD, FCCM
Professor of Anesthesiology, Surgery, and Urology, University of Southern California School of Medicine. Vice Chairman, Department of Anesthesiology, Los Angeles County–University of Southern California Medical Center. Director, Intensive Care Unit, and Chief of Anesthesia, USC/Kenneth Norris Cancer Hospital, Los Angeles, California.
Hyperthermia; Anesthesia for High-Risk Patients

ANN E. THOMPSON, MD
Professor of Anesthesiology/Critical Care Medicine and Pediatrics, University of Pittsburgh School of Medicine. Director, Pediatric Critical Care Medicine, Children's Hospital of Pittsburgh, Pittsburgh, Pennsylvania.
Caring for a Child in an Adult Intensive Care Unit

JAIME TISNADO, MD, FACR, FACC
Professor of Radiology, Cardiovascular and Interventional Radiology, and Surgery, Medical College of Virginia School of Medicine, Virginia Commonwealth University. Consultant in Cardiovascular and Interventional Radiology, H. H. McGuire Veterans Administration Medical Center, Richmond, Virginia.
Interventional Radiology for the Critically Ill Patient

MARTIN TOBIN, MD
Professor of Medicine, Loyola University of Chicago Stritch School of Medicine, Maywood, Illinois. Program Director, Division of Pulmonary and Critical Care Medicine, Loyola University Medical Center; Foster G. McGaw Hospital, Maywood; Edward Hines, Jr. Veterans Administration Hospital, Hines, Illinois.
Assessment of Pulmonary Function in Critically Ill Patients; Weaning from Respiratory Support in Airflow Obstruction States

SATORU TODO, MD
Professor and Chairman, The First Department of Surgery, Hokkaido University School of Medicine, Sapporo, Japan.
Intestinal and Multiple Organ Transplantation

GAIL T. TOMINAGA, MD, FACS
Associate Professor, Department of Surgery, John A. Burns School of Medicine. Director, Trauma Services, Queen's Medical Center, Honolulu, Hawaii.
Plasma and Blood Substitutes

TOR INGE TØNNESSEN, MD, PhD
Associate Professor, Department of Anesthesiology and Intensive Care, University of Oslo; Norwegian National Hospital, Oslo, Norway.
Intracellular pH and Electrolyte Regulation

ARTHUR L. TRASK, MD, FACS
Clinical Professor of Surgery, Uniformed Services University of Health Sciences, Bethesda, Maryland. Consultant in Trauma, INOVA Regional Trauma Center, Falls Church, Virginia.
Epidemiology of Trauma

LORRAINE N. TREMBLAY, MD, PhD
Research Fellow, University of Toronto Faculty of Medicine, Toronto, Ontario, Canada.
Constant Gas Flow and High-Frequency Ventilation

STEVEN J. TROTTIER, MD
Clinical Associate Professor of Medicine and Faculty, Critical Care Training Program, Saint Louis University School of Medicine; St. John's Mercy Medical Center, St. Louis, Missouri.
Pathophysiology of Acute Lung Injury

JEAN-LOUIS TROUILLET, MD
Assistant Director, Intensive Care Unit, Hôpital Bichat, Paris, France.
Severe Community-Acquired Pneumonia

ELAINE TUOMANEN, MD
Professor of Pediatrics, University of Tennessee, Memphis, College of Medicine. Member and Chair, Department of Infectious Diseases, St. Jude Children's Research Hospital, Memphis, Tennessee.
Pathogenesis of Gram-Positive Bacterial Infection

DAVID V. TUXEN, MD, MBBS, FRACP, DipDHM
Honorary Clinical Associate Professor, Monash University. Director, Department of Intensive Care and Hyperbaric Medicine, Alfred Hospital, Melbourne, Victoria, Australia.
Independent Lung Ventilation

GUILLERMO E. UMPIERREZ, MD, FACP
Clinical Associate Professor, Emory University School of Medicine. Director, Internal Medicine, Georgia Baptist Medical Center, Atlanta, Georgia.
Diabetic Emergencies

NICHOLAS B. VEDDER, MD
Associate Professor of Surgery, University of Washington School of Medicine, Seattle, Washington.
Neutrophil–Endothelial Cell Interactions

J. DAVID VEGA, MD
Assistant Professor of Surgery, Emory University School of Medicine. Associate Director, Adult Heart and Lung Transplant Program, Emory University Hospital, Atlanta, Georgia.
Heart Transplantation

GEORGE C. VELMAHOS, MD
Assistant Professor of Surgery, University of Southern California School of Medicine. Attending Surgeon, Division of Trauma and Critical Care, Los Angeles County–University of Southern California Medical Center, Los Angeles, California.
Common Bedside Procedures in the Intensive Care Unit; Penetrating Injuries of the Neck

GEORGE VETROVEC, MD, FACC
Professor of Medicine, Chairman, Division of Cardiology, Medical College of Virginia School of Medicine, Virginia Commonwealth University, Richmond, Virginia.
Interventional Therapies for Cardiogenic Shock

DHARMAPURI VIDYASAGAR, MD
Professor of Pediatrics, University of Illinois College of Medicine at Chicago. Director of Neonatology, University of Illinois Hospital at Chicago Medical Center, Chicago, Illinois.
Surfactant Physiology, Metabolism, Function, and Therapy

ROBERT M. WACHTER, MD
Associate Professor of Medicine and Associate Chairman, Department of Medicine, University of California, San Francisco, School of Medicine, San Francisco, California.
Management of HIV and AIDS-Related Infection in the Intensive Care Unit

JONATHAN WASSERBERGER, MD, FAACT
Professor, University of California, Los Angeles, UCLA School of Medicine, Los Angeles, California.
Medical Toxicology in Critical Care Medicine

KENNETH WAXMAN, MD, FACS
Director of Surgical Education, Santa Barbara Cottage Hospital, Santa Barbara, California.
Physiologic Response to Injury; Plasma and Blood Substitutes; The Acute Abdomen

LAWRENCE R. WECHSLER, MD
Professor of Neurology and Neurosurgery, University of Pittsburgh School of Medicine. Director, Stroke Institute, University of Pittsburgh Medical Center, Pittsburgh, Pennsylvania.
Management of Acute Ischemic Stroke

RICHARD E. WEIBLEY, MD, MPH
Pediatric Critical Care Specialist, Intensive Care Services Associates PA, Tampa, Florida.
Proximal Airway Disorders in the Pediatric Patient

FRANCIS X. WHALEN, MD
Fellow, Department of Anesthesiology/Critical Care Medicine, University of Pittsburgh School of Medicine, Pittsburgh, Pennsylvania.
Alternative Organ Donor Categories

RODNEY A. WHITE, MD
Professor of Surgery, University of California, Los Angeles, UCLA School of Medicine, Los Angeles. Chief, Vascular Surgery, and Associate Chair, Department of Surgery, Harbor-UCLA Medical Center, Torrance, California.
Diagnosis and Therapy of Emergent Vascular Diseases

GINGER SCHAFER WLODY, RN, MS, EdD, FCCM
Chair, Quality Management Department, Carl T. Hayden Veterans Administration Medical Center, Phoenix, Arizona.
Impact of Health Care and Technology Trends on Critical Care Practice

CHARLES C. J. WO, BS
Research Associate, University of Southern California, Los Angeles, California
Hemodynamic Evaluation and Management of Acute Illnesses in the Emergency Department

MARK A. WOOD, MD
Associate Professor of Medicine, Medical College of Virginia School of Medicine, Virginia Commonwealth University, Richmond, Virginia.
Cardiac Pacemakers and Implantable Defibrillators in the Intensive Care Unit Setting

VERNA YANCY, MD
Assistant Professor of Anesthesiology, University of Texas Medical Branch, Galveston, Texas.
Brain Function Monitoring

HOWARD YONAS, MD
Professor of Neurosurgery and Peter Jannette Chair of Neurosurgery, University of Pittsburgh School of Medicine, Pittsburgh, Pennsylvania.
Intracranial Hemorrhage

STUART J. YOUNGNER, MD
Professor of Medicine, Psychiatry, and Biomedical Ethics, Case Western Reserve University School of Medicine. Director, Clinical Ethics Program, University Hospitals of Cleveland, Cleveland, Ohio.
Medical Futility

MIHAE YU, MD
Professor of Surgery and Program Director, Division of Surgical Critical Care, University of Hawaii School of Medicine. Director, Surgical Intensive Care Unit, Queens Medical Center, Honolulu, Hawaii.
Trauma Care of the Elderly

GARY P. ZALOGA, MD, FCCM
Director, Critical Care Medicine, Department of Medicine, Washington Hospital Center, Washington, D.C.
Neuroendocrine Immunology in the Critically Ill Patient; Calcium, Magnesium, and Phosphorus Disorders; Enteral Nutrition; Obesity in the Critically Ill Patient

ARNO L. ZARITSKY, MD
Professor and Chairman, Department of Pediatrics, Eastern Virginia Medical School. Senior Vice-President for Academic Affairs, Children's Hospital of the King's Daughters, Norfolk, Virginia.
Pediatric Resuscitation

BARBARA J. ZAROWITZ, PharmD, FCCM
Adjunct Professor of Pharmacy, College of Pharmacy and Allied Health Professions, Wayne State University. Director, Ambulatory Clinical Pharmacy, Henry Ford Health System, Detroit, Michigan.
Alterations in Drug Disposition in the Elderly

BARBARA A. ZEHNBAUER, PhD
Associate Professor of Pediatrics and Pathology, Washington University School of Medicine. Director, Molecular Diagnostic Laboratory, Barnes-Jewish Hospital, Saint Louis, Missouri.
Regulation of Gene Expression; Genetic Influences on Critical Illness

THOMAS R. ZIEGLER, MD
Assistant Professor of Medicine and Associate Director, Nutrition and Metabolic Support Services, Department of Medicine, Emory University School of Medicine, Atlanta, Georgia.
Diabetic Emergencies

JACK E. ZIMMERMAN, MD, FCCM
Professor of Anesthesiology and Medicine, George Washington University School of Medicine and Health Sciences. Director, Intensive Care Unit Research, George Washington University Medical Center, Washington, D.C.
Benchmarking and Clinical Reengineering in the Intensive Care Unit

JANICE L. ZIMMERMAN, MD, FACP, FCCP, FCCM
Associate Professor, Department of Medicine, Baylor College of Medicine. Director, Medicine Emergency Center, Ben Taub General Hospital, Houston, Texas.
Hypertensive Crises: Emergencies and Urgencies

PREFACE

Critical care is no longer a young specialty in medicine. Essentially, it was introduced in the 1950s with respiratory care and artificial ventilation during the worldwide polio epidemics. Anesthesiologists were the most heavily involved both in Europe and North America through the 1960s and 1970s, because the need for an artificial airway, mechanical ventilation, and cardiopulmonary resuscitation were the most common problems and because these emergencies were particularly familiar to the anesthesiologists.

During the 1980s, internists and pediatricians, especially in the United States, increasingly became interested in intensive care. This interest was shared by surgeons, who initiated trauma units in the early 1960s and later, particularly in the 1990s, also have become frequent critical care specialists in the intensive care unit (ICU) setting.

Gradually, pulmonologists, cardiologists, neurologists, neurosurgeons, cardiothoracic surgeons, traumatologists, and transplant surgeons have demonstrated particular interest in the critical care management of their patients. Consequently, renowned specialists from all these fields and many others have made outstanding contributions to this new edition of our *Textbook of Critical Care.*

The first edition of this textbook was the product of a brainstorming session of a few intensivists in the early 1980s in collaboration with the newly formed Society of Critical Care Medicine (SCCM). Indeed, the first two editions were published as the Society of Critical Care Medicine Textbook of Critical Care. However, many prominent members of SCCM publish critical care textbooks, and it was considered unfair competition to have SCCM sponsor one of these. Therefore, the third and subequent editions are no longer the official product of the SCCM.

The fourth edition has been significantly reorganized. Considering the increasing trend of rapid lifesaving therapy delivered at the scene of a serious accident or in critical illness and continued during transportation to and in the emergency department of the receiving hospital with rapid pursuit of diagnosis and subsequent definitive therapy, many critically ill patients no longer need admission to the hospital if the diagnostic work-up and treatment may be completed in an emergency department short-term ICU within 24 hours. Therefore, this edition covers Resuscitation and Medical Emergencies in the first section, with a second section on Trauma. Imaging comes next, followed by Cell Injury and Cell Death. Infectious Diseases and Endocrinology, Metabolism, Nutrition, and Pharmacology are presented before more organ-specific conditions are discussed. As before, patient care issues and ethical problems are covered separately toward the end of the book. With rapidly increasing age of the population, a greater emphasis on geriatric critical care has been made, and many new chapters describing these problems have been added. Neonatal issues are no longer included, although there still are some 20 chapters throughout the text on pediatric critical care, for all of which Peter R. Holbrook, MD, remains the responsible editor.

To keep this book in one handy volume with approximately 2000 pages, we had to exclude a few excellent chapters to make room for new information. A special effort has been made to avoid redundancy among chapters. No less than 116 chapters are completely new or extensively rewritten, and 86 chapters have been revised to include up-to-date information. Thus, the fourth edition, similar to the third edition, contains just above 200 chapters. The authors, section editors, and four main editors have all carefully selected new and old information to keep this reputable textbook on the highest level, yet readily available as a reference source in the ICU not only to critical care specialists but also to all other physicians and surgeons with patients in intensive care, as well as ICU nurses, respiratory therapists, and senior medical students on ICU assignment, who wish to seek better understanding regarding optimal management of their critically ill and injured patients.

In addition to the authors and editors, a number of other professional individuals have contributed in various ways to the production of this book. Meta Buehler is greatly appreciated for her continued assistance especially related to the Cardiovascular Section. We particularly acknowledge Michael Hess, who with short notice produced excellent chapters on several topics. We are also grateful to the publishing editors at W.B. Saunders, first Beth Hatter and later Judy Spahr, for their untiring efforts in the production of this text.

All of us also greatly appreciate the hard work of those secretaries and other personnel who helped us finalize this book. We hope that this text will be useful not only for critical care physicians and nurses and other ICU specialists but also for all physicians preparing for subspecialty board examinations in critical care.

AKE GRENVIK STEPHEN M. AYRES
PETER R. HOLBROOK WILLIAM C. SHOEMAKER

NOTICE

CONTENTS

SECTION XII

CENTRAL NERVOUS SYSTEM

Section Editor: Ake Grenvik, MD, PhD, FCCM

SECTION XIII

TRANSPLANTATION

Section Editor: Ake Grenvik, MD, PhD, FCCM

SECTION XIV
ORGANIZATION AND MANAGEMENT OF CRITICAL CARE

Section Editors:
Joann I. Lamb, MA, MSN, PA-C, FCCM
Stephen M. Ayres, MD, FCCM

SECTION XV
ETHICAL DECISION MAKING IN CRITICALLY ILL PATIENTS

Section Editors: Joann I. Lamb, MA, MSN, PA-C, FCCM
Stephen M. Ayres, MD, FCCM

COLOR PLATES

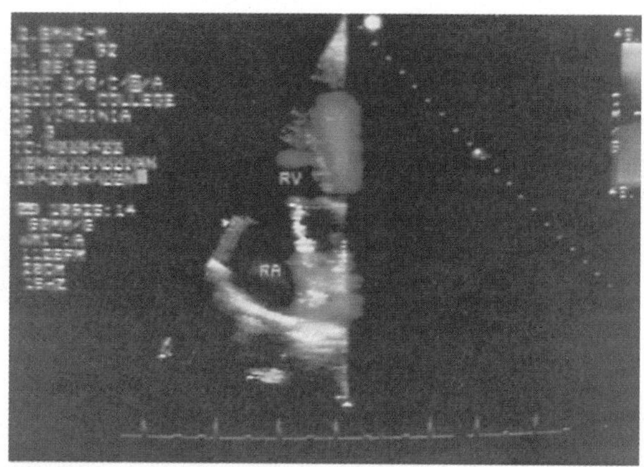

Figure 42–5. A color-flow Doppler echocardiogram in the apical four-chamber view showing tricuspid regurgitation.

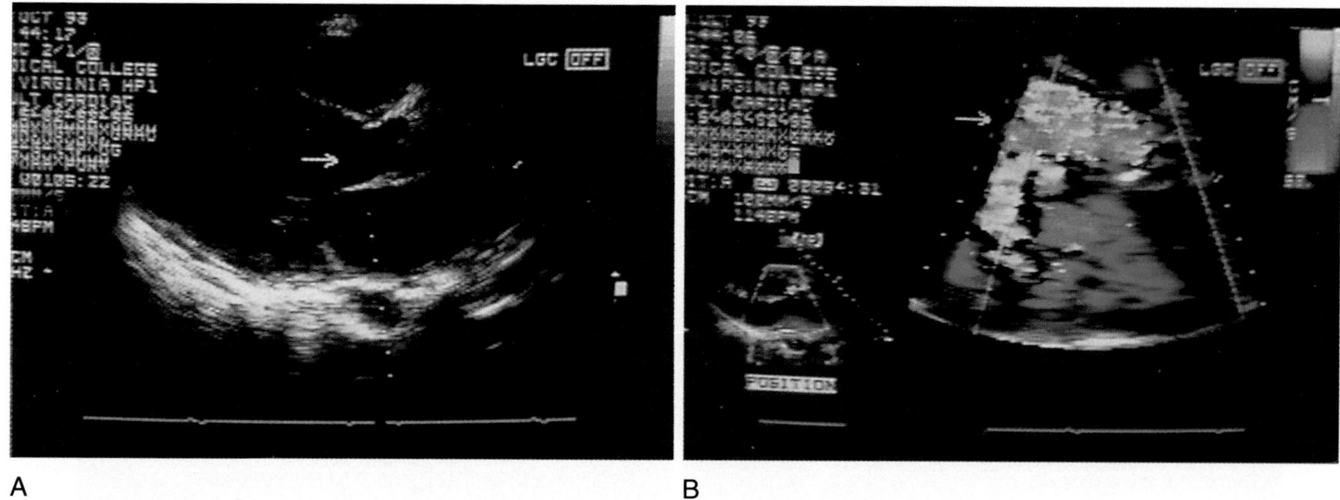

Figure 42–10. *A,* A two-dimensional echocardiogram in the parasternal long-axis view in a patient with aortic regurgitation. *B,* A color-flow Doppler echocardiogram in the parasternal long-axis view of the same patient with aortic regurgitation as in *A*.

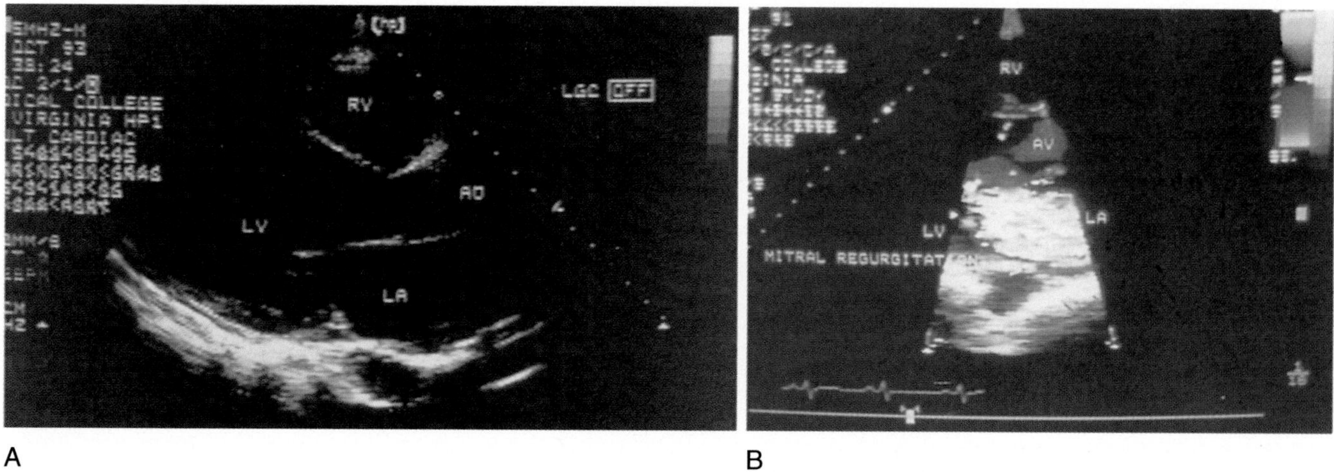

Figure 42–11. *A,* A two-dimensional echocardiogram in the parasternal short-axis view showing left atrial enlargement in a patient with severe mitral regurgitation. *B,* A color-flow Doppler echocardiogram in the parasternal short-axis view showing severe mitral regurgitation in the same patient as in *A*. AV = aortic valve.

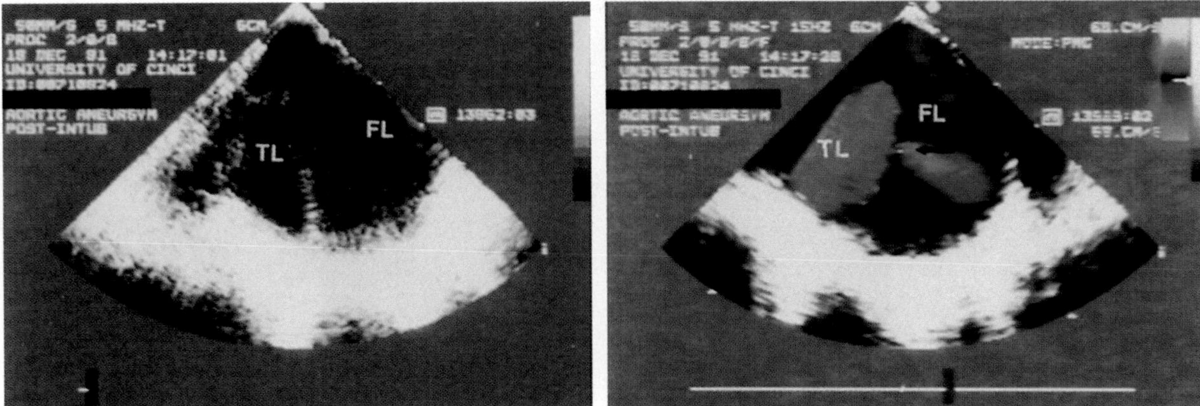

A **Figure 42–14.** Aortic dissection. *A,* Transesophageal echocardiogram (TEE), horizontal view, showing an intimal flap with a small true lumen and a larger false lumen with spontaneous echo contrast. *B,* TEE with color-flow Doppler study showing a small true lumen and a larger false lumen, with a jet through the entry site into the false lumen. B

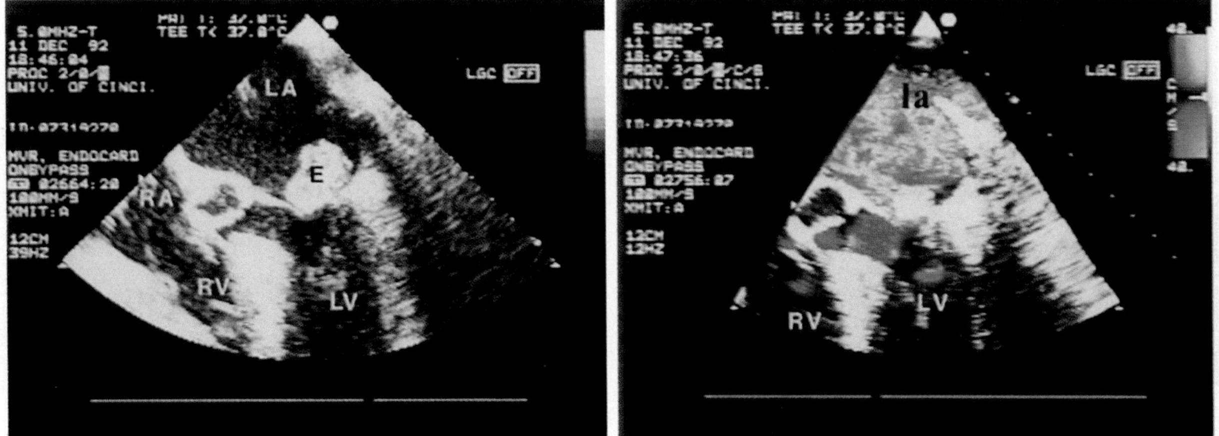

A **Figure 42–16.** *A,* A 2.8 × 1.8 cm vegetation associated with an abscess attached to the posterior mitral valve leaflet shown by transesophageal echocardiography. *B,* During the same procedure, the color-flow study shows severe mitral regurgitation. E = vegetation. B

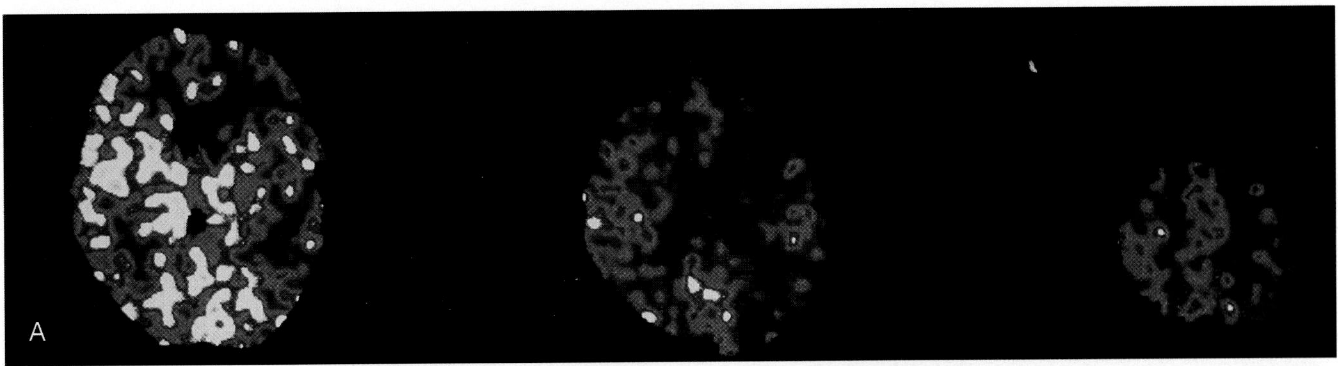

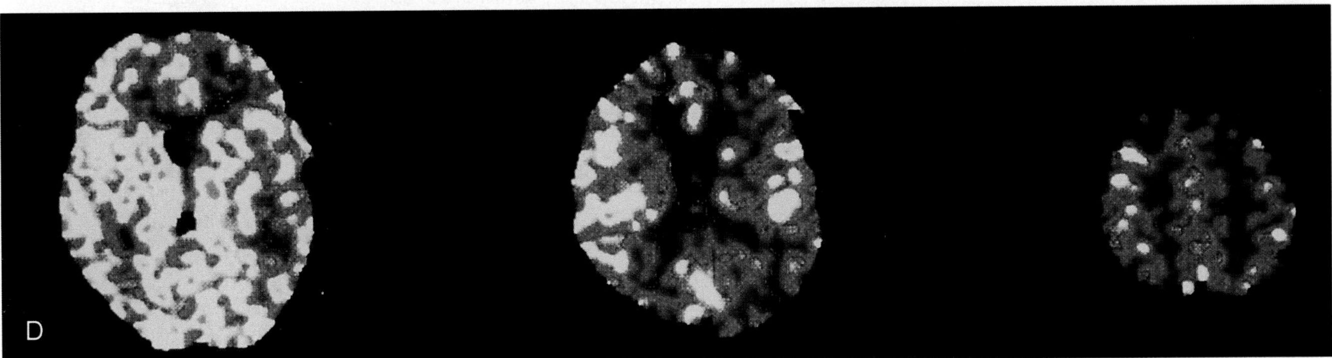

Figure 171–2. *A,* A three-level xenon/CT cerebral blood flow study obtained in a 40-year-old patient 8 days after a subarachnoid hemorrhage and 1 hour after the onset of aphasia and a new weakness of the right arm. *D,* The xenon/CT cerebral blood flow study obtained immediately after papaverine infusion revealed a dramatic improvement of perfusion within the anterior and middle cerebral territories.

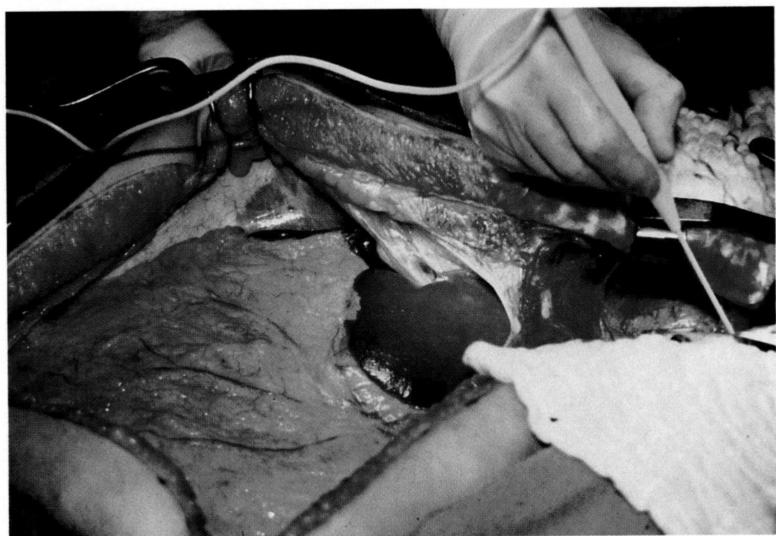

Figure 177–4. Intraoperative photograph showing the total midline incision used for multiple procurement. (Courtesy of Andreis Stieber, MD.)

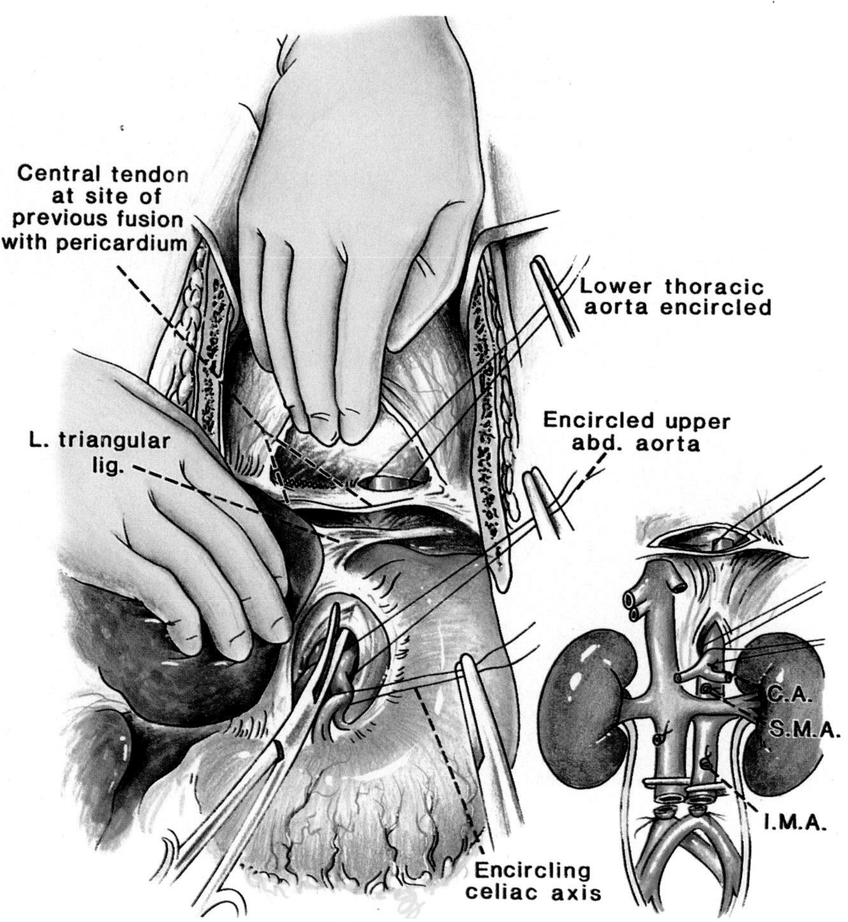

Figure 177–5. The aorta is dissected and encircled just above (or, alternatively, just below) the diaphragm. L. triangular lig. = left triangular ligament; encircled upper abd. aorta = encircled upper abdominal aorta; C.A. = celiac axis; S.M.A. = superior mesenteric artery; I.M.A. = inferior mesenteric artery.

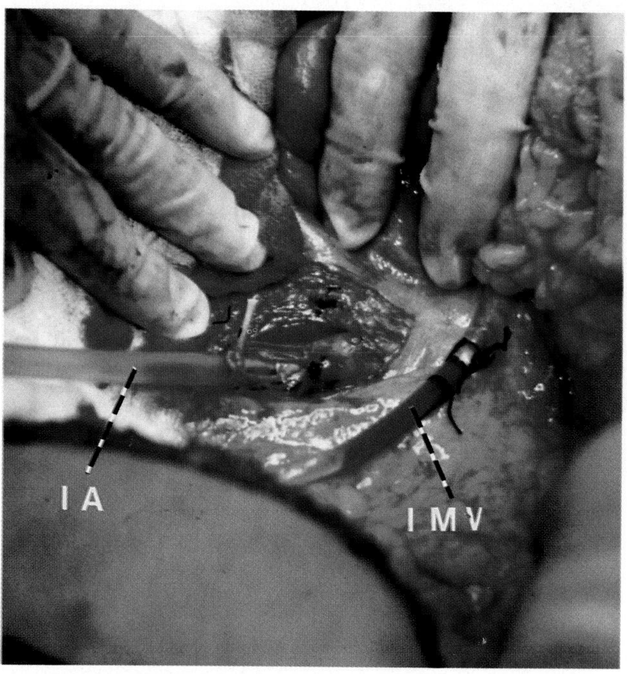

Figure 177–6. Intraoperative photograph showing cannulas for cold perfusion inserted into the dissected donor inferior mesenteric vein (IMV) and infrarenal aorta (IA). (Courtesy of Andreis Stieber, MD.)

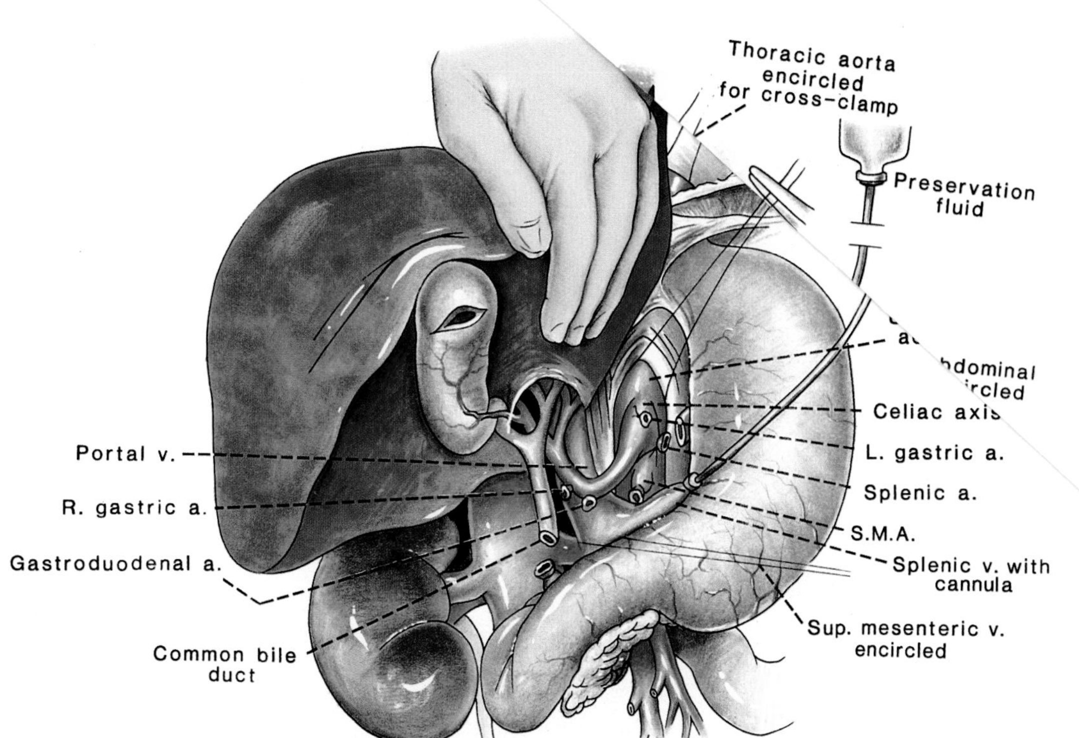

Figure 177–7. Liver hilar dissection, transection of the common bile duct, and incision of the gallbladder fundus to prevent autolysis of the mucosa of the biliary tract. In this drawing, the splenic vein is cannulated; however, the inferior mesenteric vein can be cannulated alternatively, as shown in Figure 177–6. Portal v. = portal vein; R. gastric a. = right gastric artery; Gastroduodenal a. = gastroduodenal artery; L. gastric a. = left gastric artery; Splenic a. = splenic artery; S.M.A. = superior mesenteric artery; Splenic v. with cannula = splenic vein with cannula; Sup. mesenteric v. encircled = superior mesenteric vein encircled.

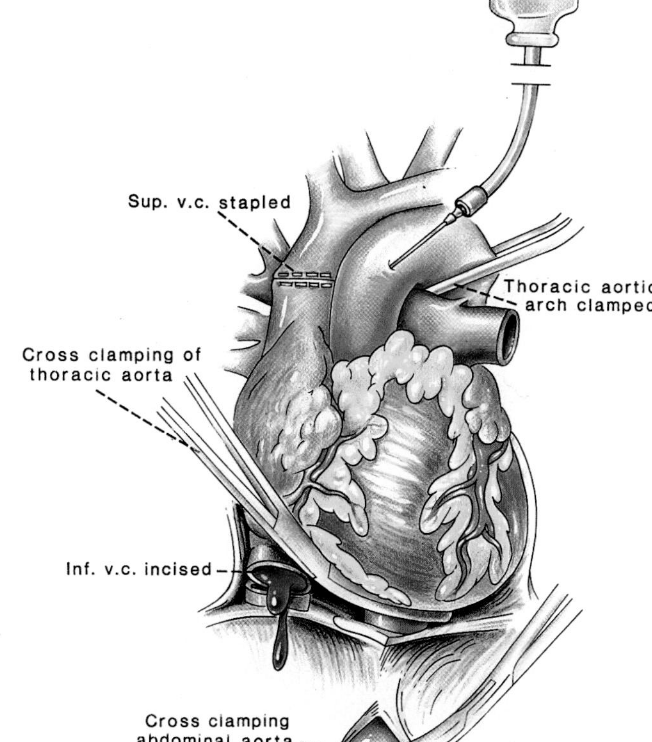

Figure 177–8. Occlusion of the superior vena cava inflow and simultaneous clamping of the aorta proximal to the innominate artery. The aorta is also simultaneously clamped just above or below the diaphragm. Cardioplegic solution infused through the ascending aorta is allowed to run only in the heart. Sup. v.c. stapled = superior vena cava stapled; Inf. v.c. incised = inferior vena cava incised.

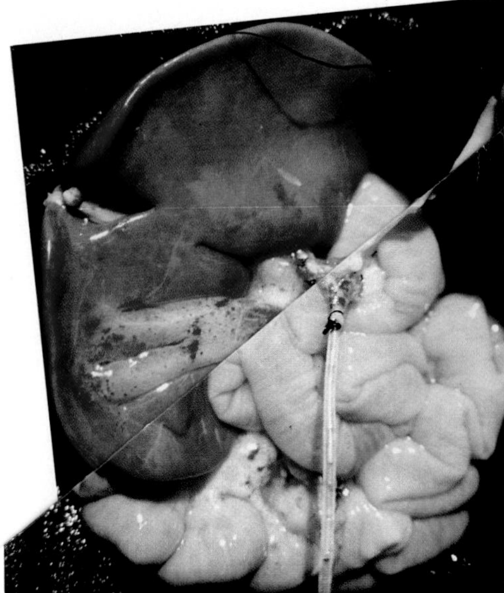

Figure 177–9. En bloc harvesting of liver and small bowel from a pediatric donor.

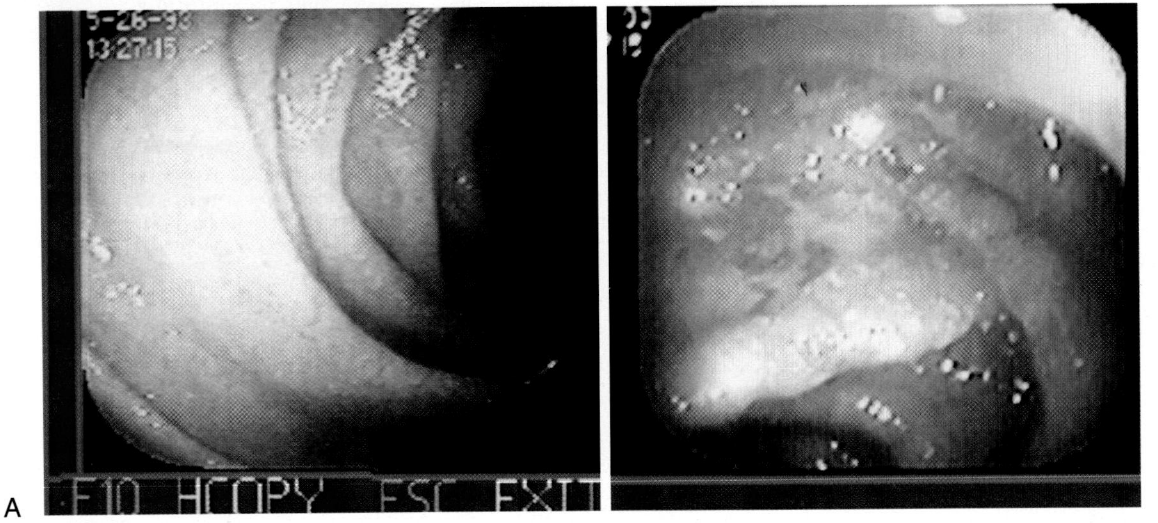

Figure 184–6. *A,* Normal endoscopic appearance of the transplanted small intestine. *B,* Moderate acute cellular rejection of an intestinal allograft demonstrating diffuse edema and focal erythema.

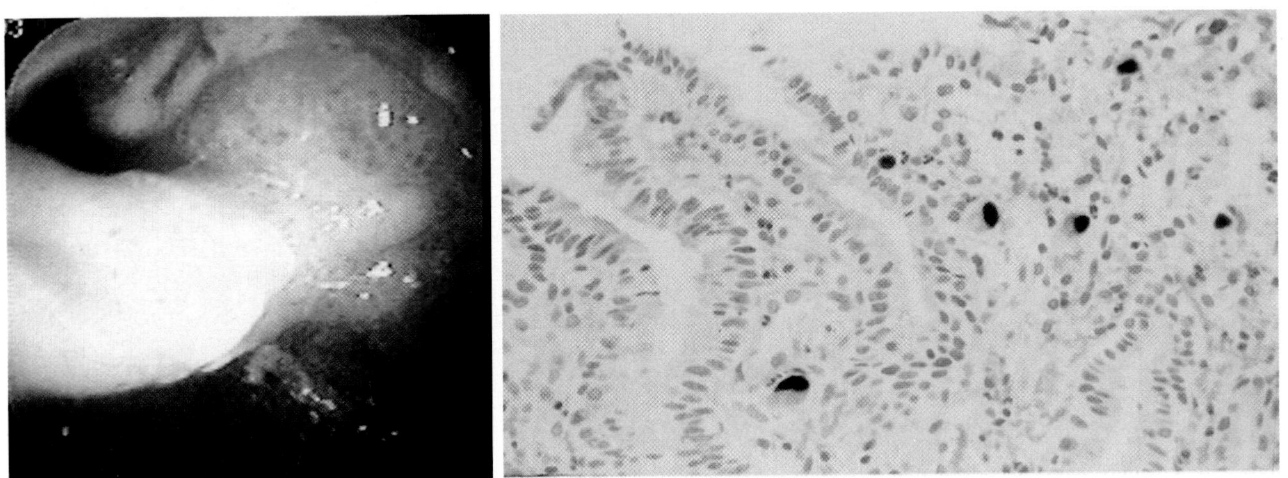

Figure 184–8. *A,* Endoscopic appearance of cytomegaloviral enteritis is characterized by hyperemic erosions. *B,* The diagnosis was confirmed histologically by the presence of characteristic inclusions, by staining for viral antigens, or both. Note the focal neutrophilic inflammation. (Immunoperoxidase for cytomegalovirus antigens, ×350.)

Introduction

Stephen M. Ayres, MD, FCCM

Critical Care Medicine (CCM) includes the life-support continuum from the scene through discharge from the intensive care unit (ICU). This requires emergency medicine (emergency department physicians, who also control prehospital resuscitation and life-support) and intensive care medicine, the topic of this book. Thus CCM requires team action by physicians with various specialty backgrounds and added expertise in resuscitation, as well as community-wide emergency medical services (EMS) systems. These Emergency and Critical Care Medicine (ECCM) systems include a continuum of life support from the scene (self-help, help from bystanders or ambulance personnel), via transport and emergency department to operating room and intensive care unit.[1]

This brief comment, made more than two decades ago at a National Institutes of Health (NIH) Consensus Development Conference, seemed more utopian than practical at the time. Today, the contentious economic forces swirling around the delivery of health care of all sorts have forced these concepts to become reality.

The authors of the third edition of the *Textbook of Critical Care*[2] warned readers that the United States was moving rapidly to dramatically change the way its health care was to be financed and delivered. Any health reform plan would certainly require physicians to act as managers of resource allocation as well as diagnosticians and caregivers. The vast amount of new information contained in this fourth edition is weighty evidence of the need for students and physicians to develop new methods of acquiring and retrieving information. Intensivists have served as resource managers and should be well prepared to take on this important new role in an expanded fashion. They have also led the way in the use of protocols and guidelines as methods for reducing reams of data into useful approaches to diagnosis and treatment.

Intensivists have several major advantages over the rest of what has become the medical marketplace. Ordinarily, the issue of medical necessity is not disputed by insurers except when patients have significant signs of impending doom. In addition, intensivists began to assess their own performance, even before they were formally organized into a new discipline. They developed severity of illness and outcome analyses systems and "benchmarked" their practice by comparing themselves to others treating the same types of critically ill patients. They built their practice on the triage principles of military medicine and showed that survival from critical illness in civilian life could be enhanced if physiologic derangements were rapidly reversed in what soon became called the moment of opportunity or the "golden period."

This introduction reviews the major shifts in the United States health policy since the failure of health care reform in 1993, the impact of managed care on the practice of intensive care medicine, and the improbable marriage of critical care medicine, emergency medicine, and managed care leaders. It attempts to turn the problem of managed care into efficient care, where the mandates of cost containment and quality care become convergent in specially organized acute care centers.

Critical care medicine has come of age during this last quarter of the 20th century. Not long ago, physicians watched helplessly as life hung in the balance between those forces promoting life and those leading to death. But at long last, during the second quarter of the 20th century, the memorable portrait of the physician sitting at the bedside of a child through the long night, waiting for either recovery or death, became replaced by vignettes of resurrection, as physicians labored actively to turn back the intrusion of the "Grim Reaper." Step by labored step, the understanding of life-promoting forces evolved, and at some moment in the very recent past an extremely ill individual could be said to profit more by medical action than by medical inaction.

Critical care in its various forms plays a central role in the access to medical care for millions of Americans who have experienced it as well as for those who may depend on it for the management of life-threatening injury or disease in the future. Because it is a dramatic display of medical intervention at its best, critical care runs the risk of being viewed in terms that would conceptualize it as an end in itself—in truth, as part of a medical system that is expected to contribute its share of service for the welfare of the entire society. As part of the fabric of medical care, critical care has all of the strengths and weaknesses, and is subject to all of the criticisms and changes, that characterize the health and medical effort in this last period of the 20th century. Simply because the stakes and costs for this sort of care are so high, ill-considered changes could seriously damage the American health care effort, whereas carefully planned and rational changes in the way such care is delivered could improve the quality and decrease the cost of medical care in general.

CRITICAL CARE AND THE RISE OF TECHNOLOGY

Critical care developed as optimism and confidence in the ability of technology to conquer almost all human problems marked the period following the Second World War. Victory had convinced many that the scientific, industrial, and technologic expertise of Americans, demonstrated so convincingly during wartime, could lead to an ever-increasing standard of life for all. Nowhere was this optimism more evident than in the belief that biomedical research could lead to the control of disease and the extension of life. Congress generously supported the NIH, and by 1994 the total appropriations had risen to $11.3 billion.[3] Leveraged by industrial investment, its share soon averaged two thirds of the total spending on research and development. In 1947, the total for all federal research spending had been only $7 million. Important discoveries quickly led to new pharmaceutical agents and expensive medical devices. The new profitability of the medical enterprise, caused in large part by the support of the federal government's Medicare program, fueled a "medical arms race." Hospitals rushed to gain the competitive edge over their rivals by purchasing the latest piece of medical equipment. Costs began to skyrocket, and although life expectancy increased, many began to question buying at great cost a few extra months of life. Critical care became known as the "high tech specialty" and was deemed the enemy by health policy planners.[4]

Hundreds of new products have appeared in the American health care market since the mid-1950s. Some of these products show their capacity to help but, unfortunately, also to injure. Some products are of unproven effectiveness, and some are ineffective and even harmful. All are expensive, and many raise serious ethical concerns over their use.

Beginning in the 1950s, life-supporting techniques (such as cardiac monitoring systems that signal an abnormal heart beat, electrical defibrillators that restore the heart beat to normal, respirators that breathe for patients who can no longer breathe unaided, and dialysis devices that substitute for damaged kidneys) appeared. In the 1960s, diagnostic techniques (such as ultrasonography, computed tomography [CT], magnetic resonance imaging [MRI], automated blood and urine testing, studies of body cells [Papanicolaou smears]) and treatment technology (such as heart valves, pacemakers that return the heart to its rhythmic beating, artificial hearts and transplanted organs) became available and dramatically changed the way medicine is practiced.

THE CALL FOR HEALTH CARE REFORM

It is not surprising that concerns over the costs of health care began in the United States, where costs were higher than in any other place in the world. In the winter of 1977, an entire issue of the journal *Daedalus*, entitled "Doing Better and Feeling Worse: Health in the United States," was devoted to health care.[5] The issue began with a call for change:

Doing Better and Feeling Worse—is this a fair appraisal of the "health system" that now prevails in the United States? Those who are openly skeptical of many features of health care in late twentieth-century America will ask whether it makes any sense even to speak of a "health care system" in a country where services are so fractionated and largely controlled by private physicians who appear almost indifferent to demands for certain kinds of attention. While the costs of medical service continue to rise dramatically—in most instances galloping ahead even more rapidly than the price of other goods in this inflationary era—new evidences of fraud and malpractice are discovered in federal programs as well as in the private sector. These revelations only provide additional fuel for the already widespread opinion that in health—as in education, justice, and welfare—things have recently gone strangely awry and only substantial reforms will set them right.

At that time, the journal editors worried that health care costs had risen from $39 billion in 1965 to $119 billion in 1976. By 1993, total expenditures had risen to more than $800 billion and serious problems still existed in access to health care. By 1996, the total cost of care health in the United States was $1 trillion, although the rate of rise had been strikingly reduced.[6]

The calls for reform were many and repeated. Harris Wofford upset the front-runner in an election for the U.S. Senate, and his victory was attributed to his support for health care changes. President William Clinton called the health care situation a major crisis and pledged to work for reform.

THE ADMINISTRATION'S HEALTH SECURITY PLAN

The presidential planners rejected the single-payer system adopted by most other countries because they knew it would be termed "socialized medicine" and had little chance of acceptance by the Congress. Instead, they chose the "managed competition" approach of the Jackson Hole think tank, led by Paul Ellwood. Many health care theorists visited Jackson Hole regularly and helped formulate the approach to managed competition.[7]

Apparently, the idea of managed competition began with H.M. and A.R. Somers in 1971, although its precise lineage is not clear. It is a significant compromise between the single-payer and managed care approaches and may yet find itself on center stage once again. Managed competition had its roots in the original Federal Employee Health Benefit Program and was based on the idea of sponsorship. The sponsor would contract with health plans concerning benefits covered, prices, enrollment procedures, nature of the medical group, and other conditions of participation. The sponsor would structure equitable rules, create price-elastic demand, and avoid uncompensated risk selection. The sponsors were called "health insurance purchasing cooperatives" and attempted to blend the competitive and regulatory features of existing health plans. They would not be governmental agencies, even though the plan was portrayed as a giant bureaucracy by its opponents.

The Clinton Plan drew heavily on the refinements of managed competition developed by Paul Starr in his book, *The Logic of Health-Care Reform*. Although many economists had believed that managed competition and global budgeting were antithetical, Starr proposed that they should be combined.[8]

President Clinton decided to incorporate Starr's concepts into his "Health Security Plan." Three key provisions of the plan, purchasing alliances, employer mandate, and global budgeting, were creative but controversial.[9] All citizens and legal residents would be guaranteed health insurance and a federally guaranteed benefit plan, and all such individuals would receive coverage through their alliance. A National Health Board would review and update the standard benefits package. The package would include benefits typically offered by employers. The benefit package would emphasize primary care and preventive services.

Each state would establish one or more regional health alliances for its residents. Workers would be required to obtain coverage through the health alliance where they live unless they worked for companies with more than 5000 employees; in that case, they would belong to a corporate alliance. Employers would be required to pay 80% of the average premium across all alliance plans (the employer mandate). Small employers would be capped at 7.9% of payroll. Sliding scale subsidies would be available to employers with 50 or fewer employees if the average wage were less than $24,000 per year. Firms with less than $12,000 average annual wage would have contributions capped at 3.5% of total payroll.

Health plans would contract with alliances and follow federal standards, including minimum benefits, enrollment practices, and termination of coverage. Premiums would be "community-rated." Every person would pay the same premium, there would be no underwriting or risk rating. Physicians could join more than one health plan. Health plans would be accountable, publish outcomes of treatment, and develop consumer grievance and appeals procedures. Premiums would be limited to the same rate of growth as the annual growth in the Consumer Price Index (CPI). The National Health Board would adjust premium targets to reflect each alliances population and characteristics such as age, gender, and health status. There would also be administrative simplification, coordination of benefits, and development of alternative resolution systems for malpractice claims.[9]

POLITICS AS USUAL

Most of the insured population were insensitive to the rising costs of care because it was paid by their employers, and the uninsured had little political weight. Some analysts suggested that major health care reform could not occur until the cost of health premiums caused real pain and reached as much as 50% of take-home pay. The lessons of 1993–1994 suggest that this may be correct. The President had originally planned to introduce health care reform as part of the first budget reconciliation bill, for which only a simple majority was needed for passage, but Senator Robert Byrd objected and scuttled the plan. It was all downhill after this strategic defeat. The budget bill, the North American Free Trade Agreement (NAFTA), and casualties in Somalia caused the White House to delay consideration until well into 1994.

Attempting to replace 1500 insurance companies with new alliances or purchasing pools was obviously going to galvanize the insurance industry into action. Equally distasteful to the insurance industry was the system of price controls on insurance premiums that would be administered through the alliances. Willis Gradison, former congressman from Ohio and previously a supporter of health reform, became president of the insurance industry trade organization, the Health Insurance Association of America (HIAA). In a political commercial, fictional characters "Harry" and "Louise" appeared on television frequently, wondering what outrages the Clinton Administration was going to visit next on the American public.

THE RESPONSE OF THE MEDICAL PROFESSION

Unlike the brutal opposition mounted by the medical profession when reforms were debated in the past, the American Medical Association (AMA) expressed qualified support. The AMA was committed to reform, it said, and now worked to persuade the Clinton Administration to make significant modifications in its plan. During its annual meeting in October 1993, the AMA announced that they could

agree with many broad aspects of the Clinton plan but opposed many details, including insurance premium ceilings and reductions in reimbursements under the existing Medicare health plan for the elderly. . . . The AMA said a letter was mailed two days earlier to 710,000 doctors. . . . The letter from senior AMA officials praised some Clinton initiatives as "good for patients," including his proposal for universal health coverage to include the estimated 37 million Americans without health insurance. But the officials expressed serious reservations about proposals that would limit patient and doctor choices, undermine quality of medical care and lead to federal controls over the medical profession.[10]

During the 103rd Congress, health care reform became mired in the sludge of upcoming congressional elections and proposals of any sort were roundly rejected. The Administration refused to compromise in its demand for universal coverage and global budgets, and even sensible and relatively modest proposals by Republicans like Senator John Chaffee were rejected. The intense political fragmentation of the 103rd Congress doomed any sort of health care reform and Congress ignored a major opportunity for providing high-quality health care to all Americans. The congressional debate was shelved and largely forgotten by most in leadership positions. Meanwhile, the private sector began to tightly control health care access of Americans.[11]

THE AFTERSHOCKS

Even though the Congress did not believe that problems within the health care system had reached crisis levels, the systemic problems of inadequate access and rising costs still remained. In the midst of party bickering and positioning, the impact of transformations and distortions of the health care system on individual patients and their physicians lay largely ignored. Physicians remained immersed in the reams of paperwork engendered by multiple insurers, multiple forms, multiple fee schedules, and multiple "rules of engagement." Physicians were so frustrated that many jumped at the reduced paper trail required of a single-payer system and preferred the comfort of a salary rather than fee-for-service with its dozens of fee schedules. Not a single health care reform bill passed, and the tiger of unregulated managed care was unleashed.

"It's very disappointing," said James Todd, executive vice president of the AMA.

Our biggest concern is the rapid consolidation of health care delivery systems under the control of giant insurance companies. . . . We're concerned patients are being bought, sold and being told to what doctor they can go, to what facility they must go to receive care, and under the present circumstances patients are becoming pawns.[12]

The failure of the federal government to act placed the burden of the uninsured on the states, while the tactics used by integrated managed care systems has raised costs and led many state employees to believe that their level of care has deteriorated. Medicaid costs consume large fractions of state governments, even though eligibility is sharply limited and many of the poor remain uninsured. Even though it is politically correct to speak of the states as laboratories, the vacuum created by federal inaction has required quick response by the states. New York State announced plans to expand coverage to tens of thousands of uninsured, using savings obtained by cuts in Medicaid. The Clinton Administration approved a demonstration project in Florida that could extend coverage to patients well above the poverty line; Oregon, Tennessee, Hawaii, Kentucky, Rhode Island, and the state of Washington will all seek waivers to implement programs aimed at those who cannot afford insurance and are not covered by Medicaid. Many of these plans will involve employees in more than one state, and most will require repeal of the Employment Retirement Income Security Act (ERISA).

THE STAKEHOLDERS IN HEALTH CARE

Physicians and their patients are but one constituency in an enterprise that is of vital concern to the corporate world and to the insurance industry. Physicians are generally apolitical but would do well to understand the forces allied against them. They might be surprised to know how different stakeholders view the vast panorama of health care in the United States. To physicians and nurses, health care is a calling; to patients, of course, it represents their best chance to restored health. To corporate America, health care becomes a business expense; and to insurers, health care becomes a profitable undertaking. Reducing health care costs increases corporate profits, and health insurance has suddenly become one of the most profitable businesses in the country. The business community has sensed the possibility of major profits. In 1981, only 18% of health maintenance organizations (HMOs) were "for-profit"; by 1995, 71% of HMOs were established as for-profit corporations. At the moment, it appears that the insurance industry and business at large—not patients or their physicians—are in the driver's seat. The insurance industry had invested heavily to defeat the Clinton proposal and reaped its rewards as it moved to tightly regulate the ability of physicians to diagnose and treat their patients. The method they picked was called "managed care"![13]

The organized management of medical problems is not new. "Case-management" is a term borrowed from the social sciences that describes the organization of health care resources in such a manner as to maximize preventive, diagnostic, and treatment efforts. Managed competition, as envisioned by Ellwood and his colleagues in the Jackson Hole group, was designed to allow consumers to pick the health plans best suited to their needs. Managed care began as a method for improving care but soon became a tool of the insurance industry to deny access to expensive health care in order to reduce costs and provide profits for insurers.

At first blush, the idea made sense. The term managed care implies that health care services are not generally well managed or coordinated. HMOs have a cohesive medical staff that work together in order to provide quality care at the lowest possible price. Because many physicians do not wish to be salaried employees of a group practice, other methods of achieving a similar goal have been developed. Networks of physicians called "independent practice associations" (IPAs) have been organized, and physicians within the network agree to reduce unnecessary utilization and keep fees as low as possible. The reward to the physician is an increased volume of patients, and the physician may trade a lesser fee than desired in return for a promise of increased patient numbers. Patients must receive care from primary care physicians belonging to the network and can receive specialty care only if the insurance plan and the physician agree that the referral is indicated and warranted. Only specialists belonging to the network can receive referred patients from general physicians within the network.

Revolutionary changes in social structure challenge the entire body politic, but the rapid shift in the method of delivering health care moved far beyond anything envisioned by the White House planners.[13] Managed care extracted the most innovative parts of managed competition and turned it into a system designed to refuse or delay care. Control of health care has shifted leadership away from practicing physicians to the insurance industry. "Harry" and "Louise" succeeded far beyond their fondest dreams and wrecked the fee-for-service payment system and much of the physician-patient relationship. Today, nearly 75% of American workers receive coverage from HMOs, Preferred Provider Organizations (PPOs), and Point of Service (POS) plans. The shift to managed care of all kinds has been incredible; it increased from 51% of all employer-based insurance plans in 1993 to 73% in 1995. Even plans aimed at companies with fewer than 50 employees are tightly managed; these plans rose from 29% in 1993 to 82% in 1995.

The rise in POS plans is particularly striking and could be important in steering critically ill people to hospitals skilled in their care. Coverage requires approval of the assigned primary care physician and is broader when subscribers stay within the plan's network. The plans also cover out-of-network services, although in some instances the approval of a primary care physician is required.

Managed care places a major burden on physicians because the insurance company closely scrutinizes their practice patterns and individual patient care decisions. In a sense, it is the price to be paid for avoiding a single-payer system. Physicians are generally participants in a PPO, which permits them to deal only with hospitals and physicians within the network. Employers have jumped to the managed care concept because it appears to reduce costs by at least 10% in comparison with conventional fee-for-service reimbursement. In 1987, 41% of employer-supported care was unmanaged; in 1990, all but 5% of workers were under some type of management.[13] In 1998, nearly all employers offered some managed care plan.

MANAGED CARE DOES REDUCE HEALTH CARE COSTS

Levit and colleagues,[6] in presenting "National Health Spending Trends in 1996" have pointed out that

Spending for personal health care services in the United States remains far higher than that in any other industrialized country. Nevertheless, in the past five years spending increases have slowed dramatically as a result of low general medical-specific inflation, as the growth of managed care enrollment, and the capacity of health plans to negotiate discounts from a provider system weakened by over capacity.

In 1996, the last year that statistics were available, total spending for health care was $1,035.1 billion, just tipping the trillion-dollar level. The percentage increase was 4.4—a striking decline from the double-digit inflation that lasted until 1990. The cost of physician services increased only 2.9%, as many physicians experienced significant reductions in income. Actual physician expenditures were $146.3 billion in 1990 and rose to $202.1 billion in 1996, whereas prescription drugs rose from $37.7 billion to $62.2 billion.

The rush to managed care has not pleased physicians, who are frustrated with the intrusion of insurance company managers into their practices and the incredible paperwork required in dealing with dozens of insurance companies, each with their own fee-schedule, rules for participation, and insurance forms. Physicians are forced to limit care for many problems and are not allowed to provide patients with complete information about their care options.

Incredibly, the technique of managed care is now being used to ration health care services. During the "grand debate" of 1993, there was great concern over the possibility of rationing health care. The state of Oregon attempted to refuse Medicaid payments for certain procedures that were not deemed cost-effective, and most people believed that rationing would begin with the very poor.[14] In contrast, the wealthy and the poor have access to health care, but middle class insured patients are now refused care on the basis of insurance company decisions. It was not meant to be that way, but the lack of regulations has allowed managed care organizations to function in any manner that would decrease costs. Their success in cutting costs through tough negotiation with providers has discouraged them from attempting more creative approaches to delivering quality care. But consumer activism and the workings of the marketplace are prodding insurers to return to the original principles and intentions of managed competition.

COST CONTAINMENT AND THE ACUTE CARE UNIT: THE 23-HOUR ACUTE UNIT

Improbably, in the 1990s, the need to continue the containment of costs in the hospital set in motion a series of events that supported two bedrock principles of critical care medicine:

1. A golden period exists immediately after the onset of serious illness or injury when appropriate treatment could prevent death or disability.
2. Intensivists broadly trained in the care of seriously ill patients provide more efficient care than a series of medical and surgical specialists.

Although considerable evidence supporting these principles existed, turf battles, the power of traditional subspecialists, and the need to fill hospital beds delayed their implementation.

In the years following the enactment of Medicare, hospital administrators constantly encouraged physicians to admit patients to the hospital and to keep them there! The per diem method of reimbursement provided little incentive for early discharge, and the constant slogan of the administrator was "fill the beds."

In addition, the concept of the golden period was constantly ignored in emergency departments of teaching hospitals. Resident physicians followed unwritten rules regarding admission to their own services and constantly tried to transfer less interesting patients to other services in the same or other hospitals. A sociologist, Terry Mizrah,[15] studying the behavior of residents in the emergency department, was led to entitle her study "Getting Rid of Patients." Resident surgeons performed differently and combed the hospital and emergency departments for patients with abdominal pain or other problems that could lead to a trip to the operating room.

Hospital administrators took note of the situation and realized that one method of reducing hospital admissions was to admit patients to a 23-hour unit that would not incur the costs of an actual admission to the hospital. At about the same time, physicians and administrators realized that the "emergency room"—now christened the "emergency department"—was the only area in the hospital where all of the resources of knowledgeable consultants and diagnostic equipment were readily at hand. The 23-hour treatment unit was entrenched as a method of cost containment. Miraculously, this approach actually improved patient care.[16]

The heart of the acute care unit is the use of clinical pathways. Clemmer and Spuhler[17] describe these pathways:

Clinical pathways or care maps are designed to focus on the logisti-

cal flow of care through a health care system by integrating various aspects of care into an efficient and seamless care plan across departments. They coordinate personnel, equipment and procedures into a logical plan or continuum of care. Although they are usually disease-specific, they tend to be general in nature and retain a lot of flexibility in order to meet the care needs over a spectrum of patient acuities. They are designed to apply to the majority of a specific type of patient, but also expect outlier to fall outside of the pathway on a regular basis. One or more guidelines or protocols may be incorporated into the pathway. Pathways are very dependent upon the institution's resources, structure, and organization and are therefore institution-specific. Although institutions share their pathways, they are almost always modified to meet the peculiarities of the institution.

Protocols are the bridge between outcomes research and practice. They guide the health care professional to the desired pathway and determine the architecture of the selected route. Protocols must be based on scientific evidence and relevance. They are usually developed by teams involving all appropriate practitioners assisted by information in the literature. They must be clear, able to be modified, and lead to cost-effective clinical practice.

THE CONVERGENCE OF INTENSIVE AND EMERGENCY MEDICAL CARE

The Importance of Triage

Two new medical disciplines, critical care and emergency medical care, evolved at the beginning of the era of cost containment. Both disciplines were initially geographically bound by a specific location; the emergency medicine physician was based in the emergency department, while the intensivist remained in the ICU. The separation was artificial and largely political.

Once again, the comments made at the NIH Consensus Conference[18] on the seamless nature of immediate care are particularly appropriate:

Critical Care Medicine (CCM) is a multi-disciplinary and multi-professional medical/nursing field concerned with patients who have sustained or are at risk of sustaining acutely life-threatening single or multiple organ system failure due to disease or injury. These conditions necessitate prolonged minute-to-minute therapy or observation in an intensive care unit (ICU) which is capable of a high level of intensive therapy in terms of quality and immediacy. In its broadest meaning, CCM includes management at the scene of onset of critical illness or injury during transportation, in the emergency department, during surgical intervention in the operating room, and finally in the ICU.

The 23-hour acute care unit is an important link in patient care that begins with the mobile ICU and stretches to the stepdown unit. These units attempt to match staffing and technology with patient need.

The first step in caring for a critically ill patient is to recognize that he or she is in serious difficulty. Patients are brought to the emergency department or to physicians' offices, but the gravity of the situation may not be apparent, even though there are serious malfunctions in one or more organ systems. A subtle change in a physical sign may be the first indication of general collapse. Early warning signs are frequently overlooked or dismissed unless physicians and nurses are constantly on the alert for harbingers of critical illness.

Similar levels of pre-hospital care should be available to all Americans. There seems to be no rational explanation for the presence of well-trained paramedics in one geographical location but not in another. Standards exist for paramedic training in some states but not in others. Minimal federal guidelines for training and certification should be developed, since the states vary widely in their commitment to the support of social services. The cost of an integrated hospital transportation system would pay for itself because inappropriate or delayed care is itself extremely expensive. The costs of a patient languishing in a coma for months following serious injury could probably pay for one or two ambulances! An untapped resource for pre-hospital care exists in the many fire departments throughout the United States. Firemen and women make ideal paramedics and should receive such training and certification.

Identifying the Critically Ill Patient

In earlier times, the intensivist could do little more than administer lifesaving techniques such as cardiopulmonary resuscitation, ventilator care, and defibrillation. While keeping patients alive is obviously essential, it is just the beginning of the intensivist's responsibility. The evaluation and interpretation of the presenting clinical signs and assignment of causal agents are of paramount importance. The evaluation of patients in special diagnostic units (see later) greatly facilitates the diagnostic process. Medical and nursing trainees must master the fine art of triage as they select appropriate "critical pathways" for the patients who enter the emergency department.

Subtle changes may be overlooked or dismissed unless the triage officer is ever aware of the possibility of serious trouble. It is easy and reassuring to the medical professional to dismiss an abnormal failure by ascribing to it an unimportant cause. The weakest link in patient care may well be the tendency of physicians or other triage officers to convince themselves that everything will be all right. Philosophically, sins of omission are frequently more common than sins of commission. Does modern cost containment pressure encourage physicians to discount potentially life-threatening signs or symptoms? How are triage professionals trained and encouraged to focus only on the patient at hand regardless of the rules established by their managed care organization?

Important signs of serious injury and illness include low-blood pressure or weak peripheral pulses, cold temperature of extremities, and peripheral cyanosis. Poor cardiac output produces constriction of cutaneous arterioles and stimulation of sweat glands, resulting in the characteristic cold, pale and clammy skin. Often the first signs of impaired oxygen delivery to the tissues are alterations in cerebral function. Although coma is an obvious sign of severe illness, subtle changes in mental status may indicate serious hemodynamic or metabolic abnormalities. Other warning signs include reduced urinary output, dyspnea or hyperpnea, high temperature, unexplained fatigue, chest pains, and tachycardia or palpitations.

Many of these signs and symptoms may be produced by one or more causal agents. Differential diagnosis requires consideration of many possible etiologic agents, including infection and sepsis, trauma, exposure to physical stressors (e.g., hypothermia, hyperthermia, emotional stress), cardiovascular dysfunction, toxic agents (e.g., poisons, carbon monoxide inhalation), immunologic disorders, and specific infectious diseases (e.g., Rocky Mountain spotted fever), insect bites, and other sources of disease.

The use of protocols greatly improves the ability of clinicians to detect critical illness. Once the critically ill patient is identified, he or she must be categorized into an appropriate pathophysiologic state and admitted to a critical pathway, such as trauma, sepsis, coma, cardiac abnormalities, overdosage, or other serious problem. Critical pathways have their own protocols that simultaneously attempt to establish diagnosis and treatment.

THE HIGH-PERFORMANCE ACUTE CARE/INTENSIVE CARE UNIT

Since the 1960s, critical care physicians and nurses have used their experience to develop the practice of their discipline. Other medical disciplines have been unwilling to evaluate their own practice until recently. Intensivists developed coordinated care systems, analysis of outcomes of treatment options, and protocols and guidelines for the care of individual patients. Knaus and associates,[19] for example, showed that ICUs with the lowest death rates used standard approaches or "protocols" and did not permit each physician to develop a completely unique treatment plan for each patient. In addition, a medical director with considerable authority for managing admission and discharge policies and coordinating the care of individual physicians was present and a high level of educational achievement was present for critical care nurses.

Other published studies are consistent with these views. A prospective pilot project organized by the American Association of Critical Care Nurses[20] studied the effects of a coordinated care in an ICU and showed that the mortality rate for 192 patients was 51% of that predicted by Acute Physiology and Chronic Health Evaluation (APACHE) scoring, new complications did not occur, and both staff and patient satisfaction was high.

The ability of specially trained critical care physicians to lower mortality rates in ICUs was shown by two studies. Reynolds and coauthors[21] reported that the mortality from septic shock decreased from 74% to 23% when specially trained physicians supervised care. Brown and Sullivan[22] found a 52% decrease in ICU deaths when a full-time critical care specialist was recruited and coordinated the care of the patient's own physician.

Continuous Quality Improvement

There is evidence that the process or manner of providing critical care is an important determinant of survival needs to be institutionalized. Although slow to be accepted in the medical arena, the continuous quality improvement (CQI) strategy, designed by Deming and detailed by Berwick[23] and his Japanese colleagues soon after the end of World War II, provides an important framework for health care organizations seeking to constantly improve the outcomes of their care. The first of Deming's Fourteen Points was the radical definition of a company's objective. Rather than making money, its mission was to stay in business and provide jobs through innovation, research, constant improvement, and maintenance. Today's profit-driven health care system is the antithesis of the Deming model.

The level of collaboration between physicians and nurses and the organization of human resources, rather than the technical capability of individual practitioners, seems to determine the outcome. The better the management of human resources, the better the outcome, independent of resources. On-site physician and nurse leaders ensure that patient needs are matched in the availability of resources by the implementations of sound admission and discharge policies. Effective clinical managers triage patients and attempt to resolve conflict among health care practitioners, particularly among physicians. In many units, physician managers are managers in name only and do not triage, make decisions, or resolve conflicts. Nurses are forced, in the absence of a working medical director, to make moment-to-moment decisions that determine patient outcome. A collaborative nurse-physician relationship usually suggests that physician leadership is present within the units on a reliable and regular basis. The most successful units seem to carefully utilize nurse resources. Clerical tasks, such as seeking laboratory reports, managing patient records, housekeeping, and making telephone calls, are performed by individuals other than nurses.

The intensivist's commitment to constantly improving the quality of care seeps through the pages of a recently published issue of "Role of Outcomes Research in the Intensive Care Setting." This scholarly document provides significant advice for all who care for the critically ill:

Improvement can be defined as attainment of an unprecedented level of performance. In health care, performance may be measured in terms of clinical outcomes, patient satisfaction, error rates, waste, costs to produce a given product, productivity, market share, and much more. Continuous improvement requires that we reject the current level of performance—the status quo. Grounded in the present, continuous improvement has its eye on the future. It is not a technique that concerns itself simply with putting out fires or solving sporadic problems. Instead its goal is better long-term performance—improving basic design to achieve a superior product.[24]

Although the principles of CQI have been but slowly accepted by organizations like HMOs, there have been exceptions. "The Prospective Study of Mortality Associated with Coronary Artery Bypass Grafting," conducted by members of the New England Cardiovascular Disease Study Group, is a fine example of CQI in a medical setting.[25] The investigators found that mortality rates among individual hospitals varied from 3.1% to 6.3% and that the variation could not be explained by differences in severity. Mortality rates for individual surgeons varied from 1.9% to 11%. Following a 5-year regional intervention to improve hospital mortality, leaning heavily on the precepts of CQI, average mortality decreased by 24%. An editorial writer, in *JAMA*, commented that this was an example of John Dewey's general model of learning: "to take action guided by theory, and then reflect on that action." The study is all the more remarkable when one considers that a group of cardiac surgeons and cardiologists admitted that their quality of care could be improved and took measures to improve it.

Other examples of CQI in action are the SUPPORT*[26] study of end-of-life decisions in seriously ill hospitalized patients and Donald Berwick's article, "Eleven Worthy Aims for Clinical Leadership of Health System Reform."[27]

The Emergence of High-Quality HMOs

The fourth edition of the *Textbook of Critical Care* prepares the intensivist to practice high-quality critical care medicine. This chapter seeks to help intensivists better navigate the maelstrom of managed care by constantly seeking the talisman of high-quality performance. The health policy theorist Robert Berenson[28] has pointed out that

The logic of managed competition suggests that within each health care market, networks with different distinct organizational characteristics and internal cultures will form and compete, initially on price and style of care and later on quality and value. Individual consumers will be able to recognize the differences among plans and make plan selection based on their own assessment of comparative value.

There are insufficient choices within individual markets; 78% of all employers offer just one plan, although there may be different options within that plan. Lack of continuity of care is common; 41% of patients who changed plans had to change their primary care provider.

There has been much less attention paid to the delivery of care than to this financing of care. Berenson[28] suggests that

---

*SUPPORT = the study to understand prognoses and preferences for outcomes and risks of treatment.

physicians believe they must strive to become high-quality providers. In addition, they must understand the power of consumer choice, capitation, risk adjustment, consumer choice,[7] vertical integration, and physician incentives.

The way a group of intensivists organizes themselves may well determine their success or failure. Teamwork may be enhanced when insurers, hospitals, and physicians are in the same corporate structure (vertical integration). Working for the common goal of quality care, such a group also helps one to understand the importance of cost-effective practice.

As discussed, intensivists have pioneered the development of predictive tools such as APACHE and other scoring systems that can measure the quality of the care they deliver. Similar levels of advanced quality assurance have rarely been implemented in other disciplines of medical practice. As the public understands that the quality of care can be measured, they will almost certainly select plans with the best track record. Discriminating consumers, who show evidence that their physicians have the best chance of producing survivors in patients with a serious illness or injury, would be likely to select those plans. Riding the banner of proven quality performance, intensivists can begin to organize networks that showcase the excellence of their parent plan. The concepts of vertical integration, capitation, provider incentives, and risk adjustment are important components of these super plans.

Whereas patients in a fee-for-service population pay only when they require services, patients (subscribers) in a capitated population pay a fee every month whether they require services or not. Most HMOs and PPOs do their best to recruit subscribers who are basically healthy. Realizing that there is a fixed amount available each year for patient care, physicians attempt to allocate expensive resources to those individuals who really need them.

Physicians may consciously or unconsciously steer healthy patients to HMOs, since the regular capitation payments come monthly, even if the subscriber never requires medical care. Sicker patients, in contrast, are frequently referred to programs who pay fee-for-service so that the physician receives maximum reimbursement for each encounter.

Risk adjustment for capitated patients attempts to compensate physicians caring for patients who may anticipate consuming more health care than other individuals. Subscribers may charge the same premium, but the medical group is capitated at a higher level. Risk adjustment is particularly important for intensivists because the patients they see are "high risk" by definition. While ethicists debate the probity of financial incentives, incentive payments that reward favorable outcome rather than those that reward cost-containment might be particularly useful in the ICU environment.

THE IMPORTANCE OF GOAL SETTING IN HEALTH CARE ORGANIZATIONS

Perhaps the greatest casualty of failed health care reform in the United States is the concept of the accountable health plan. In contrast, health care plans have hidden their activities and attempted to become as unaccountable as possible. Concepts such as capitation and vertical integration are powerful methods for containing costs if the goal of the organization is better health care. If the goal is enhanced shareholder profits, the concepts become downright dangerous. A recent study by an individual close to Columbia/Hospital Corporation of America has revealed what can happen if administrators are rewarded for economic rather than health care performance.[29]

Columbia/HCA followed a systematic program of purchasing hospitals in order to consolidate the hospital market and reduce competition. Instead of following traditional certificate of need approaches, it basically bought out the competition. The organization attempted to develop the vertical integration described earlier in order to control the practices of its physicians and to justify what was called a "continuum of care." The federal government also impounded Columbia/HCA records after raiding its offices and alleged irregularities in self-referral and billing practices. The company defended itself by arguing that it was attempting to goad the federal government into reforming the health care system. Goldsmith,[30] in discussing Kleinke's report, retorts:

> *Columbia/HCA's agenda had nothing to do with "reform." It was simply about becoming a $50 billion company. . . . It is an iconoclastic and poorly researched apology for a management that betrayed the trust of its shareholders, patients, and 260,000 workers.*

Attempts to consider patients as commodities that can be traded in the marketplace has fueled interest in returning control of medicine to health care professionals. A novel approach is to vest leadership of health care organizations to the professionals who actually deliver care. The provider group collects premiums, determines rates of capitation, and delivers care. These Provider Service Organizations (PSOs) may become popular as physicians become more frustrated with managed health care by corporations and decide to chart their own destiny.[31]

Consumer choice and adequate disclosure may be the engine that will force the shift to a much more acceptable program of managed care. Plans must disclose and advertise. Report cards on availability and attitudes of primary care physicians should be widely distributed. The education and experience of major specialists must be readily available. Details of clinical outcomes, practice methods, ways of controlling utilization, freedom of providers to fully discuss all methods of available treatment, and the use of provider incentives should be completely disclosed.

Victor Fuchs[32] is a well-known health economist who urges physicians to better understand the nature of the practice into which they are thrust. He bemoans the commercialization of medicine and the erosion of professional norms even as he emphasizes that no nation can provide its citizens with all of the health care they might be able to use with some benefit. He believes that physicians should operate health care organizations and bring their value-filled experiences to better help their patients. Why operate health care like any other corporations, he asks? He pleads with physicians to "reclaim their authority" not simply by ignoring managed care but by reforming its goals from that of profitability to public service.

For the intensivist, Fuchs states, in a letter written to President Clinton, "we must tame but not destroy technologic change because such change is the most important force behind the escalation of health expenditures." He asks: Will a market-driven system of allocating health resources be more effective at taming technology than was our traditional system of delivery and financing?[32]

The future of critical care medicine is bright because the need for its services is obvious. One can imagine the power of a group of emergency and intensive care physicians who become part of a PSO and accept risk-adjusted capitation payments. The plan requires that all patients with shock, sepsis, acute respiratory failure, severe trauma, and other serious problems be treated only by the group and in their hospital. Soon the word gets around that more people seem to leave the unit compared to the experience with other hospitals. A few years ago, publishing one's success would have been considered either in bad taste or a sure trip to litigation. In tomorrow's world, broadcasting outcomes will ensure survival.

References

1. Safar P: The critical care continuum. *In:* Major Issues in Critical Care Medicine. Parillo JE, Ayres SM (Eds). Baltimore, Williams & Wilkins, 1984, p 71.

2. Shoemaker WC, Ayres SM, Grenvik A, Holbrook PR: Textbook of Critical Care. 3rd ed. Philadelphia, WB Saunders, 1995, pp 1-6.
3. Foote SB: Managing the medical arms race: Public policy and medical device innovation. Berkeley, University of California Press, 1992, pp 56-59.
4. Relman, AS: The new medical-industrial complex, N Engl J Med 1980; 303:963.
5. Doing better and feeling worse: Health in the United States. Proceedings of the American Academy of Arts and Sciences. Daedalus 1997; 106.
6. Levit KR, Lazenby HC, et al: National health spending trends in 1996. Health Aff (Millwood) 1998; 17:35-51.
7. Enthoven, AC, Braden BR: The History and Principles of Managed Competition. Health Aff (Millwood) 1993; 12 (Suppl):24-47.
8. Starr P: The Logic of Health Care. Knoxville, Tenn, Whittle Direct Books, 1992.
9. President's health security plan: The Clinton Blueprint, the White House Domestic Policy Council. New York. Random House, 1993.
10. Clinton plan backed by doctors' group: GOP chairman attacks parts of reform. *The Wall Street Journal*, October 21, 1993.
11. Ayres SM: Health care in the United States. Chicago, American Library Association, 1996.
12. Health care: Still seeking a cure. *Washington Post*, September 28, 1994, p A6.
13. Jensen G, Morisey M, Gafney S: The new dominance of managed care: Insurance trends in the 1990s. Health Aff (Millwood) 1997; 16:125-135.
14. Eddy DM: Oregon's methods: Did cost-effectiveness fail? JAMA 1991; 266:2135-2141.
15. Mizrah, T: Getting rid of patients: Contradictions in the socialization of physicians. New Brunswick, NJ, Rutgers University Press, 1986.
16. Roberts RR, Zalenski RJ, Mensah EK, et al: Costs of an emergency department-based accelerated diagnostic protocol vs. hospitalization in patients with chest pain. JAMA 1997; 278:1670-1676.
17. Clemmer TP, Spuhler, VJ: Developing and gaining acceptance for patient care protocols. New Horiz 1998; 6:12-19.
18. Parillo J, Ayres SM (Eds). Major Issues in Critical Care Medicine. Baltimore, Williams & Wilkins, 1984, p 277.
19. Knaus WA, Draper EA, Wagner DP, et al: An evaluation of outcome from intensive care in major medical centers. Ann Intern Med 1986; 104:410-418.
20. Mitchell PH, Armstrong SA, Simpson TF, et al: American Association of Critical Care Nurses' Demonstration Project: Profile of excellence in critical care nursing. Heart Lung 1989; 18:219-237.
21. Reynolds HN, Haupt MT, Thill-Baharozian MC, et al: Impact of critical care physician staffing on patients with septic shock in a university hospital medical intensive care unit. JAMA 1988; 252:2023-2027.
22. Brown JJ, Sullivan G: Effect on ICU mortality of a full-time critical care specialist. Chest 1989; 96:127-129.
23. Berwick EM: Continuous improvement as an ideal in health care. N Engl J Med 1989; 320:53-56.
24. Kilo CM, Kabcenell AK, Berwick DM: Beyond survival: Toward continuous improvement in medical care. New Horiz 1998; 6:3-11.
25. O'Connor GT, Plume SK, Olmstad EM, et al: A regional intervention to improve the hospital mortality associated with coronary artery bypass. JAMA 1996; 275:841-846.
26. SUPPORT Principal Investigators: A controlled trial to improve care for seriously ill hospitalized patients: The study to understand prognoses and preferences for outcomes and risks of treatment (SUPPORT). JAMA 1995; 274:1591-1598.
27. Berwick DM: Eleven worthy aims for clinical leadership of health system reform. JAMA 1994; 272:797-802.
28. Berenson RA: Beyond competition. Health Aff (Millwood) 1997; 16:171-179.
29. Kleinke JD: Deconstructing the Columbia/HCA investigation. Health Aff (Millwood) 1998; 17:17-25.
30. Goldsmith J: Columbia/HCA: A failure of leadership. Health Aff (Millwood) 1998; 17:27-29.
31. Hirschfeld E: Assuring the solvency of provider-sponsored organizations. Health Aff (Millwood) 1996; 15:28-31.
32. Fuchs V: Physicians as agents of social control: The thoughts of Victor Fuchs. Health Aff (Millwood) 1998; 17:91-96.

1

Cardiopulmonary-Cerebral Resuscitation

Sten Rubertsson MD, PhD, EdICM
Peter Safar, MD, Drhc, FCCM, FCCP

For many people, cardiac arrest is a natural ending of a long and productive life. A substantial number of humans, however, are struck by this event too early in life. Failure to fully resuscitate has brought tragic consequences, including financial problems for both family and society. For the survivors, it is important to mitigate any type of cerebral insult leading to various degrees of neurologic, mental, or cognitive dysfunctions, which are not only devastating for family and friends but also torturous for conscious patients themselves.

Delivery of cardiopulmonary resuscitation (CPR) over the past 40 years through emergency medical services (EMS) and critical care medicine (CCM) has resulted in suboptimal improvement in final outcome. Spontaneous circulation has been restored in fewer than 50% of CPR attempts (outside hospitals or in hospitals but outside special care units). Half of those patients whose circulation was restored died in the hospital, primarily of heart or brain failure. Among the long-term survivors, 10% to 30% have suffered permanent brain damage.

In a recent review of in-hospital cardiac arrests, a wide variation in reported survival rate to discharge ranged from 0% to 29%, with a mean of 14%.[1] In out-of-hospital cardiac arrests, the survival to discharge is 0% to 40%, depending on subgroups.[2, 3] Unfortunately, only about 5% of all reported cardiac arrest victims have left the hospital alive and returned to productive lives. However, when CPR was initiated within 4 minutes by bystanders at the scene and spontaneous circulation was restored within 8 minutes (with defibrillation and drug therapy) by an ambulance team trained in advanced cardiac life support (ACLS), about 40% have been discharged.[3]

The reasons for the poor results are multifactorial, including the rapidity and efficacy with which resuscitation interventions are delivered. In the 1960s, CPR was extended to cardiopulmonary-cerebral resuscitation (CPCR).[4, 5] This was done to save "hearts and brains too good to die" by reversing airway obstruction (usually due to coma), hypoventilation, apnea, sudden cardiac death (usually due to coronary artery disease), exsanguinating hemorrhage (usually due to trauma), and other acute dying processes.[6] In order to improve outcome, a prompt response with initiation of effective CPR by the bystander, followed by the EMS delivery team, is needed. The outcome of CPCR attempts should be evaluated in terms of quality of life. For every victim, the EMS delivery team should estimate the duration of cardiac arrest (no blood flow), CPR (low blood flow), and severe hypoxemia and determine the quality of survival at least in terms of overall and cerebral performance categories.[5]

The CPCR system[5] consists of three phases:

- Basic life support (BLS)
- Advanced life support (ALS), including ACLS and advanced trauma life support (ATLS)
- Prolonged life support (PLS)

Each phase consists of three steps (steps A-B-C, D-E-F, and G-H-I, respectively) (see Fig. 1-1).

Therefore, the concept of the "chain of survival" has been supported by the World Federation of Societies of Anesthesiologists (WFSA),[5] the American Heart Association (AHA),[7] and the European Resuscitation Council (ERC).[8] This life support process includes:

- Early activation of the EMS system
- Early BLS, including airway control, artificial ventilation, and precordial compression (external cardiac massage, external chest compression [ECC])
- Early defibrillation
- Early ACLS, including intubation and medication

Novel therapies may mitigate secondary derangements, thereby improving survival and neurologic recovery.[9] Current research is aimed at maximizing cardiovascular resuscitation, circulatory stabilization, and the support of recovery from postischemic-anoxic encephalopathy. These attempts should achieve consistent reversibility and recovery without brain damage from at least 10 minutes of normothermic total circulatory arrest.[9] In the United States, this achievement might save an additional 100,000 lives without brain damage each year because the present average mobile intensive care unit (ICU) (ALS) ambulance response time of 8 to 10 minutes cannot be reduced further.

BASIC LIFE SUPPORT

Airway Control

The most common site of airway obstruction is the hypopharynx.[5] During coma from any cause in humans (but not in animals), when the head is in the flexed or midposition, the relaxed tongue and neck muscles cannot lift the base of the tongue and epiglottis from the posterior pharyngeal wall (see Fig. 1-1). The nasal passage is sometimes obstructed by congestion, blood, mucus, or a valve-like behavior of the soft palate that blocks exhalation, regardless of whether the patient is in the lateral, supine, or prone position.[5] Other causes of airway obstruction include foreign matter, laryngospasm, bronchospasm, bronchial secretions, mucosal edema, aspiration of gastric contents or foreign matter, and inflammatory processes.

Thus, emergency airway control (see Fig. 1-1, step A) should start with stretching of the anterior neck structures by tilting the head backward, use of chin support, and, if necessary, addition of forward displacement of the mandible and opening of the mouth (the triple airway maneuver) (see Fig. 1-2).[4, 5] An unconscious patient should be placed supine and horizontal, with the head tilted backward and aligned with the neck and chest. The patient's legs may be elevated to centralize the blood volume. The prone position makes the face inaccessible. When an unconscious patient is breathing spontaneously and adequately and the rescuer cannot keep holding the head, the stable side position is preferred, with the head maintained tilted backward. The next step should be an attempt at positive-pressure inflation of the lungs.

If foreign body obstruction is suspected, the method for loosening and expelling foreign matter in the upper air passages (back blows, abdominal thrusts, chest thrusts, finger sweep) remains controversial. Abdominal thrusts produce a weak cough effect. Back blows produce higher airway pressures than thrusts when the airway is closed, but they may either loosen the object or further impact it in a standing or

CARDIOPULMONARY – CEREBRAL RESUSCITATION
PHASE ONE BASIC LIFE SUPPORT
Emergency Oxygenation
IF UNCONSCIOUS
AIRWAY Tilt head backward
Add jaw thrust if necessary
IF NOT BREATHING
BREATHE
Inflate lungs 2 times
mouth-to-mouth, mouth-to-nose,
mouth-to-adjunct, bag-mask
MAINTAIN HEAD TILT
● Feel carotid pulse (5 – 10 sec.)
● If pulse present, continue 12 lung inflations/min
Call for help.
IF PULSE ABSENT
no breathing or gasping
deathlike appearance
CIRCULATE
● ONE OPERATOR:
Alternate 2 lung inflations with 15 sternal compressions.
● TWO OPERATORS:
Alternate 1 lung inflation with 5 sternal compressions.
Compress 80 – 100/min.
Compr./relax. time = 50/50
Activate Emergency Medical Service System.
Depress lower sternum 1½ – 2" (4 – 5 cm)
CONTINUE RESUSCITATION until spontaneous pulse returns, more qualified personnel arrive, the rescuer is exhausted after about 30 min., or the patient is pronounced dead by a physician.
PHASE TWO ADVANCED LIFE SUPPORT
Restoration of Spontaneous Circulation
DO NOT INTERRUPT CARDIAC COMPRESSIONS AND LUNG VENTILATION
INTUBATE TRACHEA WHEN POSSIBLE
DRUGS AND FLUIDS, I.V. LIFELINE
EPINEPHRINE (ADRENALINE)
0.5 - 1.0 mg I.V. repeat every 5 min. until spontaneous pulse returns
SODIUM BICARBONATE
1 mEq/kg I.V. if arrest over 5 min.
Monitor and normalize arterial pH and blood gases
I.V. FLUIDS as indicated
E.K.G. Ventricular fibrillation ? Asystole ? Bizarre complexes ?
FIBRILLATION TREATMENT
IMMEDIATE EXTERNAL DEFIBRILLATION
D.C. 200-300-360 Joules
Repeat shock as necessary
LIDOCAINE (LIGNOCAINE)
1–2 mg/kg I.V. if necessary
continue I.V. infusion
IF ASYSTOLE
repeat Epinephrine every 5 min. Vasopressors as needed.
CONTINUE RESUSCITATION until good pulse.
Restore normotension promptly
D.C. 200-360 J
PHASE THREE PROLONGED LIFE SUPPORT
Post-Resuscitative Brain-Oriented Therapy
GAUGING Determine and treat cause of arrest
Determine salvageability
HUMAN MENTATION - - CEREBRAL RESUSCITATION
INTENSIVE CARE
Immediately after restoration of spontaneous circulation and throughout coma - -
Ameliorate post-anoxic encephalopathy

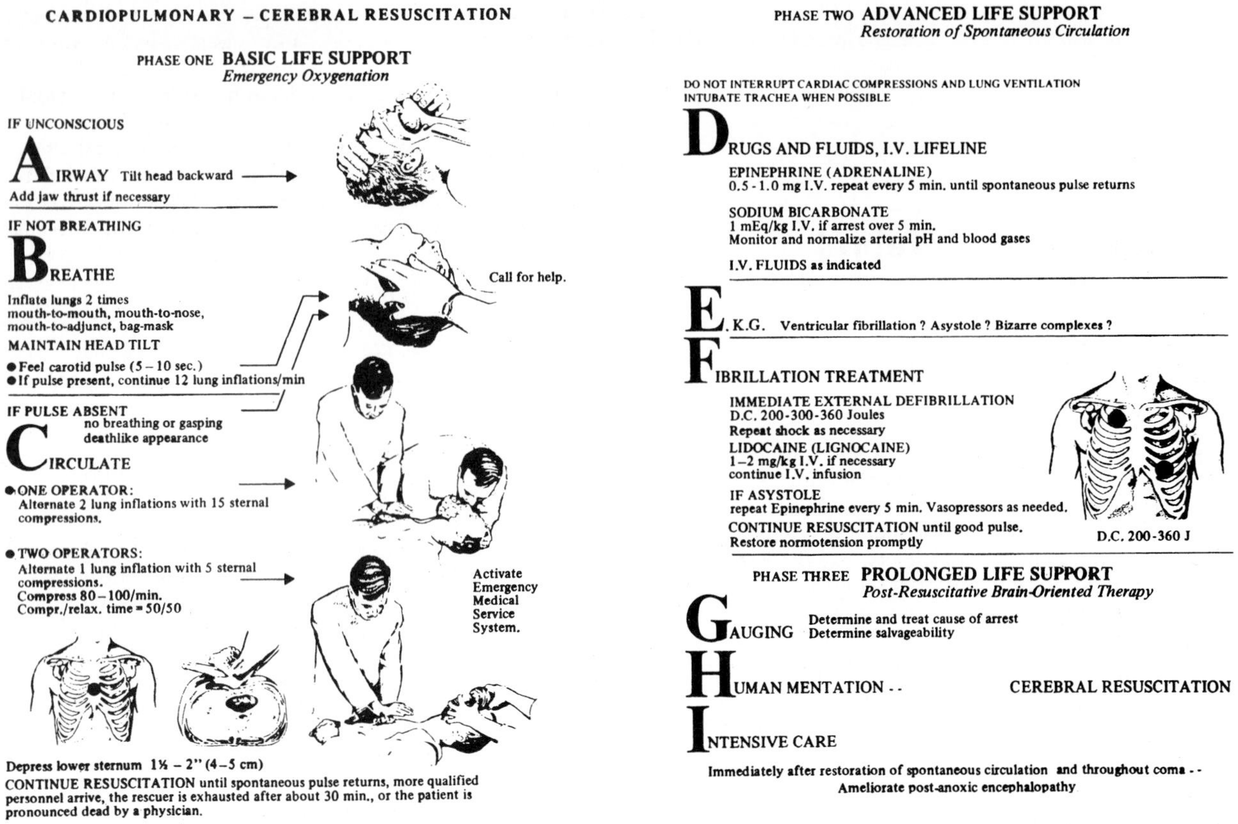

Figure 1–1. Phases and steps of cardiopulmonary-cerebral resuscitation (CPCR).

Steps A, B, and *C* constitute basic life support (BLS).

Step A, Airway control includes backward tilt of the head, forward displacement of the mandible, and separation of lips, followed by insertion of a pharyngeal or tracheal tube when indicated.

Step B, Breathing support is by intermittent positive-pressure ventilation with exhaled air, air, or oxygen.

Step C, Circulation support consists of external or internal cardiac massage. In cases of trauma, it includes control of external hemorrhage by pressure.

Steps D, E, and *F* constitute advanced life support (ALS) (i.e., restoration of spontaneous circulation and other functions).

Step D, Drugs and fluids.

Step E, Electrocardiography.

Step F, Fibrillation treatment (electric defibrillation).

Steps G–I, Prolonged life support is a combination of *Step G* (gauged [i.e., titrated]), *Step H* (humanized [i.e., brain-oriented and hypothermia]), and *Step I* (intensive care).

(From Safar P, Bircher N: Cardiopulmonary Cerebral Resuscitation: Guidelines by the World Federation of Societies of Anesthesiologists [WFSA]. 3rd ed. Philadelphia, WB Saunders, 1988.)

sitting victim. Back blows are not recommended by the American Heart Association, but they are recommended abroad.

Devices for airway control may be considered for use in BLS and ACLS. The use of nasopharyngeal and oropharyngeal tubes still requires backward tilt of the head. Use of the esophageal obturator and esophageal gastric tube airway has been accompanied by an increased risk of complications.[7] The pharyngotracheal lumen airway is inserted blindly into the oropharynx and can result in either esophageal or tracheal placement. The use of the pharyngotracheal lumen airway, the esophageal-tracheal tube, and the laryngeal mask needs further evaluation.[7]

Endotracheal intubation with a cuffed tube is preferred to control the airway. Patients who tolerate an intubation attempt need an endotracheal tube. Details of intubation techniques should be studied and practiced,[5] including (1) equipment needed, (2) orotracheal versus nasotracheal intubation, (3) rapid-sequence intubation, (4) intubating the awake patient, (5) difficulties encountered during intubation attempts, (6) tactile orotracheal intubation, (7) transillumination orotracheal intubation, (8) use of the lighted stylet, (9) fiberoptic laryngoscopic intubation, (10) special considerations for the intubation of infants and small children, (11) extubation, and (12) complications.[5] A gastric tube should be inserted as soon as feasible. An alternative to endotracheal intubation is cricothyrotomy, performed by trained personnel.[5] Tracheotomy (below the cricoid cartilage) should be an elective procedure.

Clearing the pharyngeal airway and the tracheobronchial tree may require strong suction. In massive aspiration of solid foreign matter, ventilation bronchoscopy, use of a large-bore, rigid ventilation bronchoscope rather than the popular flexible, small-bore fiberoptic bronchoscope can be a lifesaving resuscitative measure. Bronchodilation and bronchial clearing are important maneuvers in the management of status asthmaticus, severe bronchitis, near-drowning, and aspiration. Tension pneumothorax can asphyxiate a patient rapidly by lung collapse and bronchial kinking and compression due to mediastinal displacement. If tension pneumothorax is suspected, confirmation by needle puncture (in the anterior upper thorax) and insertion of a large-bore chest tube (by open or closed technique) should not be delayed until confirmation by radiography.[5]

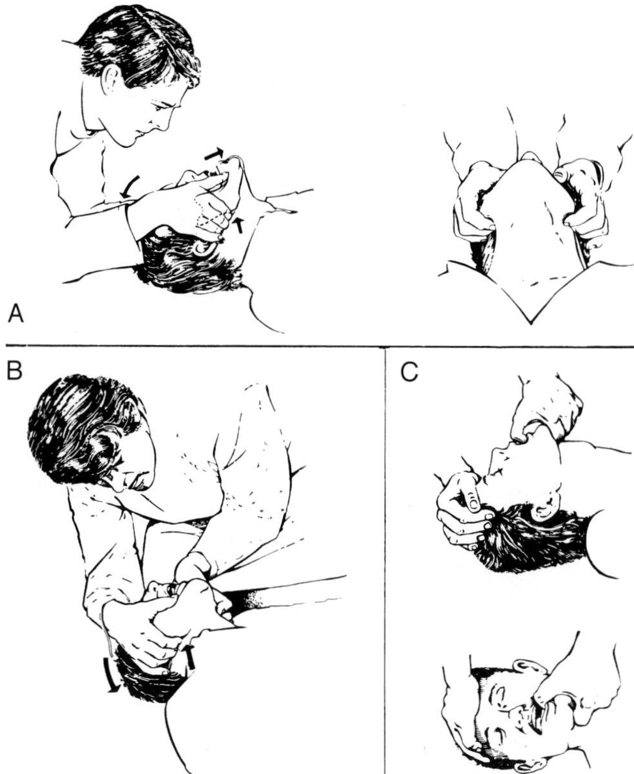

Figure 1–2. Optimal airway control maneuver without the use of equipment. The triple airway maneuver consists of tilting the patient's head backward, displacing the mandible forward, and opening the mouth. *A,* The operator is at the patient's vertex (for a spontaneously breathing patient). *B,* The operator is at the patient's side for direct mouth-to-mouth ventilation. The operator seals the patient's nose with his or her cheek for mouth-to-mouth breathing. The operator then seals the patient's mouth with his or her other cheek for mouth-to-nose breathing. *C,* Modified triple airway maneuver with the thumb-jaw lift method (for a relaxed patient only.) (From Safar P, Bircher N: Cardiopulmonary Cerebral Resuscitation: Guidelines by the World Federation of Societies of Anesthesiologists [WFSA]. 3rd ed. Philadelphia, WB Saunders, 1988. Illustration© Asmund S. Laerdal, Stavanger, Norway, 1981.)

Breathing Support

Currently recommended methods of artificial ventilation are based on intermittent inflation of the lungs with positive pressure applied to the airway, followed by passive exhalation at atmospheric pressure.[5] If direct mouth-to-mouth ventilation is impossible, one should try mouth-to-nose ventilation.[5] During ventilation via mask, which closes the mouth, nasal obstruction can be overcome with use of the triple airway maneuver (see Fig. 1–2) or insertion of an oropharyngeal or nasopharyngeal tube under the mask. Pressing the cricoid cartilage backward can counteract gastric insufflation and passive regurgitation. When high inflation pressures are needed, endotracheal intubation is preferable.

The chance that a rescuer might become infected during direct mouth-to-mouth ventilation (with hepatitis or the human immunodeficiency virus [HIV]) is minimal. No such transmission has been documented.[5, 7, 8] Although transmission of HIV via blood is a possibility, such transmission via saliva has not been documented. Laypersons should carry a saliva filter, face mask, or face shield. Health professionals should carry a valved exhaled air ventilation device that directs the victim's exhaled air away from the operator. Adjuncts for use by health professionals should include an adapter for optional oxygen enrichment. For a nonintubated patient, mouth-valve-mask ventilation with oxygen is recommended because both of the rescuer's hands are free to provide mask fit, head tilt, and jaw thrust. The self-refilling bag-valve unit, when attached to an oronasal facemask, is difficult to use; when it is attached to a tracheal tube, however, it is easy to use and highly effective.

The optimal FIO_2 during steps A-B-C and after restoration of spontaneous circulation (ROSC) remains to be determined. The reason for this is the existing evidence of reperfusion injury by partially reduced oxygen species causing microvascular and neuronal injury of the brain.[10] In comparisons of ventilation with pure oxygen to air during experimental CPR, the arterial-mixed venous oxygen content difference was approximately 25% greater with pure oxygen than with air; however, there was no difference in systemic oxygen uptake.[11] In paralyzed humans, with normal circulation and lungs, normal blood gases have been achieved with mouth-to-mask[12] or direct mouth-to-mouth ventilation.[13]

Lately, there have been conflicting reports on the importance and effectiveness of initial ventilation during CPR.[14, 15] Choosing not to perform positive-pressure ventilation may prove effective in animals, which have straight airways and do not become obstructed even in the absence of a tracheal tube when the patient is unconscious. In humans, however, the airways are kinked and always obstructed in the absence of backward tilt of the head when the patient is comatose.[13, 16] Moreover, in humans with cardiac arrest, with or without tracheal tube in place, forceful sternal compressions alone have been shown not to move significant amounts of air.[13, 16]

In conclusion, the current recommendation is to start steps A-B-C promptly, followed by intubation and ventilation with pure oxygen as soon as available, because flow of oxygenated blood is the limiting factor during CPR.

Circulation Support

Cardiac arrest is "the clinical picture of sudden cessation of circulation in a patient who was not expected to die at the time."[5] Cardiac arrest is recognized when all the following are present: (1) unconsciousness, (2) apnea or gasping, (3) death-like appearance, and (4) no pulse in the carotid and femoral arteries.

Primary cardiac arrest results from either ventricular fibrillation (VF), which may be preceded by ventricular tachycardia (VT), or asystole (e.g., from heart block or drug overdose). *Secondary* cardiac arrest results from asphyxia or exsanguination, usually in mechanical asystole (pulselessness) with electrocardiogram (ECG) complexes continuing in the form of pulseless electric activity (PEA), also called *electromechanical dissociation* (EMD); this is relatively easy to reverse. In prolonged untreated VF, however, defibrillation may change VF to electric asystole or EMD, which may be difficult to reverse. If primary VF remains untreated, it weakens and becomes electric asystole; with reperfusion, the VF pattern returns.

Pulselessness is determined by palpating the carotid artery (see Fig. 1–1). In cardiac arrest, emergency artificial circulation is most readily produced by intermittent external chest compressions (see Fig. 1–1).[17] The blood flow produced by standard external CPR is unpredictably low—between 0% and 30% of normal.[5–8, 17] Because pressing on the sternum creates right atrial pressure peaks almost as high as arterial pressure peaks, perfusion pressures are low as well. Blood flow can be optimized by a 50:50 compression-relaxation ratio and is little influenced by compression rates between 40 and 120 per minute. In adults, a rate of about 80 compressions per minute (one to two compressions per second) is recommended. The currently recommended rates and ratios of ventilations to sternal compressions (2:15 for nonintubated patients, 1:5 for intubated patients) are a compromise.[5]

During CPR, the trachea should be intubated as soon as possible without interrupting chest compressions for more than 15 seconds at a time. Once the endotracheal tube has been inserted, lung inflations during CPR need not be synchronized with chest compressions. If performed optimally, standard external CPR can sometimes preserve cerebral and myocardial viability in dogs and patients for more than 30 minutes, even after cardiac arrest (no blood flow) times of 5 to 10 minutes.[5-8, 17] Blood flow seems to be generated by variable combinations of heart-pump and chest-pump mechanisms (see later).

During CPR with steps A-B-C, the earliest possible attempts at electric defibrillation should be made. Epinephrine should be given intravenously, but if intravenous access is not readily available, epinephrine may be given intratracheally (with the dose doubled to tripled) or intraosseous (in children). CPR should be continued until a strong spontaneous pulse is restored. In asphyxial cardiac arrest (*mechanical asystole*), a spontaneous pulse may return after a few minutes of effective CPR without the need for countershock; or CPR can provoke secondary VF.[6] Precordial thumping by fist cannot be expected to terminate VF, but it can (unpredictably) transform ventricular tachycardia into either sinus rhythm or VF.[7] Repetitive thumping (once per second) and sternal compressions (as for artificial circulation), however, are effective methods of mechanical pacing.[5]

In cases of trauma, circulation support goes beyond external cardiac resuscitation, which in itself has little to offer in an exsanguinated victim. Measures that may be needed in trauma include (1) manual control of external hemorrhage, (2) airway control, (3) artificial ventilation, (4) primary and secondary survey, (5) extrication, (6) positioning for shock, (7) intravenous fluid resuscitation to prevent cardiac arrest from blood loss (not necessarily to restore normotension, which might provoke renewed bleeding), (8) use of a tourniquet, (9) control of internal hemorrhage below the diaphragm with the use of military antishock trousers (MAST), and (10) resuscitative surgery.

ADVANCED CARDIAC LIFE SUPPORT

ACLS protocols combine pharmacologic and mechanical interventions for ROSC by improving perfusion pressures and blood flows to vital organs and treating arrhythmias. The present ACLS protocol is based on four components:

- Early defibrillation
- Administration of drugs
- Ventilation (oxygenation)
- Circulatory support

Defibrillation

Without doubt, early defibrillation is the most important intervention in improving ROSC[16, 17] and, therefore, outcome.[3] At least 50% of patients in cardiac arrest are in VF when the first ECG recording is done. The amplitude of VF decreases over time to a flat line, reflecting worsening of myocardial ischemia. Minimal delay to defibrillation should improve the chance of survival. If the countershocks are delivered within 2 minutes of untreated VF, steps A-B-C may not have to precede countershock. That is realistic only in the monitored ICU patient. If untreated VF exists longer, myocardial reoxygenation with ventilation and sternal compressions should precede countershock.[17] Although appropriate drug therapy can often prevent VF, pharmacologic defibrillation has proved unreliable. Defibrillating electric shocks produce simultaneous depolarization of all myocardial fibers, after which spontaneous contractions may start if the myocardium is oxygenated and not acidotic.

Electrical therapy for life-threatening cardiac dysrhythmias consists mainly of (1) direct-current (DC) external electrical countershocks for VT or VF and (2) external or transvenous electric pacing for complete heart block (severe bradycardia) or asystole. Additional steps include (1) a simple chest thump for witnessed VT or VF, (2) repetitive chest thumps (fist pacing) for heart block with bradycardia, and (3) synchronized cardioversion for atrial fibrillation or VT with pulse.

The energy that is discharged by a defibrillator is measured in watt-seconds or joules (J). Direct-current countershock is produced by a capacitor-discharge type defibrillator, with up to 360 J delivered in about 0.01 second. Guidelines for external defibrillation[5, 7, 8] to terminate VF is to deliver a sequence of 200, 300, and 360 J external shocks (about 3 J/kg in adults and 2 J/kg in children). Patients with other dysrhythmias require less energy (e.g., 100 J for VT, atrial fibrillation, and paroxysmal supraventricular tachycardia, and 25 to 50 J for atrial flutter). External paddles should be 10 cm in diameter for adults, 8 cm for children, and 4.5 cm for infants. For open-chest CPR, energies of about 0.5 J/kg is suggested; paddles should be 6 cm in diameter for adults, 4 cm for children, and 2 cm for infants.[5]

Good electrical contact should be provided by using gel between the electrodes and the skin. One paddle should be placed to the right of the upper half of the sternum, below the clavicle; the other is placed to the left of the cardiac apex, below the left nipple. Polarity influences the ECG reading but not the success of defibrillation. Defibrillation attempts should begin with 200 J (for 70-kg adults) and a quick look at the ECG. If VT or VF continues, 300 J is applied immediately. If these attempts are unsuccessful, 360 J is applied. These three shocks should be given in rapid succession and followed by CPR steps A-B-C. Countershocks with 360 J (maximum available) should then be repeated without interrupting chest compressions more than 10 seconds at a time.

If several shocks fail to alleviate VF despite optimal chest compressions and intermittent positive-pressure ventilation (IPPV), epinephrine, lidocaine, and sodium bicarbonate ($NaHCO_3$) should be given in this sequence. If this measure is unsuccessful, bretylium is indicated. Patients have occasionally recovered after more than 1 hour of external CPR with multiple defibrillation attempts.[5, 7] Myocardial damage can be caused by excessive electric current; however, the importance of promptly restoring spontaneous circulation outweighs the risk of slight myocardial damage resulting from electric shock.

Recommendations to improve the success of defibrillation include the following:

- Repositioning the paddle electrodes, because VF may appear as asystole
- Correcting electrode placement
- Creating a close interface between the paddles and the chest wall
- Using heavy pressure on the paddle electrodes
- Pressing the paddles on the chest to expel air from the lungs
- Following the recommendations for energy
- Allowing brief intervals between a series of about three shocks, sufficient only to recharge the defibrillator
- Checking defibrillators regularly for energy delivery
- Monitoring blood gases and pH

The efficacy of automatic external electric defibrillation is well established.[18] Automatic external defibrillators (AEDs) have not brought about shock inappropriately. Over the last decade, AEDs have been more readily available for use by EMS teams and by trained lay persons. These portable defibrillators read the ECG, recognize VF, and discharge countershocks of 200 to 360 J automatically or semiautomatically (giving audio orders to the operator). AEDs use disposable stick-on chest electrodes and record the ECG for medical review, and some units also provide a programmed printout of critical ECG data. In community trials in Pittsburgh, Pa., and Rochester, Minn., automatic defibrillation by police, who usually reach the victim faster than paramedics, has significantly increased out-of-hospital CPR survivors.

Drugs

Epinephrine

During cardiopulmonary resuscitation, only a few drugs have proved useful. Since the first CPR guidelines, epinephrine (adrenaline) has been accepted as the drug of choice in the ACLS protocol.[5, 7, 8] Sympathomimetic amines that stimulate only the β receptors, such as isoproterenol, low-dose dopamine, and dobutamine, do not aid in restoration of spontaneous circulation and are not indicated during CPR.[5, 7, 8]

Several experimental studies have shown that epinephrine increases myocardial and cerebral blood flow during CPR. Epinephrine also helps to restore spontaneous normotension in cardiac arrest of more than about 1 to 2 minutes' duration, irrespective of the ECG diagnosis. These effects mainly have been attributed to (1) peripheral α-receptor stimulation, resulting in greater perfusion pressure through heart and brain, and (2) possible β-receptor effect on the coronary arteries and brain vessels, resulting in increased blood flow to both of these organs. Although epinephrine can produce VF, it can also help convert fine VF into coarse VF, which is more susceptible to termination by electrical countershock.

The current recommended dose of epinephrine is 1 mg/70 kg body weight as an IV bolus and repeated every 3 to 5 minutes until ROSC. If administered intratracheally, the dose of epinephrine should be at least doubled and diluted in 10 mL of isotonic sodium chloride. There is no agreement, however, on the optimal dose of epinephrine. Therefore, extensive experimental efforts have been made to determine whether a larger dose would result in a higher survival rate.

Several experimental studies have supported the use of "high-dose" epinephrine to improve myocardial and brain blood flow and enhance ROSC.[19, 20] These promising results initiated clinical trials with five to ten times the recommended dose of epinephrine.[21-26] Some of these studies showed enhanced ROSC rates[21, 24, 26] but no overall difference in good cerebral outcome rates. A possible explanation to the failure of high-dose epinephrine to improve cerebral outcome in clinical trials was suggested in a study whereby cortical blood flow tended to be lower and the blood flow increase of shorter duration in the group treated with high-dose compared with "standard-dose" epinephrine.[27] In addition, excessive epinephrine levels can lead to secondary circulatory deterioration after ROSC.[28]

Other Sympathomimetic Amines

One negative effect of epinephrine is the intense tachycardia often observed immediately after ROSC, which can lead to recurrent VF and myocardial ischemia. Therefore, several other drugs with primarily peripheral vasoconstrictor effects have been studied as a substitute for epinephrine during CPR. Sympathomimetic amines that primarily stimulate α receptors, such as norepinephrine, metaraminol, phenylephrine, and methoxamine, also help to restore spontaneous circulation. Their ultimate benefit, however, remains to be proven in clinical trials.

One promising drug is *vasopressin*. During CPR, this drug appears to increase systemic vascular resistance. Circulating endogenous vasopressin concentrations are very high in patients in cardiac arrest during CPR, and vasopressin levels are significantly higher in resuscitated than in nonresuscitated patients.[29] Vasopressin may increase peripheral vasoconstriction directly via the "V_1" receptor or by potentiating the vasoconstrictor effect of endogenous catecholamines.[30] Vasopressin administered during cardiac arrest to pigs receiving either open or closed-chest CPR has resulted in higher blood flow through the heart and brain when compared with epinephrine.[31] In a preliminary clinical study, a significantly larger portion of patients treated with vasopressin, in contrast to those treated with epinephrine, were resuscitated successfully and survived for 24 hours.[32]

Lidocaine and Bretylium

In persistent or refractory VF, an antifibrillatory agent should be considered even if the chance for ROSC and good neurologic outcome is low.[7] In the guidelines, lidocaine is the first choice because it is more familiar to most emergency personnel than other drugs and is faster-acting. The recommended dose of lidocaine is 1.0 to 1.5 mg/kg by IV push, which could be repeated once in 3 to 5 minutes to a total of 3 mg/kg. An additional countershock should be administered between these doses. If defibrillation and lidocaine cannot convert VF or when VF recurs despite lidocaine therapy, bretylium should be considered. The recommended dose of bretylium tosylate is 5.0 mg/kg IV bolus, after which defibrillation should be attempted. A second dose of bretylium tosylate, 10 mg/kg IV, can be repeated once within 5 minutes.

Alkaline Buffers

Acidosis during cardiac arrest is mainly a result of perfusion failure with inadequate tissue oxygenation, resulting in anaerobic metabolism with decrease in adenosine triphosphate (ATP) production and lactic acid and carbon dioxide accumulation. There is also a respiratory component attributable to failure of ventilation, resulting in further accumulation of carbon dioxide that exceeds normal buffering capacity.[33] The role of alkaline buffering during CPR has been discussed by several authors and remains unclear.[33] The administration of sodium bicarbonate in this situation may cause hyperosmolarity and increase P_{CO_2} of mixed venous and coronary sinus blood as well as cerebrospinal fluid.[33]

Reduced coronary perfusion pressure and no improvement of survival after the administration of sodium bicarbonate during CPR have also been reported. These results have led the AHA to recommend cautious use of buffering in the treatment of cardiac arrest.[7] On the other hand, it is well known that metabolic and respiratory acidemia ($pH < 7.2$) decreases myocardial contractility and inhibits the cardiovascular response to catecholamines, which can hamper resuscitation. Furthermore, recent experimental data,[34] demonstrating improved outcome with the administration of sodium bicarbonate during CPR in dogs after prolonged circulatory arrest, support the use of buffers. Another study suggested that alkaline buffers during CPR increased intracellular adenosine concentration, which is potentially beneficial as adenosine has positive metabolic effects and antiarrhythmic and cardioprotective properties.

Present recommendations by the AHA[7] and ERC[8] call for epinephrine to be administered first, followed by $NaHCO_3$, 1 mmol/kg IV once during CPR, but only when cardiac arrest (no blood flow) of at least 2 to 5 minutes' duration may have occurred. This is important to prevent the arterial pH from decreasing below pH 7.2 during the early phase after ROSC, when acids from previously ischemic tissues are washed out.

The administration of $NaHCO_3$ should be repeated no more than every 10 minutes during the low-flow state of CPR and should be titrated as soon as possible, aiming for pH values of 7.3 to 7.5 or for normalizing the calculated base deficit.

Mechanisms for Improving Blood Flow During CPR, Steps A-B-C

During the most recent decades, several investigations have focused on two major theories for the generation of blood flow during closed-chest CPR. The initial concept was the "cardiac pump" theory, which describes the heart function as a multichamber pump with competent valves.[17] The heart is squeezed between the sternum and the spine during compression of the chest, causing forward ejection of blood.[17] This has been further supported by many authors.[17, 36, 37]

The second is the "thoracic pump" theory, a consequence of the fact that all contents of the chest are subjected to the same pressure variations.[38] Thoracic compression produces global elevation of intrathoracic pressure and a resultant pressure gradient across the thoracic inlet squeezing blood from the pulmonary vascular bed through the heart and into the peripheral vessels. The heart acts like a passive conduit without significant valve function. During compression, the great systemic veins are more easily collapsed than the aorta and the systemic arteries. Functional venous valving at the thoracic inlets favor blood flow into the arterial circulation.[38–40]

Babbs and colleagues[36] and later Paradis and coworkers[41] have indicated that one or the other mechanism may predominate in different situations or in individual victims of cardiopulmonary arrest. It is likely that the cardiac pump mechanism is predominant initially in children and in broad-chested dogs, with the thoracic pump mechanism predominant later during increasing ischemic times in barrel-chested adults and in keel-chested dogs.

Interposed Abdominal Compression CPR

Abdominal compressions between sternal compressions (counterpulsations) increase venous return, elevate intrathoracic and aortic pressure, and provide retrograde aortic flow, thereby improving blood flow to the heart and brain. The interposed abdominal compressions are applied in midline, equidistant from the xiphoid process and the umbilicus of the abdomen, at a pressure of 150 to 200 mm Hg during the relaxation phase of precordial compression.[42] The abdominal compression technique was first described by Harris and Redding and was further developed by Ohomoto and associates who combined the interposed abdominal compressions along with standard closed-chest CPR.[5, 42] Animal studies have shown increased coronary perfusion pressure, cardiac output, and common carotid blood flow using interposed abdominal compression CPR[42] compared with standard closed-chest CPR. In humans, improved resuscitation rate and survival to hospital discharge have been reported with in-hospital cardiac arrests.[43] In out-of-hospital patients in cardiac arrest who were treated with interposed abdominal compression CPR compared with standard CPR, no difference in survival was found.[44] For clinical neurologic outcome studies, see Brain-Oriented Resuscitation later in the chapter.

Pneumatic Vest CPR

The pneumatic vest CPR increases intrathoracic pressure fluctuations by small circumferential changes in the dimensions of the thorax and thereby improves venous return and forward aortic flow. In a study of dogs, Halperin and coworkers[45] demonstrated improved coronary blood flow and survival when using cyclic inflations of a pneumatic vest during CPR. In a small human study, pneumatic vest CPR, compared with standard CPR, resulted in greater coronary perfusion pressure but there was no difference in survival between the two techniques[46]; there was an initial period of 11 ± 4 minutes before the patients were randomized to receive either vest CPR or to continue to receive standard closed-chest CPR. Currently, an international multicenter study in Europe and the United States is comparing the pneumatic circumferential vest with standard CPR, but results are still pending. A pneumatic vest is under development for use by ambulance personnel.

Active Compression-Decompression CPR

Active compression-decompression (ACD) CPR causes increased intrathoracic pressure fluctuations with enhanced cardiac compression and forward aortic blood flow. Venous return to the chest is improved during decompression. The concept for this technique arose from an anecdotal report that a lay rescuer had used a toilet plunger to perform chest compressions and decompressions on a cardiac arrest victim, who survived. The ACD device, consisting of a silicon rubber suction header, piston, and handle, is placed over the mid sternum; after manual compression, it permits active chest decompression.

Animal studies have shown increased cardiac output and coronary perfusion pressure[47] and greater cerebral and myocardial blood flow in contrast to standard closed-chest CPR.[48] In a preliminary study, increased ROSC and 24-hour survival, but not improved hospital discharge rate, was reported from in-hospital cardiac arrest victims treated with ACD-CPR.[49] Three studies in patients with out-of-hospital cardiac arrest reported no difference in ROSC or survival to hospital discharge when comparing this technique to standard CPR.[50–52] One of these studies also reported no improvement in survival or neurologic outcome in 773 patients with in-hospital cardiac arrest.[52]

Recently, a randomized multicenter study of ACD-CPR reported improved short-term survival and neurologic outcome at hospital discharge in out-of-hospital cardiac arrest victims.[53] In Europe, several additional studies using this technique have been performed, but a definitive clinical advantage has not yet been demonstrated.[54]

Phased Chest and Abdominal Compression-Decompression CPR

Phased chest and abdominal compression-decompression CPR[55] is a combination of ACD-CPR and interposed abdominal compression. This form of CPR is produced with a device that resembles a seesaw. One piston suction cup is positioned on the chest, and another one is on the abdomen. Chest compression is coincident with abdominal decompression, which is followed by chest decompression plus abdominal compression. In an experimental study on pigs, improved coronary perfusion pressure, ROSC, survival, and neurologic outcome were found compared to standard CPR.[55] This was a small, preliminary study, but the technique looks promising. Clinical trials are being performed, but no results have been presented so far.

Open-Chest CPR

Standard external CPR produces very low blood flow.[17, 38, 39, 55–59] Cardiac output in pigs was only 10% of normal and 20% during open-chest CPR.[56–58] Between 1900 and 1960, open-chest CPR produced high survival rates with good brain function when practiced in hospitals, usually in operating rooms.[4, 5] Even 2.5 hours of open-chest CPR led to recovery. The open-chest technique was replaced by sternal compressions (*closed-chest* CPR) in the beginning of the 1960s[17] because of a 70% survival rate seen after in-hospital cardiac arrest treated immediately with closed-chest CPR and its ability to be initiated by nonphysicians outside the hospital. Open-chest CPR is physiologically superior, producing higher perfusion pressures and blood flow than closed-chest CPR in humans[59] and a better outcome in dogs.[60]

Thus, open-chest CPR provides a better chance for sustaining cerebral and myocardial viability and restoring spontaneous circulation. In addition, open-chest CPR permits direct palpation and observation of the heart, which helps guide drug and fluid therapy and electrical countershocks in difficult, protracted CPR efforts. Finally, the open-chest method permits direct compression of a bleeding site in intrathoracic exsanguination and, in cases of intra-abdominal hemorrhage, allows temporary compression or clamping of the thoracic aorta above the diaphragm.

Unfortunately the open-chest technique has been forgotten and is now recommended only in certain situations. We consider the indications for open-chest CPR to be[5]:

1. Chest already open (in the operating room).
2. Suspected intrathoracic hemorrhage.
3. Suspected intra-abdominal exsanguination (for clamping the lower thoracic aorta).
4. Suspected massive pulmonary embolism.
5. Hypothermic cardiac arrest (open-chest CPR permits direct warming of the heart).
6. Inability of external CPR to produce a carotid or femoral pulse (as in cases with chest or spine deformities or severe emphysema with barrel chest).
7. Suspected long duration of unwitnessed cardiac arrest.
8. Inability of optimal external CPR-ALS to promptly restore spontaneous normotension within 5 to 10 minutes.

Indications 1 to 6 have been part of the national[7] and international[8] recommendations.

The technique of open-chest CPR includes endotracheal intubation and intermittent positive-pressure ventilation with positive end-expiratory pressure provided by a second operator. Mouth-to-mouth ventilation during thoracotomy is feasible but difficult. Only a scalpel (or a pocket knife) is needed for access to direct heart compression. Sterility is optional. A skin incision over the fourth or fifth left intercostal space is followed if the chest is entered bluntly and the intercostal muscles are cut. The intercostal space is pried open. A rib spreader, if available, is inserted. One should start heart compressions immediately and open the pericardium later, compressing about once per second and adjusting the compression force and rate to the filling of the heart.

The operator, standing to the patient's left, faces cephalad and places the thumb of the left hand over the left ventricle posteriorly and the second through fifth fingers over the right ventricle anteriorly. While compressing the ventricles, the operator must avoid the atria and feels for the worm-like motion of VF. Compression of the descending aorta with the other hand is optional. Heart compressions may be more effective if the heart is compressed against the sternum or if two hands are used. If the operator is uncertain about VF, the pericardium should be opened. Epinephrine may be injected into the cavity of the left ventricle. If needed, $NaHCO_3$ should be given intravenously.

Defibrillation is provided by two internal electrodes with saline-soaked gauze pads, as previously described; one is placed behind the heart over the left ventricle, and the other is placed over the right ventricle. The operator starts with 0.5-J/kg shocks. External transthoracic countershock with the chest open is also possible. In massive pulmonary thromboembolism, direct heart massage plus breaking up the clots may be effective. A mechanical open-chest cardiac compression device, such as the Anstadt cup or another mechanical means of physically pressurizing the pericardium, is effective but also requires special experience and bulky devices. In suspected cardiac tamponade, rapid needle puncture alongside the xiphoid process may obviate the need for thoracotomy.

The total switch from open-chest CPR to the noninvasive closed-chest technique in the beginning of the 1960s may have been a mistake. Newer closed-chest techniques have been tried but with no improvement in survival. If physicians had kept up the open-chest technique as a first-line intervention in hospitals instead of the now standard, closed-chest CPR, more lives might have been saved. In a study of out-of-hospital cardiac arrests, switch to open-chest CPR, after initial failure of prolonged closed-chest CPR to restart heart beat, resulted in ROSC.[61] Open-chest CPR needs to be taught again to all physicians and medical students. This requires practice on large (anesthetized) laboratory animals. New ACLS protocols should upgrade it for use not only as a last attempt.

Minimally Invasive Direct Cardiac Massage

Minimally invasive direct cardiac massage[62] utilizes a plunger-like device inserted through a small intercostal incision over the apex of the heart. Without opening the pericardium, the operator places the device directly on the ventricles of the heart, producing an artificial circulation by cyclic cardiac compression and relaxation. In two studies on pigs, this technique has resulted in cardiac output, systemic blood pressure, and coronary and cerebral perfusion similar to results produced by conventional open-chest, bimanual cardiac massage.[62] This technique, however, has been tested in only a few patients and needs further clinical investigation.

Emergency Cardiopulmonary Bypass

Emergency cardiopulmonary bypass (CPB) is the ultimate but also the most invasive method of resuscitation, even when venoarterial pumping via oxygenator is performed without thoracotomy.[63] Normal systemic and organ blood flow may be sustained for prolonged intervals without the progressive hemodynamic deterioration observed during conventional closed-chest CPR. The technique is even more efficacious than open-chest CPR because it permits control of blood pressure, flow, oxygenation, temperature, and composition as well as prolonged assisted circulation without thoracotomy.[63] CPB may also permit delivery of brain resuscitation agents that depress the cardiovascular system.[63] In dogs, ten outcome studies documented the superiority of emergency (portable) CPB over standard external CPR-ALS to achieve ROSC after up to 20 minutes of normothermic no-flow and improved cerebral recovery.[63] Between 1984 and 1991, 125 patients in 17 hospitals within the United States in whom conventional CPR was unsuccessful, showed a 20% ROSC rate after use of CPB, and 14% were alive after 30 days.[64]

A trial of CPB in the emergency department found cannulation of the femoral artery as well as placement of a catheter draining the venae cavae, technically problematic and time-consuming.[65] Procrastination in switching from CPR-ALS to CPB reduces the chance to improve outcome. Out of the hospital, a portable CPB unit approved for use in patients has been recommended[63] but is not yet available. In trauma-related cardiac arrests, for inducing and reversing "profound hypothermic suspended animation" and for prolonged assisted circulation (over days), CPB with heparin-bonded circuit, to avoid systemic heparinization (which can cause cerebral hemorrhage), may offer breakthroughs.[66, 67]

Intra-aortic Balloon Occlusion

In the past, various methods of intra-aortic (retrograde) flush infusion for ROSC from cardiac arrest have been studied by the groups of Negovsky in Moscow and Safar in Pittsburgh.[4, 5]

Intra-aortic balloon occlusion of the descending aorta is a new and promising technique. It resembles the aortic cross-clamping previously used in combination with the open-chest CPR technique.[5] Placement of an aortic balloon catheter provides unique access to the coronary and cerebral vascular bed during CPR. This aortic access opens a whole new field of possible resuscitative interventions during and after CPR.

Several studies using intra-aortic balloon occlusion during CPR have demonstrated improved coronary perfusion pressure,[68, 69] increased carotid and coronary artery blood flow,[70] greater survival,[68, 69] and better neurologic outcome.[69] Combined with intra-aortic infusion of hypertonic saline and dextran, this procedure has been shown to improve cerebral blood flow and brain oxygen supply during open-chest CPR.[71] Furthermore, intra-aortic balloon occlusion in combination with selective aortic arch perfusion with oxygenated ultrapurified polymerized bovine hemoglobin or oxygenated perflubron emulsion improved the rate of ROSC.[72, 73]

In a recent canine outcome study of exsanguination to cardiac arrest and 15 minutes no-flow, survival without brain damage was achieved after flushing brain and heart via an intra-aortic balloon catheter with 1 bolus of saline solution at 4°C at the start of arrest.[74] Intra-aortic balloon occlusion would be feasible clinically, especially in the hospital's emergency department and intensive care units (ICUs), where percutaneous insertion may be quickly employed for positioning of the balloon catheter without fluoroscopy.

BRAIN-ORIENTED RESUSCITATION

Over the past three decades, brain-oriented researchers have tried to find interventions that minimize the ischemic insult to the brain caused by cardiac arrest, that is, by temporary complete *global brain ischemia* (GBI).[9] Several deleterious mechanisms that occur during the ischemic insult and after ROSC have been suggested; many have been documented and reviewed.[9] After ROSC and hypertensive reperfusion, transient hyperemia is followed by delayed protracted cerebral hypoperfusion. The "no-reflow phenomenon," seen with hypotensive reperfusion, seems to be prevented with normotensive and hypertensive reperfusion.[9] Ischemia sets the stage for deleterious cascades of reactions affecting cerebral neurons during and after reperfusion.[9] Calcium loading, glutamate release, and release of oxygen radicals[10] and other cascades lead to lipid peroxidation and apoptosis or necrosis of selectively vulnerable neurons. These events result in disturbances that lead to the ultimate neuronal cell death. The postischemic-anoxic encephalopathy "matures" over several days of reperfusion; therefore, long-term outcome studies in large animals with intensive care life support are needed to determine brain-saving treatments.[9]

Pharmacologic Approach

After promising animal data and promising preliminary clinical data,[75] the efficacy of thiopental loading on survival and neurologic recovery was tested in the first randomized clinical CPCR outcome study, the multicenter international Brain Resuscitation Clinical Trial I (BRCT I) (1979–1984).[76] The barbiturate treatment did not statistically increase the overall proportion of patients with good cerebral outcome.[76] A subgroup of patients with severe brain insult showed numerical benefit from thiopental.[76] The calcium entry blocker lidoflazine improved cerebral outcome when it was given after cardiac arrest in a canine outcome model.[77] In the BRCT II (1984–1989),[78] again there was no statistically significant difference in the overall proportion of patients who achieved good cerebral outcome with lidoflazine versus those without lidoflazine.[78] Similarly, after the calcium entry blocker nimodipine showed benefit in monkeys after global brain ischemia,[79] no statistical overall improvement was demonstrated in a clinical trial.[80]

Discrepancy between experimental and clinical results is not unusual and might be unavoidable, particularly in resuscitation research. Large animal outcome studies permit control of insult and life support. Clinical outcome trials are plagued by numerous unknown or uncontrollable variables. Identifying patients who are within the therapeutic window is impossible. When BRCT II data[78] were retrospectively analyzed, with those patients (of both groups) excluded who had inadequate blood pressure support or cardiac rearrest after ROSC, the lidoflazine group had significantly more survivors with good cerebral outcome compared with the control group.[81]

After 15 years of experience with BRCTs,[26, 76, 78, 81] Safar suspects that such study mechanisms make the proof of "no benefit" or moderate benefit in some cases impossible and that a breakthrough effect would be so obvious that randomly withholding it raises questions of ethics. Therefore, cardiac arrest outcome studies in reproducible large animal models with intensive care life support should be accepted as "clinical trials," to be followed by studies to determine feasibility and side effects in sick humans before inclusion in treatment guidelines.[9] The ideal drug for brain resuscitation must have a positive effect on outcome after administration during CPR or after successful ROSC. Such an effect by a single drug is unlikely to be possible because the multifactorial pathogenesis of the postischemic encephalopathy requires a multifaceted treatment.

Physical Approach

In contrast to pharmacologic approaches, two physical cerebral resuscitation methods have been documented as beneficial. The first such treatment is *cerebral blood flow (CBF) promotion*.[82–88] Hypertensive reperfusion improves cerebral recovery.[82, 85] Hypertensive hemodilution during the delayed protracted cerebral hypoperfusion phase, which begins 1 to 2 hours after reperfusion and can last 12 hours, improves not only CBF[82, 83, 88] but also outcome in dogs.[84, 85] In patients, hypotensive reperfusion was associated with worse and hypertensive reperfusion with improved cerebral outcome.[86, 87] Safar suggests for the management of comatose post–cardiac arrest patients to titrate and normalize the often dangerously low cerebral venous Po_2 values after cardiac arrest[88] with hypertension by vasopressor, hemodilution by plasma substitute, and $Paco_2$ control by ventilation adjustments. Mixed cerebral venous Po_2 changes reflect global cerebral hypoperfusion not accompanied by hypometabolism (i.e., a mismatching of oxygen delivery to oxygen demand). The inhomogeneity of cerebral hypoperfusion[83] cannot be monitored in the ICU. A brief hypertensive bout during or after ROSC should be part of standard CPCR protocols.[82–88] It often happens spontaneously as the result of epinephrine given during CPR; if not, it should be induced by a vasopressor agent.

The second effective physical treatment is *mild resuscitative cerebral hypothermia* (34°C) during CPR (if possible) and immediately after ROSC. Moderate therapeutic hypothermia (30°C) to protect and preserve the brain during circulatory arrest has enabled open heart surgery since the 1950s.[89] Uncontrolled observations with resuscitative (post–cardiac arrest) moderate hypothermia were followed by abandonment of this treatment because of side effects (e.g., arrhythmias) and management problems (e.g., slow external cooling). In 1987, Safar and associates, in outcome data of canine studies, discovered that after prolonged cardiac arrest, protective-preservative accidental mild hypothermia correlated with good cerebral outcome.[90] This was followed by resuscitative (post-arrest) mild hypothermia trials that clearly documented the outcome benefit of early post-arrest mild cooling.[91-95] Simultaneously and independently, other investigators documented protective-preservative as well as resuscitative benefit from mild cerebral hypothermia in incomplete forebrain ischemia rat models.[96, 97]

Several synergistic mechanisms in mild resuscitative hypothermia are suggested, both during and after ischemia.[9] These include:

1. Preservation of adenosine triphosphate (ATP).
2. Reduced lactacidosis.
3. Reduced free fatty acid production.
4. Improved glucose utilization, mitigation of abnormal ion fluxes.
5. Decreasing oxygen demand, excitotoxicity, free radical reactions, and deleterious enzyme reactions.
6. Tightening of membranes.

Clinical studies in out-of-hospital and in-hospital cardiac arrest patients are ongoing (F. Sterz, Vienna, personal communication). For prolonged cardiac arrest, the best outcome so far achieved has been in dogs, with 11 minutes of normothermic VF no-flow.[95] Resuscitation with combination of mild hypothermia from ROSC to 12 hours plus promotion of CBF with hypertensive reperfusion, moderately low hematocrit, and normocapnea, resulted in complete functional and histologic cerebral recovery[95]—a better result than with each treatment alone in historic comparisons. Clinical feasibility trials are needed.

Accidental hypothermia with shivering, vasoconstriction, and sympathetic discharge can be deleterious, whereas mild hypothermia under poikilothermia induced by the insult or drugs, is easy to induce, safe, and clearly neuron-protective and resuscitative. For trauma patients in shock, the discrepancy between accidental uncontrolled hypothermia correlating with poor outcome and controlled therapeutic hypothermia in animal models increasing survival needs to be appreciated. Clinically, mild cooling can be achieved slowly with noninvasive external methods, faster with peritoneal cooling, and fastest with blood cooling.

WHEN NOT TO START AND WHEN TO STOP CARDIOPULMONARY-CEREBRAL RESUSCITATION

Modern CPCR has sparked dialog on many ethical dilemmas.[98] Emergency resuscitation should not be started when a patient is in the terminal stages of an incurable disease, when the order "do not attempt resuscitation" (DNAR) has been specified, or when another reason to withhold CPR is obvious.[5, 7] For initiation of emergency resuscitation, time should not be wasted on contemplation or consultation. When the rescuer is in doubt, CPCR should be initiated. When CPCR is contraindicated, prolonged life support should be discontinued.[98-100] Discontinuance of efforts to provide emergency resuscitation should be determined on the basis of cardiac death, not brain death. EMD is not proof of irreversibility. Cardiac death is evident when the heart beat cannot be restarted despite a maximum effort for at least 30 minutes.[5] As long as VF or VT is present, however, a chance to restore spontaneous circulation still exists. Emergency CPB during irreversible heart failure might in the future serve as a bridge until emergency implantation of an artificial or donor heart can be performed.

In patients with ROSC, but who are still in coma without neurologic recovery, there is no consensus on the time before one can be sure that recovery is futile and that withdrawing life support can be safely obtained. Before brain death can be certified, however, more than 24 hours of extracerebral organ stabilization is required. After initial partial neurologic recovery, dilated fixed pupils and apnea may develop. Neurologic signs of brain death are frequently associated with vasopressor-resistant hypotension. In protracted coma without brain death, the medical decision to terminate life support for persistent vegetative state (letting the patient die) is part of critical care triage, namely, determining the appropriate level of care.[100]

Irreversibility of the vegetative stage should be determined on the basis of published predictive criteria,[99] clinical judgment, and laboratory data.[5] This decision should be made by an experienced physician, who should also seek advice from consultants. Letting a patient die of natural causes should take place in a dignified setting, which can be provided even in the ICU.[100]

FUTURE PERSPECTIVES

Future CPCR research needs to focus on finding methods that are feasible not only in the hospitals but also in the field for use by ambulance services. New CPR methods should improve blood flow to vital organs and should restore spontaneous circulation with beneficial neurologic outcome. A few promising methods and interventions exist that in the future might be used not only in the laboratories but also in the clinical situation. Although these new methods or interventions are more invasive, however, it is hoped that they will improve patient outcome. Until these new methods prove beneficial in patient outcome, open-chest CPR should be taught, and, whenever possible, reinstituted as a first-line intervention, replacing the now standard closed-chest CPR.

Researchers also need to intensify brain-oriented studies to better understand how neurons die. Such study will help to find interventions, or both drugs, that can prevent cell death after ischemic-anoxic insults and improve neurologic function and quality of life. All of these measures, it is hoped, will reduce the still dismal outcome of cardiac arrest victims. Even minor improvements may have a great impact on the numbers of survivors and their quality of life.

ACKNOWLEDGMENTS

Some selections of this review have been adapted from a CPCR chapter in the previous edition of this book, by P. Safar, N. Bircher, and N. Abramson; and from a review on resuscitation by S. Rubertsson, submitted to Acta Anesth Scand. *Safar's recent research has been supported by the A.S. Laerdal Foundation, the National Institutes of Health, and the U.S. Department of Defense, Office of Naval Research.*

References

1. Ballew KA, Philbrick JT: Causes of variation in reported in-hospital CPR survival: A critical review. Resuscitation 1995; 30:203–215.
2. Weston CFM, Jones SD, Wilson RJ: Outcome of out-of-hospital cardiorespiratory arrest in South Glamorgan. Resuscitation 1997; 34:227–233.
3. Eisenberg MS, Horwood BT, Cummins RO, Reynolds-Haertle R, Hearne TR: Cardiac arrest and resuscitation: A tale of 29 cities. Ann Emerg Med 1990; 19:179–186.
4. Safar P: History of cardiopulmonary-cerebral resuscitation. *In:* Cardiopulmonary Resuscitation. Kaye W, Bircher N (Eds). New York, Churchill Livingstone, 1989, pp 1–53.
5. Safar P, Bircher N: Cardiopulmonary Cerebral Resuscitation: Guidelines by the World Federation of Societies of Anesthesiologists (WFSA). 3rd ed. Philadelphia, WB Saunders, 1988.

6. Safar P, Bircher N: The pathophysiology of dying and reanimation. *In:* Principles and Practice of Emergency Medicine. 3rd ed. Vol 1. Schwartz GR, Cayten CG, Mangelsen MA, et al (Eds). Philadelphia, Lea & Febiger, 1992, pp 3-41.
7. American Heart Association: Guidelines for cardiopulmonary resuscitation and emergency cardiac care. JAMA 1992; 268:2171-2302. [See also previous guidelines in JAMA 1966, 1974, 1980, 1985.]
8. European Resuscitation Council: Adult advanced cardiac life support: The European resuscitation guidelines. BMJ 1993; 306:1589-1593.
9. Safar P: Resuscitation of the ischemic brain. *In:* Textbook of Neuroanesthesia with Neurosurgical and Neuroscience Perspectives. Albin MS (Ed). New York, McGraw-Hill, 1997, pp 557-593.
10. Traystman RJ, Kirsch JR, Koehler RC: Oxygen radical mechanisms of brain injury following ischemia and reperfusion. J Appl Physiol 1991; 71:1185-1195.
11. Rubertsson S, Karlsson T, Wiklund L: Systemic oxygen uptake during experimental closed-chest cardiopulmonary resuscitation using air or pure oxygen ventilation. Acta Anaesthesiol Scand 1998; 42:32-38.
12. Elam J, Brown E, Elder J Jr: Artificial respiration by mouth-to-mask method: A study of the respiratory gas exchange of paralyzed patients ventilated by operator's expired air. N Engl J Med 1954; 250:749-754.
13. Safar P, Escarraga L, Elam J: A comparison of the mouth-to-mouth and mouth-to-airway methods of artificial respiration with the chest-pressure arm-lift methods. N Engl J Med 1958; 258:671-677.
14. Berg RA, Kern KB, Sanders AB, Otto CW, Hilwig RW, Ewy GA: Bystander cardiopulmonary resuscitation: Is ventilation necessary? Circulation 1993; 88:1907-1915.
15. Idris AH, Banner MJ, Wenzel V, Fuerst RS, Becker LB, Melker RJ: Ventilation caused by external chest compression is unable to sustain effective gas exchange during CPR: A comparison with mechanical ventilation. Resuscitation 1994; 28:143-150.
16. Safar P, Brown TC, Holtey WH, Wilder R: Ventilation and circulation with closed chest cardiac massage in man. JAMA 1961; 176:574-576.
17. Kouwenhoven WB, Jude JR, Knickerbocker GG: Closed-chest cardiac massage. JAMA 1960; 173:1064-1067.
18. Weil MH (Ed): CPR Wolf Creek IV Conference. New Horiz 1997; 5.
19. Brown CG, Werman HA, Hamlin RL, Davis EA, Hobson J, Ashton J: Comparative effects of graded doses of epinephrine on regional brain blood flow during CPR in a swine model. Ann Emerg Med 1986; 15:1138-1144.
20. Brown CG, Werman HA, Davis EA, Hobson J, Hamlin RL: The effects of graded doses of epinephrine on regional myocardial blood flow during cardiopulmonary resuscitation in swine. Circulation 1987; 75:491-497.
21. Goetting MG, Paradis NA: High-dose epinephrine improves outcome from pediatric cardiac arrest. Ann Emerg Med 1991; 20:22-26.
22. Linder KH, Ahnefeld FW, Prengel AW: Comparison of standard and high-dose adrenaline in the resuscitation of asystole and EMD. Acta Anaesthesiol Scand 1991; 35:253-256.
23. Stiell IG, Hebert PC, Weitzman BN, Wells GA, Sankaranarayanan R, Stark RM, Higginson LAJ, Ahuja J, Dickinson GA: High-dose epinephrine in adult cardiac arrest. N Engl J Med 1992; 327:1045-1050.
24. Brown CG, Martin DR, Pepe PE, Steuven H, Cummins RH, Gonzalez E, Jastremski M, and the multicenter high-dose epinephrine study group: A comparison of standard-dose and high-dose epinephrine in cardiac arrest outside the hospital. N Engl J Med 1992; 327:1051-1055.
25. Callaham M, Madsen CD, Barton CW, Saunders CE, Pointer JA: Randomized clinical trial of high-dose epinephrine and norepinephrine vs standard-dose epinephrine in pre-hospital cardiac arrest. JAMA 1992; 268:2667-2672.
26. Abramson NS, Safar P, Sutton-Tyrrell K, Craig MT: A randomized clinical trial of escalating doses of high dose epinephrine during cardiac resuscitation (Abstract). Crit Care Med 1995; 23(Suppl A178).
27. Gedeborg R, C:son Silander H, Ronne-Engström E, Rubertsson S, Wiklund L: Adverse effects of high-dose epinephrine on cerebral blood flow during experimental cardiopulmonary resuscitation. Submitted.
28. Neumar RW, Bircher NG, Sim KM, Xiao F, Zadach KS, Radovsky A, Katz L, Ebmeyer U, Safar P: Epinephrine and sodium bicarbonate during CPR following asphyxial cardiac arrest in rats. Resuscitation 1995; 29:249-263.
29. Lindner KH, Strohmenger HU, Ensinger H, Hetzel WD, Ahnefeld FW, Georgieff M: Stress hormone response during and after cardiopulmonary resuscitation. Anesthesiology 1992; 77:662-668.
30. Ishikawu SE, Goldberg J, Schrier DM, Aisenbrey G, Schrier RW: Interrelationship between the pressor effects of vasopressin and other vasoactive hormones in the rat: Minerva Electrolyte Metab 1984; 10:184-189.
31. Lindner KH, Prengel AW, Pfenninger EG, Lindner IM, Strohmenger HU, Georgieff M, Lurie KG: Vasopressin improves vital organ blood flow during closed-chest cardiopulmonary resuscitation in pigs. Circulation 1995; 91:215-221.
32. Lindner KH, Dirks B, Strohmenger H-U, Prengel AW, Lindner IM, Lurie KG: Randomised comparison of epinephrine and vasopressin in patients with out-of-hospital ventricular fibrillation. Lancet 1997; 349:535-537.
33. Vukmir RB, Bircher NG, Safar P: Sodium bicarbonate in cardiac arrest: A reappraisal: Am J Emerg Med 1996; 14:192-206.
34. Vukmir RB, Bircher NG, Radovsky A, Safar P: Sodium bicarbonate may improve outcome in dogs with brief or prolonged cardiac arrest. Crit Care Med 1995; 23:515-522.
35. Wiklund L, Ronquist G, Roomans GM, Rubertsson S, Waldenström A: Response of myocardial cellular energy metabolism to variation of buffer composition during open-chest experimental cardiopulmonary resuscitation in the pig. Eur J Clin Invest 1997; 27:417-426.
36. Babbs CF, Bircher N, Burkett DE, Frissora HA, Hodgkin BC, Safar P: Effect of thoracic venting on arterial pressure and flow during external cardiopulmonary resuscitation in animals. Crit Care Med 1981; 9:785-788.
37. Deshmukh HG, Weil MH, Gudipati CV, Trevino RP, Bisera J, Rackow EC: Mechanism of blood flow generated by precordial compression during CPR. Chest 1989; 95:1092-1099.
38. Rudikoff MT, Maugan WL, Effron M, Freund P, Weisfeldt ML: Mechanism of blood flow during cardiopulmonary resuscitation. Circulation 1980; 61:345-352.
39. Niemann JT, Rosborough JP, Hausknecht M, Garner D, Criley JM: Pressure-synchronized cineangiography during experimental cardiopulmonary resuscitation. Circulation 1981; 64:985-991.
40. Lesser R, Bircher N, Safar P, Stezoski W: Venous valving during standard cardiopulmonary resuscitation (CPR) (Abstract). Anesthesiology 1980; 53:S153.
41. Paradis NA, Martin GB, Goetting MG, Rosenberg JM, Rivers EP, Appleton TJ, Nowak RM: Simultaneous aortic, jugular bulb, and right atrial pressures during cardiopulmonary resuscitation in humans. Circulation 1989; 80:361-368.
42. Babbs CF, Sack JB, Kern KB: Interposed abdominal compression as an adjunct to cardiopulmonary resuscitation. Am Heart J 1994; 127:412-421.
43. Sack JB, Kesselbrenner MB, Bregman D: Survival from in-hospital cardiac arrest with interposed abdominal counterpulsation during cardiopulmonary resuscitation: JAMA 1992; 267:379-385.
44. Mateer JR, Steuven HA, Thompson BM, Aprahamian C, Darin JC: Pre-hospital IAC-CPR versus standard CPR: Paramedic resuscitation of cardiac arrests. Am J Emerg Med 1985; 3:143-146.
45. Halperin HR, Guerci AD, Chandra N, Herskowitz A, Tsitlik JE, Niskanen RA, Wurmb E, Weisfeldt ML: Vest inflation without simultaneous ventilation during cardiac arrest in dogs: Improved survival from cardiopulmonary arrest. Circulation 1986; 74:1407-1415.
46. Halperin HR, Tsitlik JE, Gelfand M, Weisfeldt ML, Gruben KG, Levin HR, Rayburn BK, Chandra NC, Jack Scott C, Kreps B, Siu CO, Guerci AD: A preliminary study of cardiopulmonary resuscitation by circumferential compression of the chest with use of a pneumatic vest. N Engl J Med 1993; 329:762-768.
47. Cohen TJ, Tucker KJ, Redberg RF, Lurie KG, Chin MC, Dutton JP, Scheinman MM, Schiller NB, Callaham ML: Active compression-decompression resuscitation: A novel method of cardiopulmonary resuscitation. Am Heart J 1992; 124:1145-1150.

48. Lindner KH, Pfenninger EG, Lurie KG, Schürmann W, Lindner IM, Ahnefeld FW: Effects of active compression-decompression resuscitation on myocardial and cerebral blood flow in pigs. Circulation 1993; 88:1254–1263.
49. Cohen TJ, Goldner BG, Maccaro PC, Ardito AP, Trazzera S, Cohen MB, Dies SR: A comparison of active compression-decompression cardiopulmonary resuscitation with standard cardiopulmonary resuscitation for cardiac arrests occurring in the hospital. N Engl J Med 1993; 329:1918–1921.
50. Lurie KG, Shultz JJ, Callaham ML, Schwab TM, Gisch T, Rector T, Frascone RJ Long L: Evaluation of active compression-decompression CPR in victims of out-of-hospital cardiac arrest. JAMA 1994; 271:1404–1411.
51. Schwab TM, Callaham ML, Madsen CD, Utecht TA: A randomized clinical trial of active compression-decompression CPR vs standard CPR in out-of-hospital cardiac arrest in two cities. JAMA 1995; 273:1261–1268.
52. Stiell IG, Hébert PC, Wells GA, Laupacis A, Vandemheen K, Dreyer JF, Eisenhauer, MA, Gibson J, Higginson LAJ, Kirby AS, Mahon JL, Maloney JP, Weitzman BN: The Ontario trial of active compression-decompression cardiopulmonary resuscitation for in-hospital and prehospital cardiac arrest. JAMA 1996; 275:1417–1423.
53. Plaisance P, Adnet F, Vicaut E, Hennequin B, Magne P, Prudhomme C, Lambert Y, Cantineau JP, Léopold C, Ferracci C, Gizzi M, Payen D: Benefit of active compression-decompression cardiopulmonary resuscitation as a prehospital advanced cardiac life support: A randomized multicenter study. Circulation 1997; 95:955–961.
54. Wik L, Mauer D, Robertson C: The first European pre-hospital active compression-decompression (ACD) cardiopulmonary resuscitation workshop: A report and a review of ACD-CPR. Resuscitation 1995; 30:191–202.
55. Tang W, Weil MH, Schock RB, Sato Y, Lucas J, Sun S, Bisera J: Phased chest and abdominal compression-decompression: A new option for cardiopulmonary resuscitation. Circulation 1997; 95:1335–1340.
56. Rubertsson S, Grenvik Å, Wiklund L: Blood flow and perfusion pressure during open vs closed-chest cardiopulmonary resuscitation in pigs. Crit Care Med 1995; 23:715–725.
57. Rubertsson S, Grenvik Å, Zemgulis V, Wiklund L: Systemic perfusion pressure and blood flows before and after administration of epinephrine during experimental CPR. Crit Care Med 1995; 23:1984–1996.
58. Rubertsson S, Wiklund L: Hemodynamic effects of epinephrine in combination with different alkaline buffers during experimental, open-chest, cardiopulmonary resuscitation. Crit Care Med 1993; 21:1051–1057.
59. Del Guercio LRM, Feins NR, Cohn JD: A comparison of blood flow during external and internal cardiac massage in man. Circulation 1965; 31(Suppl 1):171–180.
60. Bircher N, Safar P: Cerebral preservation during cardiopulmonary resuscitation. Crit Care Med 1985; 13:185–190.
61. Hachimi-Idrissi S, Leeman J, Hubloue Y, Huyghens L, Corne L: Open chest cardiopulmonary resuscitation in out-of-hospital cardiac arrest. Resuscitation 1997; 35:151–156.
62. Buckman RF, Jr, Badellino MM, Mauro LH, Aldridge SC, Milner RE, Malaspina PJ, Merchant NB, Buckman RF III: Direct cardiac massage without major thoracotomy: Feasibility and systemic blood flow. Resuscitation 1995; 29:237–248.
63. Safar P, Abramson NS, Angelos M, Cantadore R, Leonov Y, Levine R, Pretto E, Reich H, Sterz F, Stezoski SW, Tisherman S: Emergency cardiopulmonary bypass for resuscitation from prolonged cardiac arrest. Am J Emerg Med 1990; 8:55–67.
64. Hill JG, Bruhn PS, Cohen SE, Gallagher MW, Manart F, Moore CA, Seifert PE, Askari P, Banchieri C: Emergent applications of cardiopulmonary support: A multiinstitutional experience. Ann Thorac Surg 1992; 54:699–704.
65. Tisherman SA, Safar P, Abramson N, Marrone G, Kormos R, Stein K, Peitzman A, Paris P: Emergency cardiopulmonary bypass for resuscitation from CPR-resistant cardiac arrest: Preliminary report on clinical feasibility study. (Abstract) Prehosp Disaster Med 1991; 6:206.
66. Tisherman SA, Safar P, Radovsky A, Peitzman A, Marrone G, Koboyama K, Weinrauch V: Profound hypothermia (<10°C) compared with deep hypothermia (15°C) improves neurologic outcome in dogs after two hours circulatory arrest induced to enable resuscitative surgery. J Trauma 1991; 31:1051–1062.
67. Capone A, Safar P, Radovsky A, Wang Y, Peitzman A, Tisherman SA: Complete recovery after normothermic hemorrhagic shock and profound hypothermic circulatory arrest of 60 minutes in dogs. J Trauma 1996; 40:388–394.
68. Rubertsson S, Bircher NG, Alexander A: Effects of intra-aortic balloon occlusion on hemodynamics during and survival after experimental cardiopulmonary resuscitation in dogs. Crit Care Med 1997; 25:1003–1009.
69. Tang W, Weil MH, Noc M, Sun S, Gazmuri RJ, Bisera J: Augmented efficacy of external CPR by intermittent occlusion of the ascending aorta. Part 1. Circulation 1993; 88:1916–1921.
70. Rubertsson S, Gedeborg R, Wiklund L: Intra-aortic balloon occlusion of the descending aorta during experimental CPR (Abstract). Crit Care Med 1995; 23(Suppl):A177.
71. Nozari A, Rubertsson S, Gedeborg R, Nordgren A, Wiklund L: Maximization of cerebral blood flow during experimental CPR does not ameliorate post-resuscitation hypoperfusion. Submitted.
72. Paradis NA: Dose-response relationship between aortic infusion of polymerized bovine hemoglobin and return of circulation in a canine model of ventricular fibrillation and advanced cardiac life support. Crit Care Med 1997; 25:476–483.
73. Manning JE, Batson DN, Gansman TW, Murphy CA Jr, Perretta SG, Norfleet EA: Selective aortic arch perfusion using serial infusions of perflubron emulsion. Acad Emerg Med 1997; 4:883–890.
74. Woods R, Safar P, Takasu A, Prueckner S, Stezoski S, Stezoski J, Tisherman S: Hypothermic aortic arch flush for preservation of brain and heart during prolonged exsanguination cardiac arrest in dogs (Abstract). J Trauma 1998; 45:1116.
75. Breivik H, Safar P, Sands P, Fabritius R, Lind B, Lust P, Mullie A, Orr M, Renck H, Snyder JV: Clinical feasibility trials of barbiturate therapy after cardiac arrest. Crit Care Med 1978; 6:228–244.
76. Brain Resuscitation Clinical Trial I Study Group: Randomized clinical study of thiopental loading in comatose survivors of cardiac arrest. N Engl J Med 1986; 314:397–403.
77. Vaagenes P, Cantadore R, Safar P, Moosy J, Rao G, Diven W, Alexander H, Stezoski W: Amelioration of brain damage by lidoflazine after prolonged ventricular fibrillation cardiac arrest in dogs. Crit Care Med 1984; 12:846–855.
78. Brain Resuscitation Clinical Trial II Study Group: A randomized clinical study of a calcium-entry blocker (lidoflazine) in the treatment of comatose survivors of cardiac arrest. N Engl J Med 1991; 324:1225–1231.
79. Steen PA, Gisvold SE, Milde JH, Newberg LA, Scheithauer BW, Lanier WL, Michenfelder JD: Nimodipine improves outcome when given after complete cerebral ischemia in primates. Anesthesiology 1985; 62:406–414.
80. Roine RO, Kaste M, Kinnamen A, Nikki P, Sarna S, Kajaste S: Nimodipine after resuscitation from out-of-hospital ventricular fibrillation: A placebo controlled, double-blind randomized trial. JAMA 1990; 264:3171–3177.
81. Abramson N, Kelsey S, Safar P, Sutton-Tyrell K: Simpson's paradox and clinical trials: What you find is not necessarily what you prove. Ann Emerg Med 1992; 21:1480–1482.
82. Hossman KA, Lechtape-Gruter H, Hossman V: The role of cerebral blood flow for the recovery of the brain after prolonged ischemia. Z Neurol 1973; 204:281–299.
83. Leonov Y, Sterz F, Safar P, Johnson DW, Tisherman SA, Oku K: Hypertension with hemodilution prevents multifocal cerebral hypoperfusion after cardiac arrest in dogs. Stroke 1992; 23:45–53.
84. Safar P, Stezoski SW, Nemoto EM: Amelioration of brain damage after 12 minutes cardiac arrest in dogs: Arch Neurol 1976; 33:91–95.
85. Sterz F, Leonov Y, Safar P, Radovsky A, Tisherman S, Oku K: Hypertension with or without hemodilution after cardiac arrest in dogs. Stroke 1990; 21:1178–1184.
86. Martin DR, Persse D, Brown CG, Jastremski M, Cummins RO, Pepe PE, Gonzales E, Steuven H: Relation between initial post-resuscitation systolic blood pressure and neurologic outcome following cardiac arrest (Abstract). Ann Emerg Med 1993; 22:206.

87. Spivey WH, Abramson NS, Safar P, Sutton-Tyrell, Schoffstaff JM, BRCT II Study Group: Correlation of blood pressure with mortality and neurologic recovery in comatose postresuscitation patients (Abstract). Ann Emerg Med 1991; 20:453.
88. Oku K, Kuboyama K, Safar P, Obrist W, Sterz F, Leonov Y, Tisherman SA: Cerebral and systemic arteriovenous oxygen monitoring after cardiac arrest: Inadequate cerebral oxygen delivery. Resuscitation 1994; 27:141-152.
89. Dripps RD (Ed): The Physiology of Induced Hypothermia. Washington DC, National Academy of Sciences, 1956.
90. Safar P: Resuscitation from clinical death: Pathophysiologic limits and therapeutic potentials. Crit Care Med 1988; 16:923-941.
91. Leonov Y, Sterz F, Safar P, Radovsky A, Oku K, Tisherman S, Stezoski SW: Mild cerebral hypothermia during and after cardiac arrest improves neurologic outcome in dogs. J Cereb Blood Flow Metab 1990; 10:57-70.
92. Sterz F, Safar P, Tisherman S, Radovsky A, Kuboyama K, Oku K: Mild hypothermic cardiopulmonary resuscitation improves outcome after prolonged cardiac arrest in dogs. Crit Care Med 1991; 19:379-389.
93. Weinrauch V, Safar P, Tisherman S, Kuboyama K, Radovsky A: Beneficial effect of mild hypothermia and detrimental effect of deep hypothermia after cardiac arrest in dogs. Stroke 1992; 23:1454-1462.
94. Kuboyama K, Safar P, Radovsky A, Tisherman SA, Stezoski SW, Alexander H: Delay in cooling negates the beneficial effect of mild resuscitative cerebral hypothermia after cardiac arrest in dogs: A prospective, randomized, controlled study. Crit Care Med 1993; 21:1348-1358.
95. Safar P, Xiao F, Radovsky A, Tanigawa K, Ebmeyer U, Bircher N, Alexander H, Stezoski SW: Improved cerebral resuscitation from cardiac arrest in dogs with mild hypothermia plus blood flow promotion. Stroke 1996; 27:105-113.
96. Busto R, Dietrich WD, Globus MY, Ginsberg MD: Postischemic moderate hypothermia inhibits CA 1 hippocampal ischemic neuronal injury. Neurosci Lett 1989; 101:299-304.
97. Coimbra C, Drake M, Boris-Moller F, Wieloch T: Long-lasting neuroprotective effect of postischemic hypothermia and treatment with an antiinflammatory/antipyretic drug: Evidence for chronic encephalopathic processes following ischemia. Stroke 1996; 27:1578-1585.
98. Safar P: The physician's responsibility towards hopelessly critically ill patients: Ethical dilemmas in resuscitation medicine. Acta Anaesthesiol Scand Suppl 1991; 35(96):147-149.
99. Edgren E, Hedstrand U, Kelsey S, Sutton-Tyrell K, Safar P, and BRCT I Study Group: Assessment of neurological prognosis in comatose survivors of cardiac arrest. Lancet 1994; 343:1055-1059.
100. Grenvik Å, Powner DJ, Snyder JV, Jastremski MS, Babcock RA, Loughhead MG: Cessation of therapy in terminal illness and brain death. Crit Care Med 1978; 6:284-291.

2

Pediatric Resuscitation

Arno L. Zaritsky, MD

The outcome following cardiac arrest in children is poor.[1] Since pediatric cardiac arrest often follows a progressive deterioration of cardiorespiratory function, the degree of ischemia and acidosis is often severe by the time cessation of cardiac function occurs compared with acute cessation of cardiac activity in ventricular fibrillation arrest. The mortality rate following out-of-hospital cardiac arrest is 90% to 95%. The outcome following resuscitation of hospitalized children is also poor, with an 85% to 90% mortality rate. Thus, the resuscitation of the pulseless, nonbreathing pediatric victim is often frustrating. Outcome is much better following respiratory arrest.

This chapter reviews the epidemiology of pediatric cardiac arrest, techniques in basic life support, resuscitation drug therapy, and decisions regarding when to discontinue resuscitation efforts. The techniques described represent current concepts and recommendations,[2] but the reader should recognize that these concepts and recommendations may change. To help standardize subsequent research and scientific advancement, an international consensus conference developed uniform guidelines for the reporting of pediatric advanced life support data[3]; definitions and terminology in this chapter are derived from these guidelines.

Cardiac arrest refers to the clinical state characterized by the absence of *detectable* cardiac activity, with the recognition that some children with clinical cardiac arrest may have measurable aortic pressure if an arterial line is inserted (i.e., pseudo-EMD [electromechanical dissociation]). Cardiac arrest in children usually results from profound hypoxemia, hypercarbia and/or ischemia. It is less commonly based on an underlying cardiac disorder producing ventricular dysrhythmias or heart failure.

Basic cardiopulmonary resuscitation (CPR) is an attempt to restore effective circulation with external chest compressions plus expired air inflation of the lungs. Note that basic CPR is *not* limited to patients with cardiac arrest but is also used in children with severely compromised cardiac output.

Return of spontaneous circulation (ROSC) refers to the return of any spontaneous central palpable pulses, regardless of the duration. ROSC may be classified as *intermittent* or *sustained*. Sustained ROSC is defined as a duration sufficient to permit transfer of the patient from the site of arrest to the emergency department (ED) for out-of-hospital arrests or to the intensive care unit (ICU) or operating room for in-hospital arrests. For cardiac arrests within one of these "final destination" sites, ROSC for 20 minutes or more is considered sustained.

Pediatric resuscitation is challenging because of the technical demands of vascular access, airway control, and selection of pediatric equipment and drug dosages. Unfortunately, selection of equipment is often based on an imprecise estimation of the child's weight. Because of the tremendous size variation in children (from a 3-kg newborn infant to the 100-kg adolescent), therapeutic modalities that are size-dependent require some adjustment for the individual patient. This can lead to the loss of precious seconds or minutes at a time when it is most critical. In addition, equipment selection should be based on the child's size and anatomy rather than age, which can be associated with wide variations in size.

BASIC LIFE SUPPORT TECHNIQUES

Airway and Breathing

The optimal method for opening the airway consists of (1) the head tilt, (2) the chin lift procedure, or (3) the jaw thrust. The jaw thrust is preferred in children with possible cervical spine injury. Once the airway is opened, two to five resuscitation breaths are delivered, each 1 to 1.5 seconds in duration.[2] The long inspiratory time is recommended to avoid high airway pressures, which redirect gas into the stomach rather than into the lungs. Breaths are delivered at a rate of 30 to 60/min in neonates, 15 to 20/min in the toddler and child, and 12 to 15/min in the adolescent. To avoid high airway pressures, the rescuer should interrupt compressions to permit the longer inspiratory time.

Because transmission of human immunodeficiency virus

(HIV) and hepatitis is a concern, a pocket mask or similar device is recommended to protect the rescuer during resuscitation. A one-way valve is used to limit the risk of contamination with these devices. Alternatively, a bag-valve-mask device can be used. For this procedure. a selection of masks is required for children of different sizes, and more skill is needed to achieve a tight seal, open the airway, and simultaneously compress the ventilation bag.

Circulation

When introduced in 1960,[4] closed-chest compression was assumed to produce blood flow by direct cardiac compression between the sternum and vertebral bodies. Subsequent data showed that a global increase in intrathoracic pressure results in forward flow of blood ("thoracic pump" mechanism).[5] Studies using a piglet model, which more closely mimics the infant or small child, produced closed-chest, compression-induced cardiac output that was much higher than the output reported in adult animals.[6] Clinical evidence also suggests that the cardiac output during closed-chest compression in small pediatric patients and some adults is produced by direct cardiac compression.[7, 8]

The apparently disparate results supporting thoracic pump or cardiac pump mechanisms probably reflect differences in study models, particularly the duration of arrest. In most clinical studies, patients have a long arrest time prior to invasive catheter insertion. Prolonged arrest reduces vascular tone, changing the physiology of compression-induced cardiac output. With the use of transesophageal echocardiography, short arrest times with early CPR more often show direct compression-induced closure of the atrioventricular (AV) valves and opening of the semilunar valves with forward flow of blood.[8, 9] It is likely that direct cardiac compression is important in infants and children secondary to their compliant chest wall. It is not always appreciated, however, that careful attention to technique and timing are critical to achieving an optimal cardiac output. Only 33% of trained laypersons were able to perform adequate CPR; even in a pediatric ICU, the adequacy of chest compressions was often poor.[7, 10] Although the most junior member of the team is often assigned the task of chest compressions, data suggest that experience improves measured blood flow[11]; therefore, the team leader must ensure that optimal technique is being provided.

If direct cardiac compression is important, the rescuer should apply compression directly over the heart. Although compression at the intermammary line was recommended in the past, data now show that the heart is positioned over the lower third of the sternum in individuals of all ages.[12] Compression is delivered one finger width below the intermammary line, with compression depth approximately one-third the anterior-posterior diameter of the chest.[2] When possible, encircling the infant's chest and compressing with overlapping thumbs appear to produce higher cardiac outputs.[13]

The optimal rate of chest compression is uncertain. There are conflicting data regarding the rate and duty cycle of compressions. Consensus recommendations are to apply compressions for newborns at a rate of 120/min and for all other ages of children at a rate of 100/min.[2] Compressions should be interposed with ventilations in a 5:1 compression:ventilation ratio.

The quality of chest compression is assessed by (1) palpation of pulses, (2) improvement of color, and (3) possibly end-tidal carbon dioxide (CO_2) monitoring. Although palpation of femoral pulses may be reassuring, there is evidence that the pulse may represent retrograde venous flow.[14] End-tidal CO_2 monitoring reflects pulmonary blood flow during CPR and is predictive of ROSC.[15, 16]

ADVANCED LIFE SUPPORT TECHNIQUES

Unlike the focus on early use of *automated external defibrillators* (AEDs) in adults, the initial priorities in pediatric cardiac arrest are to secure the airway and provide adequate ventilation followed by vascular access and drug administration. To rapidly select equipment and calculate infrequently used drug doses, it is highly recommended that precalculated doses and equipment selection information should be in ready proximity to sites where children may arrest. The Broselow Pediatric Emergency Tape is a useful tool for accurately estimating weight and selecting equipment.[17, 18] The tape is based on the relationship between body length and body weight, providing the 50th percentile of weight for length.

Vascular Access

Rapid vascular access is often difficult to achieve in the pulseless child, but it is critical because intravenous epinephrine administration is often essential to restart the heart. The *central venous route* of drug administration is ideal but is difficult to achieve in the cardiac arrest setting. The *peripheral venous route* is used with the recognition that different peripheral venous sites may not be equivalent. Animal and adult studies suggest that injection into a peripheral vein that drains into the superior vena cava is superior to sites that drain into the inferior vena cava.[19] This presumably results from to-and-fro flow of blood in the inferior vena cava during chest compression, which is not as effectively collapsed as the superior vena cava. Limited pediatric animal studies have not shown any important effect of route of drug administration. Furthermore, a fluid bolus effectively increases the delivery of peripherally injected drugs into the central circulation.[20] When using peripheral venous routes, one should flush the catheter with *at least* 5 mL of saline to help deliver the drug to the central circulation.

Besides intravenous routes of drug administration, the *intraosseous route* is effective for rapid drug delivery.[21] The bone marrow space of long bones in children is very vascular, providing a ready means of both drug and fluid administration. Intraosseous injections are usually given in the proximal tibia, but the distal femur and anterior superior iliac spine also are used. Intraosseous needles should not be placed in fractured long bones because the administered fluids and drugs will leak from the fracture site. Similarly, one should not place a needle into a long bone where a previous needle was placed and subsequently displaced, since drugs may leak out of the previous insertion site. Although the risks are small, bilateral compartment syndromes, placement of the needle in the patella, and tibial fractures have been reported.[22–24] Any drug or fluid that can be given intravenously can be given by the intraosseous route.

Endotracheal Drug Administration

The intravenous or intraosseous route is always preferred for drug administration during cardiopulmonary arrest since each produces more reliable drug delivery. In infants and children in whom intravenous or intraosseous access is delayed, certain lipid-soluble drugs may be given by the *endotracheal route*. These drugs include *l*idocaine, *e*pinephrine, *a*tropine and *n*aloxone (a mnemonic for LEAN). Although the endotracheal route has the theoretic advantage of more rapid delivery of drugs to the arterial circulation by absorption from the pulmonary capillaries, the kinetics of drug absorption do not favor this route.

The optimal dose and method of drug delivery by the

endotracheal route are debatable. According to experimental data, the initial dose should be ten times the initial intravenous dose (i.e., 0.1 mg/kg) of epinephrine, using *1:1,000* epinephrine to limit the volume. The most efficient drug absorption occurs in the alveoli and small airways; thus, effective delivery of the drug to these absorptive surfaces is important. Although injection through a catheter positioned into the lower airway is intuitively preferable, direct endotracheal instillation of epinephrine followed by 5 mL of saline effectively disperses the drug into the lower airways.[25] It is important to follow drug administration with several deep positive pressure breaths to help distribute the drug into the lower airways. Although the kinetics for atropine and lidocaine absorption should be similar to that for epinephrine, the absence of convincing data means that no clear recommendations can be made. At least two to three times the recommended intravenous dose is a reasonable starting point for endotracheal atropine and lidocaine.

RESUSCITATION PHARMACOLOGY

The following section reviews the action, indications, dose, route, and toxicity of resuscitation drugs. These recommendations reflect current guidelines adopted by the American Heart Association in 1992.[26]

Epinephrine

Epinephrine has both α- and β-adrenergic actions, but the large doses used in cardiac arrest produce predominant α-adrenergic effects. This action increases coronary perfusion pressure and myocardial and cerebral blood flow by preventing arterial collapse of intrathoracic arteries and selectively increasing vascular resistance in the skin, muscle, and splanchnic vascular beds.[27, 28]

Epinephrine is indicated in all cardiac arrest settings (i.e., asystole, pulseless electrical activity, and ventricular fibrillation). The recommended dose is controversial. Experimental and limited clinical data suggest that a dose 10 to 20 times larger than the currently recommended dose more effectively increases cerebral and myocardial blood flow and increases the rate of restoration of spontaneous circulation.[29, 30] Three large multicentered studies in adults, however, found no beneficial effect of 7.5 to 15 mg of high-dose epinephrine compared with standard doses.[31-33]

In a model of asphyxial pediatric arrest, high-dose epinephrine increased the rate of ROSC but also increased ICU mortality, with ventricular fibrillation seen only in the high-dose epinephrine group.[34] More recent clinical data in children have not shown a beneficial effect of high-dose epinephrine.[35] The clinical implication is that high-dose epinephrine should not be given early after the onset of cardiac arrest because toxicity will be the likely result if the patient is not severely ischemic and acidotic. With prolonged arrests, however, endogenous epinephrine concentrations are 100 to 1000 times higher than normal levels and "standard" doses of epinephrine may fail to raise the concentration further.[36] Clearly, prolonged arrest represents a state with profound alteration of epinephrine pharmacodynamics.

To achieve a balance between the potential toxicity of high-dose epinephrine versus the possible benefit of more rapidly restarting the heart, the current recommendation is to initially give 0.01 mg/kg of epinephrine. If this dose is not effective in 3 to 5 minutes, use a dose 10 to 20 times larger (i.e., 0.1 to 0.2 mg/kg) of epinephrine. Repeated doses of 0.1 to 0.2 mg/kg are given every 3 to 5 minutes of continued arrest.

Acidosis in Cardiac Arrest

A combination of low blood flow and poor ventilation leads to a mixed respiratory and metabolic acidosis during a cardiac arrest. Severe acidosis depresses myocardial contractility, blunts myocardial and peripheral vascular responses to exogenous catecholamines, increases pulmonary vascular resistance, dilates systemic vascular beds, and decreases glycolytic pathway activity, thus impairing adenosine triphosphate synthesis. Correction of acidosis during an arrest is, therefore, an appropriate concern, but the optimal method is controversial.

Recent data show that the cellular acidosis noted during a cardiac arrest is poorly reflected by an arterial blood gas determination.[37] Following intubation, ventilation and chest compression the blood passing through the lungs may be well oxygenated and have a low P_{CO_2}. The total blood flow through the lungs, however, is often low. Thus, even though arterial blood gases may show a normal or high pH with a respiratory alkalosis, simultaneous mixed venous blood gases show a profound acidosis, which is secondary to a severe respiratory acidosis combined with a metabolic acidosis.[37]

The key to therapy of acidosis is to restore tissue perfusion. One can best accomplish this by restoring cardiac activity and supporting circulatory function. The latter procedure may include the administration of fluid to increase intravascular volume. A modest bolus of 5 to 10 mL/kg, repeated as needed based on examination, is often safer than rapid 20-mL/kg boluses because the latter dose may cause pulmonary edema if myocardial pumping function is markedly impaired.

Sodium Bicarbonate

Sodium bicarbonate ($NaHCO_3$) buffers the accumulated metabolic acids through the following reaction:

$$NaHCO_3 + H^+ \leftrightarrow Na^+ + H_2CO_3 \leftrightarrow H_2O + CO_2$$

Unless ventilation is adequate, the reaction cannot proceed to the right by the elimination of formed CO_2. Following intubation, ventilation is not usually the limiting factor; instead, inadequate blood flow results in poor CO_2 elimination. Administration of sodium bicarbonate increases CO_2 production, which may worsen intracellular acidosis, adversely affecting cellular function.

On the basis of concerns about the adverse effects of sodium bicarbonate, the absence of clinical data showing a beneficial effect,[38] and limited data showing that it has a beneficial effect in cardiac arrest models,[39] the American Heart Association guidelines have deemphasized its use.[26] Sodium bicarbonate in a dose of 1 mEq/kg may be infused intravenously or intraosseously only *after* (1) the airway is secured, (2) the victim is hyperventilated, (3) effective chest compressions are being delivered, and (4) epinephrine administration has been ineffective. Subsequent doses (0.5 mEq/kg; 0.5 mL/kg) may be given every 10 minutes of continued arrest. Administration of sodium bicarbonate in the post-arrest setting to correct acidosis is controversial but may be helpful as long as the previous caveats regarding effective perfusion and ventilation are remembered.

Glucose

Glucose is the major energy substrate of the brain and of the neonate's myocardium; vigorous myocardial contractility may not be possible when hypoglycemia occurs. Infants and small children are predisposed to hypoglycemia because they have limited glycogen stores. Conversely, hyperglycemia has an adverse effect on central nervous system acidosis and neurologic outcome by providing increased substrate for lactate formation during anaerobic glycolysis.[40, 41] Although this is true for *preischemia* blood glucose concentration, it seems reasonable to avoid post-arrest hyperglycemia in case ischemia recurs.

Therefore, hypoglycemia and the need for glucose should be documented when possible; if present, the dose of glucose is 0.5 to 1.0 g/kg infused as a 25% dextrose in water ($D_{25}W$) solution in older children and $D_{10}W$ in neonates. The latter solution is used to reduce the acute osmotic effect. The major side effects from glucose administration are related to local irritation from infusion of this hypertonic solution and iatrogenic glucosuria, which may increase urine output even when splanchnic perfusion remains inadequate.

Atropine

At low doses, atropine has central and peripheral parasympathomimetic actions that may produce paradoxical vagotonic effects. Through its vagolytic actions, atropine may be helpful in the treatment of bradycardia accompanied by poor perfusion and hypotension, but clinical studies have not shown a beneficial effect from atropine in asystole or EMD. Recent animal data show contradictory effects of atropine in a model of EMD.[42, 43]

If bradycardia persists despite adequate ventilation, administration of atropine is appropriate, although if the bradycardia is a manifestation of poor myocardial function and/or coronary perfusion, epinephrine administration is likely to be more effective. Atropine may be given by the intravenous, intraosseous, or endotracheal route. A minimum dose of 0.1 mg is used to avoid paradoxical bradycardia. A maximum single dose of 1.0 mg may be used and repeated to a total maximum dose of 1.0 mg in a child and 2.0 mg in an adolescent. These maximum doses produce complete vagal inhibition, and additional doses are not helpful.

Tachycardia may follow atropine administration, but it is usually well tolerated in pediatric patients. Mydriasis may obscure the neurologic examination findings, but the presence of fixed dilated pupils following an arrest should not be attributed to atropine.[44]

Calcium

Calcium is essential in excitation-contraction coupling. Normally, calcium entry into the cardiac myocyte stimulates calcium release from the endoplasmic reticulum; the increase in intracellular calcium concentration stimulates actin-myosin coupling. Contraction ceases when calcium is pumped out of the cytoplasm into the sarcoplasmic reticulum or extracellular environment. Infants demonstrate greater inhibition of cardiac contractility by calcium channel blockers, suggesting that intracellular calcium release is deficient and cardiac contractility is more dependent on extracellular calcium influx. Thus, hypocalcemia in an infant may be manifested by poor contractility and a clinical picture of cardiogenic shock.

Based on adult studies, there is no evidence to support the use of calcium in asystole and its use in EMD is questionable.[45, 46] Only limited data are available in pediatric patients. Hypocalcemia occurs in pediatric patients in cardiac arrest, but in most of these patients it was associated with septic shock.[47] Ionized hypocalcemia is relatively common in the pediatric ICU, occurring in 18% of patients in one large series.[48] More recent data suggests that calcium antagonizes the action of epinephrine and other adrenergic agents and exerts its major action on blood pressure by producing systemic vasoconstriction rather than a positive inotropic effect.[49] For these reasons, calcium is indicated only for the following:

- To correct documented ionized hypocalcemia
- To antagonize the adverse cardiovascular actions of hyperkalemia (*not* caused by digitalis toxicity) and hypermagnesemia
- To reverse the hypotension produced by calcium channel blocker toxicity

For its indicated conditions, calcium is given intravenously or intraosseously in a dose of 20 mg/kg of calcium chloride ($CaCl_2$). Repeated doses increase the risk of morbidity so the initial dose should be repeated only once in 10 minutes if needed; subsequent doses should be based on measured deficiencies of *ionized* calcium concentration.[48] Rapid calcium administration should be avoided because bradycardia or sinus arrest may occur. Calcium chloride solution is hyperosmolar and sclerosing; severe chemical burns may occur if the solution extravasates from peripheral injection sites. Because calcium forms an insoluble precipitate in the presence of sodium bicarbonate, a saline flush is essential between doses.

Lidocaine

Since ventricular fibrillation is seen in fewer than 10% of pediatric arrests,[50] lidocaine is not commonly required. When ventricular tachycardia or fibrillation is present, one should rule out metabolic causes (e.g., hyperkalemia and hypothermia), drug toxicity (e.g., digoxin and tricyclic antidepressants), and myocarditis.

Lidocaine is indicated for the unusual pediatric arrest rhythms: ventricular tachycardia and fibrillation. Lidocaine is given in an initial bolus dose of 1 mg/kg and is repeated, if needed, in 10 to 15 minutes. If a second dose is required, a lidocaine infusion is started at 20 to 50 μg/kg/min; lower infusion rates (5 to 10 μg/kg/min) are used in patients with liver disease or persistent low cardiac output states, since lidocaine clearance is depressed in these conditions. A suggested method of infusion preparation is presented in Table 2–1.

Lidocaine is rapidly redistributed from the plasma compartment following bolus injection, and the plasma concentration may transiently fall to subtherapeutic levels if a single bolus is followed by an infusion. High lidocaine plasma concentrations can depress myocardial contractility and produce hypotension through peripheral vasodilation. Additional toxicities result

TABLE 2–1. Preparation of Infusion Medications Using the "Rule of 6"

Drug	Calculation Rule
Epinephrine Norepinephrine Isoproterenol Prostaglandin E_1	0.6 × the body weight in kilograms (kg) is the number of milligrams (mg) to add to make a final volume of 100 mL (1 dL)
	Then, 1 mL/hr delivers 0.1 μg/kg/min
Dopamine Dobutamine Nitroprusside Nitroglycerine Amrinone	6 × the body weight in kg is the number of milligrams to add to make a final volume of 100 mL (1 dL)
	Then, 1 mL/hr delivers 1 μg/kg/min
Lidocaine	60 × the body weight in kilograms is the number of milligrams to add to make a final volume of 100 mL (1 dL)
	Then, 1 mL/hr delivers 10 μg/kg/min

from central nervous system effects ranging from drowsiness, disorientation, and dysarthria to muscle twitching and generalized seizures. Discontinuation of the infusion is usually effective therapy for toxicity. If necessary, diazepam, lorazepam, or phenobarbital may be given to control seizure activity.

Bretylium

Bretylium is an antidysrhythmic agent with complex pharmacology. Bretylium has a biphasic sympathetic nervous system effect: it initially increases blood pressure and heart rate by stimulating catecholamine release, followed in several minutes after a bolus injection by a fall in both blood pressure and heart rate resulting from inhibition of catecholamine reuptake, which depletes catecholamine stores.

There are no pharmacokinetic or pharmacodynamic studies of bretylium use in pediatric patients, although anecdotal reports suggest its effectiveness in treating ventricular fibrillation in children.[51] The recommended dose is 5 mg/kg, followed by another attempt at defibrillation. If a second dose is needed, 10 mg/kg may be given and the countershock repeated. The most common side effect is hypotension, which typically responds to head-down positioning and fluid administration.

Adenosine

Adenosine acts at specific myocardial receptors to produce several important effects:

- Decreased sinoatrial (SA) node and AV node automaticity
- Decreased atrial contractility
- Decreased atrial action potential duration
- Suppressed norepinephrine release

Adenosine is now the drug of choice in the treatment of supraventricular tachycardia in children. It is rapidly cleared with a half-life of only 9 seconds and thus must be administered as a rapid bolus. The site of administration affects the dose, since the closer the injection site is to the heart, the more drug will be delivered to its site of action.

Initial doses of 100 μg/kg are given and subsequently doubled if they are not effective. Within the ICU, smaller doses (50 μg/kg) are often adequate if injected through a central venous line. Maximal doses for children are uncertain, with doses up to 350 μg/kg reported[52]; the usual maximal adult dose is 12 mg.

Magnesium

Magnesium was introduced into ACLS drug regimens in the most recent guidelines because of increasing evidence of its effectiveness in the prevention of arrhythmias in patients with acute myocardial infarction, the treatment of tachyarrhythmias due to digoxin toxicity, and the treatment of torsades de pointes ventricular tachycardia.[53] The latter condition often results from drug toxicity or metabolic imbalance. Magnesium may also be useful in the treatment of ventricular tachycardia or fibrillation resistant to lidocaine.[54]

The exact mechanism of action in these settings, the precise role for magnesium in pediatric CPR, and the optimal dosage and speed of administration, when used, are all uncertain. A slow infusion of 25 to 50 mg/kg intravenously over 20 minutes is recommended in asthmatic patients since rapid administration may result in hypotension, bradycardia, and decreased cardiac contractility. It is noteworthy, however, that administration over 1 minute is recommended in adults with ventricular dysrhythmias.[53] A similar rapid rate in children in cardiac arrest seems reasonable.

Defibrillation and Cardioversion

The treatment of ventricular fibrillation and pulseless ventricular tachycardia in children is similar to the treatment used in adults.[2] The initial treatment is defibrillation with 2 J/kg, followed by 2 to 4 J/kg twice if needed. If the child does not respond, CPR is restarted and epinephrine is given. The examiner should also look for correctable causes of the arrhythmia. In general, AEDs should not be used unless the child is large because high-energy delivery may independently increase the severity of post-resuscitation myocardial dysfunction.[55]

For tachyarhythmia, such as atrial fibrillation or supraventricular tachycardia producing poor perfusion, low-energy doses of ¼ to 1 J/kg can be used. The higher-energy dose is used in the treatment of ventricular tachycardia. The largest paddles that can fit on the child should be used to increase current delivered.

POST-RESUSCITATION STABILIZATION

Following successful resuscitation, children often require additional support to maintain a stable rhythm and improve perfusion secondary to "stunning" of the myocardium.[56] The time course of improvement in myocardial function after cardiac arrest associated ischemia is unclear. In addition, after cardiac arrest, it appears that cerebral autoregulation is lost.[57] The implication of lost autoregulation is that postresuscitation hypotension impairs cerebral perfusion, whereas hypertension after resuscitation produces excessive cerebral blood flow and pressure. This portion of the chapter provides a practical approach to drug selection in the postresuscitation phase and to the general management of critically ill infants and children with cardiogenic shock.

Postresuscitation patients are often poorly perfused, hypotensive, and very acidotic. After a cardiac arrest, a common reason for persistent poor perfusion is cardiogenic shock, resulting from arrest-associated myocardial ischemia.[58] Some post-arrest patients also may have poor lung compliance because of aspiration, cardiogenic pulmonary edema, or lung contusion. Poor respiratory function complicates the ability to achieve adequate oxygenation and ventilation. In all post-arrest patients, primary attention is focused on stabilizing the airway, providing adequate oxygenation and ventilation, and restoring adequate organ perfusion. In children with poor lung compliance, application of positive end-expiratory pressure (PEEP) may help to improve oxygenation and ventilation.

Pharmacologic treatment of poor tissue perfusion is based on the patient's hemodynamic state, as reflected by physical findings. In all poorly perfused or hypotensive post-arrest patients, administration of a 10 mL/kg fluid bolus over several minutes with careful observation for signs of fluid overload is reasonable.

Epinephrine Infusion

Three vasoactive agents are commonly used in the post-arrest setting for the treatment of hypotension or very poor perfusion: (1) dopamine, (2) dobutamine, and (3) epinephrine. Although dopamine is often the drug of choice in adults with post-arrest shock, in pediatric patients epinephrine by infusion is the initial treatment of choice, particularly if the child is hypotensive. Epinephrine more effectively increases myocardial perfusion pressure. Because coronary artery disease is rare in children, there is less concern about epinephrine's dysrhythmogenic effects and the risk of myocardial ischemia resulting from increasing myocardial oxygen demand in excess of coronary artery oxygen delivery. Other common side effects of epinephrine include:

1. Hyperglycemia, which may produce an osmotic diuresis.
2. An increased serum lactate level, which impairs the value of measuring this substrate as an index of ischemia.
3. A decreased potassium concentration secondary to a β_2-adrenergic action on cells.[59]

The required infusion rate of epinephrine varies between 0.05 and 1.0 μg/kg/min; 0.2 to 0.3 μg/kg/min is typically adequate. Preparation of the drip is presented in Table 2–1. One should remember that a higher starting infusion dose may be required in the hypotensive patient.

Dobutamine Infusion

Dobutamine may be an effective agent in the *normotensive*, post-arrest patient with persistently poor perfusion secondary to diminished cardiac function. In the hypotensive patient, dobutamine may further decrease blood pressure because it often decreases systemic vascular resistance.[60] Experimental data suggest that dobutamine may be effective in reversing the myocardial dysfunction that occurs after cardiac arrest.[61] In children with cardiogenic shock, dobutamine has the beneficial effects of typically increasing cardiac output and decreasing pulmonary wedge pressure, central venous pressure, and systemic and pulmonary vascular resistances.[60] The usual infusion dose is 5 to 20 μg/kg/min (see Table 2–1).

Dopamine Infusion

Dopamine has positive inotropic and chronotropic effects and tends to increase systemic and pulmonary vascular resistance, especially at the high infusion rates often required in the post-arrest patient. The advantage of this drug, when used at low infusion rates (2 to 5 μg/kg/min), is its selective effect to enhance renal and splanchnic perfusion. Usual infusion rates are 5 to 20 μg/kg/min (see Table 2–1). Dopamine is indicated for children with persistently poor perfusion and low normal blood pressure. The decision to use dopamine over dobutamine is often arbitrary and based on personal preference.

TERMINATION OF RESUSCITATION EFFORTS

The decision to terminate resuscitation efforts in the pediatric patient is often much more difficult than in the adult because of the emotional stress associated with the death of a child. Unfortunately, the outcome of cardiac arrest in pediatric patients is poor.[1] Prolonged, aggressive resuscitative efforts may restart the heart, but they do not restore brain function. This is particularly true if the child suffers an out-of-hospital cardiac arrest and is in cardiac arrest on hospital arrival.[62–64]

There are limited outcome data to guide the clinician. Three pediatric CPR studies that examined predictors of outcome found that the number of doses of resuscitation medications was predictive of outcome.[47, 64, 65] In all three studies, children who required more than two doses of epinephrine did not survive to hospital discharge. No recent study has reexamined this relationship since high-dose epinephrine was recommended in patients who did not respond to standard doses.[26]

The following practical approach is suggested as an aid to deciding when to terminate pediatric cardiac resuscitation:

1. Ensure that adequate ventilation and oxygenation are being provided.
2. Provide effective chest compression.
3. Obtain vascular access, and give epinephrine at least every 5 minutes, if not sooner, with the second dose being 10 to 20 times larger than the first.
4. Rule out reversible causes of cardiac arrest (severe hypovolemia, tension pneumothorax, pericardial tamponade, and metabolic conditions, such as severe hypoglycemia or hyperkalemia).
5. Determine electrolytes, glucose, and an arterial blood gas level, although no electrolyte or blood gas abnormality is predictive of outcome. Recognition and correction of severe metabolic abnormalities may be helpful.

If these procedures are not effective and no correctable metabolic disorder is found, the rescuer should consider profound hypothermia and drug intoxication. The former is easy to exclude, the latter depends on the patient history and clinical suspicion. If a stable, perfusing rhythm does not develop after these procedures, it is appropriate to stop. In the child who arrives pulseless and asystolic, this approach typically takes no longer than 15 to 20 minutes.

References

1. Zaritsky A: Outcome of pediatric cardiopulmonary resuscitation. Crit Care Med 1993; 21(Suppl):S325–S327.
2. Nadkarni V, Hazinski MF, Zideman D, et al: Pediatric resuscitation: An advisory statement from the Pediatric Working Group of the International Liaison Committee on Resuscitation. Circulation 1997; 95:2185–2195.
3. Zaritsky A, Nadkarni V, Hazinski MF, et al: Recommended guidelines for uniform reporting of pediatric advanced life support: The Pediatric Utstein Style. Pediatrics 1995; 96:765–779.
4. Kouwenhoven WB, Jude JR, Knickerbocker GG: Closed-chest cardiac massage. JAMA 1960; 173:1064–1067.
5. Rudikoff MT, Maughan WL, Effron M, et al: Mechanisms of blood flow during cardiopulmonary resuscitation. Circulation 1980; 61:345–351.
6. Schleien CL, Dean JM, Koehler RC, et al: Effect of epinephrine on cerebral and myocardial perfusion in an infant animal preparation of cardiopulmonary resuscitation. Circulation 1986; 73:809–817.
7. Berg RA, Sanders AB, Milander M, et al: Efficacy of audio-prompted rate guidance in improving resuscitator performance of cardiopulmonary resuscitation on children. Acad Emerg Med 1994; 1:35–40.
8. Ma MH, Hwang JJ, Lai LP, et al: Transesophageal echocardiographic assessment of mitral valve position and pulmonary venous flow during cardiopulmonary resuscitation in humans. Circulation 1995; 92:854–861.
9. Redberg RF, Tucker KJ, Cohen TJ, et al: Physiology of blood flow during cardiopulmonary resuscitation: A transesophageal echocardiographic study. Circulation 1993; 88:534–542.
10. Berden HJ, Bierens JJ, Willems FF, et al: Resuscitation skills of lay public after recent training. Ann Emerg Med 1994; 23:1003–1008.
11. Fodden DI, Crosby AC, Channer KS: Doppler measurement of cardiac output during cardiopulmonary resuscitation. J Accid Emerg Med 1996; 13:379–382.
12. Orlowski JP: Optimum position for external cardiac compression in infants and young children. Ann Emerg Med 1986; 15:667–673.
13. Menegazzi JJ, Auble TE, Nicklas KA, et al: Two-thumb versus two-finger chest compression during CPR in a swine infant model of cardiac arrest. Ann Emerg Med 1993; 22:240–243.
14. Connick M, Berg RA: Femoral venous pulsations during open-chest cardiac massage. Ann Emerg Med 1994; 24:1176–1179.
15. Bhende MS, Karasic DG, Menegazzi JJ: Evaluation of an end-tidal CO_2 detector during cardiopulmonary resuscitation in a canine model for pediatric cardiac arrest. Pediatr Emerg Care 1995; 11:365–368.
16. Cantineau JP, Lambert Y, Merckx P, et al: End-tidal carbon dioxide during cardiopulmonary resuscitation in humans presenting mostly with asystole: A predictor of outcome. Crit Care Med 1996; 24:791–796.
17. Lubitz DS, Seidel JS, Chameides L, et al: A rapid method for estimating weight and resuscitation drug dosages from length in the pediatric age group. Ann Emerg Med 1988; 17:576–581.
18. Luten RC, Wears RL, Broselow J, et al: Length-based endotracheal tube and emergency equipment in pediatrics. Ann Emerg Med 1992; 21:900–904.

19. Dalsey W, Barsan W, Joyce S, et al: Comparison of superior vena caval and inferior vena caval access using a radioisotope technique during normal perfusion and cardiopulmonary resuscitation. Ann Emerg Med 1984; 13:881-884.
20. Gaddis GM, Dolister M, Gaddis ML: Mock drug delivery to the proximal aorta during cardiopulmonary resuscitation: Central vs peripheral intravenous infusion with varying flush volumes. Acad Emerg Med 1995; 2:1027-1033.
21. Spivey W: Intraosseous infusions. J Pediatr 1987; 111:639-643.
22. Galpin RD, Kronick JB, Willis RB, et al: Bilateral lower extremity compartment syndromes secondary to intraosseous fluid resuscitation. J Pediatr Orthop 1991; 11:773-776.
23. Glaeser PW, Hellmich TR, Szewczuga, D, et al: Five-year experience in prehospital intraosseous infusion in children and adults. Ann Emerg Med 1993; 22:1119-1124.
24. La Fleche FR, Slepin MJ, Vargas J, et al: Iatrogenic bilateral tibial fractures after intraosseous infusion attempts in a 3 month old infant. Ann Emerg Med 1989; 18:1099-1101.
25. Jasani MS, Nadkarni VM, Finkelstein MS, et al: Effects of different techniques of endotracheal epinephrine administration in pediatric porcine hypoxic-hypercarbic cardiopulmonary arrest. Crit Care Med 1994; 22:1174-1180.
26. Subcommittee on Pediatric Resuscitation, American Heart Association: Guidelines for cardiopulmonary resuscitation and emergency cardiac care: VI. Pediatric advanced life support. JAMA 1992; 268:2262-2275.
27. Otto C, Yakaitis R, Blitt C: Mechanism of action of epinephrine in resuscitation from asphyxial arrest. Crit Care Med 1981; 9:321-324.
28. Michael JR, Guerci AD, Koehler RC, et al: Mechanisms by which epinephrine augments cerebral and myocardial perfusion during cardiopulmonary resuscitation in dogs. Circulation 1984; 69:822-835.
29. Brown CG, Werman HA: Adrenergic agonists during cardiopulmonary resuscitation. Resuscitation 1990; 19:1-16.
30. Goetting MG, Paradis NA: High-dose epinephrine improves outcome from pediatric cardiac arrest. Ann Emerg Med 1991; 20:22-26.
31. Brown CG, Martin DR, Pepe PE, et al: A comparison of standard-dose and high-dose epinephrine in cardiac arrest outside the hospital. N Engl J Med 1992; 327:1051-1055.
32. Callaham M, Madsen CD, Barton CW, et al: A randomized trial of high-dose epinephrine and norepinephrine versus standard dose epinephrine in prehospital cardiac arrest. JAMA 1992; 268:2667-2672.
33. Stiell IG, Hebert PC, Weitzman BN, et al: High-dose epinephrine in adult cardiac arrest. N Engl J Med 1992; 327:1045-1050.
34. Berg RA, Otto CW, Kern KB, et al: A randomized, blinded trial of high-dose epinephrine versus standard-dose epinephrine in a swine model of pediatric asphyxial cardiac arrest. Crit Care Med 1996; 24:1695-1700.
35. Dieckmann RA, Vardis R: High-dose epinephrine in pediatric out-of-hospital cardiopulmonary arrest. Pediatrics 1995; 95:901-913.
36. Wortsman J, Paradis NA, Martin GB, et al: Functional responses to extremely high plasma epinephrine concentrations in cardiac arrest. Crit Care Med 1993; 21:692-697.
37. Weil M, Rackow E, Trevino R, et al: Difference in acid-base state between venous and arterial blood during cardiopulmonary resuscitation. N Engl J Med 1986; 315:153-156.
38. Dybvik T, Strand T, Steen PA: Buffer therapy during out-of-hospital cardiopulmonary resuscitation [see comments]. Resuscitation 1995; 29:89-95.
39. Vukmir RB, Bircher N, Radovsky A, et al: Sodium bicarbonate may improve outcome in dogs with brief or prolonged cardiac arrest. Crit Care Med 1995; 23:515-522.
40. Anderson RV, Siegman MG, Balaban RS, et al: Hyperglycemia increases cerebral intracellular acidosis during circulatory arrest. Ann Thorac Surg 1992; 54:1126-1130.
41. Nakakimura K, Fleischer JE, Drumond JC, et al: Glucose administration before cardiac arrest worsens neurologic outcome in cats. Anesthesiology 1990; 72:1005-1011.
42. DeBehnke DJ, Swart GL, Spreng D, et al: Standard and higher doses of atropine in a canine model of pulseless electrical activity. Acad Emerg Med 1995; 2:1034-1041.
43. Blecic S, Chaskis C, Vincent JL: Atropine administration in experimental electromechanical dissociation. Am J Emerg Med 1992; 10:515-518.
44. Goetting MG, Contereas E: Systemic atropine administration during cardiac arrest does not cause fixed and dilated pupils. Ann Emerg Med 1991; 20:55-57.
45. Stueven H, Thompson B, Aprahamian C, et al: The effectiveness of calcium chloride in refractory electromechanical dissociation. Ann Emerg Med 1985; 14:626-629.
46. Stueven H, Thompson B, Aprahamian C, et al: Lack of effectiveness of calcium chloride in refractory asystole. Ann Emerg Med 1985; 14:630-632.
47. Zaritsky A, Nadkarni V, Getson P, et al: CPR in children. Ann Emerg Med 1987; 16:1107-1110.
48. Cardenas-Rivero N, Chernow B, Stoiko MA, et al: Hypocalcemia in critically ill children. J Pediatr 1989; 114:946-951.
49. Zaloga GP, Strickland RA, Butterworth JF IV, et al: Calcium attenuates epinephrine's β-adrenergic effects in postoperative heart surgery patients. Circulation 1990; 81:196-200.
50. Mogayzel C, Quan L, Graves JR, et al: Out-of-hospital ventricular fibrillation in children and adolescents: Causes and outcomes. Ann Emerg Med 1995; 25:484-491.
51. Mongkolsmai C, Dove J, Kyrouac J: Bretylium tosylate for ventricular fibrillation in a child. Clin Pediatr 1984; 23:696-698.
52. Kugler JD, Danford DA: Management of infants, children, and adolescents with paroxysmal supraventricular tachycardia. J Pediatr 1996; 129:324-328.
53. Iseri LT: Role of magnesium in cardiac tachyarrhythmias. Am J Cardiol 1990; 65:47K-50K.
54. Roden DM: Magnesium treatment of ventricular arrhythmias. Am J Cardiol 1989; 63:43G-46G.
55. Xie J, Weil MH, Sun S, et al: High-energy defibrillation increases the severity of postresuscitation myocardial dysfunction. Circulation 1997; 96:683-686.
56. Kern KB, Hilwig RW, Rhee KH, et al: Myocardial dysfunction after resuscitation from cardiac arrest: An example of global myocardial stunning. J Am Coll Cardiol 1996; 28:232-240.
57. Nishizawa H, Kudoh I: Cerebral autoregulation is impaired in patients resuscitated after cardiac arrest. Acta Anaesthesiol Scand 1996; 40:1149-1153.
58. Lucking SE, Pollack MM, Fields AI: Shock following generalized hypoxic-ischemic injury in previously healthy infants and children. J Pediatr 1986; 108:359-364.
59. Brown MJ: Hypokalemia from $beta_2$-receptor stimulation by circulating epinephrine. Am J Cardiol 1985; 56:3D-9D.
60. Zaritsky AL: Catecholamines, inotropic medications, and vasopressor agents. *In:* The Pharmacologic Approach to the Critically Ill Patient. 3rd ed. Chernow B (Ed). Baltimore, Williams & Wilkins, 1994, pp 387-404.
61. Kern KB, Hilwig RW, Berg RA, et al: Postresuscitation left ventricular systolic and diastolic dysfunction: Treatment with dobutamine. Circulation 1997; 95:2610-2613.
62. Sheikh A, Brogan T: Outcome and cost of open- and closed-chest cardiopulmonary resuscitation in pediatric cardiac arrests. Pediatrics 1994; 93:392-398.
63. Ronco R, King W, Konley DK, et al: Outcome and cost at a children's hospital following resuscitation for out-of-hospital cardiopulmonary arrest. Arch Pediatr Adolesc Med 1995; 149:210-214.
64. Schindler MBB, Bohn D, Cox PN, et al: Outcome of out-of-hospital cardiac or respiratory arrest in children. N Engl J Med 1996; 335:1473-1479.
65. Nichols DG, Kettrick RG, Swedlow DB, Lee S, Passman R, Ludwig S: Factors influencing outcome of cardiopulmonary resuscitation in children. Pediatr Emerg Care 1986; 2:1-5.

3

Resuscitation of the Newborn

George A. Gregory, MD

Although neonates are significantly more resistant to the effects of asphyxia[1] (as a result in great part to preservation of heart, brain, and adrenal gland blood flow and to decreased glucose utilization and decreased central nervous system [CNS] metabolism), CNS injuries are still common following birth. Many of the injuries that occur do so prior to birth.[2-4] However, there are marked physiologic changes in the cardiovascular and respiratory systems that must occur at birth, and inability to make these changes often leads to death or to survival with CNS injury. This chapter describes the causes and effects of cardiorespiratory insufficiency at birth and the methods by which they can be corrected. Recommendations of the American Heart Association are included when possible. Knowledge of cardiopulmonary development and cardiopulmonary resuscitation of neonates is extremely important because approximately 6% of all newborns and 80% of premature neonates require some form of resuscitation at birth.[5]

CARDIORESPIRATORY PHYSIOLOGY

The lungs evolve from the foregut of the fetus by the 14th day of gestation. By the 20th week, the airways are lined with cuboidal epithelium and the pulmonary capillaries are present. By 26 to 28 weeks, the capillaries are in contact with the developing terminal airways and extrauterine life is possible for the first time in significant numbers of infants. By 30 to 32 weeks' gestation, the cuboidal epithelium is flattened and thinned, making gas transfer easier.

At 20 weeks' gestation, large quantities of surface active material are present within the alveolar lining (type II) cells.[6] By 28 to 32 weeks' gestation, some of this material is found on the surface lining of the distal airways. After 34 to 38 weeks' gestation, surface active material is present in terminal airways. Thyroxin, steroids, and catecholamines[7-9] release surface active material from type II cells in the fetus; at birth, breathing further stimulates its release.[10]

Fetal airways contain approximately 30 mL/kg of plasma ultrafiltrate, which is continuously produced in the lungs and discharged into the mouth. Some of the discharged fluid is swallowed; the remainder is expelled into the amniotic fluid.[11, 12] About 300 mL of lung fluid is produced each day.[13] Normally, the lung fluid contains no amniotic fluid. With fetal gasping, however, 30 to 60 mL of amniotic fluid is drawn into the lungs, thereby contaminating the fetal lung fluid. Removal of lung fluid is initiated during labor,[14] continued during delivery, and completed after birth (Fig. 3–1).[15] Preterm and term neonates born by cesarean section, without a trial of labor, have more lung water and more difficulty adapting to extrauterine life than do term babies born vaginally.

Infants normally breathe within 30 seconds and sustain respiration by 90 seconds after birth. The initial outward recoil of the chest at birth helps fill the lungs with air. Mild acidosis, hypercarbia, hypoxia, pain, cold, touch, noise, and umbilical cord clamping all stimulate breathing and sustain rhythmic respiration.[16, 17] Severe acidosis, hypoxia, CNS injury, and maternal use of drugs (such as narcotics, barbiturates, local anesthesia, magnesium, and alcohol) depress respiration.

The fetal circulation is in parallel; the circulation of adults is in series (Fig. 3–2).[18, 19] The fetal right ventricle ejects two thirds of the combined ventricular output, and the left ventricle ejects one third.[20] This imbalance occurs because of intracardiac and extracardiac shunts (foramen ovale and ductus arteriosus). The foramen ovale allows oxygenated blood from the placenta to enter the left atrium, from which it enters the left ventricle and aorta. Poorly oxygenated blood from the superior vena cava enters the right atrium and right ventricle and is ejected into the pulmonary artery. Ninety per cent of pulmonary artery blood bypasses the lungs and joins descending aorta blood (via the ductus arteriosus).[20] The remaining 10% of the right ventricular output perfuses the fetal lungs.

Lung expansion, breathing, increased pH, and raised alveolar oxygen tensions decrease pulmonary vascular resistance (PVR) and increase pulmonary blood flow at birth.[11, 21] Hypoxia, acidosis, hypovolemia, hypoventilation, atelectasis, and a cold environment increase the PVR.[22, 23] Combined hypoxia and acidosis increase PVR more than either of these stimuli alone.

The decrease in PVR at birth reduces pulmonary arterial pressure and increases pulmonary blood flow. At the same time, systemic vascular resistance (SVR), arterial pressure, and

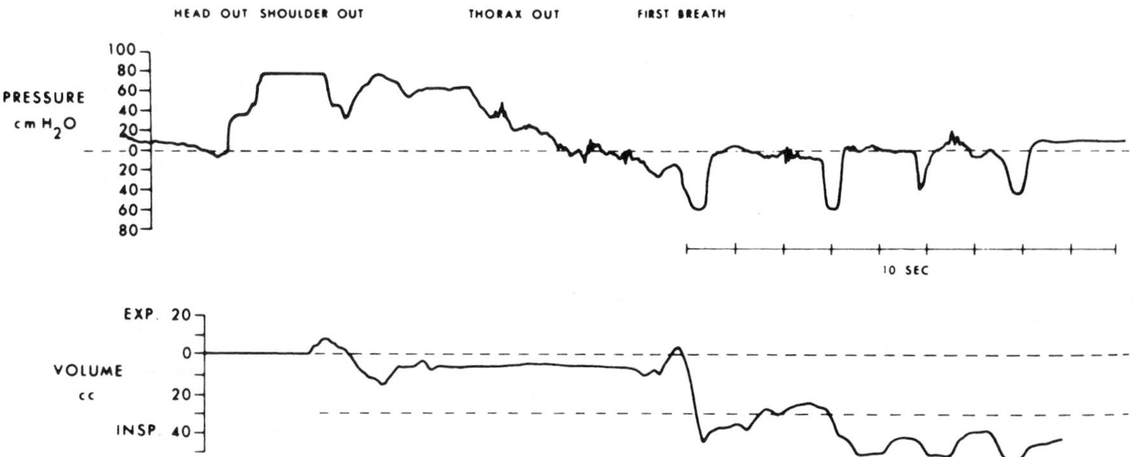

Figure 3–1. Intrathoracic pressures of the infant during delivery. Note the increased intrathoracic pressure when the mouth and head have been delivered. (From Gregory GA: Resuscitation of the newborn. Anesthesiology 1975; 43:225.)

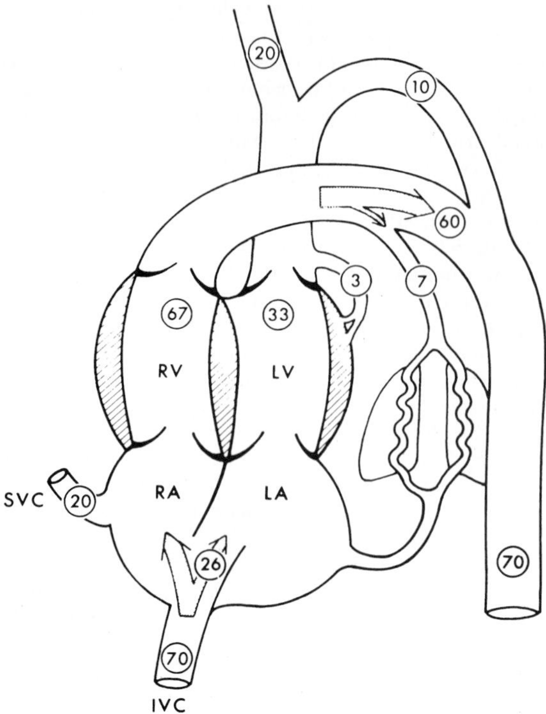

Figure 3–2. Diagram of the fetal circulation. The numbers within the circles are percentages of the combined ventricular output. (From Gregory GA: Resuscitation of the newborn. Anesthesiology 1975; 43:225.)

cardiac output increase. The combination of reduced PVR and increased SVR reduces right-to-left shunting of blood through the ductus arteriosus. The increased pulmonary blood flow augments blood return to the left atrium, thus raising left atrial pressure above right atrial pressure and closing the foramen ovale. Anatomic closure of the foramen ovale may not occur for months, if ever.

In full-term infants, the ductus arteriosus is closed by oxygen, acetylcholine, parasympathetic nerve stimulation, and prostaglandins.[24–26] A partial pressure of arterial oxygen (Pa_{O_2}) of 55 to 85 mm Hg (the Pa_{O_2} of healthy, term infants) closes the ductus arteriosus of term lambs, whereas a Pa_{O_2} of 300 to 500 mm Hg causes insignificant constriction of the ductus arteriosus in preterm lambs.[27] Complete closure of the ductus arteriosus may not occur for 10 to 14 days in term infants or for several months in preterm infants. Hypothermia, hypoxia, and acidosis may reestablish right-to-left shunting of blood through the ductus arteriosus during the first few weeks of life.

Asphyxia is common in fetuses and neonates. In fetuses, it is caused by maternal hypoxia (e.g., cyanotic congenital heart disease, congestive heart failure, or respiratory failure), reduced placental-umbilical blood flow (e.g., maternal hypotension, catecholamine secretion, or abruptio placentae), or placental diseases (e.g., calcification, infarction, or infection). In fetal asphyxia, the Pa_{O_2} decreases from a normal of 25 to 40 mm Hg to less than 5 mm Hg in 2 minutes (Fig. 3-3) because the fetus's only oxygen store is in blood. The partial pressure of arterial carbon dioxide (Pa_{CO_2}) rises rapidly because carbon dioxide (CO_2) cannot be removed. In less than 5 minutes, combined metabolic and respiratory acidosis reduce the pH to 7.0 or less.[28]

In early asphyxia, cardiac output is normal but its distribution is altered.[29] Blood flow to the liver, kidneys, gut, muscle, and skin is reduced; flow to the heart, brain, adrenal glands, and placenta is maintained at prehypoxic levels or is increased.[30] This redistribution of blood flow helps maintain the oxygenation and nutrition of these vital organs. The hearts of hypoxemic fetuses depend on stored energy reserves (glycogen) to sustain their function; when these stores are consumed, the myocardium fails and arterial pressure and cardiac output decrease. (Preterm infants have limited glycogen reserves.) The pH is usually less than 7.0 at this point. Bradycardia (<100 beats per minute) severely reduces cardiac output. Central venous pressure increases as a result of both venous constriction and myocardial failure.

Intrapartum asphyxia may increase or decrease a neonate's blood volume,[31] but hypovolemia is more frequent and occurs in the presence of one of the following:

1. Partial occlusion of the umbilical vessels (such as the umbilical cord around the neck or umbilical cord compression).
2. Hemorrhage from the fetoplacental unit (such as abruptio placenta or transection of the placenta during cesarean section).
3. Maternal hypotension (such as shock, trauma, or anesthesia).
4. Asphyxia.

ASSESSMENT OF THE FETUS AT BIRTH

The Apgar score is still a useful guide to neonatal well-being and resuscitation,[32, 33] but it is only a guide and should be used as such. This system evaluates five variables (Table 3-1) at 1, 5, and 10 minutes of age. If the Apgar score is 7 or less at 5 minutes of age, the score should be redetermined every 5 minutes for a total of 20 minutes. Each variable is given a score from 0 to 2, and the Apgar score at each time is the

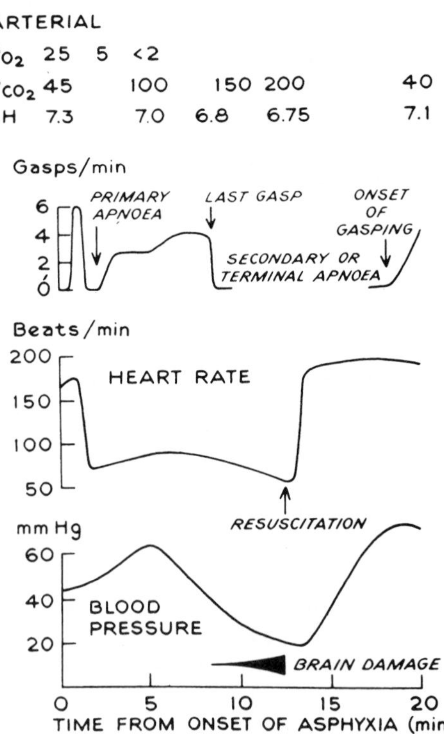

Figure 3–3. The response of newborn monkeys to asphyxia. (From Dawes GS: Foetal and Neonatal Physiology, Chicago, Year Book Medical Publishers, 1968.)

TABLE 3–1. The Apgar Scoring System*

	Apgar Score		
Variable	*0*	*1*	*2*
Heart rate	Absent	Less than 100 bpm	More than 100 bpm
Respiratory effort	Absent	Slow, irregular	Good, crying
Color	Blue, pale	Body pink, extremities blue (acrocyanosis)	Completely pink
Reflex irritability (response to insertion of a nasal catheter)	Absent	Grimace	Cough, sneeze
Muscle tone	Limp	Some flexion of extremities	Active motion

*Each variable is evaluated individually and scored from 0 to 2 at both 1 and 5 minutes of age. The score at each time period is the sum of the scores of the individual variables. A score of 10 is perfect.

bpm = beats per minute.

sum of these scores. Previously, the score at 1 minute was shown to correlate with both acidosis and survival,[34] but with better resuscitation, this no longer appears to be true. The 5-minute score may predict neurologic outcome.[35, 36] To be of value, each Apgar variable must be evaluated at both 1 and 5 minutes of age.

Resuscitation should start immediately, if indicated by inadequate heart rate or respiration. It should not be delayed until the 1-minute Apgar score is obtained.

Heart Rate

The heart rate of healthy neonates is usually 120 to 160 beats per minute. A heart rate of less than 120 beats per minute significantly reduces cardiac output and tissue perfusion. A heart rate less than 100 beats per minute severely reduces cardiac output and requires treatment.

Respiratory Effort

Healthy neonates breathe 30 to 60 times per minute and usually have no pause between inspiration and expiration, thus helping to maintain their functional residual capacity. Apnea occurs with severe acidosis, asphyxia, maternal use of drugs, infections (such as meningitis or septicemia), and CNS injury. Tachypnea (>60 breaths per minute) occurs with hypoxemia, hypovolemia, acidosis (metabolic and respiratory), CNS hemorrhage, pulmonary gas leaks, and pulmonary disease (e.g., hyaline membrane disease, aspiration syndromes, or infection).

Muscle Tone

Most infants are active at birth and respond to stimuli by moving their extremities. Asphyxia, maternal drugs, CNS injury, amyotonia congenita, and myasthenia gravis decrease a neonate's muscle tone. Flexion contractures, absent joint creases, or both suggest a lack of movement in utero and probable CNS injury.

Reflex Irritability

Infants respond to having an extremity flicked by withdrawing the extremity, and they respond to insertion of a nasal catheter by grimacing or crying. Lack of response to these stimuli suggests the presence of hypoxia, acidosis, sedation by maternal drug use, CNS injury, or congenital muscle disease.

Color

All infants have a blue-tinged cast to their skin at birth. Sixty seconds later, most infants are entirely pink, except for their hands and feet. If central cyanosis is still present at 90 seconds of age, low cardiac output, methemoglobinemia, polycythemia, congenital heart disease, and a pulmonary disorder (such as respiratory distress syndrome, airway obstruction, hypoplastic lungs, or diaphragmatic hernia) should be suspected—particularly if the neonate remains blue despite ventilation with oxygen.

Infants who are pale at birth are often asphyxiated, hypovolemic, acidotic, or anemic, or they have congenital heart disease. If heart disease is present, it is usually a left-sided obstructive lesion, such as mitral atresia, aortic atresia, or coarctation or hypoplasia of the aorta. Infants who are entirely pink at birth may be intoxicated with alcohol or magnesium, or they may be alkalotic (pH > 7.5). Those who are ruborous are usually polycythemic.

RESUSCITATION EQUIPMENT

If neonatal resuscitation is to proceed smoothly, all delivery room personnel must know the location of the resuscitation equipment and be skilled in its use. The proper function and correct calibration of this equipment should be determined daily and just before each birth.

The resuscitation bed should allow positioning of an infant's head below the body, both to aid in the removal of lung fluid and to decrease aspiration of gastric contents. A servo-controlled infrared heater maintains a neonate's temperature between 36°C and 37°C. Two suction devices are needed: one to clear secretions from the mouth and airway of the neonate and the other to evacuate a pneumothorax should this become necessary.

The equipment for tracheal intubation should include the following:

- Sizes 0 and 00 straight laryngoscope blades
- A small laryngoscope handle
- Sizes 2.5-, 3.0-, and 3.5-mm endotracheal tubes
- No. 5, 6, and 8 French suction catheters that easily pass through the endotracheal tubes

An extra light bulb and batteries for the laryngoscope should be stored in the delivery room.

The ventilation system should permit maintenance of positive end-expiratory pressure and allow ventilatory rates of 1 to 150 breaths per minute. This is most easily done with a modified Ayres T piece (Fig. 3–4). The ventilation system should not have one-way valves because they often stick, especially at high gas flows and high respiratory rates. If the valve sticks, it may prevent the neonate from exhaling, in which case hypercarbia and a pneumothorax may develop. Ambu bags can be especially dangerous if used improperly.

Blood gas and pH determinations are required during resuscitation. Blood for these determinations is most easily obtained

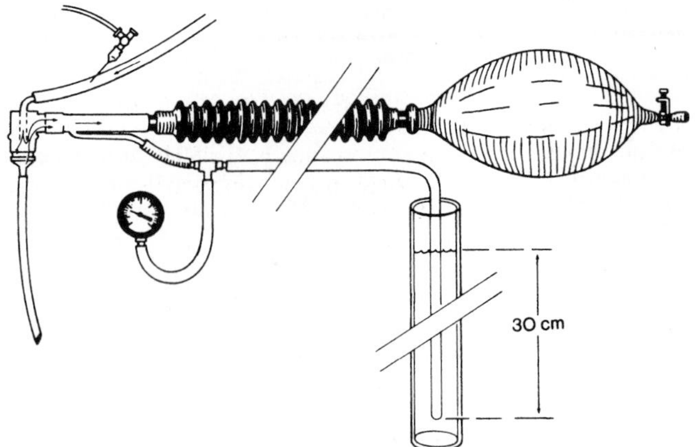

Figure 3–4. A modified Ayres T piece, which allows positive end-expiratory pressure and has a "pop-off" valve to reduce the likelihood of a pneumothorax. (From Gregory GA, Kitterman JA, Phibbs RH, et al: Treatment of the idiopathic respiratory-distress syndrome with continuous positive airway pressure. N Engl J Med 1971; 284:1333. Copyright © 1971, Massachusetts Medical Society.)

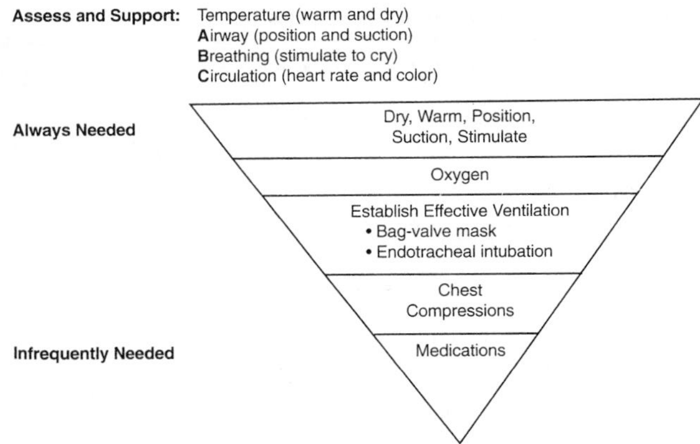

Figure 3–6. Inverted pyramid reflecting relative frequencies of neonatal resuscitation efforts for the newborn who does not have meconium-stained amniotic fluid. Note that a majority of infants respond to simple measures. (Reproduced with permission. Textbook of Pediatric Advanced Life Support, 1997. Copyright American Heart Association.)

from an umbilical artery catheter; however, while the umbilical artery catheter is being inserted, a pulse oximeter should be applied to a hand or foot to guide oxygen therapy until the catheter is in place (Fig. 3-5). If there is right-to-left shunting of blood at the ductus arteriosus, the oxygen saturation in the lower extremity may be much lower than that in the right upper extremity. If there is right-to-left shunting of blood at the foramen ovale, the oxygen saturation will be the same in all extremities. If shunting of blood is suspected through the ductus arteriosus, a pulse oximeter probe should be placed on the right hand and on one of the lower extremities. This is especially helpful in patients who are known to have or are suspected of having a diaphragmatic hernia.

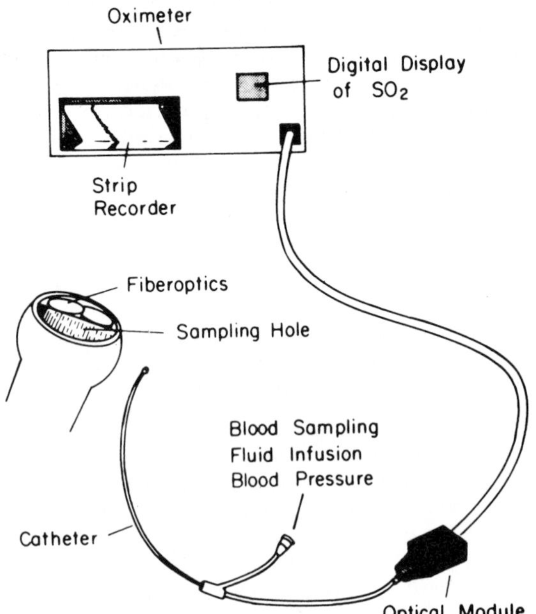

Figure 3–5. The oximetric system for measuring arterial oxygen saturation continuously. The catheter contains fiberoptics that transmit light to and from blood passing the catheter tip. (From Wilkinson AR, Phibbs RH, Gregory GA: Continuous measurement of oxygen saturation in sick newborn infants. J Pediatr 1978; 93:1016.)

The heart rate and electrocardiogram (needle electrodes) should be monitored continuously in sick neonates during resuscitation. Arterial and central venous pressures should also be monitored continuously if there is concern about the adequacy of the intravascular volume.

INITIAL EVALUATION

The inverted triangle, published by the American Heart Association, is a good guide to the care that is needed in the delivery room (Fig. 3-6). Proceeding from top to bottom is a logical way to ensure that patients obtain the care needed. Someone besides the obstetrician (e.g., an anesthesiologist, pediatrician, or neonatologist) should evaluate and resuscitate the neonate at birth. If intrauterine asphyxia is detected or strongly suspected (Table 3-2), at least two assistants are needed, one to provide ventilation and the other to insert an umbilical artery catheter and correct acid-base and blood volume abnormalities. A resuscitation plan should be developed before the infant's birth if possible.

As an infant's head is delivered, the mouth and nose should be suctioned with a bulb syringe. Once the body is delivered, the neonate should be held at the level of the introitus and dried with a towel to stimulate crying and reduce evaporative heat loss. If the neonate is held below the level of the introitus while the umbilical arteries are still pulsating, the blood volume is increased and polycythemia may develop.[31-35] Polycythemia increases the incidence of high PVR, hypoxia, acidosis, and CNS injury. Raising the neonate above the level of the introitus, especially placing him or her on the mother's abdomen, may cause hypovolemia.

Once breathing is established and the umbilical cord stops pulsating, the cord should be clamped and cut and the neonate handed to the person responsible for resuscitation. Stripping blood from the umbilical cord to the neonate may increase blood volume,[42] respiratory rate,[43] lung water,[44] pulmonary artery pressure, and Pa_{CO_2},[45] whereas lung compliance, functional residual capacity, and Pa_{O_2} may decrease.[46] Early cord clamping, on the other hand, may deprive the neonate of as much as 30 mL/kg of blood (Fig. 3-7).[40] However, if the neonate is asphyxiated (flaccid, pale, limp, or cyanotic), the umbilical cord should be clamped as soon as possible and the neonate handed to the resuscitator. Remember, *early cord clamping almost always causes hypovolemia.*

TABLE 3–2. Disorders Frequently Associated with Asphyxia at Birth

Maternal conditions
1. Older primigravida (older than 35 yr)
2. Diabetes
3. Hypertension
4. Toxemia
5. Maternal treatment with any of the following:
   a. Glucocorticoids
   b. Diuretics
   c. Antimetabolites
   d. Reserpine, lithium
   e. Magnesium
   f. Ethyl alcohol
   g. β-Adrenergic drugs (to stop premature labor)
6. Abnormal estriol levels
7. Anemia (hemoglobin <10 g/dL)
8. Blood type or group isoimmunization
9. Previous birth of child with a hereditary disease
10. Current maternal infection or infection during pregnancy with rubella, herpes simplex, syphilis
11. Abruptio placentae
12. Placenta previa
13. Antepartum hemorrhage
14. History of birth of previous infant with jaundice, thrombocytopenia, cardiorespiratory distress, congenital anomalies
15. Narcotic, barbiturate, tranquilizer, or psychedelic drug use
16. Ethyl alcohol intoxication
17. History of previous neonatal death
18. Prolonged rupture of membranes

Conditions of labor and delivery
1. Forceps delivery other than low elective
2. Vacuum extraction delivery
3. Breech presentation and delivery or other abnormal presentation
4. Cesarean section
5. Prolonged labor
6. Prolapsed umbilical cord
7. Cephalopelvic disproportion
8. Maternal hypotension
9. Sedative or analgesic drugs given intravenously within 1 hr of delivery or intramuscularly within 2 hr of delivery

Fetal conditions
1. Multiple births
2. Polyhydramnios
3. Meconium-stained amniotic fluid
4. Abnormal heart rate or rhythm
5. Acidosis (fetal scalp capillary blood)
6. Decreased rate of growth (uterine size)
7. Premature delivery
8. Amniotic fluid surfactant test negative or intermediate within 24 hr of delivery

Neonatal conditions
1. Birth asphyxia
2. Birth weight (inappropriate for gestational age)
3. Meconium staining of the skin, nails, or umbilical cord
4. Signs of cardiorespiratory distress

Consequently, the blood volume will require expansion after birth with saline, albumin, or blood. Failure to do so increases the likelihood of respiratory, cardiovascular, and CNS complications.

After the umbilical cord is cut, the neonate should be placed in a radiantly heated resuscitation bed. The airway should be cleared by gently suctioning the mouth and nose with a bulb syringe. Prolonged suctioning must be avoided because it can induce vomiting, hypoxia, and dysrhythmias (usually bradycardia).

If the respiratory pattern and color are normal at 1 minute of age (top level of triangle, Fig. 3-6), the only requirement is to dry the neonate, keep her or him warm, administer blow-by oxygen until the neonate is pink, and pass a suction catheter through each nostril into the posterior pharynx to rule out choanal atresia. The latter should be done early because choanal atresia can be lethal. Once patency of the nares is ensured, the catheter should be passed through the mouth and advanced into the stomach. Inability of the catheter to enter the stomach suggests that the patient has esophageal atresia. If the catheter enters the stomach and more than 25 mL of fluid is removed, the patient may have a small-bowel obstruction.

The 1-minute Apgar score reflects a neonate's condition at birth and may indicate the need for resuscitation; consequently, this score may be used as a guide to resuscitation. However, it is also important to carefully reevaluate the Apgar score at 5 and again at 10 minutes of age; some infants who look well at 1 minute are sick by 5 or 10 minutes of age.

Most infants (90%) have a 1-minute Apgar score of 8 to 10 and require only nasal and oral suctioning, drying of the skin, and maintenance of a normal body temperature (top level of triangle). When stable, these infants can be wrapped in a warm blanket and handed to the parents.

Infants with 1-minute Apgar scores of 5 to 7 have suffered mild asphyxia just before birth (level 2 of triangle). They usually respond to vigorous stimulation during drying and to having oxygen blown over their face. If they respond slowly, a bag and mask can be used to ventilate the lungs with 80% to 100% oxygen. With appropriate care, such infants are usually well by 5 minutes of age. Blood gases measured at 2 minutes of age usually show a Pa_{O_2} of 50 to 70 mm Hg, a Pa_{CO_2} of 40 to 50 mm Hg, a pH of 7.15 to 7.25, and a base deficit of approximately 10 mEq/L. By 10 minutes of age, the pH and base deficit of these patients usually are normal and the Pa_{CO_2} is less than 40 mm Hg.

Infants with Apgar scores of 3 to 4 at 1 minute of age are moderately depressed (level 3 of triangle). They are usually cyanotic and have poor respiratory efforts at birth. With bag-and-mask ventilation, their cardiac output improves and their skin becomes pink. If they have never breathed, it may be difficult to ventilate their lungs by bag and mask because their airway resistance exceeds that of the esophagus. In that case, gas preferentially enters the esophagus, stomach, and gut during bag-and-mask ventilation, further interfering with ventilation. Therefore, if a neonate has not breathed spontaneously, it is usually preferable to insert an endotracheal tube before assisting ventilation. Blood gas and pH measurements should

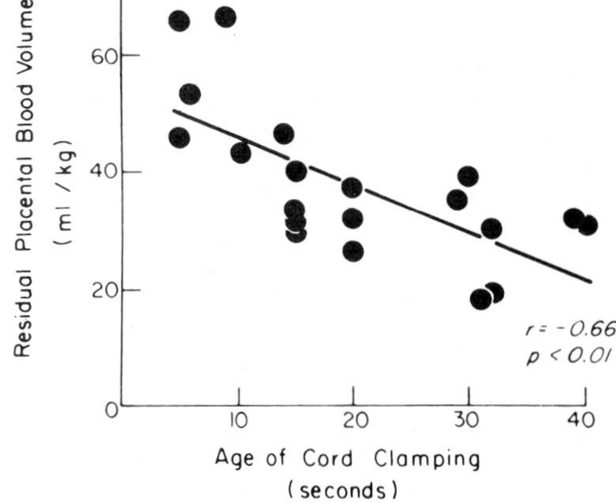

Figure 3–7. Effects of early and late cord clamping on placental blood volume. (From Ogata ES, Kitterman JA, Phibbs RH: the effect of time of cord clamping and maternal blood pressure on placental transfusion with cesarean section. Am J Obstet Gynecol 1977; 128:197.)

be obtained from a doubly clamped segment of umbilical cord as soon as possible. If the pH is less than 7.2, blood gas and pH values should be obtained from a warmed heel or preferably from a radial artery. If the patient has a base deficit greater than 10, it may be necessary to administer sodium bicarbonate ($NaHCO_3$).

PULMONARY RESUSCITATION

Infants with an Apgar score of 2 or less are severely asphyxiated and require *immediate* resuscitation (levels 4 to 6 of triangle).

The trachea should be intubated immediately, and the lungs should be ventilated 30 to 60 times per minute with 80% to 100% oxygen and enough positive pressure to expand the chest normally. Overexpansion of the lungs for even brief periods may cause severe damage to the lungs, especially to the lungs of premature infants.[47] Every fifth breath should be held for 2 to 3 seconds to expand atelectatic lungs and remove lung fluid. Maintaining a positive end-expiratory pressure of 2 to 4 cm H_2O often improves oxygenation.

Tracheal Intubation

An infant's larynx is located more anteriorly than that of an adult. Extending the head displaces the infant's larynx even more anteriorly, making tracheal intubation more difficult. If the head is placed in a neutral or "sniffing" position (Fig. 3–8), the trachea is most easily visualized. The laryngoscope should be held with the thumb and index finger of the left hand while the chin is grasped with the ring and middle fingers of the same hand. This fixes the head, hand, and laryngoscope into a single unit and reduces the incidence of pharyngeal trauma if the infant's head moves. The handle of the laryngoscope blade should be pulled up and out at 45 degrees, and pressure should be applied over the hyoid bone with the small finger of the left hand. The latter moves the larynx posteriorly and improves one's view of the larynx. The endotracheal tube should then be inserted 1 to 2 cm below the vocal cords, depending on the infant's size. A small gas leak should be present between the endotracheal tube and the trachea when 15 to 30 cm H_2O of pressure is generated. The appropriate size of endotracheal tube is usually 2.5 mm internal diameter for infants weighing less than 1.5 kg, 3.0 mm for 1.5- to 2.5-kg infants, and 3.5 mm for infants over 2.5 kg. If the endotracheal tube is the same width as the widest portion of the fingernail of the small finger, the tube fits the trachea more than 90% of the time.

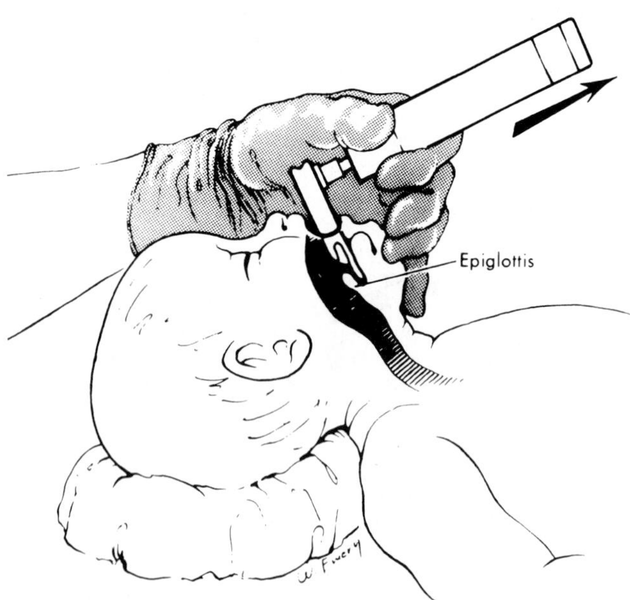

Figure 3–8. Laryngoscopy of the newborn infant. (From Gregory GA: Cardiopulmonary resuscitation of the newborn. *In* The Anesthesiologist, the Mother, and the Newborn. Baltimore, Williams & Wilkins, 1974, pp 200–209.)

The lungs should be expanded with an anesthesia bag, and the effects of ventilation must be closely monitored. If the Pa_{O_2} rises above 80 mm Hg or if the oxygen saturation exceeds 95%, the inspired oxygen concentration should be reduced in 5% to 10% decrements until the Pa_{O_2} is 50 to 70 mm Hg or until the oxygen saturation is 87% to 95%. This is especially important for preterm neonates, who may experience retinopathy of prematurity (retrolental fibroplasia) when the Pa_{O_2} is 100 to 150 mm Hg for a few hours. One should monitor the infant's heart rate continuously during endotracheal intubation in an effort to detect dysrhythmias or bradycardia.

It may be difficult to intubate the trachea of infant who has an hypoplastic mandible. If so, insertion of a No. 1 laryngeal mask usually provides and adequate airway, and this should be done earlier rather than later. Ventilation can usually be accomplished through the mask. Occasionally, it is necessary to insert an orogastric tube at the same time to prevent gastric distention with air.

Adequacy of Ventilation

The adequacy of ventilation is best assessed by physical examination and blood gas determination. Both sides of the chest should rise equally and simultaneously with inspiration. If one side rises before the other, endobronchial intubation may have occurred or the neonate may have a pneumothorax or a congenital lung anomaly.

Breath sounds are well transmitted in these small chests and may be normal despite the presence of atelectasis or a pneumothorax. The breath sounds should be heard over the stomach, but they should not be as loud as those heard over the chest. If they are as loud, the examiner determines whether esophageal intubation has occurred or whether the patient has a tracheoesophageal fistula.

With adequate ventilation, cyanosis should disappear, the heart rate should rise to normal, and the patient should establish rhythmic breathing. Most asphyxiated infants have normal lungs; therefore, it is uncommon to require more than 25 cm H_2O of pressure to expand their lungs.

Excessive airway pressure is the major cause of pulmonary gas leaks during resuscitation. Infants with stiff lungs (as found in erythroblastosis fetalis, congenital anomalies of the lung, or pulmonary edema) require high ventilation pressures and are susceptible to pulmonary gas leaks. If inadequate pressures are used to ventilate the lungs, however, hypoxia, acidosis, CNS injury, and death may occur. Therefore, one must apply sufficient pressure during inspiration to move the chest a normal amount. If pulmonary gas leaks occur, they should be drained with a thoracostomy tube.

Routine Tracheal Suctioning

Ten to 15% of women experience meconium staining of the amniotic fluid. Of the infants born to these women, 60% have meconium in their trachea at birth.[48] After birth, the infant's breathing moves meconium into the periphery of the lungs unless the meconium is removed before or immediately after the onset of breathing. Sixteen per cent of infants with meconium staining have some respiratory difficulties during the first few days of life. Ten per cent have a pneumothorax or pneumomediastinum on chest radiographs, but only one third of these infants have respiratory distress.

Because of the seriousness of the complications associated with meconium aspiration, thick particulate or "pea soup" meconium should be removed from the trachea as soon as possible after birth. Thin, watery meconium does not need to be removed. The physician can most effectively remove meconium by applying a suction device to the end of the endotracheal tube and applying negative pressure as the tube is withdrawn from the trachea. The laryngoscope should be kept in place as the endotracheal tube is removed. If meconium is suctioned from the trachea, the endotracheal tube should be reinserted immediately.

After suctioning twice, the physician gently ventilates the lungs with oxygen. Absence of meconium in the mouth and posterior pharynx does not preclude its presence in the trachea.[41] Oxygen should be blown over the infant's face, and the heart rate should be monitored continuously during laryngoscopy and tracheal suctioning. Suctioning the stomach reduces the likelihood of regurgitation and aspiration of meconium at a later time. Meconium aspiration has been reviewed elsewhere.[49] Routine tracheal suctioning is also appropriate after severe vaginal bleeding.

VASCULAR RESUSCITATION

Vascular resuscitation is the least understood and least practiced area of neonatal resuscitation. It is seldom mentioned in textbooks, even though hypovolemia is common in asphyxiated neonates at birth.

If the response to ventilation and tactile stimulation is not immediate, one should insert an umbilical artery catheter in order to determine blood gas and pH values, measure arterial pressure, expand blood volume, and administer drugs. An umbilical venous catheter (with its tip above the diaphragm) allows central venous pressure to be determined and to be used as an index of adequate volume replacement. The normal central venous pressure of neonates is 4 to 12 cm H_2O (discussed later). Care must be taken to assure that no air bubbles are injected into the vascular system, as the presence of a patent foramen ovale may permit entry of air into the left side of the circulation and cause coronary artery, cerebral arterial, or other arterial obstruction.

CORRECTION OF ACIDOSIS

Respiratory acidosis is corrected by assisting ventilation. Metabolic acidosis is improved by correcting blood volume deficits and infusing $NaHCO_3$. However, $NaHCO_3$ administration is associated with several potentially serious problems:

1. $NaHCO_3$ is very hypertonic. Therefore, $NaHCO_3$ increases the likelihood of intracranial hemorrhage occurring in preterm neonates if the $NaHCO_3$ is given rapidly and in large volumes.

2. The complete reaction of $NaHCO_3$ with hydrogen ions produces approximately 1250 mL of CO_2/50 mEq of $NaHCO_3$; some of this CO_2 is buffered. If ventilation is adequate, most of the CO_2 is immediately exhaled and the Pa_{CO_2} rises less than 4 mm Hg. On the other hand, if ventilation is inadequate (as it usually is in asphyxiated infants), the Pa_{CO_2} rises markedly and death may ensue. Hypercarbia dilates the cerebral vessels and increases cerebral blood flow, further increasing the likelihood of intracranial hemorrhage. To avoid these complications, one should give $NaHCO_3$ slowly (not faster than 1 mEq $kg^{-1} \cdot min^{-1}$) while the patient is artificially ventilated.

3. Administering $NaHCO_3$ also may induce hypotension (Fig. 3-9).

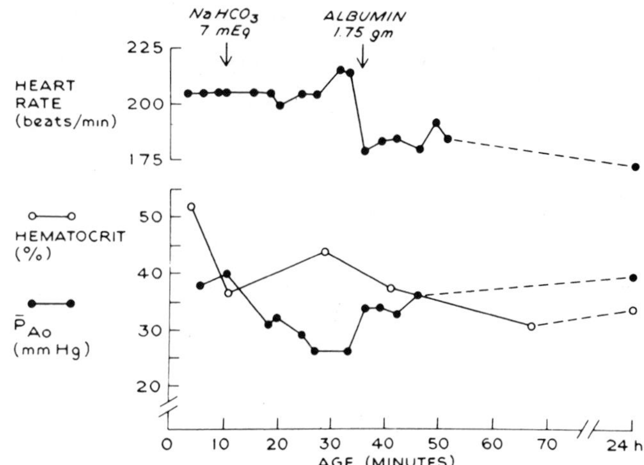

Figure 3–9. Effects of sodium bicarbonate ($NaHCO_3$) on arterial blood pressure (PAO), heart rate, and hematrocrit (Hct). Hypotension occurred followng the administration of $NaHCO_3$. The Hct decreased as fluid was pulled into the intravascular space to compensate for the hypovolemia that was present since birth. Raising pH decreased the peripheral vasoconstriction produced by the preexisting acidosis. Giving albumin increased the arterial pressure to normal. Based on the final Hct, the infant's initial blood volume was approximatley 30% less than predicted. (Illustration reprinted from Phibbs RH: What is the evidence that blood pressure monitoring is useful? *In*: Problems of Neonatal Intensive Care Units. Lucey JF [Ed]. Report of the Fifty-Ninth Ross Conference on Pediatric Research. Columbus, Ohio, Ross Laboratories, 1969, pp 81-86.)

4. $NaHCO_3$ administration does not increase the intracellular acidosis of the neonatal brain.[50] The administration of THAM instead of $NaHCO_3$ may prevent some of these problems but may induce others. For instance, there may be marked abnormalities in serum electrolytes and, because a larger volume of fluid must be administered, hypervolemia may be induced. The advantage of THAM is that it buffers both intracellular and extracellular acidosis.

If the Apgar score is 2 or less at 2 minutes of age or 5 or less at 5 minutes despite adequate ventilation and stimulation, a blood gas sample should be sent to the laboratory and 1 to 2 mEq/kg of $NaHCO_3$ is administered while the lungs are artificially ventilated. $NaHCO_3$ should not be infused into an umbilical venous catheter if the tip of the catheter is in the liver, because doing so may cause hepatic necrosis. Blood gases and pH should be monitored after giving the drug. If the pH is 7.1 or less and the Pa_{CO_2} is less than 45 mm Hg, one fourth of the base deficit can be corrected with $NaHCO_3$. If the pH is greater than 7.1, ventilation of the neonate's lungs should be continued and another blood gas measurement obtained in 5 minutes. If the repeat blood gas determination does not show an increased pH, one fourth of the base deficit should be corrected with $NaHCO_3$ while someone is continuing to ventilate the lungs.

Metabolic acidosis occurs when heart failure or hypovolemia reduces tissue perfusion. Raising the pH to 7.25 or greater usually improves cardiac output, increases liver perfusion, and decreases metabolic acid production (Fig. 3-10). If hypoglycemia is the cause of heart failure, the physician should raise the serum glucose level to 45 to 90 mg/dL by infusing 5 mL/kg of 10% dextrose solution over 3 to 5 minutes. This glucose bolus should be followed with continuous infusion of 10% glucose. However, hyperglycemia should be avoided because it may worsen neurologic outcome.[53-54]

If the heart failure is due to congenital cardiac anomalies or hypoxic myocardial depression, the cardiac output should be

TABLE 3–3. Average Systolic, Diastolic, and Mean Arterial Blood Pressures (mm Hg) During the First 12 Hours of Life in Normal Infants

	Hours											
	1	2	3	4	5	6	7	8	9	10	11	12
Body weight 1001–2000 g												
Systolic	49	49	51	52	53	52	52	52	51	51	49	50
Diastolic	26	27	28	29	31	31	31	31	31	30	29	30
Mean	35	36	37	39	40	40	39	39	38	37	37	38
Birth weight 2001–3000 g												
Systolic	59	57	60	60	61	58	64	60	63	61	60	59
Diastolic	32	32	32	32	33	34	37	34	38	35	35	35
Mean	43	41	43	43	44	43	45	43	44	44	43	42
Birth weight >3000 g												
Systolic	70	67	65	65	66	66	67	67	68	70	66	66
Diastolic	44	41	39	41	40	41	41	41	44	43	41	41
Mean	53	51	50	50	51	50	50	51	53	54	51	50

increased by an infusion of isoproterenol (one should start with 0.05 μg · kg^{-1} · min^{-1} and increase the dose as necessary). Isoproterenol usually raises the cardiac output, but the heart rate often must be increased to 160 to 190 beats per minute for this drug to be effective.

In rare instances (e.g., congenital heart block), it may be necessary to treat congenital bradycardia with a transvenous pacemaker immediately after birth. Dopamine may also improve cardiac output, but much larger doses may be required (5–100 μg · kg^{-1} · min^{-1}) to achieve normal blood pressure and normal perfusion for infants.[55] If the acidosis is due to hypovolemia, as it usually is, the blood volume should be increased.

CORRECTION OF HYPOVOLEMIA

Hypovolemia is detected by measuring arterial pressure and by physical examination. Approximately 60% of asphyxiated preterm infants are hypovolemic at birth, partly because of the appropriate early clamping of the umbilical cord (see Fig. 3-7).[46] Infants who have partial umbilical cord occlusion, abruptio placenta, or accidental placental transection during a cesarean section are usually hypovolemic.

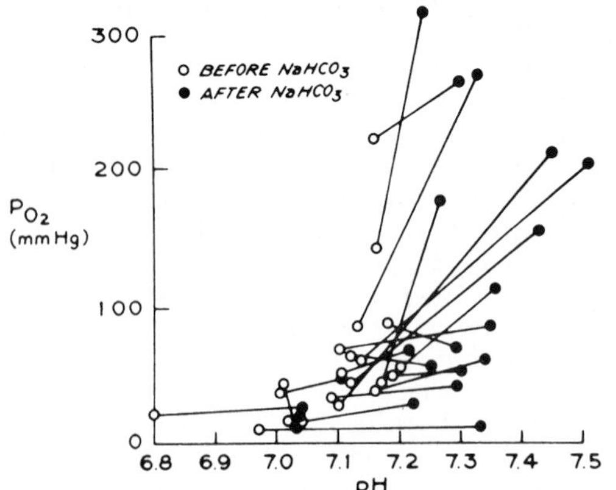

Figure 3–10. Effects of sodium bicarbonate ($NaHCO_3$) infusion on Pao_2 and pH when ventilation was held constant in asphyxiated infants. the Pao_2 rose when the pH rose above 7.10 to 7.20. (From Gregory GA: Resuscitation of the newborn. Anesthesiology 1975; 43:225.)

Arterial blood pressure can be measured with a Doppler system or an indwelling arterial catheter and strain-gauge.[56] During resuscitation, the latter is advantageous because arterial pressure is measured continuously. In the author's experience, the mean arterial pressure, which increases with increasing gestational age (Table 3-3), is more representative of a patient's condition than the systolic or diastolic pressure. However, a decrease of more than 5 mm Hg in the systolic blood pressure with each inspiration is also suggestive of hypovolemia.

Knowing the central venous pressure also helps one in deciding whether a neonate is hypovolemic. This pressure is normally 4 to 12 cm H_2O at end expiration. If it is less than 4 cm H_2O, hypovolemia should be suspected.

Hypovolemic infants are usually pale and have poor capillary filling and poor peripheral perfusion (Table 3-4). The extremities are cold, and the pulse (especially radial and posterior tibial pulses) is weak or absent. Infants intoxicated with alcohol or magnesium are usually pink, peripherally dilated, hypotensive, and often acidotic.

The key to treating hypovolemia is intravascular volume expansion with blood, plasma, or crystalloid. If one suspects that a neonate may be hypovolemic at birth, O-negative, low-titer blood should be crossmatched against the mother before birth; 1 unit of packed cells and 1 unit of whole blood should be brought to the delivery room in separate sealed plastic ice

TABLE 3–4. Relationship of Skin Color, Capillary Refill Time, Pulse Volume, and Extremity Temperature to Hypovolemia

Amount of Volume Depletion	Skin Color	Capillary Refill Time (sec)	Posterior Tibial Pulse Volume	Skin Temperature
None	Pink	<2	+ + + +	Warm
5%	Pale	3–4	+ +	Cold from midcalf and midforearm out
10%	Gray	4–5	0	Cold midthigh and upper arm out
15%	Mottled	>5	0	Entire extremity cold

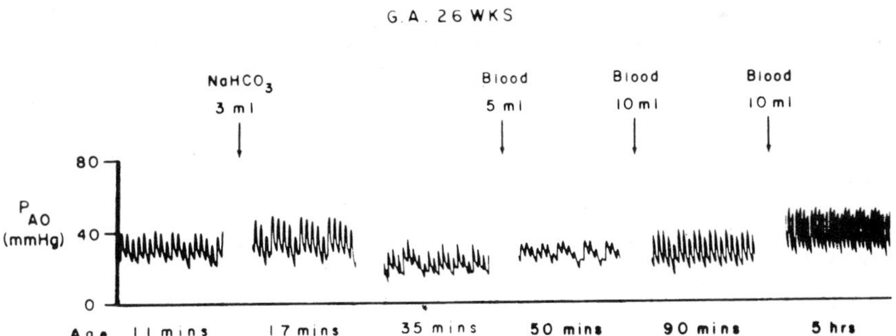

Figure 3–11. Effect of hypovolemia in a preterm infant. PAO equals mean arterial pressure. (From Gregory GA: resuscitation of the newborn. Anesthesiology 1975; 43:225.)

chests. If the blood is not used within 4 hours, it can be returned to the blood bank.

If crossmatched blood is unavailable, blood can be withdrawn in a sterile fashion from the umbilical placental arteries and veins into a syringe containing 1 to 2 units of heparin per milliliter of blood. After the blood is filtered, it can be given to the neonate. Placental blood vessels of asphyxiated babies frequently contain large amounts of blood.[46] Blood group incompatibility is not a concern because blood in the placental vessels belongs to the neonate; giving placental blood poses a small risk of infection, and it takes several minutes to obtain the blood. If blood is not available, 1 to 2 g of 25% albumin per kilogram or 10 mL/kg of plasma or lactated Ringer's solution is given. The volume of fluid required to raise the blood pressure to normal may be enormous; at times it exceeds 50% of the blood volume (85 mL/kg) (Fig. 3–11), particularly if the placenta is abrupted or if it is transected during a cesarean section.

Overexpansion of the intravascular volume and hypertension should be avoided because asphyxiated infants cannot autoregulate their cerebral circulation.[57–59] Thus, overexpansion of the blood volume and hypertension increase the likelihood of intracranial hemorrhage, especially in premature neonates.[60]

Pulmonary gas leaks or high airway pressures cause hypotension because they interfere with the venous return to the heart. Hypoglycemia, hypocalcemia, and hypomagnesemia also cause hypotension. Alcohol-induced and magnesium-induced hypotension usually respond to blood volume expansion. Hypermagnesemic neonates also may respond to an infusion of 100 mg/kg of calcium gluconate.

Polycythemia (hematocrit > 65%) occurs with delayed cord clamping, with holding the neonate below the introitus after birth, and with stripping the umbilical cord of blood. The hyperviscosity that accompanies polycythemia can reduce the pulmonary blood flow and increase the right-to-left shunting of blood through the ductus arteriosus and foramen ovale. When polycythemia is present, the hematocrit value should be reduced to 50% to 55% by an exchange transfusion with 5% plasma or albuminated saline (4 g albumin per 100 mL saline). The sequelae of polycythemia include cardiac and renal failure as well as cerebral, intestinal, and renal vein thrombosis.

CARDIAC MASSAGE

If the heart rate is less than 100 beats per minute and does not increase when the patient is ventilated with 100% oxygen by bag and mask, the trachea should be intubated, the lungs ventilated with oxygen, and closed-chest massage begun. Both thumbs should be placed at mid sternum, with the fingers encircling the chest to support the back (Fig. 3–12). The sternum is compressed 1 to 2 cm or 0.5 to 0.75 inch (about one third of the distance to the anterior vertebral column) at a rate of 100 to 150 times per minute. Ventilation of the lungs occurs 40 to 60 times per minute and is continuous during cardiac massage. The effectiveness of cardiac massage is best monitored by the arterial pressure measurement. If this is not available, the pupil size should be monitored. The pupils should be in the midposition or constricted. If they are dilated and if atropine has not been given, cerebral blood flow and oxygenation are inadequate.

Ideally, each chest compression should generate a systolic pressure of 80 mm Hg. This pressure, in conjunction with compression of about 120 times per minute, maintains diastolic pressure greater than 25 mm Hg, which is probably adequate for coronary perfusion.

All resuscitation drugs should be infused in the smallest volume possible to reduce the risk of hypervolemia (Table 3–5).[52] This means filling the dead space of the catheter and tubing with high drug concentrations, which may cause serious dysrhythmias or cardiac arrest if the drugs are flushed in rapidly. To avoid these complications, one should withdraw three times the volume of the catheter and stopcock before injecting anything into the catheter. It is preferable to infuse vasoactive drugs into a separate intravenous line. Because

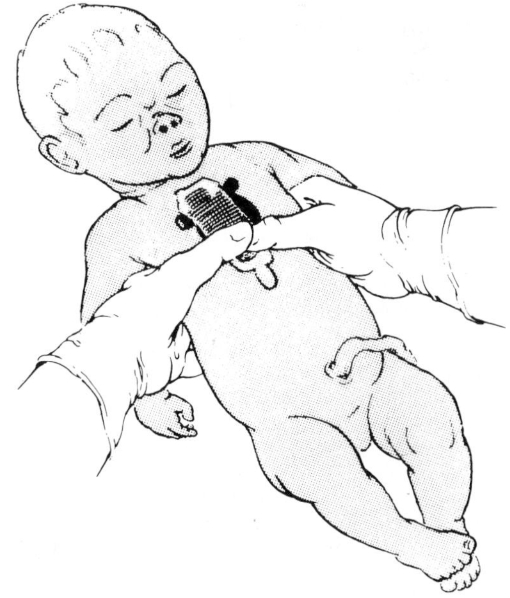

Figure 3–12. Closed-chest cardiac massage. For simplification, ventilation is not shown. (From Gregory GA: Cardiopulmonary resuscitation of the newborn. *In*: The anesthesiologist, the Mother, and the Newborn. Baltimore, Williams & Wilkins, 1974, pp 200–209.)

TABLE 3–5. Drugs Used During Resuscitation

Drug	Indication	Dose*	Route	Response	Complication
Atropine	Bradycardia	0.03 mg/kg	IV	Increased heart rate	Marked tachycardia, diminished cardiac output
Calcium gluconate	Low cardiac output	100 mg/kg over 5–10 min (ECG monitoring)	IV	Improved cardiac output	Bradycardia, dysrhythmias
Epinephrine	"Flat line" ECG	0.1 mL/kg of a 1 : 10,000 solution	IV	"Flat line" ECG converted to some rhythmic response	Hypertension, ventricular fibrillation
Isoproterenol	Bradycardia, hypotension, low cardiac output	4 mg/250 mL 5% dextrose in water; begin with 0.5 mg/kg/min, and increase until heart rate increases	IV	Increased heart rate, improved cardiac output	Dysrhythmias, low cardiac output if heart rate > 180–200 bpm

* Doses given are starting doses and may have to be increased. Most drugs tend to be more effective when pH > 7.15.
Abbreviations: ECG = electrocardiogram; bpm = beats per minute.

acidosis decreases the effectiveness of resuscitation drugs, the pH should be raised above 7.2 as soon as possible.

References

1. Glass HG, Snyder FF, Webster E: The rate of decline in resistance to anoxia of rabbits, dogs, and guinea pigs from the onset of viability to adult life. Am J Physiol 1944; 140:690.
2. Himwich HE, Alexander FAD, Fazekas JF: Tolerance of the newborn to hypoxia and anoxia. Am J Physiol 1941; 133:327.
3. Roland EH, Hill A: Clinical aspects of perinatal hypoxic-ischemic brain injury. Semin Pediatr Neurol 1995; 2:57.
4. Depp R: Perinatal asphyxia: Assessing its causal role and timing. Semin Pediatr Neurol 1995; 2:13.
5. Leuthner SR, Jansen RD, Hageman JR: Cardiopulmonary resuscitation of the newborn: An Update. Pediatr Clin North Am 41: 1994; 893.
6. Platzker ACG, Kitterman JA, Mescher EJ, et al: Surfactant in the lung and tracheal fluid of the fetal lamb and acceleration of its appearance by dexamethasone. Pediatrics 1971; 56:554.
7. Ballard PL: Hormones and lung maturation: Thyroid hormone effects and binding. *In*: Monographs on Endocrinology. Gross F, Grumbach MM, Labhart A (Eds). Heidelberg, Springer-Verlag, 1986, pp 197–230.
8. Platzker ACG, Kitterman JA, Clements JA, et al: Surfactant appearance and secretion in the fetal lamb lung in response to dexamethasone. Pediatr Res 1972; 6:406.
9. Lawson EW, Brown EB, et al: Influence of epinephrine on fetal pulmonary fluid release and surfactant production. Am Rev Respir Dis 1978; 118:1023.
10. Lawson EW, Birdwell RL, Huang PS, et al: Augmentation of pulmonary surfactant secretion by lung expansion at birth. Pediatr Res 1979; 13:611.
11. Adams FH, Moss AJ, Fagan L: The tracheal fluid of the foetal lamb. Biol Neonate 1963; 5:151.
12. Ross FB: Comparison of foetal pulmonary fluid with foetal plasma and amniotic fluid. Nature 1963; 199:1100.
13. Mescher EJ, Platzker ACG, Ballard PL, et al: Ontogenicity of tracheal fluid pulmonary surfactant and plasma corticoids in the fetal lamb. J Appl Physiol 1975; 39:1017.
14. Bland RD, McMillan DD, Bressack MA, et al: Clearance of liquid from lungs of newborn rabbits. J Appl Physiol 1980; 49:171.
15. Karlberg P: The adaptive changes in the immediate postnatal period, with particular reference to respiration. J Pediatr 1960; 56:585.
16. Chernick V, Fariday EE, Pagatakhan RD: Role of the peripheral and central chemoreceptors in the initiation of fetal respiration. J Appl Physiol 1975; 38:407.
17. Jansen AH, Chernick V: Site of chemosensitivity in fetal sheep. J Appl Physiol 1975; 39:1.
18. Dawes GS: Foetal and Neonatal Physiology. Chicago, Year Book Medical Publishers, 1968.
19. Rudolph AM, Heymann MA: Fetal and neonatal circulation and respiration. Annu Rev Physiol 1974; 36:187.
20. Rudolph AM: Congenital Diseases of the Heart. Chicago, Year Book Medical Publishers, 1974.
21. Rudolph AM, Yuen S: Response of the pulmonary vasculature to hypoxia and H^+ ion concentration changes. J Clin Invest 1966; 45:399.
22. Cassen S, Dawes GS, Mott JC, et al: The vascular resistance of the foetal and newly ventilated lung of the lamb. J Physiol 1964; 171:61.
23. Brady JP, Rigatto H: Pulmonary capillary flow in infants. Circulation 1969; (Suppl III):50.
24. Asali NS, Morris JA, Smith RW, et al: Studies on ductus arteriosus circulation. Circ Res 1963; 13:478.
25. Heymann HS, Rudolph AM: Constriction of the ductus arteriosus by acetylcholine in premature infants. Circulation 1971; 43:11.
26. Evans N: Diagnosis of patent ductus arteriosus in the preterm newborn. Arch Dis Child 1993; 68:58.
27. McMurphy DM, Heymann HA, Rudolph AM, et al: Developmental changes in constriction of the ductus arteriosus: Responses of oxygen to vasoactive agents in the isolated ductus arteriosus of the fetal lamb. Pediatr Res 1972; 6:231.
28. Dawes GS: Foetal and Neonatal Physiology. Chicago, Year Book Medical Publishers, 1968.
29. Behrman RE, Lees MH, Peterson EN, et al: Distribution of circulation in the normal and asphyxiated fetal primate. Am J Obstet Gynecol 1970; 108:956.
30. Biehl DR, Coté J, Wade JG, et al: Uptake of halothane by the foetal lamb *in utero*. Can Anaesth Soc J 1983; 30:24.
31. Yao AC, Lind J: Blood volume in the asphyxiated term neonate. Biol Neonate 1972; 21:199.
32. Apgar V: A proposal for a new method of evaluation of the newborn infant. Curr Res Anesth 1953; 32:260.
33. Apgar V, James LS: Further observations on the newborn scoring system. Am J Dis Child 1962; 104:419.
34. James LS, Weisbrot IM, Prince CE, et al: The acid-base status of human infants in relation to birth asphyxia and onset of respiration. J Pediatr 1958; 52:379.
35. Drage JS, Berendes H: Apgar scores and outcome of the newborn. Pediatr Clin North Am 1966; 13:635.
36. Lam BC, Yeung CY: Perinatal features of birth asphyxia and neurologic outcome. Acta Paediatr Jpn 1992; 34:17.
37. Yao AC, Moinain H, Lind J: Distribution of blood between infant and placenta after birth. Lancet 1969; ii:871.
38. Black VD, Lubchenco LO, Koops BL, et al: Neonatal hyperviscosity: Randomized study of effect of partial plasma exchange transfusion on long-term outcome. Pediatrics 1985; 75:1048.
39. Van der Elst CW, Molteno CD, Molan AF, et al: The management of polycythemia in the newborn infant. Early Hum Dev 1980; 4:393.
40. Hart A, Ulrich M: Late prognosis in untreated neonatal polycythemia with minor or no symptoms. Acta Pediatr Scand 1982; 71:629.
41. Black VD, Lubchenco LO, Luckey DW, et al: Developmental and neurologic sequelae of neonatal hyperviscosity syndrome. Pediatrics 1982; 69:426.
42. Gunther H: The transfer of blood between baby and placenta in the minutes after birth. Lancet 1957; i:1277.

43. Oh W, Lind J, Gessner IH: The circulatory and respiratory adaptation to early and late cord clamping in newborn infants. Acta Pediatr Scand 1966; 55:17.
44. Cassidy G: Effect of caesarean section on neonatal body water spaces. N Engl J Med 1971; 285:887.
45. Oh W, Arcilla RA, Lind J, et al: Arterial blood gases and acid balance in the newborn infant: Effects of cord clamping at birth. Acta Pediatr Scand 1966; 55:593.
46. Ogata ES, Kitterman JA, Phibbs RH: The effect of time of cord clamping and maternal blood pressure on placental transfusion with cesarean section. Am J Obstet Gynecol 1977; 128:197.
47. Bjorklund LJ, Ingimarsson J, Curstedt T, John J, Robertson B, Werner O, Vilstrup CT: Manual ventilation with a few large breaths at birth compromises the therapeutic effect of subsequent surfactant replacement in immature lambs. Pediatric Research 1997; 42:348.
48. Gregory GA, Gooding C, Phibbs RH, et al: Meconium aspiration in infants: A prospective study. J Pediatr 1974; 85:848.
49. Katz VL, Bowes WA Jr: Meconium aspiration syndrome: Reflections on a murky subject. Am J Obstet Gynecol 1992; 166:171.
50. Sessler D, Mills P, Gregory GA, et al: Effects of bicarbonate on arterial and brain intracellular pH in neonatal rabbits recovering from hypoxic lactic acidosis. J Pediatr 1987; 111:817.
51. Welsh FA, Sims RE, McKee AE: Effect of glucose on recovery of energy metabolism following hypoxia-oligemia in mouse brain: Dose-dependence and carbohydrate specificity. J Cereb Blood Flow Metab 1983; 3:486.
52. Gardiner M, Smith ML, Kagstrom E, et al: Influence of blood glucose concentration on brain lactate accumulation during severe hypoxia and subsequent recovery of brain energy metabolism. J Cereb Blood Flow Metab 1982; 2:429.
53. Ginsberg MD, Welsh FA, Budd WA: Deleterious effect of glucose pretreatment on recovery from diffuse cerebral ischemia in the cat. Stroke 1980; 11:347.
54. Sheldon RA, Partridge JC, Ferriero DM: Postischemic hyperglycemia is not protective to the neonatal rat brain. Pediatr Res 1992; 32:489.
55. Perez CA, Reimer JM, Schreiber MD, et al: Effect of high dose dopamine on urine output in newborn infants. Crit Care Med 1986; 14:1045.
56. Versmold HT, Kitterman JA, Phibbs RH, et al: Aortic blood pressure during the last 12 hours of life in infants with birth weight 610–4,200 grams. Pediatrics 1981; 67:607.
57. Lou HC, Lassen NA, Friis-Hansen B: Impaired autoregulation of cerebral blood flow in the distressed newborn infant. J Pediatr 1979; 94:118.
58. Lou HC, Lassen NA, Friis-Hansen B: Is arterial hypertension crucial for the development of cerebral hemorrhage in premature infants? Lancet 1979; i:1215.
59. Del TJ, Louis PT, Goddard FJ: Cerebrovascular regulation and neonatal brain injury. Pediatr Neurol 1991; 7:3.
60. Lou HC, Lassen NAS, Tweed WA, et al: Pressure passive cerebral blood flow and breakdown of the blood-brain barrier in experimental fetal asphyxia. Acta Pediatr Scand 1979; 68:57.
61. Burchfield DJ, Berkowitz ID, Berg RA, et al: Medications in neonatal resuscitation. Ann Emerg Med 1993; 22:435.

4

Exsanguination

Juan A. Asensio, MD, FACS • David Hanpeter, MD
Hugo Gomez, MD • Santiago Chahwan, MD
Sebastian Orduna, MD • Lisa McDuffie, MD

Yo quiero cuando me muera
sin patria pero sin amo
tener en mi tumba un ramo
de flores y una bandera.

It is my wish that upon my death
without a country but without a master
to have in my tombstone
some flowers and my beloved flag.

JOSE MARTÍ
Cuban poet and author

For many years, trauma surgeons have struggled with the concept of shock. Numerous definitions have been recorded in the literature. These definitions have ranged from simple descriptions of the clinical process to very elaborate observations made of the changes occurring at the cellular and subcellular level. Exsanguination as an entity is certainly feared but is not foreign to, trauma surgeons. The increase in violence in our society as well as the improvement of Emergency Medical Systems (EMS) now consistently allows for the rapid transport of many patients who otherwise would not have survived to reach a trauma center.[1]

Exsanguination as an entity awaits a better definition, not only as a clinical syndrome but also physiologically and biochemically. Anderson[2] has defined an exsanguinating patient as one who is "losing his entire blood volume in minutes." Trunkey[3] describes major hemorrhage within the context of flow, defining severe hemorrhage as one with rates of blood loss that surpass 150 mL/min. The American College of Surgeons Advanced Trauma Life Support Manual[4] indirectly defines exsanguination as the clinical presentation of hemorrhagic shock in patients who have lost 40% or more of their blood volume. There is no doubt that these attempts at definition clearly signal a critical situation; however, by no means is any one of these definitions complete.

Asensio[1, 5] has defined what is viewed as the worst manifestation of shock as a physiologic entity, namely the syndrome of exsanguination.

Exsanguination is the most extreme form of hemorrhage. It is usually caused by injuries to major components of the cardiovascular system, injuries to parenchymatous organs, or both. It is a hemorrhage in which there is an initial loss of 40% of the patient's blood volume with a rate of blood loss . . . exceeding 250 mL per minute. If this hemorrhage is not controlled, the patient may lose one half of his or her entire blood volume in 10 minutes.

Other injuries that may cause exsanguination are major and complex pelvic fractures as well as thoracoabdominal injuries.

Thus, exsanguination implies a rate of blood loss that clearly cannot be replaced by ordinary resuscitative measures. It mandates immediate lifesaving surgical intervention.[1, 5] An exsanguinating patient is one who will tax the most experienced trauma surgeon as well as the busiest of trauma centers. Using this proposed definition, this chapter identifies injuries prone to exsanguination and provides guidelines for the resuscitation and management of patients with this syndrome.

INCIDENCE

Little information exists that defines the true incidence of exsanguination in the literature. Even fewer data are available regarding the different injuries that are prone to cause this syndrome. The incidence of exsanguination can be estimated by analysis of multiple factors, which include the following:

- Percentage of patients arriving in the emergency department fulfilling the criteria of Advanced Trauma Life Support (ATLS)[4] Class IV Shock
- Number of units of blood transfused
- Volume of crystalloid solutions required for resuscitation
- Specific organs injured
- Intraoperative blood loss
- Early mortality rate

The incidence can also be estimated from carefully performed autopsy studies. According to Trunkey and Blaisdell,[6] up to one half of civilian trauma deaths occur from exsanguination or a disruption of the central nervous system (CNS) within 1 hour of injury. Within 2 or 3 hours after the initial injury, 30% or more civilian trauma deaths occur from major internal hemorrhage. Injuries caused by military style weapons, such as automatic rifles with high-muzzle-velocity energy, as well as close-range shotgun injuries are well known to result in exsanguination.[7] Similarly, major blunt thoracoabdominal trauma resulting in rupture of the liver is also classically known to produce this entity.

Civilian autopsy studies have identified the two leading causes of death in trauma patients. Baker and colleagues,[8] reviewing 437 autopsied trauma deaths in a 5-year period, reported a 31.2% mortality rate due to exsanguination. In this series, nearly all patients (92%) dying of penetrating injuries succumbed within the first 2 days. CNS injuries in this study were the leading cause of death and accounted for 50.1% of the mortality rate. These findings are also validated in a study by Trunkey and Lim.[9] In their autopsy study, exsanguination accounted for 35% of the deaths; similarly, CNS injury accounted for 44.9%. Both studies implicated injuries to the heart, aorta, major blood vessels, and liver as the organs most responsible for causing exsanguination.

An analysis of military data from the Vietnam Conflict reached similar conclusions in identifying causes of death in combat casualties. Of 43,601 combat deaths experienced by military personnel in Vietnam from January 21, 1961, to December 31, 1975, 88% were revealed to be casualties in action.[10] Bellamy[11] calculated that 50% of the combat personnel deaths incurred in the battlefield were due to rapid hemorrhage. Similarly, in reviewing the casualties suffered by those admitted to military hospitals, Arnold and Cutting[12] found CNS injury to be the most common cause of hospital deaths (42%), with hemorrhagic shock and exsanguination accounting for 24%.

TABLE 4–1. Organs and Organ Systems with a High Incidence of Exsanguination

Heart	Venous system
Thoracic vascular system	Inferior vena cava
Abdominal vascular system	Portal vein
Arterial system	Liver
Abdominal aorta	
Superior mesenteric artery	

From Asensio JA: Exsanguination from penetrating injuries. Trauma Q 1990; 6:1–25.

INJURIES PRONE TO EXSANGUINATION

Several organ and organ system injuries have been associated with high early mortality, most of which are directly ascribable to exsanguination. Well-known organs and organ systems associated with a high incidence of exsanguination include the heart, both the thoracic and abdominal vascular systems, and the liver (Table 4–1).[1, 5] Individual injuries to components of the thoracic and abdominal vascular system can be subdivided into the arterial and venous systems. Of the arterial system, the most notorious injuries causing exsanguination include the thoracic aorta and its major branches, the abdominal aorta, and the superior mesenteric artery. In the venous system, the inferior vena cava, in all of its anatomic locations, and the portal vein show the highest incidence of exsanguination.[1, 5]

Until recently, few data existed describing the incidence of exsanguination caused by injuries to these organs and organ systems. In an extensive review of the literature, Asensio[1, 5] generated data describing the incidence of exsanguination for these various injuries (Tables 4–2 to 4–7). The incidence is highest for injuries to the abdominal aorta, in both suprarenal and infrarenal locations. Exsanguination accounts for 52% of all mortalities secondary to these injuries.

In a review of the literature, 7454 cases of hepatic injuries were collected and analyzed. In this group were a total of 940 deaths, with an overall mortality of 12.6%. Exsanguination accounted for 503 of the 940 deaths and was responsible for 54% of all deaths from hepatic injuries (Table 4–8). Exsanguination is clearly the major cause of death for these injuries. The overall incidence of exsanguination in hepatic injuries is 7%.[1, 5]

TABLE 4–2. Incidence of Exsanguination in Penetrating and Blunt Cardiac Trauma*

First Author	Year	No. of Patients	No. of Patients Exsanguinated	Incidence of Exsanguination (%)
Bolanowski	1973	44	9	20.45
Mattox	1974†	106	22	20.75
Beach	1975	34	3	8.82
Evans	1979	46	5	10.86
Baker	1980†	168	40	23.80
TOTAL		398	79	

From Asensio JA: Exsanguination from penetrating injuries: Trauma Q 1990; 6:1–25.
*Average combined incidence, 19.84%.
†Includes blunt trauma cases.

TABLE 4–3. Incidence of Exsanguination in Penetrating Abdominal Aortic Injuries (Suprarenal and Infrarenal Aorta)*

First Author	Year	No. of Patients	No. of Patients Exsanguinated	Incidence of Exsanguination (%)
Lim	1974	30	15	50.00
Mattox	1975	28	16	57.14
Buchness	1976	5	0	0.0
Myles	1979	24	13	54.16
Brinton	1982	13	3	23.07
Millikan	1985	23	11	47.80
Accola	1987	79	51	64.55
TOTAL		202	109	

From Asensio JA: Exsanguination from penetrating injuries. Trauma Q 1990; 6:1–25.
*Average combined incidence, 53.96%.

TABLE 4–4. Incidence of Exsanguination in Penetrating Trauma to the Superior Mesenteric Artery*

First Author	Year	No. of Patients	No. of Patients Exsanguinated	Incidence of Exsanguination (%)
Perdue	1968	4	0	0.0
Fullen	1972	9	1	12.50
Graham	1978	45	12	26.60
Lucas	1981	13	3	38.46
Kashuk	1982	6	1	16.66
TOTAL		76	19	

From Asensio JA: Exsanguination from penetrating injuries. Trauma Q 1990; 6:1–25.
*Average combined incidence, 25%.

TABLE 4–5. Incidence of Exsanguination in Trauma to the Inferior Vena Cava (Penetrating and Blunt)*

First Author	Year	No. of Patients	No. of Patients Exsanguinated	Incidence of Exsanguination (%)
Turpin	1977	34	15	83.0
Graham	1973	301	91	30.0
Cohen	1980	15	2	13.3
Kudsk	1984	70	30	42.8
TOTAL		420	138	

From Asensio JA: Exsanguination from penetrating injuries. Trauma Q 1990; 6:1–25.
*Average combined incidence, 32.85%.

TABLE5 4–6. Incidence of Exsanguination in Trauma to the Portal Vein (Penetrating and Blunt)*

First Author	Year	No. of Patients	No. of Patients Exsanguinated	Incidence of Exsanguination (%)
Mattox	1974	22	9	40.90
Busuttil	1979	10	2	20.00
Petersen	1979	28	8	28.57
Stone	1982	41	10	24.39
TOTAL		101	29	

From Asensio JA: Exsanguination from penetrating injuries. Trauma Q 1990; 6:1–25.
*Average combined incidence, 28.71%.

TABLE 4–7. Overall Incidence of Exsanguination in Hepatic Trauma (Penetrating and Blunt)*

First Author	Year	No. of Patients	No. of Patients Exsanguinated	Incidence of Exsanguination (%)
Lim	1972	285	29	10.17
Trunkey	1974	811	55	6.78
Defore	1976	1,590	122	7.67
Lucas	1976	637	37	5.80
McInnis	1977	233	8	3.43
Flint	1977	178	2	1.12
Walt	1978	1,404	112	7.97
Levin	1978	546	19	3.48
Elerding	1979	225	15	6.66
Carmona	1982	443	19	4.29
Bluett	1983	102	3	2.94
Feliciano	1986	1,000	82	8.20
TOTAL		7,454	503	

From Asensio JA: Exsanguination from penetrating injuries. Trauma Q 1990; 6:1-25.
*Average combined incidence, 6.75%.

MANAGEMENT

The management of exsanguination requires quick thinking, leadership, and prompt operative intervention to achieve favorable outcomes. Because the rate of blood loss is extremely massive, immediate lifesaving surgical intervention yields the best opportunity to save the patient. Basic resuscitative maneuvers, including rapid restoration of the lost blood volume as well as prompt and effective control of hemorrhage, are of the utmost importance.[4] Figure 4-1 is a flow chart that we currently use in the management of the exsanguinating trauma patient.[1, 5]

Venous Access

Securing venous access is imperative; the presence of profound hypovolemic shock and massive systemic vasoconstriction possesses a challenging problem. Although placement of a minimum of two large-bore intravenous lines in the upper extremities is desirable, severe vasoconstriction often makes this impossible and alternate routes of venous access (e.g., subclavian, internal jugular, and femoral veins) must thus be considered.

In an exsanguinating hemorrhage, even central veins can collapse. Despite their constant anatomy, little guarantee exists that they can be cannulated under adverse hemodynamic states; one must be aware of the increased risk in placing central lines in subclavian veins and jugular veins. Well-known complications of venous access, such as inadvertent arterial cannulation, pneumothorax, hemothorax, air emboli, and inadvertent placement of these catheters within the thoracic cavity, causing hydrothorax, may occur; given the critical status of these patients, these complications may not be noticed immediately and may jeopardize outcome.

Currently, percutaneous cannulation of the femoral vein as a central line is our route of choice. Lines in the upper extremity are preferred if injury to the major abdominal venous system is suspected. Posner and coworkers[13] attempted to define the natural history of untreated inferior vena caval perforations in an animal model and to evaluate the efficacy of venous access with such injuries. They concluded that lower-extremity venous access in the presence of contained retroperitoneal hematomas from inferior vena caval injuries is both safe and efficacious. These authors suggested that this may also be true for humans with similar types of injuries, but they caution that it is dangerous to extrapolate animal model results to acutely injured patients. Usually, only patients with contained retroperitoneal hematomas survive to reach the hospital alive; however, it must be assumed that most retroperitoneal hematomas occurring from major abdominal vascular

TABLE 4–8. Exsanguination as a Factor in the Mortality of Hepatic Trauma (Penetrating and Blunt)

First Author	Year	No. of Patients	No. of Deaths	Overall Mortality (%)	No. of Patients Exsanguinated	Percentage Exsanguination Accounting Mortality
Lim	1972	285	52	18.8	29	55.7
Trunkey	1974	811	106	13.0	55	51.9
Defore	1976	1,590	209	13.0	122	58.0
Lucas	1976	637	95	15.0	37	39.0
McInnis	1977	233	26	11.2	8	30.7
Flint	1977	178	36	20.0	2	5.5
Walt	1978	1,404	179	13.0	112	62.5
Levin	1978	546	55	10.0	19	43.0
Elerding	1979	225	34	15.0	15	54.0
Carmona	1982	443	40	9.0	19	47.5
Bluett	1983	102	3	2.9	3	100.0
Feliciano	1986	1,000	105	10.5	82	78.0
TOTAL		7,454	940	12.6	503	54.0

From Asensio JA: Exsanguination from penetrating injuries. Trauma Q 1990; 6:1-25.

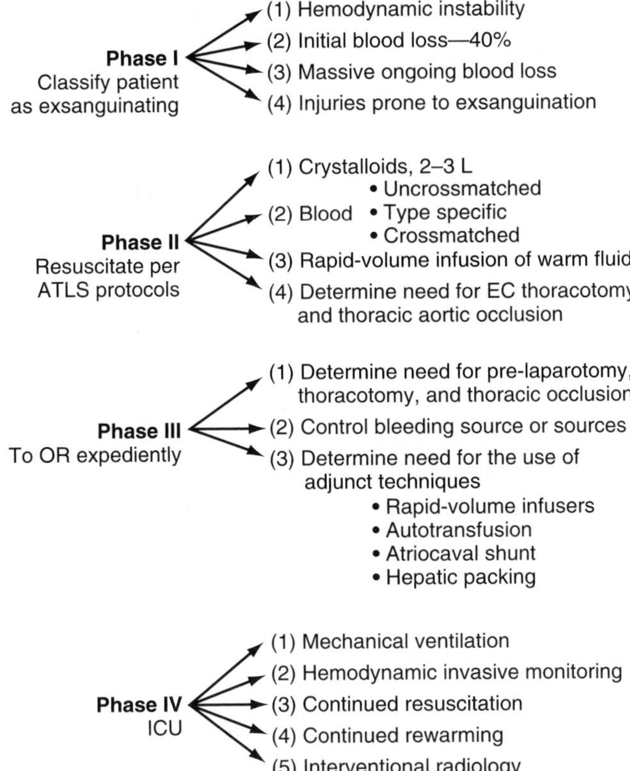
Phase I
Classify patient as exsanguinating
(1) Hemodynamic instability
(2) Initial blood loss—40%
(3) Massive ongoing blood loss
(4) Injuries prone to exsanguination
Phase II
Resuscitate per ATLS protocols
(1) Crystalloids, 2–3 L
(2) Blood • Uncrossmatched • Type specific • Crossmatched
(3) Rapid-volume infusion of warm fluids
(4) Determine need for EC thoracotomy and thoracic aortic occlusion
Phase III
To OR expediently
(1) Determine need for pre-laparotomy, thoracotomy, and thoracic occlusion
(2) Control bleeding source or sources
(3) Determine need for the use of adjunct techniques
• Rapid-volume infusers
• Autotransfusion
• Atriocaval shunt
• Hepatic packing
Phase IV
ICU
(1) Mechanical ventilation
(2) Hemodynamic invasive monitoring
(3) Continued resuscitation
(4) Continued rewarming
(5) Interventional radiology

Figure 4–1. Flow chart for the management of exsanguination. OR = operating room; ATLS = Advanced Trauma Life Support; EC = external carotid (artery); ICU = intensive care unit. (Modified from Asensio JA: Evolving issues in emergency medical serices and trauma. Exsanguination Emerg Care 1991; 7:59–75.)

injuries are no longer contained. Consequently, lower-extremity venous access may not be the method of choice for rapid intravascular volume replacement.

Variables controlling flow rates of fluids infused in exsanguinating patients include (1) catheter size and length, (2) tubing size, (3) fluid type, and (4) method of administration. Dula and coworkers[14] evaluated flow rates in intravenous catheters of different bores with different fluids: crystalloids, packed red blood cells, whole blood, and albumin. They also evaluated different methods of administration including gravity, blood pump, pressure infusion cuff, and manual push with a 50-mL syringe. They confirmed that the larger the cross-sectional area and the shorter the length of the catheter, the greater the flow. Also, flow rates were slowest when flow was administered by gravity, and flow rates were best with the addition of a pressure infusion cuff. Furthermore, whole blood demonstrated greater flow rates for any tubing size and by any infusion method compared with packed red blood cells. With the addition of a pressure infusion cuff, flow rates with both whole blood and packed red blood cells increased significantly.

Millikan and coworkers[15] studied flow rates of crystalloids and whole blood through various of intravenous (IV) catheters and tubing systems and determined that the 10-gauge IV catheter and that the No. 8 French (Fr.) pulmonary artery catheter introducer provided flow rates equivalent to IV tubing inserted directly into the vein as a cutdown. They also determined that the addition of large-bore intravenous tubing connected to these catheters in place of standard tubing could increase flow rates of crystalloids and whole blood to a range of 1200 to 1400 mL/min. At the same time, they also found that the standard 16-gauge subclavian catheters were inefficient as means for rapid infusion of fluids.

Dutky and coworkers[16] studied rapid fluid administration through the No. 8.5 Fr. pulmonary artery catheter introducer with various fluids (e.g., crystalloids, whole blood, and diluted packed red blood cells) using tubing of different sizes. The flow rate of crystalloids through blood tubing was found to be double that of the regular IV tubing. The flow rate for trauma tubing was three times that of blood tubing. These authors also noted that warm crystalloid, reconstituted packed red blood cells could be infused almost twice as fast as cold whole blood. Their data also described the effect of kinking of the catheter introducer on flow rate; when a catheter was kinked, flow rates were halved. Therefore, placement of a large-bore catheter by itself does not guarantee high flow rates. These data were also corroborated by Zorko and Polsky.[17]

These studies were instrumental in shaping the philosophy of fluid replacement as it is practiced today. The use of large-bore catheters with a large cross sections and small lengths, the use of trauma tubing, and the use of pressure to increase flow rates are the mainstays of rapid delivery of lost intravascular blood volume. One may also achieve this effect with the use of rapid-infuser technology, which infuses fluids under pressure while simultaneously heating them.

Crystalloids

The preferred fluid for resuscitation of the exsanguinating trauma patient is Ringer's lactate.[18–21] It is well known that the intravascular space is reduced by blood loss and that the red blood cell mass is rapidly reduced by close to 50% while the plasma space is reduced by approximately 35%. The interstitial space is called on to replace intravascular volume losses.[18, 21, 22] This process is known as *transcapillary refill* and is one of the endpoints of the neurohumoral response to shock.

Shires and associates have shown that in order for the resuscitation to be successful it must replace not only the lost intravascular volume losses but also interstitial space losses.[23, 24] This is best accomplished with a balanced salt solution. Ringer's lactate is the solution of choice.[23, 24] Its average pH is 6.5, and its lactate component is metabolized to bicarbonate, which helps to neutralize the acidosis produced from hypoperfusion. Similarly, its electrolyte composition most closely resembles that of the interstitial fluid. The use of normal saline as a resuscitation fluid must take into account its average pH of 5, and the propensity of normal saline to precipitate (or produce) hyperchloremic acidosis.[23–25]

Traverso and coworkers[26] developed a rapid hemorrhage model in anesthetized swine to simulate exsanguination. Four separate crystalloid solutions were investigated to evaluate their efficacy in preventing death after an otherwise induced fatal hemorrhage. These solutions consisted of (1) normal saline, (2) Ringer's lactate, (3) Plasma-Lyte A, and (4) Plasma-Lyte R. One hundred sixteen swine were exsanguinated and their shed blood replaced with a volume equal to 300% of their shed blood with the previously described solutions. Ringer's lactate resuscitation solution produced a survival of 67%; normal saline, 50%, Plasma-Lyte R, 40%; and Plasma-Lyte A, 30%. The investigators concluded that Ringer's lactate is still the best crystalloid solution because of (1) its decreased chloride load, compared with normal saline, and (2) its absence of acetate or magnesium, compared with Plasma-Lyte solution.

Using a meta-analysis, Velanovich[27]compared results generated from eight previously published randomized clinical trials comparing the efficacy of crystalloid and colloid solutions for resuscitation. This analysis revealed a 5.7% relative difference in mortality rates in favor of crystalloid therapy. A separate analysis conducted in a subset composed of trauma patients revealed a 12.3% difference in mortality rate in favor of crystalloid therapy.

The results of all these studies lend validity to the rationale of resuscitating the exsanguinating trauma patient with Ringer's lactate solution.

Blood

The first clinical use of a blood transfusion was recorded in 1828 by Blundell.[28] Blood transfusions were used for the first time in the management of combat casualties during the American Civil War.[29] Crile[30] in 1909 reported the first recorded transfusions in trauma patients. Landsteiner[31] discovered the three basic blood groups. In 1902, Von Decastello and Sturli[32] discovered the AB blood type. In 1915, the introduction of citrate anticoagulant by Lewisohn[33] made possible the development of blood storage and blood-banking techniques.

During World War II, transfusions were used routinely by military surgeons in the management of wartime casualties. It was also during this war that the universal donor protocol was developed. Extensive experience during the Korean and Vietnam Conflicts validated its safety and efficacy.[34-39] During the Vietnam Conflict, component therapy evolved so that the universal blood type could be administered as packed red blood cells.[40] The concept of blood replacement utilizing the rule of "3 in 1"—1 mL of lost blood replaced by 3 mL of crystalloids—was developed by Pruit and coworkers in 1965. These investigators demonstrated that normal subjects who lost 25% of their blood volume could be resuscitated safely with a crystalloid volume equal to 3.5 times the amount of blood lost.[40]

Current guidelines for the management of blood replacement therapy in the trauma patient originated from evidence developed by trauma surgeons. Shackford and coworkers[41] determined that packed red blood cells, when reconstituted with crystalloid solutions, had essentially the same physiologic effect as whole blood when used as blood replacement therapy for intraoperative blood losses. Gervin and Fischer[42] reported in a 3-year study, the efficacy of type-specific, crossmatched blood. From this study, in which patients were administered type-specific, uncrossmatched blood with no transfusion reactions, the authors concluded that type-specific uncrossmatched blood provides a safe alternative in the resuscitation of exsanguinating patients.

Schwab and coworkers[43] looked at the safety and efficacy of type O blood in the immediate resuscitation of severely injured hypovolemic patients. In this study, in which 83 patients received 330 units of type O uncrossmatched blood, there were no blood grouping incompatibilities and no transfusion reactions. From these data, the authors concluded that type O blood is safe and has additional advantages over type-specific blood. These advantages include immediate availability and its universal application for all recipients.

At the Los Angeles County/University of Southern California (LAC-USC) Trauma Center, the exsanguinating male patient is resuscitated with group O, Rh-positive blood initially, and type-specific blood as soon as possible. Fully typed and cross-matched blood is administered as it becomes available, but this takes 30 minutes. In females of childbearing age, the LAC-USC Trauma Center's blood bank preferentially uses group O, Rh-negative, uncrossmatched blood in the initial resuscitation.

Several blood substitutes have been developed throughout the years. They include perfluorocarbons, bovine polymerized hemoglobin, polymerized pyridoxilated hemoglobin, encapsulated hemoglobin in liposomes, and diaspirin cross-linked hemoglobin. Many of these substitutes initially appeared to be quite promising as effective oxygen carriers, but their toxicity precludes their utilization at this time. Although perfluorocarbons have an excellent oxygen-carrying capacity, their disassociation curve is linear, in contrast to the sigmoid curve of oxyhemoglobin. This necessitates that the patient to be ventilated with high fractions of inspired oxygen (FIO_2) in order for the oxygen-carrying capabilities to be effective. This may produce deleterious pulmonary changes secondary to oxygen toxicity.

Of the blood substitutes, the most promising appears to be diaspirin cross-linked hemoglobin. Preliminary studies reveal good oxygen-carrying capacity without toxicity. Although the number of units of this product transfused has been few, no long-term studies exist to document its continued safety and efficacy.[44, 45]

ADJUNCTS IN THE MANAGEMENT OF EXSANGUINATING INJURIES

Thoracic Aortic Occlusion

Thoracic aortic occlusion was first studied experimentally by Sankaran and coworkers.[46] They focused on finding a solution for the well-known cardiovascular collapse noted in patients experiencing abdominal vascular injuries once the tamponading effect created by the elevated intra-abdominal pressure would be released during laparotomy. In porcine models, they noted that animals subjected to prelaparotomy thoracotomy after the creation of a standard wound of the abdominal aorta did not experience cardiovascular collapse. On the basis of these findings, these investigators concluded that there may be a role for thoracic aortic occlusion prior to laparotomy in patients with major abdominal vascular injury.

The findings of this study were applied to the clinical arena by Ledgerwood and coworkers.[47] Hypotensive patients harboring massive hemoperitoneum secondary to exsanguinating abdominal vascular injuries underwent thoracotomy and thoracic aortic occlusion, resulting in salvage of several patients. On the basis of their findings, these authors made a case for thoracotomy and thoracic aortic occlusion prior to laparotomy in this clinical scenario and outlined a protocol for management.

This protocol includes the following:

1. Immediate endotracheal intubation.
2. Venous access with large-bore catheters.
3. Rapid infusion of 2 to 3 L of crystalloids.
4. Immediate transport to the operating room while type-specific blood is being transfused.

If the systolic blood pressure remained at 80 mm Hg or less while the patient was being prepared, an additional 2 units of blood was administered. If the systolic blood pressure rose to 100 mm Hg, the abdomen was then opened. If the patient's systolic blood pressure remained below 100 mm Hg, thoracotomy and thoracic aortic occlusion were first performed.

Many studies outlining the deleterious effects of this technique have been published. Extensive discussion of this body of literature is beyond the scope of this chapter. The spectrum of opinion ranges from those who strongly advocate never using this technique[48] to those who use it liberally.[49] What is clear is that the indiscriminate use of this technique does not yield good outcomes.[50] The technique of thoracotomy plus aortic occlusion seems to have a well-defined role as an effective weapon in the trauma surgical armamentarium.[51]

Thoracic aortic occlusion should be reserved for patients who have (1) sustained penetrating cardiac injuries, (2) arrived with some vital signs in the trauma center,[52] and (3) sustained penetrating thoracic injuries and are in need of cardiopulmonary resuscitation. Performance of this technique in the emergency department for patients sustaining abdominal vascular injuries yield as a survival rate of 5%. This technique should be performed by qualified surgeons skilled in a management of trauma.

Much higher survival rates are obtained with this technique in patients who have survived long enough to reach the operating room. Wiencek and coworkers,[53] using strict protocol, reported a 42% survival rate in patients who underwent this procedure in the operating room and who responded with systolic blood pressure greater than 90 mm Hg. These authors developed a patient profile that would be helpful in identifying patients for whom this procedure would be of no value. This profile consists of:

- A systolic blood pressure below 70 mm Hg on admission
- Four or more associated injuries
- A shock period longer than 30 minutes
- Hemorrhage in excess of 10 units of blood

The physiologic effects of emergency thoracotomy and thoracic aortic occlusion include the following:

- Preservation and redistribution of remaining blood volume
- Improvement in coronary and carotid perfusion
- Reduction of subdiaphragmatic blood loss
- An increase in left ventricular stroke work index
- Improved myocardial contractility

However, there are some deleterious effects. Blood flow to abdominal viscera and kidneys is reduced to approximately 10%, as is the blood flow to the spinal cord. The procedure induces anaerobic metabolism, hypoxia, and lactic acidosis and imposes a tremendous afterload on an already compromised left ventricle.

Little information is available regarding the length of safety for aortic cross-clamping time. One of us (JAA) has noted that greater survival rates are observed if the aortic cross-clamp can be removed in less than 15 minutes. If the aortic clamp remains in place for more than 15 to 30 minutes, most of these patients do not survive. If they do survive, they experience a significant incidence of multiple systems organ failure. This author (JAA) has treated one survivor in whom the aortic clamp remained in place for 90 minutes.

Rapid Infusers

Rapid restoration of lost blood volume is key in determining survival of the exsanguinating patient. Blood replacement must surpass the rate of ongoing blood loss. In the exsanguinating patient, the necessity of restoring lost blood volume is often hampered by the high viscosity and cold temperature of the transfused blood.[1, 5] Ideally, the characteristics of a rapid-infusion system should include[1, 5]:

1. The ability to deliver large volumes of both crystalloid and blood at rates that surpass the rate of losses.
2. The ability to overcome the high-viscosity characteristics of blood to increase its flow rate while preserving the integrity of the infused red blood cell mass.
3. The ability to warm the administered solutions to prevent hypothermia while at the same time preventing protein denaturation.

Currently, three rapid-infuser systems are on the market: the Rapid Infusion System (Haemonetics Corporation, Braintree, Mass.), the Bard 37 (CR Bard, Inc., Billerica, Mass.), and the Level I fluid warmer (Level I technologies, Inc., Plymouth, Mass.). These units can infuse between 1000 and 2200 mL of warm crystalloid solutions and 500 mL of packed red blood cells per minute.[54]

Although no data exist to demonstrate an improvement in survival in trauma patients when rapid-infuser techniques are employed, studies have proved that the technology is safe and serves as a useful adjunct in the management of exsanguinating patients by means of rapid transfusion and prevention of the development of hypothermia and its deleterious sequelae.[55-57] The policy of LAC-USC is to use rapid-infuser technology extensively in all patients needing significant blood volume replacement. This technology is used in the trauma center resuscitation area, the operating room, and the surgical intensive care unit (ICU).

Autotransfusion

Experimental autotransfusion was first described in 1818 by Blundell.[58] In 1886, Duncan[59] first used it in human subjects. The first successful infusion of collected blood from hemothoraces during World War I was reported by Henry and Elliot.[60] Brown and Debenheim[61] reported on autotransfusion in the management of civilian hemothoraces. Griswold and Ostner[62] instituted autotransfusion in patients sustaining abdominal trauma. Klebanoff[63, 64] devised a modification of the cardiotomy reservoir, which resulted in the first commercial system, called the Bentley autotransfusion system (Bentley Laboratories, Irvine, Calif.).

Autotransfusion can be used in elective vascular and cardiac surgical procedures. Von Koch and coworkers[65] reported their experience in 1977 with autotransfusion from collected hemothoraces with a Sorensen devise (Sorensen Research Co., Salt Lake City). Indications for autotransfusion in the trauma patient include injuries to the heart as well as the major thoracic and abdominal blood vessels. This technique has also been utilized for injuries involving solid organs, such as the liver and spleen. Autotransfusion is contraindicated in the presence of associated gastrointestinal injuries accompanied by massive contamination.

Some advantages of autotransfusion over banked blood include the avoidance of the risk of transmission of hepatitis and acquired immunodeficiency syndrome (AIDS), blood type incompatibility, and allergic and immune reactions. Autotransfusion results in red blood cells with higher levels of 2,3-DPG and higher resistance to osmotic stress. The hematocrit value in the prepared units for autotransfusion ranges between 60% and 65%.[1, 5] The autotransfusion process removes the free red blood cell stroma, plasma free hemoglobin, anticoagulants, activated clotting factors, and platelets.

Complications include the risk of anticoagulation, prolongation of the prothrombin (PT) and partial thromboplastin times (PTT), and hypofibrinogenemia. These potential complications become important issues in exsanguinating patients.

Despite the attractiveness of the concept, autotransfusion has not assumed a very prominent role in the management of trauma patients. Several studies have determined that autotransfusion, although a valuable adjunct technique, cannot replace the blood bank but can supplement it.[66, 67] Furthermore, the practical applications of instituting a protocol, in addition to the issues of contamination, have limited the role of autotransfusion to shed blood from chest tubes utilizing the Sorensen device.

Atriocaval Shunting

The use of the atriocaval shunt can be a valuable adjunct to the management of exsanguinating injuries from the liver. Most of these injuries involved the retrohepatic vena cava, major hepatic veins, portal vein, or combinations of these structures. The shunt was originally described by Shrock and associates in 1968[68] after extensive studies in the animal laboratory revealed that few vessels drained into the suprarenal vena cava and could be bypassed. The first successful use of this shunt was reported by Bricker and Wukasch in 1970.[69]

The technique for insertion of an atriocaval shunt is complex and time-consuming. The shunt should be considered if the performance of a Pringle maneuver fails to control hepatic bleeding. Often, this device is used very late in the intraoperative course, when the patient is already hypothermic and coagulopathic. As a technique, it is used in less than 5% of all major hepatic injuries.[70-72] The mortality rate of patients undergoing shunting ranges from 55% to 81%.[73-75]

Many trauma surgeons have become disenchanted with the use of the atriocaval shunt, preferring instead to follow a direct approach to the retrohepatic cava and major hepatic veins, as advocated by Pachter and colleagues.[76, 77] This approach employs rapid-finger fracturing of the hepatic parenchyma on Cantlie's line, which defines the major intralobar fissure separating the right and left hepatic lobes and is devoid of major vascular structures.

Hepatic Packing

Pringle[78] first described packing as an adjunct in the management of hepatic injuries. Hepatic packing remained the mainstay of treatment for all hepatic injuries from the turn of the 20th century until World War II. At that time, improved operative methods resulted in a marked reduction in mortality. During World War II, the use of packing was condemned, given the high incidence of intra-abdominal sepsis associated with its use. In 1981, hepatic packing was brought back as a valuable adjunct in the management of hepatic hemorrhage. Feliciano and coworkers[79] reported a series of 465 patients sustaining hepatic injuries, 10 of whom underwent packing (2.2%), with a mortality rate of 10%. On the basis of these data, they concluded that the pack should be utilized as a valuable adjunct with specific indications.

The currently accepted indications for the use of hepatic packing include injuries with hemorrhage not amenable to control by any other means. Packing must be performed before severe hypothermia, coagulopathy, or acidosis develops, and it must not be used in desperation before major arterial and venous structures are controlled.[79, 80]

In general, the use of hepatic packing is limited to approximately 5% of all hepatic injuries. Data from six series were reviewed.[79-84] Among 3448 patients, 162 (4.7%) required hepatic packing for control of exsanguinating hemorrhage; 93 patients (57.4%) did not survive.[79-84]

Angioembolization

During the 1990s, interventional radiology has developed rapidly. The immediate use of angioembolization for the management of major pelvic hemorrhage has been extrapolated to serve as an adjunct in the management of major hepatic injuries. The protocol used at the LAC-USC Trauma Center for dealing with major hepatic injuries includes rapid surgical intervention to control major arterial and venous bleeding, extensive use of hepatotomy and hepatorrhaphy, the use of the argon beam coagulator, and immediate hepatic packing. The patient is then transferred to the interventional radiology suite for angioembolization and subsequently brought to the surgical ICU for continued resuscitation, hemodynamic invasive monitoring, and continued warming. Further operative interventions are carried out to remove packs and to debride as soon as the patient's status is improved.[85]

CRITICAL CARE MANAGEMENT OF THE SURVIVING EXSANGUINATING PATIENT

ICU Treatment

Patients who have survived exsanguinating hemorrhage are usually admitted to the surgical ICU with severe hemodynamic instability. Many are in need of continuing resuscitation. Most are hypothermic, acidotic, and coagulopathic. They are intubated and ventilated, and many make the trip from the operating room with the help of vasopressors. In summary, this is a very critical patient population, manifesting the sequelae of profound shock. Many will have already embarked on the road toward the development of the multiple systems organ failure (MSOF) syndrome.

The hemodynamic instability exhibited by these patients is multifactorial. The fact that they survived a complex lifesaving surgical procedure does not mean that the cycle of hypothermia, coagulopathy, acidosis, and dysrhythmias has been totally interrupted. These patients need invasive hemodynamic monitoring, correction of hypothermia, restoration of intravascular volume, correction of acidosis, and restoration of tissue perfusion as lifesaving measures.

The LAC-USC protocol mandates the following:

1. Immediate implementation of invasive hemodynamic monitoring.
2. Correction of hypothermia by the utilization of warm crystalloids.
3. Blood and blood products via rapid infuser technology.

The patient is covered with a warm air mattress, and routine measurements of the following are obtained:

1. All pulmonary artery catheter–related parameters.
2. Arterial and mixed venous blood gases.
3. Blood chemistry profiles.
4. Serial monitoring of lactic acid levels coupled with hematologic measurements, including complete blood count, platelet count, and coagulation parameters inclusive of fibrinogen levels.

Patients must be monitored for the development of complications with late manifestations, such as the delayed presentation of iatrogenic pneumothorax incurred by multiple attempts at placement of central lines. This complication may not manifest immediately, however; it can present as the patient is placed on positive-pressure ventilation with increasing levels of positive end-expiratory pressure (PEEP). Similarly, the development of the abdominal compartment syndrome can occur secondary to the rapid expansion of the third space. This can cause massive visceral edema. Routine intra-abdominal pressures are monitored to identify this syndrome early. Finally, all patients are closely monitored for the possibility of a missed bleeding source, which may necessitate a return trip to the operating room.

Post-traumatic Hypothermia

Hypothermia is defined as a core temperature below 35°C. It can be divided into mild (32° to 35°C), moderate (30° to 32°C) and severe (<30°C). The multifactorial causes for the development of hypothermia in the exsanguinating trauma patient include:

1. Exposure to cold environments in the resuscitating area and operating room.
2. Volume replacement with crystalloids stored at room temperatures.
3. Banked blood stored at 4°C.

4. Having more than one body cavity exposed simultaneously.
5. Massive blood losses.

The multiple deleterious effects of hypothermia include decreases in cardiac output, depression of myocardial contractility and increased susceptibility to dysrhythmias, decreased alveolar ventilation, pulmonary edema, renal dysfunction, and cold diuresis coupled with ischemia to the gastrointestinal tract and impaired platelet function. Given the deleterious effects of hypothermia, its prevention demands the highest priority in the management of the exsanguinating patient. Prevention commences in the emergency department, where all patients must be covered with warm blankets. Patients must be transfused with warm crystalloid solutions and blood. The use of rapid-infuser technology is strongly recommended starting in the emergency department and continued throughout the patient's stay in the operating room and surgical ICU.

In the operating room, the lower extremities must be wrapped; the patient is placed on an electric blanket on the operating table and a warm air mattress should cover much of the exposed surface of the patient's body. The temperature of the ventilator cascade must be increased to 42°C. Periodically irrigating exposed cavities with warm saline and maintaining an operating room temperature at 29°C (85°F) are some of the measures undertaken to prevent hypothermia. Success is clearly related to rapid surgical control of the exsanguinating hemorrhage and rapid restoration of the lost intravascular blood volume with warm crystalloids and blood.[1, 5]

Luna and coworkers[86] studied 94 intubated trauma patients to determine the incidence and risk factors for hypothermia. The temperature in the massively transfused patients fluctuated between 32.4° and 33.9°C. The authors concluded that hypothermia is common among severely injured patients and identified risk factors such as alcohol and advanced age.

Jurkovich and coworkers[87] studied the impact of hypothermia on outcome in 71 adult trauma patients and correlated mortality with cold temperature. Of those patients with core temperatures below 34°C, 44% died. In those with temperatures below 33°C, 69% died. No survivors were found in these series when core temperatures were below 32°C.

Coagulopathies and Complications of Massive Transfusion

Massive transfusion is defined as transfusion needs exceeding 10 units of whole blood or packed red blood cells in 24 hours.[88] Massive transfusion carries numerous complications, including dilutional thrombocytopenia,[89] which is directly proportional to the number of units of blood transfused and immunosuppression. Other well-known complications of massive transfusion include hyperkalemia, which occurs in approximately 7% of patients receiving more than 10 units of blood.[90] The presence of hyperkalemia can compound dysrhythmias caused by hypothermia; however, hypokalemia occurs with greater frequency and is present in 53.6% of patients who have undergone massive transfusion.[91]

Hypocalcemia usually takes place when transfusion rates exceed 100 mL/min and is related to increased plasma citrate concentrations associated with large transfusions of stored blood.[92] Hypocalcemia and citrate toxicity occur in the settings of hypothermia and impaired hepatic function from decreased perfusion. Hypomagnesemia is also frequently seen after massive transfusion.

The concentration of coagulation factors is known to decrease during cold blood storage. The factors most seriously impaired are factors V and VIII, whose concentrations drop precipitously; the activity of factors I, II, and VII also decreases significantly. Fresh frozen plasma and platelet transfusions are optimized when the patient's core temperature reaches 34°C because the activity of both factors and platelets is improved.[88, 93, 94] Similarly, replacement of fibrinogen must be considered because the activity and concentration of this factor falls drastically.

Our guidelines call for the transfusion of fresh frozen plasma after the first 10 units of packed red blood cells. We use a formula of 30 mL/kg and transfuse until PT and PTT are normalized. Similarly, we transfuse platelets after 10 units of packed red blood cells have been administered. Cryoprecipitate is also transfused intraoperatively in exsanguinating patients, but objective measurements should be obtained to guide replacement whenever possible. If the measured fibrinogen level is less than 100 mg/dL, cryoprecipitate must be administered.

SUMMARY

Exsanguination is an ill-defined but extremely dramatic syndrome. Its management requires prompt thinking and aggressive surgical intervention within the context of the well-thought-out management plan. This plan should have as its ultimate goal rapid and definitive control of the exsanguinating bleeding source or sources.

References

1. Asensio JA: Exsanguination from penetrating injuries. Trauma Q 1990; 6:1–25.
2. Anderson KA: Pre-hospital care in traumatically induced hemorrhage and exsanguination. J Emerg Nurs 1984; 10:141.
3. Trunkey DD: Trauma. Sci Am 1983; 249:28–35.
4. Committee on Trauma, American College of Surgeons: Advance Trauma Life Support Instructor Manual. Chicago, American College of Surgeons,1993.
5. Asensio JA, Ierardi R: Exsanguination. Emerg Care Q 1991; 7:59–75.
6. Trunkey DD, Blaisdell FW (Eds). Abdominal Trauma: Trauma Management, vol 1. New York, Thieme and Stratton, 1982.
7. Sherman RT, Parrish RA: Management of shotgun injuries. J Trauma 1963; 3:76.
8. Baker CC, Oppenheimer L, Stephens V, et al: Epidemiology of trauma deaths. Am J Surg 1980; 140:144–150.
9. Trunkey DD, Lim RC: Analysis of 425 consecutive trauma fatalities: An autopsy study. J Am Coll Emerg Physician 1974; (November/December):368–371.
10. Department of Defense, Office Adjutant Defense Service (Comptroller), Directorate of Information, Operations, and Control: Table 1051. Number of Casualties Incurred by USA Military Personnel in Connection with the Conflict in Vietnam: Cumulative from 1 January 1961 Through 31 December 1975. January 1976.
11. Bellamy RF: The causes of death in conventional land warfare: Implications for combat casualty care research. Mil Med 1984; 149:55–62.
12. Arnold K, Cutting RT: Cases of death in United States military personnel in Vietnam. Mil Med 1978; 143:161–164.
13. Posner MC, Moore EE, Greenholz SK, et al: Natural history of untreated inferior vena cava injury and assessment of venous access. J Trauma 1986; 26:698–701.
14. Dula DJ, Muller HA, Donovan JW: Flow rate variance of commonly used IV infusion techniques. J Trauma 1981; 21:480–482
15. Millikan JS, Cain LT, Hansbrough J: Rapid volume replacement for hypovolemic shock: A comparison of techniques and equipment. J Trauma 1984; 24:428–431
16. Dutky PA, Stevens SL, Maull KI: Factors affecting rapid fluid resuscitation with large bore introducer catheters. J Trauma 1989; 29:856–860.
17. Zorko MF, Polsky SS: Rapid warming and infusion of packed red blood cells. Ann Emerg Med 1986; 15:907–910.
18. Carey LD, Lowery BD, Cloutier CT: Hemorrhagic shock. Curr Prob Surg 1971; 8:1048.

19. Gerrick SJ, Ledgerwood AM, Lucas CE: Post-resuscitative hypertension: A reappraisal. Arch Surg 1980; 115:1486.
20. Lobett WM, Wangensteen SL, Glenn TM, et al: Presence of myocardial depressant factor in patients with circulatory shock. Surgery 1981; 70:223.
21. Lucas CE, Ledgerwood AM: The fluid problem in the critically ill: Symposium on critical illness. Surg Clin North Am 1993; 63:439–454.
22. Lucas CE, Benishek DJ, Ledgerwood AM: A proposed mechanism for reduced pressure after shock. Arch Surg 1982; 117:675–679.
23. Shires GT, Carrico CJ, Canizard PC: Major Problems in Clinical Surgery, Vol 13. Philadelphia, WB Saunders, 1973.
24. Shires GT, Canizard PC: Fluid resuscitation in the severely injured. Surg Clin North Am 1973; 53:1341–1366.
25. Asensio JA, Barton JM, Wonsetler LA, et al: Trauma: A systematic approach to management. Am Fam Physician 1988; 38:97–112.
26. Traverso LW, Lee WP, Langford MJ: Fluid resuscitation after an otherwise fatal hemorrhage: I. Crystalloids solutions. J Trauma 1986; 26:168–175.
27. Velanovich V: Crystalloid versus colloid fluid resuscitation: A meta-analysis of mortality. Surgery 1989; 105:65–71.
28. Blundell J: Successful case of transfusion. Lancet 1828; 1:431.
29. Kuhns WJ: Blood transfusion in the civil war. Transfusion 1965; 5:92.
30. Crile GW: Hemorrhage and transfusion: Experimental and Clinical Research. New York, Appleton, 1909.
31. Landsteiner K: Zur Kenntnis der antifermentativen, lystichen and agglutinierenden Wirkungen des Blut. Zentralbl Bakteriol 1900; 27:357.
32. Von Descastello A, Sturli A: Uber die Isoagglutinive in Serum gesunder und kranker Menschen. Munch Med Wochenschr 1902; 26:1090.
33. Lewishon R: Blood transfusion by the citrate method. Surg Gynecol Obstet 1915; 21:37.
34. Barnes A: Status of the use of universal donor blood transfusions. Clin Lab Sci 1973; 4:147–160.
35. Crosby WH: The safety of blood transfusion in treatment of mass casualties. Mil Med 1955; 117:354.
36. Barnes A: Status of the use of universal donor blood transfusion. CRC Crit Rev Clin Lab Sci 1973; 4:147–160.
37. Barnes A: Transfusion of universal donor and uncrossmatched blood. Bibl Haematol 1980; 46:132–142.
38. Kendrich DB: Blood Program in World War II. Washington, DC, Medical Department, US Army, 1964.
39. Barnes A, Allen TE: Transfusion subsequent to administration of universal donor blood in Vietnam. JAMA 1968; 204:147–149.
40. Pruitt Ba, Moncrief J, Mason AD: Effect of Buffered Saline Solution upon Blood Volume of Man Acute Hemorrhage: Annual Research Progress Report. San Antonio, Institute of Surgical Research, 1965.
41. Shackford SR, Virgilio RW, Peters RM: Whole blood versus packed cell transfusions. Ann Surg 1981; 193:337–340.
42. Gervin AS, Fisher RP: Resuscitation of trauma patients with type-specific uncrossmatched blood. J Trauma 1984; 24:327–331.
43. Schwab CW, Shayne JP, Turner J: Immediate trauma resuscitation with type O uncrossmatched blood: A two-year prospective experience. J Trauma 1986; 26:897–902.
44. Cohn SM: Is blood obsolete? J Trauma 1997; 42:730–732.
45. Schultz SC, Powell CC, Burris DG, et al: The efficacy of diaspirin crosslinked hemoglobin solution resuscitation in a model of uncontrolled hemorrhage. J Trauma 1994; 37:408–412.
46. Sankaran S, Lucas C, Walt AJ: Thoracic aortic clamping for prophylaxis against sudden cardiac arrest during laparotomy for acute massive hemoperitoneum. J Trauma 1975; 15:290–296.
47. Ledgerwood AM, Kazmers M, Lucas CE: The role of thoracic aorta occlusion for massive hemoperitoneum. J Trauma 1976; 16:610–615.
48. Feliciano DV, Bitondo CG, Cruse PA, et al: Liberal use of emergency center thoracotomy. Am J Surg 1986; 152:654–659.
49. Shimazu S, Shatney C: Outcome of trauma patients with no vital signs on hospital admission. J Trauma 1983; 23:213–216.
50. Millikan JS, Moore EE: Outcome of resuscitative thoracotomy and descending aortic occlusion performed in the operating room. J Trauma 1984; 24:387–392.
51. Moore EE, et al: Post injury thoracotomy in the emergency department: A critical evaluation. Surgery 1979; 86:590–598.
52. Asensio JA, Murray J, Demetriades D, et al: Penetrating cardiac injuries: A prospective study of variables predicting outcomes. J Am Coll Surg 1998; 186:24–34.
53. Wiencek RG Jr, Wilson RF: Injuries to the abdominal vascular system: How much does aggressive resuscitation and prelaparotomy thoracotomy really help? Surgery 1987; 102:731–736.
54. Smith SJ Jr, Snider MT: An improved technique for rapid infusion of warmed fluid using a level I fluid warmer. Surg Gynecol Obstet 1989; 168:273–274.
55. Fried SJ, Satiani B, Zeeb P: Normothermic rapid volume replacement for hypovolemic shock: An in vivo and in vitro study utilizing a new technique. J Trauma 1986; 26:183–186.
56. Satiani B, Fried SJ, Falcone RE: Normothermic rapid volume replacement in traumatic hypovolemia. Arch Surg 1987; 122:1044–1047.
57. Falcone RE, Fried SJ, Zeeb P, et al: Rapid volume replacement with warmed blood and fluids. Angiology 1989; 40:964–969.
58. Blundell J: Experiments on the transfusion of blood by the syringe. Med Chir Trans 1818; 9:56092.
59. Duncan J: On reinfusion of blood in primary and other amputations. Br Med J 1886; 1:192–193.
60. Henry H, Elliot TR: The morbid anatomy of wounds of the thorax. J R Army Med Corps 1916; 27:520–555.
61. Brown AL, Debenheim MW: Autotransfusion: Use of blood from hemothorax. JAMA 1931; 96:1223–1225.
62. Griswald RA, Ostner AB: Use of autotransfusion in surgery of serous cavities. Surg Gynecol Obstet 1943; 77:167–177.
63. Klebanoff G: Early clinical experience with a disposable unit for intra-operative salvage and reinfusion of blood loss (intra-operative autotransfusion). Am J Surg 1970; 120:718–722.
64. Klebanoff G: Intra-operative autotransfusion with the Bentley ATS-100. Surgery 1978; 83:708–712.
65. Von Koch L, Defore WW, Mattox KL: A practical method of autotransfusion in the emergency center. Am J Surg 1977; 133:770–772.
66. Jurkovich GJ, Moore EE, Medina G: Autotransfusion in trauma: A pragmatic analysis. Am J Surg 1984; 148:782–785.
67. Glover JL, Broadie TA: Intra-operative autotransfusion. Surg Annu 1984; 16:39–56.
68. Schrock T, Blaisdell WF, Mathewson C Jr: Management of blunt trauma to the liver and hepatic veins. Arch Surg 1968; 96:698–704.
69. Bricker DL, Wukasch DC: Successful management of an injury to the suprarenal inferior vena cava. Surg Clin North Am 1970; 50:999–1002.
70. Yellin AE, Chaffee CB, Donovan AJ: Vascular isolation in treatment of juxtahepatic venous injuries. Arch Surg 1971; 102:566–573.
71. Fullen WD, Mc Donough JJ, Popp MJ, et al: Sternal splitting approach for mayor hepatic or retrohepatic vena cava injury. J Trauma 1974; 4:903–911.
72. Turpin I, State D, Schwartz A: Injuries to the inferior vena cava and their management. Am J Surg 1977; 134:25–32.
73. Kudsk KA, Sheldon GF, Lim RC Jr: Atrial-caval shunting (ACS) after trauma. J Trauma 1982; 22:81–85.
74. Burch J, Feliciano DB, Mattox KL: The atriocaval shunt: Facts and fictions. Ann Surg 1988; 207:555–568.
75. Rovito PF: Atrial caval shunting in blunt hepatic vascular injury. Ann Surg 1987; 205:318–321.
76. Pachter HL, Spenser FC, Hofstetter SR: Experience with the finger fracture technique to achieve intrahepatic in 75 patients with severe injuries to the liver. Ann Surg 1993; 197:771.
77. Pachter HL, Spenser FC, Hofstetter SR, et al: Significant trend in the treatment of hepatic trauma: Experience with 411 injuries. Ann Surg 1992; 215:492.
78. Pringle JH: Notes on the arrest of hepatic hemorrhage due to trauma. Ann Surg 1908; 48:541–549.
79. Feliciano DB, Mattox KL, Jordan GL Jr: Intra-abdominal packing for control of hepatic hemorrhage: A reappraisal. J Trauma 1981; 21:285–290.
80. Carmona RH, Peck D, Lim RC Jr: The role of packing and planned reoperation in severe hepatic trauma. J Trauma 1984; 24:779–784.
81. Feliciano DB, Mattox KL, Burch JM, et al: Packing for control of hepatic hemorrhage. J Trauma 1986; 26:738–743.
82. Ivatury RR, Nallathambi M, Gunduz Y, et al: Liver packing for uncontrolled hemorrhage: A reappraisal. J Trauma 1986; 26:744–753.

83. Cogbill TH, Moore EE, Juricovich GJ, et al: Severe hepatic trauma: A multi-center experience with 1335 liver injuries. J Trauma 1988; 28:1433-1438.
84. Lucas CE, Ledgerwood AM: Prospective evaluation of hemostatic techniques for liver injuries. J Trauma 1976; 16:442-451.
85. Asensio JA: Unpublished data.
86. Luna GK, Marer RV, Pavlin EG, et al: Incidence and effect of hypothermia in severely injured patients. J Trauma 1987; 27:1014-1018.
87. Jurkovich GJ, Greiser WB, Luterman A, et al: Hypothermia in trauma victims: An ominous predictor of survival. J Trauma 1987; 27:1019-1024.
88. Rutledge R, Sheldon GF, Collins ML: Massive transfusion: Critical care management of the trauma patient. Surg Ciln North Am 1986; 2:791-805.
89. Claggett GP, Olsen WR: Non-mechanical hemorrhage in severe liver injury. Ann Surg 1978; 187:369-374
90. Wilson RF, Mammen E, Walt AJ: Eight years of experience with massive blood transfusion. J Trauma 1971; 11:275.
91. Lee T, Lun K: Review of problems of massive blood transfusion in a surgical intensive care unit. Ann Acad Med Singapore 1985; 14:175-184.
92. Ludbrook J, Wynn V: Citrate intoxication. Br Med J 1958; 2:523.
93. Martin D, Lucas C, Ledgerwood A, et al: Fresh frozen plasma supplement to massive red blood cell transfusion. Ann Surg 1985; 202:505-511.
94. Reed R, Ciavarella D, Heimbach D, et al: Prophylactic platelet administration during massive transfusion. Ann Surg 1986; 203:40-48.

5

Resuscitation Algorithms in Acute Emergency Conditions

William C. Shoemaker, MD, FCCM

CLINICAL DECISIONS IN RESUSCITATION

The sudden unexpected appearance of an acute emergency may be a prelude to confusion and disaster. In contrast to nonemergency conditions, time is of the essence. High-risk emergency victims concomitantly require rapid diagnostic work-up, physiologic monitoring, and therapy of specific injuries or disease states. Confusion may occur because three simultaneous processes must proceed in different tracks:

- Diagnosis of the primary and secondary diseases
- Monitoring and correction of circulatory shock
- Therapy for the primary problem

Treatment of a patient with multiple life-threatening problems or severe associated preexisting medical conditions leaves minimal margin for error. Fluid therapy must be initiated quickly and titrated appropriately in the initial resuscitation, and must be continued in the subsequent post-shock recovery period to achieve optimal outcome. The challenge is to provide a well-organized, coherent approach prioritized according to the life-threatening aspects of each problem as the patient moves from the emergency department (ED), to the operating room (OR) or the intensive care unit (ICU). These crucial decisions involve priorities and goals best defined by branch chain decision trees or clinical algorithms.

TRADITIONAL APPROACH TO DECISION MAKING IN RESUSCITATION

In the traditional approach, well-established concepts stated in narrative form are listed for diagnostic work-up and therapy. These concepts are often supplemented by anecdotal observations, by reviews of the results of specific types of accidents or illnesses, and by information from experimental shock in anesthetized animals. Traditional approaches apply generalized principles for patients of a given diagnostic category.

Conventional clinical approaches provide lists of diagnostic and laboratory tests designed to cover most problems; obviously, some of these plans may be appropriate to some therapeutic activities but inappropriate to others[1] (Table 5-1). Lists of needed clinical and laboratory data may be problematic, because they leave the impression that perhaps all this information might be required before the important initial decisions are made. By the time one covers half the list, there are conflicting historic information, changing clinical signs, and questionable laboratory tests that delay decisions. Traditional approaches to emergency care attempt to be complete but may be difficult to apply and, because of complexities, easily lead to diagnostic tangents. Descriptions of diseases and their therapy in medical texts are organized according to diagnostic categories, which is appropriate when diagnoses are known; however, when patients arrive at the ED without specific diagnoses, the conventional approach may result in delays in diagnosis and therapy.

The algorithmic approach enfolds the diagnostic and monitoring processes into a branch chain decision tree to expedite decisions at important junctures as the process unfolds. Clinical algorithms apply similar concepts in a systematic organized fashion by progressively and successively stratifying patients by clinical criteria defined by each decision node; then algorithms define therapeutic criteria and titrate therapy to predetermined endpoints characterized by survival patterns. The advantage is that each decision may be made as soon as the criterion of each decision node is met without the need to wait until all other information required for subsequent decisions is available.

TABLE 5–1. Evaluation, Diagnosis, and Therapy of Trauma Patients

1. Withdraw blood sample for hematocrit, typing, crossmatch, electrolytes, and routine chemistries.
2. Start intravenous fluids.
3. Insert central venous pressure catheter.
4. Examine lungs; tap chest if pneumothorax or hemothorax is suspected.
5. Examine heart.
6. Insert Foley catheter and measure urine output.
7. Measure arterial blood gases.
8. Obtain electrocardiogram.
9. Measure blood volume or hemoglobin/hematocrit.
10. If cardiac tamponade suspected from rising central venous pressure, obtain echocardiogram, computed tomographic scan, or pericardiocentesis.
11. Examine abdomen; if blunt trauma with organ damage is suspected, perform diagnostic peritoneal lavage.
12. Examine the patient thoroughly for evidence of fractures, wounds, and other injuries.
13. Search for sources of obscure bleeding.
14. Search for sources of infection; perform a culture of available body fluids.
15. Hematologic evaluation: prothrombin time, partial thromboplastin time, platelet count, fibrinogen, bleeding and clotting times.

Common Problems in Resuscitation

Most preventable errors of emergency fatalities occur not because of ignorance but because of the failure to act expeditiously at crucial moments. Delays in resuscitation may result from the following:

- Disorganized activity
- Failure to recognize priorities
- Inability to appreciate the complexities of emergency problems

Although most times the correct therapeutic measures eventually are performed, often they are not done at the right time, in the right amount, or in the right order. A major difficulty in organizing priorities for emergency care is that the exigencies of emergency situations preclude carefully controlled scientific studies. Moreover, in most clinicians' minds, the urgent demand for therapy focuses on one or more key issues to the exclusion of other important considerations. Successful resuscitation depends on the following:

- Nature and extent of the primary illness or injury
- Amount of blood and fluid losses
- Patient's age and previous state of health
- Number and extent of associated medical conditions
- Time delay in instituting therapy
- Volume and rate of fluids administered
- Choice of fluids given

Experienced physicians manage emergency victims with excellent outcomes, but it is difficult to describe their approaches objectively so that students, residents, and younger clinicians might emulate them. Less experienced physicians or those in community hospitals who see limited numbers of major emergency victims may need help to organize priorities for a wide variety of generally accepted principles. The branch chain decision tree provides the vehicle to organize information and decision rules to clinical conditions.

From both organizational and scientific viewpoints, it is difficult to evaluate associated medical conditions and preexisting illnesses during emergency resuscitation. Although the general principles of resuscitation and emergency care are well known, the major difficulty operationally is to provide optimal emergency care without delay and without missing important steps. This involves evaluating the process of emergency care by specifically defined criteria and priorities at each step to achieve the best outcome.

Evaluations of these clinical problems from detailed reviews of many clinical series over several decades suggest that delays in decision making and therapy might be prevented and care improved if clinical management were organized in the context of a decision tree. Most medical activity, according to McDonald and colleagues[2] consists of simple recognition-response arcs that can be defined by decision rules that deal expeditiously with emergency problems.

BRANCH CHAIN LOGIC: THE DECISION TREE

The algorithmic approach to resuscitation is based on the premise that decision rules can be defined by clinical and physiologic criteria for the important problems. These diagnostic and therapeutic decision rules may be expressed in the format of a branch chain decision tree. This framework provides the skeleton for commonly encountered major clinical problems. This does not preclude other additional care not specified by the decision tree; it simply provides the organizational framework for most urgent decisions.

Initially, clinical algorithms were first used for paramedical personnel involved in triage,[1] for nurse clinicians and physicians' assistants,[2] and for physicians in treating acute illness and trauma in the ED.[3, 4, 9-20] The branch chain logic is ideally suited to resuscitation and fluid management in patients with shock. Prospective clinical trials have demonstrated improved outcome with resuscitation algorithms.[12, 13]

Branch chain logic is probably the process that clinicians use subconsciously to reason, and algorithms generated by careful analysis may represent formal conceptualizations of the thought processes that go into decision making. An algorithm, therefore, uses branch chain logic as a set of formalized procedure rules that are applied to a specific recurring set of conditions. Complex problems are broken down into a series of components that are characterized by specific criteria. In essence, an algorithm is a formalized set of step-by-step instructions with detailed specifications for each decision node. It is essentially a closed system, designed to accomplish a given task by precisely defined criteria, for entry, for each step, for the sequence of steps, and for specific endpoints at which to stop.

The Clinical Algorithm

Branch chain decision trees represent sets of guidelines that are less precisely and less quantitatively defined than mathematical algorithms. That is, clinical algorithms are less rigorously defined than mathematical equations or algorithms used in computer programming. On the other hand, the term "algorithm" is often misapplied to flow charts describing the number of patients who passed through decision points or the results of decisions but not the explicit criteria needed to make these decisions. The essential algorithmic features are well-defined sets of criteria that specify each sequential decision node.

The branch chain logic approach specifies the minimum information needed to make the first decision; as soon as that information is available, the decision can be made and therapy instituted. In the meantime, information is gathered for the next decision. Thus, the acquisition of the relevant data and the administration of each type of therapy are sequenced to address the most important and urgent decisions first. This approach selects from widely varied heterogeneous groups, patients of specifically defined groups in order of their life-threatening probabilities. Each successive decision node defines the problem in the order of its life-threatening capability and recommends therapy for the particular clinical subset selected; as each subset is addressed, the residual population becomes progressively more homogeneous. The stepwise process provides the organizational framework for accomplishing urgent prioritized objectives without limiting other clinical activities.

In essence, each node on the decision tree stratifies the subjects by explicit prearranged criteria and specifies the next action to be taken. This process provides a plan that shows the following at a glance:

- Specific criteria for each decision node
- Sequence of this sorting operation
- Tasks to be performed at each decision node

This method facilitates more expeditious, consistent, and complete therapy than management hastily arranged by those who happen to be present or on call at the time. Most important, it does not readily allow essential parts of the process to be neglected.

Algorithmic Conventions and Notations

By conventional notations, ovals or balloons give criteria for entrance or exit from the algorithm, decision nodes are indicated by diamonds or hexagons, and rectangles indicate diagnostic procedures or therapeutic interventions. The criteria needed for each decision are indicated by the values shown inside the hexagons. The temporal decision sequences shown by arrows indicate the order of the decision nodes.

Common clinical problems that lend themselves to this approach must have very specific and well-defined criteria for each decision. Questions that require interpretation (e.g., "How sick is the patient?") do not make good decision nodes because they are not answered by a simple "yes" or "no" based on objective data. In contrast, straightforward, routinely managed problems whose answers have been well worked out and clinically tested are more easily expressed in the algorithmic format. With these essential tasks addressed, clinicians are then free to concentrate on problems that cannot be easily defined and that require considered clinical judgment.

This chapter describes three clinical algorithms for the following:

1. Initial fluid resuscitation of emergency hypotensive patients in the ED.
2. Subsequent fluid management of the critically ill patient being monitored with a central venous pressure (CVP) catheter.
3. Management of blunt and penetrating wounds of the chest and abdomen.

The third decision tree extends the algorithmic approach from the relatively simple fluid management problem to a more comprehensive organization of diagnosis, monitoring, and therapy of trauma. A fourth algorithm for high-risk surgical patients using a pulmonary artery catheter is described in Chapter 8 (Shock).

INITIAL FLUID RESUSCITATION OF HYPOTENSIVE EMERGENCY PATIENTS

Usually, the most crucial problem in the hypotensive emergency trauma victim is unrecognized hypovolemia from delay or inadequate fluid resuscitation. Upper airway obstruction may be more urgent, but it is less common and usually readily correctable with intubation and mechanical ventilation.

Description and Strategy Conveyed by the Algorithm

A resuscitation algorithm designed for fluid therapy in the first 30 to 60 minutes of hypotensive patients entering the ED was based on the premise that hypovolemia causes most of the mortality and morbidity of trauma and other acute emergency conditions (Fig. 5-1). The emergency algorithm may be used to illustrate the therapeutic strategy for fluid resuscitation of hypotensive emergencies.

In the first decision point, the criterion for initiation of fluid therapy is mean arterial blood pressure (MAP) less than 60 mm Hg or systolic pressure less than 90 mm Hg. MAP is defined as the diastolic pressure plus one third of the pulse pressure, which is the difference between systolic and diastolic pressures. Thus, in emergency patients, hypotension is all that is needed to start the first liter of saline or lactated Ringer's solution.

The second decision point involves the choice of fluids. Patients who are younger than 45 years and who have no cardiac history may be able to tolerate more salt and water; they are given an additional liter of Ringer's lactate plus 500 mL of colloids (albumin or starch).

The third decision point is a CVP greater than 15 mm Hg, which defines criteria to slow or stop fluid administration.

The fourth decision point, hematocrit (Hct) less than 25%, defines the criteria for use of O-negative or uncrossmatched (type-specific) blood in patients with rapid exsanguinating hemorrhage.

Finally, the MAP response to therapy is used as the decision criterion to recycle or to proceed to the next section.

In essence, hypotension is the criterion for starting fluids; age, cardiac history, and Hct define the type and amount of fluids. The young, previously healthy gunshot victim may tolerate large volumes of crystalloids, whereas the elderly cardiac patient receiving a 1-g salt diet may not. The MAP response is a guide to effectiveness of the fluids, and the CVP defines the upper limits for volume therapy. The initial MAP is roughly analogous to a car's accelerator, and the CVP and MAP response are analogous to the brakes.

Effectiveness of the Resuscitation Algorithm

The algorithm was tested prospectively in all hypotensive emergency patients entering a surgical ED over 2.5 years; 50% of the patients were managed with the algorithm, and 50% were managed by the standard of care of a university-run county hospital; compliance with the algorithm was carefully documented in each patient.[12, 13] Of 6833 emergency admissions, 603 patients (9%) had hypotension either on admission to or during the stay in the ED. In addition, another 135 patients (2%) of all patients, or 22% of the hypotensive patients, normally maintained low MAP, mean 75 ± 3 (SD) mm Hg, but they did not have medical conditions that could account for this hypotension; this was more common in, but not confined to, young females.

Of the 603 hypotensive patients, 6% were admitted in full arrest, 18% in severe shock (MAP = 0 to 60 mm Hg), and 52% in moderate shock (MAP = 60 to 80 mm Hg); 24% were initially normotensive but subsequently became hypotensive during initial management in the ED. The average lowest MAP value was 53 ± 25 (SD) mm Hg. There were 114 (19%) deaths and 169 (28%) patients with complications.[12, 13] Of all in-hospital complications, 8% were related to shock; these organ failures and complications included shock lung, acute renal failure, circulatory failure, sepsis in the uncontaminated patient, and possible fluid overload.

Of the patients with shock-related organ failures, 25 (52%) died. Patients whose management was in compliance with the algorithm had the most rapid resuscitations; as the number of deviations from the algorithm increased, resuscitation times were more prolonged.[12, 13] There was an 85% survival rate in those with satisfactory compliance compared with a 64% survival rate in patients with deviations from the algorithm. Most of the delays and shock-related complications were preventable. In essence, there were significantly reduced resuscitation times and fewer shock-related organ failures, complications, and deaths when patients were resuscitated according to the algorithm.[12, 13]

There were 265 (44%) hypotensive patients in this series who had severe associated medical illnesses; these patients were more vulnerable to complications and death.

The algorithm is most useful in these emergency patients with severe associated illnesses in whom delay or unorganized therapy was more likely to lead to unsatisfactory outcomes. When the algorithm was followed in patients with severe associated illnesses, resuscitation times were more rapid, ICU stays and hospitalizations were shorter, and mortality rates were lower.

Although prolonged resuscitation may be tolerated in young patients with only mild hypotension and no other medical problems, relatively short delays or small technical problems may be lethal in patients with severe associated medical prob-

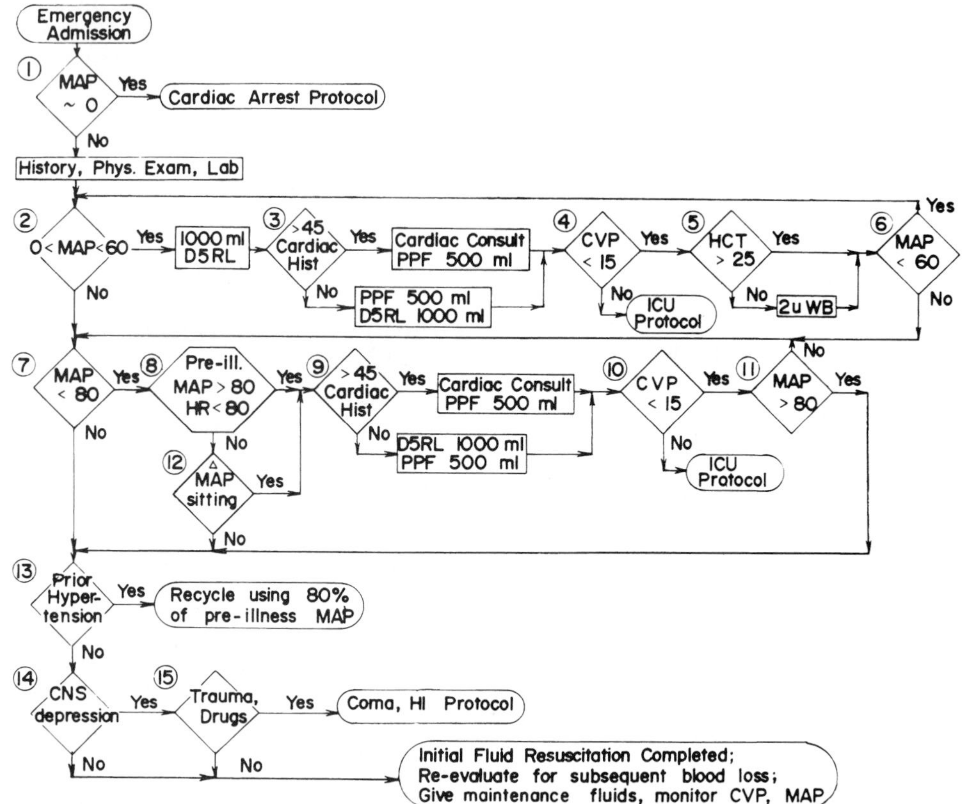

Figure 5–1. Clinical algorithm for the initial (1st hour) resuscitation of emergency admissions. This algorithm was designed for resuscitation of the acute emergency patient to restore circulatory integrity as rapidly as possible without producing fluid overload. MAP = mean arterial blood pressure; RL = lactated Ringer's solution; CVP = central venous pressure; CNS = central nervous system.

Step 1: If the MAP is zero or nearly zero, determine whether cardiac arrest has occurred and begin cardiopulmonary resuscitation immediately. If the patient has an MAP <20 mm Hg, alert personnel for a possible cardiac arrest.

Step 2: If the MAP is <60 mm Hg, immediately start administration of RL or D5RL (dextrose 5% in RL), 1000 mL, and run as rapidly as possible, especially if the MAP is <50 mm Hg.

Step 3: If the patient is <45 years old and does not have a history of cardiac disease, place a CVP line and start another infusion of D5RL, 1000 mL, plus 500 mL of plasma protein fraction (PPF) or artificial colloid through a third intravenous line.

Step 4: Monitor the CVP at frequent intervals during the rapid infusion of these three solutions so as not to exceed values >15 cm H_2O. If the CVP is >15 cm H_2O, go directly to the ICU protocol.

Step 5: If the Hct is <25%, give 2 U of O-negative or type-specific blood. When crossmatched blood becomes available, transfusions of whole blood or packed red cells should be given to maintain Hct at >33%.

Step 6: Rapid restoration of the MAP to 60 mm Hg is the titration endpoint for fluids in this section. If the MAP is <60 mm Hg, recycle from Step 2 through Step 6. If a MAP >60 mm Hg has been achieved, proceed to Step 7.

Step 7: If the MAP is <80 mm Hg, go to Step 8; if not, proceed to Step 13.

Step 8: If the MAP is <80 mm Hg, inquire from the patient or the patient's family or consult a previous hospital record to evaluate the patient's "normal" pre-illness control MAP. If the MAP is <80 mm Hg and the heart rate (HR) is >80 beat/min, measure orthostatic blood pressure (Step 12).

Step 9: As in Step 3, the cardiac patient requires less salt and water but more colloid. If the age of the patient is >45 years or if he or she has a history of cardiac disease, give 500 mL of colloid; if the patient's age is <45 years and he or she has no history of cardiac disease, give 1000 mL of D5RL plus 500 mL of colloid.

Step 10: Fluids may be given safely if the CVP is <15 cm H_2O; if this is exceeded, go to the ICU protocol and continue to give fluids as needed to restore circulatory integrity, provided wedge pressures of 18 mm Hg are not exceeded.

Step 11: If the MAP is >80 mm Hg without exceeding a CVP of >15 cm H_2O, the objective of this cycle has been achieved. If the MAP is <80 mm Hg, recycle Steps 7 through 11.

Step 12: Orthostatic blood pressure is measured. If a 10-mm Hg change in the MAP occurs on sitting or standing, this is presumptive evidence of at least 1000 mL of blood volume deficit.

Step 13: After the MAP has been restored to the normal value (>80 mm Hg), it is still necessary to be sure that the pre-illness blood pressure was normal. If a prior hypertension was observed, the patient should be recycled from Step 7 through Step 13 using 80% of the pre-illness value as the criterion for the adequacy of resuscitation.

Step 14: Examine the patient for evidence of CNS depression, drug poisoning, or drug abuse.

Step 15: Examine the patient for evidence of head injury or other trauma. If trauma is present, the patient should be treated in accordance with a coma-head injury protocol.

(Reproduced with permission from Hopkins JA, Shoemaker WC, Chang PC, et al: Results of a clinical trial on the use of an emergency resuscitation algorithm. Crit Care Med 1983; 11:621.)

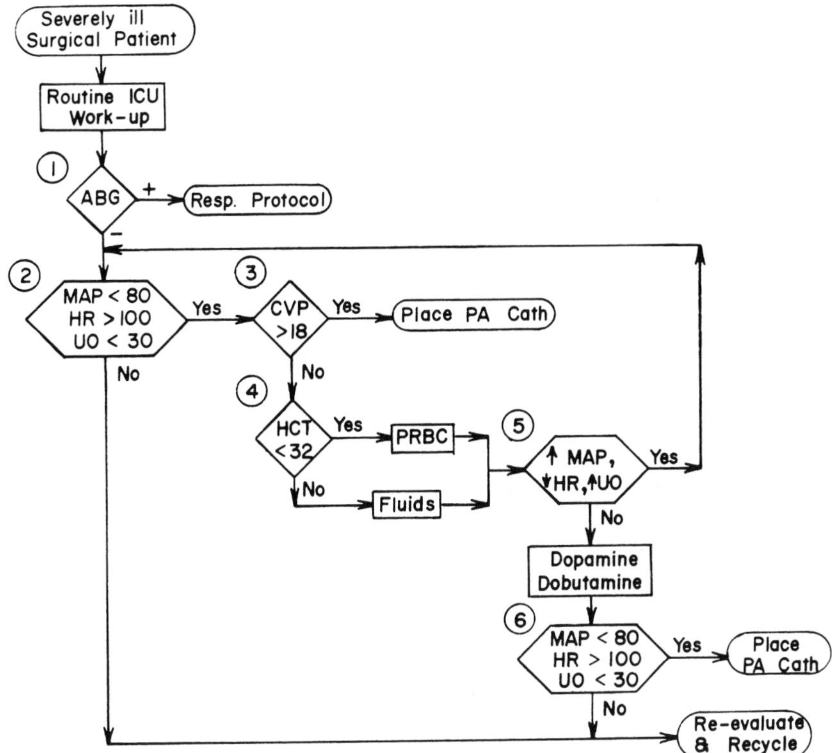

Figure 5–2. Algorithm for subsequent continuing fluid management in patients with central venous pressure (CVP) catheters. If the routine work-up has not been completed, the following should be ordered: chest radiography, complete blood count and differential, routine electrolytes and blood chemistries (M300), 12-lead electrocardiography, and urinalysis, Hct, prothrombin time, partial thromboplastin time, and platelets if significant blood loss or bleeding tendency is present, as well as other indicated radiographic and laboratory studies. If evidence of sepsis is present, culture blood, urine, or sputum, drain site, and cerebrospinal fluid if appropriate.

Step 1: Assess arterial blood gases (ABG); if abnormal, proceed with respiratory protocol.

Step 2: If mean arterial pressure (MAP) is <80 mm Hg, heart rate (HR) is >100 beats/min, or urine output (UO) is <30 mL/hr, measure CVP and proceed to Step 3, as inadequate hydration is a likely possibility. If MAP is >80 mm Hg, HR is <100 beats/min, and UO is >30 mL/hr, re-evaluate at frequent intervals.

Step 3: If CVP is >18 mm Hg, place a pulmonary artery (PA) catheter; if CVP is <18 mm Hg, measure Hct.

Step 4: If Hct is <32%, give 2 U packed red cells (PRBC) or 1 U whole blood. If Hct is >32%, give 1 L Ringer's lactate or 500 mL plasma protein fraction.

Step 5: If the fluid load given above improves MAP, HR, or UO, this is evidence of hypovolemia or dehydration; proceed to Step 2 to test adequacy of fluid load. If the criteria of Step 2 (MAP >80 mm Hg, HR <100 beats/min, UO >30 mL/hr) are met, reevaluate at intervals; if not, recycle from Steps 3 to 5. This fluid cycle may be repeated as long as (1) there is continued improvement and (2) CVP does not exceed 18 mm Hg. However, it is also necessary to search for continued fluid losses. If the fluid load given as described does not improve MAP, HR, or UO, dehydration and hypovolemia are unlikely; start administration of an inotropic agent, such as dobutamine or vasopressors in low doses, and titrate gradually to achieve the optimal result.

Step 6: If MAP is >80 mm Hg, HR is <100 beat/min, and UO is >30 mL/hr, reevaluate at frequent intervals. If these goals are not reached, place a PA catheter.

lems. With limited physiologic reserves, small problems at any stage may be life-threatening. Most patients fall somewhere between these two extremes, where moderate degrees of inadequately treated hypovolemia may limit circulatory function and outcome.

ALGORITHM FOR FLUID MANAGEMENT OF PATIENTS WITH CENTRAL VENOUS PRESSURE CATHETERS

The resuscitation algorithm covers initial intravenous fluid management for the first hour. A branch chain decision tree has been developed for the subsequent management of critically ill or hemodynamically unstable patients who are thought to have hypovolemia but who have only CVP catheters (Fig. 5-2). In this algorithm, MAP, heart rate, urine output, Hct, and CVP were used as criteria. The basic premise under these conditions is that increments of volume expanders may be used to titrate therapy to optimal responses without exceeding safe CVP pressures (<18 mm Hg) to obviate fluid overload. This algorithm is useful in managing fluid therapy after the initial resuscitation and in administering fluid challenge to patients with suspected hypovolemia.

COMPREHENSIVE BRANCH CHAIN DECISION TREE FOR TRAUMA RESUSCITATION

The two previously described algorithms were addressed to the specific problem of fluid resuscitation based on the assumption that hypovolemia is the most urgent problem in shock. Although decision rules for fluid resuscitation are rather straightforward and the decision trees are relatively simple, algorithms that attempt to address the total immediate care of the trauma victim are an order of magnitude more complex than the fluid resuscitation algorithms. Nevertheless,

TABLE 5–2. Common Problems in Blunt and Penetrating Trauma to the Thorax and Abdomen

1. Cardiac or respiratory arrest or both
2. Respiratory distress
3. Circulatory shock
4. Laceration of the heart wtih or without cardiac tamponade
5. Cardiac contusion
6. Pneumothorax, tension pneumothorax, hemothorax
7. Lacerations of the trachea, bronchus with air leak
8. Sucking chest wound
9. Fractures of ribs with or without flail chest
10. Pulmonary contusion
11. Injury to great vessels
12. Laceration or rupture of esophagus, stomach, small bowel, colon, or bladder
13. Laceration of diaphragm
14. Laceration or rupture of liver, spleen, kidney, or pancreas
15. Vascular injuries
16. Fractures of pelvis, spine, and long bones
17. Retroperitoneal, mesenteric, or omental hematomas

comprehensive decision trees for expeditious resuscitation, including monitoring, diagnosis, and therapy of penetrating and blunt trauma of the chest and abdomen, were designed and tested.

The algorithms for trauma are based on the assumption that it is imperative to (1) restore circulatory integrity, (2) establish a diagnosis, and (3) begin definitive therapy as rapidly as possible. All three of these activities need to be carried out simultaneously on separate parallel tracts. Cardiopulmonary resuscitation (CPR) for cardiac arrest and fluid therapy for shock are early subroutines.

General Principles and Concepts

Here are some guidelines for resuscitation:

1. If the patient is hypotensive or in shock, immediate resuscitation and surgical exploration are mandatory.
2. If the MAP does not immediately respond to adequate volumes of fluids ($\geq$5 L), urgent surgical exploration is mandatory to control the bleeding source. Fluid resuscitation is continued vigorously during the surgical attempts to control bleeding.
3. Gunshot wounds, except tangential or grazing wounds, should be explored.
4. Stab wounds without abdominal findings, except for localized tenderness at the wound site, may be considered for conservative (nonoperative) management to avoid negative explorations and to shorten the hospital stay.
5. Cardiac tamponade must be considered in stab wounds and gunshot wounds of the chest as well as the upper abdomen, flank, and back; about 2% of penetrating chest wounds have tamponade. Elevated CVP is usually the first monitored sign of tamponade.
6. Patients with blunt abdominal trauma and peritoneal signs should undergo urgent surgical exploration with or without diagnostic peritoneal lavage to repair lacerated solid or perforated gastrointestinal injuries.
7. Computed tomographic (CT) scans of head, chest, and abdomen may be done in hemodynamically stable patients with questionable abdominal signs and in patients with head injuries, coma, drug overdose, or ethanol intoxication.
8. Thoracoabdominal injuries require special consideration and should be explored with less rigorous indications (including hypotension, abdominal tenderness, guarding, and rebound tenderness) or CT findings.
9. Repeated physical examinations provide important information in questionable cases.
10. Penetrating abdominal wounds are often overdiagnosed and unnecessarily explored, whereas blunt trauma is more frequently underdiagnosed and explored too late.

Algorithm for Blunt and Penetrating Injuries of the Thorax and Abdomen

Figure 5-3 describes a clinical algorithm for the management of blunt and penetrating thoracic and abdominal injuries. The major decision points are presented, and criteria for each decision are suggested. Table 5-2 lists common problems associated with blunt and penetrating wounds of the thorax and abdomen. Table 5-3 lists the most common diagnostic

TABLE 5–3. Diagnostic Procedures, Monitoring Systems, and Therapy in Blunt and Penetrating Trauma of the Thorax and Abdomen

Diagnostic Procedure	Monitoring	Therapy
1. Cervical spine radiograph	1. MAP	1. CPR
2. Chest radiograph, AP and lat	2. Heart rate	2. Fluids, blood
3. Chest tap, chest tube	3. CVP	3. Oxygen by mask
4. Abdominal radiograph: upright, decubitus	4. Urine output	4. Needle thoracentesis
5. An IV urogram	5. ECG	5. Chest tube
6. Echocardiography	6. Hct	6. Tracheal intubation
7. Angiography	7. ABGs	7. Mechanical ventilation
a. Aortic arch	8. NG tube; output, volume, and Hct	8. Thoracotomy, repair of injuries
b. Celiac axis	9. Chest tube: output, volume, and Hct	9. Laparotomy, repair of injuries
c. Internal and external iliac arteries		
d. Peripheral vessels		
8. Bronchoscopy		
9. Pericardiocentesis		
10. CT scan		
11. Liver, lung scan		
12. MUGA scan		
13. Endoscopy		
14. Minilap		

MAP = mean arterial pressure; CPR = cardiopulmonary resuscitation; AP = anteroposterior; lat = lateral; CVP = central venous pressure; IV = intravenous; ECG = electrocardiogram; Hct = hematocrit; ABGs = arterial blood gases; NG = nasogastric; CT = computed tomographic; MUGA = multiple gated acquisition.

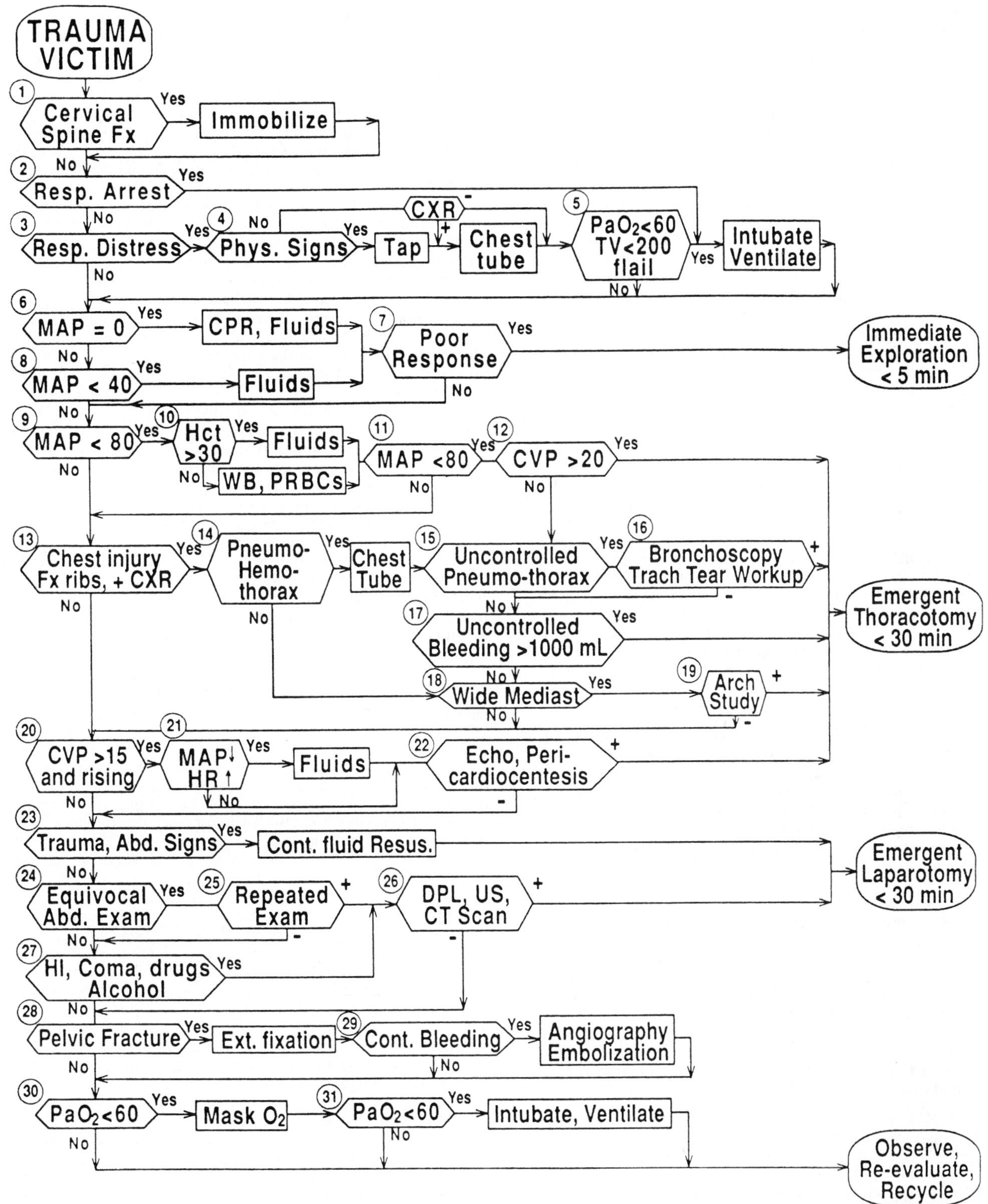

Figure 5–3. Algorithm for the clinical management of blunt and penetrating thoracic and abdominal injuries.

Step 1: If patient has any physical signs (penetrating wounds, contusions, swelling, extremity weakness, or sensory loss) of blunt or penetrating neck injury or has any neck pain, maintain external cervical immobilization, obtain lateral cervical spine radiographs to screen for major cervical injury, and continue resuscitation.

Step 2: If respiratory arrest occurs, intubate and begin mechanical ventilation.

Step 3: If respiratory distress or depressed level of consciousness is present as defined by one or more of the following criteria, proceed to Steps 4 through 8: tachypnea (respiratory rate ≥30 breaths/min), bradypnea (respiratory rate ≤8 breaths/min), sternal retraction, use of accessory breathing muscles, flaring of nasal alae during respiration, cyanosis of the lips or skin, or Glasgow Coma Scale score (GCS) ≤9.

Step 4: If physical signs of pneumothorax are present, such as hyperresonance, distant or decreased breath sounds, or open chest wounds, perform an immediate needle thoracostomy in the midclavicular line ofthe second intercostal space (ICS) of the

Legend continued on following page

Figure 5–3 *Continued*

affected side. Then place a No. 36 or No. 40 chest tube into the affected hemithorax at ICS 4–5 in the midaxillary line and proceed to Step 5. If no physical signs of tension pneumothorax are observed, obtain a portable chest radiograph (CXR). If CXR findings are normal, proceed to Step 5. If the CXR shows a hemothorax or pneumothorax, perform tube thoracostomy and go to Step 5. However, if 1000 mL of blood is immediately obtained from the tube, clamp the tube and obtain a CXR. If after the drainage of 1000 mL of blood the CXR shows an estimated 500 mL or more of blood still in the hemithorax (massive hemothorax), transport the patient to the operating room (OR) for further chest drainage and possible thoracotomy. (Letting chest drainage continue in the emergency department [ED] may precipitate a hypovolemic cardiac arrest.) Colloids (5% albumin or hydroxyethyl starch) should be infused rapidly while the patient is prepared for the OR.

Step 5: Intubate and start mechanical ventilation if one or more of the following conditions exists: $Pa{O_2}$ is <60 mm Hg on 40% facemask O_2, $Pa{CO_2}$ is >45 mm Hg, spontaneous tidal volume (VT) is <200 mL, respiratory rate is >30 breaths/min or <8 breaths/min, flail segment exists, or GCS is <9. Adjust ventilator settings to maintain arterial oxygen saturation at ≥93% or $Pa{O_2}$ ≥60 mm Hg and $Pa{CO_2}$ at ≤45 mm Hg. Proceed to Step 6.

Step 6: If the patient has a detectable pulse and blood pressure (BP), proceed to Step 8. If the patient has no detectable BP (MAP = 0), rapidly administer 3 to 5 L of fluids and 2 to 4 U of O-negative blood or packed cells while simultaneously initiating the Advanced Cardiac Life Support (ACLS) protocol. With large-bore intravenous (IV) lines, 1 L of fluid may be given in 2 to 5 minutes. Inserting IV tubing via cut downs into the greater saphenous, antecubital, or basilic vein establishes very effective resuscitation lines. Proceed to Step 7.

Step 7: If, with fluid resuscitation and ACLS, a detectable pulse returns and the MAP rises to ≥40 mm Hg, proceed to Step 9. If a response is obtained but the MAP remains <40 mm Hg, transport the patient to the OR for immediate exploration. If no detectable pulse or BP is obtained with resuscitation, proceed as follows:

1. For *penetrating truncal wounds:* If the patient had signs of life at some time in the field or the ED, perform a left anterior thoracotomy. This is done to relieve pericardial tamponade, to perform direct cardiac massage, to cross-clamp the descending thoracic aorta and increase blood flow to the coronary arteries and brain, and to stop other intrathoracic bleeding. The incision may be easily extended to a transsternal thoracotomy (if necessary) to control hemorrhage from the right hemithorax. If the penetrating injury is on the right thorax, a right anterior thoracotomy may be done first to control bleeding from the wound.
2. For *blunt injuries:* Continue maximum volume infusion; perform bilateral needle thoracostomy immediately followed by bilateral tube thoracostomy (midaxillary line, ICSs 4) to relieve tension pneumothorax; and perform pericardiocentesis to diagnose cardiac tamponade. If cardiac tamponade is present, perform left anterior thoracotomy; if either tube thoracostomy drains 1000 mL of blood and flow continues, clamp the tube, continue transfusions, and transport the patient to the OR for thoracotomy. Allowing the tube output to continue may increase intrathoracic hemorrhage and lead to rapid cardiac arrest from hypovolemia.

Step 8: If MAP is >40 mm Hg, proceed to Step 9. If the MAP is <40 mm Hg or systolic arterial pressure (SAP) is <60 mm Hg, insert two large-bore IV (≥16-gauge) catheters (either percutaneously or by cut down) and rapidly infuse 3 to 5 L of fluid. If inferior vena caval injury is suspected, use at least one upper extremity vein for volume infusion. If the MAP remains ≤40 mm Hg for >5 minutes, the patient should be transported to the OR for exploration. If the MAP rises to >40 mm Hg, continue expectant volume loading and proceed to Step 9.

Step 9: If the MAP is >80 mm Hg, proceed to Step 13. If the MAP is <80 mm Hg or SAP is <100 mm Hg, administer IV fluids and proceed to Step 10.

Step 10: Measure hemoglobin (Hgb) or Hct or both. If the Hct is >30%, continue infusing IV fluids. If Hct is <30%, administer 2 U PRBC or 2 U whole blood. Proceed to Step 11.

Step 11: If, after resuscitation, the MAP rises to >80 mm Hg, proceed to Step 13. If the MAP remains <80 mm Hg, insert a CVP catheter and go to Step 12.

Step 12: If the patient's CVP is <20 mm Hg, proceed to Step 13. If the CVP is ≥20 mm Hg, continue resuscitation and repeat both MAP and CVP measurements at 5-minute intervals. If over three consecutive measurements the CVP remains >20 mm Hg with the MAP remaining <80 mm Hg, presume cardiac tamponade is present and transport patient to the OR for exploratory thoracotomy. If the CVP is ≥20 mm Hg and the MAP has risen >80 mm Hg, reduce rate of fluid infusion by 50% and recheck both CVP and MAP at 5-minute intervals. If the CVP subsequently rises to >24 mm Hg, presume cardiac tamponade is present and transport patient to the OR for exploratory thoracotomy. Otherwise, proceed to Step 13.

Step 13: Obtain a portable CXR; if a hemothorax or pneumothorax is present, proceed to Step 14. If a "sucking" chest wound is present, cover injury with petroleum-impregnated gauze and place a chest tube on the affected side. If the CXR is normal and no other clinical signs of thoracic injury are present, proceed to Step 23.

Step 14: If a hemothorax or pneumothorax is present, place a chest tube (>36 French) in midaxillary line at ICS 4 or 5. Replace lost blood using an autotransfusion device if the tube output is >200 mL. Proceed to Step 15. If the patient has no hemothorax or pneumothorax, proceed to Step 18.

Step 15: If a pneumothorax persists despite the proper performance of tube thoracostomy or if an air leak persists, place a second chest tube and go to Step 16.

Step 16: If the pneumothorax/air leak persists after a second tube thoracostomy has been performed on the affected side, proceed with bronchoscopy to evaluate for major tracheobronchial injury. If injury is diagnosed, proceed with thoracotomy and repair. If the second tube thoracostomy controls the air leak, or if the bronchoscopy reveals no tracheobronchial injury, proceed to Step 17.

Step 17: If, after the initial hemothorax is drained, the chest tube accumulates >100 mL of blood per hour for 3 or more hours, proceed with exploratory thoracotomy. If bleeding is controlled, proceed to Step 18.

Step 18: If the mediastinum appears to be of normal width on the CXR and no other signs of a thoracic great vessel injury exist (pleural cap, indistinct aortic arch, obliteration of aortopulmonary window, displacement of nasogastric tube or mainstem bronchus), proceed to Step 20. If the mediastinum appears widened on CXR or if one or more of the other signs of great vessel injury are present, proceed to Step 19.

Step 19: Obtain an aortic and great vessel angiogram. If the angiogram demonstrates great vessel injury, proceed with emergent thoracotomy and repair. For blunt injuries and penetrating thoracoabdominal wounds, a peritoneal tap and lavage should be performed in the OR prior to thoracotomy to rule out intra-abdominal hemorrhage. For patients needing thoracotomy who are also suspected of having intracranial lesions that require operative intervention, a rapid computed tomography (CT) head scan may be obtained before thoracotomy, or diagnostic burr holes may be performed simultaneously with thoracotomy. If the great vessel angiogram has a negative result, go to Step 20.

Step 20: If the patient has clinical signs of cardiac tamponade, such as distended neck veins or distant heart sounds, or both, or has a penetrating injury in proximity to the precordial region, insert a CVP catheter in a subclavian or internal jugular vein. Perform three simultaneous CVP and MAP measurements over a 15-minute period. If the CVP is persistently <15 mm Hg, go to Step 23. If the patient's CVP is >20 mm Hg for three consecutive readings or is >15 mm Hg and rises over three successive measurements, proceed to Step 21.

Step 21: If, after the three readings in Step 20 have been performed, the MAP is <80 mm Hg or the HR is >110 beats/min, give 500 mL of 5% albumin or hetastarch (Hespan) over 10 minutes. After infusion is initiated, proceed to Step 22. If the MAP remains >80 mm Hg and the HR is <110 beats/min, proceed to Step 22 without giving an additional fluid bolus.

Step 22: Obtain echocardiogram or perform pericardiocentesis or subxyphoid window creation. If blood is present in the pericardial

Figure 5–3 *Continued*
sac, assume cardiac tamponade is present and proceed with exploratory thoracotomy or median sternotomy. Also, if at any time the patient's MAP falls >15 mm Hg over a 5-minute period, assume cardiac tamponade is present and proceed with exploratory thoracotomy or median sternotomy. If no blood is found in the pericardial sac, based on the results of echocardiography, pericardiocentesis, or subxyphoid window creation, proceed to Step 23.

Step 23: If the patient has an abdominal or thoracoabdominal gunshot wound (except one with a tangential "grazing" trajectory that could not possibly penetrate the abdominal cavity) or a stab wound with hypotension (MAP <80 mm Hg), diffuse tenderness, rebound tenderness, decreased bowel sounds, or other abdominal findings, exploratory laparotomy should be performed within 30 minutes. Patients with blunt injury and diffuse peritoneal irritation should undergo exploration. If the patient does not have diffuse peritoneal signs, proceed to Step 24.

Step 24: If the patient has a blunt injury or stab wound and has equivocal abdominal examination findings, proceed to Step 25.

Step 25: Perform at least three sequential abdominal examinations over a 15-minute period. If the patient's abdomen becomes nontender, proceed to Step 27. If equivocal examination results persist, proceed to Step 26.

Step 26: Proceed as follows:

1. If the patient has blunt injury, perform peritoneal tap and lavage or triple-contrast abdominal and pelvic CT; if either test has positive results, perform exploratory laparotomy within 30 minutes. If results are negative, proceed to Step 27.
2. If the patient has a stab wound over the rectus sheath, perform local wound exploration; if the wound extends through the anterior rectus sheath, perform either peritoneal tap and lavage or triple-contrast abdominal and pelvic CT. If either test yields positive results, perform exploratory laparotomy within 30 minutes. If the anterior rectus sheath has not been penetrated or if diagnostic test results are negative, proceed to Step 27.
3. If the patient has a stab wound between the lateral rectus sheath and the midaxillary line, either peritoneal tap and lavage or triple-contrast abdominal and pelvic CT should be performed. If either test yields a positive result, perform exploratory laparotomy within 30 minutes. If the patient has a stab wound posterior to the midaxillary line, perform triple-contrast abdominal and pelvic CT. If either test has a positive result, perform exploratory laparotomy within 30 minutes. If diagnostic test results are negative, proceed to Step 27.

Step 27: If the patient has evidence of head injury, drug ingestion, or ethanol intoxication, a normal abdominal examination may be inaccurate, and, therefore, the patient should undergo either peritoneal tap and lavage or triple-contrast abdominal and pelvic CT. If either has a positive result, proceed with exploratory laparotomy within 30 minutes; if results are negative, proceed to Step 28.

Step 28: If no pelvic fracture is present, proceed to Step 30. If the patient has a pelvic fracture, evaluate its stability. If the fracture is stable, proceed to Step 29. If the fracture is unstable, either immediately place Military Anti-Shock Trousers or emergently consult an orthopedist for external fixation.

Step 29: Perform serial Hgb/Hct measurements every 30 minutes. If the patient's Hgb/Hct drops and the patient needs >6 U PRBCs within 6 hours postadmission to maintain Hgb >10 g/dL or Hct >30%, perform pelvic vessel angiography for possible embolization. Proceed to Step 30. If Hgb/Hct remains stable, proceed to Step 30.

Step 30: Obtain measurements of arterial blood gases (ABGs). If the patient's Pa_{O_2} is <60 mm Hg on room air, administer 40% O_2 by facemask and proceed to Step 31. If, on room air, the patient's Pa_{O_2} is >60 mm Hg, observe the patient for subsequent signs of respiratory distress, hypotension, and new symptoms of thoracic or abdominal injury.

Step 31: After 40% O_2 has been administered for 10 minutes, obtain a repeat set of ABG measurements. If the Pa_{O_2} is still <60 mm Hg, intubate, ventilate, and reevaluate for thoracic or abdominal injury. If the Pa_{O_2} is >60 mm Hg, observe the patient and reevaluate him or her periodically.

MAP = mean arterial pressure; Hct = hematocrit; PRBC = packed red blood cells; HR = heart rate; CVP = central venous pressure.

procedures, monitoring systems, and therapeutic interventions in the management of trauma patients. These three activities should proceed concurrently along three parallel tracks according to the priorities described by the algorithm. This algorithm describes the clinical conditions and circumstances for the most important management decisions in blunt and penetrating trauma.

The entrance criteria include all patients with either blunt or penetrating injuries from thoracic or abdominal trauma. The general work-up includes rapid physical assessment; this step may be preempted by emergency situations, such as cardiac arrest and severe shock. In the latter circumstances, the work-up should proceed in parallel with resuscitation; treatment of shock, similar to CPR in cardiac arrest, takes precedence over diagnostic tests and other therapy. The routine minimal work-up should include blood type and crossmatch, spun Hct, complete blood count, portable chest radiograph, prothrombin time, partial thromboplastin time, serum electrolytes (sodium, potassium, chloride, bicarbonate), glucose, blood urea nitrogen, creatinine, and urinalysis. Abdominal radiography, arterial blood gas measurement, additional blood chemistries (such as calcium and amylase), and other tests may be performed if indicated.

Initial feasibility studies of this algorithm were carried out prospectively in a county hospital setting,[15, 16, 18] and, subsequently, in a prospective series of 1000 patients with possible truncal injury collected over a 13-month period. During this time, 2843 trauma patients were evaluated in the ED, 1457 were admitted to the hospital, and 326 were admitted to the surgical ICU.[19, 20] Of the 1000 patients in the study group, 338 (34%) had blunt trauma (292 accidents involving motor vehicles, 35 assaults, and 11 falls) and 662 (66%) had penetrating injuries (502 truncal gunshot wounds, 138 truncal stab wounds, 22 truncal shotgun wounds). Sixty (6%) patients (37 with penetrating injuries, 23 with blunt trauma) arrived at the ED with no signs of life and no cardiac electrical activity; these patients were pronounced dead on arrival and were excluded from analysis, leaving 940 patients in the study group. The outcomes of these study patients were evaluated in terms of type of trauma and deviations from the algorithm.

There were 135 deaths (14% mortality) in the study group of the 940 patients. One hundred (16%) of 625 patients with penetrating injuries died, and 35 (11%) of the 315 blunt trauma patients died. There were deviations from the algorithm in 58 (43%) of the 135 fatal cases in contrast to only 69 (9%) of the 805 survivors who were managed in compliance with the algorithm.

There were deviations in the management of 127 (14%) of the 940 study group patients; 58 (46%) of these 127 patients died, whereas only 77 (9%) of 813 patients whose management complied with the algorithm died ($P < .001$). The most common deviations were delayed operation (56 occurrences with 25 deaths, 45% mortality), transport of unstable patients to the radiology area (12 occurrences, six deaths, 50% mortality), and inappropriate observation instead of operation (12 occurrences, three deaths, 25% mortality).

Of the 940 patients, 105 (11%) had injury severity scores (ISS) above 50; 28 of 43 (65%) with deviations from the algorithm died, whereas 48 of 62 (77%) whose management complied with the algorithm died (not significant). Of the 264 patients with ISS scores greater than or equal to 20 and less than or equal to 50, 25 of 60 (42%) managed with deviations died, whereas only 23 of 193 (12%) whose management followed the algorithm died ($P < .001$). The remaining 571 patients had ISS scores below 20; five of 24 (21%) with deviations died, whereas only six of 547 (1%) who complied with the algorithm died ($P < .001$).

The data from this series suggest that the majority of preventable trauma deaths that occur in the periadmission period stem not from misunderstandings of the proper procedural management of trauma but from delays in intended therapy and from inadequate assessment of the patients' physiologic status, such as inappropriate transport to radiology or inappropriate observation. This is likely due to conventional approaches focusing on the diagnosis and treatment of specific injuries but not focusing on the rapid diagnosis and correction of circulatory derangements that cause early patient mortality.

These data support the hypotheses that (1) branch chain decision trees facilitate expeditious therapy and (2) therapeutic decisions based on specific, objective criteria rather than subjective clinical assessment will improve outcome when rapid executions of multiple diagnostic and interventional maneuvers are necessary for patient survival. We can conclude that patients with serious injuries are salvageable when appropriately and expediently managed and that those with ISS scores between 20 and 50 will show the greatest improvement in survival when managed by the algorithm.

PHYSIOLOGIC AND THERAPEUTIC PROBLEMS IN TRAUMA RESUSCITATION

Initial Monitoring

In emergency admissions and in the early phase of shock, circulation is initially monitored by:

- Blood pressure
- Heart rate
- Respiratory rate
- Temperature
- Hct
- CVP
- Electrocardiogram (ECG)
- Hourly urinary output with specific gravity or osmolality
- Blood gas/pH measurements

Blood pressure, heart rate, respiratory rate, and temperature ("vital signs") are used for the initial screening.

The Hct is used to diagnose and assess initial blood loss, provided there is time for extracellular water to cross the capillary membrane into the plasma volume. It usually takes 3 to 4 hours for blood losses to change the Hct significantly.

CVP is important as an endpoint during initial resuscitation to indicate plasma volume overload. CVP values of 20 mm Hg or more suggest (1) congestive cardiac failure, (2) overtransfusion or overadministration of fluids, or (3) too rapid administration of blood or fluids.[3]

The ECG is frequently used to detect and monitor suspected arrhythmias. Although it is appropriate for assessment of cardiac rhythm and electrical activity, the ECG is rarely useful in patients with hemorrhage, trauma, or sepsis, except to rule out associated cardiac problems.

Urinary output below 30 mL/hour may reflect inadequate blood volume, decreased renal blood flow, or impaired renal parenchymal function. If there is no preexisting renal damage, and if urinary specific gravity is greater than 1.018 or urine osmolality is more than 500 mOsm/L, urine output may reflect renal tissue perfusion. However, patients resuscitated with large volumes of sodium-rich fluids may have adequate urine output despite low blood volume.

The blood volume measurement, if done properly and accurately, is the most reliable means to evaluate blood volume status, particularly during unstable hemodynamic conditions.

Serial measurements of vital signs, Hct, CVP, hourly urinary output, blood volume, and blood gases provide the necessary information on which decisions for management can be based. If blood pressures fall precipitously after hemorrhage, however, fluid therapy must be started immediately and given vigorously. Subsequently, physiologic monitoring should be started as soon as possible to indicate when conservative therapy should give way to surgical intervention. A systematic record of monitored data provides a continuous evaluation of the circulatory status during initial resuscitation, subsequent therapy, operative intervention, and postoperative management.

Clinical Criteria for Fluid Therapy

The first and most important goal of the treatment of shock and its sequelae is to restore blood volume. However, criteria for achieving this goal have been poorly defined. Clinical studies in this area are often incompletely controlled with poor documentation for the degree of hypovolemia, for the extent of the blood volume correction, and for the time factors involved.

The clinical criteria most often used for adequate blood volume restoration are:

- Arterial pressure
- Heart rate
- Hct
- Urine output
- CVP
- Pulmonary arterial wedge pressures

In the initial hypotensive period, changes in these clinically monitored variables reflect physiologic compensations and decompensations for hypovolemia. In subsequent periods after the initial resuscitation, when patients become critically ill, most of these variables have been unreliable for evaluation of hypovolemia when compared with careful blood volume measurements.

Although the commonly monitored variables roughly correlate with hypovolemia in the initial hypotensive crisis, this is clearly not the case in the ICU patient in whom venous wall compliance changes compensate for blood volume alterations. Frequently, the initial resuscitation with sodium-rich solutions restores MAP and urine output without properly correcting unrecognized hypovolemia.

With massive crystalloid infusions, patients may still have suboptimal blood volume despite marked expansion of the interstitial fluid compartment and restoration of blood pressure. Furthermore, critically ill post-traumatic and postoperative patients, as well as those with malnutrition and chronic wasting diseases, often have hypovolemia with expanded extracellular water and reduced plasma protein concentrations.[24, 25]

This salt and water alteration is intensified by antidiuretic hormone and aldosterone. These fluid maldistributions are frequently unsuspected when vital signs, CVP, and urine output are the only criteria used for the assessment of volume status.

Management of the Trauma Patient Immediately After Admission to the Emergency Department

Severe hypovolemia, severe hypoxia, and upper airway obstruction are the most important and urgent problems of the emergency trauma victim, accounting for the majority of preventable trauma deaths in the early management period. These problems, although frequently life-threatening, are usually easily recognized clinically and are often readily correctable with appropriate therapy. Severe hypovolemia manifests as pallor, tachycardia, hypotension, altered mental status, oliguria, and cold, clammy skin. Hypoxia may present with cyanosis, ash-gray color, tachypnea, dilated nasal alae, suprasternal and intercostal retraction, and agitation. Upper airway obstruction presents with a wide range of symptoms; partial obstruction produces agitation, tachypnea, stridor, wheezing, and use of accessory breathing muscles, and total obstruction produces apnea, cyanosis, and altered mental status ranging from severe agitation to lethargy and collapse.

In extreme cases of these three common problems, rapid fluid administration, endotracheal intubation with mechanical ventilation, and CPR may be needed and take precedence over diagnostic and therapeutic maneuvers. After these catastrophic conditions are addressed and corrected, the other therapeutic goals should be defined and treatment prioritized according to the life-threatening capacity of each condition.

Resuscitation of the Trauma Patient Using Prospectively Tested Physiologic Goals

Approximately 50% of all trauma fatalities occur at the time of or shortly after injury. Lethal hypoxia or exsanguination occurring within 12 to 24 hours after emergency admission is responsible for another 20% of trauma deaths; a small percentage of these patients die in the operating room. In most trauma fatalities, however, patients die of multiple vital organ failures either in the early postinjury period or weeks later in the surgical ICU. These organ failures have their origins in earlier unrecognized tissue hypoxia from hypovolemia and uneven (i.e., maldistributed, microcirculatory flow). Therapy, therefore, should be directed to the major underlying pathophysiology of shock (i.e., inadequate oxygen transport from low or maldistributed flow at the organ and microcirculatory levels). The low blood volume or low oxygen consumption ($\dot{V}O_2$) in the early period and the normal or high $\dot{V}O_2$ in the middle or late period are often less than needed to meet increased metabolic requirements.

In general, therapy should be titrated to attain the optimal goals rather than given as a standardized prescribed dose. Moreover, treatment of one vital organ failure can jeopardize the function of another vital organ. In multiple vital organ failure, therapy for each impaired organ should be titrated to appropriate physiologic goals to avoid compromising the other vital organs. The major objective is to correct the life-threatening physiologic as well as physical problems. At the least, it is necessary to institute early therapy for potentially lethal circulatory problems before they become irreversible. The longer shock or perfusion deficiencies persist, the more likely an unfavorable outcome.

Supranormal Cardiac Index, Oxygen Delivery, and Volume of Oxygen Consumption Values as Therapeutic Goals in Severe Trauma

In an empirical study of a series of 90 severely traumatized patients, 60 of whom survived the initial management period but had significant (>2000 mL) blood loss, Bishop and colleagues observed that the 60 survivors had significantly higher values of cardiac index (CI), oxygen delivery, and $\dot{V}O_2$ than did the 30 nonsurvivors and that these differences were most pronounced in the first 24 hours after injury. These empirically observed survivor values were then tested as resuscitation goals in a prospective double-arm formal clinical trial and showed a significant improvement in mortality (18% versus 34%, $P < .05$) and reduction in shock-related organ failures (mean $\pm$ SD $= 0.74 \pm 0.28$ per patient versus 1.62 ± 0.45 per patient, $P < .05$) compared with conventional treatment. These data suggest that post-traumatic increases in CI, DO_2, and $\dot{V}O_2$ are primary physiologic compensations that, if inadequate, may result in organ failure and death and that timely vigorous therapy that augments these compensations will improve survival.

Therapeutic Efficacy

If hemodynamic and oxygen transport variables are measured before, during, and after the administration of a therapeutic agent with a known physiologic action, important information is often revealed about the nature of that disturbed circulation. That is, responsiveness to the action of an agent suggests that a circulatory deficiency was present and that there was also some reserve capacity that could be stimulated to improve function. Failure of response suggests one of the following:

1. The therapy was ineffective.
2. The patient had limited physiologic reserve capacity.
3. The disorder was irreversible.

A trial of therapy with agents of specific actions (e.g., plasma expanders) and agents with inotropic actions (alpha and beta agonists), such as dobutamine, dopamine, isoproterenol, and norepinephrine, may thus provide physiologic data that have diagnostic, therapeutic, and prognostic value.

Because bulk transport of oxygen is the important circulatory function, $\dot{V}O_2$ may be used to evaluate the effectiveness of a given therapeutic agent. Short-term changes in $\dot{V}O_2$ during and immediately after administration of therapeutic agents to patients in shock may reflect changes in tissue perfusion. Prompt increases in $\dot{V}O_2$ after administration of specific agents suggests that therapy improved tissue perfusion and tissue oxygenation.

Fluid Therapy of Acute Circulatory Problems

The following fluid therapy recommendations for resuscitation of acute hypotensive and hypovolemic problems are proposed:

1. Red blood cell losses should be replaced with red blood cells.
2. Water loss from dehydration should be replaced with crystalloids.
3. Plasma volume losses should be replaced with plasma or its colloidal equivalent (i.e., plasma protein fraction, 5% or 25% albumin, hydroxyethyl starch, or other artificial colloids).

Saline, glucose, and Ringer's lactate solution in various combinations are commonly used for initial resuscitation in mild degrees of shock and subsequent replacement of daily fluid losses. In general, 3 to 5 L of fluid usually replaces acute losses in mild to moderately ill patients who do not have extrarenal fluid losses and who tolerate nothing by mouth. However, patients with enteric fistulas, diarrhea, vomiting, large volumes of nasogastric suction, and other extrarenal fluid losses may require several times this volume to replace the estimated fluid losses and maintain blood pressure, heart rate, urine output, CVP, and Hct.

After the estimated extrarenal fluid losses are replaced, the optimal volume is best determined by fluid-balance studies that collect, measure, and record urinary, nasogastric suction, fecal, and enteric fistula losses; the estimated insensible losses are added to this. The intraoperative insensible losses occurring when the peritoneal or pleural cavities are opened may be 400 to 700 mL/hr (6 to 9 mL/kg/hr), depending on ambient temperature and humidity.

In the patient with severe shock, the initial resuscitation should be at least one-third colloids to maintain the administered fluids in the blood volume compartment. By the time patients reach the ICU, however, they usually have already been given excessive crystalloids; in these circumstances, fluid challenge with 25 g of concentrated (25%) albumin, 500 mL of plasma protein fraction (5% albumin), fresh frozen plasma, or starch is recommended. Whole blood or packed red blood cells should be given in sufficient quantities to maintain Hct at about 34%. The therapeutic goals of the critically ill shock and trauma patient are empirically determined by survivors' mean values for CI (5.0 L/min/m^2), $\dot{D}O_2$ (800 mL/min/m^2), and $\dot{V}O_2$ (170 mL/min/m^2).[23, 26, 27]

SUMMARY: THE ALGORITHMIC APPROACH TO DECISION MAKING

The algorithmic approach does not attempt to take away decisions from the physician or to take the art out of medicine. In a sense, algorithms resemble postoperative standing orders that specify the volume and rates for fluids or vasopressor infusions at various blood pressures. The resuscitation algorithms are not just guidelines to organize the care by serial steps; they apply clinically tested principles in a prioritized manner.

Clinical algorithms attempt to find a middle ground between the one extreme that all patients are different and must be handled individually and the other extreme that all patient care can be diagrammed and computerized. All patients are certainly different, but there are common decisions on which diagnosis and therapy are based; these decisions can be expressed in a logical format for most clinical problems, no matter how complicated.

In practice, algorithms are not meant to be followed slavishly; minor deviations will occur in the work-up because of extraneous circumstances not covered by the algorithm. However, carefully thought-out, peer-reviewed protocols that are the result of well-established, literature-supported strategies can be followed in major clinical decisions. Moreover, they are useful in structuring therapy for complex physiologic problems.

The algorithmic approach places the most common problems in a prioritized order, thereby preselecting the patients coming to each node, and then provides criteria based on decision rules for expeditious diagnosis, monitoring, and therapeutic decisions. Problems are addressed in the order of their life-threatening capability. Algorithms are particularly useful when time is of great importance, such as the resuscitation of emergency shock and trauma patients. Because of its objectivity and usefulness as a teaching tool, the algorithmic approach is of practical benefit in the training of residents and students in teaching hospitals but is also useful in community hospitals where physicians manage emergency patients less frequently.

Inadequate fluids and delays in resuscitation are clearly related to an increased incidence of shock-related complications: shock lung, acute renal failure, cardiopulmonary arrest, sepsis, cardiac failure, and fluid overload. When the algorithm is followed satisfactorily, resuscitation is faster and fewer shock-related complications occur, particularly in patients with severe associated illnesses in which the margin for error is small. The shorter surgical ICU stay, shorter hospitalization, and reduced mortality in these patients indicate cost effectiveness in this approach. Algorithms provide a potentially useful approach to complex clinical situations fraught with emotionally held opinions, anecdotal descriptions, and judgmatic pronouncements repeated in the manner of a party line.

References

1. Shoemaker WC, Bryan-Brown CW: Resuscitation and immediate care of the critically ill and injured patient. Semin Drug Treat 1973; 3:249.
2. McDonald CJ: Use of a computer to detect and respond to clinical events: Its effect on clinical behavior. Ann Intern Med 1976; 84:162.
3. Shoemaker WC: Algorithm for resuscitation: A systematic plan for immediate care of the injured or postoperative patient. Crit Care Med 1975; 3:127.
4. Shoemaker WC: Algorithm for early recognition and management of cardiac tamponade. Crit Care Med 1975; 3:59.
5. Larsen KT, Vickery MD, Collis PB, et al: A logical algorithmic alternative to a non-system. J Am Coll Emerg Physicians 1973; 2:183.
6. Slay LE, Riskin WG: Algorithm-directed triage in an emergency department. J Am Coll Emerg Physicians 1976; 5:869.
7. Greenfield S, Anderson H, Winickoff RM, et al: Nurse-protocol management of low back pain: Outcomes, patient satisfaction, and efficiency of primary care. West J Med 1975; 123:350.
8. Sox HC, Sox CH, Tompkins RK: Training of physicians' assistants by a clinical algorithm system. N Engl J Med 1973; 258:818.
9. Ellis BW: Use of logic based flow patterns in the investigation and management of surgical disorders. Br J Surg 1975; 62: 800.
10. Shoemaker WC, Hopkins JA, Greenfield S, et al: Resuscitation algorithm for management of acute emergencies. J Am Coll Emerg Physicians 1978; 7:361.
11. Eiseman B, Watkyns R: Surgical Decision Making. Philadelphia, WB Saunders, 1978.
12. Hopkins JA, Shoemaker WC, Chang PC, et al: Results of a clinical trial on the use of an emergency resuscitation algorithm. Crit Care Med 1983; 11:621.
13. Shoemaker WC, Hopkins JA: Clinical aspects of resuscitation with and without an algorithm: Relative importance of various decisions. Crit Care Med 1983; 11:630.
14. Shoemaker WC: Resuscitation of the critically ill patient: Use of branch chain decision trees to improve outcome. Emerg Med Clin North Am 1986; 4:655.
15. Shoemaker WC, Corley RD, Liu M, et al: Development and testing of a decision tree for blunt trauma. Crit Care Med 1988; 16:1199.
16. Liu M, Shoemaker WC, Kram HB, Harrier HD: Design and prospective evaluation of an algorithm for penetrating truncal injuries. Crit Care Med 1988; 16:1191.
17. Shoemaker WC, Kvetan V, Fyodora V, et al: Clinical algorithm for initial resuscitation in disasters. Crit Care Clin 1991; 7:363.
18. Bishop MH, Shoemaker WC, Jackson G, et al: An algorithm for blunt and penetrating truncal trauma. Crit Care Clin 1991; 7:383.
19. Bishop MH, Shoemaker WC, Jackson G, et al: Evaluation of a single comprehensive algorithm for the management of blunt and penetrating thoracic and abdominal trauma. Am Surgeon 1991; 57:712.
20. Bishop MH, Shoemaker WC, Shori S, et al: Evaluation of a comprehensive algorithm for the management of blunt and penetrating truncal trauma: Report of 1000 cases. J Trauma (in press).
21. Shippy CR, Appel PL, Shoemaker WC: Reliability of clinical monitoring to assess blood volume in critically ill patients. Crit Care Med 1984; 12:107.
22. Wo CJ, Shoemaker WC, Appel PL, Bishop MH: Unreliability of blood pressure and heart rate for evaluation of circulatory stability in emergency resuscitation and critical illness. Crit Care Med 1992; 21:95.
23. Shoemaker WC, Bland RD, Appel PL: Therapy of critically ill postoperative patients based on outcome prediction and prospective clinical trials. Surg Clin North Am 1985; 65:811.
24. Elwyn DH, Bryan-Brown CW, Shoemaker WC: Nutritional aspects of body water dislocations in postoperative and depleted patients. Ann Surg 1975; 182:76.
25. Shoemaker WC, Bryan-Brown CW, Quigley L, et al: Body fluid shifts in depletion and post-stress states and their correction with adequate nutrition. Surg Gynecol Obstet 1973; 136:371.
26. Bishop MH, Wo CJ, Appel PL, et al: Relationship between supranormal circulatory values, time delays, and outcome in severely traumatized patients. Crit Care Med 1993; 21:56.
27. Bishop MH, Shoemaker WC, Kram HB, et al: Prospective trial of

survivor values of cardiac index, oxygen delivery, and oxygen consumption as resuscitation endpoints in severe trauma. J Trauma 1995; 38:780–7

28. Shoemaker WC, Schluchter M, Hopkins JA, et al: Comparison of the relative effectiveness of colloids and crystalloids in emergency resuscitation. Am J Surg 1981; 142:73.

Intravenous and Intra-arterial Access

M. H. Parsa, MD • Cyrus J. Parsa, MD
Angus C. Sampath, DSc, MD

Techniques for vascular catheterization that permit long-term integrity and sterility are described based on personal experience with 22,462 catheters from May 1968 to December 1997 (Tables 6–1 to 6–3).[1–4] We believe that most line-related infections are due to fluid administration–related infections. Contamination and clinical sepsis during preparation and the handling of intravenous line connections are common dangers that lead to clinical sepsis. The infusion fluids were used as culture media at room temperature for growth of commonly encountered microorganisms. These results and precautionary recommendations against septic complications,[5, 6] as well as measures for early detection and management of complications of insertion and long-term maintenance, are outlined in Tables 6–4 and 6–5. Table 6–6 lists contraindications to subclavian and internal jugular venous catheterization.

INTRAVENOUS ACCESS

Percutaneous Insertion of Peripheral Vein Catheters

Catheterizations of readily accessible subcutaneous veins are of vital importance in critically ill patients; these veins should be utilized sparingly for essential purposes and duration. Upper-extremity veins should be sought with sterile operative technique first; then the external jugular veins and veins of the feet and ankles should be accessed.

First, the physician applies a tourniquet in the extremities to impede venous return, making the desired vein detectable visually or by palpation. The tourniquet is then temporarily released while the area is shaved and prepared with povidone-iodine solution. Skin debris is removed with a sterile gauze and firm friction motions in all directions; this aids penetration of the antiseptic preparation into the epidermis. A 5-minute interval should be allowed for povidone-iodine drying to release free iodine, the active ingredient. The tourniquet is reapplied tightly, and the skin is first pierced by the needle catheter, which is then advanced subcutaneously for 1.5 to 2 cm. The vein lumen is entered from the top or from either side.

Withdrawal of blood by the syringe confirms intravenous catheter tip placement. The needle is removed, the catheter is advanced and connected to the fluid infusion tubing, and the free flow of the fluid into the vein is confirmed by lack of extravasation. The presence of a subcutaneous bulge accompanied by slowing of the gravity drip indicates infiltration; the catheter then should be replaced. The correctly placed catheter is then fixed to the skin by tape. The skin entry/exit site is prepared again with povidone-iodine solution followed by application of 3 to 5 g of 1% silver sulfadiazine antimicrobial cream and covered with sterile gauze taped firmly in place. The extremity, preferably, should be elevated above the heart level to accelerate venous flow.

TABLE 6–1. Summary of Experience with Conventional Percutaneous Venous Catheterization Techniques (May 1968–December 1997)

Catheterization by Percutaneous Venipuncture	No.†
1. Supraclavicular subclavian or junctional*	6256
2. Infraclavicular subclavian	2323
3. Internal jugular from posterior and anterior border of sternocleidomastoid muscle	489
4. External jugular	50
5. Cephalic	50
6. Basilic	50
7. Femoral	359
8. Right brachial	3
9. Left brachial	1
Total catheterizations	9581

*Supraclavicular subclavian vein puncture at the junctional zone of the subclavian and internal jugular veins.

†Includes Swan-Ganz, subcutaneously tunneled Silastic, triple-lumen, double-lumen, venous hemodialysis, and totally implanted catheters.

Central Venous Catheters

Long intravenous catheters can be introduced through the basilic or cephalic veins for the tip to reach the superior vena cava[7]; this type of central venous (CV) catheter, however, may become thrombosed in a few days, forming a tender, hard cord along the course of the vein, and may need to be removed.

The external jugular vein on either side, which may be visible during inspiration and expiratory phases in the supine or Trendelenburg position, can be catheterized according to the previously described skin preparation followed by sterile draping with the operator using sterile gloves. Long catheters may be advanced via the external jugular vein into the superior vena cava, but the catheter may not pass through the sharp angle where the external jugular vein joins the subclavian vein. When the catheter is thin and pliable, it may be maintained in the superior vena cava for 2 to 6 weeks. Short catheters usually can be maintained in the external jugular vein for 5 to 7 days before the vein becomes thrombosed. Potential problems with internal jugular vein catheters are air embolus or bleeding from inadvertent disconnections of the tubing.[8]

When burns or skin infections preclude the use of upper-extremity and external jugular veins, the physician uses foot and ankle veins for temporary venous access with the techniques of skin preparation, catheter insertion, and dressing care as just described.

When the superficial veins cannot be catheterized by percutaneous puncture, they may be surgically exposed and catheterized by direct needle puncture or a venotomy (venous cutdown). The rate of wound and catheter infection is high if sterile technique is not observed. If intravenous therapy is required longer than 10 days, a subclavian or internal jugular vena cava catheter should be inserted from the beginning of treatment to spare superficial veins for subsequent emergency intravenous access.

TABLE 6–2. Summary of Experience in Insertion of Intravenous Catheters by Special Techniques (May 1968–June 1985)

Technique	Access Site/Vein	No. Cases	No. Catheters
Double catheter by percutaneous puncture			
Two punctures in one vein	Subclavian	185	370
	Internal jugular	13	26
	Femoral	10	20
Two punctures in adjacent veins	Internal jugular and subclavian	40	80
One puncture (two guide wires via Swan-Ganz catheter sheath, two catheters over guide wires)	Subclavian	17	34
	Femoral	2	4
Double catheters in one vein by cutdown	Internal jugular	1	2
	External jugular	4	8
	Cephalic subclavian	6	12
	External iliac	1	2
	Common iliac	1	2
	Inferior vena cava	2	4
	Gonadal	1	2
	Axillary	2	4
Single catheter by cutdown	Subclavian	24	24
	Internal jugular	20	20
	Inferior epigastric	7	7
	Lateral thoracic	6	6
	Cephalic	60	60
	Basilic	15	15
	Brachial	15	15
	External jugular	25	25
	Saphenous	100	100
Intraoperative, abdominal	Gonadal	7	7
	Portal	22	22
Thoracotomy	Greater azygos	1	1
	Right atrium	2	2
Intracostal	Anterolateral	4	4
Intrasternal	Body of sternum	1	1
Intra-arterial	Left subclavian artery	1	1
Total cases		595	
Total catheters			880

TABLE 6–3. Variety and Number of Double-Lumen and Triple-Lumen Central Venous Catheters Inserted (in Order of Preference for Safety Based on Clinical Applicability) from July 1985 to December 1997

Approach	Vein	Double Catheters		Triple Catheters		
Right supraclavicular	Subclavian	2176		20		
Left supraclavicular	Subclavian	1904		23		
Right infraclavicular	Subclavian	576		18		
Left infraclavicular	Subclavian	572		13		
Right posterior sternomastoid border	Internal jugular	148		1		
Left posterior sternomastoid border	Internal jugular	125		0		
Right supraclavicular and right posterior border	Subclavian and internal jugular	53		4		
Left supraclavicular and left posterior border	Subclavian and internal jugular	42		4		
Right supraclavicular and right infraclavicular	Subclavian	77		7		
Left supraclavicular and left infraclavicular	Subclavian	100		4		
Right infraclavicular and right posterior border	Subclavian and internal jugular	18		0		
Left infraclavicular and left posterior border	Subclavian and internal jugular	18		0		
Right groin	Femoral	41		1		
Left groin	Femoral	2		0		
Total cases		5852	+	95	=	5950*
Total catheters		11,704	+	285	=	12,001*

*Includes three cases each with four catheters (not listed in table).

TABLE 6–4. Risk Factors for Complications in Central Venous Catheterization and Long-Term Maintenance

Inadvertent Arterial Puncture

- Hypertension
- Coagulopathy
- Long and large-bore needles
- Lack of experience of the operator*
- Tortuous or aneurysmal arteries

Inadvertent Puncture of Lymphatic Ducts

- Portal hypertension
- Intravenous drug abuse (venous thrombosis increasing lymphatic flow)

Inadvertent Puncture of Lung Apex

- Apical blebs
- Emaciation
- Lung diseases (COPD, PCP, and TB)
- Old age
- Long needles (relative to the thickness of soft tissue between the skin and lung apex)
- History of iatrogenic pneumothorax consequent to central venous catheterization attempts
- Mechanical ventilation with a high PEEP and large tidal volume

Air Embolus

- Hypovolemia and low venous blood pressure
- Labored inspiratory efforts and tachypnea
- Inappropriate position of the patient (head elevated) during subclavian/internal jugular vein puncture/cannulation
- Accidental disconnection of the catheter from the intravenous tubing (patient in upright position)
- Via subclavian or internal jugular catheter tract just removed and skin site not covered by sterile bandage

Intravenous Catheter-Related Infection

- Contaminated technique of insertion and/or maintenance
- Immunocompromised state
- Terminal cancer state
- Long-term indwelling intravenous catheter or therapy

Clot Formation

- Catheter malposition and retraction/regression of the tip
- Hypercoagulability states
- Catheter infection
- Chemically and physically irritative catheters and infusion fluids
- Long-term indwelling catheters

Clogging/Obstruction of Catheter/Intravenous Tubing

- Sharp kinking of catheter/infusion tubing
- Blood reflux into the catheter after intravenous fluids run dry
- Placement of intravenous fluids bags/bottles below the heart level with the intravenous tubings open to allow blood reflux

Accidental Removal of Catheter

- Restless and uncooperative patients†
- Inexperienced patient care, including patient transport team members in protection of central venous catheters‡
- Inadequate catheter maintenance by nurses/physicians

Severity of Sequelae of Complications

- Delayed recognition
- Inappropriate and/or inadequate treatment

*Lack of experience of the operator is a risk factor for all technical complications.

†Lack of patient cooperation is a major risk factor for many of the technical and long-term maintenance complications. Restless patients should be deeply sedated and hand restrained at least during the procedure.

‡Lack of experience of long-term maintenance team members is a risk factor for all long-term maintenance complications.

COPD = chronic obstructive pulmonary disease; PCP = *Pneumocystis carinii* pneumonia; TB = tuberculosis; PEEP = positive end-expiratory pressure.

TABLE 6–5. Potential Complications of Central Venous Catheters in Percutaneous Insertion and Long-Term Maintenance

Subclavian and Internal Jugular Veins

- Puncture of the pleural dome alone
- Puncture of the pleural dome and lung apex
- Clinically or radiologically detectable pneumothorax*
- Hemothorax and/or soft-tissue and mediastinal hematoma
- Needle injury to the adjacent arteries
- Puncture of lymphatic ducts, lymphorrhagia, chylomediastinum, and chylothorax
- Catheter misplacement in pleural cavity and consequent deposition of fluids and blood infusates in the pleural space
- Venous air embolus
- Injury to vertebral vessels with possible brain stem ischemic damage

Subclavian Veins

- Injury to brachial plexus directly by the needle or indirectly by the pressure of a tense arterial origin hematoma
- Injury to the clavicle or first-rib periosteums, cartilages, or ligaments and consequent osteitis/chondritis and calcific reactions

Internal Jugular

- Needle injury to the vagus nerve, phrenic nerve, cervical sympathetic chain, stellate ganglion, and cervical plexus
- Ischemic brain infarction caused by injury or clot and air embolism via the carotid artery
- Needle injury to the trachea and esophagus
- Injury to transverse processes of the cervical vertebrae with consequent reactions and infections of periosteum and bone
- Brain infarct caused by venous thrombosis extending to intracranial venous sinuses

All Venipuncture/Cannulation Techniques and Long-Term Catheters

- Inadvertent arterial puncture and consequent soft-tissue hematoma, intracavitary and external bleeding, false aneurysm, and arteriovenous fistulas
- Detour of the catheter tip into a branch
- Catheter tip in apposition to the vein wall and consequent wall perforation/erosion
- Catheter tip advanced too far (longer catheters)
- Catheter shorter than the desirable length or retraction/regression of catheter tip back into smaller veins
- Catheter tip positioned against the blood flow
- Clot and fibrinous sleeve formation
- Thrombosis of the vein and thromboembolism
- Catheter-related infections
- Catheter shredding and catheter embolus
- Guide wire embolus
- External bleeding from catheter skin site (venous or arterial)
- Accidental removal of catheters
- Clogging of catheters

*A chest x-ray film taken at the end of the forced expiratory phase with the patient in an upright or opposite lateral decubitus position is most likely to show a minimal pneumothorax. We do not know the minimal amount of free air in the pleural space that will show as pneumothorax radiologically. A CT scan of the chest is more sensitive to show small amounts of pneumothorax. Clinically, 10% to 15% pneumothorax is necessary to sense diminished breath sounds by auscultation while the patient is breathing with normal tidal volume.

TABLE 6–6. Contraindications for Subclavian and Internal Jugular Central Venous Catheterization

Absolute and General

Conditions of severe bleeding tendency and coagulopathy states
Persistent shock
Obstruction of the superior and inferior venae cavae, innominate, subclavian, and internal jugular veins and recently failed attempts at cannulation by an experienced operator
Respiratory distress, tachypnea, and labored inspirations
Present traumatic injury to the superior vena cava, innominate, internal jugular or subclavian veins
Patient's refusal or retraction of previously given consent

Relative and Specific

In process of cardiopulmonary resuscitation (external thoracic cardiac compressions)
In restless and uncooperative patients
Infection, burns, or presence of cancerous lymph nodes in the area of planned vein puncture
Tracheostomy with copious secretions close to planned vein puncture site
Left supraclavicular subclavian or internal jugular vein puncture attempt low in the neck, in cirrhotics
Infraclavicular vein puncture attempt when costoclavicular space is very narrow
Supraclavicular vein puncture attempt when the outer end of clavicle is going steeply cephalad and the position cannot be corrected
Severe hypertension, tortuosity of the arteries, and proximity of an aneurysm to the vein
When attempt in one side has resulted in a severe complication at the time or even previously
When sterile technique cannot be observed in nonemergency intravenous access establishment
Lack of experience of the operator without direct expert supervision

Indications for Placement of Intravenous Catheters with Central Tip Location

The indications for central vein catheters are:

1. Central venous pressure monitoring.
2. Long-term infusion of medications, hypertonic, hypotonic, and other solutions irritating to the vessel.
3. Need for long-term (>10 days) intravenous access.
4. Venous hemodialysis.
5. No accessible peripheral superficial veins.
6. Pulmonary artery catheters.
7. Transvenous cardiac pacemakers.

The main deep veins accessible for percutaneous needle catheterization are (1) subclavian, (2) internal jugular, and (3) femoral. The order of preference is (1) supraclavicular approach to the subclavian vein, (2) infraclavicular approach, (3) internal jugular, and (4) femoral vein. Veins on the right side of the body are the first choice unless precluded by anatomic abnormalities, venous blockage or other pathologic conditions, and bedside obstacles.

Subclavian Vein to Superior Vena Cava Catheterization

With necessary technical skills and aseptic precautions, the subclavian vein can be catheterized from above (preferred) or below the clavicle (Fig. 6–1*A, B*). The subclavian vein has a *lateral* segment overlying the first rib and a *medial* segment overlying the pleural dome.

Catheterization of the subclavian vein in the first segment is recommended to avoid puncturing the pleural dome and lung apex. When this approach is not successful, the needle is advanced supraclavicularly and puncture of the second segment is attempted over the pleural dome (Fig. 6–2). In this approach, one should advance the needle tangentially with gentle negative pressure in the syringe in order to detect vein entry and to prevent the needle piercing the posterior vein wall into the pleural dome or lung apex.

In some patients, particularly those with contractured shoulders, the outer end of the clavicle moves cephalad, making supraclavicular approach difficult or impossible; instead, the vein may be more accessible infraclavicularly. Also in this approach, we try to enter the vein in the first segment overlying the rib, but it is hard to tell when the needle tip crosses the first rib where it may puncture the pleural dome (Fig. 6–3).

Internal Jugular Route to Superior Vena Cava Catheterization

The internal jugular runs cephalad to caudad between anterior scalene and sternocleidomastoid muscles. The vein also runs

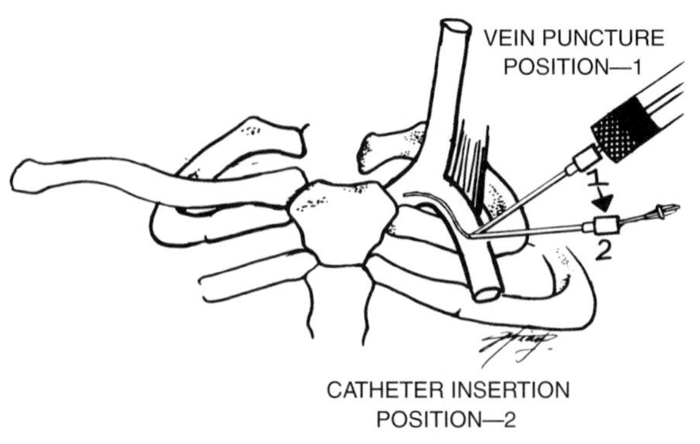

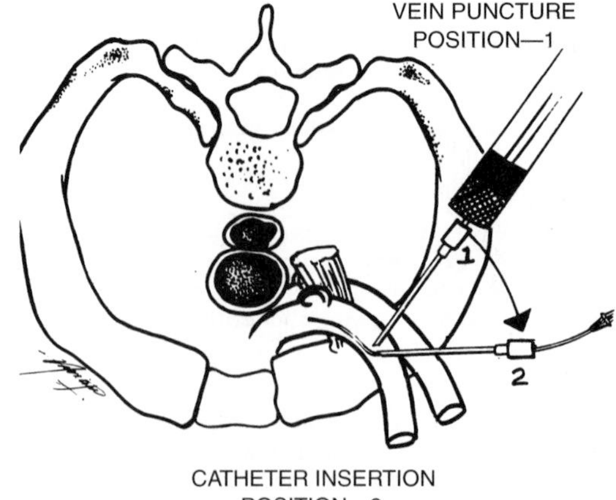

Figure 6–1. Puncture and catheterization of the left subclavian vein by the supraclavicular approach in the vein segment superimposed on the first rib. Following puncture of the vein, evidenced by aspirating blood with a free flow in the syringe (position 1), the shaft of the needle is moved in line with the course of the vein, as much as possible (position 2). The catheter is then inserted.

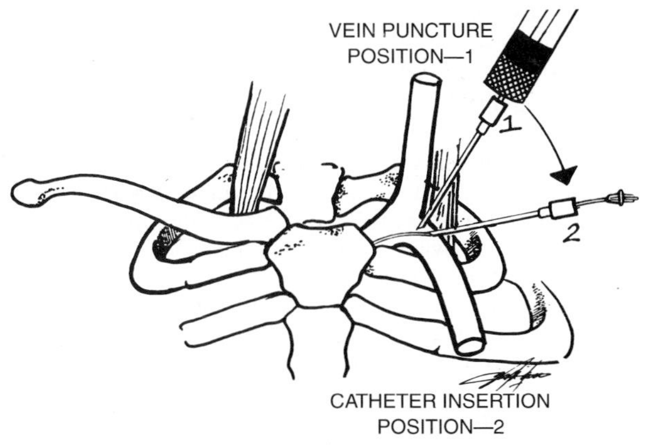

FRONTAL PLANE

Figure 6–2. Puncture and catheterization of the left subclavian vein by the supraclavicular approach in the vein segment medial to the first rib. When the subclavian vein is punctured in this segment, the puncture of the pleural dome and lung apex is more likely, especially if the needle traverses the posterior wall of the vein; this happens when the walls of the vein collapse against the pressure exerted by the needle tip.

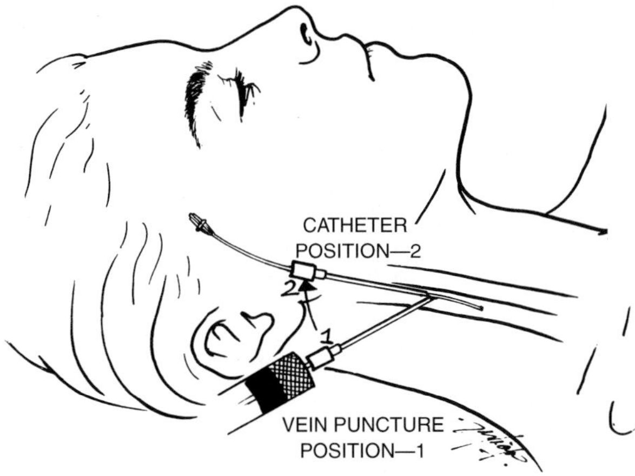

SIDE VIEW PLANE

Figure 6–4. Internal jugular puncture from the lateral border of the sternocleidomastoid muscle. The needle at 45° is advanced to the lateral border of the muscle and 45° to the frontal plane (position 1), with the patient's face turned 45° to the opposite side. Following vein puncture, the needle shaft is moved in line with the axis of the vein to insert the catheter (position 2).

in the slightly lateral to medial and anterior to posterior directions. The vein on the right side is usually larger and more distant from the common carotid artery. The vein should be punctured from the lateral border of the sternocleidomastoid muscle; this approach may be facilitated with the patient in the supine or Trendelenburg position to increase jugular venous pressure. The needle tip is advanced into the vein from the anterior wall, moving caudad rather than from the lateral wall directed medially, which may inadvertently traverse the vein and puncture the common carotid artery (Fig. 6–4).

Femoral Vein to Inferior Vena Cava Catheterization

When the previously described approaches are ineffective, femoral vein (inferior vena cava) catheters may be used, if needed, for short-term fluid therapy. In adults, the groin is shaved and prepared with antiseptic solution and the catheter is inserted under sterile technique. A pliable femoral catheter with a small diameter is safer; in patients with hypercoagulability states, thromboembolism can develop.[9, 10]

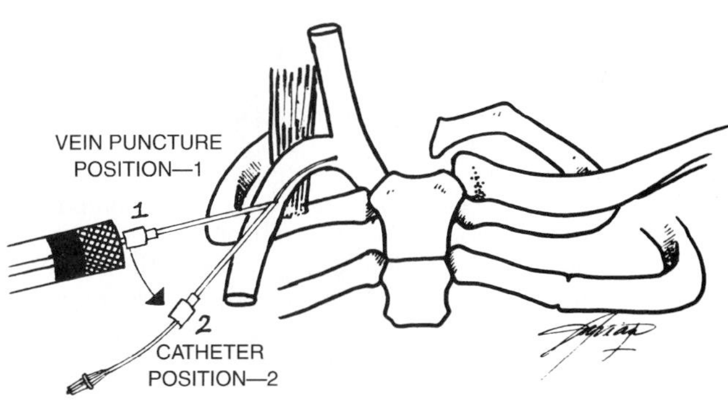

FRONTAL PLANE

Figure 6–3. Puncture of the right subclavian vein infraclavicularly in the segment over the first rib (position 1) and cannulation after the needle shaft is moved along the course of the vein (position 2).

Unusual Intravenous Access Techniques

When these techniques fail to yield intravenous access, we have used a variety of the following unusual approaches: (1) access by operative exposure of saphenous or femoral veins in patients who are pulseless and (2) exposure of the common iliac vein and inferior vena cava extraperitoneally through an oblique incision in the lower lateral abdominal wall. During intra-abdominal operations, when a previous intravenous access has been lost and no other access can be gained outside the operative field, intravenous access via the portal vein branches, the right gonadal vein, or directly into the inferior vena cava has been used.[11-13] Percutaneous translumbar catheterization of the inferior vena cava has been reported.[14, 15] In patients with no intravenous access, such as chronic intravenous drug abusers or chronic and repetitive intravenous therapy for medical management, access into the spongeous bone marrow (such as the ribs, sternum, iliac crest, or tibial plateau in children) can provide entry points into the venous circulation via a needle, but the infusate must be forced in by a pump. Insertion of a short cannula into the interspaces of the ribs subfascially and extrapleurally provides a rapid absorption area for infiltrated fluid.

If a patient without intravenous access has a cardiac arrest, an arterial access established by percutaneous puncture or cutdown can be used for intravascular medications, except for vasoconstrictors, until blood pressure is reestablished; then intra-arterially tolerated fluids can be infused only by pump. If all of these access techniques are unsuccessful, a right anterolateral thoracotomy in the fifth interspace provides access to the greater azygos vein or the right atrium after a pericardiotomy. One or two catheters may be inserted into the atrium by direct needle puncture or, preferably, by the Seldinger technique.

When the access site is exposed by cutdown, the catheter should be inserted by direct needle puncture with the Seldinger technique or through a small venotomy incision with subsequent repair of the venotomy site rather than ligation of the vein, since it is always possible that the vein will recanalize after catheter removal.

Varieties of Intravenous Catheters

The desirability of a catheter depends on low coagulogenicity. The more pliable, shorter, and smaller-diameter catheters result in less clot formation than the semirigid, longer catheters with larger diameters. When double-lumen or triple-lumen catheters are used, intravenous fluids should always be infused at safe speeds through each lumen. When any lumen has no or very slow flow, microbial contaminants may grow in the stagnant channel. The incidence of catheter-related infections is higher in indwelling catheters with no flow. Our data on the growth of microorganisms in various intravenous fluid solutions showed that undiluted heparin or 50% to 70% glucose inhibits growth of microorganisms. Therefore, channels with no flow must be filled with undiluted heparin or 50% to 70% glucose to inhibit bacterial growth.

Subcutaneously Tunneled Central Venous Catheters

These central venous catheters are utilized for long-term infusions. The catheters are inserted either by percutaneous needle puncture of the vein or by cutdown. Following advancement of the catheter tip into the lower part of the superior vena cava, the external end of the catheter is brought out 10 to 20 cm away from the insertion site through a subcutaneous tunnel that is easily accessible by the patient to provide self-care of the site. In infection prone patients, the safest environment for such catheter insertions is the operating room. When in doubt, the location of the tip should be confirmed by fluoroscopy in the operating suite where adjustments can be readily made. However, conventional untunneled central venous catheters are effective, safer, and less costly.[16]

Venous Hemodialysis Catheters

The venous hemodialysis catheter is inserted via the internal jugular or subclavian vein and the tip advanced into the superior vena cava. Occasionally when these veins are inaccessible, the femoral vein can be used; the right side is preferred. These large semirigid catheters are associated with a high incidence of infection, clot formation, mural fibrosis, venous stricture, and sometimes occlusion[17-20]; they should be limited to short-term use in patients likely to recover quickly from acute renal failure or in patients with chronic renal failure requiring an interval means of dialysis until an arterial venous fistula is ready for use. Since clot formation by fibrin sleeves around the catheter occurs, both channels should be vigorously flushed before each dialysis treatment. Free backflow of blood by syringe aspiration is needed for the outflow channel, but this is not essential for the inflow channel if fluid can be injected without resistance. In the event of clinically manifest infection, these large-diameter catheters can be cultured by endoluminal brush technique.[21]

Pulmonary Artery Catheters

The pulmonary artery catheter, preferably, should be inserted via the internal jugular or subclavian vein. When these veins are not accessible, the femoral vein may be used.[13] Chemically or osmotically irritative solutions should not be infused through the *side port*, which opens into the brachiocephalic vein, but these solutions may be infused through the *proximal port*, which opens into the superior vena cava or the right atrium. Pulmonary artery catheters should be removed as soon as possible.[22-24] Prolonged catheter use leads to increased fibrin deposition, clot formation, and catheter-related infections.[25] Mechanical injury of tricuspid and pulmonary valves by the catheter accentuated by contractile motions of the heart may erode the valves and form vegetations.[26-28] The prolonged use of the pulmonary artery catheter leads to multiple fibrin sheaves in subclavian and brachiocephalic veins and thrombosis of pulmonary artery branches. The degree of clot formation in patients as a reaction to the presence of the catheter varies with coagulation parameters. In patients in a hypercoagulability state as well as patients who are more infection-prone, these catheters should remain in place for the shortest time and reinserted, if essential, with prolonged catheter-free intervals.

The technique of insertion, complications, and incidence of related infections have been described.[13, 23] The skin entry site is widely prepared with povidone-iodine antiseptic solution, followed by application of 3 to 5 g of 1% silver sulfadiazine cream covered with a sterile gauze dressing. Gauze dressing, unlike the transparent adhesive dressings, absorbs skin perspiration and allows aeration. When securing the gauze in place with adhesive tape, we leave some areas uncovered by the tape to permit circulation of air beneath the dressing.[29] Dressings should be changed daily for the first 5 days and at least two to three times a week thereafter.

Intra-arterial Catheters

The intra-arterial catheter is inserted by percutaneous puncture into the radial, brachial, dorsalis pedis, or femoral artery. Other smaller arteries can be cannulated by operative exposure. In small children and in patients with severe hypotension, these arteries may need to be cannulated by operative exposure. In either case, the surgeon should cannulate the artery using the Seldinger technique to prevent oozing of blood from around the cannula. When a guide wire is not available, cannulation can be achieved through a small transverse arteriotomy, which is then repaired snugly around the catheter. When possible, the catheter tip should be directed along—rather than against—the arterial blood flow.

COMPLICATIONS OF ACCESS

Inadvertent Arterial Puncture

The arteries parallel or adjacent to the vein targeted for puncture, as well as the arteries crossing the vein path, may be entered by the needle tip, particularly if the operator is unfamiliar with the vascular anatomy in that area.[30-37] This complication becomes particularly dangerous when the patient is hypertensive or coagulopathic or has a nearby aneurysm. It is essential that the operator manually examine the area for aneurysmal dilatation or tortuosity to avoid such arterial injuries. Percutaneous deep venous catheterization in patients with severe coagulation defects or severe hypertension should be delayed until these abnormalities are controlled.

During subclavian venipuncture attempts, the needle attached to a syringe is advanced with a mild negative pressure to detect intravascular entry and inadvertent entry into pleural space, apex of the lung, or the trachea. In case of arterial puncture, the consequent *internal bleeding* that cannot be effectively controlled by application of direct pressure may result in massive mediastinal hematoma and hemothorax. *External bleeding* is easily controlled by fingertip pressure. When an artery is inadvertently punctured in a patient with adequate arterial pressure and oxygenation, the complication is readily recognizable by the presence of bright red blood

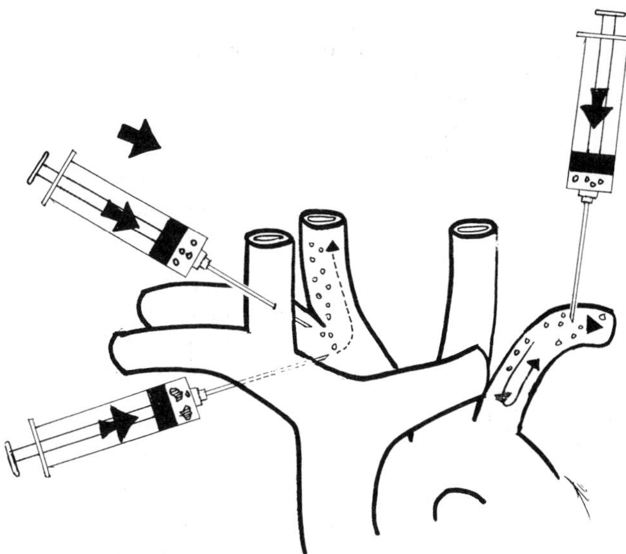

AIR OR BLOOD CLOT EMBOLISM,
CONSEQUENT TO INCIDENTAL
ARTERIAL PUNCTURES

Figure 6–5. Possible inadvertent adjacent arterial punctures that may occur during attempts to puncture the subclavian or internal jugular vein. Injection of clots or air bubbles mixed with blood in the syringe can be detrimental, particularly when they go into the carotid artery; air bubbles and blood clots accumulated in the syringe must be discarded and not injected into the vessel.

spontaneously flowing into the syringe and requiring manual counterpressure to return the blood back into the vessel. If the complication is not recognized, high-pressure pulsatile bleeding will be evident when the syringe is detached from the needle to advance the catheter. Should this catheter be connected to infusion fluid without a pump, blood reflux will be evident in the tubing. Whenever the arterial puncture is recognized, the needle or the catheter should be immediately removed and finger pressure applied until the bleeding stops. Some of the arterial punctures associated with subclavian or internal jugular vein catheterization attempts are illustrated in Figure 6–5. With inadvertent arterial punctures, the operating physician must avoid injecting air, bubbles, or clots into the artery. When hemodialysis and Swan-Ganz and other equally large-bore catheters are inserted percutaneously by the Seldinger technique, the guide wire may be mistakenly placed in an artery followed by insertion of the large-bore catheter, resulting in a large arterial injury.[35] Such an injury may need operative intervention for hemostasis by repair; in some patients, particularly the elderly, this may lead to lethal hemorrhage. Therefore, the operator should first insert a 16-gauge single-lumen catheter into the vein. After correct placement of the central venous catheter is ascertained, the guide wire is inserted or reinserted and the catheter is removed. Only over a safely and correctly placed guide wire can large-bore catheters be introduced with certainty that arterial entry will not occur.

Bleeding from the Skin Entry Site

External oozing of blood from the catheter skin site must be completely stopped before dressings are applied. Frequently, this kind of oozing is due to high venous pressure, which can be alleviated and stopped by elevating the head of the bed and applying manual pressure to the site (Tables 6–7 and 6–8). If oozing continues despite these maneuvers, a suture is passed beyond the catheter skin site and tied in a circle tightly enough to stop oozing without causing skin necrosis and infection at the site. This suture should be removed within 24 hours or after it has served its hemostatic purpose.

Inadvertent Lymphatic Duct Puncture

The thoracic duct, when enlarged in patients with hepatic portal hypertension, is most commonly injured during left supraclavicular subclavian vein or left internal jugular vein catheterization and uncommonly during left infraclavicular subclavian vein approach. If the duct is inadvertently punctured, a clear or milky fluid is aspirated in the syringe. When the duct puncture site is at the junction with the vein, the return of blood mixed with lymph fluid may obscure this complication until lymph oozes from around the catheter. Once the complication is recognized, the procedure should be abandoned at that site, the head of the bed should be elevated, and manual pressure should be applied to the site until lymphorrhagia abates. In previously undiagnosed portal hypertension, occurrence of this complication served as a clue that led to the diagnosis. Occassionally the thoracic duct joins the right subclavian vein. When lymphatic pressure is elevated and the thoracic duct is traversed by a needle entering the pleural space, chylothorax may develop subsequently.

The incidence of inadvertent puncture of the thoracic jugular and subclavian lymphatic trunks with normal lymphatic pressure is unknown. The low lymphatic duct pressure in normal states frequently does not result in spontaneous exter-

TABLE 6–7. Causes of External Fluid Leakage and Hemolymphorrhagia at the Catheter Site After Vein Puncture or Catheterization Attempts

Venous Blood

- Subclavian vein catheter traversing the external jugular vein at the supraclavicular region
- Markedly elevated venous pressure systemically or from segmental venous blockage
- Forceful coughing or straining
- Sitting or standing up immediately after femoral vein catheterization
- Severe coagulopathy
- During cardiopulmonary resuscitation (from chest compressions and/or coagulopathy)

Arterial Blood

- Needle injury to subcutaneous or deep arteries

Lymph Fluid

- Needle injury to the thoracic duct, especially in cirrhotics, and subclavian or jugular lymphatic trunks in supraclavicular, subclavian, or internal jugular puncture low in the neck in patients with thrombosis of innominate veins*

Edema Fluid

Pleural Effusion Fluid

- When pleural dome has been punctured during venipuncture attempts with the patient in supine position

***Intravenous Fluid*†**

- Backing out via the fibrinous sleeve tract
- Caused by a puncture in the extravascular soft-tissue portion of the catheter

*Puncture of a tortuous lymphatic trunk during infraclavicular subclavian vein puncture attempts is rare but possible, especially in the left side.
†Intravenous fluid leakage stops by shutting off the intravenous fluid flow.

TABLE 6–8. Causes of Internal Fluid Leakage or Hemolymphorrhagia as the Result of Subclavian or Internal Jugular Vein Puncture or Catheterization Attempts

Subcutaneous, Interstitial, or Mediastinal Collection

Seldom from venous origin unless the venous pressure is too high and the vein has sustained a major injury/tear
Frequently from inadvertent puncture of the following arteries:
- Common carotid
- Transverse cervical artery
- Suprascapular artery
- Subclavian artery
- Innominate artery
- Internal mammary artery
- Vertebral artery
- Small subcutaneous or other unnamed arteries

Lymphorrhagia from the injured thoracic duct or other lymphatic branches/trunks (jugular and subclavian trunks) with high pressure

Pleural Space as Hemothorax, Hydrothorax, or Chylothorax

In patients with coagulopathy and shock, as a result of pleural dome puncture(s)
Puncture of the subclavian or internal jugular vein into the pleural space or catheters traversing these veins into the pleural space
Puncture of the arteries into the pleural space (subclavian, common carotid, innominate, and internal thoracic)
Rupture/decompression of a mediastinal hematoma into the pleural space
Infusion of fluid and/or blood via a catheter misplaced in the pleural space
Chylothorax as a result of simultaneous needle puncture of a lymphatic duct, with high pressure, into the pleural dome space*

*Chylothorax has not been observed in this series.

nal leakage of lymphatic fluid because the soft tissue pressure exceeds that of lymphatic pressure.

Extravasation of Other Clear Fluids From the Catheter Skin Site

Pleural effusion fluid may seep out from around the catheter skin site of patients in whom the pleural dome has been inadvertently punctured during attempts for venous cannulation; this seepage usually ceases when the patient is placed in an upright or semi-upright position. Patients with anasarca may seep edema fluid that does not stop with local pressure. When the tip of the central venous catheter enters a smaller tributary vein, such as an internal thoracic vein or greater azygos vein, the small vein will thrombose in a few days and the infused intravenous fluid may leak back out through a complete fibrin sleeve formed around the catheter; this seepage will be abated by repositioning the catheter tip. Holes and cracks in the extravascular catheter segment produce seepage of intravenous fluid (see Table 6–7).

Puncture of the Pleural Dome, Lung Apex, and Trachea

Pneumothorax commonly results from puncture of the lung apex, apical blebs, or emphysematous lung. Preventive cautions include (1) advancing the needle toward the vein at the end of the expiratory phase and (2) eliminating positive end-expiratory pressure (PEEP) and reducing large tidal volumes in patients on mechanical ventilation while attempting venipuncture but temporarily compensating by increasing oxygen flow and respiratory rates.

The earliest evidence of lung apex puncture is air in the syringe in response to negative pressure created by the syringe, which has an airtight connection to the puncture needle. Air is withdrawn into the syringe after the needle tip penetrates the pleural dome when a preexisting pneumothorax is unrecognized, but this does not cause deterioration. Also, air entry into the syringe may suggest tracheal puncture when the needle tip is advanced in this direction.[38] Tracheal puncture in most cases occurs with internal jugular puncture attempts and occasionally with supraclavicular subclavian vein puncture attempts. There may be an audible hissing sound during the expiratory phase when the needle has penetrated the trachea or the cuff of an in situ endotracheal or tracheostomy tube. An immediate air leak occurs from around the tube during inspiratory phase; obviously, reinflation of the punctured cuff does not hold. Puncture of large apical blebs that communicate with bronchioles leads to rapidly increasing pneumothorax, which requires immediate decompression; pleural catheters with a one-way valve are recommended for this problem.[39, 40] Patients with puncture of apical blebs that do not communicate with bronchioles develop limited pneumothorax proportional to the size of the disrupted bleb; they do not require decompression if they remain asymptomatic.

In patients with immediately recognized puncture of the lung apex, the intended intravenous catheter should be introduced into the pleural space through the puncture needle while it is still in place. Repeated intermittent aspirations of pleural air with a large syringe may eliminate the pneumothorax in cases without continuous major air leaks (Fig. 6–6).

Puncture of apical blebs that are completely adherent to the parietal pleura may result in soft-tissue emphysema. Subcutaneous emphysema may also develop from tension pneumothorax owing to puncture of the lung apex. Puncture of the apex of the normal lung usually does not occur in infraclavicular subclavian venipuncture attempts because the apex of the normal lung, while ventilated with normal tidal volumes, usually remains caudad to the first rib. Normal lung apex may be punctured during the supraclavicular approach to the subclavian vein medial to the first rib or the internal jugular vein close to its junction with the subclavian vein, especially with long needles (>2 inches) in the average-sized adult. Needle puncture of the apex of the normal lung usually does not result in clinically detectable pneumothorax unless the patient is on positive-pressure ventilation with large tidal volumes.

It is essential to auscultate both lung fields once before and several times after the procedure for comparison of bilateral breath sounds. Patients in the supine position with intact pain sensation who develop a sudden and significant air leak into the pleural space experience pain and heaviness in the ipsilateral hemithorax anteriorly. The pain gradually dissipates while the sensing of heaviness may remain. When the pneumothorax is large and the air leak continuous, most patients manifest signs and symptoms of respiratory distress; these symptoms are undetectable in patients who are unconscious, paralyzed, or anesthetized. Such patients undergo auscultation and percussion over both lung fields in addition to blood gas analyses and chest radiographic studies to detect signs of pneumothorax. Subclavian or internal jugular punctures in patients undergoing general anesthesia should be done prior to the induction of anesthesia or postoperatively when a good-quality chest x-ray film can be obtained. When subclavian or internal jugular vein cannulation is performed during general anesthesia, frequent auscultation of breath sounds bilaterally is essential.

In about 70% of patients with puncture of the lung apex, aspiration of air in the syringe is usually the only early sign of this complication. This sign is reliable only when the connection of the needle to the syringe is airtight and the lumen of the needle has not become blocked by a clot or fatty tissue

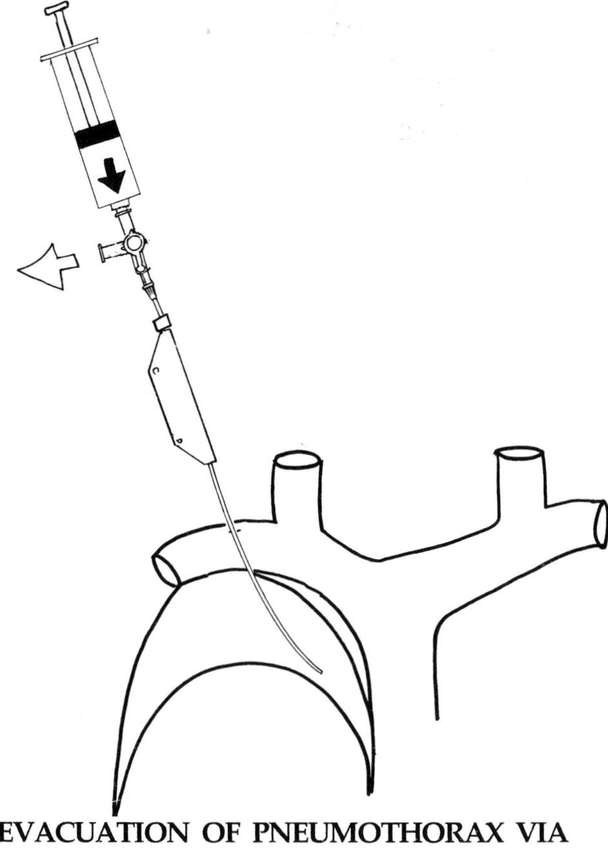

Figure 6–6. While subclavian or internal jugular venipuncture is being attempted, if air is obtained in the syringe attached airtight to the needle, the syringe is detached and the intravenous catheter is inserted via the needle into the pleural space. In the presence of adhesions of the lung apex to the pleural dome, catheter insertion may not be possible. Repeated aspirations of pleural air by a large syringe attached to a three-way stopcock via the catheter may clear the pneumothorax completely; otherwise, if the pleural cavity air is not cleared by this means, a pleural catheter tube is inserted through the second or third intercostal space.

during needle advancement. If a chest radiograph shows 10% to 25% pneumothoraces within 48 hours in an asymptomatic patient, treatment is not usually necessary unless the pneumothorax increases in size.

Isolated pleural dome punctures that do not pierce the lung may be detected if there is preexisting fluid, blood, or air in the pleural dome space or if the inserted catheter does not yield blood while it is gradually withdrawn. Punctures of the pleural dome in patients with severe coagulopathy may result in massive ipsilateral hemothorax by slow but continuous oozing of blood from the parietal pleural puncture site. When the vein or the artery is also punctured, there may be rapid bleeding into the pleural space. Intrapleural bleeding is accentuated by preexisting fibrosis of the tissues surrounding the vessels of intravenous drug-addicted patients. Needle puncture tracts through fibrotic tissues can remain patent for some time while the normal soft tissues rapidly obliterate puncture tracts. Large hemothoraces requiring drainage by a chest tube or operative intervention for hemostasis rarely occur.

Air Embolism

The audible aspiration of air into a vein via a needle with the tip in the vein while the hub is open to air during the inspiratory phase indicates air embolus. Air embolus can occur during subclavian or jugular vein catheterization in hypovolemic patients with low venous pressure in the supine or even Trendelenburg position. It can also occur in patients with adult respiratory distress syndrome (ARDS) and with strongly negative inspiratory intrathoracic force that lowers the venous pressure below atmospheric pressure; this may be clinically evidenced by collapse of the external jugular veins during the inspiration. Respiratory rates may be so rapid that the catheter cannot be advanced into the needle within the time of each expiratory phase. Air embolus occurs when patients cannot hold their breath, when the catheters are not introduced during expiration, or when the hub is not blocked by a fingertip.

When air embolus occurs, the needle hub must be immediately blocked with a fingertip. Air emboli are stopped as soon as the catheter tip is introduced into the needle hub. If cardiac arrest occurs, cardiopulmonary resuscitation must be promptly instituted. In patients with preexisting respiratory distress, the condition worsens proportionate to the amount of air embolus; in these cases, it is necessary to provide immediate ventilatory support for hypoxemia and the aggravated respiratory distress. Other patients may need prompt endotracheal intubation and ventilatory support and high-flow oxygen for as long as necessary.

Small amounts of air emboli occurring during one or two normal inspirations is usually well tolerated. Some patients, however, may experience a dry cough persisting for 10 to 30 minutes, presumably from air emboli and ischemia in the terminal branches of the pulmonary artery that irritate the visceral pleura. Of 48 patients with air emboli, 15 developed a self-limited cough, 10 required immediate vigorous respiratory support for a few hours until the respiratory distress abated, and four of these 10 patients required external chest cardiac compressions for cardiac arrest (Table 6–9).

Air embolus may occur by accidental disconnection of the intravenous catheter when the disconnected end is above the level of the right cardiac atrium.[8] Air embolus may also occur from a subclavian or internal jugular catheter tract that has been in place for several days if the site is not obliterated by a dressing immediately following removal[41]; scar tissue formed around the tract may keep it open for some time after the catheter is removed because scar tissue is persistent in intravenous drug abusers.

Subclavian and jugular vein puncture in patients with both low venous pressure and ARDS should be avoided to prevent the occurrence of air embolus. Potentially lethal air embolus in critically ill patients can be prevented by avoidance of subclavian and jugular venipuncture procedures until venous pressure during the inspiratory phase becomes positive, as evidenced by engorged external jugular veins in the supine position.

Malposition of the Catheter

When subclavian or the internal jugular vein catheterization is attempted on the side with an existing hemothorax, the catheter may be introduced into the pleural space with resultant blood return and incorrect assumption of proper intravenous placement.[42] Unlike other extravascular positions of catheters,[43] this is the only extravascular position that yields blood freely by syringe aspiration; however, this blood fails to clot. This catheter does not follow the expected anatomic course by chest radiography. After a thorocostomy tube is placed, the infusate collects in the drainage system.

An experienced operator feels when the catheter may be going in the wrong direction intravenously by sensing undue resistance during insertion that has to be overcome by greater than the usual force needed for advancement. When such a

TABLE 6–9. Technical Complications in 6110 Cases with 11,685 Catheters Inserted (July 1985–December 1997)

Complications in Decreasing Order of Frequency	No.	Percentage of Complications: Cases	Catheters
1. Inadvertent arterial puncture or catheterization	353	5.77	3.02
2. Puncture, apex of lung without subsequent clinically manifest pneumothorax	63	1.03	0.53
a. Puncture, apex of lung resulting in clinically manifest pneumothorax requiring decompression	37	0.60	0.31
b. Clinically detected isolated pleural dome puncture alone	13	0.21	0.11
c. Total punctures of pleural dome and apex of the lung	113	1.85	0.97
3. Needle injury to thoracic duct	79	1.29	0.67
a. Needle injury to other lymphatic ducts	31	0.50	0.26
b. Total clinically detected lymphatic duct injuries	110	1.80	0.94
4. Venous air embolus during cannulation	48	0.78	0.41
5. Tracheal puncture	10	0.16	0.08
6. Hemoptysis	3	0.04	0.02
7. Seizures (history of epilepsy)	2	0.03	0.01
8. Asthmatic attack and tachycardia (history of asthma)	2	0.03	0.01
Total	641	10.48	5.48

All of the above complications, except for some of the needle injuries to lymphatic ducts which manifested later on, were recognized at the time of occurrence and resolved immediately.

resistance is met, the catheter should not be forced but should be drawn back and readvanced repeatedly, if necessary, until it freely passes to the desired length. The only specific test of catheter patency and correct tip position within the vein lumen is that aspiration force applied by a small syringe freely yields blood. However, this test does not confirm the proper intravenous course of the catheter (Tables 6–10 and 6–11).

The most common malposition is the infraclavicular catheter entering into the ipsilateral internal jugular vein (Fig. 6–7). Semirigid catheters are more apt to be misdirected than soft, pliable catheters that are carried along by blood flow. Soft catheters with metal stylets make them semirigid; when resistance is met, the stylet is partially withdrawn to allow the catheter tip to regain pliability and to be carried by blood flow while being advanced.

Misdirected catheters can also be corrected with a guide wire inserted through the catheter while it is removed. The tip of the guide wire is then pulled back into the vein of entry and readvanced, repeatedly, if necessary, until it can be advanced without resistance to most of its length. The catheter is going in the right direction when advancement does not meet undue resistance. Detours of catheters into the azygos, internal mammary, ipsilateral axillary, and contralateral innominate veins are rare.[2, 4] Malpositioned catheters must be correctly positioned, replaced, or removed as soon as possible to prevent thrombosis (Table 6–12).

TABLE 6–10. Clinical Assessment of the Position of Intended Central Venous Catheters

Group	Criteria
1. Correctly placed, tip in the center of the vein or parallel to the wall	Catheter length appropriate (not short and not long) Catheter advanced, meeting no resistance Catheter stylet is straight when pulled out, and it can be reintroduced without undue resistance Catheter can be moved back partially and advanced into the vein without resistance Catheter yields blood freely, aspirating it by a syringe even when the catheter is partially withdrawn and readvanced; rapid injection of the blood aspirated in the syringe that produces no pain or sense of awareness in the patient indicates central location* Venous pressure fluctuates with respirations and central venous pressure is as expected
2. Correctly placed, but the tip is against a vein wall, needing repositioning by manipulation until blood can be aspirated freely	Blood cannot be aspirated freely by a syringe, but there is a blood reflux in the infusion tubing when the intravenous fluid bottle or bag is lowered below bed level
3. Questionable; these are the catheters that detour into the internal jugular, homolateral subclavian, opposite innominate, homolateral internal thoracic, vertebral, or greater azygos veins	There was undue resistance to catheter advancement at some point, which was overcome by force If all other criteria in group 1 are present, catheter is correctly placed but the position still needs to be verified by x-ray film If some or all criteria in group 1 do not exist, catheter is misplaced and must be repositioned or replaced before or after x-ray confirmation
4. Definitely misplaced	Advancement met with undue resistance, which is overcome by force; catheter does not yield blood; once it is partially withdrawn, it cannot be readvanced

*This is the only test indicating that the tip of the catheter is not close to and not in apposition to the wall, as long as the catheter has no side openings.

TABLE 6–11. Clinical and Radiologic Evidence of Malpositioned Catheters

Location and Position of Tip	Signs and Symptoms
Internal jugular, catheter lumen facing cephalad	No respiratory fluctuations of venous pressure Pain on that side of the neck created by rapid injection of fluids via the catheter; intravenous fluid stops running by pressing on the vein cephalad to the tip of catheter; pain and swelling on that side of the neck caused by thrombosis of the vein later on should the malpositioned catheter be left in place No blood return via the catheter after a few days with confirming x-ray evidence of malposition
Left internal mammary	X-ray film shows the catheter to the left of mediastinum and anterior in lateral projection Vague discomfort and pain, anterior chest No fluctuations of venous pressure by respirations No blood return from the catheter after a few days as a result of vein thrombosis Leakage of intravenous fluid from around the catheter skin site after a few days
Vertebral vein	X-ray film shows the catheter tip going cephalad and posteriorly Vague discomfort and patient's awareness of the presence of catheter in the back of the neck; leakage of intravenous fluids from around the skin site of catheter entry and no blood return via catheter after a few days
Greater azygos vein	X-ray film shows the catheter detouring from the superior vena cava course medially and posteriorly Vague discomfort/pain in the back of the chest Leakage of intravenous fluid from around the catheter as a result of venous thrombosis and formation of a fibrinous sleeve along or around the catheter leading the intravenous fluid to outside
Right atrium	Venous pressure 2 to 5 cm of water higher than that of the superior vena cava; x-ray evidence confirms the position
Tip of catheter against tricuspid valve leaklets	Blood can be aspirated by a syringe in diastole, whereas no blood can be aspirated in systole (intermittently)
Tip of catheter against flow of venous blood	Venous pressure 2 to 5 cm of water higher than that when the tip of catheter is in the direction of blood flow Smaller veins become thrombosed and intravenous fluid may leak out via the fibrinous sleeve around catheter
Right ventricle	Venous pressure weakly pulsatile and much higher than central venous pressure Premature ventricular contractions may appear initially or when manipulating catheter; conscious patient can feel irregular contractions associated with anxiety
Tip of catheter against wall of the vein or heart chambers	No blood return by aspiration with a syringe but present by lowering the intravenous bottle or bag below the bed level with the intravenous tubing open
Opposite innominate and subclavian vein (crossing over)	X-ray evidence; swelling of the opposite arm caused by vein thrombosis when the catheter is left in place for a few days
Homolateral axillary vein	Edema and swelling of the arm; pain and tenderness in the axilla; palpable cord-like and tender axillary vein

Intravenous Clot Formation and Catheter-Related Infection

Intravenous catheter-related infection may be described as *primary* when there is no other identifiable source of infection and *secondary* when sterile catheters are colonized by microorganisms that were present in the body at the time of catheterization. A *superimposed* catheter-related infection occurs when blood or catheter culture reveals a new microorganism with no identifiable source.

Intravascular catheters are foreign bodies that communicate to the outside; they have fibrin and blood clots inside and around them that enhance the development and persistence of infection (Tables 6–13 and 6–14). Reports in the literature indicate that most catheter infections are due to skin microorganisms that gain access to the circulation via the catheter tract.[44] However, it is likely that skin flora of patients and health care members gain access to the circulation through:

1. Unsterile technique of catheterization.
2. Disconnections and reconnections of the infusion tubing.
3. Administration of contaminated intravenous fluids.
4. Injections through the inadequately prepared injection sites of intravenous tubing.

In patients without burns or other sources of contamination close to the catheter site, gram-negative organisms and *Candida albicans* often proliferate within intravascular catheters and connecting lines. Accumulation of fibrin debris, particulate matter, and microbial slime within these catheters, and secondary to line manipulations (connections and disconnections) may result in the development of sepsis.[45, 46] Forceful flushing of the catheter with a syringe or by maximally accelerating the infusion pump at least daily minimizes the accumulation of debris within the intravascular catheter because constant slow flow or stasis may enhance microbial growth inside contaminated catheters. Nutrients of intravenous fluids support microbial growth; therefore, the duration of intravenous fluid infusion at room temperature must be limited to a safe period.

Bacterial Growth in Commonly Used Infusion Fluids

We studied the growth of seven commonly encountered microorganisms in 15 frequently used intravenous solutions to determine a safe period for each unit of these fluids to be administered to patients with little or no microbial growth at room temperature. Ten milliliters of each of 15 intravenous fluids were placed in sterile tubes in triplicates as culture media and then contaminated with 0.1 mL of prepared inoculum for each organism and kept at room temperature (25°C). The intravenous fluids and organisms tested were 10% FreAmine; 25% and 5% albumin; 6% hydroxyethyl starch; 5%,

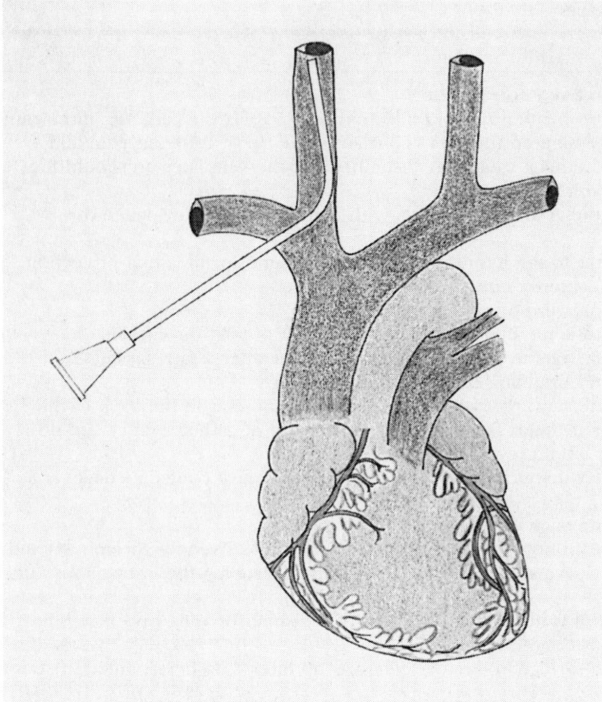

Figure 6–7. Detour of a catheter inserted via the right subclavian vein infraclavicularly into the homolateral internal jugular vein. This detour is common, but clinically detectable, and frequently preventable or correctable at the time of venous cannulation.

TABLE 6–13. Precautions That May Reduce Catheter Infection

1. Catheterize by the first or second puncture attempt.
2. Remove the needle, ordinarily retained over the catheter, by a guide wire to avoid trapping blood and microorganisms between the needle and catheter or between needle and the needle guard.
3. Keep intravenous fluid flow uninterrupted to prevent blood reflux into the catheter and intravenous tubings.
4. Flush catheter free from debris by running the intravenous fluid freely several minutes once or twice a day.
5. Avoid suturing the catheter to the skin; use tape instead.
6. Prevent pressure sore or soreness of the skin at the site of the catheter hub and intravenous tubing connection by placing a gauze pad underneath.
7. Provide antiseptic preparation and apply silver sulfadiazine cream at the catheter skin site at least daily, preferably three times daily in infection-prone patients.
8. Use chemically inert catheters with as short a length, as small a diameter, and as soft a substance as possible.
9. Remove catheters as soon as possible.
10. Change site once a week in septic patients, if possible; otherwise, exchange catheter twice a week in septic patients.
11. Avoid creation of hematoma at the site and fluid, blood, and lymph leakage from around the catheter site.
12. Leave catheter sites exposed in patients with marked perspiration or burns at the skin site.
13. Apply waterproof dressings over the catheter site when the patient is showering or when there is a nearby contamination source, and change at least daily.*
14. Create a subcutaneous tunnel to place the catheter skin exit/entry site away from the nearby source of contamination.
15. Apply dry gauze dressing over the catheter site, permitting air circulation to keep it dry.

*We use only waterproof transparent adhesive dressing for this purpose and when the patient is showering or bathing.

TABLE 6–12. Possible Detours and Malpositions of Central Venous Catheters in Order of Frequency

Vein and Site of Origin or Course of Catheter	Possible Malpositions of the Catheter Tip
Subclavian, infraclavicular	In homolateral internal jugular, axillary, and vertebral veins
Subclavian, supraclavicular	In homolateral internal mammary, opposite innominate, and axillary veins
Internal jugular (left)	In homolateral internal mammary and subclavian veins
Innominate (right)	In left innominate
Superior vena cava	In greater azygos, right atrium, coronary sinus, inferior vena cava, right ventricle, pulmonary artery
Femoral (left)	In ascending lumbar and homolateral internal iliac veins
Femoral (right)	In homolateral internal iliac vein
Inferior vena cava	In right atrium, superior vena cava, right innominate, right internal jugular, right ventricle, pulmonary artery
Internal jugular (left)	Against inferior wall of left innominate, right wall of superior vena cava
Subclavian (left)	Against right wall of superior vena cava
Subclavian (right)	Against left wall of right innominate, inferior wall of left innominate
Femoral (left)	Against superior wall of left common iliac, right wall of inferior vena cava
Femoral (right)	Against left wall of inferior vena cava

TABLE 6–14. Factors That May Lead to Intravenous Catheter-Related Infection

Multiple puncture attempts at one site at one or repeated settings
Hematoma around the catheter soft-tissue tract
Blood clots or stains allowed to remain under the dressing
Fibrin or blood clots retained within the catheter and intravenous tubing
Leakage of lymph, interstitial edema fluid, intravenous fluids, or blood and accumulation of perspiration under the dressing, which keep the catheter site moist
Blood trapped between the catheter inside the needle segment and between the needle and the needle guard
Sutures at the catheter site, especially hemostatic sutures, tied tightly
Catheters with no blood return, ball valve clot at the tip
Catheters with fibrinous sleeve
Catheters inserted close to infection or contamination sources
Short distance between the skin puncture and vein puncture sites
Catheters inserted through skin burns
Misdirected, coiled, and partially withdrawn catheters
Catheters in patients with preexisting sepsis: sepsis is perpetuated
Catheters in patients with long-term intravenous therapy (>4 mo)
Long, large-bore, rigid, and/or multiple long-term catheters
Immune deficiency states
Catheters inserted under emergency conditions, during cardiopulmonary resuscitation, and during operative interventions*
Persistent shock
Advanced cancer, renal, and/or hepatic failure
Catheters and intravenous tubings handled by unsterile technique
Unsterile intravenous fluids preparation and administration techniques
Constant moisture at the catheter skin site

*We replace all catheters considered or suspected of being contaminated after the emergency situation is averted.

10%, and 70% glucose; 12% glucose and 7% amino acids (formula 1); 25% glucose and 5% amino acids (formula 2); 47% glucose and 2.5% amino acids (formula 3); 56% glucose and 1.25% amino acids (formula 4); 10% FreAmine plus vitamins and trace elements (formula 7); and lactated Ringer's and normal saline solutions. The inocula were *Staphylococcus epidermidis, Staphylococcus aureus, Escherichia coli, Pseudomonas, Klebsiella, Serratia, and C. albicans.* Growths of microorganism in the 13 transparent fluids were measured by densitometry up to 144 hours. The growth in nontransparent 20% fat emulsion as well as tripticase soy broth was measured by quantitative subcultures on blood agar plates (kept in an incubator at 37°C) up to 24 hours with colony counts and used as controls.

S. epidermidis did not grow in any of the 13 solutions. Some or all of the six other organisms grew significantly in lactated Ringer's solution; normal saline; 5% albumin; 6% hydroxyethyl starch; 5%, 10% glucose; 25% albumin; 10% FreAmine, formula 1, and formula 2 between 6 and 96 hours. There was no detectable growth in 70% glucose, formula 3, or formula 4, but the dormant organisms inoculated in these solutions grew in quantitative subcultures on blood agar plates. Growth in 20% fat emulsion and in tripticase soy broth was quantitatively subcultured on blood agar plates using a 0.001 mL calibrated loop. Colony counts showed growth of more than 100 colonies of all organisms with the exception of *Candida*, which showed slower growth, from the time of inoculation up to 24 hours. In this study we found 20% fat emulsion to be the most supportive of microbial growth.[47-50] Because the possibility of inadvertent contamination of intravenous fluids always exists in clinical fluid therapy, we recommend that each unit of these or similar solutions be administered over less than 8-hour periods.

To identify a fluid with the maximum bacteriostatic effect for locking indwelling intermittently used catheters or lumens, we studied the effect of the six solutions that may inhibit microbial growth. These solutions were inoculated with the six listed microorganisms using 0.1 mL of the standardized inocula. The inoculated and control solutions were kept at room temperature (25°C) up to 66 hours. Immediately after inoculation and at subsequent intervals, these solutions were subcultured using 0.001 mL on blood agar plates and incubated for 24 hours at 37°C. Contrary to our expectation, organisms grew significantly in all of these solutions except for 50% glucose and undiluted heparin (1000 U/mL). Furthermore, it became apparent that undiluted heparin manifests a bactericidal property after 6 hours. Therefore, undiluted heparin is the solution of choice for locking intravascular catheters or lumens with no flow.

Catheter-enhanced infection is associated with increased blood coagulability; the greater the coagulability of blood, the greater the frequency of catheter-related infection and the earlier the venous thrombosis.[10, 19, 51-56] Hypercoagulable patients with continuous indwelling central venous catheters may thrombose percutaneously accessible veins in 3 to 4 months. Indwelling venous catheters may last 9 to 12 months in patients with hypocoagulability state and prolonged clotting time.[55] At the end stage of venous thrombosis, the veins become partially occluded by cavernous intraluminal clots but permit some venous blood flow through their irregular channels.[38] The most effective means of stopping septic conditions at this stage of venous thrombosis is to remove all intravascular catheters and administer the essential antibiotics intramuscularly or orally and via nasoenteral, gastrostomy, or jejunostomy tubes.[12]

Neurologic Injuries

Neurologic injuries directly or indirectly caused by arterial injuries or venous thrombosis have been reported.[57, 58] We found an injury to the nerve of the pectoralis major muscle consequent to an infraclavicular subclavian venipuncture that gradually led to atrophy of the muscle. In another case, temporary paresis of the upper extremity occurred in a patient with hypertension and end-stage renal disease from a large hematoma in the supraclavicular fossa due to an inadvertent arterial puncture after attempted subclavian vein puncture; the hematoma was a result of delayed application of local pressure.

Catheter Embolus

A potential complication in insertion of two or more catheters side by side in the same vein is transection of the catheter already in place with the second or the third needle puncture.[13, 38, 59] The surgeon may avoid this complication by not advancing the second or the third needle against any undue resistance of the soft tissues in front of the needle. When resistance is sensed, the needle is partially withdrawn and redirected until it passes without undue resistance.

Complications to the Operator

The inevitable consequence of working with needles is a needlestick injury at a time when the prevailing circumstances are not optimal and when the operator may be rushed or fatigued; should this happen, the procedure must be temporarily halted. We perform a 10- to 15- minute hand scrub with an antiseptic detergent soap preceded and followed by application of 2% tincture of iodine to the needlestick site. The surgeon then resumes and completes the procedure after donning sterile gloves and using new equipment.

The operator and the assistants may be sprayed with blood if the operator is not holding the hub of the needle against the syringe firmly to prevent separation while injecting the blood aspirated in the syringe back into the vessel. Blood spray can also occur while the syringe is disconnected from the needle to insert the catheter. The operator should avoid facing the hub of an intravascular needle in order to prevent a jet of blood from the veins with high pressure from arteriovenous fistula, tricuspid valve insufficiency, and unrecognized inadvertent arterial puncture. The use of eye protectors during the procedure is advisable.

If the used needles and blades are discarded by hand at the end of the procedure, they should be picked up carefully one by one; when they are picked up as a group, the sharp ends should be placed on the same side and kept under direct vision until disposed of. While one is attempting to grasp a sharp instrument manually, the hand should always approach the instrument from the tail, not the tip end. All sharp instruments must be kept under direct vision during handling and placed in a constant safe spot on the procedure field when they are not needed.

GENERAL COMMENTS

The single-lumen soft, pliable, 8-inch-long, 16- or 19-gauge catheter used in this series is one of the least costly catheters. Because of its small diameter, pliability, and inertness it is very safe, as evidenced by the results in this series. The 8-inch length, when inserted via the subclavian or jugular veins, is sufficient to reach the lower one third of the superior vena cava. In normal-sized adults, this catheter seldom reaches the atrium, hence no catheter-induced cardiac arrhythmia. There is no catheter shredding, embolus, or tip erosion, as reported by others[59-67] in this series. Two or three single-lumen catheters are not only less costly but are also better tolerated for much longer periods within a vein than the double-lumen and triple-lumen catheters. Furthermore, when two or three single-lumen catheters are necessary, they can be removed individually when one is no longer needed. Conversely, with double-lumen and triple-lumen catheters, when one lumen is no longer needed, it cannot be eliminated, and contaminants, when present, may grow in the stagnant fluid within the unused lumen.

The side-by-side catheters inserted in the same vein or adjacent veins in one region can be covered with one dressing. Application of 1% silver sulfadiazine cream to the catheter site twice weekly, at the time of dressing change, in patients with normal resistance to infection and one to three times a day in patients susceptible to catheter-related infection may help reduce infections originating from the catheter skin site.[29] Silver sulfadiazine cream is applied with two sterile, cotton-tipped applicators or a sterile tongue blade. In between dressing changes, the site may be examined by lifting the dressing partially. The lifted portion of the dressing is then turned back and taped in place. Polyglycolic acid suture, utilized to anchor the catheter to the skin or for cessation of oozing or lymph from the catheter skin site, is associated with minimal skin reaction and subsequent scar formation. The minimal skin irritation may also help prevent stitch infection. Nevertheless, we prefer affixing catheters to the skin using sterile adhesive strips.

Routine x-ray studies following unsuccessful or successful attempts for catheter insertion are not necessary. When an experienced operator does not notice "give" in the syringe during venipuncture attempts (aspiration of air into the syringe) and auscultation of breath sounds (after completion of the procedure or after unsuccessful attempts) continues to remain normal and equal bilaterally, there is no pneumothorax. When the catheter of appropriate length has been advanced easily without undue resistance, the intravenous course of the catheter is proper. When the catheter yields blood freely with syringe aspiration, the tip is properly positioned within the vein lumen away from or parallel to the vein wall.

Indications for chest radiography are as follows:

1. When air is aspirated into the syringe during venipuncture attempts. If such a patient has good breath sounds and no respiratory distress immediately following venous cannulation or unsuccessful attempts, the chest film should be taken within 24 to 48 hours. Slow air leaks into the pleural cavity may not demonstrate pneumothorax in chest films taken early after the attempts or the completed procedure. Until the chest x-ray is taken in these patients, the chest is auscultated bilaterally as often as necessary for comparing and monitoring breath sounds. Massive air leaks from the puncture of large blebs communicating with bronchioles place the patient at risk for a tension pneumothorax. Tension pneumothorax is diagnosed clinically and decompressed immediately without an initial chest film. A postdecompression chest film is necessary to confirm the complete reexpansion of the collapsed lung.
2. When the operator has experienced undue resistance to the advancement of the catheter at one point and the resistance cannot be circumvented with repeated attempts.
3. When the catheter length is shorter or longer than the distance it should traverse; an x-ray film may be needed to localize the catheter tip.
4. When there is any doubt regarding the necessity of obtaining or not obtaining an x-ray film.
5. Catheter shredding or embolus.
6. Lack of blood return via the indwelling catheter later on, with the possibility of catheter tip erosion. The radiographic study should utilize injection of radiopaque material. Infusions via catheters in which erosion of the tip is suspected should be stopped until erosion is ruled out.
7. Suspected intrapleural misplacement of catheter in the case of preexisting hemothorax. This misplacement is diagnosed clinically by the lack of clotting of the blood sample taken for this purpose. Nevertheless, if an x-ray is deemed necessary, the infusion should not be started until the x-ray is taken and catheter misplacement is ruled out.
8. Inadvertent intra-arterial catheter placement (in hypotensive patients). No vasoactive agent should be administered via such catheters until intravenous position of the catheter is confirmed.

These indications amount to fewer than 20% of all cases. Therefore, an experienced operator can indicate whether a chest film is indicated and when it should be obtained. Only in the absence of sufficient experience of the operator can routine x-ray studies after unsuccessful and successful attempts be justified.

Antiseptic bonded catheters[68] and exchange of central venous catheters over guide wires for prevention or management of catheter sepsis may not prove effective.[69] The guide wire can transmit microbial contaminants within the existing catheter to the replacement catheter. In the third edition of this textbook, we reported our experience with exchange of catheters via the existing catheter tract immediately following removal without the use of a guide wire in 103 such cases with 143 catheters.

The incidence of infection and other complications of central venous cannulation in the presence of systemic and general or local contraindications for the application of such modalities increases. We believe that existing septicemia is a contraindication for indwelling central venous catheters.

Infection-free and thrombosis-free longevity of the veins with intravenous indwelling catheters is variable and depends on:

- State of blood coagulability
- Catheter material
- Catheter size
- Intravenous catheter length
- Traumatizing motions of the catheter
- Type of intravenous fluids infused
- Sterility of the cannulation technique
- Long-term maintenance

Clot formation around all catheters occurs with varying degrees of rapidity and varying amounts in all patients, eventually resulting in complete blockage of the veins to further cannulation and recurrent or persistent sepsis. Anticoagulation therapy from the beginning of establishment of venous cannulation in patients with hypercoagulability states may increase the thrombosis-free longevity of venous accesses[70]; it may also decrease the incidence of catheter infection. Intravenous therapy must be completed within the safe period, for each patient, which falls short of thrombosing all of the accessible veins or the development of persistent or recurrent catheter-related sepsis. In patients who manifest hypercoagulability states and susceptibility to catheter-related infection, treatment by catheter jejunostomy[12, 71] or gastrostomy as alternatives to intravenous catheters may prove lifesaving.

Individual and team experience in establishment and safe maintenance of vascular accesses minimizes the number, frequency, severity, and sequelae of complications. In this experience, there were fewer complications with fewer consequences of the complications in the second part compared to those in the first part. Properly executed intravascular cannulations with safe long-term maintenance of these catheters utilized only during the essential period of management for each patient can prove lifesaving. Conversely, improperly established intravascular cannulations with improper long-term maintenance kept in place for unnecessarily long periods may become life-threatening.

References

1. Parsa MH, Ferrer JM, Habif DV, et al: Intravenous hyperalimentation: Indications, technique and complications. Bull NY Acad Med 1972; 48:920.
2. Parsa MH, Ferrer JM, Habif DV: Safe Central Venous Nutrition: Guidelines for Prevention and Management of Complications. Springfield, Ill, Charles C Thomas, 1974.
3. Parsa MH, Tabora F: Establishment of intravenous lines for long-term intravenous therapy and monitoring. Surg Clin North Am 1985; 65:835.
4. Parsa MH, Tabora F: Central venous access in critically ill patients in the emergency department. Emerg Med Clin North Am 1986; 4:709.
5. Parsa MH, Freeman HP: Precautions for long-term maintenance of central venous catheters: The need for patient and personnel education. Part I. Surg Rounds 1992; 15:967.
6. Parsa MH, Freeman HP: Precautions for long-term maintenance of central venous catheters: The need for patient and personnel education: Part II. Surg Rounds 1992; 15:1013.
7. Merrel SW, Peatross BG, Grossman MD, et al: Peripherally inserted central venous catheters: Low-risk alternatives for ongoing venous access. West J Med 1994; 160:25–30.
8. Ferrer JM, Parsa MH: Fatal air embolism via subclavian vein. N Engl J Med 1970; 282:688.
9. Shefler A, Gillis J, Lam A, et al: Inferior vena cava thrombosis as a complication of femoral vein catheterisation. Arch Dis Child 1995; 72:343–345.
10. Trottier SJ, Veremakis C, O'Brien J, et al: Femoral deep vein thrombosis associated with central venous catheterization: Results from a prospective, randomized trial. Crit Care Med 1995; 23:52–59.
11. Parsa MH, Tabora F, Freeman HP: Vascular cannulation techniques in intravenous drug addicts and patients with limited or difficult intravenous access. Contemp Surg 1987; 31:31.
12. Parsa MH, Shoemaker WC: Nutritional failure. *In*: Textbook of Critical Care. Shoemaker WC, Thompson WL, Holbrook PR, et al (Eds). Philadelphia, WB Saunders, 1984, p 664.
13. Parsa MH, Tabora F, Al-Sawwaf M: Vascular access techniques. *In*: Textbook of Critical Care. 2nd ed. Shoemaker WC, Ayres S, Grenvik A, et al (Eds). Philadelphia, WB Saunders, 1989, p 122.
14. Bennett JD, Papadouris D, Rankin RN, et al: Percutaneous inferior vena caval approach for long-term central venous access. J Vasc Interv Radiol 1997; 8:851–855.
15. Lund GB, Trerotola SO, Scheel PJ Jr: Percutaneous translumbar inferior vena cava cannulation for hemodialysis. Am J Kidney Dis 1995; 25:732–737.
16. Raad I, Davis S, Becker M, et al: Low infection rate and long durability of nontunneled Silastic catheters: A safe and cost-effective alternative for long-term venous access. Arch Intern Med 1993; 153:1791–1796.
17. Guest SS, Kirsch CM, Baxter R, et al: Infection of a subclavian venous stent in a hemodialysis patient. Am J Kidney Dis 1995; 26:377–380.
18. Schillinger F, Schillinger D, Montagnac R, et al: Post catheterisation vein stenosis in haemodialysis: Comparative angiographic study of 50 subclavian and 50 internal jugular accesses. Nephrol Dial Transplant 1991; 6:722.
19. Khanna S, Sniderman K, Simons M, et al: Superior vena cava stenosis associated with hemodialysis catheters. Am J Kidney Dis 1993; 21:278.
20. Surratt RS, Picus D, Hicks ME, et al: The importance of preoperative evaluation of the subclavian vein in dialysis access planning. Am J Roentgenol 1991; 156:623.
21. Kite P, Dobbins BM, Wilcox MH, et al: Evaluation of a novel endoluminal brush method for in situ diagnosis of catheter related sepsis. J Clin Pathol 1997; 50:278–282.
22. Rello J, Coll P, Net A, et al: Infection of pulmonary artery catheters: Epidemiologic characteristics and multivariate analysis of risk factors. Chest 1993; 103:132.
23. Parsa MH, Al-Sawwaf M, Shoemaker WC: Complications of pulmonary artery catheterization: Cost benefit analysis. Probl Gen Surg 1985; 2:133.
24. Raad I, Umphrey J, Khan A, et al: The duration of placement as a predictor of peripheral and pulmonary arterial catheter infections. J Hosp Infect 1993; 23:17–26.
25. Raad II, Luna M, Khalil SA, et al: The relationship between the thrombotic and infectious complications of central venous catheters. JAMA 1994; 271:1014–1016.
26. Kaye GC, Rodgers H, Smith DR, et al: Bacterial endocarditis of the tricuspid valve after insertion of a central venous catheter. Br J Clin Pract 1990; 44:762.
27. Bernardin G, Milhaud D, Roger PM, et al: Swan-Ganz catheter-related pulmonary valve infective endocarditis: a case report. Intens Care Med 1994; 20:142–144.
28. Soding PF, Klinck Jr, Kong A, et al: Infective endocarditis of the pulmonary valve following pulmonary artery catheterization. Intens Care Med 1994; 20:222–224.
29. Parsa MH, Lau K, Jampayas I, et al: Intravenous catheter-related infection. Infect Surg 1985; 4:789.
30. Amaral JF, Grigoriev VE, Dorfman GS, et al: Vertebral artery pseudoaneurysm: A rare complication of subclavian artery catheterization. Arch Surg 1990; 125:546.
31. Sloan MA, Mueller JD, Adelman LS, et al: Fatal brainstem stroke following internal jugular vein catheterization. Neurology 1991; 41:1092.
32. Elariny HA, Crockett D, Hussey JL: False aneurysm of the thyrocervical trunk. South Med J 1996; 89:519–521.
33. Stock U, Link J, Dutschke P: Iatrogenic vertebrojugular arteriovenous fistula. Anaesthesia 1996; 51:687–688.
34. Stewart RW, Hardjasudarma M, Nall L, et al: Fatal outcome of jugular vein cannulation. South Med J 1995; 88:1159–1160.
35. Walser EM, Crow WN, Zwischenberger JB, et al: Percutaneous tamponade of inadvertent transthoracic catheterization of the aorta. Ann Thorac Surg 1996; 62:895–896.
36. Robinson JF, Robinson WA, Cohn A, et al: Perforation of the great vessels during central venous line placement. Arch Intern Med 1995; 155:1225–1228.
37. Baldwin RT, Kieta DR, Gallagher MW: Complicated right subclavian artery pseudoaneurysm after central venipuncture. Ann Thorac Surg 1996; 62:581–582.
38. Parsa MH, Shoemaker WC: Intravascular access and long-term catheter maintenance. *In:* Textbook of Critical Care. 3rd ed. Shoemaker WC, Ayres S, Grenvik A, et al (Eds). Philadelphia, WB Saunders, 1994, pp 234–253.
39. Samelson SL, Goldberg EM, Ferguson MK: The thoracic vent: Clinical experience with a new device for treating simple pneumothorax. Chest 1991; 100:880–882.
40. Molina PL, Solomon SL, Glazer HS, et al: A one-piece unit for treatment of pneumothorax complicating needle biopsy: Evaluation in 10 patients. AJR 1990; 155:31–33.
41. Phifer TJ, Bridges M, Conrad SA: The residual central venous catheter track: An occult source of lethal air embolism: Case report. J Trauma 1991; 31:1558.
42. Kollef MH: Fallibility of persistent blood return for confirmation of intravascular catheter placement in patients with hemorrhagic thoracic effusions. Chest 1994; 106:1906–1908.
43. Clevens RA, Bradford CR: Airway obstruction secondary to central line intravenous fluid extravasation. Arch Otolaryngol Head Neck Surg 1994; 120:437–439.
44. Ray S, Stacey R, Imrie M, et al: A review of 560 Hickman catheter insertions. Anaesthesia 1996; 51:981–985.
45. Liñares J, Sitges-Serra A, Garau J, et al: Pathogenesis of catheter sepsis: A prospective study with quantitative and semiquantitative cultures of catheter hub and segments. J Clin Microbiol 1985; 21:357–360.
46. Marrie TJ, Costerton JW: Scanning and transmission electron microscopy of in situ bacterial colonization of intravenous and intraarterial catheters. J Clin Microbiol 1984; 19:687–693.
47. Mally MA, Meng HC, Schaffner W: Microbial growth in lipid emulsions used in parenteral nutrition. Arch Surg 1975; 110:1479–1481.
48. Deitel M, Kaminsky VM, Fuksa M: Growth of common bacteria and *Candida albicans* in 10% soybean oil emulsion. Can J Surg 1975; 18:531–535.

49. Gilbert M, Gallagher SC, Eads M, et al: Microbial growth patterns in a total parenteral nutrition formulation containing lipid emulsion. JPEN J Parenter Enteral Nutr 1986; 10:494–497.
50. Scheckelhoff DJ, Mirtallo JM, Ayers LW, et al: Growth of bacteria and fungi in total nutrient admixtures. Am J Hosp Pharm 1986; 43:73–77.
51. Kaye GC, Smith DR, Johnston D: Fatal right ventricular thrombus secondary to Hickman catheterisation. Br J Clin Pract 1990; 44:780.
52. Figuerola M, Tomas MT, Armengol J, et al: Pericardial tamponade and coronary sinus thrombosis associated with central venous catheterization. Chest 1992; 101:1154.
53. Dollery CM, Sullivan ID, Bauraind O, et al: Thrombosis and embolism in long-term central venous access for parenteral nutrition. Lancet 1994; 344:1043–1045.
54. Woodyard TC, Mellinger JD, Vann KG, et al: Acute superior vena cava syndrome after central venous catheter placement. Cancer 1993; 71:2621–2623.
55. Shefler A, Gillis J, Lam A, et al: Inferior vena cava thrombosis as a complication of femoral vein catheterization. Arch Dis Child 1995; 72:343–345.
56. Gould JR, Carloss HW, Skinner WL: Groshong catheter-associated subclavian venous thrombosis. Am J Med 1993; 95:419–423.
57. Pleasure JR, Shashikumar VL: Phrenic nerve damage in the tiny infant during vein cannulation for parenteral nutrition. Am J Perinatol 1990; 7:136.
58. Zeligowsky A, Szold A, Seror D, et al: Horner syndrome: A rare complication of internal jugular vein cannulation. JPEN J Parenter Enteral Nutr 1991; 15:199.
59. Parsa MH, Tabora F, Freeman HP: Techniques of insertion of double or triple IV catheters in one vein or two adjacent veins. Surg Rounds 1987; 10:43.
60. Beauregard JF, Matsumoto AH, Paul MG, et al: Venobronchial fistula: A complication associated with central venous catheterization for chemotherapy. Cathet Cardiovasc Diagn 1990; 19:49.
61. Winkler TR, Hanlin RJ, Hinke TD, et al: Unusual cause of hemoptysis: Hickman-induced cava-bronchial fistula. Chest 1992; 102:1285.
62. Rogers BB, Berns SD, Maynard EC, et al: Pericardial tamponade secondary to central venous catheterization and hyperalimentation in a very low birthweight infant. Pediatr Pathol 1990; 10:819.
63. Byard RW, Bourne AJ, Moore L, et al: Sudden death in early infancy due to delayed cardiac tamponade complicating central venous line insertion and cardiac catheterization. Arch Pathol Lab Med 1992; 116:654.
64. Parsa MH: Fatal cardiac tamponade. JAMA 1983; 249:1707.
65. Collier PE, Goodman GB: Cardiac tamponade caused by central venous catheter perforation of the heart: A preventable complication. J Am Coll Surg 1995; 181:459–463.
66. Flatley ME, Schapira RM: Hydropneumomediastinum and bilateral hydropneumothorax as delayed complications of central venous catheterization. Chest 1993; 103:1914–1916.
67. Duntley P, Siever J, Corwes ML, Marpel K, Heffner JE: Vascular erosion by central venous catheters: Clinical features and outcome. Chest 1992; 101:1633–1638.
68. Pemberton LB, Ross V, Cuddy P, et al: No difference in catheter sepsis between standard and antiseptic central venous catheters: A prospective randomized trial. Arch Surg 1996; 131:986–989.
69. Badley AD, Steckelberg JM, Wollan PC, et al: Infectious rates of central venous pressure catheters: Comparison between newly placed catheters and those that have been changed. Mayo Clin Proc 1996; 71(9):838–846.
70. Bern MM, Lokich JJ, Wallach SR, et al: Very low doses of warfarin can prevent thrombosis in central venous catheters: A randomized prospective trial. Ann Intern Med 1990; 112:423.
71. Parsa MH, Tabora F, Al-Sawwaf M: Enteral feeding. *In:* Textbook of Critical Care. 2nd ed. Shoemaker WC, Ayres S, Grenvik A, et al (Eds). Philadelphia, WB Saunders, 1989, pp 1073–1080.

7

Invasive and Noninvasive Monitoring

William C. Shoemaker, MD, FCCM • M. H. Parsa, MD

All science is measurement.

HELMHOLTZ

Monitoring, a major reason for admission to the intensive care unit (ICU), may vary from the assessment of vital signs for hospital admission, screening, and surveillance in routine cases to comprehensive circulatory monitoring of hemodynamic, respiratory, and oxygen transport functions in high-risk patients; criteria for monitoring high-risk patients are listed in Table 7–1.[1] The primary purpose of circulatory monitoring is to obtain frequent, repetitive, or continuous measurements of circulatory functions that are usually displayed at the bedside to allow prompt recognition of circulatory problems and early initiation of therapy. Monitoring differs from diagnostic methods, such as biochemical analyses or radiologic imaging, that are less frequently performed and are used to document specific diagnoses. However, the distinction between monitoring and diagnostic procedures becomes blurred when chest radiographs, arterial blood gas determinations, serum electrolyte analyses, and coagulation profiles are performed many times per day.

No single physiologic measurement or group of measurements can convey all aspects of a patient's condition. Clinical judgment, on the other hand, is subjective, is hard to define precisely, and cannot be quantitatively applied as a "yardstick." However, noninvasive hemodynamic monitoring in the emergency department and operating room and invasive hemodynamic and oxygen transport monitoring in the operating room and ICU may be used to identify correctable physiologic deficiencies in their early stages. Monitoring, like laboratory values and radiographic studies, supplements rather than supplants clinical guesswork with objective physiologic criteria; physiologic data may substantiate clinical opinions, give baseline values to judge progress, and provide criteria for titrating therapy to optimal goals. Most important, monitoring provides objective criteria for the evaluation of physiologic deficiencies separate from the diagnosed anatomic disease. This distinction is particularly important, because most people die not of their disease but of physiologic deficiencies that lead to vital organ failures.

This chapter summarizes the various circulatory parameters from routine noninvasive surveillance to invasive hemodynamic and oxygen transport monitoring methods. The monitoring of fetus and child, electrocardiography, electroencephalography, ventilation studies, arterial blood gas analysis, radiology, digital imaging, and cerebral pressure measurement are discussed in subsequent chapters.

ROUTINE SURVEILLANCE MONITORING

The patient undergoing elective surgery without complications is often monitored postoperatively simply with vital signs, electrocardiogram (ECG), urine output, central venous

TABLE 7–1. High-Risk Criteria for Surgical Patients

Preoperative Patients

1. Previous severe cardiorespiratory illness (e.g., acute MI, COPD, stroke)
2. Extensive ablative surgery planned for carcinoma (e.g., esophagectomy and total gastrectomy, or prolonged surgery [>6 hr])
3. Severe multiple trauma (e.g., involving more than three organs or more than two systems; opening of two body cavities [left side of chest and abdomen]; multiple longbone and pelvic fractures)
4. Massive blood loss (>8 units): BV >1.5 L/m^2 and Hct >20 mL/dL within 48 hr before admission
5. Age older than 70 yr and evidence of limited physiologic reserve of one or more vital organs
6. Shock: MAP <60 mm Hg; CVP <5 mm Hg; UO <20 mL/hr; cold, clammy skin
7. Septicemia: positive blood culture, WBC count >12,000/mm^3, spiking fever >101°F for 48 hr, chills
8. Evidence of septic shock (temperature >101°F, WBC count >12,000/mm^3) plus hypotension (MAP <70 mm Hg)
9. Severe nutritional problems associated with a surgical illness: weight loss >20 lb, albumin concentration <3 g/dL, osmolarity <280 mOsm/L
10. Respiratory failure (e.g., Pa_{O_2}, <60 mm Hg or FIO_2 >0.4, Qsp/Qt >30%, patient on mechanical ventilation)
11. Acute abdominal catastrophe (e.g., pancreatitis, gangrenous bowel, peritonitis, perforated viscus, and internal gastrointestinal bleeding)
12. CVP >15 mm Hg after fluid resuscitation
13. Acute renal failure: blood urea nitrogen >50 mg/dL, creatinine >3 mg/dL, C_{H_2O} >10 mL/hr
14. Acute hepatic failure (bilirubin >3 mg/dL, albumin concentration <3 g/dL, LDH >200 U/mL, alkaline phosphatase >100 U/mL, ammonia >120 μg/mL
15. Acute agitation, depressed nervous system, semicoma, or coma

Postoperative Patients

1. Acute catastrophic change, suggesting fresh MI, pulmonary embolus, or postoperative bleeding
2. Hypotension: MAP <70 mm Hg or unstable vital signs
3. Operative misadventure (e.g., use of >8 units of WB or PRBCs for estimated 4000-mL blood loss in the operating room)
4. Severe sepsis, perforated viscus, gangrenous bowel, peritonitis, pneumonia, positive blood culture, aspiration pneumonia, temperature elevation >101°F for >2 days
5. Any vital organ failure, that is, the same as in above preoperative conditions
6. Postoperative fluid-electrolyte problem requiring more than 5000 mL of fluids per day
7. Failure to respond to adequate volume therapy, which is replacement of blood losses estimated from sponge and lap counts and as judged by clinical criteria, such as arterial pressure, UO, Hct, level of consciousness, and motor responses

MI = mycocardial infarction; COPD = chronic obstructive pulmonary disease; BV = blood volume; Hct = hematocrit; MAP = mean arterial pressure, UO = urine output; WBC = white blood cell; LDH = lactate dehydrogenase; WB = whole blood; PRBCs = packed red blood cells; CVP = central venous pressure.

pressure (CVP), and occasional arterial blood gas determinations.

Vital Signs

Arterial pressure, heart rate, temperature, and respiratory rate—the vital signs—are the simplest, most easily measured, and most commonly monitored noninvasive circulatory variables. They are useful for screening and are part of routine hospital and ICU admissions, physical examinations, daily nursing routines, and preoperative and postoperative workups. Vital signs are recorded more frequently during periods of circulatory instability to provide a running graphic record of a patient's condition that may alert attendants to unexpected circulatory problems.

Arterial Pressures

Arterial blood pressure reflects overall circulatory status but lacks diagnostic specificity.[2] Arterial pressure falls in the following circumstances:

- After hypovolemia from blood or fluid loss
- During cardiac failure, acute trauma, sepsis, and anaphylactoid and vasovagal reactions
- With acute spinal cord and other neural lesions
- In the late or terminal stage of most diseases

Decreased blood pressure may also indicate circulatory decompensation or the failure of a specific therapy. Pressures increase with stress, excitement, anxiety, burns, and head injuries and in patients with hypertension or hypertensive diathesis. Increased blood pressure may indicate improved circulatory function, adrenal stress response, or excessive vasopressor therapy.

Arterial pressure measurements do not directly reflect reductions of blood flow and volume but, rather, the failure of the normal circulatory compensations, such as the adrenal stress response to hypovolemia. The interactions of blood pressure, flow, and volume are extremely complex, but hypotension simply represents failure of compensatory mechanisms after gross circulatory changes. Arterial pressure measurements are useful for screening and for rapid assessment of trends in emergency conditions, such as trauma and covert gastrointestinal bleeding; however, in and of themselves, they are of limited physiologic significance.

Normal arterial blood pressure, measured with a sphygmomanometer cuff, is approximately 120/80 mm Hg for healthy, young adults; this value increases gradually with age. As a rough estimate, the upper limit of normal for systolic pressures is 100 mm Hg plus the patient's age; systolic pressures greater than 160 mm Hg and diastolic pressures greater than 90 mm Hg suggest hypertension. Young adults, especially teenaged girls, may have blood pressures as low as 90/60 mm Hg. It is important for treatment to know the patient's preillness baseline pressures, especially if they are not within the standard range.

The pulse pressure is the difference between the systolic pressure and the diastolic pressure. Decreased pulse pressure may precede decreases in diastolic pressure in patients in whom shock is developing and is an early sign of hypovolemia.

Mean arterial pressure (MAP) is defined as the sum of the diastolic pressure and one third of the pulse pressure; alternatively, it may be expressed as one third of the sum of the systolic pressure and twice the diastolic pressure. MAP is also measured directly in various invasive and noninvasive recording systems as the dampened "electrical mean" of the systolic and diastolic pressures. MAP is frequently used in the calculation of derived hemodynamic variables, such as the systemic (peripheral) vascular resistance index, left ventricular stroke work index, and left cardiac work index.

Intra-arterial Blood Pressure

Devices for the invasive monitoring of blood pressure through the axillary, radial, ulnar, or femoral artery provide continuous display of the waveform along with measurements of systolic and diastolic pressures and of MAP. (The technique of catheter insertion, associated precautions, and its complications are discussed in Chapter 6.)

Intra-arterial pressure measured by intra-arterial catheters, pressure transducers, and a continuous recording apparatus that has been zeroed and calibrated is more accurate than cuff measurement of pressure. Under normal conditions, pressures obtained from intra-arterial catheters are about 2 to 8 mm Hg greater than cuff-measured pressures. In critically ill patients, intra-arterial pressures may be 10 to 30 mm Hg greater than cuff-measured pressures. Furthermore, cuff-measured pressures may be inaccurate in patients with severe vasoconstriction and low stroke volume.

Differences of 50 to 60 mm Hg between intra-arterial catheter-measured pressures and cuff-measured pressures have been reported. The following are indications for continuous invasive pressure recording:

- Shock
- Critical illness
- Marked peripheral vasoconstriction
- Intraoperative and postoperative monitoring of patients undergoing extensive or life-threatening operations
- Monitoring of patients with other high-risk conditions

In these cases, accurate continuous arterial pressure display is needed to observe trends and to titrate therapy. Moreover, arterial catheters allow frequent arterial blood gas measurements.[3]

Pressures should be measured in both arms early in the hospital course because specific unilateral arteriosclerotic or traumatic vascular lesions may produce differences of 10 to 20 mm Hg between the left-sided and right-sided values. Similarly, in trauma to the aorta or femoral artery, differences in cuff pressures between one leg or arm and the other may occur. Femoral arterial pressures are usually 5 to 10 mm Hg greater than brachial pressures.

Decreased arterial pressures during shock and trauma states are nonspecific and may be delayed because of the compensatory stress response; they poorly reflect deficits in blood volume or cardiac function. Pressures may be misleading in the case of falling blood volume and flow because the compensatory sympathetic adrenal stress reaction tends to maintain blood pressure, at least transiently, with declining blood flow. Hypotension occurs after compensatory mechanisms are exhausted, but this may be long after the precipitating event. Severely reduced cardiac output for periods of 40 minutes to 2 hours before a significant reduction in arterial pressure has been demonstrated.[3, 4] On the other hand, arterial pressure may be restored by fluids well before cardiac output and oxygen transport are corrected.[5]

Noninvasive Blood Pressure Monitoring

Manometric blood pressure measurements obtained by sphygmomanometry with the Korotkoff blood pressure sounds are routinely used to assess systolic and diastolic pressures. Initially, Dinamap (Critikon, Tampa, Fla.) measured only MAP, but current models display systolic, mean, and diastolic pressures. The instrument is sensitive to motion artifact, particularly muscle activity in the arm. This was the only available noninvasive method until 1970, when crystal microphones and piezoelectric crystals that employed the Doppler principle were developed. Subsequently, microprocessor-based devices such as Infrasonde (Puritan-Bennett, Carlsbad, Calif.) and Accutorr (Datascope, Paramus, N. J.), which use an oscillometric method that automatically inflates and deflates the cuff, were developed. These systems improved sensitivity, particularly in patients with low pressures and low blood flow.

The Infrasonde device is an auscultatory method for determining systolic and diastolic pressures. With its use, two crystal microphones are positioned over the bronchial artery; these microphones identify the Korotkoff blood pressure sounds. The cuff deflation rate can be selected by the operator.

Heart Rate

Indications for monitoring heart rate are the same as those for arterial pressure. Arterial pressure and heart rate are routinely measured at the same time and graphically recorded daily or twice daily on the vital signs sheet of the hospitalized patient's chart or at more frequent intervals intraoperatively, for patients in the ICU, for those receiving emergency services, and for those in special care units. Heart rate is usually determined by manual palpation of the radial artery just above the wrist for at least 30 seconds.

Tachycardia is defined as a heart rate greater than 100 beats per minute. When premature ventricular contractions or other irregularities are present, the heart rate may be determined by auscultation at the apex; the difference between apical and radial rates represents the number of dropped beats. Heart rates may also be measured automatically from either the ECG wave or the arterial pulse wave. In invasive hemodynamic monitoring, the heart rate is used to calculate stroke volume from cardiac output.

Heart rate is a nonspecific hemodynamic variable. Increased heart rate is part of an early neurohormonal stress response that also tends to increase flow in the presence of falling pressure. Its increase suggests blood flow and blood volume deficits; the faster the heart rate, the greater the hypovolemia or cardiac impairment. However, heart rate also increases with infection, anxiety, fear, fever, exercise, pain and discomfiture, and other nonspecific stresses.

Bradycardia, defined as a slow heart rate (<50 beats/min), may occur with inferior myocardial infarction when right coronary artery occlusion produces ischemia that blocks the sinoatrial node; it may also occur with other types of arteriosclerotic heart disease. Bradycardia during low cardiac output is an ominous sign suggesting markedly reduced and inadequate coronary blood flow that compromises myocardial performance. Arrhythmias associated with cardiac problems require that ECG and other methods be used to obtain specific diagnosis.

Temperature

Body temperature is measured routinely with the determination of blood pressure, pulse, and respiratory rate. It is usually measured either orally when significant elevations are not expected or rectally in ill patients. The central core temperature may be measured at the tympanic membrane or midesophagus for greater accuracy. Pulmonary arterial (PA) temperature, which also reflects core temperature, is routinely and continually measured by the PA thermodilution catheter.

Temperature elevations are most often associated with infection, the septic syndrome or systemic inflammatory response syndrome (SIRS), tissue necrosis, late-stage carcinomatosis, Hodgkin's disease, leukemia, hyperthyroidism, malignant hyperthermia, heat exhaustion, strenuous exercise, and other hypermetabolic states. Low-grade fever is also present after accidental or surgical trauma and particularly when hematomas, foreign bodies, fistulas, urinary extravasation, or stasis of urinary excretion or of bronchial secretions is present. Hypothermia may occur in some patients with septic shock, reduced metabolism associated with hypothyroidism, malnutrition, severe anemia, shock, trauma, and cold exposure. Like arterial pressure and heart rate determination, temperature measurement is a useful but nonspecific screening test.

Hematocrit

The hematocrit, a measure of the percentage of red blood cells in a sample of venous blood, has been widely used to assess blood loss after trauma and surgery. In general, hematocrit values are decreased by hemorrhage and increased by dehydration and hypovolemia; they are increased with packed red blood cell transfusions and decreased by fluid administration. The hematocrit is measured in the following situations:

- On routine admission
- In emergency conditions, including trauma and hemorrhage or suspected hemorrhage
- With fever, dehydration, or other water losses
- With suspected overtransfusion or overhydration
- With hemolysis, cell aggregation or sludging, and microthrombi
- With destruction of red blood cells after freshwater drowning, envenomation, consumption coagulopathies, and disseminated intravascular coagulation
- In high-risk postoperative patients, especially when intraperitoneal bleeding is suspected
- In patients with acute illnesses, circulatory shock, and sepsis

To measure the hematocrit, blood samples are drawn from a peripheral vein or artery; the blood is immediately injected into four or more heparinized capillary tubes, which are promptly spun for 4 minutes in a microcentrifuge. The results of replicate samples should agree to within 1%. Alternatively, 4 mL of blood is drawn into a syringe containing 0.1 mL heparin (1000 U/mL) and is immediately placed into a Wintrobe tube, which is centrifuged at 2000 *g* for 30 minutes. When blood is drawn for hematocrit measurement and allowed to stand for even brief periods, the red blood cells begin to settle and aggregate, leaving the top half of the syringe with considerably fewer cells than the bottom half; shaking the sample does not completely eliminate this problem because cell aggregates are not broken up by simple shaking. However, errors of less than 1% can be obtained when the hematocrit tubes are filled immediately after the blood is drawn.

Decreased percentage of red blood cells is an indirect effect of blood loss produced by the compensatory transcapillary refilling of plasma volume by interstitial water. This compensation takes appreciable time to occur. If a patient rapidly exsanguinates within a few minutes, the first and the last drops of blood have nearly the same hematocrit.[6] However, 500-mL blood loss in human volunteers is replaced by interstitial water during 18 hours.[6, 7] Plasma volume replacement after 600-mL blood loss occurs at about 1 mL/min for the first few hours and thereafter at successively decreasing rates. In the severely bled anesthetized dog, replacement occurs at maximum rates of 2.5 mL/min.[8] For these reasons, serial hematocrits at 2- to 4-hour intervals are recorded in the early period of traumatic or postoperative shock and when covert blood loss is suspected.

Decreases in serial hematocrits of postoperative and posttraumatic patients can signal the possibility of intra-abdominal hemorrhage, but such measurements are not specific and have severe limitations. Hematocrits represent static measurements of venous red blood cell concentrations; they are affected by gains or losses of plasma water as well as by gains or losses of red blood cells. For example, the hematocrit does not distinguish the effects of hemorrhage from those of red blood cells dropping out of the circulation by cell aggregation, microthrombi formation, or fluid retention; hematocrits do not distinguish between transfused red blood cells and newly synthesized red blood cells. Moreover, hematocrits may not be affected by fluids given intravenously that equilibrate or leak from the plasma into the interstitial space. Therefore, after a patient has been given large fluid volumes and transfusions, hematocrit changes are often misleading and difficult to interpret. Serial hematocrit measurements are a reasonably good screening test for assessing gross changes in the early stages of hemorrhage but do not reliably estimate the blood volume status.[9]

Urine Output Rate

After bladder catheterization with an indwelling urethral Foley catheter, the urine may be collected in a closed sterile system and the rate of urine output measured (usually hourly) and recorded. The catheter must be flushed with an aseptic solution at regular intervals, because the most common cause of low urine output or anuria in the hospitalized patient is a plugged catheter.

The urine output rate is a rough approximation of the perfusion to this one vital organ, provided that the patient has an adequate blood volume and no preexisting renal disease. In resuscitation from acute injury, decreased urine flow may reflect low blood volume, low cardiac output, poor perfusion of the kidney, or the onset of acute oliguric renal failure. However, urine output is not an adequate reflection of tissue perfusion in shock states, especially septic shock; good urine output has been documented up to the hour of death in patients with severe septic shock. More precise measures of renal function, such as creatinine, osmolar, and free water clearances, are presented later.

Electrocardiographic Monitoring

The ECG evaluates the electrical events of cardiac contraction by sensing voltages at the body surface. Early studies assumed the body to be a homogeneous volume conductor with uniform geometry similar to a tank of saline to accommodate the complex three-dimensional character of the body with varying distances of the heart from the recording electrodes. The Dutch physiologist Einthoven, in one model, represented the heart by two charged electrodes: a dipole with one positive pole and one negative pole; this dipole is surrounded by a hypothetical equilateral triangle. The electrical activity of the heart, represented by the equivalent dipole, changes its magnitude and orientation during the cardiac cycle. The sides of the triangle, which represent the axes of the three standard limb leads, provide a triaxial frame of reference for spatial orientation of magnitudes and directions of cardiac electrical activity. When it is combined with the chest (V lead) readings, the model can be further refined to have frontal, sagittal, and horizontal components; this approach led to considerable information on the electrophysiology of the heart (Chapters 42 and 95).

The standard three-lead ECG is recorded from the right arm (RA), left arm (LA), and left leg (LL). The standard limb leads are defined as lead I (LA-RA), lead II (LL-RA), and lead III (LL-LA); differences in electrical potential produced by the heart are measured across the designated limbs. Small electrodes corresponding to each lead are attached to the chest after application of a conductive salt paste to the skin. These electrodes pick up ECG waveforms, which are continuously displayed and, when desired, recorded on a permanent record at the patient's bedside and at a central monitor station. A 12-lead ECG is essential for cardiac patients and is useful to rule out cardiac complications in acutely injured patients, postoperative patients, and patients with sepsis. Frequently, lead II or other individual leads may be continuously monitored for arrhythmias.

The 12-lead ECG pattern is specific for diagnosis of cardiac conditions, and continuous ECG display of the lead II waveform provides the earliest indication of electrical changes associated with disorders of the cardiac muscle. Continuous ECG monitoring is essential for the patient with acute myocardial infarction because arrhythmias are the most common life-threatening complications. Although done routinely, continuous ECG monitoring of the postoperative general surgical patient is infrequently useful because the incidence of significant arrhythmias is low; we have found three acute myocardial infarctions after 8000 operations in a county hospital setting. The ECG may be overemphasized in noncardiac elective postoperative patients without high-risk criteria.[10] However, in hypovolemic and traumatic shock, arrhythmias, signs of subendocardial ischemias, and bradycardia occur with inadequate oxygen delivery to the myocardium and may suggest precardiac arrest conditions (see Chapter 8).

CHEMICAL METHODS

Assessment of Serum Electrolytes

Measurement of serum electrolyte levels is particularly important in acutely ill patients. Hypokalemia is associated with alkalosis from gastric outlet obstruction and other gastrointestinal conditions that produce severe vomiting; hyperkalemia is associated with acidosis. Hyperglycemia is associated with diabetes, stress, trauma, and head injury; hypoglycemia is associated with insulin reactions, insulinoma, or nutritional deficiency. Increasing levels of blood urea nitrogen and creatinine are associated with renal failure.

Chemical Assessment of Tissue Hypoxia

Five laboratory values suggest the presence of tissue hypoxia with anaerobic metabolism from inadequate tissue perfusion or unevenly distributed microcirculatory flow:

- Acidosis characterized by pH below 7.2
- Base deficit of more than 5 mEq and bicarbonate level below 20 mEq/L
- Anion gap of more than 8 mEq/L
- Blood lactate levels above 2 mEq/dL
- Gastric wall pH below 7.2

Routine Blood Chemistries

In acute illness, accidents, and other emergencies, serum sodium, potassium, and chlorine ion concentrations and blood glucose, lactate, blood urea nitrogen, and creatinine measurements are routinely taken. Testing of these biochemical indicators confirms or rules out various diagnoses, monitors the progress of various disease states, and assesses the efficacy of therapy in acute, rapidly progressive illnesses.

Prothrombin time, partial thromboplastin time, fibrinogen determination, fibrin split products, and platelet counts are used to monitor acute bleeding and clotting problems associated with shock, sepsis, trauma, and hemorrhage.

MINIMALLY INVASIVE MONITORING

More extensive invasive hemodynamic and oxygen transport monitoring may be used in actual or suspected acute circulatory problems, as follows:

- Perioperatively with high surgical risk
- Acute myocardial infarction or congestive heart failure
- Sepsis, septic syndrome, or SIRS
- Overt and covert blood loss
- Major trauma, head injury, or blunt injury to the chest or abdomen
- Shock or circulatory dysfunction from potentially life-threatening conditions

Invasive physiologic monitoring is done to identify circulatory deficiencies, to evaluate underlying physiologic problems, to define criteria for therapeutic goals, and to titrate therapy to achieve predetermined optimal goals.

Arterial Blood Gas and pH Measurements

Measurements of arterial blood gases and pH are useful for screening pulmonary function in critically ill patients (Table 7-2). They are essential in patients with respiratory illness and are indicated in the initial evaluation and work-up of patients with a variety of conditions[11, 12]:

- Patients with tachypnea, dyspnea, chronic obstructive pulmonary disease, and adult respiratory distress syndrome
- Those who have experienced accidental trauma, acute emergency conditions, extensive surgery, burns and smoke inhalation, and other catastrophic conditions
- Patients receiving controlled or assisted ventilation or oxygen therapy
- Critically ill patients suspected of having respiratory complications
- Preoperative evaluation and postanesthesia surveillance
- Patients with fluid and electrolyte problems
- Those with restlessness, anxiety, or mental confusion
- Those who have drug overdose
- Patients with altered mental status or who do not respond appropriately after anesthesia (see Chapter 8)

The first laboratory signs of early lung problems are usually arterial blood gas abnormalities, such as arterial partial pressure of oxygen ($Pa{O_2}$) values less than 70 mm Hg or arterial hemoglobin saturation ($Sa{O_2}$) below 90% in patients breathing room air (fractional inspired oxygen [FIO_2] = 0.2), arterial partial pressure of carbon dioxide ($Pa{O_2}$) values greater than 45 mm Hg, and pH values below 7.3 or above 7.5. Respiratory failure is suggested by $Pa{O_2}$ values of less than 50 mm Hg in the patient breathing room air or a $Pa{O_2}/FIO_2$ less than 200. The acutely ill patient is usually given supplementary oxygen by mask or nasal prongs as well as chest therapy. If these measures do not improve the blood gas values, endotracheal intubation and mechanical ventilation should be considered before $Pa{O_2}$ drops to less than 60 mm Hg. However, patients

TABLE 7–2. Blood Gas Variables and Normal Values on Room Air (FIO_2 = 0.21)

Arterial oxygen tension, $Pa{O_2}$, 80–95 mm Hg
Mixed venous oxygen tension, $P\bar{v}{O_2}$, 35–50 mm Hg
Arterial oxygen saturation, $Sa{O_2}$, 96–99%
Arterial oxygen concentration, $Ca{O_2}$, 17–20 mL/dL
Mixed venous oxygen concentration, $C\bar{v}{O_2}$, 12–15 mL/dL
Arteriovenous oxygen difference, $C(a - v)O_2$, 4–5 mL/dL
Arterial carbon dioxide tension, $Pa{CO_2}$, 35–45 mm Hg
Arterial carbon dioxide concentration, $Ca{CO_2}$, 23–27 mmol/L
Mixed venous carbon dioxide tension, $P\bar{v}{CO_2}$, 40–45 mm Hg
pH, 7.36–7.44
Bicarbonate (HCO_3^-), 22–28 mEq/L
Base excess or deficit, +3 to −3 mEq/L

with chronic respiratory insufficiency may tolerate low blood gas values but not require mechanical ventilation.

Gastric Tonometry

Gastric tonometry measures gastric and intestinal wall carbon dioxide by equilibration of partial pressure of carbon dioxide between a 2.5-mL saline-filled balloon on the end of a nasogastric tube and the gut wall layers. After 40 to 60 minutes allowed for equilibration, the balloon's saline is sampled and analyzed for P_{CO_2} in a blood gas analyzer; at the same time, an arterial blood sample is obtained for blood bicarbonate levels and the pHi is calculated from the Henderson-Hasselbalch equation.[13, 14]

The balloon carbon dioxide values are in equilibration with tissue carbon dioxide so that increases in the balloon carbon dioxide reflect increased tissue carbon dioxide production and indirectly reflect the degree of anaerobic metabolism. In shock, anaerobic metabolism generates hydrogen ions (H^+) that are then buffered by tissue bicarbonate and result in carbon dioxide production.[15-17] Normal tonometric measurement of gastric carbon dioxide establishes the adequacy of gastric circulation, whereas cellular accumulation of carbon dioxide reflects tissue hypoxia and acidosis.

Recent improvements have used an automated system that pumps air into the tonometer's balloon and then measures and records carbon dioxide by infrared analysis every 10 to 15 minutes.[17] Alternative methods being developed are balloonless fiberoptic carbon dioxide sensors directly in the gastric bubble; their utility and reliability must be determined in prospective trials.

Blood Volume Measurements

Blood volume is commonly inferred indirectly from measurements of arterial pressure, heart rate, CVP, pulmonary artery occlusion pressure (PAOP), urine output, and hematocrit. These may be useful during resuscitation of patients who are not seriously ill; however, they are notably unreliable indicators of blood volume in patients who are critically ill or in shock (Figs. 7–1 and 7–2). Blood volume measurements provide definitive therapeutic answers to hypovolemia and hypervolemia but have largely been replaced by PAOP (wedge pressure) measurements because of the hazards of radioactivity, the time required for measurement, and the cost associated with blood volume measurements.

Blood volume measurement is based on a simple concept: a known amount of a marker or indicator that mixes uniformly with the plasma or blood is injected intravenously, and its concentration or radioactivity is measured in blood samples obtained at timed intervals after injection of the indicator.[9, 18, 19] The concentration of the indicator is inversely proportional to its volume of dilution; the volume of dilution is calculated by the standard dilution formula,

$$C_1V_1 = C_2V_2$$

where C_1 and V_1 are the concentration and volume, respectively (i.e., mass of the injected indicator), and C_2 and V_2 are the concentration and volume of the indicator in its volume of distribution at the time of sampling.

Plasma volume was first measured with photometric assay of dyes, such as Evans blue (T1824), that are initially distributed in the plasma volume. This technique was replaced by radioassay of human serum albumin labeled with isotopic iodine (I 125 or I 131) and, to a much lesser extent, of erythrocytes labeled with chromium Cr 55 or phosphorus P 32. The ^{125}I- or ^{131}I-tagged albumin is available and convenient, but red blood cell labels are usually reserved for various research studies. In labeled albumin studies, two or more

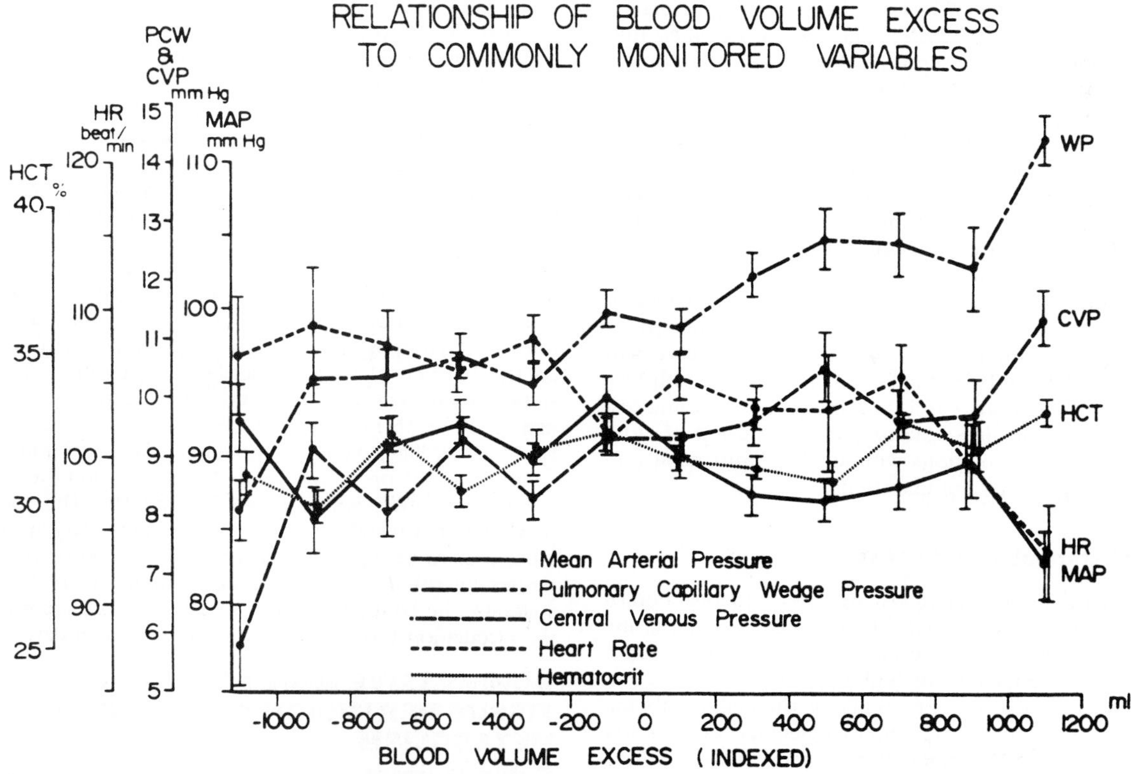

Figure 7–1. Mean ± SEM of the commonly monitored variables on the *y*-axis plotted against their corresponding blood volume excess (+) or deficit (−) indexed. Note the poor capacity of the monitored variables to predict blood volume. (From Shippy CR, Appel PL, Shoemaker WC: Reliability of clinical monitoring to assess blood volume in critically ill patients. Crit Care Med 1984; 12:107.)

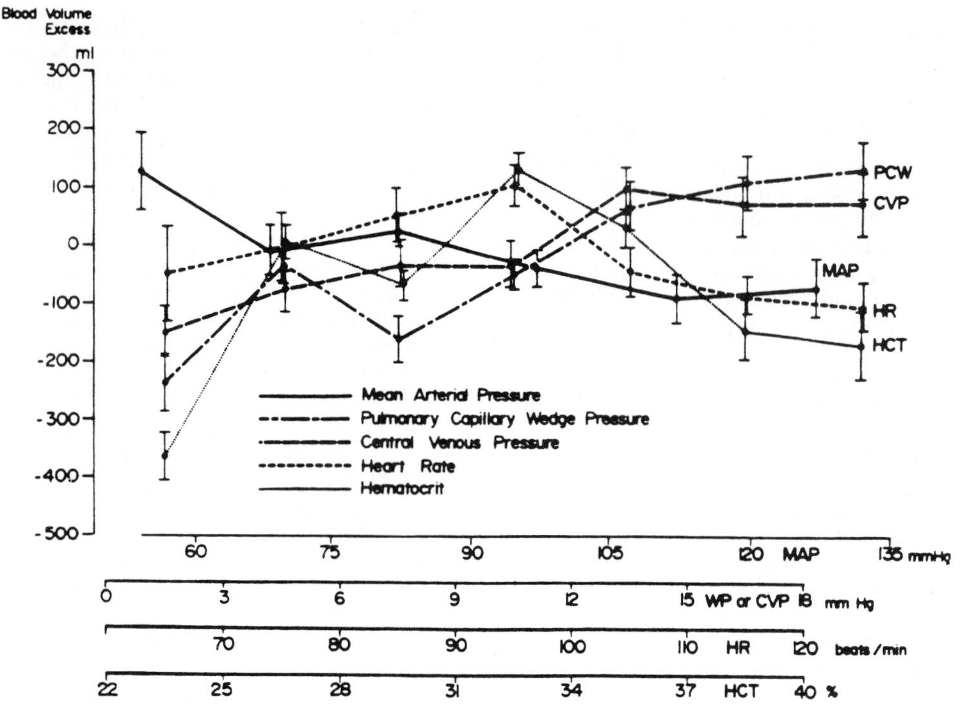

Figure 7–2. Mean ± SEM values of blood volume excess (+) or deficit (−) index on the *y*-axis plotted against their corresponding monitored variables. Note the poor capacity of the blood volume values to predict monitored variables. (From Shippy CR, Appel PL, Shoemaker WC: Reliability of clinical monitoring to assess blood volume in critically ill patients. Crit Care Med 1984; 12:107.)

preinjection control serum or plasma samples are radioassayed in duplicate and after injection of a measured dose of the labeled albumin, and three to six timed postinjection samples are similarly assayed; 4% corrections in the hematocrit measurements are made for the packing fraction of plasma, and 6% corrections are made for the difference between venous hematocrit and total body hematocrit.[20-22]

Normal blood volume is 2.74 L/m^2 or 7.5 mL/kg for males, 2.37 L/m^2 or 7 mL/kg for females. The patient in shock due to hemorrhage, trauma, and sepsis has been found empirically to do better with about 500 mL in excess of the expected norm (i.e., 3.2 L/m^2 for males and 2.9 L/m^2 for females). The extra volume compensates for maldistributions of blood volume, pooling of blood in the splanchnic area, red blood cell aggregation in the microcirculation, and red blood cell microthrombi. Accurate measurements require meticulous isotope dilution to obtain reproducible measurements with an acceptable error of 8% to 10%.

Blood volume, cardiac functional capacity, and colloidal osmotic pressure are of major importance in fluid therapy.[5-9, 18, 19] Hypovolemic patients with normal cardiac reserve can readily tolerate volume load (fluid challenge); those with low colloidal osmotic pressure, cardiac problems, and chronic respiratory conditions are less able to tolerate infusion of large volumes of crystalloid solutions without development of pulmonary edema and other complications.

Colloidal Osmotic Pressure

The plasma and interstitial fluids are two aqueous bodies separated by the capillary basement membrane, a semipermeable membrane that is freely permeable to water and electrolytes but barely permeable to high-molecular-weight compounds such as plasma proteins. Similarly, the cell membrane separates the intracellular water and extracellular water. Water migrates through each membrane to equalize the concentrations of the solutions on either side by the process of osmosis. The colloidal osmotic pressure, or oncotic pressure, is the osmotic force exerted on a membrane by macromolecules. It is a measure of the hydrostatic pressure applied to a solution of greater concentration that is just able to prevent the net movement of water across the membrane. Colloidal osmotic pressure, like osmotic pressure, is determined solely by the number of molecules in solution on each side of the membrane.

Normally, plasma water escapes from the vascular space at the arterial end of the capillary, where hydrostatic pressure is greatest. Water returns at the venous end because venous colloid osmotic pressure is greater than that of the interstitial water. The equivalent of the plasma volume (i.e., 3000 mL in the healthy 70-kg man) leaves and returns to the vascular space each minute. By contrast, about 1% of the plasma proteins, mainly albumin, also leaves the vascular space per minute; most of these proteins are returned by way of the lymphatics. About one third of the plasma water may be outside the anatomic confines of the vasculature at any given time. After hemorrhage, capillary refilling of the plasma volume occurs primarily as a result of these osmotic forces.[23]

The distribution of water between the intravascular and interstitial compartments of the systemic circulation depends on the balance of forces described by Starling.[23] The hydrostatic pressures at the arterial end of the capillary are approximately 25 to 35 mm Hg; the tissue pressure, −2 to +2 mm Hg; the capillary venous pressures, 10 to 15 mm Hg; the venous oncotic pressures, 24 to 28 mm Hg; and the interstitial oncotic pressure, about 15 to 20 mm Hg. The forces that determine net water movement across a capillary are normally close to zero or slightly negative; excess water driven into the tissues by this low net pressure is returned to the vascular space by the lymphatics. Two to 4 L of lymph are returned to the circulation through the thoracic duct each day.

NONINVASIVE MONITORING OF TISSUE PERFUSION AND OXYGEN METABOLISM

Pulse Oximetry

The development of microprocessors and light-emitting diodes has made continuous noninvasive monitoring of arterial oxygenation a routine monitoring method. In this technique, a red diode and an infrared diode are rapidly pulsed in sequence, and the amounts of light transmitted by each throughout successive heart beats are used to calculate a running average of Sa_{O_2} that is then displayed continuously on a monitoring screen.

The pulse oximeter (Nellcor, Pleasanton, Calif.) is designed to measure oxygen saturation differences in the pulse waveform; thus, without a good waveform, the instrument cannot function accurately. Moreover, it does not distinguish oxyhemoglobin level from the level of carboxyhemoglobin or that of methemoglobin, knowledge of which is needed in patients who have been exposed to carbon monoxide.

Simultaneous measurements of arterial saturation by the standard in vitro blood gas analysis (Sa_{O_2}) and pulse oximetry (Sp_{O_2}) showed reasonably good correlations ($r = 0.84$), but accuracy of pulse oximetry progressively decreased below 92% and became unreliable at values below 85%.[24] Nevertheless, it is a standard of care for early warning of hypoxemia, because early recognition of respiratory problems is more important than Sp_{O_2} accuracy at low values.

Pulse oximeters are useful during initial resuscitation of patients who have experienced trauma or other acute emergencies, during intraoperative and postoperative high-risk surgery, during anesthesia induction, and in critically ill patients with unstable hemodynamics or suspected respiratory problems. They are particularly helpful for titration of FI_{O_2} during mechanical ventilation and during weaning of patients from mechanical ventilation. The frequency of arterial blood gas measurement may be reduced with the use of pulse oximetry. This is important in children and in those with acute, rapidly changing critical illnesses. Disposable probes are used in patients with infectious conditions.

Transcutaneous Oxygen Monitoring of Tissue Perfusion

Clark[12] developed the first practical polarographic electrode in 1956 using a semipermeable polyethylene membrane–covered platinum cathode. This rapidly became the standard for blood gas analysis. Subsequently, Hüch and associates[25] and Eberhard and colleagues[26] described the use of heated Clark electrodes for continuous noninvasive transcutaneous oxygen tension (Ptc_{O_2}) measurements. On the assumption that Pa_{O_2} and Ptc_{O_2} are identical or nearly identical to their arterial blood measurements, this technology was used as a surrogate for Pa_{O_2} values in neonates and infants and to reduce the need for arterial blood sampling. When differences between Pa_{O_2} and Ptc_{O_2} occurred, they were usually attributed to failure of the Ptc_{O_2}-measuring instrument. Although Ptc_{O_2} usually reflected Pa_{O_2} when the neonate was hemodynamically stable, it was appreciably lower than Pa_{O_2} in the seriously ill neonate with circulatory problems.

In adults, Ptc_{O_2} is about 80% of the value for Pa_{O_2} during stable or normal hemodynamic conditions[27]; however, when blood flow rate limits body metabolism, Ptc_{O_2} tracks flow. In both normal and low-flow states, Ptc_{O_2} was used to track oxygen delivery ($\dot{D}_{O_2}$). In essence, Ptc_{O_2} is only indirectly related to Pa_{O_2}; it is directly related to local tissue perfusion and oxygenation.[28]

The heating of the skin by the transcutaneous electrode changes the structure of the lipoproteins in the stratum corneum from the gel to the sol state. This allows rapid diffusion of oxygen from subcutaneous tissues to the surface electrode. However, the heating affects tissue and blood by decreasing oxygen solubility, shifting the oxyhemoglobin dissociation curve to the right, and dilating the local metarterioles. An electrode temperature of 44° to 45°C increases diffusion of oxygen across the stratum corneum and avoids vasoconstriction in the local area of the skin being measured.[27-29] This allows the Ptc_{O_2} to become closer to Pa_{O_2} in hemodynamically stable patients.[28]

Ptc_{O_2} measures oxygen tension in a local segment of heated skin.[27] This is not necessarily the same in all segments of the skin or in other peripheral tissues; because the skin is most sensitive to peripheral vasoconstriction from the adrenomedullary stress response, it provides an earlier warning than Sv_{O_2} and $\dot{V}_{O_2}$.[21, 22] Limitations of Ptc_{O_2} are that the electrode placement must be changed every 4 to 6 hours to avoid first-degree skin burns, the thermal environment should be reasonably constant, and the membranes must be calibrated before each use and each change in skin site. The membrane must be changed when readings become unstable.

Early studies in the adult demonstrated the capacity of transcutaneous oxygen tension to reflect tissue oxygen tension.[27-30] Transcutaneous oxygen tension (Ptc_{O_2}) has been shown to reflect the delivery of oxygen to the local area of skin; it also parallels the mixed venous oxygen tension except under late or terminal conditions in which peripheral shunting leads to high mixed venous hemoglobin saturation ($S\bar{v}_{O_2}$) values.[27]

Because Ptc_{O_2} values are dependent on both Pa_{O_2} and local blood flow (or local $\dot{D}_{O_2}$), Ptc_{O_2} may track Pa_{O_2} when flow is adequate and track flow or $\dot{D}_{O_2}$ when Pa_{O_2} is adequate. In either case, Ptc_{O_2} reflects local $\dot{D}_{O_2}$. From a practical clinical viewpoint, the Ptc_{O_2} patterns reflect tissue perfusion and oxygenation useful for screening.[29] On room air, Ptc_{O_2} values greater than 65 mm Hg suggest satisfactory perfusion; values from 40 to 65 mm Hg suggest marginal perfusion; values from 25 to 40 mm Hg indicate impaired tissue perfusion; and values less than 25 mm Hg indicate severe shock.[24, 29]

Ptc_{O_2} and $\dot{V}_{O_2}$ values were simultaneously measured in a series of trauma patients admitted to the emergency department. The Ptc_{O_2} roughly tracked $\dot{V}_{O_2}$ at an initial baseline period, the nadir, and the postresuscitation period, but the Ptc_{O_2} nadir occurred about 12 minutes before the $\dot{V}_{O_2}$ nadir.[24] Measurement of Ptc_{O_2} is useful in the management of trauma and other emergency conditions immediately after hospital admission, in the perioperative and postanesthesia period, and in the ICU. Because it measures tissue perfusion, it is an important part of multicomponent noninvasive monitoring systems.[24, 29]

Transcutaneous Carbon Dioxide Tension

Transcutaneous carbon dioxide tension (Ptc_{CO_2}) measurement based on the use of the Stowe-Severinghaus carbon dioxide electrode was initially used in neonates to approximate Pa_{CO_2}. However, the Ptc_{CO_2} values parallel but consistently overestimate by 10 to 30 mm Hg the Pa_{CO_2} values in both hemodynamically stable neonates and adults.[30]

In shock, Ptc_{CO_2} may be greatly elevated to values above 100 mm Hg; it is inversely related to cardiac output.[30] Differences between the value of Pa_{CO_2} and Ptc_{CO_2} reflect accumulation of carbon dioxide in the tissues due to inadequate perfusion and indirectly reflect peripheral perfusion in shock states.

RENAL FUNCTION MONITORING

Urine Output Rate

Urine, which is the end product of renal excretory function, is generated by plasma filtration and subsequent volume and composition changes in the ultrafiltrate. The hourly rate of urine output obtained with the use of an indwelling urethral catheter is a rough first approximation to renal perfusion, provided that the patient has an adequate blood volume and no preexisting renal disease. Polyuria refers to daily urine output of more than 3 L, oliguria to less than 0.4 L in 70-kg persons; anuria is urine output of less than 50 mL/day. In acute injury, decreased urine flow may reflect low blood volume, low cardiac output, poor perfusion of the kidney, or the onset of acute oliguric renal failure.

Glomerular Filtration Rate

Renal function may initially be evaluated by concentrations of blood urea nitrogen, normally 10 to 20 mg/dL, and serum creatinine, normally less than 1.5 mg/dL. Abnormal values or increasing values of these two compounds suggest impaired renal function; this may be more precisely evaluated by glomerular filtration rates by creatinine clearance (normal, 90 to 140 mL/min), the standard clinical method, or inulin clearance, which is the classic "gold standard."

Plasma and Urine Osmolality; Osmolar and Free Water Clearances

The ability of the kidney to concentrate urine is its most sensitive and important function. This capacity, which conventionally has been inferred from urine output rates and specific gravity, is best evaluated by measurements of the ratio of the osmolalities of urine and plasma (Uosm/Posm) or by determinations of osmolar and free water clearances. Uosm/Posm greater than 1.7 suggests good concentrative ability, but in the presence of oliguria, this ratio may be normal even when osmolar clearance is low. Renal function is better evaluated by determination of osmolar clearances, which express the rate of solute removal from the plasma; normally, the osmolar clearance is 120 mL/hr, but it is markedly decreased in acute renal failure.

Free water clearance, which more explicitly considers osmotic clearance with respect to the rate of urine output, is a more sensitive indicator that may be used to predict the early onset of postoperative acute renal failure. Normally, it is strongly negative, ranging from −25 to −100 mL/hr. Transient positive values followed by values close to zero precede the development of acute renal failure. For example, a patient with urine osmolality of 330 mOsm/L, plasma osmolality of 300 mOsm/L, and urine output of 100 mL/hr has a relatively normal osmolar clearance (110 mL/hr); however, the high free water clearance (10 mL/hr) indicates high-output renal failure.

Osmolality of both plasma and urine is easily measured by using the freezing point depression method (with a Fiske osmometer) or the vapor pressure method. Uosm/Posm is readily calculated from these two measurements. If the rate of urinary output (V) is also measured with the same specimen, the osmolar clearance (Cosm) is

$$\text{Cosm} = \text{Uosm}/\text{Posm} \times \text{V}$$

and the free water clearance is

$$C_{H_2O} = \text{V} - \text{Cosm}$$

CEREBRAL FUNCTION MONITORING

Level of Consciousness and the Glasgow Coma Scale Score

Clinical assessment of the level of consciousness is a sensitive index of brain edema in postoperative and post-traumatic patients. This has been standardized as the Glasgow Coma Scale, which provides a semiquantitative measure of the degree of consciousness or coma.[31]

Electroencephalography

Electroencephalography may be used to noninvasively evaluate neural function intraoperatively and in critically ill patients with possible central nervous system deficits. It may be used to diagnose and localize cerebral lesions in patients with acute neurologic problems, including craniocerebral injuries. Continuous electroencephalographic monitoring is occasionally used to evaluate cerebral perfusion during the administration of anesthetics during open heart surgery, carotid endarterectomy, cerebrovascular surgery, epilepsy surgery, and induced hypotension for various surgical procedures (see Chapter 166).

Intracranial Pressure Measurement

Cerebral edema rapidly increases intracranial pressures because the brain, unlike other organs, is rigidly confined within the skull. Even small amounts of swelling may displace part of the 120 to 150 mL of cerebrospinal fluid and can result in high tissue pressures, headache, loss of consciousness, coma, and brain death. Increased intracerebral pressures are most frequently seen after closed head injury, intracranial operations, subarachnoid hemorrhage, and other vascular accidents as well as in patients with Reye's syndrome, brain tumor, meningitis, and encephalitis.

Continuous intracranial pressure measurement and recording can be obtained with a hollow, fluid-filled Richmond screw placed in the subdural space or with a cannula placed in the lateral ventricle. After local anesthesia with 1% or 2% lidocaine, the screw or the cannula is inserted through small burr holes made in the parietal region of the calvarium; the nondominant hemisphere is usually selected. The Richmond screw may be placed just beneath the dura; the screw or cannula sensor is attached to a conventional pressure transducer and recording system for measurement, graphic display, and recording of intracranial pressures. The intraventricular cannula is more accurate and less likely to become dampened than is the screw. Cerebrospinal fluid may be withdrawn for culture and chemical analyses or drained during periods of intracranial hypertension.

VENTILATORY MONITORING

Ventilation, the movement of gas in and out of the lungs, is commonly assessed by determination of the *tidal volume* (V_T), the average volume of gas inspired with each breath; the *minute volume* (MV), the mean volume of inspired gas per minute; and the *respiratory rate* (f), the mean number of breaths taken per minute. Less commonly, the *respiratory quotient* may be measured by spirometry or calculated from the rate of carbon dioxide production ($\dot{V}CO_2$) based on end-tidal carbon dioxide tensions (P_{ETCO_2}) measured by mass spectrometry. The dead space (V_{DS}/V_T) is also calculated from the P_{ETCO_2} by the Bohr equation (see Chapter 110).

INVASIVE HEMODYNAMIC MONITORING

Invasive monitoring is usually performed at the rate of four or five times the expected mortality rate to include all potentially correctable fatal deficiencies. Monitoring should be initiated as early as possible because it is more cost-effective to prevent circulatory deficiencies that lead to organ failures than to treat them after they are established. Table 7-1 lists high-risk surgi-

TABLE 7–3. Monitored Physiologic Variables

Arterial blood pressure (systolic, diastolic, and mean)
Heart rate
Temperature
Hematocrit and hemoglobin concentration
Urine output rate
Electrocardiogram (see Chapter 95)
Serum electrolytes and blood chemistries
Central venous pressure
Arterial blood gases and pH (see Chapters 110 and 120)
Pulse oximetry
Transcutaneous oxygen and carbon dioxide tensions
Blood volume, plasma volume
Plasma colloidal osmotic pressure
Plasma and urine osmolality, osmolar and freewater clearances
Electroencephalogram (see Chapter 166)
Intracranial pressure (see Chapter 166)
Pulmonary arterial and precapillary wedge pressures
Cardiac output and hemodynamic variables
Oxygen transport variables
Continuous cardiac output and oxygen consumption measurements
Ventilatory monitoring (see Chapter 112)
Noninvasive cardiac output by ultrasound method
Noninvasive cardiac output by thoracic electrical bioimpedance
Multicomponent circulatory monitoring

cal conditions appropriate for invasive monitoring that have an expected mortality rate of about 30%.[1] Hemodynamic monitoring may also be indicated when vital signs, hematocrit, blood gases, urine output, and CVP suggest the presence of circulatory problems.

About 25 monitored variables are commonly used for evaluating critically ill ICU patients (Table 7-3). They vary from vital sign measurements to the invasive assessment of hemodynamic and oxygen transport variables. Normal values of commonly monitored variables are listed in Table 7-4.

Central Venous Pressure

Following the classic work on venous pressures,[32-34] CVP and right atrial pressure monitoring were used to guide volume replacement for both medical and general surgical patients. Because it is simple and available, CVP monitoring is routinely used to guide fluid therapy after hemorrhage, surgery, accidental trauma, sepsis, and other emergency conditions with suspected blood volume deficits or excesses.

The catheters are simple to place, and the pressures are easy to read. The most important problem in accurately measuring CVP is the establishment of a consistent "zero" point that permits measurement of meaningful changes by individual attendants on different shifts. The point of entrance of the vena cava into the right atrium is located about 10 cm above the posterior surface of the back or 10 cm below the sternum in the sixth interspace in the supine position. The point selected may be marked on the patient's side with a felt-tip pen, and the pressure transducer is adjusted to this level as the bed is raised or lowered; alternatively, the effect of changes in the body position or height of the bed may be corrected electronically.

TABLE 7–4. Normal Values for the Most Commonly Monitored Variables

Variable	Normal Value	Units
Arterial blood pressure	120/80	mm Hg
Mean arterial pressure	80–95	mm Hg
Heart rate	60–80	beats/min
Temperature	36–37	degrees Celsius
Hematocrit	42–45	%
Hemoglobin concentration	13–15	g/dL
Central venous pressure	−2 to +6	mm Hg
Urine output	40–60	mL/hr
Blood volume		
Men	2.74	L/m^2
Women	2.37	L/m^2

The average CVP values during normal inspiration and expiration in healthy persons are −2 and +6 mm Hg, respectively. A healthy, ambulatory person who is lying down may have CVP values that average about 6 to 8 mm Hg; as the vascular tree accommodates, the CVP values gradually decrease. The upper limit of normal commonly used for acutely ill patients is 10 mm Hg. However, critically ill patients receiving mechanical ventilation and positive end-expiratory pressure, who require fluid volume to maintain arterial pressure, may have CVP values of 20 mm Hg. When CVP values exceed 15 to 18 mm Hg, a pulmonary arterial balloon flotation catheter may be used to measure the pulmonary artery occlusion (wedge) pressure (PAOP) for more precise titration of fluids.

CVP is increased by blood volume, impaired cardiac function, increased intrathoracic or increased intra-abdominal pressures, vasopressors, and fluid therapy. It is lowered by improved cardiac function, reduced intrathoracic pressure, vasodilators, hypovolemia, and sudden blood or fluid losses. However, CVP values and changes in CVP after therapy also depend on venous wall compliance. Large fluid infusions may produce only small transient CVP changes in hypovolemic patients, but even small fluid volumes may appreciably elevate CVP in patients with stress, chronic congestive cardiac failure, fluid overload, overtransfusion, or hypervolemia. Patients with chronic renal and cardiac failure are particularly vulnerable to either fluid overload or more fluid than they can handle; by contrast, acutely ill hypovolemic patients are particularly vulnerable to delayed or inadequate fluid therapy. This problem is overcome by careful titration of fluids and blood losses.

Although reduced CVP occurs during and immediately after acute hemorrhage, the blood volume and CVP correlate poorly after the patient has remained a day or so in the ICU, despite the presence of major blood volume deficits or excesses. This is because venous wall compliance rapidly accommodates to wide variations in blood volume; CVP and PAOP usually remain about 8 to 12 mm Hg despite carefully measured blood volume deficits of 1 L/m^2 to excesses of 2 L/m^2 (see Figs. 7-1 and 7-2). Therefore, it is seriously misleading to assess blood volume status from CVP because the correlation between CVP and blood volume according to conventional thinking is not just overly simplistic, it is relevant only in the extreme range of CVP or PAOP.

Measurement errors are caused by catheter obstruction, motion artifacts, and failure to establish consistent baseline values in patients who must be frequently repositioned or whose bed must be lowered or elevated; in the last two instances, it is absolutely necessary to make corresponding transducer changes. Methods for placing CVP lines and other vascular access problems are covered in Chapter 6.

Patients with right-sided heart failure classically have distention of the neck veins that reflects increased CVP. In many instances, right-sided heart failure is secondary to left-sided heart failure; in such cases, left atrial, end-diastolic, and, subsequently, PA wedge pressures rise; PA pressure elevations increase the work of the right side of the heart. If the PA systolic pressure is less than 40 mm Hg in chronic conditions, the right ventricle usually maintains normal flow. However, with prolonged elevation of PA pressure, the right ventricle may fail, and CVP can increase. Less commonly, right-sided heart failure occurs with right myocardial infarction and without left-sided heart failure, particularly in patients with pulmonary hypertension. Also, right-sided heart failure may occur in the presence of high pulmonary vascular resistance caused by pulmonary emboli, chronic obstructive lung disease, adult respiratory distress syndrome, and other types of respiratory failure.

Wide variation in the CVP may occur:

1. If the central line slips into the right ventricle.
2. In severe right-sided heart failure and dilation of the atrioventricular ring.
3. In cases of tricuspid insufficiency.

CVP measurements are most useful during early resuscitation from acute injury with hypotension; initially, hypovolemia occurs with low CVP. A CVP in excess of 20 to 25 mm Hg usually indicates that too much fluid has been given, that fluids were given too rapidly, or that an exaggerated stress response has occurred. Knowledge of CVP is most helpful with failure of only one organ system, such as cardiac failure, or uncomplicated blood loss. Increased CVP or wedge pressures in response to administration of a standardized volume load over a prescribed time period provide valuable information; tolerance to volume loads indicates adequate cardiac reserve capacity.

Peripheral venous pressures in the high ranges reflect CVP, but measurements of these two pressures diverge in the low ranges. The central venous system, including the right atrium and the vena cava and its major branches, acts as a unicameral system with nearly equal pressures. In hypovolemia, the extent of the unicameral behavior of the system is limited, and the peripheral venous pressures largely reflect local influences upstream from their site of measurement. By contrast, in the hypervolemic state and in right-sided heart failure, the venous tree is distended by the accumulation of blood behind the right ventricle; as this venous engorgement increases, the dimensions of the unicameral central venous pool increase along with peripheral venous pressure measurements; then high peripheral venous pressure values closely correlate with high CVP values.

Insertion of Pulmonary Artery Catheters

Description of catheter insertion and its complications are detailed in Chapter 6. The PA balloon flotation catheter is commercially available on a 100-cm double-lumen, triple-lumen, or quadruple-lumen catheter. In its simplest form, it consists of an inflatable balloon connected to the tip of the catheter's smaller (minor) lumen. The balloon may be inflated with 0.5 to 0.8 mL of air (not water), introduced with a 1- or 2-mL syringe attached to the minor lumen that is suitably marked by a red-handled, on-off valve. The bursting volume of the balloon is less than 3 mL. The major or distal lumen, which terminates at the catheter tip, should be filled with saline before insertion to avoid the small air embolus produced by infusion of fluid into an "empty" (air-filled) catheter lumen.

The quadruple-lumen PA cardiac output catheter has a yellow distal port that is used to withdraw blood samples and to record PA and PAOP measurements; the proximal blue port is for injection of iced glucose solution for cardiac output measurements.[35-37] The quadruple-lumen catheter includes a thermodilution system for cardiac output measurements and pacing electrodes.

The catheter is percutaneously introduced into the subclavian, jugular, brachial, or femoral vein; if this is not possible, it can be introduced by cutdown on a suitably sized vein in the antecubital fossa, saphenous system, or other accessible site (see Chapter 6). If the subclavian vein is used, the catheter is advanced centrally about 40 cm (indicated by the markings on the side of the catheter); the hub of the catheter is connected to a suitable pressure transducer and recording device. At this point, the patient is asked to take a deep breath or to cough; sizable pressure oscillations indicate that the tip of the catheter is in the vena cava.

Next, 0.05 to 0.8 mL of air is introduced into the minor lumen, and the catheter is further advanced gently while the attendant views the pressure waveform. The bloodstream usually carries the catheter into the right atrium, where the atrial A and V waves may be seen (Fig. 7–3). As the catheter is cautiously advanced, the characteristic right ventricular pulse waves become visible. The systolic pressure in the right ventricle usually ranges from 20 to 30 mm Hg; the diastolic pressure reading is close to the CVP or right atrial pressure. As the catheter is advanced farther, high-frequency oscillations ("ringing") indicate passage of the catheter's tip through the pulmonary valve and into the PA. At this point, the pulmonary systolic pressure is similar to that of the right ventricle, but the pulmonary diastolic pressure is considerably higher than

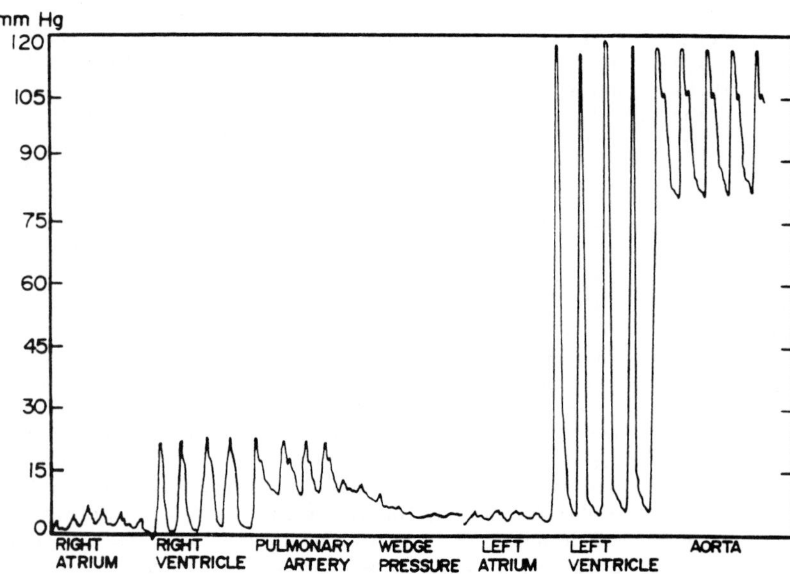

Figure 7–3. Intravascular pressure measurements at various segments of the vascular system, showing the general pattern of the various pressure waveforms from the right atrium, right ventricle, and pulmonary artery and, with the inflation of the balloon, wedge pressure; left atrial, left ventricular, and aortic pressure waveforms are then shown.

the right ventricular diastolic pressure, which is similar to the CVP or PAOP.

The inflated balloon is advanced until it reaches a PA branch. The physician deflates the balloon by removing the syringe; the barrel of the syringe is not withdrawn, because even with slight suction, the thin wall of the balloon may be forced into the catheter port and rupture. When the balloon is gradually reinflated, the pressure at the catheter's tip falls, and the pulse wave dampens; this plateau is called the *wedge pressure* because of its similarity to the pressure obtained when an ordinary cardiac catheter is "wedged" into a small PA branch. The assumption is that a static, nonflowing column of blood that extends from the catheter's lumen to the pulmonary arterioles, capillaries, and veins of the lung segment provides a measure of the pressure downstream from the catheter tip and approximates the pulmonary venous and left atrial pressures.[35-37]

Complications of cardiac catheterization include pulmonary infarction, small pulmonary embolus formation, rupture of a branch of the PA, pneumothorax, arteriovenous fistula formation, kinking or looping of the catheter in the right ventricle, knotting of the catheter, arrhythmias, infection, bacterial colonization on the catheter wall, and bleeding and local infection at the insertion site.

Pulmonary Artery and Pulmonary Artery Occlusion (Wedge) Pressures

The balloon-tipped, flow-directed PA (Swan-Ganz) catheter is commonly used to measure PA pressures and PAOP as a means to assess left ventricular filling pressures; this is similar to that of CVP values to assess right ventricular filling pressure.[35, 36] The PA catheter is frequently used to diagnose circulatory deficiencies and to differentiate acute cardiac failure from hypovolemia or hypervolemia problems.[37] It is also used with cardiac output and oxygen transport measurements to monitor the progress of therapy in patients with acute myocardial infarction or other types of cardiac problems, shock, trauma, or other critical illnesses in which the fluid and circulatory status is uncertain. For example, in acute myocardial infarction, the expected hemodynamic pattern is hypotension, low cardiac output, and increased ventricular filling pressure (i.e., PAOP), usually in combination with decreased ventricular contractility and compliance. Monitoring PA pressure and PAOP is indicated to observe the progress of the disease and to titrate various therapeutic interventions.

In normal conditions, left atrial pressure is within 2 or 3 mm Hg of right atrial pressure; but in the higher ranges or in patients with valvular lesions, the mean left atrial pressure or PAOP may be higher than the right atrial pressure or CVP. There are marked differences between CVP and PAOP with predominantly unilateral ventricular disease when pulmonary vascular resistance is elevated in acute postoperative respiratory failure.

PA hypotension is frequently seen in hypovolemic shock, but PA hypertension may occur in patients after rapid fluid resuscitation for hypovolemic and traumatic shock as well as in those with congenital intra-atrial and intraventricular defects, chronic obstructive lung disease, and primary pulmonary hypertension. Transient PA pressure increases accompany fluid and transfusion therapy, particularly in various shock syndromes.

The PAOP closely parallels left atrial and left ventricular end-diastolic pressures unless significant mitral valve stenosis or pulmonary venous resistance exists (as may be seen in patients with chronic obstructive pulmonary disease). In mitral stenosis, high PAOP cannot be taken to mean that left ventricular filling is adequate because of increased pressure gradients across the mitral valve. During and after mitral and aortic valve replacement, left ventricular filling pressures may be measured by using left atrial pressures obtained through a left atrial catheter placed intraoperatively.

PAOP is affected by the same factors that influence CVP, that is, blood volume, ventricular function, intrathoracic and intra-abdominal pressures, vasopressors, vasodilators, and fluid therapy as well as by conditions that increase cardiac afterload. PAOP, similar to CVP, is not a reliable measure of blood volume[9] (see Figs. 7-1 and 7-2). In ICU conditions, pulmonary and systemic venous wall tone accommodates to blood volume deficits or excesses; this leads to CVP and PAOP usually between 8 and 12 mm Hg in patients with either hypovolemia or hypervolemia. With fluid therapy, sudden increases in the PAOP to greater than 20 mm Hg may be due to infusion of too much intravenous fluid too rapidly, to inadequate left ventricular contractility, or to high positive end-expiratory pressure or intrathoracic pressure.

Although blood volume should not be inferred from the absolute or "static" CVP or PAOP values, these pressure measurements will indicate the capacitance for additional fluids. For example, if standardized volumes of 500 mL of colloids or 1000 mL of crystalloids are given in a 1-hour period, the increase in CVP or PAOP and the duration of this increase indicate tolerance to additional fluid therapy; a CVP or PAOP increase from 10 to 12 mm Hg that finally settles at 11 mm Hg 30 minutes after the infusion suggests that more fluids may be safely given if needed to achieve physiologic goals, but persisting increases from 10 to 17 mm Hg suggest limited tolerance for additional fluids.

Cardiac Output and Hemodynamic Variables

The important aspects of the hemodynamic system are blood pressure, volume, flow, and tissue perfusion. *Cardiac output* is the rate of blood flow pumped by the heart per minute; measurements are easy to make, readily automated, simple in concept, relatively straightforward as a technique, and with appropriate quality control may be performed by nurses and medical technologists. Volume and flow measurements should be indexed by dividing them by the patient's body surface area or body weight and expressed as cardiac index. This standardization allows comparison of hemodynamic values of patients with widely varying size and body habitus. The various hemodynamic variables may be calculated from pressure and flow data by use of standard formulas (Table 7-5).

In 1887, Fick postulated that if the oxygen content of arterial (Ca_{O_2}) and mixed venous ($C\bar{v}_{O_2}$) blood as well as oxygen consumption ($\dot{V}_{O_2}$) were known, blood flow could be calculated with use of the following equation:

$$\text{cardiac output} = \dot{V}_{O_2}/(Ca_{O_2} - C\bar{v}_{O_2})$$

The direct Fick method for estimation of cardiac output has become the physiologists' gold standard against which other methods are evaluated. Initially, the direct Fick method classically required measurement of $\dot{V}_{O_2}$ by spirometry or by timed collection of expired gas in a Douglas bag and simultaneous anaerobic sampling of blood from a systemic artery and the right ventricle or PA at the time of the $\dot{V}_{O_2}$ measurements. Oxygen concentrations were classically measured directly by manometry but are now calculated from hemoglobin concentrations and saturations measured by co-oximetry (Co-Oximeter, Radiometer, Westlake, Ohio; and Instrument Laboratories, Lexington, Mass.). Nowadays, $\dot{V}_{O_2}$ is calculated by metabolic carts that measure inspired and expired oxygen concentrations and tidal volume. This requires meticulous

TABLE 7–5. Hemodynamic Variables

Variable	Formula	Normal Value	Units
Cardiac index	CI = cardiac output/BSA	3.2 ± 0.2	$L \cdot min^{-1} \cdot m^2$
Systemic vascular resistance index	SVRI = 79.92* (MAP − CVP)/CI	2180 ± 210	$dyne \cdot s/cm^5 \cdot m^2$
Pulmonary vascular resistance index	PVRI = 79.92* (MPAP − WP)/CI	270 ± 15	$dyne \cdot s/cm^5 \cdot m^2$
Mean transit time	Direct measurement	15 ± 1.4	s
Central blood volume	CBV = MTT × CI × 16.7	830 ± 86	mL/m^2
Stroke index	SI = CI/HR	46 ± 5	mL/m^2
Left ventricular stroke work	LVSW = SI × MAP × 0.144*	56 ± 6	$g \cdot m/m^2$
Right ventricular stroke work	RVSW = SI × MPAP × .0144*	8.8 ± 0.9	$g \cdot m/m^2$
Left cardiac work	LCW = CI × MAP × .0144	3.8 ± 0.4	$kg \cdot m/m^2$
Right cardiac work	RCW = CI × MPAP × .0144	0.6 ± 0.06	$kg \cdot m/m^2$

*0.0144 and 79.92 are conversion terms.
BSA = body surface area; MAP = mean arterial pressure; CVP = central venous pressure; MPAP = mean pulmonary artery pressure; WP (or PAOP) = pulmonary artery occlusion pressure (or wedge pressure); MTT = mean transit time; HR = heart rate.

standardization and calibration (see later, Continuous Cardiac Output and Oxygen Consumption Monitoring). These measurements and their calculations require steady-state conditions and are not valid in unstable hemodynamic states and acute crises.

The indicator dilution technique for measurement of cardiac output was described by Hamilton and coworkers and is based on a concept originally proposed by Stewart. A measured amount of indicator (e.g., 2 to 4 mg of indocyanine green dye) is injected rapidly into a CVP catheter, and arterial blood is continuously sampled through a constant withdrawal syringe and assayed by a photodensitometer. The cardiac output (CO) is obtained by the formula

$$CO = \text{amount of dye injected}/\int_0^\infty c(t)dt$$

and the mean transit time (MTT) is expressed by the formula

$$MTT = tc(t)dt/\int_0^\infty c(t)dt$$

where t is time and c is dye concentration in arterial blood.

Thermodilution Method for Cardiac Output

The thermal dilution method is an application of the indicator dilution principle. In thermodilution, the indicator is a measured quantity of iced saline or 5% glucose solution; dilution of the cold solution in the bloodstream is measured by a calibrated thermocouple positioned about 10 cm upstream from the point of injection. The small amount of cold solution injected into the PA does not measurably affect the temperature of venous blood returning to the right side of the heart and therefore does not produce errors from recirculation of the indicator, as do dyes such as indocyanine green and Evans blue dye, or radioactive labels of albumin (^{125}I) or red blood cells (^{55}Cr). This obviates the problem of separating the primary washout curve from the recirculating indicator, simplifies cardiac output calculations, allows frequently repeated measurements, and does not require removal of blood for photometric or radioactivity analysis. Thermodilution used in conjunction with the PA balloon flotation catheter to obtain simultaneous PAOP has become the clinical standard for hemodynamic evaluation, particularly in early stages of acute critical illness.

Low cardiac index is characteristic of hemorrhage, myocardial infarction, cardiac tamponade, and other forms of central pump failure. Patients with septic, postoperative, and traumatic shock typically have patterns of high blood flow unless they are severely dehydrated, hypovolemic, elderly, or bedridden or have associated cardiac problems. In patients with severe sepsis or burn shock, the cardiac index may be more than twice the normal value. Similarly, stroke index, both left and right ventricular stroke work indexes, and left cardiac work index and right cardiac work index are reduced in hypovolemic and cardiogenic shock but are usually increased in septic, postoperative, and traumatic shock. Increased cardiac index, stroke work, and myocardial performance in the latter conditions may be the body's response to increased circulatory and metabolic requirements, wound healing, tissue repair, immunochemical mediators, and restoration of body metabolism after prior oxygen debt, inadequate tissue perfusion, severe stress, and failure to keep up with blood or fluid losses. In essence, normal values for the unstressed, normal volunteer subject are not appropriate as goals for the critically ill patient or the patient in shock.

Increased vascular resistance resulting from the neurohumoral adrenal stress response is an early transient compensatory response to hypotensive low cardiac output from hypovolemia and cardiogenic shock. This response maintains arterial pressures in the face of decreasing blood flow, at least for a limited time. Hypotension occurs when compensatory responses that increase blood pressure and systemic vascular resistance index values are overwhelmed, exhausted, or attenuated by acidosis and metabolic vasodilatory mechanisms. Pulmonary vascular resistance may increase with trauma, hemorrhage, lung hypoxia, high-altitude sickness, adult respiratory distress syndrome, and other forms of stress. An increased pulmonary vascular resistance index, which is also initiated by neural and other mechanisms, precedes the increased pulmonary venous admixture or shunting that occurs with postoperative and post-traumatic adult respiratory distress syndrome.

Right Ventricular Catheter

The PA catheter was modified and developed for right ventricular thermodilution cardiac output measurements by right atrial injection of cold fluid boluses.[38–40] The instrument uses a fast response thermistor mounted at the tip to rapidly measure temperature changes at the bedside; this allows additional calculations, including right ventricular ejection fraction, and both right ventricular end-diastolic volume (RVEDV) and end-systolic volume (RVESV) index.[38–40] The catheter is useful for evaluation of right ventricular functions, particularly right ventricular afterload, which is assessed by RVEDV in relation to PA pressure measurements. It is also useful for management of fluid therapy in patients with suspected right-sided heart failure or when large rapid volumes of fluid and transfusions are given to patients who sustained rapid blood losses. In trauma patients, the RVEDV index, but not PAOP, correlated with changes in the cardiac index when the patients were ventilated at different airway pressures.[41, 42] Dhainaut and colleagues[43] found only poor correlation between right atrial pressure and RVEDV in septic patients when right ventricular filling was varied by inflating and deflating MAST trousers.

Oxygen Transport Variables and Other Circulatory Functions

Cardiac output and PAOP are important hemodynamic variables that reflect cardiac function in relation to inflow. However, the primary function of the circulation is to provide for body metabolism by microcirculatory tissue perfusion. This is reflected by the bulk delivery of oxygen and nutrients and removal of carbon dioxide and other end products of metabolism, such as lactate and pyruvate, that will be recycled through hepatic intracellular metabolic pathways. Oxygen has the highest percentage of extraction of all blood components, is the most flow-dependent blood constituent, and is the constituent whose arteriovenous gradient is easiest to measure. Moreover, oxygen is essential to body metabolism; hypoxic brain death or permanent neurologic deficit occurs when cardiac arrest lasts for more than 5 minutes. For all these reasons, it is useful to monitor oxygen metabolism as early as possible to observe the complete patterns of circulatory dysfunction and failure.

At present, it is not possible to measure tissue perfusion directly. However, the functional circulatory status is evaluated by observing changes in the temporal patterns of $\dot{V}O_2$ in relation to the patterns of the cardiac index and $\dot{D}O_2$ (Table 7–6).[44, 45] Decrease in $\dot{V}O_2$ indicates reduction of the overall rate of oxidative metabolism and may be due to the following:

- Inadequate delivery of oxygen to the tissues from low flow, that is, $\dot{D}O_2$
- Low hemoglobin concentration, that is, anemia
- Low arterial blood oxygen, that is, hypoxemia
- Inadequate tissue perfusion from uneven or maldistributed microcirculatory flow
- Decreased metabolic rates resulting from specific disease states (e.g., hypothyroidism, malnutrition, vitamin deficiencies), cancericidal drug therapy, drug overdose or other metabolic poisoning, hypothermia, and terminal states

Increased $\dot{V}O_2$ indicates increased tissue metabolism from the following:

- Increased metabolic demand from sepsis, hyperthermia, post-traumatic states, burns, vigorous exercise, and hyperthyroidism
- Compensatory increases in metabolism after prior tissue hypoxia from low blood flow or uneven flow, tissue injury, hypothermia, or cardiac event
- The use of various drugs, anesthetics, adrenergic agonists that stimulate metabolism, or poisons that dissociate oxidative phosphorylation

Greater than normal $\dot{V}O_2$ does not necessarily mean that the circulation is adequate, because increased metabolic requirements associated with tissue repair or prior oxygen debt may require greater than normal metabolism to restore normal function. Patients with major trauma, sepsis, and burns require appreciable increases in $\dot{V}O_2$. If $\dot{V}O_2$ is greater than normal before therapy but does not increase with therapy, (1) tissue perfusion is already adequate, (2) therapy is ineffective, or (3) the circulatory defect is irreversible, as in the late stage of shock or after multiple vital organ failures. A low or normal $\dot{V}O_2$ before and after therapy suggests that the therapy is ineffective or that the defect is irreversible. When $\dot{V}O_2$ is low before therapy and increases afterward, either the patient's condition has spontaneously improved or the administered agent has improved tissue perfusion and oxygen metabolism.[44, 45]

Infrequent or random measurements of $\dot{V}O_2$ give limited snapshot views of the pattern of events. However, when therapeutic agents are given one at a time with $\dot{V}O_2$ monitored before, during, and after each therapy, changes in $\dot{V}O_2$ may reflect changes in metabolism or tissue perfusion produced by the therapy.[44, 45]

The PA catheter's effectiveness in critically ill patients has been challenged by Connors and associates,[46] who showed higher mortality in the initial care of a large series of critically ill medical patients with organ failure and 60% expected mortality. Similar results were reported in patients with myocardial infarction,[47–50] in randomized trials of surgical patients with organ failure on their ICU admission,[51, 52] and in a PA catheter consensus conference.[53] However, randomized trials in surgical patients performed early showed improved outcome.[54–61] These discrepant outcomes may be due to differences in the definition of the term "early" as well as to differences in the nature of circulatory problems in medical and surgical patients and the use of well-defined treatment plans. Improved outcome should not be expected in late-stage medical patients, particularly if therapy is not changed because of monitoring.

In a meta-analysis, Boyd and Bennett[61] reviewed seven prospective randomized series of patients who entered the ICU after organ failure or sepsis had occurred and had no outcome improvement with therapy; they compared these with seven other prospective randomized series that showed significant outcome improvement when early therapy was given to achieve physiologic goals in the first 8 to 12 hours postoperatively or prophylactically.[54–61] Clearly, time factors are of the essence.

Continuous Cardiac Output and Oxygen Consumption Monitoring

Historically, continuous $\dot{V}O_2$ has been directly measured by external spirometry since before the turn of the century. Because of the considerable errors and artifacts produced by the spirometers, these systems were replaced by collection of

TABLE 7–6. Oxygen Transport Variables

Variable	Formula	Normal Value	Unit
Arterial Hgb saturation	Direct measurement	96 ± 1	%
Mixed venous Hgb saturation	Direct measurement	75 ± 1	%
Arterial oxygen content	$CaO_2 = SaO_2 \times 1.36 \times Hgb + (0.0031 \times PaO_2)$	19 ± 1	mL/dL
Mixed venous oxygen content	$C\bar{v}O_2 = S\bar{v}_2 \times 1.36\ Hgb + (0.0031 \times P\bar{v}O_2)$	14 ± 1	mL/dL
Oxygen delivery	$\dot{D}O_2 = CI \times CaO_2$	520 ± 16	$mL \cdot min^{-1} \cdot m^2$
Oxygen consumption	$\dot{V}O_2 = CI\ (CaO_2 - C\bar{v}O_2)$	131 ± 2	$mL \cdot min^{-1} \cdot m^2$
Oxygen extraction	$O_2\ ext = \dot{D}O_2/\dot{V}O_2$	26 ± 1	%

Hgb = hemoglobin; CI = cardiac index.

expired gas in the Douglas bag for later gas analysis. Subsequently, Guyton[62] measured $\dot{V}O_2$ continuously in animals confined to an airtight box. Westenskow and associates[63] developed a metabolic gas monitor with which gas from the inspiratory and expiratory limbs was sampled and analyzed for oxygen concentrations with a zirconium oxide sensor and for carbon dioxide with an infrared sensor. Hankeln and colleagues[64, 65] developed a microcomputer-assisted monitoring system for the continuous, on-line, real-time calculations of cardiac output and of hemodynamic and oxygen transport variables. This system continuously displays $\dot{V}O_2$, $\dot{V}CO_2$, cardiac index, and an array of 20 or more hemodynamic variables calculated from inspired and expired oxygen and carbon dioxide concentrations, minute ventilation, temperature, ECG, heart rate, and intravascular pressures. The data are converted to digital form, processed, displayed on a monitoring screen, and stored for subsequent evaluation.

Similar systems are available on metabolic monitoring carts and in newer ventilator models (Puritan-Bennett, Carlsbad, Calif.; and Siemans, Cupertino, Calif.). A method for continuous measurement of cardiac output using frequent thermal impulses has been reported.[66]

When an oximetric PA catheter was used, continuous $S\bar{v}O_2$ and periodic SaO_2 measurements allowed calculation of continuous cardiac output.[67] This system was reported to have reasonably good agreement with the thermodilution cardiac output method and was used prospectively to evaluate predictors of outcome in a wide range of clinical conditions. Davies and coworkers[67] have continuously monitored cardiac output using the Westenskow oxiconsumeter system for continuous $\dot{V}O_2$ measurement compared with PA catheter oximetry and pulse oximetry. They reported good agreement with the thermodilution cardiac output method under ideal clinical conditions.

NONINVASIVE CIRCULATORY MONITORING

Various noninvasive systems provide continuous displays of specific cardiac, pulmonary, and tissue perfusion functions in acute circulatory problems.

Ultrasound Method for Noninvasive Cardiac Output Estimation

The Doppler ultrasound method uses frequency shifts of an ultrasound wave reflected from a moving substance to measure cardiac output. In blood flow estimations, sound is reflected from a moving column of red blood cells leaving the heart. Continuous-wave Doppler ultrasound and pulsed Doppler ultrasound systems are commercially available.[68, 69]

The continuous-wave system uses A-mode or M-mode Doppler estimation of aortic root cross-sectional area, which is usually performed before velocity measurement. Bernstein's critique[70] describes the theoretical aspects of and practical problems associated with these methods. Doppler methodology has been greatly enhanced by fast Fourier transform analysis of the Doppler frequencies. A wide variety of transducer designs have made possible greater application of this method at the bedside.

Noninvasive Cardiac Output by Impedance Measurement

Thoracic electrical bioimpedance measures the apparent changes in resistance to the flow throughout the cardiac cycle of a small-amplitude (0.2 to 4.0 mA) alternating current at 40 to 100 kHz applied to the chest.[70] Thoracic electrical bioimpedance was initiated by Nyboer[71] and developed as a medical instrument by Kubicek and colleagues.[72] In the 1970s, the original system was developed as the Minnesota Impedance Cardiograph (Surcom, Minneapolis). Subsequently, several improvements were made, including diastolic clamping of the electrical signal. Bernstein[73] developed an improved mathematical representation of the thorax and corrected for changes in body habitus. Sorba Medical Systems (Milwaukee, Wis.), has developed a modification of the Minnesota instrument based on analysis of waveforms by ensemble averaging of the impedance waveform.

Wang and coworkers[74–76] at Drexel University developed an improved thoracic electrical bioimpedance device based on recently available hardware and software innovations from aerospace industries and on major improvements in the electrode system for data acquisition. The system now has completely redesigned software for data analysis, data processing, and data management (Renaissance Technologies, Newtown, Pa.).

In the impedance method, the injecting electrodes produce an electrical field across the thorax from the base of the neck to the level of the xiphisternal junction; the electrical signals travel predominantly down the aorta rather than through aerated alveoli. Clinical evaluations under the worst-case scenario of emergency trauma in an inner-city county hospital have shown improved stability of the signal and satisfactory agreement with simultaneous thermodilution cardiac output measurements.[24, 77–79]

The Renaissance Technologies system is based on time-frequency distribution technology and uses a signal processing technique that provides high signal-to-noise ratios for measurement of mechanical functions of the heart. The device is capable of rapid signal processing with minimal computations because of its all-integer-coefficient filtering technology; it uses noninvasive disposable prewired hydrogen electrodes positioned on the skin and three ECG leads placed across the precordium and left shoulder.[76–79] A 100-kHz, 4-mA alternating current is passed through the patient's thorax by the outer pairs of electrodes, and the voltage is sensed by the inner pairs of electrodes; the voltage sensed by the inner electrodes captures the baseline impedance (Z_0), the first derivative of the impedance waveform (dZ/dt), and the ECG.[74–76]

The system allows early therapy based on continuous display of the cardiac index, which may be combined with pulse oximetry and transcutaneous oxygen and carbon dioxide pressures to assess pulmonary and tissue perfusion and oxygenation for early management of acute illnesses. In multicenter studies, this impedance device provided stable signals and reliable cardiac output estimations even under extenuating emergency conditions.[24, 77] Of 2192 simultaneous bioimpedance and thermodilution cardiac index measurements in 860 critically ill patients in the emergency department, operating room, and ICU, the correlation coefficient r was .85, r^2 was .73 ($P < .001$), and precision and bias was $-0.124 + 0.75$ L/min/m^2.

When there is extensive pulmonary edema, pleural effusion, hemothorax, massive chest wall edema, or chest tubes parallel to the aorta, electrical signals may preferentially travel through these electrolyte solutions more than the aorta and thereby reduce the impedance signal-to-noise ratio. When these conditions appreciably interfere with accuracy, they can be identified by reductions in the baseline control impedance (Z_0) lower than 15 ohms and by the height of the impedance waveform lower than 0.3 ohm. With use of these values as criteria, the correlation coefficient r was 0.93, r^2 was .87, bias and precision was $-0.14 + 0.54$ L/min/m^2, and the average difference between thermodilution and impedance measurements was 9.8% + 6.7%; this is similar to the differences between successive thermodilution measurements (9.4 ± 6.2%).[24] With Z_0 and dZ/dt values lower than 15 ohms and 0.3 ohm, respectively, impedance estimates were observed to track and trend thermodilution values but were not regarded as sufficiently reliable to be taken at face value. This is a major limitation of impedance methodology. More important, however, the impedance changes satisfactorily tracked and trended thermodilution values. The correlations of bioimpedance versus thermodilution cardiac output were equivalent to those of pulse oximetry compared with the standard blood gas analysis. No instance of spurious impedance values that would have led to incorrect or harmful therapy was observed.[24] Minor differences between thermodilution and impedance cardiac output estimations were offset by the continuous on-line display of data that allowed instant recognition of changes in the course of illness and the responses to therapy.[80-84]

In all monitoring and imaging techniques, motion, anxiety, restlessness, shivering, hyperventilation, and agitation may interfere with the measurements as well as increase physiologic responses. However, it is less important in emergency conditions to have the same accuracy required in stable ICU conditions, because the patient's baseline measurements are often unknown and optimal values for each patient may vary with comorbid conditions. In practice, a 10% to 15% difference between invasive and noninvasive cardiac output estimations would be acceptable when changes of 30% to 50% from the normal range are present. However, thermodilution also has appreciable inaccuracies in both high and low cardiac output ranges and especially when the patient has hypothermia, arrhythmias, Valsalva effects, motion artifacts, shivering, anxiety, and errors from injectate temperature calibration. Direct Fick $\dot{V}O_2$ measurements, the physiologists' gold standard, are precluded by the nonsteady states of emergency conditions.

INTEGRATED NONINVASIVE MULTICOMPONENT SYSTEM FOR HEMODYNAMIC MONITORING

Sets of noninvasively monitored data[79-85] consist of the following:

- Cardiac output measurements measured by bioimpedance
- Arterial oxygen saturations measured by pulse oximetry
- $Ptco_2$ and $Ptcco_2$
- Mean arterial blood pressure by noninvasive systems
- Heart rate and ECG

These data are used for early warning of cardiac, pulmonary, and tissue perfusion functions.

Recent reports showed lack of effectiveness of PA catheterization in critically ill medical patients and relatively late-stage surgical patients with organ failure. Because invasive monitoring requires critical care environments, the early hemodynamic patterns may have been missed. Early noninvasive hemodynamic monitoring systems can be used by themselves or as the "front end" of invasive monitoring to supply more complete descriptions of circulatory pathophysiology.

Invasive hemodynamic monitoring provides a series of snapshots at infrequent intervals. Noninvasive monitoring provides similar physiologic information that allows early recognition of low flow and poor tissue perfusion; these are represented by continuous, on-line, real-time displays that allow prompt recognition of circulatory abnormalities and early therapeutic intervention in acutely ill emergency patients when time factors are crucial. Noninvasive monitoring can be applied in about 2 minutes without interfering with the emergency patient's management. Minor differences between impedance and thermodilution measurements are offset by the advantages of continuous graphic displays of data. Noninvasive monitoring is easier, quicker, cheaper, and safer than invasive monitoring. Table 7-1 lists indications for monitoring.

Routinely monitored variables are evaluated one at a time, and each detected abnormality is then corrected; this "one-at-a-time search for a defect and then correct it" leads to an uncoordinated and sometimes contradictory therapeutic plan. Moreover, technical developments in monitoring systems have provided a wide range of invasive and noninvasive physiologic variables that allow extensive assessment of complex interacting circulatory functions. When they are combined with pulse oximetry and transcutaneous Po_2 and Pco_2, these noninvasive monitoring systems can be used for early warning of cardiac, pulmonary, and tissue perfusion functions.[22-35] This means that interactions of multiple physiologic measurements can be analyzed to define early primary events separate from secondary and tertiary events and to develop coherent integrated therapeutic plans for cardiac, pulmonary, and tissue perfusion functions.

The emergency department is the primary entry point into medical care for many acutely ill patients, and this early period provides a crucial opportunity for early assessment and rapid therapeutic interventions that may affect outcome. A major dilemma is that shock is easily diagnosed in late stages when therapy is ineffective, but early diagnosis is difficult because shock is first recognized by imprecise signs and subjective symptoms. The noninvasive systems provide early available screening methods for continuous assessment of circulatory parameters and titration of therapy to predetermined goals.

The patient who has undergone elective surgery without complications may be easily monitored with routine screening that includes assessment of vital signs, ECG, and CVP. More comprehensive hemodynamic and oxygen transport monitoring is needed in high-risk surgical patients during and after major surgery (see Table 7-1). The mortality rates after major surgical procedures are usually in the range of 1% to 2%, but the mortality rates of many high-risk patients seen in the surgical ICU may be as high as 20% to 30%. To reduce these mortality rates, it is advisable to monitor all potentially fatal cases (e.g., preoperative patients with high-risk factors as well as critically ill, medical, septic, and postoperative patients). It may be necessary to monitor at least four or five times the actual number of deaths to be sure that the optimal therapy is given to patients with potentially fatal conditions. Invasive hemodynamic monitoring may also be useful when routine screening with monitoring of vital signs, CVP, hematocrit, and blood gases suggests more extensive hemodynamic problems.

Noninvasive hemodynamic and oxygen transport monitoring can identify correctable physiologic alterations at the earliest possible moment before they become life-threatening or irreversible.[24, 80-87] Furthermore, such monitoring provides objective circulatory measurements and criteria for therapeutic decision making. In essence, such monitoring replaces clinical suspicion and guesswork with objectively determined physiologic criteria.

SUMMARY

The early period of illness provides a crucial opportunity for early assessment and rapid therapeutic interventions that may affect outcome. A major dilemma is that shock is easily diagnosed in late stages when therapy is ineffective, but early diagnosis is difficult because shock is first recognized by imprecise signs and subjective symptoms. Noninvasive systems provide early, readily available screening methods for continuous assessment of circulatory parameters and titration of therapy to predetermined goals, or they may be used as the "front end" of subsequent invasive monitoring.

The effectiveness of the PA catheter in critically ill late-stage patients with organ failures has been questioned. Boyd and Bennett,[61] in a meta-analysis of prospective randomized series, showed that improved outcome is unlikely when ICU admission for invasive monitoring is delayed until after organ failure occurs. Clearly, time factors are extremely important. Noninvasive systems provide alternatives for early monitoring because they can be applied on admission to the emergency department or in the operating room, on the hospital floor, or in the physician's office and may be used to follow the course of acute life-threatening illness.

Both invasive and noninvasive monitoring systems provide similar information that identifies episodes of hypotension, low cardiac index, arterial hemoglobin desaturation, and poor tissue perfusion shown by low P_{tcO_2}, high P_{tcCO_2}, and low $\dot{V}O_2$ before and during initial resuscitation. It is less important in emergency conditions to have the same accuracy required in stable ICU conditions, because the patient's baseline measurements are often unknown and optimal values for each patient may vary with comorbid conditions.

In practice, a 10% to 15% difference between invasive and noninvasive cardiac output estimations would be acceptable when 30% to 50% changes from the normal range are present. However, thermodilution also has appreciable inaccuracies in both high and low cardiac output ranges and especially when the patient has hypothermia, arrhythmias, Valsalva effects, motion artifacts, shivering, anxiety, and errors from injectate temperature calibration. Direct Fick $\dot{V}O_2$ measurements, the physiologists' gold standard, are precluded by the nonsteady states of acute emergency conditions.

Noninvasive monitoring systems give continuous displays of physiologic data that provide information allowing early recognition of low flow and poor tissue perfusion that are more pronounced in the nonsurvivors. Noninvasive systems are acceptable alternatives to invasive monitoring.

References

1. Shoemaker WC, Kram HB, Appel PL, et al: The efficacy of central venous and pulmonary artery catheters and therapy based upon them in reducing mortality and morbidity. Arch Surg 1990; 125:1332–1338.
2. Wo CJ, Shoemaker WC, Appel PL, et al: Unreliability of blood pressure and heart rate to evaluate cardiac output in emergency resuscitation and critical illness. Crit Care Med 1993; 21:218–223.
3. Adler DC, Bryan-Brown CW: Use of the axillary artery for intravascular monitoring. Crit Care Med 1973; 1:148–150.
4. Monson DO, Shoemaker WC: Sequence of hemodynamic events after various types of hemorrhage. Surgery 1968; 63:738–749.
5. Shoemaker WC, Kram HB: Effects of crystalloids and colloids on hemodynamics, oxygen transport, and outcome in high-risk patients. *In:* Debates in Clinical Surgery. Simmons RC, Udehuo AS (Eds). Chicago, Year Book Medical Publishers, 1990, pp 263–316.
6. Skillman JJ, Awwad HK, Moore FD: Plasma kinetics of the early transcapillary refill after hemorrhage in man. Surg Gynecol Obstet 1967; 123:983–996.
7. Moore FD: Effects of hemorrhage on body composition. N Engl J Med 1965; 273:567–577.
8. Wiggers CJ: Physiology of Shock. New York, Commonwealth Fund, 1950.
9. Shippy CR, Appel PL, Shoemaker WC: Reliability of clinical monitoring to assess blood volume in critically ill patients. Crit Care Med 1984; 12:107–112.
10. Lewis FJ, Quinn ML: Continuous electrocardiogram monitoring in a surgical intensive care unit. Crit Care Med 1977; 4:73–75.
11. Shapiro BA, Harrison RA, Walton JR (Eds): Clinical Application of Blood Gases. 4th ed. Vol 3. Chicago, Year Book Medical Publishers, 1990.
12. Clark LC Jr: Monitor and control of blood and tissue oxygen tensions. Trans Am Soc Artif Intern Organs 1956; 2:41.
13. Fiddian-Green RG, Pittenger G, Whitehouse WM: Back diffusion of CO_2 and its influence on the intramural pH in gastric mucosa. J Surg Res 1982; 33:39–48.
14. Gutierrez G, Palizas F, Doglio G, et al: Gastric intermucosal pH as a therapeutic index of tissue oxygenation in critically ill patients. Lancet 1992; 339:195–199.
15. Clark CH, Gutierrez G: Gastric intramucosal pH: A noninvasive method for indirect measurement of tissue oxygenation. Am J Crit Care 1992; 1:53–60.
16. Schlictig R, Bowles SA: Distinguishing between aerobic and anaerobic appearance of dissolved CO_2 in intestine during low flow. J Appl Physiol 1994; 76:2443–2451.
17. Gutierrez G, Brown SD: Gastrointestinal tonometry: A monitor of regional dysoxia. New Horiz 1996; 4:413–419.
18. Shoemaker WC, Bryan-Brown CW, Quigley L, et al: Body fluid shifts in depletion and poststress states and their correction with adequate nutrition. Surg Gynecol Obstet 1973; 136:371–374.
19. Shoemaker WC, Monson DO: Effect of whole blood and plasma expanders on volume-flow relationships in critically ill patients. Surg Gynecol Obstet 1973; 137:453–457.
20. Davis HA: Blood Volume Dynamics. Springfield, Ill, Charles C Thomas, 1962.
21. Albert SN: Blood Volume. Springfield, Ill, Charles C Thomas, 1963.
22. Moore FD: The Body Cell Mass and Its Supporting Environment: Body Composition in Health and Disease. Philadelphia, WB Saunders, 1963.
23. Starling EH: On the absorption of fluids from the connective tissue spaces. J Physiol 1896; 19:312.
24. Shoemaker WC, Belzberg H, Wo CCJ, et al: Multicenter study of noninvasive monitoring systems as alternatives to invasive monitoring of acutely ill emergency patients. Chest 1998; 114: 1643–1652.
25. Hüch A, Hüch R, Meinzer K, et al: Eine schnelle behizte Proberflach-electrode zur kontinuierlichen Uberwachung des P_{O_2} beim Menschen. *In:* Electrodenaufbau und Eigenschaften. Stuttgart, Proc Medizin-Technik, May 16, 1972.
26. Eberhard P, Mindt W, Hammacher K: Perkutane Messung des Sauerstoff-partialdruckes. *In:* Methodik und Anwendungen. Stuttgart, Proc Medizin-Technik, May 16, 1972.
27. Tremper KK, Shoemaker WC: Transcutaneous oxygen monitoring of critically ill adults with and without low flow shock. Crit Care Med 1981; 9:706–709.
28. Tremper KK, Waxman K, Shoemaker WC: Effects of hypoxia and shock in transcutaneous P_{O_2} values on dogs. Crit Care Med 1979; 7:526–531.
29. Shoemaker WC, Wo CCJ, Demetriades D, et al: Early physiologic patterns in acute illness and accidents. New Horiz 1996; 4:395–412.
30. Tremper KK, Shoemaker WC, Shippy CR, et al: Transcutaneous P_{CO_2} monitoring in adult patients in the ICU and operating room. Crit Care Med 1981; 9:752–755.
31. Teasdale G, Jennet B: Assessment of coma and impaired consciousness. A practical scale. Lancet 1974; 2:81–84.
32. Landis EM, Hortenstine JC: Functional significance of venous blood pressure. Physiol Rev 1950; 30:1.
33. Hughes RE, Magovern GJ: The relationship between right atrial pressure and blood volume. Arch Surg 1959; 79:238.
34. Wilson JN, Grow JB, Demong CV, et al: Central venous pressure in optimal blood volume maintenance. Arch Surg 1962; 83:563.
35. Swan HJC, Ganz W, Forrester JS, et al: Catheterization of the heart in man with use of a flow-directed balloon-tipped catheter. N Engl J Med 1970; 283:447–451.
36. Swan HJC: Role of hemodynamic monitoring in the management of the critically ill. Crit Care Med 1975; 3:83–89.
37. Forrester JS, Diamond G, Chatterjee J, et al: Medical therapy of acute myocardial infarction by application of hemodynamic subsets. N Engl J Med 1976; 295:1356–1404.
38. Kay HR, Afshari M, Barash P, et al: Measurement of ejection fraction by thermodilution techniques. J Surg Res 1983; 34:337–346.
39. Nelson LD: The new pulmonary arterial catheters: Right ventricu-

lar ejection fraction and continuous cardiac output. Crit Care Clin 1996; 12:795–818.
40. Nelson LD: The new pulmonary arterial catheters: Continuous venous oximetry, right ventricular ejection fraction, and continuous cardiac output. New Horiz 1997; 5:251–258.
41. Diebel LN, Myers T, Dulchavsky S: Effects of increasing airway pressure and PEEP on the assessment of cardiac preload. J Trauma 1997; 42:585–591.
42. Jellinek H, Krafft P, Heismayr M, Stelzer H: Measurement of right ventricular performance during apnea in patients with acute lung injury. J Trauma 1997; 42:1062–1067.
43. Dhainaut JF, Pinski MR, Nouria S, et al: Right ventricular function in human septic shock. Chest 1997; 112:1043–1049.
44. Shoemaker WC, Appel PL, Kram HB: Oxygen transport measurements to evaluate tissue perfusion and titrate therapy. Crit Care Med 1991; 19:672–688.
45. Shoemaker WC, Appel PL, Kram HB, et al: Hemodynamic and oxygen transport monitoring to titrate therapy in septic shock. New Horiz 1993; 1:145–159.
46. Connors AF Jr, Speroff T, Dawson NV, et al: The effectiveness of right heart catheterization in the initial care of critically ill patients. JAMA 1996; 276:899–907.
47. Gore JM, Goldberg RJ, Spodick DH, et al: A community-wide assessment of the use of pulmonary artery catheters in patients with acute myocardial infarction. Chest 1987; 92:721–727.
48. Guyatt G, Ontario Intensive Care Group: A randomized control trial of right heart catheterization in critically ill patients. J Intensive Care Med 1991; 6:91–95.
49. Zion MM, Balkin J, Rosenmann D, et al: Use of pulmonary artery catheters in patients with acute myocardial infarction: Analysis of experience in 5841 patients in the SPRINT registry. Chest 1990; 98:1331–1335.
50. Blumberg MS, Binns GS: Swan-Ganz catheter use and mortality in myocardial infarction patients. Health Care Financ Rev 1994; 15:91–103.
51. Hayes MA, Timmins AC, Yau EHS, et al: Elevation of systemic oxygen delivery in the treatment of critically ill patients. N Engl J Med 1994; 330:1717–1722.
52. Gattinoni L, Brazzi L, Pelosi P, et al: A trial of goal-oriented hemodynamic therapy in critically ill patients. N Engl J Med 1995; 333:1025–1032.
53. Taylor RW, and the Pulmonary Artery Catheter Consensus Conference Participants: Pulmonary Artery Catheter Consensus Conference. Crit Care Med 1997; 25:910–925.
54. Shoemaker WC, Appel PL, Kram HB, et al: Prospective trial of supranormal values of survivors as therapeutic goals in high risk surgical patients. Chest 1988; 94:1176–1186.
55. Bishop MW, Shoemaker WC, Appel PL, et al: Relationship between supranormal values, time delays and outcome in severely traumatized patients. Crit Care Med 1993; 21:56–62.
56. Boyd O, Grounds M, Bennett D: Preoperative increase of oxygen delivery reduces mortality in high risk surgical patients. JAMA 1993; 270:2699–2704.
57. Berlauk JF, Abrams JH, Gilmour IJ, et al: Preoperative optimization of cardiovascular hemodynamics improves outcome in peripheral vascular surgery. Ann Surg 1991; 214:289–297.
58. Fleming AW, Bishop MH, Shoemaker WC, et al: Prospective trial of supranormal values as goals of resuscitation in severe trauma. Arch Surg 1992; 127:1175–1181.
59. Yu M, Burchell S, Hasaniya NWMA, et al: Relationship of mortality to increasing oxygen delivery in patients > 50 years of age: A prospective randomized study. Crit Care Med 1998; 26:1011–1019.
60. Bishop MH, Shoemaker WC, Kram HB, et al: Prospective randomized trial of survivor values of cardiac index, oxygen delivery, and oxygen consumption as resuscitation endpoints in severe trauma. J Trauma 1995; 38:780–787.
61. Boyd O, Bennett D: Enhancement of perioperative tissue perfusion as a therapeutic strategy for major surgery. New Horiz 1996; 4:453–465.
62. Guyton AC: A continuous cardiac output recorder employing the Fick principle. Circ Res 1959; 7:661.
63. Westenskow DR, Cutler CA, Wallace WD: Instrumentation for monitoring gas exchange and metabolic rate in critically ill patients. Crit Care Med 1984; 12:183–187.
64. Hankeln KB, Michelsen H, Schipulle M, et al: Microcomputer-assisted monitoring system for measuring and processing cardiorespiratory variables. Crit Care Med 1985; 13:426–431.
65. Hankeln KB, Michelsen H, Kubiak V, et al: Continuous on-line, real-time measurement of cardiac output and derived cardiorespiratory variables in the critically ill. Crit Care Med 1985; 13:1071–1073.
66. Yelderman MD: Continuous measurement of cardiac output with the use of stochastic system identification technique. J Clin Monit 1990; 6:323–332.
67. Davies GG, Jebson PJR, Glasgow BM, et al: Continuous Fick cardiac output compared to thermodilution cardiac output. Crit Care Med 1986; 14:881–885.
68. Lewis JF, Kuo LC, Nelson JG, et al: Pulsed Doppler echocardiographic determination of stroke volume and cardiac output. Circulation 1984; 70:425–431.
69. Mehta N, Iyawe VI, Cummin ARC, et al: Validation of a Doppler technique for beat to beat measurement of cardiac output. Clin Sci 1985; 69:377–382.
70. Bernstein DP: Noninvasive cardiac output measurement. *In:* Textbook of Critical Care. 2nd ed. Shoemaker WC, Ayres S, Grenvik A (Eds). Philadelphia, WB Saunders, 1989, p 159.
71. Nyboer J: Impedance Plethysmography. Springfield, Ill, Charles C Thomas, 1959.
72. Kubicek WG, Karnegis JN, Patterson RP, et al: Development and evaluation of an impedance cardiac output system. Aerosp Med 1966; 37:1208–1212.
73. Bernstein DP: A new stroke volume equation for thoracic electrical bioimpedance: Theory and rationale. Crit Care Med 1986; 14:904–909.
74. Wang XA, Sun HH, Adamson D, et al: Impedance cardiograph system: A new design. Ann Biomed Eng 1989; 17:535–556.
75. Wang X, Van de Water JM, Sun H, et al: Hemodynamic monitoring by impedance cardiography with an improved signal processing technique. Proc IEEE Eng Med Biol 1993; 15:699.
76. Wang X, Sun HH, Van de Water JM: Time-frequency distribution technique in biological signal processing. Biomed Instrum Technol 1995; 29:203–212.
77. Shoemaker WC, Wo CCJ, Bishop MH, et al: Multicenter trial of a new thoracic electric bioimpedance device for cardiac output estimation. Crit Care Med 1994; 22:1907–1912.
78. Wo CCJ, Shoemaker WC, Bishop MH, et al: Noninvasive estimations of cardiac output and circulatory dynamics in critically ill patients. Curr Opin Crit Care 1995; 1:211–218.
79. Belzberg H, Shoemaker WC: Noninvasive estimation of cardiac output. Curr Opin Crit Care 1997; 3:13–18.
80. Shoemaker WC, Appel PL, Kram HB: Incidence, physiologic description, compensatory mechanisms, and therapeutic implications of monitored events. Crit Care Med 1989; 17:1277–1285.
81. Shoemaker WC, Wo CCJ, Bishop MH, et al: Noninvasive monitoring of high risk surgical patients. Arch Surg 1996; 131:732–737.
82. Shoemaker WC, Wo CCJ, Bishop MH, et al: Noninvasive hemodynamic monitoring of critical patients in the emergency department. Acad Emerg Med 1996; 3:675–681.
83. Bishop MH, Shoemaker WC, Shuleshko J, Wo CCJ: Noninvasive cardiac index monitoring in gunshot wound victims. Acad Emerg Med 1996; 3:682–688.
84. Thangathuri D, Charbonnet C, Roessler P, et al: Continuous intraoperative noninvasive cardiac output monitoring using a new thoracic bioimpedance device. J Cardiothorac Vasc Anesth 1997; 11:440–444.
85. Velmahes GC, Wo CCJ, Demetriades D, et al: Invasive and noninvasive monitoring of blunt trauma in the early period after emergency admission. World J Surg (in press).
86. Belzberg H, Rivkind A, Wo CCJ, et al: Noninvasive hemodynamic and tissue perfusion monitoring of blunt trauma patients for early recognition of shock. Crit Care Med (in press).
87. Shoemaker WC, Wo CCJ: Circulatory effects of whole blood, packed red cells, albumin, starch, and crystalloids in resuscitation of shock and critical illness. Vox Sanguinis 1998; 74(suppl 2):69–74.

8

Diagnosis and Treatment of Shock and Circulatory Dysfunction

William C. Shoemaker, MD, FCCM

Almost everyone who dies of acute illness dies *with* or *of* shock; this involves an estimated million acute deaths in the United States annually. However, shock plays a role in all fatal illnesses, because circulatory failure is a part of the final common pathway. Moreover, shock not only is central to acute nonfatal circulatory disorders but also complicates other acute severe illnesses. Understanding of stressed circulation in relation to the increased body metabolism of acute illness is essential.

WHAT ARE SHOCK, CIRCULATORY DYSFUNCTION, AND CIRCULATORY FAILURE?

Most diseases are evaluated on the basis of normal ranges of relevant measurements; values outside the normal range establish criteria for diagnosis and therapy. This approach, however, is inappropriate for circulatory disorders because circulatory function normally responds to changes in body metabolism with exercise, activity, stress, endocrine problems, acute illness, and other factors. The function of the circulation is to supply body metabolism with oxygen and oxidative substrates and to remove carbon dioxide and other metabolic end products; as such, circulatory function must vary with changes in metabolism. Although normal circulatory values are usually given for the resting baseline state, the circulation normally increases to provide for increased body metabolism with exercise, fever, and acute illnesses.

Shock results from poor tissue perfusion and tissue hypoxia from inadequate circulatory compensations needed to sustain acutely increased body metabolism. Thus, the initial precipitating problem is inadequate tissue perfusion resulting from either low blood flow or unevenly distributed microcirculatory flow that occurs early in the course of acute illness and leads to local tissue hypoxia, organ dysfunction, multiple organ failure, and death. It is helpful to view the sequential patterns of hemodynamic changes to separate early primary events from secondary responses and subsequent sequelae in order to identify and treat the main underlying problem. Second, it is essential to develop an integrated therapeutic approach based on the three major circulatory components: cardiac, pulmonary, and tissue perfusion (oxygenation) function.

HOW IS SHOCK RECOGNIZED EARLY?

The diagnosis of shock is most often made by the presence of hypotension, oliguria, acidosis, and collapse in the late stage, when therapy is frequently ineffective. It is more important to recognize shock as soon as possible because it is more easily and effectively treated in the early stages. Unfortunately, circulatory problems are first recognized clinically by subjective symptoms and imprecise signs, such as cold clammy skin, pallor, weak thready pulse, unstable vital signs, cyanosis, mottled skin, central nervous system (CNS) depression, restlessness, agitation, and altered level of consciousness; blood pressure early in the course of acute injury and other types of acute circulatory dysfunction (shock) are not reliably correlated with blood flow.[1]

The lack of objectivity and reliability of these early signs and symptoms has been a major deterrent to the understanding of underlying physiology and to successful therapy. The dilemma is that the criteria for diagnosis are not the same as the criteria for early recognition. To view the initial appearance as a "miniversion" of the late stage is to miss the evolving pattern that occurs as circulatory dysfunction deteriorates into circulatory failure, organ failure, and death.

CONVENTIONAL APPROACH TO SHOCK

Conventional early therapy is usually directed toward correction of hypotension, tachycardia, oliguria, and other superficial signs and symptoms with vasopressors, diuretics, and crystalloids as if these conditions were the primary defects; the goal is to return these superficial signs and symptoms to their normal ranges. The assumption is that shock will be ameliorated simply by "cosmetically" correcting the findings that reveal shock. However, the underlying deficits of low or uneven flow with poor tissue perfusion persist and lead to organ failure and death.

The conventional approach consists of a one-at-a-time search for specific defects, their documentation, and their correction. This approach to each specific defect, followed by its normalization, leads to fragmented, episodic, and sometimes contradictory care of patients. Therapy based on this approach, unfortunately, is not maximally effective. Most patients eventually receive all the therapy they need but not necessarily at the right time, in the right amount, or in the right order.

Therapy intuitively based on simplistic notions, anecdotal information, or inadequate monitoring is likely to be suboptimal. Moreover, if the physiology is not understood or if monitoring is not timely or adequate, death may be attributed to the patient's disease rather than to delays that lead to ineffective therapy. The danger of the conventional approach is that maintenance of normal values may limit preload and compensatory increases in cardiac function that restore tissue perfusion and oxygenation. When tissue oxygenation is not monitored and corrected early, perfusion abnormalities are not recognized until adult respiratory distress syndrome (ARDS) or other organ failure occurs.

It is crucial to develop an integrated therapeutic plan that optimizes the three major circulatory components listed earlier.

ETIOLOGIC APPROACH TO SHOCK

Traditionally, shock is classified by its etiology as hemorrhagic, postoperative, cardiogenic, traumatic, neurogenic, or septic. These etiologic categories are described by clinical signs and symptoms, laboratory findings, the presumed primary pathophysiology, and therapy recommended for each cause. This approach is simple, easily understood, and generally accepted but is seriously misleading.

These overly simplistic descriptions of complex pathophysiology suggest one-dimensional therapy; for example, hemorrhagic shock should be treated with fluids, but cardiogenic shock should be treated with inotropic agents and fluid restriction. However, most critically ill patients undergo complex etiologic events; that is, postoperative shock patients may have major cardiac problems, and cardiac patients may have unrecognized hypovolemia. Not all primary etiologic events begin and end with a single physiologic defect that, if corrected, leads to survival. Life is not that simple. Moreover, the primary precipitating event sets in motion neurohormonal compensations as well as numerous cascades that activate various biochemical mediators and inflammatory responses that become part of the shock syndromes.

The major limitation of this one-dimensional etiologic approach is that it misses the interacting changes in hemodynamics and oxygen transport patterns that lead to uneven microcirculatory flow, poor tissue perfusion, tissue hypoxia, organ dysfunction, organ failure, and death. In essence, a one-dimensional approach to etiology and therapy is suboptimal.

MYOCARDIAL PERFORMANCE: AN APPROACH TO CARDIAC PHYSIOLOGY

By convention, cardiac function is evaluated by the Starling myocardial performance curve, in which cardiac index (CI), or some function of the heart, such as cardiac output, stroke volume, stroke work, or cardiac work, is plotted against the corresponding inflow pressure (pulmonary artery [PA] occlusion or "wedge" pressure).[2, 3] This is usually simplified as a line representing the lower limit of normal CI of 2.5 L/min/m^2 and a line representing the upper limit of normal for a PA wedge pressure of 20 mm Hg. These two lines divide the field into four quadrants that define four clinical subgroups according to whether they have high or low flow as well as high or low inflow pressures. A patient's observed value is then evaluated according to these criteria, and therapy is prescribed. However, this diagnostic and therapeutic paradigm is primarily related to cardiac function; it provides information to adjust fluids, inotropes, and diuretics to cardiac goals, but it does not address the major problems of the majority of noncardiac patients in an intensive care unit (ICU), whose main problem may be peripheral tissue perfusion with tissue hypoxia. The myocardial performance curve is widely used for cardiac patients, but it has limited usefulness for patients with hemorrhagic, traumatic, septic, or postoperative shock, because death of these patients is usually due to tissue hypoxia resulting from inadequate tissue perfusion, capillary leak, and multiple organ failure.

CIRCULATORY PHYSIOLOGY OF SHOCK SYNDROMES

This portion of the chapter attempts to characterize acute circulatory dysfuction by the temporal hemodynamic and oxygen transport patterns of postoperative, traumatic, septic, and cardiogenic shock. Normally, the circulatory function increases in response to exercise or physical stress; similarly, in injury and acute illness, increased body metabolism is compensated by increased circulatory function shown by increased cardiac output and oxygen delivery. Increased circulatory function under these conditions may be a normal regulatory response. The basic assumption in exercise, injury, and acute illness is that the major function of the circulation is to provide for body metabolism, which—if suddenly increased—requires commensurate circulatory increases. On a moment-to-moment basis, the circulation responds to changes in bodily activity to maintain the "milieu intérieur" for normal cellular metabolism.

In high-risk conditions, invasive PA thermodilution catheters are used in many institutions as the "gold standard" for critically ill ICU patients,[2–15] but some recent studies have shown no advantage of the PA catheter in cardiac or other medical conditions[4–7] or in postoperative patients admitted to the ICU after organ failure.[8–10] An insightful meta-analysis by Boyd and Bennett[11] found no outcome improvement in seven prospective randomized studies of patients who entered the ICU after organ failure or sepsis had occurred. These investigators noted significant outcome improvement in seven other randomized studies when PA catheter–directed therapy was given early or prophylactically.[12–19] Clearly, time is the major unresolved issue; when early or primary events are ignored, temporal patterns are lost and therapy is then directed to the consequences of, not the causes of, circulatory dysfunction.

PA catheters with or without a therapeutic plan have not been effective after organ failure has already developed, but early optimization (in the first 8 to 12 hours postoperatively) of CI, oxygen delivery ($\dot{D}O_2$), and oxygen consumption ($\dot{V}O_2$) to supranormal goals may be effective in high-risk surgical patients.[11, 12, 19] A major problem is that most critically ill medical patients are admitted to the ICU after they already have experienced organ dysfunction or failure. An alternative approach is to use noninvasive systems earlier in the emergency department or operating room or on the hospital floor to identify and correct early circulatory problems promptly, because no amount of oxygen can prevent organ failure after it has occurred (see Chapter 7, Monitoring).

The natural history of shock produced by hemorrhage, accidental injury, surgery, sepsis, and cardiac problems has been described beginning with the time of the precipitating etiologic event. The temporal hemodynamic and oxygen transport patterns of survivors and nonsurvivors were characterized during periods remote from therapy (before therapy was begun or after the immediate direct effects of therapy were over).[12, 17–24]

Physiologic mechanisms may be elucidated by comparison of the time course of survivor and nonsurvivor patterns. The patterns of survivors represent the effects of the precipitating etiologic event and the patient's own compensations augmented by therapy. The patterns of nonsurvivors represent the overwhelming effects of the shock syndrome or inadequate compensations or both. Therapy, to be maximally effective, must be focused not on superficial signs and symptoms but on an integrated optimization of cardiac, pulmonary, and tissue perfusion functions.

HEMODYNAMIC AND OXYGEN TRANSPORT MONITORING

From the clinical viewpoint, the maximum physiologic information can be obtained by monitoring with systemic arterial and PA catheters.[12–24] This technology is expensive, time-consuming, and personnel-intensive; at present, it is the most explicit circulatory monitoring that is available shortly after admission to the ICU. It provides frequent systemic and PA and venous pressure measurements (mean arterial pressure [MAP], central venous pressure [CVP], mean PA pressure [MPAP], PA occlusion pressure [PAOP]), cardiac output, arterial and mixed venous gases, hemoglobin (Hb), and Hb saturations (SaO_2); blood gases measured within 1 or 2 minutes of cardiac output may be used to calculate $\dot{D}O_2$, $\dot{V}O_2$, oxygen extraction ratio (O_2 extr), pulmonary venous admixture or shunting (Qsp/Qt), the ratio of the arterial partial pressure of oxygen to the inspired oxygen fraction (PaO_2/FIO_2), and alveolar-arterial oxygen gradient (PAO_2/PaO_2). All flow-related and volume-related variables in this chapter are indexed to body surface area. The variables, abbreviations, units, formulas, normal values, and optimal values were defined in relation to high-risk survivors of postoperative shock (Table 8–1).

TIME: A CRUCIAL FACTOR IN PATHOPHYSIOLOGY AND THERAPY

In order to evaluate underlying circulatory mechanisms, it is necessary to describe the time course or sequence of events

TABLE 8–1. Cardiorespiratory Variables

Variable	Abbreviation	Unit	Measurement or Calculation	Normal Value	Optimal Value	Per cent Correct
Volume-Related						
Mean arterial pressure	MAP	mm Hg	Direct measurement	82-102	>84	76
Central venous pressure	CVP	cm H_2O	Direct measurement	1-9	>5	62
Stroke index	SI	mL/m^2	SI = CI ÷ HR	30-50	>48	67
Hemoglobin	Hb	g/dL	Direct measurement	12-16	>12	66
Mean pulmonary artery pressure	MPAP	mm Hg	Direct measurement	11-15	<19	68
Wedge pressure	WP	mm Hg	Direct measurement	0-12	>9.5	70
Blood volume	BV	mL/m^2	BV = PV ÷ (1 − Hct)* × surface area	Men, 2.74	>3.0	76
				Women, 2.37	>2.7	
Red blood cell mass	RCM	mL/m^2	RCM = BV − PV	Men, 1.1	>1.1	85
				Women, 0.95	>0.95	
Flow-Related						
Cardiac index	CI	L/min · m^2	Direct measurement	2.8-3.6	>4.5	70
Left ventricular stroke work	LVSW	g · m/m^2	LVSW = SI × MAP × 0.0144	44-68	>55	74
Left cardiac work	LCW	kg · m/m^2	LCW = CI × MAP × 0.0144	3-4.6	>5	76
Right ventricular stroke work	RVSW	g · m/m^2	RVSW = SI × MPAP × 0.0144	4-8	>13	70
Right cardiac work	RCW	kg · m/m^2	RCW = CI × MPAP × 0.0144	0.4-0.6	>1.1	69
Stress-Related						
Systemic vascular resistance	SVR	dyne · s/cm^5 · m^2	SVR = 79.92 (MAP − CVP)† ÷ CI	1760-2600	<1450	62
Pulmonary vascular resistance	PVR	dyne · s/cm^5 · m^2	PVR = 79.92 (MPAP − WP)† ÷ CI	45-225	<226	77
Heart rate	HR	beat/min	Direct measurement	72-88	<100	60
Rectal temperature	temp	°F	Direct measurement	97.8-98.6	>100.4	64
Oxygen-Related						
Hg saturation	Sa_{O_2}	%	Direct measurement	95-99	>95	67
Arterial carbon dioxide tension	Pa_{CO_2}	mm Hg	Direct measurement	36-44	>30	69
Arterial pH	pH		Direct measurement	7.36-7.44	>7.47	74
Mixed venous oxygen tension	$P\bar{v}_{O_2}$	mm Hg	Direct measurement	33-53	>36	68
Arterial-mixed venous oxygen content difference	$C(a - \bar{v})_{O_2}$	mL/dL	$C(a - \bar{v})_{O_2} = Ca_{O_2} - C\bar{v}_{O_2}$	4-5.5	<3.5	68
Oxygen delivery	$\dot{D}_{O_2}$	mL/min · m^2	$\dot{D}_{O_2} = Ca_{O_2} \times CI \times 10$	520-720	>550	76
Oxygen consumption	$\dot{V}_{O_2}$	mL/min · m^2	$\dot{V}_{O_2} = C(a - \bar{v})_{O_2} \times CI \times 10$	100-180	>167	69
Oxygen extraction rate	O_2 ext	%	$O_2\ ext = (Ca_{O_2} - C\bar{v}_{O_2}) \div Ca_{O_2}$	22-30	<31	69

Modified from Shoemaker WC, Appel P, Bland R: Use of physiologic monitoring to predict outcome and to assist in clinical decisions in critically ill postoperative patients. Am J Surg 1983; 146:43-50.
*Hematocrit (Hct) corrected for packing fraction and large ratio of vessel hematocrit to total body hematocrit.
†Venous pressure expressed in mm Hg.

and to differentiate primary events from secondary or tertiary events. An early event may or may not be causally related to a subsequent event, but a late event may be excluded as the cause of earlier events. For example, an initial blood loss after injury may be followed by low flow, then the adrenal stress response that restores blood pressure increases heart rate and cardiac index, but subsequently leads to oliguria and finally ARDS.

Most reports have described hemodynamic and oxygen transport variables in various etiologic types of shock in terms of their mean values and standard deviation (SD) or standard error of the mean (SEM) as if only a single time line existed[21-23]; that is, the data were expressed in terms unrelated to the time of onset of the syndrome, the temporal sequence, the progression of the syndrome, or the time of death or recovery. Only rarely are complete temporal patterns of the monitored variables presented for survivors and nonsurvivors so that these patterns can be evaluated at comparable times.

A major part of the problem is the difficulty in identifying the time of onset of shock, particularly shock resulting from sepsis and occult hemorrhage. However, even if the time of onset of shock could be identified and if this time were used as a "zero" time, the subsequent time course would not necessarily be in phase because shock may evolve rapidly or slowly, depending on the severity of the etiologic event, other associated clinical problems, and the vigorousness of therapeutic efforts.[21, 22]

Alternatively, the initial low point (nadir) of the MAP or CI values has been used to identify an early time point of the syndrome. Similarly, the highest compensatory changes, such as in CI, $\dot{D}O_2$, and $\dot{V}O_2$ values, after resuscitation are other identifiable points. The initial low and the subsequent highest CI or $\dot{V}O_2$ values define two points that partially describe a time frame that is roughly similar to that of the "peaks" and "troughs" of antibiotic levels. It may be misleading to begin monitoring and describing events after hypotension has already appeared and shock is already established. When monitoring was started at, or shortly after, the time of the precipitating event, it was found that survivors started with low flow but promptly developed compensatory hyperdynamic states, whereas nonsurvivors continued to have normal or low flow, tissue hypoxia, organ failure, capillary leak, and finally death.[12, 23]

Time is also the most important issue related to therapy and outcome. The major problem is to achieve the optimal supranormal goals in the first 8 to 12 hours postoperatively. In the initial studies, effectiveness continued to decline when patients were entered into the protocol several days postoperatively; for this reason, in the second study patients were randomized preoperatively and optimized in the first 12 hours posoperatively.[12] In severely traumatized patients, incommensurately low $\dot{V}O_2$ responses to increased $\dot{D}O_2$ in the first day after injury were associated with increased organ failure and mortality; by contrast, increased $\dot{V}O_2$ associated with increased $\dot{D}O_2$ favorably affected outcome.

HEMODYNAMIC DESCRIPTION OF SHOCK

Intraoperative Hemodynamic and Oxygen Transport Patterns of Survivors and Nonsurvivors

The surgical operation represents a controlled form of trauma and provides a unique opportunity to describe and analyze the temporal patterns of circulatory dysfunction and shock, because the exact times of the start and end of operations are well documented. By contrast, the temporal sequences are not clearly apparent in septic shock, occult hemorrhage, and incipient forms of medical shock. In high-risk surgical patients, time-related measurements may be obtained (1) in a pre-illness baseline control period, (2) during anesthesia induction, (3) throughout the surgical operation, (4) during and after a hemodynamic crisis, (5) throughout the subsequent recovery periods of survivors and nonsurvivors, and (6) during the final deterioration of nonsurvivors. This descriptive approach to the pattern of physiologic events provides the basic data for a mechanistic model of surgical shock that also serves as a model for other types of shock.

Intraoperative circulatory events associated with survival and death were evaluated in 356 high-risk elective surgical patients to identify patterns of nonsurvivors at the earliest possible time and to develop more effective measures for preventing organ failure and death.[24] The conventionally monitored MAP and heart rate remained in the normal range in both groups; in the nonsurvivors, cardiac index, stroke index, stroke work, $\dot{D}O_2$, and $\dot{V}O_2$ decreased. Low $\dot{V}O_2$ was partly compensated by increased oxygen extraction rates, and arterial pressures were maintained by increased vasoconstriction (Figs. 8–1 and 8–2).

Peripheral vasoconstriction by the adrenomedullary stress response is an initial response to blood loss that maintains pressure in the presence of falling flow; however, this vasoconstriction is uneven and leads to unevenly distributed microcirculatory flow. In nonsurvivors, these early changes preceded the development of postoperative organ failure. In the presence of continued hypovolemia, the stress response may lead to poor tissue perfusion, tissue hypoxia, covert clinical shock, organ dysfunction, ARDS and other organ failure.[25-27] Lethal circulatory dysfunction begins in the intraoperative period but becomes more apparent as organs fail in later postoperative stages.

Noninvasive monitoring provides information similar to that obtained with the PA catheter[28-32]; both approaches revealed low flow, arterial hypoxemia, and poor tissue perfusion that were worse in the nonsurvivors. The multicomponent noninvasive monitoring gives continuous on-line real-time displays of circulatory data that allow early recognition of acute circulatory dysfunction. There was no instance in which noninvasive monitoring gave information that would have led to incorrect therapy. Compared with invasive monitoring, noninvasive systems are easier, safer, less expensive, and as sensitive.

Postoperative Hemodynamic and Oxygen Transport Patterns

The temporal course of circulatory patterns in the perioperative period was observed in several large series of critically ill surgical patients in order to characterize hemodynamic and oxygen transport patterns after surgical trauma in actual time elapsed from the beginning or the end of the surgical operation.[23-27, 33-37] Many associated preoperative conditions, including age, sepsis, accidental trauma, stress, hypovolemia, cirrhosis, hypertension, prior myocardial infarction, stroke, and chronic congestive cardiac failure, may greatly affect these patterns. More important, prompt vigorous therapy readily reverses these abnormal patterns.

Comparison of the physiologic patterns of postoperative survivors and nonsurvivors provides the basis for evaluating the nature and biologic importance of circulatory compensations. Changes from the normal range in survivors reflect the effects of surgical trauma and successful compensatory responses that have survival value, whereas abnormal findings of nonsurvivors may reflect the combined effects of overwhelming trauma, inadequate compensations, and delayed or inappropriate therapy.

The circulatory effects of operative trauma, per se, may

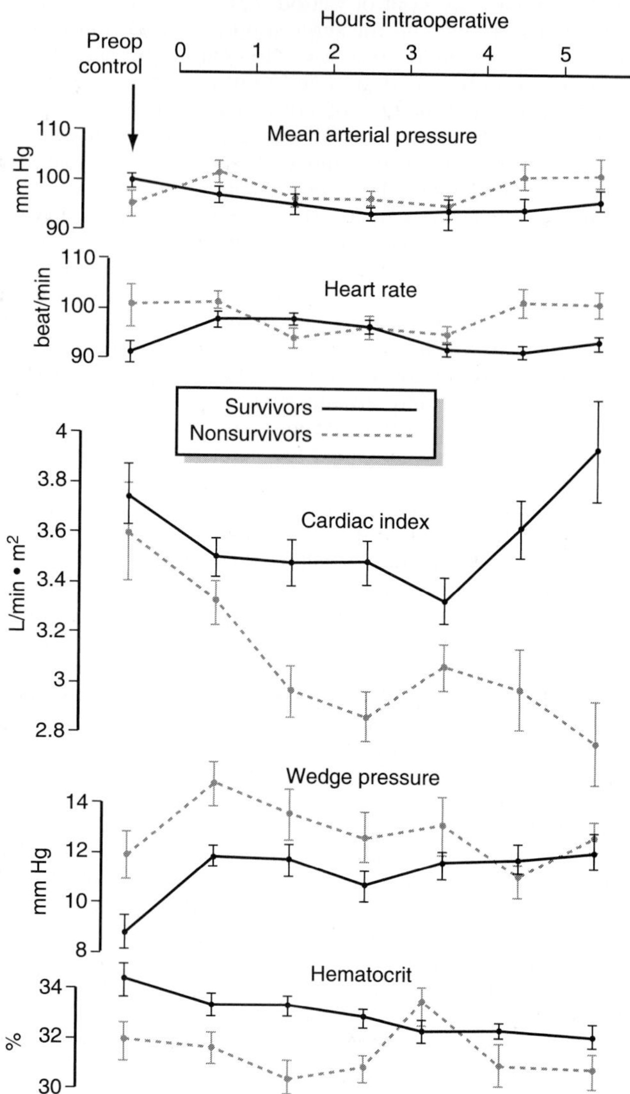

Figure 8–1. Mean hemodynamic values in a series of 356 high-risk surgical patients in the preoperative control period *(left line)* and averaged over each succeeding hour intraoperatively for mean arterial pressure, heart rate, cardiac index, pulmonary artery (PA) occlusion (wedge) pressure, and hematocrit for survivors *(solid line)* and nonsurvivors *(dotted line)*. The data show significant reductions in cardiac index especially in the nonsurvivors.

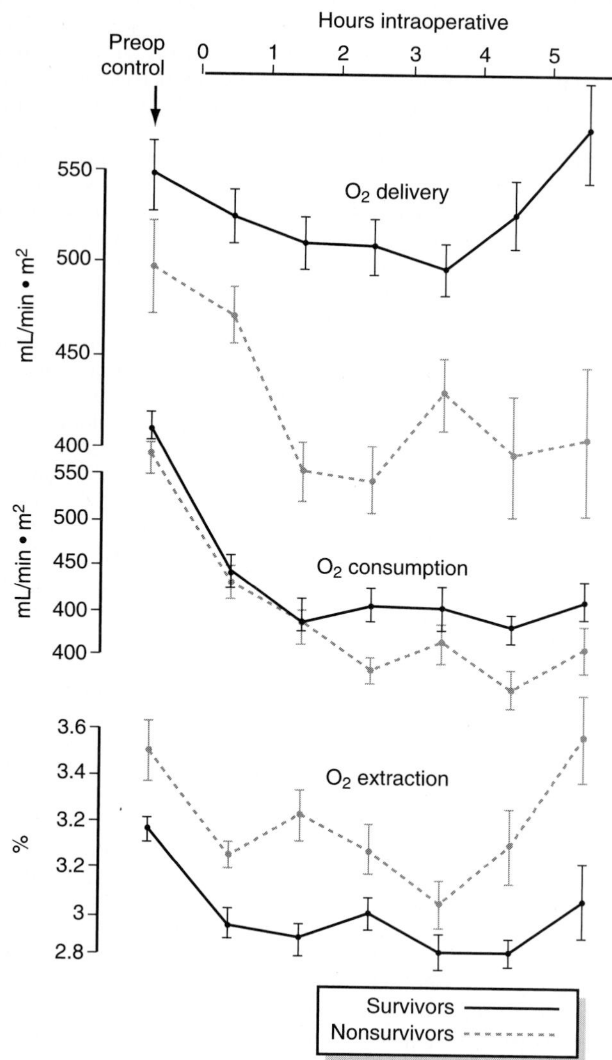

Figure 8–2. Mean oxygen transport values in a series of 356 high-risk surgical patients in the preoperative control period *(left line)* and averaged over each succeeding hour intraoperatively for survivors *(solid line)* and nonsurvivors *(dotted line)*. Note the marked reduction in oxygen delivery and oxygen consumption especially in nonsurvivors and the greater compensatory increase in oxygen extraction that tends to maintain oxygen consumption in the nonsurvivors.

be characterized by the hemodynamic and oxygen transport patterns of patients who preoperatively had normal cardiac output and no evidence of associated circulatory conditions. Intraoperatively, the mean CI, $\dot{D}O_2$, and $\dot{V}O_2$ decreased from normal preoperative values in both survivors and nonsurvivors, but the decreases were greater in the nonsurvivors.[23]

In survivors, the mean CI, $\dot{D}O_2$, and $\dot{V}O_2$ increased during the first 12 postoperative hours (Fig. 8-3). The peak postoperative values were as follows: CI greater than 4.5 L/min • m^2; $\dot{D}O_2$ greater than 600 mL/min • m^2; and $\dot{V}O_2$ greater than 170 mL/min • m^2. The nonsurvivors maintained normal or near-normal values for CI, $\dot{D}O_2$, and $\dot{V}O_2$, but these values were significantly lower than those of the survivors. Nonsurvivors' oxygen extraction ratios increased in partial compensation for inadequate tissue oxygenation. Despite normal blood gas values, nonsurvivor Qsp/Qt and PAO_2/PaO_2 values increased

Figure 8–3. Temporal postoperative patterns for mean arterial pressure, cardiac index, pulmonary artery (PA) occlusion (wedge) pressure, systemic vascular resistance, oxygen delivery, and oxygen consumption for survivors *(solid line)* and nonsurvivors *(dotted line)* among 708 high-risk surgical patients. Left time line is baseline control (BL), then intraoperative period (IO), followed by postoperative hours (e.g., 1, 2, 4, 8, 12). Note the higher mean arterial pressure, cardiac index, oxygen delivery, and oxygen consumption for survivors *(solid line)* and the slightly higher wedge pressure for nonsurvivors; systemic vascular resistance was similar in both groups.

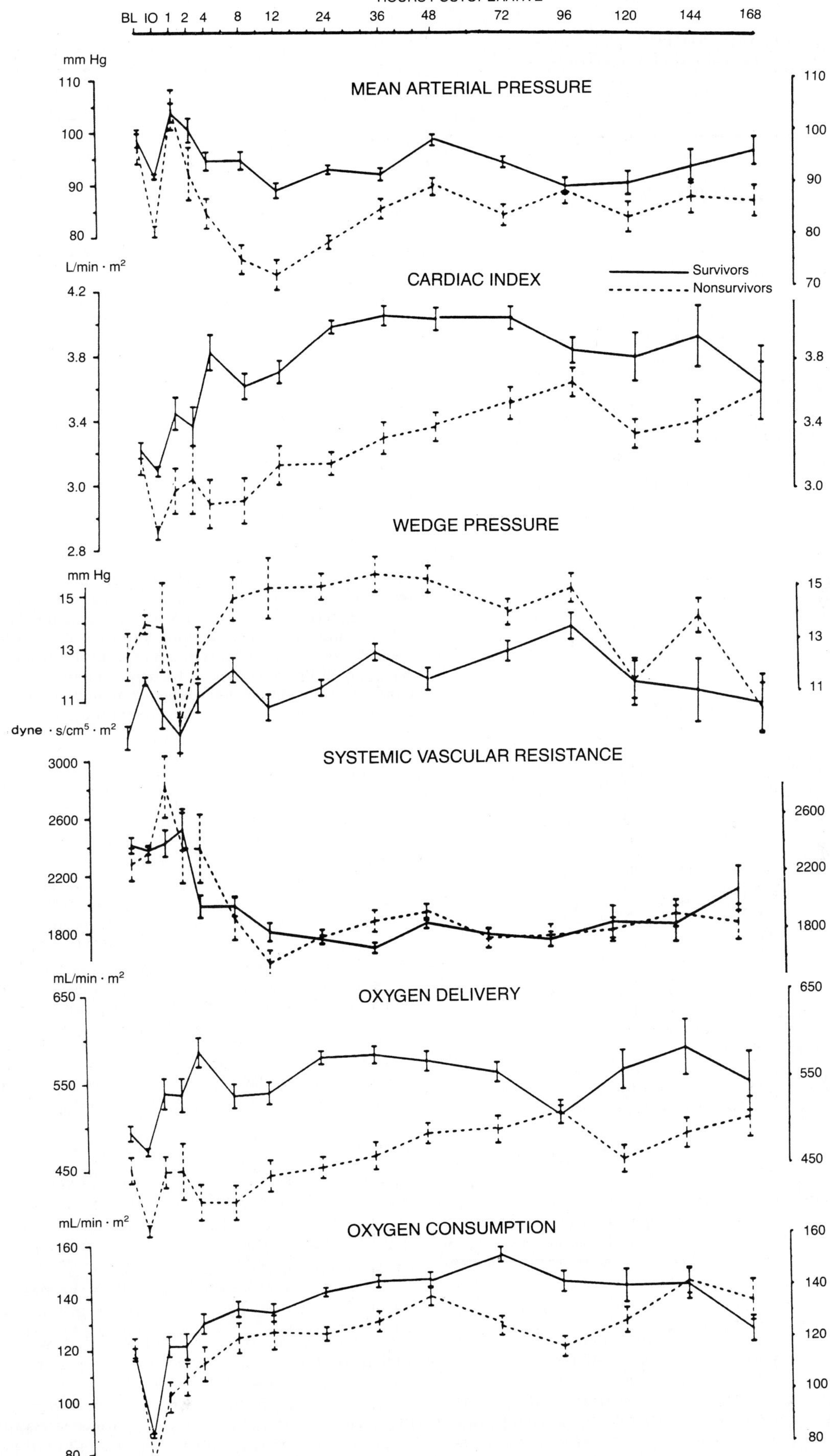

Figure 8–3 *See legend on opposite page*

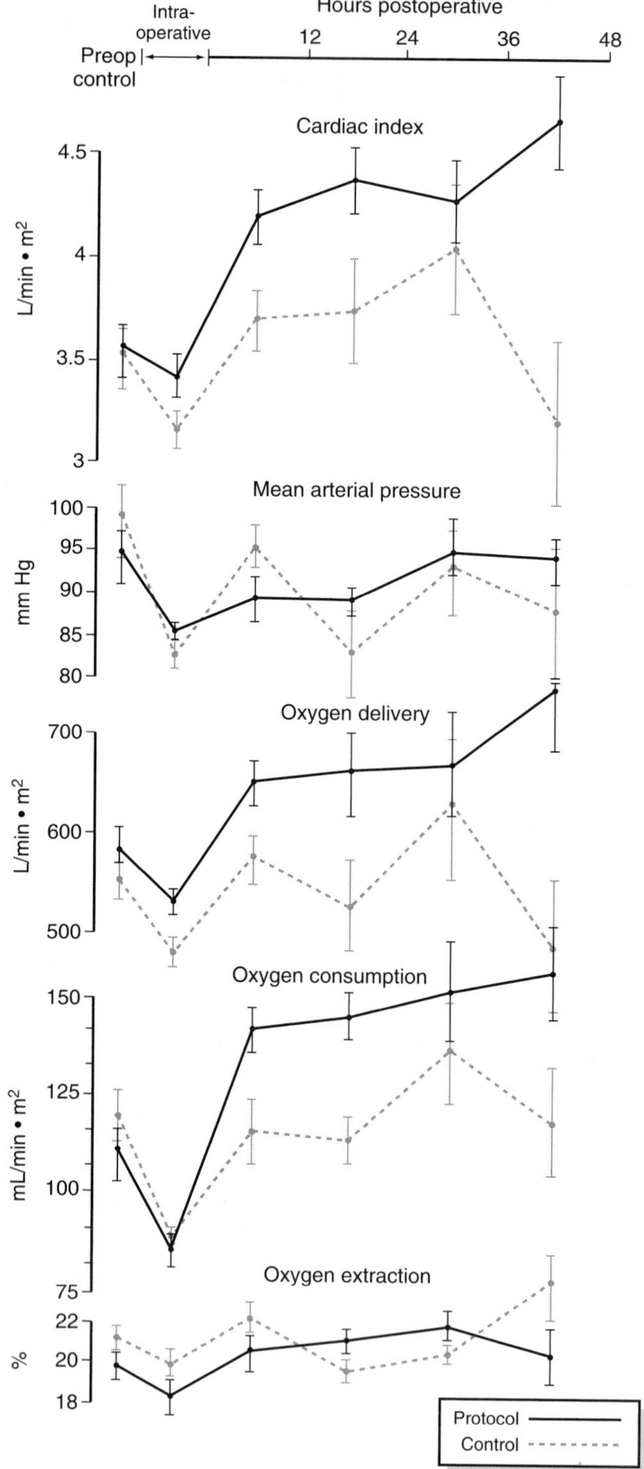

Figure 8–4. Sequential preoperative *(first time line),* intraoperative *(second time line),* and postoperative (labeled 12, 24, 36, and 48 hours) patterns for cardiac index, mean arterial pressure, oxygen delivery, and oxygen consumption for protocol *(solid line)* and control *(dotted line)* groups in a prospectively randomized trial of supranormal values as goals of therapy. Note the higher cardiac index, oxygen delivery, and oxygen consumption for the protocol group beginning in the first 12 hours postoperatively.

intraoperatively and postoperatively. Routinely recorded vital signs were similar in both groups postoperatively.[23]

Patients with low cardiac output, including elderly patients, those with congestive cardiac failure, and those with hypovolemia resulting from dehydration or hemorrhagic shock, preoperatively had high PAOP and reduced CI, $\dot{D}O_2$, and $\dot{V}O_2$. In the early postoperative period, they demonstrated compensatory increases in CI, $\dot{D}O_2$, and $\dot{V}O_2$ that were qualitatively similar to but smaller than those of patients with normal preoperative values. That is, survivor CI, $\dot{D}O_2$, and $\dot{V}O_2$ values increased in the postoperative period from their low preoperative baseline values, whereas nonsurvivors maintained lower postoperative CI, $\dot{D}O_2$, and $\dot{V}O_2$ values and high PAOP. Nonsurvivors also showed significantly greater increases in the pulmonary vascular resistance index (PVRI) and Qsp/Qt. Thus, these patients started from lower preoperative baseline cardiac output values, but differences between survivors' and nonsurvivors' postoperative patterns relative to their own preoperative baseline (control) values were similar to those of patients with normal preoperative values[23] (Fig. 8-4).

Preoperative patients with sepsis, severe stress, accidental injury, and advanced cirrhosis often had high preoperative baseline CI values.[5] Postoperatively, the survivors had increases over their own baseline values in CI, $\dot{D}O_2$, and $\dot{V}O_2$ but minimal changes in other hemodynamic variables. The nonsurviving patients had little or no increase in CI, $\dot{D}O_2$, and $\dot{V}O_2$ despite higher CVP and PAOP. The PAOP, PVRI, and Qsp/Qt were higher in nonsurvivors than in survivors. Both groups maintained mean intravascular pressures and other non–flow-related variables in their relatively normal preoperative ranges.

Similar differences in the survivor and nonsurvivor hemodynamic patterns were observed in many other conditions including severe trauma, hemorrhage, sepsis (in medical and surgical patients), acute myocardial infarction, cardiogenic shock, congestive heart failure, acute respiratory failure, cirrhosis, and head injury.[11-27, 33-55]

Early Hemodynamic and Oxygen Transport Patterns After Trauma

The hemodynamic and oxygen transport patterns after accidental trauma were similar to those described after surgery, except that after accidental injuries wider variations in the patterns occurred because of marked differences in the amount and location of injuries, associated blood loss, organ injury, and time delays to complete resuscitation.[1, 14, 15, 17, 20] In the standard Advanced Trauma Life Support (ATLS) course, the degree of shock and amount of blood loss are estimated from the systolic and diastolic blood pressure, pulse pressure, skin color, pulse rate, capillary refill, temperature, respiratory rate, and mental status. Unfortunately, blood pressure early in the course of blunt and penetrating trauma is not reliably correlated with blood flow or outcome.[1, 12]

In trauma patients with severe shock resulting from loss of more than 3000 mL of blood and with injury severity scores greater than 20, Bishop and coworkers[17, 20] observed a mortality rate of 18% when the accumulated delays were less than 24 hours from the time of injury to the time postoperatively when optimal supranormal values were achieved (Figs. 8-5 and 8-6). By contrast, when these accumulated delays were greater than 24 hours or when supranormal optimal values were not achieved, the mortality rate was 39%.

Nonsurvivors had greater initial reductions in MAP, CI, $\dot{D}O_2$, and $\dot{V}O_2$ and lesser elevations in these parameters in the first 24 hours after injury. However, after 3 to 5 days, septic complications and organ failures in nonsurvivors led to higher $\dot{V}O_2$ values associated with increased body metabolism, especially in the late stage.

Circulatory measurements with invasive PA balloon-tipped thermodilution catheters have been the gold standard for evaluation of circulatory function. Recently, use of improved noninvasive hemodynamic monitoring systems during the resuscitation of patients with blunt trauma immediately after their admission to the emergency department was found to be feasible. Results obtained with noninvasive monitoring systems that continuously display patterns of cardiac function, pulmonary function, and tissue perfusion or oxygenation were comparable to those obtained by invasive monitoring. A large series of patients with severe blunt trauma and evidence of acute circulatory dysfunction were studied shortly after admission to the emergency department.[56-58]

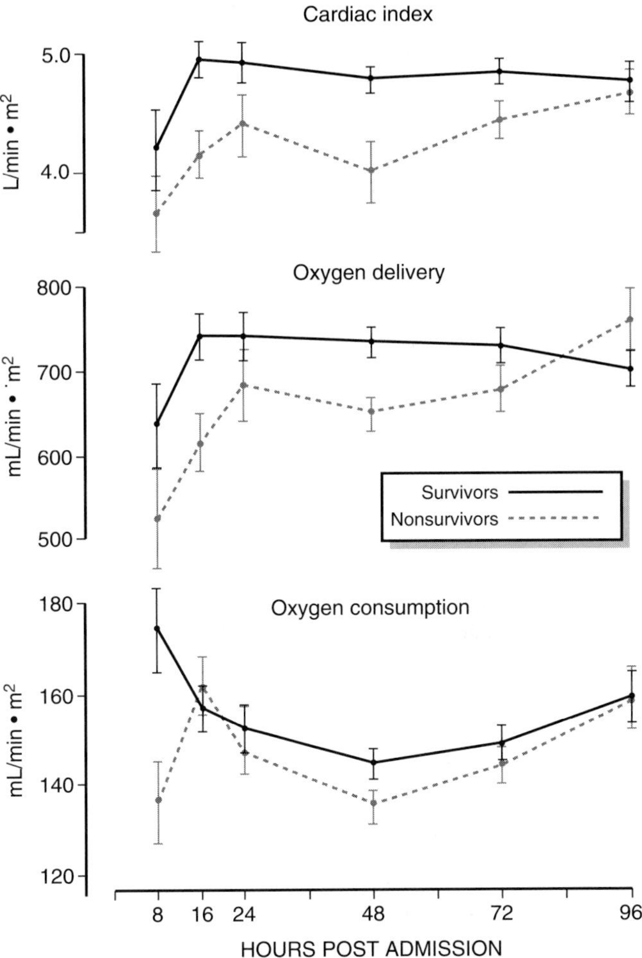

Figure 8–5. Temporal hemodynamic and oxygen transport patterns for cardiac index, oxygen delivery, and oxygen consumption for survivors *(solid line)* and nonsurvivors *(dotted line)* of blunt trauma. Time lines are hours after admission to the emergency department. (8, 16, 24, 72, and 96.). Note the higher cardiac index, oxygen delivery, and oxygen consumption for survivors *(solid line).*

Sequential Hemodynamic Patterns in Hemorrhagic Shock

With rapid blood loss, which is defined as major hemorrhage of more than 4 units that occurs in less than 4 hours, the pattern of hemorrhagic shock was characterized by reduced blood pressure, CI, CVP, PAOP, mixed venous oxygen saturation ($S\bar{v}O_2$), pH, hematocrit, $\dot{D}O_2$, and $\dot{V}O_2$ concomitant with an increased systemic vascular resistance index (SVRI) and oxygen extraction ratio.[41] With moderate degrees of hypovolemia, the initial PaO_2 values were usually normal, but in the presence of severe hypovolemia, hyperpnea and tachypnea occurred, usually with near-normal PaO_2 and pH values but low arterial partial pressure of carbon dioxide ($PaCO_2$) values, indicating respiratory alkalosis. When shock was prolonged, poor tissue perfusion and inadequate tissue oxygenation led to acidosis, increased lactate levels, and base deficits. The initial compensatory responses included increased heart rate, which increased CI by neural and neurohormonal mechanisms; increased SVRI, which tended to maintain arterial pressures in the presence of decreasing flow; and increased oxy-

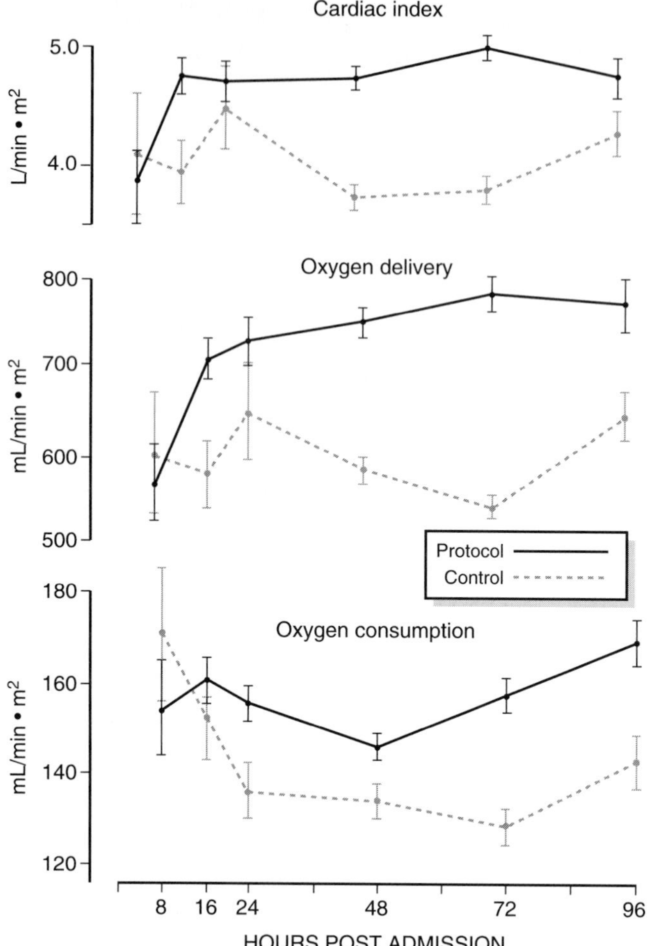

Figure 8–6. Temporal hemodynamic and oxygen transport patterns for cardiac index, oxygen delivery, and oxygen consumption for protocol *(solid line)* and control *(dotted line)* patients in a prospective randomized trial of supranormal values as goals of therapy in blunt trauma. Time lines are hours after admission to the emergency department (8, 16, 24, 72, and 96.). Note the higher cardiac index, oxygen delivery, and oxygen consumption for the protocol patients.

gen extraction ratios, which improved tissue oxygenation when blood flow was reduced.

When blood loss was slow, defined as hemorrhage that occurs for longer than 4 hours, the hemorrhagic shock pattern showed greater reductions in hematocrit and lesser reductions in MAP, CI, $\dot{D}O_2$, and $\dot{V}O_2$. Moreover, the reduced rate of $\dot{V}O_2$ was lower quantitatively but more prolonged than that occurring after rapid losses of comparable quantities of blood. After the hemorrhage was stopped and blood volume was restored with appropriate fluids, the survivors' recovery was characterized by supranormal values for CI, $\dot{D}O_2$, and $\dot{V}O_2$.

Hemodynamic and Oxygen Transport Patterns in Septic Shock

Time relationships for postoperative patients are easily marked by the time of onset or the end of the surgical operation. Sepsis, by contrast, usually has a more subtle and insidious onset. Time relationships are obscure, and progression from localized infection to generalized infection with systemic manifestations, to the septic syndrome, to septic shock, and to death may be gradual and not readily apparent. The progress of the disorder may not be recognized until advanced stages; in the fulminating form of sepsis there may be cataclysmic deterioration and rapid demise.[21, 22]

Septic shock is also difficult to understand because of the heterogeneity of patients affected; that is, widely different clinical manifestations occur in postoperative, post-traumatic, urologic, and general internal medicine patients and those with respiratory failure. Sepsis may be the primary disorder, or it may be a complication. Sepsis may also be the expected consequence in patients with obstruction of the normal flow of biologic fluids (urine, bile, or gastrointestinal fluids), immunodeficiencies, and late-stage malignancies.

Sequential hemodynamic and oxygen transport patterns of survivors and nonsurvivors were described in a series of 378 consecutive internal medicine and surgical septic shock patients to differentiate primary from secondary and tertiary events and to evaluate possible underlying mechanisms and their therapeutic implications.[21, 22] Because of the gradual transitions between the stages of septic shock and variations in the duration of each stage, specific physiologic criteria were used to define the following stages (Fig. 8–7):

1. An early period, which began with the first recorded increase in cardiac output.
2. A middle period, which was the time 48 hours before and after the maximum metabolic activity, defined as the period characterized by the highest recorded rate of oxygen consumption.
3. A late period, which was the time 48 hours before death or recovery, defined as the time when the patient had recovered sufficiently to allow discontinuation of measurements and removal of catheters.

The earliest hemodynamic changes were increases in heart rate, CI, and $\dot{D}O_2$. Early transient reductions in $\dot{V}O_2$ that preceded temperature elevations and hypotension were observed in both survivors and nonsurvivors. Subsequently, in the early and middle periods, progressive increases in CI, $\dot{D}O_2$, and $\dot{V}O_2$ were noted. These increases were greater in the survivors than in the nonsurvivors at comparable time periods.

Although 84% of the patients with sepsis were consistently hyperdynamic, transient hypodynamic episodes, defined as CI less than 2.5 L/min • m² in approximately 10% of the measurements, were seen. Also, in 8% of the nonsurvivors, transient preterminal hypermetabolic periods, defined as $\dot{V}O_2$ greater than 200 mL/min • m², were also observed; these usually occurred 18 to 72 hours before death and were followed by a progressive downhill course. In the nonsurvivors' terminal period, MAP, CI, $\dot{D}O_2$, and $\dot{V}O_2$ fell abruptly. Thus, early increases in CI and $\dot{D}O_2$ represent physiologic compensations for circulatory deficiencies that limit body metabolism and compromise survival.

Hankeln and associates[42] reported that postoperative and cardiac patients with ARDS who did survive had supranormal CI and $\dot{D}O_2$; in their series, nonsurvivors had lower values than survivors. Others also observed increased CI, $\dot{D}O_2$, and $\dot{V}O_2$ in septic shock patients.[43–52] Abraham and colleagues[43] demonstrated additional increases in $\dot{D}O_2$ and $\dot{V}O_2$ after fluid loading with colloids in patients with septic shock resulting from peritonitis. Others have corroborated the increased CI, $\dot{D}O_2$, and $\dot{V}O_2$ in patients with septic shock given fluids or inotropes.[43–52] Edwards and colleagues[51, 52] took the concept one step further by driving $\dot{D}O_2$ and $\dot{V}O_2$ to optimal supranormal values with the administration of fluids and dobutamine; using this approach, they demonstrated improved survival rates in severely ill septic shock patients. In prospective ran-

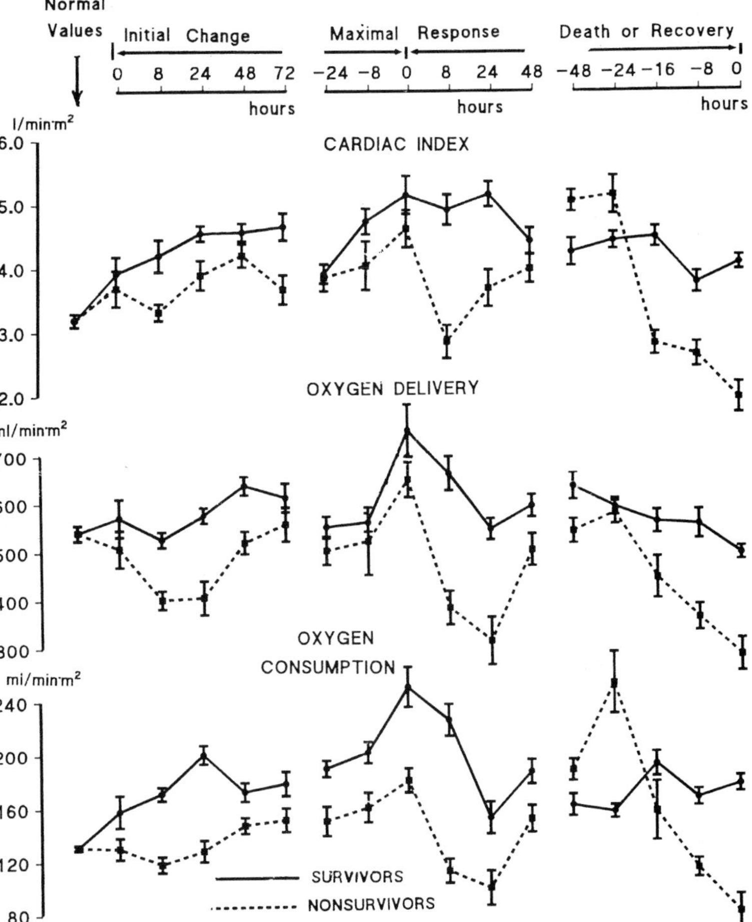

Figure 8–7. Temporal hemodynamic and oxygen transport patterns for cardiac index, oxygen delivery, and oxygen consumption for survivors *(solid line)* and nonsurvivors *(dotted line)* in a series of more than 300 patients in septic shock. Time lines normal values *(extreme left)*; "early" shock defined as the first recorded instance of increased cardiac index, "middle" stage defined as the period before and after the highest recorded rate of body metabolism, and "late" stage defined as the period before death or removal of catheter before return to the hospital floor. Note the higher cardiac index, oxygen delivery, and oxygen consumption for survivors *(solid line)*. (From Shoemaker WC, Appel PL, Kram HB: Sequence of physiologic patterns in surgical septic shock. Chest 1992; 102:208–215.)

domized studies of medical patients with septic shock, Tuchschmidt and coworkers[38] showed reduced mortality when CI was driven to 6 L/min • m² with fluids and dobutamine. In the late stage, however, this is not effective.

Figure 8–8 shows baseline control values for CI plotted against corresponding PAOP (wedge pressure) values in a series of 378 patients with septic shock during early, middle, late, and terminal stages. Also shown are changes in CI and PAOP after administration of 500 mL of 5% albumin over a 60-minute interval in each stage. The data show increased baseline CI and PAOP values in the early stage and significant responses of CI and PAOP after the fluid load. In the middle stage, there were marked significantly increases in CI but small changes in PAOP in the baseline control values and similar responses to volume therapy. In the late and terminal period, the baseline CI values decreased and the responses to treatment were minimal and insignificant. The data indicate that colloid therapy improved myocardial performance in the early and middle periods of septic shock but not in the late and terminal stages.

Figure 8–9 shows baseline control values for $\dot{V}O_2$ plotted against the corresponding $\dot{D}O_2$ values of the series of 378 patients with septic shock during early, middle, and late or terminal stages as well as changes in $\dot{D}O_2$ and $\dot{V}O_2$ after administration of 500 mL of 5% albumin over a 60-minute interval in each stage. The data show small increases in baseline $\dot{D}O_2$ and $\dot{V}O_2$ values in the early stage and significant responses of both $\dot{D}O_2$ and $\dot{V}O_2$ to the fluid load, comparable to those of nonseptic patients. In the middle stage, there were marked and significant increases in $\dot{D}O_2$ and $\dot{V}O_2$ at their baseline control period and similar responses to volume therapy. In the late or terminal period, the baseline values were very low and the responses to treatment were minimal and not significant. The data indicate that colloid therapy in the early and middle periods of septic shock produced a response similar to that of the nonseptic critically ill patients but in the late and terminal stages did not improve tissue perfusion, probably because of capillary leak.

Cardiogenic Shock

Traditionally, the Starling myocardial performance curve, defined by a CI of 2.5 L/min • m² and an arbitrary PAOP of 18 or 20 mm Hg, is used to evaluate clinical subsets of cardiogenic shock. Four quadrants described by the Starling curve and PAOP identify the physiologic impairments of these four subsets and suggest therapies appropriate to these conditions.[2, 3]

Chronic congestive cardiac failure and acute circulatory failure in patients with chronic cardiac disease have been extensively studied; reduced CI and MAP with high PAOP and SVRI were commonly found. Although numerous studies have documented these CI–venous pressure relationships, two studies of cardiogenic shock after acute myocardial infarction have reported the relationships of CI, $\dot{D}O_2$, and $\dot{V}O_2$. Da Luz and associates[53] reported oxygen transport data for seven patients,

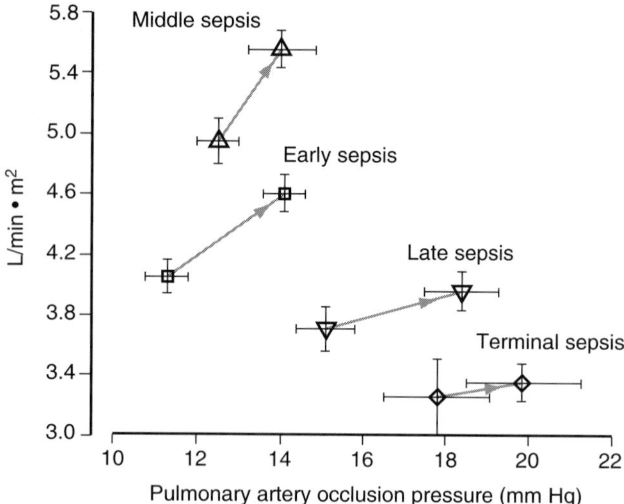

Figure 8–8. Baseline control values for cardiac index (CI) plotted against corresponding PAOP (wedge pressure) values in the series of 378 septic shock patients during early, middle, late, and terminal stages. Also shown are changes in CI and PAOP after 500 mL of 5% albumin given over a 60-minute interval in each stage. *Early stage,* Note increased baseline CI and PAOP values in and significant responses of CI and PAOP after the fluid load. *Middle stage,* Marked and significantly increased CI but small changes in PAOP and similar responses to volume therapy. *Late and terminal stages.* The baseline CI values decreased and the responses to treatment were minimal and insignificant. The data indicate that colloid therapy improved myocardial performance in the early and middle periods of septic shock but not in the late and terminal stages.

all of whom had received adrenergic drugs before the measurements were made.

Creamer and coworkers[54] reported on 19 patients in cardiogenic shock after infarction. Fourteen patients had a CI of 1.3 ± 0.5 L/min • m² before therapy; in response to therapy, they developed a CI of 2.5 ± 0.4 L/min • m² associated with pronounced increases in $\dot{D}O_2$ from 230 ± 69 to 397 ± 60 mL/min • m² and $\dot{V}O_2$ from 103 ± 31 to 124 ± 22 mL/min • m²; 13 of these 14 patients survived. Two patients with a mean CI of 0.9 ± 0.4 L/min • m² died before therapy could be given, and three patients recovered spontaneously. The authors concluded that in cardiogenic shock, supply-dependent $\dot{V}O_2$, although not elevated as in septic shock, was nevertheless an important component of both pathophysiology and therapy.[54, 55] Other goals of therapy included an increase in $\dot{D}O_2$ from 300 to 400 mL/min • m², a decrease in oxygen extraction ratio to about 30%, and an increase in $S\bar{v}O_2$ to approximately 70%. By contrast, Conners and colleagues[4] found no improvement with the PA catheter in a large series of medical patients who entered the ICU with organ failure.

The patterns of patients with septic and cardiogenic shock may be compared to those with traumatic shock.[56-58]

Hemodynamic Patterns Before and After Lowest Cardiac Index Value

Because the lowest value (nadir) of the various hemodynamic variables may occur at different times, the sequential patterns may be somewhat out of phase as each component of the patient's circulatory dysfunction may occur at a different time and may progress at a different rate. The patterns tend to become blurred when the values are related only to the time of the accident or the time of admission. Figure 8–10 illustrates the survivor and nonsurvivor patterns for MAP, heart rate, and transcutaneous oxygen values when the data for each variable were aligned in time before and after the nadir of the cardiac index measured by thermodilution. The nadir of the survivors was 17 ± 5 hours and that of the nonsurvivors 2 ± 4 hours after hospital admission.

Rationale and Experimental Basis for Monitoring

The hypothesis was that outcome would be improved if the hemodynamic and oxygen transport values of survivors were rapidly achieved by aggressive therapy within 8 to 12 hours of the onset. This was tested in a randomized series of high-risk surgical patients with the median CI, $\dot{D}O_2$, and $\dot{V}O_2$ values of survivors as therapeutic goals. The optimal goals for patients with preoperative hyperdynamic states (those with sepsis, trauma, and cirrhosis) are somewhat higher and the goals for patients with preoperative hypodynamic states (the elderly and hypovolemic and cardiac patients), are somewhat lower than those for patients with normal preoperative values.

The major premise of these clinical studies is that death in critical illness follows physiologic patterns that are independent of the clinical diagnosis and independent of the surgical operation. Although many clinicians feel that there are too many clinical differences among individual patients to develop a therapeutic plan on the basis of common physiologic patterns, we found that the similarities of sequential hemodynamic and oxygen transport patterns among patients out-

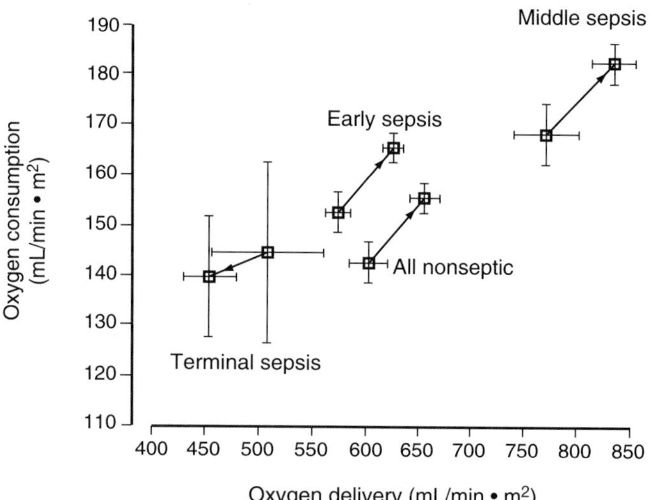

Figure 8–9. Baseline control values for $\dot{V}O_2$ plotted against the corresponding $\dot{D}O_2$ values of the series of 378 septic shock patients during early, middle, and terminal stages as well as changes in the $\dot{D}O_2$ and $\dot{V}O_2$ values after 500 mL of 5% albumin given over a 60-minute interval in each stage. There were small increases in baseline $\dot{D}O_2$ and VO_2 values in the early stage and significant responses of both $\dot{D}O_2$ and $\dot{V}O_2$ to the fluid load comparable to those of nonseptic patients. In the middle stage, there were marked and significantly increased $\dot{D}O_2$ and $\dot{V}O_2$ at their baseline control period and similar responses to volume therapy. In the terminal period, baseline values were very low and responses to treatment were minimal and not significant. Colloid therapy in the early and middle periods of septic shock produced a response similar to that of the nonseptic critically ill patients but in the late and terminal stages did not improve tissue perfusion, probably because of capillary leak.

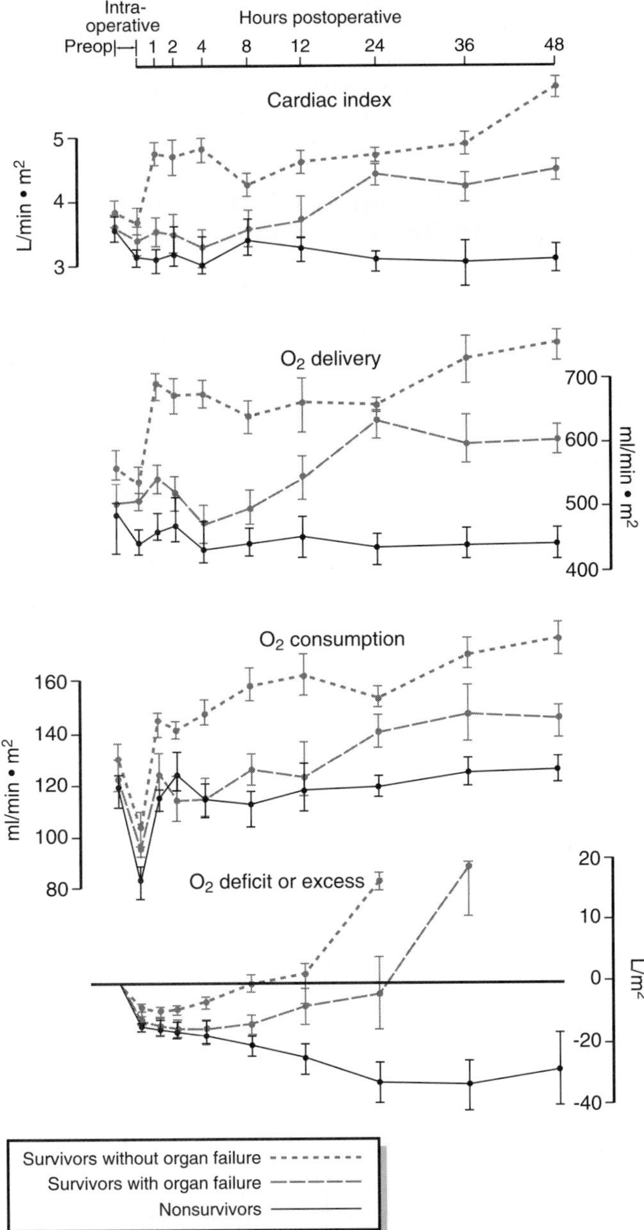

Figure 8–10. Temporal postoperative patterns for cardiac index, oxygen delivery, oxygen consumption, and calculated oxygen debt for survivors without postoperative organ failures *(dotted line)*, survivors with postoperative organ failures *(dashed line)*, and nonsurvivors *(solid line)* among 253 high-risk surgical patients. Left time line is the preoperative baseline control (BL), then intraoperative period, followed by postoperative hours (1, 2, 4, 8, 12, 24, 36, and 48 hours). Note the highest cardiac index, oxygen delivery, and oxygen consumption values for survivors without organ failures *(dotted line)*, the lowest values for nonsurvivors, and intermediate values for survivors with organ failure.

weighed individual clinical differences. This suggested that basic underlying physiologic mechanisms are reflected by common hemodynamic and oxygen transport patterns.

The second premise is that the supranormal values empirically seen in survivors reflect the effects of surgical operations, trauma, hypovolemia, sepsis, and other types of stress as well as the effects of circulatory compensations, whereas the relatively normal or subnormal values of the nonsurvivors reflect the overwhelming effects of the surgery and trauma or infection, or inadequate circulatory compensations, or both.

The important assumption is that physiologic criteria for the management of the life-threatening illness or for sepsis can be developed from the patterns of survivors. On the basis of extensive observations, it was assumed that physiologic patterns of patients who survived life-threatening illnesses provide objective criteria that may be used as the first approximation to goals of therapy.

TISSUE HYPOXIA, OXYGEN DEBT, ORGAN FAILURE, AND MORTALITY

Time Factors in Inadequately Treated Shock

When the stress or illness is excessive or there is inadequate blood flow and oxygen supply, tissue hypoxia may occur. Increasing metabolic demands of illness may overwhelm the capacity of the circulation to meet the increasing metabolic requirements for oxygen and oxidative substrates, particularly if there are preexisting cardiac, pulmonary, or other organ impairments.

The $\dot{V}O_2$ need may be estimated from the patient's own preoperative values under normal, steady-state conditions, with correction terms used to estimate "$\dot{V}O_{2(need)}$" under general anesthesia and at various body temperatures. Lowe and Ernst[59] reported $\dot{V}O_2$ under anesthesia in healthy elective patients as $\dot{V}O_{2(anesth)} = 10 \times kg^{0.72}$. This "$\dot{V}O_{2(anesth)}$" value was also corrected for temperature and was used to estimate $\dot{V}O_{2(need)}$ during the time the patient underwent general anesthesia. This value was about 100 mL/min • m². The temperature correction was based on the assumption that metabolic activity increased or decreased at a rate of 7%/°F.[25] After the anesthesia was reversed in the immediate postoperative period, the $\dot{V}O_{2(need)}$ was estimated from the patient's own preoperative baseline $\dot{V}O_2$ corrected for the effects of temperature. The temperature-corrected baseline preoperative $\dot{V}O_2$ was extrapolated as the estimated $\dot{V}O_{2(need)}$ in the immediate postoperative period. Thus, the net cumulative intraoperative and postoperative oxygen deficit was calculated from the measured $\dot{V}O_2$ minus the $\dot{V}O_{2(need)}$ estimated from the patient's own resting preoperative control values corrected for both temperature and anesthesia conditions and integrated over time.[25]

Oxygen debt was estimated in a series of 253 consecutively monitored high-risk surgical patients.[25] There were greater oxygen debts in those who died, all of whom had organ failure, than in those who survived, and oxygen debts were greater in surviving patients with organ failure than in those without organ failure (see Fig. 8–10). The calculated maximum oxygen debt for survivors who did not have organ failure was 9.2 ± 1.3 (SEM) L/m²; for survivors who had organ failure 21.6 ± 3.7 L/m²; and for nonsurvivors, all of whom had organ failure, 33.2 ± 4.0 L/m².

The average times of appearance of organ failures were as follows: ARDS, 3.6 ± 3.1 (SD) days; cardiogenic problems, 4.2 ± 4.8 days; renal failure, 5.9 ± 4.1 days; disseminated intravascular coagulation (DIC), 6.2 ± 5.6 days; and sepsis, 7.4 ± 4.9 days. Although ranges varied widely in these temporal patterns, the first organ failure began by the time of the maximum oxygen debt.

In the prospective, preoperatively randomized trial of the supranormal "optimal" oxygen transport values as goals of therapy, the protocol patients who had optimal values as therapeutic goals developed a maximum oxygen debt of 7.6 ± 3.4 L/min • m², which peaked at an average of 3 hours

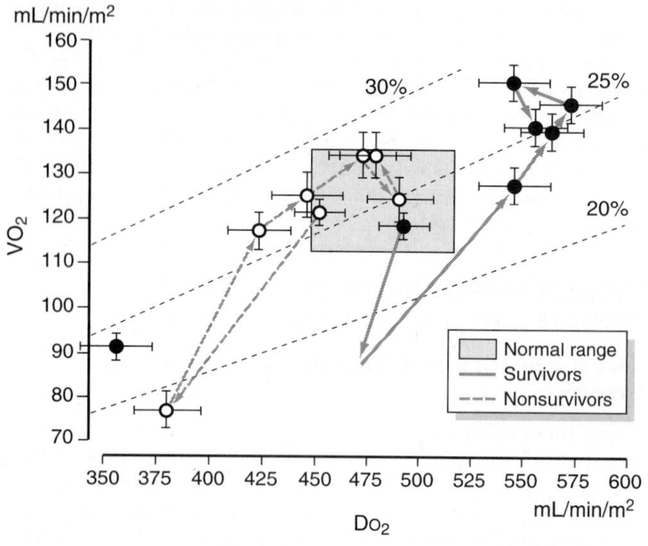

Figure 8–11. $\dot{V}O_2$ values are plotted against the corresponding $\dot{D}O_2$ for baseline control values of the series of 708 high-risk surgical patients preoperatively, intraoperatively, and postoperatively at 0 to 8 hr, 8 to 16 hr, 16 to 24 hr, 24 to 36 hr, and 36 to 48 hr for survivors *(solid line)* and nonsurvivors *(dashed lines)*. Survivors had smaller decreases intraoperatively and greater increases postoperatively than nonsurvivors. The data show marked differences between the two groups.

postoperatively and lasted an average of 13 hours postoperatively.[25] By contrast, the control patients who had normal values as therapeutic goals developed a maximum oxygen debt of 17.3 ± 6.3 L/m², which peaked at 31 hours postoperatively ($P < .05$) and lasted approximately 48 hours. There were 31 organ failures in the control group but only one in the protocol group.[12]

Clinical Significance of Oxygen Debt

There were wide differences in the amount and duration of the calculated oxygen debt between survivors and nonsurvivors as well as between the survivors with and without organ failure. When oxygen debt was prevented or rapidly repaired by increasing CI and $\dot{D}O_2$ to optimal values, the incidence of organ failure and death decreased significantly.[10] Moreover, the incidence of ARDS decreased to zero when tissue perfusion was maintained intraoperatively and in the immediate postoperative period in over 300 high-risk cancer patients per year for a 3-year period.[60] These findings indicate that tissue oxygen debt resulting from reduced tissue perfusion is the primary underlying physiologic mechanism that subsequently leads to organ failure and death

CLINICAL ASPECTS OF SHOCK AND CIRCULATORY FAILURE

Functional Circulatory Assessment

Circulatory function may be assessed by oxygen transport and oxygen metabolism values because oxygen consumption (1) is essential to life, (2) is impaired in shock states, (3) is considerably different in survivors and nonsurvivors, (4) measures overall body metabolism, and (5) is a sensitive monitored variable for outcome in acute circulatory failure. Technically, $\dot{D}O_2$ and $\dot{V}O_2$ are convenient to measure because oxygen has the highest extraction ratio of any blood constituent. Measurements of $\dot{V}O_2$ reflect the overall rate of oxidative metabolism, that is, the amount of oxygen burned per minute; this rate is not necessarily what the patient needs but is the amount of oxygen actually consumed per minute at the time of the measurement, because oxygen cannot be stored and sizable oxygen debts cannot be accumulated for appreciable periods of time without significant adverse consequences.[25-27]

Mathematical Coupling of Oxygen Delivery and Oxygen Consumption Values

There is a potential problem of mathematic coupling of $\dot{D}O_2$ values with $\dot{V}O_2$ values because CI is a common term for the calculations of both $\dot{D}O_2$ and $\dot{V}O_2$. Obviously, if CI is spuriously high or low, the calculated $\dot{D}O_2$ and $\dot{V}O_2$ will also be incorrectly high or low. Figure 8–11 illustrates the temporal patterns of $\dot{D}O_2$ values plotted against the corresponding $\dot{V}O_2$ values throughout the postoperative period of this series. To obviate this problem, the data of the series were also evaluated by plotting CI against oxygen extraction ratios (Fig. 8–12). Essentially in both approaches, the survivor and nonsurvivor patterns markedly separate.

Although this coupling is possible, it is unlikely to be a frequent or a consistent error when careful troubleshooting and quality controls are routinely used. Moreover, in a number of clinical conditions, changes in $\dot{D}O_2$ are not associated with similar changes in $\dot{V}O_2$:

1. In the middle stages of sepsis, postoperative states, and severe cardiac conditions, small $\dot{D}O_2$ changes were associated with large $\dot{V}O_2$ responses, indicating large oxygen debts.
2. Some early postoperative patients have major $\dot{D}O_2$ increases with minimum $\dot{V}O_2$ changes, suggestive of small oxygen debts.
3. Packed red blood cells in septic patients often stimulate

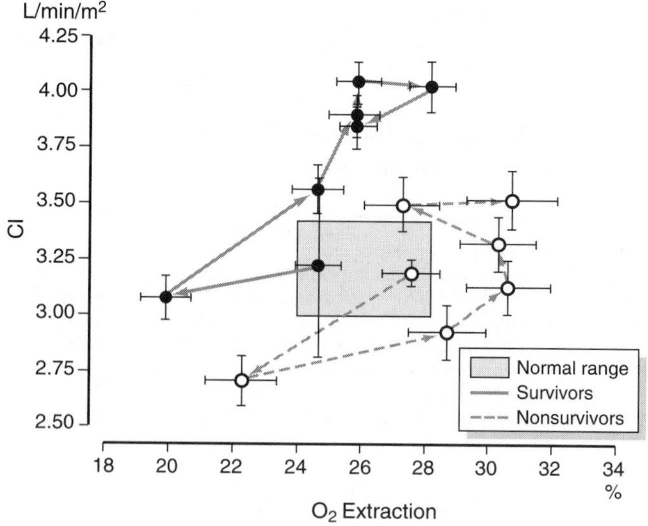

Figure 8–12. Baseline control values for cardiac index (CI) plotted against the corresponding O_2 extraction values of the series of 708 high-risk surgical patients preoperatively, intraoperatively, and postoperatively at 0 to 8 hr, 8 to 16 hr, 16 to 24 hr, 24 to 36 hr, and 36 to 48 hr for survivors *(solid line)* and nonsurvivors *(dashed lines)*. The separations between survivors and nonsurvivors of this analysis were similar to that of $\dot{V}O_2$ plotted against the corresponding $\dot{D}O_2$ values shown in Figure 8–11.

major $\dot{V}O_2$ changes with minimum or insignificant CI and $\dot{D}O_2$ changes.

4. Normal unstressed or preoperative patients may also have large $\dot{D}O_2$ increases with little or no $\dot{V}O_2$ response because there is no oxygen debt.

In essence, when $\dot{D}O_2$ and $\dot{V}O_2$ increase together, there may be supply-dependent $\dot{V}O_2$ or an error related to coupling. However, coupling cannot explain the supply-independent $\dot{V}O_2$ when increased values of $\dot{D}O_2$ are not accompanied by increased $\dot{V}O_2$ values; this relationship results in a nearly horizontal line when $\dot{D}O_2$ values are plotted against the corresponding $\dot{V}O_2$ values (see Figs. 8–11 and 8–12).

Oxygen Delivery and Oxygen Consumption Relationship in Various Etiologic Types of Shock

The patterns of $\dot{D}O_2$ and $\dot{V}O_2$ in the early compensated states of various etiologic types of acute circulatory failure illustrate various compensatory responses. Hemorrhagic and cardiac patients with progressively reduced $\dot{D}O_2$ have only moderately reduced $\dot{V}O_2$ because of increased oxygen extraction. Septic, postoperative, and trauma patients have increased $\dot{D}O_2$ and $\dot{V}O_2$ in their early compensated states. The combination of sepsis with accidental or surgical trauma further increases metabolic demands, as shown by the further increases in $\dot{V}O_2$. These data suggest that circulatory function increases when possible to compensate for increased body metabolism. When increases in $\dot{D}O_2$ are limited by hypovolemia or reduced cardiac function, an increased oxygen extraction ratio is the principal compensatory mechanism.

Supply-Dependent and Supply-Independent Oxygen Consumption

When increases in $\dot{D}O_2$ produce increased $\dot{V}O_2$, a supply-dependent $\dot{V}O_2$ exists, suggesting that oxygen deficiency is present. The increased $\dot{V}O_2$ indicates that greater than normal utilization of oxygen occurs after accumulation of a reversible oxygen debt. When the reduced $\dot{D}O_2$ appreciably lowers the $\dot{V}O_2$, it is said to be "supply-limited $\dot{V}O_2$."

Capillary Leak, Fluid Overload, and Body Water Distribution

Capillary leak occurs in the late stage of septic shock and less commonly in postoperative, traumatic, and hemorrhagic shock. It is characterized clinically by persistent hypovolemia despite adequate fluid administration and excessive peripheral edema. The leak of capillary membranes results in escape of plasma proteins and water into the interstitium. At the late stage, the edema may worsen with belated efforts to keep up with plasma volume losses.

Local tissue hypoxia and acidosis in association with biochemical mediators is thought to initiate the capillary leak. However, the precise physiologic and biochemical mechanisms and the temporal order of their interactions are not completely understood. Direct quantitative measurements of capillary leak are not available clinically, but increased capillary permeability and capillary leak can be inferred from a falloff of radiolabeled albumen and from failure of colloids and blood transfusions to maintain blood volume; as interstitial fluids expand, there is continued progression of peripheral edema. Restoration of blood volume in the early stage of shock with subsequent maintenance of intravascular volume is the best prevention; this depends on plasma oncotic pressure as well as prompt administration of adequate amounts of intravenous fluids.

Capillary leak must be differentiated from fluid overload related to excessive expansion of the interstitium with large volumes of crystalloids, which greatly expand the interstitial space but only transiently restore plasma volume. Administration of as much as 30 to 50 L of Ringer's lactate has been advocated for severe trauma by several American surgical groups.[61, 62] This volume may be tolerated in early resuscitation of young, previously healthy patients with gunshot wounds. However, elderly patients with a prior cardiac history, particularly those receiving salt-restricted diets, may not tolerate even a few liters of crystalloids; during their resuscitation, they may develop peripheral and pulmonary edema before CVP, PA wedge pressure, and intravascular volume have been restored.

The distribution of administered fluids between plasma and interstitial water during the initial crystalloid resuscitation must be considered separately from the phenomenon of capillary leak. Capillary leak, blood volume overload, and massive crystalloid infusions that expand the interstitial space may give rise to pulmonary and peripheral edema but by different mechanisms. Capillary leak occurs when increased capillary permeability allows plasma proteins to escape from the intravascular space in amounts that compromise the maintenance of plasma volume. The pulmonary edema produced by blood volume overload or cardiac failure is characterized by high PA wedge pressures (>20 mm Hg) that drive plasma water into the interstitium by hydrostatic pressure. By contrast, increased interstitial lung water may occasionally be produced after massive crystalloid infusions while wedge pressures are relatively normal, because 80% of administered crystalloids leave the intravascular space by the end of a 1-hour infusion and 40 minutes later most of the rest has left the plasma volume and entered the interstitial space.[63–65]

The presence of pulmonary edema does not necessarily mean there has been fluid overload. Pulmonary edema and peripheral edema may also be produced by cardiac failure, low protein values resulting from malnutrition, renal failure, hepatic failure, hypermetabolic states, head injuries, high-altitude sickness, anaphylactoid and drug reactions, hyperthermia, as well as carcinomatosis and other terminal states.

Falloff of Radiolabeled Albumin as a Measure of Capillary Leak

Measurements of plasma volume have been performed with iodine 131–labeled and iodine 125–labeled human serum albumin (RIHSA). Shippy and colleagues[66] described a series of more than 1700 plasma volume measurements; after two or more baseline control values were obtained, RIHSA was injected intravenously and four to six timed blood samples were obtained over the subsequent 60-minute period. The falloff of radioactivity of serial plasma samples, which indirectly reflects escape of plasma protein from the intravascular space, decreased about 1% to 2% per hour in normal preoperative conditions and 2% to 3% per hour 3 to 6 days after major life-threatening surgery. The falloff was 3% to 6% per hour in septic patients 3 to 7 days postoperatively and 5% to 9% per hour in late-stage or terminal septic patients (Fig. 8–13).

Time Relationships of Capillary Leak and Oxygen Transport Responses

Of major interest is the clinical observation that in the late stage of patients with capillary leak, there were minimal increases in $\dot{D}O_2$ and no significant improvement in $\dot{V}O_2$ with maximum fluid volume loading and inotropic stimulation. By contrast, in the early postoperative period (first 48 hours

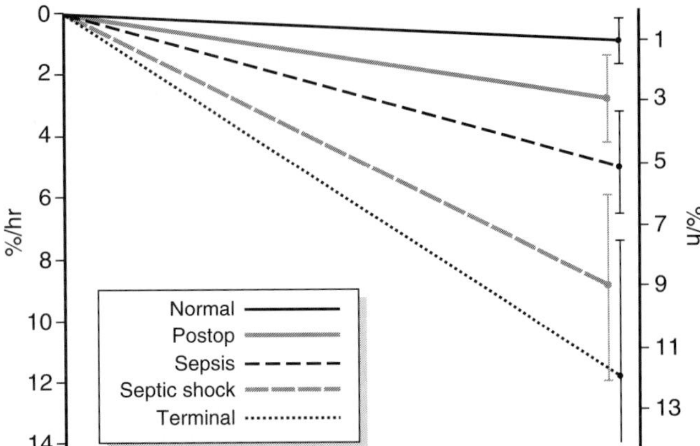

Figure 8–13. Rate of falloff of radioactivity in the plasma after intravenous injection of iodine 125-labeled albumin in normal subjects and in patients with various clinical conditions reflecting degrees of critical illness. Some of the decrease occurs as the albumin mixes with the larger extracellular pool, while some of the decrease is due to capillary leakage. Note that falloff of radioactivity increases with the degree of illness and the temporal stage, late stage septic shock having the greatest rate of decrease.

postoperatively), there were significant improvements in both variables with volume and inotropic stimulation.

Capillary leak begins in the middle period (3 to 5 days postoperatively) of some severely ill, predominantly septic, patients; it reaches its zenith in the late or terminal stage. Capillary leak is not an all-or-none phenomenon; it develops gradually over several days. Maximum therapy should be given early, before capillary leak appears, to achieve maximum effectiveness. Finally, capillary leak follows tissue hypoxia and oxygen debt and therefore is more likely to be the effect than the cause of tissue hypoxia.

Body Composition Changes in Shock

Body composition measurements in the late stage of shock revealed expanded total-body water and interstitial water with contracted plasma volume and intracellular fluid.[67, 68] These body composition abnormalities are also produced by massive crystalloid infusions that predominantly expand the interstitial fluid compartment and only minimally correct blood volume.[63–65, 68] The presence of overexpanded interstitial water and excessive total-body water does not mean that blood volume deficits have been corrected, because hypovolemia often occurs in the presence of massive peripheral edema. The increased interstitium does not contribute to circulatory function but may actually aggravate the problems of oxygen transport by increasing the diffusion pathway and the diffusion time of oxygen as it travels from the intravascular space to the cell membrane.

A Physiologic Model of Shock

A physiologic model of shock was developed on the basis of descriptions of temporal patterns of hemodynamic and oxygen transport variables of survivors and nonsurvivors in shock of various causes. These descriptions suggest that tissue hypoxia resulting from poor tissue perfusion is the basic underlying physiologic defect of all shock syndromes. Tissue hypoxia may be initiated by inadequate or maldistributed blood flow, hypovolemia, vascular occlusion, cardiac insufficiency or failure, anesthesia-induced cardiodepression, and hypoxemia. Increased metabolic demands may be caused by inflammatory responses, fever, wound healing after accidental or surgical trauma, and sepsis. Inadequate flow or increased demands may, when extensive, produce tissue hypoxia, organ dysfunction, organ failure, and death.

In this physiologic model of shock, reduction of blood flow and tissue oxygenation is the primary event, and increases in CI and $\dot{D}O_2$ are compensations that may, if sufficient and timely, correct the antecedent tissue hypoxia. The extent and duration of the antecedent tissue hypoxic event, the extent and duration of the CI and $\dot{D}O_2$ responses, and the effects of therapy must be evaluated.

Relation of Physiologic Patterns and Tissue Hypoxia to Mediators of Organ Failure

Tissue hypoxia precipitates or triggers a number of cascades yielding thromboxane, prostaglandins, and leukotrienes from the arachidonic acid cascade; histamine and other amines; serotonin; complement system; tumor necrosis factor (TNF) and other cytokines; and the continued elaboration of bacterial antigens, messengers, and oxygen free radicals by activated macrophages. These mediators, produced in hypoxic acidotic capillary beds,[69] are thought to initiate or intensify ARDS and other organ failures.

In shock syndromes, local tissue hypoxia stimulates the release of neuroendocrine peptides, hormones, and stress or "heat shock" proteins that alter T cell and B cell function as well as immunosuppressive factors. Activated T cells and other hematopoietic cells produce various cytokines, including TNF and interleukins (IL-1, IL-2, IL-6, and IL-8). The activated lymphocytes and monocytes have receptors for hormones and can simultaneously synthesize and secrete the same hormones and messengers. Activation of leukocytes by these and other biochemical mechanisms produces oxygen free radicals that, although extremely short lived, produce major tissue damage.[69–75]

The serum levels of IL-1, IL-6, IL-8, and TNF were demonstrated to rise within hours of the induction of experimental endotoxemia and the intravenous infusion of bacteria. Experimentally and clinically, activation of IL-6, IL-8, and TNF has been demonstrated in sepsis or ARDS that occurs after trauma. Increased release of each of these cytokines is associated with an acute-phase reaction and the hypermetabolic state.

The sequence of physiologic changes in relation to activation of cytokines, complement factors, and other chemical mediators needs to be elucidated. It is likely that these cytokines, the complement system, and oxygen free radicals play major roles in modulating the alterations in oxygen metabolism and hemodynamic parameters associated with shock and sepsis in affecting the metabolic responses that determine outcome in various clinical settings. The elevated plasma IL-6 and IL-8 levels reached their maxima 16 hours after posttraumatic ARDS was confirmed, but changes in hemodynamic and oxygen transport variables occurred before ARDS.[72] Antitumor necrosis factor therapy as well as free radical scavengers may be useful in approaches to the early management of septic shock.

Systemic Vascular Resistance and Distribution of Blood Flow

A commonly stated concept is that shock syndromes, particularly septic shock, result primarily from the interacting influences of vasodilatation, reduced peripheral vascular resistance index (SVRI), low blood pressure, and low blood flow. If a reduced SVRI were the pathogenic cause of shock, it would be logical to increase SVRI with vasopressors. However, a low SVRI is not well correlated with death, nor is a normal or high SVRI correlated with survival.[23] Moreover, correction of a low SVRI with vasopressors does not improve outcome. On the contrary, vasopressors tend to intensify microcirculatory maldistribution of flow by their α-adrenergic action, which produces even more uneven vasoconstriction and worsens the flow maldistributions.

A low SVRI is not a good measure of "distributive shock" because SVRI represents only the ratio of pressure to flow and not the distribution of flow. According to Ohm's law (R = e/i), resistance is the ratio of pressure to flow (MAP/CI) in direct-current circuits; it is not applicable to alternating currents or periodic functions. A high SVRI occurs when the CI is low (e.g., after hemorrhage), and a low SVRI occurs when flow is high and pressure is normal or low (e.g., after trauma, surgery, or sepsis). Because the SVRI is directly related to the CI, the total-body blood flow, it does not reflect microcirculatory flow maldistributions. Furthermore, organ vascular circuits are in parallel, and the resistance of the whole system is largely determined by the circuit with the lowest resistance. Thus, if one organ's resistance decreases while all other organ resistances increase, the calculated total resistance is decreased. Hence, the SVRI is not a good measure of either the average metarteriolar tone or the microcirculatory blood flow distribution, and it is not an appropriate criterion for therapy.

Distributive Shock

The term distributive shock has been used as a designation for a type of high-flow shock under the assumption that the flow is not normally distributed. Used in this context, it is a theoretical designation that is not defined by criteria that can be quantitatively measured at the bedside. Unevenly distributed flow has been directly observed with in vivo microscopy in experimental animals. Maldistributed blood flow has also been well documented clinically by incident light microscopy in selected accessible microscopic fields such as the scleral conjunctiva, the nail bed, and the surface of parenchymal organs (e.g., the liver during surgical operations).

Direct observations document the phenomenon, but they are not necessarily representative of all tissue beds and therefore do not quantitatively measure the extent of this problem throughout the body. Thus, flow maldistribution is a physiologic concept and a pathogenic mechanism that may be relevant in most, if not all, shock states. More explicit quantitative criteria that are clinically measurable are needed for distributive shock to qualify as a diagnostic classifier of a specific type of clinical shock.

Tissue Oxygenation as a Physiologic Cause of Organ Failure and Death

Although cardiac and respiratory functions are directly measurable, tissue perfusion and oxygenation are not quantifiable, but they are of greater consequence in terms of outcome. Inadequate tissue perfusion with either low or high flow leads to tissue hypoxia, which, when extensive in degree and protracted in time, produces organ dysfunction, multiple organ failure, and death. Most instances of death after surgery, trauma, sepsis, and other acute illnesses are preceded by multiple organ failure, the most common proximate cause of ICU deaths.

When the early manifestations of shock are alleviated by therapy that is insufficient to correct poor tissue oxygenation, the resultant oxygen debt may not be recognized until the appearance of organ failure, including ARDS, sepsis in the uncontaminated patient, acute cardiac failure or arrest, renal failure, DIC, hepatic failure, and coma.

Cardiac Depression as a Physiologic Mechanism

In septic shock, terminal states, and cardiogenic problems as well as during inhalation anesthesia, moderate degrees of cardiodepression occur. This cardiodepression may be counteracted by compensatory adrenomedullary stress responses that stimulate heart rate and cardiac contractility. The balance between the cardiodepression and the adrenal medullary stress response results in a wide range of cardiac function from hypodynamic to hyperdynamic states. This balance is also affected by the degree of shock, the presence of associated medical conditions, the capacity of the heart to compensate, blood volume status, and the temporal stage of the shock state.

The predominant physiologic effects of inotropic and fluid therapy (principally colloid therapy) are to stimulate cardiac function and increase CI. In septic shock and the late stage of postoperative and post-traumatic shock, the therapeutic action of fluids may be less effective and shorter in duration than in early nonseptic shock. Irrespective of these limitations, it is important to obtain the optimal effectiveness with fluids and inotropic agents as early as possible in order to maximize outcome despite the cardiodepressant aspects of septic or late-stage nonseptic shock.

Importance of Circulatory Variables in Outcome Prediction

Serial hemodynamic and oxygen transport measurements describe survivor and nonsurvivor temporal patterns and provide information needed to elucidate underlying circulatory mechanisms and their relevance to outcome. Each monitored variable's biologic importance may be independently evaluated by its ability to predict outcome, which is also a criterion of its usefulness for clinical decision making.

The percentages of correctly predicted outcomes for each monitored variable were calculated at each stage and for all stages in a series of postoperative patients.[76-78] The criteria are determined solely by the observed values of critically ill surgical patients who survived compared with the values of those who subsequently died.

Outcome prediction for each hemodynamic and oxygen transport variable varies from stage to stage as patients' shock syndromes evolve; that is, predictors are stage specific. $\dot{D}O_2$ and pulmonary vascular resistance index (PVRI) are good predictors in the early stage but not in the late stage, and MAP is a poor early predictor but a good late predictor. Most variables predict outcome well in the late stage, but, by this time clinical judgment is also excellent and the usefulness of predictors is minimal.

THERAPY

Goals for High-Risk Patients

Greater than normal values of CI, $\dot{D}O_2$, and $\dot{V}O_2$ were observed in survivors of high-risk surgical operations, trauma, and sepsis.[16-20] These empirically determined supernormal values were then used as objective physiologic criteria or "first approximations" to optimal physiologic goals for therapy (Table 8-2). The relatively normal or low values of the nonsurvivors' pattern serve as early warning of potentially lethal organ failure not compensated by enhanced circulatory function.

The median values of survivors of high-risk surgical opera-

TABLE 8–2. Maximum Cardiac Index (CI), Oxygen Delivery ($\dot{D}O_2$), and Oxygen Consumption ($\dot{V}O_2$) Values in Various Types of Shock*

Etiologic Type	CI (L/min · m²)	$\dot{D}O_2$ (mL/min · m²)	$\dot{V}O_2$ (mL/min · m²)
High-risk surgery	4.5 ± 0.2	600 ± 1	167 ± 18
Trauma	5.0 ± 0.3	800 ± 49	180 ± 24
Sepsis	5.5 ± 0.3	1000 ± 52	190 ± 26
Acute myocardial infarction	2.5 ± 0.4	400 ± 60	124 ± 22

*Values are mean ± SD.

tions without associated preoperative sepsis or cardiovascular problems are CI greater than 4.5 L/min • m² (normal 3.2 ± .2 L/min • m²), $\dot{D}O_2$ greater than 600 (usually 800 to 1000) mL/min • m² (normal 520 ± 57 mL/min • m²), and $\dot{V}O_2$ greater than 167 ± 18 mL/min • m² (normal 130 ± 17 mL/min • m²).[12, 17, 20–23] In patients with severe trauma, these values are CI greater than 5 L/min • m², $\dot{D}O_2$ greater than 800 mL/min • m², and $\dot{V}O_2$ greater than 180 mL/min • m². In patients with septic shock, these values are CI greater than 5.5 L/min • m², $\dot{D}O_2$ greater than 1000 mL/min • m², and $\dot{V}O_2$ greater than 190 mL/min • m². These empirically determined "supranormal" values may be used as a first approximation to physiologic goals for therapy, and relatively normal or low values of the nonsurvivors' pattern would be used as early warning of potentially lethal patterns.[23, 25–27, 33]

In patients older than 50 years of age, the CI and $\dot{D}O_2$ patterns started from lower baseline values and reached lower peak values with each successive decade; septic, traumatic, and cirrhotic patients had higher baseline values and reached higher peak values.[23] The therapeutic goals may also be modified by various diagnostic and high-risk categories, prior preoperative hyperdynamic states (trauma, stress, sepsis, recent surgery, and late-stage cirrhosis), prior hypodynamic states (hemorrhage, hypovolemia, and cardiogenic problems), time elapsed after onset of the trauma or surgical operation, terminal and preterminal states, specific postoperative organ failures (respiratory, renal, hepatic, cardiac, CNS), and postoperative complications such as sepsis, septic shock, DIC, and nutritional failure.[23, 25–27, 33]

Implications of Physiologic Compensations

Physiologic compensatory responses maintain overall circulatory function at a higher than normal level after surgery, accidental trauma, sepsis, and other types of shock. Organ failure occurs when these responses cannot compensate adequately.[18, 19] Increased cardiac output may compensate for reduced hematocrit, low PaO_2, or uneven blood flow, all of which produce inadequate tissue oxygenation.[14] Because this compensatory increase in flow has survival value, therapy should augment cardiac output; the use of β-blockers to reduce high cardiac output values in patients with traumatic or septic shock may lead to circulatory and metabolic deterioration and arrest. An understanding of physiologic responses to stress in mechanistic terms is essential in order to identify and then to augment compensatory responses that are needed for survival. If the physiology is misunderstood and the therapy is inappropriate, death may occur and attributed to the patient's disease rather than to the inappropriate therapy.

Therapeutic Plan Using a Branch Chain Decision Tree

Strategies for achieving therapeutic goals were determined empirically by evaluating the relative effectiveness of each therapy in producing the desired goals. Decision rules were generated from the patterns of survivors and nonsurvivors and from these patients' responses to specific therapeutic interventions. A branch chain decision tree was developed from these decision rules, and priorities were determined on the basis of the effects of the various therapies (Fig. 8–14).

The branch chain decision tree helps to achieve these therapeutic goals expeditiously by providing a coherent, organized management plan for patients. The plan is prophylactic in that it aims to maintain the patient in the optimal hemodynamic state and to prevent the development of tissue hypoxia, organ failure, and death from deficits in blood volume and circulatory function as determined by hemodynamic and oxygen transport patterns. It should not be necessary to wait for deficits to develop before therapy is initiated. To be optimally effective, therapy should be started as soon as possible in order to achieve the maximally compensated physiologic status before the microcirculatory defects become irreversible or before the capillary leak becomes widespread and resistant to therapy.

Blood Volume and Fluid Status

The first and most important therapeutic goal for hemorrhagic, traumatic, neurogenic, and septic shock is to restore blood volume; however, criteria for demonstrating this goal's achievement are not well defined. The use of tachycardia and reduced MAP, CVP, PAOP, urine output, and hematocrit values was based on experimental and clinical observations made immediately after sudden acute hemorrhage and the subsequent resuscitation. Although useful during acute hypovolemia, these values, including PAOP, unfortunately do not reflect the blood volume status during a patient's subsequent ICU course. Moreover, for critically ill postoperative patients, these commonly used clinical criteria were unreliable compared with careful measurements of blood volume.[63]

Contrary to the approach of many internists, surgeons are often accused of overly aggressive fluid administration in the presence of minimum clinical indications, especially in patients with surgical or accidental trauma. Medical patients, especially those with chronic cardiac, renal, pulmonary, and hepatic disorders, often have excessive amounts of salt and water and thus require diuretics and fluid restriction.

Fluid therapy controversies often arise from a common misconception: failure to diagnose deficient plasma volume clinically in the presence of excessive interstitial (extracellular) water. As an example, a patient with peripheral edema obviously has too much interstitial water but may also have hypovolemia. Frequently, patients with postoperative shock have maldistributed flow with a contracted plasma volume but increased interstitial water.[64] This is also commonly seen in inadequately resuscitated trauma patients and in patients resuscitated with massive crystalloid infusion regimens. Therapy should be aimed at improving circulatory function by restoring plasma volume, not by overloading an already expanded interstitial space.

Restoration of blood volume is the most important correctable therapeutic problem in acute circulatory shock. It is, there-

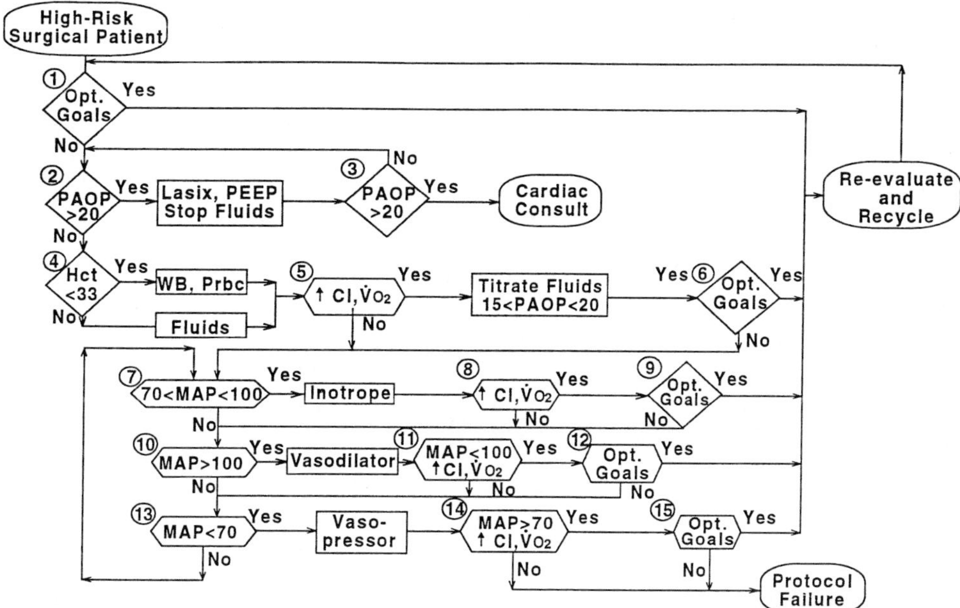

Figure 8–14. Revised branch chain decision tree.

Step 1. Determine whether the patient has reached the optimal goals. Measure cardiac index, $\dot{D}O_2$, and $\dot{V}O_2$. If cardiac index $>$ 4.5 L/min • m^2, $\dot{D}O_2$ $>$ 800 mL/min • m^2, $\dot{V}O_2$ $>$ 170 mL/min • m^2, the goals are reached, and the first objective of the algorithm has been achieved. Reevaluate and recycle at intervals to maintain these goals. If any of the preceding optimal values were not reached, proceed to step 2.

Step 2. Take pulmonary artery occlusion pressure (PAOP). If PAOP $>$ 20 mm Hg, proceed to step 3; if PAOP $<$ 20 mm Hg, proceed to step 4.

Step 3. If PAOP $>$ 20 mm Hg and there is clinical or radiographic evidence of salt and water overload or clinical findings of pulmonary congestion, give furosemide IV at increasing doses to produce diuresis and lower PAOP. If not, consider vasodilators, nitroprusside, or nitroglycerin if MAP $>$ 80 mm Hg and systolic arterial pressure (SAP) $>$ 100 mm Hg; titrate the dose needed to maintain 15 $<$ PAOP $<$ 20 mm Hg and MAP $>$ 80 mm Hg. If unsuccessful, obtain cardiology consultation and place on cardiac protocol.

Step 4. If hematocrit (Hct) $<$ 33%, give 1 U of whole blood (WB) or 2 U of packed red blood cells (Prbc). If hematocrit $>$ 33%, give a fluid load (volume challenge) consisting of one of the following (depending on clinical indications of plasma volume deficit or hydration): 5% plasma protein factor, 500 mL; 5% albumin, 500 mL; 25% albumin (25 g), 100 mL; 6% hydroxyethyl starch 500 mL; 6% dextran-60, 500 mL; lactated Ringer's solution (RL), 1000 mL.

Step 5. If the blood or fluid load improves cardiac index (CI), $\dot{D}O_2$, or $\dot{V}O_2$, continue to give appropriate fluids to increase these variables; if these are improved with adequate volume, proceed to step 8. Continue to infuse fluids until 15 $<$ PAOP $<$ 20 mm Hg; if PAOP reaches 20 mm Hg before optimal goals are reached, proceed to step 8.

Step 6. If optimal goals are reached, recycle; if not, proceed to step 8.

Step 7. If MAP $>$ 70 mm Hg and $<$ 100 mm Hg, give dobutamine by constant IV infusion to optimize cardiac index, $\dot{D}O_2$, and $\dot{V}O_2$.

Step 8. Titrate dobutamine beginning with 2 μg/min • kg and gradually increasing to 20 μg/min • kg, provided there is improvement in cardiac index (CI), $\dot{D}O_2$, or $\dot{V}O_2$ without further lowering of blood pressure (BP) until goals are met.

Step 9. If goals are reached, reevaluate and recycle. If goals are not reached or it becomes evident that higher drug doses are not more effective or that they produce hypotension, tachycardia, or dysrhythmia, continue dobutamine at its most effective dose range and proceed to step 10.

Step 10. If MAP $>$ 100 mm Hg, give vasodilator, such as nitroprusside, nitroglycerin, labetalol, or prostaglandin E_1.

Step 11. Titrate vasodilators to decrease MAP and increase cardiac index (CI), $\dot{D}O_2$, or $\dot{V}O_2$. If there is no improvement in cardiac index, $\dot{D}O_2$, or $\dot{V}O_2$ with the vasodilator, or if hypotension (MAP $<$ 80 mm Hg, SAP $<$ 110 mm Hg) occurs, reduce or discontinue the vasodilator. If there is improvement in cardiac index, $\dot{D}O_2$, or $\dot{V}O_2$, titrate vasodilator to its maximum cardiac index, $\dot{D}O_2$, or $\dot{V}O_2$ effects consistent with satisfactory pressures.

Step 12. If optimal goals are reached, reevaluate and recycle at intervals to maintain optimal goals.

Step 13. If these goals are not reached and MAP $<$ 80 mm Hg, SAP $<$ 110 mm Hg, give dopamine or other vasopressor.

Step 14. Titrate doses of vasopressor (dopamine) in the lowest dose that maintains MAP $>$ 70 mm Hg, SAP $>$ 110 mm Hg, and increases cardiac index, $\dot{D}O_2$, and $\dot{V}O_2$ to their optimal values. If pressures cannot be maintained or optimal goals reached, the patient is considered to be a protocol failure; consider reevaluation and recycling.

Step 15. If optimal goals are reached, reevaluate and recycle.

(Modified from Shoemaker WC, Appel PL, Bland RD: Use of physiologic monitoring to predict outcome and to assist in clinical decisions in critically ill postoperative patients. Am J Surg 1983; 164:43.)

fore, essential to have a reliable means of assessing this volume. Measurement of plasma volume with iodine 125-labeled albumin or of red blood cell mass with chromium 55-labeled red blood cells is time consuming, expensive, and usually performed only in research centers. The CVP and PAOP, which can be measured at frequent intervals or monitored continuously, were thought to have the needed accuracy and have largely replaced blood volume measurements for patients with most clinical conditions.

The CVP and PAOP rapidly decrease with acute hemorrhage and increase immediately after fluid therapy. High venous pressures are associated with both acute blood volume overload and cardiac failure. However, after a variable period of time in the ICU, venous pressures are notably unreliable indicators of blood volume status because of compliance changes of the walls of veins. In the postoperative ICU period, venous pressures accommodate to either high or low blood volumes with PAOP values that usually remain in the range of about 8 to 12 mm Hg. Figure 8-15 illustrates the values of over 1700 carefully measured blood volumes relative to the commonly monitored variables thought to reflect blood volume.[63] The latter fail to reflect blood volume changes over a wide range of values.

Figure 8-16 illustrates the scatter of blood volume values

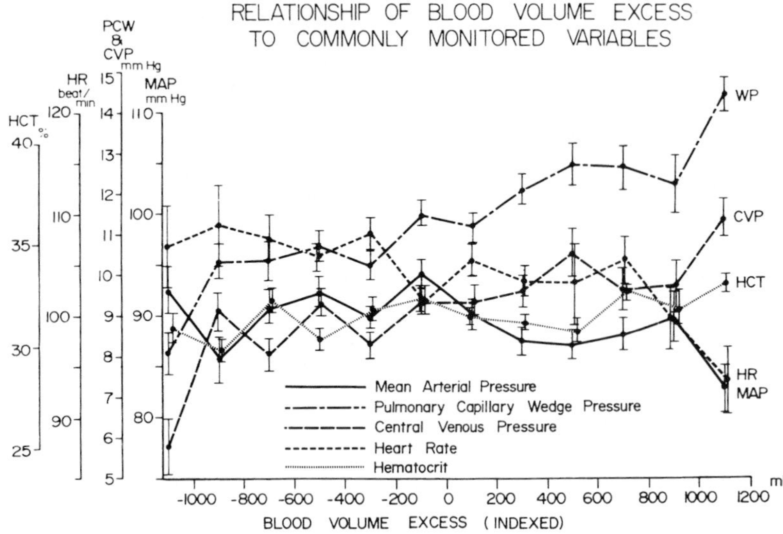

Figure 8–15. Values of blood volume (BV) indexed to body surface area (BSA) plotted against hematocrit, heart rate (HR), CVP, WP, and MAP on the *y*-axis. Blood volume values are expressed as milliliters of excess or deficit from the patient's predicted norm indexed to BSA. Note the very poor correlation of the commonly monitored variables. (From Shippy CR, Appel PL, Shoemaker WC: Reliability of clinical monitoring to assess blood volume in critically ill patients. Crit Care Med 1984; 12:107.)

relative to the corresponding CVP values. Although CVP and PAOP may accurately measure venous pressures, they do not accurately reflect blood volume in most ICU patients. However, they are useful as measures of venous wall compliance in order to determine the capacity of the vascular system to accept more volume without the production of pulmonary edema and to prevent acute blood volume overload during rapid fluid restoration. Furthermore, peripheral edema as well as pulmonary edema may result from massive crystalloid infusions that expand the interstitial space without exceeding "safe" venous pressures or fully restoring plasma volume.[75]

Daily weight assessments and fluid balance measurements are used to monitor fluid management, but both of these reflect total-body water or changes in body water, not blood volume. The distribution of body water between the plasma, interstitium, and intracellular compartments can be definitively measured only by isotopic body composition studies.

Volume Therapy

Vigorous and rapid volume loading that does not exceed PAOP values of 18 or 20 mm Hg is the first and most important therapy. It is easier to achieve the therapeutic goals with colloids, which expand the plasma volume without overexpansion of the interstitial water, than with crystalloids, which are distributed primarily in the interstitial water.[60] Plasma volume restoration cannot be assumed in the presence of pitting edema in patients who have received large volumes of crystalloids because hypovolemia frequently occurs together with expansion of interstitial water. Moreover, it cannot be assumed that one third of the extracellular water remains in the intravascular space while two thirds is distributed in the interstitium because these often cited conclusions were based on radiosulfate measurements made under normal conditions.[61] In critically ill patients, only 20% of 1000 mL of crystalloids remained in the circulation by the end of a 1-hour infusion, and 40 minutes later almost all of that had gone into the interstitial space.[60] In conditions of peripheral edema, we prefer to give concentrated (25%) albumin, which increases colloidal osmotic pressure and expands plasma volume by shifting interstitial water back into the plasma volume. Subsequently, diuretics may be used to reduce plasma volume, if this becomes a problem.

In control studies of critically ill patients, 500 mL of 5% albumin persisted for 3.5 to 4.5 hours, whereas 500 mL of hydroxyethyl starch lasted 5 to 6 hours and dextran 40 and gelatin about 1.5 to 2 hours; crystalloids lasted 40 minutes (Fig. 8–17).

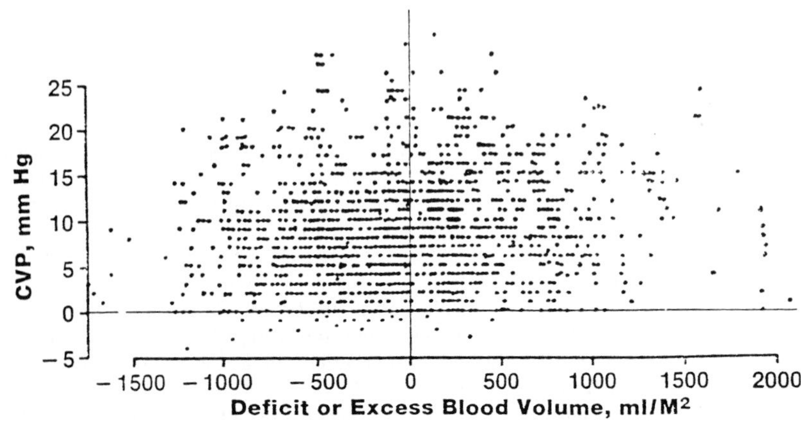

Figure 8–16. Blood volume index values plotted against simultaneously measured central venous pressure (CVP) values. (From Shippy CR, Appel PL, Shoemaker WC: Reliability of clinical monitoring to assess blood volume in critically ill patients. Crit Care Med 1984; 12:107.)

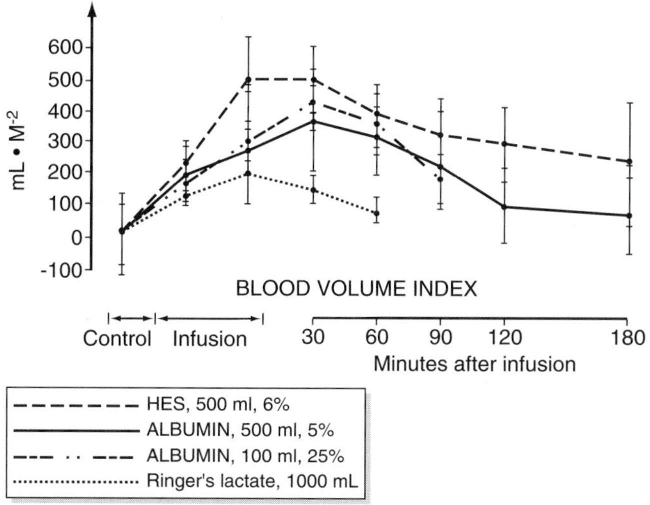

Figure 8–17. Blood volume changes documented in two prospective clinical trials by a random-order crossover design that compared the effects of 500 mL of 6% hydroxyethyl (HES) starch, 500 mL of 5% albumin, 100 mL of 25% albumin, and 1000 mL of lactated Ringer's solution in critically ill postoperative patients. The blood volume effects after starch and albumin are greater than those after the crystalloid solution. (From Hauser CJ, Shoemaker WC, Turpin I, et al: Hemodynamic and oxygen transport responses to body water shifts produced by colloids and crystalloids in critically ill patients. Surg Gynecol Obstet 1980; 150:811.)

Inotropic Agents

After the maximum effect of fluids has been obtained, administration of an inotropic agent such as dobutamine may be started at about 5 μg $kg^{-1} \cdot min^{-1}$; the appropriate dose is obtained by titration to achieve the optimal goals in terms of CI, $\dot{D}O_2$, and $\dot{V}O_2$. Dobutamine produced marked and significant increases in CI and stroke index, cardiac and stroke work, $\dot{D}O_2$, and $\dot{V}O_2$ as well as decreases in systemic and pulmonary vascular resistances and venous inflow pressures (CVP and PAOP); blood gases, pH, and Qsp/Qt were not significantly changed.[73, 74] Vasopressors, particularly in large doses, produced greater increases in blood pressure than did dobutamine but less improvement in $\dot{D}O_2$ and $\dot{V}O_2$.[74]

The effects of dobutamine were observed in a small group of patients before and after a fluid load consisting of 500 or 1000 mL of 5% albumin was given. Greater flow effects with little or no hypotension and tachycardia were observed when blood volume was adequately restored before infusion. The hypovolemic patient is extremely sensitive to vasodilators and may deteriorate rapidly if blood volume is not restored before vasodilatation. Additional fluids must be given if hypotension occurs after administration of dobutamine or other vasodilators. Stimulation of the empty heart with an inotropic vasodilator may produce severe hypotension and arrhythmias. When dobutamine produces sudden severe hypotension, this reaction may be reversed by rapid fluid administration.[73]

Vasodilator Therapy

If a patient has a normal or high MAP with a high SVRI, vasodilatation with nitroglycerin, nitroprusside, labetalol, hydralazine, or prostaglandin (alprostadil [prostaglandin E_1]) may be considered; the optimal dose is obtained by titration to achieve improved CI without production of hypotension; that is, MAP should be maintained at levels greater than 80 mm Hg and systolic arterial pressure (SAP) greater than 100 mm Hg. Intraoperatively, titrated doses of nitroglycerin were shown to maintain peripheral perfusion and prevent postoperative ARDS.[57]

Vasopressor Therapy

Vasopressor are indicated for hypotension after volume therapy has been given. *Hypotension,* defined as MAP less than 70 mm Hg and diastolic pressures less than 50 mm Hg, should be prevented because blood flow to the heart and brain is largely driven by pressure. However, the α-adrenergic effects of vasopressors also intensify the uneven vasoconstriction produced by neural mechanisms. This uneven metarteriolar constriction raises blood pressure but may further exacerbate the uneven microcirculatory flow. Because dopamine, norepinephrine, and epinephrine, in contrast to methoxamine, have inotropic actions that increase CI, the net effect on tissue perfusion and oxygenation is a balance between the favorable increase of blood flow and the unfavorable maldistribution of flow. The smallest doses of vasopressors needed to maintain the minimum satisfactory blood pressure are recommended because no administered amount of vasopressors can make up for inadequate blood volume.

Responses to a Standardized Fluid Challenge

Figures 8-8 and 8-9 illustrate the effects of 500 mL of 5% albumin given over a 1-hour period at each stage to a series of patients in various stages of septic shock. There was marked and significant improvement in myocardial performance and tissue perfusion in the early and middle stages but no significant improvement in the late and terminal stages. The trial of therapy, which dates back to Hippocrates, is a useful way to judge the effectiveness of an agent given in a standardized way for a given condition at a particular time. If the response is favorable, the agent may be repeated; if the response is unfavorable, an alternative therapy may be selected.

The data summarized before this suggest that poor tissue perfusion and tissue hypoxia in postoperative patients are due to a low CI or maldistributed peripheral blood flow in the presence of increased metabolic demands. Increased metabolism postoperatively may be augmented by proinflammatory responses, wound healing, and fever. Tissue hypoxia may also occur with accidental trauma, hypovolemia, anesthesia, sepsis, and cardiac problems. Progressively increasing tissue hypoxia may result in capillary leak and organ failure, which are widely regarded as major proximate causes of death. Outcome was improved when potentially lethal circulatory patterns were treated in the early (in the first 8 to 12 hours) postoperative period, but after the appearance of organ failure reversal of nonsurvival patterns did not improve outcome. This approach is based on the assumption that it is easier and more effective to prevent the initiators of shock (e.g., hypovolemia, hypoxemia, poor tissue perfusion, tissue hypoxia) than to treat the mediators of organ failure (e.g., cytokines, antigens, eicosanoids, heat shock proteins, and the adrenal stress response).

Strategy for Treatment of Shock

Similar underlying physiologic alterations occur in patients with severe accidental trauma, stress, and sepsis, but the optimal goals are not quantitatively the same as those for postoperative patients; that is, the underlying physiologic defects may be qualitatively similar and the metabolic requirements may be greater, but more aggressive therapy may be needed to achieve the optimal goals. The increased $\dot{D}O_2$ and $\dot{V}O_2$ in patients with severe trauma, stress, sepsis, and hypercatabolic states indicate increased metabolic requirements. However, greater than normal metabolism should not be interpreted as meaning that all metabolic needs have been met; even greater rates of $\dot{V}O_2$ may be needed. The strategy in each case is to try to open up unevenly vasoconstricted arteriolar-capillary networks by vigorous volume loading and then to increase blood flow with the use of inotropic agents and, subsequently, vasodilators to overcome vasoconstricted metarteriolar circuits.

Optimal goals can be calculated as the mean for a given etiologic type of shock or for a given population of patients. The optimal goals cannot be precisely defined for individual patients because of interpatient variations in baseline $\dot{V}O_2$ requirements, prior associated medical conditions, the amount and duration of oxygen debt, compensatory capacities, and many other factors. The optimal values after trauma and sepsis are more widely variable than those after elective surgery because the widely varying extent of injury and the virulence of the infectious agent produce wide variations in the increases of metabolic demands. A broad range of circulatory function is required to supply these increased metabolic needs.

The answer to this dilemma is an operational definition of goals. To resolve the issue of whether the patient with high $\dot{V}O_2$ has enough $\dot{V}O_2$, the $\dot{D}O_2$ is increased until no further increase in $\dot{V}O_2$ occurs (unless limited by PAOP in instances of fluid loading, by tachycardia > 130 beats/min with inotropic agents, or by hypotension with MAP < 80 mm Hg or systolic arterial pressure < 110 mm Hg with vasodilators). Thus, tissue oxygen demand is inferred indirectly by an empirical trial of therapy. If therapy increases CI, $\dot{D}O_2$, and $\dot{V}O_2$, it may be assumed that it opened up additional microcirculatory channels that perfused relatively hypoxic tissues, which then extracted more oxygen. Because tissues cannot take up more oxygen than they use, the increased $\dot{V}O_2$ after $\dot{D}O_2$ therapy indicates that an oxygen debt exists and that this debt has been at least partially satisfied. In this approach, PAOP is not used as a measure of blood volume because it clearly does not reflect blood volume.[57] Rather, PAOP is used as an upper limit for volume therapy or for the rate of volume infusion to avoid pulmonary edema.

Vasopressors are used as a last resort to maintain sufficient MAP to provide for coronary and cerebral perfusion after the maximum effects of fluids, inotropes, and vasodilators have been achieved. The hemodynamic effectiveness of each agent given separately should be established before agents are combined.

Elderly and cardiac patients have considerably different physiologic problems and different compensatory mechanisms than patients with normal hearts but multiple organ dysfunction. The heart may be the weak link in the former, but circulatory transport functions are likely to limit survival in the latter. An appropriate strategy in cardiac patients may be to stimulate cardiac function with inotropic agents and to reduce cardiac work by afterload reduction with vasodilators; preload should be augmented, but overdilation should be avoided.

The most important principles in these complex clinical conditions are:

1. Documentation of baseline hemodynamic and oxygen transport variables.
2. Measurement of changes with each appropriate agent to determine the relative effectiveness of alternative therapies.
3. Titration of the dose to achieve optimal values.

Potential Use of Monoclonal Antibodies and Free Radical Scavengers

Clinical trials of two types of monoclonal endotoxin and anti-TNF antibodies have not provided the anticipated good results or gained Food and Drug Administration (FDA) approval.[75] Additional clinical trials are being undertaken.[79] It is doubtful that any single agent will be sufficient to reverse the complex multifactorial shock state. It is likely that these and other ancillary agents, such as steroids, prostaglandins, and cyclooxygenase inhibitors, will have a role after a patient's major circulatory variables are corrected with fluids and inotropic agents. Antioxidant vitamins and antioxidant enzymes, including superoxide dismutase, catalase, and glutathione peroxidase, although not yet commercially available, may eventually be helpful in restoring and maintaining an appropriate balance between oxidants and antioxidants.

SUMMARY

The most important monitored functions are total-body blood flow reflecting cardiac function, arterial hemoglobin saturation reflecting pulmonary function, and $\dot{D}O_2$ and $\dot{V}O_2$ reflecting tissue perfusion. The temporal patterns of these interacting components characterize the physiology of surviving and nonsurviving patients. Although recognition and treatment of shock are routinely guided by subjective imprecise signs and symptoms, a more physiologic alternative is to evaluate and treat the major primary circulatory problems of (1) hypovolemia; (2) low, uneven distribution of microcirculatory flow; and (3) inadequate oxygen transport. These problems should be monitored early to identify correctable deficiencies, to give appropriate therapy early, to achieve optimal goals rapidly, and to prevent lethal organ failure.

Unless hypovolemia or impaired cardiac function was present, increases in CI and $\dot{D}O_2$ were the earliest changes in patients with trauma, elective surgery, sepsis, and other types of stress. In survivors, CI and $\dot{D}O_2$ increased earlier and the increases were greater in degree and duration than in comparable patients who subsequently died. Increased $\dot{D}O_2$, as part of the body's stress response, is the principal physiologic response to acute circulatory deficits that limit body metabolism; this increase compensates for tissue oxygen debt resulting from low or maldistributed microcirculatory flow and inadequate tissue perfusion and oxygenation. Noninvasive monitoring provides an alternative approach for describing the time course of the major circulatory components.

The results of prospective clinical trials suggest that most postoperative deaths are due to physiologic problems that can be identified, described, predicted, and prevented. For critically ill patients in various categories, therapy based on criteria of survivors should be given and monitored to obtain the optimal physiologic goals within the first 8 to 12 hours after surgery, trauma, and sepsis.

The following principles should be kept in mind:

1. *The occurrence of hypotension represents a decompensation or failure to sustain protective circulatory mechanisms.*
2. *Increases in cardiac index (CI) and oxygen delivery ($\dot{D}O_2$) usually precede the hypotensive episode and are early protective physiologic mechanisms stimulated by increased metabolic need and the adrenal-medullary stress response.*
3. *The temporal patterns of survivors of hemorrhagic, postoperative, traumatic, and septic shock syndromes indicate that CI and $\dot{D}O_2$ increase to maintain the body's metabolic needs as reflected by the oxygen consumption ($\dot{V}O_2$); these increased CI and $\dot{D}O_2$ values may be used as goals of therapy.*
4. *The equivalent noninvasive monitored variables are CI (bioimpedance), SvO_2 (pulse oximetry), transcutaneous oxygen ($PtcO_2$) and carbon dioxide ($PtcO_2$).*

5. The temporal pattern of normal or low CI, $\dot{D}O_2$, and $\dot{V}O_2$ before hypotension in nonsurvivors of the various fatal traumatic shock syndromes indicates either overwhelming etiologic events or inadequate compensations, that is, failure of the body to sustain compensatory mechanisms (decompensation).

6. Inadequate tissue oxygenation caused by inadequate perfusion is the basic pathophysiologic defect underlying shock syndromes.

7. Low flow or uneven (maldistributed) flow is the direct cause of tissue hypoxia, organ dysfunction, organ failure, and death.

8. Oxygen debt may result from increased metabolic demand or reduced oxygen supply.

9. Decreased $\dot{D}O_2$ occurs in cardiac failure, hypoxemia, respiratory failure, trauma, hemorrhage, dehydration, cardiopulmonary arrest, and other acute hypovolemic conditions.

10. Many patients with chronic disorders may insidiously experience hypovolemia and a low CI, which may be tolerated if there is no added stress, such as sepsis.

11. The most common life-threatening hypodynamic state is that of the inadequately volume-resuscitated postoperative and trauma patient.

References

1. Wo CCJ, Shoemaker WC, Appel PL, Bishop MH, et al: Unreliability of blood pressure and heart rate to evaluate cardiac output in emergency resuscitation and critical illness. Crit Care Med 1993; 21:218.
2. Swan HJC, Ganz W, Forrester JS, et al: Catheterization of the heart in man with use of a flow-directed balloon-tipped catheter. N Engl J Med 1970; 283:447.
3. Forrester JS, Diamond GA, Swan HJC: Correlation classification of clinical and hemodynamic function after acute myocardial infarction. Am J Cardiol 1977; 39:137.
4. Conners AF Jr, Speroff T, Dawson NV, Thomas C, et al: The effectiveness of right heart catheterization in the initial care of critically ill patients. JAMA 1996; 276:899.
5. Gore JM, Goldberg RJ, Spodick DH, Alpert JS, et al: A community-wide assessment of the use of pulmonary artery catheters in patients with acute myocardial infarction. Chest 1987; 92:721.
6. Guyatt G, Ontario Intensive Care Group: A randomized control trial of right heart catheterization in critically ill patients. J Intensive Care Med 1991; 6:91.
7. Zion MM, Balkin J, Rosenmann D, et al: Use of pulmonary artery catheters in patients with acute myocardial infarction: Analysis of experience in 5841 patients in the SPRINT registry. Chest 1990; 98:1331.
8. Hayes MA, Timmins AC, Yau EHS, Pallazo M, et al: Elevation of systemic oxygen delivery in the treatment of critically ill patients. N Engl J Med 1994; 330:1717.
9. Gattinoni L, Brazzi L, Pelosi P, et al: A trial of goal-oriented hemodynamic therapy in critically ill patients. N Engl J Med 1995; 333:1025.
10. Taylor RW, Pulmonary Artery Catheter Consensus Conference Participants: Pulmonary Artery Catheter Consensus Conference: Consensus statement. Crit Care Med 1997; 25:910.
11. Boyd O, Bennett D: Enhancement of perioperative tissue perfusion as a therapeutic strategy for major surgery. New Horiz 1996; 4:453.
12. Shoemaker WC, Appel PL, Kram HB, et al: Prospective trial of supranormal values of survivors as therapeutic goals in high-risk surgical patients. Chest 1988; 94:1176.
13. Boyd O, Grounds M, Bennett D: Preoperative increase of oxygen delivery reduces mortality in high risk surgical patients. JAMA 1993; 270:2699.
14. Schulz RJ, Whitfield GF, La Mura JJ, et al: The role of physiologic monitoring in patients with fractures of hip. J Trauma 1985; 25:309.
15. Fleming AW, Bishop MH, Shoemaker WC, et al: Prospective trial of supranormal values as goals of resuscitation in severe trauma. Arch Surg 1992; 127:1175.
16. Gutierrez G, Palizas F, Doglio G, et al: Gastric intramucosal pH as a therapeutic index of tissue oxygenation in critically ill patients. Lancet 1992; 339:195.
17. Bishop MH, Shoemaker WC, Kram HB, Ordog GJ, et al: Prospective randomized trial of survivor values of cardiac index, oxygen delivery, and oxygen consumption as resuscitation endpoints in severe trauma. J Trauma 1995; 38:780.
18. Tuchschmidt J, Fried J, Astiz M, et al: Supranormal oxygen delivery improves mortality in septic shock patients. Chest 1992; 102:216.
19. Berlauk JF, Abrams JH, Gilmour IJ, et al: Preoperative optimization of cardiovascular hemodynamics improves outcome in peripheral vascular surgery. Ann Surg 1991; 214:289.
20. Bishop MW, Shoemaker WC, Appel PL, et al: Relationship between supranormal values, time delays and outcome in severely traumatized patients. Crit Care Med 1993; 21:56.
21. Shoemaker WC, Appel PL, Kram HB, et al: Temporal hemodynamic and oxygen transport patterns in medical patients with sepsis and septic shock. Chest 1993; 104:1529.
22. Shoemaker WC, Appel PL, Kram HB, et al: Sequence of physiologic patterns in surgical septic shock. Crit Care Med 1993; 21:1876.
23. Shoemaker WC, Appel PL, Kram HB: Hemodynamic and oxygen transport responses in survivors and nonsurvivors of high risk surgery. Crit Care Med 1993; 21:977.
24. Shoemaker WC, Asensio JA, Wo CCJ, Thangathurai D, Velmahos G, Cornwell EE, et al: Intraoperative hemodynamic patterns of survivors and nonsurvivors of high risk elective surgery. World J Surg (in press).
25. Shoemaker WC, Appel PL, Kram HB: Role of oxygen debt in the development of organ failure, sepsis, and death in high risk surgical patients. Chest 1992; 102:208.
26. Shoemaker WC, Appel PL, Kram HB: Oxygen transport measurements to evaluate tissue perfusion and titrate therapy. Crit Care Med 1991; 19:672.
27. Shoemaker WC, Appel PL, Kram HB: Hemodynamic and oxygen transport monitoring to titrate therapy in septic shock. New Horiz 1993; 1:145.
28. Wang X, Sun H, Adamson D, et al: An impedance cardiography system: A new design. Ann Biomed Eng 1989; 17:535.
29. Wang X, Van De Water JM, Sun H, et al: Hemodynamic monitoring by impedance cardiography with an improved signal processing technique. Proc IEEE Eng Med Biol 1993; 15:699.
30. Wang X, Sun HH, Van De Water JM: Time-frequency distribution technique in biological signal processing. Biomed Instrum Technol 1995; 29:203.
31. Shoemaker WC, Wo CCJ, Bishop MH, et al: Multicenter trial of a new thoracic electric bioimpedance device for cardiac output estimation. Crit Care Med 1994; 22:1907.
32. Wo CCJ, Shoemaker WC, Bishop MH, et al: Noninvasive estimations of cardiac output and circulatory dynamics in critically ill patients. Curr Opin Crit Care 1995; 1:211.
33. Shoemaker WC, Wo CCJ, Demetriades D, Belzberg H, et al: Early physiologic patterns in acute illness and accidents. New Horiz 1996; 4:395.
34. Shoemaker WC, Wo CCJ, Bishop MH, Asensio JA, et al: Noninvasive monitoring of high risk surgical patients. Arch Surg 1996; 131:732.
35. Scalea TM, Simon HM, Duncan AO, et al: Geriatric blunt multiple trauma: Improved survival with early invasive monitoring. J Trauma 1990; 30:129.
36. Moore FA, Haemel JB, Moore EE, et al: Incommensurate oxygen consumption in response to maximal oxygen availability predicts postinjury oxygen failure. J Trauma 1992; 33:58.
37. Hankeln KB, Senker R, Schwarten JN, et al: Evaluation of prognostic indices based on hemodynamic and oxygen transport variables in shock patients with ARDS. Crit Care Med 1987; 15:1.
38. Tuchschmidt J, Fried J, Astiz M, et al: Evaluation of cardiac output and oxygen delivery improves outcome in septic shock. Chest 1992; 202:216.
39. Creamer JE, Edwards JD, Nightingale P: Hemodynamic and oxygen transport variables in cardiogenic shock secondary to acute myocardial infarction. Am J Cardiol 1990; 65:1287.
40. Rady MY, Edwards JD, Rivers EP, et al: Measurement of oxygen

consumption after uncomplicated acute myocardial infarction. Chest 1993; 103:886.
41. Bassin R, Vladick B, Kim SI, et al: Comparison of hemodynamic responses of two experimental shock models with clinical hemorrhage. Surgery 1971; 69:722.
42. Hankeln K, Senker R, Schwarten JM, et al: Evaluation of prognostic indices based on hemodynamic and oxygen transport variables in shock patients with adult respiratory distress syndrome. Crit Care Med 1987; 15:1.
43. Abraham E, Bland RD, Cobo JC, et al: Sequential cardiorespiratory patterns associated with outcome in septic shock. Chest 1984; 85:75.
44. Haupt MT, Gilbert EM, Carlson RW: Fluid loading increases oxygen delivery and consumption in septic patients with lactic acidosis. Am Rev Respir Dis 1985; 131:912.
45. Russell JA, Lockhat D, Belzberg M, et al: Oxygen delivery and consumption and ventricular preload are greater in survivors than nonsurvivors of ARDS. Chest 1988; 94:755.
46. Gilbert EM, Haupt MT, Mandanas RT, et al: The effect of fluid loading blood transfusion, and catecholamine infusion on oxygen delivery and consumption in patients with sepsis. Am Rev Respir Dis 1986; 134:873.
47. Rackow EC, Kaufman BS, Falk JL, et al: Hemodynamic response to fluid repletion in patients with septic shock. Circ Shock 1987; 22:11.
48. Packman MI, Rackow EC: Optimal left heart filling pressure during fluid resuscitation of patients with hypovolemia and septic shock. Crit Care Med 1983; 11:165.
49. Astiz ME, Rackow EC, Falk JL, et al: Oxygen delivery and consumption in patients with hyperdynamic septic shock. Crit Care Med 1987; 15:26.
50. Yu M, Levy MM, Smith P, et al: Effect of maximizing oxygen delivery on mortality and mortality rates in critically ill patients: A prospective randomized controlled study. Crit Care Med 1993; 21:830.
51. Edwards JD, Redmond AD, Nightingale P, et al: Oxygen consumption following trauma. Br J Surg 1988; 75:690.
52. Edwards JD, Brown GCS, Nightingale P, et al: Use of survivors' cardiorespiratory values as therapeutic goals in septic shock. Crit Care Med 1989; 17:1098.
53. Da Luz P, Cavanilles JM, Michaels S, Weil MH, Shubin H: Oxygen delivery, anoxic metabolism and hemoglobin-oxygen affinity (P50) in patients with acute myocardial infarction and shock. Am J Cardiol 1975; 36:148.
54. Creamer J, Edwards JD, Nightingale P: Hemodynamic and oxygen transport variables in cardiogenic shock following acute myocardial infarction and their response to treatment. Am J Cardiol 1990; 65:1297.
55. Edwards JD: Oxygen transport in cardiogenic and septic shock. Crit Care Med 1991; 19:658.
56. Shoemaker WC, Wo CCJ, Bishop MH, et al: Noninvasive hemodynamic monitoring of critical patients in the emergency department. Acad Emerg Med 1996; 3:675.
57. Bishop MH, Shoemaker WC, Schelenka J, Wo CCJ, et al: Noninvasive cardiac output monitoring of gunshot wound victims. Acad Emerg Med 1996; 3:682.
58. Velmahos GC, Wo CCJ, Murray JA, James CB, et al: Invasive and noninvasive physiologic monitoring of blunt trauma patients in the emergency department. World J Surg (in press).
59. Lowe JG, Ernst EA: The Quantitative Practice of Anesthesia: Use of the Closed Circuit. Baltimore, Williams & Wilkins, 1981, pp 146–147.
60. Thangathurai D, Charbonnet C, Wo CCJ, Shoemaker WC, et al: Intraoperative maintenance of tissue perfusion prevents ARDS. New Horiz 1996; 4:466.
61. Lucas CE, Weaver DW, Higgens RF, et al: Effects of albumin versus nonalbumin resuscitation on plasma volume and renal excretory function. J Trauma 1978; 18:564.
62. Lowe RJ, Moss GS, Jilek J, et al: Crystalloid vs colloid in the etiology of pulmonary failure after trauma. Surgery 1977; 81:676.
63. Hauser CJ, Shoemaker WC, Turpin I, et al: Hemodynamic and oxygen transport responses to body water shifts produced by colloids and crystalloids in critically ill patients. Surg Gynecol Obstet 1980; 150:811.
64. Shoemaker WC, Kram HB: Comparison of the effects of crystalloids and colloids on hemodynamic oxygen transport, mortality and morbidity. *In:* Debates in General Surgery. Simmon RS, Udeko AJ (Eds). Chicago, Year Book Medical Publishers, 1991, pp 263–316.
65. Appel PL, Shoemaker WC: Fluid therapy in adult respiratory failure. Crit Care Med 1981; 9:862.
66. Shippy CR, Appel PL, Shoemaker WC: Reliability of clinical monitoring to assess blood volume in critically ill patients. Crit Care Med 1984; 12:107.
67. Moore FD, Olesen KH, McMurrey JD, et al: Body Cell Mass and Its Supporting Environment: Body Cell Mass in Health and Disease. Philadelphia, WB Saunders, 1963.
68. Davidson I, Ottosson J, Reich J: Infusion volumes of Ringer's lactate and 3% albumin solution as they relate to survival after resuscitation of a lethal intestinal ischemic shock. Circ Shock 1986; 18:277.
69. Abraham E: Physiologic stress and cellular ischemia. Crit Care Med 1991; 19:613.
70. Bentler B: Endotoxin, tumor necrosis factor and related mediators. New Horiz 1993; 1:3.
71. McCord JM: Oxygen-derived free radicals. New Horiz 1993; 1:70.
72. Meade P, Shoemaker WC, Donnelly TJ, Abraham E, Jagels MA, Cryer HG, et al: Temporal patterns of hemodynamics, oxygen transport, cytokine, and complement activity in the development of adult respiratory distress syndrome. J Trauma 1994; 36:768.
73. Pullicino EA, Carli F, Poole S, et al: The relationship between circulating concentrations of interleukin-6, tumor necrosis factor, and the acute phase response to elective surgery and accidental injury. Lymphokine Res 1990; 9:231.
74. Van Zee KJ, DeForge LE, Fischer E, et al: IL-8 in septic shock, endotoxemia, and after IL-1 administration. J Immunol 1991; 146:3478.
75. Di Padova F, Pozzi C, Tondre MJ, et al: Selective and early increase of IL-1 inhibitors, IL-6 and cortisol after elective surgery. Clin Exp Immunol 1991; 85:137.
76. Shoemaker WC, Appel PL, Kram HB: Hemodynamic and oxygen transport effects of dobutamine in critically ill general surgical patients. Crit Care Med 1986; 14:1032.
77. Shoemaker WC, Appel PL, Kram HB: Comparison of dobutamine and dopamine in prospective crossover clinical trials in critically ill postoperative patients. Chest 1988; 96:120.
78. Luce JM: Introduction of new technology into critical care practice: A history of HA-1A human monoclonal antibiotics against endotoxin. Crit Care Med 1993; 21:1233.
79. Abraham E, Wunderink R, Silverman H, et al: Efficacy and safety of monoclonal antibody to human tumor necrosis factor alpha in patients with sepsis syndrome. JAMA 1995; 273:934.

Common Bedside Procedures in the Intensive Care Unit

George C. Velmahos, MD, PhD
Demetrios Demetriades, MD, PhD

CRICOTHYROIDOTOMY

Emergent surgical airway access is required when orotracheal intubation has failed in patients who are unable to maintain airway patency. The need for rapid initiation of assisted ventilation precludes a time-consuming procedure, such as tracheostomy, from being a reasonable alternative. Cricothyroidotomy is the procedure of choice under such strenuous circumstances.[1] The cricothyroid membrane lies directly under the skin, and its landmarks are easily identified. Although the procedure is supposed to be performed easily and quickly, it can frequently be a serious challenge even for experienced surgeons.

The procedure is as follows: The thyroid and cricoid cartilages are identified, and the larynx is stabilized between thumb and index finger of the nondominant hand. A vertical or horizontal skin incision of 3 to 4 cm is made over the cricothyroid space, and the membrane between the two cartilages is pierced. The space is dilated by a hemostatic clamp. A No. 6 French (Fr.) lubricated tracheostomy tube can be inserted through the opening. Although the choice of skin incisions depends on individual preference, a vertical midline incision is considered relatively risk-free.

Bleeding is a significant intraoperative complication, not so much for causing hemodynamic instability but because it may obstruct the surgical field and interfere with the timely insertion of the tracheal cannula. It is usually related to damage to local veins or the pyramidal lobe of the thyroid gland. Autopsy results have shown that these structures are commonly situated close to the midline.[2] Therefore, a vertical middle line incision is safer than a transverse incision which is frequently associated with hemorrhage. If bleeding occurs, direct pressure is usually effective in arresting it.

It is suggested that conversion to tracheostomy is necessary to avoid long-term complications, primarily subglottic stenosis.[3] Early reports of "high tracheostomies" noted a significant incidence of postextubation laryngeal stenosis.[4] However, Brantigan and Grow[5] found a low complication rate of 6.1% among 651 selected patients. It was soon realized that the probability of cricothyroidotomy-associated complications increased in the presence of active laryngeal infections or prolonged orotracheal intubation.[5, 6]

Sise and colleagues[7] reviewed 75 patients who had undergone cricothyroidotomy for long-term tracheal access. Morbidity was found to be similar to that in patients with tracheostomies. In view of these data and in the absence of controlled comparative studies among patients with or without conversion to tracheostomy, we can assume that conversion would be required for patients with upper airway infection or for patients who were intubated for more than 7 to 10 days prior to cricothyroidotomy. All other patients can probably be managed by cricothyroidotomy as the definitive way of accessing the airway. Early decannulation should be always pursued to reduce the risk of long-term morbidity.[8]

TRACHEOSTOMY

Tracheostomy remains the most reasonable alternative to orotracheal or nasotracheal intubation for patients who need long-term airway access. Although some authors report no adverse effects after prolonged intubation,[9] most surgeons would agree that a tracheostomy is required in such cases to avoid complications.[10–12] Even with the new low-pressure cuffs, the continuous irritation of the tracheal mucosa may lead to inflammation, granulomatous formation, and strictures.[13] Tracheostomy tubes are less prone to movement than orotracheal tubes and, therefore, less likely to produce such problems. Additionally, a tracheostomy provides a more "secure" airway because it can be safely anchored to the skin and tied around the neck.

Finally, pulmonary toilet is more effective through a short tracheostomy cannula and the dead space is reduced. As an extension of these advantages, weaning from the ventilator can be facilitated by a tracheostomy. Given these facts, tracheostomy plays an important role in the management of critically ill patients, although many issues around the timing, technique, and place of performing it are still debated.

The definition of "prolonged" intubation is not consistent in the literature but ranges from 7 to 21 days. Whited[14] compared three groups of patients prospectively. The first group received endotracheal intubation for 2 to 5 days, the second group for 6 to 10 days, and the third group for 11 to 24 days. The incidence and the character of laryngotracheal sequelae differed among the three groups. Airway stenosis was more frequent and more severe as the time of intubation was extended. Dunham and LaMonica[15] suggested that conversion to tracheostomy is not required before 2 weeks of orotracheal intubation. Rodriguez and coworkers[16] observed that patients who received tracheostomy within a week of admission spent less time on the ventilator, in the intensive care unit (ICU), and in the hospital.

It appears that complications such as airway obstruction or stenosis after removal of the tracheostomy cannula are increased if tracheostomy is performed on an inflamed or already injured trachea. For this reason, it would be beneficial to be able to predict the need for prolonged mechanical ventilation in order to offer tracheostomy in the appropriate patients at an early stage before tracheal damage is already produced. Additionally, resource utilization and bed and personnel allocation would be more effectively distributed on the basis of the anticipated duration of ventilation.

Velmahos and associates[17] introduced a simple risk score that could be used at the bedside of critically injured patients in order to predict within 48 hours of admission the need for prolonged mechanical ventilation. The score was based on four parameters derived at 48 hours after admission:

1. Presence of a pulmonary artery catheter.
2. An Injury Severity Score above 20.
3. Partial oxygen tension to fraction of inspired oxygen ratio of less than 250.
4. Fluid retention of more than 2000 mL.

The presence of all factors was associated with 100% probability of mechanical ventilation longer than 7 days, whereas the absence of all factors predicted successful extubation within the first week with 93% certainty. Similar scores that can be easily calculated during clinical rounds would also be useful in other groups of patients.

In most institutions, tracheostomy is performed in the operating room (OR). Transporting critically ill patients away from the ICU environment is associated with morbidity. A recent study showed an increased incidence of pneumonia in patients who required transport.[18] Even in the absence of complications, the safe handling of lines, endotracheal and chest tubes, monitors, and other life-support systems becomes hazardous and personnel-intensive. Further confusion is caused by the availability of an OR and an anesthesiologist, which in busy medical centers may mean significant delays. For this reason, performing tracheostomies by the ICU bedside offers multiple advantages.

Upadhay and colleagues[19] reviewed 470 elective tracheostomies done over a 4-year period. Of these procedures, 311 (60%) were performed as a bedside procedure in the ICU. No differences in complications were found between patients in the ICU and those in the OR. Another report[20] on 43 burn patients (25 in the OR, 18 in the ICU) showed that bedside tracheostomy is a safe procedure and can be performed for a substantially lower charge compared to OR tracheostomy. In a similar way, Wease and coworkers[21] reported a low incidence of complications and significant cost savings among 204 patients who underwent bedside tracheostomies.

From these data, it appears that bedside tracheostomy can be done with reasonable safety. However, it is not a procedure that should be taken lightly. Meticulous preparation, adherence to appropriate surgical principles, and provision of an adequate instrument supply and illumination are essential for the uneventful execution of such a policy.

TABLE 9–1. Studies Comparing Standard Open with the Percutaneous Dilatational Technique for Performing Tracheostomies

Study	Design	No. of Complications			
			Open		Percutaneous
Crofts et al., 1995[26]	Prospective, randomized	25	5 (25%)	28	10 (36%)
Friedman et al., 1996[27]	Prospective, randomized	26	9 (35%) (intraoperative)	27	11 (41%)
			3 (12%) (postoperative)		12 (41%)*
Graham et al., 1996[28]	Retrospective	31	12 (39%) (minor)	29	12 (41%)
			7 (23%) (major)		5 (17%)

*$P < 0.05$.

Although there are multiple variations of the open technique, the crucial steps of the procedure remain standard. Usually, a transverse neck incision exposes the pretracheal structures. The muscles are bluntly retracted off the midline, and the trachea is exposed. Anchoring sutures are placed bilaterally to assist in traction during tube insertion. The trachea is opened sharply across two to three cartilages starting from the second tracheal ring space. The surgeon should avoid the use of electrocautery while opening the trachea, particularly if the patient is ventilated at 100% of oxygen. There have been reports of ignition or explosion of the tracheal tube under such circumstances.

Variations of the tracheal incision include (1) simple vertical, (2) cross-sign, (3) vertical H, and (4) trap-door. After removal of the orotracheal tube and insertion of the tracheostomy cannula, the surgeon reapproximates the muscles around the tube in order to provide an effective seal and to accelerate the creation of a track. The anchoring sutures are exteriorized through the surgical wound and are taped to the skin. In case of tracheostomy tube dislodgment, traction by these sutures may facilitate reinsertion of an airway.

The technique of tracheostomy has changed dramatically with the advancement of the percutaneous dilatational method. Although the percutaneous technique had been described in 1957, inadequate instrumentation and associated complications prevented it from gaining popularity until 1985. At that time Ciaglia and associates[22] described the percutaneous dilatational technique using a special set of dilators (Cook Critical Care, Bloomington, Ind.). The procedure was done by the bedside and was safe and cost efficient. Many authors[23-25] favor the use of bronchoscopy in order to confirm correct placement of the needle, guide wire, and dilators. Complications associated with malplacement or inadvertent injury to the trachea have been reported, but the incidence does not seem to differ from that of the open technique.

Two prospective randomized trials[26, 27] and one retrospective study[28] have attempted a comparison between the two techniques (Table 9–1). None of these studies identified a difference in procedure-related morbidity. However, we cannot draw reliable conclusions from these results because the power of the studies was inadequate owing to a small number of patients and the lack of long-term follow-up.

Although experience is still limited with the new technique, its obvious advantages have sparked a lot of interest. An increasing body of literature provides information on technical details,[29] anesthetic considerations,[30] pathologic changes[31] and long-term outcome.[32] Law and colleagues[33] reported on the clinical, endoscopic, and pathologic findings of 41 patients who underwent percutaneous tracheostomy at least 6 months prior to examination. No patient was symptomatic. A significant (10%) tracheal stenosis was identified in four asymptomatic patients, two of whom had spirometric evidence of obstruction. A synopsis of the existing studies on percutaneous dilatational tracheostomy is shown in Table 9–2.

TABLE 9–2. Studies on Percutaneous Dilatational Tracheostomy

Study	No.	Follow-up (mos)	Mean Time (min)	Morbidity (%)
Ciaglia et al., 1985[22]	24	—	—	0
Ciaglia and Graniero, 1992[32]	165	4-60	—	4 (intraoperative) 6 (postoperative)
Toursarkissian et al., 1994[39]	141	9 ± 7	15 ± 9	11 (intraoperative) 8 (postoperative)
Winkler et al., 1994[23]	71	1-6	9 ± 3	5.5
Barba et al., 1995[25]	27	2-18	16 ± 5	—
Fischler et al., 1995[40]	17	2-36	—	—
Crofts et al., 1995[26]	25	1-3	—	25
Caldicott et al., 1995[41]	20	—	5	5
Van Heerden et al., 1996[34]	54	0.2	—	22
Van Heurn et al., 1996[31]*	12	—	—	—
Cobean et al., 1996[42]	65	7.5	14	22 (intraoperative) 9 (postoperative)
Hill et al., 1996[43]	356	72 ± 51	15 ± 8	9 (intraoperative) 7 (postoperative)
Fernandez et al., 1996[24]	162	—	—	5
Graham et al., 1996[28]	31	—	—	61
Friedman et al., 1996[27]	26	—	8 ± 5	12
Van Heurn et al., 1996[44]	150	21	—	13
Marx et al., 1996[29]	254	—	—	1.5 (major) 6.5 (minor)
Law et al., 1997[33]	41	>6	—	0 (long-term clinical)
Velmahos et al., 1998†	100	1-4	12	4

*Autopsy study.
†Unpublished data.

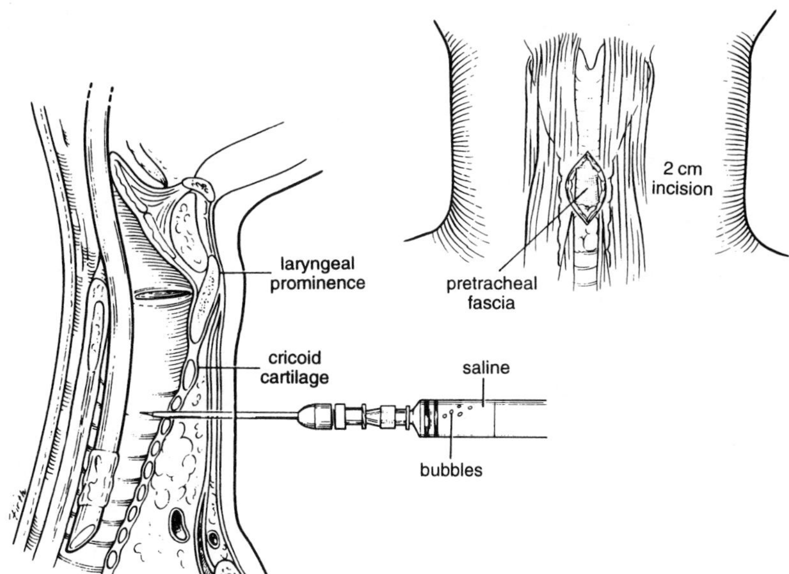

Figure 9–1. Position of a fluid-filled syringe in the trachea and aspiration of air. Note that the endotracheal tube is left in place.

In our surgical ICU, we have performed more than 100 percutaneous tracheostomies over the last 18 months. We used a commercially available kit (Cook Critical Care) and operated on all patients regardless of body habitus, need for cervical spine precautions, ventilatory requirements, or physiologic condition. Most of the procedures were performed by surgical residents in the ICU. Bronchoscopy was used only in a few selected cases. The procedure was completed in 12 minutes on average. We experienced four complications and no mortality associated with the procedure. Morbidity consisted of one case of self-limited emphysema, one case of tube dislodgment, and two cases of tracheal injury that resulted in abandoning the procedure and reestablishing orotracheal intubation. We attributed the low incidence of complications (<4%) in some important technical modifications that we introduced.

In short, our technique of percutaneous dilatational tracheostomy is as follows (Figs. 9-1 to 9-7). A 2-cm vertical incision is made in the middle of the distance between the cricoid cartilage and the suprasternal notch. The pretracheal muscles are dissected bluntly, and a finger is inserted to localize the trachea. Under digital guidance a needle is inserted to the trachea and placement is confirmed by aspirating air (bubbles in a fluid-filled syringe) (see Fig. 9-1). A guide wire is inserted into the trachea through the needle (see Fig. 9-2). The needle is withdrawn and a guiding catheter is inserted over the wire (see Fig. 9-3). Dilatation is achieved by the insertion of consecutive dilators over the guide wire–catheter complex (see Fig. 9-4). The orientation of the dilators is important. As the trachea travels toward the posterior mediastinum, it recedes from the skin. A vertical orientation of the curved dilator to the skin would result in difficult insertion into the trachea or creation of a false passage to the pretracheal space. Therefore, it is essential to place the dilator in acute angles to the skin in order to insert it vertically into the trachea. By

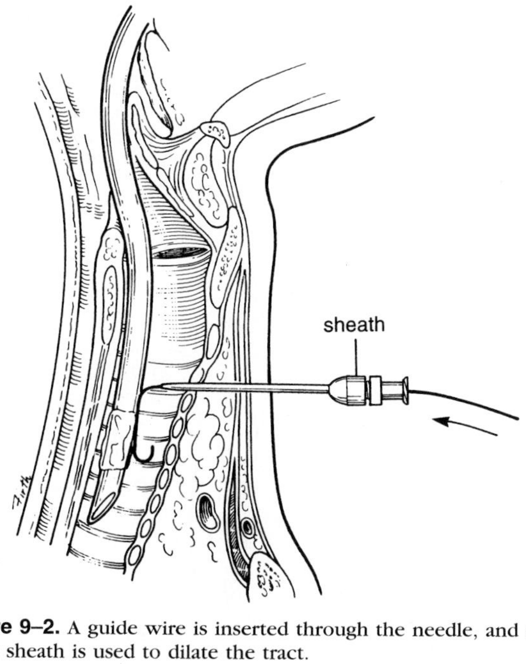

Figure 9–2. A guide wire is inserted through the needle, and a plasic sheath is used to dilate the tract.

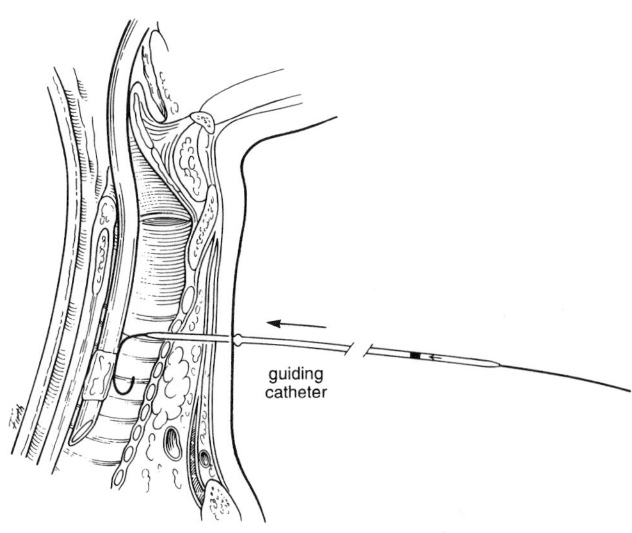

Figure 9–3. A guiding catheter is inserted over the guide wire.

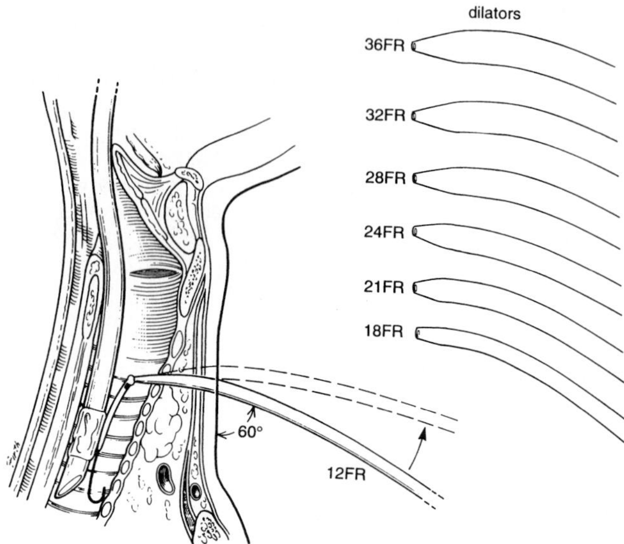

Figure 9–4. Consecutive dilatation up to a No. 36 French (FR) dilator. Note the orientation of the dilators.

directing the dilator downwards, once its tip is felt to be in the trachea, the surgeon can avoid injury to the posterior wall.

After dilation is completed up to the largest dilator, a digit is inserted through the tracheal opening (see Fig. 9-5). The endotracheal tube is withdrawn under direct palpation up to a level, right over the tracheal opening. A No. 8 tracheostomy tube is inserted over a No. 28 Fr. dilator (see Fig. 9-6). The dilator is withdrawn, and the tube is connected to the ventilator (see Fig. 9-7). The orotracheal tube is not completely removed before tracheostomy placement is confirmed.

Different instruments and techniques appear with increasing frequency as the method gains in popularity.[34] It must be emphasized that this is a surgical procedure that should not be performed without optimal conditions and experienced personnel. Just because it is done quickly and without major hazards in the majority of cases does not mean that disasters cannot occur if strict surgical principles are not kept and serious consideration is not given. It is our opinion that the patients are best served when this procedure is done by a surgeon.

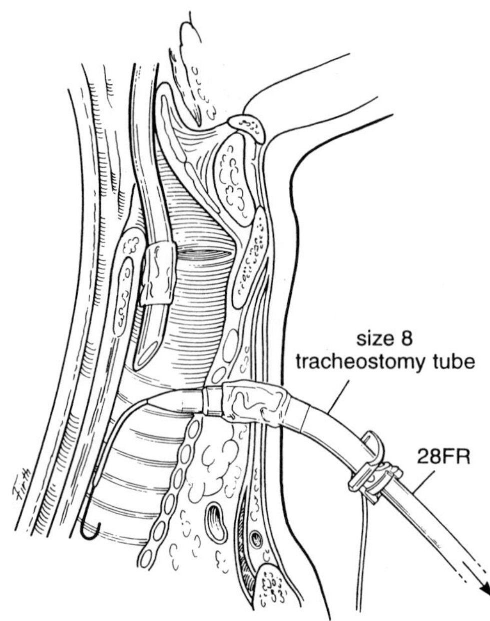

Figure 9–6. A No. 8 tracheostomy tube is inserted over a No. 28 French (FR) dilator.

Both open and percutaneous techniques are associated with short-term and long-term complications. Bleeding is, as previously described,[2] easily controlled in most instances. Malplacement of the tracheostomy tube may occur because of anatomic and technical factors. Hyperextension of the neck during insertion may mislead the surgeon as to the ideal site for tracheal puncture or incision. When the patient's head is returned to the normal position, the distance between the skin insertion and the tracheal insertion sites may increase and the tube may be pulled out inadvertently. This is particularly true for patients with thick or edematous necks. Trache-

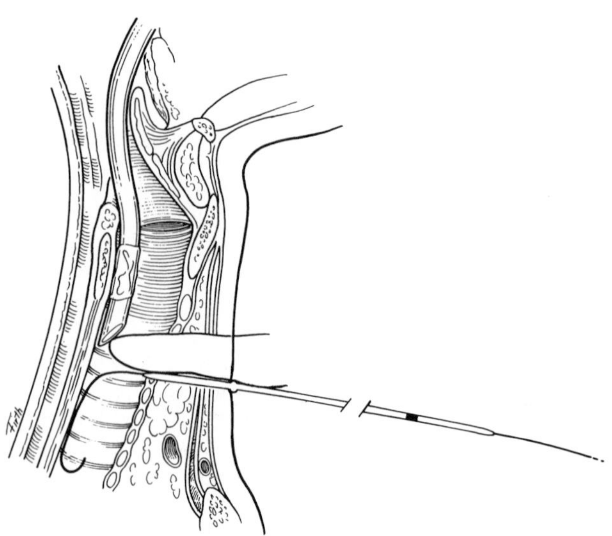

Figure 9–5. A digit is inserted to palpate the endotracheal tube and guide withdrawal over the tracheal opening.

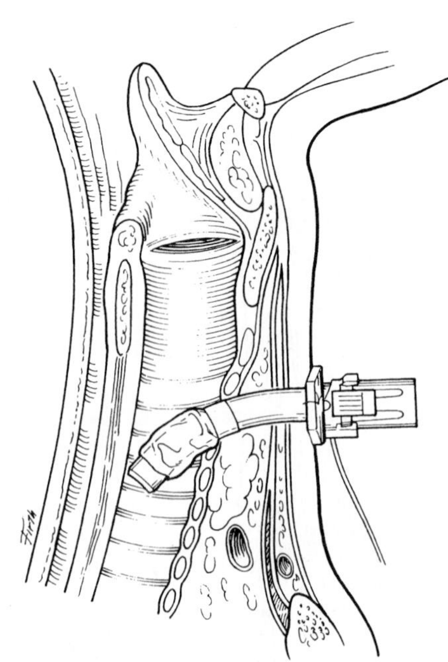

Figure 9–7. Tracheostomy in place.

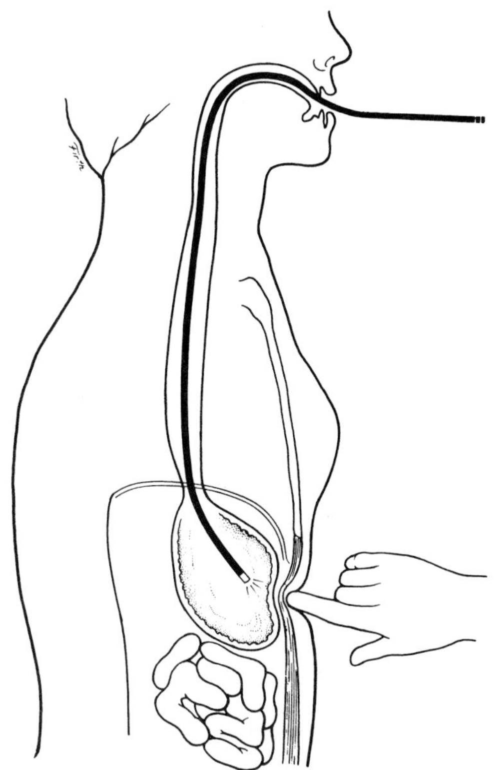

Figure 9–8. Transillumination through the abdominal wall by the gastroscope. Identification of appropriate site for gastrostomy placement.

ostomy tubes longer than standard size may be useful for extreme cases. Paratracheal placement of the tracheostomy cannula may also occur if the above-mentioned principles are not respected during percutaneous placement.

Tracheoinnominate fistula[35] is a rare but dramatic complication of tracheostomy and involves erosion through the tracheal wall and into the innominate artery. Mortality is high as a result of acute exsanguination. The complication should be suspected if a tracheostomy is pulsating or if bleeding appears through the tracheostomy tube. The surgeon can achieve immediate control by overinflating the balloon or by inserting a digit through the tracheostomy wound anterior to the trachea and compressing the innominate artery against the sternum or clavicle. These maneuvers usually allow sufficient time for emergent transport to the OR.

The most common complication after tracheostomy is obstruction of the upper airway.[13, 36] The lesions occur at mainly two places: the site of insertion to the trachea and the site of the balloon cuff. Despite the introduction of low-pressure, high-compliance cuffs, the problem has not been completely alleviated. Constant micromotion of the tube, pressure, limited blood supply due to hypotensive episodes, associated infection, poor nutrition, and the quality of the tubing material are some of many etiologic factors. Abnormalities such as subglottic stenosis, vocal cord granuloma, and scarring of previously inflamed areas are commonly seen. The trachea is more frequently involved than the subglottic area. Lesions can form even with less than 48 hours of intubation. Pathologic evidence of laryngotracheal injury occurs in as high as 90% of patients with tracheostomy, but less than 10% report clinically significant problems in the long term. Proper technique is essential to reduce the risk. Very high or very low placement, extensive destruction of tracheal rings, paramedian insertion, and inversion of cartilages toward the lumen are technical mistakes that are associated with morbidity.[37]

In summary, it seems that tracheostomy may offer significant advantages compared with prolonged oral or nasal tracheal intubation if it is performed timely and properly. If patients are predicted to require long periods of mechanical ventilation, early rather than late tracheostomy is preferred.[38] Procedures performed by the bedside are safe and cost effective and are able to avoid the adverse effects associated with transport. Although still at early stages, the percutaneous dilatational technique produces similar, if not better, results than the standard open method. Tracheostomy can be a lifesaving or life-risking procedure. Therefore, it should be performed with caution and diligence by the most specialized personnel under the best possible conditions.

PERCUTANEOUS GASTROSTOMY

Percutaneous endoscopic gastrostomy was designed as a means of achieving the benefits of enteral nutrition of critically ill patients without subjecting them to the risks of an operation. Bedside performance eliminates the additional risk of transport. The most common indication for insertion of percutaneous gastrostomies in ICU is the anticipation of the need for long-term alimentary support in patients who cannot tolerate oral diet.[45] Brain and aerodigestive tract lesions due to trauma, infection, neoplasia or other underlying conditions are the most common causes of this intolerance.

The most frequently used technique includes gastroscopy with transillumination to detect the appropriate site of insertion (Figs. 9–8 to 9–11).[46] A needle is inserted at this area and protrudes into the stomach, as seen by the scope. A wire inserted through the needle is captured by a polypectomy snare inserted through the scope. The wire is pulled back with the scope through the stomach and esophagus and exits through the patient's mouth. The gastrostomy catheter is attached to the guide wire. As traction is applied to the end of the wire that exits the abdominal wall, the gastrostomy catheter is pulled through the mouth, esophagus, and stomach

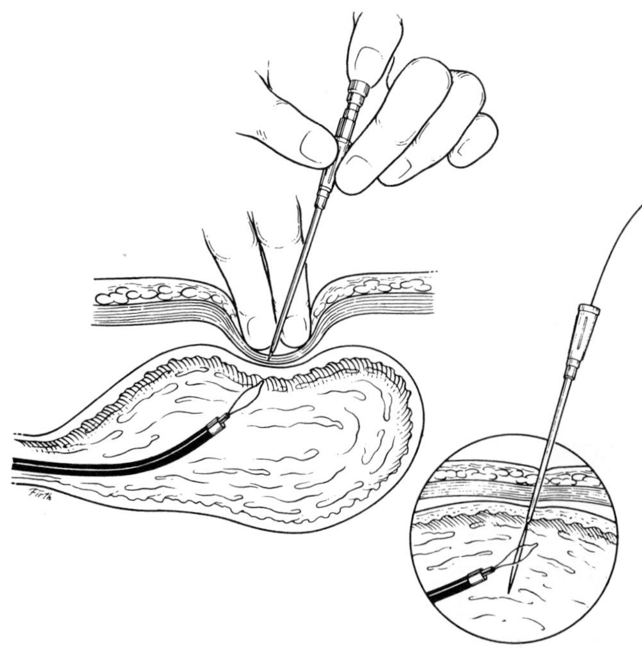

Figure 9–9. A needle is inserted percutaneously through the open loop of a biopsy snare, and a wire is captured by the snare.

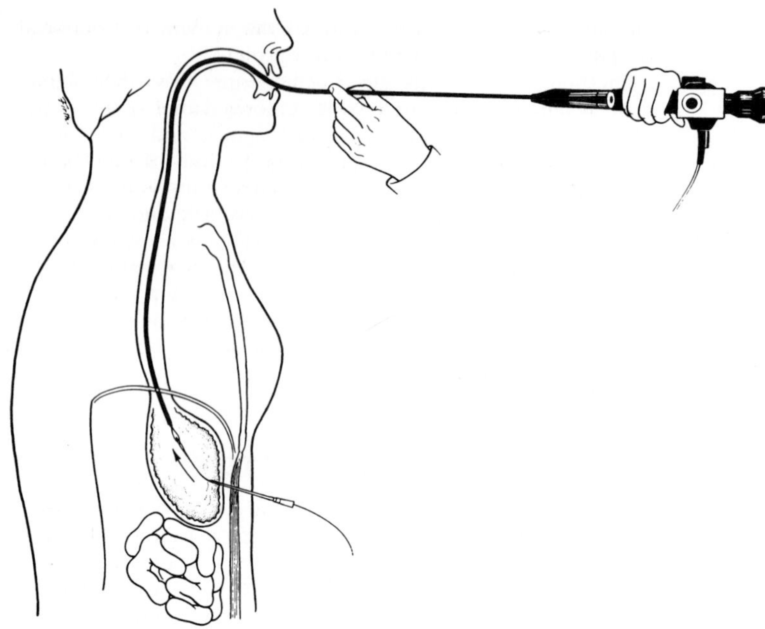

Figure 9–10. The wire and the gastroscope are withdrawn.

out to the skin. A retention crossbar immobilizes the internal part of the catheter in the stomach. Gentle pressure should be applied to the gastric wall to avoid interruption of local blood supply and necrosis.[47]

Other techniques have been described.[48, 49] Minor morbidity ranges from 4% to 13%, and major morbidity ranges from 1% to 4%.[50, 51] However, complications related directly to the procedure occur in fewer than 1% of the cases.[51]

Peritonitis following percutaneous gastrostomy placement is the most fearsome problem because it is associated with mortality, especially if it is not recognized early.[50, 52, 53] The most common cause is leakage around the catheter or injury to other organs, particularly the colon. Fluoroscopy under such circumstances is essential to image the catheter's course and position. If a leak is not identified, further evaluation by computed tomography (CT) scanning may provide information on other organ injuries. Surgical exploration is ultimately required to repair any injuries.

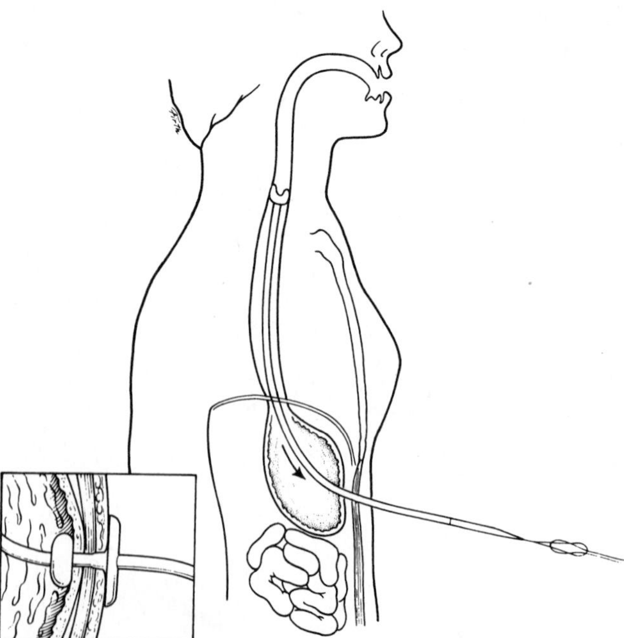

Figure 9–11. The long percutaneous gastrostomy catheter is pulled through the stomach and secured after gentle traction, which brings the internal crossbar against the stomach and the abdominal wall.

Aspiration is the most common complication.[50] Even in the presence of a cuffed endotracheal tube, the risk is not eliminated. Placing the gastrostomy tube in continuous suction for 12 hours after the procedure, careful evaluation of gastric residuals and elevation of the head of the bed to 30° during placement and during feedings may reduce such morbidity. Although delaying gastric feeding for 2 to 3 days is widely practiced to minimize leaks and aspiration episodes, early feedings have not been shown to increase morbidity rates.[54] Endoscopically assisted advancement of the feeding tube to the jejunum does not reliably reduce the risk of aspiration.[55] The procedure is more complicated and is associated with a higher incidence of tube dysfunction.[56]

Other complications include:

- Bleeding at the insertion site[50]
- Gastrocolocutaneous fistula[57]
- Local infection[58]
- Necrotizing fasciitis[59]
- Tumor implantation at the insertion site[60]
- Inadvertent removal or migration of the feeding catheter[51]

Most of these complications occur infrequently and can be prevented by meticulous technique.

Despite continuous improvement in the design of gastrostomy tubes, the devices frequently deteriorate and need to be replaced.[46, 51] A new tube should be reinserted carefully in order to avoid disruption of the existing tract. Endoscopic guidance may be useful if problems are encountered during the procedure. In general, percutaneous gastrostomy can be done safely at the ICU bedside. In combination with percutaneous tracheostomy, it may expedite the recovery and shorten the ICU stay of patients who need extended care.[61] Appropriate patient selection, strict adherence to operative principles, and administration of feedings according to protocol help in reducing complication rates and achieving the maximal benefit.

TABLE 9–3. Criteria for Diagnostic Peritoneal Lavage

Positive
Aspiration of > 10 ml of blood
Lavage fluid exits via Foley catheter or chest tube
Grossly bloody lavage return
RBC > 100,000/mL
WBC > 500/mL
Amylase > 175 U/dL
BUN > 20 mg/dL
Fibers, particulate matter in effluent
Negative
Clear fluid return
RBC < 50,000/mL
WBC < 100/mL
Amylase < 75 U/mL
Indeterminate
RBC: 50,000–100,000/mL
WBC: 100–500/mL
Amylase: 75–175 U/mL

RBC = red blood cell; WBC = white blood cell; BUN = blood urea nitrogen.

DIAGNOSTIC PERITONEAL LAVAGE

Diagnostic peritoneal lavage (DPL) was first described in 1965 and was used primarily in the evaluation of blunt abdominal trauma.[62] Its usefulness in penetrating trauma is debated.[63] As a result of the high sensitivity for detecting intraperitoneal blood, it became an important tool for the diagnosis of intra-abdominal injuries, particularly in unevaluable patients with head injuries, intoxication, or iatrogenic sedation.[64, 65] Unfortunately, some of its advantages are offset by the inherent inability to differentiate between clinically significant (requiring repair) or nonsignificant (leading to unnecessary laparotomy) injuries. Furthermore, the procedure is invasive and associated with complications.[65]

The criteria used to interpret DPL results are still unchanged (Table 9–3). According to these criteria, accuracy of 98.5% has been achieved.[65] The most difficult decision making concerns patients with indeterminate DPL results. In one study, only 4% of all patients with a DPL had indeterminate results.[66] Most of these patients had nonsignificant injuries and could have been managed successfully without an operation. Repeated DPL or CT scan can detect patients requiring exploration. In the ICU setting, DPL can be used for diagnosis of intraperitoneal bleeding or intra-abdominal infection. The use of a white blood cell (WBC) count of more than 500 cells/mm^3 is reported to carry a high accuracy rate for diagnosis of nontraumatic acute abdomen[67, 68] but has not been widely accepted in this context. The volume of lavage effluent required for reliable DPL results is estimated to be 250 mL.[69]

The open technique, as originally described by Root and coworkers,[62] is the preferred method of performing DPL in most centers. The main reason for this choice is supposedly increased safety and accuracy in placing the catheter. The technique includes a small infraumbilical incision of the skin, subcutaneous tissue, fascia, and peritoneum. After the abdominal cavity is entered, a catheter is inserted under direct visualization and directed toward the pelvis. The fascia and skin are sutured around it. A supraumbilical incision may be used if pelvic fractures, large retroperitoneal hematomas, or pregnancy is encountered. Decompression of the stomach by nasogastric suction and the bladder by catheterization is required before the procedure is started to avoid iatrogenic injuries to these organs. Even if the open DPL technique is supposed to be easy, opening the abdominal cavity through a small incision under suboptimal circumstances is time-consuming and may be fraught with pitfalls.

The method of percutaneous DPL, with the use of a trocar, has been described with the purpose of expediting and simplifying the standard procedure.[70] In 1979, a modified Seldinger technique was shown to decrease the risk of complications from the blind insertion of the trocar.[71] The percutaneous DPL was performed significantly faster in two prospective randomized studies.[72, 73] In addition, a retrospective review of 395 patients who underwent closed DPL suggested that the procedure is safe and provides high sensitivity (99%) and specificity (98%) rates.[64] On the other hand, Pachter and Hofstetter[74] reported a complication rate of 5.7% among 105 patients undergoing blind trocar placement.

In a recent prospective study of 130 trauma patients, Velmahos and colleagues[75] compared the safety and efficacy of 75 open and 55 closed DPLs. Percutaneous DPL was performed either by the trocar method,[70] in which a dialysis catheter is advanced toward the pelvis over a percutaneously placed trocar (Figs. 9–12 and 9–13), or by the Lazarus-Nelson method,[71] in which a soft catheter is advanced over a flexible J-wire that has been introduced through a percutaneously placed 18-gauge needle in a Seldinger-like technique (Figs. 9–14 to 9–17). The disadvantage of the latter technique is that the catheter of the most frequently used commercial kit

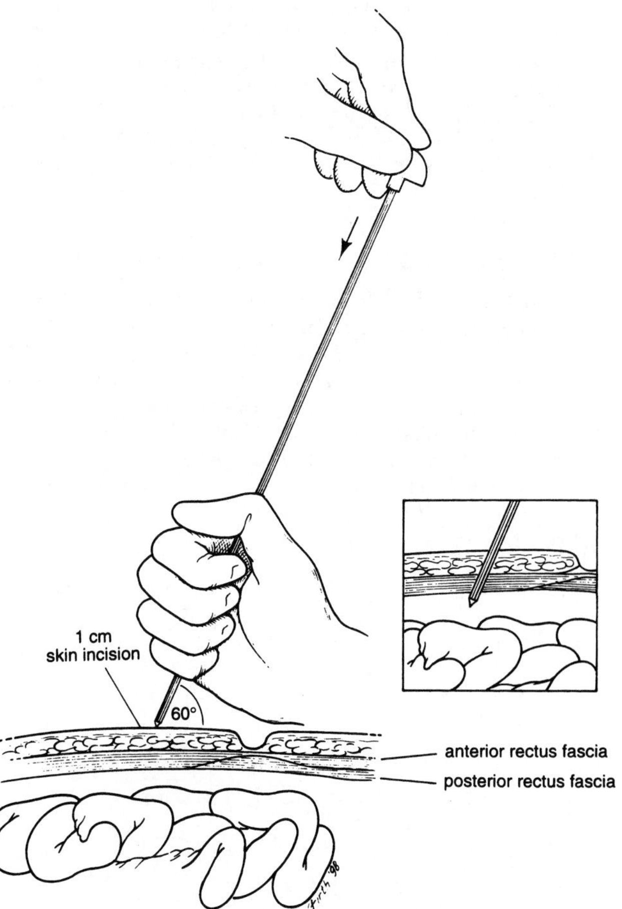

Figure 9–12. The dialysis catheter is fed over a trocar and slowly inserted through a small skin incision with direction toward the pelvis. The nondominant hand is controlling the trocar. Two characteristic "gives" are felt as the trocar travels through the anterior and posterior rectal fasciae. In this way, the trocar is barely inserted in the abdominal cavity.

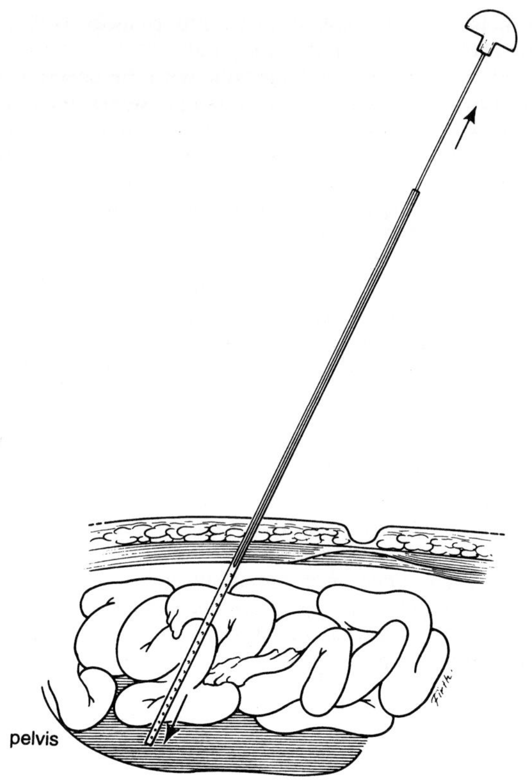

Figure 9–13. As the catheter is advanced, the trocar is withdrawn.

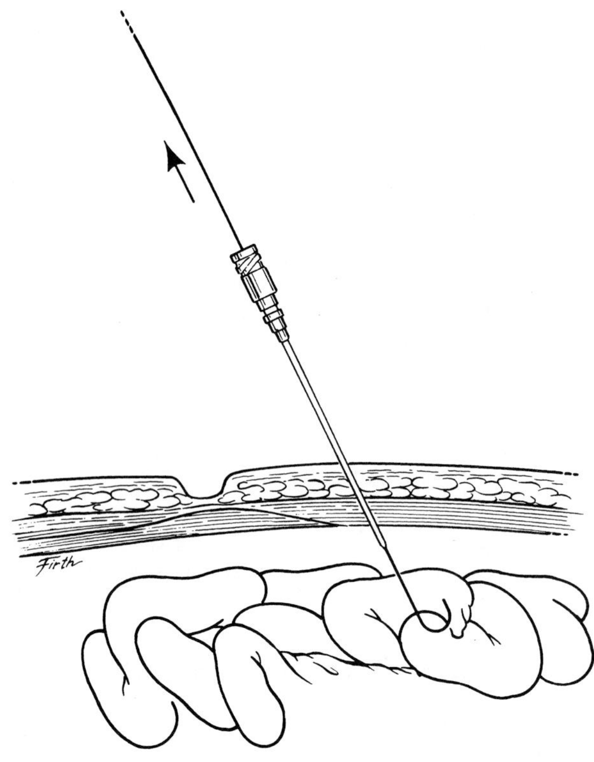

Figure 9–15. A guide wire is inserted in a Seldinger-like technique through the sheath of the needle.

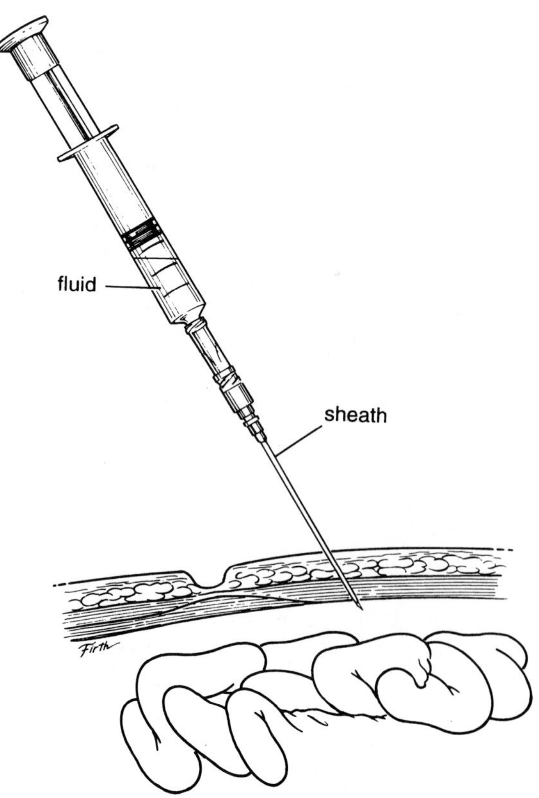

Figure 9–14. A needle is inserted through the anterior abdominal wall.

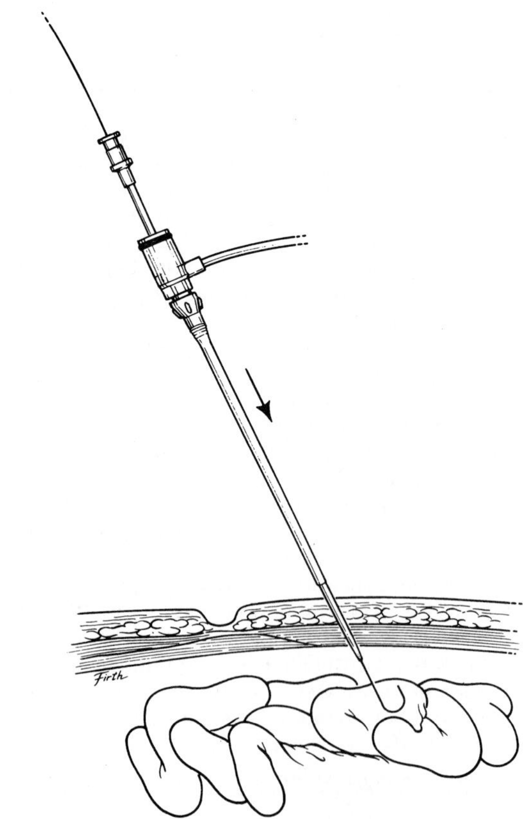

Figure 9–16. An infusion catheter and a guiding catheter are inserted over the wire.

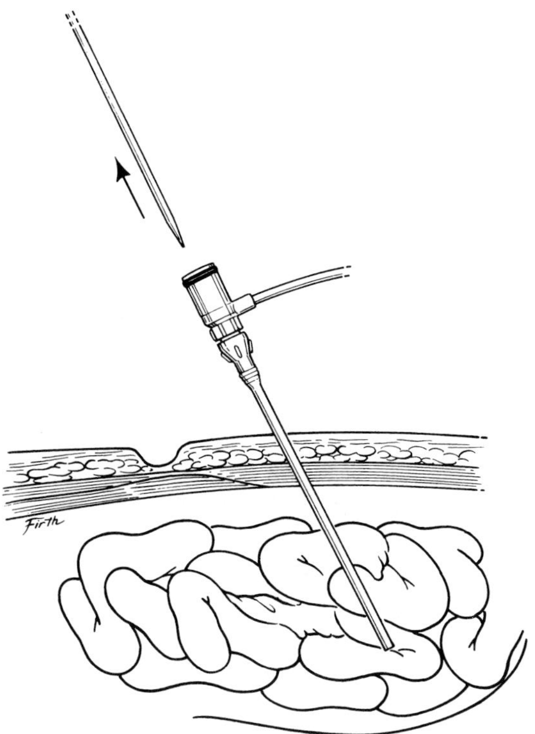

Figure 9–17. The guiding catheter is withdrawn, and the infusion catheter is left in place.

(Arrows) is soft, becomes easily blocked, and may prevent adequate lavage fluid retrieval. The sensitivity was 100% for both, and the specificity was 92% and 97%, respectively. The mean time required to perform the procedure was significantly less for the percutaneous technique (1 ± 3 versus 6.5 ± 5 min), and so were the number of cases with prolonged procedures (0 versus 13 cases). No intra-abdominal or wound complications were detected with either method, but 10 procedures (two closed, eight open) were considered failures because they could not be completed successfully. More personnel and instruments were needed for the open method. The authors concluded that although both techniques are useful and should be included in the standard surgical training, the percutaneous technique is equally safe, faster, and associated with fewer failures than the open method and should be the procedure of choice.

The recent advances of noninvasive studies have replaced DPL in many occasions. Abdominal CT scan is equally sensitive and more specific and for these reasons has become the diagnostic test of choice for hemodynamically stable patients. Abdominal ultrasonography is also used with increasing frequency for the diagnosis of intra-abdominal pathology. Although more experience is being obtained as the technique becomes widely available, it is still operator-dependent and results vary from study to study. Its noninvasive and cost effective nature, the ability for repeated examinations, and the convenience of use will most likely establish it as the diagnostic test of choice as soon as good results can be reliably reproduced. At this point, DPL can still play a significant role in the diagnosis of intra-abdominal pathology for patients who need an urgent diagnosis and who cannot be safely transported away from ICU.

THORACIC PARACENTESIS AND TUBE THORACOSTOMY

Thoracic paracentesis is used for diagnostic purposes or to drain smaller quantities of fluid that are not expected to reaccumulate.[76] Paracentesis is preferably done with the patient sitting and bending forward in order to increase the distance between ribs. A large-bore needle is inserted below the tip of the scapula over the upper border of the lower rib to avoid the intercostal vessels. Because most ICU patients cannot be placed in this position, however, paracentesis is accomplished with the patient in the recumbent position at the posterior axillary line around the fifth intercostal space. Ultrasonographic or CT scan guidance can increase the accuracy in needle placement, particularly for localized collections.[77] Close observation after the procedure by clinical and radiographic signs is essential to detect pneumothorax forming due to inadvertent lung puncture. If a pneumothorax occurs, chest tube decompression is usually necessary.

Chest tubes are inserted to drain fluid or air. Although the amounts that require drainage are arbitrary and should be correlated with the presence of related symptoms, the threshold for chest tube insertion is usually lower for ICU patients who cannot easily tolerate even minimal additional respiratory compromise. The procedure of chest tube placement should be done under strict sterile conditions. The short administration of prophylactic broad-spectrum antibiotics before the commencement of the procedure has been shown to prevent thoracostomy-related complications in trauma patients.[78]

The arm is abducted, and the lateral chest wall is exposed. A small incision over the fifth intercostal space is made. The surgeon spreads the underlying tissues by blunt dissection, creating a tunnel toward the fourth intercostal space. In a controlled fashion, the chest is entered with a hemostat over the upper border of the fifth rib. The hemostat is opened wide to increase the opening, and a digit is inserted through the hole to confirm that the lung is not at risk of injury and to dissect any preexisting adhesions. The chest tube is tunneled into the chest and directed upward. Easy advancement and twisting ensure proper placement. The tube is tied securely with skin sutures. A pursestring suture is also placed around the tube to be used to close the incision when the tube is removed. Although techniques of blind insertion by trocar have been described, the method just described is considered safer for ICU patients who may have multiple pleural adhesions and stiff lungs. Proper position should always be confirmed with a plain chest radiograph.

Barotrauma is a significant complication of positive-pressure ventilation in lungs with poor compliance.[79] The adult respiratory distress syndrome (ARDS) is the most common reason for the need of high-level respiratory support that may result in alveolar rupture from increased buildup of intrapulmonary pressures. Pneumothorax produced from barotrauma may not be readily detected in plain chest radiographs.[80] In the presence of acute hemodynamic or ventilatory compromise, the diagnosis of tension pneumothorax should be routinely ruled out. Other intrapleural pathology requiring drainage may also be missed, and evaluation by CT scan should be entertained whenever clinical suspicion arises.[80, 81] The presence of a chest tube does not preclude the formation of ipsilateral recurrent pneumothorax.[82] Sometimes multiple chest tubes are required.

Chest tubes must be removed when the clinical indications that prompted placement are no longer present. Prolonged chest tube use is an invitation to serious intrathoracic infections that outweigh the benefits of drainage.[83] The optimal method for removal has not been determined, and recurrent pneumothorax remains a problem. In a randomized trial of algorithms for discontinuing tube thoracostomy drainage, there was no difference in recurrent pneumothoraces whether tubes were removed directly off suction or after a water-seal period.[84] Arbitrary standards of practice mandate that thoracostomy tubes are removed at the time of maximal inhalation after resolution of any detectable air leak and reduction of pleural fluid output to less than 1 to 2 mL/kg/day. Follow-up chest radiographs are usually obtained within the ensuing 12 hours.[84]

References

1. Bainton CR: Cricothyrotomy. Int Anesthesiol Clin 1994; 32:95-108.
2. Goumas P, Kokkinis K, Petrocheilos J, Naxakis S, Mochoulis G: Cricothyroidotomy and the anatomy of the cricothyroid space: An autopsy study. J Laryngol Otol 1997; 111:354-356.
3. Esses BA, Jafek BW: Cricothyroidotomy: A decade of experience in Denver. Ann Otol Rhinol Laryngol 1987; 96:519-524.
4. Jackson C: High tracheotomy and other errors: The chief cause of laryngeal stenosis. Surg Gynecol Obstet 1921; 32:392-398.
5. Brantigan CO, Grow JB: Cricothyroidotomy: Elective use in respiratory problems requiring tracheotomy. J Thorac Cardiovasc Surg 1976; 71:72-81.
6. Boyd AD, Romita MC, Conlan AA, Fink SD, Spencer FC: A clinical evaluation of cricothyroidotomy. Surg Gynecol Obstet 1979; 149:365-368.
7. Sise MJ, Shackford SR, Cruikshank JC, et al: Cricothyroidotomy for long-term tracheal access. Ann Surg 1984; 200:13-17.
8. Hawkins ML, Shapiro MB, Cue JI, Wiggins SS: Emergency cricothyrotomy: A reassessment. Am Surg 1995; 61:52-55.
9. Staufer JL, Olson DE, Petty TL: Complications and consequences of endotracheal intubation and tracheotomy: A prospective study of 150 critically ill adult patients. Am J Med 1981; 70:65-76.
10. Gaynor EB, Greenberg SB: Untoward sequelae of prolonged intubation. Laryngoscope 1985; 95:1461-1467.
11. Zeitouni AG, Kost KM: Tracheotomy: A retrospective review of 281 cases. J Otolaryngol 1994; 23:61-66.
12. Manyja SL: Complications of long-term nasal and oral endotracheal intubation. J Laryngol Otol 1979; 93:369-372.
13. Grillo HC, Donahue DM, Mathisen DJ, Wain JC, Wright CD: Postintubation tracheal stenosis: Treatment and results. J Thorac Cardiovasc Surg 1995; 109:486-493.
14. Whited RE: A prospective study of laryngotracheal sequelae in long-term intubation. Laryngoscope 1984; 94:367-377.
15. Dunham CM, LaMonica C: Prolonged tracheal intubation in the trauma patient. J Trauma 1984; 24:120-124.
16. Rodriguez JL, Steinberg SM, Luchetti FA, Gibbons KJ, Taheri PA, Flint LM: Early tracheostomy for primary airway management in the surgical critical care setting. Surgery 1990; 108:655-659.
17. Velmahos GC, Belzberg H, Chan L, et al: Factors predicting prolonged mechanical ventilation in critically injured patients: Introducing a simplified quantitative risk score. Am Surg 1997; 63:811-817.
18. Kollef MH, Von Harz B, Prentice D, et al: Patient transport from intensive care increases the risk of developing ventilator-associated pneumonia. Chest 1997; 112:765-773.
19. Upadhyay A, Maurer J, Turner J, Tiszenkel H, Rosengart T: Elective bedside tracheostomy in the intensive care unit. J Am Coll Surg 1996; 183:51-55.
20. Lujan HJ, Dries DJ, Gamelli RL: Comparative analysis of bedside and operating room tracheostomies in critically ill patients with burns. J Burn Care Rehabil 1995; 16:258-261.
21. Wease GL, Frikker M, Villalba M, Glover J: Bedside tracheostomy in the intensive care unit. Arch Surg 1996; 131:552-555.
22. Ciaglia P, Firshing R, Syniec C. Elective percutaneous dilatational tracheostomy. Chest 1985; 87:15-19.
23. Winkler WB, Karnik R, Seelmann O, Havlicek J, Slany J: Bedside percutaneous dilatational tracheostomy with endoscopic guidance: Experience with 71 ICU patients. Int Care Med 1994; 20:476-479.
24. Fernandez L, Norwood S, Roettger R, Gass D, Wilkins H III: Bedside percutaneous tracheostomy with bronchoscopic guidance in critically ill patients. Arch Surg 1996; 131:129-132.
25. Barba CA, Angood PB, Kauder DR, et al: Bronchoscopic guidance makes percutaneous tracheostomy a safe, cost-effective and easy-to-teach procedure. Surgery 1995; 118:879-883.
26. Crofts SL, Alzeer A, McGuire GP, Wong DT, Charles D: A comparison of percutaneous and operative tracheostomies in intensive care unit patients. Can J Anaesth 1995; 42:775-779.
27. Friedman Y, Fildes J, Mizock B, et al: Comparison of percutaneous and surgical tracheostomies. Chest 1996; 110:480-485.
28. Graham JS, Mulloy RH, Sutherland FR, Rose S: Percutaneous versus open tracheostomy: A retrospective cohort outcome study. J Trauma 1996; 42:245-250.
29. Marx WH, Ciaglia P, Graniero KD: Some important details in the technique of percutaneous dilatational tracheostomy via the modified Seldinger technique. Chest 1996; 110:762-766.
30. Schwann NM: Percutaneous dilatational tracheostomy: Anesthetic considerations for a growing trend. Anesth Analg 1997; 84:907-911.
31. Van Heurn LWE, Van Theunissen PHMH, Ramsay G, Brink PRG: Pathologic changes of the trachea after percutaneous dilatational tracheostomy. Chest 1996; 109:1466-1469.
32. Ciaglia P, Graniero KD: Percutaneous dilatational tracheostomy: Results and long-term follow-up. Chest 1992; 101:464-467.
33. Law RC, Carney AS, Manara AR: Long-term outcome after percutaneous dilatational tracheostomy: Endoscopic and spirometry findings. Anaesthesia 1997; 52:51-56.
34. Van Heerden PV, Webb SA, Power BM, Thompson WR: Percutaneous dilational tracheostomy: A clinical study evaluating two systems. Anaesth Intensive Care 1996; 24:56-59.
35. Gelman JJ, Aro M, Weiss SM: Tracheo-innominate artery fistula. J Am Coll Surg 1994; 179:626-634.
36. McFarlane C, Denholm SW, Sudlow CLM, Moralee SJ, Grant IS, Lee A: Laryngotracheal stenosis: A serious complication of percutaneous tracheostomy. Anaesthesia 1994; 49:38-40.
37. Bennett JDC: High tracheostomy and other errors—revisited. J Laryngol Otol 1996; 110:1003-1007.
38. Consensus conference on artificial airways in patients receiving mechanical ventilation. Chest 1989; 96:178-180.
39. Toursarkissian B, Zweng TN, Kearny PA, Pofahl WE, Johnson SB, Barker DE: Percutaneous dilatational tracheostomy: Report of 141 cases. Ann Thorac Surg 1994; 57:862-867.
40. Fischler MP, Kuhn M, Cantieni R, Frutiger A: Late outcome of percutaneous dilatational tracheostomy in intensive care patients. Intens Care Med 1995; 21:475-481.
41. Caldicott LD, Oldroyd GJ, Bodenham AR: An evaluation of a new percutaneous tracheostomy kit. Anaesthesia 1995; 50:49-51.
42. Cobean R, Beals M, Moss C, Bredenberg CE: Percutaneous dilatational tracheostomy: A safe, cost-effective bedside procedure. Arch Surg 1996; 131:265-271.
43. Hill BB, Zweng TN, Maley RH, Charash WE, Toursarkissian B, Kearny PA: Percutaneous dilatational tracheostomy: Report of 356 cases. J Trauma 1996; 40:238-244.
44. Van Heurn LW, Van Geffen GJ, Brink PRG. Clinical experience with percutaneous dilatational tracheostomy: Report of 150 cases. Eur J Surg 1996; 162:531-535.
45. Mellinger JD: Percutaneous endoscopic gastrostomy: An evaluation after a decade. Gastrointest Clin North Am 1992; 2:187-194.
46. Ponsky JL, Gauderer MWL: Percutaneous endoscopic gastrostomy: A nonoperative technique for feeding gastrostomy. Gastrointest Endosc 1981; 27:9-12.
47. Klein S, Heare BR, Soloway RD: The hurried bumper syndrome: A complication of percutaneous endoscopic gastrostomy. Am J Gastroenterol 1990; 85:448-451.
48. Russell TR, Brotman M, Morris F: Percutaneous gastrostomy: A new, simplified and cost-effective technique. Am J Surg 1984; 148:132-136.
49. Will JS, Oglesby JB: Percutaneous gastrostomy. Radiology 1983; 149:449-452.
50. Foutch PG: Complications of percutaneous endoscopic gastrostomy and jejunostomy: Recognition, prevention and treatment. Gastrointest Endosc Clin North Am 1992; 2:231-248.
51. Schapiro GD, Edmundowicz SA: Complications of percutaneous endoscopic gastrostomy. Gastrointest Endosc Clin North Am 1996; 6:409-422.
52. Miller RE, Castlemain B, Lacqua FJ, et al: Percutaneous gastrostomy: Results on 316 patients and review of the literature. Surg Endosc 1989; 3:186-190.
53. Stern JS: Comparison of percutaneous endoscopic gastrostomy with surgical gastrostomy at a community hospital. Am J Gastroenterol 1986; 86:1171-1173.
54. Chaudry U, Barde CJ, Markert R, Gopalswamy N: Percutaneous endoscopic gastrostomy: A randomized prospective comparison

of early and delayed feeding. Gastrointest Endosc 1996; 44:164-167.
55. Railey DJ, Callja GA, Barkin JS: Percutaneous endoscopic jejunostomy: Indications, techniques and evaluation. Gastrointest Endosc Clin North Am 1992; 2:223-229.
56. Wolfsen HC, Kozarek RA, Ball TJ, et al: Tube dysfunction following percutaneous endoscopic gastrostomy and jejunostomy. Gastrointest Endosc 1990; 36:261-263.
57. Minocha A, Rupp TH, Jagger TL, et al: Silent gastrocolocutaneous fistula as a complication of a percutaneous endoscopic gastrostomy. Am J Gastroenterol 1994; 89:2243-2224.
58. Jain NK, Larson DE, Schroeder KW, et al: Antibiotic prophylaxis for percutaneous endoscopic gastrostomy: A prospective randomized double blind trial. Ann Intern Med 1987; 107:824-828.
59. Cave DR, Robinson WR, Brotschi EA: Necrotizing fasciitis following percutaneous endoscopic gastrostomy. Gastrointest Endosc 1986; 32:294-296.
60. Meurer MF, Kenady DE: Metastatic head and neck carcinoma in a percutaneous gastrostomy site. Head Neck 1993; 15:70-73.
61. D'Amelio LF, Hammond JS, Spain DA, Sutyak JP: Tracheostomy and percutaneous endoscopic gastrostomy in the management of the head-injured patient. Am Surg 1994; 60:180-185.
62. Root HD, Hauser CW, McKinley CR, et al: Diagnostic peritoneal lavage. Surgery 1965; 57:633-637.
63. Zappa MJ, Harwood-Nuss AL, Wears RL, Fallon WF: Objective determination of the optimal red blood cell count in diagnostic peritoneal lavage done for abdominal stab wounds. J Emerg Med 1992; 10:553-558.
64. Sherman SC, Delaurier GA, Hawkins KL, Brown LG, Treat RC, Mansberger AR: Percutaneous peritoneal lavage in blunt trauma patients: A safe and accurate diagnostic method. J Trauma 1989; 29:801-805.
65. Fisher RP, Beverlin BC, Engray LH, Benjamin CI, Perry JF Jr: Diagnostic peritoneal lavage: Fourteen years and 2,586 patients later. Am J Surg 1978; 136:701-704.
66. Demaria EJ: Management of patients with indeterminate diagnostic peritoneal lavage results following blunt trauma. J Trauma 1991; 31:1627-1631.
67. Mozingo DW, Cioffi WG, McManus WF, Pruitt BA: Peritoneal lavage in the diagnosis of acute surgical abdomen following thermal injury. J Trauma 1995; 38:5-7.
68. Richardson JD, Flint LM, Polk HC: Peritoneal lavage: A useful adjunct for peritonitis. Surgery 1983; 94:826-829.
69. Sweeney JF, Albrink MH, Bischof E, McAllister EW, Rosemurgy AS: Diagnostic peritoneal lavage: Volume of lavage effluent needed for accurate determination of a negative lavage. Injury 1994; 25:659-661.
70. Thal ER, Shires GT: Peritoneal lavage in blunt abdominal trauma. Am J Surg 1973; 125:64-69.
71. Lazarus HM, Nelson JA: A technique for peritoneal lavage without risk or complication. Surg Gynecol Obstet 1979; 149:889-892.
72. Howdieshell TR, Osler TM, Demarest GB: Open versus closed peritoneal lavage with particular attention to time, accuracy, and cost. Am J Emerg Med 1989; 7:367-371.
73. Lopez-Viego MA, Mickel TJ, Weigelt JA: Open versus closed diagnostic peritoneal lavage in the evaluation of abdominal trauma. Am J Surg 1990; 160:594-597.
74. Pachter HL, Hofstetter SR: Open and percutaneous paracentesis and lavage for abdominal trauma: A randomized prospective study. Arch Surg 1981; 116:318-319.
75. Velmahos GC, Demetriades D, Stewart M, et al: Open versus closed diagnostic peritoneal lavage: A comparison on safety, rapidity, efficacy. J R Coll Surg Edinburgh (in press).
76. Therapeutic effects of diuretics and paracentesis on lung function in patients with non-alcoholic cirrhosis and tense ascites. J Hepatol 1997; 26:833-838.
77. Van Sonneneberg E, Nakamoto SK, Mueller PR, et al: CT- and ultrasound-guided catheter drainage of empyemas after chest-tube failure. Radiology 1984; 151:349-353.
78. LoCurto JJ, Jr, Tischler CD, Swan KG, et al: Tube thoracostomy and trauma: Antibiotics or not? J Trauma 1986; 26:1067-1072.
79. Schnapp LM, Chin DP, Szaflarski N, Matthay MA: Frequency and importance of barotrauma in 100 patients with acute lung injury. Crit Care Med 1995; 23:272-278.
80. Gross BH, Spizarny DL: Computed tomography of the chest in the intensive care unit. Crit Care Clin 1994; 10:267-275.
81. Mirvis SE, Tobin KD, Kostubiak I, Belzberg H: Thoracic CT in detecting occult disease in critically ill patients. AJR 1987; 148:685-689.
82. Heffner JE, McDonald J, Barbieri C: Recurrent pneumothoraces in ventilated patients despite ipsilateral chest tubes. Chest 1995; 108:1053-1058.
83. Smith JA, Mullerworth MH, Westlake GW, Tatoulis J: Empyema thoracis: 14 year experience in a teaching center. Ann Thorac Surg 1991; 51:39-42.
84. Davis JW, Mackersie RC, Hoyt DB, Garcia J: Randomized study of algorithms for discontinuing tube thoracostomy drainage. J Am Coll Surg 1994; 179:553-557.

10

Clinical Decision Units and Acute Medical Emergencies

Nabil E. Khoury, MD • Richard Nowak, MD, MBA

BACKGROUND

Of 4945 hospital based emergency departments (EDs) in the United States, more than one third have observation units of some sort.[1] Additionally, 50% of Australian EDs and a majority of EDs in the United Kingdom and Canada have them.[2] The impact of these units in the delivery of emergent medical care is substantial. It has been estimated that 8% to 25% of all hospital admissions may be managed in a 23-hour stay unit.[3] Fully 20% to 30% of observation unit patients are admitted, indicating that a sizable proportion of these patients have serious illness requiring inpatient management.

In large part, these units are by-products of a changing economic environment and changing patient expectations. The persistent and increasing pressures for cost containment, coupled with patient demands for comfort, efficiency, and improved medical quality of care and service, have encouraged the development of observation units nationally and internationally. However, as patients become increasingly aware of their options for care, many are demanding increased choice in their venues of emergency care. The onus is on the emergency medicine community to find safe, cost effective, reliable methods to care for patients in the ED setting. Observation units may improve emergency care by facilitating patient flow and comfort in the ED and by providing aggressive early clinical interventions and more sensitive diagnosis, which may ultimately reduce morbidity and mortality, length of hospitalization, and utilization of intensive care unit (ICU) beds.

These units are variously known as *clinical decision units* (CDUs), *observation units* (OBSs), and *clinical decision and treatment units* (CDTUs), among other names. In this chapter, we refer to these units as CDUs, as this name seems to most concisely describe their purpose.

The recent proliferation of ED observation units has occurred in response to increasing pressures to limit cost while simultaneously providing optimal care for patients who might be cared for in the initial 24-hour period after presentation to the ED. More than 50% of patients observed in CDUs have diagnostic syndromes being evaluated for the possibility of serious disease. The goals of the short period of ED observation are to:

1. Improve diagnostic sensitivity and specificity in the identification of potentially serious conditions.
2. Eliminate unnecessary 1- to 2-day hospital admissions by providing standard of care, outpatient therapy to a well-defined population who present to the ED with discrete, reversible medical conditions.
3. Reduce ICU bed demands by providing protracted ED care to certain groups of patients in order to downgrade the requirement of level of intensity from that of an ICU bed to that of a stepdown unit or general patient unit bed.
4. Reduce inpatient length of stay by providing intensive ED therapy and/or diagnostic evaluations prior to patient admission.

CDUs are not critical care units in EDs. Rather, they are units of moderate care intensity providing a venue for continued care after an initial period of ED evaluation and treatment. The overall ED stay of patients admitted to a CDU is usually 24 hours or less, as determined by convention. Initial evaluation and aggressive goal-directed treatment have been shown to improve morbidity and mortality in selected critically ill ED patients.[4] The role of the CDU in subsequent patient care and its incremental impact on morbidity and mortality are not known. Furthermore, morbidity and mortality rates among patients admitted to the CDU, compared with a similar inpatient population, have not been well studied. Yet some initial data suggest that selected patients with asthma treated in the CDU rather than the inpatient ward incur lower costs and have equivalent short-term and long-term clinical outcomes, higher acceptability of treatment, and improved quality of life.[5] Obviously, more studies of this type in other diseases need to be done.

THE CDU CONCEPT

In concept, emergency department CDUs have been units with intensity of service between those of stepdown units and general inpatient wards. The nursing and physician staffing levels and the intensity of monitoring have closely resembled staffing levels on a general inpatient unit. Cardiac monitoring is frequently available, but invasive hemodynamic monitoring usually is not. Intensity of therapy (e.g., an inpatient with reactive airways disease) is greater than on a general patient unit because the CDU is responsible for delivery of total care and is not dependent on outside support, such as a respiratory therapy department. Thus, process times, from order to therapy, tend to be significantly shorter in a CDU.

CDU services are extensions of basic ED services and place additional requirements on ED staff, who are governed by extended-care rather than episodic-care principles. They require expertise different, in some respects, from that of traditional emergency medicine.[6] The American College of Emergency Physicians (ACEP) has identified goals for training physicians in the use and management of observation units. These are:

1. Familiarity with the structure, function, and staffing of observation units.
2. Education on the types of services appropriate for a CDU.
3. Understanding the characteristics of different services appropriate for a CDU.
4. Experience in the provision of such services.
5. Active involvement in the management of observation services, including billing, utilization review, and quality assurance.

Some CDUs are designed and equipped to manage a single diagnostic entity. Most commonly, these units care for patients with chest pain. As such, an extremely high degree of specialization and expertise in managing patients with a single condition develops. These specialized units, however, are limited in their contribution to the emergency services of a department. That is, only a subpopulation of patients that might appropriately be managed in observation are admitted to such units. Depending on the case mix of a particular period, such units tend to experience "boom and bust" phenomena. These units have been very extensively studied and reviewed elsewhere and have been found to provide a cost effective and efficient approach in the diagnosis and management of undifferentiated chest pain patients presenting to the ED.[7]

Less is understood about CDUs that admit patients in broader diagnostic categories. It is still unclear which groups of patients are best suited for CDU management and which criteria, if any, should be used in such determinations. Further, in many cases it is unclear which criteria should be employed in selecting specific patients for CDU admission. The idiosyncrasies of particular disease entities, the subjective component of patient conditions, and interclinician variability have so far made a broad consensus regarding admission and discharge criteria for CDU patients difficult to achieve. Furthermore, it is not clear what hospital admission and discharge rates should be from these units. Other questions include the following: (1) what is an acceptable "treatment failure rate"? and (2) what proportion of ED patients should be treated in the CDU?

Some CDUs are open units into which physicians may admit a wide clinical variety of patients for observation or short-term management of discrete entities. In some cases, a patient's private attending physician may manage cases without clinical guidelines. In other, perhaps better-defined units, clinical protocols or pathways with fairly strict entry and exclusion criteria are utilized for patients. In these units, emergency physicians tend to manage cases in consultation with primary care physicians or subspecialists, with responsibilities clearly delineated by protocol.

Until now, observation units have been used primarily in either acute diagnostic evaluations or the treatment of conditions thought to be amenable to short-term management with aggressive treatment. Characteristically, these patients are usually hemodynamically stable and thought to require only a minimum of clinical intervention to reverse the acute disease process for which the patient presented to the ED.

It is impractical to discuss the specifics of a large number of CDU diagnoses in one chapter. Instead, illustrative examples of the different conceptual roles the CDU plays in the ED evaluation and treatment process should better clarify its role.

ROLES OF THE CDU IN EMERGENCY MEDICINE

The interaction of the ED and the CDU in patient care may be summarized in four categories based on what is primarily done for patients in these two categories: observation and intervention.

Emergency Department Observation Followed by CDU Observation

The first group of CDU patients are typically observed with little or no therapeutic intervention. These patients frequently have conditions that become evident more clearly after a period of time. These diagnostic entities are amenable to CDU observation in order to improve diagnostic sensitivity.

A typical example is atraumatic abdominal pain. As recently as 25 years ago, in 41% of patients presenting to the ED with abdominal pain, no specific diagnosis was established.[8] Since that time, however, there has been a dramatic increase in availability of diagnostic and imaging capabilities, including

TABLE 10–1. Diagnoses Requiring Emergency Department and Clinical Decision Unit Observation

Atraumatic abdominal pain
Closed head injury
Rule out pneumothorax
Rule out cardiac contusion
Rule out compartment syndrome
Abdominal trauma

pregnancy testing, ultrasonography, and computed tomography (CT). Patients with undifferentiated abdominal pain constitute approximately 4.7% of all patients presenting to the ED, a figure not significantly different from that noted in 1972 at the University of Virginia Health Sciences Center.[9] However, a final diagnosis of nonspecific abdominal pain is still assigned to patients 24.9% of the time.[9]

There has clearly been a trend toward increasing specificity of diagnosis in order to decrease hospital admissions. These changes are, in part, attributable to increased availability of imaging and other testing. However, diagnosis and treatment of conditions, such as possible appendicitis, have improved with continued clinical observation. For example, in one study, the percentage of patients with nonspecific abdominal pain operated on for possible appendicitis decreased from 65% to 7%, the false-positive surgery rate declined from 15% to 1.9%, and there was no change in the perforation rate with increased observation.[10] Developing defined protocols for this and other similar entities allows a standardization of approach in a compressed clinical encounter, with the result that the clinical benefits are gained without the attendant costs of hospitalization.

Other typically "observable" CDU diagnoses are listed in Table 10–1. Patients in this category may benefit from repeated physical examination and laboratory or other diagnostic testing. Thus, observation medicine uses the extended emergency visit as an opportunity for more sensitivity in identifying patients with serious conditions that may more often manifest signs and symptoms of disease during an observation period.[11]

Emergency Department Intervention Followed by CDU Observation

Patients in this category have acute medical conditions requiring initial early ED intervention and treatment, followed by a period of observation and stabilization in the CDU. Diagnoses include disease processes such as those listed in Table 10–2.

Because some of these patients may be critically ill on arrival at the ED, in most CDUs policies have been established requiring initial stabilization of patients in the highest acuity area of the ED prior to transfer to the CDU. However, after an initial phase of hemodynamic stabilization in the ED, some patients who initially present with significant hemodynamic or metabolic derangements may become candidates for management in an observation unit. Only after a clear definition of the severity of illness can a determination for CDU transfer be made.

An example of such an entity is gastrointestinal bleeding (GIB). A well-defined protocol for nonvariceal GIB was developed at Henry Ford Hospital in 1996.[12] Algorithm-guided decisions for hospital admission, management of the GIB, and discharge are the responsibilities of the emergency medicine and gastroenterology departments. The protocol is clear in terms of defining patients according to hemodynamic stability, baseline hemoglobin, required fluid resuscitation, and comorbidities (Table 10–3). Guidelines for fluid resuscitation are implemented, and the GIB team is consulted for early assessment and emergent endoscopy as clinically indicated. Early endoscopy is performed in a substantial proportion of patients; the initial resuscitation and diagnostic phase is followed by a CDU or inpatient observation period.

TABLE 10–2. Diagnoses Requiring Emergency Department Intervention and Clinical Decision Unit Observation

Gastrointestinal bleeding
Hypoglycemia
Drug overdose

Data from the period immediately preceding the institution of the protocol have been compared with protocol data. The endpoints studied include number of hospitalizations, length of stay, and readmission rate. The number of hospitalizations decreased from 398 in 1994 to 337 in 1996 ($P < .001$). There was a decrease in length of stay, with 1994 figures showing a drop from 5.3 ± 4.3 to 3.4 ± 3.2 days ($P < .001$) in 1996. Readmission rates remained unchanged, going from 5.8% to 5.9% ($P = 0.8$) in 1994 and 1996, respectively. Such an aggressive early intervention protocol in the emergency setting was found to result in reduced hospital resource utilization while maintaining quality care for GIB patients in the ED (see Table 10–3).

Emergency Department Observation and CDU Intervention

Data concerning patients in this category have documented CDU effectiveness for chest pain. Graff and colleagues reviewed the evaluation of chest pain patients in ED chest pain units and compared these with previous studies on chest pain evaluation without the use of observation units.[13] A total of 23,407 of 444,189 patients admitted to the ED (5.3%) had chest pain as the chief complaint. In the chest pain observation units, 153/2229 patients (6.9%) were identified as having myocardial infarction (MI). Seventy-six percent of patients were discharged home from the observation units. In contrast to previous studies, MI was ruled out for a higher proportion of patients but there was a lower incidence of missed MIs, as estimated by return visits within 72 hours. Overall hospital admission rates were found to be lower, and the overall cost savings were $2.8 million at the study hospitals. The authors concluded that chest pain observation units increased the proportion of patients thoroughly evaluated for chest pain (MI rule-out), improved quality of care, and lowered overall costs of evaluation substantially.

The cost benefits of chest pain evaluation seem to be largely due to the compression of evaluation into a 9- to 12-hour rule-out, followed up by rapid ancillary testing before final disposition. In some centers, clinicians have actually noted an increased cost of management coupled with decreased CDU revenues when compared to inpatient care. Such increased costs are attributable to increased ancillary testing, such as treadmill stress testing and nuclear perfusion scanning among CDU patients.

Thus, it appears that observation medicine is shaping clinical practice by contributing to the development of ever higher standards of diagnostic sensitivity. In fact, coupled with increasingly available and utilized provocative testing, risk stratification has crept into the chest pain unit's repertoire of functions. That is, instead of merely trying to identify patients with MI, observation units are increasingly attempting to identify those patients with coronary artery disease.

TABLE 10–3. Clinical Decision Unit (CDU) Clinical Pathways: Upper and Lower Gastrointestinal Hemorrhage

Eligibility Criteria	Exclusion Criteria	Testing Prior to CDU Transfer	Treatment Prior to CDU Transfer	CDU Treatment and Observation	Discharge Criteria	Discharge Medications and Follow-up
All Patients 1. History of hematochezia or hematemesis with or without melena 2. Nasogastric aspirate clears after 2 L of saline lavage (if UGI source) ***Patients Without Renal Failure*** 1. Hb of > 8 g or a change of < 4 g of Hb from baseline (after fluid resuscitation) 2. Orthostatic vital signs should be normalized prior to CDU transfer ***Patients With Renal Failure*** 1. ≤ 2 g Hb drop from baseline 2. Orthostatic vital signs should be normalized with no more than 500 mL IVF prior to CDU transfer	1. Active UGI hemorrhage noted with gastric lavage (does not clear with 2 L of saline) 2. Coagulopathy 3. Thrombocytopenia 4. Aortic graft 5. Suspected portal hypertension 6. Other symptomatic comorbidities (i.e., ASHD, ESRD, CHF) 7. Requirement of 2 units of PRBCs or > 2 L of crystalloid to correct orthostatic hypotension and normalize BP and HR 8. Hypotension (systolic BP < 100 mm Hg) 9. Active LGI Bleed	***All Patients*** 1. CBC at presentation and after fluid resuscitation 2. Electrolytes 3. PT/PTT 4. Platelets 5. Stool hemoccult 6. IV access (2 lines where indicated) 7. *GI endoscopy will be performed prior to CDU transfer, during CDU stay, or after CDU observation in GI clinic depending on severity of patient condition* ***Selected Patients*** 1. ABG 2. Lactate 3. T & S or T & C 4. NG lavage with up to 2 L of saline 5. Orthostatic vital signs 6. Pulse oximetry (provide O_2 if Hb % sat. < 95%) 7. Foley catheter 8. ECG ≥ 50 years old or with a history of CAD 9. Tagged RBC scan	***All Patients*** 1. IV access (2 lines in patients with tachycardia, hypotension, or orthostatic hypotension) 2. NPO after midnight 3. GI notification/ consultation (consultation may be completed in A.M. for stable patients) ***Selected Patients*** 1. If patient is orthostatic, hydration as indicated. Repeat orthostatic vital signs as indicated 2. Transfusion of 1–2 units of PRBCs 3. H_2 blockers 4. Low-flow O_2 (titrate to maintain Hb % sat. > 95%) 5. NG aspirate (should clear by 2 L of NS lavage)	***RN*** 1. Vitals q 4 hr and prn 2. Review of ED record for tests, Tx, and clinical response 3. Continuation of treatment and observation a. IV hydration as indicated b. CBC q 6 hr c. H_2 blockers q 6 hr (selected patients) 4. Notify MD of any change in condition 5. Notify MD of: a. Laboratory results b. D/C criteria when met ***CDU Physician*** 1. Performs admission assessment, dictated note, and orders 2. Document condition q 6 h 3. Assess patient for symptoms, continued bleeding, etc. 4. Arrange for additional testing as indicated	1. No evidence of active UGI or LGI bleeding 2. Less than a 1 g drop in Hb unless patient is receiving continued hydration 3. Normal vital signs 4. No postural hypotension 5. No dyspnea 6. Completion of GI evaluation, including UGI endoscopy to be done either in CAT 1 or GI clinic as agreed with GI fellow* 7. If readmission is thought to be needed after endoscopy in GI clinic, the patient should be admitted from endoscopy suite. If the suite is closed (after 5 P.M.), the patient may be returned to CDU until an IPD bed is available	1. Appropriate medications, including H_2 blockers 2. Pertinent advice against use of NSAIDs, alcohol, tobacco, caffeine, etc 3. Encourage oral hydration and advancing diet as tolerated 4. Social work consultation with or without home care referral if indicated

*The GI fellow (beeper 313-705-2511) is to be notified about *all* GI bleeding.

Hb = hemoglobin; UGI = upper gastrointestinal; CAD = coronary artery disease. IVF = intravenous fluid; CHF = congestive heart failure; ESRD = end-stage renal disease; ASHD = arteriosclerotic heart disease; BP = blood pressure; LGI = lower gastrointestinal; GI = gastrointestinal; ABG = arterial blood gas; ECG = electrocardiogram; RBC = red blood cell; NPO = nothing by mouth; PRBC = packed red blood cell; ED = emergency department; MD = medical doctor; T & S = type and screen; T & C = type and crossmatch; NS = normal saline; O_2 = oxygen; CBC = complete blood count; H_2 = histamine; PT = prothrombin time; PTT = partial thromboplastin time; HR = heart rate; mm Hg = millimeters of mercury; NG = nasogastric; sat = saturation; Tx = treatment; IPD = inpatient department; D/C = discharge; CAT = category; RN = Registered Nurse; NSAIDs = nonsteroidal anti-inflammatory drugs.

TABLE 10–4. Diagnoses Frequently Admitted to Clinical Decision Units Primarily for Extended Emergency Therapy

Asthma
Cellulitis
Chronic obstructive pulmonary disease
Diabetic ketoacidosis
Congestive heart failure
Hyperemesis gravidarum
Pyelonephritis
Pancreatitis
Dehydration
Pneumonia

Emergency Department Intervention and CDU Intervention

A number of conditions necessitate both ED therapy and CDU therapy (Table 10–4). A well-studied example in this category is congestive heart failure (CHF). Treatment of this condition begins in the ED and continues through the CDU stay. CHF is the third largest cause of hospital admissions in all patients, with more than 750,000 patients admitted and more than 6 million inpatient days per year.[14] CHF is the primary cause of hospital admissions in patients over age 65 years. Approximately 35% of all patients with a diagnosis of CHF are hospitalized each year, with an average length of stay of 7.4 days.[14] In one study, aggressive treatment of CHF in an observation unit reduced the overall admission rate of this patient population from 87% to 45% and the ICU admission rate from 35% to 3%.[15]

CDU MANAGEMENT SHORTCOMINGS

Some diagnostic conditions may not be as amenable to a shortening of a diagnostic and therapeutic course. The Henry Ford Hospital CDU data base reports that during 1996–1997, 121 patients were admitted to the CDU for pneumonia, but only 43 were discharged to home, resulting in an admission rate of 61%.[14] These data appear to reflect either poor patient selection or the requirement for periods longer than 24 hours for an improvement in clinical signs and symptoms to be seen in patients with this condition. CDU stays resulting in hospital admission may have increased associated costs. What is not known is whether the intensive early intervention in the ED and CDU with antibiotic therapy, intravenous hydration, beta agonist utilization, and pulmonary toilet ultimately shorten length of stay. Thus, studies similar to the Chest Pain Evaluation Registry (CHEPER) are needed to evaluate most, if not all, clinical diagnoses admitted to CDUs to statistically assess their impact on clinical outcomes and overall health care costs.

Similarly, treatment of sickle cell anemia painful crisis in the CDU is associated with a high incidence of treatment failure. In fact, 62% of 186 patients during 1996 and 1997 were admitted to hospitals after aggressive pain control and hydration lasting an average of 12 hours and 18 minutes after ED evaluation.[16] An interesting finding in this group was that there were no clear physiologic predictive parameters of need for hospital admission versus discharge.

CDU RESEARCH

Acute care research continues to play an increasing role in the investigations of disease progression and the development of novel therapies. An attractive model for emergency medicine clinical research is the *clinical research unit* (CRU). The CRU is a dedicated area of the CDU where patients may receive cardiac monitoring, one-on-one emergency nursing, and emergency physician staffing. This approach facilitates emergency medicine clinical research in general and CDU research in particular because it controls the immediate environment of the subject, thereby facilitating clinical observations and trials. This also allows for seamless integration of the clinical and research functions of the ED. Additionally, the 24-hour window of patient care in the CDU allows patients to be treated and evaluated in a controlled setting for considerably longer periods than is typical for emergency medicine research.

It is becoming clear that management of acute disease and its resolution needs to be closely studied for a longer time than traditionally allowed in the ED. Acute disease and its resolution or progression within 24 hours need to be studied. Emergency medicine CDUs are poised to provide this research opportunity.

THE FUTURE

Major obstacles in the implementation of CDUs described in this chapter have included appropriate patient selection in terms of both the diagnosis and the severity of illness. Early investigators have used clinical guidelines in determining patient selection and enrollment into clinical pathways. Standardization of these protocols has been based primarily on clinical criteria rather than on specific physiologic scoring systems. Some efforts to validate clinical criteria for patient selection have been developed for discrete diagnoses at some centers.[16] Initial clinical criteria are established and then studied retrospectively to assess their validity.

Severity of illness is difficult to quantify in light of the myriad of conditions treated in observation units. The broadest CDUs admit patients from the ED with any number of clinical entities. As many as 32 diagnosis-based protocols are used in some centers.[16] Some centers have used clinical criteria for admission to a CDU based on the severity of presumed metabolic and physiologic abnormalities. The consensus is that some set of criteria should be employed in the selection of observation unit patients in order to provide guidelines on which ongoing assessment of treatment success and failure may be based.[17]

The *systemic inflammatory response syndrome* (SIRS) and limited cytokine measurements have been studied at ED triage as assessments of disease severity and outcomes prediction.[18, 19] Each of these, while contributing some important information, has been limited by the lack of ability to follow patients and their disease progression for a longer period than that allowed in the ED; that is, no repeated values were obtained during the remainder of the ED/CDU course.

The overall incidence of SIRS at triage was found to be 25%, and 20.6% of patients were admitted to the hospital. Patients meeting SIRS criteria at triage were 4.5 times more likely to be hospitalized than non-SIRS patients (95% confidence interval [CI] of 3.2, 6.4, $P = .001$). Furthermore, the presence of increasing numbers of SIRS criteria was associated with increasing likelihood of need for hospital admission. However, 59% of patients meeting SIRS criteria at triage were ultimately discharged home.[18, 19]

Other groups have studied SIRS for longer time periods in the inpatient setting and have suggested that the progression of disease to sepsis, severe sepsis, and septic shock can and does occur.[20] Study of SIRS criteria over the initial 24 hours after ED presentation might define patterns of SIRS criteria changes and whether these might be used more effectively as predictors for the need of ongoing or more aggressive care.

It has also been shown that limited cytokine measurements may be valuable prognostic indicators when measured at ED triage. For example, patients with detectable tumor necrosis factor-α (TNF-α) or interleukin-6 (IL-6), are significantly associ-

TABLE 10–5. Clinical Decision Unit (CDU) Clinical Pathways: Diabetic Ketoacidosis (DKA)

Eligibility Criteria	Exclusion Criteria	Testing Prior to Transfer to CDU	Treatment Prior to CDU Transfer	CDU Observation and Treatment	Discharge Criteria	Discharge Meds and Follow-up
*1. **Mild DKA*** Defined as: a. Glu = 200–1000 mg/dL b. BOHB = elevated c. pH ≥ 7.35 *2. **Moderate DKA*** Defined as: a. Glu = 200–1000 mg/dL b. BOHB = elevated c. pH = 7.20–7.35 *3. **Severe DKA*** Patients with *severe DKA* initially should be managed in CAT I until criteria of *moderate DKA* are met; at that time, they may be eligible for CDU if no other exclusion criteria are met	1. Sepsis (2 of 4 modified SIRS criteria): a. HR > 100/min b. RR > 20/min or PA_{CO_2} < 32 mm Hg c. Temperature > 38.0°C or < 36.0°C d. WBC ct. > 12,000 or < 4000 or > 10% bands 2. Hyperosmolar coma 3. Myocardial ischemia or infarction 4. Severe DKA a. Glu = 200–1200 mg/dL b. BOHB = elevated c. pH = < 7.20 5. Pregnancy	***All Patients*** 1. CBC 2. Electrolytes, including Ca, PO_4, Mg 3. BOHB 4. Initial cBG, then q 1 h if glucose < 500 g/dL 5. Urinalysis ***Selected Patients*** 1. Chest x-ray 2. ABG 3. Lactate 4. ECG 5. Serum osmolality 6. Blood culture 7. Urine culture	1. Establish IV access 2. 1 L of .9 NS should be given in first 30–60 min, then 250 mL/hr or as clinically indicated 3. Foley catheter placement prn 4. Supplemental O_2 (keep Hb % sat. ≥ 95%) 5. Oral rehydration as tolerated 6. Insulin therapy: bolus of 0.1 μ/kg regular insulin followed by a drip of 0.05–0.1 unit/kg/h IV 7. Potassium replacement: should be given if renal function is normal or near normal, good urine output, and serum potassium is in normal range 8. Antibiotic therapy for those with associated minor infections (i.e., pharyngitis, early cellulitis)	***RN*** 1. VS q 8 h or p.r.n. 2. Mental status assessment 3. Lytes profile, BOHB q 2–4 h 4. Continued therapy: a. IV hydration at 250 mL/hr or as clinically indicated b. Oral hydration c. Cont. of abx. tx. as per ED schedule d. IV insulin therapy (0.05–0.1 unit/kg/h) or per MD 5. Once glucose ≤ 250–300 mg/dL change IVF to D5NS *6. Once anion gap or BOHB is within normal range, administer regular and long-acting insulin and d/c insulin drip 2 hr thereafter* *7. Continue cBG checks q 4 h (×3) and then q 6 h with sliding scale coverage q 4 h* ***CDU Physician*** 1. Completes transfer assessment, dictated note, and orders 2. Document condition q 8 h	***Mild-Moderate DKA*** 1. Glucose ≤ 250 mg/dL 2. Normal vital signs 3. Tolerating oral fluids and medications 4. Normalization of serum electrolytes and resolution of ketosis 5. Baseline M.S. 6. Patient understands discharge instructions and can return for follow-up 7. If any of these discharge criteria are not met, admit patient ***Severe DKA*** Patients who have severe DKA at initial evaluation in CAT I should be admitted to a GPU if ketoacidosis is resolved or to ICU/IMU/Progressive care bed if not resolved	***Mild-Moderate DKA*** 1. Appropriate medications, including antibiotics and insulin or oral hypoglycemics should be provided 2. Encourage liberal oral hydration 3. Diabetes education materials should be provided prior to discharge 4. Arrange short-term follow-up with patient's PCP 5. SW consult should be initiated as needed for home care needs 6. Patients should receive information regarding diabetic teaching programs available through Division of Endocrinology and Metabolism (information is in CDU) *7. **Patients with New-Onset Diabetes*** Provide home care for Visiting Nurse Association and home support for new diabetic patients

Glu = glucose; HR = heart rate; RR = response rate; SIRS = systemic inflammatory response syndrome; WBC = white blood cell; ct. = count; CBC = complete blood count; ECG = electrocardiogram; IV = intravenous; NS = normal saline; p.r.n. = as needed; ED = emergency department; MD = medical doctor; IVF = intravenous fluid; ICU = intensive care unit; CA = calcium; Mg = magnesium; VS = vital signs; IMU = intermediate medical unit; SW = social work; PCP = primary care provider; d/c = discontinue; RN = Registered Nurse; BOHB = beta hydroxybutyrate; cBG = capillary blood glucose; PO_4 = phosphate.

ated with hospitalization.[21] In these same patients, the higher the presenting level of TNF-α, IL-6, and intercellular adhesion molecule-1 (ICAM-1), the higher the likelihood that the individual would be admitted.[22] Last, when a presenting emergency triage cytokine score—combining levels of TNF-α, IL-6, and ICAM-1—was developed, there was a significant positive association between the scoring levels and admission rates.[23]

Interestingly, in all these studies only a single sample for cytokine determination was drawn. There are fluctuations in both pro-inflammatory and anti-inflammatory cytokines over the course of disease.[24] Further study of cytokine responses during the first 24 hours of ED observation may elucidate patterns of these markers, which may contribute in predicting disease progression or potential for successful home discharge.

Thus, eligibility for CDU admission may be based on features particular to a specific disease entity or physiologic variables that cross diagnostic boundaries, such as SIRS criteria, cytokine profiles, or other objective markers. Currently, most CDU admission criteria are diagnosis-specific. Utilization of criteria such as SIRS or other physiologic scoring systems may better enable observation units to select appropriate patients and risk-stratify them irrespective of specific diagnosis. The use of scoring systems in individual patients, however, is not as reliable as in patient groups.[25] Conceptually, this approach is similar to the Acute Physiology and Chronic Health Evaluation (APACHE) or the Simplified Acute Physiology Score used in intensive care medicine.

An example of patient selection based on specific physiologic criteria is diabetic ketoacidosis (DKA). Our DKA protocol defines severity of disease in terms of severity of acidosis, modified SIRS criteria, and absence of major hemodynamic embarrassment. The Henry Ford Hospital Protocol for inclusion and exclusion of CDU DKA patients is summarized in Table 10-5.

Significant experience with a variety of scoring methods has been reported in patients admitted to the ICU.[26] Review of currently accepted scoring systems such as APACHE may help guide the emergency medicine community in developing prognostic tools for observation medicine. The APACHE system utilizes the worst values of physiologic measurements, age, and previous health status; describes illness severity for a wide range of common illnesses; and correlates these with outcome. Prospective studies have compared APACHE to other scores for specific conditions such as pancreatitis. Early on, APACHE (II) was found to be two thirds as sensitive in predicting severe pancreatitis attacks. By 48 hours after patient presentation at the ICU, its prognostic accuracy is comparable to Ranson's or Imrie's scoring systems.

For such a scoring system to be developed in the ambulatory ED/CDU population, large numbers of patients are required. Because most patients admitted to the CDU are relatively hemodynamically stable, fewer are likely to have physiologic derangements as significant as those found in patients admitted to the ICU. Also, endpoints are not mortality but, rather, morbidity and likelihood of hospitalization. Furthermore, in order to be useful, any prospective scoring method needs to be conclusive in the first few hours of a patient's ED/CDU stay. Thus, in order to validate a scoring system using multivariate analysis, we will need to study thousands of patients. Drawbacks of such a scoring system include (1) complexity, (2) computerization needs for scoring, and (3) standardization of physiologic and laboratory values and cutoffs.

It is also possible in the future that CDU patients may even be followed up longer than 24 hours for certain conditions or studies to determine resolution or ongoing control of disease. For example, we are currently involved in a leukotriene modifier study to determine the effect of these agents on acute airways obstruction throughout the ED/CDU phase. We are also following up these patients at days 10 and 28 after discharge in the CRU to see what control these agents are having on ongoing symptoms after the acute exacerbation. It is possible that this concept of CDU assessment of ongoing disease control after acute exacerbations might be applied to other conditions.

In summary, CDUs are likely to continue to evolve and develop more sophisticated and novel assessment or statification tools coupled with innovative therapies. CDUs will allow more patient-focused, economically prudent emergency care and will better integrate this care into longer-term management strategies of disease control after the acute event resolution.

References

1. Graff L: Observation Medicine. Boston, Andover Medical Publishers, 1993.
2. Wong DT, Barrow PM, Gomez M, McGuire GP: A comparison of the Acute Physiology and Chronic Health Evaluation (APACHE) II score and the Trauma-Injury Severity Score (TRISS) for outcome assessment in intensive care unit trauma patients. Crit Care Med 1996; 24:1642–1648.
3. Brillman J, Mathers-Dunbar L, Graff L, et al: Management of observation units. Ann Emerg Med 1995; 25:823–830.
4. Rivers E, Doyle D, Paul-Kagiri R, Nisenbaum R, Randall K, Tomlanovich M: Physiologic Assessment of the Critically Ill: An Outcome Evaluation of Emergency Department Intervention (Abstract). Society for Academic Emergency Medicine, 1998 Annual Meeting, May 17–20, 1998. Acad Emerg Med 1998; 59:530.
5. McDermott MF, Murphy DG, Zalenski RJ, et al: A comparison between emergency diagnostic and treatment unit and inpatient care in the management of acute asthma. Arch Intern Med 1997; 157:2055–2062.
6. Graff LG, Dunbar L, Gibler WB, et al: Observation medicine curriculum. Observation Medicine Committee, Society for Academic Emergency Medicine. Ann Emerg Med 1992; 21:963–966.
7. Graff L, Joseph L, Joseph T, et al: American College of Emergency Physician information pages: Chest pain units in emergency departments—a report from the Short-term Observation Services Section. Am J Cardiol 1995; 76:1036–1039..
8. Brewer RJ, Golden GT, Hitch DC, et al: Abdominal pain, an analysis of 1000 consecutive cases in a university hospital emergency room. Am J Surg 1976; 219–223.
9. Powers RD, Guertler AT: Abdominal pain in the ED: Stability and change over 20 years. Am J Emerg Med 1995; 13:301–303.
10. White JS, Santillana M, Holly JA: Intensive in-hospital observation: A safe way to discuss unnecessary appendectomy. Ann Surg 1975; 41:793–799.
11. Graff LG, et al: Probability of appendicitis before and after observation. Ann Emerg Med 1991; 20:503–507.
12. Podila PV, Ben-Menachem T, Oruganti NS, Fogel R: Bleeding algorithm: Specialist-driven high quality, low cost health care. Gastroenterology 1997(Suppl); 112:A35.
13. Graff LG, Dallara J, Ross M, et al: Impact on the care of the emergency department chest pain patient from the Chest Pain Evaluation Registry (CHEPER) Study. Am J Cardiol 1997; 80:563–568.
14. Graff LG: Emergency Observation Medicine: Observation for CHF and Atrial Fibrillation. September 19, 1997. (Lecture) Observation Medicine Conference, Dearborn, Mich, WSU/American College of Emergency Physicians.
15. Dunbar L: Congestive heart failure. *In:* Observation Medicine. Graff L (Ed). Boston, Andover Medical Publishers, 1993.
16. Henry Ford Hospital Clinical Decision Unit Pathways, Detroit, Henry Ford Hospital, 1998.
17. Graff L, Zun LS, Leikin J, et al: Emergency department observation beds improve patient care: Society for Academic Emergency Medicine Debate. Ann Emerg Med 1992; 21:967–975.
18. Tuttle AP, Nowak RM, Grzybowski M, et al: Systemic inflammatory response syndrome at triage: Prevalence and association with hospital admissions. Acad Emerg Med 1996; 3:478–479.

19. Tuttle AP, Nowak RM, Grzybowski M, et al: The systemic inflammatory response syndrome in the emergency department: Prevalence, association with hospital admission, and clinical utility. Crit Care Med 1997; 25:A109.
20. Rangel-Fausto MS, Pittet D, Costignan M, et al: The natural history of the systemic inflammatory response syndrome (SIRS): A prospective study. JAMA 1995; 273:117–123.
21. Nowak RM, Maliarik M, Tuttle P, et al: Non-detectable vs detectable plasma cytokines on arrival to the emergency department (ED) as predictors of hospital admission. Crit Care Med 1997; 25:A110.
22. Tuttle A, Maliarik M, Nowak RM, et al: Plasma cytokine concentrations measured at triage in the emergency department (ED) as predictors of hospital admission. Crit Care Med 1997; 25:A110.
23. Tuttle A, Nowak R, Grzybowski M, et al: A presenting emergency cytokine score measured at triage in the emergency department (ED) and admission rates. Shock 1997; 7:101.
24. Bone RC: Sir Isaac Newton, sepsis, SIRS, and CARS. Crit Care Med 1996; 24:1125–1128.
25. Beck DH, Taylor BL, Millar B, Smith GB: Prediction of outcome from intensive care: A prospective cohort study comparing Acute Physiology and Chronic Health Evaluation II and III prognostic systems in a United Kingdom intensive care unit. Crit Care Med 1997; 25:9–15.
26. Yealy DM, Dehart DA, Ellis G, et al: A survey of observation units in the United States. Am J Emerg Med 1989; 7:576–580.

11

Rapid Identification of Coronary Artery Insufficiency

Stephen M. Ayres, MD, FCCM

The defining theorem in critical care medicine is that severe pathogenic stressors, such as trauma or sepsis, initiate a series of sequential responses that lead to sepsis and multiple organ failure unless they are corrected at a very early stage.[1] Specific evidence in animal and clinical studies reveals that myocardial necrosis evolves over 24 to 36 hours after coronary vascular occlusion; mechanical or pharmacologic intervention during these "golden" moments can salvage myocardial tissue and minimize ventricular dysfunction.[2]

More than 500,000 patients die of coronary artery disease in the United States each year.[3] This chapter serves to alert the intensivist that the risk of myocardial ischemia, rather than being a primary or associated complication, is an ever-present risk in the critically ill patient. Subsequent chapters describe in detail the anatomic nature of coronary artery disease, the management of acute myocardial infarction (MI), thrombolytic therapy, and interventional therapy in coronary artery disease. The protocols for rapid diagnosis of myocardial ischemia, developed by the Division of Cardiology at the Medical College of Virginia, are found in the Appendix to this chapter.

The neurohumoral-humoral and metabolic responses to stress initially serve important adaptive purposes.[4] Although triggered by different activating systems—the neurosympathetic axis following hypoperfusion and the reticuloendothelial-macrophage system following sepsis—the subsequent responses are strikingly similar. Hypoperfusion, secondary to reduced cardiac output, hypovolemia or hypoxemia, triggers the release of adrenocorticotropic hormone (ACTH), cortisol, epinephrine, norepinephrine, and glucagon. These stress hormones attempt to provide vital organ function. Constriction of the renal and splanchnic vascular beds allows the available blood volume and flow to perfuse the heart and brain. Glycogenolysis raises blood glucose, and hormonally produced insulin resistance decreases glucose uptake in muscle and fat, redirecting the glucose flux to the brain.

Coronary artery disease is epidemic in modern Western civilization and the most common cause of death in these countries. Modern revascularization technology has led to a decrease in deaths from coronary artery disease: In Eastern Europe and in the former Soviet Union, the death rate from coronary artery disease is increasing.

The diagnosis of acute ischemic heart disease can usually be made when patients present with chest pain. When chest pain is absent or atypical, the diagnosis may be missed. The diagnosis may also be missed in the setting of other critical illness where the physician's attention is diverted by the presenting problem.

CORONARY FLOW RESPONSES TO STRESS

For many years it has been known that hypoxemia, alkalosis, and hypokalemia can lead to cardiac arrhythmias.[5] The stress response to acute respiratory failure is intense, which explains why about 25% of patients dying with acute respiratory failure have morphologic evidence of acute MI.[6] Data regarding the prevalence of myocardial ischemia during trauma are not available, but the indirect evidence cited earlier suggests that it may be significant, particularly in the individual with polytrauma and multiple transfusions.

The neurohumoral-circulatory response to stress evolved over centuries of prehistoric existence and depends on the presence of a distensible vascular system.[7] Apparently, coronary artery disease was not anticipated when the genetic templates began to evolve in humans, since a few localized areas of vascular obstruction can derail the entire organism.[8]

OXYGEN DELIVERY DURING REST AND EXERCISE

While the systemic vascular bed extracts but 25% of the oxygen delivered to it, the myocardium extracts 60% to 65% of delivered oxygen so that myocardial oxygen tension is quite low. The peripheral tissues respond to increased needs for oxygen by increasing both blood flow and oxygen extraction. Increased myocardial needs, closely related to heart rate and strength of contraction, are normally met by increasing flow, since increasing myocardial extraction would lead to dangerously low myocardial oxygen tensions.[9]

In many individuals, the coronary circulation may not be able to respond to the stress of critical illness. A group of neural, humoral, and local metabolic factors control vascular distensibility and thus regulate blood flow. Hypoxemia and hypoperfusion stimulate aortic and carotid chemoreceptors, which leads to sympathetic fiber discharge and the release of norepinephrine and epinephrine. Other factors lead to autoregulation, which requires the ability to dilate. The release of catecholamines and other stress hormones may result in cardiac arrhythmias and increased myocardial ischemia. The use of β-blockade in coronary disease, once contraindicated, may be used to attenuate the stress response. The use of β-blockade can be risky and is based on the premise that the response has overstimulated the cardiovascular system and is now counterproductive.

Emergency department (ED) experiences suggest that the occurrence of undiagnosed MI is not uncommon. Myocardial ischemia associated with another primary problem, or without chest pain, can be a challenge to any physician. Because acute interventional technology allows the immediate improvement of coronary blood flow, diagnosis of coronary insufficiency, either as a primary or secondary condition, is essential.

IDENTIFYING ISCHEMIC HEART DISEASE IN THE ACUTE CARE UNIT

The understanding of the clinical manifestations of coronary artery disease evolved in the years after the description of coronary thrombosis by Obrastzow and Straschesko[10] in Kiev in 1910 and by Herrick[11] in 1912. In Chicago, Pardee's[12] observation in 1920 that "the appearance of a Q-wave followed by ST segment elevation rising to a tall T-wave was an electrocardiographic sign of coronary artery obstruction."

Clinicians faced with patients with persistent chest pain and varying abnormalities of the ST and T segments soon realized that angina and coronary thrombosis were not the only expressions of coronary artery disease. Case reports of autopsy-proven MI without classical Q waves and ST-segment elevation appeared in the 1940s and the term "subendocardial infarction" was introduced in the belief that necrosis limited to the inner layers of the myocardium would not produce Q waves.[13] Non-Q-wave coronaries remained an imprecise diagnosis until LaDue and associates[14] reported that myocardial necrosis led to the release of the enzyme serum glutamic-oxaloacetic transaminase (SGOT) into the circulation.

Clinical studies soon showed, however, that the T-wave coronaries were not mild ones. Scheinman and Abbott[15] studied a large number of patients with "probable" or "definite" acute MIs. Surprisingly, mortality rates were 38% in patients with increased enzymes and only 19% in classic transmural infarction. Similar results were described by Lown[16] and Rigo[17] and their coauthors. Many of the patients with normal enzymes had what is now called "unstable angina."

For many years, cardiologists thought that myocardial ischemia was caused by an imbalance of myocardial oxygen delivery and demand. Even though Herrick had implicated coronary thrombosis as the causal factor, the idea had been forgotten, although warfarin (Coumadin) anticoagulants began to be used as therapy for MI. In 1971, DeWood and colleagues[18] noted that 87.3% of patients with acute transmyocardial infarction, studied angiographically within 4 hours of the onset of symptoms, showed total occlusion of a coronary artery. In patients studied 12 to 24 hours after symptoms began, the occlusion rate dropped to 64.9%. Falk[19] found that thrombosis was also a major factor in the pathogenesis of unstable angina.

A recent study emphasized the serious nature of unstable angina.[20] Boden and coworkers studied 2738 patients with non-Q-wave MIs confirmed by isoenzymes of creatine kinase with muscle and brain subunits (CK-MB); 34% of the patients were randomized to either invasive or conservative treatment. Nine per cent of the patients were excluded because of serious ischemic events in the early hours of treatment. There were 139 deaths and 291 cardiac events during the average of 23 months' follow-up, and outcomes were the same in the group receiving an invasive strategy compared with patients treated conservatively.

This new information dramatically changed medical attitudes. In the past, patients were to "rule out" an acute MI. Measurement of myocardial enzymes—first SGOT, then CK, and more recently CK-MB—became the "gold standard" for infarction and, by inference, the presence of serious coronary artery disease. If enzyme study results were negative after a few days, the patient was discharged; the infarction had been ruled out. Myoglobin is a small-molecular-weight molecule that appears in the circulating blood within several hours of infarction. The use of the myocardium-specific CK-MB and the nonspecific myoglobin molecule assist in the rapid assessment of myocardial damage. The importance of reestablishing myocardial perfusion by thrombolytic agents or angioplasty by this time made it imperative to "rule-in" patients who had acute myocardial ischemia. The need to identify evidence of myocardial ischemia in the absence of infarction led to the frequent use of angiocardiography in the early care of patients with acute symptomatology.

A less invasive approach in the evaluation of coronary perfusion is the early use of the radioisotopes, such as sestamibi. The isotope measures flow but cannot distinguish between recent and old coronary disease. This technique, together with measurement of CK-MB and myoglobin, make it possible to rule in acute myocardial ischemia with great accuracy.

THE CHEST PAIN EVALUATION UNIT

The introduction to the Fourth Edition of this text emphasized the convergence of economic and patient care imperatives that culminated in the acute care unit. An important critical pathway in the ED serves to identify patients with acute ischemic heart disease. More than 3 million patients are hospitalized yearly in the United States. Each year nearly 500,000 people die of the disease. The costs for patients found to be free of acute MI is more than $4 billion each year. The chest pain evaluation units (CPEUs) appear able to perform diagnosis of acute disease and reduce overall cost, but these units are far from perfect. There is still substantial misdiagnosis of ischemic heart disease; allegation of missed MI has become the most common cause of litigation in the ED. In a study reported by Roberts and coworkers,[21] the hospital admission rate was 45.2% in patients entered into the accelerated diagnostic protocol patients but 100% in the control group. The hospital saved $567 in total costs per patient.[20]

The need to rule in patients with either unstable angina or acute MI requires the use of chest pain protocols that use state-of-the-art techniques, such as measurement of myoglobin concentrations and radioisotopic scanning. The protocol for chest pain in the Appendix was developed by Drs. Robert Jessee (Cardiology), James Tatum (Radiology), and Joseph Ornato (Emergency Medicine) from the Medical College of Virginia, and has proved to be a rapid, sensitive, and specific way to identify myocardial ischemia.

References

1. Wiggers CA: Physiology of Shock. Chapter 51. New York, The Commonwealth Fund, 1950.
2. Sobel BE, Shell WE: Jeopardized, blighted, and necrotic myocardium. Circulation 1973; 47:215–216.
3. National Center for Health Statistics, United States, 1993. Hyattsville, Md, Public Health Service, 1994.
4. Mueller HS, Ayres SM: Propranolol decreases sympathetic nervous system activity reflected by plasma catecholamines. J Clin Invest 1980; 65:338–346.
5. Ayres SM, Grace WJ: Inappropriate ventilation and hypoxemia as causes of cardiac arrhythmias: The control of arrhythmias without antiarrhythmic drugs. Am J Med 1969; 46:495–505.
6. Karpick KM, Pratt PC, Asmundson T: Pathologic findings in respiratory failure: Goblet cell metaplasia, alveolar damage, and myocardial infarction. Ann Intern Med 1970; 72:189–197.
7. Ayres SM, Mueller HM: Hypoxemia, hypercapnia, and cardiac arrhythmias: The importance of regional abnormalities of vascular distensibility. Chest 1973; 63:981–985.
8. Smith HW: From Fish to Philosopher. Boston, Little, Brown & Co, 1973.
9. Mueller HS, Ayres SM, Gregory JJ, et al: Hemodynamics, coronary blood flow, and myocardial metabolism in coronary shock. J Clin Invest 1970; 49:1885–1902.
10. Obrastzow ND, Straschesko ND: Zur kenntnis der thrombose der

koronarterien des herzens. Z Klin Med 1910; 71:116. (Russian original in Russk Vrach, reproduced in Z Klin Med (Mosk) 1949; 27:15.
11. Herrick JB: Clinical features of sudden occlusion of the coronary artery. JAMA 1912; 59:2015.
12. Pardee HEB: An electrocardiographic sign of coronary artery obstruction. Arch Intern Med 1920; 26:244–255.
13. Levine, HD, Ford RV: Subendocardial infarction: Report of six cases and critical review of the literature. Circulation 1950; 1:246–263.
14. LaDue JS: Wroblewski F, Karmen A: Serum glutamic oxaloacetic transaminase activity in human acute transmural myocardial infarction. Science 1954; 120:497–499.
15. Scheinman MM, Abbott JA: Clinical significance of transmural versus nontransmural electrocardiographic changes in patients with acute myocardial infarction. Am J Med 1973; 55:602–607.
16. Lown B, Vassaux C, Hood WB, et al: Unresolved problems in coronary care. Am J Cardiol 1967; 20:494–508.
17. Rigo P, Taylor DR, Weisfeldt ML, et al: Hemodynamic and prognostic findings in patients with transmural and nontransmural infarction. Circulation 1975; 51:1064–1070.
18. DeWood MA, Sports J, Notske MD, et al: Prevalence of total coronary occlusion during the early hours of transmural myocardial infarction. N Engl J Med 1980; 303:897–902.
19. Falk E: Unstable angina with fatal outcome: Dynamic coronary thrombosis leading to infarction and/or sudden death—autopsy evidence of recurrent mural thrombosis with peripheral embolization culminating in total vascular occlusion. Circulation 1985; 71:699–708.
20. Boden WE, O'Rourke RA, Crawford MH: Outcomes in patients with acute non–Q wave myocardial infarction randomly assigned to an invasive and conservative management strategy. N Engl J Med 1998; 338:1785–1792.
21. Roberts RR, Zalenski RJ, Mensah EK, et al: Costs of an emergency department based-accelerated diagnostic protocol vs. hospitalization in patients with chest pain. JAMA 1997; 278:1670–1676.

APPENDIX FOR CHAPTER 11

Medical College of Virginia: Acute Care Cardiology Program

Robert Jesse, MD, PhD
James Tatum, MD
Joseph Arnato, MD
Michael Kontos, MD
F. Philip Anderson, PhD
Charlotte Roberts, RN, ACNP

CHEST PAIN PROTOCOL

Purpose

To provide a comprehensive program for the evaluation of patients presenting with chest pain or symptoms suggestive of myocardial ischemia. It is by design:

1. *Inclusive.* All patients presenting with chest pain must be included in the evaluation process. Because of the poor sensitivity and specificity of presenting symptoms and initial electrocardiogram (ECG) to accurately predict the occurrence of myocardial ischemia and/or infarction, the system begins the evaluation of all patients as potential acute MI candidates until this is ruled out and subsequent risk stratification has been assigned.
2. *Rapid.* Triage and initial treatment must be completed within 30 minutes. This goal is mandated by the need to initiate revascularization in acute MI patients in this time frame.
3. *Safe.* Current standards result in approximately 5% of acute MI patients being sent home from the ED. This is unacceptable, and the goal of this program is that no such patient should ever be permitted to escape detection and treatment.
4. *Inexpensive.* This program is designed to be both cost effective and to improve resource utilization.

It is important to recognize that the program exists as a comprehensive strategy composed of several integrated components. No one test holds significant value in and of itself; only in the context of the overall strategy does it have its full impact.

Location

The evaluation of patients presenting with symptoms suggestive of a possible ischemic cardiac etiology has been established as a cooperative program involving acute care cardiology, emergency medicine, clinical pathology, and nuclear cardiology. It is a "systems management" approach to the problem of chest pain and is, for all practical purposes, independent of venue.

Entry

The point of entry into the protocol for most patients will be the ED. However, the system is designed such that entry can be any health care environment where an initial assessment, including an ECG, can be performed. This leaves open the possibility for patients to arrive from Medical College of Virginia hospital wards and clinics as well as direct referrals from outside health care systems, such as physician offices, workplace clinics, and others.

Protocol

The evaluation of a patient's chest pain is driven by risk and probability. Upon arrival into the program, each patient is assigned into one of five levels, which are defined by the risk for occurrence of acute MI and the probability of cardiac ischemia. Track assignment triggers a "critical path," including defined order sets; then, if at any time the work-up becomes positive the level is increased to one of higher risk. When there is doubt as to the appropriate level, the rule is to err to the higher level. The goal is to have the initial assessment and track assignment completed in 30 minutes or less.

Evaluation of chest pain thus can be approached with defined goals and expectations. A full description of the entry criteria, diagnostic strategies, and treatment protocols is provided in detail in Appendix Table AP–1). Note that patients at levels 4 and 5 are evaluated solely in the ED, whereas patients at levels 1 and 2 are admitted to the critical care unit (CCU). Level 3 patients are evaluated in the CCU in a "fast-track," rule-out protocol; if results are normal, the patients can be sent home with follow-up outpatient stress testing and considered as never having been admitted.

Thus, any person presenting to the ED with chest pain ought to know within 30 minutes whether he or she is categorized as having a high, intermediate, or low risk for acute MI:

1. If considered at high risk (levels 1 and 2), the patient is admitted to the CCU with the diagnosis of acute MI or unstable angina, and appropriate therapy is initiated.
2. If judged to be at intermediate risk (level 3), the patient is placed in a fast-track, rule-out protocol. If all test results are normal, the patient can be sent home directly from the CCU in less than 23 hours.

TABLE AP11–1. Evaluation of Chest Pain

Level	Risk	Presumptive Diagnosis	Decision	Disposition
1	High	AMI	20 min	Admit to CCU
2		Unstable Angina/Probable AMI	20 min	Admit to CCU
3	Intermediate	Probable Unstable Angina/Possible AMI	<10 hr	CCU–Fast Track
4	Low	Possible Unstable Angina	<4 hr	ED evalution
5		Non-Cardiac Chest Pain	60 min	As Indicated

3. If the patient is considered at low risk (level 4), a single diagnostic procedure, resting myocardial perfusion imaging, is performed in the ED. If test results are normal, the patient goes home in approximately 3 to 4 hours. If findings are abnormal, the patient is admitted to the fast-track protocol (i.e., level 2) and scheduled for follow-up stress testing the next working day (see Rationale for the Use of Sestamibi).

A WORD ABOUT THE RULE-IN STRATEGY

The traditional practice has been to use a strategy of myocardial enzymes, including CK total and CK isozymes drawn at 8, 16, and 24 hours, and lactate dehydrogenase and its isozymes drawn each 24 hours. Both of these assays use electrophoretic techniques and are thus run as a batch once or at most twice a day, relegating this to a retrospective diagnostic tool.

We believe that systematic application of new markers allows for the detection of myocardial necrosis with essentially 100% sensitivity and specificity in 8 hours or less. Thus, we now use a reflexive testing algorithm, including myoglobin, CK-MB, and troponin I, aimed at rapid and definitive identification of myocardial necrosis with the fewest tests necessary in order to minimize costs. This allows for a prospective diagnosis, and indeed, we are finding that we can identify patients initially classified as low or intermediate risk as having myocardial necrosis in 6 hours or less.

CK-MB

The CK-MB test is now performed as a mass assay. It employs a monoclonal antibody specific to the CK-MB molecule, which is then quantitated. The units are in nanograms per milliliter (ng/mL).

Remember that skeletal muscle has a small percentage of CK-MB, usually in the range of 3% to 5%. Destruction of significant amounts of skeletal muscle may result in an elevation of CK-MB, which means that there must be a correction to the total CK. Therefore, the total CK activity, now expressed in International Units (IU), is also measured. The comparison is then made between total CK activity and CK-MB mass to give a "relative index":

$$\text{relative index} = \frac{\text{CK-MB mass (ng/mL)}}{\text{CK} - \text{total (IU)}} \times 100$$

The upper limit of normal for CK-MB is 8 ng/mL, and for the relative index it is 4 (no units). This may cause some confusion, but one can keep in mind that an isolated CK-MB elevation must be accompanied by an elevation of the relative index to be considered positive for myocardial necrosis.

We have found, in the setting of infarction, that the CK-MB mass is almost invariably detected by the 6-hour sample, if not sooner. It is interesting that these elevations are often not dramatic and that they occur in the absence of significant elevations of the total CK.

Myoglobin

Myoglobin is a protein that is present in both skeletal and cardiac muscle. Because there is no distinction between the two forms, myoglobin is not specific for myocardial necrosis. However, myoglobin is a relatively low-molecular-weight protein and is released into the systemic circulation very early following myocardial injury, often detectable within the first hour. The lack of specificity is offset by a very high level of sensitivity, and when paired with CK-MB mass, it can provide virtually 100% sensitivity and specificity.

Our experience with this strategy, both in pilot studies and through several months of clinical application, indicate that myoglobin testing is extremely accurate. It can rule in myocardial necrosis within 6 hours and, in some cases, can prospectively rule in acute MI within a few hours after onset of symptoms.

RATIONALE FOR THE USE OF SESTAMIBI

How to handle the lower-risk patient with a nondiagnostic ECG is one of the most difficult clinical decisions in the ED. Up to 5% of patients presenting to emergency departments with acute MI are sent home. These missed diagnoses account for more than 20% of the malpractice claims levied against emergency physicians. On the other hand, fewer than 20% of the patients admitted with chest pain are ultimately found to have an MI (i.e., rule-in) at a cost estimated to be from $5 billion to $13 billion annually.

We felt that some diagnostic tool was needed to discriminate among the lower-risk patients as to who needs to be admitted and who can safely be sent home. The markers for myocardial necrosis are not appropriate in this early setting, and unfortunately there are as yet no serum markers for the occurrence of an acute plaque rupture or intracoronary thrombus. We therefore decided to utilize a rest sestamibi scan as this discriminator. Injection of sestamibi is now available 24 hours a day in the ED.

The scan is performed approximately 90 minutes after injection.

1. If results are abnormal, the patient is admitted to the level 3 fast-track protocol or to level 2, depending on the clinical judgment of the attending physician.

2. If findings are normal, the patient is sent home and scheduled for the stress portion of the study the following day. The finding of a negative scan, especially if injected at the time of pain, appears to be a strong predictor of a favorable outcome.

Several caveats need to be discussed:

1. The sestamibi scan can provide three pieces of information: (a) perfusion, (b) wall motion, and (c) left ventricular ejection fraction (LVEF).
2. The scan is considered only a "rest" study. If findings are normal, this test must always be followed with a stress study in order to completely evaluate the presence of significant coronary disease.
3. If the initial scan is normal and the patient is sent home, on return for the stress portion the rest study does not need to be repeated. This markedly shortens the time spent in the nuclear medicine department at the time of the stress test.
4. If findings are abnormal, the patient will most likely need a cardiac catheterization. The knowledge of perfusion defects in advance in many cases allows the initial procedure to be staged as a percutaneous transluminal coronary angioplasty (PTCA). This measure can shorten length of stay, reduce complications, and result in significant cost savings.

The initiation of the sestamibi scan for ED evaluation of the lower-risk patients is resulting in fewer, yet more appropriate admissions to the CCU and increased throughput of patients in the ED.

Early sestamibi scans are also used in the level 3 fast-track, rule-out protocol. Here it is less a diagnostic discriminator as it is for additive data when the evaluation is positive. When the entire fast-track evaluation is negative, the rest portion of the stress test is already completed and the follow-up stress study can thus be expedited.

What about cost? If the rest study is negative, either in level 4 or along with a negative rule-out in level 3, the patient is meant to return for the stress portion of the study. In such cases, the billing should be for only a single stress sestamibi study, which is the appropriate test for completing the evaluation of these patients. Yet, the cost of the rest sestamibi study alone is far less than that of even a single day's admission to the hospital.

THE FAST-TRACK PROTOCOL

The goals of the protocol are as follows:

1. To rule in an acute MI and initiate appropriate treatment as rapidly as possible.
2. To rule in unstable angina and initiate treatment as rapidly as possible.
3. To rule out the presence of an acute coronary syndrome in under 12 hours.
4. To evaluate for the presence of significant coronary disease and its risk factors.

This is therefore a "rule-in" protocol more than a "rule-out" protocol. The structure involves the three components described before:

1. History, physical examination, and ECG.
2. Rapid biochemical assessment for myocardial necrosis using a strategy of myoglobin (early marker), CK-MB (intermediate marker), and troponin I (definitive marker).
3. Acute resting myocardial perfusion imaging to increase sensitivity for the entirety of the acute coronary syndrome.

The sestamibi scan, when positive, provides important perfusion and functional data that can guide subsequent therapy; when findings are normal, it supports the safety of early discharge and acts as the rest portion of follow-up stress myocardial perfusion imaging.

It must be kept in mind that these patients are in the intermediate-risk category. There is a small but significant risk of unstable angina and an even lower risk of acute MI. Patients at the lowest risk are evaluated in the ED; higher-risk patients must be admitted for appropriate treatment. We do not find that eliminating the presence of an acute coronary syndrome as the cause of the symptoms is sufficient in these patients. Thus, we recommend that the evaluation is not complete until the presence of significant coronary disease is also evaluated. The follow-up stress test is therefore an important part of the protocol that should not be overlooked.

SUMMARY

The acute care strategy described is novel, in that it takes a comprehensive look at each patient presenting with chest pain or related symptoms. All patients are initially considered as though they are having an MI until proven otherwise. The ensuing evaluation is dictated by the presenting clinical picture and the ECG. Triage levels are assigned on these criteria alone. The tests included in each level are meant to be diagnostic tools, not triage tools. Initial levels are assigned on clinical issues and the ECG alone, but the protocol is flexible enough to allow for change in levels as more information is available.

Each level is written as a "critical pathway" with defined order sets available for each level. The key then becomes to properly identify and triage chest pain patients in the ED, to improve the overall performance of the unit, and to markedly accelerate the appropriate initiation of treatment for the acute coronary syndromes.

12

Medical Toxicology in Critical Care Medicine

Gary J. Ordog, MD, FAACT
Jonathan Wasserberger, MD, FAACT

SOURCES OF INFORMATION: PROBLEMS

Much of the accumulated knowledge of medical toxicology has been based on case reports of single acute overdoses, chronic overexposure, epidemiologic studies, and animal experiments. Case reports demonstrate a temporal but not necessarily a causative relationship between exposure and health effects. This information is often confounded by the inability to exclude other causes of illness. Many patients with serious overdoses end up in the intensive care unit (ICU), where critical care intensivists combine their knowledge and skills with those of the medical toxicologist.

THE MEDICAL TOXICOLOGIST

Appropriate medical qualification, training, knowledge, and clinical experience are paramount to the medical toxicologist.

TABLE 12–1. Common Causes of Poisoning

	Western Europe	North America	Developing Countries
Childhood poisoning	Household products Pharmaceuticals	Household products Pharmaceuticals	Paraffin, traditional medicine products Snakebite, insect stings and bites
Childhood deaths	Carbon monoxide	Carbon monoxide	
Adolescent poisoning	Volatile substance abuse	Volatile substance abuse	
Adult poisoning (hospital admissions)	Analgesics Psychotropics Fewer barbiturates and nonbarbiturate hypnotics	Analgesics Psychotropics Fewer barbiturates and nonbarbiturate hypnotics	
Adult deaths (outside hospitals)	Carbon monoxide increasing	Carbon monoxide Petroleum distillate Pesticides Cleaning and polishing agents	Accidental and deliberate pesticide poisoning (agrochemicals)

Modified from Meredith TJ: Epidemiology of poisoning. Pharmacol Ther 1993; 59:251-256. With permission of Elsevier Science.

Vale[1] summarized areas of knowledge and areas of toxicology that are central to the work of the medical toxicologist. For those poison units that contain both treatment capability and information sources, the West Midlands Poisons Unit (in Birmingham) provides a model[1]:

1. Dedicated beds for the management of poisoned patients. The unit acts as a focus for the provision of expert critical care medical, psychiatric, and social care. The unit is staffed by physicians with a special interest in, and experience with, critical care medicine and medical toxicology. A consultant psychiatrist with a specific commitment to the poisons unit provides psychosocial assessment on a daily basis.

2. A poisons information service. Information is given to critical care medical practitioners and nursing staff and, occasionally, to veterinary practitioners (but not to members of the public) on the ingredients and toxicity of the many drugs, chemicals, household products, and plants available in present-day society. This service is available 24 hours a day, 365 days a year, and at all times physicians with extensive training in medical toxicology are available to provide expert advice to inquirers.

3. Expert clinical advice to critical care physicians on the management of specific cases of poisoning. In such cases all the available information—circumstantial, clinical, laboratory, and from other sources—has to be assessed in relationship to the substances and circumstances of exposure to determine a detailed plan for clinical management that will maximize the chances of the victim surviving and minimize the risk of short-term and long-term sequelae. This expert advice must be supplemented by a comprehensive collection of reference works and original papers. If necessary and appropriate, severely poisoned patients are transferred from other hospitals for more intensive and specialized treatment that cannot be provided locally even after advice from the critical care unit (e.g., a specialized center may deal frequently with and have extensive expertise with patients envenomated by pit vipers, thus becoming a tertiary referral center for this problem).

4. An outpatient advisory service. The medical toxicology unit has for some years offered an advisory service particularly on chronic medical problems that are alleged to have a toxicologic basis; many of these have an occupational origin. With increasing frequency, major industrial toxicological exposures are occurring, often resulting in multiple ICU admissions at once.

5. Analytic support both for the unit and the surrounding region. A close working relationship exists between the critical care medical, medical, and analytic toxicologists which strengthens and improves the quality of the overall service even further.[1]

EPIDEMIOLOGY OF POISONING

Common causes of poisoning in Western Europe, North America, and the developing countries are summarized in Table 12-1.

Exposure to Toxic Substances

There are, overall, about 4 to 5 million cases of poisoning per year in the United States. About 2 million exposures are reported each year to the American Association of Poison Control Centers (AAPCC) Toxic Exposure Surveillance System (TESS) (Table 12-2). Many cases of recognized poisoning go unreported, and many cases of poisoning are never reported. Occupational and medical examiner data are often unreported. It is estimated that between 25% and 40% of hospitalized patients are suffering from alcohol or other drug addiction. It is because of the intoxicating nature of the drugs that individuals who use them are at high risk of trauma, which brings them into hospitals and commonly into the critical care setting. In some institutions, as many as 70% of the patients presenting with trauma are intoxicated. More than 60% of spinal cord injury patients are intoxicated. More than 50% of rattlesnake bite victims are intoxicated. The most frequently reported drugs identified in the hospital setting are cocaine and other psychostimulants, opioids, alcohol and other sedative-hypnotics, volatile inhalants, hallucinogens, marijuana, and phencyclidine and other arylcyclohexylamines.[2-15]

TABLE 12–2. Human Exposures, 1988–1991

Year	Number of Participating Poison Centers	Population Served (million)	Human Exposures Reported	Cases per Million
1988	64	155.7	1,368,748	8791
1991	73	200.7	1,837,939	9200

Data taken from Litovitz TL, et al: Am J Emerg Med 1989; 7:495-545[9]; and Klein-Schwartz W, et al: J Am Geriatr Soc 1983; 31:195-199.[10]

Toxic Exposure Surveillance System

The average child presents to a health care facility about 1.5 hours after exposure. The average adult presents to a health care facility about 3.5 hours after exposure.

Fatalities

Children younger than 17 years account for most poisoning exposures but account for only about 10% of fatalities. Fatalities in children younger than 6 years are uncommon, representing about 4% of fatalities. Common toxins lethal to children and adults are listed in Table 12–3.

A total of 764 fatalities were reported in 1991 versus 545 in 1988 (United States). In adults and teenagers, an increased frequency of deaths caused by ethylene glycol, toilet bowl cleaners, monoamine oxidase inhibitors, and isoniazid was noted in 1991. Fatal exposure associated with cocaine appeared constant from 1988 to 1991. In 1980 through 1986, the rate of mortality from unintentional poisoning in the United States increased from 1.9 to 2.3 deaths per 100,000 population. This 7-year trend appears to be explained by a 49% increase in the rate of deaths from drug poisoning. In 1986, the leading causes of fatal unintentional drug poisoning were opiates and related narcotics and local anesthetics including cocaine. Most fatal poisonings caused by other solids and liquids were due to alcohol ingestion.[3, 4]

Ingestion accounted for 75.0% of exposure routes, followed in frequency by dermal exposure, inhalation, ocular exposure, bites and stings, parenteral exposure, and aspiration exposure. The overwhelming majority of human exposures were acute (95.7%); 2.1% were chronic, and 1.7% were acute on chronic. Compared with 1988, initial decontamination procedures in 1991 demonstrated some interesting trends. Activated charcoal was used in 89,026 exposures in 1988 and in 114,563 exposures in 1993. Ipecac syrup was administered in 8.4% of cases in 1988 versus 3.7% of cases in 1991. The four most frequent substances used in a poisoning in 1988 were analgesics (10.5%), cleaning substances (10.0%), cosmetics (8.1%), and plants (6.9%). By 1993, this profile had changed to cleaning substances (10.3%), analgesics (9.6%), cosmetics (8.2%), and plants (5.4%). Categories with the largest number of deaths changed (in order of frequency) from 1988 (antidepressants, analgesics, stimulants and street drugs, sedative-hypnotics) to 1993 (analgesics, antidepressants, stimulants, street drugs, sedative-hypnotics).

Poisoning Severity Score

A guide for scoring poisoning severity has been proposed by members of the European Association of Clinical Poison Centers and Clinical Toxicologists. Preliminary studies suggest that this scoring system is an effective tool for comparing data from poison centers[13] (Table 12–4).

TABLE 12–3. Common Lethal Toxins (Toxic Exposure Surveillance System)

Children	Adults
Gases, fumes, and vapors such as carbon monoxide	Gases, fumes, and vapors
Toxic alcohols	Antidepressants
Analgesics	Drugs of abuse
Iron	Cardiovascular toxins
Antidepressants	Analgesics
Cleaning substances (through aspiration)	Theophylline
Cardiovascular toxins	

Instructions

Poisoning Severity Score is a classification scheme for cases of poisoning reported to poison information centers. This scheme should be used for the classification of acute poisonings regardless of the type and number of agents involved; however, modified schemes may eventually be required for certain poisonings, and this scheme may then serve as a model.

Severity grading should take into account the overall clinical course and be applied according to the most severe signs and symptoms. Therefore, it is a retrospective process, requiring follow-up of cases. If the grading is undertaken at any other time (e.g., on admission), this must be clearly stated when the data are presented.

Severity grading should take into account only the real clinical symptoms and signs. It should not estimate risks or hazards on the basis of parameters such as amounts ingested and serum or plasma concentrations.

Treatment measures employed are not graded themselves, but the type of symptomatic or supportive treatment applied (e.g., assisted ventilation, inotropic support, hemodialysis for renal failure) may help in the evaluation of severity. Preventive use of antidotes should not influence the grading, however, but should instead be mentioned when the data are presented.

Although the scheme is in principle intended for grading of acute stages of poisoning, if disabling sequelae and disfigurement occur, they would justify a high severity grade. If a patient's past medical history is considered to influence the severity of poisoning, comment on this. Lethal cases and occurrence of sequelae should always be commented on separately when data are presented.

Regional Poison Control Centers

Since 1978, AAPCC has maintained standards for staffing, staff qualifications, data resources, and service provisions required to achieve designation as an AAPCC Regional Poison Control Center[16] (Table 12–5). Regional centers surpass nonregional centers in population served, call volume and call volume per capita, center staffing, medical direction, staff orientation, and center follow-up protocols.

Toxicity Gradations in Poisoning

Sibert and Routledge[17] have suggested a gradation of the toxicity of substances taken in accidental poisoning (Table 12–6). Henretig[18] has suggested a general approach to the poisoned patient (Table 12–7).

Medication Errors

Medication errors in and out of the hospital may result in unintentional poisoning. Such errors can be committed by both experienced and inexperienced staff, including pharmacists, physicians, nurses, and supportive-personnel (e.g., pharmacy technicians, students, clerical staff [ward clerks], administrators, pharmaceutical manufacturers, and patients and their caregivers).[19, 20]

Discontinued Drugs

A number of drugs have been discontinued because of safety problems (Table 12–8). There are inherent risks, both known and unknown, associated with the therapeutic use of drugs (prescription and nonprescription) and other pharmaceutical agents. The incidents or hazards that result from such risks have been defined as drug misadventures and include adverse drug reactions and medication errors. Medication errors follow inappropriate prescribing, patient noncompliance, dispensing errors, and medication administration errors. The rate of medication errors in neonatal and pediatric intensive care

TABLE 12–4. Poisoning Severity Score

Severity Grades

None (0)	No symptoms or signs; vague symptoms judged not to be related to poisoning
Minor (1)	Mild, transient, and spontaneously resolving symptoms or signs
Moderate (2)	Pronounced or prolonged symptoms or signs
Severe (3)	Severe or life-threatening symptoms or signs

Note that the signs and symptoms given for each grade serve as examples to assist in grading severity. Numeric values given refer to adult values.

	Minor 1	Moderate 2	Severe 3
Muscular system	Mild pain, tenderness	Pain, rigidity, cramping, and fasciculations	Intense pain, extreme rigidity, cramping, and fasciculations
	Creatine kinase (CK) ~ 250–1500 IU/L	Rhabdomyolysis, CK ~ 1500–10,000 IU/L	Rhabdomyolysis with complications, CK 10,000 IU/L Compartment syndrome
Skin	Local effects only Irritation, first-degree burns (reddening) or second-degree burns on <10% of body surface area	Second-degree burns on 10–50% of body surface (children: 10%–30%) or third-degree burns on <2% of body surface area	Second-degree burns on >50% of body surface (children: >30%) or third-degree burns on >2% of body surface area
Eye	Local effects	Irritation, redness, lacrimation, mild palpebral edema	Intense irritation, corneal abrasion
	Minor (punctate) corneal ulcers	Corneal ulcers (other than punctate), perforation	Permanent damage
Bites and stings	Local swelling, itching	Regional swelling involving the whole extremity	Extensive swelling involving the whole extremity and significant parts of adjacent areas Critical localization of swelling threatening airways
Cardiovascular system	Mild pain	Moderate pain Sinus bradycardia (HR ~ 40–50) Sinus tachycardia (HR ~ 140–180)	Extreme pain Severe sinus bradycardia (HR ~ <40) Severe sinus tachycardia (HR ~ >180)
	Isolated extrasystoles	Frequent extrasystoles, atrial fibrillation/flutter, atrioventricular block I–II, prolonged QRS and QT_c time, repolarization abnormalities Myocardial ischemia	Life-threatening ventricular arrhythmias, atrioventricular block III, asystole Myocardial infarction
	Mild and transient hypotension or hypertension	Hypotension or hypertension	Shock, hypertensive crisis
Metabolic balance	Mild acid-base disturbances (HCO_3^- ~ 15–20 or 30–40 mmol/L, pH ~7.25–7.32 or 7.50–7.59)	Acid-base disturbances (HCO_3^- ~10–14 or >40 mmol/L, pH ~7.15–7.24 or 7.60–7.69)	Severe acid-base disturbances (HCO_3^- 10 mmol/L, pH 7.15 or >7.7)
	Mild electrolyte and fluid disturbances (K^+ 3.0–3.4 or 5.2–5.9 mmol/L)	Electrolyte and fluid disturbances (K^+ 2.5–2.9 or 6.0–6.9 mmol/L)	Severe electrolyte and fluid disturbances (K^+ <2.5 or >7.0 mmol/L)
	Mild hypoglycemia (~50–70 mg/dL or 2.8–3.9 mmol/L)	Hypoglycemia (~30–50 mg/dL or 1.7–2.8 mmol/L)	Severe hypoglycemia (30 mg/dL or 1.7 mmol/L)
	Hyperthermia of short duration	Hyperthermia of longer duration	Dangerous hypothermia or hyperthermia
Liver	Minimal rise in serum enzymes (AST, ALT ~2–5 × normal)	Rise in serum enzymes (AST, ALT ~5–50 × normal) but no diagnostic biochemical (e.g., ammonia, clotting factors) or clinical evidence of liver dysfunction	Rise in serum enzymes (50 × normal) or biochemical (e.g., ammonia, clotting factors) or clinical evidence of liver failure
Kidney	Minimal proteinuria/hematuria	Hematuria Renal dysfunction (e.g., oliguria, polyuria, serum creatinine ~200–500 mmol/L)	Massive proteinuria/hematuria Renal failure (e.g., anuria, serum creatinine >500 mmol/L)

Table continued on following page

TABLE 12–4. Poisoning Severity Score *Continued*

Severity Grades

None (0)	No symptoms or signs; vague symptoms judged not to be related to poisoning
Minor (1)	Mild, transient, and spontaneously resolving symptoms or signs
Moderate (2)	Pronounced or prolonged symptoms or signs
Severe (3)	Severe or life-threatening symptoms or signs

Note that the signs and symptoms given for each grade serve as examples to assist in grading severity. Numeric values given refer to adult values.

	Minor 1	Moderate 2	Severe 3
Blood	Mild hemolysis Mild methemoglobinemia (metHb ~10–30%)	Methemoglobinemia (metHb ~ 30–50%) Coagulation disturbances without bleeding Anemia, leukopenia, thrombocytopenia	Massive hemolysis Severe methemoglobinemia (metHb >50%) Coagulation disturbances with bleeding Severe anemia, leukopenia, thrombocytopenia
Gastrointestinal tract	Vomiting, diarrhea, pain	Pronounced or prolonged vomiting, diarrhea, pain	Massive hemorrhage, perforation
	Irritation, first-degree burns, minimal ulcerations in the mouth	First-degree burns of critical localization or second- and third-degree burns in restricted areas	More widespread second- and third-degree burns
	Dysphagia	Severe dysphagia	
	Endoscopy: erythema, edema	Endoscopy: ulcerative transmucosal lesions	Endoscopy: ulcerative transmural lesions, circumferential lesions, perforation
Respiratory system	Irritation, coughing, breathlessness, mild dyspnea, mild bronchospasm	Prolonged coughing, bronchospasm, dyspnea, stridor, hypoxemia requiring extra oxygen	Manifest respiratory insufficiency (due to severe bronchospasm, airway obstruction, edema, pulmonary edema, adult respiratory distress syndrome, pneumonitis, pneumonia, pneumothorax)
	Chest film: abnormal with minor or no symptoms	Chest film: abnormal with moderate symptoms	Chest film: abnormal with severe symptoms
Nervous system	Drowsiness, vertigo, tinnitus, ataxia	Unconsciousness with appropriate response to pain	Deep coma with inappropriate response to or unresponsive to pain
		Brief apnea, bradypnea	Respiratory depression with insufficiency
	Restlessness	Confusion, agitation, hallucinations, delirium	Extreme agitation
		Infrequent, generalized, or focal seizures	Frequent, generalized seizures, status epilepticus, opisthotonos
	Mild extrapyramidal symptoms	Pronounced extrapyramidal symptoms	
	Mild cholinergic/anticholinergic symptoms		Pronounced cholinergic/anticholinergic symptoms
	Paresthesia	Localized paralysis not affecting vital functions	Generalized paralysis or paralysis affecting functions
	Mild visual or auditory disturbances	Visual and auditory disturbances	Blindness, deafness

From Mitchell L-J, Dexter EM, Bradberry SM, et al: Assessment of IPCS/CEC/EAPCTT; Dexter EM, Michell L-J, Casey PB: The role and value of phonetoxscore in cases of poisoning. Phonetoxscore by staff of the PNPIS (Birmingham Centre) (Abstract Nos. 0.83 and 0.84). *In:* Proceedings, XVIth International Congress of the European Association of Poison Centres and Clinical Toxicologists, Vienna, April 12, 1994; and Ellenhorn M: Medical Toxicology. 2nd ed. Baltimore, Williams & Wilkins, 1997.

ALT = alanine transaminase; AST = aspartate transaminase; HR = heart rate; metHb = methemoglobin.

TABLE 12–5. Regional Poison Control Center

Region	Region has comprehensive analytical toxicology services
Geographically defined	Regional transport facilities for patients
Population base 1,000,000 to 10,000,000	Regional data collection
Regional poison information service	Medical records
Continuous availability	Participation in large-scale data collection programs
Comprehensive information	Regional tabulation of experience
Written protocols	Education programs
Qualified staff	For health professionals
Regional treatment capabilities	For lay public
Knowledge of medical facilities within region	

From Geller RJ, Fisher JG III, Leeper JD, Ranganathon S: American Poison Control Centers: Still not all the same? Ann Emerg Med 1988; 17:599–603.

admissions was as high as 1 per 6.8 admissions (14.7%) in one study. Prescribing errors with potential for "severe" or "serious" adverse consequences were recently reviewed in a tertiary care teaching hospital, where 57.7% of prescribing errors were rated as having the potential to produce adverse consequences[21–33] (Table 12–9). Some look-alike or sound-alike medication pairs have been listed by Janda[34] (Table 12–10). Types of medication errors are summarized in Table 12–11.[19] Many adults and elderly patients are potential poisoning victims because of their inability to read and comprehend label instructions.[34, 35]

Ten-Times-Higher Errors

One of every four doses computed by 95 registered nurses in one study contained an error that would result in the administration of an amount that was 10 times higher or lower than the dose ordered. Eleven pediatricians given the same test made errors at the rate of one of every 26 computations attempted.[36, 37] A prospective study subsequently confirmed a 10-fold error rate in administration of drug doses.[38] Suggested solutions to this problem include (1) banning the decimal point[39] and (2) preparing a "Code Med" card that can be placed at the bedside or prominently in the chart.[40] Each institution, if it chooses, needs to prepare this type of card according to the local practice and available stock solutions. Additional suggestions include written tests for certification of all personnel involved in drug dosage preparation and administration and routine double-checking of medications with a narrow therapeutic index before their administration.[41]

BASIC APPROACH TO THE POISONED PATIENT

Decontamination of the Patient

Eye Contamination

Immediately irrigate copiously for at least 15 to 20 minutes with neutralizing solution (e.g., normal saline or water). Do not use acid or alkaline irrigating solution. The pH of the conjunctival fluid should be checked every 5 minutes and irrigation continued until the pH remains at 7.0 for 5 minutes or longer (for both acids and alkalis). Irrigating lenses, inserted into the conjunctival sacs, can aid in the irrigation process, but obtaining them should not delay the immediate initiation of irrigation. Alkali corneal burns are ophthalmologic emergencies requiring immediate consultation from an ophthalmologist.

Skin Contamination

Cutaneous absorption is a common occurrence; one in four industrial substances represents an appreciable hazard for skin absorption. Cutaneous absorption depends on several factors, such as lipid solubility, skin condition, location, caustic effect, physical conditions, and the presence of certain vehicles (dimethyl sulfoxide, methanol, defatting agents). Serious toxicity has resulted from cutaneous absorption, and health personnel should be cautious about both continuing contamination and cross-contamination with such toxic substances as parathion and other organophosphates, organic metal compounds (e.g., lead), aniline, phenol, hydrocyanic acid, and ethylene dibromide.

Treatment

1. Irrigate the area covered by a corrosive substance copiously with water or saline as soon as possible after exposure, and continue irrigating at least 15 minutes.
2. Do not use neutralizing substances.
3. Be sure to remove all contaminated clothes (e.g., diaper in bleach ingestion), because damage is related both to concentration and to duration of exposure.
4. For potentially toxic substances subject to skin absorption, health personnel should wear impermeable gloves and gowns.
5. Exposed persons should rinse with cold water and then wash thoroughly (including skinfolds, nail beds, and hair) with a nongermicidal soap. Green soap is highly effective but often not available. Repeat the rinse with cold water.
6. The process should be repeated twice more.
7. Some chemical exposures require special treatment. Lime (calcium oxide) and cement exposures are treated like alkali burns. In burns caused by flammable metals (e.g., lithium, sodium), large particles are removed and the exposed surface is covered with mineral oil. Application of polyethylene decreases tissue penetration in burns caused by phenols (cresols). Copper sulfate solution improves debridement and reduces toxicity of white phosphorus burns. For hydrofluoric acid burns, use of intradermal or intra-arterial calcium gluconate decreases tissue necrosis.
8. Chemical spills should be handled by specially trained teams (e.g., HAZMAT teams) when they are available. In contrast to human skin decontamination, water is no longer used to neutralize and wash away a spill. Priorities of cleanup have shifted to containment, absorption, and dilution.

Toxic Syndromes

The most common toxic poisoning syndrome groups likely to be encountered in an emergency department[42] are listed in Table 12–12.

The European Association of Poison Centers and Clinical Toxicologists has organized a working party to evaluate the usefulness of scales (e.g., Glasgow Coma Scale) when they are applied to poisonings.[43, 44] The following conclusions were drawn:

1. There is no merit in attempting to define individual symptoms and signs.
2. No single grading system is adequate for all situations in clinical toxicology, but this does not invalidate the benefits of a generally applicable severity grading scheme.
3. Parameters for data collection from telephone calls cannot be the same as the requirements in ICUs. Therefore, two grading schemes are necessary—one simple and one detailed—but both using the same systematic basis.
4. The grading criteria require modification for application to pediatric cases.
5. Any scale that is adopted must be applicable for longer periods than the first 24 hours.
6. Severity scales based on therapeutic intervention have

TABLE 12–6. Guide to Toxicity of Substances Taken in Accidental Poisoning

Low Toxicity

MEDICINES

- Antacids
- Antibiotics (except ciprofloxacin, sulfasalazine, and chloramphenicol)
- Calamine
- Oral contraceptives
- Vitamin preparations that do not contain iron
- Zinc oxide creams

HOUSEHOLD PRODUCTS

- Chalks and crayons
- Emulsion paints and water paints
- Fabric softeners
- Plant foods and fertilizers
- Silica gel
- Toothpaste
- Wallpaper paste
- Washing powder (except dishwasher powder)

PLANTS

- Begonia
- Cacti
- Cotoneaster
- Cyclamen
- Honeysuckle
- Mahonia
- Rowan
- Pyracantha
- Spider plant
- Sweet pea

Intermediate Toxicity

MEDICINES

- Antihistamines (most)
- Cough medicines (most)
- Fluoride
- Ibuprofen
- Laxatives
- Lignocaine gel
- Paracetamol elixir
- Salbutamol
- Thyroxine

HOUSEHOLD PRODUCTS

- Alcohol-containing colognes, aftershaves, and perfumes
- Bleach
- Detergents
- Disinfectants (most)
- Mercury thermometers
- Nail varnish remover
- Paints (oil-based)
- Pyrethrins
- Talc (if not inhaled)
- Rat or mouse poison
- Window cleaners

PLANTS

- Berberis
- Dieffenbachia (dumb cane)
- Fuchsia
- Holly
- Mistletoe
- Philodendron

Potentially Very Toxic Substances

MEDICINES

- Barbiturates
- Benzodiazepines
- Carbamazepine
- Clonidine
- Digoxin
- Diphenoxylate (Lomotil)
- Hyoscine
- Iron
- Lithium
- Mefenamic acid (Ponstan)
- Metoclopramide
- Mianserin (Bolvidon)
- Opiates (including codeine and cough medicines containing codeine)
- Paracetamol tablets
- Phenothiazines
- Phenytoin
- Quinine
- Salicylates
- Theophyllines
- Tricyclic antidepressants (including doxepin and amitriptyline) and monoamine oxidase inhibitors

HOUSEHOLD PRODUCTS

- Acids
- Alcoholic beverages
- Alkalis (including dishwasher powder and denture cleaner)
- Bottle-sterilizing tablets
- Camphor and camphorated oil
- Carbon monoxide
- Cetrimide
- Disk batteries
- Essential oils (e.g., real turpentine, pine oil, citronella, and eucalyptus)
- Ethylene glycol (antifreeze)
- Methanol
- Methylene chloride (paint stripper)
- Organochloride insecticides
- Organophosphate and carbonate insecticides
- Paradichlorobenzene mothballs
- Paraquat and other weed killers (phenoxyacetic acids)
- Petroleum distillates (white spirit, kerosene, or turpentine substitute)
- Phenolic compounds
- Slug pellets (metaldehyde)

PLANTS

- Arum lily
- Deadly nightshade
- Laburnum
- Yew

Adapted from Sibert R, Routledge PA: Accidental poisoning in children: Can we admit fewer children with safety? Arch Dis Child 1991; 66:263–266. Reprinted with permission of the BMJ Publishing Group.

TABLE 12–7. General Approach to the Poisoned Patient

Initial Life-Support Phase

Airway	Emphasis on protective reflexes
Breathing	Adequate tidal volume
	ABG?
Circulation	Early IV access
Disability	Level of consciousness
	Pupillary size, reactivity
Drugs	Dextrose (± rapid bedside test)
	Oxygen
	Naloxone
	Other ALS medications, as needed
Decontamination	
Ocular	Copious saline lavage
Skin	Copious water, then soap and water
GI	Copious saline lavage

Evaluation and Detoxification Phase

History	Brief, focused
Known toxin	Estimate amount
	Elapsed time
	Early symptoms
	Home treatment
	Significant past medical history

Suspected but unknown toxin—consider if:

Patient	Acute onset
	Age 1–5 yr
	Past history of pica ingestions
	Current household "stress"
	Multiorgan system dysfunction
	Altered mental status
	Puzzling clinical picture
	Past psychiatric history
	Past overdoses
	History of depression
	History of drug abuse
Family	Medications at home
	Recent illness (under treatment)
Social	Grandparents visiting
	Holiday parties and the like

Physical Examination

Vital signs (include core temperature)

Level of consciousness, neuromuscular status

Eyes	Pupils, extraocular movements, fundi
Mouth	Corrosive lesions, odors, hydration of mucous membranes
Cardiovascular	Rate, rhythm, perfusion
Respiratory	Rate, chest excursion, air entry, auscultatory signs
GI	Motility, corrosive effects
Skin	Color, bullae or burns, autonomic signs
Odors	Breath, clothing

Laboratory (individualize)

CBC, co-oximetry
ABG, serum osmolarity
ECG/cardiac monitor
Chest film, abdominal film
Electrolytes, BUN/creatinine, glucose, calcium, liver function tests
Rapid overdose toxicologic screen
Quantitative toxicology tests (especially acetaminophen)
Assessment of severity/diagnosis
Clinical findings
Laboratory abnormalities (anion, osmolal gaps?)
Toxidromes
Specific detoxification
Reassess ABCDs

Institute GI decontamination (if not already under way)
Antidotal therapy, if indicated
Consider excretion enhancement
Supportive care

From Henretig FM: Special considerations in the poisoned pediatric patient. Emerg Med Clin North Am 1994; 12:549–567.

ALS = advanced life support; ABG = arterial blood gas; CBC = complete blood count; ECG = electrocardiogram; BUN = blood urea nitrogen; GI = gastrointestinal; IV = intravenous.

TABLE 12–8. New Chemical Entities and New Biologic Entities Approved and Subsequently Discontinued in Light of a Safety Question in the United Kingdom, the United States, or Spain, 1974 through 1993

Drug	Trade Names*	Country	Therapeutic Class	Safety Issue
Azaribine	Triazure	U.S.	Antipsoriatic	Thromboembolism
Bendazac	Bendalina	Spain	Anti-inflammatory, for prevention of cataracts	Liver damage
Benoxaprofen	Opren, Oraflex, Bexopron	U.K., U.S., Spain	Anti-inflammatory	Liver damage, serious skin reactions
Cianidanol	Catergen	Spain	Hepatoprotector	Hemolytic anemia
Cinepazide	Vasolande, Arteripax	Spain	Vasodilator	Agranulocytosis
Dilevalol	Unicard	U.K.	β-Blocker, vasodilator	Liver damage
Encainide	Enkaid	U.K., U.S.	Antiarrhythmic	Proarrhythmic effect
Fenclofenac	Flenac	U.K.	Anti-inflammatory	Serious skin reactions, carcinogenicity in animals
Feprazone	Methrazone	U.K.†	Anti-inflammatory	Serious skin reactions, multiple problems
Flosequinan	Manoplax	U.K., U.S.	Vasodilator	Increased mortality
Gangliosides	Nevrotal	Spain	"Neurotrophic," treatment of neuritis	Acute polyneuropathy
Indoprofen	Flosint, Flosin	U.K., Spain	Anti-inflammatory	Carcinogenicity in animals, multiple problems
Isoxicam	Pacyl	Spain	Anti-inflammatory	Serious skin reactions
Nebacumab	Centoxin	U.K., Spain	Monoclonal antibody for treatment of septic shock	Increased mortality in a subgroup of patients
Nomifensine	Merital, Alival	U.K., U.S., Spain	Antidepressant	Hemolytic anemia
Perhexiline	Pexid	U.K., Spain	Vasodilator, antianginal	Peripheral neuropathy, liver damage
Pirprofen	Rengasil	Spain	Anti-inflammatory	Gastrointestinal toxicity, liver damage
Polidexide	Secholex	U.K.	Hypolipidemic	Toxic impurities
Remoxipride	Roxiam	U.K.	Antipsychotic	Aplastic anemia
Somatotropin	Crescormon, Asellacrin	U.K., U.S., Spain	Natural growth hormone	Creutzfeldt-Jakob disease
Suloctidyl	Loctidon	Spain	Vasodilator	Liver damage
Suprofen	Suprol, Supranol	U.K., U.S., Spain	Anti-inflammatory	Renal toxicity, lumbar pain
Temafloxin	Teflox	U.K., U.S.	Antibiotic	Multiorgan reactions
Terodiline	Terolin, Micturin, Uromictrol	U.K., Spain	Anticholinergic, calcium antagonist for urinary incontinence	Cardiac arrhythmias
Ticrynafen (tienilic acid)	Selacryn	U.S.	Diuretic	Liver damage
Triazolam	Halcion	U.K.‡, US	Hypnotic, anxiolytic	Amnesia, various psychiatric reactions
L-Tryptophan	Optimax, Pacitron	U.K.	Antidepressant	Eosinophilia-myalgia syndrome
Zimeldine	Zelmid	U.K.	Antidepressant	Neuropathy, convulsions, liver damage
Zomepirac	Zomax	U.K., U.S., Spain	Analgesic, anti-inflammatory	Anaphylactic shock, renal failure

From Bakke OM, Manocchia AM, de Abajo S, et al: Drug safety discontinuations in the United Kingdom, the United States, and Spain from 1974 through 1993: A regulatory perspective. Clin Pharmacol Ther 1995; 58:108–117.

*Only originator's or principal licencee's trade name is shown.

†Still marketed in Spain; not approved in the United States.

‡Still marketed in the United States and Spain.

TABLE 12–9. Sound-Alike (Often Look-Alike) Drugs

Acetohexamide/acetazolamide
Apronal label for acetaminophen/aprolidine
Azathioprine/azidothymidine
Chlorpropamide/chlorpromazine/clomipramine/clomiphene
Desipramine/disopyramide
Diamox/Diabinese
Lanoxin (digoxin)/Levoxine (brand of levothyroxine sodium)
Lasix/Losec (now known as Prilosec)
Norfloxacin (norflox)/Norflex
Quinidine/quinine
Stelazine/selegiline
Tolazamide/tolmetin

From Janda SM: Look-alike and sound-alike medication pairs. Vet Hum Toxicol 1994; 36:256. Additional data from references 21 to 32.

inherent problems that make them less satisfactory than those based on no intervention.

7. Severity should be graded according to the consequences that develop rather than those that might have occurred in the absence of treatment.

8. The Glasgow Coma Scale developed for trauma patients is inappropriate for acute poisoning. A new scale to encompass all types of impaired consciousness and disturbed behavior is required.

9. Inclusion of chronic health points in a scale for grading the severity of poisoning is irrelevant.

10. Analytic data should be used to identify cases in which specific treatment prevented the development of serious toxicity.

TABLE 12–10. Look-Alike or Sound-Alike Medication Pairs

Medication Pair	Reason for Potential Error
Amiodarone/amrinone	Used in the cardiac setting, look alike when written
Carboplatin/cisplatin	Both are chemotherapeutic agents, sound alike
Clonidine/Klonopin	Look and sound alike
Coumadin/Cardizem	Used in the cardiac setting, look alike when written
Glipizide/glycuride	Used for diabetes, look and sound alike, similar strengths
Hismanal/Ismelin	Similar strengths, sound alike
Furosemide (Lasix)/ potassium chloride	Similar strengths, often ordered in conjunction with one another
Loniten/Lotensin	Look alike when written, both used for hypertension
Mazicon/Mivacron	Both used in the anesthesia setting, sound alike (because of this similarity, Roche has changed the name of Mazicon to Romazicon)
Norvasc/Navane	Similar strengths, look alike when written
Paxil/paclitaxel (Taxol)	Sound alike
Platinol/Paraplatin	Both are chemotherapeutic agents, sound alike
Rifabutin/rifampin	Similar drug names, same strengths
Rimantadine/ranitidine	Similar drug names
Seldane/Feldene	Sound alike
Sulfadiazine/ sulfasalazine	Look alike when written
Terbinafine/terfenadine	Look and sound alike
Xanax/Zantac	Look and sound alike

From Janda SM: Look-alike and sound-alike medication pairs. Vet Hum Toxicol 1994; 36:256. Additional data from references 21 to 32.

The predictive value of these scales in overdose remains to be determined.

Other proposed scales include the Reaction Level Scale (RLS85),[45] Comprehensive Level of Consciousness Scale (CLOCS),[46] Clinical Neurological Assessment Tool (CNA),[47] Coma Recovery Scale,[48] Glasgow-Liege Scale (GLS),[49] Innsbruck Coma Scale (ICS),[50] and Glasgow Outcome Scale (GOS).[51] Details of these tests and scoring scales have been summarized by Segatore and Way.[52]

Drug-Induced Signs and Symptoms: A Systemic Review

Coma

Mechanisms of coma caused by exogenous toxins are listed in Table 12–13. Coma in narcotic users may be due to associated clinical problems (Table 12–14). The common pupillary abnormalities in coma are listed in Table 12–15. Skin changes in coma are summarized in Table 12–16. Mouth findings in coma are listed in Table 12–17. Agents that cause coma with pulmonary edema are listed in Table 12–18. Diagnostic and therapeutic actions in coma patients are presented in Table 12–19.

Seizures

Common causes of drug-induced seizures include drug withdrawal (ethanol, barbiturates, benzodiazepines) and noncompliance with prescribed and convulsant therapy by epileptic patients (Table 12–20). In one survey, the leading causes of seizure associated with poisoning were, in descending order, tricyclic antidepressants, cocaine, isoniazid, theophylline, and amphetamines.[53]

Status Epilepticus

Initial (emergent) diagnostic evaluation should include determination of antiepileptic drug levels; serum chemistry studies including glucose, sodium, calcium, and magnesium; and blood urea nitrogen determination. Urine and blood samples should be obtained for toxicologic screening. Oxygenation should be confirmed by oximetry or periodic arterial blood gas determinations. Lumbar puncture should be performed unless it is contraindicated by severe intracranial hypertension, suspected cerebral mass lesion, or obstructed cerebrospinal fluid flow (e.g., hydrocephalus). Brain imaging by computed tomography scan or magnetic resonance imaging scan is usually performed before a lumbar puncture in adults. Brain imaging is usually and eventually necessary in adults with new-onset seizures, children with nonfebrile status epilepticus, and all patients with uncontrolled epilepsy.[54] Meningitis is relatively rare in patients with status epilepticus. A second phase of diagnostic studies begins when the seizures have stopped or occur only intermittently and the patient's cardiovascular function has stabilized.[55]

Peripheral Nervous System Toxicity

Drugs reported to cause peripheral neuropathy are listed in Table 12–21.[56, 57]

Cognitive Impairment

Conditions predisposing to drug-induced cognitive impairment include age, brain disease, and addiction to alcohol or drugs. The elderly are at particular risk because of multiple diseases, multiple drug use, and age-associated alterations in drug-induced cognitive impairment. These impairments are especially evident after the use of benzodiazepines, centrally acting sympathetic antihypertensive agents, sedating antipsychotic drugs, opioids, digitalis, antiparkinsonian drugs, antidepressants, and corticosteroids.[58]

TABLE 12–11. Types of Medication Errors*

Type	Definition
Prescribing error	Inappropriate drug selection (based on indications, contraindications, known allergies, existing drug therapy, and other factors), dose, dosage form, quantity, route, concentration, rate of administration, or instructions for use of a drug product ordered or authorized by physician (or other legitimate prescriber)
Omission error†	Failure to administer an ordered dose to a patient
Unauthorized drug error‡	Administration to the patient of a dose of medication not authorized by a legitimate prescriber for the patient
Extra dose error	Administration of duplicate doses to a patient (i.e., one or more dosage units in addition to those ordered)
Wrong dose error§	Administration to the patient of a dose that is greater than or less than the amount ordered by the prescriber
Wrong route error‖	Administration to the patient of a drug by a route other than that ordered by the physician
Wrong rate error	Incorrect rate of administration of a drug product to the patient
Wrong dosage form error#	Administration to the patient of a drug product in a different dosage form than was ordered by the prescriber
Wrong time error	Failure to administer a medication dose within a predefined interval from its scheduled administration time (this interval should be established by each individual health care facility)
Wrong drug preparation error¶	Drug product incorrectly formulated or manipulated before administration
Wrong administration technique error	Inappropriate procedure or improper technique in the administration of a drug
Deteriorated drug error**	Administration of a drug for which the physical or chemical dosage form integrity has been compromised
Monitoring error	Failure to review a prescribed regimen for appropriateness, or failure to use appropriate clinical or laboratory data for adequate assessment of patient's response to prescribed therapy
Potential error	Mistake in prescribing, dispensing, or planned medication administration that is detected and corrected through intervention (by another health care provider or patient) before actual medication administration
Compliance error	Inappropriate patient behavior regarding adherence to a prescribed medication regimen
Other medication error	Any medication error that does not fall into one of the above predefined categories

Modified from ASHP Council on Professional Affairs: ASHP reports medication errors. Am J Hosp Pharm 1992; 49:640–648. Reprinted with permission of the American Society of Hospital Pharmacists, Inc.

*The categories may not be mutually exclusive because of the multidisciplinary and multifactorial nature of medication errors.

†Assumes no prescribing error. Exclusions would include patient's refusal to take the medication and failure to administer the dose because of recognized contraindications.

‡This would include, for example, a dose given to the wrong patient, unordered drugs, and doses given outside a stated set of clinical parameters or protocols.

§Exclusions would include (1) allowable deviations based on preset ranges established by individual health care organizations in consideration of measuring devices routinely provided to those who administer drugs to patients, or other factors such as conversion of doses expressed in the apothecary system to the metric system, and (2) topical dosage forms for which medication orders are not expressed quantitatively.

‖This would also include doses administered via the correct route but at the wrong site (e.g., left eye instead of right eye).

#Exclusions would include accepted protocols (established by the pharmacy and therapeutics committee or its equivalent) that authorize pharmacists to dispense alternate dosage forms for patients with special needs (e.g., liquid formulations for patients with tube feedings or those who have difficulty swallowing), as allowed by state regulations.

¶This would include, for example, incorrect dilution or reconstitution, mixing drugs that are physically or chemically incompatible, and inadequate product packaging.

**This would include, for example, use of expired drugs and improperly stored drugs.

TABLE 12–12. The Most Common Toxic Syndromes

Anticholinergic Syndromes	
Common signs	Delirium with mumbling speech, tachycardia, dry/flushed skin, dilated pupils, myoclonus, slightly elevated temperature, urinary retention, and decreased bowel sounds Seizures and dysarrhythmias may occur in severe cases
Common causes	Antihistamines, antiparkinsonian medication, atropine, scopolamine, amantadine, antipsychotic agents, antidepressant agents, antispasmodic agents, mydriatic agents, skeletal muscle relaxants, and many plants (notably jimson weed and *Amanita muscaria*)
Sympathomimetic Syndromes	
Common signs	Delusions, paranoia, tachycardia (or bradycardia if the drug is a pure α-adrenergic agonist), hypertension, hyperpyrexia, diaphoresis, piloerection, mydriasis, and hyperreflexia Seizures, hypotension, and dysrhythmias may occur in severe cases
Common causes	Cocaine, amphetamine, methamphetamine (and its derivatives 3,4-methylenedioxyamphetamine, 3,4-methylenedioxymethamphetamine, 3,4-methylenedioxyethamphetamine, and 2,5-dimethoxy-4-bromoamphetamine), and over-the-counter decongestants (phenylpropanolamine, ephedrine, and pseudoephedrine) In caffeine and theophylline overdoses, similar findings, except for the organic psychiatric signs, result from catecholamine release
Opiate, Sedative, or Ethanol Intoxication	
Common signs	Coma, respiratory depression, miosis, hypotension, bradycardia, hypothermia, pulmonary edema, decreased bowel sounds, hyporeflexia, and needle marks Seizures may occur after overdoses of some narcotics, notably propoxyphene
Common causes	Narcotics, barbiturates, benzodiazepines, ethchlorvynol, glutethimide, methyprylon, methaqualone, meprobamate, ethanol, clonidine, and guanabenz
Cholinergic Syndromes	
Common signs	Confusion, central nervous system depression, weakness, salivation, lacrimation, urinary and fecal incontinence, gastrointestinal cramping, emesis, diaphoresis, muscle fasciculations, pulmonary edema, miosis, bradycardia or tachycardia, and seizures
Common causes	Organophosphate and carbamate insecticides, physostigmine, edrophonium, and some mushrooms

From Kulig K: Initial management of ingestions of toxic substances. N Engl J Med 1992; 326:1678–1681.

TABLE 12–13. Coma Due to Exogenous Toxins: Mechanisms

Hypoxia

- Displacement of oxygen in blood and tissues
  - Carbon monoxide (carboxyhemoglobin)
  - Methemoglobinemia (ferrous [2^+] iron of hemoglobin is oxidized to ferric [3^+] iron and cannot carry oxygen), e.g., acetanilid, aniline dyes, chlorates, dinitrophenol, nitrites (At least 96 products may cause methemoglobinemia.)
- Displacement of oxygen in the atmosphere: carbon dioxide, butane, propane, methane

Depression of the Central Nervous System

- Alcohols—aliphatic, e.g., ethanol, isopropanol, methanol
- Benzodiazepines, e.g., diazepam (Valium)
- Anticholinergic drugs (rarely produce coma, usually delirium), e.g., atropine
- Anticonvulsants, e.g., phenytoin
- Antidepressants
  - Monoamine oxidase inhibitors, e.g., tranylcypromine (Parnate)
  - Tricyclic antidepressants, e.g., imipramine (Tofranil)
- Antihistamines, e.g., diphenhydramine (Benadryl)
- Barbiturates
- Bromides
- Opiate narcotics
- Tranquilizers
  - Major: phenothiazine (Thorazine), rauwolfia (Serpasil), lithium, butyrophenone (Haldol)
  - Minor
    - Chloral hydrate and derivatives: ethchlorvynol (Placidyl), methaqualone (Quaalude), paraldehyde
    - Piperidinendiones: glutethimide (Doriden), methyprylon (Noludar)

Acidosis

- Ethylene glycol (glycolic acid metabolite) antifreeze
- Isopropanol (acetic acid, formic acid)
- Methanol (formic acid)
- Paraldehyde (acetic acid)
- Salicylate (salicylic acid)

Hypoglycemic Agents

- Alcohol: ethanol
- Exogenous insulin
- Hypoglycemic drugs: sulfonylureas
- Isoniazid
- Salicylates

Enzyme Inhibitors

- Heavy metals: arsenic, cadmium, lead, mercury, thallium
- Organophosphate insecticides: parathion
- Salicylates
- Cyanide

Postictal

- Amphetamines
- Boric acid
- Camphor
- Cocaine
- Chlorinated hydrocarbons: DDT and derivatives
- Hallucinogens: LSD, phencyclidine inhalants
- Opiate narcotics: codeine, meperidine (Demerol), propoxyphene (Darvon)
- Lead
- Plants: yellow jessamine (*Gelsemium sempervirens*)
- Phenothiazines
- Tricyclic antidepressants
- Withdrawal from alcohol, sedatives, minor tranquilizers

Other Causes

- Spider bites: black widow, scorpion
- Shellfish poisoning
- Snake bites
- Food poisoning: botulism
- Mushrooms
- Organophosphate insecticides

TABLE 12–14. Clinical Problems in Narcotic Users Associated with Coma

Overdose: pure (rare); mixed and sedatives
Hypoxia: pulmonary edema, aspiration pneumonitis, pneumonia
Hypoglycemia
Postanoxic encephalopathy
Trauma
Seizure disorders
Sepsis
Hepatic encephalopathy

Dementias

Toxic disorders associated with reversible dementias are listed in Table 12–22.

Stroke

Stroke can be caused by sympathomimetic drugs (oxymetazoline, phenoxazoline, phenylpropanolamine, amphetamine, methamphetamine, ephedrine, pseudoephedrine, and cocaine).[59]

Impairment of Consciousness

Impairment of consciousness is associated with use of amphetamines, barbiturates, benzodiazepines, insulin, opiates, phenothiazines, and tricyclic antidepressants. Signs and symptoms relative to each drug are described in Table 12–23.

Benign Intracranial Hypertension

Drugs most often associated with pseudotumor cerebri (benign intracranial hypertension) include tetracycline, minocycline, nifedipine, nalidixic acid, vitamin A and retinoid analogs, co-trimoxazole, cimetidine, atenolol, and glyceryl trinitrate. This condition is characterized by a rise in cerebrospinal fluid pressure in the absence of a space-occupying lesion and with cerebral ventricles of normal or even reduced size. There may be diffuse cerebral edema. There are no localizing neurologic signs. In most cases the disorder is of unknown cause, but intracranial thrombosis and drugs are believed to be the most common precipitating factors.[60]

TABLE 12–15. The Pupil in Coma

Miosis	
Narcotics	Propoxyphene
Phenothiazine	Pentazocine
Ethanol	Oxycodone
Barbiturates	Organophosphates
Clonidine	
Mydriasis	
Usual; if deep coma, cardiorespiratory depression, cerebral hypoxia	
Sublethal coma	
Atropine	Alcohol
Glutethimide	Diphenhydramine
Imipramine	Anticholinergics
Cocaine	Scopolamine
LSD	
Normal	
Barbiturates (in stage II or III coma)	
Alcohol	
Nystagmus	
Barbiturates	
Phenytoin	
Phencyclidine	
Alcohol	

TABLE 12–16. Skin Findings and Relationship to Agents Causing Coma

Belladonna, datura, atropine	Dry, hot flushed face; low blood pressure, high temperature, high pulse
Organophosphates, arsenic, salicylates, LSD	Heavy perspiration
Bromides	Brown skin, acne
Carbon monoxide	Pink, but more often pale
Cyanide	Deep cyanosis, but good pulmonary ventilation
Heroin, phencyclidine, barbiturates, morphine, codeine, methadone	Needle marks
Barbiturates, carbon monoxide, methadone, meprobamate, imipramine, glutethimide, nitrazepam	Bullae

Headache

DURING DRUG USE. Headache occurs during use of the following drugs: amyl nitrate, atenolol, captopril, cimetidine, cocaine, diclofenac, dipyridamole, griseofulvin, indomethacin, isosorbide dinitrate, isotretinoin, metoprolol, nalidixic acid, nifedipine, nitroglycerin, piroxicam, ranitidine, and trimethoprim-sulfamethoxazole.

AFTER DRUG WITHDRAWAL. Headache occurs after withdrawal of analgesics, caffeine, ergotamine, and methysergide.

Depression

Drugs that cause depression include β-blockers, corticosteroids, fenfluramine, interferon-alfa, levodopa, methyldopa, methylphenidate, oral contraceptives, pemoline, and phenylpropanolamine. Additional anecdotes suggest an association with benzodiazepines, cimetidine, diltiazem, metoclopramide, nifedipine, ranitidine, and verapamil.[61] Depression can lead to suicidal ideation and overdosing with these same medications. Medications, drugs, and chemicals that cause dementia can also cause a reactive depression secondary to loss of function.

Odors

Odors are not often helpful in the diagnosis of poisoning. Some anecdotal reports are summarized in Table 12–24.

Eye

Nystagmus: phencyclidine, phenytoin. Downbeat nystagmus: lithium, alcohol, toluene, felbamate.

Aggression

Drugs that may induce or aggravate aggression include alcohol, amitriptyline, amphetamines, barbiturates, benzodiazepines, hallucinogens, opiates, phencyclidine, and propranolol.[62]

TABLE 12–17. Oral Findings and Relationship to Agents Causing Coma

Increased salivation	Dry mouth
Organophosphates	Atropine
Arsenic	Belladonna
Some mushrooms	Anticholinergics
	Narcotics

TABLE 12–18. Agents That Cause Coma and Pulmonary Edema

Heroin	Toxic fumes (e.g., polyvinyl chloride)
Methadone	Barbiturates
Meperidine	Glutethimide

Mania

Drug-induced mania is most often associated with steroids, levodopa and other dopaminergic agents, iproniazid, sympathomimetic amines, triazolobenzodiazepines, and hallucinogens.[63, 64]

Violence

Violence is behavior characterized by an aggressive assault or combativeness. It may be precipitated by a mental disease, situational frustration, or organic disease. Drugs inducing violent reactions include ethanol (intoxication, intolerance, and withdrawal), amphetamines, anticholinergics, aromatic hydrocarbons, cocaine, corticosteroids, LSD (lysergic acid diethylamide), phencyclidine, and sedative-hypnotics (intoxication or withdrawal). Factors contributing to violent behavior may include anemia, dementia, electrolytic abnormalities, endocrinopathies, head trauma, hypoglycemia, hypoxia, postictal states, and vitamin deficiencies.[65]

Hyperthermia: Drug-Induced Fever

Mechanisms of drug-induced fever and of drug-induced hyperthermic syndrome are summarized in Tables 12–25 and 12–26. In patients experiencing drug-induced fever, temperatures typically range from 39° to 40.6°C, and patients may appear inappropriately well. Drug-induced fever can be associated with low-grade eosinophilia and maculopapular rash. Temperature usually normalizes within 48 to 72 hours of discontinuation of the offending drug, although fever may persist for several days to weeks if the maculopapular rash presents as a component of the drug reaction. Dobutamine should be considered a cause of fever in patients being treated for heart failure.[66] In the patient with drug-induced hyperthermia, think of intoxication with phenothiazines, butyrophenones, haloperidol, cocaine, and amphetamines; alcohol abuse and alcohol withdrawal; and, uncommonly, salicylate intoxication.

Psychotic States

Psychotic states are induced by amphetamines, cocaine, and phencyclidine, although other psychotropic agents, therapeutic drugs, and occupational chemicals may be involved. Many patients who are violent may be paranoid schizophrenics.

Cardiovascular System

Adverse effects of drugs on the cardiovascular system are summarized in Table 12–27.

Hypertension

Hypertension may be caused by sympathomimetics (e.g., cocaine, amphetamines, phenylpropanolamine), anticholinergics, phencyclidine, scorpion venoms, and spider venoms. Other drugs associated with hypertension are listed in Tables 12–28 and 12–29.[67] An overview of the effects of chemical toxins on the cardiovascular system is presented in Table 12–30.[68, 69]

Cardiac Arrhythmias

Antiarrhythmic drugs (tricyclic antidepressants, phenothiazines, sedative-hypnotics [e.g., chloral hydrate]) include stimulants, hydrocarbons, phosphorus, carbon monoxide, and scorpion stings and spider bites (Table 12–31).

Hypersensitivity Myocarditis

The diagnosis of hypersensitivity myocarditis should be considered when new electrocardiographic changes, mildly elevated enzyme levels, cardiomegaly, or unexplained tachycardia is noted in a patient who has an ongoing allergic reaction to a drug, usually with evidence of eosinophilia.[70]

TABLE 12–19. Diagnostic and Therapeutic Actions in Coma Patients

Immediate Need	Drug or Cause	Diagnostic Test	Treatment
Hypoxia	Carbon monoxide	Blood—pink	Oxygen
	Methemoglobinemia	Blood—chocolate	Methylene blue
		Cyanide history	Sodium nitrite
			Sodium thiosulfate
Narcotics	Narcotics	Naloxone trial	Naloxone
Drug withdrawal	Narcotic	Methadone trial	Methadone
	Barbiturate	Nembutal trial	Nembutal (pentobarbital)
	Alcohol	Valium trial	Valium (diazepam)
Cholinergics	Organophosphates	Atropine	Atropine and pralidoxime
	Insecticides		
	Anticholinesterase drugs	Atropine	Atropine
	Parasympathomimetic agents, mushrooms, and plants		
Food poisoning	Botulism	History	Antitoxin
Spider bite	Black widow, scorpion	History	Antivenin
Snake bite	Pit viper	History	Antivenin
Uncouplers of oxidative phosphorylation	Aspirin	Ferric chloride	Pharmacologic
Anticholinergic agents	See Table 12–12	Physostigmine trial	Physostigmine
Metals	Arsenic, mercury	X-ray study of abdomen	Lavage, penicillamine
	Thallium	History	Ditiocarb
	Iron	X-ray study of abdomen	Deferoxamine
Sedative drugs	See Table 12–12	Drug screen	Pharmacologic
Methanol		History and drug screen	Ethanol
Sympathomimetic and stimulant drugs	See Table 12–12	Drug screen	Pharmacologic
Shellfish poisoning		Red tide history	Pharmacologic

TABLE 12–20. Drug-Induced Seizures

Antidepressants and Lithium Salts

Tricyclic antidepressants (frequent), including classic and "newer" antidepressants (mianserin, maprotiline, amoxapine)
Monoamine oxidase inhibitors

Antipsychotics

Phenothiazines
Butyrophenones (less frequent)

Antihistamines (H_1-receptor antagonist), more frequent in children

Antiepileptic drugs and their paradoxical proconvulsant activity

Central Nervous System Stimulants

CORTICAL STIMULANTS

Theophylline
Cocaine (hyperthermia and cardiac arrhythmias are factors); (body packer's ruptured cocaine-filled condoms)
Amphetamine (in high-dose "binge" users)

BRAIN STEM STIMULANTS

Pentatetrazol, picrotoxin (rarely used)
Spinal stimulants: strychnine
Nonprescription stimulants: caffeine, phenylpropanolamine, ephedrine)

Anesthetics

General anesthetics
Inhalation anesthetics
  Enflurane
  Isoflurane
Intravenous and nonnarcotic anesthetics
  Ketamine
  Etomidate
  Methohexital
Local anesthetics
  Lidocaine (at high doses)

Antiarrhythmic Drugs (Including Lidocaine)

Mexiletine
Tocainide
Ajmaline
Disopyramide (severe hypoglycemia)
Quinidine
Quinine (adulteration of street drugs)
Propranolol (after high doses)

Radiologic Contrast Agents

Opioids and Other Narcotic Analgesics

Morphine (at high doses in neonates and infants)
Meperidine (normeperidine)
Dextropropoxyphene
Fentanyl and sufentanyl
Partazone

Nonnarcotic Analgesics and Nonsteroidal Anti-inflammatory Drugs (NSAIDs)

Aspirin and salicylates (poisoning—depletion of brain glucose?)
Mefenamic acid (in overdose)

Antimicrobial Agents

β-Lactam antibiotics
Penicillin
Cephalosporins (rare)
Imipenem-cilastatin

Antitubercular Drugs

Isoniazid (overdose or therapeutic dose)
Cycloserine

Antifungal Agents

Amphotericin B, miconazole (rare)

Antimalarial Drugs

Chloroquine, pyrimethamine (both in overdoses)

Antineoplastic Drugs (infrequent)

Alkylating agents: chlorambucil, bisulfate, mechlorethamine
Antimetabolites: high-dose methotrexate, cytarabine
Vinca alkaloids: vincristine
Others: cisplatin, carmustine, asparaginase (infrequent)

Immunosuppressive Drugs

Cyclosporine (10% neurologic side effects)
Glucocorticoids (occasionally, more often when used with cyclosporine)

Modified from Zaccara G, Muscas GC, Messori A: Clinical features, pathogenesis and management of drug-induced seizures. Drug Saf 1990; 55:109–151; and Olson KR, Kerney TE, Dyer JE, et al: Seizures associated with poisoning and drug overdose: Changing patterns of causes and poison center consultations. Vet Hum Toxicol 1990; 32:361–366.

TABLE 12–21. Drugs Reported to Cause Peripheral Neuropathy

Drug Group	Predominantly Sensory Neuropathy	Mixed Sensorimotor Neuropathy	Predominantly Motor Neuropathy
Antimicrobial agents	Chloramphenicol Colistin Ethionamide Nalidixic acid Thiamphenicol	Chloroquine Ethambutol Isoniazid Metronidazole Nitrofurantoin Streptomycin	Amphotericin B Dapsone Sulfonamides
Anticonvulsants	Sulthiame	Phenytoin	
Antidepressants	Phenelzine Imipramine	Amitriptyline	Amitriptyline
Antimigraine drugs	Ergotamine Methysergide		
Antirheumatic drugs		Chloroquine Colchicine Penicillamine Gold Indomethacin Phenylbutazone	Gold
Cardiovascular drugs	Hydralazine	Amiodarone Clofibrate Disopyramide	
Cytotoxic drugs	Cytarabine Procarbazine Vincristine	Chlorambucil Vinblastine	
Gastrointestinal drugs		Chlorpropamide	Cimetidine
Oral hypoglycemics		Tolbutamide	Antitetanus toxin

From Morrow JI, Routledge BA: Drug-induced neurological disorders. Adverse Drug React Acute Poisoning Rev 1988; 3:105–133.

TABLE 12–22. Drugs and Chemicals Associated with Reversible Dementias

Drug or Chemical	Clinical Characteristics	Treatment
Major tranquilizers	Chronic confusional state; parkinsonism	Lower dose or discontinue medication
Antidepressants	Chronic confusional state; tremors; anticholinergic effects	Lower dose or discontinue medication
Sedative-hypnotics	Lethargy, confusional state; withdrawal syndromes	Lower dose or discontinue medication (taper dose)
Narcotics	Pupillary constriction; constipation; respiratory depression	Lower dose or discontinue; give naloxone HCl for depression; elderly, sensitivity to low doses in acute condition
Anticholinergic agents	Memory loss; confusional state; psychosis; dilated pupils; dry skin; tachycardia; wide variety of medications involved	Discontinue medication; give physostigmine in acute state
Antihypertensive agents	Psychomotor slowing, depression; methyldopa, reserpine, clonidine, propranolol	Switch to other agents for blood pressure control
Anticonvulsants	Sedation from barbiturates; possibly cerebellar signs with phenytoin use; toxic levels	Switch to another drug
Digoxin	Gastrointestinal and cardiac side effects; confusional state	Adjust dose
Antiparkinsonian agents	Use of levodopa, amantadine, bromocriptine; confusional state; psychosis	Reduce medication dose
Antibiotics	Use of penicillin, chloramphenicol; high doses, often decreased clearance in elderly	Adjust dose
Gastrointestinal agents	Chronic confusional state; cimetidine use; possibly extrapyramidal syndrome with metoclopramide	Adjust or discontinue
Antineoplastic agents	Asparaginase; intrathecal administration of methotrexate	Discontinue medication
Lead	Encephalopathy; motor neuropathy; headache; seizures, anemia; lead lines	Institute edetate chelation; eliminate exposure
Arsenic	Somnolence; sensory neuropathy; gastrointestinal symptoms; Mees' lines	Institute chelation; eliminate exposure
Organic solvents	Headache; lethargy; poor concentration; peripheral neuropathy	Eliminate exposure
Insecticides	Irritability; forgetfulness; organophosphates	Avoid exposure
Mycotoxins	Multiple signs and symptoms; molds	Avoid exposure

Modified from Mahler ME, Cummings JL, Benson DI: Treatable dementias. West J Med 1987; 146:705–712.

TABLE 12–23. Clinical Features of Impairment of Consciousness Caused by Drugs

Drug	Clinical State	Physical Signs
Amphetamines	Agitation Aggression Paranoia Hallucinations Dilated pupils Tremor Convulsions	Pyrexia Hypertension Tachycardia Arrhythmias
Barbiturates	Stupor Coma Pupils reactive Oculocephalic reflex absent Apnea Bullous lesions	Hypothermia Hypotension
Benzodiazepines	Stupor, rarely unarousable	Little respiratory depression
Insulin	Stupor Coma Tachycardia Dilated pupils Hyperreflexia and extensor plantar responses	Pallor and sweating
Opiates	Stupor Coma Pulmonary edema Skin cool and moist Pinpoint pupils (but reactive) Fasciculation	Hypotension Depressed respiration
Phenothiazines	Drowsiness Coma Dystonia	Hypotension Arrhythmias
Tricyclic antidepressants	Drowsiness Delirium Coma Warm, dry skin Hyperreflexia and extensor plantar responses Urinary retention Paralytic ileus	Hypotension Arrhythmias Dilated pupils

From Morrow JI, Routledge BA: Drug-induced neurological disorders. Adverse Drug React Acute Poisoning Rev 1988; 3:105–133.

Torsades de Pointes

Antiarrhythmic agents (e.g., quinidine, disopyramide, procainamide, lidocaine, amiodarone), psychotropics (e.g., phenothiazines, tricyclic antidepressants, tetracyclic antidepressants, maprotiline), and organophosphates are associated with torsades de pointes.

TABLE 12–24. Odors Occasionally Helpful in Diagnosis of Poisoning

Arsenic, parathion, organophosphate	Garlic
Alcohol, salicylates	Acetone
Carbon monoxide	Coal gas, petroleum exhaust
Methyl salicylate	Wintergreen
Chloral hydrate	Pear
Camphor	Camphor
Pesticides with parathion or organophosphates	Xylene or kerosene
Ethchlorvynol (Placidyl), paraldehyde	Pungent odor, aromatic paraldehyde
Solvent sniffing	Solvent
Paraldehyde	Paraldehyde, pungent
Phencyclidine (PCP)	Solvent
Ethanol	Fruity alcohol
Hydrogen sulfide—low concentration	Rotten eggs

Complete Heart Block

Class I antiarrhythmic agents (procainamide, quinidine), calcium channel blockers, β-blockers, digitalis, organophosphates, cocaine, clonidine, phenytoin, neuroleptic agents, and cyclic antidepressants may cause complete heart block.[71]

The Skin

Intravenous medications known to cause skin necrosis are listed in Table 12–32.[72] Compounds known to cause hypopigmentation are listed in Table 12–33. Chemical groups known to cause allergic contact dermatitis are listed in Table 12–34.

Note: The skin lesions noted here may not seem important in the critical care setting, but realization of the source of the problem as indicated will lead to better treatment of the critical metabolic problems. For example, identification of the contact dermatitis and its cause can lead to the reason that anaphylactic shock is developing.

Toxic epidermal necrolysis has been associated with butazones, hydantoins, sulfonamides, barbiturates, and antibiotics.[73] Pemphigus may be secondary to penicillamine, captopril, pyritinol, thiopronin, penicillin, rifampin, pyrazolone compounds, β-blockers, progesterone, heroin, piroxicam, levodopa, lysine acetyl salicylate, gold, phenobarbital, cephalexin, enalapril, pentachlorophenol, phosphatide, and hydantoin/barbiturate. Most of these drugs induce pemphigus rarely, considering their widespread use.[74]

Text continued on page 159

TABLE 12–25. Drugs That May Cause Hyperthermia*

Postulated Mechanism*	Commonly Cause Fever	Occasionally Cause Fever
Hypersensitivity reaction	Methyldopa (Aldomet) Penicillins Procainamide (Procamide, Procan, Pronestyl) Quinidine Sulfonamides Nitrofurantoin (Furadantin) Aminosalicylate sodium Rifampin (Rifadin, Rimactane) Streptomycin sulfate	Allopurinol (Lopurin, Zyloprim) Azathioprine (Imuran) Cephalosporins Hydralazine HCl (Apresoline) Iodides Isoniazid (Nydrazid)
Idiosyncratic reaction	Halothane Quinine sulfate (Quinamm, Quine, Quinite) Sulfonamides Quinidine Primaquine phosphate	
Administration-related reaction	Amphotericin B (Fungizone) Bleomycin sulfate (Blenoxane) Cephalosporins Pentazocine (Talwin) Paraldehyde	Streptokinase (Kabikinase, Streptase) Vancomycin (Vancocin, Vancoled)
Pharmacologic action	Antineoplastics Antibiotics†	
Altered thermoregulation	Cocaine (abuse) Amphetamines (abuse) Atropine sulfate Antihistamines Levothyroxine sodium (Levothroid, Synthroid)	Cimetidine (Tagamet) Amphetamines (therapeutic)
Unknown	Phenytoin sodium (Dilantin) Salicylates Barbiturates	

Adapted from Lipsky BA, Hirschmann JW: Drug fever. JAMA 1981; 245:851–854. Copyright 1981, American Medical Association.
*Some drugs may cause fever by more than one mechanism.
†During treatment of spirochetal disease.

TABLE 12–26. Drug-Induced Central Hyperthermic Syndromes*

Condition (and Common Mechanism)	Frequent Drug Causes	Possible Symptoms	Clinical Treatment†	Clinical Course
Hyperthermia (↓ heat dissipation) (↑ heat production)	Atropine, lidocaine, meperidine Nonsteroidal anti-inflammatory drug toxicity, pheochromocytoma, thyrotoxicosis	Hyperthermia, diaphoresis, malaise	Acetaminophen per rectum (325 mg every 4 h), diazepam PO or per rectum (5 mg every 8 h) for febrile seizures	Benign, febrile seizures in children
Malignant hyperthermia (↑ heat production)	Neuromuscular junction blockers (succinylcholine), halothane (1:50,000)	**Hyperthermia, muscle rigidity, arrhythmias,** ischemia,‡ hypotension, **rhabdomyolysis,** disseminated intravascular coagulation	Dantrolene sodium (1–2 mg/kg/min IV infusion)§	Familial, 10% mortality if untreated
Tricyclic overdose (↑ heat production)	Tricyclic antidepressants, cocaine	Hyperthermia, confusion, visual hallucinations, agitation, hyperreflexia, muscle relaxation, anticholinergic effects (dry skin, pupil dilation), arrhythmias	**Sodium bicarbonate** (1 mEq/kg IV bolus) if arrhythmias are present, physostigmine (1–3 mg IV) with cardiac monitoring	Fatalities have occurred if untreated
Autonomic hyperreflexia (↑ heat production)	Central nervous system stimulants (amphetamines)	Hyperthermia, excitement, **hyperreflexia**	Trimethaphan (0.3–7 mg/min IV infusion)	Reversible
Lethal catatonia (↓ heat dissipation)	Lead poisoning	Hyperthermia, intense anxiety, destructive behavior, psychosis	Lorazepam (1–2 mg IV every 4 hr); antipsychotics may be contraindicated	High mortality if untreated
Neuroleptic malignant syndrome (mixed: hypothalamic, ↑ heat dissipation, ↑ heat production)	Antipsychotics (neuroleptics), α-methyldopamine, reserpine	Hyperthermia, muscle rigidity, diaphoresis (60%), leukocytosis, delirium, rhabdomyolysis, elevated creatine phosphokinase, autonomic deregulation, extrapyramidal symptoms	**Bromocriptine** (2–10 mg every 8 hr PO or by nasogastric tube), lisuride (0.02–0.1 mg/hr IV infusion), Sinemet (carbidopa/levodopa [25/100] PO every 8 hr), dantrolene sodium (0.3–1 mg/kg IV every 6 hr)	Rapid onset, 20% mortality if untreated

From Theoharides TC, Harris RS, Weckstein D: Neuroleptic malignant-like syndrome due to cyclobenzaprine (Letter). J Clin Psychopharmacol 1995; 15:79–81.
*Boldface indicates features that may be used to distinguish one syndrome from another.
†Gastric lavage and supportive measures, including cooling, are required in most cases.
‡Oxygen consumption increases by 7% for every 1°F up in body temperature.
§Has been associated with idiosyncratic hepatocellular injury as well as with severe hypotension in one case.

TABLE 12–27. Summary of Adverse Effects of Drugs on the Cardiovascular System

Drugs Primarily Used to Treat Cardiovascular Diseases		Drugs Primarily Used to Treat Noncardiac Problems	
Drug	***Adverse Effect***	***Drug***	***Adverse Effect***
Digitalis glycosides	Various cardiac arrhythmias	Oral contraceptives	Thromboembolism Hypertension
Quinidine	Prolonged QT interval Intraventricular conduction disturbances Hypotension Quinidine syncope	Doxorubicin and daunorubicin (Adriamycin and daunomycin)	Nonspecific abnormalities of ST segment and T wave Drug-induced cardiomyopathy Endocardial fibrosis
Procainamide	Hypotension Intraventricular conduction disturbances Drug-induced lupus syndrome	Cyclophosphamide	Myocardial necrosis (in extremely high doses)
		Lithium carbonate	Various arrhythmias
Phenytoin (diphenylhydantoin)	Hypotension Arrhythmias Drug-induced lupus syndrome	Phenothiazines	Cardiac arrhythmias Nonspecific electrocardiographic abnormalities Hypotension
Propranolol	Congestive heart failure Bradyarrhythmias Hypotension (rare) Rebound angina (abrupt withdrawal in severe ischemic heart disease)	Corticosteroids	Delayed healing of infarcted myocardium
		Methylsergide	Endocardial fibrosis
		Potassium penicillin	Hyperkalemia
		Carbenicillin	Hypokalemia
Sympathomimetic amines	Tachycardia Myocardial ischemia	Lincomycin	Bradycardia, cardiac arrest (rapid infusion of large doses)
Diazoxide and hydralazine (parenterally)	Tachycardia Myocardial ischemia		
Prazosin	Postural hypotension (excessive first dose or rapid dose increment)		
Clofibrate	Various cardiac arrhythmias Elevation of aspartate transaminase, alanine transaminase, and creatine kinase levels Synergistic action with anticoagulants		

Adapted from Deglin SM, Deglin JM, Chung SK: Drug-induced cardiovascular diseases. Drugs 1977; 14:29–40; and Ellenhorn M: Medical Toxicology. 2nd ed. New York, Williams & Wilkins, 1997, p 25.

TABLE 12–28. Chemically Induced Hypertension

Ingredient	Common Use or Abuse	Notes
Steroids		
Glucocorticoids	Replacement therapy and symptomatic treatment of various diseases	Dose-dependent, sustained increase, mainly in systolic BP
Mineralocorticoids		
Black licorice	Candy, chewing gum, liquor	Dose-dependent, sustained increase in BP mimicking primary hyperaldosteronism characterized by hypokalemia, metabolic alkalosis, and suppressed plasma renin activity and aldosterone levels
Carbenoxolone	Ulcer medication	
9α-Fluoroprednisolone	Skin ointments, antihemorrhoid cream	
9α-Fluorocortisol	Ophthalmic drops and nasal sprays	
Ketoconazole	Antimycotic agent	
Estrogen	Contraception, replacement therapy, prostatic cancer	Mild, sustained BP elevation, more common in prostatic cancer premenopausal women; severe HT has been reported
Progesterone	Contraception, replacement therapy	
Androgens	Anabolic effect (abuse in athletes)	Mild, dose-dependent, sustained increase in systolic BP
Danazol (semisynthetic androgen)	Endometriosis, hereditary angioedema	
Anesthetics and Narcotics		
Cocaine	Local anesthetics; street drug	Transient severe increase in BP, especially when used with propranolol
Ketamine hydrochloride	Anesthetic agent	Transient severe increase in BP
Fentanyl citrate	Narcotic analgesic and anesthetic agent	
Scopolamine	Preanesthetic medication, motion sickness	
Naloxone hydrochloride	Opioid overdose	Transient BP elevation
Drugs Affecting the Sympathetic Nervous System		
Phenylephrine hydrochloride	Upper respiratory decongestant; ophthalmic drops	Dose-dependent, sustained increase in BP
Dipivalyl adrenaline hydrochloride	Ophthalmic drops	Severe HT has been reported; may precipitate myocardial event and therefore should be used with caution in patients with coronary disease
Epinephrine (with β-blocker)	Local anesthetic, anaphylactic reaction, bronchodilation, decongestant, antihemorrhoidal treatment	
Phenylpropanolamine	Anorexic/decongestant	
Pseudoephedrine hydrochloride	Decongestant	
Tetrahydrozoline hydrochloride	Ophthalmic vasoconstrictor drops; ophthalmic vasoconstrictor and nasal decongestant drops	

Table continued on following page

TABLE 12–28. Chemically Induced Hypertension *Continued*

Ingredient	Common Use or Abuse	Notes
Oxymetazoline hydrochloride	Decongestant drops	
Caffeine	Analgesia, vascular headache, beverages	Acute transient increase in BP
Metoclopramide	Antiemetic	Transient increase in BP in association with cancer chemotherapy
Alizapride	Antiemetic	
Prochlorperazine	Antiemetic	
Yohimbine hydrochloride	Impotence	Acute, dose-dependent increase in BP
Glucagon	Bowel spasm	Only in patients with pheochromocytoma
Physostigmine	Reverse anticholinergic syndrome	
Ritodrine hydrochloride	Inhibition of preterm labor	Hypertensive crisis has been reported
Monoamine oxidase inhibitors	Antidepressive agents	Mainly with sympathomimetic amines and with certain foods containing tyramine
Tricyclic antidepressants	Antidepressive	More common in patients with panic disorders
Buspirone	Anxiolytic	Mild dose-dependent increase in BP
Fluoxetine	Antidepressive	In combination with selegiline
Thioridazine hydrochloride	Psychotic and depressive disorders	Massive overdose may cause severe HT
Ions		
Sodium chloride	Food and drugs	In salt-sensitive subjects
Lithium	Manic depressive illness	Acute intoxication can cause severe HT
Calcium	Food and drugs	
Lead	Industry, paint	
Cadmium	Industry	
Mixed or Unknown Mechanism		
Cyclosporine	Immunosuppressive agent	Dose-dependent, mild-to-moderate increase in BP; severe HT has been reported
Alkylating agents	Neoplastic disorders	
Recombinant human erythropoietin	Anemia or renal failure	Dose-related mild increase in BP; hypertensive crisis with encephalopathy has been reported
Bromocriptine mesylate	Suppression of lactation and prolactinoma	Severe HT with stroke has been reported after use for suppression of lactation
Disulfiram	Alcoholism	Slight increase in BP; severe HT may occur in alcoholic-induced liver disease
Alcohol	Various	Dose-dependent, sustained increase in BP
Nicotine	Cigarette smoking	Acute transient increase in BP
Nonsteroidal anti-inflammatory drugs	Analgesic anti-inflammatory drugs	Mild, dose-dependent increase in BP

Modified from Grossman E, Messerli IH: High blood pressure: A side effect of drugs, poisons, and food. Arch Intern Med 1995; 155:450–460.

BP = blood pressure; HT = hypertension.

TABLE 12–29. Factors Associated with Hypertension or Hypotension

Hypertension and tachycardia	Amphetamines, cocaine, phencyclidine
Hypotension with bradycardia	Phenelzine, tranylcypromine, monoamine oxidase inhibitors, levodopa, bretylium, organophosphate insecticides, tricyclic antidepressants
Hypertension with normal or slowed pulse	Phenylpropanolamine
Malignant hypertension with intracranial hemorrhage	Amphetamine, cocaine, phencyclidine, phenylpropanolamine
Hypotension and tachycardia	Hypovolemia, shock, theophylline, cyanide, carbon monoxide poisoning
Tachycardia, little change in blood pressure	Lomotil (atropine and diphenoxylate), marijuana, thyroxine, theophylline (chronic)
Muscarinic syndrome	Organophosphate insecticides, bethanechol, pilocarpine
Clinical	Miosis, bradycardia, bronchorrhea, wheezing, hyperperistalsis, sweating

Systemic Lupus Erythematosus

As many as 10% of cases of systemic lupus erythematosus (SLE) are drug-related.[75, 76] Procainamide and hydralazine are the drugs most commonly implicated. A definite association has also been shown for isoniazid, methyldopa, quinidine, and chlorpromazine. Drugs less frequently implicated include many of the anticonvulsants, β-blockers, sulfasalazine, penicillamine, lithium, and antithyroid drugs. Drug-induced SLE usually occurs after long-term (6–12 months) high-dose therapy with the suspected drug. Clinical manifestations include arthralgias, arthritis, fever, rash, adenopathy, myalgias, pericarditis, pleuritis, pleural effusion, hepatosplenomegaly, and renal and central nervous system involvement. The antinuclear antibody (ANA) test response is positive. Rapid remission (unlike retinopathy in SLE) follows discontinuation of the drug. The ANA test response may remain positive up to 2 years.[77] Identifying and correcting the cause of a drug-induced SLE may be lifesaving in the critical care setting.

TABLE 12–30. Chemical Toxins and Cardiovascular Disease

Atherosclerotic Ischemic Heart Disease	***Arrhythmias***
Carbon disulfide (1)*	Halogenated hydrocarbons (1)
Carbon monoxide (3)	Organophosphates (1)
Combustion products (3)	Antimony (2)
Arsenic (3)	Arsenic (2)
	Arsine (1)
Nonatheromatous Ischemic Heart Disease	***Hypertension***
Organic nitrates (1)	Lead (2)
Myocardial Asphyxiants	Organic solvents (3)
	Cadmium (3)
Carbon monoxide (1)	Carbon disulfide (2)
Cyanide (1)	***Peripheral Arterial Occlusive Disease***
Hydrogen sulfide (1)	Arsenic (2)
Direct Myocardial Injury	Lead (2)
Cobalt (3)	Carbon disulfide (2)
Arsenic (1)	
Arsine (1)	
Lead (3)	
Antimony (2)	
Organic solvents (3)	

Adapted from Kirstensen TS: Cardiovascular diseases and the work environment: A critical review of the epidemiologic literature on chemical factors. Scand J Work Environ Health 1989; 15:245–264.

*Probability of causation: (1) definite, (2) probable, (3) possible.

Scleroderma

Scleroderma may follow use of carbidopa, mazindol, L-5-hydroxytryptophan, diethylpropion, pentazocine hydrochloride, local anesthetics, bromocriptine, phytonadione, cocaine, and appetite suppressants.

The Hypersensitivity Syndrome

The aromatic antiepileptic agents (phenytoin, carbamazepine, and phenobarbital) and sulfonamides are the most frequent causes of the hypersensitivity syndrome.[78] Other drugs, especially allopurinol, gold salts, and dapsone, are also associated with the syndrome. The syndrome typically develops 2 to 6 weeks after a drug is first used, later than most other serious skin reactions. With antiepileptic drugs, fever and rash are the most frequent presenting symptoms (in 87% of cases). Lymphadenopathy (in about 75%) is frequent and usually due to benign lymphoid hyperplasia. Atypical lymphoid hyperplasia and pseudolymphoma occasionally occur. Some of these cases resolve with withdrawal of the drug, but in some cases lymphoma eventually develops. Hepatitis, interstitial nephritis, and hematologic abnormalities, especially eosinophilia and mononucleosis-like atypical lymphocytosis, are also common.

Agents most often associated with vasculitis, serum sickness, and reactions resembling serum sickness are listed in Table 12–35.

Hair

Hair loss evident 2 to 4 months after beginning treatment can be caused by anticoagulants, retinol and its derivatives, interferons, and antihyperlipidemic drugs. Such loss is usually reversible on the interruption of treatment. Hirsutism may follow use of testosterone, danazol, corticotropin, metyrapone, anabolic steroids, and glucocorticoids. Hypertrichosis is observed after use of cyclosporine, minoxidil, and diazoxide.[79]

Ototoxicity

Diuretics and anti-inflammatory agents (e.g., salicylates) are associated with acute and transient impairment of hearing or tinnitus. Some antineoplastic agents and aminoglycoside antibiotics are associated with delayed and often irreversible loss of hearing. Lesions in the organ of Corti include destruction of auditory sensory cells.[80] Drug-associated causes of tinnitus and deafness occurring in the same patient can include erythromycin, aspirin, gentamicin, cisplatin, metronidazole, and naproxen. Deafness alone is occasionally observed after use of erythromycin, gentamicin, cisplatin, furosemide, metronidazole, and azithromycin. Tinnitus is more common with aspirin, quinine, indomethacin, sulindac, metoprolol, naproxen, and procaine penicillin.[81]

Rhabdomyolysis

Drugs

Koppel distinguishes a primary toxin-induced rhabdomyolysis (muscle disease caused by a direct myotoxic effect of a drug or toxin) (Table 12–36) from rhabdomyolysis secondary to muscle ischemia in drug overdose, which may be caused by local muscle compression in coma, prolonged seizures and myoclonus, and chronic intake of drugs that cause hypokalemia.[82, 83] Factors predisposing to the development of rhabdomyolysis are listed in Table 12–37. Table 12–38 proposes a differential diagnosis of rhabdomyolysis. Etiologic agents of

TABLE 12–31. Drug- or Toxin-Induced Arrhythmias

Rhythm Disturbance	Possible Cause
Sinus bradycardia or atrioventricular block	β-Blockers, calcium antagonists, cyclic antidepressants, digoxin and other cardiac glycosides, organophosphate and carbamate insecticides, phenylpropanolamine and other α-adrenergic stimulants
Sinus tachycardia	Cocaine, amphetamines, phencyclidine, antihistamines, anticholinergics, cyclic antidepressants, phenothiazines, theophylline, ethanol or sedative-hypnotic withdrawal, carbon monoxide
Prolongation of QRS interval	Cyclic antidepressants, quinidine, procainamide, disopyramide, encainide, flecainide, β-blockers, calcium antagonists, diphenhydramine (massive doses), phenothiazines (especially thioridazine)
Prolongation of QT interval (including torsades de pointes)	Cyclic antidepressants, quinidine, procainamide, disopyramide, encainide, flecainide, β-blockers, calcium antagonists, lithium, antihistamines (diphenhydramine, terfenadine, astemizole), phenothiazines, arsenic, organophosphates
Ventricular tachyarrhythmias	Cocaine, amphetamines, chloral hydrate and chlorinated hydrocarbons, theophylline, digoxin and other cardiac glycosides, tricyclic antidepressants

From Olson KR, Pentel RR, Kelley MT: Physical assessment and differential diagnosis of the poisoned patient. Med Toxicol 1987; 2:52–81.

drug- and toxin-induced rhabdomyolysis have been reviewed by Curry and colleagues[84] (Table 12–39).

Myoglobin

Myoglobin is a 17,500-D globular heme protein with a heme group identical to that of hemoglobin and the cytochromes. Myoglobin binds only one oxygen molecule and acts as an oxygen store, used when muscle is deprived of blood-borne oxygen. The normal level of myoglobin in serum is 3 to 80 μg/L. It has a volume of distribution of about 0.4 L/kg. Myoglobin in the circulation is bound to an α_2-globulin. It has a half-life of about 1 to 3 hours.

In patients with rhabdomyolysis and myocardial infarction, a rise in serum myoglobulin precedes an increase in creatine kinase. Myoglobin serum levels greater than 2000 μg/L are associated with renal complications. When urine is highly concentrated, particularly when the urine pH is low, acute renal failure after infusions of myoglobin is consistently demonstrated. At or below pH 5.6, myoglobin dissociates into ferrihemate and globulin. The ferrihemate causes a deterioration in renal function and is excreted in the urine. At high myoglobin urine concentrations (>1000 μg/mL), red discoloration of the urine or plasma is observed. Myoglobin can be detected in the urine with a dipstick for blood (hemoglobin) with a detection limit as low as 5 to 10 μg/mL. A negative test result for blood with use of a urine dipstick does not rule out rhabdomyolysis. Pink plasma with orthotoluidine-positive urine indicates that hemolysis and at least some hemoglobinemia is present. Urine that is orthotoluidine-positive for blood in the absence of pink plasma is due to myoglobinuria (in the absence of large numbers of red blood cells in the urine from bleeding into the urinary tract).[85]

Movement Disorders

Drug-induced movement disorders occur during the early phase of neuroleptic (antipsychotic, major tranquilizer) administration. Parkinsonism is clinically indistinguishable from idiopathic Parkinson's disease; it appears within the first 3 months, more often in the elderly (Table 12–40).

Akathisia

Cyclic antidepressants, monoamine oxidase inhibitors, fluoxetine, lithium, buspirone, and levodopa are the principal causes.[86]

Dystonias

Dystonias are associated principally with phenothiazines, butyrophenones, metoclopramide, and tricyclic antidepressants; with phenytoin, carbamazepine, and propranolol in high doses; and with antiemetics, cocaine, chloroquine, and hydroxychloroquine.

Chorea

Chorea is most commonly associated with the anticonvulsant drugs, especially phenytoin. Chorea has also been ob-

TABLE 12–32. Intravenous Drugs Known to Cause Skin Necrosis

Solutions and Electrolytes	*Chemotherapeutic Agents*
Dextrose 10%	Bleomycin
Mannitol	Dacarbazine
Sodium bicarbonate	Vinca alkaloids
Calcium salts	Doxorubicin
Potassium salts	Daunorubicin
Nafcillin	Dactinomycin
Vasopressors	Mitomycin
Norepinephrine	Fluorouracil
Dopamine	Streptozocin
Miscellaneous Drugs	Chlorozotocin
Radiologic dyes	Nitrogen mustard
Methylene blue	

Adapted from Dufresne RG: Skin necrosis from intravenously infused materials. Cutis 1987; 39:197–198.

TABLE 12–33. Compounds Known to Cause Hypopigmentation

o-Benzylchlorophenol (antiseptic)
p-Butylphenol (used in the manufacture of varnish and lacquer resins, as an antioxidant in soaps, and as a motor oil additive)
p-Cresol (disinfectant)
Hydroquinone and its monoethyl and monobenzyl ethers (used in black-and-white photoprocessing, in skin lighteners, and as antioxidants in synthetic rubbers)
o-Phenylphenol (used as an agricultural fungicide, as a disinfectant, and in the rubber industry)
Pyrocatechol (topical antiseptic)
p-Tertiary butylcatechol (astringent)

Adapted from Hall AH, Hogan DJ: Skin lesions and environmental exposures: Rash decisions. Case Studies in Environmental Medicine, No. 28. Atlanta, Agency for Toxic Substances and Disease Registry (ATSDR), May 1993.

TABLE 12–34. Common Causes of Allergic Contact Dermatitis

Germicides and biocides	Fragrances and perfumes
Formaldehyde-releasing compounds	Balsam of Peru
Parabens	Benzyl alcohol
Quaternary ammonium compounds	Cinnamic acid derivatives
Grains	Citronella derivatives
Barley	Metals
Oat	Chromium
Rye	Cobalt
Wheat	Nickel
Foods and spice	Organic dyes
Cardamom	*p*-Aminoazobenzene
Carrot	*p*-Phenylenediamine
Chicory	Plastic resins
Coconut	Epoxies
Coffee	Formaldehyde-based acrylics
Endive	Phenolics
Lettuce	*Rhus* plants*
Potato	Poison ivy
Radish	Poison oak
Tamarind	Poison sumac
Turmeric	Rubber products
Vanilla	Antioxidants
Medication/product ingredients	Polymerization accelerators
Preservatives	Topical medications
Lanolin	Benzocaine
Thimerosal	Neomycin

From Hall AH, Hogan DJ: Skin lesions and environmental exposures: Rash decisions. Case Studies in Environmental Medicine, No. 28, Atlanta, Agency for Toxic Substances and Disease Registry (ATSDR), May 1993.

*For a more complete listing of plants that cause dermatitis, see Adams RM: Occupational Skin Disease. 2nd ed. Philadelphia, WB Saunders, 1990, pp 507–509.

served with anabolic steroids, benzhexane, amphetamines, methylphenidate, pemoline, cimetidine, levodopa, and dopamine as well as ethanol, toluene, manganese, and cocaine.

Tardive Dyskinesia

Phenothiazines constitute the principal group of drugs associated with the disorder. Metoclopramide has also been suspect.

Tremor

Resting tremor is most pronounced at rest; it decreases with activity. Think of any cause of *toxin*-induced parkinsonism (Table 12–41).

Postural tremor is most pronounced with an outstretched hand. Think of all beta agonists, phenytoin, valproic acid, cyclic antidepressants, monosodium glutamate, lithium, arsenic, and alcohol withdrawal. Kinetic tremor is most pronounced with motion. Think of alcoholic cerebellar degeneration, mercury, lithium, and sedative-hypnotic intoxication.

Chorea tremor consists of repetitive dance-like movements. Think of anticonvulsants (phenytoin, carbamazepine), anticholinergics, dopamine agonists (amantadine, bromocriptine), ethanol, toluene, manganese, and sympathomimetics (amphetamine, cocaine).

Dystonic tremor consists of muscle group spasms (oculogyric crises, torticollis, tortipelvis, opisthotonos). Think of neuroleptics, antiemetics, cocaine, chloroquine, and hydroxychloroquine.

Myasthenic Crisis

Drug-induced myasthenic crisis may be associated with the aminoglycosides, polymyxin, penicillamine, tetracycline, quinidine, lidocaine, quinine, morphine, meperidine, curare, succinylcholine, and procainamide.[87] Recovery may occur within a few weeks of withdrawal of the toxic offender.

Myopathies

Drug-induced myopathies result from a direct toxic effect, which may be local when the drug is injected into a muscle or more diffuse when the drug is taken systemically. These myopathies also follow electrolyte disturbances, muscle compression, ischemia, and the development of an immunologic reaction directed against muscle.[88] Repeated injections of antibiotics or drugs of addiction often lead to severe muscle fibrosis and contractures.

Clofibrate and ε-aminocaproic acid cause an acute or subacute painful necrotizing myopathy with myoglobinuria and acute renal failure. Other drugs that induce toxic myopathies are the lipid-lowering agents, succinylcholine, halothane, corticosteroids, and chloroquine. Drugs that cause a hypokalemic myopathy include the thiazide diuretics, amphotericin, carbenoxolone, emetine, and alcohol. Inflammatory myopathies have followed use of D-penicillamine, procainamide, hydralazine, phenytoin, and penicillin. Environmental agents associated with myositis include foods (adulterated rapeseed oil, L-tryptophan, ciguatera toxin), occupational exposures (silica), and medical devices (collagen and silicone implants).[89]

Parkinsonism

Table 12–41 lists reported exposures associated with parkinsonism.[88] Drugs and toxins that induce parkinsonism include clebopride, MPTP (designer drug), disulfiram, lithium, organophosphates, metoclopramide, phenylpropanolamine, and antihistamines.[90] The most frequent etiologic factors are the phenothiazine or butyrophenone groups and the major tranquilizers.

Motor Neuron Disease

Excitatory amino acid neurotransmitters such as glutamate have been implicated in the pathogenesis of certain neurodegenerative disorders. Glutamate analogs such as β-methylaminoalanine, β-*N*-oxalylamino-L-alanine, and domoic acid are neurotoxic and have been linked to neurologic disorders in

TABLE 12–35. Agents Most Often Associated with Vasculitis, Serum Sickness, and Reactions Resembling Serum Sickness

Vasculitis
- Allopurinol
- Penicillin
- Aminopenicillins
- Sulfonamides
- Thiazides
- Pyrazolones
- Hydantoins
- Propylthiouracil

Raynaud's Disease or Digital Necrosis
- β-Blockers
- Ergot alkaloids
- Bleomycin

Serum Sickness
- Serum preparations
- Vaccines

Reactions Resembling Serum Sickness
- β-Blockers
- Streptokinase
- β-Lactam antibiotics

From Roujeau JC, Stern RS: Severe adverse cutaneous reactions to drugs. N Engl J Med 1994; 331:1272–1285.

TABLE 12–36. Drug-Induced Rhabdomyolysis

Syndrome	Primary Target	Pathogenetics	Clinical Features	Predisposing Factors	Typical Rise in Creatine Kinase (U/L)	Therapy	Drugs
Primary toxin-induced rhabdomyolysis	Striated muscle	Damage to membranes, metabolism	Generalized myonecrosis	Dehydration	10,000–100,000	Symptomatic	Heroin, doxylamine
Rhabdomyolysis secondary to: Muscle ischemia in drug overdose Chronic intake of drugs including hypokalemia	Microcirculation, muscle perfusion, and/or metabolism	Muscle ischemia	Local or generalized myonecrosis	Hypokalemia, hypophosphatemia, dehydration	Wide range	Symptomatic	Barbiturates Laxatives, thiazides, emetics
Malignant hyperthermia	Sarcoplasmic reticulum of striated muscle		Extreme hyperthermia, hypercapnia, muscular hypertonicity	Genetic (50%)	100,000	Dantrolene	Succinylcholine, halothane, caffeine
Neuroleptic malignant syndrome	Central nervous system		Rigor hyperthermia	Dehydration, psychiatric disease	10,000	Dantrolene (physostigmine has no effect)	Butyrophenones, phenothiazines, antipsychotics, cocaine, diphenhydramine
Central anticholinergic syndrome	Central nervous system		Rigor hyperthermia	Dehydration	<10,000	Physostigmine	
Drug-induced polymyositis/dermatomyositis	Vessels of striated muscle	Vasculitis	Pain, diffuse swelling of musculature		<10,000	Abstinence from the incriminated drug, steroids	Penicillamine, phenytoin, phenylbutazone, quinidine

From Koppel C: Clinical features, pathogenesis and management of drug-induced rhabdomyolysis. Med Toxicol Adverse Drug Experience 1989; 4:108–126. Modified by Ellenhorn M: Medical Toxicology. New York, Williams & Wilkins, 1997, p 29.

humans. Glutamate and its analogs act at *N*-methyl-D-aspartate (NMDA) receptors or neurons. Glycine, an inhibitory neurotransmitter, may also enhance NMDA-mediated neurotoxicity,[91–93] (Table 12–42).

The Kidney

Abuelo[106] has extensively reviewed potentially nephrotoxic chemicals, foods, plants, and animal venoms. Inhaled, cutaneously absorbed, and ingested nephrotoxic chemicals are listed in Tables 12–43 and 12–44. Nephrotoxic foods, nephrotoxic plants, and animals carrying potentially nephrotoxic venoms are listed in Tables 12–45 to 12–47.[107] Drugs that when given in excessive dose by the physician or misused by the patient have resulted in damage to the kidney are summarized in Table 12–48.[106] Drugs that have been associated with a hemolytic-uremic syndrome include cyclosporine, anticancer drugs (e.g., mitomycin), ticlopidine, and quinine.[108]

Incontinence

Medications that have the potential to cause incontinence are reviewed in Table 12–49.[109]

TABLE 12–37. Factors Predisposing to the Development of Rhabdomyolysis

Dehydration
Hypokalemia, hypophosphatemia, malnutrition
Psychiatric disease
Agitation, confusion, delirium
Endocrinopathies (e.g., hypothyroidism, diabetic ketoacidosis)
Shock, hypotension
Hypoxia, acidosis

Adapted from Koppel C: Clinical features, pathogenesis and management of drug-induced rhabdomyolysis. Med Toxicol Adverse Drug Experience 1989; 4:108–126.

Gastrointestinal Tract

Tongue

"Glossitis" and tongue ulceration have followed use of trimethoprim-sulfamethoxazole, diclofenac, naproxen, metronidazole, sulindac, amoxicillin, erythromycin, captopril, and piroxicam[110] (Table 12–50).

Pancreas

Drugs can cause acute pancreatitis, but with the exception of ethanol, drugs rarely cause chronic pancreatitis. Reports of acute pancreatitis are generally anecdotal.[106] Definite, probable, and questionable associations of drugs with pancreatitis are listed in Table 12–51.[107]

Esophagus

Pill-induced esophageal injury may follow use of tetracycline, doxycycline, ipratropium bromide, slow-release potassium chloride, acetylsalicylic acid, nonsteroidal anti-inflammatory drugs, and quinidine (Table 12–52). Symptoms of sudden onset of dysphagia, often accompanied by substernal chest pain and odynophagia, typically occur 4 to 12 hours after ingestion but may be delayed up to several weeks in quinidine-induced cases.[111] Iredale and George[112] have summarized causes of drug-induced gastrointestinal obstruction (Table 12–53).

Liver

The critical care physician should think of drugs as the etiology in the presence of raised aminotransferase activities, unexplained jaundice, acute hepatitis, chronic acute hepatitis, cryptogenic cirrhosis, "primary biliary cirrhosis" in the absence of antimitochondrial antibody, unexplained hepatic tumors (especially those not associated with cirrhosis), and liver disease of obscure cause.[113]

Hanson[114] has proposed the following criteria for diagnosis of drug-induced hepatitis:

TABLE 12–38. Differential Diagnosis of Rhabdomyolysis

Drug-induced rhabdomyolysis	Excessive muscle stress
Toxin-induced rhabdomyolysis	Marathon runners, military training
Rhabdomyolysis secondary to muscle ischemia in drug overdose	Status epilepticus, prolonged myoclonus or dystonia
Malignant hyperthermia	Agitation, delirium
Neuroleptic malignant syndrome	Physical damage
Central anticholinergic syndrome	Heat stroke
Drug-induced polymyositis dermatomyositis	Burns
Muscle ischemia	Infections
Crush, compartment syndrome, tourniquet shock hypokalemia, hypernatremia, hypophosphatemia	Viral (coxsackie, herpes, echo, influenza)
Sickle cell trait	Bacterial (*Clostridium, Legionella,* typhoid, staphylococci)
Shock and coma	Electrolyte and water imbalances
Occlusive arterial disease	Hyperosmolar states
Genetic defects	Endocrine dysfunction
Deficiencies of glycolytic enzymes	Neuropathy
Carnitine palmitoyltransferase deficiency	Polyneuropathy
	Motor neuron disease

Adapted from Koppel C: Clinical features, pathogenesis and management of drug-induced rhabdomyolysis. Med Toxicol Adverse Drug Exp 1989; 4:108–126.

1. Clinical and laboratory evidence of hepatocellular injury.
2. Onset of symptoms related in time to drug therapy.
3. Lack of serologic evidence for current infection with hepatitis A or B, cytomegalovirus, or Epstein-Barr virus.
4. Absence of an acute hepatic insult, such as septic shock.
5. Lack of evidence of chronic liver disease.
6. Absence of other concomitantly administered drugs, especially any known hepatotoxins.

The presence of fever, rash, eosinophilias, or lymphadenopathy is supportive but not essential.

Primary biliary cirrhosis has been associated with use of acetaminophen, chlorpromazine, phenylbutazone, tolbutamide, thiabendazole, benoxaprofen, and a compound containing glycyrrhizin, cysteine, and glycine.[115]

Colon

Cappell and Simon[116] have presented a comprehensive review of drug-associated colonic toxicity (Table 12–54).

Metabolic Disorders

Some drug-induced metabolic disorders are listed in Table 12–55.[117]

The Lungs

Noncardiogenic Pulmonary Edema

Many drugs have been associated with noncardiogenic pulmonary edema (NCPE).[118] NCPE is characterized by the simultaneous presence of severe hypoxemia, bilateral infiltrates on the chest roentgenogram, and normal pulmonary capillary wedge pressure with exclusion of other risk factors for NCPE. Agents known to cause pulmonary disease are noted in Table 12–56.[119] Agents associated with pleural effusion are listed in Table 12–57, and those associated with acute-onset pulmonary insufficiency are listed in Table 12–58. Henry[120] has suggested blockade of an oxygen cascade due to poisoning.

Asthma: Precipitators of Acute Bronchospasm and Exacerbations of Asthma

Drugs causing or exacerbating asthma are listed in Table 12–59.[121] Nonsteroidal anti-inflammatory drugs account for more than two thirds of drug-induced asthmatic reactions, with aspirin accounting for more than half of these. β-Blockers, cholinergic agonists, cholinomimetic alkaloids, chemotherapeutic agents, antibiotics, radiographic contrast agents, muscle relaxants, and intravenous anesthetic agents have also caused bronchospasm associated with systemic reactions.[121]

Chemicals That Cause Hematologic and Blood Problems

Agranulocytosis has followed exposure to analgesic anti-inflammatory drugs, antiarrhythmics, anticonvulsants, antidepressants, antihypertensive agents, antimicrobial agents, antipsychotic drugs, antithyroid drugs, diuretics, and other drugs (Table 12–60).[122] Some drugs and chemicals can induce a hemolytic anemia in persons with glucose-6-phosphate dehydrogenase deficiency[123] (Table 12–61).

Hemolysis

Hemolysis may follow exposure to arsine and stibine. It is also caused by direct erythrocyte binding (penicillin, cephalothin, streptomycin), binding to plasma protein (quinine, quinidine, sulfonylurea derivatives), and undetermined mechanisms (methyldopa, levodopa, mefenamic acid).

Drugs such as chloramphenicol may be associated with aplastic anemia. Drugs, foods, spices, and vitamins may cause abnormalities of platelet function and lead to bleeding problems[124] (Table 12–62).

Anaphylactic Reaction

Agents responsible for acute anaphylactic reactions are delineated in Table 12–63.[125, 126]

Electrolyte Disturbances

Drug-induced hyperkalemia may follow inhibition of potassium entry into cells (inhibition of Na^+,K^+-ATPase activity) observed with digitalis, β_2-adrenoceptor antagonists, and drugs that cause acidosis. Reduced potassium excretion is observed with potassium-sparing diuretics, angiotensin-converting enzyme inhibitors, nonsteroidal anti-inflammatory drugs, and agents that impair renal tubular function. Hyperkalemia follows renal Na^+ channel blockade (amiloride). Hyperkalemia is associated with abdominal pain, diarrhea, muscle pain and weakness, electrocardiographic changes (tall peaked T waves, ST-segment depression, prolonged PR interval, QRS prolongation), and cardiac arrhythmias (ventricular tachycardia, ventricular fibrillation).[133] Treat with glucose, insulin infusions, sodium bicarbonate, and calcium gluconate. Exchange resins and hemodialysis may be required.

Drug-induced hypokalemia follows enhanced potassium entry into cells (increased Na^+,K^+-ATPase activity induced by β_2-agonists, theophylline, insulin), competitive blockade of potassium channels (chloroquine, barium), gastrointestinal losses, and drug-induced metabolic alkalosis. Hypokalemia results in generalized muscle weakness, paralytic ileus, electro-

TABLE 12–39. Etiologic Agents of Drug- and Toxin-Induced Rhabdomyolysis

ε-Aminocaproic acid	Emetine	Neuroleptics
p-Aminosalicylate	Enflurane	Nitrazepam
Amitriptyline	Ethanol	Orphenadrine*
Amoxapine	Ethchlorvynol	Oxyprenolol
Amphetamines	Ethylene glycol	Palfium
Amphotericin B	Etretinate	Paraquat
Anticholinergics	Fenfluramine	Parathion*
Antidepressants	Fluoroacetate	Peanut oil
Antihistamines	9α-Fluoroprednisolone	Pemoline
Antimalarials	Gasoline sniffing	Pentamidine
Antipyrine	General anesthetics	Perphenazine
5-Azacytidine	Glutethimide	Phenazone
Barbiturates	Haff's disease	Phenazopyridine
Bee stings	Haloperidol	Phencyclidine
Benzodiazepines	Hallucinogens	Phenelzine
Benztropine*	Heroin	Phenformin
Betamethasone	Hornet stings	Phenmetrazine
Bezafibrate	Hydrocarbons	Phenobarbital
Butyrophenones	Hydrocortisone	Phenothiazines
Carbenoxolone	Hydrogen sulfide	Phenylpropanolamine
Carbon monoxide	Hydroxyzine*	Phenytoin
Carbromal	Iodoacetate	Phosphorus
Cathine	Isoflurane	Phosphine
Centipede	Isoniazid	Plasmocid
Chloral hydrate*	Isopropyl alcohol	Procainamide
Chlorazepate*	Isotretinoin	Promethazone
Chlordiazepoxide	Licorice	Propoxyphene
Chlorinated hydrocarbon insecticides	Lindane	Protriptyline
Chlormethiazole base	Lithium	Quail meat†
Chlorphenoxy herbicides	Lorazepam	Quinidine
Chlorpromazine	Lovastatin	Quinine
Chlorthalidone	Loxapine	Salicylate
Clofibrate	LSD	Sedatives
Cocaine	Marijuana	Selenium
Codeine	*p*-Mentha-1,8-diene*	Snake bite
Colchicine	Meperidine*	Strychnine
Copper sulfate	Mercuric chloride	Succinylcholine
Corticosteroids	Mescaline	Sympathomimetics
Cortisone	Metabolic poisons	Tetraethyl lead
Cyanide	Methadone	Theophylline
Dexamethasone	Methamphetamine	Thiopental
Dextromoramide	Methanol	Thiothixine
Diaminobenzene	Methaqualone*	Toxaphene
Diazepam	3,4-Methylenedioxyamphetamine	Triazolam
Diazinon*	Methylparathion*	2,4,5-Trichlorophenoxyacetic acid
2,4-Dichlorophenoxyacetic acid	Mineralocorticoids	Trimethoprim tetramine dihydrochloride
Diphenhydramine	Molindone	Trimethoprim-sulfamethoxazole
Diquat	Monoamine oxidase inhibitors	Toluene
Diuretics	Morphine	Vasopressin
Doxepin*	Moxalactam	Vitamin A derivatives
Doxylamine	Muscle relaxants	Water hemlock
	Narcotics	

Adapted from Curry SC, Chang D, Connor D: Drug- and toxin-induced rhabdomyolysis. Ann Emerg Med 1989; 18:1068–1084.
*Personally observed by the authors, but not found in review of literature.
†Quail were thought to have eaten hemlock, causing rhabdomyolysis in those who feasted on quail meat.

TABLE 12–40. Agents That Induce Movement Disorders

Compound	Manifestation
Amoxapine	Parkinsonism
Amphetamines	Hyperkinetic movements
Antihistamines	Orofacial dystonia Myoclonic jerking
Black widow spider bite	Rigidity
Butyrophenones	Parkinsonism Orofacial dystonia Opisthotonos, trismus
Caffeine	Myoclonic jerking
Carbamazepine	Orofacial dystonia
Carbon monoxide	Parkinsonism
Chloroquine	Tongue protrusion
Cocaine	Jerking, tremor
Ethylene glycol	Myoclonic jerking
Fluoride	Generalized twitching
Ketamine	Tongue protrusion
Lead (tetraethyl)	Jerking, facial grimacing
Levodopa	Facial grimacing, dystonia Head tossing, flinging extremities
Lithium	Hypertonicity, tongue dystonia, lip smacking, tremor
Metaldehyde	Twitching, hyperreflexia
Methaqualone	Rigidity, hypertonicity
Methylphenidate	Motor and verbal tics
Metoclopramide	Parkinsonism
Monoamine oxidase inhibitors	Rigidity, opisthotonos
1-Methyl-4-phenyl-1,2,3,6-tetrahydropyridine (MPTP)	Parkinsonism
Narcotics (sufentanil)	Chest wall rigidity
Nicotine	Fasciculations flaccid
Organophosphates	Fasciculations flaccid
Pethidine (meperidine)	Tremor, muscle jerking
Phencyclidine	Generalized rigidity, trismus, orofacial dystonias, twitching, athetosis
Phenothiazines	Orofacial and other dystonias
Phenytoin	Choreoathetosis
Strychnine	Rigidity, opisthotonos, trismus
Toluene (chronic)	Ataxia, jerking eye movements
Tricyclic antidepressants	Twitching, myoclonic jerking

cardiographic changes (flat or inverted T waves, prominent U waves, ST-segment depression), and cardiac arrhythmias (atrial tachycardia heart block, atrioventricular dissociation, ventricular tachycardia, ventricular fibrillation).[127] If the serum potassium level is greater than 3 mmol/L, use oral potassium. If the serum potassium level is below 3 mmol/L, replace with intravenous potassium.

Drug-induced hypernatremia follows excessive intake of sodium, salt emetics, enemas, intravenous saline solutions, excessive water loss, and drugs causing diabetes insipidus including lithium, phenytoin, and alcohol. Treatment comprises water restriction with or without loop diuretics.

Drug-induced hyponatremia follows excessive water intake and impaired water excretion by the kidney due to increased activity of antidiuretic hormone resulting from carbamazepine, chlorpropamide, and nonsteroidal anti-inflammatory drug intoxication. Treatment comprises water restriction with or without loop diuretics. If the serum sodium level is less than 120 mmol/L and cerebral symptoms are present, use hypertonic saline cautiously. Watch for central pontine myelinosis and cerebral edema.

Hypoglycemia

Browning and colleagues[128] suggest that administration of 50% glucose should be reserved for those patients in whom hypoglycemia is demonstrated. Preliminary animal and human evidence suggests that glucose-containing intravenous solutions should be avoided in patients at risk for cerebral ischemia, such as those with acute stroke, impending cardiac arrest, or severe hypotension or those receiving cardiopulmonary resuscitation.

The Elderly Population

Older patients are particularly less tolerant of drugs that act on the central nervous system. This is compounded by multiple-drug therapy and reductions in lean body mass, renal blood flow, gastric motility, and synthesis of albumin.[129]

Drug overdose in the elderly is usually due to suicidal thoughts, loneliness, chronic illness, poor eyesight, chaos in the medicine cabinet, noncompliance, suggestibility and erroneous interpretation, advertisements, gossip, poor interpretation of the physician's instructions, or confusion. Drugs commonly associated with orthostatic hypotension in the elderly are listed in Table 12–64.[130]

TOXICOLOGY SCREENS

The use of toxicology testing as a broad screen without an understanding of its limitations is hazardous. The toxicology screen has good specificity. Specificity is the percentage of patients in whom toxic substances are present but the result is reported as negative. (Good specificity means that the test gives few false-positive results.) Its sensitivity, however, is poor because many patients in whom toxic substances are present are not detected with the toxicology screen. Sensitivity is the portion of true-positive results reported as positive. (A high-sensitivity test gives few false-negative results.) The predictive value of a negative test (i.e., the portion of negative results that are truly negative) is about 40%. Improvement of the sensitivity and predictive value of the screen requires attention to the analytic methods used, good clinical communication between physician and laboratory, proper specimen collection, and understanding of the limitations and value of specific tests.

Limitations

Toxicology laboratories use several methods to screen for toxins, because there is no single, accurate, inexpensive method that detects all toxins. Each method differs in cost, accuracy, complexity, speed, and specificity. Individual test reliability depends on expertise of the analyst, equipment, method, and number of requests processed. Problems arise from the changes that occur in the storage of biologic fluids, the transfer of drugs from tube to tube, and the standards used to test drugs. Deterioration of gas-liquid chromatograph columns produces unknown residues, and ionization of gases may cause the breakdown of chemicals. In addition, labile metabolites undergo chemical changes depending on the analytic technique employed. Hence, familiarity with specific laboratory requirements, processes, and limitations is critical to the proper use of the laboratory. In the interpretation of toxicology screen results, the following questions are important:

1. For each drug category, which method is used and what is its specificity?
2. What chemicals are detected by the toxicology screen, and what varieties of screens are available (e.g., coma panel, drugs of abuse, seizure panel)?
3. What information is required on the request form?
4. Which samples are best for each specific analysis?
5. Which tests are qualitative, which are quantitative, and how quickly are the results returned?

TABLE 12–41. Agents Reported to Be Associated with Parkinsonism

Agent	Source
1-Methyl-4-phenyl-1,2,3,6-tetrahydropyridine (MPTP)	Intravenous drug abuse, occupational
Tranquilizers (flunarizine, conarazine, haloperidol, chlorpromazine, etc.)	Psychiatric medication
Antidepressants	Psychiatric medication
Lithium	Psychiatric medication
Phenothiazines	Antiemetic
Reserpine	Antihypertensive, psychiatric
Carbon monoxide	Occupational, environmental
Hydrogen cyanide	Occupational
Postanoxic injury	Environmental
Postencephalitic	Arthropod-borne infection
Carbon disulfide	Occupational (viscose rayon)
Paraquat	Herbicide
Manganese	Occupational (welding)
Mercury	Occupational
Cycad	Dietary, folk medicine (Asia)
Lathyrus	Dietary (Asia, Africa, World War II)
Rural environment: well water?	Environmental
Suspected protective factors	
Cigarette smoking	Lifestyle
Hydrazine	Lifestyle, occupational
Measles	Environmental

From Goldsmith JR, Herishanu Y, Abarband JM, Weinbaum Z: Clustering of Parkinson's disease points to environmental neurotoxins. Arch Environ Health 1990; 45:88–94. Copyright 1990. Reprinted with permission of the Helen Dwight Reid Educational Foundation. Published by Heldref Publications, Washington, DC.

Comparison of Analytical Screening Methods

Chromatography, the most frequently used analytical technique, involves a separation method based on the flow of a mobile liquid or gas over a solid or stationary phase containing the unknown. Immunoassays (enzyme multiple immunoassay technique, radioimmunoassay) are sensitive techniques less specific than chromatographic or mass spectrometry methods.

TABLE 12–42. Motor Neuron Disorders

Lathyrism[94]
Disorder of corticospinal tract: weakness, spasticity, muscle cramps, usually in legs
Chickling pea, *Lathyrus sativa,* seeds
Africa and Asia; endemic in Mysore and central India
Neurotoxin: β-*N*-oxalylanine-L-alanine (BOAA)
Parkinsonism, dementia–amyotrophic lateral sclerosis complex[95, 96]
Seeds of false sago palm, *Cyacas circinalis*
Chamorros of Guam
Neurotoxin: β-*N*-methylamino-L-alanine (BMAA)
Delay in onset? (unconfirmed association)[97, 98]
Parkinsonism in drug abusers[96]
Synthetic opiates contaminated with 1-methyl-4-phenyl-1,2,3,6-tetrahydropyridine
Selectively active against dopaminergic neurons in the substantia nigra
Mantakassa[96]
Spastic paresis
Northern Mozambique, 1981
Intake of cyanogenic glycosides from inadequate preparation of cassava
Motor neuron disease in leather workers[99]
Leather workers in United Kingdom
Solvents?
Konzo[100]
Spastic paraparesis
East Africa
Cassava (*Manihot esculenta*) insufficiently processed
Toxin: cyanogen (cyanohydrin) plus insufficient sulfur intake
Amyotrophic lateral sclerosis
Early overexposure to lead, mercury, manganese, selenium[101,102]
Doubtful association[100–104]
Anecdotal reports[105]

Thin-Layer Chromatography

A simple, inexpensive technique effective for qualitative screening, but not for quantitative measurements, is thin-layer chromatography (TLC). Separation results from absorption or partition as the mobile solvent moves across the stationary sorbent phase (usually silicic acid or aluminum oxide). For each substance, a characteristic amount of migration occurs after the test specimen is applied to the base with the liquid solvent system. Tests take 2 hours and must be interpreted carefully by experienced technicians. There are commercially available thin-layer chromatographic systems that chromatographically screen for drugs with less performance expertise than is required for standard thin-layer chromatography.

Ultraviolet Spectrophotometry

Ultraviolet spectrophotometry (UVS) is an easy, economical, and quantitative test that can detect toxic blood acetaminophen and salicylate levels as well as elevated urine phenothiazine levels. Interference by multiple-drug ingestion, however, seriously impairs its accuracy and currently restricts its use.

Gas-Liquid Chromatography

Gas-liquid chromatography (GLC) is a sophisticated but somewhat slow method that is highly accurate and specific. Liquid or dissolved solid specimens are injected into the column and vaporized by heat. Inert gases carry the specimen out of the column where chemical detectors record the emergence of the specimen as a function of time. The comparison of retention times and peak areas with known standards allows identification and quantitation. This method is effective for quantitation of blood levels of volatile liquids (methanol, ethanol, ethylene glycol).

High-Pressure (High-Performance) Liquid Chromatography

High-pressure (high-performance) liquid chromatography (HPLC) is similar in speed, specificity, and expense to gas-

TABLE 12–43. Inhaled or Cutaneously Absorbed Nephrotoxins

Probable Renal Lesion	Chemical
Chronic interstitial nephritis	Mineral spirits
Glomerulonephritis	Hydrocarbons or silicon
Hemoglobinuric acute tubular necrosis	Arsine gas
Myoglobinuric acute tubular necrosis	Carbon monoxide
Pseudoazotemia	Acetone (contaminating acetylene)
Nephrotoxic acute renal failure	Boric acid, cadmium, carbon tetrachloride, chromium, diethylene glycol, 1,2-dichloropropane, diesel fuel, dioxane, dynamite, ethylene dibromide, gasoline, Lysol (British), methyl chloride or bromide gas, methylene chloride, phenol, polyethylene glycol, povidone-iodine, tetrachloroethylene, toluene, trichloroethylene

From Abuelo JG: Renal failure caused by chemicals, foods, plants, animal venoms and misuse of drugs. Arch Intern Med 1990; 150:505–510. Copyright 1990, American Medical Association.

TABLE 12–44. Ingested Nephrotoxic Chemicals

Probable Renal Lesion	Chemical
Chronic tubulointerstitial nephritis	Cadmium, fluoride, lead
Hemoglobinuric tubular necrosis	Aniline, chlorate compounds, copper sulfate, cresol, ethylene glycol dinitrate, Lysol (British), naphthalene, *p*-phenylenediamine, potassium or sodium bromate, propylene glycol
Myoglobinuric tubular necrosis	Copper sulfate, lindane, mercuric chloride, *p*-phenylenediamine, zinc phosphide
Nephrotoxic tubular necrosis	Arsenic salts, barium chloride, carbon tetrachloride, chlordane, chloroform, 2,4-dichlorophenoxyacetic and methylchlorophenoxyacetic acids, chromium compounds, diquat, ethylene dichloride, ethylene dibromide, germanium compounds, mercury salts, methylene chloride, oxalic acid, paraquat, tartaric acid, thallium, tetrachloroethylene, trichloroethylene, turpentine, yellow phosphorus
Oxalosis	Diethylene glycol, ethylene glycol, ethylene glycol butyl ether
Pseudoazotemia	Isopropyl alcohol

From Abuelo JG: Renal failure caused by chemicals, foods, plants, animal venoms and misuse of drugs. Arch Intern Med 1990; 150:505–510. Copyright 1990, American Medical Association.

TABLE 12–45. Nephrotoxic Foods

Probable Renal Lesion	Food	Toxic Component
Chronic interstitial nephritis	Vichy water	Fluoride
	Worcestershire sauce	Unknown
Hypercalcemia (milk-alkali syndrome)	Milk	Calcium
Hemoglobinuric tubular necrosis	Fava or broad beans (*Vicia faba*)	Divicine and isouramil
Myoglobinuric tubular necrosis	Licorice	Glycyrrhizic acid (hypokalemia)
	Wild birds (chaffinch, quail, or European robin)	? Cicutoxin
Nephrotoxic tubular necrosis	Djenkol beans (*Pithecolabium lobatum*)	? Djenkolic acid
	Bile of the grass carp (*Clenopharyngodon idellus*)	? Cyprinol
Oxaloxis	Rhubarb (*Rheum rhaponticum*)	Oxalic acid

From Abuelo JG: Renal failure caused by chemicals, foods, plants, animal venoms and misuse of drugs. Arch Intern Med 1990; 150:505–510. Copyright 1990, American Medical Association.

TABLE 12–46. Nephrotoxic Plants

Plant	Scientific Name	Toxic Compound
Autumn crocus	*Colchicum autumnale*	Colchicine
Castor bean	*Ricinus communis*	Ricin and recinine
Daphne	*Daphne mezereum*	Daphnin, vesicant resin, and mezerenic acid anhydride
Herbal remedies	Exact plants unknown	Unknown
Impila	*Callilepsis laureola*	Atractyloside
Marking-nut tree	*Semecarpus anacardium*	Phenolic constituents
Poison mushrooms	*Amanita phalloides* and *Cortinarius* species	Amatoxin cyclopeptides
Rosary pea	*Abrus precatorius*	Abrin and abric acid
?	*Securidaca longipedunculata*	Methyl salicylate, saponins, tannin, and gaultherin
Water hemlock	*Cicuta maculata*	Cicutoxin

From Abuelo JG: Renal failure caused by chemicals, foods, plants, animal venoms and misuse of drugs. Arch Intern Med 1990; 150:505–510. Copyright 1990, American Medical Association.

TABLE 12–47. Animals with Potentially Nephrotoxic Venom

Common Name	Scientific Name	Location
Arthropods—arachnids		
Scorpion	*Buthus sauloci*	Iran
Brown recluse spider	*Loxosceles reclusa*	Western Hemisphere
South American house spider	*Loxosceles laeta*	Western Hemisphere
Arthropods—Hymenoptera		
Bees		
Africanized bee	*Apis mellifera scutellata*	Africa and Western Hemisphere
Wax bee	*Apis mellificus*	Worldwide
Wasps		
Indian hornet	*Vespa affinis*	Asia
Oriental hornet	*Vespa orientalis*	Asia
Yellow jacket	*Vespula germanica*	Europe
Coelenterates		
Portuguese man-of-war	*Pysalia physalis*	North Carolina
Snakes		
Australian brown snake	*Pseudonaja textilis textilis*	Australia
Black mamba	*Dendroaspis polylepis*	Southern Africa
Boomslang	*Dispholidus typus*	Southern Africa
Small-eyed black snake	*Cryptophis nigrescens*	Australia
Dugite	*Demansia nuchalis affinis*	Australia
Gwardar	*Demansia nuchalis nuchalis*	Australia
Palestinian viper	*Vipera palestinae*	Israel
Pit vipers		
Copperhead	*Agkistrodon contortix*	Western Hemisphere
Jaraca	*Bothrops jararaca*	South America
Mamushi	*Agkistrodon halys*	Japan
Rattlesnake	*Crotalus terrificus* and others	Western Hemisphere
Water moccasin (cottonmouth)	*Agikistrodon piscivorus*	Western Hemisphere
Pit viper	*Agkistrodon hypnale*	Sri Lanka
Puff adder	*Bitis arietans*	Africa
Rough-scaled snake	*Tropidechis carinatus*	Australia
Russel's viper	*Vipera russelli*	Asia
Saw-scaled sand viper	*Echis carinatus*	Africa, India, Middle East
Seasnake	*Enhydrina schistosa*	Asian waters
Small African snake	*Atracepaspis microlapidata*	Africa
Tiger snake	*Notechis scutatus*	Australia

From Abuelo JG: Renal failure caused by chemicals, foods, plants, animal venoms and misuse of drugs. Arch Intern Med 1990; 150:505–510. Copyright 1990, American Medical Association.

TABLE 12–48. Nephrotoxicity Resulting from Drugs Given in Excessive Dose by the Physician or Misused by the Patient

Renal Lesion	Drug	Circumstance of Administration
Acute interstitial nephritis	Chlorprothixene	Suicide
Acute tubular necrosis	Acetaminophen	Suicide
	Aspirin	Suicide
	Boric acid	Diaper rash
	Bismuth salts	Taken for warts
	Colchicine	Suicide
	Lead	Inadvertently self-injected with opium
	Nomifensine	Suicide
	Pennyroyal oil	Attempted abortion
	Paraldehyde	Drug overdose
	Triamterene	Suicide
	Uranium	Clinical investigation
Chronic glomerulonephritis (heroin nephropathy)	Heroin	Narcotic addiction
	Pentazocine	Narcotic addiction
Chronic interstitial nephritis (analgesic nephropathy)	Acetaminophen	Analgesic abuse
	Nonsteroidal anti-inflammatory drugs	Analgesic abuse
Hypercalcemia	Vitamin A	Acne treatment
	Vitamin D	Hypoparathyroidism* and metabolic bone disease*
Myoglobinuric tubular necrosis	Amoxapine	Suicide
	Amphetamines	Drug overdose
	Barbiturates	Drug overdose
	Cocaine	Drug overdose
	Diazepam	Drug overdose
	Doxepin hydrochloride or nitrazepam	Suicide
	Alcohol	Alcoholism
	Glutethimide	Drug overdose
	Heroin	Drug overdose
	Methadone	Drug overdose
	Phencyclidine hydrochloride	Drug overdose
	Phenylpropanolamine hydrochloride	Weight loss, drug overdose
	Strychnine	Mistaken for cocaine
Necrotizing vasculitis	Methamphetamine	Drug overdose
Obstruction (stones)	Magnesium antacid	Antacid abuse
Osmotic nephrosis	Mannitol	Excessive dose*
Oxalosis	Intravenous vitamin C	Excessive dose*

From Abuelo JG: Renal failure caused by chemicals, foods, plants, animal venoms and misuse of drugs. Arch Intern Med 1990; 150:505–510. Copyright 1990, American Medical Association.

*Prescribed by a physician.

liquid chromatography but is not restricted to volatile compounds. Complex compounds, including conjugated metabolites, are well separated by facilitating the movement of specimens with high pressures (1000 to 6000 psi).

Radioimmunoassay

Radioimmunoassay is the slowest, most expensive method, but it has good accuracy. Mixing known quantities of drug-specific antibody and known amounts of radioactively labeled drug allows analysis of the precipitate with a gamma counter. The amount of emittance inversely correlates with the presence of assayed drug. This test is excellent for detection of drugs in extremely low blood concentrations (cannabis, LSD, digoxin, paraquat).

Enzyme-Mediated Immunoassay

A fast, expensive, and simple method with intermediate accuracy and specificity, the enzyme-mediated immunoassay (EMIT) system works on the basis that the amount of drug present is proportional to the inhibition of an enzyme-substrate reaction. A known quantity of drug is labeled by chemical attachment to an enzyme. Drug-specific antibodies added to the specimen bind the drug-enzyme complex, thereby reducing enzyme activity. Free drug in the specimen competes with enzyme-labeled drug and limits the antibody-induced enzyme inactivation. Enzyme activity correlates with drug concentration in the specimen as measured by absorbance changes resulting from the enzyme's catalytic action on a substrate. EMIT is preferred over other radioimmunoassay methods in the emergency situation because of its simplicity and speed in providing information on toxic drug concentrations. EMIT eliminates the complex separation phase necessary in radioimmunoassays. The two systems are EMIT-st (single test), consisting of a compact spectrophotometer, for small laboratories, and EMIT-dau (drugs of abuse) for larger hospitals. Negative test results do not exclude the ingestion of a drug that may be present in undetectable quantities.

False-Positive Screen

Antibody cross-reactions that can produce false-positive screens include the following:

1. *Narcotics*
   a. Poppy seeds
   b. Dextromethorphan
   c. Chlorpromazine
   d. Diphenoxylate
2. *Amphetamines*
   a. Ephedrine
   b. Phenylephrine
   c. Pseudoephedrine
   d. *N*-Acetylprocainamide

TABLE 12–49. Drugs with the Potential to Cause Incontinence

Sedatives

- Diazepam (Valium), flurazepam (Dalmane), and other benzodiazepine drugs
- Alcohol

Diuretics

- Furosemide (Lasix), bumetanide (Bumex), ethacrynic acid (Edecrin)

Drugs with Potential to Weaken Bladder Contraction (Anticholinergics)

- Thorazine, Stelazine, and related antipsychotic medications
- Elavil, Sinequan, Tofranil, and related tricyclic antidepressants
- Bentyl, Pro-Banthine, Donnatal, and other antispasmodics
- Benadryl, Chlor-Trimeton, Contac, Phenergan, and other antihistamines or preparations containing them
- Morphine, codeine, meperdine, methadone, and other opiates
- Artane, Cogentin, and related drugs used for Parkinson's disease (not levo-dopa or deprenyl)
- Sominex, Unisom, and other over-the-counter insomnia medication
- Eye drops containing atropine, cyclopentolate, or tropicamide (used mainly for glaucoma)

Drugs Affecting Sympathetic Nerves

- Minipress, Catapres, Aldomet, Regitine, Yohimex, and other antagonists for sympathetic action
- Allerest, Actifed, Sudafed, Contac, Sinutab, and other preparations (including nose drops) containing phenylpropanolamine, pseudoephedrine, or other decongestants

Modified from Urinary incontinence. Harvard Med School Health Lett 1990; 15:10.

TABLE 12–50. Drug Effects on the Mouth

Dental discoloration	Fluorides, tetracycline antibiotics, chlorhexidine, liquid iron preparations
Gingival hyperplasia	Phenytoin, sodium valproate, phenobarbital, cyclosporine, nifedipine, diltiazem, verapamil, nitrendipine
Stomatitis	Cytotoxic drugs: nitrogen mustards, methotrexate, 5-fluorouracil, 6-mercaptopurine, chlorambucil, doxorubicin, daunorubicin, bleomycin; penicillamine, gold salts, locally applied aspirin, contents of chloral hydrate and valproic acid capsules, gentian violet dye
Xerostomia	Centrally acting antihypertensive agents, diuretics, antipsychotics, tricyclic antidepressants, antihistamines, anticholinergics, anticonvulsants, laxatives, muscle relaxants, narcotics, hypnotics
Sialorrhea	Pilocarpine, neostigmine, iodides
Sialadenitis	Phenylbutazone, isoproterenol, nitrofurantoin, iodine
Parotitis	Bretylium, methyldopa, clonidine, guanethidine, phenylbutazone, oxyphenbutazone, thioridazine
Erythema multiforme	Penicillins, tetracyclines, clindamycin, sulfonamides, anticonvulsants
Systemic lupus erythematosus	Procainamide, hydralazine
Pigmentation	Cisplatin, oral contraceptives, minocycline, antimalarial agents, doxorubicin
Dental caries	Drugs inhibiting flow of saliva (xerostomia), preparation with high sucrose content: vitamin syrup, antibiotics and anticonvulsant suspensions, cough syrup

Data from Kane M, Zacharczenko N: Oral side effects of drugs. Oral Health 1993; 83:29–35; and Thompson DF: Drug-induced parotitis. J Clin Pharm Ther 1993; 18:255–258. Reprinted with permission of the American Society of Health-System Pharmacists.

TABLE 12–51. Agents Associated with Acute Pancreatitis*

Definite Association	Questionable Association
Asparaginase	Acetaminophen
Azathioprine	Amiodarone
Didanosine	Ampicillin
Estrogens	Anticholinesterases
Furosemide	Carbamazepine
Mercaptopurine	Cisplatin
Pentamidine	Colchicine
Sulfonamides	Cyclosporine
Sulindac	Cytarabine
Tetracyclines	Diazoxide
Thiazides	Diphenoxylate
Valproic acid	Enalapril
Probable Association	Ergotamine
	Erythromycin
Bumetanide	Gold compounds
Chlorthalidone	Interleukin-2
Cimetidine	Isotretinoin
Clozapine	Ketoprofen
Corticosteroids	Lisinopril
Corticotropin	Mefanamic acid
ERCP† media	Metolazone
Ethacrynic acid	Nitrofurantoin
Methyldopa	Octreotide
Metronidazole	Oxyphenbutazone
Salicylates	Phenformin
Sulfasalazine	Phenolphthalein
Zalcitabine	Piroxicam
	Potassium permanganate
	Procainamide
	Ranitidine
	Roxithromycin
	Tryptophan

From Underwood TW, Frye CB: Drug-induced pancreatitis. Clin Pharm 1993; 14:440–448.

*Association is considered definite if pancreatitis developed during exposure to the agent, disappeared after withdrawal, and recurred after rechallenge. Association is considered probable if an association is thought to exist but not all of the three criteria were met. Association is considered questionable if published evidence is inadequate or contradictory.

†Endoscopic retrograde cholangiopancreatography.

   e. Chloroquine
   f. Procainamide
3. *Phencyclidine*
   a. Dextromethorphan
   b. Diphenhydramine
   c. Chlorpromazine
   d. Doxylamine
   e. Thioridazine

The most common cause of a genuinely false-positive result is antibody cross-reactivity with a substance bearing some structural similarity to the drug including poppy seeds, which may contain opium congeners, resulting in a drug screen that is positive for opiates. Also common is the ability of nasal decongestants such as ephedrine and phenylpropanolamine to produce a urine drug screen that is positive for amphetamines. Cross-reactivity may occur; phenmetrazine and L-ephedrine may produce such a positive result.

False-Negative Screen

The reasons for a false-negative test result can be divided into three general categories:

1. *Technologic shortcomings*
   a. Drug screen does not seek the drug
   b. Structural dissimilarity from drug class prototype (e.g., fentanyl)
   c. Poor laboratory quality assurance
2. *Toxicokinetic characteristics*
   a. Large volume of distribution
   b. Short elimination half-life
3. *Intentional specimen alteration or adulteration*
   a. Use of a colleague's "clean" urine
   b. Use of a fluid other than urine
   c. Drinking excessive fluids
   d. Use of a diuretic
   e. Addition of bleach, caustics, golden seal tea, lemon juice, salt, soap, or vinegar to urine

Atomic Absorption Spectrophotometry

Atomic absorption spectrophotometry is the usual method for detecting inorganic agents (e.g., lead, mercury, thallium, cadmium) but is not suitable as a screening technique. Hence, most toxicology screens do not detect heavy metals. Inductively coupled plasma atomic emission spectroscopy (ICP-AES) is a new method that allows simultaneous multielement analysis useful for the industrial workplace. ICP-AES quantitatively measures 17 elements (aluminum, barium, cadmium, chromium, copper, iron, lanthanum, lead, manganese, molybdenum, nickel, platinum, silver, strontium, tin, titanium, zinc) from a single sample.

Gas Chromatography–Mass Spectrometry

Probably the best technique with which to determine the presence of a chemical is gas chromatography-mass spectrometry (GC-MS), but the high capital equipment and operating costs limit its use to reference centers.

Quantitative Blood Levels

Drugs whose blood levels may be useful in the management of poisoning include acetaminophen, salicylates, carboxyhemoglobin, methemoglobin, methanol, ethylene glycol, lithium, iron, paraquat, digoxin, theophylline, and organophosphates.

Urine Levels

Urine samples are preferred when the blood concentration of the compound is too low for detection by conventional means. Such drugs usually either are rapidly eliminated or have large volumes of distribution. Examples are phenothiazines, barbiturates, benzodiazepines, sedative-hypnotic agents, tricyclic antidepressants, and antihistamines.

DECONTAMINATION AND ELIMINATION ENHANCEMENT TECHNIQUES

No gastrointestinal decontamination modalities have been determined to reduce morbidity and mortality by controlled clinical studies.

Recommendations for the use of methods to decontaminate the gut have traditionally relied on pharmacologic studies in animals and humans rather than on clinical studies on the efficacy and complications of these procedures. Experimental studies in the 1950s and 1960s suggested that syrup of ipecac removed more of an ingested marker (e.g., 30–40% between 30 and 60 minutes after ingestion) than did gastric lavage.[6] For example, when administered immediately, 30 minutes, and 60 minutes after ingestion, syrup of ipecac removed 60%, 40%, and 20% of an ingested dose of salicylates, respectively.[6] By comparison, gastric lavage removed 45%, 26%, and 8%, respectively, of the salicylate marker. On the basis of these and similar studies, syrup of ipecac became the method of choice for treatment of childhood poisoning in the home and the alert patient in the emergency department; however, large variation in the volumes of markers recovered from patients and the use of small-bore orogastric tubes in the animal studies raised questions about the superiority of syrup of ipecac. In human volunteers, gastric lavage recovered 45% of a nontoxic marker when lavage commenced 10 minutes after ingestion

TABLE 12–52. Drugs That Induce Esophageal Injury

Lower Esophageal Sphincter Tone	Irritate Esophageal Mucosa
α-Adrenergic antagonists	Captopril
Phentolamine	Chlorazepate
Anticholinergic agents	Clindamycin
Atropine, belladonna tincture, dicyclomine, flavoxate, methantheline, oxybutynin, propantheline	Digoxin
	Ferrous sulfate
Benzodiazepines	Lincomycin
Diazepam	Nonsteroidal anti-inflammatory drugs
β-Adrenergic agonists	Aspirin, ibuprofen, indomethacin, ketoprofen, phenylbutazone, piroxicam
Caffeine, carbuterol, isoproterenol	Penicillin
Calcium channel blocking agents	Potassium chloride
Nifedipine, verapamil	Quinidine
Dopamine	Tetracyclines
Ethanol	Doxycycline, tetracycline
Glucagon	Trimethoprim–sulfamethoxazole
Narcotic analgesics	Vitamin C
Meperidine, morphine	
Prostaglandins E_1, E_2, A_2	
Theophylline	

From Lee M, Sharfi R: Oxybutynin-induced reflux esophagitis. DICP Ann Pharmacother 1990; 34:583–585.

TABLE 12–53. Drug-Induced Gastrointestinal Obstruction

Site	Drugs
In the lumen without predisposing lesion	Barium sulfate, cholestyramine, potassium supplements, bulk laxatives, aluminum hydroxide suspension
In the lumen with predisposing lesion	Iron preparations in patients with Crohn's disease; bulk laxatives or bran in patients with renal failure, colon carcinoma, or diabetes mellitus
Within the gut wall	
Physical damage	Anticoagulants, nonsteroidal anti-inflammatory drugs, penicillamine, methylene blue in utero, alprostadil (prostaglandin E_1) infusion in neonates
Dysmotility of smooth muscle	H_1-antagonists, opiates, clonidine, calcium antagonists, dantrolene, corticosteroid withdrawal, magnesium sulfate exposure in utero, erythromycin stearate
Interference with autonomic nerve transmission	Autonomic ganglion blockers, muscarinic antagonists (e.g., atropine), anticholinergics, phenothiazines, antiparkinsonian drugs, tricyclic antidepressants, disopyramide, vincristine
Outside the gut wall	
Vascular obstruction	Oral contraceptives, corticosteroids, vasopressors, cocaine abusers
Peritoneal fibrosis	Practolol, irradiation of abdomen or pelvis, intraperitoneal antineoplastic therapy
Meconium ileus–type lesion in cystic fibrosis	Cimetidine, ipratropium bromide

From Iredale JP, George CF: Drugs causing gastrointestinal obstruction. Adverse Drug React Toxicol Rev 1993; 12:163–175. By permission of Oxford University Press.

TABLE 12–54. Drug-Induced Colon Toxicity

Toxic Effect	Drugs
Colonic ischemia	Cocaine, ergotamine, estrogen, amphetamines, digitalis, methysergide, vasopressin
Colonic pseudobstruction	Narcotics, phenothiazines, vincristine, atropine or other anticholinergics, ganglionic blocking agents, tricyclic antidepressants
Infectious or necrotizing enterocolitis	Antibiotics associated with pseudomembranous colitis, deferoxamine associated with *Yersinia* enterocolitis, chemotherapy associated with neutropenic colitis, hyperosmolar formulas in children
Allergic, inflammatory cytotoxic colitis	Gold compounds, nonsteroidal anti-inflammatory drugs, methyldopa, flucytosine, methotrexate, salicylates, sulfasalazine
Intestinal ulcers	Slow-release (wax matrices) potassium chloride
Colonic hypomotility and abdominal distention	Chronic cathartic use
Colonic structure due to retroperitoneal fibrosis	Methysergide
Toxic colitis for intrarectally administered compound	Acids, bases, other corrosives
Colitis in patients with colonic obstruction	Enemas using hypertonic radiographic contrast agents

From Cappell MS, Simon T: Colonic toxicity of administered medications and chemicals. Am J Gastroenterol 1993; 88:1684–1697. Reprinted with permission of the American College of Gastroenterology.

TABLE 12–55. Drug-Induced Metabolic Disorders and Management in the Critical Care Setting

Disorder	Offending Agents	Intervention
Fluid overload	Large carbohydrate and sodium loads; IV fluids	Monitor intake and output; maximally concentrate all fluids; restrict sodium
Hyperkalemia	Potassium-sparing diuretics; oversupplementation acidosis	Conservatively induce diuresis with loop diuretics; monitor serum and urine potassium concentration; sodium polystyrene sulfonate may be necessary
Hypernatremia	Drugs with high sodium content; blood products	Conservatively induce diuresis with "free water" replacement; avoid drugs high in sodium content; restrict sodium and dextrose; monitor serum and urine sodium concentration
Hypocalcemia	Citrate loads from blood products; aggressive phosphate replacement	Replace calcium according to serum concentration; keep calcium × phosphate product <70
Hypokalemia	Amphotericin B; corticosteroids; diuretics; alkalosis	Replace urine potassium losses; monitor serum and urine potassium concentration
Hypomagnesemia	Cisplatin therapy; cyclosporine therapy; diuretics	Replace magnesium according to serum concentration; monitor urine losses if necessary
Hyponatremia	Diuretics; nasogastric losses	Replace urine and nasogastric losses; monitor serum, urine, and nasogastric sodium concentration
Hypophosphatemia	Aluminum-containing antacids; corticosteroids; high serum insulin; aggressive calcium replacement	Replace phosphate according to serum concentration; 0.96 mmol/kg/24 hr; keep the product of calcium × phosphate <70
Metabolic acidosis	Amphotericin B; aminoglycosides	Estimate acid deficit; monitor arterial blood gases and replace deficit with acetate salts
Metabolic alkalosis	Diuretics; mineralocorticosteroids; large nasogastric losses with low pH; 140 mEq of citrate from blood replacement	Estimate base deficit; monitor arterial blood gases and replace deficit using chloride salts or HCl; use an H_2-antagonist for large nasogastric losses with low gastric pH

Modified from Driscoll DF: Drug-induced metabolic disorders and parenteral nutrition in the intensive care unit: A pharmaceutical and metabolic perspective. DICP Ann Pharmacother 1989; 23:363–371.

IV = intravenous; HCl = hydrochloride.

TABLE 12–56. Agents Known to Cause Pulmonary Disease as Seen in the Critical Care Unit

Chemotherapeutic Agents

CYTOTOXIC

- Azathioprine
- Bleomycin*
- Busulfan
- Chlorambucil
- Cyclophosphamide
- Etoposide
- Melphalan
- Mitomycin*
- Nitrosoureas
- Procarbazine
- Vinblastine
- Ifosfamide

NONCYTOTOXIC

- Methotrexate*
- Cytosine arabinoside*
- Bleomycin*
- Procarbazine*

Antibiotics

- Amphotericin B*
- Nitrofurantoin
- Sulfasalazine
- Sulfonamides
- Pentamidine

Anti-inflammation Agents

- Acetylsalicyclic acid*
- Gold
- Methotrexate
- Nonsteroidal anti-inflammatory agents
- Penicillamine*

Immunosuppressive Agents

- Cyclosporine
- Interleukin-2*

Analgesics

- Heroin*
- Methadone*
- Naloxone*
- Ethchlorvynol*
- Propoxyphene*
- Salicylates*

Cardiovascular Agents

- Amiodarone*
- Angiotensin-converting enzyme inhibitors
- Anticoagulants
- β-blockers*
- Dipyridamole
- Fibronolytic agents*
- Protamine*
- Tocainide

Inhalants

- Aspirated oil
- Oxygen*

Intravenous Agents

- Blood*
- Ethanolamine oleate (sodium morrhuate)*
- Ethiodized oil (lymphangiogram)
- Talc
- Fat emulsion

Miscellaneous Agents

- Bromocriptine
- Dantrolene
- Hydrochlorothiazide*
- Methysergide
- Oral contraceptives
- Tocolytic agents*
- Tricyclics*
- L-Tryptophan
- Radiation
- Systemic lupus erythematosus (drug-induced)*
- Complement-mediated leukostasis*

From Rosenow EC III, Myers JL, Swenson SJ, Pisani RJ: Drug-induced pulmonary disease: An update. Chest 1992; 102:239–250.
*Typically cause acute or subacute respiratory insufficiency.

TABLE 12–57. Agents Associated with Pleural Effusion

Chemotherapeutic agents
Nitrofurantoin (acute)
Bromocriptine
Dantrolene
Methysergide
L-Tryptophan
Drug-induced systemic lupus erythematosus
Tocolytics
Amiodarone
Esophageal variceal sclerotherapy agents
Interleukin-2

From Rosenow EC III, Myers JL, Swenson SJ, Pisani RJ: Drug-induced pulmonary disease: An update. Chest 1992; 102:239–250.

compared with only 28% recovery after ipecac-induced emesis. Although design factors favored the use of gastric lavage over syrup of ipecac in one study, later studies suggested that the recovery of ingested product from lavage is superior to the recovery from syrup of ipecac.[6]

Current Recommendations

There are questions regarding the prior approaches to gut decontamination such as syrup of ipecac and gastric lavage.[6] In adults, many of whom present to the emergency department only 3 to 4 hours after ingestion, a "do nothing approach" may appear to have merit. Dangers inherent in this approach center on the often unreliable history from the suicidal patient, the need for some additional controlled studies to substantiate these approaches, and the possibly distasteful medicolegal consequences of the minimalist approach. The use of activated charcoal is probably sufficient if the ingested substance is adsorbed by activated charcoal (Table 12–65). Children can be observed for about 2 hours in the emergency department without an intervention (syrup of ipecac, gastric lavage, cathartics, activated charcoal) and sent home if they are asymptomatic unless there is evidence of ingestion of substantial quantities of a toxic drug. Activated charcoal (50 to 100 g in adults; 15–30 g in children) should be administered to a patient who has ingested a substantial overdose of a toxic substance less than 1 hour before examination.

The use of repetitive doses of activated charcoal depends on specific and proved efficacy of this method in removing

TABLE 12–58. Agents Associated with Acute-Onset Pulmonary Insufficiency*

Bleomycin plus O_2	Fibrinolytic agents
Mitomycin	Protamine
Bleomycin†	Blood products‡
Procarbazine†	Fat emulsion
Methotrexate†	Hydrochlorothiazide‡
Amphotericin B	Complement-mediated leukostasis
Nitrofurantoin (acute)‡	Hyskon (dextran 70)‡
Acetylsalicylic acid‡	Tumor necrosis factor‡
Interleukin-2‡	Intrathecal methotrexate
Heroin and other narcotics‡	Tricyclic antidepressants‡
Epinephrine‡	Amiodarone plus O_2
Ethchlorvynol‡	Naloxone

From Rosenow EC III, Myers JL, Swenson SJ, Pisani RJ: Drug-induced pulmonary disease: An update. Chest 1992; 102:239–250.

*Onset at less than 48 hours.

†Associated with hypersensitivity with eosinophilia.

‡Usually reversible within 48 to 72 hours, implying noncardiac pulmonary edema rather than inflammatory interstitial pneumonitis.

TABLE 12–59. Drugs That Cause Acute Bronchospasm or Exacerbate Asthma

Types of Drugs That Cause Asthma

- Nonsteroidal anti-inflammatory drugs
- Antibiotics (nitrofurantoin, penicillins, cephalosporins, tetracycline)
- β-Adrenergic blocking agents (topical or systemic)
- Cholinergic agonists (methacholine, carbachol, bethanechol, echothiophate iodide) and cholinomimetic alkaloids (pilocarpine, muscarine)
- Corticosteroids (IV hydrocortisone in acetylsalicylic acid–sensitive asthma)
- Diuretics (triamterene/hydrochlorothiazide)
- Chemotherapeutic agents (bleomycin, podophyllotoxins, zinostatin, methotrexate, vinca alkaloids in combination with mitomycin C)

Unusual Causes of Drug-Induced Asthma

- Agents encountered by airborne exposure in pharmaceutical manufacturing or in the hospital or laboratory workplace
- Propellants or additives to inhalant medications
- Metabisulfites
- Agents inducing bronchospasm via non-immunoglobulin E mast cell activation (radiographic contrast media, opiates, polymyxin, colistin)
- Intravenous anesthetic agents and muscle relaxants
- Agents aggravating bronchospasm via local irritant effect
- Drugs causing or exacerbating gastroenteric reflex

Agents That Mimic Asthma

- Angiotensin-converting enzyme inhibitors

the drug ingested. Syrup of ipecac should now be abandoned in the hospital because there is little evidence of efficacy even in volunteer studies. Furthermore, the complications that follow the use of syrup of ipecac even in conscious patients, particularly aspiration pneumonia, combined with the diagnostic difficulties that ensue because its effects mimic those of many overdoses, are further compelling reasons to reconsider its role.[6]

Syrup of Ipecac

The lack of prospective studies on the clinical outcome of decontamination measures and the lack of efficacy of syrup of ipecac in pharmacologic studies beyond 60 to 90 minutes after ingestion have resulted in the increased use of activated charcoal as an alternative to syrup of ipecac. Endoscopic study of overdose patients indicated that neither syrup of ipecac nor lavage removes all intragastric solids, including tablets.[6] The use of syrup of ipecac often delays the administration of activated charcoal in the emergency department, but the administration of activated charcoal by nasogastric tube 10 minutes after a dose of syrup of ipecac does not alter the efficacy of ipecac in volunteers.

Indications

Administration of syrup of ipecac is recommended for alert patients who would benefit from emesis and who have no contraindication to the use of syrup of ipecac. The use of emesis to reduce absorption usually is not effective more than 4 to 6 hours after ingestion, unless the toxin itself delays absorption. Additional factors that may delay absorption include food in the stomach, other drugs (anticholinergics, narcotics, ganglionic blockers, aluminum hydroxide), and associated alterations in clinical status (e.g., pain, ulcer, ileus, acute abdomen, trauma, myocardial infarction).

Contraindications

RELATIVE. Seizure-inducing drugs, rapid coma-inducing agents, sustained-release theophylline, pregnancy, bleeding di-

TABLE 12–60. Drugs Associated with Agranulocytosis

Analgesic/Anti-inflammatory Drugs

Amidopyrine (aminopyrine)
Aminosalicylic acid
Antipyrine (phenazone)
Aspirin
Benoxaprofen
Colchicine
Fenoprofen
Gold salts
Ibuprofen
Indomethacin
Naproxen
Oxyphenbutazone
Paracetamol (acetaminophen)
Pentazocine
Phenylbutazone
Zomepirac

Antiarrhythmic Drugs

Ajmaline
Aprindine
Disopyramide
Procainamide
Propafenone
Propranolol
Quinidine
Tocainide

Anticonvulsant Drugs

Carbamazepine
Ethosuximide
Mephenytoin
Phenytoin
Primidone
Sodium valproate
Trimethadione

Antidepressant Drugs

Amoxapine
Clomipramine
Desipramine
Imipramine
Maprotiline
Mianserin

Antihypertensive Drugs

Captopril
Diazoxide
Hydralazine
Methyldopa
Nifedipine
Propranolol

Antimicrobial Drugs

Amodiaquine
Ampicillin
Carbenicillin
Cephalexin
Cephalothin
Cephradine
Chloramphenicol
Clindamycin
Cloxacillin
Co-trimoxazole
Dapsone
Doxycycline
Flucytosine
Fumagillin
Gentamicin
Griseofulvin
Hydroxychloroquine
Isoniazid
Lincomycin
Methicillin
Metronidazole
Mezlocillin
Nafcillin
Nitrofurantoin
Novobiocin
Oxacillin
Oxophenarsine
Penicillin
Pyrimethamine
Quinine
Rifampin
Ristocetin
Streptomycin
Sulfadiazine
Sulfamethoxypyridazine
Sulfapyridine
Sulfasalazine (salicylazosulfapyridine)
Sulfathiazole
Thiacetazone
Ticarcillin

Antipsychotic Drugs

Chlorpromazine
Clozapine
Fluphenazine
Mepazine
Methylpromazine
Perazine
Prochlorperazine
Promazine
Thioridazine
Trimeprazine

Antithyroid Drugs

Carbimazole
Methimazole
Methylthiouracil
Propylthiouracil
Thiouracil

Diuretics

Acetazolamide
Bumetanide
Chlorthalidone
Chlorothiazide
Ethacrynic acid
Hydrochlorothiazide
Mercurials
Methazolamide

Other Drugs

Allopurinol
Brompheniramine
Chlordiazepoxide
Chlorpropamide
Cimetidine
Diazepam
Levamisole
Levodopa
Mebendazole
Meprobamate
Methydroline
Metiamide
Penicillamine
Phenindione
Promethazine
Ranitidine
Thenalidine
Ticlopidine
Tolbutamide

From Heimpel H: Drug-induced agranulocytosis. Med Toxicol 1988; 3:449–462.

TABLE 12–61. Drugs and Chemicals That Can Induce Hemolytic Anemia in Persons with Glucose-6-Phosphate Dehydrogenase Deficiency

Acetanilid	Niridazole
Doxorubicin	Nitrofurantoin
Furazolidone	Phenazopyridine
Methylene blue	Primaquine
Nalidixic acid	Sulfamethoxazole

From Beutler E: Glucose-6-phosphate dehydrogenase deficiency. N Engl J Med 1991; 324:169–174. Massachusetts Medical Society.

athesis, excessive emesis, serious heart disease, poorly absorbed hydrocarbons, and anticipated use of whole-bowel irrigation are relative contraindications to use of ipecac. Additional relative contraindications include situations in which too much time has elapsed since the ingestion or the patient has already vomited, the substance ingested has a tendency to cause bradycardia (digitalis, β-blocker, calcium channel blockers), and the patient is very young or very old. The vomiting caused by ipecac may produce or potentiate bradycardia through vagal effects.

ABSOLUTE. Absolute contraindications include children younger than 6 months (although there are few clinical data to support this), comatose or seizing patients, corrosive substances, absent or impaired gag reflex, and coingestion of sharp solid objects. Absolute contraindications can also include nontoxic ingestions (e.g., single berry or leaf ingestions, vitamins without iron, acetaminophen ingestions less than 100 mg/kg, some antibiotics, and yellow phenolphthalein ingestion), ingestions causing altered mental status (antihistamines, opioids, benzodiazepines, ethanol, cyclic antidepressants, phenothiazines), and seizures. There are no good studies in humans either to support or to refute the use of ipecac later than 60 minutes after an ingestion.[6] Few controlled studies support the efficacy of ipecac even when it is administered within minutes of drug ingestion.

Inappropriate Use of Ipecac

The most common inappropriate use of ipecac in children was for ingestion of a nontoxic substance; in adults, the most common inappropriate use was after ingestion of a substance known to cause altered mental status. The most frequent situation in which ipecac was given inappropriately occurred when too much time had elapsed from the time of ingestion (>60 minutes).

TABLE 12–62. Drugs, Foods, Spices, and Vitamins That May Cause Abnormalities of Platelet Function

Agent*	Abnormality†
Nonsteroidal Anti-inflammatory Drugs	
Meclofenamic acid, mefenamic acid, phenylbutazone, sulfinpyrazone	Abnormal platelet aggregation in vitro
Diflunisal, piroxicam, sulindac	Abnormal platelet aggregation
Tolmetin, zompirac	Abnormal bleeding time
Indomethacin, naproxen	Abnormal platelet aggregation and bleeding time
Aspirin	Abnormal platelet aggregation and bleeding time; clinical bleeding
Diclofenac	Abnormal bleeding time; clinical bleeding
Ibuprofen	Abnormal platelet aggregation in vitro; abnormal bleeding time
β-Lactam Antibiotics	
PENICILLINS	
Carbenicillin, mezlocillin, piperacillin, ticarcillin	Abnormal platelet aggregation and bleeding time; clinical bleeding
Apalcillin, methicillin	Abnormal platelet aggregation
Ampicillin, penicillin G	Abnormal platelet aggregation and bleeding time
Sulbenicillin	Abnormal platelet aggregation in vitro
Azlocillin	Abnormal bleeding time
Nafcillin	Abnormal bleeding time; clinical bleeding
CEPHALOSPORINS	
Cephalothin	Abnormal platelet aggregation
Cefoperazone	Abnormal bleeding time
Cefotaxime	Abnormal bleeding time; clinical bleeding
Moxalactam	Abnormal platelet aggregation and bleeding time; clinical bleeding
Cardiovascular Drugs	
Dipyridamole‡	
Diltiazem, isosorbide dinitrate, isosorbide mononitrate, nimodipine, propranolol, sodium nitroprusside, verapamil	Abnormal platelet aggregation
Nifedipine, nitroglycerin	Abnormal platelet aggregation and bleeding time
Quinidine	Abnormal bleeding time; clinical bleeding
Anticoagulant, Fibrinolytic, and Antifibrinolytic Drugs	
Aminocaproic acid, heparin	Abnormal platelet aggregation and bleeding time
Protamine sulfate	Abnormal platelet aggregation in vitro
Alteplase	Abnormal bleeding time; clinical bleeding
Psychotropic Drugs	
Amitriptyline, fluphenazine, haloperidol, imipramine, nortriptyline, promazine, trifluoperazine	Abnormal platelet aggregation in vitro
Chlorpromazine	Abnormal platelet aggregation

Table continued on following page

TABLE 12–62. Drugs, Foods, Spices, and Vitamins That May Cause Abnormalities of Platelet Function *Continued*

Agent*	Abnormality†
Anesthetics and Narcotics	
Benoxinate, benzocaine, butacaine, cocaine, cyclaine, dibucaine, hydroxychloroquine, lidocaine, piperocaine, proparacaine, procaine, tetracaine	Abnormal platelet aggregation in vitro
Halothane, heroin	Abnormal platelet aggregation and bleeding time
Chemotherapeutic Agents	
Asparaginase, combination chemotherapy (cisplatin, cyclophosphamide, and either carmustine or melphalan), vincristine	Abnormal platelet aggregation
Carmustine, daunorubicin	Abnormal platelet aggregation in vitro
Plicamycin	Abnormal platelet aggregation and bleeding time; clinical bleeding
Antihistamines	
Chlorpheniramine, diphenhydramine, pyrilamine	Abnormal platelet aggregation in vitro
Radiographic Contrast Agents	
Diatrizoate meglumine (Renografin-76), diatrizoate meglumine and diatrizoate sodium (Renovist II, Urografin)	Abnormal platelet aggregation
Iopamidol, iothalamate, ioxaglate	Abnormal platelet aggregation in vitro
Other Drugs	
Clofibrate, guaifenesin, ketanserin	Abnormal platelet aggregation
Dextran, epoprostenol, nitrofurantoin	Abnormal platelet aggregation and bleeding time
Iloprost	Abnormal platelet aggregation in vitro
Ticlopidine	Abnormal platelet aggregation and bleeding time; clinical bleeding
Foods, Spices, and Vitamins	
Ginger, onion, vitamin C, vitamin E	Abnormal platelet aggregation
Cumin, turmeric, cloves	Abnormal platelet aggregation in vitro
Alcohol, n-3 fatty acids	Abnormal platelet aggregation and bleeding time
Chinese black tree fungus (Mo-er), garlic	Abnormal platelet aggregation; clinical bleeding

From George JM, Shattil SJ: The clinical importance of acquired abnormalities of platelet function. N Engl J Med 1991; 324:27–40. Massachusetts Medical Society.

*With the exception of studies demonstrating a significantly greater frequency of bleeding with aspirin, all are anecdotal observations in one or a few patients.

†"Abnormal platelet aggregation in vitro" indicates an abnormality when the agent is added to platelet-rich plasma. "Abnormal platelet aggregation" indicates an abnormality after administration of the agent to humans.

‡This drug has not been demonstrated to cause abnormal platelet function, but it has been used extensively as an antithrombotic agent.

TABLE 12–63. Mechanisms and Agents Responsible for Systemic Anaphylactic Reactions

Mechanism	Agent	Example
Immunoglobulin E-mediated reaction against native proteins	Venoms	Hymenoptera, fire ant, snake
	Airborne allergens	Pollens, molds, danders
	Foods	Peanuts, milk, egg, seafood, grains
	Enzymes	Trypsin, streptokinase, chymopapain
	Heterologous serum	Tetanus antitoxin, antilymphocyte globulin
	Human proteins	Insulin, corticotropin, vasopressin, serum and seminal proteins
	Others	Protamine, latex
Immunoglobulin E conjugates-mediated reaction against protein-hapten	Antibiotics	Penicillins, cephalosporins, sulfonamides
	Disinfectants	Ethylene oxide
Complement activation and generation of anaphylatoxins	Human proteins	Gamma globulins, other blood products
Dialysis	Contact of blood with some dialysis membranes	
Direct activation of mediator release from mast cells, basophils, or both	Hypertonic solutions	Radiocontrast medium, mannitol
	Drugs	Opiates, curare, *d*-tubocurarine, vancomycin
	Others	Dextran, fluorescein for angiography
Unknown	Nonsteroidal anti-inflammatory drugs	Aspirin, indomethacin
	Anesthetics	Lidocaine, thiopental
	Preservatives	Metabisulfites, benzoates
	Steroids	Progesterone, hydrocortisone
	Exercise	
	Exercise and food	
	Idiopathic anaphylaxis	

From Bochner BS, Lichtenstein LM: Anaphylaxis. N Engl J Med 1991; 324:1785–1790.

Gastric Lavage

A prospective controlled study of acutely self-poisoned patients by Merigian and colleagues indicates that little clinical deterioration occurs in asymptomatic patients treated without gastric emptying.[6] Gastric emptying procedures in symptomatic patients did not significantly alter the length of stay in the emergency department, mean length of time intubated, or mean length of stay in the ICU. In fact, gastric lavage was associated with a higher prevalence of medical ICU admissions and aspiration pneumonia. Studies in volunteers indicate that gastric lavage is more effective than syrup of ipecac when it is performed immediately after exposure,[6] but no statistical difference between lavage and emesis exists in the reduction of drug absorption when the markers are administered 1 hour after ingestion.

Efficacy

The efficacy of gastric lavage depends on the time elapsed between ingestion and lavage, on the amount ingested, on the inherent toxicity of the substance, and on the rate of absorption. Large amounts of unabsorbed drug will be removed from only a minority of patients who present to an emergency department after an overdose. Unfortunately, identifying the patients who will benefit the most from lavage is difficult.

Indications

Gastric lavage may be most effective for patients who ingest a life-threatening dose or who exhibit significant morbidity and who present soon (within 1 to 2 hours) after ingestion. Involvement of drugs that delay absorption, ingestion of large quantities of toxic drugs, and absence of bowel sounds on physical examination may lead to increased drug recovery at later times after ingestion. Whether these patients benefit from lavage as long as 4 to 6 hours after ingestion remains to be determined. Studies suggest that the recovery of drug at this delayed time is small. For minor to moderate ingestions of toxic substances that are adsorbed to activated charcoal, activated charcoal is probably preferred to gastric lavage.

TABLE 12–64. Drugs Commonly Associated with Orthostatic Hypotension in the Elderly

Antihypertensive Drugs	Drugs Producing Hypertension as an Adverse Effect
Diuretics	Nitrates
Calcium antagonists	Antiparkinsonian drugs
β-Blockers	(levodopa + decarboxylase inhibitors, bromocriptine, selegiline, anticholinergics)
Angiotensin-converting enzyme inhibitors	Antidepressants
Miscellaneous (prazosin, clonidine, guanfacine)	Antipsychotics (phenothiazine, butyrophenones)

From Mets TF: Drug-induced orthostatic hypotension in older patients. Drugs Aging 1995; 6:219–228.

TABLE 12–65. Adsorption of Drugs and Other Substances to Activated Charcoal In Vitro

Well Adsorbed	Poorly or Clinically Moderately Adsorbed	Inadequately Adsorbed
Aflatoxins	Aspirin and other salicylates	Cyanide
Amphetamine	DDT	Ethanol
Antidepressants	Disopyramide	Ethylene glycol
Antiepileptics	Kerosene, benzene, dichlorethane	Iron
Antihistamines	Malathion	Lithium
Atropine	Many "high-dose" nonsteroidal anti-inflammatory drugs, tolfenamic acid	Methanol
Barbiturates	Mexiletine	Strong acids and alkalis
Benzodiazepines	Paracetamol (acetaminophen)	
β-Blocking agents	Polychlorinated biphenyl compounds	
Chloroquine and primaquine	Phenol	
Cimetidine	Syrup of ipecac	
Dapsone	Tolbutamide, chlorpropamide, carbutamide, tolazamide	
Dextropropoxyphene and other opioids		
Digitalis glycosides		
Ergot alkaloids		
Furosemide		
Glibenclamide and glipizide		
Glutethimide		
Indomethacin		
Meprobamate		
Nefopam		
Phenothiazines		
Phenylbutazone		
Phenylpropanolamine		
Piroxicam		
Quinidine and quinine		
Strychnine		
Tetracyclines		
Theophylline		

From Neuvonen PJ, Olkolla KT: Oral activated charcoal in the treatment of intoxications: Role of single and repeated dose. Med Toxicol 1988; 3:33–58.

In summary, gastric lavage should not be employed routinely in the management of poisoned patients. There is no certain evidence that its use will improve outcome, and it may cause significant morbidity. Lavage should be considered only if a patient has ingested a life-threatening amount of a toxic substance within 1 hour of presentation. Even then, clinical benefit has not been confirmed in controlled studies. This will, no doubt, be modified in a subsequent publication, but it serves to indicate the present direction of thinking in the area. It does not, for the present, address the use of syrup of ipecac, activated charcoal (single or multiple dose), cathartics, or whole-bowel irrigation.

Gastric lavage followed by the instillation of activated charcoal with appropriate tracheal precautions may be useful in patients with altered mental status who present within 1 to 2 hours after ingestion. Lavage after this period may be appropriate in the presence of gastric concretions, delayed gastric emptying, or sustained-release preparations.

Cautions

1. Overall, the mortality from acute poisoning is less than 1%. The challenge for clinicians managing poisoned patients is to identify at an early stage those who are most at risk for development of serious complications and who might potentially benefit, therefore, from gut decontamination.
2. Gastric lavage is the passage of a large-bore orogastric tube and the sequential administration and aspiration of small volumes of liquid for removal of gastric contents.
3. Gastric lavage should not be considered a routine management procedure in poisoned patients.
4. Gastric emptying studies in experimental animals have shown no impressive drug recovery, particularly if lavage was delayed 60 minutes. Volunteer studies also proved no support for the use of gastric lavage. In the single clinical study in which overall benefit from lavage was demonstrated,[6] patients also received activated charcoal, which may have contributed to the apparent efficacy of lavage when this procedure was undertaken less than 1 hour after overdose.
5. Because it is known that the efficacy with which gastric lavage removes gastric contents decreases with time, lavage should be considered only if a patient has ingested a life-threatening amount of a toxic agent up to 1 hour previously.
6. Clinical and experimental studies have not confirmed the benefit of gastric lavage alone even when it is performed less than 1 hour after toxic ingestion. Drug absorption may be enhanced by its use.
7. In addition, there is no strong clinical evidence to support the view that, overall, lavage later than 1 hour after a toxic ingestion will benefit patients, including those who have ingested a tricyclic antidepressant or aspirin, although anecdotal reports indicate that impressive returns are occasionally achieved.
8. Lavage does not benefit the patient who has ingested a nontoxic agent or a nontoxic amount of a toxic agent.
9. Lavage is not useful as a deterrent to subsequent ingestions.

In conclusion, gastric emptying procedures in the emergency department are usually ineffective, may result in increased morbidity, and appear to offer no clinical advantage over charcoal alone.

Contraindications

ABSOLUTE. Lavage is absolutely contraindicated in patients with an unprotected airway, such as patients with a depressed state of consciousness, and in patients at risk of hemorrhage or perforation because of disease or recent surgery.

RELATIVE. Relative contraindications to gastric lavage are ingestion of a hydrocarbon, ingestion of an alkaline corrosive, ingestion of acid, and risk of hemorrhage or perforation because of disease or recent surgery.

Complications

Complications of gastric lavage include laryngospasm, a fall in the partial pressure of oxygen, aspiration pneumonia, sinus bradycardia, ST elevation on the electrocardiogram, and mechanical injury to the gut (rare).

Technique

1. If lavage is considered appropriate, it is essential that the staff (medical or nursing) undertaking the procedure be experienced in its execution both to reassure the conscious patient and to reduce the risk of complications.
2. If the patient is conscious, the procedure should be explained and consent obtained. A patient without previous experience of the procedure should be told, first, that a tube will be passed into her or his stomach so that the poison can be washed out and, second, that although the procedure is uncomfortable, it may lead to a faster recovery. If consent is refused for whatever reason, the procedure should not be attempted, not only because a technical assault will then be committed, but also because complications are likely to be greater.
3. Before the procedure is undertaken, it is essential to ensure that suctioning of the airway is available and functioning.
4. Endotracheal or nasotracheal intubation should precede gastric lavage in the comatose patient without a gag reflex. An oral airway should be placed between the teeth to prevent biting of the endotracheal tube if the patient recovers consciousness or convulses during the procedure.
5. The patient should be placed in the left lateral head-down position (20° tilt on the table), which has been shown to produce better lavage returns.
6. The length of tube to be inserted is measured and marked before insertion.
7. A wide-bore No. 36 to 40 French or No. 30 English gauge tube (external diameter approximately 12 to 13.3 mm) should be used in adults. The orogastric tube should be for single use only to avoid the risk of human immunodeficiency virus (HIV) and hepatitis virus transmission. The lavage tube should have a rounded end and be sufficiently firm to be passed into the passage. A nasogastric tube is of insufficient bore to produce a satisfactory lavage because particulate matter including medicines will not pass; moreover, damage to the nasal mucosa may cause severe epistaxis.
8. Force should not be used to pass the tube, particularly if the patient is struggling. Once the tube is passed, its position should be checked either by air insufflation, while listening over the stomach, or by aspiration with pH testing of the aspirate. An aliquot of this sample has traditionally been retained for toxicologic analysis, although except in the case of forensic examinations, the majority of laboratories now prefer blood or urine.
9. Lavage is carried out using small aliquots of liquid. In an adult, 200 to 300 mL of preferably warm (38°C) fluid such as saline or water should be used. In a child, 10 to 20 mL/kg body weight of warm fluid should be given. Water should preferably be avoided in young children because of the risk of inducing hyponatremia and water intoxication. Small volumes are used to minimize the risk of gastric contents entering the duodenum during lavage, because the amount of fluid affects the rate of gastric emptying. Warm fluids avoid the risk of hypothermia in the very young and very old and those receiving large volumes of lavage fluid.
10. Lavage should be continued until no further particulate matter is seen and the efferent lavage solution is clear.[6]

Activated Charcoal

Activated charcoal is emerging as a sole decontamination measure in view of the relative lack of efficacy of both syrup of ipecac and gastric lavage demonstrated in controlled clinical trials.[6] The effectiveness of several combined decontamination measures (e.g., charcoal-lavage-charcoal, charcoal 5 minutes after 60 mL of syrup of ipecac) has not been clinically evaluated in controlled studies. Serial activated charcoal can significantly reduce certain drug half-lives.[1, 6]

Precautions

The use of multiple doses of activated charcoal has been associated with several cases of intestinal obstruction, particularly in the cecum, both with and without the concomitant use of cathartics. Cathartics should not be administered with each dose of activated charcoal, particularly in infants, in whom electrolyte imbalance is likely to develop. Serious dehydration may result from such repetitive use. Multiple-dose activated charcoal should not be administered in the presence of diminished bowel sounds, proven ileus, or small bowel obstruction.

The first dose of activated charcoal can be administered through a small-bore nasogastric tube while airway control, intravenous access, blood sampling, cardiac monitoring, and other high-priority procedures are in progress. Once the patient has been stabilized, lavage with a large-bore orogastric tube can be accomplished.

Multiple-Dose Activated Charcoal

The use of repeated doses of activated charcoal, as compared with other modalities of gut decontamination, has not been subjected to controlled clinical trials and has generally not been shown to reduce morbidity and mortality. Severely poisoned adults should be given 150 to 200 g of activated charcoal through a nasogastric tube during 4 to 8 hours with the following guideline proposed: The total dose given may be more critical than the frequency of dosing. At present, multiple-dose activated charcoal is probably of value in the treatment of theophylline overdose, but it is not likely to be important in the presence of most other intoxications. It can be considered if a life-threatening amount of phenobarbital, carbamazepine, quinine, dapsone, or aspirin is ingested. Its value in the treatment of digoxin, digitoxin, phenytoin, sodium valproate, meprobamate, dapsone, carbamazepine, and cyclosporine intoxications has yet to be established by controlled studies. It does not hasten the elimination of cyclic antidepressants.[6]

Disadvantages of its use include its unpleasant taste, induction of vomiting, constipation and diarrhea, pulmonary aspiration, and gastrointestinal obstruction in patients with volume depletion. It is contraindicated in the presence of ileus or bowel obstruction and before endoscopy after corrosive ingestion unless there is a compelling need to adsorb another ingested toxin.

Dose

In children, the activated charcoal dose of 1 to 2 g/kg is not supported by clinical studies. This dose may lead to error in children because it is difficult to accurately measure 10 g of activated charcoal. Generally, 50 to 100 g is employed to fill the gut in adults. Because of mass action, large doses of activated charcoal (~1 g/kg) are necessary to promote adsorption and to prevent desorption of the drug. The continuous infusion of activated charcoal or the instillation of activated charcoal in a small nasogastric tube placed in the duodenum may improve the retention of activated charcoal in the overdose situation (e.g., theophylline) associated with protracted vomiting.

Cathartics

Mechanism of Action

The two groups of cathartics commonly used to treat patients with overdoses are (1) saline (magnesium citrate, magnesium sulfate, sodium sulfate, disodium phosphate) and (2) saccharides (e.g., sorbitol). Saline cathartics act by altering the physicochemical forces within the intestinal lumen. The osmotic retention of fluid within the gastrointestinal tract probably activates motility reflexes and enhances expulsion. Sorbitol catharsis can lead to liquid stools and abdominal discomfort.

The time to the first charcoal stool is substantially longer in overdose patients than in healthy volunteers who have been given a charcoal-sorbitol slurry, particularly when drugs with constipating effects are ingested.

Indications

Cathartics may reduce the transit time of drugs in the gut and decrease the constipating effects of multiple doses of charcoal, but they have never been shown to improve morbidity and mortality or to decrease hospital stay.

Contraindications

Contraindications to the use of cathartics include the ingestion of corrosives, severe diarrhea, adynamic or dynamic ileus, serious electrolyte imbalance, and recent bowel surgery. Cathartics should be used with caution when bowel sounds are absent.

Sorbitol

Sorbitol is now the cathartic of choice because it may be more effective than saline cathartics. In addition, sorbitol improves the palatability of activated charcoal. Whether it provides a bacteriostatic environment for the activated charcoal remains to be shown. Each milliliter of 70% sorbitol solution contains 0.9 g sorbitol. The usual dose is 1 to 2 mL of a 70% solution of sorbitol per kilogram body weight. This dose may be diluted 1:1 (i.e., 35% solution) for ambulatory adults. Sorbitol dosage in adults is 1 g/kg. Cathartics are used if indicated with only the first dose of charcoal. Patients should be carefully monitored for evidence of impaired fluid and electrolyte balance (e.g., hypernatremia) during administration of multiple doses of activated charcoal and sorbitol.

Saline Cathartics (Magnesium Citrate, Magnesium Sulfate, Sodium Sulfate)

Magnesium citrate (10% solution) is administered in a dose of 250 mL in an adult. If volume depletion is a problem, cathartics should be withheld. For more aggressive catharsis, whole-bowel irrigation should be used. Hypermagnesemia may follow excessive intake, impaired excretion, or parenteral administration of magnesium. Excessive oral intake of magnesium in the absence of either intestinal or renal disease occurs infrequently. Patients treated for overdose of drugs with frequent oral dosage of magnesium-containing cathartics may develop signs and symptoms of hypermagnesemia. Excessive oral intake of magnesium may induce diarrhea with increased levels of fecal magnesium. Fatal hypermagnesemia has followed rectal administration of magnesium preparations in cases of megacolon and bowel obstruction.[1, 6]

Whole-Bowel Irrigation

Whole-bowel irrigation is probably a useful and rapid method to empty the gut in 4 to 6 hours. It is messy and labor-intensive for patients who present to a hospital many hours after an overdose. Whole-bowel irrigation with high-molecular-weight polyethylene glycol (PEG-3350) and isosmolar electrolyte solution (PEG-ELS) is a safe and efficacious method for gut decontamination. Whole-bowel irrigation produces a more thorough cleansing of the entire intestinal tract compared with cathartics, which are agents that promote defecation rather than eliminate the whole contents of the intestines.

The previously used instillation of large volumes of isotonic saline as a means of preparing the bowel for diagnostic procedures or for gastrointestinal tract surgery was associated with electrolyte and fluid imbalance, and concern about these complications has limited the use of whole-bowel irrigation in treatment of overdoses; however, the recent development of isotonic solutions that use polyethylene glycol and sodium sulfate instead of sodium chloride has resulted in a procedure more suitable for clinical trials. This new lavage solution is available as GoLYTELY and Colyte. The use of PEG-ELS solution in whole-bowel irrigation produces no significant changes in serum electrolytes, serum osmolality, body weight, or hematocrit.

Mechanism of Action

High-molecular-weight polyethylene glycol (PEG-3350) does not produce distention of the abdomen like mannitol, which releases hydrogen in the presence of gut bacteria. The divalent sulfate ion impairs the active transport of sodium, and PEG-3350 prevents the shift of fluid across the intestinal wall by restoring the isotonicity of the solution. Both PEG-3350 and sulfate ions are poorly absorbed from the gastrointestinal tract, even in the presence of inflammatory bowel disease.

Indications

The efficacy of whole-bowel irrigation in reducing the absorption of toxins depends on the type of preparation and on the drug ingested. Activated charcoal does adsorb powdered polyethylene glycol. The concurrent administration of multiple doses of charcoal does not improve the effectiveness of whole-bowel irrigation[74]; however, in vitro data do not exclude the effectiveness of an initial dose of activated charcoal before the initiation of whole-bowel irrigation.[75] Whole-bowel irrigation does not increase the clearance of a drug already absorbed into the blood, at least in the aspirin overdose model. Potential uses for whole-bowel irrigation as a decontamination measure include ingestion of massive amounts of highly toxic drugs; ingestion of large amounts of drugs in patients presenting late (>4 hours after exposure); large overdoses of sustained-release preparations, many of which are associated with fatality or significant morbidity (Table 12–66); ingestion of drug packets by body packers or body stuffers; and ingestion of substances not adsorbed by activated charcoal. An additional possible use may be in ingestion of toxic substances that can be detected by radiography (arsenic, carbon tetrachloride, mercury, thallium). Lead has been removed by whole-bowel irrigation from the gastrointestinal tract of a patient suffering from lead toxicity.

METALS. Whole-bowel irrigation is a safe and effective decontamination procedure for potentially lethal iron ingestions, especially if the iron tablets have passed the pylorus. Activated charcoal does not adsorb iron or other metal compounds (e.g., lithium, potassium).

FOREIGN BODIES. Whole-bowel irrigation effectively removes miniature disk batteries from the gut and cocaine-filled packets in body packers and body stuffers. Iron, lead, lithium, sustained-release verapamil, and theophylline may be cleared from the gastrointestinal tract, but there is little evidence to indicate a lessening of morbidity or mortality from this procedure.

Dose

The technique for whole-bowel irrigation involves the insertion of a nasogastric tube into the stomach and the instillation of PEG-ELS solution while the patient sits on a commode. Alternatively, the solution can be ingested orally. Activated

TABLE 12–66. Drugs with Controlled-Release Preparations Associated with Fatality or Significant Morbidity

Drug	Toxic Dose	Comments
Amphetamine	>1 mg/kg	
Dexamphetamine	Variable	
Carbamazepine	>20 mg/kg	Pharmacobezoars; repeated dose of charcoal enhances clearance; charcoal hemoperfusion enhances clearance
Chlorpromazine	>10 mg/kg	Radiopaque*
Clonidine	>0.1 mg/kg	
Dextromethorphan	>10 mg/kg	
Dextropropoxyphene	>10 mg/kg	
Diltiazem	Variable	Pharmacodynamic variation†
Disopyramide	>10 mg/kg	
Felodipine	Variable	Pharmacodynamic variation†
Iron	>20 mg/kg	Radiopaque*; pharmacobezoars; does not bind to charcoal‡
Lithium	>10 mg/kg	Radiopaque*; does not bind to charcoal‡; hemodialysis enhances clearance
Meprobamate	Variable	Pharmacobezoars
Metoprolol	Variable	Pharmacodynamic variation†
Paracetamol (acetaminophen)	>150 mg/kg	
Potassium chloride	>2 mEq/kg if renal function is normal	Radiopaque*; does not bind to charcoal‡
Procainamide	>100 mg/kg	Hemoperfusion enhances clearance
Propranolol	Variable	Pharmacodynamic variation†
Quinidine	>50 mg/kg	
Salicylates	>100 mg/kg	Pharmacobezoars; radiopaque*; hemodialysis enhances clearance
Theophylline	>20 mg/kg	Pharmacobezoars; repeated dose of charcoal§ and charcoal hemoperfusion enhance clearance
Verapamil	Extremely variable	Pharmacodynamic variation†; pharmacobezoars; repeated dose of charcoal enhances clearance§

From Buckley NA, Dawson AH, Reitz DA: Controlled release drugs in overdose: Clinical considerations. Drug Saf 1995; 12:73–86.

*Radiopaque medications may lose this property with tablet dissolution. The absence of tablets on plain abdominal x-ray film does not exclude ingestion.

†Pharmacodynamic variation: toxicity from these drugs is significantly determined by factors of the patient, such as preexisting conditions and concomitant medications. It is therefore difficult to define a safe lower limit for ingestion. All such patients should receive gastrointestinal decontamination.

‡Patients poisoned by controlled-release drugs that do not bind to charcoal should be treated with whole-bowel lavage with polyethylene glycol electrolyte lavage solution (PEG-ELS).

§Increased clearance by using a repeated dose of charcoal is clinically significant. The charcoal dose may need to be increased in the presence of PEG-ELS.

charcoal may be administered before whole-bowel irrigation. The use of intravenous meoclopramide (10 mg for adults, 0.1–0.3 mg/kg body weight) may reduce the incidence of nausea and vomiting. The usual rate of fluid administration is 2 L/hour in adults. PEG-ELS solution should be given at room temperature to prevent hypothermia. The endpoint occurs when the rectal effluent is similar in appearance to the infusate. The usual infusion lasts 2 to 6 hours. This does not ensure that the toxin or foreign body is eliminated.

Precautions

Few complications occur after the use of whole-bowel irrigation for preparation of the bowel for radiographic examination or for surgery in either adults or children, even in the presence of cardiac, renal, or pulmonary disease. Complaints are usually minor and include nausea, vomiting, abdominal distention and cramps, sleep loss, and anal irrigation. Propylene glycol electrolyte lavage solution may occupy activated charcoal binding sites. It may also displace toxin from activated charcoal, leading to a substantial increase in toxin bioavailability.

Contraindications

Contraindications to the use of whole-bowel irrigation include gastrointestinal disease or dysfunction (obstruction, ileus, hemorrhage, perforation) and inadequate airway protection.

Controlled-Release Drugs

Serious effects and death may follow as late as 60 hours after overdose of sustained-release forms of drugs including verapamil, aspirin, theophylline, and lithium. Release of drug from the formulation may be further prolonged as a result of formation of a concretion of tablets in the stomach or intestine (e.g., theophylline, verapamil, carbamazepine, aspirin). Pharmacobezoars may be diagnosed by a plain abdominal radiograph (for radiopaque medications) or gastroendoscopy.

Monitoring

Treatment nomograms based on plasma concentrations calculated for standard-release formulations of some drugs (e.g., aspirin, iron, and paracetamol [acetaminophen]) are not appropriate for controlled-release formulations and their application may lead to inappropriate management. Treatment decisions need to be based on clinical toxicity and calculations of the total ingested dose. For drugs, the absolute concentration of which may indicate the need for further treatment (e.g., lithium, theophylline, procainamide), the concentration should be measured until there is a sustained decline to nontoxic levels. Poisonings with these preparations have demonstrated multiple peak concentrations indicating continuing and variable absorption for more than 24 hours. Where there is a significant risk of serious toxicity, gastric lavage should be performed on admission with an orogastric tube large enough to remove whole tablets. Patients presenting with overdose of calcium antagonists or propranolol may require pretreatment with atropine to avoid vagal stimulation, which may precipitate complete heart block or asystole.

Activated Charcoal

The role of activated charcoal in the treatment of controlled-release preparations is still being defined. Repeated doses of activated charcoal can increase the clearance of a number of drugs either by interruption of the enterohepatic circulation or by direct "dialysis" from capillaries in the gastrointestinal mucosa.

Whole-Bowel Irrigation

Use whole-bowel irrigation alone for overdose with those medications not adsorbed to charcoal. Patients with other poisonings receive a single dose of activated charcoal (to adsorb drug that is not held within the controlled-release vehicle), followed by whole-bowel irrigation. Repeated doses of activated charcoal are added only for those drugs for which it has clearly been shown to enhance clearance.

Alkaline and Acid Diuresis

Alkaline diuresis may aid in increasing renal clearance and reducing the elimination half-life of salicylates, phenobarbital, and phenoxyacetate herbicides. Complications include fluid overload, noncardiogenic pulmonary edema (salicylates), cerebral edema, and electrolyte and acid-base disturbances. Patients should be monitored frequently (plasma drug concentrations; urine pH; fluid balance; central venous pressure; electrolytes; serum sodium, potassium, calcium, magnesium). A practical role for diuresis (acid or alkaline) in the treatment of most overdoses has not been determined by controlled studies. The utility of both acid and alkaline diuresis has recently been called into question by the ability of less care-intensive methods such as repeated-dose charcoal to increase the elimination of many toxins.[6]

Extracorporeal Techniques

The efficacy of dialysis methods and hemoperfusion in acute poisoning cannot be clinically estimated easily because concomitant intestinal absorption, hepatic metabolism, and urinary excretion must be considered. With supportive treatment alone, spontaneous recovery usually occurs in 98% of the intoxications in ICUs. Extracorporeal techniques may be limited to use in salicylate, methanol, ethylene glycol, lithium, and theophylline overdose and are of limited use in sedative-hypnotic, industrial, and household poisonings. When required, such treatment should be available so that emergency hemodialysis and hemoperfusion are able to be performed within a short time[6] (Tables 12–67 and 12–68).

ANTIDOTES

Antidotes may be lifesaving. They can aid in reducing morbidity and health care costs by shortening the course of treatment. Some antidotes (e.g., naloxone, flumazenil) exhibit rapid and dramatic clinical effects. Some do not affect all the toxic effects of a particular poisoning (e.g., chelating agents), and a few are useful adjuncts to treatment without specific antidotal effects (e.g., diazepam in the treatment of organophosphate poisoning). Controlled clinical studies are limited for ethical reasons.

Antidotes are drugs and often precipitate undesirable reactions (e.g., naloxone, flumazenil). A list of antidotes and other agents useful in the treatment of poisoning appears in Table 12–69. Antidotes appear to reflect national practices (e.g., 4-dimethylaminophenol for cyanide intoxication in Germany; hydroxocobalamin for cyanide poisoning in France; silibinin for amanitin poisoning in Austria and Germany), but most antidotes, thanks to widely publicized information (medical toxicology literature, national and international meetings), have been widely used. Governmental regulations, a lack of economic incentives for manufacturers, and a paucity of controlled studies have restricted availability of a number of antidotes (e.g., hydroxocobalamin in the United States).

Special Specific Antidotes

Flumazenil

Mechanism of Action

Flumazenil antagonizes the actions of benzodiazepines by competitively inhibiting benzodiazepine activity at the γ-aminobutyric acid–benzodiazepine receptor complex. Flumazenil has little or no agonist activity in humans.

Use

Flumazenil is indicated primarily in the treatment of symptoms of benzodiazepine overdose. Flumazenil is possibly effective in improving consciousness in ethanol intoxication, in which it may aid in improving blood gas analyses and permitting extubation.[6] Patients anesthetized with 0.3 mg/kg of diazepam, or 0.03 mg/kg of flunitrazepam, or 0.3 mg/kg of midazolam with 1 mg/kg of pentazocine, nitrous oxide, and a muscle relaxant regained consciousness within 1 to 6 minutes after administration of flumazenil. Flumazenil may be useful in chronic obstructive pulmonary disease, even in patients with a therapeutic diazepam level.[6]

Cautions

1. Ventricular tachycardia, bradycardia, complete heart block, and death may follow flumazenil use.
2. Seizures and acute anxiety states may be provoked in patients dependent on benzodiazepines.
3. Seizures are more common if the patient has taken a tricyclic antidepressant, isoniazid, cocaine, or propoxyphene in addition to the benzodiazepine. Flumazenil antagonizes the anticonvulsant properties of the benzodiazepines, leaving a medication that may be epileptogenic.
4. Acute withdrawal symptoms may be seen in the benzodiazepine-dependent patient given flumazenil in an emergency facility. Because return to consciousness after a benzodiazepine overdose may be due to the development of tolerance rather than drug elimination, late use of flumazenil may lead to withdrawal symptoms.
5. Repeated doses may be required because of the short duration of action of flumazenil (<1 hour).

Dose

As a diagnostic tool in the evaluation of comatose drug overdose, flumazenil should be given as a 0.2-mg bolus intravenously, with an additional 0.1 mg/min until the patient is awake. Most patients respond to 3 mg or less. A continuous infusion of flumazenil has not been shown to be superior to a repeated bolus technique, often preferred for routine clinical use. One method of administration is to mix 2 mg of flumazenil with 1 L of normal saline intravenous fluid, starting at 100 ml/hour, and titrating based on clinical response. An intravenous dose of 5 mg may improve consciousness in alcohol intoxication but does not improve psychomotor function.

N-Acetylcysteine

Mechanism of Action

N-Acetylcysteine (NAC) may increase oxygen consumption and improve microcirculatory blood flow by stimulating the activity of endothelium-derived factor. NAC acts as a glutathione substitute that prevents the formation of an intermediate toxic substance in acetaminophen overdose.

TABLE 12–67. Drugs and Chemicals Removed with Dialysis

Barbiturates

Amobarbital
Aprobarbital
Barbital
Butabarbital
Cyclobarbital
Pentobarbital
Phenobarbital
Quinalbital
(Secobarbital)

Nonbarbiturate Hypnotics, Sedatives, Tranquilizers, Anticonvulsants

Carbamazepine
Carbromal
Chloral hydrate
(Chlordiazepoxide)
(Diazepam)
(Diphenylhydantoin)
(Diphenylhydramine)
Ethiamate
Ethchlorvynol
Ethosuximide
Galamine
Glutethimide
(Heroin)
Meprobamate
(Methaqualone)
Methsuximide
Methyprylon
Paraldehyde
Primidone
Valproic acid

Antidepressants

(Amitriptyline)
Amphetamines
(Imipramine)
Isocarboxazid
Monoamine oxidase inhibitors
(Pargyline)
(Phenelzine)
Tranylcypromine
(Tricyclics)

Alcohols

Ethanol
Ethylene glycol
Isopropanol
Methanol

Analgesics, Antirheumatic Agents

Acetaminophen
Acetophenetidin (phenacetin)
Acetylsalicylic acid
Colchicine
Methylsalicylate
(D-Propoxyphene)
Salicylic acid

Antimicrobial Agents/ Anticancer Agents

Amikacin
Dibekacin
Fosfomycin
Gentamicin
Kanamycin
Neomycin
Netilmicin
Sisomicin
Streptomycin
Tobramycin
(Vancomycin)

Bacitracin
Colistin

Ampicillin
Amoxicillin
Azlocillin
Carbenicillin
Clavulinic acid
(Cloxacillin)
(Floxacillin)
Mecillinam
Mezlocillin
(Nafcillin)
Penicillin
Piperacillin
Temocillin
Ticarcillin

(Cefaclor)
Cefadroxil
Cefamandole
Cefazolin
Cefixime
Cefmenoxime
(Cefonicid)
(Cefoperazone)
Ceforanide
(Cefotaxime)
(Cefotetan)
Cefotiam
Cefoxitin
Cefroxadine
Cefsulodin
Ceftazidime
(Ceftriaxone)
Cefuroxime
Cephacetrile
Cephalexin
Cephaloridine
Cephalothin
(Cephapirin)
Cephradine

Aztreonam
Cilastatin
Imipenem
Moxalactam

(Chloramphenicol)
Ciprofloxacin
(Clindamycin)
(Erythromycin)
Metronidazole
Nitrofurantoin
Ornidazole
Sulfonamides
Tetracycline
Tinidazole

Acyclovir
Amantadine
(Chloroquine)
Cycloserine
Ethambutol
5-Fluorocytosine
Isoniazid
Quinine

(Azathioprine)
Bredinin
Cyclophosphamide
5-Fluorouracil
(Methotrexate)

Cardiovascular Agents

Acebutolol
N-Acetylprocainamide
Atenolol
Bretylium
Captopril
(Diazoxide)
(Digoxin)
(Lidocaine)
Metoprolol
Methyldopa
(Ouabain)
Nadolol
Practolol
Procainamide
Propranolol
(Quinidine)
Sotalol
Tocainide

Metals, Inorganics

(Aluminum)*
Arsenic
(Copper)*
(Iron)*
Lead
Lithium
(Magnesium)
(Mercury)*
Potassium
Phosphate
Sodium
Strontium
(Tin)
(Zinc)

Bromide
Chloride
Iodide
Fluoride

Miscellaneous Drugs

Acipimox
Aminophylline
Aniline
Borates
Boric acid
(Chlorpropamide)
Chromic acid
Cimetidine
Dinitro-*o*-cresol
Folic acid
Mannitol
Methylprednisolone
Potassium dichromate
Sodium citrate
Theophylline
Thiocyanate
Ranitidine

Solvents, Gases

Acetone
Camphor
Carbon monoxide
(Carbon tetrachloride)
(Eucalyptus oil)
Thiols
Toluene
Trichloroethylene

Plants, Animals, Herbicides, Insecticides

Alkyl phosphate
Amanitine
Demeton sulfoxide
Dimethoate
Diquat
Methylmercury complex
(Organophosphates)
Paraquat
Snake bite
Sodium chlorate
Potassium chlorate

From Winchester JF: Poisoning: Is the role of the nephrologist diminishing? Am J Kidney Dis 1989; 13:171–183.
( ) = not well removed; ( )* = removed with chelating agent.

TABLE 12–68. Drugs and Chemicals Removed with Hemoperfusion

Barbiturates	Amobarbital Butabarbital Hexabarbital Phenobarbital Pentobarbital Quinalbital Secobarbital Thiopental Vinalbital
Nonbarbiturate Hypnotics, Sedatives, Tranquilizers	Carbromal Chloral hydrate Chlorpromazine (Diazepam) Dephenhydramine Ethchlorvynol Glutethimide Meprobamate Methaqualone Methsuximide Methyprylon Promazine Promethazine
Analgesics, Antirheumatic Agents	Acetaminophen Acetylsalicyclic acid Colchicine Methylsalicylate Phenylbutazone D-Propoxyphene Salicylic acid
Antimicrobial Agents/Anticancer Agents	(Adriamycin) Ampicillin Carmustine Chloramphenicol Chloroquine Clindamycin Dapsone Doxorubicin Gentamicin Isoniazid (Methotrexate) Thiabendazole
Antidepressants	(Amitriptyline) (Imipramine) (Tricyclics)
Plants, Animals, Herbicides, Insecticides	Amanitine Chlordane Demeton sulfoxide Dimethoate Diquat Methylparathion Nitrostigmine Organophosphates Paraquat Parathion Phalloidin Polychlorinated biphenyls
Cardiovascular Agents	*N*-acetyl-procainamide Digoxin (Disopyramide) Procainamide Quinidine
Metals, Inorganics	(Aluminum)* (Iron)*
Miscellaneous Drugs	Aminophylline Cimetidine (Fluoroacetamide) (Phencyclidine) Phenols (Podophyllin) Theophylline
Solvents, Gases	Carbon tetrachloride Ethylene oxide Trichloroethanol

From Winchester JF: Poisoning: Is the role of the nephrologist diminishing? Am J Kidney Dis 1989; 13:171–183.
( ) = not well removed; ( )* = removed with chelating agent.

Use

NAC is used for the treatment of acetaminophen overdoses. Survival improves in patients with acetaminophen-induced fulminant hepatic failure given acetylcysteine soon after acetaminophen ingestion; improvement may also be observed after encephalopathy and other signs of severe liver damage, including coagulopathy, have developed. Only the oral form of NAC is approved by the Food and Drug Administration (FDA). The intravenous form is available in the United States only through an investigational new drug (IND) protocol. Approval must be obtained through the FDA (Phone: 301-443-1479). Intravenous NAC is available in the United Kingdom and Canada.

Anecdotal Reports

Potential uses of acetylcysteine in addition to acetaminophen (paracetamol) poisoning include toxicity secondary to halogenated hydrocarbons that may deplete glutathione (chloroform-phosgene metabolite, carbon tetrachloride, bromobenzene), paraquat (in animals, conflicting data suggest diminished glutathione in liver, not lung), acrylonitrile (formation of cyanoethyacetylcysteine), naphthalene (epoxide metabolite conjugates with glutathione), sulfur mustard, and cytotoxic agents (ifosfamide—intravesical protection; bleomycin—to prevent excess lung fibrosis) and for prevention of delayed neuropsychiatric complications of carbon monoxide poisoning.

Other proposed uses include improvement of alveolar macrophage function in the bronchoalveolar lavage fluid from cigarette smoke, treatment of inflammatory joint disease, prevention of HIV expression (acquired immunodeficiency syndrome [AIDS]), use in the adult respiratory distress syndrome (free radical scavenger), potentiation of the cardiovascular effects of nitroglycerin and organic nitrites, treatment of dichromate intoxication, amanitin poisoning, and reduction of lipoprotein. No clear conclusions have emerged from these studies to provide definitive guidelines for clinical usefulness. Controlled clinical studies are required to place most of these observations in perspective.

Cautions

After repeated high doses of oral NAC, nausea, vomiting, and diarrhea may occur. Headache, hypotension, and rash rarely occur. Urticaria and hepatotoxicity are seen rarely. High-dose intravenous administration may be accompanied by anaphylactoid reactions beginning about 15 to 60 minutes after an infusion is started in 10% of patients. Asthmatic patients are especially at risk. A serum sickness–like illness has been described. Treatment is supportive and symptomatic. Activated charcoal administration before oral NAC may not diminish the hepatoprotective effect of NAC.

Naloxone

Use

A prospective, randomized, double-blind, placebo-controlled study showed that 0.4 to 1.2 mg of naloxone intravenously was no better than placebo in amelioration of hypotension in septic shock. Continuous naloxone administration may aid in suppressing opiate withdrawal symptoms in human opiate addicts during detoxification treatment. An anecdotal

TABLE 12–69. Antidotes and Other Agents Useful in Treatment of Poisoning

Antidote	Main Indication of Pathologic Condition	Other Possible Applications
Acetylcysteine	Paracetamol (acetaminophen)	Organochlorine solvents, amanitin
β-Aminopropionitrile	Caustics	
Amyl nitrite	Cyanide	Hydrogen sulfide
Ascorbic acid	Organic peroxides (osmium)	
Atropine	Cholinergic syndrome	
Aurintricarboxylic acid (ATA)	Beryllium	
Benzylpenicillin	Amanitins	
Calcium chloride or other calcium salts	HE-fluorides, oxalates	Calcium antagonists
Dantrolene	Malignant hyperthermia	Malignant neuroleptic syndrome
Deferoxamine	Iron, aluminum	Paraquat
Diazepam	Chloroquine	
Dicobalt edetate	Cyanide	
Digoxin-specific antibody fragments	Digoxin/digitoxin, digitalis glycosides	
Dimercaprol	Arsenic	Copper, gold, mercury (inorganic), lead encephalopathy
4-Dimethylaminophenol (4-DMAP)	Cyanide	Hydrogen sulfide
Ethanol	Methanol, ethylene glycol, glycol ethers	Alkoxysilanes
Flumazenil	Benzodiazepines	
Folinic acid	Folinic acid antagonists	
Glucagon	β-Blockers	
Glucose	Insulin	
Guanidine	Botulism	
Hydroxocobalamin	Cyanide	
Isoprenaline	β-Blockers	
Methionine	Paracetamol (acetaminophen)	
4-Methylpyrazole	Ethylene glycol, methanol	Coprin and disulfiram
Methylthionine chloride (methylene blue)	Methemoglobinemia	
N-Acetylpenicillamine	Mercury	
Naloxone	Opiates	
Neostigmine	Neuromuscular block (curare type) peripheral anticholinergic poisoning	
Oximes	Organophosphates	
Oxygen	Cyanide, carbon monoxide, hydrogen sulfide	
Oxygen, hyperbaric	Carbon monoxide	Cyanide, hydrogen sulfide, carbon tetrachloride
Penicillamine	Copper	Gold, lead, mercury
Pentetic acid (DTPA)	Radioactive metals	
Phentolamine	α-Adrenergic poisoning	
Physostigmine	Central anticholinergic syndrome from atropine and derivatives	Central anticholinergic syndrome from other drugs
Phytoenadione (vitamin K)	Coumarin derivatives	
Potassium hexacyanoferrate (Prussian blue C177520)	Thallium	
	Prenalterol	
Propranolol	β-Adrenergic poisoning	
Protamine sulfate	Heparin	
Pyridoxine	Isoniazid	Ethylene glycol, gyrometrine, hydrazines
Silibinin	Amanitine	
Sodium nitrite	Cyanide	Hydrogen sulfide
Sodium nitroprusside	Ergotism	
Sodium salicylate	Beryllium	
Sodium thiosulfate	Cyanide	Bromate, chlorate, iodine
Succimer (DMSA)	Lead, mercury	
Tocopherol	Carbon monoxide	Oxygen toxicity
Tolonium chloride (toluidine blue)	Methemoglobinemia	
Trientine (triethylene tetramine)	Copper	
Unithiol (DMPS)	Arsenic	Copper, nickel, lead, cadmium, mercury (methyl and inorganic)

From Meredith TJ, Jacobsen D, Haines JA, Berger J-C (Eds): International Program on Chemical Safety/Commission of the European Communities Evaluation of Antidotes Series. Vol 1. Naloxene, Flumazenil, and Dantrolene as Antidotes. EUR 14797 EN. Vol 2. Antidotes for Poisoning by Cyanide (van Heijst APVP, guest ed.). EUR 12280 EN. Cambridge, Cambridge University Press, 1993.

report suggests that intravenous naloxone, 1.6 mg, reversed the hypotension associated with a captopril overdose. Anecdotal evidence suggests that naloxone with activated charcoal may be useful in improving degree of consciousness after a valproic acid overdose.

Preliminary Studies

Naloxone induces an increase in cortisol secretion. Acute alcoholism may induce an increase in endogenous opioids in the plasma and cerebrospinal fluid. Preliminary studies tend to suggest that naloxone may reverse the effect of alcohol by its ability to increase cortisol secretion. The ultimate answer to this relationship remains to be determined. Naloxone may be an additional modality of use in the treatment of captopril-induced hypotension. The mechanism of its effectiveness in one anecdotal report is not clear. Further clinical studies are indicated.

Dose

Preliminary studies with oral naloxone administered in doses from 0.5 to 16 mg once daily indicate possible efficacy in the treatment of opioid-induced constipation. All patients should be monitored for the signs and symptoms of systemic withdrawal. Adverse reactions can be managed with single-dose reduction or lengthening of the interval. When given orally, naloxone is extensively metabolized and may have greater bioavailability at the enteric wall than systemically. Naloxone can be titrated up to 12 mg at dose intervals of 6 hours or longer, and this procedure should be used if multiple daily doses are required.

If attempts at intravenous access for naloxone injection are unsuccessful, an injection of 0.4 mg naloxone with a 22-gauge needle into the midventral surface of the tongue after aspiration with no blood return and intubation can be considered in the treatment of narcotic-induced respiratory depression. If, however, the patient has a normal blood pressure, this route may be unnecessary, because naloxone is absorbed efficiently and is rapid-acting when the patient is not in shock and an adequate dose is administered by the intramuscular route. In addition, a sublingual injection may have the potential to cause intraoral bleeding and possible airway compromise. There is also the possibility that a paramedic or other health care professional planning to use the sublingual route may be bitten by a patient who may be at high risk of having AIDS.

Continuous Infusion

A method has been determined for infusion therapy with naloxone after the bolus dose.

Step 1: Determine maintenance fluid requirements for 24 hours.
Step 2: To determine amount of naloxone (in mg) to add to the maintenance fluid for a 24-hour period, take the amount required for the initial response (in mg) × ⅔ × 24 hours.
Step 3: To determine the desired rate of naloxone infusion (in mL/hr), take the maintenance fluid (step 1) per 24 hours.

This method may reduce the risk of possible fluid overload and the potential for pulmonary edema from opioids. Naloxone should not be mixed with preparations containing bisulfite, metabisulfite, long-chain or high-molecular-weight anions, or any solution having an alkaline pH. A naloxone mixture should not be used after 24 hours from the time it was prepared.

Infusions of naloxone may be indicated when (1) repeated bolus therapy is required, (2) a large initial bolus is required, (3) a large amount of opiate or a long-acting opiate (e.g., propoxyphene, methadone) has been ingested, or (4) opioid metabolism is decreased, as in liver disease.

Naloxone is not recommended in the treatment of meperidine-induced seizures and may be detrimental.

Pathophysiology

Naloxone appears to modulate the release of catecholamines, presumably from chromaffin cells. Plasma epinephrine, norepinephrine, and dopamine concentrations were increased in a patient with pheochromocytoma after 10 mg of intravenous naloxone was administered.

NALOXONE AND MORPHINE METABOLISM. Animal studies with naloxone and morphine suggest that morphine acts mainly on the dopaminergic system in the brain, interacting with naloxone preferential receptors. Its action is also induced through the noradrenergic system in some areas of the brain. No biochemical action of morphine is apparent in the central serotoninergic system.

KAPPA RECEPTOR ACTIVATORS. Kappa receptor activators (pentazocine, butorphanol) may result in sedative and psychotomimetic effects, which are antagonized by high doses of naloxone.

TOXICOKINETICS AND CLINICAL PRESENTATION—PREGNANCY. Intravenous naloxone, 0.4 mg, may induce severe hypertension during labor in a patient with a history of previous mild hypertension. Patients with mild to moderate hypertension who receive narcotic antagonists during labor should be carefully monitored.

Drug Interactions

BUPRENORPHINE. The antagonism of buprenorphine requires large doses of naloxone and is characterized by gradual onset of the reversal effects and decreased duration of action of the normally prolonged respiratory depression.

METHOHEXITAL. The acute onset of withdrawal symptoms induced by naloxone in opiate addicts appears to be blocked by the acute action of the barbiturate methohexital. This observation requires clinical confirmation in opiate withdrawal states.

NALOXONE. Naloxone has been associated with hypertension, cardiac arrhythmias, cardiac arrest, and sudden death, all of which may be provoked by sympathetic stimulation. Seizures, by an as yet undetermined mechanism, may also follow naloxone use. Even low doses of 40 to 80 mg of naloxone may precipitate pulmonary edema in otherwise healthy young people. Large doses may induce an acute pulmonary edema in the older age groups.

For a complete discussion of the preceding topics, see the text identified in reference 6.

References

1. Vale JA: Medical toxicology: Clinical aspects. Arch Toxicol 1991; 15 (Suppl):12–13.
2. Meredith TJ: Epidemiology of poisoning. Pharmacol Ther 1993; 49:251–256.
3. Centers for Disease Control and Prevention: Unintentional poisoning mortality: United States, 1980–1986. MMWR 1989; 38:153–158.
4. Centers for Disease Control and Prevention: Unintentional ingestion of prescription drugs in children under five years old. MMWR 1987; 36:124–132.
5. Litovitz TL, Flagler SL, Manoguerra AS, et al: Recurrent poisoning among pediatric poisoning victims. Med Toxicol Adverse Drug Experience 1989; 4:381–386.
6. Ellenhorn M: Medical Toxicology, 2nd ed. New York, Williams & Wilkins, 1997.
7. Woolf AD, Lovejoy FH Jr: Epidemiology of drug overdose in children. Drug Saf 1993; 9:291–304.
8. Litovitz TL, Clark LR, Soloway RA: 1993 Annual report of the American Association of Poison Control Centers Toxic Exposure Surveillance System. Am J Emerg Med 1994; 12:546–583.
9. Litovitz TL, Schmitz BF, Holm KC: 1988 Annual report of the

American Association of Poison Control Centers National Data Collection System. Am J Emerg Med 1989; 7:495–545.
10. Klein-Schwartz W, Oderda GM, Booze L: Poisoning in the elderly. J Am Geriatr Soc 1983; 31:195–199.
11. Litovitz T, Manoguerra A: Comparison of pediatric poisoning hazards: An analysis of 3.8 million exposure incidents: A report from the American Association of Poison Control Centers. Pediatrics 1992; 89:999–1005.
12. Woolf A, Liebelt Z, Lovejoy FH Jr: Pediatric poisoning hazards (Letter; comment). Pediatrics 1993; 91:1017–1018.
13. Michell L-J, Dexter EM, Bradberry SM, et al: Assessment of IPCS/CEC/EAPCTT. Dexter EM, Michell L-J, Casey PB: The role and value of phonetoxscore in cases of poisoning. Phonetoxscore by staff of the PNPIS (Birmingham Centre) (Abstract Nos. 0.83 and 0.84). *In*: Proceedings, XVIth International Congress of the European Association of Poison Centres and Clinical Toxicologists, Vienna, April 12, 1994.
14. March AG, Bet N, Persino MG, et al: Severity grading of childhood poisoning: The Matti Center study of poisoning children (MPXC) scare. Clin Toxicol 1995; 33:223–231.
15. Koren G: Medications which can kill a toddler with one tablet or teaspoonful. Clin Toxicol 1993; 31:407–413.
16. Geller RJ, Fisher JG III, Leeper JD, Ranganathon S: American Poison Control Centers: Still not all the same? Ann Emerg Med 1988; 17:599–603.
17. Sibert R, Routledge PA: Accidental poisoning in children: Can we admit fewer children with safety? Arch Dis Child 1991; 66:263–266.
18. Henretig FM: Special considerations in the poisoned pediatric patient. Emerg Med Clin North Am 1994; 12:549–547.
19. Haslam R: Drug safety and medication systems in hospitals. Adverse Drug React Acute Poisoning Rev 1988; 3:133–146.
20. Vitillo JA, Lesar TS: Preventing medication prescribing errors. D.I.C.P. Ann Pharmacother 1991; 25:1388–1394.
21. Mayer GA: Chlorpropamide or chlorpromazine? (Letter; comment) Can Med Assoc J 1991; 144:119.
22. Hoffman JP: More on Losec or Lasix? (Letter; comment) N Engl J Med 1990; 323:1428.
23. Landis SJ. Azathioprine or azidothyridine. (Letter) Can Med Assoc J 1990; 143:611.
24. Olsen LA, Miller DR, Goswani A, McAskill AC, Newman WP: Inadvertent administration of acetohexamide instead of acetazolamide (Letter). D.I.C.P. Ann Pharmacother 1991; 25:100.
25. Pincus JM, Ike PW: Norflox or Norflex? (Letter) N Engl J Med 1992; 326:1030.
26. Garvey CW: Desipramine sent when it's disopyramide (Letter). JAMA 1989; 262:210.
27. Brierton D, Nunn-Thompson CW: Warning: Acetaminophen and aprolidine both labeled Apronal (Letter). D.I.C.P. Ann Pharmacother 1990; 24:1232.
28. Hooper PL, Tello RJ, Burstein PJ, Abrams RS: Pseudoinsulinoma: The Diamox-Diabinese switch (Letter). N Engl J Med 1990; 1323:488.
29. Fallis G: Quinine or quinidine? Can Med Assoc J 1991; 144:540–541.
30. Kurth MC, Langston JW, Tetrud WW: "Stelazine" versus "selegiline": A hazard in prescription writing (Letter). N Engl J Med 1990; 1323:1776.
31. Ahlquist DA, Nelson RL, Callaway CW: Pseudoinsulinoma syndrome from inadvertent tolazamide ingestion. Ann Intern Med 1980; 93:281–282.
32. Kramer JM: More on drug name confusion. N Engl J Med 1995; 332:753–754.
33. Lesar TS, Briceland LL, Delcoure K, et al: Medical prescribing errors in a teaching hospital. JAMA 1990; 263:2329–2334.
34. Janda SM: Look-alike and sound-alike medication pairs. Vet Hum Toxicol 1994; 36:256–259.
35. Mrvos R, Dean BS, Krenzelok EP: Illiteracy: A contributing factor to poisoning. Vet Hum Toxicol 1993; 35:466–468.
36. Perlstein PH, Callison C, White M, et al: Errors in drug computations during newborn intensive care. Am J Dis Child 1979; 133:376–379.
37. Bleyer WA, Koup JR: Medication errors during intensive care. Am J Dis Child 1979; 133:366–367.
38. Koren G, Barzilay Z, Greenwald M: Tenfold errors in administration of drug doses: A neglected iatrogenic disease in pediatrics. Pediatrics 1986; 77:848–849.
39. Bury G: Errors in drug administration (Letter). Pediatrics 1987; 79:170–172.
40. Lamont JH: Errors in drug administration. Pediatrics 1987; 79:171–177.
41. Rieder WJ, Goldstein D, Zinman H, Koren G: Tenfold errors in drug dosage. Can Med Assoc J 1988; 139:12–13.
42. Kulig K: Initial management of ingestions of toxic substances. N Engl J Med 1992; 326:1678–1681.
43. Lloyd-Thomas AP: Paediatric Glasgow Coma Scale. BMJ 1990; 301:380–382.
44. Yaeger JY, Johnston B, Sesshia SS: Coma scales in pediatric practice. Am J Dis Child 1990; 144:1088–1091.
45. Stanmark J-E, Stalhammer D, Holmgren E: The reaction level scale (RLS85): Manual and guidelines. Acta Neurochir (Wien) 1988; 91:12–20.
46. Stanczak DE, White JG, Gouview W, et al: Assessment of level of consciousness following severe neurological insult. J Neurosurg 1984; 60:955–961.
47. Crosby L, Parsons LC: Clinical neurologic assessment tool: Development and testing of an instrument to index neurologic status. Heart Lung 1989; 18:121–129.
48. Giacino JT, Kezmarsky MA, De Luca J, Cicerone KD: Monitoring rate of recovery to predict outcome in minimally responsive patients. Arch Phys Med Rehabil 1991; 72:897–901.
49. Born JD: The Glasgow-Liege Scale. Acta Neurochir (Wien) 1988; 91:1–11.
50. Benzer A, Mittershiffthaler G, Marosi M, et al: Pediatric measures of non-survival after trauma: Innsbruck Coma Scale. Lancet 1991; 338:977–978.
51. Jennett B, Bond M: Assessment of outcome after severe brain damage. Lancet 1975; 1:484–485.
52. Segatore M, Way C: The Glasgow Coma Scale: Time for change. Heart Lung 1992; 21:548–555.
53. Olson KR, Kerney TE, Dyer JE, Benowitz HL: Seizures associated with poisoning and drug overdose: Changing patterns of causes and poison center consultations. Vet Hum Toxicol 1990; 32:361–366.
54. Working Group on Status Epilepticus: Treatment of convulsive status epilepticus: Recommendations of the Epilepsy Foundation of America Working Group on Status Epilepticus. JAMA 1993; 270:854–859.
55. Zaccara G, Muscas GC, Messori A: Clinical features, pathogenesis and management of drug-induced seizures. Drug Saf 1990; 5:109–151.
56. Hoffman R: Nervous system toxicity. Personal presentation, American College of Medical Toxicology, Board Examination Review Course, September 1994.
57. Morrow JI, Routledge BA: Drug-induced neurological disorders. Adverse Drug React Acute Poisoning Rev 1988; 3:105–133.
58. Francis J, Kapoor WN: Delirium in hospitalized elderly. J Gen Intern Med 1990; 5:65–79.
59. Bruno A, Nolte KB, Chapinj J: Stroke associated with ephedrine use. Neurology 1993; 43:1313–1316.
60. Griffen JP: A review of the literature on benign intracranial hypertension associated with medication. Adverse Drug React Toxicol Rev 1992; 11:41–58.
61. Patter SB, Love EJ: Drug-induced depression: Incidence, avoidance and management. Drug Saf 1994; 10:203–219.
62. Turner P: Clinical pharmacology in criminal cases: Discussion paper. J R Soc Med 1987; 8:438–439.
63. Sulter DL, Cummings JL: Drug-induced mania-causative agents, clinical characteristics and management: A retrospective analysis of the literature. Med Toxicol Adverse Drug Experience 1989; 4:127–143.
64. Evans L: Psychological effects caused by drugs in overdose. Drugs 1980; 19:220–242.
65. Mofenson HC, Caraccio TR: The agitated, violent or acutely psychotic patient. PP/T Review. Nassau County Medical Center Regional Poison Control Center 1992; 11:301–306.
66. Chapman SA, Stephan T, Lake KD, et al: Fever induced by dobutamine infusion. Am J Cardiol 1994; 74:517.
67. Thomas SHL: Drug-induced systemic hypertension. Adverse Drug React Bull 1993; 5:559–562.

68. Kristensen TS: Cardiovascular diseases and the work environment: A critical review of the epidemiologic literature on chemical factors. Scand J Work Environ Health 1989:15:245–264.
69. Benowitz NL: Cardiotoxicity in the workplace. Occup Med 1992; 7:468–478.
70. Talieraco CP, Olney BA, Lie JT: Myocarditis related to drug hypersensitivity. Mayo Clin Proc 1985; 60:463–468.
71. Hoff JS, Syverrud SA, Tucci MA: Case conference: Complete heart block in a young man. Acad Emerg Med 1995; 2:751–756.
72. Dufresne RG: Skin necrosis from intravenously infused materials. Cutis 1987; 39:197–198.
73. Dolan PA, Flowers FP, Aranjo OE, Shuertz EF: Toxic epidermal necrolysis. J Emerg Med 1989; 7:65–69.
74. Mutasim DF, Pelc NJ, Anhalt GJ: Drug induced pemphigus. Dermatol Clin 1993; 11:463–471.
75. Krop LC: Drug-induced systemic lupus erythematosus (Letter). D.I.C.P. Ann Pharmacokinet 1991; 25:212–213.
76. Kale SA: Drug-induced systemic lupus erythematosus: Differentiating it from the real thing. Postgrad Med 1985; 77:231–242.
77. Cohen MG, Prowse MV: Drug-induced rheumatic symptoms: Diagnosis, clinical features and management. Med Toxicol Adverse Drug Experience 1989; 4:199–218.
78. Roujeau JC, Stern RS: Severe adverse cutaneous reactions to drugs. N Engl J Med 1994; 331:1272–1285.
79. Tosti A, Misciali C, Piraccini BM, et al: Drug induced hair loss and hair growth: Incidence, management and avoidance. Drug Saf 1994; 10:317–318.
80. Huang MY, Schacht J: Drug induced ototoxicity: Pathogenesis and prevention. Med Toxicol Adverse Drug Experience 1989; 4:452–467.
81. Drug-induced hearing disorders. Aust Adverse Drug React Bull 1995; 10:2.
82. Prendergast BD, George CP: Drug-induced rhabdomyolysis: Mechanisms and management. Postgrad Med J 1993; 66:333–336.
83. Koppel C: Clinical features, pathogenesis and management of drug-induced rhabdomyolysis. Med Toxicol Adverse Drug Experience 1989; 4:108–126.
84. Curry SC, Chang D, Connor D: Drug- and toxin-induced rhabdomyolysis. Ann Emerg Med 1989; 18:1068–1084.
85. Stone MJ, Willerson JT, Gomez-Sanchez CE, et al: Radioimmunoassay of myoglobin in human serum: Results in patients with acute myocardial infarction. J Clin Invest 1975; 56:1334–1339.
86. Sabaawi M, Holmes TF, Fragala MR: Drug-induced akathisias: Subjective experience and objective findings. Milit Med 1994; 159:286–291.
87. Godley PJ, Morton TA, Karboski JA, Tani JA: Procainamide-induced myasthenic crisis. Ther Drug Monit 1990; 12:411–414.
88. Mastaglia FL: Adverse effects of drugs on muscle. Drugs 1982; 24:304–321.
89. Plotz PH, Rider LG, Targoff IN, et al: Myositis: Immunologic contributions to understanding cause, pathogenesis, and therapy. Ann Intern Med 1995; 122:715–725.
90. Goldsmith JR, Herishanu Y, Abarband JM, Weinbaum Z: Clustering of Parkinson's disease points to environmental etiology. Arch Environ Health 1990; 45:88–94.
91. Ross RT: Drug-induced parkinsonism and other movement disorders. Can J Neurol Sci 1990; 17:155–162.
92. Martyn CN: Neurological clues from environmental neurotoxins. Br Med J 1987; 295:346–347.
93. Lane RJM, Dick JPR, de Belleroche J: Glycine and neurodegenerative disease. Lancet 1991; 337:732–733.
94. Feldman RG, Mayer RM, Taub A: Evidence for peripheral neurotoxic effects of trichlorethylene. Neurology 1970; 20:599–404.
95. Spencer PS, Nunn PB, Hugon J, et al: Guam amyotrophic lateral sclerosis–parkinsonism–dementia linked to a plant excitant neurotoxin. Science 1987; 237:517–522.
96. Spencer PS: Guam ALS/parkinsonism-dementia: A long-lasting neurotoxic disorder caused by "slow toxin(s)" in food? Can J Neurol Sci 1987; 14:347–357.
97. Boothby JA, de Jesus PV, Rowland LP: Reversible form of motor neuron disease: Lead "neuritis." Arch Neurol 1974; 31:18–25.
98. Stober T, Stelte W, Kunze K: Lead concentrations in blood, plasma, erythrocytes and cerebrospinal fluid in amyotrophic lateral sclerosis. J Neurol Sci 1983; 61:21–26.
99. Hawkes CH, Cavanagh JB, Fox AJ: Motoneuron disease: A disorder secondary to solvent exposure? Lancet 1989; 1:73–76.
100. Tylleskar T, Banea M, Bikangi N, et al: Cassava cyanogens and konzo, an upper motoneuron disease found in Africa. Lancet 1992; 339:208–211.
101. Roelofs-Ivenson RA, Mulder DW, Elveback LP, et al: ALS and heavy metals: A pilot case-control study. Neurology 1984; 34:393–395.
102. Conradi S, Ronnevi L-O, Nise G, Vesterberg O: Long-time penicillamine treatment in amyotrophic lateral sclerosis with parallel determination of lead in blood, plasma and urine. Acta Neurol Scand 1982; 65:203–211.
103. Yanagihara R: Heavy metals and essential minerals in motor neuron disease. *In*: Human Motor Neuron Disease. Rowland LP (Ed). New York, Raven Press, 1982, pp 233–247.
104. Garruto RM, Yanagihara R, Gajdusek DC: Cycads and amyotrophic lateral sclerosis/parkinsonism dementia (Letter). Lancet 1988; 2:1079.
105. Duncan MW, Steele JC, Kopin IJ, Markey SP: 2-Amino-3-(methylamino)-propanoic acid (BMAA) in cycad flow: An unlikely cause of amyotrophic lateral sclerosis and parkinsonism-dementia of Guam. Neurology 1990; 40:767–772.
106. Abuelo JG: Renal failure caused by chemicals, foods, plants, animal venoms and misuse of drugs. Arch Intern Med 1990; 150:505–510.
107. Underwood TW, Frye CB: Drug-induced pancreatitis. Clin Pharm 1993; 14:440–448.
108. Nelid GH: Haemolytic syndrome in practice. Lancet 1994; 334:338–340.
109. Urinary incontinence. Harvard Med School Health Lett 1990; 15:10.
110. Oral drug effects. Aust Adverse Drug React Bull 1992; 11.
111. Klegan KL, Young TL: Pill-induced esophageal injury. J Tenn Med Assoc 1992; 85:417–418.
112. Iredale JP, George CF: Drugs causing gastrointestinal obstruction. Adverse Drug React Toxicol Rev 1993; 12:163–175.
113. Committee on Safety of Medicines UK: CSM update: Adverse drug reactions and the liver (Letter). Br Med J 1985; 291:46.
114. Hanson JS: Propylthiouracil and hepatitis: Two cases and a review of the literature. Arch Intern Med 1984; 144:994–996.
115. Ishii M, Miyazaki Y, Yamamoto T, et al: A case of drug-induced ductopenia resulting in fatal biliary cirrhosis. Liver 1993; 13:227–231.
116. Cappell MS, Simon T: Colonic toxicity of administered medications and chemicals. Am J Gastroenterol 1993; 88:1684–1697.
117. Driscoll DF: Drug-induced metabolic disorders and parenteral nutrition in the intensive care unit: A pharmaceutical and metabolic perspective. DICP Ann Pharmacother 1989; 23:363–371.
118. Reed CR, Glauser FL: Drug-induced noncardiogenic pulmonary edema. Chest 1991; 100:1120–1124.
119. Rosenow EC III, Myers JL, Swenson SJ, Pisani RJ: Drug-induced pulmonary disease: An update. Chest 1992; 102:239–250.
120. Henry JA: Resuscitation from poisoning. *In*: Cardiopulmonary Resuscitation. Baskett PJF (Ed). Amsterdam, Elsevier, 1989, pp. 231–257.
121. Hunt LW, Rosenow EC III: Asthma-producing drugs. Ann Allergy 1992; 68:453–462.
122. Heimpel H: Drug-induced agranulocytosis. Med Toxicol 1988; 3:449–462.
123. Beutler E: Glucose-6-phosphate dehydrogenase deficiency. N Engl J Med 1991; 324:169–174.
124. George JM, Shattil SJ: The clinical importance of acquired abnormalities of platelet function. N Engl J Med 1991; 324:27–40.
125. DeJarnett AC, Grant JA: Basic mechanisms of anaphylaxis and anaphylactoid reactions. Immunol Allergy Clin North Am 1992; 12:501–515.
126. Lee M, Sharfi R: Oxybutynin-induced reflux esophagitis. DICP Ann Pharmacother 1990; 34:583–585.
127. Bradberry SM, Vale JA: Disturbances of potassium homeostasis in poisoning. Clin Toxicol 1995; 33:295–310.
128. Browning RG, Olson DW, Stueven HA, Mateer JR: 50% dextrose: Antidote or toxin? Ann Emerg Med 1990; 19:683–687.
129. Ghose K: Prescribing CNS drugs for elderly patients. Drugs Aging 1994; 4:275–284.
130. Mets TF: Drug-induced orthostatic hypotension in older patients. Drugs Aging 1995; 6:219–228.

13

Drug Abuse, Overdose, and Withdrawal Syndromes

Sidney H. Schnoll, MD, PhD

SCOPE OF THE PROBLEM

Drug abuse poses a significant problem for society and the health care system. Although it is a public health and medical problem, it retains by many in the public the stigma of a moral problem or lack of will by the abuser. The misconceptions about drug abuse persist despite mounting evidence from both animal and human studies that genetics play a significant role in the etiology of addiction.[1]

Health care professionals, especially physicians, tend to ignore the problem because of inadequate medical education regarding treatment of drug abuse. This lack of education has led to a fear of addiction in the patient and to more comfort dealing with the acute medical sequelae associated with addiction than with the addiction. It is estimated that drug abuse, including alcoholism, costs our society more than $140 billion a year, with some of that cost related to the admissions to critical care facilities.[2] These costs are exclusive of the costs of tobacco use. A study of intensive care unit (ICU) admissions found 28% related to substance abuse, and these admissions accounted for more than 39% of the ICU costs. This is partially due to longer lengths of stay.[3]

This chapter addresses the medical sequelae of drug addiction and abuse, with emphasis on the acute problems of intoxication and withdrawal and how they should be treated in the critical care setting. Despite this focus on the acute issues, it must be stressed that while the acute care issues are being treated, it is the time to begin to address the long-term treatment of addiction. Treatment of intoxication and withdrawal is not treatment of addiction. Addiction is a chronic problem with remissions and exacerbations like other chronic illnesses.

Several definitions are important for comprehending the scope of the problem (Table 13–1). The critical issues to remember regarding addiction are the chronicity, the consequences, and the failure to recognize the severity of those consequences. *Neuroadaptation* (physical dependence) occurs with and without addiction and is not a problem, except that the patient must be gradually withdrawn from the drugs to reduce the possibility of producing a withdrawal syndrome. Abuse of drugs can exist independently from both addiction and neuroadaptation and is more common than addiction and neuroadaptation.

When treating patients suffering the consequences of addiction or abuse, as with any other medical condition, the physician must treat the patient in a nonjudgmental and confidential atmosphere. Because of the understanding by the federal government that confidentiality must be maintained for patients to seek treatment, stringent laws have been written regarding confidentiality with drug abusers. Although we do not cover these laws here, the reader should contact the hospital attorney or a drug abuse program to learn more about these laws. Never should concern about legal issues deter a physician from adequately treating the patient. Because of the patient's fears of legal reprisals, it is often necessary to call in significant others who can provide important information. It is vital, however, to make sure that releases are signed, if possible, in order to gather the information.

Despite all the problems associated with drug abuse and the concerns about its management, it is a highly treatable disorder. As a chronic disease, addiction has no cure, but effective treatment can significantly alter its course and can result in lifestyle changes. Like any other chronic disorder, however, addiction is characterized by remissions and exacerbations; when an exacerbation occurs, treatment should be intensified and the patient should not be blamed for recurrence of the illness.

Early intervention results in better outcome. Failure to initiate treatment for the addiction results in progression of the illness which can be fatal. Many physicians erroneously assume that simply withdrawing a drug of abuse from the patient is sufficient treatment. This is treatment for the neuroadaptation but not treatment for the addiction. Treatment of the addiction is a long-term process, often quite intense in the first few weeks or months with lesser intensity over time, depending on the patient's progress.

TABLE 13–1. Terminology of Substance Abuse

Term	Definition
Abuse	Use of an illicit drug or a licit drug outside legitimate medical practice
Addiction	A chronic disorder characterized by compulsive use of drugs (craving), resulting in physical, psychologic, and social harm and continued use despite evidence of that harm (denial)
Cross-dependence	Development of dependence on a drug to which the patient has never been exposed because of exposure to a drug on which a patient has become dependent
Cross-tolerance	Development of tolerance to a drug to which the patient has never been exposed because it contains characteristics similar to those of a drug for which tolerance has developed
Dependence	Adaptation at the cellular level to drugs such that when the drug is removed, there is a characteristic set of signs and symptoms called the *withdrawal syndrome*
Detoxification	Clearance of a drug from the body through metabolic and excretory mechanisms
Multiple drug use	Use or abuse of more than one drug simultaneously, sequentially, or inadvertently
Recovery program	Action taken by an individual in the treatment of the addiction; this may include formal treatment, such as individual or group therapy, and informal treatment, such as Twelve-Step programs
Tolerance	Adaptation at the cellular level to the presence of a drug such that more drug is needed to achieve the desired effect
Withdrawal	Gradual reduction in the amount of drug given to an individual who is dependent to reduce the severity of the withdrawal syndrome *(abstinence syndrome).*

EPIDEMIOLOGY

Although the prevalence of addiction in the population is not known, a study of nearly 20,000 adults found a lifetime prevalence of alcoholism of 13.5% and a lifetime prevalence of other drug abuse of 6.1%.[4] These prevalence rates are exclusive of nicotine dependence. In hospitalized patients, at any time between 25% and 40% have problems of alcohol and other drug addiction, and their hospitalization is due to medical sequelae of the addiction.[5] These percentages may be even higher in inner-city and in Veterans Administration hospitals.

All segments of the population are at risk, and addiction is an equal opportunity disorder. Use of drugs is most prevalent in the 18- to 25-year-old age range, and then it tapers off.[6] Women are also at high risk for addiction.[7] Because genetics plays an important role in this risk, certain ethnic groups may be at higher risk than others. Individuals from Scandinavian and Irish backgrounds are at higher risk for alcoholism, as are some Native American Indians. Therefore, a history of alcohol or drug abuse in the biologic family places the patient at high risk.

Because of the intoxicating nature of the drugs, individuals who use them are at high risk for trauma. Accidents frequently bring them into hospitals, where they may wind up in critical care settings. In some institutions, as many as 70% of the patients presenting with trauma are intoxicated at the time of the traumatic event.[8] More than 60% of spinal cord injuries occur in persons who have ingested intoxicating substances.[9] Drug use is a major risk factor in human immunodeficiency virus (HIV) infection, and in some cities more than 50% of new HIV infections affect injection drug users or individuals who have had sexual relations with them. This group is also at higher risk for tuberculosis and other infectious diseases.[10]

The most common pattern is multiple drug use, which creates significant problems for the clinician because of the mixed picture of intoxications and the need to handle multiple withdrawals. Therefore, it is important to define to the greatest extent possible all the drugs that an individual has been using, including licit, illicit, and over-the-counter substances. Table 13–2 lists the most common patterns of drug use presenting in emergency departments.[11]

CLASSES OF DRUGS

Although almost any drug can be abused by an individual, the classes of drugs that cause medical or legal problems most frequently are

1. Opioids.
2. Alcohol and other sedative-hypnotics.
3. Cocaine and other psychostimulants.
4. Phencyclidine (PCP) and other arylcyclohexylamines.
5. Hallucinogens.
6. Marijuana.
7. Volatile inhalants.

TABLE 13–2. Distributions of Drug Use Patterns

Drug Group	None (%)	One (%)	Two (%)	Three or More (%)
Benzodiazepines	22.6	38.0	23.7	15.7
Narcotic analgesics	35.2	35.4	18.8	10.7
Sedative-hypnotics	34.9	35.2	15.6	14.3
Amphetamines	41.8	28.2	21.1	9.0
Hallucinogens, PCP	40.8	30.1	16.9	12.2
Alcohol in combination	—	69.2	21.2	9.6
Cocaine	42.3	42.2	11.8	3.7
Marijuana	20.0	38.1	30.8	10.7

Based on data from National Institute of Drug Abuse: Drug Abuse Warning Network. Rockville, MD, 1992.

PCP = phencyclidine.

TABLE 13–3. Classification of Narcotic Analgesics

Agonists	Mixed Agonist-Antagonists	Partial Agonists
Morphine	Pentazocine	Buprenorphine
Methadone	Butorphanol	Dezocine
Hydromorphone	Nalbuphine	
Meperidine		
Oxycodone		
Levorphanol		
Fetanyl		

Opioids

Opioids can be divided into three groups: (1) agonists, (2) agonist-antagonists and (3) partial agonists. The agonists have primary action at the mu opioid receptor, the main opioid receptor involved in analgesia, and are best characterized by morphine. Agonist-antagonist drugs have agonist actions and, as the dose increases, also display antagonist actions. The prototype drug in this category is pentazocine (Talwin). Partial agonist drugs have been developed that display agonist activity at lower doses but have a ceiling effect, in that increasing doses do not produce increasing levels of analgesia. This is in distinction to the *pure agonists,* which have no ceiling effect.[12] Examples of the three classes of opioid drugs are listed in Table 13–3.

Sedative-Hypnotics

Sedative-hypnotics are among the most widely prescribed drugs in the world. All sedative-hypnotics have a close relationship with alcohol, with which they display both cross-tolerance and cross-dependence. The oldest group of prescribed sedative-hypnotic drugs is the *barbiturates.* Barbiturates may be ultra-short-acting, short-acting, intermediate-acting, or long-acting. The ultra-short-acting, short-acting, and intermediate-acting barbiturates have a low therapeutic index, resulting in a significant chance of overdose. As tolerance develops to the therapeutic effects of the drug, tolerance does not develop to the lethal effect of the drug at the same rate; therefore, over time with continued use, the therapeutic index decreases.[13]

Barbiturates have been replaced, to a large extent, with the benzodiazepines. The benzodiazepines and their characteristics are listed in Table 13–4. As with the barbiturates, the benzodiazepines now are available in ultra-short-acting, short-acting, and longer-acting preparations. This provides greater flexibility in their use. The benzodiazepines have an extremely high therapeutic index and, therefore, are safer to use than the barbiturates and other nonbarbiturate sedative-hypnotics.[14]

Alcohol is the most widely used of all the sedative-hypnotics. Alcohol shows cross-tolerance and cross-dependence with all the other sedative-hypnotic drugs and has an extremely low therapeutic index. Other nonbarbiturate and nonbenzodiazepine sleeping pills are available but are not used widely. They all show cross-tolerance and dependence with the other sedative-hypnotic drugs.

Both the opioids and the sedative-hypnotics produce intoxication, neuroadaptation, and tolerance. When stopped abruptly, they can produce withdrawal syndromes. The *opioid withdrawal syndrome,* although uncomfortable, rarely produces discomfort beyond that of a bad case of influenza.

TABLE 13–4. Benzodiazepines

Drug	Latency	Active Metabolite	Half-Life (hr)
Alprazolam	Intermediate	Yes	12–15
Chlordiazepoxide	Intermediate	Yes	5–30
Clonazepam	Fast	No	18–50
Clorazepate	Fast	Yes	36–200
Diazepam*	Fast	Yes	20–50
Flurazepam	Intermediate	Yes	40–150
Halazepam	Intermediate	Yes	50–100
Lorazepam*	Intermediate	No	10–14
Midazolam*	Ultrafast	No	1–2
Oxazepam	Slow	No	5–10
Prazepam	Slow	Yes	36–200
Temazepam	Intermediate	Yes	8–12
Triazolam	Intermediate	No	2–5

*Available in parenteral form.

However, the sedative-hypnotic withdrawal syndrome can result in status epilepticus and a major withdrawal syndrome (DTs) that can produce severe autonomic dysfunction leading to death if not adequately treated.[15]

Psychostimulants

Epidemics of amphetamine and other psychostimulant use have occured periodically in the United States. The most recent epidemic has been related to the use of cocaine in the smokable form, known as *free base* or *crack*. Psychostimulants cause marked excitation of the central nervous system, resulting in hyperactivity, seizures, and increased blood pressure. Cocaine is unique among the psychostimulants. Besides its stimulant activity, it also has properties of a local anesthetic. All of the psychostimulants show cross-tolerance and cross-dependence with one another and, when administered in a blind fashion to users, are indistinguishable.[16]

Arylcyclohexylamines

PCP is the prototypical arylcyclohexylamine. It was developed as a general anesthetic agent but, because of its epileptogenic properties and psychotic-like sequelae, was withdrawn from the market. Although the popularity of these drugs waxes and wanes, there are still pockets of significant use of these drugs, particularly in the Los Angeles area and in Washington, D.C. PCP is often a contaminant found in other street drugs. Because of the ease with which it is manufactured, numerous analogs have been produced and are found on the street. Because of its binding to the *N*-methyl-D-aspartate (NMDA) receptor, it has become an important tool in the study of that receptor's actions.[17] Ketamine, another arylcyclohexylamine, has become increasingly popular and is known on the street as "special K" or "kitty." Its actions are similar to those of PCP.

Hallucinogens and Marijuana

The hallucinogens and marijuana and its derivatives, although popular drugs of abuse, do not cause problems that would be important in the critical care setting.

Volatile Inhalants

It was previously believed that volatile inhalants were primarily used by young preadolescents before they had access to other drugs; however, these ubiquitous compounds are used not only by preadolescents but also by adults who have become exposed to them in industrial settings. When they are used chronically, because of their toxic nature, damage to the liver, kidneys and other organs has been reported. The volatile inhalants are closely related to general anesthetics and show properties similar to those of the sedative-hypnotics.[18]

Illicit ("Street") Drugs

Because many abused drugs are sold on the illicit market, even those that may have legitimate medical use, it is not always possible to use our knowledge of the pharmacology of the pure drug when it comes to treating problems associated with street drugs. The street drug market is highly volatile and often creates its own set of problems. When purchasing a street drug, one is not always sure what is being purchased.

Over the years, analyses of street drugs have demonstrated that in more than 50% of the cases buyers may not be getting the drug they thought they were purchasing. Besides the problem of deception, there is no consistency in dose or purity. To increase their profits, drug dealers often "cut" their drugs with other substances. These can be other drugs that produce similar or different effects or inert substances added to bulk up the material. These contaminants, both drugs and nondrugs, can have their own side effects. If insoluble materials are used to bulk up drugs that are used intravenously, showers of emboli can go to the lungs and other organs. In addition, there can be significant interactions between the various drugs used to cut street drugs.[19]

The most significant factor increasing morbidity and mortality associated with drug use is route of administration. Infectious diseases are frequently associated with injection of drugs and the threat of acquired immunodeficiency syndrome (AIDS) has resulted in a move away from injection to smoking or snorting drugs.

It is important for the clinician to consider these problems associated with street drugs when treating overdose or withdrawal problems in a street drug user.

Drugs for Withdrawal or Overdose Treatment

Besides the pharmacology of the abused drugs, the pharmacology of the drugs used in the treatment of withdrawal or overdose syndromes must also be understood. During the treatment of withdrawal syndromes in the noncritical care setting, long-acting drugs are used that show cross-tolerance to the drugs on which the patient is dependent. Long-acting drugs are used because they provide more consistent blood levels, and the withdrawal syndrome associated with long-acting drugs is less severe than that seen with short-acting drugs. In the critical care setting, however, where conditions are changing rapidly, the use of a long-acting drug may prove to be detrimental if it is necessary to adjust dosages very rapidly. Therefore, it may be more appropriate to use continuous intravenous infusions of short-acting drugs so that rapid changes in drug levels can be achieved by changing the infusion rate. In addition, the first-pass effects in the liver are avoided, eliminating the development of metabolites that may be problematic. Also, when the liver is bypassed, hepatic function is not altered.

Finally, it is most important to use a drug that has few interactions with other drugs and, therefore, reducing interactions with other therapies. In our discussion of the treatment of overdose and withdrawal syndromes, these pharmacologic principles are utilized extensively.

RECOGNITION AND DIAGNOSIS OF SUBSTANCE ABUSE

Substance abuse is frequently overlooked in health care settings because clinicians are not taught how to make the diagnosis. As with any disorder, it is important to take a careful history, stressing areas that will assist in diagnosis or in recognition of patients who have a potential problem with drug use.

One of the best indicators of substance abuse problems is a previous history of drug abuse. Because addiction is a chronic disorder, it is common for a person to return to drug use during stressful situations. A family history of drug use is important because genetics may play an important role in addictive behavior. It is vital to go back at least two generations, since the problem often skips a generation. Individuals who associate with known drug abusers are also at high risk and are frequently involved with addicts because of their own use. There is no stereotypical addict. Addiction involves patients from all racial, ethnic, and socioeconomic backgrounds.

The physical examination is also critical in enabling one to make the diagnosis. We have all been taught the stigmata of cirrhosis, such as spider angiomata, rhinophyma, and palmar erythema, that can be helpful in recognizing the alcoholic. Injecting drug users may have tracks over sights of intravenous injection. When suspecting injection drug use, the physician should look not only in the antecubital fossa but also at other sites, since drug users will try to hide their use and may inject in the axilla, under the tongue, in breast veins, and in the dorsal vein of the penis. In individuals who have been unable to maintain good venous access, scars and ulcers may be present from subcutaneous injection, known as "skin-popping." To disguise track marks, drug users often draw elaborate tattoos that incorporate the tracks. These tattoos look homemade, but at times professional tattoos are used to disguise the track marks.

Other signs of heavy drug use include cigarette burns on the fingers and on the chest from "nodding off" while high from the drug use. Those who snort drugs show inflammation of the nasal mucosa, and heavy chronic users may even show perforation of the nasal septum, although this is rare. Hepatomegaly is common from alcohol use as well as from hepatitis and other problems associated with injection drug use. Murmurs also may be found from endocarditis that develops from injecting drugs.

Alterations in consciousness may also be present from drug use. Opioids and sedative-hypnotics can cause effects from sedation to coma. They also alter vital signs with decreased respirations, pulse, and blood pressure. Stimulants such as cocaine and amphetamines cause hyperactivity and paranoia. Physically, they produce hyperthermia, agitation, tachycardia, and hypertension. Ocular manifestations of drug use include nystagmus with sedatives and alcohol. Phencyclidine causes both horizontal and vertical nystagmus and sometimes rotational nystagmus. Opioids cause myosis during intoxication and mydriasis in withdrawal except for meperidine, which produces mydriasis during intoxication. On funduscopic examination, microemboli have been seen to occlude retinal vessels. Despite good studies describing the physical findings associated with drug use, the presenting signs are often difficult to interpret because of the use of multiple substances that have numerous interactions. This makes the performance of toxicologic screens critical.

One of the best ways to confirm suspicions about drug use is through laboratory findings. Because of the high rates of trauma associated with drug use, urine toxicologic screens should be performed on all patients who present for critical care from trauma. It would be wise to collect a urine sample on all patients presenting for critical care to anticipate patients who may later show withdrawal syndromes. If there is concern about alcohol use, blood alcohol levels or breath alcohol levels can be obtained. Elevations of liver enzymes, HIV infection, tuberculosis, and elevated mean corpuscular volume may all be indicators of alcohol and other drug use.

For toxicology, urine screens are superior to plasma levels because the drugs are concentrated in the urine and may be present in urine when not present in the blood. With urine toxicology, there is a window of opportunity, and a negative screen does not totally rule out that the person has not used those drugs in the recent past. Table 13–5 presents the duration of detection for various drugs in the urine.[20]

TABLE 13–5. Duration of Drug Detection in Urine and Limits of Sensitivity*

Drug	Approximate Duration of Detectability	Limits of Sensitivity
Amphetamine	48 hr	100 ng/mL
Methamphetamine	48 hr	100 ng/mL
Barbiturates		
Short-acting		
Hexobarbital		1.0 μg/mL
Pentobarbital	24 hr	100 ng/mL
Secobarbital		100 ng/mL
Intermediate-acting		
Amobarbital		1.0 μg/mL
Butabarbital	48–72 hr	0.5 μg/mL
Butalbital		1.5 μg/mL
Long-acting		
Phenobarbital	7+ days	1.0 μg/mL
Benzodiazepines	3+ days	100 ng/mL
Cocaine		
Benzoyl ecgonine	2–3 days	50 ng/mL
Ecgonine methyl ester	2–3 days	50 ng/mL
Methadone	3+ days	0.5 μg/mL
Codeine	48 hr	0.5 μg/mL
Morphine (heroin)	48 hr	100 ng/mL
Propoxyphene	6–48 hr	0.5 μg/mL
Cannabinoids	3–21 days†	19 ng/mL
Phencyclidine	±8 days‡	10 ng/mL

Adapted from Schnoll SH, Lewis DE: Drug screening in the workplace: Pros and cons. Semin Occupat Med 1986; 1:243–251. By permission of Thieme Medical Publishers.

*Interpretation of detectability must take into account many factors: metabolism, physical condition, state of hydration, route and frequency of administration, and method of detection used.

†Dependent on frequency and chronicity of use.

‡Poorly excreted in alkaline urine.

TREATMENT OF ACUTE INTOXICATION

In recent years, there has been the fortunate development of specific antagonists for some of the commonly abused drugs. The presence of these pure antagonists has provided not only rapid reversal of intoxication but also diagnosis of the intoxicating agent. In cases of coma of unknown origin, in addition to infusion of 50% glucose, naloxone (Narcan) and flumazenil (Romazicon) should be administered intravenously to determine whether coma is secondary to hypoglycemia, opioid, or benzodiazepine intoxication.

Although intoxicated patients can become extremely agitated and at times violent, physical restraints should be avoided unless all other measures fail. Placing an intoxicated patient in restraints only precipitates more agitation and aggressive behavior. Whenever possible, chemical restraints should be used to control agitation and aggressive behavior.

Opioid Intoxication

Opioid intoxication is a problem that, fortunately, can now be rapidly treated through the use of a narcotic antagonist. Naloxone has been available since the late 1970s and is an extremely safe drug that can be administered intramuscularly, subcutaneously, and intravenously in large quantities without any significant adverse effects. The signs and symptoms of opioid intoxication are listed in Table 13-6.

During administration of naloxone, two important points must be kept in mind. One, naloxone is extremely short-acting, its effects lasting 60 to 90 minutes. This is a significantly shorter time than almost all opioids except the ultra-short-acting drugs, such as fentanyl and its analogs. Because of this, naloxone must be administered repeatedly or through continuous intravenous infusion to prevent relapse into coma. The second problem is that naloxone can precipitate withdrawal in an individual who is dependent on opioids. However, this problem can be alleviated by titrating the amount of naloxone that relieves respiratory depression without precipitating withdrawal. All opioids are antagonized by naloxone, including the agonist-antagonists and the partial agonists.

Sedative-Hypnotic Intoxication

Intoxication with sedative-hypnotics in conjunction with alcohol is one of the most frequent combinations seen in the emergency department. Table 13-7 lists the signs and symptoms of overdose with sedative-hypnotic medications. The release of flumazenil has been an important addition for the treatment of benzodiazepine intoxication and overdose.[21] Like naloxone, however, flumazenil is a short-acting preparation and therefore requires either repeated dosing every 30 minutes or intravenous infusion over time to cover the longer-acting effects of most benzodiazepines. Also, like naloxone, flumazenil can precipitate a withdrawal syndrome in an individual who is dependent on benzodiazepines. This can result in seizures and a major withdrawal syndrome with severe autonomic dysfunction similar to that seen in delirium tremens.

TABLE 13–6. Opioid Intoxication and Overdose

Signs	Depressed respirations Miotic pupils (meperidine intoxication produces mydriasis) Bradycardia Hypotension Pulmonary edema Coma
Treatment	*Step 1:* Secure adequate airway, maintain cardiovascular system, perform appropriate blood studies. Do not administer stimulants. *Step 2:* Administer naloxone, 2-4 mg IV or SC, administer 50% glucose IV, and administer flumazenil 0.2-3 mg IV or SC. This administration of multiple drugs is necessary because of the frequency of multiple drug intoxications. *Step 3:* Once symptoms are relieved, give naloxone every 60-90 min, or add naloxone to IV fluids (4 mg/L), titrating a small dose over time to a desired level of consciousness. Naloxone is short-acting, requiring repeated doses to prevent patient from slipping back into coma.

TABLE 13–7. Sedative-Hypnotic/Alcohol Intoxication and Overdose

Signs	Loss of coordination Respiratory depression Nystagmus Depressed deep-tendon reflexes Hypotension Dysarthria Coma
Treatment	*Step 1:* Secure adequate airway, maintain cardiovascular system, perform appropriate blood studies. Do not administer stimulants. *Step 2:* Administer flumazenil, 0.2-3.0 mg IV or SC, administer 50% glucose IV, and administer naloxone, 2-4 mg IV or SC. This administration of multiple drugs is necessary because of multiple drug intoxications. *Step 3:* If the patient responds to flumazenil, give repeated doses every 30-60 min because most benzodiazepines are longer-acting than flumazenil. Flumazenil can be added to intravenous fluids to titrate level of consciousness. *Step 4:* Because most sedative-hypnotics are taken orally, give activated charcoal orally to prevent absorption of drug still in the gut and reduce reabsorption of active metabolites in the enterohepatic circulation. *Step 5:* For patients who do not respond to the above steps, dialysis or hemoperfusion may be necessary to reduce coma. Most sedative-hypnotic medications are extremely lipophilic and are therefore removed slowly by these methods.

Although flumazenil reverses most of the effects of a benzodiazepine overdose, it does not always reliably reverse respiratory depression. This may be due to the high frequency of intoxication with other drugs in conjunction with benzodiazepine. Flumazenil does not antagonize the effects of other sedative-hypnotics, including alcohol, barbiturates, and the nonbenzodiazepine, nonbarbiturate sleeping pills. Treatment of overdose with these drugs may require dialysis in order to clear the drug from the system because no antagonists of these drugs are available. When the drug has been taken orally, administration of activated charcoal can be important in reducing absorption of more drug into the body and preventing reabsorption of drug through the enterohepatic circulation.

With both the opioids and the sedative-hypnotics, as the intoxication clears, a withdrawal syndrome may develop. Therefore, it is important to monitor for withdrawal and treat it appropriately (see next). Failure to do this will result in more severe problems and, with sedative-hypnotics, the potential for status epilepticus and delirium.

Psychostimulant Intoxication

The most common psychostimulant intoxication occurs with cocaine. Cocaine overdoses are very common in the emergency department because, as with other street drugs, individuals taking cocaine are never aware of the purity of the drug they are buying. The signs and symptoms of the psychostimulant overdose syndrome and treatment are listed in Table 13-8. Unlike the situation of the opioids and benzodiazepines, no specific antagonist is available for the effects of cocaine or

TABLE 13–8. Psychostimulant Intoxication and Overdose

Signs	Hyperactivity Diaphoresis Mydriasis Tremor Tachycardia and arrhythmias Hypertension Hyperpyrexia Stereotypic behavior (picking at skin) Seizures Paranoia
Treatment	*Step 1:* Administer lorazepam, 2 mg, by slow IV infusion to reduce agitation and seizure potential. Give repeated doses as needed to control stimulant effects. Lorazepam has a duration of action of 90–120 minutes IV. A shorter-acting parenteral benzodiazepine, such as diazepam or midazolam, can be used if the long duration of action of lorazepam is clinically contraindicated. *Step 2:* β-Blockers may be used to treat ventricular arrhythmias. When there is evidence of ischemic injury, calcium channel blockers should be used. *Step 3:* In patients who are paranoid or violent, administer haloperidol, 5 mg IV, and repeat the dose every 30 min until symptoms subside or side effects are seen. Haloperidol and other antipsychotics may lower the seizure threshold and therefore should be used judiciously. *Step 4:* Administer ascorbic acid, 500 mg three or four times daily, to enhance excretion of amphetamine and its derivatives. Administer a diuretic when urinary pH is below 6.0. This should be done cautiously in patients with rhabdomyolysis or renal dysfunction to prevent acute renal failure.

other psychostimulants. Therefore, depending on the presenting problems, other drugs may be needed to treat specific effects of the overdose. Although cocaine itself is relatively short-acting, some of its metabolites, particularly benzoylecgonine, may produce long-acting effects after cocaine has been cleared from the system.[21] In addition, some of the cardiac effects of cocaine can occur a week to 10 days after the individual has stopped using it. Individuals who use alcohol with cocaine can synthesize cocaethylene, which may be more toxic than cocaine.[22]

One of the most difficult problems associated with severe cocaine and other psychostimulant intoxication is the psychosis that may be indistinguishable from a naturally occurring psychosis. This event is best treated with high-potency antipsychotic medications, such as haloperidol. It is best to give haloperidol intravenously because intramuscular absorption may be erratic and not rapid enough to give the desired effect. Haloperidol may lower the seizure threshold, and care should be taken when it is administered.[23]

For excessive stimulation, an intravenously administered benzodiazepine can be very useful.[24] Benzodiazepines should not be administered intramuscularly because of erratic absorption from the intramuscular injection site. Depending on the nature of the problem, there are several choices. Lorazepam intravenously has a duration of action of approximately 2 hours. Diazepam has a duration of action, when given intravenously, of about a ½ hour to 40 minutes, and if an ultra-short-acting drug is necessary, midazolam may be utilized. The choice of drug depends on the circumstances, and the availability of this range of drugs certainly is a therapeutic advantage. Because respiratory depression can occur with the use of intravenous benzodiazepines, in particular midazolam, it is best to start with a low dose and to titrate up according to the clinical picture.

Arrhythmia is associated with cocaine use and can be treated with β-blockers. If it is associated with myocardial ischemia, calcium channel blockers can also be used. Again, the choice of drug depends on the circumstance. Intravenous administration provides more precise control of medication. All psychostimulants can cause hypertension, and it may be necessary to administer antihypertensive medications if the blood pressure is at a problematic level. Hypertensive effects are usually ameliorated as the drug clears the system.[25]

Cocaine is a short-acting drug with a duration of action of several hours. However, some of the amphetamines are long-acting, and if taken in high doses, effects can persist for several days. To reduce the duration of these effects, acidification of the urine will enhance excretion of amphetamines. Acidification can be accomplished through the use of ascorbic acid, 500 mg twice or three times daily, or ammonium chloride; however, the latter may produce hepatic toxicity. Once the urinary pH is below 6.0, a diuretic should be administered to enhance drug excretion.[26] Acidification should be avoided if there are signs of muscle injury, since it can result in renal failure secondary to myoglobin precipitation in the kidney.

Phencyclidine Intoxication

Overdoses with PCP, ketamine, and other arylcyclohexylamines, although not common in all parts of the United States, can present challenging clinical problems. The signs and symptoms of PCP overdose and its treatment are presented in Table 13–9. PCP is a weak acid with a pK of 8.5. Because of this, the non-ionized drug is frequently taken up by cells where it cannot be excreted, resulting in a prolonged effect.

One of the most severe problems with PCP is *hypertensive crisis,* which needs to be addressed vigorously with potent antihypertensive medications, such as nitroprusside. Psychoses and catatonia may also result. Intoxicated individuals have also been known to become violent, some exhibiting superhuman strength in anecdotal reports. The acute psychosis and agitation can be treated, as with amphetamine overdose, through the use of intravenous haloperidol and benzodiazepines. The doses used are similar to those used for psychostimulants.[28]

Like the amphetamines, PCP is best excreted in an acid urine; this significantly decreases the duration of effects from the drug. Ascorbic acid, 500 mg twice or three times a day, or ammonium chloride can be used to acidify the urine, and it is important to try to reduce the urinary pH to 5.5 or below to enhance the excretion of the drug. There is a 100-fold difference in the rate of excretion between a pH of 5.5 and a pH of 6. Once the pH is down to 5.5, a diuretic should be administered to facilitate excretion of the drug. This significantly decreases the duration over which PCP effects persist.[28] The same caveats for acidification following amphetamine intoxication apply to treatment of PCP intoxication.

Ketamine is a much shorter-acting drug than PCP, and no significant treatment is needed except for the hypertensive crisis and seizures that can occur.

Hallucinogen Intoxication

With the recent increased use of hallucinogens, particularly on college campuses, once again acute reactions to hallucinogens are appearing in the emergency department. Of particular concern are seizures that can occur with high doses and the acute disorientation, resulting in confusion and severe anxiety known as a "bad trip." In severe cases, antipsychotic agents, such as haloperidol, are effective in reducing some of

TABLE 13–9. Arylcyclohexylamine (PCP) Intoxication and Overdose

Signs	***Low-Dose Effects***	
	Tachycardia	Distorted perception
	Numbness	Agitation
	Hypertension	Sensory isolation
	High-Dose Effects	
	Incoordination	Loss of corneal and gag reflexes
	Catatonia	Estrangement
	Nystagmus (vertical and horizontal)	Diaphoresis
	Hyperacusis	Apathy
	Hypersalivation	Aggressive behavior
	Convulsions	Coma
	Loss of sensation	
Treatment	*Step 1:* Secure adequate airway, maintain cardiovascular system, perform appropriate blood studies.	
	Step 2: Administer flumazenil: 0.2–3.0 mg IV or SC, administer 50% glucose IV and administer naloxone, 2–4 mg IV or SC. This administration of multiple drugs is necessary because PCP is often mixed with other drugs.	
	Step 3: Administer lorazepam, 2 mg by slow intravenous infusion, to reduce agitation and seizure potential. Give repeated doses as needed to control stimulant effects. Lorazepam has a duration of action of 90–120 min IV. Repeated doses may be necessary because PCP is a long-acting drug. In patients who are paranoid or violent, administer haloperidol, 5 mg IV and repeat the dose every 30 min until symptoms subside or side effects are seen. Haloperidol and other antipsychotics may lower the seizure threshold and therefore should be used judiciously.	
	Step 4: For patients with severe hypertension, administer nitroprusside or other rapidly acting antihypertensive drugs to avoid a hypertensive crisis.	
	Step 5: Administer ascorbic acid, 500 mg three or four times daily, to enhance excretion of PCP and its derivatives. Administer a diuretic when urinary pH is below 5.5. This procedure may have to be repeated for several days until the urine is clear of PCP. This should be done cautiously in patients with rhabdomyolysis or renal dysfunction to prevent acute renal failure.	

PCP = phencyclidine.

these problems, and sedation can be brought about with benzodiazepines. Problems with hallucinogens are rarely seen in the critical care setting unless the person is severely injured while intoxicated. The effects of these drugs can last up to 12 hours.[28]

In the past, hallucinogens were frequently contaminated with other drugs, resulting in unusual reactions when attempts were made to medicate these patients. When there is concern about administering drugs to these individuals, placing the person in a softly lighted room with minimal stimulation can be helpful in reducing the anxiety. Having someone present to talk to the patient, a procedure known as a "talk-down," can calm the person rapidly.

Solvent Intoxication

Although acute problems with volatile inhalants are rare, they can be serious. The most significant sequela is arrhythmia, which may result from the hydrofluorocarbons and other volatile substances that resemble some of the older general anesthetics. These arrhythmias occur from sensitization of the heart to catecholamines and have been fatal at times. Fortunately, the effects of these drugs are short-lived, and these problems are reversed rapidly. However, if arrhythmias persist, β-blockers may be effective in reducing the problems.

TREATMENT OF WITHDRAWAL SYNDROMES

For the patient in the critical care unit, withdrawal may significantly complicate care and produce new but potentially avoidable problems. Therefore, it is critical to anticipate when a withdrawal syndrome may occur and to treat it vigorously to prevent new problems. Withdrawal syndromes should not be treated on an as-needed basis because once the withdrawal syndrome occurs, it is more difficult to stop it than to maintain the patient in a state free of withdrawal signs.

When withdrawing dependency-producing drugs, it is important to gradually reduce the amount of drug the individual is taking. This can be safely done if the dose of the drug is decreased at a rate of approximately 10% of the initial dose per day, resulting in a gradual withdrawal over approximately 10 days. When an individual is more stable and if a long-acting drug is being used to effect the withdrawal, a 20% per day taper can be utilized, resulting in complete withdrawal in 5 days.

When a withdrawal schedule is being developed, the most common mistake is to increase the interval between doses of medication, often going beyond the duration of action of the drug. This results in repeated withdrawal symptoms throughout the day that may be partially relieved when the next dose of drug is administered. The more appropriate way is to maintain a dosing interval within the duration of action of the drug and to reduce the amount of drug given at each dose to get the 10% to 20% reduction per day. In most instances, because of the reduced severity of withdrawal, long-acting medications are utilized to provide a smooth withdrawal for the individual. Therefore, drugs such as methadone for opioid withdrawal and phenobarbital for sedative-hypnotic withdrawal are used in the non–critical care setting. In the critical care setting, to obtain a more precise control over the medication without accumulation and other unanticipated side effects, shorter-acting drugs may be more appropriate.

Because tolerance develops to most of the drug classes that can cause dependence, it is impossible from the patient history to determine how much drug may be needed to control the withdrawal syndrome. Therefore, it is necessary to titrate the amount of drug to the withdrawal signs of the patient. This can be most effectively and rapidly performed through intravenous administration of medication. In a tolerant individual, very high doses of medication may be necessary in order to accomplish the reduction in withdrawal signs. If short-acting drugs are used, the dose can be rapidly titrated to achieve maximum benefit without undermedicating or overmedicating, which may compromise the patient's care.

When a drug is selected to treat the withdrawal syndrome, the first choice should be one that shows cross-dependence and cross-tolerance with the drugs causing the withdrawal syndrome. Adjunctive medications can also be used, if necessary, to facilitate a smooth withdrawal (see later).

Opioid Withdrawal

Although street addicts are inordinately concerned about opioid withdrawal, rarely has anyone died from its effects. In most cases, opioid withdrawal is no more severe than a bad case of influenza, with lacrimation, rhinorrhea, nausea, vomiting, diarrhea, and piloerection. It is from the piloerection that the term "cold-turkey" was originated. The signs and symptoms of opioid withdrawal and its treatment are listed in Table 13–10. Although opioid withdrawal is not life-threatening, the patient going through it can be extremely disruptive and uncomfortable. Therefore, it is important to treat it vigorously to avoid other problems that can be very disruptive to the unit and the patient.

Traditionally, opioid withdrawal has been treated with methadone, a long-acting narcotic and, more recently, in combination with the $alpha_2$ agonist clonidine.[29] Methadone can cause problems because of its extremely long half-life and the fact that it can accumulate over time in cases of hepatic or renal impairment. If the patient's condition is rapidly changing and there is a need to rapidly alter the dose of the withdrawal medication, methadone may be inappropriate; however, if a long-acting narcotic is desired and will not interfere with the patients condition or treatment, methadone should be the treatment of choice.

TABLE 13–10. Opioid Withdrawal

Signs	Insomnia	Anxiety
	Lacrimation	Mydriasis
	Rhinorrhea	Spontaneous orgasms
	Diarrhea	Cramps
	Nausea and vomiting	Tachycardia
	Yawning	Piloerection
Treatment	***If Oral Medications Are to Be Used***	
	Step 1: Score patient on the above signs, rating 0 if absent, 1 if present mildly, and 2 if strongly present.	
	Step 2: If score is 5 or less, give no medication. If score is greater than 5, give 1 mg of methadone for each point. Repeat steps 1 and 2 every 6 hours for 24 hr. Each scoring period is independent of the previous scoring period. Patient will agitate for more medication. Scoring should be based on objective signs, not patient's subjective complaints.	
	Step 3: Add up the amount of methadone given in the 24-hr period. This is the amount of methadone necessary to prevent withdrawal in the patient. This can be given as a single daily dose or in a divided dose every 12 hr.	
	Step 4: Reduce the dose of methadone 5 mg/day. Do not tell patient the dose or the withdrawal schedule. Give medication in a fixed volume of liquid to disguise the withdrawal schedule.	
	Step 5: If patient shows signs of breakthrough withdrawal, either slow the withdrawal rate or start clonidine, 0.1 mg twice daily, and increase dose until breakthrough signs are treated. It may be necessary to give more than 1 mg of clonidine a day. Gradually reduce the clonidine dose after the withdrawal is completed to avoid rebound hypertension.	
	If Parenteral Medications Are to Be Used	
	Step 1: Score patient on the above signs, rating 0 if absent, 1 if present mildly, and 2 if strongly present.	
	Step 2: Administer morphine sulfate IV until withdrawal score is 0–5. Morphine can be increased rapidly in 1-mg increments every 5 min to reduce withdrawal signs.	
	Step 3: Once patient's withdrawal is stabilized, reduce total daily dose of morphine 10% a day. If patient is to be switched to oral medication, give oral methadone in fixed volume at a morphine-methadone conversion of 1:10. (If the patient is receiving morphine 3 mg/hr, give methadone, 30 mg/day or 15 mg every 12 hr.) Then follow Steps 3 and 4 above.	

Unlike many narcotics, methadone does not have significant first-pass metabolism and therefore is a good drug to use orally. If parenteral administration is necessary, it is preferable to use morphine intravenously, since there can be erratic absorption from subcutaneous or intramuscular injection sights.

The easiest way to deal with opioid withdrawal is to treat the signs and symptoms as they appear. A simple scoring system for determining the dose of methadone necessary is described in Table 13–10.[29] An alternative approach is to use intravenous morphine. Although a very-short-acting drug, intravenous morphine can be titrated precisely to the dose necessary to maintain the patient in a withdrawal-free state. Morphine should be increased at a minimum of 1 mg/hour or as rapidly as 1 mg every 5 minutes until signs and symptoms of withdrawal are relieved. The scoring system described in Table 13–10 can be used to determine how close the dose of morphine is to the dose necessary to relieve withdrawal.

Once the patient is stabilized with morphine, the dose can either be maintained or withdrawn at a rate of 10% of the total daily dose each day. As the patient begins to recover and can be switched to oral medication, one should remember that the oral dose of morphine is three times the parenteral dose because of significant first-pass metabolism. If there is going to be a switch from parenteral to oral medication, it may be more satisfactory to switch the patient to methadone, as described in Table 13–11. The methadone can then be reduced to 5 mg/day in a fixed volume of liquid.

Sedative-Hypnotics and Alcohol Withdrawal

The withdrawal from alcohol and other sedative-hypnotics is the only life-threatening one. If major withdrawal signs develop (e.g., delirium tremens), mortality rates can be as high as 5%, even with treatment. Therefore, major withdrawal should be treated vigorously; more important, unless the patient arrives in the hospital in major withdrawal, delerium tremens should not be permitted to occur in the hospital setting. There is no way to predict who will experience major withdrawal, but those who have undergone major withdrawal in the past are more likely to go through it in the future. There is no correlation with the amount of drug or alcohol ingested or other medical conditions. Patients with a history of chronic alcohol dependence are often vitamin-depleted, and, it is thus imperative to give thiamine and multivitamins before giving glucose to prevent the precipitation of Wernicke-Korsakoff syndrome.

Withdrawal from alcohol and other sedative-hypnotics is divided into minor or major. *Minor withdrawal* precedes major withdrawal and is more common. It is during minor withdrawal that seizures occur. The signs and symptoms of major and minor withdrawal and their treatment are listed in Table 13–11. With alcohol, an extremely short-acting drug, minor withdrawal occurs in the first 48 hours, and major withdrawal occurs 48 to 72 hours after drinking has stopped. Patients taking other sedative-hypnotic medications that are longer-acting than alcohol show a significant time shift, with minor withdrawal not appearing for 2 to 3 days after drug use has stopped and major withdrawal appearing 8 to 10 days after drug use has ceased.

In a patient who has a history of alcohol or other sedative-

TABLE 13–11. Withdrawal from Alcohol and Other Sedative-Hypnotics

Minor Withdrawal	
SIGNS	Tremors Mild diaphoresis Hallucinations Seizures Minimal disorientation Mild temperature increases Mild tachycardia Mild increases of blood pressure
TREATMENT	IF ORAL MEDICATIONS ARE TO BE USED *Step 1:* To determine level of tolerance, give pentobarbital, 200 mg PO, and wait 1 hr. Look for signs of nystagmus, ataxia, drowsiness, dysarthria, decreased blood pressure, and decreased pulse. If two or more signs are present, stop the procedure; if not, give pentobarbital, 100 mg PO, every hour until two or more signs are present or a total of pentobarbital, 600 mg, has been given. *Step 2:* Convert to phenobarbital, 30 mg for every 100 mg of pentobarbital given. Then decrease phenobarbital 10% of the initial dose per day in a fixed volume of liquid. IF PARENTERAL MEDICATIONS ARE TO BE USED *Step 1:* If a *long-acting* medication can be used, infuse phenobarbital intravenously until patient shows signs of mild intoxication as described in step 1 above. Once that dose is determined, it is the daily dose required to block withdrawal. If a *short-acting* medication is to be used, choose among midazolam, diazepam, or lorazepam, depending on rapidity of reversal of effects required. Infuse medication intravenously until signs of intoxication or reduction of withdrawal signs occurs, as in step 1 above. *Step 2:* Reduce dose 10% a day. Because phenobarbital is long-acting even when administered intravenously, it can be given as a single daily dose. For the short-acting intravenous medications, adjust frequency of administration to duration of action of the medication and reduce the total daily dose 10% a day.
Major Withdrawal	
SIGNS	Tremors Increased psychomotor activity Increased autonomic activity Marked diaphoresis Tachycardia (usually > 120 beats/min) Rapid blood pressure changes Disorientation Hallucinations No seizures
TREATMENT	*Step 1:* Administer lorazepam 4 mg IV every 5–10 min until tachycardia is reduced to less than 120 beats/min. *Step 2:* For sustained effect, continue to administer lorazepam at required dose every 2 hr and reduce total dose 10% a day or administer phenobarbital, 120 mg PO twice a day or 60 mg parenterally twice a day, and reduce at 10% a day.

hypnotic use, it is critical to begin prophylactic treatment to prevent the patient from going into sedative-hypnotic withdrawal, which can be severely disruptive to any other conditions with which the patient is presenting. In most cases, a long-acting benzodiazepine or long-acting barbiturate (phenobarbital) can be used to treat sedative-hypnotic and alcohol withdrawal. Both drugs given orally, however, can create significant problems in the critical care setting.

Phenobarbital is extremely long-acting with a half-life of more than 72 hours. It also is an enzyme inducer that may interfere with the metabolism of other medications. If it can be used, phenobarbital is the treatment of choice because of its long duration of action and because 30% is excreted unchanged in the urine. It is also available in many different dosage and delivery forms, allowing precise dosage adjustments. Phenobarbital also has a long latency, which reduces its abuse potential. Long-acting benzodiazepines are metabolized to the long-acting form on passage through the liver. Therefore, parenteral administration bypasses the liver and the long-acting metabolites are not generated.

Only three benzodiazepines can be given parenterally: midazolam, diazepam, and lorazepam. Midazolam is ultrashort-acting, and unless there is specific need for an ultrashort-acting medication, it should not be used. Diazepam intravenously has a half-life of about 30 minutes. Lorazepam intravenously has a half-life of about 2 hours. Therefore, the choice of medication will be based on specific need. Because the latency of intravenous benzodiazepines is very short (minutes), the dose can be titrated very rapidly to relieve withdrawal symptoms.

Lorazepam has a specific advantage over diazepam, in that there is less protein binding and it is excreted with only glucuronidation, which is preserved even in severe liver damage. On the other hand, diazepam has to go through multiple metabolic steps utilizing mixed oxidase systems that can be compromised in a patient with severe liver damage.

In a patient in major withdrawal, massive doses of intravenous medication may be needed. The simplest sign to monitor is tachycardia which should be brought down below 120 beats/min. The other autonomic signs and the hallucinations will respond more slowly once the patient's withdrawal state is brought under control. It is necessary to maintain a level of sedative-hypnotic drug in the system and gradually reduce the level 10% per day from the total daily dose. If the withdrawal condition is brought under control and medication is stopped, the patient will very rapidly go back into the withdrawal state.

Sometimes patients with extremely high blood alcohol levels begin to show signs of withdrawal prior to total clearance of alcohol from the system. Patients with high blood alcohol levels should be monitored closely for the development of withdrawal, and medications should be initiated when the withdrawal signs and symptoms appear. If phenobarbital is to be used, the patient should be given 30 mg of phenobarbital for each 0.05 mg/dL drop in blood alcohol level. If IV lorazepam is going to be used, 1 mg should be given for each 0.05 mg/dL drop in blood alcohol level. At this point, the total amount of medication needed can be rapidly calculated, since alcohol is metabolized by zero-order kinetics; therefore, if two blood alcohol levels are obtained at least an hour apart, the drop is linear and medications can then be appropriately timed.

Other Drug Withdrawals

The withdrawal from psychostimulants, including cocaine, is not life-threatening. During the first 24 to 48 hours after patients stop using the stimulant medication, they may be hypersomnilant for 16 to 24 hours, at which point hyperactivity and insomnia can develop. Whether or not a stimulant withdrawal syndrome actually exists is debatable. Some individuals experience depression secondary to withdrawal from psychostimulants, and this can persist for a week to 10 days after the stimulant is cut off. Should the depression persist beyond this point, a psychiatric evaluation to determine the presence of an underlying depression is warranted. Numerous medications, including antidepressants and dopamine agonists have been tried to treat the stimulant withdrawal syndrome. Many of these medications looked promising in open trials, but few have shown any significant benefit when studied in double-blind fashion. Therefore, at this time no medication is recommended.

The same lack of specific withdrawal treatment exists for PCP and the other arylcyclohexylamines, hallucinogens, marijuana, and the volatile inhalants. None of these drugs show obvious withdrawal syndromes, and there is little concern over any severe conditions developing during the withdrawal period. If medications are warranted, they should be reserved for symptomatic treatments, if at all.

SUMMARY

The problems of addiction and other drug abuse have become prominent in our society and can severely affect health care. Most important, they can have profound effects on patients who are being treated for other medical conditions, and it is often the sequelae of drug use that bring the patient to the hospital. Intoxication and withdrawal can severely complicate the treatment of a patient in the critical care setting. Therefore, it is important that physicians be aware of the signs and symptoms of both intoxication and withdrawal syndromes and the most appropriate methods to treat them. These conditions are treatable and can reduce complications that develop. However, it is critical to recognize that the treatment of intoxication or withdrawal is not the treatment of addiction. All of these patients should be referred for long-term treatment of their addiction; otherwise, they become part of the revolving-door syndrome that plagues many health care systems.

References

1. Anthenelli RM, Schuckit MA: Genetics. *In:* Substance Abuse: A Comprehensive Textbook. 2nd ed. Lowinson JH, Ruiz P, Millman RB (Eds). Baltimore, Williams & Wilkins, 1992, pp 39–50.
2. Rice DP, Kelman S, Miller LS, et al: Economic Costs of Alcohol and Drug Abuse and Mental Illness, 1985. Rockville, Md, U.S. Department of Health and Human Services, Public Health Service, Alcohol Drug Abuse, and Mental Health Administration, 1990, p 296.
3. Baldwin WA, Rosenfeld BA, Breslow MJ, et al: Substance abuse-related admissions to adult intensive care. Chest 1993; 103:21–25.
4. Regier DA, Farmer FE, Rae DS, et al: Comobidity of mental disorders with alcohol and other drug abuse: Results from the Epidemiologic Catchment Area (ECA) Study. JAMA 1990; 264:2511–2518.
5. Moore RD, Bone LR, Geller G, et al: Prevalence, detection and treatment of alcoholism in hospitalized patients. JAMA 1989; 261:403–407.
6. National Institute on Drug Abuse. National Household Survey on Drug Abuse, Main Findings, 1990. Rockville, Md, 1992.
7. Ray BA, Braude MC (Eds): Women and Drugs: A New Era for Research. Rockville, Md, National Institute on Drug Abuse, 1986.
8. Clark, RF, Harchelroad F: Toxicology screening of the trauma patient: A changing profile. Ann Emerg Med 1991; 20:151–153.
9. Heinemann AW, Mamott BD, Schnoll SH: Substance use by persons with recent spinal cord injuries. Rehabil Psychol 1990; 35:4.
10. Selwyn PA, O'Connor PG: Diagnosis and treatment of substance abusers with HIV infection. Primary Care 1992; 19:119–159.
11. National Institute on Drug Abuse: Drug Abuse Warning Network. Rockville, Md, 1992.
12. Reisine T, Pasternak G: Opioid analgesics and antagonists. *In:* Goodman and Gilman's The Pharmacological Basis of Therapeutics. 9th ed. Hardman JG, Limbird LE, Molinoff PB, Ruddon RW (Eds). New York, Pergamon Press, 1996, pp 521–526.
13. Hobbs WR, Rall TW, Verdoorn TA: Hypnotics and sedatives: Ethanol. In: Goodman and Gilman's The Pharmacological Basis of Therapeutics. 9th ed. Hardman JG, Limbird LE, Molinoff PB, Ruddon RW (Eds): New York, Pergamon Press, 1996, pp 361–398.
14. Roy-Byrne PP, Cowley DS (Eds): Benzodiazepines in clinical practice: Risks and benefits. Washington, DC: American Psychiatric Association Press, 1991.
15. Wesson DR, Smith DE, Seymour RA: Sedative-hypnotics and tricyclics. *In:* Substance Abuse: A Comprehensive Textbook. 2nd ed. Lowinson JH, Ruiz P, Millman RB (Eds). Baltimore, Williams & Wilkins, 1985, pp 271–279.
16. Gawin FH, Ellinwood EH Jr: Cocaine and other stimulants. N Engl J Med 1988; 318:1173–1182.
17. Johnson KM, Jones SM: Neuropharmacology of phencyclidine: Basic mechanisms and therapeutic potential. Annu Rev Pharmacol Toxicol 1990; 30:707–750.
18. Sharp CW, Rosenberg NL: Volatile substances. *In:* Lowinson JH, Ruiz P, Millman RB (Eds). Substance Abuse: A Comprehensive Textbook. 2nd ed. Baltimore, Williams & Wilkins, 1992, pp 303–327.
19. Schnoll SH: Pharmacological aspects of youth drug abuse. *In:* Youth Drug Abuse: Problems, Issues, and Treatment. Beschner GM, Friedman AS (Eds). Lexington, Mass, Lexington Books, 1979, pp 255–275.
20. Schnoll SH, Lewis DE: Drug screening in the workplace: Pros and cons. Seminars in Occupational Medicine 1:243, 1986.
21. Weinbroun A, Halpern P, Geller E: The use of fllumazenil in the management of acute drug poisoning: A review. Intensive Care Med 1991; 17:S32–S38.
22. Brogan WC III, Lange RA, Glaman DB: Recurrent, coronary vasoconstriction caused by intranasal cocaine: Possible role for metabolites. Ann Intern Med 1992; 116:556–561.
23. Baily DN: Plasma cocaethylene concentrations in patients treated in the emergency room or trauma unit. Am J Clin Pathol 1993; 99:123–127.
24. Ungar JR: Current drugs of abuse. *In:* Emergency Medicine: The Essential Update. Schwartz GR, Bucker N, Hanke BK, et al (Eds). Philadelphia, WB Saunders, 1989, pp 210–224.
25. Weiss RD, Mirin SM: Intoxication and withdrawal syndromes. *In:* Manual of Psychiatric Emergencies. Hyman SE (Ed). Boston, Little, Brown & Co, 1988, pp 233–244.
26. Om A, Ellaham S, DiSciascio A: Management of cocaine-induced cardiovascular complications. Am Heart J 1993; 125:469–475.
27. Caldwell J: The metabolism of amphetamines and related stimulants in animals and man. *In:* Amphetamines and Related Stimulants: Chemical, Biological, Clinical, and Social Aspects. Caldwell J (Ed). Boca Raton, Fla, CRC Press, 1980.
28. Daghestani AN, Schnoll SH: Phencyclidine abuse and dependence. *In:* Treatments of Psychiatric Disorders. 2nd ed. Gabbard GO (Ed). American Psychiatric Press, 1995, Washington, DC, pp 721–731.
29. Schnoll SH: Aiding the drug abuser. Hosp Med 1983; 19:116–155.
30. Jasinski, DR, Johnson RE, Kocher TE: Clonidine in morphine withdrawal: Differential effects on signs and symptoms. Arch Gen Psychiatry 1985; 42:1066–1076.

14

Drowning and Near-Drowning

Nick G. Anas, MD • Keith Lewis, MD

The admission of a near-drowning victim to the pediatric intensive care unit (PICU) represents an example of the most tragic and avoidable medical catastrophe in children. At the most extreme, drowning and near-drowning in children younger than 5 years of age would be nearly eliminated if all home pools were converted to playgrounds or flower gardens. At the other end of the spectrum, establishing mandatory pool safeguards, demanding responsible supervision, and providing instruction in cardiopulmonary resuscitation (CPR) for parents and caregivers would significantly reduce the incidence of drowning and near-drowning. Regardless of the path taken toward prevention, the effort would be worthwhile. In nearly every case of drowning or near-drowning, a previously healthy toddler (and the family) is forever and irreversibly damaged as the result of an entirely avoidable injury for which there is no therapy if the submersion is long enough for hypoxia to have resulted in cardiac arrest.

DEFINITIONS, INCIDENCE, AND EPIDEMIOLOGY

Drowning is defined as death by suffocation in a liquid medium. *Near-drowning* is defined as an immersion event of sufficient severity to require medical treatment and after which the patient survives for at least 24 hours, regardless of eventual outcome.[1-3] *Secondary drowning* is a phenomenon that does not occur; initially asymptomatic children who later experience respiratory distress secondary to drowning are exceedingly rare, and this complication should not be anticipated.[3]

The following epidemiologic facts and figures pertain to drowning and near-drowning[4-9]:

- Six thousand to 8000 patients per year die from water-related accidents in the United States.[10]
- Drowning is the third most common cause of accidental death worldwide.
- In California, Florida, and Arizona, drowning is the leading cause of fatal injuries in children younger than 4 years of age.[10]
- A bimodal distribution occurs in the population; that is, toddlers and adolescent males are most commonly affected.[8]
- An adolescent male participating in a boating activity while ingesting alcohol (or other drugs) and exhibiting risk-taking behavior is the prototype "older" near-drowning victim.[3]
- The incidence of water-related injuries increases on weekends, on holidays, and during the summer.
- Persons with a history of a seizure disorder[11, 17] or cardiac dysrhythmia[16] may be at higher risk for drowning if left unattended at a pool or in a bathtub.
- Other factors that increase the risk of a near-drowning or drowning episode are associated head or cervical spine injury, hypothermic conditions, and hyperventilation prior to prolonged underwater swimming.[12]
- Nonaccidental trauma (child abuse) may appear as near-drowning, particularly if it occurred in a bathtub.[13-15]
- By far, the most common site of drowning or near-drowning of a pediatric patient is a home swimming pool. In 1996, in Orange County, California, 11 of 16 (70%) of the drowning deaths occurred in a home swimming pool.[9] Furthermore, in every case, the pool was inadequately secured by proper fencing. The risk of toddler drowning or near-drowning is four times higher with an *unfenced* pool than if the pool is properly protected by four-sided fencing with entry by means of a self-closing, self-latching gate.[19] This issue is compounded by the fact that a responsible supervising adult can be identified in 84% of toddler drownings but only 18% of the events are actually witnessed.[5]
- Infant drownings occur in bathtubs 40% of the time, commonly when the child is left unattended or under the supervision of a sibling under 5 years of age.[5]
- Of children who drowned in a home pool, 42% did not receive CPR until emergency personnel arrived.
- Although the amount of money spent caring for drowning and near-drowning victims in the United States is estimated at $350 to $650 million per year, the true cost is unknown. The emotional stress placed on the family by the loss of a previously healthy child is enormous; the divorce rate among parents of drowning victims is higher than 85% in some studies.[19] Also difficult to quantitate is the cost of the number of years of productive life lost. For the long-term care of one near-drowning victim, the medical bill annually exceeds $150,000.[18]

Therefore, drowning and near-drowning represent an exceedingly important problem in the toddler and adolescent population resulting from factors related to the victims, the parents or caregivers, and the environment.

PATHOPHYSIOLOGY

The pathophysiologic consequence of near-drowning is reduced oxygen delivery to tissues, particularly the central nervous system (CNS).[20-23] It is the length of hypoxic-ischemic time as well as the body's tolerance of oxygen debt that ultimately determines the patient's chances for survival and good neurologic outcome. Furthermore, there is no support in the literature for the belief that near-drowning is different from any other hypoxic or hypoxic-ischemic insult or that the outcome is reversible or treatable. Figure 14–1 is a flow diagram that outlines the progression of events that result in life-threating CNS hypoxia in submersion incidents.

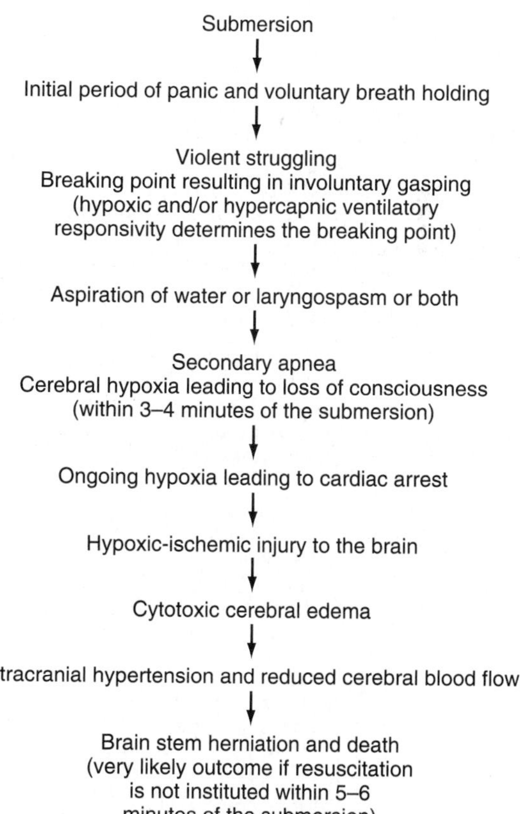
Submersion
Initial period of panic and voluntary breath holding
Violent struggling
Breaking point resulting in involuntary gasping
(hypoxic and/or hypercapnic ventilatory
responsivity determines the breaking point)
Aspiration of water or laryngospasm or both
Secondary apnea
Cerebral hypoxia leading to loss of consciousness
(within 3–4 minutes of the submersion)
Ongoing hypoxia leading to cardiac arrest
Hypoxic-ischemic injury to the brain
Cytotoxic cerebral edema
Intracranial hypertension and reduced cerebral blood flow
Brain stem herniation and death
(very likely outcome if resuscitation
is not instituted within 5–6
minutes of the submersion)

Figure 14–1. Sequence of events in drowning or near-drowning. (Data from Okada P, Levin DL: *In*: Essentials of Pediatric Intensive Care. Levin DL, Morriss FC [Eds]. St. Louis, Quality Medical Publishing, 1997, p 973[2]; and DeNicola LK et al: Crit Care Clin 1997; 13:477.[3])

The Diving Reflex

There is controversy regarding the existence of and protection afforded by the diving reflex in children.[24] Triggered by submersion of the face in cold water (<20°C), the diving reflex results in an increase in systemic blood pressure with a concomitant reduction in heart rate and preferential distribution of the cardiac output to the cerebral and coronary circulations. This mechanism tends to improve the expected outcome of near-drowning and related hypoxemia by extending oxygen (O_2) delivery over a longer period. Additionally, induced hypothermia may be protective (by reducing the cerebral metabolic rate of O_2 consumption); hypothermia is a phenomenon more likely to occur in young children because their bodies have a greater surface area and less subcutaneous fat than older children and adults.[25]

Respiratory Pathophysiology: Pulmonary Edema Formation

The gas exchange abnormalities that occur as a result of pulmonary involvement after a near-drowning event are the result of five potential mechanisms:

1. Breath holding.
2. Aspiration of fluid[26] and destruction of alveolar surfactant.[27]
3. Alveolar-capillary disruption (acute respiratory distress syndrome [ARDS]).
4. Negative pressure pulmonary edema.
5. Pulmonary hypertension.[28]

Figure 14–2 illustrates the pulmonary pathology in drowning and near-drowning.

The primary manifestation of this cascade of abnormalities is severe hypoxemia (PaO_2 < 50 mm Hg) resulting from intrapulmonary shunting. Chest roentgenograms confirm this as loss of lung volume due to generalized pulmonary edema (Fig. 14–3). Secondary pulmonary hypertension further aggravates the gas exchange derangements. Additionally, the adverse hemodynamic effect of exaggerated negative-pressure breathing (secondary to laryngospasm) may promote formation of pulmonary edema, which may be even further accentuated if hypoxic conditions have contributed to myocardial depression (e.g., cardiogenic shock).

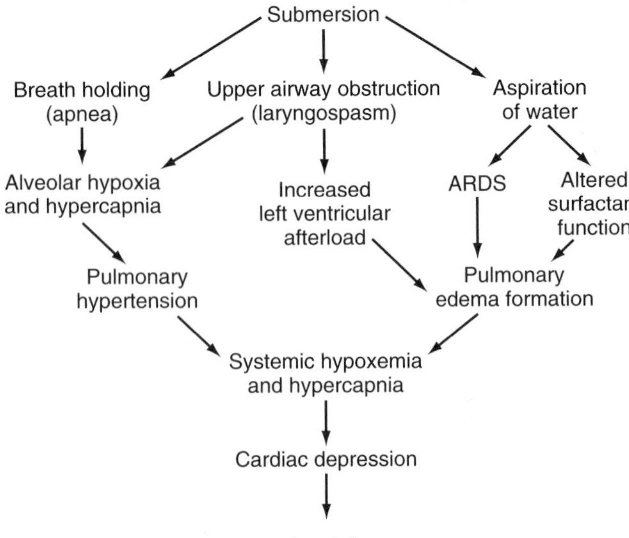

Figure 14–2. Pulmonary pathology in drowning and near-drowning. ARDS = acute respiratory distress syndrome.

Neurologic Pathophysiology

The pathophysiologic effects of an hypoxic-ischemic event (i.e., cardiopulmonary arrest) secondary to near-drowning are neurologically devastating and irreversible (see prognosis later). Details of the cellular response to hypoxia are beyond the scope of this chapter, but a few salient points are highlighted here.

Because energy stores (adenosine triphosphate [ATP]) in the brain are limited and the ability of the CNS to sustain anaerobic metabolism is minimal, interruption in oxygen delivery is not well tolerated. Two to 3 minutes of ischemia result in ATP depletion of sufficient severity to cause cytotoxic edema from disruption of cell membrane gradients. Oxygen radical production and increased intracellular calcium are central to the ongoing cellular damage; these areas are the focus of many studies and therapies aimed at disrupting this damaging cycle and reversing the effects of hypoxia and ischemia.[19]

The secondary effects of cerebral injury[33] and swelling may lead to the death of the patient. Intracranial hypertension, reduced cerebral blood flow, and altered oxygen consumption contribute to brain stem herniation and death.[29-32]

Fluid and Electrolyte Pathophysiology

Despite a great deal of study and discussion regarding electrolyte changes and compartmental fluid shift in near-drowning victims, these problems appear to be clinically undetectable and therapeutically unimportant.[34, 35] Hypervolemia and hemodilution in freshwater drownings and hypovolemia and hemoconcentration in salt water drownings have been demonstrated in the laboratory model, but these phenomena are rarely documented in the clinical model. In a study of laboratory values after near-drowning, no difference could be found between victims of freshwater and salt water events. Also, hemolysis as a result of fluid shift has not been documented to occur.

Cardiovascular Pathophysiology

The changes in cardiovascular function that occur in victims of near-drowning are predominantly secondary to the hypoxemia and acidosis of respiratory failure. Following full cardiac arrest, however, cardiac depression due to myocardial injury or infarction may lead to reduced stroke volume and increased systemic vascular resistance. The clinical manifestations are hypotension, poor peripheral perfusion, reduced mixed venous oxygen tension (PvO_2), and lactic acidosis. Additionally, the upper airway obstruction (laryngospasm) and associated exaggerated negative pleural pressure breathing due to this phenomenon can reduce cardiac output by increasing left ventricular afterload. (Often, this occurs in a patient who has not had a full cardiac arrest and who presents to the PICU neurologically intact but with evidence on chest roentgenogram of florid pulmonary edema that resolves rapidly.)

Another cardiovascular consideration in the near-drowning victim is ventricular fibrillation resulting from near-drowning in very cold water. Occasionally, a patient with an underlying cardiac dysrhythmia may have become submerged *after* the development of an abnormal rhythm resulted in inadequate cardiac output and cerebral perfusion. (This possibility should be considered in a patient known to be an adequate swimmer.)

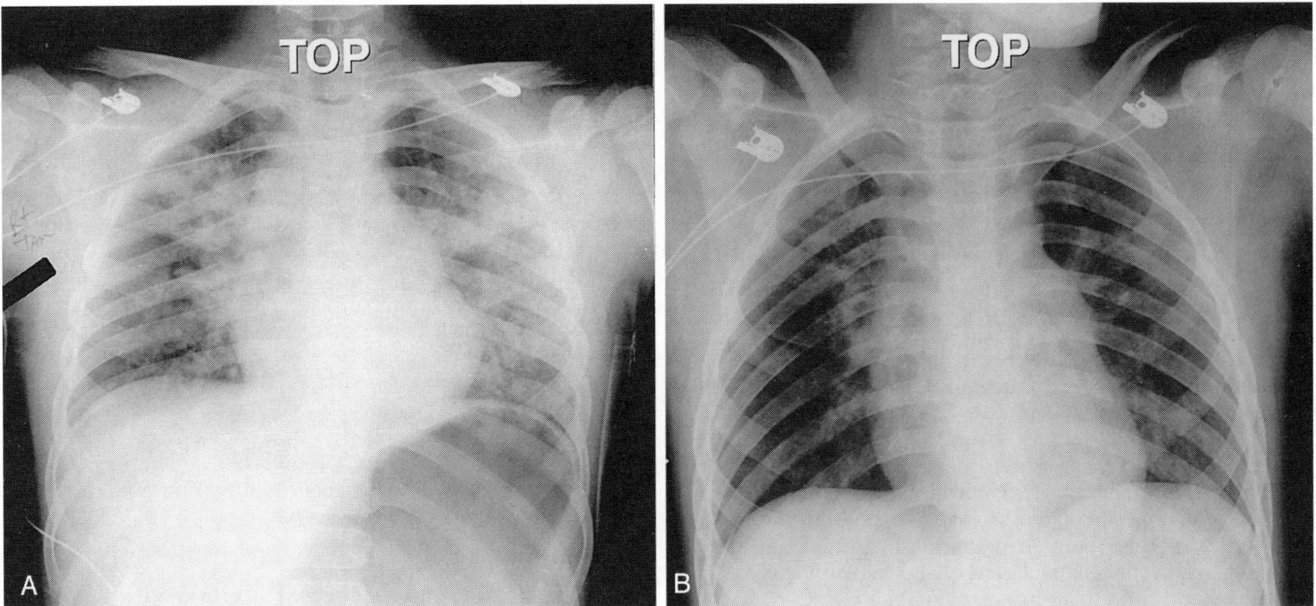

Figure 14–3. Pulmonary edema. *A*, Severe pulmonary edema in a 12-year-old near-drowning victim. *B*, Resolution of pulmonary edema within 48 hours of the submersion.

Multiple System Organ Failure

Although multiple system organ failure is an extremely uncommon outcome from a near-drowning episode, the hypoxia that occurs as the result of a full arrest may injure any major organ system. Therefore, hepatic or renal failure and disseminated intravascular coagulation (DIC) are potential pathophysiologic occurrences that need to be considered or evaluated.

MANAGEMENT

Once a near-drowning event occurs, the restoration and maintenance of oxygen delivery to the brain constitute the primary determinant of a favorable neurologic outcome or survival. Life support measures[36, 37] taken in the field and emergency department (ED) are much more likely to positively affect the outcome than intensive care therapy aimed at preventing secondary CNS injury.[39, 40]

Resuscitation in the Field

The ability and timeliness of the first responder in instituting proper CPR and thereby restoring spontaneous breathing and circulation commonly determine the quality and long-term survival of the near-drowning victim. Basic and advanced pediatric life support measures should be provided to all near-drowning patients.[36, 37] At the scene, airway opening and rescue breaths, as outlined by American Heart Association guidelines,[36] are the initial steps in resuscitation. Chest compression cannot be effectively applied with the patient still in the water.

After providing the initial airway and breathing maneuvers and extricating the patient from the water, the first responder should activate the Emergency Medical Services (EMS) system. In diving accidents or if abuse is suspected, cervical spine precautions should be applied. Other issues to rapidly consider are the presence of a foreign body or the existence of an underlying cardiac dysrhythmia or seizure disorder as the etiology of the loss of consciousness and resultant near-drowning event. Routine use of the Heimlich maneuver or abdominal thrusts to remove a foreign body is discouraged. An abdominal thrust may cause regurgitation of gastric contents with subsequent pulmonary aspiration, which may be a devastating complication.

For spontaneously breathing patients, supplemental oxygen should be provided to keep oxygen saturation (SaO_2) values above 90%; continuous oximetry should be instituted before the child is transported to the ED. In an apneic patient, the benefit of endotracheal tube versus bag-valve-mask ventilation is not established; therefore, airway management should be optimized according to the clinical setting and the technical skills of the resuscitator.

Resuscitation in the Emergency Department

All near-drowning victims should be taken to the ED for further evaluation and therapy.[40, 41] Neurologically intact patients with a normal physical examination may not require hospitalization, but this fact does not preclude the need for evaluation and a period of observation.[38]

Respiratory System

Patients with evidence of respiratory distress should be evaluated for the need for airway or ventilatory support. Endotracheal intubation for the purpose of administering high concentration of oxygen or positive end-expiratory pressure (PEEP) should be performed utilizing standard protocols and techniques.[39] The PEEP provided should begin at 4 to 6 cm H_2O and should be increased to a maximum of 12 to 14 cm H_2O, to result in an SaO_2 value greater than 90% along with a reduced fraction of inspired oxygen (FIO_2) to less than 0.5 if possible; the appropriate amount of PEEP should provide lung volume improvement as documented by chest roentgenogram to an expansion of seven to nine posterior ribs.

In addition to the application of PEEP, endotracheal intubation is indicated in patients who remain apneic despite ongoing resuscitation or who fail to maintain adequate minute ventilation because of the presence of an abnormal central respiratory pattern or, occasionally, because of respiratory muscle fatigue (more common in an infant). A nasogastric tube should be placed to remove stomach contents prior to endotracheal intubation.

Cardiovascular System

Maintenance of adequate cardiac output is critical to an optimal outcome; fluid and inotropic support may be necessary to provide sufficient oxygen delivery. Hypoglycemia and hypocalcemia may depress myocardial function and should be corrected if present.

Temperature Control

Hypothermic patients require rewarming.[42, 43] Wet clothes should be removed. Passive rewarming depends on the patient's ability to produce heat, which may be limited in a child. Therefore, active rewarming measures may be needed, such as use of heating pads or overhead warmers or lights. Core rewarming is generally not necessary but can be done safely by utilizing warmed intravenous fluids (36°C to 40°C) or warmed humidified oxygen or by placing warm fluids via gastric, bladder, or peritoneal lavage. An unusual use of extracorporeal circulation (extracorporeal membrane oxygenation [ECMO]) has also been reported to successfully heat a patient with life-threatening hypothermia.[51] Additionally, hypothermia may obscure the true neurologic status of the patient as well as contribute to ventricular irritability.

Neurologic System

Near-drowning patients with suspected or documented neurologic injury should be resuscitated in the ED unless brain death is certain. Neurologic classification based on the Conn-Barker Scoring System (Table 14–1)[44] or the Glasgow Coma Scale (GCS) (Table 14–2) may be utilized to evaluate the extent of the CNS injury.

Any patient with a Conn-Barker score of C_1 or C_2 or with a GCS value of less than 8 should be intubated and mechanically ventilated, and preparation should be made for the patient's transport to an intensive care unit (ICU). Patients with a Conn-Barker score of C_4 or a GCS value of 3 should not be resuscitated. Serial neurologic assessments may be useful in distinguishing the eventual outcome for a near-drowning victim,[45] but this process cannot be completed in the ED. Therefore, if neurologic recovery is determined to be possible, meticulous CNS management should be instituted as follows:

1. Maintain arterial blood gas tensions and pH in "physiologic" ranges: Pao_2 60 to 100 mm Hg, $Paco_2$ 40 to 50 mm Hg, and pH 7.35 to 7.45.
2. Maintain "normal" cardiac output to optimize cerebral blood flow.
3. Relax the patient by means of sedatives and, if necessary, muscle relaxants.
4. Document electrolyte balance and treat electrolyte abnormalities.
5. Perform procedures to obtain information pertinent to immediate care, such as chest roentgenography, electrocardiography, and urine toxicology screening.

Imaging of the brain with computed tomography (CT) or magnetic resonance imaging (MRI) is rarely necessary or useful, except possibly for suspected trauma and extracerebral blood. Intracranial pressure (ICP) monitoring should not be started; the presence of intracranial hypertension in this population of patients is uniformly associated with a poor outcome, and controlling ICP does not improve the chances for intact survival.[58]

Family Support

Social services or pastoral personnel should be contacted to provide emotional support for the family members. If available, the patient's pediatrician or family physician should be notified of the near-drowning event.

Conclusion

Resuscitation in the ED is directed at providing advanced life support and assessing the likelihood of a favorable neurologic outcome. Nearly all studies demonstrate an unfavorable outcome for out-of-hospital cardiac arrest secondary to hypoxia.[46–48] A study based on the experience at Children's Hospital of Orange County, California, documented an unfavorable neurologic outcome in all near-drowning patients who arrived at the ED comatose and asystolic.[49] Another study of pediatric arrest concluded that attempts at CPR for longer than 20 minutes are futile.[47]

TABLE 14–1. Neurologic Classification: Conn-Barker Scoring System for Near-Drowning Victims

Category	Description
Awake (A)	Alert, fully conscious
Blunted (B)	Obtunded or stuporous but arousable, purposeful, responsive to pain, normal respiratory pattern
Comatose (C)	Comatose and unarousable; abnormal response to pain, abnormal respiratory pattern
C_1	Decorticate with Cheyne-Stokes respirations
C_2	Decerebrate with central hyperventilation
C_3	Flaccid; apneustic or cluster breathing
C_4	Flaccid, apneic, asystolic

From Conn A, Barker G: Fresh water drowning and near drowning—an update. Can Anaesth Soc J 1984; 31:538.

Management in the PICU

By the time the near-drowning victim reaches the PICU, the neurologic outcome (i.e., maximal potential for recovery) is predetermined. The primary goal of pediatric intensive care is to ensure that no untoward event occurs that would jeopardize this potential. Therefore, the management is directed at

1. Maximizing pulmonary and cardiac function to provide adequate systemic oxygen delivery.
2. Providing excellent supportive care.
3. Continuing CNS therapies.
4. Obtaining neurologic consultation.
5. Arranging for emotional and psychologic support for the patient's parents and other family members.

Maximizing Pulmonary and Cardiac Function

The therapy described in the emergency department is continued in the PICU. (More details about promoting systemic oxygenation in disorders characterized by severe lung disease are available in other chapters and in other reviews.[52])

The goal of pulmonary management is to optimize lung volume and function in an effort to reduce the percentage of intrapulmonary shunt. It is important to realize that the pulmonary dysfunction associated with near-drowning is usually limited in time. The reversal of pulmonary edema, the regeneration of surfactant, and a reduction in capillary leak usually occur within 48 hours of the near-drowning event. Interestingly, many patients *without* neurologic injury manifest severe pulmonary involvement for 24 to 48 hours, which resolves uneventfully. Novel therapies, such as surfactant replacement,[50] nitric oxide, and the use of high-frequency oscillatory ventilation, are generally not necessary. Occasionally, fiberoptic bronchoscopy is appropriate to rule out associated foreign body aspiration.

Cardiovascular instability is similarly limited in severity and

TABLE 14–2. Glasgow Coma Scale*

Adult		Infant	
Best eye opening response (normal = 4)		Best eye opening response (normal = 4)	
Spontaneous	4	Spontaneous	4
In response to verbal stimulus	3	In response to verbal stimulus	3
In response to pain	2	In response to pain	2
None	1	None	1
Best verbal response (normal = 5)		Best verbal response (normal = 5)	
Oriented	5	Coos and babbles	5
Confused	4	Irritable crying	4
Inappropriate words	3	Vigorously cries to pain	3
Incomprehensible sounds	2	Moans to pain	2
None	1	None	1
Best motor response (normal = 6)		Best motor response (normal = 6)	
Obeys commands	6	Normal spontaneous movement	6
Localizes pain	5	Withdraws to touch	5
Withdraws to pain	4	Withdraws to pain	4
Flexion in response to pain	3	Flexion in response to pain	3
Extension in response to pain	2	Extension in response to pain	2
None	1	None	1

*Total score: 3–15; normal = 15.

time. Fluid and inotropic support to maintain blood pressure and perfusion may be employed. Occasionally, intermittent measurements of SvO_2 are useful to assess the adequacy of O_2 delivery, but rarely is pulmonary artery catheterization indicated. End-tidal CO_2 monitoring (capnography) may be used to independently assess the adequacy of cardiac output and minute ventilation.

Supportive Care

Regardless of the potential for neurologic recovery and the quality of life, providing supportive care is necessary to avoid secondary injury that would reduce the chances of a meaningful neurologic recovery. The details are not provided here, but issues related specifically to near-drowning include (1) temperature control, (2) anticonvulsant therapy for seizure activity, (3) bronchodilation or steroid treatment for bronchospasm or airway inflammation, (4) antibiotics for secondary pneumonia (rarely seen), and (5) comfort measures for pain or anxiety.

Neurologic Management

Traditionally, this section of chapters on near-drowning contained the most "therapeutic" information; now this section is the shortest. As previously stated, conservative neurologic management is advocated. Aggressive treatment of intracranial hypertension has not improved neurologic outcome.[53-59] In other words, there is no benefit from therapies directed at decreasing ICP in order to prevent secondary CNS injury after an hypoxic-ischemic insult. The cerebral edema and resultant increased ICP are direct results of the initial hypoxic condition, and the process is irreversible.

Therefore, as described in the text on ED management, neurologic therapies should be limited to providing optimal gas exchange, controlling seizure activity, and normalizing the metabolic milieu.

Consultation with Pediatric Neurology and Social Services

Because of the potential severity of the CNS injury to the near-drowning patient and the long-term implications for care, the family deserves the opinion of a neurologist. Immediate consultation should be obtained. Discussions with the neurologist and family help the intensivist to outline the plan.

Social service support is crucial because for any near-drowning case in which neurologic injury is sustained, there is tremendous tragedy. In most instances, a healthy child had breakfast with his or her family and siblings on the day of the incident, and that scene will never be entirely recreated or relived.

PROGNOSTIC EVALUATION AND OUTCOME ASSESSMENT

The Dilemma

Most physicians would agree that if intact survivors cannot be reliably differentiated from severely impaired survivors or nonsurvivors, then all patients should be treated with the full therapeutic armamentarium until the point at which prognosis can be accurately determined. Thus, today most patients are aggressively resuscitated. Then, at variable points in their course as dictated by the patient's response to therapy and the clinical circumstances, decisions regarding further interventions are made. The obvious benefit of this strategy is that initially all patients are given an equal chance to survive. The drawback is that many patients whose only fate is survival in a persistent vegetative state or death after a protracted stay in an ICU are also resuscitated.

Decisions regarding the treatment of drowning victims are based on clinical evaluation. Ideally, one would like to be able to reliably predict outcomes early on, using a simple yet thorough evaluation system. This system would need to be sensitive and specific. Few, if any, evaluation systems in medicine have proved capable of this level of certainty. The emotionally charged atmosphere that typifies drowning cases often impedes rational decision making, however, and often nothing less than absolute certainty is accepted. Furthermore, reports of miraculous recoveries are abundant in the media and only serve to further complicate the issue.

Duration of Submersion

Generally, the prognostic evaluation is based on a combination of historical information, physical examination, and results of laboratory and clinical studies. The historical information—particularly the circumstances of the incident, the timing of the rescue, and the effectiveness of CPR at the scene—is important in predicting the outcome of these patients. As previously discussed, the *water temperature* (<20°C) is important only in the rare circumstances of near-drowning in natural bodies of water in northern climates. The *immersion time* directly influences the extent of hypoxic-ischemic injury. The exact duration of submersion that is compatible with recovery is not known; however, it has been shown that irreversible CNS damage occurs after 4 to 7 minutes of submersion.[5, 14, 23, 62]

Many studies have examined the predictive value of the submersion time and clearly show a relationship to outcome. Patients with submersion times of less than 5 minutes have the best chance of a good outcome, and patients with submersion times of more than 10 minutes are more likely to suffer death or severe impairment. The outcome for submersion times between those limits is highly variable.[41, 49, 62-64] Unfortunately, an accurate submersion time is difficult to determine and so by itself is not particularly useful in decision making.

Timing of Initial Intervention

The first and best opportunity to intervene is in the prehospital setting. *Timing of the initial intervention* is crucial. Rapid restoration of adequate ventilation and circulation is imperative for preventing further damage. Studies of bystander CPR in adult cardiac arrest victims have shown beneficial effects, including less neurologic impairment.[64-71] Most data suggest a beneficial effect of immediate resuscitation for submersion victims as well.[40, 60, 61] For bystanders, CPR with mouth-to-mouth resuscitation is the best method.[37] In a study reviewing the prognostic factors in pediatric drowning and near-drowning, Orlowski[23] found that the institution of resuscitative efforts within 10 minutes of rescue was the "single most important factor influencing survival." Additionally, Quan and associates[64, 72] report 7% to 21% neurologically intact survival in submersion victims with cardiac arrest when they receive prehospital care.

Duration of Resuscitation

The *duration of CPR* indirectly relates to the immersion time and, therefore, to the extent of the hypoxic-ischemic injury.[72] The duration of CPR is also believed to reflect ongoing ischemic injury after submersion, because CPR generally provides marginal circulation at best. Thus, successful CPR reflects cardiac recovery but does not guarantee successful brain recovery. It is not uncommon for patients who are successfully resuscitated to have poor neurologic outcomes. Indeed, studies have shown that the duration of CPR required is a significant prognostic factor.[72-74] When coupled with duration of submersion, it becomes a more powerful predictor; the best outcomes are seen in patients with submersions of less than 5 minutes and no or minimal need for CPR.[42] As expected, either successful resuscitation or the presence of a pulse, spontaneous respirations, or neurologic responsiveness at the scene is associated with a higher likelihood of good outcome.[14, 41, 63, 72, 75]

Presence of a Pulse on Arrival at Emergency Department

Often resuscitation attempts in the field are unsuccessful, and patients arrive in the ED pulseless and apneic despite ongoing resuscitation. In these cases, the data are more clear: Patients who arrive in the ED *in full arrest* from all etiologic factors have a universally poor neurologic prognosis.[40, 41, 42, 60, 72, 73, 75-80] Drowning studies show that patients requiring resuscitation times longer than 25 minutes generally die or have severe neurologic impairment.[40, 49, 60, 64, 72, 73] In fact, Habib and colleagues[49] found that cardiovascular status on arrival in the ED is more predictive of abnormal outcome than initial neurologic status. The need to use cardiotonic medication is associated with similarly dismal results.[40, 41, 75]

The ED environment is the first arena in which the physician is faced with the possibility of making decisions about continuing resuscitative efforts. At some point, prolonged resuscitative efforts become futile. The data already cited suggest that 25 to 30 minutes of resuscitation in the warm-water drowning patient is reasonable and that at some point thereafter, continued efforts become futile. Some authors suggest stopping resuscitative efforts after 25 minutes in warm-water (>5°C) drowning victims.[3, 72]

Levine and associates[81] attempted to address this issue by employing end-tidal CO_2 monitoring as a means of predicting outcome in patients receiving advanced cardiac life support (ACLS) because of cardiac arrest from pulseless electrical activity (PEA). In cardiac arrest, the end-tidal CO_2 value reflects cardiac output. These researchers found that an end-tidal CO_2 value of less than 10 mm Hg after 20 minutes of CPR accurately predicted death 100% of the time.

Temperature on Arrival

The *presenting core temperature* has been evaluated as a prognostic variable. For warm-water drownings, the initial core body temperature is commonly lower in patients with poor outcomes (neurologically impaired survivors or deaths). The initial core temperature, however, has not been a reliable predictor of outcome.[37, 40, 63, 72, 74, 75] In warm-water drownings, the core temperature probably reflects the duration of submersion rather than any potential protective effect provided by hypothermia.

Neurologic Examination

Many studies have examined the *pupil response* in the ED as a prognostic variable; intact survivors are more likely to have an intact pupillary light response, whereas absence or abnormality of the pupillary response is more likely in near-drowning victims who either survive with neurologic impairment or die.[40, 41, 72-74, 78, 82]

The patient's *level of consciousness* on arrival to the hospital also correlates strongly with outcome. Patients who are awake on arrival generally have favorable outcomes. Those who are somewhat blunted often have favorable outcomes, with some exceptions. Patients who are comatose generally have poor outcomes. with mortality rates estimated to be 34% to 68%.[74, 75, 78, 83]

The GCS is a quick, easy, and reproducible assessment of CNS status (see Table 14–2). An initial GCS value below 4 to 5 appears to be highly predictive of death or severe neurologic impairment in pediatric near-drownings.[41, 45, 75, 84-86] As previously mentioned, Conn and associates developed a scoring system based on the patient's depth of coma and postural tone (see Table 14–1).[2, 44, 55] Patients are assigned to categories A, B, and C according to the depth of coma; category C is further divided into subcategories 1 through 4 on the basis of postural tone (decorticate flexion, decerebrate extension, and flaccidity). This study and others have found that patients in category C_3 or worse (flaccid and deep coma) had a dismal prognosis for recovery.[44, 49, 55, 73]

Other scoring systems that incorporate multiple factors have also been developed. Fandel and Bancalari[87] showed that all children with an arterial pH below 7.0, coma, the need for CPR, and the need for ventilatory support had a dismal prognosis. The Orlowski scoring system is based on five unfavorable prognostic factors: age less than 3 years, *estimated* maximum submersion time longer than 5 minutes, no resuscitation for 10 minutes, coma at initial presentation, and arterial pH less than 7.1. A point is given for each item present. Patients with scores of 2 or less had a 90% chance of recovery, whereas those with scores of 3 or more had just a 5% chance of recovery.[19, 23]

Laboratory Evaluation

Some laboratory studies have also had predictive value in drowning patients. Their value is limited, however, by the effects of previous treatments and the timing of the measurements. An initial arterial pH of less than 7.0 to 7.1 in the ED has been associated with a higher likelihood of an undesirable outcome.[40, 41, 49, 72-75] An initial blood glucose level greater than 400 mg/dL had been thought to be an unfavorable prognostic sign.[74, 88] A later study found, however, that the initial blood glucose level alone or in combination with the other factors was not predictive of outcome.[75]

Prediction of Outcome

The intensivist is faced with the formidable task of distinguishing, among successfully resuscitated patients, who will likely survive intact, who will likely survive severely impaired, and who will likely die. The best prognostic tool available to the intensivist has been the serial neurologic assessment, which has significantly increased predictive value over time. No improvement in the GCS value over 24 hours has been highly predictive of dismal outcome.[41, 45] In fact, a GCS value of *less* than 5 on arrival at the PICU predicts a poor outcome.[41] Similarly, inability to achieve a neurologic level above coma within 24 hours of admission to the PICU portends a similarly dismal prognosis.[41, 45]

Radiographic and Metabolic Studies

The subjective nature of clinical evaluation has prompted others to study the utility of more objective clinical studies as a means of definitively establishing prognosis in drowning patients. The utility of the cranial CT scan in predicting outcome has not been established. A favorable neurologic outcome cannot necessarily be inferred from a normal CT scan. Similarly, although an abnormal CT scan in the first 36 hours was strongly associated with poor outcome in one study, the CT finding itself does not imply irreversible damage and, hence, neurologic prognosis.[89]

Fisher and coworkers[53] looked at the usefulness of brain stem auditory evoked response (BAER) testing in predicting outcome. Serial BAER examinations in the ICU were found to be useful as an aid in assessing neurologic outcome in intact survivors and survivors who later died. However, for those who survived with neurologic deficits as well as those who survived in a vegetative state, the tests were not useful. Other drawbacks were the lack of both standardized testing methods and established normative data.[53]

Ashwal and colleagues[88] examined the prognostic implications of hyperglycemia and cerebral blood flow (measured by CT using radioactive xenon labeling) in the first 48 hours in childhood near-drowning. The predictive value of cerebral blood flow (CBF) measurement alone was found to be only 50%. CBF was significantly decreased in patients who died compared with those who completely recovered, but CBF results were not able to reliably differentiate normal from vegetative survival. Another study, by Connors and associates,[32] found no significant differences in global CBF patterns in these patients.

Global CBF, cross-brain oxygen content difference, cerebral metabolic rate for oxygen, ICP, and cerebral perfusion pressure (CPP) were assessed[32] in relation to neurologic outcome in 12 comatose drowning patients in the first 48 hours. Children who survived with functional neurologic outcome had a significantly higher cross-brain oxygen content difference at 24 hours and higher cerebral metabolic rate for oxygen at 48 hours. There were no significant differences in ICP or CPP. Other studies have documented the association of intracranial hypertension with uniformly poor outcomes.[31, 90]

In 1996, Kreis and associates[29] evaluated sequential determinations of cerebral metabolite levels in 16 near-drowning patients using magnetic resonance spectroscopy (MRS). Significant metabolite abnormalities were found in all patients compared with controls, and these changes progressed with time. A spectroscopic index was developed to distinguish between good and poor outcomes. In this study, MRS proved to be 100% specific and 90% sensitive at 48 hours and 100% sensitive by day 3 to 4.

Factors Associated with Prediction of Outcome

Although reliably predicting outcomes with an acceptable level of certainty in the acute setting is not feasible, there are factors strongly suggestive of a favorable or poor prognosis (Table 14-3). Moreover, at any point in the near-drowning patient's course, the more unfavorable factors a patient has and the more time that passes without significant recovery, the more certain it becomes that the outcome will be either survival with severe impairment or death.

For patients who survive until admission to the ICU, the rate of intact survival is reported at 40% to 80%, that of survival with neurologic impairment at 10%, and that of death at 25% to 35%.[40-42, 87, 91, 92] Few studies have looked at the long-term outcomes of survivors. Kriel and associates[93] showed that cognitive and motor outcomes strongly correlated with duration of unconsciousness. In this study of 20 near-drowning victims, the seven patients who eventually made good recoveries were all conscious within 2 weeks, but the rest remained in a persistent vegetative state.

Other Problems Resulting from Prolonged Submersion

Musculoskeletal problems, such as contractures of large muscles, hip dislocation and subluxation, and scoliosis, are com-

TABLE 14–3. Factors Associated with Prediction of Outcome in Near-Drowning

Factors Suggestive of Favorable Outcome
Submersion time <5 minutes
Immediate resuscitation
CPR given <10 minutes
Spontaneous cardiac rhythm in ED
GCS >6 on arrival at ED
Spontaneous purposeful movement and intact brain stem function at 24 hours
Factors Suggestive of Poor Outcome
Submersion time >10 minutes
No resuscitation within the first 10 minutes
CPR given >25 minutes
Use of cardiotonic medications in the field or ED
GCS score <5
No spontaneous purposeful movements 24 hours after submersion

CPR = cardiopulmonary resuscitation; ED = emergency department; GCS = Glasgow Coma Scale score.

mon in drowning survivors with hypoxic-ischemic injuries.[94] Problems with posturing and spasticity appear to be more severe and more rapidly progressive in near-drowning patients.[19, 94] Cognitive dysfunction is more commonly seen in near-drowning survivors than in patients with hypoxic-ischemic CNS injury from other causes.[19] The extent of cognitive dysfunction may not be known for an extended time.[95, 96]

Psychosocial Impact

The psychosocial impact of near-drowning on family members is tremendous and often catastrophic. The family is faced with the sudden death of a loved one or with caring for a disabled survivor. The emotions can be overwhelming, perhaps more so in drowning because of its suddenness and the intense guilt feelings associated with death or injury secondary to a preventable event. It has been suggested that loss of a child in this way more commonly leads to pathologic bereavement.[7]

There is an alarmingly high incidence of divorce after a drowning incident involving a child.[7, 96] Some studies report that 90% of marriages break up within 5 years of the death of a child.[96] Such separations are more likely to occur if the child dies from the incident.[7] In addition, the development of problems such as alcohol drinking, sleep disturbances, and significant anxiety states are common and often persistent.

Evidence suggests that disabled children have a better chance of achieving optimal development when they are cared for at home rather than in an institution. Home care of the disabled drowning survivor creates an additional set of stresses on the family and may serve as a constant reminder of the tragic event. The American Academy of Pediatrics (AAP) Task Force on Home Care of Chronically Ill Infants and Children has cited groups of factors that must be weighed in planning home care. They are environmental factors (space, water, electricity, and telephone), child factors (benefits, risks, and care needs), family factors (involvement and training of family members), and community factors (medical, social, and educational resources).[97]

The impact of drowning and near-drowning on the family cannot be minimized. The outcome for the victim becomes finalized at some point; however, the impact of the tragedy on the family is ongoing. Health care providers should ensure that the family has the necessary support and resources to give them the best chance for family survival.

PREVENTION

Because almost all drowning incidents are preventable, it is imprudent to continue to view drowning as a medical problem; rather, it is more appropriately viewed as a public health problem. It must be recognized that drowning incidents are not random events; instead, they occur in predictable patterns and circumstances. Widespread understanding of these patterns and circumstances is central to prevention. Understanding of the life-threatening consequences and devastating impact of these events underscores the need for prevention. Therefore, it is imperative that preventive efforts become the primary focus of intervention in drowning and near-drowning.

The "E's" of Drowning Prevention

The likelihood of successful prevention is increased by using a multifaceted approach.[98] The "E's" of prevention—education, engineering, enforcement, and economics—represent such a comprehensive approach (Table 14–4).[98, 99]

Preventive efforts involving the use of child car seats, seat belts, and bicycle helmets are examples of successful intervention. Drowning now outranks motor vehicle occupant death among young children precisely because of these efforts.[14]

TABLE 14–4. The "Es" of Injury Prevention

Education

- Educate caregivers, individuals, health professionals, and legislators about the risk, patterns, and circumstances of drowning
- CPR education

Engineering

- Provide protection from hazards by product and environmental design (i.e., use of isolation pool fencing)

Enforcement

- Pass and enforce laws or rules to ensure the desired behavior changes (i.e., laws mandating pool fencing, CPR instruction for pool owners)

Economics

- Provide economic incentives for adopting appropriate safety measures (i.e., insurance discounts for pool owners with isolation fencing)

CPR = cardiopulmonary resuscitation.

Education

Education is the cornerstone of drowning prevention. Studies show that most parents need education about injuries.[100-102] Health care providers are likely to be the most influential force in delivering the necessary knowledge and effecting the necessary behavior modifications in the lives of their patients.[103] Although health care providers may be more knowledgeable about injuries than the general public, there are still surprising gaps in their knowledge. Ironically, most physicians receive no formal training in injury prevention as part of their medical education.[104, 105]

An AAP survey of member pediatricians revealed that most do not provide information about drowning, even though they routinely provide guidance about other injury-related topics. Injury prevention counseling in primary care settings has been shown to increase knowledge, change behaviors, and even affect injury outcomes in children. The AAP recommends ongoing counseling about injury prevention. The AAP's The Injury Prevention Program (TIPP) is a successful approach with an age-appropriate counseling schedule.[106] The AAP Committee on Injury and Poisoning Prevention has published age-appropriate recommendations for drowning prevention (Table 14–5).[107]

Engineering

The unique developmental characteristics of toddlers and young children make them particularly vulnerable to water hazards. Potts and coworkers[108] found reliable relationships between children's risk taking and sensation seeking, and injury. Additionally, parents may overestimate the true abilities of their children. Although these factors underscore the importance of supervision in drowning prevention, it appears that supervision alone is inadequate. Even under the best of circumstances, momentary lapses in supervision are bound to occur. In fact, many studies show that in most cases, the child was reportedly being "supervised" by one or both parents at the time of the incident.[109, 110]

Pool Safety Recommendations

Because one cannot rely on supervision alone, steps must be taken to modify the environment to decrease the risk of

TABLE 14–5. American Academy of Pediatrics Recommendations for Prevention of Drowning in Infants, Children, and Adolescents

Newborn to 4 Years of Age	1. *Never* leave a child unattended in or near any body of water. 2. Remove all water from containers. 3. *Never* leave a child unattended in the bathroom. 4. Swimming lessons will not provide "drown-proofing" and may lead to a false sense of security. 5. Pool covers are *not* a substitute for four-sided fencing. 6. Parents should learn CPR and keep a telephone and approved safety equipment at the pool side.
Children 5 to 12 Years of Age	1. Children should be taught to swim. 2. Children should be taught the safety requirements for swimming in various bodies of water. 3. Never allow the child to swim without *adult* supervision. 4. Use an approved flotation device when on a boat, fishing, or playing near a river, lake, or ocean. 5. Teach the hazards of jumping or diving into water. Know the water conditions before jumping or whether diving in the water is permitted. 6. Recognize drowning risk in cold seasons. Refrain from walking, skating, or riding on weak or thawing ice. 7. Teach CPR.
Adolescents 13 to 19 Years of Age	1. Know the recommendations stated for 5- to 12-year-old children. 2. No alcohol or other drug use during aquatic activities. 3. Learn CPR.

Adapted from Committee on Injury and Poison Prevention: Drowning in infants, children and adolescents. Pediatrics 1993; 92:292. With permission of the American Academy of Pediatrics, Elk Grove Village, Ill.
CPR = cardiopulmonary resuscitation.

exposure to drowning hazards. Ideally, such steps involve instituting multiple safety barriers as "layers of protection." Four-sided pool fences, which isolate the pool on all sides, have proved to be the most effective tool in preventing swimming pool drowning. The U.S. Consumer Product Safety Commission (CPSC) and others demonstrated that complete pool fencing reduces the incidence of immersion injuries by 50% to 60%.[1, 110–112]

On the basis of identification of the key parameters that typically contribute to swimming pool drowning, the CPSC has published *Safety Barrier Guidelines for Home Pools* (Fig. 14–4).[109] It is particularly important that the barrier be at least 48 inches high, that it surround the pool on all four sides, and that it be equipped with gates that are self-latching and self-closing and with latches out of a small child's reach.

Enforcement

Despite the documented effectiveness of isolation fencing, estimates suggest that only 15% to 28% of in-ground pools in the United States may have such fencing.[110] Most swimming pool owners oppose universal barrier requirements.[113] This opposition was not even affected by a previous occurrence of a submersion event.[113] Even among those owners who endorse pool barriers, the proportion actually adopting them is smaller.[114] Thus, as with prior preventive measures such as car seats, helmets, and seat belts, legislation may be the only way to proceed. Studies from countries with pool fencing ordinances seem to support this notion.[4, 115]

Pool covers, when used alone, have not been a reliable preventive measure.[4, 29] They necessitate repetitive actions by the caregivers to be effective. They may, however, be effective when used as additional layers of protection. Pool covers tend to be more expensive than an adequate pool fence.

The CPSC states that a power safety cover may be used as an alternative to door alarms when the house forms one side of the pool barrier. If used, such a cover should meet the established standards, which require that pool covers be able to withstand the weight of two adults and a child, to allow

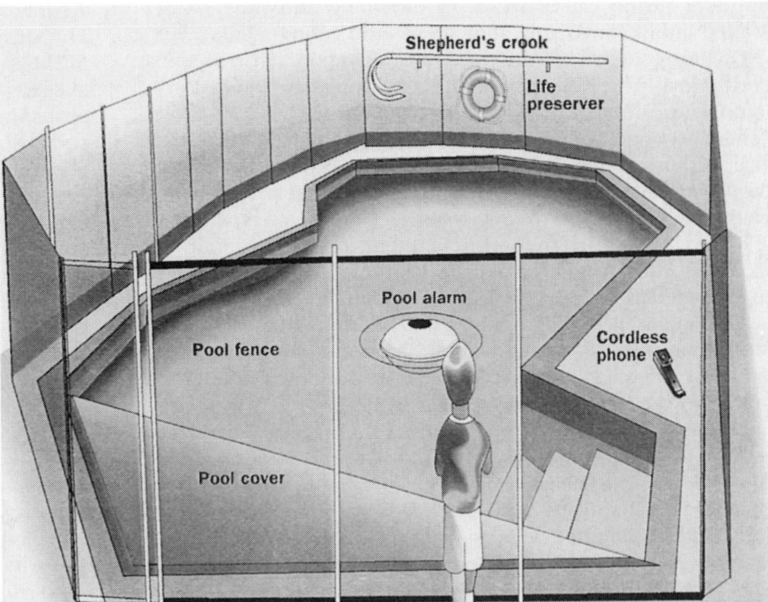

Figure 14–4. Depiction of a swimming pool equipped with the proper safety features. (From Hafer M: Playing it safe. *Los Angeles Times,* July 20, 1997.)

rescue if an individual falls onto the cover.[109, 116] Also, automatic covers are recommended, as they are easier to use and, hence, more likely to be used regularly.[117] Similarly, pool alarms have not been established as effective either, particularly for young children.[4, 107] Door alarms are indicated when the house forms one side of the pool barrier.[116] Additionally, the CPSC recommends equipping all doors giving access to the pool with audible alarms.

Recommendations for Swimming Instruction

The effectiveness of swimming instruction for children at various ages has not been determined.[107, 118, 119] The AAP does not endorse swimming instruction for children younger than 4 years of age.[107, 118, 119] Studies of 2- to 5-year-olds have shown that training improves swimming skills, including the ability to swim to the edge of the pool after jumping in.[120, 121] However, the association between swimming ability and drowning in toddlers and small children remains uncertain.[122] These studies assess abilities in a rehearsed situation in a controlled environment. Performance in a random, uncontrolled, emergency situation may be entirely different. Furthermore, opponents of early swimming instruction argue that it may blunt protective reflex responses by alleviating the initial surprise of immersion and may give parents a false sense of security.[91, 102] Also, actual swimming instruction in the very young may result in hypothermia and dangerous electrolyte imbalances due to water intoxication.[123–125] If learning to swim does help prevent drowning in toddlers and young children, the size of the effect is unknown.[122]

Finally, swimming proficiency does not make one "drown-proof"; about 25% of all young drowning victims have had swimming lessons.[126] Swimming lessons or some water safety training is generally advocated for children aged 5 years and older.[107]

Adolescent Events

The second peak in the incidence of drowning is seen in male adolescents and young adults.[14, 91, 127] Diving-related injuries are also common in this age group. The youthful exuberance, heightened risk-taking behavior, and relative lack of responsibility and maturity makes this age group particularly vulnerable. Additionally, multiple studies have implicated alcohol as a prime causal factor in drowning and other water-related injuries involving adolescents and young adults.[128–131]

Diving accidents are the third most common cause of spinal cord injury. Three fourths of all recreation-related spinal cord injuries are due to diving accidents.[132] More than 700 adolescents and young adults are involved in diving accidents each year, often resulting in significant spinal cord injuries.[133] Like drowning, these incidents are entirely preventable. The typical victim is a male between 13 and 33 years of age. Private residential pools are the most common site, and generally the victim is injured while making an ordinary dive into shallow to intermediate depths of water in an unfamiliar pool.[132–135]

Alcohol is also commonly a factor in boating accidents. More than 50% of boating fatalities are alcohol-related. Of the alcohol-related fatalities, 90% are from drowning.[136] The use of approved flotation devices has not been well evaluated, although it does appear probable that their proper use would reduce drowning morbidity and mortality. A flotation device is absolutely not a substitute for supervision, however. The U.S. Coast Guard and National Transportation Safety Board (NTSB) recommend that personal flotation devices be used by all persons in boats.[137] A review of 331 boating-related drownings in 1991 revealed that only 15% of the victims had been wearing a life vest. The NTSB estimated that 85% of the victims might have survived if they had been wearing a vest.[137] The National Center for Injury Prevention and Control recommends the use of U.S. Coast Guard–approved flotation devices for people of all ages when boating, regardless of distance traveled, size of boat, or swimming ability.[138]

As mentioned previously, there is a high incidence of abuse associated with bathtub drownings. A retrospective review of submersion incidents suggested that nearly 10% were secondary to abuse. Bathtubs are the most common site for inflicted submersion. Common findings in these cases are objective signs of abuse or incompatibilities of history with developmental stage or physical findings. These cases warrant a thorough evaluation for signs of abuse and neglect.[139]

Unfortunately, submersion injuries will continue to occur; thus, people must be prepared to promptly intervene in an emergency. It is also important to have safety equipment readily available and to know how to use it. Life preservers and a shepherd's hook should be readily available at any pool side.[107, 116] Also, a telephone with posted phone numbers for emergency services should be kept at poolside.[107, 116] Retrieving victims from the water is potentially dangerous. The American Red Cross recommends trying to retrieve victims from outside the water by reaching to them with a long object or by throwing them a device such as a ring buoy.[140]

Prehospital personnel should be trained to resuscitate the victims of submersion injuries. Communities should have triage protocols in place to ensure that patients, particularly children, are transported to the appropriate center for optimal care.[103]

The sudden drowning death or injury of a loved one should be viewed not as the end but rather as the beginning of an ongoing need for psychosocial and medical intervention.[7] Health care providers must recognize that these events exact a significant toll on the families of the victims. Thus, supportive services should be readily available to the family and should be included in the treatment of the drowning victim.

ORGAN DONATION IN NEAR-DROWNINGS

Many drowning victims are resuscitated in the ED, only to be declared brain-dead shortly thereafter. Although the brain cannot withstand the hypoxic-ischemic insult, many of the other major organs do survive this insult. Hence, drowning victims are generally excellent candidates for organ donation. The supply of donor organs is inadequate for all age groups. At the same time, the number of brain-dead individuals greatly exceeds the number of organ donors. A host of factors are probably responsible for this inequity. The disparity exists for pediatric patients as well as adults, but studies suggest that obtaining consent may be easier for pediatric patients.[19] Successful organ procurement requires a carefully coordinated multidisciplinary plan. In view of the increasing demand for donor organs and the disparity between suitable donors and actual organs donated, a more aggressive approach may also be warranted.

SUMMARY

Drowning and near-drowning are best viewed as a major public health problem rather than a medical problem. It is now well established that the problem is only minimally affected by modern medical intervention. Improved resuscitative efforts in both the prehospital and hospital settings, advanced life support measures, and refined ICU management techniques have resulted in higher numbers of survivors but have failed to appreciably increase the rate of survivors with good neurologic outcomes. There simply is nothing available now, nor on the horizon, that can reverse the neurologic devastation that the victims of these events commonly suffer. Modern medicine has little to offer the victims of drowning incidents. The fate of the drowning victim is principally determined in the water. Currently, there is no reliable way to differentiate between intact survivors and patients who will die. Furthermore, there is not even a reliable way to differentiate survivors with good outcomes from those with neurologic devastation. Thus, all patients are resuscitated to some extent, and the outcomes and resultant consequences are dealt with as they occur. This approach may seem unreasonable, but it is the reality dictated by the circumstances.

These facts make an unequivocal case for shifting the focus in drowning and near-drowning incidents from medical interventions to preventive efforts. The scope of the drowning problem demands immediate attention. The multifactorial nature of these incidents requires a comprehensive program. Prior experience with drowning prevention and other prevention programs suggests that successful intervention must be aggressive, possibly including legislative changes. A no-tolerance stance must be taken. Drownings are not random events but, rather, incidents that occur in predictable circumstances.

References

1. Wintemute G: Childhood drowning and near-drowning in the United States. Am J Dis Child 1990; 144:663.
2. Okada P, Levin DL: Drowning and near-drowning. *In:* Essentials of Pediatric Intensive Care. Levin DL, Morriss FC (Eds). St. Louis, Quality Medical Publishing, 1997, p 973.
3. DeNicola LK, Falk JL, Swensen ME, et al: Submersion injuries in children and adults. Crit Care Clin 1997; 13:477.
4. Wintemute G: Drowning in early childhood. Pediatr Ann 1992; 21:417.
5. Quan L, Gore E, Wentz K, et al: Ten year study of pediatric drowning and near-drowning in King County, Washington: Lessons in injury prevention. Pediatrics 1989; 83:1035.
6. Jumbelic M, Chambliss M: Accidental toddler drowning in a 5 gallon bucket. JAMA 1990; 263:1952.
7. Nixon J, Pearn J: Emotional sequelae of parents and siblings following the drowning or near drowning of a child. Aust N Z J Psychiatry 1977; 11:265.
8. Wintemute GJ, Kraus J, Teret J, et al: Drowning in childhood and adolescence: A population-based study. Am J Public Health 1987; 77:830.
9. Meyers H, County of Orange Health Care Agency: Orange County Drowning Death Data. Personal communication, 1996.
10. Centers for Disease Control: Fatal injuries to children—United States, 1986. MMWR 1990; 39:442.
11. Orlowski J, Rothner D, Leuders H: Submersion accidents in children with epilepsy. Am J Dis Child 1982; 136:777.
12. Waller A, Baker S, Szacka A: Childhood injury deaths: National analysis and geographic variation. Am J Public Health 1989; 79:310.
13. Griest K, Zumualt R: Child abuse by drowning. Pediatrics 1989; 83:41.
14. Brenner R, Smith G, Overpeak M: Divergent trends in childhood drowning rates: 1971 through 1990. JAMA 1994; 271:1606.
15. Shineberger C, Anderson L, Kraus J: Young children who drown in hot tubs, spas, and whirlpools in California: A 26 year survey. Am J Public Health 1990; 80:613.
16. Harris E, Knapp J, Sharma V: The Romano-Ward syndrome: A case presenting as near drowning with a clinical review. Pediatr Emerg Care 1992; 8:272.
17. Diekma D, Quan L, Holt V: Epilepsy as a risk factor for submersion injury in children. Pediatrics 1993; 91:612.
18. American Academy of Pediatrics Committee on Injury and Poison Prevention: Drowning in infants, children, and adolescents. Pediatrics 1993; 92:292.
19. Rowin M, Christensen D, Allen E: Pediatric drowning and near-drowning. *In:* Textbook of Pediatric Intensive Care. Rogers MC (Ed). Baltimore, Williams & Wilkins, 1996, p 875.
20. Pearn J: Pathophysiology of drowning. Med J Aust 1985; 142:586.
21. Craig A: Causes of loss of consciousness during underwater swimming. J Appl Physiol 1961; 16:583.
22. Siebke H, Breivek, Rod T, et al: Survival after 40 minutes submersion without cerebral sequelae. Lancet 1975; 1:1275.
23. Orlowski J: Drowning, near-drowning, and ice-water submersion. Pediatr Clin North Am 1987; 34:75.
24. Gordon BA: Drowning and the diving reflex in man. Med J Aust 1972; 2:583.
25. Conn AW: Near-drowning and hypothermia. Can Med Assoc J 1979; 120:397.
26. Colebatch HJ, Halmagyi DF: Lung mechanics and resuscitation after fluid aspiration. J Appl Physiol 1961; 16:684.
27. Giammona S, Modell J: Drowning by total immersion: Effects on pulmonary surfactant of distilled water, isotonic saline, and seawater. Am J Dis Child 1967; 114:612.
28. Colebatch HJ, Halmagyi DF: Reflex pulmonary hypertension of fresh water aspiration. J Appl Physiol 1963; 18:178.
29. Kreis R, Arcinue E, Ernst T, et al: Hypoxic encephalopathy after near drowning studied by quantitative H-magnetic resonance spectroscopy: Metabolic changes and their prognostic value. J Clin Invest 1996; 97:1142.
30. Griggs R, Arieff A: Hypoxia and the central nervous system. *In:* Metabolic Brain Dysfunction in System Disorders. Arieff A, Griggs R (Eds). Boston, Little, Brown & Co, 1992, p 39.
31. Sarnaik A, Preston G, Lieh-Lai M: Intracranial pressure and cerebral perfusion pressure in near-drowning. Crit Care Med 1985; 13:224.
32. Connors R, Frewen T, Kissoon N, et al: Relationship of cross-brain oxygen content difference, cerebral blood flow, and metabolic rate to neurologic outcome after near-drowning. J Pediatr 1992; 121:839.
33. Cohan S, Mun S, Petrite J, et al: Cerebral blood flow in humans following resuscitation from cardiac arrest. Stroke 1989; 20:761.
34. Modell J, Davis J: Electrolyte changes in human drowning victims. Anesthesiology 1969; 30:414.
35. Modell J: Serum electrolyte changes in near-drowning victims. JAMA 1985; 253:553.
36. American Heart Association: 1996 Handbook of Emergency Cardiac Care for Healthcare Providers. Hazinski MF, Cummins RO (Eds). Dallas, Mosby Lifeline, 1996.
37. Kyriacou D, Arcinue E, Peek C, et al: Effect of immediate resuscitation on children with submersion injury. Pediatrics 1994; 94:137.
38. Noonan L, Howrey R, Ginsburg C: Fresh water submersion injuries in children: A retrospective review of seventy five hospitalized patients. Pediatrics 1996; 98:368.
39. Anas N: Respiratory failure. *In:* Essentials of Pediatric Intensive Care. Levin DL, Morriss FC (Eds). St. Louis, Quality Medical Publishing, 1997, p 69.
40. Nichter M, Everett P: Childhood near drowning: Is cardiopulmonary resuscitation always indicated? Crit Care Med 1989; 17:953.
41. La Velle J, Shaw KN: Near-drowning: Is emergency department cardiopulmonary resuscitation and intensive care unit cerebral resuscitation indicated? Crit Care Med 1993; 21:368.
42. Biggart M, Bohn D: Effect of hypothermia and cardiac arrest on outcome of near-drowning accidents in children. J Pediatr 1990; 117:179.
43. Cornell HM: Accidental hypothermia. J Pediatr 1992; 120:671.
44. Conn A, Barker G: Fresh water drowning and near drowning—an update. Can Anaesth Soc J 1984; 31:538.
45. Bratton S, Jardine D, Morray J: Serial neurologic examination after near drowning and outcome. Arch Pediatr Adolesc Med 1994; 148:167.
46. Modell J: Drowning: To treat or not to treat—an unanswerable question? Crit Care Med 1993; 21:313.
47. Schindler M, Bohn D, Cox P, et al: Outcome of out-of-hospital cardiac or respiratory arrest in children. N Engl J Med 1996; 335:1473.
48. Al-Jundi S, Lubinsky P, Anas N: Duration of coma following resuscitation for cardiac arrest in children as a prognostic factor of outcome. Crit Care Med 1997; 25:A61.

49. Habib D, Tecklenburg F, Anas N: Prediction of childhood drowning and near-drowning morbidity and mortality. Pediatr Emerg Med 1996; 12:255.
50. Susuk H, Ohta J, Yamaguchi K, et al: Surfactant therapy for respiratory failure due to near drowning. Eur J Pediatr 1996; 155:383.
51. Norberg W, Agnew R, Brursvold R, et al: Successful resuscitation of a cold water submersion victim with the use of cardiopulmonary bypass. Crit Care Med 1992; 20:1355.
52. Paulson T, Spear R, Peterson B: New concepts in the treatment of children with acute respiratory distress syndrome. J Pediatr 1995; 127:163.
53. Fisher B, Peterson B, Hicks G: Use of brainstem auditory evoked response testing to assess neurological outcome following near drowning in children. Crit Care Med 1992; 20:578.
54. Conn A, Edmonds J, Barker G: Cerebral resuscitation in near drowning. Pediatr Clin North Am 1979; 26:691.
55. Conn A, Montes J, Barker G: Cerebral salvage in near drowning following neurologic classification by triage. Can J Anaesth 1980; 27:201.
56. Frewen T, Sumabat W, Hen K, et al: Cerebral resuscitation therapy in pediatric near drowning. J Pediatr 1985; 106:615.
57. Nussbaum E, Maggi J: Pentobarbital therapy does not improve neurologic outcome in nearly drowned, flaccid comatose children. Pediatrics 1988; 81:630.
58. Sarnaik A, Preston G, Lieh-Lai M, et al: Intracranial pressure and cerebral perfusion pressure in near drowning. Crit Care Med 1985; 13:224.
59. Bohn D, Biggart M, Smith C, et al: Influence of hypothermia, barbiturate therapy, and intracranial pressure monitoring on morbidity and mortality after near-drowning. Crit Care Med 1986; 14:529.
60. Quan L: Drowning issues in resuscitation. Ann Emerg Med 1993; 22:366.
61. Ornato JP: The resuscitation of near-drowning victims. JAMA 1986; 256:75.
62. Nussbaum E: Prognostic variables in nearly drowned comatose children. Am J Dis Child 1985; 139:1058.
63. Bierens JJ, van der Velde EA, van Berkel M, et al: Submersion in the Netherlands: Prognostic indicators and results of resuscitation. Ann Emerg Med 1990; 19:1390.
64. Quan L, Wentz KR, Gore EJ, et al: Outcome and predictors of outcome in pediatric submersion victims receiving pre-hospital care in King County, Washington. Pediatrics 1990; 86:586.
65. Lund I, Skulberg A: Cardiopulmonary resuscitation by lay people. Lancet 1976; 2:702.
66. Guzy PM, Morton LP, Greenfeld S: The survival benefit of bystander cardiopulmonary resuscitation in a paramedic-served metropolitan area. Am J Public Health 1983; 73:766.
67. Roth R, Stewart RD, Rogers K, et al: Out of hospital cardiac arrest: factors associated with survival. Ann Emerg Med 1984; 13:237.
68. Cummins RO, Eisenberg MS: Prehospital cardiopulmonary resuscitation—is it effective? JAMA 1985; 253:2408.
69. Ritter G, Wolfe RA, Goldstein S, et al: The effect of bystander CPR on survival of out of hospital cardiac arrest victims. Am Heart J 1985; 110:932.
70. Copley DP, Mantle JA, Rogers WJ, et al: Improved outcome for prehospital cardiopulmonary collapse with resuscitation by bystanders. Circulation 1977; 56:901.
71. Thompson RG, Hallstrom AP, Cobb LA: Bystander-initiated resuscitation in the management of ventricular fibrillation. Ann Intern Med 1979; 90:737.
72. Quan L, Kinder D: Pediatric submersions: Prehospital predictors of outcome. Pediatrics (in press).
73. Waugh JH, O'Callaghan MJ, Pitt WR: Prognostic factors and long term outcomes for children who have nearly drowned. Med J Aust 1994; 21:594.
74. Graf WD, Cummings P, Quan L, et al: Predicting outcome in pediatric submersion victims. Ann Emerg Med 1995; 26:312.
75. Christensen DW, Jansen P, Perkin RM: Outcome and acute care hospital costs after warm water near-drowning in children. Pediatrics 1997; 99:715.
76. Weinberg HD: Prognostic variables in nearly-drowned, comatose children. Am J Dis Child 1986; 140:329.
77. Peterson B: Morbidity of childhood near-drowning. Pediatrics 1977; 59:364.
78. Nagel FO, Kibel SM, Beatty DW: Childhood near-drowning—factors associated with poor outcome. S Afr J Med 1990; 78:422.
79. O'Rourke PP: Outcome of children who are apneic and pulseless in the emergency room. Crit Care Med 1986; 14:466.
80. Lewis LM, Ruoff B, Rush C, et al: Is emergency department resuscitation of out-of-hospital cardiac arrest victims who arrive pulseless worthwhile? Am J Emerg Med 1990; 8:118.
81. Levine RL, Wayne MA, Miller CC: End-tidal carbon dioxide and outcome of out-of-hospital cardiac arrest. N Engl J Med 1997; 337:301.
82. Kemp AM, Sibert JR: Outcome in children who nearly drown: A British Isles study. BMJ 1991; 302:931.
83. Modell JH, Graves SA, Kuck EJ: Near drowning: Correlation of level of consciousness and survival. Can Anaesth Soc J 1980; 27:211.
84. Spack L, Gedeit R, Splaingard M, et al: Failure of aggressive therapy to alter outcome in pediatric near-drowning. Pediatr Emerg Care 1997; 13:98.
85. Dean J, Kaufman N: Prognostic indicators in pediatric near-drowning: The Glasgow Coma Scale. Crit Care Med 1981; 9:536.
86. Beyda D, Tellez D, Liu P: Cause of pediatric submersion injuries. Crit Care Med 1990; 18:S2377.
87. Fandel I, Bancalari E: Near-drowning in children: Clinical aspects. Pediatrics 1976; 58:573.
88. Ashwal S, Schneider S, Tomasi L, et al: Prognostic implications of hyperglycemia and reduced cerebral blood flow in childhood near-drowning. Neurology 1990; 40:820.
89. Romano C, Brown T, Frewen TC: Assessment of pediatric near-drowning victims: Is there a role for cranial CT? Pediatr Radiol 1993; 23:261.
90. Dean JM, McComb JG: Intracranial pressure monitoring in severe pediatric near-drowning. Neurosurgery 1981; 6:627.
91. Levin DL, Morriss FC, Toro LO, et al: Drowning and near-drowning. Pediatr Clin North Am 1993; 40:321.
92. Shaw KN, Briede CA: Submersion injuries: Drowning and near-drowning. Emerg Med Clin North Am 1989; 7:355.
93. Kriel RL, Krach LE, Luxenberg MG, et al: Outcome of severe anoxic/ischemic brain injury in children. Pediatr Neurol 1994; 10:207.
94. Abrams RA, Mubarak S: Musculoskeletal consequences of near-drowning in children. J Pediatr Orthop 1991; 11:168.
95. Pearn J, Debuse P, Mohay H, et al: Sequential intellectual recovery after near-drowning. Med J Aust 1979; 1:463.
96. Borta M: Psychosocial issues in water-related injuries. Crit Care Nurs 1991; 3:325.
97. Coffman SP: Home care of the child and family after near-drowning. J Pediatr Health Care 1992; 6:18.
98. Stylianos S, Eichelberger MR: Pediatric trauma: Prevention strategies. Pediatr Clin North Am 1993; 6:1359.
99. Garrison HG, Fotlin GL, Becker LR, et al: The role of emergency medical services in primary injury prevention. Ann Emerg Med 1997; 30:84.
100. Rivara F, Howes D: Parental knowledge of child development and injury risk. J Dev Behav Pediatr 1982; 3:103.
101. Eichelberger MR, Gotschall CD, Feely HB, et al: Parental attitudes and knowledge of child safety: A national survey. Am J Dis Child 1990; 144:714.
102. Halperin SF, Bass JL, Mehta KA: Knowledge of accident prevention among young children in nine Massachusetts towns. Public Health Rep 1983; 98:548.
103. Hazinski MF, Francescutti LH, Lapidus GD, et al: Pediatric injury prevention: From the Pediatric Injury Prevention Panel of the National Conference on CPR and Emergency Cardiac Care. Ann Emerg Med 1993; 22:456.
104. O'Flaherty JE, Pirie PL: Prevention of pediatric drowning and near-drowning: A survey of members of the American Academy of Pediatrics. Pediatrics 1997; 99:169.
105. Bass JL, Christoffel KK, Windome M, et al: Childhood injury prevention counseling in primary care settings: A critical review of the literature. Pediatrics 1993; 92:544.
106. Bass JL: TIPP—the first ten years. Pediatrics 1995; 95:274.
107. Committee on Injury and Poison Prevention: Drowning in infants, children and adolescents. Pediatrics 1993; 92:292.

108. Potts R, Martinez IG, Dedmon A: Childhood risk taking and injury: Self-report and informant measures. J Pediatr Psychol 1995; 20:5.
109. U.S. Consumer Product Safety Commission: Safety Barrier Guidelines for Home Pools, Release No. 362. Washington, DC, U.S. Consumer Product Safety Commission, Office of Information and Public Affairs, 1997.
110. Present P: Child Drowning Study: A Report on the Epidemiology of Drownings in Residential Pools in Children Under Age Five. Washington, DC, U.S. Consumer Product Safety Commission, 1987.
111. Milliner N, Pearn J, Guard R: Will fenced pools save lives? A 10-year study from Mulgrave Shire, Queensland. Med J Aust 1980; 2:510.
112. Pearn J, Nixon J: Prevention of childhood drowning accidents. Med J Aust 1977; 1:616.
113. Wintemute GJ, Wright MA: Swimming pool owners' opinions of strategies for prevention of drowning. Pediatrics 1990; 85:63.
114. Wintemute GJ, Wright MA: The attitude-practice gap revisited: Risk of reduction beliefs and behaviors among pool owners of residential swimming pools. Pediatrics 1991; 88:1168.
115. Cass DT, Ross FL, Grattan-Smith TM: Child drownings: A changing pattern. Med J Aust 1991; 154:163.
116. Consumer Product Safety Commission: How to Plan for the Unexpected: Preventing Child Drownings. Washington, DC, Release No. 4359. CPSC Publications: CPSC Document No. 4359:1-4, 1988.
117. Gordon D: A clear and present danger. *Los Angeles Times,* June 15, 1997, p K1.
118. Committee on Pediatric Aspects of Physical Fitness, Recreation and Sports: Swimming instructions for infants. Pediatrics 1980; 65:847.
119. Committee on Sports Medicine, American Academy of Pediatrics: Policy statement: Infant swimming programs. *In:* American Academy of Pediatrics, Policy Reference Guide: A Comprehensive Guide to AAP Policy Statements Published through June 1988. Elk Grove Village, Ill, American Academy of Pediatrics, 1988, p 270.
120. Harbaugh SJ: Effects of aquatic training on swimming skill development of preschool children. Percept Mot Skills 1986; 62:439.
121. Asher KN, Rivara FP, Felix D, et al: Water safety training as a potential means of reducing risk of young children's drowning. Injury Prev 1995; 1:228.
122. Rivara FP, Grossman DC, Cummings P: Injury prevention. N Engl J Med 1997; 337:613.
123. Phillips KG: Swimming and water intoxication in infants. Can Med Assoc J 1987; 136:1147.
124. Kropp RM, Schwartz JF: Water intoxication from swimming. J Pediatr 1982; 112:947.
125. Goldberg GN, Lightner ES, Morgan W, et al: Infantile water intoxication after a swimming lesson. Pediatrics 1982; 70:599.
126. California Department of Health Services: Toddler drownings—a preventable tragedy, California Department of Health Services Press Release, 1995, p 1.
127. Baker SP, O'Neil B, Ginsburg M, et al: The Injury Fact Book. New York, Oxford University Press, 1992.
128. Howland J, Hingson R: Alcohol as a risk factor for drownings; a review of the literature (1950–1985). Accid Anal Prev 1988; 20:19.
129. Alcohol use and aquatic activities—United States, 1991. MMWR Morb Mortal Wkly Rep 1993; 42:765;681.
130. Howland J, Smith GS, Mangione T, et al: Missing the boat on drinking and boating. JAMA 1993; 270:91.
131. Smith GS, Houser J: Risk factors for drowning: A case-control study. *In:* Abstracts of the 122nd Annual Meeting of the American Public Health Association, Washington, DC, 1994.
132. Perrine MW, Mundt JC, Weiner RI: When alcohol and water don't mix: Diving under the influence. J Stud Alcohol 1994; 55:517.
133. U.S. Consumer Product Safety Commission: Warning Signs at Pools Could Prevent Accidents. Release No. 91-106. Washington, DC, U.S. Consumer Product Safety Commission, 1991.
134. Kluger Y, Jarosz D, Paul DB, et al: Diving injuries: A preventable catastrophe. J Trauma 1994; 36:349.
135. DeVivo MJ, Sekar P: Prevention of spinal cord injuries that occur in swimming pools. Spinal Cord 1997; 35:509.
136. Alcohol and Boating. Missouri Department of Public Safety, Missouri State Water Patrol, 1996, p 1.
137. Recreational Boating Safety. Safety Study NTSB/SS-93/01. Washington, DC, National Transportation Safety Board, 1993.
138. National Center for Injury Prevention and Control: Unintentional injury, fact sheet, injury prevention: Drowning. Atlanta, Division of Unintentional Injury Prevention, 1996, p 1.
139. Gillenwater JM, Quan LQ, Feldman KW: Inflicted submersion in childhood. Arch Pediatr Adolesc Med 1996; 150:298.
140. Hafer M: Playing it safe. *Los Angeles Times,* July 20, 1997, p B2.

15

Heat Stroke

Stephen M. Ayres, MD, FCCM

A silent needlessly fatal threat kills countless Americans each summertime—308 in St. Louis and 236 in Kansas City, Missouri, in 1980; 700 in Chicago in 1995; and, in July 1998, more than 50 in Texas. It is a plague that is treatable, but many health professionals do not know the treatment.

Classic heat stroke is a medical emergency that frequently eludes early diagnosis because its first symptoms may be those of sudden neurologic decompensation. Mortality rates range from 17% to 80%, depending on the awareness of local public health officials that a sustained period of high temperature and humidity is at hand. The skill of health providers is critical. Incredibly, only one of 58 patients, studied retroactively by Dematte and coworkers,[1] had adequate cooling procedures in the early moments of treatment. Instead, physicians busied themselves in evaluating organ dysfunction instead of immediately treating the cause—blistering heat!

Heat stroke is of significant interest to the intensivist for many reasons. It is a common cause of critical illness and is an important and treatable form of multiple organ failure during the summer months in many parts of the world. In addition, it is characterized by biochemically diverse alterations and evidence of multiple organ failure.

Fever in the critically ill patient is almost always considered to be a manifestation of infection and a possible harbinger of either sepsis or septic shock. Although most of the time fever encountered in the intensive care unit (ICU) is a response to microbial invasion, some fevers are due to either exposure to high temperatures or abnormalities in the thermoregulatory apparatus. Since the mid-1940s, at least seven major summer heat waves in the United States have produced large numbers of heat-related deaths and have seriously taxed the resources of physicians who were unprepared for the human ravages of high ambient temperatures. High body temperatures may be observed in certain clinical entities such as meningitis, falciparum malaria, cerebrovascular accidents near the hypothalamus, and multiple organ system failure. A body temperature of greater than 106°F (41.1°C) during a period of high ambient temperatures, combined with an early elevation of liver enzyme levels, suggests the possibility of heat stroke. Since cooling is also indicated in other patients with high temperatures, the cooling should be instituted immediately while the diagnosis is being clarified.

Human body temperature is maintained within close limits by a balance between heat production and heat dissipation. Heat is normally generated by muscular activity and metabolic reactions. It is dissipated by a mixture of radiation, convection, conduction, and evaporation. Significant heat injury can occur in athletes, military personnel working in hot environments, and workers whose occupations require vigorous activity. Experienced physicians in St. Louis have long observed that roofers in particular were exposed to heat stress and that heat injury among them could be considered an early warning sign that others in the population might soon be at risk. Heat injury can also occur in resting and unacclimated individuals who are elderly or who have abnormalities in their temperature-regulating system because of intercurrent disease.[2]

TEMPERATURE REGULATION

Radiation and convection account for about 75% of heat losses at room temperature if an individual is undressed. The wearing of clothing significantly decreases such losses. Heat loss by these mechanisms decreases as ambient temperature reaches body temperature; ambient temperatures above body temperature actually increase the heat of the body. The unique evaporative loss by sweating accounts for only 25% of heat loss at room temperature but becomes the dominant mechanism at high ambient temperatures. High humidity reduces evaporative losses, explaining why the heat syndromes are particularly common in hot, humid environments.[2]

When ambient temperatures rise, activation of hypothalamic centers leads to cutaneous vasodilation with shunting of blood away from the liver and splanchnic area in an apparent effort to contain visceral heat production to a limited region. Vasodilation enhances sweat gland activity and permits the loss of up to 1.5 L of sweat per hour in the unacclimated person. Such vasodilation increases cardiac output and stresses the heart; cardiovascular disease may limit the necessary increase in cardiac output and reduces the ability of an individual to tolerate acute heat stress. Acclimation occurs after about 1 week of prolonged heat exposure and is associated with a substantial increase in sweat volume and with a reduction in sweat sodium content of 6% to 7%. Plasma volume also increases, underscoring the need for people to increase fluid intake when in hot environments. Heart disease limits the body's adaptive response to prolonged heat exposure and increased humidity and explains the vulnerability of the sick and the elderly to heat injury.

The importance of intact hypothalamic integrating centers is demonstrated by the *neuroleptic malignant syndrome*, which is associated with the use of phenothiazines and certain other dopamine inhibitors by certain sensitive individuals. Caroff and coworkers[3] have suggested that neuroleptic malignant syndrome "may be part of a group of syndromes which, by a combination of central and peripheral mechanisms culminate in a final common pathway of skeletal muscle hypermetabolism and hyperthermia." The syndrome can usually be differentiated from the environmental heat syndromes by the associated rigidity characteristic of phenothiazine use.[3]

CONSEQUENCES OF EXPOSURE IN HOT ENVIRONMENTS

The three classic heat-related syndromes are heat cramps, heat exhaustion, and heat stroke. Heat exhaustion is found in young people during heavy exercise and appears to be related to the excessive loss of sodium chloride in the sweat. Salt losses can be considerable because the sweat content of salt is 30 to 50 mEq/L in unacclimated individuals compared with 5 mEq/L in acclimated people.

The syndromes of heat exhaustion and heat stroke are closely related; the diagnosis of heat stroke is confirmed when rectal temperature exceeds 106°F (41.1°C) and when evidence of vascular insufficiency (i.e., the "stroke" symptoms) is present. The cutoff point of 106°F is obviously arbitrary, but it is an important sign that immediate attempts at cooling are necessary because the uncoupling of oxidative phosphorylation and the failure of enzyme systems occur when the core body temperature reaches 107°C. At that temperature, cell membranes become more permeable, sodium leaks into the cells, and adenosine triphosphate (ADP) stores are depleted.[4]

Heat exhaustion follows vigorous exercise in young individuals and the failure of an appropriate cardiovascular response in older people. Diuretics (fluid loss), anticholinergics (inhibition of sweating), phenothiazines, cyclic antidepressants, monoamine oxidase inhibitors, lithium, antihistamines, sympathomimetics, hallucinogens, ethanol, salicylates, and glutethimide have all been recognized as agents that predispose to heat injury. Fluid depletion and hemoconcentration are observed in both the young and the old, although elderly patients with cardiovascular disease may have volume status that is close to normal. Individuals present with a temperature of 100° to 103°F, profuse sweating, postural hypotension, fatigue, and thirst. A relatively normal mental status distinguishes them from individuals with heat stroke. Fluid replacement with normal saline and rest in a cool place is usually sufficient to reverse the symptoms. Rest and a cool environment may be sufficient in the elderly; one should try oral fluids before resorting to the careful use of intravenous fluids.[5]

Acute neurologic abnormalities are the hallmark of heat stroke, and any individual with mental status or neurologic changes and a high body temperature should be considered to have the syndrome.[5] Other manifestations include lethargy, fatigue, dizziness, nausea, and vomiting. Body temperatures are higher than 103°F (39.4°C) and may be higher than 107°F (41.6°C). Tissue damage begins with temperatures above that level. A hot but dry skin is caused by sweat gland damage and is considered a classic sign, but many patients present with hot and moist skin. In addition to mental status and neurologic changes, there is evidence of multiple organ system dysfunction.

Liver damage is extremely common, and early elevation of the levels of liver enzymes, such as serum glutamic-oxaloacetic transaminase (SGOT) and serum glutamate pyruvate transaminase (SGPT), is a useful sign of heat stroke.[6] Pulmonary edema, disseminated intravascular coagulation (DIC), cardiovascular abnormalities, and acute renal failure are common after initial cooling and stabilization. Fluid management becomes critical because cooling results in a redistribution of blood volume from the periphery to the central organs.

Pulmonary edema due to cardiovascular dysfunction, the adult acute respiratory distress syndrome (ARDS), and a variety of pneumonias can all occur. The combination of DIC and respiratory failure suggests the diagnosis of acute ARDS and the possible development of multiple organ system failure.[7] Tek and Olshaker[5] emphasize the importance of DIC with respect to both diagnosis and outcome. The usual indicators for DIC should be monitored closely. Tek and Olshaker[5] suggest that heparin therapy, although controversial, may be useful.

Acute renal failure has been found in up to 35% of patients with heat stroke and may be caused by a "combination of direct thermal injury, hypotension, shock from cardiovascular collapse, and rhabdomyolysis."[8] Rhabdomyolysis should be treated with alkalinization and mannitol, furosemide, and fluid therapy.

Major electrolyte abnormalities are observed on hospital admission, and electrolyte shifts during treatment are commonly observed. Hypophosphatemia, hypocalcemia, hypoglycemia, and infections may occur. Calcium replacement is probably not indicated unless levels are extremely low because infused calcium may be distributed to injured muscle. Infections such as pneumonia may complicate the syndrome and may lead to a confusion in diagnosis.

RECENT HEAT EXPERIENCES IN THE UNITED STATES

St. Louis, Kansas City (Missouri), and Memphis, Tennessee

On July 1, 1980, the day that university resident staffs traditionally change hands, an incredible heat wave struck both St. Louis and Kansas City, Missouri. The ambient temperature in St. Louis was above 100°F (38.9°C) for 16 days and frequently was as high as 102° to 104°F. The humidity was high. In Kansas City, the ambient temperature was above 108°F (42.2°C) for 10 days.

Complicating the medical situation was the fact that the St. Louis City Hospital was not air-conditioned. The city had lived through disastrous heat spells in the past, but for some reason the city government officials had refused to install what had become standard hospital equipment in other hospitals throughout the United States. The inability of the aged sick—particularly patients given diuretics, antihypertensive agents, and tranquilizers—to withstand heat stress was soon to set the stage for a disaster of tragic proportions. Bodies piled up in the morgue, but patients who were fortunate enough to reach the emergency department alive survived because of vigorous cooling with crushed ice and careful attention to fluid losses. In all, 81 patients seen at St. Louis City Hospital had body temperatures greater than 105°F and were confirmed to have heat stroke. The low death rate of 7% was probably an American record. Epidemiologic study later described the magnitude of the disaster.[9]

During July 1980, there were 308 excess deaths in St. Louis and 236 in Kansas City. Death rates were 56.8% and 65.2% higher than expected in the two cities during usual conditions of ambient temperature and humidity. There were 88 heat-related deaths in nearby Memphis, Tennessee. Heat stroke rates were 10-fold to 12-fold greater in individuals over 65 years of age compared with younger people; the death rate was sixfold greater in people of low socioeconomic status who had little access to air-conditioned environments compared to more affluent individuals.[9]

Chicago, 1995

The failure of government to understand the epidemic nature of heat-related illness led to an even greater disaster in the same part of the country—in Chicago. Between July 12 and July 16, 1995, the maximal and minimal temperature readings reached unprecedented heights and the heat index remained at staggering levels for 6 days. The high temperature was accompanied by extremes of high humidity; there were more than 700 excess deaths during the period of high temperature conditions, and most deaths were heat-related. The first figure from the study documenting the situation should be enlarged and placed in a prominent location in health department offices. Within the first few days of high ambient temperatures, heat-related deaths sharply increased but the city response to the crisis appeared sluggish. A case-control study, conducted by the Centers for Disease Control and Prevention (CDC), found that frail and elderly people and those who were socially isolated were at greatest risk. The presence of air-conditioning was inversely related to the number of heat-related and cardiovascular deaths. The use of electric fans did not reduce the incidence of heat stroke, and the authors warned against wasting limited resources on a fan distribution project.[10]

The Clinical Syndrome in Chicago

O'Hara and coworkers studied 58 near-fatal patients with the classic definition of heat stroke who were admitted to hospitals between July 12 and July 20, 1995.[1] Ages of the patients ranged from 17 to 95 years (mean, 67.5); 63% were African-American. Follow-up information was available on all but one of the patients; in-hospital mortality was 21%. *Incredibly, only one of the 58 patients was adequately cooled within an acceptable time frame.* None of the patients demonstrated evidence of functional improvement during the subsequent year, and 28% died after discharge from the hospital. As discussed in this chapter, it has been known for some years that survival is maximized when the patient is rapidly cooled. Most experts agree that patients with heat stroke should be quickly cooled so that body temperature can be lowered to below 38.9°C within 30 minutes of admission. Why was this not done in the Chicago scene? Were the physicians not aware of the importance of rapid cooling, or were they so obsessed with the magnitude of the multiple organ failure that they neglected to attack the primary etiologic factor? (See Treatment later.)

The most common conditions were hypertension and alcohol abuse. Sixteen patients were taking diuretics or phenothiazines, and one was taking cocaine, an agent that increases heat production.

Thirty-three patients were comatose on admission. In addition, they exhibited a variety of neurologic abnormalities, including alterations in mental status, coma, delirium, lethargy, disorientation, and seizures. Cardiac arrhythmias were common, and 43 patients received echocardiography early in their hospital course. Thirty-five patients (60%) were intubated; 10 patients exhibited respiratory alkalosis with mixed non–anion gap acidosis. Elevated creatinine concentrations were found in 24 patients.

Infectious complications were found in 40 sites in the 33 patients. The sites included urinary tract, lungs, sinuses, skin, and colon. Bacteremia was present in 13 patients. Twenty-six patients had evidence of DIC. The clinical findings differed from those reported earlier in the severity of hematologic and renal abnormalities and the widespread incidence of infectious sequelae. Could the early failure to cool have been responsible for these continued problems?

TREATMENT

The high mortality associated with heat stroke can be reduced if patients are rapidly cooled.[11] Patients with high temperatures are covered with ice, and rectal temperatures are monitored. Intravenous fluids are administered as needed, and patients are removed from the ice baths when the rectal temperature decreases from 101° to 100°F. Neither ice water enemas nor renal dialysis is necessary, and shivering is prevented if the ice is removed before the temperature reaches normal. Shivering reduces heat loss and can be eliminated by the administration of chlorpromazine; however, Geiss and Marr[12] observed that removing a patient from the cooling tub at the prescribed temperature also prevented shivering. Most patients were not volume-depleted, and excessive fluid replacement was not needed. Specific problems (e.g., respiratory failure) were treated in the usual manner.

The medical staff at St. Louis City Hospital faced an unusual situation because the hospital was not air-conditioned. This experience illustrates the importance of the ambient temperature. It was soon noted that most of the patients who had been successfully cooled in the emergency department had heat-related complaints and high body temperatures after they were admitted to the non–air-conditioned wards. The staff responded by maintaining fluid balance with continuous intravenous infusions and by packing patients in ice water–soaked sheets, as had been done in the emergency department.

The peripheral vasoconstriction associated with immersion in ice water may have an adverse effect in individuals with cardiovascular dysfunction and has led some clinicians to consider alternative cooling methods.[13] Evaporation of 1 g of water consumes seven times as much heat as does the melting of 1 g of ice and does not produce peripheral vasoconstriction. The Makah Body Cooling Unit[14] is a refinement of the evaporative cooling method that was developed to treat the large numbers of individuals who suffered heat stroke during a pilgrimage to Mecca. Rapid cooling rates were observed, and the method is probably the best available at present; however, it may be impractical for the intermittently encountered heat stress disasters treated in hospitals throughout the United States and in other countries.[12]

PATHOGENETIC STUDIES

The Heatstroke Center of King Faisal Hospital and Al-Noor Hospital, Makah, Saudi Arabia, has long conducted clinical studies on pilgrims making the journey, or *haj*, to Mecca. Bouchama and colleagues[15] studied these patients and presented evidence of endothelial cell activation in persons with heat stroke. Studies suggested the presence of microthrombi in the microcirculation and activation of von Willebrand factor. Studies indicating the presence of DIC and respiratory distress may link its pathogenesis to other forms of ARDS. Although early cooling saves many lives, it is possible that a more fundamental understanding of the pathogenesis of heat stroke might lead to more specific and curative strategies. Levels of endotoxin, tumor necrosis factor-α, interleukins (ILα, ILβ), and interferon-γ are increased in heat stroke and decreased with cooling but are not correlated with body temperature outcomes.

Seeking early signs of heat stroke that might be predictive of outcome, Nylen and associates[16] studied 25 patients between ages 30 and 75 years who experienced heat stroke during the *haj* in 1994. Their detailed observations underscore the severity of the organ dysfunction.

The subjects were divided into three groups according to the amount of time needed to reduce rectal temperature to 38°C. Group C included all of the patients who died. Group A rectal temperatures averaged 41.7°C (108.4°F); APACHE* scores, 17. Group B rectal temperatures averaged 42.5°C (108.5°F); APACHE scores, 27. Group C rectal temperatures averaged 42.5°C (107°F); APACHE scores, 30.

Procalcitonin concentrations were measured on arrival and compared to matched controls admitted with conditions other than heat stroke. The concentration of procalcitonin was significantly higher in survivors than in nonsurvivors. The authors surmised that the inability to elicit a calcitonin response may indicate a failure in the cytokine cascade as a result of heat stress.

PREVENTION OF HEAT INJURY

Unlike the presence of epidemics caused by infectious agents, heat stroke is fundamentally a product of governmental inaction. Studies following the Chicago disaster showed that although patients with preexisting mental, pulmonary, or cardiovascular diseases were particularly at risk, socioeconomic factors were even more important. The effect of social isolation, a bedridden existence, and absence of air-conditioning seemed even more important. Spending even a few hours in an air-conditioned environment seemed protective against heat exhaustion. Some have sought to make it a political issue. Ben Lieberman of the Competitive Enterprise Institute blamed it on the high cost of air-conditioning caused by environmental regulations that raised the cost of refrigerants.[17]

Kellerman and Todd[18] described the program adopted by the city of Memphis after its experience with the heat emergency of 1980. At the beginning of the summer, health department officials begin "sentinel" visits at emergency departments to determine the presence of any heat-related admissions. When temperatures begin to rise, the print and electronic media begin informational programs emphasizing the need for air-conditioning, decreased activity, adequate hydration, and the need to seek medical help for health-related problems. Visits are made to nursing homes and residences of public assistance recipients. Individuals with air-conditioning are urged to contact any relatives without air-conditioning. People who are not able to cope with high temperatures are transported to shelters. Although formal evaluations have not been made, the median rate of heat-related deaths has been only two per year.

*APACHE = Acute Physiology and Chronic Health Evaluation.

References

1. Dematte JE, O'Mara KO, Buescher J, et al: Near fatal heat stroke during the 1995 heat wave in Chicago. Ann Intern Med 1998; 29:173–181.
2. O'Donnell TF Jr, Clowes GH: The circulatory abnormalities of heat stroke. N Engl J Med 1972; 287:734–737.
3. Caroff SN, Mann SC, Lazarus A, et al: Neuroleptic malignant syndrome: Diagnostic issues. Psych Ann 1991; 21:130–147.
4. Yarbrough BE, Hubbard RW: Heat related illness. *In*: Management of Wilderness and Environmental Emergencies. Auerbach PS, Geehr EC (Eds). St. Louis, CV Mosby, 1989, pp 119–143.
5. Tek D, Olshaker JS: Heat illness. Emerg Med Clin North Am 1991; 10:299–308.
6. Rubel CR: Hepatic injury associated with heatstroke. Ann Clin Lab Sci 1984; 14:130–136.
7. El Kassimi FA, Al-Mashadani SA, Akhtar J: Adult respiratory distress syndrome and disseminated intravascular coagulation complicating heat stroke. Chest 1986; 90:571–574.
8. Curley G, Irwin RS: Disorders of temperature control: Part 1. Hyperthermia. Intensive Care Med 1986; 1:5–14.
9. Jones TS, Liang AP, Kilbourne EM, et al: Morbidity and mortality associated with July 1980 heat wave in St. Louis and Kansas City, Mo. JAMA 1982; 247:3328–3331.
10. Semenza JC, Rubin CH, Falter KH, et al: Heat related deaths during the July 1995 heat wave in Chicago. N Engl J Med 1996; 335:84–90.
11. O'Donnell TF: Acute heatstroke: Epidemiologic, biochemical, renal and coagulation studies. JAMA 1975; 234:824–828.
12. Geiss P, Marr JJ: Management of heat injury syndromes. *In*: Critical Care: State of the Art. Anaheim, Calif, Society of Critical Care Medicine, 1982.
13. Magazanik A, Epstein Y, Udassin R, et al: Tap water: An efficient method for cooling heatstroke victims—a model in dogs. Aviat Space Environ Med 1980; 51:864–866.
14. Weiner J, Khogali M: A physiologic body cooling unit for treatment of heat stroke. Lancet 1980; ii:507–509.
15. Bouchama A, Hammami MH, Afrozul H: Evidence for endothelial cell activation/injury in heatstroke. Crit Care Med 1996; 24:1173–1178.
16. Nylen ES, Arifi AA, Becker KL, et al: Effect of classic heatstroke on serum procalcitonin. Crit Care Med 1997; 25:1362–1365.
17. Regulated to death? *Richmond Times-Dispatch*, Richmond, Va, August 27, 1995, Section F-6 (Editorial).
18. Kellerman AL, Todd KT: Killing heat. N Engl J Med 1996; 335:126–127.

16

Hyperthermia

Maged S. Mikhail, MD • Duraiyah Thangathurai, MD, FCCM

Both fever and hyperthermia may be defined as an elevation in the normal circadian fluctuations of body temperature from its normal of 36.8° ± 0.4°C. Although the distinction between the terms is somewhat arbitrary, hyperthermia usually refers to a special group of critical illnesses characterized by excessive heat production, decreased heat dissipation, and loss of thermoregulation. In contrast, most fevers are due to inflammatory processes in which the rise in body temperature is caused by circulating pyrogens that may be exogenous (microorganisms, their products, and toxins) or endogenous (cytokines—interleukins, tumor necrosis factor, and interferon).

Environmental heat exposure, several metabolic disorders, drug toxicities, and central nervous system (CNS) injuries can induce life-threatening hyperthermia. As with fever, the diagnosis of hyperthermia is not always readily apparent and requires careful evaluations of the patient and the clinical setting. Moreover, because the temperature elevations are often marked, prompt recognition and rapid treatment are necessary. Table 16–1 lists the differential diagnosis of hyperthermia and fever. Heat stroke is usually apparent from the history, whereas malignant hyperthermia is almost always related temporally to anesthesia. Unfortunately, there is considerable overlap in clinical presentation between the different hyperthermia syndromes. Regardless of the cause, marked hyperthermia (>41°C) results in serious organ dysfunction and injury, especially in the brain, liver, and kidneys.

NORMAL DEFENSE MECHANISMS AGAINST HYPERTHERMIA

Normal heat production is primarily due to metabolic activity in the liver and skeletal muscle. The trunk viscera generate most body heat at rest, but muscle becomes the major source with exercise or shivering. Heat elimination occurs by four major mechanisms. Radiation of heat from the skin to an object does not require contact. Convection heat loss results from airflow across skin. Conductive heat losses require an object to be in direct contact with skin, whereas evaporative heat loss is primarily due to sweating; evaporative heat loss from the respiratory tract is relatively unimportant. Convection and radiation are normally the most important mechanisms for heat elimination; with increased physical activity, evaporation also becomes a major mechanism for heat dissipation. Regulation of blood flow to skin and sweat gland activity are therefore critical in maintaining thermal balance.

TABLE 16–1. Differential Diagnosis of Hyperthermia and Fever

Hyperthermia
- Environmental exposure
- Malignant hyperthermia
- Neuroleptic malignant syndrome
- Thyroid storm
- Pheochromocytoma
- Serotonin syndrome
- Iatrogenic hyperthermia
- Brain stem/hypothalamic injury

Fever
- Inflammatory disorders
  - Sepsis
  - Infection
  - Trauma
  - Drug reaction
  - Transfusion reaction
  - Collagen vascular/hypersensitivity disorder
- Neoplasm
- Inherited and metabolic disease
- Factitious fever

Thermoregulation is a three-part process: (1) afferent thermal sensing, (2) hypothalamic processing, and (3) efferent responses through the sympathetic system. Unmyelinated C fibers carry heat stimuli from the skin to the spinal cord. Neural fibers responsible for temperature sensation ascend primarily in the lateral spinothalamic tract to the supraoptic nucleus and the anterior hypothalamus. Although warmth sensors in the skin appear to be most important in preventing hyperthermia, central temperature sensors in abdominal and thoracic viscera, spinal cord, and brain (primarily the hypothalamus) may also play a role.

The hypothalamus integrates all afferent temperature input. It additionally contains an area of reduced blood-brain barrier function that contains a specialized vascular network called the organum vasculosum laminae terminalis. The endothelial lining of these vessels appears to elaborate arachidonic acid metabolites, primarily prostaglandin E_2, when exposed to circulating pyrogens. The prostaglandins then diffuse into the preoptic nucleus and anterior hypothalamus, resetting core body temperature to a higher level. While the hypothalamus alters body temperature primarily by regulating vasomotor tone to the skin and sweat formation, neural output to the cerebral cortex is important in modifying behavior to compensate for changes in temperature.

The efferent hypothalamic response to heat consists of cutaneous vasodilatation, sweat formation, and inhibition of muscle tone. Sympathetically controlled changes in vasomotor tone result in cutaneous dilation and shunting of blood away from the liver and splanchnic circulation. Cutaneous vasodilatation increases cardiac output and facilitates heat transfer from viscera and muscle to skin. Sweat formation is under cholinergic sympathetic control. Important behavioral responses to heat include removal of clothing, limitation of physical activity, and movement toward cooler temperature gradients.

Acclimatization to sustained increases in body temperature is slow and requires 1 to 2 weeks for peak effect. Sweat volume can increase from 1.5 L/hour up to 4 L/hour. In addition, the threshold for sweating decreases, as does sweat sodium concentration (from 30 to 65 mEq/L to 5 mEq/L). Plasma antidiuretic hormone, growth hormone, and aldosterone levels increase. Cardiovascular mechanisms include a 10% to 25% increase in plasma volume and an increased stroke volume with a slowing of heart rate.

ENVIRONMENTAL HYPERTHERMIA

Prolonged exposure to hot, humid environments, especially with increased physical activity, can result in hyperthermia and potentially serious heat injury to vital organs. It is estimated that more than 4000 deaths due to heat stroke occur each year in the United States.[1] These injuries occur most commonly at temperatures above 32°C (90°F) and with a humidity higher than 60%. Three environmentally induced heat injury syndromes are commonly recognized: heat cramps,

TABLE 16–2. Heat Syndromes

Syndrome	Temperature	Manifestation
Heat cramps	Normal	Muscle cramps
Heat exhaustion	Normal to 39°C	Faintness, weakness
Heat stroke	>41°C	Gross neurologic impairment

heat exhaustion, and heat stroke (Table 16–2).[2] Elderly individuals as well as patients with underlying medical illnesses or who are receiving certain drug therapies are susceptible to heat injury even without physical activity.[3]

Pathophysiology

Eighty per cent of heat exposure victims are older than 65 years of age. This is likely due to impaired thermoregulation with advancing age. Older individuals appear to have decreased responsiveness of thermal sensors as well as a decreased sweat response, lower basal metabolic rate, and impaired vasoconstriction.[4] Limited cardiac reserve also impairs the ability to increase cardiac output and accelerate heat transfer from viscera and muscle to skin.

Other risk factors for environmental hyperthermia include cardiac dysfunction, schizophrenia, Parkinson's disease, alcoholism, cystic fibrosis, and paraplegia. The condition itself, the associated drug therapy, or both may impair the thermoregulatory response to heat exposure. Physically or mentally debilitated patients are not able to modify their behavior in hot weather. Table 16–3 lists drugs that may predispose to environmental hyperthermia. Drugs with anticholinergic properties reduce sweat formation, whereas diuretics and adrenergic blockers impair cardiac function. Hypokalemia impairs sweat formation as well as cardiac contractility. Alcohol predisposes to heat stroke by inhibiting antidiuretic hormone and promoting dehydration.

Heat injury can occur in otherwise healthy individuals who are engaged in strenuous physical activity in hot, humid environments. Athletes (runners and football players), hikers, military personnel, and people who have occupations that subject them to environmental exposure (miners and roofers) are at increased risk. Heat stroke is the second leading cause of deaths in athletes after head and spinal cord injuries. Evaporative heat loss accounts for most of heat elimination at temperatures above body temperature; this mechanism is markedly reduced in high humidity.

Heat Cramps

Heat cramps are the mildest and earliest form of environmental heat injury. Minimal temperature elevation is present. Symptoms are generally limited to intermittent cramping in the extremities after strenuous activity or exercise. Most patients are young, healthy individuals. Mild hypovolemia may be present and is due to sweat loss. Serum electrolyte values are usually normal. Cramping may be related to hyperventilation and a secondary respiratory alkalosis resulting in a low serum ionized calcium concentration. Treatment consists of rest, removing clothing, and oral fluid replacement with either water or an electrolyte solution.

TABLE 16–3. Drugs That Predispose to Hyperthermia

Diuretics	Antihistamines
Anticholinergics	Ethanol
Phenothiazines	Salicylates
Antidepressants	β-Adrenergic blockers
Lithium	

Heat Exhaustion

Heat exhaustion, also frequently referred to as *heat prostration*, is probably the commonest of the three syndromes. Patients are either young individuals who have been exercising or elderly patients with limited cardiac reserve. Weakness, fatigue, and dizziness are the most common complaints. Anorexia, nausea, and vomiting may also be prominent. Excessive loss of sodium chloride in sweat causes salt depletion in addition to water loss. Patients usually have mild to moderate hyperthermia (<38°C). Orthostatic hypotension and tachycardia are often present, and patients hyperventilate. The syndrome may be characterized by a predominance of either water depletion or salt depletion depending on prior water intake. Serum sodium concentration may be normal or mildly elevated. Treatment is similar to that of heat cramps if symptoms are mild. Patients with nausea or vomiting or severe volume deficits require intravenous fluid replacement.

Heat Stroke

Hyperthermia due to heat stroke is often defined as a rectal temperature above 40°C (>105°F) with acute neurologic impairment. Two variants are often distinguished depending on whether the impaired heat loss occurs with or without increased heat production (Table 16–4). Classic (nonexertional) heat stroke occurs primarily in older patients. Exertional heat stroke is more typically encountered in young, healthy individuals after strenuous activity.

Clinical Presentation

Although most definitions of heat stroke require a core temperature above 40°C, neurologic impairment may occur at lower temperatures in some patients. Neurologic manifestations include slurred speech, stupor, coma, and seizures. Seizures are more common at temperatures above 41°C. The cerebellum is especially sensitive to heat injury; consequently ataxia, dysmetria, and dysarthria may also be seen. Patients typically hyperventilate. Although profuse sweating is common, sweating may be absent, especially in the elderly; sweat glands may fail or fatigue.[5] Cardiovascular manifestations include tachycardia and an initially marked increase in cardiac output that may be limited later by dehydration or underlying cardiac disease; arterial hypotension is not uncommon. At temperatures above 42°C, direct cellular death begins to occur throughout the body as enzyme systems fail and cell membranes break down.

Laboratory findings include a high hematocrit value due to hemoconcentration and hypernatremia due to dehydration. Increased white blood cell count is not unusual. Serum potassium concentration may be low, normal, or high. Potassium

TABLE 16–4. Heat Stroke Syndromes

	Classic	Exertional
Age	Elderly	Young
Precipitating event	Heat	Heat, strenuous activity
Underlying process	Medical illness, drug therapy	None
Onset	Slow	Rapid
Sweating	Usually absent	Often present

losses are due to sweating; increases in serum potassium are due to an efflux of potassium from muscle or necrotic cells. Serum phosphate and calcium levels are low, especially with rhabdomyolysis. Hypoglycemia may occur as a result of metabolic exhaustion.[6] Elevated liver enzymes are common. Serum muscle enzyme levels may not be elevated in nonexertional heat stroke[26] but are typically high in exertional settings. Extremely high creatine kinase (CK) levels (>20,000 U/L) and hyperkalemia are suggestive of rhabdomyolysis. Cerebrospinal fluid analysis may show increased protein levels, xanthochromia, and mild lymphocytic pleocytosis.

Complications

Neurologic complications of hyperthermia include seizures, cerebral edema, and localized brain hemorrhages. Irreversible brain damage often occurs above 42°C (108°F). Cerebellar impairment may persist after recovery. Cardiac complications include tachyarrhythmias, high cardiac output, heart failure, and myocardial infarction. Pulmonary edema may be cardiogenic in patients with a limited cardiac reserve or may develop secondary to the adult respiratory distress syndrome.[7] Pulmonary aspiration can also be encountered in obtunded patients. Acute renal failure may be due to direct heat damage, renal hypoperfusion, or rhabdomyolysis. The incidence of renal failure is about 35% with exertional heat stroke, compared with 5% in classic nonexertional heat stroke, which may reflect a lower likelihood of rhabdomyolysis with classic heat stroke. Mucosal ulceration of the gastrointestinal tract is not uncommon and can lead to gastrointestinal hemorrhage. Liver damage and dysfunction are extremely common. The extent of hepatic necrosis and cholestasis may not be apparent until 48 to 72 hours after heat injury. Hematologic complications include hemolysis, thrombocytopenia, and disseminated intravascular coagulation (DIC).[7] Megakaryocytes appear to be especially sensitive to heat injury. DIC is triggered by diffuse endothelial and organ damage. Its onset is usually delayed 2 to 3 days and is associated with high mortality.

Treatment

Heat stroke is a true medical emergency because it can be associated with up to a 70% mortality rate. Modern prompt effective treatment reduces mortality to as low as 5% to 18%. Oxygen therapy, rapid cooling, and cautious hydration should be instituted immediately to avoid complications. Endotracheal intubation should be accomplished if the patient is obtunded or in respiratory distress.

Rapid cooling is accomplished by removal of clothing and either an evaporative-convective or conductive cooling technique. The former involves blowing air with fans on the patient after sponging the skin with water; cold packs are also often used. The latter technique involves either immersion in ice water or application of cooling blankets above and below the patient. Both techniques can usually reduce core temperature below 40°C in 1 hour. Immersion impairs access to the patient and may limit monitoring. Another potential disadvantage of immersion (and cooling blankets) is that intense vasoconstriction can slow the rate of heat loss.[8] However, Armstrong and colleagues[9] have reported ice-water immersion to cool hyperthermic runners almost twice as fast as convection (air exposure). Vasoconstriction may also have adverse cardiovascular effects in patients with limited cardiac reserve because it can increase cardiac afterload. Additional, more aggressive cooling measures include gastric lavage with iced saline, cold hemodialysis, and cardiopulmonary bypass. Consciousness usually returns with cooling.

Core body temperature should be monitored closely with a rectal, bladder, or tympanic temperature probe. Close monitoring of vital signs, neurologic function, and urine output and laboratory measurements, such as arterial blood gas and serum electrolyte determinations, is also mandatory. An arterial catheter facilitates blood pressure monitoring and blood gas measurements. Central venous pressure and pulmonary artery pressure monitoring can be invaluable in patients with limited cardiac reserve. Volume deficits may not be more than 2 to 3 L, especially in patients with classic heat stroke. Hypotension usually responds to intravenous fluids; however, if an inotrope is required, an agent that produces little vasoconstriction, such as dobutamine, should be used. Sodium bicarbonate therapy should be guided by serial arterial blood gas measurements.

Most clinicians do not advocate temperature correction of arterial blood gas measurements. Use of H_2-histamine blockers may decrease the incidence of gastrointestinal bleeding. Rhabdomyolysis should be treated aggressively with saline diuresis, alkalinization of the urine, and an infusion of mannitol, 0.5 g/kg, with or without furosemide. Calcium infusion may aggravate muscle damage and should generally be avoided. Seizures may be treated acutely with intravenous diazepam.

MALIGNANT HYPERTHERMIA

Although "pyrexic" anesthetic deaths were recognized in the early 1900s, malignant hyperthermia (MH) was not clearly described as a syndrome until 1960.[10] Early reports emphasized hyperthermia, muscle rigidity, and metabolic acidosis as the classic triad of MH.[11] Discovery of a similar disorder in pigs—*porcine stress syndrome*—greatly enhanced the understanding of MH.[12] Affected pigs developed an MH-like syndrome after stress or after induction of general anesthesia with halothane and succinylcholine.

Although the role of stress as a trigger in humans is not as well established, all halogenated general anesthetic gases and depolarizing muscle relaxants are now known to be potential triggering agents of MH in susceptible humans. Development of the in vitro halothane-caffeine contracture test on skeletal muscle helped to identify susceptible individuals and to establish with certainty the genetic nature of the disorder in most individuals.[13] Moreover, MH is now known to represent a group of closely related hypermetabolic disorders of skeletal muscle that can result in a sudden uncontrolled increase in intracellular calcium.

Incidence

The overall incidence of MH is between 1 in 50,000 and 1 in 100,000 patients receiving general anesthesia. The reported incidence in children is 1 in 15,000 in contrast to 1 in 40,000 adult patients. This higher incidence probably represents misdiagnosis of MH in pediatric patients who have an underlying myopathy and who experience succinylcholine-induced hyperkalemic cardiac arrest. Reports of MH vary greatly from country to country and even in different geographic localities within a country, reflecting varying gene pools. In the United States, the incidence is highest in the Midwest. The mean age of patients with a diagnosis of an MH episode is 22 years. In 80% of reported cases, both succinylcholine and a halogenated anesthetic agent were used.

Table 16–5 presents a list of drugs known to be triggers of MH. In a few rare instances, MH appears to have occurred without an exposure to a general anesthetic gas or a depolarizing muscle relaxant.[14] Chlorocresol, an additive in commercial succinylcholine preparations, may also be an additional trigger in succinylcholine-induced MH.[15]

Genetics

Although sporadic cases are described, most patients with an episode of MH have a history of relatives with a similar epi-

TABLE 16–5. Drugs Known to Trigger Malignant Hyperthermia

Halogenated General Anesthetics
Ether
Cyclopropane
Halothane
Methoxyflurane
Enflurane
Isoflurane
Desflurane
Sevoflurane
Nondepolarizing Muscle Relaxants
Succinylcholine
Decamethonium

sode or an abnormal response to the halothane-caffeine contracture test. An autosomal pattern of dominance with variable penetrance occurs in about 50% of susceptible families. The complexity of genetic inheritance patterns in families reflects the fact that MH is a heterogeneous genetic disorder; it can be caused by mutations of one or more genes on more than one chromosome.[16–18] Thus, genes on chromosomes 1, 3, 7, 17, and 19 have been linked with MH in different families.

The earliest reports linked MH with mutations in the gene for the skeletal muscle, ryanodine (Ryr1) receptor, calcium release channel on chromosome 19 in humans.[19] Subsequent reports of other families linked MH with mutations in the adult muscle, sodium channel, alpha subunit gene on chromosome 17. An autosomal recessive form of MH has been associated with the King-Denborough syndrome.[20] This syndrome occurs primarily in young boys with short stature, cryptorchidism, kyphoscoliosis, pectus deformity, slanted eyes, low-set ears, webbed neck, and winged scapulae. Other strong associations include Duchenne's muscular dystrophy[21] and central core disease.[22] Myotonia fluctuans and osteogenesis imperfecta may also increase the risk of MH.[23] Associations between MH and heat stroke or sudden death (adult or infantile) are controversial.

Pathophysiology

At least 50% of patients with an episode of MH have had a previously uneventful general anesthetic reaction when they were exposed to a triggering agent. Succinylcholine or a halogenated anesthetic agent alone may trigger an MH episode. The exact mechanism of MH and the reasons it does not occur after every exposure to a triggering agent are poorly understood. The initial focus was on an abnormal ryanodine Ryr1 receptor in patients with MH. This calcium channel receptor is responsible for calcium release from the sarcoplasmic reticulum and plays a critical role in muscle depolarization. Further studies, however, have revealed that many patients with MH have a normal ryanodine receptor and that abnormalities in secondary messengers and modulators of calcium release, such as fatty acids and phosphatidylinositol, are often present. An abnormal sodium channel in skeletal muscle may also play a role in some patients.

The final common pathway in the triggering of an MH episode is an uncontrolled increase in intracellular calcium in skeletal muscle.[24] The sudden release of calcium from sarcoplasmic reticulum removes the inhibition of troponin, resulting in intense muscle contractions. Markedly enhanced and sustained adenosine triphosphatase activity results in uncontrolled glycolysis. The hypermetabolic state rapidly progresses, producing severe lactic acidosis and hyperthermia. As muscle membranes break down, an efflux of potassium from muscle cells together with systemic acidosis produces hyperkalemia. Increased sympathetic tone, acidosis, and hyperkalemia all predispose to ventricular fibrillation and sudden death, which may occur in as little as 15 minutes.

Clinical Presentation

Although MH usually presents shortly after induction of anesthesia or at the end of surgery (Table 16–6), it may occur at any time during administration of the anesthetic agent or postoperatively in the recovery room or intensive care unit (ICU). The earliest signs reported during anesthesia are masseter muscle rigidity (MMR), tachycardia, and hypercapnia due to increased carbon dioxide production.[25] The presence of two or more signs greatly increases the likelihood of MH.[26] Isolated MMR (also called trismus or masseter spasm) occurs in only 15% to 30% of true MH episodes and may occur in up to 1% of normal patients. Moreover, fewer than 50% of patients with MMR prove to be susceptible to MH by muscle testing.[27] Tachypnea is prominent when muscle relaxants are not used. Sympathetic system overactivity produces tachycardia, hypertension, and mottled cyanosis. These signs usually precede hyperthermia, hyperkalemia, and lactic acidosis. In fact, hyperthermia may be a late sign, but when it occurs, core temperature can rise as much as 1°C every 5 minutes. Generalized muscle rigidity is not consistently present, but it occurs in up to 70% of episodes of MH in older series. Hypertension may be rapidly followed by hypotension as cardiac depression occurs. Dark urine reflects myoglobinemia and myoglobinuria.

Laboratory evaluation reveals hypercapnia, acidosis, hyperkalemia, hypermagnesemia, a marked base deficit, and a low mixed venous oxygen saturation. Serum ionized calcium concentration may initially increase before it falls. Hypoglycemia may also be present.[28] Patients also typically have increased serum myoglobin, CK, lactate dehydrogenase, and aldolase levels. Serum CK levels usually exceed 20,000 U/L. Both serum myoglobin and CK levels can increase markedly in some normal patients after succinylcholine without MH.

TABLE 16–6. Signs of Malignant Hyperthermia

Increased Metabolism
Increased carbon dioxide production
Increased oxygen consumption
Low mixed venous oxygen tension ($P\bar{v}O_2$)
Metabolic acidosis
Cyanosis
Mottling
Increased Sympathetic Tone
Tachycardia
Initial hypertension
Arrhythmias
Rigidity/Muscle Damage
Masseter muscle rigidity
Elevated serum creatine kinase
Hyperkalemia
Hypernatremia
Hyperphosphatemia
Myoglobinemia
Myoglobinuria
Hyperthermia
Fever
Sweating

Complications

Ventricular fibrillation can follow the onset of MH within minutes and is the most common cause of death. If the patient survives the first few minutes, acute renal failure and DIC can develop rapidly. Other complications of hyperthermia include cerebral edema with seizures and hepatic failure.

Treatment

The mortality rate of MH, even with prompt treatment, may still be as high as 10% to 30%.[29] Treatment is oriented at both terminating the episode and treating complications such as acidosis and hyperkalemia. The triggering agent must be stopped, and dantrolene therapy must be initiated immediately.[30] The patient must be hyperventilated with 100% oxygen until the attack is terminated. Dantrolene prevents further release of calcium from the sarcoplasmic reticulum by binding the Ryr1 receptor calcium channel.[31] The dose is 2.5 mg/kg intravenously every 5 minutes until the episode is terminated. The upper limit of dantrolene therapy is generally 10 mg/kg. Dantrolene's effective half-life is about 6 hours. After initial control, dantrolene, 1 mg/kg, intravenously is recommended every 6 hours for 24 to 48 hours to prevent relapse because MH can recur within 24 hours.[32] Dantrolene is not specific for MH; it also decreases temperature in thyroid storm and neuroleptic malignant syndrome.

Cooling measures should also be instituted immediately. Ice packs, cold air convection, and cooling blankets are used for surface cooling. Iced saline lavage of the stomach and body cavities (whenever possible) should also be instituted. Cold dialysis and cardiopulmonary bypass may also be appropriate if other measures fail.

Acidosis should be treated aggressively with intravenous sodium bicarbonate, 2 to 4 mEq/kg. Hyperkalemia should be treated with insulin and glucose infusion and diuresis. The use of intravenous calcium is generally not recommended. Calcium channel blockers should not be used with dantrolene therapy because this combination appears to promote hyperkalemia. Catecholamine vasopressors and inotropes are considered safe if used appropriately. Prophylactic procainamide 2.5 mg/kg has been recommended by some authorities to prevent ventricular fibrillation. Mannitol infusion, 0.5 g/kg, with or without furosemide should be used to establish a diuresis and prevent acute renal failure from myoglobinuria.

After a suspected episode of MH, an in vitro halothane-caffeine contracture test should be performed to confirm the diagnosis. If the test result is confirmatory, genetic counseling and testing of family members are appropriate. Baseline CK levels may be elevated chronically in 50% to 70% of people at risk for MH, but the only reliable way to diagnose MH susceptibility is by muscle testing. The halothane-caffeine contracture test may show a 10% to 20% false-positive rate, but the false-negative rate is close to zero.[33]

Both European and North American MH registries have been established to help physicians identify and treat patients with suspected MH as well as provide standardization between testing centers. There are approximately 24 muscle testing centers in Europe and 12 in North America. The Malignant Hyperthermia Association of the United States (MHAUS, telephone 1-800-98-MHAUS) operates a 24-hour hotline (1-800-MH-HYPER), an on-demand fax service (1-800-440-9990), and a Web site (www.mhaus.org).

NEUROLEPTIC MALIGNANT SYNDROME

The neuroleptic malignant syndrome (NMS) is characterized by hyperthermia, muscle rigidity with extrapyramidal signs, altered consciousness, and autonomic lability.[34] It is most commonly encountered in patients with neuropsychiatric lability.[35] The incidence of NMS has been reported to be as much as 1% of patients taking antidopaminergic drugs. The mean age of patients is 40 years, and the syndrome is twice as common in men as in women.

NMS is caused by an imbalance of neurotransmitters in the CNS. A functional dopamine deficiency results in hyperactivity of excitatory amino acids in the basal ganglia and hypothalamus.[36] The syndrome can occur either during drug therapy with an antidopaminergic agent or after withdrawal of the dopaminergic agonist in patients with Parkinson's disease. Thus, drug therapy with phenothiazines, butyrophenones, thioxanthenes, dibenzoxepines, and metoclopramide can produce NMS. Less commonly, NMS develops after abrupt withdrawal of levodopa or amantadine. NMS is not a variant of MH and usually does not recur with reexposure to an antidopaminergic agent.[36]

The onset of NMS may be within hours of drug therapy or may be delayed up to 4 weeks later; onset appears to be related more to the rate of increase in the dosage of the therapeutic agent than to the absolute dose. Most episodes of NMS occur within 2 weeks of a dose adjustment.[37] Hyperthermia generally tends to be mild and appears to be proportional to the amount of rigidity; some authors also suggest that the hypothalamus is reset to a higher temperature. The mean maximum core temperature is reported to be 40°C.[37] Extrapyramidal signs are often prominent and include akinesia, dysarthria, dysphagia, mutism, and tremor. Autonomic dysfunction results in tachycardia, labile blood pressure, diaphoresis, dyspnea, increased secretions, and urinary incontinence. Muscle rigidity can produce respiratory distress and together with the increased secretions can promote aspiration pneumonia. CK levels are typically elevated; in some patients, rhabdomyolysis may develop, resulting in myoglobinemia, myoglobinuria, and renal failure.

Even with treatment, the mortality rate of NMS may be as high as 5%. Mild forms of NMS promptly resolve after withdrawal of the causative drug (or reinstitution of antiparkinsonian therapy). Initial treatment of more severe forms of NMS should include oxygen therapy and endotracheal intubation for respiratory distress or altered consciousness. Respiratory distress requiring intubation is common (20%). Marked muscle rigidity can be controlled with muscle paralysis, dantrolene therapy, or a dopaminergic agonist, depending on the severity and acuity of the syndrome. Resolution of the muscle rigidity usually decreases body temperature. Dantrolene, 1 to 2.5 mg/kg, should be given intravenously every 6 hours. Dopaminergic agents include amantadine, 100 to 200 mg twice daily; bromocriptine, 2.5 to 10 mg three times daily; and levodopa, 100 mg three times daily. Other less effective treatments have included diphenhydramine, benztropine, and diazepam. Symptoms of NMS may last for weeks in patients receiving long-acting antidopaminergic agents such as fluphenazine.

SEROTONIN SYNDROME AND OTHER DRUG-INDUCED HYPERTHERMIAS

Hyperthermia may occur with other therapeutic drugs as well as some illicit drugs. In some cases, the hyperthermia seems to be related to increased muscle tone, tremor, or rigidity as with NMS. In other cases, increased levels of serotonin in the brain—a "serotonin syndrome"—produce hyperthermia. Manifestations of the serotonin syndrome include hyperthermia, confusion, shivering, diaphoresis, ataxia, hyperreflexia, myoclonus, and diarrhea.[38]

The serotonin syndrome occurs most commonly with psychiatric drug combinations that greatly enhance brain serotonin activity, especially at 5-HT_2 receptors. Combinations associated with the syndrome include monoamine oxidase inhibitors (MAOIs) and selective serotonin reuptake inhibitors, MAOIs and tricyclic antidepressants, MAOIs and tryptophan, and MAOIs and meperidine.[38]

Hyperthermia can also be caused by illicit drugs such as 3,4-methylenedioxymethamphetamine (MDMA or "ecstasy"). MDMA has been associated with a serotonin syndrome that has resulted in severe toxicity and deaths; hyperthermia was thought to play a major role.[38-40] Intravenous and nasal insufflation of "crack" cocaine has resulted in several deaths associated with hyperthermia, rhabdomyolysis, and renal failure.[41] The cause in these cases appears to have been multifactorial, including a direct toxic effect on muscle and adrenergic hyperstimulation.[41] Other drugs that can cause hyperthermia include amphetamine, phencyclidine (PCP), and lysergic acid diethylamide (LSD).

Most cases of the serotonin syndrome that are associated with psychiatric drugs are mild and can be managed with drug withdrawal and supportive care. If marked hyperthermia develops, the patient should be treated aggressively with external cooling and muscle paralysis similar to therapy for NMS. Some authors have also advocated methysergide and cyproheptadine for adjuvant therapy.

THYROID STORM

Thyrotoxicosis can present as hyperthermia in patients with poorly controlled or undiagnosed Graves' disease. This diagnosis is suggested by fever and tachycardia together with an enlarged thyroid gland, sweating, and anxious appearance. Thyroid storm or crisis is a medical emergency that carries a high (10%–50%) mortality rate. Factors that can precipitate acute thyrotoxicosis include induction of anesthesia, surgery, labor and delivery, severe infections, and rarely thyroiditis after radioactive iodine administration.

Early manifestations of thyrotoxicosis include heat intolerance, profuse sweating, nausea and vomiting, and diarrhea. With increasing severity, altered mental status (irritability, delirium, or coma), hyperthermia above 40°C, tachyarrhythmias, and hypotension supervene. Atrial fibrillation is especially common. Congestive heart failure may occur in up to 25% of patients. Hypokalemia is common and may be present in up to 50% of patients. Although thyroid hormone levels are high in plasma, they correlate poorly with the severity of the crisis. A sudden exacerbation of thyrotoxicosis probably represents either a rapid shift of thyroid hormone from the protein-bound to the free state or an increased responsiveness to the hormones at the cellular level.

The treatment of acute thyrotoxicosis is directed toward reversing the crisis as well as preventing its complications. Large doses of glucocorticoids (dexamethasone intravenously, 10 mg followed by 2 mg every 6 hours) inhibit the synthesis, release, and peripheral conversion of thyroxine (T_4) to triiodothyronine (T_3). Glucocorticoids may also prevent relative adrenal insufficiency secondary to the hypermetabolic state. Inhibition of thyroid hormone synthesis can be accomplished with propylthiouracil, 200 to 400 mg, followed by 100 mg every 2 hours through a nasogastric tube; an intravenous preparation is not available. Propylthiouracil is preferred over methimazole because the former also inhibits peripheral conversion of T_4. Iodide should be given to inhibit the release of thyroid hormones from the thyroid gland; intravenous sodium iodide, 1 g in 24 hours, or enteral potassium iodide, 100 to 200 mg every 8 hours, may be administered. Some clinicians prefer the x-ray contrast agent sodium ipodate, 1 g/d. Intravenous propranolol antagonizes the peripheral effects of the thyrotoxicosis and inhibits peripheral conversion of T_4. In addition, combined β_1- and β_2-blockade is preferable to selective β_1-antagonism (esmolol or metoprolol) because excessive β_2-receptor activity is responsible for the metabolic effects of thyroid hormone. β_2-Receptor blockade may also reduce muscle blood flow and reduce heat production. β-Adrenergic blockade is contraindicated in patients with low cardiac output.

Supportive measures include surface cooling with a blanket, acetaminophen (aspirin can displace thyroid hormone from plasma carrier proteins), and generous intravenous fluid replacement. Vasopressors are often necessary to support arterial blood pressure. Digoxin may be indicated in patients with atrial fibrillation to control the ventricular rate and for those with congestive heart failure. A pulmonary artery catheter greatly facilitates management in patients with signs of congestive heart failure or those with refractory arterial hypotension.

PHEOCHROMOCYTOMA

Rarely, patients with a pheochromocytoma crisis may present with significant hyperthermia (>38°C). The increase in temperature is generally thought to be due to increased heat production from catecholamine-mediated increases in metabolic rate together with decreased heat elimination from intense vasoconstriction.[42] Symptoms suggestive of pheochromocytoma are the paroxysmal nature of the tachycardia and hypertension and the severity of the hypertension. Cardiac manifestations such as arrhythmias, ischemia, or congestive heart failure may also be prominent.

Diagnosis requires measurement of urinary catecholamines or their metabolites in a 24-hour sample. Treatment is directed at antagonizing the catecholamine effects until the tumor can be removed. α-Adrenergic blockade (oral phenoxybenzamine or phentolamine infusion) should be achieved before β-adrenergic blockade (propranolol) to prevent exacerbation of hypertension. Nitroprusside and calcium channel blockers are useful in acutely controlling severe hypertension. Nitroglycerin should also be used in the presence of myocardial ischemia.

IATROGENIC HYPERTHERMIA

Iatrogenic hyperthermia is not uncommon, especially in pediatric patients. Common sources of heat in the ICU and in the operating room include humidifiers on ventilators, warming blankets, and heat lamps as well as ambient temperature. Drug therapy (see Table 16-3), especially anticholinergic agents, can also be contributory by impairing heat elimination.

HYPERTHERMIA DUE TO BRAIN STEM OR HYPOTHALAMIC INJURY

Infections, strokes, trauma, or surgery near the hypothalamus and brain stem can be associated with marked hyperthermia. Kitanaka and associates[43] reported two cases of brain stem hemorrhage associated with severe hyperthermia above 41°C, rhabdomyolysis, and renal failure. Lesser degrees of hyperthermia may be seen with CNS lesions in other areas. Reith and colleagues[44] studied body temperature after stroke and found temperature to be independently related to stroke severity, infarct size, mortality, and outcome in survivors.

Diagnosis of hyperthermia due to CNS injury requires exclusion of other causes. Although treatment should be directed at the CNS injury, prompt lowering of core temperature or even induction of mild hypothermia may preserve neurologic function and improve outcome.[44]

References

1. Clowes GHA, O'Donnel TF: Heat stroke. N Engl J Med 1974; 291:564.
2. Tek D, Olshaker JS: Heat illness. Emerg Med Clin North Am 1991; 10:299.
3. Kilbourne EM, Choi K, Jones S, Thaker SB: Risk factors for heat stroke: A case control study. JAMA 1982; 247:3332.
4. Sprung CL: Hemodynamic alterations of heat stroke in the elderly. Chest 1979; 75:361.
5. Baba N, Ruppert RD: Alteration of eccrine sweat gland in fatal heat stroke. Arch Pathol 1968; 85:669.
6. Hanson PG, Zimmerman SW: Exertional heat stroke in novice runners. JAMA 1979; 242:154.
7. El Kassimi FA, Al-Mashadani SA, Akhtar J: Adult respiratory distress syndrome and disseminated intravascular coagulation complicating heat stroke. Chest 1986; 90:571.
8. Gonzales-Alonso J, Mora Rodrigues R, Below PR, et al: Dehydration reduces cardiac output and increases systemic and cutaneous vascular resistance during exercise. J Appl Physiol 1995; 79:1487.
9. Armstrong LE, Crago AE, Adams R, et al: Whole-body cooling of hyperthermic runners: Comparison of two field therapies. Am J Emerg Med 1996; 14:355.
10. Denborough MA, Lovell RRH: Anaesthetic deaths in a family. Lancet 1960; 2:45.
11. Gronert GA: Malignant hyperthermia. Anesthesiology 1980; 53:395.
12. Topel DG, Bicknell EJ, Preston KS, et al: Porcine stress syndrome. Mod Vet Pract 1968; 49:40.
13. Rosenberg H, Reed S: In vitro contracture tests for susceptibility to malignant hyperthermia. Anesth Analg 1983; 62:415.
14. Gronett GA, Thompson RL, Onofrio BM: Human malignant hyperthermia: Awake episodes and correction by dantrolene. Anesth Analg 1980; 59:377.
15. Tegazzin V, Scutari E, Treves S, et al: Chlorocresol, an additive to commercial succinylcholine, induces contracture of human malignant hyperthermia-susceptible muscles via activation of the ryanodine receptor Ca^{2+} channel. Anesthesiology 1996; 84:1380.
16. Fletcher JE, Tripolitis L, Hubert M, et al: Genotype and phenotype relationships for mutations in the ryanodine receptor in patients referred for diagnosis of malignant hyperthermia. Br J Anaesth 1995; 75:301.
17. Wallace AJ, Wooldridge W, Kingston HM, et al: Malignant hyperthermia—a large kindred linked to the RYRI gene. Anaesthesia 1996; 51:16.
18. Serfas KD, Bose D, Patel L, et al: Comparison of the segregation of the RYR1 C1840T mutation with segregation of the caffeine/halothane contracture test results for malignant hyperthermia susceptibility in a large Manitoba Mennonite family. Anesthesiology 1996; 84:322.
19. Moroni I, Gonano EF, Comi GP, et al: Ryanodine receptor gene point mutation and malignant hyperthermia susceptibility. J Neurol 1995; 242:127.
20. McPherson EW, Taylor CA Jr: The King syndrome: Malignant hyperthermia myopathy, and multiple anomalies. Am J Med Genet 1981; 8:159.
21. Miller ED, Sanders DB, Rowlingson JC, et al: Anesthesia-induced rhabdomyolysis in a patient with Duchenne's muscular dystrophy. Anesthesiology 1978; 48:146.
22. Frank JP, Harati Y, Butler IJ, et al: Central core disease and malignant hyperthermia syndrome. Ann Neurol 1980; 7:11.
23. Rampton AJ, Kelly DA, Shanahan EC, et al: Occurrence of malignant hyperpyrexia in a patient with osteogenesis imperfecta. Br J Anaesth 1984; 56:1443.
24. MacLennan DH, Phillips MS: Malignant hyperthermia. Science 1992; 256:789.
25. Larach MG, Localio AR, Allen GC, et al: A clinical grading scale to predict malignant hyperthermia susceptibility. Anesthesiology 1994; 80:771.
26. Hackl W, Mauritz W, Schemper M, et al: Prediction of malignant hyperthermia susceptibility: Statistical evaluation of clinical signs. Br J Anaesth 1990; 64:425.
27. O'Flynn RP, Shutack JG, Rosenberg H, et al: Masseter muscle rigidity and malignant hyperthermia susceptibility in pediatric patients: An update on management and diagnosis. Anesthesiology 1994; 80:1228.
28. Bichel T, Canivet JL, Damas P, et al: Malignant hyperthermia and severe hypoglycemia after reexposure to halothane. Acta Anaesthesiol Belg 1994; 45:23.
29. Ellis FR, Halsall PJ, Christian AS: Clinical presentation of suspected malignant hyperthermia during anesthesia in 402 probands. Anaesthesia 1990; 45:838.
30. Kolb ME, Horne ML, Martz R: Dantrolene in human malignant hyperthermia: A multicenter study. Anesthesiology 1982; 56:254.
31. Nelson TE, Lin M, Zapata Sudo G, et al: Dantrolene sodium can increase or attenuate activity of skeletal muscle ryanodine receptor calcium release channel: Clinical implications. Anesthesiology 1996; 84:1368.
32. Mathieu A, Bogosian AJ, Ryan JF, et al: Recrudescence after survival of an initial episode of malignant hyperthermia. Anesthesiology 1979; 51:454.
33. Isaacs H, Badenhorst M: False-negative results with muscle caffeine-halothane contracture testing for malignant hyperthermia. Anesthesiology 1993; 79:5.
34. Caroff SN: The neuroleptic malignant syndrome. J Clin Psychiatry 1980; 41:79.
35. Caroff SN, Mann SC, Lazarus A, et al: Neuroleptic malignant syndrome: Diagnostic issues. Psych Ann 1991; 21:130.
36. Kornhuber J, Weller M: Neuroleptic malignant syndrome. Curr Opin Neurol 1994; 7:353.
37. Addonizio G, Susman VL, Roth SD: Neuroleptic malignant syndrome: Review and analysis of 115 cases. Biol Psychiatry 1987; 22:1004.
38. Sporer KA: The serotonin syndrome: Implicated drugs, pathophysiology and management. Drug Saf 1995; 13:94.
39. Ellis AJ, Wendon JA, Portmann B, et al: Acute liver damage and ecstasy ingestion. Gut 1996; 38:454.
40. Green AR, Cross AJ, Goodwin GM: Review of the pharmacology and clinical pharmacology of 3,4-methylenedioxymethamphetamine (MDMA or "ecstasy"). Psychopharmacology 1995; 119:247.
41. Daras M, Kakkouras L, Tuchman AJ, et al: Rhabdomyolysis and hyperthermia after cocaine abuse: A variant of the neuroleptic malignant syndrome? Acta Neurol Scand 1995; 92:161.
42. Allen GC, Rosenberg H: Phaeochromocytoma presenting as acute malignant hyperthermia—a diagnostic challenge. Can J Anaesth 1990; 37:593.
43. Kitanaka C, Inoh Y, Tyooda T, et al: Malignant brain stem hyperthermia caused by brain stem hemorrhage. Stroke 1994; 25:518.
44. Reith J, Jorgensen HS, Pedersen PM, et al: Body temperature in acute stroke: Relation to stroke severity, infarct size, mortality, and outcome. Lancet 1996; 347:422.

17

Injuries by Venomous and Poisonous Animals

Richard W. Carlson, MD, PhD, FCCM
Mauricio Pineda-Roman, MD • Radha Ramamrutham, MD

Numerous and varied species of poisonous and venomous animals throughout the world cause thousands of injuries each year. The severity of these poisonings ranges from minor irritation to fulminant multiple organ system failure and death. Venomous organisms have been worshipped, feared, and viewed with awe throughout history, and many misconceptions about these animals and their toxins have been perpetuated. In addition, most medical personnel have only fragmentary knowledge of venomous animals and the poisonings they cause. Many venom injuries are referred to intensive care units (ICUs) for monitoring and definitive care. It is therefore crucial for the critical care practitioner to have a fundamental understanding of venomous organisms and their toxins, priorities of management, and methods to assess and treat such poisonings. Fortunately, the vast majority of these injuries do not result in death. However, *all* envenomations should be regarded as potentially lethal. The ICU practitioner should also be able to summon expert help to identify the offending organism, secure appropriate consultation for management of specific aspects of the intoxication, and utilize unique medications, such as antivenin (antivenom).

This chapter describes clinically important venomous animals and general principles of management of envenomations. Because of the number and variety of exotic animals maintained in zoos or private collections, selected dangerous species from around the world are discussed. Additional forms native to North America are emphasized.

For more detailed information on specific envenomations, the reader is referred to texts and monographs on dangerous marine and terrestrial animals. Poison control centers can also provide assistance in the identification and management of venom injuries and may direct the clinician to consultants with special expertise. Local zoos, aquaria, universities, and colleges may also give valuable assistance. A nearby zoo may be the only local source of antivenin for management of a bite or sting by an exotic species.

PRINCIPLES OF MANAGEMENT

Priorities of management of envenomations are: (1) identification of the offending species, (2) first aid measures, (3) assessment of the severity of the injury, and (4) transport to a facility for definitive care, where (5) ongoing monitoring and (6) measures to treat local and systemic toxicity can be implemented (Fig. 17-1).

A guiding theme in treating venom injuries, as in other fields of medicine, is *do no harm*. In most instances, the patient will survive the intoxication. If significant toxicity does not develop, management should be conservative. A risk-benefit evaluation should be used for any potentially dangerous therapy, such as antivenin.

VENOMS VERSUS POISONS

The word *poison* describes a toxic substance; however, not all poisons are venoms (Table 17-1). Poisons typically cause injury when ingested, although some poisons may be administered in other ways. A *venom* is an animal poison that may or may not be toxic when ingested but causes local or systemic toxicity or both when administered parenterally.

A *venomous animal* produces a venom in a specialized group of cells or a gland and possesses a venom apparatus, such as a stinger, fang, spine, barb, or jaw, through which to deliver the toxin into the victim. *Poisonous animals* are forms that are toxic when ingested. Some animals are both venomous and poisonous.

Poisons usually consist of a single or few toxic components, whereas *venoms* are invariably mixtures of multiple substances. For example, a rattlesnake venom may contain more than 20 individual fractions, including proteins, enzymes, peptides, amines, metals, lipids, and other substances. Many of the *toxins* in a venom may affect several organ systems, so that a specific neurotropic fraction of a snake venom may also exert adverse effects on the myocardium, vascular endothelium, coagulation system, or other cells or organ systems. Poisons, in contrast, are likely to have more restricted pharmacologic properties.

Venoms from closely related forms often share certain features; however, toxins from unrelated organisms may occasionally have similar properties or chemical structures.

Finally, toxins used by an animal to capture or ingest its prey typically have different properties from those used defensively. Venoms may contain or activate mediators and inflammatory cascades within the victim, often leading to escalating autopharmacologic reactions. Mediators and systems that have been linked to venoms include bradykinin, bradykinin-potentiating peptides, slow-reacting substance of anaphylaxis (leukotrienes), angiotensin-converting enzyme (ACE) inhibitors, various cytokines, and thrombin-like enzymes. Some of these were first identified or described in association with venoms.

TABLE 17–1. Contrasts Between Poisonings and Envenomations

Poisoning	Envenomation
Single or few toxins Intoxication usually enteral Few primary target organs Primary pharmacologic effects of toxins	Multiple toxic components Parenteral administration via fang, barb, stinger (venom apparatus) Prominent secondary and tertiary responses (autopharmacologic reactions) plus reactions to therapy (antivenin)

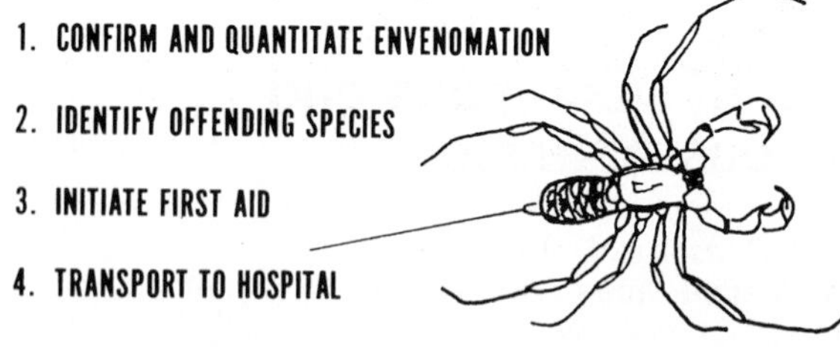

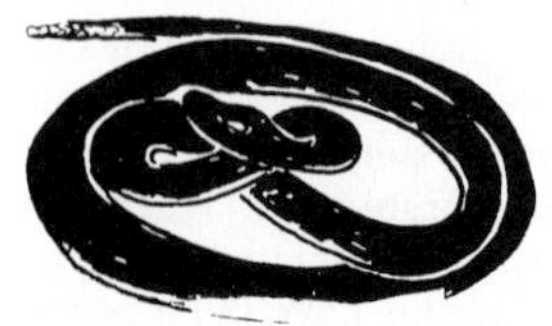
5. GENERAL &/OR SPECIFIC THERAPY:
A. REMOVE VENOM FROM WOUND
B. RETARD ABSORPTION OF VENOM
C. NEUTRALIZE VENOM (ANTIVENIN)
D. COMBAT EFFECTS OF VENOM
E. TREAT LATE OR SECONDARY EFFECTS

Figure 17–1. Principles of management of suspected venom injuries. (From Carlson RW: Injuries by venomous and poisonous animals. *In*: Principles and Practice of Medical Intensive Care. Carlson RW, Geheb MA [Eds]. Philadelphia, WB Saunders, 1993, p 1661.)

PHYLUM CHORDATA, CLASS REPTILIA, ORDER SQUAMATA, SUBORDER SERPENTES (SNAKES)

There are approximately 3000 species of snakes, of which 10% are venomous.[1-5] The venomous snakes are found in five families: Hydrophidae (sea snakes), Viperidae (vipers), Elapidae (elapids), Crotalidae (pit vipers), and Colubridae (rear-fanged snakes) (Table 17-2). Some taxonomists include the crotalids as a subfamily of the vipers.

As many as 500,000 snakebites occur each year throughout the world, with 30,000 or more fatalities, although Russell[1] suggests a somewhat smaller number. In many countries, the incidence, morbidity, and mortality of these injuries are inaccurately reported. In the United States, it is estimated that 45,000 snakebites occur each year, of which approximately one fifth are by venomous forms.[6] Only a few people (<10)

TABLE 17–2. Classification of Selected Venomous Snakes

Family	Genus/Species	Common Name
Hydrophiidae	*Laticauda, Hydrophis*	Sea snakes
Viperidae		Vipers
	Echis carinatus	Saw-scaled viper
	Echis coloratus	Carpet viper
	Vipera russelli	Russell's viper
	Bitis gabonica	Gaboon viper
	Bitis arietans	Puff adder
Elapidae		Elapids
	Ophiophagus hannah	King cobra
	Naja	Cobras
	Bungarus	Kraits
	Dendroaspis	Mambas
	Notechis scutatus scutatus	Tiger snake
	Acanthophis antarcticus	Death adder
	Oxyuranus scutellatus	Taipan
	Demansia	Brown snake
	Denisonia	Copperhead (Australia)
	Micruroides euryxanthus	Western coral snake (United States)
	Micrurus fulvius fulvius	Eastern coral snake (United States)
	Micrurus fulvius tenere	Texas coral snake
Crotalidae		Pit viper
	Crotalus	Rattlesnake
	Sistrurus	Pigmy rattlesnake, massasauga
	Agkistrodon	Cottonmouth, copperhead (United States)
	Asiatic pit vipers	
	Bothrops	Lance-headed viper
	Trimeresurus	Asiatic lance-headed viper, Habu
	Lachesis	Bushmaster
Colubridae		Rear-fanged snake (and most nonvenomous snakes)
	Dispholidus typus	Boomslang

die each year in the United States as a result of snakebite.[7] In Australia, venomous snakes outnumber nonvenomous forms, and Australia is the home of several of the most toxic snakes in the world. Approximately 3000 bites occur in the Australian subcontinent each year, and more than 200 of the victims receive antivenin. The mortality rate is less than four deaths per year because of the widespread availability of antivenin and a relatively consistent approach to the management of these injuries.[8-10]

Several factors complicate the initial evaluation of snakebites (Table 17-3). First, for at least 20% of pit viper bites and a greater percentage of elapid and sea snake injuries, there is no injection of venom.[7] The management of these "dry bites" should be conservative observation. The condition and age of the victim and the location of the wound affect the manifestations of the injury. The proportion of subcutaneous, intramuscular, or intravenous administration of toxins also influences toxicity and the balance of systemic and local deleterious effects. Finally, activity of the victim plays a role in toxicity. More physical activity favors systemic absorption of venom and greater toxicity. Although most victims do not die from snakebite, these injuries may lead to death from a variety of organ and multiorgan dysfunctions that are direct effects of the venom, from secondary or autopharmacologic responses within the victim, and from complications of therapy (Table 17-4).

Misconceptions about snake venoms have been perpetuated in medical as well as lay literature. For example, it is commonly believed that bites by cobras and other elapids are almost exclusively associated with neurologic changes. Similarly, it is widely held that bites by vipers and pit vipers invariably lead to severe local injury and that these changes

TABLE 17–3. Factors Affecting Severity of Snakebites

1. At least 20% of bites are without envenomation ("dry bites").
2. Medical status and age of patients affect the seriousness of the envenomation.
3. Size and condition of snake alter dose and quality of venom injected.
4. Localization of wound and proportion of venom given IV, SC, or IM alter the balance of local and systemic injury as well as rapidity of signs and symptoms.
5. Physical activity of patient increases absorption of toxins.
6. First aid measures may affect absorption of toxins.
7. Systemic toxicity may be life-threatening despite minimal local tissue injury.

TABLE 17–4. Potentially Lethal Conditions Associated with Snakebite and Its Treatment

Circulatory shock, cardiac dysfunction
Hemorrhage, hypovolemia
Coagulopathy, disseminated intravascular coagulation (DIC) (fibrinogenolysis, thrombocytopenia, alterations of coagulation profile, and other features similar to DIC)
Hemolysis, thrombolysis, thromboembolism
Coma, seizures, intracranial hemorrhage
Cranial nerve dysfunction
Rhabdomyolysis, renal failure, hyperkalemia
Sepsis-bactemia, secondary infection
Gastrointestinal bleeding
Respiratory failure, pulmonary edema
Anaphylaxis (to components of venom or antivenin)

TABLE 17–5. Some Components of Snake Venom

Proteins
Enzymes
Thrombin-like enzymes
Phospholipases A_2, B, and C
Collagenase
L-Amino-acid oxidase
Phosphodiesterase
Acetylcholinesterase
Proteolytic enzymes, including metalloproteinases
Prothrombin activators
Myotoxin-a
Factor V, IX, and X activators
Ribonuclease 1
5′-Nucleosidase
Peptides
Electrolytes
Carbohydrates
Lipids
Amino acids
Metals

can reliably be used to gauge the severity of the poisoning. Although these concepts have some validity when the venoms are discussed in general terms, such conclusions may lead to dangerous errors in diagnosis and management. It was also believed that the predominant cause of toxicity of snake venoms was related to their enzymatic components. It is now known that several of the lower-molecular-weight proteins and peptides, many of which have no enzymatic activity, are among the most toxic fractions.[11-13]

Quantity and Composition of Snake Venoms

Snake venoms contain toxic and nontoxic substances that are produced by glandular structures homologous to salivary glands.[14, 15] Multiple components are present in these venoms (Table 17–5). The quantity of venom yielded by a snake is usually expressed in dry weight. Toxicity is often quantitated by lethality, as milligrams of venom per kilogram of body weight that causes death of 50% of test animals given venom. This expression is the median lethal dose (LD_{50}), and the value ranges from a few micrograms to more than 10 mg/kg. The most lethal venoms (lowest LD_{50}) are found among the elapids and sea snakes, although some viper and pit viper venoms, such as those of the Mojave rattlesnake (*Crotalus scutulatus scutulatus*), are also highly toxic.

Venoms have numerous components. Many venoms contain various metalloproteinases, now believed to contribute to tissue injury at the site of the bite as well as systemic bleeding. The metalloproteinases are thought to participate in the proteolytic destruction of the extracellular matrix and basement membranes of small blood vessels and capillaries, producing myonecrosis as well as affecting coagulation. Many of the proteinases that have been studied have been from the venom of the western diamondback rattlesnake (*Crotalus atrox*); hence, they are often referred to as *atrolysins*. These proteinases cause release of tumor necrosis factor (TNF-α) from pro-tumor necrosis factor (pro-TNF-α).[16, 17]

Crotalidae (Pit Vipers)

Most snakebites in North America are due to pit vipers. These include the various rattlesnakes (genus *Crotalus*), pygmy rattlesnakes and massasauga (genus *Sistrurus*), and the cottonmouths and copperheads (genus *Agkistrodon*). Several thousand people are treated for snake venom poisoning in the United States each year.[18-22] Russell[18] estimated that an additional 1000 snakebites are not reported. Fewer than 10 deaths result annually from all of these injuries. There are several pit vipers in Asia, including the Malayan pit viper (*Agkistrodon rhodostoma*) and the sharp-nosed pit viper (*Agkistrodon acutus*).

Identification and Characteristics

Pit vipers and vipers are similar in many respects, but pit vipers have a loreal pit behind each nostril. These structures are thermosensitive organs used to localize prey and enemies. Pit vipers and most vipers have vertically elliptic pupils, whereas elapids and most nonvenomous snakes have round pupils. Crotalids and vipers have a well-developed venom apparatus consisting of long, erectile fangs and the ability to deliver a considerable dose of venom during a strike (Fig. 17–2).

There are more than 30 species of rattlesnakes, which are distributed throughout North and South America. The eastern and western diamondback rattlesnakes (*Crotalus adamanteus*

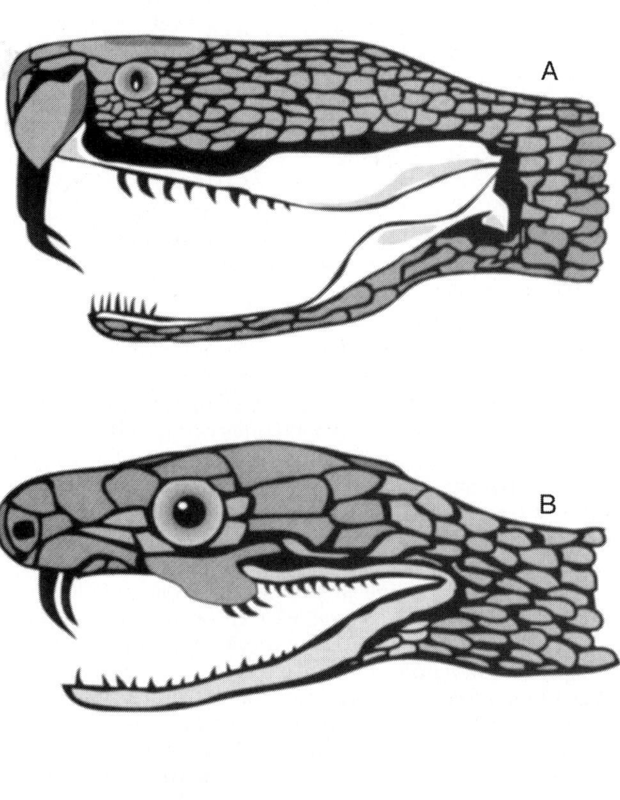

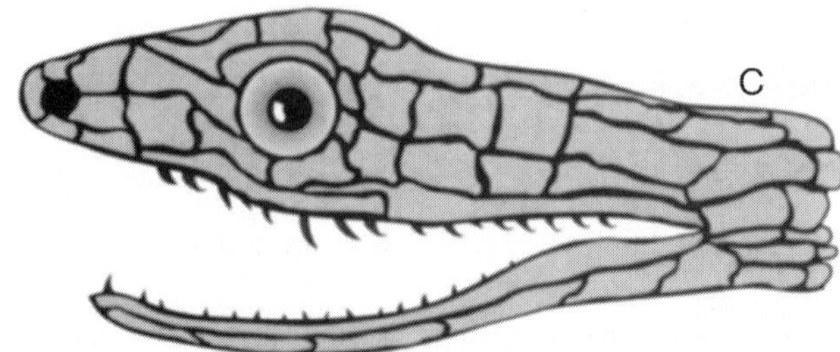

Figure 17–2. Anatomy of the mouth and fangs in pit vipers and vipers *(A)*, elapids and sea snakes *(B)*, and rear-fanged snakes *(C)*. (From Carlson RW: Injuries by venomous and poisonous animals. *In*: Principles and Practice of Medical Intensive Care. Carlson RW, Geheb MA [Eds]. Philadelphia, WB Saunders, 1993, p 1666.)

and C. atrox, respectively) are among the largest venomous snakes in the United States and account for most fatal snakebites in this country. Rattlesnakes have a triangular head and a group of horny rings at the tail that produce the rattle or buzzing noise when the snake is aroused. Like vipers, rattlesnakes are typically heavy-bodied snakes.

Clinical Features and Estimating the Severity of Crotalid and Viperid Snakebite

Bites by vipers and pit vipers produce tissue damage as well as hemostatic, cardiopulmonary, metabolic, and neuromuscular alterations. Local symptoms are typically prominent but may vary widely according to the following:

- The individual victim
- Species of the snake
- Dose of venom administered
- Proportion of subcutaneous, intramuscular, or intravenous administration of the venom

More than 20% of snakebites in humans are without envenomation, but among victims who are ultimately referred to a tertiary care center, this percentage is much lower.[7] Most injuries occur in males, usually involve a hand or a foot, and are most common in spring and summer. Many bites occur because of attempts to capture or handle a snake.

A simplified system to evaluate severity of these bites is depicted in Table 17–6. A more comprehensive method to gauge severity utilizes a score that evaluates toxicity involving six body systems: pulmonary, cardiovascular, local wound, gastrointestinal, hematologic, and central nervous. This score has been validated prospectively in 108 patients with crotalid envenomations (Table 17–7).[23] Management of such bites remains controversial. Considerations for evaluation and management are shown in Table 17–8.

The examiner should search for fang marks. Any findings involving the injured part should be described along with the time of the examination. For extremity injuries, measurements of the circumference of the extremity proximal to the bite should be made, recorded on a flow sheet, and repeated every

TABLE 17–6. Simplified Evaluation System to Grade Severity of Crotalid/Viperid Snakebites

No envenomation
Bites by venomous (or unknown) species
No local or systemic findings after several hours of observation

Minimal envenomation
Documented bite
Some local findings (edema, ecchymoses, etc.) but without progression
No systemic signs or symptoms
Victim otherwise healthy

Moderate envenomation
Documented bite
Progressive local and regional findings and/or systemic toxicity that is not life-threatening
Moderate disturbances of laboratory assays
High-risk victim (child, elderly, underlying cardiopulmonary disease, allergies)

Severe envenomation
Documented bite
Large or dangerous species or high-risk victim
Marked local and regional findings and/or serious cardiopulmonary, neurologic, metabolic, and/or hematologic derangements
Critical laboratory abnormalities
Severe reaction to antivenin

2 to 4 hours to quantitate the development of local and regional changes. This procedure is helpful for the first 12 to 24 hours to reassess local tissue injury and as a partial guide to antivenin administration.

Other features of snakebite are pain, edema, erythema, ecchymoses, and, occasionally, petechiae and blebs. Many factors, including the age and health of the patient, should be taken into account in the evaluation of these injuries and the planning of therapy.

Pain is a variable symptom after crotalid envenomation. Some patients report numbness. Pain may also be related to the development of local hemorrhage. Regional pain may involve the axilla or inguinal sites.

The venom of the Mojave rattlesnake *(C. scutulatus scutulatus)* is among the most toxic of any snake in North America.[24–26] Therefore, bites by this snake are particularly dangerous in the Southwest.[27] Injuries by the Mojave rattlesnake have been described in which local symptoms were minimal despite serious systemic neurologic toxicity. However, severe neurologic dysfunction occurs relatively infrequently.[28–30] The tropical rattlesnake, *Crotalus durissus*, also possesses an extremely potent venom, and its bites are very dangerous.

Local Changes and Infection

For other pit viper bites, local edema and hemorrhage are characteristic findings and may progress rapidly (Fig. 17–3). Edema may be accompanied by the development of blebs, which may be hemorrhagic. They usually develop within the first day. If venom is injected into a vascular structure, local findings may be minimal or absent, although serious and potentially life-threatening findings may develop quickly.[31] Paresthesias and pain may be accompanied by fasciculations. Analogous findings of muscular irritability may be manifested as cardiac arrhythmias. Some patients may complain of a rubbery or metallic taste in the mouth, which has been described after bites by the Southern Pacific rattlesnake, *Crotalus viridis helleri*, as well as the eastern diamondback (*C. adamanteus*).[5, 19]

Despite considerable local hemorrhage and edema, significant tissue necrosis is uncommon. The wound should be cleansed and maintained in a position of function. Elevation may hasten resolution of edema, although some authorities recommend keeping the injured site below heart level for the first few hours to reduce systemic absorption of venom.

Most authors conclude that fasciotomy is indicated in a very small proportion of bites. Incision and suction or excision of the wound are no longer recommended by most authorities. The indications for fasciotomy and other surgical procedures in crotalid bites have been the subject of considerable debate.[5, 32–40] When the ICU physician believes that perfusion of local structures is compromised, measurement of tissue pressure should be considered.[41–43] If the ICU physician is not a surgeon, a surgeon should be consulted to evaluate for a compartment syndrome and the need for debridement or other surgical procedures. The adequacy of vascular supply in a tense, edematous extremity is best assessed with objective measures, because in one study in which several patients exhibited marked local changes, blood flow to the region as determined by noninvasive techniques was actually normal to increased.[44] A needle, catheter, or the wick technique to measure tissue pressure is recommended when a compartment syndrome is suspected.[45]

Although multiple microorganisms are found in the mouths of snakes, the development of secondary infections is highly variable among snakebite victims. Some authorities recommend antibiotics for moderate to severe bites, but routine

TABLE 17–7. The Snakebite Severity Score (SSS) to Evaluate Crotalid Envenomation

Criterion	Points*
Pulmonary System	
No symptoms/signs	0
Dyspnea, minimal chest tightness, mild or vague discomfort, or respirations of 20 to 25 breaths/minute	1
Moderate respiratory distress (tachypnea, 26 to 40 breaths/minute; accessory muscle use)	2
Cyanosis, air hunger, extreme tachypnea, or respiratory insufficiency/failure	3
Cardiovascular System	
No symptoms/signs	0
Tachycardia (100 to 125 beats/minute), palpitations, generalized weakness, benign dysrhythmia, or hypertension	1
Tachycardia (126 to 175 beats/minute) or hypotension, with systolic blood pressure greater than 100 mm Hg	2
Extreme tachycardia (>175 beats/minute), hypotension with systolic blood pressure <100 mm Hg, malignant dysrhythmia, or cardiac arrest	3
Local Wound	
No symptoms/signs	0
Pain, swelling, or ecchymosis within 5 to 7.5 cm of bite site	1
Pain, swelling, or ecchymosis involving less than half the extremity (7.5 to 50 cm from bite site)	2
Pain, swelling, or ecchymosis involving half to all of extremity (50 to 100 cm from bite site)	3
Pain, swelling, or ecchymosis extending beyond affected extremity (more than 100 cm from bite site)	4
Gastrointestinal System	
No symptoms/signs	0
Pain, tenesmus, or nausea	1
Vomiting or diarrhea	2
Repeated vomiting, diarrhea, hematemesis, or hematochezia	3
Hematologic Symptoms	
No symptoms/signs	0
Coagulation parameters slightly abnormal; PT, <20 seconds; PTT, <50 seconds; platelets, 100,000 to 150,000/mL; or fibrinogen, 100 to 150 μg/mL	1
Coagulation parameters abnormal; PT, <20 to 50 seconds; PTT, <50 to 75 seconds; platelets, 50,000 to 100,000/mL; or fibrinogen, 50 to 100 μg/mL	2
Coagulation parameters abnormal; PT, <50 to 100 seconds; PTT, <75 to 100 seconds; platelets, 20,000 to 50,000/mL; or fibrinogen, <50 μg/mL	3
Coagulation parameters markedly abnormal, with serious bleeding or the threat of spontaneous bleeding; unmeasurable PT or PTT; platelets, <20,000/mL; or undetectable fibrinogen; severe abnormalities of other laboratory values also fall into this category	4
Central Nervous System	
No symptoms/signs	0
Clinic apprehension, headache, weakness, dizziness, chills, or paresthesia	1
Moderate apprehension, headache, weakness, dizziness, chills, paresthesia, confusion, or fasciculation in area of bite site	2
Severe confusion, lethargy, seizures, coma, psychosis, or generalized fasciculation	3

From Dart RC, Hurlburt KM, Garcia R, et al: Validation of a severity score for the assessment of crotalid snake bite. Ann Emerg Med 1996; 27:323.
*Points are assessed on the basis of manifestations caused by the venom itself (antivenom reactions not included). Ranges given are for adults; appropriate compensation should be made for age.
PT = prothrombin time; PTT = partial thromboplastin time.

prophylactic antibiotics for all bites are not indicated.[46, 47] Tetanus prophylaxis should be provided.

Unproven or Potentially Dangerous Therapy

It is important that the critical care practitioner recognize signs and symptoms of a severe envenomation but avoid unnecessary and potentially dangerous therapy, especially if envenomation is mild or absent. Restraint should also be exercised in the use of new or provocative therapies. In particular, the management of the wound and surrounding tissue injury has undergone considerable reevaluation. Several therapies, such as cryotherapy, application of high-voltage direct current to the wound, tourniquets, corticosteroids, ethylenediaminetetraacetic acid (EDTA), excision of the wound, and early extensive debridement, have been dangerous or ineffective (Table 17–9). The most efficacious initial treatment is immobilization. The patient should be kept calm and, if possible, at rest.

Cardiovascular Manifestations

In a patient with a severe bite, shock may develop. Hypovolemia, with an increase in vascular permeability to red blood cells and plasma, is the critical defect.[29, 48–51] For patients with significant intravenous administration of venom, hemoconcentration, coagulation changes, and acidemia may develop rapidly, analogous to findings in experimental models of intravenous administration of venom. Alterations in vascular resistance may also occur and aggravate hypotension; however, fluid resuscitation should be the first priority in treatment of venom shock. Furthermore, shock is neither prevented nor altered by pharmacologic agents such as corticosteroids and antivenin.[52, 53] Prompt fluid loading, particularly with colloid fluids, is the most effective method for restoring vascular volume in experimental venom shock. If crystalloid fluids are given, at least six times the volume deficit must be administered for restoration of plasma volume.[54]

Coagulation Changes, Hemostasis, and Laboratory Analyses

Coagulation assays commonly demonstrate thrombocytopenia as well as prolongation of prothrombin and partial thromboplastin times together with evidence of fibrinolysis and fibrinogenolysis.[55] In fulminant venom injuries, decreases in red

TABLE 17–8. Considerations for Evaluation and Management of Suspected Venomous Snakebite*

History

1. Identification of bite; time, location of bite, and nature of injury
2. Initial symptoms and signs (including pain, swelling, paresthesias, fasciculations, ecchymoses, weakness-paralysis, disturbances of vision, swallowing, respiratory distress, shock)
3. First aid measures and other therapy before hospital admission
4. Identify snake if possible.
5. Age and condition of patient with attention to neurologic, cardiac, hemostatic disturbances, allergies (especially horse serum), medications (cardiac, anticoagulants, antihypertensives)
6. Symptoms on admission

Physical Examination

1. Initial vital signs and cardiopulmonary assessment
2. Description of wound with attention to edema, fang marks or lacerations, ecchymoses/bullae/petechiae, local pulses and perfusion, skin color/temperature, capillary refill; consider ultrasound examination if local/regional pulses cannot be felt; regional edema, adenopathy, ecchymoses, hemorrhage
3. Complete remainder of physical exam, with attention to cardiac, neurologic (including cranial nerve function), and respiratory status
4. Record examination of wound/region, including vascular and neurologic status, as well as circumference of extremity at site and 1–2 areas proximal to bite; repeat examinations at 2–4h intervals, and document to determine extension of local findings and further evaluation such as measurement of tissue pressure

Initial Laboratory Studies (for Moderate or Severe Poisoning)

1. Complete blood count, including RBC, WBC, platelet counts, RBC morphology, and hematocrit
2. Urinalysis, including blood and microscopic examination
3. Electrolytes, BUN, creatinine, ECG
4. Creatine kinase assays

Selected Additional Procedures and Monitoring

1. Baseline coagulation profile: prothrombin and partial thromboplastin (PT, PTT) assays
2. Fibrinogen titer, fibrin-fibrinogen degradation assays (protamine, D-dimer), specific coagulation
3. Factor assays as indicated
4. Vital signs, urine output
5. Skin test for antivenin: give antivenin IV with monitoring for anaphylaxis. *Failure to improve should prompt additional antivenin therapy.*
6. Venom detection test if available
7. Type and crossmatch for blood
8. Assays for hemolysis (haptoglobin, free serum hemoglobin), complement (C50, C3)
9. Arterial blood gas; vital capacity–flow rate measurements if for suspected respiratory muscle fatigue, examination for rales (edema), wheezes, or stridor (upper airway obstruction/anaphylaxis)
10. Surgical consultation for marked local changes/debridement; measure tissue pressure if compartment syndrome is suspected
11. Tetanus prophylaxis or therapy
12. Fluids and antivenin for hypotension: titrate fluids by hematocrit and hemodynamic variables
13. Central venous or arterial catheters if needed for cardiopulmonary instability (correct hemostatic defect first if possible)
14. CT of head for altered mental status, seizures, suspected intracranial hemorrhage
15. Photographs of injury; x-ray of region to detect embedded fangs and as baseline value

*Note: No single protocol is appropriate for all snake envenomations; additional sources and references or consultants may be needed, especially for bites by exotic species or for unusual or severe injuries.

BUN = blood urea nitrogen; CT = computed tomography; ECG = electrocardiogram; RBC = red blood cell; WBC = white blood cell.

blood cell mass may be obscured by a deficit of plasma volume. The hematocrit value may not be a reliable guide to the extent of bleeding in such cases. Thrombocytopenia may develop within hours after crotalid envenomation. In one study of experimental rattlesnake venom poisoning, the degree of thrombocytopenia was related to the dose of venom.[56] Fibrinogen levels may also decline, owing in part to the fibrinogenolysis associated with the thrombin-like serine esterase venom fractions as well as to other components of venom that affect intrinsic and extrinsic clotting pathways.[57, 58] In moderate to severe poisonings, baseline measurements of fibrinogen levels, prothrombin and partial thromboplastin times, platelet count, hematocrit, and fibrin products, such as D-dimer, should be obtained and red blood cells on the peripheral smear should be examined.[59] Correction of coagulation defects with fresh frozen plasma and platelets should be considered when one is restoring volume deficits. Heparin is *not* indicated to correct the disseminated intravascular coagulation (DIC)–like picture associated with the severe hemostatic defects of crotalid envenomation.[60–62]

In general, failure of therapy to improve hemostatic disturbances should prompt consideration for additional antivenin therapy.

If arterial or central venous access is needed for monitoring or therapy, disturbances of hemostasis should be addressed, if possible, before vascular catheterization. In severe envenomations, blood gas analysis, measurements of electrolytes and creatine phosphokinase (CPK), and tests of renal function are indicated. In selected patients, radiographs of the injured part may be useful as a baseline for analysis of possible joint or bone involvement or abscesses and for the detection of embedded fangs.

Neurotropic Changes

Fasciculations, paresthesias, pain, weakness, and decreases in sensation are common after crotalid bites. These changes are probably due to local effects of venom on neuromuscular structures as well as compression of these structures. Central nervous system derangements are uncommon and usually reversible. The venom of the Mojave rattlesnake (*C. scutulatus scutulatus*) contains a fraction that affects presynaptic calcium channels, leading to a decrease in the release of acetylcholine

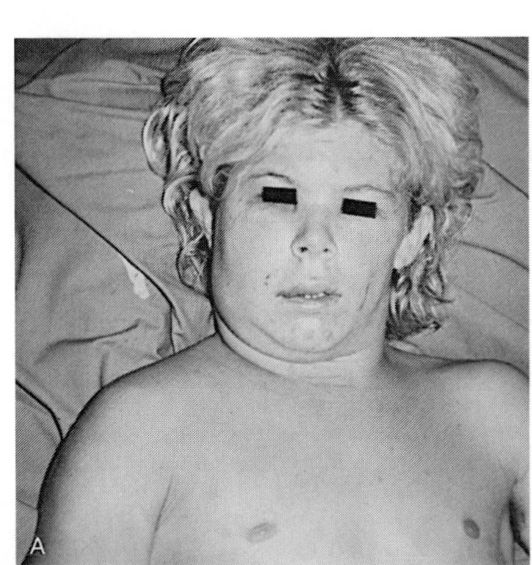

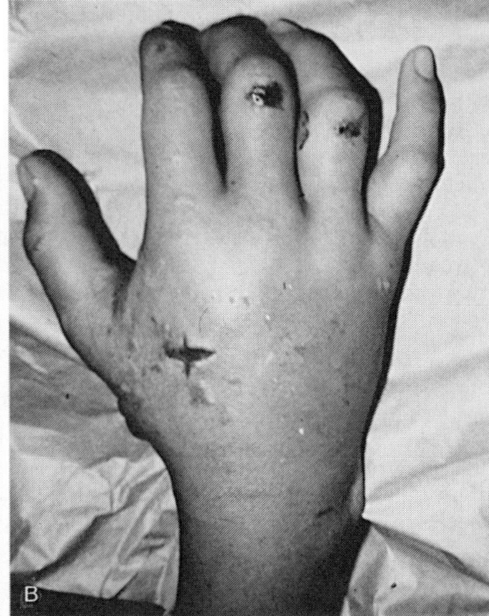

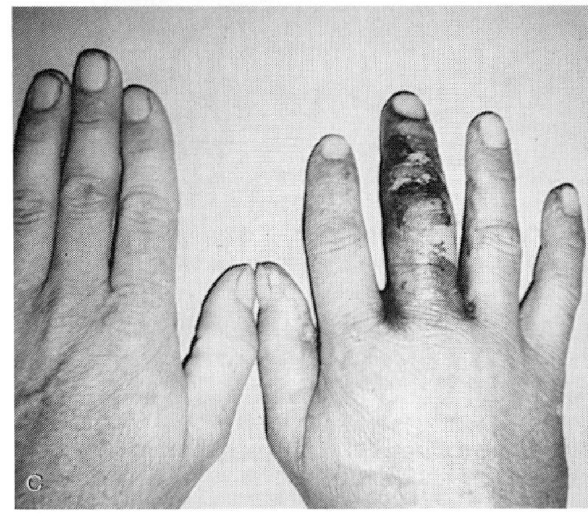

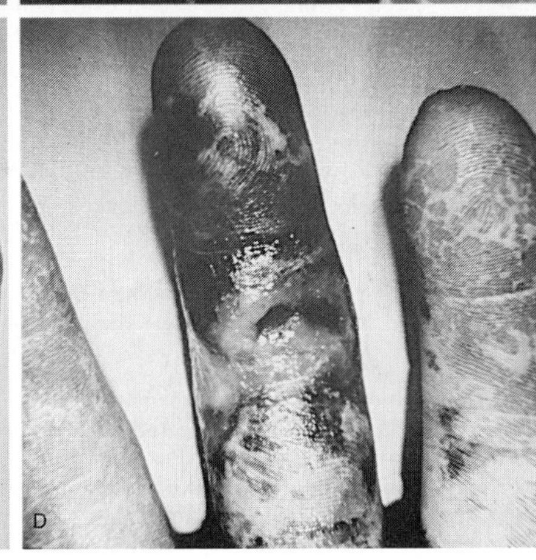

Figure 17–3. Edema, hemorrhage, and tissue injury resulting from crotalid envenomation of the face *(A)*, hand *(B)*, and finger *(C* and *D)*. (From Carlson RW: Injuries by venomous and poisonous animals. *In*: Principles and Practice of Medical Intensive Care. Carlson RW, Geheb MA [Eds]. Philadelphia, WB Saunders, 1993, p 1671.)

at the motor endpoint. This calcium channel blockade is noncompetitive.[25, 26, 63]

Antivenin

Polyvalent antivenin for American pit vipers is prepared with the use of horse serum against the venoms of four species (*C. durissus terrificus*, *Bothrops atrox*, *C. adamanteus*, and *C. atrox*). This product is the only antivenin commercially available for treatment of pit viper bites in the United States. Unfortunately, this serum has limited effectiveness against many of the lethal and other deleterious crotalid venom fractions, and its use is associated with a significant risk of acute and subacute allergic reactions, including anaphylaxis. Russell,[7] however, has observed that over a period of more than three decades, only one death in the United States has resulted from anaphylaxis from the use of antivenin for pit vipers. He suggests that fewer than 50% of all crotalid bites require antivenin. However, length of hospital stay is shorter for antivenin-treated patients than for patients not given this treatment, and antivenin is helpful in cases of moderate and especially serious envenomations.

Nevertheless, immediate hypersensitivity reactions to antivenin may be seen in as many as 25% of patients, and the incidence of delayed serum reactions appears to correlate with the dose of antivenin given.[20] Schaeffer and associates[64] found that polyvalent antivenin contains equine antibodies that bind predominantly to large (>30 kD) venom fractions but has minimal antibody titers to the smaller basic proteins and peptides in pit viper venoms. These smaller molecules are associated with many of the most deleterious properties of the venoms.

Research continues on the development of other preparations that have greater efficacy. Ovine and avian antivenins are currently under development for crotalid venoms, including the use of Fab fragments that may have greater efficacy.[65, 66] However, these products are not commercially available at this time.

Some clinicians have cautioned against the routine use of

TABLE 17–9. Ineffective or Dangerous Treatment for Snakebite

Arterial tourniquets
Corticosteroids*
Ethylenediaminetetraacetic acid (EDTA)
High-voltage electric current
Cryotherapy or application of heat
Heparin
Intra-arterial administration of antivenin
Pressure immobilization†
Early excisional therapy

*Except to treat allergic reactions to antivenin.

†Has been recommended for Australian elapid, sea snakes, and some viperid bites.

antivenin, although most authorities recommend antivenin for at least moderate to serious envenomations after a risk-benefit evaluation has been made.[21, 22, 41–44, 67, 68] Antivenin should *not* be used for trivial bites or for unconfirmed envenomations.

Recommendations as to the appropriate dose of antivenin are controversial, but up to five vials are generally recommended for moderate envenomations, up to 10 vials for more serious injuries, and up to 15 or more vials for severe envenomations. It is not uncommon for 30 to 50 vials to be given for life-threatening bites in some centers. If antivenin is given, it should be administered intravenously and as soon as practicable.[68] Pregnancy is not necessarily a contraindication to the use of antivenin.[69] The serum should *not* be injected into fingers or toes, and should *not* be used in the field. Sensitivity testing should not be omitted, although a negative skin test result may not reliably predict the lack of an acute reaction. Whenever possible, the clinician should obtain an informed consent for the use of antivenin. Delayed serum reactions occur in 10% or more of patients after antivenin therapy.[70]

Bites by other pit vipers (genus *Agkistrodon,* cottonmouths and copperheads) usually cause mild to moderate envenomations.[70–72] Therefore, fewer patients bitten by these reptiles require antivenin therapy than patients bitten by rattlesnakes.

Other crotalids of the New World are the lance-headed vipers (genus *Bothrops*), of which several dangerous species exist. These animals, characterized by a broad, flattened head, may produce a serious envenomation. *Bothrops atrox* venom is used in the preparation of Wyeth polyvalent antivenin; however, antivenin for other *Bothrops* species is prepared in Mexico or South America. The pygmy rattlesnake and massasauga (genus *Sistrurus*) are smaller snakes found in the midwestern and southeastern United States. These animals generally inflict wounds of mild to moderate severity, although the venom of the massasauga is highly toxic.

Family Viperidae (Vipers)

The family Viperidae comprises many snakes in the Old World, including all of the European and Asiatic mainlands and Africa. These snakes have large, mobile front fangs that are folded against the upper jaw at rest and are moved to the erect position for use against prey (see Fig. 17-2). The snake fully controls this process as well as the amount of venom it injects during a bite.

Some vipers are large, such as the Gaboon viper *(Bitis gabonica)*, a heavy-bodied snake that may exceed 6 feet in length. Other vipers are small but equally dangerous. The saw-scaled viper *(Echis carinatus)* and carpet viper *(Echis coloratus)* are usually less than 2 feet long but cause many serious and fatal envenomations. All vipers are dangerous to humans.

Similar to crotalid venoms, the venoms of vipers contain many enzymes and other components that alter hemostasis. Edema, tissue destruction, hemorrhage and hypovolemia, and coagulation defects are commonly observed after viper bites.[51] In some instances, the coagulopathy produced by procoagulant fractions leads to DIC. Other common causes of viperid defibrination syndromes are bites from Russell's viper *(Vipera russelli)*.

Genus *Echis* (Saw-Scaled or Carpet Vipers)

Members of the *Echis* genus account for a substantial proportion of snakebite mortalities in the Afro-Asian region. In Nigeria and other areas, thousands of people are bitten by these snakes, with considerable loss of life.[73–75] Management of *Echis* bites is controversial, and these injuries are often associated with serious local as well as life-threatening systemic complications, which often include bleeding. Antivenin is indicated for all serious envenomations, particularly when blood is incoagulable and there are progressive local findings. *Echis* bites are common and probably account for the greatest number of snake venom deaths in the world.

Clinical Features

The *Echis* bite is usually on the foot, and pain and swelling are almost universally found shortly afterward. Within the next few hours, 50% of patients experience spontaneous bleeding from remote sites, such as the gums or injection sites. Some patients experience altered consciousness, which may progress to coma and death. Hypotension and signs of hypovolemia may develop. Tissue necrosis may be massive. Hemolysis and thrombocytopenia are also observed, but incoagulable blood, together with a reliable history and evidence of local findings, predicts severe *Echis* envenomation. The use of a micro-ELISA (enzyme-linked immunosorbent assay) for detecting venom in urine, serum, aspirated fluid, or other body fluids is highly accurate for diagnosis.[76]

Despite a significant risk of anaphylaxis and the likelihood of serum sickness, antivenin treatment is indicated for *Echis* bites associated with local changes or hemostatic failure because the mortality of these bites when untreated exceeds 10%.[73, 75] Antivenin has been given several days after envenomation if systemic findings persist. Death is usually from central nervous system bleeding or hemorrhagic shock.[75] All bites should be managed in an ICU setting if possible. Progressive local signs and coagulation alterations are indications for the use of antivenin. Newer ovine Fab antivenins are now available to treat *Echis* envenomations.[77, 78]

Additional therapies may also be available in the future to counter the coagulation changes induced by these toxins. Schaeffer and associates[79] tested the effects of a synthetic inhibitor of thrombin on the coagulation and microembolic damage produced by *Echis* venom. The agent inhibited the coagulation changes as well as the hemolysis and also reduced the pulmonary microvascular damage and edema induced by the venom.[80, 81]

Bitis gabonica (Gaboon Viper) and *Bitis arietans* (Puff Adder)

Gaboon vipers and puff adders, which are native to tropical and southern Africa, are very dangerous. These large, heavy snakes possess fangs that may exceed 2 inches in length, and they produce a very toxic venom. Many bites are fatal if left untreated and account for a significant proportion of fatal snakebites in this geographic region. A large puff adder possesses enough venom to kill several humans.

Bitis venoms contain hemorrhagic components[82] as well as factors that affect both intrinsic and intrinsic coagulation pathways, leading to activation of plasminogen. Bleeding, both regional and systemic, is a common problem, as is tissue destruction. Hemorrhage is a consistent finding in experimental models using these venoms,[51, 83–86] and hemorrhagic shock is one mechanism of death. A direct cardiotoxic fraction may also contribute to shock. Our group[51] found that the venom led to perfusion failure with hypotension, hemodilution, hypoproteinemia, and marked hyperventilation in experimental subjects. Total blood volume as well as red cell and plasma volumes were critically reduced, and there was an increase in the rate of transvascular escape of albumin.

Treatment of *Bitis* bites should include prompt administration of antivenin and infusion of fluid and blood products that may include fresh frozen plasma, platelets, and red blood cells. Tissue damage may be massive.

Vipera russelli (Russell's Viper)

Russell's viper is found in a large geographic region, including northern Eurasia into and throughout Asia, as well as North

Africa and the East Indies. Bites from this snake and other venomous snakes are the fifth leading cause of death in Burma, and in Sri Lanka, Russell's viper causes five deaths per 100,000 people per year.[87, 88] Incoagulable blood is a consistent feature in patients with systemic Russell's viper envenomation. A micro-ELISA kit is available to detect venom in serum or other body fluids in victims.[76] This kit may be helpful because up to 25% of patients exhibit no evidence of envenomation; another 25% demonstrate only local findings, and 50% therefore exhibit serious toxicity, including thrombocytopenia, spontaneous bleeding, and shock.[89]

When serious toxicity is seen or the micro-ELISA demonstrates envenomation, antivenin is indicated. Several antivenins are available. Antivenin is usually effective to combat the coagulation defects and possibly exerts favorable effects on tissue damage; however, the effectiveness of different antivenin preparations varies considerably.

Renal failure is also a problem following Russell's viper envenomation. Fluid loading and correction of hemorrhagic shock may be as helpful to prevent renal failure as antivenin. Death is commonly a consequence of renal failure, hemorrhage, central nervous system hemorrhage, or shock.

Family Elapidae (Elapids)

Elapids are widely distributed, from the New World to Australia, New Guinea, Africa, southern Asia, Malay archipelago, the Philippines, and the Fiji Islands. All elapids are venomous, and the family contains some of the most lethal snakes, such as the cobras, mambas, death adders, kraits, taipans, coral snakes, and tiger snakes. The fangs of the elapids are shorter and are fixed in position (see Fig. 17–2). The king cobra (*Ophiophagus hannah*) is the largest venomous snake in the world, reaching a length of 18 feet. Elapid venoms often contain a variety of fractions that affect neuromuscular function, and envenomations often include prominent neurotropic findings; however, hemotoxic, cardiotoxic, and local tissue injury may also occur with these injuries. Elapid venoms share similarities with sea snake venoms.

Elapid neurotoxins are basic proteins and polypeptides that are devoid of enzymatic activity but act selectively on the neuromuscular junction,[90] either presynaptic or postsynaptic in action (Table 17–10). Cobra toxin and α-bungarotoxin from the krait produce an antidepolarizing block by acting on the postsynaptic end plate. Other toxins, such as β-bungarotoxin, are presynaptic and alter release of acetylcholine. Among other fractions in elapid venoms is phospholipase A, which disrupts electron transport and mitochondrial integrity.

The neurotoxin isolated from the Australian tiger snake, *Notechis scutatus*, is a presynaptic compound that inhibits release of acetylcholine and is also myonecrotic.

TABLE 17–10. Examples of Snake Venom Neurotoxins

Site and Action	Example	Effect
Postsynaptic	α-Bungarotoxin	Early paralysis
Compete for postsynaptic receptor	Tiger snake neurotoxin	Early symptoms; may be more responsive to antivenin
Presynaptic	β-Bungarotoxin	Potentially more lethal
Inhibit release of acetylcholine	Sea snake neurotoxin Taipan neurotoxin	

Modified from Minton SA: Neurotoxic snake envenoming. Semin Neurol 1990; 10:52. With permission of Thieme Medical Publishers, Inc.

Mamba (genus *Dendroaspis*) venoms are neurotoxic, myonecrotic, and anticoagulant.[91, 92] Mamba bites often lead to diaphoresis, hypotension, coma, vomiting, and respiratory arrest. Four species are found in tropical Africa. The snakes are slender and fast-moving and may be very aggressive. Mambas are extremely dangerous, and a large snake has sufficient venom to kill several people. Untreated mamba bites, therefore, are often fatal. Serial bites by one snake may occur. Death is usually due to respiratory depression or cardiac arrhythmias. Pain and local swelling are usually not prominent. Respiratory paralysis may occur within minutes. Many elapids grasp the victim and chew, introducing more venom into the wound.

There are several species of kraits (genus *Bungarus*) in Southeast Asia. These nocturnal animals may reach 7 feet in length and are usually less aggressive than mambas. However, krait bites may be fatal, and respiratory paralysis may occur within minutes. Fatalities are often associated with respiratory failure and complications of prolonged mechanical ventilation.[92] Pain and local findings are moderate to severe.

With a molecular weight of 7000, α-bungarotoxin is a competitive postsynaptic neurotoxin that causes a nondepolarizing neuromuscular block.[93, 94] Although it competes for the postsynaptic receptor, the blockade is irreversible and leads to a prolonged flaccid paralysis. The postsynaptic fractions appear to account for earlier symptoms than the presynaptic fractions and may be more responsive to the effects of antivenins. Ptosis and ophthalmoplegia seen early after envenomation, therefore, may be due predominantly to postsynaptic toxins. The presynaptic fractions inhibit release of acetylcholine and are thought to be more lethal.[90] β-Bungarotoxin and other similar toxins isolated from the tiger snake and taipan are typical presynaptic neurotoxins.

Closely related to the mambas and kraits are the cobras. At least 6 species of the genus *Naja* are widely distributed in Africa and Asia. Management of cobra bites includes antivenin as well as edrophonium (see later discussion of sea snakes).

North American Elapids

There are three species of elapids in the United States. All are brightly colored coral snakes that may be confused with several nonvenomous forms. The most dangerous is the Eastern coral snake, *Micrurus fulvius fulvius*, which may reach a length of 3 feet. This animal is found in the southern states to Mississippi. The Texas coral snake, *M. fulvius tenere,* is primarily confined to that state. The smaller Western or Sonoran coral snake, *Micruroides euryxanthus* is common in Arizona and surrounding regions of New Mexico and Mexico.

Few deaths are reported from coral snakes, although envenomation occurs in up to 75% of bites, and serious neurotoxic symptoms are common after contact with the eastern coral snake.[95] Symptoms may be delayed for up to 12 hours. Most bites occur on the hand or the foot and in the spring or fall. Local findings are seen in 40% of patients but may be mild. Neurotropic changes, including cranial nerve dysfunction and respiratory failure, may occur. These complications develop in approximately 5% of eastern coral snake bites.

Antivenin is available for eastern coral snakebite and is helpful in management, although its effectiveness in reversing or preventing severe neurotropic dysfunction has not been clarified. A significant number of patients treated with antivenin experience urticaria or serum sickness, and anaphylactic reactions are always a risk when antivenin is given. In one study, up to 15 vials of antivenin were given, although the average dose was approximately six vials.[95] Neuromuscular toxicity may be manifested as fasciculations, paresthesias, and increases in creatine kinase levels.

Bites by Sonoran and Texas coral snakes are generally less dangerous than those by the eastern coral snake. No antivenin is available for Sonoran and Texas coral snakes, and eastern coral snake antivenin is not effective for these bites.

Family Colubridae (Rear-Fanged Snakes)

Many nonvenomous snakes belong to the Colubridae family. Because all snakes have teeth, the bite of any snake can lead to local and, occasionally, systemic signs and symptoms as well as secondary infection and direct injury by the bite. The most dangerous colubrid is the boomslang (*Dispholidus typus*), a tree-dwelling snake found in tropical and southern Africa.[96, 97] The venom is extremely toxic, and bites may result in death. Marked coagulation changes typically occur, as well as other systemic effects. Antivenin is available.

Family Hydrophiidae (Sea Snakes)

Found in the Pacific and Indian oceans, sea snakes are particularly dangerous and are closely related to the elapids. Approximately 50 species reside within two subfamilies, Laticaudinae and Hydrophinae. These animals may reach lengths of more than 6 feet and are characterized by a flat tail that is used for swimming. Sea snakes are not usually very aggressive, inflicting bites usually when caught in fishing nets or otherwise handled. Their fangs are short and may not always cause envenomation. Their venom is highly toxic.

Sea snake venom contains potent fractions that affect presynaptic and postsynaptic sites. Presynaptic toxins inhibit release of the neurotransmitter acetylcholine and are somewhat more lethal than the postsynaptic neurotoxins.[90] Hemotoxic and myotoxic fractions are also present and may account in part for hemolysis and rhabdomyolysis after sea snake envenomation.[99] Tissue edema and local pain are uncommon. Pain on motion, ascending paralysis, cranial nerve dysfunction, and respiratory failure may supervene in severe envenomation. Death due to respiratory failure is a risk within the first 24 hours; subsequent fatalities are often related to renal failure and associated complications.

Management of sea snake bite is similar to that for elapid bites, beginning with immobilization and transport to a hospital. Sutherland and others have proposed use of a pressure-immobilization dressing for these poisonings to reduce systemic absorption of venom.[8, 10, 76, 100, 101] An ELISA venom detection kit may be helpful to confirm envenomation. Antivenin for sea snakes as well as tiger snake or polyvalent elapid antivenin may be used. Because skin testing is not highly predictive of acute allergic reactions, the clinician must be prepared to treat anaphylaxis after antivenin therapy. Antihistamines, epinephrine, or both, given before or concomitantly with antivenin, may reduce serious, acute systemic reactions.

Initial laboratory studies for suspected sea snake envenomation should include a venom detection assay, if available; urinalysis; complete blood count; measurements of electrolytes; blood urea nitrogen and creatinine determinations; and a coagulation profile. Assessment of respiratory and ventilatory adequacy is also indicated. During the first hours of observation, it is important to closely monitor both neurologic function and the adequacy of ventilation and oxygenation. The ability of the patient to handle secretions and to have an effective cough are important considerations. Indications for intubation and mechanical ventilation are similar to those for patients with myasthenia gravis or Guillain-Barré syndrome. Fluid therapy during the first 24 hours should be guided by hemodynamic stability, urine output, and renal function. Coagulopathies, bleeding, hemolysis, and loss of plasma volume may lead to marked changes in hematocrit. Fluid loading should utilize physiologic endpoints, such as oxygen transport, cardiac output, and cardiac filling pressures. Edrophonium hydrochloride (Tensilon), 10 mg intravenously after 0.6 mg of atropine, may be considered to treat neurotropic alterations that threaten respiratory and ventilatory function.[102] If improvement is observed with edrophonium, neostigmine may be given, 0.25 to 0.5 mg intramuscularly every 30 minutes.

SUBORDER SAURIA, FAMILY HELODERMATIDAE (VENOMOUS LIZARDS)

Heloderma horridum (Mexican beaded lizard) and *Heloderma suspectum* (Gila monster) are two venomous lizards in the Southwest United States and Mexico. These stout, slow-moving animals have grooved mandibular teeth and submandibular venom glands. When aroused, they bite and grasp their victim as venom is introduced into the wound. Fortunately, bites from these lizards are rare. Signs and symptoms resemble those of a crotalid bite, consisting of pain, edema, coagulation changes, and, in serious envenomations, cardiovascular instability.[98] There is no commercially available antivenin.

MARINE ORGANISMS AND THEIR TOXINS

Many marine organisms are toxic to humans. More than 1000 species are dangerous, ranging from unicellular protozoans to the vertebrates. Marine toxins include poisons and venoms[103, 104]; in some situations, an animal may be both poisonous and venomous. Toxic organisms are found in all of the seas and oceans of the world and in many lakes and rivers. The venomous and poisonous forms do not usually present a major problem to humans, but in some areas and under certain conditions toxic aquatic organisms may pose a risk to the local population as well as a danger to individuals.

Marine toxins are complex mixtures that vary considerably in chemical and pharmacologic properties. Some are proteins, although amines, quaternary ammonium compounds, mucopolysaccharides, lipids, and other unique chemicals have been associated with these forms. Several marine venoms contain enzymes, but these substances are less common than in many terrestrial venoms. A number of marine toxins are highly unstable. When removed from the animal, they rapidly lose many of their chemical and pharmacologic properties. Many marine toxins are heat-labile, a point that has practical importance in management of marine bite injuries.

Phylum Protozoa, Order Dinoflagellata (Paralytic Shellfish Poisoning)

Paralytic shellfish poisoning is related to the ingestion of shellfish containing toxic unicellular dinoflagellates that reach high concentrations during changes in water and weather conditions. High concentrations of these organisms (blooms) in the water cause red tide or brown water conditions. The large numbers of these protists may lead to death of fish and other marine life. The danger to humans occurs when the organisms are ingested by mollusks, echinoderms, or arthropods in which the toxins are concentrated and which are subsequently eaten by humans.

Paralytic shellfish poisoning is most common in spring and

fall months.[103-107] Sale of shellfish during these seasons may be prohibited. Bivalved mollusks, such as mussels and clams, are most commonly involved. Boiling, freezing, steaming, frying, and other techniques of preservation and cooking do *not* destroy the toxin, and many poisonings occur after consumption of the meat or broth of contaminated shellfish that have been steamed.

The genus most commonly associated with these outbreaks is *Gonyaulax.* These forms cause poisonings in North and South America and Japan and other Pacific regions, as well as several areas in the Atlantic. *Pyrodinium* and *Gymnodinium* are other genera that have been implicated in human poisonings.[107, 108]

The toxin is *saxitoxin.* A number of similar saxitoxin molecules have been identified. The structure is a tetrahydropurine derivative, and one saxitoxin has the following chemical composition: $C_{10}H_{17}N_7O_4 \cdot 2\ HCl$, with a molecular weight of 372. The material is highly toxic, and the purified toxin has an LD_{50} of approximately 3 μg/kg.[108-113]

The pharmacology of saxitoxin is similar to that of tetrodotoxin, another marine toxin. Tetrodotoxin and saxitoxin interfere with the early, transiently open channel that admits sodium ions in excitable membranes. These toxins block action potentials in nerves and muscles. Death is usually related to respiratory failure, although direct cardiotoxicity as well as hypotension caused by changes in vascular resistance may be seen.

Clinical features are primarily related to neurologic signs and symptoms. Symptoms may develop within minutes after ingestion of contaminated shellfish. Paresthesias and dysesthesias appearing initially around the mouth may progress to the limbs. Muscle paralysis may supervene, and cranial nerve dysfunction may be a prominent feature in some poisonings. Respiratory insufficiency often provokes hospital admission. Many victims may require ventilatory support. Hypotension may be seen. Mortality has decreased with aggressive ICU supportive care. Death usually occurs within the first few hours. If the patient is maintained with supportive measures, the illness subsides within 3 to 5 days.

There is no antidote or immunity for paralytic shellfish poisoning, although the diagnosis may be confirmed in some instances when the toxin is detected in gastric fluid or in the suspected food.

Ciguatera Poisoning

Ciguatera poisoning is also caused by eating seafood that has been contaminated by a dinoflagellate. In this case, the toxin (ciguatoxin) is concentrated in a variety of coral reef fish and eels. The benthic dinoflagellate *Gambierdiscus toxicus* is incorporated into the food chain from fish that feed on algae and debris around tropical reefs. These herbivores, such as the surgeonfish and parrotfish, are subsequently eaten by reef carnivores and omnivores, including moray eels, jacks and amberjacks, snappers, some tunas, groupers, and barracuda. The meat of these fish contains the toxin, which, when ingested by humans, causes the typical symptoms of the poisoning. This form of fish poisoning is termed *ichthyosarcotoxism*, as it involves the viscera, flesh, muscle, and skin of fish. The brain, intestines, liver, and gonads contain the highest concentrations of the toxin.

Ciguatera poisoning occurs in tropical and subtropical areas throughout the world. It is particularly common in the waters of the Caribbean and around Florida, the South Pacific, and Hawaii. Ciguatera poisoning is probably the most common form of marine intoxication in the United States.[109, 114-116]

There is more than one ciguatera toxin. Ciguatoxins are lipid-soluble, colorless, odorless, and heat-stable with a molecular weight of approximately 1100. They primarily affect neuromuscular transmission. Sodium permeability of excitable membranes is increased, causing depolarization. Symptoms typically include paresthesias, peripheral muscle weakness, respiratory distress, myalgias, pruritus, diaphoresis, headache, and ataxia as well as gastrointestinal symptoms, such as cramps, abdominal pain, diarrhea, nausea, and vomiting. Two commonly reported symptoms are heat-cold dysesthesia and altered taste.[116] Hypotension, tachycardia, and marked sinus bradycardia may occur. Some complaints, particularly neurologic symptoms, may persist for protracted intervals.

Treatment is supportive. For management of the more severe neurologic and cardiovascular findings, admission to an ICU is warranted. A variety of agents have been suggested to be helpful: calcium salts, mannitol, atropine, magnesium, tricyclic antidepressants, and calcium channel blockers.[117-119] Some patients report an increase in symptoms with consumption of alcohol. The toxin may be detected in contaminated fish by ELISA.[120]

Scombroid Fish Poisoning (Scombrotoxism)

Scombrotoxism is a form of ichthyosarcotoxism caused by bacteria in spoiled fish. Improperly preserved fish is the cause. Dark-meat fish, such as bonito, skipjack, mackerel, dolphin, albacore, and tuna, are most commonly implicated. Scombroid poisoning may be the most common form of fish poisoning in the world. Symptoms develop within an hour after ingestion. Flushing, nausea, diaphoresis, vomiting, diarrhea, palpitations, rash, and, occasionally, edema of the face and tongue are seen. Hypotension and respiratory distress with bronchospasm may occur.

It has now been established that this poisoning appears to be due to the production of histamine in spoiled fish.[121-124] Histamine content of affected tissues is high. Symptoms are improved by treatment with histamine H_1 and H_2 receptor antagonist drugs. Signs and symptoms may be severe and may warrant admission to an ICU, but the syndrome generally resolves within hours.

Clupeotoxism

A form of ichthyosarcotoxic poisoning, *clupeotoxism* occurs after the ingestion of herring, anchovies, bonefish, and tarpons. The cause is believed to be ingestion of dinoflagellates by these fish. The poisoning is often fatal. Signs and symptoms develop rapidly and resemble those of severe paralytic shellfish poisoning. There is no specific treatment, but the poisoning may require immediate application of life-support measures.

Phylum Porifera (Sponges)

Of the more than 5000 species of sponges, only limited numbers of tropical and subtropical forms are toxic to humans. Intoxication occurs through skin abrasions by spicules of the sponge. A variety of toxic substances have been isolated from sponges, including histamine, acetylcholine, nitrogenous bases, and steroids. Contact with some sponges may cause severe skin and local reactions as well as anaphylactoid reactions.[125-127]

Aside from management of the life-threatening allergic reactions, therapy is directly primarily at local signs and symptoms. Treatments may include soaks or application of acetic acid (5%) or isopropyl alcohol to affected parts. Topical corticosteroid preparations are also helpful. Adhesive tape applied to the region may help remove spicules. Another syndrome associated with contact with sponges is "sponge-diver's dis-

TABLE 17–11. Classification of Venomous Coelenterates

PHYLUM Cnidaria (Coelenterata)
CLASS Hydrozoa: Hydroids; stinging fire or false coral
Order Siphonophora: free-floating siphonophores
FAMILY Phyaliidae
Physalia physalis: Portuguese man-of-war, bluebottle caravelle, vissie de mer, galère
CLASS Anthozoa: Sea anemones, sea fans, corals
CLASS Scyphozoa (Scyphomedusae): jellyfish
FAMILY *Chirodropidae:* sea wasp, box jellyfish
Chironex fleckeri
Chiropsalmus quadrigatus

ease," which is caused by a coelenterate envenomation from contact with anemones attached to or near the sponge.[128]

Phylum Cnidaria (Formerly Phylum Coelenterata: Jellyfish, Anemones, and Portuguese Man-of-War)

The coelenterates comprise vast numbers of animals found throughout the seas of the world. At least 70 species are toxic to humans within three classes (Table 17–11):

- Hydrozoa (hydroids and the free-floating siphonophores or *Physalia*, commonly termed the Portuguese man-of-war)
- Anthozoa (anemones, sea fans, and corals)
- Scyphozoa or Scyphomedusae (true jellyfish)

The venom apparatus in a coelenterate is the nematocyst. Not all nematocysts are able to puncture human skin. The nematocyst is a highly sophisticated device that fires a hollow tube containing venom into a person on contact (Fig. 17–4). Activation may be induced by a variety of chemical and mechanical stimuli, a point that has clinical and therapeutic significance. There is a high concentration of nematocysts in coelenterates, particularly on the surfaces of tentacles and other structures. Hence, the dose of venom is related to the surface area of the animal in contact with the victim. In a severe exposure, literally hundreds of thousands of nematocysts may be discharged.

Interrelationships and similarities between anaphylaxis and venom injuries have been the subject of many studies, particularly of coelenterate envenomations. The original descriptions of anaphylactic and tachyphylactic responses to the venom of a sea anemone were made in the early part of this century.[129] In describing human envenomations by various cnidarians, one may find it difficult to separate allergic reactions from the primary effects of the toxins.[130] For a description of management of anaphylactic reactions, see Chapter 18.

The venom of coelenterates contains a variety of low-molecular-weight and high-molecular-weight substances. Proteins, amines, hydroxyproline, amino acids, minerals, and other substances have been isolated. The lethal components are proteins,[131, 132] some of which have enzymatic activities. Proteins with cardiotoxic properties are thought to be among the most lethal components of the dangerous cnidarians, such as the box jellyfish and the sea wasp (*Chironex fleckeri* and *Chiropsalmus quadrigatus*).[133, 134]

Envenomations range from minor skin irritation to a rapidly fatal syndrome. Immediate pain is characteristic of these injuries. Dermal reactions include pruritus, paresthesias, pain, bullae, secondary infection, local hemorrhage, desquamation, and other changes.

Attempts to remove the patient from tentacles or other parts should be accomplished quickly. Care should be exercised to avoid additional discharge of nematocysts into the patient or rescuers. Tentacles may be scraped from the wound

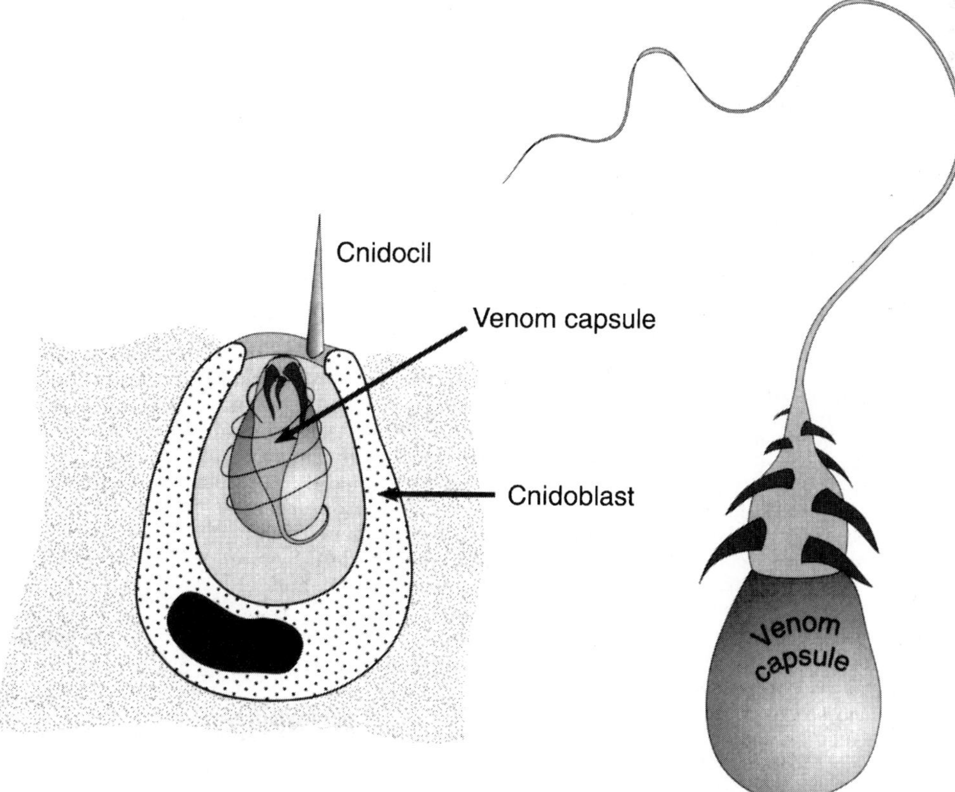

Figure 17–4. Nematocyst showing the cnidocil, cnidoblast, and venom capsule. (From Carlson RW: Injuries by venomous and poisonous animals. *In*: Principles and Practice of Medical Intensive Care. Carlson RW, Geheb MA [Eds]. Philadelphia, WB Saunders, 1993, p 1674.)

or removed with forceps. The area should be rinsed with salt water, isopropyl alcohol, acetic acid, shaving cream, a slurry of baking soda, acetic acid, or alcohol. Fresh water should *not* be used because it causes firing of nematocysts. Sea sand may be used to help remove the animal and prevent further discharge of stinging units (Table 17–12).[130, 135–140]

For contact with coral, it is important to remove tiny fragments from the wound with hydrogen peroxide and vigorous cleansing. These injuries are particularly likely to become infected and heal slowly.

Steroid cream or sprays are helpful for managing the lesions after initial treatment. Tetanus prophylaxis is indicated.

The pain associated with coelenterate stings may be excruciating and may be aggravated by movement. A cooling pack may be helpful, but ice should not touch the skin. Pain may be accompanied by systemic symptoms, such as nausea, vomiting, muscle cramps, hypotension, urticaria, bronchospasm, and respiratory distress. Hypotension and other signs, such as hemolysis, may herald a severe response to the venom. Verapamil given intravenously has been used with good results to combat life-threatening cardiotoxicity and may potentiate the effects of antivenin.[141–144]

It is possible that skin divers, swimmers, and surfers who experience repeated contact with coelenterates may develop immunoglobulin E (IgE) antibodies followed by anaphylaxis. Some reported drownings may actually have been caused by such reactions.

Hospital admission is indicated for patients with marked signs and symptoms. Observation and ICU management of life-threatening cardiopulmonary changes may be necessary.

The box jellyfish or sea wasp (*C. fleckeri*) is a scyphozoan found off the northeast coast of Australia. It has an extremely toxic venom, and cardiopulmonary collapse and death may occur within minutes after contact. Aside from first aid measures and cardiopulmonary resuscitation, an antivenin is available for intravenous use in life-threatening reactions.[144, 145]

TABLE 17–12. Emergency Treatment for Coelenterate Stings

1. Remove victim from water or exposure.
2. Evaluate for cardiopulmonary function and need for CPR.
3. Rescuers should avoid contact with tentacles or organism.
4. Disengage from tentacles or organism.
5. Gently scrape with sea sand or salt water; remove tentacles with forceps or other instruments.
6. Irrigate and cleanse affected parts.
7. Use acetic acid 5% (vinegar) or 40%–70% isopropyl alcohol for soaks or cleansing.
8. Use shaving cream and shave area to remove nematocysts.

   Do not use ammonia, fresh water, bleach, mineral spirits, or other agents—may result in further firing of nematocysts.
9. Treat local lesions:
   a. Corticosteroid cream/spray, systemic steroids for severe reactions
   b. *Pain relief:* Opiates may be required. Ice packs may be helpful (avoid contact of ice to skin).
   c. Antibiotics for abrasions or extensive injuries; secondary infection and poor healing are common.
10. Give antitetanus therapy
11. Treat systemic reactions: CPR
    a. Shock, respiratory arrest, bronchospasm: fluid loading or vasoactive agents; bronchodilators or intubation
    b. Arrhythmias: consider verapamil, 5–10 mg IV; use with caution if patient hypotensive.
    c. Gastrointestinal pain, nausea–vomiting
    d. Assess hemolysis, coagulation
    e. Assess neuromuscular status, altered sensorium, pain on motion, spasm, arthralgia, seizures, coma
    f. Fever, chills, leukocytosis
    g. Eye injuries: ophthalmology consultation
    h. Antivenin for severe reactions to *C. fleckeri*

CPR = cardiopulmonary resuscitation.

Phylum Echinodermata (Echinoderms)

Many echinoderms are venomous or poisonous. The venomous species are found in three classes:

- Asteroidea (starfish or sea star)
- Echinoidea (sea urchins)
- Holothuroidea (sea cucumbers)

Most starfish are not dangerous to humans, although contact with starfish slime or spines may lead to local and, occasionally, systemic toxicity. The only venomous starfish is the *Acanthaster planci*, found along the Great Barrier Reef of Australia. Contact with its long and sturdy spines may lead to painful wounds together with nausea, vomiting, regional muscle pain, and paralysis. There is no specific therapy.

The sea urchins possess two types of spines, primary spines and smaller secondary spines. The primary spines produce puncture wounds and often troublesome foreign body reactions. The secondary spines include the venomous, globiferous pedicellariae.[146–148]

Several toxins have been isolated from echinoderms, including steroid glycosides, serotonin, and acetylcholine-like compounds. Hemolytic and hypotensive activities as well as release of histamine and neurologic alterations have been described for these toxins.[149] The steroid molecules and attached sugars are anionic saponins that cause irreversible changes of cholinergic neuromuscular junctions. Immediate pain, edema, and other local findings may be accompanied by syncope, respiratory paralysis, and local muscle paralysis. Secondary infection of these wounds is common, and the lesions may cause considerable irritation. Therapy is supportive. Local heat may be helpful to combat pain. Pedicellariae and embedded spines should be removed if possible. There is no antivenin. The venomous sea urchins are widely distributed throughout many seas of the world.

The class Holothuroidea includes the sea cucumbers. These are free-living, bottom-dwelling echinoderms that excrete a toxin as a defensive maneuver. Toxicity may follow contact with or ingestion of a holothurian. The poison is known as *holothurin*. Holothurians may also contain intact nematocysts from ingested coelenterates. Local and/or systemic manifestations may occur from contact. Holothurin is a mixture of several closely related sulfate ester glycosides that have hemolytic and neurotropic effects. Contact may lead to a papular eruption. Therapy is similar to that for contact with other echinoderms and should include removal of slime with sea sand, vinegar, or alcohol and immersion of the affected area in hot water.

Phylum Mollusca (Mollusks)

Although there are thousands of species of mollusks, fewer than 100 may be toxic to humans. These are found in three classes of this phylum (Table 17–13):

- Gastropoda (snails, slugs, and cone shells)
- Cephalopoda (squids and octopuses)
- Pelecypoda (bivalves, including scallops, oysters, and clams)

Cone shells possess a sophisticated venom apparatus that can induce a puncture wound and injection of venom if the animal is disturbed. The most dangerous species are found in the Indo-Pacific area and are often highly sought for their

TABLE 17–13. Venomous and Poisonous Mollusks

Phylum Mollusca
- Class Gastropods: Univalve snails and slugs
  - Family Conidae: Cone shells (venomous)
- Class Pelecypoda: Bivalves (scallops, clams, oysters)—paralytic shellfish poisoning
- Class Cephalopoda: Squid, octopus, nautillus, cuttlefish
  - *Octopus maculosus* and *Octopus lunulatus:* blue-banded octopus, ringed octopus (venomous)

shells. Many toxins have been isolated from cone shells: proteins, amines, lipoproteins, and carbohydrates. Cardiovascular and neurologic effects may be life-threatening, and the venom is toxic (LD_{50}, 0.2–2.4 mg/kg).[110]

Therapy for cone shell envenomation is supportive but may include intubation, mechanical ventilation, and cardiovascular support with fluids and vasoactive agents. In addition to respiratory failure, severe envenomations may be characterized by paralysis, dysphagia, areflexia, weakness, coagulopathies, coma, hypotension, and death.[103, 104, 107] Information on the ICU management of these poisonings is limited. Some components of the venom may be heat-sensitive; local application of warm soaks may therefore be helpful.

The bites of certain cephalopods are dangerous.[150, 151] In severe cases of bites by Australian octopuses *Octopus maculosus* and *Octopus lunulatus*, the venom contains a number of small peptides that affect vascular resistance, and one component may have actions similar to those of tetrodotoxin. There is no specific therapy, and management of the wound may be difficult. Excision of the wound has been recommended in severe intoxications. Antivenin is not available.

Mollusks may be poisonous because of paralytic shellfish poisoning. In addition, mollusks may be contaminated with a variety of bacteria and viruses, including hepatitis A and various species of *Vibrio*, including *Vibrio parahaemolyticus* and *Vibrio vulnificus*. Contact with contaminated mollusks, particularly by patients who are immunocompromised, may lead to diarrheal syndromes and, with *V. vulnificus*, life-threatening bacteremic syndromes.[152, 153]

Phylum Chordata, Classes Osteichthyes and Chondrichthyes (Tetrodotoxic Fish)

One of the most interesting stories in the history of poisons was the discovery that two toxins from unrelated organisms were remarkably similar. Saxitoxin, a poison derived from a protozoa, and tetrodotoxin, an ichthyosarcotoxin, have virtually identical pharmacologic properties, despite differences in origin and chemical structure.[112] Tetrodotoxin is a perhydroquinazoline ichthyosarcotoxin found in puffer fish, ocean sunfish, and certain other fish. Saxitoxin and tetrodotoxin both affect sodium conductance of excitable membranes.[154, 155] Both compounds are extremely toxic, and only a few molecules are needed to disrupt transmission. The flesh and especially the viscera of fugu or puffer fish are poisonous, producing tetrodotoxin poisoning. The onset may be dramatic, with paresthesias about the mouth and lips within minutes, followed by salivation, marked weakness, nausea, vomiting, and progressive paralysis of systemic and respiratory muscles. Coma and seizures have been reported, and severe poisonings may be fatal.

There is no antidote; treatment is supportive. Intubation and mechanical ventilation, as well as hemodynamic support with fluids or vasoactive agents, are commonly required to manage these cases. With intensive care, however, complete recovery is possible.

Venomous Fish: Stingrays, Scorpionfish, Catfish, Weevers, and Others

More than 200 species of fish possess a venom apparatus.[13, 103, 104, 107] These animals, widely distributed among fresh and marine forms, include bony fish such as catfish, scorpionfish, stargazers, toadfish, surgeonfish, and weevers. Many elasmobranch fish, chiefly stingrays, are also venomous. The venom apparatus, except in the weevers, is used defensively. Human contact with these animals occurs through swimming, wading, fishing, or performing other activities. Injuries are either lacerations or puncture wounds (Fig. 17–5). In some cases, the wounds are life-threatening.[104]

Fish venoms are characterized by instability. Toxicity is rapidly lost when the venom or venom apparatus is exposed to heat.[103, 126, 138, 156–159] The venoms are mixtures of many compounds, although the most deleterious materials are proteins of 50 to 800 kD that are extremely heat-labile. Carlson and associates[157, 158] have found that proteins isolated from the venom of the California scorpionfish *(Scorpaena guttata)* produce marked respiratory and hemodynamic changes, including bronchoconstriction, hypotension, and alterations in heart rate (Fig. 17–6). The venom has a muscarinic action and a secondary β-adrenergic stimulating action. In experimental subjects, atropine partially counteracts the effects of acetylcholine, which is released in response to venom components.

Pain is a consistent and prominent feature of fish envenomations. The pain is excruciating and may involve an entire extremity. Other symptoms are local edema, vomiting, nausea, diaphoresis, hypotension, and bradyarrhythmias.[126, 138, 159]

The most lethal venomous fish are the stonefish, members of the genus *Synanceja,* found in the Indo-Pacific region, Australia, Indian Ocean, China Sea, and Red Sea. The venom apparatus of the stonefish, although more highly developed, is similar to that of the other scorpionfish, consisting of dorsal and pelvic spines in which an integumentary sheath covers the venom tissue located in grooves or either side of the spine. As the spine punctures the person, the integumentary

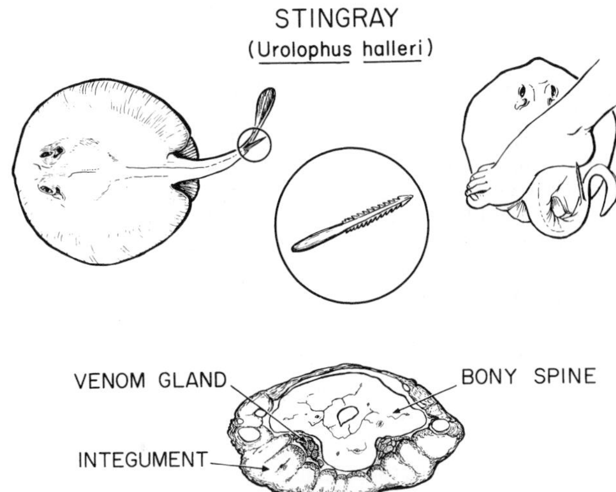

Figure 17–5. Stingray venom apparatus and mechanisms of envenomation. (From Carlson RW: Injuries by venomous and poisonous animals. *In*: Principles and Practice of Medical Intensive Care. Carlson RW, Geheb MA [Eds]. Philadelphia, WB Saunders, 1993, p 1677.)

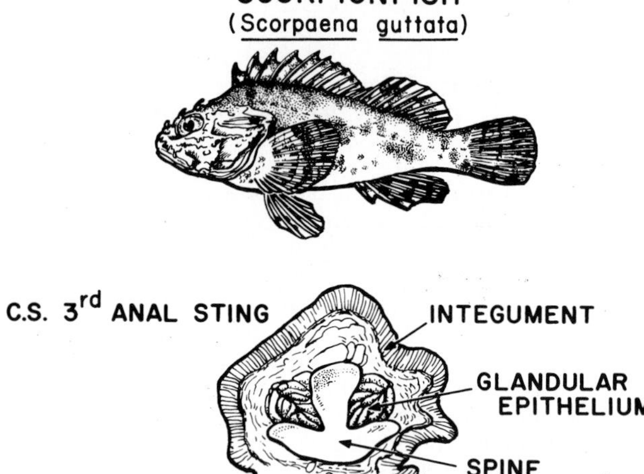

Figure 17–6. California scorpionfish *(Scorpaena guttata)* and a cross-section (C.S.) of an anal spine. (From Carlson RW: Injuries by venomous and poisonous animals. *In*: Principles and Practice of Medical Intensive Care. Carlson RW, Geheb MA [Eds]. Philadelphia, WB Saunders, 1993, p 1677.)

sheath is ruptured, and the glandular tissue in the "grooves" is introduced into the wound. Stonefish venom is extremely toxic. An antivenin to stonefish venom is available (Commonwealth Serum Laboratories, Melbourne).

Injuries by other scorpionfish are common throughout the world, because many scorpionfish are caught as food fish or maintained in aquaria. In particular, lionfish or zebra fish (genus *Pterois)* are highly prized for saltwater aquaria and result in many stings each year.[138, 160] Although large proteins are contained in lionfish venom, fluid aspirated from the blisters after a sting contains prostaglandin F_2 and small amounts of prostaglandin E_2.[161]

There are three priorities in the management of scorpionfish injuries: (1) treatment of the wound, (2) relief of pain, and (3) therapy for the systemic effects of the envenomation. For stingray injuries, the wound may be extensive and lacerated. It is important to clean the wound thoroughly and to remove any remaining portions of the venom apparatus. Debridement may be required. Secondary infection and sloughing are common. For puncture wounds by scorpionfish and other forms, the clinician must ensure that the sting has been removed. Immersion of the affected part in warm soaks is helpful to treat the pain of these injuries; application of cold may intensify the pain. Local anesthetic agents or systemic analgesic agents are often required. Lidocaine has been reported to be effective for immediate relief of pain. Stonefish antivenin is effective for these injuries and may have some effectiveness against venoms of other scorpionfish, such as lionfish and zebra fish. Patients with severe envenomations should be observed in an ICU for cardiopulmonary instability (Table 17-14). Stingray injuries are usually painful lacerations that involve the foot or hand. Stingray venom shares many chemical and pharmacologic features with scorpionfish venoms.[138, 162-165]

PHYLUM ARTHROPODA (ARTHROPODS)

There are approximately 1 million species of arthropods, and these animals cause more envenomations than any other group of animals. Several thousand venomous arthropods are dangerous to humans (Table 17-15). The spiders, scorpions,

TABLE 17–14. Principles of Treatment of Fish Stings

1. Treat the wound:
   a. Warm soaks (45°C, 113°F)
   b. Remove *ALL* components of venom apparatus and venom
   c. Laceration: debride, ensure adequate drainage; wounds heal slowly, often with secondary infection and ulceration
   d. Consider x-ray to detect embedded fang components
2. Provide relief of pain:
   a. Warm soaks
   b. Opiates may be required
   c. Local injection of xylocaine may be helpful
3. Treat secondary infection.
4. Give tetanus prophylaxis.
5. Manage cardiopulmonary crisis (severe reactions to a scorpionfish, lionfish, or for stonefish envenomation):
   a. Atropine
   b. Vasoactive agents or volume loading for hypotension
   c. Respiratory support; intubation and mechanical ventilation may be needed
   d. Antivenin for stonefish or lionfish poisoning

and the Hymenoptera account for most human injuries. Most of these envenomations are irritating but are not life-threatening. Death may result, however, from the direct effects of the venoms as well as from anaphylactic reactions to venom components. Chapter 18 presents a more complete discussion of anaphylaxis and its management.

Arthropod poisonings pose several problems in diagnosis and management. Many arthropod venoms contain substances that cause signs and symptoms resembling anaphylaxis. True anaphylactic reactions are also encountered because repeated contact with an animal may induce the production of IgE antibodies by the victim. Certain arthropod injuries, such as those by the *Loxosceles* spiders, are characterized by distinctive features, such as necrotic lesions, although other species may induce a similar response. Finally, identification of the offending animal is not possible in many cases because the animal is destroyed, not observed, or confused with another species. Therefore, the ICU physician must often provide empiric therapy for a presumed bite or sting by an arthropod. This uncertainty may create practical problems when one is contemplating specific therapy, such as antivenin or other potentially dangerous treatments.

Arthropod venoms have a wide variety of chemical and pharmacologic properties. Neurologic toxicity is common with arthropod injuries. Proteins, enzymes, peptides, amines, sugars, free bases, and alkaloids are among the many components isolated from these venoms.

TABLE 17–15. Some Medically Important Arthropods

- Phylum Arthropoda
  - Class Insecta
    - ORDER HYMENOPTERA
      - Family Apidae: bees
      - Family Bonidae: bumblebees
      - Family Vespidae: wasps, hornets, yellow jackets
      - Family Formicidae: ants
  - Class Arachnida
    - ORDER ARANEAE: Spiders
      - Family Theraphositae: tarantulas
      - Family Clubonoidae: running spiders
      - Family Salticidaei: jumping spiders
      - Family Theridiidae: comb-footed spiders (widows)
      - Family Loxoscelidae: brown (violin) spiders
      - Family Buthidae: scorpions

Class Arachnida, Order Araneae (Spiders)

Several families of spiders are of clinical importance. Virtually all spiders are venomous, but only a few have chelicerae that can inflict a bite in humans.[166, 167] Approximately 60 species of spiders in the United States cause clinically significant envenomations.

Family Theraphosidae (Tarantulas) and Family Lycosidae (True Tarantulas or Wolf Spiders)

The spiders commonly known as "tarantulas" in the United States are mygalomorphs, members of the family Theraphosidae. These large spiders are not particularly dangerous, although they bite when provoked. Envenomation leads to local pain, urticaria, edema, and other local signs and symptoms. Therapy is symptomatic. Secondary infection may occur. The wolf spiders, or true tarantulas, are also large, hairy spiders that may cause a painful bite. Necrotic lesions or systemic effects are uncommon.

Family Clubionoidae (Running Spiders), Family Salticidae (Jumping Spiders), and Family Araneidae (Golden Orb Weavers)

Running and jumping spiders are found in many gardens, yards, and fields. They account for many painful bites. A variety of reactions may occur, but the bites are usually not life-threatening. Necrotic lesions may develop on occasion.

The golden orb weavers are large, often colorful spiders that spin large webs to hunt insects. Their bites are associated with pain and local findings. Systemic toxicity is uncommon, although necrotic lesions have been reported.

Family Theridiidae (Comb-Footed or Cobweb Spiders)

The genus *Latrodectus*, in the Theridiidae family, contains the most dangerous spiders in the world. The females have large, globular bodies and long legs. They are usually black or brown and typically have distinctive red markings on the abdomen. *Latrodectus* species are found worldwide and are known by many names—black or brown widow spider, red-back spider, and shoe button spider. Several species of *Latrodectus* are found in the United States, including *Latrodectus mactans* and *Latrodectus hesperus*. The species name *mactans* means "murderer."

Latrodectus spiders are typically encountered on or close to the ground, in woodpiles, under stones or logs, and in sheds, garages, and privies. The spiders have eight eyes, and the lateral eyes are widely separated. The term "comb-footed" refers to the hind pair of legs, which are used to ensnare prey with silk. These animals are usually not aggressive but may vigorously attack anyone who disturbs their webs.

The venom contains several peptide and protein fractions ranging from 5 to more than 100 kD.[168-173] Among other properties of these fractions are neuromuscular conduction disturbances with an initial release of acetylcholine or catecholamines. Postsynaptic depolarization and morphologic changes occur at the end plate.

Clinical features of *Latrodectus* bites are distinctive.[174-177] The bite produces some initial pain, although local features are usually minimal. There may be local paresthesias. Vance and associates[178] have suggested that the area of the bite often displays characteristic features. They describe a halo lesion, consisting of a circular area of pallor surrounding an erythematous zone. There may be multiple bites by a single spider, each with this characteristic lesion. Local and regional muscle irritation develops, with fasciculations, pain, and spasms. Deep tendon reflexes are increased, and there may be marked pain and spasm of muscle groups (Fig. 17-7). When this manifestation involves the abdominal muscles, the findings may resemble those in acute abdomen.

A variety of other findings may be observed, including headache, dysesthesias with burning of plantar surfaces, diaphoresis, urinary retention, ptosis, salivation, respiratory distress, nausea, and vomiting. Sharp increases in arterial pressure may lead to a hypertensive crisis. Heart rate may be raised or lowered. The increases in blood pressure, muscle tone, and reflexes may progress to generalized seizures and coma. Intracranial hemorrhage may be found in fatal envenomations. Laboratory findings and the electrocardiogram are usually nonspecific, although high values for the white blood cell count as well as creatine kinase and other muscle enzymes, hemolysis, and the development of progressive azotemia may result.

The elderly, the young, and people with underlying cardiopulmonary or neurologic disorders are particularly prone to complications of *Latrodectus* envenomations. The venom is sufficiently toxic that the envenomation may be lethal for a small child. Accordingly, for cases of suspected *Latrodectus* envenomation, it is prudent to observe the patient in an emergency room setting for several hours. If systemic symptoms do not develop during this time, the patient may be discharged. If signs of serious toxicity develop within the first few hours, however, the patient should be admitted to an ICU.

Local therapy consists of application of an ice cube or a cooling pack over the bite. A variety of agents have been used to treat the muscle spasms and pain: intravenous calcium gluconate, diazepam, magnesium sulfate, methocarbamol, and a number of sedatives. However, none of these agents has proven efficacy, and the clinician is well advised to use conventional analgesic agents and mild sedation for those symptoms.[179] For more severe reactions, antivenin is indicated. β-Blockers or other antihypertensive agents have been used, although a pure β-blocker may cause unopposed alpha effects, with worsening of hypertension. There is no consensus on the optimal drug therapy to control the hypertensive crisis, but rapid-acting vasodilators, such as nitroprusside, intravenous calcium channel blocking agents, and hydralazine, are reasonable choices.

Caution should be exercised if the patient exhibits respiratory distress. Seizures should be managed with conventional

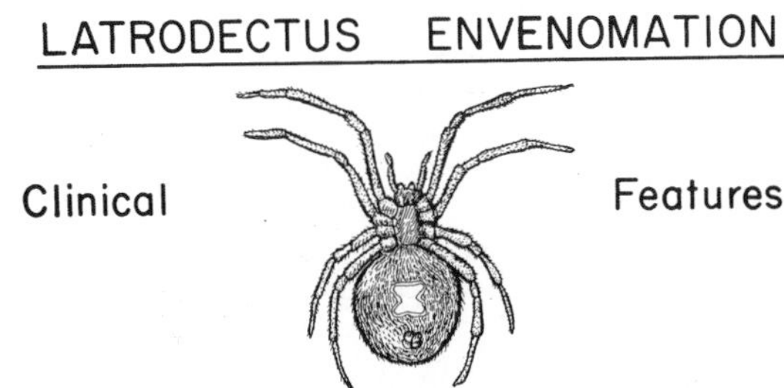

Figure 17-7. Important features of *Latrodectus* envenomation. (From Carlson RW: Injuries by venomous and poisonous animals. *In*: Principles and Practice of Medical Intensive Care. Carlson RW, Geheb MA [Eds]. Philadelphia, WB Saunders, 1993, p 1678.)

therapy: administration of a rapid-acting benzodiazepine and phenytoin (Dilantin) together with protection of the airway. It is important to monitor arterial pressure and neurologic findings closely. Dantrolene (Dantrium), a direct muscle relaxant, has also been used to treat muscle spasms[180] caused by a *Latrodectus* bite; this is not one of the indicated uses of dantrolene, which is associated with significant toxicity, including methemoglobinemia. There is no apparent benefit of the use of corticosteroids.

An antivenin (Antivenin [*Latrodectus mactans*], Merck & Co) prepared with horse serum is available and is highly effective. It may be given intravenously or intramuscularly. Administration of one vial (2.5 mL) is usually sufficient. Serum sickness and anaphylaxis are considerations that should temper use of the serum; informed consent and skin testing procedures should be performed as outlined in the package insert. Most authorities recommend antivenin for severe poisoning or in a high-risk patient.

Family Loxoscelidae (Fiddleback, Brown, Violin, and Recluse Spiders)

Spiders of the Loxoscelidae family are commonly found in North and South America and are frequently incriminated in lesions with dermal necrosis (necrotic arachnidism, also termed loxoscelism). There are several species of the genus *Loxosceles* in the United States, and all are dangerous to humans (Fig. 17–8). They are widely distributed, particularly in the South Central regions of the country. The animals are nocturnal and reclusive but bite when provoked.

These spiders may be identified as having a tan, yellowish, or gray body of 10 to 15 mm, with a violin-shaped marking on the dorsal surface of the cephalothorax, six eyes (most spiders have eight), and long, spindly legs that may be 25 mm long.

The venom has not been fully characterized but includes a number of proteins, some with enzymatic activity, such as phospholipase D (sphingomyelinase), which may be important in the development of dermonecrotic lesions, hyaluronidase, 5′-ribonuclease, and collagenase. Several lytic factors, peptides, and other components are present.[181–184] Complement activation may play a role in the dermal necrosis.

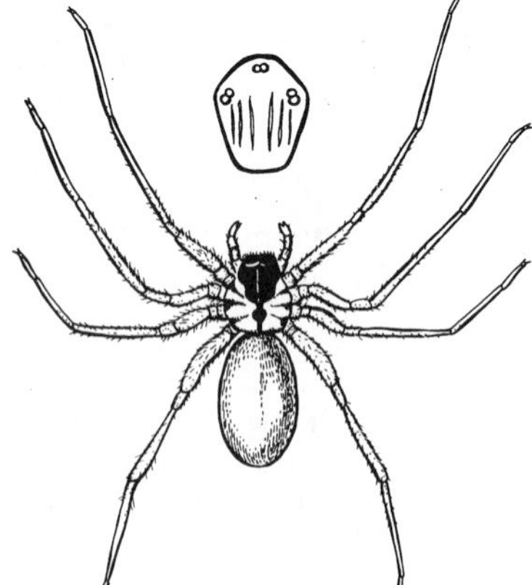

Figure 17–8. The brown recluse spider *(Loxosceles reclusa)*, showing location of three pairs of eyes and the "fiddle" on the cephalothorax. (From Carlson RW: Injuries by venomous and poisonous animals. *In*: Principles and Practice of Medical Intensive Care. Carlson RW, Geheb MA [Eds]. Philadelphia, WB Saunders, 1993, p 1679.)

TABLE 17–16. Management of Loxoscelism and Dermonecrotic Arthropod Syndromes*

1. Observe for progression of local findings.
2. Frequent examinations, especially during initial 24 hours.
3. Consider early curettage of lesion; consider dermatology/plastic surgery consultation.
4. Cleanse wound.
5. Give tetanus prophylaxis.
6. Treat secondary infection.
7. Steroids are of dubious value.
8. Some authorities recommend Dapsone, 50–200 mg/d in divided doses PO, for progressive dermonecrotic lesions, although animal studies do not confirm its efficacy.
9. Consider laboratory studies such as complete blood count, assays for hemolysis, serum electrolytes, renal function, muscle enzymes.
10. Conservative therapy indicated in most instances, including RICE (Rest, Ice, Elevation)

*Management of these lesions has been unsatisfactory in many instances. A variety of treatments have been recommended; there is currently no therapy of proven effectiveness.

The bite may be only mildly painful. Within a few hours, however, increasing pain and local findings become prominent. A central blister or bleb may develop that may have a central blue-black region surrounded by erythema. The lesion may progress with alarming speed, with an expanding area of central necrosis. This process usually begins within 12 hours, although great variations in the sequence of the local necrosis and dermal changes have been reported. Additional bullae or blebs may develop regionally. The central necrosis commonly leads to scar formation. Systemic findings may be minimal, but chills, fever, nausea, vomiting, arthralgias, coagulation changes, rash, thrombocytopenia, hemolysis, hemoglobinuria, and renal failure have been documented. Coma and seizures have also been reported, although these findings may be secondary to other systemic changes rather than primary effects of the envenomation.

Because other animal bites and stings may lead to necrotic lesions, it is important to describe an injury as cutaneous necrosis, necrotic insect bite, or presumptive, clinically typical, or documented recluse spider bite with loxoscelism.[185–188] Precise descriptions of the lesion and the spider, together with the clinical course, should be entered in the medical record. If the offending animal cannot be identified, this fact should also be noted.

Management of these lesions is often unsatisfactory, and several therapeutic techniques have been recommended to treat them (Table 17–16). There is no widely available test to confirm *Loxosceles* envenomation, nor does a commercially prepared antivenin exist for this venom. *Latrodectus* antivenin is *not* effective against *Loxosceles.*

Therapy should be directed to the local changes, which may be dramatic, as well as to systemic toxicity. The wound should be cleaned and tetanus prophylaxis administered. If the characteristic lesion is identified quickly, some authorities recommend curettage of the necrotic material within the wound.[189] Earlier reports of excision of the wound suggested that this measure helped prevent progression of the necrotic lesion. Excision is no longer recommended by most authorities, however, and may complicate the disfigurement created by these bites.[185, 190–193] Antibiotics may be needed but should not be given prophylactically. Steroids are of no proven benefit, but some authorities continue to recommend local or systemic corticosteroid preparations. In a 1997 review of 111 cases, conservative management was suggested.[194]

The α-adrenergic blocking agents and other vasodilators are

of no proven benefit, even though the necrotic lesion is in part due to intensive local vasospasm with ischemic necrosis. Heparin is not indicated. Dapsone (4,4-diaminodiphenylsulfone) has been recommended.[195] This agent is an inhibitor of white blood cell function and may limit necrosis; however, it is associated with significant side effects, such as hemolysis and methemoglobinemia. Dosage is 50 to 200 mg/day orally in divided doses. Dapsone was proposed for severe, developing dermonecrotic lesions. A variety of other treatments have been recommended, including hyperbaric oxygen and serotonin antagonists. In a study comparing dapsone, cyproheptadine, and hyperbaric oxygen in experimental subjects, however, none of these measures resulted in any significant improvement in local tissue changes.[196] The mnemonic RICE, for *r*est, *ic*e, and *e*levation, has been suggested to emphasize the conservative maneuvers that can be used in the care of patients with *Loxosceles* bites.[192, 193, 195] Monitoring of renal and hemostatic variables should be undertaken in serious envenomations. Surgical consultation is indicated for patients with marked necrotic lesions.

Class Arachnida, Family Buthidae (Scorpions)

Of the approximately 650 species of scorpions within this family, only two species within the genus *Centruroides* in North America are associated with fatal poisoning in humans. These animals, commonly termed "bark scorpions," are found in Arizona and Mexico (Fig. 17–9).[197] In tropical and subtropical regions of the world, however, including the Middle East and South America, several dangerous species of scorpions are found, and severe envenomations are common.[198–201] Life-threatening syndromes are particularly likely to occur in children or patients with cardiovascular disease. Tachycardia, seizures, hypertension, pulmonary edema, coma, vomiting, hyperreflexia, diaphoresis, cardiac injury and arrhythmias, and a variety of other findings have been documented. The venoms contain several potent protein neurotoxins, which may also affect the cardiovascular system.[202–204]

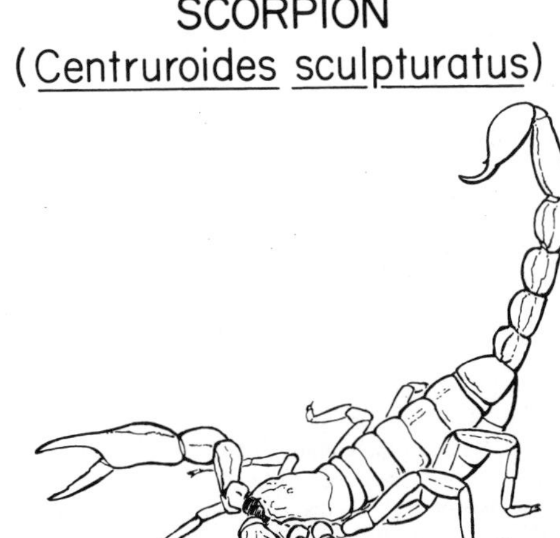

Figure 17–9. The *Centruroides* scorpion, a dangerous and common hazard in the southwestern United States and adjacent portions of Mexico. (From Carlson RW: Injuries by venomous and poisonous animals. *In*: Principles and Practice of Medical Intensive Care. Carlson RW, Geheb MA [Eds]. Philadelphia, WB Saunders, 1993, p 1680.)

The venom of *Centruroides* scorpions contains several basic proteins that are relatively resistant to proteolytic enzymes. Grading of *Centruroides* injuries should guide management. One scheme is as follows:

- Grade I: pain and local findings only
- Grade II: pain and paresthesias remote from the sting, in addition to local findings
- Grade III: cranial nerve or somatic neuromuscular dysfunction, in addition to the local changes
- Grade IV: both cranial nerve and somatic changes[205, 206]

The site of envenomation is characteristically hypersensitive, and tapping over the region may elicit severe pain. Another diagnostic clue to scorpion envenomation is that patients with this injury are typically restless and unable to remain immobile. Finally, whenever cranial nerve dysfunction is seen in arthropod envenomation, scorpion sting should be suspected. Management advice and antivenin made from goat serum are available locally (Samaritan Regional Poison Control Center, Phoenix) for serious envenomations.[205–208] Patients should be observed closely and admitted to an intensive care environment if the syndrome progresses to grade II or higher.

Although antivenin may be available for some species,[200] vasodilators such as nitroprusside, prazosin, hydralazine, and calcium channel blocking agents may be useful to combat the left ventricular failure and hypertension.[201, 209, 210] The cardiovascular manifestations of scorpion envenomation may be related to increased levels of angiotensin, renin, and catecholamines. Cardiac arrhythmias are common, and myocarditis or a picture that resembles myocardial infarction may supervene.

Class Insecta, Order Hymenoptera (Bees, Wasps, Hornets, and Ants)

The Hymenoptera comprise more than 16,000 species in the United States, but four families of this order account for the majority of insect stings: Apidae (honeybees), Bombidae (bumblebees), Vespidae (wasps, yellow jackets, and hornets), and Formicidae (fire and harvester ants). The venoms of the bees, wasps, and related forms have been studied extensively and contain a variety of proteins and low-molecular-weight substances that are toxic (Table 17–17).[211, 212] These venoms are not toxic to humans, however, unless many stings occur simultaneously. In most instances, therefore, the greatest danger from bee and wasp envenomations is anaphylaxis. Desensitiza-

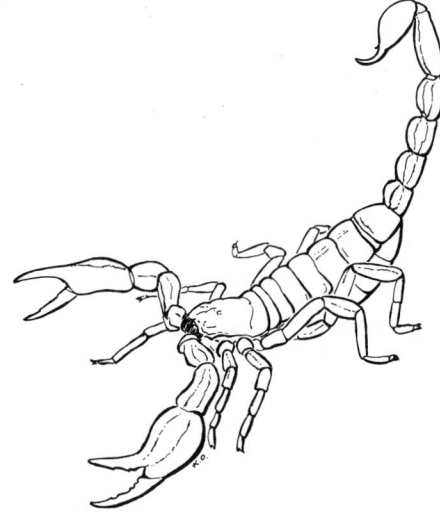

TABLE 17–17. Components of Various Hymenoptera Venoms*

Bee	Wasp, Hornet, Yellow Jacket	Fire Ant
Histamine	Histamine	Piperidines
Apamin	Kinins	Phospholipases A, B
Melittin	Serotonin	Other allergenic proteins
Mast cell degranulating substance	Phospholipases A, B	
Hyaluronidase	Other peptides that degranulate mast cells	
Acid phosphatase		
Norepinephrine		
Dopamine		
Allergen C		
Other peptides		

*Adapted from Wright DN, Lockey RF: Local reactions to stinging insects. Allergy Proc 1990; 11:23.

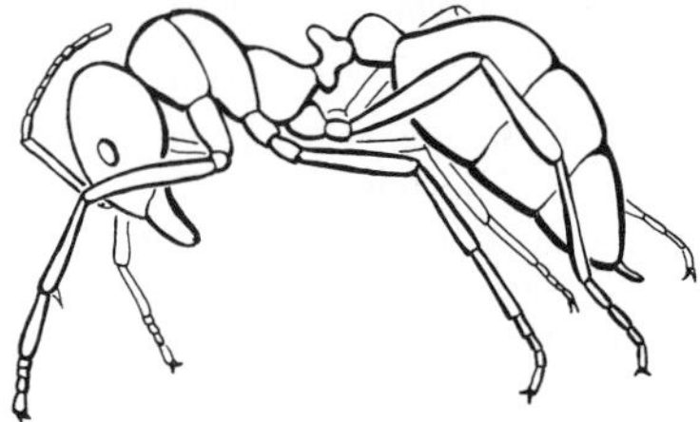

Figure 17–10. One species of the imported fire ant *(Solenopsis saevissima)*: The animal can simultaneously bite and sting. (From Carlson RW: Injuries by venomous and poisonous animals. *In*: Principles and Practice of Medical Intensive Care. Carlson RW, Geheb MA [Eds]. Philadelphia, WB Saunders, 1993, p 1681.)

tion with extracts of bee venom is indicated for patients who demonstrate marked sensitivity to it.

Many species of ants possess venoms that are painful or irritating. Formic acid, which the venoms of several ants contain in high proportion, may account for pain and local findings.

The imported red fire ant, *Solenopsis invicta*, and the imported black fire ant, *Solenopsis richteri,* have become a public health problem as well as a threat to individuals and animals in many areas of the Gulf South (Fig. 17–10).[213–215] Fatal envenomations have been described.[216, 217] These species are aggressive, and many animals are typically involved in each injury. Up to 95% of the venom is an alkaloid, although proteins and peptides are also present. The predominant alkaloids are piperidines with hemolytic, antibacterial, and cytotoxic properties.[218–220] Repeated exposure to the protein components of fire ant venom may induce IgE-mediated allergic reactions.[221–223]

A variety of skin and systemic responses may occur. Pustular and, occasionally, necrotic lesions often develop. When multiple stings occur, or if an anaphylactic reaction develops, the injury may be fatal.

Immunotherapy to fire ant extract may be useful prophylaxis for patients who have experienced serious allergic reactions. Venom is preferred to whole body extracts for desensitization. The initial treatment of the sting is empirical. No antivenin is currently available. A number of therapies have been suggested, including local agents, meat tenderizer containing papain, and other folk remedies. However, these maneuvers are probably of limited value. Corticosteroids and other agents may be helpful, particularly for late reactions. In cases of multiple stings, close observation is indicated, with monitoring of cardiopulmonary and neurologic function.

ACKNOWLEDGMENT

The authors acknowledge the assistance of Judy C. Hodgkins and the Staff of the Medical Library at Maricopa Medical Center, and appreciate the prior collaboration in toxinology with Findlay E. Russell and Richard C. Schaeffer, Jr.

References

1. Russell FE: Snake Venom Poisoning. Philadelphia, JB Lippincott, 1980.
2. Kaubert LM: Rattlesnakes: Their Habits, Life Histories and Influence on Mankind. Vol 1 and 2. Berkeley, Calif, University of California Press, 1972.
3. Minton SA, Dowling, HG, Russell FE (Eds): Poisonous Snakes of the World. 2nd ed. Washington, DC, U.S. Government Printing Office, 1968.
4. Swaroop S, Grab B: The snakebite mortality problem in the world. Bull WHO 1954; 10:35.
5. Russell FE: Snake Venom Poisoning. Great Neck, NY, Scholium International, 1983.
6. Parrish HM: Mortality from snakebite. Public Health Rep 1966; 72:1027.
7. Russell FE: AIDS, cancer and snakebite: What do these share in common? West J Med 1988; 148:84.
8. Sutherland SK, Leonard RL: Snakebite deaths in Australia 1992–1994. Med J Aust 1995; 162:616.
9. Mead HJ, Jelinek GA: Suspected snakebite in children: A study of 156 patients over 10 years. Med J Aust 1996; 164:4367.
10. Sutherland SK: Australian Animal Toxins: The Creatures, Their Toxins and Care of the Poisoned Patient. Melbourne, Oxford University Press, 1983.
11. Tu AT: Venoms, Chemistry and Molecular Biology. London, John Wiley & Sons, 1977.
12. Iwanaga S, Suzuki T: Enzymes in snake venoms. *In:* Handbook of Experimental Pharmacology. Vol 52: Snake Venoms. Lee EY (Ed). Berlin, Springer-Verlag, 1979.
13. Russell FE: Pharmacology of animal venoms. Clin Pharmacol Ther 1967; 8:849.
14. Kochva E, Gans C: Histology and histochemistry of venom glands of some crotaline snakes. Copeia 1966; 3:506.
15. Schaeffer RC Jr, Pattabhiraman T, Carlson RW, et al: The histochemistry of the venom glands of the rattlesnake *Crotalus viridis helleri*: I. Lipid and nonspecific esterase. Toxicon 1972; 110:183.
16. Moura-da-Silva A, Laing G, Paine M: Processing of pro-tumor necrosis factor-alpha by venom metalloproteinases. Eur J Immunol 1996; 16:2000.
17. Bjarnason JB, Fox JW: Hemorrhagic metalloproteinases from snake venoms. Pharmacol Ther 1994; 62:325.
18. Russell FE: Snake venom poisoning in the United States. Annu Rev Med 1980; 31:247.
19. Russell FE, Carlson RW, Wainschel J, et al: Snake venom poisoning in the United States: Experience with 550 cases. JAMA 1974; 233:341.
20. Wingert WA, Chan L: Rattlesnake bites in Southern California and rationale for recommended treatment. West J Med 1988; 148:37.
21. Gold BS, Wingert WA: Snake venom poisoning in the United States. South Med J 1994; 87:579.
22. Seiler JG, Sagerman SD, Geller RJ, et al: Venomous snakebite: Current concepts of treatment. Orthopedics 1994; 17:707.
23. Dart RC, Hurlburt KM, Garcia R, et al: Validation of a severity score for the assessment of crotalid snakebite. Ann Emerg Med 1996; 27:321.
24. Pattabhiraman TR, Russell FE: Isolation and purification of the toxic fractions of Mojave rattlesnake venom. Toxicon 1975; 13:291.
25. Valdes JJ, Thompson RG, Wolff VL, et al: Inhibition of calcium channel dihydropyridine receptor binding by purified Mojave toxin. Neurotoxicol Teratol 1989; 11:129.
26. Gopalakrishnakone P, Hawgood BJ, Holbrooke SE, et al: Sites of action of Mojave toxin isolated from the venom of the Mojave rattlesnake. Br J Pharmacol 1980; 69:421.
27. Russell FE, Puffer H: Pharmacology of snake venoms. *In:* Snake Venoms and Envenomation. Minton SA (Ed). New York, Marcel Dekker, 1971, p 87.
28. Hardy DL: Fatal rattlesnake envenomation in Arizona: 1969–1984. Clin Toxicol 1986; 24:1.
29. Hardy DL: Envenomation by the Mojave rattlesnake (*Crotalus scutulatus scutulatus*) in Southern Arizona USA. Toxicon 1983; 21:111.
30. Jansen PW, Perken RM, Van Stralen D: Mojave rattlesnake envenomation: Prolonged neurotoxicity and rhabdomyolysis. Ann Emerg Med 1991; 21:322.
31. Davidson TM: Intravenous rattlesnake envenomation. West J Med 1988; 148:45.
32. Kunkel DB, Curry SC, Vance MJ, et al: Reptile envenomations. J Toxicol Clin Toxicol 1984; 21:503.

33. Pennell TC, Babu SS, Meredith JW: The management of snake and spider bites in the Southeastern United States. Am Surg 1989; 24:128.
34. Garfin SR, Mubarak SJ, Davidson TM: Rattlesnake bites—current concepts. Clin Orthop 1979; 140:50.
35. Grace TG, Omer GE: Management of upper extremity pit viper wounds. J Hand Surg 1980; 5:168.
36. Huang TT: Surgical management of poisonous snakebite. J Miss State Med Assoc 1987; 28:656.
37. Watt CH: Treatment of poisonous snakebite with emphasis on digit dermotomy. South Med J 1985; 78:694.
38. Roberts RS, Csencitz TA, Heard CW: Upper extremity compartment syndromes following pit viper envenomation. Clin Orthop 1985; 193:184.
39. Stewart RM, Page CP, Schwesinger WH, et al: Antivenin and fasciotomy/debridement in the treatment of the severe rattlesnake bite. Am J Surg 1989; 158:543.
40. Kitchens CS: Treatment of pit viper envenomation. J Fla Med Assoc 1996; 83:174.
41. Vigsio A, Battiston B, DeFillipp OG, et al: Compartmental syndrome due to viper bite. Arch Orthop Trauma Surg 1991; 110:175.
42 Dellaero DT, Levin LS: Compartment syndrome of the hand: Etiology, diagnosis and treatment. Am J Orthop 1996; 25:404.
43. Hyde GL, Peck D, Powell DC: Compartment syndromes. Am Surg 1983; 49:563.
44. Curry SC, Kraner JC, Kunel DB, et al: Noninvasive vascular studies in management of rattlesnake envenomation to extremities. Ann Emerg Med 1985; 14:1081.
45. Garfin SR, Castiliona RR, Mubarak SJ, et al: The wick catheter technique for measurement of intramuscular pressure: A new research and clinical tool. J Bone Joint Surg (Am) 1985; 58:1016.
46. Kerrigan KR, Mertz BL, Nelson SJ, et al: Antibiotic prophylaxis for pit viper envenomation: Prospective, controlled trial. World J Surg 1997; 21:369.
47. Clark RF, Selden BS, Furbee B: The incidence of wound infection following crotalid envenomation. J Emerg Med 1993; 11:583.
48. Carlson RW, Schaeffer RC Jr, Whigham H, et al: Rattlesnake venom shock in the rat: Development of a method. Am J Physiol 1975; 229:1668.
49. Schaeffer RC Jr, Briston C, Chilton SM, et al: Hypotensive and hemostatic properties of rattlesnake venom (*Crotalus viridis helleri*) and venom fractions in dogs. J Pharmacol Exp Ther 1984; 230:393.
50. Schaeffer RC Jr, Carlson RW, Whigham H, et al: Acute hemodynamic effects of rattlesnake, *Crotalus viridis helleri*, venom. *In:* Toxins: Animal, Plant and Microbiology. Rosenberg P (Ed). Oxford, Pergamon Press, 1978, p 383.
51. Schaeffer, RC Jr, Chilton SM, Carlson RW: Puffer adder venom shock: A model of increased vascular permeability. J Pharmacol Exp Ther 1985; 233:312.
52. Schaeffer RC Jr, Carlson RW, Weil MH: Effects of antivenin and corticosteroid analogues on rattlesnake venom shock in the rat. J Pharmacol Exp Ther 1979; 211:409.
53. Schaeffer RC Jr, Carlson, RW, Puri VK, et al: The effects of colloidal and crystalloidal fluids on rattlesnake venom shock in the rat. J Pharmacol Exp Ther 1978; 206:687.
54. Haupt MT, Teerapong P, Green D, et al: Increased pulmonary edema with crystalloid compared to colloid resuscitation of shock associated with increased vascular permeability. Circ Shock 1984; 12:213.
55. Ruiz, C, Schaeffer RC Jr, Carlson RW, et al: Hemostatic changes following rattlesnake (*Crotalus viridis helleri*) venom in the dog. J Pharmacol Exp Ther 1980; 213:414.
56. La Grange RG, Russell FE: Blood platelet studies in man and rabbits following *Crotalus* envenomation. Proc West Pharmacol Soc 1970; 13:99.
57. Weiss HJ, Allan S, Davidson E, et al: Afibrinogenemia in man following the bite of a rattlesnake (*Crotalus adamanteus*). Am J Med 1969; 47:625.
58. Amaral CFS, Da Silva OA, Lopez M, et al: Afibrinogenemia following snake bite (*Crotalus durissus terrificus*). Am J Trop Med Hyg 1980; 29:1453.
59. Tu AT: Blood coagulation. *In:* Venoms: Chemistry and Molecular Biology. Tu AT (Ed). New York, John Wiley & Sons, 1977, p 329.
60. Hasiba U, Rosenbach LM, Rockwell D, et al: DIC-like syndrome after envenomation by the snake, *Crotalus horridus horridus*. N Engl J Med 1975; 292:505.
61. Simon TL, Grace TG: Envenomation coagulopathy in wounds from pit vipers. N Engl J Med 1981; 305:443.
62. Kitchens CS: Hemostatic aspects of envenomation by North American snakes. Hematol Oncol Clin North Am 1992; 6:1189.
63. Ho CL, Lee CY: Presynaptic actions of Mojave toxin. Toxicon 1981; 19:889.
64. Schaeffer RC Jr, Randall H, Resk J, et al: Enzyme-linked immunosorbent assay (ELISA) of size-selected crotalid venom antigens by Wyeth's polyvalent antivenin. Toxicon 1988; 26:67.
65. Bogdan GM, McKinney P, Porter RS, et al: Clinical efficacy of two dosing regimens of affinity purified, mixed monospecific crotalid antivenom ovine Fab (CroTab). Acad Emerg Med 1997; 4:540.
66. Cosroe P, Egen NB, Russell FE, et al: Comparison of a new ovine antivenin binding fragment (Fab) antivenin for United States Crotalidae with the commercial antivenin for protection against venom-induced lethality in mice. Am J Trop Med Hyg 1995; 53:507.
67. Weisman RS, Lizarralde SS, Thompson V: Snake and spider antivenin: Risks and benefits of therapy. J Fla Med Assoc 1996; 83:192.
68. Hostege CP, Miller MB, Wermuth M, et al: Crotalid snake envenomation. Crit Care Clin 1997; 13:889.
69. Pantanowitz L, Guidozzi F: Management of snake and spider bite in pregnancy. Obstet Gynecol Survey 1996; 51:615.
70. Weber RA, White RR: Crotalidae envenomation in children. Ann Plast Surg 1993; 31:141.
71. Lawrence WT, Giannopoulos A, Hansen A: Pit viper bites: Rational management in locales in which copperheads and cottonmouths predominate. Ann Plast Surg 1996; 36:276.
72. Randolph R, Neal GE, Williams JS, et al: Snakebite treatment at a Southeastern regional referral center. Am Surg 1995; 61:767.
73. Warrell DA, Arnett C: The importance of bites by the saw-scaled or carpet viper (*Echis carinatus*): Epidemiological studies in Nigeria and a review of the world literature. Acta Trop 1976; 33:307.
74. Pugh RNH: Bites by the carpet viper in the Niger valley. Lancet 1979; 2:625.
75. Warrell DA, Davidson NMcD, Greenwood BM, et al: Poisoning by bites of the saw-scaled or carpet viper (*Echis carinatus*) in Nigeria. Q J Med 1977; 46:33.
76. Theakson RDG, Jones MJL, Reid HA: Micro-ELISA for detecting and assaying snake venom and venom antibodies. Lancet 1977; 2:639.
77. Meyer WP, Habib AG, Onayadee AA, et al: First clinical experiences with a new ovine Fab *Echis ocellatus* snake bite antivenom in Nigeria. Am J Trop Med Hyg 1997; 56:291.
78. Laing GD, Lee L, Smith DC, et al: Experimental assessment of a new low-cost antivenin for treatment of carpet viper (*Echis ocellatus*) envenomation. Toxicon 1995; 33:307.
79. Schaeffer RC Jr, Briston C, Chilton SM, et al: Disseminated intravascular coagulation following *Echis carinatus* venom in dogs: Effect of a synthetic thrombin inhibitor. J Lab Clin Med 1986; 107:488.
80. Schaeffer RC Jr, Barnhart MI, Carlson RW: Pulmonary fibrin deposition and increased microvascular permeability to protein following fibrin microembolism in dogs: A structure-function relationship. Microvasc Res 1987; 33:327.
81. Schaeffer RC Jr, Chilton SM, Hadden TJ, et al: Pulmonary fibrin microembolism following infusion of *Echis carinatus* venom in dogs: Effects of a synthetic thrombin inhibitor. J Appl Physiol 1984; 57:1824.
82. Mebs D, Panholzer F: Isolation of a hemorrhagic principle from *Bitis arietans* (puff adder) snake venom. Toxicon 1982; 20:509.
83. Brink S, Steytler JG: Effects of puff adder venom on coagulation, fibrinolysis and platelet aggregation in the baboon. S Afr Med J 1974; 48:1205.
84. Tu AT, Honna M, Hong B: Hemorrhagic, myonecrotic, thrombotic and proteolytic activities of viper venoms. Toxicon 1969; 6:175.
85. McNally, T, Conway GS, Jackson L, et al: Accidental envenomation by a Gaboon viper (*Bitis gabonica*): The haemostatic distur-

bances observed and investigation of in vitro haemostatic properties of whole venom. Trans R Soc Trop Med Hyg 1993; 87:66.
86. Clemens R, Lorenz R, Pukrittayakamee S: Effects of antithrombin III and antivenom on procoagulant activity of Russell's viper venom in a whole blood model. Southeast Asian J Trop Med Public Health 1995; 26:143.
87. Aung-Khim: The problem of snakebites in Burma. Snake 1980; 12:125.
88. Phillips RE, Theakston RDG, Warrell DA, et al: Paralysis, rhabdomyolysis and haemolysis caused by bites of Russell's viper (*Vipera russelli*) in Sri Lanka: Failure of Indian (Haffkine) antivenom. Q J Med 1988; 68:691.
89. Myint-Lwin, Warrell DA. Phillips RE, et al: Bites by Russell's viper (*Vipera russelli*) in Burma: Haemostatic, vascular and renal disturbances and responses to treatment. Lancet 1985; 2:1259.
90. Minton SA: Neurotoxic snake envenomation. Semin Neurol 1990; 10:52.
91. Hilligan R: Black mamba bites: A report of 2 cases. S Afr Med J 1987; 72:220.
92. Looareesuwan S, Viravan C, Warrell DA: Factors contributing to fatal snake bite in the rural tropics: Analysis of 46 cases in Thailand. Trans R Soc Trop Med Hyg 1988; 82:930.
93. Narita K, Membs D, Iwanaga S, et al: Primary structure of alpha bungarotoxin from *Bungarus multicinctus* venom. J Formosan Med Assoc 1972; 71:336.
94. Endo T, Tamiya N: Current view on the structure-function relationship of postsynaptic neurotoxins from snake venoms. Pharmacol Ther 1987; 34:403.
95. Kitchens CS, Van Mierop LHS: Envenomation by the Eastern coral snake (*Micrurus fulvius fulvius*). JAMA 1987; 258:1615.
96. Aitchison JM: Boomslang bite: Diagnosis and management. S Afr Med J 1990; 78:39.
97. Du Toit DM: Boomslang (*Dispholidus typus*) bite: Case report and review of diagnosis and management. S Afr Med J 1980; 57:507.
98. Russell FE, Bogert CM: Gila monster: Its biology, venom and bite—a review. Toxicon 1981; 19:341.
99. Tu AT: Biotoxicology of sea snake venoms. Ann Emerg Med 1987; 16:1023.
100. Sutherland SK, Coulter AR, Harris RD: The rationalisation of first aid measures for elapid snakebite. Lancet 1979; 1:183.
101. Sutherland SK: Treatment of snakebite. Aust Fam Physician 1990; 19:21.
102. Watt G, Theakston RDG, Hayes CG, et al: Positive response to edrophonium in patients with neurotoxic envenomation by cobras (*Naja naja philippinensis*). N Engl J Med 1986; 315:1444.
103. Russell FE: Marine toxins and venomous and marine plants and animals. Adv Marine Biol 1984; 21:60.
104. Halstead BW: Poisonous and Venomous Marine Animals. Vols 1-3. Washington, DC, U.S. Government Printing Office, 1965–1970.
105. Provasoli L: Recent progress—an overview. *In:* Toxic Dinoflagellate Blooms. Taylor DL, Seliger HH (Eds). New York, Elsevier/North Holland, 1979, p 1.
106. Sakamoto Y, Lockey RF, Krzanowski JJ: Shellfish and fish poisoning related to the toxic dinoflagellates. South Med J 1987; 80:866.
107. Halstead BW: Dangerous Marine Animals. Centerville, Md, Cornell Maritime Press, 1980.
108. Sweeney BM: The organisms. *In:* Toxic Dinoflagellate Blooms. Taylor DL, Seliger HH (Eds). New York, Elsevier/North Holland, 1979, p 23.
109. Saunders EW Jr: Intoxication from the seas: Ciguatera, scombroid and paralytic shellfish poisoning. Infect Dis Clin North Am 1987; 1:665.
110. Russell FE, Carlson RW: Animal toxins: Marine organisms. *In:* Biology Data Book. 2nd ed. Vol II. Altman PL, Dittmer DS (Eds). Bethesda, Md, Federation of American Societies for Experimental Biology, 1973, p 726.
111. Ritchie JM: Binding of tetrodotoxin and saxitoxin to sodium channels. Philos Trans R Soc Lond Biol Sci 1975; 270:319.
112. Kao, CY: Pharmacology of tetrodotoxin and saxitoxin. Fed Proc 1972; 32:1117.
113. Narahashi T: Mechanism of action of tetrodotoxin and saxitoxin on excitable membranes. Fed Proc 1972; 31:1124.
114. Withers NW: Ciguatera fish poisoning. Annu Rev Med 1981; 33:97.
115. Morris PD, Campbell DS, Freeman JI: Ciguatera fish poisoning: An outbreak associated with fish caught from North Carolina coastal waters. South Med J 1990; 83:379.
116. Cameron J, Caupra MF: The basis of the paradoxical disturbance of temperature perception in ciguatera poisoning. Clin Toxicol 1993; 31:571.
117. Williamson J: Ciguatera and mannitol: A successful treatment. Med J Aust 1990; 153:306.
118. Pearn JH, Lewis RJ, Ruff T, et al: Ciguatera and mannitol: Experience with a new treatment. Med J Aust 1989; 15:77.
119. Calvert GM, Hryhorczuk DO, Leikin JB: Treatment of ciguatera fish poisoning with amitriptyline and nifedipine. Clin Toxicol 1987; 25:423.
120. Hokama Y, Abad MA, Kimura LH: A rapid enzyme-immunoassay for the detection of ciguatoxin in contaminated fish tissues. Toxicon 1983; 21:817.
121. Dickinson G: Scombroid fish poisoning syndrome. Ann Emerg Med 1982; 11:487.
122. Morrow JD, Margolis GR, Rowland J, et al: Evidence that histamine is the causative toxin of scombroid-fish poisoning. N Engl J Med 1991; 324:716.
123. Blakesley ML: Scombroid poisoning: Prompt resolution of symptoms with cimetidine. Ann Emerg Med 1983; 12:104.
124. Auerbach PS: Persistent headache associated with scombroid poisoning: Resolution with oral cimetidine. J Wilderness Med 1990; 1:279.
125. Sims JK, Irei MY: Human Hawaiian marine sponge poisoning. Hawaii Med J 1979; 38:263.
126. Auerbach PS: Hazardous marine animals. Emerg Clin North Am 1984; 2:531.
127. Southcott RV, Coulter JR: The effects of the Southern Australian marine stinging sponges, *Neofibularia mordens*, and *Lissodendoryx sp.* Med J Aust 1971; 2:895.
128. Zervos SG: La maladie des pécheurs d'éponges nus. Paris Med 1934; 93:89.
129. Portier P, Richet C: De l'action anaphylactique de certains vénins. CR Soc Biol Paris 1902; 54:170.
130. Togias AG, Burnett JW, Kagey-Sobotka A, et al: Anaphylaxis after contact with a jellyfish. J Allergy Clin Immunol 1985; 75:672.
131. Cobbs CS, Gaur PK, Russo AJ, et al: Immunosorbent chromatography of sea nettle (*Chrysaora quinquecirrha*) venom and characterization of toxins. Toxicon 1983; 21:385.
132. Burnett JW, Calton GJ: The chemistry and toxicology of some venomous pelagic coelenterates. Toxicon 1983; 21:385.
133. Freeman SE, Turner RJ: Cardiovascular effects of toxins isolated from the cnidarian, *Chronex fleckeri southcott.* Br J Pharmacol 1971; 41:154.
134. Martin JC, Audley I: Cardiac failure following *Irukandji* envenomation. Med J Aust 1990; 153:164.
135. Burnett JW, Calton GJ: Jellyfish envenomation syndromes updated. Ann Emerg Med 1987; 16:100.
136. Stein MR, Marraccini JV, Rothschild NE, et al: Fatal Portuguese man-o'-war (*Physalia physalis*) envenomation. Ann Emerg Med 1989; 18:312.
137. Lumley J, Williamson JA, Fenner PJ, et al: Fatal envenomation by *Chironex fleckeri,* the North Australian box-jellyfish: The continuing search for lethal mechanisms. Med J Aust 1988; 128:527.
138. Auerbach PS: Current concepts: Marine envenomations. N Engl J Med 1991; 325:486.
139. Burnett JW, Rubinstein H, Calton GJ: First aid for jellyfish envenomation. South Med J 1983; 76:870.
140. Exton DR, Fenner PJ, Williamson JA: Cold packs: Effective topical analgesia in the treatment of painful stings by *Physalia* and other jellyfish. Med J Aust 1989; 151:625.
141. Burnett JW, Gean CJ, Calton GJ et al: The effect of verapamil on the cardiotoxic activity of Portuguese man-o'-war (*Physalia physalis*) and sea nettle (*Chrysaora quinquecirrha*) venoms. Toxicon 1985; 23:681.
142. Burnett JW, Calton GJ: Response of the box-jellyfish (*Chironex fleckeri*) cardiotoxin to intravenous administration of verapamil. Med J Aust 1983; 2:192.
143. Endean R, Sizemore DJ: The effectiveness of antivenom in countering the actions of the box-jellyfish (*Chironex fleckeri*) nematocyst toxins in mice. Toxicon 1988; 26:425.

144. Burnett JW, Othman IB, Endean R et al: Verapamil potentiation of *Chironex fleckeri* (box-jellyfish) antivenom. Toxicon 1990; 218:242.
145. Williamson JA, LeRay LE, Wohlfahrt M et al: Acute management of serious envenomation by box-jellyfish (*Chironex fleckeri*). Med J Aust 1984; 141:851.
146. Baden HP, Burnett JW: Injuries from sea urchins. South Med J 1977; 70:459.
147. Cracchiolo A III, Goldberg L: Local and systemic reactions to puncture injuries by the sea urchin spine and date palm thorn. Arthritis Rheum 1977; 20:1206.
148. Strauss MB, MacDonald RI: Hand injuries from sea urchin spines. Clin Orthop 1976; 114:216.
149. Fries SL: Mode of action of marine saponins on neuromuscular tissues. Fed Proc 1972; 31:1146.
150. Sutherland SK, Lane WR: Toxins and mode of envenomation of the common ringed or blue-banded octopus. Med J Aust 1969; 1:89.
151. Edmonds CG: Non-fatal case of blue-ringed octopus bite. Med J Aust 1969; 2:601.
152. Levine WC, Griffin PM, and the Gulf Coast Vibrio Working Group: Vibrio infections on the Gulf Coast: Results of the first year of regional surveillance. J Infect Dis 1993; 167:479.
153. Pollak SJ, Parris EJ III, Barrett TJ, et al: *Vibrio vulnificus* septicemia. Arch Intern Med 1983; 143:837.
154. Oda K, Araki K, Totoki T, Shibasaki H: Nerve conduction study of human tetrodotoxication. Neurology 1989; 39:743–745.
155. Deng J-F, Tominack RL, Chung H-M, Tsai W-J: Hypertension as an unusual feature in an outbreak of tetrodotoxin poisoning. Clin Toxicol 1991; 29:71–79.
156. Schaeffer RC Jr, Carlson RW, Russell FE: Some chemical properties of the venom of the scorpionfish, *Scorpaena guttata*. Toxicon 1971; 9:69.
157. Carlson RW, Schaeffer RC Jr, La Grange RG, et al: Some pharmacological properties of the venom of the scorpionfish *Scorpaena guttata*. Toxicon 1971; 9:379.
158. Carlson RW, Schaeffer RC Jr, Whigham H, et al: Some pharmacological properties of the venom of the scorpionfish *Scorpaena guttata* II. Toxicon 1973; 10:267.
159. Kizer KW, McKinney HE, Auerbach PS: Scorpaenidae envenomation. JAMA 1985; 253:807.
160. Trestrail JH, AL-Mahasneh QM: Lionfish sting experience of an inland poison center: A retrospective study of 23 cases. Vet Hum Toxicol 1989; 31:173.
161. Auerbach PS, McKinney HE, Rees RS, et al: Analysis of vesicle fluid following the sting of the lionfish *Pterois volitans*. Toxicon 1987; 25:1350.
162. Grainger CR: Occupational injuries due to stingrays. Trans R Soc Trop Med Hyg 1980; 74:408.
163. Grainger CR: Stingray injuries. Trans R Soc Med Hyg 1985; 79:443.
164. Cross TB: An unusual stingray injury. Med J Aust 1976; 2:947.
165. Fenner PJ, Williamson JA, Skinner RA: Fatal and nonfatal stingray envenomation. Med J Aust 1989; 151:621.
166. Wong RC, Hughes SE, Voorhees JJ: Spider bites. Arch Dermatol 1987; 128:98.
167. Wilson DC, King LE Jr: Spiders and spider bites. Dermatol Clin 1990; 8:277.
168. McCrone JE, Netzolff ML: An immunological and electrophoretical comparison of the venoms of the North American *Latrodectus* spiders. Toxicon 1965; 3:107.
169. Granata F, Paggi P, Frontali N: Effects of chromatographic fractions of black widow spider venom on in vitro biological systems. Toxicon 1972; 10:551.
170. Okamoto M, Longnecker HE, Riber WF, et al: Destruction of mammalian motor nerve terminal by black widow spider venom. Science 1971; 172:733.
171. Gorio A, Mauro A: Reversibility and mode of action of black widow spider venom on the vertebrate neuromuscular junction. Nature 1970; 225:701.
172. Pinto JEF, Rothlin RP, Dagross EE, et al: Peripheral adrenergic effect of *Latrodectus mactans* venom. Toxicon 1973; 11:395.
173. Baba A, Cooper JR: The action of black widow spider venom on cholinergic mechanisms in synaptosomes. J Neurochem 1980; 34:1369.
174. Rauber A: Black widow spider bites. J Toxicol Clin Toxicol 1984; 21:473.
175. Sutherland SK, Trinca JC: Survey of 2144 cases of red-back spider bites: Australia and New Zealand 1963–76. Med J Aust 1978; 2:620.
176. Maretic Z: Latrodectism: Variations in clinical manifestations provoked by *Latrodectus* species of spiders. Toxicon 1983; 21:457.
177. Clark RF, Wethern-Kestner S, Vance VM, et al: Clinical presentation and treatment of black widow spider envenomation: A review of 163 cases. Ann Emerg Med 1992; 21:782.
178. Vance M, Curry S, Gerkin R, et al: The "target" lesion: A pathognomonic sign of black widow spider (*Latrodectus* spp) envenomation. Vet Hum Toxicol 1986; 28:485.
179. Key GF: A comparison of calcium gluconate and methocarbamol (Robaxin) in the treatment of latrodectism (black widow spider envenomation). Am J Trop Med Hyg 1981; 30:273.
180. Ryan PJ: Preliminary report: Experience with the use of dantrolene sodium in the treatment of bites by the black widow spider *Latrodectus hesperus*. J Toxicol Clin Toxicol 1984; 21:487.
181. Geren CR, Chan TK, Howell DE, et al: Isolation and characterization of toxins from brown recluse spider venom (*Loxosceles reclusa*). Arch Biochem Biophys 1976; 174:90.
182. Geren CR, Chan TK, Howell DE, et al: Partial characterization of the low molecular weight fractions of the extract of the venom apparatus of the brown recluse spider and of its hemolymph. Toxicon 1975; 13:233.
183. Wright SW, Wrenn KD, Murray L, et al: Clinical presentation and outcome of brown recluse spider bite. Ann Emerg Med 1997; 30:28.
184. Forrester LJ, Barrett JG, Campbell BJ: Red blood cell lysis induced by the venom of the brown recluse spider: The role of sphingomyelinase D. Arch Biochem Biophys 1978; 187:355.
185. Anderson PC: Spider bites in the United States. Dermatol Clin 1997; 15:307.
186. Majeski JA, Durst GG: Necrotic arachnidism. South Med J 1976; 69:887.
187. Young VL, Pin PL: The brown recluse spider bite. Ann Plast Surg 1988; 210:447.
188. Wasserman GS, Anderson PC: Loxoscelism and necrotic arachnidism. J Toxicol Clin Toxicol 1984; 21:451.
189. Hollabaugh RS, Fernandes ET: Management of the brown recluse spider bite. J Pediatr Surg 1989; 24:126.
190. Rees R, Campbell D, Rieger E, et al: The diagnosis and treatment of brown recluse spider bites. Ann Emerg Med 1987; 16:945.
191. Auer AI, Hershey FB: Surgery for necrotic bites of the brown spider. Arch Surg 1974; 108:612.
192. Rees RS, Altenbern PD, Lynch JB, et al: Brown recluse spider bites. Ann Surg 1985; 202:659.
193. Rees RS, Shack B, Withers E, et al: Management of the brown recluse spider bite. Plast Reconstr Surg 1981; 68:768.
194. Wright SW, Wrenn KD, Murray L, Seger D: Clinical presentation and outcome of brown recluse spider bite. Ann Emerg Med 1997; 3:28–32.
195. King LE Jr, Rees RS: Dapsone treatment of a brown recluse spider bite. JAMA 1985; 254:2895.
196. Phillips S, Kohn M, Baker D, et al: Therapy of brown spider envenomations: A controlled trial of hyperbaric oxygen, dapsone and cyproheptadine. Ann Emerg Med 1995; 25:363.
197. Rimsza ME, Zimmerman DR, Bergeson PS: Scorpion envenomation. Pediatrics 1980; 66:298.
198. Efrati P: Epidemiology, symptomatology and treatment of Buthidae stings. *In:* Handbook of Experimental Pharmacology. Vol 40: Arthropod Venoms. Bettini S (Ed). Berlin, Springer-Verlag, 1978, p 312.
199. Guyffon M, Vachon M, Broglio N: Epidemiological and clinical characteristics of scorpion envenomation in Tunisia. Toxicon 1982; 20:337.
200. Dehesa-Davila M, Possani LD: Scorpionism and serotherapy in Mexico. Toxicon 1994; 32:1015.
201. Freire-Maia L, Campos JA, Amaral CF: Approaches to the treatment of scorpion envenomation. Toxicon 1994; 32:1009.
202. Wang GK, Strichartz GR: Purification and physiological characterization of neurotoxins from venoms of the scorpions *Centruroides sculpturatus* and *Lenurus quinquestriatus*. Mol Pharmacol 1983; 23:519.

203. Moss J, Thoa NB, Kopin IJ: On the mechanism of scorpion toxin-induced release of norepinephrine from peripheral adrenergic neurons. J Pharmacol Exp Ther 1974; 190:39.
204. Meves H, Rubly N, Watt DD: Effect of toxins isolated from the venom of the scorpion *Centruroides sculpturatus* on the Na currents of the node of Ranvier. Pflugers Arch 1982; 393:56.
205. Curry SC, Vance MV, Ryan PJ, et al: Envenomation by the scorpion *Centruroides sculpturatus*. J Toxicol Clin Toxicol 1984; 21:417.
206. Berg RA, Tarantino MD: Envenomation by the scorpion *Centruroides exilicauda (C. sculpturatus)*: Severe and unusual manifestations. Pediatrics 1991; 87:930.
207. Bond GR: Antivenin administration for Centruroides scorpion sting: Risks and benefits. Ann Emerg Med 1992; 21:788.
208. Rachesky IJ, Banner W, Dansky J, et al: Treatment for *Centruroides exilicauda* envenomation. Am J Dis Child 1984; 138:1136.
209. Gueron M, Sofer S: Vasodilators and calcium blocking agents as treatment of cardiovascular manifestations of human scorpion envenomation. Toxicon 1990; 28:127.
210. Bawaskar HS, Bawaskar PH: Prazosin for vasodilator treatment of acute pulmonary oedema due to scorpion sting. Ann Trop Med Parasitol 1987; 81:719.
211. Habermann E: Bee and wasp venoms: The biochemistry and pharmacology of their peptides and enzymes are reviewed. Science 1972; 177:314.
212. Piek T: Neurotoxins from venoms of the Hymenoptera: Twenty-five years of research in Amsterdam. Comp Biochem Physiol (C) 1990; 96:223.
213. Stafford CT, Hutto LS, Rhoades RB, et al: Imported fire ant as a health hazard. South Med J 1989; 82:515.
214. Owens VJ, Malloy C, Schuman S, et al: Underrecognition of morbidity from stings of the red imported fire ant in the Southeastern United States. Public Health Nurs 1990; 7:88.
215. deShazo RD, Butcher BT, Banks WA: Reactions to the stings of the imported fire ant. N Engl J Med 1990; 323:462.
216. Bloom FL, Del Mastro PL: Imported fire ant death: A documented case report. J Fla Med Assoc 1984; 71:87.
217. Rhoades RB, Stafford CT, James FK Jr: Survey of fatal anaphylactic reactions to imported fire ants stings: Report of the Fire Ant Subcommittee of the American Academy of Allergy and Immunology. J Allergy Clin Immunol 1989; 84:159.
218. MacConnell JG, Blum MS, Fales HM: Alkaloid from fire ant venom: Identification and synthesis. Science 1970; 168:840.
219. MacConnell JG, Blum MS, Buren WF, et al: Fire ant venoms: Chemotaxonomic correlations with alkaloidal compositions. Toxicon 1976; 14:69.
220. Javors MA, Zhou W, Maas JW, et al: Effects of fire ant venom alkaloids on platelet and neutrophil function. Life Sci 1993; 53:1105.
221. Ford JL, Dolen WK, Feger TA, et al: Evaluation of an in vitro assay for fire ant venom-specific IgE. J Allergy Clin Immunol 1997; 100:425.
222. Moffitt JE, Barker JR, Stafford CT: Management of fire ant allergy: Results of a survey. Ann Allergy Asthma Immunol 1997; 79:125.
223. Ponder RD, Stafford CT, Kiefer CR, et al: Development of an enzyme-linked immunosorbent assay for measurement of fire ant venom-specific IgE. Ann Allergy 1994; 72:329.

18

Anaphylactic Reactions

Marilyn T. Haupt, MD • Tisha K. Fujii, DO
Richard W. Carlson, MD, PhD, FCCM

Anaphylaxis is a life-threatening, acute inflammatory, dramatic clinical response to environmental stimuli. In susceptible individuals, these stimuli elicit a complex sequence of cellular and biochemical events that produce the critical clinical sequelae that may lead to upper airway edema, bronchospasm, increases in vascular permeability, acute respiratory failure, and circulatory shock. Untreated or improperly managed reactions are likely to be fatal, but prompt recognition and early treatment may be lifesaving. Acute-care physicians must be able to identify the acute presentation of anaphylaxis and to distinguish these reactions from other acute cardiopulmonary crises. The immediate management of these events should proceed rapidly and automatically. After initial management, the critical care specialist must be prepared to treat the advanced manifestations of anaphylaxis by using a physiologic approach.

The number of agents producing anaphylaxis is extensive. Commonly implicated agents are cited in Table 18–1.

HISTORICAL BACKGROUND

The first record of anaphylaxis was believed to have been carved in wood in the form of hieroglyphics in 2641 BC (Fig. 18–1). Although the interpretation of this writing has been controversial, one theory is that King Menes of Egypt died suddenly after a wasp sting.[1–3] A more basic understanding of anaphylaxis was imparted by the work of two French investigators, Portier and Richet.[4] These physiologists demonstrated that a first injection of sea anemone venom into a dog was innocuous, although a subsequent injection was fatal. They used the term *anaphylactique*, or reverse protection, to describe this phenomenon, and contrasted these reactions with the attenuated or tachyphylactic response that commonly protects subjects from reintroduced antigens.

Subsequent laboratory experiments and clinical studies further defined the histopathologic and gross anatomic changes associated with anaphylactic reactions as well as the complex sequence of immunologic, cellular, and biochemical events. More recent landmarks in the understanding of this acute allergic emergency include (1) the identification and recognition of the role of immunoglobulin E (IgE),[5] (2) the characterization of slow-reacting substance of anaphylaxis (SRS) into a group of mediators now known to be *leukotrienes* (LTs),[6, 7] (3) the emerging knowledge of cytokines, and (4) the characterization of granule-derived and membrane-derived mediators from mast cells and basophils.[8–11]

DEFINITIONS

The *classic anaphylactic response* refers to an IgE-mediated allergic reaction, which is also referred to as a *type I reaction* according to the classification of Gell and Coombs. Type I reactions have also been referred to as reagin-dependent reactions, immediate hypersensitivity reactions, and cytotropic responses. The anaphylactic reaction has similarities to other type I reactions, such as allergic rhinitis, hives and urticaria,

TABLE 18–1. Agents Commonly Implicated in Anaphylactic and Anaphylactoid Reactions

Class	Agent
Antibiotics	Penicillin and penicillin analogs, cephalosporins, tetracyclines, erythromycin
Nonsteroidal anti-inflammatory agents	Salicylates, aminopyrine
Narcotic analgesics	Morphine, codeine, meprobamate
Local anesthetics	Procaine, lidocaine, cocaine
General anesthetics	Thiopental
Anesthetic adjuncts	Succinylcholine, tubocurarine
Blood products, antisera, and related substances	Red blood cell, white blood cell, and platelet transfusions; gamma globulin; rabies, tetanus, and diphtheria antitoxin, antilymphocyte globulin, snake and spider antivenom, protamine
Diagnostic agents	Iodinated radiographic contrast agents
Foods	Eggs, milk, nuts, legumes (peanuts, soybeans, kidney beans), fish, shellfish
Venoms	Bees, wasps, hornets, fire ants, scorpions
Enzymes and other biologicals	Acetylcysteine, pancreatic enzyme supplements, streptokinase, chymopapain, latex
Extracts of potential allergens used in desensitization	Pollen, food, venoms
Chemotherapeutic agents	Cisplatin, cyclophosphamide, daunorubicin, methotrexate
Other drugs or agents	Protamine, chlorpropamide, parenteral iron, iodides, thiazide diuretics, dialysis membranes, angiotensin-converting enzyme inhibitors

and allergic asthma. In these reactions, an immunologic sequence of events involving antigen and IgE-specific effector cells (tissue-based mast cells and circulating basophils) results in the release of inflammatory mediators. Unlike other type I reactions, however, anaphylaxis is generalized rather than restricted to local sites such as the nasal mucosa, airways, or skin. Agents that typically produce classic anaphylactic reactions include the penicillins, stings from the order Hymenoptera (bees, wasps, hornets, and fire ants), egg albumin vaccines and heterologous and homologous sera, streptokinase, and latex rubber.

Anaphylactoid, or *pseudo-allergic, reactions* have clinical manifestations identical to those of classic anaphylactic reactions. However, a non–IgE-mediated release of mast cell–derived and basophil-derived mediators is implicated in these disorders. Typical agents producing anaphylactoid reactions include radiographic contrast dyes, dialysis membranes, opiates, angiotensin-converting enzyme (ACE) inhibitors, salicylates, and other nonsteroidal anti-inflammatory agents (NSAIDs).[12] Exercise has also been associated with an anaphylactoid clinical response.[13]

Idiopathic anaphylactoid reactions may also be clinically identical to anaphylactic reactions, but neither a specific inciting agent nor immune mediation has been demonstrated. These events are rare and seldom fatal. Nighttime and postprandial occurrences are typical. Idiopathic anaphylactoid reactions typically occur in young adults who frequently have multiple allergies. Complete remissions are common.[14, 15]

Factitious anaphylaxis refers to the simulation of anaphylaxis. This illness is believed to represent a type of Munchausen's syndrome. In some instances, a patient may claim a response to an antigen such as bee venom. In other instances, the syndrome is confused with idiopathic anaphylaxis because an inciting agent is not identified.[16]

Although the severity of an anaphylactic reaction can usually be predicted by the rapidity of onset, late and recurrent manifestations may occur. These are termed "second wave" reactions, or "biophasic anaphylaxis." These responses are distinct from persistent or progressive responses.[17, 18]

INCIDENCE AND SIGNIFICANCE

The true incidence of anaphylactic and anaphylactoid reactions is difficult to determine because of their spontaneous, unpredictable nature and because of the inability to distinguish these reactions from other acute events, such as vasovagal episodes and acute cardiac, pulmonary, and metabolic crises (Table 18–2). The hospitalized patient may be at significant risk for serious allergic reactions because of the number of drugs and biologicals used in this setting. Up to 0.05% of such patients may experience these reactions. The most frequently reported anaphylactic episodes involve antibiotics, which are usually of the penicillin and cephalosporin β-lactam varieties.[19-21] Penicillin allergy is prevalent in approximately 2% of individuals, but the reported incidence of anaphylaxis is considerably variable. It is estimated that 400 to 500 deaths occur annually from penicillin anaphylaxis.[22, 23] Adults from 20 to 40 years of age are most commonly affected.[24] Most penicillin is metabolized to the penicilloyl hapten, the major determinant. Some reports suggest that 0.01% of patients have anaphylactic reactions to penicillin, and up to 9% of these reactions are fatal.

Anaphylaxis caused by the cephalosporins has also been described.[25] In patients with a history of allergic reactions to penicillin, a 3% to 7% allergic reaction rate to cephalosporin is expected. Precise information on the incidence of anaphylaxis in response to newer β-lactam antibiotics (e.g., aztreonam and imipenem) awaits additional clinical experience with these drugs; however, extensive in vivo cross-reactivity with penicillins characterizes the bicyclic carbapenem drugs, which are represented by imipenem.[21] Therefore, a significant incidence of anaphylaxis from this class of antibiotics is likely

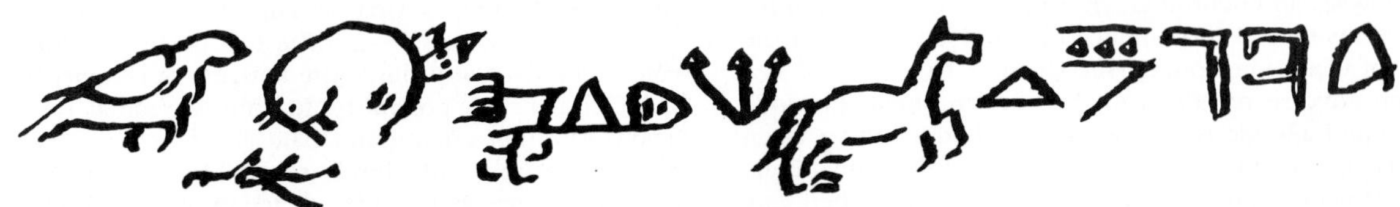

Figure 18–1. The death of the King of Egypt, Menes, is depicted in hieroglyphs carved in wood. Translation: "Fate pierced [him] by a wasp, the King of the Two Crowns of Manshu. This board tablet set up of hanging wood is dedicated [to his memory]."

TABLE 18–2. Conditions That May Resemble Anaphylactic Reactions

1. Acute cardiac events
2. Acute congestive failure induced by hyperosmolar agents (radiocontrast agents, mannitol)
3. Acute drug overdose
4. Carcinoid syndrome
5. Chinese restaurant syndrome (monosodium glutamate reaction)
6. Factitious anaphylaxis
7. Foreign body aspiration/upper airway obstruction
8. Hereditary angioedema
9. Pulmonary embolism
10. Spontaneous pneumothorax
11. Seizure disorder
12. Status asthmaticus
13. Upper airway obstruction
14. Vasovagal reaction

in patients who have had allergic reactions to penicillin. In contrast, the monocyclic β-lactam antibiotics represented by aztreonam show no cross-reactivity with penicillin.

Prior to the implementation of widespread pretreatment of sensitive individuals with corticosteroids and histamine antagonists, approximately 200 to 800 deaths per year from acute reactions to iodinated radiographic contrast agents were estimated.[26] Most of these reactions are characterized by typical symptoms of anaphylaxis.[27] Although these reactions were seen in less than 2% of individuals taking these agents, the high mortality rate was attributed to the large number of contrast agents used each year. Fortunately, the incidence of these serious and occasionally fatal reactions has been dramatically reduced by prophylaxis with steroids and antihistamines and by the increased use of non-ionic contrast material, which is associated with lower reaction rates.[28]

Insect stings account for more deaths resulting from anaphylaxis in the United States than do all other types of venoms. Up to 4% of the United States population report systemic reactions to insect stings. Annually, approximately 60 to 80 deaths are reported from insect stings, but many deaths are probably unreported or not identified as due to insect stings. Most fatal stings are caused by insects from the order Hymenoptera.[23, 24, 29, 30] Fire ants originally imported from South America to the United States have proliferated in the rural and urban portions of the southern Gulf and southwestern states. These insects have been responsible for a significant number of immediate hypersensitivity reactions. Fire ants are aggressive and in some regions sting up to 58% of residents yearly. It has been estimated that anaphylaxis occurs in up to 1% of fire ant stings.

Snake bites probably account for approximately a dozen deaths per year in the United States. Snake venom poisoning produces clinical signs and symptoms that may resemble some features of anaphylaxis, especially injuries by pit vipers (rattlesnakes, moccasins, and copperheads). However, snake bite victims experience additional problems related to the variety of enzymes, proteins, and peptides contained in the venom. These problems may include local tissue necrosis, coagulopathies, hemolysis, and neurologic transmission defects. Anaphylactic reactions may also be induced by antivenin used in the treatment of venom poisoning (see Chapter 17).

Although adverse reactions to food are frequent, the incidence of type I allergic reactions to foods is difficult to ascertain because many reported reactions are probably nonallergic in nature. However, allergic reactions to food have been estimated to characterize 1% to 2% of adverse food reactions in children.[31] Lower estimates for adult food hypersensitivity have been suggested.[32, 33] A small number of these allergic reactions may have features of systemic anaphylaxis.

Anaphylactic reactions, as well as other type I allergic reactions, are characteristically observed in susceptible, genetically predisposed individuals. The evolution of these complex IgE-mediated reactions has been a subject of considerable speculation. A popular theory is that a system of localized IgE-mediated reactions to parasitic antigens conveyed a survival advantage to individuals exposed to parasites. Several observations support this view.[34] In one study, children infected with a wide variety of helminthic parasites exhibited elevated serum IgE concentrations.[35] In another study, humans infected with *Ascaris* worms had decreased worm burdens if they produced large quantities of IgE.[36] In addition, the areas of high IgE synthesis in laboratory subjects correspond to the sites of entry of many parasites, including the lymphoid tissue of the respiratory tract, gastrointestinal tract, and skin.

These observations suggest that, when localized, IgE-mediated reactions may be important in combating parasitic antigens as well as other antigens. Anaphylaxis, a systemic reaction, may thus represent a failure to restrict the IgE-mediated reactions to local areas. This failure may be genetically determined or acquired. The resultant generalized release of mediators, triggered by the IgE interaction with antigens, mast cells, and basophils, leads to increases in vascular permeability, vasodilation, and impaired gas exchange. These effects are clearly decompensatory and threaten survival.

SEQUENCE OF EVENTS LEADING TO ANAPHYLAXIS

Immunologic Events

Following initial exposure of antigen to a susceptible individual, antigen-specific IgE molecules are elaborated. Anaphylaxis occurs when the antigen is reintroduced. A period of several weeks is typically required between the first and subsequent exposure to antigen for a clinically significant reaction to develop. The site of reintroduction may be the skin, respiratory tract, or gastrointestinal tract. Introduction of antigen by intramuscular and intravenous routes may characterize the administration of drugs or venoms.

The antigens that produce classic anaphylaxis are usually small bivalent proteins of 10 to 70 kilodaltons (kD). *Haptens*, small chemicals that combine with a host protein, may also function as antigens.[37] The reactive anhydrides or quinones found in industrial chemicals as well as the β-lactam group of the penicillins and cephalosporins appear to function as haptens by directly conjugating to protein. Penicillin may become antigenic by directly reacting with amino acid groups or by reacting with these groups after spontaneous conversion to penicillenic acid. Other drugs (e.g., acetaminophen, isonizid, and hydralazine) may become haptens after enzymatic conversion in the liver or in other organs.[38] Anaphylactic reactions to polysaccharides (e.g., dextrans and hydroxyethyl starches) have also been described but are infrequent.

For a more complete description of the subcellular events that are involved in anaphylaxis, the reader is referred to texts and monographs on immunology.[12, 39, 40] IgE, like other immunoglobulins, is composed of two identical heavy chains and two identical kappa or lambda light chains linked by disulfide bonds (Fig. 18–2). The Fab portion of the IgE molecule recognizes and binds the antigen. Specificity for antigen is located in the polymorphic amino-terminal region of the heavy and light chain pairs. The Fc or carboxy terminal portion of the molecule binds reversibly to high-affinity FcεRI receptors expressed on the surface of mast cells and basophils (Fig. 18–3). The FcεRI consists of an alpha chain that binds to the Fc portion of IgE.[40, 41]

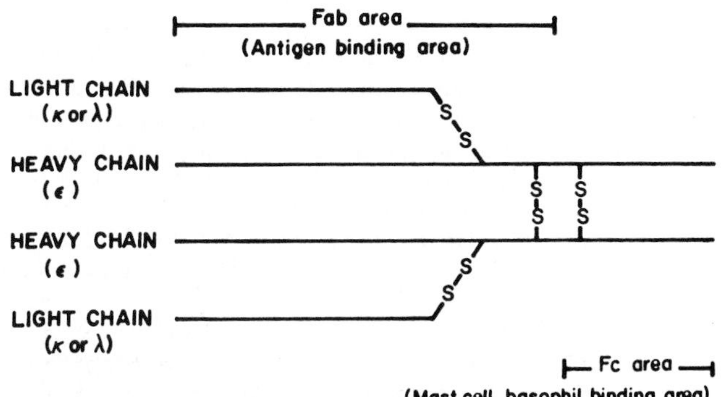

Figure 18–2. An immunoglobulin E (IgE) molecule, composed of four polypeptide chains linked by disulfide bonds, is illustrated. The heavy chains, or epsilon (ε) chains, are unique to IgE. The light chains may be kappa (κ) or lambda (λ) chains and are also characteristic of other immunoglobulins. Antigen binding takes place at the Fab area. The Fc area binds to mast cells or basophils.

The combination of IgE with antigen sets the stage for a sequence of events leading to the release of biochemical mediators that produce the clinical syndrome of anaphylaxis. The bivalent antigen, by cross-bridging of IgE and FcεRI molecules, triggers the chemical reactions that result in the release of mediators from intracellular granules and from membrane-based phospholipids. Bridging of only a few hundred IgE molecules is required to initiate cell activation and mediator release.[42]

An immunologic basis for anaphylaxis without mediation by IgE has also been described. Immunoglobulins of the IgE class may combine with antigens to produce an antigen-antibody complex, which activates complement. Activated complement results in the generation of anaphylatoxins C3a and C5a. These components affect the release of mediators from mast cells and produce clinical symptoms typical of anaphylaxis. The IgG-mediated reactions are classified as *type III reactions,* according to the classification of Gell and Coombs, and have previously been termed *Arthus' reactions*. IgA-deficient individuals may exhibit these reactions after blood transfusions. When blood is transfused, anti-IgA (of the IgG class) to the IgA in the blood product is formed. The anti-IgA–IgA combination produced after a subsequent transfusion leads to the activation of complement, generation of C3a and C5a, and anaphylactic symptoms. Approximately 1 in 700 individuals is IgA-deficient, and 40% have class-specific anti-IgA. Therefore, a considerable number of people are susceptible to anaphylactic reactions to blood transfusion.[37, 43] Anaphylaxis to protamine is also thought to be an IgG-mediated response.[44]

Anaphylaxis as well as other type I allergic reactions may be followed by *late-phase reactions*. These reactions may occur from 6 to 12 hours after the immediate reaction and are characterized by the infiltration of a variety of cells into areas of antigen introduction. The cells include polymorphonuclear cells as well as mast cells and basophils. A second wave of mediator release ensues and may lead to a recurrence or exacerbation of anaphylactic symptoms.[18]

Nonimmunologic Events

A variety of non-IgE-mediated stimuli initiate anaphylactoid reactions. The mechanisms leading to the nonimmunologic release of mediators, however, remain the subject of ongoing investigation. There is emerging evidence that several pathways from stimulus to mediator release may characterize the anaphylactoid response.

In some reactions, the surface receptors of mast cells and basophils appear to be directly activated by the offending agent. A direct stimulation of these cells is believed to initiate the anaphylactoid response to iodinated radiographic contrast agents, opiates, curare, tubocurarine, and highly charged polyanionic antibiotics. Physical stimuli (heat, cold, exercise) and hyperosmolar stimuli (radiographic contrast agents, dextran, mannitol, 50% dextrose) may also produce reactions by directly stimulating mast cells and basophils.

Aspirin and other NSAIDs are thought to produce anaphylactoid reactions through the inhibition of cyclooxygenase. It has been postulated that this inhibition facilitates the production of lipoxygenase-derived mediators. These mediators, which include the LTs and related compounds, produce bronchospasm and vascular permeability defects that are typical of anaphylaxis. Other theories accounting for aspirin sensitivity have been proposed, such as direct stimulation of mast cells, platelets, or eosinophils and activation of the complement cascade.[45] Up to 50% of patients with sensitivity to aspirin exhibit sensitivity to the yellow dye tartrazine, which is frequently used as food coloring (FD & C Yellow No. 5).[46] Al-

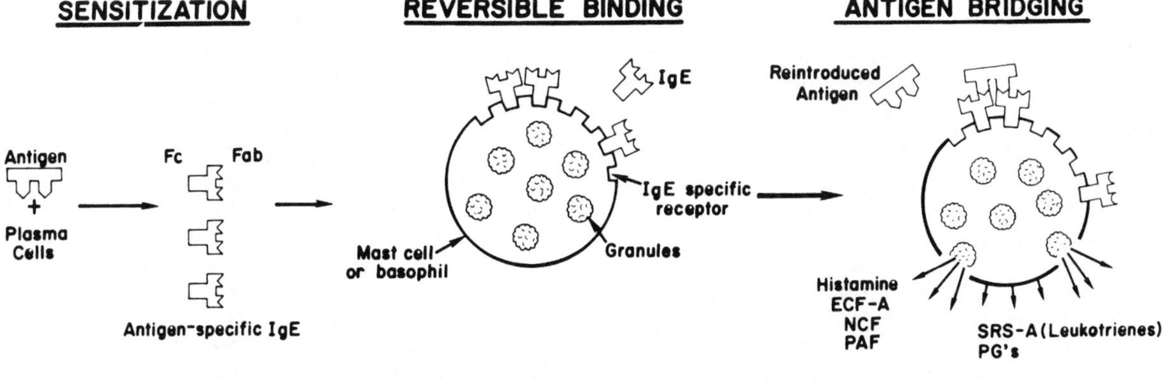

Figure 18–3. Sequence of events leading to mediator release. The initial exposure of antigen to plasma cells, termed "sensitization," leads to the synthesis of antigen-specific IgE. The Fc portion of the IgE molecule binds reversibly to receptors on mast cells and basophils. When antigen is reintroduced, it cross-links two cell-bound IgE molecules (also termed "antigen bridging"). This bridging initiates a sequence of biochemical events in the cell leading to the release of mediators from granules and from the cell wall. ECF-A = eosinophil chemotactic factor of anaphylaxis; NCF = neutrophil chemotactic factor; PAF = platelet-activating factor; SRS-A = slow-reacting substance of anaphylaxis; PG's = prostaglandins.

though the chemical structure of tartrazine is similar to that of several NSAIDs, the mechanism for anaphylaxis to this chemical also remains unclear.

Cellular Characteristics, Actions, and Interactions

Mast cells and *basophils* are important components of the anaphylactic response because of their role in the release of biochemical mediators that produce both local and systemic abnormalities.[41, 47, 48] There are characteristic differences between these cells. Mast cell precursors can be found in embryonic tissue and the thymus. Basophil precursors are found in the bone marrow. Mast cells are more abundant than basophils and reside in the connective tissue of submucosal and subcutaneous tissues. Basophils are usually found circulating in the blood but have also been identified in the nasal and bronchial mucosa in patients with hypersensitivity disease of the respiratory tract.[41, 49]

Mast cells are crucial to anaphylactic reactions. There are at least two types of mast cells: MC_T and MC_{TC}. MC_T cells are involved with the immune system and are increased in allergic and parasitic disease. These cells are decreased in patients with acquired immunodeficiency syndrome (AIDS) and chronic immunodeficiency diseases.[48] The MC_T cells also have greater levels of tryptase and are found predominantly in mucosal surfaces. Mast cells are now believed to play a major role not only in hypersensitivity reactions but also in many other *mast cell–leukocyte cytokine cascade reactions* for both acute and chronic disorders.[47]

In spite of these differences in origin and location, major functional differences between mast cells and basophils have not been identified. Both cells have many structural and biochemical similarities. In addition to specific receptors for the Fc portion of IgE, both cells have granules that bind basic dyes. These granules contain *histamine*, a major mediator in anaphylaxis, as well as histidine decarboxylase, an enzyme responsible for the synthesis of histamine. Mast cells contain up to 1 pg per cell of histamine. *Tryptase* is a major cell neutral serine protease in mast cells. This tetrameric endopeptidase is stored in a fully active form in the granules. There are two forms of tryptase: α and β. Tryptase cleaves bronchodilator peptides, vasoactive intestinal polypeptide (VIP), and peptide histidine methionine.[48] Thus, tryptase is involved in sensitization of bronchial responsiveness, kallikrein-like activity affecting collagen and fibronectin, mitogenic effects for fibroblasts and epithelial cells, granulocyte chemoattractant, and up-regulation of intercellular adhesion molecule. Heparin and other proteoglycans are also found in mast cells. Approximately 75% of the total proteoglycans in mast cells is heparin, with 25% as chondroitin sulfates. *Chymase*, another protease, is stored in an active form in granules.

The primary mediators are derived from the granules as well as from the membranes of these cells. It was previously thought that release of arachidonic acid and activation of cyclooxygenase or 5-lipoxygenase to form prostagladins (PGs) or LTs occurred primarily on the plasma membrane. However, these processes appear to occur on the nuclear membrane, so that PG and LT release is initially intracellular.

Eosinophils are bone marrow–derived leukocytes with acidophilic granules. They migrate to the site of allergen introduction in anaphylaxis as well as in other type I allergic reactions. Eosinophils dwell primarily in tissues but may also be found in the blood. A variety of chemotactic factors attract eosinophils, including mast cell–derived and basophil-derived chemotactic factors, antigen-antibody complexes, complement, and histamine. The granules of eosinophils contain a variety of mediators, including the cationic proteins, which are toxic to helminthic parasites. Eosinophils also elaborate substances that inactivate LTs and histamine.[12, 29, 41, 50] The role played by eosinophils in acute allergic emergencies remains unclear. Although the inactivation of LTs and histamine may dampen the inflammmatory response associated with anaphylaxis, the antiparasitic properties of eosinophilic granular proteins may exacerbate local tissue injury.

Platelets and *polymorphonuclear neutrophils* (PMNs) respond to the release of mast cell-derived and basophil-derived chemotactic factors as well as to the tissue injury produced during the anaphylactic response. These cells also release an abundant variety of inflammatory mediators. The significance and extent of the participation of these cells in anaphylaxis remain poorly defined, but, PMNs may be responsible, in part, for recurrent or late-phase anaphylactic episodes.

Primary Mediators of Anaphylaxis

Mediators derived from mast cell and basophils are termed *primary mediators* to distinguish them from secondary mediators. *Secondary mediators* may be defined as substances released from other leukocytes and from cascading biochemical pathways after primary mediator release. Primary mediators may be further classified into *preformed mediators*, such as tryptase, chymase, and histamine, which are stored in the intracellular granules, and *newly synthesized mediators*, such as those derived from the metabolism of arachidonic acid. The physiologic characteristics of the major primary mediators are listed in Table 18–3.

Histamine is a primary granule-derived mediator that has been studied extensively.[41, 51] It is regarded as a prototypic mediator of anaphylaxis. Histamine stimulates both histamine H_1 and H_2 receptors located on the surfaces of vascular and bronchial smooth muscle cells. Stimulation of histamine H_1 receptors causes precapillary arteriolar dilation, contraction of postcapillary venules, and the formation of intercellular gaps between capillary endothelial cells. These changes increase capillary hydrostatic pressure and permeability, encouraging movement of plasma from the intravascular space to the interstitium. Histamine H_1 receptor stimulation is associated with bronchial smooth muscle contraction. Histamine H_2 receptor stimulation is associated with vasodilation, enhanced mucus secretion, increases in heart rate and mycardial contractility, inhibition of eosinophils, increased gastric acid secretion, and inhibition of T cells. The vasoactive and cardiac effects of histamine H_2 receptor stimulation are believed to play important roles in the clinical manifestations of anaphylaxis. Arachidonic acid metabolism via the lipoxygenase pathway leads to the LTs, a family of potent mediators formerly known as "slow-reacting substances of anaphylaxis."

Additional primary mediators modulate the cellular response in anaphylaxis and have hydrolytic, proteolytic, and cytotoxic activity. Examples of these other primary mediators include tryptase, heparin, chymase, chymotryptase, kininogenase, acid hydrolases, and cathepsin G.

Newly formed primary mediators are also released during anaphylaxis. Arachidonic acid metabolism via the cyclooxygenase pathway leads to the production of PGD_2 and $PGF_{2\alpha}$, which have bronchoconstrictive effects. PGD_2 is one of the most significant products of cyclooxygenase activity of the mast cell. Lipoxygenase products include the sulfidopeptide LTs, such as LTC_4 and its derivatives LTD_4 and LTE_4. LTs may have more profound effects on bronchospasm than histamine does. Release of arachidonic acid products appears to vary for the gut, lung, or skin.[41] Platelet-activating factor (PAF) is another lipid mediator released from mast cells.

Cytokines are formed and secreted by inflammatory cells during allergic reactions. These substances modulate the im-

TABLE 18–3. Primary Mediators Produced by Mast Cells and Basophils and Their Physiologic Effects

Mediator	Physiologic Effect
Histamine	Histamine H_1 receptor stimulation
	Bronchial smooth muscle contraction
	Increased vascular permeability
	Cardiac arrhythmias
	Increased mucus secretion
	Vasoactive effects (vasodilation, vasoconstriction)
	Histamine H_2 receptor stimulation
	Increased vascular permeability
	Increased mucus and gastric acid secretion
	Activation of inhibitory lymphocytes
	Histamine H_3 receptor stimulation
	Inhibition of histamine synthesis and release
Platelet-activating factor	Increased vascular permeability
	Bronchospasm
	Aggregation and activation of platelets
	Attraction of neutrophils and eosinophils
Eosinophil chemotactic factors	Attraction of eosinophils
Neutrophil chemotactic factors	Attraction of neutrophils
Arachidonic acid metabolites (COX1, COX2)	Bronchoconstriction
Prostaglandin D_2	Potentiation of leukocyte migration
Prostaglandine E_2	Bronchodilation
Prostaglandin $F_2\alpha$	Bronchoconstriction
LTC_4, LTD_4, LTE_4	Bronchoconstriction
	Increased vascular permeability
LTB_4	Attraction of neutrophils and eosinophils
Enzymes	
Serine proteases, TAME, including tryptase chymase,	Degradation of parasitic and host tissue
carboxypeptidase A, sulfatases, exoglycosidases	Interaction with complement components, coagulation cascade, and kinin system
Oxidative enzymes	
Superoxide dismutase	Inactivation of O_2 and associated cytotoxic effects
	Inactivate cytotoxic effects of H_2O_2
Peroxidase	May inactivate LTC_4
Heparin and other proteoglycans	Anticoagulant activity
	Anticomplement activity
	Assistance in repair of injured tissues
Adenosine	Bronchospasm
	Mast cell degranulation regulation
Serotonin	Vasoactive effects
Cytokines IL-4, IL-5, IL-6, IL-8, IL-13, TNF-α, MIP-1α, basic fibroblastic growth factor	Immune and inflammatory modulation

TNF = tumor necrosis factor; LTC = leukotriene; H_2O_2 = hydrogen peroxide; O_2 = oxygen; TAME = tosyl-L-arginine methylesterase; COX = cyclooxygenase; MIP = macrophage inflammatory protein.

mune response. A variety of cytokine-related processes occur during anaphylaxis, including up-regulation of the IgE response, enhancement or induction of basophil recruitment, and mediator production. Interleukins (IL-3, IL-4, IL-5, IL-6, IL-8, IL-13), B-fibroblast growth factor (B-FGF), and tumor necrosis factor (TNF-α) and others are involved in these processes. For IgE reactions, mast cells are a significant source of TNF-α.[10, 11, 41] Accordingly, mast cells are critical for the development of the mast cell–leukocyte cytokine cascade, which serves to perpetuate tissue reactions and damage.[11, 47, 48]

Regulation of Primary Mediator Release

The release of primary mediators from mast cells and basophils is an energy-requiring process, which may be modified by intracellular levels of adenosine 3′,5′-cyclic monophosphate (cAMP), guanosine 3′,5′-cyclic monophosphate (cGMP), calcium and other bivalent cations, and agents that affect microtubular function. Pharmacologic agents that favorably alter the levels of these modulators are used in the treatment of anaphylaxis (Table 18–4). Agents that increase intracellular levels of cAMP, for example, inhibit the release of mediators and are associated with clinical improvement. These include beta$_2$ agonists, such as epinephrine and metaproterenol, which increase cAMP by stimulating adenylate cyclase. Methylxanthines, such as aminophylline and theophylline, increase intracellular cAMP levels by inhibiting phosphodiesterase, although experimental data suggest that this effect is minimal at therapeutic concentrations.[50]

Mediator release from mast cells and basophils is associated

TABLE 18–4. Pharmacologic Modulation of Mediator Release

Inhibit release
Beta-adrenergic drugs (↑ cAMP)
Phosphodiesterase inhibitors (↑ cAMP)
Anticholinergic drugs (↓ cGMP)
Glucagon (↑ cAMP)
Enhance release
β-Blockers (↓ cAMP)
α-Adrenergic drugs (↓ cAMP)
Cholinergic drugs (↑ cGMP)

cAMP = cyclic adenosine monophosphate; cGMP = cyclic guanidine monophosphate.

with an influx of calcium and may be inhibited by calcium channel blockers. Other bivalent cations, such as magnesium and manganese, may also enhance mediator release.[52]

Secondary Mediators

The release of primary mediators from mast cells and basophils sets the stage for involvement by *secondary mediators*. Secondary mediators of anaphylaxis include products of enzyme-dependent, cascading biochemical pathways. In addition, the products of neutrophils, platelets, and eosinophils activated by mast cell–derived and basophil-derived chemotactic factors may be regarded as secondary mediators.

The activated complement system generates highly reactive mediators with a variety of pathophysiologic effects. Activation of both the classic and alternative pathways has been observed in anaphylaxis. The anaphylatoxins C3a and C5a are potent mediators that contract smooth muscle; increase vascular permeability; attract neutrophils, macrophages, and monocytes; and injure cellular membranes. C3a and C5a also stimulate additional mediator release from mast cells and basophils.[53, 54] Complement components C6, C7, C8, and C9 cause further membrane damage. Additionally, C3 binds to receptors on eosinophils and may modulate the effector functions of these cells.[51, 55]

The coagulation cascade and fibrinolytic systems are activated during anaphylaxis when factor XII (Hageman's factor) is exposed to the subendothelial collagen of injured vessels. Activation of all of these cascades produces intravascular coagulation, production of oxygen radicals, and additional tissue injury. Activated factor XII also stimulates the kinin system to produce *bradykinin*, a potent mediator of vascular permeability.[56]

Approximately 6 to 12 hours after the immediate reaction, a late-phase reaction may occur. These reactions are believed to arise from an additional wave of mediator release from a variety of cells, including polymorphonuclear cells as well as mast cells and basophils. This release of mediators is believed to be triggered by the infiltration of these cells into the area of antigen introduction.[57–60]

Pathophysiologic Effects of Mediators

Although the mediators released and synthesized during an anaphylactic crisis have a variety of actions, the acute clinical presentation of this disorder suggests that the major effects are due to sudden increases in vascular permeability, systemic arteriolar vasodilation, and bronchial smooth muscle contraction. Autopsies in fatal cases of anaphylaxis reveal edema of the lungs, larynx, epiglottis, skin, and viscera. In one study, 36 of 40 fatalities exhibited gross pulmonary congestion, with fluid-filled alveoli apparent on light microscopy.[61] Another autopsy study revealed that almost one half of anaphylactic fatalities exhibited acute pulmonary emphysema with hyperdistended alveoli and thinning of alveolar septa.[62] Because of the association of acute pulmonary emphysema with upper airway edema, especially involving the larynx, these anaphylactic deaths appear to result from complete upper airway obstruction. Alveolar rupture, caused by forced exhalation against the obstruction, and inability to ventilate may thus be preterminal events.

Although cardiac dysfunction, especially dysrhythmias, reduced contractility, and myocardial ischemia and necrosis have characterized anaphylaxis in laboratory animals, evidence of cardiac abnormalities in the autopsies of fatal cases of human anaphylaxis appears to be minimal.[61, 62] Nevertheless, dysrhythmias, myocardial infarction, and coronary artery vasospasm may occur. Reduced cardiac contractility may characterize the effects of histamine and LTs on the myocardium in laboratory studies, but most patients with anaphylaxis show no evidence of impaired cardiac function as assessed by routine clinical tests.[62–64]

Laboratory Findings

Diagnosis of anaphylactic reactions is primarily based on the clinical presentation and signs and symptoms. Some laboratory studies may be helpful and may also be used to document activation of mast cells (Table 18–5); however, the clinician should never wait for confirmation by laboratory tests before initiating emergency treatment. As vascular permeability increases, the sudden loss of plasma volume may lead to marked hemoconcentration with a sharp increase in the hematocrit value.[65–67] Other blood cell counts may also increase as a result of volume contraction and other factors. The electrocardiogram (ECG) may show ST and T wave changes and other abnormalities that reflect myocardial ischemia.[68] Evidence of complement activation may be present. Histamine levels have been studied and, when elevated, help confirm activation of mast cells. These levels may be elevated for minutes after the acute episode.[69] However, histamine has a short plasma half-life because it is rapidly metabolized (within 1–2 min) by histamine-*N*-methyltransferase and diamine oxidase *(histaminase)*. These features limit use of histamine assays in many instances of anaphylactic reactions. Mast cell–derived tryptase appears to be a better marker of these reactions, as tryptase levels persist for hours.[50, 70, 71] LT products also appear in the urine after such reactions and may be used to document activation of mediators.[72, 73] Radioallergosorbent tests (RASTs), which measure antigen-specific IgE, may also help establish an IgE reaction.[74]

CLINICAL AND HEMODYNAMIC FEATURES

Although the clinical presentation of anaphylaxis is highly variable, most patients have severe, rapidly progressive symptoms. The symptoms may be modified by the portal of entry for the antigen as well as by the rate of absorption and degree of hypersensitivity to the antigen. Accordingly, gastrointestinal symptoms may precede more severe systemic symptoms after ingestion of an antigen. These symptoms may include nausea, vomiting, abdominal cramps, and diarrhea. Anaphylaxis in-

TABLE 18–5. Laboratory Studies in Anaphylaxis

Test/Assay	Comment
Chest x-ray	Hyperinflation, emphysema, ARDS in some patients
Electrocardiogram	ST-T changes are common; atrial and ventricular arrhythmias; possibly Q-wave infarction
Complete blood count	Hemoconcentration (↑ hematocrit); WBC count ↑ or ↓; eosinophils ↑
Complement	Evidence of complement consumption
Blood histamine	Levels increase within minutes; decline within 30 min
Blood tryptase	Levels increase within minutes; persist for hours
Urinary LTE_4	Increased levels for up to 12 hr; reflect lipoxygenase activation
Radioallergosorbent tests (RASTs)	Positive for IgE-mediated reactions

LTE_4 = leukotriene E_4; ARDS = acute respiratory distress syndrome; WBC = white blood cell; IgE = immunoglobulin E.

duced by peanuts, fish, shelfish, nuts, legumes, and other foods or food additives, therefore, may be serious and occasionally fatal. Inhalation of an antigen may produce nasal coryza, a sensation of tightness or a lump in the throat, hoarseness, stridor, wheezing, and dyspnea. Introduction of antigen through the skin may produce local pruritus, urticaria, and swelling before the development of systemic symptoms.

Anaphylactic reactions must be distinguished from other cardiopulmonary crises (see Table 2). Severe status asthmaticus may occasionally be associated with hemodynamic alterations, and bronchospasm is a common feature of anaphylactic reactions. Similarly, upper airway obstruction from any cause may also be confused with laryngospasm associated with anaphylaxis. In addition to anaphylactoid reactions, radiocontrast agents may produce respiratory distress, wheezing, and cardiovascular alterations caused by sudden volume expansion and acute congestive heart failure induced by the infusions of the hyperosmolar media. Vasovagal reactions may present with hypotension and other hemodynamic features. In vasovagal reactions, however, bronchospasm is absent and the patient is pale and cool, often manifesting bradycardia. Hereditary angioedema, carcinoid syndrome, and systemic mastocytosis may also be confused with anaphylactic reactions, although history and other features may allow differentiation from anaphylaxis, particularly for recurrent episodes. The so-called Chinese restaurant syndrome, a reaction to monosodium glutamate, is also a condition that may be mistaken for anaphylaxis. However, the triad of features of paresthesias and burning sensations of the neck and chest, palpitations, and weakness, together with flushing and other symptoms but no hemodynamic or respiratory distress, typifies the monosodium glutamate symptom complex.[33, 75]

Factitious anaphylaxis is a phenomenon that includes repeated episodes of "attacks" that may resemble anaphylaxis but that do not improve with conventional therapy. These episodes, however, do not involve life-threatening manifestations.[16]

Anaphylactic reactions are typically rapid in onset. In one review of 72 of 80 articles on anaphylaxis in which the time of the reaction could be identified, it occurred within 60 minutes.[76]

The most life-threatening reactions are usually explosive, typically occuring within minutes of exposure to the antigen. Patients with these reactions may describe a feeling of impending doom before more defined symptoms develop. Generalized cutaneous abnormalities may be observed and include erythema, urticaria, and flushing. Swelling of the periorbital and perioral areas is characteristic. Edema of posterior pharynx, uvula, tonsils, and the vocal cords may develop rapidly. Auscultation may reveal generalized wheezing and stridor. Auscultatory and radiographic signs of pulmonary edema may be present owing to noncardiogenic pulmonary edema.[65] Circulatory shock, oliguria, and lactic acidosis may emerge as plasma continues to escape the circulation. In some instances, such as following intravenous injection of antigen, circulatory shock may develop without preceding cutaneous and respiratory abnormalities. The clinical features of anaphylaxis may respond quickly to treatment or, in the most severe cases, may persist for several hours. Patients receiving β-adrenergic blocking agents or ACE inhibitors may have more severe and protracted reactions.[77–82] An initial favorable response to treatment may be followed by a late-phase reaction, a recurrence of symptoms approximately 6 to 12 hours after the initial reaction.[52]

Hemodynamic descriptions of human anaphylaxis are limited to the detailed studies of a few cases. The loss of circulating plasma volume is a characteristic feature and may be associated with hemoconcentration, hypotension, tachycardia, decreased cardiac filling pressures, and decreased cardiac output.[65–67] Vasodilation may contribute to the reduction in venous return and cardiac output and is associated with decreased systemic vascular resistance. Lactic acidosis emerges. Changes in myocardial contractility are minimal in human anaphylaxis when assessed in studies employing routine hemodynamic monitoring. Many patients with anaphylaxis respond favorably to fluid therapy and do not require inotropic support.[65–68] In some instances, reduced contractility may be observed in association with myocardial ischemia and infarction.[68, 83–87] Some of these adverse cardiac and other effects have been associated with overzealous epinephrine administration with attendant myocardial ischemia.[88, 89]

Hemodynamic characteristics in primate models of anaphylaxis are similar to those in humans. After antigenic challenge, a transient increase in cardiac output is observed and is followed by decreases in arterial pressure, right and left ventricular filling pressures, and peripheral vascular resistance.[86, 90] The transient increase in cardiac output has been attributed to left ventricular unloading from vasodilation and/or an increase in cardiac contractility. Elevated plasma levels of epinephrine, norepinephrine, and histamine have been observed in laboratory animals as well as humans[91–94] and may contribute to this increase in contractility. When hypotension and shock become established, cardiac output decreases because of a decrease in venous return from decreased plasma volume. In the canine model of anaphylaxis, splanchnic vasodilation and pooling of blood contributes to the decrease in venous return.[94, 95]

Pulmonary edema fluid sampled from the airway of patients with anaphylaxis is characterized by protein and oncotic levels that are virtually identical to those of plasma. An association of pulmonary edema with low pulmonary arterial wedge pressures has also been observed.[65, 93] These findings suggest that the pulmonary edema in anaphylaxis is due to increased pulmonary microvascular permeability.

In summary, the major hemodynamic characteristics of human anaphylaxis are determined by a decrease in vascular tone as well as an increase in vascular permeability. These effects lead to the venous pooling of blood and loss of circulating plasma volume.

MANAGEMENT

Initial Management

Treatment should begin immediately, with the following priorities: *A* (airway), *B* (breathing), and *C* (cardiac competence).[96] A patent airway, together with a progressive intensive approach that matches the severity of the reaction, must be established (Fig. 18-4). Removal of toxin at the site of introduction or an attempt to delay systemic absorption may be helpful. A large-bore intravenous access should be established for fluid therapy. Pharmacologic support should begin with *epinephrine*,[87] the mainstay of pharmacologic therapy. Epinephrine is of proven efficacy in reversing bronchoconstriction and hypotension associated with anaphylaxis. The β-adrenergic effects of epinephrine inhibit mediator release by increasing intracellular levels of cAMP. In addition, β-adrenergic stimulation decreases bronchospasm, increases myocardial contractility, and increases heart rate. The α-adrenergic properties of epinephrine are associated with constriction of systemic arterioles. This property of epinephrine leads to an elevation of diastolic pressure and may thus increase coronary perfusion.

Critical care staff should be familiar with the dilutions of epinephrine that are commonly available: 1:1000 and 1:10,000 (Table 18-6). Epinephrine in the 1:10,000 dilution is available

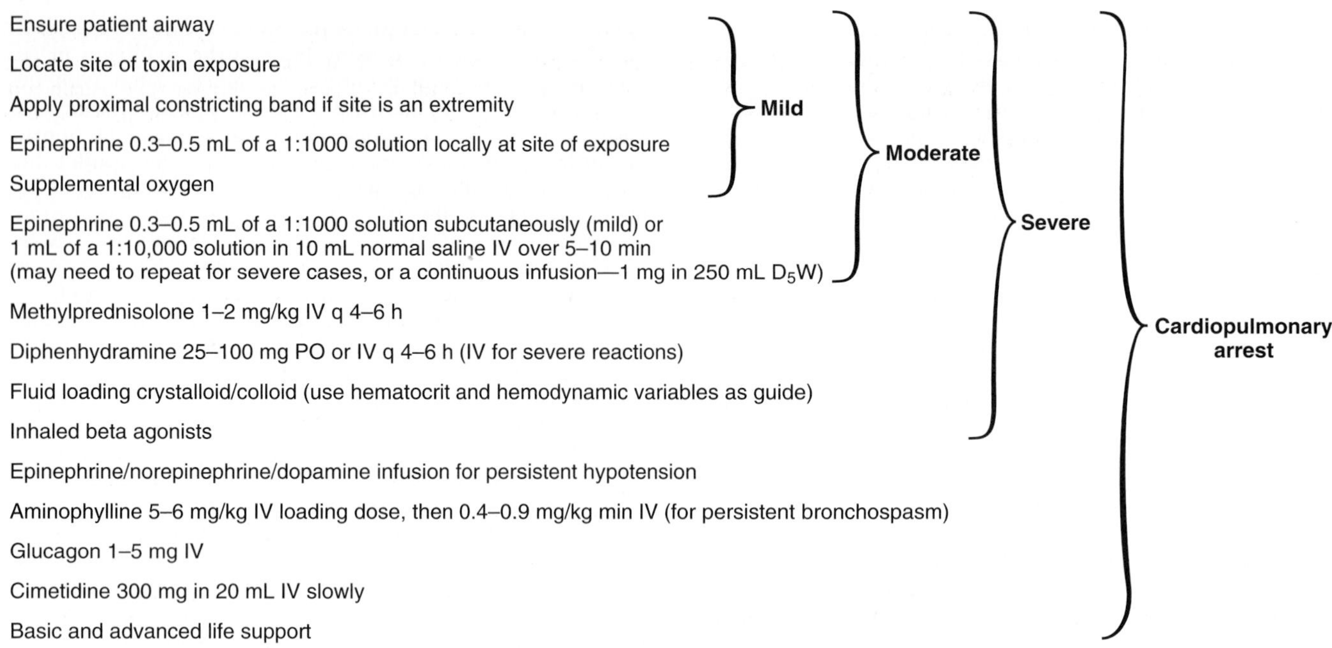

Ensure patient airway
Locate site of toxin exposure
Apply proximal constricting band if site is an extremity
Epinephrine 0.3–0.5 mL of a 1:1000 solution locally at site of exposure
Supplemental oxygen
Mild
Epinephrine 0.3–0.5 mL of a 1:1000 solution subcutaneously (mild) or
1 mL of a 1:10,000 solution in 10 mL normal saline IV over 5–10 min
(may need to repeat for severe cases, or a continuous infusion—1 mg in 250 mL D5W)
Moderate
Methylprednisolone 1–2 mg/kg IV q 4–6 h
Diphenhydramine 25–100 mg PO or IV q 4–6 h (IV for severe reactions)
Fluid loading crystalloid/colloid (use hematocrit and hemodynamic variables as guide)
Inhaled beta agonists
Severe
Epinephrine/norepinephrine/dopamine infusion for persistent hypotension
Aminophylline 5–6 mg/kg IV loading dose, then 0.4–0.9 mg/kg min IV (for persistent bronchospasm)
Glucagon 1–5 mg IV
Cimetidine 300 mg in 20 mL IV slowly
Basic and advanced life support
Cardiopulmonary arrest

Figure 18–4. Approach to management of anaphylaxis based on severity of the reaction. D_5W = 5% dextrose in water.

as prefilled syringes. Most authors recommend that for mild reactions 0.3 to 0.5 mL of the 1:1000 solution (0.3–0.5 mg) be given subcutaneously. This dose may be repeated at 5- to 10-minute intervals if symptoms do not improve. For severe reactions, a dilute solution of epinephrine should be given intravenously. When conventional intravenous access routes are difficult to obtain, alternatives for administration of epinephrine should be explored. Epinephrine may be administered intravenously through the femoral vein or through a vein in the venous plexus under the tongue. Epinephrine may also be instilled directly into the bronchopulmonary tree through an endotracheal tube or by injection through the cricothyroid membrane.

The dose of epinephrine for intravenous administration in severe anaphylaxis is controversial. Most authors recommend an initial dose of 0.3 to 0.5 mg; however, several case reports of anaphylaxis have documented cardiac ischemia, hypertensive crises, and acute myocardial infarction after epinephrine.[83–89, 92] Because of these experiences, a starting dose of 0.1 to 0.2 mg may be infused in 5 to 10 minutes at a 1:100,000 dilution (0.1–0.2 mL of a 1:1000 dilution mixed in 10 mL of normal saline or 1–2 mL of a 1:10,000 dilution mixed in 10 mL of normal saline).[87] This cautious starting dose may need to be repeated at frequent intervals if symptoms do not improve. Alternatively, a continuous infusion of epinephrine may be started after the initial doses of epinephrine. The infusion (1–2 mg in 5% dextrose in water (D_5W), 4–9 μg/mL mixed concentration: 4 mL/250 mL) is similar to the dose recommended in advanced cardiac life support protocols.[76] The infusion may be started at 1 μg/minute and increased to 4 μg/minute if symptoms of hemodynamic instability persist. Cardiac rhythm should be monitored for all patients who receive epinephrine.

A team approach is important in severe cases of anaphylaxis because initial interventions must proceed rapidly and, if possible, simultaneously.

Admission to a critical care unit is indicated for all serious cases of anaphylaxis. Hospitalization should not be precluded for patients with severe symptoms who exhibit a favorable response to initial therapy because patients are susceptible to late-phase reactions. Severe symptoms may occur up to 12 hours after the initial attack. The patient should be monitored for signs of circulatory shock and respiratory failure. Accordingly, blood pressure, urine output, and heart and respiratory rates should be evaluated at frequent intervals.

The electrocardiogram (ECG) should be monitored continuously during the initial period because of the risks of serious dysrhythmias and cardiac ischemia related to the reaction and catecholamine therapy.

When signs of circulatory shock and impaired pulmonary gas exchange develop, invasive monitoring is indicated. As with other forms of circulatory shock, fluid therapy, inotropic and vasopressor therapy, and ventilatory support should be titrated to cardiopulmonary parameters to maintain organ perfusion, pulmonary gas exchange, and systemic oxygen delivery.

Close attention to the airway is important. Frequent assessment for hoarseness, stridor, and upper airway obstruction is required for patients whose airway is not protected with an endotracheal tube. If consciousness is altered, the head and neck should be positioned so that the airway is not obstructed by the tongue. If stridor caused by laryngeal or upper respiratory tract edema develops, endotracheal intubation should be attempted. Because intubation may be difficult in the presence of laryngeal edema, personnel capable of performing an emergency cricothyrotomy or tracheostomy should be available.

TABLE 18–6. Administration Guidelines for Epinephrine

Mild reactions:
0.3–0.5 mL 1:1000 (0.3–0.5 mg) SC
May repeat q5–10 min
Consider 0.1–0.2 mL (0.1–0.2 mg) at site of sting or entry
Moderate to severe reactions:
Slow IV infusion of 0.1–0.2 mL 1:1000 in 10 mL NS or 1–2 mL of 1:10,000 in 10 mL NS (1:100,000)
For persistent hypotension consider:
Continuous infusion of 1–2 mg in 250 mL D_5W or NS (4–8 μg/mL) at 2+ μg/min

SC = subcutaneously; IV = intravenously; NS = normal saline; D_5W = 5% dextrose in water.

If spontaneous ventilation is uncertain or impaired, mechanical ventilation should be implemented. Supplemental oxygen should be provided as needed. Positive end-expiratory pressure (PEEP) may be necessary when hypoxemia, pulmonary edema, and reduced lung compliance develop. However, adverse effects of PEEP on cardiac output and arterial pressure may be aggravated by hypovolemia induced by vascular permeability defects during anaphylaxis.

If possible, the site of antigen introduction should be identified. If the patient is unconscious or unaware of the site of antigen introduction, a thorough search of skin surfaces should proceed. Retained stingers may be removed. If the site of envenomization is an extremity, a constricting band should be applied to delay the absorption of the venom. This band should be sufficiently tight to delay venous absorption of venom but should not interrupt arterial flow. A dilute solution of epinephrine (1:10,000 solution) may be injected locally to retard systemic absorption of venom through alpha-adrenergic–mediated vasoconstriction.

Vigorous fluid therapy with crystalloids and colloids is an important component of the initial treatment of anaphylaxis. Fluids effectively reverse the intravascular volume deficits produced by increased vascular permeability. They also counteract the effects of mediator-induced vasodilation by increasing venous return. One approach to fluid therapy is to replace estimated plasma losses with a plasma substitute. Colloid fluids, such as 5% human serum albumin and 6% hydroxyethyl starch, are rational choices because they mimic the oncotic properties and electrolyte concentrations of plasma. Considerably larger volumes (two to six times) of crystalloid than colloid are required to achieve comparable intravascular volume repletion. In one laboratory study of severe shock analogous to anaphylactic shock, six times more crystalloid was required to produce volume expansion similar to that in colloid-resuscitated animals.[97] Reversal of hemoconcentration is a reasonable resuscitative goal for stable patients. For unstable patients, however, fluid therapy should be titrated with the use of hemodynamic variables.

If hypotension and other signs of circulatory shock persist after the initial administration of epinephrine and fluids, inotropic support is required. In general, the continuous infusion of a catecholamine is employed. Some authorities recommend a continuous infusion of epinephrine. Norepinephrine has also been utilized (4–8 mg in 1 L of saline, infused at 4 to 8 μg/minute 0.1 μg/kg/minute). Dopamine may be given at infusions of up to 15 μg/kg/minute (400 mg/250 mL/D_5W or normal saline, 1.6 mg/mL). If infusions greater than 24 μg/kg/minute are not effective in restoring arterial pressure, epinephrine or norepinephrine should be used. In one reported case of anaphylaxis dopamine was ineffective.[98]

When faced with a patient who remains hypotensive despite ongoing catecholamine therapy, the clinician should recheck the adequacy of oxygenation and ventilation, consider additional volume infusion, assess acid-base and electrolyte status, and employ supplementary therapeutic maneuvers (discussed later). Ongoing release of mediators from a retained stinger or other mechanism should be considered. In addition, the intensive care unit (ICU) staff should determine whether during the initial phases of the reaction additional events, such as myocardial infarction, have intervened. Finally, reevaluation of the patient is indicated to substantiate the diagnosis of anaphylaxis and to exclude other cardiopulmonary crises.

Additional Therapeutic Options and Special Circumstances

When symptoms of anaphylaxis persist after initial treatment with epinephrine and fluids, other pharmacologic agents may be tried.[99, 100] The rationale for the use of these agents is based on a basic knowledge of their pharmacologic actions in the laboratory setting and in clinical conditions that usually do not include anaphylaxis. Because of the sporadic presentation of clinical anaphylaxis, most clinical experience with these drugs is anecdotal and inconclusive. When patients are responding poorly to initial treatment, however, additional therapeutic maneuvers may be considered.

Agents that block the peripheral effects of histamine are logical additions to the pharmacologic management of anaphylaxis. *Antihistamines* block the systemic effects of histamine by competitively inhibiting histamine (H_1 and H_2) receptors. These drugs may thus favorably influence histamine H_1 receptor-mediated increases in vascular permeability and bronchial smooth muscle contraction. Antihistamines may also block histamine H_2 receptors in the myocardium, which mediate increases in heart rate, dysrhythmias, atrioventricular conduction delays, and coronary vasoconstriction. Diphenhydramine, a histamine H_1-receptor antagonist, may be given intravenously at 4- to 6-hour intervals in doses of 25 to 100 mg. Three hundred milligrams of the histamine H_2 receptor blocker cimetidine (in 50 mL of normal saline) or another H_2 blocking agent in suitable dosage may be infused intravenously during 5 minutes and repeated at 6- to 8-hour intervals.[101]

Aminophylline is a methylxanthine that is frequently employed in anaphylaxis. This agent potentially inhibits phosphodiesterase and may thus decrease mediator release by increasing intracellular cAMP concentrations. However, this effect may be minimal at therapeutic concentrations. Nevertheless, aminophylline may be helpful to alleviate bronchospasm. A loading dose of 5 to 6 mg/kg is infused during 20 minutes and is followed by a continuous infusion of 0.2 to 0.9 mg/kg/hour. Caution should be used if cardiac arrhythmias develop and in patients for whom high doses of epinephrine are employed.

Corticosteroids should be administered in patients with severe reactions because they increase tissue responsiveness to beta agonists and inhibit the synthesis of histamine. These agents also prevent or attenuate late-phase reactions by inhibiting the characteristic secondary wave of mediator release. Methylprednisolone, 1 to 2 mg/kg, should be given intravenously in severe cases, repeated at 4- to 6-hour intervals for 24 hours, and rapidly tapered.

Inhalational drugs may have a role in the treatment of bronchospasm associated with anaphylaxis. One inhaled beta agonist that may be used is metaproterenol, 0.2 to 0.3 mL of a 5% solution in 2.5 mL of saline administered by nebulization and repeated every 2 to 4 hours. Ipratropium bromide is a bronchodilator with anticholinergic properties; 36 μg may be inhaled and repeated at 2- to 4-hour intervals as needed. If 12 inhalations during 24 hours is not exceeded, laryngeal edema, if mild, may respond to nebulized racemic epinephrine. It is believed that localized vasoconstriction from the α-adrenergic properties of these drugs minimizes edema formation in the laryngeal area. Racemic epinephrine, 0.5 mL of a 2.25% solution diluted in 3.5 mL of distilled water, may be administered by nebulization. Terbutaline, 0.25 mg subcutaneously or 1 mg in saline by inhalation, may also be used. For severe laryngeal edema associated with respiratory distress or stridor, intubation of the trachea should be strongly considered.

Several other agents have been used in cases of human anaphylaxis or in laboratory models of anaphylaxis with apparent success. *Glucagon*, a pancreatic hormone that increases intracellular cAMP levels through the activation of adenylate cyclase, may be considered, particularly for patients who have received β-adrenergic blockers.[77, 78, 102–105] Some clinicians, therefore, suggest 1 to 5 mg of glucagon intravenously. Because of the role of calcium in enhancing mediator release, it has been speculated that *calcium channel blockers* might be useful in anaphylaxis. Calcium channel blocking agents may prevent histamine-induced symptoms; however, these agents have proved disappointing in alleviating bronchospasm in clinical trials of asthma, and their negative inotropic effects are undesirable in severe anaphylaxis. Accordingly, these agents are generally not employed in anaphylaxis. *Opiate antagonists* reverse the inhibitory effects of endogenous opiates on the sympathetic nervous system and have been effective in laboratory models of anaphylaxis.[106] Management of persistent bronchospasm and respiratory failure may require maneuvers utilized for status asthmaticus, including adjustments of ventilator flow rate, title volume, and peak airway pressures as well as permissive hypercapnea (see Chapter 132).

Anaphylactic reactions that occur during pregnancy pose unique management problems. Priorities are identical to those for the nonpregnant patient, although measures that may affect uteroplacental blood flow deserve special consideration.[100, 107–112] *Ephedrine* in doses of 25 to 50 mg intravenously may be used as a vasoactive agent. However, if volume loading, ephedrine, and other measures are ineffective, the clinician may need to utilize agents with α-adrenergic properties. The risks of compromising fetal perfusion because of persistent hypotension must be weighed against potentially harmful effects of agents that alter uteral placental vascular tone.[110, 111]

Anaphylactic reactions may occur during a variety of procedures and diagnostic studies. Drugs and biologicals used during these procedures are the most common cause of the reaction and should be evaluated. Reactions may occur during hemodialysis and the use of ethylene oxide (ETO) to sterilize dialysis equipment may lead to the formation of haptens from serum proteins that induce the response.[113, 114] Complement activation by the dialysis membrane is another mechanism. Discontinuation of dialysis, changing cartridges, and use of other methods of sterilization as well as conventional management of the reaction may be required.

Premedication for patients at risk for a reaction to radiocontrast agents significantly reduces the incidence and seriousness of these reactions. Some authorities recommend treating all patients, whereas other authors restrict premedication for those at increased risk of having a reaction.[28, 115–118] One technique is to give two 32-mg oral doses of methylprednisolone or an equivalent dose of another corticosteroid, one dose 6 to 14 hours prior to, and the other dose 2 hours prior to, administration of contrast material.[115] Antihistamine agents may also be given as part of the premedication regimen.

Management After Anaphylactic Episode: Prophylaxis and Immunotherapy

Because of the life-threatening nature of anaphylaxis, arrangements must be made for patients who have experienced anaphylaxis to receive follow-up by a physician experienced in the management of acute allergic events. Skin testing may be required to identify the inciting agent, particularly for insect sting desensitization. Instructions in self-treatment of subsequent events is often necessary. Kits are available with self-injectable epinephrine and oral antihistamines for patients to take immediately after exposure to antigen.

Methods to desensitize individuals immediately before the administration of a drug have been described in detail, especially for penicillin,[119] aspirin,[120] and insulin;[121] however, these techniques, which involve exposure to antigen in increments of 20 to 30 minutes, may be unsuccessful and occasionally fatal.

Additional desensitization procedures may be required in selected individuals.[122, 123] Accordingly, patients who experience an anaphylactic reaction should be evaluated by an allergist.

Management of anaphylaxis, therefore, should include treatment of the acute reaction, identification of the antigen or inciting circumstances, avoidance, patient education, and possible desensitization.

ACKNOWLEDGMENT

The authors are grateful for the assistance of Judy C. Hodgkins and the staff of the Medical Library of Maricopa Medical Center.

References

1. Waddell LA: Egyptian Civilization: Its Sumerian Origin and Real Chronology and Sumerian Origin of Egyptian Hieroglyphs. London, Luzac and Co, 1930.
2. Chaffee F: Insect-sting allergy. J Allergy 1969; 45:309.
3. Cohen SG: The pharoah and the wasp. Allergy Proc 1989; 10:149.
4. Portier P, Richet C: De l'action anaphylactique de certains venins. CR Soc Biol Paris 1902; 54:170.
5. Ishizaka T: IgE and mechanisms of IgE-mediated hypersensitivity. Ann Allergy 1982; 43:313.
6. Murphy RC, Hammarstrom S, Samuelsson B: Leukotriene C: A slow reacting substance from murine mastocytoma cells. Proc Natl Acad Sci USA 1979; 76:4275.
7. Lewis RA, Austin KF, Soberman RJ: Leukotrienes and other products of the 5-lipoxygenase: Biochemistry and relation to pathobiology in human diseases. N Engl J Med 1990; 323:645.
8. Serafin WE, Austen KF: Mediators of immediate hypersensitivity reactions. N Engl J Med 1987; 317:50.
9. Stevens RL, Austen KF: Recent advances in the cellular and molecular biology of mast cells. Immunol Today 1989; 10:381.
10. Gordon JR, Burd PR, Galli SJ: Mast cells as a source of multifunctional cytokines. Immunol Today 1990; 11:458.
11. Galli SJ, Costa JJ: Mast cell–leukocyte cytokine cascades in allergic inflammation. Allergy 1995; 50:851.
12. Terr AI: Anaphylaxis and urticaria. *In*: Medical Immunology. 9th ed. Stites DP, Terr AI, and Parsloa TG (Eds). Stamford, Conn, Appleton & Lange, p 409, 1997.
13. Sheffer AI, Austin KF: Exercise-induced anaphylaxis. J Allergy Clin Immunol 1980; 66:106.
14. Wiggins CA, Dykewicz MS, Patterson R: Idiopathic anaphylaxis: A review. Ann Allergy 1988; 62:1.
15. Wong S, Dykewicz MS, Patterson R: Idiopathic anaphylaxis: A clinical summary of 175 patients. Arch Intern Med 1990; 150:1323.
16. McGrath KG, Greenberger PA, Zeiss CR: Factitious allergic disease: Multiple factitious illness and familial Munchausen's stridor. Immunol Allergy Pract 1984; 6:41.
17. Light WC, Reisma RE, Shimizu MA, et al: Unusual reactions following insect stings. J Allergy Clin Immunol 1977; 59:391.
18. Stark BJ, Sullivan TJ: Biphasic and protracted anaphylaxis. J Allergy Clin Immunol 1986; 78:76.
19. Idsoe O, Guthe T, Willcox RR, et al: Nature and extent of penicillin side-reactions with particular reference to fatalities from anaphylactic shock. Bull WHO 1968; 38:159.
20. Parker CW: Allergic drug responses-mechanisms and unsolved problems. Crit Rev Toxicol 1972; 1:261.
21. Saxon A, Beall GN, Rohr AS, et al: Immediate hypersensitivity reactions to beta-lactam antibiotics. Ann Intern Med 1987; 107:204.
22. Anderson JA: Allergic reactions to drugs and biologic agents. JAMA 1992; 268:2845.
23. DeShazo RD, Kemp SF: Allergic reactions to drugs and biologic agents. JAMA 1997; 278:1895.
24. Gadde J, Spence M, Wheeler B, Adkinson NF: Clinical experience with penicillin skin testing in a large inner-city STD clinic. JAMA 1993; 270:2456.
25. Kabins SA, Eisenstein B, Cohen S: Anaphylactoid reaction to an initial dose of sodium cephalothin. JAMA 1965; 193:165.

26. Kellerman R: Reactions to radiographic contrast media. Am Fam Physician 1981; 23:149.
27. Cohan RH, Dunnick NR, Bashore TM: Treatment of reactions to radiographic contrast media. AJR 1988; 151:263.
28. Lasser EC, Berry CC, Talner LB, Santini LC, et al: Pretreatment with corticosteroids to alleviate reactions to intravenous contrast material. N Engl J Med 1987; 317:845.
29. Barnard JH: Studies of 400 Hymenoptera sting deaths in the United States. J Allergy Clin Immunol 1973; 52:259.
30. DeShazo RD, Butcher BT, Banks WA: Reactions to the stings of the imported fire ant. N Engl J Med 1990; 323:462.
31. Bock SA: Prospective appraisal of complaints of adverse reactions to foods in children during the first three years of life. Pediatrics 1987; 79:683.
32. Metcalfe DD: Diseases of food hypersensitivity. N Engl J Med 1989; 321:255.
33. Metcalfe DD, Sampson HA, Simon RA (Eds): Food Allergy: Adverse Reactions to Foods and Food Additives. 2nd ed. Cambridge, Mass, 1997.
34. Matsuda H, Watanabe N, Kiso Y, et al: Necessity of IgE antibodies and mast cells for manifestations of resistance against larval *Haemaphysalis longicornis* ticks in mice. J Immunol 1990; 144:259.
35. Johansson SGO, Melvin T, Vahlquist B: Immunoglobulin levels in Ethiopian preschool children with special reference to high concentrations of immunoglobulin E (IgND). Lancet 1968; 1:1118.
36. Phils JA, Harrold AJ, Whiteman GV: Pulmonary infiltrates, asthma and eosinophilia due to *Ascaris suum* infestation in man. N Engl J Med 1972; 286:965.
37. Austen KF: The anaphylactic syndrome. *In*: Immunological Diseases. 4th ed. Samter M, Talmadge DW, Frank MM, et al (Eds). Boston, Little, Brown & Co, 1988, p 1119.
38. Van Arsdel PP: Diagnosing drug allergy. JAMA 1982; 247:2576.
39. Rich RR (Ed): Clinical Immunology: Principles and Practice. St. Louis, Mosby-Year Book, 1997.
40. Hudson DP: Biology of the immune system. JAMA 1997; 278:1804.
41. Costa JJ, Weller PF, Galli SJ: The cells of the allergic response: Mast cells, basophils and eosinophils. JAMA 1997; 278:1815.
42. Dembo M, Goldstein B, Sobotka AK, et al: Degranulation of human basophils. J Immunol 1979; 123:1864.
43. Vyas GN, Holmadahl L, Perkins HA, et al: Serologic specificity of human anti-IgA and its significance in transfusion. Blood 1969; 34:573.
44. Sharath MD, Metzger WJ, Richerson HB, et al: Protamine-induced fatal anaphylaxis. J Thorac Cardiovasc Surg 1985; 90:86.
45. Samter M, Stevenson DD: Reactions to aspirin and aspirin-like drugs. *In*: Immunological Diseases. 4th ed. Samter M, Talmadge DW, Frank MM, et al (Eds). Boston, Little, Brown & Co, 1988, p 1135.
46. Juhlin L, Michaelsson G, Zetterstron D: Urticaria and asthma induced by food and drug additives in patients with aspirin hypersensitivity. J Allergy Clin Immunol 1972; 50:92.
47. Galli SJ: New concepts about the mast cell. N Engl J Med 1993; 328:257.
48. Church MK, Levi-Schaffer F: The human mast cell. J Allergy Clin Immunol 1997; 99:155.
49. Schwartz LB, Huff T: Biology of mast cells and basophils. *In*: Allergy: Principles and Practice. 4th ed. Middleton E Jr, Reed CE, Ellis EF, Adkinson NF, Yunginger JW, Bussee WW (Eds). St. Louis, Mosby-Year Book, 1993, pp 135–168.
50. Weller PF: The immunobiology of eosinophils. N Engl J Med 1991; 324:1110.
51. Schwartz LB, Yuninger JW, Miller J, Bokhari R, Dull D: Time course of appearance and disappearance of human mast cell tryptase in the circulation after anaphylaxis. J Clin Invest 1989; 83:1551.
52. Kaliher M: Hypotheses on the contribution of late-phase allergic responses to the understanding and treatment of allergic diseases. J Allergy Clin Immunol 1984; 73:311.
53. Duorak AM, Lett-Brouns M, Thueson D, et al: Complement-induced degranulation of human basophils. J Immunol 1981; 126:523.
54. Hugli TE, Muller-Eberhard HJ: Anaphylatoxins C3a and C5a. Adv Immunol 1978; 26:1.
55. Frank MM, Fries LF: The role of complement in inflammation and phagocytosis. Immunol Today 1991; 12:322.
56. Rubin LE, Levi R: Protective effect of bradykinin in cardiac anaphylaxis. Circ Res 1995; 76:434.
57. Lemanski RFJ, Kaliner MA: Late phase allergic reactions. *In*: Allergy: Principles and Practice. 4th ed. Middleton E Jr, Reed CE, Ellis EF, Adkinson NF, Yunginger JW, Bussee WW (Eds). St. Louis, Mosby-Year Book. 1993, p 320.
58. Abraham WM, Saielczak MW, Ahmed A, et al: Anti-a4 integrin mediates antigen-induced late bronchial responses and prolonged airway hyperresponsiveness in sheep. J Clin Invest 1994; 93:776.
59. Smith CW: Cellular adhesion and interactions. *In*: Clinical Immunology: Principles and Practice. Rich RR, Fleisher TA, Schwartz BD, Shearer WT, Strober W (Eds). St. Louis, Mosby-Year Book, 1996, p 176.
60. Bochner BS, Schleimer RP: The role of adhesion molecules in human eosinophil and basophil recruitment. J Allergy Clin Immunol 1994; 94:427.
61. Delage C, Irey NS: Anaphylactic deaths: A clinicopathologic study of 43 cases. J Forensic Sci 1972; 17:525.
62. James LP, Austen KF: Fatal systemic anaphylaxis in man. N Engl J Med 1964; 270:597.
63. Graver LM, Robertson DA, Levi R, et al: IgE-mediated hypersensitivity in human heart tissue: Histamine release and functional changes. J Allergy Clin Immunol 1986; 77:709.
64. Burke JA, Levi R, Guzo Z-G et al: Leukotrienes C4, D4 and E4: Effect on human heart and guinea-pig cardiac preparations in vitro. J Pharmacol Exp Ther 1982; 221:235.
65. Carlson RW, Schaeffer RC, Puri VK et al: Hypovolemia and permeability pulmonary edema associated with anaphylaxis. Crit Care Med 1981; 9:883.
66. Silverman HJ, Van Hook C, Haponik EF: Hemodynamic changes in human anaphylaxis. Am J Med 1984; 77:341.
67. Hanashiro PK, Weil MH: Anaphylactic shock in man: Report of two cases with detailed hemodynamic and metabolic studies. Arch Intern Med 1967; 119:129.
68. Booth BH, Patterson R: Electrocardiographic abnormalities during human anaphylaxis. JAMA 1970; 211:627.
69. Smith PL, Kgey-Sobotka A, Bleecker ER, et al: Physiologic manifestations of human anaphylaxis. J Clin Invest 1980; 66:1072.
70. Schwartz LB, Bradford TR, Rouse C, et al: Development of a new, more sensitive immunoassay for human tryptase: Use in systemic anaphylaxis. J Clin Immunol 1994; 14:190.
71. Yuninger JW, Nelson DR, Squillace DL, et al: Laboratory investigation of deaths due to anaphylaxis. J Forensic Sci 1991; 36:857.
72. Christie PE, Tagari P, Ford-Hutchinson AW, et al: Urinary leukotriene E_4 concentrations increase after aspirin challenge in aspirin-sensitive asthmatic patients. Am Rev Respir Dis 1991; 143:1025.
73. Maltby NH, Taylor GW, Ritter JM, et al: Leukotriene C_4 elimination and metabolism in man. J Allergy Clin Immunol 1990; 85:3.
74. Patterson R: Diagnosis and treatment of drug allergy. J Allergy Clin Immunol 1988; 81:380.
75. Yang WH, Drouin MA, Herbert M, et al: The monosodium glutamate symptom complex: assessment in a double-blind placebo-controlled, randomized study. J Allergy Clin Immunol 1997; 99:757.
76. Apter AJ, LaVallee HA: How is anaphylaxis recognized? Arch Fam Med 1994; 3:717.
77. Lang DM, Alpern MB, Visintainer PF, et al: Elevated risk of anaphylactic reaction from radiocontrast media is associated with both beta-blocker exposure and cardiovascular disorders. Arch Intern Med 1993; 153:2033.
78. Javeed N, Javeed H, Javeed S, et al: Refractory anaphylactoid shock potentiated by beta-blockers. Cathet Cardiovasc Diagn 1996; 39:383.
79. Hannaway PJ, Hopper GDK: Severe anaphylaxis and drug-induced beta-blockade. N Engl J Med 1983; 308:1536.
80. Ingall M, Goldman G, Page LB: Beta-blockade in stinging insect anaphylaxis. JAMA 1984; 251:1432.
81. Toogood JH: Risk of anaphylaxis in patients receiving beta-blockers. J Allergy Clin Immunol 1988; 81:1.
82. Orfan N, Patterson R, Dykewicz MS: Severe angioedema related to ACE inhibitors in patients with a history of idiopathic angioedema. JAMA 1990; 264:1287.

83. Levine HD: Acute myocardial infarction following a wasp sting. Am Heart J 1976; 91:365.
84. Sullivan TJ: Cardiac disorders in penicillin-induced anaphylaxis. JAMA 1982; 248:2161.
85. Austin SM, Banajit B, Khim CS: Reversible acute cardiac injury during cefoxitin-induced anaphylaxis in a patient with normal coronary arteries. Am J Med 1984; 77:729.
86. Raper RF, Fisher MM: Profound reversible myocardial depression after anaphylaxis. Lancet 1988; 1:368.
87. Barach EM, Nowak RM, Lee TG, et al: Epinephrine for treatment of anaphylactic shock. JAMA 1984; 251:2118.
88. Horowitz BZ, Jadallah S, Derlet RW: Fatal intracranial bleeding associated with prehospital use of epinephrine. Ann Emerg Med 1966; 28:725.
89. Alexander R, Paggachan R, Smith GB, et al: Treatment of anaphylaxis: Avoid subcutaneous or intramuscular adrenaline. Br Med J 1995; 311:1434.
90. Smedegard G, Revenas B, Lundberg C: Anaphylactic shock in monkeys passively sensitized with human reaginic serum: I. Hemodynamic and cardiac performance. Acta Physiol Scand 1981; 111:239.
91. Moss J, Fahmey NR, Sunder N, et al: Hormonal and hemodynamic profile of an anaphylactic reaction in man. Circulation 1981; 63:210.
92. Hamberger B, Friedholm BB, Farnebo LO: Anaphylaxis and plasma catecholamine. Life Sci 1980; 26:1465.
93. Olinger GN, Becker RM, Bonchek LI: Non-cardiogenic pulmonary edema and vascular collapse following cardiopulmonary bypass: Rare protamine reaction? Ann Thorac Surg 1980; 29:20.
94. Enjeti S, Bleeker ER, Smith PL, et al: Hemodynamic mechanisms in anaphylaxis. Circ Shock 1983; 11:2197.
95. Kapin MA, Ferguson JL: Hemodynamic and regional circulatory alterations in dog during anaphylactic challenge. Am J Physiol 1985; 249:H430.
96. Guidelines for cardiopulmonary resuscitation (CPR) and emergency cardiac care (ECC). JAMA 1992; 268:2171.
97. Haupt MT, Teerapong P, Green D, et al: Increased pulmonary edema with crystalloid compared to colloid resuscitation in shock associated with increased vascular permeability. Circ Shock 1984; 12:213.
98. Sullivan TJ, Stark HJ: Drug Reactions. *In*: Current Therapy in Internal Medicine. Bayless TM, Brain MC, Cherniak RM (Eds). St. Louis, CV Mosby, 1984, p 24.
99. Perkin RM, Anas NG: Mechanisms and management of anaphylactic shock not responding to traditional therapy. Ann Allergy 1985; 54:202.
100. Anderson MW, deShazo RD: Anaphylaxis and anaphylactoid reactions. *In*: Difficult Medical Management. Taylor RB (Ed). Philadelphia, WB Saunders, 1991, p 25.
101. Mayumi N, Kimura S, Asano M, et al: Intravenous cimetidine as an effective treatment for systemic anaphylaxis and acute allergic skin reactions. Ann Allergy 1987; 58:447.
102. Zaloga GP, DeLacey WS, Holmboe E, et al: Glucagon reversal of hypotension in a case of anaphylactoid shock. Ann Intern Med 1986; 105:65.
103. Compton J: Use of glucagon in intractable allergic reactions and as an alternative to epinephrine. J Emerg Nursing 1997; 23:45.
104. Ward DE, Jones B: Glucagon and beta blocker activity. Br Med J 1976; 2:151.
105. Jacobs RL, Rake GW, Fournier DC, et al: Glucagon in anaphylaxis. J Allergy Clin Immunol 1981; 69:331.
106. Gullo A, Romano E: Naloxone and anaphylactic shock. Lancet 1983; 1:819.
107. Edmondson WC, Skilton RWH: Anaphylaxis in pregnancy: The right treatment? Anesthesia 1994; 49:454.
108. Slater RM, Bowles BJM, Pumphrey RSH: Anaphylactoid reaction to oxytoxin in pregnancy. Anesthesia 1985; 40:655.
109. Entman SS, Moise KJ: Anaphylaxis in pregnancy. South Med J 1984; 77:402.
110. Ladner C, Brinkman CR, Weston P, et al: Dynamics of uterine circulation in pregnant and non-pregnant sheep. Am J Physiol 1970; 218:257.
111. Van Nimegen D, Dyer D: The action of vasopressors on isolated uterine arteries. Am J Obset Gynecol 1974; 118:1099.
112. Belfort MA, Dildy GA, Cotton DB: Obstetrics and Gynecology in the Intensive Care Unit. *In*: Principles and Practice of Medical Intensive Care. Carlson RW, Geheb MA (Eds): Philadelphia, WB Saunders, 1993, p 1593.
113. Grammer LC: Hypersensitivity. Nephrol Dial Transplant 1994; 9S:29.
114. Kraske GK, Shinaberger JH, Klaustermeyer WB: Severe hypersensitivity reactions during hemodialysis. Ann Allergy Asthma Immunol 1997; 78:217.
115. Lasser EC, Berry CC, Mishkin MM, et al: Pretreatment with corticosteroids to prevent adverse reactions to nonionic contrast media. Am J Roentgenol 1994; 162:523.
116. Greenberger PA, Patterson R: The prevention of immediate generalized reactions to radiocontrast media in high-risk patients. J Allergy Clin Immunol 1991; 87:867.
117. Greenberger P, Patterson R, Kelly J, et al: Administration of radiographic contrast media in high-risk patients. Invest Radiol 1980; 15:S40.
118. Cohan RH, Leder RA, Ellis JH: Treatment of adverse reactions to radiographic contrast media in adults. Radiol Clin North Am 1996; 34:1055.
119. Weiss ME, Adkinson NF: Immediate hypersensitivity to penicillin and related antibiotics. Clin Allergy 1988; 18:515.
120. Pleskow WN, Stevenson DD, Mathison DA, et al: Aspirin desensitization in aspirin sensitive asthmatic patients. J Allergy Clin Immunol 1982; 69:11.
121. Mattson JR, Patterson R, Roberts M: Insulin therapy with systemic insulin allergy. Arch Intern Med 1975; 135:818.
122. van der Linden P-WG, Struyvenberg A, Kraaijenhagen RJ, et al: Anaphylactic shock after insect sting challenge in 138 persons with a previous insect-sting reaction. Ann Intern Med 1993; 118:161.
123. Imbeau SA: Selecting patients for insect venom immunotherapy. Ann Intern Med 1993; 119:438.

19

Hemodynamic Evaluation and Management of Acute Illnesses in the Emergency Department

William C. Shoemaker, MD, FCCM • Michael J. Sullivan, MD
Charles C. J. Wo, BS

Patients who enter the emergency department (ED) with acute illness usually have symptoms and findings suggesting a number of possible diagnoses. The initial effort of the physician is to evaluate the patient's condition, develop a list of differential diagnoses, and begin a definitive assessment of appropriate blood chemistry profiles, x-rays, cultures, and other tests. The objective is to establish the diagnosis so that specific therapy may be started and the patient followed up or directed to the appropriate clinic or private physician for continued care. On occasion, the primary diagnosis may be circulatory in origin, such as acute myocardial infarction, chronic congestive heart failure, or arrhythmias. More often, however, circulatory dysfunction complicates another disorder that is usually regarded as the primary problem with circulatory problems as complications (Table 19-1). More importantly, circulatory dysfunction, whether primary or secondary, may become a serious or life-threatening problem if missed or underestimated.

Even though chief complaints are vague, ill-defined, or extraneous to the real problem, circulatory dysfunction in any acute illness may be suspected from imprecise signs and sub-

TABLE 19–1. Diagnostic Categories Likely to Result in Circulatory Dysfunction

Blunt trauma	Pneumonia
Gunshot wounds	Cellulitis
Stab wounds	Sepsis
Burns	Heat exhaustion
Crushing injuries	Alcoholic cirrhosis
Hemorrhage	Hyperemesis gravidarum
Acute myocardial infarction	Drug overdose
Heart failure with or without pulmonary edema	Protracted vomiting
	Prolonged diuretic therapy
Arrhythmias	Seizures

jective symptoms (Table 19-2). Circulatory dysfunction also may be suggested by hypotension or orthostatic changes in blood pressure and heart rate (a positive tilt test). These findings are not diagnostic, but they call attention to potentially severe circulatory problems, suggesting low flow and poor tissue perfusion from partially compensated hypovolemia or impaired cardiac function (see Chapter 8). Conventionally, these problems had been evaluated and treated in the intensive care unit (ICU) using invasive hemodynamic monitoring; with recently availability of noninvasive monitoring systems, however, these problems may be appropriately evaluated and therapy started in the ED.

Our approach is to identify and noninvasively monitor patients with early acute circulatory deficiencies, beginning in the first few minutes of arrival in the ED, and then to titrate therapy to correct or optimize treatment of hemodynamic problems as soon as possible. Early or preventive therapy is easier and more effective than waiting until the patient is admitted to the ICU after organ failure occurs.

METHODS AND CONCEPTS

Relation of Circulatory Dysfunction to Anatomic Pathology

Structural and functional abnormalities are the twin components of acute disease processes; they are (1) the anatomic changes produced by the disease process and (2) the associated functional circulatory deficiencies. The functional circulatory component is usually secondary to an anatomic-pathologic disease but may be the primary process, such as in anaphylactic or septic shock and disseminated intravascular coagulopathy. Treatment should cover both aspects of the disorder. Osler pointed out that patients rarely die of their disease; rather, they die of complications. In modern parlance, irrespective of the diagnosis, patients die of circulatory dysfunction leading to multiple organ failure.

Initial Care

The emergency physician, who may be responsible for interventions that determine the level of care necessary after admission, must be fully informed about methods and concepts of early hemodynamic management in acutely ill patients. The initial focus of diagnostic, monitoring, and therapeutic strategies in the ED are geared toward the assessment of the degree, magnitude, and extent of anatomic and organ dysfunctions. Less attention is given to the assessment of circulatory function, especially in acute nonemergent conditions. In part, this is because of the unavailability of definitive and reliable methods to monitor and evaluate circulatory therapy. When the extent of circulatory function is unclear, regardless of the initial insult, emergency management should evaluate and treat each of the major cardiovascular components—volume, flow, oxygenation, and tissue perfusion.

The care of patients who must undergo emergency operation may begin in the ED with prompt vigorous resuscitation. Both circulatory function and anatomic-pathologic lesions must be corrected. The success of one is interdependent with the success of the other. The patient and the disease are approached from two interrelated and complementary goals: (1) anatomic repair of the pathologic disorder and (2) simultaneous monitoring of physiologic deficiencies, restoration of circulatory function with therapy to maintain optimal circulatory function. Intraoperative physiologic deficiencies with or without compensations occur in cardiac, pulmonary, or tissue perfusion functions regardless of initiating insults or anatomic lesions. In routine cases, these may be relatively simple; in high-risk categories, hemodynamic monitoring should be used to assess and correct circulatory dynamics as they occur.

TABLE 19–2. Signs and Symptoms Suggesting Circulatory Dysfunction

1. Listlessness, depression, muscular weakness, confusion, disorientation, inability to communicate, anxiety, or agitation
2. Dehydration, thirst, dry mucous membranes, decreased skin turgor, decreased capillary refill, or oliguria
3. Cold, pale, clammy, mottled or cyanotic skin
4. Hypotension, weak thready pulse, sinus tachycardia, premature ventricular contractions, or other arrhythmias
5. Tachypnea or hyperpnea

Assessment of Fluid Therapy

Except for pulmonary edema and acute myocardiac infarction, most acutely ill patients receive intravenous fluids, either crystalloids or colloids, during their initial resuscitation. For many acute illnesses in the ED, fluid administration is an integral part of therapy. Conventional assessment of responses to transfusions or fluid therapy consists of intermittent recording of vital signs and other rather imprecise markers of hypovolemia. Skin turgor, urinary output, capillary refill, and normalization of vital signs are indirect markers whose normalization is presupposed to signify adequate intravascular expansion. Many studies have shown that these markers have limited sensitivity and specificity to define adequacy of fluid therapy in circulatory dysfunction. The circulatory dysfunction of acute illness and the hemodynamic effects of various fluid regimens have been studied noninvasively.[1] Regardless of the type and amount of fluid therapy used, improved cardiac, pulmonary, and tissue perfusion functions are appropriate criteria that reflect improved outcome. With immediate feedback and knowledge of the effects of various fluids, fluid therapy may be more readily titrated to achieve physiologic end points.

Monitoring Methods of Evaluating Circulatory Problems

Circulatory monitoring is seldom effective in improving outcome when it is used after organ failure has already occurred.[1–9, 19] Delay in starting is the most frequent cause of ineffective therapy, and too often patients do not arrive at the ICU until they are in late irreversible shock. It is crucial to monitor and treat patients as early as possible because early shock is readily reversible, but therapy usually is ineffective in late stage shock after organ failure has already occurred. The goal is to improve outcome by earlier warning with noninvasive monitoring systems in the ED and by prompt adequate therapy. In the chronic medical outpatient with anemia, restoration of red blood cells may be straightforward, but resuscitation of acutely ill emergency patients is highly complex as well as controversial.

The crucial problems are as follows:

- What is the nature of the disorder we are treating?
- How do we describe and measure it?
- What are the early temporal hemodynamic patterns beginning in the ED that determine outcome?
- How and when do various fluids, transfusions, blood products, and plasma substitutes affect the outcome of shock and circulatory dysfunction?

Invasive Hemodynamic Monitoring

The flow-directed balloon tipped pulmonary artery catheter is the current clinical "gold standard" for circulatory monitoring and for comparisons with new technology. Cardiac output is measured by the pulmonary artery (PA) thermodilution catheter (Swan-Ganz) method at intervals. Intravascular pressures, including systemic and PA pressure, central venous pressure (CVP), and wedge pressure (PAOP) may be obtained at intervals along with thermodilution measurements. Arterial blood and PA (mixed venous) blood may be anaerobically sampled at the time of thermodilution measurement, immediately analyzed, and used to calculate oxygen delivery ($\dot{D}O_2$) and oxygen consumption ($\dot{V}O_2$) (see Chapter 7). PA catheters provide the maximum logistically feasible monitoring, but because these monitoring systems require critical care environments, they are rarely available in the ED. However, noninvasive systems can provide similar hemodynamic information in the ED more easily, cheaply, and quickly and with comparable accuracy and reliability.[1]

Noninvasive Monitoring

Advances in hardware and software have led to an improved thoracic electric bioimpedance device that provides reliable, clinically relevant, continuous measurement of cardiac function. A thoracic bioelectric impedance device (I.Q. System, Renaissance Technology, Inc., Newtown, Pa.) may be applied shortly after admission to the ED. Four pairs of disposable prewired hydrogen electrodes are appropriately positioned on the skin,[10] and three electrocardiogram (ECG) leads are placed across the precordium and left shoulder.[10, 11] A 100-kHz, 4-mA alternating current is passed through the patient's thorax by the outer pairs of electrodes, and the voltage difference is measured by the inner pairs of electrodes. Baseline impedance (Z_0) is calculated from the voltage changes sensed by the inner pairs of electrodes. The first derivative of the impedance waveform (dZ/dT) is calculated from the time-impedance curve (see Chapter 7). Earlier studies have documented satisfactory correlation between thermodilution and bioimpedance cardiac index (CI) values[1, 12-17] and have explored its application in trauma and various acute illnesses (see Chapter 7).[15-22]

Heart rate, mean arterial pressure (MAP), pulse oximetry, CI, transcutaneous oxygen tension ($Ptco_2$), transcutaneous carbon dioxide tension ($Ptcco_2$), and the fractional inspired oxygen concentration (FIO_2) may be measured and recorded at intervals with the other measurements by an interfaced personal computer and filed directly into a data base.

Arterial blood pressures may be measured with an automatic noninvasive system (Dinamap, Critikon, Tampa, Fla.) at intervals simultaneously with other monitored values.

A standard pulse oximeter (Nellcor, Pleasanton, Calif.) is placed on a finger or toe in a routine fashion to measure continuously arterial blood oxygen saturation (Sao_2).[1, 23] Pulse oximetry gives the arterial oxyhemoglobin saturation, which in turn is a good estimation for Pao_2 when Pao_2 is below 100 torr. A drop of Pao_2 from 150 torr to 100 torr, for example, does not produce significant changes in Sao_2. However, pulmonary dysfunction may be instantly recognized by hypoxemia; this is more important than Sao_2 accuracy at Pao_2 levels above 100 torr or below 60 torr.

Tissue perfusion is usually inferred from *subjective symptoms* (e.g., weak thready pulse, cold clammy skin, altered mental status) or *imprecise signs* (e.g., blood pressure, heart rate). When the circulation is normal, $Ptco_2$ averages about 80% of the arterial O_2; with low flow or shock, however, it seriously underestimates arterial blood gas because it actually measures the oxygen tension of the heated skin surface, not the arterial blood. $Ptco_2$ may be continuously monitored in both neonate and adult (Novametrics Medical Systems, Wallingford, Conn.). A major misunderstanding is that pediatricians and neonatologists have used these instruments for almost 40 years as surrogate measures of arterial blood gases. This system uses the same Clark polarographic oxygen electrode that is routinely used in the standard in vitro blood gas analysis.[24-30] Gel electrolyte is applied to the sensor, and the sensor is fixed by an adhesive ring to alcohol-prepared skin on the anterior chest wall or shoulder, depending on area of injury and surgical procedure. The manufacturer recommends 20 minutes for equilibration after application before monitoring. At 44°C, the lipopolysaccharide layer of the stratum corneum changes from a gel to a sol state, facilitating gas diffusion from the subepidermal tissue to the sensor.[25] In addition, the heating inhibits local vasoconstriction. To avoid electrode-induced first-degree skin burns, the sensor is moved to a different area of skin in the same general locale every 4 hours. $Ptco_2$ values are measured in torr, indexed to FIO_2, and expressed as a dimensionless ratio, $Ptco_2/FIO_2$.

$Ptcco_2$ of the skin surface may be monitored with the standard Stowe-Severinghaus electrode.[31, 32]

Evaluation of Tissue Perfusion

Previous studies have demonstrated, in the acutely ill adult, the ability of $Ptco_2$ to directly measure tissue oxygen tension, which in turn reflects oxygen delivery to the local area of skin.[1, 18-32] Early studies[15-17, 26-29] evaluated $Ptco_2$ and $Ptcco_2$ as direct objective measurements of skin perfusion. $Ptco_2$, measured by the Clark polarographic electrode, and $Ptcco_2$, measured by the Stowe-Severinghaus electrode, are no more or less accurate and reliable than this same technique, which is used in standard blood gas analyzers; they directly measure gases in a localized segment of the skin. Although skin is not the most important organ, it is the first to react to sympathetic-adrenal stress response and, therefore, to provide early warning of poor tissue perfusion, impending organ failure, and death. When local tissue hypoxia of vital organs, such as the heart and brain, is revealed by the same sensors, it is already late in the course of shock and organ failure. From a practical viewpoint, early warning of impending circulatory dysfunction is preferable to definitive documentation of organ failure and death.

It is effective to assess tissue oxygenation with $Ptco_2$ while pulse oximetry is used to assess arterial hemoglobin saturation (oxygenation). However, the most important question is, how well do $Ptco_2$ and $Ptcco_2$ reflect clinical outcome in acute illnesses? Recent studies[1, 18-22] demonstrated a close relationship of $Ptco_2$ and $Ptcco_2$ with tissue perfusion patterns and outcome in a large series of trauma patients. The data are consistent with the concept that low flow and poor tissue perfusion, which lead to organ failure and death, may be documented early in the resuscitation period. These variables may be used to titrate early fluid therapy to reach preset physiologic goals as a strategy to prevent subsequent lethal organ failure.[1-9, 15-22]

Indications for and Aims of Noninvasive Hemodynamic Monitoring

The indications for monitoring and therapy can be defined by diagnostic categories or by the history of disorders that compromise circulatory function or contribute to poor outcome (see Table 19–1). When the diagnosis is known, patients may profit by noninvasive hemodynamic monitoring that titrates specific therapy to optimal values. Table 19–2 lists clinical signs and symptoms that reflect unstable hemodynamic states in widely varying clinical conditions; patients usually have hypovolemia, low flow states, and poor tissue perfusion as underlying problems. Noninvasive monitoring may be undertaken in the ED for specific diagnostic conditions or for nonspecific clinical findings that suggest circulatory dysfunction. In either case, monitoring is used to measure the degree of circulatory impairment, to define therapeutic goals, and to titrate therapy to achieve these goals expeditiously.[1, 15-22]

An Integrated Approach to the Circulatory Physiology of Acute Illness

An integrated approach to monitoring involves the three major circulatory components: (1) cardiac, (2) pulmonary, and (3) tissue perfusion functions. Cardiac function is represented by CI, changes in pulmonary function are reflected by pulse oximetry, and tissue perfusion is represented by $Ptco_2/FIO_2$ concentration ratio and $Ptcco_2$ values. The temporal patterns of these primary circulatory dysfunctions may be demonstrated by monitoring these essential variables continuously over time.[15]

Figure 19–1 illustrates the CI, MAP, $Sapo_2$, and $Ptco_2/FIO_2$ data of a gunshot victim who lost an estimated 5 L of blood; he was initially resuscitated in the ED, where he was found to have normal hemodynamic values except for poor tissue perfusion, which was restored by four transfusions of red blood cells. This number dropped again in the operating room (OR), where he received four more red blood cell transfusions, 3000 mL of crystalloids and 1000 mL of starch, which finally corrected and then optimized these variables. He was ob-

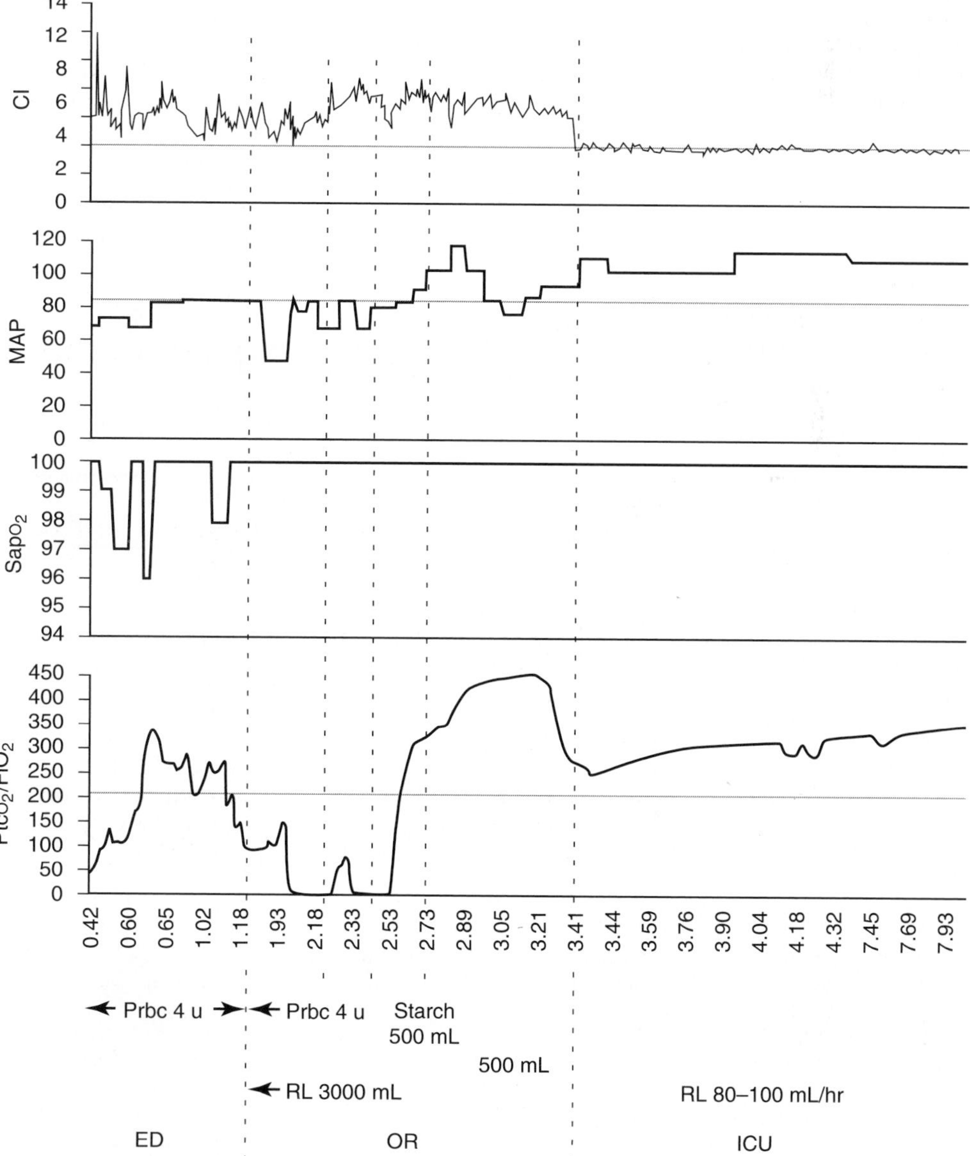

Figure 19–1. Illustrative data of a patient who had continuous monitoring from admission to the ED and initial resuscitation after an abdominal gunshot wound with lacerations of spleen, liver, and ileum that produced an estimated 5000 mL blood loss. *Upper section,* Cardiac index (CI). *Second section,* Mean arterial pressure (MAP). *Third section,* Arterial hemoglobin saturation by pulse oximetry ($Sapo_2$), *Fourth section,* $Ptco_2/FIO_2$. Time from admission to the emergency department (ED) is shown below the lowest horizontal line; therapy given during the times between the vertical lines in the ED, operating room (OR), and intensive care unit (ICU) are shown below. Prbc = packed red blood cells; RL = Ringer's lactate.

served while in the ED, OR, and ICU with continuous monitoring to provide a running account of the three important interacting circulatory components.

Figures 19–2 and 19–3 show the MAP, CI, $Sapo_2$, and $Ptco_2/FIO_2$ values of survivors and nonsurvivors of blunt trauma for the first 8 hours after ED admission. The circle diagrams in the lowest section represent the changing patterns of cardiac, pulmonary, and tissue perfusion functions.

Figure 19–4 shows the net cumulative deficit (below the horizontal line) or excess (above this line) for MAP, CI, $Sapo_2$, and $Ptco_2/FIO_2$ values of survivors and nonsurvivors of severe blunt trauma during the first 8 hours beginning at the time of admission to the ED. These data illustrate the net cumulative amount of deficit or excess of flow, arterial pressure, arterial oxygenation, and tissue perfusion in quantitative terms for those who survive and those who do not survive during their current hospitalization. The survivors during the first 8 hours after ED admission had a net cumulative excess over normal CI values of 348 L/m^2 · min; the nonsurvivors had an excess over normal of 104 L/m^2 · min. The calculated excess of MAP over normal values was 2935 mm Hg · min for survivors and 652 mm Hg · min for nonsurvivors. The calculated excess of $Sapo_2$ was +1800 torr · min for survivors, and the calculated deficit was −2200 torr · min for nonsurvivors. The calculated excess for dimensionless ratio ($Ptco_2/FIO_2$) was +33,391 for survivors, and the deficit for nonsurvivors was −72,348.

The data illustrate how relatively small changes that are tolerated over short periods may accumulate into appreciable losses over time. Furthermore, these net cumulative changes during the initial resuscitation period in the ED demonstrate major differences in survivor and nonsurvivor patterns of circulatory dysfunction. Monitoring in the ED can document low flow states and poor tissue perfusion, and it provides the means to titrate therapy to achieve the desired endpoint and maintains the appropriate values until other systems are brought into line and the patient is recovering satisfactorily.

Primary Physiologic Types of Shock: Hemorrhage, Hypoxia, and Anemia

More than 75 years ago, Barcroft classified shock as (1) *stagnant hypoxia* (low flow), (2) *anemic hypoxia* (low hematocrit), and (3) *hypoxic hypoxia* (low arterial oxygenation); later he added *tissue hypoxia* to include intracellular metabolic deterioration. Although instances of relatively pure etiologic types of shock have been described, most clinical shock conditions are combinations of the three primary types of shock and also are affected by age, prior illnesses, comorbid conditions, and differences in the reserve capacities of cardiac, pulmonary, and perfusion compensations.

In order to elucidate the possible influence of each of these three types of shock in complex clinical situations, Schwartz

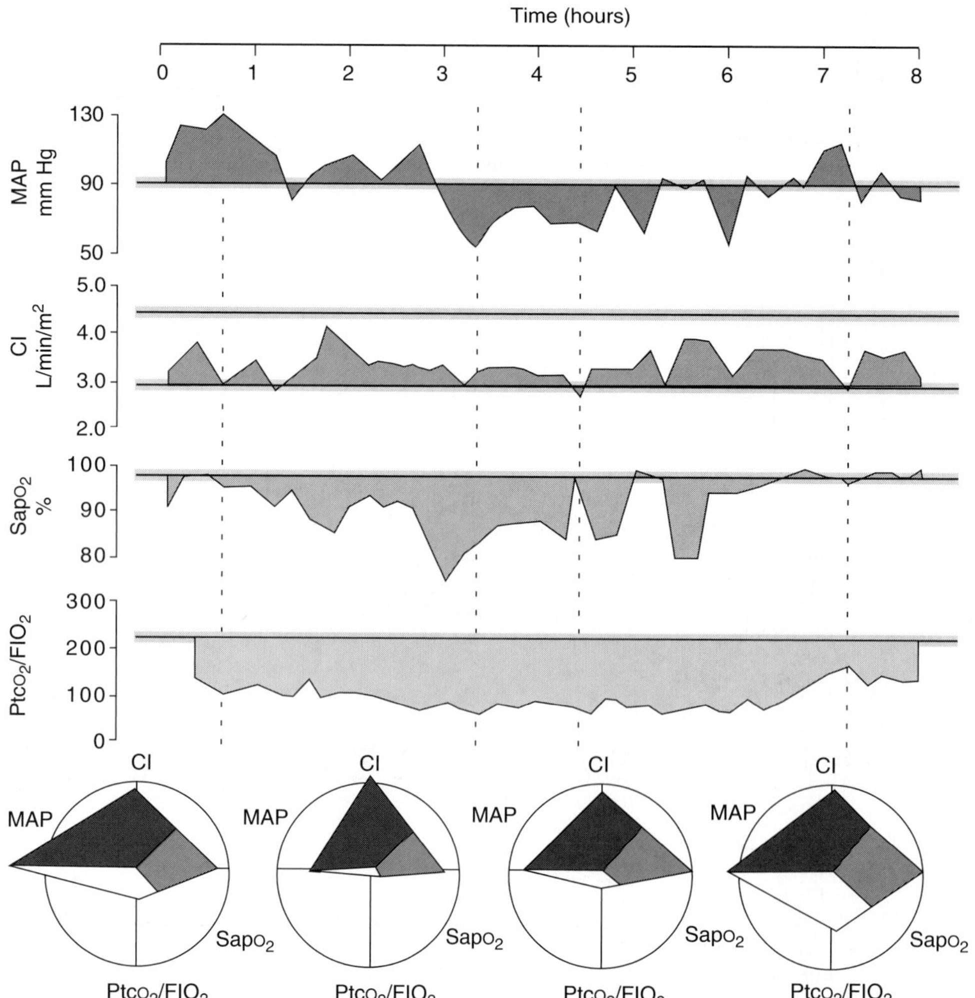

Figure 19–2. Data representing mean values of 82 consecutively monitored surviving patients with blunt truncal injury during the first 8 hours after admission to the emergency department (ED). *Top,* Time from ED admission. *First section,* mean arterial pressure (MAP). *Second section,* Cardiac index (CI). *Third section,* Arterial hemoglobin saturation by pulse oximetry ($Sapo_2$). *Fourth section,* $Ptco_2/FIO_2$. *Horizontal lines* represent normal values, and the additional *horizontal line* in the CI section at 4.5 L/min/m^2 represents the optimal goal. The *circle diagrams* at the bottom represent the interacting cardiac, pulmonary, and tissue perfusion functions at the time of each of the vertical *dashed lines*. Note the slight hypertension, the high CI that almost reaches optimal values throughout the first 8 hours of hospitalization, and the relatively normal $Sapo_2$ and $Ptco_2/FIO_2$.

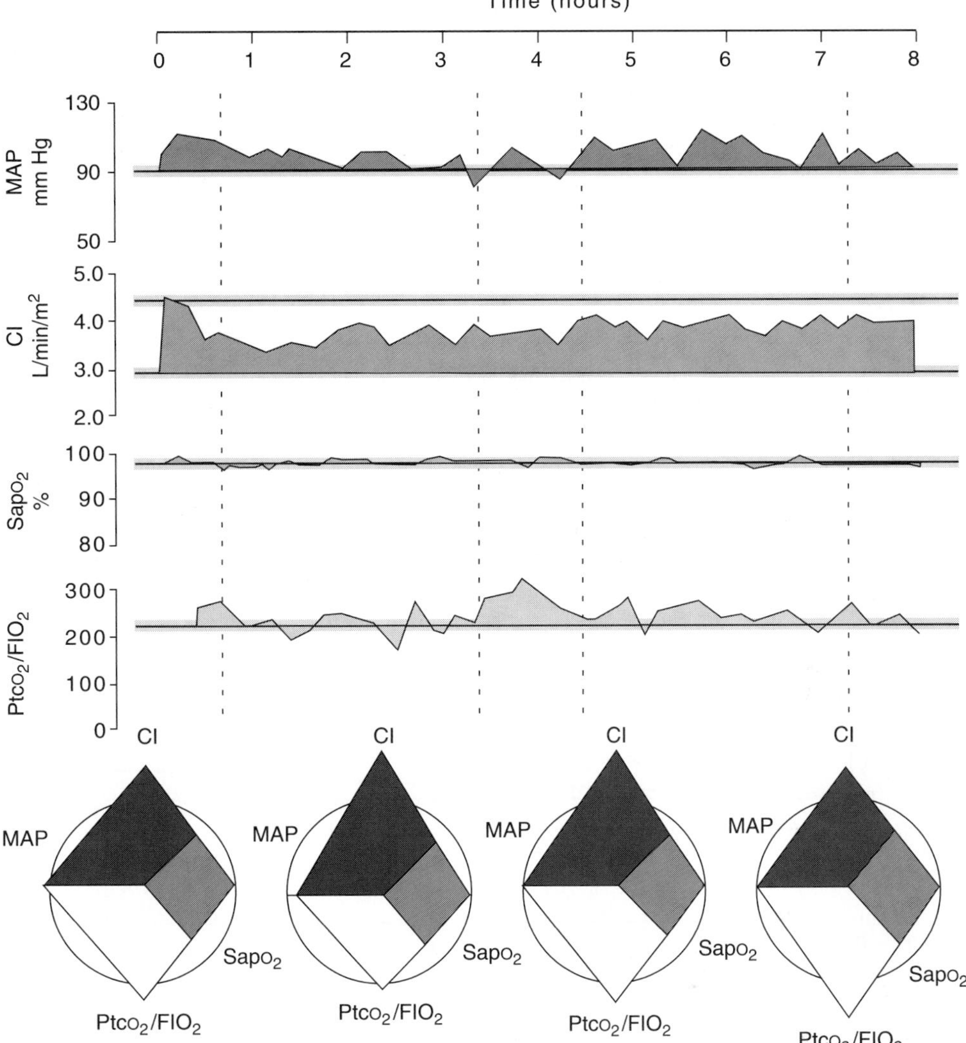

Figure 19–3. Data representing mean values of 27 consecutively monitored nonsurviving patients with blunt truncal injury during the first 8 hours after admission to the emergency department (ED). *Top,* Time from ED admission. *First section,* mean arterial pressure (MAP). *Second section,* Cardiac index (CI). *Third section,* Arterial hemoglobin saturation by pulse oximetry (Sa_{O_2}). *Fourth section:* Ptc_{O_2}/FI_{O_2}. *Horizontal lines* represent normal values, and the additional *horizontal line* in the CI section at 4.5 L/min/m² represents the optimal goal. The *circle diagrams* at the bottom represent the interacting cardiac, pulmonary, and tissue perfusion functions at the time of each of the vertical dashed lines. Note the pronounced hypertension in the first hour, relatively normal CI, the pronounced reduction of Sa_{O_2} after the first hour subsequently corrected by intubation, mechanical ventilation with high FI_{O_2} levels, and the marked and sustained reduction in tissue perfusion, reflected by Ptc_{O_2}/FI_{O_2} values, throughout the period of observation.

and colleagues[33] described in three groups of experimental animals, each of which were subjected to a single etiologic event: (1) rapid hemorrhage, (2) progressive reduction in inspired oxygen concentrations, and (3) progressive replacement of red blood cell mass with plasma. Figure 19–5 illustrates these three hemodynamic patterns. Hemorrhage progressively decreased MAP, CI, and $\dot{D}O_2$, the primary effects of hypovolemia; it increased systemic vascular resistance (SVR), O_2 content difference, and O_2 extraction ratios, which may be compensatory effects of hypovolemia that maintained the $\dot{V}O_2$ relatively normal until late in the course of events.[33] This suggests that maintenance of $\dot{V}O_2$ was a regulatory mechanism that controlled compensations to hypovolemia.

Anemia decreased SVR and $\dot{D}O_2$, and it increased CI and O_2 extraction ratios; the MAP, O_2 content difference, and $\dot{V}O_2$ remained relatively normal.[33] This suggests that reduced hemoglobin, being primary, caused reduced $\dot{D}O_2$ and compensatory increases in CI (with associated fall in SVR) to maintain $\dot{V}O_2$ as long as possible.

Hypoxia decreased arterial Pa_{O_2} and $\dot{D}O_2$, the primary effects of hypoxia, and increased O_2 extraction ratios in compensation for the hypoxemia; the increases in SVR occurred late, while the MAP, CI, O_2 content difference, and $\dot{V}O_2$ remained relatively normal until late.[33] These data are consistent with the concept that the $\dot{V}O_2$ is the controlling or regulatory mechanism that is maintained to preserve cellular metabolism by various compensations; by definition, the compensations depart from their normal range in order to preserve $\dot{V}O_2$, since the major function of the circulation is to provide for cellular oxidative metabolism.

MONITORING AND MANAGEMENT OF ACUTE ILLNESSES

Dehydration and Hypovolemia

Hypovolemia from dehydration, poor fluid intake, blood loss, diarrhea, vomiting, and excessive diuretic therapy may be easy to recognize and straightforward to treat in most instances. However, hemodynamic monitoring is particularly useful when there are associated comorbid conditions, such as cardiac history of previous infarctions, findings of early cardiac failure, arrhythmias, age over 65 years, chronic pulmonary disorders, and other complex conditions.

Blunt Trauma

Previous studies have demonstrated that increased flow is critical to survival of acutely ill trauma patients[1–9, 14–22]; Bishop and colleagues[34, 35] found early increased $\dot{D}O_2$ less than 24 hours after trauma to be associated with improved survival.

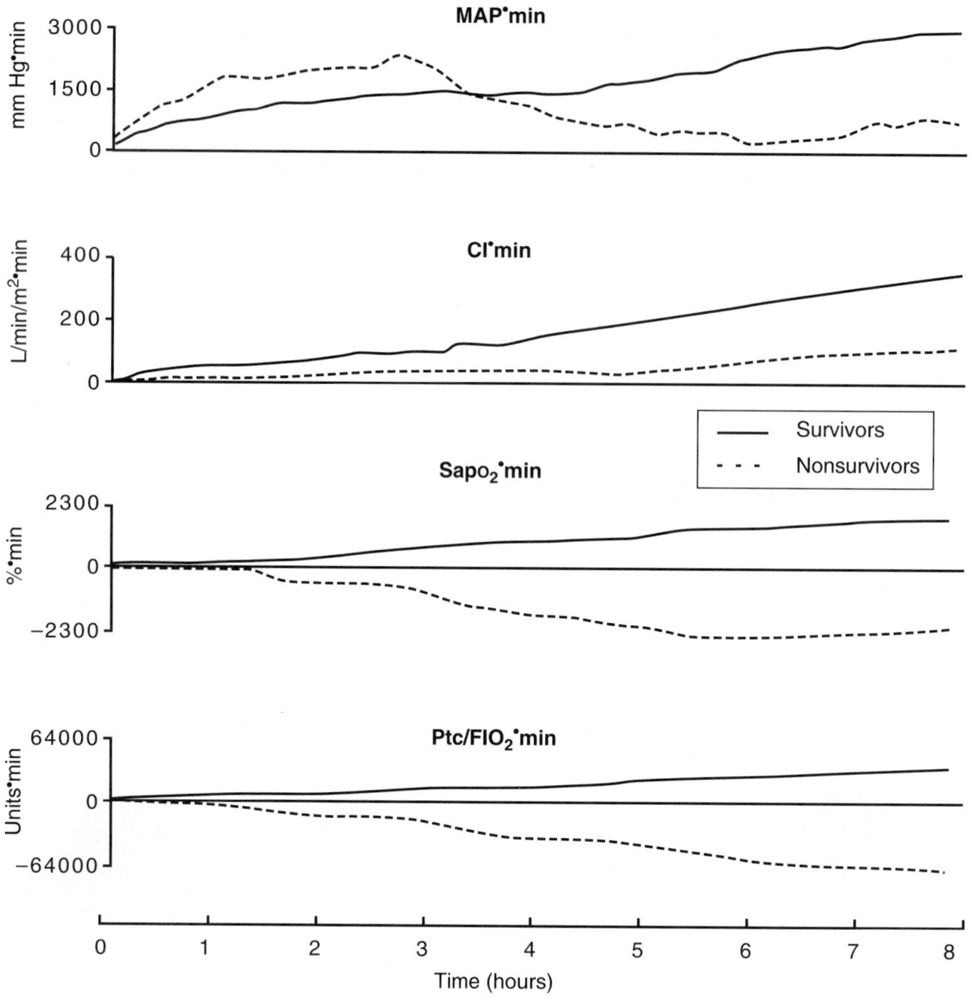

Figure 19–4. The net cumulative deficit or excess in mean arterial pressure (MAP•min), flow (cardiac index [CI]• min), and arterial hemoglobin saturation (Sa_{O_2}• min), reflected by tissue perfusion (Ptc_{O_2}/FIO_2) values, for survivors and nonsurvivors of blunt truncal trauma throughout the first 8 hours of observation. The initial high cumulative excess in MAP in nonsurvivors is followed by reduced net cumulative pressure excesses, in contrast to the sustained cumulative gains in the survivors. Note the marked and sustained cumulative increases in flow in the survivors compared with only modest cumulative gains in the nonsurvivors. Note the continued cumulative excesses in Sa_{O_2} in the survivors compared with continuing cumulative deficits in the nonsurvivors. Finally, note the sustained cumulative excess in tissue perfusion in survivors compared with the progressive cumulative deficit in nonsurvivors.

Recently, several consecutively series of acute severely injured patients were monitored in the ED. Belzberg and associates[22] prospectively compared hemodynamic patterns by simultaneous invasive and noninvasive measurements during resuscitation of 80 consecutively monitored blunt trauma patients beginning in the first few minutes after arrival in the ED through the early phase of hospitalization. Episodes of hypotension, low CI, arterial hemoglobin desaturation, low Ptc_{O_2}, high $Ptcc_{O_2}$, and low $\dot{V}_{O_2}$ were observed before and during initial resuscitation. MAP, CI, pulse oximetry, Ptc_{O_2}, Ptc_{O_2}/FIO_2 ratio, $\dot{D}_{O_2}$, and $\dot{V}_{O_2}$ were greater in the survivors; $Ptcc_{O_2}$ values were higher in the nonsurvivors.[22]

The noninvasive monitoring systems begun in the ED provided early warning with information similar to that of the invasive thermodilution method; both approaches identified initial low flow and poor tissue perfusion that were compensated by subsequent increases in flow and oxygen transport (Fig. 19-6). Noninvasive monitoring was used early in acute emergency conditions to identify hemodynamic deficiencies in patients with suspected circulatory problems. Early circulatory abnormalities were identified in 64/80 (80%) of these seriously injured blunt trauma victims; 14 (18%) of these patients with circulatory compromise died during their hospitalization.[22]

The hemodynamic response to severe blunt trauma, while not entirely uniform, demonstrated a consistent initial pattern of circulatory events with reduced flow despite normal or increased arterial pressure. This pattern was more pronounced in the patients who died, suggesting increased mortality in patients whose increased pressure failed to generate adequate flow increases. It has been shown that these pressure changes may be mediated by the production of catecholamines and other vasoactive substances, which are elements of the stress response. Other authors have demonstrated that increased flow is critical to survival of high-risk critically ill patients.[1-9, 14-22, 34-38]

The vasoconstrictive response and consequent "peripheral shunt" may be uneven in terms of the various organs affected as well as within the vascular beds of each organ. The low or uneven flow to the skin, which is often the first organ affected, is directly reflected by low Ptc_{O_2}, which is usually the first abnormality observed. The compensatory stress response may adequate, inadequate, or transiently sufficient. When the stress response becomes either overwhelmed or exhausted, there is a reduction in blood pressure in patients previously considered to be "stable." This transient nature of the stress response may be due to overwhelming injury, hypovolemia, or exhaustion of the stress response. The smaller initial transient fall in CI in survivors and the subsequent rise in flow and $\dot{D}_{O_2}$ may be a compensatory response to the initial low flow state[15-17] or may be due to lesser injury, lesser degrees of hypovolemia, greater preload, more aggressive therapy, and increased metabolic demand produced by trauma itself. The combination of increased demand and abnormal perfusion

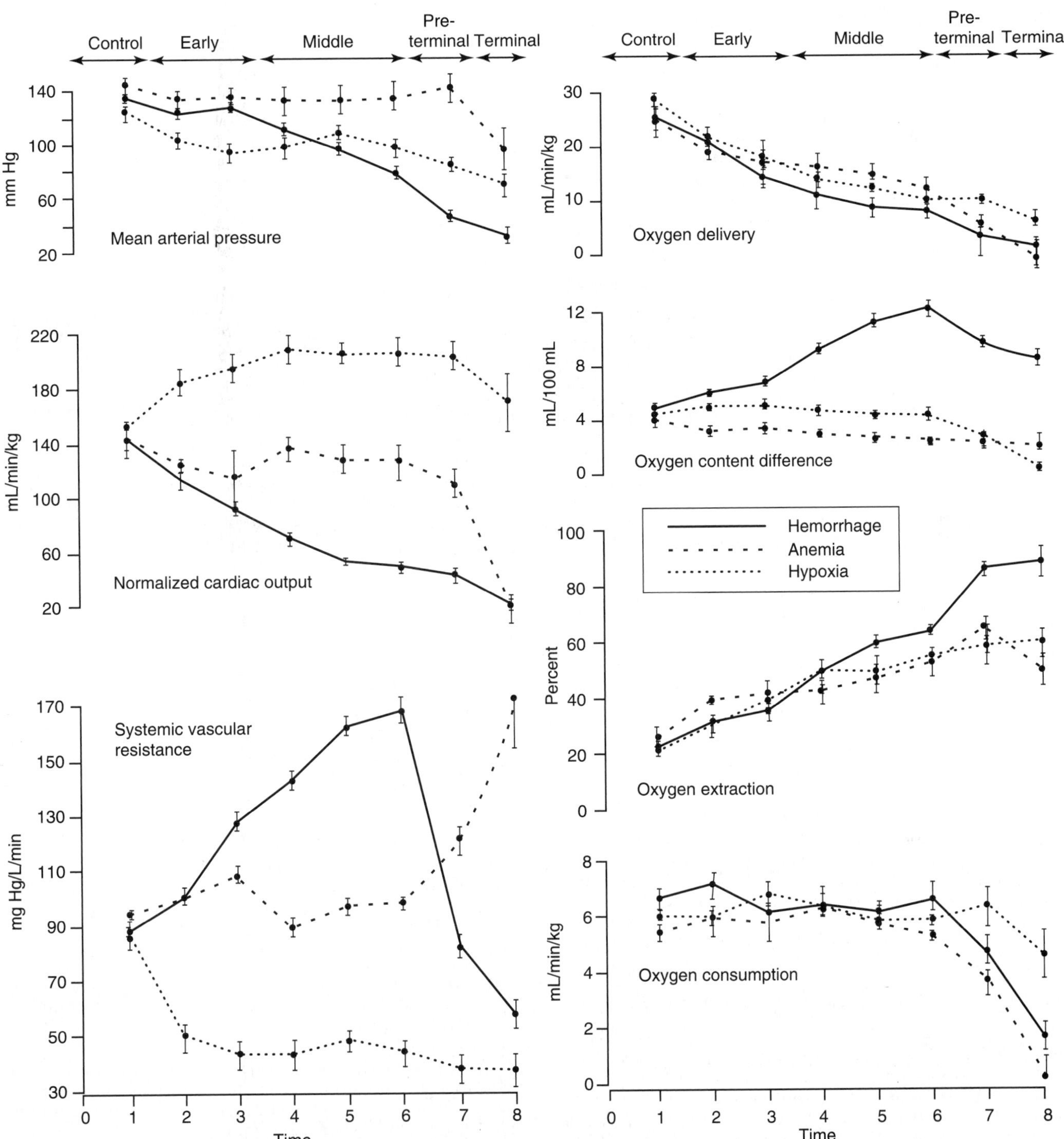

Figure 19–5. Hemodynamic patterns in three groups of experimental animals, each subjected to a single shock-producing event: (1) rapid hemorrhage, (2) reduction in inspired oxygen concentrations, and (3) replacement of red blood cell mass with plasma. Hemorrhage progressively decreased mean arterial pressure (MAP), cardiac index (CI), and oxygen delivery ($\dot{D}O_2$) (the primary effects of hypovolemia), and it increased systemic vascular resistance (SVR), O_2 content difference, and O_2 extraction ratios. Anemia decreased SVR and $\dot{D}O_2$ and increased CI and O_2 extraction ratios; MAP, the O_2 content difference, and $\dot{V}O_2$ remained relatively normal. Hypoxia decreased arterial PaO_2 and $\dot{D}O_2$ (the primary effects of hypoxia) and increased O_2 extraction ratios in compensation for the hypoxemia; the SVR increases occurred late; the MAP, CI, O_2 content difference, and VO_2 remained relatively normal until late. (From Schwartz S, Frantz RA, Shoemaker WC: Sequential hemodynamic and oxygen transport response in hypovolemia, anemia, and hypoxia. Am J Physiol (Heart Circ) 1981; 241:H864–871.)

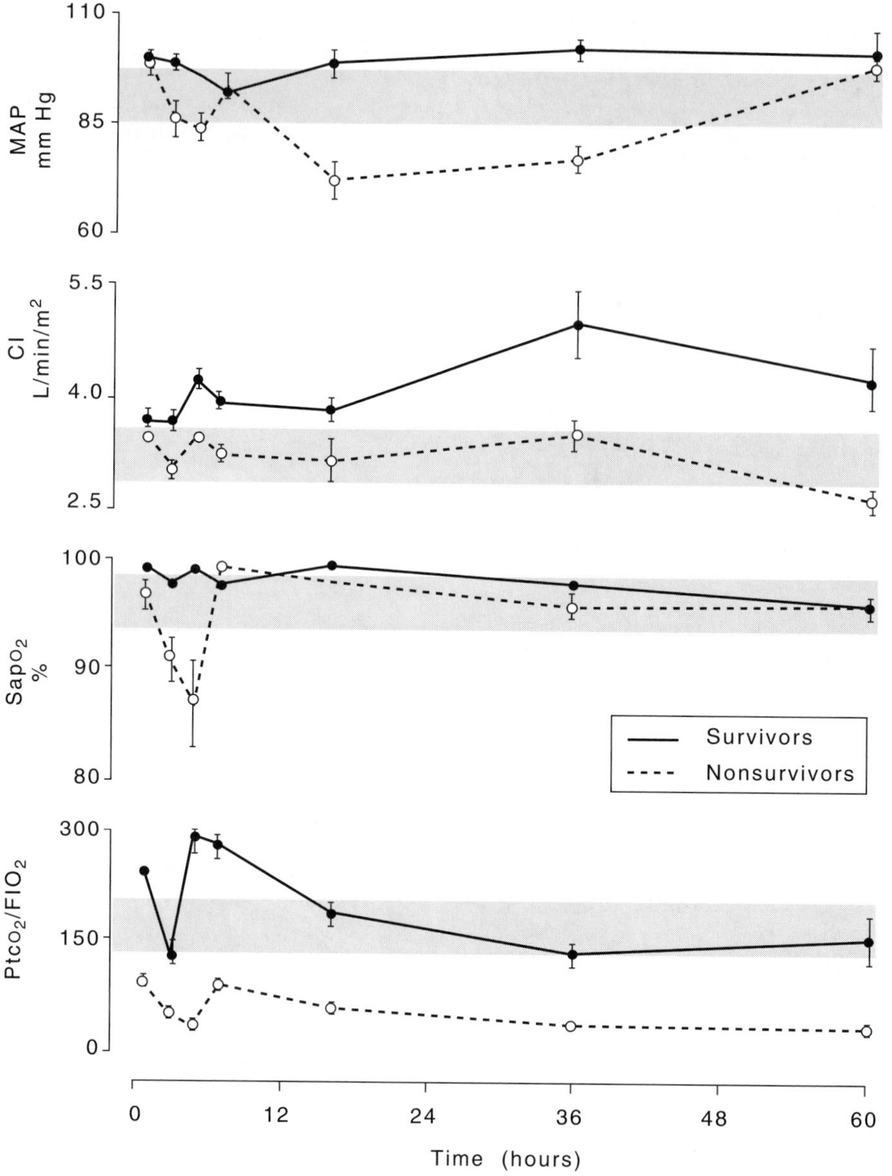

Figure 19–6. Noninvasive hemodynamic data of a consecutive series of 92 monitored blunt trauma patients from the time of admission to the emergency department for mean arterial pressure (MAP), cardiac index (CI), arterial hemoglobin saturation ($Sapo_2$), and tissue perfusion ($Ptco_2/FIO_2$). Data of survivors are shown in *solid lines*; data of nonsurvivors are shown in *dashed lines. Shaded areas* represent normal ranges. Note marked differences between survivors and nonsurvivors, particularly in CI and $Ptco_2/FIO_2$.

leads to the development of oxygen debt, which may ultimately lead to multisystem organ failure and death.[36]

Early Patterns After Penetrating Injury

Bishop and coworkers[34, 35] reported an 18% mortality rate in penetrating trauma from gunshot wounds with severe shock from blood loss of greater than 3000 mL and injury severity scores of greater than 20, when the accumulated delays were less than 24 hours from the time of injury to the time postoperatively when optimal supranormal values were achieved. By contrast, when delays were greater than 24 hours or when supranormal optimal values were not achieved, the mortality rate was 39%.

Subsequently, 65 patients with acute circulatory problems from truncal gunshot wounds were simultaneously monitored by invasive and noninvasive systems shortly after admission to the ED of a university-run county hospital.[15-17] The aim was to prospectively compare simultaneous invasive and noninvasive measurements of circulatory function during resuscitation and to describe acute hemodynamic patterns of survivors and nonsurvivors. Episodes of hypotension, low cardiac index, arterial hemoglobin desaturation, low $Ptco_2$, high $Ptcco_2$, and low $\dot{V}o_2$ were observed during initial resuscitation shortly after admission. The noninvasive monitoring systems provide early warning with information similar to that of the invasive thermodilution method; both approaches identified low flow and poor tissue perfusion that were more pronounced in the nonsurvivors. Of the 65 patients, 34 (52%) had reduced a cardiac index that averaged 1.86 ± 0.71 (SD) L/min/m² at its nadir; 33 (51%) had reduced $Ptco_2$ averaging 20.4 ± 2.9 torr; 29 (45%) had high $Ptcco_2$ averaging 69.8 ± 1.9 torr; 27 (41%) had hypotension averaging 58 ± 2 mm Hg; and 10/60 (17%) had low arterial saturations averaging 85 ± 1.5%. Fourteen of 28 patients (50%) with $\dot{V}o_2$ measurements had low values that averaged 90 ± 4 mL/min/m².[15]

The initial reductions in MAP, CI, CVP, $\dot{D}o_2$, and $\dot{V}o_2$ and elevations in heart rate were greater in nonsurvivors. With resuscitation, there were greater elevations in the first five of

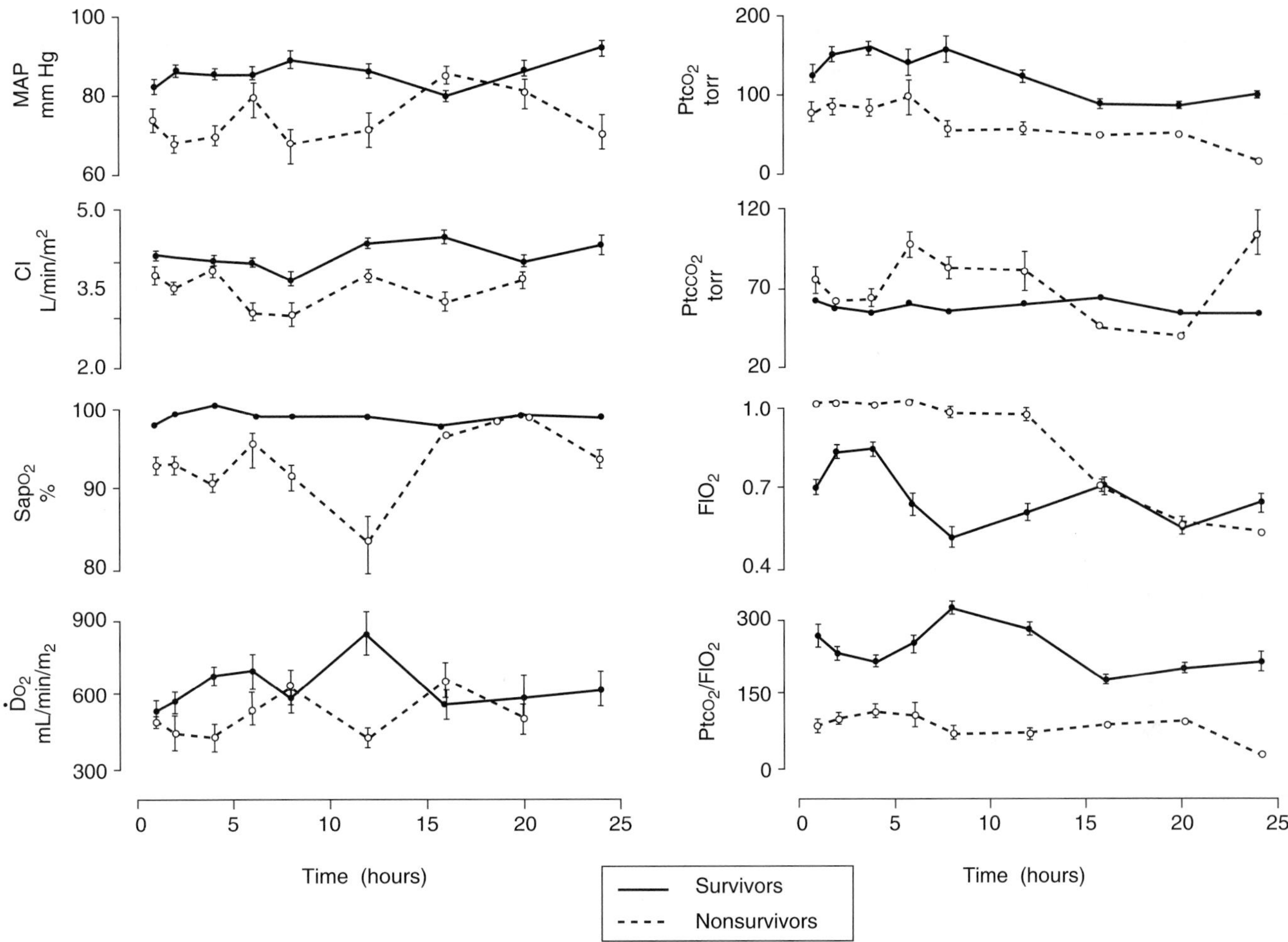

Figure 19–7. Noninvasive hemodynamic data of a consecutive series of 71 patients with gunshot wounds monitored from the time of admission to the emergency department for mean arterial pressure (MAP), cardiac index (CI), arterial hemoglobin saturation ($Sapo_2$), oxygen delivery (Do_2), $Ptco_2$, $Ptcco_2$, and tissue perfusion ($Ptco_2/FIO_2$). Survivor data are shown by in *solid lines*; nonsurvivor data are shown by *dashed lines*. Note marked differences between survivors and nonsurvivors, particularly in CI, $Sapo_2$, $Ptco_2$, and $Ptco_2/FIO_2$.

these parameters in survivors than in nonsurvivors. In some nonsurvivors after 3 or 5 days, however, septic complications and organ failures led to higher $\dot{V}o_2$ values associated with late-stage increases in body metabolism and nonphosphorylation oxidation.

The temporal patterns of invasive and noninvasive circulatory variables of survivors and nonsurvivors, beginning with the initial measurements after admission to the ED, are heart rate, MAP, CI, pulse oximetry, $Ptco_2$; $\dot{D}o_2$ and $\dot{V}o_2$ were generally higher in survivors than in nonsurvivors.

Sequential Hemodynamic Patterns in Hemorrhagic Shock

Table 19-3 shows the immediate direct effects of sudden hemorrhage of more than 4 units of blood evaluated by noninvasive methods in the ED. The table shows, for survivors and nonsurvivors, the initial baseline values on admission to the ED; the values at the nadir (or lowest recorded value) in variables that fell or the highest recorded value in the $Ptcco_2$, the only variable that rose, and the values at the initial resuscitation. There was reduced flow, MAP, and $Ptco_2$ with increased $Ptcco_2$; these effects were more pronounced in nonsurvivors. Initial $Sapo_2$ and Pao_2 values were usually close to normal, whereas tissue perfusion (reflected by reduced $Ptco_2$ and increased $Ptcco_2$) rapidly declined with moderate degrees of hypovolemia. With severe hypovolemia, hyperpnea and tachypnea occurred, usually with slightly reduced Pao_2 and pH values. With prolonged shock, poor tissue perfusion led to acidosis, base deficits, and increased lactate levels.

Rapid hemorrhage has traditionally been studied in the ICU by invasive PA monitoring and has shown reduced MAP, CI, CVP, PAOP, stroke index, stroke work, mixed venous oxygen saturation (Svo_2), pH, hematocrit, $\dot{D}o_2$, and $\dot{V}o_2$ concomitant with increased systemic vascular resistance index (SVRI) and oxygen extraction ratio.[15]

The initial compensatory responses included increased heart rate, which increased the CI by neural and neurohormonal mechanisms; increased SVRI, which tended to maintain arterial pressures in the face of decreasing flow; and increased oxygen extraction ratios, which improved tissue oxygenation when blood flow had been reduced.

With prolonged hemorrhage, the shock pattern showed greater reductions in hematocrit and lesser reductions in MAP, CI, $\dot{D}o_2$, and $\dot{V}o_2$; the reduction in $\dot{V}o_2$ was lower quantitatively but more prolonged than that occurring after rapid losses of comparable quantities of blood. After bleeding was stopped

TABLE 19–3. Noninvasive Hemodynamic Patterns in Various Acute Emergencies: Mean Values ± SEM

	Survivors			Nonsurvivors		
Variable Unit	***Baseline***	***Nadir***	***Resuscitation***	***Baseline***	***Nadir***	***Resuscitation***
			Hemorrhage			
CI, L/min/m^2	3.91 ± 0.78	2.15 ± 0.57	3.85 ± 0.83	4.42 ± 1.35	1.24 ± 0.30*	2.30 ± 0.10
MAP, mmHg	98 ± 29	65 ± 8	97 ± 13	71 ± 17	52 ± 23	88 ± 3
$Sapo_2$, %	93 ± 4	89 ± 1	95 ± 3	91 ± 4	88 ± 6*	94 ± 4
$Ptco_2$, torr	54 ± 7	32 ± 14	60 ± 15	82 ± 38	17 ± 14†	58 ± 34
$Ptcco_2$, torr	59 ± 7	65 ± 8‡	55 ± 3	83 ± 43	121 ± 61†, ‡	34 ± 23
			Cardiogenic Shock			
CI, L/min/m^2	2.93 ± 0.76	2.30 ± 0.68	3.15 ± 0.72	1.82 ± 0.66	1.41 ± 0.57*	2.37 ± 0.41
MAP, mmHg	87 ± 14	74 ± 18	92 ± 16	73 ± 18	51 ± 13*	79 ± 16
$Sapo_2$, %	97 ± 4	92 ± 6	96 ± 3	95 ± 5	91 ± 1	94 ± 4
$Ptco_2$, torr	43 ± 18	26 ± 9	43 ± 10	28 ± 18	19 ± 13	42 ± 24
$Ptcco_2$, torr	56 ± 8	65 ± 9	58 ± 9	107 ± 46	113 ± 44	109 ± 42
			Hypertension			
CI, L/min/m^2	2.85 ± 0.50	2.32 ± 0.63	3.26 ± 0.57	1.83 ± 0.48	1.52 ± 0.54	2.55 ± 0.79
MAP, mmHg	120 ± 14	134 ± 13‡	119 ± 11	122 ± 19	138 ± 12‡	127 ± 2
$Sapo_2$, %	96 ± 3	95 ± 2	96 ± 3	94 ± 3	93 ± 4	95 ± 2
$Ptco_2$, torr	45 ± 14	27 ± 9	41 ± 8	74 ± 9	20 ± 15*	38 ± 14
$Ptcco_2$, torr	61 ± 15	73 ± 17	64 ± 12	42 ± 6	64 ± 4	40 ± 6
			Early Sepsis			
CI, L/min/m^2	3.88 ± 1.03	3.03 ± 1.10	3.84 ± 1.38	3.23 ± 1.11	2.51 ± 1.11	3.72 ± 1.31
MAP, mmHg	80 ± 5	65 ± 12	86 ± 16	79 ± 15	59 ± 13*	87 ± 8
$Sapo_2$, %	96 ± 2	90 ± 9	95 ± 3	95 ± 3	84 ± 12	94 ± 3
$Ptco_2$, torr	55 ± 19	23 ± 16	56 ± 25	39 ± 17	16 ± 14*	43 ± 21
$Ptcco_2$, torr	67 ± 16	69 ± 21	61 ± 10	88 ± 5	174 ± 6‡	51 ± 6
			Drug Overdose			
CI, L/min/m^2	3.52 ± 0.90	3.30 ± 0.76	3.97 ± 0.95	2.36 ± 1.84	1.19 ± 0.76	3.14 ± 0.75
MAP, mmHg	87 ± 6	80 ± 7	85 ± 9	55 ± 3	43 ± 12*	68 ± 22
$Sapo_2$, %	95 ± 3	94 ± 4	95 ± 3	93 ± 4	68 ± 18*	92 ± 7
$Ptco_2$, torr	34 ± 6	29 ± 5	37 ± 5	9 ± 2	1 ± 3*	10 ± 11
$Ptcco_2$, torr	56 ± 6	60 ± 6	56 ± 3	85 ± 21	87 ± 31‡	73 ± 28
			Stroke			
CI, L/min/m^2	2.66 ± 0.51	2.16 ± 0.55	3.01 ± 0.61	2.14 ± 0.95	1.84 ± 0.77*	2.80 ± 1.90
MAP, mmHg	84 ± 23	68 ± 20	86 ± 11	68 ± 24	29 ± 5*	57 ± 24
$Sapo_2$, %	95 ± 3	92 ± 3	95 ± 4	96 ± 4	88 ± 6	95 ± 4
$Ptco_2$, torr	40 ± 3	29 ± 4	43 ± 7	25 ± 14	19 ± 13	35 ± 30
$Ptcco_2$, torr	55 ± 5	62 ± 2	55 ± 5	61 ± 13	65 ± 10	55 ± 12

*$P < .05$.
†$P < .01$.
‡Highest recorded value for $Ptcco_2$ and MAP in hypertension and hemorrhage.
CI = cardiac index; MAP = mean arterial pressure; $Sapo_2$ = arterial hemoglobin saturation; $Ptco_2$ = transcutaneous oxygen tension; $Ptcco_2$ = transcutaneous carbon dioxide tension.

and blood volume was restored with appropriate fluids, the recovery pattern in survivors usually consisted of normal or somewhat elevated values for CI, $\dot{D}o_2$, and $\dot{V}o_2$.

Head Injury

Early studies have characterized circulatory changes after head injury as hypertension and increased cardiac output, but several different patterns evolve over time and reflect various underlying mechanisms. The direct physiologic response to head trauma is increased cardiac output, MAP, and heart rate when fluid resuscitation is adequate. Elevation of blood pressure without elevation in heart rate—the Cushing response—occurs with cerebral hypoperfusion and is roughly correlated with high intracranial pressure (ICP). In 60 patients with head trauma noninvasively monitored on arrival to the ED, the predominant finding was the hyperdynamic state characterized by high CI, tachycardia, hypertension, normal pulmonary function, and reduced $Ptco_2/FIO_2$ values.[39] In general, the observed CI and tissue perfusion values were greater in survivors than in nonsurvivors and in patients with a high Glasgow Coma Scale (GCS) score compared with those with a low GCS score (see Chapter 27). The patterns of patients with isolated head injuries were similar to patterns of patients with head injury and associated somatic injuries; however, heart rate, CI, and $Ptco_2/FIO_2$ values in patients with isolated head injury were slightly higher. Three of 60 (5%) of the patients with isolated head injuries demonstrated early significant arterial desaturation. Increased arterial pressure and flow in survivors and those with a high GCS score may be compensatory responses to poor tissue perfusion-oxygenation mediated in part by adrenomedullary and central neural mechanisms.[39–41]

Pronounced deficiencies in peripheral tissue perfusion and oxygenation were found in trauma patients with profound hypovolemia refractory to resuscitation[36–48]; this reflects exaggerated sympathoadrenal vasoconstriction. High ICP associated with edema from closed head trauma of varying severity may interfere with cerebral perfusion and lead to ischemia, hypoxia, and hypercarbia of the brain parenchyma. Hypercarbia activates central nervous system (CNS) pH and bicarbonate sensors that profoundly stimulate the sympathetic nervous system, evidenced by increases in blood pressure (Cushing response), cardiac output, and $\dot{V}O_2$, but with minimal tachycardia.

Lack of an apparent sympathoadrenal response in patients with severe head injury suggests inability of the CNS to generate or communicate the appropriate response or the periphery's inability to respond appropriately. If the function of the periphery in the acutely traumatized patient is otherwise intact, primary or secondary neuronal injury is most likely the cause of the limited response. We should not expect mechanisms mediated by the CNS to operate predictably after head trauma. Erratic, unexpected behavior of regulatory mechanisms may result from one of the following:

- Primary damage to areas of the brain
- Cerebral hypoxia due to hypovolemia, systemic hypotension, low cerebral perfusion pressure or regional hypoperfusion
- Secondary injury from cerebral edema, hemorrhage, or inflammation

With damage or dysfunction of the areas that regulate hemodynamic function, ineffective, inappropriate, or uncontrolled attempts by malfunctioning response systems or failure of central inhibitory mechanisms may produce hemodynamic deviations from the normal, including those that can be maladaptive or detrimental to recovery.

Cardiovascular Emergencies

Cardiovascular emergencies present with a wide range of signs and symptoms. The initial history and physical examination may not differentiate between a life-threatening condition and the slow progression of an underlying disease state. Similarly, two acute life-threatening situations—acute myocardial infarction and dissecting aortic aneurysm—may be indistinguishable on initial presentation. Mistaking one for the other may lead to increased morbidity and mortality; that is, thrombolytic therapy for an aortic dissection or surgical intervention for an acute myocardial infarction may lead to avoidable mortality. A range of cardiovascular diseases may share common manifestations that make differentiation by routine assessment and monitoring difficult. Intermittent arrhythmias, congestive heart failure, and pulmonary embolism can present with a chief complaint of shortness of breath. Late in the course of disease, physiologic compensatory mechanisms may fail and unmask the underlying pathologic processes.

The ED may used for patients at risk for an ischemic cardiac event by history or by risk factors with unremarkable physical and ECG findings. Current practice is for cardiac enzyme evaluation to monitor for release of intracellular cardiac myocyte content signaling cell death. Cardiac enzymes take several hours to peak, and evaluation must be repeated to increase specificity. Regional wall-motion abnormality noted on echocardiography in the ED is an appropriate method of detecting cardiac ischemia after onset of ischemic events. Noninvasive hemodynamic monitoring is a useful approach to measure the physiologic deficiencies and to plan therapy. Unmonitored interventions targeted at supporting circulatory function may not be effective. Unsuccessful resuscitation was associated with the use of epinephrine, atropine, bicarbonate, calcium, and lidocaine for in-hospital cardiac arrest.[49]

Patients may be stratified into high-risk or low-risk categories for an ischemic cardiac event by historical and clinical risk criteria. Continuous hemodynamic monitoring of cardiac function allows instantaneous recognition of changes in hemodynamic variables secondary to an ischemic event (see Table 19-3). Physiologic monitoring of circulatory parameters to achieve endpoints targeted to specific physiologic criteria may improve outcome even when the diagnosis is unclear. Stabilization and support of circulatory functions based on defined hemodynamic goals can occur while diagnostic evaluations are undertaken. Physiologic patterns may identify circulatory dysfunction regardless of the underlying cardiac disease and may allow early appropriate therapy to be safely titrated even before the definitive diagnosis is established. Titration of therapy to targeted physiologic goals may obviate the need for heroic measures after cardiovascular collapse.

Heart Failure

Heart failure is a common medical emergency that is treated in the ED. About 400,000 new cases of heart failure are diagnosed each year. More than 2 million people suffer from heart failure, and more than 900,000 patients are hospitalized each year at an annual cost of $9 billion. A wide variety of left-sided and right-sided heart failure occurs when the ability of the heart to contract is impaired. Common symptoms in left-sided heart failure are dyspnea, diaphoresis, orthopnea, tachycardia, tachypnea, paroxysmal nocturnal dyspnea, and fatigue. Physical findings include pulmonary rales, wheezes, and an S_3 gallop. In right-sided failure, there is right upper quadrant pain with physical evidence of peripheral edema and jugular venous distention, hepatomegaly, hepatojugular reflux, and edema. However, signs and symptoms of cardiac decompensation are often unreliable and vague. Many of these patients initially find their way into the health care system through the ED, where treatment is begun.

Table 19-3 reviews our experience with cardiogenic shock in 39 patients with complicated cardiac failure and in six patients with acute myocardial infarction; since the patterns were similar, the two groups were combined. Treatment often is aimed at reducing cardiac work, controlling fluid retention, and enhancing myocardial contractility by vasodilating, diuretic, and inotropic agents. Intervention is initially based on clinical assessment, vital signs, and radiographic findings; however, overly vigorous diuresis can decrease preload and thereby reduce contractility. Because both overtreatment and undertreatment are dangerous, it is appropriate to titrate therapy to attain predetermined physiologic goals assessed by hemodynamic monitoring. In the absence of invasive monitoring, therapeutic interventions may be suboptimal and lead to increased mortality, but it is not usually feasible to place PA catheters in the busy ED. However, thoracic electrical bioimpedance monitoring provides similar information to PA catheters without the attendant risks of invasive procedures. Accurate assessment, effective treatment, and meaningful hemodynamic variables can be obtained quickly and accurately and used to titrate appropriate pharmacologic interventions.

Using thoracic impedance technology, Miltzman and colleagues[51] evaluated 294 patients entering the ED with heart failure. The admission impedance parameters, including baseline thoracic impedance (Z_0) and CI, were compared with the routine clinical admission vital signs. Patients were separated into four groups based on CI $>$ or $<$ 3.6 L/min/m^2 and Z_0 $>$ or $<$ 21 ohms; despite the marked differences in hemodynamic function, the vital signs of these four groups were not different. More important, 72% of patients showed improved hemodynamic values and dyspnea scores after treatment based on thoracic impedance monitoring. Milzman and colleagues concluded that vital signs alone are inadequate to assess and manage heart failure. However, thoracic bioimpedance technology provided objective data that could be used to classify and treat heart failure within minutes of presentation at the ED.[51] In clinical cardiogenic shock, the continuous, immediate feedback on the effects of therapy on cardiac function provides criteria for judicious use of fluids to correct low flow and hypotension, balanced with medication for preload reduction.

Other Medical Emergencies

Table 19–3 describes changes in the patterns of hypertensive crisis in 23 patients, sepsis and septic shock in 45 patients, drug overdose in 15 patients, and acute stroke in 21 patients. The table summarizes the initial baseline values on admission to the ED, the nadir or lowest recorded value in variables that fell, or highest value of MAP in hypertensive crises or $Ptcco_2$, the variables that rose at their worst, and the values after initial rescuscitation. In general, the common circulatory pattern was low pressure, flow, and tissue perfusion usually associated with evidence of hypovolemia; these abnormalities were worse in the patients who subsequently died in their current hospitalization.

EVALUATION OF FLUID THERAPY

Effects of Packed Red Cells, Colloids, and Crystalloids in Emergency Conditions

The relative effectiveness of various fluid therapies were studied in emergency patients shortly after their admission to the ED. The previously reported common hemodynamic patterns of nonsurvivors included decreased flow and tissue perfusion reflected by reduced CI, stroke index, $\dot{D}o_2$, and $\dot{V}o_2$ by invasive monitoring and reduced flow and tissue perfusion by noninvasive monitoring. More important, invasive and noninvasive monitoring was used to evaluate the earliest phase of shock as well as the initial resuscitation and subsequent therapeutic responses of various fluid regimens in the ED.

Table 19–4 describes increased CI, MAP, $Sapo_2$, $Ptco_2/FIO_2$, and $Ptcco_2$ after 2 units of packed red blood cells given in 65 instances, 500 mL of colloids (5% albumin, fresh frozen plasma, and 6% hydroxyethyl starch), and 1000 mL infusions of crystalloids (Ringer's lactate solution) to emergency trauma patients shortly after admission to the ED. These data document improved pressure, flow, and tissue perfusion after transfusions of packed red blood cells and colloids. There was significantly increased CI, MAP, and oxygen transport after administration of packed red blood cells and colloids (albumin, starch, and fresh frozen plasma); crystalloids (1000 mL of Ringer's lactate solution) minimally but not significantly improved CI but not oxygen metabolism. In these emergency conditions, continuing blood losses were present in many patients. Nevertheless, whole blood, packed red blood cells, and colloids improved these variables under comparable conditions.

SUMMARY: EARLY PHYSIOLOGICAL RESPONSES TO ACUTE ILLNESS

An appropriate basic assumption is that low flow, poor tissue perfusion, shock, and other circulatory dysfunctions can be recognized early by objective noninvasive criteria and that more promptly delivered therapy might be more efficacious. Noninvasively monitored data may be used to titrate early fluid and inotropic therapy to achieve optimal physiologic criteria to prevent development of lethal organ failures. To a large extent, circulatory findings in acute illnesses may be explained by well-documented physiologic responses to trauma. Tissue injury, hemorrhage, pain, fear, and hypovolemia activate the sympathoadrenal axis, releasing epinephrine and norepinephrine from the adrenal medullae and sympathetic effector neurons.[19, 23, 25, 26, 41] *Continued stress of hypovolemia, hypotension, tissue injury, and the sympathoadrenal response activate the hypothalamic-hypophyseal-adrenal axis via afferent neural signals. This activation causes corticotropin-releasing hormone (CRH) release by the hypothalamus and elaboration of adrenocorticotropic hormone (ACTH) by the adenohypophysis. ACTH stimulates the adrenals to secrete cortisol, which increases cardiac output and in part mediates the post-traumatic hypermetabolic state. The hypermetabolic state, which requires increased blood flow, makes tissues more susceptible to local ischemic events.*[41]

Cardiopulmonary catecholamine effects immediately after trauma include increased blood pressure, heart rate, cardiac contractility, minute ventilation, and peripheral vasomotor tone. Although these adaptive effects are usually beneficial, exaggerated but uneven peripheral vasoconstriction leads to increased but maldistributed microcirculatory flow with localized areas of hypoperfusion, tissue hypoxemia, and localized intravascular hypovolemia.[15, 25, 37] *The hypoxic acidotic endothelium of poorly perfused capillaries*

TABLE 19–4. Hemodynamic Changes after Administration of Packed Red Blood Cells (2 U), Colloids (500 mL) and Ringer's Lactate Solution (100 mL) in Emergency Patients as Indicated by Noninvasive Monitoring

Variable	Packed Red Blood Cells (n = 65)	Colloids (n = 15)	Ringer's Lactate Solution (n = 65)
CI, L/min/m^2	0.59 ± 0.15†	0.59 ± 0.10†	0.30 ± 0.21
MAP, mmHg	6.2 ± 3.7	9.2 ± 4.1*	−0.7 ± 2.1
Sao_2, %	−1.8 ± 1.44	−0.9 ± 0.4	−0.5 ± 0.4
$Ptco_2/Fio_2$	22.6 ± 15.2	40.7 ± 13.9†	9.2 ± 6.2
$Ptcco_2$	−3.1 ± 2.5	0.9 ± 1.6	0.2 ± 1.5

*P $<$ 0.5.
†P $<$ 0.1; values are mean ± SEM.
CI = cardiac index; MAP = mean arterial pressure; Sao_2 = arterial oxygen saturation; $Ptco_2/Fio_2$ = transcutaneous oxygen tension/fractional inspired oxygen concentration; $Ptcco_2$ = transcutaneous carbon dioxide tension.

activates macrophages and leukocytes and produces cytokines, platelet activating factor, eicosanoids, intravascular coagulation, and many other known and unknown immunochemical cascades; the activated macrophages and white blood cells produce oxygen free radicals and local tissue destruction that mark the systemic inflammatory response syndrome (SIRS).

With resuscitation and reperfusion of hypoxic capillaries, these activated cellular and immunochemical cascades are washed into the venous circulation and lead to the SIRS, end-organ dysfunction, multiple vital organ failures, and death.[25] *The survivors have greater physiologic reserve capacity and the ability to generate increased flow and tissue perfusion needed to provide adequate tissue oxygenation in the presence of increased metabolic need.*[2–9, 15, 25, 51] *Differences between hemodynamic patterns of survivors and nonsurvivors have motivated investigators to suggest aggressive fluid therapy titrated to reach optimal physiologic goals, defined by the survivor patterns, as a strategy to improve patient outcome.*[1–3] *Fluid therapy is titrated to maintain intravascular volume, improve tissue perfusion, and overcome regional circulatory deficiencies caused by uneven, maldistributed vasoconstriction.*

We may conclude that trauma patients can be appropriately and profitably noninvasively monitored in the ED. The changes identified during the first few minutes or hours of hospitalization demonstrate circulatory deficiencies, adequacy of physiologic responses, and effectiveness of therapeutic interventions. Patients who do not respond with adequate perfusion of the tissue beds, as manifest by skin perfusion-oxygenation have a higher likelihood of complications and death. Early hemodynamic monitoring may lead to a better understanding of survivor and nonsurvivor physiologic patterns, earlier identification of circulatory deficiencies associated with poor outcomes, and more definitive therapeutic protocols that improve outcome.

References

1. Shoemaker WC, Belzberg H, Wo CCJ, et al: Multicenter study of noninvasive monitoring as alternatives to invasive monitoring of acutely ill emergency patients. Chest 1998; 114:1643–1652.
2. Shoemaker WC, Appel PL, Kram HB, et al: Prospective trial of supranormal values of survivors as therapeutic goals in high risk surgical patients. Chest 1988; 94:1176.
3. Boyd O, Grounds M, Bennett D: Preoperative increase of oxygen delivery reduces mortality in high risk surgical patients. JAMA 1993; 270:2699.
4. Yu M, Levy MM, Smith P, et al: Effect of maximizing oxygen delivery on mortality and mortality rates in critically ill patients: A prospective randomized controlled study. Crit Care Med 1993; 21:830–838.
5. Yu M, Burchell S, Hasaniya NWMA, Takanishi DM, et al: Relationship of mortality to increasing oxygen delivery in patients ≥50 years of age: A prospective, randomized trial. Crit Care Med 1998; 26:1011–1019.
6. Scalea TM, Simon HM, Duncan AO, et al: Geriatric blunt multiple trauma: Improved survival with early invasive monitoring. J Trauma 1990; 30:129–136.
7. Tuchschmidt J, Fried J, Astiz M, et al: Evaluation of cardiac output and oxygen delivery improves outcome in septic shock. Chest 1992; 202:216.
8. Berlauk JF, Abrams JH, Gilmour IJ, et al: Preoperative optimization of cardiovascular hemodynamics improves outcome in peripheral vascular surgery. Ann Surg 1991; 214:189.
9. Moore FA, Haemel JB, Moore EE, et al: Incommensurate oxygen consumption in response to maximal oxygen availability predicts postinjury oxygen failure. J Trauma 1992; 33:58.
10. Wang X, Sun H, Adamson D, et al: An impedance cardiography system: A new design. Ann Biomed Eng 1989; 17:535–556.
11. Wang X, Van De Water JM, Sun H, et al: Hemodynamic monitoring by impedance cardiography with an improved signal processing technique. Proc IEEE Eng Med Biol 1993; 15:699.
12. Shoemaker WC, Wo CCJ, Bishop MH, et al: Multicenter trial of a new thoracic electric bioimpedance device for cardiac output estimation. Crit Care Med 1994; 22:1907.
13. Wo CCJ, Shoemaker WC, Bishop MH, et al: Noninvasive estimations of cardiac output and circulatory dynamics in critically ill patients. Curr Opin Crit Care 1995; 1:211–218.
14. Shoemaker WC, Wo CCJ, Bishop MH, et al: Noninvasive monitoring of high risk surgical patients. Arch Surg 1996; 131:732–737.
15. Shoemaker WC, Wo CCJ, Demetriades D, et al: Early physiologic patterns in acute illness and accidents. New Horiz 1996; 4:395–412.
16. Bishop MH, Shoemaker WC, Shuleshko J, Wo CCJ: Noninvasive cardiac index monitoring in gunshot wound victims. Acad Emerg Med 1996; 3:682–688.
17. Shoemaker WC, Wo CCJ, Bishop MH, et al: Noninvasive hemodynamic monitoring of critical patients in the emergency department. Acad Emerg Med 1996; 3:675–681.
18. Tatevossian RG, Wo CCJ, Velmahos GC, Demetriades D, Roth B, Asensio JA, Shoemaker WC: Transcutaneous O_2 and CO_2 monitored values as early warning signs of tissue hypoxia and hemodynamic shock in critically ill emergency patients. Crit Care Med (in press).
19. Tatevossian RG, Shoemaker WC, Wo CCJ, et al: Hemodynamic patterns that precede the development of ARDS: Use of noninvasive monitoring as early warning of ARDS in critically ill emergency patients. Intensive Care Med (submitted).
20. Velmahos GC, Wo CCJ, Demetriades D, et al: Invasive and noninvasive monitoring of blunt trauma in the early period after emergency admission. J Am Coll Surg (submitted).
21. Velmahos GC, Wo CCJ, Demetriades D, et al: Early continuous noninvasive hemodynamic monitoring after severe blunt trauma. Injury 1999; 30:209–214.
22. Belzberg H, Rivkind A, Wo CCJ, Shoemaker WC, et al: Noninvasive hemodynamic and tissue perfusion monitoring of blunt trauma patients for early recognition of shock. Crit Care Med (in press).
23. Standard application of pulse oximetry. J Clin Monit 1989; 5:37–62.
24. Lubbers DW: Theoretical basis of the transcutaneous blood gas measurements. Crit Care Med 1981; 9:721–733.
25. Tremper KK, Huxtable RF: Dermal heat transport analysis for transcutaneous O_2 measurements. Acta Anesth Scand Suppl 1978; 68:4.
26. Tremper KK, Waxman K, Shoemaker WC: Effects of hypoxia and shock on transcutaneous Po_2 values in dogs. Crit Care Med 1979; 7:526.
27. Tremper KK, Shoemaker WC: Transcutaneous oxygen monitoring of critically ill adults with and without low flow shock. Crit Care Med 1981; 9:706–709.
28. Venus B, Patel KC, Pratap KS, Konchigeri H, Vidysager D: Transcutaneous oxygen monitoring during pediatric surgery. Crit Care Med 1981; 9:714–716.
29. Tremper KK, Waxman K, Bowman R, Shoemaker WC: Continuous transcutaneous oxygen monitoring during respiratory failure, cardiac decompensation, cardiac arrest, and CPR. Crit Care Med 1980; 8:337.
30. Rowe MI, Weinberg G: Transcutaneous oxygen monitoring in shock and resuscitation. J Pediatr Surg 1979; 14:773.
31. Tremper KK, Shoemaker WC, Shippy CR, Nolan LS: Transcutaneous carbon dioxide monitoring on adult patients in the ICU and operating room. Crit Care Med 1981; 9:752–757.
32. Severinghaus JW, Peabody J, Thunstrom A, et al (eds): Workshop on methodologic aspects of transcutaneous blood gas analysis. Acta Anaesth Scand Suppl 1978; 68:1–124.
33. Schwartz S, Frantz RA, Shoemaker WC: Sequential hemodynamic and oxygen transport responses in hypovolemia, anemia, and hypoxia. Am J Physiol (Heart Circ) 1981; 241:H864–H871.
34. Bishop MW, Shoemaker WC, Appel PL, et al: Relationship between supranormal values, time delays and outcome in severely traumatized patients. Crit Care Med 1993; 21:56.
35. Bishop MH, Shoemaker WC, Kram HB, et al: Prospective randomized trial of survivor values of cardiac index, oxygen delivery, and oxygen consumption as resuscitation endpoints in severe trauma. J Trauma 1995; 38:780–787.

36. Shoemaker WC, Appel PL, Kram HB: Role of oxygen debt in the development of organ failure, sepsis, and death in high risk surgical patients. Chest 1992; 102:208-215.
37. Waxman K: Shock: Ischemia, reperfusion and inflammation. New Horiz 1996; 4:153-160.
38. Gann DS, Lilly MP: The neuroendocrine response to multiple trauma. World J Surg 1993; 7:101-118.
39. Nichols TP, Shoemaker WC, Wo CCJ, et al: Tissue oxygenation after head trauma is related to survival. Neurosurgery (in press).
40. McLeod AA, Neil-Dwyer G, Meyer CHA, et al: Cardiac sequelae of acute head injury. Br Heart J 1982; 47:221-226.
41. Popp AJ, Gottlieb ME, Paloski WH, et al: Cardiopulmonary hemodynamics in patients with serious head injury. J Surg Res 1982; 32:416-421.
42. Shoemaker WC, Appel PL, Kram HB: Hemodynamic and oxygen transport responses in survivors and nonsurvivors of high risk surgery. Crit Care Med 1993; 21:977-990.
43. Dunham CM, Siegel JH, Weireter L, et al: Oxygen debt and metabolic acidemia as quantitative predictors of mortality and the severity of the ischemic insult in hemorrhagic shock. Crit Care Med 1991; 19:231-243.
44. Schultz RJ, Whitfield GF, LaMura JJ, et al: The role of physiologic monitoring of patients with fractures of the hip. J Trauma 1985; 25:309-316.
45. Cortbus F, Jones PA, Miller JD, et al: Cause, distribution and significance of episodes of reduced cerebral perfusion pressure following head injury. Acta Neurochir 1994; 130:117-124.
46. Zornow MH, Prough DS: Fluid management in patients with traumatic head injury. New Horiz 1995; 3:488-498.
47. Bullock R, Chesnut RM, Clifton G, et al: Guidelines for management of severe head injury. J Neurosurg 1996; 11:667-709.
48. Shoemaker WC, Wo CCJ, Gruen JP, et al: Hemodynamic and oxygen metabolic patterns in brain death after head trauma: Implications for management of the organ donor. (Submitted).
49. Creamer JE, Edwards JD, Nightingale P: Hemodynamic and oxygen transport variables in cardiogenic shock secondary to acute myocardial infarction. Am J Cardiol 1990; 65:1287.
50. Rady MY, Edwards JD, Rivers EP, et al: Measurement of oxygen consumption after uncomplicated acute myocardial infarction. Chest 1993; 103:886-895.
51. Milzman DP, Samoddar R, Moscowitz L, et al: Thoracic impedance monitoring of cardiac output in the Emergency Department improves heart failure resuscitation. Ann Emerg Med 1998; 32(Suppl part 2):561.
52. Shoemaker WC, Wo CCJ: Circulatory effects of whole blood, packed red cells, albumin, starch, and crystalloids in resuscitation of shock and critical illness. Vox Sang 1998; 74(Suppl 2):69-74.

20

Epidemiology of Trauma

Arthur L. Trask, MD, FACS

Traumatic injury in the United States is, to a large extent, preventable. As in the investigation of acute diseases, the epidemiologic study of traumatic injury leads to an increased understanding of the trauma process, to the identification of potential predictors of its clinical course and outcome, and to the formulation of effective preventive strategies. However, traditional epidemiologic methods have been applied to trauma only since the 1960s.[1]

Traumatic injury is a probabilistic function of a specific population at risk, in a specific risk environment, with a specific level of risk protection. The causative agent is energy, principally kinetic, that leads to a forcible disruption of normal anatomy or physiology. Traumatic injury can be analyzed on a population as well as on an individual basis. From an epidemiologic perspective, the essential element in the assessment of trauma is the systematic collection of data. The primary data elements are the (1) severity, (2) frequency, and (3) social significance of the injury. Other important factors include who is being injured, how people are injured, where the injury is taking place, and the circumstances. Such data are indispensable for comparing local injury rates with state, regional, and national norms and for evaluating potential interventions.

This chapter discusses the epidemiology of trauma, with emphasis on the sources of data available for the study of traumatic injury, and methods available for describing more fully the medical health hazard of trauma. An understanding of the epidemiology of trauma increases the potential for optimal care of the trauma patient as well as the number of opportunities for secondary and primary prevention.

OVERVIEW

Epidemiologic assessment of traumatic injury provides the critical care specialist with the most reliable estimates of patient numbers, injury type, severity of injury, clinical outcome, and potential for complications. It also provides reliable estimates of national, regional, and local trends in the type and severity of traumatic injury, which can prove invaluable for long-term planning by a critical care facility. In addition, injury trends are essential for identifying the crucial resources for a critical care unit, such as personnel, equipment, and training requirements. With computer support available at most hospitals today, reliable projections of critical care requirements based on local trauma statistics are readily available and can be used to define local hospital priorities for optimal critical care.

TRAUMA MORTALITY

With a traumatic injury, the severity of injury and the availability of an effective trauma care system define the initial clinical course.[2] In 1983, Trunkey described the trimodal distribution of trauma death as a function of time after injury.[3, 4] The model, based on a retrospective analysis of traumatic deaths in San Francisco over 2 years, identified three distinct peaks in mortality.

The first peak, occurring within the first hour, describes fatal injuries for which provision of immediate medical care is minimally effective. These injuries include lacerations to the brain or major blood vessels. Patients in this early phase usually do not reach the hospital alive. More than 50% of all trauma deaths occur in the first phase.

The second peak from 1 to 4 hours, includes patients for whom immediate definitive medical treatment may be lifesaving. Death during this period is the result of significant head injury, severe hemorrhage, or other multiple injuries. Prevention of death in this second phase is the primary goal of an effective regional trauma care system. The development of the American College of Surgeons (ACS) Committee on Trauma's "Resources for Optimal Care of the Injured Patient"[5] and its Advanced Trauma Life Support curriculum are directed specifically at improving both prehospital and initial hospital treatment for the trauma patients at risk in this category.

The third peak occurs over 1 to 5 weeks. Sepsis and multiple organ failure predominate as causes of death for patients in this group. Early and optimal critical care for patients at risk in this third phase reduces the number of patients who die of these causes.

CLASSIFICATION OF INJURY

Trauma can range from an uncomplicated single injury to extremely complex multiple injuries. An understanding of trauma requires consideration of three essential elements of injury classification: (1) mechanism of injury, (2) severity of injury, and (3) projected clinical outcome.

Mechanism of Injury

Two classes of traumatic injury have been defined:

1. *Blunt trauma* is a distributed dissipation of kinetic energy either by concussion or by deceleration. Blunt trauma can lead to direct contusive injury, shearing, vascular disruption, and indirect lacerations secondary to skeletal fractures.
2. *Penetrating trauma* is a more focal dissipation of a projectile's kinetic energy that leads to direct-impact lacerations and fractures.

A narrower classification scheme for trauma is analysis of the mechanism of injury. Mechanism of injury describes the physical forces and the environment in which trauma occurs. For example, a motor vehicle collision refers to one mechanism of injury. However, the mechanism of injury can be further described by specifics of the injury event, such as vehicle speed and whether the vehicle's occupant was wearing a seat belt. Such microanalysis is codified by the E-Code descriptors of the International Classification of Disease (ICD)-9 convention. Mechanism of injury analysis is extremely important in identifying potential injury prevention programs.

Severity of Injury

Efforts to develop improved prognostic indicators for trauma require better clinical descriptive measures for traumatic injury. Wisner[6] has reviewed the history of the development of injury scoring. Initial scoring for triage purposes emphasized an inventory of the wounds sustained. It was thought that such an inventory would adequately describe the clinical state of the trauma patient. The *Injury Severity Score* (ISS) is a scaled measure of the anatomic injury sustained. As with burn calculations, the ISS is calculated on the basis of body parts. An international convention sponsored by the Association for Advancement of Automotive Medicine developed a scoring procedure for traumatic injury. The type and severity of injury to an organ or tissue are assigned an *Abbreviated Injury Score* (AIS). The maximal AIS for each body part is squared, and the highest three body part scores are summed to yield the ISS.[7]

Prediction of Outcome

As a measure of anatomic injury, ISS has proved to be less predictive of clinical course and outcome than two more recent measures: (1) the *Trauma Score* (TS) and (2) the *Revised Trauma Score* (RTS).[6] Both the TS and RTS rely on physiologic measures of injury rather than on anatomic disruption. The RTS has been shown to be a more reliable predictor of outcome and is based on three physiologic measures:

- The *Glasgow Coma Scale* score (a measure of neurologic status)
- Respiratory rate
- Systolic blood pressure

A third measure has been developed to relate anatomic injury (ISS) and physiologic status (RTS). The *TRISS* plot (RTS on the *y*-axis, ISS on the *x*-axis) allows a hospital to directly relate its clinical outcomes with population-based outcome statistics. A probability of survival line, calculated from data of the Major Trauma Outcome Study (MTOS), overlays the TRISS plot and identifies outlying patients; this provides a valuable quality assurance measure for trauma personnel.

In addition to these measures, a knowledge of injury "clustering" can aid the trauma physician in evaluating more fully the clinical course of an injured patient. Certain types of injuries coincide with a high frequency. Knowledge of injury clusters can significantly reduce missed injuries. An example of an injury clustering phenomenon is blunt trauma to the chest suffered during a car crash. The basic forces of impact are dissipated simultaneously on the two body regions, commonly leading to associated lower-extremity fractures.

Populations at Risk

The clinical cycle of trauma begins with the description of a population at risk. Large-scale studies of accident incidence rates, morbidity, and mortality have defined demographic, socioeconomic, behavioral, legal, and product-related factors that influence the incidence and severity of traumatic injury.[8] Figure 20–1 describes the demographic relationship between a child's age and sex and bicycle or motor vehicle–related fatalities. Age and sex were found to be major determinants of the frequency of fatal bicycle-related injuries.

Figure 20–2 relates the incidence of homicide-related mortality in young American males. Teenaged black males are 10-fold more likely to die of homicide than white males.

Figure 20–3 demonstrates the impact of personal behavior on trauma rates. In 1991, 20% of all fatal or severe injury car crashes in the United States involved alcohol as a contributing factor. The rate of alcohol involvement was threefold greater for fatal crashes than for property damage alone. Emphasis on prevention of drunk driving and raising of the legal drinking age have markedly reduced the rate of alcohol-related car crashes during the 1990s.

Figure 20–4 dramatically portrays the potential impact of laws specifically enacted to reduce trauma rates by increasing protection from injury.[9, 10] Between 1966 and 1969, 40 states passed some form of motorcycle helmet law. Motorcycle fatalities decreased in number coincidentally with passage of those laws. However, 27 states repealed or weakened those laws in the late 1970s. Motorcycle fatalities rose dramatically following repeal. These examples illustrate the wide utility of trauma epidemiology in describing the injury environment and in suggesting preventive strategies.

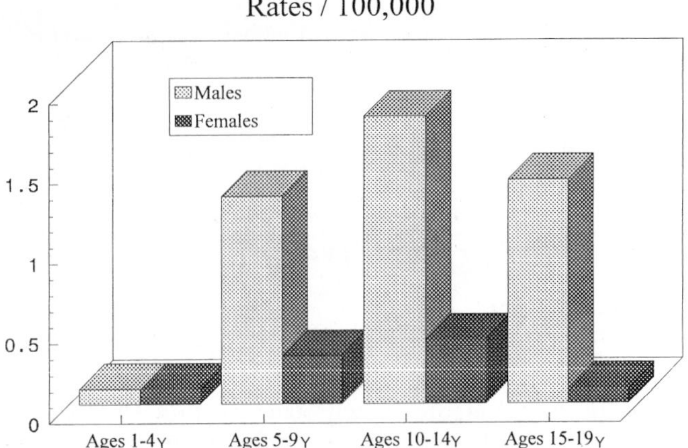

Figure 20–1. This graph describes the age and sex dependence of mortality for bicycle and motor vehicle collisions. The mortality rate for young males is fourfold greater than that for young females (per 100,000 children). (Redrawn from Children's Safety Network. [1991]: A Data Book of Child and Adolescent Injury. Washington, DC, National Center for Education in Maternal and Child Health, 1991.)

National Statistics

Until recently, national statistics on the incidence, severity, and outcome of major trauma have been difficult to abstract. Responsibility for collecting injury statistics varies according to federal agency. Statistics on motor vehicle accidents are

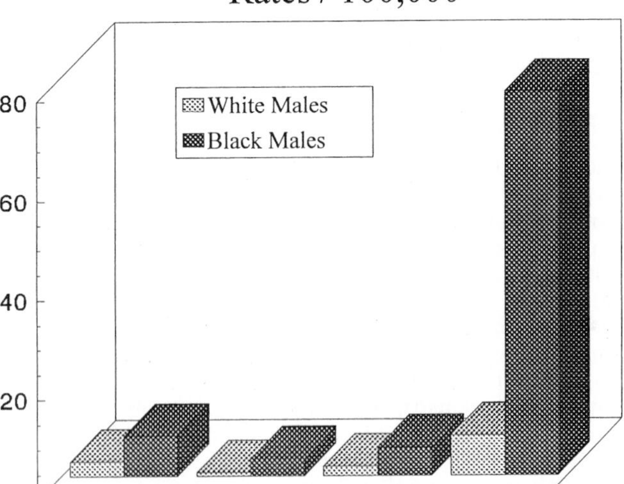

Figure 20–2. This graph compares the homicide mortality rates for young white males with those of young black males. Teenaged black males have a homicide mortality that is 10-fold greater than that of teenaged white males. (Redrawn from Children's Safety Network. [1991]: A Data Book of Child and Adolescent Injury. Washington, DC, National Center for Education in Maternal and Child Health, 1991.)

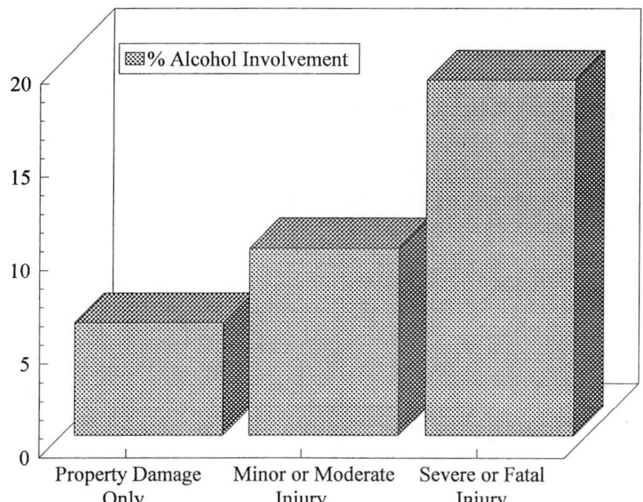

Figure 20–3. Per cent of motor vehicle crashes in 1991 in which alcohol was identified as a contributing factor. (Redrawn from General Estimates System. 1991. Washington, DC, National Highway Traffic Safety Administration, U.S. Department of Transportation publication DOT HS 807954, 1993.)

the responsibility of the U.S. Department of Transportation; occupational injuries, the U.S. Department of Labor; and home and recreation injuries, the National Safety Council. Each of these agencies publishes annual reports on the incidence, prevention, and economic cost of traumatic injury.

An excellent example of a national data base is the statistical survey of motor vehicle crashes maintained by the Department of Transportation. Statistics on the incidence of injuries due to motor vehicle crashes are available from the National Highway Traffic Safety Administration (NHTSA). NHTSA annually publishes the Fatal Accident Reporting System (FARS) report. The FARS report documents motor vehicle crash statistics on a state-by-state basis. The principal emphasis of this report is fatalities. Included are national estimates for drivers, passengers, pedestrians, and motorcyclists with respect to injury and fatality. Other data reported include seat belt use, consumption of alcohol, type of vehicle, and certain demographic information.

NHTSA has now extended the FARS data base by establishing the National Accident Sampling System (NASS), a statistically based survey of reported accidents. The NASS collects detailed information on the injuries and medical outcomes of motor vehicle crashes through its Crashworthiness Data System, which is considered essential for assessing the effectiveness of automobile design and safety regulations, such as seat belt laws. It can also provide valuable national estimates of motor vehicle injury incidence, severity, and outcome.

An important component missing from each of these reporting systems is data on the clinical course and outcome of traumatic injury. The ACS Committee on Trauma, in collaboration with hospitals in the United States and Canada, coordinated the MTOS.[11] The MTOS collected trauma registry data from more than 120 designated trauma centers and hospitals regarding injury mechanism, diagnosis, injury severity, duration of hospital stay, and clinical outcome. The MTOS data base includes more than 120,000 trauma patient records and serves as the principal population data base for developing predictive models of clinical outcome following trauma. In 1990, Champion and coworkers published the first large-scale analyses of the MTOS data.[11] These analyses form the basis for establishing the national norms of trauma care outcome. The outcome statistics from MTOS are an essential component of any trauma care quality improvement program.

With discontinuance of the large-scale data collection of MTOS, nationwide trauma statistics are now available only from disparate sources. Current federal legislation mandates a comprehensive interagency program of trauma research. The legislation further mandates that a National Trauma Registry be established to provide a continuous national statistical survey of trauma. Unfortunately, the federal government has not yet operationalized this National Trauma Registry.

The American College of Surgeons Committee on Trauma has now established National Trauma Data Bank (NTDB). This data base was designed by a collaborative group comprising trauma registry vendors, governmental agencies, emergency medical organizations, Committee on Trauma members, and other interested parties. Participation in the NTDB is voluntary but allows a trauma program to compare its outcomes with other centers across the United States.

It is important to keep in mind that national injury data bases, such as NASS, MTOS, and the NTDB, are principally of value in creating national norms. The most clinically relevant data for injury incidence, severity, and outcomes are those collected at the *local* hospital level.

Hospital-Based Trauma Registries

Hospitals that maintain a trauma registry have access to the most clinically valuable data on the epidemiology of trauma. The ability to define the local hospital experience in terms of trauma incidence and outcome is essential for proper allocation of resources, training, and quality of care improvement. Trauma registries began as isolated initiatives by interested emergency physicians and trauma surgeons using existing data base applications. With the development of trauma registry computer programs for personal computers in the 1980s, it became possible for all hospitals to collect empirical data on the local trauma experience. Most of the programs that are available also include a variety of additional features that allow the hospital to compare its local experience (incidence, outcome, complication rate) with the national results of the MTOS (Table 20–1). Unfortunately the data in the MTOS is now becoming outdated because of changes in management of trauma patients that have taken place since the study was terminated.

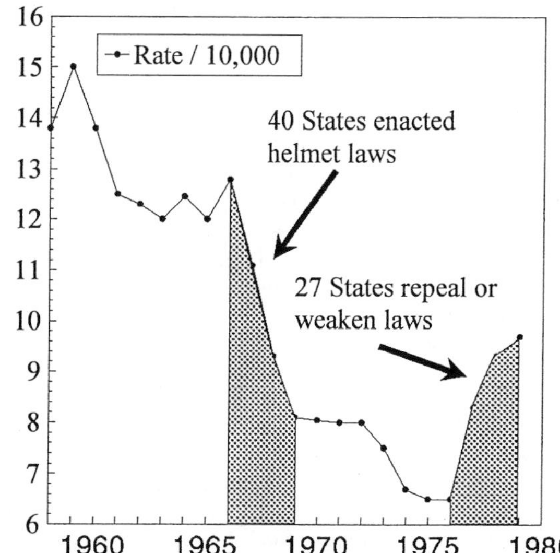

Figure 20–4. Impact of motorcycle helmet laws on motorcycle fatalities. (Redrawn from The Effectiveness of Motorcycle Helmets in Preventing Fatalities [Report and Research Note]. Washington, DC, National Highway Traffic Safety Administration, U.S. Department of Transportation publication DOT HS 807416, 1989.)

TABLE 20–1. Selected Hospital Trauma Registries: Personal Computer–Based Programs

Register	Source
TRAC	American College of Surgeons (Chicago, Ill)
Hospital Trauma Register	Richard Cales, MD (Alameda, Calif)
Trauma One	Lancet Technology (Cambridge, Mass)
Collector	Tri-Analytics, Inc. (Bel Air, Md)

National Statistics for Selected Injuries

Other chapters in this textbook provide more detailed information on the optimal assessment and management of trauma injuries. However, an overview of the magnitude of trauma's impact on health care and society is essential.

Motor Vehicle Collisions

Motor vehicle collisions represent the single most common major injury-producing mechanism. In 1991, 6.11 million motor vehicle crashes occurred in the United States. Of these, more than 2 million led to moderate, severe, or fatal injuries. Although the trend over the past several years does indicate a decrease in accident occurrence, the absolute magnitude of injury and death due to motor vehicle mishaps is staggering. In 1997 there were 7.76 million motor vehicle crashes, with 41,967 persons killed. This figure represents a decrease in the fatality rate compared with 1991.

In 1991, 3.13 million persons were injured in motor vehicles crashes. Fifteen per cent, or 470,000, of the injuries sustained were severe or fatal. Of the 3.13 million persons involved, 2.96 million were occupants of a motor vehicle. Another 170,000 pedestrians, pedicyclists, and other persons were injured. In 1991, one person was either killed or injured by a motor vehicle crash in the United States every 10 seconds. The estimated cost of motor vehicle deaths to society through lost productivity annually exceeds that for any other single cause of death.[12, 13] Fortunately, the fatality rate per 100 million vehicle miles of travel is now at its historic low of 1.7, which reflects the combined efforts of injury prevention.

Burns

Burns account for approximately 2 million injuries per year in the United States. Of those individuals who sustain injury, approximately 70,000 require some form of emergency treatment or hospitalization. Each year almost 6000 persons die of burn injuries. An important consideration is that 21,000 of those burn victims requiring hospitalization have been children and adolescents younger than age 20 years.[14] Children younger than age 5 years have a 2.5-fold greater risk of dying of a burn injury than does the population as a whole.

Falls

The National Safety Council estimates that 12 million persons are injured in falls each year.[15] Principal injuries associated with falls from height include upper-extremity and lower-extremity fractures (including heal and foot fractures), skull fractures, intracerebral hemorrhage, vertebral fractures (particularly lumbar), and lacerations.

Handguns and Violence

The increasing availability and use of handguns in America have dramatically altered the probability that a person will become a victim of penetrating trauma. Coincident with the increased availability and use of handguns is the sharp increase in urban violence associated with narcotics trafficking. Penetrating trauma by gunshot or stabbing now represents approximately 40% of the trauma cases in some urban trauma centers.[4]

SUMMARY

The application of traditional epidemiologic methods to traumatic injury can significantly improve our understanding of the mechanism, the clinical presentation, the initial and long-term clinical course, and the probability of survival afterward. Comprehensive epidemiologic data also provide the basis for quality improvement in trauma critical care. A detailed analysis of a local hospital's trauma patient experience, when compared with the national norms of the MTOS, currently provides the best available quality-of-care standard for trauma critical care.

References

1. Gordon JE: The epidemiology of accidents. Am J Public Health 1949; 39:504.
2. Shackford SR, Mackersie RC, Holbrook TL, et al: The epidemiology of traumatic death: A population-based analysis. Arch Surg 1993; 128:571.
3. Trunkey DD: Trauma. Sci Am 1983; 249:28.
4. Trunkey DD, Blaisdell FW: Epidemiology of trauma. *In*: Scientific American Medicine, Care of the Surgical Patient. Wilmore DW, Brennan MF, Harken AH, et al (Eds). New York, Scientific American, 1993.
5. American College of Surgeons (ACS) Committee on Trauma: Resources for Optimal Care of the Injured Patient. Chicago, ACS, 1990.
6. Wisner DH: History and current status of trauma scoring systems. Arch Surg 1992; 127:111.
7. Association for Advancement of Automotive Medicine: The Abbreviated Injury Scale, 1990, Revision. Des Plaines, Ill, Association for Advancement of Automotive Medicine. 1990.
8. Stylianos S, Eichelberger MR: Pediatric trauma: Prevention strategies. Pediatr Clin North Am 1993; 40:1359.
9. U.S. Department of Transportation (DOT) National Highway Traffic Safety Administration, General Estimate System, 1991. Washington, DC, U.S. DOT, 1992.
10. Cameron MH, Vulcan AP, Finch CF, et al: Mandatory bicycle helmet use following a decade of helmet promotion in Victoria, Australia: An evaluation. Accid Anal Prev 1994; 26:325.
11. Champion HR, Copes WS, Sacco WJ, et al: The major trauma outcome study: Establishing national norms for trauma care. J Trauma 1990; 30:1356.
12. U.S. Department of Transportation (DOT): National Highway Traffic Safety Administration, General Estimate System, 1991. Washington, DC, U.S. DOT, 1993.
13. U.S. Department of Transportation (DOT): National Highway Traffic Safety Administration, General Estimate System, 1997. Washington, DC, U.S. DOT, 1997.
14. Children's Safety Network: A Data Book of Child and Adolescent Injury. Washington, DC, National Center for Education in Maternal and Child Health, 1991.
15. National Safety Council: Accident Fact Book. Chicago, National Safety Council, 1986.

21

Physiologic Response To Injury

Kenneth Waxman, MD, FACS

This chapter examines the physiologic changes that occur following trauma and operations. Such consideration is important for this text because the critical illness that may follow trauma or operation can best be understood only if the usual physiologic responses to surgical and accidental trauma are appreciated. Furthermore, it is increasingly clear that the critical illness that may follow complicated trauma or operation is to a large extent mediated by exaggeration and imbalance of those physiologic compensations that normally occur. Thus, consideration of the physiologic changes that normally occur improves not only our understanding of recovery from uncomplicated trauma or operation but also our ability to provide effective treatment when complications occur.

Cuthbertson[1] defined two phases of the metabolic response to trauma, an *ebb phase* and a *flow phase*. Wilmore subsequently divided the flow phase into *catabolic* and *anabolic* stages.[2] The *ebb phase* occurs during the first several hours after injury and is characterized by hypovolemia, low blood flow, and the initial compensatory physiologic reactions to trauma and shock. Once resuscitation is complete and perfusion reestablished, the *flow phase* begins. It is characterized by a hyperdynamic stress response, fluid retention and edema, catabolism, and hypermetabolism; this *catabolic stage* may last for days to weeks, depending on the severity of injury. Once volume deficits have been eliminated, wounds have closed, and infection has been controlled, the *anabolic stage* begins. It is characterized by a return to normal hemodynamics, diuresis, the reaccumulation of protein and body fat, and the restoration of body function. The anabolic stage generally is longer than the catabolic stage and may be weeks in duration.

The initial stress responses to trauma are deeply rooted in our biologic nature. These responses are first initiated by the perception of trauma, which may be either conscious or unconscious (as during anesthesia). The experiencing of injury and pain or even the anticipation of a dangerous situation initiates protective and recovery responses, both psychologic and physiologic. The responses include protective behaviors such as immobilization, withdrawal, and antagonism. In addition, a physiologic cascade is initiated, which includes neurologic, neurohormonal, cardiovascular, immunologic, and metabolic responses to trauma. These responses are examined in this chapter.

Two general points may be made about the stress response. First, the psychologic and physiologic responses are proportionate in degree to the extent of shock and injury; they tend to be minimal for minor injury or operation and extensive for major accidental or surgical trauma. Signals that are initiated in injured or ischemic tissues communicate the extent of injury systemically. These signals are beginning to be understood and appear to be key in determining the extent of the stress response. Second, these stress responses may be necessary for recovery and are thus of survival value. When trauma is severe, however, the resultant physiologic responses are extensive and sustained. These same responses may then become injurious and contribute to a progression to critical illness and death.

STIMULI THAT INITIATE THE PHYSIOLOGIC RESPONSES TO TRAUMA

The stress response is initiated not only by injury but also by acute blood loss, shock, hypoxia, acidosis, and hypothermia. Furthermore, it can be initiated by psychologic stressors.[3-6] Fear alone initiates many aspects of the stress response, including sympathetic and neurohormonal responses, altered microcirculatory blood flow, and altered coagulation and immune function. It appears that psychologic stressors such as fear activate centrally mediated responses to trauma just as physical stressors do.

Another important stimulus that activates the stress response is pain.[7] Afferent nerve signals from injured tissues converge on the hypothalamus and stimulate the hypothalamic-pituitary axis, resulting in cortisol secretion. Pain is also a potent initiator of the sympathoadrenal axis, so that sympathetic tone and adrenal secretion of catechols are immediately activated by painful stimuli. The fact that pain is not experienced during anesthesia may be an important reason why extensive trauma of major operations is often so well tolerated, whereas a similar amount of tissue injury incurred during accidental trauma may cause a much more severe physiologic response.[8, 9] The importance of neural afferents from the site of tissue injury is confirmed in paraplegic humans, in whom the usual perioperative rise in cortisol level is not seen if the operation is carried out below the level of spinal cord damage.[3]

Hemorrhage and intravascular hypovolemia also initiate the stress response.[10, 11] Hemorrhage results in the stimulation of volume and pressure receptors, which activate the central nervous system (CNS). The response tends to be proportionate to the amount of shock; both the severity and duration of blood volume deficit are thus important determinants of the extent of physiologic response to injury. Furthermore, as hemorrhage and hypovolemia decrease cardiac output, tissue ischemia may result. Tissue ischemia is also an important activator of physiologic responses to injury, not only because it may potentiate activation of the centrally mediated stress responses but also because tissue ischemia initiates potent local responses, such as elucidation of mediators and activation of cells.

Other initiators of the stress response are hypoxemia, acidosis, and hypercarbia. Chemoreceptors located in the aorta and carotid body are activated by changes in Po_2, Pco_2, or pH.[12] In addition, decreased blood flow causes tissue hypoxia and acidosis, which result in activation of the same receptors; these chemoreceptors thus indirectly sense low blood flow. Therefore, low blood flow leads to activation of both chemoreceptors and baroreceptors, which then contribute to the initiation of central stress responses.

Hypothermia, which commonly occurs after trauma or during surgery, is sensed directly by the preoptic area of the hypothalamus and triggers the hypothalamic-pituitary axis.[13, 14] Thus, hypothermia may augment the stress response.

Another important initiator of the physiologic responses to trauma is the wound itself. Tissue injury results in the production of afferent nerve signals that stimulate the sympathoadrenal axis as well as the hypothalamic-pituitary axis.[3] Of additional importance, however, are local processes that occur within the wound or ischemic tissues. These processes are critical in initiating both local and systemic responses that affect metabolism, coagulation, inflammation, and immunity. The extent of these responses is determined by the size of the wound or by the extent of ischemic injury.

These responses to injury and ischemia act in coordination as signals that communicate systemically in a quantitative manner. Hence, the physiologic reaction is proportionate to the magnitude of injury.[15]

MEDIATORS OF THE RESPONSES TO TRAUMA

Sympathoadrenal Axis

Activation of the sympathetic nervous system occurs when afferent nerve signals reach the brain following the presentation of a number of stimuli, such as fear, pain, wounding, hemorrhage, and hypovolemia.[16–19] The adrenal medulla is stimulated whenever the sympathetic nervous system is stimulated, because release of both epinephrine and norepinephrine is triggered by splanchnic sympathetic nerves that synapse directly with adrenal medullary cells. Catecholamines exert a multitude of effects, including rises in blood pressure and heart rate, enhancement of cardiac contractility, an increase in minute ventilation, and vasoconstriction throughout the arterial and venous circulation. Catecholamines also affect pancreatic hormone release as well as metabolism of glucose, amino acid, and fat.

Although these neurogenic and circulating catecholamine effects are of immediate survival value after major injury, prolonged and excessive stimulation of the sympathoadrenal axis may lead to adverse physiologic effects. Prolonged elevation of sympathetic tone and increase in catecholamine secretion may contribute to severe and uneven arteriolar vasoconstriction. This response may, in turn, reduce microcirculatory blood flow, impairing delivery of oxygen and metabolic substrate to the tissues. Furthermore, whereas an immediate effect of an increase in sympathetic tone is the redistribution of intravascular volume from the venous capacitance vessels, which increases central blood volume, the vasoconstricting effects on postcapillary venules may subsequently result in an increase in intraluminal capillary pressure. This increase contributes to loss of intravascular volume as well as intravascular hypovolemia and edema formation. In addition, a prolonged increase in sympathoadrenal tone contributes to the catabolic metabolic state characteristic of severe trauma.

Hypothalamic-Pituitary-Adrenal Axis

Adrenal secretion of cortisol, which is central to the stress response,[2, 3, 7, 19–22] is mediated by the hypothalamic-pituitary-adrenal axis. This reflex arc is activated by stimuli, including fear, pain, hypotension, hypovolemia, and tissue injury. Neural afferent signals converge on the hypothalamus and provoke release of corticotropin-releasing factor, which stimulates secretion of adrenocorticotropic hormone (ACTH) from the anterior lobe of the pituitary gland. Other substances also may modulate the release of corticotropin-releasing factor or may have a direct effect themselves; these substances include vasopressin, angiotensin II, norepinephrine, and inhaled anesthetics. Endotoxemia also has an effect. ACTH is derived from a larger precursor called *proopiomelanocortin*. Besides ACTH, cleavage products of proopiomelanocortin include β-endorphin, β-lipotropin, and α-melanocyte-stimulating hormone. ACTH and β-endorphin are released simultaneously and in equimolar amounts from the same anterior pituitary cells.

The target organ for ACTH is the adrenal cortex, in which it stimulates synthesis and release of cortisol. The degree of hypercortisolism parallels the severity of injury and classically has been used as a marker for the extent of stress response. The effects of glucocorticoid release into the circulation include sodium retention, insulin resistance, gluconeogenesis, lipolysis, and protein catabolism. Cortisol causes demargination of leukocytes and also inhibits the activity of phospholipase A, thereby down-regulating prostaglandin synthesis. Furthermore, elevation of cortisol levels enhances the catabolic effects of tumor necrosis factor (TNF) and interleukin-6 (IL-6). Like catecholamines, cortisol is important for recovery from acute injury. However, severe trauma with an extended injury response results in prolonged cortisol secretion, which has many detrimental effects and may contribute to a progression from the adaptive stress response toward critical illness.

Antidiuretic Hormone

Loss of blood volume is sensed by atrial receptors, whereas decreased pressure is sensed by baroreceptors in the aorta as well as the carotid and pulmonary arteries; the signals are communicated to the hypothalamus. Nerve fibers from the hypothalamus directly synapse with cells in the posterior lobe of the pituitary gland, triggering release of antidiuretic hormone (ADH). ADH is a potent vasoconstrictor and thus has pressor effect. It also acts on renal collecting ducts to promote reabsorption of water, causing water retention.[23, 24]

Renin and Angiotensin

Following trauma, when blood flow through the kidneys is decreased, the juxtaglomerular cells secrete renin. Renin enzymatically cleaves a precursor protein to form angiotensin I, which is further cleaved to form angiotensin II. Angiotensin II is an extremely potent vasoconstrictor and has significant pressor effect. It also directly acts on the kidney to induce a decrease in salt and water excretion. Angiotensin II also stimulates the secretion of aldosterone, which further decreases excretion of both salt and water.[23, 25, 26]

Endogenous Opioids

Endogenous opioids are released from the pituitary gland as part of the initial stress response in an amount equimolar to that of ACTH. In addition, endorphins are released into the circulation from the adrenal glands in response to sympathetic stimulation.[27–29] The most evident role of endogenous opioids is to decrease pain.

Endogenous opioids have other actions as well. For example, opioids modulate catecholamine release from the adrenal medulla, and they may exert inhibitory feedback on pituitary activation and decrease ACTH release. Furthermore, β-endorphin directly increases the secretion of insulin. Thus, the opioids may be important as counterregulatory inhibitors of the stress response in addition to minimizing sensation of pain. The endogenous opioids may also modulate normal neutrophil and lymphocyte function (including T cell function) and activate neutrophils, thus acting as modulators of the immune system and linking CNS responses to immune responses.[30] Negative effects of endogenous opioids on circulation and immune function have been postulated, and endorphins have also been implicated as mediators that may worsen brain injury.[31]

Locally Produced Mediators

In addition to mediators that are activated centrally, important mediator substances arise from sites of tissue injury and have both local and systemic effects.

An important initiating event for the production of local mediators is endothelial disruption at sites of injury and ischemia.[32] Subendothelial collagen and basement membrane exposed by such endothelial disruption activate circulating Hageman factor (factor XII). Hageman factor initiates coagulation via the intrinsic pathway. Activation of the protein clotting system also activates the kinin and plasmin systems.[33] In addition, activated Hageman factor triggers activation of the complement cascade, which initiates inflammation.[34, 35] Another important set of processes activated by injury, ischemia, and endothelial disruption is arachidonic acid metabolism; this metabolism results in substances such as prostaglandins and leukotrienes, which are potent mediators of vascular tone and cause inflammation, cellular activation, and coagulation.[36, 37]

Another by-product of arachidonic acid release from the cell membrane is platelet-activating factor (PAF), a potent stimulator of platelet and neutrophil activation.[38, 39] Hence, PAF contributes to microvascular thrombosis at the site of injury (and perhaps systemically). Activation of neutrophils by PAF further contributes to tissue injury and inflammation.

Activation of coagulation and inflammation at sites of injury is an essential component of healing and recovery. These local processes may also amplify into systemic responses after major trauma, however, such that increased coagulation and inflammation manifest in tissues and organs distant from the sites of injury.[40] Cellular elements are fundamental to this amplification process as well. In particular, activation of monocytes and macrophages, with the resultant activation of cytokine cascades, helps to mediate many of the systemic, immunologic, and metabolic effects after trauma.[41, 42] TNF, IL-1, IL-6, and IL-8 may be particularly important as mediators of the inflammatory and metabolic processes that occur after trauma. In addition, the activation of neutrophils by local mediators at the sites of injury as well as by cytokines may contribute significantly to both local and distant capillary occlusion and inflammation.[43–45]

Another important mediator after shock and trauma may be reperfusion injury.[46] Tissues that have been ischemic because of shock or tissue injury release toxic oxygen radicals on reperfusion, which may initiate both local and systemic tissue injury. The extent of this effect is directly proportionate to the severity of shock and tissue injury. Hence, reperfusion injury may be another important mediator of the systemic manifestations of shock and injury.

The gut may play a central role in the elaboration of mediators.[46] Because the gut mucosa is highly sensitive to low blood flow following shock and trauma, it is subject to early injury. Gut ischemia may lead to the direct elaboration of inflammatory and reperfusion products. Furthermore, the barrier function of the gut mucosa may be quickly lost. As a result, bacteria and endotoxin may enter the portal circulation, possibly leading to activation of cytokine cascades within the macrophages of the mesentery and liver.

THE PHYSIOLOGIC RESPONSES

Psychologic Response

Following major trauma, patients exhibit characteristic behaviors, as follows[47, 48]:

- Immobilization, in which patients are fearful of moving or interacting
- Withdrawal, in which patients may cease being aware of their environment and become incommunicative
- Antagonism, in which patients may resist interaction and display hostility to those around them

During this time, patients experience anxiety, which tends to persist for the duration of the catabolic stage of their recovery.

Altered Vital Signs

After a trauma or major operation, vital signs are not normal; patients are typically febrile, hypertensive, tachycardiac, and tachypneic.

Fever is common in the hours and days following resuscitation from moderate to severe trauma or major operations. It may be caused by tissue inflammation and cytokine release.[49] Early fever is a normal and expected part of the physiologic response and does not indicate that infection is present; however, when fever persists for many days, infection must be suspected as part of the differential diagnosis. Fever due to a noninfectious inflammatory response or to stimulation of the CNS in patients with head injury may persist without infectious cause.

Following fluid resuscitation after trauma, blood pressure may be low, normal, or high. Blood pressure correlates poorly with either blood volume or blood flow.[50] Tachycardia is caused by sympathetic stimulation and high levels of circulating catecholamines.[51] After severe trauma, tachycardia typically persists even after hypovolemia has been corrected and pain has been controlled. This stress tachycardia may continue for days or weeks, and the return of heart rate toward the normal range often correlates with the onset of the anabolic stage of the flow phase. In severe trauma or shock, however, tachycardia may not occur, and heart rate may be normal or decreased; this may seriously impair the compensatory hyperdynamic physiologic response that is necessary for recovery.

Increased minute ventilation, which is reflected by both the presence of tachypnea and an increase in tidal volume, is also an expected response after major operation or injury.[52] It is driven by increased catecholamine levels and sympathetic tone as well as by higher oxygen consumption and carbon dioxide production following trauma. In patients with severe injury or limited pulmonary reserve, increased ventilatory demands may lead to the need for ventilatory support.

Urine output is often diminished early after trauma or operation because of hypovolemia, a decrease in renal blood flow, and a hormonal milieu that engenders sodium and water reabsorption. However, opposing factors tend to raise urine output, particularly the osmotic diuretic effects of the hyperglycemia that occurs following major trauma. In addition, resuscitation with large volumes of crystalloid solutions as well as commonly used osmotically active agents, such as radiologic contrast medium and mannitol, increase urine output. Hypothermia may also raise urine output. Interpretation of urine output may be further complicated by the possibility of the early and occult onset of oliguric or nonoliguric renal failure. Thus, urine output may be decreased, normal, or increased after trauma and may not accurately reflect the intravascular volume.[53]

Edema

The initial responses to trauma contribute to the preservation of body fluids. Vasoconstriction mediated by both the sympathetic nervous system and circulating hormones helps to reduce blood loss. Catecholamines, cortisol, aldosterone, and angiotensin II promote sodium retention, whereas ADH as well as aldosterone and angiotensin II promote water retention. Thus, after mild to moderate trauma, blood volume, interstitial volume, and intracellular volumes are preserved. With severe and prolonged trauma and stress, however, marked disturbances of the distribution of body water occur. Flux of salt and water from the intravascular space into the interstitial space results in intravascular hypovolemia, even though excesses of total body salt and water as well as edema are present.

An important cause of edema formation at the site of injury is inflammation with loss of capillary integrity. Inflammation within the wound, however, is only part of the phenomenon because edema soon becomes generalized and is present within tissues distant from the injury.[54] This systemic edema formation does not necessarily involve capillary endothelial damage and protein leakage; it may also be due to alteration of capillary physiology, which leads to salt and water loss. The presence of circulating and local vasoactive mediators and an increase in sympathetic tone for prolonged periods cause postcapillary venular vasoconstriction and a resultant rise in intraluminal capillary pressure. Hypoproteinemia also decreases intravascular oncotic pressure. These factors, in addition to inflammation, increase the egress of salt and water from the capillaries.

The magnitude of edema formation tends to be proportionate to the severity of injury and is progressive as long as the stress state persists. So that intravascular volume can be maintained during this period, large volumes of intravenous fluids must be given, and a positive fluid balance must also be maintained. In fact, the more the edema progresses, the greater the amounts of fluid required to maintain intravascular volume because the volume of distribution of salt and water into the interstitium increases. It is difficult to clinically assess the intravascular volume, and intravascular hypovolemia may be inadequately corrected in this setting.

Increased Cardiac Output

The initial stress response tends to maintain blood pressure through vasoconstriction, even if circulating blood volume is significantly reduced. The increases in heart rate and cardiac contractility tend to maintain cardiac output. However, the combination of blood loss and fluid shifts from the intravascular space into the interstitial space often results in decreased preload, so that cardiac output is reduced in the hours after the trauma. This reduction may be exacerbated during anesthesia because nearly all anesthetic agents are cardiac depressants.

As bleeding is controlled and resuscitation restores intravascular volume, cardiac output reaches supernormal levels and a hyperdynamic circulatory state obtains.[55, 56] This state is characterized by rapid heart rate and increases in blood pressure and cardiac output. The intensity of this hyperdynamic state and its duration are generally proportionate to the severity of shock and trauma or to the magnitude of the operation. The return of the circulation to normal is an important indicator that recovery is progressing and that the stress response to trauma is waning.

Impaired Oxygen Transport

Microcirculatory blood flow may be markedly altered early following trauma. Vasoconstriction, mediated by sympathetic nerves, circulating catecholamines, vasopressin, angiotensin II, and local vasoconstrictors (e.g., kinins, histamines, and prostanoids) may be pronounced. Nitrogen oxide is a potent vasodilator produced by endothelium; it is possible that a reduction in nitrogen oxide production may also decrease microcirculatory flow after trauma.[57] Within constricted capillary beds, the tendency for endothelial adherence of circulating cells is greater, particularly that of polymorphonuclear leukocytes and platelets; this tendency may be augmented by activation and an increase in the adhesiveness of these cells by such mediators as PAF, TNF, IL-1, and complement as well as by the stress hormones and neurotransmitters.[58]

The combination of microcirculatory vasoconstriction and leukocyte and platelet adhesion to the endothelium of constricted capillaries leads to a decrease in tissue perfusion in certain areas. This disturbance may be further exacerbated by the activated clotting system after trauma, particularly in areas of microcirculatory stasis; intravascular thrombosis within small vessels results.

Another factor that may contribute to impairment of oxygen transport to the cells is edema formation. A greater distance for oxygen diffusion between capillaries and cells may have an adverse effect on the delivery of both oxygen and nutritional substrate, particularly if such an increase is combined with altered microcirculatory blood flow.

Hypermetabolism

After trauma, energy demands rise to supranormal levels.[1, 2, 50, 56, 59] Metabolism, as measured by oxygen consumption, increases to supernormal levels. The extent of hypermetabolism is generally related to severity of injury. In patients undergoing major elective operations, metabolic rates may increase by 10% to 25%; in contrast, in patients who have suffered major injury, basal metabolic rates may more than double. This hypermetabolic state is closely related to the hyperdynamic circulatory state; that is, patients with very high metabolic requirements require greatly increased oxygen delivery and thus a hyperdynamic circulation with supernormal cardiac outputs. As oxygen consumption increases, so does carbon dioxide production. Therefore, an increase in minute ventilation is needed; it is achieved through increases in both tidal volume and respiratory rate mediated by sympathetic nerves and circulating catecholamines.

Inflammatory substances, such as cytokines, are important mediators of the post-traumatic hypermetabolic state. TNF, IL-1, and IL-6 have been studied best. Wilmore[2] has shown that in volunteers the creation of sterile inflammation by injection of an inflammatory agent leads to many of the components of the hypermetabolic stress response. The complete manifestation of the stress response to injury was seen, however, only when the hormones cortisol, glucagon, and epinephrine were infused in the presence of inflammation. Hence, the hypermetabolic response appears to be mediated by a combination of central stress responses and tissue inflammation.

The importance of inflammatory mediators in the post-traumatic hypermetabolic state is further suggested by a striking clinical similarity between trauma and sepsis. Fever, chills, shivering, and altered sensorium are common and expected responses to trauma, just as they are to sepsis; they may be due to many of the same mediators. As a result, making a clinical diagnosis of infection following trauma may be exceedingly difficult.

Altered Protein Metabolism

After severe trauma, marked alterations of protein metabolism occur.[59, 60] Total-body protein catabolism is increased, particularly within skeletal muscles. Total-body protein synthesis is also increased, particularly the hepatic synthesis of acute-phase proteins. The mediators of altered protein metabolism include the stress hormones, the sympathetic nervous system, and cytokines, particularly TNF, IL-1, and IL-6. In addition, growth hormone (GH) may have an important role. GH exerts potent anabolic effects to increase the incorporation of amino acids into protein. The biologic activity of growth hormone is mediated by peptides called *somatomedins*, which are produced in the liver.[61] Decreases in the production of somatomedin and somatomedin inhibitors as well as of complement and prostanoids may all interfere with GH activity after trauma.

The amino acids necessary to fuel hepatic protein synthesis are derived from peripheral protein breakdown, particularly that of skeletal muscle. The increase in protein synthesis occurs to a lesser extent than catabolism. Hence, a net loss of protein mass and a loss of nitrogen in the urine occur; the latter loss can be measured as negative nitrogen balance. After severe injury, protein breakdown results in a significant loss of muscle mass and may progress to the loss of visceral protein mass as well. The wound appears to be spared to some extent; wound inflammation and some healing tend to progress despite the existence of a catabolic state. Nonetheless, if it is severe, post-traumatic catabolism can seriously impair wound healing. With aggressive nutritional support, protein synthesis may be sufficiently enhanced to achieve nitrogen equilibrium; however, a high rate of protein breakdown persists for the duration of the stress response, regardless of nutritional support.

The nature of both protein breakdown and protein synthesis after an injury is complex. For example, following muscle protein breakdown, amino acids are not simply released into the circulation; rather, the branched-chain amino acids valine, leucine, and isoleucine are converted within the muscle into glutamate and keto acids. Glutamate may be metabolized within muscle to glutamine or alanine, whereas keto acids may be utilized by muscle for energy. The result is alteration in the concentration of amino acids released into the circulation, with relative increases in alanine and glutamine and a relative decrease in branched-chain amino acids. Glutamine is tissue trophic, particularly for the gut mucosa, and is rapidly cleared, so that in severe stress states, glutamine levels may be reduced (despite enhanced production). Greater glutamine uptake is stimulated by both TNF and IL-1.

The nature of protein synthesis is also altered following injury. Despite increased amino acid uptake by the liver, the synthesis of albumin is depressed. A large portion of the amino acids are used for energy production by gluconeogenesis, with a resultant increase in urea production. Nonetheless, an overall increase in hepatic protein synthesis, with a shift toward synthesis of acute-phase proteins (e.g., proteins of inflammation, fibrinogen, and haptoglobin). This alteration in hepatic protein synthesis is influenced by the stress hormones as well as by inflammatory cytokines.[62]

Altered Glucose Metabolism

The stress hormones cortisol, glucagon, and epinephrine increase the breakdown of glycogen to glucose; this response rapidly depletes glycogen stores following injury.[2, 59, 63, 64] Glucose is also produced by gluconeogenesis from alanine and other amino acids released by skeletal muscle breakdown. Hence, skeletal muscle breakdown in the stress state also contributes to higher glucose production. Because the wound consumes much of the available glucose, and because anaerobic metabolism predominates in injured tissue, much of the glucose is converted to lactate; lactate is recycled in the liver in the Cori cycle, fueling additional glucose production. The energy to resynthesize glucose comes primarily from fat oxidation in the liver; hence, fat stores are also depleted by processes that produce glucose. The net effect of greater glucose production is to raise extracellular glucose concentrations. The increase in glucose provides energy for wounds and the inflammatory process; macrophages and leukocytes also utilize the larger amount of glucose after injury.

Insulin levels are initially low after injury but subsequently rise to normal or supranormal levels. Nonetheless, hyperglycemia persists after severe injury. This insulin resistance may be primarily due to the persistent elevations of glucagon, cortisol, and epinephrine. Two of the major functions of insulin are inhibition of the rate of hepatic glucose production and stimulation of glucose uptake in peripheral tissues. Therefore, the insulin resistance of the stress state may be central to persistent hyperglycemia as well as to muscle, fat, and glycogen breakdown.

Altered Fat Metabolism

In health, lipids constitute more than 80% of stored fuel reserves. Most tissues can readily use fatty acids as substrates for energy metabolism, preserving glucose substrate for the brain, red blood cells, and cells of inflammation and wound healing. Following injury, fat is oxidized at an accelerated rate; this effect is mediated by sympathetic stimulation, increases in epinephrine, glucagon, and cortisol levels, and insulin resistance.[64] A high intracellular concentration of fatty acids as well as high glucagon levels inhibit fatty acid synthesis. Hence, fatty acids are released into the circulation and become available as energy substrate.

There are limitations, however, to fat mobilization following stress. For example, increased lactate stimulates reesterification within the adiposities, resulting in the futile (and energy-requiring) cycling of fat. Further, hyperglycemia may inhibit lipolysis and also may stimulate reesterification.[65] In summary, although the stress response generally results in mobilization of fat into free fatty acids, there are important limitations to this effect.

Altered Coagulation and Inflammation

Important changes of coagulation occur after injury, including activation of both clotting and fibrinolytic systems. Early after major injury, however, clotting is often impaired. After blood loss and fluid replacement with banked blood or crystalloid fluids, circulating protein clotting factors and platelets are diluted. In addition, hypothermia, which commonly occurs following injury and operation, severely affects clotting. These factors tend to impair clotting early after injury; however, the clotting system is simultaneously activated.[66] This activation is triggered by the release of tissue thromboplastin by injured tissue, which stimulates the extrinsic coagulation system. Subendothelial collagen and basement membrane exposed by trauma activate Hageman factor (factor XII) to initiate coagulation (the intrinsic pathway).

Activation of the protein clotting system also activates the kinin and plasmin systems. Activated factor XII cleaves kininogen into bradykinin, a substance that disrupts endothelium, contributing to edema, inflammation, and clotting. Activated factor XII also leads to conversion of plasminogen into plasmin.

Trauma, through its activation of factor XII and kinin, also triggers complement activation. Kinin activates complement as well. Adrenergic discharge, the stress hormones, stimulation of arachidonic acid metabolism, and activation of the clotting and complement cascades initiate and amplify coagulation and inflammation at the site of tissue damage. These processes are amplified further by platelets, monocytes, macrophages, and neutrophils.

Leukocytosis

Trauma is usually followed by leukocytosis, especially granulocytosis. Lymphocyte counts may be raised, whereas monocyte counts may be lowered. This pattern mimics that seen in sepsis but often occurs without infection. In addition to the rise in circulating neutrophil concentrations, an increase in the numbers of neutrophils within the capillary beds also appears to occur early after trauma. This effect may be initiated by the early vasoconstriction after injury and shock. In severe trauma, this effect may predominate and leukopenia may be seen. Most of the neutrophils initially trapped in the microcirculation are probably released subsequently, contributing to leukocytosis. However, a variable number of neutrophils may remain in the capillaries, particularly if resuscitation is delayed; these neutrophils may then be primed by tissue mediators and contribute to tissue ischemia and inflammation.

Altered Immunity

The immune response is markedly altered after trauma. The extent of immune disturbance is proportionate to the magnitude of injury or operation. The abnormalities seen after trauma or operation are decreases in antibody response, neutrophil chemotaxis, delayed-type hypersensitivity, fibronectin levels, and serum opsonic activity, and increases in neutrophil adherence and serum immunosuppressive factors.[67, 68] The alterations of immunity are mediated by many factors, including the central neurohormonal stress response, activation of suppressor monocytes, and substances released by the inflammatory response, such as prostaglandins and cytokines.

ANABOLIC STAGE OF THE FLOW PHASE

The second stage of the flow phase of injury represents the anabolic and recovery part of the injury response. During this stage, each physiologic alteration that occurred during the catabolic stage may be reversed.

The onset of the flow or recovery phase is heralded by a sense of well-being. Catecholamine and cortisol levels return to normal, as do temperature, heart rate, and blood pressure. Respiratory demands decrease; patients who required mechanical ventilatory support can usually be weaned from ventilators. Urine output increases, fluid balances are negative, and edema resolves. Metabolic demands decrease. Gut function improves, and appetite returns. Visceral and muscle protein is resynthesized, allowing recovery of organ function and physical rehabilitation.

This reversal process does not occur quickly. The anabolic stage of recovery generally takes longer than the acute injury and catabolic stages and thus may last many days or weeks. During this period, patients require psychologic support, nutritional support, and physical rehabilitation for complete recovery to occur. Often, the psychologic effects of trauma are the slowest to recover: A post-traumatic stress syndrome may result.[47]

SUMMARY

Trauma, either accidental or surgical, results in alteration of nearly all physiologic systems. The stress response to trauma is triggered by the psychologic and physical perception of pain, injury, and shock. The response is mediated by the CNS, circulating hormones, substances produced in response to local inflammation acting both locally and systemically, and activated circulating cells. The magnitude of this response and its duration are proportionate to the extent of injury. Anesthesia diminishes the perception of injury and may thus reduce the magnitude of the stress response to injury.

During successful recovery, all physiologic disturbances may be reversed. After severe trauma, however, the stress response may require intensive interventional support and may thus be perceived as critical illness. Because physiologic reserve is already stressed by trauma, complications superimposed on this process are of major significance and often lead to severe illness or death. Only with an understanding of the usual physiologic responses to injury can these complications be recognized, understood in context, and optimally managed.

References

1. Cuthbertson DP: Post-shock metabolic responses. Lancet 1942; i:433.
2. Wilmore DW: Homeostasis: Bodily changes in trauma and surgery. *In*: Textbook of Surgery. 13th ed. Sabiston DC Jr (Ed). Philadelphia, WB Saunders, 1986, pp 23–37.
3. Hume DM, Egdahl RH: The importance of the brain in the endocrine response to injury. Ann Surg 1959; 150:697–712.
4. Rose RM: Endocrine responses to stressful psychologic events. Psychiatr Clin North Am 1980; 3:251–277.
5. Vielacres EC, Hollifield M, Katon WJ, et al: Sympathetic nervous system activity in panic disorder. Psychol Res 1987; 21:213–221.
6. Salmon P, Pear S, Smith CC, et al: The relationship of pre-operative distress to endocrine and subjective responses to surgery: Support for Janis' theory. J Behav Mod 1988; 11:599–613.
7. Gann DS, Lilly MP: The neuroendocrine response to multiple trauma. World J Surg 1983; 7:101–118.
8. Kehlet H, Brandt MR, Rem J: Role of neurogenic stimuli in mediating the endocrine-metabolic response to surgery. JPEN J Parenter Enteral Nutr 1980; 4:152–156.
9. Zaloga GP: Catecholamines in anesthetic and surgical stress. Int Anesthesiol Clin 1988; 26:187–198.
10. DeMaria EJ, Lilly MP, Gann DS: Potential hormonal responses in a model of traumatic injury. J Surg Res 1987; 43:45–51.
11. Rea RF, Hamdan M, Clary MP, et al: Comparison of muscle sympathetic responses to hemorrhage and lower body negative pressure in humans. J Appl Physiol 1991; 70:1401–1405.
12. Cunningham DJ: Studies on arterial chemoreceptors in man. J Physiol 1987; 385:1–26.
13. Stotman GJ, Jed EH, Burchard KW: Adverse effects of hypothermia in post-operative patients. Am J Surg 1985; 149:495–501.
14. Reed HL, Chernow B, Lake CR, et al: Alterations in sympathetic nervous system activity with intraoperative hypothermia during coronary artery bypass surgery. Chest 1989; 95:616–622.
15. Bitterman H, Kinarty A, Lazarovich H, et al: Acute release of cytokines is proportional to tissue injury induced by surgical trauma and shock in rats. J Clin Immunol 1991; 11:184–192.
16. Jäättelä A, Ahlo A, Avihainen V, et al: Plasma catecholamines in severely injured patients: A prospective study on 45 patients with multiple injuries. Br J Surg 1975; 177:62.
17. Halter JB, Pflug AE, Porte D: Mechanisms of plasma catecholamines increases during surgical stress in man. J Clin Endocrinol Metab 1977; 45:936–944.
18. Maddens M, Sowers J: Catecholamines in critical care. Crit Care Clin 1987; 3:871–872.
19. Breslow MJ, Ligier B: Hyperadrenergic states. Crit Care Med 1991; 19:1566–1579.
20. Darmaun D, Matthews PE, Bier DM: Physiologic hypercortisolemia increases proteolysis, glutamine and alanine production. Am J Physiol 1988; 255:E366–E373.
21. Harris MJ, Baker RT, McRoberts JW, et al: The adrenal response to trauma, operation, and cosyntropin stimulation. Surg Gynecol Obstet 1990; 170:513–516.
22. DePadova F, Pozzi C, Tonere MJ, et al: Selective and early increase of IL-1 inhibitors, IL-6 and cortisol after elective surgery. Clin Exp Immunol 1991; 85:137–142.
23. Hilton JG, Marullo DS: Trauma-induced increases in plasma vasopressin and angiotensin II. Life Sci 1987; 41:2195–2203.
24. Judd BA, Haycock GB, Dalton RN, et al: Anti-diuretic hormone following surgery in children. Acta Paediatr Scand 1990; 79:491–496.
25. Udelsman R, Norton JA, Jelenich SE, et al: Responses of the hypothalamic-pituitary-adrenal and renin-angiotensin axes and the sympathetic system during controlled surgical and anesthetic stress. J Clin Endocrinol Metab 1987; 64:986–994.
26. Starc TJ, Staluip SA: Time course changes of plasma renin activity and catecholamines during hemorrhage in conscious sheep. Circ Shock 1987; 21:129–140.
27. Risch SC, Kalin NH, Janowsky DS, et al: Co-release of ACTH and beta-endorphin immuno-reactivity in human subjects in response to central cholinergic stimulation. Science 1983; 222:77.

28. Schadt JC: Sympathetic and hemodynamic adjustments to hemorrhage: A possible role for endogenous opioid peptides. Resuscitation 1989; 18:219-228.
29. Lloyd DA, Teich S, Rowe NI: Serum endorphin levels in injured children. Surg Gynecol Obstet 1991; 172:449-452.
30. Deitch EA, Xu D, Bridges RM: Opioids modulate human neutrophil and lymphocyte function: Thermal injury alters plasma beta-endorphin levels. Surgery 1988; 104:41-48.
31. McIntosch TK, Hayes RL, Dewitt DS, et al: Endogenous opioids may mediate secondary damage after experimental brain injury. Am J Physiol 1987; 253:E565-E574.
32. McEver RP: Role of the endothelium on the inflammatory response. *In*: Critical Care: State of the Art. Vol 12. Fullerton, Calif, Society of Critical Care Medicine, 1991, pp 121-138.
33. Ellis EF, Holt SA, Wei EP, Kontas HA: Kinins induce abnormal vascular reactivity. Am J Physiol 1988; 255:397-400.
34. Fosse E, Mollnes TE, Aasen AO, et al: Complement activation following multiple injuries. Acta Chir Scand 1987; 153:325-330.
35. Zimmerman T, Laszik Z, Nagy S, et al: The role of the complement system in the pathogenesis of multiple organ failure in shock. Prog Clin Biol Res 1989; 308:291-297.
36. Kuehl FA, Egan RW: Prostaglandins, arachidonic acid, and inflammation. Science 1980; 210:978-984.
37. Vane JR, Botting RM: Prostaglandins, prostacyclin, thromboxane and leukotrienes: The arachidonic acid cascade. *In*: Critical Care: State of the Art. Vol 12. Fullerton, Calif, Society of Critical Care Medicine, 1989, pp 1-23.
38. Feuerstein G, Siren AL: Platelet-activation factor and shock. Prog Biochem Pharm 1988; 22:181-190.
39. Feuerstein G, Jue TL, Lysko PG: Platelet-activating factor: A putative mediator in central nervous system injury. Stroke 1990; 21:90-94.
40. Nuytinck HK, Offermass XJ, Kubat K, et al: Whole-body inflammation in trauma patients: An autopsy study. Arch Surg 1988; 123:1519-1524.
41. Michie HR, Wilmore DW: Sepsis, signals, and surgical sequelae (a hypothesis). Arch Surg 1990; 125:531-536.
42. Eslcay RL, Grino M, Chen HT: Interleukins, signal transduction, and the immune system-mediated stress response. Adv Exp Med Biol 1990; 274:331-343.
43. Christou NV, Tellado JM: In-vitro polymorphonuclear neutrophil function in surgical patients does not correlate with energy but with "activity" processes such as sepsis or trauma. Surgery 1989; 106:718-722.
44. Tanaka H, Ogura H, Yokata J, et al: Acceleration of superoxide production from leukocytes in trauma patients. Ann Surg 1991; 214:187-192.
45. Leff JA, Repine JE: Blood cells and ischemia-reperfusion injury. Blood Cells 1990; 16:183-191.
46. Wilmore DW, Smith RJ, O'Dwyer ST, et al: The gut: A central organ after surgical stress. Surgery 1988; 104:917-923.
47. Weisalth L: The stressors and the post-traumatic stress syndrome after an industrial disaster. Acta Psychiatr Scand 1989; 355:25-37.
48. Achterberg J, Kenner C, Casey P: Behavioral strategies for the reduction of pain and anxiety associated with orthopedic trauma. Biofeedback Self Regulation 1989; 14:101-114.
49. Briese E, Cabana CM: Stress hyperthermia: Physiological arguments that it is a fever. Physiol Behav 1991; 49:1153-1157.
50. Shoemaker WC: Pathophysiology, monitoring, outcome prediction, and therapy of shock states. Crit Care Clin 1987; 3:307-357.
51. Bahnsor RR, Anduole GL, Clayman RJ, et al: Catecholamine excess: Probable cause of post-operative tachycardia following retroperitoneal lymph node dissection for testicular carcinoma. J Surg Oncol 1989; 42:132-135.
52. Tulla H, Takala J, Alhaoa E, et al: Respiratory changes after open-heart surgery. Intensive Care Med 1991; 17:365-369.
53. Sladen RN: Effect of anesthesia and surgery on renal function. Crit Care Clin 1987; 3:373-393.
54. Demling RH, Lalonde C, Liu YP, et al: The lung inflammatory response to thermal injury: Relationship between physiologic and histologic changes. Surgery 1989; 106:52-59.
55. Clowes GHA, Del Guerco LR, Barwinsky J: The cardiac output in response to surgical trauma. Arch Surg 1960; 81:212-222.
56. Waxman K: Hemodynamic and metabolic changes during and following operation. Crit Care Clin 1987; 3:241-250.
57. Ochoa JB, Udekwa AO, Billiar TR, et al: Nitrogen oxide levels in patients after trauma and during sepsis. Am Surg 1991; 214:621-626.
58. Davis JM, Albert JD, Tracy KJ, et al: Increased neutrophil mobilization and decreased chemotaxis during cortisol and epinephrine infusions. J Trauma 1991; 31:725-731.
59. Cipolle MD, Pasquale MD, Cerra FB: Secondary organ dysfunction: From clinical perspectives to molecular mediators. Crit Care Clin 1993; 9:261-298.
60. Ressey PQ, Jian ZM, Johnson DJ, et al: Post-traumatic skeletal muscle proteolysis: The role of the hormonal environment. World J Surg 1989; 13:465-470.
61. Hall K, Tally M: The somatomedin-insulin-like growth factors. J Intern Med 1989; 225:47-54.
62. Bankey PE, Mazuski JE, Ortiz M, et al: Hepatic acute phase protein synthesis is indirectly regulated by tumor necrosis factor. J Trauma 1990; 30:1181-1187.
63. Wolfe RR, Klein S, Herndon DN, et al: Substrate cycling in thermogenesis and amplification of net substrate flux in human volunteers and burned patients. J Trauma 1990; 30:56-59.
64. Long CL, Nelson KM, Atkin JM, et al: A physiologic basis for the provision of fuel mixtures in normal and stressed patients. J Trauma 1990; 30:1077-1085.
65. Jeevanandam M, Young DH, Schuler WR: Nutritional impact on the energy cost of fat fuel mobilization in poly-trauma patients. J Trauma 1990; 30:147-154.
66. Greenberg CS, Sane DC: Coagulation problems in critical care medicine. *In*: Critical Care Medicine: State of the Art. Vol 11. Fullerton, Calif, Society of Critical Care Medicine, 1990, pp 187-215.
67. Christou NV, Meakins JL, Gordon J, et al: The delayed hypersensitivity response and host resistance in surgical patients: 20 years later. Ann Surg 1995; 222:534-548.
68. Baxevanis CN, Papilas K, Dedousis GV, et al: Abnormal cytokine serum levels correlate with impaired cellular immune responses after surgery. Clin Immunol Immunopathol 1994; 71:82-88.

22

Anesthesia for High-Risk Patients

Duraiyah Thangathurai, MD, FCCM • Maged S. Mikhail, MD

The anesthesiologist plays a critical role in the perioperative care of high-risk trauma and emergency patients. Aggressive and appropriate management can reduce the incidence of intraoperative mortality and prevent postoperative complications. Patients presenting with arterial hypotension associated with bleeding or injury to vital organs (brain, heart, lungs, kidneys, or liver), major vessels, or the spleen may be considered at high risk for life-threatening complications in the perioperative period. Immediate causes of death in these patients include exsanguination, intracranial hemorrhage, and arterial hypoxemia[1, 2]; the most common life-threatening complications in the postoperative period are the adult respiratory distress syndrome (ARDS), acute renal failure (ARF), and multiorgan failure.

INITIAL MANAGEMENT

Initial management has three components: (1) a rapid overview, (2) the primary survey, and (3) the secondary survey. The rapid overview helps to determine whether the patient is stable. The primary survey involves evaluation of breathing, integrity of airway, and circulatory state and a brief examination of central nervous system and neck injuries. The secondary survey involves a detailed physical examination as well as diagnostic and imaging studies (e.g., computed tomography [CT], peritoneal lavage). The airway should be secured, and adequacy of ventilation must be accomplished immediately. Large-bore intravenous catheters allow rapid fluid infusion. Shock is inevitable in all high-risk patients, and time is therefore of the essence in minimizing the adverse effects of shock.

Simultaneous evaluation and resuscitation must be carried out to prevent an irreversible shock state, cerebral hypoxemia, or cardiac arrest.[3] Trauma anesthesiologists, optimally, should be involved in the management of high-risk trauma patients when they are admitted to the emergency department. Experience and familiarity in handling difficult airways allow rapid and definitive airway management. The anesthesiologist can also begin and plan further anesthetic management during the initial resuscitation. Anesthesia is often required for emergency diagnostic studies, such as CT and angiography, as well as for therapeutic procedures, such as thoracostomy, peritoneal lavage, and even thoracotomy.

Shock

Hemorrhage is the most common cause of shock and death in trauma patients. A classification system based on severity is clinically useful. Other causes that must be considered include cardiac contusion, cardiac tamponade, tension pneumothorax, hemothorax, and spinal cord injury. Delayed shock from sepsis secondary to a perforated viscus (e.g., stomach, intestine, or colon) presents several hours after the injury.

Tissue hypoxia precipitates complex interactions of cellular and humoral mediators such as cytokines, kinins, and complement. The integrity of the splanchnic circulation has recently been implicated in the liberation of cytokines and kinins.[4-6] These mediators initiate more complex interactions that may result in generalized endothelial injury, leading to a diffuse inflammatory response, the systemic inflammatory response syndrome (SIRS). Ongoing injuries provoke exaggerated cellular responses that ultimately result in multiorgan dysfunction. Delayed treatment of shock during the intraoperative period may lead to organ failures several days later.[4-10]

Previous studies have suggested that maintenance of peripheral tissue perfusion in the first 8 to 12 hours after injury or surgery reduces the incidence of organ dysfunction and operative mortality.[10] Boyd and coworkers[11] reported that optimizing oxygen transport preoperatively prevented organ dysfunction and reduced perioperative mortality. Shoemaker and colleagues[10] have shown that oxygen debt begins intraoperatively and continues to accumulate in the postoperative period. Anesthetic management, therefore, should focus on reestablishing and optimizing tissue perfusion.

Cytokines and kinins, such as tumor necrosis factor (TNF) and interleukins 1 and 6 (IL-1 and IL-6), are humoral mediators that have been implicated in endothelial damage and SIRS.[4, 5, 12] The inflammatory response leads to diffuse alterations in capillary permeability and interstitial edema that affect all organs.

The role of the splanchnic circulation has been investigated as a site of cytokine and kinin production.[6] Splanchnic circulation may have an increased sensitivity to perfusion deficits and may exhibit earlier signs of ischemia compared with other tissue beds. Splanchnic tissues may therefore become compromised sooner in the face of hypovolemia or intense vasoconstriction secondary to large doses of vasopressors that are used to maintain arterial blood pressure. Moreover, splanchnic hypoxia and cellular injury can occur in the presence of the normal parameters of hemodynamics and oxygenation (blood pressure, heart rate, pulse oximetry, and arterial and mixed venous blood gases).[13]

Perioperative hypovolemia, irrespective of the cause, results in increased catecholamine release. Normal blood flow to the heart and brain is maintained at the expense of other organs.[14] Undetected tissue hypoxia and a subsequent oxygen debt begin to occur early, but tissue vasoconstriction can be reversed with expansion of intravascular volume and the use of vasodilators such as nitroglycerin. Fluid resuscitation should begin immediately, and once systemic pressures are normalized, careful titration of nitroglycerin can help to restore or expand intravascular volume without pulmonary congestion.[15] Dopamine in low doses has the additional beneficial effect of selective splanchnic vasodilatation.

Massive Transfusion

Exsanguination from extensive injuries necessitates rapid blood transfusion. *Massive* blood transfusion may be defined as the need to replace one to two blood volumes within several hours. The procedure is commonly associated with multiple complications, including hypothermia, coagulopathy, and acid-base and electrolyte disturbances.[16] A low urine output and the continued need for vasopressors to maintain arterial blood pressure are early indicators of inadequate volume resuscitation. Massive tissue edema together with retention of crystalloid (>5 L) and poor urine output may indicate inappropriate selection of fluid during resuscitation. Either inadequate volume resuscitation or inappropriate selection of intravenous fluids may result in prolonged shock. Hypoxemia, hypotension, acidosis, inadequate urine output, and increasing airway pressures and pulmonary artery pressures are poor prognostic signs. In patients with these signs, even if they survive intraoperatively, SIRS is likely to develop, leading to postoperative ARF, ARDS, and multiorgan dysfunction.[17-19] Maintaining a normal core temperature, acid-base status, serum electrolyte levels, and coagulation function is critical in avoiding complications from massive blood transfusion.

Hypothermia

Preoperative hypothermia may be the result of prolonged hypoperfusion,[20] whereas *intraoperative* hypothermia may result from infusion of large amounts of intravenous fluids, blood products, and a cold operating room environment. Hypothermia is commonly associated with coagulopathy, cardiac arrhythmias, and refractory hypotension. It may also result in an increased incidence of postoperative wound infections.

Hypothermia should be corrected aggressively by the use of warming blankets, forced-air blankets (e.g., Bair Hugger), warm humidification of the airway, and other warming measures.[21, 22]

Acidosis

Acidosis invariably accompanies prolonged shock states. Other contributing factors are massive blood transfusion, impending ARF (renal shutdown), and ongoing hypoxia.[23-28] Acidosis improves as tissue perfusion improves. Resistant acidosis (pH < 7.20) may call for sodium bicarbonate administration. Excessive use of sodium bicarbonate has multiple deleterious effects, such as (1) worsening of tissue acidosis, (2) shifting of the hemoglobin-oxygen saturation curve to the left, leading to worsening tissue hypoxia, and (3) hypernatremia.[25] Severe hypernatremia can lead to pontine demyelination.

Hyperkalemia

Hyperkalemia results from tissue acidosis and the administration of stored blood, especially packed red blood cells.[25] The potassium concentration of a unit of packed red blood cells

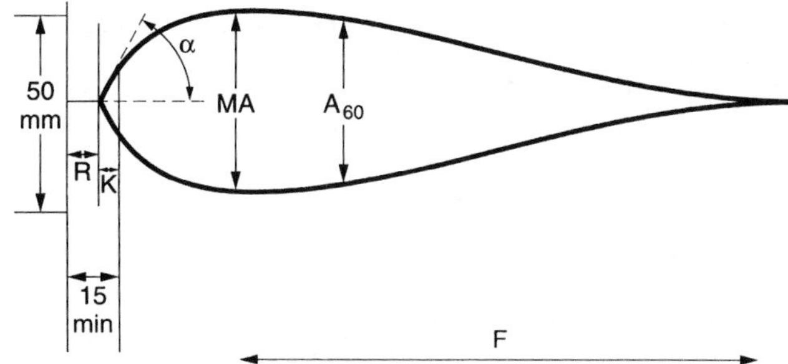

Figure 22–1. Thromboelastogram. R = time interval from blood deposition in the cuvette to an amplitude of 1 mm on the thromboelastogram; K = time interval between the end of R and a point with an amplitude of 20 mm on the thromboelastogram; MA = maximum amplitude of the thromboelastogram; α angle = slope of the external divergence of the tracing from the R value point; A_{60} = amplitude of thromboelastogram 60 minutes after maximum amplitude; F = time from MA to return to 0 amplitude (normal > 300 min). (From Capan LM, Gottlieb G, Rosenberg A: General principles of anesthesia for major acute trauma. *In*: Trauma Anesthesia and Intensive Care. Caplan LM, Miller SM, Turndorf H [Eds]. Philadelphia, JB Lippincott, 1991, p 259.)

varies with shelf life, reaching 17 to 35 mEq/L after 21 days of storage.[27, 28] Decreased urine output and tissue necrosis are often contributory. Hyperkalemia can be treated with hyperventilation, insulin and dextrose infusion, calcium chloride, and diuresis with furosemide.[29]

Coagulopathy

Coagulopathy can occur whenever several units of blood are transfused and is common after massive transfusion. Hypothermia exacerbates coagulopathy.[30] The most common cause is thrombocytopenia. Thromboelastography may be useful in confirming the cause of the coagulopathy (Fig. 22–1). Platelet transfusion is often required after transfusion of more than 10 to 15 units of packed red blood cells.[30–32] Fresh frozen plasma and cryoprecipitate are also often required.

Cardiac Arrhythmia

Cardiac arrhythmias are not uncommon in high-risk trauma patients and are due to multiple factors, such as increased sympathetic tone, hypoxemia, hypercapnia, metabolic acidosis, hyperkalemia, and hypothermia. Excessive use of inotropic drugs or an underlying myocardial contusion may also be contributory. Hypothermia is commonly associated with bradycardia and hypotension; hyperkalemia and hypoxemia together readily promote ventricular fibrillation and can rapidly produce asystole. Myocardial ischemia may present as bradycardia or ventricular tachycardia and is usually a result of ongoing shock and arterial hypotension; ischemia-induced arrhythmias may not respond to treatment until the patient is adequately volume-resuscitated.

MAJOR VISCERAL INJURIES

Intraoperative mortality has been correlated with the severity of shock as well as with the type of organ injury.[33] Table 22–1 lists factors that have been associated with increased intraoperative mortality.

Chest Injuries

Chest injuries are typically classified as *blunt* or *penetrating*. Severity is related to both the mechanism of injury and the exact anatomic site. Early cardiac or respiratory arrest is likely to develop in patients with chest injuries compared with other types of injuries.

Flail chest, pneumothorax, hemothorax, lung contusion, diaphragmatic rupture or hernia, bronchial disruption, hemoptysis, and laryngeal and tracheal injuries present with severe hypoxemia. Cardiogenic shock and hypotension are common and may be due to cardiac tamponade, cardiac contusion, rupture of the aortic or mitral valves, avulsion of the subclavian artery, traumatic dissection of the aorta, or aortic transection. Uncommon injuries include rupture of the esophagus and injury to thoracic vertebrae.

Respiratory distress from pneumothorax or hemothorax must be relieved by insertion of a chest tube. Injuries to the upper airway (larynx or trachea) necessitate fiberoptic endotracheal intubation or emergent tracheostomy. Massive hemoptysis requires isolation of the affected lung with a double-lumen endobronchial tube to prevent blood from entering the healthy lung. Bronchial injuries causing multiple fistulas require high-frequency jet ventilation or isolation of the lungs with a double-lumen tube to prevent loss of tidal volumes and severe hypoventilation. For tracheal disruption or bronchial avulsion, fiberoptic placement of the endotracheal tube or jet ventilation catheter into the unaffected bronchus is required. Lower airway pressures with jet ventilation minimize the bronchial leak. Mechanical ventilators on anesthesia machines are often incapable of sustaining adequate gas flows in patients with poor lung or chest compliance. In these situations, a more efficient intensive care unit (ICU)–type ventilator, which

TABLE 22–1. Clinical Features Associated with Increased Intraoperative Mortality

Category	Clinical Features
Mechanism of injury	Gunshot wound Pedestrian injuries
Injury severity	Mean Injury Severity Score (ISS) > 41 Mean Revised Trauma Score (RTS) > 3.0
Preoperative physiologic profile	Mean BP in the field < 50 mm Hg Mean BP on arrival to ED < 60 mm Hg Best systolic BP in the ED < 90 mm Hg Circulatory shock time > 10 min Best mean pH < 7.18 Mean preoperative crystalloid resuscitation > 3850 mL Mean red cell transfusion > 834 mL
Type of injury	Significant head, chest, abdomen, and pelvic injuries individually or in combination after blunt trauma Significant chest and abdomen injuries individually or in combination after penetrating trauma
Organ injury	Brain Liver Aortic or other major vascular injury Cardiac injury
OR resuscitation and physiologic status	Systolic BP < 90 mm Hg during first hour Systolic BP < 90 mm Hg for > 30 min Deterioration of mean pH from 7.19 to 7.01 Mean intraoperative blood loss, 5172 mL Mean blood replacement, 4541 mL Mean platelet transfusion, 784 mL Mean fresh frozen plasma, 1418 mL Mean intraoperative temperature, 32.2°C Intraoperative cardiac arrest

Data from Hoyt DB, Bulger EM, Knudson MM, et al: Death in the operating room: An analysis of a multicenter experience. J Trauma 1994;37:426.

OR = operating room; ED = emergency department; BP = blood pressure.

is capable of higher gas flows, should be used. A trial of different modes of ventilation may be necessary to optimize both oxygenation and ventilation. Reverse inspiration to expiration (I:E) ratio, sine wave gas flow, high-frequency jet ventilation, or even permissive hypercapnia may be used to provide adequate oxygenation while providing optimal conditions for the surgeon to operate. Fiberoptic bronchoscopy is often required for suctioning, lavage, and repositioning of double-lumen endobronchial tubes. Patients with hemoptysis require ongoing lavage to prevent blockage of the endotracheal or endobronchial tube.

The diagnosis of cardiac injuries can generally be confirmed by echocardiography. This modality is especially useful in the diagnosis of tamponade, rupture or dissection of the aorta, and injury to the valves.[34, 35] Cardiac tamponade can be relieved by echocardiography-guided pericardiocentesis.

Cardiac contusions may present as hypotension due to ventricular dysfunction or arrhythmias. Intraoperative transesophageal echocardiography may be useful in the diagnosis.[36, 37] Patients may require inotropic support and antiarrhythmic therapy. Pulmonary artery catheterization is useful in measuring cardiac output, mixed venous oxygen tension, and pulmonary artery pressures. Noninvasive impedance cardiac output devices are useful in trending cardiac function. Surgical and anesthetic management of injuries to the ascending aorta often necessitates cardiopulmonary bypass[37]; injuries to the aortic arch are repaired with deep hypothermic circulatory arrest.

Patients with penetrating injuries to the heart or pulmonary vessels require immediate exploration. The physician should not delay operative intervention in order to achieve optimal or stable hemodynamics. Repair of pulmonary vein injuries requires frequent lifting and manipulation of the heart. Repeated lifting and manipulation of the heart often result in intermittent episodes of bradycardia and hypotension. In penetrating injuries of the pulmonary vein or adjoining bronchi, there is an increased risk of air embolism during positive-pressure ventilation. Because air from traumatized bronchi can track down into an open pulmonary vein, the pulmonary vessel must be clamped early to prevent air entry into the pulmonary vein and to avoid systemic air embolism.

Head Injuries

Head injury is the most common cause of death from trauma. *Primary* damage is a direct consequence of the initial trauma; *secondary* damage to the brain is due to elevated intracranial pressure (ICP), hypoxemia, hypotension, and hypercapnia. The combination of hypotension and increased ICP seriously compromises blood flow to the brain. The release of excitatory amino acids, such as glutamate, as well as the formation and release of lactate, kinins, and free radicals appears to be important in the mediation of secondary damage. Free radicals cause lipid peroxidation and result in cellular damage. High serum glucose levels also exacerbate neuronal injury. Sodium influx into the cell produces neuronal swelling, and an influx of calcium results in permanent cellular death.[38]

The goal of anesthetic management is to prevent secondary injury.[39–41] Early clinical evaluation followed by radiologic imaging is necessary to arrive at the correct diagnosis and to guide the treatment.[42–44] The Glasgow Coma Scale is clinically useful in assessing the severity of and predicting outcome after head injury (Table 22–2). Scores are obtained for eye opening, verbal response, and motor response.[45] CT scanning must be done to exclude hemorrhage and evaluate the extent of damage. Accuracy of CT scans can be enhanced by the use of radiographic contrast. Magnetic resonance imaging (MRI), whenever possible, may provide additional information about the integrity of the neuronal system.

TABLE 22–2. Initial Evaluation of Consciousness: Glasgow Coma Scale (GCS)

Eye opening (E)
Spontaneous, already open and blinking
To speech
To pain
None
Verbal response (V)
Oriented
Answers but confused
Inappropriate but recognizable words
Incomprehensible sounds
None
Best motor response (M)
Obeys verbal commands
Localizes painful stimulus
Decorticate posturing (upper-extremity flexion)
Decerebrate posturing (upper-extremity extension)
No movement

GCS score ≤ 8 = deep coma, severe head trauma, poor outcome; GCS score 9–12 = conscious patient with moderate injury; GCS score > 12 = mild injury.

Initial treatment must be aimed at prevention of cerebral hypoxia. Hypoxemia must be relieved by oxygen supplementation. Mechanical ventilation may also be required. Hyperventilation to maintain $Paco_2$ between 25 and 30 mm Hg may be required to control ICP. Arterial blood pressure must be maintained at normal levels. In addition to hyperventilation, mannitol and a loop diuretic may be used to lower the ICP. A ventriculostomy catheter may be used to monitor cerebrospinal fluid pressure and to drain cerebrospinal fluid to avoid a rise in ICP.

In cases of severe head injury and refractory increases in ICP, a barbiturate coma or hypothermia may be used. Pentobarbital is commonly used. Intracranial, subdural, and extradural hematomas require prompt surgical intervention. Seizures require aggressive treatment with phenytoin therapy. Continuation of muscle relaxant or intravenous sedation is often necessary in the postoperative period to provide adequate ventilation. Frequent "bucking" on the endotracheal tube or "fighting the ventilator" acutely increases ICP and should be avoided. Positive end-expiratory pressure (PEEP) can raise ICP and therefore should be limited to 5 to 7 cm H_2O. The patient's head can also be elevated to minimize the effect of PEEP on ICP. Propofol is a short-acting sedative that provides good sedation with minimal cumulative effects. It has the additional advantage of reducing ICP, and it has a short duration that allows rapid recovery and neurologic assessment.

Abdominal Injuries

Injuries to the liver and spleen are common after major abdominal trauma. Both blunt and penetrating injuries present with signs of hemorrhage and abdominal distention. Packing of the liver, hepatorrhaphy, and hepatectomy are the methods to stop the bleeding.

Adequate resuscitation may require infusion of crystalloids, colloids, packed red blood cells, coagulation factors, and platelets. High central venous pressures are to be avoided because they increase hepatic venous pressures, produce hepatic congestion, and can increase the bleeding from the liver. Hepatic ischemia from hypotension or clamping of the portal vein (to gain temporary control of the bleeding) can produce hepatic dysfunction and can rapidly lead to citrate toxicity, acidosis, and coagulopathy.

Splenorrhaphy is currently the preferred approach for

splenic injuries. Splenectomy may be necessary, however, if the bleeding cannot be controlled or the patient is already in severe shock.

Patients with pancreatic injuries may present for debridement and irrigation. Acute pancreatitis and abdominal sepsis are the common complications after trauma. Abdominal distention, sepsis, and multiorgan dysfunction often complicate anesthetic management. It is preferable to leave these patients intubated postoperatively because persistent abdominal distention impairs spontaneous ventilation and the need for multiple debridements.

Hollow viscus injuries require removal of devitalized segments of the intestines. Fecal contamination causes peritonitis and greatly complicates anesthetic management. Bowel edema may preclude abdominal closure at the end of the procedure. Tight closures greatly increase intra-abdominal pressure and impair ventilation even with good sedation and muscle paralysis. Moreover, the increased intra-abdominal pressure can lead to an abdomen compartment syndrome that produces renal and splanchnic ischemia. Oliguria and renal shutdown are common. In such instances, the abdominal fascia is not closed until the edema subsides and until secondary closure can be undertaken at a later time.

Retroperitoneal injuries are commonly associated with pelvic fractures. Massive retroperitoneal hemorrhage involving the kidney, pancreas, or retroperitoneal vessels requires immediate operation. Multiple fractures of the kidney with an extending hematoma require exploration and nephrectomy. Aggressive fluid resuscitation is necessary to maintain the perfusion of the healthy kidney. Extravasation of urine makes intraoperative measurement of urine output difficult. Low-dose dopamine and mannitol infusion may be necessary to maintain renal perfusion and urine output.

Massive abdominal hemorrhage must be controlled immediately. In the presence of shock, it is impossible to adequately resuscitate the patient if the blood loss is uncontrolled. Temporary packing of bleeding sites or clamping of the abdominal aorta can be carried out until the anesthesiologist catches up with the blood loss. Maintaining an adequate arterial blood pressure may not be possible without clamping the aorta above the site of hemorrhage; however, the clamp should not be left for prolonged periods so that ischemic injury to the liver, kidneys, and intestines may be avoided.

Renal, splanchnic, and hepatic damage follows prolonged and repetitive cross-clamping of the aorta. Prolonged clamping of the aorta can also produce a *compartment syndrome*, especially in young patients; fasciotomy may be required. Compartment syndrome leads to rhabdomyolysis and ARF. Use of a mannitol infusion and a loop diuretic may prevent renal failure in such instances. Rapid and adequate resuscitation with fluids and blood products together with control of the bleeding sites shortens clamp time and lessens the incidence of complications.

Injuries to Inferior Vena Cava and the Abdominal Aorta

Abdominal aortic injuries are typically associated with massive hemorrhage. If the injury is above the renal and celiac arteries, mesenteric as well as renal perfusion may be seriously compromised. Hypothermia of the kidneys or use of a shunt may minimize further injury. Neurologic injuries to spinal cord may also occur if the artery of Adamkiewicz is injured. Spinal drainage may be useful in the protection of the spinal cord in such instances. Inferior vena cava (IVC) injuries are almost always associated with massive blood loss. Bleeding in the intrahepatic portion of the IVC is often uncontrollable because of difficult access. Moreover, clamping of the distal vena cava can markedly decrease venous return and lead to arterial hypotension.

SPINAL, PELVIC, AND LONG BONE FRACTURES

Spinal shock usually follows high thoracic and cervical spine injury[46] and presents with systemic hypotension. Hypotension is treated with intravenous fluids and inotropic agents if necessary. Early administration of high-dose corticosteroids and surgical intervention are necessary. Cervical spine injuries necessitate awake, fiberoptic endotracheal intubation. Succinylcholine should be avoided, especially after the first 24 hours, because patients with spinal cord injuries are at risk for succinylcholine-induced hyperkalemia.

Arterial bleeding from iliac vessels after pelvic fractures can often be stopped or controlled preoperatively by embolization; unfortunately, this procedure is not useful for control of venous bleeding. Patients with pelvic fractures are unstable hemodynamically, and the extent of the blood loss is difficult to evaluate. Inadequately resuscitated patients who undergo open reduction and fixation can be unstable intraoperatively. Central venous or pulmonary artery pressure monitoring is useful in guiding fluid therapy.

Patients with multiple long bone fractures, such as femur and tibial fractures, may be hemodynamically unstable because of occult hypovolemia. These patients also are susceptible to development of venous thromboembolism or fat embolism, which usually presents intraoperatively as acute hypoxemia or hypotension. Preexisting hypovolemia, embolic phenomenon, and intraoperative bleeding can make interpretation of central venous and pulmonary artery pressure monitoring difficult.

The occurrence of compartment syndromes after a pelvic or long bone fracture is not uncommon, especially if there is an associated vascular injury. Compartment pressures must be measured, and fasciotomy is necessary if the compartment pressures rise.

GENERAL ANESTHETIC CONSIDERATIONS

Preoperative Considerations

Preoperative evaluation of the trauma patient is complicated by an inability to obtain adequate history for the existence of coexisting diseases, previous anesthetic complications, and the last oral intake. Patients may also be in severe pain after major trauma. The administration of opioids preoperatively can produce respiratory depression and potentiate hypotension. Moreover, the combination of trauma, pain, and opioids can greatly prolong gastric emptying time and may increase the risk of pulmonary aspiration.

Induction of Anesthesia

Patients with shock are sensitive to all anesthetic induction drugs. Ketamine and etomidate may be the preferred induction agents because they have the least depressant circulatory effects. Induction requires a rapid-sequence technique with cricoid pressure. Hyperkalemia from massive trauma and spinal cord paralysis may preclude the use of succinylcholine in such instances.

Intravenous Access

Intravenous access is often limited in trauma patients because the increased sympathetic tone can cause intense peripheral venous vasoconstriction. Central venous access with a large-bore intravenous catheter, therefore, is frequently necessary. The size of the subclavian, internal jugular, and femoral veins facilitates placement of large-bore cannulas at these sites, even in the face of intense vasoconstriction. Two or more large intravenous catheters are necessary in the presence of major blood loss. Neck injuries or subclavian vein injuries preclude venous access in the neck and upper extremities, whereas IVC injuries preclude use of lower-extremity and femoral veins.

Monitoring

An arterial catheter is preferred not only for continuous blood pressure monitoring but also for frequent arterial blood gas tension measurements. Placement of arterial catheters may be difficult because of intense vasoconstriction. Noninvasive monitoring with a thoracic bioimpedance device may be useful in evaluating the cardiac output.[47] Placement of a central venous or pulmonary artery catheter is useful in accurately evaluating volume status. The anesthesiologist must be rapid in placement of these catheters in order to devote full attention to resuscitation of the patient and progress of the surgery.

Awareness

Trauma patients do not tolerate general anesthesia until they are adequately volume-resuscitated; awareness may be a serious problem that can have important psychological sequelae and medicolegal significance. Scopolamine, ketamine, and midazolam are thus useful agents in providing amnesia when volatile anesthetic agents produce hypotension. A long-acting agent, such as lorazepam, should be used sparingly in patients with head injuries to allow neurologic assessment postoperatively.

Blood Loss Measurement

It may not be possible to measure the blood loss accurately. Serial hematocrit or hemoglobin measurements may give an approximate guide for transfusion requirements.

Extubation

Extubation should be delayed in patients who are coagulopathic, acidotic, hypothermic, severely edematous, or hemodynamically unstable and in patients with poor lung compliance. Postoperative mechanical ventilation is advisable for such patients. Optimal pain management facilitates early extubation.

Pain Relief and Sedation

Pain relief techniques may include one of the following:

1. *Patient-controlled analgesia* (PCA). With this technique, the patient must be awake and cooperative.
2. *Regional anesthetic techniques*. Thoracic or lumbar epidural analgesia can be used in patients without evidence of coagulopathy. Use of dilute mixtures of a local anesthetic and an opioid in the epidural space enhances pain relief, may decrease the incidence of adverse side effects, and often improves pulmonary function. Intercostal nerve blocks may also be useful in patients with rib fractures.
3. *Continuous infusions* of opioids, benzodiazepines, or ketamine. Continuous intravenous infusions of these mixtures may be used for patients who are not candidates for PCA or regional anesthesia or for patients requiring mechanical ventilation.[48] Benzodiazepine and propofol may also be useful for sedating patients requiring mechanical ventilation.

References

1. Trunkey DD, Blaisdell FW: Epidemiology of trauma. Sci Am 1988; 4:1.
2. Sauaia A, Moore FA, Moore EE, et al: Epidemiology of trauma deaths: A reassessment. J Trauma 1995; 38:185.
3. American College of Surgeons Committee on Trauma: Initial assessment and management. *In*: Advanced Trauma Life Support Course Instructor Manual. Chicago, American College of Surgeons, 1993, p 37.
4. Malik AB: Endothelial cell interactions and integrins. New Horiz 1993; 1:37.
5. Beutler B: Endotoxin, tumor necrosis factor, and related mediators. New Horizons 1993; 1:3.
6. Biffl WL, Moore EE: Splanchnic ischaemia/reperfusion and multiple organ failure. Br J Anaesth 1996; 77:59.
7. Bigatello LM, Zapol WM: New approaches to acute lung injury. Br J Anaesth 1996; 77:99.
8. Meade P, Shoemaker WC, Donnelly TJ, et al: Temporal patterns of hemodynamic, oxygen transport, cytokine and complement activity in the development of adult respiratory distress syndrome after severe injury. J Trauma 1994; 36:651.
9. Murray JF, Matthay MA, Luce JM, et al: An expanded definition of the adult respiratory distress syndrome. Am Rev Respir Dis 1988; 138:720.
10. Shoemaker WC, Appel PL, Kram HB: Role of oxygen debt in the development of organ failure, sepsis, and death in high-risk surgical patients. Chest 1992; 102:208.
11. Boyd O, Grounds M, Bennett D: Preoperative increase of oxygen delivery reduces mortality in high risk surgical patients. JAMA 1993; 270:2699.
12. Shoemaker WC: Circulatory mechanisms of shock and their mediators. Crit Care Med 1987; 15:787.
13. Shoemaker WC, Appel PL, Kram HB: Hemodynamic and oxygen transport responses in survivors and nonsurvivors of high risk surgery. Crit Care Med 1993; 21:977.
14. Guyton AC: Textbook of Medical Physiology. 9th ed. Philadelphia, WB Saunders, 1992, p 694.
15. Thangathurai D, Charbonet C, Wo C, et al: Intraoperative maintenance of tissue perfusion prevents ARDS. New Horiz 1996; 4:466.
16. Sanchez-Capuchino A, McConachie I: Peri-operative effect of major gastrointestinal surgery on serum magnesium. Anaesthesia 1994; 49:912.
17. Ghino AJ, Elliot CT, Crapo RO, et al: Impairment after adult respiratory distress syndrome: An evaluation based on American Thoracic Society recommendations. Am Rev Respir Dis 1989; 139:1159.
18. Trottier SJ, Taylor RW: Adult respiratory distress syndrome. *In*: Textbook of Critical Care. 3rd ed. Ayres SM, Grenvik A, Holbrook PR et al (Eds). Philadelphia, WB Saunders, 1995, p 811.
19. Petty TL, Ashbaugh DG: The adult respiratory distress syndrome: Clinical features, factors influencing prognosis and principles of management. Chest 1971; 60:233.
20. Irving GA: Perioperative blood and blood component therapy. Can J Anaesth 1992; 39:1105.
21. Denlinger JK, Nahrwold ML, Gibbs PS, et al: Hypocalcemia during rapid blood transfusion in anaesthetized man. Br J Anaesth 1976; 48:995.
22. Miller RD, Brizca SM Jr: Blood, blood components, colloids and autotransfusion therapy. *In*: Anesthesia. 2nd ed. Miller RD (Ed). New York, Churchill Livingstone, 1986, p 1329.
23. Au Buchon JP: Minimizing donor exposure in hemotherapy. Arch Pathol Lab Med 1994; 118:380.
24. Brizca SM: Practical aspects of transfusion therapy. 33rd Annual Refresher Course Lectures (Chapter 125). Park Ridge, Ill, American Society of Anesthesiologists, 1982, p 1.
25. Crosby ET: Perioperative haemotherapy: II. Risks and complications of blood transfusion. Can J Anaesth 1992; 39:822.
26. Jameson L, Popic P, Harms B: Hyperkalemic death during use of a high-capacity fluid warmer for massive transfusion. Anesthesiology 1990; 73:1050.
27. Jurkovich GJ, Greiser WB, Luterman A, et al: Hypothermia in trauma victims: An ominous predictor of survival. J Trauma 1987; 27:1019.
28. Gentilello LM, Cobean R, Offner PJ, et al: Continuous arteriove-

nous rewarming: Rapid reversal of hypothermia in critically ill patients. J Trauma 1992; 32:16.
29. Gentilello LM: Advances in the management of hypothermia. Surg Clin North Am 1995; 75:243.
30. Counts RB, Haisch C, Simon L, et al: Hemostasis in massively transfused trauma patients. Ann Surg 1979; 190:91.
31. Despotis GJ, Santoro SA, Spitznagel E, et al: On-site prothrombin time, activated partial thromboplastin time, and platelet count: A comparison between whole blood and laboratory assays with coagulation factor analysis in patients presenting for cardiac surgery. Anesthesiology 1994; 80:338.
32. Lind SE: The bleeding time does not predict surgical bleeding. Blood 1991; 77:2547.
33. Hoyt DB, Bulger EM, Knudson MM, et al: Death in the operating room: An analysis of a multi-center experience. J Trauma 1994; 37:426.
34. Porembka DT, Johnson DJ, Hoyt BD, et al: Penetrating cardiac trauma: A perioperative role for transesophageal echocardiography. Anesth Analg 1993; 77:1275.
35. Helling TS, Duke P, Beggs CW, et al: A prospective evaluation of 68 patients suffering blunt chest trauma for evidence of cardiac injury. J Trauma 1989; 29:961.
36. Reif J, Prager RL: Selective monitoring of patients with suspected blunt cardiac injury. Ann Thorac Surg 1990; 50:530.
37. Buckmaster MJ, Kearney PA, Johnson SB, et al: Further experience with echocardiography in the evaluation of thoracic aortic injury. J Trauma 1994; 37:989.
38. Lam A: Anaesthetic Management of Acute Head Injury. New York, McGraw-Hill, 1995.
39. Chestnut RM: Secondary brain insults after head injury: Clinical perspectives. New Horiz 1995; 3:366.
40. Cottrell JE, Smith DS (Eds). Anesthesia and Neurosurgery. 3rd ed. St Louis, Mosby-Year Book, 1995.
41. Doberstein CE, Hovda DA, Becker DP: Clinical considerations in the reduction of secondary brain injury. Ann Emerg Med 1993; 22:993.
42. Miller J: Head injury and brain ischaemia—implications for therapy. Br J Anaesth 1985; 57:120.
43. Shackford SR, Mackerise RC, Davis JW, et al: Epidemiology and pathology of traumatic deaths occurring at a level I trauma center in a regionalized system: The importance of secondary brain injury. J Trauma 1989; 29:1392.
44. Chestnut RM, Marshall LF, Klauber MR, et al: The role of secondary brain injury in determining outcome from severe head injury. J Trauma 1993; 34:216.
45. Teasdale G, Jennett B: Assessment of coma and impaired consciousness: A practical scale. Lancet 1974; 2:81.
46. Miller SM: Management of central nervous system injuries. *In*: Trauma: Anesthesia and Intensive Care. Capan LM, Miller SM, Turndorf HR (Eds). Philadelphia, JB Lippincott, 1991, p 321.
47. Thangathurai D, Charbonnet C, Roessler P, et al: Continuous intraoperative noninvasive cardiac output monitoring using a new thoracic bioimpedance device. J Cardiothorac Vasc Anesth 1997; 11:440.
48. Mikhail M, Thangathurai D: Sedating patients in intensive care units. West J Med 1992; 157:566.

23

Acute Pain in the Intensive Care Unit

Carl Anthony Hess, MD

The management of pain from acute tissue injury has been a medical dilemma throughout history. Initial treatments were widely spiritual, and historical pain remedies reflected the current interpretation of pain pathways at the time (Fig. 23–1). Modern thinking has developed a progressive scientific approach to understanding nociceptive pathways, and pain is now accepted as a true physiologic phenomenon. The process of pain transmission is multifaceted, and research continues to yield further understanding of its mechanisms. Delineation of pain into distinct physiologic and clinical entities has provided insight into the importance of neuropathic pain in acute tissue injury.[1, 2] Central sensitization, and consequent severe pain, is now thought to occur in a significant number of postoperative patients, and this pain can be prevented in the majority of patients when analgesia is administered preemptively.

With knowledge and appreciation of the neurophysiologic basis for pain, it would seem obvious that interest in its adequate treatment would follow closely. Unfortunately, traditional bias and misconceptions have retarded the devotion of full attention to the adequate treatment of acute pain. Only since the 1980s have discovery and appreciation of the benefits of acute pain management been realized. Despite the current emphasis on acute pain treatment, there is still evidence that up to 75% of surgical patients experience severe postoperative pain.[3] In addition to the obvious emotional and psychologic benefit to the patients in pain, there is evidence of physiologic improvement, decreased morbidity, and favorable outcome with the superior control of acute pain. With this realization come scrutiny of traditionally inadequate pain

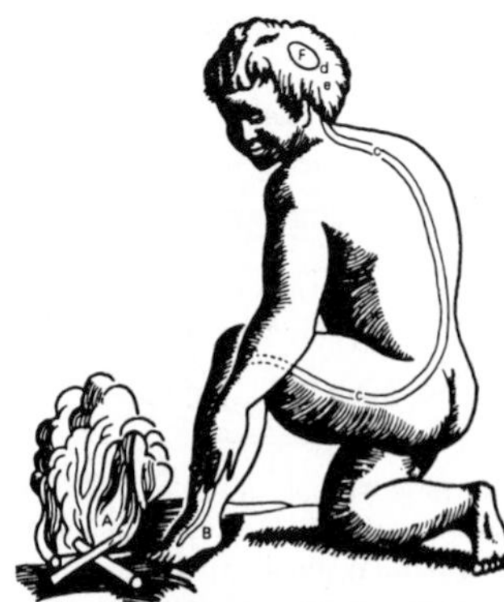

Figure 23–1. Descartes' pain concept, as illustrated by his model of a boy with his foot in a fire. His was the first theory to include the peripheral afferent nerves, spinal cord, and brain as the primary elements in pain transmission. (From Melzak R, Wall PD: Pain mechanisms: A new theory. Science 1965; 15:971. Copyright 1965, American Association for the Advancement of Science. Adapted from Descartes R: "L'Homme" [Paris, 1644], as translated by M. Foster in Lectures on the History of Physiology During the 16th, 17th, and 18th Centuries. Cambridge, England, Cambridge University Press, 1901.)

treatment regimens and motivation toward the development of better systemic and regional techniques and drug delivery technology. This chapter reviews the treatment of pain in the acute setting, emphasizing the favorable impact of adequate pain control and discussing treatment options that maximize patient benefit.

The definitions of pain are many and varied. The International Association for the Study of Pain defines *pain* as an "unpleasant sensory and emotional experience associated with actual or potential tissue damage." This definition reflects the physiologic purpose of pain—that is, survival. Pain transmission is triggered by tissue injury or the threat of tissue damage, and protective mechanisms are elicited to prevent or minimize the injury. Such mechanisms are beneficial to some extent; however, a point is reached, especially in postoperative or post-traumatic acute pain, at which these mechanisms, which are designed to protect, are ultimately detrimental to the patient. Given that pain is an emotional as well as sensory experience, it seems that other affective mechanisms combine with neurophysiologic transmission to act at the expense of outcome.

PAIN PATHWAYS AND MECHANISMS

Painful impulses are known to stimulate peripheral pain receptors, known as *nociceptors*, that transmit impulses via specialized peripheral afferent pain fibers to the spinal cord and into the brain. Subsequently, mechanisms are activated to prevent injury (behavior) and to minimize perceived pain (endogenous analgesia) (Fig. 23–2). A key element, missing in early descriptions of pain, is the role of spinal cord modulation in pain transmission, which is now considered a major focus of specialized intervention for acute pain. Modulation of pain impulses is known to occur through several dorsal horn mechanisms; these are local activation or inhibition of nociceptive impulses, release of neurotransmitters that promote pain or provide analgesia, and transmission to ascending excitatory and to descending inhibitory tracts.

Chemical modulation of pain transmission occurs via several neurotransmitter-receptor systems that have been shown to affect spinal processing of nociceptive input. Excitatory neurotransmitters (e.g., substance P) are active in the spinal cord and enhance pain transmission. The inhibitory elements are the opioids, the α_2-adrenergic fibers, γ-aminobutyric acid, and the serotoninergic and adenosinergic receptors. Endogenous neurotransmitters, like exogenously administered analgesics, work on dorsal horn neurons to inhibit excitatory transmitter release and consequently to decrease pain transmission and perception.

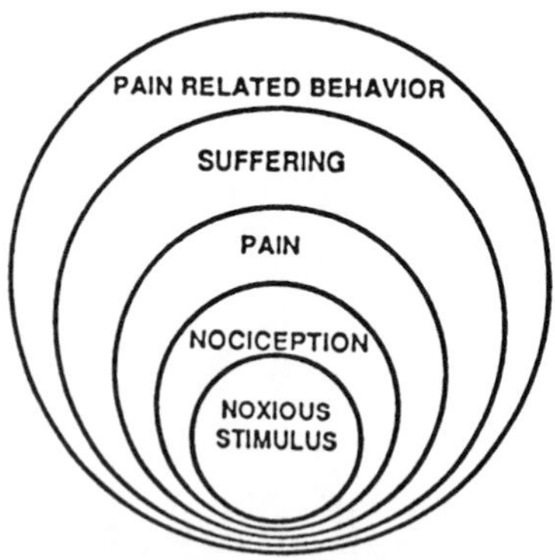

Figure 23–2. A multidimensional model of pain assessment. Evaluation and measurement are often difficult because pain is a highly subjective, multidimensional experience that combines sensory and affective components. Noxious stimuli result in pain perception, with afferent neural transmission characterizing space, time, and intensity of the stimulus. Emotional components are elicited in response to this painful experience and result in the patient's suffering, which is exhibited as pain-related behavior. Many factors affect both the sensory and emotional aspects of pain and thus affect pain behavior. Of all the components in the multidimensional model, pain-related behavior alone has potential for assessment and measurement. (From Loeser JD: Concepts of pain. *In*: Chronic Low Back Pain. Stanton-Hicks M, Boas R [Eds]. New York, Raven Press, 1982, p 124.)

Nociceptive pain, as modulated by these pathways, was once considered the sole source of acute pain. *Neuropathic pain* is now emerging as a significant factor in the severity and the longevity of postoperative pain, which possibly persists into chronic syndromes.[4] Neuropathic pain is caused by direct nerve injury or entrapment (surgical transection of small or large nerve fibers, traction, compression, positioning neuropathies, ischemia, chemicals, etc.), and exhibits clinical pain distinct from its nociceptive counterpart. Pain from nervous tissue injury is described as "burning," "shooting," and "electrical," and is associated with allodynia, hyperalgesia, hyperpathia, and increased regional sympathetic activity. These features are likely the result of central sensitization, or altered threshold of central pain neurons leading to painful response to all stimuli in an increased receptive field, which in turn is caused by the persistent neuronal barrage of neuropathia.[2] It is accepted that the *N*-methyl-D-aspartate (NMDA) receptor is involved in central sensitization, and NMDA receptor antagonists have a role in treating neuropathic pain.[5, 6]

Pathways originating in the periphery and projecting through dorsal root ganglia to dorsal horn neurons and higher centers are illustrated in Figure 23–3. Note the site of action for various pain treatment techniques. These pain treatment modalities are discussed in detail later in the chapter.

PHYSIOLOGIC CONSEQUENCES OF ANESTHESIA AND SURGERY

The importance of acute pain management is illustrated by the physical derangements brought on by acute tissue injury and their potential for improvement—most notably, pulmonary, cardiac, neuroendocrine, and vascular aberrations that can lead to greater morbidity and poor outcome. Figure 23–4 illustrates these pathophysiologic changes and their consequences.

TRADITIONAL PAIN TREATMENT REGIMENS: INADEQUACY OF ACUTE PAIN TREATMENT

Despite rapid progress in the development of new and more effective treatment techniques for acute pain, a large number of patients continue to receive traditional limited therapies consisting of *pro re nata* (prn [as needed]) intramuscular or intravenous opioid analgesia. In 1973, Marks and Sachar[7] demonstrated that 73% of medical in-patients were in moderate to severe distress even though they were receiving an analgesic regimen of prn intramuscular meperidine. Underdosing of analgesia for acute pain was emphasized, with only 1 patient of the 37 receiving doses greater than 75 mg. No adjustment of dosage for weight, increased pain frequency, or previous response was made, and physician concern about addiction and respiratory depression contributed to inadequate pain relief. In a follow-up study in 1980, Cohen[8] demonstrated a 75% rate of moderate to severe distress in surgical patients despite intramuscular narcotic regimens on a prn basis. Nursing choices reflected similar illogical concerns (e.g.,

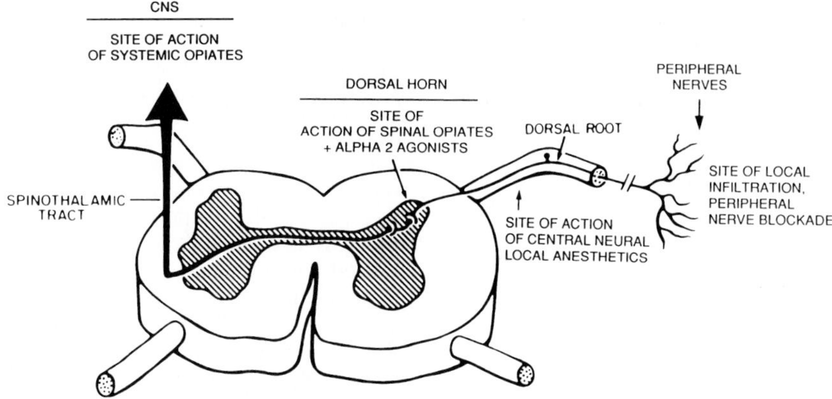

Figure 23–3. Anatomy of pain transmission and sites of analgesic action. The pain of acute tissue injury may be attenuated at many levels and by many actions. This includes blockade of peripheral nerve afferent transmission, blunting of sympathetic ganglia, dorsal root blockade by epidural or intrathecal local anesthetics, and receptor-mediated dorsal horn mechanisms (via opiates and alpha$_2$ agonists). These mechanisms result in diminution of pain transmission contralaterally to ascending spinothalamic tract neurons and, consequently, in fewer impulses traveling to higher centers in the brain. Finally, central nervous system (CNS) analgesic levels of systemic medications afford pain relief from central receptor mechanisms. (Adapted from Badner NH: Epidural agents for postoperative analgesia. Anesthesiol Clin North Am 1992; 10:322.)

no adjustment for weight or previous response), and the philosophy was that complete pain relief was not the goal.

The ineffectiveness of prn intramuscular opioids should be intuitive. Patients need to express the need for pain relief before steps leading to analgesic administration are initiated. This approach results in an excessive delay from the time of pain onset to the time of analgesia. Nursing response, patient evaluation, and preparation and administration of analgesic medications may take as long as 1 hour. Following administration, drug uptake and subsequent blood levels fluctuate dramatically and are unpredictable when the intramuscular route is used. Rapid changes in drug blood levels result in systemic analgesic levels in the subanalgesic range as well as in the excessive range, leading to adverse side effects. Clearance

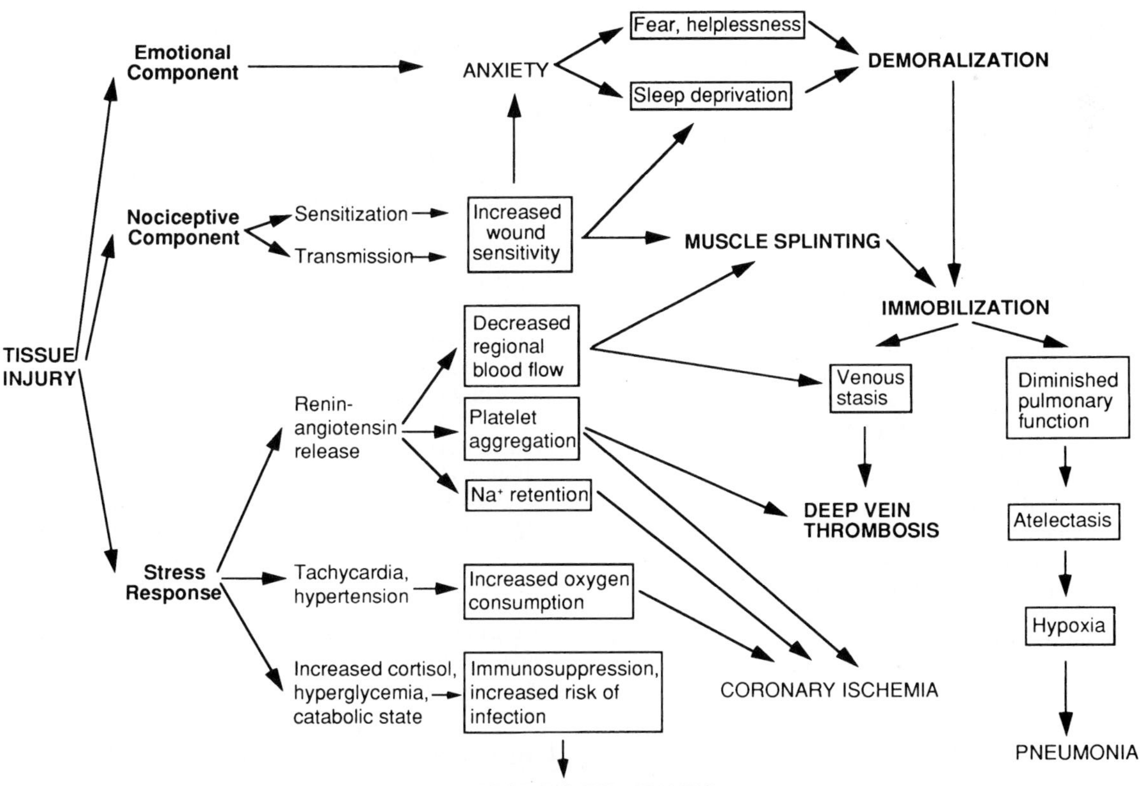

Figure 23–4. Overview of the physiologic consequences of acute tissue injury, including multisystem responses, key target organs, and contributors to morbidity, mortality, and poor outcome. (Adapted from Sinatra RS: Pathophysiology of acute pain. *In*: Acute Pain Mechanisms and Management. Sinatra RS, Hord AH, Ginsberg B, et al [Eds]. St. Louis, Mosby-Year Book, 1992, pp 44–57.)

rapidly brings drug blood levels down through the analgesic range to subtherapeutic levels, the patient experiences recurrent pain, and the cycle begins again.

The incorrect choice of medications represents a dramatic example of misconceptions that result in inadequate pain control. Specifically, paralyzing agents have been used for analgesia and sedation in critically ill patients who are ventilator dependent. Besides subjecting patients to the suffering of untreated pain, this practice produces additional emotional trauma in awake, paralyzed patients who are also in pain. In their article entitled "Paralyzed With Pain," Loper and coworkers[9] reported the prevalent misuse of paralyzing agents in an intensive care unit (ICU) setting. Their survey revealed that 5% to 10% of physicians and nurses advocated the use of pancuronium for analgesia and that a much higher percentage (50% to 70%) advocated its use for anxiolysis. Additional individuals reported that although they did not advocate the use of this agent for analgesia, they were unaware that pancuronium has no analgesic properties. Coincidentally, 80% of physicians in the survey advocated the use of diazepam for analgesia.

These results exposed a commonly held misconception that muscular paralysis represents a calm and painless state and that sedation is a good method of pain control. This is certainly not the case; neuromuscular blocking agents and benzodiazepines have no analgesic effect, and patients in the survey reported the terrifying experience of being paralyzed and not knowing why. In addition, paralyzing agents have no anxiolytic properties and should be administered with a medication properly designed for anxiety control, such as benzodiazepine, to prevent the recall of distressing experiences in the ICU—most notably, awake paralysis.

PAIN MANAGEMENT FOR ACUTE TISSUE INJURY

Systemic Opiates

Despite traditional inadequacies and the development of nonopioid pain treatment modalities, systemic opioid analgesia appropriately continues to be the mainstay of postoperative pain control. If given in regimens that consistently keep blood levels in the analgesic range, systemic opiates can be a safe and beneficial method of relieving postsurgical pain. Continuous opioid infusions or patient-controlled analgesia (PCA) regimens seem to achieve superior analgesia as well as the physical and emotional benefits inherent in adequate pain relief.

Opioid analgesics act on multiple opiate receptors in the central nervous system, spinal cord, and peripheral nervous system. Varying interactions with these receptors result in different pharmacologic profiles among the systemic opiates. The opiate receptors most often involved in supraspinal and spinal analgesia as well as in narcotic side effects are the mu and kappa receptors.

Drugs acting at opiate receptors are divided into pure agonists, agonists-antagonists, and partial agonists (Table 23–1). *Pure agonists* are used for narcotic reversal (e.g., naloxone). Examples of opioid agonists are the common systemic narcotics morphine, hydromorphone, meperidine, and methadone as well as the newer synthetic opiates fentanyl and sufentanil. *Partial agonists* include codeine and buprenorphine. *Agonists-antagonists* include pentazocine, nalbuphine, butorphanol, and the newer drug dezocine. Analgesia is most profound with the pure opioid agonists and seems to reach a plateau with partial agonists and agonists-antagonists. Opiate side effects appear to parallel the amount of agonist activity, however, and are diminished with accompanying antagonism. Table 23–1 shows commonly used narcotic analgesics with dosage equivalence and duration of action.

Side Effects of Opiates

The side effects of systemic opiates are the limiting factor in their use in critically ill patients, victims of multiple trauma, and patients undergoing extensive operations. Most notable are respiratory depression and hypotension.

Maximal respiratory depression occurs within the first 10 minutes after intravenous administration of morphine but may be delayed for 30 minutes following an intramuscular injection. An accompanying increase in arterial carbon dioxide tension and a decrease in lung volumes follow administration of an analgesic dose. In addition, morphine depresses the cough reflex, inhibiting the clearance of secretions and possibly contributing to postoperative atelectasis.

Hypotension occurs with the maintenance of therapeutic analgesic levels of morphine, likely from histamine-induced arteriolar and venous dilatation. Drugs associated with less histamine release, such as fentanyl, seem to provide analgesia with more hemodynamic stability in these patients.

Other side effects of the use of systemic narcotics are nausea and vomiting, pruritus, urinary retention, and gastrointestinal dysfunction.

Metabolism of Opiates

The metabolism of commonly used opiate analgesics is an important consideration in critically ill patients. Meperidine is broken down into a neuroexcitatory metabolite, normeperidine, which is eliminated via the renal route. Accumulation of the metabolite occurs in renal failure and with high consumption of meperidine. Normeperidine neurotoxicity manifests as fine tremor, brisk reflexes, hallucinations, and, eventually, convulsions.

With no evidence that meperidine offers better analgesia, greater patient satisfaction, or fewer side effects, the use of parenteral meperidine is declining in favor of alternative analgesics. Morphine-3-glucuronide, a metabolite of morphine, has opiate activity and can accumulate in patients with renal impairment, especially when given in continuous infusion.

Opiates for Postoperative Pain

Systemic opiate therapy may be used in an effective manner postoperatively. In patients who are critically ill, hemodynamically unstable, or unable to operate a PCA device for various reasons or in whom other techniques are unfeasible or contraindicated, the intermittent administration of systemic opiates is an effective method of postoperative pain control. Knowledge of the spectrum of postoperative pain management regimens is required to tailor treatment to each patient and to provide the most effective analgesic with a maximum of safety and a minimum of side effects.

It must be recognized, however, that some patients, despite their receiving the best possible traditional narcotic regimen, continue to experience significant postoperative pain and are therefore subject to the detriments of inadequate pain relief or to dangerous side effects of excessive doses. Extensive surgery of the upper abdomen or thorax may render a patient uncomfortable and unable to ambulate or make good respiratory effort. In such a patient, more specialized techniques, such as PCA, central neural blockade with local anesthetics or spinal opiates, peripheral nerve blocks, or intrapleural catheters, may need to be considered.

Nonsteroidal Anti-inflammatory Agents

The use of nonsteroidal anti-inflammatory agents (NSAIDs) for acute pain is controversial. Although these agents are associated with significant side effects and complications, such as gastrointestinal ulceration, renal failure, platelet dysfunction,

TABLE 23–1. Systemic Opioid Analgesics for Management of Acute Pain

	Equianalgesic Doses* (mg)	Half-Life (hr)	Peak Effect (hr)	Duration (hr)
Pure Agonists				
Morphine	10 IM	2-3	0.45-1	3-6
	20-60 PO		1.5-2	4-7
Meperidine	75 IM	2-3	0.5-1	3-4
	300 PO	—	1-2	3-6
Hydromorphone	1.5 IM	2-3	0.5-1	3-4
	7.5 PO	—	1-2	3-4
Levorphanol	2 IM	12-15	0.5-1	3-6
Methadone	10 IM	15-190	0.5-1.5	4-6
	20 PO			
Codeine	130 IM	2-3	1.5-2	3-6
	200 PO			
Partial Agonists				
Buprenorphine	0.4	2-5	0.5-1	4-6
Mixed Agonist-Antagonists				
Pentazocine	60 IM	2-3	0.5-1	3-6
	180 PO	—	1-2	3-6
Nalbuphine	10 IM	4-6	0.5-1	3-6
Butorphanol	2 IM	2-3	0.5-1	3-4

*Dose that provides analgesia equivalent to 10 mg of intramuscular morphine. Analgesic requirements and tolerance are widely variable according to patient's condition and severity of injury. Medication should be administered to low doses initially and titrated carefully to analgesic effect and to cardiovascular and respiratory status.

IM = intramuscular; PO = per os (orally).

and exacerbation of chronic obstructive pulmonary disease, their use can reduce the dosage need for strong opiate analgesics and thus diminish some opiate-related side effects.[10–18] Evidence suggests a central action of NSAIDs[19] and a potential diminution of the stress response to surgery,[20] positing a role for these agents in controlling neuropathic and nociceptive elements of acute pain. Given the increased incidence of side effects or complications with the use of NSAIDs in critically ill patients (e.g., elderly, renal failure, bleeding), however, their role in an ICU setting may be limited.

PATIENT-CONTROLLED ANALGESIA

With parenteral medications, PCA consists of a set dosage of a drug given at a set interval by patient demand, with or without an accompanying continuous infusion. PCA has been available for more than 10 years.[21] PCA technology has since developed rapidly, and its popularity has increased dramatically. Traditional agents, such as morphine and meperidine, are the most common medications used in PCA devices. Therefore, the growing use of PCA reflects recognition of the inefficiency of conventional parenteral regimens and the appreciation that more consistent, more effective drug blood levels are delivered by the PCA route of administration.[22]

Intramuscular injections lead to inconsistent plasma concentrations of medication. Onset and time to peak plasma concentration can vary up to sevenfold with repeated injections and with different patient populations. With continuous intravenous infusions or patient-controlled dosing of opioids, a more consistent opioid plasma concentration is achieved.[23] When a patient's plasma concentration of a drug falls below the minimal analgesic level, the patient begins to feel pain, administers an on-demand dose, and rapidly restores the plasma level of the drug to within the analgesic range (Fig. 23–5).

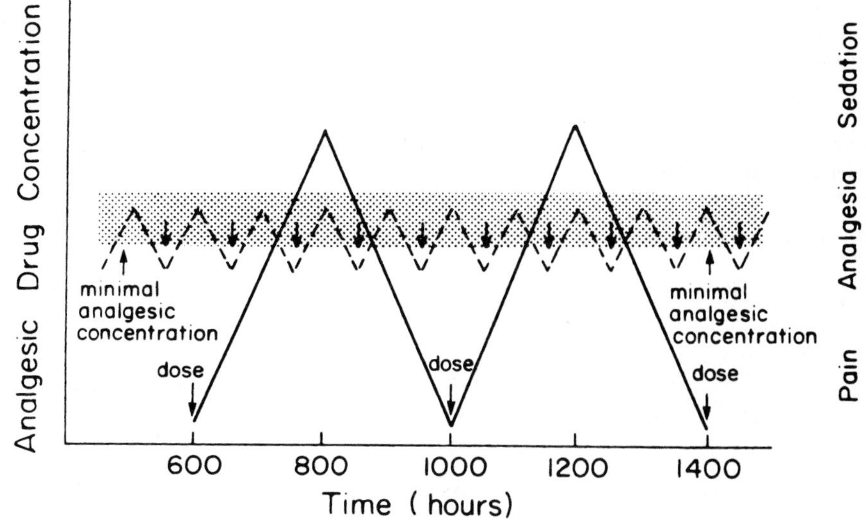

Figure 23–5. The archetypal model of patient-controlled analgesia (PCA). The comparative relation between analgesic drug concentrations, dosing intervals, and analgesic response between PCA and periodic intramuscular narcotic administration illustrates the theoretic benefit derived from PCA and the inefficiency of traditional regimens. PCA drug concentration is represented by the *dashed line*, and intramuscular opioid concentration is represented by the *solid line*. The frequent, small, and on-demand dosing of PCA affords maintenance of drug concentrations more consistently within analgesic levels. In contrast, intramuscular administration shows high variability, with the majority of concentrations in the subanalgesic or superanalgesic range; this results in unrelieved pain or side effects. (From Ferrante FM, Orav EJ, Rocco AG, et al: A statistical model for pain in patient-controlled analgesia and conventional intramuscular opioid regimens. Anesth Analg 1988; 67:457-461.)

In addition to consistent blood levels of drug, the psychologic benefit received by patients who feel some control over their pain treatment regimen cannot be underestimated. Pharmacokinetic and pharmacodynamic factors appear to be less important than psychologic considerations in a patient's decision for on-demand dosing. If a patient is an acceptable candidate for PCA, analgesia is superior to more traditional pain management techniques because the analgesia with PCA is improved and a lower overall drug dosage is needed.[22]

General Guidelines for Use

PCA devices vary in design of administration. The PCA or on-demand dose is of fixed size and is intermittently administered by the patient at a preset lockout interval. The *PCA dose* is the small quantity of analgesic given immediately upon the patient's self-evaluation and conclusion that he or she needs pain medication. The *lockout interval* is the period between PCA doses during which the device does not administer any analgesic. In addition, many PCA devices are equipped with 1-hour and 4-hour total dosage limits designed for added safety.

Many different opioids can be used in PCA regimens. Non-opioid medications are also being investigated for use in patient-controlled analgesia. Although largely empirical, guidelines for PCA administration of commonly used opioid narcotics are listed in Table 23-2.

Side Effects and Complications

Problems encountered with the use of PCA are related to side effects of the medications themselves and to mechanical or operator error. The incidence of opiate side effects with PCA does not appear to be any different from that with other methods of narcotic administration.

CENTRAL NEURAL BLOCKADE

Postoperative pain control with central neural local anesthetics has been in use since the 1940s. Unfortunately, the administration of local anesthetics in the intrathecal or epidural space, which achieve superior analgesia, is associated with dramatic cardiovascular side effects.

Clinical use of intraspinal morphine as a pain management modality began in the late 1970s. The superior analgesia provided segmentally with greater cardiovascular stability has led to the popularity of postoperative intraspinal opiates. Although less severe than those of local anesthetics, the side effects of spinal opiates are varied, the most disconcerting of which is the occurrence of late respiratory depression.

Because of this potentially fatal side effect, the use of other drugs and drug combinations has been proposed. These include opiate analgesics that are more lipid-soluble, agonist-antagonist narcotics, combinations of narcotics and local anesthetics, and non-narcotic analgesics such as the $alpha_2$ agonist clonidine. Each analgesic or analgesic combination has its merits, but no one drug or drug combination has been used without complication. The following discussion summarizes the advantages and disadvantages of the intraspinal medications commonly used for postoperative pain control.

TABLE 23–2. Guidelines for Patient-Controlled Analgesia with Various Opioid Analgesics*

Drug (Concentration)	Demand Dose	Lockout Interval (min)
Morphine (1 mg/mL)	0.5–3.0 mg	5–12
Meperidine (10 mg/mL)	5–30 mg	5–12
Fentanyl (10 μg/mL)	10–20 μg	5–10
Hydromorphone (0.2 mg/mL)	0.05–0.25 mg	5–10
Methadone (1 mg/mL)	0.5–2.5 mg	8–20
Nalbuphine (1 mg/mL)	1–5 mg	5–10

Adapted from Ferrante FM: Patient-controlled analgesia. Anesthesiol Clin North Am 1992; 10:292.

*Analgesic requirements vary widely among patients. Age, severe underlying disease, and individual response may make dosage adjustment necessary.

Central Neural Blockade with Local Anesthetics

Before the advent of indwelling catheters for intrathecal and epidural use, local anesthesia was given in single-shot injections that lasted from 3 to 4 hours in the best of circumstances. This complete neural blockade was effective for intraoperative use and proved superior in providing analgesia upon the patient's emergence from anesthesia.[24] Before catheters were used, however, the benefit could not be extended into the postoperative period, when pain control is most important.

The sites of intrathecal and epidural local anesthetic administration are in the area of the dorsal root (see Fig. 23-1). Small postganglionic sympathetic fibers are blocked first, followed by sensory fibers, and finally by motor nerve fibers. Intensity of blockade depends on the volume and concentration of the local anesthetic given. Although it provides excellent analgesia, this neural blockade often becomes problematic postoperatively because of its profound cardiovascular effects. Hypotension caused by central neural local anesthetics is of particular concern in critically ill patients and in patients undergoing major operations with ongoing blood loss and fluid shifts.

Epidural local anesthesia for postoperative pain has been reported for abdominal, thoracic, and orthopedic procedures.[24] In addition, the use of local anesthetics in thoracic epidural catheters has been shown to decrease the need for mechanical ventilation following multiple rib fractures.[25] Infusions of 0.5% bupivacaine or 1.5% lidocaine not only give superior analgesia for multiple types of surgery but also have beneficial effects on pulmonary and endocrine function. Use of epidural analgesia has been associated with shorter time to ambulation, decreased hospital stay, and lower incidence of pulmonary complications compared with treatment involving systemic pain medication.[26] Similarly, patients undergoing lower abdominal surgery were shown to have lower stress response indices with epidural anesthesia, although those undergoing upper abdominal operations did not consistently show this benefit.[27]

In light of its superior analgesia and potential physiologic benefits, local anesthetic analgesia via the epidural or intrathecal route seems ideal. The side effects, however, cardiovascular instability and motor weakness, prohibit its use in many patients. The same studies that showed beneficial effects also revealed high incidences of hypotension in patients receiving intermittent bolus or continuous infusions of local anesthetics. In addition, a high percentage of patients experienced motor blockade that precluded ambulation, even when a more dilute local anesthetic concentration was used. Because cardiovascular stability and early ambulation are emphasized as the mainstays of postoperative analgesic benefit, the use of moderate to high concentrations of local anesthetic given by bolus or infusion is not consistently practiced, especially in the ICU setting.

SPINAL OPIATE ANALGESIA

Spinal opiate analgesia refers to either intrathecal or epidural administration of a narcotic analgesic. Since the advent of its

TABLE 23–3. Spinal Opiates for the Treatment of Acute Pain

Drug	Single Dose* (mg)	Infusion Rate† (mg/hr)	Onset (min)	Duration of Single Dose‡ (hr)
Epidural				
Morphine	1–6	0.1–1.0	30	6–24
Meperidine	20–100	5–20	5	2–6
Hydromorphone	1–2	0.1–0.2	15	10–16
Fentanyl	0.025–0.10	0.025–0.10	5	2–4
Sufentanil	0.01–0.06	0.01–0.05	5	2–4
Intrathecal				
Morphine	0.1–0.5		15	8–24
Meperidine	10–30			10–24
Fentanyl	0.005–0.025		5	3–6
Sufentanil	0.004–0.0075		5	2–6

Adapted from Ready LB: Intraspinal opioid analgesia in the perioperative period. Anesthesiol Clin North Am 1992; 10:150.

*Low doses may be effective when administered to the elderly or when injected in the cervical or thoracic region.

†If combining with a local anesthetic, consider 0.0625% bupivacaine. Be wary of cardiovascular effects.

‡Duration of analgesia varies widely; higher doses produce longer duration. (Individual doses may vary, adjustment should be made according to patient physical status and pain management requirements.)

Lipid solubility: morphine < hydromorphone << meperidine << fentanyl << sufentanil.

clinical use, rapid progress has been made in management techniques that use spinal opiate analgesia, and this modality has consistently proved to provide superior analgesic efficacy and a reduction in the perioperative morbidity associated with poor pain control. The undesirable side effects associated with local anesthetics—hypotension and motor weakness—are avoided with spinal opiate therapy, but awareness of the side effects of the spinal medications is still important.

No single opiate medication has proved vastly superior to others with regard to analgesic efficacy, improvement of perioperative morbidity, and incidence of side effects. Commonly used opiate analgesics are morphine, meperidine, fentanyl, and sufentanil, and management differences are related to physicochemical properties of the drug selected (e.g., its lipid solubility), catheter placement, and dosing guidelines (Table 23–3). Nonopiate analgesics and opiate agonists-antagonists have also been used with varying degrees of success, as have opioid-local anesthetic combinations.

Morphine

Morphine, the first opiate described for spinal opiate therapy, has become the standard against which all other spinal analgesics are compared. The site of action of morphine, as with other spinal opiates, appears to be on opiate receptors in the dorsal horn of the spinal cord.[28] Epidural morphine administration has demonstrated analgesia superior to that of conventionally administered parenteral narcotics.[29] In addition, profound analgesia extends into the postoperative period.

Morphine is the least lipid-soluble of all the commonly used spinal opiates, having an octanol/water partition coefficient of 1.42. Its onset of action is therefore delayed for 45 to 60 minutes while it penetrates through the dura into the substantia gelatinosa of the dorsal horn. This drug is advantageous not only because of its extended duration of action but also because it can be administered in the low lumbar region for high abdominal or thoracic procedures. Larger doses are needed for lumbar administration (4 to 8 mg for thoracotomy versus 2 to 5 mg for lower abdominal procedures). A continuous infusion may also be used (0.1 mg/mL at a rate of 3 to 10 mL/h). Given the long duration of action afforded by morphine's lipid insolubility and pharmacokinetic profile, however, epidural infusions of the drug may be less practical than administration of the more lipid-soluble agents.

Side effects and complications of intraspinal morphine are the same as those of other commonly used spinal opiates; they are nausea and vomiting, pruritus, urinary retention, and early and late respiratory depression. Because of its persistence in the cerebrospinal fluid, the incidence and severity of side effects of morphine appear to be greater than those of more lipid-soluble opiates. Late respiratory depression has been the most dramatic side effect of intraspinally administered morphine, with early case reports of patient morbidity and mortality.

Much attention has been directed to the issue of clinical safety regarding the use of intraspinal morphine. Three large studies reviewing 15,000 patients found an incidence of late respiratory depression of less than 1%.[30–32] Numerous articles published after these studies reported similarly low rates; others have stated that intraspinal morphine can be safe despite this complication if adequate vigilance protocols are followed.[33] Late respiratory depression appears to be the result of cephalad migration of morphine in the cerebrospinal fluid, which is less likely with the more lipid-soluble opiates. Respiratory depression can occur up to 24 hours after the administration of morphine. Table 23–4 lists predisposing factors.

The other complications reported with the use of this agent are common after surgery and should not be attributed solely to intraspinal administration of morphine. Nausea and vomiting have been reported to occur in 30% to 40% of patients receiving epidural morphine. Urinary retention, which occurs in 5% to 40% of patients, is due to bladder detrusor muscle

TABLE 23–4. Factors Predisposing to the Development of Respiratory Depression Following Intraspinal Opioid Administration*

- Hydrophilic drug (e.g., morphine)
- Large or repeat doses
- Use of parenteral opioids or other central nervous system depressants
- Elderly or debilitated patients
- Coexisting respiratory disease
- Thoracic epidural analgesia
- High sensitivity to opioids (i.e., no previous exposure to opioids)
- Intrathecal administration
- Raised intrathoracic pressure (e.g., with controlled ventilation, coughing, vomiting)

Adapted from Cousins MJ, Mather LE: Intrathecal and epidural administration of opioids. Anesthesiology 1984; 61:276.

*Factors present should indicate the use of high vigilance protocols (i.e., intensive care unit admission, monitored bed, and respiratory monitoring).

dysfunction; it may be less significant in the intensive care setting because critically ill patients or those undergoing large procedures commonly have indwelling urinary catheters. Pruritus is variable, occurring in 10% to 90% of cases, and although it is not histamine-mediated, this complication responds to intravenous administration of diphenhydramine (Benadryl). If the patient's condition remains refractory, intravenous infusions of small doses of naloxone may be administered to counteract side effects independent of analgesic effect.

Meperidine

Meperidine displays the physicochemical advantages of greater lipid solubility and an octanol/water partition coefficient many times that of morphine. These features afford meperidine a quicker onset of action (15 to 30 minutes), lesser extent of cephalad spread (potentially fewer side effects), and a shorter duration of action (4 to 6 hours), which lends practicality to continuous infusion. In addition, meperidine has the distinct advantage of possessing local anesthetic properties and is the only opiate to have been used as a sole anesthetic when given intrathecally.[34] Unfortunately, this local anesthetic effect is not clinically evident when meperidine is given epidurally, and its analgesic and side effect profiles are not significantly different from those of the more lipid-soluble opiate analgesics. Nonetheless, meperidine represents a practical option in intrathecal or epidural administration, offering all the advantages of the other spinal opiates. It can be used in bolus form or as a continuous infusion and shows potential for combination with dilute local anesthetic solutions.

Fentanyl

Fentanyl, a synthetic opioid agonist that contains the same chemical nucleus as morphine, is manufactured synthetically rather than by chemical modification. Fentanyl is approximately 100-fold more potent than morphine and is 500-fold more lipid-soluble. These physicochemical properties give fentanyl a rapid onset of analgesia and a short duration of action. Its higher lipid solubility minimizes cephalad migration because of fentanyl's diffusion into the lipid layers of the dura before significant spread can occur. For this reason, larger doses need to be administered via a lumbar epidural catheter to achieve analgesia for upper abdominal and thoracic surgery (100 to 200 μg), whereas smaller doses are adequate for lower operations.

Because of its short duration of action, fentanyl is an ideal drug to be used in a continuous infusion through an epidural catheter. At a concentration between 4 μg/mL and 10 μg/mL, an infusion of 0.5 to 1.0 $\mu g \cdot kg^{-1} \cdot hr^{-1}$ is administered for postoperative pain. Epidural infusion is less likely to result in rapid or significant accumulation of systemic fentanyl levels if lumbar epidural catheters are used for low abdominal and peripheral procedures, or if thoracic epidural catheters are used for upper abdominal and thoracic procedures.

Problems encountered with epidural fentanyl infusions occur when lumbar epidural catheters are used for extensive abdominal procedures or thoracotomies, and these problems are related to the high lipid solubility of the drug. With a low epidural catheter, larger doses (1 to 1.5 $\mu g \cdot kg^{-1} \cdot hr^{-1}$) are required for analgesia, resulting in rapidly distributed systemic fentanyl concentrations similar to those required for intravenous fentanyl analgesia. It has been suggested that this analgesic regimen may be nothing more than a modified form of intravenous therapy.[35] Consistent reports of this effect indicate that epidural fentanyl infusions require insertion of the epidural catheter in close proximity to the surgical dermatomes affected.

Sufentanil

Sufentanil is a newer-generation synthetic opiate that is reported to be fivefold to sevenfold as potent as fentanyl when given systemically. Sufentanil has twice the lipid solubility of fentanyl and initially showed great promise as a successor to epidural fentanyl. Sufentanil provides excellent analgesia, a short onset of action (<15 minutes), and a duration of action longer than that of fentanyl (4 to 6 hours). Epidural dosing guidelines have revealed that sufentanil potency in the epidural space is only twice that of fentanyl; this finding is attributable to a higher degree of nonspecific uptake by lipophilic tissues.[36]

Because of its high lipid solubility and short duration of action, sufentanil has been used in intermittent bolus, in continuous epidural infusions, and even in PCA devices. Boluses of 30 to 50 μg for upper abdominal or thoracic surgery and 15 to 30 μg for peripheral procedures are required for analgesia. Epidural infusion rates of 0.15 to 0.30 $\mu g \cdot kg^{-1} \cdot hr^{-1}$ are sufficient when a dilute 1 μg/mL solution is used. Given the high lipid solubility and systemic absorption from continuous epidural infusions, the issue of plasma concentrations of sufentanil with continuous infusions has been raised. Although sufentanil has not been as extensively investigated as fentanyl, significant systemic levels have been reported and may represent a lack of true advantage of sufentanil over fentanyl in continuous infusions.[37]

Opioid–Local Anesthetic Combinations

Problems arising from the side effects and systemic absorption of spinal opiates have led to the use of narcotic–local anesthetic combinations. This practice aims to minimize the dose of spinally administered opiates and, in turn, the problems associated with their use. Also, some evidence shows that the addition of dilute local anesthetic solutions improves analgesia. Several investigations have indicated that analgesia obtained from epidural infusions of fentanyl or sufentanil was enhanced when the agent was used with dilute solutions of bupivacaine.[36] Similarly, epidural infusions of hydromorphone with more dilute bupivacaine solutions were superior to hydromorphone alone for cesarean section pain. There have been conflicting reports, however, that epidural morphine combined with bupivacaine has no advantage over epidural morphine alone in terms of analgesia, total narcotic requirement, or side effects after thoracotomy, upper abdominal surgery, and cesarean section. Similar results have been found with fentanyl-bupivacaine combinations.

Addition of local anesthetics to spinal opiate infusions or boluses may enhance analgesia without clinical signs of local anesthetic blockade. Benefit may also stem, however, from coincident sympathetic or sensory blockade achieved with a local anesthetic solution. The advantages of this combination—superior analgesia and decreased spinal opiate requirement—may be achieved at the risk of the potentially deleterious side effects of local anesthetics—hypotension, motor weakness, and inability to ambulate. The importance of the analgesic regimen therefore needs to be factored into the total plan of patient care and tailored individually to each patient's needs after acute tissue injury.

INFLUENCE ON OUTCOME

Outcome is a primary consideration in pain treatment. Patient outcome is expressed in terms of overall well-being as well as of morbidity and mortality. The goals of acute pain management should be:

1. To optimize the emotional and psychologic well-being of the patient and of his or her family (patient satisfaction).
2. To provide superior pain relief with a minimum of side effects from the medication or technique.
3. To restore or maintain preoperative physiologic function,
4. To minimize postoperative complications and thereby shorten the patient's ICU or hospital stay.

The challenge of acute pain management is to accomplish these goals in an efficient, safe, and cost-effective manner. Although no firm conclusion can be offered at present, adequate acute pain management by PCA, the use of spinal opiates, or peripheral or central neural blockade seems to show benefit over previously used regimens in postoperative recovery as well as in level of analgesia and patient satisfaction.

PCA has demonstrated outcome advantages compared to intermittent dosing in terms of decreased confusion, restoration of pulmonary function, fewer pulmonary complications, shorter time to ambulation, and shortened hospital stay.[38-40]

Since the advent of spinal opiate analgesia, the beneficial effects of spinal opiate therapy on the physiologic derangements of acute tissue injury have been consistently demonstrated. In addition to yielding favorable outcome regarding pulmonary complications,[41-43] the cardiovascular system,[44-46] neuroendocrine stress response,[27] and vascular complications,[44, 47, 48] superior analgesia with spinal opiates has demonstrated the ability to decrease the time needed for mechanical ventilation, the duration of intensive care, and the duration of hospital stay and to lower the total cost of hospitalization. Improved pulmonary outcomes and earlier extubation have also been noted with the use of spinal opiate analgesia for cardiac surgery, thoracotomy, and thoracoabdominal operations.[49, 50]

The economic impact of the benefits conferred by adequate treatment of acute pain is indicated only by the results of outcome studies. It is evident that epidural analgesia in critically ill patients has the potential to diminish morbidity and thereby to minimize the necessity for medical intervention and support. In addition to statistically significant diminution in hospital and ICU stays as well as in ventilator time, cost analyses are being presented in the literature more frequently. Adoption of more effective pain management techniques and the development of acute pain services are emerging as cost-effective alternatives to traditional parenteral narcotic techniques and represent a compassionate endeavor to optimize patient comfort.

REGIONAL BLOCKADE

Side effects such as sedation, respiratory depression, nausea, gastrointestinal dysfunction, potential cardiovascular depression, and difficulty in monitoring mental status in head-injured patients often make the use of systemic narcotics a poor option in the treatment of acute pain. Preexisting conditions (e.g., critical illness, central nervous system disease, anatomic considerations, coagulopathy) may render the use of spinal opiates impractical. As a result, many critically ill patients do not receive any pain treatment or are undertreated. If systemic opioids must be avoided, regional anesthetic techniques can be used to give excellent analgesia and help keep patients alert and cooperative. Local anesthetics can be administered for local infiltration, intravenous regional anesthesia, peripheral nerve blocks, and central neural blockade. Regional techniques exist for virtually every indication and location of pain (Table 23–5).

TABLE 23–5. Regional Blocks for Management of Acute Pain

Region	Block
Head/neck	Occipital nerve Cervical epidural Superficial cervical plexus Local infiltration
Shoulder	Interscalene plexus Local infiltration
Chest	Intercostal Thoracic epidural Interpleural
Arm	Brachial plexus IV regional Peripheral nerve (radial, median, ulnar) Local infiltration
Abdomen	Upper: Intercostal Interpleural catheter Wound infiltration Thoracic epidural Lower: Wound infiltration Thoracic/lumbar epidural
Groin (hernia)	Ilioinguinal Iliohypogastric Local infiltration Lumbar epidural
Flank (nephrectomy)	Thoracic/lumbar epidural Intercostal Paravertebral somatic
Hand	Brachial plexus Elbow/wrist (radial, median, ulnar nerves) IV regional
Fingers	Digital Wrist
Anogenital	Caudal Epidural Penile
Anterior thigh (skin graft)	Lateral femoral cutaneous
Thigh/knee	Femoral/sciatic/obturator nerve Lumbar epidural Local infiltration
Leg	Femoral/sciatic nerve Lumbar epidural Knee (saphenous, common peroneal nerves) IV regional Local infiltration
Feet	Lumbar epidural Ankle Local
Toes	Digital Ankle

IV = intravenous.

Local Infiltration

Local infiltration is perhaps the simplest means of providing extended wound analgesia. Local anesthetic can be administered by subcutaneous infiltration for analgesia of minor injuries or along the surgical edges of postoperative wounds, can be infused continuously through implanted catheters inserted at surgical sites, and can even be injected into a fracture hematoma for reduction. Fears have been expressed that injections of local anesthetics into a wound may interfere with the normal healing process; however, no evidence shows that wound healing is delayed or that infection is introduced by this technique. Bupivacaine 0.25% is the preferred local anesthetic. Epinephrine-containing local anesthetics should be avoided because of the possibility of decreased blood flow and theoretic risks of delayed wound healing.

Intravenous Regional Blockade

Although seldom used for postoperative or post-traumatic analgesia, the intravenous regional block is extremely useful for manipulation of limb fractures or for simple surgical procedures. The advantages of the technique are that it is simple, has a rapid onset and controllable duration of action, achieves some muscle relaxation, and is safe when given by experienced personnel. The procedure involves placement of a double tourniquet on the proximal extremity and the intravenous administration of large volumes of dilute local anesthetic distally (40 or 50 mL of a 0.5% lidocaine solution for an upper extremity or a lower extremity, respectively). Systemic levels of local anesthetic can result from leakage or inadvertent release of the tourniquets; for this reason, bupivacaine is not recommended for intravenous regional analgesia.

Peripheral Nerve Blockade

Peripheral nerve blockade for pain in trauma or after surgery is often not considered, either because of the inexperience of available personnel in performing the blockade or because of surgical time constraints. The techniques of peripheral nerve blockade produce effective, long-lasting analgesia with a minimum of side effects. Appropriate blocks exist for almost all areas of the body. With the use of a long-acting local anesthetic such as bupivacaine, analgesia may last up to 24 hours. Catheter techniques have been described for several peripheral blocks, including those of the intercostal space, interpleural space, femoral nerve, and brachial plexus.

Intercostal Blockade

Intercostal blockade is simple and effective and has been extensively used to provide pain relief for patients who have fractured ribs or blunt trauma or have undergone upper abdominal or thoracic surgery. Because of significant pain, these patients often have poor respiratory effort and an ineffective cough and thus risk respiratory failure, which necessitates intubation and mechanical ventilation. Systemic opioid analgesia is often problematic in these patients because of its respiratory depressant and cough suppressant actions. Consistent evidence indicates that intercostal nerve block reduces the requirements for opioids and improves pulmonary function after injury.[51]

Intercostal blockade has advantages over interpleural and thoracic epidural blockades; it is technically easier to perform and is not associated with the side effects of epidural blockade, such as hypotension, motor weakness, and urinary retention. Among the disadvantages of intercostal blocks is that multiple levels are commonly involved and, thus, multiple injection sites are needed. Furthermore, unless a continuous infusion catheter is inserted, intercostal blocks must be repeated frequently (although analgesia up to 24 hours has been obtained with bupivacaine). An inherent risk of pneumothorax, a potentially fatal complication in patients with severe respiratory compromise, also exists. Because of rapid absorption into intercostal vessels, significant systemic levels of local anesthetics may result with large or repeated doses, which can lead to profound cardiovascular or central nervous system effects.

Continuous intercostal analgesia administered via indwelling catheter has been used successfully to treat pain following upper abdominal surgery, thoracic surgery, and chest trauma, especially that caused by fractured ribs.[52] The obvious advantage is provision of prolonged analgesia without the need for multiple blocks and their associated risks. Local anesthetic administered through an indwelling catheter in a single intercostal space spreads cephalad and caudad to provide analgesia at several levels for multiple areas of injury.

Interpleural Blockade

Administration of local anesthetics via a percutaneous catheter placed between the visceral and parietal pleurae gives good unilateral thoracic dermatomal analgesia. Interpleural analgesia has been used successfully in managing various types of pain in the thorax and upper abdomen, including pain after cholecystectomy and thoracotomy that is caused by multiple rib fractures.[53] The mechanism of action of interpleural analgesia is still uncertain. Possibilities include diffusion of local anesthetic through the parietal pleura, with subsequent superficial spread to block the intercostal nerves and posteromedial spread to block nerve roots and sympathetic ganglia in the paravertebral space. Direct local anesthetic action on pleural nerve endings may also occur.

Contraindications to this block include a recent thoracic infection with pleuritis and fibrosis of the pleura. Inflammation and greater vascularity can increase absorption and the systemic toxicity of local anesthetics. Although the presence of thoracostomy tubes does not preclude use of this technique (chest tubes can actually be used to deliver the local anesthetic), it works best in situations in which no such drains are required. The degree of sensory anesthesia obtained with interpleural block is inconsistent. Frequently, pinprick sensation is well maintained, despite adequate analgesia. The greatest utility of this technique appears to be in circumstances that contraindicate the use of other regional anesthesia techniques, such as when severe vertebral injuries are present and are accompanied by multiple rib fractures.

Femoral or Sciatic Blockade

Femoral nerve blockade has been used for analgesia and muscle relaxation in femoral fractures and after total knee arthroplasty.[54] The extent of analgesia depends on the fracture site. Excellent pain relief can be obtained for midshaft fractures, good relief for lower-third fractures, and partial relief for upper-third fractures. The method can be extended to give continuous analgesia for several days with insertion of a catheter into the femoral sheath and administration of dilute local anesthetics (e.g., 0.125 to 0.25% bupivacaine solution). Increasing the volume of injectate and encouraging its cephalad spread enable the femoral nerve block to include the lateral femoral cutaneous and obturator nerves, thus achieving more complete analgesia for the upper thigh.

Except for injuries to the foot, blockade of the sciatic nerve alone is of little value in providing analgesia. Combined sciatic and femoral blocks, however, give excellent anesthesia below the knee for significant lower extremity trauma, multiple fracture sites, and dislocations around the ankle.

Brachial Plexus Blockade

Brachial plexus blockade can be performed via the axillary, infraclavicular, interscalene, and supraclavicular routes.[55] The choice of technique depends on the site of the injury and on the patient's ability to move the arm. In general, higher lesions (e.g., upper-arm injury, dislocated shoulder) require analgesia extending into the C5 dermatome, which is best achieved with an interscalene approach. The axillary approach is also very popular and has been used successfully in both adults and children.

As with other techniques, continuous infusion of local anesthetic can be used to prolong neural blockade. This is particularly useful following reimplantation procedures or other vascular injuries that result in diminished blood flow and vasospasm. The prolonged chemical sympathectomy achieved by brachial plexus blockade permits improved blood flow to the area of injury. Incomplete analgesia in the hand with these techniques can be remedied by supplemental blockade of the individual nerve (i.e., radial, median, or ulnar) at the elbow or wrist.

Other Peripheral Nerve Blocks

Multiple nerve blocks have applications in the management of acute pain for patients who have undergone surgery, have been injured, or are critically ill.[56] Ilioinguinal-iliohypogastric nerve blocks are useful after femoral groin area manipulation or hernia repair.

A wrist block is easy to perform. It involves blocking the median, radial, and ulnar nerves at the wrist. Indications for this block include lacerations or fractures of the digits and pending incision for removal of abscess of the digits.

An ankle block is likewise easy to perform; it requires blockade of five nerves at the ankle: the tibial, sural, saphenous, superficial, and deep peroneal nerves. Indications for an ankle block include the relief of pain in the sole or the dorsum of the foot.

Psoas compartment lumbar plexus blockade is another alternative for lower extremity analgesia. It is often used in conjunction with sciatic nerve blockade for complete anesthesia of the leg.

SPECIAL CASES

Patients with Multiple Trauma

Patients with varying degrees of trauma and postoperative patients suffer similarly from the pain of acute tissue injury. The management of pain in the case of uncontrolled tissue injury can be difficult and complex, and overtreatment or undertreatment of this pain can have adverse outcomes. Obviously, in the acute phase of trauma, immediate attention must be given to the stabilization of a patient's respiratory and cardiovascular status. Treatment of pain is appropriately deferred until the patient is stabilized and the extent of his or her injury is fully investigated and diagnosed. Acute pain from trauma results in profound and sustained catecholamine release that may support the blood pressure and cardiac output in a patient who has sustained large blood losses. Once respiratory and volume status has been restored, the slow titration of intravenously administered opioids for pain management is appropriate. It is performed with careful critical observation for respiratory effects, myocardial depression, and hypotension.

Acute injury causes immobility of the injured area. This inhibits movement of an injured extremity, spine, or ribs secondary to pain. Many of these injuries are so painful that a systemic narcotic must be used in doses large enough to cause potentially dangerous side effects. In this scenario, any number of regional analgesic techniques may be employed to avoid or reduce the use of systemic narcotics for pain relief. Local infiltration, peripheral nerve blockade, or central neural blockade with a local anesthetic or opiates may be employed safely alone or in combination with systemic analgesics.

Burn Patients

Patients presenting with burn injuries offer a challenge to the physicians and medical staff involved in their care. The pain from burn injuries is grossly undertreated. The primary method of pain management in burned patients should be the intravenous administration of opioids. As in acute trauma, this should be started only after a secure airway has been ensured and stable hemodynamics have been established. In general, full-thickness burns are not painful, but partial-thickness burns are extremely painful.

Patients with severe burn trauma have two types of pain. First, constant pain from the burn injury occurs at rest and with the performance of daily activities. This pain should be managed around the clock with opioid regimens. Second, procedures necessary for burn treatment, including debridement, dressing changes, hydrotherapy, and physical therapy, are associated with severe pain. This type of pain should be managed with the tailoring of a drug regimen that is specific to both the patient and the procedure.

Pain management during burn treatment procedures may consist of the use of opioids alone or in combination with anxiolytics or dissociative anesthesia with ketamine. Many clinicians use fentanyl as the opioid of choice for these procedures, with initial doses in the range of 1 to 6 μg/kg with the addition of midazolam, 0.08 mg/kg, in divided doses. Although ketamine can be given intravenously or intramuscularly, it is best to avoid intramuscular drug regimens in burn patients. Intravenous doses for ketamine can be titrated using 0.5 to 1.0 mg/kg. Because ketamine is associated with high incidences of hallucinations and excitement, it should be used in combination with anxiolytics. Although many nonpharmacologic therapeutic modalities have been tried, including hypnosis, relaxation training, biofeedback, distraction techniques, and transcutaneous electrical nerve stimulation therapy, the excruciating pain associated with burn injuries appears to require more aggressive intervention.

Patients with Major Organ Failure

Many patients suffering from major organ failure receive suboptimal pain management because of caregivers' fear that such treatment may worsen an already critical condition.[57] With major organ dysfunction, significant changes can occur in the pharmacokinetic profile of analgesic medication. Volume of distribution, clearance, and excretion are affected by organ failure, and these effects are exaggerated by drug administration. Table 23-6 summarizes the pharmacokinetics of different drugs and the pharmacodynamic changes associated with hepatic and renal failure. Acute pain management for significant, specific organ dysfunction is discussed in the following sections.

Central Nervous System

Central nervous system trauma or disease represents a challenge to the providers of acute pain control, particularly for patients who have disruption of the blood-brain barrier and increased intracranial pressure. Controversy exists as to whether these patients should receive opioid agents. The concern about opioid-induced increase in arterial carbon dioxide tension and subsequent elevation of intracranial pressure has led many clinicians to avoid the use of these agents. Use of meperidine should be avoided, because its active metabolites may induce seizure activity. Central neural blockade (epidural or intrathecal) carries the risk of dural puncture, which causes brain stem herniation. Some physicians have employed transcutaneous electrical stimulation and ketorolac as adjuvant therapy for pain relief.

Pulmonary Failure

Patients with severe pulmonary conditions (e.g., chronic obstructive pulmonary disease, restrictive lung disease, pulmonary hypertension) who sustain multiple trauma or who undergo thoracic or abdominal procedures are excellent candidates for continuous epidural opiate infusions. This technique may preserve pulmonary function postoperatively better than intravenous opioid administration. Administration of ketorolac and application of transcutaneous electrical nerve stimulation to supplement opioid therapy have had good results. Other modalities are placement of interpleural catheters,

TABLE 23–6. Pharmacokinetics of Selected Analgesic and Sedative Agents

Agent	Volume of Distribution (L/kg)	Plasma Protein Binding (%)	Hepatic Clearance ($mL \cdot kg^{-1} \cdot min^{-1}$)	Renal Excretion Free Drug (%)	Elimination Half-Life (min)	Active/Toxic Metabolites	Drug Activity*	
							Hepatic Failure	*Renal Failure*
Morphine	3.2	30	14.7	10	114	Yes	+	++
Meperidine	3.8	60	15.1	5	180–250	Yes	++	+++
Fentanyl	4.1	84	11.6	8	200	No	+	+
Sufentanil	4.5	92.5	12.7	1-2	148–164	Yes	++	+++
Methadone	6	90	2.8	5	35 hr	No	+++	+
Lidocaine	1.3	70	0.95 L/min	NA	96	Yes	++	+++
Bupivacaine	2.0	95	0.47 L/min	NA	210	No	++	++
Ketorolac	0.2	99	4.0	58	300–310	No	+	++
Diazepam	1.5	98	0.3	5	21–37	Yes	++	++
Midazolam	1.5	98	6–8	5	60–200 hr	No	++	No change

Data from Sinatra RS: Pain management in patients suffering from major organ failure. *In:* Acute Pain: Mechanisms and Management. Sinatra RS, Hord AH, Ginsberg B, et al (Eds). St. Louis, Mosby-Year Book, 1992; Stoelting RK: Opioid agonists and antagonists. *In:* Pharmacology and Physiology in Anesthetic Practice. Stoelting RK (Ed). Philadelphia, JB Lippincott, 1987; and Micaela M, Buckley T, Brogden RN: Ketorolac: A review of its pharmacodynamic and pharmacokinetic properties and therapeutic potential. Drugs 1990; 39:86.

*Key: + = mild; ++ = moderate; +++ = major potentiation of activity; NA = not available.

intercostal nerve blockade, and continuous intercostal infusions, which are used with extreme caution because of the risk of pneumothorax.

Cardiac Failure

With proper pain management, ischemic events can be avoided in patients with severe ischemic heart disease who are recovering from noncardiac surgery. Epidurally and intrathecally administered opioids suppress the catecholamine response to pain more effectively than intravenously administered opioids. Patients who receive intravenous therapy should be given intravenous opioids carefully titrated to achieve analgesia and avoid side effects. Individuals with severely depressed cardiac function who receive intravenous morphine are susceptible to hypotension. Meperidine should be used with caution in these patients because its vagolytic action may induce tachycardia, hypertension, and subsequent ischemia.

Liver Failure

In patients with liver disease, it is difficult to quantitate the extent of dysfunction in metabolism and biotransformation until the late stages of liver failure. Thus, the physician must always be concerned with analgesic overdose in these patients. The capability of the liver to synthesize may be compromised to the point that a coagulopathy develops, rendering regional analgesia impractical. If there are no contraindications to catheter placement, however, spinal opiate therapy is acceptable and provides excellent benefits for patients with hepatic failure. Intrathecal administration of morphine (0.25 to 0.5 mg) achieves superior analgesia and a duration similar to that of intravenous doses 100-fold greater and infused through a PCA device.

With epidural analgesia, when a local anesthetic is added to an opioid agent, care must be taken not to reach toxic serum concentrations of local anesthetic. If coagulopathy exists or if the surgical site does not permit the use of regional analgesia, intravenous fentanyl administered continuously or by a PCA device can be a safe alternative (see Table 23-6).

Renal Failure

Epidural or intrathecal administration of morphine in patients with renal failure offers several advantages over systemic narcotics, including superior analgesia, low dosage requirements, minimum accumulation, and absence of renal toxicity. Intravenous administration of opioids must be conducted with great care. Intravenous use of meperidine and sufentanil carries the potential for accumulation of active metabolites that are renally excreted. PCA with fentanyl represents an excellent option in patients with renal failure, because the analgesia is adequate and the renally excreted metabolites have minimal activity. The renal activity of ketorolac, although likely insignificant in the acute setting, should discourage its use in patients with renal failure (see Table 23-6).

PEDIATRIC PATIENTS

Traditional bias against treating pain in the postoperative period is exaggerated in the pediatric population because of additional misconceptions that children do not experience pain in the same manner as adults. In 1968, Swafford and Allen[58] reported that only 2 of 60 children in their surgical ward required pain medications; they stated that "pediatric patients seldom need medication for relief of pain. They tolerate discomfort well." In 1977, Eland and Anderson[59] were the first to challenge these practices and to document the extent of this bias. Their study revealed not only that many children were undertreated but also that some were not treated at all, despite their having severe injuries (e.g., traumatic amputation of the foot) or having undergone major surgeries (e.g., heminephrectomy).

Consistent disparity exists between the numbers of pain medication doses given to adults and to pediatric patients undergoing similar procedures. The undertreatment of pain in pediatric patients occurs not only in the postoperative arena; inadequate relief is given to children suffering from burn wounds, infants undergoing circumcision, and children requiring diagnostic procedures such as bone marrow aspiration. Possible explanations for inadequate pain control in pediatric patients include incorrect assumptions, traditional attitudes, the complexity of pain assessment, and the lack of research and training in this area.[60]

There is now evidence to establish that pain perception and nociception occur in neonates. Basic neural pathways develop early in fetal life, with neocorticothalamic connections forming at 20 to 24 weeks; thus, cortical perception of pain is present in even the smallest premature infant.[61] Inadequately treated pain may be more important in its long-term effects in children. Fitzgerald[62] described the basis for long-term structural and functional reorganization of the pain pathway, which results from noxious stimuli in neonates and the hyperalgesic states that result. Central sensitization may occur from greater NMDA receptor activity and from gene induction. Chronic pain states have been demonstrated in children with poor pain control after thoracotomy. Greater awareness of the need for pain control in the pediatric population as well as adequate pain assessment, correct routes of administration, and appropriate application of old and new analgesic regimens should improve the overall care of children and neonates through control of their acute pain.

Pain Management in Children

Assessment of pediatric pain can be very difficult. Children and infants may cry because of postoperative pain or because of fear, anxiety, or loneliness. Accurate interpretation of pain behavior remains the biggest challenge in properly treating pain in pediatric patients. Once the extent of pain has been established, various modalities for treatment exist. Nonpharmacologic treatment includes appropriate teaching and guidance offered in the preoperative period. Imagery, hypnosis, and distraction techniques also are helpful in treating the postoperative pain of children in various age groups. Transcutaneous electrical nerve stimulation therapy has been used alone and in combination with analgesic therapy to alleviate the pain of tissue injury.

Despite these nonpharmacologic interventions, systemic analgesic therapy is the mainstay of pediatric pain control. Management of mild to moderate forms of postoperative pain includes use of the first line of drugs, the nonopiate analgesics, such as acetaminophen and NSAIDs. Acetaminophen has a high therapeutic ratio and very few contraindications. Doses range from 10 to 15 mg/kg perorally and from 15 to 20 mg/kg rectally every 4 hours. Several of the nonsteroidal agents provide excellent pain relief. Although these medications cause platelet dysfunction, gastritis, and renal disease, side effects are rare with short-term postoperative use.

If pain persists, opioid analgesia may be required. Narcotic analgesics provide excellent relief if given in sufficient amounts at effective intervals. Table 23-7 lists the various starting doses of opioids for pediatric use. These agents may be administered by various routes, including the oral, rectal, intranasal, transdermal, intravenous, intramuscular, epidural, and intrathecal routes. Intramuscular injection is particularly distressing to pediatric patients, so much that they may deny having pain to avoid receiving an injection. PCA is now con-

TABLE 23–7. Guidelines for Postoperative Analgesia with Opioids in Children

Route	Drug	Dose*
Continuous IV	Morphine	0.05–0.06 mg · kg^{-1} · hr^{-1}
	Meperidine	0.5–0.6 mg · kg^{-1} · hr^{-1}
	Fentanyl	2–4 μg · kg^{-1} · hr^{-1}
Intermittent IV†	Morphine	0.08–0.1 mg/kg q 2 hr
	Meperidine	0.8–1 mg/kg/q 2 hr
PO	Codeine	0.5–1 mg/kg q 4 hr
	Morphine	0.3 mg/kg q 4 hr
IM‡	Morphine	0.1–0.15 mg/kg q 3–4 hr
	Meperidine	1–1.5 mg/kg q 3–4 hr

Adapted from Berde CB: Pediatric postoperative pain management. Pediatr Clin North Am 1989; 36:924.

*For nonintubated patients in the first 3 months of life, or for other patients with an increased tendency for respiratory depression, starting doses should be diminished by at least a factor of 3 to 4 from doses recommended here, and facilities for intensive observation and respiratory support should be available.

†Intravenous boluses should be administered slowly (e.g., over 15 to 20 minutes).

‡Individual response varies. Doses should be carefully titrated and adjusted according to patients' physical status and analgesic requirements.

sidered an excellent alternative to intermittent intramuscular or intravenous injection in pediatric patients. The literature suggests that if properly selected, children benefit from all the advantages of the regimen—maintenance of consistent drug levels, superior analgesia, and improved emotional status. Some centers routinely use PCA devices in patients as young as 6 years.[63]

Regional analgesia has increased the possibilities for pain treatment in children. Peripheral nerve blocks can provide perioperative analgesia and reduce total anesthetic requirements.[64, 65] Epidural and caudal use of local anesthetics with or without opiates is becoming more popular for postoperative pain control in neonates. Local anesthetic toxicity and side effects from neuraxial medications as well as complications from the regional technique must be taken into consideration.[66–75] The use of alternative caudal or epidural medications such as buprenorphine, clonidine, and midazolam has also been reported.[76–79]

Pain management in children for painful procedures, such as lumbar puncture, suturing of lacerations, bone marrow aspirations, circumcisions, and biopsies, and for pain associated with trauma and surgery are indications for the use of the regional analgesic techniques. Optimum management and outcome depend on the minimization of emotional as well as physical trauma. Psychologic and behavioral strategies combined with pharmacologic treatment modalities can be utilized successfully to accomplish a procedure without significant pain or suffering.

Children need not suffer from the pain of acute tissue injury despite the traditional inadequacy of pain management in the pediatric population. Most pain management techniques for adults are appropriate for children. As in the adult population, physiologic disturbance and poor outcome may result from inadequately treated pain in children, and the importance of adequate treatment cannot be overemphasized.

SUMMARY

In summary, inadequate acute pain relief from tissue injury can have detrimental physiologic effects that are additive to the original insult (see Fig. 23–4); they include delayed recovery from surgery or trauma, increased morbidity, and poor postoperative pulmonary function. Splinting secondary to pain, inability to clear secretions, and reactivity of the bronchial tree lead to atelectasis and pulmonary complications. Accelerated catecholamine release raises systemic vascular resistance, increases cardiac stroke work, and worsens myocardial oxygen supply-demand ratios. Hypercoagulation leads to significant thromboembolic phenomena and vascular compromise. The stress response results in excessive protein wasting and poor wound healing.

Patient anguish and suffering may lead to agitation, increasing the possibility of inadvertent extubation or disconnection of arterial and intravenous lines, and making the provision of effective nursing care more difficult. It is necessary to realize that the true importance of the adequate management of acute pain lies in outcome as well as in patient satisfaction; thus, we must use all pain treatment techniques, drugs, and drug delivery technologies at our disposal to fully treat the pain of tissue injury.

References

1. Cousins MJ, Siddall PJ: Postoperative pain: Implication of peripheral and central sensitisation. *In:* Anaesthesia 150 Years On: Proceedings of the XIth World Congress of Anesthesiologists. Sydney, 1996, pp 73–81.
2. Devor M: The pathophysiology of damaged peripheral nerves. *In:* Textbook of Pain. Wall PD, Melzack R (Eds). London, Churchill Livingstone, 1994, pp 79–100.
3. Warfield CA, Kahn CH: Acute pain management—programs in U.S. hospitals and experiences and attitudes among U.S. adults. Anesthesiology 1995; 83:1090–1094.
4. Katz J, Jackson M, Kavanagh BP, et al: Acute pain after thoracic surgery predicts long-term post thoracotomy pain. Clin J Pain 1996; 12:50–55.
5. Woolf CJ, Thompson WN: The induction and maintenance of central sensitization is dependent on *N*-methyl-D-aspartic acid receptor activation: Implications for the treatment of post-injury pain hypersensitivity states. Pain 1991; 44:293–299.
6. Ilkjaer S, Peterson KL, Brennan J, et al: Effect of systemic *N*-methyl-D-aspartate receptor antagonist (ketamine) on primary and secondary hyperalgesia in humans. Br J Anaesth 1996; 76:829–834.
7. Marks RM, Sachar EJ: Undertreatment of medical inpatients with narcotic analgesics. Ann Intern Med 1973; 78:173.
8. Cohen FL: Postsurgical pain relief: Patients' status and nurses' medication choices. Pain 1980; 9:265.
9. Loper KA, Butler S, Nessley M, et al: Clinical note: Paralyzed with pain: The need for education. Pain 1989; 37:315.
10. Clive DM, Stoff JS: Renal syndromes associated with nonsteroidal anti-inflammatory drugs. N Engl J Med 1984; 310:563–572.
11. Moote C: Efficacy of nonsteroidal anti-inflammatory drugs in the management of post-operative pain (Review). Drugs 1992; 44(Suppl 5):14–30.
12. Parker RK, Holtmann B, Smith I, et al: Use of ketorolac after lower abdominal surgery: Effect on analgesic treatment and surgical outcome. Anesthesiology 1994; 80:6–12.
13. Kavanagh BP, Katz J, Sandler AN: Pain control after thoracic surgery: A review of current techniques. Anesthesiology 1994; 81:737–759.
14. Dahl JB, Kehlet H: Non-steroidal anti-inflammatory drugs: Rationale for use in severe postoperative pain (Review). Br J Anaesth 1991; 66:703–712.
15. Claeys MA, Camu F, Maes V: Prophylactic diclofenac infusions after major orthopaedic surgery: Effects on analgesia and acute phase proteins. Acta Anaesthesiol Scand 1992; 36:270–275.
16. Pavy TJG, Gambling DR, Merrick PM, et al: Rectal indomethacin potentiates spinal morphine analgesia after caesarean delivery. Anaesth Intensive Care 1995; 23:555–559.
17. Mather LE: Do the pharmacodynamics of the nonsteroidal anti-inflammatory drugs suggest a role in the management of postoperative pain (Review)? Drugs 1992; 44(Suppl 5):1–13.
18. Fogarty DJ, Ohanlon JJ, Milligan KR: Intramuscular ketorolac following total hip replacement with spinal anaesthesia and intrathecal morphine. Acta Anaesthesiol Scand 1995; 39:191–194.
19. McCormack K: The spinal actions of nonsteroidal anti-inflamma-

tory drugs and the dissociation between their anti-inflammatory and analgesic effects (Review). Drugs 1994; 47(Suppl 5):28–45.

20. Chambrier C, Chassard D, Bienvenu J, et al: Cytokine and hormonal changes after cholecystectomy—effect of ibuprofen pretreatment. Ann Surg 1996; 224:178–182.
21. White PF: Patient-controlled analgesia: A new approach to management of postoperative pain. Semin Anesth 1985; 4:255.
22. Bollish SJ, Collins CL, Kirking DM, et al: Efficacy of patient-controlled versus conventional analgesia for postoperative pain. Clin Pharm 1985; 4:48.
23. Ferrante FM, Orav EJ, Rocco AG: A statistical model for pain in patient-controlled analgesia and conventional intramuscular opioid regimens. Anesth Analg 1988; 67:457.
24. Gregg R: Spinal analgesia: Management of postoperative pain. Anesthesiol Clin North Am 1989; 7:79.
25. Dittman M, Steenblock U, Kranzlin M, et al: Epidural analgesia or mechanical ventilation for multiple rib fractures. Intensive Care Med 1982; 8:89.
26. Buckley FP, Robinson NB, Simonowitz DA, et al: Anaesthesia in the morbidly obese. Anaesthesia 1983; 38:840.
27. Kehlet H: The stress response to anesthesia and surgery: Release mechanisms and modifying factors. Clin Anaesthesiol 1984; 2:315.
28. Yaksh TL: Spinal opiate analgesia: Characteristics and principles of action. Pain 1981; 11:293.
29. Logas WG, El-Baz N, El-Ganzouri A, et al: Continuous thoracic epidural analgesia for post-operative pain relief following thoracotomy: A randomized prospective study. Anesthesiology 1987; 67:787.
30. Rawal N, Arner S, Gustafsson LL, et al: Present state of extradural and intrathecal opioid analgesia in Sweden. Br J Anaesth 1987; 59:791.
31. Ready LB, Loper KA, Nessley M, et al: Postoperative epidural morphine is safe on surgical wards. Anesthesiology 1991; 75:452.
32. Stenseth R, Sellevold O, Breivik H: Epidural morphine for postoperative pain: Experience with 1085 patients. Acta Anaesthesiol Scand 1985; 29:148.
33. Cross DA, Hunt JB: Feasibility of epidural morphine postoperative analgesia in a small community hospital. Anesth Analg 1991; 72:765.
34. Paech MJ: Epidural pethidine or fentanyl during caesarean section: A double-blind comparison. Anaesth Intensive Care 1989; 17:157.
35. Loper KA, Ready LB, Downey M, et al: Epidural and intravenous fentanyl infusions are clinically equivalent after knee surgery. Anesth Analg 1990; 70:72.
36. Badner NH: Epidural agents for postoperative analgesia. Anesthesiol Clin North Am 1992; 10:321.
37. Cohen SE, Tan S, White PF: Sufentanil analgesia following cesarean section: Epidural versus intravenous administration. Anaesthesiology 1988; 68:129.
38. Egbert AM, Leland HP, Short LM, et al: Randomized trial of postoperative patient-controlled analgesia vs. intramuscular narcotics on frail elderly men. Arch Intern Med 1990; 150:1897.
39. Wayslak TJ, Abbott FV, English MJM, et al: Reduction of postoperative morbidity following patient-controlled morphine. Can J Anaesth 1990; 37:726.
40. Scalley RD, Berquist K, Cochran RS: Patient-controlled analgesia in orthopedic procedures. Orthop Rev 1988; 17:1106.
41. Bromage PR, Camporesi E, Chestnut D: Epidural narcotics for postoperative analgesia. Anesth Analg 1980; 59:473.
42. Cuschieri RJ, Morran CG, Howie DC, et al: Postoperative pain and pulmonary complications: Comparison of three analgesic regimens. Br J Surg 1985; 72:495.
43. Rawal N, Sjostrand UM, Christoffersson E, et al: Comparison of intramuscular and epidural morphine for postoperative analgesia in the grossly obese: Influence on postoperative ambulation and pulmonary function. Anesth Analg 1984; 63:583.
44. Yeager MD, Glass DD, Neff RK, et al: Epidural anesthesia and analgesia in high-risk surgical patients. Anesthesiology 1987; 66:729.
45. Vanstrum GS, Bjornson KM, Ilko R: Postoperative effects of intrathecal morphine in coronary artery bypass surgery. Anesth Analg 1988; 76:261.
46. El-Baz N, Goldin M: Continuous epidural infusion of morphine for pain relief after cardiac operations. J Thorac Cardiovasc Surg 1987; 93:878.
47. Modig J, Borg T, Bagge L, et al: Role of epidural and of general anesthesia in fibrinolysis and coagulation after total hip replacement. Br J Anaesth 1983; 55:625.
48. Simpson IJ, Radford SG, Forster SJ, et al: The fibrinolytic effects of anesthesia. Anesthesiology 1982; 37:3.
49. Stenseth R, Bjella L, Berg EM, et al: Effects of thoracic epidural analgesia on pulmonary function after coronary artery bypass surgery. Eur J Cardiothorac Surg 1996; 10:859–865.
50. Jayr C, Thomas H, Rey A, et al: Postoperative pulmonary complications: Epidural analgesia using bupivacaine and opioids versus parenteral opioids. Anesthesiology 1993; 78:666–676.
51. Faust RJ, Nauss LA: Post-thoracotomy intercostal block: Comparison of its effect on pulmonary function with those of intramuscular meperidine. Anesth Analg 1976; 55:542.
52. Murphy DF: Intercostal nerve blockade for fractured ribs and post-operative analgesia: Description of a new technique. Reg Anesth 1983; 8:151.
53. Covino BG: Interpleural regional analgesia. Anesth Analg 1988; 67:427.
54. Hord AJ, Roberson JR, Thompson WF, et al: Evaluation of continuous femoral nerve analgesia after primary total knee arthroplasty. Anesth Analg 1990; 70:S164.
55. Bridenbaugh LD: The upper extremity: Somatic blockade. *In:* Neural Blockade in Clinical Anesthesia and Management of Pain. 2nd ed. Cousins MJ (Ed). Philadelphia, JB Lippincott, 1988, pp 387–415.
56. Pither C, Hartrick C: Post-operative pain. *In:* Handbook in Regional Anesthesiology. Raj PP (Ed). New York, Churchill Livingstone, 1985.
57. Sinatra RS: Pain management in patients suffering from major organ failure. *In:* Acute Pain: Mechanisms and Management. Sinatra RS, Hord AH, Ginsberg B, et al (Eds). St. Louis, Mosby-Year Book, 1992, pp 399–421.
58. Swafford L, Allen D: Pain relief in the pediatric patient. Med Clin North Am 1968; 52:131.
59. Eland JM, Anderson JE: The experience of pain in children. *In:* Pain: A Source Book for Nurses and Other Health Professionals. Jacox A (Ed). Boston, Little, Brown & Co, 1977.
60. Schecter NL: The undertreatment of pain in children: An overview. Pediatr Clin North Am 1989; 36:781–794.
61. Houck CS, Troshynski T, Berde CB: Treatment of pain in children. *In:* Textbook of Pain. 3rd ed. Wall PD, Melzack P (Eds). Edinburgh, Churchill Livingstone, 1994, pp 1419–1434.
62. Fitzgerald M: Developmental biology of inflammatory pain. Br J Anaesth 1995; 75:177–185.
63. Berde CB: Pediatric postoperative pain management. Pediatr Clin North Am 1989; 36:921–940.
64. Dalens B: Peripheral nerve blockade in the management of postoperative pain in children. *In:* Pain in Infants, Children, and Adolescents. Schechter NL, Berde CB, Yaster M (Eds). Baltimore, Williams & Wilkins, 1993, pp 261–280.
65. Dalens B (Ed): Regional Anesthesia in Infants, Children, and Adolescents. London, Williams & Wilkins, 1995.
66. Weston PJ, Bourchier D: The pharmacokinetics of bupivacaine following interpleural nerve block in infants of very low birthweight. Paediatr Anaesth 1995; 5:219–222.
67. Eyres RL, Bishop W, Oppenheim RC, et al: Plasma bupivacaine concentrations in children during caudal epidural analgesia. Anaesth Intensive Care 1983; 11:20.
68. Eyres R: Local anaesthetic agents in infancy. Paediatr Anaesth 1995; 5:213–218.
69. Berde CB: Toxicity of local anesthetics in infants and children. J Pediatr 1993; 122:S14–S20.
70. Larsson BA, Olsson GL, Lonnqvist PA: Plasma concentrations of bupivacaine in young infants after continuous epidural infusion. Paediatr Anaesth 1994; 4:159–162.
71. Wood CE, Goresky GV, Klassen KA, et al: Complications of continuous epidural infusions for postoperative analgesia in children. Can J Anaesth 1994; 41:613–620.
72. Goldman LJ: Complications in regional anaesthesia (Editorial). Paediatr Anaesth 1995; 5:3–9.
73. Stratford MA, Wilder RT, Berde CB: The risk of infection from epidural analgesia in children: A review of 1620 cases. Anesth Analg 1995; 80:234–238.
74. Flandin-Blety C, Barrier G: Accidents following extradural analge-

sia in children: The results of a retrospective study. Paediatr Anaesth 1995; 5:41-46.
75. Thomas VL: Accidents following extradural analgesia in children: The results of a retrospective study (Letter). Paediatr Anaesth 1995; 5:396-397.
76. Kamal RS, Khan FA: Caudal analgesia with buprenorphine for postoperative pain relief in children. Paediatr Anaesth 1995; 5:101-106.
77. Lee JJ, Rubin AP: Comparison of a bupivacaine-clonidine mixture with plain bupivacaine for caudal analgesia in children. Br J Anaesth 1994; 72:258-262.
78. Goresky GV: The clinical utility of epidural midazolam for inguinal hernia repair in children. Can J Anaesth 1995; 42:755-757.
79. Malinovsky J-M, Lapage J-Y, Cozina A, et al: Is ketamine or its preservative responsible for neurotoxicity in the rabbit? Anesthesiology 1993; 78:109-115.

24

The Coagulopathy of Trauma

John T. Owings, MD

Coagulopathy is the pathologic process in which there is either too much or not enough clot formation. When too much clot is formed, pathologic thrombosis results; when not enough clot is formed, pathologic bleeding results. Although inadequate clot formation manifests as pathologic bleeding, excessive clot formation may manifest either as pathologic clinically apparent clotting (deep venous thrombosis [DVT] or pulmonary embolism) or paradoxically as pathologic bleeding (disseminated intravascular thrombosis).

Clotting of blood occurs as a protection from exsanguination after injury. This is true and easy to conceptualize after a major trauma, but it is equally true after a trivial injury such as tapping your elbow on a desk. Trivial insults occur continuously and so does clotting. If thrombin is viewed as the center of the coagulation cascade, the production of thrombin may be viewed as a measure of the degree of activation of the cascade. Teitel and colleagues have shown that there is constant production of thrombin; that is, clotting is a perpetually ongoing process.[1]

Given that clotting is an ongoing process, there must be forces that serve to slow the activation of clotting factors. If this were not the case, once the most minor trauma occurred, clotting would be initiated and ultimately proceed to thrombosis of the entire vascular system. Because this does not occur, there must clearly be forces that serve to decelerate (down-regulate) the coagulation cascade[2] (Table 24-1). Under normal

TABLE 24–1. Endogenous Antithrombotics and Their Function

Down-Regulator of Clotting	Prothrombotic Target
Antithrombin	Factors Xa, XIIa, XIa, thrombin
α_1-Protease inhibitor	Factor XIa, elastase
α_2-Antiplasmin	Plasmin
α_2-Macroglobulin	Kallikrein, plasmin, thrombin
C1 inhibitor	Factor XIIa, kallikrein
Heparin cofactor II	Thrombin
Protein C	Factors VIIIa, Va
Tissue factor pathway inhibitor	Factor VIIa-tissue factor complex

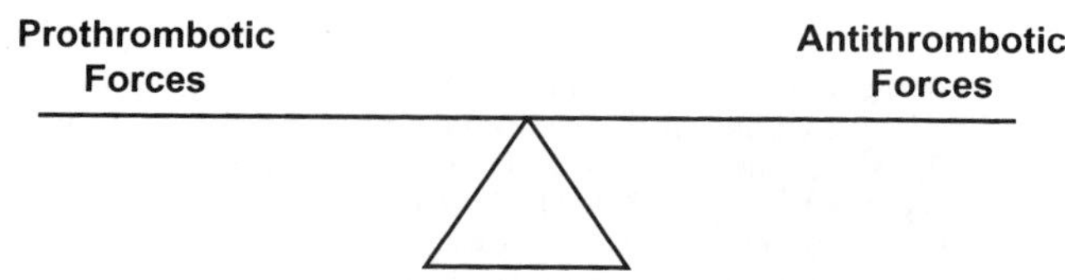

Figure 24–1. Coagulation balance.

circumstances, these antithrombotic forces have their greatest effect when they interact with substances with intact endothelium (e.g., antithrombin and endothelial glycosaminoglycans). Along the intact endothelium, the antithrombotics serve to inactivate activated clotting factors, thus protecting the vascular space from overwhelming thrombosis. Given these opposing forces, the coagulation (clotting) cascade is more appropriately viewed as a balance, a balance between prothrombotic (up-regulatory) and antithrombotic (down-regulatory) forces (Fig. 24-1).

Several conditions alter the balance between the prothrombotic and antithrombotic factors. Classic hemophilia, an inherited condition in which the patient lacks the normal amount of factor VIII, results in an increased degree of bleeding in response to minor injury. Patients with hemophilia, however, are able to form clots relatively normally with only 5% of factor VIII present. Patients who have congenital antithrombin deficiency have an increased incidence of thromboembolic events. Patients with antithrombin deficiency are at significantly increased risk for spontaneous venous thrombosis when antithrombin activity falls below 75% of normal. Within these two different conditions, it is remarkable that there is tremendous redundancy in the protection from bleeding (normal clotting with 5% of factor VIII) yet little from pathologic thrombosis (spontaneous thrombosis with antithrombin level of 75% of normal).

The degree of activation of the clotting cascade is proportional to both the quantity and potency (quality) of the clotting stimulus (thromboplastin). If a moderate clotting stimulus is provided, such as a laceration resulting in a breach in the endothelial lining, antithrombotic agents function to protect the vascular space around the site of injury against excessive clot propagation and thus pathologic thrombosis. If a massive clotting stimulus is introduced (bilateral crushed legs), it can overwhelm the antithrombotic protective mechanism. The excess activated procoagulant factors are no longer inactivated once they are outside the zone of injury, and pathologic thrombosis results.

As the quality and quantity of the clotting stimulus affect the response of the coagulation cascade, so also does the environment in which the clotting stimuli are presented. Two hundred years ago, it was thought that clotting occurred as a result of and in proportion to the exposure of the liquid blood to air. Experiments in the mid-19th century showed that in an animal " . . . bled to death by the removal of blood in successive portions, the last portions [of blood] coagulate almost instantaneously."[3] This simple study demonstrated that hypovolemia even in the absence of any injury causes a dramatic acceleration of the coagulation cascade.

Trauma alters the balance of prothrombotic and antithrombotic factors. In studies of critically injured patients, we have demonstrated a dramatic increase in the production of procoagulant factors.[4] We have also shown that trauma patients have a concurrent relative and absolute depletion of the antithrombotic protective mechanisms.[4, 5] In addition to having an increase in activated procoagulant factors and depletion of antithrombotic protectants, the trauma patient is commonly also hypovolemic (which by itself may result in hypercoagula-

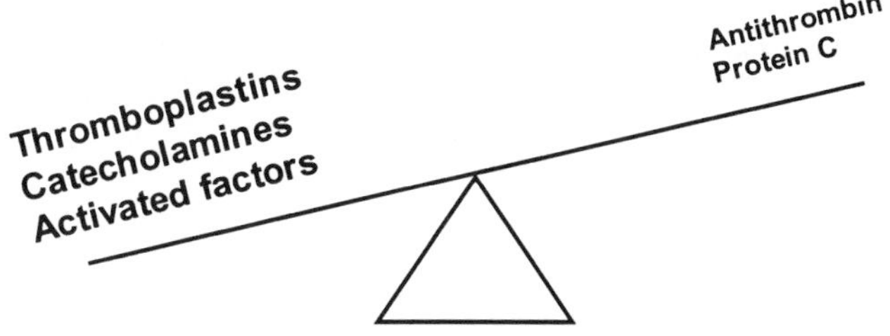

Figure 24–2. Coagulation balance after trauma.

TABLE 24–3. Causes of Post-traumatic Bleeding

Disseminated intravascular coagulation
Surgical bleeding (e.g., nonligated vessel, missed injury)
Hypothermia
Dilution
Pre-trauma medication (aspirin, warfarin)
Cirrhosis
Congenital defect

bility, probably through the release of catecholamines). So if the clotting cascade is viewed as a balance, the clotting cascade of a trauma patient after a severe injury must be viewed as being tipped strongly in favor of thrombosis (Fig. 24-2).

A strong teleologic argument can be made for why such redundancy would be built into the procoagulant side of the clotting cascade. Before the advent of modern medicine, individuals who were unable to adequately form clot would not survive childhood to pass on their genes. Survival of the severe injuries inflicted by modern transportation and weapons was unthinkable 100 years ago; as a consequence, dealing with the sequelae of these injuries (excessive activation of the coagulation cascade) is equally unthinkable for the human body.

The clinical manifestation of the imbalance between the prothrombotic and antithrombotic forces that occurs in trauma patients is pathologic thrombosis. Pathologic thrombosis can manifest on a macroscopic or microscopic level (Table 24-2). The clinical manifestation may be overt bleeding, as in severe disseminated intravascular coagulation (DIC), or none, as with most cases of DVT, which is occult. Thus, even though the manifestations are opposite, the underlying cause is the same—excessive activation of the coagulation cascade.

Not all post-traumatic bleeding is due to excessive activation of the clotting cascade. Bleeding can also occur from several other causes (Table 24-3). In this chapter, I discuss each of these causes and an approach to correcting them. The good news is that, as a rule, all causes of post-traumatic coagulopathy other than DIC are relatively easy to treat. In the *trauma* patient, however, even if another process is responsible for the acute bleeding episode, the bleeding is occurring in the hypercoagulable environment described before.

CLINICAL MANIFESTATION AS THROMBOSIS

Pathologic Macroscopic Thrombosis

When the imbalance in the coagulation cascade after trauma (hypercoagulability) results in macroscopic clot formation, the clinical manifestation is DVT. If the venous thrombus becomes dislodged and embolizes to the pulmonary vasculature, pulmonary embolism results. These topics are addressed in Chapters 101 and 139. I mention them here because it is important to recognize that they are part of the same spectrum of coagulation changes that may culminate in DIC.

TABLE 24–2. Pathologic Thrombosis

Macroscopic
Deep venous thrombosis
Pulmonary embolism
Microscopic
Disseminated intravascular coagulation
Acute respiratory distress syndrome
Multiple organ system failure

CLINICAL MANIFESTATION AS BLEEDING

Bleeding Caused by Pathologic Microscopic Thrombosis

After severe injury, the coagulation cascade has been activated to a degree seen in few other disease states. The production of thrombin may be as much as 100 times the noninjury rate. In addition to the increased circulating thrombin, the activity of two of the most important down-regulators of coagulation—antithrombin and protein C—is significantly reduced. The result is a strongly prothrombotic environment. In this hypercoagulable environment, if systemic coagulation is further stimulated, uncontrollable intravascular clotting (DIC) can occur. Once this uncontrolled microscopic intravascular clotting occurs, the fibrinolytic system is activated to prevent the microvascular circulation from becoming clogged with the circulating microthrombi.

Systemic activation of the fibrinolytic system is the final step in the progression that causes this pathologic thrombosis to manifest as bleeding. As the fibrinolytic system lyses the pathologic thrombus, it also lyses the nonpathologic thrombus that has protected the patient from uncontrolled bleeding from a closed surgical wound, intravenous (IV) site, or nasogastric tube. With this clot dissolution, the patient begins to bleed and more tissue factor is exposed where the clot has dissolved; this leads to further clot deposition and finally consumption to the point of depletion of the procoagulant factors.

In most trauma patients, even those with extensive tissue injury, DIC does not develop. The volume of clotting stimulus (thromboplastin) presented to the vascular system is not the only determinant of whether DIC will develop. The environment in which the stimulus is presented is critically important. A patient who is well hydrated and has a modest release of thromboplastin from an injury such as a femur fracture is at low risk for development of DIC. Another patient with a similar femur fracture whose injury is associated with profound prolonged shock is at high risk for DIC. A patient with a massive crush injury or one who is given mis-crossmatched blood (transfusion reaction) who has had little or no shock or hypotension is nonetheless at high risk for DIC. It is therefore the amount of thromboplastin released into the circulatory system in conjunction with the patient's vascular volume status that determines the likelihood of the development of DIC.

Several disorders are associated with DIC. Some of these are trauma-related, but many are not. Any patient can have DIC given an adequate stimulus (intravascular thromboplastin release) when he or she is in a proportionate shock. Because this is the case, to formulate a list of all the injuries and disease states that DIC is associated with is impractical. It is better to be aware that DIC can develop in any trauma patient and to be educated to its signs and diagnostic criteria.

Hematologists do not agree on a single definition of DIC. The opening of this chapter gives a description of DIC, not a definition. DIC has a spectrum of severities. In its most severe form, a clinical diagnosis with laboratory confirmation is relatively simple. In its mildest form, there may be no clinical manifestations, and although a diagnosis may be made on the basis of laboratory data, its clinical significance is nominal.

A patient with severe DIC demonstrates diffuse bleeding, including bleeding from previously hemostatic sites. A patient in this condition has gone through all of the stages outlined before. He or she has had widespread activation of the clotting cascade with depletion of procoagulant factors. This condition can be measured with the activated partial thromboplastin time (aPTT) and the International Normalized Ratio (INR) tests, which are both prolonged. The platelet count and the fibrinogen level are both decreased. As a demonstration of the final phase of DIC (the activation of the fibrinolytic system), the circulating D-dimer levels are increased. Because each of these parameters is a continuous variable, there is not a single result for any that indicates the presence of DIC. As each of these parameters becomes worse, one can infer that the degree of DIC becomes worse. Table 24–4 shows a scale that we have used in studies to grade the severity of DIC. Each parameter has been listed with a series of results of increasing adversity. If each parameter is available for a patient, the corresponding numbers (0 to 3) for the result of each laboratory value are added together. A cumulative score of 12 or greater indicates severe DIC. Surgical patients die of DIC most frequently as a result of hemorrhage. The potential diagnosis of DIC has been entertained because bleeding is present. In such a case, this scale, or any DIC panel, will help to clarify that the cause of the bleeding is indeed a consumptive coagulopathy (DIC) and not another cause, such as hypothermia (see later).

To have a rational approach to treating DIC, one should understand the forces that lead to its occurrence. Both the patient's vascular status (hypovolemia, acidemia) in which the clotting stimulus is introduced and the quality and quantity of the thromboplastin affect the response of the coagulation cascade. It is clear, therefore, that attempts to reverse the process of DIC must be aimed at both correction of the hypercoagulable state and removal of the clotting stimulus that led to the DIC.

Initially, all treatment efforts should be directed at resuscitating the patient. Large-bore IV lines with isotonic crystalloids should be inserted to correct the vascular volume deficit. All patients with severe DIC are anemic and by definition have depleted their clotting factors. Anemia should be corrected with transfusion of packed red blood cells. An ongoing repletion of clotting factors should be carried out with fresh frozen plasma, cryoprecipitate, and calcium. An alternative is administration of whole blood and calcium. In the course of these efforts, clarification of the diagnosis should be sought with a DIC panel (see Table 24–4). This helps to distinguish other potential causes of bleeding from DIC (see Table 24–3). Because all of the other causes of post-traumatic bleeding are more easily treated and require resuscitation, these efforts are warranted as an initial therapy. If the cause of bleeding is other than DIC, treatment of that cause should be undertaken.

TABLE 24–4. Laboratory Findings in Disseminated Intravascular Coagulation

Score	INR	aPTT	Platelet Count	Fibrinogen	D-dimer
0	<1.2	<34	>159,000	>200	<1000
1	1.2	>34	<150,000	<200	<2000
2	>1.4	>39	<100,000	<150	<4000
3	>1.6	>54	< 60,000	<100	>4000

Modified from Owings JT, Bagley M, Gosselin R, Romac D, Disbrow E: Effect of critical injury on plasma antithrombin activity: Low antithrombin levels are associated with thromboembolic complications. J Trauma 1996; 41:396.

INR = International Normalized Ratio; aPTT = activated partial thromboplastin time.

TABLE 24–5. Thromboplastins

Tissue factor	Amniotic fluid, fetal cells
Collagen	Endotoxin
Fragmented red blood cells	Necrotic tissue
Brain tissue	

If it appears that DIC is the cause of the bleeding, in addition to these resuscitative measures, an exhaustive search should be done to identify the source of intravascular thromboplastin release. A list of thromboplastins is shown in Table 24–5. Once found, the source of thromboplastin should be removed if possible. This effort includes amputation of dead or mangled extremities, drainage of abscesses, discontinuation of questionable transfusion material, delivery of a distressed premature infant, and abortion of abrupted placentas and nonviable products of conception.

When the DIC is not as severe as just described, the focus should be similar although less extreme. Even patients with only mild DIC should be resuscitated and should undergo replacement of depleted red blood cells and clotting proteins. Ultimately, the most important ways to prevent severe DIC in patients with mild DIC are to maintain optimal hydration and to remove the clotting stimulus.

There has been varying enthusiasm for the use of heparin in the treatment of DIC. The theory is that if enough heparin is given, the excessive clotting that has led to the depletion of the procoagulant factors and activation of the fibrinolytic system can be arrested. Once the clotting has stopped altogether, the clotting products may be replaced and the clotting stimulus removed. The heparin would then be stopped, and normal coagulation would resume. Unfortunately, patients with DIC experience dramatic reductions in antithrombin levels.[5] Because heparin acts through the potentiation of antithrombin, if little or no antithrombin is present, there will be no effective anticoagulant effect. No clinical trials have shown heparin to be of value in the treatment of DIC.

Although it is not approved by the Food and Drug Administration, clinical trials suggest that the replacement of depleted endogenous antithrombotics (antithrombin and protein C) may prove helpful in the treatment of DIC. By replacing these antithrombotics, we can lessen the imbalance in the coagulation system. These proteins are available either through purified pooled plasma (antithrombin) or by recombinant technology (protein C). Both are expensive. Our experience in a small group of patients with severe DIC was that 12 hours of antithrombin administration to a prelevel amount averaged $6000 per patient. Given the staggering expense of these agents and the lack of current studies demonstrating clear efficacy, their use cannot be recommended.

A complication often found in patients who survive DIC is the acute respiratory distress syndrome (ARDS). In an animal model, injection of fibrinogen degradation products (FDP) in the venous system causes the development of ARDS.[6] In patients with intravascular thrombosis, clotting products (e.g., D-dimers, FDP) travel through the venous system to the lungs. Once in the lungs, these substances stimulate a generalized inflammatory response through factor XII and activation of the polymorphonuclear leukocytes. In addition to the inflammatory effect of the circulating clotting products on the lungs, these stimulatory effects may be seen in the kidney (Shwartzman reaction) and manifest as renal failure or in the liver as shock liver. Each of these conditions is referable back to the derangements in the clotting cascade.

Bleeding Due to Inadequate Thrombus Formation

Bleeding in the surgical patient is not always due to DIC. In fact, it is more likely to be due to either a nonligated vessel or a primary inadequate clot formation. Table 24–3 lists a number of causes of bleeding, and all but the first (DIC) are due to inadequate clot formation. The causes of most cases of post-traumatic bleeding are fundamentally different from DIC. Because the initial supportive treatment of DIC is often definitive therapy for many of these conditions, unexpected bleeding should be managed as though it were DIC until a definitive diagnosis for the cause of bleeding has been established.

The key to the exclusion of DIC as a possible cause of excessive bleeding is a simple coagulation panel (an aPTT and INR). If aPTT and INR values are normal or nearly normal, the patient does *not* have DIC. At that time, DIC is ruled out and another diagnosis must be identified.

If aPTT and INR values are normal but the patient is bleeding diffusely, the most likely diagnosis is hypothermia (see Chapter 34). The impairment in normal coagulation occurs because the clotting enzymes function much less efficiently as body temperature decreases.[7] Laboratories warm plasma samples to 37°C as a rule in performing clotting assays. If the clotting factors are quantitatively and qualitatively normal, the aPTT and INR, when tested at 37°C, will be normal. Studies have shown that if the same sample were run at the patient's actual temperature, the aPTT and INR would both be prolonged. The treatment of hypothermic coagulopathy consists of rewarming the patient (see Chapter 34) rather than attempting to correct the prolonged clotting with plasma transfusions. In theory, continuing to transfuse cold blood products (fresh frozen plasma and packed red blood cells) into a hypothermic patient may lower the core temperature and worsen the coagulopathy.

It is critical for the operating surgeon to always consider the possibility of either a missed injury or nonligated vessel in a postoperative trauma patient. No matter how vigorous the resuscitative measures, they will be unsuccessful if ongoing bleeding is present. Further, as ongoing bleeding goes unchecked, the clotting products are consumed and the clinical picture can evolve from a simple bleeding vessel to that with a dilutional coagulopathy superimposed.

Dilution is a relatively uncommon cause of coagulopathy. Humans are able to replace clotting factors to maintain hemostasis with pure dilution (in the absence of a consumptive coagulopathy) up to the replacement of one volume of packed red blood cells. After that, if coagulation factors are not replaced, bleeding may occur simply because of inadequate concentrations of clotting factors. Pure dilutional coagulopathy, however, is rare in trauma patients because the cause of bleeding results in concurrent consumption of the clotting factors. In patients with a pure dilutional coagulopathy, the aPTT and INR are prolonged, the platelet count is low, and fibrinogen levels are extremely low. The D-dimer levels, however, may be relatively normal, given the associated derangements. Transfusion with fresh frozen plasma, cryoprecipitate, calcium, and, if needed, platelets is the appropriate treatment.

Patients with preexisting hemostatic defects, whether they are congenital, disease-related, or drug-related, pose different problems, because bleeding is one of the most common causes of death in trauma patients. When a patient has an underlying coagulation defect, it is imperative that it be identified so that corrective measures can be taken to prevent exsanguination. Table 24–6 lists a few of the most common causes of preexisting hemostatic defects in trauma patients. Clearly, this is not an exhaustive list of the causes of bleeding unrelated to trauma. Although each diagnosis has a body of literature dedicated to its treatment, I address only some of the unifying principles of both the diagnosis and treatment for the disorders within each of the two groups.

TABLE 24–6. Causes of Preexisting Hemostatic Defects

Decrease in Procoagulant Factors
Warfarin (Coumadin) therapy
Hemophilias
Cirrhosis
Inhibition of Intact Hemostatic System
Aspirin therapy
Renal failure (uremic platelets)

Patients with ineffective hemostasis due to inadequate factor levels tend to have either a prolonged INR (owing to waveform [Coumadin] therapy, cirrhosis, and the hemophilias) or aPTT (von Willebrand's disease), but not both. The fibrinogen stores are normal, and the D-dimer levels are proportional to the amount of tissue injury. In general, the treatment of these patients is relatively simple once the diagnosis is made. The missing factors, once known, should be replaced. For patients receiving warfarin or those with cirrhosis, fresh frozen plasma should be given to correct the INR. For known hemophiliacs, concentrated factor replacements should be given to correct the activity levels to normal.

Inhibition of the hemostatic process may be more difficult to confirm. There are innumerable known inhibitors of normal coagulation, but to list them or attempt to discuss them would be beyond the scope of this chapter. Both of the major conditions listed in this group in Table 24–6 are related to inhibition of the normal functioning of platelets. Both conditions may not affect the aPTT or INR, but they may manifest as oozing at the time of operation. A known history, as in most preexisting hemostatic derangements, is the best diagnostic test. In most cases, the bleeding that results from the platelet dysfunction in either case is more of a nuisance than a major issue. In neurosurgical cases, however, either condition may occasionally pose more substantial problems. In both platelet dysfunction and neurologic cases, as with von Willebrand's disease, subcutaneous injection of DDAVP frequently reduces the effects of the disorder and returns the patient to nearly normal hemostatic ability.

References

1. Teitel JM, Bauer KA, Lau HK, Rosenberg RD: Studies of the prothrombin activation pathway utilizing radioimmunoassays for the F2/F1 + 2 fragment and thrombin-antithrombin complex. Blood 1982; 59:1086.
2. Colman RW, Marder VJ, Salzman EW, Hirsh J: Plasma coagulation factors. *In:* Hemostasis and Thrombosis. Basic Principles and Clinical Practice. 3rd ed. Colman RW, Hirsh J, Marder VJ, Salzman EW (Eds). Philadelphia, JB Lippincott, 1987, p 12.
3. Gray H, Lunt LK: Factors affecting the coagulation time of blood. Am J Physiol 1914; 34:332.
4. Owings JT, Gosselin R, Battistella FD, Bagley M: Post-traumatic hypercoagulability: The role that protein C and tissue factor pathway inhibitor have in its pathogenesis. Surg Forum 1997; 48:139.
5. Owings JT, Bagley M, Gosselin R, Romac D, Disbrow E: Effect of critical injury on plasma antithrombin activity: Low antithrombin levels are associated with thromboembolic complications. J Trauma 1996; 41:396.

6. Luterman A, Manwaring D, Curreri PW: The role of fibrinogen degradation products in the pathogenesis of the respiratory distress syndrome. Surgery 1977; 82:703.
7. Johnston TD, Chen Y, Reed RL II: Functional equivalence of hypothermia to specific clotting factor deficiencies. J Trauma 1994; 37:413.

25

Transfusion Therapy

Robert C. Mackersie, MD, FACS

Ideally, the therapeutic goals of allogeneic and autologous blood transfusions should represent an extension of the general goals of resuscitation for the trauma patient: (1) restoration of circulating blood volume, (2) restoration of oxygen-carrying capacity and tissue perfusion, and (3) prevention of metabolic disturbances and complications (such as coagulopathy, acidosis, and hypothermia) and the post-resuscitation inflammatory response syndromes. Blood transfusions continue to be an important adjunct to the treatment of both major injury and a variety of critical illnesses. In the last several years, however, largely because of changes in blood banking and transfusion practices resulting from the acquired immunodeficiency syndrome (AIDS) epidemic, transfusions of red cell mass and blood components (platelets and plasma) continue to decline. Despite these recent trends and improvements in plasma and blood substitutes (see Chapter 26), allogeneic and autologous blood and blood products continue to provide the best means of improving oxygen-carrying capacity and correcting deficits and coagulation.

STORED BLOOD PRODUCTS

The earliest reported attempt at blood transfusion was in 1667, when whole animal blood was transfused into a patient. The result was a dramatic hemolytic transfusion reaction, causing the practice to be abandoned until the early 1800s, when transfusion of women hemorrhaging as a result of childbirth was again attempted. Similar incompatibility problems forestalled further progress until the discovery of ABO blood group types (Table 25–1). The subsequent development of anticoagulants, around the turn of the 20th century, permitted blood matching and preservation of donated blood for the first time. Further changes in transfusion therapy became possible when technologic developments allowed the separation of whole blood into cellular and noncellular components. The emphasis on component therapy, the most common form of transfusion today, started with several publications by the Office of Medical Applications of Research and the National Institutes of Health. The majority of donor blood collected in the United States is now separated into the red cell mass (with varying amounts of donor plasma), the platelet component, and the plasma component.

Component Procurement

A unit of full donor blood typically contains approximately 500 mL (450 mL of blood plus 50 to 60 mL of an anticoagulant preservative). Whole blood is most commonly separated into various components. Packed red blood cells (RBCs), with a hematocrit of approximately 70, are separated out by centrifugation and the extraction of platelet-rich plasma. Platelet concentrates are subsequently prepared by further centrifugation of this fraction. The remaining platelet-poor plasma frozen within 6 hours of collection becomes what is referred to as fresh frozen plasma (FFP) and contains all of the coagulation factors, including the labile factors V and VIII. Cryoprecipitate may be obtained from FFP when the insoluble protein fractions are collected at approximately 0°C. These cold, insoluble proteins include factor VIII, fibrinogen, fibronectin, and von Willebrand's factor. Plasma remaining after removal of cryoprecipitates is used to prepare a 5% albumin derivative.

Packed RBCs are stored with the goal of minimizing loss of function, hemolysis, and a number of metabolic derangements, including decreased 2,3-diphosphoglycerate (2,3-DPG), decreased adenosine triphosphate (ATP), and potassium and ammonia accumulation. Traditional agents, for instance acid citrate dextrose (ACD) and citrate phosphate dextrose (CPD), are being supplanted by newer formulations, such as Adsol (AS-1) and Nutricel (AS-3). As component separation and preservation technology improve, the amount of residual platelet and plasma transfusion associated with RBC mass transfusions has progressively decreased. It is estimated that Adsol preserved cells, for example, may contain less than 50 mL of residual donor plasma. These low-residue cell preparations may be associated with a higher incidence of coagulopathy when they are used during massive transfusions.[1]

The blood supply throughout the United States is collected and processed, for the most part, by two main networks. The

TABLE 25–1. Historical Highlights of Blood Transfusions

1665	First successful blood transfusion (dog-to-dog).
1667	Unsuccessful transfusion (lambs to humans). Transfusion outlawed.
1818	James Bondell successfully transfuses women following postpartum hemorrhage. Bondell reports 5 of 10 successful transfusions.
1900	Carl Landsteiner discovers first 3 human blood groups (ABO).
1907	Ruben Ottenberg performs first blood transfusion using ABO typing.
1912	Roger Lee develops the concept of universal donor (group O blood) and universal recipient (group AB blood).
1914	Sodium citrate is developed to allow preservation of blood.
1916	Roue and Turner introduce citrate glucose, permitting storage of blood for several days after collection.
1930	First blood bank is established in London.
1939	Lanstanner, Weiner, Levine, and Stepson discover Rh blood group system.
1940	Edward Cohn develops cold ethynyl fractionation, permitting separation of plasma into components.
1943	Loutit and Mollison discover acid citrate dextrose (ACD), permitting transfusions of greater volumes of blood.
1952	Carl Walter introduces plastic bag for blood collection.
1971	Hepatitis B screening for donating blood begins.
1979	New anticoagulant preservative, CPDA-1, extends shelf life of whole blood to 35 days.
1983–1985	Additive solutions (AS-1, AS-3) extend red blood cell shelf life to approximately 42 days.
1991	Institution of hepatitis C virus screening for blood transfusions.

AS-1 = Adsol; AS-3 = Nutricel; CPDA-1 = citrate phosphate dextrose adenine.

American Red Cross is the nation's single largest blood supplier, providing for nearly 6 million volunteer blood donations annually, and accounts for about half of the total blood supply in the United States. America's Blood Centers is currently the nation's largest network of nonprofit, independent community blood centers that collects approximately 45% of the U.S. blood supply at more than 450 blood donation sites.

Metabolic Changes in Stored Blood

A variety of metabolic changes occur, mainly in RBCs, as the result of separation and cold storage of blood products (Table 25–2). Intracellular 2,3-DPG falls in stored blood, potentially increasing the hemoglobin affinity for oxygen and reducing the P_{50} by almost 50%. It appears, however, that 2,3-DPG levels partially normalize after transfusion, and other factors governing oxygen-carrying capacity, such as acidosis and hypothermia, may be more important. Potassium leaking from stored RBCs may increase the levels in stored blood, but hyperkalemia is rarely a problem related to routine transfusion. Stored blood depends on citrate and the chelation of calcium for anticoagulation. Although citrate toxicity and hypocalcemia are theoretical possibilities, a number of clinical observations have suggested that calcium is sufficiently mobilized from bone stores to prevent clinical manifestations except under extreme (massive transfusion) situations.

Under most circumstances, modest transfusion amounts do not result in significant clinical metabolic disturbances. In the massively transfused patient, however, hyperkalemia, hypokalemia, hypocalcemia, hypomagnesemia, citrate toxicity, acidosis hyperphosphatemia, and elevations in serum ammonia have all been reported, although major clinical manifestations are relatively uncommon.

COMPONENT TRANSFUSION

Except for the patient receiving massive transfusion, in which case freshly procured whole blood may be desirable, most blood product transfusions are given as component therapy. Components in routine use include:

- "Packed" RBCs
- Leukocyte-poor RBCs
- FFP
- Platelets
- Cryoprecipitate
- Concentrates of factors VIII (for hemophilia A), VII, IX, and X and prothrombin (factor II)

Component therapy is directed at treating and minimizing the effects of preexisting or acquired coagulopathies or replacing factors lost in the course of major hemorrhage.

TABLE 25–2. Approximate Changes in CPD-Stored Red Blood Cells in 30 Days

Element	Change
2,3-DPG	+260%
ATP	−42%
Potassium	6- to 7-fold increase
Sodium	−8%
pH	7.6–6.9
Po_2	−56%
Pco_2	5-fold increase
Free hemoglobin	5- to 6-fold increase

CPD = citrate phosphate dextrose; 2,3-DPG = 2,3-diphosphoglycerate; ATP = adenosine triphosphate.

Red Blood Cells

The administration of red cell mass is directed toward maintaining oxygen-carrying capacity as well as volume expansion. The "optimal" hematocrit for purposes of resuscitation has been the subject of much debate. From a rheologic standpoint, a hematocrit of approximately 30 provides the best combination of oxygen-carrying capacity and viscosity-related flow. From a pure oxygen-carrying capacity standpoint, a hematocrit of up to 36 may be desirable and higher hematocrits may also be indicated in persons with underlying cardiac or pulmonary disease. In the healthy patient, however, a hematocrit acutely as low as 20 to 22 may be well tolerated, and the benefit of additional transfusion must be weighed against the small but real associated risks. In addition to oxygen-carrying capacity, RBCs provide an excellent means of expanding intravascular volume and may be indicated acutely in the setting of hemorrhagic shock with hypotension as a supplement to crystalloid administration.

Fresh Frozen Plasma and Coagulation Factors

With the development of the technology allowing whole blood to be separated into its various components, as previously outlined, specific indications for transfusion of FFP came under more scrutiny. Over the years, a variety of replacement formulas have been advocated in the practice of adding 1 unit of FFP and 1 unit of calcium chloride to every 4 to 5 units of banked RBCs popular in the late 1970s. Subsequent studies have suggested that neither calcium nor FFP needs to be routinely given for non–massive transfusion multiunit blood needs. Current indications for FFP include:

- Replacement of isolated factor deficiencies and various blood disorders (e.g., II, V, VIII, X, XI)
- The need for acute reversal of warfarin (Coumadin) therapy
- Massive transfusion and coagulopathy
- Treatment of thrombotic thrombocytopenic purpura

The labile coagulation factors V and VIII deteriorate fairly rapidly when they are stored in the liquid state and are often notably lacking in older whole blood. Although some deterioration in these factors occurs in the process of separation, freezing, and thawing, FFP (maintained at strictly −18°C) can be used to treat dilutional deficits in these coagulation factors. Cryoprecipitate contains principally factor VIII, von Willebrand's factor, and fibrinogen. Indications for administration include hypofibrinogenic trauma patients (fibrinogen < 100 mg/dL) in the absence of a response to FFP, von Willebrand's disease, and hemophilia A. Cryoprecipitate is typically obtained from as many as 10 individual donors and carries a proportionally greater risk for disease transmission.

Platelets

Platelets function as initiators of vasoconstriction and aggregation at the sites of injured vascular epithelium, an important component in hemostasis in trauma patients. Platelet counts above 100,000 typically are associated with normal bleeding times. Platelet counts down to 50,000 to 60,000 are generally well tolerated in otherwise healthy individuals and do not represent an indication for platelet transfusions in the absence of the need for surgical intervention. As a general rule, platelet counts below 20,000 place patients at risk for spontaneous bleeding and are a general indication for platelet transfusion, even in an otherwise asymptomatic patient.

In the trauma patient, precise endpoints for platelet transfusions have not been well defined. Current recommendations for platelet transfusion thresholds are 75,000 to 80,000 under most circumstances, with maintenance of platelet counts above 100,000 for brain or airway injuries. However, neither platelet function nor coagulation factor function is normal in the presence of hypothermia, acidosis, or severe crystalloid hemodilution. Transfusion therapy in these clinical settings must be coupled with efforts to correct underlying metabolic derangements.

TRANSFUSION RISKS AND COMPLICATIONS

Incompatibility Reactions

Major hemolytic reactions occur uncommonly after RBC transfusions and are caused principally by blood group (ABO) incompatibility; most occur as the result of clerical errors. They may also be caused occasionally by other major blood group antigens on the transfused RBCs. Clinical manifestations include chills, fever, chest or lumbar pain, and, in the unconscious patient, tachycardia, hypotension, hemoglobinuria, and sudden, otherwise unexpected diffuse microvascular bleeding. In the massively transfused patient, symptoms in the unconscious (anesthetized) patient are difficult to distinguish from the manifestations of shock and major injury. Treatment consists of the immediate cessation of the transfusion, therapy for associated shock, and confirmation of a suspected incompatibility reaction through a direct Coombs' test performed by the blood bank. Urine and plasma for free hemoglobin and renal function tests may serve as monitors of severity.

Nonhemolytic (febrile) blood transfusion reactions occur at the rate of approximately 1% to 2% and consist of relatively mild symptoms of chills and fevers. These reactions are typically caused by antibody-antigen reactions to white blood cells (WBCs) in the transfused blood and may be minimized by the use of leukocyte-poor packed RBCs.

Transmission of Blood-borne Infection

Perhaps the most concerning risk of blood transfusion is the inadvertent transmission of blood-borne viral infections. To reduce the risk of transfusion-related infections, screening tests are routinely performed on all units donated in the United States and typically include hepatitis B virus (HBV) surface antigen (HBsAg), HBV core antibodies (anti-HBc), hepatitis C virus (HCV) antibodies (anti-HCV), antibodies to the human immunodeficiency virus (anti-HIV1, anti-HIV2), the HIV-1 P24 antigen, the human T-lymphotropic virus type I (HTLV-I), and syphilis. Approximate risks for various reported and theoretically transmitted diseases are shown in Table 25–3. The highest risks are currently associated with hepatitis C transmission. This risk has been dropping steadily since routine screening began for HCV and is currently less than 0.1% of transfusion recipients.

Despite the development of HCV screening and rigorous testing of the blood supply, a small risk of contracting blood-borne viral disease from blood donated during the time between infection and seroconversion reamins. In a study of the risk of transfusion-transmitted viral infection, Schreiber and colleagues[2] evaluated more than 2 million allogeneic blood donations in more than 500,000 patients to calculate the incidence rates of seroconversion in this group. Among donors whose units passed all the routine screening tests, the risks of donating blood during an infectious "window" were estimated as follows: HIV, 1 in 493,000; HTLV, 1 in 641,000; HCV, 1 in 103,000; HBV, 1 in 63,000. The authors concluded that the risk of transmitting viral infections, given the current screening tests, is small and that development of additional screening tests should shorten the latent periods for these viruses and could reduce subsequent risks by 27% to 72%.

Immunosuppression

The potential risk of immunosuppression after blood transfusion has received much interest in a variety of areas. The initial observation that renal transplant patients enjoyed improved graft survival when given previous blood transfusions has suggested the possible relationship between blood transfusion and immunosuppression in the trauma patient. Several studies have demonstrated, largely retrospectively, that patients transfused in the course of elective oncologic operations fared less better overall than patients who were not transfused.[3]

Similar effects have been examined in trauma patients with varying results. In a study of transfusion-related infection, Agarwal and coworkers[4] demonstrated that the amount of blood transfused and an injury severity score were the two principal variables predicting post-injury infection. Unfortunately, it is frequently difficult to distinguish the immunosuppression effects of transfusion from the immunosuppressive effects of injury and shock, and this area is likely to remain controversial.

An additional complication of blood transfusions, termed *transfusion-related lung injury*, appears similar to adult respiratory distress syndrome (ARDS) and is probably indistinguishable from ARDS in the trauma population. It was originally thought to be related to microaggregate embolization to the pulmonary circulation, but subsequent experience has shown that reduction in microaggregate embolization through the use of filters is of no value in reducing the incidence of pulmonary dysfunction associated with massive transfusion.

TABLE 25–3. Transmission-Related Infection

Transmitted Disease	Approximate Risk (Per Screened Unit of Blood)
Human immunodeficiency virus (HIV)	1/450,000 to 1/660,000
Human T-lymphotropic virus (HTLV-I, II)	—
Cytomegalovirus	Requires leukocyte-poor red blood cell mass for a patient at high risk
Malaria	No significant risk
Toxoplasmosis	Risk not assessed, probably not significant
Chagas' disease	Four reported cases in the United States and Canada to date
Leishmaniasis	No documented transmission in the United States
Lyme disease	No transfusion-related cases reported
Creutzfeldt-Jakob	No reported transmission
Hepatitis A virus (HAV)	Occasional reports in the United States of transfusion-related HAV
Hepatitis B virus (HBV)	1/200,000
Hepatitis C virus (HCV)	1/4,000

Transfusion-related lung injury (or, rather, *transfusion-associated lung injury*) is now thought to be possibly related to the transfusion of leukocyte antibodies and the priming of polymorphonuclear leukocytes (PMNs) in transfused patients. A study of this process demonstrated significantly more PMN-priming activity present in post-transfusion patients exhibiting transfusion-related lung injury or febrile transfusion reactions. Whether this PMN priming by transfused leukocyte antibodies is a significant predisposing factor to ARDS or multiple organ dysfunction syndrome remains to be determined.[5]

TRANSFUSION IN THE TRAUMA PATIENT

The trauma patient may present unique demands on institutional blood resources given the emergent, unanticipated need for a variety of blood products, often in large quantities. Massive transfusion needs, although occasionally applicable to hepatic transplantation or cardiac surgery patients, occur on a regular basis at major trauma centers. For these reasons, it is important to establish institutional and practice management guidelines for these challenging clinical situations.

Pretransfusion Recipient and Donor Matching

Shortly after collection, a typical donor blood unit is analyzed to determine ABO and Rh groups and screen for the presence of RBC antibodies and any markers for blood-borne infection, as previously indicated. Recognizing the occasional need for immediate transfusion in the severely injured, rapidly bleeding trauma patient, three major options exist for donor screening before blood transfusion. Patients presenting to the emergency department in extremis from blood loss require the immediate transfusion of either whole blood or red cell mass and components.

Typical clinical indications for immediate blood transfusion include:

1. Initial arrival systolic blood pressure below 70 mm Hg and clinical evidence of hypovolemic shock.
2. Persistent or recurrent systolic blood pressure below 90 mm Hg after the initial rapid administration of 2 L of crystalloid solution.
3. An initial hematocrit of less than 25 with hypotension or evidence of ongoing hemorrhage.

The observation that mortality is correlated to shock plus an initial hemoglobin level below 8 g/dL lends support for this particular indication.[6] For immediate transfusion requirements in the trauma resuscitation area, type O blood (universal donor) may be administered until initial blood typing is completed. In general, O-negative blood is administered to women of childbearing age or younger and O-positive or O-negative blood is administered to male patients. Under these circumstances, it is probably important to limit the number of untyped blood (type O) transfused units to less than 4 or 5 if type specific blood is to be used subsequently.

The second option, under less dire circumstances, involves the administration of type-specific blood, without antigenic crossmatching. This process typically allows blood to be made available, after procurement of a recipient specimen, within 10 to 15 minutes. Formal typing and complete crossmatching should be reserved for the elective administration of blood and has no place in the acute setting. Inexperienced physicians, particularly members of the house staff, should be discouraged from asking the blood bank to "type and cross" blood for administration to trauma patients under urgent or emergent circumstances. The principal determining factor dictating the blood bank process for releasing allogeneic blood should be the time needed to transfusion. Immediate transfusion mandates type O, uncrossmatched. Emergent transfusion needs may be met by using type-specific (ABO) uncrossmatched blood, and urgent needs may allow typing and major antigen screening. Elective or planned transfusions should permit sufficient time for complete typing and crossmatching.

Concerns regarding hemolytic incompatibility reactions associated with the use of uncrossmatched blood in the emergent setting have been addressed in several prospective and retrospective clinical studies.[6–10] The consistent conclusion, based on a large number of observations, is that the routine administration of either type-specific (ABO) or type O uncrossmatched blood has not been associated with observed complications related to blood incompatibilities. Although ARDS, disseminated intravascular coagulation, and other coagulopathies occurred, none was attributable to major incompatibility reactions.

A more detailed evaluation of minor crossmatching compatibilities performed retrospectively examined the incidence of unexpected antibodies found during major crossmatch.[11] This study suggested that although weak crossmatch reactions were found, mostly in the Kell, Kidd, or Rh blood groups, the risk for significant clinical manifestations from these weak incompatibilities was low.

Transfusion Monitoring

Patients likely to require immediate, early, or massive transfusion can generally be identified at the time of arrival on the basis of physiologic changes (profound, recurrent, or persistent hypotension) or less severe clinical shock coupled with major anatomic markers (multiple or unstable pelvic fractures, gross hemoperitoneum by ultrasonography or diagnostic peritoneal lavage). Clinical and laboratory monitoring of anticipated ongoing transfusion should be started early and involve the serial assessment of hematocrit, prothrombin time (PT), partial thromboplastin time (PTT), fibrinogen, and platelets. In patients requiring massive transfusions, the assessment of electrolytes, including ionized calcium, and the close monitoring of temperature and the degree of acidosis (by arterial pH) are also important in identifying correctable factors that may affect coagulation.

Whereas laboratory assessment of coagulation is important, the threshold for laboratory detection of abnormal clotting normally requires that a given clotting factor be reduced to less than 20% of its normal activity. For this reason it is important, in addition to the laboratory monitoring of PT, PTT, and platelet count, for the clinicians involved in the management of massively transfused patients to also carefully monitor the presence or absence of microvascular bleeding at surgical sites, intravenous sites, or wounds.

Massive Transfusion Protocols

The anticipation, procurement, and balanced administration of blood products and the monitoring of transfusion and coagulation in patients requiring massive (in excess of one circulating blood volume) transfusion constitute one of the more formidable challenges in clinical medicine. An optimal institutional response to massive transfusion needs requires the coordinated efforts of anesthesiologists, surgeons, nurses, and laboratory and blood bank technical staff. Trauma centers and those institutions with the periodic need to administer large quantities of blood would benefit from the development of protocols and clinical management guidelines to help facilitate and coordinate massive transfusions. A typical protocol guiding massive transfusion in the trauma patient is shown in Table 25–4.

Ideally, the initiation of a massive transfusion protocol should occur in the trauma resuscitation area but it may also occur in the operating room. The appropriate "trigger" for a massive transfusion protocol may be based on physiologic derangements or anatomic markers, as discussed previously. General indications for initiating the massive transfusion protocol are the admission of a patient anticipated to need more than one circulating blood volume transfusion in the first 24 hours. This works out, in an average-sized patient, to about 10 or 11 units of blood. Most of these patients also have indications for immediate transfusions of O-negative or O-positive uncrossmatched blood in the trauma resuscitation area.

Rapid, early communication with blood bank personnel is an essential component of a massive transfusion protocol, particularly in regard to the timing for initial transfusions. As discussed earlier, there are few data to suggest that the 45 to 60 minutes required for crossmatching blood results in any improvement in blood incompatibility reactions, and crossmatching should probably be routinely avoided for massive transfusions. Other blood products, including platelets and FFP, also require a degree of advanced notice before clinical need. The principal limiting step in the rapid availability of frozen blood products (FFP) has been the time required to thaw the product. The use of water-bath FFP thawing devices has shortened the availability lag time to less than 20 minutes.

The overall mortality in massively transfused patients, as expected, varies considerably in the literature. One study reported 25% mortality in patients receiving 20 to 40 units of blood with 52% mortality of those receiving less than 40 units.[12] Another study reported an overall survival of 39% with a 77% mortality in coagulopathic patients.[13] The presence of shock on admission, closed head injury, and advanced age appear to be significant predictors of mortality in the population of massively transfused patients.[14]

TABLE 25–4. Massive Transfusion Protocol (Suggested Example)

Activation

General indications for activation of MTP

- Recurrent or persistent BP < 90 mm Hg after 2 U packed cells
- Anticipated *total* blood requirement ≥ 1 circulating blood volume

General indications for *immediate* (O-negative or O-positive) transfusion and MTP activation

Any clinical evidence of shock state *and*

- Initial ED BP < 70 mm Hg
- Recurrent or persistent BP < 90 mm Hg after ≥ 2 L crystalloid
- Initial Hct < 25

Coagulation Monitoring

- ED arrival blood draw to include CBC with platelets, PT, PTT, fibrinogen, blood for typing to blood bank
- Hct, PT, PTT, fibrinogen, platelets every 30 min until MTP is ended

Transfusion Thresholds

- Hct < 30
- PT > 17 s, most circumstances
- PT > 15 s, eye, brain, airway hemorrhage or factor VIII, IX deficiency
- Platelets < 75,000 for most circumstances
- Platelets < 100,000 for eye, brain, airway injury
- Fibrinogen < 100 mg/dL

Transfusion Administration

- Cells: Give recent-procurement whole blood (preferred) or PRCs to Hct = 30
- FFP: Give initial bolus 1 unit/1000 mL estimated blood volume; reevaluate.
  Continue FFP + RBCs in a 1:1 ratio until PT controlled
- Platelets: Give as bolus 1 pk/1000 mL estimated blood volume to increase count to 25,000 to 50,000; reevaluate.
  Continue platelets + RBCs in a 1:1 ratio until threshold is reached

BP = blood pressure; CBC = complete blood count; ED = emergency department; FFP = fresh frozen plasma; MTP = massive transfusion protocol; PRCs = packed red blood cells; PT = prothrombin time; PTT = partial thromboplastin time; RBCs = red blood cells; Hct = hematocrit.

Acute Coagulopathy

Coagulopathy occurring in association with massive transfusion continues to be one of the most serious problems after major injury. The precise relationship between coagulopathy and the transfusion of blood and blood products has not been determined. A large number, perhaps the majority of severely injured trauma patients, with severe coagulopathies present with clotting deficits at the time of admission. This is most likely due to the presence of circulating tissue thromboplastin produced by blood injury to either the brain or the liver, with each organ rich in this substance. Resulting coagulopathy can be profound and difficult to correct and may exacerbate hemorrhage from other injuries.

Coagulopathy in head-injured patients is a particularly notable problem reported with fairly high incidence. These patients may be identified early by alterations in platelet count, PT, or fibrinogen activity, and the coagulopathy in this group appears to be distinct to the head injury in contrast to elective neurosurgical patients.[15] The overall incidence of coagulopathy in the more severely head-injured group has been reported to be as high as 81% of those patients with a Glasgow Coma Scale (GCS) score of 6 or below and 100% of those with a GCS score on admission of 3 or 4.[16]

The most commonly cited cause of transfusion-related coagulopathy in the trauma patient is dilutional thrombocytopenia. Severe hemodilution, created by the unbalanced administration of large volumes of crystalloid solutions, may also dilute coagulation factors as well as decrease blood viscosity and further exacerbate the effects of existing thrombocytopenia. In extreme cases, severe dilutional coagulopathy, commonly associated with the observation that "the blood looks like Kool-Aid," may be extraordinarily difficult to correct and is associated with gross abnormalities in clotting studies and a high mortality.

The prevention, to the extent possible, of transfusion-related coagulopathy and the treatment of any injury (e.g., tissue thromboplastin or shock-related) coagulopathy depend on careful coagulation monitoring, as previously discussed.

A number of formulaic approaches to platelet and factor administration have been developed with the goal of preventing transfusion-related coagulopathy.[17–24] Most of these studies, however, involved the empirical administration of FFP and platelets as opposed to administration based on transfusion triggers. Studies such as one by Mannucci and colleagues[25] suggest that the administration of platelet concentrates or FFP in the absence of evaluation of hemostasis was not helpful in reducing abnormalities of coagulation.

Most studies of prophylactic administration of either FFP or platelets[26] suggest that a blind prophylactic administration is neither efficacious nor warranted in the absence of specific laboratory-based criteria. Studies also reinforce the notion that microvascular bleeding is a complex process and may be due to other factors (hypothermia, acidosis) in addition to simple transfusion.

Other studies of the correlation between actual clotting factor levels and the presence of microvascular bleeding (the ultimate test of coagulopathy) suggest that commonly used replacement formulas, in the absence of careful monitoring of coagulopathy, do not reliably account for correct clotting factor deficiencies.[27] For these reasons, it is imperative that patients receiving massive transfusions be monitored extremely closely with serial determinations of PT, hematocrit, fibrinogen, and platelet count and that appropriate transfusion triggers for RBCs, FFP, platelets, and other factors be established (see Table 25-3).

Routine administration of calcium (factor IV) as a means of preventing transfusion-related coagulopathy was once thought necessary to compensate for massive blood loss. In reality, calcium is mobilized rapidly enough from bone that it has been estimated that an otherwise well-perfused adult may tolerate 1 unit of transfused blood administered every 5 minutes without major coagulation deficits.[28] In addition, some of the newer blood preservatives, such as Nutricel, contain approximately one third of the sodium citrate that is in a traditional blood preservative, making calcium binding even less of a problem.

Transfusion thresholds developed as part of a massive transfusion protocol and based on coagulation monitoring may provide guidelines for the administration of blood or blood components. Once coagulation thresholds have been exceeded in the setting of massive transfusion, blood components may be given in approximately the following ratios: (1) FFP with packed RBCs in a ratio of 1:2 and (2) platelets with packed RBCs in a ratio of 1:1. Although these ratios are approximate, in the massively transfused patient with established coagulopathy, administration of components along with RBCs (in the absence of whole blood) may be helpful in preventing further dilutional effects by the ongoing administration of crystalloid solutions. In addition, the use of FFP should help to maintain intravascular colloid osmotic pressure, ultimately resulting in less fluid extravasation and less generalized edema.

Hypothermia and acidosis continue to be principal predictive factors in massively transfused patients of both mortality and severe coagulopathy[29, 30] and may directly and adversely affect coagulation. Both temperature and blood gases should be carefully monitored and corrected to the extent possible. Hypothermia in particular (core temperature < 35°C) has a variety of effects on the coagulation cascade and is a common accompaniment to massive transfusion. These effects include:

- Temperature-related inhibition of clotting factor enzymes
- Increased fibrinolysis
- Decreased platelet counts
- Decreased platelet function

Every attempt should be made, at the outset of resuscitation, to prevent or treat hypothermia. One major source of thermal loss is the infusion of chilled or ambient-temperature blood and blood products. Devices capable of rapidly infusing blood warmed to the patient's ambient temperature should be used routinely in large-volume resuscitations both in the emergency department and the operating room. The treatment and the prevention of hypothermia are discussed in more detail in Chapter 34.

AUTOTRANSFUSION

The ability to salvage unprocessed autologous blood from either the chest or peritoneal cavity offers a potentially attractive alternative to the donor blood transfusions. Preservation of clotting factors and platelets and the decreased risk of infectious disease transmission make either intraoperative or resuscitation-phase blood salvage a potentially viable adjunct for the severely injured patient. Experience with these techniques has been limited, however, because of the small number of eligible patients and the lack of large-volume blood salvage equipment in many centers. Experimental reports of massive autotransfusion and hemorrhagic shock models have noted significant pulmonary congestion and edema in association with fibrin thrombi.[31] Studies by the same group have also demonstrated thrombocytopenia, decreased fibrinogen, and elevated PT and PTT.

In clinical studies, the greatest experience with autotransfusion has occurred in the population of cardiopulmonary bypass patients. A number of these studies, however, have reported adverse effects of large amounts of autotransfused blood on subsequent coagulation.[32-34] From the available data, it appears that although the autotransfusion of modest amounts (1000 to 3000 mL) is perhaps well tolerated, the routine use of autotransfusion in the massively transfused patient should probably be reserved until further studies document the safety and efficacy.

For patients requiring smaller amounts of autotransfused blood, concern has been repeatedly expressed regarding the potential contamination by early use of blood from the peritoneal cavity. Several studies of this phenomenon examining blood salvaged from the peritoneal cavity that was subsequently washed and reinfused have not demonstrated any significant clinical effects.[35-37]

SUMMARY

The transfusion of RBCs, pending the development of equivalent, large-volume hemoglobin solutions (see Chapter 26), remains the optimal method of rapidly improving oxygen-carrying capacity and restoring lost red cell mass. With modest transfused amounts and appropriate screening, the risks associated with blood transfusion are acceptably low.

The transfusion of noncellular blood products should be directed at correcting specific clotting factor deficiencies and should occur in conjunction with appropriate coagulation monitoring. The massively transfused patient presents the greatest challenge in this regard and is best approached by use of established institutional guidelines and transfusion triggers built around a massive transfusion protocol.

Coagulopathy in the trauma patient is a complex event influenced by the dilutional effects of thrombocytopenia and clotting factor washout, progressive acidosis, and hypothermia. The first line of treatment involves minimizing the shock state through vigorous monitored resuscitation, avoidance of crystalloid hemodilution, and the correction of acidosis. The reflex or automatic replacement of blood factors during massive transfusion is unlikely to effectively prevent or correct coagulopathy in the absence of coagulation monitoring and directed coagulation factor therapy.

References

1. Faringer PD, Mullins RJ, Johnson RL, Trunkey DD: Blood component supplementation during massive transfusion of AS-1 red cells in trauma patients. J Trauma 1993; 34:481–485.
2. Schreiber GB, Busch MP, Kleinman SH, Korelitz JJ: The risk of transfusion-transmitted viral infections: The Retrovirus Epidemiology Donor Study. N Engl J Med 1996; 334:1685–1690.
3. Collins JA: Recent developments in the area of massive transfusion. World J Surg 1987; 11:75–81.
4. Agarwal N, Murphy JG, Cayten CG, Stahl WM: Blood transfusion

increases the risk of infection after trauma. Arch Surg 1993; 128:171–176.
5. Silliman CC, Paterson AJ, Dickey WO, Stroneck DF, Popovsky MA, Caldwell SA, Ambruso DR: The association of biologically active lipids with the development of transfusion-related acute lung injury: A retrospective study. Transfusion 1997; 37:719–726.
6. Schwab CW, Shayne JP, Turner J: Immediate trauma resuscitation with type O un-crossmatched blood: A two-year prospective experience. J Trauma 1986; 26:897–902.
7. Lefebre J, McLellan BA, Coovadia AS: Seven years experience with group O unmatched packed red blood cells in a regional trauma unit. Ann Emerg Med 1987; 16:1344–1349.
8. Schwab CW, Civil I, Shayne JP: Saline-expanded group O uncrossmatched packed red blood cells as an initial resuscitation fluid in severe shock. Ann Emerg Med 1986; 15:1282–1287.
9. Gervin AS, Fischer RP: Resuscitation of trauma patients with type-specific uncrossmatched blood. J Trauma 1984; 24:327–331.
10. Blumberg N, Bove JR: Un-cross-matched blood for emergency transfusion: One year's experience in a civilian setting. JAMA 1978; 240:2057–2059.
11. Oberman HA, Barnes BA, Friedman BA: The risk of abbreviating the major crossmatch in urgent or massive transfusion. Transfusion 1978; 18:137–141.
12. Riska EB, Bostman O, von Bonsdorff H, Hakkinen S, Jaroma H, Kiviluoto O, Paavilainen T: Outcome of closed injuries exceeding 20-unit blood transfusion need. Injury 1988; 19:273–276.
13. Phillips TF, Soulier G, Wilson RF: Outcome of massive transfusion exceeding two blood volumes in trauma and emergency surgery. J Trauma 1987; 27:903–910.
14. Wudel JH, Morris JA Jr, Yates K, Wilson A, Bass SM: Massive transfusion: Outcome in blunt trauma patients. J Trauma 1991; 31:1–7.
15. Kearney TJ, Bentt L, Grode M, Lee S, Hiatt JR, Shabot MM: Coagulopathy and catecholamines in severe head injury. J Trauma 1992; 32:608–611.
16. May AK, Young JS, Butler K, Bassam D, Brady W: Coagulopathy in severe closed head injury: Is empiric therapy warranted? Am Surg 1997; 63:233–236.
17. Noe DA, Graham SM, Luff R, Sohmer P: Platelet counts during rapid massive transfusion. Transfusion 1982; 22:392–395.
18. Hewson IR, Neame PB, Kumar N, et al: Coagulopathy related to dilution and hypotension during massive transfusion. Crit Care Med 1985; 13:387–391.
19. Counts RB, Haisch C, Simon TL, et al: Hemostasis in massively transfused trauma patients. Ann Surg 1979; 190:91–99.
20. Kravans JR, Jackson DP: Hemorrhagic disorder following massive whole blood transfusion. JAMA 1955; 159:171–176.
21. Lim RC, Olcott C, Robinson AJ, et al: Platelet response and coagulation changes following massive blood replacement. J Trauma 1973; 13:577–582.
22. Miller RD, Robbins TO, Tong MJ, et al: Coagulation defects associated with massive blood transfusions. Ann Surg 1971; 174:794–801.
23. Wilson RF, Mammen E, Walt AJ: Eight years of experience with massive blood transfusions. J Trauma 1971; 11:275–285.
24. Lucas CE: Resuscitation of the injured patient: The three phases of treatment. Surg Clin North Am 1977; 57:3–15.
25. Mannucci PM, Federici AB, Sirchia G: Hemostasis testing during massive blood replacement: A study of 172 cases. Vox Sang 1982; 42:113–123.
26. Reed RL 2d, Ciavarella D, Heimbach DM, Baron L, Pavlin E, Counts RB, Carrico CJ: Prophylactic platelet administration during massive transfusion: A prospective, randomized, double-blind clinical study. Ann Surg 1986; 203:40–48.
27. Ciavarella D, Reed RL, Counts RB, Baron L, Pavlin E, Heimbach DM, Carrico CJ: Clotting factor levels and the risk of diffuse microvascular bleeding in the massively transfused patient. Br J Haematol 1987; 67:365–368.
28. Collins JA, Knudson MM: Metabolic effects of massive transfusion. *In*: Principles of Transfusion Medicine. Rossi EC, Simon TL, Moss GS (Eds). Baltimore, Williams & Wilkins, 1991.
29. Morris JA Jr, Wilcox TR, Reed GW, Hunter EB, Wallas CH, Steane EA, Shotts SD, Vitsky JL: Safety of the blood supply: Surrogate testing and transmission of hepatitis C in patients after massive transfusion. Ann Surg 1994; 219:517–525; discussion 219:525–526.
30. Ferrara A, MacArthur JD, Wright HK, Modlin IM, McMillen MA: Hypothermia and acidosis worsen coagulopathy in the patient requiring massive transfusion. Am J Surg 1990; 160:515–518.
31. Moore EE, Dunn EL, Bess R, Clark D. Amelioration of the pulmonary effects of massive autotransfusions with corticosteroids in the dog. Surg Gynecol Obstet 1981; 152:649–652.
32. Vertrees RA, Conti VR, Lick SD, Zwischenberger JB, McDaniel LB, Shulman G: Adverse effects of postoperative infusion of shed mediastinal blood. Ann Thorac Surg 1996; 62:717–723.
33. de Haan J, Boonstra PW, Monnink SH, Ebels T, van Oeveren W: Retransfusion of suctioned blood during cardiopulmonary bypass impairs hemostasis. Ann Thorac Surg 1995; 59:901–907.
34. de Haan J, Schonberger J, Haan J, van Oeveren W, Eijgelaar A: Tissue-type plasminogen activator and fibrin monomers synergistically cause platelet dysfunction during retransfusion of shed blood after cardiopulmonary bypass. J Thorac Cardiovasc Surg 1993; 106:1017–1023.
35. Boudreaux JP, Bornside GH, Cohn I Jr: Emergency autotransfusion: Partial cleansing of bacteria-laden blood by cell washing. J Trauma 1983; 23:31–35.
36. Timberlake GA, McSwain NE Jr: Autotransfusion of blood contaminated by enteric contents: A potentially life-saving measure in the massively hemorrhaging trauma patient? J Trauma 1988; 28:855–857.
37. Ozmen V, McSwain NE Jr, Nichols RL, Smith J, Flint LM: Autotransfusion of potentially culture-positive blood (CPB) in abdominal trauma: Preliminary data from a prospective study. J Trauma 1992; 32:36–39.

26

Plasma and Blood Substitutes

Gail T. Tominaga, MD, FACS
Kenneth Waxman, MD, FACS

Plasma expansion is attained through intravenous infusion of blood or its components or of blood and plasma substitutes. Crystalloids (electrolyte solutions containing sodium) have been shown to be effective but relatively inefficient plasma volume expanders. Once infused intravascularly, crystalloids distribute throughout the entire extracellular fluid space, of which only a relatively small portion is the plasma volume. Hence, large volumes of crystalloid fluids need to be infused to result in effective plasma volume expansion.

More effective plasma expansion can be attained with colloid fluids, which contain larger molecules that diffuse relatively slowly across the semipermeable capillary membranes. The first colloid plasma substitutes were tested around the turn of the century, when a carbohydrate exudate from acacia trees was used as a volume expander. This substance was used clinically during World War I and proved to be highly antigenic. Another colloid solution developed in the early 1900s is gelatin. Gelatins are used clinically in Europe but are unavailable in the United States. Problems with these solutions include rapid urinary excretion, which causes a short duration of plasma expansion, as well as antigenicity and anaphylaxis.

One of the major disadvantages of colloid solutions is that they are unable to transport oxygen. Two types of oxygen-carrying solutions have undergone investigation—perfluorochemical (PFC) emulsions and hemoglobin solutions. Attempts to develop hemoglobin-based red blood cell (RBC) substitutes have spanned many decades. Hemoglobin in solution has many characteristics of a potentially ideal plasma expander, as follows:

- Colloid osmotic effects
- Oxygen-carrying and oxygen-releasing capacity
- Stability exceeding that of whole blood
- Absence of type-specific RBC antigens
- Absence of viral contaminants of plasma

Blood, however, has several disadvantages; it (1) requires typing and crossmatching, (2) has a short half-life, (3) poses a risk of disease transmission, and (4) cannot be used as a perfusate for organ preservation because of its higher viscosity at low temperatures.

This chapter reviews two currently available synthetic plasma substitutes, dextran solutions and hydroxyethyl starch (HES), and two types of oxygen-carrying solutions, PFC emulsions and hemoglobin solutions. Hemoglobin solutions currently undergoing clinical investigation are reviewed.

DEXTRAN

Dextrans are polysaccharides produced by the conversion of sucrose into long glucose polymers by the bacterial enzyme dextransucrase. Clinically used dextrans are produced by the bacterium *Leuconostoc mesenteroides.* The molecules produced by the bacteria are very large, with molecular weights of several million daltons. For intravenous infusion, partial acid hydrolysis produces dextran fractions within specific molecular weight ranges. Two dextran solutions are most widely used, a 6% solution with an average molecular weight of 70,000 (dextran 70) and a 10% solution with an average molecular weight of 40,000 (dextran 40, or low-molecular-weight dextran). The dextrans can be efficiently produced in large quantities and stored for many years at room temperature either in powdered form or in solution.

Dextran is mainly secreted unchanged in the urine. The rate of renal excretion depends on the molecular size, with smaller dextran molecules being excreted rapidly and larger molecules excreted very slowly. In patients with normal renal function, approximately 60% of infused dextran 40 is excreted into the urine within 6 hours, and almost 70% within 24 hours.[1] Tubular absorption of dextran is negligible. Dextran molecules that are not excreted in the urine diffuse slowly into the interstitium, where uptake into the reticuloendothelial cells and slow metabolism to carbon dioxide occur. Reticuloendothelial cell dysfunction due to this uptake has been postulated, but its clinical implication remains undetermined.

Rapid renal excretion of dextran particles of molecular weight less than 50 kD, along with tubular resorption of water, produces highly viscous urine. Urine specific gravity may increase to extremely high levels (i.e., 1.088) in patients receiving dextran 40 infusions. In patients with severe dehydration or impaired renal perfusion, the risk of acute renal failure is increased secondary to obstruction of the renal tubules by the highly viscous filtrate.[2] This complication can be avoided by concurrent administration of noncolloidal fluids.

The plasma half-life of dextran solutions depends on their molecular size. Dextran 40 is excreted more rapidly than dextran 70, but dextran 40 solutions have a higher oncotic effect per gram infused and thus produce a more pronounced plasma volume expansion.

Dextrans are effective plasma expanders with efficacy equal or superior to that of albumin. A number of studies have demonstrated this plasma volume expansion, with subsequent hemodynamic improvement.[3-5]

In addition to plasma volume expansion, dextran solutions have antithrombotic effects. These effects are probably mediated by inhibition of platelet and leukocyte aggregation as well as augmentation of blood flow in the microcirculation. Because a major pathophysiologic deficit after shock is decreased microcirculatory blood flow, administration of dextrans to patients in shock may offer a therapeutic advantage. This effect may be mediated by decreased blood viscosity by hemodilution[6] or inhibition of RBC and platelet aggregation within the capillaries by low-molecular-weight dextran,[7] which may reverse or prevent intravascular sludging.

Anaphylactic reactions to dextran occur in 0.03% to 0.07% of patients and may be severe or even fatal.[8] These reactions usually occur during infusion of the first 100 mL. Close monitoring during the initiation of dextran infusion is suggested. Isolated reports in the literature have described fetal deaths due to dextrans given maternally before or during delivery.[9]

Dextran affects normal coagulation in a dose-related fashion. Low doses of dextran (<1.5 g/kg body weight) are not associated with clinical bleeding, but platelet adhesiveness and plasma levels of clotting factors are decreased. Larger doses of dextran have been associated with significant bleeding complications.[10] Such consideration limits the use of dextran in perioperative or bleeding patients to 1000 to 1500 mL in 24 hours. Precipitation of acute renal failure has been associated with significant bleeding complications, although this issue is controversial. Usually, reports of renal failure after dextran use involve patients in whom renal perfusion has reduced or who had preexisting renal damage. Hence, dextran administration is not recommended in patients with renal insufficiency.

Another potential problem reported with dextran infusion is subsequent difficulty in blood crossmatching. This problem may be due to the adherence of the dextrans to antigens on the RBC membrane. It can be avoided by obtaining a blood specimen for crossmatching before dextran infusion.

Low-molecular-weight dextran has also been used effectively as a plasma substitute for priming in extracorporeal circulation. In addition, dextrans have been studied and used as possible effective modalities in treating patients with myocardial ischemia, cerebral ischemia, and peripheral vascular disease and in maintaining vascular graft patency.

HYDROXYETHYL STARCH

Starch, the energy storage polysaccharide of plants, is analogous functionally and structurally to glycogen, the energy storage polysaccharide molecule of animals. Starch is composed of two types of glucose polymers: amylose, a linear molecule, and amylopectin, a highly branched molecule that structurally resembles glycogen. Amylopectin is well tolerated when infused intravascularly into animals but is rapidly hydrolyzed enzymatically, with a half-life of only 20 minutes. Modification of the starch molecule by hydroxyethylation, creating HES, has made it less susceptible to amylase hydrolysis and hence more stable within the plasma.[11]

There are several types of HES solutions, characterized by their average molecular weight and level of hydroxyethyl substitution. The first-developed solution, hetastarch, has a high mean molecular weight (69,000; range 10 to 100 kD) with a wide range. This feature has implications for the elimination of HES from the vascular space. Smaller molecules are excreted unchanged into the urine, whereas larger molecules slowly diffuse into the interstitium, where slow enzymatic degradation occurs. In normal subjects, HES is almost completely cleared from the plasma within 2 days (half-life is 17 hours), yet only about 50% of the HES is eliminated from the body. The remaining HES is eliminated very slowly, and a majority of the initial dose persists in the reticuloendothelial cells for weeks after infusion.[11]

HES appears to be extremely well tolerated, with relatively uncommon and mild side effects. Allergic reactions to HES are uncommon; unlike dextran, HES is not antigenic. In one large series, the incidence of allergic reactions to HES was 0.085% in 16,405 infusions, compared with 0.011% in 60,048 infusions for albumin infusion.[12] No fatal anaphylactic reactions to HES were reported in this study.

The only clinically important adverse effect of HES infusion appears to be some impairment of coagulation, which appears to be dose related. Low doses have no effect on coagulation, whereas moderate doses (20 mL/kg) may transiently decrease platelet counts, decrease fibrinogen levels, and prolong prothrombin time and partial thromboplastin time.[13] Platelet function, including adhesiveness, remains intact. Although these effects may be measured, there is no evidence of clinical bleeding problems with HES infusions of as much as 20 mL/kg.[14] There have been no controlled human studies of larger infusions with HES, but studies of animals have shown increased incisional bleeding, greater intraoperative blood loss, and spontaneous serosal bleeding when very large doses of HES are infused.[15]

A problem of undetermined significance with HES infusion is occasional elevation of the serum amylase level. It is unclear whether (1) this hyperamylasemia is a result of subclinical pancreatitis, (2) HES acts as a physiologic stimulant to pancreatic amylase secretion, or (3) HES causes amylase aggregation.[16] It is known that amylase-starch complexes form and can increase serum amylase to more than twice the normal values during a period of several days. Unlike dextrans, HES does not interfere with blood crossmatching, and it has no apparent adverse effect on renal function.

The most commonly used HES is hetastarch, which is available as a 6% solution in physiologic salt solution and contains 60 g/L colloid and 154 mEq/L sodium and chloride. It has an osmolarity of 310 mOsm/L, pH of 5.5, and colloid oncotic pressure of 30 mm Hg.

Pentastarch, a modification of the hetastarch formulation, has a lower average molecular weight, more homogeneous particle size, and less hydroxyethyl substitution. These changes allow for a more predictable, more rapid excretion of pentastarch compared with hetastarch. Pentastarch theoretically poses less risk of reticuloendothelial impairment. In addition, larger volumes may have less effect on coagulation parameters.[17] Pentastarch is available as a 10% solution and has a colloid osmotic pressure of 40 mm Hg.

HES has been well studied for its efficacy as a plasma volume expander. Hetastarch (6% solution in saline) increases plasma volume by an amount from 71% to 230% of the volume of hetastarch infused.[18, 19] The colloid osmotic pressure is increased significantly after hetastarch infusion, thus explaining its ability to expand the plasma volume by more than the infused volume. The colloid osmotic pressure remains elevated for 2 to 5 days after HES infusion, corresponding to the plasma half-life of HES. In addition, pentastarch has a greater degree of volume expansion than either albumin or 6% hetastarch.[19]

In comparative studies of fluid therapy, infusing 6% HES solutions has increased central venous pressure, pulmonary capillary wedge pressure, cardiac output, and ventricular stroke work with efficacy equivalent to that of 5% albumin infusion.[14, 20] No bleeding problems were reported in these studies, which included perioperative patients. HES, in particular pentastarch, has also been successfully used as a priming solution for cardiopulmonary bypass.[21]

HES has similarities to and differences from dextran. Both dextran and HES effectively raise colloid osmotic pressure and plasma volume, although the plasma volume increase may be greater and somewhat more sustained after infusion of higher-molecular-weight dextrans. Dextrans are more useful agents in decreasing blood viscosity and increasing microcirculatory blood flow and thus have advantage as antithrombotic agents and as therapy for microcirculatory flow disturbances. HES, however, appears to be associated with fewer adverse effects, including a lower incidence of anaphylaxis, fewer bleeding problems, and no adverse renal effects.

PERFLUOROCHEMICAL EMULSIONS

Fluoridation of hydrocarbons generates a biologically inert liquid with high oxygen solubility. Oxygen is dissolved in PFC emulsions, which thus supply oxygen by simple diffusion after their delivery. The potential use of PFC as a blood substitute has been delayed because it requires suspension in an emulsion suitable for intravascular infusion.

In 1965, Clark and Gollan[22] demonstrated that a mouse could survive when completely submerged in a PFC liquid equilibrated with oxygen at 1 atmosphere. In 1967, Sloviter and Kamimoto[23] made a PFC emulsion with albumin and successfully used it to perfuse isolated brain preparations. In 1968, Geyer[24] performed the first successful total exchange transfusions with rats, using a PFC emulsion made from perfluorotributylamine (FC47). Significant problems occurred with these early emulsions, including prolonged tissue retention times (half-life of 895 days) and pulmonary and hepatic toxicity.

During the 1970s, an improved emulsion, Fluosol-DA 20% (Fluosol), was developed.[25] This emulsion is 20% PFC by weight and contains seven parts perfluorodecalin for short tissue dwell time and three parts perfluorotripropylamine for improved emulsion stability. Poloxamer 188 (Pluronic F-68) and egg yolk phospholipid are added as emulsifying agents, and HES is added to increase oncotic pressure. Fluosol must be stored frozen and must be infused within 24 hours of thawing.

PFC emulsions are eliminated unchanged through the airways. The particles of Fluosol emulsion have a mean diameter of 0.1 μm. This small size allows elimination through the alveolar membrane. Some uptake of PFC emulsions occurs in the reticuloendothelial cells. The half-life of Fluosol is dose-dependent. At a dose of 10 mL/kg, the circulatory half-life is approximately 8 hours; at a dose of 20 mL/kg, the plasma half-life is about 17 hours. Trace amounts of Fluosol are present in the liver and spleen for as long as 80 days after treatment. Accumulation of perfluorocarbons occurs on repeated administration. Therefore, administration of Fluosol more than once every 6 months is not recommended.

Because the oxygen dissolved in PFC emulsions is not bound as it is to hemoglobin, the amount of oxygen transported depends on the partial pressure of oxygen in the arterial blood (Pa_{O_2}). Although PFCs have about 20 times the solubility for oxygen compared with plasma, significant volumes of oxygen are still dissolved only at high Pa_{O_2} values. Thus, the clinical use of PFC emulsions requires good pulmonary function and high inspired oxygen concentrations. An advantage of this relatively low "affinity" of PFC for oxygen is that nearly all oxygen dissolved in PFC at arterial oxygen tensions is released to peripheral tissues at tissue oxygen tensions. In addition, carbon dioxide dissolves in the fluorocarbon, which carries it to the lung for excretion.

PFC emulsions improve peripheral blood flow by plasma volume expansion and possibly by improved microcirculatory flow. The small PFC emulsion particles (1/70 the size of RBCs) may flow through constricted areas of the microcirculation not accessible to RBCs. This characteristic may improve peripheral tissue oxygenation both by delivering oxygen dissolved in the PFC and by increasing plasma flow and delivery of the oxygen dissolved in plasma.

Fluosol was given to normal volunteers and tested in clinical trials in Japan in 1978.[26] It was first used in the United States in 1979, and limited trials have been performed, largely in anemic and bleeding patients who refused blood on religious grounds. Mitsuno and coworkers[27] reported that Fluosol infusion resulted in significant plasma volume expansion. Tremper and associates[28] and Waxman and colleagues[29] have reported improvement in oxygen delivery and oxygen consumption after administration of Fluosol to anemic patients.

Because of adverse side effects, the randomized clinical trial of Fluosol in the treatment of severe anemia was stopped in the mid-1990s. A number of adverse effects have possibly been related to administration of PFC emulsion; they include transient leukopenia, elevated results of liver function tests, increased pulmonary arterial pressures, transient hypotension, and pulmonary failure.[29, 30] It appears that an emulsifying agent in Fluosol, poloxamer 188, may be responsible for some of these adverse effects via activation of the complement system.[31]

A number of limitations of these solutions have prevented PFCs from playing a significant role in transfusion therapy. First, the volumes of PFC emulsion that have been infused have been limited, and with these volumes, only a relatively small amount of oxygen can be dissolved. Therefore, the oxygen-transporting capability is limited. Second, the plasma half-life is relatively short. Third, the stability of the current emulsion limits its shelf life, even when it is stored frozen. Fourth, in order to dissolve significant volumes of oxygen in Fluosol, very high PaO_2 must be achieved, and adequate pulmonary function and high inspired oxygen concentrations are necessary. Finally, a number of possible adverse effects of Fluosol administration have been reported.

There are potential therapeutic uses for PFC emulsions other than as blood substitutes. The most promising of these has been the use of PFC emulsion as a coronary artery angioplasty perfusate. Anderson and colleagues[32] demonstrated significantly prolonged time to onset of angina, reduced duration of chest pain, and improved subjective evaluation of chest pain when Fluosol was infused through the angioplasty catheter in 29 patients with single-vessel disease and good cardiac function. Cowley and associates[33] obtained favorable results from the use of Fluosol in 38 high-risk cardiac patients; cardiac output declined less in Fluosol-treated patients than in controls, and no adverse side effects attributable to Fluosol were noted. Other workers have demonstrated attenuation of myocardial ischemia when Fluosol is infused locally as an intracoronary infusion near the area of ischemia.[34] In view of these and other studies, the U.S. Food and Drug Administration (FDA) approved the clinical use of Fluosol only for coronary artery balloon angioplasties.

Other potential applications of PFCs are their use as: (1) radiation therapy enhancers, (2) drug delivery solvents, (3) radiologic contrast media in ultrasound, computed tomography, and magnetic resonance imaging, (4) acute treatments of myocardial or cerebral ischemia, and (4) liquid ventilation solutions to improve oxygen delivery and blood gas exchange.[35]

Second-generation PFC preparations based on perfluorocytlbromide (Oxygent) and perfluorodichoroctane (Oxyfluor) have been developed. Higher concentrations of these new PFCs can be used to increase oxygen-carrying capacity, although the dose is limited at 0.9 g/kg for use in humans.[36] The problem of complement activation has been solved by substituting egg yolk lecithin as surfactant.

Safety clinical trials of Oxygent (Alliance Pharmaceutical Corp., San Diego) have shown no adverse effects with increasing doses until administration of 1.8 g/kg.[37, 38] At this dose, there is a transient febrile response starting 4 hours after injection and subsiding after 14 hours. In addition, a decrease in platelet count is noted that returns to normal by day 7. Similar symptoms of fever, chills, and nausea have been reported with high doses of Oxyfluor (HemoGen, St. Louis).[39]

In phase II clinical trials of Oxygent, surgical patients receiving 100% oxygen have demonstrated a decreased need for 1 to 2 units of blood when given 0.9 g/kg Oxygent.[40] Potential continues to exist for these improved solutions as effective resuscitation fluids.

STROMA-FREE HEMOGLOBIN

The development of an ideal hemoglobin-derived blood substitute has eluded investigators for more than a century. A persistent problem has been the inability to develop hemoglobin solutions that provide adequate oxygen and carbon dioxide exchange while avoiding toxicity that precludes clinical safety and long-term survival.

Investigators in the 1940s and 1950s found hemoglobin solutions to be nephrotoxic and to cause alterations of blood coagulation and vasoconstriction. In the late 1960s, Rabiner and associates[41] reported that these toxic effects occurred because of contaminants derived from the red blood cell membrane. The term *stroma-free hemoglobin* (SFH) was introduced by these researchers to describe the more highly purified hemoglobin solutions they had prepared. Although a misnomer, because some stroma is present, the name SFH has since become the standard term for stroma-removed hemoglobin solutions. On the basis of results of these studies, Savitsky and associates[42] conducted a phase I clinical trial in 1978, in which 250 mL of stroma-free hemoglobin, containing 1.2% stroma, was administered to eight healthy volunteers. These researchers found that the nearly complete removal of stromal contaminants reduced but did not completely prevent the development of toxic reactions. They also reported that hemoglobinuria, which was previously considered innocuous, was associated with decreases in urine volume and creatinine clearance. They stressed that this deterioration in kidney function was transient and was not associated with permanent renal damage. Nevertheless, these results had a negative impact on further clinical research.

One of the major problems with the SFH preparations is increased affinity for oxygen compared with that of RBCs. The oxygen half-saturation (P_{50}) of SFH solutions varies from 12 to 16 mm Hg, compared with 26 to 27 mm Hg for fresh blood. This increased oxygen affinity, depicted by the left-shifted oxygen dissociation curve, is due to the loss of tetrameric hemoglobin, lack of 2,3-diphosphoglycerate (2,3-DPG), and a higher pH compared with the intracellular RBC pH. The higher affinity of SFH solutions for oxygen could lead to inadequate release of oxygen in the tissues, despite adequate circulating volumes of oxygen. The solutions to this problem that have evolved include reacting hemoglobin with pyridoxal-5′-phosphate, and encapsulating hemoglobin with 2,3-DPG into liposomes.

Another problem with SFH solutions is their relatively rapid clearance from the vascular space, which is due to uptake by the reticuloendothelial system and to renal excretion. In experimental studies, SFH solutions have a plasma half-life of 2 to 4 hours. Rapid loss of hemoglobin is also associated with significant osmotic diuresis, resulting in depletion of intravascular volume. To counter these effects, hemoglobin has been complexed to form larger-molecular-weight species.

The concern about renal toxicity has been one of the major obstacles preventing the clinical use of prior SFH blood substitutes. In addition, vasomotor effects and gastrointestinal symptoms are common. The mechanism of these toxicities appears to involve the extravasation of tetrameric hemoglobin. The extravasated tetrameric hemoglobin interacts with endo-

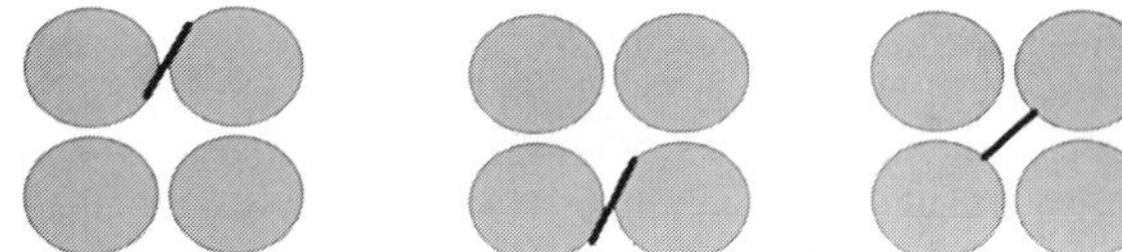

Figure 26–1. Cross-linked hemoglobin. Intramolecularly cross-linked alpha (α) and beta (β) chains within the hemoglobin tetramer. *Dark lines* are the cross-links.

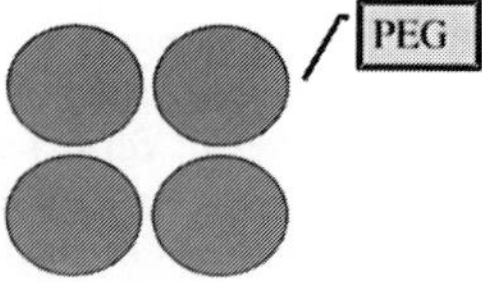

Figure 26–3. Conjugated hemoglobin. Hemoglobin tetramers are conjugated to a macromolecule, such as polyethylene glycol (PEG).

thelially derived relaxing factor, leading to unopposed vasoconstriction.[43]

To overcome these problems with SFH, hemoglobin modifications have been developed. Such modifications include cross-linked hemoglobin, which is subdivided into intramolecularly cross-linked, conjugated, and polymerized hemoglobins; and microencapsulated or liposome-encapsulated hemoglobin (LEH).

Intramolecularly cross-linked hemoglobin involves an intramolecular chemical link to stabilize the native hemoglobin molecule (Fig. 26–1). The intramolecular cross-linking agents studied are: (1) pyridoxal phosphate (PLP), (2) 2-nor-2-formylpyridoxal 5′-phosphate (NF-PLP), (3) bis-pyridoxal tetraphosphate (bis-PLP), and (4) 3,5-dibromosalicyl-bis-fumarate (DBBF). These modifications result in a reduction in oxygen affinity (i.e., increase in P_{50}) and an increase in circulatory half-life ($t^{1}/_{2}$).

Polymerization of hemoglobin involves intermolecular cross-linking of tetramers, which results in polymers of various molecular weights (Fig. 26–2). The most common polymerizing agent used is glutaraldehyde. Characteristics of a polymerized pyridoxylated hemoglobin solution (Poly SFH-P) are as follows[44]:

- Hemoglobin concentration 14 to 16 g/dL
- P_{50} 16 to 20 torr
- COP 20 to 25 mm Hg
- $t^{1}/_{2}$ 38 hours

The efficacy of Poly SFH-P has been studied in baboons. Seven adult baboons underwent a total exchange transfusion with Poly SFH-P, with 100% survival at a hematocrit value of 0. Further studies in baboons have demonstrated maintenance of baseline hemodynamics and oxygen consumption at a hematocrit value of 0 with Poly SFH-P.

Conjugation of hemoglobin involves the binding of a macromolecule to the hemoglobin tetramer to form a larger molecule (Fig. 26–3). The use of soluble polymers, such as polyethylene glycol (PEG), has resulted in conjugated hemoglobin with good circulation times. A pyridoxalated hemoglobin-polyoxyethylene conjugate (PHP) has been shown to support animals with lethal anemia by effectively transporting needed oxygen to tissues.[45] Physiologic assessments in exchange transfusion studies revealed no untoward effects on hepatic, renal, or coagulation functions.

A unique modification of hemoglobin has been the formation of artificial red blood cells. Liposome-encapsulated hemoglobin (LEH) with 2,3-DPG has a normal hemoglobin dissociation curve and an increased half-life (15–24 hours).[46] Inclusion of carbohydrate components such as gangliosides into the liposomal bilayer prolongs circulation times. As a result, these ganglioside-containing liposomes may exhibit reduced impact on the reticuloendothelial system. Acute thrombocytopenia has been reported after the intravenous injection of empty liposomes to miniature pigs and rats.[47] The manner in which liposomes induce thrombocytopenia is unclear. The LEH solutions have been shown to increase plasma half-life and can carry sufficient oxygen to sustain life,[48] but their safety has not yet been proven.

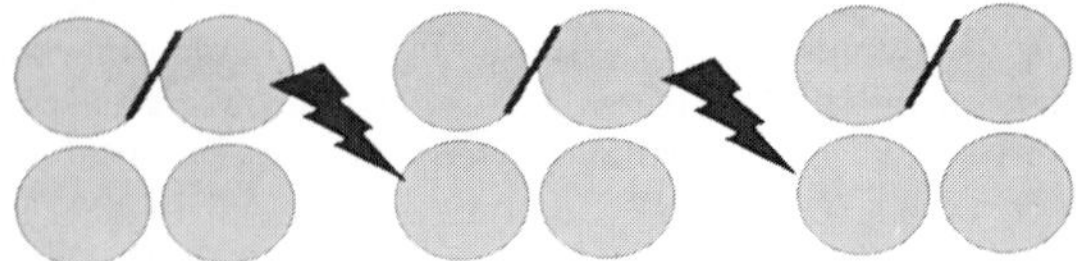

Figure 26–2. Polymerized hemoglobin. Intermolecularly linked hemoglobin tetramers. *Dark lines* and *jagged lines* are the cross-links.

Nanotechnology to prepare biodegradable hemoglobin nanocapsules or microencapsulated hemoglobin with diameters between 80 and 200 nm are being studied.[49] Superoxide dismutase, catalase, and the methemoglobin reductase system can be incorporated into these nanocapsules, decreasing the problem of methemoglobin formation and avoiding lipid peroxidation. The potential effects of reticuloendothelial system uptake is avoided, because the polylactide membrane is degraded into lactic acid and then water and carbon dioxide. Another advantage of the nanocapsules is that the hemoglobin content can be made to match that of red blood cells. This new generation of encapsulated hemoglobin appears very promising.

SOURCES OF HEMOGLOBIN

Human Hemoglobin

Traditionally, investigators have focused on human hemoglobin solutions. The preparation of hemoglobin solutions generally consists of hemolysis of washed, outdated human red blood cells, purification by crystallization and washing, and reconstitution for storage in solution or in dry form. Although these preparations are relatively stable, they gradually break down to methemoglobin when they are stored at room temperature. Shelf life is greatly prolonged if stroma-free hemoglobin is stored frozen.

Problems with the use of outdated banked blood or pedigree human donor blood as a hemoglobin source are the risks of disease transmission and the limited supply. Alternative sources of hemoglobin have therefore been investigated. Bovine hemoglobin, in particular, has been extensively studied. In addition, advances in recombinant gene techniques make recombinant human hemoglobin a viable alternative.

Bovine Hemoglobin Solutions

Bovine hemoglobin has several unique characteristics. The main attractions of bovine hemoglobin solutions are the almost limitless supply, potentially lower cost as raw materials, and avoidance of human viral disease transmission. An additional physiologic advantage of bovine hemoglobin is that it does not require 2,3-DPG to lower its oxygen affinity. Human hemoglobin must be modified by pyridoxylation to allow it to release oxygen in a stroma-free, 2,3-DPG–free environment, thus raising the risk of contamination during preparation. In contrast, bovine hemoglobin does not require modification because it uses chloride ion to lower its oxygen affinity. Fortunately, the chloride ion concentration of human plasma is adequate to decrease the oxygen affinity of bovine hemoglobin to a satisfactory level (P_{50} = 28 mm Hg) before polymerization.

One disadvantage of bovine hemoglobin is the possibility of transmission of occult animal infectious agents, such as the bovine spongiform encephalopathy prion (BSE), which causes "mad cow disease." Animal-source hemoglobin must be subject to rigorous purification procedures because of contamination with other animal-derived proteins, which may cause allergic reactions in humans.

In 1983, Feola and colleagues[50] reported that bovine hemoglobin, polymerized as well as unmodified, was an effective carrier of oxygen capable of sustaining life in animals that had severe hemorrhage. Subsequent studies showed that intravenous administration of bovine hemoglobin was safe if the hemoglobin was pure, selectively polymerized, and complemented with antioxidants or radical scavengers.[51, 52] In addition, in 1988, Feola and associates demonstrated that bovine hemoglobin with these characteristics could be safely administered to humans. In 1992, they performed a clinical trial in Zaire. Nine children with sickle cell anemia were transfused with a bovine hemoglobin solution to 25% blood volume. No adverse reactions were reported. In addition, five patients with aplastic crisis had reticulocytosis in response to transfusion. These initial studies make bovine hemoglobin solutions a potentially promising blood substitute.

Recombinant Hemoglobin Solutions

The explosion in technology for cloning and expressing genes permits seemingly unlimited opportunities for the development of protein products that are engineered for biomedical application. This approach should enable production of a hemoglobin solution that obviates the problems of purity, oxygen affinity, plasma retention, stability, and antigenicity. It also may be possible to tailor the properties of the hemoglobin through gene manipulation. Nagai and coworkers[54] were the first to produce human hemoglobin via recombinant methods.

Human hemoglobin can be synthesized in *Escherichia coli*[55] and *Saccharomyces cerevisiae*,[56] whose genomes have been modified to contain globin genes. These hemoglobins cannot be used as blood substitutes, however, for the following reasons:

1. Oxygen affinity is high, owing to the absence of 2,3-DPG, thereby precluding sufficient oxygen unloading to the tissues.
2. The hemoglobins dissociate into α-β dimers that are cleared rapidly by renal filtration or are rapidly oxidized to the nonfunctional methemoglobin form.

Soluble hemoglobin injected into the circulatory system cannot interact with 2,3-DPG in RBCs, making its oxygen affinity too high to support oxygen transport. Appropriate mutations in the globin genes that result in the expression of a synthetic hemoglobin with low oxygen affinity, resembling that of normal blood, can be produced. The coexpression of β-globin chains and α-globin subunits linked by a peptide bond results in the direct synthesis of stabilized and fully functional hemoglobin tetramers.[57] Fusion of the two α-globin subunits increases the half-life of this hemoglobin molecule in vivo by preventing its dissociation into α-β dimers. Unlike hemoglobins that have been chemically cross-linked, genetically fused di-α-hemoglobin can be produced by simple microbial fermentation and purified without further modification.[58]

During the last decade, a full understanding of globin gene regulation has been achieved. The discovery of upstream enhancer elements that are necessary for high-level, erythrocyte-specific globin gene expression has enabled the preparation of transgenic mice in which a large proportion of the hemoglobin is human.[59] This strategy has been applied to the preparation of pigs in which transgenes express human hemoglobin.[60] This approach would enable the production of large quantities of human hemoglobin, which like the bovine preparation would be free of human pathogens. Considerable problems must be solved before hemoglobin from transgenic livestock could provide a practical way to produce a safe and effective blood substitute. Although the development of such recombinant hemoglobin is very exciting, a significant challenge lies in progressing from the small-scale expression of limited amounts of recombinant protein to an economically viable production process.

CLINICAL TRIALS OF BLOOD SUBSTITUTES

Several blood substitute products are currently being investigated[61] (Table 26–1). The products under investigation have the following characteristics:

- Oxygen-unloading characteristics similar to those of blood
- Short circulation times (12–24 hours)
- Long shelf lives (1 year frozen)
- No renal toxicity
- Low risk of blood-borne viral or bacterial transmission
- No requirement for type and crossmatch

PolyHeme (Northfield) is a tetramer-free form of polymerized pyridoxylated hemoglobin (Poly SFH-P). This feature is intended to prevent extravasation of tetramers from the capillary to bind to nitric oxide, avoiding the problems related to vasoconstriction and gastrointestinal side effects. PolyHeme has been proven safe in phase I and phase II clinical trials. Its clinical safety has been reported with infusion of up to 6 units (300 g hemoglobin) PolyHeme as a blood substitute after acute trauma and emergency surgery.[62] A nonrandomized study demonstrated the ability of PolyHeme to effectively support hemodynamics and oxygen transport, maintain hemoglobin concentration, and decrease the need for allogeneic blood transfusions.[62] These findings were confirmed in a randomized trial in 44 trauma and emergency surgical patients.[63]

TABLE 26–1. Current Blood Substitutes Under Clinical Investigation

Company	Product	Modifications of Hemoglobin	Source	Trial Phase(s)
Northfield	PolyHeme™	Glutaraldehyde polymerized	Human	I, II, III
Biopure	Hemopure™	Glutaraldehyde polymerized	Bovine	I, II
Hemosol	HemoLink™	o-Raffinose polymerized	Human	I, II
Baxter	HemAssist™	Diaspirin cross-linked (DCLHb)	Human	I, II, III suspended
Baxter, Somatogen	Optro™	Recombinantly cross-linked	Recombinant	I, II
Enzon	PEG-Hb	Polyethylene glycol conjugated	Bovine	I
Ajinomoto, Apex	PHP-Hgb	Polyoxyethylene conjugated	Human	I

Phase III studies of this human polymerized hemoglobin in elective surgery are under way.

Hemopure (Biopure Corp., Cambridge, Mass.) is a glutaraldehyde polymerized bovine hemoglobin with one third the viscosity of human blood. No clinically significant adverse effects have been reported in more than 350 patients who have received Hemopure in clinical trials to a maximum dose of 250 g.[64] The hemodynamic effects of Hemopure were assessed during general anesthesia in 37 patients sustaining blood losses of at least 500 mL. Minimal elevations in mean arterial pressure were reported in the 37 patients receiving up to 1.2 g/kg Hemopure compared with 21 patients receiving lactated Ringer's solution.[65] Hemopure has unique oxygen-unloading characteristics owing to its reduced oxygen affinity and lacks the pressor effects found with other human hemoglobin solutions.

During 1998, six Phase II clinical trials were implemented in the United States. The clinical trials encompass coronary artery bypass grafting, orthopedic surgery, and the treatment of anemia.

HemoLink (Hemosol, Inc., Etobicoke, Ontario, Canada) is an o-raffinose, intermolecularly cross-linked polyhemoglobin produced from outdated human blood. Its safety was confirmed by its administration to 33 healthy volunteers, who received up to 600 mg/kg solution; mild gastrointestinal discomfort was reported at the higher doses.[66] HemoLink has been approved for Phase II evaluation in surgical patients.

HemAssist (Baxter HealthCare Corp.) is a diaspirin intramolecularly cross-linked hemoglobin solution (DCLHb) based on outdated human blood with one half the viscosity of human blood. In humans, DCLHb has been found to produce a dose-dependent increase in mean arterial pressure without significant adverse effects.[67, 68] This increase in vasomotor tone is thought to be due to nitric oxide binding. Later studies, however, have demonstrated that an increase in plasma endothelin-1 by DCLHb may be more important than nitric oxide in causing the increase in vasomotor tone.[69] The pressor effect of DCLHb has been evaluated in hemodialysis patients, surgical patients, and critically ill patients in intensive care units. Along with the pressor effect of DCLHb, volume expansion properties were demonstrated. The first safety evaluations in humans were performed on 130 patients in hemorrhagic shock at ten sites in the United States and Europe. DCLHb was safe at the doses tested. A surgical trial of HemAssist in more than 200 cardiac patients has been completed in Europe. Two multicenter trials, one in Europe and one in the United States, were initiated. During 1998, enrollment of patients into Baxter's Phase III clinical trials was stopped. After acquiring Somatogen, Inc., in May 1998, Baxter Healthcare announced that research and development would focus on second-generation hemoglobin substitutes, such as recombinant hemoglobin.

Optro is a recombinant human hemoglobin product developed by Somatogen, Inc., Boulder. It is an intramolecularly cross-linked recombinant di-α-hemoglobin produced in *E. coli.* Phase I clinical trials reported no major organ system toxicity with up to 11 g/kg of Optro infusion given over 0.8 hours.[70] Initial studies reported gastrointestinal side effects at high doses, which in later studies were avoided by proper premedication with oral ibuprofen. Phase II clinical trials of this agent started in 1994. Trials have been initiated in patients with intraoperative blood loss and in patients with end-stage renal failure as well as in patients with refractory anemia, who received Optro in conjunction with exogenous erythropoietin. Optro appears to stimulate erythropoiesis synergistically with erythropoietin. A large North American multicenter trial is ongoing.

Iwashita and colleagues,[71] at Ajinomoto Co., Inc., Tokyo, have developed a pyridoxalated hemoglobin conjugated to polyoxyethylene, a derivative of polyethylene glycol. In cooperation with Apex Bioscience, USA, they have carried out a phase I clinical trial in which doses up to 7 g were given with no significant toxicity. The primary application is focusing on septic shock and on using PHP as a nitric oxide scavenger.

PEG-Hb (Enzon, Inc., Piscataway, N.J.) consists of PEG cross-linked to bovine hemoglobin to form polyethylene glycol hemoglobin. One property unique to this agent is that it oxygenates hypoxic tumor tissue and dramatically increases sensitivity to radiation therapy in laboratory models. In addition, initial phase IA studies in healthy male volunteers demonstrated that PEG-Hb remains in circulation long enough to be consistent with weekly dosing and current fractionated radiation therapy practice. Because of these two observations, PEG-Hb has been tested as an adjuvant to radiation therapy in human cancer patients in phase IB studies.[72]

SUMMARY

Colloid fluid solutions are often used as plasma volume expanders in critically ill patients. Individual agents, including dextran and hydroxyethyl starch solutions, have unique advantages and disadvantages. These solutions, however, lack the ability to carry oxygen.

Perfluorocarbon emulsions dissolve oxygen, but concerns about their inadequate oxygen-carrying capacity and toxicity have dampened the initial enthusiasm for these agents. Two second-generation perfluorochemicals are now being investigated and show promising results.

Several hemoglobin solutions have been formulated, each with unique properties beyond its oxygen-carrying capability that can be utilized clinically. These solutions have been modified to avoid the earlier problems of renal dysfunction and gastrointestinal distress. Expanded clinical trials will achieve a better understanding of unanticipated problems with these agents. Although these blood substitutes are promising, their effects on short- and long-term survival have not been determined. Despite the many challenges encountered over the past few decades, these blood substitutes may become available for clinical use in the near future. These products, once approved by the FDA, have the potential to revolutionize transfusion medicine.

References

1. Arturson G, Granath K, Thoren L, et al: The renal excretion of low molecular weight dextran. Acta Chir Scand 1964; 127:543–548.
2. Matheson NA, Diomi P: Renal failure after the administration of dextran 40. Surg Gynecol Obstet 1970; 131:661–668.
3. Thoren L: Dextran as a plasma volume substitute. Prog Clin Biol Res 1978; 19:265–282.
4. Gelin LE, Solvell L, Zeederfeldt B: The plasma volume expanding effect of low viscous dextran and macrodex. Acta Anaesthesiol Scand 1961; 122:309–323.
5. Shoemaker WC: Comparison of the relative effectiveness of whole blood transfusions and various types of fluid therapy in resuscitation. Crit Care Med 1976; 4:71–78.
6. Dormandy JA: Influence of blood viscosity on blood flow and the effect of low molecular weight dextran. Br Med J 1971; 4:716–719.
7. Bygdeman S, Eliasson R: Effect of dextran on platelet adhesiveness and aggregation. Scand J Clin Lab Invest 1967; 20:17–23.
8. Ring J, Messmer K: Incidence and severity of anaphylactoid reactions to colloid volume substitutes. Lancet 1977; 1:466–469.
9. Barbier P, Jonville AP, Autret E, et al: Fetal risks with dextrans during delivery. Drug Safety 1992; 7:71–73.
10. Karlson KE, Garson AA, Shafton GW, et al: Increased blood loss associated with administration of certain plasma expanders: dex-

tran 75, dextran 40, and hydroxyethyl starch. Surgery 1967; 62:670–678.

11. Waxman K, Tremper KK, Mason GR: Blood and plasma substitutes: Plasma expansion and oxygen transport properties. West J Med 1985; 143:202–206.
12. Ring J, Messmer K: Incidence and severity of anaphylactoid reactions to colloid volume substitutes. Lancet 1977; 1:466–469.
13. Korttila K, Grohn P, Gordon A, et al: Effects of hydroxyethyl starch and dextran on plasma volume and blood hemostasis and coagulation. J Clin Pharmacol 1984; 24:273–282.
14. Puri VK, Paidipaty B, White L: Hydroxyethyl starch for resuscitation of patients with hypovolemia and shock. Crit Care Med 1981; 9:833–837.
15. Karlson KE, Garzon AA, Shafton GW, et al: Increased blood loss associated with administration of certain plasma expanders. Surgery 1967; 62:670–678.
16. Kohler H, Kirch W, Horstmann HJ: Formation of high molecular aggregates between serum amylase and colloidal plasma substitutes. Anaesthesist 1977; 26:623–627.
17. Strauss RG, Stansfield C, Henriksen RA, et al: Pentastarch may cause fewer effects on coagulation than hetastarch. Transfusion 1988; 28:257–260.
18. Killian JP: The effect of 6% HES, 4.5% dextran 60 and 5.5% oxgel on blood volume. Anaesthesist 1977; 24:193–197.
19. Kohler H, Zschiedrich M, Clasen R, et al: The effects of 500 ml 10% hydroxyethyl starch 200/0.5 and 10% dextran 40 on blood volume, colloid osmotic pressure and renal function in human volunteers. Anaesthesist 1982; 31:61–67.
20. Lazrove S, Waxman K, Shippy C, et al: Hemodynamic, blood volume and oxygen transport responses to albumin and hydroxyethyl starch infusion in critically ill postoperative patients. Crit Care Med 1980; 8:302–306.
21. London MJ, Franks M, Verrier ED, et al: The safety and efficacy of ten per cent pentastarch as a cardiopulmonary bypass priming solution: A randomized clinical trial. J Thorac Cardiovasc Surg 1992; 104:284–296.
22. Clark LC Jr, Gollan F: Survival of mammals breathing organic liquids equilibrated with oxygen at atmospheric pressure. Science 1966; 152:1755–1756.
23. Sloviter HA, Kamimoto T: Erythrocyte substitute for perfusion of brain. Nature 1967; 216:458–460.
24. Geyer RP: Whole animals perfusion with fluorocarbon dispersions. Fed Proc 1970; 29:1758–1763.
25. Yokoyama K, Yamanouchi K, Watanabe M, et al: Preparation of perfluorodecalin emulsion, an approach to the red cell substitute. Fed Proc 1975; 34:1478–1483.
26. Markowski H, Tenschev P, Frey R: Tolerance of an oxygen-carrying colloid plasma substitute in humans. *In:* Proceedings of the 4th International Symposium on Perfluorochemical Blood Substitutes, Kyoto, Japan, October 1978. Amsterdam, Excerpta Medica, 1979, pp 47–50.
27. Mitsuno T, Ohyanagi H, Naito R: Clinical studies of a perfluorochemical whole blood substitute (Fluosol-DA)—summary of 186 cases. Ann Surg 1982; 195:60–69.
28. Tremper KK, Friedman AE, Levine EM, et al: The preoperative treatment of severely anemic patients with a perfluorochemical oxygen-transport fluid, Fluosol DA. N Engl J Med 1982; 307:277–283.
29. Waxman K, Tremper KK, Cullen BF, et al: Perfluorocarbon infusion in bleeding patients refusing blood transfusions. Arch Surg 1984; 119:721–724.
30. Police AM, Waxman K, Tominaga G: Pulmonary complications in three patients receiving Fluosol DA-20% following life-threatening blood loss. Crit Care Med 1985; 13:96–98.
31. Vercellotti GM, Hammerschmidt DE, Craddock PR, et al: Activation of plasma complement by perfluorocarbon artificial blood: Probable mechanism of adverse pulmonary reactions in treated patients and rationale for corticosteroid prophylaxis. Blood 1982; 59:1299–1304.
32. Anderson HV, Leimgruber PP, Roubin GS, et al: Distal coronary artery perfusion during percutaneous transluminal coronary angioplasty. Am Heart J 1985; 110:720–726.
33. Cowley MJ, Snow FR, DiSciascio G, et al: Perfluorochemical perfusion during coronary angioplasty in unstable and high-risk patients. Circulation 1990; 81 (Suppl 3):IV27–IV34.
34. Kent KM, Guman MW, Cowley MJ, et al: Reduction in myocardial ischemia during percutaneous transluminal coronary angioplasty with oxygenated fluosol. Am J Cardiol 1990; 66:279–284.
35. Sakai DE, Whittaker MB, Browell NM, Zerves NT: Perfluorocarbons: Recent developments and implications for neurosurgery. J Neurosurg 1996; 85:248–254.
36. Spence RK: Perfluorocarbons in the twenty-first century: Clinical applications as transfusion alternatives. Artif Cells Blood Substit Immobil Biotechnol 1995; 23:367–380.
37. Keipert PE, Faithfull NS, Roth DJ, et al: Supporting tissue oxygenation during acute surgical bleeding using perfluorochemical-based oxygen carrier. Adv Exp Med Biol 1996; 388:603–609.
38. Cernaianu AC, Spence RK, Vassilidze MD, et al: A safety study of a perfluorochemical emulsion, Oxygent™, in anesthetized surgical patients. Anesthesiology 1994; 81:A397.
39. Goodin TH, Grossbard EB, Kaufman RJ, et al: A perfluorochemical emulsion for prehospital resuscitation of experimental hemorrhagic shock: A prospective, randomized controlled study. Crit Care Med 1994; 22:680–689.
40. Wahr JA, Trouwborst RK, Spence RK, et al: A pilot study of the efficacy of an oxygen carrying emulsion, Oxygent™, in patients undergoing surgical blood loss. Anesthesiology 1994; 80:A397.
41. Rabiner SF, Helbert JR, Lopas H, et al: Evaluation of stroma-free hemoglobin solution for use as a plasma expander. J Exp Med 1967; 126:1127–1142.
42. Savitsky JP, Doczi J, Black J, et al: A clinical safety trial of stroma-free hemoglobin. Clin Pharmacol Ther 1978; 23:73–80.
43. Gould SA, Sehgal LR, Sehgal HL, Moss G: The development of hemoglobin solutions as red cell substitutes: Hemoglobin solutions. Transfus Sci 1995; 16:5–17.
44. Hedlund BE, Drayton CP, Alsop DS, et al: Polymerized hemoglobins. *In:* Transfusion Medicine: Recent Technological Advances. Murasaki K, Peetoom F (Eds). New York, Alan R Liss, 1986, pp 39–48.
45. Matsushita M, Yabuki A, Nasu M, et al: Oxygen transport by pyridoxalated-hemoglobin-polyoxyethylene conjugate. ASAIO Trans 1987; 33:352–355.
46. Rabinovici R, Rudolph AS, Ligler FS, et al: Liposome-encapsulated hemoglobin: An oxygen-carrying fluid. Circ Shock 1990; 32:1–17.
47. Reinish LW, Bally MB, Loughrey HC, et al: Interactions of liposomes and platelets. Thromb Haemost 1988; 60:518–523.
48. Rabinovici R, Rudolph AS, Vernick K, et al: A new salutary resuscitative fluid: Liposome-encapsulated hemoglobin/hypertonic saline solution. J Trauma 1993; 35:121–127.
49. Chang TMS: Recent and future developments in modified hemoglobin and microencapsulated hemoglobin as red blood cell substitutes. Artif Cells Blood Substit Immobol Biotechnol 1997; 25:1–24.
50. Feola M, Gonzalez H, Canizaro PC, et al: Development of a bovine stroma-free hemoglobin solution as a blood substitute. Surg Obstet Gynecol 1983; 157:399–408.
51. Feola M, Simoni J, Dobke M, et al: Complement activation and the toxicity of stroma-free hemoglobin solutions in primates. Circ Shock 1988; 25:275–290.
52. Simoni J, Feola M, Canizaro PC: Generation of free oxygen radicals and the toxicity of hemoglobin solutions. Biomater Artif Cells Artif Organs 1990; 18:189–202.
53. Feola M, Simoni J, Angelillo R, et al: Clinical trial of a hemoglobin based blood substitute in patients with sickle cell anemia. Surg Gynecol Obstet 1992; 174:379–386.
54. Nagai K, Thogersen HC: Generation of beta-globin by sequence-specific proteolysis of a hybrid protein produced in *Escherichia coli.* Nature 1984; 309:810–812.
55. Hoffman SJ, Looker DL, Roehrich JM, et al: Expression of fully functional tetrameric human hemoglobin in *Escherichia coli.* Proc Natl Acad Sci U S A 1990; 87:8521–8525.
56. Ogden JE, Coghlan D, Jones G, et al: Expression and assembly of functional human hemoglobin in *S. cerevisiae.* Biomater Artif Cells Immobil Biotechnol 1992; 20:473–475.
57. Looker D, Abbott-Brown D, Cozart P, et al: A human recombinant haemoglobin designed for use as a blood substitute. Nature 1992; 356:258–260.
58. Looker D, Mathews AJ, Neway JO, et al: Expression of recombinant human hemoglobin in *Escherichia coli.* Methods Enzymol 1994; 231:364–374.

59. Behringer RR, Ryan TM, Reilly MP, et al: Synthesis of functional human hemoglobin in transgenic mice. Science 1989; 245:971-973.
60. O'Donnell JK, Martin MJ, Logan JS, et al: Production of human hemoglobin in transgenic swine: An approach to a blood substitute. Cancer Detect 1993; 17:307-312.
61. Greenburg AG, Kim HW: Current status of stroma-free hemoglobin. Adv Surg 1998; 31:149-165.
62. Gould SA, Moore EE, Moore FA, et al: Clinical utility of polymerized hemoglobin as a blood substitute after acute trauma and surgery. J Trauma 1997; 43:325-332.
63. Gould SA, Moore EE, Hoyt DB, et al: The first randomized trial of human polymerized hemoglobin as a blood substitute in acute trauma and emergent surgery. J Am Coll Surg 1998; 187:113-122.
64. Jacobs E Jr, Hughes GS: Update on clinical aspects of polymerized bovine hemoglobin (HBOC-201). Artif Cells Blood Substit Immobil Biotechnol 1996; 24:357A.
65. Wahr JA, Levy JH, Kindsher J, et al: Hemodynamic effects of bovine hemoglobin based oxygen carrying solution in surgical patients. Anesthesiology 1996; 85:A347.
66. Cohn SM: The current status of haemoglobin-based blood substitutes. Ann Med 1997; 29:371-376.
67. Przybelski RJ, Kisicki E, Daily M, et al: Diaspirin cross-linked hemoglobin: Phase I clinical safety assessment in normal healthy volunteers. Crit Care Med 1994; 22:A231.
68. Przybelski RJ, Daily EK, Kisicki JC, et al: Phase I study of the safety and pharmacologic effects of diaspirin cross linked hemoglobin solutions. Crit Care Med 1996; 24:1993-2000.
69. Gullet A, Seen A, Sharma AC, et al: Role of ET and NO in resuscitative effect of dispirin cross-linked hemoglobin after hemorrhage in rat. Am J Physiol 1997; 273:H827-836.
70. Shoemaker S, Gerber M, Evans G, et al: Initial clinical experience with a rationally designed genetically engineered recombinant human hemoglobin. Artif Blood Substit Immobil Biotechnol 1994; 22:457-465.
71. Iwashita Y: Relationship between chemical properties and biological properties of pyridoxalated hemoglobin-polyoxyethylene. Biomater Artif Cells Immobil Biotechnol 1992; 20:299-307.
72. Shorr RG, Viau AT, Abuchowski A: Phase IB safety evaluation of PEG hemoglobin as an adjuvant to radiation therapy in human cancer patients. Artif Cells Blood Substit Immobil Biotechnol 1996; 24:407.

27

Management of Traumatic Brain Injury in the Intensive Care Unit

Gabrielle F. Morris, MD • William R. Taylor, MD
Lawrence F. Marshall, MD

Traumatic brain injury is a leading cause of mortality in patients younger than 45 years, accounting for more than a third of all injury-related deaths in this country. Each year in the United States, 52,000 people die and another 80,000 suffer morbidity from traumatic brain injury.[1] Although more severe injuries are associated with poorer outcomes, the moderately injured patients also are at risk.

Closed head injury is the result of a variety of mechanisms, including motor vehicle and motorcycle accidents, falls from heights, assaults, and pedestrians being struck by motor vehicles. Penetrating injury is most often due to gunshots, but sometimes, other types of blunt objects can violate the skull. Brain injury may result from blast effect of proximal missile wounds or, rarely, as a thermal complication in burn patients. Most commonly, traumatic brain injury occurs in the presence of additional injuries to the other major organ systems, but it can occur in isolation. In particular, the coexistence of spinal injuries with head injury is well recognized.[2]

TABLE 27–1. Glasgow Coma Scale*

Modality	Patient's Best Response	Score
Eye opening (E)	Spontaneously	4
	To voice	3
	To painful stimuli	2
	None	1
Verbal (V)	Oriented and conversant	5
	Disoriented, yet conversant	4
	Inappropriate responses	3
	Incomprehensible sounds	2
	None	1
Motor (M)	Obeys commands	6
	Localizes	5
	Withdraws from pain	4
	Abnormal flexion	3
	Abnormal extension	2
	Flaccid/unresponsive	1
Total score	E + V + M	3-15

*The GCS score is calculated by adding together the patient's best response in the three modalities.

BACKGROUND

Head injuries span the spectrum of severity, ranging from minimal with only a transient loss of consciousness to the complete unresponsiveness of coma. Neurologic examination assesses three major components: level of consciousness, lateralization of motor response, and pupillary reactivity.

Perhaps the most widely recognized method of initial evaluation is the Glasgow Coma Scale (GCS).[3] This simple method is reproducible and allows accurate communication among caregivers. Patients are evaluated in three ways: eye opening, verbal response, and motor response. The total possible scores range from 3 to 15, reflecting totally flaccid unresponsive, through progressively improving, to fully normal level of consciousness. Table 27–1 demonstrates the breakdown of GCS component score values. The GCS does have its limitations, however. It does not include pupillary assessment or readily identify abnormal lateralization of motor findings, both of which are signs highly suggestive of intracranial mass lesion.

A GCS score of 3 to 8 describes severe brain injury. Patients with such scores are in coma and thus unable to interact with their environment. These patients are critically ill and usually require at least several days of maximal therapy in modern intensive care units. The patient with a GCS score of 9 to 12 has a moderate head injury; the patient who has additional systemic injuries may require an intensive level of therapy to ensure maximal neuronal function and recovery. Table 27–2 summarizes the relationship between injury severity and GCS score.

TABLE 27–2. Assessing the Glasgow Coma Scale (GCS) Score Quantifies the Severity of Traumatic Brain Injury (TBI)

GCS	Severity of TBI
13-15	Mild
9-12	Moderate
3-8	Severe

Stabilization and resuscitation of the head-injured patient are a priority,[4] which must then be followed by diagnostic neurologic imaging. Computed tomography (CT) scanning is the diagnostic imaging modality of choice.[2, 5] It can be performed within a matter of minutes and is noninvasive. The cost is acceptable. Computerized reconstruction of the CT slices allows visualization of the skull, brain, and components with sufficient anatomic detail to initiate therapy. The various brain regions are detailed with CT, allowing detection of hematomas, fractures, shift of the midline structures, evaluation of the basilar cisterns, and quantification of any mass effect.[6, 7]

Initial laboratory studies should include evaluation of the arterial blood gases and coagulation parameters in addition to the standard complete blood count, electrolyte quantification, and drug screening.[3]

PATHOPHYSIOLOGY

Primary brain injury is the direct result of the disruptive forces that are transmitted during impact. Hematomas can occur in any intracranial space or potential space. Alternatively, axons can be sheared. Unfortunately, the best therapy for brain injury is prevention. Subsequently, treatment may encompass medical rather than surgical management.[8]

Secondary brain injury is a term used to encompass all of the events after the actual traumatic event that exacerbate the brain injury and combine to worsen patient outcome. The injured brain has been repeatedly shown to be far more intolerant of secondary insults than the uninjured brain. Within the last decade, particular emphasis has been placed on the potentially treatable conditions of hypotension and hypoxia. Clinical studies have demonstrated that as little as one episode of hypotension can determine whether the ultimate outcome will be a persistent vegetative state, death, or a meaningful quality of life.[9] Thus, these insults must be continuously prevented and aggressively treated if they occur. It is in this realm where the critical care specialist has the potential to make the greatest impact on the long-term outcome of brain-injured patients.

Traumatic injury can occur to a focal brain region or more diffusely, affecting both hemispheres and the brain stem. The severity and distribution of injury are related to the traumatic mechanism, force vectors, and brain anatomy. *Diffuse axonal injury* is a form of global injury and occasionally is of sufficient severity to render patients immediately comatose. In such severe cases, it is caused by shearing forces affecting axons that traverse large areas of the brain stem, leading to dysfunction of the reticular activating system. Affected patients have a high mortality and, if they survive, a high morbidity, often improving only to a persistent vegetative state.[2, 3, 5] In clinical practice, however, diffuse axonal injury and focal brain injury often coexist. Cerebral edema and brain swelling are additional examples of pathologic diffuse injuries that increase intracranial pressure (ICP) and alter consciousness (Fig. 27–1).[10]

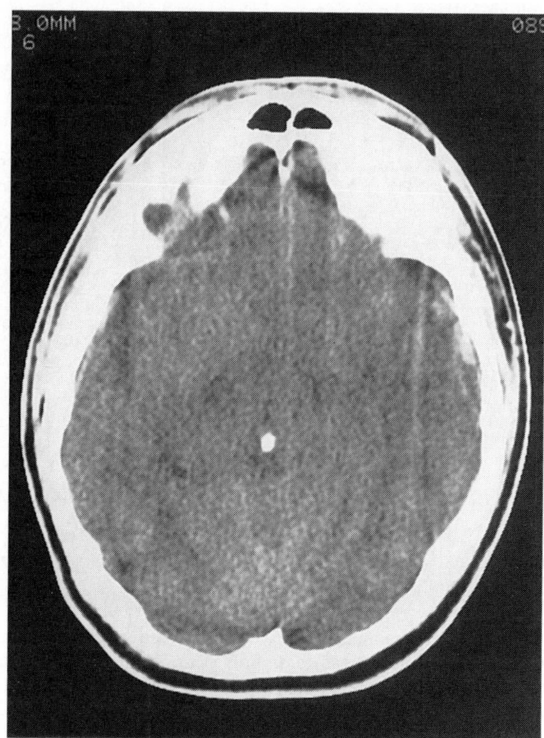

Figure 27–1. Severe diffuse axonal injury. The brain is markedly edematous and has lost all definition of its internal architecture. The patient was rendered comatose at the time of impact.

Intracranial hemorrhage occurs commonly in association with moderate and severe head injuries and usually produces mass lesions. Therapy often is surgical, directed at removing the hematoma and thereby decreasing intracranial volume. In general, masses greater than 20 to 25 mL require evacuation.[2, 3, 5, 11] Regional occurrence and distribution of the hemorrhage influence management. Thus, there are cases in which smaller lesions may be excised but larger ones may be observed.[20]

Epidural hematomas, occurring on the outer surface of the brain's protective coverings in association with skull fractures, are usually of arterial origin. With prompt evacuation of epidural hematomas, patients often have a relatively favorable outcome. With subdural hematomas, however, the force of impact is often transmitted to the brain itself. In approximately 80% of subdural hematomas, it is the underlying brain injury that determines the patient's course and outcome. Hematoma can also accumulate within the brain substance as intraparenchymal hemorrhage or a contusion. The management of these mass lesions is the most controversial. Understandably, many neurosurgeons are reluctant to traverse normal brain tissue in order to reach and remove these lesions (Fig. 27–2).[11-14]

Initially recognized years ago, traumatic subarachnoid hemorrhage (tSAH) is currently enjoying resurgent interest. Widespread availability of today's improved CT scanners has resulted in better detection of this type of intracranial bleeding. Traumatic subarachnoid hemorrhage is not a true mass lesion; rather, it is more diffuse layering of blood collecting in the subarachnoid space. Thus, it does not lend itself to surgical evacuation. The higher morbidity and mortality associated with tSAH, seen as a worse neurologic prognosis, have been clearly shown. This is not related to the volume of blood per se; rather, prognosis is determined by the distribution of subarachnoid hemorrhage and by accompanying mass lesions.[15-17]

The presence of a skull fracture implies that a large amount of force was transmitted to the patient's head. Fractures of the cranial vault can be linear or comminuted and may occur in combination with skin disruption. The skull base itself can be fractured. When such fractures occur, they may be associated with external cerebral spinal fluid (CSF) leakage (rhinorrhea or otorrhea), hearing loss, or facial palsy.[2, 3, 5]

The osseous skull is a solid vault that cannot expand. It has only three contents: brain, blood, and CSF. For the accommodation of additional volume, such as a post-traumatic hematoma, there must be compression of one of these components. The volume increase results in a rise in ICP, as described by

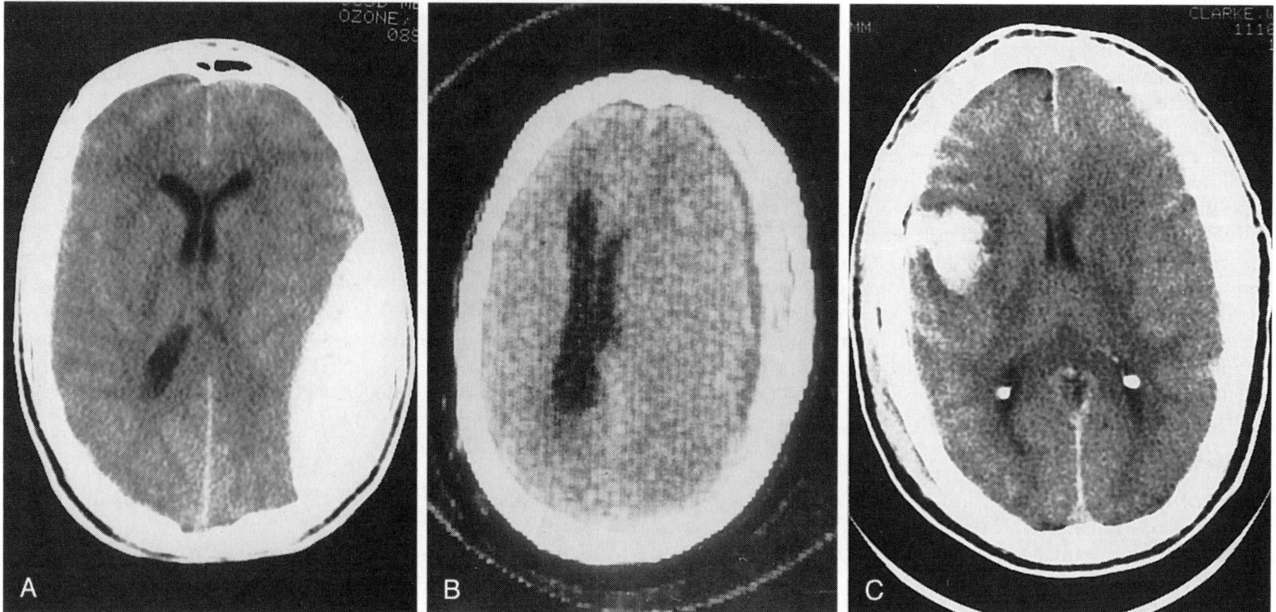

Figure 27–2. Focal traumatic brain injury as seen on the CT scans of three different patients. *A*, Characteristic biconvex shape of an epidural hematoma, a lesion that most commonly occurs with a skull fracture. *B*, This subdural hematoma is associated with significant underlying brain injury and an impressive shift of the midline structures resulting from the mass effect. *C*, A parenchymal contusion is behaving like a mass lesion coexisting with traumatic subarachnoid hemorrhage in the sulci of the brain's surface.

the Monro-Kelly doctrine: ICP is proportionally equal to the sum of the volume of the intracranial contents.[18]

Initially, this relationship is linear; masses can be compensated for either by the displacement of CSF through the foramen magnum into the lumbar cistern or by a hyperventilation-induced decrease in cerebral blood flow. Once these compensatory mechanisms are overwhelmed, the pressure-volume curve dramatically changes to an exponential relationship, as shown in Figure 27–3. The increased ICP causes shifting of the brain itself, known as *herniation*. It is imperative to identify patients at risk for herniation prior to this occurrence.[19]

Depression of the level of consciousness results from (1) extensive areas of hemispheric injury, (2) direct brain stem compression during herniation, or (3) actual brain stem injury diffusely affecting the reticular activating system. [20]

The normal brain has an exquisite ability to maintain cerebral blood flow over the range of mean arterial blood pressures. This phenomenon is known as *autoregulation*. Acute injury impairs the brain's ability for accurate autoregulation. The result is an increase in the brain's sensitivity to blood pressures that might otherwise be acceptable. Hypotension is potentially dangerous in patients with defective autoregulation and warrants immediate treatment.[21]

NEUROCHEMISTRY OF BRAIN INJURY

A number of biochemical substances have been postulated to play a major role in the propagation of neural injury. The release of these substances initiates a deleterious cascade of continued cell membrane breakdown and ionic shifts that further harm the injured brain. These substances include cytokines and free radicals. Additionally, excessive activity of the excitatory amino acids glutamate and aspartate have been implicated as etiologic agents in neural injury. Obviously, many neurochemical derangements occur simultaneously, and it is likely that the further progression of brain injury is due to a combination of these processes, which may adversely interact. A common pathway for some of these processes is calcium ion entry into the cell, a well-known mechanism of cell death in ischemia.[22-23]

CRITICAL CARE MANAGEMENT

The treatment of head injury must emphasize prevention of secondary insults to the already compromised brain tissue. All interventions must take into account the potential side effects of treatment on the patient's overall physiologic status. The severity of the primary injury, the presence of associated

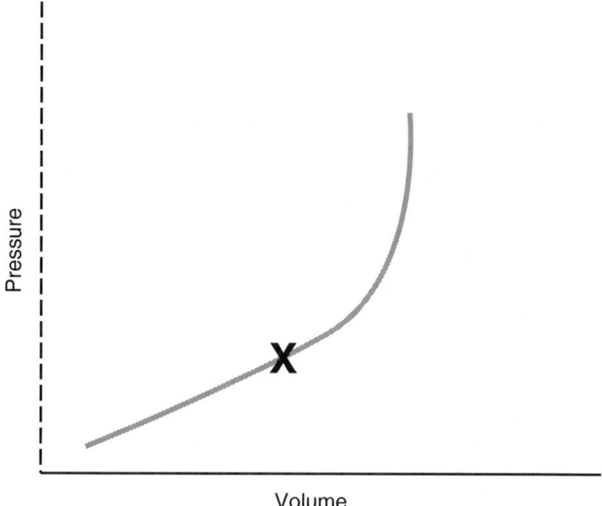

Figure 27–3. This graph of the intracranial pressure-volume relationship demonstrates the two phases of the brain's reaction to intracranial masses. Initially, compensatory mechanisms are effective; this portion of the curve is linear. When these mechanisms are overwhelmed, the curve becomes exponential in its contour, indicating that small changes in volume result in dramatic changes in intracranial pressure and, hence, significant neurologic deterioration.

injuries, and the patient's age are all pertinent to clinical decision making. The goal is to prevent all instances of secondary injury. With a high index of suspicion and consistent surveillance, prevention is optimized, and any insults can be rapidly corrected.[24]

Severely head-injured patients with GCS scores of 8 or less are by definition in a coma and require both airway protection and intensive care therapy to treat intracranial hypertension. Moderately head-injured patients (GCS score 9–12) often also need these modalities, particularly in the presence of CT scan abnormalities indicating raised ICP. For both groups, the course of treatment in the intensive care unit (ICU) can be prolonged.

The initial resuscitation and stabilization of a patient with head injury begin with attention to the "ABCs" of trauma common to all acutely injured patients: *a*irway, *b*reathing, and *c*irculation. The modifications for brain trauma are judicious use of intravenous fluids, and maintaining the cervical spine in alignment while securing the airway. Neurologic examination and diagnostic imaging are performed for classification of head injury and to initiate appropriate treatment.[4] At this time, the decision must be made for immediate intracranial surgical intervention or initial medical management. In general, surgical indications are

- Mass lesions greater than 20 to 25 mL
- Epidural hematomas, in most cases
- Open, depressed skull fractures

In the presence of contusions or intraparenchymal hematomas, the ICP is an additional guiding factor.[2, 3, 13, 14]

When intracranial surgery is elected, preparation of the patient must include an assessment of coagulation parameters and availability of blood products for transfusion. Clear communication with the anesthesia team will help prevent incidences of secondary injury, such as hypotension and hypoxia. For the injured brain, it is preferable to maintain the following parameters[3, 8]:

- Hematocrit value above 30%
- Normal prothrombin and partial thromboplastin times
- Platelet count greater than 70,000
- Arterial oxygen tension above 80 mm Hg
- Arterial carbon dioxide tension at 35 to 40 mm Hg (unless an individualized decision for hyperventilation is made by the operating neurosurgeon; see next)

These concepts are incorporated into the ICU admitting orders. Laboratory evaluation of head injury requires special emphasis on serum sodium and arterial blood gas values, coagulation parameters, and the hemogram. The blood glucose level should be tightly controlled to between 80 and 200 mg/dL, as both hypoglycemia and hyperglycemia may be associated with worse neurologic outcome. Dextrose-containing intravenous (IV) fluids are avoided. Particular attention must be paid to the patient's blood pressure; specifically, the systolic pressure should be maintained at a minimum of 100 mm Hg, and the mean arterial pressure (MAP) above 80 mm Hg if possible, to ensure adequate cerebral perfusion (detailed in subsequent discussion). The injured brain tends to absorb free water disproportionately from hypotonic solutions; thus, only isotonic fluids, such as normal saline or lactated Ringer's solution, can be used safely. Prophylaxis for peptic ulceration and deep venous thrombosis should be given in accordance with accepted protocols. Standard nursing care for invasive lines and monitors decreases the risk of subsequent infection. Early nutritional support is routine.[3, 8]

ICP monitoring is instituted in patients with severe head injuries and in those with moderate head injuries who manifest abnormal CT scans suggestive of raised ICP. Monitoring can be accomplished with either a fiberoptic intraparenchymal monitor of the Camino type or a ventriculostomy. The latter, although more invasive, has the notable advantage of providing a route for CSF aspiration, a therapeutic modality for ICP elevations. Treatment is instituted for ICP of 20 mm Hg or higher and may involve a combination of modalities, such as sedation, pharmacologic paralysis, mannitol, barbiturates, and cautious hyperventilation.

ICP is optimized in order to maximize cerebral perfusion. Cerebral perfusion pressure (CPP) is calculated by subtracting the ICP value from the MAP value. Studies suggest that it may be beneficial to treat the two parameters in concert, with the goal of keeping ICP less than 20 mm Hg while maintaining the CPP at more than 65 to 70 mm Hg. This goal can usually be attained through fluid resuscitation and careful supplementation with small quantities of vasopressors.[3, 8]

Initial therapy to lower elevated ICP includes nursing patients with the head of bed elevated 30° and ascertaining that the cervical collar is well-fitting and is not obstructing venous drainage.[25] Pharmacologic therapy begins with the use of sedatives. These can be supplemented by intermittent paralytic agents only if they are clearly needed. Persistent intracranial hypertension refractory to these measures requires intermittent, targeted therapy.[26, 27]

External drainage of CSF is a direct maneuver to treat intracranial hypertension. Decreasing the intracranial volume by even a few milliliters causes an exponential decrement in ICP. This result can be effective for a variable period, with some limitation due to continuous recirculation and production of CSF.

Mannitol is an osmotic diuretic that effectively reduces ICP. It must be used cautiously, with strict attention to the patient's volume status and electrolyte balance. Intermittent boluses appear to be more effective than continuous infusions. Prolonged use of mannitol leads to elevations in serum osmolarity and hypernatremia, both of which may limit this therapy. The patient also must have an adequate starting intravascular volume, lest the mannitol cause precipitous decreases in blood pressure and secondary brain injury. Note that any correction of serum sodium abnormalities needs to be performed slowly in order to prevent central pontine myelinolysis, an intracranial complication.[3, 8]

Hyperventilation reduces the arterial carbon dioxide tension ($Paco_2$), leading to vasoconstriction of the cerebral vessels. The vasoconstriction diminishes intracranial volume and, correspondingly, the ICP. Formerly a mainstay of ICP management, hyperventilation is used today on a more limited basis. It is not an appropriate modality for prophylaxis of ICP problems in the first 24 hours after injury. Rather, during this time, patients are managed with a $Paco_2$ target goal of 35 to 40 mm Hg, low normal. If elevated ICP is a problem requiring intervention, the treatment range should be to a $Paco_2$ of 32 to 35 mm Hg, and only in very exceptional circumstances are lower levels acceptable. Therapy should be guided by the results of ICP monitoring. In fact, lower $Paco_2$ values are deleterious, particularly in elderly patients.[8]

Barbiturates are used in selected instances for ICP reduction and perhaps for brain protection. These agents also induce hypothermia and decrease brain metabolic demands. Pentobarbital is the long-acting agent utilized for this purpose. The drug is not benign, and a thorough familiarity with its side effects is mandatory for any physician ordering its administration. Potent vasodilatation and cardiac depression occur, for which Swan-Ganz catheter monitoring is helpful in management. Pneumonia and other respiratory complications are common.[28]

Propofol, a sedative-hypnotic agent, reduces cerebral metabolism, cerebral blood flow, and ICP. This compound has been increasingly utilized for brain protection and as adjuvant ICP treatment in severe head injury. The expense of this agent may be a limiting factor in its use. The lipid load to the patient must also be considered.[29]

Intractable ICP should raise the suspicion that there has been an alteration in intracranial pathology. Repeat CT scanning may be needed to rule out interval enlargement of existing hematomas or the delayed development of new lesions. If any of these changes occurs, surgical therapy may become necessary. Repeat imaging at regular intervals is routine in postoperative patients and in patients with parenchymal contusions. It is less commonly revealing in the patient with diffuse axonal injury or whole brain edema.[2, 3, 13]

The utilization of anticonvulsants has evolved in the last few years. For severe and moderate head injuries, seizure prophylaxis is recommended for concurrent intracranial hematomas and immediately perioperatively. Duration of therapy today is shorter. In the absence of documented or suspected seizure activity, seizure medications are then tapered off.[8]

A number of trials have failed to show any benefit to head-injured patients from the use of corticosteroids. Thus, at this time, glucocorticoids have no role in the management of traumatic brain injury.[2, 3, 8]

During the last 10 years, there have been several disappointing international clinical trials of experimental pharmaceutical agents for the therapy of head injury. Free-radical scavengers, aminosteroids, and *N*-methyl-*D*-aspartate (NMDA) receptor antagonists were evaluated.[30-32] These three studies may have suffered from a common methodologic problem, the lack of ability to classify patients on the basis of known poor prognostic variables. However, it remains an accurate statement that currently, there is no single medical therapy for brain injury.

Evidence-Based Recommendations for Care in Traumatic Brain injury

The Brain Trauma Foundation, in collaboration with the Joint Section on Neurotrauma, in 1995 published evidence-based recommendations for the care of patients with brain trauma, entitled *Guidelines for the Management of Severe Head Injury*.[8] Many of their recommendations are reflected in the foregoing discussion. This booklet is an invaluable resource for the neurotraumatologist or critical care practitioner charged with treatment of acute head injuries.

PROGNOSIS AND OUTCOME

The extent of recovery from traumatic brain injury varies with the patient's age, the severity of the injury, and the type of intracranial disorder. In general, recovery is slow. More severely injured patients often benefit from in-patient rehabilitation and can then be gradually reintegrated with day school programs. Participation in such programs requires recovery to the point of being able to follow commands.

Outcome is usually assessed 6 months after injury and is based on the patient's cognitive function, independence, ability to care for self, and motor coordination. Detailed neuropsychologic testing can be used in the higher-functioning patient; it often illustrates subclinical deficits that are pertinent and can interfere with the patient's ability to successfully return to employment.[33, 34]

SUMMARY

The recent decades have brought technologic advances that have improved the delivery of health care. Patients who arrive at modern-day trauma centers are more critically ill than before. Rapid stabilization and accurate diagnostic assessment have become routine. Despite these impressive changes in the delivery of trauma care, the outcome of severe traumatic brain injury remains less than ideal. Currently, there are no definitive pharmacologic agents for therapy. Prevention is the only truly effective therapy for both primary and secondary brain injuries. The key factor for head-injured patients is secondary injury, which must be prevented whenever possible and aggressively treated if it does occur.

References

1. Sosin DM, Sniezek JE, Waxweiler RJ: Trends in death associated with traumatic brain injury, 1979 through 1992. JAMA 1995; 22:1778–1780.
2. Becker DP, Gudeman SK: Textbook of Head Injury. Philadelphia, WB Saunders, 1989.
3. Marshall SB, Marshall LF, Vos HR, et al: Neuroscience Critical Care: Pathophysiology and Patient Management. Philadelphia, WB Saunders, 1990.
4. American College of Surgeons Committee on Trauma: Advanced Trauma Life support Course for Physicians, 1993 Instructor Manual. Chicago, American College of Surgeons, 1993.
5. Cooper PR (Ed). Head Injury. 3rd ed. Baltimore, Williams & Wilkins, 1993.
6. Osborn AG: Diagnostic Neuroradiology. St. Louis, Mosby-Year Book, 1994.
7. Marshall LF, Marshall SB, Klauber MR, et al: A new classification of head injury based on computerized tomography. J Neurosurg 1991; 75:S14–S20.
8. Bullock R, Chesnut RM, Clifton G, et al: Guidelines for the Management of Severe Head Injury. Park Ridge, Ill, American Association of Neurological Surgeons, 1995.
9. Chesnut RM, Marshall SB, Piek J, et al: Early and late systemic hypertension as a frequent and fundamental source of cerebral ischemia following severe brain injury in the Trauma Coma Data Bank. Acta Neurochir Suppl (Wien) 1993; 59:121–125.
10. Ito J, Marmarou A, Barzo P, et al: Characterization of edema by diffusion-weighted imaging in experimental traumatic brain injury. J Neurosurg 1996; 84:97–103.
11. Wilkins RH, Rengachary SS: Neurosurgery. 2nd ed. New York, McGraw-Hill, 1996.
12. Eisenberg HM, Gary HE Jr, Aldrich EF, et al: Initial CT findings in 753 patients with severe head injury: A report from the NIH Traumatic Coma Data Bank. J Neurosurg 1990; 73:688–698.
13. Servadei F, Nanni A, Nasi MT, et al: Evolving brain lesions in the first 12 hours after head injury: Analysis of 37 comatose patients. Neurosurgery 1995; 37:899–906.
14. Solonuik D, Pitts LH, Lovely M, et al: Traumatic intracerebral hematomas: Timing of appearance and indications for operative removal. J Trauma 1986; 26:787–794.
15. Greene KA, Marciano FF, Johnson BA, et al: The impact of traumatic subarachnoid hemorrhage on outcome in non-penetrating head injury: Part I. A proposed CT grading scale. J Neurosurg 1995; 83:445.
16. Martin NA, Doberstein C, Zane C, et al: Posttraumatic cerebral arterial spasm: Transcranial Doppler ultrasound, cerebral blood flow, and angiographic findings. J Neurosurg 1992; 77:57.
17. Morris GF, Marshall LF: A new, practical classification of traumatic subarachnoid hemorrhage (Abstract). Acta Neurochir Suppl (Wien) 1998; 71:382.
18. Monro A: Observations on the Structure and Function of the Nervous System. Edinburgh, Creech and Johnson, 1783.
19. Miller JD, Pickard JD: Intracranial volume/pressure studies in patients with head injury. Injury 1974; 5:265–268.
20. Andrew BT, Chiles BW, Olsen WL, et al: The effect of intracerebral hematoma location on the risk of brain-stem compression and on clinical outcome. J Neurosurg 1988; 69:518–522.
21. Bouma GJ, Muizelaar JP: Relationship between cardiac output and cerebral blood flow in patients with intact and with impaired autoregulation. J Neurosurg 1990; 73:368–374.
22. Marshall LF, Marshall SB: Pharmacologic therapy: Promising clinical investigations. New Horiz 1995; 3(3):573–580.
23. Siesjo BK: Pathophysiology and treatment of focal cerebral ischemia. J Neurosurg 1992; 77:169–184.
24. Chesnut RM, Marshall LF, Klauber MR, et al: The role of secondary

brain injury in determining outcome from severe head injury. J Trauma 1993; 34:216–222.
25. Hulme A, Cooper R: The effects of head position and jugular vein compression ion intracranial pressure. *In:* Intracranial Pressure: III. Beks J, et al (Eds). Berlin, Springer-Verlag, 1976, pp 259–263.
26. Chiolero RL, de Tribolet N: Sedatives and antagonists in the management of severely head-injured patients (Review). Acta Neurochir Suppl (Wien) 1992; 55:43–46.
27. Hsiang JK, Chesnut RM, Crisp CB, et al: Early, routine paralysis for intracranial pressure control in severe head injury: Is it necessary? Crit Care Med 1994; 22:1471–1476.
28. Marshall LF, Smith RW, Shapiro HM: The outcome with aggressive treatment in severe head injuries: Acute and chronic barbiturate administration. J Neurosurg, 1979; 50:26.
29. Ravussin P, Strebel S: Propofol for neuroanesthesia. Anaesthesist 1995; 44:405–409.
30. Young B, Runge JW, Waxman KS, et al: Effects of pegorgotein on neurologic outcome of patients with severe head injury: A multicenter, randomized controlled trial. JAMA 1996; 276:538–543.
31. Maas A, Willis GN, Largarigue J, et al: A multicenter trial on the efficacy of tirilazad mesylate in cases of head injury. J Neurosurg 1998; 89:519–525.
32. Morris GF, Bullock R, Marshall SB, et al: Failure of the competitive NMDA antagonist selfotel (CGS 19755) in the management of severe head injury. J Neurosurg (in press).
33. Marshall LF, Smith RW, Shapiro HM: The outcome with aggressive treatment in severe head injuries. Part I. J Neurosurg 1979; 50:20.
34. Marshall LF, Smith RW, Shapiro HM: The outcome with aggressive treatment in severe head injuries. Part II. J Neurosurg 1979; 50:26.

28

Modern Management of Acute Spinal Cord Injury

Gabrielle F. Morris, MD • William R. Taylor, MD

Spinal cord injury (SCI) results in immediate, traumatic, and often permanent change in lifestyle and occupation. The most common cause is traumatic instability of the spinal column. The cost to the individual patient and society is enormous. The incidence of SCI has diminished recently to approximately 50 injuries per 1 million patients, almost a 25% reduction in the last 10 to 15 years. Despite this reduction, this remains a costly and permanently debilitating injury with roughly 250,000 survivors each year.[1]

Assessment and treatment of spine-injured patients warrant concerted attention directed to the spinal column and, specifically, the spinal cord. Manipulation of one can directly affect the other. Maintaining the structural integrity of the spinal column, which provides osseus foundation, allows both protection and structural support. Articulation supplemented by ligaments and muscles, both anteriorly and posteriorly, enables the multiple planes of motion while maintaining spinal cord integrity.[2, 3] The question of stability relates to this articulation and is defined as the ability of the spine to tolerate physiologic loads without the development of neurologic deficit, deformity, or progressive pain.[4] The neural elements include the spinal cord, nerve roots, and integrity of the dura common.

DIAGNOSIS AND EVALUATION

Complete examination assesses the patient's neurologic function and can define the integrity of the spinal column. With the patient adequately immobilized, physical and radiographic evaluations are performed. The extent of injury varies; patients with *complete* injury have no neurologic function distal to the level of injury; patients with *incomplete* injury have partial preservation of spinal cord function. Incomplete injuries tend to occur in characteristic syndromes (see later).[5]

Plain radiographs are the ideal screening tests. Computed tomographic (CT) scanning, commonly accompanied by sagittal reconstructions, is useful for further delineation of known pathology and is particularly demonstrative for bony definition. Magnetic resonance imaging (MRI) is more commonly used now in SCI than in past years. Rapid-sequence scanning provides detailed soft-tissue information concerning the ligaments, substance of the spinal cord, and disk protrusions to facilitate clinical decision making. These modalities are used in coordination with each other and thus help in treatment planning.[6, 7]

Two noncontiguous injuries of the spine occur in up to 15% of patients. Thus, the presence of one spine injury mandates a full radiographic evaluation of the entire spinal axis from occiput to sacrum.[8] In addition, the coexistence of head injury and SCI is a common sequela of modern transportation.[9] It is mandatory to screen spine-injured patients for head injury and to screen head-injury patients for SCI.

TYPES OF INJURY

Neurologic Injury

Neurologic injury may be permanent or transient, and sequential examinations are mandatory. Absence of any modality of function below the level of injury defines the completeness of that SCI. In the mature adult, such injury has little chance for significant recovery, and all treatment must be directed toward preventing progression or avoiding complications secondary to the injury.[10]

Incomplete SCI demonstrates variable degrees of expected recovery, and tends to occur in specific patterns. The *central cord syndrome* is well delineated and occurs commonly in the upper cervical spine in the older patient with known spinal cord stenosis. This injury delineates a much worse upper-extremity than lower-extremity function and weakness greatest in the distal upper extremity. The injury is often accompanied by painful dysesthesias of the hands, which may remain a significant residual sequela.

The *anterior spinal artery syndrome* is thought to occur secondary to disruption of the blood supply to the anterior spinal artery and can occur in a patient of any age. The debilitating nature of this injury is predicted by the spinal cord anatomy because the anterior spinal artery supplies all functions save for the dorsal column functions, which are supplied by the posterior spinal artery. The result is significant motor deficits with sparing only of the posteriorly carried sensory functions.

A hemisection of the cord, or *Brown-Séquard syndrome*, is the classic diagnosis in which a contralateral pain and temperature loss are found with ipsilateral motor dysfunction. In the lower spinal cord around the conus medullaris, an injury often presents with a significant bowel and bladder abnormality with an intermediate prognosis for recovery. A better prognosis is seen in injuries related to isolated nerve roots or that involve the cauda equina.[10, 11]

Spinal Axis

When injured, any of the musculoskeletal components—bone, ligament, or disk—may result in spinal instability and injury. Osseous injuries tend to heal well with immobilization. Ligamentous injury often confers abnormal motion and deformity, and operative stabilization is generally required. External orthoses in these cases may be required for supplementation of support postoperatively.[5] Until definitive surgical or nonoperative management can be rendered, the patients are nursed in the supine position in axial alignment. The Roto-Rest bed[12] is one commonly available adjunct specifically designed for patients with a SCI. This bed allows accompanying external traction that maintains axial stability while maximizing pulmonary function and skin integrity and allows continued nursing care to proceed unimpeded in the patient.[9]

PHYSICAL EXAMINATION

In the presence of significant SCI, clinicians must have an elevated index of suspicion for additional injuries. Patients whose neural injuries render them asensate cannot complain of the pain associated with distal extremity fractures or the development of an acute abdomen.[8] Specific concern is addressed with upper cervical SCIs and the respiratory system. The loss of accessory musculature for respiratory support can cause a rapid deterioration in the pulmonary status of the patient. This loss occasionally forces rapid intubation in the setting of cervical SCI. Thus, any change in the pulmonary status must be anticipated rather than reacted to.[9] Fiberoptic intubation or nasotracheal airway management is often required.

PATHOPHYSIOLOGY

Most of the energy delivered to the spinal cord occurs at the time of impact. This energy is then translated into spinal cord damage, which further continues with spinal cord swelling and loss of function. The cord itself can be involved both with disruption of the axonal or myelin tracts and by damage to the vascular supply resulting in hemorrhage within the cord. In the setting of acute injury, it remains paramount to maintain cord perfusion and to maintain normal parameters in the other organ systems. The pulmonary status is adversely affected by the injury. The loss of the accessory muscle function increases the work of breathing. In addition, diminished strength of cough increases problems with mucous plugging and increases susceptibility to infection. This can cause further deterioration by lowering oxygen-delivering capacity to the injured spinal cord.

The cardiovascular system is affected as it pertains to the imbalance of the sympathetic and parasympathetic outflow from the spinal cord. Unopposed parasympathetic activity results in hypotension and bradycardia, producing spinal shock, and perfusion problems can result. Autonomic dysreflexia as it affects the cardiovascular system is also not uncommon in the acute setting. The patient's temperature must also be maintained as normal as possible to avoid further energy wasting through shivering and to allow improved function of remaining organ systems.[9, 10]

MANAGEMENT

Spinal Cord

Because there is no cure available to reverse the devastation of acute and chronic SCI, medical management must focus on preventing secondary injury to the spinal cord and maintaining organ systems to prevent pulmonary, gastrointestinal, and cardiovascular complications. The first response is initiated by the team in the field as it pertains to immobilization. This immobilization should continue as the patient is brought into the emergency department and then transferred to the intensive care unit (ICU).[8] At this time, pending the type of injury, x-ray examination is often performed in the emergency department, and the patient is then placed into traction and on a Roto-Rest bed[12] to maintain pulmonary status and axial immobilization.

Perfusion to the spinal cord is enhanced to help rescue those neurons in the ischemic penumbra (partially injured neurons that may have a chance for functional recovery). To maintain this cord perfusion, the physician maintains mean arterial blood pressure above 80 to 85 mm Hg. This is initially accomplished with volume resuscitation; in most cases, this is all that is required. In a subset of patients, especially those maintaining spinal shock for a prolonged time, pharmacologic pressors or vagolytic agents must be judiciously used. The alpha agonists remain a secondary choice in this setting because of the interruption of the sympathetic chain.[13]

High-dose corticosteroids have been beneficial in long-term functional outcome of spine-injured patients. Treated patients have shown improvement to a level of one or two dermatomes in both the sensory and motor examinations. The 24-hour methylprednisolone protocol remains the standard of care and is the most common drug used. The initial dose is given as a bolus of 30 mg/kg during 15 minutes, no infusion is given for 45 minutes, and then a continuous infusion is given at a rate of 5.4 mg/kg/hour for the next 23 hours. The sooner the protocol is initiated after injury, the better the likelihood of improvement. If there is a delay of more than 8 hours after injury, the methylprednisolone protocol should not be used because it worsens outcome and results in increased complications.[14]

Systemic Medical Issues

Because SCI affects multiple organ systems, invasive monitoring is usually required. The patient should have a Foley catheter, large-bore intravenous access, and central venous pressure monitoring. In older patients, a pulmonary artery catheter may be substituted. An arterial line should be placed for optimal blood pressure management and for assessment of arterial blood gases. [15] The patient with an upper cervical spinal injury is at specific risk for pulmonary complications, namely, mucous plugging and pneumonia. Antibiotic treatment and bronchoscopy should be initiated rapidly. [16]

Attention to nitrogen balance and the institution of nutritional supplementation are necessary immediately. Most patients can be provided with nasogastric or oral feedings. Although it is not usually necessary to include the use of parenteral nutrition, in some patients the interruption of the spinal cord causes severe gastrointestinal dysfunction; in these patients, the use of total parenteral nutrition at the earliest possible time is mandatory.[17]

Meticulous care of the skin is crucial because skin breakdown and decubitus ulcer formation are very common in SCI patients, with substantial resultant morbidity. It is particularly important to assess the skin under and around external orthoses. High priority must also be given to the prevention of both peptic ulcers and deep venous thrombosis. Parenteral H_2 blockers are instituted early. Sequential pneumatic compression devices are often used in conjunction with subcutaneous heparin therapy. This measure can be supplemented with low-molecular-weight dextran or vena caval umbrella devices in high-risk patients. As with all interventional procedures, one must consider the risk-benefit ratio.[18]

Spinal Axis and Surgical Treatment

In the presence of a spinal axis injury, immobilization continues until definitive management occurs. If surgical stabilization is required, it should be performed in the most expeditious manner available that will preclude further damage to the spinal cord. Deterioration after the initial injury is the only absolute indication for early intervention; however, in most studies early surgical intervention has allowed the patient to have fewer hospital complications and to be transferred to rehabilitation sooner. There is no difference in overall outcome between the early and late surgical patient because intraoperative complications are substituted for hospital-acquired complications. In most SCI centers, in patients without acute neurologic deterioration, surgery is performed either before 24 to 36 hours or 3 to 5 days after injury.[2, 5, 19]

PROGNOSIS AND OUTCOME

In the mature adult, a patient with a complete SCI has little chance for recovery; in the younger population, however, even presentation with a complete injury does not preclude a significant improvement at 1 to 2 years. Approximately 25% of the younger population show marked functional improvement after presenting with a complete injury.[20]

An patient with an incomplete SCI has a much improved prognosis. Partial to full recovery is certainly possible, and the majority of patients tend to improve over time.

Central cord syndrome routinely shows early motor improvement, yet residual deficits of hand weakness and fine motor movements may preclude return to usual activities and occupation. Conus lesions and cauda equina and nerve root injuries have an improved prognosis for recovery of full function but may take months to years before reaching a final plateau.

Vascular injuries, such as of an anterior spinal artery, tend to show poor recovery, and the prognosis for a Brown-Séquard injury is mixed. Even partial improvements are beneficial in the long term for this devastating injury. An improvement of a dermatome level in a patient may signal the return of hand function. Often, patchy sensory recovery can allow the patient to avoid many skin integrity complications and sepsis. Every effort should be made toward placing the patient in an appropriate rehabilitation setting as early as possible.[10, 11]

FUTURE DIRECTIONS

Current research in the area of SCI remains active. The role of growth factors and neurotrophic factors is only beginning to be recognized and becoming clinically applicable. There is early promise with nerve regeneration technique in animal models. To date, transplantation results have been disappointing, yet efforts are continuing in that direction.[21-23]

Experimental protocols for pharmacologic treatment are proceeding with various classes of agents, such as free radical scavengers, excitatory amino acid inhibitors, and others. Results of these trials should be available in the near future.

SUMMARY

The last several years have delivered significant improvements in the management of SCI. These include foremost prevention along with improved emergency diagnosis and treatment. Improved surgical stabilization techniques have facilitated early mobilization of the patient, which has reduced hospital-acquired complications and allowed patients to begin rehabilitation earlier. At this time, however, prevention remains the only effective therapy and should be actively supported by organized medicine.

References

1. Sosin DM, Sniezek JE, Waxweiler RJ: Trends in death associated with traumatic brain injury, 1979 through 1992. JAMA 1995; 22:1778–1780.
2. Rothman RH, Simeone FA: The Spine. 3rd ed. Philadelphia, WB Saunders, 1992.
3. Menezes AH, Sonntag VKH: Principles of Spinal Surgery. New York, McGraw-Hill, 1996.
4. White AA, Panjabi MM: Clinical Biomechanics of the Spine. 2nd ed. Philadelphia, JB Lippincott, 1990.
5. Rea GL, Miller CA: Spinal Trauma: Current Evaluation and Management. Park Ridge, Ill, American Association of Neurological Surgeons, 1993.
6. Osborn AG: Diagnostic Neuroradiology. St Louis, Mosby, 1994.
7. Chakeres DW, Flickinger F, Bresnahan JC, et al: MR imaging of acute spinal cord trauma. Am J Neuroradiol 1987; 8:5–10.
8. American College of Surgeons Committee on Trauma: Advanced Trauma Life Support Course for Physicians: Instructor Manual. Chicago, American College of Surgeons, 1993.
9. Marshall SB, Marshall LF, Vos HR, Chesnut RM: Neuroscience Critical Care: Pathophysiology and Management. Philadelphia, WB Saunders, 1990.
10. Wilkins RH, Rengachary SS: Neurosurgery. Vol II, Part VIII, Section C: Spine Trauma. New York, McGraw-Hill, 1996.
11. Morris GF, Marshall LF: Traumatic central nervous system injury. *In*: Adult Neurology. Corey-Bloom J (Ed). St Louis, Mosby, 1998, pp 251–266.
12. McGuire RA, Green NBA, Eismont FJ, et al: Comparison of stability provided to the unstable spine by the kinetic therapy table and the Stryker frame. Neurosurgery 1988; 22:842–845.
13. Dolan EJ, Tator CH: The effect of blood transfusion, dopamine, and gamma hydroxybutyrate on posttraumatic ischemia of the spinal cord. J Neurosurg 1982; 56:350–358.
14. Bracken MB, Shepherd MJ, Collins WF, et al: A randomized, controlled trial of methylprednisolone or naloxone in the treatment of acute spinal cord injury: Results of the Second National Acute Spinal Cord Injury Study. N Engl J Med 1990; 322:1405–1411.
15. Green BA, Callahan RA, Klose KJ, de la Torre J: Acute spinal cord injury: Current concepts. Clin Orthop 1981; 154:125–135.
16. Levin AB: Intensive care. *In*: Neurosurgery. Wilkins RH, Rengachary SS (Eds). New York, McGraw-Hill, 1996, pp 425–436.
17. Clifton GL: Nutrition and parenteral therapy. *In*: Neurosurgery. Wilkins RH, Rengachary SS (Eds). New York, McGraw-Hill, 1996, pp 471–476.
18. Casas ER, Sanchez MP, Arias CR, et al: Prophylaxis of venous thrombosis and pulmonary embolism in patients with acute traumatic spinal cord lesions. Paraplegia 1976; 14:178–183.
19. Marshall LF, Knowlton SL, Garfin SR, et al: Deterioration following spinal cord injury: A multicenter study. J Neurosurg 1987; 66:400–404.
20. Menezes AH, Osenbach RK: Spinal cord injury. *In*: Pediatric Neurosurgery: Surgery of the Developing Nervous System. Cheek WR (Ed). Philadelphia, WB Saunders, 1994.
21. Schwab ME, Bartholdi D: Degeneration and regeneration of axons in the lesioned spinal cord. Physiol Rev 1996; 76:319–370.
22. Nichols J: Regeneration of immature spinal cord after injury. Trends Neurosci 1996; 19:229–234.
23. Cheng H, Cao Y, Olson L: Spinal cord repair in adult paraplegic rats: Partial restoration of hind limb function. Science 1996; 273:510–513.

29

Penetrating Injuries of the Neck

Demetrios Demetriades, MD, PhD
George C. Velmahos, MD, PhD
Juan. A. Asensio, MD, FACS

Penetrating injuries of the neck are notorious for their complexity with regard to their evaluation and management. There is no other body area with such dense concentration of vital structures—vascular, aerodigestive, spinal cord, and a plethora of cranial and peripheral nerves. This crowded anatomy makes the possibility of significant injury to vital structures after penetrating trauma very high. The clinical evaluation of many important structures is considered by some to be difficult, and delaying the diagnosis and management may result in significant morbidity and mortality. The surgical exposure of some neck structures, such as the upper part of the internal carotid artery, the vertebral artery, and the subclavian vessels, may challenge even the most experienced trauma surgeon. This chapter provides guidelines for the initial evaluation and management of patients with penetrating neck injuries and discusses some of the major controversies in the field.

PREHOSPITAL MANAGEMENT

In an urban environment, "scoop and run" to the nearest trauma center offers the best chances for survival to patients with severe bleeding or airway problems. Airway management in the prehospital setting can be a difficult task with potentially lethal complications. The presence of a large hematoma or edema or laryngotracheal trauma may make the endotracheal intubation a dangerous procedure. If the intubation is attempted without pharmacologic paralysis, there is significant risk of aggravating the bleeding and increasing the size of the hematoma by dislodging a containing clot. Pharmacologic paralysis is even more dangerous, however, because of the potentially lethal consequences of a failed intubation. A cricothyrotomy in the presence of a neck hematoma is extremely difficult, even in the most optimal environment, and it should not be attempted in the field. Bag-valve-mask (BVM) respiration is another option, but it can also be dangerous in the presence of laryngotracheal trauma. The positive pressure generated by BVM respiration may cause massive subcutaneous emphysema or air embolus if there is an associated venous injury.

In the presence of a large hematoma, application of a neck collar may aggravate any respiratory compromise. There is no need for spinal protection in knife injuries. Even in gunshot injuries, an unstable fracture is extremely unlikely. In a series of 1300 patients with gunshot injuries of the spine, Meyer and associates[1] found no case with an unstable fracture.

EMERGENCY ROOM MANAGEMENT

Airway

The initial management should be based on Advanced Trauma Life Support (ATLS) protocols: Airway is the most critical priority, and in penetrating injuries of the neck, it can be a challenging problem. Airway problems may be due to direct trauma to the larynx or to outside compression by a large hematoma (Fig. 29-1). Small injuries to the larynx or trachea inflicted by a knife rarely cause respiratory problems unless there is a significant transection of these structures. On the contrary, high-velocity gunshot injuries are more likely to cause acute airway problems. In a study of 223 patients with penetrating injuries of the neck, 6 patients (2.7%) had major laryngotracheal trauma, and 29 (13%) had a large hematoma.[2] Gunshot injuries were associated with a significantly higher incidence of large hematomas than knife wounds (20.6% vs. 6.7%).

The presence of respiratory distress or a large hematoma is a strong indication for intubation in the emergency room. Endotracheal intubation under these circumstances can challenge the skills and judgment of even the most experienced physician. The route for endotracheal intubation should be individualized according to the:

1. Local injury (i.e., size and site of hematoma, presence or absence of an open laryngotracheal wound, extent of tissue destruction).
2. Severity of respiratory distress.
3. Hemodynamic condition of the patient.
4. Experience of the physician.

In a stable patient with a large hematoma, fiberoptic intubation with the patient lightly sedated is probably the best approach, provided that an expert physician is immediately available; this is the preferred approach at the University of Southern California Trauma Center. This route is not advocated for the severely distressed or apneic patient. If this technique is not available, orotracheal intubation is the next preferred modality. The most experienced physician should attempt the intubation, and preparations should be made for a possible cricothyrotomy.

Pharmacologic paralysis to facilitate intubation should be used with great caution because of the associated risks. Inability to intubate after neuromuscular paralysis in a patient with an obstructive airway can be a potentially lethal situation. Ketamine at an IV dose of 2 mg/kg is an excellent medication for intubation of patients with large neck hematomas because it maintains the respiratory drive.

A cricothyrotomy is usually easy to perform as long as

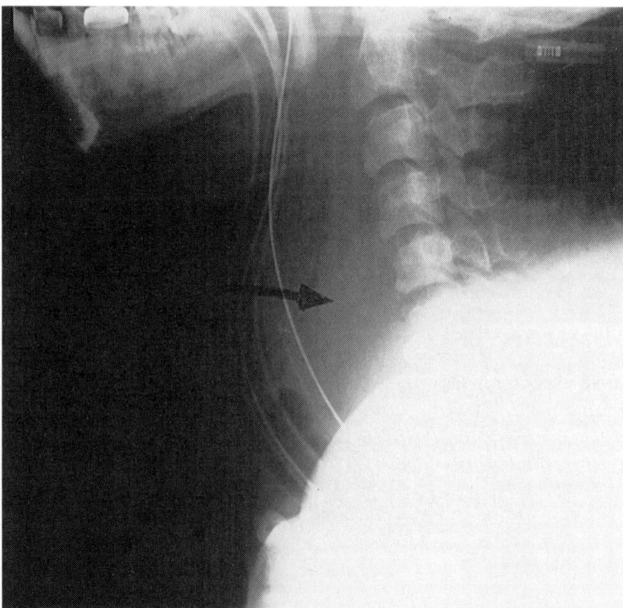

Figure 29–1. Large hematoma *(arrow)* with laryngotracheal displacement. Early intubation is indicated.

there is no central hematoma. In the presence of a central hematoma, a cricothyrotomy should be avoided, because it is a difficult procedure and because catastrophic hemorrhage may occur. In the patient with a large open tracheal wound or a complete airway transection, intubation of the distal segment of larynx or trachea is an effective way of securing the airway. Finally, insertion of a nasogastric tube before anesthesia should be avoided, because gagging and coughing may precipitate bleeding and expansion of a hematoma.

Conclusions

- Establishment of the airway in some patients with penetrating injuries to the neck can be a difficult and potentially dangerous task. The most experienced physicians in the trauma team should undertake this procedure.
- The route of intubation should be individualized according to the conditions in the neck, the presence or absence of respiratory distress, and the experience of the trauma team.

External Bleeding

External bleeding is best controlled by direct pressure, with the patient in the Trendelenburg position to avoid air embolism. In some situations, such as bleeding from subclavian vessels or high internal carotid artery injuries, direct pressure is often not effective. For these situations, we have successfully used balloon tamponade as follows[3, 4]:

1. A Foley catheter is inserted into the wound and advanced as far as it can go.
2. The balloon is then inflated with water until the bleeding stops or moderate resistance is felt (Fig. 29-2).
3. If the bleeding continues after this maneuver, the balloon is deflated, and the catheter is slightly withdrawn and reinflated. Blood flowing through the lumen of the Foley catheter is suggestive of distal bleeding, and repositioning may be required.

For supraclavicular wounds with intrathoracic bleeding, a combination of two Foley catheters may be helpful. The first catheter is inserted into the thoracic cavity through the wound, the balloon is inflated, and the catheter is pulled back firmly in order to compress the bleeding vessels against the first rib or clavicle. If external bleeding continues, a second Foley catheter is inserted in the wound tract and inflated.

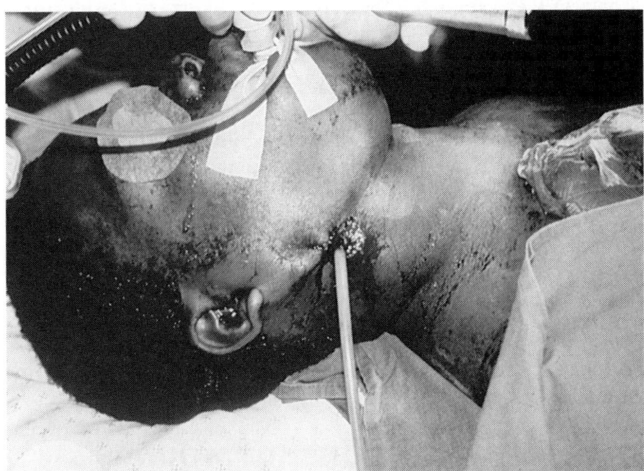

Figure 29–2. Balloon tamponade for temporary bleeding control of a high internal carotid injury.

Intravenous lines should be avoided in the arm on the side of a neck wound because of the risk of extravasation of the infused fluids from a proximal venous injury.

Cardiac arrest or imminent cardiac arrest in the emergency room is a strong indication for immediate resuscitative thoracotomy. After bleeding control by direct pressure, the right ventricle should be aspirated for air embolism, because it is a common complication in venous injuries.

DEFINITIVE MANAGEMENT

Following the primary survey according to ATLS protocols, a decision should be made about the definitive management of the patient. Patients with obvious signs or symptoms of major vascular or aerodigestive tract injuries need surgical exploration without delay. Most patients, however, present with no signs or with "soft" signs of significant injuries. The management of these patients is controversial, and there are two major schools of thought, as follows:

- Some trauma surgeons practice a policy of routine operation for all injuries that have penetrated the platysma. The proponents of this policy suggest that physical examination is not reliable and significant injuries may be missed.[5, 6] The policy of mandatory operation has the advantage of no need for specialized diagnostic investigations. In addition, nontherapeutic operations are not associated with higher incidence of complications or increased costs.[5] Most centers have not adopted this practice because of the high rate of unnecessary operations for penetrating neck injuries, which ranges from 30% to 89%.[5-7] In order to reduce this problem, some centers routinely perform operation only for zone II (between the cricoid and the angle of the mouth) injuries, reserving a selective nonoperative policy for the rest of the injuries. Asensio and colleagues,[8] in an extensive review of the literature, compared mandatory with selective surgical exploration in zone II injuries and concluded that neither approach is clearly superior.
- The more commonly practiced approach to penetrating neck trauma is a policy of selective conservative management based on clinical examination and a variety of diagnostic investigations. The criteria for operation or observation and the indications and methods of vascular assessment, however, are matters of controversy.

Physical Examination as Triage Modality

Although some surgeons hold that clinical examination alone is unreliable in identifying vascular or esophageal injuries,[5, 6] others believe that a carefully performed physical examination is highly reliable in detecting significant injuries that require treatment.[2, 3, 9-11] In a prospective study from Johannesburg, South Africa, Demetriades and colleagues[9] clinically evaluated 335 patients with penetrating injuries of the neck according to a written protocol. Angiography was performed on only 7 patients (2%). Eighty per cent (269 patients) were selected for nonsurgical management. Only two of the observed patients required subsequent operation for vascular injuries identified during the same hospitalization; no complications were found in the rest of the observed patients. Early follow-up (mean, 16 days) of 192 observed patients and late follow-up (mean, 48 days) of 111 observed patients did not reveal any significant complications.

In another study from Los Angeles, 223 patients were clinically evaluated according to a written protocol based on detailed physical examination.[2] The 176 patients judged to be hemodynamically stable were further investigated by four-vessel angiography. In the group of patients with no clinical signs of vascular injury (no active bleeding, no significant hematoma, no bruit, normal radial pulses), none had serious trauma requiring treatment, although routine angiography diagnosed 11 minor injuries not requiring treatment. The presence of "hard" signs of vascular injury (large expanding hematoma, severe active bleeding, unexplained shock not responding to intravenous fluids, diminished radial pulse, bruit) was highly diagnostic of major vascular trauma, and 28 of 29 patients with these signs had significant injuries. The presence of soft signs (small to moderate hematoma, minor bleeding, mild shock responding to fluid resuscitation) was not diagnostic of significant vascular trauma. Of 34 patients with soft signs, eight had angiographically diagnosed lesions, only one of which required intervention.

Signs or symptoms suggestive of aerodigestive injuries are subcutaneous emphysema, hoarseness, dyspnea, hemoptysis, air leak through the wound, and painful swallowing. The absence of these signs reliably excludes significant injury. In a prospective study of 152 asymptomatic patients evaluated by radiologic or endoscopic studies, Demetriades and colleagues[2] found no significant injuries (negative predictive value, 100%). Of another group of 64 symptomatic patients, 10 (15.6%) had aerodigestive injuries requiring repair. These researchers concluded that contrast swallow radiographic studies and endoscopy should be reserved only for symptomatic patients and for proximity injuries in obtunded patients in whom clinical examination is not possible.

Conclusions

- There is good evidence that physical examination performed according to a written protocol is highly reliable in detecting or raising suspicion of significant vascular or aerodigestive tract trauma.
- The patient without signs or symptoms suggestive of vascular or aerodigestive injuries is highly unlikely to have a significant injury requiring treatment.

The clinical examination protocol and the algorithm for evaluation of penetrating neck injuries shown in Figures 29-3 and 29-4 are currently in place in the Division of Trauma and Critical Care at the University of Southern California, Los Angeles.

Role of Angiography and Color-Flow Doppler Ultrasonography

Routine angiography for all proximity penetrating injuries of the neck has been advocated for the evaluation of major neck arteries.[12, 13] Such a policy eliminates unnecessary operations without missing any vascular trauma. The invasive character and costs of angiography are significant disadvantages, however. In addition, some authors suggest that angiography does not change the management.[14] In a prospective study from Los Angeles, 127 asymptomatic patients with penetrating neck injuries underwent angiography; 11 patients (8.3%) were shown to have vascular injuries on angiography, but no patient required any type of treatment.[2]

Some surgeons recommend routine angiography for injuries in zones I and II only, because these areas are hard to evaluate clinically and their surgical exploration is usually difficult.[15] The angiographic yield is still very low.[2, 9]

Other studies suggested that color-flow Doppler (CFD) ultrasonography is a reliable alternative to angiography.[2, 16, 17] In a prospective study from Los Angeles, 83 hemodynamically stable patients were examined clinically according to a strict protocol and subsequently underwent angiography and CFD.[16] Physical examination alone detected or raised suspicion of all the significant vascular injuries but missed six minor injuries not requiring treatment. CFD correctly identified all normal vessels and 10 of the 11 angiographically detected injuries; one small intimal tear not requiring treatment was missed. The combination of physical examination and CFD had sensitivity, specificity, and a negative predictive value of 100%.

Evaluation of Neck Injuries: Conclusions

The initial evaluation of penetrating neck injuries should be individualized for each medical center according to the available facilities and experience:

- A policy of mandatory surgical exploration has very little or no role in trauma centers, but it might have a place for evaluation of zone II injuries in small centers without angiographic or CFD facilities.
- A selective nonsurgical management policy is the recommended approach for organized trauma centers.

A careful physical examination according to a written protocol is the most important part of the evaluation of a patient with a penetrating neck injury; principles are as follows:

- Asymptomatic patients may be observed without any other investigation or with the addition of CFD.
- Patients with soft signs of vascular injury should be evaluated by means of CFD; if this modality is not available, an angiogram should be performed.
- Angiography is preferred over CFD in patients with a bruit, because of the potential therapeutic value — embolization or stenting can then be performed.
- A widened mediastinum in a patient with a shotgun injury and an inconclusive CFD study in a symptomatic patient should also be indications for angiography.

As previously mentioned, Figure 29-4 shows the algorithm currently used at the Division of Trauma and Critical Care at the University of Southern California, Los Angeles, for the evaluation of patients with penetrating neck injuries.

GUNSHOT WOUNDS VERSUS STAB WOUNDS

Firearms are responsible for about half of all penetrating injuries of the neck in American urban trauma centers.[2] In one prospective study of 223 patients, gunshot wounds were three times more likely to cause a large hematoma than stab wounds (20.6% versus 6.7%), twice as likely to be associated with shock (13.4% versus 7.9%), twice as likely to result in a vascular injury (26.8% versus 14.6%), twice as likely to cause aerodigestive tract injuries (7.2% versus 3.4%), and 13 times as likely to cause spinal cord trauma (13.4% versus 1.1%).[2] For these reasons, it has been suggested that a mandatory operation for gunshot wounds is a reasonable approach.[18] Such a policy, however, would be associated with an unacceptably high rate of unnecessary operations, because only 16.5% of gunshot injuries actually require operation (rate for stab wounds is 10.1%).[2]

Conclusions

Gunshot injuries should be evaluated like knife injuries, and a policy of selective nonoperative management is recommended.

TRANSCERVICAL GUNSHOT WOUNDS

Transcervical gunshot wounds are significantly more likely to injure vital neck structures than wounds that do not cross the

A. Site of Injury:

☐ Anterior neck triangle (anterior to SMS muscle)
☐ Posterior neck triangle (posterior to SMS muscle)
☐ Zone I (between clavicles and cricoid)
☐ Zone II (between cricoid and angle of mandible of skull)
☐ Zone III (between angle of mandible and base of skull)

Wound Tract:

☐ Toward midline
☐ Toward clavicle
☐ Away from midline or
☐ Can't assess

B. Vascular Structures:

1. Active bleeding: ☐ None, ☐ Minor, ☐ Moderate, ☐ Severe
2. Hypovolemia: BP > 100, ☐ BP 60–90, ☐ BP < 60
3. Hematoma: None, ☐ Small, ☐ Moderate, ☐ Large, ☐ Expanding, ☐ Pulsatile
4. Peripheral pulses (compare with contralateral):
   Distal carotid: ☐ Normal, ☐ Diminished, ☐ Absent
   Superficial temporal: ☐ Normal, ☐ Diminished, ☐ Absent
   Brachial or radial: ☐ Normal, ☐ Diminished, ☐ Absent
5. Bruit: No, ☐ Yes (if so, where ________)

C. Larynx/Trachea, Esophagus:

1. Hemoptysis (ask patient to cough): ☐ Yes, ☐ No
2. Air bubbling through wound? ☐ Yes, ☐ No (ask patient to cough)
3. Subcutaneous emphysema: ☐ Yes, ☐ No
4. Hoarseness: Yes, ☐ No
5. Pain on swallowing sputum: ☐ Yes, ☐ No
6. Hematemesis: Yes, ☐ No

D. Nervous System:

1. GCS: ☐ Eye response, ☐ Verbal response, ☐ Motor response
   Total GCS ________
2. Localizing signs:
   Pupils:
   Limbs:
   Cranial nerves:
   Facial n.: ☐ Normal, ☐ Abnormal
   Glossopharyngeal n. (check midline portion of soft palate): ☐ Normal, ☐ Abnormal
   Recurrent laryngeal n. (hoarseness, effective cough): ☐ Normal, ☐ Abnormal
   Accessory n. (lift the shoulder): ☐ Normal, ☐ Abnormal
   Hypoglossal n. (check midline position of tongue): ☐ Normal, ☐ Abnormal
   Spinal cord: ☐ Normal, ☐ Abnormal (specify)
   Horner's syndrome (myosis, ptosis): ☐ Yes, ☐ No
   Brachial plexus: median n. (fist): ☐ Normal, ☐ Abnormal
   radial n. (wrist extension): ☐ Normal, ☐ Abnormal
   ulnar n. (abduction/adduction of fingers): ☐ Normal, ☐ Abnormal
   musculocutaneous n. (flexion of forearm): ☐ Normal, ☐ Abnormal
   axillary n. (abduction of arm): ☐ Normal, ☐ Abnormal

Figure 29–3. Physical examination protocol for penetrating injuries of the neck, Division of Trauma and Critical Care, University of Southern California. GCS = Glasgow Coma Scale; BP = blood pressure; SMS = sternomastoid. (From Demetriades D, Asensio J, Velmahos G, Thal E: Complex problems in penetrating neck trauma. Surg Clin North Am 1996; 76:661–683.)

midline. In a prospective study of 97 patients with gunshot injuries, 34% of the wounds were transcervical. The incidence of significant injuries in transcervical wounds was 73%, compared with only 31% for gunshot injuries not crossing the midline.[19] Because of this high incidence of significant injuries, it has been suggested that transcervical gunshot wounds should be routinely explored surgically.[20] Demetriades and colleagues[19] reached a different conclusion; despite the high incidence of injuries to vital structures in their series of transcervical gunshot wounds, only 21% of the patients required an operation. The researchers concluded that a selective nonsurgical management policy based on a careful physical examination combined with the appropriate diagnostic investigations (angiography or CFD, esophagography, endoscopy) is a safe approach.

Conclusions

There is good evidence that transcervical gunshot wounds do not need routine surgical exploration. A selective nonsurgical management policy is safe and avoids unnecessary operations.

SPECIFIC INJURIES

Carotid Artery Injuries

Carotid artery injuries are found in about 6% of penetrating injuries of the neck.[2] Although the hospital mortality ranges from 10% to 20%, the overall mortality is very high, with some series reporting rates up to 66%.[21] Many factors influence the selection of survivors: the weapon of injury, prehospital time, site and size of injury, presence of neurologic signs, and other associated injuries. Injury to the common carotid artery is associated with a significantly higher mortality than injury to the internal carotid artery, probably because of the higher incidence of associated internal jugular vein trauma in common carotid artery injuries.[21]

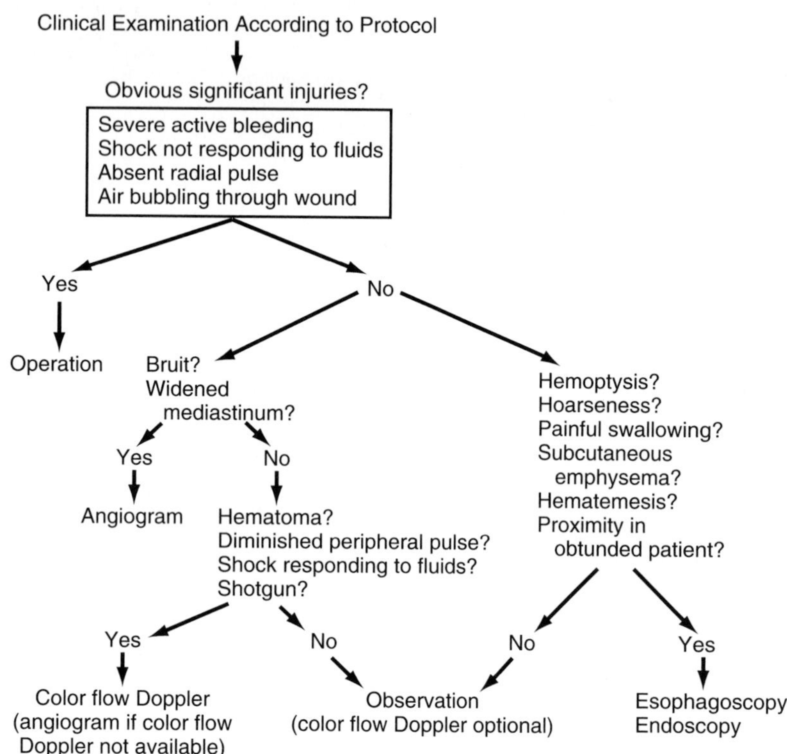

Figure 29–4. Algorithm for evaluation of penetrating neck injuries, Division of Trauma and Critical Care, University of Southern California. (From Demetriades D, Asensio J, Velmahos G, Thal E: Complex problems in penetrating neck trauma. Surg Clin North Am 1996; 76:661–683.)

Operative Exposure of Carotid Artery

The standard incision is made along the anterior border of the sternocleidomastoid muscle. For proximal injuries, addition of a median sternotomy may be necessary for better exposure. For high internal carotid artery injuries, the exposure is difficult and may challenge the skills of even the most experienced surgeon. Anterior subluxation of the mandible may provide additional exposure of about 2 cm. If this maneuver is still not adequate, a vertical osteotomy of the ramus of the mandible may be necessary (Fig. 29–5). The trauma surgeon should manage such cases jointly with a maxillofacial or neurologic surgeon.

Controversies in the Management of Carotid Artery Injuries

Repair or Ligation

In the absence of neurologic signs, every effort should be made to repair a common carotid or internal carotid injury, provided that the repair is technically possible. If there is significant loss of tissue, an interposition venous graft or transposition of the external carotid artery may be necessary. For high carotid artery injuries with active bleeding, ligation is usually necessary.

The management of the injured carotid artery in the presence of neurologic signs has been an unresolved controversial issue. In the 1970s, some authors cautioned against reestablishment of carotid artery flow in the presence of neurologic signs because of the risk of converting an anemic infarction to a hemorrhagic infarction, which has a worse prognosis.[22, 23] Later studies suggested that the risk of hemorrhagic infarction was exaggerated and recommended liberal repair.[24] Currently, the majority of authors recommend reestablishment of blood flow in most patients in whom onset of neurologic deficits is recent (less than 3 or 4 hours), provided that (1) CT scanning demonstrates no established anemic infarction or brain edema and (2) there is good backflow from the distal carotid artery (Fig. 29–6). In these conditions, ligation is advocated.[3] A similar approach is recommended for patients in coma, although the prognosis is grave irrespective of the type of operation. The diagnosis of neurologic coma should be made with caution, especially in patients in shock or with alcohol or illicit drug intoxication.

Temporary Shunts During Carotid Artery Repair

Minor carotid artery injuries can be repaired easily, and there is no need for shunting. In complex injuries, however, the repair may involve a venous graft or debridement and an end-to-end anastomosis. The role of temporary shunts in these cases is not clear, and some recommendations have been extrapolated from elective carotid artery surgery for atherosclerotic disease. It seems sensible to use shunts for complex graft reconstruction, especially in the presence of preoperative neurologic signs of severe hypotension.[3]

Minor Carotid Artery Injuries

The clinical significance of asymptomatic, radiologically detected minor arterial injuries (i.e., small intimal tears or small aneurysms) is not clear. Although some authors believe that these lesions have a benign prognosis,[25] others express concern about potential catastrophic complications, especially with carotid arteries. Our preference is surgical repair for accessible injuries and nonoperative management for high internal carotid injuries. The nonoperatively managed injuries should be closely monitored clinically and angiographically or by CFD. Low-dose aspirin is recommended for a few months, although there is no clinical evidence for its effectiveness.

Vertebral Artery injuries

The incidence of vertebral artery injuries in penetrating neck trauma is about 9% for gunshot injuries and 5% for stab

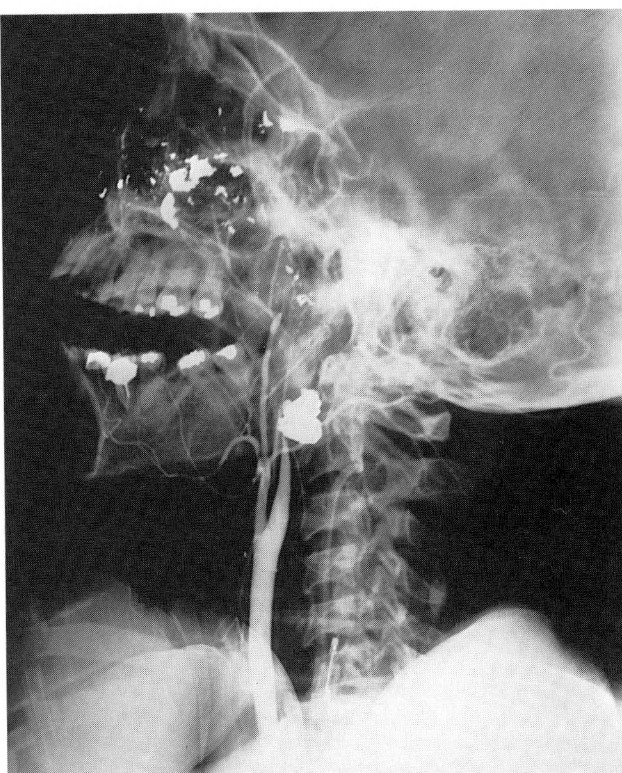

Figure 29–5. High internal carotid artery injury. Anterior subluxation or division of the mandible is necessary for surgical exposure.

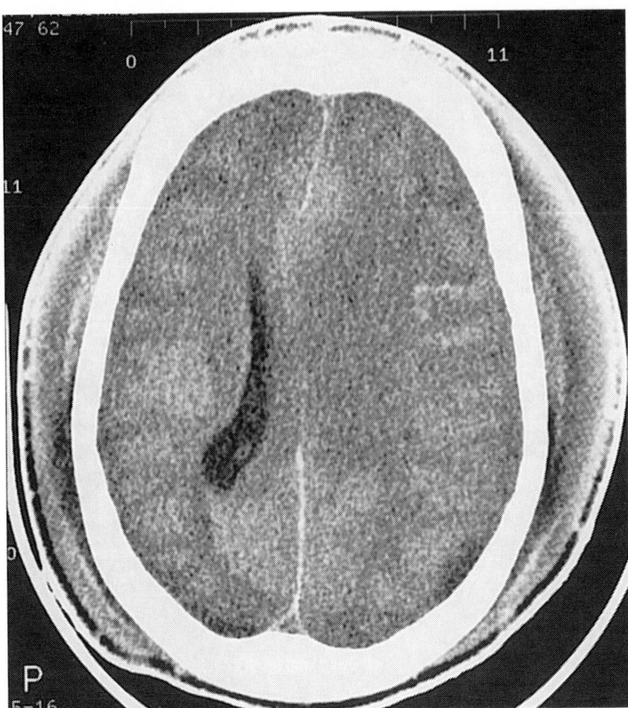

Figure 29–6. Severe brain edema with midline shift following gunshot injury and occlusion of the internal carotid artery. Revascularization should be avoided.

wounds.[2] Many of these injuries remain asymptomatic and are confirmed angiographically or by CFD. Thrombosed arteries do not require any type of treatment. Patients with false aneurysms or arteriovenous fistulas are best managed with angiographic embolization (Fig. 29–7). Because surgical exposure of the vertebral artery is difficult, it is recommended that operation be reserved for patients who have severe active bleeding or in whom embolization fails.[3, 26]

Subclavian Vascular Injuries

The subclavian vessels are injured in about 4% of all patients with penetrating neck trauma. The hospital mortality ranges from 5% to 30%, but many patients die before they reach medical care. The overall mortality for venous injuries is significantly higher than that for arterial injuries, most probably owing to (1) the inability of veins to contract and control exsanguination and (2) air embolism.[27]

Surgical exposure is difficult, and excellent knowledge of the regional anatomy is critical to the successful management of these injuries. A clavicular incision with division and possible excision of the medial third of the clavicle is usually satisfactory for distal subclavian injuries. For proximal injuries, addition of a median sternotomy provides good exposure. The old-fashioned "book thoracotomy" or "trap-door incisions" or left subclavian injuries have been abandoned by most experts.

Arterial injuries should be repaired. Ligation should be reserved for patients in critical condition because of the risk of claudication or subclavian steal syndrome for ligations proximal to the vertebral artery. Subclavian venous injuries should be repaired only if the repair can be done easily and without significant stenosis. Ligation is well-tolerated, and there are no long-term sequelae.

Endovascular Stented Grafts

The development of stents in combination with vascular grafts has opened a new field in vascular trauma. These grafts can be inserted percutaneously or through open arteriotomies away from the site of vascular trauma. They are composed of balloon-expandable steel stents covered with polytetrafluoroethylene grafts. The ideal injuries for this application are false aneurysms or arteriovenous fistulas, especially in anatomically difficult areas such as the subclavian artery and the internal carotid artery at the base of the skull (Fig. 29–8). The preliminary reports are encouraging,[28, 29] although the long-term

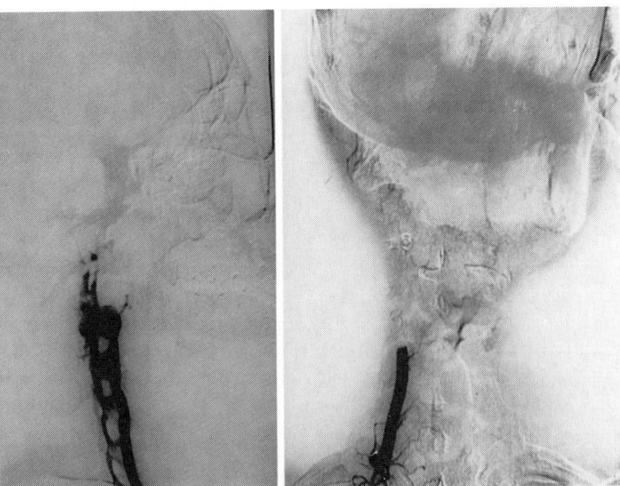

Figure 29–7. Post-traumatic vertebral artery false aneurysm and arteriovenous fistula before and after successful embolization. (From Demetriades D, Theodorou D, Asensio J, et al: Management options in vertebral artery injuries. Br J Surg 1996; 83:83–86.)

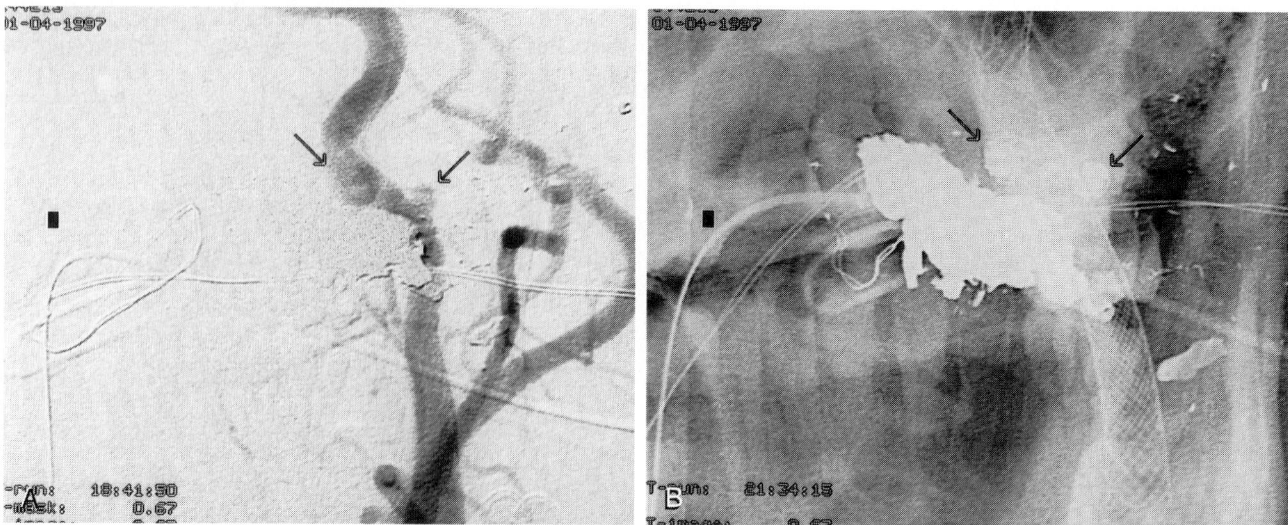

Figure 29–8. *A*, Two false aneurysms of the internal carotid artery near the base of the skull. Surgical exposure is extremely difficult. *B*, Percutaneous angiographic placement of a metal stent and embolization of the aneurysms through the stent *(arrows)*.

safety and effectiveness of endovascular stented grafts have not been documented.

Aerodigestive Tract Injuries

The incidence of aerodigestive tract injuries in penetrating injuries of the neck is about 6% (~7% in gunshot injuries; 3.5% in knife injuries).[2] As discussed earlier, the diagnosis is usually made from or strongly indicated by a meticulous clinical examination performed according to a written protocol.[2, 3] Esophagography or endoscopy is required in symptomatic patients or for proximity injuries in unevaluable patients.

Small laryngotracheal injuries can safely be managed with primary repair without tracheostomy. Extensive injuries with tissue loss should be reinforced with surrounding musculofascial flaps and protected by a tracheostomy. Esophageal injuries should be identified and repaired as early as possible. Delays in repair of such injuries of more than 12 to 15 hours are associated with significant septic complications, although the complications in cervical esophageal injuries are not as severe as those in thoracic esophageal injuries.

Thoracic Duct Injuries

The thoracic duct is usually injured in penetrating injuries at the base of the left side of the neck. Thoracic duct injuries are often missed at the initial operation, manifesting postoperatively as a milky fluid coming from the drain or the thoracostomy tube. Sometimes, the fluid does not have the characteristic milky appearance, and the diagnosis is confirmed by laboratory evaluation, which reveals a total protein level greater than 3 g/dL, a total fat content higher than 0.4 g/dL, a triglyceride level of more than 200 mg/dL, and lymphocytic predominance. These chylous leaks respond very well to conservative treatment with low-fat diet or total parenteral nutrition. It is rare that conservative management fails; when it does, open exploration or thoracoscopic ligation of the duct may be necessary.

References

1. Meyer PR, Apple DF, Bohlman HH, et al: Symposium: Management of fractures of the thoracolumbar spine. Contemp Orthop 1988; 27:90.
2. Demetriades D, Theodorou D, Cornwell E, et al: Evaluation of penetrating injuries of the neck: Prospective study of 233 patients. World J Surg 1997; 21:41–48.
3. Demetriades D, Asensio J, Velmahos G, et al: Complex problems in penetrating neck trauma. Surg Clin North Am 1996; 76:661–683.
4. Gilroy D, Lakhoo M, Charalambides D, et al: Control of life threatening hemorrhage from the neck: A new indication for balloon tamponade. Injury 1992; 23:557–559.
5. Apffedstaedt JP, Muller R: Results of mandatory exploration for penetrating neck trauma. World J Surg 1994; 18:917–920.
6. Walsh MS: The management of penetrating injuries of the anterior triangle of the neck. Injury 1994; 18:917–920.
7. Holuoke PJ, Goldstein AS, Sclafani SJ, et al: Routine versus selective exploration of penetrating neck injuries: A radiological prospective study. J Trauma 1984; 24:1010–1014.
8. Asensio JA, Valenzeano CP, Falcone RE, et al: Management of penetrating neck injuries: The controversy surrounding zone II injuries. Surg Clin North Am 1991; 71:267–296.
9. Demetriades D, Charalambides D, Lakhoo M: Physical examination and selective conservative management in patients with penetrating injuries of the neck. Br J Surg 1993; 80:1534–1536.
10. Gerst PH, Sharma PK: Selective management of penetrating neck trauma. Ann Surg 1990; 56:553–555.
11. Stein A, Kalk F: Selective conservatism in the management of penetrating wounds of the neck. S Afr J Surg 1974; 12:31–39.
12. Sclafani SJ, Caraliere G, Atweh N, et al: The role of angiography in penetrating neck trauma. J Trauma 1991; 31:557–562.
13. Weigelt JA, Thal ER, Snyder WH, et al: Diagnosis of penetrating cervical esophageal injuries. Am J Surg 1987; 154:619–622.
14. Timberlake GA, Rice JC, Kerstein MD, et al: Penetrating injury to the carotid artery: A reappraisal of management. Am Surg 1989; 55:154–157.
15. Rao PM, Ivatury RR, Sharma P, et al: Cervical vascular injury: A trauma center experience. Surgery 1993: 114:527–531.
16. Demetriades D, Theodorou D, Cornwell E, et al: Penetrating injuries of the neck in stable patients: Physical examination, angiography or color-flow Doppler. Arch Surg 1995; 130:971–979.
17. Fry WR, Dort JA, Smith RS, et al: Duplex scanning replaces arteriography and operative exploration in the diagnosis of potential cervical vascular injury. Am J Surg 1994; 168:693–696.
18. Shenk WG: Neck injuries. *In*: Principles of Trauma Surgery. Moylan JA (Ed). New York, Gower, 1992, pp 1550–1565.
19. Demetriades D, Theodorou D, Cornwell E, et al: Transcervical gunshot injuries: Mandatory operation is not necessary. J Trauma 1996; 40:758–760.
20. Hirshberg A, Wall MJ, Johnston RH, et al: Transcervical gunshot injuries. Am J Surg 1994; 167:309–312.
21. Demetriades D, Skalkides J, Sofianos C, et al: Carotid injuries: Experience with 124 cases. J Trauma 1989; 29:91–94.

22. Bradley E: Management of penetrating carotid injuries: An alternative approach. J Trauma 1973; 13:245–255.
23. Cohen A, Brief D, Matheson C: Carotid artery injuries: An analysis of eighty-five cases. Am J Surg 1970; 120:210–214.
24. Ledgerwood A, Mullins R, Lucas C: Primary repair vs ligation for carotid injuries. Arch Surg 1980; 115:488–493.
25. Stain S, Yellin A, Weaver F, et al: Selective management of nonocclusive arterial injuries. Arch Surg 1989; 124:1136–1141.
26. Demetriades D, Theodorou D, Asensio JA, et al: Management options in vertebral injuries. Br J Surg 1996; 83:83–86.
27. Demetriades D, Rabinowitz B, Pezikis A, et al: Subclavian vascular injuries. Br J Surg 1987; 74:1001–1003.
28. Marin ML, Yeith FJ, Panetta TF, et al: Transluminally placed endovascular stented graft repair for arterial trauma. J Vasc Surg 1994; 20:466–472.
29. Patel AV, Marin ML, Veith FJ, et al: Endovascular graft repair of penetrating subclavian artery injuries. J Endovasc Surg 1996; 3:382–388.

30

Thoracic Injuries

Juan A. Asensio, MD, FACS • David Hanpeter, MD
Hugo Gomez, MD • Santiago Chahwan, MD
Sebastian Orduna, MD • Bradley Roth, MD

No me pongan en lo oscuro
a morir como un traidor.
Yo soy bueno, y como bueno
morire de cara al Sol

Do not place me in the darkness
to die like traitors do.
I am good, and as a brave man
I will die facing the sun

JOSE MARTÍ
Cuban Poet and Liberator

INTRODUCTION

Thoracic injuries account for approximately 25% of all trauma deaths in the United States.[1–4] Most patients sustaining severe thoracic injuries succumb at the scene of the traumatic incident. Many of these patients die of blunt ruptures of the thoracic aorta, heart, and its chambers, and massive exsanguinating intrathoracic hemorrhage. Other important causes of death are associated injuries such as central nervous system (CNS) and exsanguinating abdominal vascular injuries.[5]

Thoracic injuries are estimated to occur with a frequency of 12 patients per million/population. Of these, four will require hospitalization and be temporarily disabled and absent from the work force.[6] In the United States, it is estimated that approximately 16,000 deaths occur from thoracic injuries every year.[2] Thus, the cost to society in health care dollars is staggering.

With blunt or penetrating injury, the basic principles of resuscitation are:

- Rapid restoration of airway
- Supplemental oxygen
- Needle decompression of a suspected tension pneumothorax
- Coverage of open wounds resulting in an open pneumothorax

Intravascular volume should be rapidly restored after placement of large intravenous lines if immediate transport of these patients to a level I trauma center is not delayed. Ideally, intravenous (IV) lines should be started during the transport.

Most thoracic injuries can be managed by closed chest tube thoracostomy.[5] It is estimated that fewer than 10% of all blunt chest injuries require thoracotomy. This rate rises to between 15% and 30% for penetrating chest injuries.[7–9] The mortality of patients sustaining chest injuries rises significantly if the patient arrives with either respiratory difficulties or shock at the trauma center. In one series, Freedland and colleagues[10] reported that 11% of thoracic trauma patients required endotracheal intubation on arrival at the trauma center; 58% of these patients died. If shock was present in addition, the mortality rose to 73%.

INITIAL ASSESSMENT AND MANAGEMENT

Trauma Center

All patients admitted to a trauma center should be resuscitated according to advanced trauma life support (ATLS) protocols.[5] Rapid establishment of an airway takes priority. Orotracheal intubation remains the route of choice with cervical in-line immobilization. Whenever an underlying cervical spine injury is suspected, fiberoptic intubation is an excellent alternative. If the patient cannot be intubated, trauma center personnel should always be prepared to perform an emergency cricothyroidotomy, which can be fraught with pitfalls, especially if there are associated penetrating neck or extensive thoracic inlet hematomas. The tamponading effects of these hematomas can be released as the incision to access the cricothyroid membrane is made.

In the rare case in which cricotracheal separation has occurred, it should be suspected and the diagnosis confirmed by the mechanism of injury. This injury usually results from direct blows to the neck, causing a fracture or separation of the cricotracheal junction. The injury is characterized by the inability to pass an endotracheal tube and by the presence of massive subcutaneous emphysema. This is the only case in which tracheostomy will prove to be lifesaving.

As with all trauma patients, a rapid and thorough physical examination must be carried out. Potentially life-threatening conditions must be identified and addressed immediately. Patients identified with a tension pneumothorax during the pre-hospital scene and who have undergone needle decompression should be immediately reevaluated, as needle decompression is not always reliable. These patients must undergo definitive chest decompression with a chest tube. Although an airway may be patent and secured by intubation, it does not guarantee the effective air exchange in patients in whom pleuropulmonary relationships have been distorted by the pneumothorax. These patients require immediate placement of a chest tube at the fifth intercostal space, mid-axillary line, under sterile conditions so that air and blood can be evacuated from the affected hemithoracic cavity.

The amount of blood egressing from the chest tube may indicate the need for an urgent thoracotomy, but the chest tube output may not always provide a reliable indicator of intrathoracic bleeding. A clotted hemothorax may not be evacuated through the chest tube. Similarly, active bleeding may not necessarily originate from the chest but may originate within the abdomen and egress into the thoracic cavity via a large diaphragmatic laceration. A displaced intra-abdominal organ may be the source of bleeding in the thoracic cavity, usually the spleen through a diaphragmatic rupture or laceration.[11]

Avoidance of iatrogenic injuries during chest tube placement is of the utmost importance. The pleural cavity should always be entered over, and not under, the ribs to avoid laceration to the intercostal vessels. It must be remembered that these vessels are fixed in position by ligaments and cannot retract. The arteries can be the source of massive bleeding, as they are branches of the thoracic aorta. Open pneumothoraces should be covered with a partial occlusive dressing, followed with simultaneous insertion of a chest tube in an area remote from the chest wall defect.

Impaled objects must not be removed in the emergency department (ED). Patients who have been impaled are often transported on their side; this poses a challenge in terms of securing an airway and inserting chest tubes. The patient must be rapidly transported to the operating room, and the patient may need to be positioned between two operating tables to allow the impaled object to dangle free for removal after appropriate surgical control has been obtained.

Patients who have incurred a penetrating thoracic injury and arrive in cardiopulmonary arrest need to undergo a thoracotomy in the ED. This procedure must be performed expeditiously, as it is fraught with pitfalls and demands rapid and skillful performance. The goals are as follows:

- Control intrathoracic hemorrhage
- Initiate cardiopulmonary massage
- Restore an effective cardiac rhythm
- Decompress cardiac tamponade
- Repair penetrating cardiac injuries

Other goals include (1) rapid cross-clamping of the descending thoracic aorta to redirect the remaining intravascular volume to perfuse the coronaries as well as the carotid arteries and (2) control of any major pulmonary injuries that may produce air emboli, either directly or by cross-clamping the pulmonary hilum.

A resuscitative thoracotomy begins with a left anterolateral thoracotomy. The patient's left arm is displaced cephalad while an incision is made at the fifth left intercostal space from the left parasternal border to the posterior axillary line. In females, the breast is retracted cephalad to avoid iatrogenic injury. The incision is rapidly extended through the skin and subcutaneous tissues as well as the intercostal muscles. A Finochietto rib retractor is placed, and the accumulated blood is removed. Any areas of bleeding are identified and either digitally controlled or clamped. The left lung is retracted medially and out of the thoracic cavity. The descending thoracic aorta is located at the diaphragmatic hiatus. It is digitally palpated, sharply and bluntly dissected until it can be encircled; it is then occluded with an aortic clamp.[12]

The pericardium is opened longitudinally, anterior to the phrenic nerve, and the heart is visualized. Any areas of laceration are rapidly repaired. If the injury is deemed to be in the right hemithoracic cavity, the surgeon carries an extension of this incision through the sternum by sharply transecting and extending the incision into a right anterolateral thoracotomy to provide ample exposure of the contents of both hemithoracic cavities and pericardium.

Any pulmonary injuries that are discovered are clamped to prevent air emboli. In cases of pulmonary hilar injuries, an aortic cross-clamp can be used to occlude the hilum. The survival rate for patients sustaining exsanguinating abdominal-vascular injuries undergoing an ED thoracotomy is 5%, but the survival rate for patients undergoing ED thoracotomy after cardiopulmonary arrest from blunt trauma is 1%.[13, 14]

When rapid restoration of intravascular volume is deemed necessary, placement of large-bore lines utilizing an 8.5 French (Fr.) introducing catheter in the femoral vein provides an excellent route. The use of trauma tubing should be encouraged because it facilitates the rapid transfusion of crystalloid solutions and blood. Rapid infusor technology should be used for two reasons: (1) its ability to rapidly restore lost intravascular volume and (2) its ability to warm transfuse warm solutions and prevent hypothermia. The crystalloid solution of choice is lactated Ringer's.[13, 14]

Physical Examination

The physical examination of the patient with a thoracic injury should be both thorough and systematic. Initial observation should include inspection of the entire thoracic cavity, and the examiner should note whether there is adequate air exchange by observing thoracic excursions. Is one hemithoracic cavity moving better than the other? Is the patient able to inspire deeply, or is the patient using the accessory muscles of respiration? Inspection should encompass the following:

- Looking for deformities
- Locating hematomas in the thoracic inlet
- Determining whether they are pulsatile
- Identifying any open wounds
- Detecting any paradoxical movement of the chest

The examiner must palpate the entire thorax, looking for the presence or absence of fractured clavicles, sternum, scapulae, ribs, or thoracic spine. The examiner can estimate the excursion of the thorax by asking the patient to take a deep breath while placing one's hands at each side of the thorax. The diagnosis of a flail chest can be clinically demanding and often may remain undetected for hours to days. Even more difficult to detect is the presence of a central flail chest in which sternocostal cartilage disarticulations are present and the sternum is freely moveable. Physical examination should include palpation of the sternum to detect pain and fractures. While palpating the thorax, the examiner should note the presence of subcutaneous emphysema or crepitus.

Palpation of the pulses at the base of the neck, particularly the carotid arteries, is important. Palpation of the supraclavicular fossa may detect thrills. The examiner should also palpate the pulses of the brachial, radial, and ulnar arteries bilaterally and compare them with the pulses in the lower extremities to note any discrepancies. The trachea should be palpated and tenderness elicited. The use of the ankle-brachial index may detect the presence of vascular injuries.

The chest is then auscultated for bruit. The presence or absence of breath sounds, their intensity, and their quality should be documented, and the presence or absence of rales and rhonchi should be detected. Air in the mediastinum usually produces a systolic "crunch" known as *Hamman's crunch*. Pneumopericardium may present as a "bruit de Moulin" or windmill bruit, described by Brichetaeu.[15]

Beck's triad, consisting of jugular venous distention, hypotension, and muffled heart tones, should be diligently searched for. However, the classical triad is not a common finding until late in the course. Similarly, *Kussmaul's sign* (jugular-venous distention on inspiration) should be searched for, although it is also infrequently present. Both of these signs indicate pericardial tamponade. The examiner should also recognize that the lower thoracic cage actually provides protection for intra-abdominal organs, chiefly liver and spleen. For left-sided lower rib fractures, there is a 20% incidence of associated splenic injuries; for right-sided lower rib fractures, there is a 10% incidence of associated hepatic injuries.[16]

DIAGNOSTIC INVESTIGATIONS

The chest is perhaps one of the easiest cavities to initially assess. A plane anteroposterior (AP) radiograph, preferably upright, can provide diagnosis of injuries to the structural components of the thoracic cavity as well as bleeding within each hemithorax. The radiograph allows visualization of fractures of the clavicles, ribs, and occasionally the sternum. Similarly, the integrity of the thoracic spine can also be assessed. The mediastinum is also evaluated by a plain radiograph. Often the initial supine film shows a wide mediastinum, but often the widening noted in the initial film disappears in a better upright film. If the mediastinum still appears to be widened (>8 cm), further investigation is warranted. A widened mediastinum may occur with bleeding from pulmonary veins, thoracic spinal fractures, and, most important, from a ruptured thoracic aorta.

Associated radiographic findings from a ruptured thoracic aorta include obliteration of the aortic knob, deviation of the trachea to the right, pleural cap, and an associated left hemothorax. Other findings include fractures of the first and second ribs with associated clavicular fractures, elevation and rightward shift of the right mainstem bronchus, depression of the left mainstem bronchus, obliteration of the aorticopulmonary window, and deviation of the nasogastric tube to the right. This last radiographic finding is least frequently seen but is the most reliable finding.[5]

A chest x-ray can also be used for diagnosis of injury to the diaphragm. The presence of a coiled nasogastric tube in the left hemithoracic cavity is pathognomonic for blunt rupture of the left hemidiaphragm.[5] Hemothorax can easily be detected on a radiograph. diagnosis of a pneumothorax, however, should be confirmed based on clinical findings obtained during the initial physical examination.

For exclusion of thoracic aortic injuries, the aortogram remains the "gold standard." Thoracic aortography reliably establishes the diagnosis of ruptured thoracic aorta. This injury is usually distal to the ligamentum arteriosum. Occasionally, a rupture of the thoracic aorta can extend into the ostium of the left subclavian artery, the left common carotid artery, and the aortic arch. It is frequently stated that out of 100 thoracic aortograms performed, 90 will be negative.[17]

The use of the helical computed tomography (CT) scan has recently come into vogue. Although it is a relatively new investigational tool, its diagnostic accuracy appears to be approximately 75%. With time and experience, this modality may be able to reduce the need for thoracic aortography. It is currently being used as a screening tool at various trauma centers across the United states.[17] A ruptured thoracic aorta can occur even in the presence of a normal chest x-ray in approximately 5% of all cases.[17] Thoracic aortography or CT scans have been used to study the thoracic aorta based purely on the mechanism of injury. Clearly well-documented acceleration-deceleration mechanisms, if found in association with radiographic findings, demand investigation. We recommend initial screening with CT if the mediastinum cannot be cleared with an upright chest radiograph and if there are no other associated radiographic findings. If the CT scan is positive, we proceed to aortography. We still consider thoracic aortography to be the gold standard and use it liberally if the chest radiograph shows a widened mediastinum and the patient has either mechanism or other positive associated findings on chest x-ray. Similarly, lateral impacts, which have now been documented to cause rupture of the thoracic aorta, also merit investigation.

If a persistent air leak develops after placement of a chest tube, two etiologic factors must be excluded—ruptured bronchus and ruptured esophagus. In such an event, bronchoscopy is required to detect any bronchial tears. In the case of the esophagus, either an esophagogram with dilute barium and/or esophagoscopy should be performed. Classically, rigid esophagoscopy has been the investigational tool of choice; however, this method necessitates general anesthesia and carries the risk of cervical esophageal rupture at Killian's triangle. Recently, flexible esophagoscopy has proved a valuable tool in the diagnosis of these injuries.[15, 18]

The acute diagnosis of penetrating diaphragmatic injuries can be difficult. Diagnostic peritoneal lavage is not very reliable because the diaphragm does not bleed much. Thoracoscopy has been used to confirm the diagnosis of these injuries, but this method requires positioning the patient, double-lumen intubation, and placement of a chest tube after the completion of the procedure. Many patients harboring penetrating diaphragmatic injuries, particularly in the left side, do not have an associated hemothorax.[19] Diagnostic laparoscopy is the method of choice. Murray and coworkers[20] have reported a 42% incidence of diaphragmatic injuries after penetrating left thoracoabdominal trauma. In many of these cases, the radiograph was entirely normal.

The use of the hand-held Doppler probe is valuable. One can use this equipment to hear the subclavian, axillary, and carotid arteries. This probe can detect bruits and continuous murmurs consistent with arteriovenous fistulas. Similarly, color flow Doppler studies can be used to diagnose injuries to these vessels without the need for invasive angiograms.

PRINCIPLES OF SURGICAL MANAGEMENT

The trauma surgeon must rethink the anatomic conceptualization of the thoracic cavity. The thoracic cavity is divided into right and left hemithoracic cavities, pericardium, anterior, and posterior mediastinum. Consequently, not every single organ within these cavities is accessible through a single incision. The choice of which thoracic cavity and incision must be given careful thought. Given the acute condition of these patients, the wrong incision does not often allow one to reconsider after a choice has been made.

Five incisions are used for the management of thoracic injuries:

1. Anterolateral thoracotomy.
2. Bilateral anterolateral thoracotomies.
3. Median sternotomy.
4. Posterolateral thoracotomy.
5. Open book thoracotomy.

Anterolateral Thoracotomy

The left anterolateral thoracotomy is the incision of choice for the patient arriving in cardiopulmonary arrest. This incision can be rapidly performed and allows access to the left hemithoracic cavity for aortic cross-clamping and open cardiopulmonary massage. The surgeon can extend this incision into *bilateral* anterolateral thoracotomies, should the need arise, by transecting the sternum. When this is done, both internal mammary arteries must be ligated. The anterolateral thoracotomy is also the incision of choice for a patient who is hemodynamically unstable and harbors an injury to either the right or the left thoracic cavities. The degree of hemodynamic instability often precludes placement of the patient in the right or left posterolateral position. Endotracheal intubation with a double-lumen tube is the ideal method of intubation. This method allows for selective collapse of the affected lung to facilitate surgical exposure.

For patients sustaining thoracoabdominal trauma that requires simultaneous abdominal exploration, anterolateral thoracotomy combined with a *midline laparotomy* is the incision of choice. Bilateral anterolateral thoracotomies allows for exposure of most thoracic organs in both hemithoracic cavities as well as the pericardium and anterior mediastinum.

Median Sternotomy

Median sternotomy is reserved for patients sustaining penetrating cardiac injuries or injuries to the origins of the great vessels of the chest. This incision can be extended into the anterior border of the sternocleidomastoid for the management of carotid arterial injuries. The right posterolateral thoracotomy is used for the management of patients sustaining penetrating right-sided pulmonary injuries or esophageal injuries. The rare azygos or hemiazygos vein injuries can also be managed by this incision. The left posterolateral thoracotomy is used for the management of left-sided pulmonary injuries and is also the incision of choice for the management of blunt ruptures of the thoracic aorta. The rare distal esophageal injury can also benefit from this incision.

Book Thoracotomy

The book thoracotomy is a complex incision, which requires a left anterolateral thoracotomy, complete or partial median sternotomy and a supraclavicular incision. Originally, this incision was described for the management of injuries to the origins of the left subclavian artery. Because the book thoracotomy is cumbersome and difficult to perform, it should be reserved for exsanguinating thoracic vascular injuries involving the origin of the left subclavian artery of a patient admitted in cardiopulmonary arrest. In these cases, a left anterolateral thoracotomy with digital occlusion of the origin of the left subclavian artery, aortic cross-clamping, and open cardiopulmonary massage may salvage some of these patients.

MANAGEMENT OF SPECIFIC INJURIES

Six thoracic injuries and clinical scenarios are lethal immediately. We have dubbed them "the six that will kill you now." They are (1) airway obstruction, (2) tension pneumothorax, (3) open pneumothorax, (4) massive hemothorax, (5) flail chest, and (6) cardiac tamponade. Prompt surgical intervention is required if the patient is to survive.

In contradistinction, six other thoracic injuries and clinical scenarios can be just as lethal but they exert their lethality on a delayed bases. They are: (1) pulmonary contusion, (2) myocardial contusion, (3) aortic disruption, (4) diaphragmatic injury, (5) tracheobronchial tree disruptions, and (6) esophageal injuries. Prompt therapeutic interventions is also required in these instances, but more time is allowed for diagnostic investigations.

Chest Wall and Pleural Injuries

Flail Chest

Flail chest occurs when there is discontinuity of a segment of the thoracic wall. A flail chest usually develops after the patient has sustained multiple rib fractures. The injury consists of at least two breaks in three separate ribs in continuity, resulting in paradoxical chest wall movement. Whereas paradoxical thoracic wall movement in the past was considered the predominant causative factor for the patients hypoxemia, it is the underlying pulmonary contusion that plays the greater role in the patient's inability to oxygenate and ventilate. The contused pulmonary tissue becomes hemorrhagic and is unavailable for gas exchange.

The multiple trauma outcome study (MTOS) of the American College of Surgeons consists of a data base of 50,000 trauma patients. Of these patients, 31% sustained thoracic injuries; of this group 5% were noted to have flail chest.[2] In the European literature, the incidence of flail chest is reported to be between 8 and 13% in studies encompassing greater than 3000 thoracic injury patients.[21]

Flail chest, as a rule, occurs not as an isolated injury but in association with other equally severe injuries. Mackersie[22] reported that in patients sustaining isolated thoracic injuries, flail chest occurred with a frequency of 20% and was associated with multiple rib fractures in 39% and pulmonary contusion in 25% of the cases. Similarly, in patients with a closed head injury, the incidence of flail chest was 52%. In patients sustaining abdominal injury, the incidence was 39%. In patients sustaining pelvic or extremity injuries, the incidence was 42%.

Physical examination of a thoracic wall by palpation may often miss the presence of flail chest secondary to splinting of the injured chest wall. Central flail chest, in which sternocostal disarticulations occur, can also be difficult to detect by physical examination. Shackford and colleagues[23, 24] reported that of 36 patients admitted with blunt thoracic injuries, five (14%) experienced a 14- to 75-hour delay in diagnosis of flail chest. Landercasper and coauthors[25] reported that of 99 patients admitted with blunt thoracic injuries, 22 (22%) experienced a delay in diagnosis ranging from 1 to 10 days. The management of flail chest should take into account the underlying injury to the lung that may render it sensitive to fluid underload and overload.

The modern-day era of flail chest management began with a study reported by Avery and coworkers.[26] They described a new method for treatment of flail chest with continuous mechanical hyperventilation to produce alkalotic apnea and internal pneumatic stabilization of the thoracic chest wall. This remained the preferred method of treatment until Trinkle and associates[27] questioned mandatory intubation and mechanical ventilation of these patients and proposed a more selective approach. In this study, a first group of patients was treated with early mechanical ventilation and subsequent tracheostomy. A second group was managed selectively and intubated only if they were unable to oxygenate or ventilate well, despite supplemental oxygen. This group was treated with fluid restriction, steroids, albumin, intensive chest physiotherapy, and a liberal regimen of pain medication. There were significant differences between these two groups. In the mechanically intubated group, patients experienced a 21% mortality rate and a 100% complication rate with a prolonged hospital course. In the selectively managed group, the patients experienced 0% mortality and a 20% complication rate and had significantly shortened hospital lengths of stay (average, 9 days).

The concept of selective endotracheal intubation and mechanical ventilation is also supported by Shackford and coworkers.[23, 24] They prospectively treated 36 patients sustaining flail chest according to a strict protocol. They reported an 85% incidence of pulmonary related complications in intubated patients along with a 69% incidence of pneumonia. Richardson and coworkers[28] treated 427 patients with severe blunt chest trauma. Their protocol included selective endotracheal intubation and mechanical ventilation, avoidance of fluid overload, and vigorous chest physiotherapy. Of this group, 328 patients were not intubated and only 10 were not benefited and required intubation for a 97% successful outcome. In the second group, 99 patients initially required intubation and mechanical ventilation. Flail chest and pulmonary contusions without flail chest occurred in 95 of these patients. Of the flail chest patient population, 50% were intubated but 70% were intubated for less than 3 days. The authors were thus able to extend the principle of selective endotracheal intubation and mechanical ventilation to patients sustaining not only flail chest but also pulmonary contusions.

Key in the management of flail chest is pain relief. All

patients with multiple rib fractures, associated chest wall contusions, and hemothoraces and pneumothoraces requiring chest tube insertion have severe pain with limited chest wall excursions. Pain relief allows the patient to maintain effective ventilation and oxygenation and to preserve the cough mechanism necessary to eliminate pulmonary secretions. Pain can be managed by analgesia, multiple rib blocks, and placement of epidural catheters; we currently favor epidural catheters. Mackersie and coworkers,[22] evaluating the safety and efficacy of continuous epidural fentanyl analgesia in 40 patients who sustained multiple rib fractures and flail chest after blunt thoracic injury, noted that this methodology yielded significant improvements in vital capacity and the ability to generate a negative inspiratory force.

Numerous methods for stabilization of the chest wall have been described, including sandbags to towel clips connected to a complicated system of weights and pulleys. These systems were ineffective and have been abandoned. The concept of surgical reduction and internal fixation may be an attractive alternative for eliminating prolonged mechanical intubation, preventing pulmonary related complications, lessening pain, facilitating physical activity, enabling the patient to return to an active life, and correcting chest wall deformities.

Paris and colleagues,[29] describing a study of 29 patients in which Frammer struts were used, were able to decrease the period of mechanical ventilation and recovery time. Moore[30] described a series of 112 patients who underwent intramedullary pinning, and demonstrated the ability to avoid tracheostomy and reduced the time spent in mechanical ventilation while lessening the chest wall deformities. Thomas and coworkers,[31] reporting a study of four patients in which Jergensen plates were used, measured pulmonary function tests after surgical reduction and stabilization. Results, however, were inconclusive. Menard and coauthors,[32] using Judet's plates, surgically stabilized 18 patients and were able to demonstrate a shorter duration of mechanical ventilation, decreasing the functional sequelae in these patients. Despite these reports, proposed benefits from surgical reduction and internal fixation of flail chest have not been conclusive.

Although literature outside the United States certainly seems to support this concept of operative stabilization, the American experience is very limited and consists of two case reports by Haasler[33] and Landreneau et al.[34] Recently there has been renewed interest in surgical techniques for chest wall stabilization. Nagaie and colleagues[35] reported a novel method for surgical stabilization of the chest using plastic straps and a tie gun. Other authors in the European surgical literature have reported good results utilizing different techniques. Reber and coinvestigators[36] reported on 11 patients stabilized by means of the Swiss external fixation (AO) technique and demonstrated improved ventilatory mechanics and decreased ventilator and intensive care unit (ICU) requirement of surgical fixation.

Ahmed and coauthors[37] compared internal fixation versus endotracheal intubation and ventilation and two patient groups. In the first group 26 patients underwent internal fixation, and in the second group 38 patients were managed with intubation and mechanical ventilation. Patients undergoing surgical fixation were weaned from the ventilator in a mean of 1.3 days, 11% required tracheostomy, and only 15% had pulmonary-related complications. The question still remains: Does the risk of a thoracotomy and a complex chest wall reconstructive procedure outweigh the benefits of surgical reduction and internal stabilization? Certainly, this issue is not clear.

Kishikawa and associates[38] prospectively studied pulmonary function of 18 patients after blunt chest trauma for 6 months. Nine of the patients had flail chest, and 12 had pulmonary contusion. Pulmonary function tests, arterial blood gases, chest radiographs, and CT scans were reviewed. It was found that functional residual capacity (FRC) remained significantly reduced throughout the 6 months of the study period in patients with sustained pulmonary contusions. The ability of the patients to oxygenate decreased when they changed from a sitting to a supine position. The patients were all documented to have fibrotic changes in the contused lung, demonstrated by CT scan 6 months after injury. These findings were also supported by an additional study of another 20 patients who had sustained pulmonary contusions 1 to 4 years previously. This study demonstrates that the reduction in lung volumes in flail chest patients is due to pulmonary fibrosis that develops after pulmonary contusion rather than chest wall deformity. Also, although flail chest may cause short-term (4 months) respiratory dysfunction, it does not cause long-term dysfunction despite the thoracic wall deformity.

How, then, can we reconcile the findings of these studies? The answers have yet to be formulated. It appears that after flail chest and pulmonary contusion, both static and dynamic compliances are altered. It follows that restoration of continuity of the chest wall and pleuropulmonary relationships, and eventually healing of the pulmonary tissue, should improve both compliances.

A provocative study that sheds some light on the role of both chest deformity and pulmonary function was reported by Gyhra and coworkers.[39] They studied the effective ventilatory function of a flail segment in both the internal and external positions in a canine model. Tidal volumes decreased, and respiratory rates increased from control to flail conditions and also when the flail segment was placed internally; both parameters improved when the flail segment was placed in the external position. Minute volumes were also decreased from flail conditions and when the flail segment was placed externally. The authors concluded that a flail segment in an internal position is deleterious for respiratory mechanics but that restoration of the flail segment to an external position significantly improved ventilatory parameters.

Rib Fractures

The ribs are the most commonly injured component of the thoracic cage. There is a correlation between impact velocity and severe chest wall trauma. There also appears to be somewhat of a linear relationship between the number of ribs fractured and the degree of impact. The most significant physiologic impairment caused by rib fractures is a decrease in dynamic compliance. Coupled with the underlying pulmonary contusion and chest wall pain usually present, fractured ribs can create a significant problem for multiply injured, infirm, and elderly patients.

Rib fractures can be confirmed by a chest radiograph, although it is said that approximately 40% of rib fractures, particularly those located in the anterior and lateral positions of the first four ribs, may not be visualized for at least 1 to 2 weeks after the original injury.[40] Positive clinical findings, despite the absence of radiologic confirmation, support the diagnosis.

The pathophysiology of rib fractures is intimately associated with the underlying pulmonary contusion. Both dynamic and static compliances of the chest wall and pulmonary tissue are altered. The underlying pulmonary contusion renders a portion of the pulmonary parenchyma unavailable for effective oxygenation and ventilation, resulting in a decrease in alveolar ventilation causing hypoxemia and hypercapnia leading to ventilatory failure.

The upper three ribs are protected by the bony framework and musculature of the upper extremity. Consequently, it takes great force to produce their fracture. The presence of these fractures constitutes a marker for severe associated injuries, including a ruptured thoracic aorta. Wilson and coworkers[41] reported on 120 patients admitted with first and second rib fractures. Major vascular trauma was documented in 6%. These findings let the authors to recommend angiography whenever these fractures are detected. Similarly, Albers et al.,[42] Fisher et al.,[43] and others[44-47] have also documented a high frequency of associated vascular injuries if upper ribs are fractured or if there are multiple fractured ribs.

The middle ribs (fourth through ninth) sustain the majority of blunt trauma. The application of an anteroposterior force causes compression of the thoracic cage with subsequent outward bowing of the ribs, fracturing their shaft. Direct impact applied to these ribs not only may result in a fracture but also may cause displacement of the fractured segment inward, which can pierce the parenchyma lacerating the lung and causing a pneumothorax or hemothorax.[5]

Fractures of the lower ribs (10th through 12th), which protect solid abdominal viscera, are known to have an associated incidence of injuries to the liver and spleen. In the right side, fracture of these ribs is associated with 10% incidence of hepatic injury; in the left side, they are associated with a 20% incidence of splenic injuries.[16] In a series reported by Bassett and coworkers[48] consisting of 783 patients with fractured ribs, 71% of the patients admitted in shock sustained an associated intra-abdominal injury.

Sternal Fractures

Sternal fractures generally occur secondary to direct impact. The impact must be of high energy and generally cause compression of the thoracic cage. Most sternal fractures involve the upper or mid portions.[49] Sternal fractures account for approximately 5% to 10% of all thoracic injuries.[16] Comminuted fractures account for less than 10% of the cases.[49, 50] Sternal fractures are generally associated with significant injuries 50% to 60% of the time. These injuries include rib fractures in approximately 40% of the patients, long bone fractures in 25%, and closed head injuries in 18%.[49, 50] Occasionally, costochondral cartilage fractures or disarticulations occur, resulting in a central flail chest.

The diagnosis of sternal fractures is established by physical examination that consistently reveals tenderness over the sternum. Deformities may also be observed. The examiner should palpate the sternocostal junctions to detect fractures and disarticulations. If the sternum is freely mobile, the diagnosis of central flail chest is certain. Physical findings should be confirmed with a plain radiograph, as well as a cross-table lateral film of the sternum; this film excludes displacement of the sternum.

Associated myocardial contusion has been reported to occur with sternal fractures. Buckman and coworkers[49] observed electrocardiographic (ECG) changes in 62% of patients with sternal fractures. Wojcik and Morgan,[50] however, utilizing ECG changes, elevation of cardiac enzyme levels, and abnormal echocardiographic findings as diagnostic criteria for myocardial contusion, could establish this diagnosis in only 18% of 66 patients. Harley and Mena[51] noted abnormal findings on radionuclide angiography in 91% of patients with sternal fractures.

The treatment of sternal fractures consists of pain relief and—in rare instances if the external fracture is displaced and impinging on the right ventricle—surgical intervention. In this case, an incision is made directly over the fracture and the fragments are elevated and fixed in a neutral position by means of sternal wires. Brookes, Hills, and Jackson and their colleagues[52-54] reported on the benign nature of isolated sternal fractures. Brookes and associates[52] reported a 6.8% incidence of cardiac dysrhythmias in 124 patients with isolated sternal fractures. The overall mortality of 272 patients with these injuries in the Brooks series was 0.74% and zero in the 124 patients with isolated fractures.

Scapular and Clavicular Fractures

Scapular Fractures

Because the scapula is well protected by a large muscular mass, scapular fractures are relatively uncommon. If the diagnosis of a fractured scapula is established, the trauma surgeon must assume that a large amount of energy has been dissipated onto the thoracic wall. According to McGahan, Thompson, and Wilber and their colleagues,[55-57] most fractures of the scapula involve the body and neck of this bone. Fractures in the glenoid, coracoid, and acromion are even less frequent. The presence of a scapular fracture serves as a marker for possible development of respiratory failure.[58] It is rare to find an isolated scapular fracture, since there is a 80% to 98% incidence of associated fractures.[55, 56]

According to Thompson and coauthors,[56] there is a 54% incidence of associated pulmonary contusions and rib fractures and a 27% incidence of associated clavicular fractures. Other significant associated injuries include a 13% incidence of brachial plexus injury and an 11% incidence of associated vascular injuries. The diagnosis of a scapular fracture can be made on the basis of clinical findings, which include local pain, edema and crepitus. Harris and Harris[58] reported that 88% of all scapular fractures are visible on the initial chest radiograph but may be overlooked in 35% of the patients. Treatment consists of shoulder immobilization and pain control. Rarely are open reduction and internal fixation necessary.

Scapulothoracic disassociation usually occurs from a hyperextension mechanism of the upper extremity. Generally, it results in musculoskeletal injuries, which may involve the clavicle, scapula, upper rib fractures, brachial plexus, and associated vascular injuries. There is a high incidence of disability when this syndrome occurs secondary to the brachial plexus injury. Axillosubclavian thrombosis secondary to intimal flaps demands immediate surgical intervention; however, there is no guarantee that functionality can be restored to the affected extremity.[59]

Clavicular Fractures

Clavicular fractures, in contrast to scapular fractures, usually occur as isolated injuries; 75% of these fractures occur in the middle third and the rest occur in the proximal and the distal thirds of this bone.[60] Clinical findings include local pain and deformity. Chest radiographs usually confirm clinical findings. Injuries to the subclavian artery have been reported.[47]

Treatment consists of pain control and immobilization with a figure-of-8 sling. Rarely are open reduction and internal fixation indicated. The outcome is generally positive, although most fractures heal with some degree of deformity. In rare cases of non-union, open reduction and internal fixation are indicated but the outcome is often failure of union. Rarely, clavicular fractures are associated with blunt injury of the axillary and subclavian vessels.[47] Thrombosis of these vessels is usually caused by an intimal flap that requires resection and repair.

Traumatic dislocation of the sternoclavicular junction occurs when a significant force has been applied to this area. Neer and Rockwood[61] report that anterior dislocations occur much more frequently than posterior dislocations. Buckerfield and Castle[62] report a significant number of associated injuries occurring with posterior sternoclavicular dislocations. These injuries affect the brachial plexus and trachea as well as both subclavian vessels. Although the absence of palpable pulses clearly points to a thrombosis of the subclavian artery, the presence of a pulse does not exclude an intimal flap in the subclavian artery that may later lead to thrombosis. In our opinion, posterior dislocation of the sternoclavicular junction demands an arteriogram as well a venous-phase study to exclude both subclavian arterial and venous injuries. Treatment consists of close reduction of either type of dislocation. Open reduction and internal fixation are reserved for failure of closed reduction.

Pneumothorax (Simple, Tension, and Open)

Pneumothorax, defined as an accumulation of air within the thoracic cavity, occurs when the normal pleuroparietal relationships are disturbed by either blunt or penetrating trauma. This results in violation of both the parietal and visceral pleurae as well as the pulmonary parenchyma, producing an escape of air into the thoracic cavity. Gray and coworkers[63] reported an 8% incidence of pneumothorax and a 42% incidence of hemopneumothorax in a series of 2917 cases of penetrating trauma. Harrison and coworkers[64] reported a 24% incidence of pneumothorax and a 55% incidence of hemopneumothorax in a series of 203 patients sustaining blunt thoracic trauma.

There are three types of pneumothorax: simple, tension, and open.

Simple Pneumothorax

The pathophysiology of pneumothorax is based on the compression effect imposed on the affected lung by the escaped air. This causes a reduction in tidal and total lung volumes, thus effectively reducing the lung's capability for oxygenation and ventilation. A pneumothorax may be caused by both blunt and penetrating trauma. Several mechanisms may produce pleuropulmonary disturbances, such as (1) fractured ribs piercing the pulmonary parenchyma, (2) deceleration and crush injuries, which may tear the lung, and (3) lacerations of the pulmonary parenchyma by stab wounds and missile injuries and by sudden increases in intrathoracic pressures.

The clinical findings include shortness of breath, chest pain, jugular venous distention, decreased breath sounds, and hyperresonance of the affected hemithoracic cavity. Treatment consists of evacuating the escaped air by the insertion of a chest tube.

Tension Pneumothorax

Tension pneumothorax results once an air leak develops from a pulmonary injury, which allows air to escape from the lung but not exit the thoracic cavity. Consequently, air is forced into the thoracic cavity without any means of escape, thus progressively increasing intrathoracic pressure and resulting in the complete collapse of the affected lung. Similarly, the mediastinum and trachea are displaced to the contralateral side, compressing the unaffected lung. This renders ventilation ineffective while at the same time decreasing venous return, since the vena cava is twisted in its axis.

The patient with a tension pneumothorax requires immediate decompression either by needle thoracostomy, often performed in the pre-hospital setting, or insertion of a chest tube. Because clinical signs may not be easily detectable in the noisy environment of a trauma center, any suspicion should mandate immediate placement of a chest tube. Similarly, the presence of bilateral tension pneumothoraces may be lethal. In these cases, the inexperienced trauma surgeon may not suspect this condition. Clinical findings may be misleading, as the patient appears to have breath sounds. The sounds transmitted are those of the heart. Tension pneumothorax should be suspected when there are penetrating injuries to both hemithoracic cavities or massive blunt trauma to the thoracic cavity.

Management consists of immediate placement of chest tubes. In a series of 287 patients incurring thoracic injuries, Mattox and coworkers[65] reported eight tension pneumothoraces and 54 bilateral pneumothoraces.

Open Pneumothorax

Blast injuries or large defects of a chest wall, which remain open, create an open pneumothorax, also described as a sucking chest wound. The opening in the chest wall allows for equilibration between the positive atmospheric and the negative intrathoracic pressure causing immediate collapse of the ipsilateral lung. Similarly, if the chest wall defect is greater than two thirds of the diameter of the trachea, air will flow preferentially through the defect, immediately rendering ventilation and oxygenation ineffective and leading to hypoxia and pulmonary arrest.

Management consists of covering the defect with a sterile occlusive dressing, which is taped securely on three sides. As the patient inspires, the dressing adheres to the thoracic wall; as the patient expires, air flows freely from the untaped corner. Chest tubes should be placed in an area remote from the defect. Immediate surgical intervention is necessary for reconstruction of the chest wall defect.

Hemothorax

A hemothorax is defined as an accumulation of blood within the thoracic cavity. It results from a disturbance of normal pleuropulmonary relationships either from blunt or penetrating trauma. Generally, penetrating trauma is the most frequent cause. The resulting hemorrhage and associated air escaping from the injured pulmonary parenchyma cause a reduction of both tidal and total lung volumes, impairing oxygenation and ventilation. Gray and coworkers[63] reported a 28% incidence of hemothorax in a series of 2917 cases of penetrating chest trauma. Harrison et al.[64] reported a 21% incidence of hemothorax in a series of 203 patients sustaining blunt chest injury.

Frequent causes include (1) fractured ribs that lacerate the lung, (2) lacerated intercostal vessels and internal mammary arteries, and (3) torn adhesions between the pleura and the lung. Clinical presentations are similar to those of pneumothorax, except that dullness of percussion is also noted. A delayed hemothorax usually occurs after blunt trauma; radiologic findings may appear between 1 and 3 days after the initial injury.

Treatment consists of the evacuation of blood from the affected hemithoracic cavity with a chest tube. If the initial volume output is less than 1000 mL, the patient should be observed, because in most cases operative intervention is not necessary. For a hemothorax that continues to incur a blood loss of 200 mL/hour during 4 hours, operative intervention is required.

Massive hemothorax has been defined as accumulation between 1000 to 1500 mL of blood in a thoracic cavity. It generally results from penetrating injuries that have extensively damaged pulmonary parenchyma, hilar pulmonary vessels, or other thoracic vascular structures. The patient may present in profound shock with neck veins that may either be flat secondary to the rapid loss of intravascular volume or distended if the hemothorax produces a mechanical compressive effect.

This condition is managed by the immediate insertion of a No. 36 to 40 Fr. chest tube. If the initial volume of blood from the thoracic cavity is greater than 1000 mL, most trauma surgeons proceed to immediate thoracotomy. Others cite the figure of 1500 mL.[65, 66] Upon initial placement of the chest tube, a large quantity of blood may egress and its flow may be continuous. If this is the case, the chest tube should be clamped and the patient immediately transferred to an operating room. However, if a large volume of blood is evacuated and suddenly stops, this may not mean that the initial hemorrhagic event has ceased; it may indicate that the bleeding has been so rapid and massive that blood has clotted within the affected hemithoracic cavity. This may produce a tension hemothorax. This situation can be deceiving and can be detected by a chest film. An immediate thoracotomy is warranted.

Traumatic Asphyxia

In 1837, the entity known as traumatic asphyxia was described as the *masque ecchymotique*, a syndrome including craniocervical and thoracic cyanosis, facial edema, petechiae, and subconjunctival hemorrhage.[67] Patients look as if they are moribund.[68] Occasionally, neurologic symptoms and chest wall and thoracic injuries may be present. This syndrome occurs when the thoracic cage has been either crushed or subjected to direct pressure transmitted by a large weight load. The pathophysiology involves sudden increases in intrathoracic and superior vena caval pressures, which are transmitted retrograde to the venous circulation. This causes reversal of blood flow and capillary rupture. This mechanism is responsible for the patient's physical appearance.

Treatment is supportive and involves securing proper oxygenation and ventilation and dealing with any associated injuries. If neurologic symptoms are present, other causes must be excluded; elevation of the head of the bed is recommended. The outcome is generally favorable but is related to the extent and duration of the asphyxia and to the severity of the associated injuries. Neurologic manifestations usually resolve in 24 to 72 hours without long-term sequelae.[70]

Pulmonary Injuries

Pulmonary injuries result from both blunt and penetrating trauma. Blunt mechanisms can cause pulmonary lacerations and intraparenchymal hematomas. Penetrating mechanisms include stab wounds and missile injuries. The low pulmonary arterial pressures, coupled with the high concentration of lung thromboplastin, generally limit hemorrhage from lung parenchyma. Approximately 10% to 15% of these patients require thoracotomy for continuous bleeding.[65, 66]

McNamara and coworkers[71] reported that 63% of Vietnam combat casualties sustaining penetrating trauma had significant lung injuries. Graham and coworkers,[72] in a series of 666 patients with thoracic injuries, reported an incidence of 56% (373) penetrating pulmonary injuries, 91 of which required thoracotomy. High-velocity missiles usually cause considerable damage with significant hemorrhage and devitalized tissue. These patients are much more likely to require early thoracotomy and pulmonary resection. For these cases, Zakharia[73] recommend a much more aggressive approach.

Massive hemothorax that can result from pulmonary parenchymal injuries can be managed by a pulmonary tractotomy. This procedure entails opening the pulmonary parenchyma directly approaching and selectively ligating the bleeding intraparenchymal vessels. This also allows the trauma surgeon to repair or ligate small transected bronchioles or bronchi.

Asensio and coworkers[74] have described the technique of stapled pulmonary tractotomy. A stapler is placed through the entrance and exit sites within the pulmonary parenchyma; this step separates the parenchyma rapidly to allow ligation of bleeding vessels. The pulmonary parenchyma can then be reconstructed after hemorrhage has been controlled. Pulmonary resections are infrequently needed to manage these injuries.

Indications for pulmonary resections[8, 72, 75, 76] include:

- Uncontrollable hemorrhage
- Extremely severe contusions
- Air embolism
- Destructive hilar injuries
- Massive intraparenchymal bleeding

Robinson and coworkers[77] reported that pulmonary resections were needed in 2% to 3% of gunshot wounds and in 1.1% of stab wounds of 168 patients sustaining lung injuries. Extensive pulmonary resections and pneumonectomies are indicated in only a few patients sustaining penetrating trauma.[78, 79] Richardson and coworkers[15] reported 34 patients (13%) undergoing lobectomy and nine patients (4%) undergoing pneumonectomies in a series 259 patients subjected to urgent thoracotomy for penetrating trauma. The vast majority of patients subjected to pneumonectomy are those with hilar injuries. The mortality rate for these patients is between 30% and 50%.[75, 77-80] Death is usually due to uncontrolled hemorrhage and air embolism.[81]

A patient with a pulmonary contusion may present with the entire clinical spectrum, ranging from benign to extremely severe and with hypoxia and respiratory failure. Initial findings on the chest radiograph reveal areas of opacification, which may progress for the very first 48 hours. Afterward, radiographic findings generally improve. For patients who cannot adequately maintain oxygenation and ventilation, early intubation and mechanical ventilation are indicated.

Airway Obstruction and Injury to the Trachea and Tracheobronchial Tree

Airway obstruction may occur when trauma victims may become unconscious, with the tongue falling backward, occluding the airway. Obstruction can also result from foreign bodies within the airway and direct structural damage to the larynx or trachea from either blunt or penetrating injury. The simplest way to relieve airway obstruction is the chin lift or jaw thrust maneuver.[5] Foreign bodies can be removed when they are visualized during laryngoscopy. If the causative agent airway obstruction is visualized and found to be located above the vocal cords, the surgeon may perform needle cricothyroidotomy, directing the needle cephalad and insufflating air under pressure. This procedure often dislodges foreign bodies.

If airway obstruction results from direct injury to the larynx or trachea, an airway may be secured with endotracheal intubation, aided by fiberoptic bronchoscopy. In some cases, immediate surgical access of the airway via cricothyroidotomy may be needed. In the extremely uncommon case of cricotracheal separation, securing an airway requires immediate performance of a lifesaving tracheostomy. Cricothyroidotomy is the procedure of choice for securing an airway, which cannot be secured by endotracheal intubation. Tracheostomy should not used for these purposes.

Overall, a patient with a fracture of the larynx generally presents with hoarseness, subcutaneous emphysema, and crepitus. There may also be total airway obstruction. In this case, immediate surgical access of the airway is lifesaving. In patients presenting with less acute symptomatology, diagnostic work-up should include CT scans of the neck and larynx to detect fractures.

Tracheal and tracheobronchial tree ruptures are uncommon. Bertelsen and Howitz[82] reported 33 cases of 1178 (2.8%) autopsied patients; of the 33 patients, 27 died instantly. Kemmerer and colleagues[83] reported five cases in 585 patients dying of vehicular accidents. De La Rocha and Kayler[84] reported six survivors of 327 patients admitted to the trauma unit in a 2-year period. Angood and coauthors[85] reported nine cases of 2000 (1%) patients treated for multiple blunt trauma (1% incidence).

Direct trauma to the trachea, including the mainstem bronchi, may be blunt or penetrating.[86, 87] Penetrating injuries to the tracheobronchial tree generally occur in association with major intrathoracic vascular, esophageal, or pulmonary injuries. Patients often present with severe respiratory distress secondary to airway compromise. Occasionally, few signs or symptoms are present, even with severe injuries. The earliest indication that an injury may exist occurs when the patient presents with a pneumothorax relieved by chest tube insertion. The presence of a large and persistent air leak, requiring multiple chest tubes to expand the lung, should point to the diagnosis. These patients should undergo immediate bronchoscopy to detect the bronchial tear. Most of these tears occur within 1 cm of the carina.

Treatment consists of immediate surgical intervention and primary repair. Missed tracheobronchial tree injuries carry a huge mortality.

Cardiac and Thoracic Vascular Injuries

Cardiac tamponade most often results from penetrating injuries of the heart. Such injuries pose a tremendous challenge, even for the most experienced trauma surgeons. Often the patient arrives *in extremis* and undergoes emergency thoracotomy. The mortality rate associated with penetrating cardiac injuries is extremely high. Beck's triad represents classic findings in a patient arriving with tamponade. This triad as well as Kussmaul's sign is the exception rather than the rule[5] (see Chapter 100, Pericardial Tamponade).

In general, penetrating cardiac injuries can be extremely deceptive in their clinical presentation. The heart may be injured by precordial as well as non-precordial injuries. Thoracoabdominal injuries can also involve the heart. The clinical presentation of penetrating cardiac injuries can range from hemodynamic stability to cardiopulmonary arrest. Many factors are at play, including the wounding agent and the time lapsed from injury to arrival in the trauma center in determining survival rates. Patients may present with exsanguination into the left hemithoracic cavity.[88]

Some authorities believe that pericardial tamponade provides a protective effect in these patients,[89] but others believe that it does not play a role.[88, 90] The truth may lie in between. Pericardial tamponade may provide its protective effect for a limited time, after which this effect becomes deleterious as the heart is unable to fill and accept venous return resulting in drastically reduced cardiac output.[88]

A contracting heart presents a moving target for the trauma surgeon to suture. Cardiac muscle does not easily lend itself to be repaired, particularly if it has sustained a gunshot wound. The muscle fibers have a propensity to continue contracting and separating from the blast effect caused by the missile. An additional challenge is presented by injuries adjacent to coronary arteries whose luminal integrity must be preserved during repair. Cardiac injuries are generally repaired with monofilament nonabsorbable sutures and, on occasion, bioprosthetic material such as polytef (Teflon) strips to buttress the repair.[12, 88]

Cardiac arrhythmias may develop immediately after the repair or may begin during the repair (i.e., ventricular fibrillation). Intraoperative cardioversion with a lower charge is required, generally consisting of 10 to 30 joules.[12, 88]

Because the heart muscle has been injured and repaired, it may not necessarily pump effectively. As a result, many patients need vasoactive drugs in order to maintain cardiac contractility, intraoperatively and postoperatively. It is recommended that these patients undergo hemodynamic invasive monitoring for effective management of preload, afterload, and myocardial contractility.

Asensio and coworkers[91] have reported a large 1-year preliminary prospective experience with penetrating cardiac injuries. In their series of 60 patients, 35 sustained gunshot wounds (58%) and 25 sustained stab wounds (42%), with an overall survival of 37%. Emergency thoracotomy was performed in 37 of 60 (62%), with a 16% survival rate.

Myocardial contusion is not usually difficult to diagnose, although in rare cases it may be lethal. Numerous controversies exist in the literature regarding its existence. Suffice it to say that patients sustaining massive blunt chest trauma and ECG abnormalities, such as multiple premature ventricular contractions (PVCs), atrial fibrillation, and ST-segment abnormalities, should be investigated to exclude myocardial contusion. According to Sutherland[92] and McLean[93] and their coworkers, myocardial contusion causing dangerous arrhythmias or impaired cardiac function occurs in 10% to 20% of cases.

Routine ECG monitoring and serial cardiac enzyme determinations are not warranted. This diagnosis is best established by two-dimensional echocardiography. Significant wall motion abnormalities demand intensive ECG monitoring. Occasionally, myocardial infarction may develop and patients may need vasoactive drugs and hemodynamic invasive monitoring.

The first ruptured the thoracic aorta was reported by Vesalius.[94] Bahnson[95] reported the first surgical repair of a posttraumatic thoracic aortic aneurysm and repair the aorta with a graft. The first successful repair of an acute thoracic aortic injury was performed by DeBakey and coauthors[96] and by Pasaro and Pace.[97] Thoracic aortic injuries may occur from penetrating and blunt mechanism. Most patients with penetrating aortic injuries exsanguinate and die at the scene of the trauma, or they arrive *in extremis* at the trauma center to undergo emergency department thoracotomy; the survival rate is very low.

Blunt traumatic ruptures of the aorta are perhaps one of the most common causes of sudden death after blunt chest trauma or a fall from great height.[5, 17] Most patients succumb at the scene of the traumatic incident and never arrive at the trauma center. Those who arrive alive usually survive because the wall rupture of the aorta is contained by the adventitia.

Although most of the patients who sustain blunt rupture of the thoracic aorta present with multiple associated injuries, approximately 30% show little or no external evidence of chest trauma.[65] Strong suspicion that a blunt rupture of the thoracic aorta may have occurred is usually raised by the history of a high-impact collision, an acceleration-deceleration mechanism, or a fall from great height. Recently, lateral impacts have also been found to rupture the thoracic aorta.[17]

Clinical findings that suggest the presence of this injury include external evidence of chest trauma, sternal fracture, thoracic inlet hematoma, and a systolic murmur in the precordium or intrascapular area. Upper extremity hypertension and decreased lower extremity pulses are also important findings. Voice change secondary to pressure in the recurrent laryngeal nerve is an infrequent finding, whereas hypotension and hemodynamic instability usually signal an impending rupture. Signs of a pericardial tamponade may be present if a retrograde rupture in the pericardium has taken place.

Patients sustaining blunt chest trauma from well-known mechanisms associated with aortic disruption and patients manifesting previously outlined radiographic findings should be investigated aggressively, either with CT or aortography. In patients with positive findings, surgical intervention is mandated as soon as feasible to prevent exsanguination from free rupture of the damaged thoracic aortic wall.

There are multiple approaches to the repair of these injuries. These include:

- Cardiopulmonary bypass, either by atriofemoral or femoro-femoral routes

- Use of a Gott shunt
- The "clamp and saw" technique

Because the patient often incurs multiple injuries, anticoagulation needed for cardiopulmonary bypass can present problems, especially if there are associated closed head injuries or pelvic fractures. With the advent of heparin-coated tubing, surgical intervention is possible without full heparinization.

Regardless of the surgical technique used to effect the repair, prolonged ischemic time of the spinal cord must be avoided at all costs. It is well known that if 30 minutes of cross-clamping time is exceeded in the absence of extracorporeal circulation, a 5% to 10% incidence of paraplegia results.[17] The preferred method of repair of rupture thoracic aortas is an aortoaortic bypass with a Dacron graft, as most of these injuries cannot be repaired primarily. The most frequent complications from surgical repair of these injuries are paraplegia, renal failure, and the pseudocoarctation syndrome, in which blood pressure in the upper extremities is significantly elevated, usually resolving in a few days.

For injury to the major thoracic vascular structures, proximal and distal control is necessary. Injuries to the innominate artery can be primarily repaired or bypassed with the use of prosthetic material, such as polytetrafluoroethylene (PTFE) or a Dacron graft. If the injury is located at the origin of the vessel, the vessel may be transected, the ostium closed, and the vessel reimplanted in the arch of aorta.[98-100] The same technique can be used for the carotid arteries.

The management of subclavian arterial injuries is challenging, given the difficult approach to these vessels. In general, if the vessels are transected, a bypass graft is usually indicated.[98, 101, 102] Injury to the origin of their most important branches (internal mammary and vertebral arteries) can be managed by ligation of these vessels. For venous injuries, primary repair or ligation may be indicated. In desperate situations, subclavian veins can be ligated. If possible, the innominate vein should be repaired. Similarly, injuries to the intrapericardial portions of the superior and inferior vena cava demand primary repair.

Esophageal Injuries

Thoracic esophageal injuries are rare. The vast majority are caused by penetrating trauma. Blunt rupture of the thoracic esophagus is extremely rare. Failure to establish the diagnosis of a thoracic esophageal injury can be lethal to the patient because the resulting spillage into the thoracic cavity and mediastinum leads to mediastinitis and thoracic sepsis.[103]

Esophageal injuries should be considered in any patient who presents with a hemothorax or pneumothorax without any associated rib fractures or a patient who has sustained a severe blow to the lower sternum or epigastrium and presents with pain or shock out of proportion to the clinical findings. Finally, this injury should be excluded if particulate matter appears in the chest tube or if radiographs reveal the presence of mediastinal air. The diagnosis can be confirmed by contrast study or esophagoscopy.[74, 103]

Treatment includes immediate thoracotomy and direct repair of the esophageal injury if it has been detected early. Wide drainage of the pleural space and the mediastinum is necessary. In these patients, the diagnosis has been established late. Primary repair of the esophagus may not be feasible and may necessitate esophageal diversion, wide drainage of the pleural and mediastinal spaces, and continuous irrigation of the thoracic cavity. The mortality for these injuries is high and rises to astronomical levels when these injuries are detected late.

Diaphragmatic Injuries

Injury to the diaphragm is most commonly seen on the left side because the liver generally occludes the defect on the right side. Generally, the appearance of hollow viscera in the left hemithoracic cavity as well as a coiled nasogastric tube easily establishes the diagnosis. Blunt trauma generally produces large diaphragmatic tears, whereas penetrating trauma usually results in small perforations. Rarely is the liver displaced into the right hemithoracic cavity.[19]

The diagnosis can be difficult, since the initial radiographic findings may be deceiving. The trauma surgeon should exercise caution while inserting chest tubes in patients in whom there is an unexplained opacification in the left hemithoracic cavity in order to prevent inadvertent perforation of displaced intra-abdominal organs.[19]

An upper gastrointestinal study generally identifies a displaced stomach into the left hemithoracic cavity. Similarly, a small-bowel follow-through or a barium enema may reveal small bowel or colon displaced into the left hemithoracic cavity. CT is not often diagnostic. Magnetic resonance imaging has been an excellent diagnostic tool in locating diaphragmatic injury, although the experience remains limited.[19]

Management of an acute diaphragmatic rupture entails surgical intervention to reposition the displaced organs to the abdominal cavity. At the same time, surgery allows for repair of the diaphragm and restores its normal continuity and motion. More important, it prevents incarceration and strangulation of displaced intra-abdominal viscera, events that carry a high mortality. Acute diaphragmatic injuries can present years after this complication.[19]

References

1. Baker CC, Oppenheimer L, Stephens B, et al: Epidemiology of trauma deaths. Am J Surg 1980; 140:144.
2. LoCicero J III, Mattox KL: Epidemiology of chest trauma. Surg Clin North Am 1989; 69:15.
3. Shorr RM, Crittenden M, Indeck M, et al: Blunt thoracic trauma: Analysis of 515 patients. Ann Surg 1987; 206:200.
4. Tonge JI, O'Reilly MJJ, Davison A, et al: Traffic crash fatalities (1968–1973): Injury pattern and other factors. Med Sci Law 1977; 17:9.
5. American College of Surgeons (ACS), Committee on Trauma: Advance Trauma Live Support Instructor Manual. Chicago, ACS, 1993.
6. Beeson A, Saegesser F: Color Atlas of Chest Trauma and Associated Injuries. Oradell, NJ, Medical Economics Books, 1983.
7. Pickard LR, Mattox KL; Thoracic Trauma: General considerations and indications for thoracotomy. *In:* Trauma. Moore EE, Mattox KL, Feliciano DB (Eds): Norwalk, Conn, Appleton & Lange, 1991, pp 319–326.
8. Richardson JD: Indication for thoracotomy in thoracic trauma. Curr Surg 1985; 42:361.
9. Washington B, Wilson RF, Seiger Z, et al: Emergency thoracotomy: A four-year review. Ann Thorac Surg 1985; 40:188.
10. Freedland M, Wilson RF, Bender JS, et al: The management of flail chest injury: Factors affecting outcome. J Trauma 1990; 12:1460.
11. Asensio JA: Discussion of: Hirschberg A, Wall MJ, Allen MK, Mattox KL: Double jeopardy: Thoracoabdominal injuries requiring surgical intervention in both chest and abdomen. J Trauma 1995; 39:231.
12. Asensio JA, Voystock J, Khatri VJ, et al: Toracotomia en el centro de urgencias. *In:* Procedimientos en el Paciente Critico. 2nd ed. Gutierrez-Lizardi P (Ed). Monterrey, Mexico, Ediciones Cuellar, 1993, pp 337–341.
13. Asensio JA: Exsanguination from penetrating injuries. Trauma Q 1990; 6:1–25.
14. Asensio JA, Ierardi R: Exsanguination. Emerg Care Q 1991; 7:59–75.
15. Richardson JD, Frank B, Miller B, et al: Complex thoracic injuries. Surg Clin North Am 1996; 76:725–748.

16. Trunkey DD: Chest wall injuries. *In:* Cervicothoracic Trauma. 2nd ed. Blaisdel FW, Trunkey DD (Eds). New York, Thieme, 1994.
17. Fabian TC, Richardson JD, Croce MA; et al: Prospective study of blunt aortic injury: Multicenter Trial of the American Association for the Surgery of Trauma. J Trauma 1997; 42:374–383.
18. Asensio JA, Berne J, Demetriades D, at al: Penetrating esophageal injuries: Time interval of safety for preoperative evaluation—how long is safe? J Trauma 1997; 43:319–324.
19. Asensio JA, Demetriades D, Rodriguez A: Injuries to the diaphragm. *In:* Trauma. Feliciano DV, Moore EE, Mattox KL (Eds). Norwalk, Conn, Appleton & Lange, 1995, pp 461–485.
20. Murray JA, Demetriades D, Cornwell EE, et al: Penetrating left thoracoabdominal trauma: The incidence and clinical presentation of diaphragm injuries. J Trauma 1997; 43:624–626.
21. Balan G, Penalver JC, Paris F, et al: Blunt chest injuries in 1696 patients. Eur J Cardiothorac Surg 1992; 6:284.
22. Mackersie RC: Chest wall injuries: New trends in analgesia. Adv Trauma Crit Care 1992; 7:115–131.
23. Shackford SR, Virgilio RW, Peters RM: Selective use of ventilatory therapy in flail chest injury. J Thorac Cardiovasc Surg 1981; 81:194.
24. Shackford SR, Smith DE, Zarins CK, et al: The management of flail chest—a comparison of ventilatory and nonventilatory treatment. Am J Surg 1976; 132:759.
25. Landercasper J, Cogbill TH, Strutt PJ: Delayed diagnosis of flail chest. Crit Care Med 1990; 18:611.
26. Avery EE, Morch ET, Benson DW: Critically crushed chests: A new method of treatment with continuous mechanical hyperventilation to produce alkalotic apnea and internal pneumatic stabilitation. J Thorac Surg 1956; 32:291.
27. Trinkle JK, Richardson JD, Franz JL, et al: Management of flail chest without mechanical ventilation. Ann Thorac Surg 1975; 19:355.
28. Richardson JD, Adams L, Flint LM: Selective management of flail chest and pulmonary contusion. Ann Surg 1982; 196:481.
29. Paris F, Tarazona V, Blasco E, et al: Surgical stabilization of traumatic flail chest. Thorax 1975; 30:521.
30. Moore BP: Operative stabilization of nonpenetrating chest injuries. J Thorac Cardiovasc Surg 1975; 70:619.
31. Thomas AN, Blaisdell FW, Lewis RF, et al: Operative stabilization for flail chest after blunt trauma. J Thorac Cardiovasc Surg 1978; 75:793.
32. Menard A, Testart J, Phillipe JM: Treatment of flail chest with Judet's struts. J Thorac Cardiovasc Surg 1983; 86:300.
33. Haasler GB: Open fixation of flail chest after blunt trauma. Ann Thorac Surg 1990; 49:993.
34. Landreneau RJ, Hinson JM, Hazelrigg SR, et al: Strut fixation of an extensive flail chest. Ann Thorac Surg 1991; 51:473.
35. Nagaie T, Tateishi H, Minagawa S: New method for the internal stabilization of flail chest. Eur J Surg 1992; 158:613.
36. Reber P, Ris HB, Inderbitzi B, et al: Osteosynthesis of the injured chest wall. Scan J Thorac Cardiovasc Surg 1993; 27:137–142.
37. Ahmed Z, Mohyndden Z: Management of flail chest injury: Internal fixation versus endotracheal intubation and ventilation. J Thorac Cardiovasc Surg 1995; 110:6, 1676.
38. Kishikawa M, Yoshioka T, Shimazu T, et al: Pulmonary contusion cases long-term respiratory dysfunction with decreased functional residual capacity. J Trauma 1991; 31:1203.
39. Gyhra A, Torres P, Pina P, et al: Experimental flail chest: Ventilatory function with fixation of flail segments in internal and external position. J Trauma 1996; 40:977–979.
40. Freed HA, Chields NN: Most frequently overlooked radiographically apparent fractures in a teaching hospital emergency department. Ann Emerg Med 1984; 13:900.
41. Wilson JM, Thomas AN, Goodman PC, Lewis FR: Severe chest trauma: Morbidity implication of first and second rib fracture in 120 patients. Arch Surg 1978; 113:846.
42. Albers JE, Rath RK, Glaser RS, Poddar PK: Severity of intrathoracic injuries associated with first rib fractures. Ann Thorac Surg 1982; 33:614.
43. Fisher RG, Ward RE, Ben-Menachem Y, et al: Arteriography and the fractured first rib: Too much for too little? AJR 1982; 138:1059.
44. Lazrobe S, Harley DP, Grinnel VS, et al: Should all patients with first rib fracture undergo arteriography? J Thorac Cardiovasc Surg 1982; 83:532.
45. Phillips EH, Rogers WF, Gaspar MR: First rib fractures: Incidence of vascular injury and indications for angiography. Surgery 1981; 89:42.
46. Woodring JH, Fried AM, Hartfield DR, et al: Fractures of first and second ribs: Predictive value for arterial and bronchial injury. AJR 1982; 138:211.
47. Poole GV: Fracture of the upper ribs and injury to the great vessels. Surg Gynecol Obstet 1989; 169:275.
48. Bassett JS, Gibson RD, Wilson RF: Blunt injuries to the chest. J Trauma 1968; 8:418.
49. Buchman R, Trooskin SZ, Flancbaum L, Chandler J: The significance of stable patients with sternal fractures. Surg Gynecol Obstet 1987; 164:261.
50. Wojcik JB, Morgan AS: Sternal fractures—the natural history. Ann Emerg Med 1988; 17:912.
51. Harley DP, Mena I: Cardiac and vascular sequelae of sternal fractures. J Trauma 1986; 26:553.
52. Brookes JG, Dunn RJ, Rogers IR: Sternal fractures: A retrospective analysis of 272 cases. J Trauma 1993; 35:46.
53. Hills MW, Delprado AM, Deane SA: Sternal fractures: Associated injuries and management. J Trauma 1993; 35:55.
54. Jackson M, Walker WS: Isolated sternal fracture: A benign injury? Injury 1992; 23:535.
55. McGahan JP, Rab GT, Dublin A: Fractures of the scapula. J Trauma 1980; 20:880.
56. Thompson DA, Flynn TC, Miller PW, at al: The significance of scapular fractures. J Trauma 1985; 25:974.
57. Wilber MC, Evans EB: Fractures of the scapula: An analysis of forty cases and a review of the literature. J Bone Joint Surg 1977; 59A:358.
58. Harris RD, Harris JH: The prevalence and significance of missed scapular fracture in blunt chest trauma. AJR Am J Roentgenol 1988; 151:747.
59. Sampson LN, Britton JC, Eldrup-Jorgensen J, et al: The neurovascular outcome of scapulothoracic dissociation. J Vasc Surg 1993; 17:1083.
60. Costa MC, Robbs JV: Nonpenetrating subclavian artery trauma. J Vasc Surg 1988; 8:71.
61. Neer CS, Rockwood CA: Fracture and dislocations of the shoulder. *In:* Fractures of Adults. Rockwood CA, Green DP (Eds). Philadelphia, JB Lippincott, 1984, p 910.
62. Buckerfield CT, Castle ME: Acute traumatic retrosternal dislocation of the clavicle. J Bone Joint Surg 1984; 66A:379.
63. Gray AR, Harrison WH, Couves CM, et al: Penetrating injuries to the chest. Am J Surg 1954; 100:709.
64. Harrison WH Jr, Gray AR, Couves CM, et al: Severe non-penetrating injuries to the chest. Am J Surg 1960; 100:715.
65. Mattox KL: Approaches to trauma involving the major vessels of the thorax. Surg Clin North Am 1989; 69:77.
66. Mansour MA, Moore EE, Moore FA, et al: Exigent postinjury thoracotomy analysis of blunt versus penetrating trauma. Surg Gynecol Obstet 1992; 175:97.
67. Williams JS, Minken SL, Adams JT: Traumatic asphyxia reappraised. Ann Surg 1968; 167:384.
68. Rosato RM, Shapiro MJ, Keegan MJ, et al: Cardiac injury complication asphyxia. J Trauma 1991; 31:1387.
69. Jongewaard WR, Cogbill TH, Landercasper J: Neurologic consequences of traumatic asphyxia. J Trauma 1992; 32:28.
70. Landercasper J, Cogbill TH: Long-term follow-up after traumatic asphyxia. J Trauma 1985; 25:838.
71. McNamara JJ, Messersmith JK, Dunn RA, et al: Thoracic injuries in combat casualties in Vietnam. Ann Thorac Surg 1970; 10:398.
72. Graham JM, Mattox KL, Beall AC Jr: Penetrating trauma of the lung. J Trauma 1979; 19:665.
73. Zakharia AT: Cardiovascular and thoracic battle injuries in the Lebanon War. J Cardiovasc Thorac Surg 1985; 89:723.
74. Asensio JA, Demetriades D, Berne J, et al: Staple pulmonary tractotomy: A rapid way to control hemorrhage in penetrating pulmonary injuries. J Am Coll Surg 1997; 185:486–487.
75. Fisher RP, Geiger JP, Guernsey JM: Pulmonary resection for severe pulmonary contusion secondary to high velocity missile wounds. J Trauma 1974; 14:293.
76. Scannel JG: Pulmonary resection—anatomy and techniques. *In:*

Thoracic and Cardiovascular Surgery. 4th ed. Glenn WWL (Ed). Norwalk, Conn, Appleton-Century-Crofts, 1983.
77. Robinson PD, Harmon DL, Trinkle JK, et al: Management of penetrating lung injuries in civilian practice. J Thorac Cardiovasc Surg 1988; 95:184.
78. Tominaga GT, Waxman K, Scannel G, et al: Emergency thoracotomy with lung resection following trauma. Am Surg 1993; 59:834.
79. Wienceck RJ, Wilson RF: Central lung injuries: A need for early vascular control. J Trauma 1988; 28:1418.
80. Carrillo EH, Block EFJ, Zeppa R, et al: Urgent lobectomy and pneumonectomy after penetrating thoracic trauma. Eur J Emerg Med 1994; 1:126.
81. Estrera AS, Pass LJ, Platt MR: Systemic arterial air embolism in penetrating lung injury. Ann Thorac Surg 1990; 50:257.
82. Bertelsen S, Howitz P: Injuries of the trachea and bronchi. Thorax 1972; 27:188.
83. Kemmerer WT, Eckert WG, Cathright JB, et al: Patterns of thoracic injuries in fatal traffic accidents. J Trauma 1961; 1:595.
84. De La Rocha AG, Kayler D: Traumatic rupture of the tracheobronchial tree. Can J Surg 1965; 28:68.
85. Angood PB, Attia EL, Brown RA, et al: Extrinsic civilian trauma to the larynx and the cervical trachea: Important predictors of long-term morbidity. J Trauma 1986; 26:869.
86. Symbas PN, Hatcher CR Jr, Vlasis SE: Bullet wounds of the trachea. J Thorac Cardiovasc Surg 1982; 83:235.
87. Symbas PN, Hatcher CR Jr, Boehm GAW: Acute penetrating tracheal trauma. Ann Thorac Surg 1976; 22:473.
88. Asensio JA, Stewart BM, Murray J, et al: Penetrating cardiac injuries. Surg Clin North Am 1996; 76:685.
89. Moreno C, Moore EE, Majune JA, et al: Pericardial tamponade: A critical determinant for survival following penetrating cardiac wounds. J Trauma 1994; 36:229-300.
90. Buckman RF, Badellino MM, Mauro LH, et al: Penetrating cardiac wounds: Prospective study of factors influencing initial resuscitation. J Trauma 1993; 34:717-727.
91. Asensio JA, Murray J, Demetriades D, et al: Penetrating cardiac injuries: A prospective study of variables predicting outcome. J Am Coll Surg 1998; 186:24.
92. Sutherland GR, Driedger AA, Holliday RL, et al: Frequency of myocardial injuries after blunt chest trauma as evaluated after radionuclide angiography. Am J Cardiol 1983; 52:1099.
93. McLean RF, Devitt JH, Dubbin J, et al: Incidence of abnormal of RNA studies and dysrhythmias in patients with blunt chest trauma. J Trauma 1991; 31:968.
94. Vesalius A: *In:* Sepulchretaum sive Anatomia Practica ex Cad a veribus Morbo. Beonetus T (Ed).
95. Bahnson HT: Definitive treatment of saccular aneurysms of the aorta with excision of sac and aortic suture. Surg Gynecol Obstet 1953; 96:383.
96. DeBakey MD, Cooley DA, Morris GC, et al: Arteriovenous fistula involving the abdominal aorta: Report of four cases with successful repair. Ann Surg 1958; 147:646.
97. Pasaro E, Pace WG: Traumatic rupture of the aorta. Surgery 1959; 41:787.
98. Mattox KL: Approaches to trauma involving the major vessels of the thorax. Surg Clin North Am 1989; 69:77.
99. Murray GF, Brawley RK, Gott VL: Reconstruction of the innominate artery by means of a temporary heparin-coated shunt bypass. J Thorac Cardiovasc Surg 1971; 62:34.
100. Johnston RH Jr, Wall MJ Jr, Mattox KL: Innominate artery trauma: A thirty-year experience. J Vasc Surg 1993; 17:134.
101. Graham JM, Feliciano DV, Mattox KL, et al: Management of subclavian vascular injuries. J Trauma 1980; 20:537.
102. Graham JM, Feliciano DV, Mattox KL: Innominate vascular injury. J Trauma 1982; 22:647.
103. Asensio JA, Berne J, Demetriades D: Penetrating esophageal injury: The time interval of safety of preoperative evaluation—how long is safe? J Trauma 1997; 43:319-324.

31

Abdominal Trauma

Edward E. Cornwell III, MD • James A. Murray, MD

Inasmuch as the hallmark of critical care is the rapid diagnosis and treatment of conditions that may adversely affect organ perfusion and function, the critically injured patient suffering from abdominal trauma presents special challenges to the trauma surgeon and the surgical intensivist. Diagnostic challenges are presented by the fact that the patient with potentially lethal abdominal injuries may present in what appears to be a clinically stable fashion on initial examination. Comorbid conditions, such as distracting thoracic and extremity injuries, and altered mental status due to shock, head trauma, or ingestion of alcohol or other drugs may impair the effectiveness of physical examination.

Once the need for surgical intervention is confirmed, strategies must be employed that address the unique intraoperative challenges that occur in the patient with major abdominal trauma. Specifically, ongoing fluid shifts from the intravascular to the interstitial compartment present difficulties in (1) achieving adequate serum levels of antibiotics administered to patients with intra-abdominal visceral injuries, (2) maintaining adequate intravascular volume and near-normal body temperature, coagulation profile, and acid-base status, and (3) securing abdominal wall closure at the completion of the operation without creating elevated intra-abdominal pressure.

Postoperatively, continued fluid shifts represent unique challenges to the ongoing goal of maintaining adequate intravascular volume, flow, and blood-carrying capacity to support organ perfusion and cell function. Accordingly, this chapter reviews abdominal trauma in the critically injured patient, with an emphasis on special considerations in the areas of (1) diagnosis, (2) operative strategies, and (3) postoperative care and monitoring.

DIAGNOSIS

Abdominal trauma should be classified according to mechanism of injury as *penetrating* trauma (i.e., gunshot wound, stab wound, shotgun wound) or *blunt* trauma (secondary to motor vehicle accidents, falls). The diagnostic implications are such that patients with blunt abdominal trauma commonly have associated injuries to other organ systems and anatomic regions, whereas patients with penetrating trauma frequently require surgical intervention. The frequency of intra-abdominal injuries that require surgical intervention is sufficiently variable that some degree of selectivity must be practiced in patients with both blunt and penetrating abdominal trauma.

Physical examination in the patient with obvious peritonitis is frequently the only test employed in some patients with major abdominal trauma. Complete exposure and inspection of the abdominal wall for ecchymoses, lacerations, and abrasions as well as for evisceration of omentum or other viscera or the presence of impaled objects is an important first step in the physical examination. Entry and exit wounds of bullets in victims of gunshot wounds may yield important information, although we should remember that bullets may be deflected by bone and other tissue. A straight line may not necessarily connect the entry wound and the exit wound.

Palpation is undertaken to assess for tenderness away from

the site of obvious wounds as well as rebound tenderness, involuntary guarding, or rigidity. Auscultation should be performed to assess for the presence and character of bowel sounds. Auscultation should extend to the chest because thoracic and abdominal injuries frequently occur together. Bowel sounds heard in the chest suggest a diaphragmatic injury. Rectal examination is undertaken to assess for tone and presence of gross blood, and a nasogastric tube and Foley catheter are important diagnostic as well as therapeutic maneuvers. Abdominal distention from a dilated stomach or full bladder may be treated by these catheters, and the return of gross blood would constitute important diagnostic information.

The need for serial abdominal examination in the patient with an initial "negative examination" cannot be overemphasized. Ongoing bleeding at a slow rate and disrupted hollow viscera may not be initially suspected in a young, healthy patient with significant cardiorespiratory reserve. Failure to perform serial examination in these patients frequently leads to the finding that these patients have "acutely deteriorated," when a more accurate description may be that there was acute recognition of a potentially lethal condition by a clinician with inadequate clinical suspicion.

Even when the abdominal examination has been thoroughly performed, it may be compromised by the presence of alcohol, other drugs, or concomitant injuries to the head and other regions. Therefore, other diagnostic modalities are frequently employed in critically injured patients with abdominal trauma.

Since its introduction by Root[1] in 1967, the *diagnostic peritoneal lavage* (DPL) had been accepted for a quarter-century as the diagnostic procedure of choice for assessing intra-abdominal hemorrhage in the hemodynamically unstable trauma patient. Although DPL can be used to identify the presence of ongoing intra-abdominal bleeding within minutes of admission, its use will continue to decrease as more trauma centers routinely employ abdominal ultrasonography in the evaluation of the injured patient.

When DPL is employed, the lavage catheter is inserted by open, semiopen, or closed technique after the stomach and bladder are decompressed by nasogastric tubes and Foley catheters. Aspiration of gross blood, bile, or intestinal contents (a "positive tap") is typically considered an indication for emergent abdominal exploration. In the absence of a positive tap, patients with blunt trauma are considered to have a positive lavage when their red blood cell (RBC) count is 100,000/mm^3. Patients with penetrating trauma have criteria for positivity that vary from institution to institution, from as low as 1000 to as high as 100,000/mm^3.[2] Employing the lower number increases the chances for performing nontherapeutic laparotomies, whereas raising the threshold for positivity runs the risk of missed or delayed diagnosis of injuries requiring surgical intervention.

DPL is advantageous in its ability to be employed in the early minutes after admission and in its high sensitivity in identifying intraperitoneal hemorrhage. Its drawbacks are its inability to assess the retroperitoneum and its occasional oversensitivity in patients with blunt abdominal trauma who may have had initial bleeding that subsequently stopped, allowing them to otherwise be candidates for nonoperative observation. In this regard, the more stable patient who requires diagnostic adjuncts for abdominal trauma may be better served with an abdominal CT scan.

Computed tomography (CT) has a proven track record in its ability to evaluate patients with blunt abdominal trauma.[3, 4] CT can reliably detect hemoperitoneum, injuries to solid organs, retroperitoneal hemorrhage, and thickening of the bowel wall. Its disadvantage is the requirement that patients be transported to the radiology suite, making it an inappropriate test for the hemodynamically unstable or under-resuscitated patient. With the wide use of spiral CT scanners and their ability to image rapidly, patients with multisystem injuries can quickly undergo CT scanning of other regions (e.g., head and chest) in addition to the abdomen.

Having been employed in Europe for more than two decades, *abdominal ultrasonography* has become particularly useful in the trauma setting[5] and is rapidly becoming the procedure of choice in the early assessment for hemoperitoneum. In some centers, it has all but supplanted the DPL, particularly because of its ability to rapidly and noninvasively detect intra-abdominal hemorrhage in the unstable patient.[6, 7] In addition, it is portable and allows real-time imaging and repeated examinations.

The *focused abdominal sonogram for trauma* (FAST) has been described as a rapid survey to assess for blood in the hepatorenal recess of Morison, the pericardial sac, the perisplenic region, and the pelvis around the bladder.[5, 8] In a study of 371 patients, Rozycki and coworkers[5] found the ultrasound examination to have an 84% sensitivity and 97.4% specificity. Several studies have affirmed that abdominal ultrasonography for trauma is a diagnostic modality that is lower cost, less invasive, and more rapidly performed than DPL.

Diagnostic laparoscopy is another modality that has made advances in recent years in the evaluation of abdominal trauma. Although laparoscopy is too insensitive to rule out hollow viscus injuries, it is an excellent modality to detect diaphragm injuries and hemoperitoneum.[9] In a prospective study of 106 consecutive patients with penetrating left thoracoabdominal trauma performed at the Los Angeles County–University of Southern California Medical Center (LAC + USC), diaphragmatic injuries were present in 60% (30/50) of the patients who had clear-cut indications for surgery (hemodynamic instability or peritonitis).[10] More important, 27% (15/56) of the patients presenting in a clinically occult fashion (hemodynamically stable, soft abdomen, normal or nonspecific findings on chest radiography) who therefore underwent diagnostic laparoscopy also had diaphragmatic injuries. These patients may well have been discharged in the absence of the protocol. Given the well-described phenomena of the delayed diaphragmatic hernia and the potential lethality of gangrenous incarcerated viscera in the thorax, there clearly is a larger role for diagnostic laparoscopy in stable patients with penetrating left thoracoabdominal trauma.

Special Considerations

Selective Management

Selective nonoperative observation has become widely accepted for patients with blunt abdominal trauma and stab wounds. Recent reports have supported the feasibility of this approach in patients with abdominal gunshot wounds.[11] Interest in initial observation of selected patients with abdominal gunshot wounds, until recent years a concept that was equivalent to surgical heresy, has grown with the increasing recognition of morbidity of a nontherapeutic celiotomy for trauma.[12–15] Demetriades and colleagues[11] described a series of 309 patients with gunshot wounds to the anterior abdomen. Ninety-two patients (29.8%) were successfully managed nonoperatively, and the overall nontherapeutic laparotomy rate was 10.8%.

The prerequisites for selective observation of patients with abdominal gunshot wounds must be carefully emphasized, lest this policy be inappropriately adopted. Patients should be in an area that permits serial evaluation and rapid transport to the operating room in the event of a change in the initial negative findings of the clinical examination. Institutions that do not have 24-hour, in-house, experienced clinicians are better served by a standard policy of mandatory exploration for patients with abdominal gunshot wounds.

"Seat Belt" Sign

Special mention is made of transverse abdominal wall ecchymosis (seat belt sign) in patients involved in motor vehicle crashes whose lap belt had been positioned above the pelvic inlet. Increasing enforcement of seat belt laws has seen a shift in the patterns of injuries, such that patients who would have previously been lethally injured at the scene from head and thoracic vascular injuries are presenting to trauma centers with intra-abdominal injuries secondary to compression by lap belts. The challenge of managing visceral injury secondary to seat belts lies in the fact that patients frequently have clinical examination findings that are equivocal or distracting injuries that compromise the abdominal evaluation. Published experience with the seat belt sign suggests an increased incidence of hollow viscus injuries and lumbar fractures.[16, 17]

Our policy is to employ mandatory abdominal CT in all stable patients admitted with a seat belt sign. Surgical intervention is employed in those patients who have suggestive findings, such as (1) free pelvic fluid in the absence of injuries to solid viscera, which may explain the finding, and (2) bowel wall thickening with or without pneumatosis.

OPERATIVE MANAGEMENT

The hallmark of surgical therapy for critically injured patients with abdominal trauma is rapid operative intervention and hemorrhage control. Aggressive fluid resuscitation is no substitute for rapid triage and achievement of hemostasis. Studies have given new perspectives on this seemingly obvious and well-established dictum.

Bickell and associates[18] in Houston performed a prospective, randomized study of hypotensive patients with penetrating torso injuries. When aggressive fluid resuscitation was delayed until operative intervention began, patient outcomes were superior to results in patients who received rapid fluid infusion on first contact with paramedics. Operating room availability led to inordinately long time intervals between injury and surgery for some of the patients, highlighting the inability of aggressive fluid resuscitation before hemostasis to improve outcome.

A retrospective study from LAC + USC involving more than 5700 patients suggested that major trauma victims transported by private means had significantly lower mortality than those transported by Emergency Medical Services (EMS), even when controlled for age, mechanism, injury severity, and injury pattern.[19] The authors hypothesized that time differences accounted for observed differences in outcome, again pointing to rapid triage and therapy as the most crucial intervention available to the clinician caring for the unstable patient with abdominal trauma.

One manifestation of the concept of the critical nature of time in treating patients with potentially lethal abdominal injuries is the increasing use of *"damage control"* techniques during therapeutic laparotomy.[20] This concept, which employs liberal use of abdominal packing to achieve cessation of ongoing major hemorrhage, rapid control of leaking intestinal injuries, and deferral of gastrointestinal anastomoses and definitive abdominal wall closure until subsequent operations, exemplifies the concept of a coordinated approach and the seamless transition of patients from the emergency department to the operating room to the intensive care unit. The goal of damage control laparotomy is to avoid the lethal triad of hypothermia, coagulopathy, and acidosis. The control of hemorrhage allows aggressive intraoperative resuscitation to begin and continue into the intensive care unit (ICU), with the return of the patient to the operating room typically occurring 24 to 48 hours later when the physiologic parameters (body temperature, coagulation status, acid-base status) have normalized.

There has been increased recognition of the effects of large fluid shifts and hyperdynamic physiologic responses in patients with major abdominal trauma prescribed prophylactic antibiotic regimens. A prospective study by Ericsson and colleagues[21] suggested that high doses of prophylactic antibiotics are more effective than long courses in reducing infections in patients undergoing laparotomy for abdominal trauma. The concept is most easily demonstrated with the aminoglycosides, for which antibiotic effectiveness is most correlative with serum drug level.[22]

Fabian and associates[23] identified a decreased postoperative infection rate in patients with penetrating abdominal trauma receiving aztreonam/clindamycin compared with those receiving gentamicin/clindamycin and attributed the differences to relative underdosing of gentamicin. Clear consensus is emerging that a distinction needs to be made between effectiveness of early and adequate doses of antibiotics in patients with major abdominal trauma and the tempting but ineffective practice of prolonged postoperative dosing.

A Consensus Development Conference held by the National Institutes of Health (NIH) in 1988 generated currently accepted guidelines regarding the use of blood and blood products to restore intravascular volume and oxygen-carrying capacity and correct coagulation abnormalities.[24] Blood products remain a vital and limited resource. The current use of blood remains at about 14 million units of blood components per year. There has been extensive research activity aimed at the development of new products and increasing the use of existing stores.

One technique available to clinicians is the use of autotransfusion devices to return shed blood to the patient. Cell-saver technology has been employed in the operating room, most commonly in elective operations. Patients with massive hemothoraces are the most common recipients of autotransfused blood in the trauma setting, although experience is mounting with abdominal trauma. The addition of an anticoagulant to the collection chamber is required. Excessive infusion of autotransfused blood (typically, >1500 mL) can lead to a coagulopathy from the administration of activated products. A time limit of 4 hours is also recommended between the time of collection and time of infusion.

POSTOPERATIVE MANAGEMENT

The first order of emphasis in a discussion of postoperative management of patients with major abdominal trauma is to highlight an all too common practice that proceeds without scientific validation and is potentially harmful. Evaluation of the literature suggests that a short course of antibiotic therapy for patients with major abdominal trauma (duration of 24 hours or less) is as effective as a long course in preventing postoperative septic complications.[25-28] Although an increasing incidence of postoperative infections can be correlated with increasing numbers of organs injured, an increasing Penetrating Abdominal Trauma Index (PATI), and a higher number of units of blood transfused, there is no evidence that prolonging the duration of "prophylactic" antibiotic regimens will decrease these established risks.[29-32]

The literature notwithstanding, many patients continue to receive longer prophylactic courses of antibiotics when they are thought to be at high risk for septic complications.[33] Prolonged courses of postoperative prophylactic antibiotics are associated with increased expense, potential side effects, toxicity, and antibiotic resistance. Studies at LAC + USC have documented long-term antibiotic therapy as a risk factor in the emergence of an increasing incidence of fungal infections and strains of *Xanthomonas* among critically injured surgical patients.[34, 35] Although the difficulty one may perceive in discontinuing antibiotic therapy after 24 hours in a patient with severe injuries is understandable, current evidence supports a practice of doing just that, with close postoperative surveillance for infections and institution of appropriate antibiotic therapy at that time. Surgical intensivists who are charged with administrative responsibilities in ICUs must take seriously the role of helping their colleagues appreciate the potential hazards of prolonged postoperative antibiotic prophylaxis in terms of cost, toxicity, and emergence of resistant strains.

Abdominal Compartment Syndrome/ Open Abdomen

Intra-abdominal hypertension (IAH) is an increasingly recognized clinical entity after severe abdominal trauma. The factors that contribute to the increase in intra-abdominal pressure are bowel edema, retroperitoneal hematoma, intra-abdominal bleeding, and massive fluid resuscitation. The presence of intra-abdominal packing may also contribute to IAH by producing mesenteric venous obstruction, further worsening bowel edema. Attempts to close an abdomen in the presence of these factors often lead to an array of organ dysfunction (renal, respiratory, cardiac) that comprises the abdominal compartment syndrome.

Evaluation of intra-abdominal pressure can be performed by *direct* introduction of a catheter into the peritoneal cavity or by *indirect* methods that use the bladder or stomach. We prefer to use a water manometer transducing the bladder pressure through a Foley catheter. This technique, first described by Kron and colleagues,[36] has been validated to accurately reflect intra-abdominal pressure.[37] Continuous monitoring can be obtained by using a transducer connected to the Foley catheter. One should keep in mind that conversion of 1 mm Hg is equal to 1.36 cm H_2O.

The pressure at which IAH becomes clinically significant is not constant. As a guide, we use 30 cm H_2O, at which point intervention must be strongly considered. The clinical status of the patient and organ function dictate whether or not a decompressive celiotomy should be performed.

Elevation of intra-abdominal pressures not only affects the abdominal viscera but also is associated with cardiac, pulmonary, and neurologic complications. The cardiac effects include a decrease in stroke volume, tachycardia, and elevation of central venous and pulmonary artery pressures. An elevated venous pressure may not reflect the true intravascular volume in the presence of elevated abdominal pressure. As intra-abdominal pressure increases, pulmonary compliance decreases, leading to elevation of intra-thoracic pressures and hypercapnia.

Oliguria is an early manifestation of IAH and is due to compression of the renal vasculature, most likely the venous system, as well as of the renal parenchyma.

Adverse effects of IAH on splanchnic blood flow have been demonstrated in animal models. This response is directly proportional to the elevation in abdominal pressure in the presence of a constant blood pressure and cardiac output. Eleftheriadis and coworkers[38] demonstrated intestinal hypoperfusion and an increase in bacterial translocation with use of a pneumoperitoneum model. After decompression of the abdomen, bacteria were absent from the lymph nodes but were still present in the liver and spleen.

Recent work has demonstrated the effect of IAH on intracranial pressure (ICP) and cerebral perfusion pressure (CPP). During laparoscopic insufflation of the abdomen, an elevation in ICP has been demonstrated[39] and has been shown to exacerbate rises in ICP in a head-injury model. An intra-abdominal pressure of 25 mm Hg produced a significant decrease in CPP and an associated increase in ICP, findings that were reversed with decompression of the abdomen.

Because of the complex problems that arise from uncontrolled elevations in abdominal pressure and the systemic effects of abdominal compartment syndrome, we have adopted a liberal policy in not closing the abdomen primarily if the risk factors for the development of abdominal compartment syndrome exist. These include patients who have sustained major trauma and cannot undergo closure primarily because of extensive bowel edema, massive retroperitoneal edema or hematoma, or abdominal packing. We prefer to use a sterile intravenous (IV) bag for our initial coverage of the bowel.

If the abdomen is closed at the initial operation, we monitor the abdomen closely with physical examination and bladder pressures and correlate these findings with clinical evidence of abdominal compartment syndrome. The severity of the clinical symptoms in conjunction with the abdominal pressure determines whether a decompressive celiotomy is required.

Noninvasive Hemodynamic Monitoring

The evaluation of circulatory function with invasive techniques, such as the pulmonary artery catheter, has been the "gold standard." Newer technology using thoracic electrical bioimpedance allows continuous measurement of cardiac output noninvasively.[40] When these modalities, are applied with pulse oximetry and transcutaneous oxygenation assessment of tissue perfusion, the patient's status can be assessed. These newer modalities of monitoring also provide continuous measurements that enable early detection of responses to intervention or hemodynamic deterioration.

References

1. Root HD: Abdominal trauma and diagnostic peritoneal lavage revisited. Am J Surg 1990; 159:363.
2. Thompson JS, Moore EE: Peritoneal lavage in the evaluation of penetrating abdominal trauma. Surg Gynecol Obstet 1981; 153:861.
3. Matsubara TK, Fong HMT, Burns CM: Computed tomography of abdomen (CTA) in the management of blunt abdominal trauma. J Trauma 1990; 30:410.
4. Federle MP, Goldberg HI, Kaiser JA, et al: Evaluation of abdominal trauma by computed tomography. Radiology 1981; 138:637.
5. Rozycki GS, Ochsner MG, Schmidt JA, et al: A prospective study of surgeon performed ultrasound as the initial diagnostic modality for injured patient assessment. J Trauma 1995; 39:492.
6. Wherrett LJ, Boulanger BR, McLellan BA, et al: Hypotension after blunt abdominal trauma: The role of emergent abdominal sonography in surgical triage. J Trauma 1996; 41:815.
7. Kimura A, Otsuka T: Emergency center ultrasonography in the evaluation of hemoperitoneum: A prospective study. J Trauma 1991; 31:20.
8. Boulanger BR, Brenneman FD, McLellan BA, et al: A prospective study of emergent abdominal sonography after blunt trauma. J Trauma 1995; 39:325.
9. Ivatury RR, Simon RJ, Stahl WM: A critical evaluation of laparoscopy in penetrating abdominal trauma. J Trauma 1993; 34:822.
10. Murray JA, Demetriades D, Cornwell EE III, et al: Penetrating left thoracoabdominal trauma: The incidence and clinical presentation of diaphragm injuries. J Trauma 1997; 43:624.
11. Demetriades D, Velmahos G, Cornwell EE III, et al: Selective nonoperative management of gunshot wounds of the anterior abdomen. Arch Surg 1997; 132:178.
12. Nance ML, Nance FC: It is time we told the emperor about his clothes. J Trauma 1996; 40:185.
13. Henderson VJ, Organ CH, Smith RS: Negative trauma celiotomy. Am Surg 1993; 59:365.

14. Renz BM, Feliciano DV: Unnecessary laparotomies for trauma: A prospective study of morbidity. J Trauma 1995; 38:350.
15. Demetriades D, Vandenbossche P, Ritz M, et al: Non-therapeutic operations for penetrating trauma: Early morbidity and mortality. Br J Surg 1993; 80:860.
16. Chandler CF, Lane JS, Waxman KS: Seatbelt sign following blunt trauma is associated with increased incidence of abdominal injury. Am Surg 1997; 63:885.
17. Rutledge R, Thomason M, Oiler D, et al: The spectrum of abdominal injuries associated with the use of seat belts. J Trauma 1991; 31:820.
18. Bickell WH, Wall MJ Jr, Pepe PE, et al: Immediate versus delayed fluid resuscitation for hypotensive patients with penetrating torso injuries. N Engl J Med 1994; 331:1105.
19. Demetriades D, Chan L, Cornwell EE III, et al: Paramedic vs. private transportation of trauma patients: Effect on outcome. Arch Surg 1996; 131:133.
20. Rotondo MF, Schwab CW, McGonigal MD, et al: "Damage control": An approach for improved survival in exsanguinating penetrating abdominal injury. J Trauma 1993; 35:375.
21. Ericsson CD, Fischer RP, Rowlands BJ, et al: Prophylactic antibiotics in trauma: The hazards of underdosing. J Trauma 1989; 29:1356.
22. Moore RD, Smith CR, Lietman PS: The association of aminoglycoside plasma levels with mortality in patients with gram-negative bacteremia. J Infect Dis 1984; 149:443.
23. Fabian TC, Hess MM, Croce MA, et al: Superiority of aztreonam/clindamycin compared with gentamicin/clindamycin in patients with penetrating abdominal trauma. Am J Surg 1994; 167:291.
24. National Institutes of Health Consensus Conference: Perioperative red blood cell transfusion. JAMA 1988; 260:2700.
25. Dellinger EP: Antibiotic prophylaxis in trauma: Penetrating abdominal injuries and open fractures. Rev Infect Dis 1991; 13(Suppl 10):S847.
26. Oreskovich MR, Dellinger EP, Lennard ES, et al: Duration of preventive antibiotic administration for penetrating abdominal trauma. Arch Surg 1982; 117:200.
27. Dellinger EP, Wertz MJ, Lennard ES, et al: Efficacy of short-course antibiotic prophylaxis after penetrating intestinal injury: A prospective randomized study. Arch Surg 1986; 121:23.
28. Fabian TC, Croce MA, Payne LW, et al: Duration of antibiotic therapy for penetrating abdominal trauma: A prospective trial. Surgery 1992; 112:788.
29. Nichols RL, Smith JW, Klein DB, et al: Risk of infection after penetrating abdominal trauma. N Engl J Med 1984; 311:1065.
30. Moore EE, Dunn EL, Moore JB, et al: Penetrating abdominal trauma index. J Trauma 1981; 21:439.
31. Nelken N, Lewis F: The influence of injury severity on complication rates after primary closure or colostomy for penetrating colon trauma. Ann Surg 1989; 209:439.
32. Moore FA, Moore EE, Sauaia A: Blood transfusion: An independent risk factor for postinjury multiple organ failure. Arch Surg 1997; 132:620.
33. Hadjiminas D, Cheadle WG, Spain DA, et al: Antibiotic overkill of trauma victims? Am J Surg 1994; 168:288.
34. Cornwell EE III, Belzberg H, Berne TV, et al: The pattern of fungal infections in critically ill surgical patients. Am Surg 1995; 61:847.
35. Cornwell EE III, Willey P, Belzberg H, et al: Characteristics of *Xanthomonas* infections in critically ill surgical patients. Am Surg 1996; 62:478.
36. Kron IL, Harman PK, Nolan SP: The measurement of intra-abdominal pressure as a criterion for abdominal re-exploration. Ann Surg 1984; 199:28.
37. Iberti TJ, Kelly KM, Gentili DR, et al: A simple technique to accurately determine intra-abdominal pressure. Crit Care Med 1987; 15:1140.
38. Eleftheriadis E, Kotzampassi K, Botsios D, et al: Splanchnic ischemia during laparoscopic cholecystectomy. Surg Endosc 1996; 10:324.
39. Josephs LG, Este-McDonald JR, Birkett DH, Hirsch EF: Diagnostic laparoscopy increases intracranial pressure. J Trauma 1994; 36:815.
40. Wang X, Van De Water JM, Sun HH, et al: Hemodynamic monitoring by impedance cardiography with an improved signal processing technique. Proc IEEE Eng Med Biol 1993; 15:699.

32

Intensive Care Management of the Injured Child

Matthew L. Moront, MD • Martin R. Eichelberger, MD

The next millennium will undoubtedly bring many advances in science and medicine; a cure for the acquired immunodeficiency syndrome (AIDS) or cancer may occur within our lifetimes. Despite these lofty expectations, the number one killer of our nation's children continues. Injury is responsible for more deaths in the pediatric population than all other diseases combined.[1, 2] This realization is even more staggering when one considers that each year nearly 150,000 children will become permanently disabled and 15,000 or more will die as a result of intentional and unintentional injury.[3, 4] Focus on the priorities of the initial resuscitation phase of care and the development of a strategy for critical care can mitigate preventable death of injured children.

MECHANISM OF INJURY

An analysis of the mechanisms of injury among children encourages action to develop strategies for prevention. The motor vehicle is the predominant cause of injury and death in children. Despite passenger restraint laws for infants and children in all 50 states and the District of Columbia, thousands of children are killed each year as motor vehicle occupants. Lack of appropriate restraint use contributed to many of these fatalities. Motor vehicles are also implicated in a number of injuries involving bicycles.[3, 5] Each year, nearly 300 children are killed and more than 300,000 are injured in bicycle-related incidents.[6] Analysis of the experience at Children's National Medical Center (CNMC) with more than 7800 consecutively admitted children age 14 years or younger reveals that motor vehicle–related injuries comprised nearly 25% of all trauma admissions, with an overall mortality of 3%.[7, 8]

Falls constitute another common mechanism of injury among children. Injury severity is related to the height of the fall and the type of surface. Falls occur more frequently in urban areas and during the summer months as a result of open windows. The mean age of children with this mechanism of injury at CNMC is 5.4 years. Despite its prevalence, children who fall are rarely killed and carry a mortality rate of less than 1% at CNMC.[7, 8]

Children suffering burns or inhalation injuries represent the third leading cause of admission at CNMC. Burn injuries can be *flame* injury or *scald* injury. Although scald injuries are more common and occur more frequently in toddlers, they are associated with a low mortality. In contrast, victims of flame burns are generally older children who have a greater severity of injury and a significant mortality rate.[7, 8] Most deaths from fires occur as a result of smoke inhalation. Heated toxic by-products that are inhaled include carbon monoxide, cyanide, and sulfur compounds, which result in hypoxia, severe pneumonitis, and direct parenchymal injury. Burn injuries are responsible for the longer lengths of hospitalization and higher charges per child than any other mechanism of injury.[7, 8, 10]

Intentional injury is the leading cause of death in children under 1 year of age.[7, 8, 11] Child abuse is frequently underrecognized and often goes unreported. It is estimated that more than 1.6 million children are abused or neglected each year and that for every fatality, there are nearly 100 nonfatal assaults. Child abuse is difficult to prove, and recurrent injury is common.[11] Clues to the diagnosis are delayed presentation, a history that does not correspond with the injuries found on physical examination, and unusual behavior from either the parents or the child.

Children in the adolescent age group are increasingly the victims of intentional injury; urban African American males aged 15 to 18 incur risk five times that of white males of the same age. Firearms are responsible for nearly half of the deaths in males and one third of deaths in females.[12, 13]

INITIAL RESUSCITATION

Initial resuscitation of the injured child proceeds based on principles and priorities appropriate for children. A systematic approach to resuscitation requires focus on securing an airway ventilation and circulation.

Medical care begins with the activation of the Emergency Medical Service (EMS) system. Paramedics assess the injured child and establish an airway. In route, they attempt intravenous access and alert the receiving trauma center as to the child's condition and estimated arrival time. The trauma center then activates a designated team that assembles in the resuscitation area in preparation for the arrival of the injured child. Prearrival preparations for an injured child include selecting the necessary equipment based on the approximate weight or age of the child, obtaining O-negative blood, and notifying consultants, radiology, and the operating room of the impending arrival. It is important to have available customized equipment for children and to educate team members familiar with the use of the instruments.

Optimal care for an injured child requires an organized and well-trained team ready to carry out preassigned tasks quickly and efficiently. The team is most often led by a pediatric surgeon or a trauma surgeon knowledgeable in the care of injured children. Other team members include representatives from anesthesia, emergency medicine, critical care, and nursing. Prior to arrival, the team leader is given information concerning the mechanism of injury, prehospital intervention, and the child's present condition. On arrival, the child is rapidly assessed by a *primary survey,* designed to quickly identify any life-threatening injuries or conditions.[14] The primary survey is followed by a short transition period and a more detailed *secondary survey.* Airway is the initial priority in the primary survey, followed by *B*reathing and *C*irculation (ABCs), *N*eurologic *D*isability, and *E*xposure.[15]

AIRWAY

Establishment of a secure airway is the highest priority in the care of injured children. Protection of the cervical spine through proper immobilization is essential until an injury is excluded. Assessment of the airway begins prior to the child's arrival in the resuscitation area. Information concerning the mechanism of injury, physical examination, and field vital signs can alert the clinician to signs of potential compromise. On arrival, the clinician begins the primary survey by visually assessing the child's color, respiratory rate, mental status, and chest wall movement. All children receive supplemental oxygen and placement of an electrocardiogram (ECG) and pulse oximetry monitors. A child's ability to answer simple questions confirms the presence of a patent airway and gives insight as to the level of consciousness. Next, the mouth and nares are inspected for blood, secretions, or a foreign body. Signs of severe maxillofacial or laryngeotracheal trauma should alert the physician to the potential for airway instability and the need for additional airway support.

Interventions to open the airway progress from a simple jaw thrust technique or placement of an oral airway to endotracheal intubation; rarely is establishment of a surgical airway necessary because in most instances simple maneuvers will be successful. Children who cannot maintain a secure airway despite simple interventions require endotracheal intubation. Appropriate candidates for intubation include children with an arrival Glasgow Coma Scale (GCS) score of 8 or less, severe maxillofacial trauma, and respiratory distress.[15-17] The assurance of a secure airway can be difficult in children with an altered level of consciousness as a result of traumatic brain injury. They frequently respond appropriately during the primary survey but then become progressively obtunded as external stimulation decreases. Careful monitoring and repeated reassessment prior to the resuscitation bay are necessary to prevent airway compromise. Children with altered mental status due to shock from blood loss or hypoxia must also be carefully evaluated. These children often rapidly improve after adequate fluid resuscitation or simple airway interventions. The team leader must work in concert with other team members to ensure that all children maintain a secure airway throughout resuscitation.

When the security or patency of a child's airway is in question, definitive control is provided by endotracheal intubation. This is best performed in a controlled setting by personnel experienced with pediatric airway management. Medications to provide sedation and muscle relaxation are essential and must be readily available. Short-acting barbiturates (thiopental, 2 to 5 mg/kg) or benzodiazepines (midazolam, 0.1 mg/kg) are often used to induce amnesia and sedation. In hypotensive children, the dosage must be adjusted to avoid enhancement of hypotension. Muscle relaxation is accomplished with either a short-acting nondepolarizing agent (rocuronium, 0.1 mg/kg) or a rapid-acting depolarizing agent (succinylcholine, 2 mg/kg). Children often manifest an intense vagal response during airway manipulation, resulting in elevated intracranial pressure (ICP) and profound bradycardia; pretreatment with atropine (0.1 mg/kg) in children 10 years of age and younger blunts these cardiac effects. Avoidance of increased ICP is essential in children with traumatic brain injury. Lidocaine (1 mg/kg) minimizes ICP elevations during airway manipulation.[18, 19]

Determination of appropriate endotracheal tube size is possible using the formula (age + 16)/4 or selecting an endotracheal tube with the same diameter as the nail on the child's fifth finger. Uncuffed endotracheal tubes are used in children younger than 8 years of age because the subglottic is the narrowest portion of a child's airway.[20] An orogastric tube is placed following endotracheal intubation to decompress the stomach and to reduce the possibility of aspiration. Intubated trauma victims require continuing doses of sedation and analgesia with paralytic agents to prevent unintentional extubation.

BREATHING

After definitive airway control, evaluation of respiratory mechanics to ensure that adequate gas exchange is the next priority. Assessment begins with observation for symmetric chest wall movement and for signs of increased work of breathing, such as intercostal retractions or nasal flaring. The chest is then auscultated for symmetry of breath sounds and for normal heart tones. Percussion reveals hyperresonance or dullness, indicating intrapleural air or fluid, respectively. The chest of a child is more pliable than that of an adult. The ribs are more cartilaginous and possess less protective musculature, allowing underlying parenchymal injury to occur in the absence of rib fracture or chest wall contusion. The mediastinum is less well fixed, making deceleration injury to the great vessels extremely rare but increasing the incidence of tension pneumothorax.

The diagnosis of a tension pneumothorax is suggested by respiratory distress, absent or decreased breath sounds, hyperresonance to percussion, and tachypnea. In the clinically stable child, x-ray confirmation is valuable; however, needle or thoracostomy tube decompression should be immediately performed if the clinical condition deteriorates. Needle decompression is accomplished by inserting a large (18-gauge) needle in the third or fourth intercostal space in the midclavicular line. A thoracostomy tube is best placed at or above the nipple line, in the midaxillary line posteriorly and superiorly. Children with hemothorax apparent on chest x-ray frequently require thoracostomy tube drainage. An initial output of greater than 20 mL/kg or sustained output greater than 2 mL/kg/hour requires surgical exploration for hemostasis.[14–16]

Thoracic injury in children is usually the result of a large transfer of kinetic energy to a relatively small surface area. In one study, the presence of a significant thoracic injury increased mortality more than 10-fold compared with children without these injuries.[21, 22] Multisystem trauma was common and occurred in more than 80% of children with thoracic injuries.

Concomitant head injuries increased mortality to 36% and were seen in more than half of the children studied. Although an isolated rib fracture rarely is associated with death, the presence of multiple rib fractures increased mortality to 42%, and children sustaining head and multiple rib fractures had a staggering 71% mortality rate.[21–23]

CIRCULATION

After airway control and adequate gas exchange are established, perfusion is evaluated and shock is reversed. Signs of inadequate tissue perfusion include altered mental status, delayed capillary refill, cool mottled extremities, and decreased peripheral pulses in proportion to central pulses. The presence of tachycardia, tachypnea, and a narrowed pulse pressure also suggests the need for volume resuscitation. Unlike adults, children will commonly maintain a normal systolic blood pressure despite the loss of up to 25% of their blood volume. It is essential to recognize that blood pressure is not a sensitive indicator of hypoperfusion in injured children.[16, 17, 19, 20]

Once all sites of serious hemorrhage are controlled by direct pressure, intravenous access is required. Placement of two large-bore catheters into peripheral veins is optimal but is frequently difficult in infants or children with vascular collapse. No more than 90 seconds is spent attempting peripheral access before progressing to direct visualization of the vein by surgical cutdown; direct access is best accomplished at the greater saphenous vein, located 1 cm medial and superior to the medial malleolus. If intravenous access cannot be provided by either of these methods, percutaneous central vein cannulation by the Seldinger technique at the femoral vein should be considered. The femoral vein's location away from the head and chest allows insertion while procedures above the diaphragm occur simultaneously. Additionally, complications from attempted femoral line placement are less likely to be as life-threatening as those from either a subclavian or an internal jugular vein injury.

In life-threatening situations and when attempts at peripheral access are unsuccessful, an intraosseous infusion device is placed.[16, 24, 25] Preferred sites include the medial aspect of the anterior tibial plateau, medial malleolus, and distal femur. The thin bony cortex of children younger than 7 years of age facilitates placement, but the intraosseous route can be used in any age group with infusion rates comparable to the peripheral route. The intraosseous infusion route is safe for all medications administered during resuscitation.[24–26]

Fluid resuscitation begins with the rapid administration of 20 mL/kg of warmed lactated Ringer's solution. Reassessment of the clinical indicators of hypoperfusion will guide the clinician as to the need for an additional fluid bolus. If further volume resuscitation is required after two bolus infusions of 20 mL/kg crystalloid, transfusion with 10 mL/kg of the most type-specific packed erythrocytes available is initiated through a warming device.[16, 20, 27] Persistent blood or fluid requirements indicate ongoing hemorrhage necessitating surgical exploration for hemostasis. Although control of life-threatening hemorrhage is clearly the priority during the primary survey, small lacerations in the scalp, mouth, or extremities can bleed profusely and result in shock.[14, 16, 17]

DISABILITY

Central nervous system (CNS) injury occurs in the majority of children with multisystem trauma. Rapid assessment and appropriate management are essential in preventing secondary injury to the brain. The CNS evaluation begins after control of the airway, after revision of adequate ventilation, and after restoration of perfusion. Hypoxia and hypotension are linked to secondary brain injury.[28, 29] Children suspected of traumatic brain injury (TBI) require oxygenation to a $Pa{O_2}$ near 100, hyperventilation to a $P{CO_2}$ between 30 and 35, and normovolemia.[28, 30, 31]

The child's neurologic status is often evident by simple observation of the child on arrival to the resuscitation area. Evidence of unconsciousness, decerebrate or decorticate posture, seizure, or asymmetry of limb movement alerts the clinician to the possibility of serious neurologic injury. In children older than 1 year of age, the GCS is a useful tool for assessing CNS damage; children with a GCS score of 8 or below require immediate intubation. Because paralytic agents are frequently useful during airway control, documentation of neurologic states is helpful before intubation. When the diagnosis is in doubt, the child with a head injury should be intubated.

A rapid, thorough physical examination follows the initial visual assessment. The scalp should be checked quickly for any obvious discontinuity or protruding brain matter. The pupils are examined for size, symmetry, responsiveness to light, and consensuality. The cervical spine is palpated while alignment is maintained to detect any stepoff or significant point tenderness. The ability to respond to voice commands or stimuli is assessed along with extremity movement, muscle strength, and sensation. Signs of severe neurologic injury, such as a GCS score of 8 or less, lateral gaze deviation, abnormal posture, or an enlarged, asymmetric pupil suggests focal neurologic injury and requires endotracheal intubation and radiographic evaluation by computed tomography (CT) scan once stable. There is rarely a need to perform bur hole cranial decompression in the resuscitation area. The use of mannitol during the resuscitation of the brain is useful for impending herniation, but maintenance of normovolemia is essential despite the excessive urine output this osmotic diuretic creates.[31, 32]

After initial resuscitation efforts are completed, radiographic assessment is begun. In children with suspected neurologic injury, CT is imperative. It is a sensitive and reliable modality widely used to assess the presence of extra axial blood. Several recent reports describe a 10% to 20% incidence of an abnormal CT scan in children with mild head injury.[33–35] These children arrived without documented loss of consciousness but an initial GCS score of 12 to 14 or reported loss of consciousness but a GCS score of 15 in the resuscitation area. Accordingly, all children with either documented loss of consciousness or a GCS score of less than 15 undergo a head CT or overnight observation.

EXPOSURE

Although exposure is the final step in the primary survey, it is actually initiated by EMS personnel prior to arrival. Clothing that covers the extremities is cut or removed to obtain blood pressure and pulse measurements, to place intravenous lines, and to expose and splint obvious extremity fractures. The process is continued in the resuscitation area in order to facilitate a thorough physical examination. Visualization of all areas of the body is imperative, including those temporarily covered by arm boards, splints, collars, and dressings. Areas difficult to inspect in the prone position, such as the back, flanks, and perineum must not be neglected. Although this type of visualization is difficult during resuscitation of a severely injured child, it must be completed before the patient leaves the resuscitation area. Failure to accomplish this increases the risk of missed injury and morbidity in the injured child.

Although complete exposure of the child is helpful, maintenance of core body temperature is important. *Hypothermia,* defined as a core temperature below than 36°C, has a number of adverse effects. A low temperature significantly increases oxygen consumption, perpetuates ongoing acidosis, and decreases the effectiveness of the blood coagulation by reducing the efficiency of the cascade enzymes.[36, 37] Failure to prevent or rapidly reverse hypothermia results in a troublesome coagulopathy and an increase in fluid requirements and subsequent hemodilution.[36–38]

Injured children are especially vulnerable to the complication of hypothermia. They have an increased body surface area to weight ratio, causing significant heat loss during exposure. Intravenous fluids are frequently not warm, further reducing core temperature. Finally, severely injured children frequently require numerous radiologic studies that are conducted in areas maintained well below core body temperature.

Treatment of hypothermia depends upon careful monitoring of core temperature, administration of warm intravenous fluids, conservation of body warmth using a blanket and heat lamps, and increase in ambient temperature. Injured children who arrive with a core temperature of less than 36.5°C should immediately be rewarmed by means of a preestablished hypothermia protocol. Early intervention reduces further heat loss and prevents many of the complications associated with hypothermia-induced coagulopathy.[37, 38]

TRANSITION

Completion of the primary survey signals team members to begin the transition phase of resuscitative care. The evaluation and treatment of life-threatening injuries occur simultaneously over a very short period of time, usually 5 to 10 minutes in most cases. The transition phase is the time between the primary and secondary survey in which other necessary tasks are completed, such as trauma radiographs of the lateral cervical spine, chest, and pelvis. Seriously injured children often require additional intravenous access, a urinary catheter, and gastric decompression. All intubated children and those with suspected maxillofacial injury require orogastric tube placement. Blood and urine specimens are obtained for analysis and crossmatch. Medications, including antibiotics, an analgesic, and a sedative, are administered as needed. During this time, thoracostomy tubes are secured, fractures are splinted, and consultants are notified. If evacuation to a facility with additional capabilities is required, contact is initiated during this phase. Further diagnostic testing must not delay transfer of the injured child to the receiving facility.

SECONDARY SURVEY

The secondary survey begins with a detailed and systematic examination of the child to uncover any injury not addressed during the primary survey. It includes a head-to-toe physical examination, any additional radiographic studies, and continuous respiratory, neurologic, and hemodynamic assessment. The physical examination is commonly started at the head, where the scalp is checked for laceration, hematoma, or bony crepitus. The tympanic membranes are visualized, the pupils are reexamined, and the facial bones are palpated for tenderness, instability, or deformity. The mouth is inspected for loose teeth, lacerations, or malocclusion. The cervical spine is once again carefully palpated to assess for signs of stepoff or tenderness and to ensure no injury has been hidden by the cervical collar. The thorax and abdomen are again palpated, including the flanks, back, and perineum. All extremities are inspected, with each joint tested through its normal range of motion. Finally, peripheral pulses are confirmed, and a neurologic and rectal examination is performed.

Although this survey can be conducted any time after the primary survey, it is best performed when the patient and the examiner are not distracted by other activities. In many instances, the primary survey, transition phase, and secondary survey can be completed within 15 minutes, allowing the injured child to move expeditiously and safely to the operating room or radiology suite for additional studies. In radiology, extremities suspected of fracture are evaluated after appropriate abdominal, thoracic, or cranial CT scans are obtained. Children suffering blunt injury to the abdomen require a CT scan without oral contrast.[39, 40]

Diagnostic peritoneal lavage (DPL) is rarely indicated in children because the majority of solid organ injuries in this age group are treated without operation using the information provided by CT.[41, 42] Children suspected of having an epidural or subdural hematoma requiring emergency evacuation are logical candidates for DPL; however, all of these children require a head CT prior to surgery. The addition of an abdominal CT for a child already on the table adds very little time.

Hemodynamically unstable children suspected of concomitant head and thoracoabdominal trauma represent a unique challenge. Exsanguinating hemorrhage in the chest or abdomen must be surgically controlled as soon as possible, but life-threatening head injury also requires expeditious treatment. Surgically correctable life-threatening head injuries are infrequent in children; diffuse axonal injury is the most common cause of death from head trauma. Although the information provided by a head CT would be useful to rule out these injuries, the potential delay from transport to the CT scan is a risk in children with severe ongoing hemorrhage. Maintenance of circulating blood volume and rapid surgical hemostasis reduce secondary brain injury caused by hypotension.

STABILIZATION IN THE INTENSIVE CARE UNIT

Once the initial priorities of resuscitation and evaluation have been fulfilled, attention is directed toward physiologic homeostasis. Effective care requires a multidisciplinary team approach and meticulous attention to detail. Management necessitates continuous reassessment to detect changes signifying physiologic derangement and recognition of the unique needs of children.

AIRWAY MANAGEMENT

The appropriate evaluation and management of the airway is the initial priority in case of an injured child. Significant differences in anatomy, physiology, and airway techniques in children challenge any clinician responsible for providing pediatric life support. Airway compromise is one of the most common causes of pediatric cardiac arrest.

The anatomy of the pediatric airway is a challenge to properly manage. Infants and small children possess relatively large posterior oropharyngeal structures and a proportionately smaller mouth, making control of the tongue and visualization of pharyngeal structures during intubation difficult. A larger occiput in infants increases the angle between the oral and tracheal axis and also contributes to airway obstruction in children with altered mental status. In young children, the larynx occupies a more cephalad position, usually at the C-3 to C-4 level. As a child matures, it descends to a position at C-6 to C-7. This also results in an increased angle between the base of the tongue and glottis. Additionally, the larynx of a child is cone-shaped, with the narrowest portion below the vocal cords at the level of the cricoid cartilage. This differs from the adult larynx, which is more cylindrically shaped and less distensible, with the smallest diameter easily visualized during intubation. This anatomic difference necessitates uncuffed endotracheal tubes in children younger than 8 years of age.[14, 16, 20, 43]

Visualization of the cord structures is facilitated by use of a straight laryngoscope blade instead of the curved blade commonly used in intubation of adults. The epiglottis is shorter and shaped similar to an omega, which makes manipulation during intubation more difficult.

Infants and children also demonstrate several important differences in respiratory physiology and mechanics that must be considered during evaluation and treatment. The metabolic rate and oxygen consumption of children is two or three times higher than that of adults. Airway obstruction or inadequate ventilation results in hypoxia and hypercarbia much sooner than in an adult. Infants are obligate nose breathers until approximately 6 months of age.[43] Any device, such as a nasogastric tube, that may compromise nasal airway patency should be avoided; this is especially true in premature infants. Attempts to correct hypoxia with supplemental oxygen are best made via the nasal route with the child in a comfortable position.

The ribs, chest wall, and intercostal muscles of infants are extremely compliant and provide minimal thoracic support, causing tidal volume to approach airway closing volume and decreasing functional residual capacity. The poorly developed intercostal muscles contribute little to the work of breathing in infants. This causes alveolar ventilation to be almost totally dependent on diaphragmatic movement. Unfortunately, the infant diaphragm has a predominance of fast-twitch muscle fibers and does not reach muscular maturity until the child is approximately 2 years of age, making it far more susceptible to fatigue than in an older child or adult. Additionally, any process that interferes with diaphragmatic excursion, such as aerophagia, intra-abdominal hemorrhage, or the increased intrathoracic pressure of tension pneumothorax, can severely compromise respiratory function.[43, 44]

One of the most significant differences between adults and children is the relatively small size of the upper airway. Minimal amounts of edema or fluid in infants can cause life-threatening obstruction and airway compromise. As a child grows and develops, the airway diameter increases with a corresponding decrease in airway resistance until the child is approximately 8 years of age. Resistance to laminar airflow is inversely proportional to the fourth power of the radius. It is easy to see that even a 1- or 2-mm reduction in lumen diameter is associated with nearly a 75% reduction in airway cross-sectional area. Turbulent flow from crying, edema, laryngospasm, or a foreign body must be avoided.[44, 45]

MANAGEMENT OF RESPIRATORY FAILURE

Respiratory failure is generally defined as the inability to provide adequate alveolar ventilation or to support requisite alveolar oxygen requirements for a given clinical situation. There are many causes and contributing factors that predispose an injured child to respiratory compromise, including altered mental status, copious airway secretions or edema secondary to infection or systemic inflammatory response syndrome (SIRS), craniofacial or cervical trauma, pulmonary contusion, flail chest, aspiration, pneumonia, sepsis, and abdominal distention. Airway control and mechanical ventilatory support restore alveolar oxygenation and ventilation to acceptable levels and reverse ongoing hypoxia, acidosis, or atelectasis.

Initiating mechanical ventilation support reduces the work of breathing, increases lung volume through alveolar recruitment, and minimizes the stress of respiratory failure. Associated physiologic benefits include an overall reduction in oxygen consumption, greater latitude in the use of narcotics and sedatives, and the ability to transiently reduce intracranial pressure by judicious hyperventilation (P_{CO_2} 30 to 35).[46, 47]

After airway control, appropriate ventilatory support depends on the technique. Modern ventilators accomplish gas exchange by introducing oxygen at a predetermined concentration using positive pressure. Carbon dioxide is removed by expanding the lungs a reproducible amount by controlling either pressure or volume at a preset number of times per minute. In children, ventilatory support is commonly initiated with a volume-cycled ventilator at an oxygen concentration of 100% and a tidal volume of 8 to 12 mL/kg at 15 to 25 times per minute. Synchronized intermittent mandatory ventilation (SIMV) is used for the injured child who cannot spontaneously initiate an adequate respiratory effort because of sedation or head injury that requires hyperventilation or decrease in work of breathing. Positive end-expiratory pressure (PEEP) is applied in an effort to reduce airway resistance and work of breathing, improve functional residual capacity, and increase oxygenation. PEEP is usually initiated between 5 and 10 cm H_2O and increased as oxygenation or compliance decreases. Although possible complications of PEEP include increased mean airway pressure, increased intracranial pressure, and decreased venous return, some studies in adults suggest that PEEP less than 10 cm has little effect on these parameters.[16, 47, 48]

The *assist control* mode of ventilation is used in children who are able to spontaneously initiate an adequate number of breaths but require assistance generating an acceptable tidal volume. In the assist control method, each respiratory effort causes a preset tidal volume to be delivered, allowing the child some control over minute ventilation. Assist control is best used to provide active wean from the ventilator or in a spontaneously breathing child who is "fighting the ventilator." Volume-cycled ventilators maintain a relatively constant tidal volume using varying amounts of pressure. Flow rate is constant throughout the inspiratory phase, so that airway pressures increase and peak at the end of inspiration. Reduced airway compliance is manifest by changes in peak inspiratory pressure (PIP), increased PEEP, a higher oxygen flow rate, and shortened inspiratory time. One must avoid prolonged peak inspiratory pressure greater than 35 to 40 cm H_2O to prevent barotrauma and the respiratory distress syndrome (RDS).[47–49]

Several important aspects of RDS require comment. Whereas inspection of chest radiographs reveals a diffuse generalized parenchymal process, evidence suggests that there is considerable heterogeneity among lung units. This coexistence of healthy lung units in close proximity to compromised lung units has been implicated as a major contributing factor in the progressive deterioration characteristic of RDS. The substantial PIP and PEEP required for gas exchange in volume control–ventilated children with RDS cause overdistention, barotrauma, and scarring in the uncompromised alveoli.[47-49] To mitigate this process, one may apply of pressure control ventilation (PCV). Initially used to treat premature infants with hyaline membrane disease, PCV utilizes high flow rates delivered in a square waveform through a variable tidal volume. A pressure limit and rate are set, with the tidal volume determined by both static and dynamic compliance. This high flow rate achieves peak pressure rapidly, allows increased alveolar recruitment, and improves gaseous diffusion at lower peak airway pressures, which reduces overdistention and barotrauma to healthy lung units.

Results from several studies in adults and children have shown that a ventilator strategy consisting of PCV, FIO_2 less than 0.5, PEEP less than 15 (including auto-PEEP), and PIP less than 40 with tidal volumes 5 to 7 mL/kg (permissive hypercapnia) improves survival and decreases the total number of ventilator days.[48-51] Permissive hypercapnia utilizes the buffering capability of the kidney to compensate for the hypercarbia that develops as a result of the reducing tidal volume to minimize PIP. This reduction in tidal volume allows greater amounts of PEEP to be used to improve oxygenation without increasing PIP to levels that would be injurious.

Children who have been intubated for prolonged periods require weaning of ventilator support prior to extubation. Weaning is necessary if the injured child's mental status is such that the child cannot fully protect the airway or handle secretions. Occasionally, the diaphragm and other respiratory muscles have undergone some degree of atrophy or there is significant underlying parenchymal disease. Effective ventilator weaning requires a strategy that allows a child to initiate a breath and contribute a variable amount to the inspiratory effort. Pressure support ventilation (PSV) enables children who can initiate spontaneous breaths to contribute to the tidal volume goal without having to move the entire tidal volume.

PSV utilizes pressure limits to achieve a desired spontaneous tidal volume (4 to 6 mL/kg). Each time the child inspires, a preset pressure delivers the desired tidal volume, which varies as the child's effort and compliance change. As the child's mental or respiratory status improves, a gradual reduction of the amount of support is possible by decreasing the pressure applied to maintain a given tidal volume is. In this way children can control much of the minute volume, remain intubated, and be as comfortable as possible without risking the disuse atrophy associated with assist control ventilation.[52]

Criteria for safe extubation include the ability to initiate an adequate number of spontaneous breaths, handle secretions, and to achieve a PCO_2 below 55 and a PaO_2 greater than 60 on supplemental oxygen. If this is questionable; a trial with a T piece or continuous positive airway pressure (CPAP) can be administered for a short time as an interim challenge. Although a variety of formulas and numeric criteria have been suggested as guides to determine who will successfully tolerate extubation, clinical judgment is widely regarded as the best predictor of success or failure.

UNCONVENTIONAL MODALITIES

High-frequency ventilation (HFV) was first used in the early 1980s to treat children with severe respiratory failure using either high-frequency jet ventilation (HFJV) or high-frequency oscillation (HFO). High-frequency ventilation accomplishes gas exchange by instilling very small tidal volumes under low pressure at high respiratory rates ($>$120 breaths/min). A variety of mechanisms are thought to be responsible for gaseous mixing during high-frequency ventilation, including Taylor dispersion forces, bulk convection, and pendelluft. Taylor dispersion occurs most often at anatomic branch points, where turbulent flow causes an interaction between gases exhibiting laminar flow and those undergoing random diffusion. Pendelluft refers to the exchange of gas between lung units with differing degrees of disease.[47, 53]

HFOV permits application of a small tidal volume that maintains PIP just above mean airway pressure (MAP). Because arterial oxygen content (PaO_2) is directly related to MAP, HFO raises PaO_2 without increasing PIP to levels that induce barotrauma. Few studies exist describing the use HFV in nonneonatal pediatric patients with severe respiratory failure.

Arnold and coworkers[54] published a report on seven children with severe respiratory failure who were responding poorly to conventional ventilation therapy and were subsequently switched to HFO. Six of the seven children survived with no worsening of their barotrauma and little or no change in cardiac output. HFO is initiated by selecting a MAP 2 to 3 cm higher than the MAP on conventional volume ventilation. The MAP is then adjusted to achieve chest expansion such that the diaphragm is at the level of the ninth or 10th rib; further increases in MAP pose a risk for barotrauma and compromise of cardiac output. Oxygenation can also be increased by the use of higher concentrations of inspired oxygen. Removal of carbon dioxide (CO_2) is achieved by manipulating the amplitude (ΔP) of the oscillating diaphragm and the speed at which the diaphragm moves (Htz). Children with respiratory failure who weigh more than 15 kg are usually started on 8 to 12 Htz and a ΔP between 30 and 50, depending on the level of CO_2 retention present. Frequent blood gas determinations, chest radiographs, and central venous monitoring assist in management.

Extracorporeal membrane oxygenation (ECMO) is a technique applied to neonates and children with severe respiratory failure who are unresponsive to conventional ventilation as a result of a reversible cause. It is a rare salvage therapy for children with refractory respiratory failure. Although anecdotal reports and small series have been reported, further investigation is necessary before ECMO gains widespread acceptance in the pediatric population.[55, 56]

HEMODYNAMIC MONITORING AND STABILIZATION

The ability to continuously and accurately measure blood pressure, monitor oxygen kinetics, and assess the benefits of therapeutic interventions is essential for optimal care of the injured child. This process begins early during the resuscitation phase and continues seamlessly to the critical care unit. Assessment of adequate tissue perfusion and of circulating volume is essential. Altered mental status, cool or mottled extremities, tachycardia, tachypnea, and hypotension are all indicators of inadequate tissue perfusion. Children who are not stable after repeated fluid bolus or who require inotropic drug infusion require placement of an intra-arterial catheter to assess ongoing hemodynamic instability, to monitor inotropic support, and to measure arterial blood gases.

Noninvasive blood pressure monitoring using a sphygmomanometer should always be used in conjunction with indwelling arterial lines. Selecting an appropriate cuff size is essential for an accurate blood pressure measurement. The cuff is placed at the midpoint of the limb, with the length approximately 40% of the circumference of the extremity being used.[57] Occasionally, there is a significant discrepancy between the cuff and arterial catheter pressures. Although cuff pressures are an indirect measurement of blood pressure and vary in relation to cuff size, direct readings from indwelling arterial catheters can also be inaccurate because of resonance overshoot, waveform dampening from air in the tubing, catheter tip thrombus, or calibration error.[58] When a discrepancy occurs between the cuff and indwelling line, improved accuracy is possible by placing the cuff above the limb with the arterial catheter and inflating the cuff while simultaneously observing the arterial trace. Inflating the cuff until the arterial trace becomes flat and reading the cuff pressure when the first arterial trace spike appears improve accuracy. Peripherally obtained systolic and diastolic blood pressures can be higher and lower, respectively, than the actual aortic pressure. The mean arterial pressure, obtained by adding one third of the systolic pressure to the diastolic pressure, is the most reliable value and should be used whenever possible.[59]

Appropriate sites for arterial cannulation include radial, dorsalis pedis, posterior tibial, femoral, and axillary arteries. Complications resulting from arterial cannulation are relatively rare and include vessel thrombosis, distal embolization, and tissue loss.[60] Evidence in adults reveals that nearly 30% of adult radial arteries are thrombosed at the time of decannulation.[61] A study examining the incidence of systemic infection from arterial cannulation in children reported this occurrence in less than 1% of the cohort.[62] Complications resulting from the placement of femoral arterial catheters include limb length discrepancies and distal ischemia. If distal perfusion becomes compromised after the insertion of an arterial catheter, removal is imperative.[63]

Central venous catheters are commonly placed in critically injured children requiring significant volume replacement, hemodynamic monitoring, vasopressor administration, hyperalimentation, and reliable venous access. Most seriously injured children have normal cardiac function and demonstrate intravascular volume depletion. Using central venous pressure to assess intravascular volume status is frequently as reliable as measurements from a pulmonary artery catheter.[64] Complications do occur and include hematoma, thrombosis, vessel injury, air embolism, and infection. The risk of infectious complications tends to rise with the length of time the catheter has been in place. Central venous catheters left in position less than 72 hours carry an infection rate of less than 2%.[65, 66] Venous access in injured children is safest by cannulation of the internal jugular or femoral vein. This allows unimpeded access to the chest and avoids many of the life-threatening complications possible with a subclavian vein cannulation. The right subclavian vein may be connected, but the complication rate is higher. The tip of the catheter is best placed in the superior vena cava; catheter tip placement should be avoided in the right atrium. Arrhythmias caused by infusions of fluids at suboptimal temperatures, by right atrial perforation, or by inadvertent right ventricular placement are all potential complications of venous catheters.

Pulmonary artery catheters are not normally required for assessment of cardiopulmonary status in children. Indications for placement include children with cardiac failure requiring inotropic support, significant renal or pulmonary dysfunction in which preload cannot be accurately measured, or inadequate tissue perfusion despite appropriate volume resuscitation. Common sites for cannulation include the right internal jugular, femoral, or subclavian veins. In children younger than 2 years of age or weighing less than 10 kg, the femoral approach may be the easiest. Pediatric pulmonary artery catheters are supplied in No. 5 French and 7 French sizes, with the 5 French recommended for children weighing less than 30 kg.[64] Placement is performed with distal port pressures and waveforms as the catheter tip passes through the heart and into the pulmonary artery. If difficulty is encountered, fluoroscopy or bedside echocardiography may be helpful.

One advantage of placing a pulmonary artery catheter is the ability to measure mixed venous oxygen saturation (Svo_2). Adequate tissue oxygenation is a balance between oxygen supply and oxygen demand. The ability to measure changes in the oxygen saturation of the venous blood returning to the lungs allows assessment of the adequacy of oxygen delivery in relation to oxygen consumption, which is especially valuable when interpreting the usefulness of a therapeutic intervention. Optimal mixed venous saturation ranges between 65% and 75%. A reduction below 65% or a sudden change of 5% to 10% should prompt a reevaluation of cardiac index, hemoglobin, and oxygen saturation. The accuracy of Svo_2 may be decreased by the arteriovenous shunting seen in sepsis, technical problems associated with the catheter tip, or faulty connections.

SHOCK AND OXYGEN KINETICS

The ability to recognize and treat shock is essential in the case of an injured child. Historically, the definition and classification of shock have undergone a variety of modifications. As our understanding of pathophysiology increases, the description of shock has changed from the level of the organism, to the level of the organ system, and, finally, to the level of the organelle. Shock is now defined as an imbalance between oxygen supply and oxygen demand resulting in a failure of perfusion to meet the metabolic needs of the cell. Inherent in this definition is that inadequate perfusion can be a result of decreased supply, increased demand, or some combination of both. Attempts at reversing the deleterious effects of shock are aimed at improving oxygen delivery (Do_2) and reducing oxygen consumption (Vo_2).

Oxygen delivery can be calculated by the following equation:

$$Do_2 = CO \times (1.36 \times Hb \times Sao_2) + (0.003 \times Pao_2)$$

where Hb is the concentration of hemoglobin, Sao_2 is the saturation of arterial hemoglobin, and Pao_2 is the partial pressure of arterial oxygen. Using a hemoglobin concentration of 15 g/dL and assuming the ability to fully saturate the available hemoglobin, Do_2 is calculated to be 12 to 15 mL/kg/min, by body surface area or 500 to 600 mL/m^2/min. The contribution of dissolved oxygen in the blood ($0.003 \times Pao_2$) is minimal and can be excluded to provide ease in calculations in most instances.[64, 67]

Vo_2 is more difficult to measure and requires either a closed-circuit rebreathing volumetric analysis or mixed expired gas analysis. Both methods are limited by technical problems in obtaining accurate clinical data. Oxygen consumption can also be obtained with the Fick method, but a pulmonary artery catheter is necessary and this is the least accurate of the three methods described.[68] Factors increasing Vo_2 include sepsis, agitation, fever, muscular activity, cytokine production, and excess catecholamine levels. Normal Vo_2 in adults is 3 mL/kg/min or 120 mL/m^2/min. Children have a greater surface area to mass ratio, increasing Vo_2 to as much as 8 mL/kg/min.[64, 67, 68] In a normal state, the ratio of Do_2 to Vo_2 is approximately 4:1, allowing consumption to remain independent of delivery. In severely injured children, decreased Do_2 caused by hemorrhage and hypoxia can reduce this ratio.

These same factors also raise consumption by causing increases in circulating catecholamines, in the work of breathing, and in cytokine production. If this process continues, the Do_2:Vo_2 ratio decreases to an extent that Vo_2 becomes dependent on oxygen delivery. Clinical studies have estimated this critical point to be a ratio of about 3. Below this, the diminished supply cannot meet metabolic needs, resulting in anaerobic metabolism, increased lactate production, and metabolic acidosis.[64, 67]

The initial compensatory response to a reduction in DO_2 is an increase in cardiac output. The exact feedback mechanism by which this occurs is poorly understood. One study suggests that sensory cells similar to those of the carotid body exist in the pulmonary arteries and respond to alterations in either CO_2 levels or venous oxygen saturation (SvO_2). If alterations in the cardiac output are unable to restore adequate DO_2, the remaining deficits are met with an increase in the amount of oxygen extracted at the cellular level. It is this increased extraction that can be seen when mixed SvO_2 is measured.

Oxygen delivery must be increased by careful evaluation of each component in the equation. Hemoglobin is measured and, if necessary, transfusion of blood occurs. Cardiac output, which is the product of heart rate and stroke volume, can be maximized by sequential assessment of preload, contractility, and afterload using central venous, pulmonary artery, or oximetric analysis. SaO_2 is evaluated by blood gas values or pulse oximetry and is improved by oxygen, intubation, and controlled ventilation in a stepwise approach. The contribution of the oxygen dissolved in the blood to delivery is minimal and can be ignored during clinical assessments.

MANAGEMENT OF CRANIOCEREBRAL INJURY

Estimates describing the incidence of traumatic brain injury range between 100 and 200 per 100,000 children.[69, 70] Brain injury is the leading cause of death in injured children, with 75% of all deaths attributed to craniocerebral trauma.[14, 16, 17] Unfortunately, injury to the central nervous system is quite common, occurring in approximately 50% of all injured children.[16, 17] Those children who survive severe neurologic injury often require expensive rehabilitation and account for many years of lost productivity in society.[16, 32, 70]

The brain of a child is different from that of an adult. The mass of the head represents nearly 15% of the total body in a infant compared with only 3% in an adult. By age 6 years, a child's brain has reached more than 90% of its final mass. Young children have less well developed neck musculature and flatter cervical facets, making cranial stabilization more difficult. The skull of an infant is soft and pliable, with open fontanelles and sutures. As the child ages, the bony cortex becomes thicker and more brittle until approximately 3 years of age, when it resembles that of an adult. The immature brain has a greater water content and has undergone less myelination than in the adult. The majority of myelination occurs between 2 and 6 years of age and is accompanied by increasing synaptic and dendritic arborization. The spaces containing cerebrospinal fluid (CSF) both intraventricular and subarachnoid, are proportionately smaller, providing less of a cushioning effect and a smaller reservoir for removal during periods of increased ICP. The net result is a softer and more easily injured brain with a greater susceptibility to shear injury than in adults.[16, 17, 71, 72]

The mechanisms of injury responsible for most pediatric brain injury are age-related and distinct from those occurring in adults. In children under 2 years of age, child abuse and injuries sustained as a motor vehicle occupant make up the majority of cases. Falls are also prevalent in this age group and are frequently given as the mechanism of injury when abuse is suspected. As children become toddlers and enter preschool, falls and injuries due to motor vehicles continue to predominate, with a greater percentage in this group injured as pedestrians struck by motor vehicles. As older children become more independent, they are frequently injured as bicyclists and pedestrians.[7, 8, 14, 20]

The pathophysiology of traumatic brain injury that begins at the moment of impact is termed *primary injury;* fracture, contusion, and laceration all fall into this category. The most common primary injury in children is due to shearing stress, which occurs during sudden deceleration or rotation. Disruptions in the myelin sheath and minute vascular hemorrhage, typically in the corpus callosum, internal capsule, and cerebellar peduncles, can cause severe and permanently disabling neurologic injury known as diffuse axonal injury. Secondary injuries occur subsequent to the initial insult and can be the result of increased ICP, hypoxia, ischemia, hypotension, seizures, or space-occupying lesions. Besides prevention, little can be done about primary injury. The treatment strategy of craniocerebral trauma is aimed at reducing or preventing secondary injury.[72–74]

Blood flow to the brain is tightly controlled by autoregulation. Regional cerebral blood flow remains independent of MAP over a wide range. Oxygen and glucose must be immediately available to sustain the brain's high metabolic needs. Interruption of this process results in hypoxia and ischemia. Autoregulation is designed to maintain cerebral perfusion pressure (CPP). This can further be defined by the equation,

$$CPP = MAP - ICP$$

where ICP is intracranial pressure and MAP is mean arterial pressure.

Increased ICP results from expansion of one or more components within the cranium. These are venous and arterial blood volume, brain volume, space-occupying lesions (hematoma), or increased volume of CSF spaces. Normal ICP in adults and children is recognized to be less than 10 mm Hg. MAP usually ranges between 60 and 80 mm Hg in all but very young children, in which it is less. CPP is considered adequate at levels above 50 mm Hg.[16, 71, 72]

The decision to place an intracranial pressure monitor in a child with traumatic brain injury is based on a number of factors. In general, any child with an admission GCS score of 8 or less as a result of craniocerebral trauma should be monitored. Children frequently sustain diffuse axonal injury that is not apparent on the initial CT scan. Severe cerebral edema after occurs in these children anywhere from 6 to 36 hours after injury and must be carefully monitored so that treatment adjustment is salutary. Children with a GCS score of above 8 rarely exhibit significant increases in ICP, and monitoring in the group is unnecessary.

In many institutions, a ventriculostomy catheter is the preferred monitoring device for head-injured children. It has the advantage of being both diagnostic and therapeutic in that CSF can be directly drained, reducing the ICP and improving the cerebral blood flow. If preexisting cerebral edema is present, ventriculostomy placement can be difficult because of compression of the ventricles. The catheter can also become obstructed, which registers as an acute rise in ICP. One must avoid malfunction of the monitoring device to prevent spurious elevation of ICP and resultant unnecessary intervention. Fiberoptic devices have gained popularity because malfunction is less common. These devices can be placed in the intraventricular, subarachnoid, and subdural spaces but cannot be used to remove fluid.

The treatment of severe head injury is directed by the general principle of preventing or reducing secondary brain injury. The avoidance of hypoxia, hypotension, and decreased cerebral pressure are all important steps in achieving this goal. Hypoxia is alleviated by intubation, positive pressure ventilation, and ensuring an arterial PaO_2 of 65 of better.

Hypotension is treated in a stepwise fashion by first volume infusion with isotonic fluids to normovolemia. Next, vasopressors such as dopamine or phenylephrine (Neo-Synephrine) are added to raise MAP so that the difference between MAP and ICP (CPP) is greater than 50. Finally, treatment is directed at reducing ICP in an effort to maintain CPP greater than 50.

Reducing ICP can be accomplished in a variety of ways. Adequate sedation and pain control are essential in minimizing secondary injury after traumatic brain injury. Head-injured children frequently require significant amounts of sedation after intubation. Children with head injury also respond well to administration of analgesia even in the absence of other painful injuries. Seizures, work of breathing, and fever all increase cerebral oxygen utilization and should be controlled.

One technique involves continuous infusions of midazolam and fentanyl to achieve sedation and analgesia without causing hypotension. In some instances, paralysis in the form of a continuous vecuronium drip is used. As cerebral edema resolves, the paralysis is reversed and the sedation is titrated to allow daily neurologic examinations. For rapid reduction of ICP, hyperventilation is the easiest method; reducing the serum P_{CO_2} to between 28 and 35 causes a concomitant decrease in the CSF pH, which results in cerebral vasoconstriction. The net result is a decrease in the hyperemia associated with the abnormal function of the blood-brain barrier characteristic of children with severe head injury.

P_{CO_2} must be carefully monitored and maintained above 28 mm Hg, or the resulting vasoconstriction may actually decrease CPP to worsen secondary injury. Unlike the case in adults, this effect is not transient and causes vasoconstriction despite prolonged hypocarbia.

Children with evidence of severe intracranial hypertension or sudden cerebral deterioration often benefit from the administration of mannitol. The mechanism of action is that of an osmotic diuretic, drawing fluid from the interstitium into the central circulation, causing a reduction in ICP. Mannitol also appears to lower blood viscosity and may alter the flow characteristics of the microcirculation in the brain. One additional theory is that mannitol acts as an oxygen radical scavenger, which reduces cellular damage and prevents further secondary injury. The initial dose of mannitol for a child suspected of having elevated ICP or signs of herniation is 1 g/kg given in the resuscitation area. Urine output must be carefully monitored and replaced to avoid hypovolemia and hypotension. Additional doses of mannitol (0.25 to 1 g/kg) can be administered every 6 to 12 hours to treat persistent ICP elevation, but serum osmolality should not exceed 320 mOsm/L.[16, 32, 75]

MANAGEMENT OF COAGULATION DISORDERS

The diagnosis of the many different types of coagulation disorders is a challenging aspect of care for the severely injured child. Although there are many children with inherited coagulation abnormalities, most pediatric trauma victims have no antecedent disorder. Despite this, initial evaluation requires specific questions regarding abnormal bleeding; bruisability, hematuria, or blood in the gastrointestinal (GI) tract or joints suggests coagulopathy, which requires further investigation. Diseases of the liver or kidney suggest the potential for disorders of coagulation.

The initial physical examination of an injured child is often not helpful in elucidating evidence of preexisting coagulopathy. Excessive bleeding during routine venipuncture combined with hematuria or blood from the endotracheal tube may indicate clotting abnormalities.

Dilutional coagulopathy in severely injured children most often occurs following large volume replacement for blood loss. Replacement of greater than one blood volume requires rapid restoration of intravascular volume to improve oxygen-carrying capacity, usually with packed red blood cells (PRBCs). Failure to replace the platelets and clotting factors not contained in PRBCs results in a quantitative dilutional coagulopathy. Platelet counts decrease an average of 40% after one blood volume replacement, 60% after two, and 70% after three. Children with a normal platelet count prior to injury do not require platelet transfusions despite blood volume replacement. Platelets are required if the measured platelet count is less than 50,000/mm^3 or if further bleeding is expected and the platelet count is less than 100,000/mm^3.[76, 77] Transfusions of 0.1 to 0.2 units/kg of pooled platelets can be used as a guide to initiate therapy. Frequent reassessment and clinical observation are mandatory because the degree of dilutional thrombocytopenia is directly related to the number of blood volumes transfused and the initial platelet count.

Coagulopathy resulting from the dilution of clotting factors occurs with as little as one blood volume transfusion and is recognized by prolongation of the prothrombin time (PT) and partial thromboplastin time (PTT) to levels 1.5 to two times the control values. Fresh frozen plasma (FFP) is administered in 10 mL/kg increments until coagulation studies approach normal levels or clinical signs of bleeding resolve. Fibrinogen levels below 100 mg/dL require replacement with cryoprecipitate. One unit of cryoprecipitate raises the plasma fibrinogen 5 to 7 mg/dL and must be administered within 6 hours of thawing.[78, 79]

Consumptive coagulopathy occurs when tissue injury, tissue ischemia, or acidosis causes the release of tissue thromboplastin and the subsequent activation of the clotting cascade. This causes platelet activation, excess thrombin production, and accelerated fibrinolysis, resulting in premature clot dissolution, continued bleeding, and increasing consumption of clotting factors. Fibrin thrombi form in the microvasculature, trapping platelets and red blood cells (RBCs). This process, disseminated intravascular coagulation (DIC), leads to thrombocytopenia, hypofibrinogenemia, prolongation of PT and PTT, and increased fibrin degradation products (FDPs).[80, 81] The extent of coagulopathy is related to the duration and severity of the underlying insult. Rapid restoration of circulating blood volume, normothermia, and adequate tissue perfusion is essential in preventing and reversing this type of consumptive coagulopathy.

Complications from massive transfusion include electrolyte disturbances, transfusion reactions, and hypothermia. Hypocalcemia occurs when the citrate used to maintain anticoagulation binds ionized calcium.[82] Although rapidly metabolized by the liver and kidney, clearance is impeded by hypotension, hypothermia, and hepatic and renal dysfunction. Hypocalcemia causes myocardial depression and arrhythmia and can exacerbate existing coagulopathy. FFP contains four times the amount of citrate in PRBCs and poses the greatest risk when rapidly infused in infants and small children.

A small child requires less than 30 ml/min, of FFP for hypocalcemia to develop, especially if FFP is administered via a central catheter, where there is less time for dilution and metabolism.[82] Frequent monitoring of the ionized calcium and judicious calcium administration are required for severely injured children undergoing massive resuscitation. Calcium chloride contains three times the available calcium gluconate compared per milligram and does not require hepatic metabolism.[82, 83]

Hyperkalemia occurs as a result of a shift in potassium from RBCs into the plasma during prolonged storage. Plasma potassium concentrations in stored blood may double after 3 to 4 weeks and may reach levels of 8 mEq/100 mL. Acidosis, hypocalcemia, and rapid infusion increase the likelihood of clinically significant hyperkalemia and life-threatening arrhythmia. Neonates or children with impaired renal function should receive fresh blood or washed RBCs. Hypokalemia is more common during large volume resuscitation and occurs as a result of alterations in catecholamines, aldosterone, and antidiuretic hormone (ADH).[84–86]

Acute hemolytic transfusion reactions do occur and are largely a result of ABO incompatibility. Clinical manifestations include fever, chills, tachycardia, and hemoglobin after transfusion of as little as 10 to 15 mL of blood. Anaphylactic reactions occur when blood containing gamma A immunoglobulin (IgA) antigens is transfused to IgA-deficient patients with IgA antibodies. Symptoms include immediate bronchospasm, shock, and wheezing and may quickly progress to total vascular collapse and arrest.

METABOLIC RESPONSE AND NUTRITION DURING CRITICAL ILLNESS

Restoration of positive nitrogen balance through appropriate nutritional support is essential to optimal care in the severely injured child. Providing the necessary substrates to meet metabolic requirements has been shown to shorten hospital stay, to improve wound healing, and to reduce the risk of infection.[87] The formulation of an individual nutritional plan involves a number of variables, including age, weight, preexisting nutritional status, and severity and type of injury.

A variety of methods exist to measure and monitor the energy needs of adults and children. Serum albumin is a widely used biochemical marker with a 20-day half-life and a high rate of extravascular exchange. It is associated with increased mortality and prolonged hospitalization when low.[88, 89] Albumin's long half-life and variability after large volume resuscitations make it more indicative of injury severity than current nutritional status. Transferrin is an exclusively intravascular transport protein for iron, with an 8-day half-life that correlates with nutritional status.[90] Prealbumin provides the best correlation to nitrogen balance in clinical use today. It has a half-life of only 2 days and rapidly responds to both albumin restriction and increase in nitrogen balance. Indirect calorimetry uses direct volumetric spirometry to measure oxygen consumption and CO_2 production and calculate metabolic energy expenditure. This can be combined with resting expenditure calculations derived from the Harris-Benedict equation, which is more accurate for children over 10 years of age. Technical difficulties assessing severely injured children make this an accurate but cumbersome method of obtaining a nutritional profile.[89–91]

Significant differences in the metabolic needs of children from those of adults include a 50% higher basal metabolic rate and the additional energy requirements of growth. Children sustaining severe injuries require an additional 50% to 100% increase above baseline values.[91, 92] The stress response is initiated when injury stimulates the production of cortisol, epinephrine, and norepinephrine. These humoral changes increase the circulating levels of glucose, free fatty acids, and ketones and decrease the number of amino acids in the blood. Protein catabolism from skeletal muscle and decreased protein synthesis cause increased mobilization of amino acids and significant urinary nitrogen losses.

Children with protein energy malnutrition often exhibit reduced T and B cell function, delayed complement activation, and neutrophil dysfunction. Certain amino acids are involved in the modulation of immune function. Arginine is a nonessential amino acid precursor for nitric oxide that promotes wound healing and increases the activity of natural killer and helper T cells in humans. Glutamine is also a nonessential amino acid found primarily in skeletal muscle and involved in the synthesis of nucleic acids. Recent evidence suggests glutamine may be the preferred fuel for enterocytes and lymphocytes during a stress response. Although glutamine and arginine make up approximately 6% of the available amino acids, they constitute more than 50% of the amino acids mobilized during metabolic stress.

We can construct nutritional plan by first calculating the fluid and caloric requirements of the injured child. The age, weight, prior nutritional status, and nature of the injury affect these calculations. Maintenance fluid requirements are determined by weight and consist of 100 mL/kg/day for children under 10 kg, 1 L plus 50 mL/kg/day for every kilogram over 10 kg in children between 10 and 20 kg, and 1.5 L plus 20 ml/kg/day for children greater than 20 kg. Children with significant ongoing losses, such as gastric fluid, bile, or stool, require these losses to be replaced. This can easily be accomplished with the use of fluid infusion of the most appropriate crystalloid solution available. Careful assessment of daily urine output, blood urea nitrogen (BUN) and urine specific gravity allow adjustment of the total daily fluids to maintain euvolia.

Baseline caloric requirements are as follows:

- Infants, 90 to 120 kcal/kg/day
- Toddlers, 75 to 90 kcal/kg/day
- Children, 60 to 75 kcal/kg/day
- Adolescents, 30 to 60 kcal/kg/day

Adjustments to these guidelines are made for body type and circumstances that increase caloric requirements. Children with major trauma, sepsis, or burns often require 30% to 60% more calories to maintain positive nitrogen balance.[93]

Parenteral nutrition allows the relative proportions of protein, fat, and carbohydrates to be individualized. Baseline *protein* requirements are highest in infants (2 to 3 g/kg/day) and decrease as the child grows (1.5 to 2.0 g/kg/day). Protein calories should not exceed 25% of the total calories, with essential amino acids constituting approximately 30% of the total protein administered.

Intravenous *fats* are a concentrated isotonic source of calories that prevent essential fatty acid deficiency and provide 20% to 40% of the total caloric input. Fats in the form of a 10% or 20% solution of intralipids are started at a rate of 0.5 g/kg/day and advanced 0.5 to 1.0 g/kg/day until 3 to 4 g/kg/day is reached.

Carbohydrates in the form of 10% to 30% solutions of dextrose are used to supply the remainder of the caloric requirements. Parenteral nutrition is commonly initiated with a 10% to 15% solution and advanced 2.5% to 5% daily until the total carbohydrate calories are reached. Dextrose solutions greater than 25% are to be avoided because they increase the risk of vascular damage.

Vitamins, minerals, and trace elements are added to improve wound healing, restore immunocompetence, and maintain a normal electrolyte profile. Young children require additional calcium and phosphorus supplementation to meet the needs of skeletal growth.

Laboratory assessment and daily adjustments are an essential part of providing total parenteral nutrition in the injured child. Serum glucose levels are checked daily in the form of chemical strips and during routine electrolyte analysis. Protein levels are observed by weekly urine nitrogen testing or monitoring of albumin, prealbumin, or transferrin levels. Biweekly triglyceride levels are helpful for following intralipid concentrations. Weight gain should average 20 to 25 g/day in the infant and 0.5% of the total body weight in kg/day for children. Other indicators of adequate nutrition include improved muscle strength and wound healing, decreasing need for respiratory support, and the ability to overcome systemic infection.

Nutritional support can be delivered enterally or intravenously. The use of the GI tract is preferable to the parenteral route when possible. Data from both the adult and pediatric literature have shown a reduction in complications from infection when compared with matched controls receiving parenteral nutrition. Enteral nutrition stimulates enterocytes and mucous secretion and is thought to reduce the incidence of bacterial translocation. Children requiring prolonged nutritional support have a greatly reduced risk of hepatic damage associated with chronic parenteral nutrition if administration of nutrition occurs through the intestine. Enteral feedings also provide a significant cost savings estimated to be more than $400 a day.

Occasionally, the GI tract is not available and parenteral nutrition is the only alternative. Situations that may preclude enteral feeds include infection, abdominal surgery, pelvic trauma, and a variety of metabolic disturbances. The small intestine rarely becomes completely dysfunctional, with peristalsis evident even during abdominal surgery. The stomach and colon undergo a greater degree of ileus, making the passage of a transpyloric feeding tube essential in many cases. Even small amounts of enteral feedings can have a beneficial effect on mucosal atrophy and intestinal immunocompetence. Feedings are initiated at approximately 20% to 30% of the desired goal and advance slowly over 48 hours, depending on gastric residuals and lack of abdominal distention. Full-strength feedings are routinely well tolerated and preferable unless the child requires increased amounts of free water, which can then be added to the enteral feeds in divided doses. Enteral feeds stimulate the GI tract to produce stool, but delays of 5 to 7 days are common. If a child receiving enteral feeds has not produced stool after 1 week, a rectal examination is performed to ensure that there is no distal impaction.

MANAGEMENT OF PAIN AND ANXIETY

Severely injured children require analgesia and frequently benefit from sedation to alleviate the anxiety that commonly accompanies endotracheal intubation, invasive procedures, and loss of autonomy. Inadequate sedation and pain control impairs respiratory excursion and vital capacity, increases oxygen consumption, and prolongs the stress response associated with serious injury.[16] The ideal agent for sedation and analgesia is one with rapid onset and dissipation, minimal cardiorespiratory effects, and a wide therapeutic index. Although no one drug fulfills all of these criteria, several are useful.[94]

After the initial evaluation, pain control and sedation therapy are carefully instituted. Children with extremity fractures or significant soft-tissue injury require analgesia and sedation prior to reduction or debridement. If a head injury is suspected, small amounts of a short-acting analgesic can be titrated to comfort without compromising the neurologic examination. Intravenous fentanyl at a dose of 1 to 2 μg/kg every 20 to 40 minutes to achieve a level of comfort is preferable. The short half-life of this drug allows neurologic examination after 30 to 40 minutes if small doses are used. Sedation is added for intubated children or those without neurologic injury.

Opioids are the most commonly used agents for analgesia in an intensive care setting. Although all narcotics provide analgesia, none of them provide the amnesia necessary for children receiving neuromuscular blocking agents or undergoing painful procedures while awake. A variety of narcotics are available that can be administered intravenously, orally, or subcutaneously. Transdermal fentanyl patches have been used in children requiring continuous analgesia but are not indicated for children under 12 years of age because of serious respiratory depression in young children.[94] Subcutaneous administration of narcotics is a consideration when drug incompatibilities exist or when intravenous access is limited. Bruera and coworkers[95] described the use of 25-gauge butterfly needles to inject narcotics subcutaneously in the anterior abdominal wall of 13 patients for a total of 60 patient-days. There were no infectious complications and minimal local effects at the injection site.

Despite an increasing array of alternatives, the intravenous route is still the most commonly used method for administration of narcotics and sedation for critically injured children. Continuous infusion with intermittent bolus dosing is superior to time interval or on-demand dosing. Narcotics are administered in micrograms per kilogram per hour with a starting dose between 50 and 100 μg/kg/hour of morphine for children with fractures or thoracoabdominal incisions. Fentanyl, a potent synthetic narcotic with minimal cardiovascular effects and a short half-life, is an acceptable alternative. It is given by continuous infusion, with starting doses between 2 and 4 μg/kg/hour. Reports of increased ICP limit its use to patients without head injuries.[94, 96] Adverse effects are similar to morphine, with rare cases of chest wall rigidity, reversible with naloxone or neuromuscular blocking agents being reported. Hydromorphone (Dilaudid) causes less histamine release and is an alternative to morphine when pruritus and nausea occur. Fentanyl also causes minimal histamine release and can be used in this situation. Meperidine (Demerol) offers few advantages and causes seizures, dysphoria, and CNS toxicity. The CNS toxicity is due to the prolonged half-life (15 to 20 hours) of the active metabolite normeperidine, which is dependent on renal excretion and which is seldom the drug of choice. Methadone (Dolophine) is an infrequently used narcotic with a long plasma half-life (18 hours) and excellent bioavailability when taken orally. One study reported improved pain control with less supplemental narcotic doses with methadone compared with morphine in children 3 to 7 years old. Methadone is also useful in tapering narcotics in children previously requiring large prolonged doses.[97]

Sedation is also an essential component in the critical care management of injured children. Benzodiazepines are the most commonly used drugs for sedation in pediatric intensive care units. This class of drugs works through its effects on the inhibitory neurotransmitter γ-aminobutyric acid (GABA) and causes antegrade amnesia without significant retrograde amnesia. The two most commonly used agents are midazolam (Versed) and lorazepam (Ativan). Midazolam has a rapid onset, short elimination half-life, and wide therapeutic index. It is commonly used for invasive procedures in conjunction with an analgesic at doses ranging from 0.1 to 0.2 mg/kg. Midazolam is also effective as a continuous infusion at rates of 100 to 250 μg/kg/hour. Hepatic or renal dysfunction may increase the free fraction of midazolam to two to three times the normal level.[94, 98, 99] Drugs that interfere with protein binding, such as heparin, also increase the plasma concentration. Despite its short half-life (2 to 4 hours), extensive residual sedation in children without renal or hepatic dysfunction has been reported with prolonged use.[94] This effect is most likely due to its active hydroxyl metabolite. Lorazepam has a similar mechanism of action to midazolam but a longer half-life (4 to 8 hours) and is metabolized by glucuronyl transferase, in contrast to midazolam's elimination via the P_{450} system. It is also half as expensive per day for a continuous infusion.

Ketamine is a dissociative anesthetic with both amnesic and analgesic properties, a rapid onset of action, and a short elimination half-life that was first used clinically in 1965. Unlike benzodiazepines and opioids, ketamine produces a dose-related increase in heart rate and blood pressure via the release of endogenous catecholamines from the sympathetic nervous system. There is also a direct negative inotropic effect that is generally overshadowed, except in situations of maximal sympathetic stimulation or preexisting decreased myocardial contractility.[100] Ketamine has little effect on respiratory drive but can increase pulmonary vascular resistance and should be avoided in children with pulmonary hypertension. Additional respiratory effects include relief of bronchospasm and increased secretions.

Ketamine may also raise intracranial pressure and has been associated with a hallucinogenic emergence phenomenon. This effect is dose-related and is more common in older children. Pretreatment with a small amount of midazolam is effective in preventing this adverse effect. Initial dosing consists of an intravenous bolus of 2 to 4 mg/kg, although ketamine can also be given orally.[94, 100, 101]

The parenteral nonsteroidal anti-inflammatory drug ketorolac (Toradol) is used in adults and has also been shown effective in children for postoperative analgesia.[102] Contraindications include patients with platelet or clotting abnormalities, with renal dysfunction, or those at risk for GI bleeding. Although not currently approved for intravenous administration, clinical experience has demonstrated the safety of this route. Ketorolac is given every 6 hours at a dose of 0.5 mg/kg, not to exceed 30 mg/day.

Controlling the pain and anxiety of an injured child requires facility and a variety of agents, routes of administration, and techniques. Every effort must be made to optimize analgesia and sedation, with frequent reassessments and a low threshold to increase support.

Critical care of injured children requires application of techniques to guarantee adequate oxygenation and maintenance of circulating blood volume. Homeostasis is the goal of effective treatment of physiologic derangement. A multifaceted, comprehensive approach to management results in increase in survival from injury to children.

References

1. Buckly J: The shame of emergency medicine: Kids at risk. U.S. News World Rep, January 1992.
2. Allshouse MJ, Rouse T, Eichelberger MR: Childhood injury: A current perspective. Pediatr Emerg Care 1993; 9:159–164.
3. Baker SP, O'Neak B, Ginsburg MJ, et al: The Injury Fact Book. 2nd ed. New York, Oxford University Press, 1992.
4. Durch JS, Lohr KW (Eds): Emergency Medical Services for Children. Washington, DC, Institute of Medicine, National Academy Press, 1993.
5. Guyers B, Elers B: The causes, impact and preventability of childhood injuries in the United States: The magnitude of the problem—an overview. Am J Dis Child 1990; 144:627–646.
6. Fingerhut LA: Data from the National Vital Statistics System: Office of Analysis and Epidemiology. Hyattsville, Md, National Center for Health Statistics. July 1993.
7. Peclet MH, Newman KD, Eichelberger MR, et al: Patterns of injury in children. J Pediatr Surg 1990; 25:85–91.
8. Moront ML, Gotschall CS, Eichelberger MR, et al: Resource allocation for childhood injury control: The importance of trauma registry data (Poster). American Pediatric Surgical Association program, May 1997, Naples, Fla, 164
9. Hall JR, Reyes HM, Horvat M, et al: The mortality of childhood falls. J Trauma 1989; 29:1273–1275.
10. Finkelstein JL, Schwartz SB, Madden MR, et al: Pediatric burns: An overview. Pediatr Clin North Am 1992; 39:1145–1163.
11. U.S. Department of Health and Human Services: Study findings: Study of national incidence and prevalence of child abuse and neglect. Report of Contract 105-85-1702. Washington, DC, 1988.
12. Fingerhut LA, Ingram DD, Feldman JJ: Firearm homicide among black teenage males in metropolitan counties: Comparison of death rate in two periods, 1983 through 1985 and 1987 through 1989. JAMA 1992; 267:3054–3058.
13. McGonigal MD, Cole J, Schwab CW, et al: Urban firearm deaths: A five year perspective. J Trauma 1993; 35:532–537.
14. Eichelberger MR: Pediatric Trauma-Prevention, Acute Care, Rehabilitation. 1st ed. St. Louis, Mosby-Year Book, 1993.
15. American College of Surgeons, Committee on Trauma: Advance Trauma Life Support Course. Chicago, American College of Surgeons, 1993.
16. Moront ML, Williams JA, Eichelberger MR, et al: The injured child: An approach to care. Pediatr Clin North Am 1994; 41:1201–1225.
17. Schafermeyer R: Pediatric trauma. Emerg Med Clin North Am 1993; 11:187–205.
18. Nakayama DK, Gardner MJ, Rowe MI: Emergency endotracheal intubation in the pediatric population. Ann Surg 1990; 211:218–223.
19. Oldham K, Colombani P, Foglia R: Surgery of Infants and Children: Approach to the Pediatric Trauma Patient. Philadelphia, Lippincott-Raven, 1997, pp 391–416.
20. American Heart Association: Textbook of Pediatric Advanced Life Support. Dallas, American Heart Association, 1994.
21. Peclet MH, Newman KD, Eichelberger MR, et al: Thoracic trauma in children: An indicator for increased mortality. J Pediatr Surg 1990; 25:961–966.
22. Beaver BI, Laschinger JC: Pediatric thoracic trauma. Semin Thorac Cardiovasc Surg 1992; 4:233–262.
23. Reilly JP, Brant ML, Mattox KL: Thoracic trauma in children. J Trauma 1993; 34:329–331.
24. Guy J, Haley K, Zuspan S: Use of intraosseous infusion in the pediatric trauma patient. J Pediatr Surg 1993; 28:158–161.
25. Neufeld JD, Marx Ja, Moore EE, et al: Comparison of intraosseous, central, and peripheral routes of crystalloid infusion for resuscitation of hemorrhagic shock in a swine model. J Trauma 1993; 34:422–428.
26. Glaeser PW: Five year experience in pre-hospital intraosseous infusions in children and adults. Ann Emerg Med 1993; 22:1119–1124.
27. Pollack CV: Prehospital fluid resuscitation of the trauma patient: An update on controversies. Emerg Med Clin North Am 1993; 11:61–70.
28. Chesnut RM, Marshall LF: The role of secondary brain injury in determining outcome from severe head injury. J Trauma 1993; 43:216–222.
29. Ong LC, Selldurai BM, Dhillon MK, et al: The prognostic value of the Glascow Coma Scale, hypoxia, and computerised tomography in outcome prediction of pediatric head injury. Pediatr Neurosurg 1996; 24:285–291.
30. Michaud LJ, Rivera FP, Grady MS, et al: Predictors of survival and severity of disability after severe brain injury in children. Neurosurgery 1992; 32:254–264.
31. Kaufman BA, Darcey JR: Acute care management of closed head injury in childhood. Pediatr Ann 1994; 23:18–28.
32. Luersson TG, Klauber MR, Marshall LF: Outcome from head injury related to a patient's age: A longitudinal prospective study of adult and pediatric injury. J Neurosurg 1988; 68:409–416.
33. Jeret JS, Mandell M, Anziska B, et al: Clinical predictors of abnormality disclosed by computed tomography after mild head trauma. Neurosurgery 1993; 32:916.
34. Harad FT, Kerstein MD: Inadequacy of bedside clinical indicators in identifying significant intracranial injury in trauma patients. J Trauma 1992; 32:359–363.
35. Deitrich AM, Bowman MJ, Ginn-Pease ME, et al: Pediatric head injuries: Can clinical factors reliably predict an abnormality on computed tomography? Ann Emerg Med 1992; 22: 1535–1540.
36. Harrigan C, Lucas CE, Ledgerwood AM: The effect of hemorrhagic shock on the clotting cascade in injured patients. J Trauma 1989; 29:1416–1422.
37. Ferrara A, MacArthur JD, Wright HK, et al: Hypothermia and acidosis worsen coagulopathy in the patient requiring massive transfusion. Am J Surg 1990; 160:515–518.
38. Pratt A, McCroskey BL, Moore EE: Hypothermia-induced coagulopathies in trauma. Surg Clin North Am 1988; 68:775–785.
39. Taylor GA, Eichelberger MR, O'Donnell R, et al: Indications for computed tomography in children after blunt trauma. Ann Surg 1991; 213:121–126.
40. Freshman SP, Wisner D: Secondary survey following blunt trauma: A new role for abdominal CT. J Trauma 1993; 34:337–341.

41. Drew R, Perry JF, Fisher RP: The expediency of peritoneal lavage for blunt trauma in children. Surg Gynecol Obstet 1977; 145:885–888.
42. Perry JF, Strate RG: Diagnostic peritoneal lavage in blunt: abdominal trauma. Indications and results. Surgery 1972; 71:898–901.
43. Coté CJ, Todres ID: The pediatric airway. *In:* A Practice of Anesthesia for Infants and Children. 2nd ed. Coté CJ, Ryan JF, Todres ID, Groudsouzian NG (Eds). Philadelphia, WB Saunders, 1993.
44. Mansell A, Bryan C, Levinson H: Airway closure in children. J Appl Physiol 1972; 33:711–714.
45. Wittenborg MH, Gyepes MT, Crocker D: Tracheal dynamics n infants with respiratory distress, stridor, and collapsing trachea. Radiology 1967; 88:653–662.
46. Downes JJ, Fulgencio T, Raphaely RC: Acute respiratory failure in infants and children. Pediatr Clin North Am 1972; 19:423–445.
47. Ring JC, Stidham GL: Novel therapies for acute respiratory failure. Pediatr Clin North Am 1994; 41:1325–1363.
48. Paulson TE, Spear RM, Peterson BM: Improved survival using high-frequency pressure control ventilation with high PEEP in children with ARDS. Crit Care Med 1993; 21:S290–296.
49. Davis SL, Furman DP, Costarino AT Jr: Adult respiratory distress syndrome in children: Associated disease, clinical course and predictors of death. J Pediatr 1993; 123:35–43.
50. Rappaport SH, Shpiner R, Yoshihara G, et al: Randomized, prospective trial of pressure-limited ventilation in severe respiratory failure. Crit Care Med 1994; 22:22–35.
51. Abraham E, Yoshihara G: Cardiorespiratory effects of pressure controlled ventilation in severe respiratory failure. Chest 1990; 98:1445–1459.
52. Esteban A, Frutos F, Tobin MJ, et al: A comparison of four methods of weaning patients from mechanical ventilation. N Engl J Med 1995; 332:345–358.
53. Cogbill CH, Haywood JL, Chatburn RL, et al: Neonatal and pediatric high-frequency ventilation: Principles and practice. Respir Care 1991; 36:598–608.
54. Arnold JH, Truog RD, Thompson JE, et al: High-frequency oscillatory ventilation in pediatric respiratory failure. Crit Care Med 1993; 21:272–279.
55. O'Rourke PP, Stolar CJH, Zwischenberger JB, et al: Extracorporeal membrane oxygenation: Support for overwhelming pulmonary failure in the pediatric population—collective experience from the Extracorporeal Life Support Organization. J Pediatr Surg 1993; 28:523–528.
56. Bartlett RH: Extracorporeal life support for cardiopulmonary failure. Curr Probl Surg 1990; 27:621–640.
57. Perloff D, Grim C, Flack J, et al: Human blood pressure determination using sphygmomanometry. Circulation 1993; 88:2460–2468.
58. McIntyre KM, Lewis AJ (Eds): Textbook of Advanced Cardiac Life Support. Dallas, American Heart Association, 1983, pp 166–167.
59. Abrams JH, Cerra F, Holcroft JW: Cardiopulmonary monitoring. Sci Am 1989; Vol. 1.
60. Bedford RF, Wollman H: Complications of percutaneous radial artery cannulation. An objective prospective study in man. Anesthesiology 1973; 38:228–236.
61. Mandel Ma, Darchot PJ: Radial artery cannulation in 1,000 patients: Precautions and complications. J Hand Surg (Am) 1977; 2:482–485.
62. Furfaro S, Gauthier M, Lacroix J, et al: Arterial catheter-related infections in children: A 1-year cohort analysis. Am J Dis Child 1991; 145:1037–1042.
63. Cilley RE: Arterial access in infants and children. Semin Pediatr Surg 1992; 1:174–178.
64. Hirschl RB, Heiss K: Cardiopulmonary critical care and shock. *In:* Surgery of Infants and children: Scientific Principles and Practice. Oldham KT, Colombani PM, Foglia RP (Eds). Philadelphia, Lippincott-Raven, 1977.
65. Malatinsky J, Faybik M, Samel M, et al: Surgical infection and thromboembolic complications of central venous catheterization. Resuscitation 1983; 10:271–281.
66. Swanson RS, Uhlig PN, Gross PL, et al: Emergency intravenous access through the femoral vein. Ann Emerg Med 1984; 13:244–247.
67. Hirschl RB: Oxygen delivery in the pediatric surgical patient. Curr Opin Pediatr 1994; 6:341–346.
68. Rasanen J: Continuous breathing circuit flow and tracheal tube cuff leak: Sources of error during pediatric indirect calorimetry. Crit Care Med 1992; 20:1335–1340.
69. Goldsteim FC, Levin HS: Epidemiology of pediatric closed head injury: Incidence, clinical characteristics, and risk factors. Learn Disabil 1987; 20:518–527.
70. Kraus JF, Black MA, Hessol N, et al: The incidence of acute brain injury and serious impairment in a defined population. Am J Epidemiol 1984; 119:186–192.
71. Freide RL: Developmental Neuropathology. New York, Springer-Verlag, 1975.
72. Ward JD: Craniocerebral injuries. *In:* Management of Pediatric Trauma. Buntain WL (Ed). Philadelphia, WB Saunders, 1995.
73. Adams JH, Graham DI, Scott G, et al: Brain damage in non-missile head injury. J Clin Pathol 1980; 33:1132–1145.
74. Adams JH, Graham DI, Murry LS, et al: Diffuse axonal injury due to non-missile head injury in humans: An analysis of 45 cases. Ann Neurol 1982; 12:557–562.
75. Pollay M, Fullenwider C, Roberts PA, et al: Effect of mannitol and furosemide on blood-brain osmotic gradient and intracranial pressure. J Neurosurg 1983; 59:945–950.
76. NIH Consensus Conference: Platelet transfusion therapy. JAMA 1987; 257:1777–1780.
77. Coté CJ, Liu LMP, Szyfelbein SK, et al: Changes in serial platelet counts following massive blood transfusion in pediatric patients. Anesthesiology 1985; 62:197–201.
78. NIH Consensus Conference: Fresh frozen plasma: Indications and risks. JAMA 1985; 253:551–553.
79. Coté CJ, Coté MA: Changes in prothrombin and partial thromboplastin times during massive blood loss in children undergoing Harrington rod instrumentation. Presented at Spring Session, Section on Anesthesiology, American Academy of Pediatrics, New York, June 4, 1988.
80. Bell WR: The pathophysiology of disseminated intravascular coagulation. Semin Hemato 1994; 31:19–25.
81. Bick RL: Disseminated intravascular coagulation: Objective criteria for diagnosis and management. Med Clin North Am 1994; 78:511–544.
82. Coté CJ, Drop LJ, Hoaglin DC, et al: Ionized hypocalcemia after fresh frozen plasma administration to thermally injured children: Effects of infusion rate, duration, and treatment with calcium cloride. Anesth Analg 1988; 67:152–160.
83. Coté CJ, Drop LJ, Daniels AL, et al: Calcium cloride versus calcium gluconate: Comparison of ionization and cardiovascular effects in children and dogs. Anesthesiology 1987; 66:465–470.
84. Brown KA, Bissonnette B, MacDonald M, et al: Hyperkalemia during massive blood transfusion in pediatric craniofacial surgery. Can J Anesthesiol 1990; 37:401–408.
85. Hall TL, Barnes A, Miller JR, et al: Neonatal mortality following transfusion of red cells with high plasma potassium levels. Transfusion 1993; 33:606–609.
86. Luban NLC, Strauss RG, Hume HA: Commentary on the safety of red cells preserved in extended-storage media for neonatal transfusions. Transfusion 1991; 31:229–235.
87. Merritt RJ, Suskind RM: Nutritional survey of hospitalized pediatric patients. Am J Clin Nutr 1979; 32:1320–1325.
88. Dark DS, Pingleton SK: Nutrition and nutritional support in critically ill patients. J Intensive Care Med 1993; 8:16–33.
89. Burritt MF, Anderson CF: Laboratory assessment of nutritional status. Hum Pathol 1984; 15:130–133.
90. Roza AM, Tuitt D, Shizgal HM: Transferrin: A poor measure of nutritional status. J Parenter Enteral Nutr 1984; 8:523–528.
91. Baker JP, Detsky AS, Wesson DE, et al: Nutritional assessment: A comparison of clinical judgment and objective measurements. N Engl J Med 1982; 306:969–972.
92. Pollach MM, Wiley JS, Kanter R, et al: Malnutrition in critically ill infants and neonates. J Parenter Enteral Nutr 1982; 6:20–24.
93. Wesley JR, Coran AG: Intravenous nutrition for the pediatric patient. Semin Pediatr Surg 1992; 1:212–230.
94. Tobias JD, Rasmussen GE: Pain management and sedation in the pediatric intensive care unit. Pediatr Clin North Am 1994; 41:1269–1292.
95. Bruera E, Gibney N, Stollery D, et al: Use of the subcutaneous route of administration of morphine in the intensive care unit. J Pain Symptom Manage 1991; 6:263–265.

96. Sperry RJ, Bailey PL, Reuchman MV, et al: Fentanyl and sufentanil increase intracranial pressure in head trauma patients. Anesthesiology 1992; 77:416–420.
97. Berde CB, Beyer JE, Bournaki MC, et al: Comparison of morphine and methadone for prevention of postoperative pain in children. J Pediatr 1991; 119:136–141.
98. Trouvin JH, Farinotti R, Haberer JP, et al: Pharmacokinectics of midazolam in anesthetized cirrhotic patients. Br J Anaesth 1988; 60:762–767.
99. Vinik HR, Reves JG, Greenblatt DJ, et al: The pharmacokinetics of midazolam in chronic renal failure patients. Anesthesiology 1983; 59:390–394.
100. Wayman K, Shoemaker WC, Lippman M: Cardiovascular effects of anesthetic induction with ketamine. Anesth Analg 1980; 59:355–358.
101. White PR, Way WL, Trevor AJ: Ketamine: Its pharmacology and therapeutic uses. Anesthesia 1982; 56:119–136.
102. Watcha MF, Jones MB, Lagueruela R, et al: Comparison of ketoralac and morphine as adjuvants during pediatric surgery. Anesthesiology 1992; 76:368–372.

33

Burn Care and Inhalation Injury

William R. Schiller, MD, FACS

Thermal injury produces intense and multifaceted physiologic responses that have been the subject of considerable study for the past 50 years. These responses begin shortly after injury and, presumably, allow survival of minimally treated individuals with small burns. Nevertheless, early and complex intervention by the burn team is required for salvage of patients with large burns in the modern intensive care setting.

Accurate evaluation of the burn victim must include assessment of severity factors, such as:

- Age
- Burn extent and depth
- Presence of inhalation injury
- Influence of associated illnesses
- Mechanisms of the burn
- Elapsed time to treatment

A paper by Slattery and colleagues[1] has shown that both pre-hospital personnel and burn teams have inherent inaccuracy in their efforts to quantify burn size. This is clearly an area where improved technology to measure burn size would facilitate care. Methodical resuscitative management of burns, such as described in the Advanced Burn Life Support course, includes attention to airway protection, adequate ventilation, and aggressive fluid resuscitation based on body weight and burn extent.[2] A search for concomitant blunt or penetrating injuries in addition to the burn is appropriate in some cases. Care of the burn wound and early eschar excision has some limiting effect on infectious complications. Multidisciplinary burn teams have become the prototype to carry out the critical care necessary to optimize the chances of survival for the burn victim.

RESUSCITATION

Loss of body fluids through an acutely "leaky" capillary bed into the extracellular space is a well-known phenomenon in burn patients. Although much of the resultant burn edema is confined to the injured body parts, with burns involving less than 20% of the body surface area (BSA), larger burns tend to produce edema involving the whole body, including uninjured areas. Direct effects on the microcirculation, including increased hydrostatic pressure, venous outflow compromise, and changes in the extracellular space, have all been documented. In addition, while histamine is the prime mediator of increased capillary permeability in smaller burns, multiple mediators have been demonstrated in larger burns.[3, 4] Such additional molecules as bradykinin, products of arachidonic acid metabolism, and oxygen free radicals may be involved.[5]

Fluid replacement in recent experience has been guided by a family of volume restoration formulas derived from clinical observation and experimental data.[6–9] The most extensively used of these burn resuscitation guidelines is the *Parkland formula*, which prescribes 4 mL of lactated Ringer's solution per percentage burn per kilogram body weight. Burn surgeons recognize that the formula is only a guide from which deviation may be indicated to normalize blood pressure, pulse, and urine output. Other techniques, such as the modified Brooke and hypertonic saline solutions, have also been used with success.[10, 11] Some studies, however, have demonstrated no special advantage of hypertonic saline compared with Parkland formula.[12] One report even expressed concern that use of hypertonic saline may carry additional risk and produce poor outcome in some cases.[13]

Resuscitation Goals

Dries and Waxman,[14] however, have documented that urine output, blood pressure, and pulse provide inaccurate and insensitive information concerning adequacy of burn resuscitation. This is of particular concern because using traditional circulatory endpoints may significantly increase the likelihood that unrecognized underresuscitation will result from the Parkland formula as presently practiced. The effort to improve the circulatory quality of burn resuscitation began to emerge with the report by Aikawa and associates[15] in 1978 of their experience with 39 severely burned patients who were resuscitated with the aid of pulmonary artery catheters. Although only 19 of 25 patients with greater than 40% burns had undergone pulmonary artery catheterization within 12 hours of injury, the authors were able to gather some interesting preliminary data, including graphic information related to heart filling pressures during the early post-burn period. They illustrated low cardiac index and left ventricular stroke work index that gradually reached supranormal levels within 48 to 72 hours. There was an inverse relationship of cardiac output to systemic vascular resistance that decreased as cardiac index rose. The most notable observation was a normal blood pressure in the face of low cardiac output and high resistance, indicating the insensitivity of blood pressure readings as a monitoring tool. Even though catheter tip cultures were positive in 33% of the patients, most infections occurred in patients in whom the catheter had been in place for more than 3 days. Aikawa's group also demonstrated poor correlation between right-sided and left-sided heart filling pressures, especially in older patients and in those with preexisting cardiopulmonary disease. The beneficial effect of dopamine in improving the stroke work index was mentioned. Overall, conclusions concerning usefulness of invasive monitoring were not possible, however, because 28 of the 39 patients died.

In 1981, a follow-up of 21 additional patients with a mean burn size of 60% total body surface area (TBSA) was reported by Aikawa and coworkers.[16] Although resuscitation was unsuccessful in only two, 13 additional patients did not survive their burns. This may have been due to inadequate circulatory endpoints because it appeared that values for unstressed individuals and mean infused fluid volumes of less than 4 mL per percentage burn per kilogram body weight were used. Both of the reports by Aikawa and coworkers reported events that were interpreted as depression of myocardial contractility by the authors. Aikawa's group also mentioned a beneficial effect of low-volume colloid infusion 6 to 18 hours after the burn. The authors concluded that information from invasive monitoring offered the potential to optimize many circulatory factors not appreciated by traditional monitoring.

Miller and coworkers[17] attempted to derive hemodynamic parameters from burn patients that would provide resuscitation goals by delineating the circulatory performance curves of survivors and nonsurvivors. Unfortunately, because only five of their 22 patients survived, they were unable to achieve statistical significance between the outcomes of the two groups. In 1995, however, Schiller and associates[18] reported hemodynamic data from 53 patients, 37 survivors and 16 nonsurvivors, who had been resuscitated with use of circulatory endpoints proposed by Shoemaker and colleagues[19] in non-burn patients. Their study demonstrated significant differences between the two groups including higher values for cardiac index, left ventricular stroke work index, and oxygen consumption in survivors. Nonsurvivors illustrated higher values for infused fluid volumes, higher heart filling pressures, and greater use of both colloids and cardiotonic drugs. In addition, they confirmed the observation that in nonsurvivors, increases in cardiac output were of lesser magnitude as the systemic vascular resistance decreased in response to fluid resuscitation compared with cardiac output responses in survivors. Blood pressure, pulse, and urine values did not discriminate between survivors and nonsurvivors during the first 3 days post burn.

A follow-up study in 1997 by the same group reported an increased survival in burn patients when hyperdynamic circulatory endpoints were used during the initial resuscitation.[20] In addition, they demonstrated that the Parkland formula was a relatively accurate resuscitation guideline in smaller burns but became less accurate as the burns involved larger surface areas greater than 20% or when inhalation injury was present. They also illustrated in the control group that inconsistent use of the pulmonary artery catheter during the resuscitation failed to improve survival.

Another report, published at the same time by Barton and coworkers,[21] illustrated the effects of hyperdynamic resuscitation on oxygen delivery and consumption in nine burn patients. These authors produced hyperdynamic circulatory endpoints but were uncertain because of the nature of their small study whether their technique would improve survival. They compared their oxygen delivery and consumption data with those published by Demling and associates,[22] who demonstrated that oxygen consumption was consistently related to delivery in burned sheep with inhalation injury but became independent of delivery in those with burns alone. The Barton data showed a similar relationship at oxygen deliveries below 800 mL/min/m^2, but any correlation was lost at higher deliveries. Because of a small number of their study patients, the authors were uncertain whether consumption could be made independent of delivery in the setting of a severe burn and the extent to which outcome could be improved if such an event were achieved. The Barton study also demonstrated the phenomenon of depressed myocardial function during early resuscitation.

Specific Physiologic Issues

Questions concerning the mechanism of myocardial depression have been the subject of numerous studies. Although a distinct myocardial depressant factor has not been identified, numerous physiologic events have been shown to produce compromised myocardial function. Experimentally, the association of increased vasopressin levels in canine burns with vasoconstriction and depressed myocardial function has been noted.[23]

Another study in burned rats illustrated poor myocardial contractility as a result of low myocardial adenosine triphosphate (ATP) levels.[24] The problem of diminished contractility was limited by aggressive fluid resuscitation, but large fluid volumes did not reverse this defect if significant delays in treatment occurred.

Horton and associates[25] have contributed to the understanding of post-burn myocardial depression. Using experimentally burned guinea pigs, they demonstrated that blockade of tumor necrosis factor (TNF) action in myocardium prevented or diminished myocardial dysfunction. Because plasma levels of TNF were not elevated, they proposed a paracrine function of TNF within the heart tissue as the mechanism of this observation. Horton[26] also demonstrated in burned rats that oxygen free radical production could be implicated as a factor resulting in myocardial depression. This finding may be related to a previously described dysfunction of calcium flux across cell membranes as a possible cause of myocardial depression in burn victims. Vaughan and coworkers also showed that both allopurinol and pentoxifylline attenuated the severity of myocardial depression.[27]

A paper by Schnarrs and coworkers[28] in 1986 described the use of plasma exchange in the failing resuscitations of seven patients with a mean burn size of 65% TBSA and a mean age of 42 years, half of whom had sustained inhalation injury. These patients had been resuscitated with modified Brooke formula plus at least 100% additional infused calculated volumes and still had urine volumes less than 0.5 mL/kg/hour and a mean cardiac index of approximately 2.9 L/min/m^2. While demonstrating an increase in cardiac index of approximately 50% as a result of plasma exchange, all of the patients ultimately died. This study suggested that although plasma exchange might be useful as a means to attempt salvage of unsuccessful resuscitations, the question arises as to whether these patients as a group were underresuscitated to inadequate circulatory endpoints.

Supplementary endpoints that may enhance the quality of burn resuscitation include (1) rapid resolution of hypothermia, (2) possible use of gastric tonometry to assess splanchnic microcirculatory perfusion, and (3) aggressive treatment of lactic acidosis. Rewarming of the patient by body heat production was shown by Shiozaki and coworkers[29] to be significantly less effective in nonsurvivors than in those who survived large burns.

Two studies by Gutierrez[30] and Ivatury[31] and their coworkers documented experience with gastric tonometry in critically ill patients. Gutierrez and associates studied 260 ICU patients with various forms of organ failure, prospectively compartmentalizing them as intramucosal pH either greater or less than 7.35. Each group was then further subdivided into control or protocol groups. Protocol groups received prompt, intense efforts to improve hypotension, hypoxia, anemia, acidosis, respiratory hypercapnia, and hypothermia. Control patients received a variety of treatments by individual physicians following their own policies. Patients with intramucosal pH below 7.35 had similar poor outcomes whether or not they were treated by the protocol. Conversely, protocol patients with treatment-normalized intramucosal pH above 7.35 had a significantly higher survival rate than did control patients.

The study of seriously traumatized patients, published in 1996 by Ivatury and associates, compared use of intramucosal pH greater than 7.3 with optimization of oxygen delivery and consumption as resuscitation endpoints. Intramucosal pH values seemed to be a more useful predictor of survival than optimization of hemodynamic values.

In summary, the two studies by Gutierrez and Ivatury[30, 31] suggested that use of gastric tonometry in conjunction with optimization of circulatory endpoints in trauma patients improved the quality of resuscitation. This technique also might allow better control of fluid volume infusion, thus limiting the fluid overload syndrome that is common during the diuresis phase of hyperdynamic resuscitation.

Finally, a study by Jeng and coworkers[32] demonstrated the persistence of elevated lactic acid levels and increased base deficit in burn patients resuscitated with use of the Parkland formula. Standard resuscitation guidelines of urine output greater than 30 mL/hour and mean arterial pressure of more than 70 mm Hg were employed. Abnormally high lactate levels were recorded in 70% of the data points, suggesting inadequate tissue perfusion. They speculated that current resuscitation endpoints are inadequate and may contribute to organ failure in severe burns.

Pooled data from 95 patients in our series of burn resuscitations guided by the pulmonary artery catheter confirmed that cardiac index, left ventricular stroke work index, and oxygen consumption achieved statistically significant values allowing discrimination of survivors and nonsurvivors.[33] On the basis of this experience, use of the survivor means of a cardiac index of 5.5 L/min/m², left ventricular stroke work index of greater than 50 g • m/m², oxygen consumption of 200 mL/min/m², and oxygen extraction ratios between 20% and 30% as circulatory resuscitation goals seems appropriate.

One must remember, however, that the magnitude of the hemodynamic responses is related to multiple factors, including (1) severity of the burn, (2) presence of inhalation injury, and (3) age of the patient. Circulatory responses and physiologic resistance to burn injury significantly differ from the norm in older patients and in children, especially the very young. Elderly burn victims generally exhibit definite limitations in their ability to accept fluid loading, thereby curtailing the hemodynamic responses, which results in increased mortality.[34, 35] Children, in contrast, require additional fluid, as documented by Merrell and associates.[36] In their report, adults, in the first 24 hours after a burn, were documented to require 4 mL per percentage burn per kilogram body weight, whereas children required 5.8 mL per percentage burn per kilogram body weight. These increased fluid requirements may be provided by use of this formula, by use of the fluid regimen published by Carvajal,[37] or in some centers by use of the traditional Parkland formula plus maintenance fluids.

Resuscitation of burns from mechanisms such as exposure to chemicals or electric current is dependent on the physician's assessment of injury severity and the patient's response to fluid replacement. Protection of organ function often becomes a dominant issue, especially in electrical burns, in which myoglobinuria may result in renal failure. Provision of enough replacement fluid to ensure brisk urine output is a commonly used and frequently successful strategy.[38]

Fluid resuscitation techniques in burn patients continue to evolve, especially in situations in which severe burn injury has occurred. We have recently been able to construct computerized resuscitation curves based on hemodynamic responses of 150 patients in whom pulmonary artery catheters were used to enhance circulatory responses as much as possible (Fig. 33–1). These images consistently demonstrate larger than Parkland-predicted volumes being necessary to produce what are believed to be optimal responses. They also provide a more realistic guideline than the Parkland step curve for management of adequate fluids to the volume-dependent burn patient while attempting to control excess fluid administration after the acute shock phase of the first 24 hours begins to subside during the subsequent 48-hour period.

Although much remains to be learned, attempts to improve the quality of resuscitation as a means to protect cell function and integrity seem justified. Further developments of technology to monitor tissue perfusion and response to injury may allow improved understanding of burn pathophysiology and increase survival of patients.

INHALATION INJURY

Pathophysiology

Inhalation of noxious materials may occur as part of the burn injury complex, especially as a result of structure fires, fuel ignition secondary to motor vehicle accidents, and incidents resulting from flaming substances such as gasoline, propane, and natural gas. Inhalation injury may affect primarily the upper airway as a thermal insult or the lung parenchyma secondary to inhalation of toxic substances such as smoke, or a combination of the two mechanisms of injury may be present. Smoke inhalation routinely produces systemic pathologic changes as manifested by increased fluid requirements and significantly greater mortality. It is made inordinately worse by the presence of cutaneous thermal burn.[39]

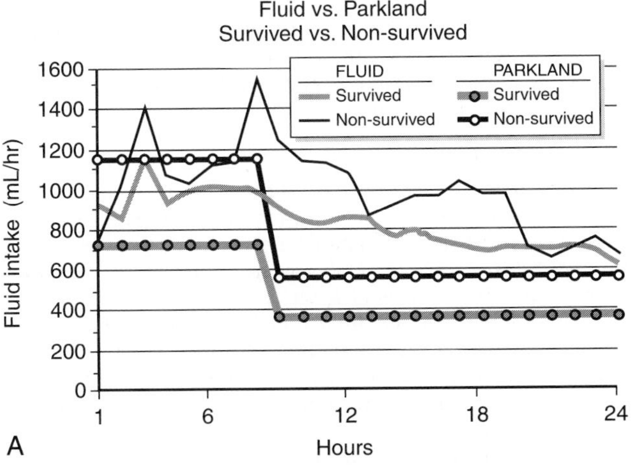

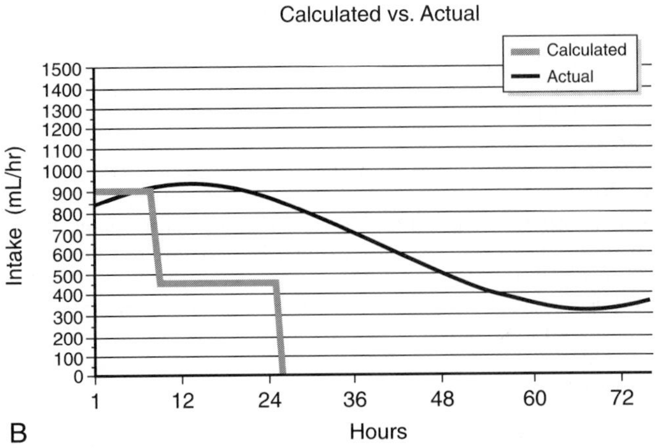

Figure 33–1. *A*, A summary of fluid volumes given to those patients who lived or died compared with Parkland-derived fluid volumes. *B*, Comparison of Parkland-calculated resuscitation volumes in a 40% total body surface area (TBSA) burn with inhalation injury to the actual fluid volume curve required to produce hyperdynamic circulatory endpoints in burn survivor.

In general, severity of inhalation is related to four factors:

1. Heat of the inhaled gases is a prime determinant of its pathologic potential.
2. Composition of the gas, including presence and size of particles, and toxic products such as carbon monoxide are important.
3. Concentration of toxic agents.
4. Duration of exposure plays a key role in the ultimate severity of the inhalation component of the injury. In addition, burn size and patient factors such as age and pre-injury state of health will influence the final outcome.

Upper airway thermal injury produces tissue edema, which threatens airway patency and is routinely managed by intubation and ventilator support to maintain respiratory function. When edema subsides, rapid weaning from the ventilator and extubation often conclude the critical management of upper airway thermal injury. A spectrum of injury severity exists such that injured individuals either may be slow to proceed to extubation or may develop late airway stenosis or both.[40]

Specific Inhalation Toxins

Parenchymal inhalation injury, however, is much more complex and life-threatening. A large number of metabolic toxins produced as a result of incomplete combustion, especially of synthetic or natural building materials, may initially produce profound organ and cellular hypoxia. Prominent among these volatile chemicals are carbon monoxide, cyanide, and a considerable number of mucosal and mitochondrial poisons. Carbon monoxide may aggravate whatever hypoxic events exist from the injurious incident by binding to the hemoglobin molecule and thereby limiting oxygen transport. In addition, significant exposure to carbon monoxide may also affect other biochemical systems, such as myoglobin and cytochrome function. A broad spectrum of body dysfunction resulting from increasing intensity of hemoglobin saturation by carbon monoxide has been documented. Use of 100% inhaled oxygen as part of the resuscitation regimen facilitates off-loading of carbon monoxide by competitively displacing it from the oxygen-binding transport site on the hemoglobin molecule.[41] Hyperbaric oxygen is potentially useful but rarely practical in the burn unit setting or indicated in the patient's overall treatment.

Treatment of presumed cyanide poisoning can be much more of a problem for a variety of reasons. Although a profound inhibitor of mitochondrial oxidative processes, effective resuscitation enhances a body enzyme system termed *rhodanese.* Contained in the liver, rhodanese can transform cyanide to thiocyanate, destined for urinary excretion.[42] Second, in most hospitals, timely determination of cyanide levels is not available, thus making decisions regarding treatment uncertain. Third, use of sodium nitrate to produce methemoglobin and subsequent cyanide off-loading in itself aggravates hypoxic situations, especially in regard to myocardial function.

In general, specific treatment for cyanide inhalation should not proceed unless there are overt signs of cellular respiratory compromise, such as inordinately low oxygen consumption. Also, newer modalities for treatment of cyanide toxicity, such as intravenous hydroxocobalamin, may be equally effective and less toxic than traditional methods.[43] Other toxic inhalants produce nonspecific lung damage in large part by conversion to acids and by their propensity for activation of inflammatory mediators. Specific inhalants, such as superheated steam, apparently produce lung damage solely on the basis of thermal injury to both airways and lung parenchyma.[44] Chlorine vapors may cause severe pulmonary compromise both in its elemental form and by conversion to toxic metabolites such as hydrochloric acid. Furthermore, chlorine gas is one of the few inhalants to produce a pathologic state that is responsive to steroid administration.[45]

In the pathologic panoply of adverse pulmonary reactions secondary to inhalation injury, several events seem consistent. Presence of particles, their size, total dose, and distribution within the lungs are important in production of the resultant inhalation injury. One study illustrated that filtering particles from smoke breathed by anesthetized sheep greatly diminished the severity of inhalation injury. Conversely, the presence of particles less than 3 μm in diameter decreased lung compliance, increased lung lymph flow, increased oxygen consumption, and produced severe histologic alveolar damage. Oxidant activity in airway fluid was documented.[46] Mucosal damage may decrease ciliary activity and increase the production of mucus. Consequently, normal clearance of bacterial and inhaled particulates is diminished and increased pulmonary secretions may occlude small airways.

While mechanical ventilation may be lifesaving, bacterial colonization and secretion production may be intensified by vulnerability of the body's defense mechanisms secondary to the inhalation damage. Furthermore, the pulmonary circulation is affected, and abnormalities such as increased bronchial blood flow produce narrowing of airways and lung edema. Lung lymphatic function is impaired, also contributing to pulmonary edema. Alveolar instability and diffuse collapse occur as a result of surfactant inactivation, which may produce significant arterial oxygen desaturation secondary to profound ventilation-perfusion mismatch, generally referred to as intrapulmonary shunting. Activation of inflammatory mediators such as superoxide radicals and cytokines apparently intensifies the deranged physiologic processes after inhalation injury.[47] Furthermore, experimental evidence indicates that impaired alveolar macrophages from smoke-damaged animals produce less than optimal interactions with neutrophils, thereby increasing the likelihood of bronchopneumonia.[48]

When the above-described events are manifested in the clinical scenario, several identifiable stages have been described.[49] First is the initial asphyxia and cellular hypoxia, seen during the early resuscitation period. Next, respiratory insufficiency may develop during the 48 to 72 hours after admission, requiring extraordinary ventilatory efforts that persist for variable lengths of time and may themselves produce mortality. This stage may be complicated by the onset of the next clinical phase of bacterial proliferation producing bronchopneumonia. Finally, if the patient is fortunate enough to survive these pathologic challenges, a gradual recovery phase begins. At this time, withdrawal from the necessity of ventilator support occurs with degrees of complexity, and pulmonary repair progresses to return of function. Residual defects, such as airway stenosis, pulmonary fibrosis, and constrictive airway overreactivity, have been documented.[50]

Inhalation Management

Clinical evaluation of patients thought to have inhalation injury begins with the history and physical findings at the time of hospital admission. Situations in which the patients are injured in closed, smoke-filled spaces, when large burns are produced by flames, especially if the face and neck are involved and when known inhalation of toxic chemicals has occurred, are responsible for the majority of patients with inhalation injury. Admission chest radiography findings are typically normal; nonspecific infiltrates of varying severity gradually develop during the next 2 or 3 days. Xenon lung scanning to demonstrate areas of diminished ventilation shortly after admission has been shown to be the most sensitive method of confirming the diagnosis of inhalation injury.[51]

Bronchoscopy, in addition, may provide valuable positive information early in the clinical course of burn victims because bronchoscopic damage indicates a more serious injury than do positive findings on xenon scanning alone.

Both Masanes and coworkers[52] and Khoo and coworkers[53] have documented the usefulness of this technique if careful evaluation of bronchoscopic mucosal appearance and mucosal cell characteristics is done. In the Khoo report, 200 tracheal and bronchial cells were bronchoscopically recovered per patient and scored for six normal characteristics. Using a total cellular score of greater or less than 500 as the defining breakpoint of a severe pathologic process, the authors concluded that mortality in patients with a score below 500 was 42.6%, whereas mortality in patients with a score above 500 was only 8.3%.

Overall accuracy of present modalities for diagnosis of inhalation injury is cited in a review by Shirani and associates.[5] They found that accuracy was 85% for bronchoscopy alone and 87% for xenon scan alone but reached 93% when both modalities were used. Prediction of the clinical development of inhalation injury by Shirani and Pruitt[54] has resulted in a formula that has received some independent validation by other workers. Shirani and Pruitt proposed such factors as injury in a closed space, presence of a facial burn, TBSA burn, and age as predictors of severe inhalation injury (Fig. 33–2). When Darling and coworkers[55] described 100 consecutive patients with inhalation injury, the overall mortality was 47%, and Pruitt values were predictive of death with a *P* value of less than .0001.

The question of volume of fluid resuscitation in the presence of inhalation injury remains unresolved. The proceedings of the National Institutes of Health (NIH) Workshop on Burn Management state that the ideal volume of fluid for burn resuscitation will normalize circulatory variables while minimizing organ dysfunction such as pulmonary edema.[56] This guideline clearly implies the desirability of fluid restriction in the face of combined burn and inhalation injury, a concept that continues to be supported in contemporary literature.[57] Unfortunately, the uniform experience in burn centers is that inhalation significantly increases fluid requirements for adequate resuscitation compared with patients with burn injury alone. Furthermore, several authors have documented that underresuscitation aggravates pulmonary dysfunction and adversely affects survival in burn patients with inhalation injury.[58, 59] The problem remains, therefore, how to optimize these specialized resuscitation issues, thereby protecting organ function while avoiding pulmonary edema to whatever extent is feasible. These questions lie at the heart of efforts to enhance resuscitation by invasive monitoring and organ system–specific monitoring, such as gastric tonometry and measurement of lung water.[31, 60]

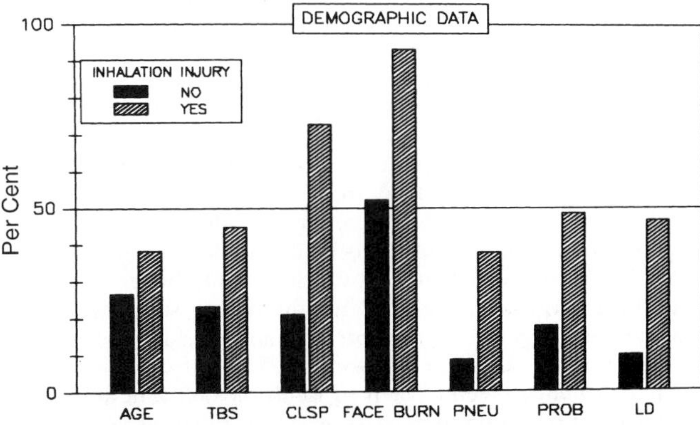

Figure 33–2. Data on patients with and without inhalation injury. In patients with inhalation injury, age and total burn size (TBS) were slightly higher; more patients had injury in closed spaces (CLSP), and there was a higher incidence of facial burns and pneumonia (PNEU). Age and burn size–adjusted probability of death (PROB) and observed mortality (LD) per 100 patients were also higher in that group. (From Shirani KZ, Pruitt BA Jr, Mason AD Jr: The influence of inhalation injury and pneumonia on burn mortality. Ann Surg 1987; 205:82–87.)

Concurrent with the efforts to optimize resuscitation have been exploratory attempts to blunt the pathologic effects of inhalation on body homeostasis. Demling and associates,[61] using sheep as experimental subjects in which to study controlled inhalation injury, reported on lung oxidant activity plus distant organ involvement after smoke exposure. Although evidence of parenchymal oxidant activity was minimal, they documented substantial oxidants at airway surfaces in association with severe pulmonary damage. Furthermore, they found evidence of oxidant activity in liver and kidneys but not gut. A previous study had produced similar results with the additional finding that a cutaneous burn plus smoke inhalation increased the magnitude of lung parenchyma lipid peroxidation.[62] Unfortunately, these changes did not correspond well in their study with the clinical development of lung dysfunction that appeared later.

A paper by LaLonde and coworkers[63] indicated that although 4-hour postexposure airway changes did not correlate with lung dysfunction, there was a high degree of correlation with the 24-hour changes, the increased fluid requirements, and the oxygen consumption associated with lung dysfunction. These pathologic events were thought to be due to systemic oxidant effects.

Inhalation Management

In an attempt to control lung inflammatory changes, Demling and associates[64] used aerosolized deferoxamine in the sheep smoke inhalation model. When it was used as a pentastarch complex, they observed significant airway protection, presumably by chelating iron-based oxidants. The pentastarch was thought to increase the effective half-life and to enhance mucosal adherence of deferoxamine. This study appeared to confirm the pathologic role of oxidants in the development of lung dysfunction after smoke inhalation.

A study that supports this concept was reported by Wolyniec and coworkers[65] in a mouse oxygen toxicity model. In this model, the investigators blocked adverse oxidant effects by use of human manganese superoxide dismutase instilled into the affected airways.

Other attempts at blocking airway and pulmonary oxidants have been reported with use of different chemical pathway blockers. For example, two studies from the same institution used BW-755C, a combined cyclooxygenase and lipoxygenase inhibitor, to reduce lung injury after acrolein smoke inhalation in sheep. It was found that pulmonary hypertension, increased airway resistance, and pulmonary edema were diminished. By use of selective inhibitors, the authors postulated that increased airway resistance and pulmonary artery pressures were mediated by the effects of thromboxane production, whereas pulmonary edema seemed to be mediated by leukotriene B_4.[66, 67]

Another thromboxane-blocking study using a different protocol also demonstrated that both increased pulmonary vascular and airway resistance were prevented, but pulmonary edema was not, indicating an etiologic mechanism for edema other than thromboxane.[68] Pentoxifylline has improved ventilation-perfusion mismatch in the smoke inhalation sheep model, probably by multiple mechanisms of action.[69] Other studies have demonstrated protection of lung from inhalation injury by use of phenytoin,[70] oxygen free radical scavengers,[71] 21-amino steroids,[72] and hyperbaric oxygen.[73] At present, most of these studies report the results from experimental animals and none has been validated for routine clinical use in humans.

Ventilator support in patients with severe inhalation injury can be extremely challenging. Although standard-volume ventilation with positive end-expiratory pressure (PEEP) may suffice in some individuals with markedly decreased compliance, the usual tidal volumes of 10 to 15 mL/kg body weight result in elevated peak pressures and subsequent barotrauma. Furthermore, inability to clear secretions effectively by conventional ventilation, coupled with the trauma of focal alveolar overdistention and oxygen toxicity, exacerbates the situation. This pathologic ventilation scenario results in failure to sustain viable gas exchange and subsequent mortality of approximately 30% to 60% of severe inhalation-injured patients who experience respiratory failure.[74]

Several techniques have been proposed to cope with this type of respiratory failure:

1. Pressure-controlled, low-volume ventilation with permissive hypercapnia and inverse inspiratory to expiratory ratios have met with some success.[75]
2. High-frequency jet ventilation held promise as a means of lowering mortality, but further study suggests minimal, if any, superiority over conventional ventilation.[76, 77]
3. Use of extracorporeal membrane oxygenation (ECMO) has resulted in some encouraging anecdotal data, but this modality is both effort-intensive and technology-intensive without clear-cut evidence of producing improved survival.[78]

In one study of non-burn patients with respiratory failure in whom conventional ventilation, high-frequency jet techniques, or low-volume ventilation was not successful, with a resulting historical mortality of 91%, ventilation with low volumes and carbon dioxide removal was evaluated.[79] Mortality in this group was reduced to 51.2%, and those who improved did so within 48 hours. No similar confirmatory information is available for patients with inhalation injury.

Use of intravenous devices to control carbon dioxide levels in patients with severe inhalation injury managed by low-volume ventilation and permissive hypercapnia holds some promise.[80] Another report documented the feasibility of a technique termed *airway pressure release ventilation* in non-burn patients.[81] Although it offers some low-pressure ventilatory advantages, only five of 18 patients with severe acute respiratory failure survived. No data exist regarding its use with patients suffering from inhalation injury.

Use of volumetric diffusive ventilation has been reported in both pediatric and adult burn patients with respiratory failure.[82, 83] Compared with conventional ventilation, gas exchange and hemodynamic variables were improved by use of the volumetric diffusive ventilation technique. Preliminary information suggests that this mode of ventilation may have value in patients with severe inhalation injury and possibly in those failing conventional ventilation. Use of inhaled nitric oxide as an adjunct to ventilatory management has been shown in experimental animals and in humans to decrease pulmonary artery hypertension and to improve oxygenation while producing no effect on pulmonary inflammatory responses.[84, 85] Exogenous surfactants have been investigated as a means of opening alveoli. With proper delivery techniques, some forms of surfactant have been effective whereas others have not.[86, 87] Use of tracheostomy in the clinical management of thermal respiratory injury has gone through phases of enthusiasm and rejection. A paper documenting successful use of percutaneous tracheostomy techniques illustrated potential for considerable benefit to those patients with respiratory compromise.[88] Large controlled trials using these ventilatory techniques will be required before effective and sophisticated management strategies can be devised that are capable of producing consistently improved survival in patients with inhalation injury.

INFLAMMATORY MEDIATORS AND IMMUNE RESPONSE

The burn wound itself is the source of many early inflammatory mediators, which may explain why prompt excision significantly improves outcome from severe thermal injuries.[89] Reports indicate the presence of cytokines in blister fluid and skin donor sites. Interleukin-1 (IL-1) activity has been documented in blister fluid of burned humans by Kupper and coworkers.[90] This finding may account for some of the metabolic changes seen in burn patients, including individual acute-phase protein responses by hepatocytes, as well as its being an immune system stimulant. Acute-phase proteins such as α_1-acid glycoprotein and α_2-macroglobulin are known to increase after burn injury, whereas albumin and transferrin levels decrease, all in response at least in part to the effects of IL-1. Other data that support the probable immune system–stimulating role of IL-1 in burns include experimental studies of sepsis in burned mice wherein IL-1 administration improved survival from 13% in control animals to 60% in treated animals.[91] Cytokine level increases have also been detected in the wound beds of autograft donor sites in experimental situations. These include growth factors such as epidermal growth factor, fibroblast growth factor, and platelet-derived growth factor. Cytokines such as IL-1 and TNF have also been reported. Studies in human burn patients have validated many of these findings and suggest a healing and inflammation-mediating function within the wound itself.[92]

Burn Suppression of Immune Function

Immunosuppression may also be initiated by events within the wound, specifically by substances residing in the subeschar fluid space and perhaps producing systemic effects by means of lymphatic transport from the wound. Two papers by Ferrara and coworkers[93, 94] documented immune suppressive tissue fluid from a canine burn model that was validated by a similar finding in human burn victims. Fluid samples had a consistent suppressive effect on cell-mediated immunity in both situations. Other studies have demonstrated such burn-derived substances as prostaglandins, complement fragments, and "suppressor active peptides" that diminish immune function.[95, 96]

A report by Matsuo and associates[97] has defined multiple suppressor T cells derived from splenic cells of thermally injured mice. These mice were susceptible to a spectrum of post-burn infections, and this vulnerability was able to be transferred to normal mice by infusion of these suppressor cells. Furthermore, increased numbers of T suppressor cells have been detected in burn patients and are likely to have an adverse effect on immune responses.[98]

Burn injury is well known to inhibit T cell function.[99] The mechanism is incompletely understood, but several possibilities have received investigative support. Prostaglandins may be responsible for some but not all of these effects.[100]

A report by Huribal and associates[101] has illustrated increased levels of endothelin-1 and monocyte-derived prostaglandin E_2 in patients with large burns. Although mediation of adverse outcome was postulated, no such correlation was possible in their small series of burn victims. Inadequate production of IL-2 in response to burn injury or IL-2 function inhibition may be present. One such IL-2 stimulatory function known to be decreased in burn victims is natural killer (NK) cell activity. In some experimental situations, this defect can be reversed by means of exogenous IL-2. Attenuation of IL-2 dysfunction may be related to such entities as circulating endotoxin, cell-free IL-2 receptors found in serum, and excess IL-6 levels.[102] Serum levels of inflammatory mediators are time-dependent. Both burned and unburned skin have been identified as sources of IL-6.[103, 104] Although IL-6 is the most consistently elevated cytokine in burn patients, increased levels of IL-1 and TNF are known to occur (Fig. 33–3).

A paper by Endo and coworkers[105] concerning 42 burn patients demonstrated that although individuals with burns in the 20% to 39% TBSA range exhibited minimal plasma TNF levels, those with greater than 60% TBSA burns had significant but delayed plasma level elevations. Endotoxin and TNF levels seemed unrelated. Overall, these mediators have most persistent expression in burn patients who ultimately succumb to the effects of sepsis.[106]

It has been postulated that elevated levels of IL-6 produce an effect on protein metabolism by stimulation of liver macrophages (Kupffer cells), which have a known potential to affect hepatocyte biosynthetic function.[107] It has been shown that cytokine production by Kupffer cells themselves may effect some of the post-burn changes in liver-derived serum proteins.[108] These cytokines apparently stimulate messenger ribonucleic acid (mRNA) mechanisms, resulting in complex changes in liver protein synthesis. Although Kupffer cell–derived IL-6 may be partially responsible for elevated serum IL-6 levels, other sources, such as enterocytes, have been shown in burned guinea pigs to produce large amounts of inflammatory mediators, including IL-6.[109]

Inhibition of B cell responses may result from less than optimal levels of interferon-γ (IFN-γ), one of the primary cytokines that stimulates immunoglobulin production. An experimental study involving treatment of septic burned mice with IFN-γ resulted in significant improvement in survival, thought to have been due to stimulation of B cell function.[110] IFN-γ also regulates the interaction between macrophages and T lymphocytes whereby antigens are presented to helper

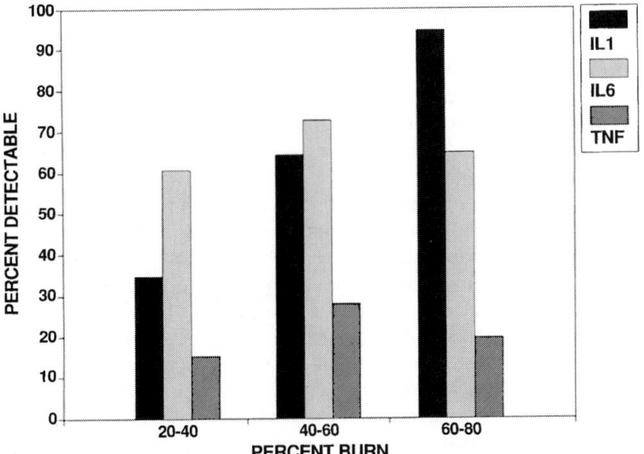

Figure 33–3. Plasma cytokines in surviving burned patients and area of total body surface burn. Cytokine values were grouped by burn size as displayed. Bars represent the percentage of samples with detectable levels of cytokine. IL = interleukin; TNF = tumor necrosis factor. (From Drost AC, Burleson DG, Cioffi WG, Jordan BS, Mason AD Jr, Pruitt BA Jr: Plasma cytokines following thermal injury and their relationship with patient mortality, burn size, and time postburn. J Trauma 1993; 35:335–339.)

lymphocytes. These activated lymphocytes then stimulate B lymphocytes by means of IL-2 to produce antibodies.[98] Low levels of immunoglobulin G and fibronectin have been demonstrated in burn patients, including correlation of mortality with severity of depletion.[111, 112] However, attempts to replenish these proteins have not led to increased survival.

Impairment of granulocyte and macrophage function after burns is well known. Gamelli and associates[113] have defined the inhibitory role of macrophages in response to serum endotoxin. They showed that use of recombinant human granulocyte colony-stimulating factor (G-CSF) in burned mice prevented marrow suppression by inhibitory macrophages. The authors postulated that G-CSF may act by inhibiting prostaglandin production or TNF-α secretion. TNF-α has the ability to inhibit binding of G-CSF to its macrophage receptor sites. The report cautioned, however, that therapeutic use of this modality is likely to be dose-dependent, and excess amounts may actually increase mortality.

In addition, Ogle and associates[114] studied immunoactive substances derived from bone marrow macrophages of burned guinea pigs. Although these macrophages produced increased amounts of TNF and prostaglandin E_2 within the first 24 hours after the burn, there was no such increase in IL-1 levels. These macrophages were also reported to exhibit increased cytotoxicity toward experimental target cells. Leukopenia has been reported as a transient complication of topical silver sulfadiazine. Whether this poses an actual threat to survival of the patient or incidence of infection remains unclear.[115] At present, we temporarily change to an alternative topical agent if the white blood cell (WBC) count falls below 2000 cells/mm^3. Silver sulfadiazine cream can usually be resumed once the counts begin to rise.

The source of post-burn TNF activity is gradually becoming better understood. TNF secretion is apparently a local tissue phenomenon, especially in lung and skin. As reported by Rodriguez and coworkers,[103] IL-8 was also produced in the lung, especially in burn patients with inhalation injury. They also proposed that IL-8 might be a marker for severity of injury because the production of IL-8 was quantitatively related to burn size. Somewhat surprisingly, liver production of TNF was not documented early after burn injury but was increased after subsequent exposure to endotoxin.[116]

Efforts to alter levels of TNF will require considerable refinement. Although suppression of TNF is apparently effective in improving survival in septic experimental animals, clinical use has not verified efficacy in humans.[117, 118] Dosage and timing appear to be important for improving clinical outcome when supervening sepsis develops in a critically ill patient. Prostaglandin blockade, especially by means of ibuprofen administration, may also lead to adverse outcomes because prostaglandins normally exert an inhibitory effect on TNF-α production. In one experimental study, inhibition of prostaglandins resulted in excess production of TNF-α by Kupffer cells, peritoneal macrophages, and neutrophils from burned animals.[119] Conversely, indomethacin may restore macrophage sensitivity to prostaglandin inhibition of TNF secretion and thus contribute to survival of patients.[120]

METABOLISM

Catabolic Mediators

Burns produce a characteristic metabolic response, probably first described by Cuthbertson[121] in 1930 as ebb and flow phases during and after resuscitation from major nonthermal injury. These alterations include increased cardiac output, high oxygen consumption, hypermetabolism characterized by enhanced glucose production, protein wasting, and requirements for heat production exaggerated by calorie expenditure. If not treated, the catabolic response may result in severe protein depletion and loss of muscle mass. These events are predominantly, but not exclusively, hormone-mediated.

In 1974, Wilmore[122] suggested that human metabolic response to burns is primarily mediated by catecholamines, especially epinephrine. By use of selective blockade of hormone action, it was confirmed that the mechanism of this metabolic burn response is mediated by β-adrenergic effect. Wilmore's studies also demonstrated a direct linear relationship between the extent of burn and the magnitude of the metabolic response up to about 40% TBSA burn. Additional metabolic increments then become smaller with larger burn size and reach a plateau response at about twice normal energy expenditure.

Wilmore also illustrated that burn victims reestablish their thermogenic homeostasis at a higher than normal level (~38°C). Environmental temperatures much warmer than those selected by normal individuals are preferred by burn patients. Allowing the patient to function below the equilibrium level results in a measurable increase in catecholamine response. Conversely, inability to achieve a normothermic state or inadequate catecholamine response represents an early indication of nonsurvival.[122]

Subsequent studies by Bessey and associates[123] in 1984 used intravenous infusions of epinephrine, glucagon, and cortisol to approximate the plasma levels of each hormone seen in catabolic burn patients. Using this triple-hormone technique, these investigators were able to reproduce many, but not all, of the metabolic changes of burn patients in normal volunteers. These changes included a hypermetabolic state, negative nitrogen and potassium balance, glucose intolerance, hyperinsulinemia with insulin resistance, sodium retention, and peripheral leukocytosis. The magnitude of these responses, however, did not reach the same levels as those seen in burn patients. Interestingly, growth hormone (GH) and thyroid hormone do not become elevated in burn victims. Although triiodothyronine (T_3) levels become elevated, thyroid-stimulating hormone (TSH) levels remain low, producing the so-called "sick euthyroid syndrome." Failure of GH to respond may account for a relative inability to effectively mobilize fats as an energy source in this situation.[124, 125]

Other stimuli of post-injury hypermetabolism may include several cytokines and bacterial components. Both IL-1 and TNF-α produce the clinical metabolic changes in question. Although most studies have been unable to demonstrate significant plasma levels of IL-1 and TNF-α in the immediate post-burn resuscitation period, it is possible that these messenger proteins exert paracrine or apocrine effects on local tissues. Furthermore, endotoxin, presumably translocated from the gastrointestinal tract, may directly or indirectly stimulate metabolic changes. A study of burn patients who received polymyxin B to block the effects of endotoxin revealed a much improved trend toward positive nitrogen balance, although neither mortality nor incidence of organ failure was different from that of control subjects.[126]

Catabolism of lean body mass to produce large quantities of intermediate metabolites coincident with massive gluconeogenesis appears to be the genetically preprogrammed response to stress by mammalian metabolism. Studies by Brown and associates[127] reported arterial and venous levels of amino acids taken from the leg of burn patients. They documented that glutamine constituted more than 50% of all amino acids mobilized from the leg; alanine represented 7% to 8%; and as a group, lysine, glycine, and valine represented approximately 22%. In spite of these findings, systemic mixed venous levels of most amino acids are low, suggesting massive organ uptake as a response to critical burn or trauma stress.[128]

In an effort to clarify some of the post-burn metabolic changes, Jahoor and coworkers[129] blocked the production of insulin and glucagon by means of intravenous somatostatin and then restored insulin to its previous level by exogenous insulin infusion. They illustrated that insulin availability was necessary to allow alanine flux; insulin resistance and high serum insulin levels seen in burn victims resulted in increased mobilization of alanine from skeletal muscles. The authors also concluded that glucagon, when unopposed by high insulin levels, was at least partially responsible for glucose production in large magnitude. Furthermore, although massive glucose synthesis is associated with high alanine levels, infusion of alanine does not increase glucose production.[130] This suggests that the glucose production is being driven by a mechanism separate from mere high alanine levels. When glucose is infused into burn patients, gluconeogenesis is not effectively inhibited as in normal individuals, and approximately five times the insulin levels of normal volunteers is required to normalize glucose to basal levels.[131] The presence of insulin resistance and its importance in post-burn metabolism seem confirmed by these studies.

Post-burn Metabolic Changes

The deranged glucose and protein metabolism seen in burn patients has been the subject of much experimental and clinical investigation. Further understanding of underlying mechanisms for these changes is slowly being described. An animal study involved in situ perfusion of livers from rats subjected to a 20% TBSA burn.[132] The study attempted to document isolated liver reactions to burn injury without any influence from other metabolic sources in the body. Glucose production increased during the perfusion period but did not differ from that in non-burn control animals. Production of urea and ketone bodies, however, was significantly increased in the livers of burned animals. Oxygen consumption by the liver from burned rats was increased compared with that in control animals. Branch chain amino acids were released by the liver, whereas the remainder of amino acids were taken up by the liver. The authors interpreted changes in arginine, ornithine, and citrulline levels as representing enhancement of urea production by the liver. These results indicate that although the liver from burned rats exhibits a hypermetabolic state and urea production is up-regulated, stimuli for gluconeogenesis do not originate from the liver itself.

Other experimental studies by Fang and coworkers[133] on skeletal muscle from burned rats have demonstrated several energy-dependent proteolytic pathways. They identified ubiquitin, a 76–amino acid peptide, as an important ATP-dependent cofactor in degradation of muscle protein. Both lysosomal and nonlysosomal mechanisms seem to be involved in protein breakdown after thermal injury. However, energy-dependent nonlysosomal mechanisms predominated as a source of skeletal muscle proteolysis in their study.

Lipid metabolism in burn patients is characterized by "futile cycling."[134] Lipolysis after burn injury is mediated by lipase sensitive to the action of β-adrenergic agonists. Although fat mobilization is blunted compared with that in fasted control subjects, fatty acids are largely reesterified to triglycerides in primarily cytosol reactions in burn patients. There is a fivefold increase of lipid cycling in burn victims.[135] Energy-producing reactions in cell mitochondria are blunted, possibly because of decreased availability of carnitine, which is necessary for fatty acids to gain access to the mitochondria.[136] When fatty acids are fed as an energy source to patients with acute burns, reesterification and peripheral storage as fat are common. Furthermore, feeding as fat does not spare protein.[137] Some fat feeding may enhance glucose oxidation and prevent essential fatty acid deficiency.[138]

Estimation of nutritional requirements has traditionally been accomplished by means of several formulas based on burn size and body weight.[139, 140] The simplest of these formulas was proposed by Curreri and coworkers.[141] The formula states that 25 calories per kilogram body weight and 40 calories for each per cent of the BSA involved by the burn should be provided daily for most adult patients. In addition, 1.5 to 2.0 g protein plus multivitamins and trace minerals should be given. No more than 20% to 30% of the calorie intake should be provided as fat. It has been the general experience, however, that all of the available formulas overestimate nutritional needs. Therefore, direct measure by means of the metabolic cart seems to be the most accurate method of evaluating appropriate nutritional requirements.[142]

Nutrition Support Strategies

Whenever possible, the gastrointestinal tract should be the primary route for nutrients. Not only do enteral techniques enhance the nutritional effect of prescribed feedings, but use of the gut most likely limits translocation of bacteria and their toxic products.[143] Furthermore, integrity of mucosal immune protective mechanisms may be preserved by use of enteral feedings as opposed to parenteral feedings through a central vein.

Experimental studies by Gianotti and coauthors[144] have demonstrated specific beneficial effects of enteral feeding components, such as fiber content, while confirming the superiority of enteral feeding over total parenteral nutrition (TPN). Fiber apparently stimulates gut secretion of trophic hormones, thus partially protecting the burned individual from translocation of bacteria. Attempts at nutritional enhancement by formulation of so-called modular feedings or hormonal supplementation have been reported during the past decade. Glutamine supplementation may be beneficial because it is a specific energy substrate for intestine and some inflammatory cells.[145] This amino acid stimulates protein synthesis and elevates the plasma GH levels. Specific benefit in burn patients remains to be confirmed.

One recent evaluation compared a high-protein, low-fat tube feeding enriched by omega-3 fatty acids, vitamins A and C, zinc, and amino acids (including arginine, histidine, and cysteine) with another popular enhanced feeding formula. Reduction of wound infection and length of the patient's stay were reported.[146] Another study compared immune system–enhancing enteral feedings with standard feedings; no advantage was found, but the specialized formula was twice the cost.[147]

The role of customized feeding formulations remains to be defined. Dietary additions to reduce activity of lipid peroxides after burns have been reported. Copper, zinc, and selenium are trace elements with potential antioxidant activity. A study of trace element feeding using urinary malondialdehyde as an indicator of overall lipid peroxidation suggested that these trace elements may limit undesirable oxidant activity, although the results did not achieve statistical significance.[148]

Hormone additives have also received attention. A study using the beta agonist cimaterol to increase the anabolic effects of feedings was performed in burned guinea pigs. When the recovering animals were killed on day 14, post-burn treated animals exhibited greater muscle and total body weight with increased total protein content compared with control animals.[149]

Human GH supplementation, which has been studied in burn victims, exhibits protein-sparing and wound-healing properties. Hyperglycemia, possibly due to insulin resistance, was, however, a consistent adverse by-product thought to seriously limit its use in severe burns as an anabolic agent.[145]

Insulin-like growth factor-1 (IGF-1) has been used in burn patients and experimental animals.[150] This hormone is found in decreased levels immediately after a burn and gradually increases during recovery. When given to burn victims, IGF-1 acts to preserve lean body mass. However, most of these patients exhibit inhibition of insulin secretion, potentially an undesirable side effect.[151] In addition, clinical safety issues remain to be resolved.[152]

Insulin infusions also hold some promise, but large doses are required for effective protein sparing, provoking comments of concern from many clinicians.[153] Testosterone derivatives may facilitate early return to the anabolic state.[145] Hepatotoxicity is a concern with some of the long-acting compounds. Oxandrolone may have some clinical usefulness in the recovery phase although clinical trials are still in progress.

Last, obesity in itself may be a factor leading to increased morbidity. In a study by Gottschlich and coworkers,[154] 15 obese patients were compared for the incidence of morbidity with nonobese control subjects. Obese patients required more ventilator days and received antibiotics twice as long as nonobese control subjects.

Efforts to provide sufficient energy support to burn patients to avoid more than 10% to 15% loss of pre-injury weight should be started during the resuscitation phase soon after hospital admission. Continuing efforts to modify dietary intake and suppress catabolism with resultant metabolic improvement show promise as a means of increasing post-burn survival.

INFECTION IN BURN PATIENTS

Skin barrier compromise to infectious invasion has always been a constant threat to survival of the patient after burn injuries. Development of microbiologic culturing techniques provided information that a large number of burn victims succumbed to *Streptococcus pyogenes* infections in the preantibiotic era. Efforts to forestall these infections by stimulation of eschar formation were unsuccessful. Arrival of the antibiotic era in the form of penicillin provided early protection from streptococcal infections followed by subsequent death due to other bacterial infections. Finally, development of effective antibacterial topical agents has allowed better control of post-burn infections. Use of silver sulfadiazine cream now provides the bulwark of protection from bacterial invasion of burn eschar.[155] Concomitantly, other investigators developed 0.5% silver nitrate solution and mafenide cream for clinical use in suppressing bacterial growth in burn eschar.[156, 157] Since then, several studies have confirmed that prophylactic antibiotics provide no advantage in burn care.

The origin of bacteria in burn eschar has been the source of considerable study. Although such mechanisms as patient-to-patient transfers due to poor hand-washing techniques, organisms from respiratory equipment, and airborne contaminants have been implicated, the majority of organisms originate from the patient—from the gastrointestinal tract, lungs, or skin.[158]

The identity of these organisms has been relatively constant over time. Approximately 45% are gram-positive, an equal number represent a spectrum of gram-negative bacteria, and 8% to 10% are *Candida* species.[159] Viral infections have been reported, especially attributed to herpes simplex virus and cytomegalovirus.[160] Monitoring of burn wound bacterial flora has evolved as overall eschar management has shifted to early excision. Originally, aggressive culturing of burn eschar that was treated with topical antimicrobial agent until spontaneous separation was the standard practice. Quantitative bacterial counts greater than 10^5 per gram of tissue were documented as indicating significant invasive infection and were ultimately predictive of mortality.[161] At present, however, with rapid surgical removal of eschar, this tactic seems to have a more limited usefulness. Studies of burn wound infection monitoring indicate that limited numbers of specimens from the wounds poorly reflect the bacterial status of the wound as a whole.[162]

The controversy over swab or biopsy specimens continues. Steer and associates[163] studied 141 paired culture specimens in 74 patients and found recovery of the same set of species in 54%. They also reported that burn wound cultures could not predict the onset of sepsis or graft failure.

Ultimately, control of burn wound infection resides in early surgical eschar removal and provision of a biologic covering to the wound. In large burns, in which donor sites are limited, temporary measures, such as use of a homograft or xenograft, allow sequential harvesting of available autograft donor sites. Use of newer techniques, such as cultured keratinocytes and dermal replacement, may be helpful in selected situations.

Non-burn wound infections constitute a formidable array of threats to the survival of burn victims. A surveillance study reported 90 nosocomial infections per 100 discharges and deaths. This figure transposes to 32.3 infections per 1000 patient-days. Pneumonias were most common by a factor of 2, followed by urinary tract infections, bacteremias, wound infections, and cellulitis.[164] Invasive procedures, such as endotracheal intubation, central venous catheterization, and urinary catheterization, were implicated as contributing to these infections. This information suggests that the earliest possible removal of invasive devices should be a goal of the care team.

Most burn centers practice aggressive culturing of vulnerable sites, especially in response to febrile episodes. Although the practice is controversial, routine changing of central venous lines over a wire guide as a means of monitoring the bacterial status of essential central lines is widely practiced.[165, 166] A common protocol involves changes every 3 to 5 days with complete line removal only in response to positive cultures. This policy is an admitted compromise with either complete, and often unnecessary, removal with every febrile episode or an arbitrary indication for removal of asymptomatically infected lines, thus prolonging exposure of the patient to infectious risk.

ANCILLARY ISSUES

During the course of recovery from critical burn wounds, a plethora of potentially severe complicating factors may arise. One of the most time-intensive and skill-intensive issues is that of restoring the burned individual to a functional status. Dedicated expertise of physical, occupational, and speech therapists is required to coax and retrain often reluctant burn victims back to a meaningful life. These efforts may be hampered by psychologic barriers of many origins, residual medical problems, and occasional reticence of third-party payers to undertake these complex tasks.

Additional medical problems may revolve around such issues as slow weaning from the ventilator, closure of focal areas of residual open wounds, persistent fever, and pain management. Deep venous thrombosis is a well-known complication of severe burns, and the team should be alert to its development.[167] Prophylaxis by means of low-dose heparin, low-molecular-weight heparin, and lower-extremity compression garments is commonly practiced in many burn centers. Development of heterotopic ossification in burned extremities, especially involving elbows and knees, can seriously compromise efforts at rehabilitation.[168] In some patients, peripheral nerve palsies may also develop, with or without heterotopic ossification.[169]

Underlying causes and potential methods of prevention of these troublesome problems remain unresolved issues in burn care. On occasion, nutrition efforts are hampered by the development of ileus of various causes and by the appearance of elevated serum pancreatic enzyme levels. These enzyme elevations are usually nonspecific and resolve spontaneously, although post-burn pancreatitis is a well-known entity.[170] Support of family involvement in the patient's care is a necessary but rewarding requirement for the burn team. Positive interactions can help smooth out the serious and predictable life-threatening crises seen in care of burned individuals. Finally, some patients will not survive, and humane management of a patient's demise is greatly enhanced by strong cooperative bonds between the family and the burn team.

References

1. Slattery DE, Schiller WR, Pollack CV Jr: A prospective comparison of direct measurement of burn size to estimates by prehospital providers, emergency physicians and burn surgeons (Abstract). J Burn Care Rehabil 1997; 18:S93.
2. Advanced Burn Life Support Course. 2nd ed. Lincoln, Neb, Nebraska Burn Institute, 1994.
3. Arthurson G: Microvascular permeability to macromolecules in thermal injury. Acta Physiol Scand 1979; 463:111.
4. Warden GD: Burn shock resuscitation. World J Surg 1992; 16:16.
5. Shirani KZ, Vaughan GM, Mason AD Jr, et al: Update on current therapeutic approaches in burns. Shock 1996; 5:4.
6. Cope O (Ed): Management of the Cocoanut Grove burns at the Massachusetts General Hospital. Philadelphia, JB Lippincott, 1943.
7. Evans EI, Purnell OJ, Robinett PW, et al: Fluid and electrolyte requirements in severe burns. Ann Surg 1952; 135:804.
8. Baxter CR, Shires GT: Physiological response to crystalloid resuscitation in severe burns. Ann N Y Acad Sci 1968; 150:874.
9. Muir IFK, Barclay TL, Settle JAD: Burns and Their Treatment. 3rd ed. London, Butterworth, 1987.
10. Moncrief JA: Effect of various fluid regimens and pharmacologic agents on the circulatory hemodynamics of the immediate post-burn period. Ann Surg 1966; 164:723.
11. Monafo WW: The treatment of burn shock by the intravenous and oral administration of hypertonic lactated saline solution. J Trauma 1970; 10:575.
12. Gunn ML, Hansbrough JF, Davis JW, et al: Prospective, randomized trial of hypertonic sodium lactate versus lactated Ringer's solution for burn shock resuscitation. J Trauma 1989; 29:1261.
13. Huang PP, Stucky FS, Dimick AR, et al: Hypertonic sodium resuscitation is associated with renal failure and death. Ann Surg 1995; 221:543.
14. Dries DJ, Waxman K: Adequate resuscitation of burn patients may not be measured by urine output and vital signs. Crit Care Med 1991; 19:327.
15. Aikawa N, Martyn JAJ, Burke JF: Pulmonary artery catheterization and thermodilution cardiac output determination in the management of critically burned patients. Am J Surg 1978; 135:811.
16. Aikawa N, Ishibiki K, Naito C, et al: Individualized fluid resuscitation based on haemodynamic monitoring in the management of extensive burns. Burns 1981; 8:249.
17. Miller JG, Bunting P, Burd DAR, et al: Early cardiorespiratory patterns in patients with major burns and pulmonary insufficiency. Burns 1994; 20:542.
18. Schiller WR, Bay RC, McLachlan JG, et al: Survival is predicted by early response to Swan-Ganz resuscitation in major burn injuries. Am J Surg 1995; 170:696.
19. Shoemaker WC, Appel PL, Kram HB, et al: Prospective trial of supranormal values of survivors as therapeutic goals in high risk surgical patients. Chest 1988; 94:1176.
20. Schiller WR, Bay RC, Garren RL, et al: Hyperdynamic resuscitation improves survival in patients with life-threatening burns. J Burn Care Rehabil 1997; 18:10.
21. Barton RG, Saffle JR, Morris SE, et al: Resuscitation of thermally

injured patients with oxygen transport criteria as goals of therapy. J Burn Care Rehabil 1997; 18:1.
22. Demling RH, Knox J, Youn Y, et al: Oxygen consumption early postburn becomes oxygen delivery dependent with the addition of smoke inhalation injury. J Trauma 1992; 32:593.
23. Hilton JG, McPherson MB, Marullo DS: The relationship between postburn increases in peripheral resistance and vasopressin. Burns 1986; 12:410.
24. Mueller M, Sartorelli K, DeMeules JE, et al: Effects of fluid resuscitation on cardiac dysfunction following thermal injury. J Surg Res 1988; 44:745.
25. Giroir BP, Horton JW, White DJ, et al: Inhibition of tumor necrosis factor prevents myocardial dysfunction during burn shock. Am J Physiol 1994; 267:H118.
26. Horton JW: Oxygen free radicals contribute to postburn cardiac cell membrane dysfunction. J Surg Res 1996; 61:97.
27. Vaughan WG, Horton JW, White DJ: Burn induced cardiac dysfunction is reduced by pentoxifylline. Surg Gynecol Obstet 1993; 176:459.
28. Schnarrs RH, Cline CW, Goldfarb IW, et al: Plasma exchange for failure of early resuscitation in thermal injuries. J Burn Care Rehabil 1986; 7:230.
29. Shiozaki T, Kishikawa M, Hiraide A, et al: Recovery from postoperative hypothermia predicts survival in extensively burned patients. Am J Surg 1993; 165:326.
30. Gutierrez G, Palizas F, Doglio G, et al: Gastric intramucosal pH as a therapeutic index of tissue oxygenation in critically ill patients. Lancet 1992; 339:195.
31. Ivatury RR, Simon RJ, Islam S, et al: A prospective randomized study of end points of resuscitation after major trauma: Global oxygen transport indices versus organ-specific gastric mucosal pH. J Am Coll Surg 1996; 183:145.
32. Jeng JC, Lee K, Jablonski K, et al: Serum lactate and base deficit suggest inadequate resuscitation of patients with burn injuries: Application of a point-of-care laboratory instrument. J Burn Care Rehabil 1997; 18:402.
33. Schiller WR, Bay RC: Hemodynamic and oxygen transport monitoring in management of burns. New Horiz 1996; 4:475.
34. Agarwal N, Petro J, Salisbury RE: Physiologic profile monitoring in burned patients. J Trauma 1983; 23:577.
35. Horton JW, Baxter CR, White DJ: Differences in cardiac responses to resuscitation from burn shock. Surg Gynecol Obstet 1989; 168:201.
36. Merrell SW, Saffle JR, Sullivan JJ, et al: Fluid resuscitation in thermally injured children. Am J Surg 1986; 152:664.
37. Carvajal HF: A physiologic approach to fluid therapy in severely burned children. Surg Gynecol Obstet 1980; 150:379.
38. Sances A Jr, Larson SJ, Myklebust J, et al: Electrical injuries. Collective review. Surg Gynecol Obstet 1979; 149:97.
39. Zawacki BE, Jung RC, Joyce J, et al: Smoke, burns and the natural history of inhalation injury in fire victims: A correlation of experimental and clinical data. Ann Surg 1977; 185:100.
40. Gaissert HA, Lofgren RH, Grillo HC: Upper airway compromise after inhalation injury. Complex strictures of the larynx and trachea and their management. Ann Surg 1993; 218:672.
41. Reisdorff EJ, Wiegenstein JG: Carbon monoxide poisoning. In: Emergency Medicine. 4th ed. New York, McGraw-Hill, 1996.
42. Westley J, Adler H, Westley L, et al: The sulfur transferases. Fundam Appl Toxicol 1983; 3:377.
43. Houeto P, Borron SW, Sandouk P, et al: Pharmacokinetics of hydroxocobalamin in smoke inhalation victims. J Toxicol Clin Toxicol 1996; 34:397.
44. Balakrishnan C, Tijunelis AD, Gordon DM, et al: Burns and inhalation injury caused by steam. Burns 1996; 22:313.
45. Weiss SM, Lakshminarayan S: Acute inhalation injury. Clin Chest Med 1994; 15:103.
46. LaLonde C, Demling R, Brain J, et al: Smoke inhalation injury in sheep is caused by particle phase, not the gas phase. J Appl Physiol 1994; 77:15.
47. Bidani A, Wang CZ, Heming TA: Early effects of smoke inhalation on alveolar macrophage functions. Burns 1996; 22:101.
48. Herlihy JP, Vermeulen MW, Joseph PM, et al: Impaired alveolar macrophage function in smoke inhalation injury. J Cell Physiol 1995; 163:1.
49. Demling RH: Smoke inhalation injury. New Horiz 1993; 1:422.
50. Wright JL: Inhalational lung injury causing bronchiolitis. Clin Chest Med 1993; 14:635.
51. Agee RN, Long JM III, Hunt JL, et al: Use of 133-xenon scan in early diagnosis of inhalation injury. J Trauma 1976; 16:218.
52. Masanes MJ, Legendre C, Lioret N, et al: Fiberoptic bronchoscopy for the early diagnosis of subglottal inhalation injury: Comparative value in the assessment of prognosis. J Trauma 1994; 36:59.
53. Khoo AKM, Lee ST, Poh WT: Tracheobronchial cytology in inhalation injury. J Trauma 1997; 42:81.
54. Shirani KZ, Pruitt BA Jr, Mason AD Jr: The influence of inhalation injury and pneumonia on burn mortality. Ann Surg 1987; 20:82.
55. Darling GE, Keresteci MA, Ibañez D, et al: Pulmonary complications in inhalation injuries with associated cutaneous burn. J Trauma 1996; 40:83.
56. Pruitt BA Jr: Fluid resuscitation for extensively burned patients. Second conference on supportive therapy in burn care sponsored by the National Institute of General Medical Sciences. J Trauma 1981; 21:690.
57. Scheulen JJ, Munster AM: The Parkland formula in patients with burns and inhalation injury. J Trauma 1982; 22:869.
58. Navar P, Saffle J, Warden GD: Effect of inhalation injury on fluid resuscitation requirements after thermal injury. Am J Surg 1985; 150:716.
59. Herndon DN, Traber DL, Traber LD: The effect of resuscitation on inhalation injury. Surgery 1986; 100:248.
60. Mitchell JP, Schuller D, Calandrino FS, et al: Improved outcome based on fluid management in critically ill patients requiring pulmonary artery catheterization. Am Rev Respir Dis 1992; 145:990.
61. Demling RH, LaLonde C, Picard L, et al: Changes in lung and systemic oxidant and antioxidant activity after smoke inhalation. Shock 1994; 1:101.
62. Demling RH, Picard L, Campbell C, et al: Relationship of burn-induced lung lipid peroxidation on the degree of injury after smoke inhalation and a body burn. Crit Care Med 1993; 21:1935.
63. LaLonde C, Picard L, Youn YK, et al: Increased early postburn fluid requirements and oxygen demands are predictive of the degree of airways injury by smoke inhalation. J Trauma 1995; 38:175.
64. Demling R, LaLonde C, Ikegami K: Fluid resuscitation with deferoxamine hetastarch complex attenuates the lung and systemic response to smoke inhalation. Surgery 1996; 119:340.
65. Wolyniec WW, Raymond EL, Souza DJ, et al: Topical administration of manganese superoxide dismutase (MnSOD) inhibits pulmonary oxygen toxicity in mice (Abstract). Am J Respir Crit Care Med 1994; 149:A460.
66. Janssens SP, Musto SW, Hutchison WG, et al: Cyclooxygenase and lipoxygenase inhibition by BW-755C reduces acrolein smoke-induced acute lung injury. J Appl Physiol 1994; 77:888.
67. Hales CA, Musto S, Hutchison WG, et al: BW-755C diminishes smoke-induced pulmonary edema. J Appl Physiol 1995; 78:64.
68. Loick HM, Traber LD, Tokyay R, et al: Thromboxane receptor blockade with BM 13,177 following toxic airway damage by smoke inhalation in sheep. Eur J Pharmacol 1993; 248:75.
69. Ogura H, Cioffi WG, Okerberg CV, et al: The effects of pentoxifylline on pulmonary function following smoke inhalation. J Surg Res 1994; 56:242.
70. Nishida K, Matsumoto N, Kikuchi Y, et al: Effect of phenytoin on smoke inhalation injury in sheep. Shock 1995; 4:211.
71. Cox CS Jr, Zwischenberger JB, Traber DL, et al: Heparin improves oxygenation and minimizes barotrauma after severe smoke inhalation in an ovine model. Surg Gynecol Obstet 1993; 176:339.
72. Wang S, Lantz RC, Chen GJ, et al: The prophylactic effects of U75412E pretreatment in a smoke-induced lung injury rabbit model. Pharmacol Toxicol 1996; 79:231.
73. Stewart RJ, Mason SW, Taira MT, et al: Effect of radical scavengers and hyperbaric oxygen on smoke-induced pulmonary edema. Undersea Hyperb Med 1994; 21:21.
74. Rue LW, Cioffi WG, Mason AD Jr, et al: The risk of pneumonia in thermally injured patients requiring ventilatory support. J Burn Care Rehabil 1995; 16:262.
75. Tharratt RS, Allen RP, Albertson TE: Pressure controlled inverse ratio ventilation in severe adult respiratory failure. Chest 1988; 94:755.

76. Carlon GC, Howland WS, Ray C, et al: High-frequency jet ventilation: A prospective randomized evaluation. Chest 1983; 84:551.
77. Nieman GF, Cigada M, Paskanik AM, et al: Comparison of high-frequency jet to conventional mechanical ventilation in the treatment of severe smoke inhalation injury. Burns 1994; 20:157.
78. Lessin MS, El-Eid SE, Klein MD, et al: Extracorporeal membrane oxygenation in pediatric respiratory failure secondary to smoke inhalation injury. J Pediatr Surg 1996; 31:1285.
79. Gattinoni L, Pesenti A, Mascheroni D, et al: Low-frequency positive-pressure ventilation with extracorporeal CO_2 removal in severe acute respiratory failure. JAMA 1986; 256:881.
80. Zwischenberger JB, Nguyen TT, Tao W, et al: IVOX with gradual permissive hypercapnia: A new management technique for respiratory failure. J Surg Res 1994; 57:99.
81. Cane RD, Peruzzi WT, Shapiro BA: Airway pressure release ventilation in severe acute respiratory failure. Chest 1991; 100:460.
82. Rodeberg DA, Housinger TA, Greenhalgh DG, et al: Improved ventilatory function in burn patients using volumetric diffusive respiration. J Am Coll Surg 1994; 179:518.
83. Cioffi WR, Rue LW, Graves TA, et al: Prophylactic use of high-frequency percussive ventilation in patients with inhalation injury. Ann Surg 1991; 213:575.
84. Ogura H, Saitoh D, Johnson AA, et al: The effect of inhaled nitric oxide on pulmonary ventilation-perfusion matching following smoke inhalation injury. J Trauma 1994; 37:893.
85. Sheridan RL, Hurford WE, Kacmarek RM, et al: Inhaled nitric oxide in burn patients with respiratory failure. J Trauma 1997; 42:629.
86. Nieman GF, Paskanik AM, Fluck RR, et al: Comparison of exogenous surfactants in the treatment of wood smoke inhalation. Am J Respir Crit Care Med 1995; 152:597.
87. Feldbaum DM, Wormuth D, Nieman GF, et al: Exosurf treatment following wood smoke inhalation. Burns 1993; 19:396.
88. Caruso DM, Al-Kasspooles MF, Matthews MR, et al: Rationale for "early" percutaneous dilational tracheostomy in burn patients. J Burn Care Rehabil 1997; 18:424.
89. Janzekovic Z: A new concept in the early excision and immediate grafting of burns. J Trauma 1975; 15:42.
90. Kupper TS, Deitch EA, Baker CC, et al: The human burn wound as a primary source of interleukin-1 activity. Surgery 1986; 100:409.
91. Silver GM, Gamelli RL, O'Reilly M, et al: The effect of interleukin-1 alpha on survival in a murine model of burn wound sepsis. Arch Surg 1990; 125:922.
92. Grayson LS, Hansbrough JF, Sirvent-Zapata RL, et al: Quantitation of cytokine levels in skin graft donor site wound fluid. Burns 1993; 19:401.
93. Ferrara JJ, Dyess DL, Luterman A, et al: The suppressive effect of subeschar tissue fluid upon in vitro cell-mediated immunologic function. J Burn Care Rehabil 1988; 9:584.
94. Ferrara JJ, Dyess DL, Luterman A, et al: Transportation of immunosuppressive substances produced at the site of burn injury into the systemic circulation. The role of lymphatics. J Burn Care Rehabil 1990; 11:281.
95. Hoyt DB, Ozkan AN: Immunosuppression in trauma patients. J Intensive Care Med 1991; 6:71.
96. Kravitz M: Immune consequences of burn injury. AACN Clin Issues Crit Care Nurs 1993; 4:399.
97. Matsuo R, Herndon DN, Kobayashi M, et al: $CD4^-$ $CD8^-$ TCRα/β suppressor T cells demonstrated in mice 1 day after thermal injury. J Trauma 1997; 42:635.
98. Hultman CS, Yamamoto H, deSerres S, et al: Early but not late burn wound excision partially restores viral-specific T lymphocyte cytotoxicity. J Trauma 1997; 43:441.
99. O'Riordain DS, Mendez MV, O'Riordain MG, et al: Molecular mechanisms of decreased interleukin-2 production after thermal injury. Surgery 1993; 114:407.
100. Holzheimer RG, Molloy RG, O'Riordain DS, et al: Long-term immunotherapeutic intervention with pentoxifylline in a mouse model of thermal injury and infection. J Trauma 1995; 38:757.
101. Huribal M, Cunningham ME, D'Aiuto ML, et al: Endothelin-1 and prostaglandin E_2 levels increase in patients with burns. J Am Coll Surg 1995; 180:318.
102. Gibran NS, Heimbach DM: Mediators in thermal injury. Semin Nephrol 1993; 13:344.
103. Rodriguez JL, Miller CG, Garner WL, et al: Correlation of the local and systemic cytokine response with clinical outcome following thermal injury. J Trauma 1993; 34:684.
104. Kawakami M, Kaneko N, Anada H, et al: Measurement of interleukin-6, interleukin-10, and tumor necrosis factor-alpha levels in tissues and plasma after thermal injury in mice. Surgery 1997; 121:440.
105. Endo S, Inada K, Yamada Y, et al: Plasma tumour necrosis factor α (TNF-α) levels in patients with burns. Burns 1993; 19:124.
106. Drost AC, Burleson DG, Cioffi WG, et al: Plasma cytokines following thermal injury and their relationship with patient mortality, burn size and time postburn. J Trauma 1993; 35:335.
107. DeBandt JP, Chollet-Martin S, Hernvann A, et al: Cytokine response to burn injury: Relationship with protein metabolism. J Trauma 1994; 36:624.
108. Wu J, Ogle CK, Fischer JE, et al: The mRNA expression and in vitro production of cytokines and other proteins by hepatocytes and Kupffer cells following thermal injury. Shock 1995; 3:268.
109. Ogle CK, Mao J, Hasselgren P, et al: Production of cytokines and prostaglandin E_2 by subpopulations of guinea pig enterocytes: Effect of endotoxin and thermal injury. J Trauma 1996; 41:298.
110. Hershman MJ, Sonnenfeld G, Logan WA, et al: Effect of interferon-gamma treatment on the course of a burn wound infection. J Interferon Cytokine Res 1988; 8:367.
111. Munster AM, Moran KT, Thupari J, et al: Prophylactic intravenous immunoglobulin replacement in high-risk burn patients. J Burn Care Rehabil 1987; 8:376.
112. Liu X, Luo Z, Yang Z, et al: Clinical significance of the changes in serum fibronectin in severely burned patients. Burns 1996; 22:295.
113. Gamelli RL, He L, Liu H: Recombinant human granulocyte colony-stimulating factor treatment improves macrophage suppression of granulocyte and macrophage growth after burn and burn wound infection. J Trauma 1995; 39:1141.
114. Ogle CK, Guo X, Alexander JW, et al: The activation of bone marrow macrophages 24 hours after thermal injury. Arch Surg 1993; 128:96.
115. Zapata-Sirvent RL, Hansbrough JF: Cytotoxicity to human leukocytes by topical antimicrobial agents used for burn care. J Burn Care Rehabil 1993; 14:132.
116. Clancy KD, Lorenz K, Hahn E, et al: Down-regulation of tissue specific tumor necrosis factor-α in the liver and lung after burn injury and endotoxemia. J Trauma 1997; 42:169.
117. O'Riordain MG, O'Riordain DS, Molloy RG, et al: Dosage and timing of anti–TNF-α antibody treatment determine its effect on resistance to sepsis after injury. J Surg Res 1996; 64:95.
118. Natanson C, Hoffman WD, Suffredini AF, et al: Selected treatment strategies for septic shock based on proposed mechanisms for pathogenesis. Ann Intern Med 1994; 120:771.
119. Dong Y, Herndon DN, Yan TZ, et al: Blockade of prostaglandin products augments macrophage and neutrophil tumor necrosis factor synthesis in burn injury. J Surg Res 1993; 54:480.
120. Molloy RG, O'Riordain M, Holzheimer R, et al: Mechanism of increased tumor necrosis factor production after thermal injury. J Immunol 1993; 151:2142.
121. Cuthbertson DP: The disturbance of metabolism produced by bone and non-bony injury, with notes on certain abnormal conditions of bone. Biochem J 1930; 24:1244.
122. Wilmore DW: Nutrition and metabolism following thermal injury. Clin Plast Surg 1974; 1:603.
123. Bessey PQ, Watters JM, Aoki TT, et al: Combined hormonal infusion simulates the metabolic response to injury. Ann Surg 1984; 200:264.
124. Vaughan GM, Pruitt BA Jr: Thyroid function in critical illness and burn injury. Semin Nephrol 1993; 13:359.
125. Jeffries MK, Vance ML: Growth hormone and cortisol secretion in patients with burn injury. J Burn Care Rehabil 1992; 13:391.
126. Cone JB, Wallace BH, Lubansky HJ, et al: Manipulation of the inflammatory response to burn injury. J Trauma 1997; 43:41.
127. Brown JA, Gore DC, Jahoor F: Catabolic hormones alone fail to reproduce the stress-induced efflux of amino acids. Arch Surg 1994; 129:819.
128. Jeevanandam M, Young DH, Ramias L, et al: Aminoaciduria of severe trauma. Am J Clin Nutr 1989; 49:814.
129. Jahoor F, Herndon DN, Wolfe RR: Role of insulin and glucagon

in the response of glucose and alanine kinetics in burn-injured patients. J Clin Invest 1986; 78:807.
130. Wolfe RR, Jahoor F, Herndon DN, et al: The glucose alanine cycle: Origin of control. JPEN J Parenter Enteral Nutr 1985; 9:107a.
131. Wolfe RR, Durkot MJ, Allsop JR, et al: Glucose metabolism in severely burned patients. Metabolism 1979; 28:1031.
132. Yamaguchi Y, Yu Y, Zupke C, et al: Effect of burn injury on glucose and nitrogen metabolism in the liver: Preliminary studies in a perfused liver system. Surgery 1997; 121:295.
133. Fang C, Tiao G, James H, et al: Burn injury stimulates multiple proteolytic pathways in skeletal muscle, including the ubiquitin-energy-dependent pathway. J Am Coll Surg 1995; 180:161.
134. Wolfe RR, Herndon DN, Jahoor F, et al: Effect of severe burn injury on substrate cycling by glucose and fatty acids. N Engl J Med 1987; 317:403.
135. Wolfe RR, Herndon DN, Peters EJ, et al: Regulation of lipolysis in severely burned children. Ann Surg 1987; 206:214.
136. Gottschlich MM, Alexander JW: Fat kinetics and recommended dietary intake in burns. JPEN J Parenter Enteral Nutr 1987; 11:80.
137. Long JM, Wilmore AD, Mason AD, et al: Effect of carbohydrate and fat intake on nitrogen excretion during total intravenous feeding. Ann Surg 1977; 185:417.
138. Gollaher CJ, Fechner K, Karlstad M, et al: The effect of increasing levels of fish oil-containing structured triglycerides on protein metabolism in parenterally fed rats stressed by burn plus endotoxin. JPEN J Parenter Enteral Nutr 1993; 17:247.
139. Harris JA, Benedict FG: A Biometric Study of Basal Metabolism in Man. Publication 279. Washington, DC, Carnegie Institute of Washington, 1919.
140. Allard JP, Pichard C, Hoshino E, et al: Validation of a new formula for calculating the energy requirements of burn patients. JPEN J Parenter Enteral Nutr 1990; 14:115.
141. Curreri PW, Richmond D, Marvin J, et al: Dietary requirements of patients with major burns. J Am Diet Assoc 1974; 65:415.
142. Garrel DR, deJonge L: Thermogenic response to feeding in severely burned patients: Relation to resting metabolic rate. Burns 1993; 19:467.
143. Mainous MR, Block EFJ, Deitch EA: Nutrition support of the gut: How and why. New Horiz 1994; 2:193.
144. Gianotti L, Nelson JL, Alexander JW, et al: Post injury hypermetabolic response and magnitude of translocation: Prevention by early enteral nutrition. Nutrition 1994; 10:225.
145. Demling RH, DeSanti L: Use of anticatabolic agents for burns. Curr Opin Crit Care 1996; 2:482.
146. Gottschlich MM, Jenkins M, Warden GD, et al: Differential effects of three enteral dietary regimens on selected outcome variables in burn patients. JPEN J Parenter Enteral Nutr 1990; 14:225.
147. Saffle JR, Wiebke G, Jennings K, et al: Randomized trial of immune-enhancing enteral nutrition in burn patients. J Trauma 1997; 42:793.
148. Berger MM, Chiolero R: Relations between copper, zinc and selenium intakes and malondialdehyde excretion after major burns. Burns 1995; 21:507.
149. Nelson JL, Chalk CL, Warden GD: Anabolic impact of Cimaterol in conjunction with enteral nutrition following burn trauma. J Trauma 1995; 38:237.
150. Fang C, Li BG, Wang JJ, et al: Insulin-like growth factor 1 stimulates protein synthesis and inhibits protein breakdown in muscle from burned rats. JPEN J Parenter Enteral Nutr 1997; 21:245.
151. Rennert NJ, Caprio S, Sherwin RS: Insulin-like growth factor 1 inhibits glucose-stimulated insulin secretion but does not impair glucose metabolism in normal humans. J Clin Endocrinol Metab 1993; 76:804.
152. Cioffi WG, Gore DC, Rue LW III, et al: Insulin-like growth factor-1 lowers protein oxidation in patients with thermal injury. Ann Surg 1994; 220:310.
153. Jahoor F, Shangraw RE, Miyoshi H, et al: Role of insulin and glucose oxidation in mediating the protein catabolism of burns and sepsis. Am J Physiol 1989; 257:E323.
154. Gottschlich MM, Mayes T, Khoury JC, et al: Significance of obesity on nutritional, immunologic, hormonal, and clinical outcome parameters in burns. J Am Diet Assoc 1993; 93:1261.
155. Stanford W, Rappole BW, Fox CL Jr: Clinical experience with silver sulfadiazine: A new topical agent for control of *Pseudomonas* infections in burns. J Trauma 1969; 9:377.
156. Moyer CA, Brentano L, Gravens DL, et al: Treatment of large human burns with 0.5% silver nitrate solution. Arch Surg 1965; 90:812.
157. Moncrief JA, Lindberg RB, Switzer RE, et al: The use of a topical sulfonamide in the control of burn wound sepsis. J Trauma 1966; 6:407.
158. Kagan RJ, Warden GD: Management of the burn wound. Clin Dermatol 1994; 12:47.
159. Weber JM, Tompkins DM: Improving survival: Infection control and burns. AACN Clin Issues Crit Care Nurs 1993; 4:414.
160. Kagan RJ, Naraqi S, Matsuda T, et al: Herpes simplex virus and cytomegalovirus infections in burned patients. J Trauma 1985; 25:40.
161. Pruitt BA Jr, Foley FD: The use of biopsies in burn patient care. Surgery 1973; 73:887.
162. Steer JA, Papini RPG, Wilson APR, et al: Quantitative microbiology in the management of burn patients. II. Relationship between bacterial counts obtained by burn wound biopsy culture and surface alginate swab culture, with clinical outcome following burn surgery and change of dressings. Burns 1996; 22:177.
163. Steer JA, Papini RPG, Wilson APR, et al: Quantitative microbiology in the management of burn patients. I. Correlation between quantitative and qualitative burn wound biopsy culture and surface alginate swab culture. Burns 1996; 22:173.
164. Wurtz R, Karajovic M, Dacumos E, et al: Nosocomial infections in a burn intensive care unit. Burns 1995; 21:181.
165. Gregory JA, Schiller WR: Subclavian catheter changes every third day in high risk patients. Am Surg 1985; 51:534.
166. Sheridan RL, Weber JM, Peterson HF, et al: Central venous catheter sepsis with weekly catheter change in paediatric burn patients: An analysis of 221 catheters. Burns 1995; 21:127.
167. Rue LW, Cioffi WG Jr, Rush R, et al: Thromboembolic complications in thermally injured patients. World J Surg 1992; 16:1151.
168. Evans EB: Heterotopic bone formation in thermal burns. Clin Orthop 1991; 263:94.
169. Dagum AB, Peters WJ, Neligan PC, et al: Severe multiple mononeuropathy in patients with major thermal burns. J Burn Care Rehabil 1993; 14:440.
170. Ryan CM, Sheridan RL, Schoenfeld DA, et al: Postburn pancreatitis. Ann Surg 1995; 222:163.

34

Accidental Hypothermia

David Heimbach, MD • Gregory J. Jurkovich, MD
Larry M. Gentilello, MD

Because humans are homeotherms, they attempt to maintain a constant body temperature despite changes in environmental temperature. Normal body temperature is 37°C under the tongue, 38°C in the rectum, 32°C at the skin, and 38.5°C deep in the liver, and we are uncomfortable and inefficient with much deviation from normal.[1] Because humans evolved in the tropics, they do not adapt well to the cold. The ideal or "neutral" environmental temperature (no thermogenesis or heat dissipation necessary) for a naked person is 28°C (82.5°F).[2] Humans have a uniquely high capacity to dissipate heat at the cost of evaporating body water and a relatively poor capacity to increase heat production. Thus, outside the tropics, people must rely heavily on environmental thermoregulation by wearing clothes, living in shelters, and burning fuel for heat.

DEFINITIONS

Hypothermia is generally defined as a core body temperature below 35°C (95°F).

Primary accidental hypothermia occurs in patients with normal thermoregulation who become cold because of overwhelming environmental cold stress (e.g., immersion, lost in the wilderness).

Secondary accidental hypothermia occurs in patients with abnormal heat production or thermoregulation who become cold despite only mild cold stress (e.g., hypothyroidism, stroke, hypoadrenalism, trauma, hypoglycemia, drug overdose).

"Urban" hypothermia is the term sometimes used to describe the hypothermia of the homeless, typically found in those predisposed to cooling by drugs, alcoholism, age, debilitating diseases, poverty, or some combination of these factors.[1, 3, 4]

Induced hypothermia is produced in a medical environment for therapeutic purposes.

Chronic hypothermia develops in patients with impaired heat generation (i.e., the elderly and infirm) who live in nonheated apartments, are under continual cold stress, and after a while are found to always have a low temperature, as if they have autoregulated to a new set temperature.

Although there is some uniformity of the definition of hypothermia as a core body temperature below 35°C (95°F), the literature is replete with various definitions of profound, severe, moderate, and mild hypothermia. The published literature on accidental hypothermia generally defines mild hypothermia between 35°C and 32°C, moderate hypothermia between 32°C and 28°C, and severe hypothermia below 28°C.[5] However, the physiologic response to hypothermia is one of transitional changes, with few exact temperature-dependent responses. Beginning at a core temperature of about 34°C, the regulatory portion of the hypothalamus is impaired, and at 29°C, it is lost completely.[6] As a result, at a temperature of about 30°C, humans become poikilothermic and rapidly cool to the ambient temperature. At a core temperature of about 29°C, cardiac arrhythmias occur; at 23°C, apnea is common; and asystole will generally occur at a core temperature of 21°C.

The body has a number of adaptations to compensate for a decrease in core temperature down to about 33°C. Vasomotor adjustments regulate the blood flow from the body core to the surface and extremities but can compensate for changes in environment temperature over a range of no more than 4°C. *Shivering* is the involuntary rapid contraction of large muscle masses and can increase heat production by a factor of about 3 above resting levels. A fivefold increase has been postulated as the theoretical maximum, but only a heavily muscled endurance athlete can sustain that level of oxygen consumption for more than a few minutes. Unfortunately, shivering is relatively ineffective as a warming mechanism because most of the heat is produced near the body surface, and about 75% is lost to the environment.

Shivering occurs from just below 37°C to 31°C. Below this temperature, shivering thermogenesis ceases, and some authors have therefore identified 32°C to be a level of severe or profound hypothermia.[7] A temperature of 32°C does appear to be clinically important in the patient with associated injuries, with survival being unlikely if core temperature falls below this level.[8] Broadly speaking, the transition from a "safe zone" of hypothermia (where physiologic adaptations are working) to a "danger zone" of hypothermia (no defenses) occurs between 33°C and 30°C.[2]

A number of confounding factors can further impair temperature control. Intoxicants, medications, extremes of age, and the general state of health exaggerate heat loss, as can dehydration and fatigue.

Hypothermia occurs in a variety of clinical settings from a number of causes. "Accidental" hypothermia is defined as a spontaneous decrease in core temperature, usually in a cold environment and associated with an acute problem but without any primary disorder of the temperature-regulatory center. This is most commonly seen in neonates; the elderly; the unconscious, immobile, or drugged person; and the person who becomes exhausted while working in a cold environment. Mortality rates for accidental hypothermia have generally ranged from 30% to 80%, although a multicenter review of 428 cases of accidental hypothermia reported an overall mortality of only 17%.[7] Underlying illness or infection is generally thought to contribute to the majority of fatalities.

Although the protective effects of hypothermia are routinely employed in cardiac and transplant surgery, accidental hypothermia alters homeostasis in a variety of ways, including reducing cardiac output, renal blood flow, and cerebral metabolism and inducing cardiac irritability and, in severe cases, ventricular fibrillation. In addition, it induces platelet dysfunction, coagulopathy, acidosis, pancreatitis, disorientation, and coma.[2, 9–11] The temperature ranges listed before are somewhat artificial but are based on the fact that as core temperature reaches 32°C, cardiac conduction disturbances become apparent, and at 28°C, the risk of arrhythmias rises rapidly.[12]

In reality, the physiologic effects of hypothermia vary not only according to its depth but also with its duration, rapidity of onset, and a variety of other factors. For example, a temperature of 32°C arrived at during several days in a person lost in the wilderness has implications different from an acute temperature of 28°C in a victim of cold-water immersion, and treatment strategies must vary accordingly. In the first case, the patient will be exhausted and the energy stores needed for spontaneous rewarming will be absent; the acute hypothermia victim will be capable of shivering and spontaneous rewarming. The patient with a 32°C temperature who is not shivering is probably in greater danger than the patient with a 28°C temperature who is shivering vigorously.[13]

MECHANISMS OF HEAT LOSS OR TRANSMISSION

The physical principles that govern heat loss or gain are important in preventing hypothermia and in developing effective rewarming strategies. There are four primary means of heat loss or transmission.

Conduction

Conduction is the transfer of heat between two masses in contact with one another. The rate of heat transfer is dependent on the temperature gradient at the interface and the size of the contact area. It is also determined by the "thermal conductivity" of the materials, which describes their resistance to heat flow, or insulating properties. Metals and liquids are most conductive, and gases are most insulating. Conductive heat transfer is also inversely proportional to the distance the heat must travel, that is, to the "thickness" of the material being heated.

The ability of conductive warming techniques to raise core body temperature is inversely related to the thickness of the skin and subcutaneous tissue. The dissipation of heat to other parts of the body is directly related to the blood supply through the heated tissue. Because of the poor cutaneous circulation in hypothermic individuals, burns have been caused with levels of external heat that would not be uncomfortable to a normothermic patient. To prevent thermal injury, the temperature of an external heat source must be within several degrees of skin temperature. Because metals and liquids have high thermal conductivity, lying on a metallic or wet surface can dramatically increase the rate of heat loss from the body. Water is some 25 to 30 times more conductive than air, and lying on a wet surface is one of the fastest ways to lose body heat.

Convection

Convection is the transfer of heat due to the flow of liquids or gases over a surface. When warm air overlying a patient is continuously swept away, convective heat loss to the environment occurs. The forces governing convective heat transfer are extremely complex owing to the lack of laminar flow across irregular bodies. Convective heat loss is proportional to the body surface area, the temperature difference between the body and the air flowing over the surface, and the air velocity.

The greatest risk of convective heat loss occurs during movement or transport of the patient. Helicopter evacuation of a trauma victim has the potential to cause enormous convective heat losses especially at the landing site because of the enormous wind-chill factor generated by propeller downdraft.[14] Transport of the patient into the hospital and even from one part of the hospital to another can cause convective heat loss if the patient is not adequately covered.

Radiation

Transfer of radiant energy is due to electromagnetic transmission and is proportional to the fourth power of the temperature difference between the body and its surroundings. The fourth power relationship explains the fact that much of the heat loss that occurs in fully exposed patients is by this route.

Evaporation

The rate of heat loss by evaporation of water from the surface of the body is proportional to the change in vapor pressure from the surface to ambient air and the velocity of air movement.

At usual room temperature and humidity, approximately one third of evaporative heat loss occurs in the lung during the process of saturating inspired air, and the rest is from the skin surface. Evaporation usually accounts for 10% to 15% of total body heat loss. This increases with high minute ventilation, particularly on breathing of dry room air gas. Because the vaporization of water requires 0.577 kcal of heat per milliliter, leaving as little as 30 mL of water to vaporize on the skin can result in a heat loss of 18 kcal, nearly half of an anesthetized patient's hourly heat production.

PATHOPHYSIOLOGY

Cardiovascular

Initially, a sympathetic response increases myocardial oxygen consumption and causes tachycardia and peripheral vasoconstriction. This is followed by bradycardia, which becomes severe by 32°C. Caused by a decrease in spontaneous depolarization of pacemaker cells, it is atropine refractory.[15] Mean arterial pressure, myocardial contractility, and cardiac output dramatically fall. These changes often persist during rewarming.[16, 17]

Electrocardiographic (ECG) findings are inconsistent but include a classic J wave (following the QRS complex) as hypothermia becomes more severe. Although J waves can occur in other pathologic conditions (central nervous system lesions and sepsis), they are important diagnostic features, and to the unwary they can be confused with ECG findings in myocardial infarction. There are no classic arrhythmias, but atrial and ventricular fibrillation are not uncommon and unidirectional blocks facilitate serious arrhythmias. Anything that can further irritate the myocardium, such as Swan-Ganz catheter placement, can be particularly dangerous at this time.

Respiratory System

Respiratory rate falls, and although carbon dioxide production decreases with each degree in temperature drop, hypoventilation and carbon dioxide retention produce hypoxia and severe respiratory acidosis, compounding the accumulating metabolic acidosis.

Central Nervous System

The brain cools inconsistently, but the electroencephalogram becomes abnormal below 34°C and becomes flat at 19 to 29°C.[18] Cerebral vascular autoregulation protects the brain to levels of 25°C, although mentation and motor function are variably abnormal. Some patients can converse normally at a temperature of 25°C, but subtle changes are invariably present in speed of reasoning, and sometimes dysarthria and ataxia can mimic stroke. Hyperreflexia is usually present to temperatures of 32°C, but hyporeflexia generally occurs below 32°C. Behavior changes are inconsistent, but preexisting psychoses may resurface, and judgment often suffers, sometimes signaling the death knell for expeditions when leaders use risk-taking behavior.

Coagulation

A particular worry, especially in the hypothermic injured patient, is a bleeding propensity. Because coagulation tests, such as prothrombin time, are performed at 37°C in the laboratory, test results may not reflect the abnormalities clinically present. Thrombocytopenia and platelet dysfunction are common. On the other hand, a syndrome similar to disseminated intravascular coagulation (DIC) can occur with an increased propensity to thromboembolism, although fibrin split products are not usually elevated.[19, 20]

TREATMENT

One of the earliest references to rewarming was described in the Bible:

> *Now King David was old and stricken in years: and they covered him with clothes, but he gat no heat. Wherefore his servants said, let there be sought a young virgin: and let her stand before the king, and let her cherish him, and lie in thy bosom, that my lord the king may get heat. And the damsel was very fair and cherished the King and ministered to him: but the King knew her not.*
>
> 1 Kings 1:1–4

Hypothermia is still difficult to treat, and early attention to the mechanisms of heat loss outlined before remains the best form of therapy. Once it occurs, our current state of knowledge suggests that every effort should be made to minimize cold stress and to aggressively rewarm the victim. This may be particularly true as core body temperature approaches 32°C, a temperature fairly well tolerated in primary accidental hypothermia but virtually fatal in the trauma victim.

Pre-hospital Treatment

Hypothermia is often combined with mental and physical exhaustion. Once energy stores are depleted, an extremely cold environment is no longer necessary to rapidly lower body temperature. Judgment is impaired, and patients may have slurred speech and confusion. Coma is not irreversible. When a patient is found down, cold, stiff, and cyanotic, he or she is not necessarily dead. Like head-injured patients who are not "brain-dead until they are warm and brain-dead," the hypothermia victim may ultimately make a remarkable recovery even when signs of life are initially absent. Rescuers should generally be aggressive in rescuing even patients who seem to be dead at the scene. Absence of peripheral pulses may just represent intense vasoconstriction and decreased cardiac output, although there may be enough circulation to sustain life.

Estimation of body temperature is often unreliable because thermometers calibrated to body temperature are inaccurate in very cold environments. Further, estimates based on shivering, mental status, and "feel of the skin" are unreliable.

Comatose patients should be handled with extreme care. Ventricular fibrillation or asystole may be induced by any noxious stimuli (endotracheal intubation, chest compression, insertion of a central line). Even bumps in moving the patient or during transport can be initiating factors; ambulance running with sirens and lights should be avoided.

The hallmark of rescue is to avoid further temperature loss. Dry insulating covers attenuate all of the mechanisms of heat loss mentioned before. Obviously, wet clothing should be replaced with dry blankets, pads, coats, or sleeping bags. The patient must not further exert himself or herself and should be kept horizontal to minimize hypotension and sympathetic discharge. Vigorous rubbing is detrimental because it only induces vasodilation and may further suppress shivering.

As with any victim, the ABCs (airway, breathing, and circulation) are paramount. Supplemental oxygen should be given if it is available. Peripheral veins may be difficult to find. Intravenous (IV) fluids containing 5% dextrose warmed to body temperature should be given if possible. Even if available, hot-water bottles or heat packs should be used cautiously because they may burn the poorly perfused skin in a surprisingly brief period. Rescuers may have mechanisms to warm inspired air, a demonstrated safe and effective method of beginning rewarming.[21, 22]

Aluminized space blankets are often used during transport of the patient to reduce radiant heat loss. With any air movement, the space blanket begins to "flap," allowing cold air to circulate between it and the patient, which can offset any benefits it may have in reducing radiant losses. Careful wrapping or placement of an additional blanket on top of the space blanket is therefore necessary. In several studies in which aluminized space blankets were used to prevent intraoperative heat loss, no significant effects on conservation of body heat were demonstrated; patients arrived to the recovery room with the same core temperature whether or not these devices were used.[23, 24] These studies were performed on patients undergoing neurosurgical and head and neck procedures, in which much of the body surface was available for wrapping. As much as 50% of radiant heat loss from patients occurs from the neck up, because vessels in the scalp do not significantly vasoconstrict even in hypothermic conditions. The head should be covered to minimize radiant losses, particularly in the patient with alopecia.

In-Hospital: Emergency Department and Intensive Care Unit

An ECG, Doppler pulses, and temperature monitoring are indicated. Tympanic monitoring with the newer infrared devices is noninvasive and nonirritating, but the accuracy of these devices has not been assessed in the severely hypothermic patient. Esophageal monitoring is useful after tracheal intubation, but in proximity to the trachea with heated gases, its reliability is inconstant.

General laboratory studies include electrolyte determinations; complete blood count; clotting studies (prothrombin time, partial thromboplastin time, and platelet count); and blood urea nitrogen, creatinine, amylase, calcium, and magnesium concentrations. A toxicology screen is important for obtunded patients. Radiologic examinations are similar to those for the obtunded trauma patient—cervical spine, chest, abdomen as indicated. Peripheral intravenous lines and a central line proximal to the right atrium may be useful, as might an arterial line for monitoring. A nasogastric tube and Foley catheter complete the initial survey.

Hypothermic patients are likely to be dehydrated. Intravenous replacement of normal saline should begin with a rapid infusion of about 1000 mL. Bolus administration containing glucose should be used cautiously, because it may cause significant hyperglycemia; hypothermic patients are insulin-resistant and may already be hyperglycemic. Giving them more glucose will worsen this and may cause osmotic diuresis in these patients who are already probably dry. It is important to not give insulin to the hyperglycemic hypothermic patient. The insulin has little effect while the patient is cold but then becomes active during rewarming, which can lead to severe hypoglycemia.

Rewarming

Intravenous Crystalloid Fluids

Patients become hypothermic at a rate proportional to their fluid requirements if unwarmed fluids are given.[25] When given a 1-L infusion of room-temperature (21°C) crystalloid, the patient must generate 16 kcal of heat to raise the temperature of the water to 37°C. Four liters of room-temperature crystalloid consumes 64 kcal, the equivalent of 1 hour's total body heat production. If the patient is unable to provide this additional heat, a decrease in body temperature would be inevitable. The loss of 64 kcal would decrease the body temperature of a 70-kg patient by roughly 1.1°C, which is enough to cause vigorous shivering.

Although warm IV fluids are important in preventing heat loss, they are not an effective means of treating hypothermia because of the small difference in temperature and large difference in mass between the body and the infused fluid. Warm IV fluids equilibrate with body temperature, liberating heat in the process. One liter of 40°C crystalloid infused into a 32°C patient would be equivalent to transfusing 8 kcal into the patient, which will increase body temperature by only 0.14°C. When fluid requirements are massive, however, a significant quantity of heat can be transfused into the patient with IV fluids. Twenty-five liters of 40°C fluid infused into a 32°C patient would be equivalent to 25 × 8 kcal = 200 kcal. (The actual amount of heat transfer would be somewhat less. As body temperature increases, the temperature difference between the body and the IV fluid decreases, and less heat contained in the fluid is dissipated in the body.)

The colder the patient, the more effective is warmed IV fluid. If the patient receives a liter of 42°C fluid and the temperature is 33°C, the patient receives 9 kcal; but if the temperature is 28°C, the patient receives 14 kcal. A cold patient with a decreased oxygen consumption may be producing only 30 kcal. Thus, 2 L of fluid provides 28 kcal, nearly doubling the patient's spontaneous rewarming rate. Based on the specific heat of the body, it takes 58 kcal to raise the body temperature of a 70-kg person by 1°. So, 28 kcal increases temperature by one half of a degree (keep in mind that airway rewarming provides only 8 kcal per hour). In fact, temperature increases more because of compartmentalization. The body shuts down perfusion to skin, muscles, and extremities when it is very cold and perfuses only the core, which is about 20% of body mass. Whereas it takes 58 kcal to raise the temperature of a 70-kg person 1°, raising the temperature of the core, which is about 20% of 70 kg, requires only about 12 kcal. Thus, the important core organs can be effectively rewarmed with warm fluid if the patient is very cold and vasoconstricted.

Storing emergency department fluids in a warm cubicle is advisable in the absence of an effective warming device. However, 40°C fluid decreases to about 32°C if it is left at room temperature for just 10 minutes. Thus, unless fluid is given rapidly under pressure, the patient still receives hypothermic fluid, which will worsen the hypothermia. An in-line warmer should be used whenever possible.

Microwave warming of crystalloid solutions is an alternative but has several limitations. One liter of crystalloid at room temperature can be heated to 40°C in 2.5 minutes in an ordinary microwave oven; however, considerable variability exists in the heating capacity of different microwave ovens, and each institution should experiment with times on their own appliance. Overheating fluids can potentially cause a problem, and because of the known uneven tendencies of microwave heating, solutions should be shaken vigorously before administration. Glucose-containing solutions cannot be microwaved because glucose caramelizes at 60°C.[9, 26] Microwave warming can be performed only on solutions stored in plastic bags. Glass bottles contain metal caps that cannot be used in microwave ovens. Some people are using very hot fluids (67°C) for warming. If these fluids are given slowly, there seems to be little damage to the blood elements.

Having solved numerous technical problems, a microwave in-line blood warmer has been approved that may be the way of the future. A central line that emits microwaves for warming is being developed. Microwaves are better controlled now than in the past.

Warmed Blood

The previous recommendation of the American Association of Blood Banks that blood not be heated above 40°C has been increased to 42°C. Microwave blood warming should not be performed, because this results in morphologic changes in red blood cells and increases in intracellular adenosine triphosphate and 2,3-diphosphoglycerate. This is probably due to the uneven nature of microwave warming and the fact that heating blood to temperatures above 46.3°C results in hemolysis.

Airway Rewarming

Airway rewarming is another means of transferring heat to the patient. The large amount of heat liberated by water as it condenses is used during this process. Two mechanisms are at work here. The first occurs because the inspired air borders on saturation, and its temperature is higher than that of the patient. This temperature difference results in condensation of the humidity in the airways on contact with the relatively cold lung surface. The amount of water vapor capable of being held by air depends on the temperature of the air.

At 41°C, fully saturated air can hold 0.054 mL H_2O per liter of air. At 30°C, air can hold only 0.030 mL H_2O per liter. When a 30°C patient inspires the saturated 41°C air, the temperature of the air equilibrates with that of the body, and 0.024 mL H_2O per liter of air condenses. With a minute ventilation of 10 L/min, or 600 L/hour, 14 mL H_2O per hour condenses within the respiratory tract. Because the heat of vaporization of water is 0.577 kcal/per milliliter of H_2O, the amount of heat liberated equals

$$0.577 \text{ kcal/mL } H_2O \times 14 \text{ mL } H_2O\text{/hour} = 8.0 \text{ kcal/hour}$$

The actual amount of heat transfer is somewhat less because humidifiers are not 100% efficient, cooling of the air in the ventilator circuit leads to condensation of water in the tubing, and the temperature of the inspired air may not fully equilibrate with body temperature before it is exhaled. When a patient is breathing dry, cold air, the amount of heat lost through the airways is considerable because the patient must warm the air to body temperature and fully saturate it.

Body Cavity Lavage

In comparative studies, however, pleural or peritoneal lavage results in significantly greater heat transfer than does airway rewarming.[2] Body cavity lavage is a process whereby warm fluid is circulated in the thoracic or abdominal cavities to try to warm the patient's core. The temperature of the water entering the patient exceeds the temperature of the body cavity and on exiting should be close to the patient's temperature. The amount of heat transferred is dependent on the difference between the inlet and outlet water temperature and the mass flow rate per unit time.

If 1 L of 40°C water is infused into a body cavity and exits at 35°C, 5 kcal of heat will have been left in the body. The rate of rewarming is *indirectly* dependent on the body cavity used, because the water exits at a colder temperature if it flows through a well-perfused area such as the pleural space. There are limits to the efficiency of this technique, since the only way to increase the difference between inlet and outlet temperature is to increase the dwell time. Attempts at increasing heat exchange by increasing the flow rate result in a higher outlet temperature. Also, as the body temperature rises, rewarming becomes progressively more inefficient, as a longer dwell time is then needed to maintain the same difference in inlet and outlet temperature, or less heat will be transferred per unit time.

The observed rewarming rates with body cavity lavage have varied greatly because most studies fail to take into account the patient's own contribution to the warming process. Otto and Metzler[2] found pleural and peritoneal lavage to be equivalent. Pleural irrigation is more likely to result in cardiac rewarming than is peritoneal lavage and may be the preferred method if an arrhythmia is present. Peritoneal lavage is more likely to rewarm the liver and will perhaps restore its synthetic and metabolic properties more quickly. Because the surface area for heat exchange is small, stomach, colon, and bladder are poor sites for body cavity lavage.

Conductive Rewarming

Conductive rewarming with heating blankets is inefficient because the dimensions in contact with the blanket are only the occiput, shoulders, presacral region, and heels, which equal only 20% to 30% of the body surface area. According to English and colleagues,[27] a fluid-circulating heating blanket can transmit 55 kcal/hour to an average-sized patient. However, these observations were made in a warm room in normothermic individuals with well-perfused skin and subcutaneous tissues. During hypothermia, the thermal conductivity of the skin has been found to be roughly equivalent to cork.[5] In hypothermic individuals, studies based on observed rewarming rates indicate that transmission of only 2.7 to 5.2 kcal/hour per degree temperature difference between blanket and skin occurs. Although studies have repeatedly failed to show a significant contribution to body heat from heating blankets, the heating blanket may contribute to heat savings by diminishing ongoing heat losses.[28]

External rewarming has been implicated as a cause of vasodilatation, hypotension, and the "afterdrop" phenomenon. The *afterdrop* is defined as a continual decline in core temperature after removal from the cold. In a study comparing heating blankets with internal rewarming by peritoneal lavage or cardiac bypass, the externally rewarmed group required two to three times the amount of crystalloid as well as repeated injections of bicarbonate, epinephrine, atropine, and dopamine.[29] In some settings, a potentially adverse effect of external rewarming is cessation of shivering. External rewarming can provide a sensation of warmth to cutaneous thermoreceptors without actually transmitting a significant amount of heat. Shivering will then be inhibited, the patient's own heat generation will diminish, and the duration of hypothermia may be prolonged.

Immersion Rewarming

Because water has a much greater specific heat than air, warm-water immersion can transmit a significant amount of heat. The hydrostatic squeeze that occurs during immersion may offset any vasodilator effects, and removal from the tank can result in a precipitous drop in venous return and blood pressure.[30] Because heat is applied externally, circulation to the skin surface is required for effective heat transfer, and failure of rewarming may occur when there is absent or diminished circulation.[10] This method is probably contraindicated in severely traumatized patients because it limits access to the patient, and it is electrically hazardous when patients are intubated and invasively monitored. In the event of ventricular fibrillation, the patient must be removed from the tank and thoroughly dried. Defibrillating a wet patient is ill-advised; the charge merely runs over the wet body surface and is ineffective, and it may short to the ground and cause burns.[31]

Radiant Rewarming

Radiant warmers can be helpful but can produce intense local heat if the circulation to the skin is poor, and they can cause thermal injury. A blanket can be placed over the patient so that a burn is less likely. However, a blanket interposed between the patient and the warmer traps a pocket of warm air between the blanket and the patient. Radiant heat is then supplied only to the blanket, and the patient is warmed in a relatively inefficient manner by conduction and convection from the overlying air. On the basis of observed rewarming rates in hypothermic patients, Henneberg and colleagues[11] have calculated an approximate heat transfer of 17.7 kcal/hour with the use of an overhead radiant warmer. An additional effect of radiant warming is rapid cessation of shivering due to its effects on peripheral thermal receptors.

Increasing Ambient Temperature

Most surgeons and anesthesiologists attempt to combat hypothermia by increasing the operating room (OR) temperature because the cold OR environment provides significant thermal stress to the patient. The thermoneutral zone is the temperature at which an awake, naked patient can maintain body temperature without increasing energy expenditure, and it is about 28°C. When the patient is lying naked in usual OR ambient temperatures of 18 to 20°C, the heat lost because of convection and radiation alone is estimated to be as high as 284 kcal/hour.[5] Although it may appear logical to increase the OR temperature, studies have not shown that patients undergoing surgery in warm ORs (>21°C) are significantly warmer on arrival in the recovery room than are patients in cold ORs.[32, 33] This may be due to the fact that any marginal benefit from changes in room temperature are not apparent because of the massive heat losses that are occurring.

Cardiopulmonary Bypass and Arteriovenous Rewarming

Cardiopulmonary bypass is gaining support as the preferred method of rewarming the victim of severe primary accidental hypothermia. A Swiss multicenter trial studied the long-term effects of cardiopulmonary bypass rewarming in otherwise healthy individuals with accidental hypothermia leading to cardiac arrest.[34] Of 232 hypothermic patients, 32 were treated; of the 15 who became long-term survivors, 14 had full recovery. This nearly 50% recovery compares favorably with the 8% to 10% recovery from cardiopulmonary resuscitation after normothermic cardiac arrest. Bypass provides the fastest method of rewarming; it provides adequate and immediate circulatory support; and it rewarms the heart before the rest of the body, avoiding hypovolemic shock from peripheral vasodilatation. This technique is complex and not available in many institutions, and in the patient with additional trauma, the need for systemic heparinization is an absolute contraindication to its use. Heparinless cardiopulmonary bypass made possible by centrifugal pumps has been used to rewarm hypothermic pigs, with no thromboembolic sequelae or changes in coagulation.[35]

Another option is the technique of *continuous arteriovenous rewarming*. This technique uses femoral arterial and venous catheters and the patient's own blood pressure to create a circulatory fistula that drives blood through a heparin-bonded compact countercurrent heat exchanger.[36] The flow rate of blood through the heat exchanger is less than that achieved with full bypass, but with a systolic blood pressure of 80 mm Hg or more, flow rates of 150 to 300 mL/min are achieved. This exceeds the rate of fluid exchange obtained with body cavity lavage, and because the reinfused blood fully equilibrates with body temperature, much more heat is donated to the patient. In preliminary studies, warming rates similar to those of cardiac bypass have been achieved, without the need for heparin or pump assistance.

Treatment Summary

Mild Hypothermia (Above 32°C)

Noninvasive passive external rewarming is all that is necessary. The patient can be covered with dry insulation in a warm environment. With proper monitoring and fluid replacement, rewarming rates between 0.5 and 1°C per hour can be achieved. Caution should be exercised in the elderly patient or in a patient who is hypoxic or has cardiac disease. The onset of dramatic shivering will markedly increase oxygen consumption, and the patient's catecholamine level will be extraordinarily high. Myocardial infarction is not uncommon in the elderly at this temperature.

Moderate Hypothermia (28° to 32°C)

Active rewarming is indicated along with extensive monitoring that does not risk increased cardiac irritability. Rewarming to the skin includes plumbed garments, hot-water bottles, heating pads and blankets, and radiant heat sources. A commercially available Bair Hugger circulates forced hot air through a blanket. Care must be used to avoid cutaneous burns, especially in vasoconstricted skin. Immersion in a 40°C bath has been advocated, but if cardiac irritability occurs, resuscitation becomes nearly impossible.

Active core rewarming with use of heated, humidified air has been well studied and may be of value. Heated fluid infusions have a limited role, and body cavity warming with fluids is more adaptable to the patient who will undergo surgery for associated injuries.

Severe Hypothermia (Below 28°C)

Cardiopulmonary bypass or continuous arteriovenous rewarming should be considered the treatment of choice in addition to the measures listed before.

References

1. Luna GK, Maier RV, Pavlin EG, Anardi D, Copass MK, Oreskovich MR: Incidence and effect of hypothermia in seriously injured patients. J Trauma 1987; 27:1014–1017.
2. Otto RJ, Metzler MH: Rewarming from experimental hypothermia: Comparison of heated aerosol inhalation, peritoneal lavage, and pleural lavage. Crit Care Med 1988; 16:869–875.
3. Severinghaus JW: Temperature gradients during hypothermia. Ann N Y Acad Sci 1962; 80:515–521.
4. English MJM, Farmer C, Scott WAC: Heat loss in exposed volunteers. J Trauma 1990; 30:422–424.
5. Maclean D, Emslie-Smith D: Accidental Hypothermia. Edinburgh, Blackwell Scientific Publications, 1977.
6. Steen PA, Soule EH, Michenfelder JD: The detrimental effect of prolonged hypothermia in cats and monkeys with and without regional cerebral ischemia. Stroke 1979; 10:522–529.
7. Fox RH, Brooke OG, Collins JC, Bailey CS, Healey FB: Measurement of deep body temperature from the urine. Clin Sci Mol Med 1975; 48:1–7.
8. Millikan JC, Cain TL, Hansbrough J: Rapid volume replacement for hypovolemic shock: A comparison of techniques and equipment. J Trauma 1984; 24:428–431.
9. Werwath DL, Schwab CW, Scholten JR, Robinett W: Microwave ovens: A safe new method of warming crystalloids. Am Surg 1984; 50:656–659.
10. Jessen K, Hagelson JO: Peritoneal dialysis in the treatment of profound accidental hypothermia. Aviat Space Environ Med 1978; 49:426–429.
11. Henneberg S, Eklund A, Joachimsson PO, et al: Effects of a thermal ceiling on postoperative hypothermia. Acta Anaesth Scand 1985; 29:602–606.
12. Virtue RW: Hypothermic Anesthesia. Springfield, Ill, Charles C Thomas, 1955.
13. Lloyd EL: Hypothermia and Cold Stress. Rockville, Md, Aspen, 1986.
14. Fox JB, Thomas F, Clemmer TP, Grosman M: A retrospective analysis of air-evacuated hypothermia patients. Aviat Space Environ Med 1988; 59:1070–1075.
15. Preston BR: Effect of hypothermia on systemic and organ system metabolism and function. J Surg Res 1976; 20:49.
16. Tveita T, Mortensen E, Henry O, et al: Hemodynamic and metabolic effects of hypothermia and rewarming. Arctic Med Res 1991; 50:48–52.
17. Harari A, Regnier B, Rapin M, et al: Haemodynamic study of prolonged deep accidental hypothermia. Eur J Intensive Care Med 1975; 1:65–70.
18. Ehrmantraut WR, Ticktin HE, Fazekas JF: Cerebral hemodynamics and metabolism in accidental hypothermia. Arch Intern Med 1957; 99:57.
19. Mahajan AL, Myers TJ, Baldini MG: Disseminated intravascular coagulation during rewarming following hypothermia. JAMA 1981; 245:2517–2518.
20. Sabapathi R, Ridley C, Yen MC: Complete recovery from profound hypothermia associated with DIC. Md Med J 1986; 35:203–204.
21. Lloyd EL, Croxten D: Equipment for the provision of airway rewarming in the treatment of accidental hypothermia in patients. Resuscitation 1981; 9:61–65.
22. Lloyd EL, Frankland JC: Accidental hypothermia: Central rewarming in the field. Br Med J 1984; 4:717.
23. Radford P, Thurlow AC: Metallized plastic sheeting in prevention of hypothermia during surgery. Br J Anaesth 1979; 51:237–239.
24. Bourke DL, Wurm H, Rosenberg M, Russell J: Intraoperative heat conservation using a reflective blanket. Anesthesiology 1984; 60:151–154.
25. Slotman GJ, Jed EH, Burchard KW: Adverse effects of hypothermia in postoperative patients. Am J Surg 1985; 149:495–500.
26. Staples PJ, Griner PF: Extracorporeal hemolysis of blood in a microwave blood warmer. N Engl J Med 1971; 285:317–319.
27. English MJM, Farmer C, Scott WAC: Heat loss in exposed volunteers. J Trauma 1990; 30:422–424.
28. Morrison RC: Hypothermia in the elderly. Int Anesth Clin 1988; 26:124–133.
29. Moss JF, Haklin M, Southwick HW, et al: A model for the treatment of accidental severe hypothermia. J Trauma 1986; 26:68–74.
30. Golden F StC: Problems of immersion. Br J Hosp Med 1980; 24:371–374.
31. Marcus P: The treatment of acute accidental hypothermia: Proceedings of a symposium held at the RAF Institute of Aviation Medicine. Aviat Space Environ Med 1979; 50:834–843.
32. Joachimsson PO, Hedstrand U, Tabow F, et al: Prevention of intraoperative hypothermia during abdominal surgery. Acta Anesth Scand 1987; 31:330–337.
33. Roizen MF, Sohn YJ, L'Hommedieu CS, et al: Operating room temperature prior to surgical draping: Effect on patient temperature in recovery room. Anesth Analg 1980; 59:852–855.
34. Walpoth BH, Walpoth-Aslan BN, Mattle HP, et al: Outcome of survivors of accidental deep hypothermia and circulatory arrest treated with extracorporeal blood warming. N Engl J Med 1997; 337:1500–1505.
35. DelRossi AJ, Cernainu AC, Vertrees RA, et al: Heparinless extracorporeal bypass for treatment of hypothermia. J Trauma 1990; 30:79–82.
36. Gentilello LM, Cortes V, Moujaes S, et al: Continuous arteriovenous rewarming: Experimental results and thermodynamic model simulation of treatment for hypothermia. J Trauma 1990; 30:1436–1449.

35

Trauma to the Pregnant Patient

Susan I. Brundage, MD, MPH • Jill K. Davies, MD
Gregory J. Jurkovich, MD

INCIDENCE AND DEMOGRAPHICS

The pregnant patient in the trauma intensive care unit (ICU) is an unusual occurrence. Although there were almost 4 million births recorded in 1996 in the United States,[1] the overall incidence of trauma during pregnancy has been reported to be only 7%.[2] Most of these injuries are minor, as evidenced by a 1983 study reporting that 0.04% of pregnant women were hospitalized secondary to trauma.[3] Nonetheless, trauma is still the leading cause of death in women of reproductive age, and maternal trauma is reported to be the leading cause of nonobstetric fetal death.[4] Motor vehicle collisions are the leading cause of injury during pregnancy, followed by falls and direct assaults to the abdomen.[5] Perhaps even more troubling is a study estimating a 20% prevalence of physical abuse during pregnancy.[6]

MATERNAL AND FETAL OUTCOMES

Injuries in the pregnant patient do not result in a higher maternal mortality compared with the similarly injured nonpregnant patient. However, significant injury is associated with an increased incidence of preterm labor, spontaneous abortion, abruptio placentae, and intrauterine fetal death. Minor trauma can also result in an increased incidence of fetomaternal hemorrhage, abruptio placentae, and preterm delivery. A meta-analysis of seven studies evaluating maternal and fetal outcome after trauma reported a fetal death rate of 41% for pregnant patients who sustained any of the following life-threatening injuries: maternal hypotension, perforated viscera, emergent laparotomy, severe head injury, or severe thoracic injuries. A fetal death rate of only 1.6% was reported for non–life-threatening injuries.[7] A study by Rothenberger and colleagues[8] confirms the prognostic significance of maternal hypotension, with the authors reporting an 80% fetal mortality rate.

Fetal mortality is significantly higher than maternal mortality in the traumatically injured gravida. Kissinger and associates[9] retrospectively evaluated 93 traumatically injured patients admitted to three level I trauma centers from 1985 to 1990. The maternal mortality was 3% compared with a fetal mortality rate of 15%. Fetal heart rate at admission was also not an accurate predictor of fetal outcome. Not surprisingly, more severely injured patients, as determined by their Injury Severity Score (ISS), had a higher incidence of nonviable pregnancies (mean viable pregnancy maternal ISS = 6.2; mean nonviable pregnancy maternal ISS = 21.6). Also, Glasgow Coma Scale (GCS) scores differed significantly in viable (GCS = 14.5) and nonviable pregnancies (GCS = 12.0). Specific injuries resulting in an increased incidence of fetal death included direct uteroplacental injury, pelvic fracture, and severe head injury plus any injury resulting in maternal shock or hypoxia. Although the figure was less than the 80% fetal mortality associated with maternal hypotension reported by Rothenberger, Kissinger's study reported a 67% fetal death rate associated with maternal hypotension. Maternal hypoxemia was associated with a 33% fetal death rate. The study concluded that maternal physiologic and laboratory values did not predict fetal outcome and that maternal monitoring by standard noninvasive methods is inadequate to ensure fetal welfare.

Appropriate care of the severely injured pregnant patient requires cooperation among the disciplines of general surgery, obstetrics and gynecology, and critical care. Depending on the specific injuries of the pregnant patient, the coordinated efforts of surgical subspecialties and anesthesia may also be required. This chapter addresses recommendations for the initial evaluation and management of the pregnant trauma patient.

INITIAL EVALUATION

The use of diagnostic tests and procedures should not be altered in the pregnant patient. As for any traumatically injured patient, establishing the status of the ABCs—airway, breathing, circulation—is the first priority. The Advanced Trauma Life Support (ATLS) protocol of the American College of Surgeons should be followed.[10] An obstetrician should be included in the trauma team. If the fetus has an estimated gestational age of greater than 24 weeks, the team should also include a pediatrician or neonatologist in case of an emergent cesarean section delivery. Maintaining adequate fetal oxygenation through establishment and support of the maternal airway is crucial, including supplemental 100% oxygen by mask and endotracheal intubation. The patient should be placed in the left lateral decubitus position on a backboard with spinal precautions maintained by immobilization to prevent the supine hypotensive syndrome. Patients require at minimum two large-bore intravenous lines (18-gauge or greater) for resuscitation with crystalloid and blood products as recommended by ATLS protocol.

The presence of hypotension or tachycardia in the mother requires immediate administration of fluids plus a search for a site of bleeding. Sites at which an adult can lose enough blood to cause hypotension include the chest, abdomen, retroperitoneum, soft-tissue injuries, and large scalp lacerations. Because the gravid uterus receives 30% of the cardiac output (~500 to 700 mL/min), placental abruption can also result in hemorrhage and hypotension.[11] Up to 2 L of intrauterine blood may accumulate. As in any traumatically injured patient, tachycardia and oliguria (defined as a urine output of less than 30 mL/hour) may be a better sign of early compromise than the later sign of hypotension.[12]

The initial trauma radiology series that consists of chest, pelvic, and lateral cervical spine radiographs should be obtained immediately. Pneumothorax or hemothorax detected by either physical examination or chest radiography is an indication for immediate tube thoracostomy. The use of trocars to place chest tubes is generally contraindicated. Awareness of the upward displacement of the diaphragm and intra-abdominal contents during pregnancy is important, and a chest tube should be placed at the third or fourth intercostal space with careful confirmation of intrapleural position by digital examination.

Urinary and gastric intubation is indicated in the pregnant trauma patient. Gastric intubation for decompression is particularly important in the gravid patient. The functional gastrointestinal changes associated with pregnancy include a dilated, hypomotile stomach, which places the patient at greater than usual risk for aspiration. A full physical examination is part of the secondary survey of the injured patient. Of note, the abdominal examination of every female patient of reproductive age should include palpation of the suprapubic area to determine the presence of a palpable uterus. This has been termed the "mother's maneuver" and consists of palpation over the umbilicus to detect a pregnant uterus. A vaginal examination is an essential part of the physical examination. Evaluation for rupture of the membranes can be determined by using phenaphthazine (Nitrazine) paper. Amniotic fluid is relatively alkaline, with a pH of 7; the pH of normal vaginal fluid is less than 4.5. A sterile speculum examination is indicated as long as the patient is hemodynamically stable and there is no contraindication to proper positioning, such as lower-extremity, pelvic, or spinal fractures. A rectal examination is a fundamental component of the evaluation of any trauma patient and should also be performed.[13]

In addition to standard physical examination of the abdomen, many injured patients require a more definitive diagnostic test to assess for the presence of intra-abdominal pathology. Use of diagnostic adjuncts to evaluate the abdomen is essential in the intubated patient. In the nonintubated patient, many factors can interfere with the quality of the physical examination. Other painful injuries can distract the patient from more subtle visceral-parietal pain. The stretching of the peritoneum that occurs during pregnancy can lessen the sensitivity of the parietal nerve fibers. Altered GCS score and presence of alcohol or drugs can also interfere with the physical examination findings. Patients who appear hemodynamically stable but have major injuries, an altered GCS score, or injuries that require lengthy orthopedic or neurosurgical procedures should undergo diagnostic evaluation of the abdomen despite an unremarkable abdominal examination. The abdomen can be quickly evaluated in the emergency department (ED) for presence of hemoperitoneum by use of ultrasonography or *diagnostic peritoneal lavage* (DPL), depending on the expertise available. DPL has been documented to be a safe and accurate examination during pregnancy. Use of the open technique above the umbilicus and above the level of the fundus is recommended. DPL has the advantage of being fast, highly sensitive, and relatively inexpensive, and the patient is under the direct observation of the physician.

Ultrasonography can provide important information regarding the presence or absence of hemoperitoneum or free fluid from perforated abdominal viscera. In addition, ultrasound examination can provide information regarding placental abruption, fetal movement, and the presence of fetal heart motion (Fig. 35-1). Ultrasonography is an excellent diagnostic study because it is noninvasive, involves minimal risk of iatrogenic injury, and involves no radiation exposure. Use of ultrasonography does require the presence of an expert to perform

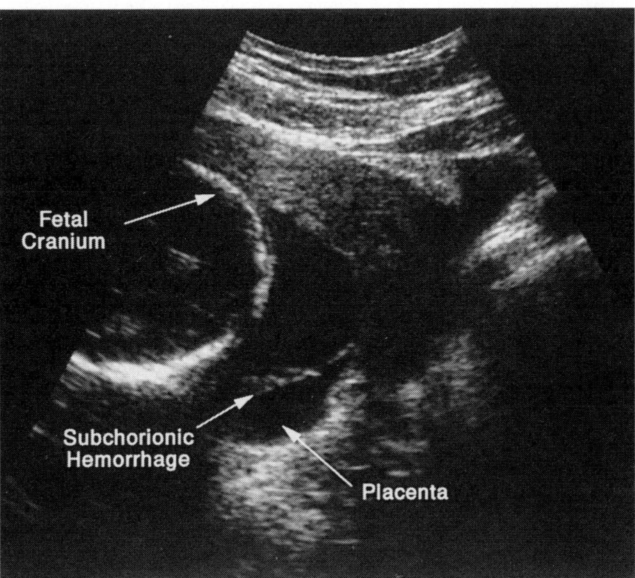

Figure 35–1. Transabdominal ultrasound of the abdomen in a pregnant trauma patient demonstrating the fetal cranium and placenta. The hyperechoic area represents subchorionic hemorrhage, which is characteristic of placental abruption. (Courtesy of Sara Shaves, M.D., Department of Radiology, University of Washington, Harborview Medical Center.)

the examination and interpret results in the emergency setting.

Use of computed tomography (CT) has gained popularity in evaluation of the traumatically injured patient. CT is also noninvasive and accurate, and it affords better visualization of the retroperitoneum and intrauterine structures of the fetus and placenta (Fig. 35–2). Placental injuries, such as hemorrhage and abruption, may be noted on CT scan; however, obtaining a CT scan places the injured patient in the radiology suite, which is not the ideal circumstance for adequate monitoring. Hemodynamically unstable patients are poor candidates for CT scan evaluation. In addition, CT does not provide accurate information regarding injuries to the diaphragm and bowel.

The greatest risk for radiation exposure occurs during the 2nd to 10th weeks of pregnancy, which is the time of organogenesis. By the 20th week of pregnancy, fetal abnormalities secondary to radiation are unlikely. The maximum recommended dose by the National Council on Radiation Protection during pregnancy is 0.5 cGy, although teratogenicity occurs between 5 and 15 rad. Approximately 30% of the dose absorbed by the mother is assimilated by the fetus. Chest and lateral cervical spine films expose the mother to 0.002 cGy, and a pelvic radiograph exposes the mother to 0.36 cGy.[14] Pregnancy should not deter clinically indicated radiographic studies such as abdominal CT scan, intravenous pyelography, and angiography. Protective shielding of the pelvis during radiographic examinations is appropriate.

Intra-abdominal injuries should be managed as in any trauma patient. Immediate laparotomy is indicated for a gunshot wound to the abdomen, for stab wounds with evidence of penetration of the peritoneum, and for evidence of maternal hemoperitoneum combined with hemodynamic instability after blunt trauma. Immediate laparotomy for cesarean section is indicated for signs of fetal distress, depending on fetal age (see Emergent Cesarean Section next).

Pelvic fractures can be a source of massive hemorrhage and have been associated with a 57% fetal death rate.[9] The use of pneumatic antishock garments is controversial in any trauma patient, and inflation of the abdominal compartment is contraindicated in pregnancy. Inflation of the lower-extremity compartments can lead to further bleeding from pelvic veins and should be used with great caution. Angiography and embolization of bleeding pelvic arteries and application of an external fixator to control venous bleeding are modalities used to treat significant bleeding associated with pelvic fracture. Immobilizing the pelvis by a sling, sheet, or beanbag is a readily available alternative and should be employed in all cases while awaiting angiography or placement of an external fixator.

EMERGENT CESAREAN SECTION

Cesarean section may be indicated for fetal distress, placental abruption, uterine rupture, fetal malpresentation in labor, an unstable pelvic fracture, a lumbosacral fracture, and inadequate exposure at the time of trauma laparotomy. To be considered potentially viable, the fetus should weigh at minimum 500 g and be at least of 24 weeks' gestation.[15]

A 1996 study by Morris and coworkers[16] reviewed 441 pregnancies in 114,952 admissions to nine level I trauma centers. Thirty-two of these 441 pregnant patients required emergency cesarean sections. All of these procedures were performed for fetal distress, maternal distress, or both. Fetal distress was defined by bradycardia, decelerations, or lack of fetal heart tones. Maternal distress was defined by a systolic blood pressure less than 90 mm Hg or acute decompensation. Fetal survival was 45% (n = 15), and maternal survival was 72% (n = 23). The absence of fetal heart tones predicted a 100% mortality. If fetal heart tones are absent, treatment should be entirely directed toward maternal survival. An estimated gestational age greater than 26 weeks and presence of fetal heart tones combined gave a 75% fetal survival rate. Infant survival was independent of maternal distress or maternal ISS. In fact, with a maternal ISS above 25, maternal survival was 44% compared with fetal survival of 78%, illustrating the success of immediate recognition of the need for cesarean section.[16] Figure 35–3 illustrates the algorithm recommended by Morris and colleagues for emergent and perimortem cesarean section.

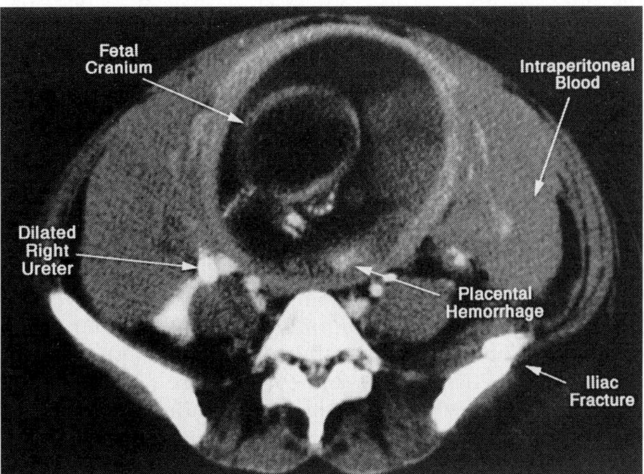

Figure 35–2. CT scan of the abdomen in a pregnant trauma patient depicting free intraperitoneal blood, a dilated right ureter with extravasation of contrast, the enlarged uterus of pregnancy with the fetal cranium visible, and an area of high intensity in the placenta representing hemorrhage. (Courtesy of Frederick Mann, M.D., Department of Radiology, University of Washington, Harborview Medical Center.)

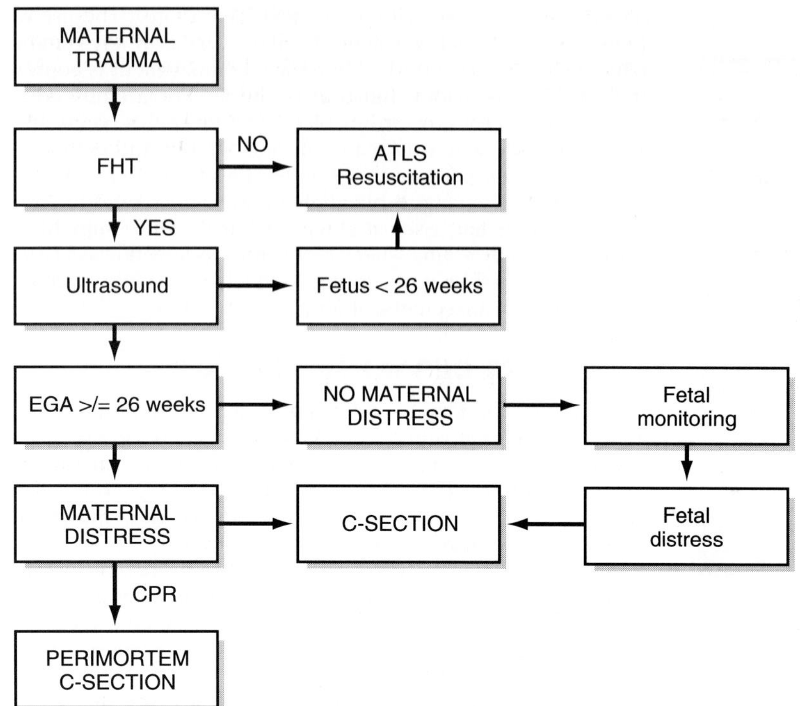

Figure 35–3. Clinical algorithm for emergency cesarean section (C-section) and perimortem cesarean section. EGA = estimated gestational age; FHT = fetal heart tone; ATLS = Advanced Trauma Life Support; CPR = cardiopulmonary resuscitation. (Redrawn from Morris JA, Rosenbower TJ, Jurkovich GJ, et al: Infant survival after cesarean section for trauma. Ann Surg 1996; 223:481–491.)

Approximately 200 successful postmortem cesarean sections have been reported in the literature.[17] The interval between maternal death and cesarean section is crucial. The prognosis for an infant delivered by cesarean section less than 5 minutes after maternal death is excellent, but fetal survival is unlikely if cesarean section is performed 20 minutes after maternal death.[18] Cardiopulmonary resuscitation (CPR) should be continued throughout delivery and maintained after delivery because there have been reports of maternal survival after CPR and cesarean section, presumably secondary to increased venous return and preload after delivery of the fetus.[12]

Patients with devastating neurologic injuries who are brain-dead but who remain hemodynamically stable can have a viable fetus. Emergency cesarean section is not indicated in this situation. The mother should be maintained in the ICU with ventilatory and circulatory support to await further fetal maturation and a more optimal situation for delivery.[19]

PHYSIOLOGY OF THE PREGNANT PATIENT

Overview

Care of the injured pregnant patient requires an understanding of the physiologic changes the body undergoes during pregnancy. The changes that occur in the cardiovascular, respiratory, gastrointestinal, genitourinary, musculoskeletal, endocrine, and hematologic systems during pregnancy are summarized in Tables 35-1 and 35-2. Figure 35-4 illustrates the location of the uterine fundus by gestational age in weeks. Detailed descriptions of the physiologic changes to the cardiovascular and respiratory systems that are most pertinent to the trauma patient follow.

Cardiovascular System

During pregnancy, the total blood volume of the patient increases by approximately 55%. Normal vital signs may be sustained with loss of up to 35% of blood volume.[20] Hence, maternal hemodynamic stability does not guarantee that the fetus is well perfused. In fact, maternal hypotension is a late and ominous sign. Cardiovascular changes create a high-output, low-resistance state. The placenta functions as a modified arteriovenous shunt.

During the first 10 weeks of gestation, cardiac output increases by approximately 40%. This hyperdynamic state is maintained throughout the remainder of the pregnancy. Starting at 10 weeks, the plasma volume increases, reaching 50% by 28 weeks. However, the hematocrit increases by only approximately 20%, resulting in a greater increase in plasma relative to red blood cells, hence the "physiologic anemia of pregnancy." Consequently, the hematocrit decreases from approximately 40% to 32% by the 34th week. Both heart rate and stroke volume increase while blood pressure decreases slightly as a result of increased capacitance. By term, approximately 30% of maternal cardiac output is dedicated to perfusion of the uterus.[21]

The uterus lacks circulatory autoregulation. Catecholamine release prompted by maternal hypovolemia results in decreased perfusion to the peripheral, splanchnic, and uterine circulation and shunting of blood to more vital maternal organs. Maintenance of uterine blood flow is reliant on maternal blood pressure. A decrease of up to 35% of blood volume may have no measurable effect on maternal blood pressure. In this circumstance, the fetus is underperfused despite apparent hemodynamic stability of the mother. Thus, relying on maternal hemodynamic stability as evidence of sufficient fetal perfusion is a grave error. Once maternal hemodynamic instability is noted, the fetus may already have been severely compromised. As previously noted, maternal hypotension has been associated with fetal mortality ranging from 67% to 80%.[8, 9]

Tachycardia, hypotension, and a decrease in central venous pressure are classic evidence of mild hypovolemia, yet they are normal changes of pregnancy. Differentiating normal changes of pregnancy from traumatically induced alterations is a challenge. Positional hypotension may develop when the patient is supine. Compression of the inferior vena cava (IVC)

TABLE 35–1. Anatomic and Functional Alterations of Pregnancy

System	Alteration
Cardiovascular	Increased plasma volume Heart displaced cephalad and rotated Increased heart rate Increased cardiac output Decreased blood pressure Decreased peripheral vascular resistance Decreased central venous pressure
Respiratory	Diaphragm displaced approximately 4 cm cephalad Increased chest circumference Increased tidal volume Decreased functional residual capacity
Gastrointestinal	Increased salivation Increased gastroesophageal reflux Decreased gastroesophageal sphincter competency secondary to progesterone Delayed gastric emptying Decreased gastrointestinal motility Increase in gallbladder volume Decrease in gallbladder emptying Cephalad displacement of intraperitoneal contents by gravid uterus
Genitourinary	Uterus becomes largest intraperitoneal organ Displacement of urinary bladder Dilatation of ureters and renal pelvices Glomerular filtration rate increases by 50%
Musculoskeletal	Symphysis pubis widens Sacroiliac joints widen Unstable gait develops secondary to shift of center of gravity
Endocrine	Pituitary gland doubles in size Increase in parathormone Increase in calcitonin
Hematologic	Mild leukocytosis "Physiologic anemia of pregnancy" Hypercoagulable state

by the gravid uterus decreases preload and results in a decrease in cardiac output. Supine hypotension may be relieved by placing the patient in the left lateral decubitus position. This positioning can be attained while full spinal precautions are maintained by elevating the right side of the patient's backboard to 30°. However, this syndrome occurs in only 10% of pregnant patients, and hemorrhage as the underlying cause of hypotension must be the first assumption until it is vigilantly eliminated. The supine hypotensive syndrome significantly affects the patient's hemodynamic status during the induction of general, epidural, and spinal anesthesia.

The IVC compression syndrome, coupled with hypercoagulability secondary to elevation in fibrinogen and coagulation factors VII, VIII, IX, X, and XII, is a relative contraindication to routine use of lower-extremity intravenous lines. Pregnant patients immobilized in the ICU are at increased risk for development of deep venous thrombosis. Thromboembolic disease (TED) stockings and sequential compression devices should be used for prophylaxis. Subcutaneous heparin prophylaxis and intravenous heparin may be safely used in patients without contraindications to anticoagulation. Low-molecular-weight heparin has not been well studied in pregnancy, but research has demonstrated that an increased dose (40 mg twice daily) is needed. Neither unfractionated nor low-molecular-weight heparin crosses the placenta.[22]

Fluid resuscitation is the mainstay of care of any traumatically injured patient, and the pregnant patient is no different. Lactated Ringer's solution is the most appropriate choice for crystalloid resuscitation. Administration of normal or hypertonic saline can lead to an undesirable hyperchloremic acidosis. As with any nonpregnant trauma patient, vasopressors and inotropes should not be used to elevate blood pressure at the expense of adequate organ perfusion. In the pregnant patient, vasopressors should also be avoided because they further diminish uterine blood flow and are inclined to provoke fetal distress. The only acceptable indications for use of vasopressors are neurogenic spinal shock and significant cardiac contusion with associated cardiac dysfunction. In these cases, invasive monitoring by pulmonary artery catheter should be employed.

Maternal blood volume and hemoglobin oxygen-carrying capacity should always be optimized. Anemia is not well tolerated in the pregnant trauma patient. Transfusion is indicated for blood loss of 1 L or more. Although transfusion of Rh-compatible blood is preferable, type-specific or O-negative blood may be transfused if crossmatched blood is not immediately available and postponing transfusion would result in compromised perfusion. Administration of $Rh_O(D)$ immune globulin is indicated if an Rh-negative mother is exposed to Rh-positive blood or if fetomaternal hemorrhage occurs.

Respiratory System

Placental progesterone stimulates the medullary respiratory center, resulting in a slight increase in respiratory rate. Tidal volume and minute ventilation both increase by 40% beginning in the first trimester. An increase in tidal volume and minute ventilation results in a decreased $Paco_2$ and an elevated serum bicarbonate level, resulting in a chronic compensated respiratory alkalosis. A $Paco_2$ of 40 mm Hg is greatly elevated

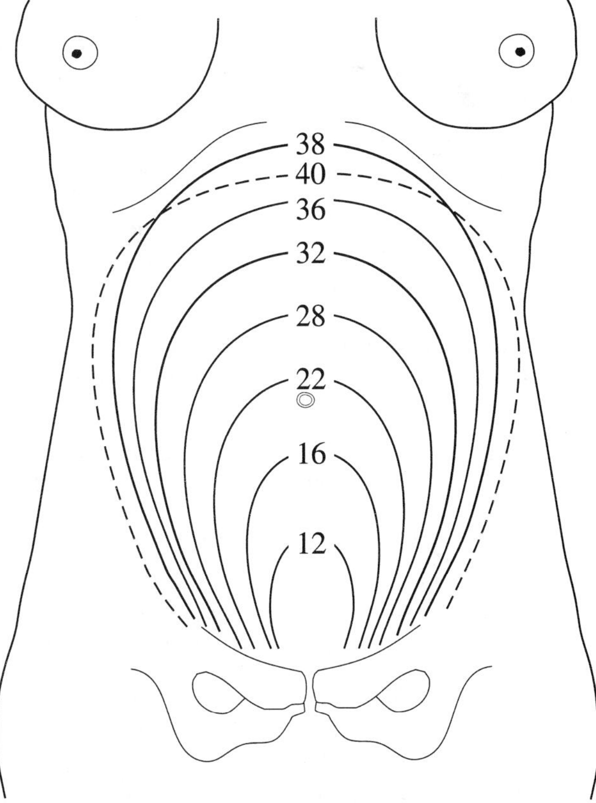

Figure 35–4. Approximate location of the uterine fundus by gestational week.

TABLE 35–2. Physiologic Alterations of Pregnancy

System	Nonpregnant Physiology	Pregnant Physiology	Significance
Cardiovascular			Supine position can decrease venous return by compression of the inferior vena cava Loss of 30% blood volume before hypotension is evident
Heart rate	70–80 bpm	80–95 bpm	
Cardiac output	4.5 L/min	6 L/min	
Stroke volume		Increased	
Systolic blood pressure	110 mm Hg	102–108 mm Hg	
Diastolic blood pressure	70 mm Hg	50–65 mm Hg	
Central venous pressure		Decreased when supine	
Electrocardiogram		Flattened T waves in III, V_1, and V_2 Q waves in III and aVF	
Respiratory			Shorter induction for inhalation anesthetics Chronic respiratory alkalosis
Tidal volume	500 mL	700 mL	
Residual volume	1200 mL	720–960 mL	
Respiratory rate	12–20 bpm	Increased	
pH	7.38–7.44	7.41–7.46	
Po_2	95–100 mm Hg	100–108 mm Hg	
Pco_2	35–45 mm Hg	27–32 mm Hg	
HCO_3	24–30 mm Hg	19–25 mm/L	
Base excess		3–4 mEq/L	
Hematologic			"Physiologic anemia of pregnancy" Elevated white blood cell count may be misinterpreted Hypercoagulable state
Blood volume	4000 mL	5200–6000 mL	
Plasma	2400 mL	3700 mL	
Red blood cells	1600 mL	1900 mL	
Hemoglobin	12–16 g/dL	10–14 g/dL	
Hematocrit	35–48%	32–42%	
White blood cells	4500–10,000/mm^3	5000–14,000/mm^3	
Platelets	150,000–350,000/mm^3	Normal or ≥150,000/mm^3	
Fibrinogen	300 mg/100 mL	600 mg/100 mL	
Coagulation factors		Increased fibrinogen and factors VII, VIII, IX, X, XII	

bpm = beats per minute.

in advanced pregnancy and indicates inadequate ventilation and a probable underlying acidosis. Decreased maternal bicarbonate levels have been correlated with an adverse fetal outcome. A retrospective study of maternal bicarbonate level as an indicator for maternal and subsequent fetal hypoperfusion evaluated 51 injured gravid patients.[23] The mean maternal bicarbonate level was 20.3 ± 2.2 mEq/L with fetal survival compared with 16.4 ± 3 mEq/L with fetal death. Maternal mortality was zero for the higher bicarbonate level compared with 56% for the lower level.

A decrease in functional residual capacity of 20% combined with an increase of 15% in oxygen consumption during pregnancy may result in critical fetal hypoxemia with mild maternal hypoxemia. These alterations in respiratory physiology also result in a shorter induction time for inhalation anesthetics. The fetal oxyhemoglobin dissociation curve is shifted to the left compared with the adult dissociation curve, indicating the greater affinity of fetal hemoglobin for oxygen. This shift of the oxyhemoglobin curve also results in decreased oxygen reserve in the fetus. A low fetal Pao_2 maintains a constant oxygen gradient from placenta to the fetus.[24] Thus, the fetus has little oxygen reserve and quickly becomes hypoxemic if inadequately supplied with oxygen.

Supplemental 100% oxygen should be administered by mask regardless of apparent hemodynamic stability. Whereas monitoring with pulse oximetry provides useful information regarding maternal oxygen saturation, determination of arterial blood gases is essential to evaluate for oxygen content and detrimental acidosis. Early intubation is preferable to placing the fetus at risk for hypoxemia. Aggressive control of the airway and continual maintenance of adequate fetal oxygenation are essential.

INTENSIVE CARE MANAGEMENT OF THE PREGNANT PATIENT

Monitoring

The basic measures of fetal monitoring are fetal heart tones and fetal movement. Monitoring can be performed by either continuous cardiotocographic monitoring (CTM) or interval Doppler evaluation of fetal heart tones every 15 minutes. Use of CTM is preferable to interval Doppler monitoring.

Fetal distress is characterized by decreased variability of fetal heart rate, decelerations after contractions, tachycardia greater than 160 beats per minute, or bradycardia less than 110 beats per minute. The fetus is considered potentially viable at 24 weeks with a weight of at least 500 g. Any fetus of greater than 24 weeks' gestation that is considered viable requires monitoring for at least 4 hours after the traumatic event. In a study by Pearlman and coauthors,[25] all cases of placental abruption were detected within the first 4 hours of monitoring. This minimum of 4 hours should be extended to 24 hours if any clinical signs of abruption, such as vaginal bleeding, are present. Also, if more than one uterine contraction every 15 minutes is noted and still present at 4 hours, monitoring should continue for 24 hours. Some trauma centers mandate a 24-hour protocol for CTM after trauma.[16] When placental disruption is noted and fetal distress is present, cesarean section is required. Small placental disruptions with

TABLE 35–3. Maternal and Fetal Effects of Medications Commonly Employed in the Intensive Care Unit

Medication	Significance
Alpha agonists (i.e., epinephrine)	Uteroplacental vasoconstriction Mild oxytocics
Atropine	No known teratogenicity Minimal effects on fetal heart rate
Benzodiazepines	Possible neonatal CNS depression
Bretylium	Minimal effect, safe
β-Blockers	Fetal bradycardia Intrauterine growth restriction Hypoglycemia
Calcium channel blockers	Maternal hypotension Uterine atony Fetal hypoxemia and acidosis
Dopamine	No known adverse effects Effects on uterine blood flow unknown
Dobutamine	No known adverse effects
Local anesthetics (i.e., lidocaine)	Maternal seizures Fetal acidosis Fetal cardiovascular depression Fetal CNS depression
Narcotics (i.e., morphine, meperidine, and fentanyl)	No teratogenic effects Respiratory depression Decreased FHR variability
Neuromuscular blocking agents	Teratogenicity unknown Neonatal respiratory depression and apnea
Nitroprusside	Transient fetal bradycardia Monitoring of maternal cyanide and methemoglobin levels suggested
Propofol	Increased maternal death and offspring mortality in animal studies No human studies

Data from Briggs GG, Freeman RK, Yaffe JJ: Drugs in Pregnancy and Lactation. 3rd ed. Baltimore, Williams & Wilkins, 1990.
CNS = central nervous system; FHR = fetal heart rate.

no associated fetal distress do not necessarily require cesarean section and can result in viable term pregnancies.

Fetal and Maternal Complications

Premature Labor

The most common obstetric issue after trauma is uterine contractions caused by prostaglandins released by the myometrium and decidual cells. Ninety per cent of contractions after trauma stop spontaneously.[25] Contractions that do not stop usually have an underlying pathologic process, such as a placental abruption. An ultrasound examination or a CT scan should be obtained immediately to evaluate for placental abruption. The use of tocolytics in these cases is generally contraindicated.[25]

Abruptio Placentae

Abruption is a separation of the placenta from the uterine wall that occurs with deceleration forces. Placental abruption is the most common cause of fetal loss in injured patients. Placental abruption occurs in 1% to 5% of minor traumas and in from 30% to 50% of major traumas. Maternal mortality from abruption is less than 1%, but fetal death ranges from 30% to 70%.[7] Abruption can occur with minimal external evidence of trauma. Loss of placental surface for gas exchange can result in fetal hypoxia and carbon dioxide accumulation, leading to fetal distress and death. In addition, abruption can result in disseminated intravascular coagulopathy (DIC) in the mother.

The clinical signs of vaginal bleeding, abdominal cramping, uterine tenderness, amniotic fluid leakage, maternal hypovolemia, an enlarging uterus, and alterations in fetal heart rate are concerns for placental abruption. Fetal distress is more common than vaginal bleeding as an indicator of placental abruption. Confirmation of abruption can be difficult. The sensitivity of transabdominal ultrasonography in detecting small amounts of placental hemorrhage depends on the skill of the operator and the resolution of the equipment. Evidence of retroplacental hematoma or subchorionic hemorrhage is diagnostic of placental abruption.[26, 26a] Fetal heart rate monitoring is more sensitive in identifying placental injury than ultrasound examination.[7]

Uterine Rupture

Much less common than abruptio placentae is uterine rupture. This event has been noted in approximately 1% of pregnant women injured in motor vehicle collisions.[20, 24] Uterine rupture should be suspected when there are easily palpable fetal parts because the fetus has been extruded from the uterus. Fetal heart tones are also often absent. If an unusually large amount of amniotic fluid is found at the time of DPL, suspicion for uterine rupture should be high. Cesarean section may be lifesaving for the fetus if it is still viable.

Fetomaternal Hemorrhage

Fetomaternal hemorrhage is the transplacental hemorrhage of fetal blood into the maternal circulation. This condition has been reported to occur in 28% to 31% of pregnant trauma patients and is unrelated to the severity of injury. Transfusion can lead to maternal Rh sensitization, fetal anemia, exsanguination, or fatal fetal cardiac arrhythmias. The Kleihauer-Betke acid elution test can be used to determine the presence of fetomaternal hemorrhage.

The Kleihauer-Betke test allows an estimate of transfusion volume by identifying fetal red blood cells in maternal peripheral blood smears. Fetal cells stain darkly secondary to hemoglobin F concentrations; maternal cells stain lightly. The sensitivity of the test, 5 fetal red blood cells per 1000 maternal red blood cells, is not sufficient to identify all cases of fetomaternal hemorrhage. Up to 70% of women may be sensitized by only 1 mL of fetal blood.[27] However, this test is potentially useful in known Rh-negative women to assist in quantification of the amount of Rh_O(D) immune globulin (RhoGAM) required. All Rh-negative women who are injured should receive at least 1 ampule of RhoGAM to prevent Rh isoimmunization. One 300-mg ampule of RhoGAM should cover a fetomaternal hemorrhage of up to 15 mL of fetal red blood cells or 30 mL of fetal whole blood. If the estimation of fetomaternal hemorrhage is greater, the dose of Rh immune globulin should be adjusted on the basis of the Kleihauer-Betke test results.

Amniotic Fluid Embolism

Although extremely rare after trauma, amniotic fluid embolism is a noteworthy obstetric condition. Amniotic fluid embolism usually occurs during labor (70%), with cesarean section (19%), or after vaginal delivery (11%), but it has also been reported after pelvic trauma.[28] It is responsible for 10% of maternal deaths in the United States. Maternal mortality is quoted at 60% to 80%. Only 15% of maternal survivors are neurologically intact. Fetal survival is only 39%. DIC develops in 30% of patients with amniotic fluid embolism. Chest radiographs resemble those seen in adult respiratory distress syndrome (ARDS). The clinical and hemodynamic sequelae are similar to those seen with septic shock. A 1995 article by Clark and associates[28] suggests that amniotic fluid embolism is actually an anaphylactic reaction.

ICU care is supportive, and cesarean section should be considered immediately if the fetus is potentially viable, as determined by estimated gestational age and presence of fetal heart tones.

Medications

Numerous medications are useful in caring for the critically injured patient in the ICU. Although commonly used in the ICU, neuromuscular blocking agents (e.g., succinylcholine, vecuronium bromide, pancuronium bromide, and etomidate) have unknown teratogenic effects. However, these paralytic agents do cross the placenta and can cause respiratory depression and apnea in the neonate. Overall, inhaled general anesthetic agents are safe in the pregnant patient.[13]

Several inotropes commonly used in the ICU have significant effects on the gravid patient and the fetus. Following the central tenet that care of the mother is the primary concern, if these pharmacologic agents are necessary, they should be used. An awareness of possible detrimental effects to the pregnancy is important but should not deter their use if they are deemed clinically required. Table 35-3 reviews the effects of these medications on the pregnant patient and fetus.

Administration of prophylactic antibiotics for open fractures or prevention of wound infections in laparotomies is acceptable. Without a significant left shift indicating infection, the upper limit of white blood cell count considered normal during pregnancy is 15,000 and would not require antibiotic therapy. Penicillins and cephalosporins have no reported adverse effects. Aminoglycosides have the potential to cause maternal and fetal nephrotoxicity and ototoxicity. Trimethoprim is a folic acid antagonist and consequently should be avoided in the first trimester. Sulfonamides are contraindicated in late pregnancy because they compete for bilirubin-binding sites on albumin and can cause neonatal kernicterus. Chloramphenicol is contraindicated because of bone marrow toxicity and the "gray baby syndrome." Tetracyclines and quinolones are contraindicated throughout pregnancy secondary to their effects on teeth, bone, and cartilage.[13]

Tetanus toxoid can be administered at any time during pregnancy.[10]

Cardioversion

Elective cardioversion for arrhythmias has been safely performed in all trimesters of pregnancy. Maternal cardioversion with 80 and 200 joules has been shown to have no effect on the fetal heart rhythm.[29] The fetal heart should be monitored during cardioversion although the amount of energy reaching the heart is minimal.

INJURY PREVENTION

Motor vehicle collisions are the most common cause of injury during pregnancy. Properly positioned seat belts do not increase the risk of fetal loss. The lap belt should be placed across the bony pelvis, not the dome of the uterus. Two major studies support the use of seat belts in preventing both maternal and fetal injury in motor vehicle collisions.

In 1971, Crosby and Costiloe[30] retrospectively reviewed 208 pregnant women involved in motor vehicle collisions to ascertain the impact of lap belts; 28 patients were restrained and 180 were unrestrained. There was no evidence that lap belts caused an increase in maternal or fetal mortality. Significantly, mortality for ejected occupants was 33% and was 5% for those occupants not ejected. The associated fetal death rate was 47% when the mother was ejected and 11% when the mother was not ejected.

In 1993, Wolf and colleagues[31] retrospectively reviewed 1243 restrained and 1349 unrestrained pregnant women involved in motor vehicle collisions to examine the impact of lap belts and lap-plus-shoulder harnesses versus no restraining system. Unrestrained drivers were 1.9 times more likely to have a low-birth-weight baby and 2.3 times more likely to give birth within 48 hours after the crash. On the basis of these studies, the American College of Obstetricians and Gynecologists advises use of three-point restraint systems during pregnancy.[32]

Intentional violence does not spare the pregnant woman. The prevalence of domestic violence during pregnancy has been estimated at 8% to 20%.[6] One article noted that 22% of injuries sustained by pregnant patients were caused by abuse.[33] Battered women are more likely to be pregnant or to have recently miscarried than are nonbattered women.[34] Recognition of the high prevalence of domestic abuse as a significant hazard to both the mother and fetus should result in vigilance on the part of the health care professional during both emergency care and routine prenatal care.

Screening for domestic abuse should be a basic component of prenatal care. Medical professionals providing emergency care to the injured pregnant patient should have a high index of suspicion for abuse as the underlying cause. Because violence during pregnancy tends to be recurring, early intervention can positively affect the health of both the mother and child.

References

1. Births and deaths: United States, 1996. Monthly Vital Statistics Report, Vol 46, Supplement 2. Washington, DC, US Department of Health and Human Services, Public Health Service, National Center for Health Statistics, 1996.
2. Peckham C, King R: A study of intercurrent conditions observed during pregnancy. Am J Obstet Gynecol 1963; 87:609.
3. Lavin JP, Polski S: Abdominal trauma during pregnancy. Clin Perinatol 1983; 10:423.
4. Fildes J, Reed L, Jones N, et al: Trauma: The leading cause of maternal death. J Trauma 1992; 32:643.
5. Williams JK, McClain L, Rosemurgy AS: Evaluation of blunt trauma in the third trimester of pregnancy: Maternal and fetal considerations. Obstet Gynecol 1990; 75:33.
6. Peterson R, Gazmararian JA, Spitz AM, et al: Violence and adverse

pregnancy outcomes: A review of the literature and directions for future research. Am J Prev Med 1997; 13:366.
7. Pearlman MD, Tintinalli JE: Evaluation and treatment of the gravida and fetus following trauma during pregnancy. Obstet Gynecol Clin North Am 1991; 18(Suppl 2):371.
8. Rothenberger D, Quattlebaum FW, Perry JF, et al: Blunt maternal trauma: A review of 103 cases. J Trauma 1978; 18:173.
9. Kissinger DP, Rozycki GS, Morris J, et al: Trauma in pregnancy: Predicting pregnancy outcome. Arch Surg 1991; 126:1079.
10. American College of Surgeons Committee on Trauma: Advanced Trauma Life Support Manual. Chicago, American College of Surgeons, 1997.
11. Assali NS, Douglas RA, Baird WW: Measurement of uterine blood flow and uterine metabolism. Am J Obstet Gynecol 1953; 66: 248.
12. Clarke SL: Trauma in pregnancy. *In:* Critical Care Obstetrics. Boston, Blackwell Scientific Publications, 1991, p 498.
13. Esposito TJ: Trauma during pregnancy. Emerg Med Clin North Am 1994; 12:167.
14. Chatterjee MS: Physiology of pregnancy. *In:* Trauma and Pregnancy. Haycock CE (Ed). Littleton, Mass, PSG Publishing Company, 1985, p 78.
15. Amon E: Limits of fetal viability. Obstet Gynecol Clin North Am 1988; 15:321.
16. Morris JA, Rosenbower TJ, Jurkovich GJ, et al: Infant survival after cesarean section for trauma. Ann Surg 1996; 223:481.
17. Katz VL, Potters DJ, Droegemueller W: Perimortem cesarean section. Obstet Gynecol 1986; 68:571.
18. Weber CE: Postmortem cesarean section: Review of the literature and case reports. Am J Obstet Gynecol 1971; 110:158.
19. Anderet NB, Cohen I, Abramowicz JS: Traumatic coma during pregnancy with persistent vegetative state: Case report. Br J Obstet Gynaecol 1984; 91:939.
20. Mighty H: Trauma in pregnancy. Crit Care Clin 1994; 10:623.
21. Neufeld JD, Moore EE, Marx JA, et al: Trauma in pregnancy. Emerg Med Clin North Am 1987; 5:623.
22. Barbour LA: Current concepts of anticoagulant therapy in pregnancy. Obstet Gynecol Clin North Am 1997; 24:499.
23. Scorpio RJ, Esposito TJ, Smith LG, et al: Blunt trauma during pregnancy: Factors affecting fetal outcome. J Trauma 1992; 32:213.
24. Neufield JD: Trauma in pregnancy, what if . . .? Emerg Med Clin North Am 1993; 11:207.
25. Pearlman MD, Tintinalli JE, Lorenz RP: A prospective controlled study of outcome after trauma during pregnancy. Am J Obstet Gynecol 1990; 162:1502.
26. Cunningham FG, MacDonald PC, Gant NF (Eds). Obstetrical hemorrhages. *In:* Williams Obstetrics. 19th ed. Norwalk, Conn, Appleton & Lange, 1997, p 750.
26a. Nyberg DA, Mack LA, Benedetti TJ, et al: Placental abruption and placental hemorrhage: Correlations of sonographic findings with fetal outcome. Radiology 1987; 164:357.
27. Lavery JP, Staten-McCormick M: Management of moderate to severe trauma in pregnancy. Obstet Gynecol Clin North Am 1995; 22:69.
28. Clark SL, Hankins GD, Dudley DA, et al: Amniotic fluid embolism: Analysis of the national registry. Am J Obstet Gynecol 1995; 172:1158.
29. Cullhead I: Cardioversion during pregnancy. Acta Med Scand 1983; 214:169.
30. Crosby WM, Costiloe JP: Safety of lap-belt restraint for pregnant victims of automobile collisions. N Engl J Med 1971; 384:632.
31. Wolf ME, Alexander BH, Rivara FP: A retrospective cohort study of seatbelt use and pregnancy outcome after a motor vehicle crash. J Trauma 1993; 34:116.
32. American College of Obstetricians and Gynecologists (ACOG): Trauma during pregnancy—November 1991. Technical Bulletin No. 161.
33. Connolly AM, Katz VL, Bash KL, et al: Trauma and pregnancy. Am J Perinatol 1997; 14:331.
34. Helton AS, McFarlane J, Anderson ET: Battered and pregnant: A prevalence study. Am J Public Health 1987; 77:1337.
35. Briggs GG, Freeman RK, Yaffe SJ: Drugs in Pregnancy and Lactation. 3rd ed. Baltimore, Williams & Wilkins, 1990.

36

Trauma Care of the Elderly

Mihae Yu, MD

Trauma is no longer a problem inflicting primarily the young; it is the fifth most common cause of death in people above 65 years of age. With the population aging, the U.S. Census Bureau estimates that 52 million Americans will be 65 years old or more by the year 2040 and will make up 23% of the population. The oldest old (>85 years) are the fastest-growing portion of the population, with an estimated contribution of 12.2 million lives in the year 2040. One half of the population in an intensive care unit (ICU) is over age 65 years.[1] Although 12.7% of the population is 65 years or older, 29% of trauma-related deaths are in this older age group.[2] Critical care of the older trauma patient is a reality, and ethical issues regarding life expectancy and quality of life are dilemmas in the era of cost containment.

Increasing age may be associated with higher mortality in the injured[3-6] but may not be as important as severity of injury[7-9] or physiologic reserve of the patient[10]; age, degree of injury, and premorbid condition may each contribute to both acute and long-term prognosis.[4, 11] This chapter reviews the goals of acute resuscitation and treatment of the critically injured elderly patients, with special emphasis on early hemodynamic monitoring and support.

PHYSIOLOGIC CHANGES AND CONCURRENT MORBIDITY WITH AGE

Although the general definition of a geriatric population begins at age 65, the physiologic changes with aging are a gradual and individual process. With age, the myocardium demonstrates decreased numbers of myocytes and sinus node cells, and there is a higher incidence of atrial dysrythmias and sick sinus syndrome.[12, 13] Cardiac output diminishes over the years, with only half of the cardiac output decline explained by decreased oxygen (O_2) demands.[14] Early diastolic filling diminishes with age, and ventricular filling or preload becomes more dependent on atrial contraction.[12] Reduced left ventricular filling may be a normal aging phenomenon.[15] Exercise-induced maximum heart rate response[16] and increment in ejection fraction decrease with senescence,[17] although chronic exercise seems to attenuate this response to aging.[12, 17] Less arterial distensibility and baroreceptor reflex and lack of homeostatic mechanisms make older people more susceptible to hemodynamic changes.[12]

The prolongation of relaxation time of the myocardium, in combination with increased stiffness of the ventricle, leads to higher left ventricular end-diastolic pressure with increased susceptibility to pulmonary edema and congestive heart failure despite normal systolic function.[12] The incidence of congestive heart failure increases with age, and it is important to differentiate systolic from diastolic dysfunction because treatment differs.[12] Vasodilating and inotropic agents, digoxin, and diuretics are effective for treatment of systolic dysfunction, whereas diastolic dysfunction requires maintenance of preload, calcium channel blockers, angiotensin-converting enzyme inhibitors, and β-adrenergic antagonists.[12]

With increasing years, the pulmonary system manifests a

lower Pao_2, reduced chest wall compliance, respiratory muscle strength, and altered immune response.[18] The mortality rate with respiratory failure is reported to be higher in patients above 60 years old than in younger patients.[19] Older patients demonstrate decreased blood flow to the liver and kidneys despite normal liver function test results and serum creatinine levels with increased susceptibility to ischemia.[20] The kidneys are less able to concentrate with age.[21, 22] Unrecognized liver and renal dysfunction, despite normal biochemical parameters, may lead to overdosing of medications.

Immunosuppression with less antibody production, T-lymphocyte dysfunction, and inability to clear bacteria have been reported with age,[23, 24] resulting in higher mortality due to compromised immune response.[24] A sharp increase in nosocomial infection, including bacteremia and pneumonia after age 49, is seen.[23, 25, 26] Fever in response to infection or inflammation may be absent in the elderly,[23] and inability to mount a febrile response (hypothermia) may be associated with a worse prognosis.[19]

The incidence of diabetes mellitus increases over the years.[27] Hormonal imbalance, such as hypothyroidism[28] and adrenal response to stress, need to be assessed and monitored, especially during a prolonged course in the ICU.[27, 29] The general nutritional state of the patient and the inability to mount a protein response in the elderly[30] should be considered when nutritional support is planned.

The incidence of preexisting morbidities in older trauma victims is well documented,[4, 10] and the prevalence of cardiopulmonary disease may be as high as 70% or more, depending on the study group.[11, 31] Concomitant use of aspirin and coumadin for underlying cardiovascular disease may cause relatively minor injuries to become major sources of bleeding. Use of calcium channel blockers and β-blockers as well as intrinsic cardiac disease may block the normal response to stress and hemorrhage. Chronic diuretic use with volume contraction increases susceptibility to blood volume loss.[29] Inability to accomplish vasoconstriction in response to the cool environment make the elderly susceptible to hypothermia with its devastating complications of bleeding. Acute care of the traumatized elderly patients continues to be a challenge.

EARLY RESUSCITATION AND TREATMENT

After the initial peak in mortality due to head injury and hemorrhage, the most common cause of death in older trauma victims is multisystem organ failure and sepsis.[10, 32] Preventable deaths may contribute to a third of all deaths, and more than half of the deaths related to multisystem organ failure may be due to lack of timely cardiopulmonary support.[32]

There are two fundamental principles of resuscitation: (1) early recognition of shock and (2) maintenance of tissue perfusion. Early (<12 to 24 hr) treatment of shock, payment of oxygen debt, and prevention of inflammatory mediator response to ischemia are vital for patient survival.[33, 34]

Although it is agreed that early treatment of shock is desirable, tissue ischemia may not be clinically evident until multisystem organ failure process has already been initiated. Shoemaker and colleagues[35] have demonstrated the pitfalls of relying on vital signs, urine output, pH, and Po_2 and reported no differences between survivors and nonsurvivors. A common error is to wait for patients to demonstrate hemodynamic instability before inserting a pulmonary artery catheter with treatment to a physiologic endpoint. Because there seems to be a short time interval when treatment is most effective in having an impact on survival, selection of high-risk patients by the disease process and comorbid conditions is a practical approach.

Older patients may demonstrate deceptively normal vital signs despite a low cardiac output and mixed venous oxygen saturation (Svo_2).[36] Scalea and colleagues[36] demonstrated an improved survival rate of 53% in patients older than 65 years of age with diffuse blunt trauma with early (<2.2 hr) hemodynamic monitoring and augmentation of cardiac output. Historical controls averaged 5.5 hours before invasive monitoring and treatment with a survival rate of only 7%. Expeditious placement of pulmonary artery catheter and treatment to augment oxygen delivery, as necessary, to meet oxygen consumption has been demonstrated to improve survival in trauma victims[37] as well as in high-risk surgical patients[35, 38–40] Intensive care medicine has to be preventive medicine because delay of treatment until after development of multisystem organ failure results in high mortality rates.

The second principle of resuscitation is to deliver sufficient oxygen to meet the metabolic demands of the tissues and to maintain a healthy balance between oxygen delivery (Do_2) and volume of oxygen consumption (Vo_2):

$$\begin{gathered}O_2 \text{ delivery (mL/min/m}^2) = \\ [(\text{hemoglobin g/dL} \times 1.36 \text{ mL } O_2/\text{g hemoglobin} \times Sao_2) \\ + (0.0031 \text{ mL } O_2/100 \text{ mL blood/mm Hg} \times Pao_2 \text{ mm Hg})] \\ \times (\text{cardiac index L/min/m}^2 \times 10)\end{gathered}$$

Oxygen delivery relies on maintenance of three major components: (1) hemoglobin, (2) cardiac index, and (3) arterial saturation. Oxygen consumption may be derived by two techniques: (1) the reverse Fick equation and (2) indirect calorimetry.[41] The reverse Fick equation requires measurement of mixed venous O_2 saturation from the pulmonary artery:

$$\begin{gathered}O_2 \text{ consumption (mL/min/m}^2) = \\ (\text{arterial content of oxygen} - \text{mixed venous content of } O_2) \\ \times \text{cardiac index} \times 10\end{gathered}$$

Indirect calorimetry requires a metabolic gas monitor to calculate the amount of oxygen consumed from gas measurements at the patient's mouthpiece. Problems with each technique and relevance to the clinical area have been discussed previously.[41] The normal oxygen extraction ratio (O_2 ER), calculated as Vo_2/Do_2, is 0.25 in a nonexercising subject.[42]

HEMODYNAMIC GOALS

With the stress of trauma and/or hemorrhagic shock, metabolic demands are higher. In younger patients, the cardiopulmonary system may respond appropriately by augmenting cardiac output with increased heart rate, stroke volume, or both. Older subjects have demonstrated an inability to respond to exercise with the same degree of stroke volume as younger subjects.[14] Yu and associates[40] reported that critically ill patients requiring pulmonary artery catheterization and age 50 years or older had a 83% probability of not self-generating a Do_2 above 600 mL/min/m² or more in the first 24 hours of resuscitation. Inability of the cardiopulmonary system to rise to the occasion to compensate for higher metabolic demands or payment of oxygen debt increases the risk of multisystem organ failure and death.[34]

The quantity of oxygen delivery necessary to meet the tissue demands varies with the patient's age, sex, and premorbid condition as well as the disease process. Shock and colleagues[43] observed that Vo_2 remained constant in healthy males aged 20 to 97 years until age 45, then decreased with every decade. The exercise-trained elderly subjects demonstrated less decline in Vo_2 compared to the sedentary subjects.[16] This finding implies that the exercise-trained elderly may need higher Do_2 than their sedentary colleagues, but the conditioned heart should be able to respond by increasing cardiac output proportionately. Other factors affecting Vo_2 are (1) sex, with women generally consuming less oxygen,[16] and (2) stress hormone levels.[44] Older women with a sedentary lifestyle and a lower baseline oxygen consumption may require less oxygen delivery compared with active younger men.

Differences in hemodynamic variables with age were demonstrated by Shoemaker and colleagues[45] in 708 high-risk surgical patients. Although higher increases in oxygen transport variables were observed after surgery in survivors than in nonsurvivors, careful analysis revealed that preoperative baseline cardiac index, Do_2, Vo_2, and postoperative augmentation of these parameters decreased with age, hemorrhage, hypovolemia, and cardiac impairment and increased with cirrhosis, sepsis, and other types of trauma. This study demonstrated the difference in cardiac index between survivors and nonsurvivors and its relationship to age in decades above age 50 years. As age increased, the absolute values of cardiac index decreased, although survivors continued to demonstrate higher levels compared with nonsurvivors.

The minimum standard of care in the resuscitation of critically ill patients of all ages is as follows:

- Achievement of normal vital signs (based on the individual's premorbid values)
- Urine output of greater than 30 to 50 mL/hr (based on the patient's size and renal function)
- Svo_2 above 65% (preferably $\geq$70%)
- O_2 delivery to meet the O_2 demands of the tissues

Literature reports variations of the same theme in the hemodynamic goals used. In trauma victims, Fleming and colleagues[37] aimed to achieve cardiac index above 4.5 L/min, Vo_2 above 166 mL/min/m^2, and Do_2 above 670 mL/min/m^2. In "high-risk" surgical patients[38] and in a heterogenous group of patients, including those with hemorrhagic shock,[39, 40] a Do_2 goal of 600 mL/min/m^2 or higher was used. Improved survival was found in patients who were able to attain a higher Do_2 level; however, these studies[37-40] included patients of all ages, although the median patient age in the study by Boyd and colleagues[38] was 70 years.

A prospective randomized trial, assessing patients 50 years of age or older who were unable to generate Do_2 $\geq$600 mL/min/m^2, with sepsis, septic shock, systemic inflammatory response syndrome (SIRS), and acute respiratory distress syndrome (ARDS), demonstrated improved survival in patients between ages 50 and 70 years in whom cardiac output was augmented to Do_2 600 mL/min/m^2 or more within the first 24 hours of pulmonary artery catheter insertion.[46] The control group was treated in order to attain normal vital signs and urine output as well as Do_2 of 450 to 550 mL/min/m^2. Survival benefit was not demonstrated in patients older than 75 years of age. The O_2 ERs of patients above 75 years of age were below 0.20 in both the treatment and control groups, suggesting that the lower Do_2 level of 450 to 550 mL/min/m^2 was adequate to meet the demands of the tissues. Although this study was not restricted to only trauma victims, it assessed the older population separately and demonstrated that the very old (>75 years of age) may not need as high a Do_2 level because the baseline metabolic rate may be lower.[16, 43]

Since the normal O_2 ER is below 0.25 in a nonexercising subject, ratios above 0.25 imply inadequate reserve in Do_2 to meet the tissue demands.[42] Weissman and colleagues[47] described different responses to increased oxygen demand according to the hemodynamic state of critically ill patients; patients a with high Do_2 and an O_2 ER at 0.20 or lower increased their O_2 ER whereas those with a lower DO_2 and an O_2 ER at 0.20 or above increased their cardiac output. Placing patients at a higher Do_2 level and a lower O_2 ER state may enable tissues to extract more oxygen in response to stress, since spontaneous increases in cardiac output may not be a luxury available to older and diseased hearts. Association between improved survival and lower O_2 ER has been reported in high-risk patients[38] and in patients with sepsis, ARDS, SIRS, and septic shock between 50 and 75 years of age.[46] In the latter study, the O_2 ER at 24 hours of resuscitation was 0.23 $\pm$ 0.06 in the treatment group and 0.26 $\pm$ 0.05 in the control group (statistically significant). No prospective randomized trials treating patients to reach an O_2 ER goal of less than 0.25 have been reported, although clinical trials are being initiated.

If the balance between Do_2 and Vo_2 is essential, decreasing the oxygen demands in patients with poor cardiopulmonary reserve may be an important aspect of treatment. Manthous and colleagues[48] estimated a 9.7% $\pm$ 3.4% decrease in Vo_2 with every degree in centigrade cooling. Sedation[49] and good pain control[50] are valuable aspects of acute treatment, and improvements in arterial saturation, Svo_2 and cardiac output may be observed with relief of nociceptive stimuli. Although the benefits of heavy sedation and paralyzing agents in acute resuscitation of patients with marginal cardiopulmonary status has not been confirmed, it may help to divert the limited oxygen delivery to vital organs rather than to an active skeletal muscle system. As a result of rapid onset of muscle atrophy, the need for sedatives and paralyzing agents should be reassessed frequently and weaning should take place as soon as physiologic parameters allow.

OXYGEN DELIVERY GOALS

Because achievement of higher levels of oxygen delivery has been repeatedly shown to be related to survival,[34-40, 45] it is important to review the therapy aimed to optimize oxygen delivery in patients with severe injury of all types and all ages, since the principles are similar. The three components of oxygen delivery are:

- Arterial saturation
- Hemoglobin
- Cardiac output

Optimizing Arterial Saturation

As a result of pulmonary changes with age (see earlier) and the high incidence of concomitant cardiopulmonary disease,[4, 10] the threshold for intubation should be lower in older patients before irreversible hypoxic damage of vital organs (e.g., myocardial infarction) occurs. Clinicians need to look for subtle signs of distress, such as an inappropriately normal $Paco_2$ despite a metabolic acidosis or use of accessory respiratory muscles despite a normal respiratory rate. Attributing a high $Paco_2$ to a patient's history of smoking or of chronic obstructive pulmonary disease is dangerous unless such a history is clearly documented in previous medical records.

The goal of ventilator support is to achieve arterial saturation of 90% or above on a nontoxic FiO_2 (<50–60%) while minimizing the work of breathing. Each increase in ventilator support leading to higher intrathoracic pressure must be followed by a reassessment of the cardiac system to ensure stability. The threshold for pulmonary artery catheter insertion should be lower for elderly patients. Nonpulmonary causes of a decrease in Pao_2 can be determined only by sampling Svo_2. A decrease in cardiac output, increased oxygen consumption, or a falling hemoglobin level will result in a lower Svo_2, leading to a decrease in arterial Po_2 in patients with a moderate amount (>20%) of intrapulmonary shunt. Increasing ventilator support when the cause of a Pao_2 decline is nonpulmonary may result in further compromise of cardiac output and worsening of the Svo_2 and Pao_2. The safest approach is to increase FiO_2 until individual components of the cardiopulmonary system have been assessed by measuring hemoglobin, cardiac output, and arterial blood gas and by evaluating factors that increase oxygen consumption. Changes and therapy of the pulmonary system must be done in conjunction with cardiac assessment and treatment.

Optimizing Hemoglobin

Blood transfusions should be administered on an individual basis, depending on the patient's age, underlying cardiopulmonary disease, symptoms, life expectancy, and expected future blood loss. Hemoglobin is an important variable in the oxygen delivery equation. It is estimated that for every 1 g of hemoglobin decrease, cardiac output must increase by 9% in order to maintain same oxygen delivery.[51] Although an appropriate increase in cardiac output in response to anemia has been documented in younger patients,[52] patients with myocardial problems—whether due to traumatic contusion or inherent myocardial disease—may not mount an appropriate response.[53]

Under normal conditions, myocardial tissue is at maximum extraction. As hemoglobin levels fall, coronary blood must increase either by coronary vasodilatation or by increasing cardiac output in order to maintain the same oxygen delivery to the myocardium. Canine models have demonstrated that animals with coronary artery stenosis are less able to tolerate lower hemoglobin levels than control animals with normal coronary arteries.[54, 55] A lower left ventricular stroke work index[54] and compromised oxygen transport to specific organs have been demonstrated.[55] Fan and colleagues[56] observed the best hematocrit value for oxygen transport in dogs differed for individual organs, with the optimum hematocrit value being 45% for the body as a whole.

Older patients unable to bring about augmented cardiac output and oxygen delivery in response to increased tissue demands may be at risk for myocardial damage and multisystem organ failure. Myocardial damage should be considered in older patients with hemodynamic instability. Routine screening of a heterogeneous group of surgical ICU patients reported 11 of 89 patients (12%) to have myocardial infarction (MI) at the time of ICU admission.[40] Similar screening of patients 50 years and older with hemorrhagic shock who were unable to mount a Do_2 600 mL/min/m^2 or above demonstrated a surprisingly high incidence of myocardial damage in 19 of 37 patients at time of ICU entry.[57] Another study of patients aged 50 to 75 years with sepsis, ARDS, SIRS, and septic shock reported 10 of 66 patients to have an MI at time of ICU admission.[46]

An increased incidence of MI and mortality has been reported in patients with a cardiac history with either lower hemoglobin levels[58] or fewer red blood cell transfusions.[59] A retrospective study of trauma victims older than 60 years of age demonstrated that survivors had higher hemoglobin levels (12.1 g/dL) and higher Do_2 than did nonsurvivors.[10] A prospective randomized trial infusing red blood cells liberally to maximize oxygen delivery to 600 mL/min/m^2 or above resulted in a significantly greater hemoglobin level of 13.5 ± 1.5 g/dL, a higher Do_2 and better survival in the treatment group than in the control group, with an average hemoglobin level of 12.3 $\pm$ 1.1 g/dL and Do_2 of 450 to 550 mL/min/m^2.[46] Red blood cells should be administered more liberally in patients with known coronary artery disease or myocardial dysfunction and should be titrated to a normal Svo_2 and desired Do_2. A higher hematocrit level than the traditional value of 30% may improve oxygen transport and reduce mortality in subjects with coexisting cardiac dysfunction.

Optimizing Cardiac Output

Cardiac output is dependent on preload, afterload, and contractility. Optimization of preload is the first step in augmenting cardiac output. Higher filling pressures are observed in the older age group with exercise because of stiffer ventricles secondary to deposition of collagen.[14] The "optimum" pulmonary artery occlusion pressure (PAOP) is a constantly changing value that is dependent on the patient's myocardial compliance and valvular function. Mitral valve dysfunction may cause elevated PAOP readings despite lower left ventricular end-diastolic pressures. Myocardial compliance may decrease with acute ischemia from coronary artery disease, contusion from trauma, and high intrathoracic pressure transmitted by positive-pressure ventilation, and a higher PAOP may be necessary to generate an optimum stroke volume. Increased intra-abdominal pressures from surgery and third spacing of fluids may cause elevation of diaphragm and high intrathoracic pressures. Intra-abdominal compartmental syndrome may cause elevated PAOP readings despite hypovolemia, and this syndrome needs to be recognized and treated with surgical decompression when necessary.[60]

Although some clinicians fear fluid resuscitation, especially in patients with pulmonary contusion, hypovolemia and tissue ischemia may aggravate pulmonary dysfunction and ARDS by stimulating mediator release.[61] Blood volume deficit may be a major contributor to development of ARDS.[61] There were no differences in fluid balance between survivors and nonsurvivors in patients 50 years of age or older with ARDS, SIRS, sepsis, and septic shock.[46] Even in situations of extreme capillary leak (septic models), large amounts of volume were not associated with worsening pulmonary shunt when oxygen delivery was maintained.[61] Euvolemia should be the goal of fluid resuscitation. High PAOP ($>$18 mm Hg) may lead to high-pressure pulmonary edema, and most clinicians give fluids up to a PAOP of 15 to 18 mm Hg as clinically indicated.

Afterload manipulation may not be an option in hypotensive patients. Hypertension is more common in the elderly despite hypovolemia, and careful initiation of vasodilators may augment cardiac output. After every therapeutic maneuver—whether it be volume infusion or changing dosages of vasoactive agents—reassessment of preload, afterload, and cardiac output is mandatory. Preload is expected to decrease after initiation of vasodilating agents, and volume infusion may be needed to place the heart on the optimum filling pressure point of the ventricular function curve. If the goals of cardiac output, Svo_2, and oxygen delivery are not achieved with adequate preload and afterload reduction, blood or inotropic agents should be considered.

Augmenting contractility with inotropic agents is a controversial area. Although inotropic agents increase myocardial oxygen consumption, simultaneous improvement of oxygen delivery to the coronary arteries may compensate for higher oxygen demand. Although some practitioners are reluctant to use inotropic agents in older patients for fear of increasing myocardial ischemia, routine screening of patients who have undergone augmentation to a Do_2 of 600 mL/min/m^2 or higher with inotropic therapy have not demonstrated an increased incidence of MI [38, 40, 46] Most patients with an MI died of multisystem organ failure rather than a cardiac event.[40, 46] The benefits of maintaining tissue perfusion (including the myocardial tissue) seem to outweight the risks of inotropic agents.

Our prospective randomized trial of older patients, between 50 and 75 years of age with ARDS, SIRS, sepsis, and septic shock, enrolled more patients who arrived with an MI into the high Do_2 group and significantly more patients were treated with inotropic agents. Improved survival was demonstrated in patients treated to a $Do_2 \geq 600$ mL/min/m^2 compared to the control group treated to a Do_2 between 450 and 550 mL/min/m^2.[46] The dangers of using vasoactive drugs in older patients with an MI was not confirmed. The current treatment of patients with cardiac disease is to decrease myocardial oxygen consumption with β-blockers and afterload reduction—the antithesis of augmenting cardiac output. The short-term goals of inotropic support in the acute phase of resuscitation are different from the long-term goals of preserving a diseased myocardium. Owing to the high mortality (≥40%) once organ failure occurs and the hospital charges averaging more than $200,000 per patient,[39, 40, 46] the benefits of Do_2 augmentation with vasoactive agents may outweigh the risks. The very old (>age 75 years) may not need the same degree of Do_2 augmentation, and careful consideration of patient requirements by monitoring Svo_2 and O_2 ER is a practical approach.

Weaning Support

The goal of acute resuscitation aims for a higher Do_2 level than the patient's premorbid state to satisfy increased metabolic demands. When reversal of tissue ischemia is achieved as best as can be assessed clinically, it is important to withdraw active support and allow a return to baseline hemodynamic states. Weaning the patient from vasoactive, sedating, and paralyzing agents is done in a stepwise fashion with frequent reassessments. Clinical judgment is used to determine the optimal hemodynamic parameters in relation to the state of the disease process. A patient requiring a PAOP of 20 mm Hg to maintain normal blood pressure during the first 24 hours of injury caused by a noncompliant myocardium may do equally well with lower filling pressures as cardiac compliance improves with time. A lower hemoglobin level may be tolerated after the acute shock state is over. The goals of treatment and acceptable hemodynamic parameters should change with the patient's disease state and time course.

CONSIDERATIONS AFTER INTENSIVE CARE

The stress of acute trauma may unmask a previously unknown disease, such as a cardiac problem, or may aggravate a known condition, such as renal dysfunction or diabetes mellitus. Close communication with the primary physician is important for long-term follow-up of chronic diseases. Initiation of a cardiac workup should be done in patients with documented myocardial ischemia or damage when they are stable enough to undergo diagnostic and therapeutic interventions.

The elderly are more tolerant of disability and have a more positive attitude than the younger cohorts with the same functional diasbility.[8] Physicians' personal views on quality of life should not be imposed.[1] Post-hospital follow-up studies on the elderly injured have demonstrated good results. Eighty-nine per cent of blunt trauma survivors aged 65 years or over ultimately returned home. Two-year follow-up found no differences in functional recovery between those aged 60 years old or more or younger with an Injury Severity Score 16 or above.[6] Specific groups of patients may not have such a good outcome. Only 49% of patients 65 years of age or older with proximal femur fractures returned home.[31] Early involvement of geriatric experts and aggressive rehabilitation measures may improve functional outcome.[63]

Preventive measures to avoid trauma in the elderly would be cost-effective.[3, 4] Older trauma victims consume one third of the trauma expense. Reimbursement by Diagnosis-Related Groups (DRGs) grossly underestimates true cost, since length of hospital stay in patients 65 years of age or older is twice as long as expected.[3] As the patient ages, the most frequent cause of geriatric trauma in patients above 80 years of age is falls, followed by motor vehicle accidents, then automobile versus pedestrian accidents. For patients under 80 years old, the frequency of motor vehicle accidents surpasses falls.[5] With an aging population, prevention of falls is important, and society needs to address these safety issues for homes as well as public institutions.[5]

It is evident that literature does not support resource allocation based on age alone. Although the elderly may have higher hospital mortality rates either due to comorbidity or higher severity of injury,[3, 4, 6, 7] the decision to withdraw life support should be based on the severity of illness, comorbidities, and quality of life acceptable to the patient rather than on age.

References

1. Adelman RD, Berger JT, Macina LO: Critical care for the geriatric patient. Clin Geriatr Med 1994; 10:19.
2. Melton SM, Patton JH, Lyden SP, et al: Care of the geriatric trauma patient. Tenn Med 1996; 89:291.
3. Finelli FC, Jonsson J, Champion HR, et al: A case control study for major trauma in geriatric patients. J Trauma 1989; 29:541.
4. Gubler KE, Davis R, Koepsell T, et al: Long-term survival of elderly trauma patients. Arch Surg 1997; 132:1010.
5. Schwab CW, Kauder DR: Trauma in the geriatric patient. Arch Surg 1992; 127:701.
6. van der Sluis CK, Klasen HJ, Eisma WH, et al: Major trauma in young and old: What is the difference? J Trauma Injury Infect Crit Care 1996; 40:78.
7. Shabot MM, Johnson CL: Outcome from critical care in the "oldest old" trauma patients. J Trauma Injury Infect Crit Care 1995; 39:254.
8. Rockwood K, Noseworthy TW, Gibney RTN, et al: One-year outcome of elderly and young patients admitted to intensive care units. Crit Care Med 1993; 21:687.
9. Mahul PH, Perrot D, Tempelhoff G, et al: Short and long term prognosis, functional outcome following ICU for the elderly. Intensive Care Med 1991; 17:7.
10. Horst HM, Obeid FN, Sorenson VJ, et al: Factors influencing survival of elderly trauma patients. Crit Care Med 1986; 14:681.
11. DeMaria EJ, Kenney PR, Merriam MA, et al: Aggressive trauma care benefits the elderly. J Trauma 1987; 27:1200.
12. Wei JY: Age and the cardiovascular system. N Engl J Med 1992; 327:1735.
13. Olivetti G, Melissari M, Capasso MJ, et al: Cardiomyopathy of the aging human heart: Myocyte loss and reactive cellular hypertrophy. Circ Res 1991; 68:1560.
14. Granath A, Jonsson B, Strandell T: Circulation in healthy old men, studied by right heart catheterization at rest and during exercise in supine and sitting position. Acta Med Scand 1964; 176:425.
15. Sartori MP, Quinones MA, Kuo LC: Relation of Doppler-derived left ventricular filling parameters to age and radius/thickness ratio in normal and pathologic states. Am J Cardiol 1987; 59:1179.
16. Ogawa T, Spina RJ, Martin WH: Effects of aging, sex, and physical training on cardiovascular responses to exercise. Circulation 1992; 86:494.
17. Wei JY, Li YX, Lincoln T, et al: Chronic exercise training protects aged cardiac muscle against hypoxia. J Clin Invest 1989; 83:778.
18. Meyer KC, Ershler W, Rosenthal NS, et al: Immune dysregulation in the aging human lung. Am J Respir Crit Care Med 1996; 153:1072.
19. Gee MH, Gottlieb JE, Albertine KH, et al: Physiology of aging related to outcome in the adult respiratory distress syndrome. J Appl Physiol 1990; 69:822.
20. Van Dam J, Zeldis JB: Hepatic diseases in the elderly. Gastroenterol Clin North Am 1990; 19:459.
21. Demarest GB, Osler TM, Clevenger FW: Injuries in the elderly: Evaluation and initial response. Geriatrics 1990; 45:36.
22. Pesola GR, Akhavan I, Carlon GC, et al: Urinary creatinine excretion in the ICU: Low excretion does not mean inadequate collection. Am J Crit Care 1993; 2:462.
23. Smith PW: Nosocomial infections in the elderly. Infect Dis Clin North Am 1989; 3:763.

24. Smith PW, Roccaforte JS, Daly PB: Infection and immune response in the elderly. Ann Epidemiol 1992; 2:813.
25. Haley RW, Hooton TM, Culver DH, et al: Nosocomial infections in U.S. hospitals, 1975–1976. Am J Med 1981; 70:947.
26. Gross PA, Rapuano C, Adrignolo A, et al: Nosocomial infections: Decade-specific risk. Infect Control 1983; 4:145.
27. Desai D, March R, Watters JM: Hyperglycemia after trauma increases with age. J Trauma 1989; 29:719.
28. Van den Berghe G, de Zegher F: Anterior pituitary function during critical illness and dopamine treatment. Crit Care Med 1996; 24:1580.
29. Santora TA, Schinco MA, Trooskin SZ: Management of trauma in the elderly patient. Surg Clin North Am 1994; 74:163.
30. Jeevanandam M, Young DH, Ramias L, et al: Effect of major trauma on plasma free amino acid concentrations in geriatric patients. Am J Clin Nutr 1990; 51:1040.
31. Sartoretti C, Sartoretti-Schefer S, Ruckert R, et al: Comorbid conditions in old patients with femur fractures. J Trauma Injury Infect Crit Care 1997; 43:570.
32. Pellicane JV, Byrne K, DeMaria EJ: Preventable complications and death from multiple organ failure among geriatric trauma victims. J Trauma 1992; 33:440.
33. Moore FA, Haenel JB, Moore EE, et al: Incommensurate oxygen consumption in response to maximal oxygen availability predicts post injury multiple organ failure. J Trauma 1992; 33:58.
34. Bishop MH, Shoemaker WC, Appel PL, et al: Prospective randomized trial of survivor values of cardiac index, oxygen delivery, and oxygen consumption as resuscitation endpoints in severe trauma. J Trauma 1995; 38:780.
35. Shoemaker WC, Appel PL, Kram HB, et al: Prospective trial of supranormal values of survivors as therapeutic goals in high-risk surgical patients. Chest 1988; 94:1176.
36. Scalea TM, Simon HM, Duncan AO, et al: Geriatric blunt multiple trauma: Improved survival with early invasive monitoring. J Trauma 1990; 30:129.
37. Fleming A, Bishop M, Shoemaker W, et al: Prospective trial of supranormal values as goals of resuscitation in severe trauma. Arch Surg 1992; 127:1175.
38. Boyd O, Grounds M, Bennett ED: A randomized clinical trial of the effect of deliberate perioperative increase of oxygen delivery on mortality in high-risk surgical patients. JAMA 1993; 270:2699.
39. Yu M, Levy MM, Smith P, et al: Effect of maximizing oxygen delivery on morbidity and mortality rates in critically ill patients: A prospective, randomized, controlled study. Crit Care Med 1993; 21:830.
40. Yu M, Takanishi D, Myers SA, et al: Frequency of mortality and myocardial infarction during maximizing oxygen delivery: A prospective, randomized trial. Crit Care Med 1995; 23:1025.
41. Yu M: Invasive and noninvasive oxygen consumption and hemodynamic monitoring in elderly surgical patients. New Horizons 1996; 4:443.
42. Barlett RH: Oxygen kinetics: Pitfalls in clinical research. J Crit Care 1990; 5:77.
43. Shock NW, Grevlich RC, Costa PT, et al: Normal human aging: The Baltimore longitudinal study of aging. Chapter V. Cross Sectional Studies of Aging in Men. Washington, DC, U.S. Department of Health and Human Services, 1984.
44. Bessey PQ, Watters JM, Aoki TT, et al: Combined hormonal infusion simulates the metabolic response to injury. Ann Surg 1984; 200:264.
45. Shoemaker WC, Appel PL, Kram HB: Hemodynamic and oxygen transport responses in survivors and nonsurvivors of high-risk surgery. Crit Care Med 1993; 21:977.
46. Yu M, Burchell SA, Hasaniya WMA, et al: The relationship of mortality to increasing oxygen delivery in patients ≥50 years of age: A prospective randomized trial. Crit Care Med 1998; 26:1011.
47. Weissman C, Kemper M, Harding J: Response of critically ill patients to increased oxygen demand: Hemodynamic subsets. Crit Care Med 1994; 22:1809.
48. Manthous CA, Hall JB, Olson D, et al: Effect of cooling on oxygen consumption measured in febrile critically ill patients. Am J Respir Crit Care Med 1995; 151:10.
49. Harding J, Kemper M, Weissman D: Midazolam attenuates the metabolic and cardiopulmonary responses to an acute increase in oxygen demand. Chest 1994; 106:194.
50. Rady MY, Little RA, Edwards JD, et al: The effect of nociceptive stimulation on the changes in hemodynamics and oxygen transport induced by hemorrhage in anesthetized pigs. J Trauma 1991; 31:617.
51. Greenburg AG: New transfusion strategies. Am J Surg 1997; 173:49.
52. Laks H, Pilon RN, Klovekorn WP, et al: Acute hemodilution: Its effect on hemodynamics and oxygen transport in anesthetized man. Ann Surg 1974; 180:103.
53. Baxter BT, Minion DJ; McCanoe CL, et al: Rational approach to postoperative transfusion in high-risk patients. Am J Surg 1993; 166:720.
54. Case RB, Berglund E, Sarnoff SJ: Ventricular function: VII. Changes in coronary resistance and ventricular function resulting from acutely induced anemia and the effect theron of coronary stenosis. Am J Med 1955; March, p 397.
55. Levy PS, Quigley RL, Gould SA: Acute dilutional anemia and critical left anterior descending coronary artery stenosis impairs end organ oxygen delivery. J Trauma Injury Infect Crit Care 1996; 41:416.
56. Fan FC, Chen RYZ, Schuessler GB, et al: Effects of hematocrit variations on regional hemodynamics and oxygen transport in the dog. Am J Physiol 1980; 23:H545.
57. Nelson AH, Fleisher LA, Rosenbaum SH: Relationship between postoperative anemia and cardiac morbidity in high-risk vascular patients in the intensive care unit. Crit Care Med 1993; 21:860.
58. Hebert PC, Wells G, Tweeddale M, et al: Does transfusion practice affect mortality in critically ill patients? Am J Respir Crit Care Med 1997; 155:1618.
59. Yu M, Burchell SA, Hasaniya NW, et al: Incidence of myocardial damage in surgical patients age ≥50 years with hemorrhagic shock. J Trauma Injury Infect Crit Care 1997; 43:199.
60. Yu M, Takiguchi SA, Takanishi D, et al: Evaluation of the clinical usefulness of thermodilution volumetric catheters. Crit Care Med 1997; 23:681.
61. Shoemaker WC, Appel P, Czer LSC, et al: Pathogenesis of respiratory failure (ARDS) after hemorrhage and trauma: I: cardiorespiratory patterns preceding the development of ARDS. Crit Care Med 1980; 8:504.
62. Yu M, Hasaniya NW, Takanishi DM, et al: High-volume vs. standard fluid therapy in a septic pig model. Arch Surg 1997; 132:1111.
63. Goldstein FC, Strasser DC, Woodard JL, et al: Functional outcome of cognitively impaired hip fracture patients on a geriatric rehabilitation unit. J Am Geriatr Soc 1997; 45:35.

37

Critical Care Imaging of the Chest

Howard Jolles, MD • Daniel A. Henry, MD
Lynn Coppage, MD • Timothy J. Cole, MD

The portable chest radiograph (PCXR) remains an integral part of the evaluation of critically ill patients. New findings or changes in findings are reported in as many as 65% of studies.[1] Even more significantly, a study of 200 intensive care unit (ICU) patients[1] reported these findings to directly affect decision making in patient care, leading to therapeutic changes in 66% of intubated patients and 23% of nonintubated patients. Most often this resulted in the treatment of pulmonary edema, in the repositioning of an endotracheal tube, or in the detection of a new airspace process. Atelectasis, pleural air or fluid, and catheter malpositions were also noted.

Although the literature supports the routine use of daily chest radiographs in ICU patients,[1-3] these bedside examinations are one of the most frequently performed, labor-intensive radiologic studies with variable image quality. The clinical demand for PCXRs has made it an increasingly important radiology service, accounting for up to 40% to 50% of all chest examinations ordered.[2] Thus, special attention to these "routine" studies is necessary to ensure that (1) the highest image quality is maintained, (2) guidelines are developed to prioritize these examinations on a case-by-case basis, (3) appropriate clinical information is provided to the radiologist, and (4) a mechanism for prompt, accurate communication of interpretations is in place. Morning radiology ICU rounds are conducted daily with the patient management team at our institution (Medical College of Virginia) such that significant findings may be communicated and a treatment plan discussed.

To facilitate optimal use of resources, we have developed a patient-driven priority system for PCXR so that the appropriate response by the portable radiography team is predicated on well-defined indicators; in this way, the most critically ill patients are imaged in a clinically relevant time frame. Clinical indicators were established by consensus of the ICU directors and thoracic radiologists that stratified patients into four levels of service, in descending order of acuity. With continued shift toward outpatient health care management and proportional increase in severity of inpatient illness, the demand for bedside portable chest radiography can be expected to increase. Given the current limitations of budgets and personnel, priority strategies such as these can improve both our efficiency and quality of care for patients.

TECHNICAL CONSIDERATIONS

Conventional Radiography

Portable radiography of the chest is generally obtained with 75 to 80 kV (peak), the exposure adjusted by varying milliamperage. A wide-latitude film-screen combination minimizes errors in exposure. The radiographs are obtained in the anteroposterior projection with the patient upright whenever possible. Because of space limitations in the ICU, a minimum film-tube distance of 40 inches is used rather than the 72 inches preferred in the radiology department.

By its very nature, portable chest radiography suffers from several disadvantages, some technical and others related to the patient. The kilovoltage and milliamperage are limited, so that exposures are relatively long, and image contrast may be excessive.[4] Antiscatter grids markedly improve the quality of bedside chest radiographs by limiting the blurring and distortion caused by scatter radiation. Because the grid is frequently misaligned, however, a mechanical or optical alignment system is necessary to avoid the technical problem of grid cutoff. For this reason, together with the requirement of mandatory film-tube distances and the increased radiation dose, grids are not always practicable. Automatic exposure devices are commercially available and provide an improvement in film consistency. However, they are cumbersome and difficult to position and, as a result, seldom used. The illness of the patient together with multiple associated life-support devices and problems in controlling respiratory and body motion are added obstacles to good image quality. (When the patient is on mechanical ventilation, exposing the radiograph during a "sigh" breath may yield better quality, more consistent films.) Considering that portable chest examinations make up about 50% of all chest films in large institutions,[5] the importance of dedicated, competent, portable radiograph technologists and an effective quality-assurance program cannot be overemphasized.

Digital Radiography

In addressing these technical and patient-related problems encountered in portable chest radiography, digital image technology has shown promising results. Digital, or computed, radiography uses a phosphor plate rather than film to store the radiographic image and has the advantages of consistent film density, flexible image processing, and lower radiation dose. The diagnostic accuracy and confidence level of these systems are similar to those obtained with conventional film-screen radiography.[6]

Digital image processing identifies the portion of the dynamic range containing the diagnostic information and then adjusts the final output for display at a consistent, optimized contrast and density. It is this compensatory control that obviates repeated examinations because of errors in exposure or the necessity to interpret films of marginal diagnostic quality. These advantages, however, do not obviate the need for accurate positioning of the patient and alignment of the beam, and there is no time saving for each portable examination. Slight delays in waiting for image processing, spontaneous downtime, and the costs of hardware and service fees should be taken into consideration. Nevertheless, not only does digital radiography have the immediate advantages of improved image consistency and the option of image processing (selection of window and level settings), but more important, it provides sharing of images on a digital network.

Teleradiography and the Picture Archiving and Communications System

Immediate access to portable chest images is particularly useful in the ICU, where information is desired without delay. The electronic transmission of radiologic images (teleradiography) is typically performed together with image storage on a digital medium, a picture archiving and communications system (PACS). One can enter PCXRs into a PACS by recording

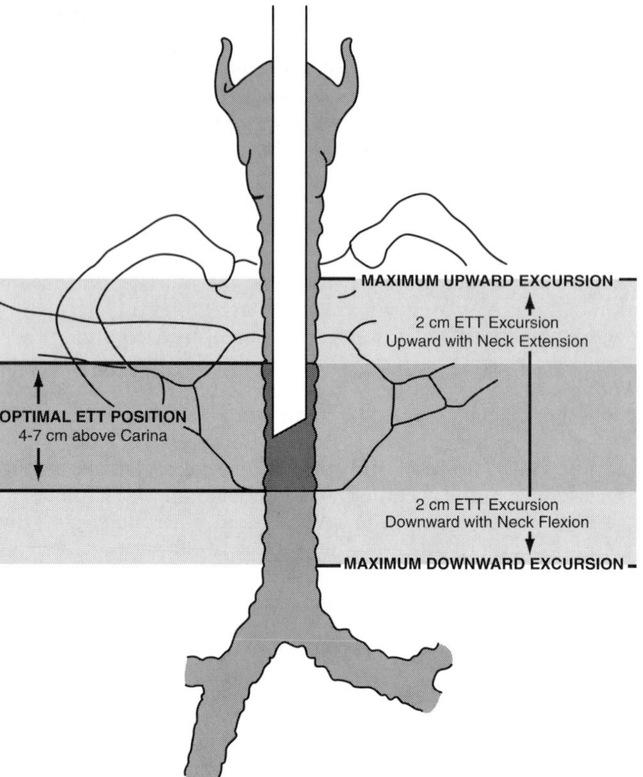

Figure 37–1. Illustration demonstrating the zone of optimal endotracheal tube (ETT) position and maximum safe excursion *(shaded areas)* from the zone boundaries with neck movement. ETT excursion outside these areas may be problematic.

them initially in a digital format or digitizing an analog image generated by the imaging device to a digital signal. In this way, medical images can be transmitted over a digital network for display at other locations, such as an ICU, within minutes of their acquisition.[7]

LIFE-SUPPORT CATHETERS AND TUBES

A significant percentage of clinically unsuspected findings on PCXR in the ICU setting relate to malposition or complications of life-support catheters and tubes.[8] Bekemeyer and colleagues[9] found that 27% of newly placed catheters or tubes were improperly positioned and that 6% resulted in a radiographically visible complication of the intervention. Although many such abnormalities are not immediately life-threatening, some require rapid correction to avoid clinical deterioration in patients with marginal cardiopulmonary reserve.

Endotracheal Tubes

Significant malpositioning of the endotracheal tube has been demonstrated in 12% to 15% of chest radiographs obtained in intubated patients.[10] An analysis of the position of the tube tip as it relates to the carina and the degree of neck flexion or extension should be routinely performed on each radiograph. Most endotracheal tubes have a dense radiopaque strip and a somewhat less dense but still visible side wall. Optimally, in an adult patient the tube tip should rest 4 to 7 cm above the carina, with the patient's head in a neutral position (i.e., with the mandible, if visible, projecting over the fifth or sixth cervical vertebral body). One can establish the location of the carina in most cases by following the inferior wall of the left mainstem bronchus proximally. Because the tube is secured at the nose or mouth, there is up to 4 cm of excursion of the tube tip, downward with neck flexion or upward with extension[11] (Fig. 37–1). In addition, rotation of the head augments this excursion. Attention should also be paid to the inflated cuff, which should not cause bulging of the tracheal walls, because this may produce ischemia, predisposing to tracheostenosis or tracheoesophageal fistula (Fig. 37–2). These complications are less likely, however, with the almost exclusive use of large-diameter, large-volume cuffs with soft, moderately compliant, thin walls.

The most common complication detected on the first postintubation PCXR is endotracheal tube malposition. Because of the less acute angle of the right mainstem bronchus to the trachea, bronchial intubation occurs here more frequently[12]

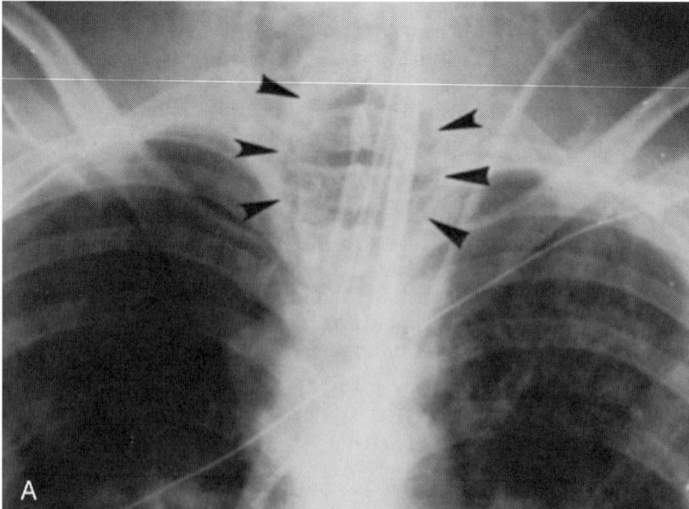

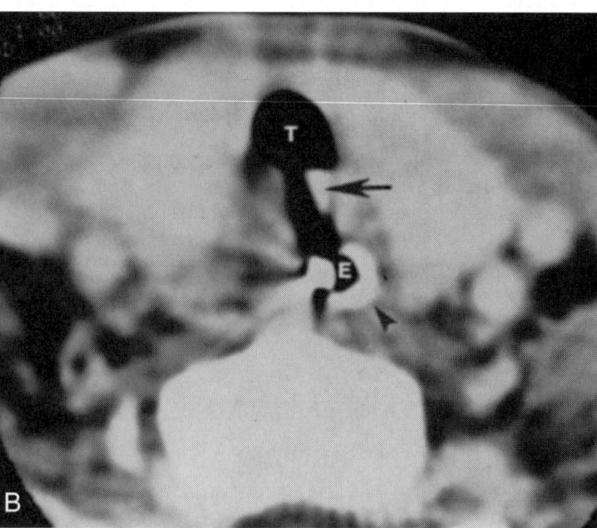

Figure 37–2. *A*, A coned-down anteroposterior view of the upper chest demonstrates overdistention of the radiolucent endotracheal tube cuff *(arrowheads)* that exceeds the diameter of the normal trachea. *B*, The patient subsequently developed signs and symptoms of recurrent aspiration, which prompted CT evaluation. A transaxial image at the level of the thyroid gland reveals a fistulous communication *(arrow)* between the posterior wall of the trachea (T) and the esophagus (E). Note the nasogastric tube *(arrowhead)*.

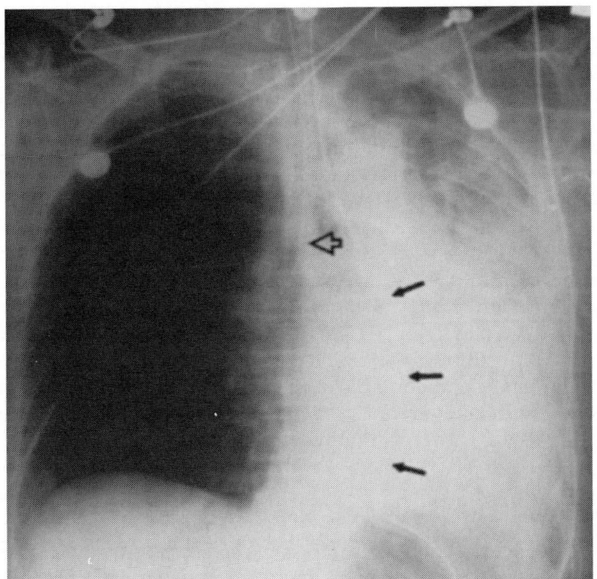

Figure 37–3. The tip of the endotracheal tube *(open arrow)* extends into the right mainstem bronchus, and hyperinflation of the right lung is present. Signs of volume loss of the left lung include increased opacity of the hemithorax with ipsilateral shift of the heart and mediastinal structures. Note the leftward displacement of the radiopaque nasogastric tube *(arrows)*.

(Fig. 37–3). If this malposition goes undetected, the subsequently underaerated left lung may become more atelectatic and possibly progress to complete collapse. The hyperinflation of the right lung may result in pneumothorax.[13] Esophageal intubation, although usually apparent clinically, may be first suggested on the chest radiograph by visualization of the endotracheal tube lateral to the tracheal wall, gaseous distention of the stomach or esophagus, and displacement of the trachea by the inflated cuff. The optimal radiographic examination to distinguish between tracheal and esophageal intubation is the 25° right posterior oblique projection with a nasogastric tube in place and the patient's head turned to the right.[14] This position allows clear separation between the trachea and esophagus and is diagnostic in 96% of patients.

Mechanical ventilation may alter the appearance of the PCXR considerably.[15] The institution of positive pressure, particularly positive end-expiratory pressure (PEEP), improves lung volumes and may result in an apparent radiographic improvement. Whenever possible, serial radiographs should be interpreted with knowledge of current ventilatory settings or at least with the recognition that ventilatory pressures have been changed.

Tracheostomy Tubes

Patients requiring long-term assisted ventilation may require placement of a tracheostomy tube. Post-placement radiographs, including a lateral film when feasible, should be assessed for proper tracheostomy tube alignment and position (i.e., the tube should overlie the air column and run parallel to the tracheal walls). Ideally, the tracheostomy tube tip should lie between one-half and two-thirds the distance from the stoma to the carina, although the stoma itself is usually difficult to localize. The tracheostomy tube width should be approximately two-thirds the tracheal width.[11] Persistent acute angulation can damage the tracheal walls and erode into the mediastinum. Overdistention of the cuff may cause mucosal ulceration with pressure necrosis, leading to tracheostenosis or tracheomalacia.

Pneumomediastinum on the first post-placement radiograph requires close follow-up because a persistent pneumomediastinum may be the result of malposition or an ongoing air leak. A widened mediastinum suggests the possibility of hemorrhage. Pneumothorax in the setting of recent tracheostomy tube placement is seen most commonly after inadvertent puncture of the apical pleura.

Central Venous Pressure Catheters

Single-lumen and double-lumen central venous pressure (CVP) catheters are used routinely in the ICU setting. Insertion may be by either the subclavian or the internal jugular vein; less commonly, the external jugular vein may be accessed. For accurate CVP readings, the catheter tip should rest beyond the most distal venous valves of the large central veins and optimally in one of the brachiocephalic veins or in the superior vena cava (Fig. 37–4). In a retrospective study of 500 subclavian catheter placements,[16] 68% were properly placed, 21.4% were in the right atrium, and 0.4% were in the right ventricle. Complications of catheter placement in the right side of the heart include arrhythmias, endocardial damage, and an increased incidence of cardiac perforation with hemopericardium and tamponade.[11] An unusual-appearing catheter course may indicate an extravascular position, an arterial location (Fig. 37–5), or cannulation of a smaller venous vessel such as the internal thoracic or left superior intercostal vein. Knowledge of vascular anatomy is important because normal

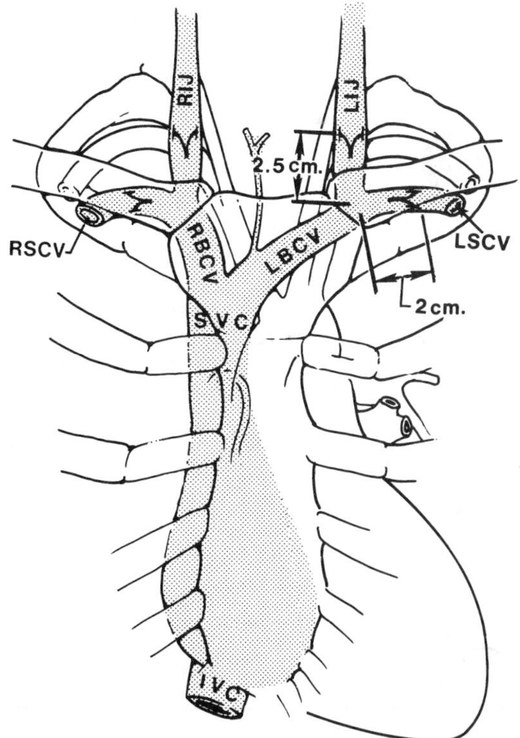

Figure 37–4. Diagram illustrating central venous anatomy. The most proximal venous valves (V) are located 2 to 2.5 cm from the origin of the left and right brachiocephalic veins (LBCV and RBCV, respectively), in the left and right internal jugular (LIJ and RIJ, respectively), and in the left and right subclavian veins (LSCV and RSCV, respectively). Central venous catheter tips should rest distal to these valves, optimally in the superior vena cava (SVC).

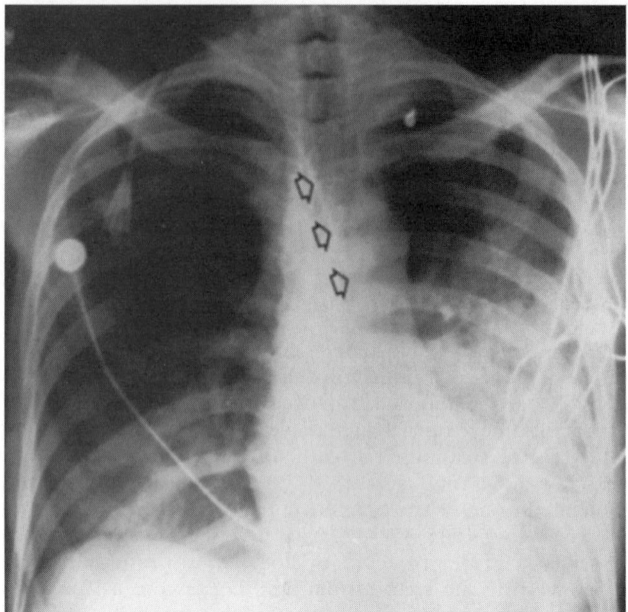

Figure 37–5. Portable chest radiograph following central line placement, presumably through the right internal jugular vein, shows the catheter extending across the midline *(open arrows)* in a course more medial than expected. Although an extravascular location could not be excluded, arterial catheterization was confirmed by pressure readings.

variations may result in a seemingly peculiar appearance, such as placement into a persistent left superior vena cava.

Other complications related to CVP catheter placement (Fig. 37–6) are cited in Table 37–1, with pneumothorax present on as many as 6% of the PCXRs immediately after insertion.[17]

Swan-Ganz Catheters

The Swan-Ganz catheter is used routinely to provide physiologic data regarding cardiac function. It is used to measure right atrial, right ventricular, and pulmonary artery wedge pressures while estimating left atrial and left ventricular end-diastolic pressures. Such measurements aid in distinguishing between cardiac and noncardiac causes of pulmonary edema.[18] The catheter may also be used to determine cardiac output by the thermodilution technique.

To achieve the most accurate pulmonary arterial wedge pressure reading, the catheter should be "floated" into the dependent, posterior lower lobe arterial branches, where it will lie at or below the level of the left atrium in the supine position (zone III).[19] Catheters directed into more anterior branches of the upper lobes or middle lobe (zones I and II) may reflect alveolar pressures and thereby give less precise readings (Fig. 37–7). Increasing PEEP recruits a greater percentage of the pulmonary capillary bed to zones I and II, adding increased importance to this catheter position. When the balloon is deflated after a reading, the catheter tip should be retracted into a more central, large-caliber vessel or a central pulmonary artery. An inflated balloon should never be observed on the PCXR, indicating that the catheter has been left in the wedged position for an extended time.

The use of the Swan-Ganz catheter is not without risk. Complications include those mentioned in Table 37–1 and also problems that are unique to this particular device. If the catheter is left in a peripheral position, perforation and distal hemorrhage may result[20] (Fig. 37–8). Excess catheter coiled in the sinus portion of the right ventricle predisposes to cardiac arrhythmias and sudden distal migration of the tip. Pulmonary artery pseudoaneurysm has been reported as a complication of Swan-Ganz catheter monitoring.[21]

TABLE 37–1. Radiographically Visible Complications of Central Catheter Placement

Malposition
Pneumothorax
Venous or arterial perforation with extrapleural, pleural, or mediastinal hemorrhage or ectopic infusion
Cardiac perforation
Retained introducer wire or catheter fragment
Knotted catheter
Air embolus

Intra-aortic Counterpulsation Balloon

The intra-aortic balloon pump is a cardiac assist device used in patients with cardiogenic shock, after myocardial infarction, and in some cases after cardiac surgery. The balloon (~26 cm in length) is inflated with helium during diastole, reducing afterload and augmenting coronary artery perfusion.[22] Generally introduced through the common femoral artery, its radiopaque distal tip should be visible in the proximal descending thoracic aorta distal to the aortic knob and above the level of the left mainstem bronchus. If the PCXR is exposed during diastole, the tubular radiolucency of the gas-filled balloon may be visible in the descending aorta (Fig. 37–9). When the tip extends more proximally into the aortic arch or into the left subclavian artery (Fig. 37–10), there is an increased risk of vascular complications. Dissection of the aortic wall has been described and reported as a subtle loss of definition of the descending thoracic aorta on the PCXR.[23] An intramural loca-

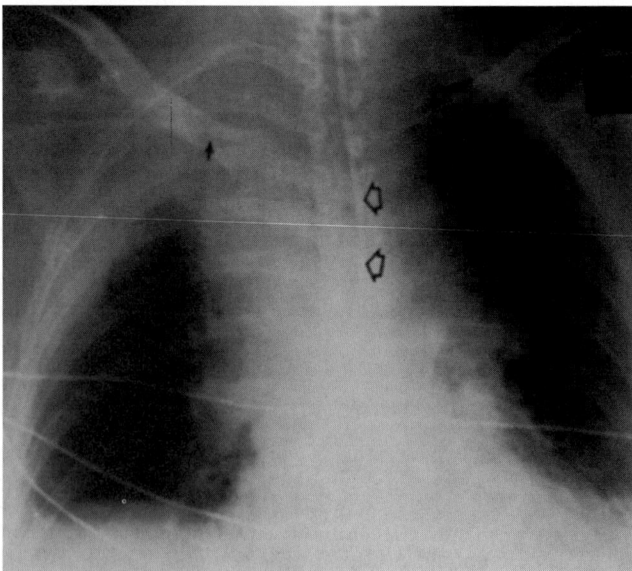

Figure 37–6. The tip of a right subclavian cordis sheath *(small arrow)* is faintly seen projecting over the medial right clavicle. Hemorrhage into the extrapleural space and mediastinum results in abnormal soft-tissue density along the right lateral chest wall and lung apex as well as in marked mediastinal widening. Mass effect in the mediastinum is suggested by leftward deviation of the nasogastric tube *(open arrows)*.

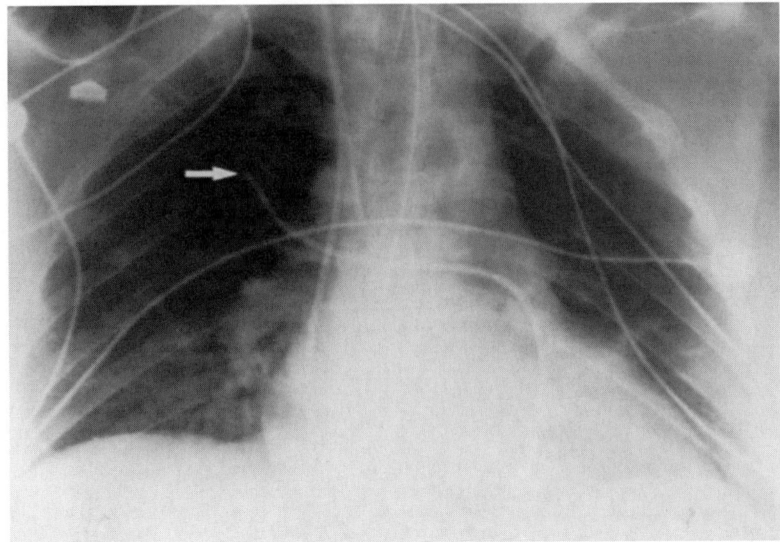

Figure 37–7. A Swan-Ganz catheter directed into an upper lobe branch of the right pulmonary artery *(arrow)* lies above the level of the left atrium and is, therefore, a less accurate predictor of left ventricular end-diastolic pressure in this position.

tion can be confirmed with computed tomography (CT) or, if necessary, angiography.

Percutaneous Intravascular Central Catheter

One new device gaining widespread acceptance is the percutaneous intravascular central catheter (PICC). This catheter is only 2 to 5 French (Fr.) in size and is placed into the superior vena cava through the antecubital, basilic, or brachial vein. Having a low complication rate compared with other central access lines, PICCs may be difficult to visualize radiographically because of their small size and faint radiographic density (Fig. 37-11). Attention is needed in detecting the PICC on follow-up films because it may be more frequently displaced than conventional central venous lines owing to its increased flexibility.[24]

CRITICAL PATHWAYS FOR CRITICAL CARE

The foregoing text discussed technical issues and various intensive care appliances common to a broad spectrum of critical care situations. The following sections focus on specific clinical entities, their radiographic presentation, their course, and the critical care circumstances in which they frequently occur. These pathways include neurologic, cardiovascular, pulmonary, gastrointestinal, and immune-challenged clinical entities as the more common indicators for admission to a critical care unit. The role of chest imaging in diagnosis and decision making is stressed.

Neurologic Disorders

Here we focus on the clinical entities and their radiographic counterparts that occur in patients with head injury, seizure,

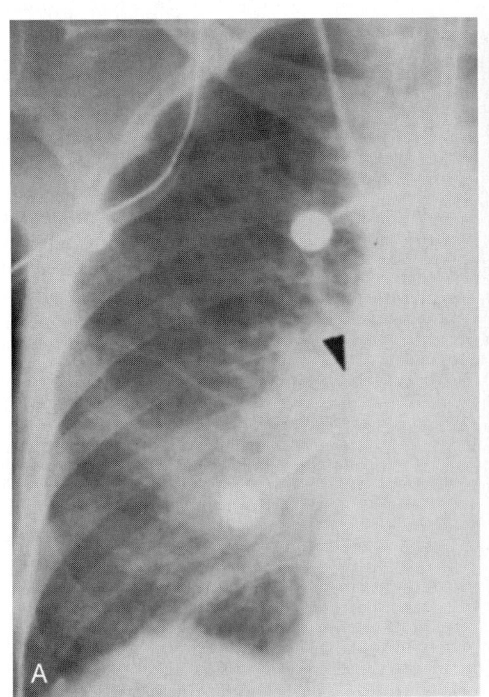

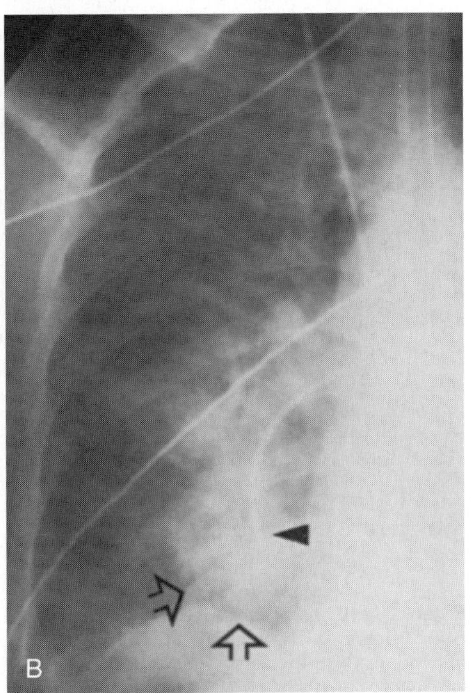

Figure 37–8. *A*, This coned-down view of the right hemithorax in a patient with cardiogenic pulmonary edema reveals vascular indistinctness and perihilar haze. The tip of the Swan-Ganz catheter *(arrowhead)* is faintly visible in the right pulmonary artery, above an overlying electrocardiograph electrode wire. *B*, One day later in this same patient, the Swan-Ganz catheter migrated peripherally *(arrowhead)*, resulting in an area of hemorrhage that is seen as a new opacity *(open arrows)* in the cardiophrenic angle.

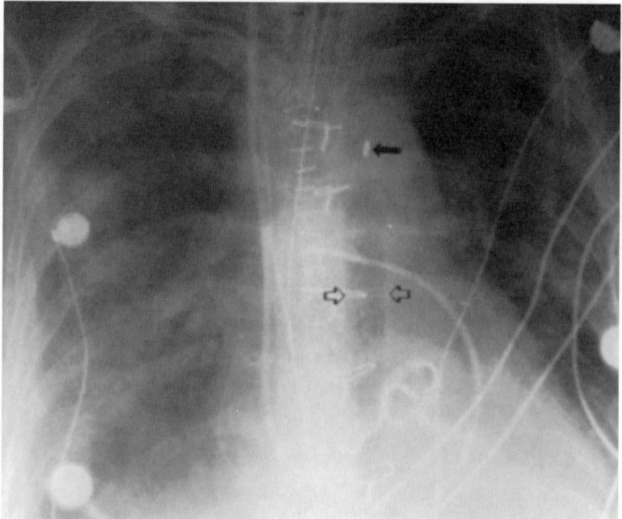

Figure 37–9. The radiopaque tip of the intra-aortic counterpulsation balloon *(arrow)* in the proximal descending thoracic aorta is in appropriate position. Because the film was exposed during diastole, the inflated balloon can be seen as an elliptic lucency projecting to the left of the dorsal spine behind the cardiac silhouette *(open arrows)*.

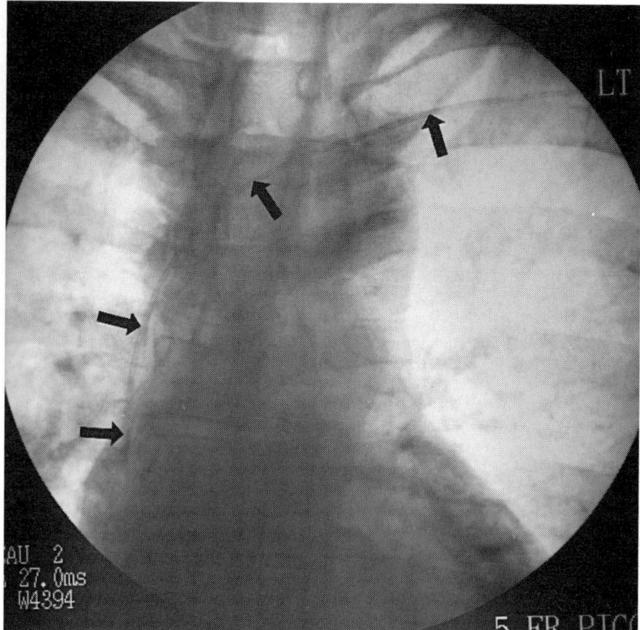

Figure 37–11. Digital subtraction image enhances visibility of a No. 5 French percutaneous intravenous central catheter (PICC) placed through the left arm with tip in the caval-atrial junction *(arrows)*.

and stroke. These patients frequently present with reduced consciousness and impaired neurologic function. They are frequently intubated and sometimes suffer prolonged immobility and recumbency.

Neurogenic Pulmonary Edema

Impaired pulmonary function is a common but poorly understood complication of head injury. Shanahan,[25] who observed 11 patients with clinical evidence of postictal pulmonary edema, first described neurogenic pulmonary edema (NPE). NPE may occur in up to 50% of serious head injuries.[26] The association of NPE with head injury was reported by Simmons and colleagues,[27] who observed alveolar edema, hemorrhage, and congestion in the lungs in soldiers dying of isolated head wounds. The "blast" theory postulates that the initial central nervous system insult results in a massive sympathetic discharge with severe systemic and pulmonary hypertension, leading to edema through increased pulmonary blood volume and pressure as well as pulmonary endothelial damage. Another theory proposes that NPE is caused by a neurally induced increase in capillary permeability.[28]

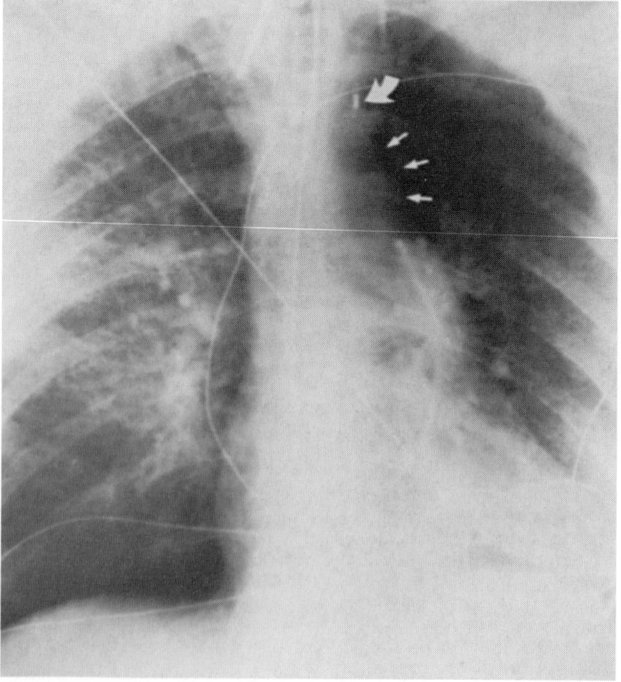

Figure 37–10. Suboptimal position of an intra-aortic counterpulsation balloon with the radiopaque tip *(curved arrow)* projecting above the aortic knob *(small arrows)* into the proximal left subclavian artery.

CRITICAL PATHWAY. The clinical syndrome of NPE can manifest in one of two distinct forms: acutely, within minutes to hours of the central nervous system insult, or more insidiously during several days.

The *acute* form is heralded by dyspnea and may be accompanied by hemoptysis; physical findings include rales, tachypnea, and tachycardia. On the initial PCXR (Fig. 37–12), NPE causes acute, homogeneous, bilateral airspace disease with prominent air bronchograms. It is frequently asymmetric in distribution, with normal heart size and a narrow vascular pedicle. A predilection for abnormality of the upper lobes has been noted; in one series, a patchy, peripheral distribution was present in 50% of patients.[26] Kerley's lines, peribronchial cuffing, and pleural effusions are conspicuously absent, findings commonly seen in hydrostatic edema. It has been suggested that patients with PaO_2:FIO_2 ratios less than 300 mm Hg and diffuse pulmonary abnormalities on the initial PCXR may be considered to have NPE.[28] Remarkable clearing in 48 hours is typical and suggestive of the diagnosis.[29]

The *delayed* form occurs anywhere from 12 hours to several days after the central nervous system insult; it is more insidious in onset, with gradual development of tachypnea and rales. The PCXR findings are the same as in the acute variety; the differential diagnosis includes aspiration, noncardiogenic edema associated with septic and hypovolemic shock, and acute cardiogenic edema while the heart is still of

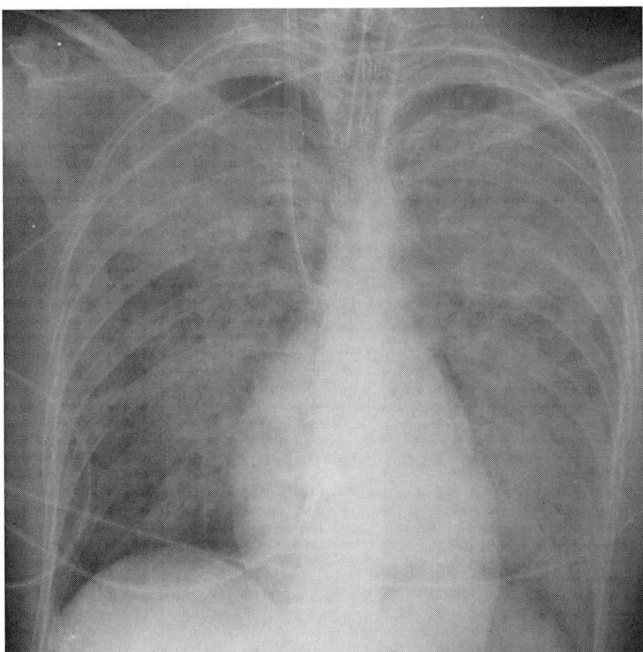

Figure 37–12. Neurogenic pulmonary edema in a 42-year-old woman with subarachnoid hemorrhage. A portable chest radiograph demonstrates bilateral airspace disease with predominance in the upper zones. Note normal heart size and the presence of air bronchograms. These findings, together with the absence of Kerley's lines and pleural effusions, are consistent with noncardiogenic edema.

normal size. Difficulties in diagnosis of the delayed form may arise because it is more commonly seen in trauma victims who may have other forms of noncardiogenic pulmonary edema.[29] The diagnosis is sometimes ascertained retrospectively, because the rapid radiographic clearing in 24 to 72 hours excludes other diagnoses such as massive aspiration, pneumonia, and adult respiratory distress syndrome (ARDS); absence of electrocardiographic and enzyme changes militate against acute cardiogenic edema.

Aspiration Pneumonia

Stroke complicated by the need for mechanical ventilation is a common admitting diagnosis to the ICU. The majority of patients present within 24 hours after the onset of coma or are admitted secondarily after initial treatment in medical or neurologic services. In one series,[30] 15.3% of patients succumbed to respiratory failure including pneumonia and pulmonary embolism. The incidence of microbiologically confirmed pneumonia in comatose ICU patients is about 40%, as reported by Sirvent and associates,[31] occurring in their series on the average of 4.4 ± 2.1 days after institution of mechanical ventilation. The widely accepted pathophysiologic mechanism of early pneumonia in the stroke patient is the aspiration of oropharyngeal contents secondary to glottic dysfunction.[32]

CRITICAL PATHWAY. Massive aspiration of acid gastric contents can lead to hemorrhagic tracheobronchitis and diffuse lung injury. Patients present with sudden apnea, hypotension, cyanosis, and fever. The degree of lung injury increases significantly as the volume and acidity of the aspirate increase.[33]

The clinical course generally follows one of three patterns: (1) rapid improvement in clinical and radiographic abnormalities; (2) rapid progression of radiographic abnormalities and decline in clinical status with death ensuing within days; and (3) transient stabilization of clinical and radiographic abnormalities followed by a protracted period of worsening secondary to pneumonia due to bacterial superinfection, onset of ARDS, or both.[34] In most of the patients (85%), airspace disease secondary to aspiration is apparent on the initial radiograph, usually bilateral and asymmetric in distribution[32] (Fig. 37–13).

Two distinct radiographic patterns of distribution are described, including (1) a predominance of central or perihilar abnormalities and (2) a predominance of lower zone abnormalities. Because most patients are supine when aspiration occurs, most disease is posterior in location and favors the right side because of the more vertical course of the right main bronchus from the trachea. The extent of abnormality on the initial chest radiograph does not necessarily correlate with the clinical outcome.[35] Acute airway obstruction may accompany aspiration and produce atelectasis of varying severity or hyperinflation due to a check-valve mechanism.

Cardiovascular Disorders

Cardiovascular disease may be manifest as chest pain in the acute-care setting, and cardiac ischemia, aortic dissection, and pulmonary embolism are important diagnostic considerations. Radiographic imaging is an integral part of the initial clinical evaluation, the subsequent course of treatment, and the assessment of complications.

Acute Myocardial Infarction: Cardiogenic Pulmonary Edema

The PCXR is the most commonly used noninvasive technique for assessing abnormalities of lung water in critically ill patients[36]; it is sensitive in the detection of pulmonary edema, even before the onset of cardiorespiratory symptoms. In three series of patients with acute myocardial infarction, the radiographic findings of left-sided cardiac failure were present in 24% to 38% of patients when the diagnosis was not yet clinically apparent.[37] Disagreement exists over the ability of the PCXR to reliably differentiate between cardiogenic, permeability, and renal/overhydration forms of edema; nevertheless,

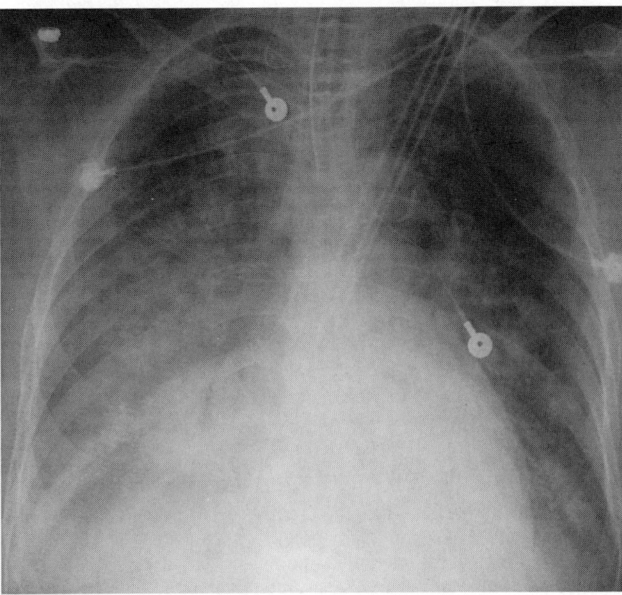

Figure 37–13. A 63-year-old woman was admitted to the intensive care unit with history of ethanol abuse, seizures, and stroke. Three days after admission, there is bilateral, asymmetric airspace disease secondary to aspiration pneumonia. Note the basilar and right-sided predominance, typical of aspiration.

several characteristics are recognized that can be objectively interpreted and yield clinically valuable information.[36-39]

CRITICAL PATHWAY. Cardiogenic pulmonary edema (congestive heart failure) may complicate the clinical course in patients with acute myocardial infarction, mitral valve disease, cardiomyopathy, and arrhythmias. A careful examination of the PCXR has shown significant correlations between pulmonary venous pressures and radiographic findings of pulmonary vascular congestion and edema.[37]

On the initial PCXR, cardiomegaly may or may not be present, depending on the acuity of the event and past history of cardiovascular disease. In acute left ventricular decompensation, pulmonary artery wedge pressures between 12 and 20 mm Hg have been associated with *redistribution* of pulmonary blood flow, resulting in dilatation of upper lobe vessels and shrinking of lower zone vessels. Detection of this early finding, however, is dependent on the examination of the patient in the upright position, usually not feasible in the ICU because of the patient's critical status. Interstitial pulmonary edema and pleural effusions are evident, however, when the wedge pressure rises into the range of 20 to 30 mm Hg, heralded by the presence of the following signs (Fig. 37–14):

1. Haziness of the hila, which are increased in size and density.
2. Septal (Kerley's) lines.
3. Peribronchovascular haze.
4. Subpleural edema with fissural thickening.
5. Pleural effusion.

A correlation between azygous vein width and mean right atrial pressure has been reported on upright chest radiographs and may serve as an additional radiographic indicator of cardiogenic edema.[37] When the wedge pressure exceeds 30 mm Hg, alveolar flooding generally occurs; in this instance, cardiogenic edema sometimes presents as a "batwing" pattern in the perihilar regions with relative sparing of the periphery. Unlike the case with permeability edema, air bronchograms are less commonly seen in the cardiogenic variety.

In the first days after acute myocardial infarction, the PCXR should be monitored for assessment of heart size, changes in the severity and distribution of pulmonary edema, pleural effusion, placement of life-support lines and tubes, and presence of complications such as pneumonia or changes suggestive of pulmonary embolism.

In general, 1.5- to 2-cm differences in heart size are not considered significant in order to allow for systolic and diastolic phases of cardiac activity. A rapid increase in heart size necessitates the exclusion of pericardial effusion. When pericardial tamponade occurs, pulmonary edema, if present, will suddenly decrease because of the relative obstruction to venous return. A patient in whom there is a sudden increase in edema suggests the possibility of a ruptured papillary muscle or acute ventricular septal defect. Correlation of the radiographic findings and clinical picture is necessary; changes in edema may reflect not only cardiac function but also fluid

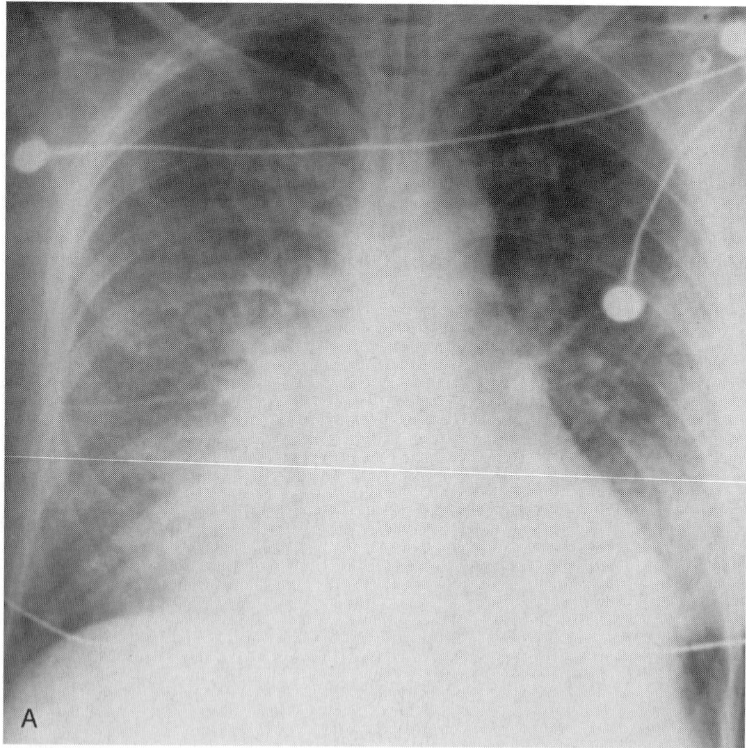

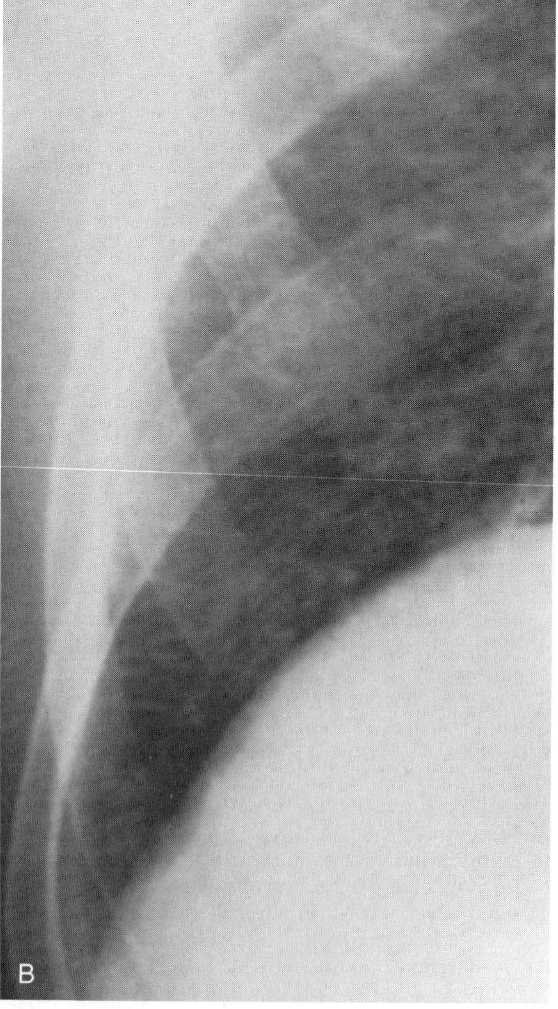

Figure 37–14. *A*, Portable chest radiograph in a patient with cardiogenic pulmonary edema reveals mild cardiomegaly and signs of interstitial edema, including vascular indistinctness and perihilar haze. Subpleural edema fluid results in apparent thickening of the minor fissure. *B*, Fluid in the interlobular septa (Kerley's lines).

balance (i.e., volume overload, status after cardiac catheterization and large osmolar radiographic contrast loads, or renal insufficiency). Rapid shifts in parenchymal abnormality are typical of pulmonary edema, which usually has a bilaterally symmetric appearance. Asymmetry in the parenchymal abnormality may reflect an underlying pneumonia or aspiration event. Pneumonia is usually focal and clears more slowly than pulmonary edema; occasionally, however, bland aspiration may mimic the appearance of congestive heart failure.

In the patient with chronic obstructive pulmonary disease and centrilobular emphysema, asymmetric distribution of pulmonary edema is common, occurring predominantly in the lower lobes where an intact vascular bed is present. Pulmonary edema may also be unevenly distributed in the patient with congestive heart failure and acute pulmonary embolism, in which the involved portions of lung are "protected" from edema by occlusion of the feeding vessels.

One should be cognizant of a source of discrepancy between the central hemodynamics and the PCXR: the "post-therapeutic phase lag"[37] (i.e., those instances when a fall in pulmonary wedge pressure is not accompanied by a concomitant clearing of edema from the chest radiograph). Because a considerable amount of extravascular lung water can be accommodated in the interstitial space, it may behave like a sequestered pool and be removed in a relatively slow fashion. In these instances, the PCXR must be regarded as a more accurate index of extravascular fluid than the actual hemodynamic parameters, and this distinction should be taken into account for therapeutic planning.

Aortic Dissection

The characteristics to distinguish the chest discomfort associated with cardiac ischemia from that of aortic dissection are sometimes lacking, and some clinical overlap may occur. Clinical manifestations of aortic dissection depend on its path as it courses through the aorta.[40] Acute aortic dissection is a relatively common catastrophic illness, even though great strides have been made in the diagnosis and treatment of this highly lethal disease. The diagnosis is confirmed by an imaging study.

CRITICAL PATHWAY. The chest radiograph in aortic dissection is generally nonspecific. However, comparison to previous chest radiographs may reveal an enlarging or more tortuous aorta, an enlarging cardiac shadow related to congestive heart failure or pericardial hemorrhage, or additional signs of congestive heart failure. Displacement of intimal calcification of the aorta is an additional sign that must be viewed with caution, considering the patient's position and rotation as well as aortic anatomy.

Chest CT or magnetic resonance imaging (MRI) is ideal for the noninvasive diagnosis and assessment of aortic dissection (Fig. 37–15). They are well-established and definitive imaging modalities for studying thoracic aortic disease and rival aortography.[41] Both are capable of determining the thoracic and abdominal extent of the process, detecting pericardial or periaortic hematoma, and visualizing false and true lumens as well as intimal flaps. Aortic MRI has some advantages, in that it does not employ radiation or require contrast media. It can be performed in virtually any anatomic plane, is useful to evaluate aortic valve integrity and cardiac function, and can be viewed in cine mode to better understand flow dynamics and branch patency.

Acute Pulmonary Embolism

In the patient with suspected pulmonary embolism, the initial imaging evaluation should begin with the chest radiograph. Several plain film findings have been described in association with pulmonary embolism, most commonly atelectasis or parenchymal foci of increased opacity. Other radiographic signs include local oligemia (Westermark's sign), prominent central pulmonary arteries (Fleischner's sign), pleura-based area of increased opacity (Hampton's hump), vascular redistribution,

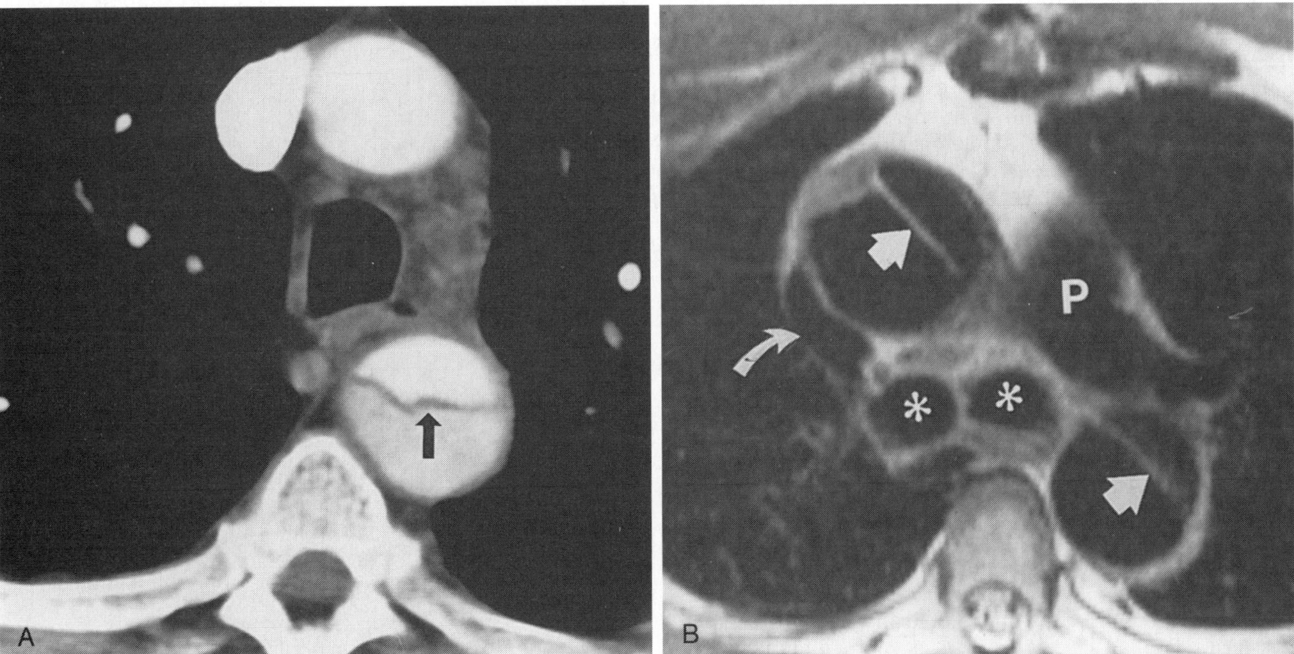

Figure 37–15. Aortic dissection. *A*, Aortic dissection in a 72-year-old man. Spiral CT just below the level of the aortic arch demonstrates an intimal flap in the proximal descending aorta *(arrow)*. Note the differential enhancement of the true lumen anteriorly in contrast to the false lumen posteriorly. *B*, Turbo spin-echo, black blood MRI of aortic dissection in a 34-year-old man. The axial image shows an intimal flap involving both the ascending and descending portions of the aorta *(straight arrows)*. Note also the right and left main bronchi *(asterisks)*, the superior vena cava *(curved arrow)*, and the main and left pulmonary arteries (P).

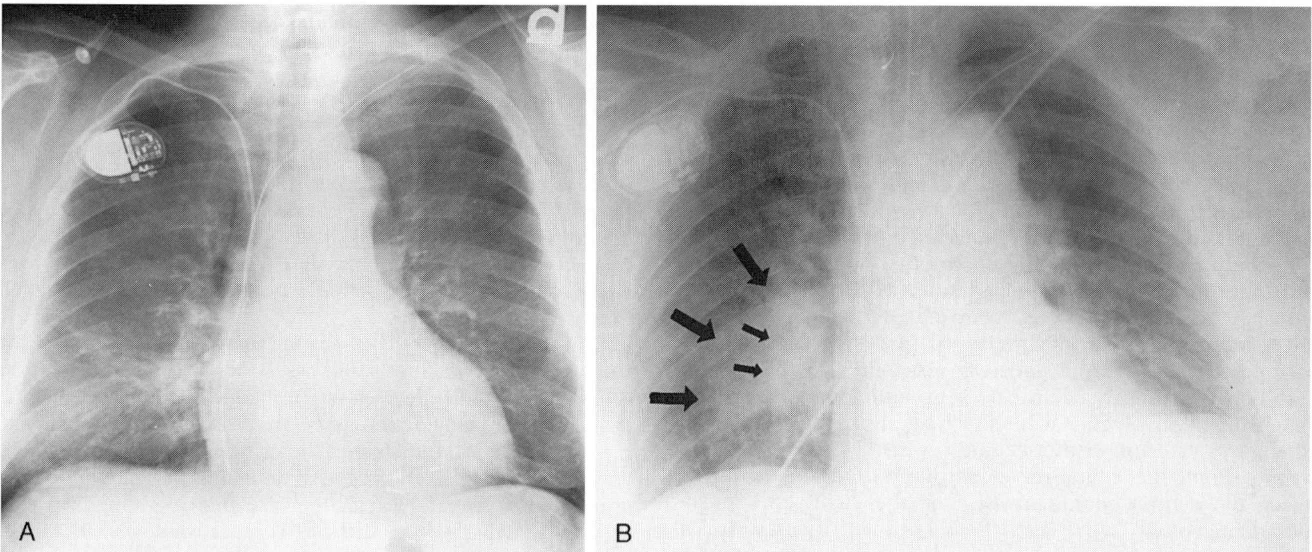

Figure 37–16. *A*, Baseline posteroanterior chest radiograph in 70-year-old man with pacemaker infection demonstrates a right atrioventricular sequential pacemaker and amputated left pacing wire with tip in the right ventricle. Cardiomegaly and tortuous aorta are present with clear lung fields. *B*, Portable chest radiograph 3 days later shows enlargement of the right interlobar pulmonary artery secondary to pulmonary embolism *(small arrows)* with perihilar airspace disease resulting from parenchymal hemorrhage *(large arrows)*.

pleural effusion, elevated hemidiaphragm, and enlarged hilum (Fig. 37-16).

Although suggestive of pulmonary embolism, these findings often require confirmation; thus, the main value of chest radiography is to exclude diagnoses that may clinically mimic pulmonary embolism and to complement the interpretation of the ventilation-perfusion (V/Q) lung scan.[42] V/Q scanning is frequently the next imaging study, and the utility may be limited by the presence of pleuroparenchymal abnormalities; in the Prospective Investigation of Pulmonary Embolism Diagnosis (PIOPED) study, only 12% of patients with pulmonary embolism had normal findings on chest radiography.[42] Thus, in the population of ICU patients, the likelihood of a false-positive V/Q scan is high and that of a true negative is lower. Ventilation-perfusion scintigraphy is most valuable in those patients having a normal study result (14% to 40% of patients) or when a high probability of pulmonary embolism is present (10% to 20% of patients).[43] In these instances, the diagnostic work-up is completed. For those with nondiagnostic (i.e., low probability, indeterminate) findings, however, additional information is frequently needed.

Traditionally, pulmonary angiography is the next recommended test and the recognized gold standard for the detection of pulmonary embolism. Despite this fact, it has been shown that fewer than 50% of patients with nondiagnostic V/Q scintigraphy actually undergo angiography.[43] For these reasons, a less invasive yet specific imaging test is needed in the diagnostic armamentarium to assess this most difficult and challenging population of patients.

During the past several years, spiral CT angiography has emerged as a useful modality in making the diagnosis of pulmonary embolism. Specificity and sensitivity are reported in excess of 90%, approaching the results of the gold standard, pulmonary angiography.[44] Spiral CT enables direct visualization of thrombus within the lumen of main, lobar, and segmental arteries (Fig. 37-17). Diagnosis is more difficult at the subsegmental level, where isolated clot has been reported on pulmonary angiography in 5% to 36% of patients. Recent advances in technique and instrumentation allow visualization of slightly more than 60% of subsegmental vessels, markedly improving the ability of this technique to assess for small clots.[44] Given the number of patients with suspected pulmonary embolism and nondiagnostic V/Q scan, or compromise of the diagnostic utility of the V/Q scan by the presence of pleuroparenchymal abnormality, spiral CT can play a significant role.

CRITICAL PATHWAY. In patients with suspected pulmonary embolism, the initial PCXR is scrutinized to exclude other etiologic factors, such as pneumonia, collapse, pneumothorax, and pulmonary edema, which may provide the explanation for the symptoms. If this is not helpful, further investigation is necessary, and two major imaging strategies have been advocated:

1. Obtain V/Q scan and duplex Doppler ultrasonography as the initial imaging studies. Patients with nondiagnostic V/Q scan and negative Doppler study results should next undergo spiral CT.[45]
2. Goodman and colleagues[46] suggest a diagnostic algorithm with cost-effective features using spiral CT and lower-extremity Doppler ultrasonography to proceed as follows. In patients with symptoms of pulmonary embolism, spiral CT should be done; if a clot is detected, the work-up is completed. If the findings are normal, Doppler ultrasonography is recommended because spiral CT may be falsely negative in the case of subsegmental emboli, and this study provides assurance that no large clot in the femoropopliteal system is present. In patients with symptoms of both pulmonary embolism and deep venous thrombosis, the evaluation should begin with Doppler ultrasonography; if a clot is detected, imaging ceases. If findings are normal, the patient next undergoes spiral CT. Abnormal results lead to treatment, whereas further imaging would cease with a normal CT result. In either strategy, angiography could be reserved for patients whose initial work-up findings are normal but for whom high clinical suspicion remains.

Detection of pulmonary embolism by spiral CT is an exciting advance that needs further study over time to assess its final role in our diagnostic armamentarium. MRI as yet falls short in spatial resolution and conspicuity of clot compared with spiral CT.[47] However, it holds the promise of diagnosing pulmonary embolism without ionizing radiation or need for

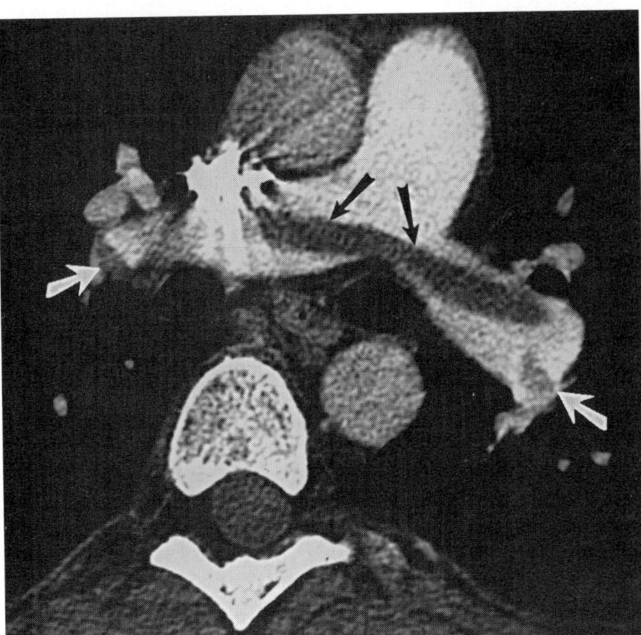

Figure 37–17. Non-Hodgkin's lymphoma and dyspnea on exertion in a 37-year-old man. Spiral CT demonstrates a saddle embolus at the bifurcation of the pulmonary artery *(black arrows)* with smaller clots in the left and right pulmonary arteries *(white arrows)*.

contrast material while simultaneously imaging the deep veins for thrombosis.

Acute Respiratory Failure

High mortality rates are common for patients with acute respiratory failure, even in ICUs specializing in modern critical care techniques. In an international multicenter study, only 55.6% survived their hospitalization whereas 44.4% died in the hospital.[48] In this study, survival rates were higher in patients with acute respiratory failure caused by pneumonia (63%) or post-shock lung injury (status after surgery or trauma) (67%) and lower in patients with sepsis (46%). Advanced or life-threatening pneumonia can evolve from a community-acquired or hospital-acquired source. Both types of pneumonia continue to be significant clinical problems and account for a substantial number of hospital admissions or prolonged hospitalizations and deaths.

CRITICAL PATHWAY. The PCXR is of value in narrowing the differential diagnosis of a wide spectrum of disorders, including problems in the following:

1. Oxygenation (i.e., pulmonary edema, pneumonia, pneumothorax, pulmonary embolism, atelectasis, ARDS).
2. Ventilation (i.e., neuromuscular abnormalities, drug overdose).
3. Combined causes (i.e., asthma, ARDS, chronic obstructive pulmonary disease).[49]

Community-Acquired Pneumonia

Community-acquired pneumonia may be typical or atypical. Typical pneumonias are pulmonary parenchymal infections thought to arise from microorganisms that inhabit the human nasopharyngeal airway. Infection results when normal host defense mechanisms fail to combat organisms occultly aspirated during sleep.[50] Organisms commonly identified include *Streptococcus pneumoniae, Staphylococcus aureus, Haemophilus influenzae,* and other gram-negative rod organisms as well.[50]

Atypical pneumonia differs in that the infection is thought to be acquired through inhalation of organisms from an environmental reservoir rather than by aspiration of airway secretions. *Legionella pneumophila* and influenza virus are common organisms producing this type of life-threatening pneumonia.[50]

CRITICAL PATHWAY. The chest radiograph is an early diagnostic tool in the patient with the clinical signs of pneumonia. It confirms the clinical appraisal and provides additional information to weigh the severity of the pulmonary infection while excluding other conditions. Certainly, the chest radiograph does not provide organism-specific information, but it can yield important clues in developing a therapeutic plan.

The radiographic presentation of pneumonia is well established for its generic appearance as an airspace-filling opacity. The specific radiographic details depend on several factors, including:

- Pulmonary architectural substrate
- Immune status of the patient
- Previous therapy and course of illness
- Virulence of the organism
- Presence or absence of coexisting cardiopulmonary conditions

The geography of pulmonary involvement is important. Focal airspace opacities confined to a single lobe or lung zone are more commonly seen with typical community-acquired pneumonias. The presence of more widespread or bilateral involvement should raise the suspicion of an atypical pneumonia or immune compromise (Fig. 37–18). The radiographic appraisal of what portions of lung are not involved is almost as important as determining the anatomic extent of the pneumonia.

Once therapy is begun, gradual clearing should be observed. Volume loss is a common observation in the ICU patient and may or may not be related to the ongoing infection. However, an endobronchial process should be considered with a focal process and accompanying volume loss. The presence or development of pleural fluid may be a sign of a

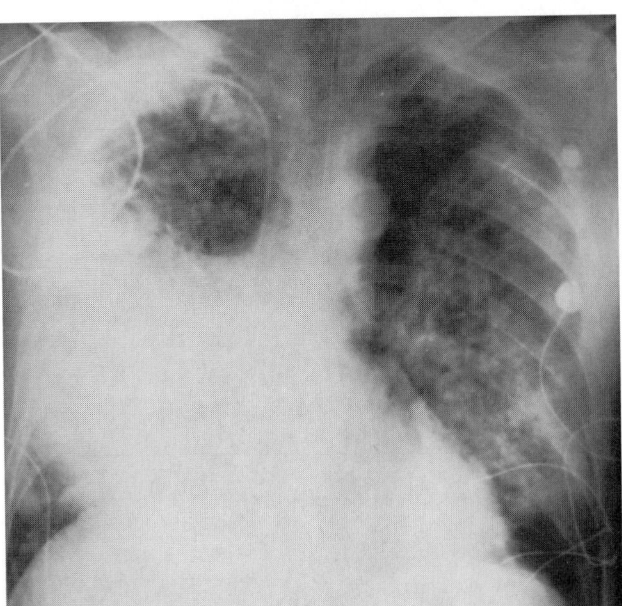

Figure 37–18. In this patient with fulminant pneumonia due to *Legionella*, an initial focus of airspace disease in the right lung progressed to dense consolidation with spread to the contralateral lung within a period of days.

pleural complication. As the parenchymal or pleural involvement grows more complicated, the sensitivity of the PCXR declines in defining the extent of disease. Chest CT provides benefit in detecting subtle complications such as empyema, abscess, and cavitation and in better defining the geographic pulmonary parenchymal burden.

Nosocomial Pneumonia

Nosocomial pneumonia is associated with the highest fatality rate among nosocomial infections.[51] It is most often associated with mechanical ventilation in patients hospitalized in the ICU, seen in anywhere from 9% to 21% of patients with varying causes of respiratory failure.[52] Risk factors for the development of ventilator-associated pneumonia include[51]:

- Intracranial pressure monitoring
- Prophylaxis with gastric acid inhibitors
- Chronic lung disease
- Depressed consciousness
- Endotracheal intubation
- Aspiration of stomach contents
- Thoracoabdominal surgery

The most important pathogens are *S. aureus, Pseudomonas aeruginosa, Acinetobacter* species and other gram-negative bacilli, *Haemophilus, S. pneumoniae, Branhamella catarrhalis, Neisseria* species, and other species of streptococci and coagulase-negative staphylococci. The cause of ventilator-associated pneumonia is polymicrobial in 21% to 42.3% of cases. The rate of nosocomial pneumonia varies, depending on the diagnostic criteria used. Experience has shown, however, that application of clinical and radiographic criteria only can lead to an overdiagnosis of pneumonia in the patient with respiratory failure, except for patients with ARDS.[51] Using clinical, radiographic, and laboratory data, physicians in the study of Fagon and colleagues[53] were able to accurately confirm the diagnosis of pneumonia in less than two thirds of cases.

CRITICAL PATHWAY. The radiographic diagnosis of pneumonia is suggested by the presence of airspace opacity, in particular asymmetric focal abnormalities that are new, worsening, or persistent (Fig. 37–19). It is agreed that ventilator-associated pneumonia can be accurately diagnosed by rapid cavitation of a pulmonary infiltrate or a pulmonary infiltrate adjacent to an empyema.[51] On PCXR, however, other disorders, such as atelectasis, bland aspiration, pulmonary hemorrhage, atypical pulmonary edema, asymmetric ARDS, and neoplasms, can appear similar to pneumonia, yielding a diagnostic accuracy of 52%.[52]

Asthma

Most asthmatic patients never experience a life-threatening acute exacerbation of their disease. Most patients who experience an episode of fatal or life-threatening asthma have a history of at least moderately severe disease. Previously intubated and mechanically ventilated patients are generally considered at high risk for life-threatening attacks.[54]

CRITICAL PATHWAY. The asthmatic patient may be seen initially in the emergency department, where the chest radiograph will probably be obtained to exclude other causes of diffuse wheezing, such as emphysema, bronchiectasis, chronic bronchitis, and major airway obstruction.[55] The radiograph may show hyperinflation, signs of transient pulmonary hypertension, and at times varying degrees of atelectasis. Pulmonary vascular patterns may be altered with diffuse narrowing, redistribution, and subpleural oligemia in the outer 2 to 4 cm of the lung.[55]

After intubation, ventilator-related complications are monitored with periodic chest radiography. Atelectasis, mucous plugging, pneumonia, air leak, and malpositioned endotracheal tube may be encountered.[54] Signs of atelectasis include a local increase in density that may be discoid ("plate-like") or segmental or that may involve an entire lobe (Fig. 37–20). Elevation of the hemidiaphragm and mediastinal shift occur when volume loss is present in lobes adjacent to these structures. Hilar displacement, compensatory overinflation, and rib approximation are additional indirect signs of atelectasis. When caused by mucous plugging, atelectasis commonly occurs and clears rapidly, particularly after pulmonary toilet or bronchoscopy. On occasion, plugs may move out of one lobe or segment into another, giving a shifting picture of atelectasis over time.

Air leak causing pneumomediastinum and pneumothorax occasionally occurs. The cardinal radiographic sign of pneumothorax is visualization of a fine linear opacity paralleling

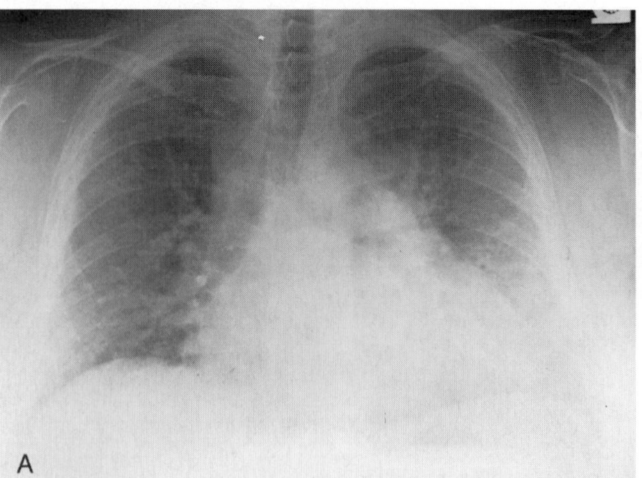

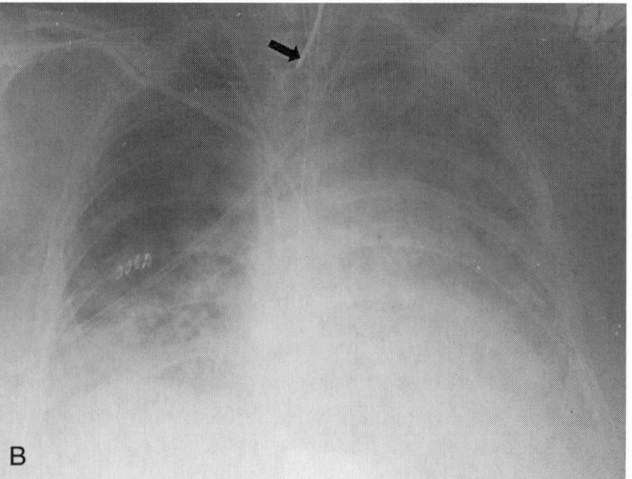

Figure 37–19. Nosocomial pneumonia. *A*, Baseline chest radiograph in 42-year-old woman with a history of pulmonary fibrosis demonstrates cardiomegaly and a diffuse, fine interstitial abnormality. *B*, The patient was admitted to the intensive care unit in respiratory failure following thoracoscopic lung biopsy (note surgical staples over the right mid zone) that revealed desquamative interstitial pneumonitis. One week later, there are clinical findings of pneumonia and bilateral airspace disease on the portable chest radiograph. The right upper lobe is relatively spared. Bronchoscopic cultures were positive for *Staphylococcus aureus*. Note the malpositioned feeding tube tip in the upper esophagus *(arrow)*.

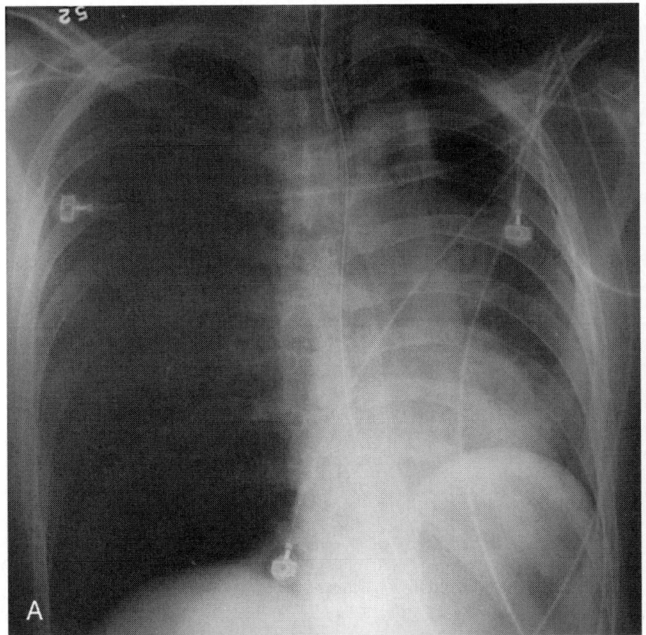

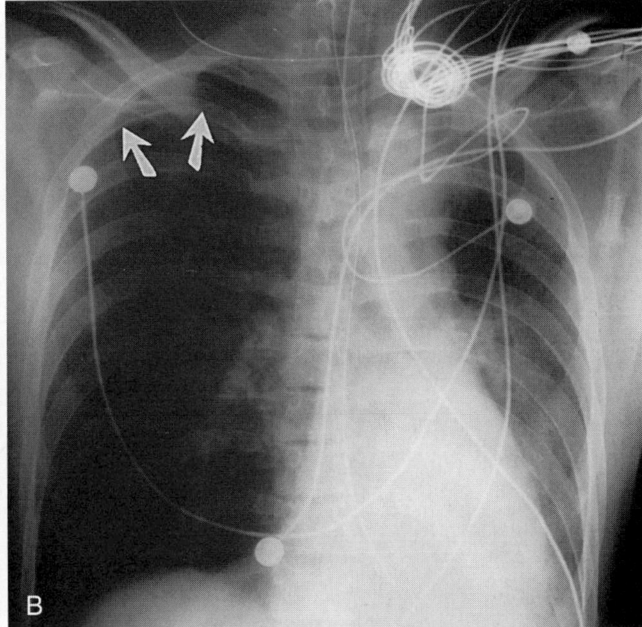

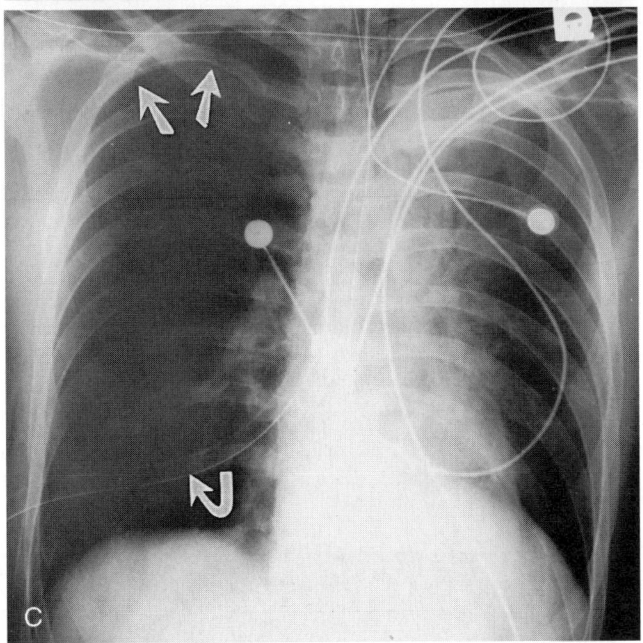

Figure 37–20. Respiratory failure in a 23-year-old patient with asthma. *A*, After intubation, there is partial collapse of the left upper and lower lobes by mucous plugging. The right lung is hyperinflated, and the cardiomediastinal silhouette is shifted to the left secondary to the collapse. *B*, Same patient, next day. Image shows complete collapse of the left lower lobe and partial left upper lobe collapse secondary to shifting plugs. Pneumothorax is now present in the right apex (seen to better advantage in *C*) *(arrows)* with the majority at the right base, causing a deep costophrenic sulcus. *C*, Later, same day. A right thoracostomy tube has been inserted *(curved arrow)*. The right apical pneumothorax persists *(straight arrows)*, although the deep right costophrenic sulcus is no longer present following partial evacuation of the pneumothorax. In the interval, the left lower lobe has partially reexpanded but there is persistent collapse in the left upper lobe.

the chest wall representing the visceral pleura outlined by intrapleural air on one side and aerated lung on the other. In the ICU, where radiographs are obtained with patients in the supine or semierect position, air collects along the lateral chest wall at the lung bases or medially, where it may simulate pneumomediastinum.[56] Hyperlucency of the hemidiaphragm and a deep costophrenic angle ("deep sulcus" sign) on the side of the pneumothorax may provide clues to the diagnosis (see Fig. 37–20*B*). Radiographic signs of tension include:

1. Contralateral shift of the heart and mediastinal structures.
2. Total or near-total collapse of the ipsilateral lung (although this may not be observed in the patient with a densely consolidated, noncompliant lung).
3. Flattening or inversion of the ipsilateral hemidiaphragm.

Skinfolds and large bullae can be confused with pneumothorax. If the diagnosis cannot be made with certainty on the supine PCXR, a lateral decubitus or upright PCXR can be obtained.

Drug Overdose

Cocaine and heroin are among the most commonly abused substances in the United States, and both drugs are associated with the development of respiratory insufficiency and pulmonary edema. Overdose of tricyclic antidepressants is an important cause of death from drug ingestion and is associated with respiratory complications.[57]

CRITICAL PATHWAY. After the intravenous administration of heroin, patients who present with altered state of consciousness, pupillary constriction, and respiratory depression frequently have pulmonary edema. Pulmonary edema may occur anytime within the first few hours, or it can be delayed up to 24 hours later. On PCXR (Fig. 37–21), diffuse, symmetric, perihilar airspace opacity is noted, noncardiogenic in nature

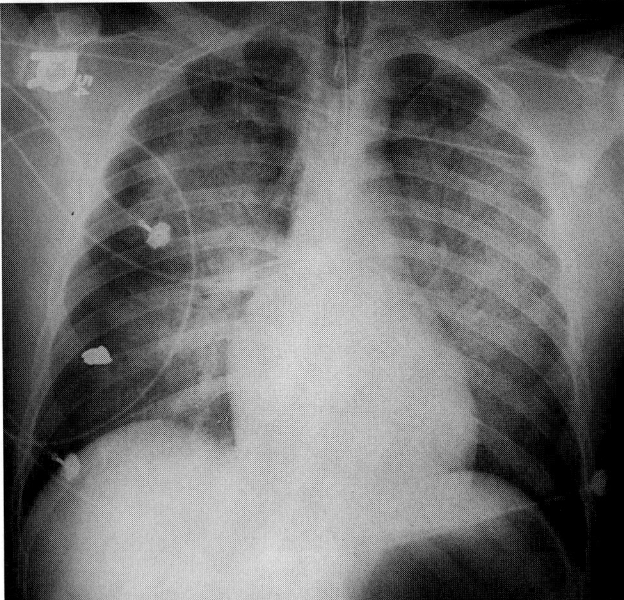

Figure 37–21. Heroin overdose and respiratory failure in a 38-year-old man. Portable chest radiography demonstrates dense bilateral airspace disease with normal heart size and absence of pleural effusion. Findings are consistent with opiate-induced noncardiogenic pulmonary edema. Note bullet fragment over the right lower zone from a previous gunshot wound.

(i.e., normal heart size, absent pleural effusions), secondary to hypoxia or transient elevation of intracranial pressure. In general, if improvement does not occur in the next 24 to 48 hours, survival is unlikely. Airspace disease persisting in excess of 5 days suggests the possibility of a superimposed process or complication such as pneumonia.[57]

Cocaine may also produce noncardiogenic pulmonary edema, regardless of the route of administration, secondary to direct alveolar capillary injury or tissue ischemia. As in heroin overdose, the PCXR demonstrates symmetric, bilateral airspace disease. Rarely, patients smoking freebase cocaine ("crack") may present with hemoptysis and airspace disease secondary to diffuse alveolar hemorrhage[58, 59]; pneumopericardium, pneumomediastinum, and pneumothorax have also been reported.[60] In addition to pulmonary abnormalities, cocaine may also cause myocardial infarction, dilated cardiomyopathy, valvular heart disease, myocarditis, arrhythmia, sudden death, and aortic rupture[60] (Fig. 37–22).

Tricyclic overdose has been associated with the complications of cardiac arrhythmias, seizures, respiratory depression, and coma. The PCXR may demonstrate opacities consistent with alveolar pulmonary edema, and these patients have clinical ARDS. The noncardiogenic pulmonary edema of tricyclic-induced ARDS is thought to be secondary to increased capillary permeability as a direct toxic effect of the drug.[57] One must take into account the state of hydration in assessing changes in the parenchymal abnormality or the presence of pleural effusion. As for any patient with altered state of consciousness, the PCXR should be monitored for the possibility of aspiration pneumonia.

Adult Respiratory Distress Syndrome

The sudden emergence of tachypnea, obvious respiratory distress with use of accessory muscles of respiration, diffuse and usually symmetric pulmonary infiltrates on PCXRs, and refractory hypoxemia were first described[61] in patients with a unique form of acute respiratory failure, all requiring mechanical ventilatory assistance. The PCXR is useful in the course of ARDS for the following:

1. To exclude the presence of other or coexistent processes (i.e., pneumonia, pneumothorax).
2. To assess the position of life-support and monitoring devices during the acute phase.
3. To evaluate for complications in the later stages of treatment (barotrauma, pneumonia, abscess).

CRITICAL PATHWAY. Three pathologic stages have been described[62] that in the absence of preexisting disease broadly correlate with the radiographic findings:

- *Stage I* (0–24 hours) is an initial exudative phase in which sloughing of the alveolar epithelium and capillary endothelium occurs. There are few if any radiographic correlates to this early phase, referred to as a radiographically latent stage. During this time interval, other causes of hypoxemia, such as pulmonary embolism, are included in the differential diagnosis.
- *Stage II* (24–36 hours) ushers in the appearance of dense airspace consolidation because of fluid leakage into the interstitium and alveolar spaces with alveolar collapse. The PCXR may show a ground-glass opacification initially, followed by patchy, frequently peripheral consolidation with prominent air bronchograms. These radiographic findings have been reported to have an accuracy of 84% in the diagnosis of ARDS.[52]
- *Stage III* (72 hours onward) is characterized by fibroproliferation and hyperplasia of type II alveolar pneumocytes. Airspace consolidation slowly decreases, but there may be evidence of residual reticular and ground-glass opacity (Fig. 37–23). Uncommonly, signs of air leak including pneumomediastinum, subcutaneous emphysema, and pneumothorax may appear (Fig. 37–24), related to the severity of the lung injury.[63] Even a seemingly small pneumothorax may have dramatic clinical impact because the lungs are noncompliant and unable to fully collapse. CT evaluation of the lungs in ARDS[64] has demonstrated that most pulmonary opacities are bilateral (92%), gravity-dependent (86%), and basilar (68%) (Fig. 37–25). In only 25% of patients are the findings homogeneous, the remainder having patchy consolidation or mixed airspace/

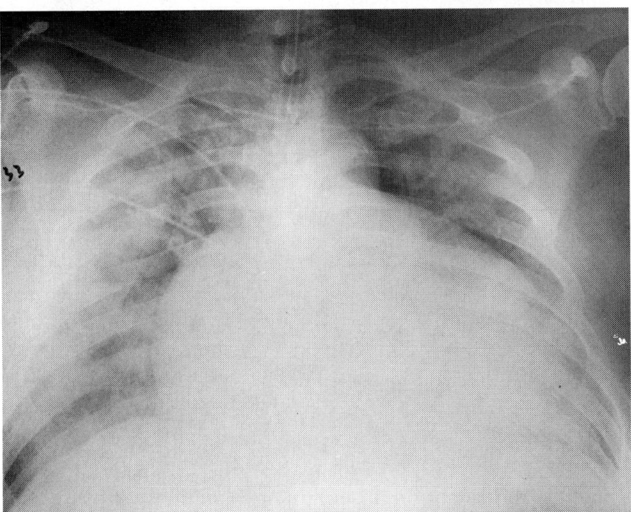

Figure 37–22. The patient is a 37-year-old chronic cocaine abuser with respiratory and cardiac failure. Portable chest radiograph demonstrates a massively enlarged heart secondary to cocaine-induced cardiomyopathy as well as widespread pulmonary edema.

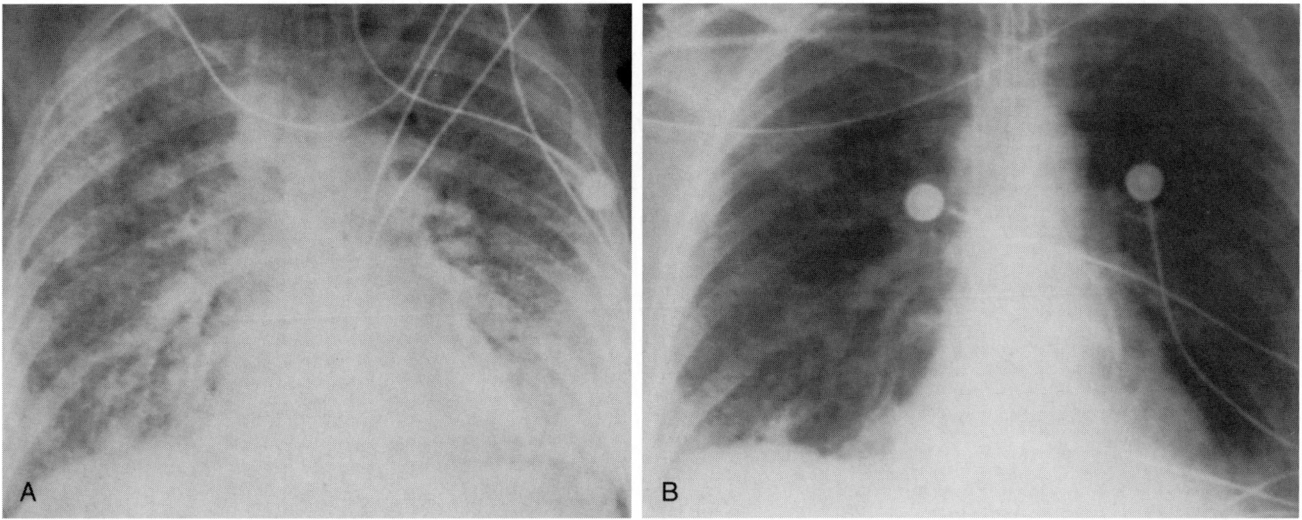

Figure 37–23. *A*, Portable chest radiograph of a patient with clinical signs and symptoms of adult respiratory distress syndrome demonstrates bilateral airspace disease with extensive involvement of the lung periphery. Note the prominent central air bronchograms, normal heart size, and absence of pleural fluid. *B*, A film taken 1 week later with the patient still intubated shows residual interstitial opacities, particularly at the right lung base.

ground-glass opacity with air bronchograms. Small pleural effusions are seen in about 50% of patients. CT evidence of pneumonia, abscess, and barotrauma (interstitial emphysema, subpleural air cysts, pneumomediastinum, and pneumothorax), undetected on the PCXR, may be discovered, which can clarify unexplained deterioration in respiratory status.

The use of partial liquid ventilation during extracorporeal life support in patients with acute severe respiratory failure may result in complete or subtotal opacification of the lung fields by perfluorocarbon agents that improve pulmonary gas exchange and lung compliance[65] (Fig. 37–26).

Gastrointestinal Bleeding

The patient presenting with massive gastrointestinal blood loss is rapidly assessed to determine hemodynamic status, activity of bleeding, and underlying medical conditions that complicate management. The first priority is to determine the extent of blood loss and whether perfusion is compromised.[66] Radiographic investigations are centered on emergency angiography for diagnosis and hemostasis of bleeding sites or placement of a transjugular intrahepatic portosystemic shunt.

CRITICAL PATHWAY. The PCXR is obtained early in the course of massive gastrointestinal bleeding to assess for the presence of aspiration, especially in the presence of hepatic encephalopathy (Fig. 37–27). During the course of volume resuscitation, the cardiopulmonary status is evaluated for the possibility of fluid overload; radiographic signs include the presence of a widened vascular pedicle, interstitial pulmonary edema with Kerley's lines, and pleural effusions. Appropriate positioning of central venous lines, Swan-Ganz pulmonary artery catheter, and life-support tubes is also confirmed, and the complication of a pneumothorax is excluded.

Pneumomediastinum can occur secondary to esophageal rupture *(Boerhaave's syndrome)* or perforation during endos-

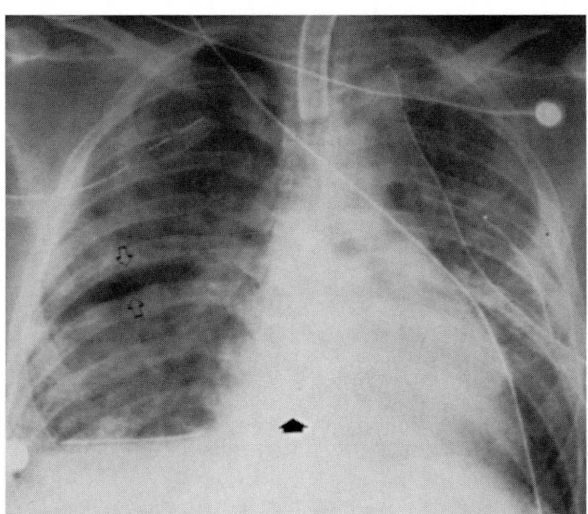

Figure 37–24. Bilateral chest tubes were required in this patient with adult respiratory distress syndrome and barotrauma. Note the presence of intrafissural air *(open arrows)* and of residual intrapleural air at the right lung apex. The right basilar chest tube was nonfunctional, and the tip projected across the midline *(arrow)*.

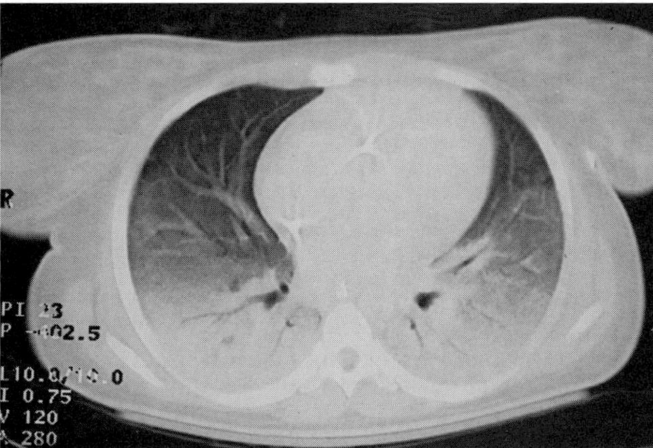

Figure 37–25. Chest CT in a 15-year-old female with molar pregnancy and adult respiratory distress syndrome. Note the homogeneous airspace disease with air bronchograms in the dependent portions of both lungs. On other images, peripheral nodules secondary to metastatic disease were also present.

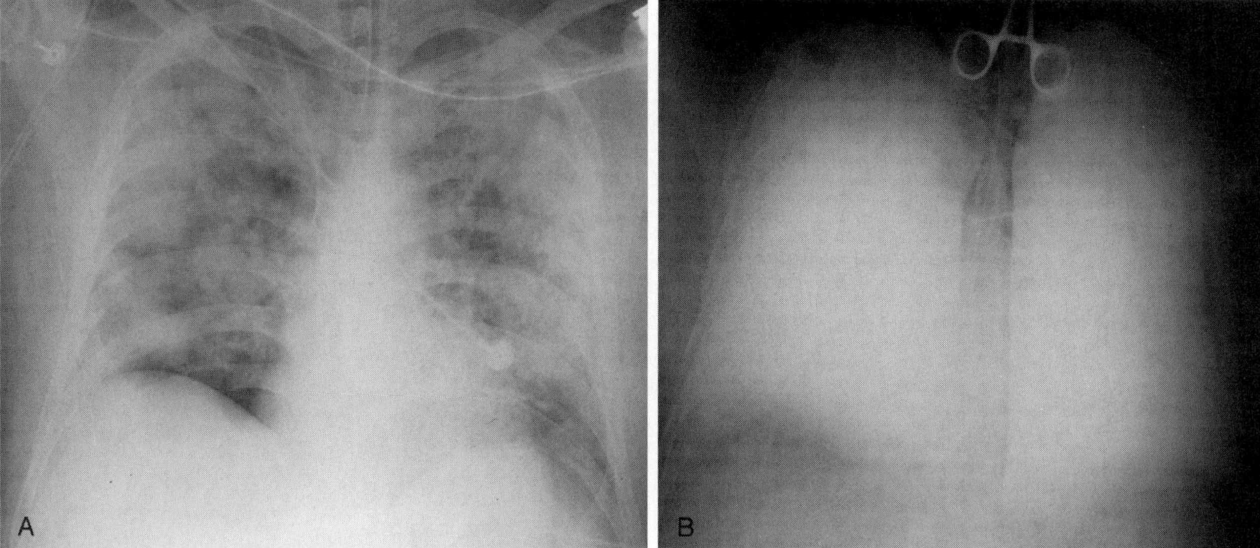

Figure 37–26. *A*, The patient is a 43-year-old man with a gunshot wound to the abdomen and subsequent laparotomy, sepsis, and respiratory failure. Portable chest radiograph demonstrates bilateral airspace disease extending to the lung periphery and the presence of air bronchograms consistent with adult respiratory distress syndrome. *B*, Two days later, after administration of perfluorocarbon liquid ventilation through the endotracheal tube. The lungs are densely opacified and increased in volume.

copy, most often appearing as a linear lucency along the cardiomediastinal border. It may be associated with soft-tissue emphysema in the supraclavicular region and neck and eventuate in pneumothorax. Widening and increased density of the mediastinum are suggestive of a periesophageal hematoma or fluid collection from esophageal leak and mediastinitis. Patients undergoing esophagogastroduodenoscopy (EGD) are at increased risk for aspiration secondary to (1) premedication and topical anesthesia that impair the gag reflex, (2) mechanical impairment of swallowing during the procedure, and (3) active bleeding and gastric lavage during the EGD. In one study of ICU patients with upper gastrointestinal bleeding,[67] new left lower lobe parenchymal disease secondary to aspiration developed in six of 24 (25%) nonintubated patients after EGD was performed with the patient in the left lateral decubitus position. Fever or leukocytosis with oxygen desaturation subsequently developed in five patients with airspace disease; the sixth patient experienced collapse of the left lower lobe without symptoms.

The balloon tamponade of varices is associated with a 30% incidence of complications that may be evaluated radiographically, including aspiration pneumonia, esophageal rupture, and airway obstruction.[68]

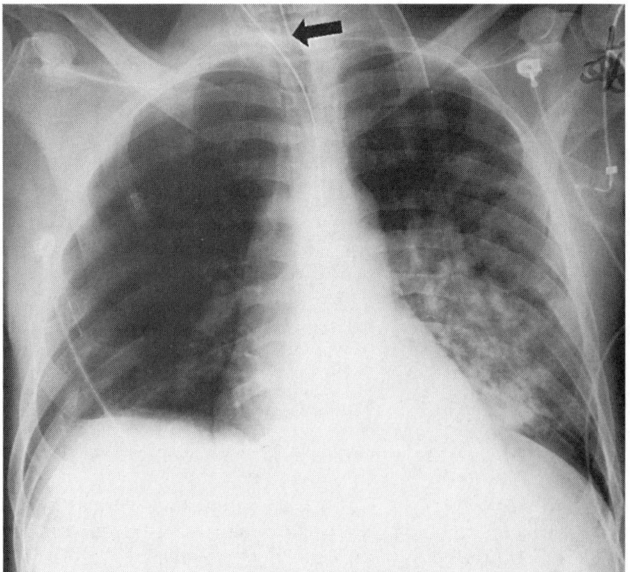

Figure 37–27. Portable chest radiograph in a 52-year-old man after massive upper gastrointestinal bleeding and endoscopy. There is extensive airspace disease in the left lower lobe secondary to aspiration of blood. Note the high position of the endotracheal tube *(arrow)*.

The Immunocompromised Host in the Intensive Care Unit

Acquired Immunodeficiency Syndrome

Thoracic complications are a major cause of morbidity and mortality in patients with the acquired immunodeficiency syndrome (AIDS). In one series, 51% died of respiratory insufficiency; 76% of the total had opportunistic infections, and 37% had neoplasms.[69] *Pneumocystis carinii* pneumonia occurs in the clinical course of many patients with AIDS and is a frequent cause of death.

CRITICAL PATHWAY. Signs and symptoms of *P. carinii* pneumonia are nonspecific, including nonproductive cough, increasing dyspnea, and variable fever. Malaise and constitutional symptoms may be the main initial complaint.[70]

On the PCXR, *P. carinii* pneumonia initially appears as a diffuse, bilateral, symmetric, finely granular or reticular abnormality that may be interstitial or airspace in nature (Fig. 37–28). Typically, adenopathy and pleural effusions are absent. Not uncommonly, this pattern may progress to frank homogeneous airspace disease. A less common presentation consisting of multiple nodular opacities may be confused with a fungal or malignant cause. An increased incidence of predominantly upper lobe involvement is reported with the use of aerosolized pentamidine, which is poorly distributed to the upper zones and therefore less effective in preventing reactivation in this area.[71] Thin-walled pneumatoceles, often multiple and reaching diameters of up to 10 cm, may occur (Fig.

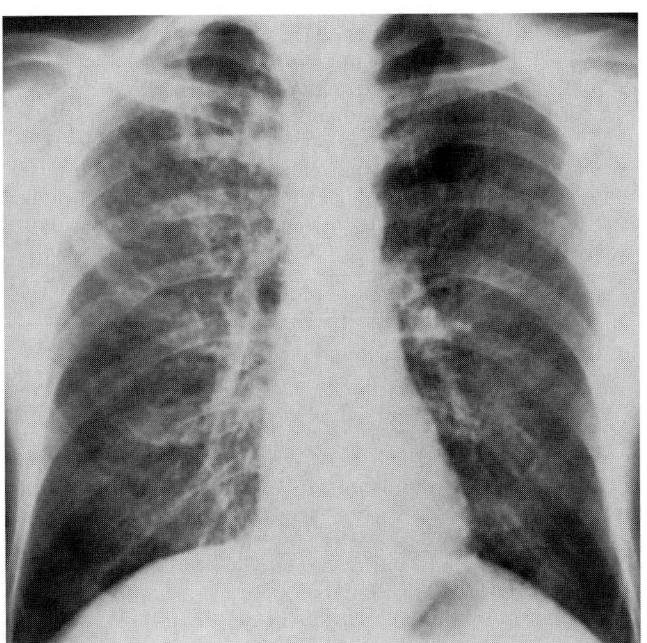

Figure 37–28. Typical radiographic appearance of *Pneumocystis carinii* pneumonia presenting as a diffuse interstitial pneumonia. Note the absence of adenopathy and pleural effusion.

37-29). Spontaneous pneumothorax (Fig. 37-30), frequently but not always seen in association with visualized pneumatoceles or bullae, may result in persistent air leak and require multiple pleural drainage catheters.[72] On chest CT, ground-glass attenuation is seen that may be diffuse and homogeneous or patchy in distribution. High-resolution CT is useful in the symptomatic patient with a normal or equivocal PCXR to confirm or exclude significant parenchymal lung disease and accelerate more aggressive diagnostic approaches in confirmed cases. On the average, pneumonia may be seen on high-resolution CT about 5 days before the PCXR findings become diagnostic in the immunocompromised host.[73]

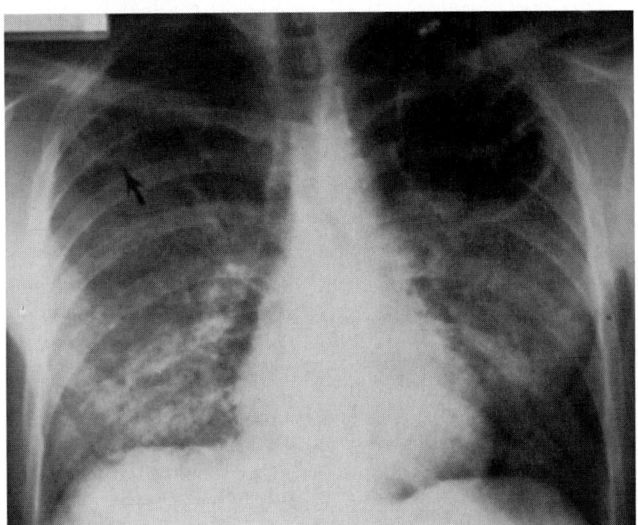

Figure 37–29. Chest radiograph of a young man with acquired immunodeficiency syndrome and *Pneumocystis carinii* pneumonia demonstrates bilateral interstitial and airspace disease. A large pneumatocele is present in the left upper lung zone, and a smaller cystic cavity is visible on the right *(arrow)*.

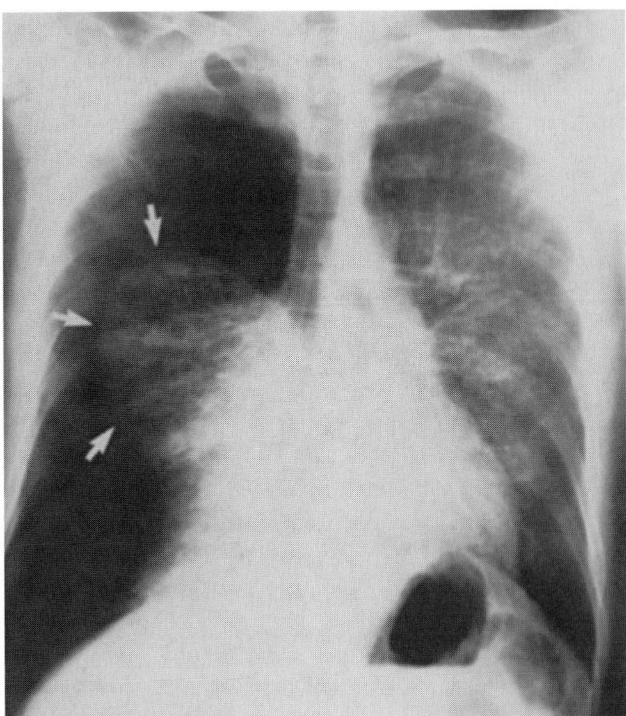

Figure 37–30. Same patient as in Figure 37-28. The course of pneumonia was complicated by a right tension pneumothorax *(arrows)*. Signs of tension seen here include contralateral shift of the heart and the mediastinum as well as depression of the right hemidiaphragm.

In uncomplicated cases of *P. carinii* pneumonia, radiographic improvement is generally noted in 7 to 10 days. If initial clinical response is followed by an apparent relapse on PCXR in 3 to 4 days, the possibility of volume overload secondary to the large quantity of fluid delivered with trimethoprim-sulfamethoxazole should be considered. Recognition of pleural effusion and intrathoracic adenopathy is of practical importance in the radiographic differential diagnosis of AIDS-related thoracic diseases. Although rare in cases of isolated *P. carinii* pneumonia, pleural fluid or adenopathy should suggest another superimposed neoplastic or inflammatory process, such as lymphoma or mycobacterial infection. In these instances, CT may again be helpful in refining the differential diagnosis.[74]

Lung Transplantation

Patients undergoing single or double lung transplantation are subject to several unique complications, including (1) reperfusion edema (the reimplantation response), (2) acute rejection, and (3) infection.

Reperfusion Edema

Reperfusion edema occurs in almost all transplanted lungs. In the series of Anderson and coworkers,[75] it occurred in 98% of patients, and it is evident in virtually all patients within 48 hours of transplantation.

CRITICAL PATHWAY. Reperfusion edema appears as perihilar or basilar interstitial or airspace disease that is frequently present on the first postoperative PCXR and peaks in severity by day 4 (Fig. 37-31); in general, there is a poor correlation between radiographic severity and physiologic parameters. It is important to exclude other conditions, such as fluid overload, left ventricular failure, rejection, infection, and atelectasis. However, any process beginning or worsening after day 5

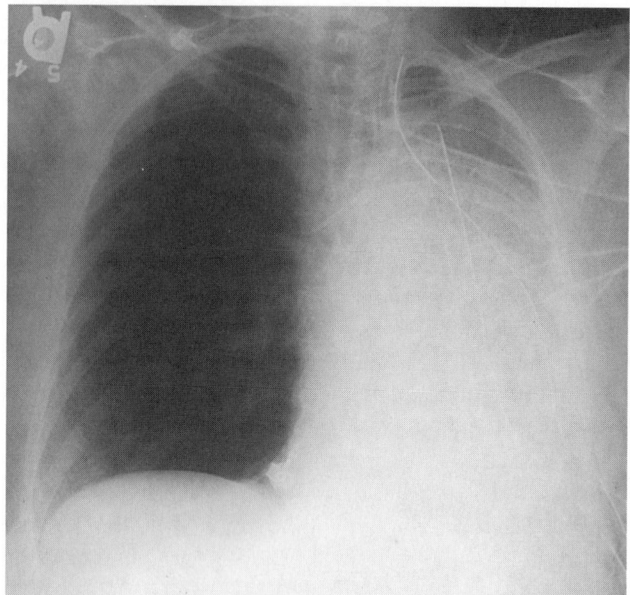

Figure 37–31. Portable chest radiograph on the first postoperative day following left lung transplant for emphysema in a 52-year-old woman. Note the diffuse airspace disease in the left lung secondary to reperfusion pulmonary edema. The right lung is overexpanded and hyperlucent owing to the underlying emphysema.

following lung transplantation is unlikely to represent this entity and should be investigated accordingly.[76]

Acute Rejection

Acute lung rejection may cause radiographic abnormalities generally seen between 5 and 10 days after transplantation. It is suggested clinically on the basis of fever and decreased oxygen saturation in the absence of infection, airway obstruction, or volume overload.

CRITICAL PATHWAY. The diagnosis is suggested by the presence of septal lines and new or increasing pleural effusions, without evidence of increased cardiac or vascular pedicle size; these findings are 68% sensitive and 90% specific for acute rejection. Worsening or persistent radiographic abnormality after postoperative day 5 (when reperfusion edema would be expected to improve) was predictive of acute rejection in 14 of 15 patients in Murray's study.[77]

Infection

Infection occurs in up to 75% of patients after lung transplantation, more often in the transplanted lung because of denervation with loss of the cough reflex and impaired mucociliary clearance.[77] The time course may be helpful in that bacterial infections are most commonly seen in the first month, whereas fungal and viral pneumonias appear 2 to 3 months later.

CRITICAL PATHWAY. On the PCXR, bacterial infections are suggested by the presence of airspace consolidation in the setting of cough, fever, and dyspnea. Nodular or cavitary disease may be caused by necrotizing infections such as disease due to *P. aeruginosa.*

Cytomegalovirus (CMV) is the most common opportunistic pulmonary pathogen,[78] causing diffuse or focal hazy opacity or reticular or reticulonodular interstitial abnormality, often associated with small effusions (see Fig. 37–34). Clinically, CMV infection peaks at 4 months postoperatively; patients present with dyspnea, fever, and cough. Radiographic abnormality occurs almost exclusively in the transplanted lung; however, it may be visualized in only one third to two thirds of cases.[78]

Candidiasis and invasive aspergillosis are the most common fungal infections in this population; both occur more commonly in lungs that have been previously traumatized by past infections, acute rejection, or other post-transplant complication.[79] Invasive aspergillosis may have a distinctive radiographic picture of one or more nodular opacities with lucent crescents or a surrounding "halo" due to hemorrhage (see Fig. 37–33).[80, 81] The radiographic manifestations of these infections are nonspecific, however, and CT may be useful in directing bronchoscopy or percutaneous needle biopsy.[79]

Bone Marrow Transplantation

Respiratory complications are a major cause of morbidity and mortality after bone marrow transplantation (BMT) and are reported in 40% to 60% of patients.[82] This population is susceptible not only to diseases common to other immunosuppressed patients (i.e., adverse reactions to chemotherapy, total-body radiation, opportunistic pneumonias, noninfectious pneumonitis) but also to graft-versus-host disease. The BMT patient is unique in that the onset of pulmonary complications is temporally related to the sequence of (1) the regimen of chemotherapy and radiation before transplantation, (2) the impairment of immune functions after BMT, and (3) the onset of graft-versus-host disease.[83]

CRITICAL PATHWAY. In the first 30 days after BMT (before engraftment), most pulmonary abnormalities are noninfectious in etiology and include pulmonary edema, diffuse alveolar hemorrhage, and drug reactions. Bacterial pneumonia secondary to neutropenia and aspiration in patients with severe mucositis receiving narcotic analgesics may occur, as may fungal (*Aspergillus* and *Candida)* and viral (herpes simplex, respiratory syncytial, and parainfluenza) infections.[84] Because the clinical presentations of these infectious complications may be indistinguishable from noninfectious causes, the PCXR findings remain a key factor in diagnosis and follow-up.

Pulmonary Edema. This complication is reported in anywhere from 11% to 65% of patients during the first weeks after BMT.[85] Patients present with tachypnea, dyspnea, hypoxia, and sometimes fever. Combined overhydration, cardiogenic edema, renal insufficiency, and hypoalbuminemia are among the many causes.[84] Diffuse, ground-glass opacity associated with Kerley's lines is characteristic of edema and not commonly seen with interstitial pneumonia. It may have a somewhat protracted course and resolve slowly during 8 to 17 days. Any patient presenting in the first 2 weeks after BMT with Kerley's lines should be regarded as having a transient process that does not require biopsy. CT should be reserved for patients with atypical clinical and radiographic findings.[82]

Diffuse Alveolar Hemorrhage. Usually occurring within the first few weeks of BMT, this complication is associated with a prevalence of up to 14%. Risk factors include age older than 40 years; prior radiation to the chest, mediastinum, or total body; BMT for solid tumors; and renal insufficiency.[86] Although most patients have cough, dyspnea, and hypoxemia, hemoptysis is uncommon. Radiographic abnormalities usually appear within the first 2 weeks after BMT in the form of bilateral interstitial and airspace opacity in the mid and lower zones, indistinguishable from edema or opportunistic infection (Fig. 37–32). On occasion, the process is unilateral, leading to confusion with pneumonia.[87] The course is usually fulminant with development of severe, widespread airspace consolidation, and mortality is reported in up to 100% of patients.[83, 88]

Drug Reaction. Pulmonary drug toxicity develops in as many as 31% of patients after autologous BMT; a reaction may occur in the early period or as long as 12 weeks later. Pulmonary symptoms are nonspecific and include dry cough, fever, and dyspnea.[89] PCXR findings of drug toxicity are nonspecific,

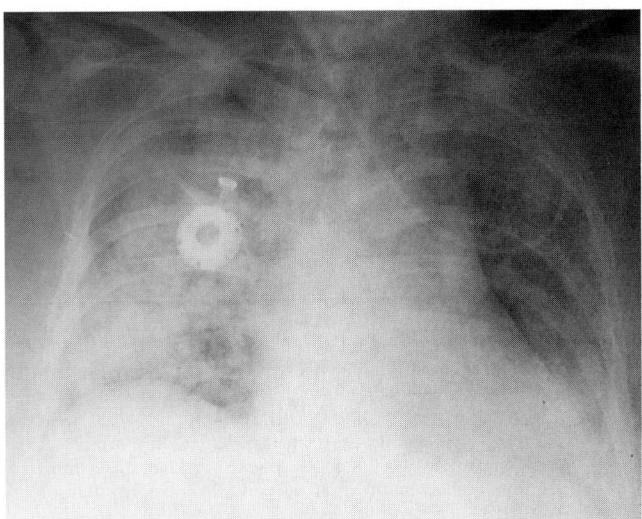

Figure 37–32. Portable chest radiograph in a 50-year-old woman 6 weeks after allogeneic related bone marrow transplant for chronic myeloid leukemia. Bilateral airspace disease, asymmetric in distribution and secondary to pulmonary hemorrhage, is present.

demonstrating bilateral, diffuse, or patchy airspace opacities,[90] which may proceed to consolidation and ARDS. On CT scan, clues to the presence of drug reaction include peripheral, ill-defined airspace or nodular opacities, random in distribution, with dependent involvement of the lower lobes.[89] High-resolution CT may show ground-glass attenuation in addition to ill-defined nodules and coarse reticular densities.[91, 92]

Pneumonia. Bacterial pneumonia occurs in 20% to 50% of patients in the neutropenic period immediately after BMT,[86] including both gram-positive and gram-negative organisms. Anaerobes from aspiration secondary to severe mucositis and narcotic analgesia may also play a role. On PCXR, airspace consolidation is seen that may be segmental, lobar, or patchy in distribution; diffuse or focal cavitary diseases are also reported.[93] CT may demonstrate ground-glass opacity from early pneumonia before visualization on PCXR[85]; thus, this modality may be helpful when pneumonia is suspected but the radiograph is still normal. *P. carinii* pneumonia is unusual in the early transplant period because of trimethoprim-sulfamethoxazole prophylaxis, generally given for 100 days after BMT.[86] Perihilar interstitial abnormality progressing to bilateral airspace consolidation during 3 to 5 days is characteristic of *P. carinii* pneumonia. The absence of adenopathy and pleural effusion and the sparing of previously irradiated lung are additional clues to the diagnosis.[94] On CT, ground-glass attenuation is seen most commonly, with miliary pattern, small nodules, reticular opacities, septal thickening, and cystic lesions also reported.[91]

Fungal pneumonias usually appear in the early post-transplant period when patients are severely neutropenic and almost all are febrile.[95] *Aspergillus* and *Candida* are the most common pathogens, with *Cryptococcus*, *Histoplasma*, and *Coccidioides* reported. *Aspergillus* infection occurs in as many as 4% to 13% of all patients; the infection is life-threatening.[83, 84] On PCXR, focal airspace opacities or nodular densities are highly suggestive of fungal infection. Crescent-shaped lucencies within the nodules are characteristic of invasive pulmonary aspergillosis (Fig. 37–33). This sign, however, is a relatively late finding, appearing on the average of 41 days after BMT. On CT, a characteristic halo may be seen around the nodules earlier in the course of the disease, about 15 days after BMT. This finding is most suggestive of invasive aspergillosis,[95] although the sign has also been reported in association with *Candida,* CMV, and herpes simplex pneumonias.[96] Unlike invasive aspergillosis, *Candida* pneumonia has nonspecific features on PCXR, consisting of bilateral airspace disease or, rarely, a miliary pattern.[82] On CT, pulmonary nodules, ground-glass attenuation, and airspace disease may be seen; in 60% of patients with nodules, the halo sign is evident.[96, 97] Low-attenuation lesions in the liver, spleen, and kidneys may be seen on CT in patients with either invasive aspergillosis or *Candida* infection.

Viral pneumonias are among the most common infections during the first 3 weeks after BMT. The radiographic appearance is that of a progressive, mixed interstitial and airspace process that is diffuse and symmetric, either linear or nodular in nature.[93] Herpes simplex virus is one of the most frequent pathogens[86]; the diagnosis is suggested by the presence of

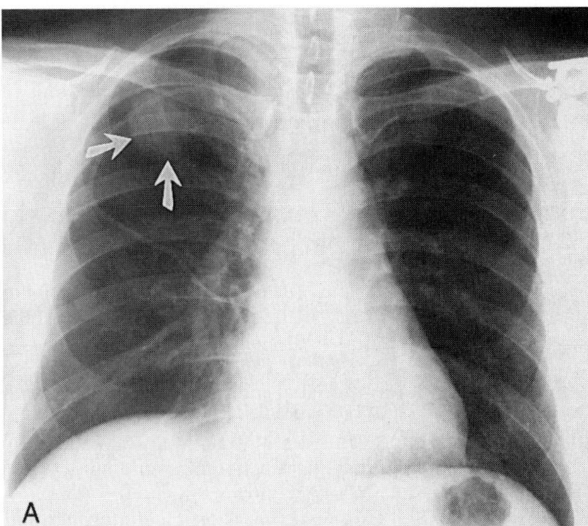

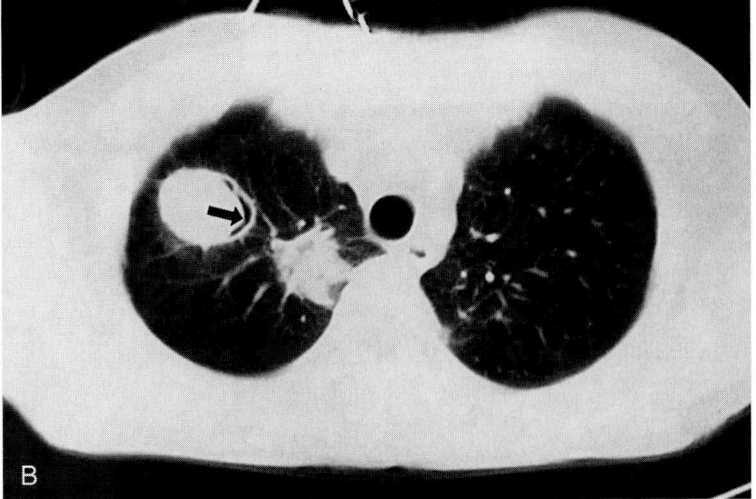

Figure 37–33. Invasive aspergillosis. *A*, The patient is a 48-year-old man with Hodgkin's lymphoma and bone marrow transplant 3 years previously. He presented with fever, neutropenia, and cough. Chest radiograph demonstrates a poorly defined nodular density in the right upper lobe *(arrows)*. A crescentic lucency was faintly visible along the inferomedial aspect of the nodule. *B*, CT demonstrates the nodular density in the right upper lobe with lucent crescent secondary to invasive aspergillosis *(arrow)*. A second nodule is present adjacent to the spine.

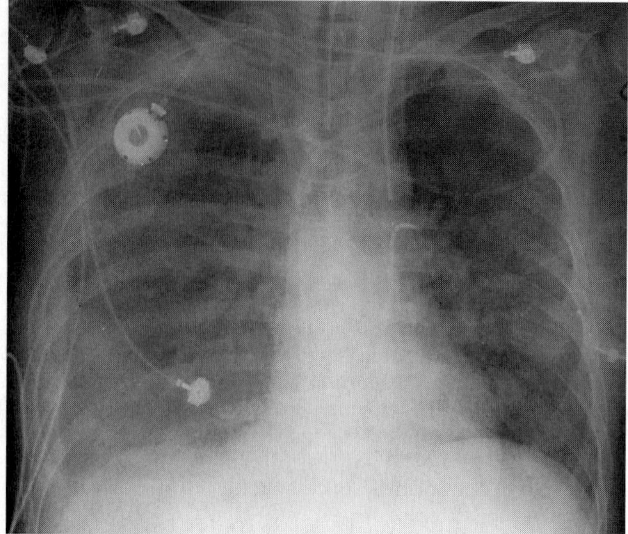

Figure 37–34. Cytomegalovirus pneumonia in a 54-year-old woman with chronic myelomonocytic leukemia 103 days following bone marrow transplantation. Diffuse reticular interstitial abnormality is present with areas of confluence and nodularity. Right pleural effusion is also seen.

cutaneous, oral, or esophageal involvement.[96] On PCXR, nonspecific bilateral airspace consolidation is seen, typically beginning in the lower lobes peripherally and progressing superiorly and centrally.[93] On CT, patchy ground-glass opacity and diffuse nodules with ill-defined margins may be seen.[91] In the first 10 days after BMT, respiratory syncytial virus has also been identified as a common pathogen, the pneumonia typically preceded by an upper respiratory infection. The findings on PCXR are nonspecific, consisting of focal or diffuse abnormalities; the diffuse abnormality is associated with a poor outcome.[98]

Cytomegalovirus pneumonia typically occurs later, between 2 and 6 months after BMT. The prevalence of and mortality associated with this infection are decreasing as a result of prophylaxis with ganciclovir and use of cytomegalovirus immune globulin.[99] Radiographic findings include widespread reticular opacities, small nodules, airspace consolidation, or a combination of these patterns (Fig. 37–34). CT is more sensitive than PCXR for the early detection of the interstitial pneumonia. Small nodules with ground-glass attenuation proceed to airspace consolidation; fine reticular opacities, septal thickening, and nodules of various sizes have been reported[86, 99] (Fig. 37–35).

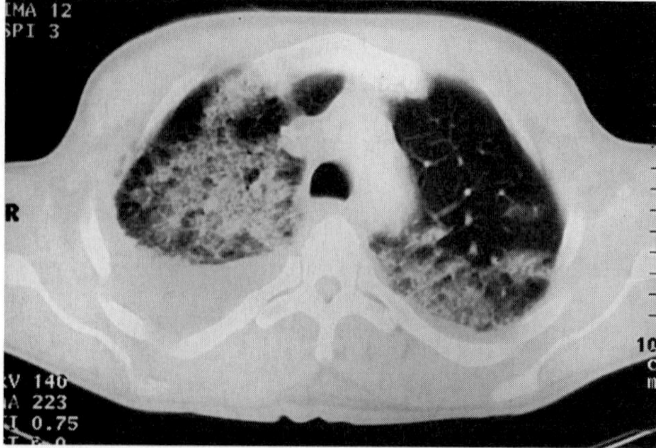

Figure 37–35. Non-Hodgkin's lymphoma and cytomegalovirus pneumonia in a different patient. CT demonstrates mixed interstitial and airspace opacity with bilateral pleural effusions. On other images, small, ill-defined nodules were also present.

References

1. Marik PE, Janower ML: The impact of routine chest radiography on ICU management decisions: An observational study. Am J Crit Care 1997; 6:95.
2. Wandtke J: Bedside chest radiography. Radiology 1994; 190:1.
3. Cascade PN, Kazerooni EA: Aspects of chest imaging in the intensive care unit. Crit Care Clin 1994; 10:247.
4. Marglin SI, Rowberg AH, Godwin JD: Preliminary experience with portable digital imaging for intensive care radiography. J Thorac Imaging 1990; 5:49.
5. Niklason LT, Heang-Ping C, Cascade PN, et al: Portable chest imaging: Comparison of storage phosphor digital, asymmetric screen-film, and conventional screen-film systems. Radiology 1993; 186:387.
6. Sagel SS, Jost RG, Glazer HS, et al: Digital mobile radiography. J Thorac Imaging 1990; 5:36.
7. MacMahon H, Giger M: Portable chest radiography techniques and teleradiology. Radiol Clin North Am 1996; 34:1.
8. Hall JB, White SR, Karrison T: Efficacy of daily routine chest radiographs in intubated, mechanically intubated patients. Crit Care Med 1991; 19:689.
9. Bekemeyer WB, Crapo RO, Calhoun S, et al: Efficacy of chest radiography in a respiratory intensive care unit: A prospective study. Chest 1985; 88:691.
10. Henschke CI, Yankelevitz DF, Wand A, et al: Accuracy and efficacy of chest radiography in the intensive care unit. Radiol Clin North Am 1996; 34:21.
11. Zarshenas Z, Sparschu RA: Catheter placement and misplacement. Crit Care Clin 1994; 10:417.
12. Brunel SW, Coleman DL, Schwartz DE, et al: Assessment of routine chest roentgenograms and the physical examination to confirm endotracheal tube position. Chest 1989; 96:1043.
13. Zwillich CW, Pierson DJ, Creagh CR, et al: Complications of assisted ventilation: A prospective study of 354 consecutive episodes. Am J Med 1974; 57:161.
14. Smith GM, Reed JC, Choplin RH: Radiographic detection of esophageal malpositioning of endotracheal tubes. Am J Roentgenol 1990; 154:23.
15. Zimmermann JE, Goodman LR, Shahvari MBG: Effect of mechanical ventilation and positive end expiratory pressure (PEEP) on chest radiograph. Am J Roentgenol 1979; 133:811.
16. Conces DJ, Holden RW: Aberrant locations and complications in initial placement of subclavian vein catheters. Arch Surg 1984; 119:293.
17. Gibson RN, Hennessy OF, Collier N, et al: Major complications of central venous catheterization: A report of five cases and a brief review of the literature. Clin Radiol 1985; 36:205.
18. Brandstetter RD, Gitler B: Thoughts on the Swan-Ganz catheter. Chest 1986; 89:5.
19. West J, Dollery C, Naimack A: Distribution of blood flow in isolated lung: Relation to vascular and alveolar pressures. J Appl Physiol 1964; 19:713.
20. Sise MJ, Hollingsworth P, Brimm JE, et al: Complications of the flow-directed pulmonary artery catheter: A prospective analysis of 219 patients. Crit Care Med 1981; 9:315.
21. Dieden JD, Friloux LA III, Renner JW: Pulmonary artery false aneurysms secondary to Swan-Ganz pulmonary artery catheters. Am J Roentgenol 1987; 149:901.
22. Dunkman WB, Leinbach RC, Buckley MJ, et al: Clinical and hemodynamic results of intra-aortic balloon pumping and surgery for cardiogenic shock. Circulation 1972; 46:465.
23. Hyson EA, Ravin CE, Kelly MJ, et al: Intra-aortic counterpulsation balloon: Radiographic considerations. Am J Roentgenol 1977; 128:115.
24. Cascade PN, Kazerooni EA: Aspects of chest imaging in the intensive care unit. Crit Care Clin 1994; 10:247.
25. Shanahan WI: Acute pulmonary edema as a complication of epileptic seizures. N Y State J Med 1908; 87:54.

26. Ell SR: Neurogenic pulmonary edema. Invest Radiol 1991; 26:499.
27. Simmons R, Martin A, Heisterkamp C, et al: Respiratory insufficiency in combat casualties (pulmonary edema following head injury). Ann Surg 1969; 170:39.
28. Rogers FB, Shackford SR, Trevisani GT, et al: Neurogenic pulmonary edema in fatal and nonfatal head injuries. J Trauma 1995; 39:860.
29. Bekemyer WB, Pinstein ML: Neurogenic pulmonary edema: New concepts of an old disorder. South Med J 1989; 82:380.
30. Burtin P, Bollaert PE, Feldmann L, et al: Prognosis of stroke patients undergoing mechanical ventilation. Intensive Care Med 1994; 20:32.
31. Sirvent JM, Torres A, El-Ebiary M, et al: Protective effect of intravenously administered cefuroxime against nosocomial pneumonia in patients with structural coma. Am J Respir Crit Care Med 1997; 155:1729.
32. Shifrin RY, Choplin RH: Aspiration in patients in critical care units. Radiol Clin North Am 1996; 34:83.
33. Exarhos ND, Logan WD Jr, Abbott OA, et al: The importance of pH and volume in tracheobronchial aspiration. Chest 1965; 47:167.
34. Bynum LJ, Pierce AK: Pulmonary aspiration of gastric contents. Am J Respir Crit Care Med 1976; 114:1129.
35. Landay MJ, Christensen EE, Bynum LJ: Pulmonary manifestations of acute aspiration of gastric contents. Am J Roentgenol 1978; 131:587.
36. Aberle DR, Wiener-Kronish JP, Webb WR, et al: Hydrostatic versus increased permeability pulmonary edema: Diagnosis based on radiographic criteria in critically ill patients. Radiology 1988; 168:73.
37. Pistolesi M, Miniati M, Milne ENC, et al: The chest roentgenogram in pulmonary edema. Clin Chest Med 1985; 6:315.
38. Aberle DR, Smith RC, Mann H, et al: Radiographic differentiation between different etiologies of pulmonary edema. Invest Radiol 1987; 22:859.
39. Miniati M, Pistolesi M, Pailetti P, et al: Objective radiographic criteria to differentiate cardiac, renal and injury lung edema. Invest Radiol 1988; 23:433.
40. Eagle K, DeSanctis RW: Diseases of the aorta. *In:* Heart Disease: A Textbook of Cardiovascular Medicine. 4th ed. Braunwald E (Ed). Philadelphia, WB Saunders, 1992, p 1535.
41. Higgins C: Thoracic aortic disease. *In:* Essentials of Cardiac Radiology and Imaging. Higgins C (Ed). Philadelphia, JB Lippincott, 1992, p 185.
42. Worsley DF, Alavi A, Aronchick JM, et al: Chest radiographic findings in patients with acute pulmonary embolism: Observations from the PIOPED study. Radiology 1993; 189:133.
43. Van Rossum AB, Pattynama PMT, Ton ERTA, et al: Pulmonary embolism: Validation of spiral CT angiography in 149 patients. Radiology 1996; 201:467.
44. Remy-Jardin M, Remy J, Artaud D, et al: Peripheral pulmonary arteries: Optimization of the spiral CT acquisition protocol. Radiology 1997; 204:157.
45. Ferretti GR, Bosson JL, Buffaz PD, et al: Acute pulmonary embolism: Role of helical CT in 164 patients with intermediate probability at ventilation-perfusion scintigraphy and normal results at duplex US of the legs. Radiology 1997; 205:453.
46. Goodman LR, Lipchik RJ, Kuzo RS: Acute pulmonary embolism: The role of computed tomographic imaging. J Thorac Imaging 1997; 12:83.
47. Woodard PK, Sostman HD, MacFall JR, et al: Detection of pulmonary embolism: Comparison of contrast-enhanced spiral CT and time-of-flight MR techniques. J Thorac Imaging 1995; 10:59.
48. Vasilyev S, Schaap RN, Mortensen JD: Hospital survival rates of patients with acute respiratory failure in modern respiratory intensive care units. Chest 1995; 107:1083.
49. Kreit JW, Rogers RM: Approach to the patient with acute respiratory failure. *In:* Textbook of Critical Care. 3rd ed. Shoemaker WC, Ayres SM, Grenvik A, Holbrook PR (Eds). Philadelphia, WB Saunders, 1995, p 684.
50. Gleeson K, Reynolds H: Life-threatening pneumonia. Clin Chest Med 1994; 15:581.
51. Mayhall CG: Nosocomial pneumonia. Infect Dis Clin North Am 1997; 11:427.
52. Winer-Muram HT, Rubin SA, Ellis JV, et al: Pneumonia and ARDS in patients receiving mechanical ventilation: Diagnostic accuracy of chest radiography. Radiology 1993; 188:479.
53. Fagon J, Chastre J, Hance AJ, et al: Evaluation of clinical judgment in the identification and treatment of nosocomial pneumonia in ventilated patients. Chest 1993; 103:547.
54. Leatherman J: Life-threatening asthma. Clin Chest Med 1994; 15:453.
55. Fraser R, Paré J, Paré P, Fraser R, Genereux G: Diagnosis of Diseases of the Chest. Philadelphia, WB Saunders, 1990, pp 2062, 2066.
56. Tocino IM, Miller MH, Fairfax WR: Distribution of pneumothorax in the supine and semirecumbent critically ill adult. Am J Roentgenol 1985; 144:901.
57. Aronchik JM, Gefter WB: Drug induced pulmonary disorders. Semin Roentgenol 1995; 30:18.
58. Heffner JE, Harley RA, Schabel SI: Pulmonary reactions from illicit substance abuse. Clin Chest Med 1990; 11:151.
59. Murray RJ, Albin RJ, Mergner W, et al: Diffuse alveolar hemorrhage temporally related to cocaine smoking. Chest 1988; 93:427.
60. Boxt LM, Katz J, Reagan K: Drug-induced changes in the radiographic appearance of the heart. Semin Roentgenol 1995; 30:49.
61. Ashbaugh DG, Bigelow DB, Petty TL, Levine BE: Acute respiratory distress in adults. Lancet 1967; 2:319.
62. Desai SR, Hansell DM: Lung imaging in the adult respiratory distress syndrome: Current practice and new insights. Intensive Care Med 1997; 23:7.
63. Weg JG, Anzueto VA, Balk RA, et al: The relation of pneumothorax and other air leaks to mortality in the acute respiratory distress syndrome. N Engl J Med 1998; 338:341.
64. Goodman LR: Congestive heart failure and adult respiratory distress syndrome: New insights using computed tomography. Radiol Clin North Am 1996; 34:33.
65. Kazerooni EA, Pranikoff T, Cascade PN, et al: Partial liquid ventilation with perflubron during extracorporeal life support in adults: Radiographic appearance. Radiology 1996; 198:137.
66. Lieberman D: Gastrointestinal bleeding: Initial management. Gastroenterol Clin North Am 1993; 22:723.
67. Lipper B, Simon D, Cerrone F: Pulmonary aspiration during emergency endoscopy in patients with upper gastrointestinal hemorrhage. Crit Care Med 1991; 19:330.
68. Conn HO, Simpson JA: Excessive mortality associated with balloon tamponade of bleeding varices: A critical reappraisal. JAMA 1967; 202:587.
69. Kang E-Y, Staples CA, McGuiness G, et al: Detection and differential diagnosis of pulmonary infections and tumors in patients with AIDS: Value of chest radiography versus CT. AJR Am J Roentgenol 1996; 166:15.
70. Kuhlman JE: Pneumocystic infections: The radiologist's perspective. Radiology 1996; 198:623.
71. Conces DJ, Kraft JL, Vix VA, et al: Apical *Pneumocystis carinii* pneumonia after inhaled pentamidine prophylaxis. Am J Roentgenol 1989; 152:1192.
72. Feuerstein IM, Archer A, Pluda JM, et al: Thin walled cavities, cysts and pneumothorax in *Pneumocystis carinii* pneumonia: Further observations with histopathologic correlation. Radiology 1990; 174:697.
73. Heussel C, Kauczor HU, Heussel GE, et al: Early detection of pneumonia in febrile neutropenic patients with high-resolution CT: What is time gain compared with chest radiography? Chicago, Radiological Society of North America Scientific Program, December 2, 1996.
74. Hartman TE, Primack SL, Müller NL, et al: Diagnosis of thoracic complications in AIDS: Accuracy of CT. AJR Am J Roentgenol 1994; 162:547.
75. Anderson DC, Glazer HS, Semenkovich JW, et al: Lung transplant edema: Chest radiography after lung transplantation—the first 10 days. Radiology 1995; 195:275.
76. Kundu S, Herman SJ, Winton TL: Reperfusion edema after lung transplantation: Radiographic manifestations. Radiology 1998; 206:75.
77. Murray JG, McAdams HP, Erasmus JJ, et al: Complications of lung transplantation: Radiologic findings. Am J Roentgenol 1996; 166:1405.
78. Shreeniwas R, Schulman LL, Berkmen YM, et al: Opportunistic bronchopulmonary infections after lung transplantation: Clinical and radiographic findings. Radiology 1996; 200:349.
79. Herman SJ: Radiologic assessment after lung transplantation. Radiol Clin North Am 1994; 32:663.

80. Primack SL, Hartman TE, Lee KS, et al: Pulmonary nodules and the CT halo sign. Radiology 1994; 190:513.
81. Kuhllman JE, Fishman EK, Burch PA, et al: Invasive pulmonary aspergillosis in acute leukemia. Chest 1987; 92:95.
82. Winer-Muram HT, Gurney JW, Bozeman PM, et al: Pulmonary complications after bone marrow transplantation. Radiol Clin North Am 1996; 34:97.
83. Ettinger NA, Trulock EP: State of the art: Pulmonary considerations of organ transplantation. Part 2. Am Rev Respir Dis 1991; 144:213.
84. Dichter JR, Levine SJ, Shelhammer JH: Approach to the immunocompromised host with pulmonary symptoms. Hematol Oncol Clin North Am 1993; 7:887.
85. Graham NJ, Müller NL, Miller RR, et al: Intrathoracic complications following allogeneic bone marrow transplantation: CT findings. Radiology 1991; 181:153.
86. Chan CK, Hyland RH, Hutcheon MA: Pulmonary complications following bone marrow transplantation. Clin Chest Med 1990; 11:323.
87. Witte RJ, Gurney JW, Robbins RA, et al: Diffuse pulmonary alveolar hemorrhage after bone marrow transplantation: Radiographic findings in 39 patients. Am J Roentgenol 1991; 157:461.
88. Jules-Elysee K, Stoiver DE, Yahalom J, et al: Pulmonary complications in lymphoma patients treated with high dose therapy and autologous bone marrow transplantation. Am Rev Respir Dis 1992; 146:485.
89. Patz EF Jr, Peters WP, Goodman PC: Pulmonary drug toxicity following high-dose chemotherapy with autologous bone marrow transplantation: CT findings in 20 cases. J Thorac Imaging 1994; 9:129.
90. Krowka MJ, Rosenow EC: Pulmonary complications of bone marrow transplantation. Chest 1985; 87:237.
91. Brown MJ, Miller RR, Müller NL: Acute lung disease in the immunocompromised host: CT and pathologic examination findings. Radiology 1994; 190:247.
92. Padley SPG, Adler B, Hansell DM, et al: High-resolution computed tomography of drug induced lung disease. Clin Radiol 1992; 46:232.
93. McLoud TC, Naidich DP: Thoracic disease in the immunocompromised patient. Radiol Clin North Am 1992; 30:525.
94. Forest JV: Radiographic findings in *Pneumocystis carinii* pneumonia. Radiology 1972; 103:539.
95. Mori M, Galvin JR, Barloon TJ, et al: Fungal pulmonary infections after bone marrow transplantation: Evaluation with radiography and CT. Radiology 1991; 178:721.
96. Primack SL, Müller NL: High-resolution computed tomography in acute diffuse lung disease in the immunocompromised patient. Radiol Clin North Am 1994; 32:731.
97. Janzen DL, Padley SPG, Adler BD, et al: Acute pulmonary complications in immunocompromised non-AIDS patients: Comparison of diagnostic accuracy of CT and chest radiography. Clin Radiol 1993; 47:159.
98. Hertz MI, Englund JA, Snover D, et al: Respiratory syncytial virus-induced acute lung injury in adult bone marrow transplants: A clinical approach and review of the literature. Medicine (Baltimore) 1989; 68:269.
99. Nomura F, Shimokata K, Sakai S, et al: Cytomegalovirus pneumonitis occurring after allogeneic bone marrow transplantation: A study of 106 recipients. Jpn J Med 1990; 29:595.

38

Chest Imaging in Pediatric Intensive Care

Stephanie E. Spottswood, MD, MSPH • Lakshmana Das Narla, MD • Elizabeth Hingsbergen, MD

Radiologic imaging of the pediatric chest contributes significantly to prompt diagnosis and appropriate management of infants and children with life-threatening cardiopulmonary disorders. Respiratory distress in the neonate can result from problems of prematurity, adverse perinatal events, and congenital malformations of the lung and heart. Respiratory distress in the older infant or child is most commonly due to acute airway disease or traumatic injury; chronic illness and surgical conditions are less commonly responsible.

New treatment modalities and advances in ventilator design and monitoring technology have led to the survival of progressively younger neonates. Sophisticated imaging techniques can provide important insight into thoracic pathologic processes. Ultrasonography, although limited by the poor transmission of sound waves through the air-filled chest, is useful for delineating fluid collections or evaluating the integrity of the diaphragm. Occasionally, computed tomography (CT) or magnetic resonance imaging may be used for further clarification of the cause or location of certain chest processes, whereas echocardiography is invaluable in the evaluation of congenital heart disease.

Critical to the successful management of these patients are the careful radiographic evaluation of the chest and the positioning of intrathoracic life-support devices. In most cases, the frontal projection radiograph and an adequate clinical history are sufficient to establish the diagnosis, so that clinical treatment can be initiated and life-threatening complications monitored. In other cases, the radiologist can assess the need for additional radiologic evaluation and guide the intensivist in selecting the most appropriate study.

This chapter describes some of the more significant medical and surgical disorders of the chest in infants and children.

PEDIATRIC MONITORING: CATHETERS AND TUBES

Central Venous Catheters: Malpositions and Complications

Intravenous catheter malposition or prolonged catheter placement may result in several complications, including intrathoracic infusion of fluids, intra-arterial placement, venous thrombosis, and thromboembolism. Consequently, regular monitoring of proper catheter positioning is important.

In infants, a small amount of arm movement or chest rotation can significantly distort catheter position or result in considerable dislocation of central venous catheters on sequential films. Figure 38–1*A, B* shows how a catheter may "travel" from the medial aspect of the subclavian vein to the internal jugular vein. The mechanism for this phenomenon is probably positional; it occurs frequently, and the clinician should be alert to the possibility.

Sometimes a catheter may appear to be intravenous when, in fact, it is not. When the catheter position is not clearly

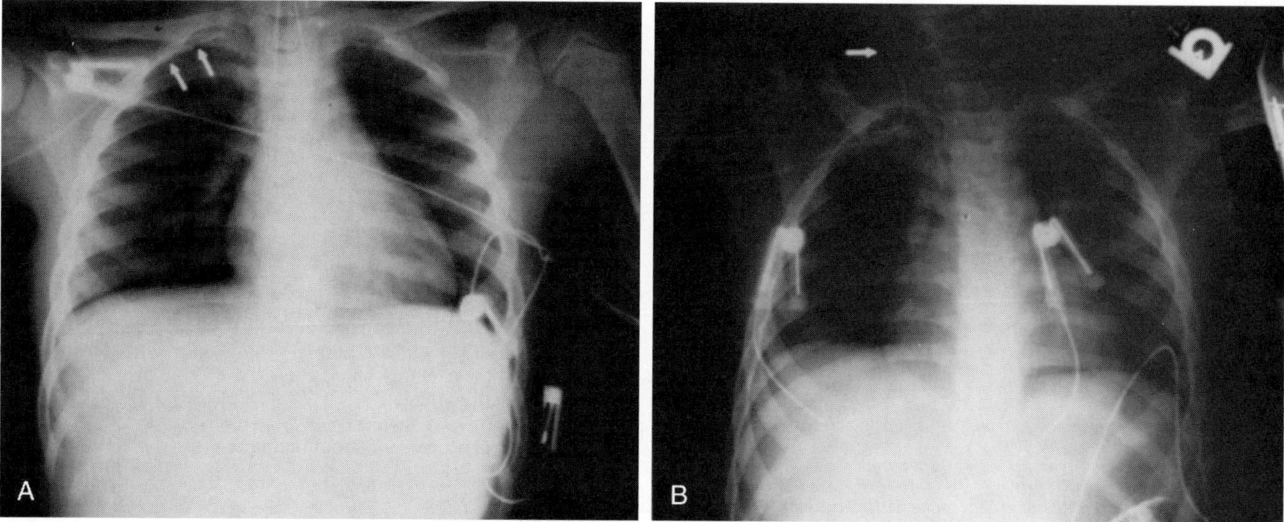

Figure 38–1. Migration of a subclavian catheter. *A,* A right subclavian catheter is in place *(arrows)* with its tip at the proximal margin of the superior vena cava. *B,* A follow-up radiograph shows the catheter in internal jugular vein *(arrow).* No interim manipulation of the catheter occurred.

defined on the chest radiograph, a contrast study may be indicated (Fig. 38–2). Alternatively, a catheter may penetrate a vascular wall and enter the mediastinum, with extravasation of infused fluid into the mediastinal space.

Prolonged catheter placement can lead to venous thrombosis or thromboembolism. The thrombus may calcify and become visible radiographically (Fig. 38–3). Thrombus formed from central venous catheters may also travel intravascularly, from the superior vena cava into the internal jugular vein and as far cephalad as the transverse sinus.

Chest Tubes

Chest tubes require appropriate positioning to function properly. If the purpose is to evacuate a pneumothorax, the tube tip should be directed anteriorly and superiorly. If the function is to drain pleural fluid, the tube should be directed posteriorly and inferiorly. In all cases, the most distal side port of the tube must be positioned within the thoracic cavity. Inadvertent placement of a chest tube in the lung parenchyma occasionally occurs and may produce a bronchopleural fistula (Fig. 38–4).

RESPIRATORY DISORDERS MANIFESTING ACUTELY DURING THE FIRST FEW DAYS OF LIFE

Neonatal respiratory distress has numerous causes.[1] The more commonly encountered, requiring management in the neonatal intensive care unit (ICU), are listed in Table 38–1.

Common causes of neonatal respiratory distress include *primary pulmonary processes*, such as respiratory distress syndrome, neonatal pneumonia, transient tachypnea of the newborn, and meconium aspiration syndrome. *Congenital*

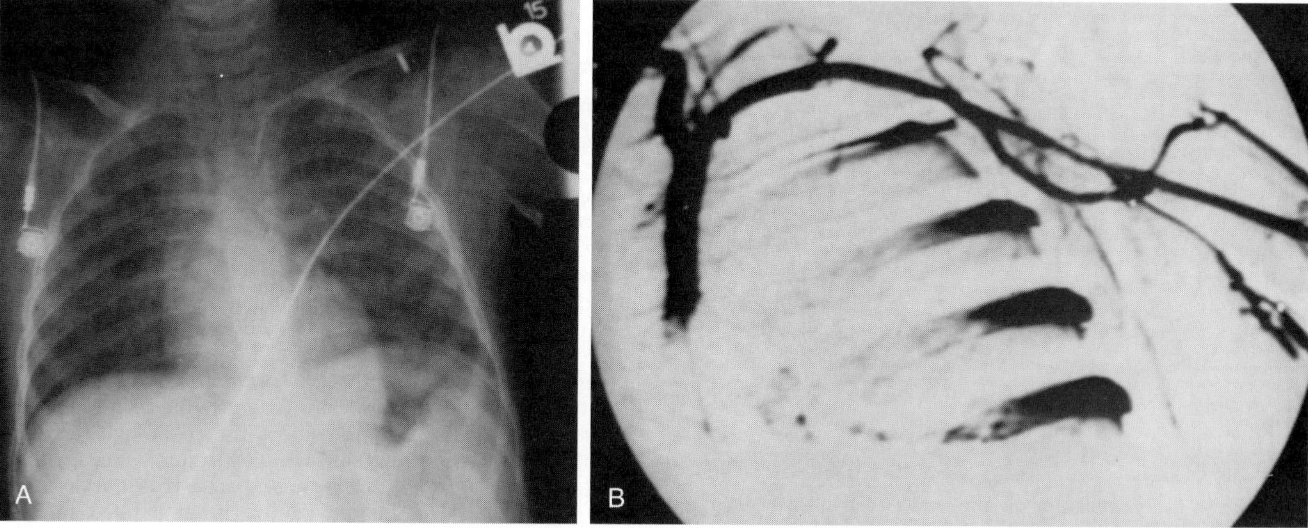

Figure 38–2. Malposition of a subclavian catheter. A subclavian catheter was placed intraoperatively for vascular access and was presumably positioned in the left subclavian vein. Postoperatively, the patient experienced a tingling sensation in the left arm, and a chest radiograph was obtained. *A,* The chest radiograph suggested intra-aortic placement of the catheter. *B,* Contrast injection through the catheter shows opacification of the left subclavian artery, innominate artery, and descending aorta.

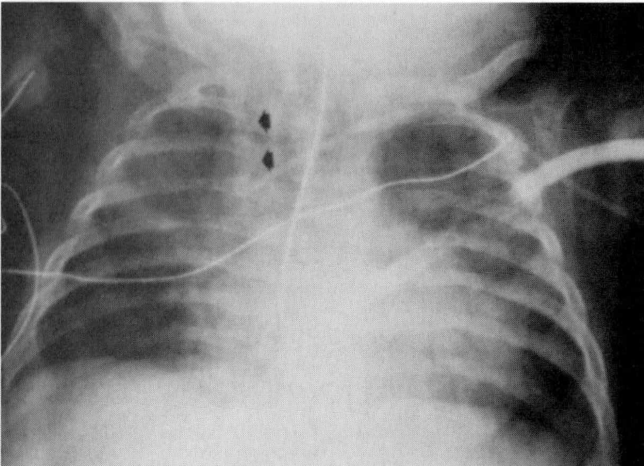

Figure 38–3. Calcified thrombus in the superior vena cava. This is a patient with prolonged catheter placement in the right internal jugular vein. Note the thickly calcified serpiginous structure outlining the superior vena cava. The thrombus propagated intravascularly, extending from the superior vena cava into the internal jugular vein, and intracranially, passing into the transverse sinus.

pulmonary anomalies make up another category of problems that compromise respiration as a result of mass effect or secondary pneumonitis. *Cardiovascular anomalies* usually cause respiratory distress from either cyanosis or congestive heart failure. Persistent pulmonary hypertension causes respiratory distress when, in the absence of cardiac anomalies, there is unrelenting hypoxemia despite aggressive oxygen therapy and ventilatory support.

Many extrathoracic problems can produce neonatal respiratory distress, such as congenital malformations of the oral cavity, upper airway, and neck. Central nervous system lesions and metabolic derangements can lead to respiratory compromise. These processes have no specific chest-radiographic findings and are not discussed in this chapter.

The initial chest radiograph of the infant with respiratory distress is obtained to assist with the diagnosis, but it may not be specific. Serial films, however, are most helpful in recognizing improvement or deterioration of lung conditions and in identifying complications. The following discussion reviews the clinical, pathophysiologic, and radiographic manifestations of some of the more important pulmonary processes manifesting acutely in the neonatal period.

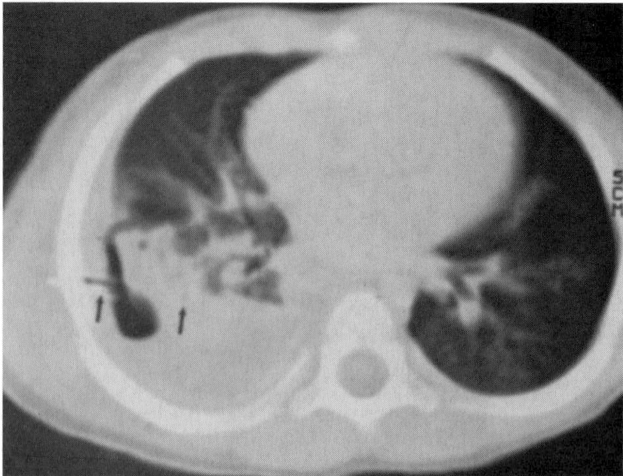

Figure 38–4. Malposition of a chest tube in a 16-month-old infant with right upper lobe pneumonia and right pleural effusion. The chest tube was unable to bring about drainage of the pleural fluid. CT of the chest reveals the intraparenchymal location of the tube *(arrows)* and the resultant bronchopleural fistula. Note the abnormal air collection in the right lateral hemithorax.

TABLE 38–1. Causes of Neonatal Respiratory Distress

Airway Obstruction
Choanal atresia
Macroglossia, micrognathia
Congenital subglottic stenosis
Laryngeal web or stenosis
Tracheomalacia
Primary Lung Disorders
Respiratory distress syndrome
Neonatal pneumonia
Transient tachypnea of the newborn
Meconium aspiration syndrome
Congenital Pulmonary Anomalies
Congenital diaphragmatic hernia
Congenital lobar emphysema
Pulmonary hypoplasia
Tracheoesophageal fistula
Congenital cystic adenomatoid malformation
Bronchogenic cyst
Neurenteric cyst
Pulmonary sequestration
Pulmonary agenesis
Jeune syndrome (asphyxiating thoracic dystrophy)
Congenital Cardiovascular Anomalies
Pulmonary atresia/severe pulmonic stenosis
Ebstein's anomaly
Tricuspid atresia
D-transposition of the great arteries
Hypoplastic left-heart syndrome
Critical aortic stenosis
Severe coarctation of the aorta
Interrupted aortic arch
Total anomalous pulmonary venous return, with obstruction
Other complex congenital heart lesions
Nonpulmonary Disorders
Metabolic derangement: acidosis, hypothermia, hypoglycemia
Central nervous system lesions: ischemia, hemorrhage
Other
Persistent pulmonary hypertension (persistent fetal circulation)

Primary Lung Disorders

Respiratory Distress Syndrome

Respiratory distress syndrome (RDS) affects premature infants as a result of inadequate pulmonary surfactant. The major phospholipid component of surfactant, phosphatidylcholine, has begun to be synthesized and stored at 20 weeks' gestation.[2] It is not clear, however, when these lipids are secreted as surfactant and when surfactant is available in quantities sufficient for successful ventilation after birth. Absence of adequate amounts of surfactant causes neonatal respiratory distress, manifested pathologically as diffuse atelectasis, edema, and cellular injury, with leakage of protein and fluid into the alveoli that coalesces to form hyaline membranes.

The radiographic findings reflect the pathologic features, with hypoexpansion, and diffuse, fine reticulogranularity of the lungs, usually with air bronchograms. It is important to interpret as air bronchograms only those air-filled bronchi seen beyond the cardiac margins; those confined within the margins of the heart are seen normally because of the relative translucency of the neonatal mediastinum. If severe, the reticulogranular pattern may obscure the margins of the cardiac

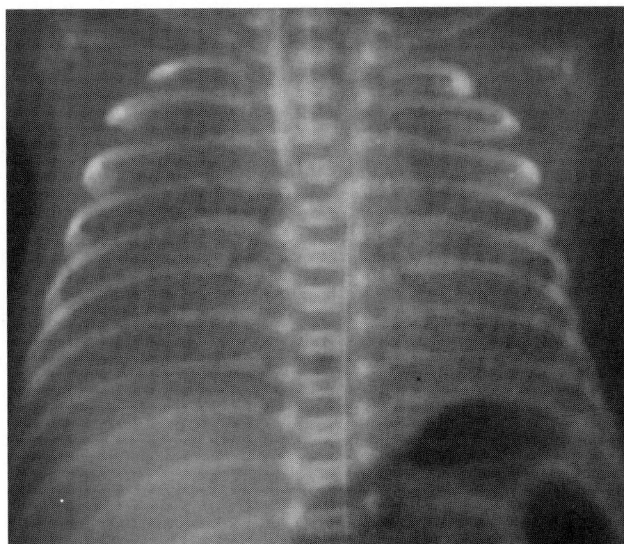

Figure 38–5. Respiratory distress syndrome in a premature newborn. The characteristic findings, diffuse granular infiltrate and air bronchograms, are visualized.

silhouette (Fig. 38–5). In severe cases, the radiographic findings usually appear immediately after birth. In less severe cases, there may be as much as a 24-hour delay before the radiograph becomes diagnostic.

If the disease is mild to moderate in severity, it usually resolves within 4 to 7 days. Traditional treatment regimens include oxygen delivery with continuous positive airway pressure and mechanical ventilation with positive end-expiratory pressure. Newer treatment, used in conjunction with mechanical ventilation, consists of surfactant replacement therapy. With the advent of this modality, the frequency and severity of RDS have significantly decreased by both clinical and radiographic criteria.[3] Studies have shown that prophylactic surfactant therapy in newborns younger than 30 weeks' gestation results in a higher survival rate (75%) compared with rescue surfactant therapy (52%).[4]

Neonatal Pneumonia

Bacterial infections are a major cause of morbidity and mortality in the newborn. The agent most responsible for neonatal pneumonia is the group B β-hemolytic streptococcus (GBS). Infection with GBS is usually early in onset, most often resulting from the neonate's exposure to infected amniotic fluid either in utero or during vaginal transit. Maternal risk factors include premature labor and premature rupture of membranes. Histopathologic changes in the lungs bear some similarity to those seen in RDS, with patchy hyaline membrane formation but without the severe atelectasis seen with RDS. This finding is accompanied by inflammatory exudate mixed with cocci.[5]

Radiographically, patients with GBS pneumonia exhibit features indistinguishable from those of RDS, with reticulogranularity and air bronchograms. Commonly, however, the lungs are normally expanded, and there may be a pleural effusion with GBS pneumonia, which helps to distinguish it from RDS. In a retrospective study of infants who died of GBS pneumonia, chest radiographs demonstrated pleural effusions in 67%; pleural fluid was uncommon in a comparison group of infants with RDS and a group with positive blood cultures for organisms other than GBS.[6]

Treatment of neonatal pneumonia consists of broad-spectrum antibiotics and supportive care. Patients may have associated pulmonary hypertension. Survivors commonly have severe sequelae from septic shock and hypoxemia.

Transient Tachypnea of the Newborn

Transient tachypnea of the newborn (TTN), also known as "wet lung disease" and "retained fetal fluid," is a common, self-limited condition. It is characterized by tachypnea and mild cyanosis during the first several hours to days of life and is caused by delayed resorption of fetal lung fluid. Predisposing factors include cesarean section, maternal diabetes, significant maternal sedation, precipitous delivery, and asphyxia. It is believed that the lack of the usual uterine squeeze that occurs in normal vaginal delivery is responsible for the delayed clearing of fluid from the lungs into the bronchial tree.

The radiographic findings are typically streaky, linear densities emanating from the hila and extending to the lung periphery, representing prominent vascular markings with hazy margins, which are caused by excessive perivascular interstitial fluid. These markings are often accompanied by a fluid-filled minor fissure or small pleural effusions, usually seen at the costophrenic sulcus (Fig. 38–6). The cardiac silhouette is normal in size. The chest film usually shows clearing within 48 to 72 hours. If these findings persist beyond 72 hours with normal heart size, the differential diagnosis should include neonatal pneumonia, obstructive total anomalous pulmonary venous return, and patent ductus arteriosus. Because the radiographic changes of TTN mimic those of other, more severe processes, it should be considered a diagnosis of exclusion.

Treatment of TTN is supportive, with oxygen and parenteral fluids. The prognosis is excellent.

Meconium Aspiration

Fetal distress can result in passage of meconium in utero; gasping respirations can then cause aspiration of meconium with bronchial obstruction, followed by postnatal interference with gas exchange and severe respiratory distress. This disorder occurs in as many as 62% of neonates born with meconium-stained amniotic fluid[7] and is seen in term and postmature infants who have experienced some degree of intrapartum hypoxia. Pulmonary hypertension may follow the meconium aspiration, contributing to the hypoxia.

The chest radiograph usually reveals hyperexpansion of the lungs with bilateral, coarse, patchy densities reflecting obstructive atelectasis and probable associated pneumonitis (Fig. 38–7). Complications of air-block phenomena (pneumothorax, pneumomediastinum, and so on) occur in approximately 25%

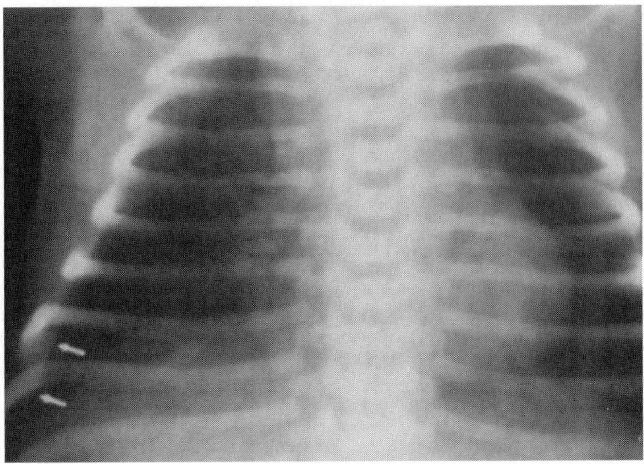

Figure 38–6. Transient tachypnea in a near-term neonate with increased respiratory rate. Note the prominent, hazy vascular markings and small right pleural effusion *(arrows)*.

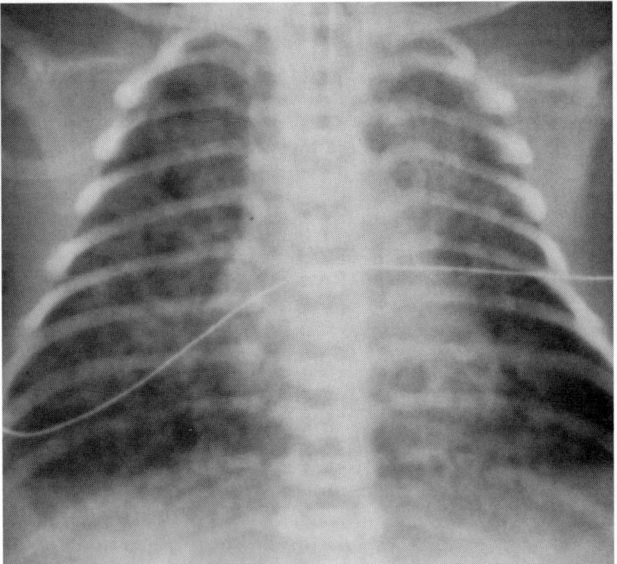

Figure 38–7. Meconium aspiration syndrome. This chest radiograph reveals coarse, asymmetric, and patchy bilateral opacities and hyperinflation.

of cases and cause greater morbidity and possible mortality. The risk of these complications is raised with the barotrauma of mechanical ventilation.

Therapy with oxygen and mechanical ventilation is traditional. Drug therapy using pulmonary vasodilators and high-frequency ventilation can also be used. Failure of noninvasive methods of treatment, as judged from the predetermined parameters of arterial-alveolar gradients and other such formulas, can logically lead to the use of extracorporeal membrane oxygenation (ECMO), a form of cardiopulmonary bypass that may improve survival and reduce long-term morbidity (see later). Patients with persistent progressive pulmonary hypertension and severe right-to-left shunting who are not responding to ventilator and pharmacologic manipulation may benefit from ECMO.

Persistent Pulmonary Hypertension

Persistent pulmonary hypertension, also known as "persistent fetal circulation," is sustained, elevated pulmonary arterial pressure with right-to-left shunting through a patent foramen ovale, a patent ductus arteriosus, or an extrathoracic shunt. The shunting occurs because pulmonary vascular resistance exceeds systemic vascular resistance after transition to neonatal circulation. This disorder may be an isolated, idiopathic process, or it may be secondary to other pathophysiologic events, such as meconium aspiration, perinatal asphyxia, neonatal sepsis (including GBS pneumonia), and congenital diaphragmatic hernia.

The chest radiograph may show a variety of abnormalities, including the presence of interstitial fluid densities with or without cardiomegaly, or it may appear completely normal.

Inhaled nitric oxide (iNO) for persistent pulmonary hypertension rapidly increases oxygenation without causing systemic hypotension and reduces the requirement for ECMO. The mechanism appears to be secondary to increased levels of the endothelium-1 (ET-1) and cyclic guanosine monophosphate (CGMP).

Selected Congenital Pulmonary Anomalies

Pulmonary Hypoplasia

Pulmonary hypoplasia involves a spectrum of lung abnormalities that are characterized by pulmonary underdevelopment due to a variety of in utero insults. The process can be unilateral or bilateral. *Unilateral* pulmonary hypoplasia occurs when lung development is arrested; rudimentary pulmonary tissue is evident on pathologic study. Patients with unilateral pulmonary hypoplasia are usually asymptomatic. The chest radiograph reveals a small, radiodense affected hemithorax caused by reduced aeration.

Bilateral pulmonary hypoplasia most commonly occurs secondary to intrauterine compression of the fetal thorax, which is usually caused by oligohydramnios resulting from either severe bilateral renal disease or urinary outflow tract obstruction. Bony dysplasias of the thoracic cage (e.g., asphyxiating thoracic dystrophy), which restrict fetal respiratory movements, can also limit pulmonary growth, leading to bilateral hypoplasia. Intrathoracic masses that directly compress the lung, such as congenital diaphragmatic hernia and congenital cystic adenomatoid malformation, may be etiologic factors. Primary pulmonary hypoplasia, although less common, can also occur.

Clinically, patients with bilateral pulmonary hypoplasia have severe respiratory distress and are prone to complications such as pneumothorax and pneumomediastinum. The chest radiograph in bilateral hypoplasia demonstrates clear but small lungs. Spontaneous pneumothorax may be present at birth (Fig. 38–8).

Congenital Diaphragmatic Hernia

The cephalad migration of abdominal viscera through a defect in the diaphragm results in congenital diaphragmatic hernia (CDH). The incidence is 1 in 4000 live births. The potential sites for herniation are the substernal space (foramen of Morgagni), the posterolateral region (foramen of Bochdalek), and the esophageal hiatus. The term CDH typically refers to the posterolateral form.

A peritoneal sac is present 10% to 20% of the time and is believed secondary to membranous closure of the canal with incomplete muscularization. Most hernias occur on the left. Hernia contents can include bowel, stomach, spleen, liver, or omentum. The herniated abdominal structures exert considerable mass effect on the lungs, leading to long-standing compression and mediastinal shift in utero and resultant bilateral pulmonary hypoplasia. Both lungs are diminished in size, but the process is more marked on the ipsilateral side.

Clinically, the newborn may have a scaphoid abdomen, and

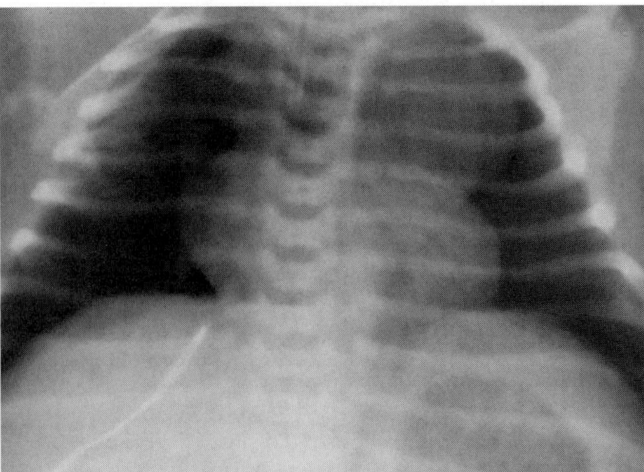

Figure 38–8. Pulmonary hypoplasia resulting from renal dysplasia. A chest radiograph obtained after intubation in this neonate with respiratory distress reveals bilateral pneumothoraces (lungs are collapsed medially). Note the small size of the thoracic cage.

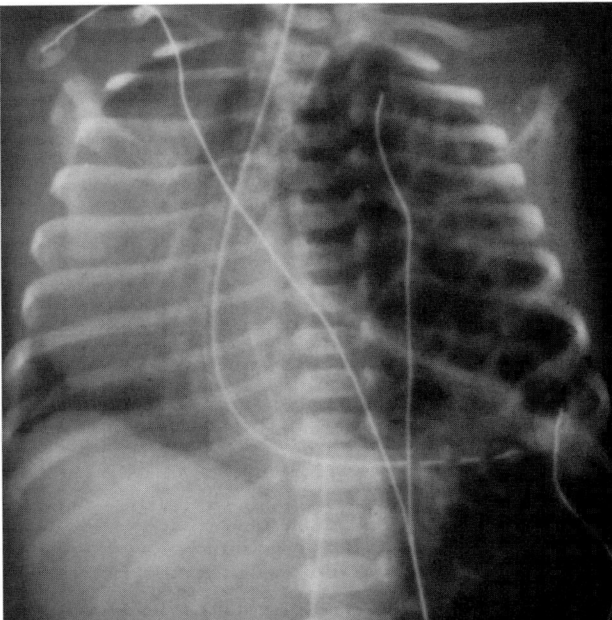

Figure 38–9. Congenital diaphragmatic hernia in a newborn infant with respiratory distress and a scaphoid abdomen. Multiple cystic lucencies are seen in the left side of the chest; the cysts exhibit mass effect and cause mediastinal shift to the right. Note the abnormal position of the nasogastric tube, with the tip returning to the chest.

bowel sounds may be auscultated in the chest. Large hernias cause severe and immediate respiratory distress because of respiratory compromise from pulmonary compression and hypoplasia.

The chest radiograph classically demonstrates multiple, bubbly-appearing lucencies representing loops of intestine in the affected hemithorax, with pulmonary compression and shift of the mediastinum to the contralateral side (Fig. 38–9). Immediately after birth, before the infant has swallowed air into the gut, the herniated structures may be radiopaque, representing fluid-filled or collapsed bowel. There is usually a paucity or complete absence of abdominal bowel gas, depending on the size of the hernia. This finding may be very important to the diagnosis if the bowel in the chest is gasless. Dilated, gas-filled, intra-abdominal bowel suggests bowel entrapment and obstruction.

In the newborn infant, the intrathoracic changes of CDH are radiographically similar to those seen in cystic adenomatoid malformation.[8] In the latter condition, however, the normal component of abdominal gas should be present.

The infant is resuscitated and stabilized before surgical correction, with measures such as nasogastric intubation to relieve trapped air and positive-pressure ventilation. If there is relentless respiratory deterioration, the patient may benefit from the use of high-frequency (jet) ventilation or ECMO.

Treatment options for CDH include permissive hypercapnia, intratracheal pulmonary ventilation (ITPV), surfactant at the time of birth followed by partial liquid ventilation (PLV), and iNO used during PLV to reduce pulmonary vascular resistance. In utero tracheal occlusion in affected fetuses has been successfully performed at two centers and has resulted in acceleration of lung growth.

Between 1981 and 1995, centers using ECMO reported a survival in CDH of 65% (range, 44% to 70%). Long-term follow-up of patients with CDH is essential because morbidity from chronic lung disease may be quite high.

Congenital Lobar Emphysema

Congenital lobar emphysema is characterized by progressive hyperinflation and air trapping in one or more pulmonary lobes. The usually single hyperinflated lobe causes compression and atelectasis of the adjacent lobes or contralateral lung. Proposed causes include an obstructing lesion or congenitally insufficient bronchial cartilage leading to bronchial collapse. This results in a focal, ball-valve obstruction with air trapping, most commonly affecting the left upper lobe. The right middle and right upper lobes are next most commonly affected.

Clinically, there is acute or subacute respiratory distress in the newborn infant. Some neonates, however, are asymptomatic until older and then present with multiple respiratory infections and wheezing. Breath sounds are usually diminished over the involved lung.

The chest radiograph may initially demonstrate a large, radiopaque mass occupying one lobe and compressing adjacent aerated lobes. This mass is initially radiopaque because of delayed clearance of fetal lung fluid from the abnormal lobe.[9] Later, after the fluid evacuates, the affected lobe becomes hyperlucent and hyperexpanded (Fig. 38–10*A*). There is compressive atelectasis of the adjacent lung parenchyma and mediastinal shift to the contralateral side. Similar findings are demonstrated on chest CT images (Fig. 38–10*B*).

If the child is acutely symptomatic, surgical removal of the overinflated lobe with or without prior bronchoscopy is usually performed. However, there can be long-term improvement with conservative management. In one retrospective study of 12 children so treated, there was both symptomatic and radiologic improvement during an average follow-up of approximately 3 years.[10] Nonsurgical therapy can be anatomically assessed with both serial chest radiographs and CT, which can demonstrate a reduction of the emphysematous lobe. Gradual improvement in pulmonary function can be evaluated with nuclear medicine ventilation-perfusion imaging.

Esophageal Atresia and Tracheoesophageal Fistula

Esophageal atresia and tracheoesophageal fistula are congenital malformations in a spectrum of anomalies that may exist independently or in various combinations. The malformations occur secondary to defective separation of the primitive trachea and esophagus. The result is (1) an abnormal fistulous connection to the trachea either from an atretic segment of esophagus or from a nonatretic esophagus or (2) complete atresia of the esophagus with no fistulous connection.

The most common variation is proximal atresia with distal tracheoesophageal fistula (85%). Saliva and feedings may pass into the trachea from above and gastric contents may reflux into the trachea from below, passing through the fistula and inciting a severe aspiration pneumonitis.

In the case of esophageal atresia with or without a fistula, there is difficulty handling normal secretions, with drooling and choking. Resistance is encountered proximally during attempted passage of a nasogastric tube.

The appearance on chest radiographs varies with the specific type of anomaly. With esophageal atresia, a dilated, gas-filled proximal esophageal pouch may be present. If this is an isolated finding with no fistula, no gas is present within the abdominal bowel loops (Fig. 38–11). When a fistula is present from the trachea to the distal esophagus, the abdominal bowel loops are gas-filled and distended; there may be evidence of aspiration pneumonitis.

Selected Congenital Cardiovascular Anomalies

Cardiovascular anomalies usually manifest as cyanosis or congestive heart failure and can be so classified. Table 38–2 lists

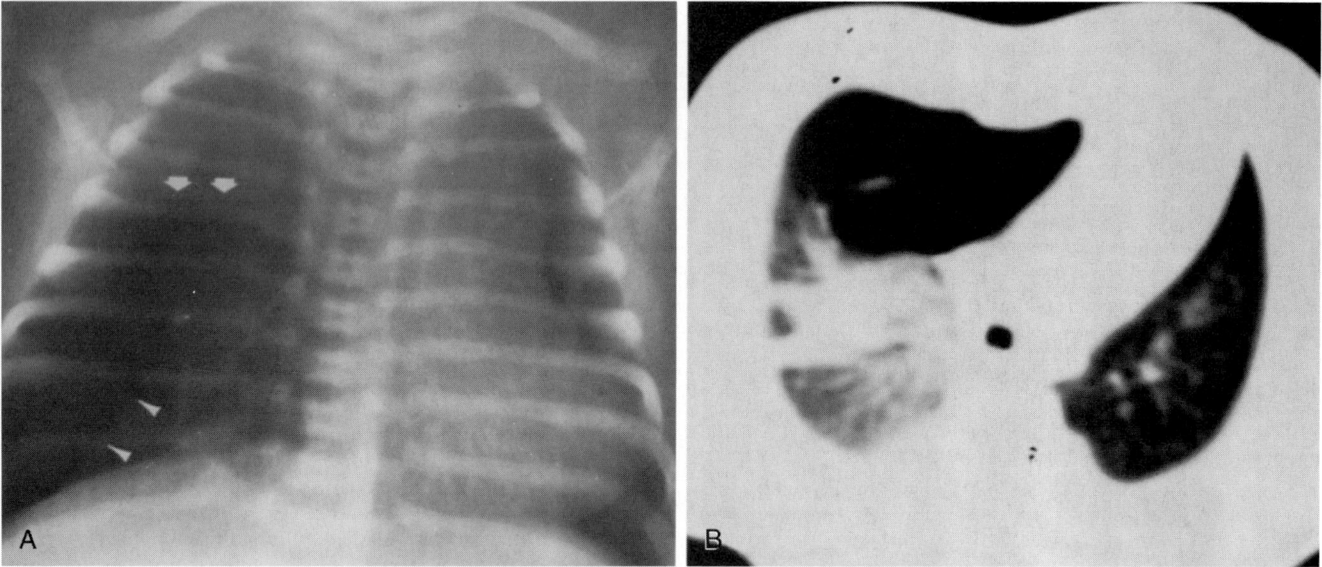

Figure 38–10. Congenital lobar emphysema. *A,* The right middle lobe is hyperlucent and hyperinflated, with resultant compression of the upper and lower lobes. Note the minor fissure *(arrows)* and the margin of right lower lobe *(arrowheads)*. *B,* A CT image demonstrates hyperexpansion of the middle lobe with vessel attenuation and compression of adjacent lung parenchyma. Note the shift of the heart to the left.

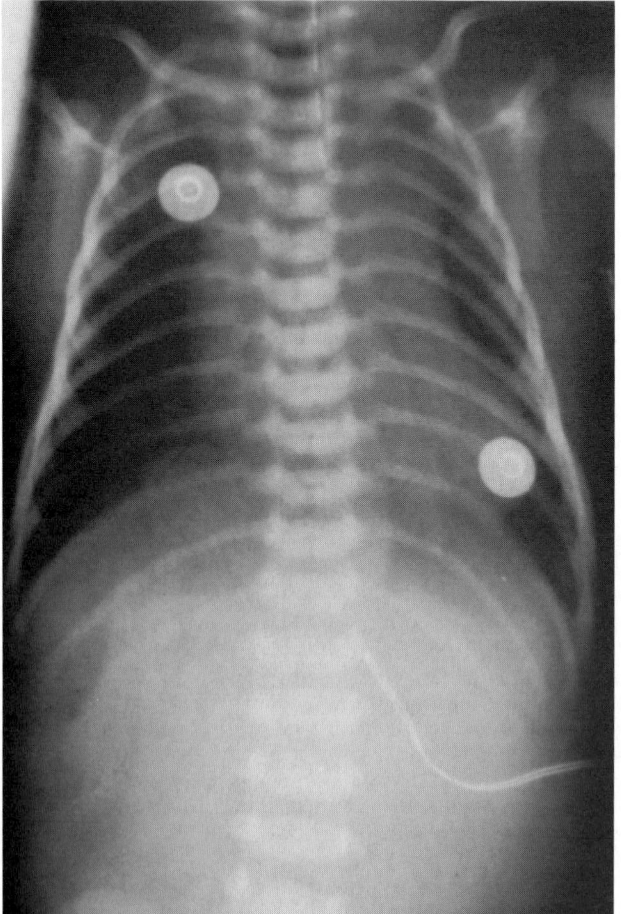

Figure 38–11. Esophageal atresia in a newborn with drooling and choking. The nasogastric tube could not be passed (note the tip at the T3 vertebral level). No gas is present in the abdomen; this is consistent with esophageal atresia without fistula.

TABLE 38–2. Congenital Heart Disease in Neonates by Clinical Presentation

Diseases Presenting with Cyanosis
Pulmonary atresia/severe pulmonary stenosis with intact pulmonary septum
Pulmonary atresia/severe pulmonary stenosis with ventricular septal defect
Ebstein's anomaly
Tricuspid atresia
D-transposition of the great arteries
Diseases Presenting with Congestive Heart Failure
Hypoplastic left-heart syndrome
Critical aortic stenosis
Coarctation of the aorta: severe
Coarctation syndrome
Interrupted aortic arch
Total anomalous pulmonary venous return, with obstruction
Truncus arteriosus

Data from Gyepes MT, Vincent WR: Severe congenital heart disease in the neonatal period: A functional approach to emergency diagnosis. Am J Roentgenol 1971, 116:490.

TABLE 38–3. Congenital Heart Disease in Neonates by Radiographic Presentation

Decreased Pulmonary Vascularity
Pulmonary atresia/severe pulmonary stenosis with intact pulmonary septum
Pulmonary atresia/severe pulmonary stenosis with ventricular septal defect
Ebstein's anomaly
Tricuspid atresia
Pulmonary Venous Obstruction
Hypoplastic left-heart syndrome
Coarctation of the aorta: severe
Critical aortic stenosis
Coarctation syndrome
Interrupted aortic arch
Total anomalous pulmonary venous return, with obstruction
Initially Normal and Then Increased Pulmonary Vascularity
D-transposition of the great arteries
Atrioventricular canal
Truncus arteriosus
Single ventricle

congenital cardiac anomalies that occur during the neonatal period according to this classification, which is adapted from a functional approach to diagnosis developed by Gyepes and Vincent.[11] The selected lesions are seen in patients who are symptomatic at or shortly after birth.

Neonatal cardiovascular anomalies can also be characterized according to the features visualized on the chest radiograph.[12] The cardiac configuration is usually abnormal in patients with congenital heart disease, but the heart can also appear completely normal with severe cardiac disease. Certain cardiac configurations are characteristic of certain congenital anomalies, as follows:

1. The oval or "egg-on-a-string" appearance is seen in D-transposition of the great arteries. The "string" represents the narrow superior mediastinum and results from the radiographically invisible thymus and the anteroposterior relationship of the transposed aorta and main pulmonary artery (the pulmonary artery lies directly behind the aorta).
2. A boot-shaped heart is seen with tetralogy of Fallot and is produced by the prominent, laterally displaced cardiac apex (caused by right ventricular hypertrophy) and the concave main pulmonary artery segment seen just superiorly.
3. Marked cardiomegaly in the neonate is usually caused by right atrial enlargement (prominent rounded border of the right side of the heart) and should suggest either Ebstein's anomaly or pulmonary atresia or severe stenosis with an intact ventricular septum.

Although these characteristic configurations may be helpful, a more useful radiologic clue to the cause of the cardiac anomaly can be derived from the appearance of the pulmonary vascular markings (Table 38-3). Decreased pulmonary vascularity denotes diminished volume of blood flowing through the lungs with right-to-left shunting and clinical cyanosis. Decreased pulmonary blood flow is evident in obstructive lesions of the right side of the heart, such as pulmonary atresia or severe stenosis, tricuspid atresia, and Ebstein's anomaly (Fig. 38-12). Tetralogy of Fallot, which is usually detected later in infancy, can manifest in the newborn if the associated pulmonary stenosis is severe. Pulmonary venous obstruction indicates passive congestion of the pulmonary venous bed with transudation of fluid into surrounding perivascular interstitial tissues. This pattern is characterized radiographically by prominent vessels with indistinct margins. Pulmonary venous

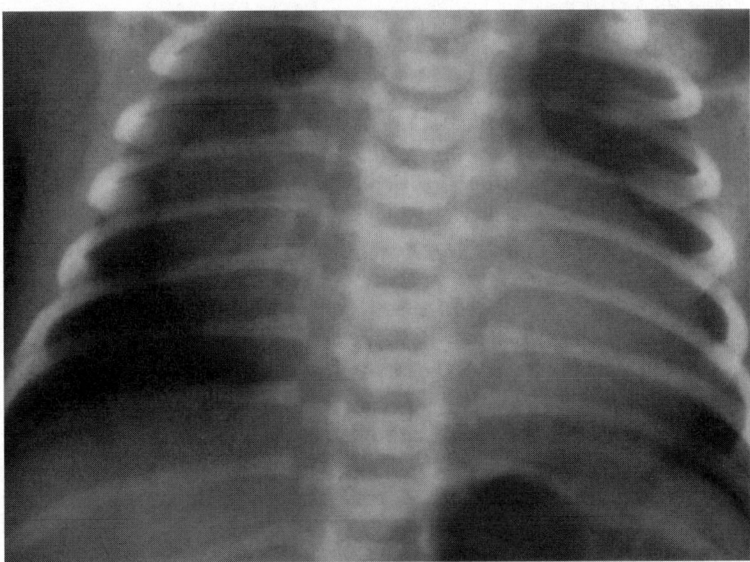

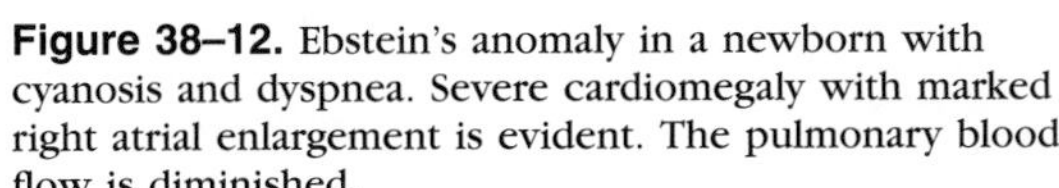

Figure 38–12. Ebstein's anomaly in a newborn with cyanosis and dyspnea. Severe cardiomegaly with marked right atrial enlargement is evident. The pulmonary blood flow is diminished.

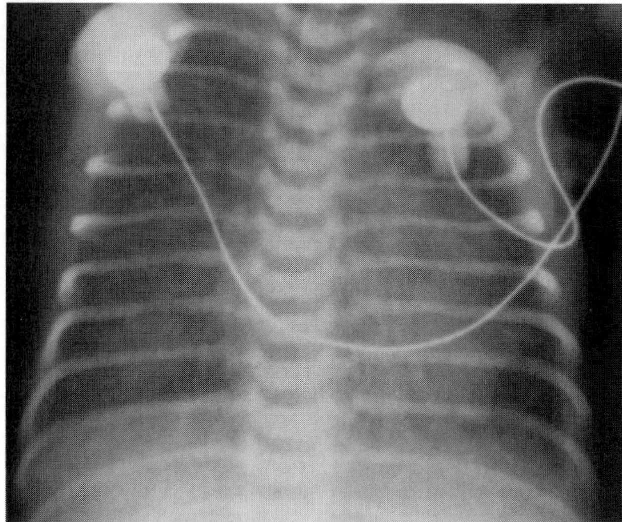

Figure 38–13. Hypoplastic left-heart syndrome in a newborn infant with grunting, poor systemic perfusion, and hepatomegaly. Cardiomegaly and marked pulmonary venous congestion are present. Note the small, bilateral pleural effusions.

hypertension is associated with obstructive lesions of the left side of the heart, such as hypoplastic left-heart syndrome (Fig. 38–13), critical aortic stenosis, severe coarctation of the aorta, and total anomalous pulmonary venous return with obstruction (Fig. 38–14). The clinical presentation in these disorders is usually congestive heart failure and diminished systemic perfusion.

Congestive heart failure can also manifest in the newborn secondary to perinatal events affecting the heart. Such events are transient myocardial ischemia due to perinatal asphyxia, myocarditis caused by perinatal infection, tachyarrhythmias, and conduction disturbances. Additional noncardiac causes of congestive heart failure in the neonate include (1) high-flow states, as seen with arteriovenous malformations (vein of Galen malformation, hemangioendothelioma), and severe anemia; (2) metabolic abnormalities, such as hypoglycemia and acidosis; (3) severe infection; and (4) hydrops.

Increased pulmonary vascularity, seen when more than the normal volume of blood is flowing through the lungs, is present in conditions with left-to-right shunts. This radiographic finding is rarely present within the first few days of life, because the amount of shunted blood is initially restricted by the high pulmonary vascular resistance in the transition period from fetal to neonatal life. Gradually, however, the neonate's pulmonary vascularity increases over time and appears excessive in patients with left-to-right shunts. At least a two-to-one shunt is required for radiographic recognition. Patients with admixture lesions such as tricuspid atresia, truncus arteriosus, and single ventricle usually present at birth because of severe cyanosis. Although not strictly considered an admixture lesion, D-transposition of the great arteries should be included in this group; it is the most common cause of cyanotic congenital heart disease in the newborn.

During the first few days of life, the pulmonary vascularity on the normal neonate's chest radiograph is normal to slightly diminished because of high pulmonary vascular pressures. If there is also a cyanotic lesion, the pulmonary blood flow is markedly diminished, usually because of pulmonic stenosis. Later, as pulmonary vascular resistance decreases, shunting can occur across a patent foramen ovale, patent ductus arteriosus, or septal defect, and increased pulmonary blood flow is visualized (Fig. 38–15). Other left-to-right shunt lesions, including atrioventricular canal defects and large ventricular septal defects, manifest later in infancy as either a murmur or congestive failure from markedly increased pulmonary vascular flow. Patients with atrial septal defects rarely have severe cardiopulmonary problems during the first 30 days of life.

Another important consideration in the category of left-to-right shunts is the premature neonate with RDS who has persistent patency or reopening of a partially closed ductus arteriosus. The chest radiograph is often key to the diagnosis when the clinical picture is uncertain. Poor definition of pulmonary vessels caused by interstitial edema and diffuse air space haziness due to florid alveolar edema are the hallmarks

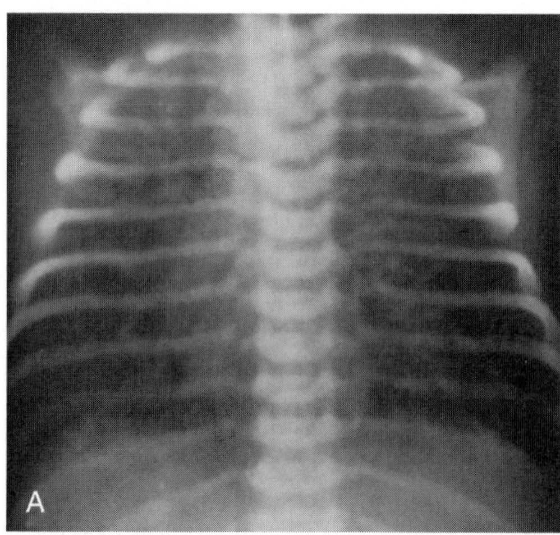

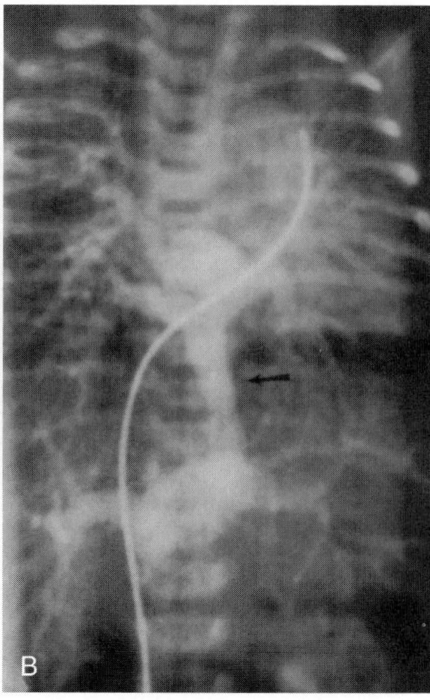

Figure 38–14. Total anomalous pulmonary venous return with subdiaphragmatic obstruction. *A,* This initial chest radiograph demonstrates prominent pulmonary vessels with indistinct margins, a finding consistent with venous congestion. The heart is of normal size; this is typical for type III total anomalous pulmonary venous return. *B,* Venous phase of the pulmonary angiogram shows pulmonary veins converging to form an anomalous vessel *(arrow)* that travels subdiaphragmatically to enter the portal vein.

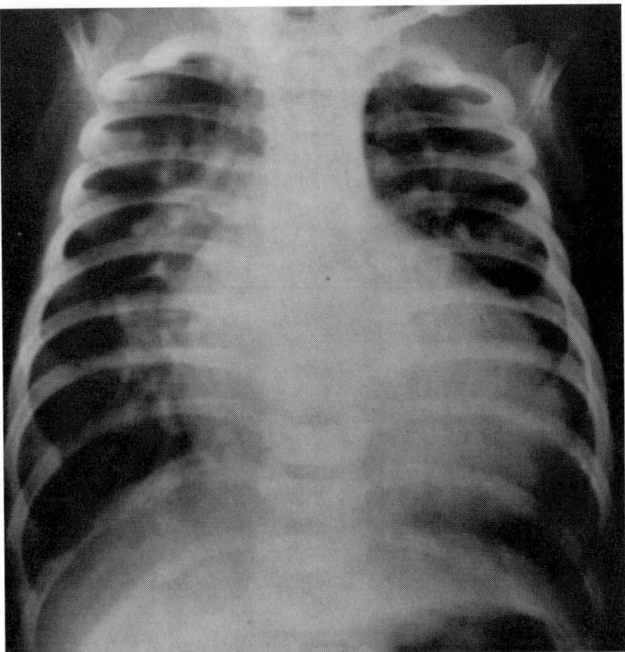

Figure 38–15. D-transposition of the great vessels. This chest radiograph of an older infant illustrates markedly increased pulmonary blood flow. Note "egg-on-a-string" appearance of the cardiac silhouette, which occurs secondary to a narrow cardiac waist, enlarged heart, and inapparent aorta. The aorta and pulmonary artery are aligned more anteroposteriorly than usual, giving the appearance of a narrow mediastinum.

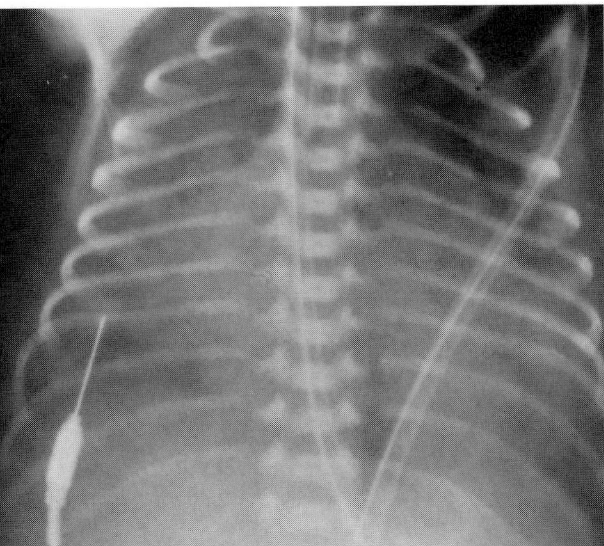

Figure 38–16. Patent ductus arteriosus in a premature neonate with respiratory distress syndrome (RDS). The initial chest radiograph demonstrated a mild granular infiltrate, a finding consistent with RDS. Six days later, the patient became tachypneic. This follow-up chest radiograph reveals the development of cardiomegaly, indistinct pulmonary vascular margins, and diffuse lung opacity; these signs are consistent with pulmonary edema occurring secondary to patent ductus arteriosus.

(Fig. 38–16). Enlargement of the cardiac silhouette often occurs but is not always evident. Visualization of blood flow through the patent ductus arteriosus by means of color-flow Doppler ultrasonography is used to confirm the diagnosis.

Air-Block Phenomena in the Neonate

Air-block phenomena occur with high-pressure ventilation. Air escapes from the terminal airspaces and dissects into the interstitial or pleural space, creating fixed areas of abnormal inflation. Such processes occur commonly in the ventilated neonate when "excessive" or uneven ventilation exerts prolonged tension on alveolar walls. Other inciting conditions are the infant's own forceful, initial respiratory efforts, resuscitation procedures, and generalized or localized air trapping. The resulting pathologic air collections include pulmonary interstitial emphysema, pneumomediastinum, pneumothorax, pneumopericardium, pneumoperitoneum, and intravascular air embolism.

Pulmonary Interstitial Emphysema

Pulmonary interstitial emphysema occurs when air dissects from a ruptured alveolus into the interstitium and becomes trapped. Lung compliance is significantly reduced, and chest excursion may be decreased. Radiographically, the affected area is hyperinflated, and branching radiolucencies that extend from the hila to the lung periphery do not collapse on expiration and do not resemble air in branching bronchi. These lucencies can be linear or rounded and cyst-like in appearance (Fig. 38–17).

Conservative management of unilateral pulmonary interstitial emphysema is sometimes effective; the patient is positioned with the overinflated lung in the dependent position in an effort to decompress it through decreased ventilation. When more aggressive treatment is needed, selective intubation of the contralateral mainstem bronchus or selective balloon occlusion of the ipsilateral bronchus may be attempted. Alternative therapies for severe, diffuse pulmonary interstitial emphysema include high-frequency (jet) ventilation and ECMO. Pulmonary interstitial emphysema may secondarily produce pneumomediastinum or pneumothorax.

Pneumomediastinum

Pneumomediastinum occurs when interstitial air from a ruptured alveolus escapes into the mediastinum. In the neonate, this follows barotrauma and traumatic intubation or occasionally can be seen spontaneously. Pneumomediastinum is seen most reliably on the lateral chest radiograph, which can

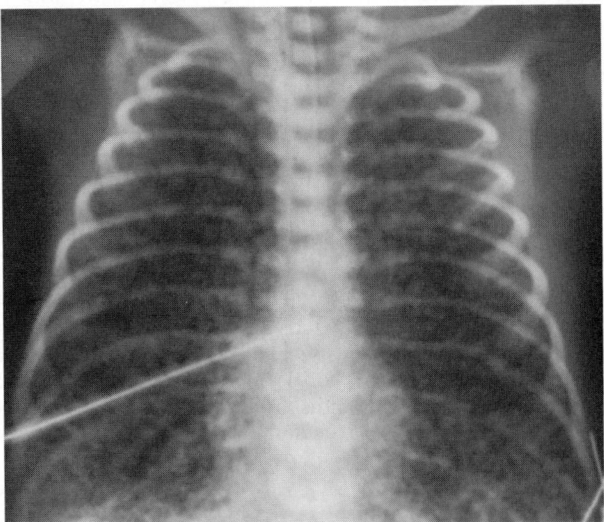

Figure 38–17. Pulmonary interstitial emphysema in a premature infant treated with mechanical ventilation for respiratory distress syndrome. Both lungs are severely hyperexpanded, with linear and circular lucencies radiating from the hila to the periphery.

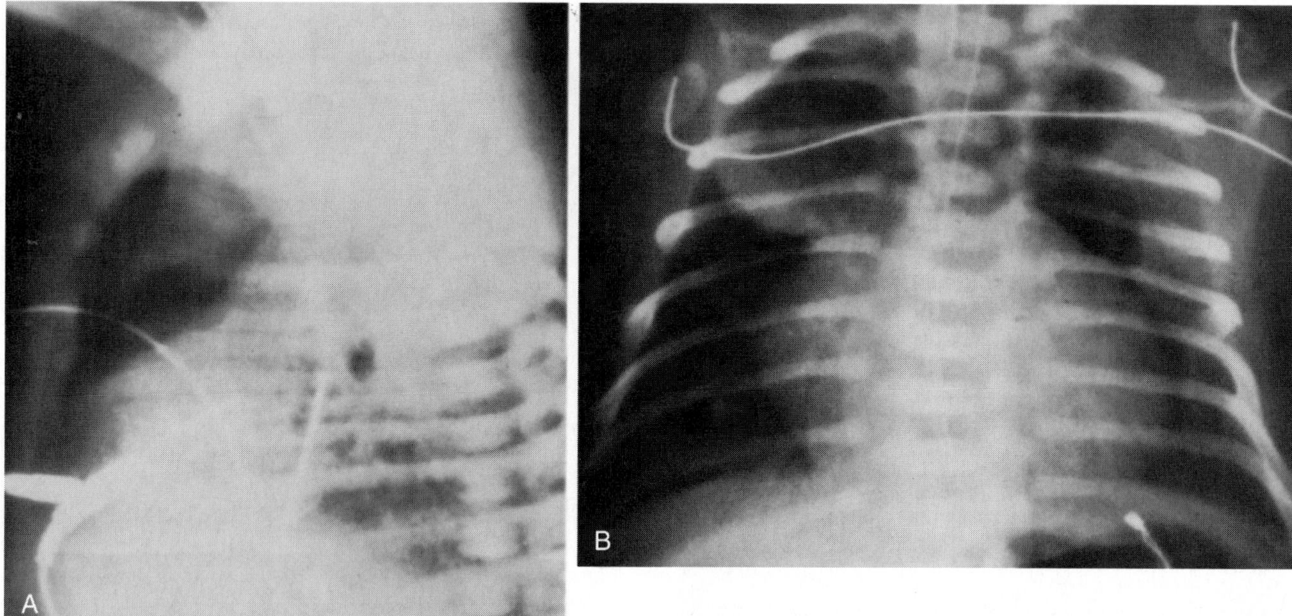

Figure 38–18. Pneumomediastinum. Lateral *(A)* and frontal *(B)* chest radiographs reveal lucency centered over the mediastinum superiorly and lifting of the thymus ("spinnaker sail" sign).

be obtained in the cross-table lateral projection. The abnormal air collection is anterior to the heart in the mediastinal space (Fig. 38–18*A*). The frontal view of the chest may also demonstrate elevation of the thymus by the air collection, creating the thymic "spinnaker sail" sign (Fig. 38–18*B*). A linear area of radiolucency along the cardiac border or outlining the edge of the descending aorta is more subtle evidence of mediastinal air. Subcutaneous emphysema in the neck may be noted. Occasionally, a medially located pneumothorax may mimic pneumomediastinum. They can be differentiated with a lateral decubitus film; a pneumothorax moves along the elevated portion of the thorax, whereas the pneumomediastinum does not.

Mediastinal air collections may decompress by dissecting into the fascial planes of the neck, with subcutaneous emphysema, or by tracking through the esophageal hiatus into the abdomen, leading to free retroperitoneal or intraperitoneal air. Collections can also be seen subpulmonically, loculated by or within the inferior pulmonary ligaments. Serious complications include rupture into the pericardial sac, with pneumopericardium or disruption of the pulmonary venous system, and systemic air embolism.

There is no specific therapy for pneumomediastinum. It is important, nevertheless, to observe the neonate with pneumomediastinum for the potentially serious complications mentioned previously.

Pneumothorax

Pneumothorax occurs when air dissects from a ruptured alveolus into the interstitium and escapes into the pleural space. Several risk factors for development of pneumothorax are well-known: meconium aspiration, pulmonary hypoplasia caused by renal dysplasia, endotracheal intubation, resuscitation, and positive-pressure ventilation. The infant may exhibit signs of sudden deterioration, with severe respiratory distress. Breath sounds are diminished over the affected hemithorax.

The chest radiograph usually demonstrates lung collapse with an expanded pleural space on the ipsilateral side. If the pneumothorax is under tension (Fig. 38–19), there is associated mediastinal shift to the contralateral hemithorax. More subtle signs of pneumothorax include widened rib interspaces and depression of the ipsilateral hemidiaphragm, giving a "deep sulcus" sign.

Occasionally, the air in pneumothorax can accumulate medial to the lung. In this instance, if the diagnosis is not straightforward, a lateral decubitus view, with the suspected side up, often reveals the abnormality.

Placement of a chest tube is required in patients with tension pneumothorax, in patients with progressive accumulation of intrapleural air, and in patients receiving positive-pressure ventilation. Tube position is confirmed on frontal and lateral chest radiographs. When optimally placed, the tube is directed into the anterior pleural space, with the side port projecting within the confines of the chest wall.

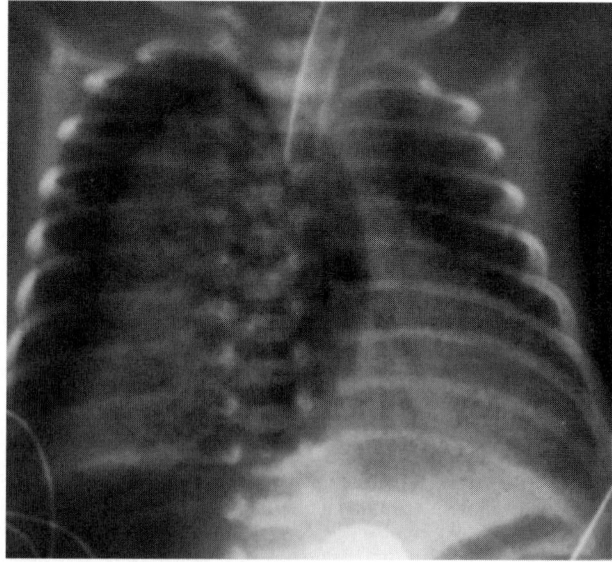

Figure 38–19. A right-sided tension pneumothorax in neonate treated for respiratory distress syndrome.

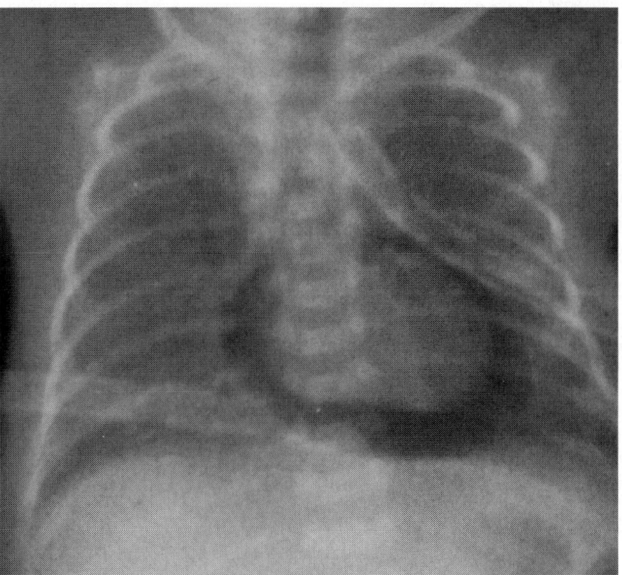

Figure 38–20. Pneumopericardium in an infant with respiratory distress syndrome. Note the presence of radiolucent air encircling the heart that has occurred secondary to barotrauma. The endotracheal tube is high in position at the thoracic inlet.

Pneumopericardium

Pneumopericardium occurs when air ruptures into the pericardial sac. This abnormal air collection is less common than those previously described, but because it has potentially severe consequences, accurate and rapid diagnosis is important. Symptomatic patients often have acute onset of hypotension, cyanosis, and reduced pulse pressure, and decreased breath sounds are detected on auscultation. The chest radiograph reveals a well-defined radiolucency encircling the heart (Fig. 38–20). The cardiac silhouette may be diminished in size if the process is under significant tension, with restricted venous return to the heart. Clinical signs of impaired cardiac output or cardiac tamponade require pericardiocentesis, sometimes with placement of a pericardial drainage catheter.

Pneumoperitoneum

Pneumoperitoneum follows the decompression of intrathoracic air, such as pneumomediastinum, into the abdomen. The presumed mechanism is extension through a diaphragmatic hiatus into the retroperitoneum, into the bowel mesentery, and through the subserosal surface of the bowel with subsequent leak into the peritoneal cavity.[13] The importance of making this diagnosis is to differentiate the process from a ruptured viscus or from necrotizing enterocolitis with perforation. A ruptured viscus demonstrates free intraperitoneal air without associated abnormal collection of air in the chest. The hallmark of necrotizing enterocolitis is linear or circular lucencies within the bowel wall, sometimes accompanied by portal venous gas. If the pneumoperitoneum is sufficiently large, it may limit diaphragmatic movement and compromise respiration.

Intravascular Air Embolism

Intravascular air embolism is a rare but serious complication of positive-pressure assisted ventilation. It often follows pulmonary interstitial emphysema and is usually massive. Air can be seen filling the heart and large vessels on the chest radiograph. The finding usually represents a terminal event in the treatment of RDS.

RESPIRATORY DISORDERS PRESENTING IN THE OLDER INFANT AND CHILD

Severe respiratory distress in children is a common indication for admission to the pediatric ICU. The causes are many, but the mechanisms of lung injury are frequently similar. The most common pediatric respiratory problems requiring ICU management are acute airway disease and various types of trauma. Surgical conditions and complications of chronic illnesses make up the remainder. Current critical care management of these problems can be assisted by multiple imaging modalities, including plain films, ultrasonography, CT, and nuclear medicine scintigraphy.

Airway Disease

Bronchiolitis

Bronchiolitis is an acute inflammatory process of the respiratory epithelium in infants and small children, whose airways are relatively small and highly susceptible to inflammatory narrowing. Pathophysiologically, edema and secretions obstruct the small bronchioles, creating airway narrowing, areas of irregular aeration, air trapping, and atelectasis. Affected children experience sudden onset of wheezing, caused by turbulent expiratory airflow traveling through narrowed air passages. Fever, cough, tachypnea, and tachycardia are common. Infants and children up to 2 years of age are usually affected. Children with bronchopulmonary dysplasia, congenital heart disease, or immunodeficiency syndromes especially are at increased risk for bronchiolitis and commonly need treatment in an acute care setting. *Respiratory syncytial virus* (RSV) is the most common etiologic agent, although a number of other viral pathogens have been incriminated. Hospitalization for RSV pneumonia is rarely required, but of those patients who are hospitalized, 11% may require intensive care and 8% may need intubation and ventilation.[14]

The chest radiograph typically demonstrates generalized hyperinflation of the lungs as a result of air trapping (Fig. 38–21). Areas of focal hyperinflation alternate with patchy zones of atelectasis. As the disease develops, the areas of atelectasis may progress to complete segmental or lobar collapse. There may be perihilar linear opacities, caused by bronchial wall thickening, and peribronchial cuffing, which represents peribronchial inflammatory edema.

In 1996, the U. S. Food and Drug Administration (FDA) approved intravenous RSV immunoglobulin (RSVIGIV) (RespiGam) for use in high-risk infants younger than 2 years to protect them from the most serious consequences of RSV infection. Recommendations for use include the administration of RSVIGIV in five monthly doses beginning in November of each year. More recently, the FDA has approved a synthetic monoclonal antibody (IgG) called SYNAGIS (Medi-493). It is administered intramuscularly in children monthly during the RSV season. Candidates for this new treatment include children under 3 years of age, premature infants younger than 32 weeks, and children with bronchopulmonary dysplasia or cystic fibrosis. Preliminary studies have shown significant reductions in RSV patient admissions.

Sudden-onset wheezing can also occur with foreign body aspiration, an important differential diagnostic consideration in suspected bronchiolitis. In foreign body aspiration, there is air trapping on the affected side, which is exaggerated on lateral decubitus views.

Asthma

Asthma is a chronic, intermittent, obstructive pulmonary process characterized by airway hyperactivity in response to a

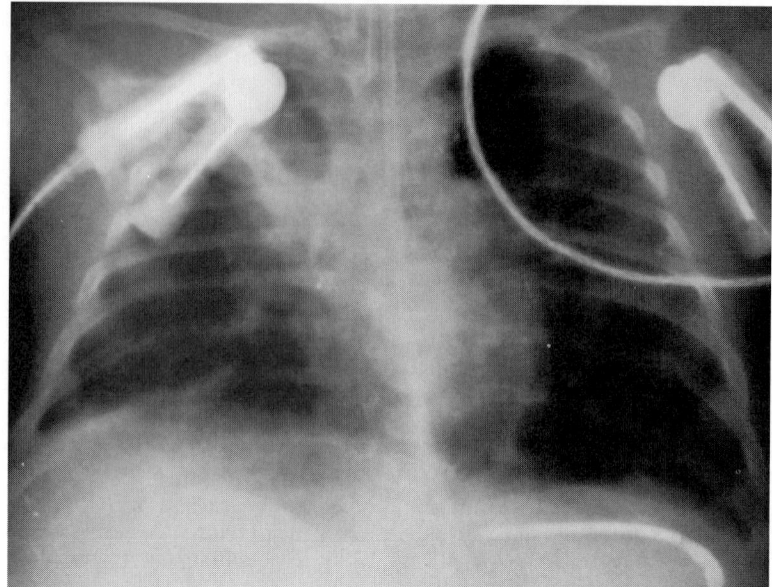

Figure 38–21. Bronchiolitis in an infant with fever and wheezing who was intubated for hypoxia. This chest radiograph shows the typical findings of airways pneumonia (bronchiolitis). Frequently, as in this patient, bronchiolitis is caused by respiratory syncytial virus. Visualized on this film are generalized hyperinflation, peribronchial thickening, and focal areas of hyperlucency (caused by air trapping) that alternate with areas of increased density occurring secondary to atelectasis or pneumonitis.

number of stimuli. Airway narrowing along with smooth muscle spasm and inflammatory edema causes airflow obstruction and air trapping. The increased resistance to airflow leads to wheezing and hypoxemia. There is no specific cause, although allergens, emotional stress, and exercise seem to be common precipitating factors. Asthma behaves clinically like bronchiolitis, except that unless it is complicated, there is no specific infectious agent. Usually, the two diseases are distinguished clinically by the age of presentation. Bronchiolitis occurs in children younger than 2 years; recurrent wheezing after this age is usually asthma.

The chest radiograph may be normal, or it may demonstrate increased aeration with increased perihilar markings and peribronchial cuffing. Patchy areas of atelectasis or infiltrate may be present, indicating complicated asthma. Atelectasis results from mucus plugging of the airway. Occasionally, the mucus-plugged bronchus can be visualized radiographically (Fig. 38–22). Patchy infiltrate may represent infection, which is usually viral. The main pulmonary arteries may be enlarged, with normal-caliber peripheral vessels, reflecting transient pulmonary hypertension.[15]

The chest radiograph is obtained primarily to exclude other diagnoses and to look for complications, such as atelectasis due to mucus plugging, obstructive emphysema, air-block phenomena, and secondary pneumonia.

Pulmonary Insults Secondary to Accidental Injury

Near-Drowning

Drowning is defined as a death by suffocation after submersion in a liquid medium; the term *near-drowning* is used when the patient recovers, at least temporarily, from the submersion episode. Patients who are initially resuscitated following submersion but who expire within 24 hours are ultimately classified as drowning victims. It is estimated that 6000 to 8000 patients a year die of drowning in the United States. Of all drowning deaths, 40% occur in children younger than 5 years, with another 15% to 20% of drowning victims between the ages of 5 and 20 years (see Chapter 10). Drowning or near-drowning occurs in a wide variety of locations, including bathtubs, hot tubs, pails of water, swimming pools, lakes, streams, rivers, and oceans.

Lung injury is secondary to aspiration of either the submersion medium or stomach contents. Some researchers believe that seawater aspiration is more likely to produce pulmonary edema, whereas freshwater aspiration causes more damage to the pulmonary structures.[16–18] In a review of 20 cases of near-drowning, however, the composition of the aspirated fluid had no bearing on the biochemical changes occurring in the lung.[19] Of more practical importance in preventing secondary injury is the promptness with which treatment is initiated at the scene or during transport to a hospital.

Clinically, near-drowning victims are hypoxic with a metabolic acidosis, and pulmonary edema soon develops. The

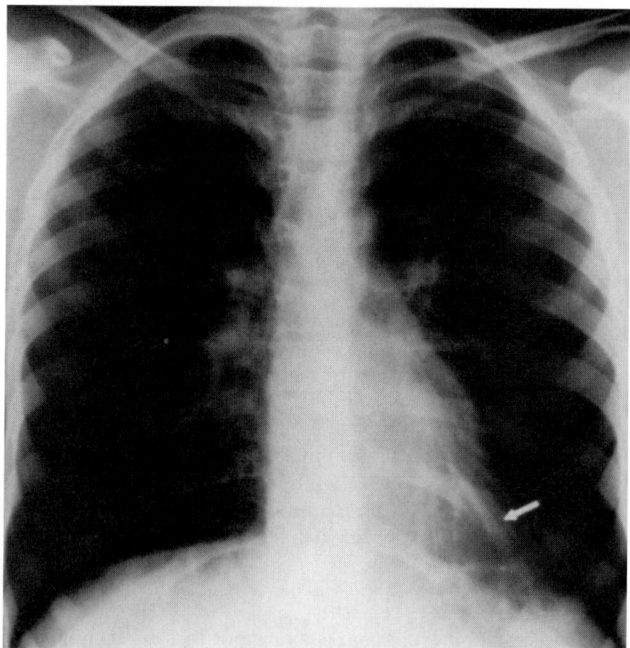

Figure 38–22. A 12-year-old boy with asthma. The chest radiograph demonstrates the typical findings of lung hyperinflation, peribronchial thickening, and increased perihilar markings. Note the thick, linear, obliquely oriented band of opacity in the left lower lobe that is consistent with a mucus-filled bronchus *(arrow)*.

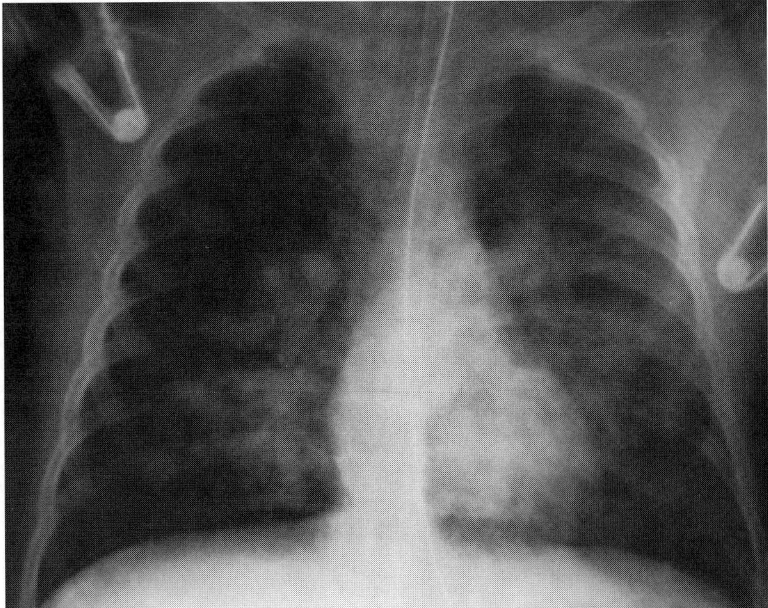

Figure 38–23. Near-drowning. A 5-year-old child was found facedown in a swimming pool containing chlorinated water. The child was intubated for hypoxia and acidosis. This chest film shows bilateral central "fluffy" alveolar infiltrates and a heart of normal size, findings typical for pulmonary edema and early acute respiratory distress syndrome (ARDS) resulting from near-drowning.

initial chest radiograph may be nonrevealing. Within 24 to 48 hours, however, there are usually bilateral alveolar densities in a pattern reflecting noncardiogenic pulmonary edema (Fig. 38–23). Pulmonary edema results from greater permeability of the alveolocapillary membrane secondary to hypoxic injury. These changes may progress to diffuse airspace consolidation, pneumonia, abscess formation, or, rarely, acute respiratory distress syndrome (ARDS) (Fig. 38–24).[20] If the child survives, chronic pulmonary sequelae are uncommon.

Hydrocarbon Aspiration

Hydrocarbon pneumonia occurs when hydrocarbon-based materials, such as kerosene and gasoline, are accidentally ingested. Because of their low viscosity and surface tension, these materials are readily aspirated into the tracheobronchial tree. Table 38–4 lists hydrocarbon compounds that are commonly stored within the reach of young children and accidentally ingested. The aspiration of hydrocarbons incites an inflammatory reaction in the lung, with destruction of surfactant, bronchial wall edema, and necrosis.

The chest radiograph reveals patchy airspace disease in the medial, basilar portions of the lungs that somewhat resemble pulmonary edema (Fig. 38–25). The radiographic changes are usually slow to resolve. Complications include pneumatocele formation, pleural effusion, air-block phenomena, and even frank necrosis.

Smoke Inhalation

Smoke inhalation is a major cause of death in fires. The lung injury is believed to be produced primarily by the irritant

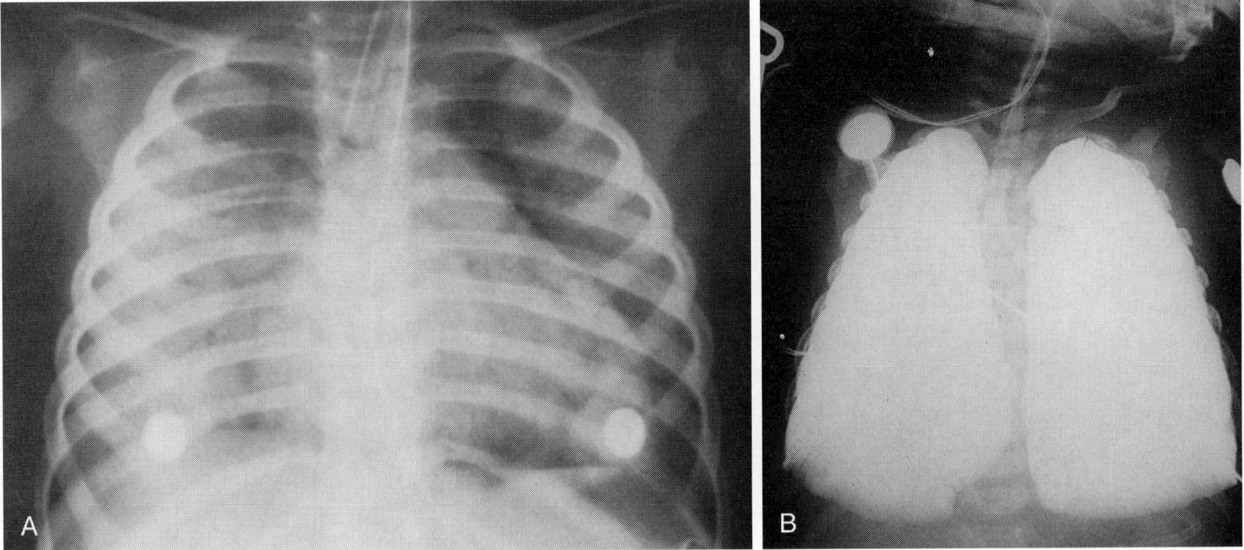

Figure 38–24. *A,* Acute respiratory distress syndrome (ARDS) in a 15-month-old infant who was admitted to the emergency department with seizures, anemia, and shock of unknown etiology. He underwent massive volume resuscitation, and ARDS then developed. The ARDS subsequently cleared. This chest radiograph shows a diffuse alveolar process and air bronchograms. Note the relative sparing of the medial aspects of the lungs, which is typical for ARDS. *B,* The patient is an 8-month-old infant with ARDS after respiratory syncytial viral pneumonitis being treated with liquid ventilation.

TABLE 38–4. Hydrocarbon Compounds Accidentally Ingested by Children

Gasoline
Kerosene
Floor wax
Furniture polish
Lighter fluid
Paint thinner
Acetone
Turpentine

effect of the combusted material inhaled and secondarily by upper airway burns. Airway irritation produces mucosal edema and sloughing, increases capillary permeability and extravascular lung water, reduces ciliary function, and alters surfactant production. These changes correlate well with the radiographic findings: airway obstruction, pulmonary interstitial edema, atelectasis, lung consolidation, and respiratory failure from ARDS (see Fig. 38–24).[21]

Chest Trauma

Chest trauma in children is rare (see Chapter 159). When chest injuries occur, the cause is usually nonpenetrating or blunt trauma, primarily from motor vehicle accidents. Blunt trauma to the chest can produce severe damage to intrathoracic organs without evidence of bony trauma to the thoracic cage. The ribs and other skeletal structures of the pediatric chest are often spared because of their extreme pliability. Even in a child without recognizable fractures, however, a CT scan may reveal unsuspected intrathoracic injuries.

In acute trauma, the head and abdomen are routinely evaluated with CT. Portable chest radiographs alone may underestimate or fail to demonstrate significant chest injuries. In a retrospective study of 512 children examined with CT after blunt abdominal trauma, in which several sections of the lower chest were included in the scanning, more than one third of the chest abnormalities seen on CT had been underestimated or missed on the most recent chest radiographs.[22] Consequently, it is recommended that at least three or four images of the lower chest be included in the abdominal CT scan to assist in the early recognition of unsuspected intrathoracic injury.

When bony trauma is evident, the location can indicate other potential sites of injury. Fractures of the first three ribs are commonly associated with injury to the great vessels, trachea, and major bronchi. Posterior rib fractures in infants and toddlers, especially in several stages of healing, suggest the possibility of child abuse. Fractures of the lower ribs may indicate injury to the liver, spleen, or diaphragm. Sternal fractures may portend the presence of cardiac contusion or tamponade.

Common Pulmonary Injuries

Nonpenetrating chest trauma results most commonly in three types of pulmonary injury: (1) pulmonary contusion, (2) pulmonary hematoma, and (3) traumatic pneumatocele. The basic mechanism for each is severe force applied to the chest wall, which is secondarily compressed, with transmission of the force to the underlying lung parenchyma.

Pulmonary contusion is the most common injury from blunt chest trauma. It follows exudation of fluid and blood into the lung parenchyma. Chest radiographic findings, usually present soon after trauma, typically are either ill-defined, patchy areas of airspace consolidation or diffuse, homogeneous consolidation (Fig. 38–26). Contusions generally resolve within 24 to 48 hours, with complete clearing by 3 to 4 days.

Pulmonary hematoma is secondary to traumatic hemorrhage into the lung parenchyma from ruptured capillaries. It usually occurs after severe blunt trauma, as in motor vehicle accidents. Children and young adults are susceptible to this injury because of the greater flexibility of their chest walls. Pulmonary hematoma may be recognized soon after trauma; however, it can be first seen several hours to several days later. It is commonly masked by surrounding pulmonary contusion; once the contusion resolves, the radiographic features of the hematoma become evident.

On chest radiographs, hematomas are usually homogeneous, well-circumscribed, radiodense masses occasionally containing air-fluid levels. In contrast to pulmonary contusions, pulmonary hematomas heal slowly, usually resolving gradually over several months.

Traumatic pneumatoceles are acute, primary lesions resulting from laceration of the lung. The rupture of alveolar walls leads to dissection of air into a cavity, which assumes a spheric contour (see Fig. 38–26). Pneumatoceles may be round or oval, ranging in size from 2 to 14 cm. They can be

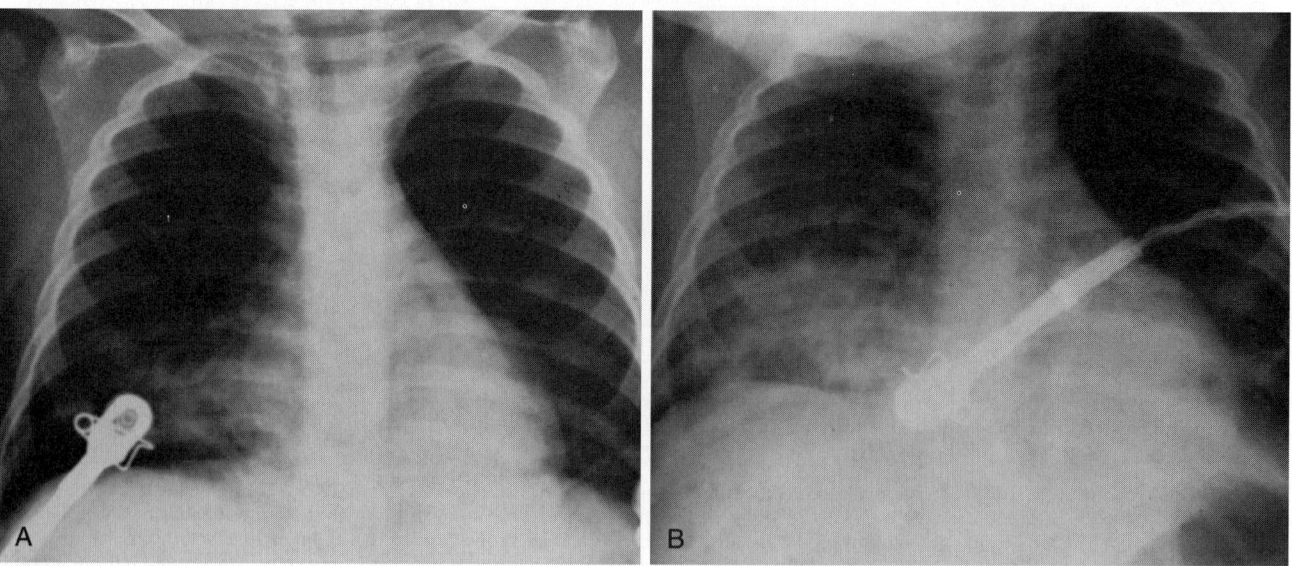

Figure 38–25. Hydrocarbon aspiration in an 8-month-old infant who ingested furniture polish. *A*, An early film demonstrates basilar, patchy alveolar infiltrates. *B*, A film obtained 4 days later shows more extensive consolidation at the lung bases.

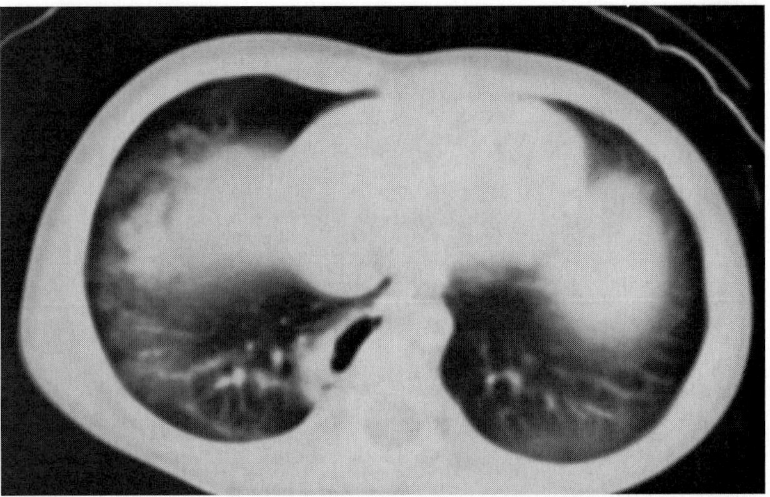

Figure 38–26. Chest trauma in a 2-year-old child run over by a car. This axial CT image demonstrates a right-sided radiopacity (representing lung contusion), a wedge-shaped radiolucency abutting the right margin of the heart (representing a right pneumothorax), and an oblong radiolucency in the right paraspinal area (consistent with a traumatic pneumatocele). Note the absence of rib fractures.

single or multiple and may contain blood, often with an air-fluid level. When filled with blood, they may be characterized as pulmonary hematomas. They may not be recognized as cystic lesions until the blood is evacuated, a process that may take up to 12 hours.[23] The patient may experience hemoptysis for several days as the blood is expectorated. Although some pneumatoceles may persist for several weeks, most clear completely in 2 to 3 weeks.

Less Common Pulmonary Injuries

Additional, less common chest injuries produced by blunt trauma in children are (1) tracheobronchial fracture, (2) diaphragmatic rupture, (3) aortic rupture, and (4) lung torsion.

Traumatic *fractures of the trachea and bronchi*, although relatively uncommon, represent serious intrathoracic injuries from severe compression injury of the chest or a sharp blow to the anterior neck. Radiographic features include mediastinal and subcutaneous cervical emphysema and persistent segmental lung collapse; tension pneumothorax may be present. Often there is persistent air leak despite optimal positioning of a chest tube. Approximately 10% of children demonstrate no radiographic or physical evidence of intrathoracic injury.[24]

Traumatic *diaphragmatic rupture* is a difficult diagnosis. It must be differentiated from more common injuries, such as hemothorax, diaphragmatic hemiparesis, and eventration. The latter two can be excluded with prior radiographs, if available. Rupture occurs more commonly on the left side, primarily because of the protective effect of the liver on the right. Radiographic diagnosis can be made through recognition of an elevated hemidiaphragm and gas-filled bowel above the diaphragm with mediastinal shift to the contralateral hemithorax. Pleural fluid may be present if there is strangulated bowel. Confirmation of rupture can be made through radiographic confirmation of the distal portion of a nasogastric tube high in the left chest within herniated stomach or on an upper gastrointestinal study. If there is persistent doubt about the diagnosis, ultrasonography, CT, or a nuclear medicine liver-spleen scan should confirm or refute it.

Traumatic *aortic rupture* is exceedingly rare in children. Radiographic findings are the same as those identified in adults: mediastinal widening, poor visualization of the aortic knob, tracheal deviation, and hemorrhagic apical pleural fluid. Spouge and coworkers[25] recommend aortography for patients in whom these findings are present in concert with additional signs of significant chest trauma. CT is useful in distinguishing a large thymus or vascular anomaly from traumatic vascular injury when no other signs of thoracic trauma are present.

Traumatic *torsion of the lung* is a rare complication of chest trauma that occurs predominantly in children. Children are believed to be susceptible to this injury because of their easily compressible thoracic cages. The lung is rotated 180°, displacing the lung base superiorly into the upper hemithorax and the lung apex inferiorly into the lower thorax. The chest radiograph reveals reversal of the pulmonary arterial markings. The injury results in compromise of the vascular supply, with airspace edema and hemorrhage. This diagnosis is considered a surgical emergency and is suggested clinically by the unilateral absence of breath sounds.

Pneumonia in the Pediatric Critical Care Patient

Pneumonia in the ICU setting can be classified as either community-acquired or hospital-acquired (nosocomial). *Community-acquired* infections can be transmitted by respiratory shedding from patients admitted to the ICU. The responsible organisms are either viral or bacterial. *Nosocomial infections* occur at a high rate in the ICU partly because the patients have severe underlying disease and partly because so many invasive and therapeutic procedures are performed. Such infections are responsible for a high rate of morbidity among pediatric ICU patients. Lower respiratory tract infections are greatest in frequency and occur secondary to multiple pathogens, such as *Klebsiella* species, *Pseudomonas aeruginosa, Staphylococcus aureus, Candida* species, and *Escherichia coli.*[26] Sources of respiratory infection in the ICU include transmission of organisms from contaminated personnel or equipment and aspiration pneumonia in obtunded patients, who have difficulty handling oral secretions.

Chest radiographic features vary according to the responsible organism. Staphylococcal pneumonia is a particularly virulent bronchopneumonia seen commonly in infants. The organism can secondarily invade the airways after influenza, and it is a relatively common agent in nosocomial infections. Staphylococcal pneumonia initially affects the airways and then progresses to segmental consolidation (Fig. 38–27*A*), often complicated by pleural effusion, empyema, or lung abscess. Pneumatocele formation, relatively common with pediatric staphylococcal pneumonia, can occur during the healing phase (Fig. 38–27*B*).

Streptococcus pneumoniae causes pneumonia in children with underlying illness, particularly those with sickle cell disease or immune deficiency. The usual radiographic pattern is homogeneous lobar consolidation, sometimes accompanied by pleural effusion or empyema (Fig. 38–28*A*). Ultrasonography may be of value in distinguishing between mobile effusion and loculated empyema (Fig. 38–28*B*).[27] Additionally, it provides an assessment of the amount of fluid present and may be used to localize an anatomic point for thoracentesis.

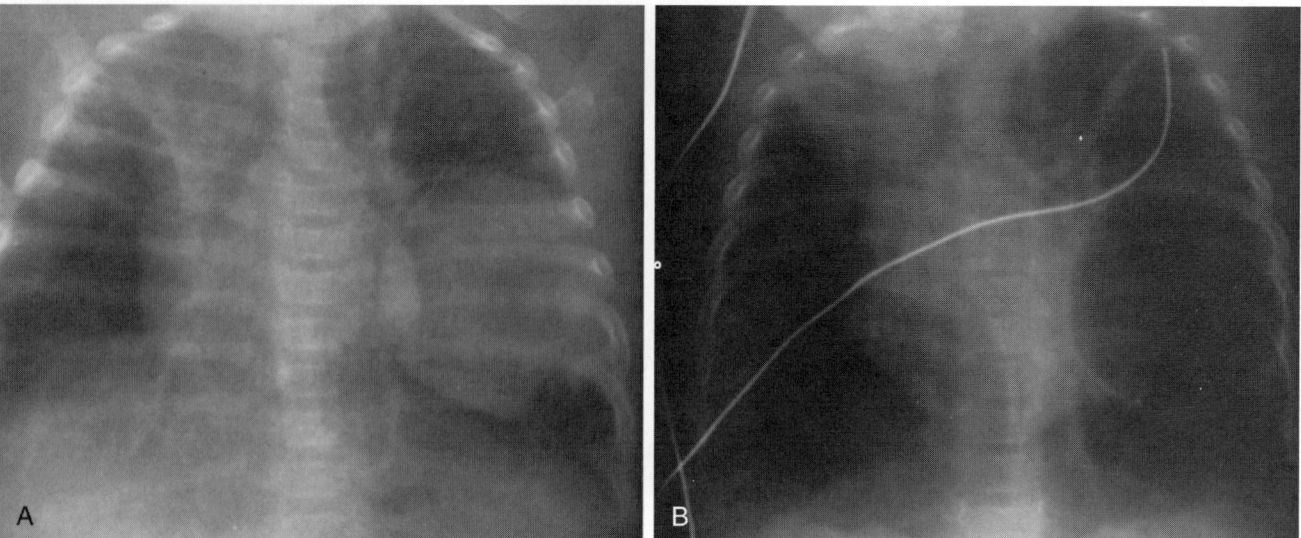

Figure 38–27. Staphylococcal pneumonia with pneumatocele formation. *A,* An initial supine radiograph shows a large, mass-like area of consolidation in the left lower lobe and a central area of rounded radiolucency, findings consistent with abscess formation. Bilateral upper lobe atelectasis is present. *B,* A follow-up radiograph obtained 2 weeks later reveals a large, thin-walled, cystic area of radiolucency, representing pneumatocele formation in the prior region of consolidation. Note the generalized hyperinflation and the patchy areas of atelectasis bilaterally.

Gram-negative organisms are also virulent agents that can cause dense lobar consolidation, bulging fissures, and abscess formation because of large amounts of inflammatory exudate. Abscess formation is characterized radiographically as air-fluid levels in cavitary lesions.

Pulmonary Problems Secondary to Systemic Diseases

Pneumonia in the Immunocompromised Host

Several underlying medical problems can place children at greater risk for opportunistic infection of the lungs; some of these are listed in Table 38–5. Children with malignancies are at great risk for the development of pneumonia and may require hospitalization in the ICU. The cause of pneumonia in such a child differs, depending on whether the patient is neutropenic. In both neutropenic and non-neutropenic hosts, there is loss of cellular and humoral immunity, which leaves the child at risk for infection by both gram-positive and gram-negative pathogens (e.g., *S. pneumoniae, Haemophilus influenzae*). Neutropenic patients are additionally at risk for infection by opportunistic *(S. aureus, Staphylococcus epidermidis)* or enteric gram-negative organisms as well as fungal agents. Notably, neutropenic patients cannot mount a normal inflammatory response, and the usual signs of infection may not be present. Patients who have leukemia or have undergone bone marrow transplantation are also at risk for viral (e.g., cytomegalovirus) and fungal (e.g., *aspergillus*) infections.[28]

Children with human immunodeficiency virus (HIV) are at risk for a number of opportunistic pulmonary infections; the

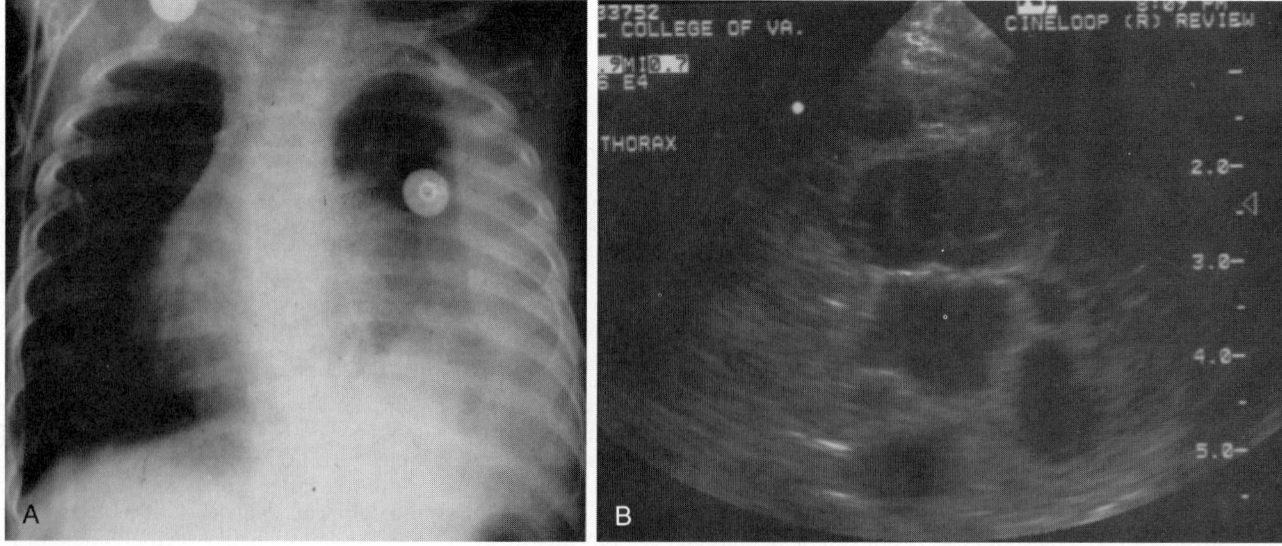

Figure 38–28. Streptococcal pneumonia with empyema. *A,* This chest radiograph demonstrates a large, homogeneous opacity along the left lateral chest wall that extends into the lower hemithorax; mediastinal shift to the right is also apparent. *B,* This sonogram of the left hemithorax reveals the loculated configuration of the empyema, with both cystic and solid components well visualized.

TABLE 38–5. Conditions Predisposing to Opportunistic Lung Infection

DiGeorge syndrome
Agammaglobulinemia
Immunoglobulin A deficiency
Severe combined immunodeficiency syndrome
Ataxia telangiectasia
Wiskott-Aldrich syndrome
Chronic granulomatous disease
Cystic fibrosis
Immotile cilia syndrome
Alpha-antitrypsin deficiency
Scimitar syndrome
Swyer-James syndrome
Organ transplantation with immunosuppressant therapy
Cancer chemotherapy
Steroid therapy

most common is *Pneumocystis carinii* pneumonia, which occurs in some 40% to 50% of pediatric patients with acquired immunodeficiency syndrome.[29, 30] *P. carinii* has been classified as either a protozoal parasite or a fungus (Ascomycetes). This organism invades the type I alveolar cells of the lung, inciting the development of foamy material within the alveoli and interstitial edema. Hypoxemia and decreased pulmonary compliance result, along with fever, dyspnea, and tachypnea. Symptoms can become severe enough to require ventilatory support. The majority of pediatric HIV infections are acquired either through transplacental exposure or by exposure to maternal blood during delivery.[31] Other, less common means of transmission are contaminated blood products and sexual abuse.

The initial chest radiograph may be normal. Soon after presentation, however, patchy, localized or diffuse interstitial infiltrates appear. This appearance usually progresses to diffuse, patchy opacities that may rapidly coalesce, becoming more homogeneous. Secondary complications, including pneumomediastinum and pneumothorax, are not uncommon. It is not clear whether these air-block complications result from mechanical ventilation or the disease process itself.

Other common pulmonary processes in children with HIV are lymphocytic interstitial pneumonitis, various recurrent bacterial infections, and a host of viral pneumonias, the most common being cytomegalovirus and RSV.[32, 33]

Sickle Cell Anemia: Acute Chest Syndrome

Acute chest syndrome is one of the vaso-occlusive crises seen in sickle cell disease. It is characterized by fever, pleuritic chest pain, cough, tachypnea, and hypoxemia. Radiographically, a focus of atelectasis or infiltrate is usually seen, sometimes accompanied by a pleural effusion (Fig. 38–29). Up to 25% of hospital admissions and deaths in sickle cell patients can be attributed to this syndrome.[34] The exact cause is not clear, but several theories have been proposed. Bacterial pneumonia is identified in 25% of patients[35] and was previously accepted by many as the cause. In those patients in whom bacterial infection is not found, however, alternative explanations have been considered for the pulmonary infiltrate.

Pulmonary infarction, although not always diagnosed from radiographic or scintigraphic criteria, has been accepted by many as the logical cause of the clinical syndrome of pain and pulmonary infiltrate.[36–38]

Rib infarction is another proposed mechanism. Rucknagel and coworkers[39] have suggested that rib infarction with associated bone pain causes pleuritis and splinting, leading to hypoventilation, atelectasis, and radiographic changes resembling those seen in pneumonia. These researchers found that in each of their 10 patients with sickle cell disease who had chest pain and radiographic infiltrate, radionuclide bone scans showed evidence of rib infarction. Rucknagel and coworkers[39] have recommended that prevention of hypoventilation as well as control of pain be considered as therapeutic goals. Their findings, although convincing, await further confirmation.

Another possible mechanism, proposed by Bhalla and colleagues,[40] is microvascular pulmonary occlusion without overt infarction. Using thin-section CT scanning, these researchers were able to detect, with high sensitivity and specificity, areas with a deficiency of visible arterioles and venules indicating hypoperfusion. Parenchymal consolidation was the chest radiographic correlate of this finding. Bhalla and colleagues[40] suggested that timely diagnosis of acute chest syndrome using thin-section CT would permit early and appropriate treatment to improve perfusion. These findings also await corroboration.

Pneumococcal pneumonia, although not specifically associated with acute chest syndrome, is often seen in sickle cell disease and has serious consequences when not treated.[41]

On the basis of current understanding of the molecular pathogenesis of sickle cell disease, three approaches have undergone thorough laboratory and clinical investigation: (1) chemical inhibition of hemoglobin S polymerization, (2) reduction of the intracellular hemoglobin concentrations, and (3) pharmacologic induction of hemoglobin F using hydroxyurea.

The current recommendations for treatment of acute chest syndrome consist of antibiotics, intravenous hydration, analgesia, oxygen, and simple blood or exchange transfusion. Incentive spirometry may help prevent or decrease the manifestation of acute chest syndrome in patients with thoracic cage bone infarctions.

Acute Respiratory Distress Syndrome

ARDS is an acute, severe progressive inflammatory process that can occur secondary to a variety of underlying pulmonary and nonpulmonary conditions (Table 38–6). The name of the syndrome, first described in adults, was derived from its similarity to neonatal RDS, the pathologic features being acute alveolar damage and formation of hyaline membranes. ARDS does occur in children, but the incidence is not known.

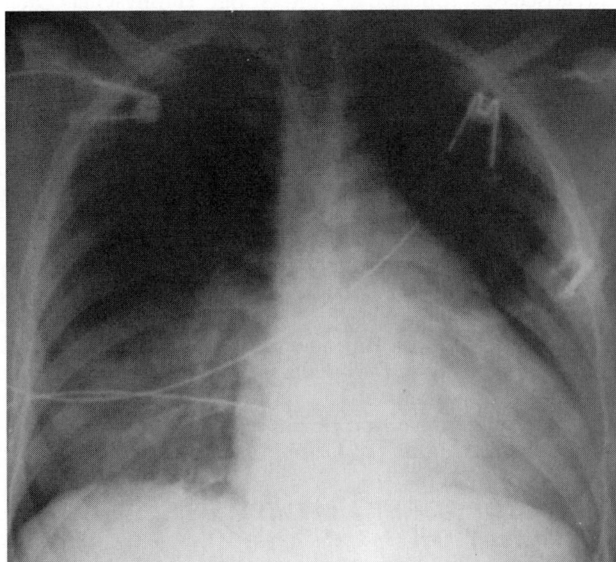

Figure 38–29. Acute chest syndrome in a 13-year-old girl with sickle cell anemia who presented with chest pain, fever, and tachypnea. This chest radiograph reveals cardiomegaly and infiltrate in the right lower lobe and the medial left lower lobe.

TABLE 38–6. Adult Respiratory Distress Syndrome: Predisposing Conditions

Pneumonia
Sepsis
Pulmonary embolism: air, fat
Disseminated intravascular coagulation
Drug overdose
Trauma
Inhalation of noxious substances

Pathologically, the inciting condition causes injury to the alveolocapillary membrane, promoting fluid leakage and pulmonary edema. Three stages have been described.[42]

Stage I reveals minimal fluid leakage confined to the interstitial space. The lungs at this stage may be radiographically normal, or lung volumes may be diminished as a result of microatelectasis and minimal interstitial edema.

Stage II is a period of extensive fluid leakage, fibrin deposition, and hyaline membrane formation, causing ill-defined, patchy opacities on chest radiographs. These patchy areas of opacity coalesce rapidly to form large areas of alveolar consolidation (see Fig. 38–24). The appearance is commonly the reverse of the typical "bat's wing" pulmonary edema pattern, in that the process begins more peripherally and progresses centrally, eventually becoming indistinguishable from that seen in cardiogenic pulmonary edema, with the exception that the heart size is usually normal. Pleural effusion is not characteristically present.

Stage III is typified histologically by alveolar cell hyperplasia and collagen deposition, with a less dense, more ground-glass radiographic appearance. Radiolucencies are believed to represent areas of ischemia that are ventilated but poorly perfused.

Radiographic evidence of healing can be seen 5 to 7 days after the onset of respiratory failure, with the homogeneous consolidation diminishing.[43] The lungs remain abnormal for a variable period thereafter, with a reticular appearance reflecting fibrosis.

CT scanning is increasingly utilized in patients with ARDS for detection of complications not usually seen on chest radiography. The location of the chest tubes can be confirmed, and abscesses, pulmonary interstitial emphysema, pneumomediastinum, and pneumothorax can be better visualized, on CT.

Treatment options for ARDS, both currently used and undergoing investigation, include conventional ventilation, pressure-controlled inverse-ratio ventilation, permissive hypercapnia, surfactant replacement, high-frequency oscillatory ventilation, nitric oxide, liquid ventilation (total or partial), and ECMO. A multicenter prospective, randomized study of the use of propofol and permissive hypercapnia is currently under way.

The significance of distinguishing ARDS from any underlying causative condition is that the patient may die of ARDS in spite of successful resolution of the underlying condition. The mortality rate for ARDS in adults is greater than 50%.[44] An estimated mortality rate in pediatric patients is 59%.[45, 46] Despite the high mortality, studies in adults have shown that for those who do survive, the prognosis for recovery of pulmonary function is good.

EXTRACORPOREAL MEMBRANE OXYGENATION

ECMO is a type of arteriovenous cardiopulmonary bypass that provides support for patients with respiratory failure resulting from a potentially reversible cause. Criteria for pediatric candidates for ECMO are as follows:

- Persistent respiratory failure despite therapy with 100% oxygen, high-pressure ventilation, and appropriate pharmacologic agents
- Birth weight greater than 2 kg
- Gestational age more than 34 weeks
- Assisted ventilation for fewer than 10 days

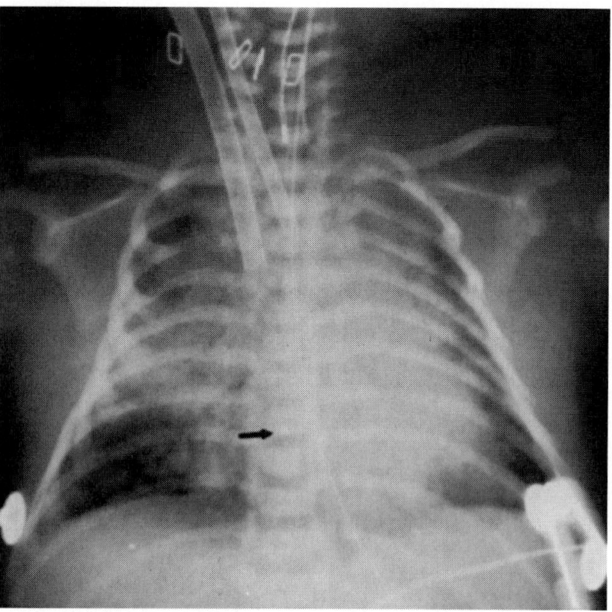

Figure 38–30. This patient was treated with extracorporeal membrane oxygenation for meconium aspiration. The arterial cannula tip is in the aortic arch. A radiopaque marker demonstrates the tip of the venous cannula in the right atrium *(arrow)*. Note the high position of the endotracheal tube.

Neonatal disease processes most commonly treated with ECMO are listed in Table 38–7. Also included are patients who have undergone surgical correction of congenital heart anomalies and who cannot be removed from acute cardiopulmonary bypass.

The process usually involves cannulation of the right internal jugular vein and right common carotid artery. Venous blood is removed from the right atrium via the superior vena cava and the internal jugular cannula, and oxygenated blood is returned to the thoracic aorta via the common carotid cannula. The flow bypasses the heart and lungs, giving them a chance to heal. Gas exchange is provided, and the potential for oxygen toxicity and barotrauma is minimized. ECMO also alleviates right-to-left shunting in patients with persistent pulmonary hypertension.

The initial chest radiographs of patients undergoing ECMO usually demonstrate diffuse lung opacification with air bronchograms and a variable amount of basilar atelectasis (Fig. 38–30). The subcutaneous tissues may be expanded because of edema from an accumulation of fluid in the extravascular spaces. Clinical improvement in the lungs may proceed faster

TABLE 38–7. Neonatal Disease Processes Treated with Extracorporeal Membrane Oxygenation

Meconium aspiration syndrome
Congenital diaphragmatic hernia
Perinatal asphyxia
Sepsis
Congenital pneumonia
Pulmonary hypoplasia
Persistent pulmonary hypertension from a variety of causes
Primary cardiac failure

than radiographic improvement. Daily radiographs are obtained to monitor the position of the ECMO cannulas and the other catheters and tubes and to monitor any complications, such as air-block phenomena.

ECMO is discontinued when the patient's lung function has recovered or when there is evidence of a serious complication, the most common being intracranial hemorrhage, which is monitored with cranial sonography. Cerebral infarction can also occur. ECMO results in improved survival and a lower incidence of chronic lung disease.[47, 48]

With the advent of the double-lumen catheter, a venovenous approach may decrease the morbidity of ECMO by sparing the carotid artery and enhancing oxygenation of the lungs and coronary circulation via return of oxygenated blood to the right side of the heart.[49]

References

1. Wood BP: The newborn chest. Radiol Clin North Am 1993; 31:667.
2. Jobe AH: The respiratory system: Part 1. The developmental biology of the lung. *In:* Neonatal-Perinatal Medicine—Diseases of the Fetus and Infant. 5th ed. Fanaroff AA, Martin RJ (Eds). St. Louis, Mosby-Year Book, 1992, p 790.
3. Wood BP, Sinkin RA, Kendig JW, et al: Exogenous lung surfactant: Effect on radiographic appearance in premature infants. Radiology 1987; 165:11.
4. Kendig JW, Notter RH: A comparison of surfactant as immediate prophylaxis and as rescue therapy in newborns of less than 30 weeks' gestation. N Engl J Med 1991; 324:865.
5. Ablow RC, Driscoll SG, Effmann EL, et al: A comparison of early onset group B streptococcal neonatal infection and the respiratory distress syndrome of the newborn. N Engl J Med 1976; 294:65.
6. Weller MH, Katzenstein AA: Radiological findings in group B streptococcal sepsis. Radiology 1976; 118:385.
7. Wiswell TE, Tuggle JM, Turner BS: Meconium aspiration syndrome: Have we made a difference? Pediatrics 1990; 85:715.
8. Hernanz-Schulman M: Cysts and cystlike lesions of the lung. Radiol Clin North Am 1993; 31:631.
9. Cleveland RH, Weber B: Retained fetal lung fluid in congenital lobar emphysema: A possible predictor of polyalveolar lobe. Pediatr Radiol 1993; 23:291.
10. Kennedy CD, Habibi P, Mathew DJ, et al: Lobar emphysema: Long term imaging follow-up. Radiology 1991; 180:189.
11. Gyepes MT, Vincent WR: Severe congenital heart disease in the neonatal period: A functional approach to emergency diagnosis. Am J Roentgenol 1971; 116:490.
12. Crowley JJ, Oh KS, Newman B, et al: Telltale signs of congenital heart disease. Radiol Clin North Am 1993; 31:573.
13. Leonidas JC, Berdon W: The neonate and young infant. *In:* Caffey's Pediatric X-Ray Diagnosis. 9th ed. Silverman FN, Kuhn JP (Eds). St. Louis, Mosby-Year Book, 1993, p 1987.
14. Green M, Brayer AF, Schenkman KA, et al: Duration of hospitalization in previously well infants with respiratory syncytial virus infection. Pediatr Infect Dis J 1989; 8:601.
15. Blair DN, Coppage L, Shaw C: Medical imaging in asthma. J Thorac Imaging 1986; 1:23.
16. Modell J, Moya F, Newby EJ, et al: The effects of fluid volume in seawater drowning. Arch Intern Med 1967; 67:68.
17. Yamamoto K, Yamamoto Y, Kikuchi H: The effects of drowning media on the lung water content: An experimental study on rats. Z Rechtsmed 1983; 90:1.
18. Orlowski JP, Abulleil MM, Philips JM: Effects of tonicities of saline solutions on pulmonary injury in drowning. Crit Care Med 1987; 15:126.
19. Putnam CE, Tummillo AM, Myerson DA, et al: Drowning: Another plunge. Am J Roentgenol 1975; 125:543.
20. Fine NL, Myerson DA, Myerson PJ: Near-drowning presenting as adult respiratory distress syndrome. Chest 1974; 65:347.
21. Spurrier EA, Spear RM, Munster AM: Burns, inhalational injury, and electrical injury. *In:* Textbook of Pediatric Intensive Care. 2nd ed. Rogers MC (Ed). Baltimore, Williams & Wilkins, 1992, p 1510.
22. Sivit CJ, Taylor GA, Eichelberger MR: Chest injury in children with blunt abdominal trauma: Evaluation with CT. Radiology 1989; 171:815.
23. Fagan CJ, Swischuk LE: Traumatic lung and paramediastinal pneumatoceles. Radiology 1976; 120:11.
24. Mahboubi S, O'Hara AE: Bronchial rupture in children following blunt abdominal trauma. Pediatr Radiol 1989; 10:133.
25. Spouge AR, Burrows PE, Armstrong D, et al: Traumatic aortic rupture in the pediatric population. Pediatr Radiol 1991; 21:324.
26. Merritt WT, Stephens M: Nosocomial infections in the pediatric intensive care unit. *In:* Textbook of Pediatric Intensive Care. 2nd ed. Rogers MC (Ed). Baltimore, Williams & Wilkins, 1992, p 30.
27. Ben-Ami TE, O'Donovan JC, Yousefzadeh DK: Sonography of the chest in children. Radiol Clin North Am 1993; 31:517.
28. Gordon JB, Yeager AM: Management of the child with malignant disease in the pediatric intensive care unit. *In:* Textbook of Pediatric Intensive Care. 2nd ed. Rogers MC (Ed). Baltimore, Williams & Wilkins, 1992, p 1412.
29. Caldwell MB, Rogers MF: Epidemiology of pediatric HIV infection. Pediatr Clin North Am 1991; 38:1.
30. Sanders-Laufer D, DeBruin W, Edelson PJ: *Pneumocystis carinii* infections in HIV-infected children. Pediatr Clin North Am 1991; 38:69.
31. Ambrosino MM, Genieser NB, Krasinski K: Opportunistic infections and tumors in immunocompromised children. Radiol Clin North Am 1992; 30:639.
32. Goodman PC: Pulmonary disease in children with AIDS. J Thorac Imaging 1991; 6:60.
33. Berdon WE, Mellins RB, Abramson SJ, et al: Pediatric HIV infection in its second decade: The changing pattern of lung involvement—clinical, plain film, and computed tomographic findings. Radiol Clin North Am 1993; 31:453.
34. Bhalla M, Abboud MR, McLoud TC, et al: Acute chest syndrome in sickle cell disease: CT evidence of microvascular occlusion. Radiology 1993; 187:45.
35. Davies SC, Luce PJ, Win AA, et al: Acute chest syndrome in sickle cell disease. Lancet 1984; 1:36.
36. Barrett CE: Acute pulmonary disease in sickle cell anemia. Am Rev Respir Dis 1971; 104:159.
37. Sprinkle RH, Cole T, Smith S, et al: Acute chest syndrome in children with sickle cell disease. Am J Pediatr Hematol Oncol 1986; 8:105.
38. Poncz M, Kane E, Gill FM: Acute chest syndrome in sickle cell disease: Etiology and clinical correlates. J Pediatr 1985; 107:861.
39. Rucknagel DL, Kalinyak KA, Gelfand MJ: Rib infarcts and acute chest syndrome in sickle cell diseases. Lancet 1991; 337:831.
40. Bhalla M, Abboud MR, McLoud TC, et al: Acute chest syndrome in sickle cell disease: CT evidence of microvascular occlusion. Radiology 1993; 187:45.
41. Young RC, Castro O, Baxter RP, et al: The lung in sickle cell disease: A clinical overview of common vascular, infectious, and other problems. J Natl Med Assoc 1981; 73:19.
42. Greene R: Adult respiratory distress syndrome: Acute alveolar damage. Radiology 1987; 163:57.
43. Paré JAP, Fraser RG: Pulmonary hypertension and edema. *In:* Synopsis of Diseases of the Chest. Fraser RS, Paré JAP, Fraser RG, et al (Eds). Philadelphia, WB Saunders, 1983, p 515.
44. Royal JA, Levin DL: Adult respiratory distress syndrome in pediatric patients: I. Clinical aspects, pathophysiology, pathology, and mechanisms of lung injury. J Pediatr 1988; 112:169.
45. Lyrene RK, Troug WE: Adult respiratory distress syndrome in a pediatric intensive care unit: Predisposing conditions, clinical course, and outcome. Pediatrics 1981; 67:790.
46. Effmann EL, Menten DF, Kirks DR, et al: Adult respiratory distress syndrome in children. Clin Pediatr 1983; 22:401.
47. Bartlett RH, Andrews AF, Toomasian CCP, et al: Extracorporeal membrane oxygenation for newborn respiratory failure: Forty-five cases. Surgery 1982; 92:2.
48. Krummel TM, Greenfield LJ, Kirkpatrick BV: Extracorporeal membrane oxygenation in neonatal pulmonary failure. Pediatr Ann 1982; 11:11.
49. Finer NN, Tierney AJ, Ainsworth W: Venovenous extracorporeal membrane oxygenation: The effects of proximal internal jugular cannulation. J Pediatr Surg 1996; 31:1391.

39

Computed Tomography and Magnetic Resonance Imaging of the Abdomen in the Critical Care Patient

Ann S. Fulcher, MD • Richard A. Szucs, MD

Technologic advances in computed tomography (CT) and magnetic resonance (MR) imaging during the past few years have further enhanced the usefulness of these modalities in imaging the critically ill patient. Faster spiral CT scanners acquire each image in 1 second or less, which allows imaging of the entire abdomen in a single breath hold. The faster scan times make the patient's movement and respiratory motion much less of a problem and eliminate breathing misregistration. Useful diagnostic information can be obtained even in patients who cannot suspend respiration.[1, 2] The advances in MR imaging have been even greater, with scan times reduced from minutes to seconds. Stronger, high-performance gradients and technical improvements in software have led to the development of faster MR sequences. Gradient-echo and fast spin-echo sequences permit imaging during a single breath hold.[3, 4] As with CT, useful images can be obtained with some sequences even without suspended respiration. MR uses no ionizing radiation, has no known risks in the pregnant patient, and can image directly in multiple planes (Fig. 39–1). Standard patient monitoring and life-support devices are not compatible with the high magnetic field of the MR scanner and in the past limited the utility of MR imaging in critical care patients. However, the development of MR-compatible devices allows monitoring of critically ill patients; patients can be safely imaged even on a ventilator or under general anesthesia.

Patients in the intensive care unit (ICU) frequently have signs or symptoms that require imaging evaluation. These include sepsis, unexplained abdominal pain, abdominal distention, diarrhea, and occult blood loss. CT of the abdomen plays an important role in the evaluation of these patients because it can assess the gastrointestinal tract and solid organs of the abdomen as well as the mesentery and retroperitoneum. CT can establish the diagnosis or further direct the diagnostic work-up and is helpful in distinguishing between conditions that require surgical intervention and those that can be managed medically. For example, when CT demonstrates a mass or adenopathy, cells or tissue for diagnosis can be obtained from CT-guided aspiration or core biopsy. If an abscess is identified on CT, CT-guided catheter drainage can be therapeutic. In cases of gastrointestinal perforation, when a pneumoperitoneum is identified on CT, the CT findings may suggest the likely source of perforation and help direct the surgical approach.

MR imaging provides an alternative for imaging patients who cannot receive the iodinated intravenous contrast agents used for CT because of a history of reaction to the contrast agent or impaired renal function. The contrast material used for MR imaging, gadolinium, can be safely administered to these patients.

A recently introduced MR technique, magnetic resonance cholangiopancreatography (MRCP), is a noninvasive method of imaging the biliary and pancreatic ducts[4] (Fig. 39–2). Because MRCP can image the entire biliary tract and pancreatic duct in 5 to 10 minutes and does not require the use of contrast material or sedation, it is particularly useful in evaluating the critically ill patient with suspected pancreaticobiliary disease. The sensitivity and specificity of MRCP are comparable to those of endoscopic retrograde cholangiopancreatography (ERCP) in determining the presence, level, and cause of obstruction.

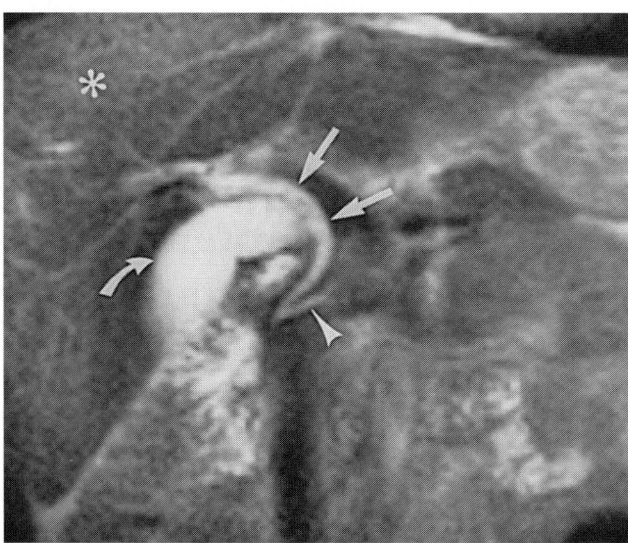

Figure 39–1. Abdominal MR image. Coronal T2-weighted MR image of the abdomen obtained during breath holding demonstrates the liver *(asterisk)*, extrahepatic bile duct *(arrows)*, pancreatic duct *(arrowhead)*, and gallbladder *(curved arrow)*.

Transport of critically ill patients to the CT or MR suite is not without potential risk. Indeck and colleagues[5] reported that in 68% of their patients, transportation from the ICU to the radiology department resulted in a change in physiologic status that required therapeutic intervention, and in only 25%

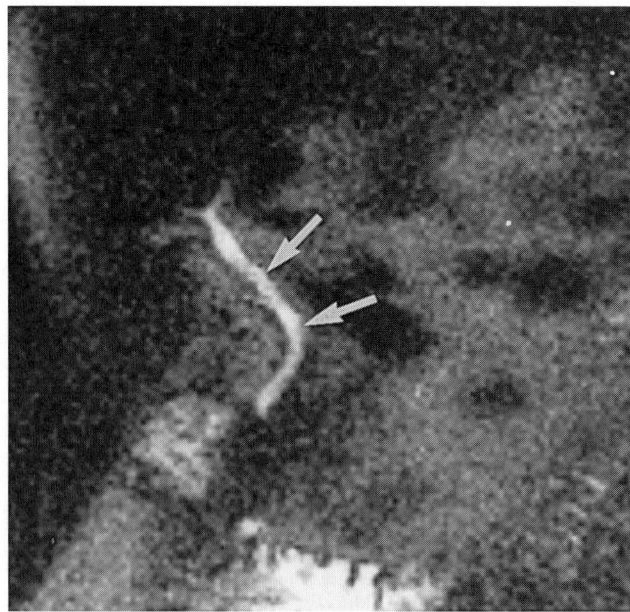

Figure 39–2. Magnetic resonance cholangiogram (MRC). Coronal MRC shows the extrahepatic bile duct *(arrows)* without the use of contrast material.

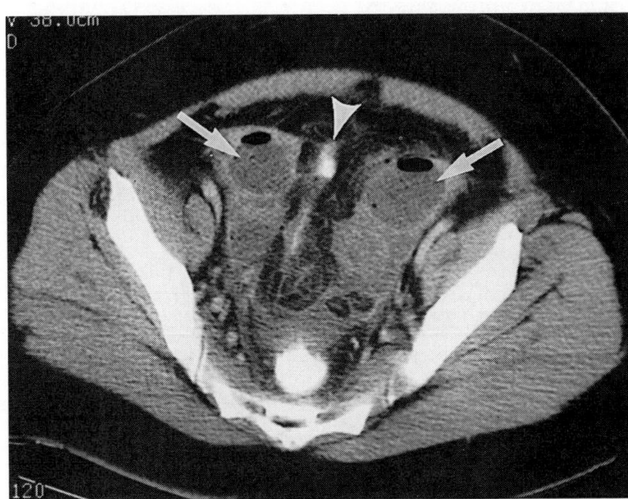

Figure 39–3. Postoperative abscesses. A 40-year-old woman after hysterectomy presented with pelvic pain, fever, and leukocytosis. An axial CT scan reveals multiple pelvic abscesses *(arrows)* that contain air-fluid levels. The collapsed sigmoid colon *(arrowhead)* lies between the abscesses.

of patients did the results of diagnostic testing alter management of the patient. Evens and Winslow[6] reported that 53% of their critically ill, mechanically ventilated adults had clinically important changes in arterial oxygen saturation, heart rate, or systolic blood pressure during intrahospital transport. Both authors stressed that the risks versus benefits should be carefully evaluated before it is decided to transport the critically ill patient and that intensive monitoring and care of these patients should be maintained during transport.

A more recent prospective study comparing patients transported outside the ICU with matched control patients who did not leave the ICU concluded that intrahospital transport of critically ill patients is safe and carries a low risk of complications.[7] Numerous studies have documented that the information gained may result in significant changes in management of the patient. Patients should always be accompanied by critical care personnel for monitoring and support during transport and examination.

It is imperative that an optimal CT examination be performed in these patients. The entire abdomen and pelvis should be examined. Adequate bowel opacification with oral contrast material is particularly important in patients thought to have an abscess. Many of these patients have adynamic ileus with fluid-filled loops of bowel. Without proper oral contrast enhancement, it may be impossible to distinguish an extraluminal fluid collection from fluid-filled bowel loops. Intravenous contrast material is also important, particularly to demonstrate focal abnormalities of the solid organs, such as abscesses or infarcts, and to define the enhancing wall of an intra-abdominal abscess.

INTRA-ABDOMINAL ABSCESS

The most common indication for abdominal CT in the critically ill patient is the detection of an abscess. Patients with abscesses may present with fever, leukocytosis, or sepsis. Most abscesses in this population occur after surgery (Fig. 39–3); other abscesses are enteric related, representing complications of diverticulitis, appendicitis, or Crohn's disease. Still other abscesses may be confined to the solid organs, such as the liver and spleen, and may be pyogenic, fungal, or amebic in etiology. The importance of prompt diagnosis and treatment is underscored by mortality rates of up to 30% for surgically drained abscesses and up to 100% for undrained abscesses.[8]

The high accuracy of CT (>95%) in the detection of abscesses and its ability to guide therapeutic intervention in the form of percutaneous drainage make CT the modality of choice in the evaluation of a suspected abscess.[9] Abscesses typically appear as collections of fluid or soft-tissue density, which contain air in only 30% to 50% of cases. Although some abscesses demonstrate rim enhancement after intravenous administration of contrast material, in many instances needle aspiration is the only means of differentiating an abscess from a noninfected collection, such as a resolving hematoma or loculated ascites. Because unopacified, fluid-filled bowel loops may mimic an abscess, complete opacification of the bowel with contrast material is imperative to firmly diagnose an abscess.

Microabscesses of the liver, spleen, and kidneys in immunocompromised patients may be due to hematogenous dissemination of infection. These opportunistic infections are most commonly caused by *Candida*, *Aspergillus*, and *Cryptococcus*. On CT, microabscesses appear as multiple, well-defined, low-attenuation foci usually measuring less than 2 cm in diameter[10] (Fig. 39–4). In addition to detecting microabscesses, CT

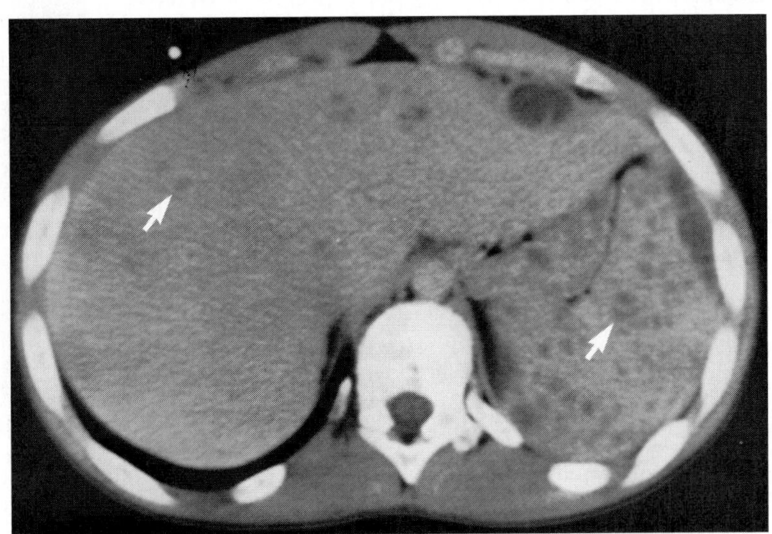

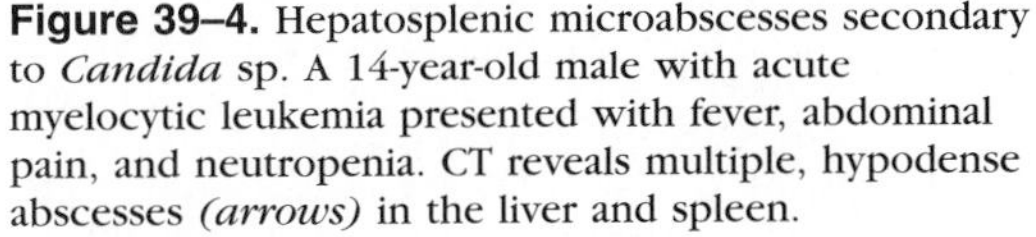

Figure 39–4. Hepatosplenic microabscesses secondary to *Candida* sp. A 14-year-old male with acute myelocytic leukemia presented with fever, abdominal pain, and neutropenia. CT reveals multiple, hypodense abscesses *(arrows)* in the liver and spleen.

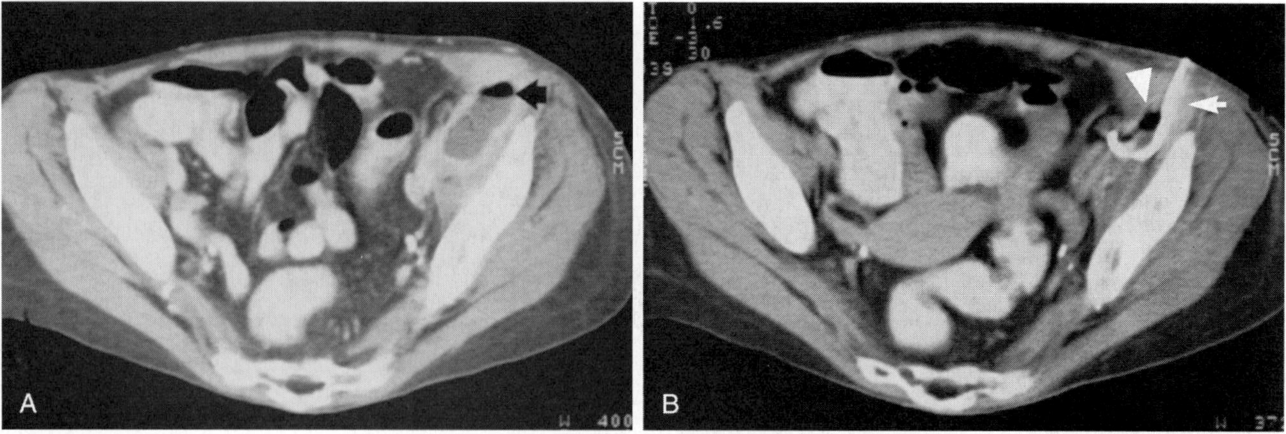

Figure 39–5. Diverticular abscess before and after percutaneous drainage. A 57-year-old woman with Crohn's disease presented with left lower quadrant pain, fever, and leukocytosis. *A*, An abscess containing an air-fluid level *(arrow)* and demonstrating an enhancing rim lies adjacent to the left iliacus muscle. *B*, A percutaneous drainage catheter *(arrow)* is noted in the evacuated abscess cavity. Only a small amount of air *(arrowhead)* remains in the cavity.

is useful in guiding percutaneous biopsy of the involved organs to determine the causative organism. Although CT is sensitive in detecting microabscesses, the absence of visible microabscesses does not exclude the presence of infection in a given organ.

The therapeutic efficacy of percutaneous abscess drainage in conjunction with intravenous antibiotics is well established (Fig. 39-5). Percutaneous drainage may be used as a temporizing measure in some instances, whereas it may serve as definitive therapy in others, obviating the need for surgery. Reported success rates for abscess drainage include 71% to 82% for postoperative abscesses,[11, 12] 90% to 93% for periappendiceal abscesses,[13-15] 90% for diverticular abscesses,[16, 17] and 91% for primary pyogenic hepatic abscesses.[18]

PANCREATITIS

Pancreatitis is an important entity in critical care patients, not only as a primary cause of ICU admission but also because of the susceptibility of ICU patients to the development of pancreatitis secondarily. Cholelithiasis, surgery, hypotension with ischemia, drug therapy, and ulcer formation are among the causes of pancreatitis in the critical care setting.[19]

In most cases, the diagnosis is established on clinical grounds when patients have abdominal pain with elevated lipase and amylase levels. Sonography has traditionally been performed in patients with a first episode of pancreatitis to assess for gallstones as a cause. Although the sensitivity of sonography is high for the detection of gallbladder calculi, neither sonography nor CT has a consistently high sensitivity for the detection of common bile duct stones. Specifically, the sensitivity for the detection of choledocholithiasis ranges from 23% to 75% for sonography[20-23] and from 23% to 90% for CT.[24, 25] Until the advent of MRCP, ERCP was required to evaluate for the presence of common duct calculi (Fig. 39-6). However, studies have shown that the sensitivity, specificity, accuracy, positive predictive value, and negative predictive value of MRCP at least equal those of ERCP in the diagnosis of choledocholithiasis.[26, 27] The importance of MRCP in the evaluation of choledocholithiasis as a cause of pancreatitis lies in its high negative predictive value. If MRCP excludes common bile duct calculi, the patient may be spared an invasive procedure such as ERCP. No further imaging may be necessary if a patient responds to conservative management.

Cross-sectional imaging is reserved for patients with clinically severe pancreatitis to identify and evaluate the extent of local complications.[28] CT is the method of choice because the entire abdomen and retroperitoneum can be evaluated. The major complications of acute pancreatitis include pancreatic necrosis, development of fluid collections, hemorrhage, and infection. These, along with other complications such as biliary obstruction, vascular thrombosis, and pseudoaneurysm formation, can be detected with CT. CT grading systems based on the CT appearance and presence or absence of necrosis have been used along with Ranson's criteria to determine prognosis in severe pancreatitis.[29, 30]

Pancreatic necrosis is an important complication to recognize because of its association with increased morbidity and mortality. Areas of necrosis may lead to development of fluid collections or pancreatic ascites and have a high risk for subsequent infection (Fig. 39-7*A-C*). CT with rapid infusion

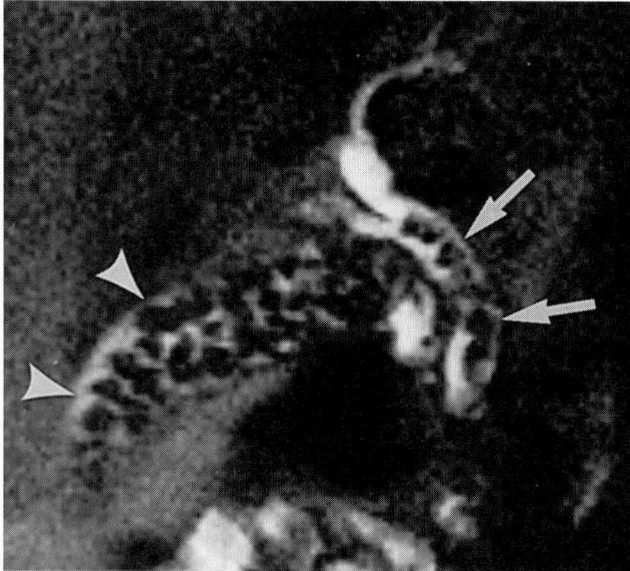

Figure 39–6. Choledocholithiasis and cholelithiasis. A 35-year-old pregnant woman presented with abdominal pain and elevated amylase level. A coronal magnetic resonance cholangiogram (MRC) shows multiple calculi in the common bile duct *(arrows)* and in the gallbladder *(arrowheads)*.

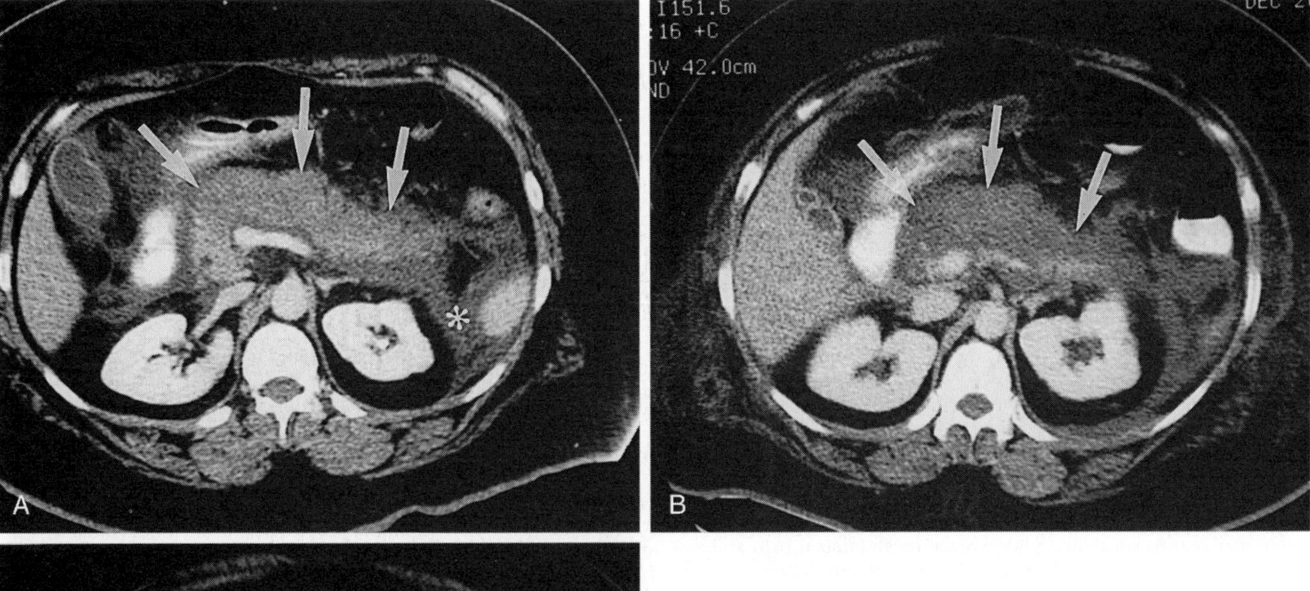

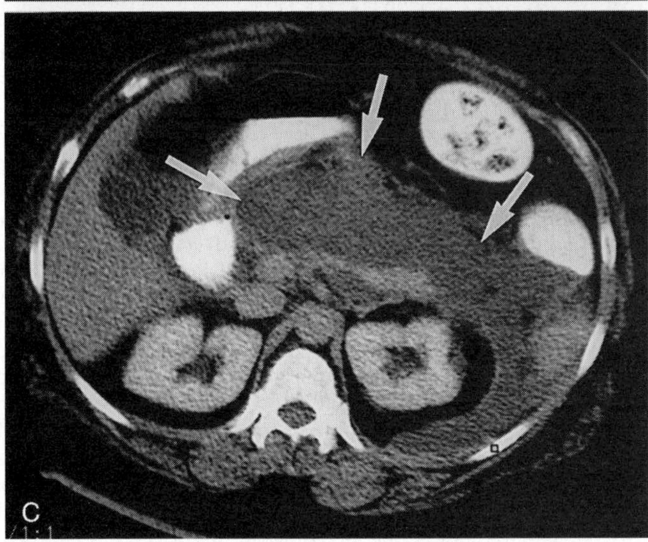

Figure 39–7. Evolution of acute necrotizing pancreatitis. A 45-year-old woman presented with abdominal pain and elevated amylase and lipase levels. *A*, Enhanced CT obtained 1 day after onset of pain shows an enlarged pancreas *(arrows)* and retroperitoneal fluid *(asterisk)*. *B*, Enhanced CT obtained 4 days after presentation reveals minimal enhancement of the pancreas *(arrows)* indicative of necrosis. *C*, Enhanced CT performed 2 weeks after presentation shows near-complete replacement of the pancreas *(arrows)* with fluid density material.

of intravenous contrast material is the best method to identify pancreatic necrosis.[31] Necrotic areas are seen as regions of nonenhancement within the gland. Infected necrosis requires surgical debridement.

Hemorrhagic pancreatitis usually appears as diffuse hemorrhage into a pancreatic phlegmon. Inflammation can result in formation of pseudoaneurysms of the splenic artery or other vessels. Rupture of a pseudoaneurysm or erosion into a large vessel may lead to formation of a large focal hematoma (Fig. 39–8). These patients usually become hypotensive, and emergency transcatheter embolization of the bleeding vessel can be lifesaving.[32] Inflammatory changes can also lead to splenic vein thrombosis with development of gastric varices or arterial thrombosis with resultant bowel ischemia that may progress to bowel perforation.

The development of fluid collections in pancreatitis is common, occurring in up to 50% of patients in some series.[33] Most of these fluid collections, particularly if less than 6 cm in diameter, resolve spontaneously. It is estimated that fewer than 10% become infected.[34] The accurate and early diagnosis of infection is crucial because of the high morbidity and mortality associated with suppurative pancreatitis. The presence of infection cannot be reliably confirmed with imaging criteria alone. Identification of gas within a collection is highly suggestive of infection but is not specific because gas may enter a collection through a communication with the gastrointestinal tract. Therefore, CT-guided fine-needle aspiration plays an important role in detection of infection in patients with fluid collections. It is a safe and reliable method with a low false-negative rate.[35]

The discovery of infection warrants immediate intervention by either percutaneous or surgical drainage. It is important to distinguish infected fluid collections from infected pancreatic necrosis because the latter usually requires surgical debridement. The term *pseudocyst* should be reserved for chronic fluid collections that have an enhancing rim or remain unchanged for a prolonged period. Pseudocysts may require percutaneous or surgical intervention if they become infected, are larger than 10 cm, or cause symptoms as a result of mass effect on adjacent structures. CT-guided percutaneous drainage of pancreatic abscesses and chronic pseudocysts plays an important part in the management of complicated pancreatitis. The success rate is higher for pseudocysts (90%) than for abscesses or complex collections (47%).[36, 37]

INTRAPERITONEAL AND RETROPERITONEAL HEMORRHAGE

Intraperitoneal or retroperitoneal hemorrhage may be suspected in patients with decreasing hematocrit, abdominal

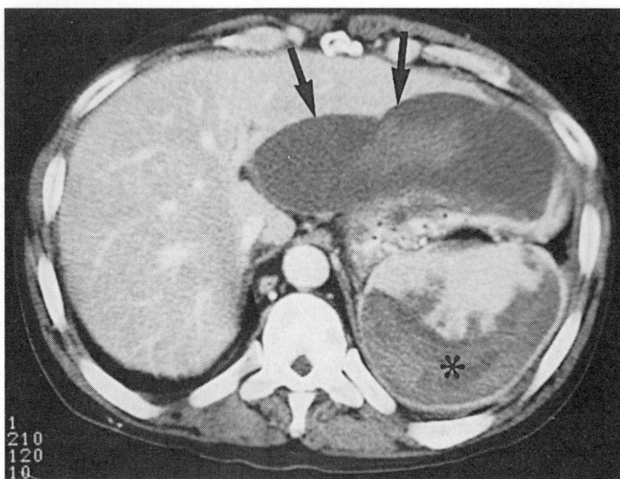

Figure 39–8. Subcapsular splenic and hepatic hematomas secondary to hemorrhage into preexisting pseudocysts. A 50-year-old man with acute pancreatitis presented with worsening abdominal pain and a decreasing hematocrit. An enhanced CT scan demonstrates subcapsular hematomas of the spleen *(asterisk)* and liver *(arrows)*, which contain acute and subacute hemorrhage.

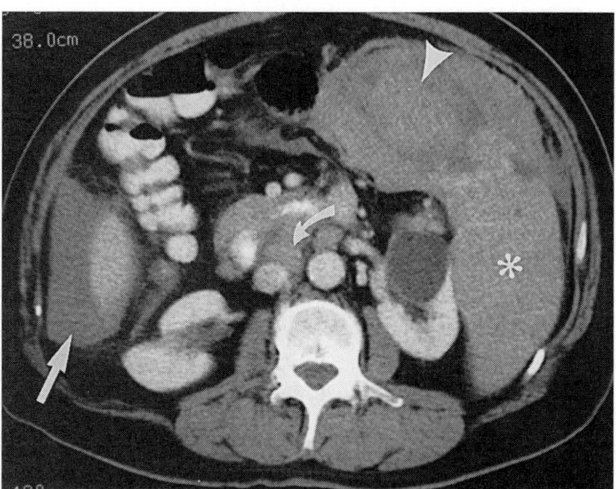

Figure 39–9. Intraperitoneal and intrasplenic hemorrhage. A 71-year-old man with lymphoma presented with abdominal pain, hypotension, and decreased hematocrit. An axial CT scan shows high-attenuation blood *(arrow)* adjacent to the liver tip. The spleen *(asterisk)* is enlarged and contains both acute *(arrowhead)* and subacute hemorrhage. Retroperitoneal lymphadenopathy is present *(curved arrow)*.

pain, or hypotension and no known bleeding source. Although some patients have an underlying coagulopathy related to conditions such as renal failure, hemophilia, or systemic lupus erythematosus, many experience bleeding because of anticoagulation or after interventional procedures such as cardiac catheterization.

Because of the often emergent need to image patients with suspected hemorrhage, CT scanning is usually conducted without the use of intravenous or oral contrast material. CT is useful not only in documenting the presence of hemorrhage but also in determining its extent. The CT appearance of blood varies with the age of the hemorrhage. *Acute* hemorrhage is manifested as high-attenuation material ranging from 30 to 50 Hounsfield units; *subacute* hemorrhage is lower in density and may demonstrate an in vivo hematocrit effect related to separation of components of blood. When intraperitoneal hemorrhage occurs, blood preferentially collects in the pelvic cul de sac and in the hepatorenal fossa, the most dependent regions of the pelvis and abdomen. With more severe hemorrhage, blood enters the paracolic gutters and perihepatic and perisplenic spaces, often resulting in pain related to irritation of the diaphragm (Fig. 39–9).

Acute retroperitoneal hemorrhage is depicted on CT as high-attenuation fluid that results in fat stranding, displacement of adjacent organs, and infiltration of the psoas muscles. Such hemorrhage may originate in the retroperitoneum, as in the case of a ruptured abdominal aortic aneurysm (Fig. 39–10), or may occur in the inguinal region and dissect cephalad to secondarily involve the retroperitoneum, as may occur after cardiac catheterization[38, 39] (Fig. 39–11). Postcatheterization hemorrhage is more common after interventional procedures that require large sheaths and postprocedure anticoagulation therapy.

In addition to intraperitoneal and retroperitoneal hemorrhage, bleeding may occur into the abdominal wall musculature (Fig. 39–12), most commonly involving the rectus abdominis muscles within the rectus sheath. This type of hemorrhage often presents clinically as an abdominal wall mass.

SMALL-BOWEL AND COLON PATHOLOGY

Small-Bowel Obstruction

Small-bowel obstruction is usually suspected on clinical grounds when patients manifest crampy abdominal pain, abdominal distention, nausea, vomiting, and obstipation. Abdominal plain films are usually the first study obtained and often confirm the diagnosis. Plain films are diagnostic in only 50% to 60% of cases; equivocal in 20% to 30%; and normal, nonspecific, or misleading in 10% to 20%.[40] Closed loop obstruction occurs when a loop or loops of small bowel twist on the mesentery or become incarcerated in an internal hernia and is particularly difficult to detect on plain films because the obstructed loops are often fluid-filled. Closed loop obstruction can progress to strangulation with resultant ischemia, infarction, and perforation. If findings on plain films are normal or equivocal or if it is important to determine the cause of the obstruction, additional imaging may be needed. A contrast-enhanced small-bowel series has traditionally been the next study obtained. The small-bowel series is most helpful in low-grade or partial obstruction. With high-grade or complete obstruction, a small-bowel series may take hours to perform

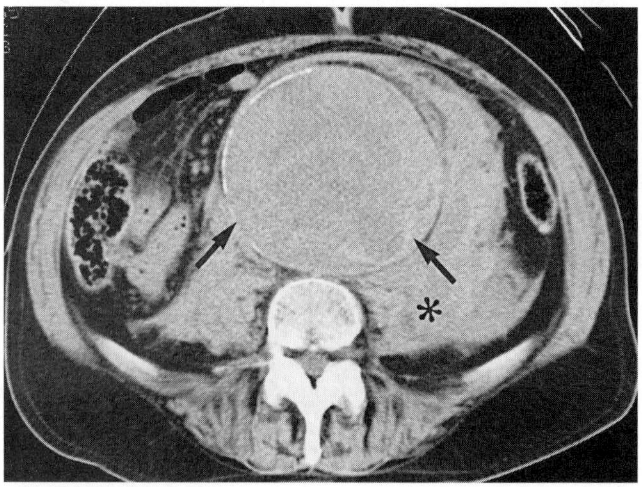

Figure 39–10. Ruptured abdominal aortic aneurysm. A 75-year-old man presented with abdominal pain and hypotension. An unenhanced CT shows a ruptured, 11-cm aortic aneurysm *(arrows)* and acute blood *(asterisk)* in the retroperitoneum.

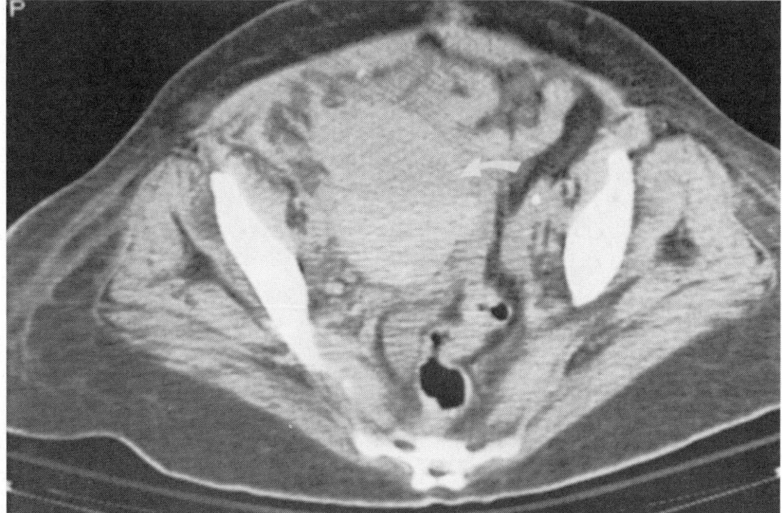

Figure 39–11. Pelvic hematoma. A 65-year-old man demonstrated a decreasing hematocrit following coronary artery angioplasty. An unenhanced CT scan reveals a hematoma *(curved arrow)* adjacent to the right pelvic side wall. More cephalad images (not shown) revealed that the hematoma extended into the retroperitoneum to the level of the kidneys. The hematoma occurred as a result of a lacerated femoral artery that had been punctured above the inguinal ligament.

and may not determine the cause or reveal the presence of strangulation.[41]

Some reports have documented an increasingly important role for CT in the evaluation of intestinal obstruction. Early reports in patients with high-grade obstruction showed a sensitivity of 90% to 96%, specificity of 96%, and accuracy of 95%.[42, 43] The sensitivity and specificity are lower with partial obstruction.[44] CT can distinguish small-bowel obstruction from adynamic ileus and determine the level, severity, and cause of the obstruction[45] (Fig. 39–13). Obstruction secondary to neoplastic or inflammatory disease can be differentiated from simple obstruction due to adhesions. The diagnosis of adhesive obstruction is made when there is a transition from dilated to nondilated loops without a mass. CT can detect strangulation or ischemia by demonstrating bowel wall thickening, edema or enhancement, pneumatosis intestinalis, and mesenteric changes. With bowel perforation, CT reveals pneumoperitoneum or free intraperitoneal fluid. It can both expedite surgery when signs of strangulation, ischemia, or perforation are detected and avoid unnecessary surgery when nonoperative management of adhesive obstruction is considered. CT is recommended when plain film findings are nonspecific or equivocal, when malignant or inflammatory etiology is suspected, and to exclude strangulation when nonoperative management is contemplated.[46] The short examination time and ability of CT to establish the diagnosis and cause of obstruction make it particularly valuable in the critical care patient.

Small-Bowel Ischemia

The types of acute small-bowel ischemia include

- Occlusive arterial ischemia secondary to emboli or thrombi

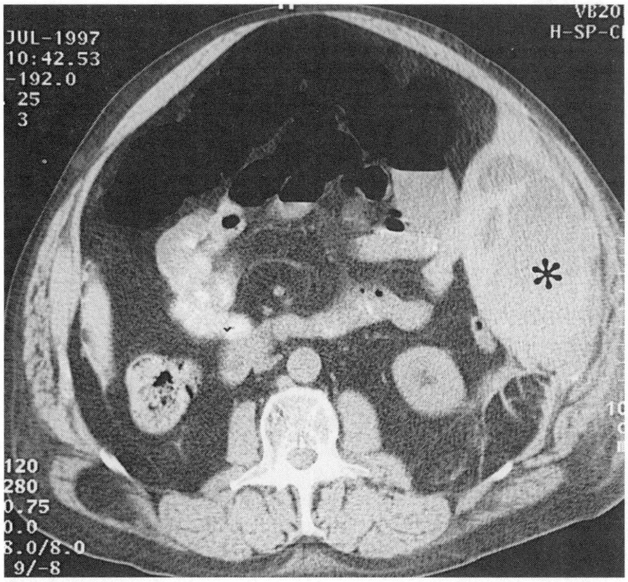

Figure 39–12. Abdominal wall hematoma. A 68-year-old man receiving anticoagulant therapy for atrial fibrillation presented with an abdominal mass. An unenhanced CT scan demonstrates a lateral abdominal wall hematoma *(asterisk)*.

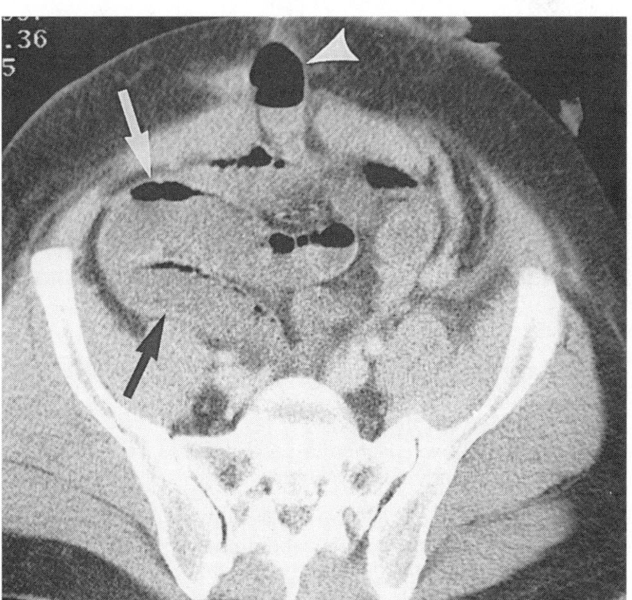

Figure 39–13. Small-bowel obstruction. A 39-year-old man was experiencing abdominal pain, nausea, and vomiting 2 days after abdominal surgery. CT demonstrates dilated, air-filled, and fluid-filled small bowel loops *(arrows)* due to a midline incisional hernia that contains a small bowel loop *(arrowhead)*.

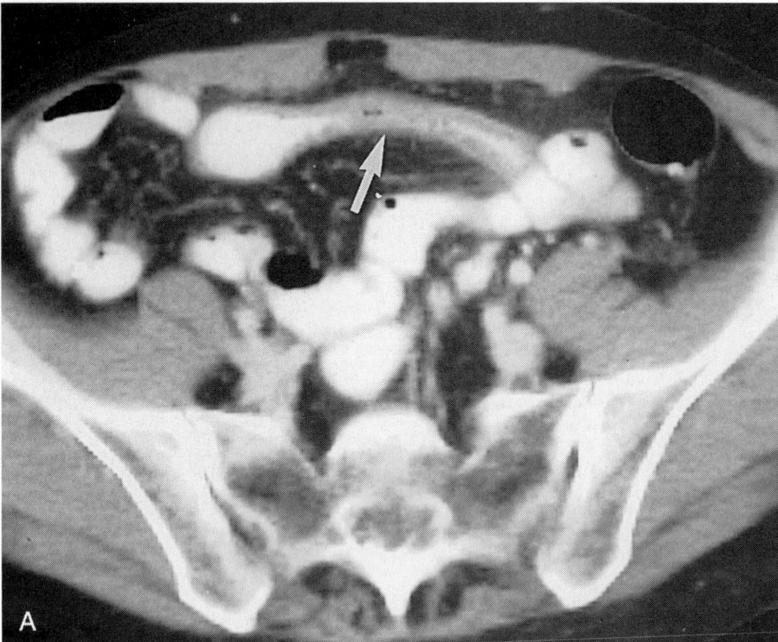

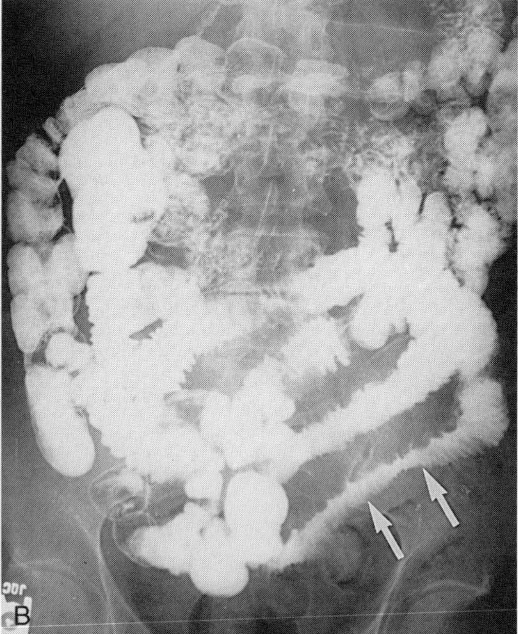

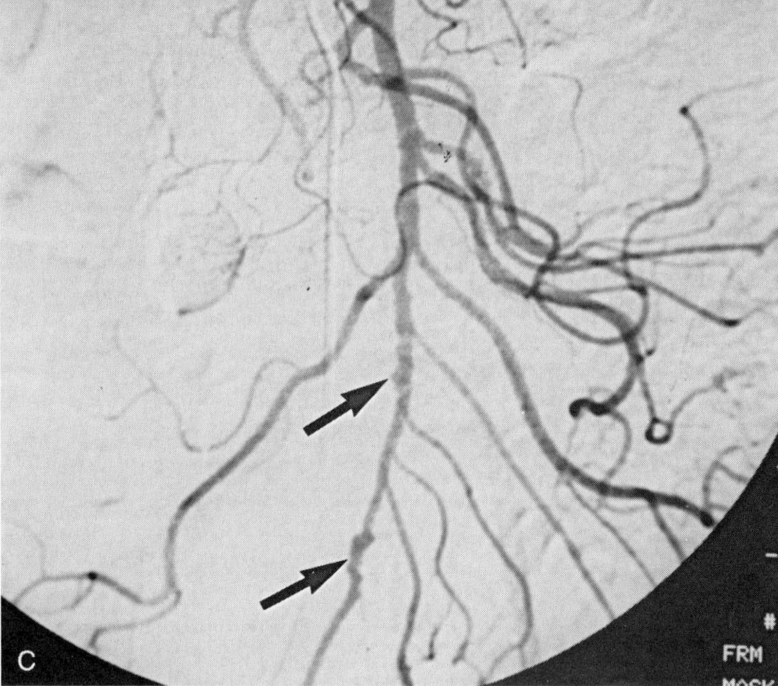

Figure 39–14. Small-bowel ischemia caused by vasculitis. A 52-year-old woman with rheumatoid arthritis presented with severe abdominal pain. *A*, Enhanced CT scan shows a thickened loop of ileum *(arrow)* indicative of ischemia. *B*, Upper gastrointestinal series and small-bowel followthrough demonstrates narrowed, thickened ileum *(arrows)*. *C*, Mesenteric angiogram reveals irregularity *(arrows)* of the ileocolic branch of the superior mesenteric artery due to vasculitis.

- Nonocclusive ischemia due to conditions such as cardiac dysfunction and hypotension
- Mesenteric vein thrombosis
- Focal small-bowel ischemia secondary to vasculitis (Fig. 39–14), cocaine, and mesenteric tears

Because patients with small-bowel ischemia may demonstrate nonspecific symptoms, such as abdominal pain, diarrhea, anorexia, and sepsis, ischemia often presents a diagnostic dilemma.

Although angiography remains the standard of reference for the diagnosis of intestinal ischemia, conventional radiographs and CT provide noninvasive means of evaluating patients with suspected ischemia. Conventional radiographs of the abdomen may demonstrate bowel distention and wall thickening, pneumatosis intestinalis, a gasless abdomen, and portal vein gas. Lund and associates[47] noted that although conventional radiographs may detect findings suggestive of ischemia, CT more reliably demonstrates these findings as well as additional abnormalities, such as mesenteric engorgement and mesenteric vein gas. In addition, CT may detect arterial and venous thrombi.[47, 48] The early findings of ischemia, such as bowel dilatation, are nonspecific. Unfortunately, the more specific findings, such as portal and mesenteric vein gas, are not present until the bowel has infarcted (Fig. 39–15).

Pseudomembranous Colitis

Pseudomembranous colitis (PMC) is an infectious colitis that is usually associated with overgrowth of *Clostridium difficile*

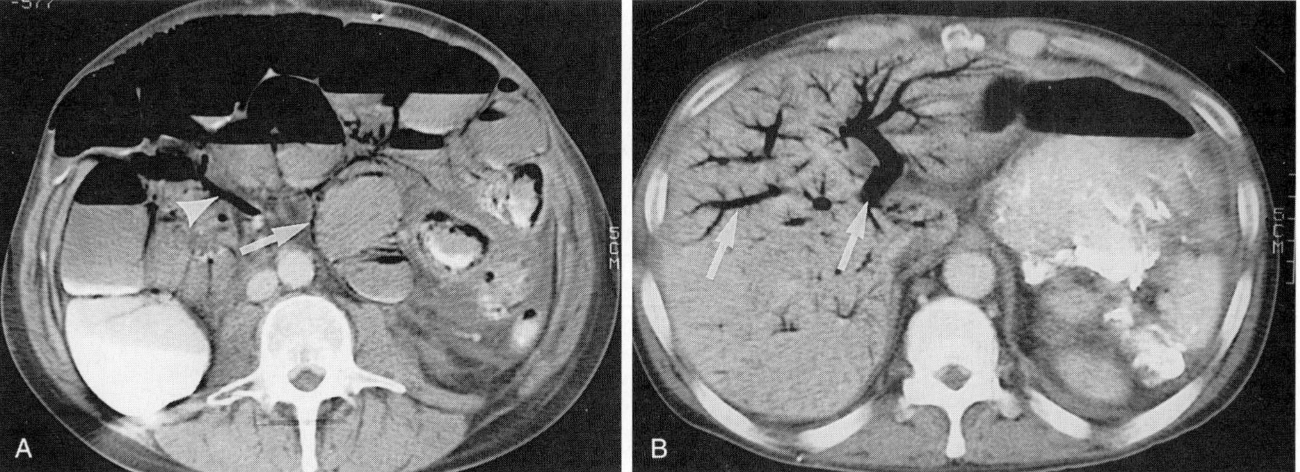

Figure 39–15. Small-bowel infarction. A 65-year-old man underwent CT examination because of abdominal distention, pain, and hypotension. *A*, Enhanced CT scan shows bowel dilatation, pneumatosis intestinalis *(arrow)*, and gas in a mesenteric vein branch *(arrowhead)*. *B*, Enhanced CT scan of the upper abdomen demonstrates extensive portal vein gas *(arrows)*.

after antibiotic use. Less commonly, PMC occurs in the setting of prolonged hypotension or hypoperfusion of the bowel, intestinal surgery, bowel ischemia, and debilitating diseases.[49, 50] Because the patient often presents with nonspecific findings, such as fever, elevated white blood cell count, and diarrhea, the diagnosis may first be suggested on the basis of CT findings.

In a study of 26 patients with PMC who underwent CT, bowel wall thickening was noted in 88%, and trapping of contrast material between thickened colonic folds resulting in the "accordion" sign was noted in 19%[49] (Fig. 39–16). Additional findings include bowel wall edema, pericolonic stranding, and ascites. The involvement of the colon with PMC is diffuse in as many as 70% of cases but may be segmental.[50] Although the CT findings associated with PMC are nonspecific, they suggest the diagnosis of PMC in the appropriate clinical setting.

Typhlitis

Typhlitis, also known as *neutropenic colitis*, is an inflammatory process of undetermined pathogenesis that involves the cecum, ascending colon, and terminal ileum. Although typhlitis was originally described in leukemic children treated with chemotherapy, this condition has been reported in patients with lymphoma, aplastic anemia, the acquired immunodeficiency syndrome (AIDS), and organ transplants.[51, 52] If it is left untreated, transmural necrosis develops, predisposing patients to perforation.

The importance of CT in the setting of typhlitis lies in the early detection of this process. The CT findings of typhlitis include bowel wall thickening, pericolonic fluid and fat stranding, and pneumatosis intestinalis[52, 53] (Fig. 39–17). Although similar findings may be seen in association with conditions such as appendicitis, diverticulitis, ischemia, pseudomembranous colitis, and leukemic infiltration, these findings suggest typhlitis when they are seen in neutropenic patients with malignant neoplasms or other debilitating diseases.

Opportunistic Infections of the Small Bowel and Colon

Immunocompromised patients, such as those with AIDS and those receiving chemotherapy or immunosuppression, are predisposed to the development of opportunistic infections.[54] The small bowel and colon are frequently involved by these

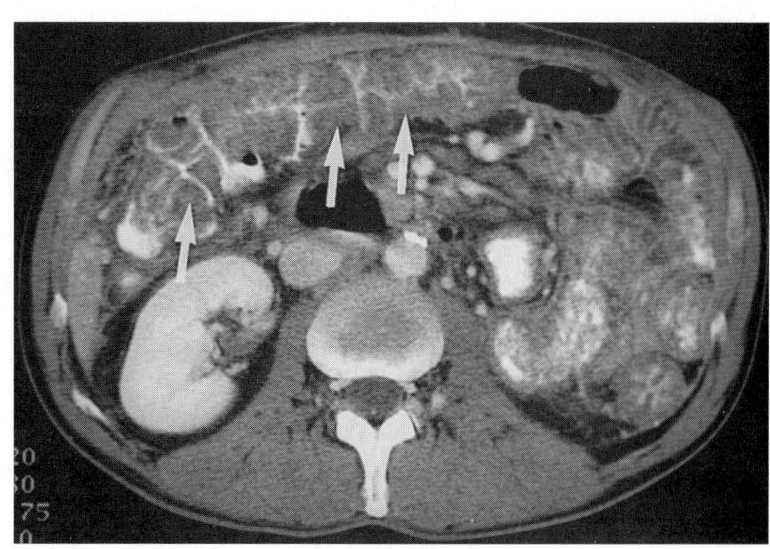

Figure 39–16. Pseudomembranous colitis. A 45-year-old man presented with diarrhea following antibiotic therapy. Enhanced CT scan demonstrates a thickened, hypodense colon wall *(arrows)*. Oral contrast material trapped between the thickened haustra represents the "accordion" sign.

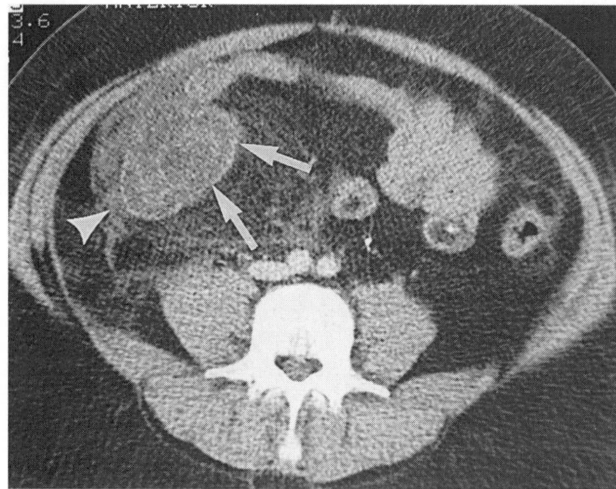

Figure 39–17. Typhlitis. A 34-year-old man with lymphoma presented with neutropenia, right lower quadrant pain, and hypotension. CT shows a thickened, hypodense cecum *(arrows)* and stranding of the pericolic fat *(arrowhead)*.

infections. In general, these patients present with fever, wasting, and diarrhea that may be profuse. CT is useful in depicting the features of such infections, which may include focal or diffuse bowel wall thickening (Fig. 39–18), fluid-filled bowel loops, and associated findings such as lymphadenopathy and hepatosplenomegaly.

Colonic involvement by cytomegalovirus is manifested as marked wall thickening that may be focal or diffuse.[55] When focal involvement occurs, the cecum and ascending colon are preferentially involved; associated extension into the terminal ileum may be noted. *Cryptosporidium* and *Mycobacterium avium-intracellulare* usually involve the small bowel and result in fold thickening.[56] CT scans of patients with *Cryptosporidium* often demonstrate not only bowel wall thickening but also fluid-filled bowel. Lymphadenopathy may be seen with *M. avium-intracellulare* but occurs less commonly than with *Mycobacterium tuberculosis. M. tuberculosis* characteristically involves the cecum and terminal ileum and is often associated with regional lymphadenopathy.[57, 58] Mycobacterial infections often result in caseation of lymph nodes seen as central areas of low attenuation on CT. CT-guided aspiration of lymphadenopathy may assist in distinguishing mycobacterial infections from AIDS-related malignant neoplasms such as Kaposi's sarcoma or lymphoma.

References

1. Brink JA, Heiken JP, Wang G, et al: Helical CT: Principles and technical considerations. Radiographics 1994; 14:887–893.
2. Brink JA: Technical aspects of helical (spiral) CT. Radiol Clin North Am 1995; 33:825–841.
3. Reiderer SJ: Recent technical advances in MR imaging of the abdomen. J Magn Reson Imaging 1996; 6:822–832.
4. Mitchell DG: Fast MR imaging techniques: Impact in the abdomen. J Magn Reson Imaging 1996; 6:812–821.
5. Indeck M, Peterson S, Smith J, et al: Risk, cost and benefit of transporting ICU patients for special studies. J Trauma 1988; 28:1020–1025.
6. Evans A, Winslow EH: Oxygen saturation and hemodynamic response in critically ill, mechanically ventilated adults during intrahospital transport. Am J Crit Care 1995; 4:106–111.
7. Szem JW, Hydo LJ, Fischer E, et al: High-risk intrahospital transport of critically ill patients: Safety and outcome of the necessary "road trip." Crit Care Med 1995; 23:1660–1666.
8. Gerzof SG, Oates E: Imaging techniques for infections in the surgical patient. Surg Clin North Am 1988; 68:147–165.
9. Roche J: Effectiveness of CT in the diagnosis of intra-abdominal abscess. Med J Aust 1981; 25:85–88.
10. Chew FS, Smith PL, Barboriak D: Candidal splenic abscesses. AJR Am J Roentgenol 1991; 156:474.
11. Lambiase RE, Cronan JJ, Dorfman GS, et al: Postoperative ab-

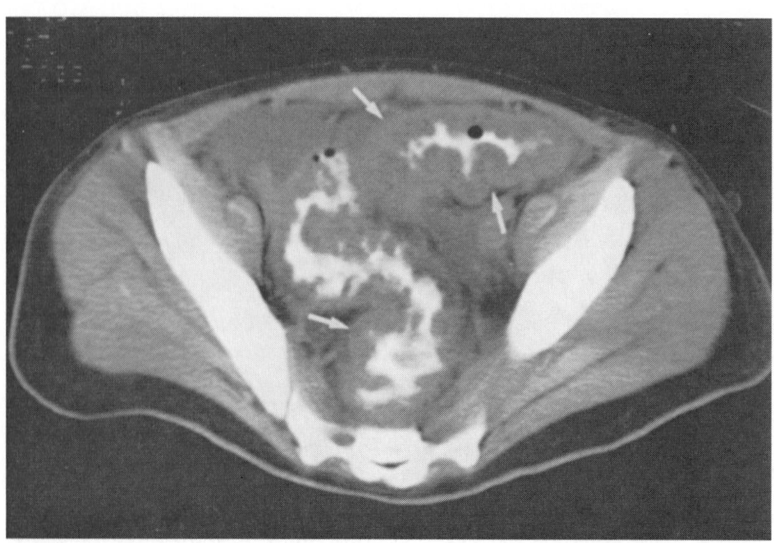

Figure 39–18. Cytomegalovirus colitis. A 36-year-old man with AIDS presented with a 1-week history of fever and watery diarrhea. CT demonstrates marked thickening of the sigmoid colon *(arrows)*. Culture of a rectal biopsy specimen revealed cytomegalovirus.

scesses with enteric communication: Percutaneous treatment. Radiology 1989; 171:497-500.
12. Schechter S, Eisenstat TE, Oliver GC, et al: Computerized tomographic scan-guided drainage of intra-abdominal abscesses: Preoperative and postoperative modalities in colon and rectal surgery. Dis Colon Rectum 1994; 37:984-988.
13. Jeffrey RB Jr, Federle MP, Tolentino CS: Periappendiceal inflammatory masses: CT-directed management and clinical outcome in 70 patients. Radiology 1988; 167:13-16.
14. Jeffery RB Jr, Tolentino CS, Federle MP, et al: Percutaneous drainage of periappendiceal abscesses: Review of 20 patients. AJR Am J Roentgenol 1987; 149:59-62.
15. vanSonnenberg E, Wittich GR, Casola G, et al: Periappendiceal abscesses: Percutaneous drainage. Radiology 1987; 163:23-26.
16. Mueller PR, Saini S, Wittenberg J, et al: Sigmoid diverticular abscesses: Percutaneous drainage as an adjunct to surgical resection in 24 cases. Radiology 1987; 164:321-325.
17. Neff CC, vanSonnenberg E, Casola G, et al: Diverticular abscesses: Percutaneous drainage. Radiology 1987; 163:15-18.
18. Johnson RD, Mueller PR, Ferrucci JT, et al: Percutaneous drainage of pyogenic liver abscesses. AJR Am J Roentgenol 1985; 144:463-467.
19. Greenberger NJ, Toskes PJ, Isselbacher KJ: Acute and chronic pancreatitis. *In:* Harrison's Principles of Internal Medicine. Isselbacher KJ (Ed). New York, McGraw-Hill, 1994, pp 1520-1532.
20. Pasanen P, Partanen K, Pikkarainen P, et al: Ultrasonography, CT, and ERCP in the diagnosis of choledochal stones. Acta Radiol 1992; 33:53-56.
21. Laing FC, Jeffrey RB Jr: Choledocholithiasis and cystic duct obstruction: Difficult ultrasonographic diagnosis. Radiology 1983; 146:475-479.
22. Laing FC, Jeffrey RB, Wing VW: Improved visualization of choledocholithiasis by sonography. AJR Am J Roentgenol 1984; 143:949-952.
23. Cronan JJ: US diagnosis of choledocholithiasis: A reappraisal. Radiology 1986; 161:133-134.
24. Jeffrey RB, Federle MP, Laing FC, et al: Computed tomography of choledocholithiasis. AJR Am J Roentgenol 1983; 140:1179-1183.
25. Baron RL: CT diagnosis of choledocholithiasis. Semin Ultrasound CT MR 1987; 8:85-102.
26. Fulcher AS, Turner MA, Capps GW, et al: Half-Fourier RARE magnetic resonance cholangiopancreatography: Experience in 300 patients. Radiology 1998; 207:21-32.
27. Guibaud L, Bret PM, Reinhold C, et al: Bile duct obstruction and choledocholithiasis: Diagnosis with MR cholangiography. Radiology 1995; 197:109-115.
28. Moulton JS: The radiologic assessment of acute pancreatitis and its complications. Pancreas 1991; 6(Suppl 1):S13-S22.
29. Balthazar EJ, Ranson JHC, Naidich DP, et al: Acute pancreatitis: Prognostic value of CT. Radiology 1985; 156:767-772.
30. Balthazar EJ, Robinson DL, Meigbow AJ, et al: Acute pancreatitis: Value of CT in establishing prognosis. Radiology 1990; 174:331-336.
31. London NJ, Leese T, Lavelle JM, et al: Dynamic computed tomography in acute pancreatitis: A prospective study. Br J Surg 1991; 78:1452-1456.
32. Mauro MA, Jaques P: Transcatheter management of pseudoaneurysms complicating pancreatitis. J Vasc Interv Radiol 1991; 2:527-532.
33. Kourtesis G, Wilson SE, Williams RA: The clinical significance of fluid collections in acute pancreatitis. Am Surg 1990; 56:796-799.
34. Stiles GM, Berne TV, Thommen VD, et al: Fine needle aspiration of pancreatic fluid collections. Am Surg 1990; 56:764-768.
35. Gerzof SG, Banks PA, Robbins AH, et al: Early diagnosis of pancreatic infection by computed tomography-guided aspiration. Gastroenterology 1987; 93:1315-1320.
36. Lee MJ, Rattner DW, Legemate DA, et al: Acute complicated pancreatitis: Redefining the role of interventional radiology. Radiology 1992; 183:171-174.
37. VanSonnenberg E, Wittich GR, Casola G, et al: Percutaneous drainage of infected and noninfected pancreatic pseudocysts: Experience in 101 cases. Radiology 1989; 170:757-761.
38. Quint LE, Holland D, Korobkin M, et al: Role of femoral vessel catheterization and altered hemostasis in the development of extraperitoneal hematomas: CT study in 44 patients. AJR Am J Roentgenol 1993; 160:855-858.
39. Trerotola SO, Kuhlman JE, Fishman EK: CT and anatomic study of postcatheterization hematomas. Radiographics 1991; 11:247-258.
40. Lo AM, Evans WE, Carey LC: Review of small bowel obstruction at Milwaukee County General Hospital. Am J Surg 1966; 111:884-887.
41. Maglinte DD, Balthazar EJ, Kelvin FM, et al: The role of radiology in the diagnosis of small bowel obstruction. AJR Am J Roentgenol 1997; 168:1171-1180.
42. Meigbow AJ, Balthazar EJ, Cho KC, et al: Bowel obstruction: Evaluation with CT. Radiology 1991; 180:313-318.
43. Fukuya T, Hawes DR, Lu CC, et al: CT diagnosis of small bowel obstruction: Efficacy in 60 patients. AJR Am J Roentgenol 1992; 158:765-769.
44. Maglinte DD, Gage SN, Harmon BH, et al: Obstruction of the small intestine: Accuracy and role of CT in diagnosis. Radiology 1993; 188:61-64.
45. Taourel PG, Fabrer JM, Pradel JA, et al: Value of CT in the diagnosis and management of patients with suspected acute small bowel obstruction. AJR Am J Roentgenol 1995; 165:1187-1192.
46. Balthazar EJ: CT of small bowel obstruction. AJR Am J Roentgenol 1994; 162:255-261.
47. Lund EC, Han SY, Holley HC, et al: Intestinal ischemia: Comparison of plain radiographic and computed tomographic findings. Radiographics 1988; 8:1083-1108.
48. Alpern MB, Glazer GM, Francis IR: Ischemic or infarcted bowel: CT findings. Radiology 1988; 166:149-152.
49. Fishman EK, Kavuu M, Jones B, et al: Pseudomembranous colitis: CT evaluation of 26 cases. Radiology 1991; 180:57-60.
50. Ros PR, Buetow PC, Pantograg-Brown L, et al: Pseudomembranous colitis. Radiology 1996; 198:1-9.
51. Wagner ML, Rosenberg HS, Fernbach DJ, et al: Typhlitis: A complication of leukemia in childhood. AJR Am J Roentgenol 1980; 109:341-350.
52. Merine DS, Fishman EK, Jones B, et al: Right lower quadrant pain in the immunocompromised patient: CT findings in 10 cases. AJR Am J Roentgenol 1987; 149:1177-1179.
53. Frick MP, Maile CW, Crass JR, et al: Computed tomography of neutropenic colitis. AJR Am J Roentgenol 1984; 143:763-765.
54. Smith PD, Quinn TC, Strober W, et al: Gastrointestinal infections on AIDS. Ann Intern Med 1992; 116:63-77.
55. Teixidor HS, Honig CL, Norsoph E, et al: Cytomegalovirus infection of the alimentary canal: Radiologic findings with pathologic correlation. Radiology 1987; 163:317-323.
56. Nyberg DA, Federle MP, Jefferey RB, et al: Abdominal CT findings of *Mycobacterium avium-intracellulare* in AIDS. AJR Am J Roentgenol 1985; 145:297-299.
57. Balthazar EJ, Gordon R, Hulnick D: Ileocecal tuberculosis: CT and radiologic evaluation. AJR Am J Roentgenol 1990; 154:499-503.
58. Radin DR: Intraabdominal *Mycobacterium tuberculosis* vs *Mycobacterium avium-intracellulare* infections in patients with AIDS: Distinction based on CT findings. AJR Am J Roentgenol 1991; 156:487-491.

40

Interventional Radiology for the Critically Ill Patient

Jaime Tisnado, MD, FACR, FACC
Janice M. Newsome, MD

Establishing a diagnosis and initiating temporary or definitive treatment of a life-threatening process in a critically ill patient must proceed as rapidly as possible. Diagnosis and treatment, which usually require several days, must be done in a few hours. Because in critically ill patients surgery can be hazardous, use of cross-sectional imaging modalities—ultrasonography, computed tomography (CT), and magnetic resonance imaging (MRI)—has permitted rapid diagnosis as well as safe and effective intervention by radiologists. Recent improvements in technology, such as power Doppler ultrasonography, spiral (helical) CT, CT angiography (CTA), and MR angiography (MRA), have diminished the need for invasive diagnostic imaging. Thus, in many instances invasive radiology is directly aimed at treatment rather than at diagnosis.

Improvements in radiographic equipment, guide wire and catheter technology, and newer pharmaceuticals have resulted in high rates of success and low rates of complications. The availability of special (hydrophilic) guide wires, micropuncture sets, and microcatheter systems (e.g., Tracker, glide catheters) and numerous interventional devices has greatly facilitated the procedures.

Extensive diagnostic and interventional procedures can be performed via percutaneously introduced catheters, without surgery and its attendant complications and with minimal invasion of tissue organs. A protracted convalescence is thus avoided. Many lesions that are difficult to approach surgically can be accessed rapidly and easily with interventional techniques. Sometimes an interventional procedure is only temporary, to buy time until a more definitive (surgical or medical) procedure can be performed when the patient's condition has improved. At other times, the radiologic procedure is the definitive one.

This chapter reviews our experience in interventional radiologic diagnosis and management of critically ill patients. We provide a brief and practical discussion of the most frequently performed interventional procedures, many of which are simple and easy to perform, and can be learned in a short time.

A team approach by clinicians, surgeons, and radiologists must be fostered to achieve a successful outcome. We must emphasize that a serious commitment of time and resources is required. Specialist nurses, ideally with critical care experience, and radiologic technologists with special training in interventional procedures offer support to physicians. Other ancillary personnel, if available, would be ideal to improve team efforts: nurse practitioners, physician's assistants, and nurse clinicians, among others.

Specialized radiographic angiographic laboratories with state-of-the-art equipment are needed to facilitate interventional procedures. A single-plane (or a "biplane") 14 × 14 inch or 16 × 16 inch image intensifier with digital subtraction angiography (DSA) is ideal. A 100-mm spot camera device enhances the capabilities of the room. Today, large-format (14 × 14 inch) cut filming has been almost completely replaced by DSA. A liberal supply of pharmaceuticals, catheters, guide wires, and needles and numerous interventional devices must be available. Most of these devices are very expensive; thus, careful management of the material inventory is imperative.

ACUTE GASTROINTESTINAL HEMORRHAGE

Acute gastrointestinal (GI) bleeding is classified into three basic categories:

- Upper GI bleeding from gastroesophageal (GE) varices
- Upper GI bleeding of arterial or arteriolocapillary origin
- Lower GI bleeding

Upper GI bleeding *(hematemesis)* originates from sites proximal to the ligament of Treitz, and lower GI bleeding *(melena* or *hematochezia)* originates from sites distal to the ligament.

Successful management of GI hemorrhage requires the joint efforts of the medical, surgical, and radiologic teams. In the initial work-up, the rate and quantity of blood loss are assessed and the patient is stabilized as quickly as possible. Sources of bleeding are then localized to the upper or lower GI tract. In general, as many as 75% to 80% of patients usually respond to conservative management.[1, 2] Angiographic diagnosis and transcatheter therapy become the management of choice only when most conservative medical treatments fail.

In the work-up of these patients, endoscopy, scintigraphy, and selective arteriography are used to identify GI bleeding sites. Endoscopy must be the initial procedure for upper GI bleeding. Radionuclide scans are important screening tests for lower GI bleeding. Either technetium 99m-sulfur colloid (^{99m}Tc-SC) or ^{99m}Tc-labeled red blood cells (^{99m}Tc-RBCs) are administered intravenously. The diagnosis of acute bleeding is confirmed when the radionuclide extravasates and subsequently accumulates and moves through the GI tract (Fig. 40–1). Radionuclide scanning is much more sensitive than arteriography for detecting GI bleeding.

Arteriographically, acute GI bleeding is demonstrated by extravasation of contrast material into the stomach or bowel lumen that persists and increases as the arterial phase progresses into the venous phase. A single site is usually identified, but multiple small sites of extravasation may be seen. Thus, a complete arteriographic study should be done and correlated with the bleeding scan. Arteriography is sensitive and specific for localizing bleeding sites when the rate of hemorrhage is at least 0.5 mL/min.[3] Therefore, patients with a persistent bloody nasogastric (NG) aspirate despite adequate lavage and patients who require continuing transfusions to maintain stability are most likely to have positive arteriograms. On the other hand, arteriography is not indicated after active bleeding has stopped; however, an emergent angiographic intervention may be indicated after an initial severe bleeding episode subsides and the patient's ability to tolerate subsequent bleeding episodes is low. In these cases, angiography is used for either (1) transcatheter therapy of an endoscopically visualized bleeding lesion when the bleeding cannot be controlled or treated endoscopically, or (2) therapy of a pharmaceutically induced bleed.

Transcatheter Therapy

Two types of transcatheter therapy for GI bleeding lesions are available: (1) intra-arterial vasopressin infusion and (2) embolization. Vasopressin controls hemorrhage by arteriocapillary vasoconstriction and by contraction of the muscle walls of the GI tract.[2, 4] Embolization controls hemorrhage by occluding the bleeding vessels.

For upper GI bleeding, the catheter is advanced, if possible, superselectively into the bleeding artery, most often the left gastric or gastroduodenal artery. Other frequent sources are short gastric, pancreatic, and splenic arteries. For lower GI bleeding, placement of the catheter into the superior or inferior mesenteric artery is usually adequate. The initial intra-arterial dose of vasopressin is 0.2 unit per minute. Arteriography is repeated after 20 to 30 minutes of infusion. The arteriographic endpoint is cessation of bleeding with mild to moderate vasoconstriction. The dose of vasopressin may be increased to a maximum of 0.4 unit/min, if the initial dose of 0.2 unit/min does not control the bleeding. If bleeding persists, after 0.4 unit/min, embolization or surgery must be considered. When the bleeding is controlled, the infusion of vasopressin is gradually tapered in decrements of 0.1 unit/min every 6 to 12 hours. However, resumption of therapy may be necessary should bleeding recur during this "weaning." Care must be taken to make sure the catheter is not dislodged from the artery being infused, as this is the most common cause of treatment failure.

For embolotherapy, the catheter must be positioned as close

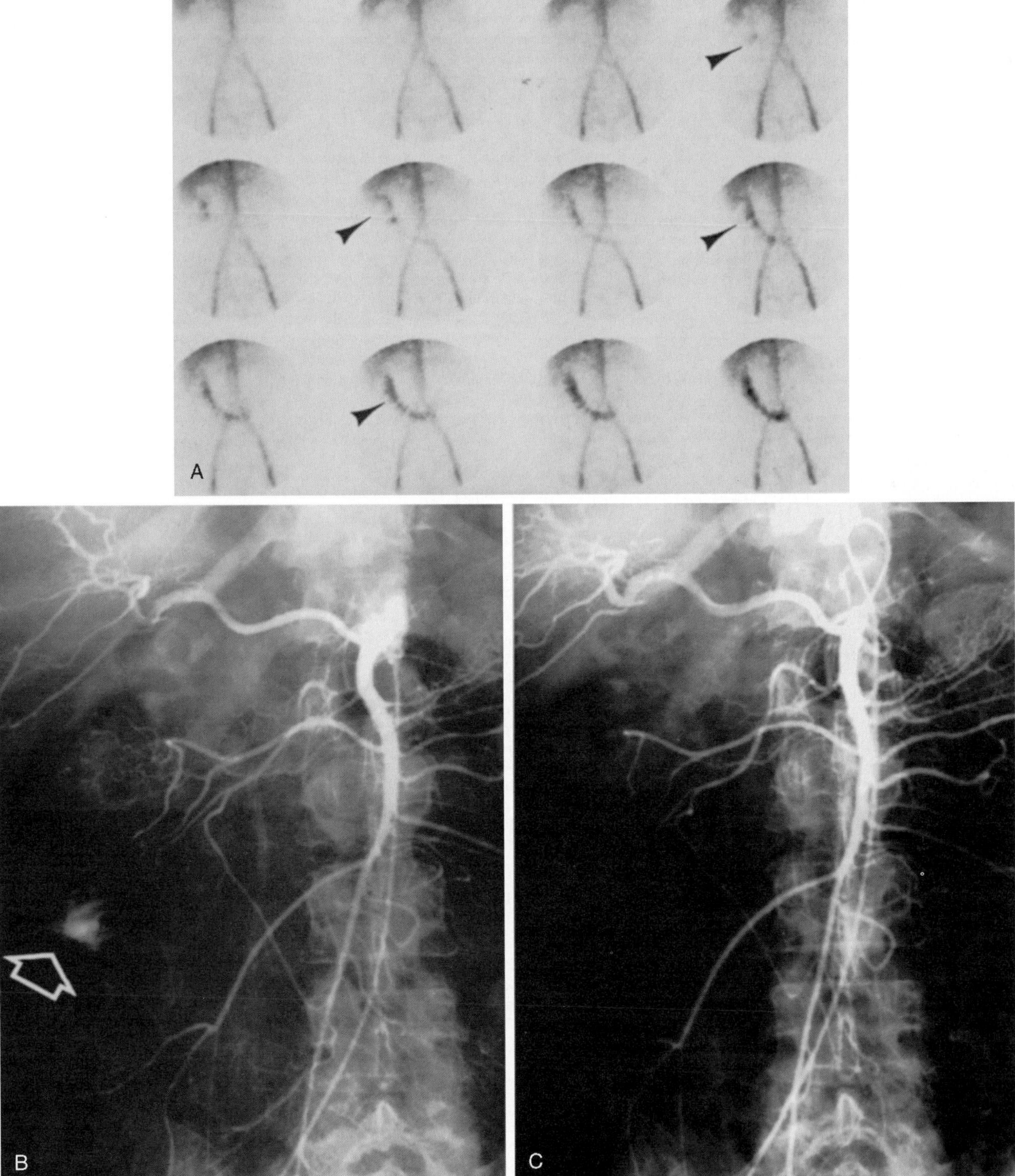

Figure 40–1. The patient is a 60-year-old woman with lower gastrointestinal bleeding. *A,* A ^{99m}Tc-labeled-red blood cell radionuclide scan demonstrates colonic bleeding in the hepatic flexure *(arrowheads). B,* A superior mesenteric artery arteriogram demonstrates extravasation from a right colic branch *(arrow). C,* Arteriography after 20 minutes of vasopressin infusion at 0.2 unit/min demonstrates cessation of bleeding and mild vasoconstriction. At surgery, multiple colonic diverticula were found.

as possible to the bleeding site, and the artery is occluded with an embolic agent. Small particles of absorbable gelatine sponge (Gelfoam) are most often used. Gelfoam, a temporary embolization agent, is resorbed in a few weeks or months, allowing for recanalization of occluded arteries, after the bleeding site has healed. Small stainless steel coils or platinum microcoils are used for permanent occlusion. Polyvinyl alcohol sponge (Ivalon) particles are preferred for permanent control of tumor-related GI bleeding. In these cases, recanalization is not desirable and permanent occlusion is preferable.

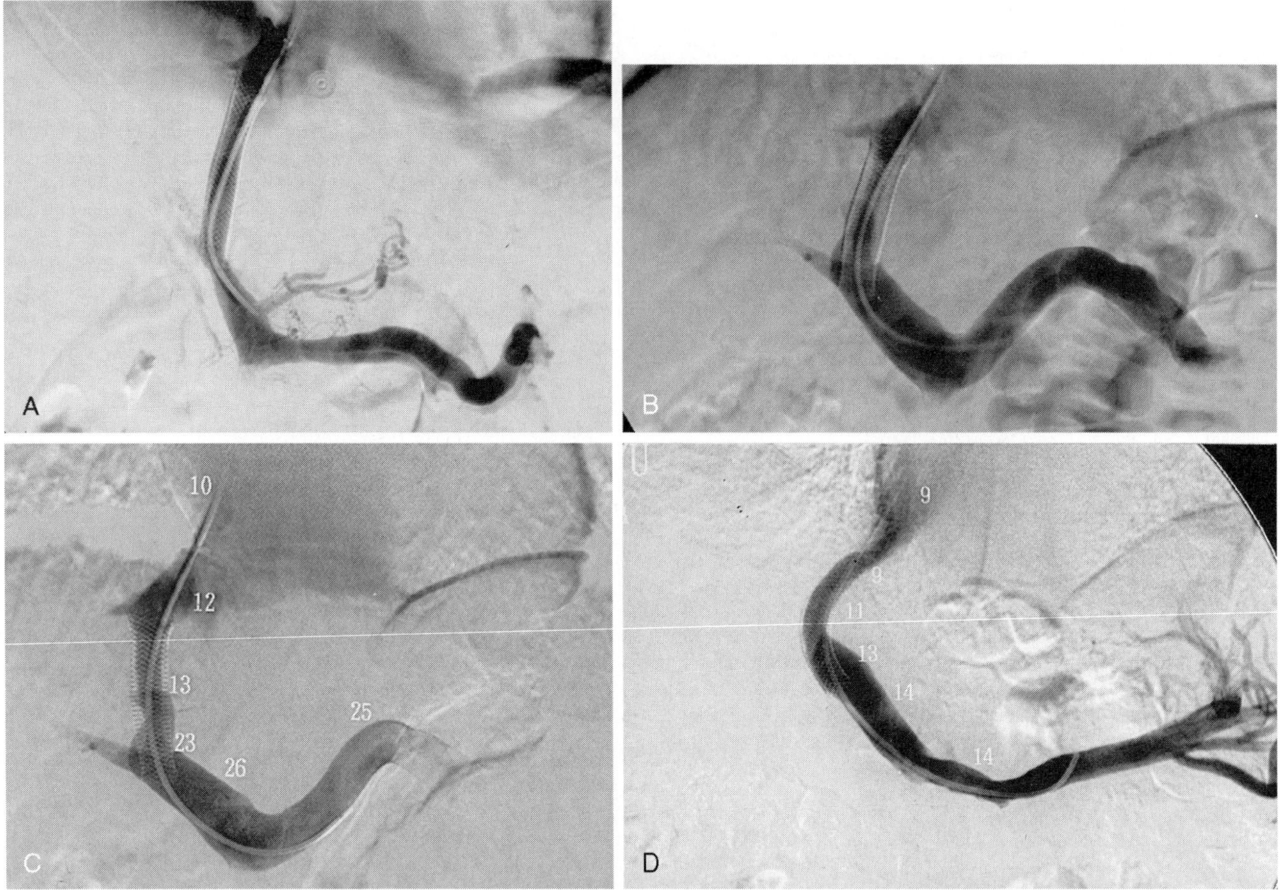

Figure 40–2. The patient, a middle-aged man, presented with alcoholic cirrhosis and variceal bleeding. Sclerotherapy failed to stop the bleeding. *A,* After a transjugular intrahepatic portosystemic shunt (TIPS) procedure, there is excellent flow through the newly created shunt, from right hepatic vein to the right portal vein. *B,* Follow-up 6 months later showed a gradient of 15 mm Hg. After dilatation, the gradient decreased to 8 mm Hg. The patient did well. *C,* One year later, there is significant narrowing of the shunt due to neointimal proliferation, as reflected by the pressures. *D,* After redilatation, there is excellent flow through the shunt. The neointimal tissue is no longer present.

Variceal Hemorrhage

When bleeding from varices due to portal hypertension is suspected, endoscopy is the primary diagnostic and therapeutic modality. It is useful for demonstrating GE variceal bleeding and for ruling out other sources of bleeding, since extravariceal causes account for more than 30% of bleeding episodes in this group of patients. Intravenous vasopressin infusion and endoscopic sclerotherapy of bleeding esophageal varices are the therapeutic mainstays for variceal bleeding. Sometimes tamponade with a Sengstaken-Blakemore tube can be used as a temporary (24- to 48-hour) measure to control bleeding or stabilize the patient's condition until definitive therapies are instituted, such as surgical portosystemic shunts of diverse configurations and transjugular intrahepatic portosystemic shunt (TIPS). Because the surgical mortality for acutely bleeding patients is high (at least 50%), surgical options are now rarely used to manage acute variceal bleeding.

In the past, when sclerotherapy or vasopressin infusion failed, percutaneous transhepatic catheterization of the portal vein and embolization of coronary and short gastric varices was an alternative therapy. Because of its association with mortality and rebleeding, the procedure was only temporary, to control bleeding until a surgical shunt or liver transplantation could be performed. Currently, the procedure is obsolete.

TIPS has become the treatment of choice for nonsurgical, radiologic control of variceal bleeding.[5,6] Briefly, from a jugular vein approach, a long, curved needle is placed into a hepatic vein (usually the right one) and advanced through the liver parenchyma into the right (usually) or left portal vein. The intrahepatic tract is then dilated with a balloon catheter, and a metallic mesh stent (Wallstent) is placed in the newly created shunt to maintain patency of the channel. The result is a portosystemic shunt that allows decompression of varices and a dramatic decrease in portal pressures (Fig. 40–2). Furthermore, TIPS does not preclude eventual liver transplantation.

At present, the procedure is effective and safe for controlling acute variceal hemorrhage, even when sclerotherapy has failed. Mortality with the procedure is <1%, and major complications are uncommon. TIPS placement also improves or controls ascites. Patients with intractable ascites can benefit greatly from this procedure. At this time, we are participating in a national study to assess the value of TIPS for ascites. Technical success of TIPS is almost 95%, and its long-term efficacy is excellent and comparable to that of surgical shunt procedures. Unfortunately, the procedure is not definitive, and frequent revisions and redilatations of the shunt are needed (every 6 to 12 months). The restenosis rate is almost 50% at 1 year. Thus, close follow-up and manipulation are necessary to keep the shunts patent and functional. Complete occlusion of the shunt is uncommon but may require placement of a second shunt (Fig. 40–3).

Upper Gastrointestinal Bleeding of Arterial or Arteriolocapillary Origin

Arteriography is indicated when endoscopy localizes a bleed that is not controlled by conservative or invasive endoscopic

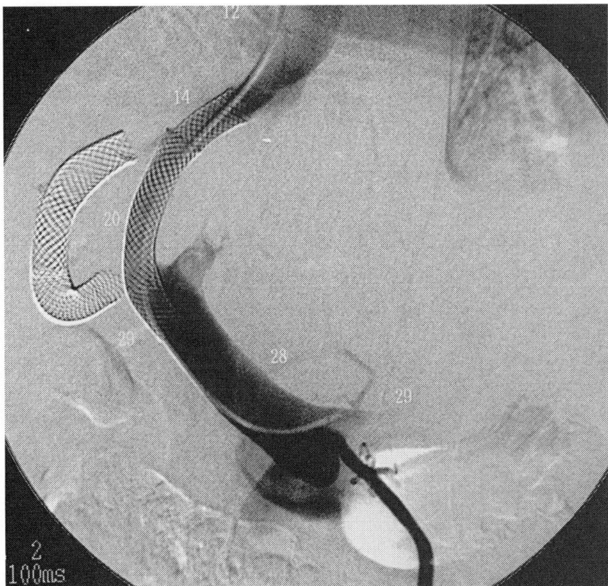

Figure 40–3. A middle-aged man had transjugular intrahepatic portosystemic shunt (TIPS) placement for massive gastrointestinal bleeding. One week, later, he experienced another bleeding episode. Doppler ultrasonography demonstrated occlusion of the shunt. Therefore, a new shunt was created. Note the original shunt on the left.

management or when endoscopic findings are negative or inconclusive and significant GI bleeding persists. Initially, selective celiac arteriography is performed, followed by superselective left gastric or gastroduodenal arteriography. On occasion, superior mesenteric, pancreatic, splenic, or hepatic arteriography is needed.

Hemorrhage of a Mallory-Weiss tear is treated successfully with vasopressin infusion into the left gastric artery or with embolization. Embolization controls more than 95% of cases. Hemorrhagic gastritis and gastric stress ulcers respond to vasopressin in more than 80% of cases. Pyloroduodenal ulcer bleeding is much less effectively controlled by vasopressin: success rates are of only 30% to 50%. Embolization should be the initial transcatheter therapy for duodenal hemorrhage.[7, 8]

Aneurysms, pseudoaneurysms, and arteriovenous fistulas (AVF) of the visceral arteries are uncommon sources of serious upper and lower GI hemorrhage.[9, 10] The most common sites, in decreasing order, are the splenic, gastroduodenal, hepatic, and pancreatic arteries. In the past, surgery was the principal treatment of visceral aneurysmal bleeding; currently, embolotherapy with stainless steel coils, platinum microcoils, or Gelfoam or Ivalon particles has become the initial therapy of choice (Fig. 40–4).[9, 10]

Lower Gastrointestinal Bleeding

Only about 10% of acute GI bleeds originate distal to the ligament of Treitz. Once rectal or anal causes have been ruled out by proctosigmoidoscopy, radionuclide scanning and arteriography are indicated for management. Endoscopy usually is not helpful because visualization is poor in an unprepared colon owing to retained blood and feces. Thus, for massive continuous hemorrhage arteriography is the initial study. Patients with only moderate or intermittent bleeding can undergo a radionuclide scan before arteriography. If the scan is not diagnostic or is negative, arteriography is delayed until active bleeding recurs, or is performed electively in the hope of finding another underlying lesion (tumor, angiodysplasia, arteriovenous malformation [AVM]) that could be causing the hemorrhage. If the radionuclide scan is positive, selective superior and inferior mesenteric arteriography is performed according to information obtained from the scan. Because scintigraphy is more sensitive than arteriography and GI bleeding is often intermittent, a positive scan may be followed by a negative arteriogram. In these cases, the need for further work-up is based on the clinical situation.

The major causes of colorectal bleeding are diverticulosis and angiodysplasia. Inflammatory or ischemic colitis, ulcers, tumors, and AVMs are less common causes. It must be empha-

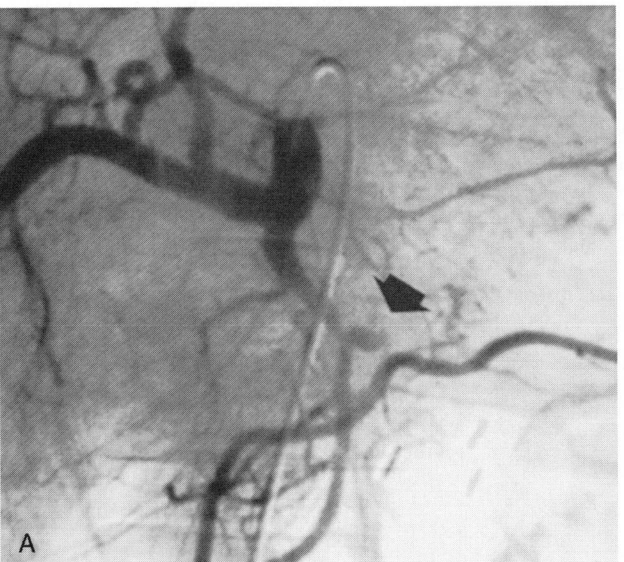

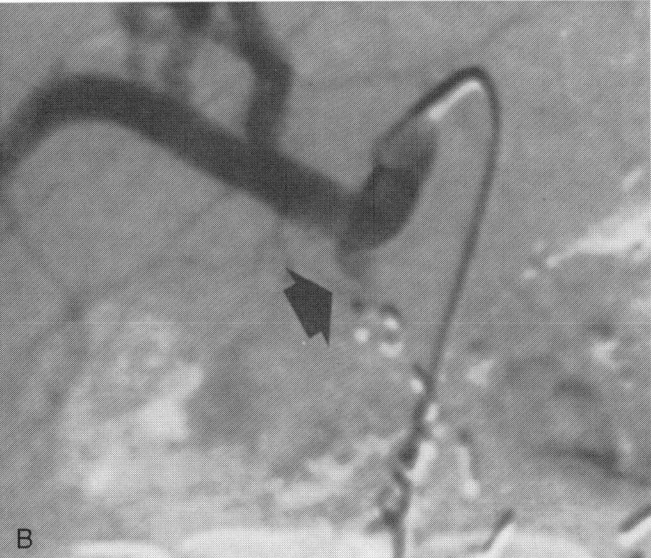

Figure 40–4. A 36-year-old man presented with severe pancreatitis and recurrent upper gastrointestinal hemorrhage. *A,* Celiac arteriography demonstrates a small pseudoaneurysm arising from the gastroduodenal artery *(arrow). B,* Absorbable gelatin sponge (Gelfoam) particles and stainless-steel coils were placed proximal and distal to the pseudoaneurysm neck. Arteriography after embolization demonstrates occlusion of the gastroduodenal artery *(arrow).* No further bleeding occurred.

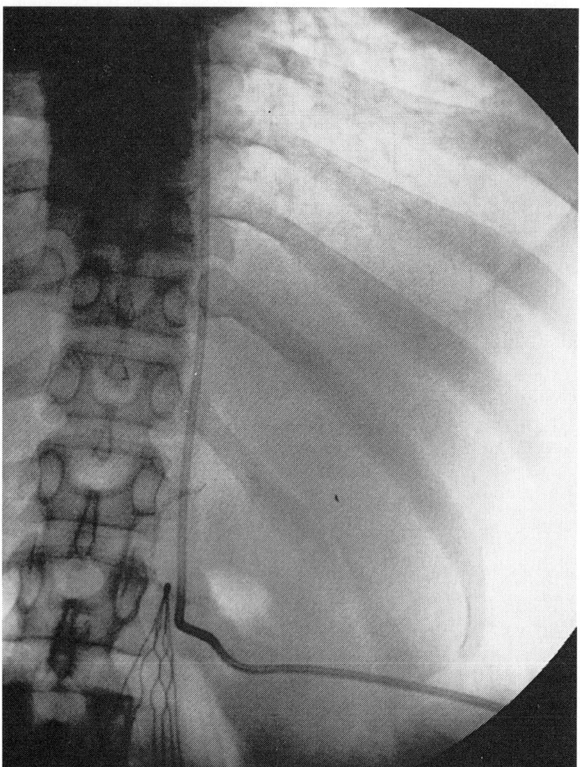

Figure 40–5. In this patient, an 18-year-old boy, numerous central catheters were placed for total parenteral nutrition. Eventually, all the central venous accesses were depleted. Therefore, a percutaneous, translumbar catheter was inserted in the inferior vena cava (IVC), with the tip in the right atrium. The filter in the IVC was used as a reference to puncture the IVC. Care was taken not to disturb the filter. (Image in prone position.)

sized that, although colonic diverticula are more common in the left colon, the most diverticular hemorrhages occur in the right colon (see Fig. 40–1).

The radiologic intervention for lower GI bleeding is vasopressin infusion into either the superior or inferior mesenteric artery (or both simultaneously when both are involved). The doses are usually the same as those described for upper GI bleeding. Diverticular bleeding is controlled in as many as 90% of cases, but it recurs in 20% to 30% of cases. Embolization with small Gelfoam particles is an alternative if vasopressin therapy fails. The rectum can be safely embolized because of its rich collateral blood supply. Embolization of jejunal, ileal, and colonic bleeding sites can be done successfully, but the approach is controversial because of increased risks of infarction and other ischemic complications. Embolization should be done as selectively and peripherally as possible to avoid complications. Tracker catheters or another microcatheter system can be helpful in negotiating tortuous vessels. Several reports of successful embolization of small intestine and colon lesions are available.

CENTRAL AND PERIPHERAL VENOUS ACCESS

Venous access is routinely required for critically ill patients. In the past, the role of interventional radiologists has been angiographic diagnosis of malfunctioning catheters, mapping of venous anatomy before catheter placement, retrieval of embolized catheter fragments, unknotting of catheters, and repositioning of malpositioned catheters.[11]

The role of the radiologist has expanded greatly. Long-term central venous catheters and ports are now readily placed by radiologists the same day or within 24 hours, thus avoiding surgery for critically ill patients. In addition, peripherally inserted central catheters (PICCs) are placed routinely by the radiology team. With the aid of digital fluoroscopy and duplex color Doppler ultrasonography, radiologists are very successful at difficult central catheter placements.[12] Image-guided catheter placements are frequently more successful than anatomy-guided ones. Puncture complication rates are much lower, and infection complication rates are comparable to those for surgically established access. When all the usual central access sites have been depleted, an inferior vena cava catheter can be placed by the percutaneous translumbar approach; alternatively, an intrahepatic vein catheter can be placed by the percutaneous transhepatic approach (Fig. 40–5).

Interventional radiologic techniques are also helpful in reestablishing vascular access in critically ill patients. Thrombosed dialysis AVFs and grafts can be lysed with urokinase infusion or with numerous available mechanical devices introduced through vascular sheaths into the thrombosed grafts, to break and pulverize clots mechanically (Fig. 40–6). After lysis and recanalization, underlying stenoses are found and dilated with angioplasty, thereby extending the longevity of the graft. Because central venous stenoses often respond poorly to balloon dilatation, metallic mesh Wallstents and other stents are successfully placed across stenoses or recanalized venous occlusions to maintain patency (Fig. 40–7).[13, 14] Every effort must be made to maintain the access as long as possible.

Because central venous stenoses are frequent causes of graft failure in critically ill patients with AVFs, these stenoses must be corrected to preserve the life of the AVF. In patients with catheter-induced venous thromboses, local infusion of urokinase into the clot may restore venous patency without remov-

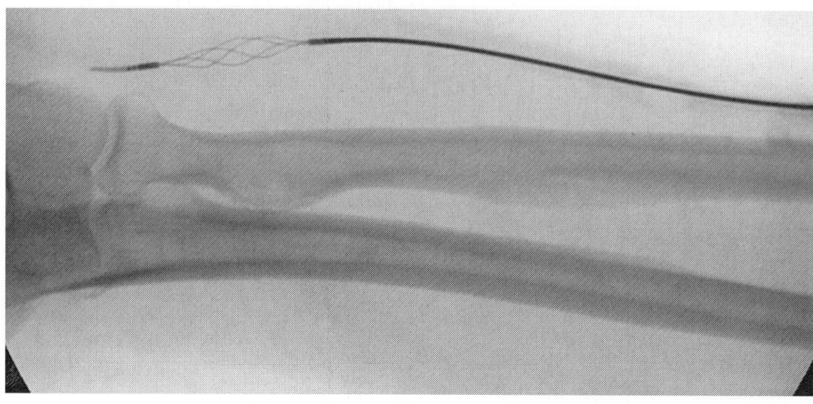

Figure 40–6. A mechanical device to fragment clot is noted in the venous side of an arteriovenous fistula (AVF). Mechanical recanalization of the AVF was successful.

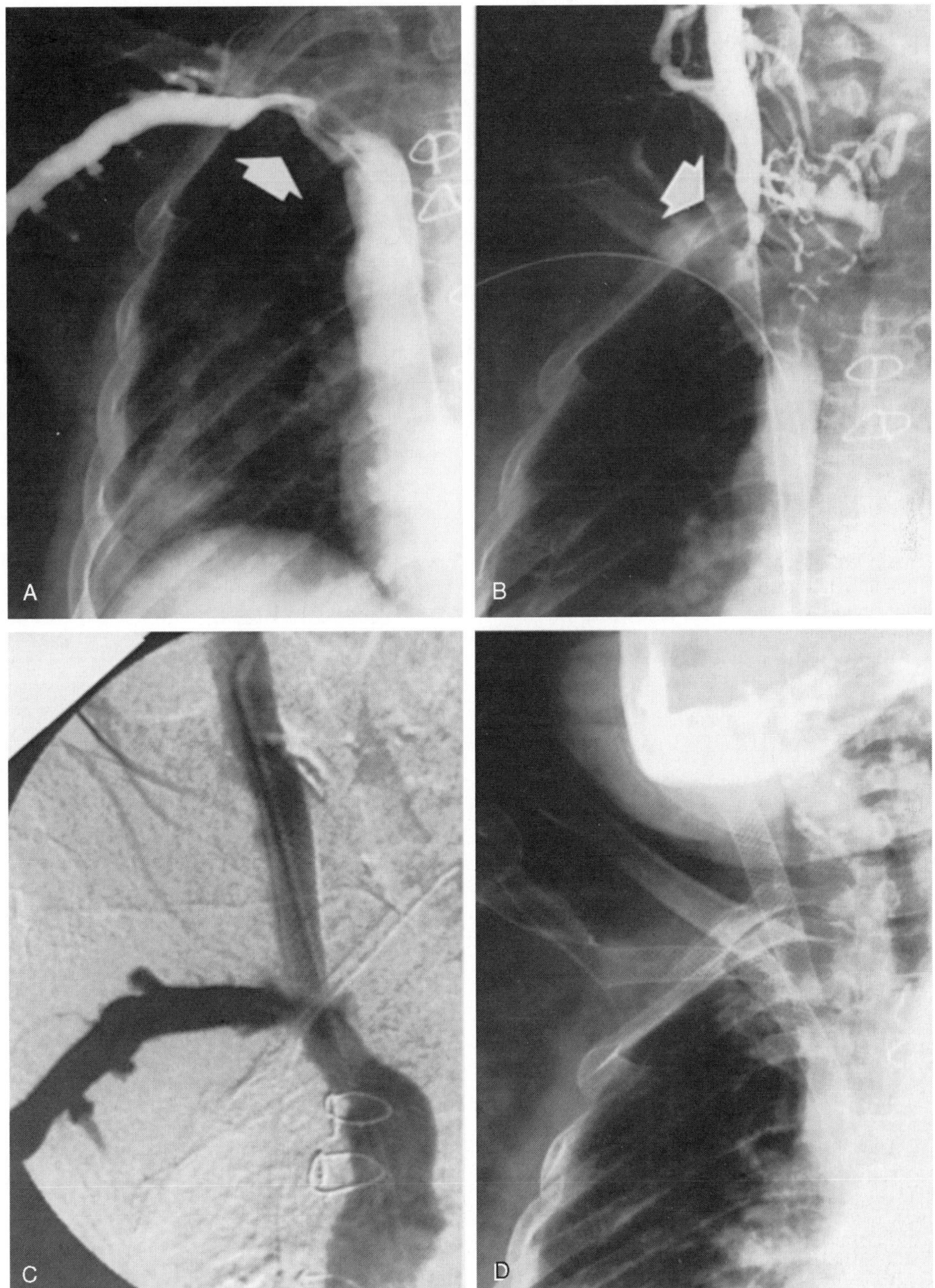

Figure 40–7. Multiple dialysis catheter placements in the central veins were unsuccessful in the patient, a 77-year-old woman. *A* and *B,* Marked stenoses are present in the right internal jugular and subclavian veins at their confluence *(arrows).* Because the stenoses were not adequately recanalized by percutaneous transluminal angioplasty alone, metallic Wallstents were placed. *C,* At 6 months' follow-up, the stented central veins remained patent, with excellent flow through the subclavian and internal jugular veins. *D,* Unopacified stents in place.

ing the catheter. When thrombolysis fails to restore patency, percutaneous fibrin sheath stripping of catheters is used. A loop snare advanced through a femoral venous approach is used to tightly encircle the catheter and strip the encasing fibrin sheath from the tip of the catheter. Thus, the central catheters for hemodialysis do not need to be changed in these patients with limited and depleting venous access sites.

UROLOGIC INTERVENTIONS

Percutaneous nephrostomy placement is the principal extravascular procedure performed on critically ill patients. The most common indications are supravesical urinary tract obstruction causing hydronephrosis or pyonephrosis, and urinary diversion to heal urinary tract leaks or fistulas. Emobolization of the ureters is sometimes necessary to divert the urine completely. This procedure is easily done in the angiographic laboratory (Fig. 40–8).

Access can be gained to the collecting system using fluoroscopy or ultrasonography. Ultrasound has the advantage of providing rapid localization and real-time imaging without radiation. Some sonographic transducers have built-in needle slots that allow directing the needle within the plane of the transducer. When fluoroscopy is used, the renal anatomy is defined by direct injection of contrast material into the upper collecting system. With the patient positioned prone or prone oblique, a 21- or 22-gauge Chiba needle is inserted from a posterolateral flank approach, along Brödel's line (near the posterior axillary line) into an appropriate calyx or infundibulum. After guide-wire placement and tract dilatation, a No. 8 to 10 French nephrostomy drainage catheter with a self-retaining locked loop is inserted and positioned in the renal pelvis to prevent catheter displacement. Before percutaneous nephrostomy placement, any coagulopathy present must be corrected and antibiotic therapy initiated, if pyonephrosis is suspected or if the patient has heart disease that requires endocarditis prophylaxis.[15, 16] Unilateral or bilateral nephrostomy tubes are placed, depending on the circumstances.

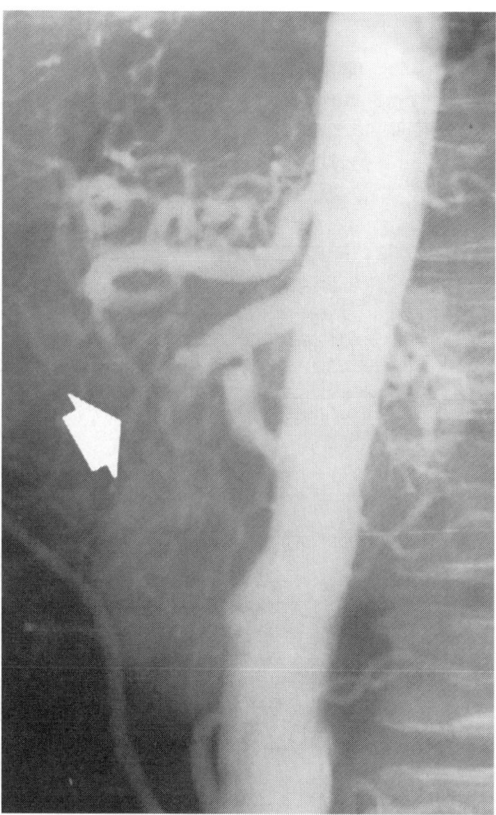

Figure 40–9. Lateral aortogram reveals an embolus in the proximal superior mesenteric artery *(arrow)*.

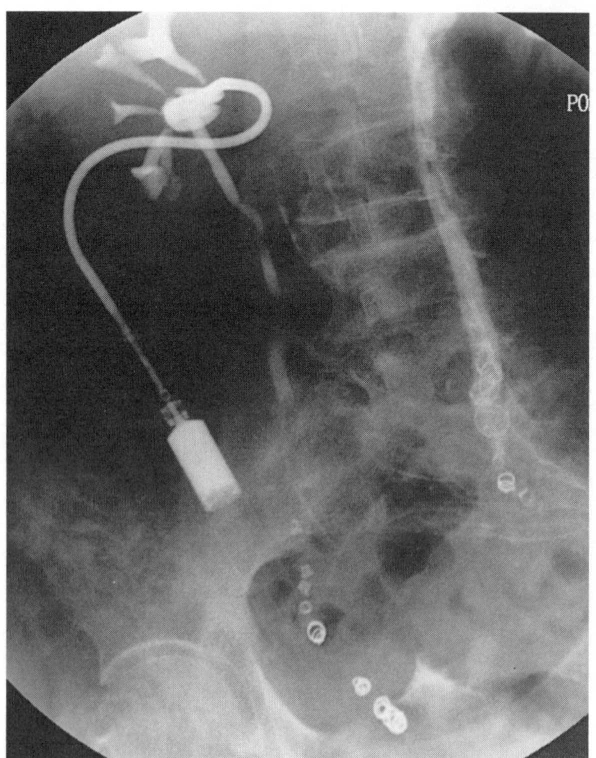

Figure 40–8. Urinary fistulas developed in the pelvis of an elderly woman with diffuse pelvic malignancy. Therefore, bilateral ureteral embolization was performed using numerous stainless steel coils intermixed with alternating pieces of absorbable gelatin sponge (Gelfoam). Complete diversion of urine was accomplished, resulting in closure of urinary fistulas.

In conclusion, the interventional radiologist can contribute significantly to the care of these critically ill patients. A team effort, with urologists, nephrologists, and other clinicians, is necessary for successful patient management.

VASCULAR INTERVENTIONS

Mesenteric Ischemia

Mesenteric ischemia can be *acute* or *chronic* and *occlusive* or *nonocclusive*. It is usually considered only after other causes of acute abdominal disease have been excluded. Patients are usually elderly and often have multiple medical problems. They may present with abdominal pain of acute onset out of proportion to physical findings, nausea, vomiting, and diarrhea, with or without blood. Rapid clinical deterioration, with sepsis, acidosis, hypotension, and death, may ensue. Unfortunately, the problem is so serious that even when mesenteric ischemia is properly diagnosed and treated, the mortality rate may be as high as 70%.[17] Occlusive ischemia is due to either arterial embolism (60% to 80%) or thrombosis (20% to 30%). Nonocclusive ischemia, related to a low-flow state such as cardiogenic shock, occurs in about 20% of cases.

Arteriography must be done before any barium contrast studies, lest residual barium in the GI tract obscure angiographic findings. Biplanar aortography must be done. The lateral view is used to evaluate the origins of the celiac, superior mesenteric, and inferior mesenteric arteries, since these visceral vessels originate anteriorly from the aorta (Fig. 40–9). The frontal view shows the distal visceral branches. Selective arteriography is frequently necessary for an accurate diagnosis.

The treatment of occlusive ischemia varies according to the clinical situation. The presence of peritoneal signs usually demands immediate exploratory surgery and bowel resection for gangrene, if present. Otherwise, the interventional radiologic management consists of fragmentation of the thrombus into smaller pieces with guide wires and catheters, transcatheter thrombolysis with urokinase, suction thromboembolectomy, or balloon thromboembolectomy followed by thrombolytic therapy.[18, 19] Lytic therapy is with urokinase, 4000 units/min for 2 hours, then 2000 units/min for 2 hours, followed by a smaller dose (usually 100,000 units/hour for several hours or days, as necessary). The patients are monitored carefully for peritoneal signs and for clotting and electrolyte disturbances. When significant stenoses involving two or more mesenteric arteries are found, transluminal balloon angioplasty may be performed.

Angioplasty and vascular reconstruction with metallic stents is successful in selected patients. Dramatic results have been obtained (Fig. 40–10). Although the long-term results of percutaneous transluminal angioplasty (PTA) are inferior to those of surgical bypass grafting, the lower morbidity and mortality and ease of repetition offer an attractive alternative in these critically ill patients. Together, radiologists, surgeons, and other clinicians must manage these patients.

For nonocclusive mesenteric ischemia, intra-arterial infusion of papaverine into the superior mesenteric artery is usually effective. The dose of papaverine is 1 mg/min for 12 to 24 hours or more. Nifedipine can be given for its additive vasodilating effect. The therapy should be discontinued only when significant clinical improvement is observed. If bowel infarction is suspected, surgical exploration may become necessary. Papaverine is an antispasmodic drug used during, between, and after operations. Underlying medical problems such as heart failure, hypovolemia, and cardiogenic shock must also be corrected. Despite significant improvements in surgical and radiographic techniques, nonocclusive mesenteric ischemia remains a major management problem.

For severe chronic mesenteric ischemia, surgical revascularization is indicated. Surgery is successful in 70% of cases and has a 3% to 8% mortality rate.[18] Focal stenotic lesions can be treated successfully with PTA and placement of stents.[20]

Peripheral Ischemia

Acute lower or upper extremity ischemia usually results from thrombotic or embolic occlusion of native arteries or bypass grafts. Prompt arteriography provides the definitive diagnosis and allows for transcatheter therapy with urokinase, followed by PTA and stenting, according to the particular situation. Thrombolysis or PTA can restore perfusion to the ischemic limb and permit a semielective surgical intervention, thus reducing morbidity and mortality (Fig. 40–11). Shorter-lived, and therefore safer, large-dose urokinase infusion protocols are now being used.[21] The choice of thrombolysis or surgery depends on the degree of limb ischemia. Success rates of 100% and 84%, respectively, can be achieved in viable and threatened limbs; however, with irreversible ischemia the success rate is only about 50%, and a higher rate of major complications is expected. Thrombolysis also permits identification of an underlying flow-limiting stenosis that may have precipitated the thrombosis. Once antegrade flow is reestablished, PTA and stenting may be performed (Fig. 40–12).[22]

Complications of catheter-directed low-dose thrombolysis are uncommon and certainly easier to manage than those of systemic thrombolysis. Major bleeding complications occur in only 2% to 4% of patients, most at the puncture site.[21] Possible complications of central nervous system hemorrhage or distal embolization should not preclude lytic therapy. Absolute con-

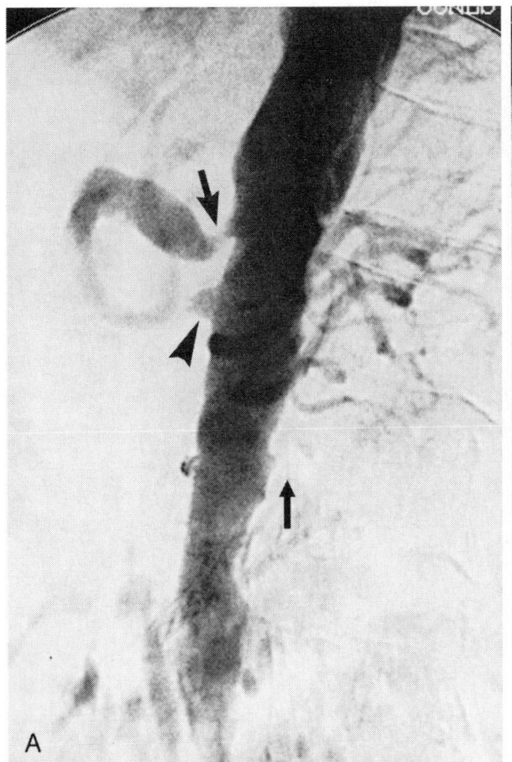

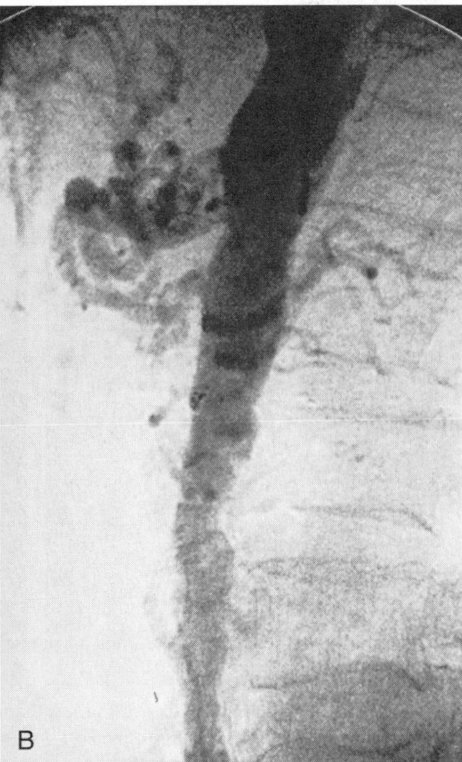

Figure 40–10. An elderly man with diffuse and advanced arteriosclerosis presented with chronic mesenteric ischemia. *A,* The lateral aortogram shows marked stenosis of the celiac axis *(arrow).* There is complete occlusion of the superior mesenteric artery *(arrowhead)* and complete occlusion of the inferior mesenteric artery. After percutaneous transluminal angioplasty and stenting of the celiac axis *(B),* there is excellent flow and the stenosis is no longer present.

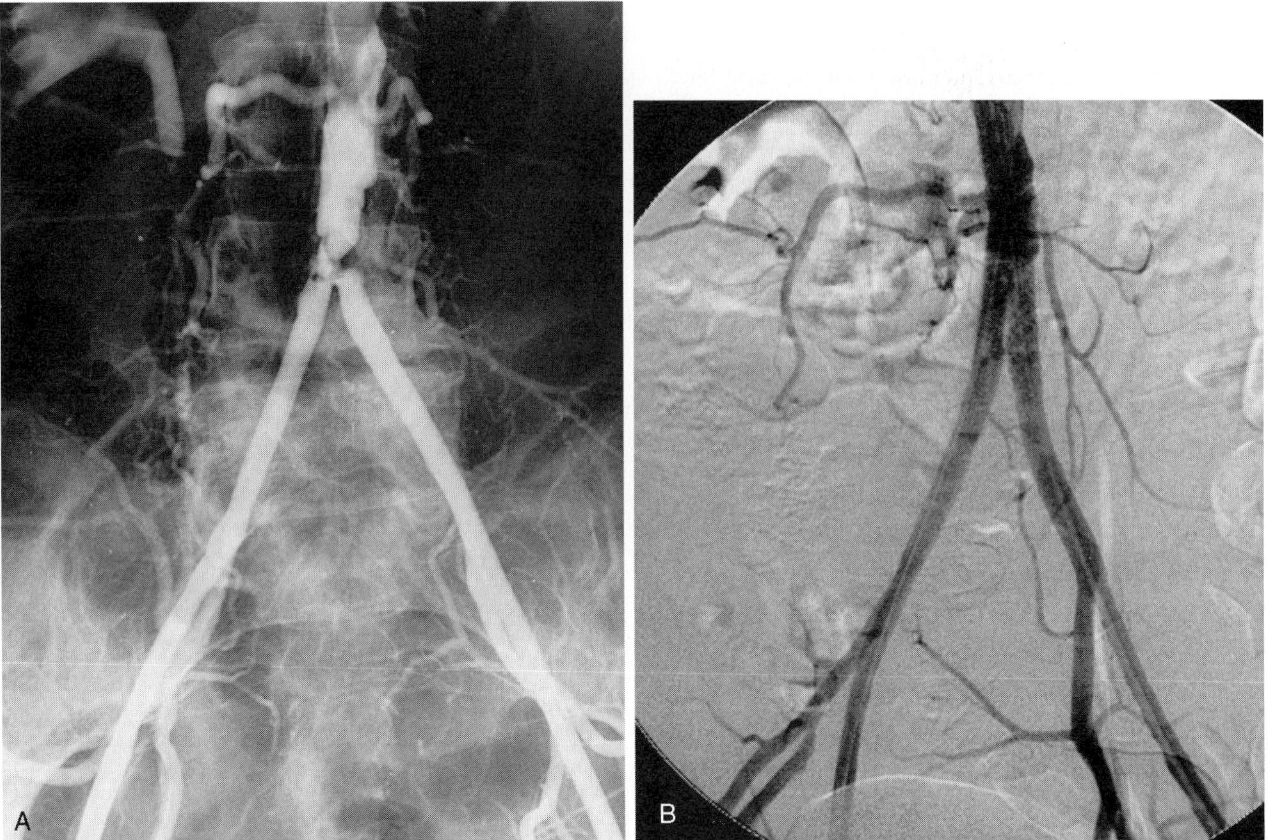

Figure 40–11. The patient, a middle-aged woman who was a chronic smoker, presented with long-standing ischemic claudication of both lower extremities. *A,* An aortogram demonstrated marked stenosis of the distal aorta and both common iliac arteries. *B,* After percutaneous transluminal angioplasty and stenting, there is excellent reconstitution of luminal diameter. The patient became asymptomatic and was advised to stop smoking.

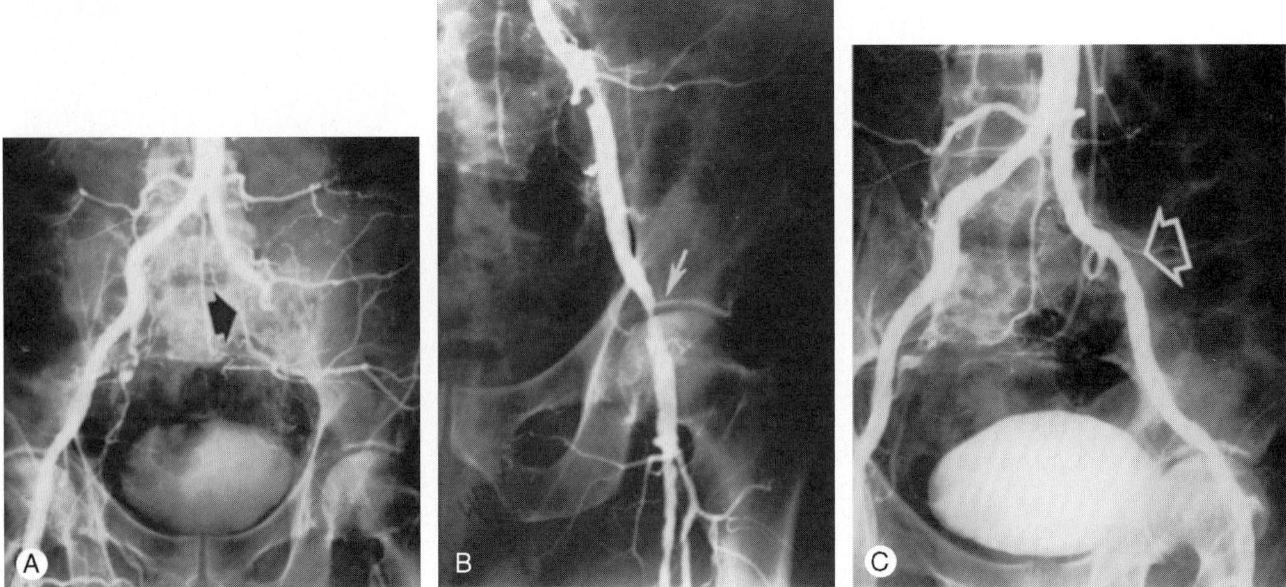

Figure 40–12. *A,* Acute thrombosis of the left external iliac artery *(arrow)* and common femoral artery. *B,* After flow was restored, the primary stenosis is visible. *C,* Another area of stenosis was identified and dilated *(arrow).* The left external iliac artery remained patent a few years later.

traindications include active GI or genitourinary (GU) tract bleeding, recent stroke or craniotomy (within 3 to 6 months), intracranial neoplasm, and irreversible ischemia with gangrene (because of the risk of "postperfusion syndrome" and its serious consequences). Shorter, large-dose infusion methods have significantly reduced the bleeding complications; furthermore, lytic therapy can be performed in the postoperative period in special circumstances. Concomitant intravenous heparinization, which is needed to avoid pericatheter thrombosis, is responsible for some of the major complications associated with thrombolysis. Therefore, very careful monitoring of heparin administration is strongly recommended.

PTA provides recanalization of stenotic or occluded vessels by controlled injury to the arterial wall. An initial technical success rate of 85% to 96% and a slightly lower rate of clinical improvement are expected.[23] Vascular stenting further improves the success of these procedures, both angiographically and hemodynamically (see Figs. 40–11 and 40–12). Currently, lesions in the iliac arteries and in the abdominal aorta are routinely treated with stents. Long-term patency as high as 90% to 93% at 5 years is expected.[24] Lesions in the superficial femoral arteries are not yet amenable to definitive PTA and stenting, because of high rates of recurrence; however, several reports of successful PTA and stenting of the superficial femoral arteries are available.

Placement of stent-grafts (i.e., stents covered with graft such as Dacron and Gore-Tex, among others) is just being developed in most large medical centers. The procedure is considered semi-investigational at this time. The procedure holds promise for nonsurgical treatment of patients with abdominal or thoracic aortic aneurysms who would not tolerate extensive emergency surgery, particularly in cases of ruptured aneurysms.[24a] Furthermore, stent-grafts may be used to repair, temporarily or permanently, traumatic injuries to major arteries of the upper and lower extremities and the aorta. It is anticipated that stent-grafting will become a routine procedure in the next 2 to 3 years.

Acute upper extremity ischemia is a rare but serious clinical problem. Major causes include embolism, thrombosis, trauma, or underlying collagen vascular disorders. On occasion, the so-called thoracic outlet syndrome may be responsible. Selective small dose infusions of thrombolytic agents are very effective, even for the most severe and diffuse occlusions. Because surgical alternative therapy is of limited use in upper extremity ischemia, angiographic management is the treatment of choice.[25] Adjunctive vasodilators and anticoagulation with heparin and coumadin have very important roles in the management of vasospastic and organic occlusive disorders of the upper extremities.

Renal Ischemia

Renal ischemia, usually due to acute arterial occlusion by thrombi or emboli, results in loss of renal function. The treatment options include surgical bypass or endarterectomy, PTA, thrombolysis, stenting, and medical therapy. PTA has a technical success rate of 80% to 97% and is clinically beneficial in 75% to 90% of cases, depending on the cause, location, and severity of the stenoses as well as on the patient's underlying clinical condition (Fig. 40–13).[26] Ostial stenoses, previously believed to respond poorly to PTA alone, have shown good long-term results since the routine placement of stents.[27] On the other hand, with rapidly deteriorating or acute renal failure the clinical success of PTA is much more modest, in the range of 30% to 50%, which is still considered reasonable because of the minimal invasiveness of PTA and stenting as compared with surgery. The overall complication rates for PTA are 5% to 10%, lower than for surgery (reported complication rate, 20%). We believe that PTA is the ideal first choice for recanalization of renal arteries.[28] Some unusual clinical situations are stenosis in solitary kidneys and in horseshoe kidneys in critically ill patients (Figs. 40–13 and 40–14).

Thrombolysis of acute renal artery thrombosis has not been widely implemented. Only scattered reports are available in the literature. It is generally accepted that improvement in renal function is less likely in this clinical situation, and that

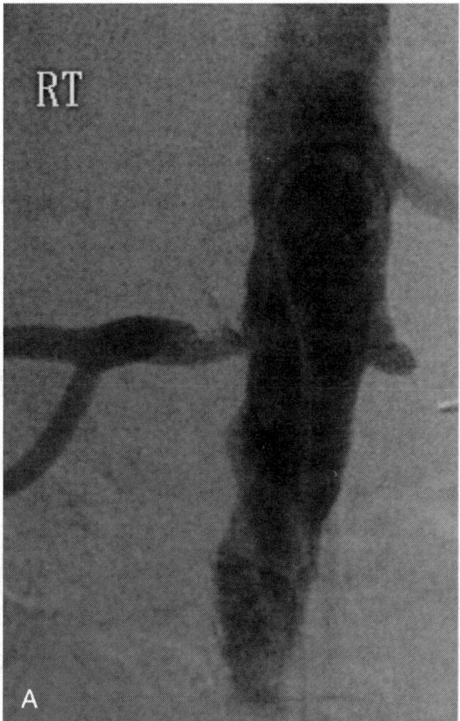

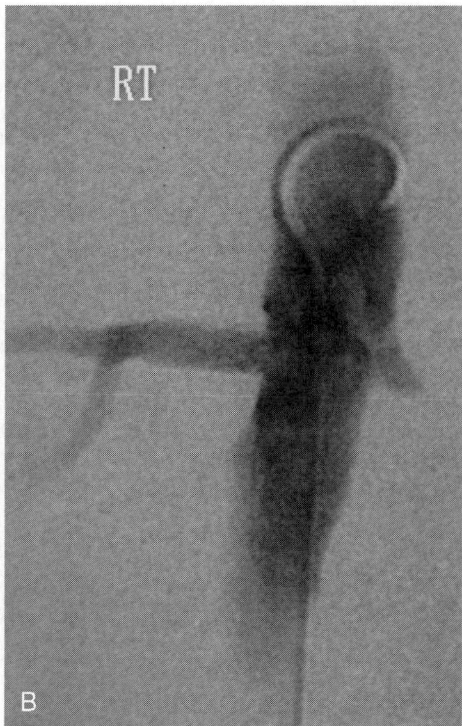

Figure 40–13. Abdominal aortogram before *(A)* and after *(B)* percutaneous transluminal angioplasty and stenting of the renal artery of a solitary right kidney. The left kidney had been resected a long time ago.

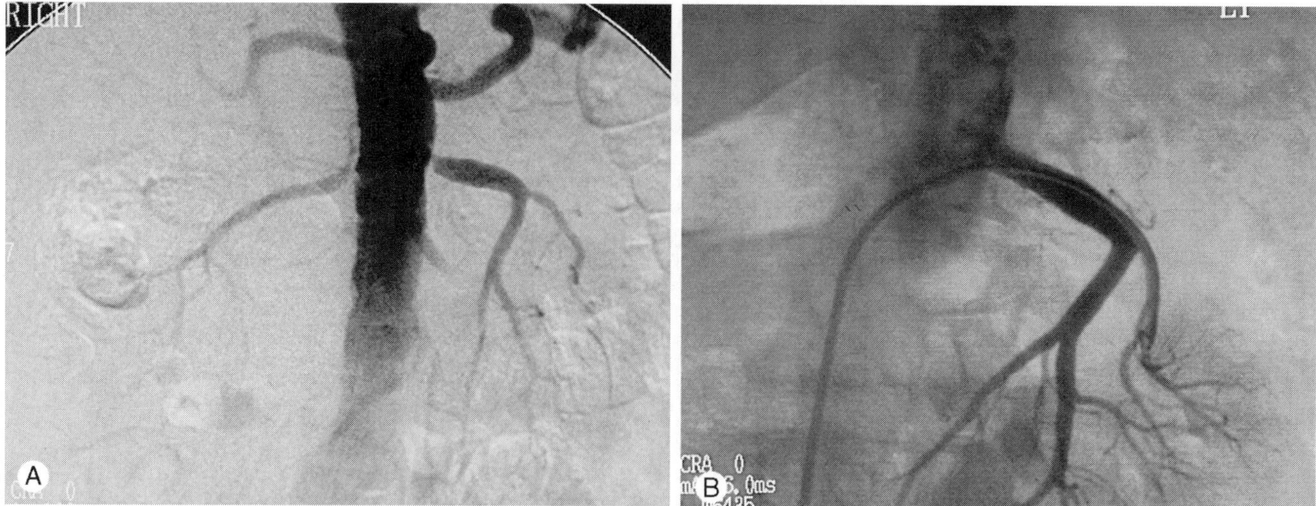

Figure 40–14. A middle-aged man presented with deteriorating renal function and hypertension. Imaging studies demonstrated a mass in the right side of a horseshoe kidney. *A,* An abdominal aortogram showed marked stenosis and almost complete occlusion of the left renal artery. The right renal artery is almost completely occluded. *B,* Successful percutaneous transluminal angioplasty and stenting of the left renal artery was done prior to resection of the right kidney.

the infusion of urokinase must be instituted as early as possible if one expects clinical improvement.

PERCUTANEOUS NEEDLE BIOPSY

Percutaneous needle biopsy yields samples for either cytologic or histologic diagnosis. Percutaneous imaging-guided biopsy is now widely accepted and has largely replaced exploratory laparotomy for tissue diagnosis. If a safe pathway to the organ or lesion is available, as determined by cross-sectional imaging (CT, ultrasonography, MRI), a small-caliber Chiba needle (20- to 23-gauge) is used, to obtain cells and tissue samples.[29] A 14-gauge cutting needle may be used to obtain core samples for histologic diagnosis. The Chiba needle may safely traverse the stomach, bowel, or other organs to sample deep solid lesions. The overall accuracy of the procedure ranges from 79% for 1-cm or smaller lesions to 98% for 2-cm or larger ones.[30]

Complications are variable but, overall, are estimated to be less than 2%.[29] Major complications include hemorrhage, infection, inadvertent organ injury, pneumothorax, bile leakage, peritonitis, and pancreatitis. Very rarely, needle track seeding of tumor cells can occur.

Liver biopsy in patients with acute, semiacute, or fulminant hepatic failure may be performed either percutaneously or by the transjugular venous route. The transjugular access is preferred in patients with coagulopathy or ascites. Immediate diagnosis is frequently necessary in patients with a liver transplant to establish prompt therapy, as the clinical picture of rejection and occlusion of hepatic arteries can mimic each other. Some patients may need immediate thrombolysis or surgery of thrombosed hepatic artery anastomoses, and others may need liver cell transplantation or aggressive pharmacotherapy.

INTERVENTIONS IN LIVER FAILURE

Liver cell transplantation is a procedure now being developed and investigated to help patients with acute, subacute, or fulminant liver failure. The procedure supplements the function of the diseased liver, thereby sustaining life until an organ becomes available or until the liver function recovers from the acute insult.[31] Briefly, the splenic artery is catheterized selectively from a femoral arterial approach, or the portal vein is catheterized by percutaneous puncture of the liver, after which hepatocytes previously isolated from excess donor liver tissue that was not used for transplantation are injected into the spleen or liver.[31, 31a] Preliminary reports suggest that these transplanted hepatocytes provide metabolic support in these critically ill patients, "bridging" life and buying time until an organ becomes available. Dramatic recovery has been observed in some of our patients. Since liver cell transplantation is usually done on very short notice, involved health care providers and interventional radiologists must be service-ready (Fig. 40–15).

A new technique for liver transplantation is under evaluation at our institution: *related living donor* or *nonrelated living donor.* In these procedures, part of the liver of a living person is removed and implanted in the recipient. The introduction of this technique has provided another treatment option for patients with liver disease.

Other interventions in the liver for critically ill patients include PTA and stenting of stenotic or occluded hepatic veins in patients with Budd-Chiari syndrome. Sometimes the angiographic treatment is the definitive one. At other times, it is a temporizing one until definitive shunting or liver transplantation is done (Fig. 40–16).

PERCUTANEOUS ASPIRATION OR DRAINAGE OF FLUID COLLECTIONS

Some critically ill patients may present with fluid collections anywhere in the body, mainly the abdomen and pelvis. Surgical drainage in these conditions may be associated with a prohibitive rate of complications and even a high mortality rate. The availability of CT, ultrasonography, and MRI, and the development of special catheters and guide wire systems have allowed percutaneous drainage of collections such as abscesses, cysts, hematomas, bilomas, urinomas, pseudocysts, lymphoceles, necrotic tumors, and loculated ascites, among others (Fig. 40–17).

Two types of drainage can be performed: (1) Seldinger's technique with a needle, guide wire, and catheter; and (2) trocar technique with catheter-trocar systems. The choice depends on the circumstances and the experience of the opera-

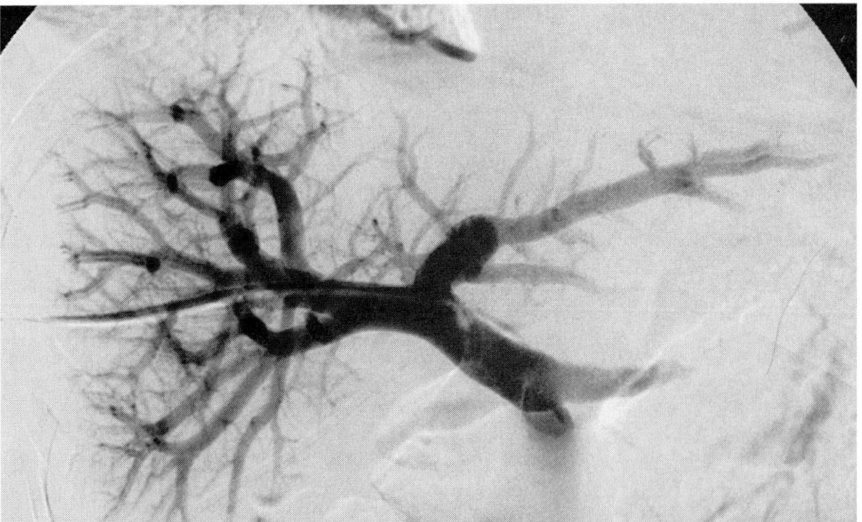

Figure 40–15. Percutaneous transhepatic catheterization of the right portal vein was performed in this young woman with fulminant liver failure. A 5 French catheter was placed in the portal vein just proximal to its bifurcation to infuse hepatic cells. Three infusions of hepatocytes were made. The patient improved dramatically, and returned home without need for additional therapy. Serial transjugular biopsy specimens were taken, showing recovery of hepatic necrosis.

tor. The rates of success of percutaneous drainage are 70% to 90%, and of death 1% to 13%.[32, 33] The average reported complication rate of 10% is much lower than that for surgical drainage, particularly in these very sick patients who could not tolerate surgery. The risks of general anesthesia and extensive surgery are thus avoided. Furthermore, aspiration of fluid, tissue, or debris allows for immediate Gram staining. Drainage catheters, which may range in size from No. 8 to 36 French, also allow for injection of specific agents into the cavities. Cysts, either single or loculated, may be ablated with alcohol, and infected, loculated hematomas can be lysed with thrombolytic agents. In addition to drainage, aggressive antibiotic therapy must be continued until the infection has completely disappeared.

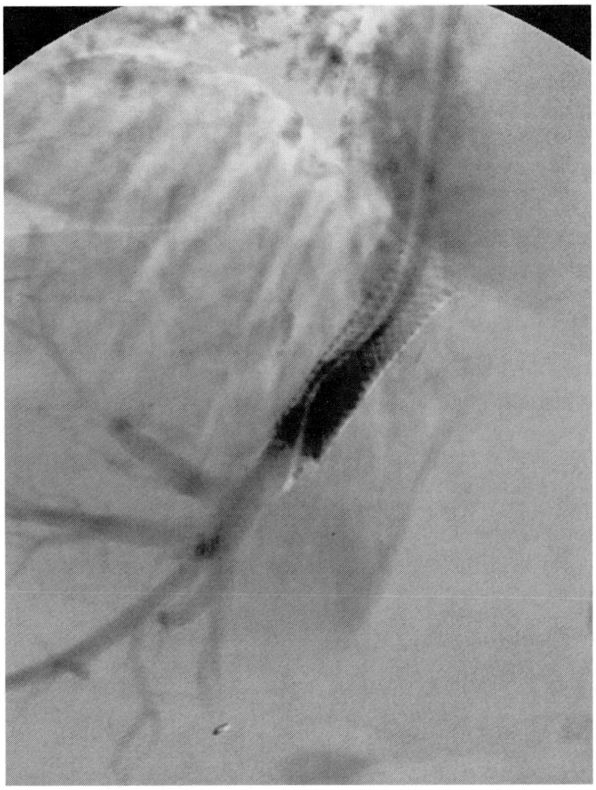

Figure 40–16. The patient, a young woman taking oral contraceptives for a long time, presented with abdominal pain, ascites, and hepatomegaly. Angiography demonstrated extensive occlusion of hepatic veins. Percutaneous transluminal angioplasty and stenting of hepatic veins were performed. Significant clinical improvement was accomplished.

In most patients, the placement of a PICC is necessary for long-term antibiotic administration. The evolution of the collection is best evaluated with serial CT and gentle injections of contrast material under fluoroscopy ("abscessography"). Imaging methods are very important for placement or repositioning of the drainage catheters, which may need to be moved or repositioned frequently as the cavity changes in size or disappears completely (Fig. 40–18).

The only absolute contraindication to percutaneous drainage is the absence of a safe access route to the collection, as demonstrated by imaging methods. Traversal of contaminated organs such as small bowel or colon should be avoided, when possible.

Major complications include septicemia; contamination of

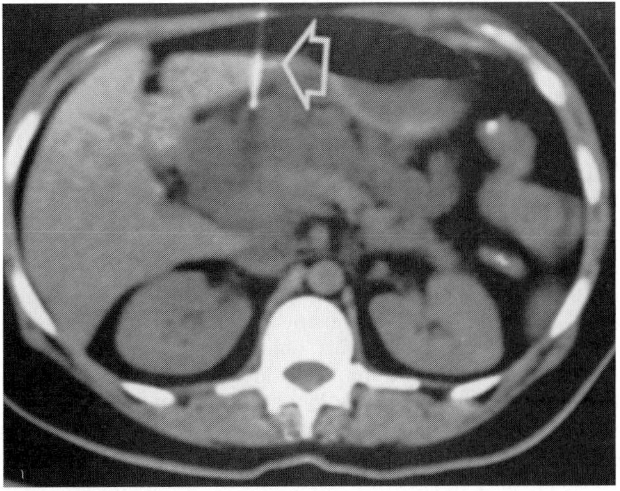

Figure 40–17. Transgastric aspiration and drainage of a lesser sac fluid collection. A Chiba needle *(arrow)* traverses the fluid-filled gastric antrum.

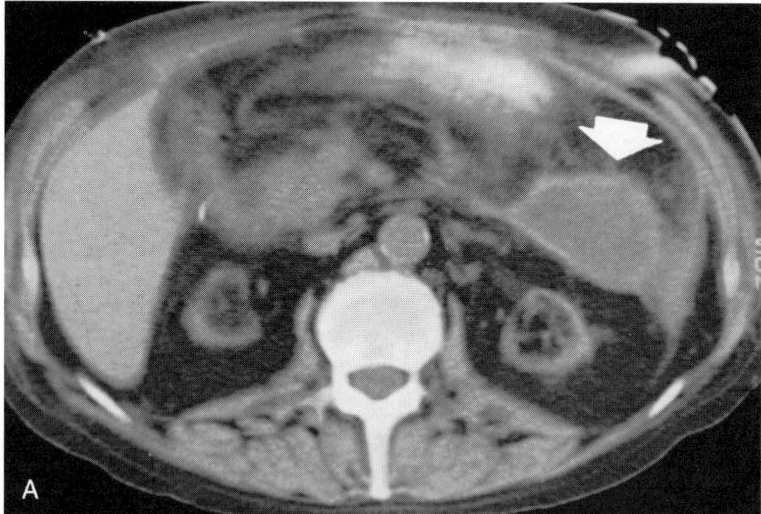

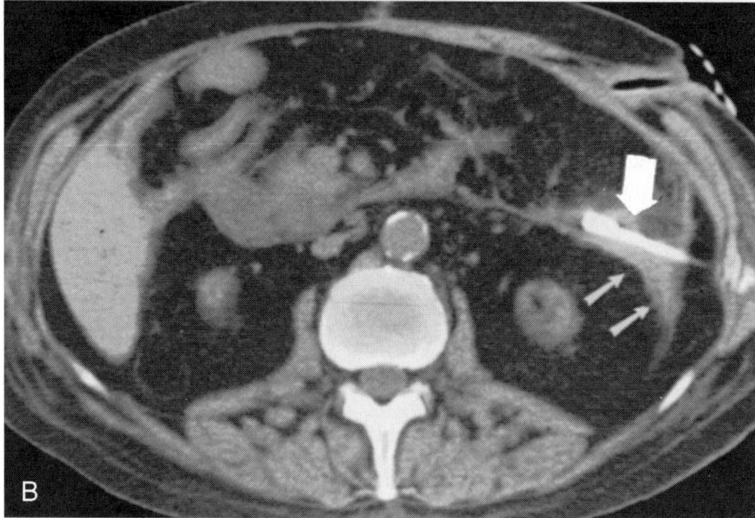

Figure 40–18. *A,* A fluid collection in the left anterior pararenal space is noted on the initial CT scan *(arrow). B,* Two months after percutaneous drainage, the cavity had disappeared. Fatty inflammation *(thin arrows)* and the drainage catheter *(thick arrow)* are evident.

an initially sterile collection or organ; fistula to the small bowel, colon or rectum; hemorrhage; traversal of the pleural space; pneumothorax; and infection at the puncture site. Despite the high success rates for percutaneous drainage of fluid collections, surgical drainage is the only viable alternative when percutaneous drainage fails. Moreover, drainage by either method must be done as soon as possible, because excessive delay of surgery and persistent sepsis can lead to multiple organ failure and, eventually, death.

BILIARY TRACT INTERVENTIONS

Cholangitis with associated sepsis is one of the main reasons for biliary decompression in critically ill patients with obstructive biliary tract disease. Infection may be present in about one third of malignant obstructions and two thirds of benign ones.[34] Percutaneous transhepatic cholangiography (PTC) followed by percutaneous biliary drainage and stent placement, is an effective, safe, and minimally invasive approach. Percutaneous biliary drainage is usually performed through a transhepatic route. The goal of drainage is stabilization of the critically ill patient until definitive treatment can be provided, either endoscopically or surgically. The success rate for establishing access to the biliary system by percutaneous interventional techniques is greater than 95% in patients with ductal dilatation, as demonstrated by imaging methods.[34, 35]

Immediate major complications occur in 10% to 54% of cases and are due to pericatheter bile leak, hemorrhage, or sepsis. Delayed major complications include cholangitis, peritonitis, pancreatitis, pneumothorax, hemobilia, biliopleural fistula, intrahepatic or perihepatic abscess, and skin infection. Percutaneous biliary drainage is contraindicated in the context of diffuse liver metastases, less than 2 to 4 weeks of life expectancy, or asymptomatic jaundice.

The conventional treatment of acute cholecystitis or gallbladder empyema is cholecystectomy, which has an associated mortality rate of 0.5% to 1.8%; however, the mortality rate for emergency cholecystectomy in elderly patients is about 13%, approximately 10 times higher.[36] Thus, at least in critically ill patients, percutaneous cholecystostomy is an attractive alternative and is as effective as surgical or laparoscopic cholecystectomy and the ideal procedure for acalculous cholecystitis.[37] The procedure is usually a temporary measure to stabilize septic patients until definitive surgical cholecystectomy can be done. Percutaneous cholecystostomy can also be used as access for percutaneous interventions such as retrieval of gallstones, dilation and stenting of benign or malignant strictures, implantation of radioisotopes, and even endoluminal biopsy (Fig. 40–19).

Biliary stones can be crushed with special baskets or crushing devices and retrieved after dilation of the tract. Alternatively, the stones may be dislodged and pushed into the duode-

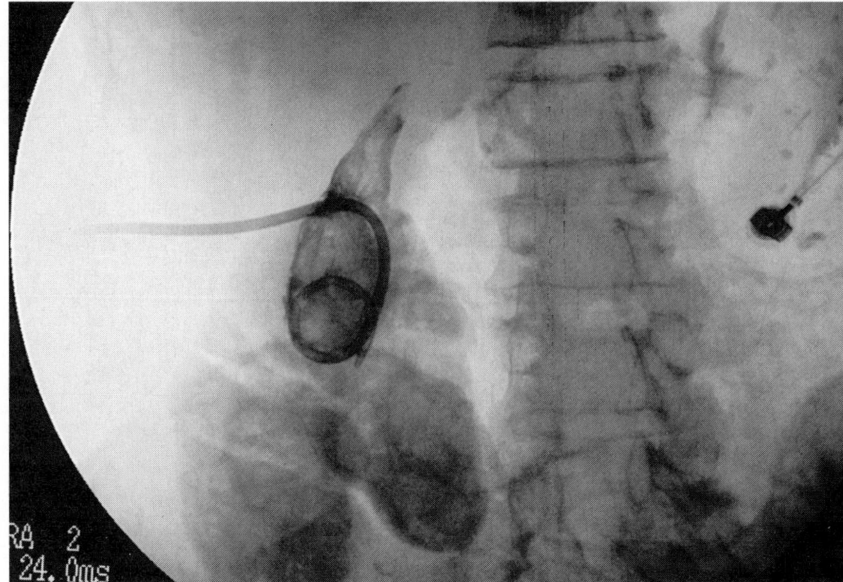

Figure 40–19. An elderly man presented with acute right upper quadrant abdominal pain, fever, sepsis, and jaundice. The diagnosis of acalculous cholecystitis was confirmed by ultrasonography. Therefore, percutaneous cholecystostomy was easily done under ultrasonographic and fluoroscopic guidance. Large amounts of infected bile were drained. The infection defervesced, and the patient recovered. The catheter was removed.

num with an occlusion balloon catheter or another device. Retained common duct stones can be removed through a T-tube tract after 4 to 6 weeks wait for the tract to mature. The overall success of percutaneous stone removal is between 90% and 95%.

Biliary strictures are best treated surgically; in critically ill patients, however, this may not be possible and balloon dilation and stent placement should thus be performed. The long-term patency of the biliary ducts after dilation is excellent and the rate of major complications low. Both surgery and balloon dilation are successful in 70% to 80% of cases. If neither procedure can maintain patency, an internal plastic endoprosthesis may be used. Metallic stents remain patent longer than plastic ones, but they cannot be removed; thus, their use must be carefully planned (Fig. 40–20). In addition, covered Wallstents are just now being used, with variable success.[38, 39]

In conclusion, percutaneous approaches to the biliary system in critically ill patients are a safe and effective means of providing the same temporizing effects as surgical approaches, but in a much less invasive manner.

PERCUTANEOUS GASTROSTOMY AND PLACEMENT OF ENTERAL FEEDING TUBES

Radiologic placement of gastrostomy and gastrojejunostomy feeding tubes is now increasing. General anesthesia is not required, so the associated morbidity is eliminated. Many ICU patients will need nutritional support (supplemental or complete) to recover from their disease or injuries. Some patients have impaired swallowing function, neurologic disorders, head and neck lesions, or esophageal lesions that require supplemental or complete nutritional support. Short-term nutritional needs usually are met with NG and nasoenteric tube feedings or total parenteral nutrition (TPN), which can be administered via temporary or permanent central catheters placed by interventional radiologists.[40]

Surgical gastrostomy is associated with morbidity and mortality rates of 6% and 1%, respectively.[41] Although endoscopic insertion of gastrostomy tubes is now routine, it is relatively expensive and requires general sedation and major cooperation from patients. It may also result in poor gastric emptying, thus delaying feedings. Since TPN requires an indwelling catheter, infection, catheter-induced thrombosis, and venous complications are common problems that render catheters nonfunctional.

Gastrostomy or transgastric jejunal tube feeding are alternatives for long-term feeding. These tubes are tolerated well by the patients, and the procedures are associated with a low complication rate. Peritonitis, hemorrhage, and aspiration secondary to GE reflux are the most serious complications. The risk of aspiration is greatly reduced by placing a percutaneous gastrojejunal (PGJ) tube.

Fluoroscopically guided percutaneous placement of gastrostomy, gastrojejunostomy, and jejunostomy tubes is more attractive (Fig. 40–21). The stomach is inflated with air via a NG tube until adequate gastric distention is achieved. Alternatively, intragastric fluid-filled balloons can be used for gastric distention and support of the stomach wall. Percutaneous puncture of the abdominal wall and stomach is done with a Seldinger needle in large patients or a 22-gauge needle in small, cachectic patients. A No. 10 to 30 French tube can be placed in a very short time, with a success rate of about 95%. Numerous tubes are available of different configurations and materials. The choice depends on the operator. The tube can be replaced once the tract has matured, in about 2 weeks. For placement of a gastrojejunal tube, a curved catheter is advanced into the pylorus and proximal jejunum. A gastrostomy tube can be converted to a gastrojejunostomy tube successfully in more than 95% of cases. Major complications are rare and include retrogastric hematoma, perforation of colon or small bowel, wound site infection, and hemorrhage from the gastrostomy site; however, treatment is required for only about 3% of these complications.[41, 42]

In conclusion, percutaneous placement of a gastrostomy or gastrojejunostomy feeding tube is important for the nutrition of critically ill patients. This approach is safe, simple, cost effective, and highly successful. It offers a safe and convenient alternative to surgery.

PULMONARY THROMBOEMBOLISM AND DEEP VENOUS THROMBOSIS

Pulmonary embolism (PE) is the great simulator of other diseases and one of the leading causes of death in the United

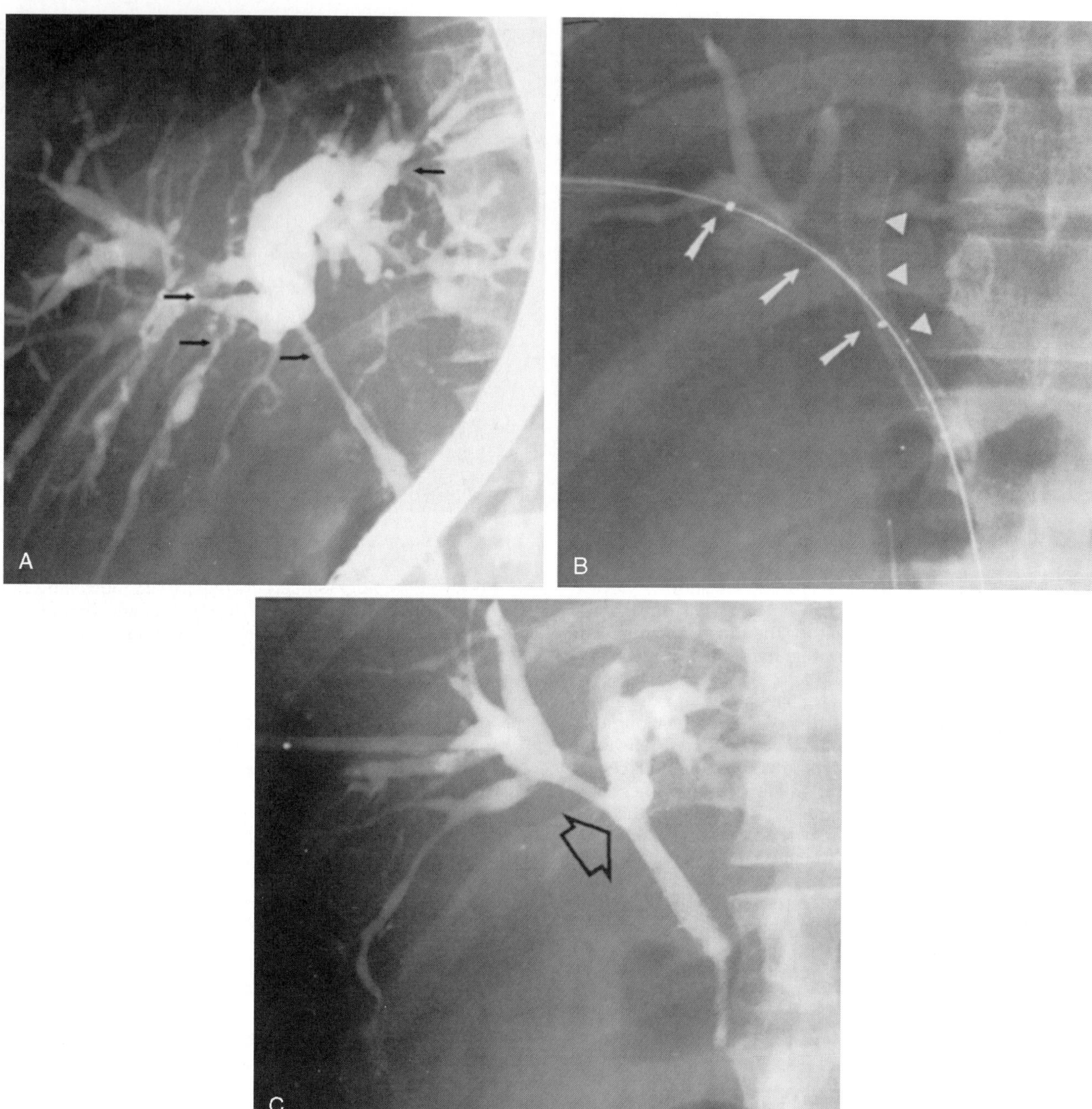

Figure 40–20. *A,* The cholangiogram reveals diffuse areas of narrowing and dilatation of the biliary ducts *(arrows). B,* After percutaneous transhepatic access was established, a partially opened Wallstent is noted during deployment into one of the right biliary ducts *(arrows).* Another completely opened Wallstent is in one of the left ducts *(arrowheads). C,* A cholangiogram following stenting shows widely patent ductal lumens *(arrow).*

States. Previous reports have estimated a yearly incidence of 600,000 new cases. Furthermore, one fourth to one third of patients with PE die if the diagnosis is not made and treatment instituted. The clinical diagnosis is often difficult; the accuracy of clinical diagnosis is 50% at best. Laboratory tests are not helpful. The vast majority of patients have an abnormal chest radiograph, but the radiographic findings are nonspecific.

For many years, pulmonary arteriography has been the definitive diagnostic procedure for PE. With the advent of new-generation CT scanners and improvements in technology, including spiral (helical) CT and CT angiography, the initial diagnosis is now being made with these noninvasive imaging methods. CT is rapidly becoming the initial imaging modality of choice to screen for suspected PE.[43–45] CT is highly successful in demonstrating large and medium-sized emboli in the main pulmonary arteries and the lobar branches (Fig. 40–22). Small segmental or subsegmental emboli are not as easily detected with the current technology, but it is anticipated that newer CT technology will improve their detection. The value of MRI in the evaluation of PE remains controversial at this time.

Previously it had been estimated that 90% of PES originate from deep venous thrombosis (DVT) of the lower extremities and pelvis and the remaining 10% from the superior vena cava and central veins. With widespread and "routine" placement

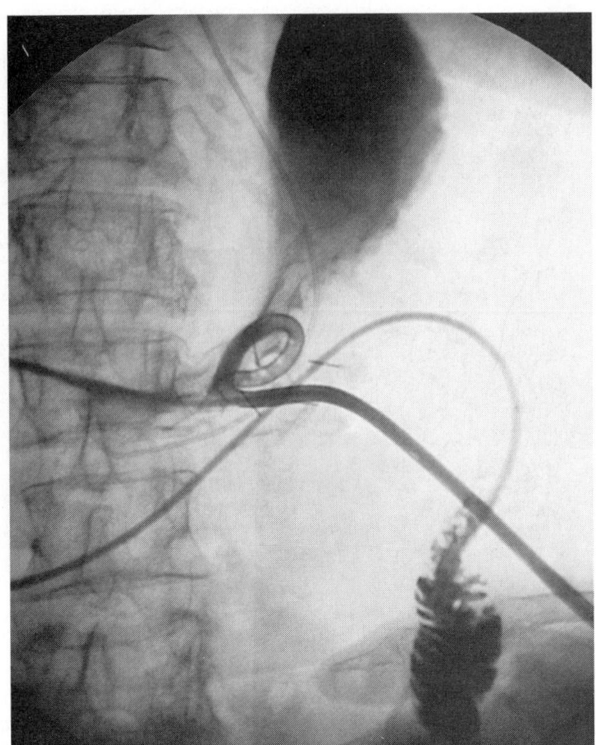

Figure 40–21. The patient is an elderly cachectic man who was unable to eat. Therefore, a percutaneous gastrostomy was done. The stomach was insufflated, punctured, and dilated, and a No. 14 French tube was easily inserted in the fundus. The patient was discharged.

of central catheters, however, the incidence of massive DVT of the upper extremities has increased. Therefore, the incidence of PE from sources other than the lower extremities and pelvis must be increasing as well.

DVT is associated with significant morbidity and mortality and is an important cause of chronic disability. Venography is still the "gold standard" for definitive diagnosis of DVT but is rarely needed now, as duplex color Doppler ultrasonography has become the study of choice for detection of DVT of the lower extremities. Venography is, therefore, used only when ultrasonography is inconclusive or when calf DVT is suspected. Ultrasound is not accurate in DVT of the calves. This is important only if DVT of the calves is going to be treated.

Pulmonary scintigraphy has been the traditional screening test for PE. The accepted concept is that a high-probability ventilation-perfusion (V/Q) scan showing multiple segmental defects of perfusion and normal ventilation is very suggestive of PE. In this category, about 87% of patients have PE confirmed at pulmonary arteriography. Furthermore, a normal V/Q scan virtually rules out PE; however, it has been reported that 5% to 10% of patients in this category have PE at pulmonary arteriography. Thus, the majority of patients undergoing lung scanning have either indeterminate or intermediate scan findings. The incidence of PE at pulmonary arteriography in this group of patients is about 30%. Finally, about 10% to 20% of patients with low-probability scans are found by pulmonary arteriography to have PE.[46–49]

The conventional treatment of DVT (and its complication, PE) has been systemic heparin therapy for 7 to 10 days followed by anticoagulation with oral warfarin (Coumadin) for 3

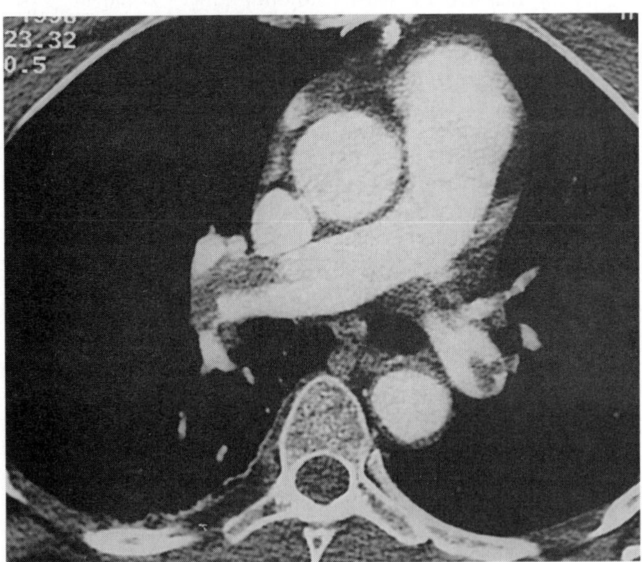

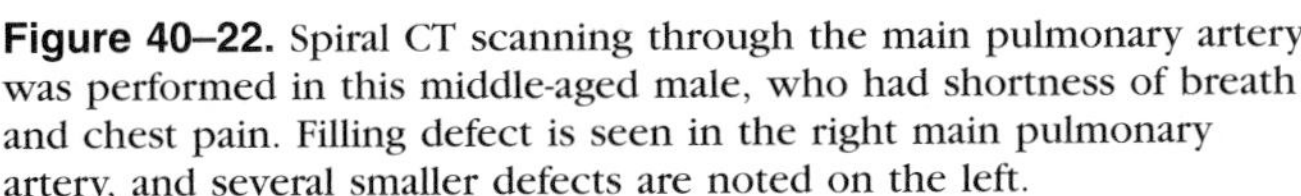

Figure 40–22. Spiral CT scanning through the main pulmonary artery was performed in this middle-aged male, who had shortness of breath and chest pain. Filling defect is seen in the right main pulmonary artery, and several smaller defects are noted on the left.

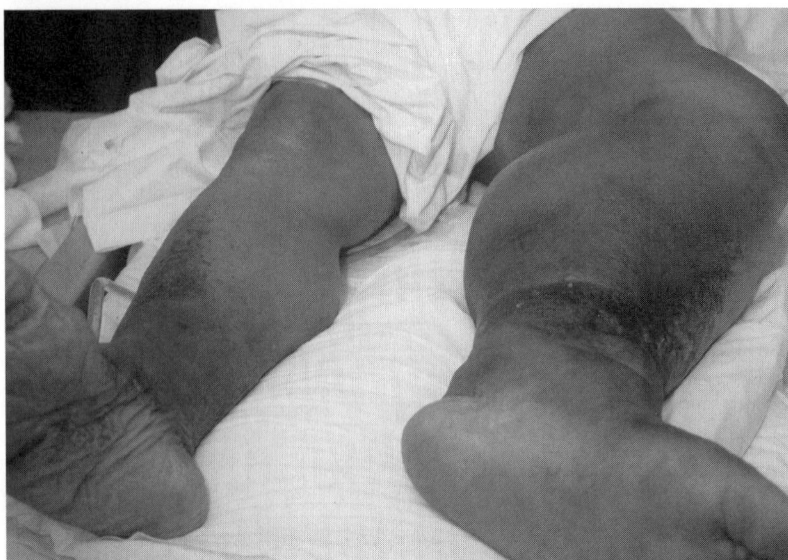

Figure 40–23. A young African American man presented with acute, severe, diffuse, painful swelling and discoloration of the left lower extremity. The diagnosis of phlegmasia cerulea dolens was made. Aggressive transcatheter fibrinolytic therapy resulted in eventual salvage of the leg.

months or more. More recently, low-molecular-weight heparin is being used successfully in a selected group of patients. The treatment of DVT has not changed significantly since the 1960s, and even though it is still the treatment of choice, as many as two thirds of patients with iliofemoral DVT eventually have a post-thrombotic syndrome leading to chronic disability. An uncommon but serious emergency of iliofemoral DVT is phlegmasia cerulea dolens (Fig. 40–23), compromise to the arterial supply of the limb secondary to venous disease. Interventional radiologists have a critical role in the management of this entity, as catheter-directed fibrinolytic therapy is now the treatment of choice (Fig. 40–24). Dramatic results have been obtained in this serious complication of DVT.

Complications of heparin therapy occur in as many as 10% to 20% of patients. Oral anticoagulation with warfarin is also associated with a significant rate of complications, increasing in proportion to the duration of the therapy (i.e., the longer the therapy, the higher is the risk of complications). Hemorrhagic complications occur in about 30% of patients who take Coumadin for 2 years or longer.

In addition to heparin therapy, surgical thrombectomy, embolectomy with suction catheter devices and balloon catheters, and local and systemic fibrinolysis are accepted treatments for massive PE with cardiopulmonary collapse. More recently, multiple mechanical thrombectomy instruments have been added to the armamentarium of the radiologist. The Amplatz thrombectomy device is now approved by the U.S. Food and Drug Administration and is safe to be used in native vessels such as the pulmonary arteries. Other instruments are being developed for the same purposes.

In treating DVT, anticoagulation prevents new thrombus formation or stops the progression of existing thrombi, but it does not eradicate already formed thrombi. Thrombolytic therapy with urokinase, on the other hand, either systemically or locally lyses the existing clot. Local low-dose fibrinolytic therapy has been used in a selected group of patients with massive PE, with spectacular results. Systemic fibrinolytic therapy is also effective, but is associated with a significant rate of hemorrhagic complications; thus, it is no longer administered (Fig. 40–25).

The placement of filters in the inferior vena cava (IVC) is a well-established procedure to manage or prevent PE.[50] It is well known that for many patients anticoagulation is contraindicated. In addition, some patients develop recurrent PE despite adequate anticoagulation. Others who are critically ill are at risk for DVT and PE, and prophylaxis against PE is desirable. Therefore, interruption of the IVC is the procedure of choice to manage these patients (Fig. 40–26). Furthermore, most patients being treated with heparin for massive DVT still require interruption of the IVC, as heparin does not lyse already formed thrombus and the risk of PE is high.

Other vascular problems can be managed successfully with interventional radiologic techniques. Effort thrombosis of central veins can be lysed with urokinase followed by PTA. Sometimes stents can be placed in residual stenoses. In the future, perhaps stent-grafts may be used in some cases, but venous thrombosis of the stent-graft is a problem that needs to be solved. At this time, the use of stent-grafts for venous disease remains controversial. Other vascular lesions such as AVMs and AVFs cause serious disability in critical patients and are lesions that can be managed by interventional radiologists (Fig. 40–27).[51]

In conclusion, prevention of PE is the goal of management of DVT. Early diagnosis and treatment of DVT prevent serious consequences. Vascular and interventional radiologists have major roles in the management of critically ill patients with DVT and PE.

BRONCHIAL ARTERY EMBOLIZATION FOR MASSIVE HEMOPTYSIS

Massive hemoptysis (defined as bleeding of 300 to 600 mL in 24 hours) is a rare but life-threatening condition that requires emergent management. Mortality is 50% to 80%, usually as a result of asphyxiation rather that exsanguination. A single expectoration can contain 500 mL of blood. Hemoptysis almost always originates from hypertrophy of the bronchial arteries (90% of the cases). Rupture of the bronchial arteries into the lung parenchyma results in massive hemoptysis. Rupture of a mycotic aneurysm of a pulmonary artery is occasionally the cause. Pulmonary AVMs and AVFs are rare causes of massive hemoptysis.[52-55] The most common underlying causes are tuberculosis and other granulomatous diseases, cystic fibrosis (especially in young patients), and bronchiectasis. Carcinoma of the lung and fungal infections are causes in older persons.

Most patients with massive hemoptysis have poor respiratory reserve and so are very poor surgical candidates. Furthermore, surgery requires lung resection, making the borderline

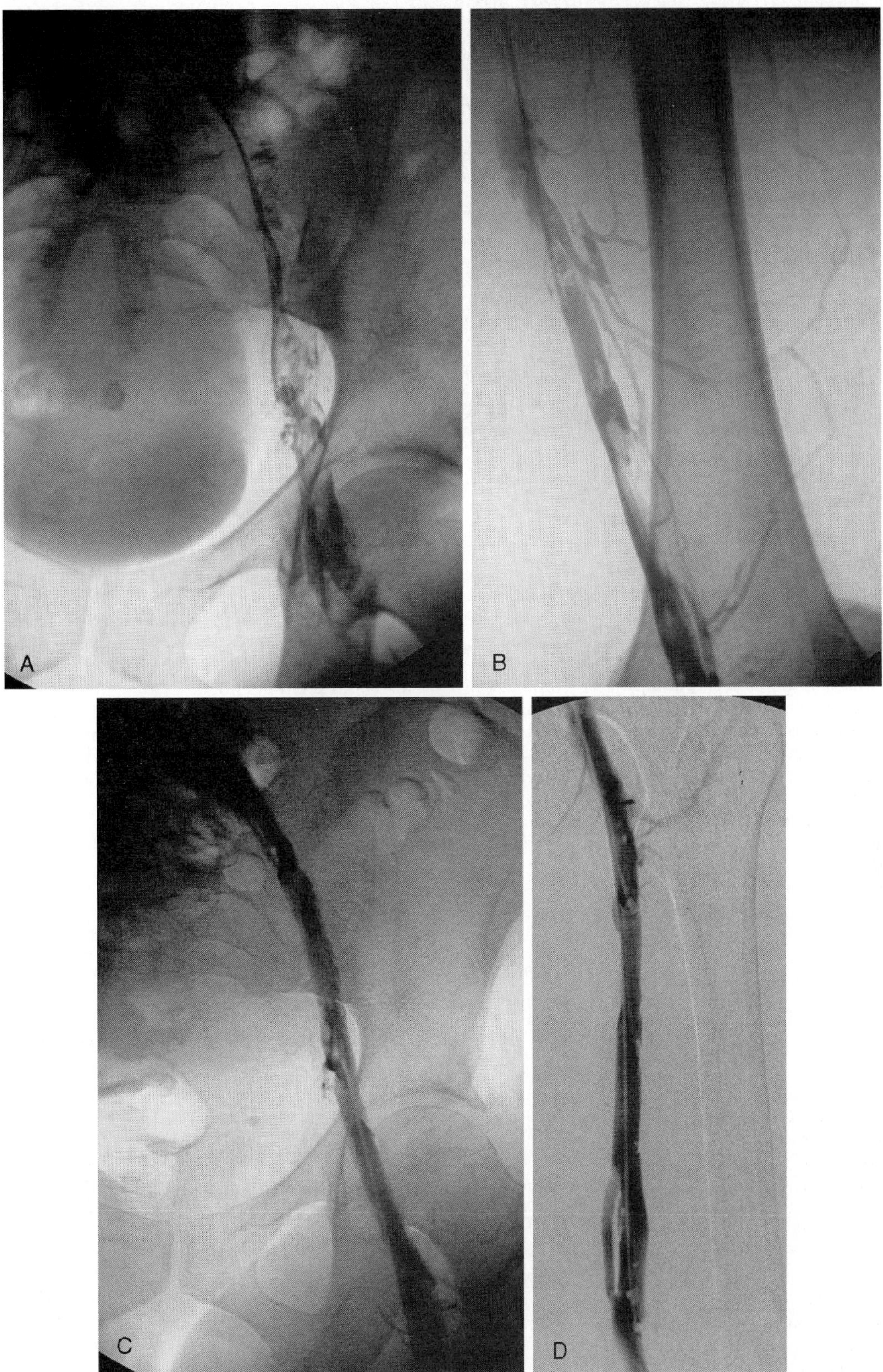

Figure 40–24. This young man presented with acute, severe, diffuse, painful swelling of the left lower extremity. *A* and *B,* A venogram was performed by insertion of a catheter in the extensive thrombus of the entire left lower extremity. A contralateral right common femoral vein approach was used to insert a No. 5 French infusion catheter. Full recovery was obtained after 48 hours of urokinase infusion. *C* and *D,* The venogram shows spectacular resolution of extensive deep venous thrombosis.

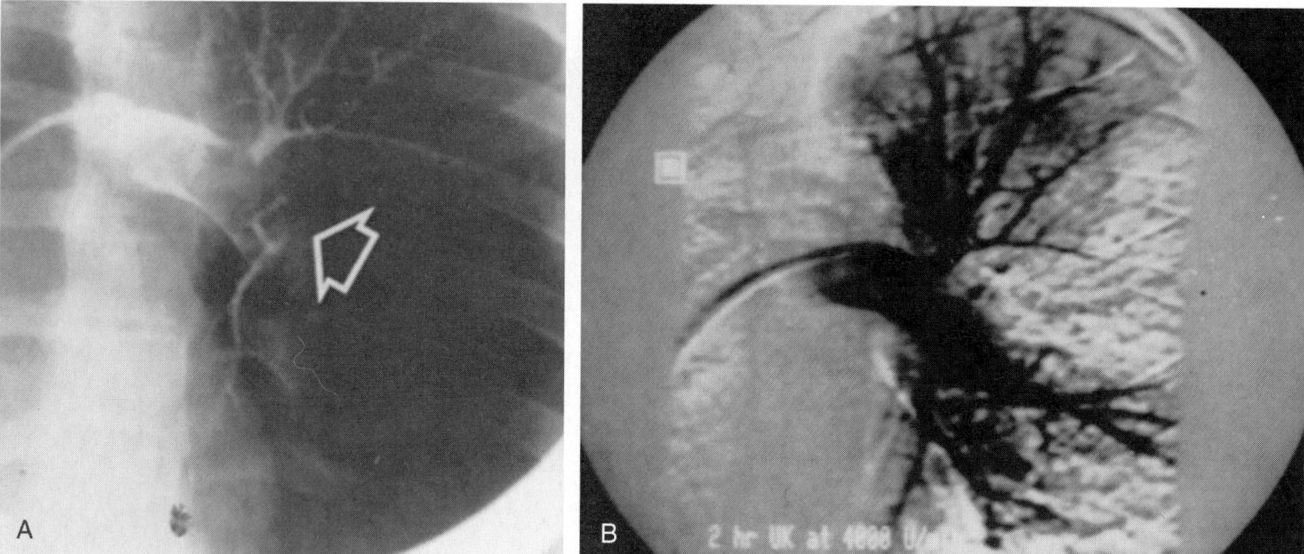

Figure 40–25. A young woman presented with shortness of breath and severe cardiorespiratory deficit. *A,* Complete occlusion of the left main pulmonary artery due to massive embolism is noted *(arrow). B,* Excellent recanalization was achieved after 2 hours of local, low-dose infusion of urokinase through a catheter placed in the emboli.

respiratory reserve even worse. Therefore, bronchial artery embolization is the ideal therapy for these critically ill patients.

In the work-up of patients with massive hemoptysis, the initial imaging study is chest radiography, followed by CT. Frequently this suffices to localize bleeding to a lobe. Bronchoscopy is mandatory, unless it is unavailable or is unfeasible because of the patient's condition. In addition, balloon occlusion of the uninvolved bronchus can be performed as a lifesaving procedure, to prevent asphyxiation.

Interventional radiologic management consists of selective bronchial arteriography followed by embolization of the bronchial arteries. The authors prefer Gelfoam and Ivalon particles to embolize peripheral arteries. Very rarely, stainless steel coils or platinum microcoils are used to occlude the arteries proximally (Fig. 40–28); however, this proximal occlusion may preclude future embolization, should rebleeding occur, and thus is not recommended.

Thorough knowledge of bronchial arterial anatomy is important, as there are many variations. Arteriography usually begins with thoracic aortography with the aim of identifying the origins of the bronchial arteries and enlargement, if any, of other systemic arteries supplying the affected areas. The

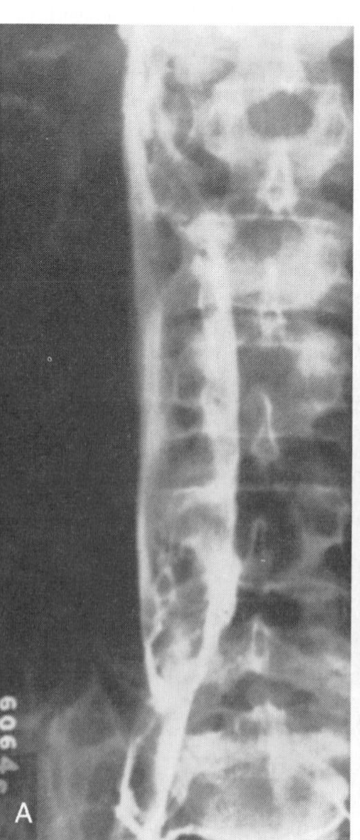

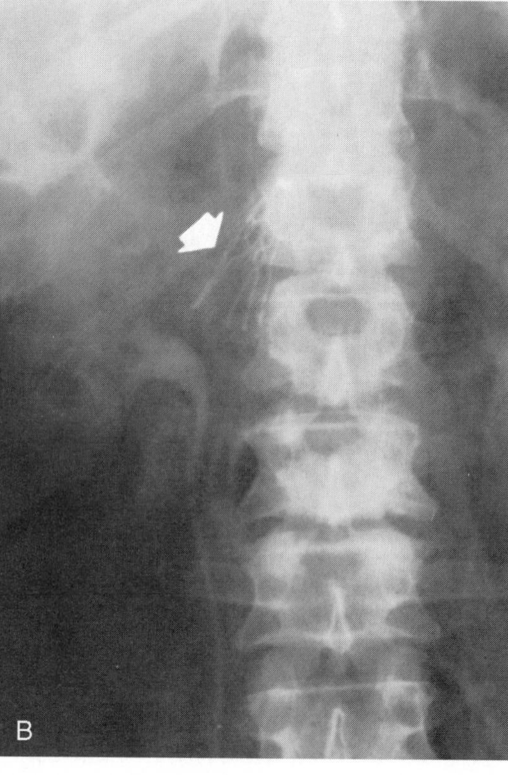

Figure 40–26. *A,* Massive thrombosis of the inferior vena cava to the level of the renal veins is demonstrated. *B,* A Greenfield filter was placed in the suprarenal portion of the inferior vena cava *(arrow).*

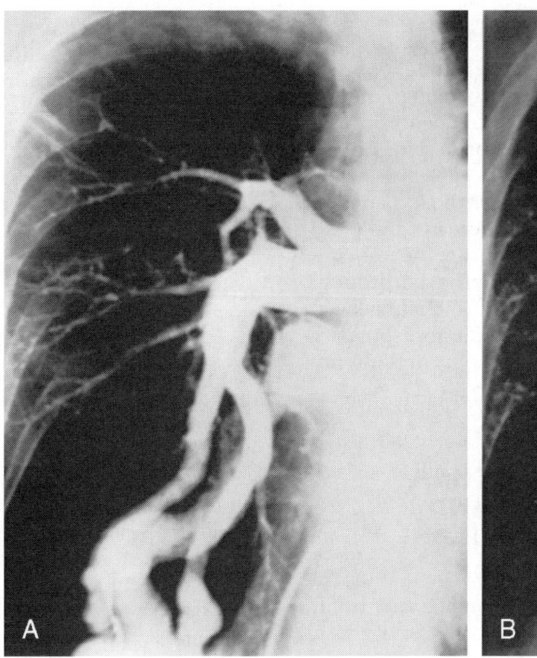

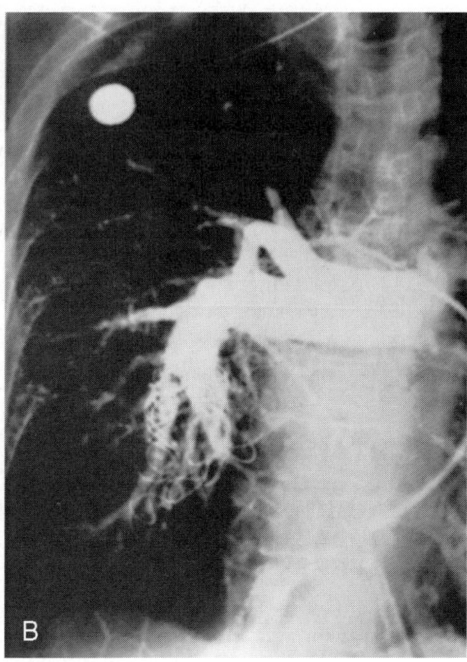

Figure 40–27. An elderly woman presented with severe cyanosis, which had been present since childhood. *A,* A pulmonary arteriogram shows a huge arteriovenous malformation (AVM) fed by two large arteries and drained by a dilated vein. *B,* Embolization with about 30 stainless steel coils, ranging from 5 to 10 mm in size, resulted in complete obliteration of the AVM. Recovery was uneventful. The cyanosis subsided immediately.

bronchial arteries originate from the anterior or anterolateral aspect of the thoracic aorta at the level of T3 to T8 vertebrae. There are four common anatomic variations: (1) two left and one right, prevalence (41%); (2) one right and one left (21%); (3) two left and two right (21%), and (4) one left and two right (10%). The bronchial arteries can originate together with the intercostal arteries in some patients. The artery of Adamkiewicz can originate from the left bronchial arteries or the intercostal arteries at the level of T5 to L3 and usually takes a hairpin turn. Identification of this artery is critical, as, on occasion, embolization is contraindicated because of the high risk of permanent spinal cord injury.[55]

Gelfoam particles are the most frequently used agent for embolizing benign lesions. For malignant processes, permanent materials such as Ivalon are preferred. Other agents—powders, liquids (alcohol), glues—should not be used because of the high risk of peripheral bronchial necrosis. Embolization is highly effective, controlling hemoptysis in 80% to 90% of patients; recurrence rates are 10% to 15%. Technical success of the procedure is about 98% to 99% in the authors' experience (see Fig. 40–28).

The major complications include permanent spinal cord injury (about 1% of cases). Bronchial infarction is rare. Peripheral embolization can be avoided with careful technique. Transient myelitis is uncommon and usually subsides with conservative treatment.

In conclusion, bronchial artery embolization is a safe and highly successful procedure to control life-threatening hemoptysis in critically ill patients and is associated with few complications.

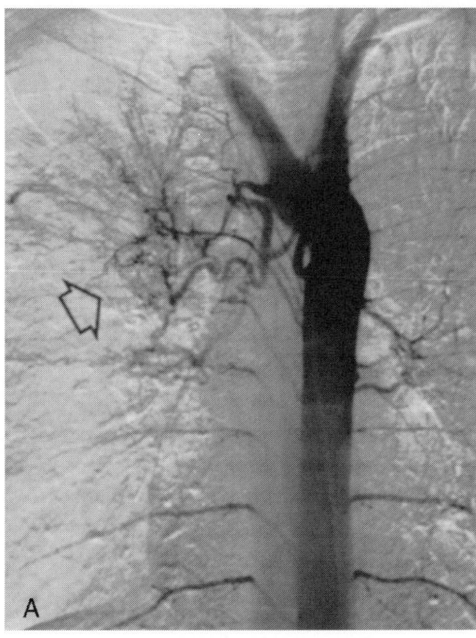

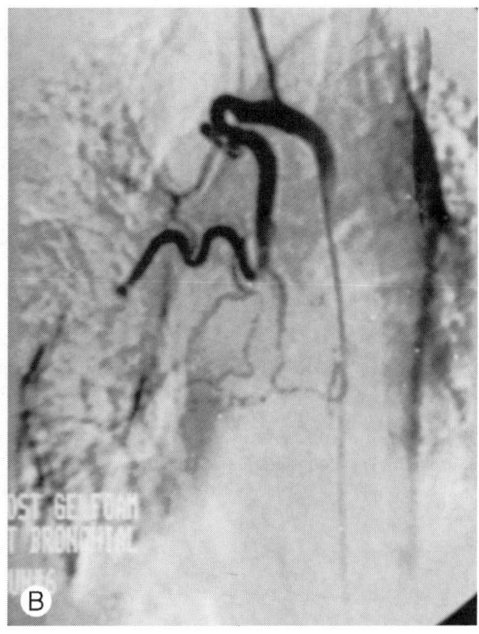

Figure 40–28. A young man with cystic fibrosis presented with massive hemoptysis. Bronchoscopy showed right-sided bleeding. *A,* A thoracic aortogram shows marked enlargement of right bronchial arteries *(arrow).* A selective right bronchial arteriogram (not shown) demonstrated marked tortuosity and hypertrophy of bronchial artery branches. *B,* After embolization with gelatin sponge (Gelfoam) and polyvinyl alcohol particles, there is complete obliteration of the arteries. The hemorrhage stopped and did not recur.

TRACHEOBRONCHIAL STENTING

Critically ill patients with severe disability due to tracheobronchial stenoses and dyskinesias secondary to malignancies, chronic fibrotic diseases, or restenosis at the tracheobronchial anastomoses are very difficult to manage. Shortness of breath is very incapacitating and can result in death.

With the advent of metallic stents some of those patients, particularly those with stenoses due to carcinoma of lung and postoperative stenoses after lung transplant, are now being treated with placement of Wallstents in the affected bronchi or trachea. We have treated patients with tracheomalacia, with spectacular results. Dramatic improvement in respiratory symptoms is immediate. In many patients our preliminary results are very encouraging (Fig. 40–29).

PERCUTANEOUS RETRIEVAL OF CATHETER FRAGMENTS AND OTHER IATROGENIC FOREIGN BODIES AND MANIPULATION OF INTRAVASCULAR CATHETERS

Rupture and embolization of catheter fragments and other intravascular foreign bodies, such as filters, stents, and wires, and formation of knots in catheters, thrombus formation, and catheter malpositioning are serious complications of percutaneous catheterization techniques. Significant morbidity and a mortality rate as high as 75% have been reported when embolized catheters are not removed. Major complications include thrombosis, sepsis, arrhythmias, myocardial necrosis, myocardial perforation, pericardial tamponade, endocarditis, and pulmonary thromboembolism. If the catheter fragments are removed, however, full recovery is expected (Fig. 40–30).[10]

In the past, surgery was the only way to remove embolized catheters or intravascular foreign bodies. Because embolized catheters usually become lodged in the cardiac chambers or pulmonary arteries, removal by surgical means involves a major operation. With advances in angiographic techniques, removal of embolized catheter fragments and other intravascular foreign bodies, repositioning of malpositioned catheters, unknotting of knotted catheters, and stripping of clotted catheters are relatively simple procedures, done with low risk, on an outpatient basis, in a short time.[57] In the authors' experience, they can be accomplished in 10 to 15 minutes.[11]

Continuous electrocardiographic and pulse oximetry monitoring, and vital signs assessments are mandatory during attempts at retrieval. Arrhythmias, perforation of vessels or cardiac chambers, and myocardial or endothelial damage may occur during retrieval. A variety of instruments can be used. The authors have used many combinations of nitinol gooseneck loops, retrieval baskets, Curry loop snares, deflector wires, different types of angiographic catheters, grasping and alligator forceps, and others.

Migration of the fragments or foreign bodies peripherally into the pulmonary arteries makes removal almost impossible. Cardiac arrhythmias are common and can be prevented with intravenous lidocaine. Perforation of major vessels or cardiac chambers is a serious but rare complication.

In conclusion, vascular and interventional radiologists use different techniques to retrieve intravascular catheter fragments and other iatrogenic foreign bodies, unknot catheters, and reposition and strip central venous catheters. A major operation that could include open-heart surgery is avoided. These procedures are quick, simple, safe, and highly effective.

ACUTE TRAUMA

Trauma is the third most frequent cause of death in young people in the United States. It is the most common cause of death in those aged 15 to 45 years. In the United States, more than 100,000 people die of trauma-related causes every year. More people die of trauma in 1 year than died in the Vietnam and Korean Wars together, yet little emphasis has been placed on the diagnostic and interventional aspects of trauma.

The authors' institution is a level I trauma center, which requires the presence of emergency medicine physicians, an-

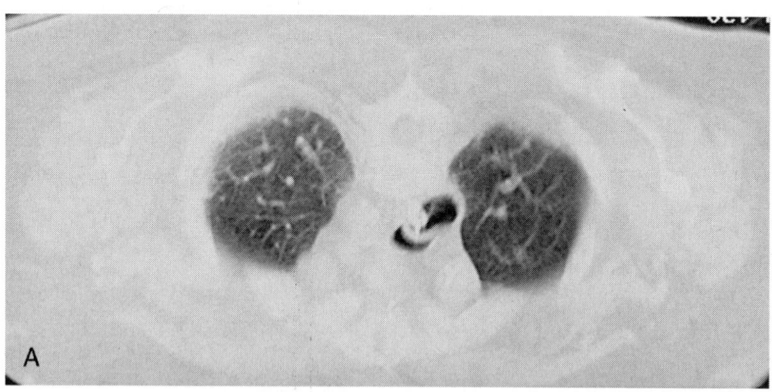

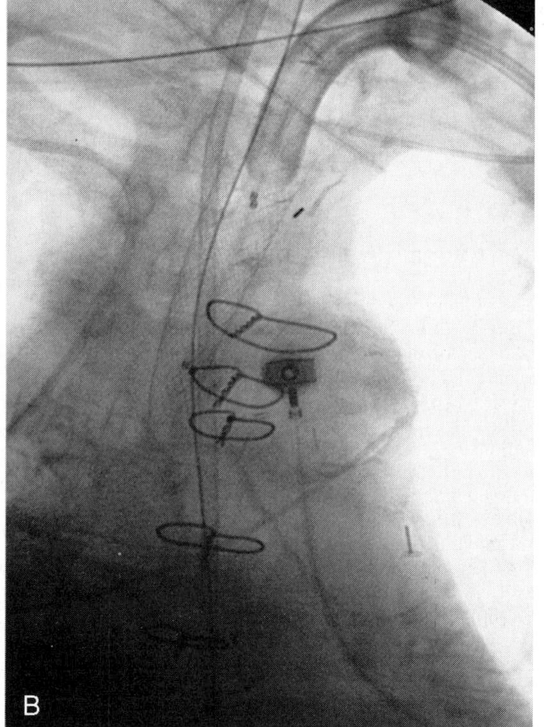

Figure 40–29. An elderly woman presented with acute respiratory distress. At bronchoscopy, significant tracheomalacia was found. *A,* A CT scan of the chest showed marked functional narrowing of the trachea; therefore, tracheal stenting was performed. *B,* A wire was inserted in the trachea, and a 24 × 70 mm Wallstent was released. Extreme care was taken to avoid placement of the stent over the vocal cords. Note the basket-weave appearance to the stent just below the tracheostomy tube.

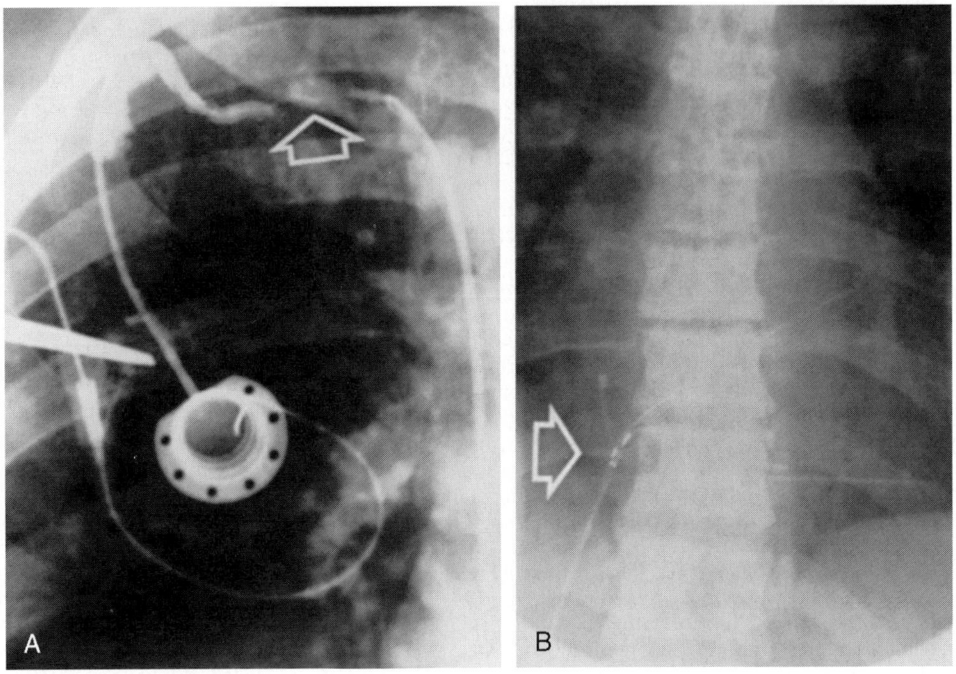

Figure 40–30. A portable catheter was placed in the subclavian vein for chemotherapy in a young woman. *A,* A few weeks later, the catheter became broken at its entrance into the subclavian vein *(arrow).* The fragment embolized to the right atrium. *B,* During catheter retrieval, the foreign body was snared with a retrieval basket and removed in less than 10 minutes *(arrow).*

esthesiologists, and trauma surgeons 24 hours a day, 7 days a week. In addition, radiologists must be available for immediate diagnostic and therapeutic consultation. Technologists experienced in diagnostic radiology, angiography, neuroradiology and body imaging (CT, ultrasonography) must be readily available. Equipment required includes CT, ultrasonography, radionuclide scanning, and vascular and interventional radiology laboratories. This novel method of management of acutely traumatized patients has resulted in significant decreases in morbidity and mortality and faster recovery, despite the increasing rate and severity of the trauma.

Only three or four radiographs, including lateral cervical spine, chest, abdomen, and pelvis views, are necessary in the emergency department for the initial assessment and triage of acutely and severely traumatized patients. Thereafter, patients may undergo CT scanning in the emergency department. The availability of spiral CT in emergency radiology departments has enhanced greatly the work-up of trauma patients. We can now perform full-body CT in a few minutes in the emergency department, with minimal transfer of patients. Thereafter, patients may go to the radiology department for an emergency radiologic or angiographic exploration or to the operating room for emergency surgical exploration.[58, 59]

In some institutions, ultrasonography is used for triage purposes in lieu of spiral or conventional CT, but the accuracy of ultrasonography is limited, and sometimes findings are misleading. Rapid and appropriate triage is important for reduction of morbidity and mortality.[58, 59] A new specialty, emergency radiology is being developed in a few major trauma centers in the United States. In addition, the emergency department is now staffed by physicians with special training in emergency medicine, a relatively new specialty with a bright future.

Angiographic intervention is the definitive treatment for severe injuries in some instances. On other occasions, a necessary operation can be postponed until a later date, when the patient's clinical condition has stabilized. The angiographic intervention is frequently adjunctive to surgery and enables a major operation to be replaced by a minor or at least a less extensive one. It is the authors' belief that an operation performed only to control hemorrhage in a severely traumatized patient is unnecessary and even contraindicated or detrimental to their well-being, when the bleeding can be controlled with an angiographic intervention. Moreover, surgical intervention frequently involves ligation of major arterial branches to control bleeding, thus precluding future angiographic interventions, as the access routes may already be occluded.[58, 59]

Head and Neck Trauma

The diagnostic and interventional management of traumatic vascular lesions of the head and neck is evolving continuously. The topic is mentioned here only because it is the domain of interventional neuroradiologists and is not relevant to this chapter. A new subspecialty, interventional neuroradiology or surgical neuroradiology, is being developed. We hope that, as more people are trained in newer techniques, they will have major roles in treating victims of head and neck trauma, with its devastating consequences. It is well-known that thousands of victims are affected by a true epidemic costing billions of dollars for health care and rehabilitation.

Chest Trauma

About 25% of patients sustaining acute trauma die of chest injuries. Acute traumatic rupture of the thoracic aorta and brachiocephalic arteries is a catastrophic automobile accident injury. Although about 80% to 90% of patients die at the scene of the accident, some 10% to 20% survive the initial episode and present in the emergency department for radiologic evaluations. Only 5% of undiagnosed patients are alive 4 months later, and eventually a chronic pseudoaneurysm occurs. A chest radiograph is usually obtained in the emergency department to seek signs of mediastinal bleeding. Unfortunately, the vast majority of chest radiographs obtained in the emergency department are of suboptimal quality and show many abnormalities that are nonspecific or misleading. Furthermore, the chest radiograph may appear normal in 5% to 10% of patients with aortic rupture.

Spiral CT is emerging as the study of choice for screening blunt trauma to the chest. Its current role is to evaluate for mediastinal hematoma. If CT is negative (i.e., does not show mediastinal bleeding) aortography may not be necessary. If CT is "positive," aortography should be performed immediately. This protocol has significantly decreased the number of negative aortograms. Some clinicians also use transesophageal echocardiography (TEE) to check for mediastinal blood. It is important to emphasize that neither CT nor TEE has been shown to be an adequate substitute for aortography. Furthermore, the nature of the injury must dictate the need for aortography. Finally, aortography is very simple, quick, and safe and must be used without reservation when rupture of the aorta needs definitively to be ruled out.

The most common site of rupture is the aortic isthmus (Fig. 40–31).[58, 60] Ruptures of the ascending aorta are usually fatal and, therefore, are not seen at arteriography. Rupture of the brachiocephalic arteries occurs in about 15% of patients in our experience. With good-quality studies, false-positive results are extremely rare.

Penetrating injuries to the chest are common in the authors' patient population. Total or partial transection to the brachiocephalic, internal mammary, and intercostal arteries, among others, can occur. Emergent arteriography usually demonstrates occlusion of the vessel lumen, pseudoaneurysms, or AVF. Extravasation of contrast material is not commonly seen, owing to spasm and retraction of the vessel. Interventional radiologic management with embolization prevents possible catastrophic bleeding as soon as the thrombus lyses or the spasm subsides and obviates difficult operations. Routinely, embolization of the involved arteries utilizes Gelfoam, stainless steel coils, or platinum microcoils.[58, 61]

Abdominal Trauma

Both blunt and penetrating trauma to the abdomen are frequent in this era of high-speed, sometimes drunken, driving, gunshot trauma, and other violent behavior. The spleen is the solid organ most often injured; often the liver is injured as well (Fig. 40–32). Injuries to hollow viscera are less common. Usually, patients are taken to surgery for exploratory laparotomy. Then, they may be returned to Radiology for exploratory arteriography (Fig. 40–33). Embolization is very effective in controlling arterial bleeding from solid and hollow organs and in stopping the (very rare) lumbar arterial bleeding, which is very difficult to detect at exploratory laparotomy. Major operations to control hemorrhage must be avoided (Fig. 40–34).[56, 58, 62]

Pelvic Trauma

Blunt pelvic trauma is a common result of high-speed, aggressive, or drunken driving. Pelvic fractures can lead to life-threatening bleeding because of the proximity of pelvic arteries to the bony pelvis. Pelvic arteriography and embolization of the bleeding arteries (usually branches of the internal iliac arteries) is the management of choice for pelvic trauma. It is impossible to predict the presence or degree of pelvic hemorrhage based on plain radiography. CT is emerging as a screening method for pelvic lesions; however, it is well known that the severity of the fractures does not predict the character of the hemorrhage. Patients with severe pelvic fractures can have minor pelvic bleeding and, conversely, those with minor fractures can have life-threatening hemorrhage.

Control of pelvic bleeding must be achieved with angiography rather than surgery. Surgery usually involves ligation of the internal iliac arteries and does not control bleeding, because the hemorrhage usually originates from small peripheral branches, and collateral circulation is extensive, particularly in young patients. Furthermore, ligation of the internal iliac

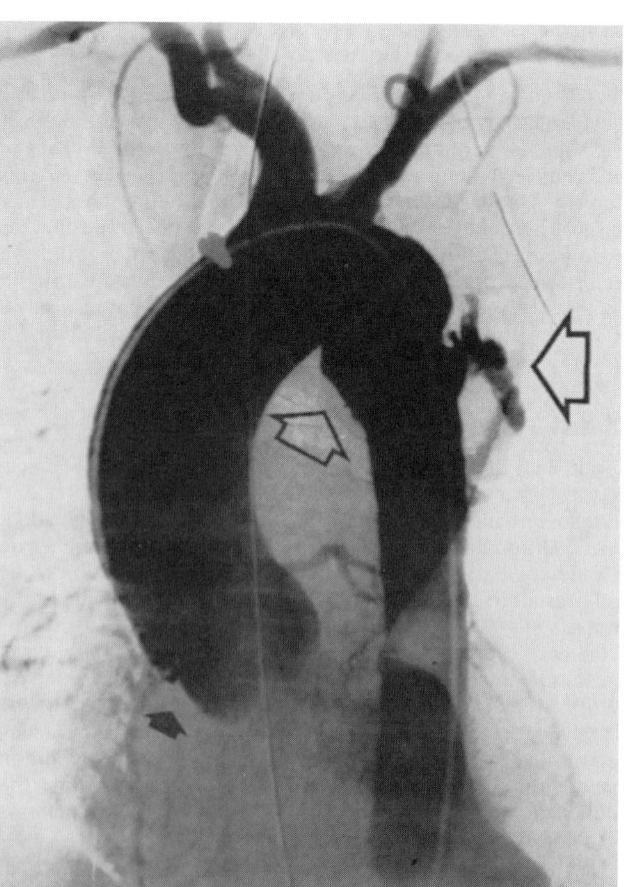

Figure 40–31. Thoracic aortogram of a middle-aged man involved in a head-on car collision shows a pseudoaneurysm at the level of the aortic isthmus. Extravasation of contrast material *(arrows)* as well as an intimal injury in the ascending aorta *(small arrow)* is also noted. Subsequently, the patient died.

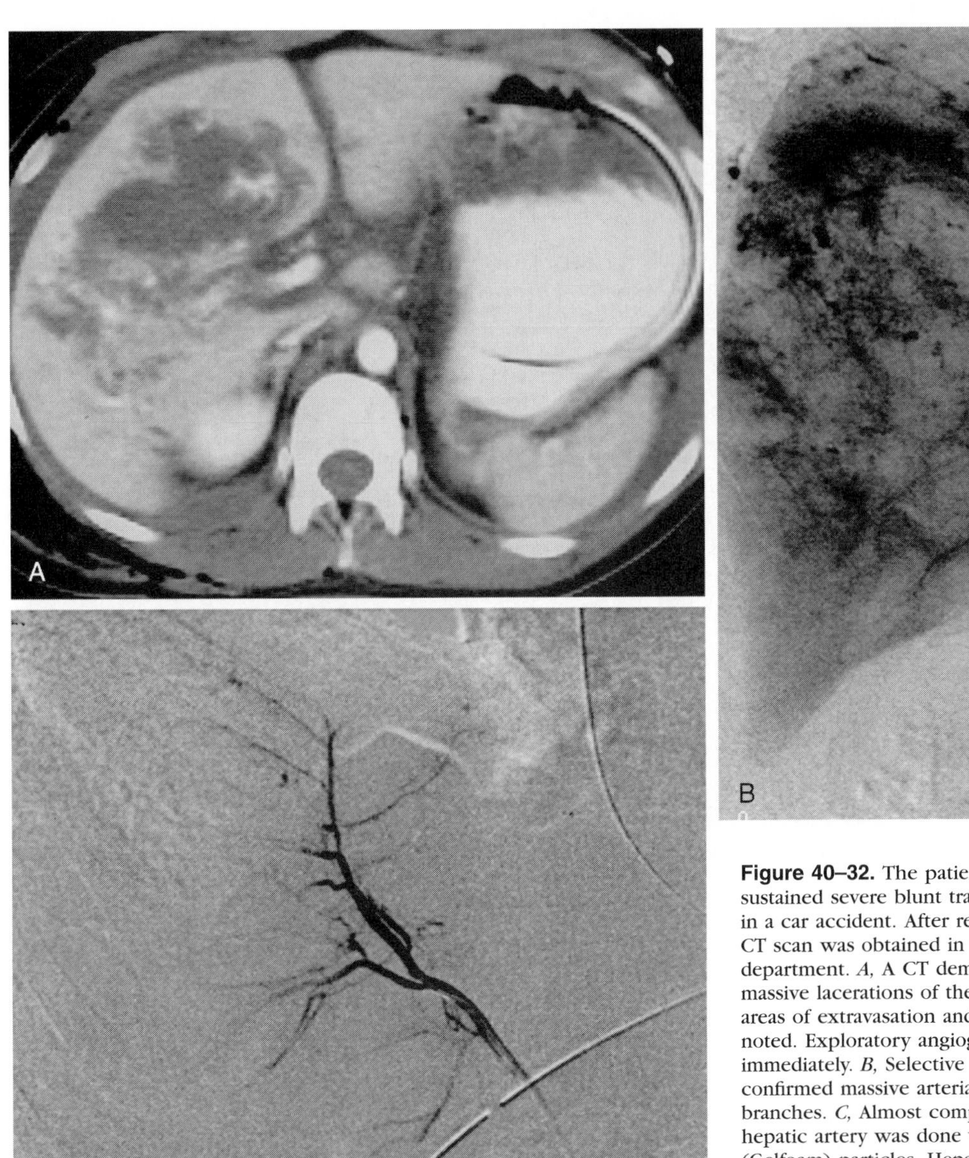

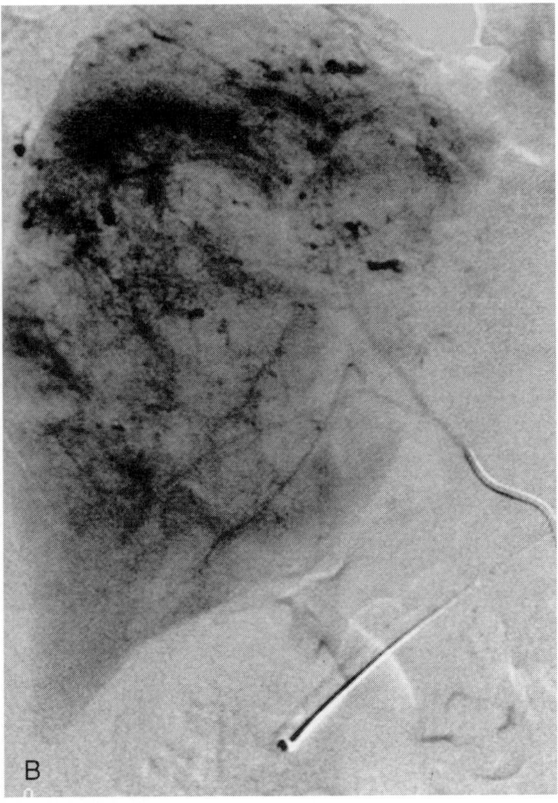

Figure 40–32. The patient is a young woman who sustained severe blunt trauma to the abdomen and pelvis in a car accident. After resuscitation, an emergency spiral CT scan was obtained in the emergency radiology department. *A,* A CT demonstrates hemoperitoneum and massive lacerations of the right lobe of the liver. Several areas of extravasation and intraparenchymal hematoma are noted. Exploratory angiography was performed immediately. *B,* Selective right hepatic arteriography confirmed massive arterial bleeding from myriad small branches. *C,* Almost complete embolization of the right hepatic artery was done with absorbable gelatin sponge (Gelfoam) particles. Hepatic bleeding stopped immediately. Because the patient's condition was extremely unstable for surgery, exploratory angiography was the ideal management.

arteries precludes future angiographic intervention. Thus, in this situation surgery is detrimental rather than therapeutic.[63] Gelfoam is the preferred agent for embolization because it is temporary and recanalization occurs in a few weeks or months. On occasion, the authors have used stainless steel coils for central occlusion after achieving peripheral embolization with Gelfoam. We prefer not to embolize the trunks of the internal iliac arteries, so that repeat embolization can be performed, if necessary (Fig. 40–35).

Extremity Trauma

Blunt and penetrating trauma to the limbs are frequent and can injure arteries that lie close to bony structures. The brachial and popliteal arteries are more prone to injury. Duplex color Doppler ultrasonography is the noninvasive method used to evaluate these patients when they exhibit none of the classic signs of arterial injury. Arteriography is necessary with expanding hematoma, bruit or thrill, acute bleeding from the wound, and diminished pulses or none. Arteriography is frequently positive in this setting. Arteriography performed only to determine "proximity" of a vessel to the site of injury yields very few useful findings.

Arteriographic management of extremity vascular injuries is safe and effective. Operations performed specifically to control hemorrhage are unnecessary and must be abandoned. In this situation, transcatheter embolotherapy of bleeding arteries is the management of choice.[64]

At the present time the role of stent-grafts in the management of acute traumatic injuries to peripheral arteries is evolving. A very promising role for stent-grafts in trauma to major arteries is anticipated. AVFs and pseudoaneurysms can readily be controlled with embolization. Furthermore, arteriography can be used to screen suspected vascular injuries not detected by noninvasive methods. Surgical exploration is avoided when arteriographic findings are negative and surgical exploration can be guided by the angiographic findings.[65]

In conclusion, vascular and interventional radiologists are

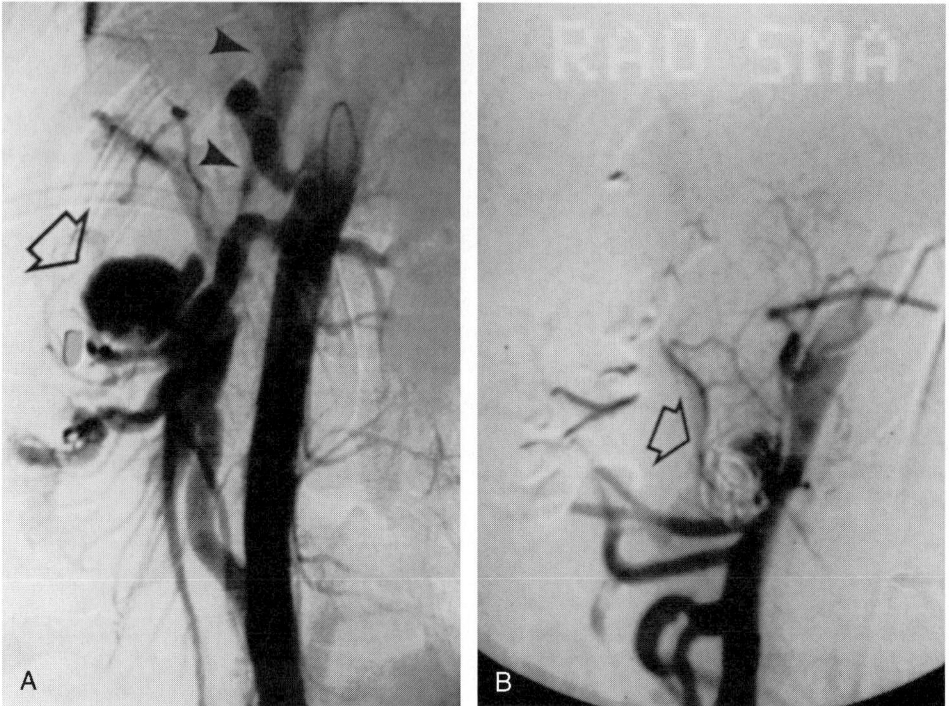

Figure 40–33. A young man sustained a bullet wound to the abdomen. *A,* An abdominal aortogram obtained 2 weeks after surgical exploration shows a large pseudoaneurysm from the superior mesenteric artery *(arrow)* associated with an arteriovenous fistula with the superior mesenteric vein and early opacification of the portal vein *(arrowheads)*. *B,* After embolization with absorbable gelatin sponge (Gelfoam) particles and several stainless-steel coils, a superior mesenteric arteriogram shows obliteration of the arteriovenous fistula and pseudoaneurysm *(arrow)*.

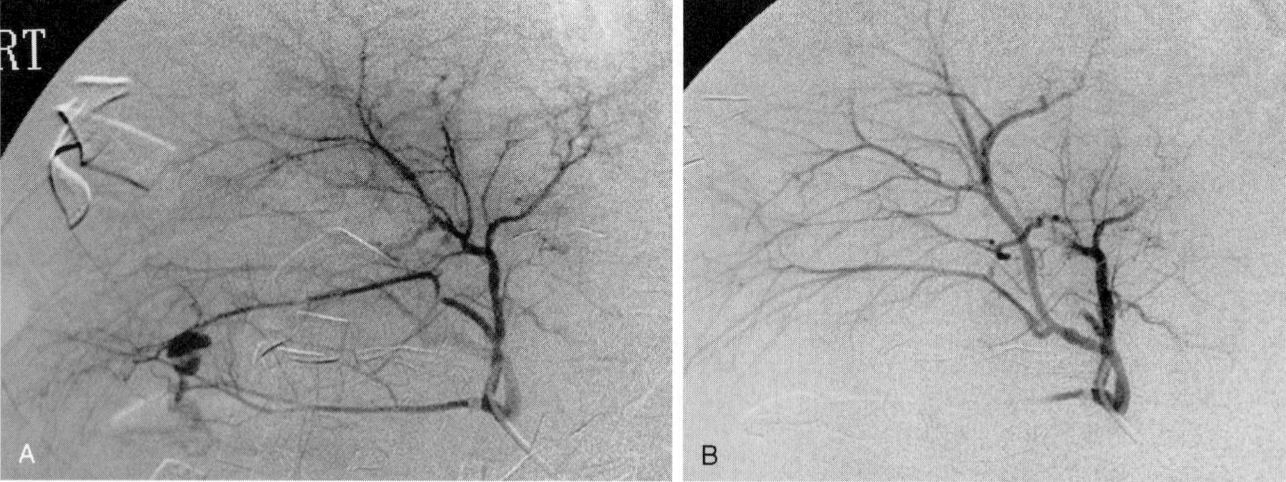

Figure 40–34. The patient, a young man who was stabbed in the abdomen, underwent exploration, and several lacerations were sutured. Despite this measure, bleeding continued. *A,* Hepatic arteriography demonstrated significant bleeding from one of the branches to the inferior segment of the right lobe. *B,* Selective embolization with absorbable gelatin sponge (Gelfoam) controlled the bleeding. The patient became stable and recovered.

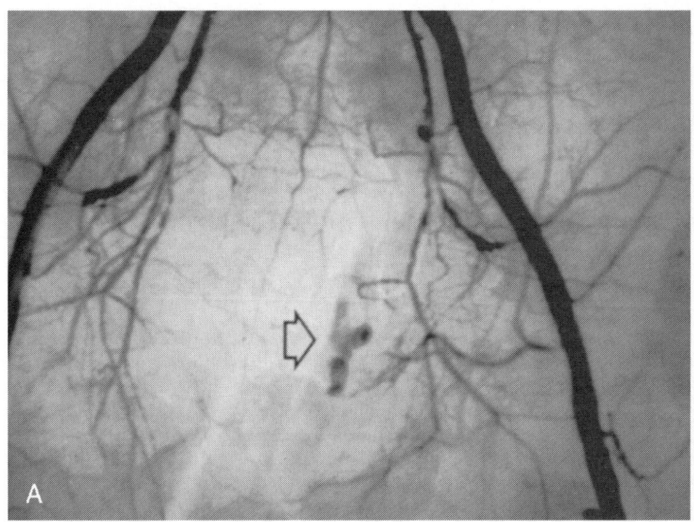

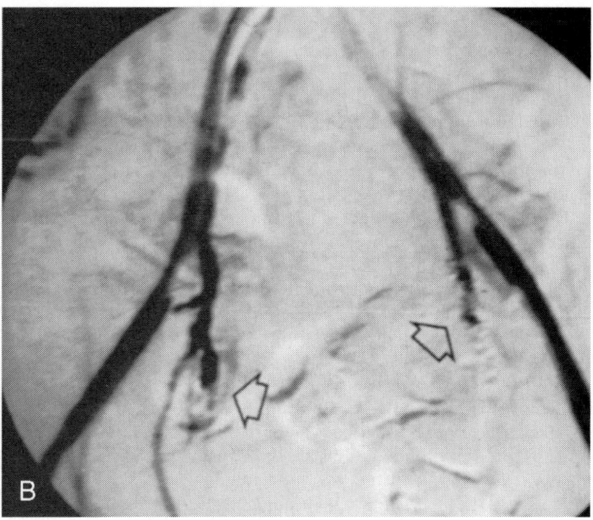

Figure 40–35. Pelvic arteriogram of a young woman involved in a severe automobile accident. *A,* Extravasation of contrast material from branches of the internal iliac arteries is evident *(arrows). B,* Both internal iliac arteries were embolized with several absorbable gelatin sponge (Gelfoam) particles *(arrows).* The patient recovered fully after a protracted hospitalization.

very important members of the management team for polytrauma patients who have arterial injuries to their extremities. In selected patients, angiographic management improves the outcomes. Severely traumatized patients must be cared for in level I trauma centers.

References

1. Kollef MH, Canfield DA, Zuckerman GR: Triage considerations for patients with acute gastrointestinal hemorrhage admitted to a medical intensive care unit. Crit Care Med 1995; 23:1048–1054.
2. Kadir S, Ernst CB: Current concepts in angiographic management of gastrointestinal bleeding. Curr Probl Surg 1983; 20:287–343.
3. Winzelberg GC, McKusick KA, Froelich JW, et al: Detection of gastrointestinal bleeding with ^{99m}Tc-labeled red blood cells. Semin Nucl Med 1982; 12:139–146.
4. Rahn NH, Tishler JM, Han SY, et al: Diagnostic and interventional angiography in acute gastrointestinal hemorrhage. Radiology 1982; 143:361–366.
5. Chau TN, Patch D, Chan YN, et al: "Salvage" transjugular intrahepatic portosystemic shunt: Gastric fundal compared with esophageal variceal bleeding. Gastroenterology 1998; 114:981–987.
6. Haskal ZJ, Scott M, Rubin RA, et al: Intestinal varices: Treatment with the transjugular intrahepatic portosystemic shunt. Radiology 1994; 191:183–187.
7. Bell SD, Lau KY, Sniderman KW: Synchronous embolization of the gastroduodenal artery and inferior pancreaticoduodenal artery in patients with massive duodenal hemorrhage. J Vasc Interv Radiol 1995; 6:531–536.
8. Toyoda H, Nakano S, Takeda I, et al: Transcatheter arterial embolization for massive bleeding from duodenal ulcers not controlled by endoscopic hemostasis. Endoscopy 1995; 27:304–307.
9. Messina LM, Shanley CJ: Visceral artery aneurysms. Surg Clin North Am 1997; 77:425–442.
10. Stambo GW, Hallisey MJ, Gallagher JJ Jr: Arteriographic embolization of visceral artery pseudoaneurysm. Ann Vasc Surg 1996; 10:476–480.
11. Cho SR, Tisnado J, Beachley MC, et al: Percutaneous unknotting and repositioning of intravascular catheters and percutaneous retrieval of embolized catheter fragments and other iatrogenic foreign bodies. *In:* Emergency Interventional Radiology. Neal MP, Tisnado J, Cho SR (Eds). Boston, Little, Brown & Co, 1989, pp 249–278.
12. Denny DF: Placement and management of long-term central venous access catheters and ports. AJR Am J Roentgenol 1991; 161:385–393.
13. Dake MD, Semba CP, Enstrom RJ, et al: Percutaneous treatment of venous occlusive disease with stents. J Vasc Interv Radiol 1993; 4:42–46.
14. Hood DB, Yellin AE, Richman MF, et al: Hemodialysis graft salvage with endoluminal stents. Am Surg 1994; 10:733–737.
15. Leroy AJ: Percutaneous nephrostomy: Techniques and instrumentations. *In:* Clinical Urology. Pollack HM (Ed). Philadelphia, WB Saunders, 1990, pp 2725–2738.
16. Farrell TA, Hicks ME: A review of radiologically guided percutaneous nephrostomies in 303 patients. J Vasc Interv Radiol 1997; 8:769–774.
17. Newman TS, Magnuson TH, Ahrendt SA, et al: The changing face of mesenteric infarction. Am Surg 1998; 64:611–616.
18. Wojtowycz M: Interventional Radiology and Angiography. St. Louis, Mosby-Year Book, 1990, pp 110–112.
19. Mathias K: Angiographic management of intestinal ischemia. *In:* Interventional Radiology. Dondelinger RF, Rossi P, Kurdziel JC, et al (Eds). New York, Thieme, 1990, pp 645–652.
20. Yamkado K, Takeda K, Nomura Y, et al: Relief of mesenteric ischemia of Z-stent placement into the superior mesenteric artery compressed by the false lumen of an aortic dissection. Cardiovasc Intervent Radiol 1998; 21:66–68.
21. McNamara TO, Bomberger RA, Merchant RF: Intra-arterial urokinase as the initial therapy for acutely ischemic lower limbs. Circulation 1991; 83(Suppl I): I-106–I-119.
22. Clouse ME, Stokes KR, Perry LJ, et al: Percutaneous intraarterial thrombolysis: Analysis of factors affecting outcome. J Vasc Interv Radiol 1994; 5:93–100.
23. Wojtowycz M: Percutaneous angioplasty, recanalization, and vascular stents. *In:* Interventional Radiology and Angiography. St. Louis, Mosby-Year Book, 1990, pp 162–188.
24. Palmaz JC, Laborde JC, Rivera FJ, et al: Stenting of the iliac arteries with the Palmaz stent: Experience from a multicenter trial. Cardiovasc Interv Radiol 1992; 15:291–297.

24a. Uflacker R, Robinson JG, Brothers TE, et al: Abdominal aortic aneurysm treatment: Preliminary results with the Talent Stent-graft system. J Vasc Interv Radiol 1998; 9:51–60.

25. Tisnado J, Bartol DT, Cho S-R, et al: Low-dose fibrinolytic therapy in hand ischemia. Radiology 1984; 150:375–382.
26. Tegtmeyer CJ, Kellum CD, Ayers C: Percutaneous transluminal angioplasty of the renal artery: Results and long-term follow-up. Radiology 1984; 153:77–84.
27. Rundback JH, Gray RJ, Rozenblit G, et al: Renal artery stent placement for the management of ischemic nephropathy. J Vasc Interv Radiol 1998; 9:413–420.
28. Hennequin LM, Joffre FG, Rousseau HP, et al: Renal artery stent placement. Radiology 1994; 191:713–719.
29. Smith EH: Complications of percutaneous fine-needle biopsy. Radiology 1991; 178:253–258.
30. Charboneau JW: US-guided biopsy. *In:* A Categorical Course in Diagnostic Radiology. Interventional Radiology, Syllabus, Radiological Society of North America, December 1–6, 1991. Mueller PR,

van Sonnenberg E, Becker GJ (Eds). Oak Brook, Ill, Radiological Society of North America, 1991, pp 9–16.

31. Strom SC, Fisher RA, Thompson MT, et al: Hepatocyte transplantation as a bridge to orthotopic liver transplantation in terminal liver failure. Transplantation 1997; 63:559–569.
31a. Schumacher IK, Okamoto T, Kim BH, et al: Transplantation of conditionally immortalized hepatocytes to treat hepatic encephalopathy. Hepatology 1996; 24(2):337–343.
32. Kurdziel JD, Dondelinger RF: Intraperitoneal fluid collections. *In:* Interventional Radiology. Dondelinger RF, Rossi P, Kurdziel JC, et al (Eds). New York, Thieme, 1990, pp 102–130.
33. Picus D, Marx MV: Peritoneal cavity, percutaneous drainage of intra-abdominal abscesses and fluid collections. *In:* Current Practice of Interventional Radiology. Kadir S (Ed). Philadelphia, BC Decker, 1991, pp 572–577.
34. Wojtowycz M: Interventional Radiology and Angiography. St. Louis, Mosby-Year Book, 1990, pp 309–340.
35. Wittich GR, van Sonnenberg E, Simeone JF: Results and complications of percutaneous biliary drainage. Semin Intervent Radiol 1985; 2:39–49.
36. Malone DE: Interventional radiologic alternatives to cholecystectomy. Radiol Clin North Am 1990; 28:1145–1156.
37. Hashizume M, Sugimachi K, MacFayden BV: The clinical management and results of surgery for acute cholecystitis. Semin Laparosc Surg 1998; 5:69–80.
38. Born P, Rosch T, Bruhl K, et al: Long-term results of endoscopic treatment of biliary duct obstruction due to pancreatic disease. Hepatogastroenterology 1998; 45:833–839.
39. Hausegger KA, Thurnher S, Bodendorfer G, et al: Treatment of malignant biliary obstruction with polyurethane-covered Wallstents. AJR Am J Roentgenol 1998; 170:403–405.
40. Kandarpa K: Percutaneous gastrostomy and gastrojejunostomy tube placement. *In:* Handbook of Cardiovascular and Interventional Radiologic Procedures. Kandarpa K (Ed). Boston, Little, Brown, & Co., 1989, pp 125–130.
41. Ho C-S, Gray RR, Goldfinger M: Percutaneous gastrostomy for jejunal feeding. Radiology 1985; 156:349–351.
42. McLoughlin RF, So B, Gray RR: Fluoroscopically guided percutaneous gastrostomy: Current status. J Can Assoc Radiol 1996; 47:10–15.
43. Garg K, Welsh CH, Feyerabend AJ, et al: Pulmonary embolism: Diagnosis with spiral CT and ventilation-perfusion scanning—correlation with pulmonary angiographic results or clinical outcome. Radiology 1998; 208:201–208.
44. Cross JJ, Kemp PM, Walsh CG, et al: A randomized trial of spiral CT and ventilation perfusion scintigraphy for the diagnosis of pulmonary embolism. Clin Radiol 1998; 53:177–182.
45. Mago JR, Remy-Jardin M, Muller NL, et al: Pulmonary embolism: Prospective comparison of spiral CT with ventilation-perfusion scintigraphy. Radiology 1997; 205:447–452.
46. Gurney JW: No fooling around: Direct visualization of pulmonary embolism. Radiology 1993; 188:169–620.
47. Gresham CL: Deep venous thrombosis. South Med J 1993; 86:438–440.
48. Dalen JE, Alpert JS: Natural history of pulmonary embolism. Prog Cardiovasc Dis 1975; 17:259–270.
49. Alderson PO, Martin EC: Pulmonary embolism: Diagnosis with multiple imaging modalities. Radiology 1987; 164:297–312.
50. Greenfield LJ, Proctor MC: Endovascular methods for caval interruption. Semin Vasc Surg 1997; 10:310–314.
51. Coldwell M, Stokes KR, Yakes WF: Embolotherapy: Agents, clinical applications, and techniques. RadioGraphics 1994, 14:623–643.
52. Mauro MA, Jaques PF, Morris S: Bronchial artery embolization for control of hemoptysis. Semin Intervent Radiol 1992; 9:45–51.
53. Najarian KE, Morris CS: Arterial embolization in the chest. J Thorac Imaging 1998; 13:93–97.
54. Hartnell CG: Embolization in the treatment of acquired and congenital abnormalities of the heart and thorax. RadioGraphics 1993; 13:1349–1362.
55. Uflacker R, Keammerer A, Neves C, et al: Management of massive hemoptysis by bronchial artery embolization. Radiology 1983; 146:627–634.
56. Ben-Menachem Y, Coldwell DM, Young JWR: Hemorrhage associated with pelvic fractures: Causes, diagnosis and emergent management. AJR Am J Roentgenol 1991; 157:1005–1014.
57. Egglin TK, Dickey KW, Rosenblat M, et al: Retrieval of intravascular foreign bodies: Experience in 32 cases. AJR Am J Roentgenol 1995; 164:1259–1264.
58. Ben-Manachem Y: Angiography in diagnosis of vascular trauma. *In:* Radiology: Diagnosis, Imaging, Intervention. Vol 2. Taveras JM, Ferrucci JJT (Eds). Philadelphia, JB Lippincott, 1988, pp 1–14.
59. Ben-Menachem Y: Logic and logistics of radiography, angiography and intervention in blunt trauma. Radiol Clin North Am 1981; 19:171–186.
60. Symbas PJ, Horsley WS, Symbas PN: Rupture of the ascending aorta caused by blunt trauma. Ann Thorac Surg 1998; 66:113–117.
61. Smith DC, Senal MO, Bailey LL: Embolotherapy of a ruptured internal mammary artery secondary to blunt chest trauma. J Trauma 1982; 22:333–335.
62. Hagiward A, Yukioka T, Ohta S, et al: Nonsurgical management of patients with blunt splenic injury: Efficacy of transcatheter embolization. Radiology 1991; 167:159–166.
63. Ben-Menachem Y: Radiology. *In:* Early Care of the Injured Patient. Moore EE (Ed). Philadelphia, BC Decker, 1990, pp 84–90.
64. Ohki T, Veith, EJ, Kraas C, et al: Endovascular therapy for upper extremity injury. Semin Vasc Surg 1998; 11:106–115.
65. Modrall JG, Weaver FA, Yellin AE: Diagnosis and management of penetrating vascular trauma and the injured extremity. Emerg Med Clin North Am 1998; 16:129–144.

41

Imaging of the Central Nervous System in the Critical Care Patient

Fred J. Laine, MD

MODALITIES

Plain Radiographs

Plain radiographs are rapid, inexpensive, and accurate but are of limited value in studies of the central nervous system (CNS). Although they are very useful in evaluating soft tissue abnormalities of chest, abdomen, and pelvis, plain radiographs are inadequate for evaluating the soft tissues of the head and spine. Their main usefulness, with respect to the CNS, lies in their accuracy in evaluating osseous integrity and alignment. Therefore, the plain radiograph is typically the first study obtained in the evaluation of traumatic injuries of the spine. Radiographs of the skull of a patient with head injury can demonstrate fractures, but they do not provide significant information about intracranial injury.

Computed Tomography

Computed tomography (CT) represents the most widely used imaging modality for evaluation of critical care patients with CNS disorders. It is widely available, rapid, and accurate and has relatively no contraindications in the acute setting. The clinical utility of CT is increased by multiple modifications, including contrast administration, window techniques, and various reconstruction techniques. Iodinated contrast agents are available for intravenous injection with CT. With their use, lesions that cause a breakdown in the blood-brain barrier as well as vascular structures, both normal and abnormal, enhance or "light up" on CT scans. Varying the gray-scale "window levels" permits evaluation of osseous structures with a wide window and soft tissue structures with a narrow window. Reconstructed images allow merger of easily obtained axial images to be reproduced in coronal or sagittal planes. Three-dimensional (3D) reconstructed CT images can be produced and rotated in any plane.

For a xenon-CT scan, the patient inhales xenon gas while sequential CT "cuts" are obtained; subsequently, xenon uptake is calculated. This technique is not widely available but is becoming an important diagnostic tool for measuring cerebral blood flow. CT angiography (CTA) eliminates the background tissue and allows visualization of vascular structures. Reconstruction of these images enables a noninvasive evaluation to be made of vascular structures.

Magnetic Resonance Imaging

Magnetic resonance (MR) imaging utilizes magnetic field gradients and radiofrequency pulses rather than the ionizing radiation employed by other imaging modalities. Continuous refinements in MR imaging sequence techniques have drastically reduced imaging time and improved conspicuity of pathologic changes. A gadolinium-based contrast agent can also be intravenously injected to enable better visualization of intracranial and intraspinal disease. MR angiography (MRA) sequences use the property of flowing spins to create an angiographic image. The methods available create greater signal intensity in flowing blood than in the surrounding stationary tissues. The images can be "reconstructed" in three dimensions to simulate a standard angiogram.

A wide variety of MR sequences are being investigated that are based on physiologic changes rather than anatomic changes. Functional MR imaging techniques are showing promise in (1) the detection and assessment of cerebral pathophysiology and (2) the characterization and regional mapping of distinct human cognitive functions, such as vision, motor skills, language, and memory.[1] Diffusion-perfusion MR imaging has the capability of measuring molecular diffusion and capillary flow and perfusion.[2]

The disadvantages of obtaining MR imaging for the evaluation of critical care patients rest on the preprocedural preparation and screening.[3] The modality is contraindicated in patients with pacemakers, certain cardiac valves, and intraocular metal fragments. Careful screening for the presence of cerebral aneurysm clips and other metallic devices, stents, and surgical devices is necessary to determine their compatibility with MR imaging. In addition, respirators and physiologic monitors must be MRI-compatible. Only oxygen and nitrogen tanks composed of aluminum can enter the MRI suite. Commonly, patients must be switched from an MRI-incompatible respirator to an MRI-compatible respirator before the procedure can take place. All of these precautions and modifications can significantly delay imaging in the acute setting. In addition, such basic medical instruments as stethoscopes, hemostats, and scissors must remain outside the MRI suite.

Angiography

Percutaneous transfemoral catheterization is used to evaluate the anatomy and integrity of the cerebral and spinal vasculature. Cerebral angiography is an invasive procedure and imposes some risk. The overall complication rate is 2% to 4%, with the majority of complications, such as groin hematoma, subintimal injections, and minor allergic reactions, being minor and transient.[4] The more severe complications, such as cerebral infarction, seizure, and death, are uncommon.

Although Doppler ultrasonography and MRA have made a significant impact on evaluation of cerebrovascular diseases, especially atherosclerotic disease, cerebral angiography is still considered the standard technique for this indication. In the acute setting, with intracranial hemorrhage, angiography is necessary to establish the presence of vascular malformations or aneurysms. In cases of trauma, angiography is used to evaluate vascular integrity.

Interventional neuroradiology has made great strides in the treatment of a variety of neurovascular lesions. Safer microcatheters and development of a wide variety of treatment options enable neuroradiologists to gain access to a lesion through preexisting vascular paths. Therapeutic neuroradiologic techniques that are now available include the following:

- Embolization of vascular tumors, aneurysms, and arteriovenous malformations (AVMs)
- Placement of stents
- Angioplasty
- Thrombolysis

IMAGING OF THE BRAIN

Patterns of Disease

Edema

Cerebral edema or brain swelling is caused by a localized or diffuse abnormal accumulation of water and sodium. It differs from cerebral engorgement, which is caused by vasodilatation or obstructed venous outflow. Both conditions lead to an increase in brain volume and are difficult to distinguish with routine imaging studies. Newer methods, such as xenon-CT and MR imaging with diffusion-weighted imaging (DWI), are useful in distinguishing between the two.

Three types of edema have been described:

1. *Vasogenic edema* is the result of increased capillary permeability and involves mainly the white matter. This type is most often associated with tumor, abscess, or trauma but can also be seen with infarct and ischemia.
2. *Cytotoxic edema* is the result of cellular swelling and involves both gray matter and white matter. Ischemia, anoxia, and hypo-osmolar states are the primary considerations.
3. *Interstitial edema* is the result of the migration of cerebrospinal fluid (CSF) into the periventricular white matter. This form of edema is secondary to conditions that impede CSF absorption, such as hydrocephalus.

Except for location, the imaging appearance of edema is similar for all types. On CT scans, increased water is seen as a decrease in density and appears dark. On MR images, an increase in water is seen as an area of decreased signal on T1-weighted images but as an area of increased signal on T2-weighted images. The three types appear as follows on MR images:

1. Vasogenic edema extends along the fingers of white matter interposed between areas of normal gray matter (Fig. 41-1); this pattern is in a nonvascular distribution and is often associated with mass effect.
2. Cytotoxic edema involves gray matter and white matter, and the decreased density extends uniformly to the calvarium; typically, this edema follows a vascular distribution and produces less mass effect for its size (Fig. 41-2).
3. Interstitial edema involves the periventricular white matter and appears as a fairly symmetric, low-density rim in the periventricular regions that masks the ventricular wall and gradually fades into the surrounding white matter.

Hemorrhage

Intracranial hemorrhage may be identified as parenchymal or extra-axial (epidural, subdural, and subarachnoid spaces) in location. Parenchymal hemorrhage can be traumatic in origin, but it is more likely to have nontraumatic origins in underlying disease, such as hypertension, neoplasm, or a vascular anomaly. Epidural and subdural extra-axial hemorrhage is most often a result of trauma. Subarachnoid hemorrhage is most com-

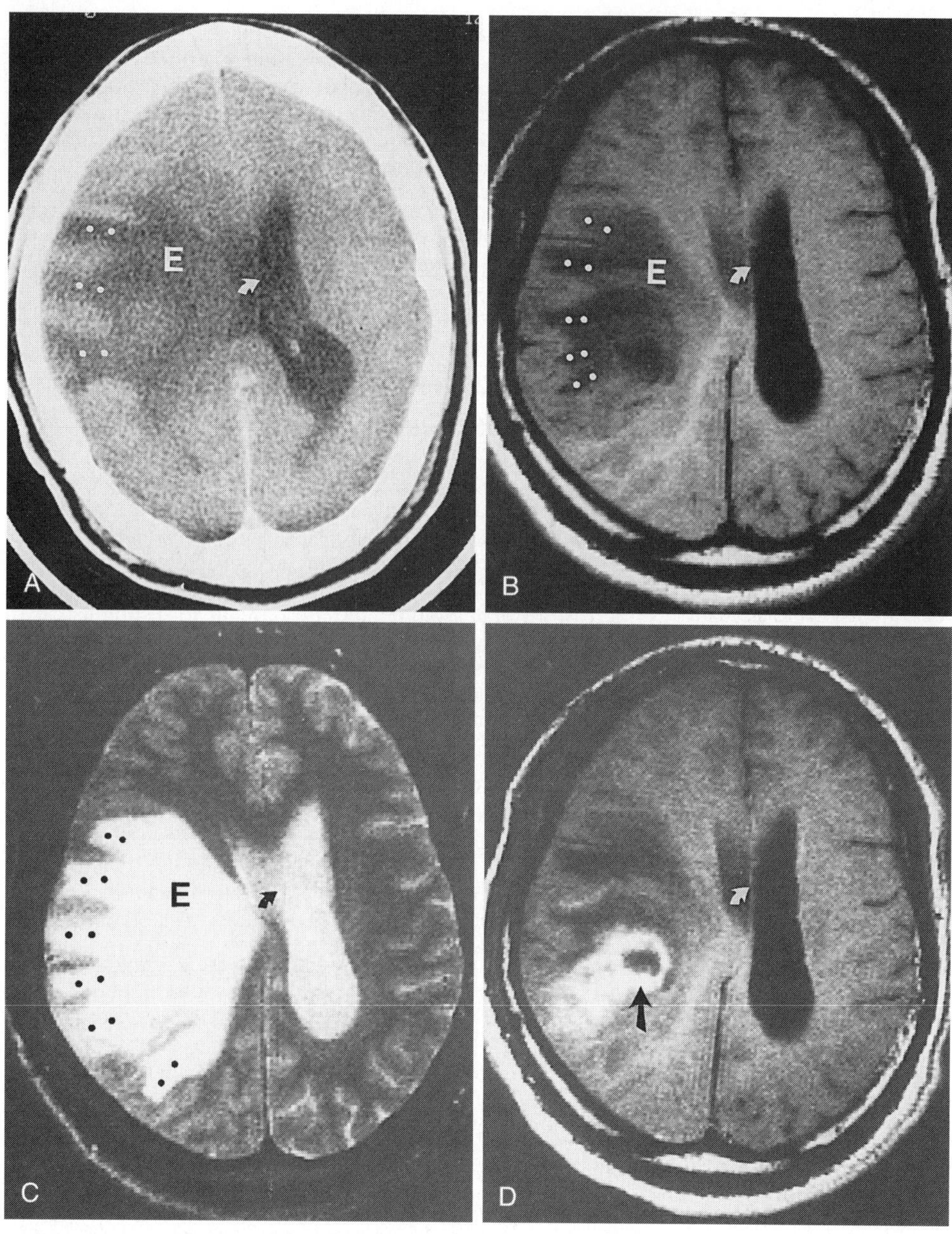

Figure 41–1. Vasogenic edema, glioblastoma. Noncontrasted axial CT image *(A)*, axial T1-weighted MR image *(B)*, and axial T2-weighted MR image *(C)* demonstrate an area of edema (E) on all images. The edema extends along the white matter fibers *(dots)* with normal gray matter interposed. *D*, Axial T1-weighted MR image following contrast enhancement demonstrates the enhancing tumor nidus *(arrow)* distinct from the surrounding edema. Subfalcine herniation is also demonstrated on these images *(curved arrows)*.

monly secondary to trauma but is also associated with a ruptured congenital aneurysm.

The appearance of hemorrhage on the image depends on the age of the hemorrhagic event with respect to the time of imaging. On CT, acute hemorrhage typically appears hyperdense because of the high hematocrit and globin component[5] (Fig. 41–3). This pattern may vary, however, with different clinical situations. Acute hematomas may be isodense with brain in patients who are anemic and whose hemoglobin level drops below 10 g/dL[6, 7] and in patients with a coagulopathy in whom clot retraction cannot be produced.[8] As hemorrhage resolves, the CT appearance also changes. Initially, as the clot retracts, the CT density may rise for 2 to 3 days after the initial event. Thereafter, the clot begins to liquefy and then resorb. The CT appearance demonstrates continuously decreasing density through an isodense stage between 1 and 6 weeks (depending on size) after the event, and finally reaches a hypodense stage. The final appearance of resolved hemorrhage on CT scanning may show no residual abnormality or may demonstrate a focus of low attenuation or calcification.[9]

The appearance of hemorrhage on the MR image is more complicated because of the varying paramagnetic properties of blood breakdown products. As hemorrhage resolves, fibrinolysis, leukocyte infiltration, hemoglobin denaturation, and changes in red blood cell (RBC) morphology interact to alter the MR appearance of hemorrhage at different stages.[10] The progression of resolution represents a continuum of changing intensity values and is not an all-or-none phenomenon. It progresses through the following stages (during resolution, these stages may be present simultaneously):

1. During the first 24 hours following parenchymal hemorrhage, intact RBCs containing oxyhemoglobin accumulate. Because the oxyhemoglobin is diamagnetic, it appears slightly hypointense to isointense on T1-weighted images and isointense to hyperintense on T2-weighted images.
2. Within 3 to 5 days, the hemoglobin becomes deoxygenated. The deoxyhemoglobin is paramagnetic and appears similar to oxyhemoglobin on T1-weighted images, but it is hypointense with brain on T2-weighted images (see Fig. 41–3*B* and *C*).
3. Between 3 and 7 days, intracellular methemoglobin be-

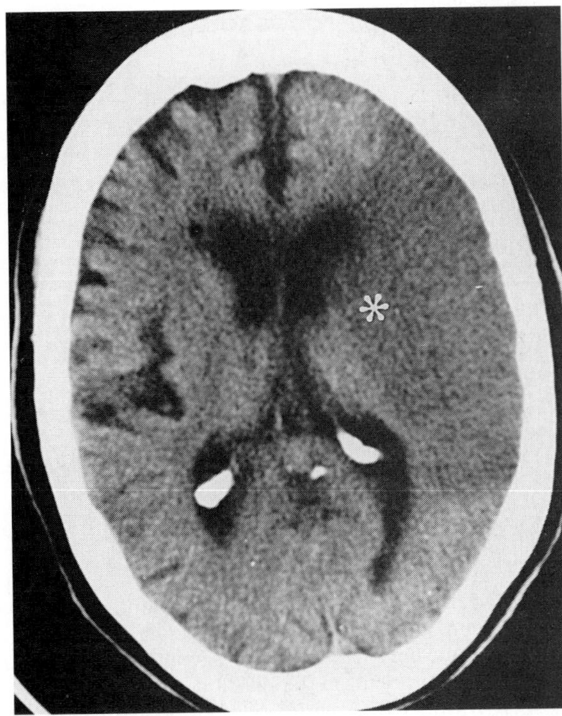

Figure 41–2. Cytotoxic edema, acute infarct. Axial noncontrasted CT image demonstrates an area of decreased density *(asterisk)* involving the left middle cerebral artery territory. Gray and white matter structures are involved, and there is little mass effect.

gins to accumulate, beginning peripherally and advancing toward the center of the clot. On T2-weighted images, the intracellular methemoglobin behaves similar to deoxyhemoglobin and remains hypointense, but now the T1 values begin to increase, causing the periphery of the clot to become hyperintense (see Fig. 41–3*B* and *C*).

4. Between 7 days and 2 to 3 months, the RBCs lyse and release methemoglobin into the extracellular space. During this stage, signal intensities on both T1-weighted and T2-weighted images increase. Hence, the hemorrhage is bright on both sequences (see Fig. 41–3*B* and *C*).

5. During the final stage, which may begin within 2 weeks and last for years, conversion of methemoglobin to hemosiderin occurs as a result of phagocytic degradation. Iron is removed from the hematoma and deposited at the periphery. Signal intensities again decrease, giving rise to hypointense signal on both T1-weighted and T2-weighted images.

Most hematomas are associated with a surrounding area of edema that can be misinterpreted as an additional area of hemorrhage. Like oxyhemoglobin, edema is hypointense to isointense in comparison with brain on T1-weighted images and hyperintense on T2-weighted images. The signal characteristics of edema remain constant, however, and gradually fade over time.

Mass Effect, Shift, and Herniation

Lesions that increase intracerebral mass may eventually cause brain herniation.[11] This may be the direct result of an enlarging lesion such as a tumor or the indirect result of a lesion such as the edema caused by a tumor. Two relatively fixed dural partitions within the skull create compartments across which brain substance may herniate. The falx cerebri separates the cerebral hemispheres, and the tentorium separates the cerebral hemispheres from the posterior fossa structures. Herniation is described in terms of location as follows:

Subfalcine herniation occurs when the medial surface of a hemisphere, usually the cingulate or supracingulate gyrus, is compressed against or displaced beneath the falx. With CT or MR imaging, early signs may be seen as compression or distortion of the lateral ventricles (see Fig. 41–1). Later stages are recognized from deviation of the falx and identification of the hemispheric structures that are crossing the midline.

Transalar herniation occurs when a mass, located in the frontal or temporal lobes, displaces brain tissue across the sphenoid ridge. When the mass arises in the temporal lobe

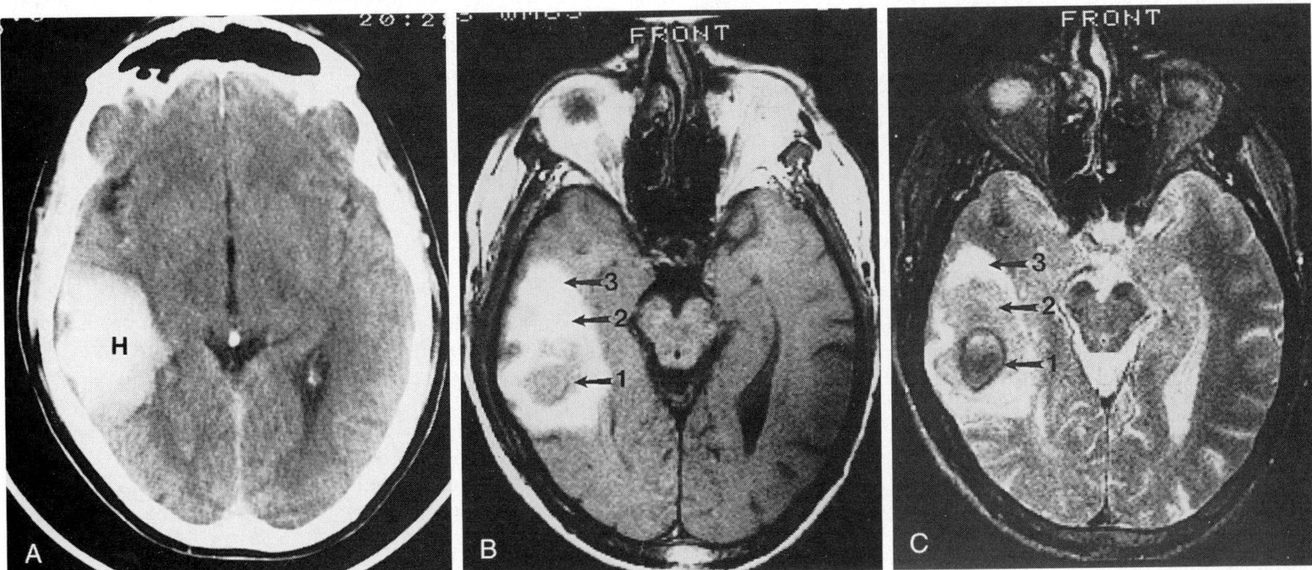

Figure 41–3. Hemorrhage. Axial CT image *(A)* demonstrates large area of hemorrhage in the right temporal lobe (H). T1-weighted MR image *(B)* and T2-weighted MR image *(C)* demonstrate the hemorrhage in various stages of breakdown. The center of the lesion is dark on the T1-weighted and T2-weighted images, indicating the oxyhemoglobin (1). The intermediate zone is bright on T1-weighted image and gray on the T2-weighted image, indicating intracellular methemoglobin (2). The outer rim is bright on both the T1-weighted and T2-weighted images, indicating extracellular methemoglobin (3).

and brain is displaced above the sphenoid ridge into the anterior cranial fossa, the result is termed *ascending* transalar herniation. When the mass arises in the frontal lobe and displaces brain inferiorly into the middle cranial fossa, the result is termed *descending* transalar herniation. With CT or MR imaging, the herniated brain can be identified directly or indirectly by detecting displacement of the sylvian portion of the middle cerebral artery.

Transtentorial herniation occurs when a mass arising on either side of the tentorium results in brain herniation through the tentorial incisura. *Descending* transtentorial herniation is caused by a supratentorial mass that displaces the medial temporal lobe through the incisura. On CT or MR imaging, the herniated brain pushes against and rotates the brain stem. This produces widening of the ipsilateral brain stem cistern and effacement of the contralateral cistern (Fig. 41-4). Associated findings include dilatation of the contralateral temporal horn secondary to ventricular trapping. *Ascending* transtentorial herniation is caused by an infratentorial mass that displaces the pons, vermis, and adjacent portions of the cerebellar hemispheres upward through the incisura. On CT and MR imaging, the brain stem cisterns are symmetrically effaced as the cerebellar vermis bulges up through the incisura. There is often associated acute hydrocephalus, caused by compression of the sylvian aqueduct.

Tonsillar herniation occurs when the cerebellar tonsils are pushed through the foramen magnum. This process results in medullary compression and dysfunction of the vital respiratory and cardiac control centers. Sagittal MR imaging is the primary modality for demonstrating tonsillar herniation and the secondary effects on the brain stem.

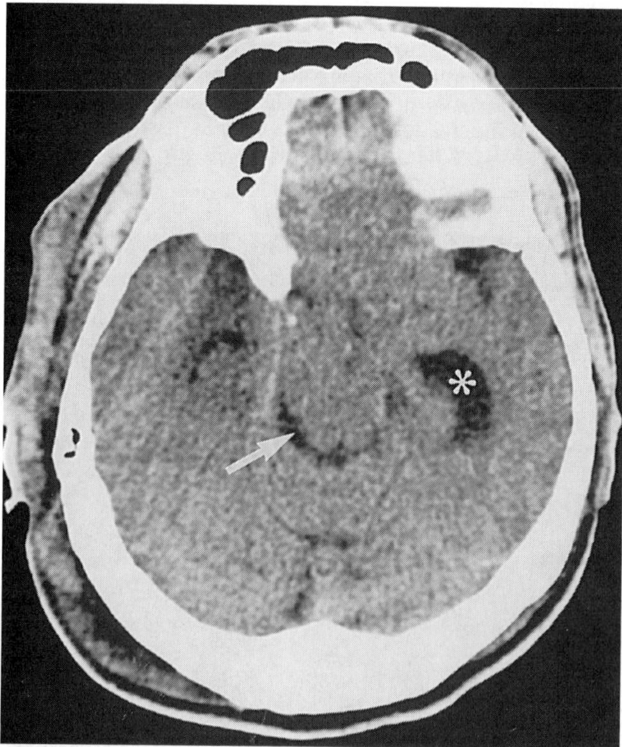

Figure 41–4. Right descending transtentorial herniation. Axial noncontrasted head CT scan at the level of the midbrain in a patient with a large right parietal subdural hematoma. The ipsilateral subarachnoid cistern is widened *(arrow),* and the contralateral subarachnoid cistern is obliterated because of brain stem rotation. The left temporal horn is also dilated *(asterisk),* indicating trapping of the left lateral ventricle.

Specific Disease Processes

Head Trauma

In patients with acute head injury, management decisions must be made rapidly. The critical issue is rapid, accurate detection of potentially treatable or surgically correctable lesions. In this regard, CT continues to be the primary modality in the initial evaluation of patients with head injury.[12] The advantages of CT include short examination time, wide availability, detection of fractures, lack of contraindications, and high accuracy.[13] Although MR imaging is more sensitive in detecting intracranial traumatic lesions, it is limited by longer examination time, lesser visualization of hyperacute hematomas, and difficulty of monitoring patients.[13]

For evaluation of chronic head injury, MR imaging is the modality of choice. It can be used to identify small foci of old hemorrhage and gliosis and to evaluate the presence and extent of diffuse axonal injury (shear injury) with greater sensitivity than CT.[14, 15]

Injury to brain parenchyma may result in contusion, axonal injury (shear), or hematoma. The imaging appearance of hematomas was described previously. *Contusions* are caused by the impact of parenchyma directly against bone and are most commonly seen along the gyral surface of the frontal and temporal lobes. *Shear injuries* are secondary to rotational forces that produce tears in axonal fibers and are most commonly seen within white matter tract (subcortical white matter, corpus callosum, internal capsule, and brain stem).

Except for location, the imaging characteristics of nonhemorrhagic contusions and shear injuries are similar. Initial studies may be normal or may simply demonstrate small foci of edema. Shear injuries may remain nonvisible on CT but are more apparent on MR imaging. Larger contusions may contain petechial hemorrhage and appear as ill-defined heterogeneous lesions with little or no mass effect. Edema and mass effect may increase in the first 48 hours following trauma, making these lesions more evident on imaging studies.

Damage to the brain coverings may lead to hemorrhage into intraventricular, subarachnoid, subdural, or epidural spaces. Their appearances on CT are as follows:

- *Intraventricular* and *subarachnoid hemorrhages* are identified as replacements of the normal low-density CSF by the high-density blood. When subtle, subarachnoid hemorrhage can be mistaken for generalized edema with loss of the basal cisterns.
- *Subdural hematomas* typically appear as crescentic, mixed, or hyperdense collections that cross suture lines but not dural attachments (Fig. 41-5*A*).
- *Epidural hematomas* appear as biconvex, hyperdense collections that cross dural attachments but not suture lines (Fig. 41-5*B*).

With rapid accumulation of blood in such hemorrhages, unretracted semiliquid clot may be present. In this situation, the CT scan demonstrates hypodense areas within the hyperdense hematoma, the so-called swirl sign.[16] Distinction between these two collections is important, because the epidural hematoma is due to arterial bleeding and is a surgical emergency. Without surgery, subdural and epidural hematomas resolve through a gradual decrease in density and appear hypodense at about 3 weeks' time.

Vascular Lesions

Ischemia, Occlusive Disease, and Infarct

Although CT demonstrates only about half of infarcts within the first 48 hours, it remains the imaging modality of choice in evaluating patients with symptoms of transient ischemic attack (TIA), reversible ischemic neurologic deficit (RIND), or

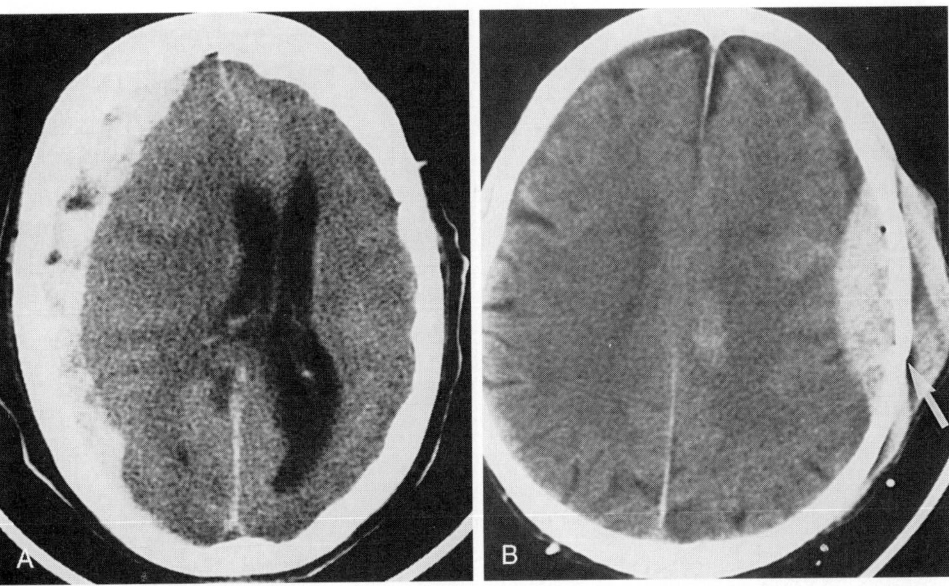

Figure 41–5. Subdural and epidural hematoma. *A,* Axial head CT scan demonstrates a mixed-density *subdural* hematoma along the right frontoparietal lobes. The mixed-density appearance is most likely due to the presence of unretracted semiliquid clot. *B,* Axial head CT scan demonstrates a left biconvex hyperdense collection that is classic for *epidural* hematoma. The presence of a fracture *(arrow)* can also be identified.

completed stroke.[17] In the acute setting, CT can (1) identify the location and extent of infarction, (2) distinguish ischemic stroke, hemorrhagic infarction, and primary intracerebral hemorrhage, and (3) effectively exclude lesions that mimic stroke.

The CT appearance depends on the age of the infarct, as follows:

- In the *hyperacute stage* (first 24 hours), the CT scan may be normal or may demonstrate a subtle decrease in density and loss of gray-white differentiation (Fig. 41-6).
- During the *acute stage* (within the first week), the infarct becomes more pronounced on CT, owing to the decreased density produced by cytotoxic edema (see Fig. 41-2). The infarct is better defined, involves both gray matter and white matter, and corresponds to a known vascular territory.
- The *subacute stage* may persist for 1 to 3 weeks, during which time the edema and mass effect begin to resolve.
- *Chronic infarcts* demonstrate parenchymal replacement with well-defined, sharply marginated zones of cystic encephalomalacia and gliosis. The infarct behaves as a contracting, rather than expanding, mass.

The MR appearance reflects the changes of cytotoxic edema (Fig. 41-7).

Treatment of acute embolic infarct with intra-arterial thrombolysis has been gaining momentum and is changing the role of imaging. Thrombolysis has a very narrow therapeutic window for the initiation of treatment (0 to 3 hours). Any delay decreases the likelihood of positive outcome. Because of this time frame, many newer methods are being studied as replacements for CT as the initial imaging modality.[18] Newer

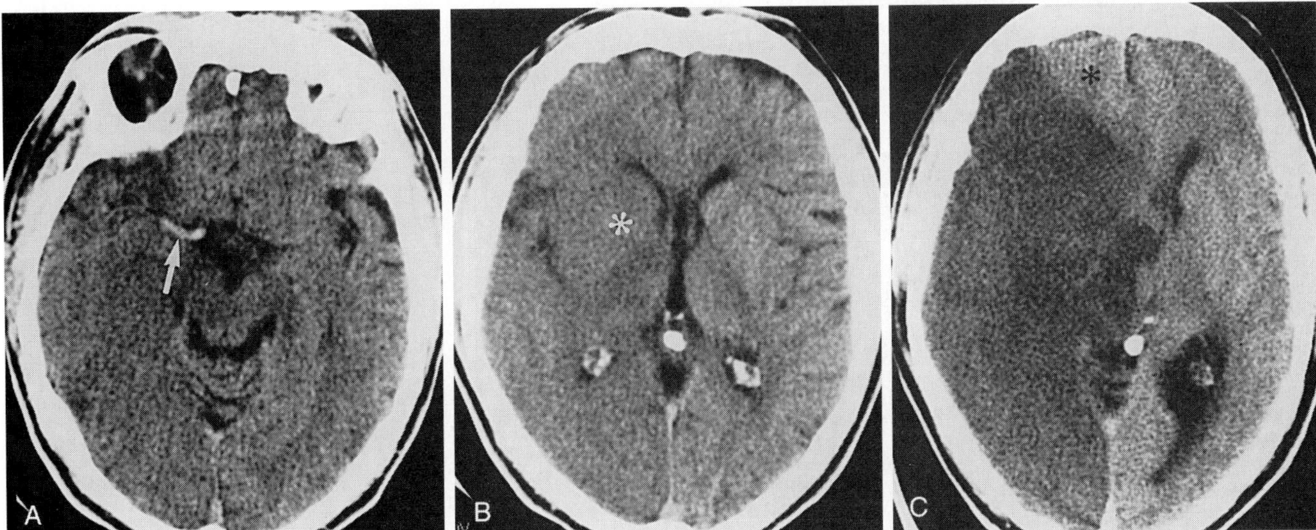

Figure 41–6. Acute infarct. Axial noncontrasted CT images obtained at the level of the temporal lobe *(A)* and through the level of the basal ganglia *(B)* demonstrate an area of low density involving the gray and white matter of the right hemisphere. There is loss of gray-white matter differentiation, especially noticeable in the region of the basal ganglia *(asterisk, B)*. Compare the right and left sides. High density is identified within the right middle cerebral artery *(arrow, A)* representing clot. *C,* Axial noncontrasted CT image obtained 48 hours later demonstrates marked edema involving the territories of the right middle and posterior cerebral arteries. Note the sparing of the right anterior cerebral artery territory *(asterisk, C)*.

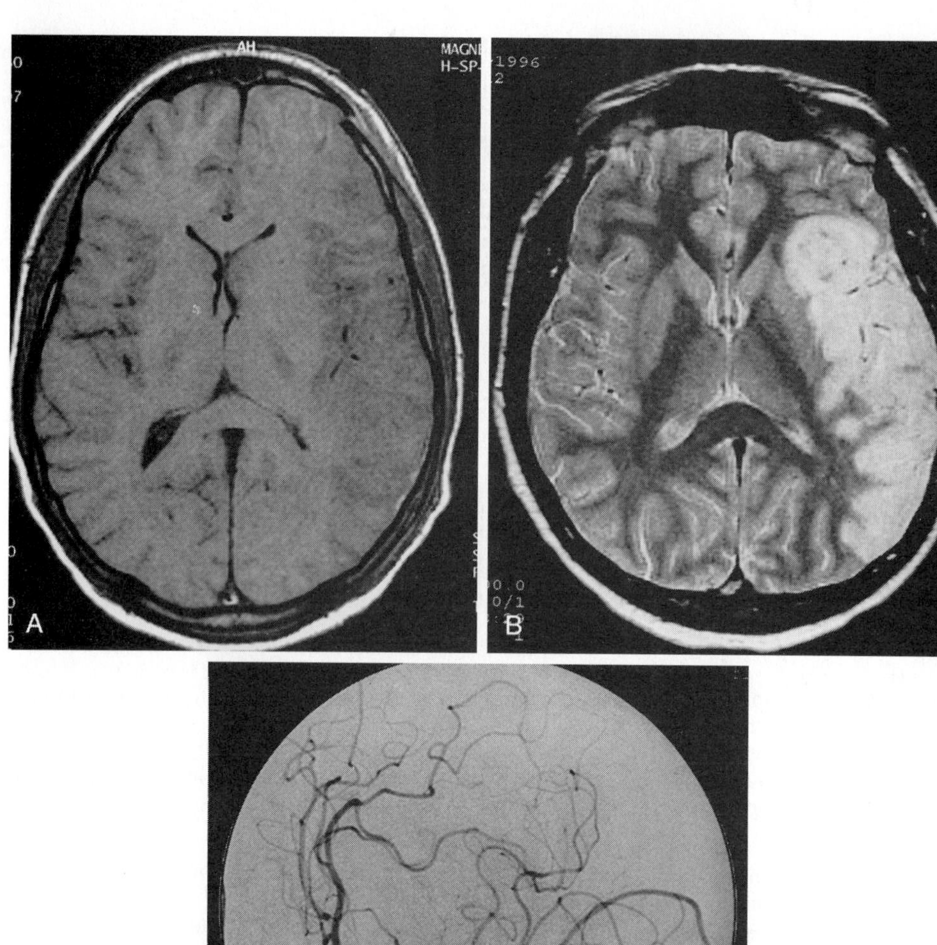

Figure 41–7. Infarct. Axial T1-weighted MR image *(A)* and axial T2-weighted MR image *(B)* in a patient being evaluated for stroke. The initial CT scan (not shown) was normal. MR images demonstrate an area of cytotoxic edema involving the distal left middle cerebral artery territory. The edema is hypointense to brain on the T1-weighted image and hyperintense to brain on T2. *C,* Left internal carotid artery angiogram demonstrated the occluded branch of the left middle cerebral artery *(arrow).* Within the proper time frame, intra-arterial thrombolysis would be a method of management for this patient.

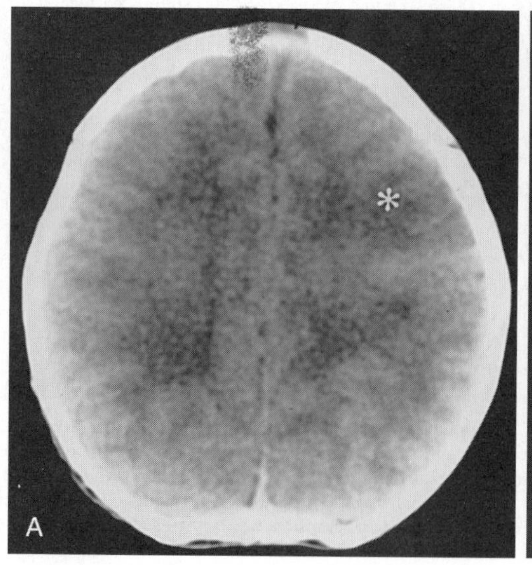

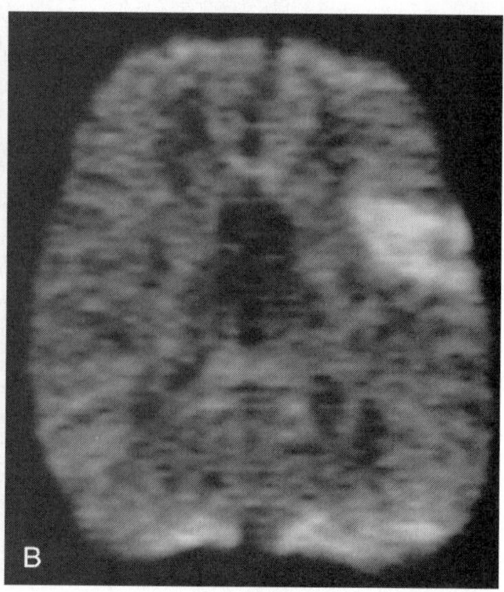

Figure 41–8. Acute infarct. *A,* Axial CT scan of a young child with a coagulopathy. The study demonstrates a vague area of low density involving a portion of the left frontal lobe *(asterisk). B,* Diffusion-weighted axial MR image clearly demonstrates this focal area of infarct.

MR imaging techniques can provide significant information regarding acute cerebral infarction[18]; they can reveal changes in gross anatomy, metabolic alterations (MR spectroscopy), water movement restrictions (diffusion-weighted MRI) (Fig. 41-8), and vasculature status (MR angiography). During the hyperacute and early acute stages, when the CT appearance is most commonly normal, MR imaging can readily demonstrate the zone of infarction. In addition, patterns of contrast enhancement in acute ischemia may have prognostic implications with regard to the completeness or reversibility of the ischemic insult.[19] Other methods being utilized are xenon-CT, single photon emission computed tomography (SPECT), Doppler ultrasonography, and positron-emission tomography (PET).[17] The advantages and disadvantages of these techniques and their future roles in stroke therapy are still under investigation.

Congenital Aneurysm and Subarachnoid Hemorrhage

Evaluation of a patient for a suspected ruptured cerebral aneurysm should begin with CT without contrast enhancement to demonstrate subarachnoid hemorrhage (Fig. 41-9). If the result is positive and the patient is a surgical candidate, a cerebral angiogram is performed to (1) identify the aneurysm, (2) detect additional aneurysms, (3) determine which aneurysm has ruptured in the patient with multiple aneurysms, and (4) determine the presence or absence of associated vasospasm (see Fig. 41-9). MRI and MRA are playing increasingly important roles in the evaluation of aneurysms, although primarily in the nonacute setting, when screening is needed for patients considered to be at high risk for aneurysms and for patients with focal cranial nerve deficits.[20]

Therapy for congenital aneurysms is undergoing significant changes. The ability to treat certain aneurysms with intravascular techniques using detachable coils or balloons now plays an important role in the management of ruptured and nonruptured aneurysms. The technique of endovascular occlusion of intracranial aneurysms using detachable platinum coils (GDC coils) now provides a therapeutic alternative, especially in patients with aneurysms that are considered to be technically difficult or are associated with a high surgical risk.[21, 22]

For the patient with the clinical suspicion of vasospasm, imaging modalities other than angiography have proved helpful. Xenon-CT has been demonstrated to be useful in assessing regional blood flow in patients with symptomatic vasospasm.[23] Transcranial Doppler ultrasonography provides an additional noninvasive method of measuring flow velocities and indirectly assessing vessel diameter.[24, 25] Treatment of symptomatic vasospasm is also undergoing changes. Percutaneous transluminal balloon angioplasty and intra-arterial papaverine infusion have been effective in treating patients with vasospasm.[26]

Vascular Malformations

Four types of vascular malformations are described: (1) AVMs, (2) capillary telangiectasias, (3) cavernous angiomas, and (4) venous angiomas.

AVMs are the most common type. The unruptured AVM either may not be apparent on CT scans without contrast enhancement or may appear as a subtle, hyperdense region. After administration of contrast agent, large, linear, tortuous, high-density structures, representing the serpentine vessels, are identified (Fig. 41-10). On MR imaging, these abnormal vessels appear as areas of signal absence (flow void), which are caused by rapid flow of blood through the normal vessels. Angiography is performed for evaluation of these lesions, because it demonstrates the feeding arteries and draining veins and can establish whether the supply is pial, dural, or mixed (see Fig. 41-10). Intravascular embolization of all or a portion of the AVM may also be performed as a treatment option.[27]

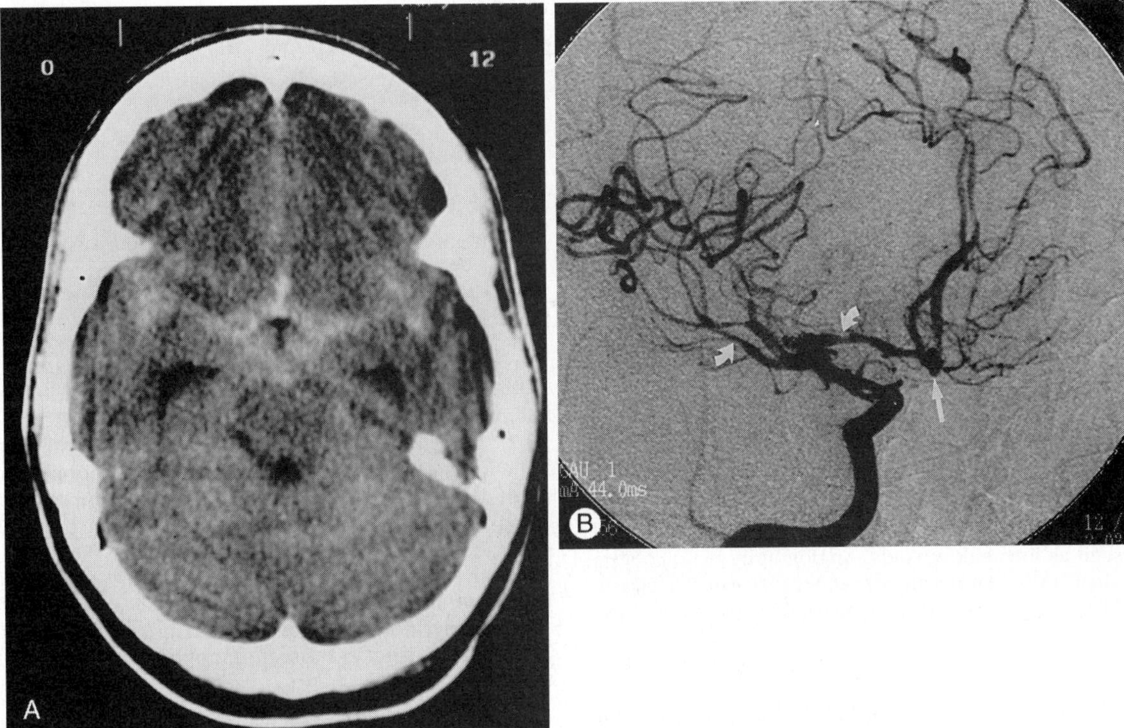

Figure 41–9. Subarachnoid hemorrhage and aneurysm. *A,* Axial noncontrasted head CT scan reveals high density (blood) replacing the normal low density of cerebrospinal fluid within the suprasellar cistern and subarachnoid spaces. This indicates subarachnoid hemorrhage. *B,* Right internal carotid artery angiogram demonstrates presence of a congenital anterior communicating artery aneurysm *(arrow)* as well as the presence of vasospasm *(curved arrows).*

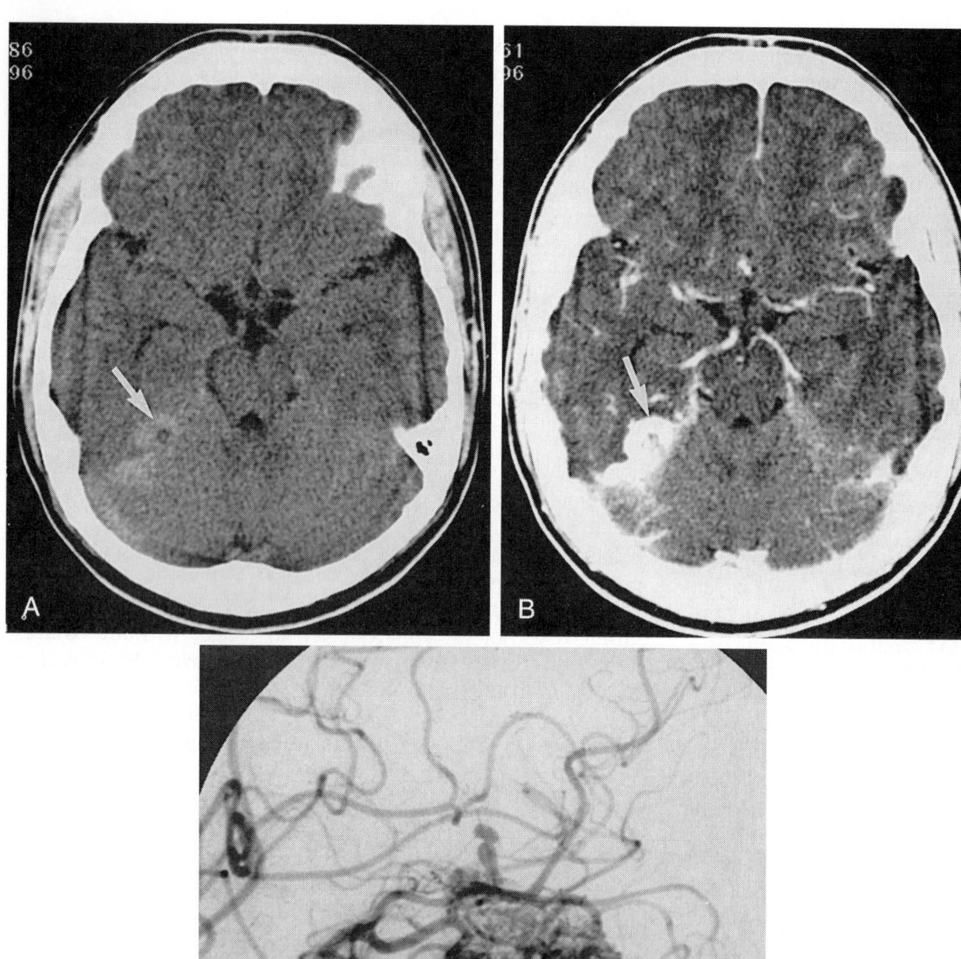

Figure 41–10. Arterial venous malformation. *A,* Axial noncontrasted head CT scan reveals a vague area of hyperdensity in the posterior right temporal region *(arrow). B,* Contrast-enhanced CT image demonstrates linear enhancement of this lesion *(arrow). C,* Internal carotid artery angiogram demonstrates an arterial venous malformation being fed by the posterior cerebral artery.

With rupture of an AVM, the imaging characteristics are those of hemorrhage, as described previously.

Capillary telangiectasias and *cavernous angiomas* are best evaluated by MR imaging; angiography typically has normal results, and CT is insensitive. The MRI signal characteristics are variable because of the presence or absence of blood products.

Venous angiomas are typically not apparent on CT without contrast enhancement, but the large transcortical vein can be identified following administration of contrast agent. The "caput medusa," or smaller feeding veins, are commonly seen as well and are diagnostic. On MR imaging, the large vein and caput are seen as linear flow voids. Angiography is not necessary for evaluation of venous angiomas because of their classic CT and MRI appearances and the untreatable nature of these lesions.

Neoplasm

Neoplasms are typically grouped according to location. This method helps narrow the differential diagnosis, because tumors vary widely in imaging characteristics according to their internal components. Knowledge of the imaging characteristics of specific tumors, the age and sex of the patient, clinical presentation, and lesion location help narrow the differential diagnosis and often provide a specific diagnosis.[28]

The CT characteristics of some tumor types are as follows:

1. Low-grade gliomas may appear as subtle nonenhancing masses, but higher-grade gliomas often demonstrate heterogeneous enhancement with large areas of necrosis and vasogenic edema (see Fig. 41–1).
2. Metastatic lesions may be low-density and therefore enhance, as seen with lung or breast carcinomas, or may be high-density secondary to hemorrhagic components, as seen with melanoma and thyroid and renal cell carcinomas (Fig. 41–11).
3. Cystic tumors, such as cystic astrocytomas, may be composed of large CSF-density cysts.
4. Epidermoid and dermoid tumors commonly contain areas of fat density and therefore appear very hypodense (lower than CSF density).

MR imaging has high sensitivity but low specificity in evaluation of neoplasms because most tumors appear similar. Tumors are typically low-intensity on T1-weighted images and high-intensity on T2-weighted images (see Fig. 41–1). There are a few notable exceptions because the signal characteristics

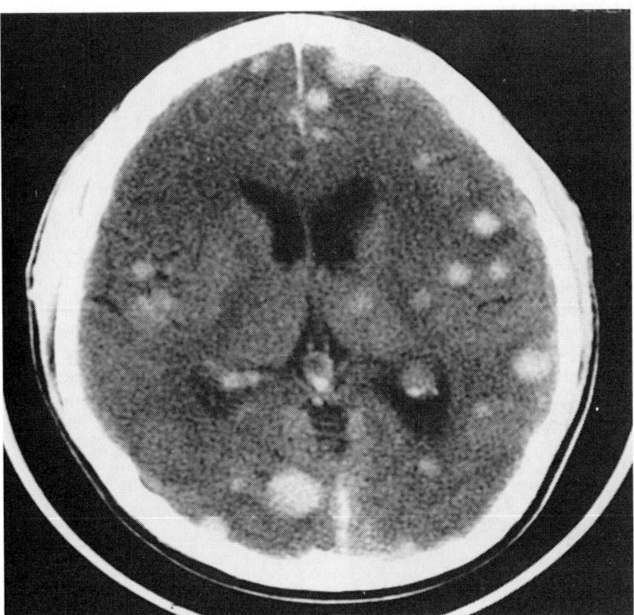

Figure 41–11. Intracranial metastatic disease. Axial postcontrasted head CT scan reveals multiple enhancing nodules throughout the gray and white matter structures consistent with metastatic disease.

reflect tumor composition. For example, meningiomas, owing to their homogeneous cellular make-up, tend to be isointense with brain on T1-weighted and T2-weighted images. Epidermoid tumors appear bright on T1-weighted images and less bright on T2-weighted images, reflecting their high fat content.

Infection and Inflammation

Infectious and inflammatory processes may be considered according to their primary site of involvement, either parenchymal or extra-axial.

Parenchymal Infections

Parenchymal infections are encephalitis, cerebritis, and cerebral abscess.

Encephalitis, a diffuse inflammation of the brain, is often viral or toxic in origin. MR imaging, which is more sensitive and demonstrates the changes earlier than CT, is the modality of choice when encephalitis is clinically suspected. On CT, encephalitis appears as vague areas of low density, typically involving the temporal lobes, and subtle gyral enhancement occurs after administration of contrast agent. On MR imaging, affected brain typically appears hypointense on T1-weighted images and hyperintense on T2-weighted images.

Cerebritis, an early phase of abscess formation, appears similar to encephalitis but is more focal in nature.

Cerebral abscess results from liquefactive necrosis, which produces a localized collection of pus or caseous material in a cavity surrounded by a fibrous capsule. On CT, an abscess cavity demonstrates central hypodensity (necrotic cavity), a thin isodense wall (capsule), and surrounding low density (edema). Following administration of contrast agent, there is enhancement of the capsule. Unlike the shaggy, irregular walls of a tumor, the wall of an abscess is typically smooth, well-defined, and uniform in thickness. These are important differential features. MRI findings in cerebral abscess are similar to CT findings. The central cavity has variable signal characteristics, depending on the contents. The capsule is isointense to hyperintense on T1-weighted images, is hypointense on T2-weighted images, and enhances after contrast agent is administered.

Extra-axial Infections

Extra-axial infections include ventriculitis, meningitis, and subdural or epidural empyemas. MR imaging is usually the modality of choice for extra-axial infections. In general, with CT or MRI, use of a contrast agent is necessary to establish the diagnosis of extra-axial infection.

On CT or MR imaging, *ventriculitis* is characterized only by enhancement of the involved ventricular wall.

In *meningitis*, CT and MR imaging may be normal or may demonstrate diffuse enhancement of the meningeal surfaces after administration of a contrast agent. The diagnosis of meningitis is made on clinical grounds and CSF studies. Imaging is performed to exclude associated abscess or empyema and to evaluate for complications such as hydrocephalus and vascular thrombosis.

Subdural and epidural *empyemas* are collections of pus that most often occur as complications of sinusitis, otitis, surgery, or trauma. On CT, the collections commonly have a density intermediate between CSF and acute hemorrhage. On MR imaging, the collections are typically hypointense to brain on T1-weighted images and hyperintense on T2-weighted images.

White Matter Disease

White matter diseases are classified as *dysmyelinating* (improper formation or maintenance of myelin) or *demyelinating* (normal myelin destroyed by exogenous or endogenous agents). Dysmyelinating disorders include the leukodystrophies and storage diseases. Demyelinating disorders can be:

- Idiopathic (multiple sclerosis)
- Postinfectious (progressive multifocal leukoencephalopathy) (Fig. 41–12)
- Toxic-degenerative
- Vascular

MR imaging is much more sensitive than CT and is the study of choice for the evaluation of presence and extent of white matter disease. On T1-weighted images, these lesions appear as vague regions of low intensity. On T2-weighted images, white matter lesions appear hyperintense. Newer T2-weighted imaging sequences have the ability to suppress the bright signal produced by the CSF and increase the visualization of white matter lesions.[29, 30] Although the majority of white matter diseases are similar on imaging studies, the pattern of white matter involvement occasionally can lead to a more limited or specific diagnosis.

White matter diseases uncommonly manifest acutely. More typically, they appear as a slow progression of neurologic deficits. In acute manifestations, toxic and vascular diseases are the primary considerations. Vascular disorders have been considered earlier in this chapter.

Toxic demyelination results from interaction of a chemical compound with the brain and may occur acutely. Radiation therapy and chemotherapeutic agents, such as cyclosporin A and methotrexate, may result in acute transient leukoencephalopathy. MR imaging demonstrates white matter lesions involving the deep white matter with sparing of the cortex and underlying subcortical arcuate fibers.[31]

Central pontine myelinolysis (CPM) occurs in alcoholic or malnourished patients and in patients who have undergone rapid correction of hyponatremia. On MR imaging, the white matter abnormalities are seen in the pons with sparing of the corticospinal tracts.

Acquired hepatocerebral degeneration occurs with many types of chronic liver disease, such as alcoholic cirrhosis, hepatitis, and portosystemic shunts.[32] MR imaging commonly

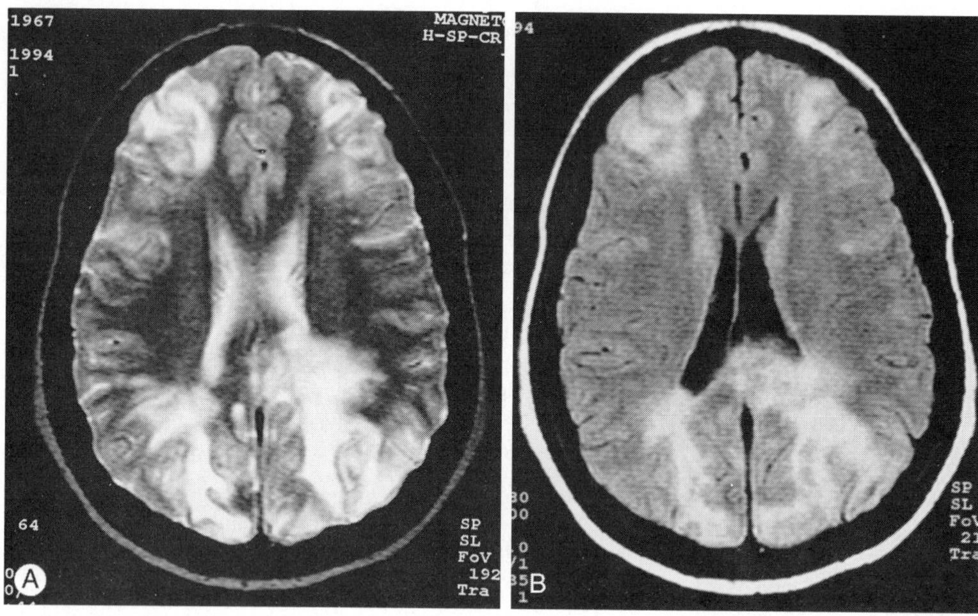

Figure 41–12. Progressive multifocal leukoencephalopathy (PML). Axial T2-weighted image *(A)* and FLAIR MR image *(B)* in a patient positive for the human immunodeficiency virus. Multiple areas of white matter disease are identified. The FLAIR image increases conspicuity. These findings in this patient population indicate a postinfectious demyelinating process of PML.

demonstrates bilateral basal ganglia hyperintensities on T1-weighted images.

IMAGING OF THE SPINE

Patterns of Disease

It is often useful to classify spinal canal disease according to location in three spaces: intramedullary, extramedullary-intradural, and extradural (Fig. 41–13). Certain pathologic lesions occur with greater frequency in specific spaces. Therefore, the diagnostic considerations can be significantly narrowed if a lesion can be localized to one of these spaces. In most instances, MR imaging is the modality of choice for evaluating spinal disorders, especially in the acute setting. The modality's high degree of tissue contrast and spatial resolution can localize most lesions to a specific compartment, determine extent of disease, and offer an accurate differential diagnosis. The only exception would be in acute trauma, in which bony alignment and stability are best demonstrated by plain radiographs, and fracture evaluation and detection of fragment displacement are best accomplished with CT.

Intramedullary Lesions

Intramedullary lesions expand the spinal cord as they enlarge, gradually thinning the subarachnoid space, usually symmetrically (see Fig. 41–13*A*). If of sufficient size, the intramedullary expansion may produce changes of the bony spinal canal, including posterior scalloping of the vertebral bodies, flattening of the spinous processes, widening of the interpeduncular distances, and overall widening of the canal. Intramedullary disease is most often secondary to a variety of neoplasms, most commonly gliomas (ependymoma, astrocytoma, and glioblastoma). Other tumors are dermoid cysts, sarcomas, hemangioblastomas, and intramedullary metastases. In the acute setting, infectious processes, such as transverse myelitis, granulomas (sarcoidosis, tuberculosis), and abscesses, must be considered. Traumatic injuries, such as cord contusion and hematomas, can also produce an intramedullary pattern.

Extramedullary-Intradural Lesions

Extramedullary-intradural lesions are contained within the subarachnoid space but are external to the cord (see Fig. 41–13*B*). These lesions displace the arachnoid layer of the meninges but leave the dura in place. On imaging studies, the subarachnoid space flares out to form a "cap" at its interface with the lesion. Tumors, mostly benign, represent the largest proportion of lesions in this space. The majority are meningiomas and nerve sheath tumors. Other much less common disorders occurring in this space are arachnoid cysts, drop metastases, lymphomas, and dermoid and epidermoid tumors.

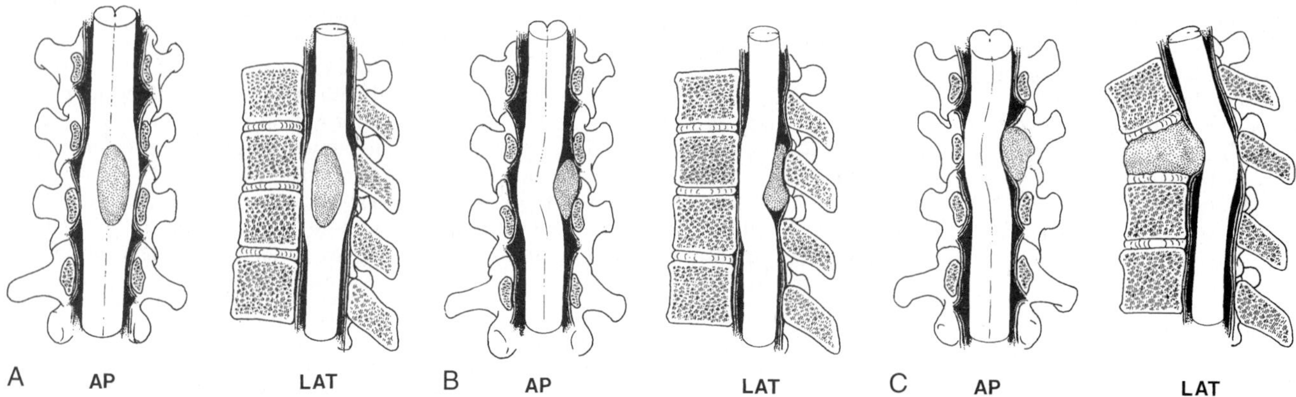

Figure 41–13. *A–C,* Spinal compartments. Anteroposterior (AP) and lateral (LAT) views of the spinal cord and canal demonstrate the appearance of an intramedullary lesion *(A),* an extramedullary intradural lesion *(B),* and an extradural lesion *(C).*

Extradural Lesions

Extradural lesions lie outside the subarachnoid space. Except for the absence of the subarachnoid cap at the interface with the lesion, the imaging pattern of extradural lesions may be indistinguishable from that of extramedullary-intradural lesions. Extradural lesions typically produce a more gradual displacement of the subarachnoid space and spinal cord (see Fig. 41–13*C*). Excluding disk disease, the most common extradural disorder is metastatic disease with epidural extension. Pathologic fractures of the involved vertebrae are common and are often associated with spinal cord compression. Primary tumors of the spine and direct extension from paraspinal neoplasms make up the other malignant lesions of the extradural compartment; they include lymphoma, myeloma and plasmacytoma, sarcoma, and vertebral body chordomas.[33] Benign lesions, which are uncommon in this compartment, are nerve sheath tumors, meningiomas, lipomas, and primary bone lesions, such as osteoblastomas, giant cell tumors, and aneurysmal bone cysts. Diskitis or osteomyelitis with epidural abscess is an additional consideration.

Specific Disease Processes

Spinal Cord Injury

The sequence in obtaining and using the various imaging modalities for evaluating spine injury remains controversial and is usually based on the availability of these modalities at the individual trauma center. Initial evaluation usually involves a plain film series. Plain radiography is rapid, accurate, and widely available, and allows a confident distinction between stable and unstable injuries. Only bony injury is directly seen with this technique, however; soft tissue injury is indirectly inferred from plain films by identifying changes in bone alignment (Fig. 41–14*A*). Commonly, in a patient with a cervical spine injury, a single lateral view of the spine is obtained first. If it shows normal alignment, a complete series is obtained, including oblique and odontoid views. For suspected thoracic and lumbar injuries, lateral and anteroposterior films suffice, but oblique views can be added if questionable areas are identified.

Indications for CT of the spine are (1) for further evaluation of detected fractures, (2) for further evaluation of suspected fractures or confusing plain film findings, and (3) for evaluation of areas not well visualized on standard plain film.[34] The sensitivity of CT for fracture detection is between 78% and 100%.[34] Higher resolution and sagittal and coronal re-formations aid in the sensitivity (see Fig. 41–14*B* and *C*). Meticulous attention to technique is needed, however, because subtle alignment abnormalities suggesting ligamentous injury may be missed. Because of the high sensitivity of CT for most types of bony injury, some studies suggest CT as the primary modality in patients with suspected cervical spine injury.[35, 36]

MR imaging is the only method that can directly visualize intrinsic spinal cord injury and soft tissue injury (see Fig. 41–14*D*). MR imaging enables the identification of and distinction between cord hematoma and contusion (edema), which affect the prognosis. Cord hematoma has a poor prognosis and indicates a complete lesion, whereas localized edema has a better prognosis for recovery of motor function.[37] Traumatic disk herniations can be readily identified. Detection of the presence of disk herniation with cord compression can change a patient from a nonsurgical candidate to a surgical candidate or a planned posterior stabilization surgical approach to a combined anterior and posterior approach.

MR imaging is also useful in detecting ligamentous injury through visualization of edematous changes or discontinuity in the ligaments. Although these findings are usually secondary, detection of isolated ligamentous injury may identify patients at risk for delayed instability. Epidural hematoma and the extent to which it is compressing the spinal cord are also identified with MR imaging. Finally, although fractures are

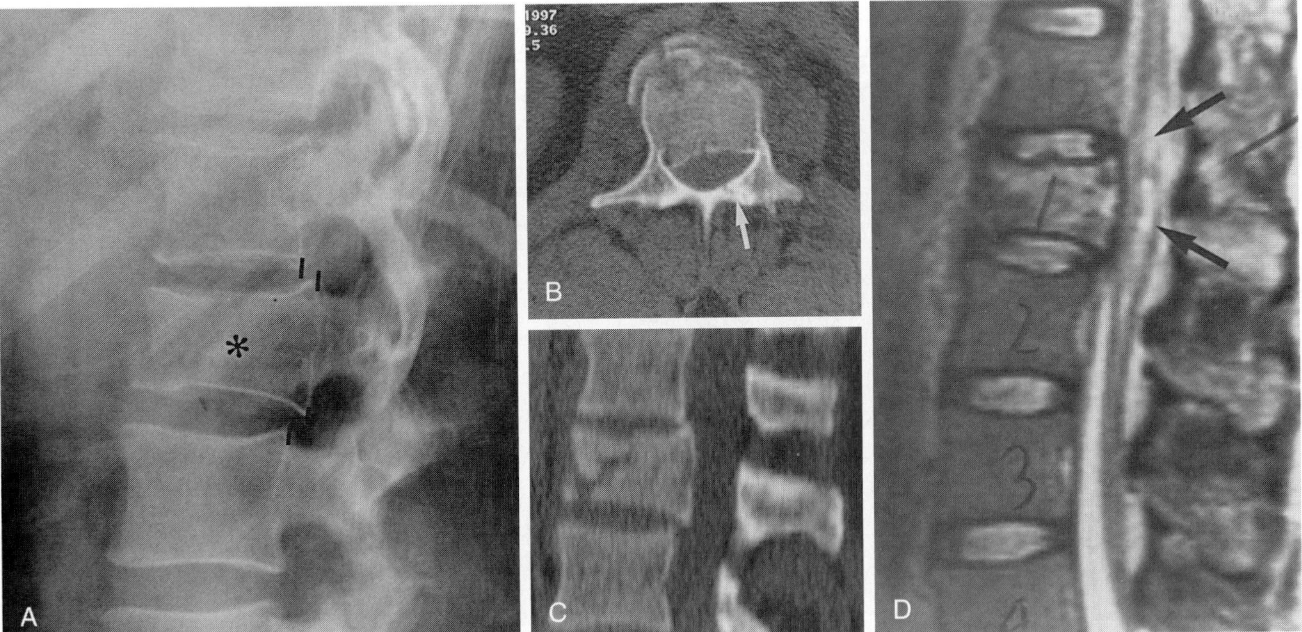

Figure 41–14. Post-traumatic vertebral body compression fracture. *A,* Lateral plain film of the thoracolumbar junction reveals compression fracture involving the L1 vertebral body *(asterisk).* The decreased height of the vertebral body and the inferior anterior corner fracture are well seen. The retropulsed body can also be seen when compared to the outline of the adjacent vertebral bodies *(lines).* Axial CT scan *(B)* and sagittal reconstructed CT study *(C)* of the same patient add substantial detail about the degree of canal narrowing secondary to the retropulsed fragment. A left laminar fracture *(arrow, B)* that was not apparent on the plain films is also seen. *D,* Sagittal T2-weighted MR image demonstrates the compression fracture of L1 and the retropulsed posterior body. The image also demonstrates contusion and swelling of the conus *(arrows)* as a direct result of the compression fracture.

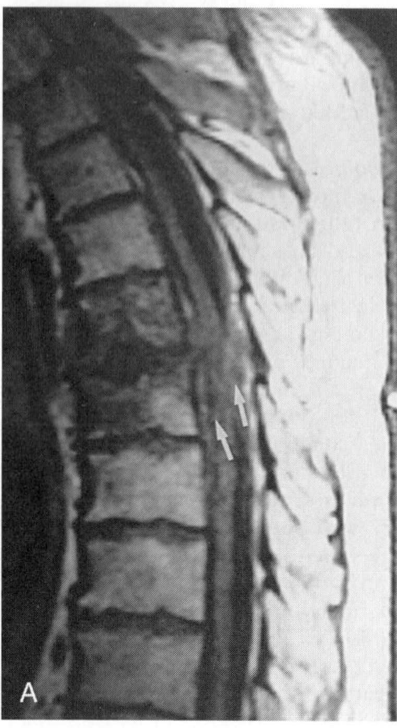

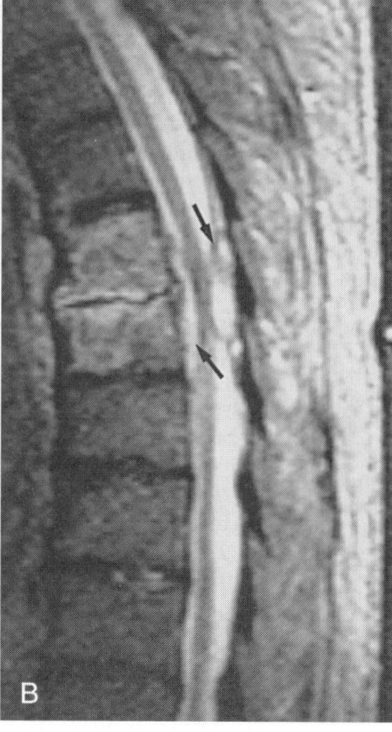

Figure 41–15. Diskitis with epidural abscess. Sagittal T1-weighted *(A)* and T2-weighted *(B)* MR images demonstrate features of diskitis and adjacent osteomyelitis. The vertebral bodies and disk space are low signal on T1-weighted and bright signal on T2-weighted images. The presence of an epidural abscess *(arrows)* surrounding and compressing the cord is also identified.

difficult to detect with MRI, the effect of bony fragment displacement and alignment abnormalities on the cord or nerve roots is elegantly seen with this modality (see Fig. 41–14*D*).

Principles for the evaluation of spinal cord injury can be summarized as follows:

- Plain films are a useful screening modality for identifying bony fractures and alignment abnormalities.
- CT further defines identified or suspected fractures as well as areas that are difficult to see clearly on plain films.
- MR imaging is useful to identify intrinsic cord injuries and extrinsic soft tissue and bone abnormalities along with their effects on the spinal cord.
- Occasionally, all three modalities are necessary to establish the appropriate treatment plan.

Spinal Infection

Infections that involve the spine include diskitis, epidural and subdural infections, myelitis, and cord abscess. In the management of spine infections, delay in treatment can in-

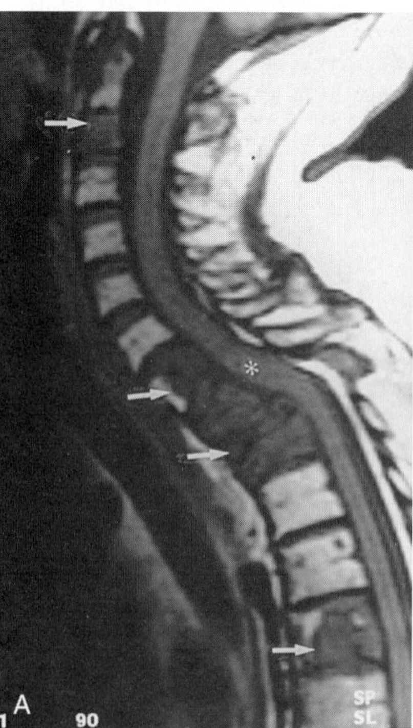

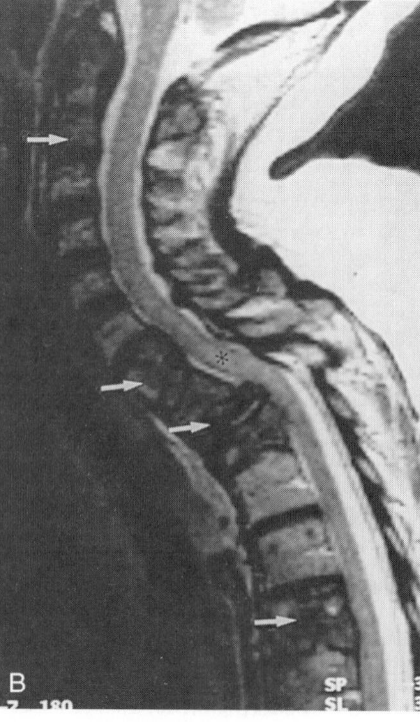

Figure 41–16. Metastatic disease. Sagittal T1-weighted *(A)* and T2-weighted *(B)* MR images of the spine in a patient with metastatic disease. The metastatic lesions *(arrows)* can be readily seen as low-intensity areas on T1-weighted images, replacing the normal bright marrow. The high signal within the uninvolved vertebral bodies represents postradiation changes. The hypointense lesions on the T2-weighted image, rather than the more typical hyperintense character, reflects the post-treatment appearance. Multiple compression fractures are identified within the upper thoracic spine with collapse, retropulsed fragments, and cord compression. Edematous changes within the cord secondary to the compression *(asterisk)* are also identified.

crease morbidity and mortality.[38] Early diagnosis is therefore critical. MR imaging has become the primary imaging modality in all forms of spinal infections because of its higher sensitivity and its ability to detect changes earlier than plain films and CT. MR findings in diskitis are characteristic (Fig. 41-15). T1-weighted images show a narrowed disk space and hypointensity in the adjacent vertebral bodies. T2-weighted images show high signal in the affected disk space and vertebral bodies. Post-contrast studies show enhancement of the infected disk space and osteomyelitic bone. Paraspinal abscess, epidural extension, meningeal involvement, and any compression on the cord are also readily seen with MR imaging.

Although MR imaging is sensitive in defining areas of myelitis, the findings are nonspecific and resemble those in other noninfectious and demyelinating disorders. Typically, focal or diffuse areas of hyperintensity are seen within the cord on T2-weighted images. Contrast enhancement is variable.

Neoplasm

Neoplasms involving the spinal axis typically manifest as progression of myelopathic or cord compression symptoms. MR imaging is the primary modality in any suspected spinal tumor. It demonstrates the location, extent, and nature of most tumors regardless of the compartment of origin. Primary tumors of the bony elements and direct extension from paraspinal neoplasms are also easily identified with MR imaging.

In the evaluation of metastatic disease, MR imaging has been shown to be more sensitive than bone scintigraphy.[39] Epidural and paraspinous soft tissue involvement and cord compression are also easily evaluated with MR imaging. Diffuse metastatic disease is recognized as heterogeneous or homogeneous hypointensity on T1-weighted images and hyperintensity on T2-weighted images (Fig. 41-16). MR imaging has become valuable in identifying compression fractures and associated cord compression and commonly enables the distinction between benign (osteoporotic) and pathologic (metastatic) fractures. Benign fractures have marrow intensity that is isointense on all sequences with the marrow of uninvolved vertebral bodies, whereas pathologic fractures demonstrate the signal changes described previously for metastatic disease.[40]

References

1. Moseley ME, Glover GH: Functional MR imaging: Capabilities and limitations. Neuroimaging Clin North Am 1995; 5:161-192.
2. Le Bihan D: Diffusion/perfusion MR imaging of the brain: From structure to function. Radiology 1990; 177:328-329.
3. Shellock FG, Morisoli S, Kanal E: MR procedures and biomedical implants, materials, and devices: 1993 update. Radiology 1993; 189:587-599.
4. Hankey GJ, Warlow CP, Sellar RJ: Cerebral angiographic risk in mild cerebrovascular disease. Stroke 1990; 21:209-222.
5. Brooks RA, DeChiro G, Patronas N: MR imaging of cerebral hematoma at different field strengths: Theory and applications. J Comput Assist Tomogr 1989; 13:194-206.
6. Smith WP Jr, Batnitzky S, Rengachary SS: Acute isodense subdural hematomas: A problem in anemic patients. AJR 1981; 136:543-546.
7. Stein SC, Ross SE: Moderate head injury: A guide to initial management. J Neurosurg 1992; 77:562-564.
8. Kirkpatrick JB, Hayman LA: Pathophysiology of intracranial hemorrhage. Neuroimaging Clin North Am 1992; 2:11-23.
9. Kreel L, Kay R, Woo J, et al: The radiological (CT) and clinical sequelae of primary intracerebral hemorrhage. Br J Radiol 1991; 64:1096-1100.
10. Blackmore CC, Francis CW, Bryant RG, et al: Magnetic resonance imaging of blood and cells in vitro. Invest Radiol 1990; 25:1316-1324.
11. Laine FJ, Shedden AI, Dunn MM, et al: Acquired intracranial herniations: MR imaging findings. AJR Am J Roentgenol 1995; 165:967-973.
12. Brocker B, Rabin M, Levin A: Clinical and surgical management of head injury. Neuroimaging Clin North Am 1991; 1:387-396.
13. Gentry LR: Primary neuronal injuries. Neuroimaging Clin North Am 1991; 1:411-432.
14. Zimmerman RA, Bilaniuk LT, Hackney DB, et al: Head injury: Early results of comparing CT and high-field MR. AJR 1986; 147:1215-1222.
15. Gentry LR, Godersky JC, Thompson B, et al: Prospective comparative study of intermediate-field MR and CT in the evaluation of closed head trauma. AJNR 1988; 9:91-100.
16. Greenberg J, Cohen WA, Cooper P: The "hyperacute" extra-axial intracranial hematoma: Computed tomographic findings and clinical significance. Neurosurgery 1985; 17:48-56.
17. Weingarten K: Computed tomography of cerebral infarction. Neuroimaging Clin North Am 1992; 2:409-419.
18. Castillo M: Prethrombolysis brain imaging: Trends and controversies. AJNR Am J Neuroradiol 1997; 18:1830-1834.
19. Crain MR, Yuh WTC, Greene GM, et al: Cerebral ischemia: Evaluation with contrast-enhanced MR imaging. AJNR Am J Neuroradiol 1991; 12:631-639.
20. Heiserman JE, Bird CR: Cerebral aneurysms. Neuroimaging Clin North Am 1994; 4:799-822.
21. Guglielmi G: Endovascular treatment of intracranial aneurysms. Neuroimaging Clin North Am 1992; 2:269-278.
22. Bryan RN, Rigamonti D, Mathis JM: The treatment of acutely ruptured cerebral aneurysms: Endovascular therapy versus surgery. AJNR Am J Neuroradiol 1997; 18:1826-1830.
23. Yonas H, Sekhar L, Johnson SW, et al: Determination of irreversible ischemia by xenon-enhanced computed tomographic monitoring of cerebral blood flow in patients with symptomatic vasospasm. Neurosurgery 1989; 22:368-372.
24. Lupetin AR, Davis DA, Beckman I, et al: Transcranial Doppler sonography: 1. Principles, technique, and normal appearances. RadioGraphics 1995; 15:179-191.
25. Burch CM, Wozniak MA, Sloan MA, et al: Detection of intracranial internal carotid artery and middle cerebral artery vasospasm following subarachnoid hemorrhage. J Neuroimaging 1996; 6:8-15.
26. Eskridge JM, Song JK: A practical approach to the treatment of vasospasm. AJNR Am J Neuroradiol 1997; 18:1653-1660.
27. Graves VB, Duff TA: Intracranial arteriovenous malformations: Current imaging and treatment. Invest Radiol 1990; 25:952-960.
28. Osborn AG, Rauschning W: Brain tumors and tumorlike masses: Classification and differential diagnosis. *In*: Diagnostic Radiology. Osborn AG (Ed). St. Louis, Mosby-Year Book, 1994, pp 401-528.
29. Hajnal JV, Bryant DJ, Kasuboski L, et al: Use of fluid attenuated inversion recovery (FLAIR) pulse sequences in MRI of the brain. J Comput Assist Tomogr 1992; 16:841-844.
30. De Coene B, Hajnal JV, Gatehouse P, et al: MR of the brain using fluid-attenuated inversion recovery (FLAIR) pulse sequences. AJNR Am J Neuroradiol 1992; 13:1555-1564.
31. Ball WS Jr, Prenger EC, Ballard ET: Neurotoxicity of radio/chemotherapy in children: Pathologic and MR correlation. AJNR Am J Neuroradiol 1992; 13:761-776.
32. Kulisevsky J, Ruscalleda J, Grau JM: MR imaging of acquired hepatocerebral degeneration. AJNR Am J Neuroradiol 1991; 12:527-528.
33. Weinstein JN, McLain RF: Primary tumors of the spine. Spine 1987; 12:843-851.
34. Cornelius RS, Leah JL: Imaging evaluation of cervical spine trauma. Neuroimaging Clin North Am 1995; 5:451-463.
35. Kirshenbaum K, Nadimpalli S, Fantus R, et al: Unsuspected upper cervical spine fractures associated with significant head trauma: Role of CT. J Emerg Med 1990; 8:183-198.
36. Lindsey R, Diliberti T, Doherty B, et al: Efficacy of radiographic evaluation of the cervical spine in emergency situations. South Med J 1993; 86:1253-1255.
37. Schaefer D, Flanders A, Osterholm J, et al: Prognostic significance of magnetic resonance imaging in the acute phase of cervical spine injury. J Neurosurg 1992; 76:218-223.
38. Sklar EML, Post MJD, Lebwohl NH: Imaging of infection of the lumbosacral spine. Neuroimage 1993; 3:577-590.
39. Algra PR, Bloem JL, Tissing H, et al: Detection of vertebral metastases: Comparison between MR imaging and bone scintigraphy. RadioGraphics 1991; 11:219-232.

40. Baker LL, Goodman SB, Perkash I, et al: Benign versus pathologic compression fractures of vertebral bodies: Assessment with conventional spin-echo chemical-shift and STIR MR imaging. Radiology 1990; 174:495–502.

42

Echocardiography in Critical Care

Michael C. Kontos, MD • J. V. Nixon, MD

Echocardiography has matured into a powerful and portable diagnostic and prognostic tool. Using high-frequency sound waves, the echocardiogram can image the structures of the heart and the great vessels and provide anatomic and physiologic information about myocardial performance. Because dilemmas in a critical care unit revolve around issues of hypotension and shock, echocardiography may differentiate cardiac and noncardiac causes of hypotension and provide a way to monitor therapeutic interventions (Table 42–1). In addition to anatomic information, through the use of Doppler and color-flow imaging, important physiologic data about valvular and myocardial function can be obtained. Because studies can be carried out at the bedside without significant risk to patients, echocardiography is convenient, may be performed serially, and avoids the inconvenience of transporting critically ill patients to other departments.

This chapter explores the uses and limitations of transthoracic (TTE) and transesophageal (TEE) Doppler echocardiography in the critical care setting. Echocardiography is approached within the framework of (1) the basic working principles of echocardiography, (2) the *diagnostic* utility of TTE and TEE in assessing critically ill patients, and (3) the use of TTE and TEE in *managing* critically ill patients with specific disorders.[1, 2]

GENERAL PRINCIPLES

Echocardiography is unique among medical imaging techniques because it uses reflected high-frequency sound waves to produce the picture. Unlike radiographic, magnetic resonance, and nuclear imaging, which depend on backprojection, ultrasonography relies on the operator to direct the beam to the target of interest. Because sound waves are attenuated by tissue, image quality can vary greatly between patients and between operators. Therefore, echocardiography requires skilled personnel to perform the procedure and, more important, an experienced echocardiographer to interpret the study.

Two-dimensional (2-D) echo images are the result of computer processing of reflected signals from a multiple phased array of vibrating piezoelectric crystals. Various frequencies can be selected, with the general rule that higher-frequency transducers have better resolution at the expense of penetration. For adults, 2.5- to 3.5-MHz transducers are usually used for TTE imaging and 5-MHz frequency transducers for TEE imaging. A new imaging innovation, *second-harmonic imaging,* can enhance TTE imaging. During harmonic imaging, the ultrasound signal is transmitted at one frequency and received at a multiple of the transmission frequency.[3] Typical imaging frequencies used are a transmission (fundamental) frequency of 1.5 to 2 MHz and a receiving signal of 3 to 4 MHz.

TABLE 42–1. Causes of Hypotension

Cardiac	Noncardiac
Tamponade	Hypovolemia
Acute LV dysfunction—MI	Septic
Acute RV dysfunction—MI	Neurologic
Pulmonary embolism	
Pulmonary embolism and RV failure	

LV = left ventricle; MI = myocardial infarction; RV = right ventricle.

Doppler echocardiography uses the principle that the frequency of waves changes in relation to changing distance. The target of Doppler echocardiography is red blood cells. Because red blood cells are much smaller than the wavelength of ultrasound, backscatter waves (the impedance difference between red blood cells and plasma) are the subject of interrogation.[4]

Two forms of Doppler echocardiography are available: continuous-wave and pulsed-wave Doppler. *Continuous-wave* is the older form and is useful for detecting high-velocity jets typically seen with stenosed valves. Because two different transducers are used, one for projection and one for reception, the continuous-wave type is not subject to any limits in velocity but has range ambiguity (Fig. 42–1). The *Pulsed-wave* type uses the same transducer for sending and receiving the signal. Because the rate at which the transducer alternates between sending and receiving the signal is known, localization of the Doppler shift at a specific point is possible (range specificity). The operator can place the pulsed Doppler probe onto the 2-D image and "listen" for the presence of increased flow (Fig. 42–2). Both continuous-wave and pulsed-wave Doppler data may be displayed as a plot of velocity against time (*x*-axis) with the signal intensity reflected in the gray scale and the direction of flow on the ordinate (*y*-axis). Pulsed-wave Doppler is used for detecting the extent of valvular regurgitation and the presence of abnormal blood flow. Pulsed-wave Doppler is limited by its inability to record high-velocity jets where signal aliasing occurs.[5] When the Doppler shift frequency exceeds one half of the pulse repetition frequency (the Nyquist limit), the signal can wrap around itself

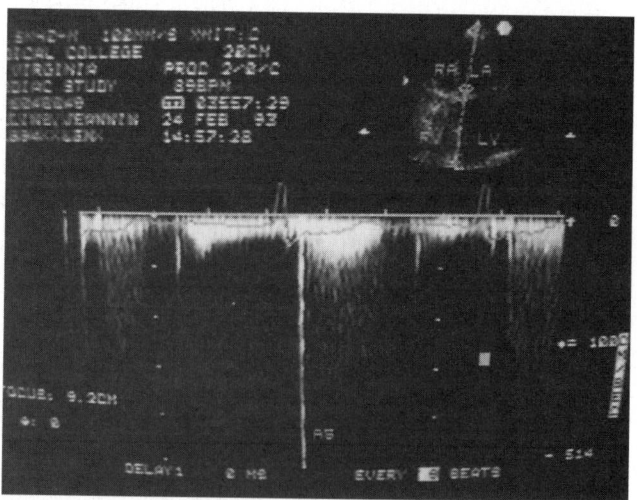

Figure 42–1. Continuous-wave Doppler echocardiography of a patient with severe aortic stenosis demonstrates the range ambiguity of the continuous-wave signal and its ability to detect high-velocity flows. RA = right atrium; RV = right ventricle; LA = left atrium; LV = left ventricle.

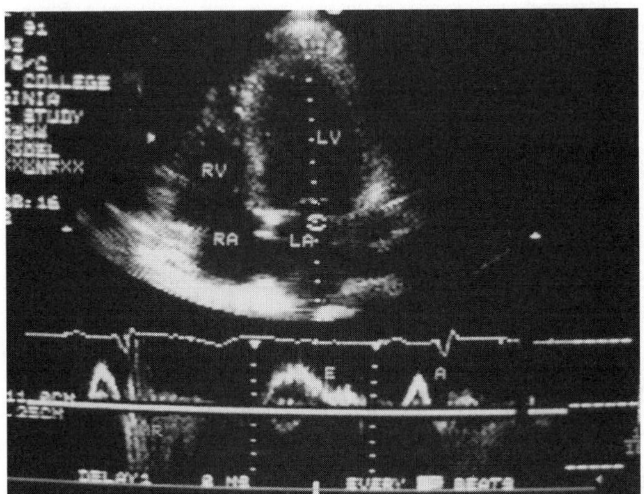

Figure 42–2. Pulsed-wave Doppler echocardiography of a patient with moderate mitral regurgitation demonstrates the range specificity of the pulsed-wave signal in detecting the presence of flow in a specific location. E = early left ventricular filling velocity; A = atrial systolic filling velocity.

and appears to change direction ("aliasing"). Aliasing is an important clue that higher velocities are present.

Through computer quantification, blood flow patterns in the 2-D images can be displayed as a colored map. In Doppler color-flow imaging or mapping, the pulsed Doppler signal is color-encoded with respect to velocity and direction.[6] The degree of color saturation quantifies velocity, and the direction of motion is reflected by different colors. These images are semiquantitative estimates of blood flow. The presentation of flow data with respect to anatomy provides a graphic map of the heart and blood flow. Confirmation with pulsed Doppler within these regions of color flow adds to sensitivity and specificity of detecting and quantifying the presence of valvular abnormalities. Doppler color-flow imaging is also bound by the Nyquist limit and cannot display the full Doppler spectrum.

TRANSTHORACIC ECHOCARDIOGRAPHY

TTE can be rapidly and serially performed at the bedside of critically ill patients. An average study can take from 10 to 30 minutes depending on the question being asked and the extent of information desired. Because infinite tomographic cuts can be made through selected windows, a standard approach is taken using five to six views (see later). The American Society of Echocardiography has devised a guide for quantifying left ventricle (LV) dimensions and wall motion on the basis of a 16-segment model (Fig. 42–3).[7] Standardization has made reproducible measurements and comparable studies between centers and operators possible.

Parasternal long-axis views of the heart are usually obtained first (Fig. 42–4). The right ventricle (RV) is seen anteriorly, and the whole of the septum is visualized with the LV below the septum. The aortic root and valve are on the right, with the left atrium (LA) below. The mitral valve is seen in cross section. The posterior wall of the LV is imaged along its length. This view is the basis of measuring the LV, LA, and aortic root dimensions.

The *parasternal short-axis* view is obtained by rotating the transducer 90° (see Fig. 42–4*B*). At the base of the heart, the aortic valve is seen in cross section along with the RV outflow tract and the pulmonic valve. By sliding the transducer toward the apex, one can obtain successive short-axis views of the LV. The mitral valve orifice is observed below the aortic valve (see Fig. 42–4*C*). Sliding the transducer more to the apex results in a cross section of the LV at the level of the papillary muscles. This level is important in assessing regional wall motion because all three coronary arteries supply this area.

When the transducer is shifted to the apex, *four-chamber* (RV, LV, right atrium [RA], RV) and *two-chamber* (LV, LA) views are obtained. The apical views are used to assess global function and to determine the integrity of valvular function. Although the intra-atrial and intraventricular septa are seen, dropout is often observed because these structures are parallel to the ultrasound beam. Intracardiac masses may be detected in this view (see Fig. 42–4*D*). The four-chamber view provides optimal Doppler studies of the mitral, tricuspid, and aortic valves. Color Doppler mapping can quantify the extent of mitral regurgitation. Aortic valve area may be estimated from Doppler studies of the aortic flow in the four-chamber view. Foreshortening and a more medial positioning of the transducer in the apical four-chamber view result in better images of the tricuspid valve and the RV. The presence of tricuspid regurgitation can be used to estimate pulmonary artery systolic pressures. Rotation of the transducer by 90° provides the two-chamber apical long-axis view and is important in assessing true anterior and posterior wall motion (see Fig. 42–4*E*).

The subcostal view is used consistently for critically ill patients and may be the only viable acoustic window (see Fig. 42–4*F*). For patients who have emphysema or who are using high-volume, positive-pressure ventilators, hyperflation of the

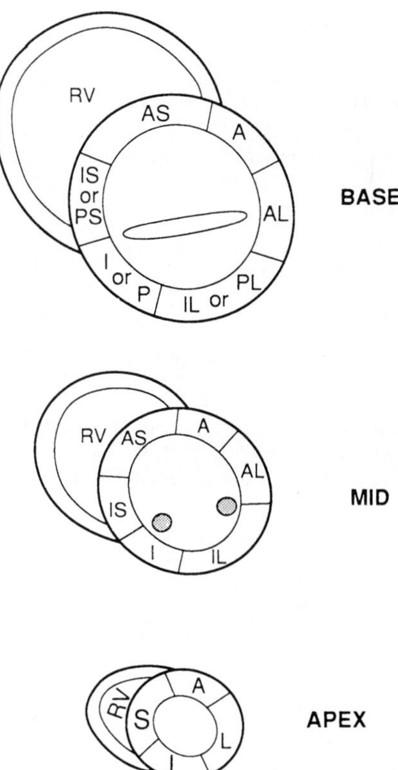

Figure 42–3. Sixteen-segment model for left ventricular wall motion analysis advocated by the American Society of Echocardiography. A = anterior; AL = anterolateral; IL = inferolateral; I = inferior; IS = inferoseptum; AS = anterior septum; PL = posterior lateral; P = posterior; PS = posterior septum; L = lateral wall; S = septum. (From Schiller NB, Shah PM, Crawford M, et al: Recommendations for quantitation of the left ventricle by two-dimensional echocardiography. J Am Soc Echocardiogr 1989; 2:358.)

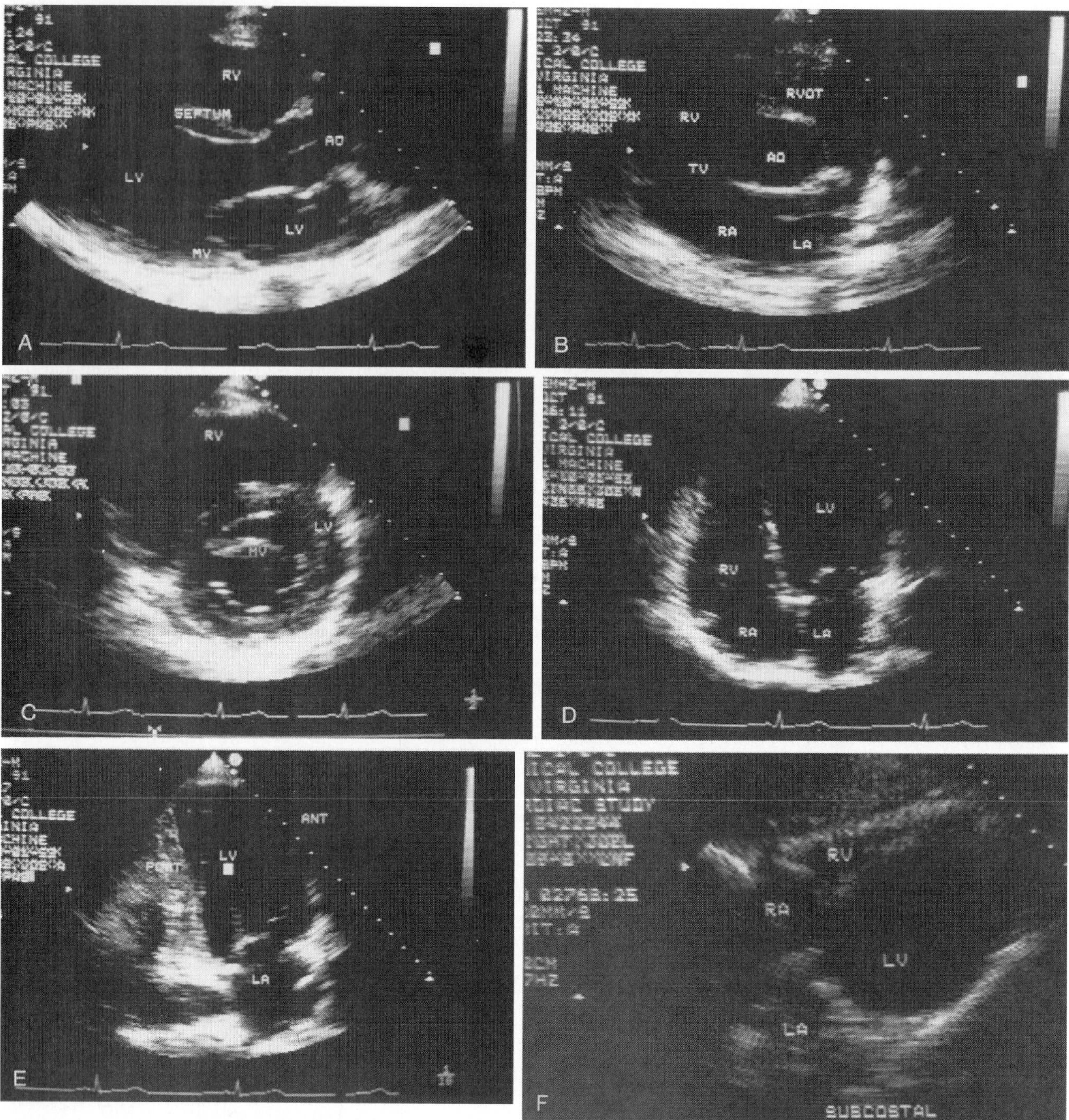

Figure 42–4. *A,* A normal echocardiogram in the parasternal long axis. MV = mitral valve; AO = aortic root. *B,* A normal two-dimensional echocardiogram in the parasternal short-axis view at the level of the aortic root. TV = tricuspid valve; RVOT = right ventricular outflow tract. *C,* A normal two-dimensional echocardiogram in the parasternal short-axis view at the level of the tips of the mitral valve leaflets. *D,* A normal two-dimensional echocardiogram in the apical four-chamber view. *E,* A normal two-dimensional echocardiogram in the apical two-chamber view. ANT = anterior. *F,* A normal two-dimensional echocardiogram in the subcostal view.

lungs results in poor parasternal and apical windows. The transducer is placed slightly right of the epigastrium, and the heart is imaged through the diaphragm. Four-chamber images can be obtained, and clockwise rotation by 90° results in short-axis views of the LV. The subcostal view is optimal for examining the intra-atrial septum by Doppler imaging for the presence of atrial septal defects. The inferior vena cava, hepatic veins, and abdominal aorta can be imaged from this location.

The suprasternal position of the transducer allows visualization of the aorta, the aortic arch, and the origin of the brachiocephalic vessels and the descending aorta. The LA, the right pulmonary artery, and the aortic arch in cross section can be seen by rotating the transducer. Doppler assessment of the aortic valve may also be performed in this position.

TRANSESOPHAGEAL ECHOCARDIOGRAPHY

TEE involves the echocardiographic evaluation of the heart and adjacent structures utilizing an ultrasonic transducer attached to the end of an esophageal-gastric flexible and steerable endoscope. TEE in an intensive care unit (ICU) is indicated as follows:

1. To assess valvular function (prosthetic and native).
2. To search for intracardiac shunts, masses (thrombus and tumor), endocarditis and its complications, and possible mediastinal or thoracic bleeding that may result in tamponade.
3. To evaluate patients for aortic pathology including aortic dissection.[8-11]
4. To evaluate hypotension of unknown cause.

TEE is also indicated when TTE images are suboptimal or not obtainable. This is frequently the situation in patients who are mechanically ventilated or who have chest wall bandages or chest tubes.

A comprehensive TEE examination incorporates a sequence of transducer positions and tomographic planes of imaging.[12] Initially TEE probes were limited to monoplane imaging, allowing only views of the short-axis and frontal views of the heart. Development of the biplane probe made it possible to view the heart in the longitudinal plane. Multiplane probes are now standard in most echocardiography laboratories and can sequentially image the heart and aorta throughout 180° of rotation, allowing systematic examination of all cardiac and aortic structures.

Absolute and relative contraindications for TEE include a history of esophageal pathology, such as previous esophageal surgery, strictures, varices, systemic sclerosis, esophagitis, or chest wall radiation. Upper gastrointestinal bleeding, dysphagia, and odynophagia are also contraindications.[8-12] Patients having elective TEE should fast for 6 hours before the procedure to avoid the possibility of aspiration.

Complications of the TEE examination are rare (<1.0%).[13, 14] In a multicenter study of 10,419 TEE examinations, intubation was unsuccessful only 1.5% of the time.[14] After TEE placement, fewer than 1% of the examinations had to be interrupted because of the patient's intolerance. One death occurred as a result of hematemesis caused by unsuspected lung carcinoma that had eroded into the esophagus.[14] Other described complications include arrhythmias, angina, congestive heart failure, laryngospasm, bronchospasm, hypoxia, and temporary vocal cord dysfunction.[14] Other mechanical complications include Mallory-Weiss tear,[15] transtracheal placement, bronchial obstruction, and aortic compression, particularly in children. In patients thought to have esophageal disease, the incidence of esophageal perforation complicating flexible esophageal gastroscopy is as low as 0.02% to 0.03%.[16] Only two esophageal tears or perforations have been reported with TEE.[14] Mechanical malfunction of the TEE probe, with buckling of its tip, was described in four patients. Resistance to movement of the probe was the only initial sign.

TEE has been successfully performed in critically ill patients without a significant increase in the incidence of complications.[2, 10, 11] In patients with an endotracheal tube, esophageal intubation may be difficult, and introduction of the probe under direct laryngoscopy may be necessary. A paralytic agent may also be necessary to ensure adequate sedation.

Currently, routine antibiotic prophylaxis is not required for TEE. Several studies have confirmed the low incidence of bacteremia on which these recommendations are based.[17-19] However, in some high-risk patients, such as those with previous episodes of endocarditis or having prosthetic valves, antibiotic prophylaxis is often administered before TEE.[12]

HEMODYNAMIC USES OF ECHOCARDIOGRAPHY

Acutely ill patients often present with life-threatening hypotension. Clinical assessment gives clues to the etiology (see Table 42-1). In complicated cases, such as hypotension associated with gastrointestinal bleeding complicated by myocardial infarction (MI) in an older patient, echocardiography can provide important diagnostic information. The presence of normal wall motion and a hyperdynamic left ventricle indicates that volume resuscitation is the initial treatment of choice. In contrast, the presence of severe left ventricular dysfunction with significant regional wall motion abnormalities would indicate that pump failure is an important contributor to the hypotension. In addition, Doppler echocardiography offers the potential for obtaining information similar to that obtained with pulmonary artery catheterization but in a significantly shorter time without the risk of complications inherent in any invasive procedure. Two-dimensional echocardiography is most helpful in guiding radically different therapies in patients presenting with hypotension and similar clinical findings.[20]

Estimation of Pulmonary Artery Pressures

In addition to providing anatomic data, Doppler echocardiography yields hemodynamic information previously gained only by invasive Swan-Ganz monitoring. This includes estimates of right-sided pressures, such as pulmonary artery systolic and diastolic pressures as well as right atrial pressure. Pulmonary artery systolic pressure is estimated as the sum of the estimated right atrial pressure and the gradient between the RV and RA.[21] This gradient is estimated by application of the modified Bernoulli equation (Table 42-2, Equation 1) using the peak velocity of the continuous-wave Doppler signal across the tricuspid valve. Color-flow Doppler imaging can help to guide the placement of the continuous-wave beam; however, the presence of detectable tricuspid regurgitation on color-flow Doppler is not a prerequisite for obtaining measurable regurgitant signals.[22] Similarly, estimates of pulmonary artery diastolic pressure can be obtained using continuous-wave Doppler across the pulmonary valve when pulmonary regurgitation is present.[23] A number of different methods can be used to estimate the RA pressure; these include measuring the inferior vena cava diameter, taking into account the percentage change with respiration, and determining the ratio of the peak systolic and diastolic hepatic vein flows.[24, 25] Alternatively, RA pressure can be estimated as 5 to 10 mm Hg and added to the RV systolic pressure to yield the pulmonary artery systolic pressure.[26] Addition of these estimates of the RA pressure to the gradient derived by the continuous-wave imaging results in an accurate measurement of PA systolic pressure (Fig. 42-5) (see Color Plate).[27, 28] Newer, more sensitive technology and use of a focused examination allow estimation of PA systolic pressure in more than 80% of patients, making this method applicable to the majority of patients.[22]

Estimation of Pulmonary Capillary Wedge and Left Atrial Pressure

As with the methods of determining pulmonary artery systolic pressure, the velocity of mitral regurgitation can be used to

TABLE 42–2. Equations for Calculating Hemodynamic Data from the Echocardiogram

Equation 1. Bernoulli's equation
change in pressure = 4 × (instantaneous velocity)^2

Equation 2. Estimation of cardiac output
pulmonary artery cross-sectional area or aortic valve area × velocity flow integral = stroke volume

cardiac output (L/min) = stroke volume (mL) × heart rate (beats/min)

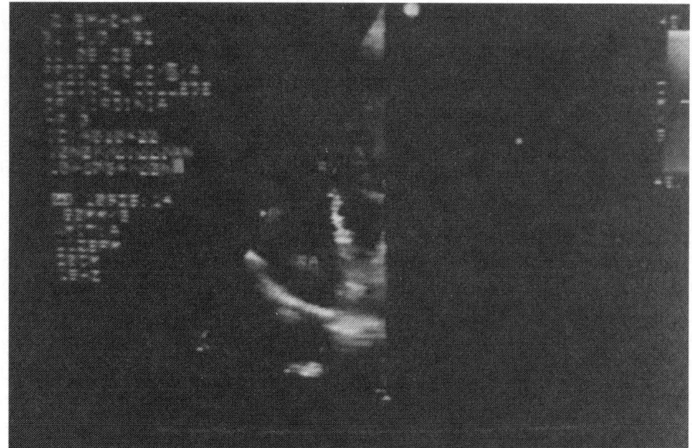

Figure 42–5. A color-flow Doppler echocardiogram in the apical four-chamber view showing tricuspid regurgitation. (See Color Plate.)

assess LA pressure and has been shown to have a high correlation with invasively determined pressures in patients with congestive heart failure ($r^2 = 0.88$) (Fig. 42-6).[29] One limitation of this technique is the requirement of mitral regurgitation. Also, because the velocities are squared, small errors can result in significant overestimates of LA pressure. Because brachial sphygmomanometry cuff pressure was used to estimate LV systolic pressure, mitral regurgitation cannot be used to estimate LA pressure by this method in patients with aortic stenosis, LV outflow tract obstruction, or subclavian artery diseases.

Other means of estimating LA pressure include measuring mitral valve inflow velocities and pulmonary vein flow patterns. A restrictive pattern (increased E-wave, decreased A-wave, E/A ratio ≥ 2) is associated with increased left ventricular end-diastolic pressure (LVEDP) and wedge pressures.[20] Both the E-wave deceleration time and the deceleration rate have high correlations with pulmonary wedge pressures.[30] It is important, when measuring mitral valve velocities, to make all measurements at the tips of the mitral valve leaflets, as measuring more proximal to the annulus results in significantly lower peak velocities.[31] Accurate measurements when the heart rate is above 100 to 120 beats/min may be difficult, as the E and A waves begin to blend together. Use of this method is limited in patients with normal systolic function, as the E-wave deceleration time correlates poorly with left ventricular diastolic pressure.[32] In this situation, the difference between the pulmonary A-wave duration and the mitral A-wave duration has a high correlation with LVEDP. A difference of 0 ms had a sensitivity of 100% and specificity of 76% for predicting an LVEDP greater than 19 mm Hg.

Studies have demonstrated that measurement of mitral valve inflow velocities provides important prognostic information in addition to the ability to estimate left ventricular pressures. A deceleration time less than 124 ms was the strongest predictor of hospital admission and cumulative cardiac events in both symptomatic and asymptomatic patients with congestive heart failure (CHF).[33] It also provided important incremental predictive information over and above that of ejection fraction, age, and functional class. Measurement of deceleration time has been shown to separate patients with ejection fractions less than 30% into those with short-term and long-term survival.[34]

The feasibility of obtaining these measurements was demonstrated in a study of echocardiography in 112 intensive care patients. Measurements could be obtained in approximately two thirds of them.[35] If the various methods described here are used, measurement of cardiac hemodynamics in a patient with advanced CHF may obviate the need for right-sided heart catheterization.[36]

Estimation of Cardiac Output

Doppler echocardiography is a readily available technique for accurately determining cardiac output. The aortic valve is the valve to use and the most commonly used, as there appears to be less variability in determining the outflow tract area than with other valves, but any visible valve without significant stenosis or regurgitation can be used.[37] The flow-velocity integral (area under the spectral Doppler velocity plot) multiplied by the outflow tract area yields stroke volume. Cardiac output is the product of stroke volume and heart rate, and thus instantaneous right and left cardiac outputs can be measured and have been validated.[38, 39]

These measurements have been shown to correlate well with thermodilutional measurements. One study found a higher correlation with thermodilutional measurement of cardiac output using a regression equation involving mean left ventricular outflow tract velocity rather than the foregoing conventional technique. The inaccuracies of the traditional method were primarily related to errors in measuring the left ventricular outflow tract area and resulted in the highest intraobserver and interobserver error.[40]

PERICARDIAL DISEASE

Standard clinical techniques used to confirm the presence of pericardial fluid, such as electrocardiography and chest

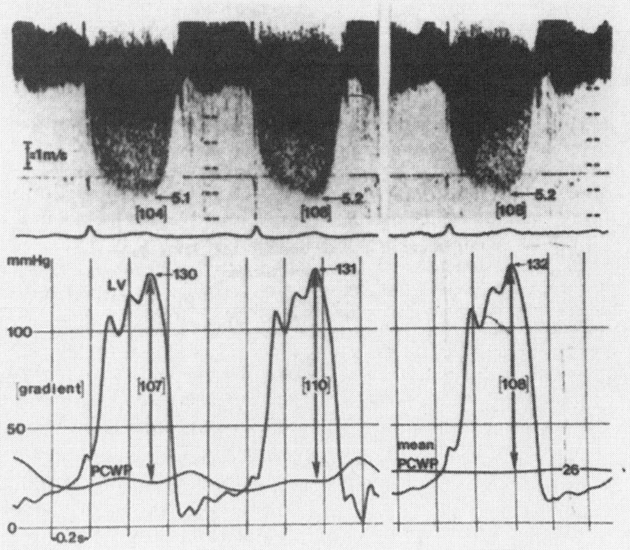

Figure 42–6. Simultaneous continuous-wave Doppler recordings of a mitral regurgitation jet and catheter recordings from the left ventricle and pulmonary capillary wedge positions in a patient with mitral regurgitation and mild mitral stenosis. The use of mild regurgitant flow velocity to estimate left atrial pressure is illustrated. Pressure gradients are shown in brackets. Simultaneous measurement of systolic blood pressure by cuff gave 132 mm Hg; this value corresponds to an estimated left atrial pressure of 24 mm Hg, which correlates closely with the recorded mean pulmonary capillary wedge pressure (PCWP) at end-expiration of 26 mm Hg. (From Gorcsan J III, Snow FR, Paulsen W, et al: Noninvasive estimation of left atrial pressure in patients with congestive heart failure and mitral regurgitation by Doppler echocardiography. Am Heart J 1991; 121:858–863.)

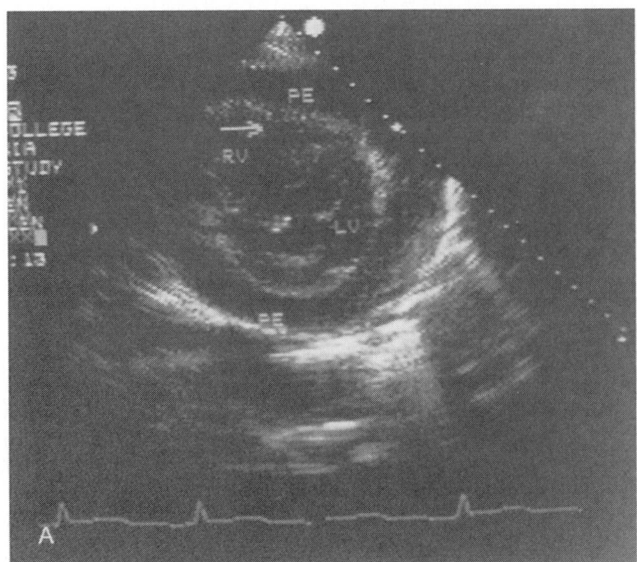

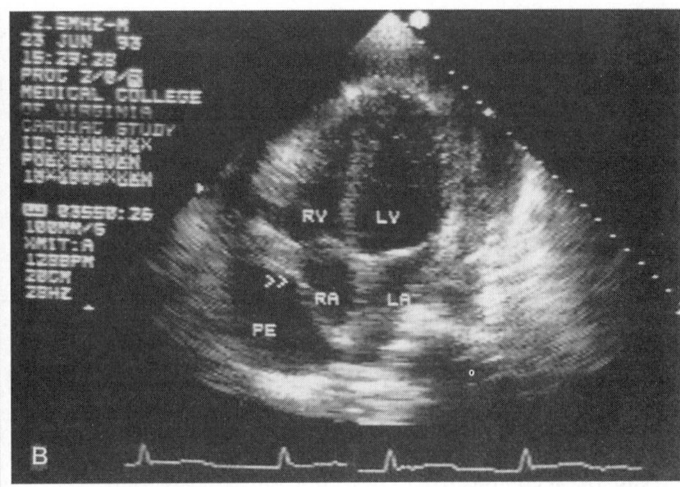

Figure 42–7. *A,* A two-dimensional echocardiogram in the parasternal short-axis view showing a circumferential pericardial effusion. *B,* A two-dimensional echocardiogram in the apical four-chamber view showing right atrial free-wall late diastolic collapse *(arrows)*, which is characteristically associated with cardiac tamponade. PE = pericardial effusion.

radiography, have limited sensitivity and specificity for predicting either moderate or large pericardial effusions.[41, 42] In contrast, echocardiography is optimal for detecting and diagnosing pericardial effusion. The pericardium is a fibroserous membrane composed of anisotropic collagen fibrils that unite the heart into a working unit. Normally, as much as 50 mL of serous fluid can be present in the pericardial sac. Echocardiography may detect as little as 12 mL. Increasing pericardial effusion can develop as a response to injury, and its impact on myocardial performance is dependent on the amount of fluid and its rapidity of accumulation. Echocardiography not only confirms pericardial effusion but also assists in pericardiocentesis. Not all echo-free space represents pericardial effusion, because epicardial fat and fibrocalcific pericardial disease are indiscernible by echocardiography (Fig. 42–7*A*).[43]

Pericardial tamponade is a life-threatening condition. It is defined hemodynamically as elevation of intrapericardial pressure with progressive limitation of diastolic filling that results in reduced stroke volume and ultimately systemic hypotension. The classic profile includes pulsus paradoxus, equalization of the LV and RV diastolic pressures, and depression of cardiac output. Tamponade may be occult, especially in medical patients who do not present with Beck's classic triad of decline in blood pressure, elevated central venous pressure, and a small, quiet heart.[44] Rather, nonspecific signs and symptoms, such as dyspnea, tachycardia, and pulsus paradoxus, are more common.[45]

ECHOCARDIOGRAPHIC FEATURES OF CARDIAC TAMPONADE

Cardiac tamponade is now recognized as a continuum rather than a rigid "all-or-none" phenomenon. Tamponade is characterized by progressive increase in intrapericardial pressures. The first echocardiographic evidence of tamponade is RA collapse, which occurs as pericardial pressure exceeds RA pressure. The specificity of this sign increases as the duration of RA collapse increases and is high if RA collapse persists for at least one third of the cardiac cycle.[46] As pericardial pressure increases, RV filling is impaired and systolic collapse becomes evident (Fig. 42–7*B*).[47] If RV collapse is present, longer duration of RV collapse in diastole may signify worsening hemodynamic compromise.[48] Ultimately, impaired LV filling results in decreased cardiac output and systemic hypotension.[49] These signs are preload-dependent and can be absent in patients with significant RV hypertrophy (those with chronic obstructive pulmonary disease, left ventricular hypertrophy, or pulmonary hypertension) or in patients who have undergone a pericardiectomy and uncoupling of the RV and LV.[50] In patients with LV dysfunction, RA and RV collapse can occur with smaller pericardial pressures and absent pulsus paradoxus.[51]

A number of other echocardiographic features are associated with cardiac tamponade (Table 42–3). Abnormal respiratory variation in tricuspid and mitral flow velocities may be present in pericardial constriction, obstructive airway disease, and right ventricular infarction.[52] Dilatation of the inferior vena cava (IVC) with lack of inspiratory collapse indicates increased RA pressure.[53] Other uncommon signs of cardiac tamponade include pseudohypertrophy of the LV and a right-to-left shunt across a patent foramen ovale.[54–57]

For patients with clear-cut echocardiographic and clinical evidence of tamponade, the decision to perform pericardiocentesis is relatively straightforward. In many cases, however, echocardiographic evidence of tamponade is present without obvious clinical sequelae. This occurs when pericardial pressure increases to the point at which it equals or surpasses RA

TABLE 42–3. Echocardiographic Features of Cardiac Tamponade

Abnormal respiratory changes in ventricular dimensions
Right atrial compression
Right ventricular diastolic collapse
Abnormal respiratory variation in tricuspid and mitral flow velocities
Absent *y* descent on superior vena cava and hepatic vein flow patterns
Dilated inferior vena cava with lack of respiratory collapse
Left atrial compression
Left ventricular diastolic compression
Movement of the interventricular septum toward the left ventricle during inspiration
Swinging heart

pressure, resulting in RA collapse before there is significant impairment in cardiac output. The decision to perform pericardiocentesis should be made primarily on clinical grounds rather than on the basis of echocardiographic evidence of tamponade. Sometimes, however, the diagnosis of tamponade can be confirmed retrospectively, when symptom improvement is noted after removal of the effusion. The yield of diagnostic information from pericardiocentesis for patients without evidence of tamponade is low.[58]

Once a pericardial effusion has been detected and the decision to perform pericardiocentesis has been made, TTE can guide placement of the drainage catheter. Because the location of the largest collection of fluid can be visualized, echocardiography-guided pericardiocentesis has become a safe procedure, with few complications. The operator usually notes the depth to pericardial fluid and the necessary angle and approach. Confirmation of the pericardial location of the catheter can be accomplished by injection of agitated saline (or echo contrast) into the pericardial space. The most common location for a pericardiocentesis is the apex, followed by the subcostal approach.[59] Infrequent complications include pneumothorax, bleeding, and right ventricular perforation. Serious complications occurred in only 1% of patients.[59]

No particular combination of echocardiographic signs is characteristic of constrictive pericarditis. Increased pericardial thickness behind the posterior wall may suggest thickening, but these measurements are not readily reproducible and are subject to gain error.[60] Some findings include mild LA enlargement with normal LV size, dilatation of the vena cava, flattening of LV endocardial motion during middle and late diastole, and premature opening of the pulmonic valve.[61, 62] Septal motion and Doppler flow of the mitral and tricuspid valves are abnormal during inspiration and expiration.[63, 64]

ACUTE PULMONARY EMBOLISM

In a patient who presents with dyspnea, hypoxia, and a clear chest radiograph, pulmonary embolism is one of the most important differential diagnoses. Signs of RV failure include RV dilatation and hypokinesis,[65] pulmonary hypertension, and increased RV afterload stress.[66] RV dilation and hypokinesis can result from both acute failure secondary to pulmonary embolism and chronic pulmonary hypertension. Regional dysfunction, with akinesia of the middle free wall with normal apical wall motion, has been reported to be a highly specific sign that indicates RV failure secondary to pulmonary embolism.[67] Other echocardiographic features of pulmonary embolism occasionally seen include abnormal septal position and paradoxical septal motion (compatible with increased right ventricular pressure and volume overload) and pulmonary artery dilatation. An embolus can rarely be seen in the pulmonary artery outflow tract or crossing the atrial septum owing to increased right heart pressures.[68]

When TTE is inadequate, TEE allows visualization of the RV and proximal pulmonary arteries. In a serial TEE study of patients with pulmonary emboli, eight of 24 patients (33%) had thrombi in the pulmonary artery.[69] If the diagnosis of pulmonary embolism can be made by TEE, an unstable patient may avoid the risks associated with pulmonary arteriography.[70] In patients with circulatory shock, the embolism was seen in the pulmonary artery with TEE in 58% of 60 patients with pulmonary embolism.[71]

A number of studies have documented that evidence of RV failure demonstrated by TTE identifies a group of patients with pulmonary embolism at increased risk for complications and mortality.[66, 72, 73] One study found that clinically stable patients with pulmonary embolism having pulmonary hypertension or RV dilatation were high-risk patients for whom thrombolytic therapy was beneficial.[74] The mobility and expediency of 2-D echocardiography in precluding other causes of hypotension can be important in the treatment of patients with pulmonary embolism. Because it can be performed at the bedside, echocardiography is becoming increasingly relied on as the diagnostic procedure for many patients with pulmonary embolism, especially hemodynamically unstable patients.[75]

RIGHT VENTRICULAR MYOCARDIAL INFARCTION

An important cause of hypotension in patients with inferior myocardial infarction (MI) is RV infarction. Autopsy studies have shown an incidence of RV involvement from 1% to 43%, with variability attributed to diverse definitions of RV infarction, different pathologic techniques, and different population samples.[76] When hemodynamic criteria are used, 15% to 20% of inferior wall MIs have RV involvement with severe hemodynamic derangement in 3% to 8% of the cases.[77] In patients with acute MI and hypotension, recognition of RV infarction is critical and needs to be differentiated from other conditions that can present similarly, such as pericardial tamponade, pericardial constriction, and pulmonary embolism, all of which may involve diastolic pressure equalization. These conditions may all involve jugular venous distention, right-sided CHF, clear lungs, and low cardiac output.[78-80] Echocardiography is useful in rapidly differentiating these three clinical entities.

Echocardiographic recognition of RV infarction includes RV enlargement along with inferior LV wall-motion abnormalities. The RV dilates with ischemic injury, and the RV free wall may show diminished motion.[81, 82] Because minor hypokinesis is difficult to determine, right ventricular akinesis or dyskinesis is often required to make the diagnosis of RV infarction.[83-85] Right ventricular akinesis is a sensitive sign of RV infarction and is demonstrable in almost all patients with clinical or hemodynamic evidence of RV infarction. The greater the amount of RV involvement demonstrated by echocardiography, the more common the presence of hemodynamic abnormalities. Other echocardiographic signs of RV dysfunction include caudal motion of the tricuspid annulus of less than 1.5 cm,[82] paradoxical septal motion, and reversed peak velocities of the tricuspid valve (normally early E greater than A atrial filling velocities).[86] It is important to note that the echocardiographic signs of RV infarction are nonspecific and any condition that increases RV afterload provokes these signs. Besides estimation of RV function, determination of tricuspid regurgitation is also important. These patients often have significant hemodynamic dysfunction and may not respond to inotropic infusion.[87]

The preferred views for assessment of RV wall motion are the four-chamber and subcostal views. When massive RV dilatation is present, the RV free wall may not be readily seen on the apical four-chamber view. Medial positioning of the transducer so that the apex is formed by the RV allows visualization of the free wall.

If both RV infarction and pericardial tamponade coexist, the RV appears dilated and has less tendency to exhibit diastolic collapse. RA and RV collapse requires higher pericardial pressures and larger pericardial effusions and occurs later in diastole.[88] In addition to inferior LV infarction, anteroseptal MI can cause RV dysfunction owing to the commonly shared septum.[89, 90] LV dysfunction eventually causes RV dilatation and dysfunction. In patients with chronic heart failure, RV dilatation may be an independent predictor of mortality.[91]

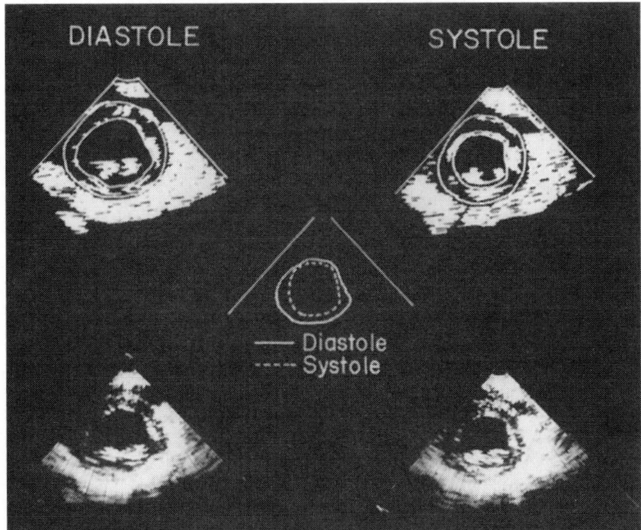

Figure 42–8. Two-dimensional echocardiograms in the parasternal short-axis views showing hypokinesia in the anterolateral segment in a patient with acute anterior myocardial infarction. (From Nixon JV, Narahara KA, Smitherman TC: Estimation of myocardial involvement in patients with acute myocardial infarction by two-dimensional echocardiography. Circulation 1980; 62:1248–1255.)

ISCHEMIC HEART DISEASE

Regional wall motion develops in the left ventricle within seconds of coronary occlusion (Fig. 42–8).[92–94] Diastolic dysfunction with thinning of the myocardium and bulging is seen on TTE with acute coronary occlusion. However, 2-D echocardiography is more conventionally used in this setting to determine the prognosis and identify complications of acute MI (Table 42–4).

Echocardiography has been used extensively for acute imaging in both the coronary care unit (CCU) and the emergency department (ED). Sabia and colleagues[95] performed echocardiography on 180 patients within 4 hours of presentation to the ED. Technically adequate studies were obtained in 169 (94%). Sensitivity for detecting MI by TTE was high (93%), but specificity was limited, attributable in part to the 31 patients with prior MI. If only patients having either ST-segment elevation or regional wall-motion abnormalities were admitted, the number of hospital admissions could have been reduced by 32% and charges by 34%.

Echocardiography is also useful for identifying patients with ischemia without infarction. Nixon and coworkers[94] studied 19 patients without prior MI who presented with chest pain. Echocardiograms were obtained at the time of admission and before discharge. Patients who had no improvement or worsening of wall-motion scores from the admission echocardiogram to the discharge one were more likely to have a complicated postdischarge course, with more frequent and severe episodes of angina. Peels and colleagues[96] studied 43 patients with no prior history of MI or coronary disease who were admitted after presenting to the ED with chest pain. The sensitivity of regional wall-motion abnormalities for diagnosis of significant coronary disease was 88%, the specificity was 78%, and the positive predictive value was 85%.

TABLE 42–4. Mechanical Complications of Acute Myocardial Infarction

Mitral regurgitation
Papillary muscle dysfunction
Papillary muscle rupture
Chordal rupture
Cardiac rupture
Papillary muscle rupture (5%)
Ventricular septal rupture (10%)
Free-wall rupture (85%)
LV aneurysm
LV pseudoaneurysm
LV thrombus
Infarct expansion

LV = left ventricle.

Kontos and colleagues[97] obtained echocardiograms in the ED for 260 patients with possible cardiac ischemia. Wall-motion abnormalities were demonstrated in 22 of the 23 (96%) patients with MI. Among the 166 patients with negative echocardiography, only one patient had MI, and three others underwent revascularization. The sensitivity for predicting either infarction or revascularization was 91%, with a negative predictive value of 97%, compared with a sensitivity of the electrocardiogram (ECG) of only 40%.

Echocardiography can provide important prognostic information on patients admitted for possible MI. Kan and associates[98] were able to obtain adequate two-dimensional echocardiograms for 345 of 370 (93%) patients prospectively studied within 12 hours of admission for acute MI. Patients with wall-motion scores of 10 or higher had a 1-year mortality of 61%, compared with 3% for those with wall-motion scores less than 10.

Berning Steensgaard,[99] studying 201 consecutive patients admitted with acute MI, found that the echocardiographic wall-motion score index was more predictive of in-hospital and 1-year mortality than the Killip classification. Overall mortality within Killip classes I and II was closely correlated with the degree of wall-motion abnormalities.

Sabia and coworkers[100] found that 32% of the patients initially evaluated in the ED for possible cardiac ischemia suffered cardiac complications over the ensuing 2 years. The presence of systolic dysfunction was an independent prognostic variable in predicting both short-term and long-term adverse cardiac events. When combined with clinical, historical, and ECG variables, systolic dysfunction significantly improved the prediction of late events.

Fleischmann and colleagues[101] investigated the prognostic utility of two-dimensional and Doppler echocardiography in 513 patients studied within 1 month of presentation to the ED for possible cardiac chest pain. After adjusting for clinical and ECG variables, left ventricular systolic dysfunction and moderate to severe mitral regurgitation independently predicted mortality. After exclusion of the 107 patients who had MI at the time of initial evaluation, left ventricular systolic dysfunction and mitral regurgitation remained independent predictors of mortality.

TTE has a number of limitations for evaluating chest pain in the acute setting. Echocardiography may be normal in patients with small or nontransmural infarctions. Poor echocardiographic windows may limit imaging of some patients, although with technologic improvements, adequate images have been obtained in more than 95% of subjects.[100, 102] False-positive echocardiograms related to wall-motion abnormalities may occur as a result of abnormal septal motion in patients with right ventricular volume overload or left bundle branch block. Wall-motion abnormalities, both segmental and global, may also be present in patients with myocarditis.[103]

Important mechanical complications of acute MI include acquired ventricular septal defect, LV thrombi, ischemic mitral regurgitation, and LV rupture. TTE is ideally suited for detecting ventricular thrombi and is more sensitive than angio-

TABLE 42–5. Echocardiography and Stenotic Valvular Heart Disease

Mitral stenosis
Abnormally high wedge values in patients with good LV ejection fraction and frequent pulmonary edema
Aortic stenosis
Whether to institute vasodilator therapy in patient with congestive heart failure

LV = left ventricle.

graphic ventriculography.[104] Echocardiographic morphology of the thrombus can predict the possibility of systemic embolism. For example, thrombi that protrude into the LV cavity and that are mobile during the cardiac cycle have a higher risk of causing systemic embolization than thrombi that are sessile.[105–107]

Papillary rupture is often catastrophic. It is secondary to disruption of the necrosed head of the papillary muscle and occurs in 1% of all MIs.[108] Massive mitral regurgitation is usually associated with a flail leaflet. Because of its size and blood supply, the posterior medial papillary muscle is often ruptured. The size of the infarction does not predict the propensity for papillary rupture, because 50% of patients have small or non-Q wave MIs.[109] In acute mitral regurgitation, the murmur may be absent, and color Doppler assessment can be falsely negative because of a poor acoustic window or a rapid heart rate. Increased early mitral inflow velocity or a hyperdynamic LV wall may be the only echocardiographic sign. In these cases, TEE is necessary for diagnosis. Prompt recognition with surgical intervention may be lifesaving. Mortality remains elevated, however, with 50% survival at 24 hours and 16% survival at 8 weeks.

Ischemic mitral regurgitation is a marker of adverse prognosis and is usually a consequence of LV dysfunction and annular dilatation rather than of isolated papillary ischemia.[110] The murmur of mitral regurgitation is often absent on physical examination.[111] On 2-D echocardiography, incomplete closure of the mitral valve is associated with ischemic regurgitation.[112] Recognition is important, because future management with angiotensin-converting enzyme inhibitors and closer monitoring for heart failure may improve survival.

Free-wall rupture occurs in 1.5% of all heart attacks and accounts for 8% to 24% of infarct-related deaths.[113] Patients usually present with hypotension, distended neck veins, and electromechanical dissociation. Pericardial tamponade is invariably present, and this constellation of symptoms in a patient on the seventh or eighth day of infarction should prompt heroic measures if the patient is to survive. Rarely, a patient may present subacutely, and corrective surgery is undertaken if the clinician is astute.

VALVULAR HEART DISEASE

Doppler echocardiography allows physiologic assessment of valvular function in conjunction with structural function. In hemodynamically compromised patients, significant valvular abnormalities can influence inotropic and hemodynamic management. For example, in elderly patients with heart failure and hypotension, the presence of aortic stenosis significantly affects the hemodynamic management and the choices of diuretic and vasodilator therapy. If sepsis develops in these patients, they may have a low cardiac output and artificially raised systemic vascular resistance even though they may be systemically vasodilated. In this case, they benefit from both dobutamine and dopamine inotropic therapy.

TTE can assess the valves for congenital anomalies, calcification, vegetations, and masses. Doppler mapping and color mapping graphically illustrate the results of any morphologic abnormality. Valvular stenosis (Tables 42–5 and 42–6) creates higher velocities of blood flow that can be detected by Doppler studies. Valvular regurgitation (Tables 42–7 and 42–8) produces reversed flow compared with the cardiac cycle. For aortic and mitral stenosis (see Table 42–5), Doppler estimation of instantaneous gradients and calculated mean gradients correlate well with similar measurements obtained during cardiac catheterization.[114] The peak instantaneous gradient is linearly related to the mean gradient (two thirds of peak instantaneous gradient = mean gradient). Alternatively, the mean gradient

TABLE 42–6. Obstruction of the Left Ventricular Outflow Tract

Valvular—aortic stenosis
Dynamic outflow obstruction
Interventricular—hypertrophic cardiomyopathy
Subaortic—discrete subaortic stenosis
Supravalvular
Aortic arch interruptions
Coarctation of the aortic isthmus

TABLE 42–7. Aortic Regurgitation

Chronic
Rheumatic fever
Healed infective endocarditis
Degenerative calcified disease
Bicuspid aortic valve
Aortic root dilatation
Hypertension
Marfan's syndrome
Cystic medial degeneration
Annuloaortic ectasia
Atherosclerosis
Syphilis
Systemic lupus erythematosus
Acute
Acute infective endocarditis
Traumatic rupture of aortic leaflet
Rupture of myxomatous valve
Aortic dissection

TABLE 42–8. Mitral Regurgitation

Congenital
Cleft mitral valve
Atrioventricular cushion defect
Myxomatous degeneration
Mitral valve prolapse
Rheumatic
Infectious endocarditis
Ischemic
Calcific
Degenerative with mitral annular degeneration
Renal or hyperparathyroid diseases
Traumatic
Chordal rupture caused by nonpenetrating chest trauma
Cardiomyopathy
Dilated
Hypertrophic
Restrictive
Myocarditis
Severe aortic regurgitation

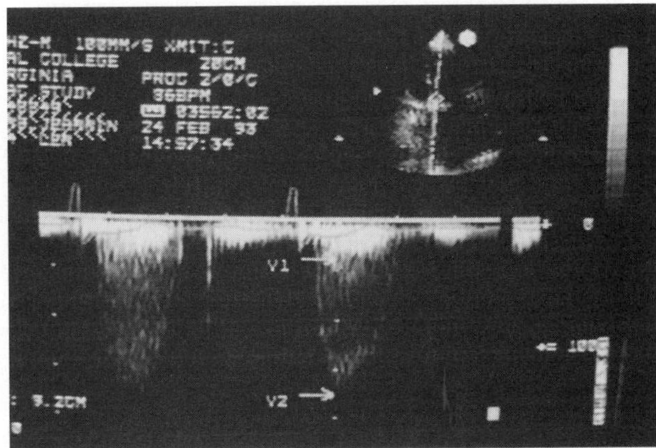

Figure 42–9. Continuous-wave Doppler echocardiographic recording of a patient with severe aortic stenosis. V1 = flow velocity in left ventricular outflow tract; V2 = maximal flow velocity recorded along the cursor line, which reflects postvalvular velocity in the ascending aorta.

can be derived from the integral of the spectral Doppler velocity envelope (Fig. 42–9). Because gradients are a function of the driving force (i.e., the cardiac output), the aortic valve area is calculated from the continuity equation, which compares the velocity of blood proximal and distal to the valve (see Table 42–2). The aortic valve area calculations are usually within 10% of cardiac catheterization–derived aortic valve areas.[115]

With aortic regurgitation, color mapping demonstrates a regurgitant jet that is usually central, streaming into the LV during diastole (Fig. 42–10; see Color Plate and Table 42–7). The severity of aortic regurgitation may be quantitatively assessed. The width, length, and area of the regurgitant jet, the slope of the spectral Doppler map, and reversal of flow in the descending aorta have been used to quantify the degree of regurgitation.[116, 117] In the authors' experience, reversal of flow in the descending aorta and width of the regurgitant jet greater than 60% of the LV outflow tract correlate most closely with severe aortic regurgitation.

Mitral regurgitation is detected by color Doppler mapping of the LA (Fig. 42–11*A* and *B*; see Color Plate and Table 42–8). Pulsed Doppler recordings may be used to confirm the presence of retrograde flow of blood during systole (see Fig. 42–2). Severe mitral regurgitation is present when flow retrograde to the pulmonary vein is seen by pulsed Doppler and when the regurgitant jet area is greater than 40% of the LA area.[118] However, eccentric jets that impinge on the LA wall are underestimated by color Doppler imaging by as much as 40%.[119] These eccentric regurgitant jets can cause asymmetric pulmonary edema when selectively engaging the right pulmonary vein.[120]

The degree of mitral stenosis can be quantified by planimetry of the mitral valve orifice in the parasternal short-axis view (see Table 42–5).[121] The pressure gradient during diastole is independent of cardiac output and is prolonged in the presence of mitral stenosis. Because flow across a stenotic valve is turbulent, color-flow mapping demonstrates a narrow candle-like jet. Color mapping can guide the optimal position of the Doppler probe for estimating the mitral valve area (MVA). Doppler interrogation of transmitral flow can measure the pressure half-time (time taken for the initial maximum diastolic gradient to drop to one half) and the mitral valve area calculated from the relationship MVA = 220/pressure half-time in milliseconds (Fig. 42–12).[122] Compared with the MVA derived by cardiac catheterization using the Gorlin formula, the pressure half-time MVA derived by continuous-wave Doppler is in agreement within 0.2 cm^2.[123]

AORTIC DISEASE

The proximal ascending aorta is well seen by TTE. Most of the aorta can be seen by combining the left and right parasternal, suprasternal, supraclavicular, and subcostal windows in 80% of patients.[124] Aortic root diseases, such as sinus of Valsalva aneurysms and annuloaortic ectasia, can be observed by echocardiography, and aortic root enlargement of greater than 6 cm has been used as a criterion for aortic root replacement.[125]

Dissection of the ascending aorta is a life-threatening condition in which early mortality can be as high as 1% per hour.[126] Prompt diagnosis and treatment are lifesaving. Surgical therapy benefits patients with ascending aortic involvement (standard A or DeBakey I and II), and distal type III or Stanford B can usually be managed medically.[127, 128] Echocardiography is well suited for evaluating patients with possible aortic dissection, as it is a widely available, noninvasive technique that can be performed at the bedside. TTE is useful for identifying proximal dissection and identifies other potential complications, such as aortic regurgitation and pericardial effusion (Fig. 42–13*A* and *B*). The sensitivity of TTE in identifying the ascending aorta ranges from 78% to 100%, although for the descending aorta it is only 55% to 31%.[129, 130]

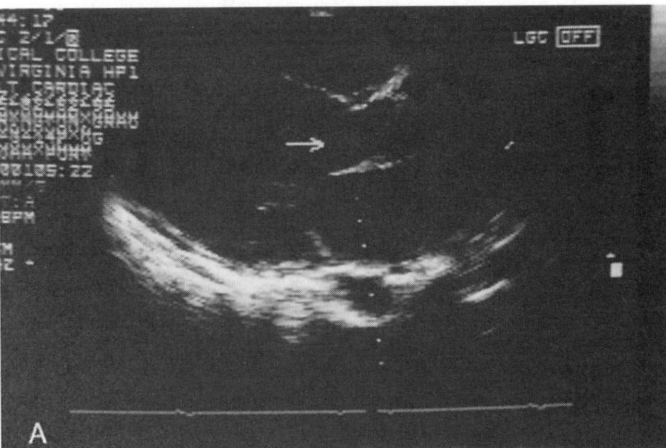

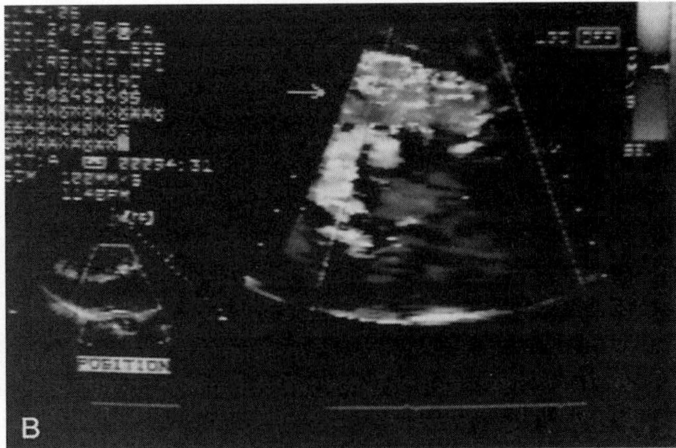

Figure 42–10. *A*, A two-dimensional echocardiogram in the parasternal long-axis view in a patient with aortic regurgitation. *B*, A color-flow Doppler echocardiogram in the parasternal long-axis view of the same patient with aortic regurgitation as in *A*. (See Color Plate.)

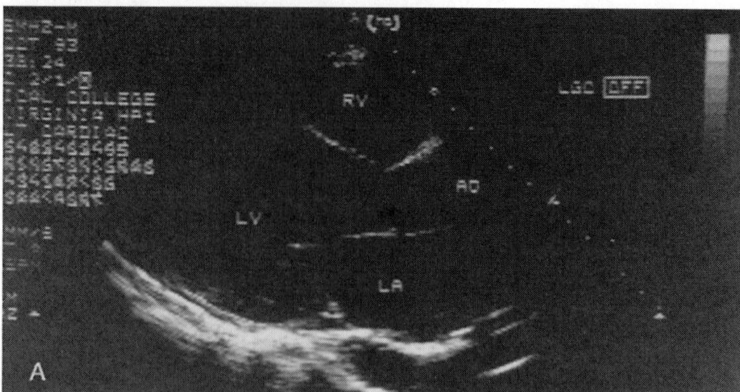

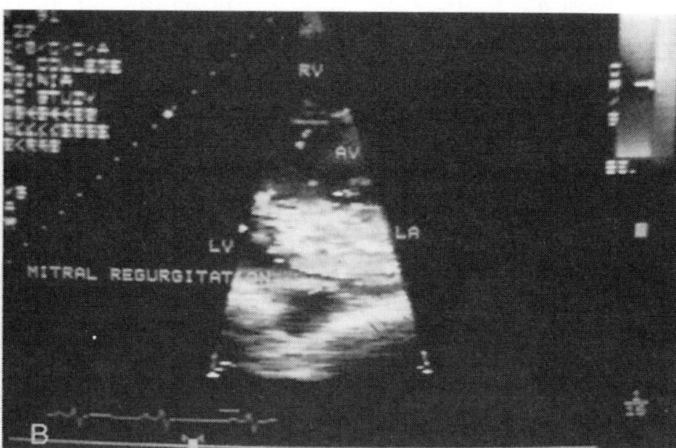

Figure 42–11. *A,* A two-dimensional echocardiogram in the parasternal short-axis view showing left atrial enlargement in a patient with severe mitral regurgitation. *B,* A color-flow Doppler echocardiogram in the parasternal short-axis view showing severe mitral regurgitation in the same patient as in *A*. AV = aortic valve. (See Color Plate.)

In contrast, TEE has a sensitivity that exceeds 95% and specificity greater than 90% in most studies[129-139] (Fig. 42–14 [see Color Plate] and Table 42–9). Correct identification of an acute aortic tear or dissection can be lifesaving.[133, 137, 138] Erbel and colleagues,[131] in the European Cooperative Study, evaluated the efficacy of TEE for detecting acute aortic dissection compared with standard methods of computed tomography (CT) and angiography. The diagnosis of aortic dissection was confirmed by surgery or autopsy. The sensitivity was 99% and the specificity 98% for TEE, compared with 88% and 94% for angiography and 83% and 100% for CT. In addition to identification of the dissection flap, TEE can identify other important diagnostic findings, including the entry and exit points.

Hashimoto and coworkers,[132] using TEE assessment for the diagnosis of dissecting aortic aneurysm, showed correct detection of the entry and intimal flap in all cases, compared with a 42% detection rate using conventional modalities. As with TTE, the presence of pericardial effusion as well as the presence and severity of aortic insufficiency can be identified. TEE can also determine the presence or absence of coronary artery involvement with high sensitivity and specificity.

Ballal and associates[134] found that TEE correctly identified the dissection in 29 of 34 patients with a sensitivity of 97%, a specificity of 100%, and positive and negative predictive values of 100% and 96%, respectively. TEE also correctly precluded aortic dissection in all 27 patients without dissection. Of particular importance was the echocardiographic identification of coronary artery involvement with the aortic dissection in six of seven patients.

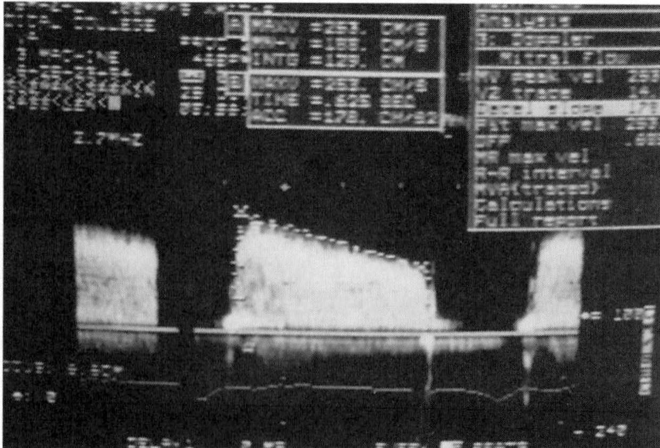

Figure 42–12. The spectral display of a continuous-wave Doppler echocardiogram in a patient with significant mitral stenosis. Quantification of the mitral stenosis may be performed with a number of spectral Doppler variables, including the deceleration slope.

Several large studies have compared TEE with magnetic resonance imaging (MRI) for diagnosis of aortic dissection.[129, 130] The sensitivities for both TEE and MRI were 100%. Of concern was the low specificity of TEE (68.2%) compared with that of MRI (100%). The false-positive results primarily involved evaluation of the ascending aorta and arch. In addition, false-positive results may occur with secondary extensive plaque formation and echo reverberations in the ectatic vessel.[130] Thrombus formation in the false lumen of the aortic arch and the descending segments of the thoracic aorta was more easily and consistently identified by MRI. The frequency of identification of aortic regurgitation, pericardial effusion, and entry site of the dissection was the same with the two techniques. A follow-up study of aortic dissection compared MRI, TEE, TTE, and CT.[130] The sensitivities of TTE, TEE, MRI, and CT were 59.3%, 97.7%, 98.3%, and 93.8%, respectively. The specificities were similar to these in the earlier study, with 83%, 76.9%, 97.8%, and 87.1%, respectively, for TTE, TEE, MRI, and CT.

TEE is useful for assessment of repaired type A aortic dissection.[135] Patients have a higher survival rate (90%) when no flow is detected in the false lumen, easily assessed by TEE. As with CT, TEE identifies prosthetic false aneurysms, sinus of Valsalva aneurysms, and aortic valve involvement.

The decision on which imaging technique to use for the initial evaluation of patients with potential aortic dissection depends on the expertise of the center, underlying characteristics of the patients, and information that is desired. Sensitivities of TEE, MRI, and CT (when helical CT is used) are comparable, although each offers certain advantages and disadvantages. TEE can be used to identify entry and exit points,

TABLE 42–9. Transesophageal Echocardiographic Identification of Acute Aortic Dissection: Typical Findings

Small true lumen
Large false lumen
Entry site
Communication between the lumina demonstrated by color-flow Doppler
Intimal flap with undulating motion
Thrombus in the false lumen and spontaneous echoes

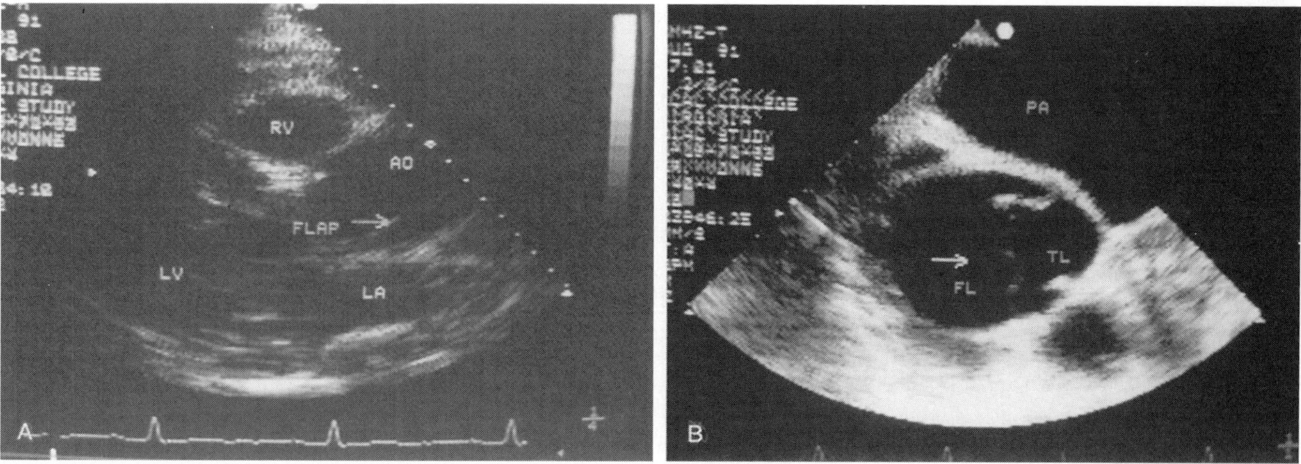

Figure 42–13. *A,* A transthoracic two-dimensional echocardiogram showing the flap in a type 1 dissection of the ascending aorta. *B,* A transesophageal two-dimensional echocardiogram of the same patient as in *A* showing the true lumen (TL) and the false lumen (FL) of this type 1 aortic dissection. AO = aorta; PA = pulmonary artery.

coronary artery involvement, pericardial effusion, and aortic regurgitation, most of which are not identifiable by CT. Although pericardial effusion and aortic regurgitation, most of which are not identifiable by CT. Although pericardial effusion and aortic regurgitation are also identified if cine-MRI is used, an additional 15 to 30 minutes is needed and coronary artery involvement is not revealed. The primary disadvantages of TEE include inability to limit the aortic arch, difficulty in determining branch vessel involvement, and difficulty in determining distal extension of the dissection in patients with descending aorta involvement. However, because TEE can be performed at the bedside, it is clearly the imaging technique of choice in unstable patients. For patients without dissection, TEE can be particularly helpful in delineating other causes of hemodynamic instability that mimic aortic dissection.[134]

Intramural hemorrhage or localized hematoma forming in the aortic wall is an entity that may be a precursor of dissection.[140] Intramural hemorrhage may result from spontaneous rupture of the vasa vasorum resulting in aortic wall disintegration or intimal fracture of an atherosclerotic plaque, allowing propagation of blood into the aortic media. Diagnostic characteristics of intramural hemorrhage are splitting of the multiple layers of the aortic wall with increased wall thickness, increased distance from the aortic lumen to the esophagus, and a periaortic echo-free zone secondary to fluid extravasation.[139] Identification of this condition is important, as it frequently progresses to aortic dissection or rupture or cardiac tamponade.[140]

The technique has proved useful in evaluating the aorta for thrombus and atherosclerotic debris. TEE is capable of identifying the amount and extent of atheromatous debris in the aorta.[141] Atherosclerotic debris is associated with coronary artery and cerebrovascular disease. The incidence of embolic events is increased when a mobile or pedunculated plaque is visualized.[137, 142] A significant increase in postoperative stroke is noted in patients with a mobile atheroma undergoing cardiac surgery.[143] TEE can be used to identify debris in the ascending aorta and to alter the site of aortic cannulation and cross-clamping, in order to limit the extent of a cerebral event after cardiac surgery.[144–146]

INFECTIVE ENDOCARDITIS

The diagnosis of infective endocarditis is a clinical one based on history and physical examination, blood cultures, and serologic tests. Echocardiography has increasingly gained impor-

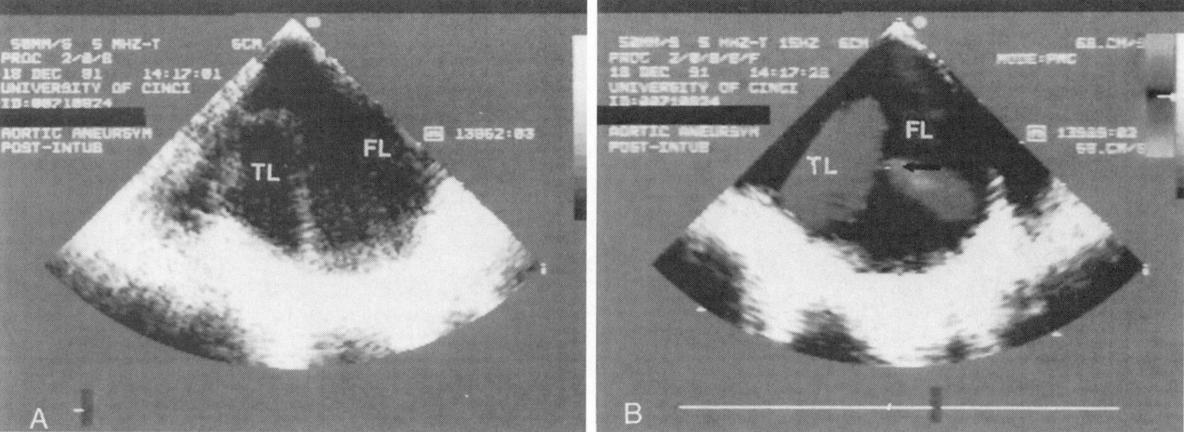

Figure 42–14. Aortic dissection. *A,* Transesophageal echocardiogram (TEE), horizontal view, showing an intimal flap with a small true lumen and a larger false lumen with spontaneous echo contrast. *B,* TEE with color-flow Doppler showing a small true lumen and a larger false lumen, with a jet through the entry site into the false lumen. (See Color Plate.)

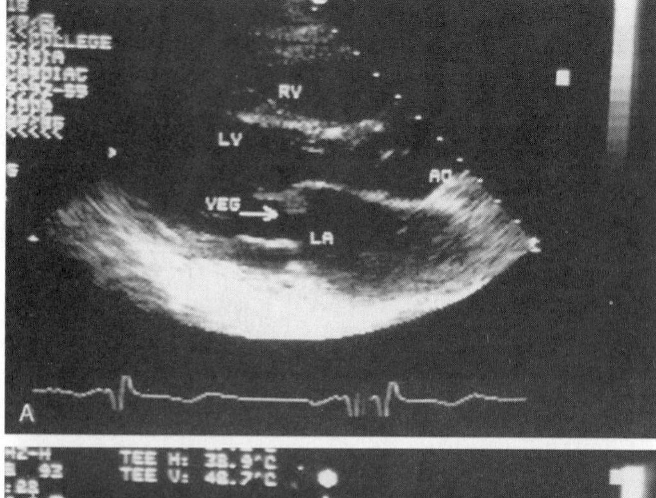

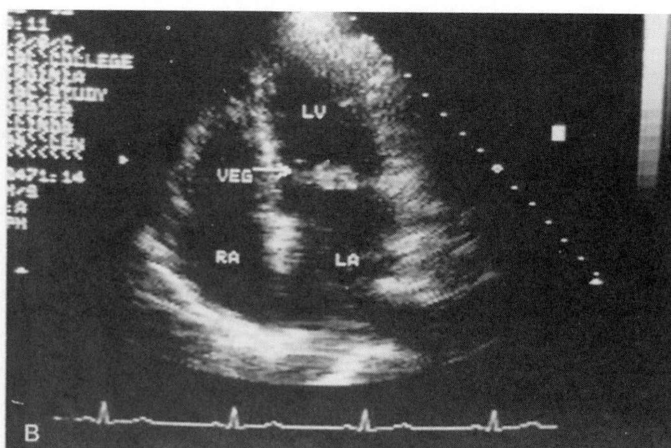

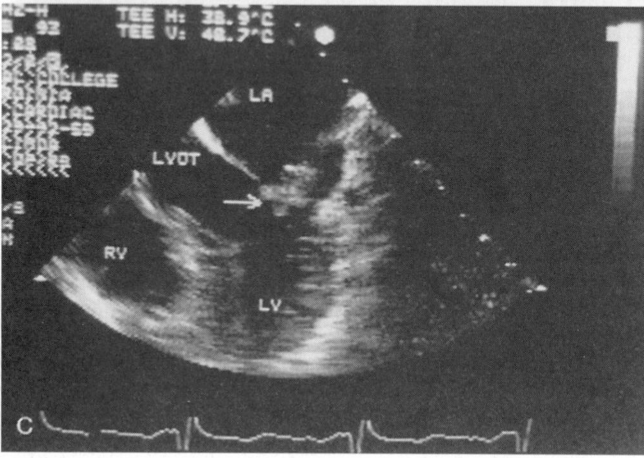

Figure 42–15. *A,* A transthoracic two-dimensional echocardiogram in the parasternal long-axis position of a vegetation attached to the anterior mitral leaflet of a patient with endocarditis. *B,* A transthoracic two-dimensional echocardiogram in the apical four-chamber view of the same patient as in *A* with endocarditis. *C,* A transesophageal two-dimensional echocardiogram showing the vegetation on the anterior leaflet of the mitral valve *(arrow)* in the same patient as in *A* and *B.* VEG = vegetation on the anterior leaflet of the mitral valve; LVOT = left ventricular outflow tract.

tance for the diagnosis of endocarditis, with approximately 60% sensitivity for detecting vegetations (Figs. 42–15 and 42–16) (see Color Plate).[147] Vegetations as small as 2 to 5 mm may be detected with TTE. In contrast, the sensitivity of TEE for identifying patients with endocarditis exceeds 90% and vegetations as small as 1 to 2 mm can be visualized.[148, 149] Although the sensitivity is not perfect, the absence of echocardiographic evidence of endocarditis is predictive of a low incidence of complications. In patients with a high suspicion of endocarditis in whom the initial TEE is negative, repeated TEE after 5 to 7 days may useful for identifying an additional 5% of patients with endocarditis.[150] If clinical suspicion of endocarditis is low, an adequate TTE for possible native valve endocarditis may be sufficient to exclude the diagnosis.[151, 152] However, in patients who have a suboptimal window or prosthetic valves, TEE is indicated. In patients with right-sided endocarditis, TTE and TEE have similar sensitivities, although the image quality may be somewhat improved with TEE.[153]

The important role that echocardiography, both TTE and TEE, plays in the diagnosis of endocarditis is recognized in

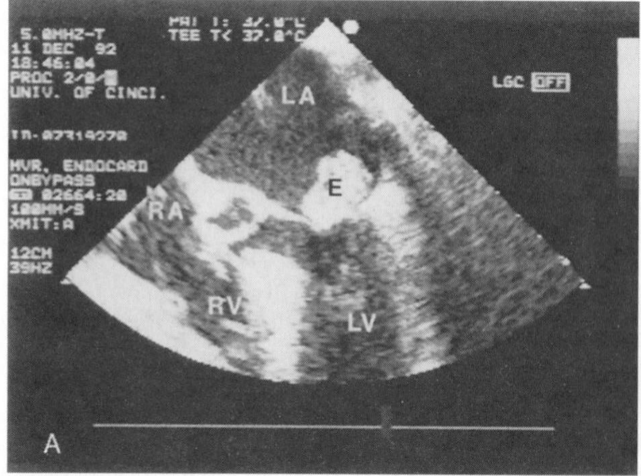

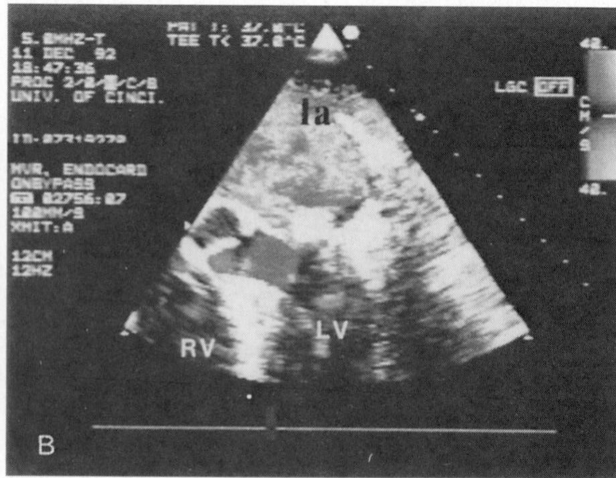

Figure 42–16. *A,* A 2.8 × 1.8 cm vegetation associated with an abscess attached to the posterior mitral valve leaflet shown by transesophageal echocardiography. *B,* During the same procedure, the color-flow study shows severe mitral regurgitation. E = vegetation. (See Color Plate.)

the Duke criteria for the diagnosis of endocarditis.[154] Specific echocardiographic findings, including visualization of an oscillating intracardiac mass, presence of an abscess, partial dehiscence of a prosthetic valve, or new valvular regurgitation, are considered major criteria for diagnosis of endocarditis.

The size, extent, and mobility of vegetations are significant predictors of complications in patients with endocarditis.[155] A vegetation size exceeding 10 mm on TEE is associated with an increased rate of complications, including a 47% incidence of an embolic event.[147] Embolic events are more common in patients with mitral valve endocarditis.

Two-dimensional echocardiography may be useful in monitoring the clinical course, especially in patients with left-sided endocarditis. Vegetation size exceeding 10 mm and aortic valve involvement correlate with a need for valve replacement and a worse outcome.[156] A decrease in vegetation size on repeated echocardiography after 4 to 8 weeks of therapy has been associated with an improved outcome compared with those in whom the vegetation was either unchanged or increased in size.[157]

Vegetations can be difficult to visualize in prosthetic valve endocarditis owing to the metallic struts. With bioprosthetic valves, although the cusps can be seen, the quality of the images is poorer than with native valves. TTE is of limited usefulness because of the acoustic shadowing from the prosthetic devices. TTE detects only 33% of endocarditis cases, whereas the sensitivity of TEE exceeds 80%.[158] In patients with both mitral and aortic prosthetic valves, imaging of the mitral valve may be limited by shadowing from the aortic valve. Detection of vegetations is lower in patients with prosthetic valve endocarditis; visualization of periprosthetic leaks, abscess formation, valvular obstruction or dehiscence offers indirect evidence of the diagnosis.

An important complication of endocarditis is valve ring abscess. The presence of abnormal prosthetic valve rocking motion, thickening of the aortic root, and sinus of Valsalva aneurysm can signal a ring abscess.[155, 159] Valve ring abscess is more common with aortic valve endocarditis and is associated with increased morbidity and mortality.[160] The sensitivity of TTE for identifying abscesses is less than 30%, compared with a sensitivity of 87% for TEE, making it the imaging modality of choice for patients with suspected abscess formation.[161]

Recommendations for when TEE should be performed for patients with possible endocarditis are evolving. In patients for whom the diagnosis is considered, TTE should be performed. In patients with a high suspicion of endocarditis who have a prosthetic valve or suboptimal TTE images, TEE is indicated. Whether to perform TEE in patients with evidence of endocarditis from TTE depends on the clinical scenario. In clinically stable patients with an organism of low virulence, involving the mitral or tricuspid valve, TTE may be adequate. Because of the high morbidity and mortality and the increased incidence of abscess formation associated with endocarditis caused by *Staphylococcus aureus,* TEE is often recommenced. In patients with aortic valve endocarditis, TEE is indicated because of the high incidence of associated paravalvular abscess formation.[161] Finally, in the patient who is not responding to treatment, TEE may be useful for excluding potential complications.

TRAUMATIC DISEASES

Cardiac trauma can have a variety of causes. Chest wall injury can cause cardiac damage by compressing the heart or causing ischemic injury by damaging a coronary artery. Deceleration can result in tearing injuries, often to the aorta, the pulmonary veins, or the venae cavae, related to the heart swinging as it is suspended from the great vessels. Finally, valvular injury can result from a sudden increase in intrathoracic pressures. The most common causes of cardiac trauma are motor vehicle accidents, falls, and blows from nonpenetrating objects.

Penetrating trauma to the heart can involve the RV, LV, RA, and LA in order of greatest frequency.[162] Hemopericardium with tamponade leads to death unless the problem is quickly recognized. Echocardiography can be immensely helpful in identifying this problem and in assisting with emergency drainage of tamponade. One study found that introduction of echocardiography in a trauma ED resulted in a significant improvement in survival of patients with penetrating cardiac injury, because of a significant decrease in the time to diagnosis and intervention.[163]

The majority of cardiac injuries resulting from blunt trauma involve damage to the myocardium with resulting myocardial contusion. If the trauma is severe enough, cardiac rupture can occur. Echocardiographic signs found in animal models of blunt cardiac trauma include increased end-diastolic wall thickness (resulting from myocardial edema), increased echo brightness (from cell damage and hemorrhage), and segmental wall-motion abnormalities.[163] In patients, the hallmark of cardiac contusion is visualization of regional wall-motion abnormalities.[164] Less commonly, ventricular or atrial septal defects may occur.

Most studies have demonstrated that echocardiography is a more sensitive identifier of cardiac contusion than the ECG or myocardial markers.[165] However, routine use of echocardiography as a screening tool in all patients with chest trauma is not indicated. The presence of abnormalities on echocardiography is not predictive of morbidity or mortality.[166, 167] In most cases, clinically important complications of myocardial contusion rarely occur in patients who are hemodynamically stable.[168] Echocardiography is indicated for patients who are hemodynamically unstable or who have significant arrhythmias, progressive dyspnea, or ischemic patterns on the ECG.[169] In these patients, timely echocardiography is mandated to preclude important pericardial and valvular abnormalities.

Valvular injury can result from two mechanisms. Tricuspid and mitral insufficiency can result from rupture of the papillary muscles, chordae tendineae, or from direct rupture of the valve leaflets. Aortic valve injury can result from a sudden increase in intrathoracic pressure during diastole.[170] In some cases, the degree of damage may not be apparent for days after the injury.

TEE is frequently required for cardiac imaging of patients after chest wall trauma, because TTE imaging may be suboptimal in up to 60% of patients.[171, 172] TEE is also useful for evaluating the aorta after a traumatic chest injury. Aortography has the disadvantages of being invasive, time-consuming, and unable to exclude cardiac injury. A number of studies have demonstrated that TEE is an accurate imaging technique for diagnosis of traumatic aortic rupture or tear or a periaortic hematoma.[173, 174] As with aortic dissection, the inability to image the aortic arch is a disadvantage; however, most aortic tears occur at the aortic isthmus distal to the origin of the left subclavian artery. TEE also cannot be performed in patients who have cervical neck injuries or significant orofacial injuries. Another limitation is that small arterial injuries resulting in a limited flap may be apparent. Many of these regress spontaneously, and early operative intervention is not warranted.[175]

Because patients with significant trauma often have multiple chest tubes in place or are intubated, the echocardiographic window is often limited. In these cases, TEE can be performed.

INTRACARDIAC AND EXTRACARDIAC MASSES

The cause of intracardiac masses can be either thrombus material or neoplastic tissue, associated with obstruction or systemic embolization.[176-179] TEE is particularly helpful when TTE evaluation is inconclusive, such as with small tumors and thrombi, laminated thrombi, thrombi limited to the left or right atrial appendage, or poor images.[178]

TTE may be inconclusive in detecting a mass in the presence of prosthetic valves.[176] TEE overcomes this dilemma by having imaging ability posterior to the mechanical device (see Fig. 42-16). Left atrial thrombus can be seen by TEE in patients who have mitral stenosis or atrial fibrillation. A thrombus is occasionally visualized adjacent to central lines. TEE should be used for assessing the atrial appendage, particularly if a patient has signs and symptoms of systemic embolization and is undergoing cardioversion or mitral valve repair or replacement.[180] During percutaneous mitral balloon valvulotomy, TEE has also helped in guiding insertion of the balloon catheter through the stenotic orifice of the mitral valve and evaluating the residual mitral regurgitation and intracardiac shunt. TEE has also been useful for identifying RA thrombi located on the tips of catheters.[181]

INTRACARDIAC SHUNTS

Intracardiac shunts, acquired and congenital, are occasionally noted in critically ill patients.[182] TEE correctly identifies patent foramen ovale, ostium secundum, and ostium primum defects. In comparison with that of cardiac catheterization, the calculated shunt flow volume and pulmonary-to-systemic blood flow ratio showed a close correlation with TEE.

Paradoxical embolism is a concern for critical care physicians. Estimates of the prevalence of patent foramen ovale (PFO) defined by postmortem studies are 25% to 35%.[183] At basal in vivo conditions, the patency is 5% to 10% but increases to 18% to 22% after augmentation of the pressure differential in the atria by the Valsalva maneuver, coughing, or sudden release of positive intrathoracic pressure.[184-186] Detection of a PFO by contrast imaging by TEE is superior to detection by TEE.[187] A Valsalva maneuver enhances the value of this test. This is particularly important in assessment of patients with cardiac conditions and individuals with unexplained strokes. Hausmann and colleagues[185] detected a PFO in 50% of patients who were younger than 40 years and who had an unexplained ischemic stroke. Chen and associates[188] found a PFO in 44% of patients during normal breathing and 63% during a Valsalva maneuver with contrast TEE during cardiac catheterization.

PFO may allow a paradoxical embolic event leading to neurologic impairment or death. The possibility of creating a right-to-left shunt in patients with refractory hypoxemia exists. TEE is useful in searching for an intracardiac cause. The unidirectional flap-valve nature of the PFO permits shunt flow even with a transient interatrial pressure gradient or reversal of the normal left-to-right pressure differential.

CRITICALLY ILL PATIENTS

For critically ill patients, echocardiography, especially TEE, can provide important diagnostic information. Patients are often intubated or have bandages or chest tubes in place that severely limit the ability to obtain adequate TTE images. Indications for TEE in critically ill patients include:

1. Unexplained hypotension or hemodynamic instability.
2. Suspicion of endocarditis or significant valvular disease in a native or prosthetic valve.
3. Possible aortic dissection.
4. Diagnosis of possible complications of myocardial infarction.
5. Cardiac tamponade.

TEE has also been used for evaluation of cardiac arrest.[189, 190] Important information obtained includes the presence of a dilated RV, indicating pulmonary embolism or RV infarction, and small localized hemorrhage causing tamponade of the RA in postsurgical patients. In patients with unexplained hypotension, demonstration of a small hypercontractile LV with a normal pulmonary venous inflow pattern (predominant systolic wave) indicates that the likely etiologic mechanism of the hypotension is volume depletion.[191] Aggressive volume repletion can rapidly reverse the hypotension, allowing discontinuation of vasopressors.

A number of studies have shown that TEE often provides diagnostic information that was not suspected, resulting in a change of therapy in a significant minority of patients. These changes include addition or removal of pharmacologic treatments and referral for cardiac surgery.[10, 11, 192, 193] In some of these studies, the information provided by echocardiography was more accurate than that obtained using pulmonary artery catheters to determine the cause of the hypotension.[191] TEE can also provide important prognostic information. Demonstration of a nonventricular limitation to cardiac output was associated with improved survival in patients in intensive care compared with patients with ventricular disease or hypovolemia.[193]

SUMMARY

Although echocardiography is a powerful diagnostic tool, a working understanding of the background principles is necessary to apply this imaging technology in clinical practice. Because technical expertise is needed to perform a thorough study, and because a detailed understanding of cardiac anatomy and physiology is a prerequisite to interpreting the examination, familiarity with echocardiography is likely to enhance care of patients. Echocardiography is useful in evaluating patients with shock because it demonstrates myocardial performance and can help distinguish cardiac from noncardiac causes of hypotension. Because multisystem failure and sepsis syndrome influence myocardial function, echocardiography may enable one to make decisions about inotropic therapy. Echocardiography is diagnostic of effusive pericardial diseases and significant valvular abnormalities. Echocardiography has the potential to provide hemodynamic data equivalent to those obtained with a Swan-Ganz catheter in determinations of cardiac output and pulmonary artery systolic pressures. Because echocardiography is easily performed at the bedside, critically ill patients do not have to be transported out of the ICU. Echocardiography will be increasingly used in all critical care areas as more specialists become familiar with the wealth of data that can be obtained.

ACKNOWLEDGMENT

The authors wish to thank Ms. Cecilia Delacruz Lindsey for her assistance in the preparation of this chapter.

References

1. Fili EO, Labovitz AJ: Transesophageal echocardiography: Expanding indications for ICU use. J Crit Illness 1992; 7:85.
2. Pearson AC, Castello R, Labovitz AJ, et al: Safety and utility of transesophageal echocardiography in the critically ill patient. Am Heart J 1990; 119:1083.
3. Burns PN, Powers JE, Simpson DH, et al: Harmonic imaging: Principles and preliminary results. Clin Radiol 1996; 51(Suppl I):50.
4. Cannon SR, Richards KL: Principles and physics of Doppler. *In:*

Cardiac Imaging. Marcus ML, Schelbert HR, Skorton DJ, et al (Eds). Philadelphia, WB Saunders, 1991, pp 365–373.
5. Hatle L, Angelsen B (Eds): Doppler Ultrasound in Cardiology: Physical Principles and Clinical Applications. 2nd ed. Philadelphia, Lea & Febiger, 1985.
6. Sahn DJ: Real time two-dimensional Doppler echocardiographic flow mapping. Circulation 1985; 71:849.
7. Schiller NB, Shah PM, Crawford M, et al: Recommendations for quantitation of the left ventricle by two-dimensional echocardiography. J Am Soc Echocardiogr 1989; 2:358.
8. Seward JB, Khandheria BK, Oh JK, et al: Transesophageal echocardiography: Technique, anatomic correlations, implementation and cardiac applications. Mayo Clin Proc 1988; 63:649.
9. Porembka DT, Hoit BD: Transesophageal echocardiography in the intensive care patient. Crit Care Med 1991; 19:826.
10. Oh JK, Seward JB, Khandheria BK, et al: Transesophageal echocardiography in critically ill patients. Am J Cardiol 1990; 66:1492.
11. Foster E, Schiller NB: The role of transesophageal echocardiography in critical care: UCSF experience. J Am Soc Echocardiogr 1992; 5:368.
12. Seward JB, Khandheria BK, Oh JK, et al: Biplanar transesophageal echocardiography: Anatomic correlations, image orientation and clinical applications. Mayo Clin Proc 1990; 65:1193.
13. Geibel A, Kasper W, Behroz A, et al: Risk of transesophageal echocardiography in awake patients with cardiac disease. Am J Cardiol 1988; 62:337.
14. Daniel WG, Kasper W, Erbel R: Safety of transesophageal echocardiography: A multicenter survey of 10,419 examinations. Circulation 1991; 83:817.
15. Dewhirst WE, Stragand JJ, Fleming BM: Mallory-Weiss tear complicating intraoperative transesophageal echocardiography in a patient undergoing aortic valve replacement. Anesthesiology 1990; 73:777.
16. Dawson J, Cockrel R: Esophageal perforation at fiberoptic gastroscopy. Br Med J 1981; 283:583.
17. Pongratz G, Henneke K, von der Grun M, et al: Risk of endocarditis in transesophageal echocardiography. Am Heart J 1993; 125:190.
18. Erbel R, Engberding R, Daniel W, et al: Echocardiography in the diagnosis of aortic dissection. European Cooperative Study Group for Echocardiography. Lancet 1989; i:457.
19. Shyu KG, Hwang JJ, Lin SC, et al: Prospective study of blood culture during transesophageal echocardiography. Am Heart J 1992; 125:1541.
20. Appleton CP, Gallowa JM, Gonzalez MS, et al: Estimation of left ventricular filling pressures using two dimensional and Doppler echocardiography in adult patients with cardiac disease: Additional value of analyzing left atrial size, left atrial ejection fraction and the difference in duration of pulmonary venous and mitral flow velocity at atrial contraction. J Am Coll Cardiol 1993; 22:1972.
21. Pai RG, Shah PM: Echocardiographic and other noninvasive measurements of cardiac hemodynamics and ventricular function. Curr Probl Cardiol 1995; 20:681.
22. Borgeson DD, Seward JB, Miler FA, et al: Frequency of Doppler measurable pulmonary artery pressures. J Am Soc Echocardiogr 1996; 9:832.
23. Masuyama T, Kodama K, Kitabatake A, et al: Continuous wave Doppler echocardiographic detection of pulmonary regurgitation and its application to noninvasive estimation of pulmonary artery pressure. Circulation 1986; 74:484.
24. Kircher BJ, Himmelman RB, Schiller NB, et al: Noninvasive estimation of right atrial pressure from the inspiratory collapse of the inferior vena cava. Am J Cardiol 1990; 66:493.
25. Nagueh SF, Kopelen HA, Zoghbi WA: Relation of mean right atrial pressure to echocardiographic and Doppler parameters of right atrial and right ventricular function. Circulation 1996; 93:1160.
26. Yock PG, Popp RL: Non-invasive estimation of right ventricular systolic pressure by Doppler ultrasound in patients with tricuspid regurgitation. Circulation 1984; 70:657.
27. Laaban JP, Diebold B, Zelinski R, et al: Noninvasive estimation of systolic pulmonary artery pressure using Doppler echocardiography in patients with chronic obstructive pulmonary disease. Chest 1989; 6:1258.
28. Seppanen MP, Kappa PO, Kero PO, et al: Doppler derived systolic pulmonary artery pressure in acute neonatal respiratory distress syndrome. Pediatrics 1994; 93:769.
29. Gorcsan J III, Snow FR, Paulsen W, Nixon JV: Noninvasive estimation of left atrial pressure in patients with congestive heart failure and mitral regurgitation by Doppler echocardiography. Am Heart J 1991; 121:858.
30. Pazzoli M, Capomolla S, Pinna G, et al: Doppler echocardiography reliably predicts pulmonary artery wedge pressure in patients with chronic heart failure with and without mitral regurgitation. J Am Coll Cardiol 1996; 27:883.
31. Gardin JM, Dabestani A, Takenaka K, et al: Effect of imaging view and sample volume location on evaluation of mitral flow velocity by pulsed Doppler echocardiography. Am J Cardiol 1986; 57:1335.
32. Yamamoto K, Nishimura RA, Chaliki HP, et al: Determination of left ventricular filling pressure by Doppler echocardiography in patients with coronary disease: Critical role of left ventricular systolic function. J Am Coll Cardiol 1997; 30:1819.
33. Giannuzzi P, Temporeeli PL, Bosomini E, et al: Independent and incremental prognostic value of Doppler-derived mitral deceleration time of early filling in both symptomatic and asymptomatic patients with left ventricular dysfunction. J Am Coll Cardiol 1996; 28:383.
34. Nishimura RA, Schwartz RS, Tajik AJ, et al: Noninvasive assessment of left ventricular relaxation by Doppler echocardiography: Validation with simultaneous cardiac catheterization, Circulation 1993; 88:146.
35. Nagueh SF, Kopelen HA, Zoghbi WA: Feasibility and accuracy of Doppler echocardiographic estimation of pulmonary artery occlusive pressure in the intensive care unit. Am J Cardiol 1995; 75:1256.
36. Stein JH, Neumann A, Preston LM, et al: Echocardiography for hemodynamic assessment of patients with advanced heart failure and potential heart transplant recipients. J Am Coll Cardiol 1997; 30:1765.
37. Lewis JF, Kuo LC, Nelson JG, et al: Pulsed Doppler echocardiographic determination of stroke volume and cardiac output: Clinical validation of two new methods using the apical window. Circulation 1984; 70:425.
38. Gardin JM, Burn CS, Childs WJ, et al: Evaluation of blood flow velocity in the ascending aorta and main pulmonary artery of normal subjects by Doppler echocardiography. Am Heart J 1984; 107:310.
39. Huntsmann LL, Stewart DK, Barnes SR, et al: Noninvasive Doppler determination of cardiac output in man—clinical validation. Circulation 1983; 67:593.
40. Evangelista A, Garcia-Dorado D, Garcia H, et al: Cardiac index quantification by Doppler ultrasound in patients without left ventricular outflow tract abnormalities. J Am Coll Cardiol 1995; 25:710.
41. Eisenberg MJ, Dunn MM, Kanth N, et al: Diagnostic value of chest radiography for pericardial effusion. J Am Coll Cardiol 1993; 22:588.
42. Eisenberg MJ; de Romeral LM, Heidenreich PA, et al: The diagnosis of pericardial effusion and cardiac tamponade by 12-lead ECG: A technology assessment. Chest 1996; 110:318.
43. Clark JG, Berberich SN, Zager JR, et al: Echocardiographic findings of pericardial effusion mimicked by fibrocalcific pericardial disease. Echocardiography 1985; 2:467.
44. Beck CS: Two cardiac compression triads. JAMA 1935; 104:714.
45. Guberman BA Fowler NO, Engel PJ, et al: Cardiac tamponade in medical patients. Circulation 1981; 64:633.
46. Gilliam LD, Guyer DE, Gibson TC, et al: Hydrodynamic compression of the right atrium: A new echocardiographic sign of cardiac tamponade. Circulation 1983; 68:294.
47. Armstrong WF, Schilt BF, Helper DJ, et al: Diastolic collapse of the right ventricle with cardiac tamponade: An echocardiographic study. Circulation 1982; 65:1491.
48. Gaffney FA, Keller AM, Peshock RM, et al: Pathophysiologic mechanisms of cardiac tamponade and pulsus alternans shown by echocardiography. Am J Cardiol 1984; 53:1662.
49. Reddy PS, Curtis E, Uretsky B: Spectrum of hemodynamic changes in cardiac tamponade. Am J Cardiol 1990; 66:1487.
50. Freeman GL: The effect of the pericardium on function of normal and enlarged hearts. Cardiol Clin 1990; 8:579.

51. Hoit BD, Gabel M, Fowler NO: Cardiac tamponade in left ventricular dysfunction. Circulation 1990; 82:1370.
52. Appleton CP, Hatle LK, Popp RL: Cardiac tamponade and pericardial effusion: Respiratory variation in transvalvular flow velocities studied by Doppler echocardiography. J Am Coll Cardiol 1998; 11:1020.
53. Himmelman RB, Kircher B, Rockey DC, et al: Inferior vena cava plethora with blunted respiratory response: A sensitive echocardiographic sign of cardiac tamponade. J Am Coll Cardiol 1988; 12:1470.
54. Segnni ED, Beker B, Arbel Y, et al: Left ventricular pseudohypertrophy in pericardial effusion as a sign of cardiac tamponade. Am J Cardiol 1990; 66:508.
55. Thompson RC, Finck SJ, Leventhal JP, et al: Right-to-left shunt across a patent foramen ovale caused by cardiac tamponade: Diagnosis by transesophageal echocardiography. Mayo Clin Proc 1991; 66:391.
56. D'Cruz IA, Constantine A: Problems and pitfalls in the echocardiographic assessment of pericardial effusion. Echocardiography 1993; 10:151.
57. Fowler NO: Cardiac tamponade: A clinical or an echocardiographic diagnosis? Circulation 1993; 87:1738.
58. Alio-Bosch J, Candell-Riera J, Monge L, et al: Intrapericardial echocardiographic images and cardiac constriction. Am Heart J 1991; 121:207.
59. Callahan JA, Seward JB: Pericardiocentesis guided by two dimensional echocardiography. Echocardiography 1997; 14:497.
60. Pandian NG, Skorton DJ, Kieso RA, et al: Diagnosis of constrictive pericarditis by two-dimensional echocardiography: Studies in a new experimental model and in patients. J Am Coll Cardiol 1984; 4:1164.
61. Tei C, Child JS, Tanaka H, et al: Atrial systolic notch on the interventricular septal echocardiogram: An echocardiographic sign of constrictive pericarditis. J Am Coll Cardiol 1983; 1:907.
62. Wann LS, Weyman AE, Dillon JC, et al: Premature pulmonary valve opening. Circulation 1977; 55:128.
63. Hatle LK, Appleton CP, Popp RL: Differentiation of constrictive pericarditis and restrictive cardiomyopathy by Doppler echocardiography. J Am Coll Cardiol 1988; 11:757.
64. Oh JK, Hatle LK, Seward JB, et al: Diagnostic role of Doppler echocardiography in constrictive pericarditis. J Am Coll Cardiol 1994; 23:154.
65. Kaul S: Doppler echocardiography in critically ill cardiac patients. Cardiol Clin 1991; 9:711.
66. Kasper W, Konstantidines S, Geibel A, et al: Right ventricular afterload stress detected by echocardiography in patients with clinically suspected pulmonary embolism. Heart 1997; 77:346.
67. McConnell MV, Solomon SD, Rayan ME, et al: Regional right ventricular dysfunction detected by echocardiography in acute pulmonary embolism. Am J Cardiol 1996; 78:469.
68. Nelson CW, Snow FR, Barnett M, et al: Impending paradoxical embolism: Echocardiographic diagnosis of an intracardiac thrombus crossing a patent foramen ovale. Am Heart J 1991; 122:859.
69. Wittlich N, Erbel R, Todt M, et al: Detection of pulmonary artery thrombi in transesophageal echocardiography in patients with pulmonary embolism. Eur Heart J 1989; 10(Suppl):21.
70. Yee LL, Williams GP, Gaitner NS, et al: Diagnosis of acute intraoperative pulmonary thromboembolism by transesophageal echocardiography. Am Heart J 1993; 135:262.
71. Wittlich N, Erbel R, Eichler A, et al: Detection of central pulmonary artery thromboemboli by transesophageal echocardiography in patients with severe pulmonary embolism. J Am Soc Echocardiogr 1992; 5:515.
72. Kasper W, Meinhertz T, Henkel B, et al: Echocardiographic findings in patients with proved pulmonary embolism. Am Heart J 1986; 112:1284.
73. Wolfe MW, Lee RT, Feldstein ML, et al: Prognostic significance of right ventricular hypokinesis and perfusion lung scan defects in pulmonary embolism. Am Heart J 1994; 127:1371.
74. Konstantinides S, Geibel A, Olschewski M, et al: Association between thrombolytic treatment and the prognosis of hemodynamically stable patients with major pulmonary embolism. Circulation 1997; 96:882.
75. Kasper W, Konstantinides S, Geibel A, et al: Management strategies and determinants of outcome in acute major pulmonary embolism. J Am Coll Cardiol 1997; 30:1165.
76. Nixon JV: Right ventricular myocardial infarction. Arch Intern Med 1982; 142:945.
77. Cohn JN, Guiha NJ, Broder MI, et al: Right ventricular infarction: Clinical and hemodynamic features. Am J Cardiol 1974; 33:209.
78. Lorell B, Leinbach RC, Pohost GM, et al: Right ventricular infarction: Clinical diagnosis and differentiation from cardiac tamponade and pericardial constriction. Am J Cardiol 1979; 43:465.
79. Lee WH, Fisher J: Right ventricular diastolic disorders. Arch Intern Med 1983; 143:332.
80. Williams JF: Right ventricular infarction. Clin Cardiol 1990; 13:309.
81. Jaffe CC, Weltin G: Echocardiography of the right side of the heart. Cardiol Clin 1992; 10:41.
82. Kaul S, Tei C, Hopkins JM, et al: Assessment of right ventricular function using two-dimensional echocardiography. Am Heart J 1984; 107:526.
83. Dell'Italia LJ, Starling MR, Crawford MH, et al: Right ventricular infarction: Identification by hemodynamic measurements before and after volume loading and correlation with noninvasive techniques. J Am Coll Cardiol 1984; 4:931.
84. D'Arcy B, Nanda NC: Two dimensional echocardiographic features of right ventricular infarction. Circulation 1982; 65:167.
85. Lopez-Sendon J, Garcia MA, Coma-Conella I, et al: Segmental right ventricular function after acute myocardial infarction: Two dimensional echocardiographic study of 63 patients. Am J Cardiol 1983; 51:390.
86. Joseph G, Jose VJ: Right ventricular filling abnormalities in acute inferior wall myocardial infarction—a pulsed Doppler study. Indian Heart J 1990; 42:437.
87. Dhainaut JF, Ghannad E, Villemant D, et al: Role of tricuspid regurgitation and left ventricular damage in the treatment of right ventricular infarction–induced low cardiac output syndrome. Am J Cardiol 1990; 66:289.
88. Hoit BD, Fowler NO: Influence of acute right ventricular dysfunction on cardiac tamponade. J Am Coll Cardiol 1991; 18:1787.
89. Anderson HR, Falk E, Nielsen D: Right ventricular infarction: Frequency, size and topography in coronary heart disease: A prospective study comprising 107 consecutive autopsies from a coronary care unit. J Am Coll Cardiol 1987; 10:223.
90. Chuttani K, Sussman H, Pandian NG: Echocardiographic evidence that regional right ventricular dysfunction occurs frequently in anterior myocardial infarction. Am Heart J 1991; 122:850.
91. Lewis JL, Webber JD, Sutton LL, et al: Discordance in degree of right and left ventricular dilation in patients with dilated cardiomyopathy: Recognition and clinical implications. J Am Coll Cardiol 1993; 21:649.
92. Tennant R, Wiggers CJ: The effect of coronary occlusion on myocardial contraction. Am J Physiol 1935; 112:351.
93. Nixon JV, Narahara KA, Smitherman TC: Estimation of myocardial involvement in patients with acute myocardial infarction by two-dimensional echocardiography. Circulation 1980; 62:1248.
94. Nixon JV, Brown CN, Smitherman TC: Identification of transient and persistent segmental wall motion abnormalities in patients with unstable angina by two-dimensional echocardiography. Circulation 1982; 65:1497.
95. Sabia, PJ, Afrookteh A, Touchstone DA, et al: Value of regional wall motion abnormalities in the emergency room diagnosis of acute myocardial infarction. Circulation 1991; 84:I-85.
96. Peels CH, Visser A, Kupper AJ, et al: Usefulness of two dimensional echocardiography for immediate detection of myocardial ischemia in the emergency room. Am J Cardiol 1990; 65:687.
97. Kontos MC, Arrowood JA, Paulsen WH, Nixon JV: Early echocardiography can predict cardiac events in emergency department patients with chest pain. J Emerg Med 1998; 315:550.
98. Kan G, Visser CA, Koolen JJ, et al: Short and long term predictive value of admission wall motion score in acute myocardial infarction: A cross sectional echocardiographic study of 345 patients. Br Heart J 1986; 56:422.
99. Berning J, Steensgaard F: Early estimation of risk by echocardiographic determination of wall motion index in an unselected population with acute myocardial infarction. Am J Cardiol 1990; 65:567.
100. Sabia PJ, Abbott RD, Afrookteh A, et al: Importance of two dimensional echocardiographic assessment of left ventricular

systolic function in patients presenting to the emergency room with cardiac related symptoms. Circulation 1991; 84:1615.

101. Fleischmann KE, Goldman L, Robiolio PA, et al: Echocardiographic correlates of survival in patients with chest pain. J Am Coll Cardiol 1994; 23:1390.
102. Nishimura RA, Tajik AJ, Shub C, et al: Role of two dimensional echocardiography in the prediction of in-hospital complications of acute myocardial infarction. J Am Coll Cardiol 1984; 4:1080.
103. Medina R. Panadis IP, Morganroth J, et al: The value of echocardiographic regional wall motion abnormalities in detection coronary artery disease in patients with or without a dilated left ventricle. Am Heart J 1985; 109:799.
104. Meltzer RS, Guthaner D, Rakowski J, et al: Diagnosis of left ventricular thrombi by two-dimensional echocardiography. Br Heart J 1979; 42:261.
105. Stratton JR, Lighty GW Jr, Pearlman AS, et al: Detection of left ventricular thrombus by two-dimensional echocardiography: Sensitivity, specificity, and causes of uncertainly. Circulation 1982; 66:156.
106. Visser CA, Kan G, Meltzer RS, et al: Embolic potential of left ventricular thrombus after myocardial infarction: A two dimensional echocardiographic study of 119 patients. J Am Coll Cardiol 1985; 5:1276.
107. Nihoyannopoulous P, Smith GC, Maseri A, et al: The natural history of left ventricular thrombus in myocardial infarction: A rationale in support of masterly inactivity. J Am Coll Cardiol 1989; 14:903.
108. Nishimura RA, Schaff HV, Shub C, et al: Papillary muscle rupture complicating acute myocardial infarction: Analysis of 17 patients. Am J Cardiol 1983; 51:373.
109. Wei JV, Hutchins GM, Bulkley BH: Papillary muscle rupture in fatal myocardial infarction. Ann Intern Med 1979; 90:149.
110. Kaul S, Spotnitz WD, Galsheen WP, et al: Mechanism of ischemic mitral regurgitation: An experimental evaluation. Circulation 1991; 84:2167.
111. Lehmann KG, Francis CK, Doodge HT, et al: Mitral regurgitation in early myocardial infarction: Incidence, clinical detection and prognostic implications. Ann Intern Med 1992; 177:10.
112. Goodley RW, Wann S, Rogers EW, et al: Incomplete mitral leaf closure in patients with papillary muscle dysfunction. Circulation 1981; 63:565.
113. Rasmussen S, Leth A, Kjoller E, et al: Cardiac rupture in acute myocardial infarction: A review of 72 consecutive cases. Acta Med Scand 1979; 205:11.
114. Currie PJ, Seward JN, Redder GS, et al: Continuous-wave Doppler echocardiographic assessment of severity of calcific aortic stenosis: A simultaneous Doppler-catheter correlative study in 100 adult patients. Circulation 1985; 71:1162.
115. Oh JK, Taliercio CP, Holmes DR, et al: Prediction of the severity of aortic stenosis by Doppler aortic valve area determination: Prospective Doppler catheterization correlation in 100 patients. J Am Coll Cardiol 1988; 11:1227.
116. Teague SM, Heinsime JA, Anderson JL, et al: Quantification of aortic regurgitation utilizing continuous wave Doppler ultrasound. J Am Coll Cardiol 1986; 8:592.
117. Takenaka K, Dabestani A, Gardin JM, et al: A simple Doppler echocardiographic method for estimating severity of aortic regurgitation. Am J Cardiol 1986; 57:1340.
118. Abbasi AS, Allen MW, Decristofaro D, et al: Detection and estimation of the degree of mitral regurgitation by range-gated pulsed Doppler echocardiography. Circulation 1980; 61:143.
119. Chen C, Thomas JD, Anconian J, et al: Impact of impinging wall jet on color Doppler quantification of mitral regurgitation. Circulation 1991; 84:712.
120. Gurney JW, Goodman LR: Pulmonary edema localized in right upper lobe accompanying mitral regurgitation. Radiology 1989; 171:397.
121. Henry WL, Griffith JM, Michaelis LL, et al: Measurement of mitral valve orifice area in patients with mitral valve disease by real-time, two-dimensional echocardiography. Circulation 1975; 51:827.
122. Hatle L, Angelsen B, Tromsdal A: Noninvasive assessment of atrioventricular pressure half-time by Doppler ultrasound. Circulation 1979; 60:1096.
123. Motro M, Neufeld HN: Should patients with pure mitral stenosis undergo cardiac catheterization? Am J Cardiol 1980; 46:515.
124. Ewy GA, Appleton CP, De Maria AN, et al: ACC/AHA Guidelines for the clinical application of echocardiography: A report of the American College of Cardiology/American Heart Association Task Force on assessment of diagnostic and therapeutic cardiovascular procedures (Subcommittee to develop guidelines for the clinical application of echocardiography). J Am Coll Cardiol 1990; 16:1505.
125. Gott VL, Pyeritz RE, Magovern GJ Jr, et al: Surgical treatment of aneurysms of the ascending aorta in the Marfan syndrome: Results of composite-graft repair in 50 patients. N Engl J Med 1986; 314:1070.
126. Hirst AE Jr, Johns VL Jr, Kime SW Jr: Dissecting aneurysm of the aorta: A review of 505 cases. Medicine (Baltimore) 1958; 37:217.
127. Daily PO, Trueblood HW, Stinson EB, et al: Management of acute aortic dissection. Ann Thorac Surg 1970; 10:237.
128. DeBakey ME, Henly WS, Cooley DA, et al: Surgical management of dissecting aneurysms of the aorta. J Thorac Cardiovasc Surg 1965; 49:130.
129. Nienaber CA, Spielmann RP, von Dkodolitsch Y, et al: Diagnosis of thoracic aortic dissection: Magnetic imaging versus transesophageal echocardiography. Circulation 1992; 85:434.
130. Nienaber CA, von Kodolitsch Y, Nicolas V, et al: The diagnosis of thoracic aortic dissection by noninvasive imaging procedures. N Engl J Med 1993; 328:1.
131. Erbel R, Engberding R, Daniel W, et al: Echocardiography in the diagnosis of acute dissection: European Cooperative Study Group for Echocardiography. Lancet 1989; i:457.
132. Hashimoto S, Kumada T, Osakada G, et al: Assessment of transesophageal Doppler echocardiography in dissecting aortic aneurysm. J Am Coll Cardiol 1989; 14:1253.
133. Adachi H, Kyo S, Takamoto S, et al: Early diagnosis and surgical intervention of acute aortic dissection by transesophageal color flow mapping. Circulation 1990; 82:IV-19.
134. Ballal RS, Nanda NC, Gatewood R, et al: Usefulness of transesophageal echocardiography in assessment of aortic dissection. Circulation 1991; 84:1903.
135. Roudaut RP, Marcaggi XL, deVille C, et al: Value of transesophageal echocardiography combined with computed tomography for assessing repaired type A aortic dissection. Am J Cardiol 1992; 70:1468.
136. Cigarroa JE, Isselbacher EM, DeSanctis RW, et al: Diagnostic imaging in the evaluation of suspected aortic dissection: Old standards and new directions. N Engl J Med 1993; 328:35.
137. Goarin JP, Le Bret F, Riou B, et al: Early diagnosis of traumatic aortic rupture by transesophageal echocardiography. Chest 1993; 103:618.
138. Goldstein SA, Mintz GS, Lindsay J, et al: Comprehensive evaluation by echocardiography and transesophageal echocardiography. J Am Soc Echocardiogr 1993; 6:634.
139. Erbel R, Oelert H, Meyer J, et al: Effect of medical and surgical therapy on aortic dissection evaluated by transesophageal echocardiography. Circulation 1993; 87:1604.
140. Nienaber CA, Kodolitch Y, Petersen B, et al: Intramural hemorrhage of the thoracic aorta: Diagnostic and therapeutic implications. Circulation 1995; 92:1465.
141. Coy KM, Maurer G, Goodman D, et al: Transesophageal echocardiographic detection of aortic atheromatosis may provide clues to occult renal dysfunction in the elderly. Am Heart J 1992; 123:1684.
142. Katz ES, Tunick PA, Rusinek H, et al: Protruding aortic atheromas predict stroke in elderly patients undergoing cardiopulmonary bypass: Experience with intraoperative transesophageal echocardiography. J Am Coll Cardiol 1992; 20:70.
143. Horowitz DR, Tuhrim S, Budd J, et al: Aortic plaque in patients with brain ischemia: Diagnosis by transesophageal echocardiography. Neurology 1992; 42:1602.
144. Albeis GW, Comess KA, DeRook FA, et al: Transesophageal echocardiographic findings in stroke subtypes. Stroke 1994; 25:23.
145. Karalis DG, Chandrasekaran K, Victor MF, et al: Recognition and embolic potential of intraortic debris. J Am Coll Cardiol 1991; 17:73.
146. Porembka DT, Johnson DJ, Fowl RJ, et al: Descending thoracic aortic thrombus as a cause of multiple system organ failure: Diagnosis by transesophageal echocardiography. Crit Care Med 1992; 20:1184.

147. Mugge A, Daniel WG, Frank G, et al: Echocardiography in infective endocarditis: Reassessment of prognostic implications of vegetation size determined by the transthoracic and the transesophageal approach. J Am Coll Cardiol 1989; 14:631.
148. Khandheria BK, Freeman WK, Sinak LJ: Infective endocarditis: Evaluation by transesophageal echocardiography. *In:* Transesophageal Echocardiography. Freeman WK, Seward JB, Khandheria BK, et al (Eds). Boston, Little, Brown and Co, 1994, p 307.
149. Erbel R, Rohman S, Drexler M, et al: Improved diagnostic value of echocardiography in patients with infective endocarditis by transesophageal approach: A prospective study. Eur Heart J 1988; 9:43.
150. Sochowski RA, Kwan LC: Implications of negative results on a monoplane transesophageal echocardiographic study in patients with suspected infective endocarditis. J Am Coll Cardiol 1993; 21:216.
151. Irani WN, Grayburn PA, Afridi I: A negative transthoracic echocardiogram obviates the need for transesophageal echocardiography in patients with suspected native valve active infective endocarditis. Am J Cardiol 1996; 78:101.
152. Lindner JR, Case RA, Dent JM, et al: Diagnostic value of echocardiography in suspected endocarditis: An evaluation based on the pretest probability of disease. Circulation 1996; 93:730.
153. Shively Bk, Gurule FT, Roldan CA, et al: Diagnostic value of transesophageal compared with transthoracic echocardiography in infective endocarditis. J Am Coll Cardiol 1991; 18:391.
154. Durack DT, Lukes A, Bright DK: New criteria for diagnosis of infective endocarditis: Utilization of specific echocardiographic findings. Am J Med 1994; 96:200.
155. Sanfilippo AJ, Picard MH, Davidoff R, et al: Prediction of risk for complications in patients with left sided infectious endocarditis. J Am Coll Cardiol 1991; 18:1191.
156. Stewart JA, Silimperi D, Harris P, et al: Echocardiographic documentation of vegetative lesions in infective endocarditis: Clinical implications. Circulation 1980; 61:374.
157. Rohmann S, Erbel R, Darius H, et al: Prediction of rapid versus prolonged healing of infective endocarditis by monitoring vegetation size. J Am Soc Echocardiogr 1991; 4:465.
158. Daniel WG, Mugge A, Grote J, et al: Comparison of transthoracic and transesophageal echocardiography for detection of abnormalities of prosthetic and bioprosthetic valves in the mitral and aortic positions. Am J Cardiol 1993; 71:210.
159. Arnett EN, Roberts WC: Prosthetic valve endocarditis: Clinicopathological analysis of 22 necropsy patients with comparison of observations in 74 necropsy patients with active infective endocarditis involving natural left-sided cardiac valves. Am J Cardiol 1976; 38:281.
160. Rohmann S, Erbel R, Mohr-Kahaly S, et al: Use of transesophageal echocardiography in the diagnosis of abscess in infective endocarditis. Eur Heart J 1995; 16B:54.
161. Daniel WG, Mugge A, Martin RP, et al: Improvement in the diagnosis of abscesses associated with endocarditis by transesophageal echocardiography. N Engl J Med 1991; 324:795.
162. Kissane RW: Traumatic heart disease. Circulation 1952; 6:421.
163. Plummer D, Brunette D, Asinger R, et al: Emergency department echocardiography improves outcome in penetrating injury. Ann Emerg Med 1992; 21:709.
164. Hiatt JR, Yeatman LA Jr, Child JS: The value of echocardiography in blunt chest trauma. J Trauma 1988; 28:914.
165. Jesse RL, Kontos MC: Evaluation of chest pain in the emergency department. Curr Prob Cardiol 1997; 22:149.
166. Miller FB, Shumate CR, Richardson D: Myocardial contusion: When can the diagnosis be eliminated? Arch Surg 1989; 124:805.
167. Wisner DH, Reed WH, Riddick RS: Suspected myocardial contusion: Triage and indications for monitoring. Ann Surg 1990; 212:82.
168. Christensen MA, Sutton KR: Myocardial contusion: New concepts in diagnosis and management. Am J Crit Care 1993; 2:28.
169. Pretre R, Chilcott M: Blunt trauma to the heart and great vessels. N Engl J Med 1997; 336:626.
170. Pandian NG, Skorton DJ, Doty DB, et al: Immediate diagnosis of acute myocardial contusion by two dimensional echocardiography: Studies in a canine model of blunt chest trauma. J Am Coll Cardiol 1983; 2:488.
171. Chi S, Blair TC, Gonzalez LL: Rupture of the normal aortic valve after blunt chest trauma. Thorax 1977; 32:619.
172. Chirillo F, Totis O, Cavarzerani A, et al: Usefulness of transthoracic and transesophageal echocardiography in recognition and management of cardiovascular injuries after blunt chest trauma. Heart 1996; 75:301.
173. Smith MK, Cassidy JM, Souther S, et al: Transesophageal echocardiography in the diagnosis of traumatic rupture of the aorta. N Engl J Med 1995; 332:356.
174. Brooks SW, Young JC, Cmolik B, et al: The use of transesophageal echocardiography in the evaluation of chest trauma. J Trauma 1991; 31:841.
175. Frykberg ER, Crump J, Dennis JW, et al: Non-operative observation of clinically occult arterial injuries: A prospective examination. Surgery 1991; 109:85.
176. Aschenberg W, Schluter M, Kremer P, et al: Transesophageal echocardiography for the detection of left atrial appendage thrombus. J Am Coll Cardiol 1986; 7:163.
177. Felner JM, Churchwell AL, Murphy DA: Right atrial thromboemboli: Clinical, echocardiographic and pathophysiological manifestations. J Am Coll Cardiol 1984; 4:1041.
178. Reeder GS, Khandheria BK, Seward JB, et al: Transesophageal echocardiography and cardiac masses. Mayo Clin Proc 1991; 66:1101.
179. Faletra F, Ravini M, Moreo A, et al: Transesophageal echocardiography in the evaluation of mediastinal masses. J Am Soc Echocardiogr 1992; 5:187.
180. Hwang JJ, Kuan P, Lin SC, et al: Reappraisal by transesophageal echocardiography in the significance of left atrial thrombi in the prediction of systemic arterial embolization in rheumatic mitral valve disease. Am J Cardiol 1992; 70:769.
181. Gilon D, Schechter D, Rein AJJT, et al: Right atrial thrombi are related to indwelling central venous catheter position: Insights into time course and possible mechanism of formation. Am Heart J 1998; 135:457.
182. DeBelder MA, Tourikis L, Griffith M, et al: Transesophageal contrast echocardiography and color flow mapping: Methods of choice for the detection of shunts at the atrial level. Am Heart J 1992; 124:1545.
183. Hagan PT, Scholz DG, Edwards WD: Incidence and size of patent foramen ovale during the first ten decades of life: An autopsy study of 965 hearts. Mayo Clin Proc 1984; 59:17.
184. Stoddard MF, Keedy DL, Dawkins PR: The cough test is superior to the Valsalva maneuver in the delineation of right to left shunting through a patent foramen ovale during contrast transesophageal echocardiography. Am Heart J 1993; 125:185.
185. Hausmann D, Mugge A, Becht I, et al: Diagnosis of patent foramen ovale by transesophageal echocardiography and association with cerebral and peripheral embolic events. Am J Cardiol 1992; 70:668.
186. LeChat PH, Mas JL, Lascault G, et al: Prevalence of patent foramen ovale in patients with stroke. N Engl J Med 1988; 318:1148.
187. Stollberger C, Schneide B, Abzieher F, et al: Diagnosis of patent foramen ovale by transesophageal contrast echocardiography. Am J Cardiol 1993; 71:604.
188. Chen WJ, Kuan P, Lien WP, et al: Detection of patent foramen ovale by contrast transesophageal echocardiography. Chest 1992; 101:1515.
189. van der Wouw PA, Koster RW, de le Marre BJ, et al: Diagnostic accuracy of transesophageal echocardiography during cardiopulmonary resuscitation. J Am Coll Cardiol 1997; 30:780.
190. Porter TR, Ornato JP, Guard C, et al: Transesophageal echocardiography to assess mitral valve function and flow during cardiopulmonary resuscitation. Am J Cardiol 1992; 70:1056.
191. Reichert CI, Visser CA, Koolen JJ, et al: Transesophageal echocardiography in hypotensive patients after cardiac operations. J Cardiovasc Surg 1992; 104:321.
192. Heidenreich PA, Stainback RF, Redberg RF, et al: Transesophageal echocardiography predicts mortality in critically ill patients with unexplained hypotension. J Am Coll Cardiol 1995; 26:152.
193. Chan KL: Transesophageal echocardiography for assessing cause of hypotension after cardiac surgery. Am J Cardiol 1988; 62:1142.

43

Intracellular pH and Electrolyte Regulation

Tor Inge Tønnessen, MD, PhD

In clinical practice, the most commonly ordered laboratory tests are measurements of electrolytes and pH because of the great importance of these parameters to the function of the body. Unfortunately, they largely reflect the extracellular milieu, and what happens intracellularly is not known to the clinician. There is, however, a huge body of knowledge on the regulation of *intracellular* pH and electrolytes. Because most of the studies have been carried out in vitro, the functions of these mechanisms in vivo have not been fully elucidated. Fortunately, with the increasing utilization of magnetic resonance imaging (MRI) and positron-emission tomography (PET) scanning for real-time measurements of intracellular parameters in vivo, a lot of this basic knowledge has been applied to the understanding of whole-body physiology and pathophysiology. In order for the knowledge to expand further, however, the clinician and clinical scientist need to have an appreciation of these basic processes. It is the intent of this chapter to give the clinician some insight into this topic.

The widespread writing on pH and electrolyte disturbances in the clinical literature has given rise to certain assumptions about their treatment, such as:

- Bicarbonate is an *extracellular* buffer and is not effective to treat *intracellular* pH disturbances.
- Administration of bicarbonate gives rise to intracellular acidification.
- Acidosis must be corrected in order to optimize cellular function.

This chapter addresses these questions and others on the basis of current knowledge that clearly disputes their validity. Also, future treatment of acid-base disorders in the form of drugs to specifically inhibit or stimulate intracellular regulatory mechanisms and thereby normalize the disturbances is discussed. Thus, exciting new treatment for diverse disorders such as cerebral edema, myocardial stunning, ischemia, inflammation, and cancer might be available through the application of current basic knowledge about how cells regulate their cytosolic pH and electrolytes.

MECHANISMS INVOLVED IN THE REGULATION OF CYTOSOLIC pH

As a result of metabolism, approximately 20,000 mmoles of carbon dioxide (CO_2), approximately 1500 to 4500 mmoles lactic acid, and approximately 100 to 200 mmoles of other nonvolatile acids are formed each day. Also, alkaline compounds, although to a lesser extent, are end products of catabolism. The large acid load makes the effective regulation of pH in the body vital, because a number of cellular processes are highly pH-sensitive.

Intracellular pH is not uniform throughout the cells. The pH of the cytosol (pH_i) is in most cells somewhat lower (0.02 to 0.3 pH units) than extracellular pH (pH_o),[1, 2] but many cells have higher pH_i than this.[3] pH_i is not a static value; it changes according to the activation of the cell. The pH of cell organelles is markedly different from the cytosolic pH. Thus, lysosomes are very acidic (pH 4.5–5.5), and endosomes and Golgi apparatus somewhat more alkaline (pH 5.5 to 6.5), whereas the nucleus is only slightly more acidic than the cytosol.

The four main defense mechanisms enabling the body to precisely regulate pH despite a very heavy acid load due to cellular metabolism are as follows:

1. Physiochemical buffers both in the extracellular fluid (ECF) and intracellular fluid (ICF).
2. Transport of acid and base across the cell membrane via specific mechanisms.
3. Removal of volatile acid by respiration.
4. Removal of nonvolatile acid and absorption of base by the kidneys.

Physiochemical Buffering

Extracellular Buffering

The main buffers in the blood and interstitial fluid are proteins, phosphate, and bicarbonate (i.e., weak acids and their conjugate base). Even though the bicarbonate buffer system has a pK value of 6.1, it is quantitatively the most important extracellular physiologic buffer, owing to its high concentration (~25 mM) and the fact that the "weak acid" CO_2 (carbon dioxide) is effectively removed by respiration. The extracellular phosphate concentration is 1 to 2 mmol, and this buffer is therefore much less important. The total extracellular protein concentration is 2 to 4 mmol, but each protein has many buffering residues, making them important buffers.

The extracellular buffering of nonvolatile acids (hydrogen ion [H^+]) is very effective. Because the bicarbonate/CO_2 complex is the dominating system, however, buffering of excess CO_2/H_2CO_3 is rather ineffective extracellularly, and relatively small variations of CO_2 caused by alteration of respiration may markedly influence the pH of the blood plasma. Thus, the main buffering of CO_2/H_2CO_3 takes place *intracellularly* in red blood cells and tissue cells.

Intracellular Buffering

Protein concentrations inside most cells are 20 to 25 g/dL (in erythrocytes, 30 g/dL); in blood plasma, 5 to 7 g/dL; and in the interstitial space, 3 to 5 g/dL.[4] This accounts for the much more powerful buffering capacity within the cell compared with extracellular compartments. At physiologic concentrations, the bicarbonate ion (HCO_3^-) constitutes approximately half of the buffering capacity. In red blood cells, hemoglobin is a particularly effective buffer because of its high concentration and its many residues of histidine, which is the only amino acid with significant buffering power near neutral pH. Importantly, deoxygenated hemoglobin has a higher affinity for protons than its oxygenated counterpart (Haldane effect).

Contrary to common belief, the concentration of HCO_3^- inside the cells is not very different from the concentration in the extracellular space and blood plasma.[2] CO_2 is, in practical terms, freely cell membrane–permeant. The transmembrane HCO_3^- gradient must, by necessity, be equal to the transmembrane pH gradient. The intracellular pH of most cells is 0.05 to 0.3 pH unit lower than the extracellular pH,[1, 2] but in a sizable number of cells, cytosolic pH is higher than extracellular pH.[3] Accordingly, intracellular bicarbonate is between 12 and 30 mmol under normal physiologic conditions. In studies of cultured cells, the intracellular buffering power is twice as effective in the presence of bicarbonate as in its absence.[5-7] Because the plasma membranes of all cells are highly permeable to CO_2, intracellular CO_2 concentration is, under most circumstances, equal to the extracellular concentration. The removal of CO_2 by respiration effectively regulates the intracellular carbonic acid concentration. Therefore, every HCO_3^- ion can buffer two to four times better than any other physiologic buffer. Not only does CO_2 effectively diffuse across the cell membrane; there are also specific transporters for HCO_3^-. The intracellular concentration of HCO_3^- can therefore be regulated independent of CO_2, making this buffering system remarkably effective for both intracellular and extracellular buffering.

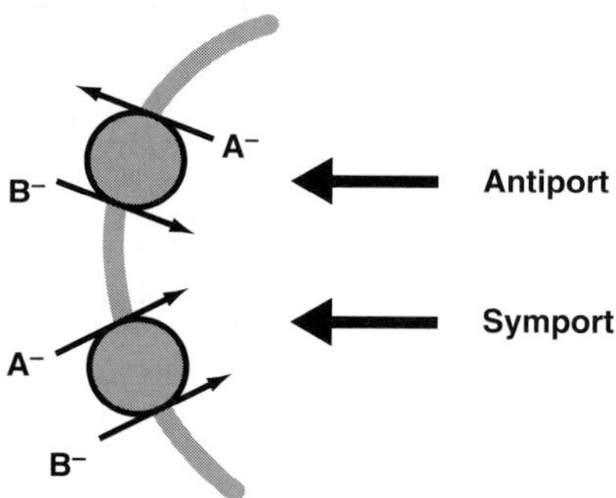

Figure 43–1. Difference in direction of transport for antiport and symport.

Transmembrane Transport of Acid and Base

The Importance of Transmembrane Transport for Cellular Function

Because of its hydrophobic interior, the lipid bilayer of the plasma membrane is highly impermeable to most polar molecules, thereby preventing most of the water-soluble contents from escaping. In order to transport these molecules in a controlled manner, cells have evolved very specialized *membrane transport proteins.* These are large proteins that span the entire membrane by having their α-helices cross the plasma membrane several times. This arrangement creates an interior of the protein that shields the transported molecules from the hydrophobic lipid membrane.

There are two major classes of membrane transport proteins, carrier proteins and channel proteins. *Carrier proteins* (also called *carriers* or *transporters*) bind the specific solute to be transported and undergo a conformational change in order to transfer the solute across the membrane. *Channel proteins* form water-filled "pores" that extend across the lipid bilayer. These channels can be closed or open; once they are open, electrolytes traverse the channels according to both the specificity of the channel and the transmembrane gradient of the solute.

All channel proteins and many carrier proteins allow only *passive transport,* facilitated diffusion (i.e., the direction of transport is determined by the electrochemical gradient). Transport of a solute against its electrochemical gradient occurs only with carrier proteins and is either *primary active transport* (i.e., requires metabolic energy most often by the hydrolysis of adenosine triphosphate [ATP]) or *secondary active transport* (meaning that the transport of the solute is coupled to the simultaneous or sequential transfer of another solute with a more favorable electrochemical gradient). Secondary active transport can be achieved either as a *symport,* whereby both solutes are transported in the same direction, or as an *antiport* whereby the solutes are exchanged in opposite directions (Fig. 43–1). Antiport in the literature is often called *exchanger* or *exchange mechanism.*

All of these mechanisms depend on the sodium ion (Na^+)/potassium ion (K^+) "pump" for their proper function. This pump is a transmembrane carrier protein with an ATPase function, that is, it hydrolyzes ATP as a part of the transport mechanisms to harness energy, enabling an active transport of electrolytes against their electrochemical gradient. Because three Na^+ are transported out of the cell in exchange for two K^+, the mechanism is *electrogenic,* and a transmembrane potential is built up. The direct effect of the pump, however, seldom contributes more than 20% of the membrane potential. The rest of the membrane potential emanates from an indirect effect of the pump by building up an outward-directed K^+ gradient, which, because of this ion's ability to permeate the membrane, builds up the membrane potential. This permeability is achieved by a K^+ leak channel protein. Most channel proteins have the ability to close and open in response to stimuli. If they are regulated by the electrical status of the cell, they are called *voltage-gated* channels; if humoral mediators determine their activity, they are *ligand-gated.*

Mechanisms of Transmembrane Acid and Base Transport

Charged molecules like H^+, hydroxide ion (OH), and HCO_3^- cannot readily cross lipid membranes. In order to be transported across the cell membrane, they need specific carrier proteins (Table 43–1).

Apart from the primary active processes, which are H^+/K^+-ATPase in gastric parietal cells and H^+-translocating ATPase (which directly utilizes ATP), the cell's transport processes are secondary active (i.e., dependent on the ion gradients to carry out their transport of acid and base equivalents).

Figure 43–2 depicts the different mechanisms for regulation of cytosolic pH (pH_i). Mechanisms for elevation of pH_i are found on the left side, and mechanisms that decrease pH_i on the right. As is evident from the figure, electrolyte transport is an integrated part of pH regulation. Consequently, these mechanisms regulate not only pH_i but also intracellular ion concentrations, cell volume, and transcellular transport of electrolytes. Thus, the cells use a small set of transmembrane transport mechanisms to carry out several different tasks. Needless to say, these mechanisms must be precisely regulated for them to occur in a controlled manner.

Na^+/H^+ Antiport

Na^+/H^+ antiport catalyzes the entry of extracellular Na^+ in exchange for intracellular H^+, eliciting a rise in pH_i (Fig. 43–3). The exchange process is secondary active, driven by the chemical gradients of Na^+ and H^+, and therefore depends on

TABLE 43–1. Mechanisms of Transmembrane Acid and Base Transport

Electroneutral Processes	Electrogenic Processes
1. Na^+/H^+ antiport	1. Na^+/HCO_3^- symport
2. Na^+-coupled Cl^-/HCO_3^- antiport	2. Proton-translocating ATPase
3. Na^+-independent Cl^-/HCO_3^- antiport	
4. H^+/K^+-ATPase	
5. H^+/lactate$^-$ symport	

ATPase = adenosine triphosphatase; Cl^- = chlorine ion; H^+ = hydrogen ion; HCO_3^- = bicarbonate; K^+ = potassium ion; NA^+ = sodium ion.

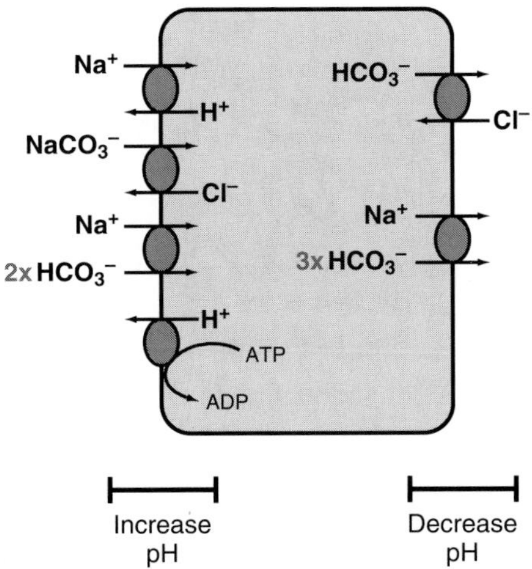

Figure 43–2. The most common mechanisms for transmembrane transport of acid and base.

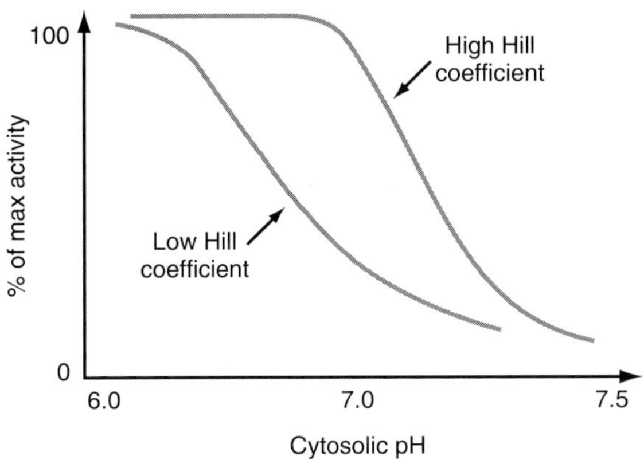

Figure 43–4. Activity of Na^+/H^+ antiport as a function of cytosolic pH.

the operation of the Na^+/K^+-ATPase. The Na^+/H^+ antiport is found in nearly every cell studied. It has been cloned and thoroughly characterized. Three different types of the antiports have been found, designated NHE-1, NHE-2, and NHE-3. NHE-1 is the ubiquitous form found in most cells, whereas the other isoforms are found in specialized cells like kidney cells and have different kinetic and physiologic characteristics.[8]

The Na^+/H^+ antiport has an internal pH "sensor"; that is, its activity is regulated by the intracellular pH.[1] Thus, the antiport is activated by decreasing pH_i[1] (Fig. 43–4). Cells with steeply regulated antiports (with a so-called high Hill coefficient) are thus very sensitive to relatively small changes in pH_i.[9] The dynamics of this antiport in different cells varies greatly, and a 30-fold difference in its activity has been found in various cells.[10]

The pH sensor on the cytosolic side of the antiport is also important to shut off the activity of the antiport at normal pH_i, protecting the cell from undue alkalinization. Because the $Na^+_{outside}/Na^+_{inside}$ ratio is greater than 10, pH_i would exceed 8.0 if the Na^+/H^+ antiport were active at a pH_i higher than the resting pH_i.[11]

The *extracellular pH* (pH_o) may also greatly influence the transport activity of the antiport. In most cells, extracellular protons may severely reduce the rate of Na^+/H^+ exchange, indicating that this antiport also has an *external* pH sensor.[12] Thus, when the cells produce acids that acidify the cytosol and the extracellular milieu is neutral because of an effective perfusion, the removal of H^+ from the cell is very effective. If, however, perfusion is marginal (i.e., under ischemic conditions), reducing the removal of extracellular acid, the transport of acid via the Na^+/H^+ antiport is markedly inhibited. Also, a systemic low pH decreases the effectiveness of Na^+/H^+ antiport in cells throughout the body, and correction of extracellular pH, which can be achieved clinically, increases pH_i to some extent.

It is beyond doubt that Na^+/H^+ exchange is of major importance in the normalization of pH_i after extensive acidification of the cytosol. Evidence indicates that this antiport in various cells does not contribute to the maintenance of steady-state cytosolic pH at neutral pH_o.[13] In other types of cells, however, the Na^+/H^+ antiport is active at a more alkaline pH and appears to be important for the maintenance of steady-state pH_i.

Na^+-Coupled Cl^-/HCO_3^- Antiport

The Na^+-coupled chlorine ion (Cl^-/HCO_3^- antiport most likely exchanges extracellular sodium bicarbonate ($NaCO_3^-$) with intracellular Cl^- (Fig. 43–5). $NaCO_3^-$ is formed by one Na^+ and two bicarbonate molecules. This antiport transports two base equivalents for every Na^+ (i.e., $CO_3^- + 2H^+ \leftrightarrow H_2CO_3 \leftrightarrow CO_2$ + water [H_2O]) and thus neutralizes two protons.[14, 15]

The role of the Na^+-coupled Cl^-/HCO_3^- antiport in the regulation of pH_i varies among cells. Unlike the Na^+/H^+ antiport, it does not appear to be an omnipresent transport mechanism, although it is found in many of the cells in which pH_i regulation has been studied in the presence of HCO_3^-.[10] Different isoforms of this transport mechanism have been found.[16] Like the Na^+/H^+ antiport, the Na^+-coupled Cl^-/HCO_3^- antiport increases in activity as pH_i is decreased, suggesting a cytosolic pH_i-sensitive site on the transport protein.[13, 15, 17] Also, pH_o appears to regulate the activity of the antiport. Some studies show a marked inhibition of its activity when pH_o is decreased.[18] In some cells studied, the system is quiescent around neutral pH_i and is activated only when pH_i is lowered.[19] This observation contrasts with findings in other cells, in which the antiport is also active at higher pH_i values. Moreover, in some cells, the antiport appears to be constitutively active—that is, not fully down-regulated even at high pH_i.[13] The activity of the Na^+-coupled Cl^-/HCO_3^- antiport is often higher than that of the Na^+/H^+ antiport at pH_i near neutrality, but not at lower pH_i values.[13] Thus, in many cells,

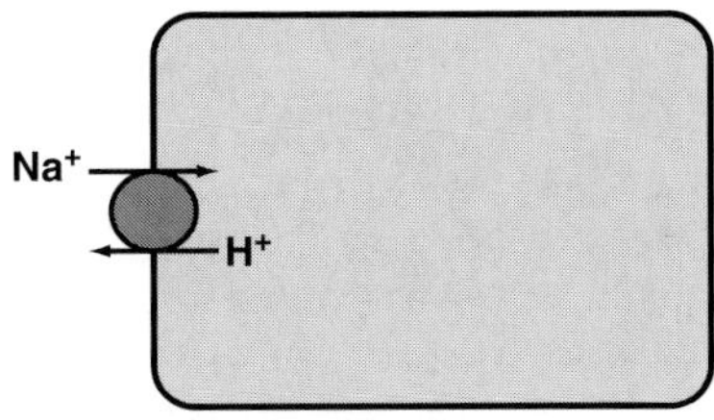

Figure 43–3. Na^+/H^+ antiport.

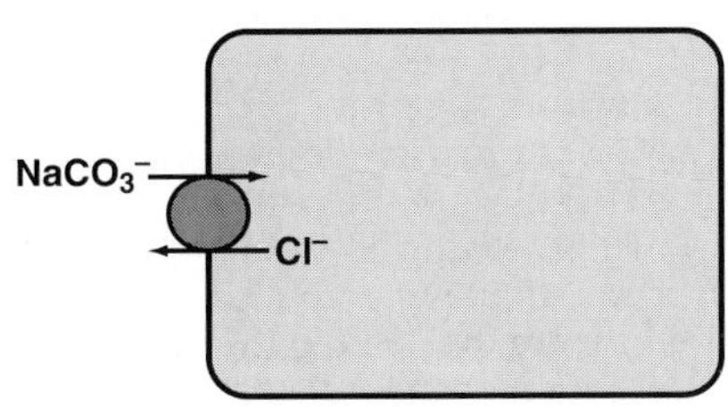

Figure 43–5. Na^+-coupled Cl^-/HCO_3^- antiport.

the Na^+-coupled Cl^-/HCO_3^- antiport is the most important mechanism to keep pH_i at a physiologic level.

Na^+/HCO_3^- Symport

The Na^+/HCO_3^- symport transports Na^+ and HCO_3^- undirectionally, apparently without exchange of other ions. The transport is electrogenic because of the transport of more than one HCO_3^- per Na^+. The Na^+ to HCO_3^- gradient directs transport of these ions *into* the cells if the interior is acidic compared with the extracellular space (Fig. 43–6); thus, under such conditions, this symport functions as an alkalinizing mechanism.[20]

A similar symport has been identified in the basolateral (serosal) membrane of proximal tubular cells in the kidneys. Its function appears to be the main mechanism for HCO_3^- *exit* across the basolateral membrane in this nephron segment and probably also in the thick ascending loop of Henle[21] (see Fig. 43–6). A coupling ratio of HCO_3^- to Na^+ of 3:1 is sufficient to transport HCO_3^- outward. The transport is energized by the negative membrane potential and the outward gradient of HCO_3^-, thus overcoming the opposing inward gradient for Na^+.

H^+/Lactate$^-$ Symport

Undissociated lactic acid is noncharged and can therefore to some extent penetrate membranes by non-ionic diffusion. The vast majority of lactic acid, however, is dissociated even under ischemic conditions. In cardiac muscle cells, skeletal muscle cells, and the placenta, a H^+/lactate$^-$ symport has been identified.[22-24] These cells produce large amounts of lactic acid, which needs to be transported rapidly out of the cells. The H^+/lactate$^-$ symport is extremely effective in increasing cytosolic pH in these cells during a lactic acid load. It is several times more effective to increase cytosolic pH than to increase activity of the Na^+/H^+ antiport, which is also found in these cells. The driving force for export of lactate from the cells is the concentration gradient.[23, 24] Thus, extracellular accumulation of lactic acid caused by insufficient blood flow to transport lactic acid away severely decreases the ability of the cells to counteract intracellular acidification.

Proton-Translocating ATPases

Proton-translocating ATPases ("proton pumps") utilize ATP directly as an energy source to pump protons either into intracellular vesicles (endosomes, lysosomes) (so-called V-type ATPase) or across the plasma membrane (P-type ATPase). These processes increase the cytosolic pH by pumping protons out of the cells or into these vesicles (Fig. 43–7). Subsequently, many of the vesicles fuse with the plasma membrane by exocytosis, and the protons are expelled. It may appear illogical to hydrolyze ATP to get rid of protons, inasmuch as hydrolysis of one ATP molecule liberates approximately 0.8 H^+ equivalents into the cytoplasm. For the proton ATPases studied, however, the stoichiometry is 2 or 3 H^+ transported per ATP molecule hydrolyzed,[25] making it a cost-effective process. Because the transport of H^+ is electrogenic, it is accompanied

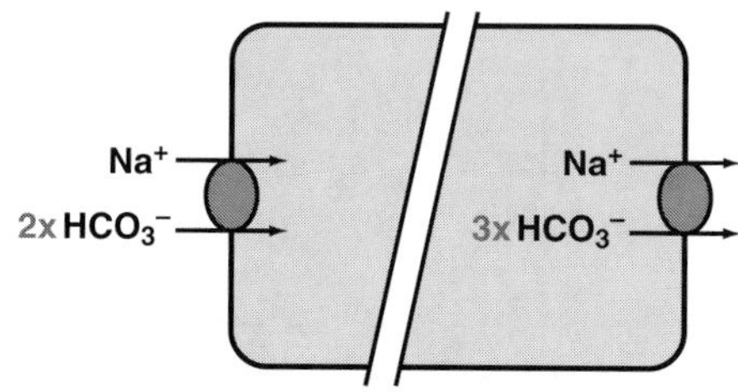

Figure 43–6. The two types of Na^+/HCO_3^- symport.

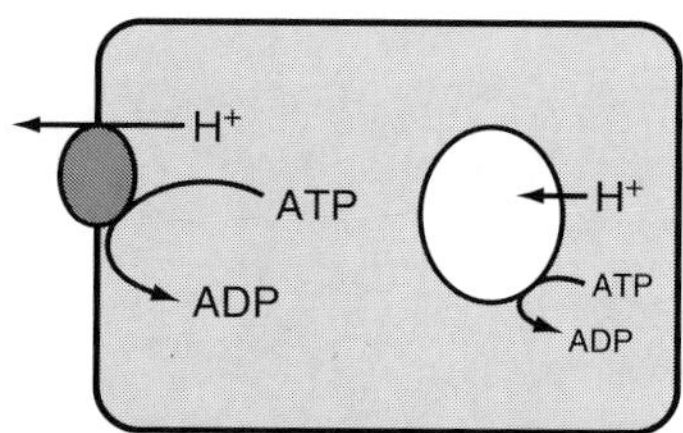

Figure 43–7. H^+-Translocating ATPases.

by transport of Cl^- through a separate channel to preserve electroneutrality.

Plasma membrane proton pumps have been identified in mammalian renal cells, pancreatic and biliary duct cells, human macrophages and neutrophils, type II pneumocytes, and osteoclasts. In many other cells studied, no evidence of plasma membrane H^+ pumps has been found.

The proton pump possessed by type II pneumocytes and alveolar epithelial cells might explain the low pH in epithelial lining fluid. Osteoclasts secrete protons through this mechanism to produce an acidic environment that resorbs bone.

Na^+-Independent Cl^-/HCO_3^- Antiport

Under physiologic conditions, the Na^+-independent Cl^-/HCO_3^- antiport exchanges external Cl^- for internal HCO_3^-, eliciting a decrease in pH_i (Fig. 43–8). Thus, this antiport decreases pH_i by extruding base (HCO_3^-), which in turn elevates pH_o. This increase in pH_o may be important in the regulation of extracellular acidosis (see later discussion of metabolic acidosis). Also, the regulation of cytosolic Cl^- and cell volume appears to be markedly influenced by the activity of the Na^+-independent Cl^-/HCO_3^- antiport. Furthermore, the antiport is of great importance for the transcellular transport of Cl^- and HCO_3^- in epithelial cells.

This transport system has been most extensively studied in erythrocytes, in which the Cl^-/HCO_3^- exchange (often called the Hamburger shift) is mediated by the so-called band 3, one of the most abundant proteins in the red cell membrane.[26] Subsequently, similar anion exchangers have been found in a number of nucleated cells,[5, 20, 27, 28] and they appear to be nearly ubiquitous proteins in the plasma membrane. Thus, in a study of more than 20 different cell lines, a Na^+-independent Cl^-/HCO_3^- antiport was found in all but one.[10]

An important property of the Na^+-independent Cl^-/HCO_3^- antiport is its ability to respond to alterations in cytosolic pH[27] (Fig. 43–9). Thus, at higher pH_i, the activity of the antiport increases. The pH_i dependence is present in most cells, although in some cell lines, it is presumably absent.[10] The antiport seems to have an internal pH sensor, which is sensitive to small alterations in proton-base concentrations and allows a precise regulation of pH_i by the Na^+-independent Cl^-/HCO_3^- antiport. The pH_i value for transition from low to high activity is different in different cells,[10, 13, 15, 27, 28] and it is regulated by physiologic ligands, temperature, and drugs.[29-32]

Equally important as the *activation* of the Na^+-independent Cl^-/HCO_3^- antiport at high pH_i is its *deactivation* at lower

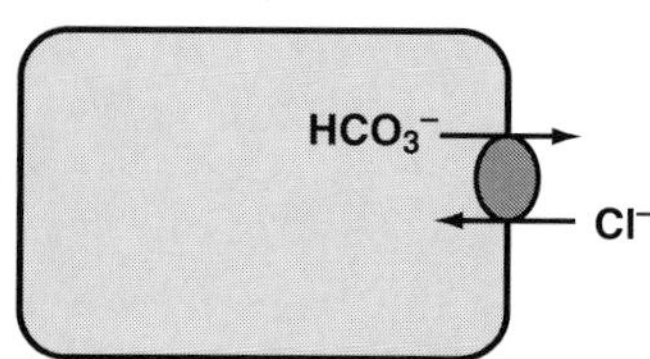

Figure 43–8. Na^+-Independent Cl^-/HCO_3^- antiport.

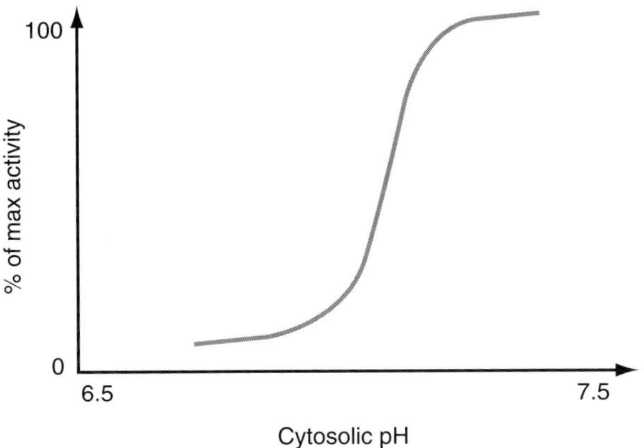

Figure 43–9. Activity of antiport as a function of cytosolic pH.

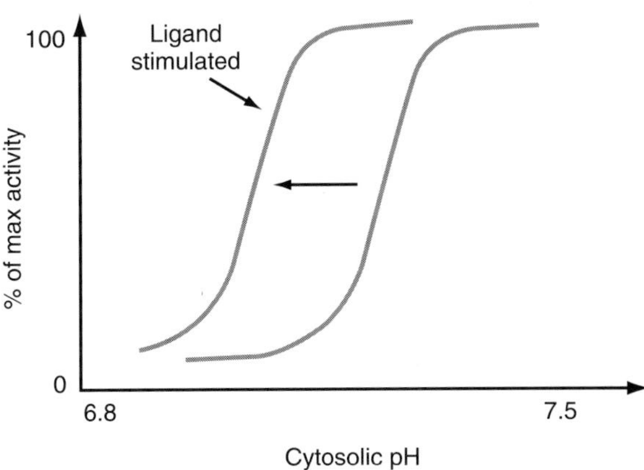

Figure 43–11. Modification of the activity of Na^+-independent Cl^-/HCO_3^- antiport by ligands.

pH_i values. If its activity were not severely decreased at pH_i less than 7.1, the antiport would acidify the cytosol to nonphysiologic values.[5] Thus, the regulation of the antiport to a low-activity state prevents an acidification that would otherwise occur if the antiport continued to work at a high rate.

Physiologic Control of pH-Regulating Mechanisms

In recent years, a large number of reports have appeared on the regulation of the activity of ion transport mechanisms by growth factors, hormones and other physiologic ligands, and several drugs. A detailed discussion of the different receptors and second messenger mechanisms involved in these regulations is beyond the scope of this chapter. It is noteworthy, however, that all known second messenger systems have been found to participate. More than one system may take part in the same cell.

The common short-term effect of physiologic ligands is a modification of the pH dependence of involved antiports. Thus, most factors activating the Na^+/H^+ antiport or the Na^+-coupled Cl^-/HCO_3^- antiport shifts the pH_i value for activation to a more alkaline level (for review, see Grinstein and colleagues[11]) (Fig. 43–10). Therefore, at physiologic pH_i, the antiports become active, eliciting a rise in pH_i. Activation of the Na^+-independent Cl^-/HCO_3^- antiport makes it active at a lower pH_i value than normal (Fig. 43–11), tending to decrease the pH_i. Thus, depending on which antiport is stimulated, stimulation by a ligand may either increase or decrease pH_i.

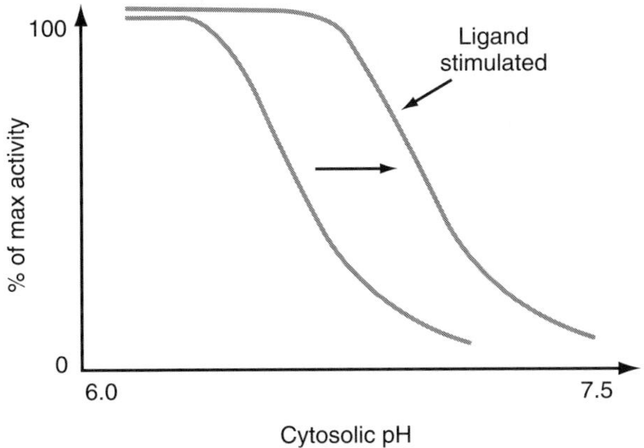

Figure 43–10. Modification of the activity of Na^+/H^+ antiport by ligands.

In many cases, more than one antiport is stimulated by the same ligand. Vasopressin, for instance, has been found to stimulate the Na^+/H^+ antiport, the Na^+-coupled Cl^-/HCO_3^- antiport, and the Na^+-independent Cl^-/HCO_3^- antiport in mesangial cells.[17] The resting pH_i does not change, but the cells are more able to withstand acid and base challenges. There are literally hundreds of papers describing different effects of physiologic ligands and drugs on these antiports; a few of these effects are listed in Table 43–2.

Several pathologic conditions and numerous ligands appear to alter the activity of antiports on a long-term basis (i.e., several hours to days). In many cases, the activation of the Na^+/H^+ antiport appears not to be a modification of its pH_i sensitivity but rather an alteration in the maximal transport velocity (V_{max}).[33]

Drug Effects on pH_i-Regulating Mechanisms

The diuretic drug amiloride, at concentrations obtained in vivo, inhibits Na^+-conducting channels in kidney cells. In

TABLE 43–2. Effects of Drugs and Physiologic Ligands on Antiports

Compound	Na^+/H^+ Antiport	Na^+-Coupled Cl^-/HCO_3^- Antiport	Na^+-Independent Cl^-/HCO_3^- Antiport
Epinephrine	↑		
Isoproterenol			↑
Vasopressin	↑		↑
Angiotensin II	↑		
Dopamine	↓		↓
Serotonin	↑		↑
Endothelin	↑		
Interleukins 1, 2, 3	↑		
Interferon	↑		
Prolactin	↑		
Parathyroid hormone	↓		
Thyroid hormone	↑		
NSAIDs	↓	↓	↑
Pathway			
cAMP	↓ ↑	↑	↑ ↓
Ca^{2+}	↑		
Protein kinase C	↑		↑ ↓

Ca^{2+} = calcium ion; cAMP = cyclic adenosine monophosphate; Cl^- = chlorine ion; H^+ = hydrogen ion; HCL_3^- = bicarbonate; Na^+ = sodium ion; NSAIDs = nonsteroidal anti-inflammatory drugs.

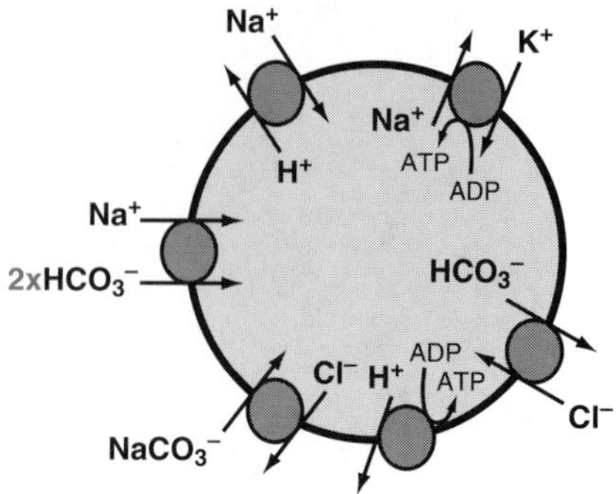

Figure 43–12. Cooperation between the most common mechanisms for regulation of cytosolic pH.

higher concentration, however, it is a strong inhibitor of the Na^+/H^+ antiport. It is being used extensively as a research tool to inhibit the Na^+/H^+ antiport in cell experiments. Newer derivatives of amiloride have a more specific inhibitory effect on the Na^+/H^+ antiport without interfering with the Na^+-conducting channel and may be used in vivo to inhibit the Na^+/H^+ antiport.

Diuretic drugs like bumetanide and furosemide exert their action by inhibiting the $Na^+/K^+/2\ Cl^-$ symport in the ascending part of Henle's loop. In higher concentration, they also inhibit the Na^+-independent Cl^-/HCO_3^- antiport, but it is unknown whether this finding has a clinical consequence. Drugs for relatively specific inhibition of Cl^-/HCO_3^- antiports are also available.

Nonsteroidal anti-inflammatory drugs (NSAIDs) have strong effects on the Na^+-coupled Cl^-/HCO_3^- antiport and the Na^+-independent Cl^-/HCO_3^- antiport. At presumably pharmacologic concentrations, the drugs stimulate the activity of the Na^+-independent Cl^-/HCO_3^- antiport, whereas they inhibit the Na^+-coupled Cl^-/HCO_3^- antiport in several cell lines.[29] The net effect is a decrease in pH_i. At higher drug concentrations, which are found in the gastrointestinal tract after oral intake and systemically with overdoses, NSAIDs inhibit both Cl^-/HCO_3^- antiports by competitive inhibition, probably through interaction with the transport site for the anions.[30] This may be part of the "local erosive effect" of these drugs (see text on gastric cells) and may also be related to acid-base disturbances in case of salicylic acid intoxication.

Drugs such as catecholamines, dopamine, and vasopressin also modify the action of these mechanisms (see Table 43–2).

Cooperation Among pH_i-Regulating Mechanisms

All cells possess more than one pH_i-regulating mechanism. pH_i therefore is determined by the relative activity of these mechanisms.[13] Figure 43–12 shows the quantitatively most important mechanisms. Each cell type differs, and no known cell possesses all the depicted mechanisms.

The *Na^+/H^+ antiport* is present in all cells. In many cell types, it is the main pH-regulating antiport to increase pH_i after an acid load, whereas in other cell types, the bicarbonate-dependent antiports are the most important. Thus, in certain cells, the Na^+/H^+ antiport is decisive for steady-state pH, whereas in other cells, its activity is required not to keep pH_i normal under resting conditions but only to normalize pH_i after an acid load.

There are two bicarbonate-dependent mechanisms which are able to increase pH_i, namely the *Na^+-coupled Cl^-/HCO_3^- antiport* and *Na^+/HCO_3^- symport.* One or the other of these mechanisms is present in the majority of cells. The *Na^+-coupled Cl^-/HCO_3^- antiport* seems to consist of $NaCO_3^-$ exchanged with Cl^-. This mechanism carries one Na^+ and two bicarbonate equivalents into the cells. The carbonate may bind two protons and thereby increase the pH_i in an efficient way with less osmotic load on the cell (i.e., less Na^+ influx per buffering equivalent) than the Na^+/H^+ antiport. The Na^+/HCO_3^- symport increases pH_i in certain cells when pH_i is lower than pH_o. (As mentioned previously, in kidney cells, a basolateral Na^+/HCO_3^- symport is the major mechanism for extrusion of HCO_3^- and carries a stoichiometry of 1 Na^+:3 HCO_3^-.) All these mechanisms increase their activity as pH_i is lowered and increase pH_i. At low extracellular pH, however, the effectiveness of these mechanisms is reduced to a different extent in different organs, underlining the necessity of regulating pH_o to increase pH_i. pH_i is not, however, merely a passive consequence of pH_o, because these mechanisms still have a certain activity even at low pH_o.

Certain cells, such as macrophages, neutrophils, kidney cells, and pneumocytes, have a proton pump (H^+-translocating ATPase) that extrudes H^+. These cells also possess a Na^+/H^+ antiport and, in many cases, a Na^+-coupled Cl^-/HCO_3^- antiport as well. Why do they need two or three mechanisms to fight acidosis? The reason appears to be that because the Na^+/H^+ antiport and the Na^+-coupled Cl^-/HCO_3^- antiport decrease their activity markedly at low extracellular pH (even if they are stimulated by low pH_i), these mechanisms do not suffice under extreme circumstances of acidity, whereas the proton pumps maintain a high activity even in very acidic environments by overcoming an enormous transmembrane gradient of protons (1:1000, ~pH_o 4.5). Thus, macrophages and neutrophils in the acidic milieu in an abscess probably depend on a proton pump to function satisfactorily.

The mechanisms just mentioned all increase pH_i. When a critical pH_i level is reached, the Na^+-independent Cl^-/HCO_3^- antiport is activated. At pH_i above neutrality, intracellular HCO_3^- is exchanged for extracellular Cl^-; as a result, the pH_i is reduced. A prerequisite for this to occur in a controlled manner is the striking pH_i dependence for the activation of this antiport. Thus, in most cells, the antiport is idle at pH_i below 7.1 and is then sharply activated at pH 7.2 to 7.4. It should be noted, however, that this transition value is different in various cells and also depends on the activation of the cells by various physiologic ligands.

Figure 43–13 shows an example of the activity of the $Na^+/$

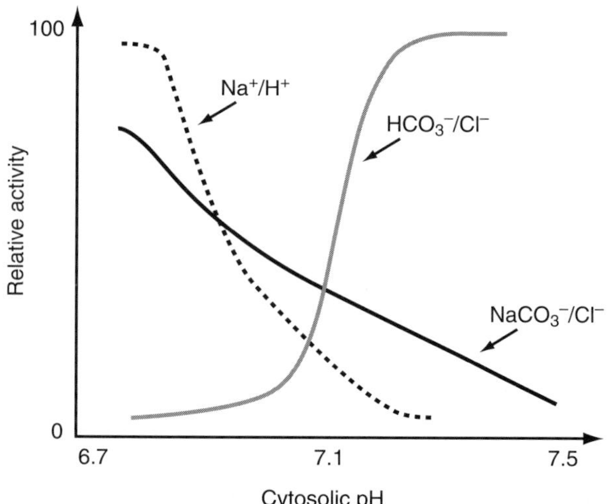

Figure 43–13. Relative activity of different antiports as a function of cytosolic pH.

H^+ antiport, the Na^+-coupled Cl^-/HCO_3^- antiport, and the Na^+-independent Cl^-/HCO_3^- antiport at different pH values, demonstrating how these mechanisms vary in significance according to the acid load of the cell. Also the activity of these mechanisms is significantly changed by many growth factors, other physiologic ligands, and certain drugs (see Table 43–2). Thus, pH_i (or at least the ability to withstand an acid or base load) varies with the activity state of the cell.

To elucidate the effect of *bicarbonate-dependent* mechanisms on intracellular pH, experiments in vitro can be carried out in the presence or absence of HCO_3^-. From these experiments, the following conclusions can be drawn:

1. The intracellular buffering power is approximately doubled in the presence of HCO_3^-.
2. The resting pH in most cells is *higher* in the presence of bicarbonate,[34] because of both the higher buffering power and the activity of the Na^+-coupled Cl^-/HCO_3^- antiport or Na^+/HCO_3^- symport, which will increase pH_i. In a number of cells, however, pH_i has been found to be lower in the presence of HCO_3^-, owing to a high activity of the Na^+-independent Cl^-/HCO_3^- antiport, which acidifies the cytosol.[13]
3. The recovery from both an acid load and an alkali load is faster in the presence of bicarbonate than in its absence because of buffering power plus the activity of HCO_3^--dependent mechanisms.
4. Bicarbonate is therefore of major importance for the regulation of intracellular pH and is readily transported across the plasma membrane by specific carrier mechanisms. *Thus, it is incorrectly stated in many textbooks that HCO_3^- is not important for regulation of cytosolic pH.*

Should metabolic acidosis be treated with bicarbonate? With administration of bicarbonate, an immediate increase in extracellular HCO_3^-, P_{CO_2} (depending on the ability of the respiratory system to ventilate), and pH is found. Because CO_2 is freely membrane-permeable, an immediate intracellular acidification takes place if extracellular P_{CO_2} is increased. This acidification is very short-lived because the bicarbonate treatment has increased the extracellular pH, making the conditions very favorable for a high activity of the Na^+/H^+ antiport and the Na^+-coupled Cl^-/HCO_3^- antiport. Thus, within minutes, the cytosolic pH is higher than before treatment with bicarbonate. Therefore, despite a short-lived acidification, bicarbonate treatment is effective to increase pH_i in cases of metabolic acidosis.

Role of pH_i-Regulating Mechanisms in Excretion of Acid by Respiration

A prerequisite for the functioning of the bicarbonate buffer system is the excretion of CO_2 by the lungs. Some 13,000 to 20,000 mmoles of CO_2 are produced daily as the result of oxidative metabolism, generating H^+ that must be eliminated in order to prevent acidosis. Because of the high intracellular content of carbonic anhydrase, CO_2 is processed much more rapidly to H^+ and HCO_3^- inside the erythrocytes than in the blood plasma. Simultaneously with CO_2 entering the cells, O_2 leaves and hemoglobin is deoxygenated. Deoxygenated hemoglobin has a higher pK than its oxygenated counterpart, so it can buffer more acid (Haldane effect), providing an effective buffering of protons. Also counteracting acidification is the formation of carbamino-hemoglobin from CO_2 and hemoglobin (Fig. 43–14). Hence, relatively large amounts of CO_2 can be added to the blood (1.3 mmoles CO_2 per liter) without eliciting a decrease in pH of more than 0.05 pH units. The Haldane effect enables the body to double the amount of CO_2 transported.

The majority (~80%) of CO_2 is transformed to HCO_3^-,

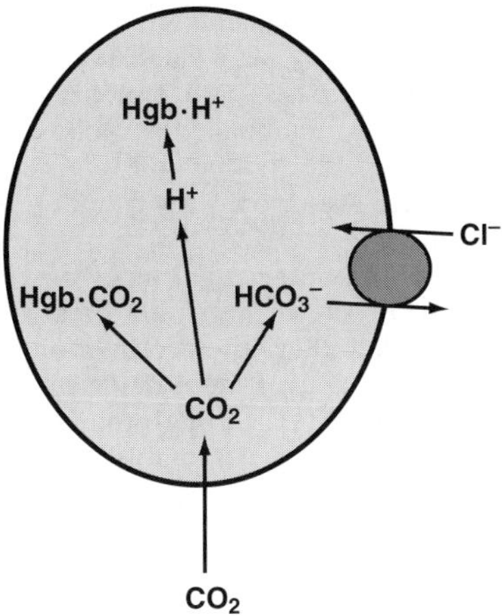

Figure 43–14. Mechanisms of carbon dioxide transport by red blood cells.

which is exported from the erythrocytes into the blood plasma. Bicarbonate must be transported across the erythrocyte membrane very rapidly to assure an effective transport of CO_2 by the blood. An Na^+-independent Cl^-/HCO_3^- antiport (band 3) is capable of handling this matter. The antiport protein is abundant in erythrocytes, where it constitutes about 25% to 30% of the total membrane protein[35] with about 106 molecules per cell.

Several lines of evidence indicate that the transport of bicarbonate across the red cell membrane is a rate-limiting step in the elimination of CO_2 by the lungs during physical exercise and in other situations of hyperdynamic circulation, but not at rest. At rest, about 1.9 mmoles of CO_2 per minute, yielding 1.5 mmoles of HCO_3^-, is transported by the blood. The capillary passage time in the lungs is about 0.7 seconds under these conditions. This is sufficient time for Cl^-/HCO_3^- exchange to reach 99% equilibrium.[26, 36] With strenuous exercise, however, about 6 mmol of CO_2 is transported, and the capillary passage time is decreased to 0.3 second because of the increased cardiac output. During this short passage time, Cl^-/HCO_3^- exchange attains only 90% of equilibrium and therefore limits the elimination of CO_2 by the lungs. Severe anemia and severe salicylate intoxication (which inhibits Cl^-/HCO_3^- exchange) might limit the elimination of CO_2 by the lungs because there is simply not enough antiport activity to carry out this increased transport.[37, 38] In the peripheral tissues, Cl^-/HCO_3^- exchange would be rate-limiting, decreasing the ability of the tissues to get rid of CO_2. There would be higher CO_2 *tension* in the interstitial fluid, but the *amount* transported by the blood would be limited because of the decreased capacity of the Cl^-/HCO_3^- antiport. An arterial blood gas measurement would not reveal any abnormalities despite a tissue "respiratory" acidosis.

Disturbances in pH can influence the oxygen (O_2) dissociation curve of hemoglobin. Thus, acidosis shifts the curve to the right, increasing the unloading of oxygen, whereas alkalosis has the opposite effect. Erythrocytes have a considerable ability to keep their intracellular pH near normal despite systemic alkalosis or acidosis. Therefore, hemoglobin per se is surrounded by a pH value higher than we measure in arterial blood. The effect of pH on the oxygen dissociation curve is therefore moderately less than expected.

Handling of Acid-Base Balance by Renal pH_i-Regulating Mechanisms

In addition to the production of 13,000 to 20,000 mmoles of the volatile acid CO_2, there is a daily production of 40 to 200 mmol of nonvolatile acids, mainly from the metabolism of food. During muscular exercise, a substantial amount of lactic acid is also produced (up to 4500 mmol a day). This lactic acid is to a large extent metabolized and does not need to be excreted, whereas the other nonvolatile acids are excreted by the kidneys. From this standpoint, the function of the kidneys is to excrete H^+ and absorb HCO_3^-.

Preservation of bicarbonate involves two renal processes: (1) the reabsorption of virtually all bicarbonate filtered through the glomeruli and (2) the reclamation of bicarbonate consumed in the buffering of fixed acids in the blood. The latter process is accomplished through the excretion of equivalent amounts of protons as "titratable acid" in the urine. Approximately 4500 mmol of HCO_3^- is filtered each day, and more than 99.9% is reabsorbed. Of this, 80% to 90% is reabsorbed in the proximal tubules, about 5% in the loop of Henle, 3% in the distal tubules, and 1% to 2% in the collecting ducts.

The mechanism of reabsorption of bicarbonate appears to vary in the different nephron segments. The Na^+/H^+ antiport appears to be the major mechanism for export of H^+ across the luminal membrane in the proximal tubule, but at least in the S3 segment of the proximal tubule and in the distal tubule, a proton-translocating ATPase is capable of transporting a major part of the H^+[39] (Fig. 43–15). The exported H^+ reacts with the filtered HCO_3^- to form CO_2 and H_2O. CO_2 diffuses readily across the luminal membrane to form H^+ and HCO_3^- inside the cells. The protons are again exported via the Na^+/H^+ antiport or H^+-ATPase and then reutilized.

The basolateral exit of bicarbonate can be mediated by a $Na^+/3\ HCO_3^-$ symport or an Na^+-independent Cl^-/HCO_3^- antiport.[21, 40] The former mechanism is dominant in the proximal tubule and appears to account for 70% to 80% of the HCO_3^- exit; the latter mechanism seems to be dominant in the more distal part of the nephron. There is a correlation between increased activity of the Na^+/HCO_3^- symport and Na^+-independent Cl^-/HCO_3^- antiport and increased systemic acid load. The Na^+/H^+ antiport on the luminal side and the Na^+/HCO_3^- symport on the basal side are both stimulated by angiotensin II, which thereby increases bicarbonate absorption.[41] Parathyroid hormone (PTH) inhibits the reabsorption and reclamation of HCO_3^-, by increasing cyclic adenosine monophosphate (cAMP) and thereby inhibiting the Na^+/H^+ antiport.[42]

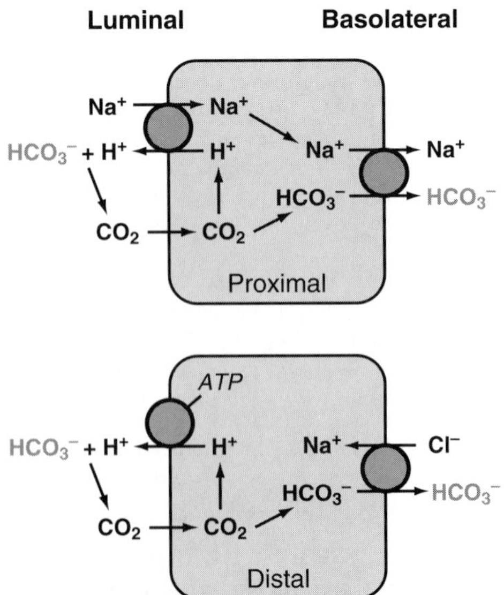

Figure 43–15. Mechanisms for the reabsorption of bicarbonate in the proximal and distal tubule.

The activity of the Na^+/H^+ antiport has been demonstrated to inhibit renin release.[43] Angiotensin II has been found to stimulate the Na^+/H^+ antiport in renal tubular membranes via a phospholipase A_2-mediated mechanism.[44] Consequently, the inhibitory effect of angiotensin II on renin release appears to be mediated by stimulation of the Na^+/H^+ antiport, because an amiloride analog has been shown to inhibit this effect.[43] Hyperosmolarity also inhibits the secretion of renin; this effect depends on the Na^+-independent Cl^-/HCO_3^- antiport.

REGULATION OF CELL VOLUME AND ELECTROLYTE CONCENTRATION

The cellular volume is strictly regulated. The plasma membrane of most cells is highly permeable to water, and the cell volume is therefore determined by the intracellular and extracellular content of osmotically active solutes. The cells contain impermeant macromolecules (mainly proteins) that will induce a colloid-osmotic swelling as a result of the entry of diffusible ions and water, which occurs because of the Gibbs-Donnan equilibrium. This swelling is counteracted by ion-extruding pumps (mainly the Na^+/K^+-ATPase) and other ion transport mechanisms.

In addition to the effort involved in maintaining a constant volume under resting conditions, many cells are challenged by anisotonic conditions under physiologic and pathophysiologic conditions. For example, renal cells are exposed to both hypertonic and hypotonic urine, blood cells traversing the kidney face areas with high osmolarity, and intestinal cells are exposed to anisotonic solutions. In absorbing and secreting epithelia, the large transcellular transport of ions and water requires effective mechanisms to maintain a normal cell volume. For instance, in kidney proximal tubule cells, the transcellular transport of water each minute is four times the cell volume; in pathophysiologic conditions, such as dehydration, hyperglycemic acidosis, and edema, the cells are exposed to conditions that may severely change the cell volume.

In order to counteract the shrinking or swelling in anisotonic media, cells have volume regulatory processes. Swollen cells tend to reduce their volume by loss of potassium chloride (KCl) and accompanying water (regulatory volume decrease [RVD]). Shrunken cells increase their volume by net uptake of sodium chloride (NaCl). Na^+ is then exchanged with K^+ by Na^+/K^+-ATPase, eliciting a net gain of KCl that results in a concomitant uptake of water (regulatory volume increase [RVI]). The ability to recover the initial volume varies between different cells. Both RVD and RVI are due to activation of ion transport systems, some of them also involved in the regulation of pH_i.

Regulatory Volume Decrease

The following three transport mechanisms have been found to mediate RVD after swelling of the cells:

- Separate conductive K^+ and Cl^- transport pathways (Fig. 43–16)
- An electroneutral K^+/Cl^- symport
- Electroneutral functionally coupled exchange K^+/H^+ and Cl^-/HCO_3^- antiports

The first process appears to be the main mechanism operating in human cells.

Because RVD is elicited in situations in which the hypotonicity is due to hyponatremia, there is often a decrease in pH_i, because both the Na^+/H^+ antiport and the Na^+-coupled Cl^-/HCO_3^- antiport have less favorable gradients under these conditions.[45]

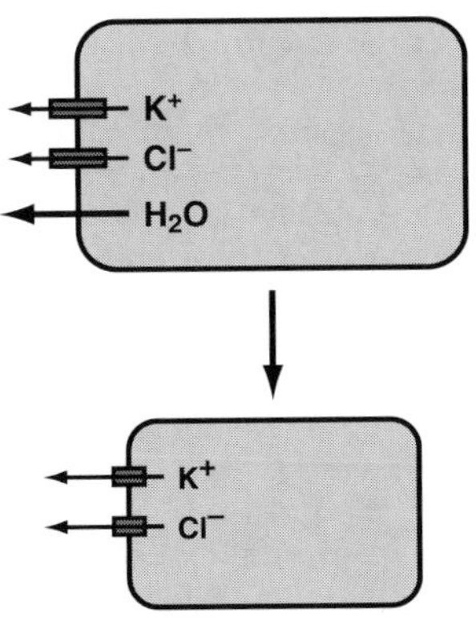

Figure 43–16. Regulatory volume decrease.

Regulatory Volume Increase

The transport systems involved in increasing cell volume are as follows:

- $Na^+/K^+/2\ Cl^-$ symport (Fig. 43-17)
- Na^+/Cl^- symport
- Electroneutral Na^+/H^+ antiport functionally coupled to Cl^-/HCO_3^- antiport (Fig. 43-18)

A sizable number of cells use both $Na^+/K^+/2\ Cl^-$ symport and Na^+/H^+ exchange functionally coupled to Cl^-/HCO_3^- exchange.

Cells also increase their volume prior to cell division. Growth factor–induced stimulation of $Na^+/K^+/2\ Cl^-$ symport, Na^+/H^+ exchange, and Na^+-independent Cl^-/HCO_3^- antiport has been reported to elicit these changes.[46, 47]

REGULATION OF INTRACELLULAR ION CONCENTRATION

The regulation of ion concentration is closely related to the regulation of cell volume. The dominating intracellular cation is K^+, and its concentration appears to be mainly controlled by the activity of the Na^+/K^+-ATPase. Thus, even if the concentration of Na^+ is increased by activation of Na^+/H^+ exchange, Na^+ is pumped out of the cells again in exchange with K^+. Therefore, in most if not all human cells, K^+ is the predominant intracellular cation, and its concentration does not vary much from one cell type to another.

As far as anions are concerned, the cytosolic concentration varies greatly in different cells. This fact is not well recognized, because it is repeatedly stated in textbooks that the transmembrane distribution of Cl^-, and thereby the cytosolic concentration of Cl^-, is determined by the membrane potential. The concentration of $[Cl^-]_i$ varies, however, from approximately 4 mmol in excitable cells (neurons and muscle) to more than 100 mmol in nucleated blood cells.[47] Other cell types contain intermediate concentrations of 40 to 60 mmol. Even in cells with high Cl^- concentration, the membrane potential is 30 to 60 mV. Thus, the internal Cl^- concentration is far above its electrochemical equilibrium; this is due to activity of the $Na^+/K^+/2\ Cl^-$ symport, which because of the ion gradients will transport considerable amounts of Cl^- *into* the cells.

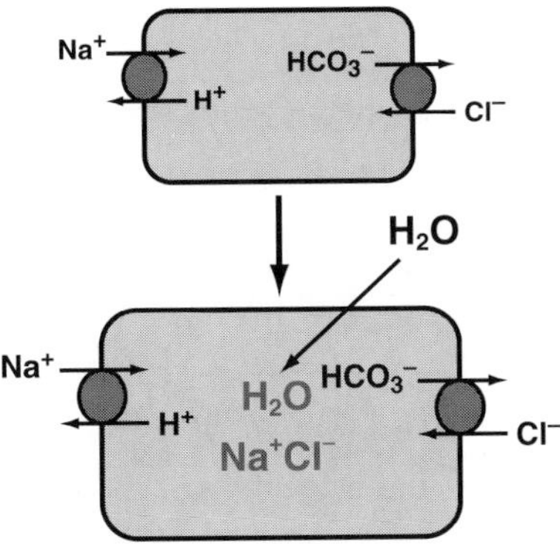

Figure 43–17. Regulatory volume increase.

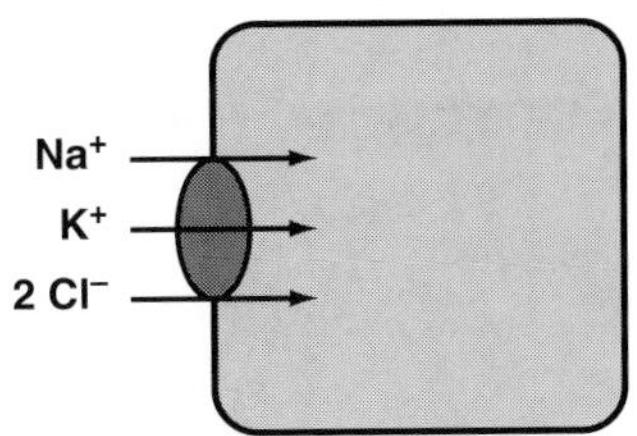

Figure 43–18. $Na^+/K^+/2\ Cl^-$ symport.

The internal concentration of HCO_3^- depends on pH_i, because CO_2 is highly membrane-permeable. Conversely, altering the concentration of HCO_3^- changes pH_i. Because this is achieved by a Cl^-/HCO_3^- exchange, the internal Cl^- concentration is also influenced by pH.

Many cells possess Na^+-independent Cl^-/HCO_3^- antiports, Na^+-coupled Cl^-/HCO_3^- antiports, $Na^+/K^+/2\ Cl^-$ symport, and Na^+/H^+ antiports. As discussed previously, all these processes are involved in the regulation of intracellular ion concentrations. Therefore, the dynamic interaction among them determines the concentration of cations and anions.

TRANSCELLULAR TRANSPORT

Transcellular transport is a property of polarized epithelial cells. Such cells (e.g., renal tubular cells and intestinal epithelial cells) have a different milieu at the apical (luminal) membrane compared with the basolateral (serosal) membrane therefore, these cells transport some solutes in one direction and others in the opposite direction. In order to accomplish this, the type of transmembrane transport molecules (antiports, symports) have to be different on the luminal and serosal sides.

Gastric Cells

In gastric *parietal* (oxyntic) cells, K^+/H^+-ATPase pumps protons out of the cells at the apical membrane into the gastric lumen in exchange for extracellular K^+ (Fig. 43-19). Protons are accompanied by chlorine ions, which leave the cells through Cl^--conductive channels. An Na^+-independent Cl^-/HCO_3^- antiport is found in the basolateral membrane.[48] This antiport is highly pH_i-dependent, because its activity increases with rising pH_i.[49] The Na^+-independent Cl^-/HCO_3^- antiport fulfills two purposes: (1) influx of Cl^- to substitute for the apical Cl^- efflux and (2) basolateral export of HCO_3^- to decrease pH_i, which is markedly increased by export of H^+ via the apical K^+/H^+-ATPase. Also, Na^+/K^+-ATPase and Na^+/H^+ antiport are found in the basolateral membrane. The Na^+/H^+ antiport is stimulated by secretagogues (histamine and related compounds), thus elevating pH_i to a value at which the Na^+-independent Cl^-/HCO_3^- antiport is active. The mechanism of action for the antiulcer drug omeprazole is to specifically inhibit the H^+/K^+-ATPase.

In *mucosal* cells of the stomach and duodenum, export of HCO_3^- takes place at the apical membrane in order to protect the cells against the gastric acid. Bicarbonate reacts with H^+

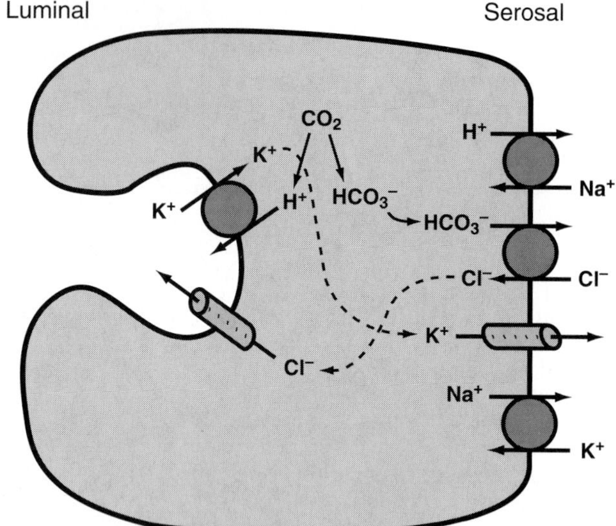

Figure 43–19. Mechanisms for transmembrane transport of electrolytes, acid, and base in the parietal cell.

to form water and CO_2, the latter of which escapes through the mucus barrier secreted by the mucosal cells (Fig. 43–20). By this mechanism, the pH at the luminal surface of the mucosa is near neutral. An Na^+-independent Cl^-/HCO_3^- antiport is situated in the apical membrane and is partly responsible for the HCO_3^- secretion. In the basolateral membrane, an Na^+-dependent HCO_3^- influx takes place. This transport may occur through an Na^+-coupled Cl^-/HCO_3^- antiport, and the transcellular transport of HCO_3^- would therefore depend on the operation of two different Cl^-/HCO_3^- antiports. Interestingly, mucosal cells are protected against luminal acid by supplying HCO_3^- on the serosal side, in accordance with the previously mentioned notion of transcellular transport of HCO_3^-. An Na^+/H^+ antiport is located in the basolateral (serosal) membrane; if pH_i decreases because of an influx of H^+ at the luminal membrane, this antiport is activated to increase pH_i. The activity of this Na^+/H^+ antiport increases also in the presence of a high pH of the blood on the serosal side. Interestingly, it has been found that high systemic bicarbonate concentration and pH value are associated with a lower incidence of stress ulcers.

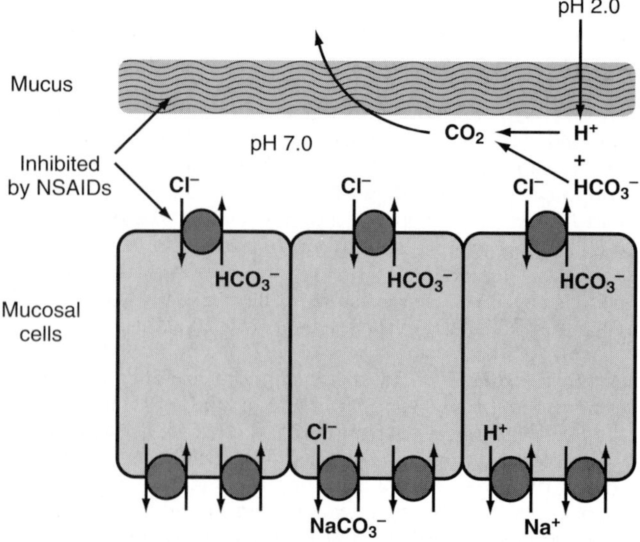

Figure 43–20. Secretion of bicarbonate by gastric mucosal cells.

The NSAIDs often cause peptic ulcer. This process is partly due to a local erosive effect and partly to a systemic effect, but the precise mechanisms of action are not established. High concentrations of NSAIDs strongly inhibit both the Na^+-coupled and the Na^+-independent Cl^-/HCO_3^- antiports.[30] The inhibition of bicarbonate transport reduces the concentration of bicarbonate available to neutralize the gastric acid at the apical surface of the cells and thereby imposes an acid load on the cells. The increased acidification of cells exposed to NSAIDs may be toxic and cause peptic ulcer. Also, when the transport of bicarbonate to the external surface of the cells is reduced by an NSAID, extracellular pH decreases, and the NSAID picks up protons to be de-ionized. Under these conditions, the drug easily penetrates the cell membrane by nonionic diffusion, accumulates inside the cells, and may therefore be toxic to the cells.

Kidney

The transcellular transport of bicarbonate is described earlier in this chapter.

In salt-absorbing tubular cells, both the Na^+/H^+ antiport and the Na^+-independent Cl^-/HCO_3^- antiport have been identified on the *apical* side. Evidence has been presented that a part (30% to 50%) of the NaCl absorption is mediated by a parallel activity of these two antiports[50] (Fig. 43–21). In this case, H^+ and HCO_3^- are transported out of the cells by these two antiports and immediately enter the cells again as CO_2, thus taking part in a catalytic cycle. In other organs as well (intestines, gallbladder, salivary glands), such parallel exchange is an important part of the transcellular transport of salt.

Low dietary NaCl intake increases the activity of Na^+/H^+ antiport to effectively absorb Na^+ and prevent hyponatremia. High intake of NaCl, however, down-regulates this antiport. Dopamine, working via DA_1 receptors, increases the concentration of cAMP and thereby inhibits the Na^+/H^+ antiport, leading to natriuresis.[51] Atrial natriuretic peptide appears to have a similar effect.

ROLE OF pH_i-REGULATING MECHANISMS IN PATHOPHYSIOLOGIC CONDITIONS

Acid-Base Disturbances

It should be noted that the definitions of acid-base disturbances are based on measurements of pH and CO_2 and on calculations of HCO_3^- and base excess in blood plasma, which does not necessarily reflect the intracellular conditions. Also, most blood gases are measured arterially, which reflects tissue conditions to a lesser extent than venous measurements. The body is remarkably tolerant to changes in acidity. Because we use the logarithmic pH scale to measure acidity, we often forget that at pH 7.1, the amount of free protons is *double*

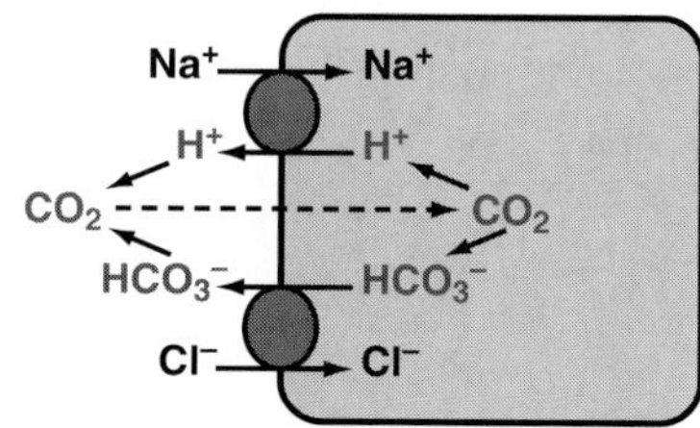

Figure 43–21. Absorption of salt in renal tubule.

that at pH 7.4 (Table 43–3). Imagine what would happen if Na^+ or K^+ concentration were doubled!

Metabolic Acidosis

Metabolic acidosis is caused by several disorders. In many cases, nonvolatile acids, either endogenous (e.g., lactic acid, ketoacids in diabetes mellitus) or exogenous (salicylate and other intoxications) bring about the pH disturbance.

Under normal conditions, lactic acid production is approximately 15 to 30 mmol/kg/day. The maximum capacity of the liver to convert lactic acid to glucose via gluconeogenesis or to CO_2 via the citric acid cycle is 3.5 mol/day. If this capacity is exceeded, lactic acidosis ensues. In the setting of severe liver failure, lactic acidosis occurs with normal production of lactic acid.

Under conditions of aerobic metabolism, the glycolytic pathway goes via pyruvate to the Krebs cycle and then to oxidative phosphorylation. Under anaerobic conditions, however, the NADH (reduced form of nicotinamide adenine dinucleotide [NAD]) formed from the glycolytic pathway builds up, because it is not used in Krebs' cycle. The cells are depleted of NAD^+, and the glycolytic pathway is halted. In order to regain NAD^+ to be able to produce ATP, lactic acid is formed according to the following reaction: $Pyr^- + NADH + H^+ \leftrightarrow$ Lactic acid $+ NAD^+$. This anaerobic pathway generates 2 moles of H^+ per mole of glucose. Thus, a considerable amount of acid is produced. The enzyme catalyzing the formation of a lactate, lactate dehydrogenase (LDH), is regulated by the pH_i such that an acidosis tends to decrease LDH activity whereas an alkalosis increases it. Respiratory alkalosis decreases the elimination of lactate by decreasing its clearance by 40% and thereby increasing its half-life (from ~15 to ~45 minutes). Thus, eliciting alkalosis with treatment under these conditions may increase the lactic acid content.

Lactate production may markedly increase also under conditions in which the cell apparently is not hypoxic. This is the case in some septic models.

Lactic acid and ketoacids are synthesized intracellularly, increasing the intracellular acid load. The cytosolic buffering power (proteins, phosphate, bicarbonate) attenuates the fall in pH_i. The acids are membrane-permeant in their protonated form and, to some extent, leave the cells by non-ionic diffusion. There is, however, evidence that a H^+/lactate$^-$ symport markedly increases the transmembrane transport of protons and lactate in heart and muscle cells. Also, Na^+/H^+ antiport and probably the Na^+-coupled Cl^-/HCO_3^- antiport elevate pH_i in cases of intracellular lactic acidosis, but H^+/lactate$^-$ symport appears to be the most efficient mechanism when lactic acid is effectively removed extracellularly. If extracellular lactic acid is not removed by a sufficient blood circulation, an extracellular acidosis ensues. Further removal of lactic acid from the cells, as well as the Na^+/H^+ and Na^+-coupled Cl^-/HCO_3^- antiports is inhibited. Thus, in cases of systemic acidosis, the removal of lactic acid from the cells is inhibited. Also, in cases of local lactic acidosis due to hypoperfusion, a severe intracellular acidosis develops as a result of the dissipation of the inside:outside gradient of lactic acid. Bicarbonate reacts with H^+ to form CO_2, which is not removed and can give rise to an intracellular P_{CO_2} above 300 mm Hg.

Interestingly, a disease has been detected in which the lactate transporter is absent in skeletal muscle cells. After muscle exercise, lactate is therefore removed slowly from the intracellular space, and patients experience muscle pain and fatigue.

In cases of systemic metabolic acidosis, bicarbonate in the blood and interstitial fluid buffers the acids by forming CO_2, which is eliminated by respiration. Hence, the concentration of HCO_3^- decreases considerably. This decrease in HCO_3^- strongly affects the bicarbonate gradient across the cell membrane. HCO_3^-, therefore, tends to leave the cells because of a reversed inside:outside gradient, predominantly by the Na^+-independent Cl^-/HCO_3^- antiport, lowering pH_i and elevating pH_o. This is functionally equivalent to a net transport of H^+ into the cells. Thus, even though the cell membranes are poorly permeable to H^+ per se, an effective *intracellular* buffering of *extracellular* acidosis may be accomplished by the operation of the Na^+-independent Cl^-/HCO_3^- antiport.[2] The intracellular space of the body is more than twice the extracellular space, and the intracellular buffering power per volume unit is much higher than the extracellular power. Therefore, indirectly importing H^+ by exporting HCO_3^- via the Na^+-independent Cl^-/HCO_3^- antiport is probably an important defense mechanism in systemic acidosis. Thus, the body compensates for metabolic acidosis not only through hyperventilation and slow compensation by the kidneys but also through transport of acid equivalents across the cell membranes to buffer the acid intracellularly. The Na^+/H^+ and Na^+-coupled Cl^-/HCO_3^- antiports counteract this increased cytosolic acid load. Because of the decreased extracellular HCO_3^- and low extracellular pH in metabolic acidosis, pH_i is not fully normalized.

TABLE 43–3. pH and Hydrogen Ion (H^+) Concentrations

pH	H^+ Concentration (nmoles/L)
7.70	20
7.40	40
7.10	80
7.00	100

Respiratory Acidosis

In cases of respiratory acidosis, P_{CO_2} is increased, resulting in a decreased pH. This acid load cannot be buffered effectively extracellularly by bicarbonate, which is usually the main buffer system. Buffering, albeit insufficient, is achieved by extracellular proteins and phosphate. Because it is highly membrane-permeable, CO_2 quickly enters the cells and yields H^+ and HCO_3^-. H^+ is buffered by proteins and phosphate to some extent, but nevertheless, an intracellular acidosis ensues. This activates the Na^+/H^+ antiport and, depending on the cell type, also the Na^+-coupled Cl^-/HCO_3^- antiport. Thus, pH_i increases but attains a lower value than in situations of lower P_{CO_2}. This means that a portion of the protons formed by the increased P_{CO_2} are quickly buffered intracellularly. Because (1) the extracellular buffering is slight, (2) H^+ is exported out of the cells by the Na^+/H^+ antiport and (3) HCO_3^- is imported into the cells via the Na^+-coupled Cl^-/HCO_3^- antiport, the extracellular pH is not effectively normalized. Thus, the decrease in pH_o is more pronounced than the fall in pH_i.

Slower defense mechanisms against respiratory acidosis than those already discussed are the elimination of acids and the reabsorption of HCO_3^- by the kidneys. Particularly important in this context is that long-standing acidosis itself may interfere with the response of pH_i-regulating mechanisms. Thus, the Na^+/H^+ antiport, the Na^+/HCO_3^- symport and the Na^+-independent Cl^-/HCO_3^- antiport, which are all important for reabsorption of HCO_3^- by the kidneys, increase their maximal velocity in response to the increased acid load, so that they are able to eliminate acid and absorb HCO_3^- more efficiently. The mechanisms involved in this regulation are not well characterized, but at least in the case of the Na^+-independent Cl^-/HCO_3^- antiport, an increased synthesis of antiports is involved.

Metabolic Alkalosis

Metabolic alkalosis is clinically separated into chloride-responsive and chloride-unresponsive types. Chloride-responsive metabolic alkalosis is due to excess loss of chloride (vomiting, nasogastric suctioning, diuretic therapy), whereas the chloride-unresponsive type may be due to excess alkali load or excess mineralocorticoid effect. The chloride-responsive type illustrates the close coupling between concentration of Cl^-, $[Cl^-]$, and concentration of HCO_3^-, $[HCO_3^-]$.

The generation of metabolic alkalosis in cases of Cl^- loss from the stomach may be partly explained by the action of the Na^+-independent Cl^-/HCO_3^- antiport in the parietal cells. In short, for the parietal cells to secrete large amounts of hydrochloric acid (HCl), Cl^- must be imported across the basolateral membrane, and the HCO_3^-, which is generated when H^+ is formed, must be exported across the basolateral membrane. This is accomplished by a pH_i-regulated Na^+-independent Cl^-/HCO_3^- antiport (see Fig. 43-19). For each H^+ and Cl^- lost by vomiting or nasogastric suction, one HCO_3^- is exported from the parietal cell and elicits an alkalosis. Usually, the kidneys are able to excrete HCO_3^- rapidly, but in the case of dehydration, which often occurs as a result of the gastrointestinal fluid loss, the kidneys reabsorb almost all Na^+ and water to compensate for the fluid loss. An anion must accompany the reabsorption of Na^+. Because $[Cl^-]$ is low, bicarbonate instead is reabsorbed and the alkalosis persists. Some of the reabsorbed Na^+ is electrically balanced by the excretion of H^+ or K^+. Because H^+ is reduced in metabolic alkalosis, K^+ is excreted, inducing a hypokalemia, which is often found in metabolic alkalosis.

The cells compensate for an intracellular alkalosis by exporting HCO_3^- in exchange for Cl^- via the Na^+-independent Cl^-/HCO_3^- antiport. This antiport is activated at alkaline pH and is driven by the anion gradients. Thus, if the inwardly directed Cl^- gradient is greater than the HCO_3^- gradient, pH_i decreases. With increasing systemic alkalosis, the gradient for HCO_3^- and Cl^- is more unfavorable, and the regulation of pH_i is less effective. Thus, the intracellular compartment buffers an extracellular alkalosis. Because the buffering capacity is higher intracellularly than extracellularly, pH_i remains lower than pH_o.

Respiratory Alkalosis

Because of the high membrane permeability for CO_2, the cytosolic pH is rapidly elevated in respiratory alkalosis. The cells to some extent counteract this elevation by activating the Na^+-independent Cl^-/HCO_3^- antiport, as described previously. Because of the higher buffering power inside the cells, the intracellular pH deviation is less than the extracellular change.

In chronic respiratory alkalosis, the $[HCO_3^-]$ is lowered as a result of the increased excretion of bicarbonate by the kidneys. The Na^+/HCO_3^- symport, which is one of the main mechanisms for reabsorption of HCO_3^- in the proximal tubule, has a greater transport capacity in patients with chronic alkalosis.

Cardiovascular Function

Effect of pH on Cardiac Function

Studies examining the effect of acidification on muscle contractility have shown that a relatively small acidification of heart muscle (~0.2 pH units) has a severe negative inotropic effect, reducing the contractility by 40% to 50%. This is due to (1) a decreased sensitivity of troponin C for calcium (Ca^{2+}), (2) interference of H^+ with cross-linking of actin and myosin, and possibly (3) inhibition of Na^+/Ca^{2+} exchange in the plasma membrane.[52] These studies were done in isolated hearts or myocardial cells (i.e., devoid of sympathetic innervation). In vivo, the activation of the sympathetic nervous system by acidosis compensates for the direct negative inotropic effect of the acid, so the cardiovascular effects of a moderate acidosis are minor in normal hearts; this is accomplished by the inotropic effect of the sympathetic transmitters, but stimulation of the Na^+/H^+ antiport via an α receptor also plays a role.[52] Even relatively mild acidosis (pH 7.25), however, has been found to decrease the stimulatory effect of norepinephrine,[53] and at pH_o 7.00, virtually no stimulatory effect of epinephrine is found.

β-Blockers decrease the activity of the Na^+/H^+ antiport. The negative inotropic effect of Ca^{2+} channel blockers is markedly increased by acidosis. In situations in which the sympathetic nervous system is activated to keep the cardiac output sufficient when pH is normal (i.e., congestive heart failure), an acidosis might severely decrease cardiac function. Thus, the arbitrary pH value 7.2, which is often cited in textbooks as a cutoff value at which to start treating an acidosis, might be satisfactory for the patient with a normal heart but devastating for a patient with cardiac failure. Furthermore, with low pH, the effects of catecholamines are tachycardia and peripheral vasoconstriction rather than increased inotropy, thereby jeopardizing myocardial oxygenation and increasing intramyocardial acidosis. Therefore, the decision concerning treatment should be based on cardiovascular parameters of the patient in question and not on a fixed pH value.

During rapid contractions of the heart, lactic acid accumulates. The lactic acid is transported out from the cardiac muscle fibers, to a large extent, by the H^+/lactate$^-$ symport. To effectively transport lactic acid out of the cells, the extracellular acid must be rapidly removed by perfusion in diastole. In cases of cardiac ischemia due to hypoperfusion, lactic acid rapidly accumulates intracellularly and causes a myocardial acidosis (see later discussion of ischemia).

Apart from the lactic acid transporter, the Na^+/H^+ antiport and a Na^+-coupled Cl^-/HCO_3^- antiport appear to provide the main mechanisms for fighting acidosis in cardiac cells.[54] The Na^+/H^+ antiport is regulated by the Ca^{2+}/calmodulin system, ATP, angiotensin, α receptors, and probably β receptors. The Na^+-independent Cl^-/HCO_3^- antiport appears to be the main mechanism for extruding base. Evidence has been presented that this antiport is highly pH_i-sensitive and increases its activity with increasing pH_i in cardiac cells much like it does in other cells.

Reperfusion after an ischemic event involves a rapid normalization of the acidic intracellular pH developed during the ischemic event. This involves a massive activation of the Na^+/H^+ antiport,[55] which might theoretically have two side effects: (1) a large transport of Na^+ into the cell, resulting in cell swelling, and (2) reversal of Na^+/Ca^{2+} antiport, which usually transports Ca^{2+} out of the cells. Thus, the result is an increased intracellular content of Ca^{2+}, which will result in contracture. Thus, inhibition of Na^+/H^+ antiport could actually protect the heart during reperfusion. It has indeed been found to be the case in many studies[56, 57] and will probably be exploited in future treatment of reperfusion injury.

Vascular Function

In vascular smooth muscle cells, an Na^+/H^+ antiport, an Na^+-coupled Cl^-/HCO_3^- antiport (or, possibly, an Na^+/HCO_3^- symport in some preparations), and an Na^+-independent Cl^-/HCO_3^- antiport have all been found to participate in pH_i regulation. In several studies, the bicarbonate-dependent mechanisms appear to be quantitatively more important than the Na^+/H^+ antiport. Thus, pH_i was found to be higher in the presence of bicarbonate than in its absence.[58]

Also, there seems to be a link in vascular smooth muscle between contractility and pH_i. Vascular smooth muscle is regulated by several ligands with vasoconstricting or vasodilatory effects. Many of the vasoconstrictor agents (e.g., norepinephrine, epinephrine, serotonin, endothelin, vasopressin) stimulate the Na^+/H^+ antiport and increase pH_i in the absence of HCO_3^-. In the presence of physiologic concentrations of bicarbonate, no change in pH_i by these ligands was found, ruling out the proposed "second messenger role" of pH_i. The reason for the lack of change in pH_i despite the activation of the Na^+/H^+ antiport is that at least serotonin and vasopressin also activate the Na^+-independent Cl^-/HCO_3^- antiport, which counteracts the alkalinization. Also the Na^+-coupled Cl^-/HCO_3^- antiport is stimulated by vasopressin. The results of these actions are that the cells are more able to withstand acid or base loads. Nevertheless, significant acidosis or alkalosis might interfere with the actions of these physiologic ligands. Thus, alkalosis (pH 7.6) can increase the vasoconstrictive action of norepinephrine, serotonin, and prostaglandin $F_{2\alpha}$. Conversely, acidosis inhibits their action, particularly the effect of norepinephrine. Consequently, the most common effect of in vivo acidosis is dilation of vessels in the systemic circulation, whereas alkalosis is associated with vasoconstriction. It is important to realize, however, that these effects depend on which ligands are present. The reactivity of pulmonary vessels to acidosis might be vasoconstriction. Thus, acidosis may give rise to pulmonary hypertension. This is particularly evident in the newborn, in whom acidosis that elicits pulmonary hypertension can convert the circulatory system to a fetal pattern (persistent fetal circulation). There are, however, contradictory findings in the literature concerning the effect of pH disturbances on the reactivity of pulmonary vessels. Interestingly, alkalosis was found to inhibit hypoxic vasoconstriction of pulmonary vessels by stimulating the production of vasodilatory prostacyclin (prostaglandin I_2).

Central Nervous System

In the patient with diabetic ketoacidosis, *cerebral edema* may develop after the extracellular acidosis is corrected.[59] Thus, at the time that systemic pH is normalized, the mental condition of the patient may be severely disturbed. It has been found that cerebral edema is mainly an intracellular swelling. Ketoacidosis elicits a decrease in pH_i that should activate the Na^+/H^+ antiport. When the extracellular pH is low, however, the Na^+/H^+ antiport is inhibited.[59] When pH_o is normalized because of treatment, the Na^+/H^+ antiport functions at maximal speed to increase cytosolic pH, and the cells gain Na^+ in considerable amounts. It has been found in vitro that this process results in intracellular swelling. The concomitant action of the Na^+-independent Cl^-/HCO_3^- antiport increases the intracellular salt and water gain. Therefore the action of these pH_i-regulating antiports may give rise to intracellular edema. In most cells of the body, intracellular edema may not have serious negative effects, but intracranially, a moderate swelling may be life-threatening. The combined action of the Na^+/H^+ and Na^+-independent Cl^-/HCO_3^- antiports may also increase cell volume in other cases of cerebral edema (e.g., after ischemia and trauma). In vitro inhibition of these antiports abolishes intracellular edema. Effective inhibitors of antiports to be used in vivo will soon be tested for their efficacy in cases of cerebral edema.

Ischemia

Ischemia not only jeopardizes the supply of oxygen but also severely inhibits the removal of products of metabolism, such as lactic acid, CO_2, and protons. With the decreased supply of O_2, the cells revert to anaerobic metabolism, which they may sustain for varying periods without damage, depending on cell type. In cells where phosphocreatine is abundant, such as muscle cells, ATP is still present for several hours of complete ischemia if the muscle is resting. Myocardial cells also contain phosphocreatine, but because of constant activity, they cannot tolerate more than 10 to 20 minutes of complete ischemia without severe energy failure. The brain cells contain less phosphocreatine and can be irreversibly damaged by 5 minutes of severe ischemia.

Under purely ischemic conditions, there is anaerobic metabolism and no oxidative phosphorylation. Because the respiratory chain can no longer oxidize NADH to NAD^+, NADH accumulates (i.e., the cell is in a more reduced state). NADH has a negative feedback effect on glycolysis, and NAD^+ must be regenerated in order for glycolysis to continue.[60] Conversion of pyruvate to lactate uses NADH as a cofactor and is therefore a way for the cells to get rid of the excess of reduced substances. A side effect of lactic acid generation is metabolic acidosis.

The hydrolysis of ATP also yields free protons.[61] An average ATP concentration of the cell is 4 to 6 mmol,[62] and for every ATP molecule hydrolyzed, approximately 0.8 proton is liberated.[61] Thus, hydrolysis of ATP can contribute to acidification. In one study, acidification occurring shortly after initiation of ischemia correlated with the decrease in ATP.[63]

Other nucleotide breakdown products (undine 5′-monophosphate, inosine 5′-monophosphate) (UMP, IMP) plus the generation of free fatty acids from breakdown of membrane phospholipids can also contribute to acidification, but to a minor extent. The production of lactic acid, however, is quantitatively the most important contributor to acidification. Lactic acid concentrations higher than 40 mmol have been found in the tissue during ischemia.[64, 65] Lactic acid has a pKa of 3.8 and therefore, at close to neutral pH inside the cells, is nearly fully dissociated (i.e., the free protons acidify the cells[66] and the intracellular pH decreases considerably). pH values below 5 have been found in ischemic tissue.[67]

Weak bases inside the tissue immediately buffer a large proportion of protons formed during the aforementioned processes. The major buffers are proteins and bicarbonate, whereas inorganic phosphate buffers to a a lesser extent. Under physiologic conditions, the only amino acid in proteins with a pK_a near physiologic pH is histidine. Thus, the amount of histidine in a protein correlates highly with its buffering power at close to physiologic pH.[68] As intracellular pH decreases, the buffering power of proteins increases as a result of the protonation of side groups with lower pK_a, somewhat limiting severe intracellular acidification.[69]

Protons formed during anaerobic metabolism to a large extent react with HCO_3^- to form CO_2 and water. Buffering by HCO_3^- in the tissue gives rise to a high P_{CO_2} (30 to 80 kPa, 200 to 600 mm Hg). Thus, during tissue metabolic acidosis, large quantities of "respiratory acid" (i.e., CO_2) are formed. Because the blood supply is severely limited under these conditions, CO_2 is not transported away, but accumulates in the tissue. The idea of using P_{CO_2} to detect an ischemic condition is based on the accumulation of CO_2 in the tissue as a result of a primary intracellular metabolic acidosis buffered by bicarbonate.[70–73]

During ischemia, the acidosis starts intracellularly. Nevertheless, pH_i has been found to be higher than pH_o, indicating that the cells are able to export H^+ also under ischemic conditions.[74] This finding is not surprising, because the Na^+/H^+ antiport, the Na^+-coupled Cl^-/HCO_3^- antiport, and the Na^+/HCO_3^- symport are not primary active ATP-dependent mechanisms. Thus, for a limited period, the cells are able to withstand severe acidification. With continued export of protons and lactic acid, these metabolites accumulate extracellularly. This accumulation decreases the effectiveness of pH_i-

regulating mechanisms because of both their inhibition by low extracellular pH and the dissipation of the Na^+ gradient across the plasma membrane due to energy failure and, therefore, loss of Na^+/K^+-ATPase activity. The cytosolic pH strongly depends on the removal of extracellular acids and CO_2 to regulate pH_i. Therefore, with zero-flow ischemia, the decrease in pH_i is much more pronounced than, for instance, with hypoxia and normal flow.

Low pH_i per se, as found in ischemic tissue, can lethally damage cells.[67] Interestingly, a reproducible study has found that injury following ischemia in brain cells is more severe if the research animal or the patient is hyperglycemic at the time of ischemia and thereby has an increased lactic acidosis.[75] However, many cell types sustain extended periods of low pH_i and still survive. Rather than being the major cause of injury, the acidosis is more likely to facilitate the effects of free oxygen radicals, calcium, and so on.

Complicating this concept are in vitro experiments that surprisingly indicate that acidosis in certain instances may *protect* the cells against hypoxic or ischemic injury.[76] Acidosis slows down the activity of most intracellular enzymes and possibly also that of enzymes involved in the generation of harmful substances such as free radicals. As long as the cell is not too acidotic, this slowdown of activity might be beneficial under ischemic conditions. This theory, however, is applicable to cell types whose low activity during acidosis can be tolerated by the body, such as liver and kidney, but, in most cases, not to myocardial cells.

During reperfusion, the extracellular protons and CO_2 are rapidly removed. The cells then have a low pH_i and high pH_o, the most favorable situation for a rapid regulation of pH_i back to normal. In fact, the regulation of pH_i is so rapid that only 5 to 10 minutes are required for normalization. The whole metabolism of the cells suddenly changes to high activity, including generation of free radicals and other potentially harmful substances. The cells swell as a result of the rapid influx of Na^+ via the Na^+/H^+ antiport, which might be detrimental intracranially. Thus, it might theoretically be beneficial to inhibit the rapid regulation of pH_i back to normal on reperfusion. Indeed, several papers support this view by showing improvements in function and cell survival when Na^+/H^+ antiport is inhibited by amiloride or its derivatives.[76, 77] This approach is also feasible clinically and might be an important way to influence cell survival in ischemic conditions.

Inflammation

Polymorphonuclear neutrophils and lymphocytes possess an Na^+/H^+ antiport, an H^+-translocating ATPase, and an Na^+-independent Cl^-/HCO_3^- antiport.[78] The activity of the Na^+-independent Cl^-/HCO_3^- antiport in lymphocytes is strongly pH_i-dependent.[79] Basophilic cells possess an Na^+/H^+ antiport and an Na^+-coupled Cl^-/HCO_3^- antiport.[78]

The extracellular pH (interstitial pH) is often markedly acidic in inflammatory exudates, sometimes because of the increased production of acid by polymorphonuclear neutrophils and, at other times, because of the production of acid by bacteria. In order to function properly, the inflammatory cells must withstand this external acid load. Under these circumstances, the Na^+/H^+ antiport is inhibited by the low pH_o, whereas the H^+-translocating ATPase still works very effectively and is able to counteract the acidification to a large extent. *Bacteroides* produces large amounts of succinic acid.[80] This acid is excreted from the bacteria and, because of the high membrane permeability at acidic pH_o, gains access to the cytosol of the polymorphonuclear neutrophils, causing a strong cytosolic acidification. This acidification inactivates the polymorphonuclear neutrophils. Thus, the excretion of organic acid by bacteria may be a defense mechanism against the immunologic system to considerably increase the virulence of the bacteria.

Almost all NSAIDs are weak acids. They bind strongly to serum albumin, but at low pH, a considerable part of the drug is released from the protein. Thus, in acidic inflammatory exudates, these drugs are accumulated and therefore exert a strong action on the inflammatory cells. It has been found that NSAIDs decrease pH_i in certain kidney cells by stimulating the Na^+-independent Cl^-/HCO_3^- antiport and inhibiting the Na^+-coupled Cl^-/HCO_3^- antiport.[81] It is not known whether the same action is present in leukocytes.

Cancer

The metabolism of cancer cells deviates from that of normal cells in several ways, among which is higher production of lactic acid due to anaerobic metabolism. This increase is caused both by the preferential use of this pathway by cancer cells and by the hypoxic conditions that often develop inside tumors. Numerous measurements of tumor pH have been published, and the results show considerable variation. The average pH in tumors appears to be 0.5 to 1.5 pH units lower than that in normal tissues, although in some studies, a higher than normal pH has been found.[82, 83] The low pH is caused both by increased lactic acid and by protons released in the hydrolysis of ATP.

In accordance with the idea that an increased pH_i is necessary or at least permissive for proliferation, some transformed cell lines have been found to have a higher pH_i in vitro than their nontransformed parental cells measured at neutral pH_o.[84] Significantly, in vivo mutant malignant cells lacking the Na^+/H^+ antiport either fail to form tumors or form tumors that grow at a considerably slower rate than the corresponding cells possessing the antiport.[85] This finding implies a key role for Na^+/H^+ antiport for tumor growth in vivo. It is tempting to speculate that because of the lactic acidosis in the tumor, $[HCO_3^-]$ is very low and the cells therefore depend on the Na^+/H^+ antiport to keep their pH_i at a value permissive for growth. Thus, the increased activity of the Na^+/H^+ antiport that is found in some malignant cells may not be necessary to increase pH_i to a value higher than that found in normal cells but may be necessary to withstand the greater acid load found in tumors.

From a therapeutic point of view, the idea of exploiting a low pH to kill cells has attracted much attention.[83, 86] Thus, acidic cytostatic drugs gain greater access to cells at low pH_o, whereas alkaline drugs are excluded from the cells. The knowledge of tumor pH measured by phosphorus 31 (^{31}P) nuclear magnetic resonance spectroscopy could therefore influence the choice of cytostatic drugs. The cells in the acidic interior of the tumor are probably in a nonproliferative state. Because most cytostatic drugs interfere with cell division, these cells may be able to survive and start proliferating later, when the majority of the other cells have been killed by the treatment. Therefore, drugs that could further decrease pH_i in nonproliferating cells to a value incompatible with survival are highly needed.

SUMMARY

During the last decade, we have witnessed a revolution in our understanding of intracellular regulation of pH and electrolytes. A short summary of our current understanding is as follows:

1. All cells have several transmembrane transport mechanisms (most notably Na^+/H^+ antiport, Na^+-coupled Cl^-/HCO_3^- antiport, Na^+/HCO_3^- symport, H^+ ATPases, and Na^+-independent Cl^-/HCO_3^- antiport) to keep intracellular pH near normal levels despite a heavy acid or base load.

2. These transmembrane transport mechanisms are highly regulated in their activity by both intracellular and extracellular pH, natural ligands (e.g., paracrine and endocrine hormones, growth factors, vasoactive substances), and many drugs.

3. The bicarbonate system is the most important buffer system, both extracellular and intracellular. The other major buffer system is protein. Prerequisites for the efficacy of the bicarbonate system are the removal of CO_2 by respiration and the transmembrane transport of HCO_3^- via Na^+-coupled Cl^-/HCO_3^- antiport, Na^+/HCO_3^- symport, or Na^+-independent Cl^-/HCO_3^- antiport.

4. These mechanisms are also involved in the regulation of intracellular electrolytes, cell volume, transcellular transport, and membrane potential. As in a network, disturbances in one of the processes markedly influence the others.

5. These processes are obviously involved in acid-base disturbances and are important to correct pH deviations. Equally important, these processes appear to be involved in the pathophysiology of ischemia and reperfusion, cerebral edema, kidney failure, peptic ulcer, heart failure, hypovolemic and septic shock, inflammation, and cancer.

6. With the current detailed knowledge of the molecular biology of these processes, new drugs that interfere with their activity will be discovered. In fact, several drugs in current use, such as amiloride, furosemide, NSAIDs, dopamine, and epinephrine, have been shown to alter the activity of these mechanisms in vitro. Thus, in the future drug treatment of these disorders will be available, providing a rational approach to their management instead of our current guessing about the beneficial or detrimental effect of bicarbonate administration.

References

1. Frelin C, Vigne P, Ladoux A, Lazdunski M: The regulation of the intracellular pH in cells from vertebrates. Eur J Biochem 1988; 174:3–14.
2. Tønnessen TI: Regulation of Cytosolic pH in Mammalian Cells. Oslo, The Norwegian Cancer Society, 1990.
3. Chen LK, Boron WF: Intracellular pH regulation in epithelial cells. Kidney Int Suppl 1991; 33:S11–S17.
4. Lowenstein J: Acid and Basics. New York, Oxford University Press, 1993.
5. Olsnes S, Ludt J, Tonnessen TI, Sandvig K: Bicarbonate/chloride antiport in Vero cells: II. Mechanisms for bicarbonate-dependent regulation of intracellular pH. J Cellular Physiol 1987; 132:192–202.
6. Boron WF: Intracellular pH regulation in epithelial cells. Ann Rev Physiol 1986; 48:377–388.
7. Boron WF, Boyarsky G, Ganz M: Regulation of intracellular pH in renal mesangial cells. Ann NY Acad Sci 1989; 574:321–332.
8. Demaurex N, Grinstein S: Na^+/H^+ antiport: Modulation by ATP and role in cell volume regulation (Review). J Exp Biol 1994; 196:389–404.
9. Aronson PS, Nee J, Suhm MA: Modifier role of internal H^+ in activating Na^+/H^+ exchanger in renal microvillus membrane vesicles. Nature 1982; 299:161–163.
10. Reinertsen KV, Tønnessen TI, Jacobsen J, Sandvig K, Olsnes S: Role of chloride/bicarbonate antiport in the control of cytosolic pH. Cell-line differences in activity and regulation of antiport. J Biol Chem 1988; 263:11117–11125.
11. Grinstein SD, Rotin D, Mason MJ: Na^+/H^+ exchange and growth factor-induced cytosolic pH changes: Role in cellular proliferation. Biochim Biophys Acta 1989; 988:73–97.
12. Hoffmann EK, Simonsen LO: Membrane mechanisms in volume and pH regulation in vertebrate cells. Physiol Rev 1993; 69:315–382.
13. Tønnessen TI, Sandvig K, Olsnes S: Role of Na(+)(−)H^+ and Cl(−)-HCO_3− antiports in the regulation of cytosolic pH near neutrality. Am J Physiol 1990; 258:C1117–C1126.
14. Boron WF: Intracellular pH-regulating mechanism of the squid axon: Relation between the external Na^+ and HCO_3^- dependences. J Gen Physiol 1985; 85:325–345.
15. Tønnessen TI, Ludt J, Sandvig K, Olsnes S: Bicarbonate/chloride antiport in Vero cells: I. Evidence for both sodium-linked and sodium-independent exchange. J Cell Physiol 1987; 132:183–191.
16. Little PJ, Neylon CB, Farrelly CA, Weissberg PL, Cragoe EJ Jr, Bobik A: Intracellular pH in vascular smooth muscle: Regulation by sodium-hydrogen exchange and multiple sodium dependent HCO_3^- mechanisms. Cardiovasc Res 1995; 29:239–246.
17. Tønnessen TI, Aas AT, Ludt J, Blomhoff HK, Olsnes S: Regulation of Na^+/H^+ and Cl^-/HCO_3^- antiports in Vero cells. J Cell Physiol 1990; 143:178–187.
18. Boron WF, Knakal RC: Na^+-dependent Cl^-/HCO_3^- exchange in the squid axon: Dependence on extracellular pH. J Gen Physiol 1992; 99:817–837.
19. Ladoux A, Krawice I, Cragoe EJ Jr, Abita JP, Frelin C: Properties of the Na^+-dependent Cl^-/HCO_3^- exchange system in U937 human leukemic cells. Eur J Biochem 1987; 170:43–49.
20. Jentsch TJ, Janicke I, Sorgenfrei D, Keller SK, Wiederholt M: The regulation of intracellular pH in monkey kidney epithelial cells (BSC-1): Roles of Na^+/H^+ antiport, Na^+-HCO_3(−)-($NaCO_3^-$) symport, and Cl^-/HCO_3^- exchange. J Biol Chem 1986; 261:12120–12127.
21. Boron WF, Boulpaep EL: The electrogenic Na/HCO_3 cotransporter. Kidney Int 1989; 36:392–402.
22. Balkovetz DF, Leibach FH, Mahesh VB, Ganapathy V: A proton gradient is the driving force for uphill transport of lactate in human placental brush-border membrane vesicles. J Biol Chem 1988; 263:13823–13830.
23. Roth DA, Brooks GA: Lactate pyruvate transport is dominated by a pH gradient-sensitive carrier in rat skeletal muscle sarcolemmal vesicles. Arch Biochem Biophys 1990; 279:386–394.
24. Khandoudi N, Bernard M, Cozzone P, et al: Mechanisms of intracellular pH regulation during postischemic reperfusion of diabetic rat hearts. Diabetes 1995; 44:196–202.
25. Swallow CJ, Grinstein S, Rotstein OD: Cytoplasmic pH regulation in macrophages by an ATP-dependent and N, N′-dicyclohexylcarbodiimide-sensitive mechanism: Possible involvement of a plasma membrane proton pump. J Biol Chem 1988; 263:19558–19563.
26. Wieth JO, Andersen OS, Brahm J, Bjerrum PJ, Borders CL Jr: Chloride-bicarbonate exchange in red blood cells: Physiology of transport and chemical modification of binding sites. Philos Trans R Soc Lond B Biol Sci 1982; 299:383–399.
27. Olsnes S, Tønnessen TI, Sandvig K: pH-regulated anion antiport in nucleated mammalian cells. J Cell Biol 1986; 102:967–971.
28. Olsnes S, Tønnessen TI, Ludt J, Sandvig K: Effect of intracellular pH on the rate of chloride uptake and efflux in different mammalian cell lines. Biochemistry 1987; 26:2778–2785.
29. Tønnessen TI, Aas AT, Sandvig K, Olsnes S: Effect of anti-inflammatory analgesic drugs on the regulation of cytosolic pH by anion antiport. J Pharmacol Exp Ther 1989; 248:1197–1206.
30. Tønnessen TI, Aas AT, Sandvig K, Olsnes S: Inhibition of chloride/bicarbonate antiports in monkey kidney cells (Vero) by non-steroidal anti-inflammatory drugs. Biochem Pharmacol 1989; 38:3583–3591.
31. Ludt J, Tonnessen TI, Sandvig K, Olsnes S: Evidence for involvement of protein kinase C in regulation of intracellular pH by Cl^-/HCO_3^- antiport. J Membr Biol 1991; 119:179–186.
32. Vigne P, Breittmayer JP, Frelin C, Lazdunski M: Dual control of the intracellular pH in aortic smooth muscle cells by a cAMP-sensitive HCO_3^-/Cl^- antiporter and a protein kinase C-sensitive Na^+/H^+ antiporter. J Biol Chem 1988; 263:18023–18029.
33. Preisig PA, Alpern RJ: Chronic metabolic acidosis causes an adaptation in the apical membrane Na/H antiporter and basolateral membrane $Na(HCO_3)_3$ symporter in the rat proximal convoluted tubule. J Clin Invest 1988; 82:1445–1453.
34. Bierman AJ, Cragoe EJ Jr, de Laat SW, Moolenaar WH: Bicarbonate determines cytoplasmic pH and suppresses mitogen-induced alkalinization in fibroblastic cells. J Biol Chem 1988; 263:15253–15256.
35. Passow H: Molecular aspects of band 3 protein-mediated anion transport across the red blood cell membrane. Rev Physiol Biochem Pharmacol 1986; 103:61–203.
36. Crandall ED, Bidani A: Effects of red blood cell HCO_3(−)/Cl^- exchange kinetics on lung CO_2 transfer: Theory. J Appl Physiol Respir Env Exercise Physiol 1981; 50:265–271.

37. Crandall ED, Winter HI, Schaeffer JD, Bidani A: Effects of salicylate on HCO_3^-/Cl^- exchange across the human erythrocyte membrane. J Membr Biol 1982; 65:139–145.
38. Wieth JO, Brahm J: Inhibitory effect of salicylate on chloride and bicarbonate transport in human red cells: A possible explanation for the stimulatory effect of salicylate on respiration [Danish]. Ugesk Laeger 1978; 140:1859–1865.
39. Kurtz I: Apical Na^+/H^+ antiporter and glycolysis-dependent H^+-ATPase regulate intracellular pH in the rabbit S3 proximal tubule. J Clin Invest 1987; 80:928–935.
40. Nakhoul NL, Chen LK, Boron WF: Intracellular pH regulation in rabbit S3 proximal tubule: Basolateral Cl-HCO_3 exchange and Na-HCO_3 contransport. Am J Physiol 1990; 258:F371–F381.
41. Geibel J, Giebisch G, Boron WF: Angiotensin II stimulates both Na(+)-H^+ exchange and Na^+/HCO_3^- cotransport in the rabbit proximal tubule. Proc Natl Acad Sci USA 1990; 87:7917–7920.
42. Hensley CB, Bradley ME, Mircheff AK: Parathyroid hormone-induced translocation of Na-H antiporters in rat proximal tubules. Am J Physiol 1989; 257:C637–C645.
43. Kurtz A, Della Bruna R, Scholz H, Baier W: Amiloride enhances the secretion but not the synthesis of renin in renal juxtaglomerular cells. Pflugers Arch 1991; 419:32–37.
44. Morduchowicz GA, Sheikh-Hamad D, Dwyer BE, Stern N, Jo OD, Yanagawa N: Angiotensin II directly increases rabbit renal brush-border membrane sodium transport: Presence of local signal transduction system. J Membr Biol 1991; 122:43–53.
45. Madshus IH, Tønnessen TI, Olsnes S, Sandvig K: Effect of potassium depletion of Hep 2 cells on intracellular pH and on chloride uptake by anion antiport. J Cell Physiol 1987; 131:6–13.
46. Mason MJ, Smith JD, Garcia-Soto JJ, Grinstein S: Internal pH-sensitive site couples $Cl^-(-)HCO_3^-$ exchange to Na^+-H^+ antiport in lymphocytes. Am J Physiol 1989; 256:C428–C433.
47. Grinstein S: Intracellular chloride concentration: Determinants and consequences. Prog Clin Biol Res 1987; 254:31–43.
48. Muallem S, Burnham C, Blissard D, Berglindh T, Sachs G: Electrolyte transport across the basolateral membrane of the parietal cells. J Biol Chem 1985; 260:6641–6653.
49. Muallem S, Blissard D, Cragoe EJ Jr, Sachs G: Activation of the Na^+/H^+ and Cl^-/HCO_3^- exchange by stimulation of acid secretion in the parietal cell. J Biol Chem 1988; 263:14703–14711.
50. Preisig PA, Rector FC Jr: Role of Na^+-H^+ antiport in rat proximal tubule NaCl absorption. Am J Physiol 1988; 255:F461–F465.
51. Jadhav AL, Liu Q: DA1 receptor mediated regulation of Na(+)-H^+ antiport activity in rat renal cortical brush border membrane vesicles. Clin Exp Hypertens, Part A: Theory Pract 1992; 14:653–666.
52. Gambassi G, Spurgeon HA, Lakatta EG, Blank PS, Capogrossi MC: Different effects of alpha- and beta-adrenergic stimulation on cytosolic pH and myofilament responsiveness to Ca^{2+} in cardiac myocytes. Circ Res 1992; 71:870–882.
53. Achike FI, Dai S: Influence of pH changes on the actions of verapamil on cardiac excitation-contraction coupling. Eur J Pharmacol 1991; 196:77–83.
54. Grace AA, Kirschenlohr HL, Metcalfe JC, Smith GA, Weissberg PL, Cragoe EJ Jr, Vandenberg JI: Regulation of intracellular pH in the perfused heart by external HCO_3^- and Na(+)-H^+ exchange. Am J Physiol 1993; 265:H289–H298.
55. Vandenberg JI, Metcalfe JC, Grace AA: Mechanisms of pH_i recovery after global ischemia in the perfused heart. Circ Res 1993; 72:993–1003.
56. Maddaford TG, Pierce GN: Myocardial dysfunction is associated with activation of Na^+/H^+ exchange immediately during reperfusion. Am J Physiol 1997; 273:H2232–H2239.
57. Scholz W, Albus U, Counillon L, Gogelein H, Lang HJ, Linz W, Weichert A, Scholkens BA: Protective effects of HOE642, a selective sodium-hydrogen exchange subtype 1 inhibitor, on cardiac ischaemia and reperfusion. Cardiovasc Res 1995; 29:260–268.
58. Putnam RW: pH regulatory transport systems in a smooth muscle-like cell line. Am J Physiol 1990; 258:C470–C479.
59. Van der Meulen JA, Klip A, Grinstein S: Possible mechanism for cerebral oedema in diabetic ketoacidosis. Lancet 1987; 2:306–308.
60. Alberts B, Bray D, Lewis J, Raff M, Roberts K, Watson JD: Molecular Biology of the Cell. New York, Garland Publishing, Inc, 1994.
61. Swallow CJ, Rotstein OD, Grinstein S: Mechanisms of cytoplasmic pH recovery in acid-loaded macrophages. J Surg Res 1989; 46:588–592.
62. Stryer L: Biochemistry. New York, WH Freeman, 1988.
63. Terrier F, Lazeyras F, Posse S, Aue WP, Zimmermann A, Frey BM, Frey FJ: Study of acute renal ischemia in the rat using magnetic resonance imaging and spectroscopy. Magn Res Med 1989; 12:114–136.
64. Katsura K, Ekholm A, Siesjo BK: Tissue P_{CO_2} in brain ischemia related to lactate content in normo- and hypercapnic rats. J Cereb Blood Flow Metab 1992; 12:270–280.
65. Katsura K, Ekholm A, Asplund B, Siesjo BK: Extracellular pH in the brain during ischemia: Relationship to the severity of lactic acidosis. J Cereb Blood Flow Metab 1991; 11:597–599.
66. Mizock BA, Falk JL: Lactic acidosis in critical illness. Crit Care Med 1992; 20:80–93.
67. Kraig RP, Petito CK, Plum F, Pulsinelli WA: Hydrogen ions kill brain at concentrations reached in ischemia. J Cereb Blood Flow Metab 1987; 7:379–386.
68. Nunn JF: Carbon dioxide. *In*: Applied Respiratory Physiology. Nunn JF (Ed). Oxford, Butterworth-Heinemann Ltd, 1993, pp 207–221.
69. Chen LK, Boron WF: Acid extrusion in S3 segment of rabbit proximal tubule: I. Effect of bilateral CO_2/HCO_3^-. Am J Physiol 1995; 268(Pt 2):F179–F192.
70. Tønnessen TI: Biological basis for P_{CO_2} as a detector of ischemia (Review) (79 refs). Acta Anaesthesiol Scand 1997; 41:659–669.
71. Rozenfeld RA, Dishart MK, Tønnessen TI, Schlichtig R: Methods for detecting local intestinal ischemic anaerobic metabolic acidosis by P_{CO_2}. J Appl Physiol 1996; 81:1834–1842.
72. Schlichtig R, Bowles SA: Distinguishing between aerobic and anaerobic appearance of dissolved CO_2 in intestine during low flow. J Appl Physiol 1994; 76:2443–2451.
73. Tønnessen TI, Kvarstein G: PCO_2 electrodes at the surface of the kidney detect ischemia. Acta Anaesthesiol Scand 1996; 40:510–519.
74. Yan GX, Kleber AG: Changes in extracellular and intracellular pH in ischemic rabbit papillary muscle. Circ Res 1992; 71:460–470.
75. Siesjo BK: Pathophysiology and treatment of focal cerebral ischemia: Part II. Mechanisms of damage and treatment. J Neurosurg 1992; 77:337–354.
76. Currin RT, Gores GJ, Thurman RG, Lemasters JJ: Protection by acidotic pH against anoxic cell killing in perfused rat liver: Evidence for a pH paradox. FASEB J 1991; 5:207–210.
77. Meng HP, Lonsberry BB, Pierce GN: Influence of perfusate pH on the postischemic recovery of cardiac contractile function: Involvement of sodium-hydrogen exchange. J Pharmacol Exp Ther 1991; 258:772–777.
78. Swallow CJ, Grinstein S, Sudsbury RA, Rotstein OD: Cytoplasmic pH regulation in monocytes and macrophages: Mechanisms and functional implications. Clin Invest Med 1991; 14:367–378.
79. Mason MJ, Smith JD, Garcia-Soto JJ, Grinstein S: Internal pH-sensitive site couples $Cl^-(-)HCO_3^-$ exchange to Na^+-H^+ antiport in lymphocytes. Am J Physiol 1989; 256:C428–C433.
80. Rotstein OD, Nasmith PE, Grinstein S: The *Bacteroides* by-product succinic acid inhibits neutrophil respiratory burst by reducing intracellular pH. Infect Immun 1987; 55:864–870.
81. Tonnessen TI, Aas AT, Sandvig K, Olsnes S: Effect of anti-inflammatory analgesic drugs on the regulation of cytosolic pH by anion antiport. J Pharmacol Exp Ther 1989; 248:1197–1206.
82. Newell KJ, Tannock IF: Reduction of intracellular pH as a possible mechanism for killing cells in acidic regions of solid tumors: Effects of carbonylcyanide-3-chlorophenylhydrazone. Cancer Res 1989; 49:4477–4482.
83. Tannock IF, Rotin D: Acid pH in tumors and its potential for therapeutic exploitation. Cancer Res 1989; 49:4373–4384.
84. Gillies RJ, Martinez-Zaguilan R, Martinez GM, Serrano R, Perona R: Tumorigenic 3T3 cells maintain an alkaline intracellular pH under physiological conditions. Proc Natl Acad Sci USA 1990; 87:7414–7418.
85. Lagarde AE, Franchi AJ, Paris S, Pouyssegur JM: Effect of mutations affecting Na^+:H^+ antiport activity on tumorigenic potential of hamster lung fibroblasts. J Cell Biochem 1988; 36:249–260.
86. Rotin D, Wan P, Grinstein S, Tannock I: Cytotoxicity of compounds that interfere with the regulation of intracellular pH: A potential new class of anticancer drugs. Cancer Res 1987; 47:1497–1504.

44

Cellular Effectors of the Septic Process

Randeep S. Jawa, MD • Gina A. Quaid, MD
Joseph S. Solomkin, MD

Our understanding of the architecture of the cellular response to infection has undergone considerable change in the past decade, primarily as a consequence of the discovery of new families of cytokines and other messengers for intercellular communication. This knowledge helps define avenues for manipulation of the inflammatory response and amelioration of the unwanted consequences of sepsis.

The inflammatory response can be divided into at least five phases:

1. Recognition of microbial contamination or tissue injury.
2. Release of signaling molecules.
3. Recruitment of cellular effectors.
4. Destruction of invading microbes and metabolism of injured tissue.
5. Restoration of tissue integrity (wound healing).

ARCHITECTURE OF THE INFLAMMATORY RESPONSE

A vast array of mediators and cell types are involved in inflammation. The interaction between an inflammatory mediator (termed a *ligand*) and its cellular receptor provides a differential cellular response to varying ligand concentrations, which results in exquisitely sensitive intercellular communication. Ligand-receptor interactions provide multiple levels of regulation of the inflammatory response, such as production of inflammatory mediators, regulation of their receptors, and production of receptor agonists and antagonists. Ultimately, these mediators affect cell activities. A schematic of some of these events is provided in Figure 44–1.

Multiple levels of mediators, receptors, and activation states at both cellular and molecular levels afford precise regulation of a response that is primarily intended to flood a site of microbial contamination or tissue injury with highly efficient effector cells. Inflammation is "tailored" to deal with a range of tissue injury states, from single cell death to extensive infections such as peritonitis; however, this highly potent system can overwhelm the host and can result in death from multisystem organ failure.

Redundancy is another key characteristic of this system. Multiple mediators with overlapping activities are generated that alter cell activities during the inflammatory event.

Cytokines

It is probable that the cytokine system arose, at least partially, through gene duplication. The idea of gene duplication is based on the structural and receptor similarities between cytokines. For example, the interleukins IL-2, IL-3, IL-4, IL-5, IL-6, IL-7, and IL-13 and granulocyte macrophage-colony-stimulating factor (GM-CSF) cytokines share significant structural homology and belong to the *short-chain* 4-α helix subfamily.[6]

Numerous other cytokines are not uniquely proinflammatory or anti-inflammatory. At a given time, they can have stimulatory effects on certain mediators and inhibitory effects on other mediators. In some cases, the cytokine regulation of mediators can be very different between cell populations, depending on the dose and the presence of other stimuli (Fig. 44–2). Cytokines also have the ability to regulate themselves.

Receptors

Cytokine receptors regulate the cellular response. Like cytokines, cytokine receptors share several structural and functional features. Structurally, these receptors are generally high-molecular-weight proteins located on the cell membrane and they share three major components: (1) an extracellular binding site for specific ligands, (2) a transmembrane, lipophilic domain that orients and provides structure to the receptor, and (3) an intracellular domain that transduces signals. Extracellular domains of receptors may bind multiple cytokines secondary to the consensus sequences between them. Receptors in general share many components. These shared structural features have led to classification of receptors into several families and subfamilies, whose members often share intracellular signaling pathways and functions.

The type and number of receptors present on the cell surface determine the capability of the interleukin to control cell function. One mechanism for controlling cell function via receptors involves differing affinities for ligand. At different concentrations, ligands bind different receptors and induce different cell functions. Changing the conformation of the receptor or internalizing the ligand with receptor can regulate signal transduction itself.

Another avenue for controlling cell function is expression of the receptor on cell surface. Up-regulation of the receptor can occur by multiple mechanisms, an example being exocytosis of receptors from storage pools. Mechanisms for rapid down-regulation of cell surface receptors include (1) internalization, (2) endoproteolytic release of transmembrane proteins, and (3) glycolipid cleavage of select proteins.[7] Endoproteolytic cleavage of a receptor is another form of cell regulation, owing to its ability to be a soluble form of an agonist or antagonist.[7]

Adhesion Molecules

Adhesion molecules can also regulate the septic response. These molecules allow the adhesion of leukocytes to endothelium and interstitial matrix proteins. A variety of adhesion molecules are expressed on endothelial cells and leukocytes. "Addressins" are forms of these molecules that allow leukocytes to "home in" on a target location. For example, selective neutrophil attachment to postcapillary venule endothelium is directed by a addressin molecule.[8, 9] Adhesion molecules can also transduce signals and activate leukocytes.[10]

Many mediators regulate the expression of adhesion molecules. Mediators target messenger ribonucleic acid (mRNA) synthesis or exocytosis of cell granules to increase cell expression of adhesion molecules in some cell lines. In a variety of cell lines, these molecules are constitutive and, therefore, "insensate" to this type of regulation. Modulation of cell surface expression and selective cell surface localization of these molecules constitute important mechanisms for differential leukocyte responses in inflammation.

Cells

The primary circulating cells that participate in the septic response are mononuclear phagocytes and neutrophils; how-

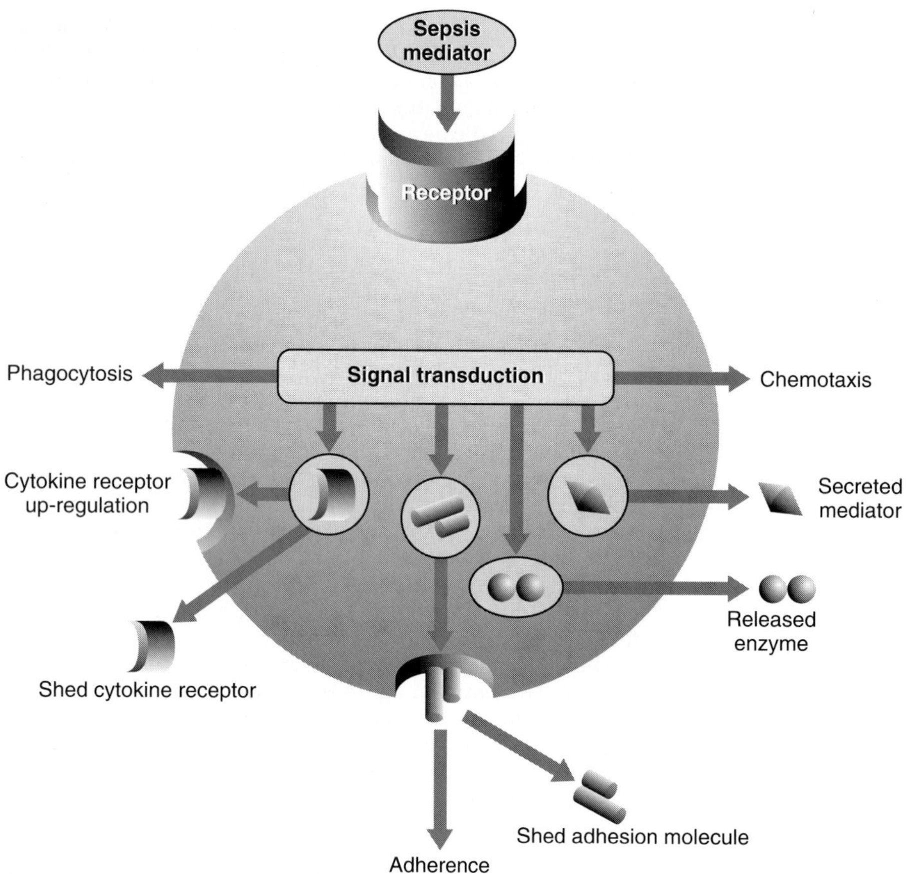

Figure 44–1. General cellular response in sepsis. Not all functions apply to all cells.

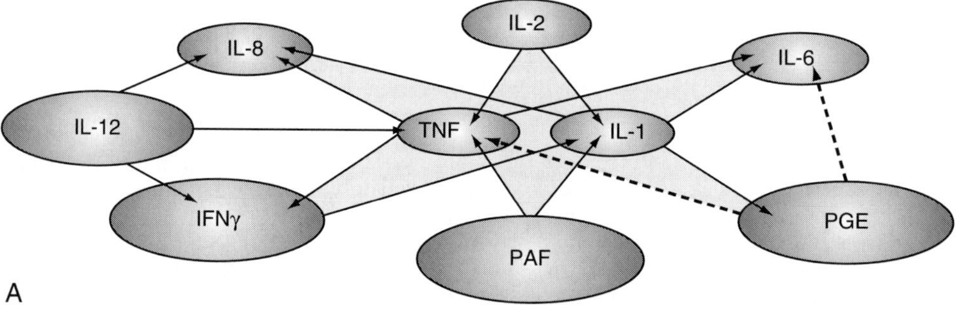

Figure 44–2. *A,* Examples of stimulatory cytokine interactions. *B,* Examples of inhibitory cytokine interactions. *Dashed lines* in both diagrams represent interactions that can be stimulatory or inhibitory, depending on associated stimuli. IL, interleukin; PGE, prostaglandin; IFN, interferon; PAF, platelet-activating factor.

ever, work in vitro supports a role for T cells, B cells, and natural killer (NK) cells as well. They produce an array of proinflammatory and anti-inflammatory mediators and growth factors. Growth factors, specifically, help to expand the pool of effector cells. Some of the possible interactions among these cell types are shown in Figure 44–3. Specific mediators and their cellular sources are detailed in Table 44–1.

Perhaps the key recognition cells in the inflammatory response are mononuclear phagocytes, also known as *interstitial macrophages* or *macrophage-like cells.* They are widely distributed in all tissues. Mononuclear phagocytes are recruited into an area of tissue injury after the initial wave of neutrophil infiltration. On arrival they release an array of cytokines,[11–14] including:

- IL-1α, IL-1β, IL-6, IL-8, IL-10, and IL-12
- Tumor necrosis factor-α (TNF-α)
- GM-CSF
- Granulocyte colony-stimulating factor (G-CSF)
- Monocyte chemoattractant protein-1 (MCP-1)
- Monocyte inhibitory protein-α (MIP-1α)

These molecules play major roles in the pathogenesis of septic shock.[11, 13, 14]

In turn, multiple cytokines, including IL-1α, IL-1β, IL-3, IL-4, IL-10, IL-13, TNF-α, transforming growth factor-β (TGF-β), interferon-γ (IFN-γ), and GM-CSF regulate mononuclear phagocyte activity and cytokine secretion.[13] Other immune cells also produce, and are regulated by, cytokines. For example, neutrophils produce TNF-α, IL-3, and IL-8 and are highly responsive to TNF-α, IL-1β, IL-6, and IL-8.[12, 15–21]

Some "nonimmune" cells also play a crucial role in the pathogenesis of sepsis, including endothelial cells, platelets, and vascular smooth muscle cells. Endothelial cells produce IL-1β, IL-6, IL-8, TNF, endothelin-1, prostaglandins, nitric oxide, and platelet-activating factor (PAF).[9, 22–24] They can also produce adhesion molecules that play a key role in leukocyte-endothelial cell binding interactions. Once bound, activation or transendothelial migration of leukocytes occurs. Platelets mediate the septic process by producing PAF, platelet-derived growth factor (PDGF), TGF-β, serotonin, prostaglandins, thromboxane A_2 (TXA_2), and nitric oxide, and they can also interact with neutrophils to generate the anti-inflammatory molecule, lipoxin A_4 (LXA_4).[12, 22, 25–27] Vascular smooth muscle cells also participate in the septic process by secreting chemokines, specifically IL-8.

RECOGNITION SYSTEMS OF THE SEPTIC CASCADE

Initiation of the septic response requires the interaction of a "foreign" substance with host proteins and cell surface receptors. Once activated, the inflammatory response is channeled through a controlled and selected set of mediators. Immunoglobulins are known to activate this system, but there are other major systems that can also activate inflammation: lipopolysaccharide (LPS), lipopolysaccharide-binding protein (LBP), and CD14 group and the complement system.

Lipopolysaccharide, Lipopolysaccharide-Binding Proteins, and CD14

The lipid A portion of LPS on gram-negative organisms has been studied extensively as a non–complement-mediated activator of the inflammatory response. This molecule interacts with monocytes and other cell types via the CD14 receptor.[25] Once combined with the LBP, macrophages are activated and production of TNF-α, IL-1, IL-6, GM-CSF, prostaglandin E_2 (PGE_2), and nitric oxide begins.[25, 28–30] LPS-mediated cytokine production can also be regulated by other mediators of inflammation, such as IFN-γ and IL-10.[31] The response can be completely blocked by the binding of LPS-LBP complex with bactericidal permeability-increasing protein (BPI).[31] LPS has also been shown to have immunosuppressive effects. For ex-

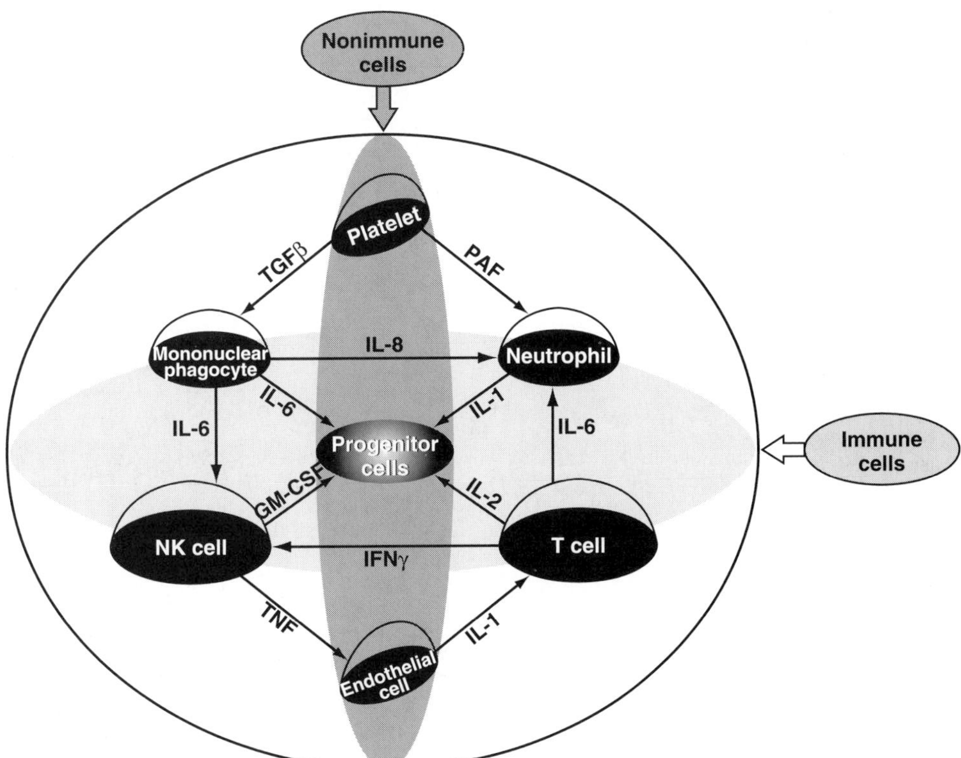

Figure 44–3. Examples of intercellular communication. B cells and vascular smooth muscle cells are not shown. NK, natural killer; IL, interleukin; TGFβ, transforming growth factor beta; PAF, platelet-activating factor; GM-CSF, granulocyte-macrophage colony-stimulating factor; TNF, tumor necrosis factor; IFN, interferon.

TABLE 44–1. The Interleukins and Tumor Necrosis Factor

Mediator	Source	Inducer of Mediator	Inhibitor of Mediator	Induced by Mediator	Inhibited by Mediator	Actions
IL-1	Monocytes/macrophages T cells NK cells Most nucleated cells	TNF GM-CSF M-CSF IFN-γ PAF TGF-β C5a	IL-4 IL-10 IL-13 IFN-γ PGE$_2$	IL-6 IL-8 TNF IFN-γ PAF MCP-1 Eicosanoids	N/A	Stimulates cellular proliferation Activates resting T cells Enhances TNF cytotoxicity Supports B cell proliferation Supports B cell antibody production Promotes cellular adherence Increases endothelial adhesion molecule expression Produces procoagulant state Induces hypotension Acute phase response activation (via IL-6) Induces fever Induces weight loss
IL-2	T cells NK cells	IL-12 PAF	IL-10 PGE$_2$ Elevated cAMP	IL-1 TNF PGI$_2$	N/A	T cell growth factor Induces capillary leakiness Decreases arterial pressure
IL-3	T cells Neutrophils	IL-12	IL-12	N/A	N/A	Stimulates hemopoiesis Regulates progenitor cell growth
IL-4	T cells NK cells	PGE$_2$	IL-12	LXA$_4$ 15-s-HETE	IL-1 IL-6 IL-8 IL-10 IL-12 TNF MIP-1α	Stimulates B and T cell growth Stimulates hemopoiesis Stimulates macrophages Enhances lymphocyte-endothelial adhesion Increases MHC I and II expression
IL-5	T cells	N/A	N/A	N/A	N/A	Induces B cell differentiation
IL-6	Monocytes/macrophages B cells T cells Endothelial cells Fibroblasts Endocrine tissue	IL-1 TNF IFN-γ PDGF Viruses	IL-4 IL-10 IL-13 PGE$_2$	N/A	N/A	Signal in T cell activation Induces B cell antibody secretion Activates PMNs Activates NK cells Induces acute phase response Induces hyperglobulinemia Pyrogen
IL-7	Bone marrow stromal cells Spleen stromal cells Thymus stromal cells	N/A	N/A	TNF IL-1 IL-6	N/A	Induces B cell precursor proliferation Induces thymocyte proliferation
IL-8	Macrophages Neutrophils Hepatocytes Endothelial cells Fibroblasts	TNF IL-1 IL-12	IL-4 IL-10 IL-13	N/A	N/A	Neutrophil chemoattractant Activates neutrophils Enhances neutrophil transendothelial migration Induces fibroblast collagen production Induces angiogenesis
IL-9	T cells	TNF	N/A	N/A	N/A	Lymphoid cell growth factor Myeloid cell growth factor
IL-10	Monocytes/macrophages B cells Helper T cells	N/A	IL-4 IL-13	N/A	IL-1 IL-2 IL-6 IL-8 IL-12 TNF IFN-γ	Suppresses inflammatory response Inhibits macrophage activation Inhibits macrophage cytokine release Inhibits macrophage antigen presentation Increases IL-1 receptor antagonist
IL-11	Bone marrow stromal cells	N/A	N/A	N/A	N/A	Shortens G0 phase of progenitor cells Stimulates B cell antibody production
IL-12	Monocytes/macrophages B cells Skin Langhans cells	N/A	IL-4 IL-10 IL-13	IL-2 IL-3 IL-8 IL-10 TNF IFN-γ GM-CSF	IL-4 IL-3	T cell growth factor Stimulates proinflammatory cytokine release

TABLE 44–1. The Interleukins and Tumor Necrosis Factor *Continued*

Mediator	Source	Inducer of Mediator	Inhibitor of Mediator	Induced by Mediator	Inhibited by Mediator	Actions
IL-13	Helper T cells	N/A	N/A	N/A	IL-1	Inhibits monocyte inflammatory cytokine production
					IL-6	Inhibits monocyte & endothelial cell procoagulant activity
					IL-8	Induces 15-lipoxygenase pathway
					IL-10	Immunomodulatory effects on B cells
					IL-12	
					TNF	
					GM-CSF	
					MIP-1α	
IL-14	B cells	N/A	N/A	N/A	N/A	B cell growth factor
IL-15	Mononuclear cells	N/A	N/A	N/A	N/A	T cell growth activator
	Epithelial cell line					T cell chemoattractant
	Fibroblast cell line					Stimulates B cell proliferation
	Nonlymphoid cells					Induces B cell antibody production
						Stimulates NK cells
TNF	Monocytes/macrophages	TNF	IL-4	IL-1	N/A	Activates neutrophils
	Lymphocytes	IL-1	IL-10	IL-6		Stimulates macrophages
	NK cells	IL-2	IL-13	IL-8		Stimulates endothelial cell proliferation
	Kupffer cells	IL-12	TGF-β	IL-9		Direct endothelial cell toxicity
	Neutrophils	PAF	Elevated cAMP	IL-10		Induces MHCI expression
	Mast cells	C5a	β agonists	PAF		Increases microvascular permeability
	Endothelial cells	PGE_2	PGE_2	MCP-1		Induces hypotension
	Keratinocytes	Enterotoxin		Eicosanoids		Stimulates angiogenesis
	Smooth muscle cells	Viruses				Induces intravascular coagulation
	Astrocytes	Fungi				Induces gut mucosal damage
		Parasites				Decreases gastrointestinal blood flow
						Decreases lipoprotein lipase activity
						Induces anorexia
						Induces hyperglycemia
						Induces fever

N/A = not available; IL = interleukin; NK = natural killer; TNF = tumor necrosis factor; GM-CSF = granulocyte macrophage colony-stimulating factor; M-CSF = monocyte colony-stimulating factor; IFN = interferon; PAF = platelet-activating factor; TGF = transforming growth factor; PDGF = platelet-derived growth factor; MCP = monocyte chemotactic protein; PG = prostaglandin; LX = lipoxin; MHC = major histocompatibility complex; HETE = hydroxyeicosatetraenoic acid; MIP = macrophage inflammatory protein.

ample, when humans are given an infusion of LPS or, endotoxin IL-2 production is suppressed, reducing T cell proliferation and inducing partial immunosuppression.[32]

The Complement System

The complement system is composed of a series of proteins whose ordered polymerization results in the release of inflammatory molecules, opsonization of microorganisms, induction of microbial and host cell lysis, activation of a variety of cells, and activation of the coagulation system (Fig. 44–4). Activation of the complement cascade occurs through stabilization of C3b bound to a foreign surface via electrostatic interactions provided by factor B. Once the bound complex becomes enzymatically active, it is able to cleave subsequent complement components, forming a membrane attack complex and releasing soluble proinflammatory mediators C3a, C5a, and C4a, appropriately dubbed *anaphylatoxins*. Circulating carboxypeptides rapidly degrade anaphylatoxins to markedly less potent desArg forms.

Complement molecules have a multitude of effects on the immune system and the human body. Foreign particle surfaces coated with C3 increase phagocytosis and clearance of immune complexes by leukocytes.[24] Released C5a induces polymorphonuclear cell activation (enhanced responsiveness to subsequent stimuli), migration, adherence, and aggregation.[22] It also increases pulmonary vascular resistance and induces hypoxemia.[33] All the anaphylatoxins can increase vascular permeability, decrease systemic vascular resistance, induce leukopenia, and indirectly enhance leukocyte aggregation.[22, 34] The complement system also interacts in cytokine networks. For example, C5a can induce the production of TNF-α, IL-1, and IL-6 by monocytes.[34] Hemorrhagic necrosis, a hallmark of sepsis, results when the complement system interacts with cytokines; specifically, it acts synergistically with TNF.[24]

Four major complement receptors have been identified. Their functions are diverse, ranging from enhancing phagocytosis to serving as adhesion molecules.

Complement receptor 1 (CR1) recognizes C3b, and it has a variety of functions in different cells.[24] This receptor enhances the ability of mononuclear and polymorphonuclear phagocytes to phagocytose particles coated with immunoglobulin G (IgG) and C3b.[24] On erythrocytes, it binds C3b-fixed immune complexes and aids in their disposal by transporting them to the liver for clearance by Kupffer cells.[24] CR1 functions as a membrane-linked inhibitor of complement activation on erythrocytes and leukocytes.[24]

CR2 binds to C3bi and to C3dg/C3d and is expressed principally on B cells, thymocytes, transformed B- and T-cell lines, and certain nonimmune cells.[24] Ligands of CR2 function as B-cell growth factors and enhance proliferation of activated B cells.[24]

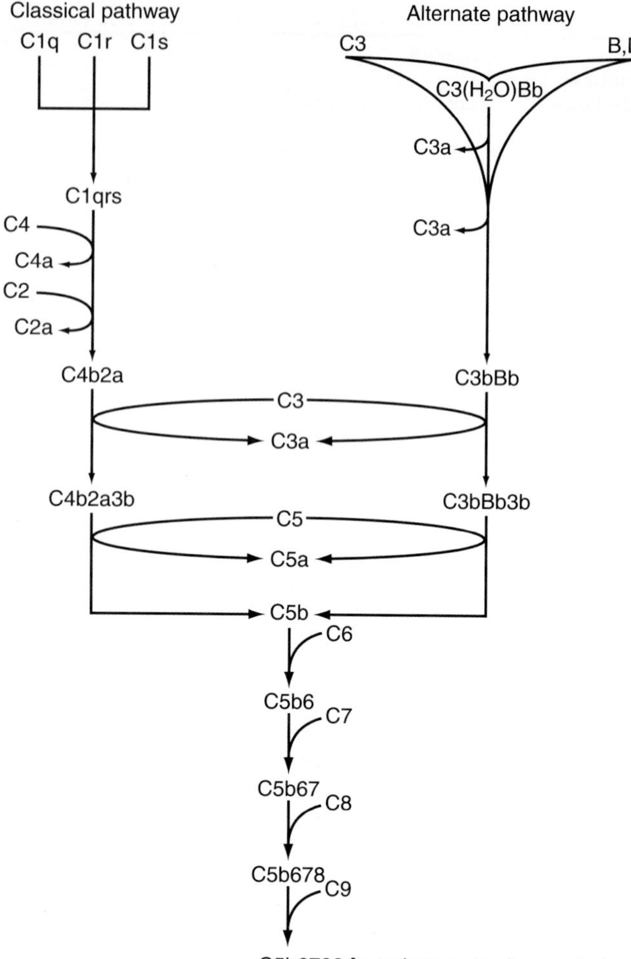

Figure 44–4. The complement system. (Redrawn by permission from Muller-Eberhard H: Complement: Chemistry and pathways. *In* Inflammation: Basic principles and clinical correlates. Gallin J, Goldstein I, Snyderman R (Eds). New York, Raven Press, 1988, p 22.[194])

Both CR3 and CR4 can function as adhesion molecules. CR3 binds to C3bi and C3d and is expressed on neutrophils, monocytes, cytotoxic T cells, NK cells, and (weekly) on macrophages.[24] CR3 binding to particles coated with C3bi induces phagocytosis and subsequent respiratory burst activity in leukocytes.[24] This receptor is also involved in lymphocyte-mediated, complement-dependent, and antibody-dependent cytotoxicity.[24] CR4 is structurally and functionally similar to CR3 and also binds to C3bi.[24] CR4 mediates macrophage phagocytosis, respiratory burst activity, and adhesion.[24]

MEDIATORS OF THE INFLAMMATORY CASCADE

Cytokines are the major mediators of the inflammatory response. There are four overlapping categories of cytokines:

1. Proximal mediators.
2. Proinflammatory cytokines induced by the proximal mediators.
3. Anti-inflammatory cytokines.
4. Growth factors for immune and nonimmune cells.

A fifth category of cytokines, dubbed *other mediators,* focuses on cytokines other than TNF and the interleukins. Identified mediators are also divided according to the available evidence for their contributions to the septic response. Strong experimental evidence in vitro and in vivo supports the role of many mediators in sepsis. Many additional messengers may play a role in this response, based on their activities in vitro; however, they lack in vivo experimental support. Participation of these molecules may be indirect. They may induce growth and proliferation or recruit new cells to fuel the septic response. Brief summaries of the mediators are provided in Tables 44–1 and 44–2.

Proximal Mediators

Tumor Necrosis Factor-α

TNF has global effects on the body and the immune system. There are two subtypes of TNF, TNF-α and TNF-β. They share about 30% amino acid homology, bind to the same receptor, and elicit similar responses.[38] TNF-α is produced as a 26-kD prohormone, which is processed to a single peptide of 17 kD.[16] Mature TNF-α molecules are composed of three of these 17-kd peptides.[16] TNF-α is secreted primarily by macrophages and monocytes but can also be secreted by T cells, NK cells, neutrophils, endothelial cells, keratinocytes, smooth muscle cells, and astrocytes.[15, 16]

Immunologically, TNF-α can govern the responses of other cytokines and can have direct actions at a cellular level of many different systems. A complex system of checks and balances regulates its production and effects. TNF-α is the first cytokine released by endotoxin action on monocytes/macrophages.[29] It is a central regulator of interactions between cytokines (see Fig. 44–2). TNF induces production and/or release of IL-1, IL-6, IL-8, IL-9, IL-10, PAF, MCP-1, eicosanoid, IL-1 receptor antagonist, and soluble TNF receptor.[12, 16, 22, 35] TNF synthesis and release can be up-regulated by IL-1, IL-2, IL-12, TNF-α itself, IFN-γ PAF, and C5a.[16, 29, 37] Inhibition of TNF production or release is controlled by IL-4, IL-10, IL-13, TGF-β cortisol, and agents that increase intracellular cyclic adenosine monophosphate (cAMP).[14, 16, 36-39] The cAMP-elevating agents include PGE_2, phosphodiesterase inhibitors (pentoxifylline, amrinone), and β-adrenergic agonists.[36, 37] Interestingly, while PGE_2 stimulates TNF production from resting monocytes, it inhibits TNF production by activated macrophages.[22] In vivo, TNF-α has also been shown to stimulate macrophage and neutrophil functions, activate neutrophil production, and induce major histocompatibility complex I (MHC-I) molecule expression.[22, 40]

Of note, pre-formed mRNA levels of TNF are constitutively present in a variety of healthy tissues, and levels of TNF-α mRNA increase minimally, if at all, during endotoxemia.[36] It is thought that the presence of pre-formed mRNA shortens the lag time between cell stimulation and TNF release.

TNF-α can directly affect many organ systems. In the vascular system, TNF-α stimulates and inhibits different endothelial cell activities, such as inducing endothelial cell proliferation and IL-1β secretion[12, 40]; however, TNF-α can also be directly toxic to vascular endothelial cells.[22] Through a complex series of actions, TNF-α induces vasodilatation (and thus hypotension) during an inflammatory response. The pulmonary vascular tree, in particular, becomes highly permeable, leading to interstitial edema.[12, 40] In the lung parenchyma, TNF-α induces neutrophil accumulation.[12]

Gastrointestinal (GI) and metabolic effects of TNF-α are multiple. On the GI tract, it induces anorexia thought to be mediated by intestinal blood flow, inhibits gastric emptying, and induces gut mucosal damage.[12, 22] TNF-α specifically affects lipid and glucose metabolism during sepsis. Lipid metabolism is inhibited when exposed to TNF-α by decreasing lipoprotein lipase activity.[12, 22] Glucose production and secretion

TABLE 44–2. Other Mediators in the Septic Process

Mediator	Source	Inducer of Mediator	Actions
IFN-γ	T cells NK cells	TNF IL-1 IL-12	Activates B cells Encourages PMN activation Activates macrophages Modulates inflammatory cytokine secretion Augments production of adhesion molecules
Complement	Hepatocytes Mononuclear cells	LPS	Anaphylaxis Increases vascular permeability Decreases systemic vascular resistance Induces leukopenia Stimulates IL-1, IL-6, an TNF-α production
TGF-β	Platelets Monocytes	N/A	Inhibits B and T cell proliferation Monocyte chemoattractant Stimulates monocytes
PAF	Platelets Neutrophils Basophils Endothelial cells	TNF	Induces platelet aggregation Promotes neutrophil aggregation Bronchoconstriction Increases vascular permeability Hypotension
MCP-1	Lymphocytes Fibroblasts Activated monocytes	TNF IL-1 IL-4 PDGF LPS	Monocyte chemoattractant
MIP-1α	Mononuclear phagocytes	N/A	Monocyte chemoattractant B cell chemoattractant Chemokinetic for neutrophils
MIP-1β	Monocytes Lymphocytes Fibroblasts	N/A	Mediates T cell chemotaxis Mediates T cell adherence
GM-CSF	Monocytes T cells NK cells Megakaryocytes	N/A	Stimulates monocyte/macrophage functions Myeloid cell growth factor
PGE	Macrophages Epithelial cells Fibroblasts Most cells	IL-1 IL-6 TNF LPS Complement	Inhibits B and T cell proliferation Inhibits T cell IL-2 production Inhibits T cell IL-2 receptor expression Inhibits B cell activation events Inhibits IgM and IgG3 synthesis Inhibits monocyte MHCII expression Stimulates T cell GM-CSF secretion
LTB4	Mononuclear cells Neutrophils	N/A	Increases vascular permeability Chemoattractant
LXA_4	Mononuclear cells	N/A	Decreases leukocyte-endothelial adhesion Inhibits NK cell cytotoxicity
15-s-HETE	Mononuclear cells	N/A	Decreases leukocyte-endothelial adhesion Antagonizes LTB4 effects on neutrophils

N/A = not available; IFN = interferon; TGF = transforming growth factor; PAF = platelet-activating factor; MCP = monocyte chemotactic protein; MIP = macrophage inflammatory protein; GM-CSF = granulocyte macrophage colony-stimulating factor; PG = prostaglandin; LT = leukotriene; LX = lipoxin; HETE = hydroxyeicosatetraenoic acid; TNF = tumor necrosis factor; IL = interleukin; LPS = lipopolysaccharide; PDGF = platelet-derived growth factor; Ig = immunoglobulin; MHC = major histocompatibility complex; NK = natural killer.

are increased via glycolysis after exposure to TNF-α.[12, 22] Lactic acid levels also increase as a consequence of TNF-α.[12]

The coagulation system and the hypothalamus are directly altered by TNF-α in sepsis. On the coagulation system, it is pivotal in inducing coagulopathy through up-regulation of tissue factor (TF) and down-regulation of thrombomodulin and protein C activities.[41] Further perpetuation of coagulopathy via TNF-α takes the form of counteracting fibrinolysis by down-regulating of tissue plasminogen activator (tPA) and up-regulating of plasminogen activation inhibitor 1 (PAI-1).[41] Finally, TNF-α induces fever by direct stimulation of the hypothalamus.[22]

Interleukin-1

Like TNF, IL-1 not only affects the cytokine interactions but can also affect different organ systems. It is the other central regulator in cytokine interactions. IL-1 exists in two forms, IL-1α and IL-1β. Both have a molecular weight (MW) of 175 kD in humans, and they bind to the same receptors and appear to have similar functions.[42] IL-1 is produced by mononuclear cells, but virtually every nucleated cell can produce it in response to injury.[12] Many of its actions are similar to and can be synergistic with TNF-α.[22]

Synthesis and secretion of IL-1 are regulated at multiple levels, from IL-1 production to IL-1 receptor antagonism. Its production is induced by TNF-α, GM-CSF, monocyte colony-stimulating factor (M-CSF), IFN-γ, TGF-β, and perhaps the teichoic acid component of the cell walls of gram-positive bacteria.[17, 22, 43–45] Inhibition of IL-1 production is regulated by IL-4, IL-10, IL-13, PgE_2, and also IFN-γ (depending on associated conditions).[14, 22, 45] Other agents that can modulate production of IL-1 include corticosteroids, prostaglandins, and cAMP.[45]

IL-1 helps to mobilize the immune system in response to

inflammation. It stimulates the release of cytokines: IL-6, IL-8, TNF-α, IFN-γ, PAF, MCP-1, CSFs, and a variety of eicosanoids.[12, 17, 22] Lymphocytes are activated and stimulated to proliferate and mature in the presence of IL-1.[22] IL-1 also supports polymorphonuclear and mononuclear phagocyte activation and their subsequent inflammatory cytokine release.[22, 46] In addition, it promotes leukocyte–endothelial cell adherence by increasing expression of adhesion molecules on endothelial cells.[17, 22, 36, 47]

As with TNF-α, IL-1 activation in sepsis results in a procoagulant state by inducing TF and PAI-1 synthesis while decreasing thrombomodulin secretion.[29] Additional effects of IL-1 include fever (via direct stimulation of the hypothalamus), hypotension, natriuresis, anorexia, acute-phase response induction (via IL-6), suppression of lipoprotein lipase activity, and stimulation of adrenocorticotrophic hormone (ACTH) release.[12, 22]

IL-6, IL-8, and IL-12: Tumor Necrosis Factor and IL-1-Induced Proinflammatory Mediators

Interleukin-6

IL-6 is produced by monocytes/macrophages, B cells, T cells, thymic stromal cells, megakaryocytes, endothelial cells, keratinocytes, and fibroblasts in response to inflammatory stimuli.[48, 49, 55, 56] The hypothalamus, anterior pituitary, and adrenal cortex also produce IL-6.[51] Production of IL-6 is induced by IL-1, TNF-α, IFN-γ, PDGF, and viruses.[12] Its synthesis and release can be inhibited by IL-4, IL-10, and IL-13.[14]

In the liver, IL-6 regulates the production of the acute-phase proteins in response to inflammation.[48, 49] Specifically, it stimulates production of C-reactive protein (CRP), fibrinogen, and serum amyloid A protein.[48, 49] IL-6's ability to induce the synthesis of acute-phase proteins is associated with pyrexia and with increased corticosteroid production.[12] Protein breakdown in skeletal muscle is also activated in the presence of IL-6.[50]

IL-6 has a variety of immune-mediated effects as well. It acts as a signal in T cell activation, proliferation, and differentiation.[49, 51] Interactions with IL-1 and TNF-α augment T cell proliferation.[22] B cell secretion of antibody and differentiation into plasma cells are induced by IL-6.[49, 51] Like IL-12, IL-6 requires IL-2 to augment immunoglobulin secretion from B cells.[52] In conjunction with IL-4 and IL-5, IL-6 can help in the development of humoral immunity.[53] IL-6 itself can activate NK cells and polymorphonuclear leukocytes (PMNs), specifically accumulation of neutrophils.[22, 54]

Interleukin-8

Chemokines are the family of proteins to which IL-8 belongs. These are cationic proteins of 70 to 100 amino acid residues that share four conserved cysteine residues involved in two disulfide bonds. Chemokines can be sorted into two groups according to the spacing of the two amino-terminal cysteines, either CC (the cysteine molecules are side by side) or CXC (spaced by an amino acid). The latter primarily affect neutrophils and include NAP-2, GRO-α, and IL-8.

IL-8 is produced by macrophages, neutrophils, T cells, endothelial cells, fibroblasts, and hepatocytes.[12, 17, 21, 57] IL-8 production can be induced by IL-1, IL-12, and TNF-α; inhibition is controlled by IL-4, IL-10, and IL-13.[12, 14, 58] Chemoattraction for neutrophils is the most important function of IL-8.[17, 59] It can also activate neutrophils by inducing enzyme release, priming them for enhanced superoxide production, up-regulating their adhesion molecules, and enhancing transendothelial migration.[17, 59, 60] Additionally, IL-8 has some chemotactic activity on lymphocytes.[12]

Interleukin-12

IL-12 is produced by human peripheral blood mononuclear cells (PBMCs), B cells, and Langerhans cells in the skin.[58] It is a heterodimeric cytokine composed of disulfide-bonded 35-kD (p35) and 40-kD (p40) subunits.[61] The p35 subunit exhibits partial homology to IL-6 and G-CSF, and the p40 subunit exhibits extensive homology to the extracellular domain of the IL-6 receptor.[52] In vitro experiments indicate that while the heterodimeric IL-12 induces intracellular signal transduction, a homodimer composed of the IL-12 p40 subunit inhibits IL-12 activity.[62]

The main function of IL-12 is to stimulate NK and T cells, including cytotoxic T cells.[63, 64] A T cell growth factor, it exhibits properties similar to those of IL-2.[65] It can also induce proliferation of B cells and peripheral blood mononuclear cells (PBMCs) synergistically with IL-2, but IL-2 must be present for this to occur.[52, 61] In T and NK cells, IL-12 induces the production of IL-2, IL-3, IL-8, IL-10, TNF-α GM-CSF, M-CSF, and IFN-γ.[58, 66] Inhibition of IL-12 itself can be controlled via IL-4, IL-10, and IL-13.[14] Interestingly, IL-12 has been shown to antagonize the expression and function of IL-4. IL-12 is also known to affect hematopoiesis, but it is unclear at this time whether the effect is inhibitory or stimulatory.[66]

IL-4, IL-10, and IL-13: Major Down-regulators of Cytokine Production

Interleukin-4

The first major interleukin that inhibits cytokine production, and thus the inflammatory response, is IL-4. It is synthesized principally by helper T cells.[12] The main target of inhibition of IL-4 is the production and release of cytokines in monocytes (IL-1, IL-6, IL-8, IL-10, IL-12, TNF-α and MIP-1α).[13, 14, 67] It can also down-regulate monocyte cell surface TNF receptor-55/75 expression.[46] IL-4 indirectly down-regulates the inflammatory response by increasing production of the anti-inflammatory arachidonic acid metabolites, such as 15-5-hydroxyeicosatetraenoic acid (15-s-HETE) and LXA-4, by stimulating 15-lipoxygenase, and by increasing production of IL-1 receptor antagonist.[46, 68] IL-4 itself is regulated by PGE_2 (stimulation) and IL-12 (inhibition).[66, 67]

IL-4 can also act as proinflammatory mediator. For example, B and T cell growth and differentiation depend on IL-4.[12, 69] Lymphocytes require it for the production of IL-3, IL-5, IL-6, IL-9, IL-10, GM-CSF, and IL-4 itself.[67, 70] It can enhance lymphocyte–endothelial cell adhesion as well.[22] On macrophages, IL-4 stimulates induction of macrophage antigen expression.[22, 69] Expression of MHC I and MHC II antigens is also enhanced by IL-4.[69]

Interleukin-10

IL-10 is another suppressor of the inflammatory response.[11, 67] It is generated by B cells, helper T cells, and monocytes/macrophages.[67, 71] It directly affects B cells, T cells, NK cells, and macrophages.[11, 12, 72] Like IL-4, IL-10 inhibits IL-6, IL-8, IL-12, IFN-γ, and MIP-1α production and increases IL-1 receptor antagonist (IL-1ra) production.[14, 39, 75, 78, 79] It can also inhibit IL-2 production.[39] Experiments in vitro with monocytes/macrophages reveal that IL-10 inhibits IFN-γ stimulation, cell activation, production of mediators (TNF-α, IL-1, and nitric oxide), MHC II, and antigen expression.[47, 73-75] Experiments on monocytic and lymphoblastic cell lines also indicate that IL-10 inhibits leukocyte adhesion to IL-1–stimulated endothelial cells.[47] Indirectly, IL-10 inhibits cytokine synthesis by activated T cells and NK cells.[73]

IL-10 has proinflammatory effects similar to those of IL-4. In synergy with IL-2, it acts as a growth factor for B and T cells.[76, 77] IL-10 itself is regulated via gene expression. TNF and IL-12 up-regulate deoxyribonucleic acid (DNA) production, whereas IL-4 and IL-13 inhibit it[14, 22, 66]

Interleukin-13

The third major inhibitor of the inflammatory process is IL-13. It shares 25% to 30% amino acid–sequence homology, and significant functional homology, with IL-4.[80, 81] Like IL-4 and IL-10, IL-13 inhibits inflammatory cytokine production by monocytes.[68, 82] The major cytokines it inhibits in monocytes are IL-1, IL-6, IL-8, IL-10, IL-12, and TNF production.[14] In other cells, IL-13 can inhibit production of GM-CSF, G-CSF, and MIP-1α production.[14] Like IL-4, IL-13 indirectly inhibits the inflammatory response via the 15-lipoxygenase pathway, directly inhibits the procoagulant activity of monocytes and endothelial cells that have been exposed to inflammatory mediators, down-regulates monocytic expression of CD14, up-regulates monocytic expression of some adhesion molecules, and induces B cell proliferation and immunoglobulin production.[14, 68, 82-84] Unlike IL-4, however, IL-13 cannot stimulate T cells.[85] Simultaneously, IL-13 up-regulates IL-1 receptor agonist production.[81]

IL-2, IL-3, IL-5, IL-7, IL-9, IL-11, IL-14, and IL-15: Growth Factors

Interleukin-2

IL-2 is an important cytokine growth factor. Its targets of execution are T cells, B cells, NK cells, and monocytes.[32, 86] Activated T cells produce IL-2, and proliferation of these cells requires its presence.[12, 22] IL-2 can also act in synergy with other interleukins to promote T-cell growth. Other immunologic effects of IL-2 include stimulation of TNF, IL-1, and prostaglandin I_2 (PGI_2) release as well as activation of serum complement.[29, 87, 88] Apart from the immune system, IL-2 can affect the cardiovascular system by reducing arterial pressure, systemic vascular resistance, and ejection fraction.[22] It also increases cardiac output and capillary leakiness.[12, 22] IL-2 itself is stimulated for release by IL-12 and PAF and inhibited by IL-10.[25, 39, 58] Similar to TNF and IL-1, its gene transcription is down-regulated by PGE_2 and other cAMP-elevating events.[89]

Interleukin-3

Acting synergistically with IL-6 and erythropoietin, IL-3 helps regulate growth and differentiation of progenitor cells of several lineages, including granulocytes, monocytes, lymphocytes, erythrocytes, and megakaryocytes.[12, 18] Some experiments also indicate that IL-3 stimulates transcription of endothelial adhesion molecule genes.[18] IL-3 is produced by activated T cells, neutrophils, mast cells, eosinophils, and megakaryocytes. It can be stimulated or inhibited by IL-12.[58, 66]

Interleukin-5

IL-5 induces B cells to differentiate into plasma cells after antigenic stimulation.[12] It is produced by T cells. IL-5 is structurally comparable to IL-2, IL-4, and GM-CSF in that it is composed of two domains, each of which is composed of four helical bundles with two beta sheets.[90]

Interleukin-7

IL-7 is a bone marrow, thymic, and splenic stromal cell factor capable of inducing the growth and proliferation of B cell precursors and mature T cells, including cytotoxic T cells.[12, 13, 91, 92] It may or may not act with IL-2 to induce T cell proliferation.[91] Synergistically with IL-12, IL-7 induces helper T and cytotoxic cells to proliferate.[92] NK cell cytotoxicity is regulated by IL-7.[91] Some findings in vitro indicate that IL-7 may also stimulate secretion of IL-1α, IL-1β, TNF-α, and IL-6.[13, 93]

Interleukin-9

IL-9 is a growth factor for lymphoid and myeloid lineage cells.[12] IL-9 targets include human T cells, B cells, fetal thymocytes, and erythroid progenitor cells.[94] It is produced by T cells.[95]

Interleukin-11

IL-11 is a T cell–dependent stimulator of B cell growth and immunoglobulin production.[96, 100] It also synergizes with IL-3 to shorten the G0 period of progenitor cells, similar to IL-6 and G-CSF.[98] It can enhance megakaryocyte and platelet formation, and it may play a role in macrophage maturation and activation.[99, 101] IL-11, like IL-6, stimulates hepatocytes to produce acute-phase proteins.[101] It can be produced by bone marrow and lung stromal cells in response to inflammatory cytokines, histamine, and specific respiratory tract viruses.[96, 97] In vitro experiments suggest that recombinant IL-1 and recombinant TGF-β can stimulate IL-11 production.[96] IL-4 inhibits the secretion of IL-11 in pulmonary stromal cells.[96]

Interleukin-14 and Interleukin-15

IL-14 is a B lymphocyte growth factor, and IL-15 is an "IL-2–like" T lymphocyte growth factor.[65, 100, 102] IL-15 can also act as a chemoattractant for T cells, and it stimulates NK cells to proliferate and secrete cytokines, such as IFN-γ and TNF-α.[65, 102] The most abundant sources of IL-15 are nonlymphoid tissues, specifically muscle and placental tissues.[104] Interestingly, many cell types transcribe IL-15 genes, but the cytokine is translated into protein at a very slow rate.[103, 104]

Other Mediators of Acute Inflammation and the Septic Response

A variety of noncytokine mediators participate in the inflammatory response. Represented here are IFN-γ, eicosanoids, transforming growth factor β (TGF-β), PAF, monocyte chemotactic protein 1 (MCP-1), MIP-1, and GM-CSF. These molecules can act directly or indirectly on an array of cell types, coordinating with the cytokines to regulate inflammation.

Interferon γ

IFN-γ is a T cell lymphokine that has immunomodulatory effects on several cell lines. Production of these molecules is induced by viruses, bacterial antigens, TNF, IL-1, and IL-12.[12, 58] In B cells, IFN-γ helps to activate them to increase antibody production.[22] PMNs become activated, can accumulate, and have enhanced phagocytic activity after being exposed to IFN-γ.[22] IFN-γ also activates monocytes and macrophages and promotes proinflammatory cytokine release from them.[46, 105] IFN-γ also promotes expression of TNF-α receptors on macrophages.[22] Adhesiveness between monocytes and endothelial cells is enhanced with IFN-γ.[106] It can also augment production of adhesion molecules on leukocytes and endothelial cells, which activates leukocyte–endothelial cell adhesion.[22, 107] Endothelial cells exhibit marked morphologic changes after exposure to IFN-γ.[22] Cytokine release and production can be modulated by IFN-γ.[22] For example, IFN-γ promotes the release of IL-1 and IL-6, and it can act synergistically with IL-2 to increase TNF-α release.[22]

Eicosanoids

Although an extensive review of the eicosanoids is provided in another chapter, they are briefly reviewed here because of their importance in the septic response. Eicosanoids are a family of polyunsaturated 20-carbon fatty acids that are synthesized from arachidonic acid by most cells in the body.[108] Arachidonic acid metabolism by an alternative 15-lipoxygenase pathway (not the 5-lipoxygenase pathway) leads to the generation of 15-s-HETE and thereby LXA_4 or LXB_4.[68, 109] The 15-lipoxygenase pathway operates principally in leukocytes, but it has also been detected in reticulocytes and airway epithelial cells.[27] Lipoxin synthesis can also occur by transformation of leukocyte-generated LTA_4 by either 15-lipoxygenase or 12-lipoxygenase in adjoining mesangial cells or platelets.[27]

PGE series eicosaonids are secreted by several cell types, including fibroblasts, follicular dendritic cells, macrophages, and epithelial cells.[110] PGE synthesis is induced by IL-1, IL-6, TNF-α, complement components, and cross-linking of Fc receptors.[110] They mediate a variety of lymphocytic activities, including inhibition of B and T cell proliferation, IL-2 secretion and IL-2 receptor expression in T cells, B cell activation, and IgM and IgG3 synthesis.[110] PGE_2 can interfere with interactions between monocytes and T cells in vivo. It can also inhibit monocyte expression of MHC II molecules and suppress antigen presentation to T cells.[89]

Monocytes increase the production of PGE_2, and concomitant increases in serum levels are observed in response to inflammation.[89] Elevations in these eicosanoids cause global immunosuppressive effects (e.g., reduction of TNF-α and IL-1 production and decreased thymocyte responsiveness to IL-1).[22, 111] Eicosanoids also can enhance the immunosuppressive effects of TGF-β and IL-6.[67] Kupffer cells in the liver can limit production of IL-6 and TNF-α by concurrently producing PGE_2.[112] PGE also has some proinflammatory effects: for example, it can stimulate GM-CSF production in T cells.[110]

Leukotriene-generated B_4 (LTB_4) is another important proinflammatory molecule. It is the first chemoattractant generated by macrophages after LPS stimulation, and it can be synthesized by neutrophils.[114, 115] LTB_4 is a potent chemoattractant for neutrophils that increases neutrophil adhesion to endothelium.[68, 113] LTB_4 can increase vascular permeability via direct or indirect mechanisms.[22] In addition, LTB_4 can up-regulate IL-6 and TNF-α production.[111]

LXA_4 and 15-s-HETE are molecules whose main job is to inhibit the inflammatory response. 15-s-HETE decreases LTB_4 generation by leukocytes, antagonizes LTB_4-mediated neutrophil chemotaxis, and suppresses leukocyte activation in response to ionophores or other activators.[68] LXA_4 and 15-s-HETE diminish the respiratory burst activity of neutrophils.[27] They also inhibit NK cell cytotoxicity and decrease leukocyte–endothelial cell adhesion.[68]

Transforming Growth Factor β

TGF-β is released from platelets in response to inflammation.[12] It is a monocyte chemoattractant, and following chemotaxis it activates them to produce TGF-β1 (in an "autocrine" manner), IL-1, TNF, and PDGF.[12, 22] TGF-β can also be immunosuppressive by decreasing IL-1 and TNF-α–mediated neutrophil adhesion and inhibiting B and T cell proliferation.[12, 116] In other cells, however, TGF-β1 promotes cell growth, repair, and metabolism.[22]

Platelet-Activating Factor

PAF is a potent mediator of anaphylaxis and hyperactivity. It is thought to be a key contributor to circulatory shock.[25] Several animal shock model studies have shown that PAF infusion mimics the shock state, levels are markedly increased in shock, and antagonists provide significant protection against diverse forms of shock such as shock- or sepsis-induced organ dysfunction.[25]

PAF is produced in neutrophils, macrophages, NK cells, platelets, endothelial cells, and epithelial cells.[22, 25, 26] It has global effects on the body. PAF has direct effects on different organ systems. The pulmonary bronchi constrict in its presence. It has negative inotropic effects on the heart, causes hypotension, and increases vascular permeability.[22, 25] At the cellular level, PAF can induce platelet aggregation and promotes leukocyte activation and subsequent free radical formation.[22]

Inflammatory messenger networks are also modulated by PAF. For example, it induces IL-1, IL-2, TNF-α, leukotriene, and TXA_2 production.[22, 25] It can also proximally mediate many toxicities associated with endotoxin, TNF, or IL-1 infusion.[118] Production of PAF itself can be stimulated by TNF-α.[117] A mechanism for IL-1 PAF–induced activity may be associated with lipoxygenase metabolite.[25] Experimental studies in animals suggest that PAF may be the greatest stimulus for eicosanoid release in endotoxemia.[113]

Monocyte Chemotactic Protein-1 and Macrophage Inflammatory Protein-1

MCP-1 is a 76 amino acid polypeptide that induces monocyte chemotaxis and activation.[12] It is produced by lymphocytes and fibroblasts.[12] It can be produced by monocytes after stimulation with TNF-α, IL-1, PDGF, and/or LPS.[12]

MIP-1α is a C-C chemokine. It is produced by mononuclear phagocytes. MIP-1α is a chemotactic molecule for T cells and monocytes and is chemokinetic for neutrophils.[119] In studies in vitro MIP-1β is produced in large amounts by monocytes, fibroblasts, and lymphocytes early after activation, and it mediates both T cell chemotaxis and adhesion.[120] MIP-1β also augments adhesion of $CD8^+$ T cells.[119, 120]

Granulocyte-Macrophage Colony–Stimulating Factor

GM-CSF is produced by mononuclear phagocytes, T cells, megakaryocytes, and thymic stromal cells.[56, 57, 121] Apart from its growth factor activity, GM-CSF also stimulates PMN phagocytosis, degranulation, and cytotoxicity.[22] It can promote macrophage activity.[22]

CELL SURFACE RECEPTORS FOR TUMOR NECROSIS FACTOR AND THE INTERLEUKINS

Interleukins can elicit many cellular responses similar to inflammation as a result of shared receptor components that activate similar intracellular pathways. Receptors also share mechanisms for up- or down-regulation, and thus serve as other mechanisms for altering the cellular response to a mediator. For example, the production of soluble receptors for IL-4, IL-7, IL-10, and TNF inhibit biologic activity of the cognate ligands, but soluble receptors for IL-6 augment ligand activity.[39, 122, 123]

Examination of these receptors is simplified when they are grouped according to their shared structural and/or functional features. For example, the *hematopoietin* receptor family is made up of IL-2, IL-3, IL-4, IL-5, IL-6, IL-7, IL-9, IL-12, and GM-CSF receptors.[58, 99, 104, 124, 125] The defining features of this family are found primarily in the extracellular domains, which include four conserved cysteine residues, a series of alternating hydrophobic and polar residues, and a Trp-Ser-X-Trp-Ser amino acid motif.[99] As with most cytokine receptors, the cytoplasmic domain transduces the signal and contains a large number of serine and proline residues.[94] This domain is believed to be the target of kinases. Protein phosphorylation by various tyrosine or serine kinases is a well-recognized mechanism for initiating transduction of a binding stimulus into an intracellular effect. In the hematopoietin receptor family intrinsic tyrosine kinase activity does not exist. Members of this family associate with and activate members of several other kinase families, such as the *Jak* kinases.[125] Tyrosine kinase–associated receptors often require ligand-induced receptor dimerization for signaling.[126] Many interleukins that signal via *Jak* kinases, such as IL-6, IL-9, and IL-12, can activate other common intracellular mediators, such as the STAT (signal transducers and activators of transcription) proteins.[125, 127] Receptors that are classified separately include TNF, IL-1, IL-8, and IL-10.

Receptors for Tumor Necrosis Factor

There are two types of TNF receptors that are found in most cells: type I (TNF-R55) and type II (TNF-R75).[15, 128] All biologic activities attributed to TNF-R75 can also exerted by TNF-R55 but usually at much lower densities of receptors. Both receptor types can activate sphingomyelinase with concurrent formation of ceramide and activation of NF-κB, but only TNF-

R55 is responsible for cytotoxicity and expression of adhesion molecules on endothelial cells.[128]

TNF-R75 has a higher affinity and dissociation rate than TNF-R55, preferentially binding TNF at low concentrations. After binding TNF-α, TNF-R75 passes the ligand to neighboring TNF-R55.[128] Some studies suggest TNF-R75 plays an accessory role to enhance or synergize TNF-R55 effects. These findings have led some researchers to label TNF-R55 an *omnipotent receptor.*[128] In cells transfected with the TNF receptors, signaling of TNF-R75 seemed to be highly dependent on receptor density as compared with TNF-R55.[128]

TNF-R55 and TNF-R75 lack any inherent kinase activity. It is postulated that following clustering of the TNF-α receptors, the associated protein kinases, TNF-R–associated factors (TRAFs), TNF-R55–associated death domain protein (TRADD), and receptor-interacting protein (RIP), may become activated. This may lead to downstream stimulation of several intracellular signal transduction pathways and transcription factors.[128]

Both TNF receptors can be found in a soluble form in the circulation of healthy individuals, and their numbers can increase in many noninfectious and infectious disease states.[16] Soluble components of these receptors represent shed portions from the cell surface.[16] Soluble TNF receptors (sTNF-R) bind TNF-α, rendering it incapable of agonist activity, but increase its half-life, especially at low levels.[40, 129] Shedding soluble TNF-R modulates the immune response by rendering cells less sensitive to TNF-α. In experimental human models of endotoxemia, TNF-α receptors are transiently down-regulated, shed, and desensitized to TNF-α on circulating monocytes and granulocytes.[16]

Receptors for Interleukin-1

There are two receptors for IL-1, and they belong to the immunoglobulin superfamily.[44] IL-1α and IL-1β bind to both receptors and appear to have identical functions.[42] The p80 (80-kD) IL-1 receptor is called IL-1RtI, and the p68 (68-kD) IL-1 receptor is called IL-1RtII.[44] IL-1RtI is expressed in T cells, fibroblasts, keratinocytes, and hepatocytes.[44] It has two domains: an extracellular ligand-binding domain and a cytosolic domain.[44] Once the receptor has bound its ligand, both domains are internalized.[44] Type 1 receptor expression is stimulated by IL-2 and is inhibited by IL-1.[44] In fibroblasts, expression of this receptor appears to be mediated by PDGF's increasing gene expression.[44]

IL-RtII is expressed on B cells, neutrophils, and bone marrow cells.[44] IL-RtII and IL-1RtI have 28% amino acid homology.[44] One major difference between these receptors is the highly truncated cytosolic domain of IL-RtII.[44] IL-RtII also has a different binding affinity and transduces a different signal than does IL-1RtI.[44] IL-1 also down-regulates type II receptor.[44] Signal transduction pathways for both IL-1 receptors are unclear.[44] In general, IL-1α binds best to the type I receptor and IL-1β binds best to the type II receptor.[44]

There is a naturally occurring IL-1 receptor antagonist (IL-1 ra). It is a 22-kD protein that shares 14% to 26% sequence homology with IL-1β.[16, 118] IL-1 ra can bind to the IL-1 receptor with no demonstrable IL-1 activity.[118] IL-1ra is produced in response to bacterial infection, and its production is thought to protect against the deleterious effects of bacterial toxins in animals.[41]

Receptors for IL-2, IL-4, IL-7, IL-9, IL-13, and IL-15

Except for IL-13, this group of interleukin receptors shares a common γ-chain subunit. The γ-chain has been designated γ_c.[101, 104, 134] These receptors also have α and β chains. The α chain is unique to each receptor binding a specific cytokine.[101]

An example of this group is the IL-2 receptor. IL-2 has three receptors: high-, intermediate-, and low-affinity ones.[65, 103] The high-affinity IL-2 receptor has at least three subunits: α (p55), β (70/75-kD), and γ (64-kD) chains.[104, 130] There are combinations of these chains that produce IL-2 receptors with lower affinities. The intermediate-affinity IL-2R is a heterodimer composed of β and γ chains, whereas the low-affinity IL-2R consists of a solitary α chain.[103, 131] The low-affinity receptor can bind IL-2 but is unable to transduce signal.[104, 130]

The β chain is shared with the IL-15R and has significant sequence homology to the gp130 subunit of the IL-6 receptor.[104, 132, 133] On its own, this β chain has minimal to no binding activity and requires either the IL-2R α or γ chain to bind to IL-2.[132, 133] It is necessary, however, for IL-2 internalization and signal transduction.[104, 130] The γ_c chain is also required for IL-2 internalization and signal transduction.[104, 130, 135] This chain is capable of very weakly binding IL-2, but only in the presence of the other components.[133, 136]

Components of the high-affinity IL-2 receptor are shared with most of the other members of this group. These shared components are likely responsible for shared interleukin-receptor signal transduction mechanisms and functions. For example, IL-2R, IL-4R, and IL-7R share different receptor components with each other, increasing the receptor's affinity for its ligand.[104, 130, 135] Heterodimerization of the β and γ chains is necessary for signaling by IL-2R and may be necessary for signaling by IL-4R and IL-7R.[126, 137] They also share functional similarities. To illustrate this point, IL-2R, IL-4R, and IL-9R all transduce signal via JAK kinases, and IL-2, IL-4, and IL-7 can transduce signal via *src* kinase families.[86, 104, 127, 138] Another function shared by IL-2, IL-4, and IL-7 is activation of intracellular phosphotidylinositol 3 kinase.[138] Additionally, IL-4R and IL-9R both transduce signal via insulin receptor substrate 1 protein (IRS-1).[127] An exception to the general principle of unshared α chains involves IL-4R and IL-13R. This shared structural component explains their similar functional responses.[80, 134, 139]

Receptors for IL-3 and IL-5

IL-3, IL-5, and GM-CSF receptors have a common β subunit, which has been designated β_c.[131] These receptors also have differing α chains with low affinity and subsequently can interact with a common β (gp140) chain, which generates high-affinity receptors capable of signal transduction.[99] The β subunit does not associate with any of these ligands unless *they* have first associated with the α subunit.[6, 18, 140]

Receptors for IL-6 and IL-11

Receptors for IL-6 and IL-11 are composed of α and β subunits.[141–143] The α subunits are specific for IL-6 and IL-11.[142] The common β (gp130) subunit is a membrane glycoprotein, also known as the *affinity converter* or *signal transducer,* because of its ability to transduce signal.[142, 144–146] The intracellular portion of this protein potentiates gene-modulatory and antiproliferative effects of IL-6 in vitro.[145]

The IL-6Rα (gp80) subunit recognizes IL-6 with low affinity ($10-^{9}$ M), but binding with the β subunit generates high-affinity IL-6-binding sites.[147] The extracellular binding between these subunits occurs through a disulfide-linked homodimerization but only when the α chain is bound to ligand.[143, 145] Once receptor-ligand binding has occurred, in vitro models have shown that the receptor is internalized and down-regulated.[27]

Neither the IL-6Rα or IL-6Rβ subunit, has any inherent

tyrosine kinase activity.[142] Tyrosine kinases, specifically the *Jak* kinases, do associate with the dimerized IL-6Rβ.[145, 148] After the kinase has been activated, it initiates a phosphorylation cascade, in which the kinase appears to phosphorylate the kinases themselves, IL-6Rβ, and other specific cytosol proteins, including STAT proteins.[148]

Like the TNF receptor, IL-6 has a soluble receptor. This is a 50- to 55-kD protein and is the extracellular α subunit of the membrane anchored receptor.[129] These receptors can bind to IL-6 and then interact with cellular gp 130 to elicit an IL-6 response.[143] The β component does not need to bind α subunit for this reaction to occur. In contrast to sTNFR, sIL-6r seems to stimulate the biologic activity of IL-6.[129]

Receptors for IL-8

IL-8 has two receptors, IL-8RA and IL-8RB,[149-151] which belong to a "serpentine" type of receptor superfamily. Members of this superfamily include pheromone, cAMP, and secretin-like and metabotropic glutamate receptors. Although their activating ligands vary much in structure and character, the amino acid sequences of the receptors are very similar and are believed to adopt a common structural framework comprising seven transmembrane helices. These receptors are also members of a class of receptors for peptides involved in the proinflammatory response, including two receptors for *N*-formylpeptides (FPR1, FPR2), one homologue of these (FPRL2) and the receptor for complement fragment C5a (C5aR).[152] The RB is a "promiscuous" receptor, because it binds a number of chemokines, such as Gro-α and NAP-2. The genes encoding IL-8RA and IL-8RB are located on human chromosome 2.[152]

The IL-8 receptors are G protein–coupled receptors, in contrast to other cytokine receptors that are tyrosine kinase–coupled.[153] These G protein–coupled receptors, which are rhodopsin-like, represent a widespread protein family that includes receptors for hormones, neurotransmitters, and light. They transduce extracellular signals through interaction with guanine nucleotide–binding (G) proteins and subsequent phosphotidylinositol phospholipase C activation.[153] This results in activation of various protein kinases and, finally, in a cellular response.

Receptors for IL-10

The IL-10 receptors, along with the IFN receptors, belong to the class II cytokine receptor family.[72] The characteristic that defines class II receptors is the extracellular domains that exist alone in a monomeric form but oligomerize in the presence of ligand.[39] Motifs in this family have little resemblance to hematopoietin receptor and tyrosine kinase–receptor families,[72] although, in a specific human B-cell line, there are some high-affinity IL-10 receptors.[71]

Receptors for IL-12

IL-12 receptor shares homology with the IL-4, IL-6, IL-12, and G-CSF receptors.[58, 154, 155] Specifically, the β component of this receptor shares significant homology with the IL-6β component.[154, 155] There are three binding sites of the IL-12 receptor, which, respectively, have high, medium, and low affinity.[154] The low-affinity binding sites are made up of disulfide-linked IL-12Rβ dimers or oligomers.[155] Once IL-12 is bound to its receptor, tyrosine-mediated phosphorylation transduces the signal that directs cell function.[125]

INTRACELLULAR MESSENGERS

Following binding of a mediator to its receptor, activation of a sequence of enzymes results in a cell response. Examples of these enzymes are tyrosine and serine kinases and phospholipases. Once activated, a variety of so-called second messengers are released. These are small molecules that propagate or inhibit functional responses. Common second messengers include calcium, cAMP, cyclic guanosine monophosphate (cGMP), and adenosine. Each is now discussed individually.

Calcium

Calcium homeostasis is very important to the survival and function of cells. The "final common pathway" to toxic cell death is calcium overload.[158] It is high levels of calcium that activate proteases, phospholipases, endonucleases, and other enzymes that cause degradation of intracellular proteins, cellular membranes, and nuclear DNA.[157]

Disturbances in calcium homeostasis may also contribute to many pathological states seen clinically. For example, patients with systemic inflammatory response syndrome (SIRS) exhibit alterations in early signal transduction secondary to changes in intracellular calcium.[156] In trauma patients, T cells display an attenuation in intracellular calcium mobilization as compared with that in healthy volunteers.[89] In patients with sepsis, there is indirect evidence that intracellular calcium is elevated while the plasma ionized calcium concentration is decreased.[157] This may explain the mechanism for sepsis-related inhibition of T cell activation.[89]

Normal changes in calcium levels modulate a variety of activities in immune cells. For example, in neutrophils an elevated calcium level triggers superoxide generation, enzyme secretion, actin gel-sol transitions, and locomotion.[156] In T lymphocytes, stimulated receptors cause immediate elevation of intracellular calcium.[89]

Cyclic Adenosine Monophosphate

Several inflammatory mediators alter cAMP levels to effect cellular responses in inflammation. For example, PGE_2 increases intracellular cAMP levels, which may inhibit T cell proliferation.[89] β-Adrenergic agonists may suppress LPS-induced transcriptional activation of the TNF-α gene by stimulating adenylate cyclase activity and thus increasing cAMP synthesis.[160] The adenosine receptors may also affect TNF-α levels by inhibiting or stimulating adenylate cyclase.[159]

Cyclic AMP is also a potent regulator of TNF-α synthesis in monocytes. This has been proven with cell membrane–permeable analogues of cAMP. These agents are known to increase intracellular cAMP by upregulating adenylate cyclase (PGE_2, PGI_2), or by inhibition of phosphodiesterase (pentoxifylline). Pentoxifylline is known to inhibit TNF-α synthesis as well.[159] This has led to considerable work with pentoxifylline and its derivatives as potential modifiers of the response to sepsis. Similar to pentoxifylline, cAMP can inhibit TNF-α synthesis. It blocks transcription of TNF-α-specific mRNA in LPS-stimulated macrophages.[159]

Adenosine

Adenosine's ability to effect cell function depends on its concentration. Experiments have shown that at low concentrations adenosine stimulates PMN adherence, phagocytosis, and superoxide anion production, whereas at higher concentrations adenosine inhibits these effects.[144, 159] These opposing effects are attributed to two different adenosine receptors, contrasted in affinity for adenosine and effects on adenylate cyclase.[159] The A1 receptor has high affinity for adenosine and inhibits adenylate cyclase activity, but the A2 receptor has low affinity for adenosine and activates adenylate cyclase, which inhibits TNF-α production.[159]

Adenosine also appears to exert a profound effect on leukocyte mobility. One mechanism of inhibiting migration is preventing endothelial cell retraction, which occurs when leukocytes attempt to extend their pseudopodia into the intercellular junctions.[161] Another is its ability to inhibit (1) actin polymerization and (2) activation-dependent shape change of neutrophils, which can enhance cell flexibility.[145] These may decrease pulmonary neutrophil sequestration and are possible clinical targets to be explored in the future for preventing acute respiratory distress syndrome (ARDS).[145]

LEUKOCYTE AND ENDOTHELIAL CELL ADHESION MOLECULES

Three major adhesion molecule families mediate endothelial cell–leukocyte adhesion. These families include members of the (1) *immunoglobulin* family, which are located principally on endothelial cells, (2) the integrin family, mainly located on leukocytes, and the (3) selectin family, whose constituents are located on endothelial cells or leukocytes. A summary of the adhesion molecules is provided in Table 44–3.

Immunoglobulin Family Adhesion Molecules on Endothelial Cells

There are three major types of immunoglobulin adhesion molecules in this family: intercellular adhesion molecule 1 (ICAM-1, CD54); intercellular adhesion molecule 2 (ICAM-2, CD02); and vascular cell adhesion molecule 1 (VCAM-1, INCAM-110). Their structures share similar immunoglobulin domains. ICAM-1 allows endothelial cells to bind monocytes, neutrophils, and T cells.[162, 163] Its expression is increased by lipopolysaccharide, IL-1, TNF-α, and IFN-γ, but in some cells it is constitutively present.[8, 162, 163] Its ligands on the leukocyte are CD11A/CD18 and CD11B/CD18.[8, 162]

ICAM-2 (CD102) facilitates binding between endothelium and monocytes, neutrophils, and T cells.[162, 163] It is constitutively present on a variety of different cell types, including endothelial cells.[8, 162, 163] Compared to ICAM-1, it possesses only two of the five immunoglobulin domains.[8] ICAM-2 ligand on the leukocyte is CD11A/CD18.[162]

VCAM-1 facilitates binding between endothelium and lymphocytes or monocytes, similar to ICAM-1 and ICAM-2, but it is also expressed on extravascular tissues such as follicular dendritic cells.[8, 9, 162] Neutrophils cannot bind to VCAM-1, because they lack VLA-4.[8] It is expressed in two forms: six- or seven-immunoglobulin domains.[8] VCAM-1 ligand on the leukocyte is very late antigen 4 (VLA-4).[9] Its expression is increased by LPS, TNF-α, IL-1, and IL-4, but not by IFN-γ.[8, 162]

Integrin Family Adhesion Molecules on Leukocytes

The integrins consist of α and β components, which form noncovalent heterodimers in the cell membrane.[8] To become adhesive, leukocyte integrins need to be activated, but the molecular mechanisms involved in activation are incompletely understood.[163] It is known that quantitative and qualitative changes occur in these receptors after activation, and their activity is dependent on the presence of divalent cations.[163, 164] Two integrin subfamilies important in leukocyte–endothelial cell interactions are the β_2- and α_4-integrins.[8] As an example, with ICAM-1, β_2-integrin attachment to the cytoskeleton is mediated by α-actinin.[165] Talin, another cytoskeletal protein, has also been shown to interact with the cytoplasmic domain of integrin heterodimers.[165]

TABLE 44–3. Leukocyte and Endothelial Cell Adhesion Molecules

Adhesion Molecule	Ligand	Stimulators
Leukocyte expression		
CD11A/CD18 (LFA-1)	ICAM-1 ICAM-2 ICAM-3	N/A
CD11B/CD18 (CR-3, MAC1)	ICAM-1 LPS C3bi C3dg L-selectin Fibrinogen	LTB_4 C5a TNF PDGF
CD11C/CD18 (CR4, p150,95)	C3bi Fibrinogen	N/A
VLA-4(α4β1)	VCAM-1 Fibronectin	N/A
α4β7	VCAM-1 MAdCAM-1	N/A
L-Selectin (Mel-14)	Sialylated Lewis a Sialylated Lewis x CD34 GlyCam-1 MAdCAM-1 CD11B/CD18	N/A
Endothelial cell expression		
ICAM-1(CD54)	CD11A/CD18 CD11B/CD18	IL-1 TNF IFN-γ
ICAM-2	CD11A/CD18	Constitutively expressed
VCAM-1(INCAM-110)	VLA4	IL-1 IL-4 TNF LPS
E-selectin (ELAM-1)	Sialylated Lewis a Sialylated Lewis x ESL-1 CD34 PSGL-1	IL-1 TNF LPS IFN-γ Substance P
P-selectin (GMP-140)	Sialylated Lewis a Sialylated Lewis x PSGL-1	Histamine Thrombin LTC_4 Hydrogen peroxide

Modified by permission from Pober J, Cotran R: The role of endothelial cells in inflammation. Transplantation. 1990; 50: 537–544.

N/A = not available; ICAM = intercellular adhesion molecule; LPS = lipopolysaccharide; VCAM = vascular cell adhesion molecule; VLA = very late antigen; PSGL = P-selectin glycoprotein ligand; LT = leukotriene; TNF = tumor necrosis factor; IFN = interferon; PDGF = platelet-derived growth factor; IL = interleukin.

β_2-Integrins

The β_2-integrins include three distinct but related α-chain polypeptides—CD11A, CD11B, and CD11C—that associate with the common β_2 subunit CD18.[8] They are concentrated on the nonvillous planar cell body.[166] The avidity of β_2-integrins for their ligands can be regulated by cellular activation.[168] In addition to adhesion, they play a role in transducing signals that enhance leukocyte activation and proliferation.[167]

CD11A/CD18 (lymphocyte functional-associated antigen 1,

LFA-1) is expressed in the majority of leukocytes, including monocytes, NK cells, neutrophils, and some T cells. It binds to ICAM-1, ICAM-2, and ICAM-3.[8, 9, 163]

CD11B/CD18 (CR-3, CR3bi, MAC1) is found on monocytes, granulocytes, NK cells, and certain subclasses of lymphocytes.[8, 9, 169] It binds to ICAM-1, LPS, soluble B glucan, factor X, C3bi, C3dg, fibrinogen and L-selectin.[163, 170, 171] It is involved in neutrophil homotypic aggregation, adherence, chemotaxis, phagocytosis, and cytotoxicity.[171] It can also promote release of both reactive oxygen intermediates and proteolytic enzymes from neutrophils.[172] Expression of CD11B/CD18 can be up-regulated by LTB_4, C5a, TNF-α, PDGF, and cross-linking of L-selectin molecules.[168, 169, 171]

CD11B/CD18 molecules are expressed in small numbers on unactivated neutrophil surfaces.[168] They are up-regulated and become functionally active upon neutrophil stimulation.[168] During locomotion, CD11B/CD18 expression is up-regulated as CD11B/CD18 granules fuse with the plasma membrane near the lamellipodia.[173] CD11B/CD18 can increase TNF-α secretion and, under appropriate conditions, can mediate adhesion-dependent hydrogen peroxide production in some cells.[167, 168]

CD11C/CD18 (CR-4, P150,95) is expressed by monocytes, granulocytes, NK cells, and certain subclasses of lymphocytes.[8, 9] It binds to C3bi, possibly fibrinogen, and at least one counterreceptor on the surface of endothelial cells.[163] Both CD11B/CD18 and CD11C/CD18 are stored in intracellular vesicles in neutrophils that are brought to the surface from intracellular pools on stimulation with chemoattractants such as LTB_4 and C5a.[163, 164] TNF-α and PDGF can also increase expression of CD11C/CD18.[163, 164]

α_4-Integrins

Lymphocytes and monocytes express α_4-integrin $\alpha_4\beta_1$, and lymphocytes express $\alpha_4\beta_7$.[106, 162, 174] The $\alpha_4\beta_1$ molecules (VLA-4, CD49D/CD29) are found in lymphocytes and monocytes,[162] and they bind to VCAM-1 and fibronectin.[8, 166] $\alpha_4\beta_7$ integrins bind to VCAM-1 and MAdCAM-1, a mucosal vascular addressin, selectively expressed by venules involved in lymphocyte trafficking to mucosal tissues.[166]

Experiments indicate that these integrins initiate primary leukocyte–endothelial cell contact and, subsequently, support transient interactions between them, including rolling, activation-enhanced firm adhesion, and arrest in lymphocytes.[166] $\alpha_4\beta_7$ also appears to be concentrated on the microvillous projections of leukocytes.[166] These projections represent the initial site of cell contact under flow.[166]

Selectin Family Adhesion Molecules on Endothelial Cells and Leukocytes

The main function of selectins is leukocyte-endothelial adhesion. Selectins are calcium-dependent glycoprotein receptors that have a common molecular structure characterized by an amino-terminal calcium-dependent (C-type) lectin domain, an epidermal growth factor (EGF) domain, a series of complement-regulatory domains, a transmembrane domain, and a short cytoplasmic tail.[8, 175, 176] The lectin domain is essential for cell adhesion.[8] The EGF domain appears to have a regulatory role.[8] Selectins exhibit considerable homology in their extracellular regions, but no homology exists between the cytoplasmic domains; this suggests that distinct functions are encoded within these regions.[165] There are three members of this family: E-selectin, P-selectin, and L-selectin.[8] They are named after the cell types on which they are primarily found: E (endothelial cell), P (platelet), and L (leukocyte).

The ligands for the selectins are carbohydrates.[8] All selectins can bind sialylated Lewis x with varying affinities.[166, 177] Sialylated Lewis x is a sialylated and fucosylated structure on carbohydrate groups of both glycoproteins and glycolipids.[161, 177] Selectins can also bind certain carbohydrate determinants on some glycoproteins or proteoglycans with much higher avidity.[177] They are susceptible to proteolytic cleavage and can also exist in the circulation in soluble form.[178]

E-selectin (ELAM-1) is found exclusively on endothelial cells. It is activated by TNF-α, IL-1β, LPS, IFN-γ, and substance P.[8, 177] E-selectin allows endothelial cells to bind to neutrophils, monocytes, certain memory T cells, basophils, and eosinophils.[9, 162, 173, 174] Its expression is up-regulated by IL-1 and TNF-α.[162] Expression of Lewis x and sialylated Lewis a on neutrophils correlates with their ability to bind E-selectin.[8] It can bind to a glycoprotein E-selectin ligand, ESL-1, which is a variant of a receptor for fibroblast growth factor.[177] E-selectin also binds to CD34, a component of a peripheral node addressin.[179]

P-selectin is constitutively found in the α and dense granules of platelets, as well as in endothelial Wiebel palade bodies.[8, 9, 162, 177] It allows binding between endothelial cells and neutrophils or monocytes and between platelets and monocytes or neutrophils.[162, 177] Endothelial cell stimulation with thrombin, histamine, LTC_4, and/or hydrogen peroxide increases P-selectin expression.[8, 9, 162, 177] The P-selectin ligand on neutrophils and monocytes is known to have Lewis x as at least part of its structure.[8] Both P- and E-selectin can bind to a glycoprotein ligand on myeloid cells called *P-selectin glycoprotein ligand-1* (PSGL-1).[177] Observations have suggested that P- and E-selectins recognize two categories of glycoprotein ligands, one class being mononuclear phagocyte specific and the second being common for both endothelial selectins.[177]

L-selectin is expressed by hematopoietic progenitor cells, immature thymocytes, neutrophils, monocytes, certain lymphocytes, and some NK cells.[7, 162, 177] It is concentrated and functional on the microvilli projections of unstimulated neutrophils, and it is functional on many leukocytes.[168, 177] In the mouse, the L-selectins bind with high avidity to at least three heavily glycosylated mucinlike proteins in vitro: GlyCAM-1, CD34, and MAdCAM-1.[177] Each of these three molecules bears sulfated, sialylated, and fucosylated O-linked carbohydrate side chains that appear to be essential for L-selectin binding.[7, 177]

Unlike the other two selectins, L-selectin is constitutively made on the cell surface.[9] It is shed from the surface of lymphocytes and neutrophils following cellular activation.[9] The mechanism of release of L-selectin from the cell surface results from activation-induced changes in the conformation of L-selectin, which expose nascent epitopes near the membrane-spanning region that are immediately susceptible to cleavage by an endogenous, perhaps ubiquitous, endoprotease.[177] This soluble selectin is functionally active and in high concentrations can inhibit leukocyte attachment to endothelium.[178] In vitro, soluble L-selectin can inhibit leukocyte binding to endothelium by allowing leukocyte detachment after the initial event.[7, 9] Shedding of L-selectin may also affect lymphocyte migration, as L-selectin appears to play a key role in their homing to lymph nodes.[7, 9]

Down-regulation of L-selectin can be induced in vitro by a variety of chemoattractants and in vivo after diapedesis of leukocytes surface L-selectin expression is reduced.[180, 181] Neutrophil activation through L-selectin and CD11B/CD18 molecules may also result in the production and release of mediators such as LTB_4 and proteases, which also down-regulate L-selectin surface expression.[168] Conformational changes in the receptor itself also decrease functional ability of this molecule.

L-selectin plays a role in signal transduction. Experiments have demonstrated that cross-linking of L-selectin molecules on the surface of human peripheral blood neutrophils initiates a dose-dependent increase in intracellular calcium which activates the respiratory burst and induces superoxide anion generation.[168, 182] Other experiments on isolated human neutrophils have shown L-selectin–induced mitogen-activated protein (MAP) kinase activation.[182] It can also enhance TNF-α and IL-8 gene expression.[182] L-selectin may also be involved in activation-induced neutrophil aggregation.[176]

A Model of Leukocyte Recruitment and Adhesion to Injured Endothelial Surfaces

Experimental observations suggest that chemoattractants diffuse into the lumens of microvessels and act on chemoattractant receptors on leukocytes. Then, they increase their adhesiveness and attach to vascular endothelial cells.[8, 70] Most of the work that has been done with this model studied neutrophils, but similar models exist for mononuclear phagocytes and helper T cells.[172]

There are three stages in the neutrophil model: (1) rolling, (2) activation, and (3) adhesion. The first stage, rolling, involves transition of the leukocyte from the circulating state to tumbling along the wall.[172] In the lumen the leukocyte is moving at speeds of 1000 μm/second, with erythrocytes in the center of the lumen of the capillary or venule.[172] Once the leukocyte hits the wall, it tumbles along the vessel at much slower speed (30 μm/second).[172] This rolling along affected venule segments occurs within minutes after tissue injury, as neutrophils begin to interact loosely with the walls of venules.[183] Rolling leukocytes can either adhere firmly to the vessel wall or roll along the entire vessel's length, but the majority of rolling leukocytes frequently detach and return to the mainstream of flowing blood.[161] Rolling also appears to involve the selectins.[172] In vitro studies suggest that L-selectin mediates rolling partly by presenting neutrophil carbohydrate ligands to the vascular E- and P-selectins.[183]

Leukocyte margination has been attributed to red blood cells. Normally, red blood cells pile up behind the larger leukocytes in capillaries. Once the diameter of the vessel becomes 50% larger than the diameter of the leukocyte, the red cells overtake the white cell and push it toward the venular wall.[161] This theory is supported in rat studies showing that very little leukocyte margination occurs when mesenteric venules perfused with leukocyte suspensions are devoid of red blood cells.[161] The level of leukocyte rolling and firm adhesion can be extrapolated from the prevailing wall shear rate in postcapillary venules.[161] It also dictates the contact area between rolling leukocytes and the endothelial cell surface.[161] Because this has been studied only in traumatically injured vessels, it is unclear whether leukocyte rolling is normally present in postcapillary venules.[161]

The second event, activation, is mediated by chemotactic agents that are released from or are attached to the endothelial surface.[172] Neutrophils activated by chemoattractants rapidly shed L-selectin from their surface, and simultaneously, leukocyte surface expression of the activation-dependent adhesion molecule CD11B/CD18 is increased.[183] This activation enables the third stage of firm adhesion and transendothelial migration to occur by promoting the function of integrin adhesion molecules on the leukocyte surface.[172] Subsequent neutrophil transmigration to the extravascular space is then mediated by adherence via the leukocyte integrins CD11A/CD18 and CD11B/CD18.[172] It stands to reason that the circulating neutrophils contain a high level of L-selectin and low level of integrin, but the converse is true once the neutrophil has migrated.[172] Studies are now being done to further elucidate leukocyte adhesion and migration.

A CLINICAL MODEL OF CYTOKINE INTERACTIONS: THE ACUTE RESPIRATORY DISTRESS SYNDROME

ARDS is a clinical consequence of these molecular and cellular events. It can accompany sepsis, severe trauma, pancreatitis, and other proinflammatory disorders. Cells of the respiratory system produce an array of inflammatory mediators whose actions can result in pathologic changes. In response to infection or injury, stromal or epithelial respiratory cells can secrete IL-1, IL-6, IL-8, GM-CSF, G-CSF, and M-CSF.[26] Alveolar macrophages can also produce several regulatory and chemotactic cytokines, including TNF-α, IL-1, IL-6, IL-8, PAF, PDGF, TGFα, TGFβ, prostaglandins, and leukotrienes.[111, 184] Hypoxia itself can initiate the release of TNF-α and IL-1β.[185]

Excess production of these cytokines (TNF-α, IL-1, IL-6, and IL-8) and complement component dysregulation has been linked to the pathologic consequences of ARDS.[33, 184] As currently envisioned, alveolar epithelial cells are induced by interstitial macrophage secretion products (TNF-α and IL-1) to produce IL-8 and other chemokines such as proinflammatory lipids like PAF and various leukotrienes. These mediators cause neutrophil attachment to the local endothelium and subsequent transendothelial migration into the alveolar space.[186–189] Other cytokine-mediated effects on neutrophils include up-regulation of adhesion molecules, enhancement of transendothelial migration, stimulation of the respiratory burst, and induction of degranulation.[60] Neutrophils are believed to be the key to the genesis of ARDS because of their ability to cause cell and matrix injury through oxidant production and protease release.[60] Major supportive evidence for this theory is observed in trauma, burn, and sepsis patients. Histologic examination of the lungs from patients who succumb to ARDS reveals a neutrophilic infiltrate in the alveolar interstitium.[190, 191] Bronchoalveolar lavage fluid from patients with ARDS contains a large number of neutrophils and neutrophil-derived enzymes and oxidants.[192, 193] As this lesion evolves, fibrosis, with thickening of the alveolar-capillary junction, occurs.

SUMMARY

This chapter demonstrates that the inflammatory response encountered in sepsis depends on many mediators. Structural and functional characteristics of these mediators are redundant, to act as checks and balances for the response. The inflammatory response is regulated at multiple levels, from cytokine production to adhesion molecule shedding. Clinical pathology can be understood from a thorough comprehension of the molecular and cellular changes that occur secondary to trauma or sepsis. Understanding the components of the inflammation can also help physicians to design better pharmaceutical regimens to prevent severe pathologic conditions secondary to the septic process.

ACKNOWLEDGMENT

The authors wish to acknowledge John F. Valente, MD (Clinical Instructor in Surgery, Department of Surgery, University of Cincinnati College of Medicine) and Cynthia M. Cave (Laboratory Assistant, Department of Surgery, University of Cincinnati College of Medicine) for their excellent assistance in preparing this manuscript.

References

1. Clark R, Malech H, Gallin J, et al: Genetic variants of chronic granulomatous disease: Prevalence of deficiencies of two cyto-

solic components of the NADPH oxidase system. N Engl J Med 1989; 321:647–652.
2. Lomax K, Leto T, Nunoi H, Gallin J, Malech H: Recombinant 47-kilodalton cytosol factor restores NADPH oxidase in chronic granulomatous disease. Science 1989; 245:409–412.
3. Campbell E, Senior R, McDonald J, Cox D: Proteolysis by neutrophils: Relative importance of cell-substrate contact and oxidative inactivation of proteinase inhibitors in vitro. J Clin Invest 1982; 70:845–852.
4. Kanofsky J: Singlet oxygen production by biological systems. Chem Biol Interact 1989; 70:1–28.
5. Plow E: Leukocyte elastase release during blood coagulation: A potential mechanism of activation of the alternative fibrinolytic pathway. J Clin Invest 1982; 69:564–572.
6. Nicola NA: Structural aspects of cytokine/receptor interactions. Ann NY Acad Sci 1995; 766:253–262.
7. Chen A, Engel P, Tedder TF: Structural requirements regulate endoproteolytic release of the L-selectin (CD62L) adhesion receptor from the cell surface of leukocytes. J Exp Med 1995; 182:519–530.
8. Williams TJ, Hellewell PG: Adhesion molecules involved in the microvascular inflammatory response. Am Rev Respir Dis 1992; 146:545–550.
9. Bevilacqua MP: Endothelial-leukocyte adhesion molecules. Annu Rev Immunol 1993; 11:767–804.
10. Shaw S: Regulation of T-cell adhesion to endothelium. Semin Hematol 1993; 30:56–65.
11. Lin R, Astiz M, Saxon J, Saha D, Rackow E: Relationships between plasma cytokine concentrations and leukocyte functional antigen expression in patients with sepsis. Crit Care Med 1994; 22:1595–1602.
12. Bellomo R: The cytokine network in the critically ill. Anaesth Intensive Care 1992; 20:288–302.
13. Alderson MR, Tough TW, Ziegler SF, Grabstein KH: Interleukin 7 induces cytokine secretion and tumoricidal activity by human peripheral blood monocytes. J Exp Med 1991; 173:923–930.
14. de Waal Malefyt R, Figdor CG, Huijbens R, Mohan-Peterson S, Bennett B, Culpepper J, Dang W, Zurawski G, de Vries JE: Effects of IL-13 on phenotype, cytokine production, and cytotoxic function of human monocytes: Comparison with IL-4 and modulation by IFN-γ or IL-10. J Immunol 1993; 151:6370–6381.
15. Cerami A: Inflammatory cytokines. Clin Immunol Immunopathol 1992; 62:s3–s10.
16. van der Poll T, Lowry S: Tumor necrosis factor in sepsis: Mediator of multiple organ failure or essential part of host defense? Shock 1995; 3:1–12.
17. Van Zee KJ, DeForge LE, Fischer E, et al: IL-8 in septic shock, endotoxemia, and after IL-1 administration. J Immunol 1991; 146:3476–3482.
18. Brizzi MF, Garbarino G, Rossi PR, et al: Interleukin 3 stimulates proliferation and triggers endothelial-leukocyte adhesion molecule 1 gene activation of human endothelial cells. J Clin Invest 1993; 91:2887–2892.
19. Chollet-Martin S, Montravers P, Gibert C, et al: Relationships between polymorphonuclear neutrophils and cytokines in patients with adult respiratory distress syndrome. Ann NY Acad Sci 1994; 725:354–366.
20. Kita H, Ohnishi T, Okubo Y, Weiler D, Abrams JS, Gleich GJ: Granulocyte/macrophage colony-stimulating factor and interleukin 3 release from human peripheral blood eosinophils and neutrophils. J Exp Med 1991; 174:745–748.
21. Elliot MJ, Finn AHR: Interaction between neutrophils and endothelium. Ann Thorac Surg 1993; 56:1503–1508.
22. Bone RC: The pathogenesis of sepsis. Ann Intern Med 1991; 115:457–469.
23. Luscher TF: Endothelin: Systemic arterial and pulmonary effects of a new peptide with potent biologic properties. Am Rev Respir Dis 1992; 146:s56–s60.
24. Deitch EA, Mancini MC: Complement receptors in shock and transplantation. Arch Surg 1993; 128:1222–1226.
25. Zellweger R, Ayala A, Schmand J, Morrison M, Chaudry I: PAF-antagonist administration after hemorrhage-resuscitation prevents splenocyte immunodepression. J Surg Res 1995; 59:366–370.
26. Adler KB, Fischer BM, Wright DT, Cohn LA, Becker S: Interactions between respiratory epithelial cells and cytokines: Relationships to lung inflammation. Ann NY Acad Sci 1994; 725:128–145.
27. Badr KF: Leukotrienes and 15-lipoxygenase products in glomerulonephritis. Adv Nephrol 1995; 24:19–31.
28. Harbrecht B, Wang S, Simmons R, Billiar T: Cyclic GMP and guanylate cyclase mediate lipopolysaccharide-induced Kupffer cell tumor necrosis factor-α synthesis. J Leukoc Biol 1995; 57:297–302.
29. Salgado A, Boveda JL, Monasterio J, Segura RM, Mourelle M, Gomez-Jimenez J, Peracaula R: Inflammatory mediators and their influence on haemostasis. Haemostasis 1994; 24:132–138.
30. Cebon J, Layton JE, Maher D, Morstyn G: Endogenous haemopoietic growth factors in neutropenia and infection. Br J Haematol 1994; 86:265–274.
31. Molijn G, Spek J, van Uffelen J, de Jong F, Brinkmann A, Bruining H, Lamberts S, Koper J: Differential adaptation of glucocorticoid sensitivity of peripheral blood mononuclear leukocytes in patients with sepsis or septic shock. J Clin Endocrinol Metab 1995; 80:1799–1803.
32. Gough DB, Jordan A, Mannick JA, Rodrick ML: Impaired cell-mediated immunity in experimental abdominal sepsis and the effect of interleukin 2. Arch Surg 1992; 127:859–863.
33. Donnelly TJ, Meade P, Jagels M, et al: Cytokine, complement, and endotoxin profiles associated with the development of the adult respiratory distress syndrome after severe injury. Crit Care Med 1994; 22:768–776.
34. Dofferhoff A, De Jong H, Bom V, et al: Complement activation and the production of inflammatory mediators during the treatment of severe sepsis in humans. Scand J Infect 1992; 24:197–204.
35. Christman J, Holden E, Blackwell T: Strategies for blocking the systemic effects of cytokines in the sepsis syndrome. Crit Care Med 1995; 23:955–963.
36. Giroir B: Mediators of septic shock: New approaches for interrupting the endogenous inflammatory cascade. Crit Care Med 1993; 21:780–789.
37. Sevem A., Rapson N, Hunter C, Liew F: Regulation of tumor necrosis factor production by adrenaline and β-adrenergic agonists. J Immunol 1992; 11:3441–3445.
38. Spooner C, Markowitz N, Saravolatz L: The role of tumor necrosis factor in sepsis. Clin Immunol Immunopathol 1992; 62:s11–s17.
39. Tan JC, Braun S, Rong H, et al: Characterization of recombinant extracellular domain of human interleukin-10 receptor. J Biol Chem 1995; 270:12906–12911.
40. Suter P, Suter S, Girardin E, Roux-Lombard P, Grau G, Dayer J: High bronchoalveolar levels of tumor necrosis factor and its inhibitors, interleukin-1, interferon, and elastase, in patients with adult respiratory distress syndrome after trauma, shock, or sepsis. Am Rev Respir Dis 1992; 145:1016–1022.
41. Gardlund B, Sjolin J, Nilsson M, Roll M, Wickerts C, Wretlind B: Plasma levels of cytokines in primary septic shock in humans: Correlation with disease severity. J Infect Dis 1995; 172:296–301.
42. Leon P, Redmond HP, Shou J, Daly JM: Interleukin 1 and its relationship to endotoxin tolerance. Arch Surg 1992; 127:146–151.
43. Sullivan JS, Kilpatrick L, Costarino AT Jr., Lee SC, Harris MC: Correlation of plasma cytokine elevations with mortality rate in children with sepsis. J Pediatrics 1992; 120:510–515.
44. Dinarello CA: Interleukin-1 and interleukin-1 antagonism. Blood 1991; 77:1627–1652.
45. Ghezzi P, Dinarello CA, Bianchi M, Rosandich ME, Repine JE, White CW: Hypoxia increases production of interleukin-1 and tumor necrosis factor by human mononuclear cells. Cytokine 1991; 3:189–194.
46. Joyce DA, Gibbons DP, Green P, Steer JH, Feldmann M, Brennan FM: Two inhibitors of pro-inflammatory cytokine release, interleukin-10 and interleukin-4, have contrasting effects on release of soluble p75 tumor necrosis factor receptor by cultured monocytes. Eur J Immunol 1994; 24:2699–2705.
47. Krakauer T: IL-10 inhibits the adhesion of leukocytic cells to IL-1 activated human endothelial cells. Immunol Lett 1995; 45:61–65.
48. Green R, Whiting J, Rosenbluth A, Beier D, Gollan J: Interleukin-6 inhibits hepatocyte taurocholate uptake and sodium-potas-

sium-adenosinetriphosphatase activity. Am J Physiol 1994; 267:G1094–G1100.
49. Buck C, Bundschu J, Gallati H, Bartmann P, Pohlandt F: Interleukin-6: A sensitive parameter for the early diagnosis of neonatal bacterial infection. Pediatrics 1994; 93:54–58.
50. Quinn LS, Haugk KL, Grabstein KH: Interleukin-15: A novel anabolic cytokine for skeletal muscle. Endocrinology 1995; 136:3669–3672.
51. Zhou D, Kusnecov AW, Shurin MR, DePaoli M, Rabin BS: Exposure to physical and psychological stressors elevates plasma interleukin 6: Relationship to the activation of hypothalamic-pituitary-adrenal axis. Endocrinology 1993; 133:2523–2530.
52. Jelinek DF, Braaten JK: Role of IL-12 in human B lymphocyte proliferation and differentiation. J Immunol 1995; 154:1606–1613.
53. de Waal Malefyt R, Abrams JS, Zurawski SM, et al: Differential regulation of IL-13 and IL-4 production by human $CD8^+$ and $Cd4^+$ ThO, Th1 and Th2 T cell clones and EBV-transformed B cells. Int Immunol 1995; 7:1405–1416.
54. Friedland JS, Suputtamongkol Y, Remick DG, et al: Prolonged elevation of interleukin-8 and interleukin-6 concentrations in plasma and of leukocyte interleukin-8 mRNA levels during septicemic and localized *Pseudomonas pseudomallei* infection. Infect Immun 1992; 60:2402–2408.
55. Ertel W, Krombach F, Kremer JP, et al: Mechanisms of cytokine cascade activation in patients with sepsis: Normal cytokine transcription despite reduced CD14 receptor expression. Surgery 1993; 114:243–251.
56. Wickenhauser C, Lorenzen J, Thiele J, et al: Secretion of cytokines (interleukins-1α, -3, and -6 and granulocyte macrophage colony-stimulating factor) by normal human bone marrow megakaryocytes. Blood 1995; 85:685–691.
57. Wolf SS, Cohen A: Expression of cytokines and their receptors by human thymocytes and thymic stromal cells. Immunology 1992; 77:362–368.
58. Trinchieri G: Interleukin-12: A proinflammatory cytokine with immunoregulatory functions that bridge innate resistance and antigen-specific adaptive immunity. Annu Rev Immunol 1995; 13:251–276.
59. Solomkin JS, Bass RC, Bjomson HS, Tindal CJ, Babcock GF: Alterations of neutrophil responses to tumor necrosis factor alpha and interleukin-8 following human endotoxemia. Infect Immun 1994; 62:943–947.
60. Biffl WL, Moore EE, Moore FA, Carl VS, Franciose RJ, Banerjee A: Interleukin-8 increases endothelial permeability independent of neutrophils. J Trauma 1995; 39:98–103.
61. DeSai B, Quinn PM, Wolitzky AG, Mongini PKA, Chizzonite R, Gately MK: IL-12 receptor: II. Distribution and regulation of receptor expression. J Immunol 1992; 148:3125–3132.
62. Mattner F, Fischer S, Guckes S, et al: The interleukin-12 subunit p40 specifically inhibits effects of the interleukin-12 heterodimer. Eur J Immunol 1993; 23:2202–2208.
63. Chizzonite R, Truitt T, Desai BB, et al: IL-12 Receptor: I. Characterization of the receptor on phytohemagglutinin-activated human lymphoblasts. J Immunol 1992; 148:3117–3124.
64. Mehrotra PT, Wu D, Crim JA, Mostowski HS, Siegal JP: Effects of IL-12 on the generation of cytotoxic activity in human $CD8^+$ T lymphocytes. J Immunol 1993; 151:2444–2452.
65. Munger W, DeJoy SQ, Jeyaseelan Sr. R: Studies evaluating the antitumor activity and toxicity of interleukin-15, a new T cell growth factor: Comparison with interleukin-2. Cellular Immunol 1995; 165:289–293.
66. Eng VM, Car BD, Schnyder B, et al: The stimulatory effects of interleukin (IL)-12 on hematopoiesis are antagonized by IL-12-induced interferon γ in vivo. J Exp Med 1995; 181:1893–1898.
67. Ayala A, Lehman DL, Herdon CD, Chaudry IH: Mechanism of enhanced susceptibility to sepsis following hemorrhage: Interleukin-10 suppression of T-cell response is mediated by eicosanoid-induced interleukin-4 release. Arch Surg 1994; 129:1172–1178.
68. Nassar GM, Morrow JD, Roberts II LJ, Lakkis FG, Badr KF: Induction of 15-Lipoxygenase by Interleukin-13 in human blood monocytes. J Biol Chem 1994; 269:27631–27634.
69. Shou J, Motyka LE, Daly JM: Intestinal microbial translocation: Immunologic consequences and effects of interleukin-4. Surgery 1994; 116:868–876.
70. Tunon de Lara JM, Okayama Y, McEuen AR, Heusser CH, Church MK, Walls AF: Release and inactivation of interleukin-4 by mast cells. Ann NY Acad Sci 1994; 725:50–58.
71. Tan JC, Indelicato SR, Narula SK, Zavodny PJ, Chou C-C: Characterization of interleukin-10 receptors on human and mouse cells. J Biol Chem 1993; 268:21053–21059.
72. Carson WE, Lindemann MJ, Baiocchi R, et al: The functional characterization of interleukin-10 receptor expression on human natural killer cells. Blood 1995; 85:3577–3585.
73. Liu Y, Wei SH-Y, Ho AS-Y, Malefyt Rd-W, Moore KW: Expression cloning and characterization of a human IL-10 receptor. J Immunol 1994; 152:1821–1829.
74. Marchant A, Deviere J, Byl B, De Groote D, Vincent J-L, Goldman M: Interleukin-10 production during septicaemia. Lancet 1994; 343:707–708.
75. Napolitano LM, Campbell C: Polymicrobial sepsis following trauma inhibits interleukin-10 secretion and lymphocyte proliferation. J Trauma 1995; 39:104–111.
76. Ding L, Shevach EM: IL-10 inhibits mitogen-induced T cell proliferation by selectively inhibiting macrophage costimulatory function. J Immunol 1992; 148:3133–3139.
77. Fluckiger A-C, Garrone P, Durand I, Galizzi J-P, Banchereau J: Interleukin 10 (IL-10) upregulates functional high affinity IL-2 receptors on normal and leukemic B lymphocytes. J Exp Med 1993; 178:1473–1481.
78. Zurawski G, de Vries JD: Interleukin 13, an interleukin 4-like cytokine that acts on monocytes and B cells, but not on T cells. Immunol Today 1994; 15:19–26.
79. Cassatella MA, Meda L, Gasperini S, Calzetti F, Bonora S: Interleukin 10 (IL-10) upregulates IL-1 receptor antagonist production from lipopolysaccharide-stimulated human polymorphonuclear leukocytes by delaying mRNA degradation. J Exp Med 1994; 179:1695–1699.
80. Obiri NI, Debinski W, Leonard WJ, Puri RK: Receptor for interleukin 13: Interaction with interleukin 4 by a mechanism that does not involve the common γ chain shared by receptors for interleukins 2, 4, 7, 9, and 15. J Biol Chem 1995; 270:8797–8804.
81. Vita N, Lefort S, Laurent P, Caput D, Ferrara P: Characterization and comparison of the interleukin 13 receptor with the interleukin 4 receptor on several cell types. J Biol Chem 1995; 270:3512–3517.
82. Derocq J-M, Segui M, Poinot-Chazel C: Interleukin-13 stimulates interleukin-6 production by human keratinocytes: Similarity with interleukin-4. FEBS Lett 1994; 343:32–36.
83. Yano S, Sone S, Nishioka Y, Mukaida N, Matsushima K, Ogura T: Differential effects of anti-inflammatory cytokines (IL-4, IL-10, and IL-13) on tumoricidal and chemotactic properties of human monocytes induced by monocyte chemotactic activating factor. J Leukocyte Biol 1995; 57:303–309.
84. Cosentino G, Soprana E, Thienes CP, Siccardi AG, Viale G, Vercelli D: IL-13 down-regulates CD14 expression and TNF-α secretion in normal human monocytes. J Immunol 1995; 155:3145–3151.
85. Smerz-Bertling C, Duschi A: Both interleukin 4 and interleukin 13 induce tyrosine phosphorylation of the 140-kDa subunit of the interleukin 4 receptor. J Biol Chem 1995; 270:966–970.
86. Taniguchi T, Miyazaki T, Minami Y, et al: IL-2 signaling involves recruitment and activation of multiple protein tyrosine kinases by the IL-2 receptor. Ann NY Acad Sci 1995; 766:235–244.
87. Rabinovici R, Sofronski MD, Borboroglu P, et al: Interleukin-2-induced lung injury: The role of complement. Circ Res 1994; 74:329–335.
88. Cinat M, Waxman K, Vaziri ND, et al: Soluble cytokine receptors and receptor antagonists are sequentially released after trauma. J Trauma 1995; 39:112–120.
89. Choudhry M, Ahmad S, Sayeed M: Role of Ca^{2+} in prostaglandin E_2-induced T-lymphocyte, proliferative suppression in sepsis. Infect Immun 1995; 63:3101–3105.
90. Wells TNC, Graber P, Proudfoot AEI, et al: The three-dimensional structure of human interleukin-5 at 2.4-angstroms resolution: Implication for the structures of other cytokines. Ann NY Acad Sci 1994; 725:118–127.
91. Costello R, Brailly H, Mallet F, Mawas C, Olive D: Interleukin-7 is a potent co-stimulus of the adhesion pathway involving CD2 and CD28 molecules. Immunology 1993; 80:451–457.
92. Mehrotra PT, Grant AJ, Siegal JP: Synergistic effects of IL-7 and IL-12 on human T cell activation. J Immunol 1995; 154:5093–5102.

93. Pandrau-Garcia D, de Saint-Vis B, Saeland S, et al: Growth inhibitory and agonistic signals of interleukin-7 (IL-7) can be mediated through the CDw127 IL-7 receptor. Blood 1994; 83:3613–3619.
94. Renauld J-C, Houssiau F, Louahed J, Vink A, Van Snick J, Uyttenhove C: Interleukin-9. Ad Immunol 1993; 54:79–97.
95. Renauld J-C, Kermouni A, Vink A, Louahed J, Van Snick J: Interleukin-9 and its receptor: Involvement in mast cell differentiation and T cell oncogenesis. J Leukocyte Biol 1995; 57:353–360.
96. Einarsson O, Geba GP, Zhou Z, et al: Interleukin-11 in respiratory inflammation. Ann NY Acad Sci 1995; 762:89–101.
97. Adunyah SE, Spencer GC, Cooper RS, Rivero JA, Ceesay K: Interleukin-11 induces tyrosine phosphorylation, and c-jun and c-fos mRNA expression in human K562 and U937 cells. Ann NY Acad Sci 1995; 766:296–299.
98. Suen BY, Chang M, Lee SM, Buzby JS, Cairo MS. Regulation of Interleukin-11 protein and mRNA expression in neonatal and adult fibroblasts and endothelial cells. Blood 1994; 84:4125–4134.
99. Clardy CW: Complement activation by whole endotoxin is blocked by a monoclonal antibody to factor B. Infect Immun 1994; 62:4549–4555.
100. Ford R, Tamayo A, Martin B, et al: Identification of B-cell growth factors (interleukin-14; high molecular weight-B-cell growth factors) in effusion fluids from patients with aggressive B-cell lymphomas. Blood 1995; 86:283–293.
101. Cherel M, Sorel M, Lebeau B, et al: Molecular cloning of two isoforms of a receptor of the human hematopoietic cytokine interleukin-11. Blood 1995; 86:2534–2540.
102. Wilkinson PC, Liew FY: Chemoattraction of human blood T lymphocytes by interleukin-15. J Exp Med 1995; 181:1255–1259.
103. Carson WE, Giri JG, Lindemann MJ, et al: Interleukin (IL) 15 is a novel cytokine that activates human natural killer cells via components of the IL-2 receptor. J Exp Med 1994; 180:1395–1403.
104. Giri JG, Anderson DM, Kumaki S, Park LS, Grabstein KH, Cosman D: IL-15, a novel T cell growth factor that shares activities and receptor components with IL-2. J Leukocyte Biol 1995; 57:763–766.
105. Redmond HP, Chavin KD, Bromberg JS, Daly JM: Inhibition of macrophage-activating cytokines is beneficial in the acute septic response. Ann Surg 1991; 214:502–508.
106. Wang J, Beekhuizen H, Furth RV: Surface molecules involved in the adherence of recombinant interferon-γ (rIFN-γ)-stimulated human monocytes to vascular endothelial cells. Clin Exp Immunol 1994; 95:263–269.
107. Soilu-Hanninen M, Salmi A, Salonen R: Interferon-β downregulates expression of VLA-4 antigen and antagonizes interferon-γ-induced expression of HLA-DQ on human peripheral blood monocytes. J Neuroimmunol 1995; 60:99–106.
108. Renauld J-C, Vink A, Louahed J, Snick VJ: Interleukin-9 is a major anti-apoptotic factor for thymic lymphomas. Blood 1995; 85:1300–1305.
109. Rowley AF, Lloyd-Evans P, Barrow SE, Serhan CN: Lipoxin biosynthesis by trout macrophages involves the formation of epoxide intermediates. Biochemistry 1994; 33:856–863.
110. Roper R, Brown D, Phipps R: Prostaglandin E_2 promotes B lymphocyte Ig isotype switching to IgE. J Immunol 1995; 154:162–170.
111. Thivierge M, Rola-Pleszczynski M: Involvement of both cyclooxygenase and lipoxygenase pathways in platelet-activating factor–induced interleukin-6 production by alveolar macrophages. Ann NY Acad Sci 1994; 725:213–222.
112. Callery MP, Kamei T, Mangino MJ, Flye MW: Organ interactions in sepsis. Arch Surg 1991; 126:28–32.
113. Fletcher J: Eicosanoids: Critical agents in the physiological process and cellular injury. Arch Surg 1993; 128:1192–1196.
114. Rankin JA, Sylvester L, Smith S, Yoshimura T, Leonard EJ: Macrophages cultured in vitro release leukotriene B_4 in response to stimulation with lipopolysaccharide and zymosan. J Clin Invest 1990; 86:1556–1564.
115. Feinmark SJ: The role of the endothelial cell in leukotriene biosynthesis. Am Rev Respir Dis 1992; 146:s51–s55.
116. Moser R, Olgiati L, Patarroyo M, Fehr J: Chemotoxins inhibit neutrophil adherence to and transmigration across cytokine-activated endothelium: Correlation to the expression of L-selectin. Eur J Immunol 1993; 23:1481–1487.
117. Thompson WA, Coyle S, Van Zee K, et al: The metabolic effects of platelet-activating factor antagonism in endotoxemic man. Arch Surg 1994; 129:72–79.
118. Cendan JC, Souba WW, Copeland EM III, Lind DS: Cytokines regulate endotoxin stimulation of endothelial cell arginine transport. Surgery 1994; 117:213–219.
119. Lukacs NW, Strieter RM, Elner VM, Evanoff HL, Burdick M, Kunkel SL: Intercellular adhesion molecule-1 mediates the expression of monocyte-derived MIP-1α during monocyte-endothelial cell interactions. Blood 1994; 83:1174–1178.
120. Tanaka Y, Adams DH, Hubscher S, Hirano H, Siebenlist U, Shaw S: T-cell adhesion induced by proteoglycan-immobilized cytokine MIP-1β. Nature 1993; 361:79–83.
121. Hart PH, Ahem MJ, Smith MD, Finlay-Jones JJ: Regulatory effects of IL-13 on synovial fluid macrophages and blood monocytes from patients with inflammatory arthritis. Clin Exp Immunol 1995; 99:331–337.
122. Stasi R, Zinzani PL, Galieni P, et al: Detection of soluble interleukin-2 receptor and interleukin-10 in the serum of patients with aggressive non-Hodgkin's lymphoma. Cancer 1994; 74:1792–1800.
123. Armitage RJ, Ziegler SF, Friend DJ, Park LS, Fanslow WC: Identification of a novel low-affinity receptor for human interleukin-7. Blood 1992; 79:1738–1745.
124. Chua AO, Chizzonite R, Desai BB, et al: Expression cloning of a human IL-12 receptor component: A new member of the cytokine receptor superfamily with strong homology to gp130. J Immunol 1994; 153:128–136.
125. Bacon CM, Petricoin EF III, Ortaldo JR, et al: Interleukin 12 induces tryosine phosphorylation and activation of STAT4 in human lymphocytes. Proc Natl Acad Sci U S A 1995; 92:7307–7311.
126. Nakamura Y, Russell SM, Mess SA, Adelstein S, Leonard WJ: Heterodimerization of the IL-2 receptor β and γ chain cytoplasmic domains is required for signalling. Nature 1994; 369:330–332.
127. Yin T, Keller SR, Quelle FW, Yang Y-C: Interleukin-9 induces tyrosine phosphorylation of insulin receptor substrate-1 via JAK tyrosine kinases. J Biol Chem 1995; 270:20497–20502.
128. Vandenabeele P, Declercq W, Beyaert R, Fiers W: Two tumour necrosis factor receptors: structure and function. Trends Cell Biol 1995; 5:392–399.
129. Frieling JTM, van Deuren M, Wijdenes J, et al: Circulating interleukin-6 receptor in patients with sepsis syndrome. J Infect Dis 1995; 171:469–472.
130. Burton JD, Bamford RN, Peters C, et al: A lymphokine, provisionally designated interleukin T and produced by a human adult T-cell leukemia line, stimulates T-cell proliferation and the induction of lymphokine-activated killer cells. Proc Natl Acad Sci U S A 1994; 91:4935–4939.
131. Noguchi M, Nakamura Y, Russell SM, et al: Interleukin-2 receptor γ chain: A functional component of the interleukin-7 receptor. Science 1993; 262:1877–1822.
132. Ward LD, Howlett GJ, Discolo G, et al: High affinity interleukin-6 receptor is a hexameric complex consisting of two molecules each of interleukin-6, interleukin-6 receptor, and gp130. J Biol Chem 1994; 269:23286–23289.
133. Nakarai T, Robertson MJ, Streuli M, et al: Interleukin 2 receptor γ chain expression on resting and activated lymphoid cells. J Exp Med. 1994; 180:241–251.
134. He Y-W, Malek TR: The IL-2 receptor γ_c chain does not function as a subunit shared by the IL-4 and IL-13 receptor: Implication for the structure of the IL-4 receptor. J Immunol 1995; 155:9–12.
135. Kawahara A, Minami Y, Taniguchi T: Evidence for a critical role for the cytoplasmic region of the interleukin 2 (IL-2) receptor γ chain in IL-2, IL-4, and IL-7 signaling. Mole Cell Biol 1994; 14:5433–5440.
136. He Y-W, Adkins B, Furse RK, Malek TR: Expression and function of the γ_c subunit of the IL-2, IL-4, and IL-7 receptors. J Immunol 1995; 154:1596–1605.
137. Nelson BH, Lord JD, Greenberg PD: Cytoplasmic domains of the interleukin-2 receptor β and γ chains mediate the signal for T-cell proliferation. Nature 1994; 369:333–336.
138. Venkitaraman AR, Cowling RJ: Interleukin-7 induces the association of phosphatidylinositol 3-kinase with the α chain of the interleukin-7 receptor. Eur J Immunol 1994; 24:2168–2174.

139. Zurawski SM, Chomarat P, Djossou O, et al: The primary binding subunit of the human interleukin-4 receptor is also a component of the interleukin-13 receptor. J Biol Chem 1995; 270:13869–13878.
140. Ihle JN, Witthuhn BA, Quelle FW, Yamamoto K, Silvennoinen O: Signaling through the hematopoietic cytokine receptors. Annu Rev Immunol 1995; 13:369–398.
141. Sehgal PB, Wang L, Rayanade R, Pan H, Margulies L: Interleukin-6-type cytokines. Ann NY Acad Sci 1995; 762:1–14.
142. Nakajima K, Matsuda T, Fujitani Y, et al: Signal transduction through IL-6 receptor. Involvement of multiple protein kinases, STAT factors, and a novel H7-sensitive pathway. Ann NY Acad Sci 1995; 762:55–70.
143. Egawa M, Maeno M, Kung H-F, Schwabe M: Expression of the human interleukin 6 receptor α-chain in *Xenopus laevis* oocytes. Cytokine 1995; 7:83–88.
144. Goldie A, Fearon K, Ross J, Barclay R, Jackson R, Grant I, Ramsay G, Blyth A, Howie J: Natural cytokine antagonists and endogenous antiendotoxin core antibodies in sepsis syndrome. JAMA 1995; 274:172–177.
145. Firestein GS, Boyle D, Bullough DA, et al: Protective effect of an adenosine kinase inhibitor in septic shock. J Immunol 1994; 152:5853–5859.
146. Schwabe M, Zhao J, Kung H-F: Differential expression and ligand-induced modulation of the human interleukin-6 receptor on interleukin-6–responsive cells. J Biol Chem 1994; 269:7201–7209.
147. Salvati AL, Lahm A, Paonessa G, Ciliberto G, Toniatti C: Interleukin-6 (IL-6) antagonism by soluble IL-6 receptor γ mutated in the predicted gp130-binding interface. J Biol Chem 1995; 270:12242–12249.
148. Wang Y, Fuller GM: Biosynthetic and glycosylation events of the IL-6 receptor β-subunit, gp130. J Cell Biochem 1995; 57:610–618.
149. Leong S, Kabakoff R, Herbert C: Complete mutagenesis of the extracellular domain of interleukin-8 (IL-8) type A receptor identifies charged residues mediating IL-8 binding and signal transduction. J Biol Chem 1994; 269:19343–19348.
150. Horuk R: The interleukin-8–receptor family: From chemokines to malaria. Immunol Today 1994; 15:169–174.
151. Holmes W, Lee J, Kuang W, Rice G, Wood W: Structural and functional expression of a human interleukin-8 receptor. Science 1991; 253:1278–1280.
152. Alvares V, Coto E, Setien F, Lopez-Larrea C: A physical map of two clusters containing the genes for six proinflammatory receptors. Immunogenetics. 1994; 40:100–103.
153. Knall C, Worthen GS, Buhl AM, Johnson GL: IL-8 signal transduction in human neutrophils. Ann NY Acad Sci 1995; 766:288–295.
154. Chua AO, Wilkinson VL, Presky DH, Gubler U: Cloning and characterization of a mouse IL-12 receptor-β component. J Immunol 1994; 155:4286–4294.
155. Gillessen S, Carvajal D, Ling P, et al: Mouse interleukin-12 (IL-12) p40 homodimer: A potent IL-12 antagonist. Eur J Immunol 1995; 25:200–206.
156. Burke PA, Murray-Canning C, Chartier S, et al: Alterations in Ca^{2+} signal transduction in critically ill surgical patients. Surgery 1994; 116:378–387.
157. Song S, Karl IE, Ackerman JJ, Hotchkiss RS: Increased intracellular Ca^{2+}: A critical link in the pathophysiology of sepsis? Proc Nat Acad Sci U S A 1993; 90:3933–3937.
158. Todd III J, Mollitt D: Effect of sepsis on erythrocyte intracellular calcium homeostasis. Crit Care Med 1995; 23:459–465.
159. Thiel M, Chouker A: Acting via A2 receptors, adenosine inhibits the production of tumor necrosis factor-α of endotoxin-stimulated human polymorphonuclear leukocytes. J Lab Clin Med 1995; 126:275–282.
160. McAllister SK, Bland LA, Arduino MJ, Aguero SM, Wenger PN, Jarvis WR: Patient cytokine response in transfusion-associated sepsis. Infect Immun 1994; 62:2126–2128.
161. Granger DN, Kubes P: The microcirculation and inflammation: Modulation of leukocyte–endothelial cell adhesion. J Leukocyte Biol 1994; 55:662–673.
162. Pober JS, Cotran RS: The role of endothelial cells in inflammation. Transplantation 1990; 50:537–544.
163. Li R, Xie J, Kantor C, et al: A peptide derived from the intercellular adhesion molecule-2 regulates the avidity of the leukocyte integrins CD11b/CD18 and CD11c/CD18. J Cell Biol 1995; 129:1143–1153.
164. Stacker SA, Springer TA: Leukocyte integrin P150,95 (CD11c/CD18) functions as an adhesion molecule binding to a counter-receptor on stimulated endothelium. J Immunol 1991; 146:648–655.
165. Pavalko FM, Walker DM, Graham L, Goheen M, Doerschuk CM, Kansas GS: The cytoplasmic domain of L-selectin interacts with cytoskeletal proteins via α-actinin: Receptor positioning in microvilli does not require interaction with α-actinin. J Cell Biol 1995; 129:1155–1164.
166. Berlin C, Bargatze RF, Campbell JJ, et al: α4 Integrins mediate lymphocyte attachment and rolling under physiologic flow. Cell 1995; 80:413–422.
167. Fan S-T, Edgington TS: Integrin regulation of leukocyte inflammatory functions: CD11b/CD18 enhancement of TNF-α responses of monocytes. J Immunol 1993; 150:2972–2980.
168. Crockett-Torabi E, Sulenbarger B, Smith CW, Fantone JC: Activation of human neutrophils through L-selectin and Mac-1 molecules. J Immunol 1995; 154:2291–2302.
169. Monk PN, Banks P: The role of protein kinase C activation and inositol phosphate production in the regulation of cell-surface expression of Mac-1 by complement fragment C5a. Biochim Biophys Acta 1991; 1092:251–255.
170. Wright SD, Weitz JI, Huang AJ, Levin SM, Silverstein SC, Loike JD: Complement receptor type three (CD11b/CD18) of human polymorphonuclear leukocytes recognizes fibrinogen. Proc Natl Acad Sci USA 1988; 85:7734–7738.
171. Monk PN, Barker MD, Partridge LJ: Multiple signaling pathways in the C5a-induced expression of adhesion receptor Mac-1. Biochim Biophys Acta 1994; 1221:323–329.
172. Finn A, Strobel S, Levin M, Klein N: Endotoxin-induced neutrophil adherence to endothelium: Relationship to CD11b/CD18 and L-selectin expression and matrix disruption. Ann NY Acad Sci 1994; 725:173–182.
173. Smith CW: Endothelial adhesion molecules and their role in inflammation. Can J Physiol Pharmacol 1993; 71:76–87.
174. Luscinskas FW, Ding H, Lichtman AH: P-selectin and vascular cell adhesion molecule 1 mediate rolling and arrest, respectively, of $CD4^+$ T lymphocytes on tumor necrosis factor α–activated vascular endothelium under flow. J Exp Med 1995; 181:1179–1186.
175. Rinder HM, Tracey JL, Rinder CS, Leitenberg D, Smith BR: Neutrophil but not monocyte activation inhibits P-Selectin mediated platelet adhesion. Thromb Haemost 1994; 71:750–756.
176. von Andrian UH, Chambers JD, Berg EL, et al: L-selectin mediates neutrophil rolling in inflamed venules through sialyl $Lewis^x$-dependent and -independent recognition pathways. Blood 1993; 82:182–191.
177. Tedder TF, Steeber DA, Chen A, Engel P: The selectins: Vascular adhesion molecules. FASEB J 1995; 9:866–873.
178. Donnelly SC, Haslett C, Dransfield I, et al: Role of selectins in development of adult respiratory distress syndrome. Lancet 1994; 344:215–219.
179. Puri KD, Finger EB, Gaudemack G, Springer TA: Sialomucin CD34 is the major L-selectin ligand in human tonsil high endothelial venules. J Cell Biol 1995; 131:261–270.
180. Abbassi O, Kishimoto TK, McIntire LV, Smith CW: Neutrophil adhesion to endothelial cells. Blood Cells 1993; 19:245–260.
181. Kishimoto TK, Wamock RA, Jutila MA, et al: Antibodies against human neutrophil LECAM-1 (LAM-1/Leu-8/DREG-56 antigen) and endothelial cell ELAM-1 inhibit a common CD18–independent adhesion pathway in vitro. Blood 1991; 78:805–811.
182. Waddell TK, Fialkow L, Chan CK, Kishimoto TK, Downey GP: Signaling functions of L-selectin. J Biol Chem 1995; 270:15043–15411.
183. Butcher E: Leukocyte–endothelial cell recognition: Three (or more) steps to specificity and diversity. Cell 1991; 67:1033–1036.
184. Thomassen MJ, Meeker DP, Antal JM, Connors MJ, Wiedemann HP: Synthetic surfactant (exosurf) inhibits endotoxin-stimulated cytokine secretion by human alveolar macrophages. Am J Respir Cell Molec Biol 1992; 7:257–260.
185. Roumen RMH, Hendriks T, van der Ven-Jongekrijg J, et al: Cyto-

kine patterns in patients after major vascular surgery, hemorrhagic shock, and severe blunt trauma. Ann Surg 1993; 218:769-776.
186. Lo S, Van Seventer G, Levin S, Wright S: Two leukocyte receptors (CD11a/CD18 and CD11b/CD18) mediate transient adhesion to endothelium by binding to different ligands. J Immunol 1989; 143:3325-3329.
187. Lo S, Detmers P, Levin S, Wright S: Transient adhesion of neutrophils to endothelium. J Exp Med 1989; 169:1779-1793.
188. Smith C, Marlins S, Rothlein R, Toman C, Anderson D: Cooperative interactions of LFA-1 and MAC-1 with intercellular adhesion molecule-1 in facilitating adherence and transendothelial migration of human neutrophils in vitro. J Clin Invest 1989; 83:2008-2017.
189. Smith C, Kishimoto T, Abbassi O, et al: Chemotactic factors regulate lectin adhesion molecule 1 (LECAM-1)-dependent neutrophil adhesion to cytokine-stimulated endothelial cells in vitro. J Clin Invest 1991; 87:609-618.
190. Bachofen M, Weibel E: Alterations of the gas exchange apparatus in adult respiratory insufficiency associated with septicemia. Am Rev Respir Dis 1977; 116:589-614.
191. Schnells G, Voigt W, Redi H, Schlag G, Glatzl A: Electron microscopic investigation of lung biopsies in patients with posttraumatic respiratory insufficiency. Acta Chir Scand 1980; 499(Suppl):9-20.
192. Campbell EJ, Senior RM, Welgus HG: Extracellular matrix injury during lung inflammation. Chest 1987; 92:161-167.
193. Cochrane C, Spragg R, Revak S: Pathogenesis of the adult respiratory distress syndrome: Evidence of oxidant activity in the bronchoalveolar lavage fluid. J Clin Invest 1983; 71:754-761.
194. Muller-Eberhard H: Complement: Chemistry and pathways. *In* Inflammation: Basic Principles and Clinical Correlates. Gallin J, Goldstein I, Snyderman R (Eds). New York, Raven Press, 1988, p 22.

45

Hematopoietic Colony-Stimulating Factors

Amal M. Abu-Ghosh, MD • Francisco Bracho, MD
Ivan Kirov, MD • Mitchell S. Cairo, MD, FAAP

Colony-stimulating factors (CSFs) are a family of glycoprotein hormones that regulate production and differentiation of hematopoietic cells. Many individual CSFs have now been identified, cloned, and characterized. The CSFs are a complex family of cytokines, often referred to as hematopoietic growth factors (HGFs). The term CSF was coined because these factors stimulated the formation of clonal colonies within in vitro culture systems. The study of hematopoietic growth factors has now evolved from the laboratory into an expanding number of clinical applications. The clinical utility of these CSFs is based on their extremely potent biologic activity in stimulating primitive and mature hematopoietic cells.

Specific erythroid, myeloid, thrombopoietic, and lymphoid hematopoietic growth factors have now been cloned and used in experimental systems to help enhance our understanding of normal hematopoiesis as well as hematopoietic diseases. The American Society of Clinical Oncology (ASCO) has established guidelines and recommendations for the use of hematopoietic CSFs (granulocyte CSF [G-CSF], granulocyte-macrophage CSF [GM-CSF]) on the basis of the results of several clinical trials. The use of CSFs has been recommended after chemotherapy to decrease the incidence of febrile neutropenia, after autologous and allogeneic stem cell transplantation (bone marrow and peripheral stem cells), and for mobilization of peripheral stem cell donors.[1, 2] Clinical trials have also shown the efficacy of using other HGFs, such as thrombopoietin (TPO) and interleukin-11 (IL-11) in enhancing platelet recovery and erythropoietin (EPO) in improving the chronic anemia associated with renal failure and anemia secondary to chemotherapy. This review focuses on the biology of these HGFs as well as their current and future clinical applications in the treatment of hematologic and other disorders.

BIOLOGY OF HEMATOPOIESIS

Hematopoiesis is a complex process that begins with an uncommitted pluripotent hematopoietic stem cell (PPSC). This cell can self-renew, proliferate, and differentiate into all of the hematopoietic lineages. Figure 45-1 illustrates our current understanding of the complex interaction of the hematopoietic growth factors at many different stages in hematopoiesis. The final result of this hematopoietic physiologic process is a mature, lineage-restricted effector cell that circulates in the bloodstream. The less mature forms of blood cells, known as *progenitor cells,* can differentiate into different lineages, depending on their exposure to individual and combinations of HGFs. Primitive progenitor cells maintain their multipotent potential, whereas more mature progenitor cells become committed as they differentiate into specific lineages.

The schematic diagram of hematopoiesis (see Fig. 45-1) is derived from in vitro culture systems in which progenitor cells have been identified and induced with specific growth factors, resulting in differentiated progeny in various culture systems. Early progenitors are called colony-forming units (CFUs) and are named for the lineages that are derived from a specific colony. Thus, a CFU-GM is capable of giving rise to granulocytes and macrophages, whereas a CFU-MK can give rise only to megakaryocytes. One of the earliest primitive CFUs studied in colony assays is the CFU-GEMM (granulocyte, erythrocyte, macrophage, and megakaryocyte), which does not contain lymphoid cells or their progenitors and has no ability for self-renewal. The PPSC that expresses CD34 represents the most primitive hematopoietic stem cell that can be identified by immunophenotyping.[3] These cells represent 0.5% to 2% of the mononuclear cells of the bone marrow and less than 0.1% of the mononuclear cells of the peripheral blood.[3] The hematopoietic growth factors interact with specific receptors on primitive stem cells and stimulate their proliferation and differentiation into committed lineages.[3]

Currently, on the basis of multiple in vitro studies, the HGFs have been subdivided into three groups. Early-acting cytokines include stem cell factor (SCF) (c-*kit* ligand), Flt-3 ligand (FL), interleukin-6 (IL-6), IL-11, and (FL)TPO; intermediate-acting cytokines include interleukin-3 (IL-3), GM-CSF, and interleukin-4 (IL-4); and late-acting cytokines include interleukin-5 (IL-5), erythropoietin, and G-CSF.[4] The in vivo process of hematopoiesis is far more complex, with many other local microenvironmental factors influencing blood cell development. These include many nonhematopoietic cells such as fibroblasts and endothelial cells, which come into contact with hematopoietic progenitors during their maturation and circulation in the bone marrow and blood. In addition, the human PPSC has yet to be identified by immunophenotyping, although small populations of progenitor cells can be isolated that contain stem cells, as demonstrated by their ability to engraft in lethally irradiated animals after stem cell transplantation (bone marrow transplantation [BMT]).[5]

Each hematopoietic growth factor is coded for by a unique gene, as shown in Table 45-1. Many of these genes are located on chromosome 5, which has also been shown to be involved

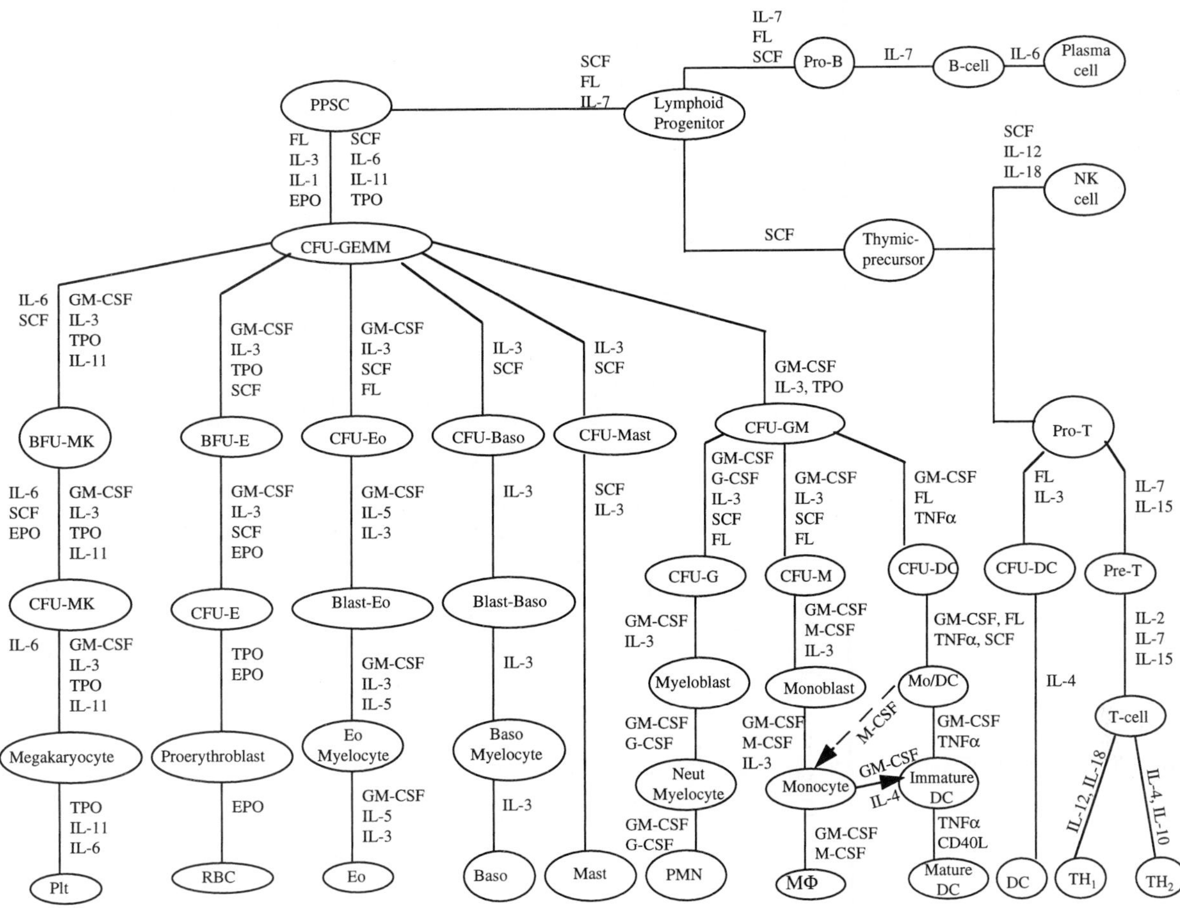

Figure 45–1. Colony-stimulating factors in hematopoiesis. PPSC = pluripotent stem cell; CFU = colony-forming unit; BFU = burst-forming unit; GEMM = granulocyte, erythrocyte, macrophage, and megakaryocyte; GM = granulocyte-macrophage; E = erythroid; MK = megakaryocyte; Eo = eosinophil; Baso = basophil; G = granulocyte; M = macrophage; DC = dendritic cell; Mo = monocyte; NK = natural killer; IL = interleukin; CSF = colony-stimulating factor; SCF = stem cell factor; FL = Flt 3 ligand; EPO = erythropoietin; TPO = thrombopoietin; L = ligand; TNFα = tumor necrosis factor α; TH = T helper; MΦ = macrophage; RBC = red blood cell; PMN = polymorphonuclear neutrophil leukocyte; Plt = platelet; Neut = neutrophil.

in various hematopoietic disorders such as myeloid leukemia and myelodysplastic syndromes. Each growth factor is produced by a variety of cells and has specific target cells, which are also described in Table 45–1.

Regulation of the production of hematopoietic growth factors is a complex process that is only partially understood at this time. As illustrated in Figure 45–1, growth factors exert their influence at various stages of differentiation, affecting multiple lineages. Regulation of specific CSF receptors, through either positive or negative cellular and microenvironmental influences, also plays a part in the regulation of normal hematopoiesis. In vitro culture systems have confirmed the important role of the microenvironment as well as exogenous and endogenously produced growth factors in regulating the hematopoietic process. Abnormal conditions and disease processes, such as severe anemia and sepsis, result in the production of multiple cytokines and growth factors that participate in biologic cascade processes, which regulate the production of growth factors and their receptors in a process known as transmodulation. The important role of cytokines in sepsis is discussed in the individual sections on specific CSFs. It is clear that the CSFs play a major role both in specific diseases and in the body's response to specific diseases.

GRANULOCYTE-MACROPHAGE COLONY-STIMULATING FACTOR

GM-CSF is a cytokine produced by activated T lymphocytes, macrophages, mast cells, fibroblasts, and other mesenchyme-derived cells that stimulate the production, differentiation, and maturation of myeloid hematopoietic precursors. GM-CSF also enhances the function of mature myeloid cells, including neutrophils, monocytes, and eosinophils. The gene encoding GM-CSF is located on chromosome 5q21.32, and it encodes a protein that contains 127 amino acids with a molecular weight of 14 to 35 kD, depending on the degree of glycosylation.[6] GM-CSF is an intermediate-acting cytokine (see earlier), and it can act on relatively early hematopoietic progenitors (see Fig. 45–1) of multiple cell lineages and can act in concert with other CSFs to influence the proliferation of these cells. Low concentrations of GM-CSF are required for viability of neutrophils and monocytes (and their progenitors).[7]

Two classes of GM-CSF receptors have been identified, and they are distinguished by their high-affinity or low-affinity binding to GM-CSF. The receptors are found on hematopoietic cells as well as on endothelial cells and some solid tumor cells.[7]

GM-CSF enhances the effector function of mature neutrophils, eosinophils, and monocyte/macrophages. These effects, which have been shown in vitro and in vivo, include augmentation of neutrophil oxidative metabolism, chemotaxis, phagocytosis, leukotriene release, degranulation, and antibody-dependent cellular cytotoxicity (ADCC).[8] Similar effects are found in monocyte/macrophages as well as in enhanced intracellular killing, potentiation of antigen processing, and increased production of tumor necrosis factor (TNF), IL-1, and monocyte colony-stimulating factor (M-CSF). Eosinophil func-

TABLE 45–1. Hematopoietic Growth Factors

Cytokine	Chromosome Location	Protein (kD)	Cellular Source	Progenitor Cell Target	Mature Effector Cell Target
G-CSF	17q11.22	18–22	Monocytes, fibroblasts, endothelial cells	CFU-GEMM, CFU-GM, CFU-G	Neutrophil
GM-CSF	5q21.32	14–35	T lymphocytes, monocytes, fibroblasts, endothelial cells, osteoblasts, smooth-muscle cells, mast cells	CFU-GEMM, CFU-GM, CFU-G, BFU-E, BFU-Eo	Neutrophil, eosinophil, monocyte
M-CSF	1p13-31	47–90	Fibroblasts, monocytes, endothelial cells, placenta	CFU-GM, CFU-M	Monocyte, neutrophil, eosinophil, basophil
SCF	12q14.3qter	26	Fibroblasts, stromal cells, endothelial cells, visceral yolk sac	BFU-E, CFU-E, CFU-MK, CFU-GEMM, PPSC	?NK ?DC
IL-3	5q23.31	28	T lymphocytes, monocytes	CFU-GEMM, CFU-GM, CFU-M, CFU-G, CFU-Baso, CFU-MK, CFU-Eo, BFU-E, CFU-E, PPSC	Eosinophil, neutrophil, basophil, monocyte
IL-6	7p15	19–26	Monocytes, T and B lymphocytes, fibroblasts, endothelial cells	PPSC, CFU-GEMM, CFU-GM, BFU-E	B cell, T cell, hepatocyte
IL-11	19q13.3	20	Fibroblasts, endothelial cells	CFU-GM, CFU-E, BFU-E, CFU-GEMM, CFU-MK	
FL	19q13.3-13.4	30	Bone marrow stroma	PPSC, CFU-GEMM, CFU-GM, CFU-Eo, primitive thymocyte pro-B cell	DC
TPO	3q27-28	70	Liver, kidney	CFU-MK, megakaryocytes, CFU-GM, CFU-GEMM, BFU-E	Platelets
EPO	7q21.3-q22.1	14–39	Interstitial cells of peritubular capillary bed of kidney, hepatocytes	CFU-GEMM, BFU-E, CFU-E, Proerythroblasts	

CSF = colony-stimulating factor; SCF = stem cell factor; G = granulocyte; M = macrophage; IL = interleukin; EPO = erythropoietin; TPO = thrombopoietin; FL = Flt 3 ligand; BFU = burst-forming unit; CFU = colony-forming unit; GEMM = granulocyte, erythrocyte, macrophage, megakaryocyte; PPSC = pluripotent hematopoietic stem cell; Baso = basophilic; MK = megakaryocyte; E = erythrocyte; Eo = eosinophil; DC = dendritic cell; NK = natural killer.

tion is similarly enhanced by GM-CSF, especially eosinophil viability and protozoal killing.

Human studies have demonstrated transient leukopenia with a decrease in circulating neutrophils, eosinophils, and monocytes as well as pulmonary neutrophil sequestration after GM-CSF administration.[9] This is followed by leukocytosis secondary to neutrophil demargination, increased marrow neutrophil production, and increased half-life of circulating neutrophils. Phase I and II trials have shown that GM-CSF is well tolerated at doses from 8 to 16 μg/kg/day, with fever and rash occurring at doses of 32 μg/kg/day or more.[10] Toxicities included bone pain, myalgias, fever, elevation of transaminases, rash, and facial flushing. Dose-limiting toxicities (16 to 32 μg/kg) have included a capillary leak syndrome with generalized edema and pleural and pericardial effusions.[11] Comparisons of the different formulations of GM-CSF have shown differences between the clinical activities and toxicities of the glycosylated (yeast-derived sargramostim or Chinese hamster ovary cell–derived regramostim) and nonglycosylated (*Escherichia coli*–derived molgramostim and ecogramostim) forms. The glycosylated form regramostim was characterized by a longer serum half-life, greater neutrophil-stimulating activity, and less leukotriene production.[12] Sargramostim was associated with less prominent fluid retention, dyspnea, fever, myalgias and bone pains, and first-dose phenomenon compared with the nonglycosylated forms.[13, 14]

GM-CSF has been studied in very-low-birth-weight (VLBW) neonates in both a phase I and a phase II trial.[15] These newborns have an increased susceptibility to infection related to both quantitative and qualitative neutrophil defects. In particular, neonates respond to infection with neutropenia and have decreased numbers of neutrophil progenitors in bone marrow compared with adults. Because of its ability to increase marrow production and increase circulating neutrophils, GM-CSF was evaluated as an agent to enhance neonatal phagocytic immunity and, it was hoped, to decrease the incidence of neonatal nosocomial infections. Between 1992 and 1994, 20 neonates (500 to 1500 g) younger than 3 days of age were given either placebo or escalating intravenous (IV) doses of GM-CSF once or twice daily for 7 days. No reported grade III or IV toxicities were attributable to GM-CSF administration. Increases in absolute neutrophil count (ANC), absolute monocyte count, and platelet counts were demonstrated at doses of 10 μg/kg/day. Numbers of late bone marrow neutrophil progenitors (postmitotic pool) were increased without a depletion of early progenitors (premitotic pool).[15]

We have completed a multicenter, double-blind, randomized, and placebo-controlled pilot phase II trial of *prophylactic* GM-CSF in VLBW (501 to 1000 g) neonates ($n = 61$).[16] Subjects were randomized within the first 3 days of life to receive either placebo or GM-CSF (8 μg/kg/day) as a 2-hour IV infusion for 28 days. There was a significant (61%) reduction in the proportion of confirmed nosocomial infections in the GM-CSF versus placebo group with a parallel significant reduction in the incidence of positive cultures in the GM-CSF cohort compared with placebo-treated neonates. This study suggests that the enhancement of neonatal phagocytic immunity by GM-CSF, when initiated in the first 72 hours of life, may reduce the incidence of nosocomial infection within the first month of life. A larger, double-blind, randomized, placebo-controlled phase III trial is ongoing.

GM-CSF has been used in the treatment of severe aplastic anemia (SAA) in children and adults. Clinical trials have evaluated the role of GM-CSF as a single agent and in combination with other more traditional therapies. A phase I and phase II trial of recombinant human GM-CSF (rhGM-CSF) in children with SAA showed a transient response that was not sustained after withdrawal of the cytokine.[10] Patients suffering from long-standing, severe, treatment-resistant aplastic anemia with complete myelopoietic failure did not benefit from rhGM-CSF therapy.[17] Also, early administration of rhGM-CSF before the initiation of immunosuppressive therapy did not enhance myelopoietic responses.[18] However, concomitant administration of rhGM-CSF with immunosuppressive therapy has been beneficial in children and adults with SAA, resulting in fewer days of hospitalization and less infections.[19, 20] The use of GM-CSF after allogeneic transplantation for SAA has also been evaluated, and the results indicated a possible role in accelerating marrow recovery.[21]

The potential role of CSFs, particularly G-CSF and GM-CSF, in patients with acute myelocytic leukemia (AML) has been studied in several phase III trials that evaluated the effects of CSFs on the duration of neutropenia, the differentiation of myeloblasts, and the enhancement of leukemic cell proliferation with increased response to cycle-specific chemotherapy.

Geller[22] and Schiffer[23] analyzed and reviewed the results of several phase III trials. These analyses showed a modest and significant reduction in the duration of severe neutropenia compared with that in the placebo-treated groups. There was no reduction in the incidence of severe infections, antibiotic use, or duration of hospitalization. There was no improvement in the complete response (CR) rate or overall survival.[24] GM-CSF was well tolerated with no increased toxicity, and there was no increase in leukemia relapse. ASCO[1] has recommended that CSF be used after induction therapy in patients 55 years of age or older, and there may be a similar effect on younger patients in reducing the duration of neutropenia. The use of CSFs before or during induction for priming effects outside clinical trials is not recommended at present.

GM-CSF has also been used in patients with myelodysplastic syndrome, either alone[25, 26] or in combination with IL-3,[27] with improvement in the neutrophil count and reduction in the number of patients experiencing infections. The effect lasted as long as GM-CSF was administered, and there was no effect on the other hematopoietic cell lineages.

The use of GM-CSF after standard-dose chemotherapy has been found to reduce significantly the duration and severity of neutropenia in patients with non-Hodgkin's lymphoma (phase III trial).[28] Trials in pediatric patients with solid tumors undergoing intensive chemotherapy have also shown a beneficial reduction in the incidence of infection and days of neutropenia.[29] However, the use of GM-CSF for patients receiving chemoradiotherapy for small-cell lung cancer (SCLC) resulted in more toxic deaths, severe thrombocytopenia, and nonhematologic toxicities.[30] The use of GM-CSF in patients with germ cell tumors or after vincristine, ifosfamide, carboplatin, and etoposide (V-ICE) chemotherapy in patients with SCLC did not show any benefit in reduced complications of myelosuppression from aggressive therapy.[31, 32]

GM-CSF has been used after ablative chemotherapy to augment hematopoietic engraftment after BMT. In a randomized placebo-controlled study in patients undergoing autologous BMT for hematologic malignancies, GM-CSF shortened the duration of neutropenia, antibiotic therapy, and hospitalization.[33] This study led to U.S. Food and Drug Administration (FDA) approval of use of GM-CSF in this clinical setting. The use of GM-CSF after allogeneic BMT significantly decreased the duration of neutropenia, decreased infections and days of hospitalization, and this therapy was well tolerated.[34] The use of GM-CSF for mobilization of peripheral blood progenitor cells (PBPCs) resulted in efficient collection of PBPCs and rapid restoration of hematopoietic function after high-dose chemotherapy.[35]

GM-CSF has also been studied in patients with acquired immunodeficiency syndrome (AIDS) in an attempt to circumvent the myelosuppression that results from the retroviral infection as well as the myelotoxicity of antiviral chemotherapy. GM-CSF increased peripheral myeloid blood counts in patients with AIDS.[11, 36] Patients who were neutropenic as a result of azidothymidine (AZT) or interferon therapy were subsequently able to receive these medications once they began taking GM-CSF. Clinical trials have also evaluated the role of GM-CSF after chemotherapy for AIDS-related Kaposi's sarcoma and non-Hodgkin's lymphoma.[37, 38] The use of GM-CSF in this setting was associated with decreased severity and duration of neutropenia and decreased days of hospitalization for fever and neutropenia.

GM-CSF has also been explored for the ex vivo expansion of hematopoietic progenitor cells. Of particular interest is the use of GM-CSF in combination with other cytokines, such as TNF-α or IL-4, to enhance the ex vivo generation of dendritic cells.[39, 40] Dendritic cells are professional antigen-presenting cells (APCs) and are believed to be the initiators of both cellular and humoral immune responses. In the presence of GM-CSF, both $CD34^+$ hematopoietic progenitors and peripheral blood monocytes differentiate into dendritic cells.[41, 42] Dendritic cells generated ex vivo are being explored for their potential to heighten the immune response in traditionally poorly immunogenic diseases including human immunodeficiency virus (HIV) infection and malignancy.[43, 44]

Extensive research on animal tumor models has shown that GM-CSF gene–transfected tumors can become immunogenic and can elicit tumor-specific immunity in vivo.[45, 46] When injected into mice, GM-CSF–transfected B16 melanoma cells became more immunogenic and murine GM-CSF gene–transfected AML cells were more potent than B7.1-transfected tumor cells in producing tumor-specific immunity. Phase I clinical trials using GM-CSF gene–transfected melanoma or sarcoma cell vaccines are under way to evaluate acute and long-term toxicities associated with this form of gene therapy.[47] Phase I trials in patients with stage IV melanoma using GM-CSF–transfected autologous melanoma cells have been completed. No grade II to grade IV toxicities were reported, and the vaccination site showed local reactions that were dose dependent. Biopsy of the vaccination sites demonstrated T cells, dendritic cells, macrophages, and eosinophils. Preexisting melanoma lesions showed infiltration with T cells, plasma cells, and eosinophils with necrotic tumor cells. Cytotoxic T lymphocytes (CTLs) with autologous tumor cytotoxicity were also isolated from the tumor sites. Further trials are needed to assess the long-term effects of GM-CSF tumor vaccines on tumor regression and long-term survival.[48, 49]

GRANULOCYTE COLONY-STIMULATING FACTOR

G-CSF is a hematopoietic growth factor that exerts its effect on cells of the neutrophil lineage by stimulating proliferation and differentiation of granulocytes and their committed precursors (see Fig. 45–1). G-CSF is considered a late-acting CSF because of its relative lineage specificity. G-CSF also enhances mature neutrophil function. Human G-CSF was first identified after the purification of murine G-CSF by Nicola and colleagues in 1983.[50] In 1985, Welte and coworkers[51] purified human G-CSF from the bladder carcinoma cell line 5637. The gene for G-CSF was subsequently cloned in 1986[52] and was mapped to chromosome 17q11.22.[53] G-CSF is a single polypeptide chain consisting of 201 amino acids, with 177 making up the mature molecule and 30 in the leader sequence. The protein can be heavily glycosylated and therefore has a variable molecular mass of 18 to 22 kDa. Recombinant G-CSF has been produced in *E. coli* and has been shown to have activity similar to that of the native protein.[54] Endogenous G-CSF is produced primarily by mature macrophages but is also produced by endothelial cells, fibroblasts, and mesothelial cells. G-CSF production can be stimulated in these cells by TNF-α, lipopolysaccharide (LPS), IL-1, IL-3, IL-6, and SCF (see Fig. 45–1).[54] The significance of G-CSF receptors expressed on nonhematopoietic cells is unknown.

The role of G-CSF in steady-state hematopoiesis is unknown; however, during stressed conditions (e.g., in sepsis, after cytotoxic chemotherapy, in congenital neutropenia), endogenous G-CSF levels increase markedly and are inversely proportional to the circulating ANC.[54, 55] G-CSF stimulates the proliferation of committed progenitor cells, shortens bone marrow transit time, reduces neutrophil storage pool, and increases peripheral neutrophil counts.[56] G-CSF gene inactivation in mice results in chronic neutropenia and failure to increase the neutrophil count during experimental *Listeria monocytogenes* sepsis.[13]

Cairo and colleagues[57] demonstrated that endogenous G-CSF production correlates with myeloid engraftment after autologous and allogeneic BMT. Experimental data have shown that G-CSF can produce a rapid release of bone marrow neutrophils into the circulation and reduce granulocyte maturation time. Multiple animal studies have documented that G-CSF can cause neutrophilia with little toxicity.[58] Furthermore, G-CSF can enhance the effector function of mature neutrophils by priming oxidative metabolism, promoting chemotaxis and phagocytosis, and augmenting antibody-dependent cellular cytotoxicity.[13, 59] These studies have led to many clinical trials using G-CSF in a variety of conditions and are summarized in the following paragraphs. Of note, toxicity associated with G-CSF has been minimal, with the most common side effect being bone pain, which subsides on discontinuation of the drug.

Bodey and coworkers[60] first demonstrated that the risk of infection in cancer patients receiving myelosuppressive chemotherapy correlates with the depth and duration of neutropenia. Several phase II studies of G-CSF after chemotherapy have demonstrated clinical efficacy in ameliorating the hematologic and infectious toxicity of intensive treatment regimens.

Crawford and associates[61] published the results of a double-blind phase III study of patients with SCLC who were randomized to receive prophylactic G-CSF after chemotherapy cycles. The G-CSF group had a reduced duration and severity of neutropenia as well as a lower incidence of febrile neutropenia, infections, hospitalizations, and antibiotic use.[61] Similar results were reported with G-CSF use in children with solid tumors.[62]

The results of a phase I study evaluating the efficacy of G-CSF after cycles of chemoradiotherapy in patients with SCLC have been published. G-CSF use did not allow chemotherapy dose escalation but shortened the duration of neutropenia at the maximal tolerated dose and reduced the need for dose reduction.[63]

Use of G-CSF as an adjunct to induction chemotherapy in adults with acute lymphoblastic leukemia (ALL) was evaluated in a phase III trial. Administration of G-CSF on day 2 of chemotherapy resulted in a decrease in the duration and severity of neutropenia, febrile neutropenia, and documented infection.[64] A similar trial in children with ALL resulted in a reduction in the duration of neutropenia but did not lower the number of severe infections or rate of hospitalization for febrile neutropenia and did not affect the overall event-free survival.[65] The use of G-CSF for severe febrile neutropenia (absolute neutrophil count $< 500/mm^3$) after chemotherapy was associated with a reduced duration of neutropenia but did not provide any other clinical benefit.[66] Patients with metastatic germ cell tumors with a poor prognosis benefited from the use of G-CSF during intensive chemotherapy and had a reduction in the incidence of toxic deaths compared with the control group, but there were no effects on overall survival.[67] The ASCO guidelines support the use of hematopoietic growth factors when the incidence of febrile neutropenia is 40% or higher after chemotherapy or for patients at increased risk for chemotherapy-induced infections.[1]

The use of G-CSF after completion of induction therapy in patients with AML decreased the duration of neutropenia and the risk of infection in phase III clinical trials.[68, 69] The 1996 ASCO recommendations support the use of HGF after induction in older patients but do not support the use of growth factors for a priming effect before or during induction in patients with AML.[1] G-CSF can also increase the absolute neutrophil counts in patients with myelodysplastic syndrome (MDS),[70] and the ASCO guidelines support intermittent administration to patients with severe neutropenia and recurrent infections.[1]

The use of G-CSF after autologous BMT shortens the duration of neutropenia, duration of hospitalization, and number of days of protracted fever.[71-73] G-CSF use has also been effective in reducing the duration of neutropenia after allogeneic BMT and PBPC transplantation.[74] The role of G-CSF in mobilization of PBPCs has also been extensively studied.[75] G-CSF can induce up to a 100-fold increase of circulating progenitor cells in patients with various malignancies.[76] The use of G-CSF in combination with other early-acting growth factors, such as IL-3 and SCF, can result in a synergistic effect on peripheral blood stem cell mobilization.[77, 78] The mobilization of PBPCs by the combination of G-CSF and GM-CSF was not significantly better than mobilization using G-CSF alone.[79]

G-CSF has also been used to mobilize donors of PBPCs for allogeneic transplantation.[73, 80, 81] The use of G-CSF before bone marrow harvest for autologous transplantation in patients with lymphoma resulted in hematopoietic recovery similar to that of recipients of G-CSF–mobilized PBPCs.[82]

Use of G-CSF to decrease the morbidity and mortality of neonatal infections has been explored. Toxic human neonates with neutropenia who received G-CSF had significant fivefold increases in ANC compared with similar untreated neonates. This increase was sustained for 3 days, and a twofold increase was still observed after 7 to 10 days. A similar increase in ANC was noted when neutropenia was associated with maternal pregnancy-induced hypertension.[83] Another noted hematopoietic effect was an increase in the absolute monocyte count (AMC).[84, 85]

We have also reported the results of a randomized, placebo-controlled trial of G-CSF in human neonates with sepsis.[86] Forty-two patients younger than 3 days of age with clinically presumed sepsis, most critically ill and receiving ventilation, were enrolled to receive either IV placebo or G-CSF on various dose schedules. There was no evidence of G-CSF–induced toxicity or of increased pulmonary toxicity in any of the neonates studied. In these newborns with presumed sepsis, dose-dependent increases in the marrow neutrophil storage pool (postmitotic) were seen without a change in the bone marrow neutrophil proliferative pool (premitotic). A trend for increased numbers of CFU-GM and CFU-GEMM was also noted after G-CSF administration.

With respect to long-term sequelae of G-CSF use in the neonatal period, we also completed follow-up of 21 of 28 surviving neonates enrolled at our institution 2 years after receiving G-CSF and did not note any long-term adverse hematologic, immunologic, or developmental effects in this cohort of patients.[87] Only a larger, multicenter, blind, placebo-controlled trial can determine whether the use of G-CSF in presumed septic, young (<3 days old) neonates is associated with a decrease in mortality, morbidity, and cost of care in this clinical setting.

Treatment of patients with congenital neutropenia (Kostmann's syndrome) with G-CSF has resulted in a significant increase in neutrophil counts; an improved clinical response, as demonstrated by decreased infections, antibiotic use, and hospital stay[88, 89]; and an improvement in general health perceptions.[90] G-CSF has also been used in patients with cyclic neutropenia to decrease cycling time and increase the neutrophil nadir[91] and has been effective in infants with autoimmune neutropenia, inducing a temporary increase in neutrophil counts.[92]

Patients with aplastic anemia have also benefited from G-CSF therapy, with increases in neutrophil counts but without effects on red blood cells or platelets.[93] G-CSF has been used to treat HIV-associated neutropenia and has been associated with a significant increase in total lymphocytes, T cells, $CD8^+$ T cells, $CD4^+$ T cells, and natural killer cells.[94]

G-CSF has been used in combination with other HGFs for ex vivo expansion of hematopoietic progenitors to enhance myeloid and platelet engraftment and reduce the morbidity associated with delayed engraftment. The addition of G-CSF to a combination of SCF, IL-3, and IL-6 resulted in a one-log increase in total cell expansion and a twofold increase in CFU-GM expansion.[95] Ex vivo expansion of umbilical cord blood has also been extensively studied. Combinations of SCF, FL, IL-3, IL-6, and EPO in addition to G-CSF have been used.[96] The best conditions and cytokine combinations have yet to be determined and are under investigation.

INTERLEUKIN-6

IL-6 is a 184-amino-acid, 26-kD glycoprotein that was originally cloned from T lymphocytes as a molecule that induced immunoglobulin production by B lymphocytes.[97] It is produced by monocytes, T cells, B cells, fibroblasts, and endothelial cells as well as by several tumor cell lines.[98] It has a broad range of activity in many hematopoietic and nonhematopoietic cell types, including induction of acute-phase proteins, immunoregulation, neural differentiation, and hematopoiesis.[98, 99] IL-6 gene expression is stimulated by LPS, interferon-γ, platelet-derived growth factor, and various viruses, including HIV.[100]

IL-6 is a potent mitogen for B cells[101] and can induce resting T cells and up-regulate IL-2 production.[100] Because of T cell stimulatory activity, IL-6 has been studied for antitumor effects. Although in several preclinical animal models IL-6 reduced the mortality rate associated with malignant disease, this has not been borne out in human studies. IL-6 has not had an appreciable effect in renal cell cancer, advanced adult malignancies,[102] or pediatric solid tumors.[103] Moreover, IL-6 has been implicated as an autocrine or paracrine growth factor for multiple myeloma. Many myeloma cell lines are IL-6–dependent. IL-6 and its soluble receptor are elevated in multiple myeloma and other paraproteinemias. Therefore, several strategies for blocking IL-6 action have been employed for the treatment of multiple myeloma, including anti–soluble IL-6 receptor antibodies. Dexamethasone and all-*trans* retinoic acid may modify myeloma proliferation through inhibition of the IL-6 autocrine loop.

IL-6 plays a major role in the inflammatory response. Elevated levels are observed in serum during bacterial sepsis, in synovial fluid in arthritic conditions, in amniotic fluid of infected neonates, and in spinal fluid during meningitis.[104] IL-6 is thought to be the major cytokine in the induction of the acute-phase protein response. Patients with autoimmune and collagen vascular disease show increased serum levels of IL-6, including Castleman's disease and the related syndrome of polyneuropathy, organomegaly, endocrinopathy, M protein, and skin changes (POEMS syndrome).

IL-6 has significant thrombopoietic activity in vitro and in vivo. IL-6 appears to have synergistic activity with other cytokines, including IL-3, GM-CSF, and G-CSF in stimulating bone marrow and peripheral blood CFUs in mice[105-107] and in vitro cultures of human cells. IL-6 can increase platelet counts in normal mice and primates.[108, 109] In addition, IL-6 has been shown to decrease the duration of the platelet nadir and to prevent severe thrombocytopenia in irradiation- or chemotherapy-induced myelosuppression in animals.[110-112] Therefore, IL-6 has been tested in myelosuppressed patients to decrease chemotherapy-related thrombocytopenia and in patients with aplastic anemia or MDS to increase platelet counts.

In several phase I trials in adults, IL-6 resulted in an increased platelet count and had variable effects on the white blood cell (WBC) count.[113-115] Anemia has been consistently observed but has been shown to be dilutional in nature. These studies also demonstrated no change in megakaryocyte numbers or in CFU-Meg; however, changes in megakaryocyte ploidy and platelet function in patients receiving IL-6 have been reported.[116] IL-6 was therefore thought to act principally on committed platelet progenitors. In patients receiving myelosuppressive chemotherapy, IL-6 appeared to shorten the duration of the platelet nadir and allow dose intensification. However, translation to human clinical use has been hampered by the systemic toxicity of IL-6. In patients with MDS or aplastic anemia (AA),[117] the beneficial effects of increased platelet numbers were usually abrogated by the increase in anemia and need for red blood cell transfusions. In addition, all studies have found frequent constitutional toxicities, including headache, fever, chills, and myalgia.[102] Biochemical signs of inflammation were also present with a significant increase in C-reactive protein, fibrinogen, and serum amyloid A.[118] In children, these constitutional toxicities were dose-limiting at 2.5 μg/kg/day.[119] In adults, constitutional symptoms at low doses were controlled with antipyretics. Dose-limiting toxicities in adults at doses greater than 20 μg/kg/day included cardiac arrhythmias, hyperbilirubinemia, reversible hemiplegia, hallucinations, and confusion. IL-6 is not likely to continue to be useful in vivo, but its use for ex vivo expansion of stem or immune cells is still promising.

Leary and colleagues[107] demonstrated that IL-6 combined with IL-3 can act synergistically to support multilineage progenitor cells. Several investigators demonstrated that this combination can induce quiescent stem cells to cycle and proliferate in vitro. Others have used IL-6 in combination with other cytokines to expand hematopoietic progenitor cells in ex vivo systems.

ERYTHROPOIETIN

EPO is a sialoglycoprotein hormone that has been identified as the CSF that regulates red blood cell production (erythropoiesis). During the 1950s, investigators were able to demonstrate the transfer of an erythropoietic stimulus from hypoxic rats[120] and anemic rabbits.[121] EPO was first isolated and purified in 1977 by Miyake and coworkers,[122] and the gene was cloned in 1985 by two separate groups.[123, 124] The gene has been mapped to chromosome 7.[125] The protein has a molecular mass of 14 to 39 kD, depending on the degree of glycosylation.

The liver is the primary site of EPO production in the fetus. EPO production is switched to the kidneys by 120 to 140 days and is completed by 40 days after birth.[126, 127] Studies of animal models suggest that the interstitial cells of the peritubular capillary bed are the site of EPO production in humans[128] and the hepatocytes surrounding central veins in the liver are the site of EPO production in the fetus.[129] EPO production is increased in response to anemia or subtle changes in oxygen tension that are sensed by the interstitial cells of the peritubular capillary bed of the kidneys.[130, 131] EPO binds to specific receptors on the cell surface of erythroid cells.[132] The burst-forming unit erythroid (BFU-E) is the earliest cell in the erythroid lineage. The BFU-E is mostly unresponsive to EPO and has a low number of EPO receptors. The more mature CFU erythroid (CFU-E) has more EPO receptors and is the primary target cell for EPO. More EPO receptors are present on the more mature cells between CFU-E and the proerythroblasts.[133, 134] No EPO receptors are found on mature erythrocytes or reticulocytes.

EPO interacts with IL-3, IL-1, GM-CSF, and SCF in stimulating erythroid progenitors and promoting erythropoiesis.[135, 136] In addition, EPO can act in concert with other cytokines to stimulate myeloid, monocyte, and megakaryocytic cells in vitro and in vivo.

The clinical applications of EPO were first studied after the production of recombinant human EPO in 1985. Recombinant EPO was first used in patients with end-stage renal disease who were undergoing dialysis and was found to decrease transfusion requirements and enable the patients to become transfusion-independent.[137] Improvements in appetite, activity level, sense of well-being, uremic coagulopathy, and pruritus have also been reported.[138, 139] Recombinant human EPO therapy has also improved anemia in renal transplant recipients with chronic graft failure.[140]

Other clinical trials[141] have studied the effects of EPO in ameliorating anemia of cancer. Children with sarcoma who were receiving chemotherapy were treated with EPO at a starting dose of 150 U/kg/day and iron supplementation. A significant reduction in red blood cell transfusions compared with the control group was reported, and a decrease in platelet transfusion was also noticed.[142] Also, patients with multiple myeloma or non-Hodgkin's lymphoma benefited from EPO therapy. Patients with low EPO levels inappropriate to the degree of anemia were more likely to respond to EPO therapy.[143] EPO therapy was also effective in improving anemia and the quality of life and in reducing red blood cell transfusions in cancer patients with or without chemotherapy.[144] However, the use of EPO in combination with G-CSF for children with Hodgkin's and non-Hodgkin's disease undergoing autologous BMT was not effective in reducing red blood cell or platelet transfusion requirements.[145] The use of EPO in combination with G-CSF in patients with AIDS receiving zidovudine therapy resulted in a significant increase in $CD4^+$ cells, neutrophil count, and hemoglobin levels compared with patients treated with zidovudine alone.[146, 147]

EPO has been well tolerated by children and adults. It has been used to augment the presurgical blood collection from anemic patients undergoing elective surgery. The use of EPO enhanced erythropoiesis, permitted the storage of more autologous blood, and reduced the risk of allogeneic transfusion.[148, 149] Although EPO increased erythropoiesis and total red blood cell production in nonanemic patients, it did not increase the number of donated autologous units[150] or the need for allogeneic blood transfusions.[151]

EPO therapy has also been investigated for the treatment of anemia in premature infants. Randomized clinical trials of EPO in very-low-birth-weight infants have shown that giving 250 IU/kg/day three times a week from day 3 to day 42, in addition to iron supplementation starting on day 14, resulted in reduced red blood cell transfusion requirements compared with the control group receiving iron therapy alone.[152] Other randomized trials have shown that early therapy with EPO before 7 days of age resulted in improved hemoglobin and reticulocyte counts but did not decrease transfusion needs, but EPO starting after 21 days did decrease transfusion requirements.[153] Early administration of EPO to very sick preterm infants was not effective in decreasing transfusion needs compared with the need of less sick infants.[154, 155]

The toxicity of EPO has been minimal, hypertension being the most significant side effect in patients with renal failure.[156] It is believed that hypertension is exacerbated by a rapid rise in hematocrit and can usually be prevented by careful monitoring of blood counts with appropriate EPO dose modification.[11] Iron deficiency may accompany anemia of chronic disease, cancer, or renal failure, and iron supplementation may improve the response to EPO.[157, 158] Predictors of response to EPO therapy include a low EPO level, usually less than 100 mU/mL, which is considered inadequate for the degree of anemia in cancer patients.[159] More accurate predictions can be made if one uses the ratio of the observed EPO level (O) to the expected EPO level (E), as seen in patients with an equivalent degree of anemia caused by iron deficiency or blood loss. Seventy per cent of patients with an O/E ratio less than 0.9 respond to EPO therapy.[160] Response can also be predicted with a higher degree of accuracy (>90%) when, after 2 weeks of EPO therapy, there is a hemoglobin increase of more than 0.5 g/dL and a serum EPO level less than 100 mU/mL.[161]

MACROPHAGE COLONY-STIMULATING FACTOR

M-CSF was the first myeloid CSF to be identified and was originally called CSF-1. M-CSF is produced by fibroblasts, endothelial cells, macrophages, and placental tissue.[100] M-CSF, unlike other myeloid CSFs, is not produced by T cells. The M-CSF gene was cloned[162] and the gene mapped to chromosome 1p13.21,[163] which encodes a protein with a molecular weight of 14.5 kD. However, the biologically active protein exists as a homodimer that is variably glycosylated and has a molecular weight of 47 to 90 kD.

M-CSF induces the proliferation and differentiation of committed monocyte/macrophage progenitor cells. M-CSF also enhances the function of mature monocyte/macrophages, which continue to express receptors for this relatively lineage-specific cytokine. The M-CSF is the product of the *fms* proto-oncogene.[164] Mutations in this receptor can lead to dysregulated growth of cells and oncogenesis.

The effects of M-CSF on mature monocytes have been well studied. M-CSF enhances intracellular killing of *Mycobacterium avium-intracellulare* and *Candida albicans* as well as ADCC and tumoricidal activity of macrophages.[165] M-CSF stimulates the production and release of IL-1, TNF, G-CSF, interferon, ferritin, plasminogen activator, thromboplastin, prostaglandins, and superoxide dismutase.[166] M-CSF also enhances the expansion of a $CD16^+$ monocyte phenotype in patients with metastatic cancer, which was greater than the response seen in normal volunteers.[167] The effects of M-CSF on erythropoiesis have been studied in patients with chronic renal failure and severe anemia.[168] Compared with healthy adult volunteers, patients had higher M-CSF levels. In vitro cultures of bone marrow progenitors showed no difference between the BFU-E counts in patients and control subjects; however, the CFU-E number was significantly lower in patients. The addition of M-CSF to cell cultures suppressed both BFU-E and CFU-E cells in patients but enhanced cell growth in control subjects. The in vivo effects of M-CSF on erythroid progenitors are not yet clear, but M-CSF may increase the existing decreased sensitivity of erythroid progenitors to EPO.

Clinical trials utilizing M-CSF are lagging behind those using G-CSF and GM-CSF. Komiyama and coworkers[169] reported an increase in leukocyte and neutrophil counts in neutropenic children treated for 7 days with purified urinary M-CSF. Motoyoshi and associates[170] treated 24 patients with urinary M-CSF after chemotherapy and demonstrated a decrease in the duration of the neutrophil nadir compared with that after albumin treatment, although fever was a significant side effect in the M-CSF group. Nemunaitis and coworkers[171] reported the results of a phase I trial of recombinant human M-CSF in patients with invasive fungal infections who received BMT. Analysis of the long-term outcome of 46 patients treated with M-CSF and standard antifungal therapy has shown that thrombocytopenia was the only toxicity and was seen with higher doses. M-CSF was well tolerated at doses up to 2000 $\mu g/m^2/d$. Overall survival was increased to 39% but less than 20% in the historical control population. However, survival correlated with the score of Karnofsky performance and the specific type of fungal infection. A score of 20% or higher was associated with improved survival, and patients with *Candida* infection and a Karnofsky performance of 20% or higher had better survival (50%) than patients with *Aspergillus* infection (20%).

M-CSF has also been evaluated in a phase I trial in combination with R24, a mouse monoclonal antibody against GD3 ganglioside that has been shown to localize to melanoma tumors.[172] Monocytosis occurred in all patients, with increased expression of human leukocyte antigen HLA-DR and decreased expression of CD14, a subtype active in ADCC. Some patients had tumor regression and improved survival, but further trials are needed to investigate this potential cellular immune application.[172]

INTERLEUKIN-11

IL-11 is a multifunctional growth factor initially cloned in 1990 from the primate stromal cell line PU-34.[173] It is characterized as a 199-amino acid polypeptide, encoded by a 7-kb gene that contains five exons and four introns and is located on chromosome 19q13.3.[174] In synergy with other early and late growth factors, IL-11 stimulates in vitro proliferation of primitive stem cells and multipotent and committed progenitor cells from different sources, including cord blood,[175] bone marrow,[175, 176] and peripheral blood.[177] It appears to exert its effect by increasing the number of cells entering into active cell cycle[178] and by shortening the cell cycle time.[179]

In combination with IL-3, TPO, or SCF, IL-11 stimulates various stages of megakaryocytopoiesis and thrombocytopoiesis, including both the production and maturation of megakaryocytes.[180–182] In combination with SCF, IL-11 enhances CFU-GM formation from $CD34^+$ cells isolated from cord blood and adult bone marrow.[175] IL-11 can stimulate erythroid progenitors in vitro in combination with IL-3, even in the absence of EPO.[183] IL-11 and its receptor are also expressed on epithelial cells of the gastrointestinal tract.[184, 185] In vitro studies showed that IL-11 can reversibly inhibit the proliferation of intestinal crypt cell lines.[185, 186]

Cairo and colleagues[187] showed that the administration of IL-11 to newborn rats before experimental group B streptococcal sepsis resulted in a significant increase in the circulating platelet count without affecting red or white blood cell counts and was associated with a decreased mortality rate. Cairo and coworkers[188] also demonstrated that the combination of IL-11 and G-CSF acts synergistically in increasing the circulating neutrophil count while maintaining an increase in the circulating platelet count.

IL-11 accelerates platelet and myeloid recovery and decreases mortality and morbidity resulting from experimental *Pseudomonas aeruginosa* sepsis in mice after myeloablative therapy and bone marrow transplantation.[189, 190] Du and coworkers[189, 191] reported that in transplanted mice, rhIL-11 decreased the time of platelet and ANC recovery from 18 to 14 days and from 15 to 10 days, respectively. Lethally irradiated mice transplanted with syngeneic bone marrow cells infected with a retrovirus expressing the human IL-11 complementary DNA (cDNA) demonstrated accelerated recovery of circulating platelets and red and white blood cells.[192] One study has shown that ectopic expression of murine IL-11 via a retrovirus vector accelerated platelet and ANC recovery in secondary and tertiary BMT mice and that IL-11 expression in vivo appears to enhance maintenance of primitive hematopoietic stem cells.[193]

In animal studies in which IL-11 was used after radiation- or chemotherapy-induced gastrointestinal mucosal damage, pretreatment of mice with IL-11 followed by irradiation was associated with significant increases in the survival of intestinal crypt stem cells.[194] This effect may be due to inhibition of crypt cell proliferation, which was demonstrated in vitro.[185] In mice receiving 5-fluorouracil (5-FU) and sublethal radiotherapy, IL-11 therapy significantly decreased morbidity and mortality related to sepsis by endogenous gut organisms and enhanced the recovery of small intestinal mucosal cells; these findings suggest that IL-11 may also stimulate the epithelial cell after cytotoxic therapy. In a hamster model of oral mucositis, IL-11 decreased the severity and duration of mucositis in a dose-dependent fashion.[195]

The ability of IL-11 to attenuate acute inflammatory processes was demonstrated in several animal models.[196-198] In a mouse model of endotoxemia, pretreatment with rhIL-11 blocked elevated TNF-α, IL-1β, and interferon-γ (INF-γ) serum levels in a dose-dependent manner after LPS administration. The anti-inflammatory effect of IL-11 on both murine and rabbit models of endotoxemia appears to be due to down-regulation of proinflammatory cytokine production and nitric oxide release through effects on macrophages.[199]

In children undergoing myeloablative therapy, Cairo and colleagues[197] demonstrated a significant inverse correlation between circulating platelet counts and IL-11 levels.[197] In a phase I trial in adults receiving cyclophosphamide and doxorubicin for stage 3B or stage 4 breast cancer, rhIL-11 administered subcutaneously once daily was well tolerated at doses of 10, 25, and 50 μg/kg/day.[200] Higher doses were associated with grade II constitutional symptoms (fatigue, myalgia, or arthralgia). Other adverse effects of rhIL-11 were reversible, including mild edema and dilutional anemia. At doses of 25 μg/kg/day, rhIL-11 appeared to reduce the degree of chemotherapy-induced thrombocytopenia.[200]

A randomized, placebo-controlled phase II trial of rhIL-11 at 25 and 50 μg/kg/day in adult cancer patients with a history of severe thrombocytopenia secondary to chemotherapy was performed.[175] Patients had a variety of malignancies and received a variety of chemotherapy regimens. RhIL-11 or placebo was administered daily subcutaneously beginning 1 day after completion of chemotherapy and continuing for 14 to 21 days or until the platelet count reached more than 100,000/mm^3. The most significant side effects were transient atrial arrhythmias, edema, and headache. This pivotal study demonstrated that rhIL-11 significantly increases the likelihood of avoiding platelet transfusion during the subsequent cycle of chemotherapy. Thirty per cent of the patients randomized to receive rhIL-11 at 50 μg/kg/day avoided a platelet transfusion, compared with 4% of the patients randomized to receive placebo.[175]

In another randomized, placebo-controlled study of women with breast cancer receiving dose-intensive cyclophosphamide and doxorubicin plus G-CSF, rhIL-11 was administered subcutaneously at a dose of 50 μg/kg/day for 10 to 17 days or until the platelet count was more than 50,000/mm^3.[201] The patients were given transfusions for platelet count below 20,000/mm^3. The rhIL-11 was generally well tolerated and produced mild to moderate adverse effects, most likely related to fluid retention. Sixty-eight per cent of the patients randomized to receive rhIL-11 did not require platelet transfusions, compared with 41% of the patients randomized to receive placebo. The study demonstrated that rhIL-11 accelerates platelet recovery and significantly decreases the number of platelet transfusions after dose-intensive chemotherapy, allowing maintenance of planned doses over repeated cycles.[201]

Preliminary results of an ongoing phase I and phase II study of rhIL-11 plus G-CSF following ifosfamide, carboplatin, and etoposide (ICE) chemotherapy in pediatric patients with solid tumors or lymphoma have been reported.[202] IL-11 was administered subcutaneously once a day at escalating doses of 25, 50, 75, and 100 μg/kg/day. This first pediatric clinical trial demonstrated that rhIL-11 was well tolerated, and there was no evidence of grade III or grade IV toxicity at double (100 μg/kg/day) the recommended adult dose of 50 μg/kg/day. In comparison with the historical control administration of G-CSF (5 μg/kg/day) alone, the combination of IL-11 (100 μg/kg/day) and G-CSF appeared to decrease the median time for platelet and ANC recovery after ICE chemotherapy from 27 to 19 days and 22 to 17 days, respectively.[203, 204] The percentage of patients whose platelets recovered by day 21 and the median number of platelet transfusions after ICE chemotherapy also compared favorably with the historical control with G-CSF alone: 67% versus 25% and six versus two platelet transfusions.

The study also demonstrated that the combination of rhIL-11 and G-CSF increased significantly the subsets of early (CD34$^+$, CD34$^+$/38$^+$, CD34$^+$/38$^-$, CD34$^+$/DR$^+$) and committed (CD34$^+$/41$^+$) progenitor cells, as well as the cells expressing IL-3 and GM-CSF receptors in peripheral blood at the time of myeloid recovery after ICE chemotherapy, compared with baseline values. The levels of proinflammatory cytokines IL-1α, IL-1β, IL-6, TNF-α, and IFN-γ did not increase after the administration of rhIL-11 in this pediatric trial. We speculated that the combination of IL-11 plus G-CSF may enhance earlier platelet recovery and decrease platelet transfusion by inducing both early and committed subsets of progenitors along the megakaryocytic lineage and potentially induce a subset of cells that respond to other endogenous cytokine stimulation.[202]

The FDA has approved rhIL-11 (Neumega) for the prevention of chemotherapy-induced severe thrombocytopenia and reduction of the need for platelet transfusions after myelosuppressive chemotherapy in patients with nonmyeloid malignancies who are at risk for severe thrombocytopenia. The manufacturer's recommended adult dose is 50 μg/kg/day and the pediatric dose 75 to 100 μg/kg/day.

THROMBOPOIETIN

The ligand for the c-*mpl* receptor, a critical regulator of megakaryopoiesis, was cloned in 1994 by five different groups.[205-209] Thrombopoietin is also known as c-*mpl* ligand, megapoietin, and megakaryocyte growth and developmental factor (MGDF) (truncated version of thrombopoietin). The cDNA for human TPO encodes a molecule containing 322 amino acids; the carboxy-terminal domain is important in stabilizing the molecule in the circulation and the amino-terminal domain is 23% identical to EPO. The gene for TPO is located on chromosome 3q27-28.[210]

TPO is the primary hematopoietic growth factor that supports the growth of megakaryocytic colonies. Preclinical experiments have shown that TPO supports the growth of murine and human megakaryocytes,[211-213] causing an increase in the size of cultured megakaryocytes, increased ploidy, and increased expression of glycoprotein Ib and IIb/IIIa on the cell surface.[182] Platelets cultured in vitro demonstrated normal function in the presence of adenosine diphosphate (ADP) or thrombin.[214] Other investigators have compared the effects of TPO with those of other thrombopoietic cytokines such as IL-3, IL-11, and IL-6 on the growth of megakaryocytes. TPO was the only growth factor found to be crucial for the development of megakaryocytes and platelets. Neutralizing TPO by the addition of a soluble Mpl resulted in failure of development of mature megakaryocytes when IL-3, IL-6, and IL-11 were added to the culture, which suggests that the in vivo effects of those cytokines are TPO-dependent.[215]

The effects of TPO on the growth of other hematopoietic cells were also studied. Yoshida and coworkers[216] reported that when TPO was used as a single agent in serum-free cultures of cord blood CD34+ cells, TPO alone supported the generation of megakaryocyte colonies as well as of blast colonies that differentiated into CFU-GM, BFU-E, and CFU-GEMM when IL-3, IL-6, SCF, EPO, GM-CSF, and TPO were added on day 7 of culture. Other investigators have reported on the synergistic effect between TPO and early-acting cytokines, such as SCF, IL-3, IL-11, and G-CSF, in in vitro hematopoiesis.[217–219]

The role of TPO in the regulation of megakaryopoiesis has been studied in patients with different hematologic conditions compared with normal control subjects.[197, 220] TPO levels were found to be considerably elevated in patients with thrombocytopenia secondary to bone marrow hypoplasia undergoing myeloablative therapy for BMT or patients with severe AA. However, TPO levels in patients with immune thrombocytopenia characterized by increased platelet destruction were not elevated compared with those in the control group. Patients with idiopathic thrombocytopenic purpura (ITP) have increases in megakaryocyte progenitor cells, megakaryocytes, and platelet production, with an increase in the total number of cells expressing Mpl receptors, resulting in increased binding of TPO and lower levels in the circulation.[197]

Several clinical trials have investigated the in vivo effects of TPO. Two preparations of TPO have been developed:

- Peg-rHuMGDF (Amgen), in which polyethylene glycol is added to a truncated form of Mpl-L to increase in vivo stability
- rhTPO, a full-length recombinant human form of mpl-L

Clinical phase I trials evaluating the effects of MGDF after chemotherapy have been completed.[221] MGDF, in combination with G-CSF, was administered to patients after myelosuppressive chemotherapy. MGDF resulted in an elevation in platelet counts without an adverse effect on red blood cells or white blood cells. The response to MGDF was dose-related, with an earlier increase in platelet counts when higher doses of MGDF were used. Patients who received MGDF before chemotherapy and after chemotherapy had more rapid platelet recovery. The rise in platelet count was seen in 8 to 10 days and maximum levels were seen at 12 to 18 days.

Fanucchi and colleagues[222] reported the results of a double-blind, placebo-controlled dose escalation trial of MGDF in 53 patients with lung cancer treated with carboplatin. Higher platelet nadirs and earlier platelet recovery (14 versus 21 days) were observed in the MGDF group compared with the control group. MGDF has been well tolerated with no reported adverse effects.

The effects of MGDF on mobilization of bone marrow progenitor cells have also been studied. MGDF causes an increase in the number of bone marrow megakaryocytes without affecting other bone marrow progenitors. In contrast, there was a dose-dependent increase in the peripheral blood progenitor cells, including CFU-GM, BFU-E, and CFU-Meg.[223] Maximum mobilization occurred at day 12, with the earliest increase seen by day 8. Further studies are required to determine the optimal dose and schedule of administration of MGDF or TPO in combination with G-CSF.

The use of MGDF to stimulate donors for plateletpheresis and enhanced platelet function and survival is also under investigation. Ex vivo expansion of megakaryocyte progenitors has deen studied in a clinical trial of autologous PBPC transplantation.[224] MGDF was used in combination with SCF, IL-3, IL-6, IL-11, FL, and macrophage inflammatory protein 1α. The expanded product was well tolerated by patients and contained an increased percentage of megakaryocyte progenitors. Further trials are needed to evaluate the appropriate dose of Mpl ligand to decrease platelet transfusions and enhance ex vivo expansion in recipients of allogeneic BMT or cord blood transplants. Another potential clinical application that warrants investigation is the use of TPO or MGDF after allogeneic BMT to enhance platelet recovery.[225]

INTERLEUKIN-3

IL-3 was first purified from the WEHI-3B cell line[226] and is a monomeric glycoprotein with a molecular weight of 28 kD.[227] The gene was cloned in 1986[228] and mapped to chromosome 5q23.31 near the GM-CSF gene.[229] Unlike other CSF genes, the murine and human IL-3 genes have only minimal homology (29%), which explains the protein's relative species specificity despite the similarity of biologic properties. IL-3 has an extremely broad range of target cells, including neutrophil, eosinophil, basophil, monocyte, megakaryocyte, and erythrocyte precursors (see Fig. 45–1). IL-3 is produced by activated T cells, monocytes, and natural killer cells. The IL-3 receptor is part of the cytokine receptor family. Overexpression of IL-3 in an experimental murine gene transfer model leads to a myeloproliferative disorder, raising questions about the importance of IL-3 gene regulation during normal hematopoiesis.

IL-3 acts on a broad range of target cells and their progenitors (see Fig. 45–1), and synergism with other growth factors is well documented in murine and human models of hematopoiesis. The combination of IL-3 and GM-CSF has been shown to stimulate megakaryocyte progenitors.[230] Other IL-3 combinations can stimulate T and B lymphocyte growth as well as mast cell and eosinophil function.[166] IL-3 can affect mature cell function in a manner similar to that of other CSFs. IL-3 has been shown to increase monocyte tumoricidal activity via increased TNF-α production, IL-1 activity, ADCC, and antigen expression.[100]

Several reports of IL-3 activity in animals have demonstrated the effects of IL-3 in ameliorating myelosuppressive toxicity of chemotherapy, increasing progenitor cells in peripheral blood, and augmenting multiple hematopoietic lineages after prolonged IL-3 treatment.[231] The combination of IL-3 and IL-6 stimulates stem cell cycling in the mouse[232] as well as in humans in in vitro assays.[233] Thrombopoiesis in primates was increased after sequential administration of IL-3 and IL-6 compared with IL-3 treatment alone.[234] Sequential IL-3 followed by GM-CSF led to a doubling of leukocyte counts in monkeys compared with control animals. These experiments suggest that IL-3 can act by priming multipotential progenitors for late-acting CSFs.

Clinical trials evaluating the postchemotherapeutic effects of IL-3 have been completed. A phase II trial investigating the role of IL-3 after chemotherapy in patients with SCLC showed that IL-3 significantly increased the platelet count nadir, shortened the duration of thrombocytopenia ($<$75,000/mm^3), and reduced the mean time to platelet recovery ($>$100,000/mm^3) compared with the control group.[235] The neutrophil nadir was increased and the time of neutropenia ($<$1000/mm^3) was significantly reduced.[235] The use of IL-3 in combination with G-CSF or GM-CSF after autologous BMT has also been evaluated. Sequential administration of IL-3 and GM-CSF resulted in neutrophil engraftment (ANC $\geq$ 1000/mm^3) by day 16, which was faster than the recovery after either GM-CSF or IL-3 alone. Platelet recovery time was also enhanced with a median time to platelet engraftment (≥20,000/mm³) of 15 days, which was significantly improved compared with the use of G-CSF, GM-CSF, or IL-3 as single therapy after autologous BMT. Lower IL-3 doses (2.5 μg/kg) are better tolerated than higher doses (5 μg/kg).[236]

Another clinical trial evaluated the use of IL-3 in combination with G-CSF after autologous BMT for malignant lymphoma. The addition of IL-3 resulted in enhanced neutrophil recovery (11 days for ANC ≥ 500/mm³), enhanced platelet recovery (15 days for platelets ≥ 20,000/mm³), lower transfusion requirements, and decreased infections and hospitalization time.[237]

The combination of IL-3 and G-CSF after chemotherapy has been used to mobilize patients who were extensively pretreated. The combination has been well tolerated, with adequate collection of numbers of CD34⁺ cells and early hematopoietic recovery.[238] The use of IL-3 as a single agent for patients with severe aplastic anemia had limited benefit, with only transient increases in the neutrophil count in 9 of 15 of patients treated.[239] The toxicity data from IL-3 trials show side effects similar to those of other CSFs, including headache, fever, bone pain, and myalgia.

IL-3 has also been used in combination with other hematopoietic growth factors during ex vivo expansion of hematopoietic progenitors to facilitate engraftment after transplantation. IL-3 was used in combination with SCF, IL-6, and EPO for the expansion of bone marrow progenitors and maintenance of long-term culture initiating cells (LTC-ICs).[95] Ex vivo expansion of human umbilical cord blood to increase the number of progenitors available for transplantation has also been studied using different combinations of cytokines IL-3, IL-6, SCF, FL, EPO, and G-CSF.[240] Expansion of megakaryocytic progenitors ex vivo to enhance platelet recovery has been studied using IL-3, MGDF, SCF, IL-6, G-CSF, and IL-11.[224] The optimal conditions for expansion of hematopoietic progenitors are still under investigation and need to be determined, and clinical trials evaluating the safety of these products are under way.

STEM CELL FACTOR

SCF is the ligand for the c-*kit* proto-oncogene.[241] This CSF is also known as mast cell growth factor, Kit ligand, and steel factor because it has been shown to be the product of the steel locus in the mouse.[242] It is a 26-kD protein that maps to chromosome 12q14.3-qter and 12q22-24.[243, 244] The gene locus for its receptor, c-*kit*, is located on chromosome 4q31-34.[245, 246]

SCF is produced by fibroblasts, marrow stromal cells, fetal liver cells, and other mesenchyme-derived cells. Mice with genetic mutations in the steel locus or c-*kit* gene (the SCF receptor) have a distinct abnormal phenotype characterized by macrocytic anemia, mast cell deficiency, and defects in melanocytosis and gametogenesis. The c-*kit* gene is expressed in a small percentage of myeloid and monocytic cells[247-250] but is highly expressed in erythroid and erythroleukemia cell lines,[247-249, 251] mast cells, and most megakaryocytic cells.[247, 249, 251] It is not expressed on lymphoid cells, lymphoma cells (B or T), lymphoid leukemia cells (pre-B, B, T), or myeloma cells. The c-*kit* receptor is also expressed on the blasts in acute myelogenous leukemia[252-260] and is seen on most cells of chronic myelogenous leukemia (CML) during blast crisis.[259]

The in vivo effects of SCF on mast cells have shown that SCF regulates the migration, maturation, proliferation, and activation of mast cells in vivo.[261] SCF promotes the growth of early erythroid progenitor cells (BFU-E) and, to a lesser extent, the more mature CFU-Es.[262-266] The effects of SCF on BFU-E require costimulation with EPO[135, 267-269] or combination with IL-6 and soluble IL-6 receptor.[270] SCF synergizes with TPO to regulate megakaryocyte and platelet production[271] and to stimulate multilineage hematopoietic stem cell growth.[218, 219, 272-274] In combination with IL-7, it can stimulate the development of B cell progenitors in murine models.[275-277] SCF, when combined with IL-7, IL-3, or IL-12, can enhance the growth of primitive (CD3⁻ CD4⁻ CD8⁻) thymocytes but not the more mature thymocyte populations.[278] SCF can enhance the development of natural killer cells from human bone marrow when used in combination with IL-2, IL-7, or IL-15 in in vitro studies.[279-281] Dendritic cell production from human CD34⁺ bone marrow or cord blood cells is enhanced when SCF and TNF-α are used with GM-CSF.[282-284]

Phase I and phase II clinical trials with rhSCF have been completed. Patients with advanced non–small-cell lung carcinoma (NSCLC) were given rhSCF for 14 days before chemotherapy, followed by an additional 14 days after chemotherapy. The most frequent adverse effects secondary to rhSCF were local skin reactions at the injection site, with edema, erythema, pruritus, skin hyperpigmentation, and urticaria, and, less frequently, systemic anaphylactoid reactions.[285] These effects are mostly related to the induction of mast cell hyperplasia by SCF and endogenous inflammatory mast cell mediator release.[286] The hematologic effects after rhSCF include a modest increase in the white blood cell and platelet counts. No changes in bone marrow cellularity, but at higher doses an increase in circulating BFU-E and CFU-GM has been seen after rhSCF.[285] The use of SCF in combination with G-CSF for PBPC mobilization in breast cancer patients was evaluated in a phase I and phase II trial. The use of SCF alone for mobilization resulted in a 10-fold decrease in CD34⁺ cell yield compared with the G-CSF group. There was a significant decrease in ANC and platelet recovery. However, the combination of SCF with G-CSF resulted in an enhanced mononuclear cell yield, a two- to threefold increase in CD34⁺ cell yield, and an increase in the CFU-GM and BFU-E compared with the G-CSF group. Both groups showed early ANC and platelet recovery.[287] Other clinical trials have reported similar results,[288, 289] with an increase in the more primitive progenitor cells (CD34⁺/CD38⁻) when SCF was used with G-CSF as compared with G-CSF alone.[290]

The use of SCF in combination with other HGFs during ex vivo expansion of hematopoietic progenitors has also been extensively studied. For optimal expansion, combinations of SCF with IL-1, IL-3, IL-6, GM-CSF, G-CSF, and EPO have been used.[271, 291, 292] SCF has also been used in combination with IL-3 and IL-6 as a promoter of retroviral transduction in human hematopoietic progenitor cells, resulting in efficient gene transfer to committed and primitive progenitors.[293-295]

FLT-3 LIGAND

Flt-3 ligand (FL) is the cognate ligand for the *fms*-like tyrosine kinase receptor 3 (flt-3).[296] FL is a 235-amino-acid glycoprotein and exists as either a membrane-bound or soluble protein isoform. The gene is located on chromosome 19q13. FL messenger RNA (mRNA) can be found in many tissue types including bone marrow stroma.[297] The receptor flt-3 is expressed principally on hematopoietic cells and has structural homology to the receptors for M-CSF (c-*fms*) and SCF (c-*kit*). In vitro FL, like SCF, has little hematopoietic activity of its own but synergizes with both early-acting and late-acting HGFs for cell survival and growth. FL acts on early hematopoietic activity including lymphoid progenitors.[298] FL has been shown to increase the growth of CFU-GM, CFU-GEMM, CFU-Meg, thymic precursors, and pro-B cells but not BFU-E or mast cells. Synergism can be dramatic, with fivefold to 30-fold expansions during in vitro cultures when FL is added to other cytokines.[299-301]

In vivo mouse models have shown that FL has hematopoi-

TABLE 45–2. Clinically Approved and Investigational Usage of Hematopoietic Growth Factors

HGF	Approved Clinical Indication	Investigational Therapies
G-CSF	Chemotherapy-induced febrile neutropenia Shorten the duration of neutropenia after myeloablative therapy Mobilization of PBSCs	SAA Ex vivo expansion of hematopoietic stem cells Neonatal sepsis
GM-CSF	After myeloablative therapy After induction chemotherapy in AML patients (phase III) Mobilization of PBSCs	HIV infection SAA MDS Tumor vaccines (phase I–II) Neonatal sepsis (phase III)
TPO	Pending	Mobilization of PBSC Post chemotherapy Post myeloablative therapy Mobilization of platelet donors Ex vivo expansion of stem cells
IL-11	After chemotherapy-induced severe thrombocytopenia in nonmyeloid malignancies	AML MDS GVHD Ex vivo expansion of stem cells Mucositis
EPO	Anemia of end-stage renal disease Cancer chemotherapy HIV infection Preoperative collection of autologous blood	Anemia of chronic disease (rheumatoid arthritis) Anemia of prematurity Post myeloablative chemotherapy Anemia of pregnancy MDS Perioperatively
FL	Pending	Mobilization of PBSCs Mobilization of DCs Ex vivo expansion of PBSCs and DCs

HGF = hematopoietic growth factor; G-CSF = granulocyte colony-stimulating factor; GM-CSF = granulocyte-macrophage CSF; TPO = thrombopoietin; IL-11 = interleukin-11; EPO = erythropoietin; FL = Flt 3 ligand. PBSC = peripheral blood stem cell; DC = dendritic cell; SAA = severe aplastic anemia; MDS = myelodysplastic syndrome; GVHD = graft-versus-host disease; HIV = human immunodeficiency virus; AML = acute myelocytic leukemia.

etic activity as a single agent and can synergize with other cytokines. FL increases the peripheral blood white blood cell count, monocyte count, and subpopulations of dendritic cells. Spleen and marrow cellularity is also increased. Spleen and marrow studies showed increases up to 123-fold in CFU-GEMM and CFU-GM. When combined with G-CSF, FL increased peripheral blood CFU-GM 100-fold.

Because of the noted increases in the otherwise rare dendritic cell lineage, FL has been explored as an adjuvant to immunotherapy for cancer. When injected within 4 days before a tumor challenge, FL can protect mice from tumor or leukemic growth; when the tumor cells are genetically engineered to express FL, the mice become immune to all subsequent tumor challenges.[302, 303] Although FL and flt-3 can be found on malignant hematopoietic cells and can induce in vitro cell growth in select AML cells, FL also protects mice against a leukemic challenge. Notably, malignant B cells express high levels of FL and flt-3 and are not responsive to FL-induced proliferation.[304]

Human phase I trials have been initiated and preliminary data show increases in peripheral blood dendritic cells and monocytes.[289] The only adverse effects noted to date have been enlarged lymph nodes. Future trials are needed to determine whether FL can act as a mobilizer of peripheral blood stem cells, an ex vivo expander of stem and immune cells, and/or an immunotherapeutic agent.

SUMMARY

The use of hematopoietic growth factors has been extensively studied over the past few years. FDA approval for the use of G-CSF, GM-CSF, IL-11, and EPO has been achieved (Table 45–2). G-CSF and GM-CSF are currently recommended for use after chemotherapeutic regimens with increased risk of febrile neutropenia or after myeloablative chemotherapy for BMT. The use of GM-CSF and G-CSF for mobilization of peripheral blood stems and bone marrow donors is also recommended to enhance hematopoietic recovery and decrease morbidity after transplantation. Beneficial effects of GM-CSF and G-CSF have also been shown in patients with severe aplastic anemia and in patients with AIDS undergoing therapy. The use of GM-CSF and G-CSF in neonates has also been investigated in phase I and phase II trials. Increased neutrophil counts and function were demonstrated, with a reduced incidence of nosocomial infections with GM-CSF use.

Thrombopoietin, a cloned growth factor, has been tested in phase I and phase II clinical trials. Early platelet recovery with higher nadirs was achieved. TPO has also been used for mobilization of bone marrow progenitors and in donors before plateletpheresis. IL-11 has been approved by the FDA for severe thrombocytopenia secondary to chemotherapy, and EPO has been approved for amelioration of the anemia of end-stage renal disease, after cancer chemotherapy, for AIDS patients, and to enhance autologous blood collections.

Several phase I and phase II trials evaluating the use of FL, M-CSF, IL-3, and TPO are still ongoing. The optimal HGF combination for mobilization or ex vivo expansion of stem cells needs to be determined. Use of hematopoietic growth factors in cancer immunotherapy and development of tumor vaccines is still under extensive investigation. Recommendations regarding the use of hematopoietic growth fac-

tors in specific hematologic and nonhematologic diseases have been established. More clinical research is required to evaluate the possible clinical applications of newly discovered hematopoietic growth factors and new clinical indications for currently approved CSFs.

ACKNOWLEDGMENTS

The authors would like to thank Linda Rahl for her editorial assistance in the preparation of the manuscript. We also thank Elizabeth S. Dodson for her help in preparing the tables and figure. Supported in part by the Pediatric Cancer Research Foundation and the Walden W. and Jean Young Shaw Foundation.

References

1. Update of recommendations for the use of hematopoietic colony-stimulating factors: Evidence-based clinical practice guidelines. J Clin Oncol 1996; 14:1957.
2. American Society of Clinical Oncology recommendations for the use of hematopoietic colony-stimulating factors: Evidence-based, clinical practice guidelines. J Clin Oncol 1994; 12:2471.
3. Glaspy J, Davis MW, Parker WR, et al: Biology and clinical potential of stem-cell factor. Cancer Chemother Pharmacol 1996; 38:53.
4. Ogawa M, Johnson R: Differentiation and proliferation of hematopoietic stem cells. Blood 1993; 81:2844.
5. Spangrude GJ, Heimfeld S, Weissman IL: Purification and characterization of mouse hematopoietic stem cells. Science 1988; 241:58.
6. Furman WL, Crist WM: Potential uses of recombinant human granulocyte-macrophage colony-stimulating factor in children. Am J Pediatr Hematol Oncol 1991; 13:388.
7. Gasson JC: Molecular physiology of granulocyte-macrophage colony-stimulating factor. Blood 1991; 77:1131.
8. Weisbart RH, Golde DW: Physiology of granulocyte and macrophage colony-stimulating factors in host defense. Hematol Oncol Clin North Am 1989; 3:401.
9. Devereux S, Linch DC, Campos Costa D: Transient leucopenia induced by GM-CSF. Lancet 1987; ii:1523.
10. Guinan EC, Sieff CA, Oette DH, et al: A phase I/II trial of recombinant granulocyte-macrophage colony-stimulating factor for children with aplastic anemia. Blood 1990; 76:1077.
11. Groopman JE, Molina JM, Scadden DT: Hematopoietic growth factors: Biology and clinical applications. N Engl J Med 1989; 321:1449.
12. Denzlinger C, Tetzloff W, Gerhartz HH, et al: Differential activation of the endogenous leukotriene biosynthesis by two different preparations of granulocyte-macrophage colony-stimulating factor in healthy volunteers. Blood 1993; 81:2007.
13. Lieschke GJ, Grail D, Hodgson G: Mice lacking granulocyte colony stimulating factor have chronic neutropenia, granulocyte and macrophage progenitor cell deficiency, and impaired neutrophil mobilization. Blood 1994; 84:1737.
14. Dorr RT: Clinical properties of yeast-derived versus *Escherichia coli*-derived granulocyte-macrophage colony-stimulating factor. Clin Ther 1993; 15(1):19.
15. Cairo MS, Christensen R, Sender LS: Results of a phase I/II trial of recombinant human granulocyte-macrophage colony-stimulating factor in very low birthweight neonates: Significant induction of circulatory neutrophils, monocytes, platelets and bone marrow neutrophils. Blood 1995; 86:2509.
16. Cairo MS, Seth T, Fanaroff A, et al: A double blinded, randomized, placebo (P) controlled pilot study of RhGM-CSF (GM) in low birth weight neonates (LBWN): Preliminary results demonstrate a significant reduction in nosocomial infections with RhuGM-CSF. Pediatr Res 1996; 39:294a.
17. Nissen C, Tichelli A, Gratwohl A, et al: Failure of recombinant human granulocyte-macrophage colony-stimulating factor therapy in aplastic anemia patients with very severe neutropenia. Blood 1988; 72:2045.
18. Doney K, Storb R, Appelbaum FR, et al: Recombinant granulocyte-macrophage colony stimulating factor followed by immunosuppressive therapy for aplastic anaemia. Br J Haematol 1993; 85(1):182.
19. Hord JD, Gay JC, Whitlock JA, et al: Long-term granulocyte-macrophage colony-stimulating factor and immunosuppression in the treatment of acquired severe aplastic anemia. J Pediatr Hematol Oncol 1995; 17(2):140.
20. Lopez-Karpovitch X, Ulloa-Aguirre A, von Eiff C, et al: Treatment of methimazole-induced severe aplastic anemia with recombinant human granulocyte-monocyte colony-stimulating factor and glucocorticosteroids. Acta Haematol 1992; 87(3):148.
21. Bunin N, Leahey A, Kamani N, et al: Bone marrow transplantation in pediatric patients with severe aplastic anemia: Cyclophosphamide and anti-thymocyte globulin conditioning followed by recombinant human granulocyte-macrophage colony stimulating factor. J Pediatr Hematol Oncol 1996; 18(1):68.
22. Geller RB: Use of cytokines in the treatment of acute myelocytic leukemia: A critical review. J Clin Oncol 1996; 14:1371.
23. Schiffer CA: Hematopoietic growth factors as adjuncts to the treatment of acute myeloid leukemia. Blood 1996; 88:3675.
24. Lowenberg B, Suciu S, Archimbaud E, et al: Use of recombinant granulocyte-macrophage colony-stimulating factor during and after remission induction chemotherapy in patients aged 61 years and older with acute myeloid leukemia (AML): Final report of AML-11, a phase III randomized study of the Leukemia Cooperative Group of European Organisation for the Research and Treatment of Cancer (ORTC-LCG) and the Dutch Belgian Hemato-Oncology Cooperative Group (HOVON). Blood 1997; 90:2952.
25. Gradishar WJ, Le Beau MM, O'Laughlin R, et al: Clinical and cytogenetic responses to granulocyte-macrophage colony-stimulating factor in therapy-related myelodysplasia. Blood 1992; 80:2463.
26. Yoshida Y, Nakahata T, Shibata A, et al: Effects of long-term treatment with recombinant human granulocyte-macrophage colony-stimulating factor in patients with myelodysplastic syndrome. Leuk Lymphoma 1995; 18:457.
27. Nand S, Sosman J, Godwin JE, et al: A phase I/II study of sequential interleukin-3 and granulocyte-macrophage colony-stimulating factor in myelodysplastic syndromes. Blood 1994; 83:357.
28. Gerhartz HH, Engelhard M, Meusers P, et al: Randomized, double-blind, placebo-controlled, phase III study of recombinant human granulocyte-macrophage colony-stimulating factor as adjunct to induction treatment of high-grade malignant non-Hodgkin's lymphomas. Blood 1993; 82:2329.
29. Burdach SE, Muschenich M, Josephs W, et al: Granulocyte-macrophage-colony stimulating factor for prevention of neutropenia and infections in children and adolescents with solid tumors. Results of a prospective randomized study. Cancer 1995; 76:510.
30. Bunn PA, Crowley J, Kelly K, et al: Chemoradiotherapy with or without granulocyte-macrophage colony-stimulating factor in the treatment of limited-stage small-cell lung cancer: A prospective phase III randomized study of the Southwest Oncology Group. J Clin Oncol 1995; 13:1632.
31. Bajorin DF, Nichols CR, Schmoll HJ, et al: Recombinant human granulocyte-macrophage colony-stimulating factor as an adjunct to conventional-dose ifosfamide-based chemotherapy for patients with advanced or relapsed germ cell tumors: A randomized trial. J Clin Oncol 1995; 13:79.
32. Steward WP, von Pawel J, Gatzemeier U, et al: Effects of granulocyte-macrophage colony-stimulating factor and dose intensification of V-ICE chemotherapy in small-cell lung cancer: A prospective randomized study of 300 patients. J Clin Oncol 1998; 16:642.
33. Nemunaitis J, Rabinowe SN, Singer JW, et al: Recombinant granulocyte-macrophage colony-stimulating factor after autologous bone marrow transplantation for lymphoid cancer. N Engl J Med 1991; 324:1773.
34. Nemunaitis J, Rosenfeld CS, Ash R, et al: Phase III randomized, double-blind placebo-controlled trial of rhGM-CSF following allogeneic bone marrow transplantation. Bone Marrow Transplant 1995; 15:949.
35. Bishop MR, Anderson JR, Jackson JD, et al: High-dose therapy and peripheral blood progenitor cell transplantation: Effects of

recombinant human granulocyte-macrophage colony-stimulating factor on the autograft. Blood 1994; 83:610.
36. Groopman JE, Mitsuyasu RT, DeLeo MJ, et al: Effect of recombinant human granulocyte-macrophage colony-stimulating factor on myelopoiesis in the acquired immunodeficiency syndrome. N Engl J Med 1987; 317:593.
37. Kaplan LD, Kahn JO, Crowe S, et al: Clinical and virologic effects of recombinant human granulocyte-macrophage colony-stimulating factor in patients receiving chemotherapy for human immunodeficiency virus–associated non-Hodgkin's lymphoma: Results of a randomized trial. J Clin Oncol 1991; 9:929.
38. Gill PS, Mitsuyasu RT, Montgomery T, et al: AIDS Clinical Trials Group Study 094: A phase I/II trial of ABV chemotherapy with zidovudine and recombinant human GM-CSF in AIDS-related Kaposi's sarcoma. Cancer J Sci Am 1997; 3(5):273.
39. Hart DNJ: Dendritic cells: Unique leukocyte populations which control the primary immune response. Blood 1997; 90:3245.
40. Bracho F, van de Ven C, Qian JX, et al: The use of autologous plasma to ex vivo generate allostimulatory dendritic cells (DC) from cord blood (CB) mononuclear cells stimulated with Flt3-ligand, GM-CSF, TNFa, IL-4. Proc Am Assoc Cancer Res 1998; 39:354.
41. Romani N, Reider D, Heuer M, et al: Generation of mature dendritic cells from human blood: An improved method with special regard to clinical applicability. J Immunol Methods 1996; 196:137.
42. Kiertsher S, Roth M: Human CD14[+] leukocytes acquire the phenotype and function of antigen-presenting dendritic cells when cultured in GM-CSF and IL-4. J Leukoc Biol 1996; 59:208.
43. Shurin MR: Dendritic cells presenting tumor antigen. Cancer Immunol Immunother 1996; 43:158.
44. Mayordomo JI, Zorina T, Storkus WJ, et al: Bone marrow–derived dendritic cells pulsed with synthetic tumour peptides elicit protective and therapeutic antitumour immunity. Nat Med 1995; 1:1297.
45. Dunussi-Joannopoulos K, Dranoff G, Weinstein HJ, et al: Gene immunotherapy in murine acute myeloid leukemia: Granulocyte-macrophage colony-stimulating factor tumor cell vaccines elicit more potent antitumor immunity compared with B7 family and other cytokine vaccines. Blood 1998; 91:222.
46. Wang J, Yang WK, Yang Y, et al: Paradoxical effect of GM-CSF gene transfer on the tumorigenicity and immunogenicity of murine tumors. Int J Cancer 1998; 75:459.
47. Mahvi DM, Sondel PM, Albertini MR, et al: Phase I/IB study of immunization with autologous tumor cells transfected with the GM-CSF gene by particle-mediated transfer in patients with melanoma or sarcoma. Hum Gene Ther 1997; 8:875.
48. Soiffer R, Lynch T, Mihm M: Effects of interleukin-3 fusion protein on chemotherapy-induced multi-lineage myelosuppression in patients with sarcoma. J Clin Oncol 1994; 12:715.
49. Rankin EM, Kremers B, Gallee M: Immunomodulation following vaccination with autologous, GM-CSF transduced and irradiated tumor cells in patients with advanced melanoma (Abstract). Proc Am Soc Clin Oncol 1997; 16:489.
50. Nicola NA, Metcalf D, Matsumoto M, et al: Purification of a factor inducing differentiation in murine myelomonocytic leukemia cells: Identification as granulocyte-colony-stimulating factor. J Biol Chem 1983; 258:9017.
51. Welte K, Platzer E, Lu L, et al: Purification and biochemical characterization of human pluripotent hematopoietic colony-stimulating factor. Proc Natl Acad Sci U S A 1985; 82:1526.
52. Nagata S, Tsuchiya M, Asano S, et al: Molecular cloning and expression of cDNA for human granulocyte colony-stimulating factor. Nature 1986; 319:415.
53. Simmers RN, Webber LM, Shannon MF, et al: Localization of the G-CSF gene on chromosome 17 proximal to the breakpoint in the t(15;17) in acute promyelocytic leukemia. Blood 1987; 70:330.
54. Lieschke GJ, Burgess AW: Granulocyte colony-stimulating factor and granulocyte-macrophage colony-stimulating factor. N Engl J Med 1992; 327:28.
55. Demetri G, Griffin J: Granulocyte colony-stimulating factor and its receptor. Blood 1991; 78:2791.
56. Pajkrt D, van Deventer SJH: Is G-CSF safe and useful in the treatment of infectious diseases in the non-neutropenic host? Intensive Care Med 1997; 23:1.
57. Cairo MS, Suen Y, Sender L, et al: Circulating granulocyte colony-stimulating factor (G-CSF) levels after allogeneic and autologous bone marrow transplantation: Endogenous G-CSF production correlates with myeloid engraftment. Blood 1992; 79:1869.
58. Welte K, Bonilla MA, Gillio AP, et al: Recombinant human granulocyte colony-stimulating factor effects on hematopoiesis in normal and cyclophosphamide-treated primates. J Exp Med 1987; 165:941.
59. Lopez AF, Nicola NA, Burgess AW, et al: Activation of granulocyte cytotoxic function by purified mouse colony-stimulating factors. J Immunol 1983; 131:2983.
60. Bodey G, Buckley M, Sathe YS, et al: Quantitative relationship between circulating leukocytes and infection in patients with acute leukemia. Ann Intern Med 1966; 64:328.
61. Crawford J, Ozer H, Stoller R, et al: Reduction by granulocyte colony-stimulating factor of fever and neutropenia induced by chemotherapy in patients with small-cell lung cancer. N Engl J Med 1991; 325:164.
62. Weinthal J, Gillan E, Hodder F, et al: G-CSF significantly reduces the nadir of neutropenia, hospitalizations, and costs during intensive chemotherapy in children with solid tumors (Abstract). Proc Am Soc Clin Oncol 1992; 11:362.
63. Glisson B, Komaki R, Lee JS, et al: Integration of filgrastim into chemoradiation for limited small cell lung cancer: A phase I study. Int J Radiat Oncol 1998; 40:331.
64. Geissler K, Koller E, Hubmann E, et al: Granulocyte colony-stimulating factor as an adjunct to induction chemotherapy for adult acute lymphoblastic leukemia—a randomized phase III study. Blood 1990; 90:590.
65. Pui C-H, Boyett JM, Hughes WT, et al: Human granulocyte colony-stimulating factor after induction chemotherapy in children with acute lymphoblastic leukemia. N Engl J Med 1997; 336:1781.
66. Hartmann LC, Tschetter LK, Habermann TM, et al: Granulocyte colony-stimulating factor in severe chemotherapy-induced afebrile neutropenia. N Engl J Med 1997; 336:1776.
67. Fossa SD, Kaye SB, Mead GM, et al: Filgrastim during combination chemotherapy of patients with poor-prognosis metastatic germ cell malignancy. J Clin Oncol 1998; 16:716.
68. Heil G, Hoelzer D, Sanz MA, et al: A randomized, double-blind, placebo-controlled, phase III study of filgrastim in remission induction and consolidation therapy for adults with de novo acute myeloid leukemia: The International Acute Myeloid Leukemia Study Group. Blood 1997; 90:4710.
69. Goodwin JE, Kopecky KJ, Head DR, et al: A double blind placebo controlled trial of G-CSF in elderly patients with previously untreated acute myeloid leukemia: A Southwest Oncology Group Study (Abstract). Blood 1994; 86(Suppl 1):434a.
70. Greenberg P, Taylor K, Larson R, et al: Phase II randomized multicenter trial of G-CSF vs observation for myelodysplastic syndromes (MDS) (Abstract). Blood 1993; 82:196a.
71. Stahel RA, Jost LM, Cerny T, et al: Randomized study of recombinant human granulocyte colony-stimulating factor after high-dose chemotherapy and autologous bone marrow transplantation for high-risk lymphoid malignancies. J Clin Oncol 1994; 12:1931.
72. Linch DC, Scarffe H, Proctor S, et al: Randomised vehicle-controlled dose-finding study of glycosylated recombinant human granulocyte colony-stimulating factor after bone marrow transplantation. Bone Marrow Transplant 1993; 11:307.
73. Schmitz N, Dreger P, Zander AR, et al: Results of a randomised, controlled, multicentre study of recombinant human granulocyte colony-stimulating factor (filgrastim) in patients with Hodgkin's disease and non-Hodgkin's lymphoma undergoing autologous bone marrow transplantation. Bone Marrow Transplant 1995; 15:261.
74. Klumpp TR, Mangan KF, Goldberg SL, et al: Granulocyte colony-stimulating factor accelerates neutrophil engraftment following peripheral-blood stem-cell transplantation: A prospective, randomized trial. J Clin Oncol 1995; 13:1323.
75. Sheridan WP, Begley CG, Juttner C, et al: Effect of peripheral-blood progenitor cells mobilised by filgrastim (G-CSF) on platelet recovery after high-dose chemotherapy. Lancet 1992; 1:640.
76. Duhrsen U, Villeval JL, Boyd J, et al: Effects of recombinant human granulocyte colony-stimulating factor on hematopoietic progenitor cells in cancer patients. Blood 1988; 72:2074.

77. Engel H, Korbling M, Palmer J, et al: Randomized trial of G-CSF alone versus sequential interleukin-3 (IL-3) and G-CSF treatment to peripheralize progenitor cells for apheresis and blood stem cell autotransplantation in patients with advanced stage breast cancer (Abstract). Blood 1994; 84:108a.
78. Begley CG, Basser R, Mansfield R, et al: Randomized prospective study demonstrating a prolonged effect of SCF with G-CSF (filgrastim) on PBSC in untreated patients: Early results (Abstract). Blood 1994; 84:25a.
79. Spitzer G, Adkins D, Mathews M, et al: Randomized comparison of G-CSF + GM-CSF vs G-CSF alone for mobilization of peripheral blood stem cells: Effects on hematopoietic recovery after high-dose chemotherapy. Bone Marrow Transplant 1997; 20:921.
80. Dreger P, Haferlach T, Eckstein V, et al: G-CSF–mobilized peripheral blood progenitor cells for allogeneic transplantation: Safety, kinetics of mobilization, and composition of the graft. Br J Haematol 1994; 87:609.
81. Bensinger WI, Weaver CH, Appelbaum FR, et al: Transplantation of allogeneic peripheral blood stem cells mobilized by recombinant human granulocyte colony-stimulating factor. Blood 1995; 85:1655.
82. Damiani D, Fanin R, Silvestri F, et al: Randomized trial of autologous filgrastim-primed bone marrow transplantation versus filgrastim-mobilized peripheral blood stem cell transplantation in lymphoma patients. Blood 1997; 90:36.
83. La Gamma EF, Alpan O, Kocherlakota P: Effect of granulocyte colony-stimulating factor on preeclampsia-associated neonatal neutropenia. J Pediatr 1995; 126:457.
84. Bedford Russell AR, Davies EG, Ball SE, et al: Granulocyte colony stimulating factor treatment for neonatal neutropenia. Arch Dis Child 1995; 72:F53.
85. Kocherlakota P, La Gamma EF: Human granulocyte colony-stimulating factor may improve outcome attributable to neonatal sepsis complicated by neutropenia. Pediatrics: electronic pages 1997; 100(1):e6.
86. Gillan ER, Christensen RD, Suen Y, et al: A randomized, placebo-controlled trial of recombinant human granulocyte-colony stimulating factor administration in newborn infants with presumed sepsis: Significant induction of peripheral and bone marrow neutrophilia. Blood 1994; 84:1427.
87. Rosenthal J, Healey T, Ellis R, et al: A two-year follow-up of neonates with presumed sepsis treated with recombinant human granulocyte colony-stimulating factor during the first week of life. J Pediatr 1996; 128:135.
88. Welte K, Zeidler C, Reiter A, et al: Differential effects of granulocyte-macrophage colony-stimulating factor and granulocyte colony-stimulating factor in children with severe congenital neutropenia. Blood 1990; 75:1056.
89. Mempel K, Pietsch T, Menzel T, et al: Increased serum levels of granulocyte colony-stimulating factor in patients with severe congenital neutropenia. Blood 1991; 77:1919.
90. Cleary PD, Morrissey G, Yver A, et al: The effects of rG-CSF on health-related quality of life in children with congenital agranulocytosis. Qual Life Res 1994; 3:307.
91. Hammond WP, Price TH, Souza LM, et al: Treatment of cyclic neutropenia with granulocyte colony-stimulating factor. N Engl J Med 1989; 320:1306.
92. Bux J, Behrens G, Jaeger G, et al: Diagnosis and clinical course of autoimmune neutropenia in infancy: Analysis of 240 cases. Blood 1998; 91:181.
93. Kojima S, Fukuda M, Miyajima Y, et al: Treatment of aplastic anemia in children with recombinant human granulocyte colony-stimulating factor: A phase I-II trial. Blood 1991; 77:937.
94. Strickler RB, Goldberg B: Increase in lymphocyte subsets following treatment of HIV-associated neutropenia with granulocyte colony-stimulating factor. Clin Immunol Immunopathol 1996; 79:194.
95. Poloni A, Giarratana MC, Firat H, et al: The ex vivo expansion capacity of normal human bone marrow cells is dependent on experimental conditions: Role of the cell concentration, serum and CD34[+] cell selection in stroma-free cultures. Hematol Cell Ther 1997; 39(2):49.
96. Fietz T, Hilgenfeld E, Berdel WE, et al: Ex vivo expansion of human umbilical cord blood does not lead to co-expansion of contaminating maternal mononuclear cells. Bone Marrow Transplant 1997; 20:1019.
97. Hirano T, Yasukawa K, Harada H, et al: Complementary DNA for a novel human interleukin (BSF-2) that induces B lymphocytes to produce immunoglobulin. Nature 1986; 324:73.
98. Weber J: Interleukin-6: Multifunctional cytokine. *In*: Biologic Therapy of Cancer Updates. Vol 3. Devita VT, Hellman S, Rosenberg SA (Eds). Philadelphia, JB Lippincott, 1993.
99. Olencki T, Budd GT, Murthy S, et al: Immunoregulatory and hematopoietic effects of interleukin-6 (rhIL-6) in cancer patients (Abstract). Proc Am Soc Clin Oncol 1993; 12:292.
100. Holbrook ST, Christensen R: Hematopoietic growth factors. Adv Pediatr 1991; 38:23.
101. Muraguchi A, Hirano T, Tang B, et al: The essential role of B-cell stimulatory factor-2 (BSF-2/IL-6) for the terminal differentiation of B cells. J Exp Med 1988; 167:332.
102. Weber J, Yang J, Topalian S, et al: Phase I trial of subcutaneous interleukin-6 in patients with advanced malignancies. J Clin Oncol 1993; 11:499.
103. Bouffet E, Phillip T, Negrier CI, et al: Phase I study of interleukin-6 in children with solid tumors in relapse. Eur J Cancer 1997; 33:1620.
104. Damas P, Ledoux D, Nys M, et al: Cytokine serum level during severe sepsis in human IL-6 as a marker of severity. Ann Surg 1992; 215:356.
105. Ishibashi T, Kimura H, Shikama Y, et al: Interleukin-6 is a potent thrombopoietic factor in vivo in mice. Blood 1989; 74:1241.
106. Koike K, Nakahata T, Kubo T, et al: IL-6 enhances murine megakaryocytopoiesis in serum free culture. Blood 1990; 75:2286.
107. Leary AG, Ikebuchi K, Hirai Y, et al: Synergism between interleukin-6 and interleukin-3 in supporting proliferation of human hematopoietic stem cells: Comparison with interleukin-1α. Blood 1988; 71:1759.
108. Ishibashi T, Shikama Y, Kimura H, et al: Thrombopoietic effects of interleukin-6 in long-term administration in mice. Exp Hematol 1993; 21:640.
109. Ryffel B, Car BD, Woerly G, et al: Long-term interleukin-6 administration stimulates sustained thrombopoiesis and acute-phase protein synthesis in a small primate—the marmoset. Blood 1994; 83:2093.
110. Herodin F, Mestries J-C, Janodet D, et al: Recombinant glycosylated human interleukin-6 accelerates peripheral blood platelet count recovery in radiation-induced bone marrow depression in baboons. Blood 1992; 80:688.
111. Burstein SA, Downs T, Friese P, et al: Thrombocytopoiesis in normal and sublethally irradiated dogs: Response to human interleukin-6. Blood 1992; 80:420.
112. Takatsuki F, Okano A, Suzuki C, et al: Interleukin 6 perfusion stimulates reconstitution of the immune and hematopoietic systems after 5-fluorouracil treatment. Cancer Res 1990; 50:2885.
113. D'Hondt V, Humblet Y, Guillaume T, et al: Thrombopoietic effects and toxicity of interleukin-6 in patients with ovarian cancer before and after chemotherapy: A multicentric placebo-controlled, randomized phase Ib study. Blood 1995; 85:2347.
114. van Gameren MM, Willemse PH, Mulder NH, et al: Effects of recombinant human interleukin-6 in cancer patients: A phase I-II study. Blood 1994; 84:1434.
115. Veldhuis GJ, Willemse PHB, Sleijfer DT, et al: Toxicity and efficacy of escalating dosages of recombinant human interleukin-6 after chemotherapy in patients with breast cancer or non–small-cell lung cancer. J Clin Oncol 1995; 13:2585.
116. Oleksowicz L, Puszkin E, Mrowiec Z, et al: Alterations in platelet function in patients receiving interleukin-6 as cytokine therapy. Cancer Invest 1996; 14:307.
117. Schrezenmeier H, Marsh J, Stromeyer P, et al: A phase I/II trial of recombinant human interleukin-6 in patients with aplastic anaemia. Br J Haematol 1995; 90:283.
118. Banks RE, Forbes MA, Storr M, et al: The acute phase protein response in patients receiving subcutaneous IL-6. Clin Exp Immunol 1995; 102:217.
119. Shen V, Bergeron S, Krailo M, et al: Enhanced hematological recovery but a high incidence of grade (GD) III/IV toxicities attributed to interleukin-6 (IL-6) in children with recurrent/refractory solid tumors treated with rIL-6 and G-CSF following ifosfamide, carboplatin, and etoposide (ICE). Proc Am Soc Clin Oncol 1997; 16:110a.
120. Reissmann KR: Studies of the mechanism of erythropoietic stimulation in parabiotic rats during hypoxia. Blood 1950; 5:372.

121. Erslev A: Humoral regulation of red cell production. Blood 1953; 8:349.
122. Miyake T, Kung CK-H, Goldwasser E: Purification of human erythropoietin. J Biol Chem 1977; 252:5558.
123. Jacobs K, Shoemaker C, Rudersdorf R, et al: Isolation and characterization of genomic and cDNA clones of human erythropoietin. Nature 1985; 313:806.
124. Lin FK, Suggs S, Lin CH, et al: Cloning and expression of the human erythropoietin gene. Proc Natl Acad Sci U S A 1985; 82:7580.
125. Law ML, Cai F-Y, Lin F-K: Chromosomal assignment of the human erythropoietin gene and its DNA polymorphism. Proc Natl Acad Sci U S A 1986; 83:6920.
126. Zanjani ED, Ascensao JL, McGlave PB, et al: Studies on the liver to kidney switch of erythropoietin production. J Clin Invest 1981; 67:1183.
127. Zanjani ED, Poster J, Burlington H, et al: Liver as the primary site of erythropoietin production in the fetus. J Lab Clin Med 1977; 89:640.
128. Fisher JW, Koury S, Ducey T, et al: Erythropoietin (Epo) production by interstitial cells of hypoxic monkey kidneys. Br J Haematol 1996; 95:27.
129. Semenza GL: Regulation of erythropoietin production—new insights into molecular mechanisms of oxygen homeostasis. Hematol Oncol Clin North Am 1994; 8:863.
130. Lucarelli G, Porcellini A, Carnevali C, et al: Fetal and neonatal erythropoiesis. Ann N Y Acad Sci 1968; 149:544.
131. Clemons GK, Fitzsimmons SL, Demanicor D: Immunoreactive erythropoietin concentrations in fetal and neonatal rats and the effects of hypoxia. Blood 1986; 68:892.
132. Ueno M, Seferynska I, Beckman B, et al: Enhanced erythropoietin secretion in hepatoblastoma cells in response to hypoxia. Am J Physiol 1989; 257:C743.
133. Sawyer ST, Koury MJ: Erythropoietin requirement during terminal erythroid differentiation: The role of surface receptors for erythropoietin (Abstract). J Cell Biol 1987; 105:1077.
134. Sawada K, Krantz S, Dai C-H, et al: Purification of human blood burst-forming units-erythroid and demonstration of the evolution of erythropoietin receptors. J Cell Physiol 1990; 142:219.
135. McNiece ID, Langley KE, Zsebo KM: Recombinant human stem cell factor synergizes with GM-CSF, G-CSF, IL-3 and Epo to stimulate human progenitor cells of the myeloid and erythroid lineages. Exp Hematol 1991; 19:226.
136. Migliaccio G, Migliaccio AR, Adamson JW: In vitro differentiation of human granulocyte/macrophage and erythroid progenitors: Comparative analysis of the influence of recombinant human erythropoietin, G-CSF, GM-CSF and IL-3 in serum depleted and serum deprived cultures. Blood 1989; 72:1452.
137. Winearls CG, Oliver DO, Pippard MJ, et al: Effects of human erythropoietin derived from recombinant DNA on the anaemia of patients maintained by chronic haemodialysis. Lancet 1986; ii:1175.
138. Eschbach JW, Egrie JC, Downing MR, et al: Correction of the anemia of end-stage renal disease with recombinant human erythropoietin: Results of a combined phase I and II clinical trial. N Engl J Med 1987; 316:73.
139. Evans RW, Rader B, Manninen DL: The quality of life of hemodialysis recipients treated with recombinant human erythropoietin: Cooperative Multicenter EPO Clinical Trial Group. JAMA 1990; 263:825.
140. Lezaic V, Djukanovic L, Pavlovic-Kentera V: Recombinant human erythropoietin treatment of anemia in renal transplant patients. Ren Fail 1995; 17:705.
141. Miller CB, Jones RJ, Piantadose S, et al: Decreased erythropoietin response in patients with the anemia of cancer. N Engl J Med 1990; 322:1689.
142. Porter JC, Leahey A, Polise K, et al: Recombinant human erythropoietin reduces the need for erythrocyte and platelet transfusions in pediatric patients with sarcoma: A randomized, double-blind, placebo-controlled trial. J Pediatr 1996; 129:656.
143. Cazzola M, Messinger D, Battistel V, et al: Recombinant human erythropoietin in the anemia associated with multiple myeloma or non-Hodgkin's lymphoma: Dose finding and identification of predictors of response. Blood 1995; 86:4446.
144. Ludwig H, Sundal E, Pecherstorfer M, et al: Recombinant human erythropoietin for the correction of cancer associated anemia with and without concomitant cytotoxic chemotherapy. Cancer 1995; 76:2319.
145. Chao NJ, Schriber JR, Long GD, et al: A randomized study of erythropoietin and granulocyte colony-stimulating factor (G-CSF) versus placebo and G-CSF for patients with Hodgkin's and non-Hodgkin's lymphoma undergoing autologous bone marrow transplantation. Blood 1994; 83:2823.
146. Zuccotti GV, Plebani A, Biasucci G, et al: Granulocyte-colony stimulating factor and erythropoietin therapy in children with human immunodeficiency virus infection. J Int Med Res 1996; 24(1):115.
147. Perrella O, Finelli E, Perrella A, et al: Combined therapy with zidovudine, recombinant granulocyte colony stimulating factors and erythropoietin in asymptomatic HIV patients. J Chemother 1996; 8(1):63.
148. Price TH, Goodnough LT, Vogler WR, et al: The effect of recombinant human erythropoietin on the efficacy of autologous blood donation in patients with low hematocrits: A multicenter, randomized, double-blind, controlled trial. Transfusion 1996; 36(1):29.
149. Goodnough LT, Rudnik S, Price TH, et al: Increased preoperative collection of autologous blood with recombinant human erythropoietin therapy. N Engl J Med 1989; 321:1163.
150. de Pree C, Mermillod B, Hoffmeyer P, et al: Recombinant human erythropoietin as adjuvant treatment for autologous blood donation in elective surgery with large blood needs (> or = 5 units): A randomized study. Transfusion 1997; 37:708.
151. Goodnough LT, Price TH, Friedman KD, et al: A phase III trial of recombinant human erythropoietin therapy in nonanemic orthopedic patients subjected to aggressive removal of blood for autologous use: Dose, response, toxicity, and efficacy. Transfusion 1994; 34(1):66.
152. Maier RF, Obladen M, Scigalla P, et al: The effect of epoetin beta (recombinant human erythropoietin) on the need for transfusion in very-low-birth-weight infants: European Multicentre Erythropoietin Study Group. N Engl J Med 1994; 330:1173.
153. Doyle JJ: The role of erythropoietin in the anemia of prematurity. Semin Perinatol 1997; 21(1):20.
154. Obladen M, Maier RF: Recombinant erythropoietin for prevention of anemia in preterm infants. J Perinat Med 1995; 23(1-2):19.
155. Soubasi V, Kremenopoulos G, Diamandi E, et al: In which neonates does early recombinant human erythropoietin treatment prevent anemia of prematurity? Results of a randomized, controlled study. Pediatr Res 1993; 34:675.
156. Abraham PA, Marces MG: Blood pressure in hemodialysis during amelioration of anemia with erythropoietin. J Am Soc Nephrol 1991; 2:927.
157. Tasaki T, Ohto H, Noguchi M, et al: Iron and erythropoietin measurement in autologous blood donors with anemia: Implications for management. Transfusion 1994; 34:337.
158. Biesma DH, Van de Wiel A, Beguin Y, et al: Erythropoietic activity and iron metabolism in autologous blood donors during recombinant human erythropoietin therapy. Eur J Clin Invest 1994; 24:426.
159. Erslev AJ: Erythropoietin. N Engl J Med 1991; 324:1339.
160. Barosi G: Inadequate erythropoietin response to anemia: Definition and clinical relevance. Ann Hematol 1994; 68:215.
161. Ludwig H, Fritz E, Leitgeb C, et al: Prediction of response to erythropoietin treatment in chronic anemia of cancer. Blood 1994; 84:1056.
162. Kawasaki E, Ladner M, Wang A, et al: Molecular cloning of a complementary DNA encoding human macrophage-specific colony-stimulating factor (CSF-1). Science 1985; 230:291.
163. Morris SW, Valentine MB, Shapiro DN, et al: Reassignment of the human CSF-1 gene to chromosome 1p13-p21. Blood 1991; 78:2013.
164. Sherr CJ, Rettenmier CW, Sacca R, et al: The c-*fms* proto-oncogene product is related to the receptor for the mononuclear phagocyte growth factor, CSF-1. Cell 1985; 41:665.
165. Ralph P, Nakoinz I: Stimulation of macrophage tumoricidal activity by the growth and differentiation factor CSF-1. Cell Immunol 1987; 105:270.
166. Robinson BE, Quesenberry PJ: Hematopoietic growth factors:

Overview and clinical applications: Part II. Am J Med Sci 1990; 300:237.

167. Saleh MN, Goldman SJ, LoBuglio AF, et al: CD16+ monocytes in patients with cancer: Spontaneous elevation and pharmacologic induction by recombinant human macrophage colony-stimulating factor. Blood 1995; 85:2910.
168. Kawano Y, Takaue Y, Minakuchi J, et al: Effects of monocyte-macrophage colony-stimulating factor (M-CSF) on in vitro erythropoiesis of marrow progenitor cells from patients with renal anemia. Eur J Haematol 1995; 54:147.
169. Komiyama A, Ishiguro A, Kubo T, et al: Increases in neutrophil counts by purified human urinary colony-stimulating factor in chronic neutropenia of childhood. Blood 1988; 71:41.
170. Motoyoshi K, Takaka F, Kusumoto K, et al: Phase I and early phase II studies on human urinary colony-stimulating factor. Jpn J Med 1991; 21:185.
171. Nemunaitis J, Meyers JD, Buckner CD, et al: Phase I trial of recombinant human macrophage colony-stimulating factor in patients with invasive fungal infections. Blood 1991; 78:907.
172. Minasian LM, Yao TJ, Steffens TA, et al: A phase I study of anti-GD3 ganglioside monoclonal antibody R24 and recombinant human macrophage-colony stimulating factor in patients with metastatic melanoma. Cancer 1995; 75:2251.
173. Paul SR, Bennett F, Calvetti JA, et al: Molecular cloning of a cDNA encoding interleukin 11, a stromal cell–derived lymphopoietic and hematopoietic cytokine. Proc Natl Acad Sci U S A 1990; 87:7512.
174. McKinley D, Wu Q, Yang-Feng T, et al: Genomic sequence and chromosomal location of human interleukin-11 gene (*IL11*). Genomics 1992; 13:814.
175. Trepicchio WL, Bozza M, Dorner AJ: Recombinant human interleukin-11 attenuates the proinflammatory response through regulation of cytokine gene expression. Exp Hematol 1996; 24:1099.
176. Du XX, Williams DA: Interleukin-11: A multifunctional growth factor derived from the hematopoietic microenvironment. Blood 1994; 83:2023.
177. Sato N, Sawada K, Koizumi K, et al: In vitro expansion of human peripheral blood CD+34 cells. Blood 1993; 82:3600.
178. Leary AG, Zeng HQ, Clark SC, et al: Growth factor requirements for survival in G_0 and entry into the cell cycle of primitive human hemopoietic progenitors. Proc Natl Acad Sci U S A 1992; 89:4013.
179. Tanaka R, Katayama N, Ohishi K, et al: Accelerated cell-cycling of hematopoietic progenitor cells by growth factors. Blood 1995; 86:73.
180. Broudy VC, Lin NL, Kaushansky K: Thrombopoietin (c-*mpl* ligand) acts synergistically with erythropoietin, stem cell factor, and interleukin-11 to enhance murine megakaryocyte colony growth and increases megakaryocyte ploidy in vitro. Blood 1995; 85:1719.
181. Kaushansky K, Broudy VC, Lin N, et al: Thrombopoietin, the Mpl ligand, is essential for full megakaryocyte development. Proc Natl Acad Sci U S A 1995; 92:3234.
182. Kaushansky K, Lok S, Holly RD, et al: Promotion of megakaryocyte progenitor expansion and differentiation by the c-Mpl ligand thrombopoietin. Nature 1994; 369:568.
183. Quesniaux VFJ, Clark SC, Turner K, et al: Interleukin-11 stimulates multiple phases of erythropoiesis in vitro. Blood 1992; 80:1218.
184. Du XX, Doerschuk CM, Orazi A, et al: A bone marrow stromal-derived growth factor, interleukin-11, stimulates recovery of small intestinal mucosal cells after cytoablative therapy. Blood 1994; 83:33.
185. Peterson R, Trepicchio W, Bozza MM, et al: GI growth arrest and reduced proliferation of intestinal epithelial cells induced by rhIL-11 may mediate protection against mucositis (Abstract). Blood 1995; 86:311.
186. Booth C, Potten CS: Effects of IL-11 on the growth of intestinal epithelial cells in vitro. Cell Prolif 1995; 28:528.
187. Cairo MS, Plunkett JM, Schendel P, et al: The combined effects of interleukin-11, stem cell factor, and granulocyte colony-stimulating factor on newborn rat hematopoiesis: Significant enhancement of the absolute neutrophil count. Exp Hematol 1994; 22:1118.
188. Cairo MS, Plunkett JM, Nguyen A, et al: Effect of interleukin-11 with and without granulocyte colony-stimulating factor on in vivo neonatal rat hematopoiesis: Induction of neonatal thrombocytosis by interleukin-11 and synergistic enhancement of neutrophilia by interleukin-11 + granulocyte colony-stimulating factor. Pediatr Res 1993; 34(1):56.
189. Du XX, Neben T, Goldman S, et al: Effects of recombinant human IL-11 on hematopoietic reconstitution in transplanted mice: Acceleration of recovery of peripheral blood neutrophils and platelets. Blood 1993; 81:27.
190. Du XX, Keller D, Maze R, et al: Comparative effects of in vivo treatment using interleukin-11 and stem cell factor on reconstitution in mice after bone marrow transplantation. Blood 1993; 82:1016.
191. Du XX, Keller D, Goldman S, et al: Functional effects of interleukin-11 treatment in vivo following bone marrow transplantation and combined modality therapy in mice (Abstract). Exp Hematol 1992; 20:768.
192. Paul S, Goldman S, Muench M, et al: IL-11 expression in donor bone marrow cells improves hematological reconstitution in lethally irradiated recipient mice (Abstract). Blood 1991; 78:260.
193. Hawley RG, Hawley TS, Fong AZC, et al: Thrombopoietic potential and serial repopulating ability of murine hematopoietic stem cells constitutively expressing interleukin-11. Proc Natl Acad Sci U S A 1996; 93:10297.
194. Potten CS: Interleukin-11 protects the clonogenic stem cells in murine small intestinal crypts from impairment of their reproductive capacity by radiation. Int J Cancer 1995; 62:356.
195. Sonis S, Muska A, O'Brien J, et al: Alteration of the frequency, severity and duration of chemotherapy-induced mucositis in hamsters by interleukin-11. Eur J Cancer 1995; 31B:261.
196. Barton BE, Shortall J, Jackson JV: Interleukins 6 and 11 protect mice from mortality in staphylococcal enterotoxin–induced toxic shock model. Infect Immunol 1996; 64:714.
197. Chang M, Suen Y, Meng G, et al: Differential mechanisms in the regulation of endogenous levels of thrombopoietin and interleukin-11 during thrombocytopenia: Insight into the regulation of platelet production. Blood 1996; 88:3354.
198. Misa BR, Ferranti TJ, Keith JCJ, et al: Recombinant human interleukin-11 prevents hypotension in LPS-treated anesthetized rabbits. J Endotoxin Res 1996; 3:297.
199. Tepler I, Elias L, Smith JW, et al: Recombinant human interleukin-11 in cancer patients with severe thrombocytopenia due to chemotherapy. Blood 1996; 87:3607.
200. Gordon MS, Nemunaitis J, Hoffman R, et al: A phase I trial of recombinant human interleukin-6 in patients with myelodysplastic syndromes and thrombocytopenia. Blood 1995; 85:3066.
201. Isaacs C, Robert N, Bailey A, et al: Randomized placebo-controlled study of recombinant human interleukin-11 to prevent chemotherapy induced thrombocytopenia in patients with breast cancer receiving dose-intensive cyclophosphamide and doxorubicin. J Clin Oncol 1997; 15:3368.
202. Kirov I, Goldman S, Blazar B, et al: Recombinant human interleukin 11 (Neumega) is tolerated at double the adult dose and enhances hematopoietic recovery following ifosfamide, carboplatin, and etoposide (ICE) chemotherapy in children: Correlation with rapid clearance, lack of induction of inflammatory cytokines and mobilization of early progenitor cells (Abstract). Blood 1997; 90(10 Suppl 1):581a.
203. Cairo MS, Shen WP, Miser J, et al: A randomized trial of two doses of G-CSF (5.0 vs 10.0 mcg/kg/d) following ifosfamide, carboplatin, and etoposide (ICE) chemotherapy in children with recurrent solid tumors (RST): Significant clinical activity but no improvement in hematopoietic recovery (HR) with increased dose of G-CSF (Abstract). Proc Am Soc Clin Oncol 1995; 14:255.
204. Ali-Nazir A, Davenport V, Reaman G, et al: A phase I/II trial of rh IL-11 following ifosfamide, carboplatin, and etoposide (ICE) chemotherapy in pediatric patients (pts) with solid tumors (ST) or lymphoma (L): Enhancement of hematological reconstitution (Abstract). Proc Am Soc Clin Oncol 1996; 15:274.
205. Bartley TD, Bogenberger J, Hunt P, et al: Identification and cloning of a megakaryocyte growth and development factor that is a ligand for the cytokine receptor Mpl. Cell 1994; 77:1117.
206. de Sauvage FJ, Hass PE, Spencer SD, et al: Stimulation of megakaryocytopoiesis and thrombopoiesis by the c-Mpl ligand. Nature 1994; 369:533.

207. Kuter DJ, Beeler DL, Rosenberg RD: The purification of megapoietin: A physiological regulator of megakaryocyte growth and platelet production. Proc Natl Acad Sci U S A 1994; 91:11104.
208. Lok S, Kaushansky K, Holly R, et al: Cloning and expression of murine thrombopoietin cDNA and stimulation of platelet production in vivo. Nature 1994; 369:565.
209. Sohma Y, Akahori H, Seki N: Molecular cloning and chromosomal localization of the human thrombopoietin gene. FEBS Lett 1994; 353:57.
210. Marsh JC, Gibson FM, Prue RL, et al: Serum thrombopoietin levels in patients with aplastic anaemia. Br J Haematol 1996; 95:605.
211. Broudy V, Lin N, Kaushansky K: Thrombopoietin (c-*mpl* ligand) acts synergistically with erythropoietin, stem cell factor, and interleukin-11 to enhance murine megakaryocyte colony growth and increases megakaryocyte ploidy in vitro. Blood 1995; 7:1719.
212. Papayannopoulou T, Brice M, Kaushansky K: The influence of Mpl-ligand on the development of megakaryocytes from CD34⁺ cells isolated from bone marrow, peripheral blood (Abstract). Blood 1994; 84:32.
213. Wendling F, Maraskovsky E, Debill N, et al: c-Mpl ligand is a humoral regulator of megakaryocytopoiesis. Nature 1994; 369:571.
214. Choi ES, Nichol JL, Hokom MM: Platelets generated in vitro from proplatelet-displaying human megakaryocytes are functional. Blood 1995; 85:402.
215. Zucker-Franklin D, Kaushansky K: Effect of thrombopoietin on the development of megakaryocytes and platelets: An ultrastructural analysis. Blood 1996; 88:1632.
216. Yoshida M, Tsuji K, Ebihara Y, et al: Thrombopoietin alone stimulates the early proliferation and survival of human erythroid, myeloid and multipotential progenitors in serum-free culture. Br J Haematol 1997; 98:254.
217. Itoh N, Katayama N, Kato T, et al: Activity of the ligand for c-*mpl*, thrombopoietin, in early haemopoiesis. Br J Haematol 1996; 94:228.
218. Ku H, Yonemura Y, Kaushansky K, et al: Thrombopoietin, the ligand for the Mpl receptor, synergizes with steel factor and other early acting cytokines in supporting proliferation of primitive hematopoietic progenitors of mice. Blood 1996; 87:4544.
219. Sitnicka E, Lin N, Priestley GV, et al: The effect of thrombopoietin on the proliferation and differentiation of murine hematopoietic stem cells. Blood 1996; 87:4998.
220. Usuki K, Tahara T, Iki S, et al: Serum thrombopoietin level in various hematological diseases. Stem Cells 1996; 14:558.
221. Basser RL, Rasko JEJ, Clarke K, et al: Thrombopoietic effects of pegylated recombinant human megakaryocyte growth and development factor (PEG-rHuMGDF) in patients with advanced cancer. Lancet 1996; 348:1279.
222. Fanucchi M, Glaspy J, Crawford J, et al: Effects of polyethylene glycol–conjugated recombinant human megakaryocyte growth and development factor on platelet counts after chemotherapy for lung cancer. N Engl J Med 1997; 336:404.
223. Rasko JE, O'Flaherty E, Begley CG: Mpl ligand (MGDF) alone and in combination with stem cell factor (SCF) promotes proliferation and survival of human megakaryocyte, erythroid and granulocyte/macrophage progenitors. Stem Cells 1997; 15(1):33.
224. Bertolini F, Battaglia M, Pedrazzoli P, et al: Megakaryocytic progenitors can be generated ex vivo and safely administered to autologous peripheral blood progenitor cell transplant recipients. Blood 1997; 89:2679.
225. Ishida A, Miyakawa Y, Tanosaki R, et al: Circulating endogenous thrombopoietin, interleukin-3, interleukin-6 and interleukin-11 levels in patients undergoing allogeneic bone marrow transplantation. Int J Hematol 1996; 65(1):61.
226. Ihle JN, Keller T, Henderson L, et al: Procedure for the purification of interleukin-3 to homogeneity. J Immunol 1982; 129:2431.
227. Ihle JN, Keller J, Oroszalan S, et al: Biologic properties of homogeneous interleukin 3. I. Demonstration of WEHI-3 growth factor activity, mast cell growth factor activity, p cell–stimulating factor activity, colony-stimulating factor activity, and histamine-producing cell–stimulating factor activity. J Immunol 1983; 131:282.
228. Yang Y-C, Ciarletta AB, Temple PA, et al: Human IL-3 (multi-CSF): Identification by expression cloning of a novel hematopoietic growth factor related to murine IL-3. Cell 1986; 47:3.
229. Yang Y-C, Kovacic S, Kriz R, et al: The human genes for GM-CSF and IL-3 are closely linked in tandem on chromosome 5. Blood 1988; 71:958.
230. Bruno E, Hoffman R: Effect of interleukin 6 on in vitro human megakaryocytopoiesis: Its interaction with other cytokines. Exp Hematol 1989; 17:1038.
231. Donahue R, Seehra J, Metzger M, et al: Human IL-3 and GM-CSF act synergistically in stimulating hematopoiesis in primates. Science 1988; 241:1820.
232. Bodine D, Karlsson S, Nienhuis A: Combination of interleukins 3 and 6 preserves stem cell function in culture and enhances retrovirus-mediated gene transfer into hematopoietic stem cells. Proc Natl Acad Sci U S A 1989; 86:8897.
233. Nolta JA, Kohn DB: Comparison of the effects of growth factors on retroviral vector–mediated gene transfer and the proliferative status of human hematopoietic progenitor cells. Hum Gene Ther 1990; 1:257.
234. Gessler K, Valent P, Bettelheim P: In vivo synergism of recombinant human interleukin-3 and recombinant human interleukin-6 on thrombopoiesis in primates. Blood 1992; 79:1155.
235. Kudoh S, Sawa T, Kurihara N, et al: Phase II study of recombinant human interleukin 3 administration following carboplatin and etoposide chemotherapy in small-cell lung cancer patients: SDZ ILE 964 (IL-3) Study. Cancer Chemother Pharmacol 1996; 38:S89.
236. Fay JW, Bernstein SH: Recombinant human interleukin-3 and granulocyte-macrophage colony-stimulating factor after autologous bone marrow transplantation for malignant lymphoma. Semin Oncol 1996; 23(2):22.
237. Lemoli RM, Rosti G, Visani G, et al: Concomitant and sequential administration of recombinant human granulocyte colony-stimulating factor and recombinant human interleukin-3 to accelerate hematopoietic recovery after autologous bone marrow transplantation for malignant lymphoma. J Clin Oncol 1996; 14:3018.
238. Kolbe K, Peschel C, Rupilius B, et al: Peripheral blood stem cell (PBSC) mobilization with chemotherapy followed by sequential IL-3 and G-CSF administration in extensively pretreated patients. Bone Marrow Transplant 1997; 20:1027.
239. Bargetzi MJ, Gluckman E, Tichelli A, et al: Recombinant human interleukin-3 in refractory severe aplastic anaemia: A phase I/II trial. Br J Haematol 1995; 91:306.
240. Gehling UM, Ryder JW, Hogan CJ, et al: Ex vivo expansion of megakaryocyte progenitors: Effect of various growth factor combinations on CD34⁺ progenitor cells from bone marrow and G-CSF–mobilized peripheral blood. Exp Hematol 1997; 25:1125.
241. Zsebo K, Wypych J, McNiece I, et al: Identification, purification, and biological characterization of hematopoietic stem cell factor from buffalo rat liver–conditioned medium. Cell 1990; 63:195.
242. Zsebo KM, Williams DA, Geissler EN, et al: Stem cell factor is encoded at the Sl locus of the mouse and is the ligand for the c-*kit* tyrosine kinase receptor. Cell 1990; 63:213.
243. Geissler EN, Liao M, Brook JD, et al: Stem cell factor (SCF), a novel hematopoietic growth factor and ligand for c-*kit* tyrosine kinase receptor, maps on human chromosome 12 between 12q14.3 and 12qter. Somat Cell Mol Genet 1991; 17:207.
244. Anderson DM, Williams DE, Tushinski R, et al: Alternate splicing of mRNAs encoding human mast cell growth factor and localization of the gene to chromosome 12q22-q24. Cell Growth Differ 1991; 2:373.
245. Qiu F, Ray P, Brown K, et al: Primary structure of c-*kit*: Relationship with the CSF-1/PDGF receptor kinase family—Oncogenic activation of v-*kit* involves deletion of extracellular domain and C terminus. EMBO J 1988; 7:1003.
246. Yarden Y, Kuang WJ, Yang-Feng T, et al: Human proto-oncogene c-*kit*: A new cell surface receptor tyrosine kinase for an unidentified ligand. EMBO J 1987; 6:3341.
247. Hu ZB, Ma W, Uphoff CC, et al: c-*kit* expression in human megakaryoblastic leukemia cell lines. Blood 1994; 83:2133.
248. Andre C, d'Auriol L, Lacombe C, et al: c-*kit* mRNA expression in human and murine hematopoietic cell lines. Oncogene 1989; 4:1047.
249. Da Silva N, Hu ZB, Ma W, et al: Expression of the *FLT3* gene in human leukemia-lymphoma cell lines. Leukemia 1994; 8:885.
250. Wang C, Curtis JE, Geissler EN, et al: The expression of the proto-oncogene C-*kit* in the blast cells of acute myeloblastic leukemia. Leukemia 1989; 3:699.

251. Morita S, Tsuchiya S, Fujie H, et al: Cell surface c-*kit* receptors in human leukemia cell lines and pediatric leukemia: Selective preservation of c-*kit* expression on megakaryoblastic cell lines during adaptation to in vitro culture. Leukemia 1996; 10:102.
252. Ikeda H, Kanakura Y, Tamaki T, et al: Expression and functional role of the proto-oncogene c-*kit* in acute myeloblastic leukemia cells. Blood 1991; 78:2692.
253. Lerner NB, Nocka KH, Cole SR, et al: Monoclonal antibody YB5.B8 identifies the human c-*kit* protein product. Blood 1991; 77:1876.
254. Kubota A, Okamura S, Shimoda K, et al: The c-*kit* molecule and the surface immunophenotype of human acute leukemia. Leuk Lymphoma 1994; 14:421.
255. Reuss-Borst MA, Buhring HJ, Schmidt H, et al: AML: Immunophenotypic heterogeneity and prognostic significance of c-*kit* expression. Leukemia 1994; 8:258.
256. Kanakura Y, Ikeda H, Kitayama H, et al: Expression, function and activation of the proto-oncogene c-*kit* product in human leukemia cells. Leuk Lymphoma 1993; 10:35.
257. Lauria F, Bagnara GP, Rondelli D, et al: Cytofluorimetric and functional analysis of c-*kit* receptor in acute leukemia. Leuk Lymphoma 1995; 18:451.
258. Carlesso N, Pregno P, Bresso P, et al: Human recombinant stem cell factor stimulates in vitro proliferation of acute myeloid leukemia cells and expands the clonogenic cell pool. Leukemia 1992; 6:642.
259. Goselink HM, Williams DE, Fibbe WE, et al: Effect of mast cell growth factor (c-*kit* ligand) on clonogenic leukemic precursor cells. Blood 1992; 80:750.
260. Valverde LR, Matutes E, Farahat N, et al: c-*kit* receptor (CD117) expression in acute leukemia. Ann Hematol 1996; 72:11.
261. Galli SJ, Zsebo KM, Geissler EN: The kit ligand, stem cell factor. Adv Immunol 1994; 55:1.
262. Broudy VC, Lin N, Zsebo KM, et al: Isolation and characterization of a monoclonal antibody that recognizes the human c-*kit* receptor. Blood 1992; 79:338.
263. Ashman LK, Cambareri AC, To LB, et al: Expression of the YB5.B8 antigen (c-*kit* proto-oncogene product) in normal human bone marrow. Blood 1991; 78:30.
264. Papayannopoulou T, Brice M, Broudy VC, et al: Isolation of c-*kit* receptor–expressing cells from bone marrow, peripheral blood, and fetal liver: Functional properties and composite antigenic profile. Blood 1991; 78:1403.
265. Uoshima N, Ozawa M, Kimura S, et al: Changes in c-Kit expression and effects of SCF during differentiation of human erythroid progenitor cells. Br J Haematol 1995; 91:30.
266. Briddell RA, Broudy VC, Bruno E, et al: Further phenotypic characterization and isolation of human hematopoietic progenitor cells using a monoclonal antibody to the c-*kit* receptor. Blood 1992; 79:3159.
267. Broxmeyer HE, Hangoc G, Cooper S, et al: Influence of murine mast cell growth factor (c-*kit* ligand) on colony formation by mouse marrow hematopoietic progenitor cells. Exp Hematol 1991; 19:143.
268. Broxmeyer HE, Cooper S, Lu L, et al: Effect of murine mast cell growth factor (c-*kit* proto-oncogene ligand) on colony formation by human marrow hematopoietic progenitor cells. Blood 1991; 77:2142.
269. Xiao M, Leemhuis T, Broxmeyer HE, et al: Influence of combinations of cytokines on proliferation of isolated single cell-sorted human bone marrow hematopoietic progenitor cells in the absence and presence of serum. Exp Hematol 1992; 20:276.
270. Sui X, Tsuji K, Tajima S, et al: Erythropoietin-independent erythrocyte production: Signals through gp130 and c-kit dramatically promote erythropoiesis from human CD34$^+$ cells. J Exp Med 1996; 183:837.
271. Carow CE, Hangoc G, Cooper SH, et al: Mast cell growth factor (c-*kit* ligand) supports the growth of human multipotential progenitor cells with a high replating potential. Blood 1991; 78:2216.
272. Ramsfjell V, Borge OJ, Cui L, et al: Thrombopoietin directly and potently stimulates multilineage growth and progenitor cell expansion from primitive (CD34$^+$CD8$^-$) human bone marrow progenitor cells: Distinct and key interactions with the ligands for c-kit and flt3, and inhibitory effects of TGF-β and TNF-α. J Immunol 1997; 158:5169.
273. Ramsfjell V, Borge OJ, Veiby OP, et al: Thrombopoietin, but not erythropoietin, directly and potently stimulates multilineage growth of primitive murine bone marrow progenitor cells in synergy with early acting cytokines: Distinct interactions with the ligands for c-kit and FLT3. Blood 1997; 88:4481.
274. Kobayashi M, Laver JH, Kato T, et al: Thrombopoietin supports proliferation of human primitive hematopoietic cells in synergy with steel factor and/or interleukin-3. Blood 1996; 88:429.
275. Hirayama FL, Lyman SD, Clark SC, Ogawa M: The flt3 ligand supports proliferation of lymphohematopoietic progenitors and early B-lymphoid progenitors. Blood 1995; 85:1762.
276. Hirayama F, Shih JP, Awgulewitsch A, et al: Clonal proliferation of murine lymphohemopoietic progenitors in culture. Proc Natl Acad Sci U S A 1992; 89:5906.
277. Ball TC, Hirayama F, Ogawa M: Lymphohematopoietic progenitors of normal mice. Blood 1995; 85:3086.
278. Godfrey DI, Kennedy J, Gately MK, et al: IL-12 influences intrathymic T cell development. J Immunol 1994; 152:2729.
279. Shibuya A, Nagayoshi K, Nakamura K, et al: Lymphokine requirement for the generation of natural killer cells from CD34$^+$ hematopoietic progenitor cells. Blood 1995; 85:3538.
280. Silva MR, Hoffman R, Srour EF, et al: Generation of human natural killer cells from immature progenitors does not require marrow stromal cells. Blood 1994; 84:841.
281. Mrozek E, Anderson P, Caligiuri MA: Role of interleukin-15 in the development of human CD56$^+$ natural killer cells from CD34$^+$ hematopoietic progenitor cells. Blood 1996; 87:2632.
282. Saraya K, Reid CD: Stem cell factor and the regulation of dendritic cell production from CD34$^+$ progenitors in bone marrow and cord blood. Br J Haematol 1996; 93:258.
283. Rosenzwajg M, Canque B, Gluckman JC: Human dendritic cell differentiation pathway from CD34$^+$ hematopoietic precursor cells. Blood 1996; 87:535.
284. Szabolcs P, Moore MS, Young JW: Expansion of immunostimulatory dendritic cells among the myeloid progeny of human CD34$^+$ bone marrow precursors cultured with c-*kit* ligand, granulocyte-macrophage colony-stimulating factor, and TNF-α. J Immunol 1995; 154:5851.
285. Crawford J, Lau D, Erwin R, et al: A phase I trial of recombinant methionyl human stem cell factor (SCF) in patients with advanced non–small cell lung carcinoma (NSCLC) (Abstract). Proc Am Soc Clin Oncol 1993; 12:135.
286. Costa JJ, Demtri GD, Hayes DF, et al: Increased skin mast cells and urine methyl histamine in patients receiving recombinant methionyl human stem cell factor (Abstract). Proc Am Assoc Cancer Res 1993; 34:211.
287. McNiece I, Glaspy J, LeMaistre F, et al: Effects of recombinant methionyl human stem cell factor (rhSCF) and filgrastim (rhG-CSF) on mobilization of peripheral blood progenitor cells: Preliminary laboratory results from a phase I/II study (Abstract). Blood 1993; 82:84.
288. Glaspy JA, Shpall EJ, LeMaistre C, et al: Peripheral blood progenitor cell mobilization using stem cell factor in combination with filgrastim in breast cancer patients. Blood 1997; 90:2939.
289. Moskowitz CH, Stiff P, Gordon MS, et al: Recombinant methionyl human stem cell factor and filgrastim for peripheral blood progenitor cell mobilization and transplantation in non-Hodgkin's lymphoma patients—results of a phase I/II trial. Blood 1997; 89:3136.
290. Weaver A, Ryder D, Crowther D, et al: Increased numbers of long-term culture–initiating cells in the apheresis product of patients randomized to receive increasing doses of stem cell factor administered in combination with chemotherapy and a standard dose of granulocyte colony-stimulating factor. Blood 1996; 88:3323.
291. Migliaccio G, Migliaccio AR, Druzin ML, et al: Long-term generation of colony-forming cells in liquid culture of CD34$^+$ cord blood cells in the presence of recombinant human stem cell factor. Blood 1992; 79:2620.
292. Brandt J, Briddell RA, Srour EF, et al: Role of c-*kit* ligand in the expansion of human hematopoietic progenitor cells. Blood 1992; 79:634.
293. Nolta JA, Smogorzewska EM, Kohn DB: Analysis of optimal conditions for retroviral-mediated transduction of primitive human hematopoietic cells. Blood 1995; 86:101.

294. Nolta JA, Crooks GM, Overell RW, et al: Retroviral vector-mediated gene transfer into primitive human hematopoietic progenitor cells: Effects of mast cell growth factor (MGF) combined with other cytokines. Exp Hematol 1992; 20:1065.
295. Dunbar CE, Cottler-Fox M, O'Shaughnessy JA, et al: Retrovirally marked CD34-enriched peripheral blood and bone marrow cells contribute to long-term engraftment after autologous transplantation. Blood 1995; 85:3048.
296. Lyman SD, Jacobsen SEW: c-*kit* ligand and Flt3 ligand: Stem/progenitor cell factors with overlapping yet distinct activities. Blood 1998; 91:1101.
297. Lisovsky M, Braun SE, Ge Y, et al: Flt3-ligand production by human bone marrow stromal cells. Leukemia 1996; 10:1012.
298. Namikawa R, Muench MO, de Vries JE, et al: The FLK2/FLT3 ligand synergizes with interleukin-7 in promoting stromal-cell–independent expansion and differentiation of human fetal pro-B cells in vitro. Blood 1996; 87:1881.
299. Molineux G, McCrea C, Qiang Yan X, et al: Flt-3 ligand synergizes with granulocyte colony-stimulating factor to increase neutrophil numbers and mobilize peripheral blood stem cells with long-term repopulating potential. Blood 1997; 89:3998.
300. Sudo Y, Shimizaki C, Ashihara E, et al: Synergistic effect of FLT-3 ligand on the granulocyte colony-stimulating factor–induced mobilization of hematopoietic stem cells and progenitor cells into blood in mice. Blood 1997; 89:3186.
301. Brasel K, McKenna HJ, Morissey PJ, et al: Hematologic effects of flt3 ligand in vivo in mice. Blood 1996; 88:2004.
302. Esche C, Subbotin VM, Maliszewski C, et al: FLT3 ligand administration inhibits tumor growth in murine melanoma and lymphoma. Cancer Res 1998; 58:380.
303. Chen K, Braun S, Lyman S, et al: Antitumor activity and immunotherapeutic properties of Flt3-ligand in a murine breast cancer model. Cancer Res 1997; 57:3511.
304. Drexler HG: Expression of FLT3 receptor and response to FLT3 ligand by leukemic cells. Leukemia 1996; 10:588.

46

Receptor Physiology

Frederick J. Ehlert, PhD

The idea of a "receptor" was first introduced by Ehrlich and Langley around the beginning of the 20th century in an attempt to explain the remarkably selective and potent effects that some natural and synthetic chemicals had on biologic tissues. They argued that pharmacologic agents must interact specifically with macromolecular components in tissue to produce physiologic effects. This idea, of course, is now a readily demonstrable fact. Researchers have identified hundreds of receptors and determined the primary sequence of many of these proteins through gene cloning. The precision with which we now think about a receptor is perhaps most spectacularly illustrated with the nicotinic acetylcholine receptor. Electron micrographic analysis of crystallized nicotinic acetylcholine receptors from the electric ray, *Torpedo,* has produced pictures of high resolution showing a channel-like structure with a central pore, presumably representing the microscopic tunnel through which positive cations flow when the receptor binds its neurotransmitter, acetylcholine.[1]

The identification of receptors as the target for many drugs has an important corollary. It implies that drugs do not create new responses in tissues but that, rather, they start, stop, or modulate natural physiologic functions. For example, synthetic muscarinic agonists are able to elicit contractions of intestinal smooth muscle, because they bind with muscarinic receptors and trigger a signaling cascade that results in the mobilization of calcium and an activation of contractile proteins in the muscle. Obviously, this signaling pathway evolved to respond not to synthetic drugs but to the neurotransmitter acetylcholine. The idea that drugs use physiologic mechanisms applies not only to readily quantifiable responses in peripheral tissues but also to responses that are somewhat more complex. The sensation of euphoria and well-being produced by opiate drugs, such as morphine and heroin, implies the existence of reward pathways in the brain whose natural function is to provide positive reinforcement to the organism under appropriate conditions.[2]

Within this general context, one can define many classes or types of receptors. There are the so-called physiologic receptors, which mediate the effects of a variety of neurotransmitters, peptide and steroid hormones, biogenic amines, and eicosanoids. In addition, enzymes, transport proteins, and ion channels are also important receptors for a variety of drugs that usually, but not always, block the function of these proteins. Finally, the cytoskeleton and deoxyribonucleic acid (DNA) itself may constitute the "receptor" for some agents.

The aims of this chapter are to review some of the quantitative aspects of drug-receptor interactions and to provide a brief survey of the major families of the physiologic receptors and their signaling mechanisms.

RELATIONSHIP BETWEEN RECEPTOR OCCUPANCY AND RESPONSE

Receptor Theory

The binding of a reversible drug to a receptor usually obeys the following scheme:

$$D + R \leftrightarrow DR \qquad \text{[Equation 1]}$$

in which *D* denotes the drug, *R* denotes the receptor, and *DR* denotes the drug-receptor complex.

At equilibrium, the relationship between the drug-receptor complex and the drug concentration is as follows:

$$[DR] = \frac{[D]R_T}{[D] + K_D} \qquad \text{[Equation 2]}$$

in which R_T denotes the total concentration of receptors and K_D denotes the equilibrium dissociation constant of the drug-receptor complex.

The K_D has units of concentration (e.g., molar), and is equivalent to the concentration of drug required for half-maximal receptor occupancy. The K_D is a measure of the affinity of a drug for a receptor; the lower the K_D, the higher the affinity. Equation 1 is usually called the law of mass-action. Its consequences adequately reflect the manner in which a variety of drugs bind with receptors under physiologic conditions.

The size of the response elicited by a drug depends on its intrinsic efficacy and the percentage of receptors that it occupies. It is easier to understand the property of intrinsic efficacy if we consider how the drug-receptor complex behaves in the absence of other ligands or endogenous neurotransmitters. In the absence of drugs, most native receptors are silent. An agonist is a drug that binds to the receptor, turns it on, and triggers a response. The property that enables the agonist to turn on the receptor is called *intrinsic efficacy.* An antagonist is a drug that lacks intrinsic efficacy but is capable of binding to the receptor. Such agents have no effects by themselves but are capable of antagonizing the action of an agonist, whether it be an exogenous drug or an endogenous neurotransmitter. The amount of intrinsic efficacy can vary widely among different drugs, and drugs having a small or intermediate level of intrinsic efficacy are called *partial agonists*.

Inverse Agonists

This general framework may not be entirely sufficient to account for the behavior of all receptor systems. For example, the guanosine triphosphatase (GTPase) activity elicited by opiate receptors is already active in the absence of agonists when this function is measured in brain homogenate in a hypotonic buffer.[3] Under these conditions, the addition of agonists causes a further increase in the GTPase activity, whereas antagonists either have no effect or inhibit the ongoing basal GTPase activity. In other words, if the receptor is already turned on in the absence of agonists, some antagonists (known as "inverse agonists") will actually turn it off. To what extent constitutively active receptors exist in vivo is unknown. Most of the few native receptors that behave in this fashion have been shown to do so under nonphysiologic conditions. However, some mutated forms of receptors have been shown to be constitutively active.[4]

Spare Receptors Concept

Figure 46–1 shows the relationship between occupancy and response for a highly efficacious agonist (Fig. 46–1*A*), a less efficacious agonist (Fig. 46–1*B*), and a partial agonist (Fig. 46–1*C*). In Figure 46–1*A*, the concentration-response curve for the agonist lies to the left of the occupancy curve, indicating that it requires only a low level of receptor occupancy to produce a maximum response; this behavior is typical for a highly efficacious agonist. In Figure 46–1*B*, there is closer agreement between the two curves, so the response is proportional to receptor occupancy. Although this less efficacious agonist is capable of eliciting a maximum response, it can do so only at a much higher level of receptor occupancy compared with the more efficacious agonist shown in Figure 46–1*A*. In Figure 46–1*C*, the agonist has little intrinsic efficacy, so it is incapable of eliciting a maximum response even when the receptors are fully occupied; consequently, the agonist is designated a partial agonist.

When an agonist is capable of eliciting a maximum response at a submaximal level of receptor occupancy (e.g., Fig.46–1*A*), the situation is referred to as *spare receptors*. Unfortunately, this term has created considerable confusion in the pharmacologic literature. The term does not imply that some of the receptors are extra or unnecessary; rather, it simply means that only a small fraction of the total functional receptor population needs to be occupied by the agonist to elicit a maximum response. The presence of spare receptors enhances the potency of the agonist because lower concentrations of the agonist can produce effective responses.

The functional activity of the total receptor population can be appreciated by considering what happens when some of the receptors are inactivated. After partial receptor inactivation, the concentration-response curve of a highly efficacious agonist shifts to the right without a decrease in the maximum response. The loss in potency associated with inactivation of some of the receptors illustrates that spare receptors are functional and maintain the sensitivity of the receptor system. Another important point is that the presence of spare receptors does not imply that there is an excess of receptors in comparison with effectors. In fact, the converse is usually the case. In many signaling cascades, there is divergence along every step in the pathway; that is, one receptor may interact with several effector molecules, and each effector generates several second messenger molecules, and so forth. This divergence leads to amplification and thereby enables a relatively small number of agonist-receptor complexes to generate a significant physiologic response.

Antagonist Dissociation Constant

Because antagonists lack intrinsic efficacy, all that is necessary to describe their interaction with a receptor at equilibrium is the equilibrium dissociation constant. This parameter can be estimated by measuring an agonist concentration-response curve in the absence and presence of the competitive antagonist. A competitive antagonist shifts the log concentration-response curve of an agonist to the right in a parallel fashion without causing a decrease in the maximum response.

The K_D of the antagonist can be estimated from the shift in the concentration-response curve using the following equation:

$$CR - 1 = [A]/K_D \qquad \text{[Equation 3]}$$

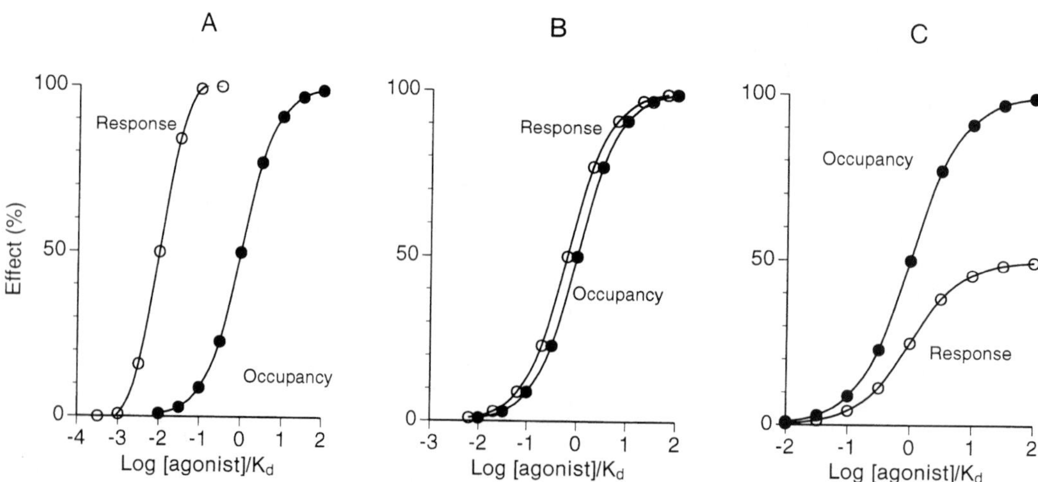

Figure 46–1. Relationship between receptor occupancy (○) and response (●) for a highly efficacious agonist *(A)*, a less efficacious agonist *(B)*, and a partial agonist *(C)*. Both occupancy and response are expressed as percentages of their maximum values and are plotted on the ordinate scale. The concentration of the agonist is expressed on the abscissa as a log of the ratio of the agonist concentration divided by its K_d.

in which *CR* (concentration ratio) denotes the EC_{50} value of the agonist (concentration of agonist causing a half-maximal response) measured in the presence of the antagonist divided by the EC_{50} value measured in the absence of the antagonist, and *[A]* denotes the concentration of the antagonist.

Secondary Allosteric Sites

The relationships just described are adequate to account for the interactions of agonists and antagonists with the primary recognition site of a receptor. Some receptors have secondary allosteric sites where drugs can also bind and modify the ability of primary ligands to activate the receptor. One such example is the gamma-aminobutyric acid-A ($GABA_A$) receptor.[5] This receptor is a chloride channel that is regulated by the neurotransmitter GABA. The binding of GABA to its site on the $GABA_A$ receptor causes the chloride channel to open. In addition to the primary GABA site, there are secondary allosteric sites, including one for benzodiazepine-like drugs. A tranquilizing benzodiazepine, like diazepam, binds to the allosteric site and increases the affinity of GABA for its site on the channel, thereby enhancing the effects of GABA. This allosteric effect can account for the pharmacologic properties of benzodiazepines, which include relief from anxiety, sedation, and protection against seizures.

In contrast, some β-carboline derivatives bind to the allosteric site and inhibit the binding of GABA. These compounds have been called *inverse agonists* because they elicit responses that are opposite to those of benzodiazepines (i.e., anxiety, convulsions). They are more appropriately referred to, however, as allosteric GABA antagonists because they produce their effects by antagonizing GABA. In addition, some compounds bind to the allosteric site and have no effect on the binding of GABA. These compounds (e.g., Ro 151788) are called benzodiazepine antagonists, and although they have no effects by themselves, they antagonize both the tranquilizing effects of benzodiazepines and the convulsant effects of β-carbolines.

RECEPTOR FAMILIES

Physiologic receptors can be divided into four families on the basis of their structural and functional properties[6]:

- Ligand-regulated gene regulatory proteins
- Ligand-regulated enzymes
- Ligand-gated ion channels
- G protein–linked receptors

Each family has a distinct overall structure and a general function that is shared by all members of the same family. Within each family, there is usually, but not always, a considerable amount of sequence homology. Regions of high homology within a given family have enabled molecular biologists to use low-stringency hybridization techniques to identify additional members of the same family. In some instances, the endogenous ligands for the cloned receptor protein have not been identified, leading to their designation as "orphan receptors." A cursory survey of these four receptor families is given next.

Ligand-Regulated Gene Regulatory Proteins

The ligand-regulated gene regulatory protein superfamily comprises a large group of soluble receptors that bind to DNA and regulate the activity of specific genes in a ligand-dependent manner.[7] This family contains receptors for thyroid hormone, retinoids, vitamin D, and the various steroid hormones, including glucocorticoids, mineralocorticoids, androgens, progesterone, and estrogen. Most of these receptors are located in the nucleus. Not surprisingly, the ligands for these receptors can readily penetrate the plasma membrane, and their access to the receptor is controlled by hormone-binding proteins and by enzymatic processing of the ligand itself.

Receptors belonging to the steroid superfamily all share a similar structure having three major domains.[7] Near the center of the sequence is a highly conserved domain of 66 to 68 amino acids that constitutes the *DNA-binding region* of the receptor. In this domain, the sequence forms two loops held in place by a zinc atom that interacts with cysteine residues on opposite sides of the loop. Each of the two loops is called a "zinc finger," and many proteins that bind with DNA have a zinc finger-like structure.

The second major domain of this family of receptors is the *carboxy-terminal region*, which functions as the ligand-binding domain. This region of the receptor also shows considerable sequence homology, particularly among the androgen, glucocorticoid, mineralocorticoid, and progesterone receptors, which have structurally similar ligands (i.e., steroids).

The third major domain is the *amino-terminal region*, which shows the greatest variation in size and the least conservation in sequence. This domain of the receptor is thought to mediate transcriptional activation.

A variety of evidence supports the existence of these distinct functional domains on steroid receptors. Perhaps the most dramatic evidence of this sort comes from studies on chimeric receptors in which a domain from one receptor is replaced with the corresponding domain from another. For example, when the 66–amino acid DNA-binding region of the estrogen receptor is replaced with that of the glucocorticoid receptor, a chimeric receptor is formed that turns on a glucocorticoid-inducible gene in the presence of estradiol.[8] Truncated receptors have also yielded clues about functional domains as well as the mechanism of ligand-induced activation. For example, glucocorticoid receptor mutants lacking most of the ligand-binding domain demonstrate constitutive activity[9]; that is, the truncated receptor binds to DNA and causes transcriptional activation in the absence of hormone. Apparently, the ligand-binding domain of the glucocorticoid receptor normally prevents DNA binding and transcriptional activation, whereas the binding of the hormone relieves this tonic inhibition. Finally, several cases of hormonal resistance have been attributed to point mutations in the ligand-binding domain that resulted in diminished hormone binding.[7]

Although the details are unclear, the binding of hormone to its receptor triggers the formation of receptor dimers that subsequently bind to DNA.[7] The sites on DNA where binding occurs are called the *hormone response elements* (HREs). These sites are located in the regulatory regions of steroid-induced genes, and several have been identified. The consensus sequences of HREs exhibit dyad symmetry, which is consistent with the idea that a receptor dimer interacts with the HRE.

Ligand-Regulated Enzymes

The ligand-regulated enzymes represent a huge family of cell surface receptors. The unifying structural feature of these receptors is the presence of an extracellular ligand-binding domain that regulates an intracellular domain that either has intrinsic enzymatic activity or associates with an enzyme. In most instances, the two domains of the receptor are connected by a single transmembrane domain. There are five classes within the ligand-regulated enzyme family:

- Receptor tyrosine kinases (RTKs), which phosphorylate signaling proteins on tyrosine residues
- Tyrosine kinase-associated receptors, which associate with enzymes having tyrosine kinase activity
- Receptor tyrosine phosphatases, which cleave phosphotyrosine ester groups on signaling proteins
- Receptor serine/threonine kinases, which phosphorylate signaling proteins containing serine and threonine residues
- Receptor guanylyl cyclases, which catalyze the formation of cyclic guanosine-3′,5′-monophosphate (GMP) within the cytosol

The RTKs and receptor guanylyl cyclases are discussed here in detail.

Receptor Tyrosine Kinases

The receptor tyrosine kinase family contains receptors for numerous growth factors, including insulin, fibroblast growth factor (FGF), epidermal growth factor (EGF), and platelet-derived growth factor (PDGF). The structural and functional properties of these receptors have been reviewed elsewhere[10, 11]; a brief description is given here.

As mentioned previously, members of this family of receptors have an extracellular ligand-binding domain, an intracellular tyrosine kinase domain, and a transmembrane domain (Fig. 46–2). Most growth factor receptors are formed from a single polypeptide chain; however, the class II RTKs, which include receptors for insulin and insulin-like growth factor, are heterotetrameric, consisting of two α and two β subunits connected by disulfide bonds (see Fig. 46–2). The two α subunits contribute to the ligand-binding domain, whereas the two β subunits traverse the membrane and possess the tyrosine kinase activity. The class I and II RTKs, which include the EGF receptor and the insulin receptor, have cysteine-rich regions in their extracellular ligand-binding domains. The class IV RTKs, which include the FGF receptor, has three immunoglobulin-like (Ig-like) domains in the extracellular, ligand-binding portion of the receptor.

The tyrosine kinase domain is the most highly conserved domain among the different classes of RTKs. This domain contains an ATP-binding site and a tyrosine acceptor site. In the class III RTKs, these two functional regions of the kinase domain are separated by a hydrophilic, proline-rich sequence of 77 to 107 amino acids. The results of studies on chimeric receptors constructed from heterologous ligand-binding and kinase domains provide further support for the existence of autonomous functional domains. In each case, the hybrid receptors have displayed the appropriate ligand specificity and kinase activity.

Ligand binding to monomeric RTKs results in dimerization, which is a prerequisite for growth factor-dependent kinase activation. Interestingly, the kinase activity of the tetrameric insulin receptor, which is analogous to an EGF receptor dimer, is much greater than that of the dimeric αβ form of the insulin receptor. The results of ligand-binding studies have demonstrated that growth factors bind to dimeric receptors with higher affinity compared with monomers, suggesting that the tighter binding of the growth factor to the dimer provides the drive for receptor aggregation. Once made active by their respective ligands, all growth factor receptors autophosphorylate on several tyrosine residues. This autophosphorylation triggers a complex signaling pathway that is characterized by a series of protein-protein interactions and the phosphorylation of signaling proteins on tyrosine residues. The details of the signaling pathway can vary according to the receptor and the cell type.

When a growth factor triggers the autophosphorylation of its receptor, various signaling proteins bind to the receptor and become activated. These signaling proteins typically contain SH-2 (src homology region 2) domains that have high affinity for specific phosphotyrosine residues on the receptor. A myriad of intracellular signaling proteins contain SH-2 domains, which are thought to mediate the effects of growth factors by binding to specific phosphotyrosine residues on the receptor.[12] These target proteins include the phosphoinositide-specific phospholipase Cγ (PLCγ), GTPase-activating protein (GAP), and members of the Src family of tyrosine kinases.

In addition, several adapter proteins have been identified that lack enzymatic activity but contain both SH-2 and SH-3 domains. These adapter proteins are thought to bind to phosphotyrosine on the receptor via their SH-2 domain and to other signaling proteins via their SH-3 domain. Examples of adapter proteins are Grb2 and SHC, which enable mSOS to associate with the growth factor receptor–complex. The docking of mSOS to the receptor via adapter proteins enables mSOS to interact with the intracellular guanosine triphosphate (GTP) binding protein, Ras, and cause it to give up its bound guanosine diphosphate (GDP) and to take up GTP. Once bound with GTP, Ras initiates a protein kinase signaling cas-

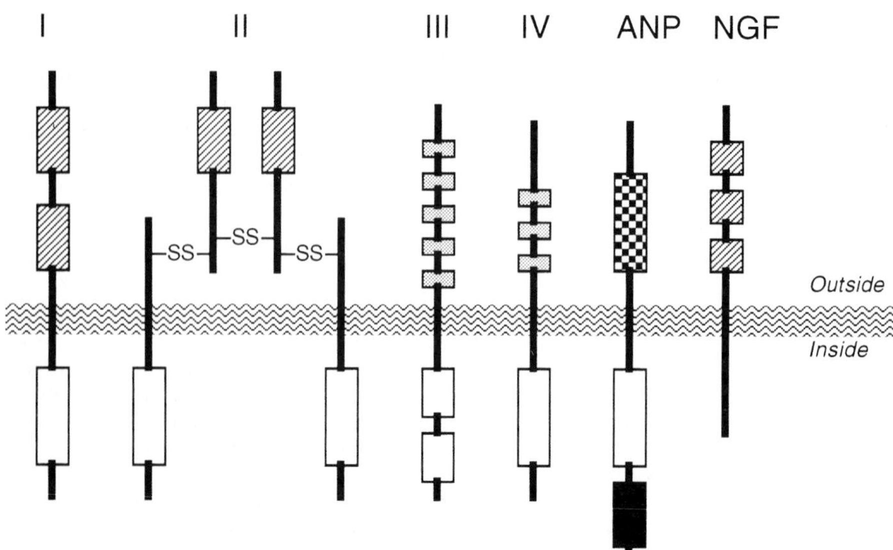

Figure 46–2. Structure of different members of the ligand-regulated enzyme superfamily of receptors. The transmembrane topography of the primary sequences of the receptor tyrosine kinases (I, II, III, and IV), the receptor for atrial natriuretic peptide (ANP), and the receptor for nerve growth factor (NGF) are shown. *Boxes* indicate the various functional domains of the receptor and are shaded according to the following scheme: *diagonal lines* = cysteine-rich domain; *shaded* = Ig domain; *checkered* = ANP-binding domain; *open* = tyrosine kinase domain; and *black* = guanylyl cyclase domain.

cade that results in the activation of mitogen-activated protein kinase (MAP kinase). This kinase triggers a variety of events associated with cellular growth and differentiation. The activity of Ras is inhibited by GAP, which increases the intrinsic GTPase activity of Ras, thereby converting it from the active GTP-bound form to the inactive GDP-bound form.

Receptor Guanylyl Cyclases

Another member of the ligand-regulated enzyme superfamily is the receptor for atrial natriuretic peptide (ANP).[13, 14] This receptor contains an extracellular ligand-binding domain for ANP, a single transmembrane domain, and an intracellular domain that has guanylyl cyclase activity (see Fig. 46-2). The binding of ANP to this receptor causes an increase in the concentration of cyclic GMP inside the cell. This second messenger activates a cyclic GMP-dependent protein kinase, which ultimately triggers a variety of responses, including diuresis, natriuresis, and vasorelaxation. Interestingly, the extracellular domain of the ANP receptor is homologous with an ANP-binding protein that is thought to have a role in the clearance of ANP from the circulation. The proximal portion of the intracellular domain is homologous to the kinase domain of the RTKs, although no ANP-induced kinase activity has been detected. The most distal portion of the intracellular domain represents the catalytic domain, and it is homologous to the soluble form of guanylyl cyclase.

Ligand-Gated Ion Channels

The ligand-gated ion channels represent a large superfamily that includes receptors for acetylcholine (nicotinic acetylcholine receptor), GABA ($GABA_A$ receptor), glycine, and various excitatory amino acids (e.g., glutamate and aspartate).[6] As their name implies, members of this superfamily are ion channels that open up and conduct an ionic current when an agonist binds upon them. In the case of the nicotinic acetylcholine receptor of the neuromuscular junction and the *Torpedo* electric organ, the ionic current is carried by positive monovalent cations, primarily sodium, whereas neuronal nicotinic receptors carry a rapidly desensitizing current of primarily calcium.[15] In the case of excitatory amino acid receptors, the ionic current is carried by both sodium and calcium, whereas inhibitory amino acid receptors (i.e., GABA and glycine receptor) carry a chloride current.

The ligand-gated ion channels have a characteristic oligomeric structure. The nicotinic acetylcholine receptor of the neuromuscular junction has a pentameric structure, consisting of two α subunits and one each of β_1, γ, and δ subunits. These subunits are arranged like the staves in a barrel-like structure having a central pore that is thought to be the channel of the receptor.[1] Although the precise subunit structure of neuronal nicotinic receptors and the other ligand-gated ion channels is unknown, it is thought to be analogous to that of the neuromuscular nicotinic acetylcholine receptor.[16, 17] For example, when expressed in *Xenopus* oocytes, α_4 and β_2 neuronal nicotinic receptor subunits form functional ligand-gated ion channels having a pentameric structure composed of two α_4 and three β_2 subunits.

It has also been shown that α_7, α_8, and α_9 subunits form functional homomeric channels in *Xenopus* oocytes, presumably consisting of five identical subunits. Whether these homomeric channels are formed in native α_7, α_8, and α_9 containing receptors is unknown. Moreover, recombinant homomeric $GABA_A$ receptors have been formed by injecting only messenger ribonucleic acid (mRNA) for the α subunit into *Xenopus* oocytes, indicating that functional, GABA-regulated ion channels can be formed from only α subunits.[18] These homomeric channels do not, however, retain all of the complex allosteric interactions characteristic of native $GABA_A$ receptors, and it is entirely possible that homomeric channels do not occur naturally.

Several different subtypes of the individual subunits have been cloned for both the nicotinic and $GABA_A$ receptors, raising the possibility of a staggering number of channel subtypes based on combinations of different types of subunits. These different subtypes of channels could have different pharmacologic and functional properties and unique developmental profiles. Although this potential diversity represents a colossal task to sort out, it also increases the likelihood that more selective drugs can be developed.

The overall structure of the ligand-gated ion channels shows homology with many of the voltage-regulated ion channels, like the sodium channel and the L type calcium channel.[6] Although the ligand-gated ion channels are primarily chemosensitive, their gating characteristics are modified by the potential of the membrane. Conversely, although the voltage-gated ion channels are primarily potential-sensitive, they are also modified by a variety of agonistic and antagonistic ligands that bind at different sites on the channel that are often allosterically linked to one another. When considered from this viewpoint, the ligand- and voltage-gated ion channels form a large superfamily of receptors.

The overall three-dimensional structure and transmembrane topography of the various types of ligand-gated cation and anion channels show considerable homologies, and a description of their general features is given here.[6] The ligand-binding domain of the nicotinic and glycine receptor appears to be on an extracellular domain of the α subunit. In the case of the neuromuscular nicotinic receptor, two molecules of acetylcholine bind to the channel and cause it to open. This scheme is consistent with the subunit structure of the channel (i.e., $\alpha_2\beta\gamma\delta$) and with the positive cooperativity that is characteristic of the binding of acetylcholine to the channel.[6] Clusters of residues having a charge opposite to that of the permiant ion are located at that channel opening in both the nicotinic and $GABA_A$ receptors, and perhaps these amino acids determine the ionic selectivity of the channel.

Ligand-gated ion channels are widespread throughout the central and peripheral nervous systems and are responsible for rapid synaptic neurotransmission, characterized by synaptic delays of less than half a millisecond. The nicotinic acetylcholine receptor is present at the neuromuscular junction, where it is responsible for eliciting skeletal muscle contraction in response to impulse flow from a motor neuron. These receptors are the targets for the neuromuscular blocking agents used as adjuncts to general anesthesia.[19] The $GABA_A$ receptor represents the major inhibitory neurotransmitter receptor in the brain, and it is an important target for a variety of drugs used to treat anxiety, convulsions, and insomnia.[20] Excitatory amino acid receptors are also abundant in brain, and inhibitors of these ion channels may have use in preventing the neuronal damage associated with brain ischemia following stroke.

G Protein–Linked Receptors

Structure

The G protein–linked family of receptors is perhaps the largest, and it comprises receptors for a variety of endogenous neurotransmitters, including acetylcholine (muscarinic acetylcholine receptor), catecholamines, histamine, serotonin, eicosanoids, and some peptides.[6] These receptors trigger responses by binding with heterotrimeric G proteins, which in turn activate various effectors, including ion channels and enzymes that generate second messengers (see later).

Not only are G protein–linked receptors involved in neurotransmission at a variety of synapses and junctions throughout the brain and peripheral autonomic nervous system, but members of this family are also involved in the special sensory functions of vision, taste, and olfaction.[21] For example, the light receptor in the retina, rhodopsin, consists of a tightly bound complex between a protein called opsin and a photoactive ligand, 11-*cis*-retinal.[22, 23] When light shines on 11-*cis*-retinal, it isomerizes to the *trans* isomer (11-*trans*-retinal), which induces a conformational change in rhodopsin, causing it to activate a G protein called *transducin* (G_T). Ultimately, transducin initiates a cascade of events leading to a hyperpolarizing response in the retinal ganglion cell. This signaling pathway is so highly amplified that a single photon of light has a 50% probability of triggering a response in the retinal ganglion cell. G protein–linked receptors are also involved in olfaction to a remarkable extent. The results of cloning studies on genomic and complementary DNA (cDNA) libraries prepared from the olfactory epithelium indicate that there may be more than 100 different types of odorant receptors in the nose, each of which may be receptive to a different spectrum of odorants.[24]

Receptors belonging to the G protein–linked class all have a similar structure, consisting of seven highly conserved, transmembrane domains of α-helix that are connected to the less conserved amino-terminal, carboxy-terminal, and intracellular and extracellular loops. It is generally assumed that the three-dimensional structure of G protein–linked receptors conforms to that of bacteriorhodopsin, which has been determined by x-ray diffraction.[25] In bacteriorhodopsin, the transmembrane (TM) domains run perpendicular to the plane of the membrane and circumscribe a central pore. Retinal and the neurotransmitters for muscarinic and catecholamine receptors are thought to bind at a site within the pore. Accordingly, point mutations in a highly conserved aspartic acid residue in the third TM domain cause a loss in agonist binding at muscarinic receptors[26] and β-adrenergic receptors.[27]

Not surprisingly, the part of the receptor involved in G protein coupling is a relatively large, hydrophilic domain that projects into the cytoplasm, namely, the third cytoplasmic (i3) loop. The strongest evidence for the coupling role of the i3 loop comes from studies on chimeric receptors in which the i3 loop of one receptor is replaced with that from another. For example, when the i3 loop of the muscarinic receptor is switched with that of the β-adrenergic receptor, the chimeric receptor triggers β-adrenergic effects in response to muscarinic agonists.[28] Analogous results have been observed in studies on chimers constructed from a variety of other G protein–linked receptors. Interestingly, the i3 loops of several receptors are constitutively active by themselves.[29] Thus, the ligand-binding domain (seven TM segments) of G protein–linked receptors probably exerts a tonic inhibitory effect on the i3 loop, and the binding of neurotransmitter relieves this inhibition.

G Proteins

The G proteins involved in receptor signaling are heterotrimeric, consisting of α, β, and γ subunits.[30, 31] The βγ subunits form a tightly bound complex that functions as a unit. The α subunits of heterotrimeric G protein are close relatives of many other low-molecular-weight G proteins that lack βγ subunits, like the Ras protein mentioned earlier. These small G proteins participate in numerous metabolic processes within the cell, including some that have little to do with transmembrane signaling at the cell surface. The basic function that G proteins accomplish at the expense of GTP hydrolysis is one of transportation between two destinations. In the case of the low-molecular-weight G protein elongation factor Tu, there is a transport of aminoacyl transfer RNA (tRNA) complexes on the ribosome, whereas in the case of heterotrimeric G proteins, the G protein shuttles between the receptor and its effector. Thus, nature uses G proteins for a variety of roles, and the involvement of heterotrimeric G proteins in receptor signaling at the cell membrane probably represents a highly specialized function.

The α subunit of heterotrimeric G proteins shows the greatest diversity, and more than 20 different types of α subunits have been cloned.[21] By contrast, the βγ subunits seem to be fewer in subtypes, and it appears that more than one type of α subunit can associate with the same dimer of βγ subunits. The α subunit confers selectivity for different receptors as well as effectors; however, the degree of selectivity is not absolute (see later discussion). For example, the M_2 subtype of the muscarinic receptor can interact with more than one type of G protein (e.g., G_o and $G_{i1\text{-}3}$[32]), and a single G protein of the G_i family can interact with more than one type of receptor (e.g., M_2-muscarinic and D_2-dopamine). Receptors that interact with G_i and G_o, however, are usually ineffective at interacting with G_s, and vice versa.[21]

There is also selectivity at the level of the G protein–effector interaction. For example, members of the G_i family can mediate an inhibition of adenylyl cyclase activity; however, these G proteins are much less effective at coupling receptors to PLCβ. The α subunit of G proteins binds GTP, resulting in activation and a dissociation of the GTP-α complex from the βγ subunits. In addition, the α subunit has GTPase activity that hydrolyzes GTP to GDP, causing the inactive GDP-α complex to coalesce with the βγ subunits.

The α subunits of some G proteins are also substrates for bacterial toxins that catalyze the adenosine diphosphate (ADP) ribosylation of the α subunit. For example, cholera toxin causes an ADP-ribosylation of the α subunit of G_s, the G protein that stimulates adenylyl cyclase activity. This ADP-ribosylation causes an inhibition of the GTPase activity, resulting in an irreversible activation of G_s and, consequently, adenylyl cyclase. In contrast, pertussis toxin causes the ADP-ribosylation of G_i and G_o, which prevents receptor-mediated activation of G_i and G_o. Transducin (G_T) is a substrate for both cholera toxin and pertussis toxin.

GTPase Cycle

Figure 46–3 shows what happens inside the cell when an agonist activates a G protein–linked receptor:

1. Initially, the G protein is in its trimeric form with GDP tightly bound to it. This inactive form of the G protein is a prerequisite for receptor interaction, because the agonist-receptor complex can interact only with the trimeric complex, not with free α or βγ subunits. Although the cell contains high concentrations (approximately 0.1 mM) of GTP, this nucleotide cannot displace GDP from the G protein because the dissociation rate of GDP from the α subunit is negligible.
2. The binding of agonist to its receptor causes a conformational change so that the i3 loop can interact with the G protein. This interaction allows the agonist to increase the rate of dissociation of GDP, making it possible for GTP to bind to the G protein.
3. The binding of GTP causes a dissociation of the GTP-α subunit from both the βγ subunits and the receptor, resulting in activation.
4. The GTP-α subunit complex is then free to turn its effector on and ultimately trigger the cell's response to the agonist. In some instances, it appears that the βγ subunits elicit the response.
5. The turn-off mechanism is the GTPase activity of the α subunit, which hydrolyzes GTP. The resulting GDP-α subunit then coalesces with the βγ subunits to form the trimeric complex, which is inactive.

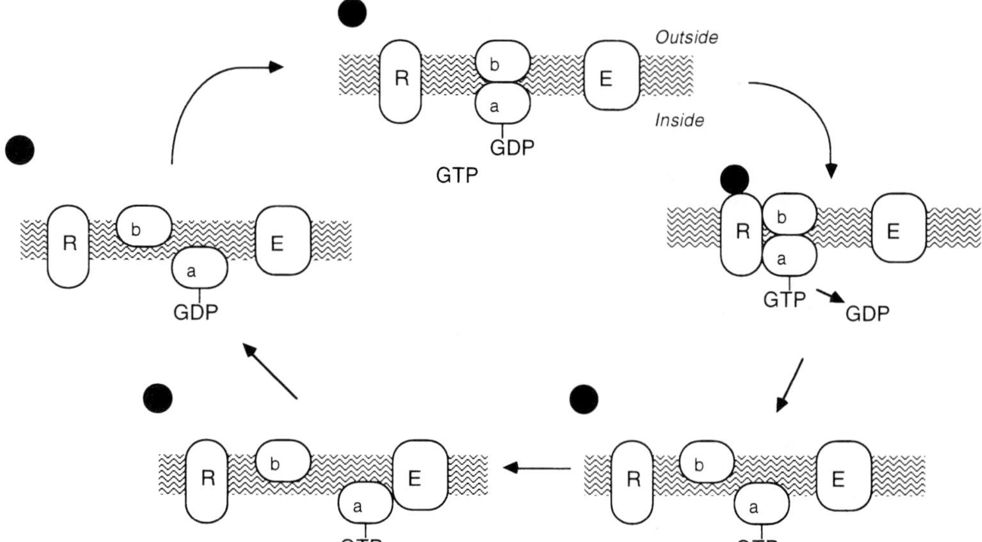

Figure 46–3. Receptor-activated GTPase cycle. Schematic diagram of the interaction of an agonist *(solid circle)* with its receptor (R) and the α (a) and βγ (b) subunits of a G protein. The effector is denoted by "E." See text for further details.

6. The cycle can then repeat itself, provided that agonist is occupying the receptor.

Several experimental observations support the scheme just described, a few of which are mentioned here. Muscarinic agonists cause the M_2 receptor to form a stable complex with G_i that can be identified on Western blots with antibodies to G_i or the M_2 receptor.[32] In contrast, antagonists do not promote the formation of a receptor–G protein complex. Moreover, the ability of the ligand to promote the ternary complex (agonist-receptor–G protein complex) is proportional to the intrinsic efficacy of the agonist.[33] This relationship is shown in Figure 46–4 for M_2-muscarinic receptors in the heart. The propensity of the agonist to generate the ternary complex can be measured in a binding assay, and this parameter is denoted by "Receptor-Gi Cooperativity" in Figure 46–4*A*. It can be seen that the cooperativity is proportional to intrinsic efficacy for a number of agonists.

Another conspicuous feature of most G protein–linked receptors is that the binding of ligands to the receptor is modified by GTP in a manner that is proportional to the intrinsic efficacy of the ligand. Both GTP and GDP cause a reduction in agonist-binding affinity, but not in antagonist affinity. The relationship between intrinsic efficacy and the inhibitory effect of GTP (GTP-shift) on ligand binding to M_2-muscarinic receptors in the heart is shown in Figure 46–4*B* for a number of ligands. The proportional relationship between the negatively cooperative effects of GTP on agonist binding and the intrinsic efficacy of the agonist is readily apparent from the plot.

The relationships shown in Figure 46–4 provide insight into the mechanism of how the receptor works. In considering Figure 46–4, it is important to note that GDP as well as GTP inhibits agonist, but not antagonist, affinity. This effect is allosteric because the agonist and the guanine nucleotide act at different sites. Therefore, the nature of the interaction between the two types of ligands is called *negative heterotropic cooperativity.* One of the properties of allosteric interactions is that they are reciprocal; that is, if GDP or GTP reduces the affinity of the agonist, then the agonist must reduce the affinity of the guanine nucleotide to precisely the same extent.[34] This agonist-mediated reduction in the affinity of GDP causes it to dissociate from the G protein more rapidly, allowing GTP to displace it from the G protein.

Although this increase in the dissociation kinetics of GDP is achieved at the cost of reducing the affinity of GTP, it does not result in a decrease in the binding of GTP, because GTP is maintained at saturating concentrations inside the cell. For example, the K_D of GTP analogs for the G protein is in the nanomolar (10^{-9} M) range, whereas the concentration of GTP inside the cell is in the millimolar (10^{-3} M) range. Thus, it can be seen that the agonist-receptor complex works by increasing the dissociation kinetics of GDP from the G protein

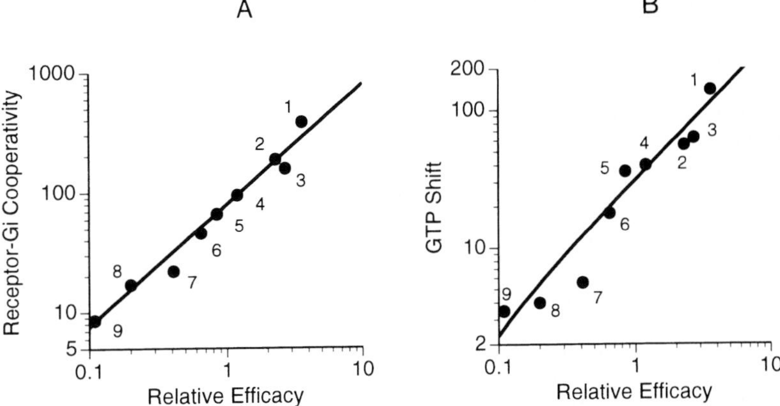

Figure 46–4. Correlation between relative efficacy and agonist-binding properties at M_2 muscarinic receptors. *A,* The positive heterotropic cooperativity between the binding of the agonist and G_i is plotted against the relative efficacy of the agonist, as determined by inhibition of adenylyl cyclase activity. *B,* The ratio of the concentration of the agonist in the presence and absence of GTP is plotted against the relative efficacy of the agonist. 1 = oxotremorine-M; 2 = carbachol; 3 = *cis*-dioxolane; 4 = oxotremorine; 5 = (+)-aceclidine; 6 = (−)-aceclidine; 7 = *N*-methylaceclidine; 8 = BM5; 9 = BOK1. (Data from Ehlert FJ: The relationship between the muscarinic receptor occupancy and a denylate cyclase inhibition in the rabbit myocardium. Mol Pharmacol 1985; 28:410.)

and that this effect is mediated by negative heterotropic cooperativity.

SIGNALING MECHANISMS OF G PROTEIN–LINKED RECEPTORS

G protein–linked receptors mediate a myriad of responses at the level of the whole tissue; however, at the subcellular level, these responses seem to be triggered by a relatively small number of transduction mechanisms. This situation illustrates that diversity is achieved through divergence in the signaling pathway, and that the factors that determine the intermediate and distal parts of the signaling mechanism are tissue-specific. Thus, calcium mobilization resulting from activation of a PLCβ-linked receptor in smooth muscle may cause contraction[35]; however, in an exocrine gland, the same transduction mechanism may cause secretion. Some of the major transduction mechanisms of G protein-linked receptors are summarized here and listed in Table 46–1.

Calcium Mobilization

Perhaps the most universal mechanism for triggering a response is to increase the concentration of calcium within the cell.[36] Not surprisingly, several different signaling mechanisms ultimately affect the levels of calcium within the cytoplasm. One common mechanism for elevating calcium is through activation of PLCβ, an enzyme that hydrolyzes the phospholipid phosphatidylinositol 4,5-bisphosphate (PIP_2) into inositol 1,4,5-trisphosphate (IP_3) and diacylglycerol (DAG).[37] This membrane-bound enzyme is activated by numerous receptors that signal through the G_q family of G proteins (see Table 46–1). The two hydrolysis products, IP_3 and DAG, act as second messengers within the cell.[38] IP_3 causes a release of calcium from the endoplasmic reticulum, and DAG activates protein kinase C. IP_3 is phosphorylated in some cells to inositol 1,3,4,5-tetrakisphosphate (IP_4), which appears to have a role in helping IP_3 mobilize calcium.[39] Both IP_3 and IP_4 are unstable and are sequentially hydrolyzed by phosphatases back to inositol, which is then recycled for synthesis of new PIP_2.

The final phosphatase in the sequence, myoinositol-1-phosphatase, is inhibited by lithium. Ultimately, this inhibition leads to an accumulation of inositol 1-phosphate (IP_1) and a depletion in inositol and inositol-containing phospholipids (e.g., PIP_2) within the brain. This depletion can lead to a dampening in receptor signaling through the PLCβ pathway, and it has been suggested that this dampening is the mechanism by which lithium attenuates the symptoms of manic-depressive psychosis.[40]

Once calcium is elevated in the cell, it can mediate a variety of effects by binding to calmodulin and activating a variety of kinases and phosphatases. The protein kinase C that is activated by DAG also mediates numerous effects, and it is the target for some tumor promoting phorbol ester derivatives.

TABLE 46–1. Signaling Mechanisms of G Protein–Linked Receptors

Representative Receptors	G Protein Family	Effector
β_1- and β_2-adrenergic	G_s	Stimulate adenylyl cyclase
D_1-dopamine		Open calcium channels
H_2-histamine		
M_2- and M_4-muscarinic	G_i and G_o	Open potassium channels
D_2-dopamine		Close calcium channels
α_2-Adrenergic		Inhibit adenylyl cyclase
M_1-, M_3-, and M_5-muscarinic	G_q	Stimulate phospholipase Cβ
α_1-Adrenergic		
Angiotensin II		
Rhodopsin	G_T	Stimulate cyclic guanosine-3′,5′-monophosphate phosphodiesterase

Data from Helper JR, Gilman AG: G proteins. Trends Biochem Sci 1992; 17:383.

Adenylyl Cyclase System

Another important signaling mechanism within the cell is the adenylyl cyclase system. G protein-linked receptors that affect adenylyl cyclase can be divided into two categories, depending on whether they stimulate or inhibit the enzyme.[21] G_s mediates the stimulation, whereas G_i mediates inhibition through a distinct group of receptors. Several different types of adenylyl cyclases have been identified, and all of these are activated by the α subunit of G_s (i.e., α_s).[40] The mechanism for inhibition of the enzyme is not entirely clear; it appears that both α_i and the βγ subunits may be involved, depending on the type of adenylyl cyclase. Once cyclic adenosine monophosphate (AMP) rises within the cell, it can mediate a variety of effects through activation of cyclic AMP–dependent protein kinase (protein kinase A). The turn-off mechanism for cyclic AMP is phosphodiesterase, which rapidly hydrolyzes cyclic AMP into AMP.

Receptor Cross-Talk

There are several possibilities for crosstalk between receptors that stimulate adenylyl cyclase and those that activate PLCβ. For example, the type I adenylyl cyclase, which is abundant in brain, is activated by calcium.[41] Also, calcium stimulates phosphodiesterase in some tissues. Moreover, the stimulation of adenylyl cyclase caused by G_s-linked receptors is enhanced by activation of protein kinase C in some tissues. Finally, α_s subunit-mediated stimulation of the type II and type IV adenylyl cyclases has been shown to be greatly potentiated by the βγ subunits, providing yet another mechanism for receptor crosstalk.

Ion Channels

In addition to the second messenger systems described previously, G protein–linked receptors can also affect a variety of ionic conductances.[42] In several instances, these effects are mediated indirectly by second messengers, whereas in other cases, there is direct coupling of G proteins to ion channels. One such example is in the heart, where muscarinic receptors and β-adrenergic receptors cause reciprocal changes in the conductivity of inwardly rectified potassium channels. These effects are mediated by G_i and G_s, respectively, and represent the mechanisms by which the vagus nerve slows heart rate and the cardiac sympathetic nerves increase heart rate.

CELLULAR SIGNALING AND CANCER

Most cancer cells contain mutations in their DNA that presumably cause tumorigenesis.[43] These mutations are of two general forms:

- *Recessive*, which result in a loss of function of tumor suppressor genes
- *Dominant*, which result in a gain in function

The genes that contain these dominant mutations are designated *oncogenes*, and their normal counterparts are referred to as *proto-oncogenes*.

Invariably, proto-oncogenes code for proteins that are part of normal receptor signaling cascades within the body; for example, truncated forms of the EGF receptor lacking the ligand-binding domain are constitutively active and cause tumorigenesis.[10] Relatively small changes in signaling proteins are oncogenic in numerous instances; for example, point mutations in G_i have been implicated in carcinoma of the ovary and adrenal gland, whereas point mutations in G_s are present in adenomas of the pituitary gland and carcinoma of the thyroid.[44] Interestingly, these point mutations result in a loss of the GTPase activity of these G proteins, causing them to become constitutively active. There are many other examples of oncogene products that are mutated signaling proteins, such as ligand-regulated gene regulatory proteins, RTKs, G protein–linked receptors, and low-molecular-weight G proteins (including Ras). Thus, in numerous instances, tumorigenesis is caused by overactive, unregulated receptor signaling.

DIVERSITY AND REDUNDANCY

In considering the diverse mechanisms by which information is transmitted throughout the body by way of receptor signaling, one is struck by two seemingly opposite principles of nature, diversity and redundancy.[45] Nature is redundant in the sense that only four different types of mechanisms can account for the function of what may turn out to be more than a thousand different types of physiologic and sensory receptors. Also, the same general GTPase cycle is harnessed for innumerable functions within the cell, ranging from protein synthesis, secretion, and neurotransmission to taste, olfaction, and vision. To accomplish these diverse tasks, nature modifies a given mechanism in an extraordinary number of ways. An appreciation of the diversity and redundancy of nature will aid in the future unraveling of biologic mechanisms and in the development of therapeutic agents to treat disease.

ACKNOWLEDGMENTS

Portions of the author's work cited in this chapter were supported by National Institutes of Health Grants NS30882 and NS26511.

References

1. Unwin N, Toyoshima C, Kubalek E: Arrangement of the acetylcholine receptor subunits in the resting and desensitized states determined by cryelector microscopy of crystallized *Torpedo* postsynaptic membranes. J Cell Biol 1988; 107:1123.
2. Stein L, Belluzzi JD: Reinforcement and neurochemical substrates. *In*: Encyclopedia of Neuroscience. Vol II. Adelman G (Ed). Boston, Birkhauser, 1987, pp 1043–1045.
3. Costa T, Herz A: Antagonists with negative intrinsic activity at delta opioid receptors coupled to GTP-binding proteins. Proc Natl Acad Sci U S A 1989; 86:7321.
4. Allen LF, Lefkowitz RJ, Caron MG, et al: G-protein-coupled receptor genes as protooncogenes: Constitutively activating mutation of the α_{1B}-adrenergic receptor enhances mitogenesis and tumorigenicity. Proc Natl Acad Sci U S A 1991; 88:11358.
5. Ehlert FJ: "Inverse agonists," cooperativity and drug action at benzodiazepine receptors. Trends Pharmacol Sci 1986; 7:28.
6. Taylor P, Insel PA: Molecular basis of drug action. *In*: Principles of Drug Action. 3rd ed. Pratt WB, et al (Eds). New York, Churchill Livingstone, 1990, pp 103–200.
7. Fuller PJ: The steroid receptor superfamily: Mechanisms of diversity. FASEB J 1991; 5:3092.
8. Green S, Chambon P: Oestradiol induction of a glucocorticoid-responsive gene by a chimaeric receptor. Nature 1987; 325:75.
9. Godowski PJ, Rusconi S, Miesfeld R, et al: Glucocorticoid receptor mutants that are constitutive activators of transcriptional enhancement. Nature 1987; 325:365.
10. Yarden Y, Ullrich A: Growth factor receptor tyrosine kinases. Ann Rev Biochem 1988; 57:443.
11. Jaye M, Schlessinger J, Dionne CA: Fibroblast growth factor receptor tyrosine kinases: Molecular analysis and signal transduction. Biochim Biophys Acta 1992; 1135:185.
12. Malarkey K, Belham CM, Paul A, et al: The regulation of tyrosine kinase signalling pathways by growth factor and G-protein-coupled receptors. Biochem J 1995; 309:361.
13. Chinkers M, Garbers DL, Chang M-S, et al: A membrane form of guanylate cyclase is an atrial natriuretic peptide receptor. Nature 1989; 338:76.
14. Garbers DL: Guanylate cyclase receptor family. Recent Prog Hormone Res 1990; 46:85.
15. Clarke PB: The fall and rise of neuronal alpha-bungarotoxin binding proteins. Trends Pharmacol Sci 1991; 13:407.
16. Luetje CW, Patrick J: Both alpha- and beta-subunits contribute to the agonist sensitivity of neuronal nicotinic acetylcholine receptors. J Neurosci 1991; 11:83.
17. Anand R, Conrow WG, Schoepfer R, et al: Neuronal nicotinic acetylcholine receptors expressed in *Xenopus* oocytes have a pentameric quaternary structure. J Biol Chem 1991; 266:11192.
18. Verdoorn TA, Draguhn A, Ymer S, et al: Functional properties of recombinant rat $GABA_A$ receptors depend upon subunit composition. Neuron 1990; 4:919.
19. Taylor P: Agents acting at the neuromuscular junction and autonomic ganglia. *In*: The Pharmacological Basis of Therapeutics. 8th ed. Gilman GG, Rall TW, Nies AS, et al (Eds). New York, Pergamon Press, 1990, pp 166–186.
20. Rall TW, Schleifer LS: Drugs effective in the therapy of the epilepsies. *In*: The Pharmacological Basis of Therapeutics. 8th ed. Gilman GG, Rall TW, Nies AS, et al (Eds). New York, Pergamon Press, 1990, pp 436–462.
21. Hepler JR, Gilman AG: G proteins. Trends Biochem Sci 1992; 17:383.
22. Stryer L: The molecules of visual excitation. Sci Am 1987; 256:42.
23. Schnapf JL, Baylor DA: How photoreceptor cells respond to light. Sci Am 1987; 256:40.
24. Birdsall NJ: Wheel on the sweet smell of success. Trends Pharmacol Sci 1991; 12:283.
25. Findlay JBC, Pappin DJC: The opsin family of proteins. Biochem J 1986; 238:625.
26. Fraser CM, Wang CD, Robinson DA, et al: Site-directed mutagenesis of M1 muscarinic acetylcholine receptors: Conserved aspartic acids play important roles in receptor function. Mol Pharmacol 1989; 36:840.
27. Strader CD, Sigal IS, Candelore MR, et al: Conserved aspartic acid residues 79 and 113 of the *beta*-adrenergic receptor have different roles in receptor function. J Biol Chem 1988; 263:10267.
28. Wong SK, Parker EM, Ross EM: Chimeric muscarinic cholinergic: Beta-adrenergic receptors that activate G_s in response to muscarinic agonists. J Biol Chem 1990; 265:6219.
29. Lefkowitz RJ, Cotecchia S, Samamama P, et al: Constitutive activity of receptors coupled to guanine nucleotide regulatory proteins. Trends Pharmacol Sci 1993; 14:303.
30. Bourne HR, Sanders DA, McCormick F: The GTPase superfamily: Conserved structure and molecular mechanism. Nature 1991; 349:117.
31. Bourne HR, Sanders DA, McCormick F: The GTPase superfamily: A conserved switch for diverse cell functions. Nature 1990; 348:125.
32. Matesic DF, Manning DR, Luthin GR: Tissue-dependent association of muscarinic acetylcholine receptors with guanine nucleotide-binding regulatory proteins. Mol Pharmacol 1991; 40:347.
33. Ehlert FJ: The relationship between muscarinic receptor occupancy and adenylate cyclase inhibition in the rabbit myocardium. Mol Pharmacol 1985; 28:410.
34. Weber G: Energetics of ligand binding to proteins. Adv Prot Chem 1975; 29:1.
35. Thomas EA, Baker SA, Ehlert FJ: Functional role for the M2 muscarinic receptor in smooth muscle of the guinea pig ileum. Mol Pharmacol 1993; 44:102.
36. Rasmussen H: The cycling of calcium as an intracellular messenger. Sci Am 1989; 261:66.

37. Cockcroft S, Thomas GM: Inositol-lipid-specific phospholipase C isoenzymes: Their differential regulation by receptors. Biochem J 1992; 288:1.
38. Berridge MJ: The molecular basis of communication within the cell. Sci Am 1985; 255:142.
39. Irvine RF: How do inositol 1,4,5-trisphosphate and inositol 1,3,4,5-tetrakisphosphate regulate intracellular Ca2+? Biochem Soc Trans 1989; 17:6.
40. Berridge MJ, Downes CP, Hanley MR: Neural and developmental actions of lithium: A unifying hypothesis. Cell 1989; 59:411.
41. Tang WJ, Gilman AG: Adenylyl cyclases. Cell 1992; 70:869.
42. Brown AM: Regulation of heartbeat by G protein-coupled ion channels. Am J Physiol 1990; 259:H1621.
43. Bishop MJ: Molecular themes in oncogenesis. Cell 1991; 64:235.
44. Lyons J, Landis CA, Harsh G, et al: Two G protein oncogenes in human endocrine tumors. Science 1990; 249:655.
45. Koshland DE: The two-component pathway comes to eukaryotes. Science 1993; 262:532.

47

Neutrophil-Endothelial Cell Interactions

Nicholas B. Vedder, MD • John M. Harlan, MD

The adherence of neutrophils to endothelium is a critical early event in host defense against microorganisms and in the repair of injured tissue. Under certain circumstances, however, the same mechanisms that mediate these normal processes can contribute to vascular and tissue injury. Neutrophil-mediated endothelial injury has been implicated as central to the pathogenesis of disorders produced by tissue ischemia and reperfusion as well as acute inflammatory diseases. Elucidation of the molecular basis of neutrophil-endothelial interactions, therefore, not only is important for understanding the acute inflammatory response but may also suggest new approaches to therapy of a wide range of human disease processes.[1-5]

NEUTROPHIL-MEDIATED INJURY

To carry out their normal functions in host defense and repair, neutrophils are armed with a diverse array of potent effector mechanisms.[2] In response to a spectrum of inflammatory stimuli such as cytokines, activated complement components, platelet-activating factor (PAF), bacterial peptides, and endotoxin, neutrophils are capable of generating and releasing a plethora of inflammatory mediators. These include reactive oxygen species, proteases, peptides, lipid mediators, and vasoactive substances.[3] When activation and release are appropriately controlled and regulated, the toxic substances act on bacteria or other material brought into the neutrophil by phagocytosis, resulting in efficient clearance of pathogens or diseased tissue. More than a century ago, Metchnikoff alluded to a process whereby phagocytic leukocytes could cause tissue injury as a result of uncontrolled release of toxic substances.[6] Neutrophil-mediated vascular and tissue injury with damage to otherwise viable host tissues and organs may result if regulatory mechanisms fail or if activation is initiated in response to diffuse or systemic inflammatory stimuli. The body, of course, has an abundance of endogenous tissue-based and plasma-based anti-inflammatory mechanisms to protect itself against such processes.[7] It is abundantly clear, however, that these endogenous mechanisms can become overwhelmed and that neutrophil-mediated vascular and tissue injury can contribute to the pathogenesis of a wide variety of clinical disorders.

Neutrophil adherence to endothelium plays a pivotal role in both neutrophil-mediated defense and repair as well as neutrophil-mediated vascular injury (Fig. 47-1). Observations of the microcirculation with intravital microscopy have elucidated a sequence of events involved in neutrophil-endothelial adhesive interactions at the site of inflammation.[1, 8-10] In response to inflammatory stimuli, signals are generated that act on both the neutrophil and the endothelial cell to initiate a sequence of events, an early step of which is increased neutrophil and endothelial cell adhesiveness.

Neutrophils are first seen leaving the laminar flow stream and rolling along the endothelial wall of postcapillary venules at the site of inflammation. This step is then followed by firm adherence to the endothelium, which arrests the neutrophil, followed subsequently by diapedesis and emigration. Once firmly adherent to the endothelium, a protected microenvironment develops beneath the adherent neutrophil in which its proteases, oxidants, or other toxic products can cause injury to the endothelium, inaccessible to circulating anti-inflammatory agents.[7] This direct endothelial injury by activated neutrophils can result in loss of microvascular integrity with edema, hemorrhage, or thrombosis, and, ultimately, organ dysfunction. Increased neutrophil adhesiveness can also cause tissue injury through homotypic adhesion or aggregation. Aggregates of neutrophils adherent to each other can occlude the microcirculation, resulting in tissue hypoperfusion and further ischemic damage.[11]

Finally, once they emigrate, neutrophils can continue to release toxic products that directly injure tissue and provoke organ damage. It is apparent, therefore, that understanding the cellular and molecular mechanisms that mediate neutrophil adherence to endothelium is central to understanding and potentially modulating neutrophil-mediated injury.

MECHANISMS OF ADHESION

Since the time of Cohnheim[12] and Metchnikoff,[6] it was a matter of debate whether alterations in the neutrophil or in the endothelial cell were responsible for the critical adhesive interaction. Not surprisingly, it is now clear that both cell types are involved. In just the past decade, more than a dozen of proteins involved in this interaction have been immunologically identified and molecularly cloned and their functions defined in vivo as well as in vitro.[8-10] These adherence molecules are currently classified into three major categories (Fig. 47-2):

- Selectins
- Integrins
- Members of the *immunoglobulin superfamily* (IgSF)

The *selectin receptors* are lectin-containing proteins that recognize specific carbohydrate counterstructures.[13] Selectin-mediated adhesion involves a rapid on-off interaction and is observed under conditions of flow, whereas integrin-dependent adhesion is sensitive to shear and is optimal under static conditions.[14] Thus, selectin receptors appear to be responsible for the initial transient adhesion of neutrophils that occurs at sites of inflammation, manifested as "rolling."

The *leukocyte integrin receptors* interact with ligands on the endothelial cell, including members of the third major class of adhesion molecules, members of IgSF. The integrin-IgSF ligand interaction mediates firm adhesion of neutrophils to endothelium at sites of inflammation as well as subsequent diapedesis and emigration. Together, these distinct adhesion

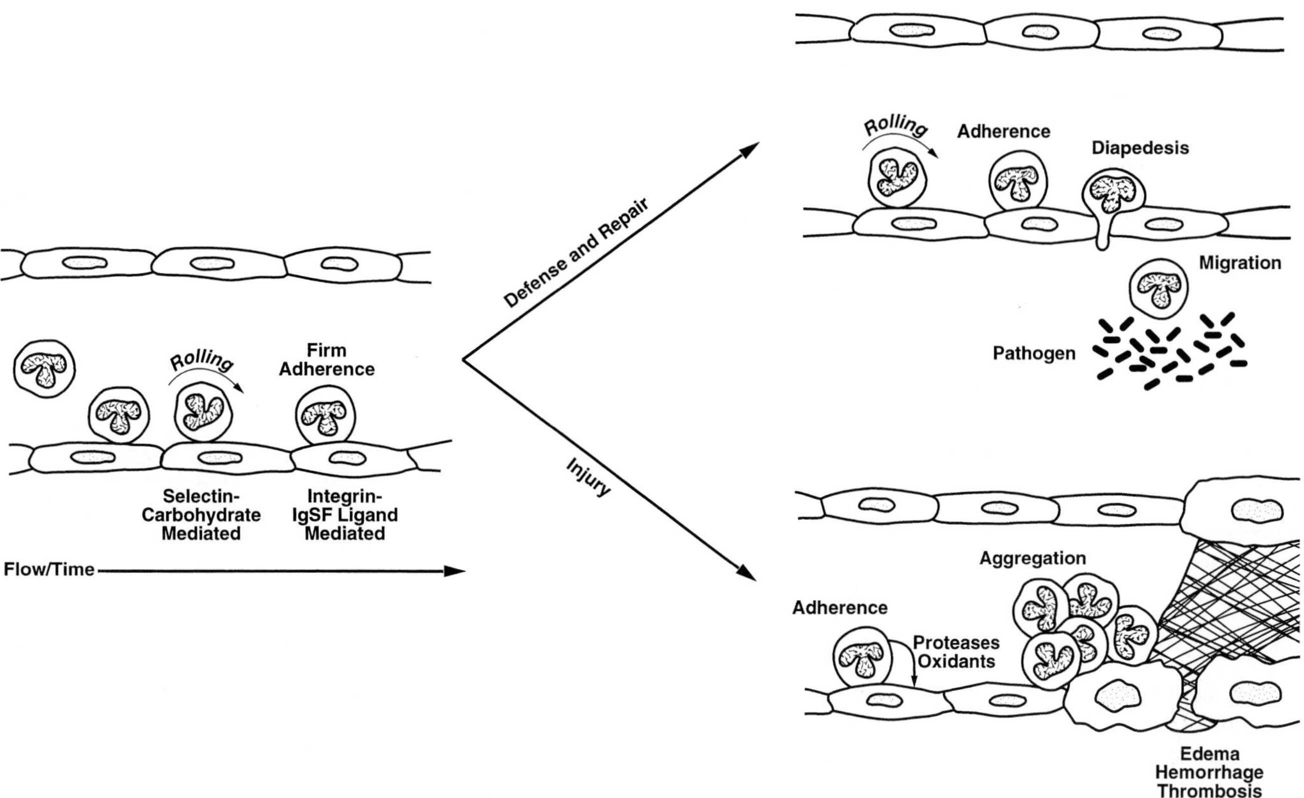

Figure 47–1. Diagrammatic representation of the sequential events that occur at a site of inflammation as neutrophils leave the laminar flow stream of a postcapillary venule. Initial selectin-mediated and carbohydrate-mediated rolling, along the surface of the endothelium, and tethering of neutrophils where local agonists then stimulate integrin and immunoglobulin superfamily (IgSF) ligand-mediated firm adherence. These two events are required either for neutrophil emigration in the setting of defense and repair or for neutrophil-mediated endothelial injury in pathologic conditions.

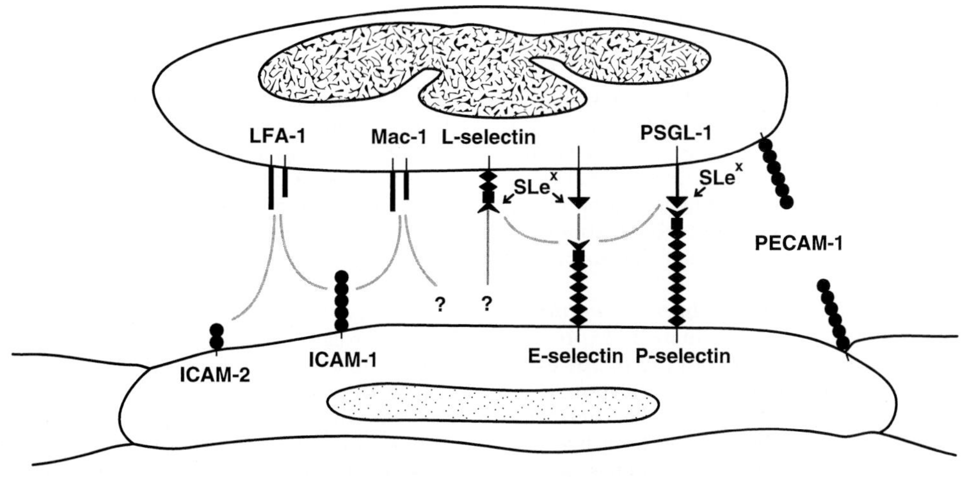

Figure 47–2. Diagrammatic representation of the known neutrophil-endothelial adhesion receptors. The β_2 integrin receptors on neutrophils, LFA-1 (CD11a/CD18) and Mac-1 (CD11b/CD18; both represented as α/β dimers), bind to intercellular adhesion molecules (ICAMs). CD11a/CD18 binds to ICAM-1 and ICAM-2; CD11b/CD18 binds to ICAM-1 and, perhaps, to other, as yet unidentified ligand(s) on the endothelial cell. Endothelial E-Selectin (CD62E) and P-selectin (CD62P; represented with their N-terminal lectin domain, epidermal growth factor domain, multiple complement regulatory repeat sequences, transmembrane domain, and cytoplasmic domain) bind to carbohydrate ligands, particularly sialyl Lewis X antigen (SLe^x; CD15s), expressed on glycoproteins of neutrophils, with P-selectin glycoprotein ligand (PSGL-1) being the primary ligand for P-selectin. L-selectin (CD62L) on neutrophils binds to an as yet unidentified carbohydrate ligand(s) on endothelium in systemic vasculature and also presents SLe^x to E-selectin and P-selectin.

systems result in a process whereby neutrophils in flowing blood are initially slowed and "tethered" to endothelium by selectin-carbohydrate interactions; then, once tethered, local inflammatory stimuli act to increase the affinity and avidity of integrins, producing firm integrin-immunoglobulin adhesion, allowing subsequent diapedesis and neutrophil-mediated injury. Flow may also have direct effects on neutrophil function by reducing pseudopod projection and deformability of circulating leukocytes while reduction of shear stress leads to pseudopod projection and spreading of leukocytes on the endothelium.[15]

Selectin/Carbohydrate-Mediated Adhesion

Selectin receptors and their carbohydrate counterstructures mediate the first step in neutrophil-endothelial cell adhesion. In vitro and in vivo evidence suggests that selectin-mediated adhesion is relatively resistant to shear forces and plays an important role in the initial rolling and tethering of neutrophils along the endothelium at sites of inflammation.[13] This ability to mediate rolling of neutrophils is due to the rapid-on/rapid-off nature of selectin adhesion as well as the localization of the receptor or its ligands at the microvillus tips and distinguishes selectin-mediated adhesion from the firm integrin/IgSF ligand-mediated adhesion that occurs under static conditions.[16] The three selectin receptors are:

- *L-selectin* (CD62L)
- *E-selectin* (CD62E)
- *P-selectin* (CD62P)

L-selectin is expressed only on leukocytes, E-selectin is localized to endothelial cells, and P-selectin is found on platelets as well as endothelial cells.

The selectin molecules consist of an amino-terminal lectin domain, an epidermal growth factor (EGF) domain, a variable number of complement regulatory repeat sequences, a transmembrane domain, and a carboxy-terminal cytoplasmic domain. Binding occurs between the lectin domain and the specific carbohydrate counterstructure on either the neutrophil (in the case of E-selectin and P-selectin) or the endothelial cell (in the case of L-selectin). For E-selectin and P-selectin receptors, the sialyl Lewis X (SLe^x; CD15s) antigen and related sialylated, fucosylated glycoconjugates are major counterstructures. Sialyl Lewis X is expressed on a number of glycolipids and glycoproteins. P-selectin glycoprotein ligand (PSGL-1) is a mucin-like molecule that presents SLe^x to P- and E-selectin[16] and functions as the primary ligand for P-selectin.[16, 17] Sulfation of PSGL-1 is necessary for P-selectin binding.[16] Although it may bind to SLe^x presented on L-selectin, the predominant glycoprotein ligands for E-selectin on human neutrophils is uncertain.[17]

P-selectin is not expressed on cultured *human umbilical vein endothelial cells* (HUVECs) and is minimally expressed on the surface of unstimulated endothelium in vivo; however, it is rapidly inducible within minutes after stimulation with thrombin, histamine, or hydrogen peroxide. This increased surface expression does not require de novo synthesis because P-selectin is stored within the Weibel-Palade bodies and is quickly translocated to the cell surface in response to stimulation. P-selectin may also have a role in later, cytokine-mediated adhesion, as these have been shown to increase levels of P-selectin messenger ribonucleic acid (mRNA) with peak levels at 3 to 4 hours.[13] It is likely, however, that the primary role of selectins is in the setting of acute inflammation and that other adhesion pathways predominate in more subacute and chronic settings.[18]

In vitro experiments have demonstrated that purified P-selectin bound to plates is capable of mediating neutrophil rolling at physiologic shear stress rates without causing firm adhesion, even with cessation of flow.[14] In contrast, an isolated integrin/IgSF ligand system does not support rolling or adherence at physiologic flow rates but can produce firm adherence once rolling is first induced by P-selectin. P-selectin–mediated adhesion, then, provides an ideal mechanism for initially slowing neutrophils at sites of inflammation. Once tethered, stimulation leads to firm, integrin-mediated adhesion and subsequent diapedesis or, under some conditions, to direct endothelial injury.

Unlike P-selectin, L-selectin is constitutively expressed on the neutrophil in the basal state and is rapidly shed from the surface in response to stimulation.[13] L-selectin binds to a cytokine-induced ligand on HUVEC in vitro as well as to high endothelial venules of lymph nodes. Although Gly-CAM-1 and CD34 have been identified as ligands for L-selectin on high endothelial venules in the mouse, the ligands for L-selectin on systemic endothelium are unknown.[13] Like E-selectin and P-selectin, L-selectin recognizes sialylated, fucosylated moieties like SLe^x, but these glycoconjugates have not been clearly identified on the surface of basal or stimulated HUVEC. The importance of L-selectin in neutrophil recruitment at sites of inflammation in vivo is supported by intravital microscopy studies that have demonstrated that blocking monoclonal antibodies, SLe^x oligosaccharides, or soluble forms of L-selectin can effectively inhibit neutrophil rolling and subsequent emigration at sites of early inflammation.[4, 13]

Although E-selectin shares the same binding properties as the other selectins, its time-course of induction in vitro is notably different. In contrast to P-selectin, E-selectin requires de novo protein synthesis and, therefore, does not reach peak surface expression for 4 to 6 hours. The agents responsible for inducing E-selectin expression are also somewhat different, being primarily cytokines, such as interleukin-1β (IL-1β), tumor necrosis factor-α (TNF-α), and lipopolysaccharide (LPS). Although the duration of expression of E-selectin on HUVEC in vitro is much longer than P-selectin, it declines gradually with much reduced but detectable levels observed at 24 hours after stimulation. In vitro studies suggest that the rapid decline results from both a decrease in transcription and from rapid internalization. In contrast to the relatively transient expression of E-selectin observed in vitro, E-selectin persists at inflammatory sites in vivo. The identification of markedly increased expression of E-selectin in sepsis and at sites of chronic inflammation, such as rheumatoid joints and delayed-type hypersensitivity reactions, supports this role for E-selectin and suggests that E-selectin may be involved in subacute and chronic inflammatory or immune reactions as well as more acute processes.[4, 19]

Through the technique of *gene targeting*, a number of mice with deficiencies of selectin receptors have been generated. These selectin "knockouts" have confirmed and further elucidated the roles of the various selectin receptors, both individually and in combination. In general, the phenotypic defects seen in these animals have been consistent with the results obtained with blocking monoclonal antibodies (Table 47–1).

There are several important caveats with respect to this model of selectin-mediated adhesion and its role in the adhesion cascade. First, rolling may not be required for adhesion and emigration under conditions of stasis as might occur in ischemic or shock states. Furthermore, although selectin-mediated rolling appears to be important for neutrophil emigration in the postcapillary venules of the systemic circulation, it does not appear to be necessary for emigration in other beds, such as hepatic sinusoids or pulmonary capillaries.[20, 21] Finally, two patients with a leukocyte adhesion deficiency (LAD) syndrome (designated *LAD type 2*) have a generalized

TABLE 47–1. Anti–adhesion Therapy in Experimental Models of Vascular and Tissue Injury*

Ischemia/Reperfusion	Inflammatory/Immune
Intestinal ischemia[45]	Inflammatory skin lesions[29]
Tissue reperfusion injury[44, 46, 60]	Edema in meningitis[57]
Shock/resuscitation[50, 51, 61, 62]	Endotoxic shock[54, 55]
Myocardial ischemia[63–65]	Allergic asthma[66]
Skeletal muscle ischemia[67]	Autoimmune diabetes[68]
Central nervous system ischemia[69]	NSAID-induced gastric injury[70]
	Burns[71]
	Graft rejection[72]
	Inflammatory lung injury[73, 74]
	Inflammatory bowel disease[75]

*Selected experimental models in which monoclonal antibodies that block neutrophil-endothelial adhesion molecules have been effective at attenuating injury. These studies fall into two major groups: (1) processes of an inflammatory or immune origin and (2) processes involving ischemia-reperfusion. See reviews 1, 4, 8, and 53 for extensive references on anti-adhesion therapy.

defect in fucose metabolism and are unable to form SLe^x or any other fucosylated structures. They exhibit mild defects in neutrophil emigration in vivo, and neutrophils from these patients are unable to bind to E-selectin or P-selectin in vitro. In comparison to severely affected patients with deficiency of β_2 integrins (*LAD type 1*), the clinical manifestations of this defect in selectin-mediated adhesion are mild, suggesting that selectin-mediated adhesion is not required for host defense under all conditions.[8]

Integrin/IgSF Ligand-Mediated Adhesion

The recent explosion of knowledge in the field of neutrophil-endothelial cell adhesion originated from studies of a genetic deficiency syndrome known as LAD type 1, in which patients manifest recurrent bacterial infections and an inability to suppurate.[22] The neutrophils in these patients demonstrate defective adherence functions both in vitro and in vivo as a result of a deficiency of the leukocyte adhesion receptor complex, CD11/CD18.

The CD11/CD18 complex consists of three heterodimeric glycoprotein subunits. Each heterodimer consists of a light or β_2-chain polypeptide (CD18), common to all three heterodimers, and distinct heavy or α-chain polypeptides, designated α_L (CD11a), α_M (CD11b), α_X (CD11c), or α_d (CD11d).[23] These heterodimers are also commonly known as

- LFA-1 ($\alpha_L\beta_2$; CD11a/CD18)
- Mac-1, Mo1, or CR3 ($\alpha_M\beta_2$; CD11b/CD18)
- p150,95 ($\alpha_X\beta_2$; CD11c/CD18)

LFA-1 is found on all leukocytes, whereas Mac-1 and p150,95 are found on phagocytes and natural killer cells but not on most lymphocytes. CD11d/CD18 ($\alpha_d\beta_2$) is found on some macrophages. The CD11 α-chains as well as the CD18 β_2-chain have been cloned and have been shown to be members of the integrin family of adhesion receptors, comprising the β_2 subclass, which is unique to leukocytes.

The molecular basis of the CD11/CD18 deficiency syndrome has been demonstrated to be heterogeneous mutations in the common β_2-chain, resulting in a deficient or abnormal β_2-chain that fails to associate with the normal α-chain into heterodimers.[22] Without heterodimer formation neither α-chain nor β_2-chain polypeptides are inserted into the plasma membrane. This leads to a severe defect in neutrophil emigration at sites of inflammation because without functional CD11/CD18 the critical steps of adherence to and diapedesis across endothelium cannot occur.[24] The defect in adhesion-dependent functions of the LAD type 1 neutrophils can be reproduced in normal neutrophils by the addition of monoclonal antibodies directed to function-related epitopes of the CD11/CD18 complex.

Studies with HUVEC demonstrate that normal neutrophils exhibit a very low level of basal adherence to HUVEC. With stimulation of neutrophils using TNF-α, C5a, IL-8, PAF, LPS, or bacterial chemotactic peptide there is a dramatic increase in neutrophil adhesiveness to endothelium—and with many of these substances, an increase in homotypic neutrophil adhesion (i.e., aggregation as well). Addition of monoclonal antibodies directed to functional epitopes of CD11b or CD18 essentially eliminates this increased adhesiveness and, in so doing, effectively blocks neutrophil-mediated endothelial injury. Inhibition of tight adherence prevents formation of a closed interface between the adherent neutrophil and the endothelium in which proteases and oxidants released by the activated neutrophil can cause injury to the endothelium.[7] This approach to inhibiting neutrophil-mediated injury, therefore, has a potential significant advantage over antiproteases or antioxidants, which are ineffective once adherence has created a protected microenvironment.

For neutrophils, CD11b/CD18 (Mac-1) appears to be the heterodimer most responsible for firm adhesion, although CD11a/CD18 (LFA-1) is also involved and is sufficient for emigration.[25] The mechanism by which CD11b/CD18 augments neutrophil adhesiveness in response to stimulation is not entirely clear. In unstimulated neutrophils, the CD11b/CD18 heterodimer exists on the cell surface and, in greater quantities, within the secondary or tertiary granules. After stimulation, the contents of these granules are translocated to the cell surface, resulting in a threefold to 10-fold increase in surface-associated CD11b/CD18. This increase in surface expression, however, is neither necessary nor sufficient to cause increased adhesiveness.[26] Instead, the primary mechanism appears to be an activation of surface receptors that produces a conformational change resulting in a high-avidity binding to ligand through what is known as "inside-out" signaling.[27] The molecular basis for avidity modulation of the β_2 integrin receptor has not been fully defined, but it is dependent on interactions of integrin cytoplasmic domains with adaptor molecules and the cytoskeleton.[28] This activation process and avidity modulation are logical targets for manipulating neutrophil adhesion and neutrophil-mediated injury in inflammation.

The endothelial counterstructures for the CD11/CD18 complex[8, 9, 23] include these IgSF members:

- Intercellular adhesion molecule-1 (*ICAM-1*) (CD54)
- *ICAM-2* (CD102)

CD11a/CD18 binds to both ICAM-1 and ICAM-2. CD11b/CD18 binds to ICAM-1, although there may be other as yet unidentified endothelial ligands for CD11b/CD18. ICAM-2 is expressed constitutively and is not regulated by most stimuli. ICAM-1 is expressed at low levels on resting endothelium in vitro and in vivo, and it is upregulated by de novo synthesis over a period of hours in response to inflammatory stimuli, such as LPS, IL-1β, and TNF-α, within peak expression after 12 to 24 hours. Monoclonal antibodies to ICAM-1 inhibit neutrophil adherence to endothelium after inflammatory stimulation in vitro, although generally to a lesser extent than monoclonal antibodies to CD11a, CD11b, or CD18.

The importance of integrin/IgSF ligand-mediated adhesion to the process of neutrophil-mediated inflammation and injury in vivo is illustrated by animal models of acute inflammation that have used monoclonal antibodies to CD11b, CD18, or ICAM-1. The first such study used intravital microscopy to examine neutrophil-endothelial adhesion and neutrophil-mediated injury in response to superfusion of a chemoattractant.[29] It was shown that a blocking CD18 monoclonal antibody effectively abolished neutrophil adherence to endothelium at the site of inflammation. With blockade of adherence, neutrophil emigration and endothelial injury, as evidenced by plasma leakage, were also effectively inhibited. Similar findings have also been noted with monoclonal antibodies to CD11b and ICAM-1, further demonstrating the central role of the CD11/CD18-ICAM-1 interactions in neutrophil-mediated inflammation and injury.[4]

Another IgSF member, *platelet-endothelial cell adhesion molecule-1* (PECAM-1 [CD31]) is involved in neutrophil-endothelial interactions.[30] PECAM-1 is found on the surface of platelets, at endothelial intercellular junctions, and on certain cells of myelomonocytic lineage. It plays an important role in transendothelial emigration of phagocytes and their migration through the subendothelial matrix. This process utilizes CD11a/CD18 interaction with ICAM-1 as well as homophilic binding of phagocyte and endothelial PECAM-1. Diapedesis also involves signaling of the endothelial cell by the leukocyte, triggering a disruption of junctional integrity.[31]

As with the selectins, knockout of CD11a, CD11b, CD18, and ICAM-1 genes in mice has confirmed the roles of these adhesion molecules with results that are, in general, consistent with those obtained with blocking monoclonal antibodies (see Table 1). However, there have been some notable discordances, raising the question whether redundant pathways develop in the knockout animals or whether the antibodies have effects apart from adherence blockade.[32]

Coordination of Neutrophil-Endothelial Cell Interactions

It is evident that the mechanisms involved in neutrophil adherence to endothelium and subsequent neutrophil-mediated endothelial injury are complex and may vary, depending on the vascular bed, the degree and nature of the inflammatory stimulus, and the time course involved. In the healthy state, there is minimal interaction between circulating neutrophils and the vascular endothelium. In response to an extravascular inflammatory stimulus, there is an initial rapidly induced selectin-mediated rolling and tethering at the site of inflammation, likely involving either P-selectin or L-selectin, or later through the induction and synthesis of E-selectin. Factors released as part of the early inflammatory process (e.g., thrombin, histamine, oxidants) can initiate P-selectin expression and thereby promote leukocyte rolling, whereas cytokines generated later (e.g., IL-1, TNF-α) can induce the L-selectin ligands or E-selectin. Rolling allows the neutrophils to come in contact with the endothelium of the inflamed vessels where subsequent activation of the integrin receptors by various agonists produces firm adherence.[14]

PAF factor or chemotactic peptides, such as IL-8, may be important in initiating β_2-integrin/ICAM-1–mediated adhesion.[33] In vitro, PAF is expressed on the endothelial surface along with P-selectin in response to thrombin, histamine, and oxidizing agents, and PAF can, in turn, result in upregulation and activation of neutrophil integrins, leading to the second step of firm adhesion. This effect can be blocked by either inhibiting P-selectin or the PAF receptor, suggesting that a coordinated or "juxtacrine" process is involved. IL-8 is a potent neutrophil chemoattractant that is a member of the cys-cys (C-C) subfamily of chemokinetic proteins. It is produced by endothelial cells and diverse other cell types in response to TNF-α, IL-1, or LPS. Endothelium-derived IL-8 expressed on luminal villi or deposited in subendothelial tissue may promote integrin-dependent adherence and diapedesis.[34, 35] This highlights the importance of local signals at the site of inflammation in directing leukocyte traffic.[9]

Additional mechanisms are also involved in the regulation of neutrophil adherence to endothelium. Other cytokines (e.g., TNF-α), infectious agents (*N*-formyl-methionyl-leucyl-phenylalanine [fMLP], LPS) and chemotaxins (e.g., leukotriene B_4 [LTB_4], C5a) can all increase the surface expression of β_2-integrin (CD11/CD18) receptors, which may be an important factor in augmenting adhesion. As mentioned previously, however, increased surface expression of integrin receptors of itself is insufficient to cause adhesion and receptor "activation" is required, resulting in a conformational change of the receptor that increases adhesiveness. The precise biochemical basis of this "inside-out" signaling continues to be elucidated.[28] There is also growing evidence that integrin-mediated adhesion triggers an "outside-in" signaling with cytoskeletal rearrangement leading to further cellular activation, triggering of oxidative pathways and the generation of a variety of biochemical signals.[36]

Many of the stimuli that cause upregulated surface expression and increased avidity of CD11b/CD18 also produce shedding of L-selectin (i.e., the integrin and selectin receptors are inversely regulated). Loss of L-selectin, with activation of neutrophils in the vascular lumen, has also been proposed as a mechanism to limit neutrophil recruitment at sites of inflammation. L-selectin may also play a role in outside-in signaling as cross-linking of L-selectin can potentiate CD11b/CD18-mediated adhesion in the presence of agonists, such as IL-8 and PAF, through the activation of kinases and changes in cytosolic calcium.[37]

Amplification of leukocyte recruitment may also occur through the process of cell-cell capture. In the presence of flow, a PSGL-1/L-selectin interaction has been shown to mediate adhesion between rolling and already adherent neutrophils.[38] Similarly, tethering of neutrophils on platelet ICAM-2 via LFA-1 has been demonstrated as a mechanism to facilitate CD11b/CD18-dependent adhesion and arrest at sites of vascular injury.[39]

Although an increase in the avidity of integrin receptors is important for firm adherence, neutrophil migration requires that there also be mechanisms to decrease avidity (i.e., to "turn off" the receptor). Indeed, avidity regulation by sequential activation-deactivation of the receptor is essential for movement. "Freezing" integrin receptors in the high avidity state enhances adherence but markedly inhibits transendothelial migration in vitro.[40] The mechanisms involved in deactivation of integrin receptors in neutrophils are not yet defined. Other mechanisms for terminating leukocyte recruitment include receptor endocytosis (E-selectin and P-selectin) and decay of local chemoattractants. Locally generated mediators (e.g., nitric oxide, TGF-β, C-reactive protein) also act to inhibit leukocyte adhesion to endothelium.[20, 41]

There are, therefore, numerous factors involved in the regulation of neutrophil-endothelial adhesive interactions. As our knowledge and understanding of the molecular basis of neutrophil adherence to endothelium increases, the tools for manipulating these processes will continue to expand, allowing more detailed analysis of neutrophil-mediated injury processes and their role in human disease.

IN VIVO MODELS OF NEUTROPHIL-MEDIATED INJURY

There are two general approaches to limiting neutrophil-endothelial adherence and neutrophil-mediated injury. One involves direct blockade of the receptor-ligand interaction through the use of monoclonal antibodies, oligosaccharides, soluble receptors, peptides, or small molecules. The other is to modify the intracellular signaling processes involved in controlling the expression and/or activation of neutrophil or endothelial adhesion molecules through compounds such as adenosine, leumedins, nitric oxide agonists, corticosteroids, and nonsteroidal anti-inflammatory agents (NSAIDs).[42] Although only a few limited human clinical trials evaluating the efficacy of specific agents to inhibit neutrophil-endothelial cell adhesion have been completed to date, there have been numerous studies using monoclonal antibodies to various adhesion receptors to examine the role of neutrophil-mediated injury in a wide variety of animal models (see Table 47–1). These studies fall into two major groups: (1) processes of an inflammatory or immune origin, and (2) processes involving ischemia–reperfusion.[1, 4]

Ischemia-Reperfusion Injury

Ischemia-related cellular, tissue, and organ injury forms the basis of many important clinical disorders, including myocardial infarction, stroke, peripheral vascular disease, and circulatory shock. Although much progress has been made in the area of early restoration of perfusion, there is evidence that in some settings a significant proportion of the tissue damage triggered by ischemia may be a consequence of events associated with reperfusion of ischemic tissues (i.e., *reperfusion injury*). Oxygen-derived free radicals generated at the time of reperfusion have been identified as potentially important mediators of this reperfusion injury.[43] Another significant source of free radicals is the neutrophil, which can also cause injury through the release of proteases and phospholipase products. An important role for neutrophils in ischemia-reperfusion injury is suggested by studies showing a close association between neutrophil accumulation and tissue injury in this setting and by studies demonstrating reduction of injury by depletion of circulating neutrophils.[4]

Adherent, activated neutrophils can cause direct endothelial injury, resulting in loss of vascular integrity and producing edema, hemorrhage, and thrombosis (see Fig. 47–1). Another possible mechanism of injury involves adherence of neutrophils to the endothelium of the microvasculature and aggregation of neutrophils within the vessel lumen, leading to occlusion and further ischemia.[11] Thus, a progressive downward spiral may result in which reperfusion induces neutrophil activation and adherence, leading to leukocyte accumulation and endothelial injury which then results in further ischemia and eventually complete cessation of flow. This may be the basis of what in the past has been called the *no-reflow phenomenon,* which more precisely might be called a *diminishing reflow phenomenon.*[44]

The mechanisms by which neutrophil adherence and injury are initiated in the setting of ischemia-reperfusion are not entirely clear. However, there is good evidence that oxygen-derived free radicals are generated at the time of reperfusion. These can initiate the process of P-selectin–mediated adhesion, release of PAF, and subsequent β_2-integrin–mediated adhesion.[33] The important role of oxygen free radicals in initiating this process has been demonstrated both in vitro and in vivo.[43]

The use of monoclonal antibodies directed against specific adhesion proteins has been extremely effective at inhibiting neutrophil accumulation and neutrophil-mediated reperfusion injury in a number of animal models. The first such study examined the role of neutrophils in reperfusion injury of feline gut and demonstrated that a CD18 monoclonal antibody effectively attenuated the increase in plasma leakage that normally occurs after intestinal ischemia and reperfusion.[45]

Studies using the isolated rabbit ear, based on its vascular pedicle, also showed that blocking neutrophil adherence functions with a CD18[44] or anti–P-selectin[46] monoclonal antibody markedly reduced reperfusion-associated edema formation as well as tissue necrosis. In these particular studies, the degree of protection was the same whether monoclonal antibody was administered before ischemia or after ischemia but immediately before reperfusion. This result provided strong evidence that neutrophil-mediated injury in the setting of ischemia and reperfusion occurs at the time of reperfusion as activated neutrophils flood the vascular bed, causing diffuse endothelial and tissue injury. In this sense, the injury is in fact a true "reperfusion injury." Time-course studies have shown, however, that in the setting of reperfusion injury, adhesion blockade must be initiated early after reperfusion in order to be effective.[47]

Inhibition of CD18/ICAM-mediated or selectin/carbohydrate-mediated adherence has subsequently been shown to be effective at attenuating reperfusion injury in numerous animal models of reperfusion injury of a variety of organs and tissue beds (Table 47–2) (reviewed in Cornejo et al.[4] and Thiagarajan et al.[48]). Even remote effects of neutrophil-mediated reperfusion injury can be potentially inhibited in this way, as with the reduction of remote lung injury after hind limb ischemia-reperfusion.[49]

Hemorrhagic shock followed by resuscitation is another important form of ischemia-reperfusion injury, representing a global or generalized ischemia-reperfusion injury. In this regard, inhibition of CD18-mediated neutrophil adherence and injury reduces organ injury, attenuates the generalized microvascular injury, and improves survival in both small animal and subhuman primate models of hypovolemic shock.[50, 51] These findings also suggest that neutrophil-mediated injury may play an important role in the development of multiple organ injury and the multiple organ failure syndrome, which are a frequent and devastating consequence of severe traumatic shock. Clinical trials are ongoing in this area, and pilot studies suggest that the pharmacology and safety are reasonable in this setting.[52]

TABLE 47–2. Functional Defects Seen in Adhesion Molecule–Deficient Mice*

Deficiency	Findings
CD18	Leukocytosis, reduced dermal but intact peritoneal emigration[76]
ICAM-1	Leukocytosis, impaired neutrophil emigration, decreased contact hypersensitivity[77]; reduced renal ischemic injury[78] and cerebral reperfusion injury[79]; protection from septic shock[80]
E-selectin	No abnormalities in leukocyte counts or emigration; defect in neutrophil emigration with addition of P-selectin mAb[81]
P-selectin	Leukocytosis, reduced neutrophil rolling and early emigration[82]
L-selectin	No abnormalities in leukocyte counts, reduced neutrophil rolling; reduced early neutrophil emigration[83, 84]; resistance to endotoxic shock[85]
P-selectin plus ICAM-1	Absent trauma-induced neutrophil rolling[86]; absent neutrophil emigration into inflamed peritoneum but normal emigration into inflamed alveoli[87]
E-selectin plus P-selectin	Extreme leukocytosis, susceptibility to bacterial infection, altered hematopoiesis[88]

*Selected experimental models utilizing adhesion molecule-deficient mice generated through gene targeting techniques. For additional references, see 89–91.

Inflammatory and Immune Processes

Monoclonal antibodies to adherence molecules have also been used in a variety of models of inflammatory or immune disease processes. A number of studies have shown that CD18 monoclonal antibodies effectively inhibit neutrophil accumulation and permeability edema in inflammatory skin lesions. In addition, both CD18 and anti-ICAM-1 antibodies as well as selectin antagonists have been shown to be effective at attenuating injury associated with bacterial meningitis, endotoxic shock, allergic asthma, autoimmune diabetes, NSAID-induced gastric mucosal injury, thermal burns, and attenuating cardiac and renal allograft rejection (see Table 47-2 references and references 1, 4, 8, and 53).

There is evidence that inhibiting neutrophil adherence in the setting of overt sepsis may actually improve outcome under certain circumstances. CD18 blockade has been shown to improve hemodynamics, reduce fluid requirements, and improve survival in rabbit models of both gram-negative and endotoxic shock.[54] Treatment with a CD11b monoclonal antibody increased survival in endotoxic shock in mice.[55] Although these studies seem to challenge the evidence from the LAD type I syndrome that neutrophil adherence and emigration are necessary for host defense, because severely deficient patients often die of sepsis, they support the concept that uncontrolled inflammation can be equally deleterious.

THERAPEUTIC POTENTIAL

Given the diverse array of important disease processes in which anti-adhesion therapy has shown striking protective effects in animal models, it is exciting to speculate about the clinical therapeutic potential of such an approach. At this time, a number of clinical trials are either ongoing or planned that will examine the efficacy and safety of anti-adhesion therapy. These studies will employ either murine or humanized monoclonal antibodies directed to CD11/CD18, ICAM-1, or the selectins, or they will use small molecules to inhibit either integrin/ICAM-1 or selectin-mediated adhesion.

In contemplating such an approach, however, one must keep in mind that by inhibiting neutrophil adherence functions, one essentially recreates the LAD syndromes. The risk of infection must be carefully weighed against any potential benefit of this form of therapy. Blocking CD18 does not increase mortality or infectious complications in models of bacterial peritonitis[56] and can actually improve outcome in certain septic models, such as bacterial meningitis[57] and gram-negative sepsis,[54] as described previously. It has also been shown, however, that with extremely high inocula of subcutaneous *Staphylococcus aureus* there can be an increase in infectious complications and mortality even after a single dose of CD18 monoclonal antibody, although this effect is not seen with lower, clinically relevant inocula of bacteria.[58] With *Escherichia coli,* however, CD18 blockade can seriously increase the risk of infection, even with clinically relevant inocula.[59]

Although these studies suggest that it may be safe to inhibit neutrophil adherence functions for a limited period of time in a carefully defined setting, they also must raise a significant note of caution about completely inhibiting such a basic physiologic process. It stands to reason that the more acute disease processes, such as those related to ischemia-reperfusion, may be more amenable to and, perhaps, more appropriate for controlled, transient inhibition of adherence.

SUMMARY

The adhesive interaction between neutrophils and the endothelium is a fundamental event in the acute inflammatory response. Recent in vitro and in vivo studies have yielded important new insights into the basic cellular and molecular mechanisms that mediate these interactions and have provided tools to manipulate them. The result is an increased understanding of the contribution of neutrophils to vascular and tissue injury in acute inflammation and a potential new approach to the treatment of human disease processes.

References

1. Harlan JM, Winn RK, Vedder NB, et al: In vivo models of leukocyte adherence to endothelium. *In*: Adhesion: Its Role in Inflammatory Disease. Harlan JM, Lui D (Eds). New York, WH Freeman and Co, 1992, pp 117-150.
2. Malech HL, Gallin JI: Current concepts: immunology. Neutrophils in human diseases. N Engl J Med 1987; 317:687-694.
3. Weiss SJ: Tissue destruction by neutrophils. N Engl J Med 1989; 320:365-376.
4. Cornejo CJ, Winn RK, Harlan JM: Anti-adhesion therapy. Adv Pharmacol 1997; 39:99-142.
5. Menger MD, Vollmar B: Adhesion molecules as determinants of disease: From molecular biology to surgical research. Br J Surg 1996; 83:588-601.
6. Metchnikoff E: Sur lallutte des cellules de l'organisme contre l'invasion des microbes. Ann Inst Pasteur 1887; 1:321.
7. Harlan JM: Neutrophil-mediated vascular injury. Acta Med Scand Suppl 1987; 715:123-129.
8. Carlos TM, Harlan JM: Leukocyte-endothelial adhesion molecules. Blood 1994; 84:2068-2101.
9. Springer TA: Traffic signals for lymphocyte recirculation and leukocyte emigration: The multistep paradigm. Cell 1994; 76:301-314.
10. Schleiffenbaum B, Fehr J: Regulation and selectivity of leukocyte emigration. J Lab Clin Med 1996; 127:151-168.
11. Schmid-Schönbein GW: Capillary plugging by granulocytes and the no-reflow phenomenon in the microcirculation. Fed Proc 1987; 46:2397-2401.
12. Cohnheim J: Lectures in General Pathology. Vol 1. London, New Sydenham Society, 1889, pp 242-382.
13. Tedder TF, Steeber DA, Chen A, et al: The selectins: Vascular adhesion molecules. FASEB J 1995; 9:866-873.
14. Lawrence MB, Springer TA: Leukocytes roll on a selectin at physiologic flow rates: Distinction from and prerequisite for adhesion through integrins. Cell 1991; 65:859-873.
15. Moazzam F, DeLano FA, Zweifach BW, et al: The leukocyte response to fluid stress [see comments]. Proc Natl Acad Sci U S A 1997; 94:5338-5343.
16. McEver RP, Cummings RD: Role of PSGL-1 binding to selectins in leukocyte recruitment. J Clin Invest 1997; 100:485-491.
17. Varki A: Selectin ligands: will the real ones please stand up? J Clin Invest 1997; 99:158-162.
18. Johnston B, Walter UM, Issekutz AC, et al: Differential roles of selectins and the $alpha_4$ integrin in acute, subacute, and chronic leukocyte recruitment in vivo. J Immunol 1997; 159:4514-4523.
19. Bevilacqua MP: Endothelial-leukocyte adhesion molecules. Annu Rev Immunol 1993; 11:767-804.
20. Karsan A, Harlan JM: The blood vessel wall. *In*: Hoffman R, et al: Hematology: Basic Principles and Practice. 3rd ed. Philadelphia, Churchill Livingstone (in press).
21. Wong J, Johnston B, Lee SS, et al: A minimal role for selectins in the recruitment of leukocytes into the inflamed liver microvasculature. J Clin Invest 1997; 99:2782-2790.
22. Anderson DC, Springer TA: Leukocyte adhesion deficiency: An inherited defect in the Mac-1, LFA-1, and p150,95 glycoproteins. Annu Rev Med 1987; 38:175-194.
23. Gahmberg CG, Tolvanen M, Kotovuori P: Leukocyte adhesion-structure and function of human leukocyte $beta_2$-integrins and their cellular ligands. Eur J Biochem 1997; 245:215-232.
24. Harlan JM, Killen PD, Senecal FM, et al: The role of neutrophil membrane glycoprotein GP-150 in neutrophil adherence to endothelium in vitro. Blood 1985; 66:167-178.
25. Lu H, Smith CW, Perrard J, et al: LFA-1 is sufficient in mediating neutrophil emigration in Mac-1-deficient mice. J Clin Invest 1997; 99:1340-1350.

26. Vedder NB, Harlan JM: Increased surface expression of CD11b/CD18 (Mac-1) is not required for stimulated neutrophil adherence to cultured endothelium. J Clin Invest 1988; 81:676–682.
27. Stewart M, Hogg N: Regulation of leukocyte integrin function: Affinity vs. avidity. J Cell Biochem 1996; 61:554–561.
28. Shattil SJ, Ginsberg MH: Integrin signaling in vascular biology. J Clin Invest 1997; 100:1–5.
29. Arfors K-E, Lundberg C, Lindbom L, et al: A monoclonal antibody to the membrane glycoprotein complex CDw18 (LFA), inhibits PMN accumulation and plasma leakage in vivo. Blood 1987; 69:338–340.
30. Newman PJ: The biology of PECAM-1. J Clin Invest 1997; 99:3–8.
31. Del Maschio A, Zanetti A, Corada M, et al: Polymorphonuclear leukocyte adhesion triggers the disorganization of endothelial cell-to-cell adherens junctions. J Cell Biol 1996; 135:497–510.
32. Kumasaka T, Quinlan WM, Doyle NA, et al: Role of the intercellular adhesion molecule-1 (ICAM-1) in endotoxin-induced pneumonia evaluated using ICAM-1 antisense oligonucleotides, anti-ICAM-1 monoclonal antibodies, and ICAM-1 mutant mice. J Clin Invest 1996; 97:2362–2369.
33. Zimmerman GA, McIntyre TM, Prescott SM: Adhesion and signaling in vascular cell-cell interactions. J Clin Invest 1996; 98:1699–1702.
34. Huber AR, Kunkel SL, Todd RF III, et al: Regulation of transendothelial neutrophil migration by endogenous interleukin-8. Science 1991; 254:99–102.
35. Middleton J, Neil S, Wintle J, et al: Transcytosis and surface presentation of IL-8 by venular endothelial cells. Cell 1997; 91:385–395.
36. Clark EA, Brugge JS: Integrins and signal transduction pathways: The road taken. Science 1995; 268:233–239.
37. Tsang YT, Neelamegham S, Hu Y, et al: Synergy between L-selectin signaling and chemotactic activation during neutrophil adhesion and transmigration. J Immunol 1997; 159:4566–4577.
38. Walcheck B, Moore KL, McEver RP, et al: Neutrophil-neutrophil interactions under hydrodynamic shear stress involve L-selectin and PSGL-1: A mechanism that amplifies initial leukocyte accumulation of P-selectin in vitro. J Clin Invest 1996; 98:1081–1087.
39. Weber C, Springer TA: Neutrophil accumulation on activated, surface-adherent platelets in flow is mediated by interaction of Mac-1 with fibrinogen bound to alpha$_{II}$-beta$_3$ and stimulated by platelet-activating factor. J Clin Invest 1997; 100:2085–2093.
40. Kuijpers TW, Mul EP, Blom M, et al: Freezing adhesion molecules in a state of high-avidity binding blocks eosinophil migration. J Exp Med 1993; 178:279–284.
41. Zouki C, Beauchamp M, Baron C, et al: Prevention of in vitro neutrophil adhesion to endothelial cells through shedding of L-selectin by C-reactive protein and peptides derived from C-reactive protein. J Clin Invest 1997; 100:522–529.
42. Berton G, Yan SR, Fumagalli L, et al: Neutrophil activation by adhesion: Mechanisms and pathophysiological implications. Int J Clin Lab Res 1996; 26:160–177.
43. Korthuis RJ, Granger DN: Reactive oxygen metabolites, neutrophils, and the pathogenesis of ischemic-tissue/reperfusion. Clin Cardiol 1993; 16:I19–I26.
44. Vedder NB, Winn RK, Rice CL, et al: Inhibition of leukocyte adherence by anti-CD18 monoclonal antibody attenuates reperfusion injury in the rabbit ear. Proc Natl Acad Sci U S A 1990; 87:2643–2646.
45. Hernandez LA, Grisham MB, Twohig B, et al: Role of neutrophils in ischemia-reperfusion–induced microvascular injury. Am J Physiol 1987; 253:H699–H703.
46. Winn RK, Liggitt D, Vedder NB, et al: Anti-P–selectin monoclonal antibody attenuates reperfusion injury to the rabbit ear. J Clin Invest 1993; 92:2042–2047.
47. Sharar SR, Mihelcic DD, Han KT, et al: Ischemia reperfusion injury in the rabbit ear is reduced by both immediate and delayed CD18 leukocyte adherence blockade. J Immunol 1994; 153:2234–2238.
48. Thiagarajan RR, Winn RK, Harlan JM: The role of leukocyte and endothelial adhesion molecules in ischemia-reperfusion injury. Thromb Haemost 1997; 78:310–314.
49. Seekamp A, Mulligan MS, Till GO, et al: Role of beta$_2$ integrins and ICAM-1 in lung injury following ischemia–reperfusion of rat hind limbs. Am J Pathol 1993; 143:464–472.
50. Vedder NB, Winn RK, Rice CL, et al: A monoclonal antibody to the adherence-promoting leukocyte glycoprotein, CD18, reduces organ injury and improves survival from hemorrhagic shock and resuscitation in rabbits. J Clin Invest 1988; 81:939–944.
51. Mileski WJ, Winn RK, Vedder NB, et al: Inhibition of CD18-dependent neutrophil adherence reduces organ injury after hemorrhagic shock in primates. Surgery 1990; 108:206–212.
52. Vedder N, Harlan J, Winn R, et al: Pilot phase 2 clinical trial of a humanized CD11/CD18 monoclonal antibody in hemorrhagic shock. *In*: The Immune Consequences of Trauma, Shock and Sepsis. Fiast E (ed). Bologna, Monduzzi Editore, 1997, pp 941–943.
53. Korthuis RJ, Anderson DC, Granger DN: Role of neutrophil-endothelial cell adhesion in inflammatory disorders. J Crit Care 1994; 9:47–71.
54. Thomas JR, Harlan JM, Rice CL, et al: Role of leukocyte CD11/CD18 complex in endotoxic and septic shock in rabbits. J Appl Physiol 1992; 73:1510–1516.
55. Burch RM, Noronha-Blob L, Bator JM, et al: Mice treated with a leumedin or antibody to Mac-1 to inhibit leukocyte sequestration survive endotoxin challenge. J Immunol 1993; 150:3397–3403.
56. Mileski WJ, Winn RK, Harlan JM, et al: Transient inhibition of neutrophil adherence with the anti-CD18 monoclonal antibody 60.3 does not increase mortality rates in abdominal sepsis. Surgery 1991; 109:497–501.
57. Tuomanen EI, Saukkonen K, Sande S, et al: Reduction of inflammation, tissue damage, and mortality in bacterial meningitis in rabbits treated with monoclonal antibodies against adhesion-promoting receptors of leukocytes. J Exp Med 1989; 170:959–969.
58. Sharar SR, Winn RK, Murry CE, et al: A CD18 monoclonal antibody increases the incidence and severity of subcutaneous abscess formation after high-dose *Staphylococcus aureus* injection in rabbits. Surgery 1991; 110:213–219.
59. Talbott GA, Sharar SR, Paulson JC, et al: Antibiotic therapy determines subcutaneous *E. coli* abscess formation after CD18 inhibition in rabbits. J Burn Care Rehabil 1998; 19:284–291.
60. Vedder NB, Bucky LP, Lopez I, et al: Inhibition of neutrophil adherence improves survival of random flaps in rabbits. Plast Surg Forum 1991; 14:373–374.
61. Ramamoorthy C, Sharar SR, Harlan JM, et al: Blocking L-selectin function attenuates reperfusion injury following hemorrhagic shock in rabbits. Am J Physiol 1996; 271:H1871–H1877.
62. Winn RK, Paulson JC, Harlan JM: A monoclonal antibody to P-selectin ameliorates injury associated with hemorrhagic shock in rabbits. Am J Physiol 1994; 267:H2391–H2397.
63. Simpson PJ Todd RF III, Fantone JC, et al: Reduction of experimental canine myocardial reperfusion injury by a monoclonal antibody (Anti-Mol, Anti-CD11b) that inhibits leukocyte adhesion. J Clin Invest 1988; 81:624–629.
64. Ma XL, Tsao PS, Lefer AM: Antibody to CD-18 exerts endothelial and cardiac protective effects in myocardial ischemia and reperfusion. J Clin Invest 1991; 88:1237–1243.
65. Weyrich AS, Ma XL, Lefer DJ, et al: In vivo neutralization of P-selectin protects feline heart and endothelium in myocardial ischemia and reperfusion injury [see comments]. J Clin Invest 1993; 91:2620–2629.
66. Wegner CD, Gundel RH, Reilly P, et al: Intercellular adhesion molecule-1 (ICAM-1) in the pathogenesis of asthma. Science 1990; 247:456–459.
67. Carden DL, Smith JK, Korthuis RJ: Neutrophil-mediated microvascular dysfunction in postischemic canine skeletal muscle: Role of granulocyte adherence. Circ Res 1990; 66:1436–1444.
68. Hutchings P, Rosen H, O'Reilly L, et al: Transfer of diabetes in mice prevented by blockade of adhesion-promoting receptor on macrophages. Nature 1990; 348:639–642.
69. Clark WM, Madden KP, Rothlein R, et al: Reduction of central nervous system ischemic injury in rabbits using leukocyte adhesion antibody treatment. Stroke 1991; 22:877–883.
70. Wallace JL, Arfors KE, McKnight GW: A monoclonal antibody against the CD18 leukocyte adhesion molecule prevents indomethacin-induced gastric damage in the rabbit. Gastroenterology 1991; 100:878–883.
71. Bucky LP, Vedder NB, Hong HZ, et al: Reduction of burn injury by inhibiting CD18-mediated leukocyte adherence in rabbits. Plast Reconstr Surg 1994; 93:1473–1480.
72. Cosimi AB, Conti D, Delmonico FL, et al: In vivo effects of

monoclonal antibody to ICAM-1 (CD54) in nonhuman primates with renal allografts. J Immunol 1990; 144:4604-4612.
73. Mulligan MS, Polley MJ, Bayer RJ, et al: Neutrophil-dependent acute lung injury: Requirement for P-selectin (GMP-140). J Clin Invest 1992; 90:1600-1607.
74. Mulligan MS, Paulson JC, De-Frees S, et al: Protective effects of oligosaccharides in P-selectin-dependent lung injury. Nature 1993; 364:149-151.
75. Podolsky DK, Lobb R, King N, et al: Attenuation of colitis in the cotton-top tamarin by anti-alpha 4 integrin monoclonal antibody. J Clin Invest 1993; 92:372-380.
76. Mizgerd JP, Kubo H, Kutkoski GJ, et al: Neutrophil emigration in the skin, lungs, and peritoneum: Different requirements for CD11/CD18 revealed by CD18-deficient mice. J Exp Med 1997; 186:1357-1364.
77. Sligh JE Jr, Ballantyne CM, Rich SS, et al: Inflammatory and immune responses are impaired in mice deficient in intercellular adhesion molecule 1. Proc Natl Acad Sci U S A 1993; 90:8529-8533.
78. Kelly KJ, Williams WW Jr, Colvin RB, et al: Intercellular adhesion molecule-1-deficient mice are protected against ischemic renal injury. J Clin Invest 1996; 97:1056-1063.
79. Connolly ES Jr, Winfree CJ, Springer TA, et al: Cerebral protection in homozygous null ICAM-1 mice after middle cerebral artery occlusion: Role of neutrophil adhesion in the pathogenesis of stroke. J Clin Invest 1996; 97:209-216.
80. Xu H, Gonzalo JA, St Pierre Y, et al: Leukocytosis and resistance to septic shock in intercellular adhesion molecule 1-deficient mice. J Exp Med 1994; 180:95-109.
81. Labow MA, Norton CR, Rumberger JM, et al: Characterization of E-selectin-deficient mice: Demonstration of overlapping function of the endothelial selectins. Immunity 1994; 1:709-720.
82. Mayadas TN, Johnson RC, Rayburn H, et al: Leukocyte rolling and extravasation are severely compromised in P selectin-deficient mice. Cell 1993; 74:541-554.
83. Arbon'es ML, Ord DC, Ley K, et al: Lymphocyte homing and leukocyte rolling and migration are impaired in L-selectin-deficient mice. Immunity 1994; 1:247-260.
84. Ley K, Bullard DC, Arbon'es ML, et al: Sequential contribution of L- and P-selectin to leukocyte rolling in vivo. J Exp Med 1995; 181:669-675.
85. Tedder TF, Steeber DA, Pizcueta P: L-selectin-deficient mice have impaired leukocyte recruitment into inflammatory sites. J Exp Med 1995; 181:2259-2264.
86. Kunkel EJ, Jung U, Bullard DC, et al: Absence of trauma-induced leukocyte rolling in mice deficient in both P-selectin and intercellular adhesion molecule 1. J Exp Med 1996; 183:57-65.
87. Bullard DC, Qin L, Lorenzo I, et al: P-selectin/ICAM-1 double mutant mice: Acute emigration of neutrophils into the peritoneum is completely absent but is normal into pulmonary alveoli [see comments]. J Clin Invest 1995; 95:1782-1788.
88. Frenette PS, Mayadas TN, Rayburn H, et al: Susceptibility to infection and altered hematopoiesis in mice deficient in both P- and E-selectins. Cell 1996; 84:563-574.
89. Ley K: Gene-targeted mice in leukocyte adhesion research. Microcirculation 1995; 2:141-150.
90. Frenette PS, Wagner DD: Insights into selectin function from knockout mice. Thromb Haemost 1997; 78:60-64.
91. Hynes RO: Targeted mutations in cell adhesion genes: What have we learned from them? Dev Biol 1996; 180:402-412.

48

Cytokines in Disease

Leland Shapiro, MD, FACP • Jeffrey A. Gelfand, MD

Cytokines are intercellular messenger polypeptides that modulate many biologic responses. They are small, with molecular mass between 8 and 30 kilodaltons (kD), and are biologically active at low concentrations (picomolar or less).

Cytokines differ from classic endocrine hormones in that they (1) are produced by many cell types rather than by discrete organs, (2) are primarily produced de novo in response to stimuli, (3) have little documented significant role in normal homeostasis, (4) are often induced in response to exogenous (not endogenous) stimuli, and (5) commonly have autocrine and paracrine effects. It is clear from these qualities that distinctions among cytokines, neurotransmitters, and hormones are mainly functional.

The nomenclature of cytokines is confusing. They are variously subdivided into "interleukins," "interferons," "growth factors," "stimulating factors," "pro-inflammatory factors," "inhibitory factors," "activating factors," and so on. These terms have usually been generated descriptively on the basis of physiologic function, target cell type, or order of discovery. Examples include the following:

- Interleukins (ILs), which currently number 18
- Macrophage-activating factor (MAF)
- Macrophage inflammatory proteins (MIP-1α and MIP-1β)
- Tumor necrosis factor (TNF)
- Granulocyte/macrophage colony-stimulating factor (GM-CSF)
- Granulocyte colony-stimulating factor (G-CSF)
- Erythropoietin

In addition, there are binding proteins and soluble cytokine receptors.

It is clear that cytokines are involved directly or indirectly in the pathogenesis of many diseases, especially those associated with inflammation or cell proliferation. Some of these are:

- Systemic inflammatory response syndrome (SIRS) or sepsis
- Human immunodeficiency virus (HIV) infection and acquired immunodeficiency syndrome (AIDS)
- Acute respiratory distress syndrome (ARDS)
- Cachexia
- Meningitis
- Atherosclerotic coronary artery disease
- Herxheimer reaction
- Congestive heart failure syndrome
- Organ fibrosis
- Kawasaki syndrome
- Solid and hematologic malignancies
- Alcoholic hepatitis
- Glomerulonephritis
- Graft rejection
- Many "collagen vascular" diseases, including rheumatoid arthritis
- Granulomatous diseases

A partial list of conditions associated with increased cytokine production is presented in Table 48-1.

TABLE 48–1. Selected Conditions Associated with Increased Cytokine Production

Condition	Example
Infectious disease	Infection due to gram-positive or gram-negative bacteria, fungi, protozoa, viruses, and mycobacteria; Jarisch-Herxheimer reaction
Trauma	Burn injury
Autoimmunity	Rheumatoid arthritis, systemic lupus erythematosus, vasculitides
Neoplasia	Many solid and hematologic malignancies
Circulating drugs/ medications	Amphotericin B
Cryptogenic inflammatory disease	Sarcoidosis, Kawasaki syndrome, inflammatory bowel disease
Cardiac disease	Acute myocardial infarction, congestive heart failure syndrome
Production of endogenous substances	Cytokines, activated complement components, immune complexes

It is often difficult to determine whether cytokines associated with a particular disease represent an epiphenomenon or whether they are causally linked to disease pathophysiology. Prospective, randomized, double-blind controlled clinical trials have established a role for TNF in rheumatoid arthritis and Jarisch-Herxheimer reaction.[1–3] In the case of rheumatoid arthritis, TNF blockade through the use of either monoclonal antibodies or soluble TNF receptors was effective in alleviating disease manifestations, thus strengthening the results. As well, a cogent case can be made for a causal role for IL-1 and TNF in sepsis or, more generally, SIRS. Three lines of evidence support a functional role for cytokines in disease pathophysiology; proceeding from weakest to strongest, they are as follows:

1. Studies demonstrate a correlation between clinical status and cytokine concentrations in body fluids or biopsy specimens.
2. Administration of cytokines to animals or humans replicate many if not all manifestations of certain diseases or syndromes.
3. Selective blockade of specific cytokines leads to diminution of disease phenomena in animals or humans.

Knockout mice, which lack functional genes for individual cytokines or cytokine receptors, are the latest-developed means of abrogating specific cytokine activity. These animals are powerful tools for evaluating the role of individual cytokines in vivo.

In addition to their direct causal role in disease pathophysiology, cytokines can serve as markers of disease activity. This feature has been shown in clinical studies involving many diseases and various body fluids and secretions. In general, concentrations of IL-6, the anti-inflammatory cytokine interleukin-1 receptor antagonist (IL-1Ra), and the inhibitory soluble TNF receptors have correlated better with disease activity than have the concentrations of circulating pro-inflammatory cytokines (see later).

Newer exciting developments include the demonstration of complex interactions between host and microorganism involving cytokines. For example, several viruses produce soluble receptors to pro-inflammatory cytokines that have immunomodulatory activity and serve as virulence factors in in vivo animal models of inflammatory diseases. Certain strains of virulent bacteria have been found to use cytokines directly as growth factors or to bind cytokines at their surfaces to enhance phagocytic cell entry and virulence.[4, 5] It has also been demonstrated that *Schistosoma mansoni* utilizes host TNF to facilitate egg-laying in a murine model.[6] The human immunodeficiency virus has been shown to gain access to mammalian cells by using chemokine receptors in association with cell-surface CD4 in a coreceptor mechanism; individuals lacking certain chemokine receptors are highly resistant to infection with HIV.

CYTOKINES AND SEPSIS (SYSTEMIC INFLAMMATORY RESPONSE SYNDROME)

Sepsis is currently the 13th leading cause of death in the United States, and it is on the rise. A 1997 study of eight academic centers documented the incidence of sepsis syndrome as 2 cases per 100 admissions, with a 34% mortality seen at 28 days.[7] Factors thought to account for this increase include an aging population, increased use of invasive therapies and devices, improved survival of individuals with debilitating illnesses, and nosocomial infections pursuant to longer hospitalization of chronically ill patients. All of these factors increase susceptibility to infection. The prevalence of community-acquired bacteremia rose from 7 cases to 13 cases per 1000 hospital admissions between the mid-1960s and the mid-1970s; greater risk was associated with extremes of age. Some important predisposing factors for the development of bacteremia or sepsis are as follows:

- Advanced age
- Use of intravenous (IV) lines and invasive devices
- Granulocytopenia
- Prior antibiotic therapy
- Severe burn injury
- Functional asplenia
- HIV infection

Septic shock has been associated with a mortality of about 50% in many studies. Quartin and colleagues,[8] in analyzing a cohort study of 1505 patients with various degrees of sepsis who had been studied between 1984 and 1985, noted a 57% mortality for those in shock. In addition to the mortality in the acute stage, data from this study indicate a persistently poor prognosis for patients with sepsis who survive the acute (30-day) event. Over a period of 5 years, the average life span in sepsis survivors was significantly shorter, 4.08 years compared with 8.03 years in controls. This difference remained even when the analysis was controlled for comorbidity. These data suggest significant residual organ dysfunction after acute episodes of sepsis.

DEFINITION

A plethora of terms associated with "sepsis" abound and need definition[9]:

Bacteremia: presence of bacteria in the blood, confirmed by culture.

Septicemia: bacteremia with significant clinical manifestations.

Sepsis: evidence of infection with a systemic response.

Sepsis syndrome: clinical evidence of infection with a systemic response sufficient to produce compromise of organ function, such as respiratory insufficiency, renal dysfunction, acidosis, and altered mental function.

Septic shock: the sepsis syndrome with documented hypotension (systolic blood pressure < 90 mm Hg or a decrease in mean arterial blood pressure greater than 40 mm Hg from the baseline).

Refractory septic shock: septic shock lasting more than 1 hour that does not respond to intervention with IV fluids or pharmacologic agents.

It has been proposed that the more general term *systemic inflammatory response syndrome* (SIRS) be used to describe clinical manifestations of systemic inflammation.[10] The gradations of SIRS correspond to the severity of sepsis beyond and including sepsis syndrome, but SIRS does not merely imply the presence or suspicion of infection. It therefore describes the clinical consequences of inflammatory endothelial activation regardless of cause.[11]

Historical Background

At the turn of the 20th century, the focus of physicians was entirely on the microorganisms responsible for producing overwhelming infections, and the prevailing hypothesis was that either "pyogenic" or toxin-producing organisms were required. In the late 1920s, the description of the Shwartzman reaction focused the attention of investigators on the state of the host for the first time. By the 1950s, the endotoxin component of gram-negative bacteria was thought to be a major pathogenic factor of sepsis. By the 1970s, complement activation and the "activated neutrophil" were thought to play major roles in the pathogenesis of sepsis. The importance of the host response was further suggested by the observed consistency of the stereotyped "septic response" to many different kinds of inciting factors and many types of infecting organisms.

The 1980s were notable for the elucidation of a number of critical endogenous pathogenic mediators, notably the cytokines and arachidonic acid–derived metabolites. It was found that (1) sepsis could be replicated in animal models by exogenous cytokine administration in the absence of bacteremia and (2) septic pathophysiology could be ameliorated by cytokine blockade. An illuminating series of experiments was performed with C3H/Hej mice, which have a mutation rendering their mononuclear leukocytes incapable of producing TNF in response to lipopolysaccharide (LPS, endotoxin) under most conditions. Such mice were found to be nearly refractory to endotoxin toxicity, indicating the primacy of the cytokine response in producing the septic state.[12]

An interesting fact concerning the mortality rate associated with septic shock is that it has not changed significantly over the past 30 years, although the types of patients in whom this syndrome develops probably have. It is remarkable that modern technology has contributed minimally to the survival statistics in this condition. Technologic advances have included invasive monitoring equipment, better diagnostic modalities, more effective vasopressors and inotropes, more powerful antibiotics, and combination antibiotic therapy. Another factor of import is the rapidly rising cost per life saved (or lost) in the face of little added benefit in ultimate outcome. A fair assumption is that improved antibiotics are not the answer to significant improvement in therapy for septic shock.

Mechanism/Process

Although microorganisms can produce exotoxins, these substances do not appear to be directly responsible for the majority of damage produced during bacterial sepsis (though there are toxin-mediated diseases, such as tetanus, toxic shock syndrome, and staphylococcal scalded skin syndrome).

The sequence of events leading to sepsis presumably begins with bacteremia. The outer membranes of all gram-negative bacteria contain LPS, or endotoxin, which interacts with the reticuloendothelial system in such a way as to produce the septic state. Lipid A appears to be the key conserved piece of the endotoxin molecule involved in this interaction.[13, 14]

Not all is known about the details of events leading to sepsis, but a model is emerging, as follows (Fig. 48–1):

1. Endotoxin binds to receptors found on mononuclear leukocytes (monocytes and macrophages).
2. This interaction results in the secretion of several cytokines. When produced in excess, the primary cytokines initiating adverse effects are IL-1 and TNF.[15, 16]
3. IL-1 and TNF orchestrate the physiology of the septic state by their effects on the temperature set point (fever induction, (?) hypothermia), vascular resistance and permeability, cardiac function and inotropic state, bone marrow effects (e.g., increased white blood cells), and effects on many enzymes, such as lactate dehydrogenase and lipoprotein lipase, that alter energy usage by many tissues. All of this morbid physiology can proceed in the absence of inciting endotoxin, as occurs in gram-positive septic shock or after clearance of endotoxin from the circulation. This finding further supports the notion that cytokines, and not the endotoxins themselves, are essential mediators of the multiple effects of sepsis.
4. Many of the effects of cytokines are mediated at the target tissues by nitric oxide (NO), arachidonic acid metabolites (prostaglandins, eicosanoids, platelet-activating factor [PAF]), and lipoxygenase derivatives.
5. IL-1 and TNF stimulate the elaboration of other cytokines, producing a cascade effect with the multiple functions of amplification and modulation (both up-regulation and down-regulation) as cytokines beget cytokines. Of special import may be the local production of IL-8 and other chemokines by cells at various organs, which have the function of recruiting and activating polymorphonuclear leukocytes and monocytic leukocytes, which can then cause tissue damage and organ dysfunction. In vitro data have documented significant IL-8 production in response to minute concentrations of IL-1 or TNF; this finding suggests an amplification role for IL-8 in the induction of sepsis after local production of IL-1 or TNF at sites of inflammation.
6. The complement, coagulation, and kinin cascades are also activated and play important roles in the septic state.[17–22]
7. Specific and nonspecific anticytokine substances are concomitantly produced, including glucocorticoids, interleukin-1 receptor antagonist (IL-1Ra), and soluble cytokine and endotoxin receptors (see later). Also, some liberated cytokines (IL-4, IL-6, IL-10, and transforming growth factor-β [TGF-β]) have anti-inflammatory effects, such as decreasing mononuclear cell synthesis of IL-1 and TNF in response to endotoxin.[23–26]

Of clinical relevance, antibiotics may exacerbate the inflammatory response to microorganisms by lysing them, releasing larger quantities of free endotoxin. This process may result in greater contact of endotoxin with cytokine-producing cells and subsequently may augment production of IL-1, TNF, and IL-8.

INTERLEUKIN-1 AND TUMOR NECROSIS FACTOR AS A SYNERGISTIC SEPTIC COMBINATION

Given the preceding discussion, there has been some controversy as to which cytokine constitutes *the* shock protein. The seminal work of Beutler and Cerami has made a strong case for TNF as *the* shock cytokine.[15] In support of their theory, it has been shown that[11]:

1. IV endotoxin infusion can produce septic shock while increasing circulating levels of TNF.
2. TNF infusions can replicate all of the physiologic effects of septic shock.

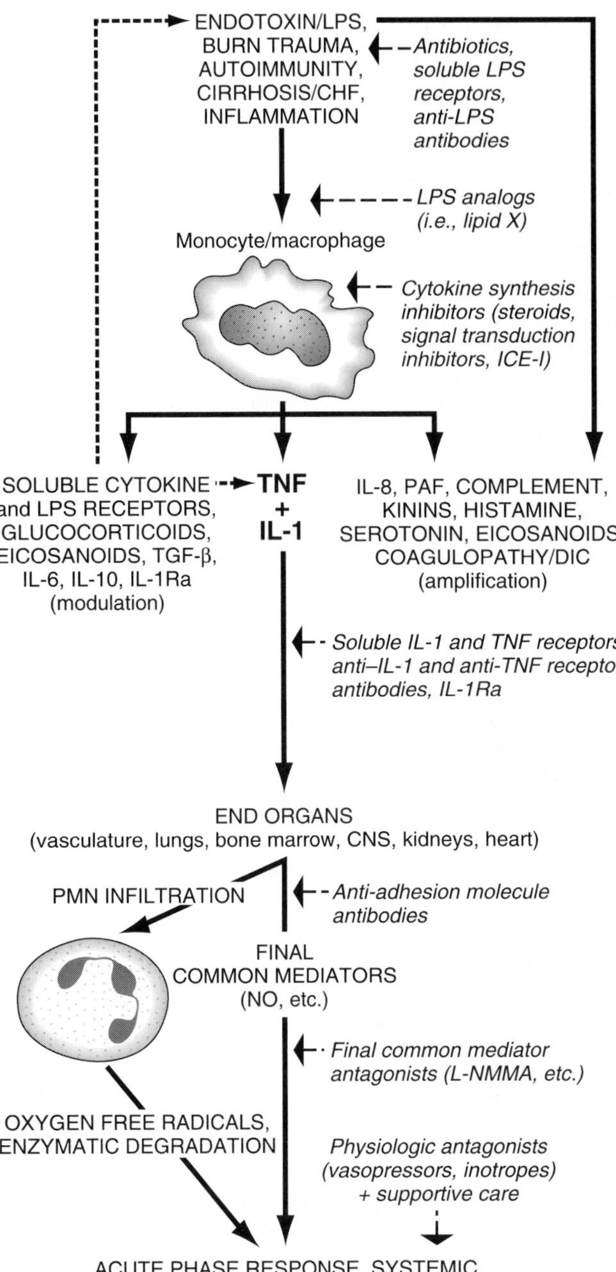

Figure 48–1. Any of a number of initiating factors can interact with mononuclear leukocytes and other cells to stimulate secretion of the key pro-inflammatory cytokines tumor necrosis factor (TNF) and interleukin-1 (IL-1). In sufficiently high circulating concentrations, these two cytokines synergistically orchestrate all the phenomena of the systemic inflammatory response syndrome by proceeding to various end organs and inducing specific final common mediators of organ dysfunction. Additionally, adhesion molecules are induced with subsequent recruitment and activation of polymorphonuclear leukocytes (aided by the chemotactic cytokine IL-8) contributing to tissue damage. Amplification and diminution of the inflammatory responses proceed concomitantly with TNF and IL-1 production as shown. Also shown are possible targets for therapeutic intervention. CHF = congestive heart failure; CNS = central nervous system; ICE-I = interleukin-1 converting enzyme inhibitor; IL = interleukin; IL-1Ra = interleukin-1 receptor antagonist; L-NMMA = L-N-monomethylarginine; LPS = lipopolysaccharide (endotoxin); NO = nitric oxide; PAF = platelet activating factor; PMN = polymorphonuclear neutrophil; TGF-β = transforming growth factor-β; TNF = tumor necrosis factor; *solid line* = pro-inflammatory response induction; *broken line* = naturally occurring down-regulatory responses; *shorter broken line with larger arrowhead* = possible areas of therapeutic intervention (italic type).

3. TNF serum levels correlate with degree of sepsis in humans (quantitated by the Acute Physiology and Chronic Health Evaluation score).

4. anti-TNF antibodies can prevent mortality as well as abrogate septic physiology after endotoxin infusion in animals.

There is much in vivo and in vitro evidence, however, to support a crucial role for IL-1 as a comediator of the sepsis syndrome. IL-1 has been shown to have effects nearly identical to those of TNF when administered to animals or humans. Specifically, TNF or IL-1 infusion into animals results in fever ("endogenous pyrogen"); anorexia; sleep ("hypnotoxin"); hypotension; metabolic acidosis; neutrophilia or neutropenia (depending on dose); increased serum levels of ACTH, IL-6, and GM-CSF; decreases in serum iron, zinc, hepatic cytochrome P_{450} activity (hence decreased metabolism of many drugs), thyroxin (possible origin of nonthyroid illness), and albumin levels; greater hepatic synthesis of acute-phase proteins (i.e., serum amyloid A protein); capillary leak (possible origin of ARDS); and death. The TNF receptor knockout mouse is resistant to lethality after administration of low doses of endotoxin.[27, 28] In the current consensus, there is little doubt about the importance of TNF and IL-1 as comediators of sepsis.

The kinetics of IL-1 may be relevant to the possibility of therapeutic cytokine modulation in sepsis. In animal models of bacteremia or endotoxemia, a rapid rise in TNF level occurs that peaks at 60 to 90 minutes, followed by a delayed increase in IL-1 level that peaks at 180 minutes; similar observations have been made in humans. Experiments have shown that TNF induces IL-1 in vivo.[29] These observations are important evidence that any attempt to treat sepsis by modulating TNF may have to be made very early in the course of sepsis; if IL-1 modulation is the target, however, intervention later in the disease process may be possible. Evidence of the importance of IL-1 in septic shock is highlighted by experiments showing that blocking IL-1 activity with the specific inhibitory molecule IL-1Ra in animal models of septic shock decreases morbidity and mortality.[30, 31]

Thus, IL-1 or TNF given intravenously can reproduce the elements of the sepsis syndrome, and blocking the activities of either experimentally can abrogate the septic state. From the clinical standpoint, the arguments about which cytokine is most important in sepsis are secondary to the fact that IL-1 and TNF appear to act synergistically in producing septic physiology. In animal models of SIRS, injections of either TNF or IL-1 produce no significant hemodynamic disarray, but these two cytokines can produce hemodynamic shock when infused together.[32] Similar experiments have documented synergistic effects of TNF and IL-1 on increasing plasma lactate, glucose, and triglycerides in animals.

The teleology of this cytokine redundancy is uncertain, but the clinical implications are not. We may not need to block all of the pro-inflammatory elements of the cytokine cascade; blocking only one or a few of them may have significant clinical benefit. As alluded to previously, there are many other mediators of sepsis (i.e., complement components, PAF, kinins, prostaglandins), but the extant data implicate IL-1 and TNF as crucial triggers in the initiation of sepsis. For this reason, most clinical trials in sepsis have targeted TNF or IL-1 blockade by pharmacologic intervention.

Platelet-Activating Factor

Platelet-activating factor is a phospholipid produced by platelets, endothelium, and mononuclear and polymorphonuclear leukocytes that has been implicated in the pathophysiology of sepsis. The evidence supporting such a role for PAF is similar to that described for IL-1 and TNF. In fact, some PAF effects are probably mediated by IL-1 and TNF production, and some TNF effects are mediated through PAF.[33] Currently, the relative contribution of PAF to the septic state is uncertain; a prospective randomized clinical study of a PAF antagonist has failed to demonstrate benefit.[34]

ROLE OF CYTOKINES IN PROTECTING THE HOST

It appears that some (as yet undefined) levels of some cytokines are beneficial, but excessive levels are detrimental. One experiment evaluated the role of exogenous IL-1Ra in a neonatal rat model of lethal bacteremic sepsis.[35] Blocking IL-1 activity with the receptor antagonist decreased lethality in this model compared with control rats, whereas very high doses of IL-1Ra promoted lethality. The adverse outcome with more complete suppression of IL-1 suggests that some quantity of IL-1 is beneficial. Murine models have demonstrated exacerbation of infection following blockade of IL-1 activity, and pretreatment with low doses of IL-1 or TNF conferred protection from the effects of subsequent infection.[36] Mice lacking one of the TNF receptors demonstrated a markedly enhanced magnitude of infection and susceptibility to death from the intracellular bacterium *Listeria monocytogenes*.[27, 28] Until we know more, the answer to the question of what critical levels of cytokines in disease traverse the boundary of helpful to harmful will have to remain "Enough, but not too much."

Following the failure of several large clinical trials of anticytokine strategies to treat sepsis, a provocative hypothesis has been put forward. It suggests that the endogenous anti-inflammatory response to sepsis (e.g., generation of corticosteroids, IL-1Ra, soluble TNF receptors) becomes predominant and that administration of anticytokine agents may be detrimental at this stage (see Fig. 48–1). During this "compensatory anti-inflammatory response syndrome" (CARS), this hypothesis suggests, pro-inflammatory agents may improve outcome. Scant clinical data support this hypothesis, and it remains speculative at this time.[37, 38]

Employing anticytokine strategies to combat infectious and inflammatory conditions is not unprecedented; this strategy occurs naturally in the course of disease in vivo. The natural control of inflammation has been shown to involve greater production of "down-regulating" or "negative feedback" substances, including soluble receptors to endotoxin, TNF, and IL-1. IL-6, IL-10, and TGF-β, which have anti-inflammatory effects, and IL-1Ra are produced. In the course of overwhelming inflammation or infection, however, these natural anticytokine mediators are thought to be produced in insufficient quantities to contain such insults. Hence, one proposed therapeutic strategy is to administer large parenteral doses of these agents (produced by recombinant DNA technology) and to employ pharmacologic blockade of multiple stages of the pro-inflammatory cascade simultaneously.

INFLAMMATORY VERSUS ANTI-INFLAMMATORY CYTOKINES

Although more than 30 cytokines have been described, they may be characterized by broad functional categories. Cytokines may have activities that are growth-promoting, pro-inflammatory, or anti-inflammatory (Table 48–2).

The primary pro-inflammatory cytokines are IL-1, TNF, and IL-8. IL-1 and TNF have nearly identical effects when injected intravenously in animal models of sepsis. As previously discussed, infusion of TNF or IL-1 into animals results in the manifestations of sepsis.

Interleukin-8 is a small cytokine with a molecular mass of about 8 kD and the functions of neutrophilic chemotaxis and activation as well as angiogenesis. Studies imply an important role for this cytokine in neutrophilic recruitment and activation at sites of inflammation, resulting in amplification of the local inflammatory response as well as tissue damage. IL-8 is secreted by many cell types, including fibroblasts, endothelium, and peripheral blood mononuclear cells. IL-8 secretagogues include endotoxin, IL-1, and TNF. In vitro, significant amounts of this cytokine are produced in response to minute concentrations of these stimuli; 1 to 10 pg/mL IL-1 or TNF can induce significant IL-8 production in human endothelial or fibroblast cells.

Interleukin-6 is also produced by many different cell types in response to various stimuli, including endotoxin, IL-1, and TNF.[39] Circulating in plasma at concentrations higher than those of most other cytokines, IL-6 is one of the best cytokine markers of inflammatory disease activity in humans. It has both anti-inflammatory and pro-inflammatory activities as a result of its functions as suppressor of pro-inflammatory cytokine induction, its role as an endogenous pyrogen, and its initiation of the acute-phase response (a property shared by IL-1 and TNF, but not IL-8). Unlike IL-1 or TNF, the presence of IL-6 in animals does not appear to be causally related to SIRS, and IL-6 knockout mice show enhanced susceptibility to *Escherichia coli*–induced lethality.[40, 41]

IL-1Ra is also a marker of disease activity. Clinical studies have found that levels of the anti-inflammatory cytokines are better markers of inflammatory disease activity than are levels of the pro-inflammatory cytokines, probably because of the greater magnitude of production or the prolonged half-lives of the former.

TABLE 48–2. Pro-inflammatory Cytokines, Anti-inflammatory Cytokines, and Soluble Tumor Necrosis Factor Receptors

	Cytokine (kD)	Major Sources	Principal Activities
Pro-inflammatory cytokines	IL-1 (17.5)	Monocyte/macrophage, lymphocyte, neutrophil, endothelium, fibroblast, keratinocyte	Activation of T cells, B cells, NK cells, neutrophils, osteoblasts, and endothelium Induces fever, sleep, anorexia, ACTH release, and hepatic acute-phase protein synthesis Leads to myocardial depression, hypercoagulability, hypotension/shock, and death Stimulates production of TNF, IL-8, and IL-6 Suppression of cytochrome P_{450}, thyroglobulin, and lipoprotein synthesis
	TNF (17.5)	Monocyte/macrophage, lymphocyte, neutrophil, endothelium, fibroblast, keratinocyte	Activation of T cells, B cells, NK cells, neutrophils, osteoblasts, and endothelium Tumoricidal activity Induces fever, sleep, anorexia, catabolism, ACTH release, hepatic acute-phase protein synthesis Leads to myocardial depression, hypercoagulability, hypotension/shock, and death Stimulates production of IL-1, IL-8, and IL-6 Suppression of cytochrome P_{450}, thyroglobulin, and lipoprotein lipase
	IL-8 (8)	Monocyte/macrophage, lymphocyte, endothelium, fibroblast, keratinocyte	Recruitment and activation of neutrophils Chemotactic for lymphocytes Angiogenesis
Anti-inflammatory cytokines	IL-10, TGF-β (35, 12.5)	T cell, fibroblast	Suppression of B cell and T cell proliferation Inhibition of endotoxin-induced monocyte IL-1 and TNF production Induction of IL-1Ra
	IL-6 (21–28)	Monocyte/macrophage, T cell, endothelium, fibroblast, keratinocyte	Induction of fever and the hepatic acute-phase response Stimulates cortisol production Decreases IL-1 and TNF production Participates in activation and proliferation of B cells and T cells Facilitates Ig production by B cells
	IL-1Ra (17.5)	Monocyte/macrophage, fibroblast	Specifically inhibits IL-1 effects, including SIRS due to endotoxin or *Escherichia coli* in animal models
Soluble TNF receptors	Derived from TNF receptors p55 and p75 (30 and 40, respectively)	Unknown, but monocyte/macrophage and neutrophils are likely	Specifically inhibits TNF effects, including SIRS due to endotoxin or *E. coli* in animal models

ACTH = adrenocorticotropic hormone; IL = interleukin; IL-1Ra = IL-1 receptor agonist; NK = natural killer; SIRS = systemic inflammatory response syndrome; TGF-β = transforming growth factor-β.

IL-6, IL-10, TGF-β, and IL-1Ra have anti-inflammatory activities. All can decrease the endotoxin-induced production of IL-1 and TNF in several in vitro and in vivo systems.

SELECTED ANTICYTOKINE STRATEGIES

The most important of many potential advantages of anti-cytokine approaches to infectious or inflammatory diseases are as follows:

1. *Applicability* to many such diseases, because therapy is directed toward the final common pathway of inflammation and not to its specific proximate cause; thus, in the case of SIRS due to infection, these approaches should be applicable to gram-positive and fungal infections as well as to gram-negative infections.

2. The *margin of safety* is likely to be great and the risk of immunogenicity small for many contemplated anticytokine agents because they are naturally occurring substances, such as IL-1Ra and soluble cytokine receptors.

3. *Specificity* of some possible anticytokine agents; for instance, soluble cytokine receptors typically demonstrate a 100- to 1000-fold greater affinity for their respective cytokines than monoclonal antibodies raised against these same cytokines.

Specific Strategies

Intracellular production of pro-inflammatory cytokines can be targeted. Signal transduction following exposure to pro-inflammatory substances leading to elaboration of TNF and IL-1 can be blocked pharmacologically.[42] Corticosteroids decrease TNF and IL-1 production and have so far demonstrated some therapeutic efficacy, especially in patients with bacterial meningitis. Thalidomide and pentoxifylline each can decrease TNF production, and administration of TGF-β, IL-6, or IL-10 has been shown to decrease induction of TNF and IL-1.

A new molecular target is the IL-1β-converting enzyme, which cleaves the biologically inactive pro-IL-1β within cells into the mature, bioactive IL-1β molecule. An IL-1-converting enzyme inhibitor (ICE-I) has been found to down-regulate the inflammatory response; ICE-I substances are now under investigation as potential therapeutic agents.[43, 44] It is instructive that the ICE knockout mouse is highly resistant to endotoxin-induced sepsis. This resistance may be due to the fact that several pro-inflammatory molecules are processed and activated by ICE; in addition to IL-1β, these molecules include the pro-inflammatory cytokine IL-18 and possibly IL-16 (of uncertain role in inflammation). For unclear reasons, secretion of IL-1α (which does not require cleavage to an active form) is also impaired in ICE knockout animals. Better survival in a rat sepsis model was seen after blockade of both IL-1 and TNF than after inhibition of either cytokine individually[45]; this finding implies greater effect of the inhibition of multiple pro-inflammatory cytokines, as is seen in the ICE knockout mouse.

After IL-1 or TNF has been produced, interventions designed to neutralize these cytokines or block their interaction with cell surface receptors are possible. Anti-TNF antibodies have been shown to significantly decrease mortality and ameliorate adverse physiologic changes in animal models of sepsis. This passive immunization treatment for adverse TNF effects has proved effective when administered up to 30 minutes after the septic challenge.

IL-1Ra is a natural product of monocytes and fibroblasts that binds to and blocks IL-1 receptors, preventing IL-1 activity. It is a unique substance, in that it is the only natural competitive antagonist of a cytokine/hormone/neurotransmitter described to date. IL-1Ra has reduced mortality by as much as 70% in rabbit, mouse, and primate models of septic shock.[30, 46, 47] An important finding of these studies is that IL-1Ra was efficacious even when administered after the onset of septic shock. This finding has clear clinical implications, because it extends the window of opportunity for treating sepsis.

Fisher and associates[48] performed a phase III double-blind trial in 893 patients with SIRS given IL-1Ra. Overall mortality rates were 34% in patients in the placebo (standard care) group and 29% in patients administered high-dose IL-1Ra by continuous intravenous infusion (2 mg/kg/hour for 72 hours) in addition to standard care. Although the difference in overall mortality rates was not statistically significant ($P = .22$), retrospective analysis demonstrated a statistically significant reduction in mortality in those patients who had a higher predicted mortality on the basis of a clinical predictive index. In a group of 595 patients with a predicted mortality of 24% or greater, a 22% reduction in mortality was obtained in those patients given IL-1Ra compared with controls ($P = .03$).

The same researchers conducted a follow-up phase III study of IL-1Ra infusion in patients with sepsis, targeting individuals with the higher predicted mortality identified in the previous study (the subgroup who benefited in the first IL-1Ra study). This second study was terminated prior to completion, however, because interim data analysis determined that significant benefit of IL-1Ra infusion was unlikely.[49]

This lack of repeatability has been a general theme in the large randomized trials of anticytokine therapy for sepsis in patients. As another example, an attempt was made to replicate the positive data collected from a retrospectively defined subset of patients from an early trial of the anti-endotoxin antibody HA-1A; this follow-up study also failed.[50] In both of these cases, the repeat studies *prospectively* evaluated the subgroups of patients who benefited in the earlier trials. In general, study groups as a whole have not benefited in the initial trials, but one or more subgroups have been shown to benefit in post hoc analysis. One must evaluate such efficacy data with great caution. Inspection of a large number of possible subgroups can easily result in false-positive findings of efficacy simply from chance alone (reviewed by Oxman and Guyatt[51]). To emphasize this point, all major sepsis trials to date that have enrolled patients with characteristics associated with benefit from therapy in post hoc analysis have failed.

Tumor Necrosis Factor Receptors

Soluble receptors to TNF (also called TNF-binding proteins [TBPs]) are found naturally in the circulation. Wallach's group and others isolated two proteins from human urine in 1989 and 1990 that specifically bound and inactivated TNF biologic activity.[52–55] These proteins have also been isolated from the supernatants of cultured peripheral blood mononuclear cells, polymorphonuclear neutrophils, and fibroblasts. Subsequent experiments demonstrated that the two TBPs are the extracellular portions of the two types of TNF receptors, probably generated by proteolysis. Current nomenclature designates the extracellular soluble portion of the type 1 (55 to 60 kD, 455 residue) TNF receptor as TNFsRp55, and the extracellular soluble portion of the type 2 (75 to 80 kD, 461 residue) TNF receptor as TNFsRp75. TNFsRp55 and TNFsRp75 are each about half the mass of their respective receptors, with masses of about 30 kD and 40 kD, respectively.

TNF receptors are found on almost all cell types except red blood cells. Large clinical trials have evaluated TNF blockade using anti-TNF antibodies or soluble TNF receptors to treat sepsis. Considered together, these trials have shown benefit in subgroups of patients studied, but definitive reduction in mortality in the study group as a whole has yet to be demonstrated.

Interleukin-1 Receptors

There are two IL-1 receptors. The type 1 IL-1 receptor (80 kD) is present on T cells and fibroblasts. The type 2 receptor (65 kD) is present on B cells and mononuclear cells. Investigations have documented the presence of both types of soluble IL-1 receptors in the circulation.

Some experimental in vivo activities of soluble IL-1 receptors are as follows:

- Prolongation of survival of allogeneic heart transplants in mice
- Decreased ipsilateral lymph node enlargement in mice administered irradiated allogeneic splenocytes in the footpad
- Reduced IL-1–assisted B-cell proliferation
- Decreased experimental allergic encephalomyelitis in rats
- Reduced joint inflammatory response in a rat antigen–induced arthritis model (synergy of anti-inflammatory effects with TNFsRp55 noted)

No definite functional role has been demonstrated in vivo for any of these naturally occurring soluble receptors to date.

End-Organ Intervention

The final common mediators of cytokine-induced damage at the multiple end organs may be antagonized. For example, it has been established that nitric oxide is a major inducer of peripheral vasodilation and decreased vascular resistance during inflammation. *N*-Monomethyl arginine (an inactive substrate for the enzyme NO synthase, the enzyme that synthesizes NO) can reverse some elements of sepsis physiology. Knockout mice lacking the inducible NO synthase gene are resistant to death from endotoxin under anesthesia.[56, 57]

SUMMARY

The 1980s and 1990s have seen the discovery of potent new antimicrobial agents and more sophisticated supportive care without substantial improvement in the outcome of septic shock. Mortality from septic shock has remained disappointingly high. New efforts have focused on the host's responses to inflammatory stimuli, such as endotoxin, with the hypothesis that the generation of endogenous mediators that constitute this response may provide a point of therapeutic attack in sepsis as well as many other disease states. Despite much promise, interventions specifically designed to modulate cytokine activity in sepsis have yet to produce definitive clinical benefit in humans.

There is no more eloquent description of the septic response to infection than that of Thomas Lewis,[58] who wrote in *The Lives of a Cell*:

We are likely to turn on every defense at our disposal; we will bomb, defoliate, blockade, seal off, and destroy all the tissues in the area. Leukocytes become more actively phagocytic, release lysosomal enzymes, turn sticky, and aggregate together in dense masses, occluding capillaries and shutting off the blood supply.... Pyrogen is released from leukocytes, adding fever to hemorrhage, necrosis, and shock. It is a shambles.

Eventually, attempts will be made to evaluate the efficacy of therapies designed to simultaneously inhibit the multiple elements of the pro-inflammatory cytokine cascade. Currently, therapeutic interventions focus on the synergistic toxicity of the cytokines and other mediators, which paradoxically gives us the opportunity to gain a therapeutic effect by disarming even one major component of this catastrophic response. Current therapies focusing on the inhibition or antagonism of TNF and IL-1 do just that.

References

1. Fekade D, Knox K, Hussein K, et al: Prevention of Jarisch-Herxheimer reactions with antibodies against tumor necrosis factor α. N Engl J Med 1996; 335:311.
2. Moreland LW, Baumgartner SW, Schiff MH, et al: Treatment of rheumatoid arthritis with a recombinant human tumor necrosis factor receptor (p75)-Fc fusion protein. N Engl J Med 1997; 337:141.
3. Elliott MJ, Maini RN, Feldmann M, et al: Randomized double-blind comparison of chimeric monoclonal antibody to tumour necrosis factor α (cA2) versus placebo in rheumatoid arthritis. Lancet 1994; 344:1105.
4. Luo G, Niesel DW, Shaban RA, et al: Tumor necrosis factor alpha binding to bacteria: Evidence for a high-affinity receptor and alteration of bacterial virulence properties. Infect Immun 1993; 61:830.
5. Porat R, Clark BD, Wolff SM, et al: Enhancement of growth of virulent strains of *Escherichia coli* by interleukin-1. Science 1991; 254:852.
6. Amiri P, Locksley RM, Parslow TG, et al: Tumor necrosis factor α restores granulomas and egg-laying in schistosome-infected SCID mice. Nature 1992; 356:604.
7. Sands KE, Bates DW, Lanken PN, et al: Epidemiology of sepsis syndrome in 8 academic medical centers. JAMA 1997; 278:234.
8. Quartin AA, Schein RMH, Kett DH, et al: Magnitude and duration of the effect of sepsis on survival. JAMA 1997; 277:1058.
9. Bone RC: Sepsis, the sepsis syndrome, multi-organ failure: A plea for comparable definitions. Ann Intern Med 1991; 114:332.
10. Bone RC: Toward an epidemiologic and natural history of SIRS (systemic inflammatory response syndrome). JAMA 1992; 268:3452.
11. Dinarello CA, Gelfand JA, Wolff SM: Anticytokine strategies in the treatment of the systemic inflammatory response syndrome. JAMA 1993; 269:1829.
12. Michalek SM, Morre RN, McGhee JR, et al: The primary role of lymphoreticular cells in the mediation of host responses to bacterial endotoxin. J Infect Dis 1980; 141:55.
13. Proctor RA, Will JA, Burhop KE, et al: Protection of mice against lethal endotoxemia by a lipid A precursor. Infect Immun 1986; 52:905.
14. Golenbock DT, Will JA, Raetz CR, et al: Lipid X ameliorates pulmonary hypertension and protects sheep from death due to endotoxin. Infect Immun 1987; 55:2471.
15. Beutler B, Cerami A: Cachectin: More than a tumor necrosis factor. N Engl J Med 1987; 316:279.
16. Dinarello CA: Biologic basis for interleukin-1 in disease. Blood 1996; 87:2095.
17. Groopman JE, Molina J-M, Scadden DT: Hematopoietic growth factors. N Engl J Med 1989; 321:1449.
18. McCabe WR: Serum complement levels in bacteremia due to gram-negative organisms. N Engl J Med 1973; 288:21.
19. Poll TVD, Buller HR, Cate HTT, et al: Activation of coagulation after administration of tumor necrosis factor to normal subjects. N Engl J Med 1990; 322:1622.
20. Suffredini AF, Harpel PC, Parrillo JE: Promotion and subsequent inhibition of plasminogen activation after administration of intravenous endotoxin to normal subjects. N Engl J Med 1989; 320:1165.
21. Reid RR, Prodeus AP, Khan W, et al: Endotoxin shock in antibody-deficient mice. J Immunol 1997; 159:970.
22. Fischer MB, Prodeus AP, Nicholson-Weller A, et al: Increased susceptibility to endotoxin shock in complement C3- and C4-deficient mice is corrected by C1 inhibitor replacement. J Immunol 1997; 159:976.
23. Barton BE, Jackson JV: Protective role of interleukin-6 in the lipopolysaccharide-galactosamine septic shock model. Infect Immun 1993; 61:1496.
24. McCartney FN, Mizel D, Wong H, et al: TGF-beta regulates production of growth factors and TGF-beta by human peripheral blood monocytes. Growth Factors 1990; 4:27.
25. Howard M, O'Garra A, Ishida H, et al: Biological properties of interleukin-10. J Clin Immunol 1992; 12:239.
26. Vannier E, Miller LC, Dinarello CA: Coordinated anti-inflammatory effects of interleukin 4: Interleukin 4 suppresses interleukin 1 production but up-regulates gene expression and synthesis of interleukin 1 receptor antagonist. Proc Natl Acad Sci U S A 1992; 89:4076.
27. Pfeffer K, Matsuyama T, Kundig TM, et al: Mice deficient for the p55 kd tumor necrosis factor receptor are resistant to endotoxic shock, yet succumb to *L. monocytogenes* infection. Cell 1993; 73:457.
28. Rothe J, Lesslauer W, Loetscher H, et al: Mice lacking the tumour necrosis factor receptor 1 are resistant to TNF-mediated toxicity but highly susceptible to infection by *Listeria monocytogenes*. Nature 1993; 364:798.
29. Dinarello CA, Cannon JG, Wolff SM, et al: Tumor necrosis factor (cachectin) is an endogenous pyrogen and induces production of interleukin-1. J Exp Med 1986; 163:1433.
30. Ohlsson K, Bjork P, Bergenfeldt M, et al: Interleukin-1 receptor antagonist reduces mortality from endotoxic shock. Nature 1990; 348:550.
31. Wakabayashi G, Gelfand JA, Burke JF, et al: A specific receptor antagonist for interleukin-1 prevents *Escherichia coli*-induced shock. FASEB J 1991; 5:338.
32. Okusawa S, Gelfand JA, Ikejima T, et al: Interleukin-1 induces a shock-like state in rabbits: Synergism with tumor necrosis factor and the effect of cyclooxygenase inhibition. J Clin Invest 1988; 81:1162.
33. Sun X, Hsueh W: Bowel necrosis induced by tumor necrosis factor in rats is mediated by platelet-activating factor. J Clin Invest 1988; 81:1328.
34. Dhainault JF, Tenaillon A, Tulzo YL: Platelet-activating factor receptor antagonist BN 52021 in the treatment of severe sepsis: A randomized, double-blind, placebo-controlled, multicenter clinical trial. Crit Care Med 1994; 22:1720.
35. Mancilla J, Garcia P, Dinarello CA: The interleukin-1 receptor antagonist can either reduce or enhance the lethality of *Klebsiella pneumoniae* sepsis in newborn rats. Infect Immun 1993; 61:926.
36. van der Meer JWM: The effects of recombinant interleukin-1 and recombinant tumor necrosis factor on non-specific resistance to infection. Biotherapy 1988; 1:19.
37. Docke W-D, Randow F, Syrbe U, et al: Monocyte deactivation in septic patients: Restoration by IFN-γ treatment. Nature Med 1997; 3:678.
38. Bone R: Sir Isaac Newton, sepsis, SIRS, and CARS. Crit Care Med 1996; 24:1125.
39. Kishimoto T: The biology of interleukin-6. Blood 1989; 74:1.
40. Dalrymple SA, Slattery R, Aud DM, et al: Interleukin-6 is required for a protective immune response to systemic *Escherichia coli* infection. Infect Immun 1996; 64:3231.
41. Libert C, Vink A, Coulie P, et al: Limited involvement of interleukin-6 in the pathogenesis of lethal septic shock as revealed by the effect of monoclonal antibodies against interleukin-6 or its receptor in various murine models. Eur J Immunol 1992; 22:2625.
42. Lee JC, Laydon JT, McDonnell PC, et al: A protein kinase involved in the regulation of inflammatory cytokine biosynthesis. Nature 1994; 372:739.

43. Cerretti DP, Kozlosky CJ, Mosley B, et al: Molecular cloning of the interleukin-1β converting enzyme. Science 1992; 256:97.
44. Thornberry NA, Bull HG, Calaycay JR, et al: A novel heterodimeric cysteine protease is required for interleukin-1 beta processing in monocytes. Nature 1992; 356:768.
45. Russell DA, Tucker KK, Chinookoswong N, et al: Combined inhibition of interleukin-1 and tumor necrosis factor in rodent endotoxemia: Improved survival and organ function. J Infect Dis 1995; 171:1528.
46. Alexander HR, Doherty GM, Buresh CM, et al: A recombinant human receptor antagonist to interleukin-1 improves survival after lethal endotoxemia in mice. J Exp Med 1991; 173:1029.
47. Fischer E, Marano MA, Zee KJV, et al: Interleukin-1 receptor blockade improves survival and hemodynamic performance in *Escherichia coli* septic shock, but fails to alter host responses to sublethal endotoxemia. J Clin Invest 1992; 89:1551.
48. Fisher CJ, Dhainaut J-FA, Opal SM, et al: Recombinant human interleukin 1 receptor antagonist in the treatment of patients with the sepsis syndrome. JAMA 1994; 271:1836.
49. Opal SM, Fisher CJ, Dhainaut J-FA, et al: Confirmatory interleukin-1 receptor antagonist trial in severe sepsis: A phase III, randomized, double-blind, placebo-controlled, multicenter trial. Crit Care Med 1997; 25:1115.
50. McClosky R, Straube RC, Sanders C, et al: Treatment of septic shock with human monoclonal antibody HA-1A. Ann Intern Med 1994; 121:1.
51. Oxman AD, Guyatt GH: A consumer's guide to subgroup analysis. Ann Intern Med 1992; 116:78.
52. Engelmann H, Aderka D, Rubenstein M, et al: A tumor necrosis factor-binding protein purified to homogeneity from human urine protects cells from tumor necrosis factor toxicity. J Biol Chem 1989; 264:11974.
53. Lantz M, Gullberg U, Nilsson E: Characterization *in vitro* of a human tumor necrosis factor binding protein: A soluble form of a tumor necrosis factor receptor. J Clin Invest 1990; 86:1396.
54. Seckinger P, Isaaz S, Dayer J-M: Purification and biologic characterization of a specific tumor necrosis factor α inhibitor. J Biol Chem 1989; 264:11966.
55. Olsson I, Lantz M, Nilsson E, et al: Isolation and characterization of a tumor necrosis factor binding protein from urine. Eur J Haematol 1989; 42:270.
56. Petros A, Bennett D, Vallance P: Effect of nitric oxide synthase inhibitors on hypotension in patients with septic shock. Lancet 1991; 338:1557.
57. MacMicking JD, Nathan C, Hom G, et al: Altered responses to bacterial infection and endotoxic shock in mice lacking inducible nitric oxide synthase. Cell 1995; 81:641.
58. Lewis T: The Lives of a Cell. New York, Viking Press, 1974, p 92.

49

Cellular Signaling and Cell Death

David J. McConkey, PhD • Richard J. Bold, MD

Programmed cell death (*apoptosis*) is the physiologic process through which tissue balance is maintained by appropriately balancing cell division with cell elimination.[1] Relatively unheralded until recently, work over the past few years has led to an explosion of information about the biochemical and molecular mechanisms that control apoptosis, and it has become evident that alterations in apoptotic pathways are intimately involved in a variety of disease processes, including critical illnesses such as sepsis and end-organ ischemia. This chapter introduces the key components of the apoptotic pathway and discusses how they appear to be regulated by cellular signaling. Subsequently, we provide an example for how these mechanisms are clinically relevant by explaining their potential involvement in tissue damage due to ischemia.

BIOCHEMICAL AND MOLECULAR MECHANISMS OF APOPTOSIS

Despite recent advances, the biochemical events involved in the apoptotic pathway are still under intense investigation.[1, 2] Some of the central components of the pathway were identified in studies of programmed cell death in the nematode *Caenorhabditis elegans*,[3] and additional contributors were defined through analysis of the effects of oncogenes and tumor suppressors on cell survival.[4] This part of the chapter describes what we now think of as the core "effector machinery" for cell death and how it is regulated by other gene products as a function of cell cycle control.

Morphology of Apoptosis

The term "apoptosis" was first coined in 1972 to describe a series of morphologic alterations associated with cell death in experimental models of ischemia and hormonal withdrawal.[5] These changes were largely detected by electron microscopy and include cell shrinkage, plasma and nuclear membrane blebbing, organelle relocalization and compaction, chromatin condensation, and production of membrane-enclosed particles containing intracellular material known as "apoptotic bodies" (Table 49–1). The morphology of apoptosis is distinct from the alterations observed in cells exposed to high doses of cytotoxic agents or other conditions that lead to rapid cellular disintegration (*necrosis*), in which cellular swelling, organelle dysfunction, mitochondrial collapse, and the spillage of cellular contents into the extracellular milieu are observed (see Table 49–1). Thus, apoptosis is characterized by the loss of contact with neighboring cells in tissues and usually occurs in isolated single cells. This contrasts with most examples of necrotic cell death, where tracts of contiguous dying cells collapse without loss of contact with neighboring cells.

Apoptotic cells display no obvious change in plasma membrane integrity, even while drastic biochemical alterations are under way. This allows for their clearance by professional phagocytic cells and neighboring cells in tissues, which recognize apoptotic cells by at least two specific mechanisms. The best studied involves changes in plasma membrane phospholipid asymmetry, whereby phosphatidylserine (PS) (normally concentrated on the cytoplasmic surface) "flips" to the outside, apparently serving as a ligand for specific PS receptors expressed by macrophages and other cell types.[6] The other involves poorly defined changes on the apoptotic cell that allow for binding to thrombospondin and subsequent recognition and uptake by monocyte vitronectin receptors.[7] Rapid

TABLE 49–1. Comparison of Cellular Changes Associated with Apoptosis and Necrosis

Apoptosis	Necrosis
Physiologic, regulated	Pathologic, unregulated
Cell shrinkage	Cell swelling
Chromatin condensation	Irregular chromatin clumping
Preservation of intracellular organelles	Dysfunction and destruction of organelles
Membrane blebbing, apoptotic bodies	Disruption of cellular membranes
Organized chromatin digestion to small fragments ("DNA ladders")	Nonspecific and random degradation of DNA ("DNA smears")

uptake of apoptotic cells by this mechanism prevents leakage of proinflammatory intracellular contents, thereby avoiding an inflammatory response.[7]

Effector Machinery for Apoptosis

Evolutionarily Conserved Components of the Pathway

Studies in the nematode *C. elegans* have been crucial to the identification of the central components of the apoptotic pathway.[3] Early work provided a complete cell lineage analysis of the organism, which revealed that of the 1090 cells produced during development, 131 die with precise timing. Mutagenesis identified two genes—*ced-3* and *ced-4*—that are required for all but one of these cell deaths,[8] and a third—*ced-9*—that acts upstream of *ced-3* and *ced-4* to prevent cell death (Fig. 49–1).[9] Soon after they were cloned mammalian homologs for *ced-3* and *ced-9* were identified: CED-3 is structurally similar to interleukin-1β–converting enzyme (ICE),[10] a cysteine protease that cleaves the precursor form of IL-1β at aspartate residues to produce the bioactive cytokine, and *ced-9* is homologous to human *bcl-2,*[11] an oncogene identified at the t(14;18) chromosomal translocation in follicular B lymphoma. In mammalian cells, the CED-3/ICE and BCL-2 families consist of several members, all of which have now been implicated in the regulation of apoptosis. For purposes of standardization, members of the CED-3/ICE family have been renamed *caspases* because they are *c*ysteine proteases which cleave their substrates at *asp*artate residues. The fact that shared gene products are required for cell death in *C. elegans* and human cells indicates that the central components of the pathway are evolutionarily conserved.

Although it is known that caspases participate in apoptosis, precisely how they contribute to cell death is not clear. Caspase substrates include deoxyribonucleic acid (DNA) repair proteins (i.e., poly [ADP-ribose] polymerase, DNA-dependent protein kinase), cytoskeletal elements (i.e., nuclear lamins, fodrin, gelsolin), cell cycle regulators (i.e., the retinoblastoma protein and p21), and signal transduction intermediates (protein kinase C-δ), but in no case is it clear that cleavage directly contributes to apoptosis. Furthermore, studies in "knockout" mice to date have been unable to identify a caspase that is required for all pathways of apoptosis, which contrasts with the situation in *C. elegans.* For example, even though caspase-3/CPP32 is considered a central component of the mammalian apoptotic pathway,[12] thymocytes from animals lacking caspase-3 undergo apoptosis normally when exposed to glucocorticoids or other stimuli.[13] Rather, defective apoptosis in the caspase-3 knockouts is most obvious in the brain, suggesting tissue-selective involvement of the protease in apoptosis. Other such examples are likely to emerge.

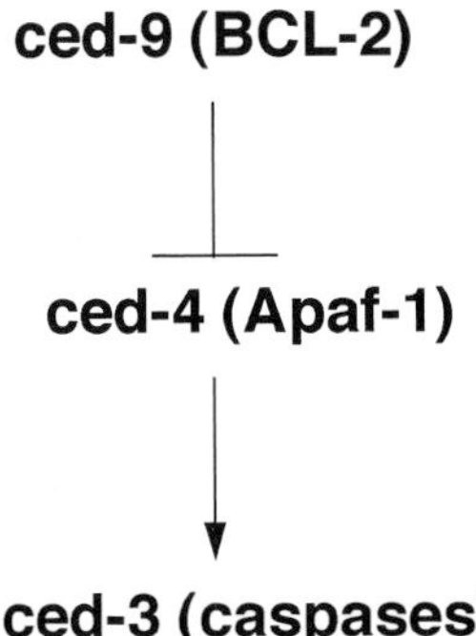

Figure 49–1. Elements of an evolutionarily conserved pathway for cell death. Pathway hierarchy of the cell death (ced) genes required for apoptosis in the nematode *Caenorhabditis elegans* is shown. The corresponding mammalian homologues are indicated in parentheses.

TABLE 49–2. BCL-2 Family Members Involved in the Control of Programmed Cell Death

Pro-apoptotic (Promotion of Cell Death)	Anti-apoptotic (Prevention of Cell Death)
BAX	BCL-2
BAK	BCL-XL
BAD	MCL-1
BCL-Xs	A1
BIK	BHRF-1
BID	

Finally, it is not clear that caspase activation is even required for cell death in most examples of apoptosis. Although caspase antagonists promote clonogenic survival in cells exposed to certain stimuli (i.e., Fas receptor engagement),[14] they merely prolong the kinetics of death in many cases.[15] It is likely that the mitochondrial alterations implicated in apoptosis (see later) are sufficient to commit the cell to death,[16] with or without caspase activation.

Identifying the biochemical mechanism of the CED-9/BCL-2 family has, if anything, been even more enigmatic.[2] The BCL-2 family in mammalian systems is more complex than it is in *C. elegans* and consists of proteins that can either prevent cell death ("anti-apoptotic," e.g., BCL-2, BCL-xL) or promote cell death ("pro-apoptotic," e.g., BAX, BAK, BAD) (Table 49–2).[2] Precisely how they do so is uncertain, but they can sometimes form homodimers or heterodimers with one another, which may allow for mechanistic fine-tuning. Early work suggested that BCL-2 might regulate a redox-sensitive anti-apoptotic pathway, and more recent work has shown that BCL-2 critically regulates mitochondrial function.[2, 16] Prompted by structural analysis demonstrating that BCL-xL is similar to certain bacterial pore-forming proteins,[17] other work suggests that the BCL-2 family can form ion channels, the properties of which may be dictated by particular protein composition.[2] Supporting this notion, several groups have now shown that BCL-2 affects intracellular Ca^{2+} compartmentalization at the level of the endoplasmic reticulum and nucleus.[18] Finally, these proteins can also function as adaptor or docking proteins.[2] Additional efforts are required to determine how each of these functions is relevant to control of cell death.

While both the CED-3/ICE and CED-9/BCL-2 homologies were defined by computer data base searches, the mammalian homologue of the nematode *ced-4* gene was identified by a classic biochemical approach. Searching for cytosolic components required for caspase-3 activation, Wang and colleagues isolated three factors from the human HeLa cell line.[19] Unexpectedly, the first was found to be the reduced form of cytochrome c (an intermediate in the mitochondrial electron transport chain).[19] The second factor purified was termed Apaf-1 (*a*poptosis *p*rotease *a*ctivating *f*actor-1), which turned out to be a novel gene product that possesses a domain near its N-terminus that is homologous to *ced-4.*[20] The third factor identified was a caspase (caspase-9).[21] A model for how these factors activate downstream processes in apoptosis is presented schematically in Figure 49–2 and described in more detail later.

Mitochondrial Control of Caspase Activation

Although it is highly likely that all intracellular compartments are dismantled simultaneously during apoptosis and that multiple organelle-based signals are involved, recent work has

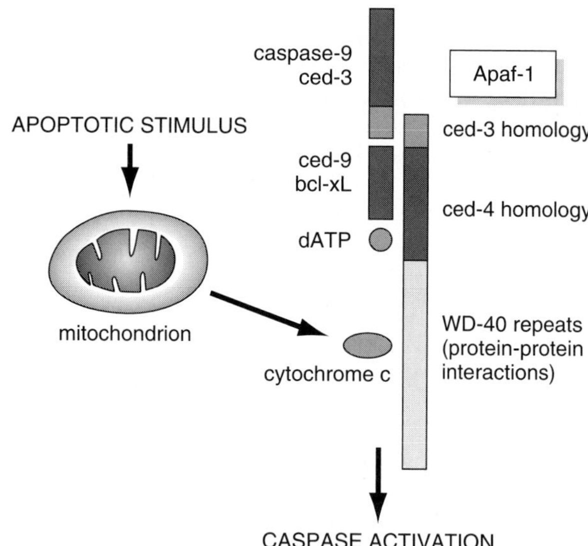

Figure 49–2. Current model for mitochondrial control of caspase activation. Once released from mitochondria, cytochrome c can form a complex with Apaf-1 (CED-4), deoxyadenosine triphosphate (dATP), and caspase-9, which then leads to activation of caspase-9 via an unknown mechanism. Given its homology to CED-4 and the fact that CED-4 can physically interact with CED-9, it is conceivable that activation of caspase-9 is also regulated by a physical interaction between BCL-2/BCL-xL and Apaf-1, although this mechanism has not been demonstrated. Apaf-1 = apoptosis protease activating factor-1.

shown that biochemical events within mitochondria play a central role.[16] The first clue implicating mitochondria in apoptosis came from a study by Hockenbery and coworkers demonstrating that the BCL-2 protein accumulates in the organelle.[22] Subsequent work by Kroemer's group demonstrated that a drop in mitochondrial membrane potential ($\Delta\Psi$) is a common, early event in diverse examples of apoptosis and that the drop in $\Delta\Psi$ is blocked by BCL-2.[16] Furthermore, apoptotic mitochondria release the electron transport chain intermediate, cytochrome c,[19] an event that is also blocked by BCL-2.[23] Precisely how all of these events are mechanistically coupled is not yet clear, although a simple explanation would be that the loss of mitochondrial membrane potential directly promotes release of cytochrome c. In support of this notion, it is known that loss of mitochondrial membrane potential can lead to the opening of large transmembrane pores in mitochondria, an event known as the *permeability transition* (PT), which might allow for leakage of cytochrome c and possibly other pro-apoptotic factors from mitochondria into the cytosol.[16] Indeed, agents that block the PT pore also block apoptosis, and agents that promote PT promote apoptosis.[16] However, this model has been undermined somewhat by recent work suggesting that the drop in $\Delta\Psi$ might occur after release of cytochrome c. These results might be reconciled if PT channel opening can occur transiently or within a subset of mitochondria prior to the global changes that occur when the drop in $\Delta\Psi$ can be detected experimentally.

The coupling of these mitochondrial alterations to caspase activation appears to involve Apaf-1, the recently cloned human homologue of the *C. elegans ced-4* gene. Previous work with CED-3, CED-4, and CED-9 indicated that CED-4 can directly bind to both of the other cell death regulators and that it was this binding that dictated whether or not CED-3 underwent proteolytic activation. Likewise, Apaf-1 appears to serve as a scaffold capable of assembling the components required for activation of caspase-9 (and possibly other caspases) in mammalian cells. Once released from mitochondria, cytochrome c can directly bind to Apaf-1, and deoxyadenosine triphosphate (dATP) binds Apaf-1 at another site on the molecule (see Fig. 49–2). Once both molecules are present, caspase-9 can also bind Apaf-1, and this promotes its enzymatic activation. Because caspases are substrates for one another and are activated by cleavage at aspartic acid residues, activation of caspase-9 may be sufficient to trigger activation of caspase-3 and other downstream caspases.

Chromatin Cleavage

Endonuclease activation is another important biochemical event in apoptosis.[24] Early work demonstrated that the chromatin in apoptotic cells is fragmented nonrandomly into integer multiples of 180 to 200 base pairs (bp) suggestive of cleavage between nucleosomes, and these "DNA ladders" remain a standard means of demonstrating apoptotic cell death. However, more recent work has shown that the formation of larger DNA fragments, most notably of 300 kilobases (kb) and 50 kb in size,[25] precedes oligonucleosomal DNA fragmentation in all systems investigated and, in some cases, cells may die by apoptosis without forming DNA ladders at all. The biochemical mechanisms underlying this stepwise chromatin cleavage remain unclear, but it appears that chromatin topology rather than sequence specificity of the endonuclease is involved.[25] It is possible that the discrete fragment sizes are generated as particular chromatin-associated proteins (topoisomerase II, lamin B, and histone H1) are sequentially cleaved by the caspases and perhaps other proteases during apoptosis, thereby exposing these regions of chromatin to endonuclease action.

Recent work indicates that caspases can directly regulate endogenous endonuclease activation during apoptosis. The first evidence of this came from studies with peptide caspase inhibitors, which block DNA fragmentation in whole cells.[26] Because the lamins can serve as caspase substrates, these effects may be explained in part by the proteolytic removal of chromatin-bound proteins, as discussed earlier. However, caspase activation also leads to the proteolytic processing and activation of DNA fragmentation factor (DFF), a heterodimeric (40-kD and 45-kD) complex that can directly promote endonuclease activation in isolated nuclei.[27] In parallel efforts, Nagata's group has identified an endonuclease, termed caspase-activated deoxyribonuclease (CAD), which is directly activated by caspases.[28] The nuclease is normally retained in the cytosol of viable cells by an inhibitor (ICAD) that binds to and blocks its nuclear localization signal.[28] However, ICAD possesses two consensus caspase cleavage sites and is clipped by caspases and removed from its association with CAD on induction of apoptosis.[29] Intriguingly, mouse ICAD is highly homologous (76% identical) to the 45-kD subunit of human DFF. The observation that overexpression of ICAD blocks DNA fragmentation in response to diverse signals for apoptosis provides strong evidence for the general involvement of this mechanism in DNA fragmentation.[29] However, there is also strong (albeit more indirect) evidence that nuclear, Ca^{2+}-dependent enzymes can also promote characteristic DNA fragmentation.[24, 25] Identification of the components of the latter is needed to determine whether there are multiple, possibly redundant pathways to endonuclease activation and DNA fragmentation in apoptosis.

Apoptosis Requires Adenosine Triphosphate

Although the morphologic alterations associated with each response are by definition distinct, the biochemical mechanisms underlying apoptosis and necrosis may in some cases be very similar. Early work with hepatocytes exposed to oxidative stress demonstrated that low to moderate levels induced endonuclease activation typical of apoptosis, whereas higher doses actually suppressed DNA fragmentation.[30] Similarly, endonuclease activation and apoptosis in response to calcium ionophore treatment in thymocytes and other cell types is dose-dependent, with apoptosis occurring at low to moderate concentrations and necrosis occurring at higher concentrations.[31]

More direct evidence for overlap comes from studies on necrotic cell death in experimental models of ischemia-reperfusion injury. Hypoxia resulting from ischemia can induce a steep decline in ATP levels due to inhibition of oxidative phosphorylation. This effect can be mimicked in vitro by incubation of cells in medium lacking glucose (or any other glycolytic energy source) plus an inhibitor of mitochondrial respiration. This "chemical hypoxia"[32] ultimately results in necrotic cell death characterized by rapid (within 60 min) and nearly complete ATP depletion, a drop in $\Delta\Psi$, mitochondrial swelling, and loss of plasma membrane integrity. The cellular swelling and plasma membrane rupture observed during chemical hypoxia clearly distinguish the response from classic models of apoptosis.

However, recent studies indicate that the biochemical mechanisms involved in cell death from chemical hypoxia overlap substantially with those involved in apoptosis. This is probably due to the fact that mitochondria serve as an important target for cell death mechanisms in both processes, as demonstrated by the precipitous drop in $\Delta\Psi$ observed in each. Strikingly, chemical hypoxia-induced cell death can be blocked by overexpression of BCL-2 or BCL-xL or with peptide or viral caspase inhibitors.[33, 34] These results challenge the notion that apoptosis and necrosis are distinct, nonoverlapping molecular pathways.

Two independent studies have provided the first direct evidence that levels of intracellular ATP dictate whether cell death occurs via apoptosis or necrosis.[34, 35] Cells incubated with either anti-CD95/Fas antibody or the protein kinase antagonist staurosporine (a "universal" trigger for apoptosis) in normal growth medium underwent rapid apoptosis that was not preceded by an early drop in ATP level. In contrast, cells treated with either stimulus under conditions of chemical hypoxia underwent necrosis and cell death was preceded by several hours by a dramatic drop in ATP levels. Analysis of the biochemical events involved in cell death demonstrated that phosphatidylserine exposure, DNA fragmentation, and caspase activation were suppressed under conditions of ATP depletion[35]; interestingly, necrosis was slower than apoptosis. Thus, ATP is required for protease and endonuclease activation and the catabolic processes activated during apoptosis directly facilitate cell death.

It should be stressed that the relative levels of other cell death intermediates can also dictate the mode of cell death, as demonstrated by the examples (Ca^{2+} and oxidative stress) already cited. These observations may help to explain why cell death in tissue injury often appears to be a mixture of necrosis and apoptosis.

Cell Cycle Regulators and Cell Death

It appears that signals for proliferation sensitize most cells to apoptosis.[36] The first strong evidence for this link came from studies on the *myc* oncogene, which was shown by two groups to simultaneously promote cell division, inhibit growth arrest, and induce apoptosis.[37, 38] Although the mechanisms involved remain unclear, myc-mediated apoptosis in some cases appears to require p53[39] and/or expression of Fas and Fas ligand.[40] Subsequent work has shown that deregulated expression of other cell cycle intermediates (i.e., the cyclins, the cyclin-dependent kinases, the phosphatase CDC25, and the transcription factor E2F1) can also sensitize cells to apoptosis and that, conversely, cell cycle inhibitors (i.e., the retinoblastoma protein and p21 WAF-1/CIP-1) are in most cases inhibitors of cell death.[36] Although at the surface these observations may seem paradoxical, the coupling of cell cycle progression to apoptosis may serve as a safeguard against uncontrolled proliferation owing to viral infection or mutagenesis. Furthermore, experience in cancer therapy provides indirect support for the idea, as it is well known that therapeutic windows exist allowing regimens that target cycling cells to exert tumor-selective cell killing.

If cell cycle entry predisposes a cell to death, how is efficient cell division ever achieved? In most cases, cells seem to require specific extracellular signals, delivered by cytokines or surface adhesion molecules that may have little to no effect on cell cycle progression but act fairly selectively to inhibit apoptosis. An excellent example is the effects of nerve growth factor (NGF), which is not directly mitogenic to neurons but possesses potent survival properties. Insulin-like growth factor-1 (IGF-1) appears to be a more general survival factor, as it has been shown to suppress apoptosis in a number of different tissue types.[4] Particular signal transduction pathways and transcription factors have been implicated in suppression of apoptosis by these receptors, as discussed later.

The tumor suppressor protein p53 has been termed the "guardian of the genome" because of its role in surveillance of DNA damage, regulation of the cell cycle, and regulation in apoptosis.[41] The p53 protein has DNA-binding and transcriptional regulatory function, and these activities have been clearly implicated in the effects of p53 on cell cycle. The cyclin-dependent kinase and cell cycle inhibitor p21 has a p53 consensus element within its promoter, and p53 can directly induce its expression, leading to cell cycle arrest.[41] If the level of DNA damage is manageable, this arrest allows time for repair; if the damage cannot be repaired, apoptotic cell death is triggered.[41] There is some evidence that this distinction is made by relative cellular content of p53 or duration of the p53 signal; when p53 content is low to moderate, cells undergo cell cycle arrest and DNA repair, whereas when p53 content is high, cells progress to apoptosis.[42] Both transcriptional activation and repression have been implicated in p53-mediated apoptosis: The death-promoting *bax* and *fas* genes as well as a number of genes implicated in the response to oxidative stress are induced by p53.[43] The identification of particular p53-suppressed survival genes requires further investigation.

Viral Regulation of Apoptosis

In order to replicate effectively, DNA viruses usurp the host's DNA replication machinery by inducing an "S-phase like" state in the cell. As noted above, however, cell cycle progression also sensitizes the cell to apoptosis, and viral infection is no exception to this rule.[44] Definitive evidence for this was first obtained in experiments on the products of the adenovirus E1A and E1B gene products.[45] The former acts much like myc to promote cell cycle progression via its ability to bind to host cell cycle regulatory proteins (p300 and the Rb protein), whereas the two proteins encoded by the E1B locus act specifically to block apoptosis. One (E1B 55 kD) acts by binding to and inactivating p53, thereby silencing p53-dependent apoptosis. The other (E1B 19 kD) possesses some homology to BCL-2, and like it can block multiple (p53-dependent and p53-independent) apoptotic pathways. Thus, viruses possessing inactivating mutations in E1B do not replicate effectively because they trigger rapid host cell apoptosis and viral genome destruction by DNA fragmentation.

Other work has demonstrated that many viral strategies for specific suppression of apoptosis exist.[44] Some viruses express soluble "decoy" versions of surface cell death receptors, which can bind to and inactivate their death-inducing ligands. Others express proteins that bind the cytoplasmic signaling domains of these receptors, preventing their coupling to the effector machinery for apoptosis. Many viruses express proteins with significant structural and functional homology to BCL-2.

Finally, some viruses contain specific caspase inhibitors, the most notable of which are the cowpox virus crmA protein, which inhibits caspase-1/ICE and caspase-8/FLICE, and the baculovirus p35 protein, which inhibits most caspases, including caspase-3/CPP32. Both appear to serve as "decoy" substrates and are cleaved in the process of caspase inhibition. Furthermore, other recent work suggests that a group of viral and cellular proteins that are homologous to the baculovirus *i*nhibitor of *ap*optosis proteins, Op-IAP and Cp-IAP, are also caspase inhibitors,[46] although the biochemical mechanisms underlying these effects are less clear and it is possible that they may affect other apoptotic mechanisms as well.

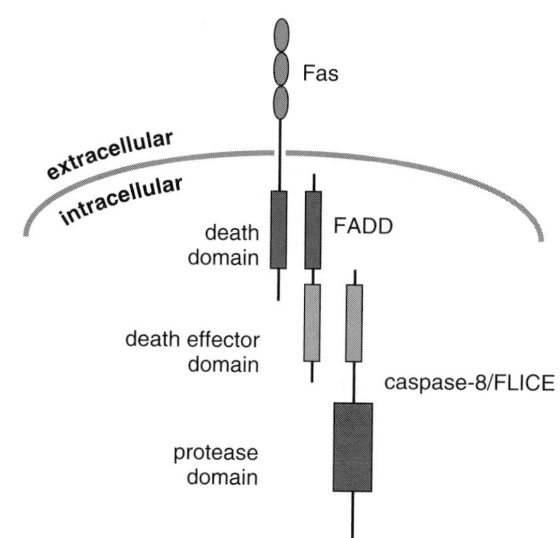

Figure 49–3. Current model for Fas-mediated caspase activation. The carboxy terminus of CD95/Fas contains an amino acid sequence element known as the "death domain" (DD) that can physically interact with a corresponding DD in an adaptor protein, FADD. In turn, FADD via its death effector domain (DED) can interact with caspase-8, which also possesses a DED. Upon binding Fas ligand or tumor necrosis factor (which most likely exist as trimers or multimers), caspase-8 molecules are brought into close proximity with one another, and it is thought that this clustering is sufficient to promote intermolecular cleavage and activation.

CELLULAR SIGNALING IN APOPTOSIS

Cell Surface Death Receptors

The type I receptor for tumor necrosis factor (TNF) and the CD95/Fas antigen are the two most familiar members of a growing family of receptors that appear to be more directly "hard-wired" to the effector machinery for cell death.[47] TNF is a monocyte-derived cytokine that was first isolated from the serum of endotoxin-treated mice and that is cytotoxic to certain activated and transformed cells, and it plays an important role in macrophage-mediated immunity. Fas was originally identified as the antigen recognized by cytotoxic antibodies that were raised independently by Yonehara's and Krammer's groups.[47a, 47b] The TNF receptor and Fas are both members of the larger receptor superfamily; unlike most of the other members, however, they possess a domain within their cytoplasmic tails (the "death domain") that directly couples these receptors to the biochemical machinery for apoptosis (Fig. 49–3).[47] The death domain can bind to adapter proteins (TRADD and FADD), which directly recruit caspase-8 to the receptor complex, and on oligomerization by their ligands, Fas and TNF-RI, promote activation of caspase-8.[48] Importantly, most evidence indicates that BCL-2 has little effect on this pathway, consistent with the idea that BCL-2 blocks caspase activation at the level of mitochondria. Fas and TNF-RI are common targets for viral inactivation, supporting the idea that they play crucial roles in antiviral immune surveillance.

Reactive Oxygen Species

Several lines of evidence indicate that oxidative stress serves as an important signal for apoptosis.[49] Early work with xenobiotics whose metabolism leads to the production of superoxide as well as with direct oxidants, such as hydrogen peroxide and tert-butylperoxide, demonstrated that low to moderate levels of oxidative stress can trigger the response. Subsequent work showed that elevated levels of oxygen radical production are also associated with other examples of apoptosis, as are precipitous drops in levels of reduced protein thiols and thiol antioxidants (i.e., glutathione). Antioxidants such as *N*-acetylcysteine, ascorbate, and α-tocopherol can block apoptosis. Furthermore, suppression of apoptosis by BCL-2 may be thiol-dependent, as we have shown that depletion of intracellular glutathione can overcome BCL-2-mediated inhibition of apoptosis.[50] Indeed, we have shown that BCL-2 directly promotes energy-dependent uptake of glutathione into the nucleus, where it can directly block caspase activation.[51]

The regulated production of reactive oxygen species is also an important host defense system against bacterial and viral infection. Macrophages, neutrophils, and other proinflammatory cells generate and release copious amounts of hydrogen peroxide, which can diffuse across lipid bilayers and directly promote apoptosis in target cells. Furthermore, in addition to its direct effects on caspases, TNF also dramatically enhances production of superoxide radicals in target cells, and overexpression of manganese superoxide dismutase (Mn-SOD) blocks TNF cytotoxicity.

Finally, it has been shown that neutrophils can produce nitric oxide (NO), which may also participate in cytotoxicity.[52] In addition to its many other physiologic effects,[53] high levels of NO (generated by the type II, or Ca^{2+}-independent, inducible NO synthase) can promote apoptosis. NO may be capable of directly triggering apoptosis in the cells that produce it, or it may combine with superoxide to form the reactive compound peroxynitrite, which has a longer biologic half-life and may be capable of limited diffusion. Importantly, NO chemistry is complex, and NO can serve as a pro-oxidant or an antioxidant, depending on levels of available superoxide, reducing agents, and other factors.

Role of Calcium

Alterations in intracellular Ca^{2+} almost invariably accompany loss of mitochondrial membrane potential and oxidative stress in various models of cell death.[54] Several lines of evidence indicate that Ca^{2+} has direct effects on both upstream and downstream components of the apoptotic pathway, serving as a signal for cell death and possibly a cofactor for protease and endonuclease activation. Early studies demonstrated that early, sustained Ca^{2+} increases are observed in numerous examples of apoptotic cell death, and agents that prevent these increases also prevent endogenous endonuclease activation.[18] Both second messenger–mediated and damage-mediated mechanisms can be involved in promoting Ca^{2+} increases in apoptotic cells.[18] In an example of the former, T cell receptor engagement on thymocytes leads to a sustained increase in the cytosolic Ca^{2+} concentration that involves protein tyrosine kinase activation, phosphorylation of the γ-isoform of phospholipase C, phosphoinositide hydrolysis leading to the production of inositol triphosphate (IP_3), and mobilization of Ca^{2+} from the endoplasmic reticulum and extracellular milieu that promote cell death. Similarly, surface antigen receptor engagement on B cells leads to Ca^{2+} increases that promote cell death. Thus, in these examples of apoptosis, Ca^{2+} increases occur via a controlled, physiologic mechanism that is also utilized in alternative responses such as cellular activation leading to proliferation.

Reactive oxygen species can also promote sustained cytosolic Ca^{2+} increases in apoptotic cells. Early work in the biochemical mechanisms underlying the cytotoxicity of agents that generate reactive oxygen species in cells (oxidative stress) indicated that the Ca^{2+} transport systems localized to the endoplasmic reticulum, mitochondria, and plasma membrane can be damaged by oxygen radicals.[55] This leads to diffusion of Ca^{2+} down its concentration gradient, a disruption of intracellular Ca^{2+} homeostasis, and sustained Ca^{2+} increases. We and others have shown that oxidative stress mediates the glucocorticoid-induced Ca^{2+} increase observed in thymocytes, probably via disruption of mitochondrial Ca^{2+} stores.[18]

Several downstream targets for Ca^{2+} have been identified in apoptotic cells. As a signal transduction intermediate, Ca^{2+} can promote activation of the serine-threonine phosphatase, calcineurin, which is the target for immunosuppressant (i.e., cyclosporine) action in lymphoid cells. Calcineurin can promote apoptosis, possibly by dephosphorylating and activating the proapoptotic BCL-2 family member, BAD (J. Reed, personal communication), and its activity is apparently regulated by direct physical binding to BCL-2.[2] Other work has shown that BCL-2 regulates Ca^{2+} fluxes in mitochondria, the endoplasmic reticulum, and the nucleus.[18] Calcium can directly disrupt plasma membrane phospholipid asymmetry, leading to exposure of PS, and the relationship between this mechanism and caspase-mediated effects is currently under investigation.[6] Calcium-activated proteases, such as calpain and the nuclear scaffold protease, may also participate with the caspases in the cleavage of important substrates during the effector phase of apoptosis.[18] Finally, several lines of evidence indicate that nuclei from a number of tissue sources possess a Ca^{2+}-activated nuclease that may participate in chromatin cleavage during apoptosis.[24]

Intracellular Acidification

Oxidative stress, Ca^{2+} mobilization, and intracellular acidification are all known causes and consequences of the mitochondrial permeability transition,[54] and it is therefore not surprising that the latter has been implicated in apoptosis. Early work by Barry and colleagues' laboratory showed that changes in pH (and not Ca^{2+}) preceded cell death induced by a variety of anticancer agents in Chinese hamster ovary (CHO) cells, and the group went on to present evidence that an acid-sensitive endonuclease activity was involved.[56] Subsequent work demonstrated that a drop in pH precedes endonuclease activation in many models of growth factor withdrawal and that BCL-2 blocks both these changes and cell death. The recent suggestion that BCL-2 and its relatives form transmembrane pores is strong indirect support for a role for acidification in apoptosis because low pH is known to promote their pore-forming abilities,[17] and H^+ fluxes, especially across the mitochondrial inner membrane, may certainly be affected. Finally, Jarvis and associates suggest that an acid sphingomyelinase is responsible for ceramide production and ceramide-mediated apoptosis in a number of different cell types,[57] and it is certainly conceivable that alterations in intracellular pH regulate its activity.

Role of Cyclic Adenosine Monophosphate

Some of the first evidence for a role for cyclic adenosine monophosphate (cAMP) in cell death came from studies by Pratt and Martin[57a] on programmed cell death in epithelial cells during fusion of the secondary palate, and other early work demonstrated that cAMP is cytotoxic to many different leukemic lymphoid cells.[58] More recently, it has been shown that cAMP has a more general role in promoting apoptosis.[58] We and others showed that E series prostaglandins and pharmacologic agents that elevate cAMP induce endogenous endonuclease activation in T lymphocytes and certain tumor cells, responses that involve cAMP-dependent protein kinase (PKA). Because cAMP often exerts its effects via changes in gene transcription and the effects of cAMP on thymocytes are blocked by inhibitors of messenger ribonucleic acid (mRNA) or protein synthesis, it is possible that alterations in gene expression are ultimately responsible for triggering apoptosis in the cells. Supporting this notion, Harrigan and colleagues showed that treatment of lymphoid cell lines with cAMP-raising agents or glucocorticoids to induce apoptosis results in overlapping patterns of mRNA expression in the dying cells, and Dowd and Miesfeld have shown that the pathways share overlapping distal elements in their cytolytic mechanisms.[58] Glucocorticoids and cAMP can also act synergistically to promote apoptosis, and we have presented evidence that the cAMP pathway of apoptosis requires glucocorticoid receptor function. Ongoing efforts are aimed at defining the signaling and transcriptional targets for cAMP-mediated apoptosis in these and other cell types.

Role of Ceramide

Some receptors stimulate sphingomyelinase and subsequently cause the hydrolysis of sphingomyelin upon ligand binding, leading to the release of diacylglycerol (DAG) and ceramide.[59] Each of these hydrolysis products of sphingomyelin appears to have separate signal transduction pathways through activation of distinct protein kinase cascades. A great deal of work has demonstrated that ceramide is a fairly common trigger for the apoptosis.[59] Ongoing efforts are aimed at identifying the downstream targets for ceramide in apoptotic cells. Ceramide activates a protein serine-threonine kinase, called *k*inase *s*uppressor of *R*as (KSR),[60] setting off a signaling cascade that ultimately leads to inhibition of the survival kinase, AKT/PKB (see later). In addition, ceramide stimulates the stress-activated protein kinases (see later).[61] Crosstalk between the ceramide pathway and protein kinase C is likely to determine the outcome of ceramide signaling, as phorbol esters and diglycerides are potent inhibitors of ceramide-induced apoptosis.[62]

Stress-Activated Protein Kinases

Mitogen-activated protein (MAP) kinases are signal transduction intermediates implicated in a vast number of intracellular responses. The first members of this family identified were extracellular signal regulated kinases 1 and 2 (ERK1/2) which have been implicated in mitogenesis mediated by growth factors that activate the H-Ras signal transduction pathway.[63] Another prototype member of this family, Jun N-terminal kinase (JNK), otherwise known as stress-activated protein kinase (SAPK), phosphorylates and activates the c-Jun proto-oncogene's DNA binding activity.[63] Exciting recent work suggests that these subfamilies of the MAP kinases mediate opposing effects on the apoptotic pathway. Apoptosis stimulated by extracellular stress (irradiation, oxidative stress, or growth factor withdrawal) involves activation of JNK,[64] a response that may require production of ceramide.[61] On the other hand, parallel activation of the ERKs blocks JNK-mediated apoptosis,[64] suggesting that a dynamic balance exists between the growth factor–activated and stress-activated MAP kinases. Ongoing investigation is aimed at identifying the downstream targets for these kinases in the apoptotic pathway.

SURVIVAL SIGNALS

Protein Kinase C

Many physiologic responses to surface receptor engagement involve the early activation of polyphosphoinositide-specific phospholipase C, resulting in the activation of two important second messengers, IP_3 and DAG. The primary action of IP_3 is to promote Ca^{2+} mobilization, whereas DAG exerts its effects via binding to and activating a family of serine-threonine kinases known collectively as protein kinase C (PKC). Activation of PKC appears to be important for the initiation of events that lead to cell proliferation, and PKC has also been implicated in tumor promotion and differentiation.

Most of the evidence for a role for PKC in apoptosis comes from work with phorbol esters, a class of tumor-promoting agents that mimic the effects of DAG to activate the enzyme. Chronic treatment of thymocytes or certain solid tumor cell lines (i.e., prostatic carcinomas) results in apoptosis, responses that can be blocked by PKC inhibitors, indicating that kinase activation is required for these responses. Curiously, however, endonuclease activation in thymocytes does not occur immediately but involves a lag period of several hours, during which phorbol esters can be removed and the cells recover. This delay is not observed in thymocytes induced to undergo apoptosis in response to treatment with various other agents. Although the biochemical basis for the lag period is not known, it may be related to special transcriptional and/or translational requirements or, perhaps more likely, to the known ability of phorbol esters to downregulate PKC protein expression after prolonged exposure of cells to the agents in culture.

Physiologic and pharmacologic activators of PKC can also block apoptosis in thymocytes and other cell types. Of particular significance is the observation that PKC activators can totally suppress ceramide-induced apoptosis,[62, 65] and perhaps as a result phorbol esters can block Fas-mediated and TNF-mediated apoptosis in a variety of model systems. Phorbol esters can also block Ca^{2+} or cAMP-mediated apoptosis, perhaps in part by suppressing Ca^{2+}-dependent endonuclease activity in nuclei.[66] Other targets for PKC include the Na^+/H^+ antiporter,[67] components of the Ras pathway, kinases responsible for activating the survival-associated transcription factor NFκB, and possibly members of the BCL-2 family (Fig. 49–4). We have proposed that apoptosis in many cases may result from imbalanced signal transduction and that activation of PKC (or other survival pathways) restores balance and possibly promotes other cellular responses (proliferation, differentiation).

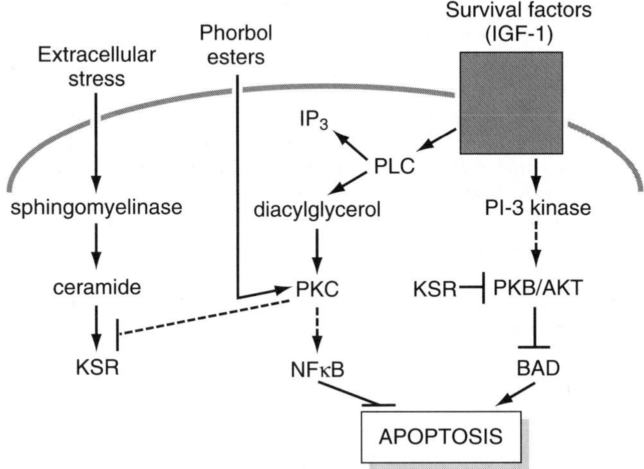

Figure 49–4. Survival factor signal transduction. Stimulation is indicated by *arrows* and inhibition by *blocked lines.* IGF-1 = insulin-like growth factor-1; PI-3 kinase = phosphatidylinositol 3-kinase; PLC = phospholipase C; PKB = protein kinase B; KSR = kinase suppressor of Ras; IP_3 = inositol triphosphate; KSR = kinase suppressor of *Ras*; PKC = protein kinase C.

Protein Kinase B/AKT Oncogene

Withdrawal of essential growth factors has long been known to induce apoptosis, yet the coupling of receptor-mediated events to survival signals has not been well elucidated. Recently, however, several independent lines of research have demonstrated the importance of the protein kinase B/*akt* oncogene pathway.[68] The oncogene *akt* was isolated from a rodent T cell lymphoma virus at the same time a novel protein kinase was identified and named protein kinase B (PKB); later these two genes were found to be, in fact, the same gene.[68] Several survival factors, including IL-2 and IGF-1 employ this signal transduction pathway. An intermediary kinase, phosphatidylinositol 3-kinase (PI-3 kinase), is activated upon receptor binding and phosphorylates the various lipid substrates, including phosphatidylinositol (PtdIns). The phosphorylated forms of PtdIns recruit PKB/AKT to the cell membrane as well as activate the kinase activity. Furthermore, the triphosphate form of PtdIns (PtdIns-P3) also directly activates another kinase, PtdIns-P3-dependent kinase-1 (PDK-1), which in turn phosphorylates PKB/AKT, which further increases the kinase activity.

PKB/AKT had been demonstrated to be involved in insulin signaling and regulation of cellular metabolism, although the downstream targets of its kinase activity and the role this kinase plays in cell survival and apoptosis are unclear. Recently, two independent groups have demonstrated that PKB/AKT is capable of phosphorylating the protein product of the *bad* gene, a proapoptotic member of the *bcl-2* gene family.[69, 70] This phosphorylation renders BAD incapable of dimerization with BCL-2 or BCL-xL. Therefore, on stimulation of the PKB/AKT cascade, the regulatory balance of apoptosis is shifted toward cell survival. These are the first pieces of evidence that have clearly demonstrated a direct route from cell surface receptors through a signal transduction pathway to the regulation of the core effector machinery for cell death.

Nuclear Factor Kappa B (NFκB)

NFκB was first identified by Baltimore's laboratory as a transcription factor that regulates immunoglobulin kappa chain expression.[71] It is actually a family of transcription factors composed of heterodimers of five different members of the Rel family of polypeptides, although the most common form of NFκB is composed of a heterodimer of two subunits termed p50 and p65.[71] Their mechanism of activation is quite interesting, inasmuch as the proteins are constitutively expressed in most cell types but are trapped within the cytosol by an inhibitory protein, IκBα, which binds to a nuclear localization signal in the Rel proteins and prevents their import. Upon cellular activation, IκB is phosphorylated and degraded, allowing NFκB to migrate to the nucleus, where it can regulate gene expression.

The first hint that NFκB might promote survival came from studies on B cell lines, where pharmacologic inhibitors of NFκB induced apoptosis.[72] Subsequently, Baltimore's group showed that livers from Rel knockout mice demonstrated fulminant apoptosis,[73] and three independent reports confirmed that NFκB is a potent inhibitor of apoptosis in diverse cell types.[74-76] Phorbol esters and a variety of cytokines are known to activate NFκB,[71] and their pro-survival effects may therefore be related to this mechanism. Candidate downstream survival genes regulated by NFκB include BCL-xL and mammalian homologs of the bacterial IAP proteins. Although NFκB has broad anti-apoptotic activity, it is likely that other transcription factors also promote cell survival, perhaps in a more tissue-specific fashion.

REGULATION OF APOPTOSIS IN ISCHEMIA-REPERFUSION INJURY

With the identification of apoptosis as a distinct mechanism of cell death, many clinical entities in which necrosis had traditionally been presumed to be responsible for cellular destruction have been reexamined. Apoptosis is now known to be involved in a vast array of diseases, from cancer to infection and autoimmunity.[1] A more comprehensive overview of the occurrence of apoptosis in situations relevant to critical care is the subject of Chapter 56. However, as the model system used by Kerr in 1972 to define the morphologic alterations of apoptosis in the liver, ischemia–reperfusion not only represents a historically significant example of the response but also is one of the more interesting from a mechanistic point of view. Therefore, we focus on this one example of cell death to show how some of the mechanistic considerations already described might be relevant.

Cardiac Myocyte Apoptosis

Recent evidence has suggested that apoptosis is the primary mode of cell death following ischemia or hypoxia in the heart,[77, 78] although both apoptosis and necrosis are independent contributing variables to infarct size in experimental models.[79] Central to this work have been technical advances that allow for sensitive measurements of rates of apoptosis in paraffin-embedded and frozen whole tissues, the most notable of which is known as terminal deoxynucleotidyl transferase (TdT)-uridine nick end labeling (TUNEL). With this approach, apoptotic myocytes can be identified as early as 2 hours after an ischemic insult.[80] Detailed analyses indicated that apoptosis was localized to regions of hypoxia,[81] and mechanistic studies demonstrated that cell death is associated with alterations in p53, BCL-2, BAX, and Fas expression.[82-84] Interestingly, enforced overexpression of BCL-2 in the heart substantially reduced cell death following an ischemic event.[85] Other evidence suggests hypoxia-mediated accumulation of ceramide mediates apoptosis during ischemia and reperfusion,[86] although whether this ceramide is produced by Fas engagement or by a more direct (possibly acidic) pathway remains to be determined.

Reperfusion, although essential for tissue salvage, paradoxically can worsen cell death. Reperfusion is especially important in cardiac function in three clinical scenarios:

- Recovery from an acute coronary arterial occlusion (whether pharmacologic, mechanical, or surgically mediated relief of acute ischemia)
- After cardiac arrest during coronary artery bypass grafting
- After cardiac transplantation

Studies by Umansky and colleagues[87] and Fliss and Gattinger[80] have demonstrated that reoxygenation accelerates the kinetics of apoptosis in myocytes but decreases the total fraction of cells that will ultimately die.

Central Nervous System Apoptosis

Hypoxic and ischemic neuronal cell death also involves both apoptosis and necrosis.[88] Utilizing a model of transient aortic ligation to induce spinal cord ischemia, Mackey and associates demonstrated neuronal cell death in the intermediate and ventral areas of the spinal cord as early as 24 hours following ischemia.[89] These findings correlated with standard histologic examination of the ischemic spinal cord, which demonstrated neuronal degeneration, and are in concordance with the results from a variety of studies examining cerebral ischemia.[90] Most of these investigations have examined ischemic regions of the cortex in animal models through ligation of the middle cerebral artery. Biochemically, elevations in Ca^{2+} are centrally involved neuronal apoptosis both as a consequence of direct damage to the cells and as a consequence of excitatory (glutamate-mediated) toxicity.[91] The molecular events are consistent with those observed in the heart in that both p53 and *bax* are upregulated in the central regions of the ischemic areas.[92] Furthermore, although these neurons are fully differentiated after mitosis, they exhibit gene expression consistent with acute DNA damage and reentry into the cell cycle. These events require new protein synthesis and preliminary data have demonstrated that blockade of protein synthesis in the ischemic regions can limit the extent of cell death and the size of the resultant infarct.[93]

Ischemia–reperfusion is a pathologic condition that illustrates the difficulty in demonstrating the distinctions between apoptosis and necrosis. Because mitochondrial respiration requires oxygen, hypoxia is a direct trigger for disruption of mitochondrial function, leading to a drop in membrane potential, and this loss of mitochondrial function is thought to be the principal mechanism underlying cytotoxicity. As already explained, loss of membrane potential is also central to current models for apoptosis; this suggests that ischemia sets the stage for such events as release of cytochrome c, oxidative stress, intracellular Ca^{2+} mobilization, acidification, and ceramide production. This also explains why BCL-2 and BCL-xL are especially effective in preventing hypoxia-induced cell death, since these proteins are known to preserve mitochondrial membrane potential in the face of stress. The metabolic characteristics of the cell type in question also affect the outcome; more drastic effects of hypoxia on ATP levels and necrosis would be expected in cells that rely on mitochondrial respiration rather than glycolysis for ATP synthesis, a consideration that may dictate relative apoptotic rates in heavily glycolysis-dependent tissues, such as the brain. Thus, a tissue oxygen tension threshold specific for each tissue probably exists, whereby a smaller loss of oxygenation serves as a direct apoptotic stimulus and a more major drop actually blocks apoptosis and leads to necrosis due to excessive depletion of ATP. Indeed, since reoxygenation leads to a sudden burst in cellular energy levels, this model predicts that reperfusion would hasten apoptosis, a prediction that is in fact borne out by the experimental data obtained to date.

SUMMARY

Enormous progress has been made over the past several years in defining the central components of the biochemical and molecular machinery for apoptosis in mammalian cells. Starting from a morphologic description of cell death and aided by genetic studies in lower organisms such as the nematode, we now know that mitochondrial alterations and the caspase proteases lie at the center of the pathway and that a number of cellular signaling processes regulate caspase activation. However, a huge number of unanswered questions remain. Although recent efforts have generated a wealth of information about the role of mitochondria in apoptosis, other organelles are also affected in parallel, and almost nothing is known about the biochemical and molecular mechanisms relevant to apoptosis regulation at these other sites. In addition, much remains unknown about how the mitochondrial alterations are induced or what leads to release of cytochrome c. Furthermore, the biochemical functions of BCL-2 and its homologues remain unclear, and little is known about how viral proteins, such as the IAPs, regulate the response. Finally, much additional effort is required to determine how apoptosis contributes to tissue biology under both physiologic and pathologic conditions.

As we compile more information about the basic mechanisms involved in apoptosis, the question of how the information might be exploited in the design of new strategies for clinical intervention also emerges. Efforts to use rates of apoptosis as prognostic factors for disease staging in acquired immunodeficiency syndrome (AIDS) and cancer are under way, and it is certainly possible that apoptotic (and necrotic) indices may prove prognostic in critical care scenarios as well. In addition, strategies to interfere with apoptosis through the use of caspase antagonists, Ca^{2+} channel blockers, antioxidants, or other modulators may prove effective in preventing or limiting secondary tissue damage due to ischemia-reperfusion and other pathologic entities. Given the pace of recent research in the area, the anticipated translation of the basic science into therapy should prove to be very exciting.

References

1. Hetts SW: To die or not to die: An overview of apoptosis and its role in disease. JAMA 1998; 279:300–307.
2. Reed JC: Double identity for proteins of the BCL-2 family. Nature 1997; 387:773–776.
3. Hengartner MO, Horvitz HR: Programmed cell death in *Caenorhabditis elegans.* Curr Opin Genet Dev 1994; 4:581–586.
4. Harrington EA, Fanidi A, Evan GI: Oncogenes and cell death. Curr Opin Genet Dev 1994; 4:120–129.
5. Kerr JFR, Wyllie AH, Currie AR: Apoptosis: A basic biological phenomenon with wide-ranging implications in tissue kinetics. Br J Cancer 1972; 26:239–257.
6. Zwaal RFA, Schroit AJ: Pathophysiologic implications of membrane phospholipid asymmetry in blood cells. Blood 1997; 89:1121–1132.
7. Savill J, Fadok V, Henson P, Haslett C: Phagocytic recognition of cells undergoing apoptosis. Immunol Today 1993; 14:131–136.
8. Ellis HM, Horvitz HR: Genetic control of programmed cell death in the nematode *C. elegans.* Cell 1986; 44:817–829.
9. Hengartner MO, Ellis RE, Horvitz HR: *Caenorhabditis elegans* gene ced-9 protects cells from programmed cell death. Nature 1992; 356:494–499.
10. Yuan J, Shaham S, Ledoux S, Ellis HM, Horvitz HR: The *C. elegans* cell death gene ced-3 encodes a protein similar to mammalian interleukin-1β-converting enzyme. Cell 1993; 75:641–652.
11. Hengartner MO, Horvitz HR: *C. elegans* cell survival gene ced-9 encodes a functional homolog of mammalian proto-oncogene bcl-2. Cell 1994; 76:665–676.
12. Nicholson DW, Ali A, Thornberry NA, et al: Identification and inhibition of the ICE/ced-3 protease necessary for mammalian apoptosis. Nature 1995; 376:37–43.
13. Kuida K, Zheng TS, Na S, et al: Decreased apoptosis in the brain and premature lethality in CPP32-deficient mice. Nature 1996; 384:368–372.
14. Longthorne VL, Williams GT: Caspase activity is required for commitment to Fas-mediated apoptosis. EMBO J 1997; 16:3805–3812.
15. McCarthy NJ, Whyte MKB, Gilbert CS, Evan GI: Inhibition of Ced-3/ICE-related proteases does not prevent cell death induced by oncogenes, DNA damage, or the BCL-2 homologue BAK. J Cell Biol 1997; 136:215–227.
16. Kroemer G, Zamzami N, Susin SA: Mitochondrial control of apoptosis. Immunol Today 1997; 18:44–52.
17. Muchmore SW, Sattler M, Liang H, et al: X-ray and NMR structure of human BCL-XL, an inhibitor of programmed cell death. Nature 1996; 381:335–341.
18. McConkey DJ, Orrenius S: The role of calcium in the regulation of apoptosis. Biochem Biophys Res Commun 1997; 239:357–366.
19. Liu X, Kim CN, Yang J, Jemmerson R, Wang X: Induction of the apoptotic program in cell-free extracts: Requirement for dATP and cytochrome c. Cell 1996; 86:147–157.
20. Zou H, Henzel WJ, Liu X, Lutschg A, Wang X: Apaf-1, a human protein homologous to *C. elegans* ced-4, participates in cytochrome c-dependent activation of caspase-3. Cell 1997; 90:405–413.
21. Li P, Nijhawan D, Budihardjo I, et al: Cytochrome c and dATP-dependent formation of Apaf-1/caspase-9 complex initiates an apoptotic protease cascade. Cell 1997; 91:479–489.
22. Hockenbery DM, Nunez G, Milliman C, Schreiber RD, Korsmeyer SJ: BCL-2 is an inner mitochondrial membrane protein that blocks programmed cell death. Nature 1990; 348:334–336.
23. Yang J, Liu X, Bhalla K, et al: Prevention of apoptosis by bcl-2: Release of cytochrome c from mitochondria blocked. Science 1997; 275:1129–1132.
24. Arends MJ, Morris RG, Wyllie AH: Apoptosis: The role of the endonuclease. Am J Pathol 1990; 136:593–608.
25. Filipski J, Leblanc J, Youdale T, Sikorska M, Walker PR: Periodicity of DNA folding in higher order chromatin structures. EMBO J 1990; 9:1319–1327.
26. Henkart PA: ICE family proteases: Mediators of all apoptotic cell death? Immunity 1996; 4:195–201.
27. Liu X, Zou H, Slaughter C, Wang X: DFF, a heterodimeric protein that functions downstream of caspase-3 to trigger DNA fragmentation during apoptosis. Cell 1997; 89:175–184.
28. Enari M, Sakahira H, Yokoyama H, Okawa K, Iwamatsu A, Nagata S: A caspase-activated DNase that degrades DNA during apoptosis, and its inhibitor ICAD. Nature 1998; 391:43–50.
29. Sakahira H, Enari M, Nagata S: Cleavage of CAD inhibitor in CAD activation and DNA degradation during apoptosis. Nature 1998; 391:97–99.
30. McConkey DJ, Hartzell P, Nicotera P, Wyllie AH, Orrenius S: Stimulation of endogenous endonuclease activity in hepatocytes exposed to oxidative stress. Toxicol Lett 1988; 42:123–130.
31. McConkey DJ, Hartzell P, Nicotera P, Orrenius S: Calcium-activated DNA fragmentation kills immature thymocytes. FASEB J 1989; 3:1843–1849.
32. Lemasters JJ, DiGuiseppi J, Nieminen AL, Herman B: Blebbing, free Ca^{2+} and mitochondrial membrane potential preceding cell death in hepatocytes. Nature 1987; 325:78–81.
33. Shimizu S, Eguchi Y, Kamiike W, et al: BCL-2 blocks loss of mitochondrial membrane potential while ICE inhibitors act at a different step during inhibition of death induced by respiratory chain inhibitors. Oncogene 1996; 13:21–29.
34. Eguchi Y, Shimizu S, Tsujimoto Y: Intracellular ATP levels determine cell death fate by apoptosis or necrosis. Cancer Res 1997; 57:1835–1840.
35. Leist M, Single B, Castoldi AF, Kuhnle S, Nicotera P: Intracellular adenosine triphosphate (ATP) concentration: A switch in the decision between apoptosis and necrosis. J Exp Med 1997; 185:1484–1486.
36. Evan GI, Brown L, Whyte M, Harrington E: Apoptosis and the cell cycle. Curr Opin Cell Biol 1995; 7:825–834.
37. Askew DS, Ashmun RA, Simmons BC, Cleveland JL: Constitutive c-myc expression in an IL-3-dependent myeloid cell line suppresses cell cycle arrest and accelerates apoptosis. Oncogene 1991; 6:1915–1922.
38. Evan GI, Wyllie AH, Gilbert CS, et al: Induction of apoptosis in fibroblasts by c-myc protein. Cell 1992; 69:119–128.

39. Hermeking H, Eick D: Mediation of c-Myc-induced apoptosis by p53. Science 1994; 265:2091-2093.
40. Hueber AO, Zornig M, Lyon D, Suda T, Nagata S, Evan GI: Requirement for CD95 receptor-ligand pathway in c-Myc-induced apoptosis. Science 1997; 278:1305-1309.
41. Levine AJ: p53, the cellular gatekeeper for growth and division. Cell 1997; 88:323-331.
42. Ronen D, Schwartz D, Teitz Y, Goldfinger N, Rotter V: Induction of HL-60 cells to undergo apoptosis is determined by high levels of wild-type p53 protein whereas differentiation of the cells is mediated by lower p53 levels. Cell Growth Differ 1996; 7:21-30.
43. Polyak K, Xia Y, Zweier JL, Kinzler KW, Vogelstein BA: A model for p53-induced apoptosis. Nature 1997; 389:300-305.
44. Teodoro JG, Branton PE: Regulation of apoptosis by viral gene products. J Virol 1997; 71:1739-1746.
45. White E: Function of the adenovirus E1B oncogene in infected and transformed cells. Semin Virol 1994; 5:341-348.
46. Devereaux QL, Takahashi R, Salvesen GS, Reed JC: X-linked IAP is a direct inhibitor of cell-death proteases. Nature 1997; 388:300-304.
47. Nagata S, Golstein P: The Fas death factor. Science 1995; 267:1449-1455.
47a. Yonehara S, Ishii A, Yonehara M: A cell-killing monoclonal antibody (anti-Fas) to a cell surface antigen co-downregulated with the receptor for tumor necrosis factor. J Exp Med 1989; 169:1747-1756.
47b. Trauth BC, Klas C, Peters AM, Matzku S, Moller P, Falk W, Debatin KM, Krammer PH: Monoclonal antibody-mediated tumor regression by induction of apoptosis. Science 1989; 245:301-305.
48. Muzio M, Chinnaiyan AM, Kischkel FC, et al: FLICE, a novel FADD-homologous ICE/CED-3-like protease, is recruited to the CD95 (Fas/APO-1) death-inducing signaling complex. Cell 1996; 85:817-827.
49. Buttke TM, Sandstrom PA: Oxidative stress as a mediator of apoptosis. Immunol Today 1994; 15:7-10.
50. Mirkovic N, Voehringer DW, Story MD, McConkey DJ, McDonnell TJ, Meyn RE: Resistance to radiation-induced apoptosis in BCL-2-expressing cells is reversed by depleting cellular thiols. Oncogene 1997; 15:146-147.
51. Voehringer D, McConkey DJ, McDonnell T, Brisbay S, Meyn RE: BCL-2 expression causes redistribution of glutathione to the nucleus. Proc Natl Acad Sci U S A 1998; 95:2956-2970.
52. Eiserich JP, Hristova M, Cross CE, et al: Formation of nitric oxide-derived inflammatory oxidants by myeloperoxidase in neutrophils. Nature 1998; 391:393-397.
53. Moncada S, Higgs A: The L-arginine-nitric oxide pathway. N Engl J Med 1993; 329:2002-2012.
54. Richter C: Pro-oxidants and mitochondrial Ca^{2+}: Their relationship to apoptosis and oncogenesis. FEBS Lett 1993; 325:104-107.
55. Orrenius S, McConkey DJ, Bellomo G, Nicotera P: Role of Ca^{2+} in toxic cell killing. Trends Pharmacol Sci 1989; 10:281-285.
56. Barry MA, Reynolds JE, Eastman A: Etoposide-induced apoptosis in human HL-60 cells is associated with intracellular acidification. Cancer Res 1993; 53:2349-2357.
57. Jarvis WD, Kolesnick RN, Fornari FA, Traylor RS, Gewirtz DA, Grant S: Induction of apoptotic DNA damage and cell death by activation of the sphingomyelin pathway. Proc Natl Acad Sci U S A 1994; 91:73-77.
57a. Pratt RM, Martin GR: Epithelial cell death and cyclic AMP increase during palatal development. Proc Natl Acad Sci U S A 1975; 72:874-877.
58. McConkey DJ, Nicotera P, Orrenius S: Signalling and chromatin fragmentation in thymocyte apoptosis. Immunol Rev 1994; 142:343-363.
59. Hannun YA, Obeid LM: Ceramide: an intracellular signal for apoptosis. Trends Biochem Sci 1995; 20:73-77.
60. Zhang Y, Yao B, Delikat S, et al: Kinase suppressor of Ras is ceramide-activated protein kinase. Cell 1997; 89:63-72.
61. Verheij M, Bose R, Lin XH, et al: Requirement for ceramide-initiated SAPK/JNK signalling in stress-induced apoptosis. Nature 1996; 380:75-79.
62. Jarvis WD, Fornari FA Jr, Browning JL, Gewirtz DA, Kolesnick RN, Grant S: Attenuation of ceramide-induced apoptosis by diglyceride in human myeloid leukemia cells. J Biol Chem 1994; 269:31685-31692.
63. Su B, Karin M: Mitogen-activated protein kinase cascades and regulation of gene expression. Curr Opin Immunol 1996; 8:402-411.
64. Xia Z, Dickens M, Raingeaud J, Davis RJ, Greenberg ME: Opposing effects of ERK and JNK-p38 MAP kinases on apoptosis. Science 1995; 270:1326-1331.
65. Obeid LM, Linardic CM, Karolak LA, Hannun YA: Programmed cell death induced by ceramide. Science 1993; 259:1769-1771.
66. McConkey DJ, Hartzell P, Jondal M, Orrenius S: Inhibition of DNA fragmentation in thymocytes and isolated thymocyte nuclei by agents that stimulate protein kinase C. J Biol Chem 1989; 264:13399-13462.
67. Rajotte D, Haddad P, Haman A, Cragoe EJ Jr, Hoang T: Role of protein kinase C and the Na^+/H^+ antiporter in suppression of apoptosis by granulocyte macrophage colony-stimulating factor and interleukin-3. J Biol Chem 1992; 267:9980-9987.
68. Hemmings BA: AKT signalling: Linking membrane events to life and death decisions. Science 1997; 275:628-630.
69. Peso LD, Gonzalez-Garcia M, Page C, Herrera R, Nunez G: Interleukin-3-induced phosphorylation of BAD through the protein kinase AKT. Science 1997; 278:687-689.
70. Datta SR, Dudek H, Tao X, et al: AKT phosphorylation of BAD couples survival signals to the cell-intrinsic death machinery. Cell 1997; 91:231-241.
71. Baeuerle PA, Baltimore D: NFκB: Ten years after. Cell 1996; 87:13-20.
72. Wu M, Lee H, Bellas RE, et al: Inhibition of NFκB/Rel induces apoptosis of murine B cells. EMBO J 1995; 15:4682-4690.
73. Beg AA, Sha WC, Bronson RT, Ghosh S, Baltimore D: Embryonic lethality and liver degeneration in mice lacking the RelA component of NFκB. Nature 1995; 376:167-170.
74. Antwerp DJV, Martin SJ, Kafri T, Green DR, Verma IM: Suppression of TNFα-induced apoptosis by NFκB. Nature 1996; 274:787-789.
75. Beg AA, Baltimore D: An essential role for NFκB in preventing TNFα-induced cell death. Nature 1996; 274:782-784.
76. Wang CY, Mayo MW, Baldwin AS: TNF- and cancer therapy-induced apoptosis: Potentiation by inhibition of NFκB. Nature 1996; 274:784-787.
77. Bromme HJ, Holtz J: Apoptosis in the heart: When and why? Mol Cell Biochem 1996; 163/164:261-275.
78. MacLellan WR, Schneider MD: Death by design: Programmed cell death in cardiovascular biology and disease. Circ Res 1997; 81:137-144.
79. Kajstura J, Cheng W, Reiss K, et al: Apoptosis and necrotic myocyte cell deaths are independent contributing variables of infarct size in rats. Lab Invest 1996; 74:86-107.
80. Fliss H, Gattinger D: Apoptosis in ischemic and reperfused myocardium. Circ Res 1996; 79:949-956.
81. Bialik S, Geenen DL, Sasson IE, et al: Myocyte apoptosis during acute myocardial infarction in the mouse localizes to hypoxic regions but occurs independently of p53. J Clin Invest 1997; 100:1363-1372.
82. Long X, Boluyt MO, Cirielli C, Capogrossi MC, Lakata EG, Crow MT: Enhanced expression of p53 in hypoxia-induced apoptosis of cultured rat cardiomyocytes. Cell Death Differ 1995; 9:235-241.
83. Misao J, Hayakawa Y, Ohno M, Kato S, Fujiwara T, Fujiwara H: Expression of BCL-2 protein, an inhibitor of apoptosis, and BAX, an accelerator of apoptosis, in ventricular myocytes of human hearts with myocardial infarction. Circulation 1996; 94:1506-1512.
84. Tanaka M, Ito H, Adachi S, et al: Hypoxia induces apoptosis with enhanced expression of Fas antigen messenger RNA in cultured neonatal rat cardiomyocytes. Circ Res 1994; 75:426-433.
85. Sawa Y, Bai HZ, Suzuki K, Tsujimoto Y, Matsuda H: Overexpression of bcl-2 gene improves the myocardial tolerance to ischemia-reperfusion by preventing DNA fragmentation. Circulation 1995; 92:I-772.
86. Bielawska AE, Shapiro JP, Jiang L, et al: Ceramide is involved in triggering of cardiomyocyte apoptosis induced by ischemia and reperfusion. Am J Pathol 1997; 151:1257-1263.
87. Umansky SR, Cuenco CM, Khutzian SS, Barr PJ, Tomei LD: Post-ischemic apoptotic death of rat neonatal cardiomyocytes. Cell Death Differ 1995; 9:235-241.
88. Rosenblum WI: Histopathologic clues to the pathways of neuronal death following ischemia/hypoxia. J Neurotrauma 1997; 14:313-326.

89. Mackey ME, Wu Y, Hu R, et al: Cell death suggestive of apoptosis after spinal cord ischemia in rabbits. Stroke 1997; 28:2012–2017.
90. Choi DW: Ischemia-induced neuronal apoptosis. Curr Opin Neurobiol 1996; 6:667–672.
91. Choi DW: Calcium: Still center-stage in hypoxic-ischemic neuronal cell death. Trends Neurosci 1995; 18:58–60.
92. Li Y, Chopp M, Powers C, Jiang N: Apoptosis and protein expression after focal cerebral ischemia in rat. Brain Res 1997; 765:301–312.
93. Shigeno T, Yamasaki Y, Kato G, et al: Reduction of delayed neuronal death by inhibition of protein synthesis. Neurosci Lett 1990; 120:117–119.

50

Prostaglandins, Thromboxanes, Leukotrienes, and Other Products of Arachidonic Acid

James A. Cook, PhD • Perry V. Halushka, PhD, MD

The first report of the biologic activity of what were subsequently identified as prostaglandins was in 1930,[1] when it was found that extracts of seminal fluid contracted uterine tissue. von Euler[2] attributed the activity of the extract to lipid substances, which he named *prostaglandins* because he thought that they came from the prostate. The structures of two of the prostaglandins (PGE_2 and $PGF_{1\alpha}$) were subsequently elucidated by use of gas chromatography–mass spectrometry, and with this discovery, research in the field rapidly grew.[3] Thromboxane B_2 (TXB_2) was isolated by Samuelsson and colleagues[4] in 1978 from human platelets. It was the stable metabolite of TXA_2, whose structure was deduced at the time and subsequently proved to be correct. The name *thromboxane* was chosen because it causes platelet aggregation (thrombosis) and has an oxetane ring system. It was ultimately shown that rabbit aorta-contracting substance was TXA_2.[5] Prostacyclin (PGI_2) was discovered in 1976.[6]

The next major group of arachidonic acid metabolites to be discovered and characterized were the leukotrienes. They derived their name from the observations that they were made by leukocytes and had triene structures.[7] The sulfidopeptide leukotrienes were shown to be the active principles of slow-reacting substance of anaphylaxis, released from mast cells and neutrophils.[7] Arachidonic acid, dihomo-γ-linolenic acid, and eicosapentaenoic acid are precursors of prostaglandins, thromboxanes, and leukotrienes. The first two are also known as *eicosatetraenoic acid* and *eicosatrienoic acid*, respectively; thus, the name *eicosanoids* is used generically to name the products of these fatty acids.

NOMENCLATURE

The products of fatty acid cyclooxygenase and lipoxygenase pathways are all named with a letter and a number. The letters for the cyclooxygenase pathway metabolites refer to the substitutions on the cyclopentane ring; in the leukotriene pathway, the letters refer to the amino acids coupled to the fatty acid.[7] The numbers refer to the number of double bonds present on the side chains.

SITES OF SYNTHESIS AND PHARMACOLOGIC ACTIVITY OF THE EICOSANOIDS

Fatty Acid Cyclooxygenase Products

The pathway for the metabolism of arachidonic acid is shown in Figure 50–1. PGA, PGB, and PGC are nonenzymatic dehydration products of PGE_2 and are considered artifacts of the extraction procedures. However, PGA is a vasodilator. PGD_2 is synthesized in large quantities by mast cells, being the major cyclooxygenase metabolite in this cell. It and its major metabolite, $9\alpha,11\beta,PGF_{2\alpha}$, are potent bronchoconstrictors and are overproduced in mastocytosis.[8] Depending on the vascular bed, it may be either a vasoconstrictor or vasodilator. Vasodilation usually occurs at the lower doses; however, it constricts only the pulmonary artery. It is also synthesized by platelets and inhibits platelet aggregation by increasing intraplatelet cyclic adenosine monophosphate (cAMP) levels. It has yet to be determined whether its synthesis is increased in shock.

PGE_2 is synthesized mainly by the kidneys, platelets, and blood vessels, but it is also synthesized by many other tissues in smaller amounts. It is a vasodilator, natriuretic, and diuretic; it inhibits gastric acid secretion and contracts uterine tissue. Four subtypes of receptors (EP) have been identified for PGE_2. They are associated with either stimulation or inhibition of adenylate cyclase and stimulation of phospholipase C.[8] PGE_2 synthesis is significantly increased in shock syndromes (discussed later).

$PGF_{2\alpha}$ is synthesized in many tissues in variable amounts. It is a bronchoconstrictor and venoconstrictor, and it contracts uterine smooth muscle. All these actions are mediated by FP receptors. Its synthesis is also increased in sepsis.

PGI_2 is made in large quantities by endothelial cells, macrophages, the lungs, and the kidneys. It is a vasodilator and antiaggregatory substance with a half-life of about 10 minutes and spontaneously hydrolyzes to form the stable metabolite 6-keto-$PGF_{1\alpha}$. The major urinary metabolite of 6-keto-$PGF_{1\alpha}$ is 2,3-dinor-6-keto-$PGF_{1\alpha}$. PGI_2 is a potent stimulator of adenylate cyclase. To date, only one class of receptors (IP) has been identified for it.[8]

TXA_2 is synthesized in large quantities by platelets, macrophages, monocytes, and the lungs. It is unstable and has a half-life of only 30 seconds and spontaneously hydrolyzes to form the stable but inactive TXB_2. The major plasma metabolite of TXB_2 is 11-dehydro-TXB_2. The major urinary metabolites are 11-dehydro-TXB_2 and 2,3-dinor-TXB_2. TXA_2 is a potent vasoconstrictor, bronchoconstrictor, and proaggregatory substance. At least two subtypes of receptors have been identified for TXA_2, the platelet and the vascular smooth muscle cell receptors.[8] Its synthesis is markedly increased in shock syndromes.

Leukotriene B_4 (LTB_4) is synthesized by white blood cells, macrophages, and synovial cells. It is a potent chemotactic substance for white blood cells.

LTC_4 is synthesized by white blood cells, lung parenchymal tissue, and macrophages. It is converted to LTD_4, the active metabolite of LTC_4. It is a vasoconstrictor and bronchoconstrictor, and it increases capillary permeability and bronchial mucus secretion. Its synthesis is increased during sepsis and adult respiratory distress syndrome (ARDS).[9] The urinary excretion of *N*-acetyl LTE_4, a metabolite of LTD_4, is increased in ARDS and shock.[10]

Arachidonic Acid Release

Release of arachidonic acid from membrane phospholipids is the rate-limiting step in the formation of eicosanoids in nonpathologic states.[11] Stimulation of cells by hormonal and

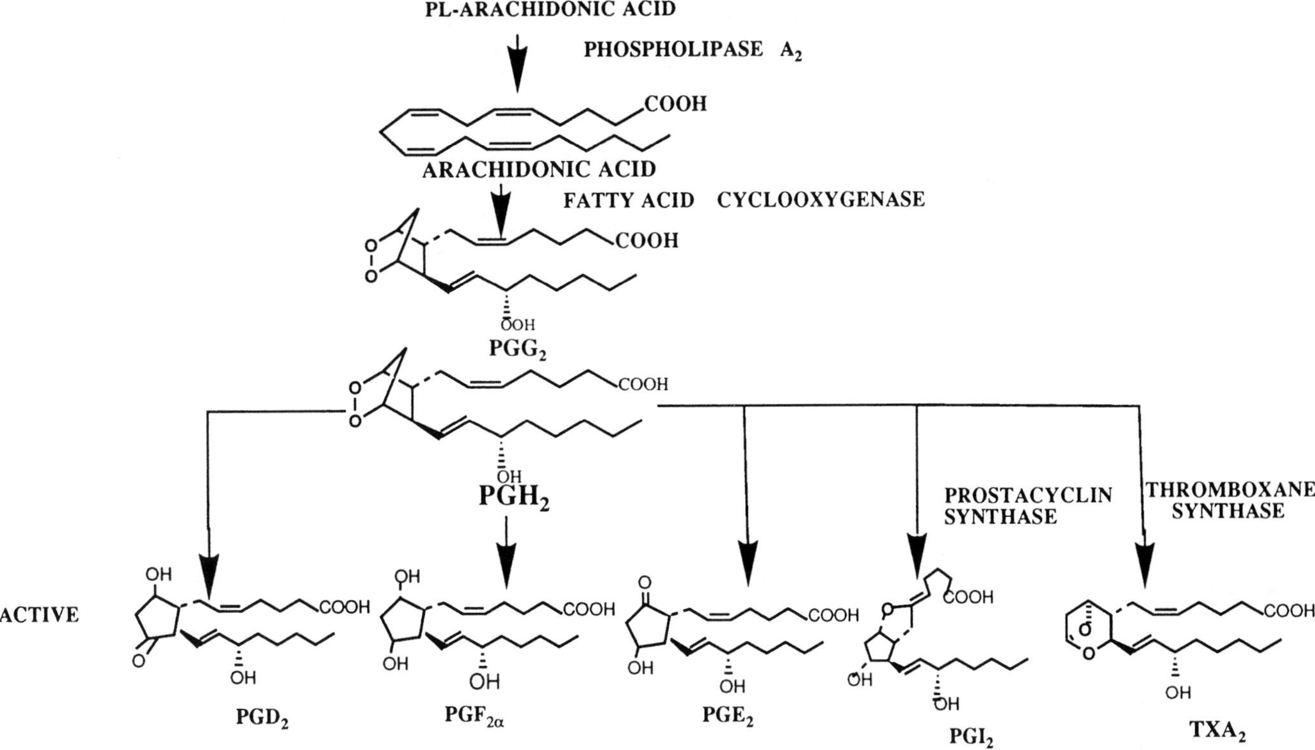

Figure 50–1. Metabolism of arachidonic acid. PG = prostaglandin; PGI_2 = prostacyclin; TXA_2 = thromboxane A_2. (From Wagner TR, Halushka PV, Cook JA: Cyclooxygenase products in septic and endotoxic shock. *In:* Handbook of Mediators in Septic Shock. Neugebauer EA, Holaday JW [Eds]. Boca Raton, Fla, CRC Press, 1993, pp 395–418.)

nonhormonal agonists results in activation of phospholipases A_2, C, or D. Activation of phospholipase A_2 results in the release of arachidonic acid from the *sn*-2 position of phosphatidylcholine and phosphatidylethanolamine.[12] Isozymes of phospholipase A_2 have been demonstrated to have specificity for catalyzing the release of arachidonic acid preferentially from either phosphatidylcholine or phosphatidylethanolamine.[13] In the other pathway, phospholipase C cleaves phosphatidylinositol 4,5-bisphosphate, resulting in inositol 1,4,5-trisphosphate and 1,2-diacylglycerol, both of which function as intracellular second messengers.[14-17] Diglyceride lipase then releases the arachidonic acid from the diacylglycerol.[18, 19]

A variety of agonists can stimulate phospholipase D.[20] Both guanine nucleotide–regulatory proteins and kinases are coupled to receptor-mediated regulation of phospholipase D. Phospholipase D activation requires a cofactor, phosphatidylinositol 4,5-bisphosphate. The metabolite phosphatidic acid produced by phospholipase D may play a role in growth regulation, activation of Ca^{2+}-independent forms of protein kinase C, neutrophil respiratory burst activity, and vesicle trafficking.[21]

The particular phospholipid substrate providing arachidonic acid in response to a specific stimulus may influence whether lipoxygenase or fatty acid cyclooxygenase products are formed. Resident murine macrophages in response to stimuli that activate the lipoxygenase pathway demonstrate dependence on the phospholipase C-diglyceride lipase pathway,[22] whereas endotoxin or phorbol myristate acetate–induced prostaglandin formation is independent of the phospholipase C-diglyceride lipase pathway.

Prostaglandin H Synthase (Fatty Acid Cyclooxygenase)

PGH synthase catalyzes the committed step in the conversion of arachidonic acid to the prostaglandin endoperoxides PGG_2 and PGH_2.[23] PGH_2 is the direct precursor for the primary prostaglandins and TXA_2. PGH synthase has been found in most of the organs of all mammalian species but not in all cell types.[22] Subcellular studies demonstrate that PGH synthase is an integral membrane protein concentrated in the endoplasmic reticulum as well as in the nuclear envelope and the plasma membrane.[24, 25] PGH synthase is approximately 68,000 daltons; species variations are attributed to different amounts of *N*-glycosylation and mannose carbohydrate side chains.[26] Two sites of enzymatic activity have been proposed,[27] and heme binding sites are conserved.[28]

PGH synthase possesses two enzymatic activities.[29] The first activity cyclizes an oxygen molecule in a bis-dioxygenase configuration at carbon-9 (C-9) and C-11, converting arachidonic acid to PGG_2. PGH synthase then uses another oxygen molecule to peroxidize this unstable metabolite at C-15, converting PGG_2 into PGH_2. The bound heme of PGH synthase is believed to act as the electron transfer site in these reactions. PGH_2 is the substrate for the enzymes responsible for the synthesis of prostaglandins D_2, E_2, $F_{2\alpha}$, and I_2 and TXA_2, the final product profile being dependent on the specific cell type.

Many fatty acids are substrates for PGH synthase, but arachidonic acid is the most common in vivo.[21] PGH synthase is inhibited by aspirin and all the nonsteroidal anti-inflammatory drugs (NSAIDs). Aspirin irreversibly inhibits the enzyme by covalently acetylating a serine residue. In platelets, the inhibition lasts for the life of the platelet (7 to 10 days) because platelets are not capable of synthesizing new enzyme.

Until recently, it was thought that there was a single cyclooxygenase enzyme. Two isoforms of cyclooxygenase (COX-1 and COX-2) have been extensively characterized. COX-1 is the constitutive, continuously expressed form that is thought to play a role in normal homeostatic processes in the kidneys and the gastrointestinal tract. COX-2 is the inducible form.[30] Its synthesis is stimulated by inflammatory stimuli such as lipopolysaccharide and interleukin-1 and growth factors.[30, 31] Both enzymes are inhibited by aspirin, indomethacin, and other NSAIDs. Several selective COX-2 inhibitors have recently been synthesized. Because they have the potential to be devoid of the side effects of the NSAIDs that inhibit COX-1,[30, 32] they may prove beneficial in the treatment of sepsis.

Lipoxygenase

The lipoxygenase pathways of arachidonic acid metabolism involve three species of lipoxygenases: 5-lipoxygenase, 12-lipoxygenase, and 15-lipoxygenase.[33-35] These enzymes insert a molecule of oxygen into arachidonic acid, respectively, at C-5, C-12, and C-15, forming the 5-, 12-, and 15-hydroxyeicosatetraenoic acids (HETEs).

5-Lipoxygenase demonstrates several unique characteristics compared with the other human lipoxygenases. It is dependent on adenosine triphosphate and Ca^{2+} for activation as well as three additional components.[36, 37] One of these components is an 18-kD protein that is required for both the translocation and activation of 5-lipoxygenase.[36, 38] This protein has been named *5-lipoxygenase-activating protein*. The 5-lipoxygenase metabolizes arachidonic acid to 5-hydroperoxyeicosatetraenoic acid (5-HPETE). 5-HPETE is further metabolized to 5-HETE and LTA_4. LTA_4 is an unstable intermediate that is rapidly metabolized to LTB_4 by LTA_4 hydrolase, to LTC_4 by LTC_4 synthase, and to other metabolites by nonenzymatic reactions. LTC_4 consists of glutathione covalently bound to arachidonic acid at the C-6 position (a sulfidopeptide leukotriene). The glutamic acid moiety of glutathione is cleaved by a γ-glutamyltranspeptidase to produce LTD_4. LTD_4 is further metabolized by a peptidase or a cysteinylglycinase to form LTE_4. LTE_4 can be *N*-acetylated and subsequently excreted in the urine.

12-Lipoxygenase metabolizes arachidonic acid to 12-HPETE and the subsequent metabolites di-HETE and tri-HETE. 12-Lipoxygenase is found in platelets and is the predominant lipoxygenase in brain tissue.

15-Lipoxygenase is approximately 70 kD.[39] Its activity is preferentially expressed only in certain cells,[40] but the biologic role of 15-lipoxygenase in these cell types is not fully understood.[41]

Other Metabolites

Cytochrome P_{450} isoforms can also oxygenate arachidonic acid at various sites.[42] This results in the production of a multitude of epoxides that have diverse biologic properties. These metabolites are usually synthesized in large quantities by the liver and kidneys. Whether these products are increased in sepsis remains unknown.

Isoprostanes are a novel group of nonenzymatically generated arachidonic acid metabolites.[43] They are formed directly by free radical oxidation of arachidonic acid while still esterified to the 2 position of membrane phospholipids. Isoprostanes are structurally similar to prostaglandins and may exert some of their effects through the activation of TXA_2 receptors. They cause vasoconstriction, change in platelet shape, and increase in pulmonary permeability.[44] Because they are generated under oxidative stress, isoprostanes may play a role in ARDS and sepsis.

INCREASED SYNTHESIS OF EICOSANOIDS IN ENDOTOXEMIA AND SEPSIS

The seminal observation that eicosanoids may be involved in the pathogenesis of endotoxic shock was made by Northover and Subramanian[45] in 1962. They demonstrated that dogs treated with aspirin before exposure to endotoxin had an improved survival compared with control animals. At that time, it was not known that aspirin inhibited prostaglandin synthesis. In 1976, Herman and Vane[46] demonstrated increased levels of PGE-like material in the renal vein of dogs given endotoxin. Taken together, these two observations suggested the possibility that eicosanoids were important in the pathogenesis of septic shock.

Increased synthesis of eicosanoids in response to endotoxemia and sepsis occurs in several animal species and in humans. Increases in plasma levels of TXB_2 and 6-keto-$PGF_{1\alpha}$ can be demonstrated in rats with experimental endotoxemia and sepsis.[33, 47-49] Similar profiles of TXB_2 and 6-keto-$PGF_{1\alpha}$ in plasma are observed in endotoxemic or septic sheep,[50, 51] pigs,[47, 52-56] and baboons.[57, 58] The relative amounts of TXB_2 and 6-keto-$PGF_{1\alpha}$ are influenced by the experimental route of endotoxin administration[59] and the frequency of endotoxin administration.[60]

5-Lipoxygenase products are also increased in endotoxemic animals and in patients with sepsis and ARDS.[61] In endotoxemic rats, Hagmann and colleagues[62] reported increases in biliary *N*-acetyl LTE_4, a stable metabolite of sulfidopeptide leukotrienes. LTC_4 levels are increased in the lungs of rats with experimental endotoxemia.[63] Increased LTB_4 levels are found in bronchoalveolar lavage fluid of endotoxemic pigs[64] and in lung lymph in endotoxemic sheep.[65] Increases in sulfidopeptide leukotrienes and LTB_4 have been demonstrated in the bronchoalveolar lavage fluid of patients with ARDS, a complication associated with sepsis.[10, 66-70]

EFFECT OF EICOSANOID SYNTHESIS INHIBITORS AND RECEPTOR ANTAGONISTS

More direct evidence that eicosanoids mediate endotoxin-induced sequelae is provided by observations that inhibition of eicosanoid synthesis or blockade of specific receptors protects animals from endotoxic shock sequelae. Numerous NSAIDs have been evaluated for potential therapeutic benefit in endotoxemia and sepsis in animal models.[33] These compounds, when used in experimental sepsis or endotoxemia, have generally been found to improve survival or survival time and to reduce cardiopulmonary dysfunction and indices of tissue injury.[33, 47-49] Among the most extensively studied prototype NSAID is ibuprofen. In various species with endotoxemia and sepsis, ibuprofen has been shown to improve systemic hypotension, pulmonary hypertension, protein and fluid extravasation, lung water flux, airway resistance, and oxygen delivery.[33, 49, 54, 59, 71-73] In some studies, however, ibuprofen did not improve shock sequelae.[73] Ibuprofen also alters neutrophil function, including inhibition of neutrophil aggregation responses, organ influx, and adherence.[71, 73] As with other NSAIDs, it is likely that some of these salutary actions are the result of pharmacologic actions of ibuprofen other than inhibition of fatty acid cyclooxygenase. These actions include potential inhibition of LTB_4 production,[73] superoxide anion production,[73] scavenging of hydroxyl radicals,[74] and burn-induced inhibition of fibrinolysis.[75]

A major concern in the use of NSAIDs is their side effects on renal and gastrointestinal function. By inhibiting endogenous prostaglandin synthesis in those organs, NSAIDs can render septic animals more susceptible to renal failure[76, 77] and gastrointestinal ulceration. The renal effects of NSAIDs can be reversed, at least in part, by the use of dopamine.[78] These side effects are due to the fact that NSAIDs inhibit both COX-1, the enzyme responsible for homeostasis in the kidneys and gastrointestinal tract, and COX-2, which is induced by lipopolysaccharide and probably mediates the increase in prostaglandin synthesis in sepsis. COX-2–selective drugs are emerging and may prove more protective in the treatment of sepsis. NS-398, a selective COX-2 inhibitor, blocks inflammatory prostaglandin synthesis but does not inhibit gastric prostaglandin production and does not produce gastric erosion.[79] L-745,337, also a COX-2–selective inhibitor, has been found to reduce the increase in core body temperature induced by lipopolysaccharide in rats.[80] Whether these inhibitors have effects on renal function and are protective in sepsis remains to be determined.

Pretreatment with TXA_2 synthase inhibitors or TXA_2 receptor antagonists improves survival time or attenuates certain shock sequelae in endotoxemic animals. The pathophysiologic events ameliorated by these pharmacologic agents include pulmonary hypertension,[81, 82] reduction in cardiac output, hypotension,[83, 84] decreased renal blood flow, decreased glomerular filtration rate,[82, 84, 85] thrombocytopenia,[81–86] renal glomerular fibrin deposition,[87] and renal glomerular microthrombi.[84] Most studies have shown that the beneficial effect of these drugs was not obtained if they were given after endotoxin. Other studies did not demonstrate improved outcome in sepsis and endotoxic shock.[88] Presumably, in these experiments, mediators other than TXA_2 dominate to produce pathophysiologic sequelae contributing to the development of shock and mortality. Use of TXA_2 receptor antagonists in endotoxemia may have several advantages over use of TXA_2 synthase inhibitors. TXA_2 receptor antagonists block the effects of both PGH_2 and TXA_2 to activate TXA_2 receptors but do not produce shunting of PGH_2 to PGI_2 synthesis.

The 5-lipoxygenase inhibitor diethylcarbamazine improved survival of mice in endotoxic shock,[64] and CGS8515 attenuated endotoxin-induced hemoconcentration and hypotension in rats.[89] AA-861, a 5-lipoxygenase inhibitor, attenuated endotoxin-induced neutropenia and concomitant oxygen radical synthesis in rats[90] and improved survival in endotoxemic mice.[91] L-651,392, another 5-lipoxygenase inhibitor, blocked endotoxin-induced pulmonary hypertension and bronchoconstriction and increased arterial-alveolar oxygen difference and lung microvascular permeability in sheep.[65]

Further evidence for the role of lipoxygenase products in endotoxin-induced shock sequelae is provided by studies using specific leukotriene receptor antagonists in experimental endotoxemia. The sulfidopeptide leukotriene receptor antagonist FPL57231 attenuated endotoxin-induced bronchoconstriction and pulmonary hypertension in sheep and cats.[92, 93] The LTD_4 receptor antagonist SKF104353 prevented endotoxin-induced hemoconcentration and thrombocytopenia and improved survival time in rats.[94] The LTD_4/E_4 receptor antagonist LY171883 improved endotoxin-induced hypotension, hemoconcentration, and leukopenia in rats. Both compounds were shown to prevent acute splanchnic permeability changes induced by endotoxin in rats[95] and mesenteric ischemia in pigs.[47] The LTB_4 receptor antagonist LY233978 has been shown to attenuate endotoxin-induced leukopenia, hemoconcentration, and hypotension in rats.[96] Another LTB_4 receptor antagonist, LY255283, however, only transiently attenuated endotoxin-induced hypotension and hemoconcentration.

Some studies have used combination therapy with cyclooxygenase inhibitors and leukotriene receptor antagonists or lipoxygenase inhibitors. Young and Passmore[97] examined the effect of combined therapy with ibuprofen and LY171883 in canine endotoxic shock. Combined blockade was more effective in maintaining blood pressure and cardiac output but provided no greater protection of renal blood flow or glomerular filtration rate. Turner and colleagues[98] demonstrated good protection with a combined cyclooxygenase and lipoxygenase inhibitor (SKF86002) in a rat model of endotoxin-induced ARDS. The inhibitor blocked the increase in lung wet-dry ratio, total bronchoalveolar lavage protein, hemoconcentration, and thrombocytopenia. Other combination therapies have been shown to be successful. Byrne and associates[99] demonstrated increased survival after delayed cyclooxygenase and histamine blockade in a porcine model of severe sepsis-induced lung injury.

CLINICAL SIGNIFICANCE OF EICOSANOIDS IN PATIENTS

Several studies reported increased TXB_2, 6-keto-$PGF_{1\alpha}$, PGE_2, and $PGF_{2\alpha}$ levels in patients with septic shock.[100–102] Oettinger and colleagues[102] evaluated the relationship of plasma TXB_2 and 6-keto-$PGF_{1\alpha}$ levels with the severity of organ dysfunction in 106 patients with gram-negative septic shock. As in other studies, TXB_2 and 6-keto-$PGF_{1\alpha}$ levels were elevated during the whole course of sepsis but were highest during the early phases. TXB_2 levels were higher in hypodynamic patients than in hyperdynamic patients, whereas the opposite was observed for 6-keto-$PGF_{1\alpha}$. Patients in the hyperdynamic group had improved lung and kidney function as determined by alveolar-arterial P_{O_2} gradient and creatinine clearance. Collectively, these studies demonstrate increased thromboxane and prostacyclin synthesis in septic patients and suggest a deleterious role for thromboxane during the septic response.

Leukotriene levels are also increased in several clinical situations. Seeger and coworkers[70] reported increased LTB_4 metabolites in the bronchoalveolar lavage fluid of patients with ARDS. Elevated sulfidopeptide leukotriene levels have also been reported in the bronchoalveolar lavage fluid, blood, and urine of patients with trauma or ARDS.[66, 68, 103] Higher leukotriene levels correlated with poor prognosis. Acutely ill patients with elevated plasma LTB_4 levels were at increased risk for development of ARDS than were those with lower levels.[69] Urinary excretion of LTE_4 was higher in trauma patients in whom ARDS later developed than in those who did not have ARDS.[103]

The NSAIDs may have beneficial effects in the treatment of patients with trauma or sepsis. Faist and coworkers[104] studied the effect of indomethacin in a randomized prospective study in 43 patients undergoing major surgical trauma. The cellular immune status was evaluated preoperatively and up to a week after surgery. In contrast to untreated patients, patients receiving indomethacin exhibited improved delayed-type hypersensitivity responses, mitogen-induced lymphocyte transformation, and a lower rate of opportunistic infections. The results suggest that NSAIDs, by preventing impairment of cell-mediated immunity, may reduce susceptibility to sepsis after surgery.

Bernard and associates[105] conducted a double-blind, placebo-controlled trial of intravenous ibuprofen (10 mg/kg) (maximum dose, 800 mg) given every 6 hours for eight doses in 455 patients with a diagnosis of sepsis. The ibuprofen-treated group did not experience any increased incidence of renal dysfunction, gastrointestinal bleeding, or other adverse effects. Short-term treatment with ibuprofen did not affect the duration of shock or 30-day survival rate. However, ibuprofen did produce significant declines in urinary 6-keto-$PGF_{1\alpha}$ and TXB_2 excretion, temperature, heart rate, oxygen consumption, and lactic acidosis. Whether more prolonged or even prophylactic treatment with NSAIDs will alter the course of septic shock remains to be determined.

These studies provide the impetus for more extensive studies of NSAIDs in trauma, sepsis, and ARDS. Combination therapy approaches with NSAIDs may also prove to be beneficial. Experimentally, combinations of drugs with NSAIDs have been more effective than single-drug treatments.[106–111] Of particular interest, in view of the demonstrated increases of lipoxygenase products in patients with ARDS, is the potential application of lipoxygenase inhibitors or leukotriene receptor antagonists.

ACKNOWLEDGMENTS

This work was supported in part by NIH GM27673. The secretarial assistance of Ms. Sybil Moore is gratefully acknowledged.

References

1. Kurzok R, Lieb CC: Biochemical studies of human semen: The action of semen on the human uterus. Proc Soc Exp Biol Med 1930; 28:268-272.
2. von Euler US: Zur Kenntnis der pharmakologischen Wirkungen von nativ Sekreten und Extrakten mannlicher accessorischer Geschlechtsdrusen. Naunyn Schmeidebergs Arch Exp Pathol Pharmacol 1934; 175:78-84.
3. Bergstrom S, Sjovall J: The isolation of prostaglandin E from sheep prostate glands. Acta Chem Scand 1960; 14:1701-1705.
4. Samuelsson B, Goldyne M, Granstrom E: Prostaglandins and thromboxanes. Annu Rev Biochem 1978; 47:997-1029.
5. Piper PJ, Vane JR: Release of additional factors in anaphylaxis and its antagonism by anti-inflammatory drugs. Nature 1969; 223:29-33.
6. Moncada S, Gryglewski R, Bunting S: An enzyme isolated from arteries transforms prostaglandin endoperoxides to an unstable substance that inhibits platelet aggregation. Nature 1976; 263:663-665.
7. Samuelsson B, Borgeat P, Hammarstrom S: Introduction of a nomenclature: Leukotrienes. Prostaglandins 1979; 17:785-787.
8. Coleman RA, Smith WL, Narumiya S VII: International Union of Pharmacology Classification of Prostanoid Receptors: Properties, distribution, and structures of receptors and their subtypes. Pharmacol Rev 1994; 46:205-229.
9. Bernard GR, Reines HD, Halushka PV, et al: Prostacyclin and thromboxane A_2 formation is increased in human sepsis syndrome: Effects of cyclooxygenase inhibition. Am Rev Respir Dis 1991; 144:1095-1101.
10. Bernard GR, Korley V, Chee P, et al: Persistent generation of peptido-leukotrienes in patients with the adult respiratory distress syndrome. Am Rev Respir Dis 1991; 144:263-267.
11. Irvine RF: How is the level of free arachidonic acid controlled in mammalian cells? Biochem J 1982; 204:3-16.
12. Lapetina EG: Regulation of arachidonic acid production: Role of phospholipases C and A_2. Trends Pharmacol 1982; 3:115-118.
13. Tanaka Y, Amano F, Kishi H, et al: Degradation of arachidonyl phospholipids catalyzed by two phospholipases A_2 and phospholipase C in a lipopolysaccharide-treated macrophage cell line, RAW264.7. Arch Biochem Biophys 1989; 272:210-218.
14. Berridge MJ, Irvine RF: Inositol trisphosphate, a novel second messenger in cellular signal transduction. Nature 1984; 312:315-321.
15. Berridge MJ: Inositol trisphosphate and diacylglycerol as second messengers. Biochem J 1984; 220:345-360.
16. Majerus PW, Connolly TM, Deckmyn H, et al: The metabolism of phosphoinositide-derived messenger molecules. Science 1986; 234:1519-1526.
17. Prpic V, Weiel JE, Somers SD, et al: Effects of bacterial lipopolysaccharide on the hydrolysis of phosphatidylinositol-4,5-bisphosphate in murine peritoneal macrophages. J Immunol 1987; 139:526-533.
18. Bell RL, Kennerly DA, Stanford N, et al: Diglyceride lipase: A pathway for arachidonate release from human platelets. Proc Natl Acad Sci USA 1979; 76:3238-3241.
19. Moscat J, Herrero C, Garcia BP, et al: Phospholipase C-diglyceride lipase is a major pathway for arachidonic acid release in macrophages. Biochem Biophys Res Commun 1986; 141:367-373.
20. Lisovitch M: Phospholipase D: Role in signal transduction and membrane traffic. J Lipid Mediat Cell Signal 1996; 14:215-221.
21. Exton JH: Phospholipase D: Enzymology, mechanisms of regulation and function. Physiol Rev 1997; 77:303-320.
22. Wightman PD, Dallob A: Regulation of phosphatidylinositol breakdown and leukotriene synthesis by endogenous prostaglandins in resident mouse peritoneal macrophages. J Biol Chem 1990; 265:9176-9180.
23. Smith WL, Marnett LJ: Prostaglandin endoperoxide synthase: Structure and catalysis. Biochim Biophys Acta 1991; 1083:1-17.
24. Smith WL: Prostaglandin synthesis and its compartmentation in vascular smooth muscle and endothelial cells. Annu Rev Physiol 1986; 48:251-262.
25. Smith WL, DeWitt DL, Allen MA: Bimodal distribution of the prostaglandin I_2 antigen in smooth muscle cells. J Biol Chem 1983; 258:5922-5926.
26. Mutsaers JH, van Halbeek H, Kamerling JP, et al: Determination of the structure of the carbohydrate chains of prostaglandin endoperoxide synthase from sheep. Eur J Biochem 1985; 147:569-574.
27. Smith WL, DeWitt DL, Kraemer SA, et al: Structure-function relationships in sheep, mouse, and human prostaglandin endoperoxide G/H synthases. Adv Prostaglandin Thromboxane Leukot Res 1990; 20:14-21.
28. Lambier AM, Markey CM, Dunford HB, et al: Spectral properties of the higher oxidation states of prostaglandin H synthase. J Biol Chem 1985; 260:14894-14896.
29. Marnett LJ, Chen YN, Maddipati KR, et al: Localization of the peroxidase active site of PGH synthase. Adv Prostaglandin Thromboxane Leukot Res 1989; 19:458-461.
30. Smith WL, DeWitt DL: Biochemistry of prostaglandin endoperoxide H synthase-1 and synthase-2 and their differential susceptibility to nonsteroidal anti-inflammatory drugs. Semin Nephrol 1995; 15:179-194.
31. Xie WL, Chipman JG, Robertson DL, et al: Expression of a mitogen-responsive gene encoding prostaglandin synthase is regulated by mRNA splicing. Proc Natl Acad Sci USA 1991; 88:2692-2696.
32. Seibert K, Zhang Y, Leahy K, et al: Pharmacological and biochemical demonstration of the role of cyclooxygenase 2 in inflammation and pain. Proc Natl Acad Sci USA 1994; 91:12013-12017.
33. Cook JA, Halushka PV: Arachidonic acid metabolites in septic shock. *In*: Multiple Organ Failure. Bihari DJ, Cerra F (Eds). Fullerton, Calif, Society of Critical Care Medicine, 1989, pp 101-124.
34. Handerson W Jr: Products of 12- and 15-lipoxygenase. *In*: Mediators of the Inflammatory Process. Henson PM, Murphy RC (Eds). New York, Elsevier, 1989, pp 45-75.
35. Shimizu T, Wolfe LS: Arachidonic acid cascade and signal transduction. J Neurochem 1990; 55:1-15.
36. Rouzer CA, Shimizu T, Samuelsson B: On the nature of the 5-lipoxygenase reaction in human leukocytes: Characterization of a membrane-associated stimulatory factor. Proc Natl Acad Sci USA 1985; 82:7505-7509.
37. Rouzer CA, Thornberry NA, Bull HG: Kinetic effects of ATP and two cellular stimulatory components on human leukocyte 5-lipoxygenase. Ann N Y Acad Sci 1988; 524:1-11.
38. Rouzer CA, Ford HA, Morton HE, et al: MK886, a potent and specific leukotriene biosynthesis inhibitor blocks and reverses the membrane association of 5-lipoxygenase in ionophore-challenged leukocytes. J Biol Chem 1990; 265:1436-1442.
39. Sigal E, Craik CS, Dixon RA, et al: Cloning and expression of human arachidonate 15-lipoxygenase. Trans Assoc Am Physicians 1989; 102:176-184.
40. Nadel JA, Conrad DJ, Ueki IF, et al: Immunocytochemical localization of arachidonate 15-lipoxygenase in erythrocytes, leukocytes, and airway cells. J Clin Invest 1991; 87:1139-1145.
41. Ford HA: Arachidonate 15-lipoxygenase: Characteristics and potential biological significance. Eicosanoids 1991; 4:65-74.
42. McGiff JC: Cytochrome P-450 metabolism of arachidonic acid. Annu Rev Pharmacol Toxicol 1991; 31:339-369.
43. Roberts LJ, Morrow JD: The generation and action of isoprostanes. Biochim Biophys Acta 1997; 1345:121-135.
44. Vacchiano CA, Tempel GE: Role of nonenzymatically generated prostanoid, 8-iso-$PGF_{2\alpha}$, in pulmonary oxygen toxicity. J Appl Physiol 1994; 77:2912-2917.
45. Northover BJ, Subramanian G: Analgesic-antipyretic drugs as an-

tagonists of endotoxin shock in dogs. J Pathol Bacteriol 1962; 83:463–468.
46. Herman AG, Vane JR: Release of renal prostaglandins during endotoxin-induced hypotension. Eur J Pharmacol 1976; 39:79–90.
47. Fink MP, Rothschild HR, Deniz YF, et al: Systemic and mesenteric O_2 metabolism in endotoxic pigs: Effect of ibuprofen and meclofenamate. J Appl Physiol 1989; 67:1950–1957.
48. Petrak RA, Balk RA, Bone RC: Prostaglandins, cyclo-oxygenase inhibitors, and thromboxane synthetase inhibitors in the pathogenesis of multiple systems organ failure. Crit Care Clin 1989; 5:303–314.
49. Bone RC: Phospholipids and their inhibitors: A critical evaluation of their role in the treatment of sepsis. Crit Care Med 1992; 20:884–890.
50. Morel DR, Huttemeier PC, Skoskiewicz MJ, et al: Dose-dependent effects of a pyridoquinazoline thromboxane synthetase inhibitor on arachidonic acid metabolites and hemodynamics during *E. coli* endotoxemia in anesthetized sheep. Prostaglandins 1987; 33:879–902.
51. Demling RH, Smith M, Gunther R, et al: Pulmonary injury and prostaglandin production during endotoxemia in conscious sheep. Am J Physiol 1981; 240:H348–H353.
52. Hardie EM, Olson NC: Prostaglandin and thromboxane levels during endotoxin-induced respiratory failure in pigs. Prostaglandins Leukot Med 1987; 28:255–265.
53. Schrauwen E, Vandeplassche G, Laekman G, et al: Endotoxin shock in the pig: Release of prostaglandins and beneficial effects of flurbiprofen. Arch Int Pharmacodyn Ther 1983; 262:332–334.
54. Nishijima MK, Breslow MJ, Miller CF, et al: Effect of naloxone and ibuprofen on organ blood flow during endotoxic shock in pig. Am J Physiol 1988; 255:H177–H184.
55. Zellner JL, Cook JA, Reines DH, et al: Hemodynamic effects of leukotriene (LT) D_4 and LTD_4 receptor antagonist in the pig. Eicosanoids 1990; 3:219–224.
56. Zellner JL, Cook JA, Reines HD, et al: Effect of a LTD_4 receptor antagonist in porcine septic shock. Eicosanoids 1991; 4:169–175.
57. Harris RH, Zmudka M, Maddox Y, et al: Relationships of TXB_2 and 6-keto-$PGF_{1\alpha}$ to the hemodynamic changes during baboon endotoxic shock. *In*: Advances in Prostaglandins and Thromboxane Research. Samuelsson B, Ramwell RW, Paoletti R (Eds). New York, Raven Press, 1980, pp 843–850.
58. Casey LC, Fletcher JR, Zmudka MI, et al: Prevention of endotoxin-induced pulmonary hypertension in primates by the use of a selective thromboxane synthetase inhibitor, OKY 1581. J Pharmacol Exp Ther 1982; 222:441–446.
59. Demling RH, Wenber H, Hechtman H, et al: Role of subcutaneous tissue endotoxin in the production of prostanoid-induced lung injury: Comparison with intravenous endotoxin response. Circ Shock 1985; 17:147–161.
60. Klosterhalfen B, Hörstmann-Jungemann K, Vogel P, et al: Time course of various inflammatory mediators during recurrent endotoxemia. Biochem Pharmacol 1992; 43:2103–2109.
61. Keppler D, Guhlmann A, Huber M, et al: Leukotrienes in shock syndromes: Metabolism and detection in vivo. Adv Prostaglandin Thromboxane Leukot Res 1990; 20:179–186.
62. Hagmann W, Denzlinger C, Keppler D: Production of peptide leukotrienes in endotoxin shock. FEBS Lett 1985; 180:309–313.
63. Chang SW, Westcott JY, Pickett WC, et al: Endotoxin-induced lung injury in rats: Role of eicosanoids. J Appl Physiol 1989; 66:2407–2418.
64. Olson NC, Salzer WL, McCall CE: Biochemical, physiological and clinical aspects of endotoxemia. Mol Aspects Med 1988; 10:511–629.
65. Coggeshall JW, Christman BW, Lefferts PL, et al: Effect of inhibition of 5-lipoxygenase metabolism of arachidonic acid on response to endotoxemia in sheep. J Appl Physiol 1988; 65:1351–1359.
66. Matthay MA, Eschenbacher WL, Goetzl EJ: Elevated concentrations of leukotriene D_4 in pulmonary edema fluid of patients with adult respiratory distress syndrome. J Clin Immunol 1984; 4:479–483.
67. Stephenson AH, Lonigro AJ, Hyers TM, et al: Increased concentrations of leukotrienes in bronchoalveolar lavage fluid of patients with ARDS or at risk for ARDS. Am Rev Respir Dis 1988; 138:714–719.
68. Antonelli A, Bufi M, De Blasi RA, et al: Detection of leukotriene B_4, C_4 and their isomers in arterial, mixed venous blood and bronchoalveolar lavage fluid from ARDS patients. Intensive Care Med 1989; 15:296–301.
69. Davis JM, Meyer JD, Barie PS, et al: Elevated production of neutrophil leukotriene B_4 precedes pulmonary failure in critically ill surgical patients. Surg Gynecol Obstet 1990; 170:495–500.
70. Seeger W, Grimminger F, Barden M, et al: Omega-oxidized leukotriene B_4 detected in the bronchoalveolar lavage fluid of patients with non-cardiogenic pulmonary edema, but not in those with cardiogenic edema. Intensive Care Med 1991; 17:1–6.
71. Rinaldo JE, Pennock B: Effects of ibuprofen on endotoxin-induced alveolitis: Biphasic dose response and dissociation between inflammation and hypoxia. Am J Med Sci 1986; 29:29–38.
72. Ward PH, Maldonado M, Moreno M, et al: Oxygen-derived free radicals mediate the cutaneous necrotizing vasculitis induced by epinephrine in endotoxin-primed rabbits. J Infect Dis 1990; 161:1020–1022.
73. Wagner TR, Halushka PV, Cook JA: Cyclooxygenase products in septic and endotoxic shock. *In*: Handbook of Mediators in Septic Shock. Neugebauer EA, Holaday JW (Eds). Boca Raton, Fla, CRC Press, 1993, pp 395–418.
74. Hamburger SA, McCay PB: Spin trapping of ibuprofen radicals: Evidence that ibuprofen is a hydroxyl radical scavenger. Free Radic Res Commun 1990; 9:337–342.
75. Rockwell WB, Ehrlich HP: Ibuprofen in acute-care therapy. Ann Surg 1990; 211:78–83.
76. Hulton NR, Johnson DJ, Wilmore DW: Limited effects of prostaglandin inhibitors in *Escherichia coli* sepsis. Surgery 1985; 98:291–297.
77. Cryer HM, Unger LS, Garrison RN, Harris PD: Prostaglandins maintain renal microvascular blood flow during hyperdynamic bacteremia. Circ Shock 1988; 26:71–88.
78. Fink MP, Nelson R, Roethel R: Low-dose dopamine preserves renal blood flow in endotoxin shocked dogs treated with ibuprofen. J Surg Res 1985; 38:582–591.
79. Masferrer JL, Zweifel BS, Manning PT, et al: Selective inhibition of inducible cyclooxygenase 2 in vivo is anti-inflammatory and nonulcerogenic. Proc Natl Acad Sci USA 1994; 91:3228–3232.
80. Chan CC, Boyce S, Brideau C, et al: Pharmacology of a selective cyclooxygenase-2 inhibitor, L-745,337: A novel nonsteroidal anti-inflammatory agent with an ulcerogenic sparing effect in rat and nonhuman primate stomach. J Pharmacol Exp Ther 1995; 274:1531–1537.
81. Taneyama C, Sasao J, Senna S, et al: Protective effects of ONO 3708, a new thromboxane A_2 receptor antagonist, during experimental endotoxin shock. Circ Shock 1989; 28:69–77.
82. Cirino M, Morton H, MacDonald C, et al: Thromboxane A_2 and prostaglandin endoperoxide analogue effects on porcine renal blood flow. Am J Physiol 1990; 258:F109–F114.
83. Svartholm E, Bergqvist D, Hedner U, et al: Thromboxane A_2-receptor blockade and prostacyclin in porcine *Escherichia coli* shock. Arch Surg 1989; 124:669–672.
84. Fukumoto S, Tanaka K: Protective effects of thromboxane A_2 synthetase inhibitors on endotoxin shock. Prostaglandins Leukot Med 1983; 11:179–188.
85. Badr KF, Kelley VE, Rennke HG, et al: Roles for thromboxane A_2 and leukotrienes in endotoxin-induced acute renal failure. Kidney Int 1986; 30:474–480.
86. Olanoff L, Cook JA, Eller T, et al: Protective effects of trans-13-APT, a thromboxane receptor antagonist, in endotoxemia. J Cardiovasc Pharmacol 1985; 7:117–120.
87. Westwick J, Fletcher MS, Kakkar VV: Inhibition of thromboxane formation prevents endotoxin-induced renal fibrin deposition in jaundiced rats. *In*: Advances in Prostaglandin and Thromboxane Research. Samuelsson B, Paoletti R, Ramwell P (Eds). New York, Raven Press, 1983, pp 83–91.
88. Furman BL, McKechnie K, Paratt JR: Failure of drugs that selectively inhibit thromboxane synthesis to modify endotoxin shock in conscious rats. Br J Pharmacol 1984; 82:289–294.
89. Matera G, Cook JA, Hennigar RA, et al: Beneficial effects of a 5-lipoxygenase inhibitor in endotoxic shock in the rat. J Pharmacol Exp Ther 1988; 247:363–371.

90. Suematsu M, Miura S, Suzuki M, et al: 5-Lipoxygenase inhibitor (AA-861) attenuates neutrophil-mediated oxidative stress on the venular endothelium in endotoxemia. J Clin Lab Immunol 1988; 25:41-45.
91. Ogata M, Matsumoto T, Kamochi M, et al: Protective effects of a leukotriene inhibitor and a leukotriene antagonist on endotoxin-induced mortality in carrageenan-pretreated mice. Infect Immun 1992; 60:2432-2437.
92. Ahmed T, Wasserman MA, Muccitell R, et al: Endotoxin-induced changes in pulmonary hemodynamic and respiratory mechanics. Am Rev Respir Dis 1986; 134:1149-1159.
93. Pacitti N, Bryson SE, McKechnie K, et al: Leukotriene antagonist FPL 57231 prevents the acute pulmonary effects of *Escherichia coli* endotoxin in cats. Circ Shock 1987; 21:155-168.
94. Smith EF III, Kinter LB, Jugus M, et al: Beneficial effects of the peptidoleukotriene receptor antagonist, SK&F 104353, on the responses to experimental endotoxemia in the conscious rat. Circ Shock 1988; 25:21-31.
95. Cook JA, Li EJ, Spicer KM, et al: Effect of leukotriene receptor antagonists on vascular permeability during endotoxic shock. Circ Shock 1990; 32:209-218.
96. Li EJ, Cook JA, Wise WC, et al: Effect of LTB_4 receptor antagonists in endotoxic shock in the rat. Circ Shock 1991; 34:385-392.
97. Young JS, Passmore JC: Hemodynamic and renal advantages of dual cyclooxygenase and leukotriene blockade during canine endotoxic shock. Circ Shock 1990; 32:243-255.
98. Turner CR, Quinlan MF, Schwartz LW, et al: Therapeutic intervention in a rat model of ARDS: I. Dual inhibition of arachidonic acid metabolism. Circ Shock 1990; 32:231-242.
99. Byrne K, Sielaff TD, Michna B, et al: Increased survival time after delayed histamine and prostaglandin blockade in a porcine model of severe sepsis-induced lung injury. Crit Care Med 1990; 18:303-308.
100. Reines HD, Halushka PV, Cook JA, et al: Plasma thromboxane concentrations are raised in patients dying with septic shock. Lancet 1982; 2:174-175.
101. Halushka PV, Reines HD, Barrow SE, et al: Elevated plasma 6-keto-prostaglandin $F_{1\alpha}$ in patients in septic shock. Crit Care Med 1985; 13:451-453.
102. Oettinger W, Berger D, Beger HG: The clinical significance of prostaglandins and thromboxane as mediators of septic shock. Klin Wochenschr 1987; 65:61-68.
103. Fauler J, Tsikas D, Holch M, et al: Enhanced urinary excretion of leukotriene E_4 by patients with multiple trauma with or without adult respiratory distress syndrome. Clin Sci 1991; 80:497-504.
104. Faist E, Ertel W, Cohnert T, et al: Immunoprotective effects of cyclooxygenase inhibition in patients with major surgical trauma. J Trauma 1990; 30:8-17.
105. Bernard G, Wheeler AP, Russel MD, et al: The effects of ibuprofen on the physiology and survival of patients with sepsis. N Engl J Med 1997; 336:912-953.
106. Ogletree ML, Begley CJ, King GA, et al: Influence of steroidal and nonsteroidal anti-inflammatory agents on the accumulation of arachidonic acid metabolites in plasma and lung lymph after endotoxemia in awake sheep. Measurements of prostacyclin and thromboxane metabolites and 12-HETE. Am Rev Respir Dis 1986; 133:55-61.
107. Olson NC, Brown TT Jr, Anderson DL: Dexamethasone and indomethacin modify endotoxin-induced respiratory failure in pigs. J Appl Physiol 1985; 58:274-284.
108. Sielaff TD, Sugerman HJ, Tatum JL, et al: Treatment of porcine *Pseudomonas* ARDS with combination drug therapy. J Trauma 1987; 27:1313-1322.
109. Wise WC, Halushka PV, Knapp DR, et al: Ibuprofen, methylprednisolone, gentamicin as conjoint therapy in septic shock. Circ Shock 1985; 17:59-71.
110. Goto M, Zeller WP, Hurley RM: Dexamethasone and indomethacin treatment during endotoxicosis in the suckling rat. Circ Shock 1990; 32:113-122.
111. Butler RR Jr, Wise WC, Halushka PV, et al: Gentamicin and indomethacin in the treatment of septic shock: Effects on prostacyclin and thromboxane A_2 production. J Pharmacol Exp Ther 1983; 225:94-101.

51

Macrophage Function

Tomas Ganz, PhD, MD

Macrophages and their secretory products have a central role in host defense against pathogenic microbes, in the development of protective immunity, in the pathogenesis of septic shock and of acute and chronic infections, and in the pathophysiologic processes of wound healing, tissue remodeling, and fibrosis.[1] In their role as scavenger cells, macrophages sequester and degrade particulates that enter the body by inhalation, trauma, or parenteral injection; they break down accumulated deposits of metabolites and dispose of senescent cells.

MORPHOLOGY AND DEVELOPMENT

Macrophages are mononuclear phagocytes, that is, cells with a single nonsegmented nucleus and the ability to ingest particles into cytoplasmic membrane-lined vacuoles. Some macrophages are freely motile (e.g., alveolar macrophages, peritoneal macrophages); others are fixed in tissues (e.g., liver and colon macrophages). The characteristic ultrastructural features of free macrophages include a ruffled membrane, sometimes with a prominent trailing extension (pseudopod), and a cytoplasm with abundant vacuoles. Some of these vacuoles (pinosomes) contain ingested fluid; others (phagosomes) contain ingested particles; yet others (lysosomes) are acidic vacuoles with digestive enzymes (hydrolases) capable of degrading proteins, complex carbohydrates, nucleic acids, and lipids. Of necessity, most of what we know about macrophages was learned from cells washed free from the pulmonary alveoli or body cavities or released from disaggregated tissues. Critical readers of the literature should be aware that crucial aspects of macrophage behavior may depend on the animal species and strain, the organ from which the macrophages were harvested, and the time and conditions ex vivo.

Most macrophages originate from bone marrow precursors that develop into blood monocytes, which, after a few days in the circulation, enter tissues and mature into macrophages.[2] Macrophages can divide, and this process contributes substantially to maintaining resident macrophage populations. The number of monocytes and macrophages is controlled by hematopoietic hormones,[3] especially interleukin-3 (IL-3), multi-colony-stimulating factor (CSF), granulocyte-macrophage CSF (GM-CSF), and macrophage CSF (M-CSF, CSF-1). IL-3 is produced by lymphocytes, and GM-CSF by macrophages, lymphocytes, endothelial cells, and fibroblasts. Inflammatory or immune stimuli, acting in part by increasing the levels of IL-1 and tumor necrosis factor-α (TNF-α), increase the production of all three CSFs, ultimately generating more monocytes and macrophages.

Morphologic and biochemical studies of macrophages have described many tissue-specific adaptations that resulted in a confusing nomenclature—for example, *Kupffer's cells* for liver macrophages and *microglia* for brain macrophages. Studies of macrophage-specific marker antigens in mice[4] revealed that all tissues contain macrophages, with particularly high concentrations in bone marrow and lymph nodes. However, when the weight of the organs is taken into account, the largest total numbers of macrophages are found in the liver, small bowel, and colon. The factors that control the differentiation of macrophages into tissue-specific subtypes are not yet understood.

MACROPHAGE RECEPTORS

Macrophages sense their environment by various membrane-associated receptor molecules. Some receptors are exposed to the extracellular fluid, span the macrophage cell membrane, and immerse their intracellular end into the cytoplasm of the macrophage. For other receptors, the functional equivalent of the cytoplasmic tail is generated by transducer and adapter proteins that are associated with the receptor.

Occupancy of receptors by their agonists results in transmission of a signal into the cytoplasm and activation of a cascade of biochemical reactions that constitutes the specific response of the cell to each agonist. The responses include (1) cellular movement toward the source of a substance (chemotaxis), (2) localized movement of the membrane in the area of receptor contact (adhesion, spreading, phagocytosis), (3) rearrangement of internal organelles (e.g., fusion of phagocytic vacuoles with lysosomes), (4) synthesis and assembly of systems required for antimicrobial activity (macrophage activation), (5) alteration in the amount or nature of substances released into the extracellular milieu (regulated secretion), and (6) initiation of cell division or cellular remodeling (mitogenesis, differentiation).

MICROBICIDAL FUNCTION AND CYTOTOXICITY

Unlike other phagocytes (i.e., neutrophils, eosinophils, monocytes), macrophages are resident in noninflamed tissues and thus are likely to interact with microbes during the earliest stages (first few hours) of infection. The response of motile macrophages to microbial invasion consists of the following:

- Movement toward the microbes (chemotaxis)
- Recognition and ingestion of microbes (phagocytosis)
- Killing and digestion of the microbes
- Recruitment of additional effector cells to the site of infection

Chemotaxis

Macrophages initiate movement toward microbes when their chemotactic receptors are occupied by (1) substances emitted by the invader (e.g., formylated peptides characteristic of prokaryotic organisms), (2) reaction products resulting from the encounter of microbes with extracellular fluids (e.g., complement fragment C5a), or (3) products released by other cells, including other macrophages, engaged in host defense activity (e.g., leukotriene B_4; small chemoattractant proteins, "chemokines"). Each chemotactic substance interacts with its own specialized receptor. Movement of macrophages to the site of invasion is induced by a gradient of concentration of the chemotactic substance that results in higher occupancy of the receptors on the leading edge of the macrophage than on its trailing end. Clearly, fixed macrophages cannot actively reach their targets and must instead entrap them. In the liver, lymph nodes, or spleen, macrophages are located near fluid channels that carry lymph or blood, and there they may contribute to removing microbes from these fluids.

Phagocytosis

Once a macrophage reaches its target, it recognizes friend from foe by another set of receptors[5-8] that detect (1) specific antibody covering the invader (recognized by Fc receptors), (2) complement fragments covalently bound to the surface of the invader (recognized by C3b or C3bi receptors), or (3) oligosaccharide moieties not present in the host (recognized by lipopolysaccharide [LPS] receptors and oligosaccharide receptors, also known as *lectins*). The contact of these receptors with ligands on the surface of the target triggers a local rearrangement of the cytoskeleton. The resulting movement of the membrane causes additional receptors to come in contact with ligands on the target, until the whole target is invaginated into the cell (the "zipper" mechanism). The connection to the outside of the cell is then pinched off to form a closed vacuole (phagosome).

Killing

Engagement of phagocytic receptors (especially Fc receptors) activates the microbicidal and digestive machinery of the macrophage, so that reactive oxygen intermediates, microbicidal and cytotoxic proteins, and hydrolytic enzymes are released into the phagocytic vacuole. In addition to these toxins, the microbe sequestered in the vacuole is also exposed to low pH and nutrient deprivation. This arrangement creates a highly biotoxic environment for the microbe while limiting the exposure of surrounding host cells to these potentially injurious influences.

The microbicidal mechanisms activated by phagocytosis include an enzyme system in the phagosomal membrane (NADPH oxidase) that transports electrons from NADPH (the reduced form of nicotinamide adenine dinucleotide phosphate) on the cytoplasmic "outside" of the phagosome to molecular oxygen inside the phagosome. The reduction of molecular oxygen yields superoxide, which is then converted to microbicidal hydrogen peroxide.[9] Another enzyme system, characterized extensively in murine macrophages, generates nitric oxide and related metabolites, some of which are microbicidal or cytotoxic. The role of this system in human macrophages is a subject of much interest but not yet well understood. Vesicles containing lysozyme, other digestive enzymes, and microbicidal and cytotoxic proteins fuse to the phagosome and deliver their contents. The pH of the vacuole, initially neutral, becomes acidic and may reach less than 5. The concentration of iron and perhaps other nutrients essential for microbes may decrease to a point at which the metabolic function of the microbe is compromised. The combined damage from these changes usually results in the death and digestion of the microbial invader.

Tissue Injury

Several proposed mechanisms would expose host tissues ("innocent bystander cells") to macrophage-derived cytotoxins. These include:

- Extracellular leakage of phagosomal contents
- Secretion of macrophage products in response to stimulation of macrophage plasma membrane in the absence of phagosome formation
- Release of preformed cytotoxins by injured or dying macrophages

In cell culture and certain animal models, macrophages can also exert selective cytotoxicity toward tumor cells by both antibody-dependent and antibody-independent mechanisms.[10] The extent to which these mechanisms contribute to tissue injury during infections or to host defense against human neoplasia is not known.

Microbial Countermeasures

Some microbes have evolved mechanisms that allow them to avoid destruction by macrophages. Certain fungi and bacteria are coated with materials that inhibit phagocytosis, others have cell walls or enzyme systems that help resist the macrophage toxins, and others somehow prevent the delivery of microbicidal and digestive proteins to the phagosome. A few species of bacteria can lyse the phagosomal membrane and escape into the cytoplasm (e.g., *Listeria*) and eventually leave the cell to infect its neighbor. Some bacteria (and perhaps all pathogenic ones), after entering the host, begin to synthesize new proteins that appear to be essential to their survival inside the macrophage and other host tissues. Certain pathogens have perfected all these survival mechanisms to the point that the macrophage is the predominant site of their multiplication (e.g., *Legionella, Histoplasma capsulatum*, some mycobacteria). The ability of macrophages to resist these intracellular pathogens is enhanced when they are exposed to various macrophage-activating factors, substances that include interferon-γ and TNF-α.

Recruitment of Additional Effector Cells

When stimulated by phagocytosis or certain soluble substances, macrophages release products that attract neutrophils (leukotriene B_4, IL-8) and lymphocytes (IL-8) to the site of infection or inflammation.

SCAVENGING FUNCTION

The ability of macrophages to break down senescent or necrotic cells and foreign particulate matter was appreciated even before their microbicidal role was known. Macrophages remove or degrade dust in the lungs, necrotic cells in wounds, injected particulates impacted in the pulmonary vasculature, and devolving structures during embryonic development. Specialized macrophages (osteoclasts) remodel bones, and other macrophages in the spleen recognize and destroy aging erythrocytes. Macrophages in atherosclerotic plaques ingest lipids and cholesterol, forming foam cells. Other macrophages participate in the lysis and degradation of blood clots and hematomas. Foreign body giant cells seen in areas of chronic antigenic or particulate stimulation are terminally differentiated forms of macrophages.

SECRETORY FUNCTION

Macrophages secrete various substances[11] that serve signaling or effector functions (Table 51–1). Some of these substances contribute to the acute response to microbial invasion by recruiting neutrophils to the site (leukotriene B_4, IL-8), generating a systemic febrile response and stimulating the synthesis of acute-phase proteins by the liver (IL-1, IL-6, TNF-α). Other secreted substances can kill microbes (lysozyme), tumor cells (TNF-α), or both (hydrogen peroxide, nitric oxide). Specialized enzymes (tissue metalloproteinases, fibrinolytic enzymes, and others) are secreted to degrade extracellular matrix and blood clot in areas of trauma or infection.[12] Yet other proteins may initiate or promote wound healing by stimulating fibroblast proliferation[12] and the formation of new capillaries[13] (transforming growth factor [TGF], basic fibroblast growth factor, platelet-derived growth factor). In animals selectively depleted of monocyte-macrophages, wound healing is impaired.

The macrophages also secrete substances that act on other host defense cells. They increase macrophage microbicidal activity (TNF-α) or decrease it (TGF-β), activate T lymphocytes (IL-1), or increase the production of neutrophils in the bone marrow (G-CSF, GM-CSF). The list of active substances secreted by macrophages is continually expanding, and only selected examples are listed in Table 51–1.

TABLE 51–1. Substances Secreted by Macrophages

Activity	Substances (Examples)
Chemotactic for neutrophils	Leukotriene B_4, IL-8
Growth factors (wound healing)	TGF-β, platelet-derived growth factor
Angiogenic factors	Basic fibroblast growth factor, TGF-β
Growth factors (hematopoietic)	GM-CSF, G-CSF
Acute-phase response, fever, signs of sepsis	TNF-α, IL-1, IL-6
Microbicidal substances	Lysozyme, hydrogen peroxide
Cytotoxic substances	TNF-α, hydrogen peroxide, nitric oxide
Macrophage-regulatory factors	TNF-α, TGF-β
Lymphocyte-regulatory factors	IL-1, IL-6
Lytic enzymes	Plasminogen activator, collagenase, elastase
Enzyme inhibitors	α_2-Macroglobulin, α_1-antitrypsin

G-CSF = granulocyte colony-stimulating factor; GM-CSF = granulocyte-macrophage colony-stimulating factor; IL = interleukin; TGF-β = transforming growth factor-β; TNF-α = tumor necrosis factor-α.

ANTIGEN-PRESENTING FUNCTION

Although macrophages are prominent effector cells, they also have an important initiating role in immune responses.[14, 15] When hosts immune to a pathogenic microbe are rechallenged with it, T lymphocytes that recognize the antigens respond by undergoing "activation": they (1) multiply and (2) release various *lymphokines*. Lymphokines are substances that regulate the function of other host defense cells, including macrophages and T and B lymphocytes. When the activation response was studied in vitro with purified populations of lymphocytes, it was found to be dependent on the presence of nonlymphocyte cells, termed *antigen-presenting (accessory) cells* (APCs). Cells that can act as APCs include macrophages, dendritic cells, and endothelial cells. Dendritic cells, the most potent APCs, are especially important in immune responses after primary exposure to a pathogen. These cells are now thought to be closely related to macrophages[16] and, like macrophages, may arise from blood monocytes under the influence of specific cytokines. They can be considered macrophages that are highly specialized for antigen presentation.

After phagocytosis by macrophages, microbes are killed and undergo proteolytic digestion. From the microbial proteins, small peptide fragments are generated. Some of these peptide fragments associate with newly synthesized carrier molecules, termed *major histocompatibility complex* (MHC) class II. The MHC class II and its associated peptide are transported to the macrophage membrane and displayed. When the macrophage makes contact with a T lymphocyte possessing receptors that recognize the peptide–MHC II combination, the T cell receptor binds to the peptide–MHC II combination and the T lymphocyte becomes activated. It has been suggested that this mode of antigen presentation prevents T cell receptors from being flooded by excess antigen because most antigens do not bind to the T cell receptor without prior processing and interaction with MHC molecules.

MACROPHAGE ACTIVATION

Previous exposure of the host to certain microbial pathogens (e.g., mycobacteria) subsequently produces an enhanced microbicidal response by macrophages. This response extends not only to the original microbial species but also, at least in part, to other microbes. The morphologic and biochemical changes that accompany the enhanced microbicidal response are defined as *activation*. Activated macrophages display increased plasma membrane ruffling, increased content of hydrolytic enzymes, enhanced production of reactive oxygen intermediates, and increased numbers of MHC class II molecules. The activation response can be reproduced by incubating macrophages with the secretory products of lymphocytes (T and natural killer cells) that have been challenged with certain microbes or microbial products.[17, 18]

Interferon-γ and TNF-α are the most important of the several activating factors purified from lymphocyte secretions. Genetically altered mice that lack interferon-γ or its receptor show poor macrophage activation in response to infection and are highly susceptible to intracellular parasites.

Macrophage activation is temporary. Specific factors that can deactivate macrophages have been identified (e.g., TGF-β and macrophage-deactivating factor).

MACROPHAGES AND ENDOTOXIN

Entry of gram-negative bacteria into the bloodstream elicits a well-known sequence of responses ranging from rigors and fever to hypoxemia and hypotension. Many, if not most, of these responses are generated by secretory products released by macrophages that interact with an LPS component of bacteria (LPS, endotoxin). Specifically, exposure of macrophages to LPS induces secretion of IL-1β, TNF-α, and IL-6, factors that can reproduce nearly all of the manifestations of endotoxemia.

Macrophages possess several sets of receptors for endotoxin, of which CD14 appears to be the main signaling receptor.[8] CD14 recognizes LPS bound to a serum factor, LPS-binding protein (LBP), and the ligation of CD14 by this complex activates the secretion of macrophage mediators. The multifunctional receptors include C3bi (CD11a/CD18), lymphocyte function–associated antigen 1 (CD11b/CD18), and p150,95 (CD11c/CD18), which interact with various surfaces, fibrinogen, adhesion molecules on other cells, and complement fragments. In relation to LPS, CD18 receptors may be important for nonopsonic (complement and antibody-free) phagocytosis of gram-negative bacteria and for removal and degradation of LPS from the bloodstream and tissues.

The third receptor type that may be important in the metabolism of LPS is the *scavenger receptor*, best known as the receptor that internalizes acetylated low-density lipoprotein. This receptor takes up various anionic ligands and transports them to lysosomes for degradation. The macrophages are particularly rich in scavenger receptors in the liver, where they may function to remove endotoxin from portal blood.

MACROPHAGES AND "MICROPHAGES"

The ability of macrophages to ingest and kill microbes was first described at the end of the 19th century by Ilya Mechnikoff, who distinguished them from the smaller "microphages," phagocytic cells today known as *granulocytes*. Although the cells overlap in some of their activities, they differ in many other respects (Table 51-2).

TABLE 51–2. Comparison of Macrophages and Granulocytes

Property	Macrophages	Granulocytes
Differ by organs and tissues	Yes	No
Mature cells can divide	Yes	No
Life span in tissues	Days to weeks	About 1 day
Phagocytosis	Yes	Yes
Generate reactive oxygen intermediates	Yes	Yes
Contain microbicidal proteins	Few known	Yes
Preformed cytoplasmic granules	Unusual	Abundant
Constitutive secretion	Yes	No
Secretion by degranulation	Limited	Prominent
Protein synthesis	Very active	Minimal
Deoxyribonucleic acid synthesis	Moderate	Inactive
Present antigen to T lymphocytes	Yes	Unknown

What is the evolutionary advantage of having two sets of phagocytes? It appears that the numerous granulocytes kept ready in several reserve compartments are rapid-deployment, "disposable" phagocytes, particularly well suited for time-limited and massive response to microbial invasion. The short life span and limited synthetic repertoire of granulocytes may make them inhospitable to intracellular parasites that would readily survive and multiply in macrophages. In contrast, the longer-lived and adaptive macrophages are better suited for tissue-specific patrol duties and prolonged response to chronic low-level infections.

SUMMARY

Macrophages, ubiquitous phagocytic and secretory cells, have a central role in host defense, inflammation, systemic response to infections, scavenging, and wound repair.

References

1. Johnston RB Jr: Monocytes and macrophages. N Engl J Med 1988; 318:747–752.
2. van Furth R: Development and distribution of mononuclear phagocytes. *In*: Inflammation: Basic Principles and Clinical Correlates. 2nd ed. Gallin JI, Goldstein IM, Snyderman R (Eds). New York, Raven Press, 1992, pp 325–339.
3. Golde DW, Baldwin GC: Myeloid growth factors. *In*: Inflammation: Basic Principles and Clinical Correlates. 2nd ed. Gallin JI, Goldstein IM, Snyderman R (Eds). New York, Raven Press, 1992, pp 291–301.
4. Lee SH, Starkey PM, Gordon S: Quantitative analysis of total macrophage content in adult mouse tissues. J Exp Med 1985; 161:475–489.
5. Raghavan M, Bjorkman PJ: Fc receptors and their interactions with immunoglobulins. Annu Rev Cell Dev Biol 1996; 12:181–220.
6. Brown EJ: Complement receptors and phagocytosis. Curr Opin Immunol 1991; 3:76–82.
7. Stahl PD: The mannose receptor and other macrophage lectins. Curr Opin Immunol 1992; 4:49–52.
8. Ulevitch RJ, Tobias PS: Receptor-dependent mechanisms of cell stimulation by bacterial endotoxin. Annu Rev Immunol 1995; 13:437–457.
9. Klebanoff SJ: Oxygen metabolites from phagocytes. *In*: Inflammation: Basic Principles and Clinical Correlates. 2nd ed. Gallin JI, Goldstein IM, Snyderman R (Eds). New York, Raven Press, 1992, pp 541–588.
10. Adams DO, Hamilton TA: Macrophages as destructive cells in host defense. *In*: Inflammation: Basic Principles and Clinical Correlates. Gallin JI, Goldstein IM, Snyderman R (Eds). New York, Raven Press, 1992, pp 637–662.
11. Nathan CF: Secretory products of macrophages. J Clin Invest 1987; 79:319–326.

12. DiPietro LA: Wound healing: The role of the macrophage and other immune cells. Shock 1995; 4:233–240.
13. Sunderkotter C, Steinbrink K, Goebeler M, Bhardwaj R, Sorg C: Macrophages and angiogenesis. J Leuk Biol 1994; 55:410–422.
14. Harding CV: Pathways of antigen processing. Curr Opin Immunol 1991; 3:3–9.
15. Unanue ER: Cellular studies on antigen presentation by class II MHC molecules. Curr Opin Immunol 1992; 4:63–69.
16. Peters JH, Gieseler R, Thiele B, Steinbach F: Dendritic cells: From ontogenetic orphans to myelomonocytic descendants. Immunol Today 1996; 17:273–278.
17. Bancroft GJ, Schreiber RD, Unanue ER: Natural immunity: A T-cell-independent pathway of macrophage activation, defined in the scid mouse. Immunol Rev 1991; 124:5–24.
18. Doherty TM: T-cell regulation of macrophage function. Curr Opin Immunol 1995; 7:400–404.

52

Regulation of Gene Expression

Timothy G. Buchman, PhD, MD, FACS, FCCM
Barbara A. Zehnbauer, PhD

This chapter consists of four parts. The first two parts are a brief, conventional overview of the programmed mechanisms regulating gene expression. The perspective is that of the research scientist and it reflects the reductionist approach to the field, emphasizing the progressively fine resolution to which the regulatory processes have been determined. The third part is an analysis of systems of genes illustrating regulatory effects which arise from linking the product of one gene to the expression of another. This fourth perspective is one of a clinician attempting to make sense of the complex interactions that characterize multiple, parallel, interacting pathways of signals and messages.

GENES: A HISTORICAL, REDUCTIONIST APPROACH[1]

Genes were originally defined in the context of the science of genetics as loci of developmental information associated with heritable characteristics. A relationship between genetic defects and metabolic abnormalities was first proposed by Garrod in 1909 after he realized that alkaptonuria (subsequently proven to be an error in tyrosine metabolism resulting in the excretion of homogentisic acid) was inherited by mendelian rules. The nature of the relationship between genes and metabolism remained obscure until the 1940s, when Beadle and Tatum demonstrated that each gene was responsible for one enzyme. Enzymes were already recognized to be catalytic proteins, but the genetic material had yet to be identified.

In 1944, Avery, MacLeod, and McCarty showed that a newly purified enzyme, deoxyribonuclease (DNA), selectively destroyed developmental information otherwise transferable between bacteria, implying that the enzyme's substrate, DNA, was in fact the bacterial "transforming principle." In 1952, Hershey and Chase reported that only the DNA portion of a bacterial virus—and not its protein coat—entered a (bacterial) cell, and this DNA was both necessary and sufficient to program viral replication. In 1953, Watson and Crick proposed a biophysical structure, the double helix, which not only accounted for the characteristic composition of DNA but also suggested a basis for semiconservative replication using each parental strand of the double helix as template from which a daughter strand was synthesized.

Gene Expression

Although ribonucleic acid (RNA) had been recognized as the link between DNA and protein by the 1950s, it remained for Nirenberg and colleagues to confirm the nature of that link. They prepared cell-free extracts containing ribosomes, transfer RNA molecules, adenosine triphosphate (ATP), and guanosine triphosphate (GTP)—everything except the RNA molecules that would later be termed messenger RNA (mRNA) molecules. When synthetic mRNA molecules (consisting of polymers of a single nucleotide) were added to these extracts, polypeptides consisting of a single amino acid were formed. Using these RNA homopolymers and simple heteropolymers, these investigators proved that RNA was the intermediate between DNA and protein and "cracked the second genetic code" by showing that addition of amino acid residues to a nascent polypeptide was programmed for by particular RNA triplets.

If gene expression reflects the number and activation state of protein molecules corresponding to a specific gene, then Nirenberg's work and that of his predecessors unequivocally separated gene expression into distinct and potentially regulatable steps. These include (1) transcription of RNA from a DNA template by a DNA-dependent RNA polymerase, (2) post-transcriptional modification of RNA into messenger form capable of being translated into polypeptide, (3) translation of mRNA into polypeptide by ribosomes, and (4) post-translational modification of the polypeptide chain into active protein.

Signals

The definition of a signal is also an operational one: Any environmental change leading to change in gene expression is a signal. The environmental change is typically a change in the local (extracellular) concentration of a particular molecule. Although signal molecules have traditionally been classified according to the distance between site of synthesis and site of action (i.e., endocrine, paracrine, and autocrine), a more useful classification divides signals according to their ability to penetrate the cytoplasmic membrane. Lipophilic thyroid and steroid hormones readily penetrate the cytoplasmic membrane. Receptors for these hormones are intracellular and therefore can have direct roles in the regulation of gene expression. Ligand binding causes these particular receptors to undergo a conformational change, thereby exposing a hidden portion of the receptor that binds promoter regions of DNA in a sequence-specific fashion.

Two points are important:

1. The receptor itself is capable of regulating gene expression according to occupancy of its binding site.
2. Such regulation occurs as a DNA sequence-specific interaction between the receptor protein and a portion of the promoter.

Because these receptors can bind both ligands and particular DNA sequences, transduction of the lipophilic hormone signals requires only this single messenger.

Other signals that are either large (e.g., proteins) or hydrophilic cannot penetrate the cytoplasmic membrane and therefore must be transduced through a receptor molecule extracellularly displayed at the cytoplasmic membrane. Such receptors are typically large, specialized protein molecules that are tightly anchored in (and therefore unable to leave easily) the cytoplasmic membrane. Although signal transduction begins by binding of the signal to this receptor at the cell surface, additional (second) messengers are required to transmit information from the inner aspect of the cytoplasmic membrane through the cell to points where gene expression is regulated. Although some cells (such as antigen-recognition cells) likely have thousands of unique receptors, receptors and their second messengers are amenable to mechanistic classification.

Seven-Pass Transmembrane Receptors

Gene Proteins

The largest family of cell-surface receptors are functionally linked to a specific class of intracellular molecules called G proteins. The cell-surface receptors are members of the seven-pass transmembrane protein family, so called because their amino acid sequence codes include a distinctive pattern of alternating hydrophobic and hydrophilic regions that serve to anchor the protein in the cell membrane: When inserted into the cell membrane, the protein snakes back and forth across the membrane seven times, creating extracellular and intracytoplasmic loops. The variable extracellular segments that determine their unique interactions respond to particular signals, such as peptide hormones. The third intracytoplasmic loop is the most variable and appears to select for the particular G protein that will ultimately generate a second messenger.

G Protein Structure and Mechanism

G proteins are heterotrimers consisting of α, β, and γ subunits. The β and γ subunits appear to be common to all G proteins, and thus it is the specific α subunit that defines precisely the activity of a G protein. Alpha subunits also characteristically bind guanylyl nucleotides and hydrolyze GTP into guanosine diphosphate (GDP). Quiescent G proteins are heterotrimers in which the α subunit has GDP in its binding site. Binding of a ligand to a seven-pass transmembrane receptor stimulates the G protein to partially liberate the α subunit from the β/γ complex, which in turn allows replacement of the resident GDP by GTP. Such replacement facilitates full dissociation of the α subunit, freeing it to activate other effector molecules, commonly adenylyl cyclase. The degree of signal amplification (e.g., how much cyclic adenosine monophosphate [cAMP] is generated) is variable and dependent at least in part on the half-life of the GTP residue on the particular α subunit. Hydrolysis of this GTP to GDP causes the α subunit to dissociate from the effector molecule and reassociate with the β/γ complex. Some α subunits ($G\alpha_s$) stimulate their effector, and others ($G\alpha_i$) inhibit it.

Intensivists practicing in developing nations are especially familiar with a regulatory error involving this second-messenger system because it is a leading cause of death among children: cholera. Cholera toxin attacks $G\alpha_s$ after GTP binding and prevents hydrolysis to GDP. This particular G protein stimulates adenyl cyclase. The massive diarrhea associated with cholera infection is directly attributable to the consequent sustained high levels of cAMP in intestinal epithelium. Receptor-linked G proteins also regulate the activity of phospholipase Cβ. The second messengers most closely associated with the latter enzyme are diacylglycerol (DAG), which activates protein kinase C, and inositol triphosphate (IP_3), which binds to intracellular receptors on the endoplasmic reticulum, which in turn release calcium ions into the cytosol.

Subtle mutations in the G protein system may have substantial impact on human critical illness. Studies of a group of hypertensive patients showed increased activity of a sodium-potassium transporter in blood cells. Transgenic mice overexpressing this protein retained salt and became hypertensive. A G_i-related signaling abnormality was then demonstrated in lymphoblasts, which also had increased sodium-potassium transporter activity, suggesting a genetic defect that was subsequently related to a polymorphism in four G_i genes. One of these G protein genes, *GNB3,* contains a single base polymorphism in which a C-to-T switch has occurred (C825T), and this allele has been shown to be overrepresented in a population of hypertensive patients in contrast to representation in normal controls. If the association of this allele with hypertension is substantiated by further studies, it may account for a substantial minority of cases of "idiopathic" hypertension.[5]

Tyrosine Kinases

The second important family of cell-surface receptors includes those hormone receptors that phosphorylate the aromatic hydroxyl group of tyrosine residues embedded in polypeptides. These *tyrosine kinases* transduce various polypeptide growth factors, including insulin and platelet-derived growth factors (PDGFs). These receptors are more varied in their structure than the seven-pass transmembrane receptors, yet all highly conserve the domain within the cytoplasmic region that catalyzes the phosphorylation of intracellular proteins.

Generally, these receptors are activated by a conformational change induced by ligand binding; the conformational change causes dimerization between like or similar receptor subunits. This dimerization results in cross-phosphorylation between these two tyrosine kinase molecules, a characteristic feature of this receptor family. The intracellular substrates for these tyrosine kinase enzymes are numerous, and it has been difficult to prove which ones are most physiologically important. Several tyrosine kinase receptors have been shown to activate phospholipase Cγ, which (like phospholipase Cβ) generates DAG and IP_3.

Other Receptors

A large class of injury-relevant membrane receptors is neither coupled to G proteins nor appears to possess intrinsic tyrosine kinase activity. These include receptors for growth hormone, prolactin, and many lymphokines and cytokines. For example, the interleukin-2 (IL-2) receptor has no intrinsic tyrosine kinase activity but interacts with an independent protein kinase when activated by IL-2. The binding of the activated IL-2 receptor to this protein kinase ($p56^{lck}$) results in changes in gene expression due to subsequent kinase reactions.

Many second messengers appear to converge through messenger-specific protein kinases toward protein phosphorylation as a final common regulatory mechanism.

Cyclic Adenosine Monophosphate

Historically, the first and most well-described second messenger is cAMP. Cyclic AMP acts as an allosteric regulator via activation of the cAMP-dependent protein kinase A (PKA). Cyclic AMP binds to a regulatory subunit of PKA, causing dissociation of another active catalytic subunit. This catalytic subunit then phosphorylates target proteins on serine-threonine residues using ATP as a cosubstrate. PKA activation is well known to regulate metabolic pathways acutely by phosphorylating target enzymes such as those that catalyze glycolysis. In addition to these metabolic and biochemical effects, however, PKA regulates gene expression by phosphorylation of DNA binding proteins that act as transcription factors. By this pathway, cAMP acts as a mediator between cell surface events and transcriptional activity.

Inositol Triphosphate-Calcium

The IP_3 mechanism that augments intracellular calcium concentration has already been suggested. Endotoxin is a familiar activator of this system. This newly released calcium then binds to calmodulin, a highly conserved cytoplasmic protein that can accommodate at least four calcium ions. This activated calmodulin has two primary effects. First, activated calmodulin regulates cAMP levels through activation of cyclic nucleotide phosphodiesterase, which degrades cAMP. Second, activated calmodulin itself activates a multifunctional protein kinase, calmodulin kinase.

Diacylglycerol

DAG, formed by the phospholipase C-catalyzed cleavage of phosphatidylinositol biphosphate (PIP_2), mediates an effect on gene expression by activation of protein kinase C, a calcium-dependent protein kinase.

MECHANISMS REGULATING GENE EXPRESSION

Initiation of Transcription

The expression of many genes is transcriptionally controlled through mechanisms that regulate the initiation of transcription. Although some nontranslated genes (e.g., genes coding for ribosomal RNA) are transcribed by RNA polymerases I and III, genes that code for proteins are transcribed by RNA polymerase II. Initiation of RNA synthesis by this enzyme requires several steps that involve binding of both regulatory and synthetic proteins to DNA sequences in the promoter and enhancer regions of genes.

Nucleosomes

Access to DNA is not trivial, because within the nucleus DNA is ordinarily compacted into nucleosomes. These globular structures are complexes of DNA and histone proteins. Histone proteins surround and charge-neutralize the DNA in a sequence-independent fashion. Each nucleosome includes about 180 base pairs of DNA and forms a structure that resembles beads (histone proteins) on a string (DNA). Although this arrangement is very efficient for close packing of DNA, transcription cannot begin until the nucleosomes are displaced to reveal the DNA sequences.

At least two distinct strategies exist for eukaryotic cells to displace nucleosomes and thereby allow RNA polymerase II to effect gene transcription: persistent displacement and induced displacement. A very few persistent nucleosome-free regions are sustained through the tight, sequence-specific binding of nonhistone proteins to the DNA. This arrangement is crucial to heat shock gene expression, which is the archetypal intracellular stress gene response. In the more common induced displacement mechanism, histones are initially displaced by the actions of nonspecific activator proteins. The displacement zones, which must include the promoter, are then occupied by sequence-specific DNA binding proteins (e.g., the activated thyroid hormone receptor). These sequence-specific binding proteins that regulate transcription are collectively called *nuclear factors.*

The promoter has at least two functional regions where the nucleosomes have to be displaced promptly. The first region is the *core promoter region,* which serves as the scaffolding on which RNA polymerase II and general initiation factors will bind to form the so-called transcription complex. This region contains the TATA box (see later), and without a TATA box, multiple transcription start sites are often active. The second functional region includes *DNA sequences* that are the target site of specific nuclear factors that are not required for initiation of transcription per se but regulate the rate at which RNA polymerase II initiates additional rounds of transcription at the core promoter region.

Transcription Complex

Initiation of transcription from the core promoter is a multistage process requiring the action of at least five initiation factor proteins and an ATP cofactor. The first stage of the process is site selection, which culminates in RNA polymerase II locating and binding selectively to the core promoter. First, an initiation protein called the TATA factor (also known as TFIID) locates a highly conserved DNA sequence called the TATA box. This TATA box, a TA-rich region of DNA, is absolutely required for transcription by RNA polymerase II. Binding of TATA factor to the TATA box forms an initial complex. Additional factors (α, TFIIB) and finally RNA polymerase II bind productively to complete the site selection process. However, the complex is not yet stable. Additional factors bind to stabilize protein-DNA contacts and anchor the proteins firmly to the DNA. Only then is the preinitiation complex complete. Subsequent activation of this complex appears to require hydrolysis of a molecule of ATP, which is not incorporated into the nascent RNA chain.

Regulatory Factors

The rate at which initiation of transcription occurs is modulated by the other promoter-enhancer DNA sequences or, more precisely, by the binding of "factors" (regulatory proteins) to those sequences. The target sequences, also known as *regulatory elements,* typically are stretches of DNA that are 6 to 20 base pairs in length and that often have dyadic symmetry. The proteins that bind to those elements have highly conserved DNA-binding domains that can be recognized on the basis of the secondary structures predicted by their amino acid sequences. These conserved DNA-binding domains have colorful names reflecting conserved structural features: the *zinc finger,* the *helix-turn-helix,* the *leucine zipper,* and the *basic helix-loop-helix.* It is the minor changes in protein structure adjacent to these regions that account for each factor's specificity with respect to its target element.

The interaction of a regulatory element with its nuclear factor can be envisioned as turning on a switch. The rate of initiation of transcription of a particular gene is regulated by the state of several such switches (i.e., a set of regulatory elements that bind specific nuclear factors). This combinatorial approach allows for tissue specificity in gene expression. It also allows for the alteration in the expression of multiple genes on transduction of a single signal.

Clearly, the activation of nuclear factors to initiate binding to regulatory elements must be very fast and tightly controlled. Three general mechanisms are operative.[5, 6] The first is *compartmentalization*; the factor can be sequestered in the cytoplasm and maintained inactive through lack of access to the regulatory elements. Second, the factor can be covalently modified to affect the DNA-binding site. Third, the factor can be covalently modified distant from the DNA-binding site in the region where it interacts with the initiation complex, the so-called *transactivation domain.* Interestingly, all of these mechanisms have been observed in nuclear factors relevant to injury/critical care. An example, but by no means a prototype, is NF-κB.

The nuclear factor NF-κB is a heterodimeric protein. Although it was originally identified in association with B cell–specific transcription factors, it is now recognized to regulate gene expression in response to phorbol esters, antigens, cytokines, ultraviolet irradiation, and virus infection. This heterodimer consists of two subunits, p50 and p65, which themselves are ordinarily bound in the cytoplasm by a third inhibitor protein molecule, IκB. The general mechanism requires that the inhibitor disassociate from the p50-p65 heterodimer so that the latter can translocate to the nucleus.

The biology of IκB has recently come into clearer focus to reveal a series of enzymes which regulate the phosphorylation state, and thereby the activity, of the inhibitor. This is important because it points to no fewer than four distinct mechanisms by which this nuclear factor itself is regulated:

- Expression of the component proteins
- Activation state of at least one component protein
- Translocation from the cytoplasm to the nucleus
- Binding to target DNA sequences

The web of mechanisms regulating the activity of this factor is unlikely to be unique and suggests that while the activation state of any factor may provide limited insight into the state of that web, the activity of even several factors may be insufficient to describe the activation state of the cell as a whole.

Enhancers and Locus Control Regions

All genes have *promoters.* Initiation of transcription of some genes is further regulated by enhancers and by locus control regions. Enhancers differ from promoters by virtue of the great distance (up to 40,000 nucleotides) over which they can influence a particular gene. Enhancers escape not only the adjacency requirement but also the directionality requirement of promoters; that is, they can be flipped end over end and reinserted into the DNA sequence, and they work perfectly well. Enhancers typically contain several regulatory elements that can bind activating (or suppressing) factors. Many such factors are cell type–specific. Multimerization of enhancers characteristically potentiates transcription.

Locus control regions are similar to enhancers but typically regulate the expression of multiple gene loci during normal growth and development. They are functionally distinguished from enhancers in that multimerization does not potentiate transcription. The β-globin locus is an example of a locus regulated by such a control region.

Promoters, enhancers, and locus control regions all have regulatory elements, and all appear to regulate initiation of transcription by element-specific binding of regulatory proteins.

Transcript Elongation

Conspicuous by its absence from this discussion is any mention of the rate of elongation of transcripts after initiation. With one notable exception (heat shock; see later), this potential regulatory mechanism appears to be unrealized or at least unrecognized. RNA polymerase II adds about 50 nucleotides per second to nascent transcripts, retarded nonspecifically by the requirement to free DNA from nucleosomes.

Transcript Processing: Appearance of Messenger Ribonucleic Acid

Soon after transcription begins, the free 5′ end of the transcript undergoes the first of three modifications required for the transcript to function as mRNA. This first modification is the addition of a methylated cap structure that requires the catalyzed formation of a unique 5′-5′ guanylyl-nucleotidyl phosphodiester bond followed by methylation of guanylyl residue at nitrogen-7. This capping event, although catalyzed, is not considered an important control point in the regulation of gene expression.

The second modification is the addition of a characteristic polyadenylylate (polyA) tail to the 3′ end of the just completed transcript. This modification is also a two-step process requiring site-directed cleavage of the primary transcript to expose a 3′-hydroxyl group to which polyA is promptly added. Interestingly, the only eukaryotic transcripts that escape this tailing requirement are those that code for histone proteins.

The third modification is splicing of the RNA molecule. Splicing is required for many, but not all, eukaryotic RNAs (heat shock RNA is an important exception) and involves site-specific excision of RNA sequences with resealing of the parent molecule. The process often occurs in defined organelles (spliceosomes). The time required for splicing reactions varies from seconds to a half hour. This splicing time is probably transcript specific but appears to be not subject to acute regulation. Only after all three of these modifications are completed can the transcript be properly identified as mRNA and be transported to the cytoplasm.

Stability of Messenger Ribonucleic Acid

None of the modifications catalogued in the preceding paragraphs appear to be acutely regulated by external signals; these modifications, however, do strongly affect the stability of the newly synthesized mRNA molecule. Degradation of mRNAs is a highly regulated process that can determine the level of expression of a gene, and the mere existence of highly unstable mRNAs allows for tight titration against transcription rates to precisely fix specific transcript levels.

At least seven different destabilizing elements have been found in mRNAs. No structure has yet been identified as conferring special stability on mRNAs: They are intrinsically stable molecules within the cell cytoplasm and remain stable until translated unless one or more of the destabilizing elements is present. Some of the destabilizing elements are nonspecific. For example, as mRNAs age, their polyA tail is progressively shortened. When the polyA tail length falls below a critical level of about 10 residues, degradation of the message occurs quickly.

Other destabilizing elements are message-specific and sequence-specific. An example is the UA-rich motif, also called the *AU-rich element* (ARE). This motif was initially identified as a repeating octamer in the 3′ untranslated region of mRNA molecules encoding many cytokines, including interferon-γ and tumor necrosis factor-α. It was shown to accelerate degradation of these cytokine mRNAs by creating chimeric genes in which the UA-rich sequences were coded into other RNA molecules. These chimeric transcripts became unstable.

Translation: Overview

Translation of mRNA into protein is a complex process that consists of three stages:

1. Initiation of translation.
2. Elongation of the nascent polypeptide chain.
3. Termination/release of the protein from the ribosome.

The rate-limiting step in the process, in nearly all cases, occurs during the initiation stage. This stage comprises two steps: (1) an mRNA among many available mRNAs is selected for translation, and (2) the ribosome identifies the initiator codon in the message and begins translation.

Elongation is a cyclic process in which transfer RNA molecules add additional amino acid residues to the C-terminal end of the nascent polypeptide chain. Termination is the release of the completed polypeptide from the ribosome. Initiation involves at least 10 polypeptide cofactors (eIFs), elongation requires at least four polypeptide cofactors, and termination requires polypeptide release factor.

Global Regulation of Translation

Global regulation of translation is well characterized and occurs primarily through changes in the phosphorylation state of initiation factors, particularly eIF-2. Cofactor eIF-2 is a cytoplasmic G protein (see earlier) that ordinarily cycles through

GTP hydrolysis and GDP binding. When elF-2 is bound to GDP, it becomes accessible to a particular kinase; if phosphorylated, it becomes inactive. Moreover, this inactive form traps another factor (G elongation factor [GEF]) crucial for initiation. This trapping mechanism is so powerful that phosphorylation of only 25% of the elF-2 pool essentially abolishes protein synthesis. It is unclear whether a global decline in translation actually constitutes a specific regulatory mechanism.

Regulation of Specific Messenger Ribonucleic Acid Translation

Very few examples of mRNA-specific proteins regulating translation in eukaryotic cells can be cited. The example that most closely affects injury and critical care concerns iron homeodynamics. Iron is essential to nearly all mammalian cells. Within the cell, bound iron is present in heme and in iron-sulfur clusters, and it is directly associated with a number of proteins catalyzing such essential functions as respiration and DNA synthesis. Free iron is toxic, producing the highly damaging hydroxyl radical via Fenton chemistry. Intracellular iron levels control the expression of key proteins. The control is exerted through specific mRNA-protein interactions in the cytoplasm, not the nucleus (this is *post-transcriptional,* not *transcriptional* regulation).

The key players are the iron regulatory proteins, IRP-1 and IRP-2. They are cytoplasmic regulators which share 79% homology and act to bind conserved mRNA stem-loops, which are the iron-responsive elements (IRE). This binding controls mRNA translation or stability itself. When the iron supply to cells is increased, IRP-1 is post-translationally inactivated while IRP-2 is degraded. Thus, the IREs are left unbound when iron is in excess. The physiologic consequence of being left unbound is that the two ferritin chains are translated at maximal rates, as are erythroid 5-ALA synthase and several enzymes of the citric acid cycle including mitochondrial aconitase. The unbound IRE of the transferrin receptor mRNA makes the latter highly unstable. As a consequence, the receptor concentration falls rapidly and iron is not absorbed by this mechanism into the cell.[6]

Small Molecules: Nitrosative and Oxidative Stress Effects on Gene Expression

Continuing with the iron example, iron metabolism is also highly regulated by nitrosative and oxidative stress. Regarding nitrosative stress, macrophages stimulated with interferon-γ and endotoxin induce both nitric oxide (NO) synthesis and binding of IREs by both IRPs. The activation is NO-dependent. Moreover, some cells do not even require the cytokine stimulation; NO-releasing drugs turn on the IREs in erythroid lineage cells, fibroblasts, and even brain slices. (The transferrin receptor mRNA synthesis falls because the inflammatory cytokine-based suppression outweighs the NO stimulation—anti-inflammatory cytokines IL-4 and IL-13 reverse the suppression.) Moreover, iron in the presence of inflammatory cytokine stimulation shuts down transcription of the inducible NO synthase (iNOS). Thus, inflammatory cytokines turn on both NO synthesis and iron accumulation; then the iron accumulation can shut off NO synthase—a tight feedback loop.

The link between iron and oxidative stress exists in both bacterial and eukaryotic cells but via different mechanisms. In eukaryotic cells, IRP-1 responds to hydrogen peroxide by losing its aconitase activity (NO also inactivates aconitase at acid pH) but increasing its IRE-binding activity; transferrin receptor expression increases while ferritin synthesis falls. Thus hydrogen peroxide tends to increase the pool of free iron, facilitating Haber-Weiss reactions. This process takes under an hour, in contrast to the NO effects which can take 15 hours. Moreover, although NO has to be continuously present to exert its effects, hydrogen peroxide exposure need only be brief; the rise in IRP-1/IRE binding and effect continues after the hydrogen peroxide is withdrawn.

Superoxide and NO combine to form peroxynitrite. The effect of peroxynitrite on IRP function and gene expression is presently contested.

Reinitiation of Translation as a Regulatory Mechanism

Reinitiation of translation in a different reading frame is a complex mechanism that has been observed so far only in yeast. It is of particular interest to intensivists because this regulatory mechanism is triggered by starvation. The mechanism involves the biosynthesis of a yeast-specific transcription factor, GCN4. Although transcripts of GCN4 are made constitutively and ribosomes bind to the message, no protein is made. Apparently, the ribosomes start to scan the message, looking for open reading frames (translation start sites), and get stuck in two small open reading frames upstream from the real coding portion of the message. When the yeasts are starved, the ribosomes scan past through the upstream regions and translate the GCN4 protein. This GCN4 protein is intrinsically active, functioning as a nuclear factor to promote transcription of 30 to 40 genes coding for enzymes required for amino acid biosynthesis.

Termination of Protein Synthesis

Termination of protein synthesis, formerly considered a general and fundamental event culminating in release of the protein product, is increasingly regarded as a pause signal regulating gene expression. The regulatory mechanisms affecting bacterial stop signals have only begun to be recognized; the role of this mechanism in eukaryotic cells remains indeterminate at present.

BOTTOM-UP AND TOP-DOWN APPROACHES

The scholar should know; one builds science with the facts just like a house can be built of stones; but an accumulation of facts is not a science just like a pile of stones is not a house.

HENRI POINCARÉ

Neither does a collection of regulatory mechanisms help the clinician understand why the patient is not responding to therapy. For this reason, it is important to examine the regulation of gene expression from a different vantage point using a "top-down" instead of a "bottom-up" view.

Gene Expression in the Intensive Care Unit

The spectrum of processes and interventions managed in the intensive care unit ranges from those mechanical problems and solutions that are clearly unrelated to gene expression (e.g., pneumothorax and tube thoracostomy) to those that have an unequivocal genetic basis and therapy (e.g., sickle cell crisis and exchange transfusion). Rather than classify all possible patient presentations and therapies according to the extent to which gene expression might play a part, it is more practical to begin by classifying abnormalities in gene expression and discuss familiar examples.

Congenital Errors

Congenital errors are primarily inherited but may not become clinically significant until childhood or even adulthood; thus, pediatric and adult intensivists confront congenital errors. One common series of error affects the β-globin gene, including sickle cell anemia and β-thalassemia (Cooley's anemia). Although sickle cell anemia had long been recognized as an inherited disease, identification of the molecular error dates only to 1956, when Ingram isolated globin from the blood of patients with sickle cell, cleaved the protein with sequence-specific proteases, and separated the peptide fragments by a combination of electrophoresis and chromatography to create a two-dimensional fingerprint. Ingram showed that a single amino acid substitution in a single gene was sufficient to account for the entire pathologic presentation of sickle cell anemia; subsequent investigators would prove that this substitution was caused by a point mutation in the DNA coding for β-globin.

The electrophoretic techniques used by Ingram were subsequently applied to β-thalassemia. The amino acids all were correct, but the amount of β-globin protein produced was insufficient. The fact that β-thalassemia also followed a recessive pattern of mendelian inheritance was proof that genes had two functional domains: a structural domain and a regulatory domain. In other words, the gene encoded not only the amino acid sequence of its protein product but also regulatory information that controlled the rate at which that protein was produced.

Congenital errors include inherited errors as well as sporadic mutations affecting germline DNA. Treatment has primarily focused on inherited errors and particularly on recessively inherited errors. The reason for this treatment focus is that correction of recessive errors can be accomplished in three distinctly different ways:

1. By replacement of a defective gene by a gene.
2. By replacement of a cell carrying the "correct" gene and its product (e.g., exchange transfusions for sickle cell anemia).
3. By replacement of the correct gene product itself (e.g., the administration of factor VIII for hemophilia).

Another feature of correction of recessive errors is that replacement typically need not be complete; restoration of a gene product to 1% to 10% of normal levels is often sufficient to correct the biochemical defect. Dominant heritable errors typically cause minimal physiologic disturbances. This is both understandable and fortunate—understandable in that a severe physiologic disturbance alleviates reproductive success and the mutation would therefore be expected to die out, and fortunate in that correction of a dominant error theoretically requires interventions aimed at every cell with faulty gene expression. Such intervention is now confined to animal research strategies aimed at the fertilized ovum and is beyond the current scope of clinical care.

Acquired Errors in Genes

Acquired errors in genes are common but are almost always silent for two reasons. First, effective immune surveillance identifies and eradicates affected cells. One familiar example of acquired error is the acquisition of new viral genes associated with acute infection. That human viruses commonly produce thousands of progeny per infected cell stands as mute testimony to the efficiency of a normal immune system in eradicating cells that are recognized as having acquired such errors. Second, acquired errors in genes and their expression generally are clinically insignificant because most errors are either insignificant or adversely affect the cell that has acquired the error. It is the uncommon but clinically significant error acquired by a single cell that affects a regulatory protein and either enhances cell replication or prolongs cell survival.

Either way, the result is a malignancy. Although a detailed review of the affected genes is more appropriately the province of molecular oncology, these genes are also of interest to intensivists precisely because their products regulate expression of many other genes. They fall into two classes. *Tumor suppressor genes* (also known as *anti-oncogenes*) are genes expressed in normal cells whose products typically regulate key steps in cell replication. *Oncogenes* are abnormal homologues of normal cellular genes whose products have key roles in the regulation of signal transduction or gene expression.

Abnormal Expression of Normal Genes

Abnormal expression of normal genes is perhaps the error most commonly encountered by intensivists. Examples include the hypoadrenalism and hypothyroidism associated with pituitary ablation, the disseminated inflammatory process that precedes development of the multiple organ dysfunction syndrome, and the rejection of a transplanted allograft. The common theme is that the regulatory failure is due to neither the regulatory nor the structural domain of the affected gene but, rather, to the insufficiency or excess of regulatory signals such as hormones and cytokines. In other words, the activation state of the regulatory web should be sufficient to define the subsequent pattern of gene expression.

We observe that the smooth and seemingly continuous signal-response behavior of a tissue (group of cells) is a purely statistical phenomenon; individual cells in a population have idiosyncratic signal-response patterns governed by the activation state of other genes and products in each specific cell. Ko and colleagues[7] demonstrated that clonally derived cells, each carrying a single copy of a beta-galactosidase reporter gene driven by a promoter consisting of one type of steroid-responsive element, had idiosyncratic responses to exposure to the steroid in their environment. Since each cell in a particular clone had experienced an identical life history, the Ko experiment demands a probabilistic interpretation for regulation of gene expression analogous to the use of statistical mechanics to explain continuous behavior of quantized atoms.

From the standpoint of the intensivist dealing with critical illness, the design of regulatory interventions should alter the probability that the genetic network of a cell will assume a particular state as opposed to "turning on" or "turning off" a single node in that regulatory web. Given that every human cell contains a hundred thousand genes, and of those genes several thousand are active at any particular moment, the rational manipulation of gene expression appears impossible at first glance. The strategies emerge only when a model system is examined.

The NK System

A useful model system is the NK system, described by Kauffman,[2] which consists of N genes each regulated by $K < N$ genes in the model network. In this system, each gene is allowed to be either active or quiescent (on or off, 1 or 0) at each time step, and the activity of each gene at time T signifies the influence of that gene product on other genes at time $T + 1$. For the sake of simplicity, we consider here only the simplest of NK systems, namely one of several systems of $N = 3$ genes whose activity is exclusively regulated by each of the other $K = 2$ gene products. In this system, the activity of each gene at time $T + 1$ is completely determined by the activity of the two other genes at time T. The determination follows the random assignment of Boolean operators to each of the N genes (Figs. 52–1 and 52–2).

Kauffman has shown for NK networks with $K = 2$, the

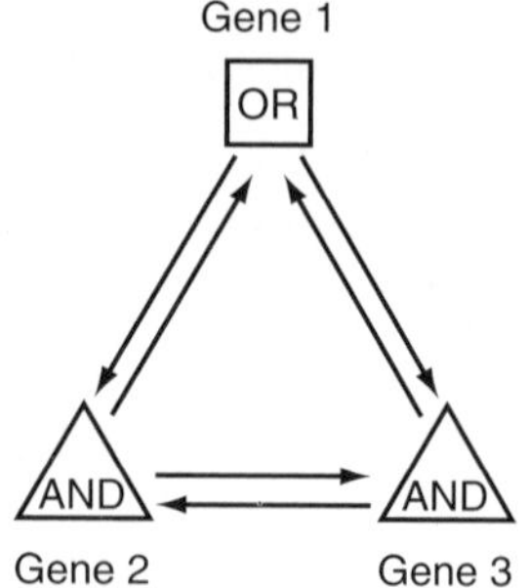

"Rules" of the network

1. Time passes in discrete steps.

2. The state of each gene at time "T" determines the state of each gene at time "T + 1."

3. There are no external influences.

Figure 52–1. A genetic network. N=3; K=2. If the three genes in the network were independent of one another, the network could exist in $2 \times 2 \times 2 = 2^3 = 2^N$ states. The number of stable states for a connected network is always smaller. The "transition table" for this connected network is as follows.

number of stable states is approximately $N^{1/2}$. If each of the 100,000 genes of the human cell was influenced by approximately two other gene products, the number of stable states would be 200 to 300, approximately the number of distinct cell types in human beings. This implies that each cell type had only a few stable states.

Returning to the N = 3, K = 2 model, it is instructive to observe that transitions among the states occur only when an external force acts on the network (Fig. 52–3). This external force could be (1) the binding of a ligand transduced through a second messenger, (2) a direct effect on a gene product or transcription factor such as heat, or (3) a mutation in the gene itself. It is even more instructive to consider what happens to this particular network if we introduce the slightest stochastic component to the state of any particular gene. Suppose that any of the three genes has a low level probability (e.g., 1:100 time steps) of changing itself from "on" to "off" or "off" to "on" at any given moment. Further consider that the "on" to "off" probability is slightly greater (1:199) than the "off" to "on" probability (1:201). Inspection of the transition diagram (see Fig. 52–3) shows that even this slight stochastic component in an otherwise deterministic system is sufficient to guarantee return of this gene network to the least activated state once the external force is removed. This model lends credence to the notion that our major role as intensivists in manipulation of gene expression is to nullify the external force and allow the activated network to return to a basal state. This model also suggests that any additional interventions should be aimed toward facilitating the transition from an activated to a basal state (see Fig. 52–3).[4]

AUTHOR'S PERSPECTIVE

Whereas management of congenital or acquired errors in gene structure or expression can be directed at a single gene, abnormal expression, particularly that due to signal excess, rarely affects individual genes. No "shock" or "injury" gene has been identified; rather, hundreds of them exist. Although the tools of molecular biology provide unique insight into the mechanisms regulating expression of these genes, it may well be insufficient to explain (much less suggest therapeutic approaches to) critical illnesses such as multiple organ dysfunction syndrome. Basic and clinical investigators, therefore, have focused on identifying signals transduced at the cell membrane, predicated on the view that neutralization of categorically harmful signals is sufficient to alter adverse gene expression and improve outcome. Unfortunately, individual signals and the genes they ultimately regulate cannot be as easily categorized or manipulated. More sophisticated approaches certainly are required to affect outcome in a predictable and salutary way.

A more intricate view of signaling and regulation of gene expression in critical illness—one that explicitly accounts for the interactions among multiple genes and multiple programs of gene expression—may ultimately prove even more useful to clinicians. This view predicts that gene expression is a self-organizing process.[2, 3] In particular, not all combinations of gene expression are possible, and cells are afforded surprisingly few stable metabolic states. This view predicts that signals and their intracellular second messengers converge not merely to regulate changes in gene expression but, rather, to facilitate transitions among metabolic states characterized according to expression of representative genes. By extension, these regulatory mechanisms would establish an implicit priority among metabolic states, and the collection of signals impinging on each cell would determine the probability of transitions between particular states.

ACKNOWLEDGMENT

Supported in part by award GM 48095 from the National Institutes of Health.

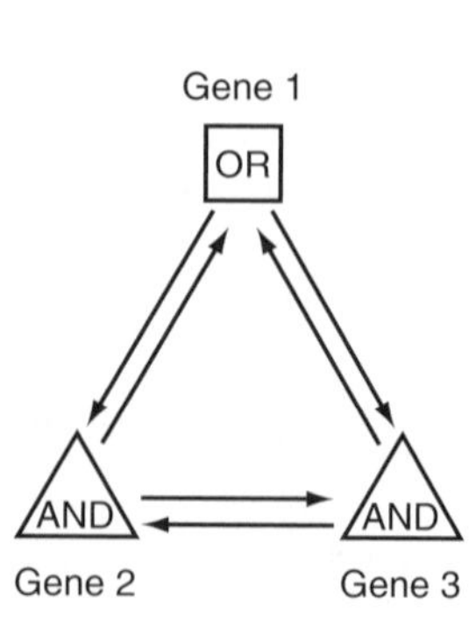

If the genes have this activity at time "T" . . .			. . .then the genes have this activity at time "T + 1"		
G1	G2	G3	G1	G2	G3
0	0	0	0	0	0
0	0	1	1	0	0
0	1	0	1	0	0
0	1	1	1	0	0
1	0	0	0	0	0
1	0	1	1	1	0
1	1	0	1	0	1
1	1	1	1	1	1

Figure 52–2. Transitions of the network. Inspection shows that this connected network has only three stable states.

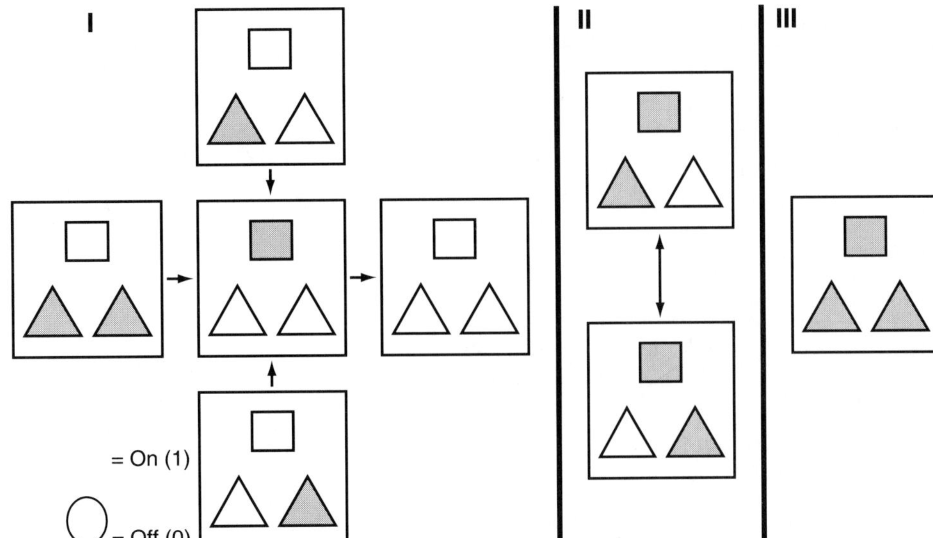

Figure 52–3. State cycles of the genetic network.

References

The first reference is a superb introduction to molecular cell biology and the regulation of gene expression. The second reference remains one of the most thought-provoking works on biologic organization ever written. The third expands the notion of states to approach concepts of increasing relevance to intensivists. The fourth is a pointer to an expanded presentation on the distinction between stability and state from which the sample NK network was derived.

1. Lodish H, Baltimore D, Berk A, Zipursky L: Molecular Cell Biology. 3rd ed. New York, Scientific American, 1995.
2. Kauffman SA: The Origins of Order: Self-Organization and Selection in Evolution. New York, Oxford University Press, 1993.
3. Chauvet GA: La Vie dans la Matière: Le Rôle de l'Espace en Biologie. Paris, Flammarion, 1995.
4. Buchman TG: Physiologic stability and physiologic state. J Trauma 1996; 41:599–605.
5. Siffert W, Rosskopf D, Siffert G, et al: Association of human G-protein beta 3 subunit variant with hypertension. Nature Genet 1998; 18:45–48.
6. Hentze MW, Kühn LC: Molecular control of vertebrate iron metabolism: mRNA based regulatory circuits operated by iron, nitric oxide and oxidative stress. Proc Natl Acad Sci USA 1996; 93:8175–8182.
7. Ko MS, Nakauchi H, Takahashi N: The dose dependence of glucocorticoid-inducible gene expression results from changes in the number of transcriptionally active templates. EMBO J 1990; 9:2835–2842.

53

Genetic Influences on Critical Illness

Barbara A. Zehnbauer, PhD • Marjorie Romkes, PhD
Joseph A. Carcillo, Jr., MD

Epidemiology models hold that a combination of environmental, genetic, and social factors contribute to disease outcomes. Recent advances in molecular genetics have enabled investigation of the role of genetic influences on disease outcomes in critically ill patients. This chapter (1) outlines genetic principles that account for inter-individual differences in susceptibility and response to disease and (2) illustrates some documented examples of genetic variations associated with differences in patient response to disease and therapy. The examples herein represent only a short list of known genetic influences in critical illness.

GENETIC PRINCIPLES

Genetic predispositions to a variety of inherited single-gene disorders from errors of metabolism to cancer have been characterized. Predisposing genetic variations or *polymorphisms* also contribute to the incidence of complex, multigene disorders. Common clinical diseases not recognized as heritable in *incidence* may have features of heritable *risk,* which influence disease severity or outcome. This increased risk, conferred by a polymorphic predisposition in susceptible individuals, may be subtle; unlike patients with inborn errors of metabolism, individuals with susceptibility or resistance to the effects of external agents are usually clinically well until the eliciting environment or substance is encountered. The adverse response may involve a time lag between the exposure and clinical manifestations in such a way that the link may be difficult to establish. Familial inheritance of the predisposing condition may be difficult to ascertain unless several family members are similarly exposed.

Human genetic markers have evolved from blood group types, electrophoretic mobility variants of serum proteins, and human leukocyte antigen (HLA) types to deoxyribonucleic acid (DNA) sequence polymorphisms. DNA polymorphisms define two or more alternative genotypes in a population, each at a frequency greater than that which could be attributed to mutation.[4] Usually, polymorphic alleles are present in a population at a frequency of at least 1%. These markers exhibit mendelian inheritance patterns and are widely distributed throughout the genome. Since the late 1970s, DNA polymorphisms have become increasingly important in the construction of human genetic maps and are relatively easy to localize on the physical map of the human genome.

Several types of polymorphic DNA markers are in use (Table 53–1), including:

- Restriction fragment length polymorphisms (RFLP)
- Variable number of tandem repeats (VNTRs) or minisatellites
- Dinucleotide, trinucleotide, or tetranucleotide (or microsatellite) repeats

TABLE 53–1. Polymorphic Genetic Markers

Marker	No. of Alleles	Size of Repeat	% Heterozygosity	No. of Loci in Genome	Example
RFLP (restriction fragment length polymorphism)	2	1 bp change (site)	30–50	$>10^5$	TNF genes, Nco1 sites
VNTR (variable number tandem repeats)	2–20	14–20 bp consensus	33–94	$>10^4$	pYNZ22.1
Minisatellite repeats	>50	9–45 bp consensus	90–99	$>10^2$	D1S7
Microsatellite repeats	>10	2, 3, or 4 bp	>90	$>10^4$	CA_n, AAT_n, $GATA_n$

bp = base pair; TNF = tumor necrosis factor.

In general, polymorphic alleles at each location must be easily distinguishable from one another in order to trace their inheritance patterns in a genetic map. RFLPs are site polymorphisms resulting from variations in DNA sequence that create or destroy specific cleavage sites for restriction endonucleases. This variability is detected as a change in the size of DNA fragments produced by cutting with restriction enzymes (Fig. 53-1*A*). This site alteration results in two different versions or alleles for the marker region.

Three different patterns are possible for a site polymorphism:

- Two copies with the site (+/+)
- Two copies without the site (−/−)
- Heterozygote (+/− or −/+) for one copy of each allele

VNTRs and microsatellites are length polymorphisms that differ by varying the number of repeated copies of a consensus DNA sequence (see Fig. 53-1*B* and 53-1*C*) between two consistent restriction enzyme sites. As the number of repeated copies varies, many different-sized polymorphic alleles result and generate genetic heterozygosity with high frequency. The diversity or informativeness of a polymorphism is based in its ability to distinguish the DNA from individuals in the population as different; thus, the potential to generate many different patterns is key to the marker's utility. Polymerase chain reaction (PCR) techniques using primer sequences that flank the polymorphism make mapping and diagnostic screening with microsatellite markers relatively quick and straightforward.

Gene-disease correlations may be made between the clinical symptoms of the disease (phenotype) and the polymorphic marker pattern or length (genotype) by linkage analysis in family studies or by statistical association in population studies (Table 53-2). *Linkage analysis* reveals a physical proximity between the disease gene and the marker locus within a specific kindred. Genetic association studies do not examine familial inheritance patterns but are case-control studies comparing unrelated affected and unaffected individuals from a population. *Positive association* is a concurrence between disease and marker alleles within a population that is greater than predicted by chance.[1] Association studies using polymorphic DNA markers are most significant when the genetic variations have functional significance and are related to the biology of the disorder. This approach may provide insight into susceptibility and pathogenesis of a disease thereby identifying genetic factors of the disease. Examples of genetic association are resistance to malaria with the sickle cell anemia allele, the increased incidence of ankylosing spondylitis in unrelated individuals with the B27 HLA type, and the incidence of diabetes mellitus in persons with the A type of the ABO blood group.[2]

Marker and disease gene associations are usually not equivalent to *physical* linkage (Fig. 53-2). Occasionally, linkage disequilibrium may be observed when there is a nonrandom association of marker and disease alleles caused by physical linkage of both loci, as observed with HLA-H C282Y marker and the gene for hemochromatosis.[5] A key component of the strength of statistical association in population studies is the composition of the healthy control population, which must represent the same composition as the population from which the patients are drawn. The healthy group must be typical of the patient population to avoid artifacts due to different allele frequencies inherent in different ethnic subgroups (founder effects).[1] A study of the genotypes of the affected individuals and their parents provides an artificial internal control that is well matched for ethnic ancestry. Genetic association within a population is a method for ascertaining genetic influences on disease phenotype when family studies are neither available nor feasible.

THE INFLAMMATORY RESPONSE

DNA polymorphisms in several genes for inflammatory functions produce stable variations in cytokine production that are positively associated with susceptibility to sepsis and multiple organ system failure. Genetic variation within the tumor necrosis factor (TNF) locus, one of the best-studied, polymorphic genes in inflammatory responses, has been important in determining susceptibility to, or severity of, a significant number of critical illnesses, including infectious diseases and septic shock.[6]

The pathophysiology of sepsis may be elicited in both animals and humans by the direct infusion of TNF alone. The TNF-α and TNF-β gene cluster contains two polymorphic sites for the restriction enzyme Nco 1 (RFLPs): one located in the promoter region for TNF-α and another in the first intron of TNF-β.[7] A single base change (G → A at base pair −308 in TNF-α and A → G at base pair [bp] 1069 within the first intron of TNF-β) creates or destroys the polymorphic scission site for this enzyme. The polymorphisms define two alternative alleles at each of these positions (TNF-α A1 and A2 plus TNF-β B1 and B2). Each allele with loss of an Nco 1 site (TNFA2 and TNFB2) correlates with increased synthesis of TNF and exacerbation of inflammatory responses.[7] This does not imply that the polymorphism itself causes increased TNF expression; however, it may be used as a marker to trace the occurrence of the allele and its possible correlation with specific clinical manifestations.[1]

McGuire and colleagues[9] hypothesized that although cerebral malaria occurred in a small fraction of malaria patients, a critical determinant was thought to be an elevated level of TNF-α associated with disease severity. Previous studies had shown a 10-fold higher plasma TNF-α concentration in children with cerebral malaria compared to those with mild malaria. These workers molecularly characterized the presence

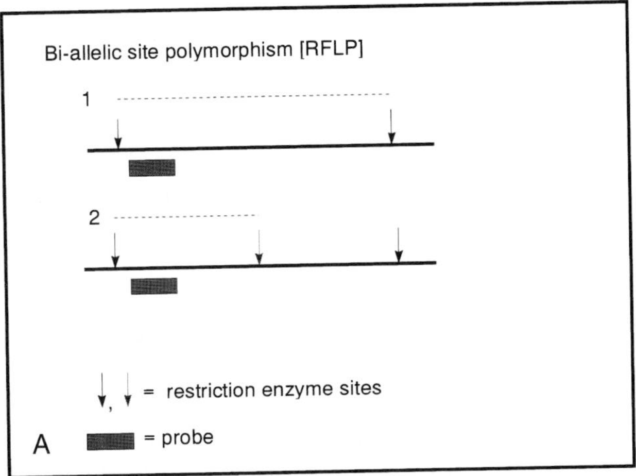

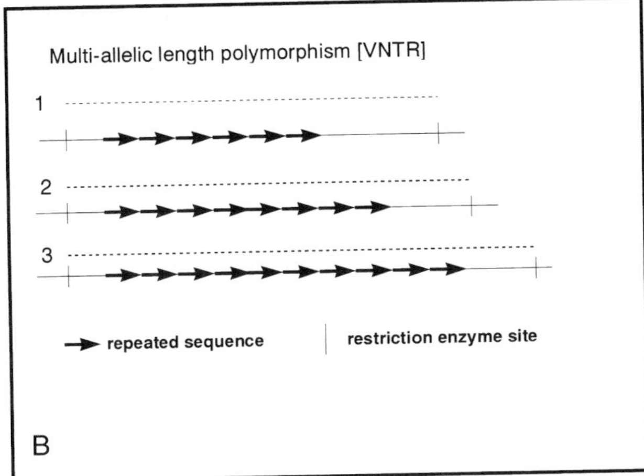

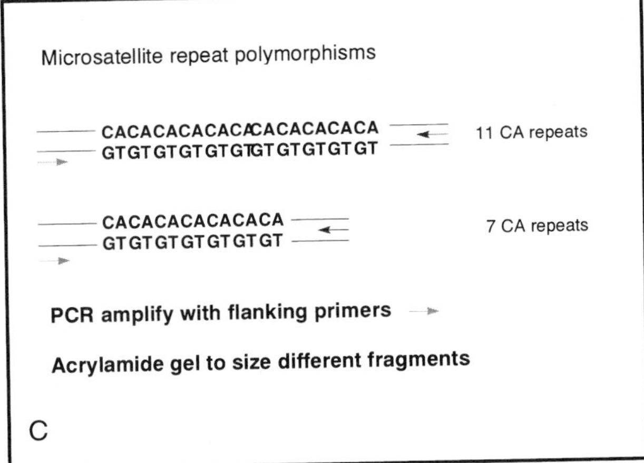

Figure 53–1. *A,* Restriction fragment length polymorphisms (RFLP) differ in size due to the presence or absence of additional restriction endonuclease sites within fragments produced by invariant enzyme sites. *B,* Variable number tandem repeats (VNTR) generate diverse restriction fragment sizes by varying the number of copies of small repeated sequences within two constant enzyme sites. *C,* Microsatellite markers also have variable number of copies of di-, tri-, or tetranucleotide repeats which are detected as polymerase chain reaction (PCR) products of varying size.

TABLE 53–2. Methods of Assessing Genetic Factors in Disease

Linkage Analysis	Association Studies
Genetic mapping of markers to locate causative gene	Tests whether genetic allele occurs more often than by chance in affected patients
Family studies with multiple generations and multiple affected relatives	Case-control population studies
Requires closely linked polymorphic markers	Requires that a candidate gene is known
Most suitable for single gene disorders	Polymorphic markers have functional significance to the biology of the disease
Markers are physically linked to the disease gene and crossing over during meiosis is low	Not usually equivalent to the physical linkage of the markers and the disease-causing gene

and frequency of the TNFA2 allele in severely affected malaria patients and compared them to the allele frequency in both normal and mild malaria control patient populations. The frequency of A1/A2 heterozygotes was similar (0.16) in each of these groups. However, the frequency of TNFA2 homozygotes was severalfold higher in the subgroups of malaria patients exhibiting severe clinical symptoms. The data were consistent, with an increased relative risk (RR) of 4 for cerebral malaria and 7 for death or severe neurologic damage in TNFA2 homozygous individuals. This regulatory polymorphism of the TNF-α gene affected the outcome of a severe infection.

Increased levels of TNF-α also correlated with the severity of meningococcal disease (MD). Nadel and coworkers[10] investigated the distribution of the TNF-α A1 and A2 alleles in children with fulminant MD. About 10% to 15% of patients with MD have meningococcal septicemia with mortality rates of 20% to 60%. In this study, TNFA1/A2 heterozygotes had an associated 2.5-fold increased risk of death from MD relative to children who did not possess the TNFA2 allele. The frequency of the TNFA2 allele in all populations was the same because TNFA2 did not alter the risk of acquiring the infection. Individuals with the TNFA2 allele had a genetic predisposition to secrete higher levels of TNF-α. The presence of the TNFA2 allele increased their risk for a more severe clinical course.

Increased levels of TNF are also observed with the TNFB2 polymorphic allele. The presence of this marker correlated with an increased risk for multiple organ failure in patients

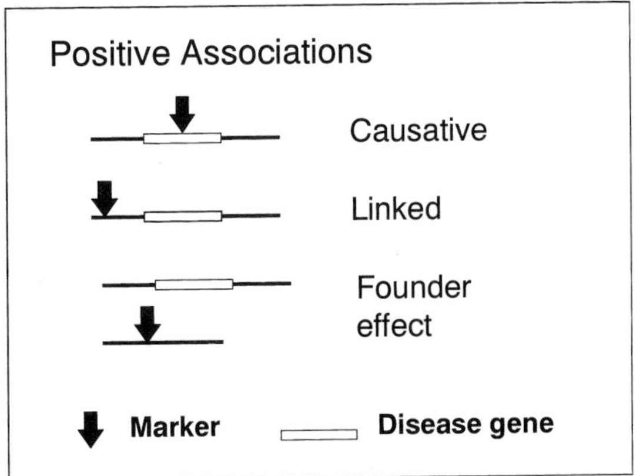

Figure 53–2. Positive gene associations. *Top,* The variant marker allele may reside in the gene that is the cause of the disease. *Middle,* The variant marker allele may be in linkage disequilibrium (i.e., physically linked) to the causative gene. *Bottom,* Within a heterogeneous population resides a subgroup of affected individuals who share many common features in addition to the marker allele and the disease phenotype because there is a common ethnic origin (founder effect).

with severe sepsis in the intensive care unit (ICU), as described by Stuber and coworkers.[8, 11] The allele frequency of TNFB2 in all ICU patients was the same as in the normal control population but was positively associated with nonsurvival in ICU patients with severe sepsis (RR, 2.1). Thus, the TNFB2 genotype predisposed these critically ill patients to a high risk for severe systemic inflammation and a poor outcome. These investigators also determined the possible association of polymorphic alleles of two other inflammation genes, interleukin-1 (IL-1β) and interleukin-1 receptor antagonist (IL-1ra), in these same patients.[11] They concluded that the IL-1β A2 allele, which correlates with high IL-1β secretion, was not a poor prognostic indicator because IL-1β A2 did not differ in incidence between patients in the ICU and normal controls or between survivors and nonsurvivors. A relatively uncommon polymorphic allele, IL-1ra A2, related to high production of the IL-1ra protein, also showed significantly higher frequency in patients with severe sepsis compared to normal controls (Fig. 53–3). Patients who were homozygous for both TNFB2 and IL-1ra A2 were exclusively nonsurvivors. The findings suggest that all polymorphic genetic variants that confer increased inflammation gene expression do not confer poor prognosis. IL-1ra A2 may contribute to susceptibility to sepsis while TNFB2 predicts high risk for poor outcome in severe sepsis.

In sarcoidosis with Lofgren syndrome, an acute form of systemic granulomatous disease, the TNFA2 genotype is more prevalent than in healthy patients or patients with other sarcoidosis disorders.[12] Again, genetic predisposition for increased TNF production and TNF-α genetic variation significantly influenced the clinical course and pathogenesis of this disease.

In clinical population association studies of cerebral malaria, meningococcal disease, severe sepsis in ICU patients, and an acute form of sarcoidosis an increased frequency of the variant TNF alleles associated with increased cytokine expression were demonstrated in affected patients when compared to matched, unaffected individuals. In each study, possession of the TNF allele, which correlated with higher gene expression, increased the risk of a poor prognosis in the most severely affected patients. Specific predisposing genetic variations in the TNF genes were implicated in the pathogenesis of these diseases.

Human immunoglobulin G (IgG) receptors are very heterogeneous. Polymorphisms have been identified for all three Fc gamma R classes. The Fc gamma RIIa polymorphism is now considered a risk factor for autoimmune, infectious disease, including severe meningococcal disease, and cytokine release during rejection treatment.[13]

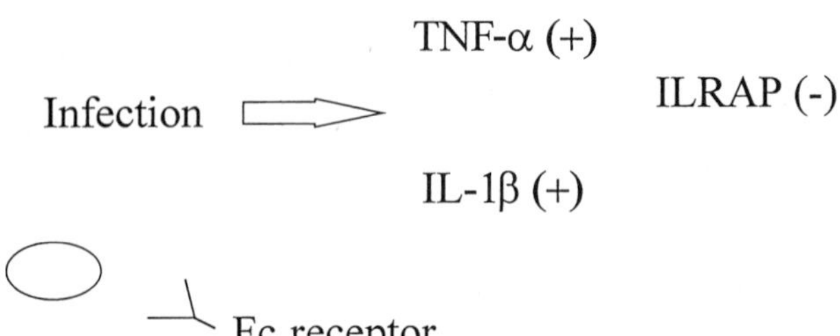

Figure 53–3. Inflammatory response. Infection results in the production of proinflammatory and anti-inflammatory cytokines. The Fc receptor aids in clearance of bacteria. Tumor necrosis factor-α (TNF-α) and interleukin-1β (IL-1β) are proinflammatory (+) cytokines and ILRAP is an anti-inflammatory (−) cytokine that inhibits IL-1β production. Poor outcomes have been observed in patients with polymorphisms associated with increased TNF-α and IL-ra protein (ILRAP) production, as well as reduced Fc receptor activity.

RESPONSES TO DRUG THERAPY

Pharmacogenetics is the study of the role of inheritance in individual variations in drug response and in the occurrence of adverse drug reactions. Interindividual differences in drug metabolism and disposition are well known. To facilitate elimination, drugs are often metabolized, undergoing *phase I* reaction, which generally involves oxidation, reduction, or hydrolysis, or a *phase II* conjugation reaction (Fig. 53–4).

Phase I metabolism is most commonly mediated by the cytochrome P450 (CYP) enzyme superfamily. More than 30 human CYPs have been characterized. These differ in their patterns of regulation, expression, and substrate specificity. The human CYPs considered to be important in drug and xenobiotic metabolism belong to families 1, 2, and 3, and some of these appear to be inducible. Large pharmacokinetic variations, ranging in magnitude from fourfold to 40-fold, often exist among members of a given population. The parent compound or its metabolites may be the active chemical.

Phase II metabolism is mediated by an extensive family of transferase enzymes. Conjugation or transfer of moieties to the substrate leads to increased solubility and ultimate biliary excretion of detoxified compounds.

Interindividual differences in metabolism can be illustrated in population curves. The presence of a bimodal distribution of drug metabolism in a population suggests that the enzyme activity variability may be attributable to genetic differences mediated at the DNA, ribonucleic acid (RNA), or protein level. Initially, genetic polymorphisms were discovered after observation of adverse drug reactions in patient populations. Single nucleotide transitions or transversions, deletions, or insertions or even gene deletion mutations can result in enzyme variants with higher, lower, or no activity (absent enzyme). A polymorphism can result in the separation of a population into at least two phenotypes: extensive metabolizer (EM) and poor metabolizer (PM). PMs have little or no activity. Genetic polymorphisms have been identified for a significant number of phase I and phase II enzymes important to drug metabolism and detoxification of toxic oxygen radical and reactive compounds.

Interindividual variability in CYP1A2 has long been recognized, but only recently has a genetic polymorphism been characterized involving a single nucleotide change in intron 1. CYP1A2 enzyme metabolizes acetaminophen, caffeine, haloperidol, and theophylline. Investigators are currently conducting studies to determine whether the polymorphism is correlated with interindividual differences in inducibility of CYP1A2.[14]

The CYP2C9 genetic polymorphisms result in reduced metabolism of phenytoin, tolbutamide, warfarin, phenytoin (Dilantin), and the nonsteroidal anti-inflammatory drugs (NSAIDs). Several genetic polymorphisms have been reported for *CYP2C9*. The most common allelic variant, *CYP2C9*3* (R144C), results in the substitution of cysteine for arginine at residue 144 and appears to reduce enzyme activity threefold in contrast to wild type. A second less common allelic variant, *CYP2C9*3* (1359L), results in activity 1/20 of wildtype. Other variants include Tyr358Cys and Gly417Asp.[15, 16]

The CYP2C19 genetic polymorphisms result in reduced metabolism of a number of drugs, including S-mephenytoin, hexobarbital, omeprazole, diazepam, imipramine, and cyclophosphamide. The PM phenotype shows interracial heterogeneity, occurring in 2% to 5% of Caucasians and 13% to 23% of Asians. Two single base pair mutations resulting in either an aberrant splice site (CYP2C19*2) or premature stop codon

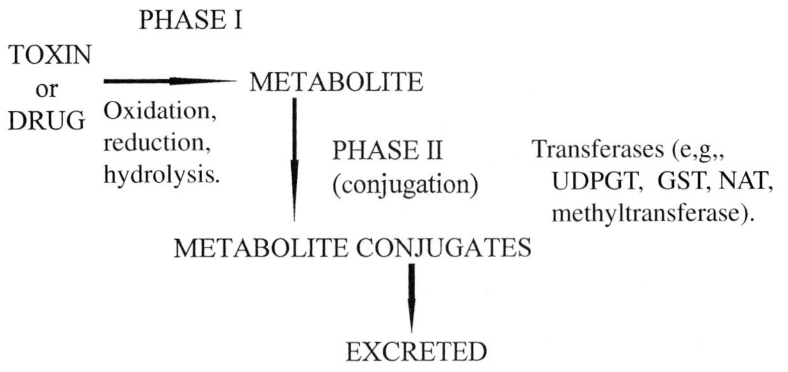

Figure 53–4. Drugs and toxins are metabolized by phase I and phase II (transferase enzymes). Genetic polymorphisms in these metabolic enzymes can lead to increased or decreased metabolism of drugs and toxins. GST = glutathione-S-transferase; NAT = *N*-acetyltransferase; UDPGT = uridine diphosphoglucuronyl transferase.

(CYP2C19*3) account for approximately 87% of Caucasian and more than 99% of Asian PM alleles. A study reported a new allelic variant, CYP2C19*4, which contains a mutation in the initiation codon and also contributes to the PM phenotype.[17-19]

Perhaps the most well characterized polymorphic CYP enzyme is CYP2D6. More than 17 allelic variants have been identified and are associated with a PM, EM, or ultrarapid metabolizer phenotype. The CYP2D6 enzyme catalyzes the oxidation of many drugs, including debrisoquine, sparteine, dextromethorphan, β-blockers, antidepressants, encainide, flecainide, and codeine. The PM phenotype was first noted in Britain, where physicians observed a significant hypotensive response to debrisoquine (a sympathetic antihypertensive drug) secondary to markedly reduced metabolism, and in Germany, where physicians noticed increased side effects associated with decreased metabolism of sparteine (antiarrhythmic drug). This PM phenotype can also lead to lack of analgesic effect with codeine because CYP2D6 metabolizes the parent compound to its active narcotic metabolite. Approximately 7% to 10% of Caucasians, 1% to 2% of Asians, and 2% of African Americans are CYP2D6 PMs.

Three allelic variants account for more than 95% of Caucasian PMs; *CYP2D6*3, CYP2D6*4,* and *CYP2D6*5*. The most common variant allele, *CYP2D6*4 (variant B),* is due to a guanine-to-adenine transition in the last nucleotide of intron 3, resulting in an aberrant 3′ splice site. The *CYP2D6*3* allele *(variant A)* results from a single nucleotide deletion in exon 5; the *CYP2D6*5* allele results from a complete deletion of the CYP2D6 gene. Each of these variants is readily identified by RFLP PCR. The ultrarapid phenotype arises from a gene duplication event where 2, 3, 4, 5, or 13 copies of the *CYP2D6*2 (variant L)* are observed occurring in approximately 5% to 7% of Caucasians.[20-24]

The ethanol-inducible CYP2E1 metabolizes isoniazid, phennylbutazone, acetaminophen, cocaine, and inhaled anesthetic agents. The gene for CYP2E1 has been mapped to chromosome 10 and spans 11.4 kilobase (kb) of genomic DNA. Several RFLPs for the CYP2E1 locus have been identified. A Dra I polymorphism in intron 2 (*CYP2E1*4*) was the first to be reported and was detected by Southern blotting. It has since been noted that the polymorphic site is in intron 6. Because the polymorphism occurs in the intron of the gene, the mutation may not affect gene expression; however, it may be linked to another mutation in this gene. The distribution of the 4* allelic frequency is 9% in Caucasians, 9% in African Americans, and 31% in Japanese.

A PstI or RsaI polymorphism (*CYP2E1*3*) in the 5′ untranslated region of the *CYP2E1* gene has also been identified. This set of polymorphisms, linked with each other, leads to a 10-fold increase in transcription. The variant allele is associated with higher transcriptional activity, although some reports do not show a functional consequence of the polymorphism. This polymorphism is therefore of interest because an increase in transcription of the gene may lead to increased metabolic activation of certain drugs. Ethnic differences in allelic frequencies for these RFLPs have also been described ranging from 2% to 27%.[25-32]

Conjugation of electrophilic and oxygen reactive compounds to glutathione by glutathione S-transferase enzymes is the major pathway for detoxification of reactive metabolites and protection against oxidative stress. The genes for glutathione S-transferase mu (*GSTM1*) and theta (*GSTT1*) are polymorphic with absence of the gene, causing a deficiency in activity. The *GSTM1* null genotype(0/0) (*GSTM1*2*) occurs in 40% to 60% of Caucasians, whereas the *GSTT1* gene is absent in approximately 40% (*GSTT*2*). GSTM1 represents 50% of glutathione S-transferase activity in the human liver.[33-36]

The *N*-acetyltransferase genetic polymorphism involves the phase II enzyme, which is responsible for individual variation in metabolism of isoniazid, sulfonylurea based drugs, procainamide, amrinone, dapsone, and caffeine. More than 50% of the Caucasian population are homozygous for this recessive trait and are of the slow acetylator phenotype. Significant frequency differences for the slow acetylator phenotype are observed among ethnic groups (e.g., 5% of Canadian Eskimos, 80% of Egyptians, 90% of Moroccans, 40% to 70% of Caucasian Europeans and North Americans, and 10% to 20% of Asians). The *NAT2** gene is associated with this polymorphism, although human *NAT1*,* which was previously thought to be genetically invariant, also displays allelic variation. Both genes have been mapped to chromosome 8. The number of allelic variants identified continues to increase. For *NAT2**, two mutant alleles—M1 (*NAT2*5B*) and M2 (*NAT2*6A*)—account for more than 90% of the alleles associated with the slow acetylator phenotype in Causcasians. The *NAT2*14A* allele appears to be of African origin, occurring in 9% of African Americans and no Caucasians. The importance of this drug metabolism polymorphism was established when patients receiving isoniazid for tuberculosis were found to have increased liver toxicity associated with the slow acetylator phenotype.[37-42]

Pharmacologic outcomes can be influenced by pharmacogenetics. Evolving genotyping techniques, including microchip arrays, optical detection of microspheres, and matrix-assisted laser desorption time of flight mass spectrometry (MALDI-TOF), will allow multiple polymorphisms to be analyzed in the clinical laboratory setting. Adjustment of medication choice or dosing in patients with identified polymorphisms should reduce adverse drug reactions and improve drug efficacy in critically ill patients.

THE THROMBOTIC RESPONSE

Endogenous anticoagulants have been identified as important to clinical hemostatic homeostasis in health and disease.

Thrombomodulin on the endothelial surface interacts with protein S to activate protein C and inhibit thrombin formation. Antithrombin III also inhibits formation of thrombin from prothrombin (Fig. 53–5). Genetic polymorphisms of the anti-coagulant proteins can increase the incidence of thrombophilia in critically ill patients.[43, 44]

Antithrombin III deficiency has been associated with more than 79 mutations. Heterozygotes have been identified in 4% of patients with inherited thrombophilia, 1% of patients with a first-time deep vein thrombosis (DVT) and 0.02% of healthy individuals.[45] Protein C deficiency has been associated with more than 160 mutations. Heterozygotes have been identified in 6% of patients with inherited thrombophilia, 3% of first-time DVT patients, and 0.3% of healthy individuals.[46–48] Protein S deficiency has been associated with 70 mutations. Heterozygotes are found in 6% of inherited thrombophilia patients and 1% to 2% of patients with a first-time DVT.[49]

Activated protein C (APC) resistance has been attributed to the factor V R506Q mutation. Replacement of Arg506 by Gln inhibits inactivation of factor Xa (cofactor activity) by activated protein C. Heterozygotes for this factor V Leiden mutation account for 19% of first-time DVT patients, 50% of patients with recurrent DVT, and 3% of healthy individuals. In some Caucasian populations, the incidence of factor V Leiden deficiency is 13% in healthy individuals. The mutation is extremely rare in Africans, Southeast Asians, Chinese, Japanese, American Indians, and Greenland Inuits.[50, 51]

A genetic polymorphism in the prothrombin gene, a G to A transition in the position 20210 of the A allele, is associated with increased prothrombin production. Heterozygotes represent 18% of inherited thrombophilia patients, 6.2% of first-time DVT patients, and 1% to 2% of healthy individuals. There is a higher than expected incidence of factor V Leiden mutation in patients with the prothrombin polymorphism, predisposing these patients to a greater tendency toward thrombophilia.[52]

The recent availability of protein C and antithrombin III concentrate provides the potential for therapies in patients with anticoagulant deficiency. Thrombotic complications (including myocardial infarction, cerebrovascular accident, pulmonary embolus and sepsis-induced disseminated intravascular coagulation and purpura fulminans) have been reported in patients with anticoagulant deficiencies. Knowledge of individual genetic polymorphisms for coagulation proteins may some day allow directed prophylactic therapies to reduce the incidence of these complications in critically ill patients.

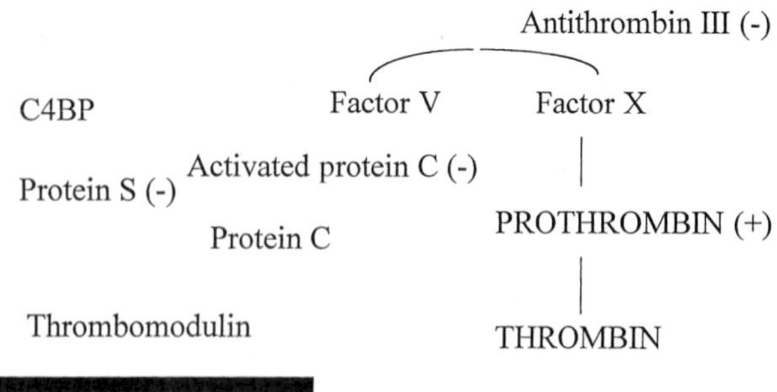

Figure 53–5. Endogenous anticoagulation. Thrombomodulin interacts with protein C and protein S to form activated protein C, which inhibits factor V participation in coagulation. Polymorphisms in protein C, protein S, or factor V can inhibit this process and may lead to increased thrombin formation. Antithrombin III also inhibits thrombin formation, whereas prothrombin increases thrombin formation. Genetic polymorphisms in these proteins are associated with increased thrombin formation.

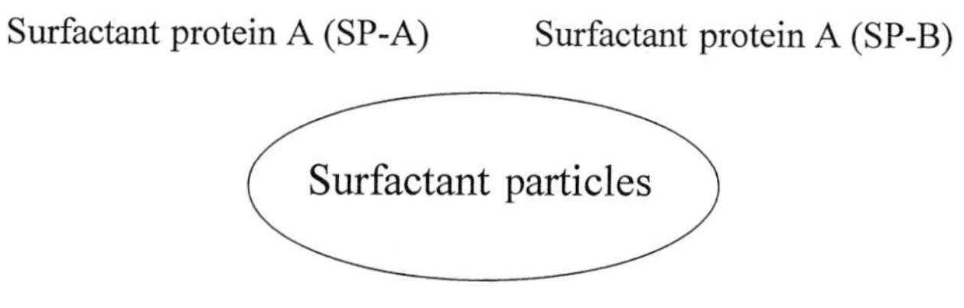

Figure 53–6. Surfactant-associated proteins. Surfactant function depends on the interaction of phospholipids and associated proteins. Genetic polymorphisms in surfactant-associated protein may contribute to poor surfactant function.

PULMONARY SURFACTANT COMPOSITION

Recent investigation of surfactant associated proteins (Fig. 53–6) may provide insight into variable susceptibility of individuals to surfactant-associated respiratory failure. Surfactant protein A (SP-A) is a collectin with important endogenous antimicrobial functions. The SPA-1 locus and SPA-2 locus show heterozygosity of 0.63 and 0.50, respectively. Nineteen of 20 haplotypes have been identified, and segregation of two haplotypes (6A2/1A0 and 6A4/1A) without recombination has been verified in a family.[53, 54] Surfactant protein B gene mutation with SP-B deficiency is associated with fatal respiratory failure in the first year of life. Variable numbers of composite repetitive motifs in intron 4 have been identified with allele E and H higher in Caucasians than African Americans or Nigerians.[55]

The recent availability of synthetic surfactant with varying concentrations of surfactant-associated protein A or B provides the opportunity to direct therapies to patients with polymorphisms for deficient production of these important protective molecules. In addition, lung transplantation has been successful for children with surfactant-associated protein B deficiency. Molecular epidemiology research will be necessary to determine the effect of heterozygous polymorphisms in surfactant-associated proteins on the pathogenesis of respiratory failure.

SUMMARY

Genetic polymorphisms of importance to critical illness are rapidly being identified. For illustrative purposes, we have examined only a limited number of these mutations. We have shown polymorphisms associated with inflammation, metabolism, coagulation, surfactant-associated protein, and endogenous antimicrobial gene products. Patients with combinations of these polymorphisms exist and are likely to be more severely affected than patients with one polymorphism. Rapid throughput and minimal blood sample requirements for PCR-based assays will likely allow clinicians to investigate the effects of interindividual genetic differences on critical illness. Genetic polymorphism analysis may improve understanding of pathogenesis and may aid in efficient design of clinical trials, reducing intensive care morbidity and mortality. Research continues on the effect of genetic variability on predisposition to critical illness. In this regard, the National Institutes of Health is establishing a major multi-institutional program, the Environmental Genome Project, to investigate how genetic polymorphisms confer increased risk of susceptibility or resistance to disease on exposure to environmental agents. A similar initiative in critical care medicine is warranted.

ACKNOWLEDGMENT

Supported in part by Grant 3M01RR0056GCRC.

References

1. Lander ES, Schork NJ: Genetic dissection of complex traits. Science 1994; 265:2037–2048.
2. Sparkes RS Human gene mapping, linkage, and association. *In:* The Genetic Basis of Common Diseases. King RA, Rotter JI, Motulsky AG (Eds). New York, Oxford University Press, 1992.
3. Hodge SE: What association studies can and cannot tell us about the genetics of complex disease. Am J Med Genet 1994; 54:318–323.
4. Thompson MW, McInnes RR, Willard HF: Genetics in Medicine. 5th ed. Philadelphia, WB Saunders, 1991.
5. Feder JN, Gnirke A, Thomas W, et al: A novel MHC class I-like gene is mutated in patients with hereditary hemochromatosis. Nat Genet 1996; 13:399–408.
6. Kunkel SL, Lukacs N, Streiter RM: Cytokines and inflammatory disease. *In:* Cellular and Molecular Pathogenesis. Sirica AE (Ed). Philadelphia, Lippincott-Raven, 1996, pp 23–35.
7. Wilson AG, di Giovine FS, Duff GW: Genetics of tumor necrosis factor-α in autoimmune, infectious, and neoplastic diseases. J Inflamm 1995; 45:1–12.
8. Stuber F, Petersen M, Bokelmann F, et al: A genomic polymorphism within the tumor necrosis factor locus influences plasma tumor necrosis factor-α concentrations and outcome in patients with severe sepsis. Crit Care Med 1996; 24:381–384.
9. McGuire W, Hill AVS, Allsopp CEM, et al: Variation in the TNF-promoter region associated with susceptibility to cerebral malaria. Nature 1994; 371:508–511.
10. Nadel S, Newport MJ, Booy R, et al: Variation in the tumor necrosis factor-α gene promoter region may be associated with death from meningococcal disease. J Infect Dis 1996; 174:878–880.
11. Stuber F, Fang X-M, Putensen C, et al: Genomic polymorphisms of interleukin-1 RA and tumor necrosis factor define an extended haplotype for risk assessment in severe sepsis (Abstract). Crit Care Med 1998; 26(Suppl):A29.
12. Seitzer U, Swider C, Stuber F, et al: Tumor necrosis factor-α promoter gene polymorphism in sarcoidosis. Cytokine 1995; 9:787–790.
13. Rascu A, Repp R, Westerdaal NA, et al: Clinical relevance of Fc gamma polymorphisms. Ann N Y Acad Sci 1997; 15:282–295.
14. MacLeod SL, Tang YM, Yokoi T, et al: The role of a recently discovered genetic polymorphism in the regulation of the human CYP1A2 gene. Proc Am Assoc Cancer Res 1998; 39:396.
15. Daly AK, Cholerton S, Gregory W, et al: Metabolic polymorphisms. Pharmacol Ther 1993; 57:129–160.
16. Bhasker CR, Miners JO, Coulter S, et al: Allelic and functional variability of cytochrome P4502C9. Pharmacogenetics 1997; 7:51–58.
17. Goldstein JA, Ishizaki T, Chiba K, et al: Frequencies of the defective CYP2C19 alleles responsible for the mephenytoin poor metabolizer phenotype in various Oriental, Caucasian, Saudi Arabian and American black populations. Pharmacogenetics 1997; 7:59–64.
18. de Morais SMF, Wilkinson GR, Blaisdell J, et al: The major genetic defect responsible for the polymorphism of S-mephenytoin in humans. J Biol Chem 1994; 269:15419–15422.
19. deMorais SM, Wilkinson GR, Blaisdell J, et al: Identification of a new genetic defect responsible for the polymorphism of (S)-mephenytoin in Japanese. Mol Pharmacol 1994; 46:594–598.
20. Gough AC, Miles JS, Spurr, NK, et al: Identification of the primary gene defect at the cytochrome P450 *CYP2D6* locus. Nature 1990; 347:773–776.
21. Hanioka N, Kimura S, Meyer UA, et al: The human CYP2D locus associated with a common defect in drug oxidation: A G1934. A base change in intron 3 of a mutant CYP2D6 allele results in aberrant 3′ splice recognition site. Am J Hum Genet 1990; 47:994–1001.
22. Heim M, Meyer UA: Genotyping of poor metabolizers of debrisoquine by allele-specific PCR amplification. Lancet 1990; 336:529–532.
23. Gonzalez FJ, Meyer UA: Molecular genetics of the debrisoquine-sparteine polymorphism. Clin Pharmacol Ther 1991; 50:233–238.
24. Agundez JAG, Martinez C, Ladero JM, et al: Debrisoquine oxidation genotype and susceptibility to lung cancer. Clin Pharm Ther 1994; 55:10–14.
25. Uematsu F, Kikuchi H, Motomiya M, et al: Association between restriction fragment length polymorphism of the human cytochrome P4502E1 gene and susceptibility to lung cancer. Jpn J Cancer Res 1991; 82:254–256.
26. Kato S, Shields PG, Caporaso NE, et al: Cytochrome P4502E1 genetic polymorphisms, racial variations and lung cancer. Cancer Res 1992; 52:6712–6715.
27. Raucy JL, Curley G, Carpenter SP: Use of lymphocytes for assessing ethanol mediated alterations in the expression of hepatic cytochrome P4502E1. Alcoholism: Clin Exp Res 1995; 19:1369–1375.
28. Guengerich FP, Kim DH, Iwasaki M: Role of human cytochrome P4502E1 in the oxidation of many low molecular weight cancer suspects. Chem Res Toxicol 1991; 4:168–179.
29. Umeno M, McBride OW, Yang CS, et al: Human ethanol inducible P450IIEI: Complete gene sequence, promoter characterization, chromosome mapping, and cDNA expression. Biochemistry 1988; 27:9006–9013.
30. Ingelman-Sundberg M, Johannson M, Perrson I, et al: Genetic polymorphism of cytochromes P-450: Interethnic differences and relationship to incidence of lung cancer. Pharmacogenetics 1992; 2:264–271.
31. Kato S, Shields PG, Caporaso NE, et al: Analysis of cytochrome P4502E1 genetic polymorphisms in relation to human lung cancer. Cancer Epidemiol Biomarkers Prev 1994; 3:515–518.
32. Kim RB, Yamazaki H, Chiba K, et al: In vivo and in vitro characterization of CYP 2E1 activity in Japanese and Caucasians. J Pharmacol Exp Ther 1996; 279:4–11.
33. Seidegard J, Vorachek WR, Pero RW, et al: Hereditary differences in the expression of the human glutathione transferase active in trans-stilbene oxide are due to a gene deletion. Proc Natl Acad Sci USA 1988; 85:7293–7297.
34. Bell DA, Thompson CL, Taylor J, et al: Genetic monitoring of human polymorphic cancer susceptibility genes by polymerase chain reaction: Application to glutathione S-transferase μ. Environ Health Perspect 1992; 98:113–117.
35. Pembles S, Schroeder KR, Spencer SR, et al: Human glutathione S-transferase theta (GSTT1): cDNA cloning and characterization of a genetic polymorphism. Biochem J 1994; 300:271–276.
36. Brockmoller J, Kerb R, Drakoulis N, et al: Glutathione S-transferase M1 and its variants A and B as host factors of bladder cancer susceptibility: A case control study. Cancer Res 1994; 54:4103–4111.
37. Blum M, Demierre A, Grant DM, et al: Molecular mechanisms of slow acetylation of drugs and carcinogens in humans. Proc Natl Acad Sci USA 1991; 8:5237–5241.
38. Grant DM: Molecular genetics of the *N*-acetyltransferases. Pharmacogenetics 1993; 3:45–50.
39. Vatsis KP, Weber WW, Bell DA, et al: Nomenclature for *N*-acetyltransferases. Pharmacogenetics 1995; 5:1–17.
40. Bell DA, Taylor JA, Butler MA: Genotype/phenotype discordance for human arylamine *N*-acetyltransferase locus. Carcinogenesis 1993; 14:1689–1692.
41. Doll MA, Jiang W, Dietz AC, et al: Identification of a novel allele at the human NAT1 acetyltransferase locus. Biochem Biophys Res Comm 1997; 233:584–591.
42. Katoh T, Bell DA: The role of *N*-acetylation polymorphisms (NAT1 and NAT2) in gastric and colorectal carcinoma. Proc Am Assoc Cancer Res 1997; 38:619.
43. DiMinno G, Grandone E, Margaglione M: Clinical relevance of polymorphic markers of arterial thrombosis. Thromb Haemost 1997; 78:462–466.
44. Ohlin AK, Norlund L, Marlar RA: Thrombomodulin gene variations and thromboembolic disease. Thromb Haemost 1997; 78:396–400.
45. Type I antithrombin deficiency: Five novel mutations associated with thrombosis. Blood Coagul Fibrinolysis 1996; 7:139–143.

46. Ireland H, Thompson E, Lane DA: Gene mutations in 21 unrelated cases of phenotypic heterozygous protein c deficiency and thrombosis: Protein C Study Group. Thromb Haemost 1996; 76:867-873.
47. Soria JM, Morell M, Estivill X, et al: A novel polymorphism (6376 G/T) in intron 7 of the human protein C gene. Hum Genet 1995; 96:243-244.
48. Spek CA, Koster T, Rosendaal FR, et al: Genotypic variation in the promoter region of the protein C gene is associated with plasma protein C levels and thrombotic risk. Arterioscler Thromb Vasc Biol 1995; 15:214-218.
49. Duchemin J, Gandrille S, Borgel D, et al: The Ser 460 to Pro substitution of the protein S alpha (PROS1) gene is a frequent mutation associated with free protein S (type Iia) deficiency. Blood 1995; 86:3436-3443.
50. Rees DC: The population genetics of factor V Leiden (Arg506Gln). Br J Hematol 1996; 95:579-586.
51. Jeffery S, Leatham E, Zhang Y, et al: Factor V Leiden polymorphism (FVQ506) in patients with ischemic heart disease, and in different populations groups. J Hypertens 1996; 10:433-434.
52. Kapur RK, Mills LA, Spitzer SG, et al: A prothrombin gene mutation is significantly associated with venous thrombosis. Arterioscler Thromb Vasc Biol 1997; 17:2875-2879.
53. Floros J, DiAngelo S, Koptides M, et al: Human SP-A locus: Allele frequencies and linkage disequilibrium between the two surfactant protein A genes. Am J Respir Cell Mol Biol 1996; 15:489-498.
54. Krizkova L, Sakthivel R, Olowe SA, et al: Human SP-A: Genotype and single-strand conformation polymorphism analysis. Am J Physiol 1994; 266(5 Pt 1):L519-L527.
55. Veletza SV, Rogan PK, TenHave T, et al: Racial differences in allelic distribution at the human pulmonary surfactant protein B gene locus (SP-B). Exp Lung Res 1996; 22:489-494.

54

Pathogenesis of Gram-Positive Bacterial Infection

Jerry L. Shenep, MD • Elaine Tuomanen, MD

In 1884, Christian Gram, a Danish physician working in Berlin and building on the previous work of Paul Ehrlich, published a new method for staining bacteria.[1] This original staining method came to be known as *Gram's stain* even though it was not a new stain per se. In effect, Gram's stain distinguished two broad structural categories of bacteria. Members of the bacterial genera with a single cell membrane stained avidly with crystal violet (*gram-positive*). Members of bacterial genera with a cell wall sandwiched between an inner and outer cell membrane did not bind crystal violet but did stain with safranin counterstain (*gram-negative*). Of clinical consequence, the outer membrane contains lipopolysaccharide (endotoxin), a unique bacterial component that has remarkably broad and potent bioactivity in trace quantities. Virtually without exception, endotoxin is lacking in gram-positive bacteria and present in gram-negative bacteria. It is this momentous discrimination of structure, which could not have been fully appreciated in Gram's time, that has underlain the clinical preeminence of Gram's staining method for more than a century. A comparison of key features of gram-negative and gram-positive bacteria is presented in Table 54–1.

Gram-positive bacterial infections are a major cause of admission to and an important complication of stay in the critical care unit. Sepsis alone accounts for roughly 10% of admissions to the intensive care unit.[2, 3] Gram-positive bacterial infections account for slightly more than half of these sepsis episodes[2, 3] (Table 54–2). For reasons that are poorly understood, in recent years the incidence of gram-positive bacterial infections has increased relative to gram-negative bacterial infections in cancer patients,[4, 5] in patients with indwelling vascular catheters,[6] in patients with sepsis,[7] and consequently in critically ill patients in general. Moreover, during the past two decades, the emergence of antibiotic resistance among gram-positive bacterial species (Table 54–3) has acutely elevated the importance of gram-positive bacteria relative to gram-negative bacteria. Emerging antibiotic resistance may partially explain the unanticipated increase in morbidity and mortality attributable to infections of all causes observed in the United States during the last decade, impressions and predictions to the contrary notwithstanding.[8]

Sepsis, meningitis, pneumonia, endocarditis, and other serious infections caused by gram-positive bacteria give rise to clinical manifestations that are generally indistinguishable from corresponding infections caused by gram-negative bacteria. Both categories of bacteria induce inflammatory responses with myriad features in common. Nonetheless, in the laboratory, the pathogenic mechanisms operative in gram-positive bacterial infections are readily distinguishable from those of gram-negative bacterial infections.

The shared and unique features of gram-positive and gram-negative bacterial organisms and their pathogenic mechanisms

TABLE 54–1. Comparison of Key Characteristics of Gram-Positive and Gram-Negative Bacteria

Characteristic	Gram-Positive Bacteria	Gram-Negative Bacteria
Capsule	+	+
Outer membrane	−	+
Lipopolysaccharide	−	+
Peptidoglycan	+	+
Teichoic and lipoteichoic acids	+	−
Adhesins	+	+
Pore-forming hemolysins	+	+
Product binds to serum protein	?	+
Product binds to CD14	+	+
Product binds to platelet-activating factor receptor	+	+
Activates NF-κB	+	+
Induces tumor necrosis factor, interleukin-1, nitric oxide	+	+

TABLE 54–2. Etiology of Gram-Positive Bacterial Sepsis

Pathogen	Incidence (%) United States[2]	France[3]
Gram-positive bacteria	39.5	47.7
Staphylococcus aureus	16	19.8
Coagulase-negative staphylococci	10.2	6
Enterococcus sp.	5.5	3.6
Streptococcus pneumoniae	4.1	8.7
Viridans streptococci	2	N/A
Other gram-positive bacteria	1.7	9.6
Gram-negative bacteria	35	45.8
Polymicrobial sepsis	11	
Nonbacterial pathogens	12	6.0
Anaerobes	2.4	

Data from Sands KE, et al: JAMA 1997; 278:234-240[2]; and Brun-Buisson C, et al: Am J Respir Crit Care Med 1996; 154:617-624.[3]

TABLE 54–3. Clinically Important Antibiotic Resistance Patterns Among Common Gram-Positive Bacterial Infections in the Critical Care Unit

Pathogen	Antibiotic Resistance	Mechanism of Resistance
Staphylococcus aureus	Methicillin Vancomycin	Decreased binding to PBP Altered cell wall structure
Coagulase-negative staphylococci	Methicillin	Decreased binding to PBP
Streptococcus pneumoniae	Penicillin Cephalosporin	Decreased binding to PBP Decreased binding to PBP
Enterococcus sp.	Penicillin Aminoglycosides Vancomycin	Decreased binding to PBP; β-lactamase Aminoglycoside *O*-phosphotransferase Altered cell wall structure
Viridans streptococci	Penicillin	Decreased binding to PBP
Streptococcus pyogenes	None	

PBP = penicillin-binding protein.

have important therapeutic implications. For instance, in the case of antimicrobial therapy, the usefulness of some antibiotics extends across both categories of bacteria (e.g., third-generation cephalosporins); others are generally restricted to members of one category or the other (e.g., vancomycin for gram-positive bacteria and aminoglycosides for gram-negative bacteria). Similarly, it is probable that as adjuvant anti-infective therapies (those in addition to antibiotics) are developed, the utility of some will be restricted according to bacterial category, whereas others may be effective for infections caused by either category of bacteria. Examples of adjuvant agents that may have restricted or extended activities by bacterial category can be found in the critical care unit in clinical trials of investigational agents for sepsis[9, 10] (Table 54–4). Knowledge of the common and distinctive aspects of the pathogenesis of infection caused by gram-positive and gram-negative bacteria will provide a rational basis for development of new adjuvant therapies and their appropriate application in clinical practice.

COLONIZATION VERSUS DISEASE

Understanding of the pathogenesis of an infection begins with knowledge of the source of the offending pathogen. In the case of coagulase-negative staphylococci, the source is usually the host's resident skin flora. In contrast, *Enterococcus* species, especially antibiotic-resistant enterococci, are often nosocomially acquired, passed from one patient to another by hospital personnel. *Staphylococcus aureus* may be part of the resident skin or nasal flora or may be nosocomially acquired. *Streptococcus pyogenes* and *Streptococcus pneumoniae* may be acquired through contact with symptomatic or asymptomatic carriers, spread by inhalation of droplets into the nasopharynx.

Gram-positive bacteria colonize the host asymptomatically using surface adhesive proteins to recognize and bind to human cell-surface determinants, usually complex carbohydrates. The simple presence of these potential pathogens in a host does not necessarily elicit disease. Symptomatic infection requires either risk factors on the part of the host or deployment of additional virulence determinants on the part of the pathogen.

TABLE 54–4. Experimental Adjuvant Therapies for Septic Shock[9, 10]

Experimental Therapy	Targeted for: *Gram-Positive Bacteria*	Targeted for: *Gram-Negative Bacteria*
Nitric oxide inhibitors	+	+
Bactericidal permeability-increasing protein	−	+
Interleukin-1 receptor antagonist	+	+
Intravenous immune globulin (toxic shock syndrome)	+	−

Data From Lynn WA, et al: Clin Infect Dis 1995; 20:143–158[9]; and Perez CM, et al: Am J Med 1997; 102:111–113.[10]

HOST FACTORS PREDISPOSING TO GRAM-POSITIVE BACTERIAL INFECTION

Although healthy individuals without recognizable risk factors do become infected with gram-positive bacteria, a predisposing host factor often facilitates invasion. In many instances, there is a predictable pattern of infecting bacterial species according to the risk factor (Table 54–5). Patients with compromised epithelium are especially predisposed to gram-positive bacterial infection. Trauma, including surgery and minor abrasions, increases susceptibility to infection with gram-positive bacterial species, especially *S. aureus*, *S. pyogenes* (group A β-hemolytic streptococci), and *Enterococcus* species. Patients with burns or varicella are especially predisposed to development of *S. pyogenes* or *S. aureus* sepsis. Although prediction of the infecting species is often accurate, caution should be exercised until the infecting organism is identified. Broad empirical antimicrobial coverage (including coverage for gram-negative bacteria) may be warranted in patients with life-threatening infection. For example, although varicella predictably predisposes to gram-positive bacterial infection, varicella lesions may also occur throughout the alimentary tract, occasionally leading to sepsis with gram-negative enteric organisms, especially in the infant or immunosuppressed host. Short-term and long-term indwelling intravascular catheters, urinary catheters, central nervous system shunt catheters, dialysis catheters, and other indwelling catheters predispose to infection with coagulase-negative staphylococci and *S. aureus*. Less commonly, streptococci, *Enterococcus* species, *Corynebacterium* species, *Bacillus* species, or gram-negative bacteria may cause catheter-related infections.

Patients with congenital or acquired cardiac valvular disease are predisposed to gram-positive bacterial infection, most often involving viridans streptococci and less commonly other streptococci, *S. aureus*, coagulase-negative staphylococci, or *Enterococcus* species. The prominent role of viridans strepto-

TABLE 54–5. Host Susceptibilities and Associated Gram-Positive Bacterial Infections

Host Susceptibility	Gram-Positive Bacterial Infection
Trauma	*Staphylococcus aureus* *Streptococcus pyogenes* (group A streptococcus) *Enterococcus* sp.
Burn	*S. pyogenes* *S. aureus*
Varicella	*S. pyogenes* *S. aureus*
Intravascular catheter	Coagulase-negative staphylococci *S. aureus* *Streptococcus* sp. *Enterococcus* sp. *Corynebacterium* spp. *Bacillus* sp.
Cardiac valvular disease	Viridans streptococci Coagulase-negative staphylococci *S. aureus* Other *Streptococcus* spp. *Enterococcus* sp.
Chronic respiratory disease	*Streptococcus pneumoniae* *S. aureus*
Asplenia	*S. pneumoniae*
Sickle cell disease	*S. pneumoniae*
Meningeal defects	*S. pneumoniae* Coagulase-negative staphylococci *S. aureus*
Newborns	*Streptococcus agalactiae* (group B streptococcus)
HIV infection	*S. pneumoniae*
Neutropenia	Viridans streptococci Coagulase-negative staphylococci *S. aureus*
Hospitalization	*Enterococcus* sp. Methicillin-resistant *S. aureus*
Tampons	TSST-producing *S. aureus*

HIV = human immunodeficiency virus; TSST = toxic shock syndrome toxin.

coccal species in endocarditis is explained by the fact that these species are the major organism colonizing the oral cavity and are by far the most common organisms found in cultures of blood obtained immediately after dental procedures.[11] Prosthetic heart valves are particularly susceptible to infection with coagulase-negative staphylococci, a species adept at binding to valvular materials.[12, 13]

Patients with splenectomy, congenital asplenia, or splenic dysfunction (e.g., sickle cell disease) are predisposed to sepsis with encapsulated organisms, most notably *S. pneumoniae*. The relatively high risk of post-splenectomy pneumococcal sepsis suggests that transient bacteremia with *S. pneumoniae* may occur occasionally in many normal hosts and that the spleen has a critical role in clearing the bacteremia before sepsis is established.

Acquired or congenital breaks in the meninges most commonly predispose to infection with *S. pneumoniae*. Less frequently, infection with coagulase-negative staphylococci, *S. aureus*, or viridans streptococci may occur in this setting. Congenital dermal sinus tracts frequently lead to cellulitis or meningitis with coagulase-negative staphylococci or *S. aureus*.

Extremes of age are a major risk factor for infection. Neonates and young infants are at special risk for *Streptococcus agalactiae* (group B streptococcus) sepsis and meningitis. The aged are at risk for a variety of bacterial infections, including those due to *S. pneumoniae, S. aureus*, and *S. pyogenes.*

In the setting of successful prophylaxis against *Pneumocystis carinii* and *Mycobacterium avium-intracellulare, S. pneumoniae* has become the most common organism causing serious infection in human immunodeficiency virus (HIV)–infected children cared for at St. Jude Children's Research Hospital and is a major pathogen in HIV-infected adults as well.[14] The possibility of pneumococcal sepsis, therefore, must be considered in any HIV-infected patient in whom sepsis is a consideration. Conversely, our recent experience has led us to have a heightened index of suspicion for HIV infection in any patient with *S. pneumoniae* infection.

Neutropenic patients with cancer are especially predisposed to gram-positive bacterial infection.[4, 5, 15–17] Although coagulase-negative staphylococci are most commonly seen, usually associated with indwelling intravascular catheters, viridans streptococci are more likely to cause infection leading to the intensive care unit. Infection with viridans streptococci can be associated with profound hypotension and the occurrence of adult respiratory distress syndrome (ARDS), complications that are not typically seen with viridans streptococcal endocarditis. Mucositis from any chemotherapy agent predisposes to viridans streptococcal sepsis, but ara-C is especially associated with this infection for reasons that have not been delineated.[16–18]

Predisposing factors should especially be considered for less common infections. Vancomycin or broad-spectrum antibiotic use is a major risk factor for the occurrence of vancomycin-resistant enterococcal infections.[19, 20] Toxic shock syndrome is most likely to occur in a setting of menstruation combined with prolonged use of tampons. Diphtheria and tetanus occur almost exclusively in the unimmunized host.

MICROBIAL FACTORS PREDISPOSING TO GRAM-POSITIVE BACTERIAL INFECTION

A number of potential virulence factors have been recognized in gram-positive bacteria[21–23] (Fig. 54–1). The most prominent are the inert polysaccharide capsules that help the organisms evade host detection and defenses (Table 54–6). Immunoglobulin A (IgA) proteases that inactivate secretory antibodies are present in all major gram-positive bacterial pathogens. Leukocidins are specifically lethal for neutrophils and macrophages. Lipases facilitate penetration of the skin, and hemolysins damage host cells and tissue. Bacterial neuraminidases and glycosyltransferases can modify host carbohydrates, presumably to facilitate microbial adherence and invasion. Deoxyribonuclease may be a virulence factor, although the mechanism of enhanced virulence is poorly understood. Catalase, which is absent from streptococci, protects bacteria such as staphylococci from hydrogen peroxide generated by host neutrophils and macrophages.

Gram-positive bacteria also share mechanisms for extensive interactions with extracellular matrix. These mechanisms include a large number of binding proteins, proteases, and hyaluronidases, which may be instrumental in allowing invasion of tissues by lysing extracellular matrix (ground substance). Binding proteins for fibronectin, laminin receptor, collagen, sialoprotein receptor, and other extracellular matrix components facilitate adherence to injured epithelium, bone

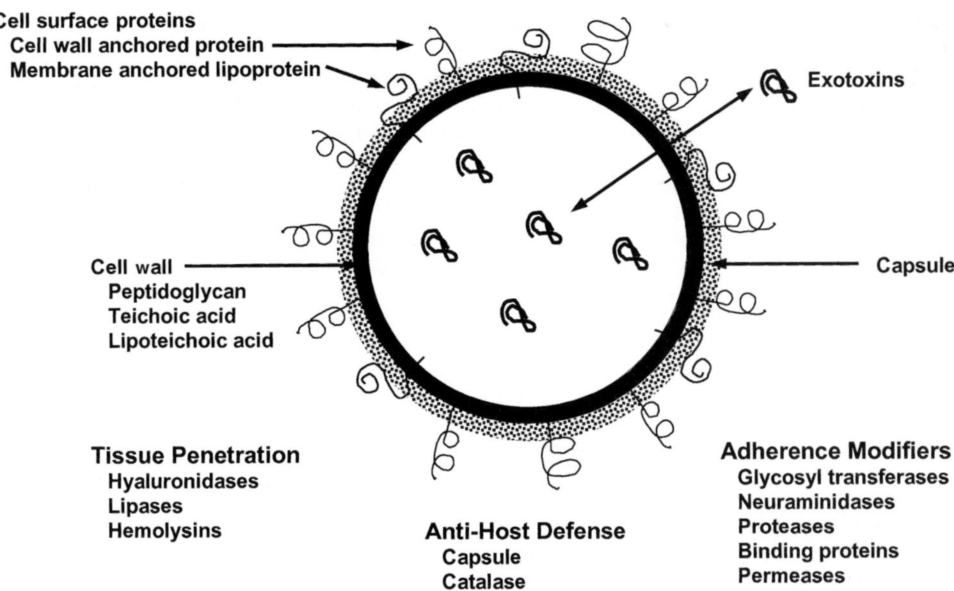

Figure 54–1. Gram-positive bacterial virulence factors. Virulence factors include those involved in adherence to host cells, those that act to counter host defenses, and those directed at tissue penetration and invasion. IgA = immunoglobulin A.

and joints (which contain sialoprotein receptor), and foreign bodies (which become coated with fibronectin and collagen). These binding proteins may particularly come into play in secondary infections after tissue injury such as may occur during a viral pneumonia.

The importance of these virulence factors should not be underestimated. For example, unencapsulated mutants of pathogenic bacteria are usually rendered nonpathogenic. The presence of surface binding proteins for sialoprotein receptor helps explain the propensity of *S. aureus* to cause bone and joint infections relative to other gram-positive bacteria. Viridans streptococci produce IgA proteases favoring colonization of oral mucosa[24] and produce extracellular dextran that facilitates binding to cardiac valves, accounting for this organism's preeminence in endocarditis. Our limited knowledge of bacterial virulence factors may be reflected in the fact that there are well above 300 surface proteins for each species. Although many are noncovalently attached to cell wall, a large group are covalently bound to the cell wall by a shared "LPXTGX" linker motif.[25, 26] Among these cell wall–linked proteins are protein A and fibronectin-binding protein of *S. aureus* and M proteins, fibronectin-binding protein, proteins G and T, and IgA-binding protein of *S. pyogenes*. These proteins facilitate adherence or, as in the case of protein A and M proteins, avoidance of phagocytosis.

TABLE 54–6. Capsular Production Among Common Gram-Positive Bacterial Pathogens

Pathogen	Capsular Production and Types
Staphylococcus aureus	11 serotypes described; unencapsulated or limited capsule formation is common
Coagulase-negative staphylococci	Unencapsulated or limited capsule formation
Streptococcus pneumoniae	90 serotypes described; types 19, 6, 23, 14, 3, 9, 11, 18 are most prevalent pathogens in the United States
Streptococcus agalactiae	6 serotypes
Streptococcus pyogenes	Most strains have hyaluronic acid capsule
Enterococcus sp.	Capsule present in some strains
Viridans streptococci	Capsule present in some strains

In addition to the cell wall–associated proteins, a class of proteins with a consensus sequence indicative of membrane anchoring are capable of interacting with the host despite their subsurface anchoring. These lipoproteins include two classes of peptide permeases that transport peptides or ions and influence a wide variety of aspects of microbial physiology, including adherence, deoxyribonucleic acid (DNA) transformation, and invasion. One such adhesin/permease, FimA of viridans streptococcus, appears to be critical for virulence in an animal model of endocarditis.[27] Other examples of lectin-like binding to eukaryotic cells include binding of the cell wall structure (peptidoglycan and lipoteichoic acid) itself or its associated structures to eukaryotic surface receptors; an example of this interaction is the binding of the phosphorylcholine of pneumococcal teichoic acid to the platelet-activating factor (PAF) receptor of eukaryotic cells.[28] Because more than 20 carbohydrate determinants can be recognized by gram-positive bacteria, many host receptors apparently remain to be discovered.[29]

EARLY HOST-MICROBE INTERACTIONS IN GRAM-POSITIVE BACTERIAL INFECTION

Once contact with the host is established, disease may result from direct invasion, as in catheter-related bacteremia; after colonization and toxin absorption, as in toxic shock syndrome; or after adherence and penetration of epithelium, as in the case of *S. pneumoniae* bacteremia. This last mechanism is an interesting example of how microorganisms have evolved to evade host defenses.

Infection develops in only a small fraction of hosts who become colonized with *S. pneumoniae*. In the asymptomatic state, the pneumococcus uses several potential binding sites on nasopharyngeal epithelial cells, including at least two classes of glycoconjugates. If inflammation of the mucous membrane occurs, new receptors are induced on the epithelial cell surface, including those that participate in the acute-phase defense response. One such receptor is the PAF receptor, which appears to be a critical binding site for pneumococci (Fig. 54-2). Both binding and *penetration* of pneumococci are significantly enhanced after the appearance of PAF receptors.[28] With the use of fluorescent markers, the PAF receptor together with bound pneumococcus has been observed to internalize into the host cell. In addition, PAF receptor antagonists significantly reduce pneumococcal invasion of host cells, indicating that the PAF receptor is an important factor in invasion.

Phosphorylcholine is common to PAF (the natural ligand for the PAF receptor) and to teichoic acid on the cell wall of pneumococci. The presence of phosphorylcholine on pneumococci suggests that this species has evolved a novel mechanism to subvert host defense responses to its advantage. This is but one of many facets of interaction between pneumococci and human host epithelium, which in concert present a highly complex and orchestrated dance between the suitor microbe and its reluctant host. That these interactions occur in concert is corroborated by the fact that single regulatory genes have been shown to coordinate expression of numerous molecules involved in adhesion and persistence.[30]

Just as colonization does not imply infection, host invasion by gram-positive bacteria does not intimate symptomatic disease in most instances. The array of host defenses directed against gram-positive bacteria[31] must be on a par with the collective array of bacterial factors aimed at evasion. Unlike many strains of gram-negative bacteria, gram-positive bacteria are not serum-sensitive; that is, complement deposition does not lead to bacteriolysis. However, neutrophils, macrophages, and the reticuloendothelial system clear nearly all invading bacteria with the assistance of acellular defenses. *Cellular* defenses are especially important in repelling invasion by *S. aureus*, coagulase-negative staphylococci, and viridans streptococci, the major gram-positive bacterial pathogens seen in the neutropenic cancer patient. *Acellular* defenses, which are particularly important for protection against *S. pneumoniae*, include the innate defenses of the complement system, acute-phase reactants, the defense collagens, and the delayed acquired protection mediated by antibody. Although the capsule of *S. pneumoniae* is relatively resistant to complement deposition, patients with isolated complement deficiencies, especially deficiencies of the early components of complement, are at increased risk of pneumococcal infection.

Thus, complement is of relevance in defense against pneumococci. Collagen binding to bacteria facilitates their uptake by macrophages. Defense collagens, such as mannose-binding protein, macrophage scavenger receptor, C1q, pulmonary surfactant protein D, and other collectins, bind to the teichoic acid phosphate determinants of most gram-positive pathogens but, notably, not to pneumococcus.[32, 33] C-reactive protein (a pentraxin) binds pneumococcal teichoic acid, which enhances opsonization and clearance from the bloodstream.

Antitoxin antibodies are highly protective against certain toxins elaborated by gram-positive bacteria, including tetanus and diphtheria toxins. Antibodies to the surface structures of some gram-positive bacteria are also protective. For example, antibodies to the capsular polysaccharide of *S. pneumoniae* are moderately protective, but the diversity and poor immunogenicity of capsular types have impeded development of a highly effective pneumococcal vaccine. In contrast, *Haemophilus influenzae* infections, virtually all caused by strains possessing a single capsular type (type b), have been nearly eliminated by development of highly immunogenic capsular polysaccharide-protein conjugate vaccines.

MECHANISMS OF CELL INJURY AND DEATH IN GRAM-POSITIVE BACTERIAL INFECTION

Some have marveled that bacteria have evolved complex mechanisms to invade their hosts, ultimately leading to destruction of both. The blood and tissues of the human host are potentially a vast, rich, virgin source of nutrition for bacterial growth. It should not be surprising, therefore, that bacterial evolution may in some species drift toward pathogenicity, with the associated bursts of replication, which we recognize as infections such as pneumonia, sepsis, meningitis, and endocarditis. Gram-positive bacteria cause cell and tissue injury through a variety of mechanisms. Some injuries are derived directly from the bacteria, and others result from the host response to infection. Knowledge of the mechanisms of host injury is the key to past and future development of effective therapeutic intervention.

Biologically Active Components of Gram-Positive Bacteria

In the case of gram-negative bacteria, lipopolysaccharide (endotoxin) has been identified as the major common mediator of host injury for nearly all pathogenic species. Endotoxin binds to lipopolysaccharide-binding protein in the serum, and this complex binds to cellular or soluble serum CD14, signaling initiation of the cytokine responses driving inflammation. This basic story is operative in all gram-negative bacteria from *Escherichia coli* to *Neisseria meningitidis*. In contrast, gram-

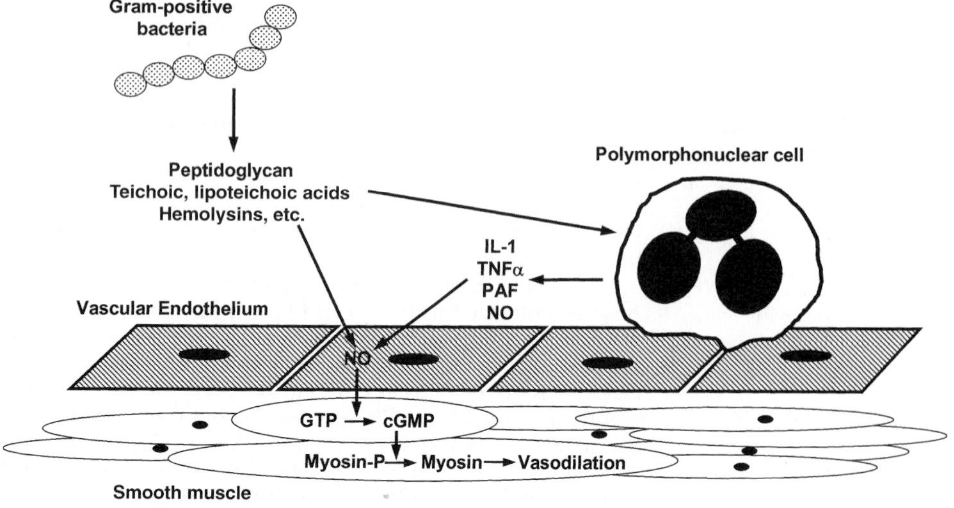

Figure 54–2. Interaction of *Streptococcus pneumoniae* with host epithelial cells. *S. pneumoniae* up-regulates platelet-activating factor (PAF) receptors in the host cells. *S. pneumoniae* then specifically binds to PAF receptors via choline binding protein A and cell wall choline. Binding of pneumococci to PAF receptors enhances invasion and transmigration of the epithelium. IL = interleukin; TNF = tumor necrosis factor; NO = nitric oxide; GTP = guanosine triphosphate; cGMP = cyclic guanosine monophosphate.

positive bacteria harbor a teichoic acid–containing cell wall, five to 10 times thicker than in gram-negative bacteria. These cell wall components are the functional noxious equivalent of endotoxin, in some cases sharing the CD14 signaling system as a target to initiate inflammation. Some of the bioactivities of gram-positive bacteria are listed in Table 54–7.

Capsule

The capsules of gram-positive bacteria, like those of gram-negative bacteria, are generally regarded as relatively inert polysaccharides. Large quantities can be injected into tissues with minimal damage, satisfying at least one criterion for an ideal immunogen. Injection of pneumococcal polysaccharide into the cerebrospinal fluid or lung does not induce inflammation.[34, 35] One study indicates that under some conditions capsular polysaccharides can stimulate murine macrophages to produce tumor necrosis factor-α (TNF-α).[36]

Peptidoglycan

Although repeating *N*-acetylglucosamine-*N*-acetylmuramic acid forms the backbone of the cell walls of all gram-negative and gram-positive bacteria, biochemical differences in the fine structures of peptidoglycan have been described for each bacterial species studied, the differences arising in the peptide cross-links connecting the polysaccharide chains. Thus, each bacterial cell wall is formed from a slightly different library of approximately 20 glycopeptides, with each glycopeptide having an individually characteristic bioactivity. Peptidoglycan from gram-positive bacteria induces a number of cytokines, including interleukin 1 (IL-1), IL-6, and TNF-α.[37, 38] Specific disaccharide peptides also induce sleep, trigger the coagulation cascade, and induce blood-brain barrier permeability.[39–41] The specific activity of peptidoglycan rivals endotoxin, and CD14 has been clearly indicated as one receptor initiating cellular responses to peptidoglycan.[42] Like endotoxin, peptidoglycan is less bioactive when it is presented on an intact bacterium. Cell wall–active antibiotics may liberate peptidoglycan and other cell wall products, augmenting inflammatory responses.

TABLE 54–7. Bioactivities of Gram-Positive Bacteria

Binding to human cells
- Neutrophils
- Macrophages
- Platelets
- Respiratory epithelial cells
- Nasopharyngeal epithelial cells
- Vascular endothelial cells
- Squamous epithelial cells of skin

Known cell-surface receptors or binding proteins
- CD14
- PAF receptor
- Mannose-binding protein
- Macrophage scavenger receptor
- Surfactant protein D

Induction of inflammatory mediators
- TNF
- IL-1β
- IL-6
- IL-8
- IL-12
- Arachidonate metabolites
- PAF
- Tissue factor
- Nitric oxide
- Alternative complement cascade

Tissue injury
- Hemolysins
- Hyaluronidases
- Lipases

IL = interleukin; PAF = platelet-activating factor; TNF = tumor necrosis factor.

Lipoteichoic Acid

Teichoic acids and lipoteichoic acids are polymers of polyribitol or polyglycerol that are covalently linked to the peptidoglycan backbone. These molecules are unique to gram-positive bacteria.[43] Several studies indicate that lipoteichoic acid induces inflammation, although its activity seems to be generally less potent and more restricted compared to that reported with lipopolysaccharide. Lipoteichoic acid has been reported to induce IL-1, IL-6, IL-8, IL-12, TNF-α, and nitric oxide.[37, 44–48] Lipoteichoic acid and peptidoglycan are also reported to act synergistically to induce inflammation.[38]

Hemolysins

S. aureus produces four types of hemolysins, known as α-, β-, γ-, and δ-toxins. Most strains of *S. aureus* produce α-toxin, a potent protein toxin. In 1928, in one of the worst disasters in vaccine history, fever, rash, and shock developed in 21 Australian children receiving a diphtheria toxoid vaccine contaminated with *S. aureus*. Twelve children died a few hours after vaccination.[49] *S. aureus* α-toxin, a known potent inducer of nitric oxide,[50] has been implicated in that tragedy.

Streptococci possess two types of hemolysins: *oxygen-stable* (S) hemolysins and *oxygen-labile* (O) hemolysins. *S. pyogenes* generally possesses both types of hemolysins; however, it is the hemolysin S that accounts for the β (clear) hemolysis seen on aerobic incubation of colonies on blood agar. The effect of the *S. pyogenes* hemolysin O (known as *streptolysin* or *streptolysin O*) can be demonstrated only under anaerobic conditions, being inactive in the presence of oxygen. *S. pneumoniae* produces only O hemolysins, one of which is pneumolysin.[51] Viridans streptococci, which typically are α-hemolytic, also produce O hemolysins.[51] The α-hemolysis produced by viridans streptococci (and presumably by *S. pneumoniae* as well) has been attributed to this organism's production of hydrogen peroxide in the absence of catalase.[52]

Hemolysin molecules insert randomly into eukaryotic cell membranes, forming pores, a property explaining their broad toxicity to many cell types.[53] These molecules appear to have potent and clinically important activities. For example, streptolysin has been reported to induce production of TNF and IL-1.[54] Pneumolysin activates complement and appears to have an important role in the development of septic shock and cell injury.[55, 56] Of particular note, pneumolysin has been proposed to be a major mediator of eighth nerve damage on the basis of cochlear cytotoxicity after intracisternal challenge with purified pneumolysin.[57] Moreover, this damage appears to be mediated by nitric oxide production because it can be blocked by inhibitors of nitric oxide formation.

Exotoxins

Endotoxin is viewed by some as a highly toxic molecule, but its toxicity wanes in comparison to some of the toxins produced by gram-positive bacteria. These include tetanus toxin, diphtheria toxin, and botulinum toxin, each capable of inducing death in trace quantities. Tetanus toxin acts to inhibit acetylcholine release at neuromuscular junctions; selective blocking of inhibitory synapses in the spinal cord accounts for tetany. Diphtheria toxin inactivates elongation factor 2 of the 60S ribosomal unit. Botulinum toxin inhibits acetylcholine release at neuromuscular junctions. Botulinum toxin is the most potent toxin known; 25 pg is lethal for mice, and 0.3

ng causes disease in humans. Curiously, the function of these potent toxins has not been determined.

Pyrogenic exotoxins include the following[58]:

- Staphylococcal enterotoxins A to E; responsible for food poisoning
- Staphylococcal toxic shock syndrome toxin 1 (TSST-1); responsible for most cases of toxic shock syndrome associated with menses and two thirds of nonmenstrual cases
- Streptococcal pyrogenic exotoxin types A (SpeA) to C (SpeC)

These exotoxins are a set of low-molecular-weight proteins that are functionally related and, except for TSST-1, structurally related as well. These exotoxins act as superantigens, activating T cells by direct interaction with the Vβ chain on T cell receptors and the major histocompatibility complex (MHC) class II molecule.[59] This interaction can induce massive stimulation of T cells, with concomitant overproduction of cytokines, and associated clinical manifestations. SpeA, SpeB, or SpeC mediates streptococcal toxic shock syndrome, associated with *S. pyogenes* infection.[60]

Host Responses to Gram-Positive Bacterial Infection

Bacteria can double every 30 minutes or so under ideal growth conditions. Were it not for an array of host defenses, human blood and tissues would be ideal conditions for many bacterial pathogens. As a consequence, host defenses must ultimately be virtually perfect. If one organism among billions acquires a mechanism to elude the defenses, the host will not survive. Most host defenses that compose the first line of defense, including epithelial and endothelial barriers, phagocytes, and antibodies, appear to be fairly innocuous to the host. In contrast, host responses to deep infections such as sepsis and meningitis may result in host cell injury and death. It is these mechanisms that are focused on herein.

CD14 and Platelet-Activating Factor Receptors

Purified cell walls of pathogenic gram-positive bacteria produce acute inflammation, indicating that the immune system recognizes the gram-positive cell wall somewhat analogously to its universal recognition of endotoxins. Endotoxin liberated from gram-negative bacteria into the blood first binds with a circulating protein, lipopolysaccharide-binding protein (LBP). The endotoxin-LBP complex subsequently binds to CD14 present on neutrophils, macrophages, endothelial cells, and other cell types. Gram-positive bacterial cell walls are also known to bind to CD14, although a molecule equivalent to LBP has not yet been found for gram-positive bacteria.[61] Signal transduction leading to the cytokine cascade is initiated by binding of any bacterial product to CD14.[42] In addition to CD14, some of these responses may involve the PAF receptor.[62] *S. pneumoniae* can induce inflammation through other as yet unknown receptors binding to the PAF receptor.[63] The cellular response to ligation of the PAF receptor is distinct from that induced by CD14 binding.[42]

NF-κB

NF-κB is a nuclear transcription factor that can be activated by gram-negative or gram-positive bacteria and signals a broad host response through induction of various cytokines. Because gram-negative bacterial lipopolysaccharide and gram-positive bacterial exotoxins and cell walls can activate this transcription factor, convergence of pathogenic pathways was once anticipated.[42, 64] However, disruption of NF-κB renders experimental mice hypersusceptible to *S. pneumoniae* but not to gram-negative bacteria, suggesting that multiple pathogenic pathways may be concurrently operative.[65]

Interleukins

The discovery that an endogenous pyrogen mediated the febrile response to infection opened a new era in our understanding of host-parasite interactions. Endogenous pyrogen, now known as IL-1, was shown to act on the hypothalamus to reset the body's temperature.[66] IL-1 is stimulated by lipopolysaccharide and gram-positive cell wall and can itself induce production of IL-6, IL-8, TNF-α, and nitric oxide; in turn, these cytokines may lead to inadequate blood perfusion of the tissues (i.e., septic shock).[67–73] These cytokines have clear beneficial effects when they are viewed at the level of the cell, but from the perspective of the host, they may be detrimental. Nonsurvivors of gram-positive bacterial sepsis have had significantly elevated levels of IL-1.[74] Lipoteichoic acid induces production of IL-8.[44] This interleukin is a potent chemotactic factor and is elevated in patients with gram-positive and gram-negative bacterial sepsis.[75]

Tumor Necrosis Factor-α

Tumor necrosis factor-α promotes production of IL-1, IL-6, and IL-8 and is clearly an important mediator of septic shock, meningitis, and other deep infections caused by gram-negative and gram-positive bacteria.[68–70, 76–78] Somewhat naively, septic shock was at one point almost equated with the presence of elevated levels of TNF-α. This distortion is based on observations that TNF-α can produce virtually all of the clinical manifestations of septic shock. Nonetheless, the multifaceted nature of septic shock is currently widely recognized, and TNF-α has been more properly relegated to its role as one among several important inflammatory mediators.

Platelet-Activating Factor

PAF is a phospholipid that not only induces aggregation of platelets and adhesion of leukocytes but also activates the cytokine cascade, resulting in hypotension. Inflammation induced by *S. pneumoniae* is mediated in part by PAF.[62] However, although *S. pneumoniae* binds to PAF receptor, this binding does not directly induce G protein signaling characteristic of the natural ligand binding.

Nitric Oxide

In the brief interval since nitric oxide was named "molecule of the year" by *Science* in 1992,[79] more than 14,000 publications have added to our knowledge of this key signaling molecule.[80–85] Nitric oxide is produced in vivo by cleavage from arginine. This cleavage is primarily mediated by a family of enzymes, nitric oxide synthases (NOSs). Neuronal NOS (nNOS) and endothelial cell NOS (cNOS) are calcium-dependent enzymes that produce nitric oxide constitutively in small amounts. In contrast, the inducible form of the enzyme (iNOS) is present in macrophages and endothelial cells. When activated, iNOS produces large quantities of nitric oxide. Lipopolysaccharide is the most widely recognized inducer of iNOS, but gram-positive organisms are potent inducers of iNOS as well. In addition, IL-1 and TNF-α, which are produced in response to both gram-negative and gram-positive infections, can also induce iNOS.

Nitric oxide has many biologic activities from microbial killing to vascular contractility regulator to neurotransmitter. Nitric oxide exists in vivo as a dissolved gas that navigates through membranes effortlessly. Since its half-life is on the order of 6 seconds, its signal can be rapidly adjusted. When produced in the vascular endothelium, nitric oxide diffuses into vascular smooth muscle cells, where it activates guanylate cyclase, producing cyclic guanosine monophosphate (GMP).

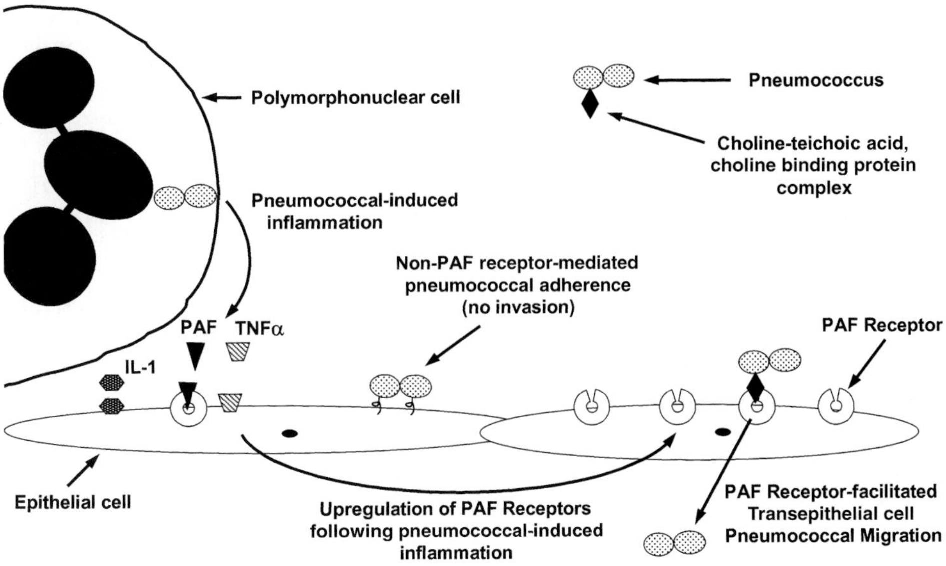

Figure 54–3. Cytokine-mediated vasodilation in gram-positive bacterial sepsis. Gram-positive cell walls and toxins induce inflammation. Production of nitric oxide (NO), the most potent vasodilator known, is stimulated directly by gram-positive bacterial products as well as indirectly through inflammatory mediators. TNF = tumor necrosis factor; PAF = platelet-activating factor; IL = interleukin.

Cyclic GMP phosphorylates myosin, leading to muscle relaxation. Clinically, excessive production of nitric oxide in response to sepsis may lead to poor vascular tone and septic shock (Fig. 54–3).

Administration of nitric oxide inhibitors can reverse hypotension within minutes in patients with septic shock.[86–88] However, vascular blood flow remains dysregulated, and to date no survival benefit has been shown from inhibition of nitric oxide.[89, 90] In fact, decreased perfusion has been noted after inhibition of nitric oxide production in some models.[91]

Complement

Cell walls of gram-positive bacteria are potent activators of both the classical and alternative pathways of complement.[92] Elevated levels of complement have been associated with fatal outcome in patients with gram-negative and gram-positive bacterial sepsis.[75] Complement activation on endothelial surfaces leads to leukocyte recruitment, resulting in cytokine release, cell injury, and capillary leakage.

Leukocytes

Chemoattractants and adhesion molecules are responsible for the localization of neutrophils to endothelial cell surfaces activated by microbial products. These leukocytes are an important source of eukaryotic cell injury.

Leukocyte adhesion is a complex process involving slowing of leukocyte trafficking mediated by selectins, adhesion mediated by CD18 β_2 integrins, and transmigration mediated by platelet–endothelial cell adhesion molecule 1 (PECAM-1). Leukocyte recruitment during pneumococcal pneumonia is the one instance in which a non–CD18-dependent mechanism is operative in parallel with CD18-dependent processes.[93] Inhibition of leukocyte adhesion at the level of selectin has not been beneficial in animal models of sepsis,[9] whereas prevention of margination of leukocytes at the level of CD18 has been protective in one study of gram-positive bacterial infection.[94] Inhibition at the level of PECAM has not been studied for gram-positive infection, but inhibition at the level of intracellular adhesion molecule (ICAM-1) has produced mixed results with protection against staphylococcal enterotoxin B[95] but increased susceptibility to pneumococcal sepsis.[96]

MANAGEMENT OF THE CRITICALLY ILL PATIENT WITH GRAM-POSITIVE BACTERIAL INFECTION

As we have become more adept at controlling or eradicating infecting bacteria with use of antimicrobial therapy, we have come to recognize that at least in the setting of effective antibiotic therapy, certain host responses to infection may be detrimental to the host. The use of corticosteroid therapy to prevent hearing loss and neurologic sequelae in gram-negative bacterial meningitis is one of the first successful applications of knowledge in this regard.[97] The principle behind the approach is the knowledge that antibiotics induce massive fragmentation of the bacterial cell wall, releasing a sudden burst of highly bioactive glycopeptides. This iatrogenic inflammatory response enhances tissue damage, and the concomitant administration of anti-inflammatory agents with antibiotics down-modulates the excess inflammation. The development of more targeted adjunctive therapies based on the mediators of gram-positive inflammation can be reasonably expected to further improve outcome.

For the 1990s, molecular biologists have set their sights on dissecting the molecular pathophysiology of sepsis, pneumonia, and meningitis.[98] Consequently, as we come to understand more fully the pathophysiology of gram-positive and gram-negative bacterial infections, an armamentarium of therapeutic interventions based on the host-to-parasite response will gain entry into clinical practice, many of which will be targeted for use in the critical care unit. Classes of agents with promise in gram-positive bacterial infections are listed in Table 54–8.

EMERGING DISEASES

With the advent of HIV infection, the concept of emerging infectious diseases has become widely appreciated. Gram-positive bacterial infections are an important class of emerging infections. Existing pathogens such as staphylococci and pneu-

TABLE 54–8. New Adjunctive Agents for Gram-Positive Bacterial Sepsis Under Investigation

- Nonsteroidal anti-inflammatory agents
- Low-molecular-weight heparin
- Antagonists of cytokine receptors
- Antagonists of leukocyte migration
  - Selectins: antibodies, carbohydrate ligand analogs, peptides
  - Chemokines: antagonists
  - Integrins: antibodies, peptides
  - Cell adhesion molecules: antibodies

mococci have become increasingly antibiotic resistant. Figures from the Centers for Disease Control and Prevention estimate that 30% of staphylococci are resistant to methicillin and 40% of pneumococci are resistant to penicillin. These resistant pathogens circulate in the community. These statistics represent dramatic and steady increases in prevalence, suggesting that antibiotic therapy for these major pathogens is increasingly complex and difficult. Enterococci are perhaps the most difficult to treat in that strains resistant to all existing antimicrobials have emerged during the past few years. Fortunately, these multiply resistant strains are usually hospital-acquired. Not only changes in antibiotic practices but also changes in vaccine practices can lead to reemerging infections. A decrease in the rate of immunization to diphtheria has led to outbreaks of this infection, particularly in countries of the former Eastern bloc.

In addition to widespread antibiotic resistance, new virulence determinants have caused major shifts in the course of infection. This is illustrated by group A streptococcal infections that evolve into the aggressive stage of necrotizing fasciitis and staphylococcal infections that produce toxic shock. In both cases, acquisition of new toxins on mobile genetic elements leads to the increased virulence. This process of continual evolution of disease is particularly virulent in gram-positive bacteria, suggesting that these infections will continue to be a challenge to the intensivist in the foreseeable future.

ACKNOWLEDGMENTS

This work was supported by National Institute of Allergy and Infectious Diseases, Grant AI27913, by National Cancer Institute Cancer Center CORE Support Grant P30 CA 21765, and by the American Lebanese Syrian Associated Charities.

References

1. Bullock W: The History of Bacteriology. New York, Dover Publications, 1979, pp 215-217.
2. Sands KE, Bates DW, Lanken PN, et al: Epidemiology of sepsis syndrome in 8 academic medical centers. JAMA 1997; 278:234-240.
3. Brun-Buisson C, Doyon F, Carlet J: Bacteremia and severe sepsis in adults: A multicenter prospective survey in ICUs and wards of 24 hospitals. Am J Respir Crit Care Med 1996; 154:617-624.
4. Rubio M, Palau L, Vivas JR, et al: Predominance of gram-positive micro-organisms as a cause of septicemia in patients with hematological malignancies. Infect Control Hosp Epidemiol 1994; 15:101-104.
5. Rubin M, Hathorn JW, Marshall D, et al: Gram-positive infections and the use of vancomycin in 550 episodes of fever and neutropenia. Ann Intern Med 1988; 108:30-35.
6. Salzman MB, Rubin LG: Intravenous catheter-related infections. Adv Pediatr Infect Dis 1995; 10:337-368.
7. Sriskandan S, Cohen J: The pathogenesis of septic shock. J Infect 1995; 30:201-206.
8. Pinner RW, Teutsch SM, Simonsen L, et al: Trends in infectious disease mortality in the United States. JAMA 1996; 275:189-193.
9. Lynn WA, Cohen J: Adjunctive therapy for septic shock: A review of experimental approaches. Clin Infect Dis 1995; 20:143-158.
10. Perez CM, Kubak BM, Cryer HG, et al: Adjunctive treatment of streptococcal toxic shock syndrome using intravenous immunoglobulin: Case report and review. Am J Med 1997; 102:111-113.
11. Speck WT, Spear SS, Krongrad E, et al: Transient bacteremia in pediatric patients after dental extraction. Am J Dis Child 1976; 130:406-407.
12. Hogt AH, Dankert J, Hulstaert CE, et al: Cell surface characteristics of coagulase-negative staphylococci and their adherence to fluorinated poly(ethylenepropylene). Infect Immun 1986; 51:294-301.
13. Christensen GD, Simpson WA, Bisno AL, et al: Adherence of slime-producing strains of *Staphylococcus epidermidis* to smooth surfaces. Infect Immun 1982; 37:318-326.
14. Janoff EN, Rubins JB: Invasive pneumococcal disease in the immunocompromised host. Microb Drug Resist 1997; 3:215-232.
15. Elting LS, Bodey GP, Keefe BH: Septicemia and shock syndrome due to viridans streptococci: A case-control study of predisposing factors. Clin Infect Dis 1992; 14:1201-1207.
16. Bochud PY, Calandra T, Francioli P: Bacteremia due to viridans streptococci in neutropenic patients: A review. Am J Med 1994; 97:256-264.
17. Bochud PY, Eggiman P, Calandra T, et al: Bacteremia due to viridans streptococcus in neutropenic patients with cancer: Clinical spectrum and risk factors. Clin Infect Dis 1994; 18:25-31.
18. Richard P, Amador Del Valle G, Moreau P, et al: Viridans streptococcal bacteraemia in patients with neutropenia. Lancet 1995; 345:1607-1609.
19. Edmond MB, Ober JF, Weinbaum DL, et al: Vancomycin-resistant *Enterococcus faecium* bacteremia: Risk factors for infection. Clin Infect Dis 1995; 20:1126-1133.
20. Tornieporth NG, Roberts RB, John J, Hafner A, Riley LW: Risk factors associated with vancomycin-resistant infection or colonization in 145 matched case patients and control patients. Clin Infect Dis 1996; 23:767-772.
21. Rogolsky M: Nonenteric toxins of *Staphylococcus aureus.* Microbiol Rev 1979; 43:320-360.
22. Tuomanen EI, Autrian R, Masure HR: Pathogenesis of pneumococcal infection. N Engl J Med 1995; 332:1280-1284.
23. Gemmell CG: Virulence determinants of *Staphylococcus epidermidis.* Med Microbiol 1986; 22:287-289.
24. Cole MF, Evans M, Fitzsimmons S, et al: Pioneer oral streptococci produce immunoglobulin A1 protease. Infect Immun 1994; 62:2165-2168.
25. Yother J, White JM: Novel surface attachment mechanism of the *Streptococcus pneumoniae* protein PspA. J Bacteriol 1994; 176:2976-2985.
26. Fischetti VA, Pancholi V, Schneewind O: Conservation of a hexapeptide sequence in the anchor region of surface proteins from gram-positive cocci. Mol Microbiol 1990; 4:1603-1605.
27. Burnette-Curley D, Wells V, Viscount H, Munro CL, Fenno JC, Fives-Taylor P, Macrina FL: FimA, a major virulence factor associated with *Streptococcus parasanguis* endocarditis. Infect Immun 1995; 63:4669-4674.
28. Cundell DR, Gerard NP, Gerard C, et al: *Streptococcus pneumoniae* anchor to activated human cells by the receptor for platelet-activating factor. Nature 1995; 377:435-438.
29. Geelen S, Bhattacharyya C, Tuomanen E: The cell wall mediates pneumococcal attachment to and cytopathology in human endothelial cells. Infect Immun 1993; 61:1538-1543.
30. Cheung AL, Eberhardt KJ, Chung E, et al: Diminished virulence of a *sar−/agr−* mutant of *Staphylococcus aureus* in the rabbit model of endocarditis. J Clin Invest 1994; 94:1815-1822.
31. Bruyn GAW, Zegers BJM, van Furth R: Mechanisms of host defense against infection with *Streptococcus pneumoniae*. Clin Infect Dis 1992; 14:251-262.
32. Dunne DW, Resnick D, Greenberg J, Krieger M, Joiner KA: The type I macrophage scavenger receptor binds to gram-positive bacteria and recognizes lipoteichoic acid. Proc Natl Acad Sci USA 1994; 91:1863-1867.
33. Polotsky VY, Fischer W, Ezekowitz AB, Joiner KA: Interactions of human mannose-binding protein with lipoteichoic acids. Infect Immun 1996; 64:380-383.
34. Tuomanen E, Liu H, Hengstler B, Zak O, Tomasz A: The induction of meningeal inflammation by components of the pneumococcal cell wall. J Infect Dis 1985; 151:859-868.
35. Tuomanen E, Rich R, Zak O: Induction of pulmonary inflammation by components of the pneumococcal cell surface. Am Rev Respir Dis 1987; 135:869-874.
36. Simpson SQ, Singh R, Bice DE: Heat-killed pneumococci and pneumococcal capsular polysaccharides stimulate tumor necrosis factor-α production by murine macrophages. Am J Respir Cell Mol Biol 1994; 10:284-289.
37. Mattsson E, Verhage L, Rollof J, Fleer A, Verhoef J, van Dijk H: Peptidoglycan and teichoic acid from *Staphylococcus epidermidis* stimulate human monocytes to release tumour necrosis factor-α,

interleukin-1β and interleukin-6. FEMS Immunol Med Microbiol 1993; 7:281–288.
38. De Kimpe SJ, Kengatharan M, Thiemermann C, et al: The cell wall components peptidoglycan and lipoteichoic acid from *Staphylococcus aureus* act in synergy to cause shock and multiple organ failure. Proc Natl Acad Sci USA 1996; 92:10359–10363.
39. Toth LA, Krueger JM: Effects of microbial challenge on sleep in rabbits. FASEB J 1989; 3:2062–2066.
40. Geelen S, Bhattacharyya C, Tuomanen E: Induction of procoagulant activity on human endothelial cells by *Streptococcus pneumoniae.* Infect Immun 1992; 60:4179–4183.
41. Spellerberg B, Prasad S, Cabellos C, Burroughs M, Cahill P, Tuomanen E: Penetration of the blood-brain barrier: Enhancement of drug delivery and imaging by bacterial glycopeptides. J Exp Med 1995; 182:1037–1044.
42. Pugin J, Heumann ID, Tomasz A, et al: CD14 is a pattern recognition receptor. Immunity 1994; 1:509–516.
43. Jennings H, Lugowski C, Young N: Structure of the complex polysaccharide C-substance from *Streptococcus pneumoniae.* Biochem J 1980; 19:4712–4719.
44. Standiford TJ, Arenberg DA, Danforth JM, Kunkel SL, VanOtteren GM, Strieter RM: Lipoteichoic acid induces secretion of interleukin-8 from human blood monocytes: A cellular and molecular analysis. Infect Immun 1994; 62:119–125.
45. Longchamp MO, Auguet M, Delaflotte S, Goulin-Schulz J: Lipoteichoic acid: A new inducer of nitric oxide synthase. J Cardiovasc Pharmacol 1992; 20(Suppl 12):S145–S147.
46. Auguet M, Longchamp MO, Delaflotte S, Goulin-Schulz JG, Chabrier PE, Braquet P: Induction of nitric oxide synthase by lipoteichoic acid from *Staphylococcus aureus* in vascular smooth muscle cells. FEBS Lett 1992; 297:183–185.
47. Cleveland MG, Gorham JD, Murphy TL, Tuomanen EI, Murphy KM: Lipoteichoic acid preparations of gram-positive bacteria induce interleukin-12 through a CD14-dependent pathway. Infect Immun 1996; 64:1906–1912.
48. English BK, Patrick CC, Orlicek SL, McCordic R, Shenep JL: Lipoteichoic acid from viridans streptococci induces the production of tumor necrosis factor and nitric oxide by murine macrophages. J Infect Dis 1996; 174:1348–1351.
49. Goodman JS: Toxic-shock syndrome and the Bundaberg disaster (Letter). N Engl J Med 1980; 303:1417.
50. Suttorp N, Fuhrmann M, Tannert-Otto S, Grimminger F, Bhadki S: Pore-forming bacterial toxins potently induce release of nitric oxide in porcine endothelial cells. J Exp Med 1993; 178:337–341.
51. Canvin JR, Paton JC, Boulnois GJ, Andrew PW, Mitchell TJ: *Streptococcus pneumoniae* produces a second haemolysin that is distinct from pneumolysin. Microb Pathog 1997; 22:129–132.
52. Barnard JP, Stinson MW: The alpha-hemolysin of *Streptococcus gordonii* is hydrogen peroxide. Infect Immun 1996; 64:3853–3857.
53. Braun V, Focareta T: Pore-forming bacterial protein hemolysins. Crit Rev Microbiol 1991; 18:115–158.
54. Hackett SP, Stevens DL: Streptococcal toxic shock syndrome: Synthesis of tumor necrosis factor and interleukin-1 by monocytes stimulated with pyrogenic exotoxin A and streptolysin O. J Infect Dis 1991; 165:879–885.
55. Berry AM, Alexander JE, Mitchell TJ, Andrew PW, Hansman D, Paton J: Effect of defined point mutations in the pneumolysin gene on the virulence of *Streptococcus pneumoniae.* Infect Immun 1995; 63:1969–1974.
56. Rubins JB, Charboneau D, Paton JC, Mitchell TJ, Andrew PW, Janoff EN: Dual function of pneumolysin in the early pathogenesis of murine pneumococcal pneumonia. J Clin Invest 1995; 95:142–150.
57. Amaee FR, Comis SD, Osborne MP: N^G-Methyl-L-arginine protects guinea pig cochlea from the cytotoxic effects of pneumolysin. Acta Otolaryngol (Stockh) 1995; 115:386–391.
58. Bohach GA, Fast DJ, Nelson RD, Schlievert PM: Staphylococcal and streptococcal pyrogenic toxins involved in toxic shock syndrome and related illnesses. Crit Rev Microbiol 1990; 17:251–272.
59. Herman A, Kappler JW, Marrak P, Pullen AM: Superantigens: Mechanism of T-cell stimulation and role in immune responses. Annu Rev Immunol 1991; 9:745–772.
60. Norrby-Teglund A, Holm SE, Norgren M: Detection and nucleotide sequence analysis of the speC gene in Swedish clinical group A streptococcal isolates. J Clin Microbiol 1994; 32:705–709.
61. Heumann D, Barras C, Severin A, Glauser MP, Tomasz A: Gram-positive cell walls stimulate synthesis of tumor necrosis factor alpha and interleukin-6 by human monocytes. Infect Immun 1994; 62:2715–2721.
62. Cabellos C, MacIntyre DE, Forrest M, Burroughs M, Prasad S, Tuomanen E: Differing roles for platelet-activating factor during inflammation of the lung and subarachnoid space. J Clin Invest 1992; 90:612–618.
63. Cauwels A, Wan E, Leismann M, Tuomanen E: Coexistence of CD14-dependent and independent pathways for stimulation of human monocytes by gram positive bacteria. Infect Immun 1997; 65:3255–3260.
64. Spellerberg B, Rosenow C, Sha W, Tuomanen E: Pneumococcal cell wall activates NF-κB in human monocytes: Aspects distinct from endotoxin. Microb Pathog 1996; 20:309–317.
65. Sha WC, Liou H-C, Tuomanen EI, Baltimore D: Targeted disruption of the p50 subunit of NF-κB leads to multifocal defects in immune responses. Cell 1995; 80:321–330.
66. Dinarello CA, Cannon JG, Wolff SM: New concepts on the pathogenesis of fever. Rev Infect Dis 1988; 10:168–189.
67. Waage A, Espevik T: Interleukin 1 potentiates the lethal effect of tumor necrosis factor alpha/cachectin in mice. J Exp Med 1988; 167:1987–1992.
68. Weinberg JR, Wright DJ, Guz A: Interleukin-1 and tumour necrosis factor cause hypotension in the conscious rabbit. Clin Sci 1988; 75:251–255.
69. Calandra T, Baumgartner JD, Grau GE, et al: Prognostic values of tumor necrosis factor/cachectin, interleukin-1, interferon-alpha, and interferon-gamma in the serum of patients with septic shock. Swiss-Dutch J5 Immunoglobulin Study Group. J Infect Dis 1990; 161:982–987.
70. Damas P, Reuter A, Gysen P, et al: Tumor necrosis factor and interleukin-1 serum levels during severe sepsis in humans. Crit Care Med 1989; 17:975–978.
71. Dinarello CA, Wolff SM: The role of interleukin-1 in disease. N Engl J Med 1993; 328:106–113.
72. Isner JM, Dietz WA: Cardiovascular consequences of recombinant DNA technology: Interleukin-2. Ann Intern Med 1988; 109:933–935.
73. Hack CE, De Groot ER, Felt-Bersma RJ, et al: Increased plasma levels of interleukin-6 in sepsis. Blood 1989; 74:1704–1710.
74. Wenzel RP, Pinsky MR, Ulevitch RJ, Young L: Current understanding of sepsis. Clin Infect Dis 1996; 22:407–413.
75. Hack CE, Hart M, Strack van Schindel RJM, et al: Interleukin-8 in sepsis: Relation to shock and inflammatory mediators. Infect Immun 1992; 60:2835–2842.
76. Waage A, Halstensen A, Espevik T: Association between tumour necrosis factor in serum and fatal outcome in patients with meningococcal disease. Lancet 1987; 1:355–357.
77. Michie HR, Manogue KR, Spriggs DR, et al: Detection of circulating tumor necrosis factor after endotoxin administration. N Engl J Med 1988; 318:1481–1486.
78. Silva AT, Appelmelk BJ, Buurman WA, et al: Monoclonal antibody to endotoxin core protects mice from *Escherichia coli* sepsis by a mechanism independent of tumor necrosis factor and interleukin-6. J Infect Dis 1990; 162:454–459.
79. Koshland DE Jr: The molecule of the year (Editorial). Science 1992; 258:1861.
80. Kilbourn RG, Griffith OW: Overproduction of nitric oxide in cytokine-mediated and septic shock. J Natl Cancer Inst 1992; 84:827–831.
81. Palmer RM: The discovery of nitric oxide in the vessel wall. A unifying concept in the pathogenesis of sepsis. Arch Surg 1993; 128:396–401.
82. Moncada S, Higgs A: The L-arginine–nitric oxide pathway. N Engl J Med 1993; 329:2002–2012.
83. Vallance P, Moncada S: Role of endogenous nitric oxide in septic shock. New Horizons 1993; 1:77–86.
84. Bradley JR, Wilks D, Rubenstein D: The vascular endothelium in septic shock. J Infect 1994; 28:1–10.
85. Schmidt HH, Lohmann SM, Walter U: The nitric oxide and cGMP signal transduction system: Regulation and mechanism of action. Biochim Biophys Acta 1993; 1178:153–175.
86. Petros A, Bennett D, Vallance P: Effect of nitric oxide synthase inhibitors on hypotension in patients with septic shock. Lancet 1991; 338:1557–1558.

87. Lorente JA, Landin L, De Pablo R, et al: L-Arginine pathway in the sepsis syndrome. Crit Care Med 1993; 21:1287-1295.
88. Petros A, Lamb G, Leone A, et al: Effects of a nitric oxide synthase inhibitor in humans with septic shock. Cardiovasc Res 1994; 28:34-39.
89. Nava E, Palmer RM, Moncada S: Inhibition of nitric oxide synthesis in septic shock: How much is beneficial? Lancet 1991; 338:1555-1557.
90. Klabunde RE, Ritger RC: N^G-Monomethyl-L-arginine (NMA) restores arterial blood pressure but reduces cardiac output in a canine model of endotoxic shock. Biochem Biophys Res Commun 1991; 178:1135-1140.
91. Robertson FM, Offner PJ, Ciceri DP, et al: Detrimental hemodynamic effects of nitric oxide synthase inhibition in septic shock. Arch Surg 1994; 129:149-155.
92. Winkelstein JA, Tomasz A: Activation of the alternative pathway by pneumococcal cell wall teichoic acids. J Immunol 1978; 120:174-178.
93. Doerschuk CM, Winn RK, Coxson HO, Harlan JM: CD18-dependent and -independent mechanisms of neutrophil emigration in the pulmonary and systemic microcirculation of rabbits. J Immunol 1990; 144:2327-2333.
94. Tuomanen EI, Saukkonen K, Sande S, Cioffe C, Wright SD: Reduction of inflammation, tissue damage, and mortality in bacterial meningitis in rabbits treated with monoclonal antibodies against adhesion-promoting receptors of leukocytes. J Exp Med 1989; 170:959-968.
95. Xu H, Gonzalo JA, St Pierre Y, et al: Leukocytosis and resistance to septic shock in intercellular adhesion molecule 1-deficient mice. J Exp Med 1994; 180:95-109.
96. Tan TQ, Smith CW, Hawkins EP, Mason EO, Kaplan SL: Hematogenous bacterial meningitis in an intercellular adhesion molecule-1-deficient infant mouse model. J Infect Dis 1995; 171:342-349.
97. Odio CM, Faingezicht I, Paris M, et al: The beneficial effects of early dexamethasone administration in infants and children with bacterial meningitis. N Engl J Med 1991; 324:1525-1531.
98. Johnson J: Molecular science sets its sights on septic shock. J NIH Res 1991; 3:61-65.

55

Nitric Oxide in Critical Illness

José A. Lorente, MD, PhD • Luis Landín, MD, PhD
Andrés Esteban, MD, PhD

Few advances in medicine have contributed to our understanding of the pathophysiology of shock to the same extent as has the discovery of nitric oxide (NO) and its roles in vascular physiology and cell function.

NO is a highly reactive radical with a half-life in aqueous solution of 5.6 seconds and in blood of as short as 0.46 msec.[1] NO is synthesized by a family of enzymes called nitric oxide synthases (NOSs). The neuronal isoform (nNOS) plays a role in central nervous system functions and nonadrenergic, noncholinergic neurotransmission; the endothelial isoform (eNOS) modulates vascular tone; and the inducible isoform (iNOS) is involved in immune defense. Both nNOS and eNOS are constitutively expressed (being referred to as cNOS), whereas iNOS is expressed only under inflammatory conditions in numerous cell types, including macrophages and endothelial and vascular smooth muscle cells. Despite being called constitutive and inducible, eNOS and nNOS may also be induced under different physiologic conditions, such as shear stress or nerve injury, and conversely, iNOS may function as a "constitutive" isoform under certain physiologic conditions in some cells.[2] In general, cNOS is important in mediating normal physiologic effects, whereas iNOS is involved in host defense mechanisms and cytotoxicity.

The different NOS isoforms share a common catalytic scheme, involving the five-electron oxidation of the terminal guanidino nitrogen of the amino acid L-arginine to form NO and L-citrulline, in a complex reaction involving molecular oxygen and the reduced form of nicotinamide adenine dinucleotide phosphate (NADPH) as cosubstrates. Numerous other redox cofactors include enzyme-bound heme, reduced thiols, flavin adenine dinucleotide, flavin mononucleotide, and tetrahydrobiopterin.

For all isoforms, NO synthesis depends on binding the calcium-regulatory protein calmodulin. For eNOS and nNOS, increases in intracellular calcium concentrations are required for calmodulin binding and consequent activation to produce NO (Fig. 55-1). In contrast, iNOS binds calmodulin with a high affinity even at low calcium concentrations. Thus, iNOS activity is not regulated by calcium; rather it is regulated at the transcriptional level and is active for hours or days after being expressed, it is not agonist regulated and produces NO at 100-fold to 1000-fold greater amounts than does cNOS.

L-Arginine is the substrate for NOS. Cellular sources of L-arginine include transmembrane uptake by the y^+ channel (shared by other amino acids such as lysine and ornithine) and, to a limited extent, intracellular proteolysis. The fate of L-arginine depends on the cell type and includes:

1. Conversion to urea through the action of arginase in the urea cycle.
2. Conversion to ornithine for polyamine synthesis.
3. Incorporation into newly synthesized proteins.
4. Conversion to NO by the enzyme NOS.

It has been shown that citrulline produced by NOS can be recycled into arginine in endothelial cells[3] in a functional arginine-citrulline cycle (or modified urea cycle) (Fig. 55-2). Although dietary arginine is an obvious source of circulating arginine for metabolic utilization, endogenous production of arginine by this cycle may play a significant role in providing L-arginine for endothelial cells under conditions associated with decreased food intake and increased L-arginine utilization, such as sepsis and inflammation.

The modified urea cycle is regulated by L-glutamine,[4] the most abundant free amino acid in the body. Glutamine inhibits the conversion of L-citrulline to L-arginine in vitro,[3, 4] L-citrulline membrane transport,[5] and agonist-stimulated NO release.[3] It is possible that a decreased glutamine concentration in sepsis may lead to an increased NO release (by relieving the inhibitory effect on NO synthesis). Indeed, an increase in extracellular glutamine concentration attenuated the increase in endothelial NO synthesis induced by substance P and other inflammatory mediators,[6] thereby increasing blood pressure, as reported for the rabbit pulmonary artery.[7]

NO formed in the endothelial cell rapidly diffuses to the underlying vascular smooth muscle cell or to the vessel lumen. In plasma, NO is converted to nitrite and *S*-nitrosothiols (RSNOs). Nitrite is rapidly oxidized by hemoglobin (Hb) to nitrate and is excreted in the urine as nitrate. Also, NO may enter the erythrocyte. In this case, oxyhemoglobin ($Hb[FeII]O_2$) scavenges NO, producing nitrate and methemoglobin (Hb[FeIII]), whereas deoxyhemoglobin (Hb[FeII]) binds NO to form Hb[FeII]NO (Fig. 55-3).[8] Because no direct method for NO detection is available, most studies have relied on the determination of nitrite plus nitrate (NOx) to assess endogenous NO production in vivo. It is thought that nitrate represents the final (albeit unspecific, for it is interfered with by several other factors, such as renal function and nitrate intake) end product, whereas nitrite is specific but unstable.

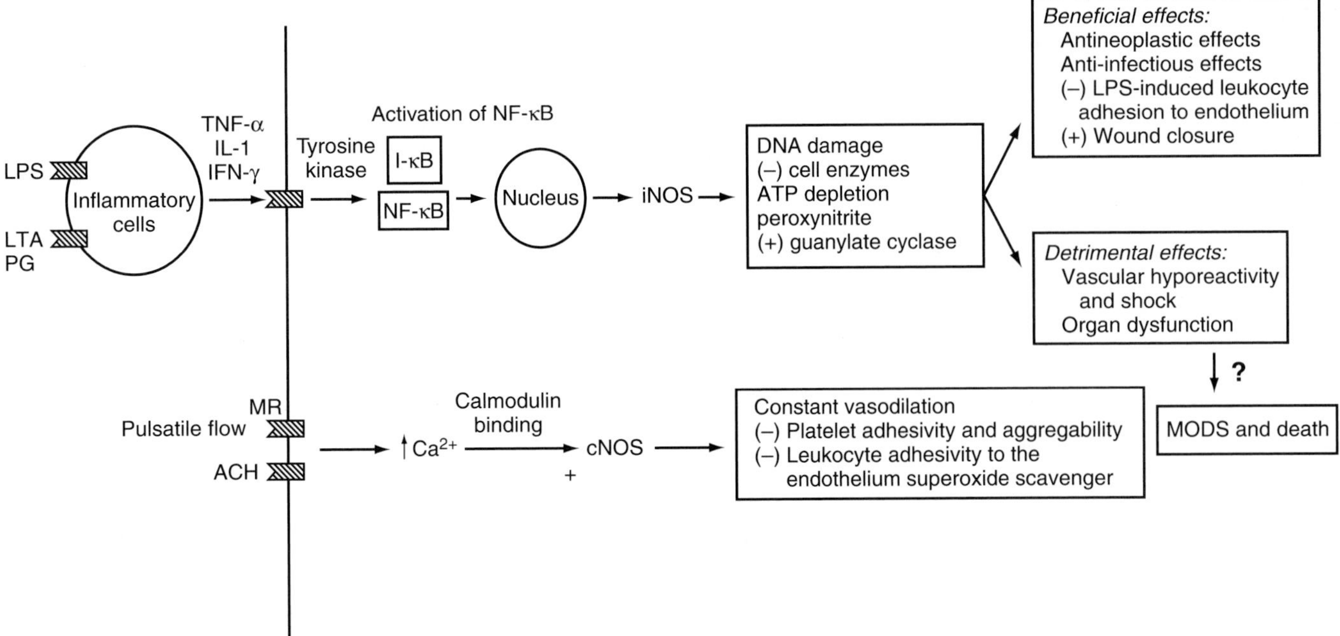

Figure 55–1. Schematic representation of the regulation and some of the effects of constitutive (cNOS) and inducible (iNOS) isoforms of the enzyme nitric oxide synthase (NOS). Gram-negative and gram-positive bacteria induce the expression of iNOS. Endotoxin (LPS) and lipoteichoic acid (LTA) or peptidoglycan (PG) trigger the release of inflammatory mediators, which bind to specific receptors, resulting in the activation of protein-tyrosine kinase, subsequent phosphorylation of intracellular proteins, and proteolytic cleavage of the inhibitory factor I-κB from the transcription factor NF-κB. Once activated, NFκ-B induces the expression of iNOS gene. NO formed by iNOS is beneficial in the host response against bacteria, parasites and tumor cells, and certain inflammatory conditions. However, its effects may also be cytotoxic for host cells and cause hemodynamic compromise, possibly contributing to multiple organ dysfunction syndrome (MODS) and death. cNOS is activated by increases in intracellular calcium, mediated by shear stress that operates through membrane mechanoreceptors (MR) or by different agonists, such as acetylcholine (ACH). By activating soluble guanylate cyclase and scavenging superoxide, NO from cNOS plays important physiologic roles. + = activation; − = inhibition. ATP = adenosine triphosphate; IFN = interferon; TNF = tumor necrosis factor; IL = interleukin.

Both oxyhemoglobin and deoxyhemoglobin rapidly deplete the amount of NO available to exert vasodilatory effects (see Fig. 55–3). Kinetic modeling predicts that most NO in the vasculature should be scavenged by hemoglobin.[8] Thus, NO levels may fall below the K_m for target enzymes (guanylate cyclase), raising the question of how NO exerts its biologic activity. One answer may be found in the formation of RSNOs,

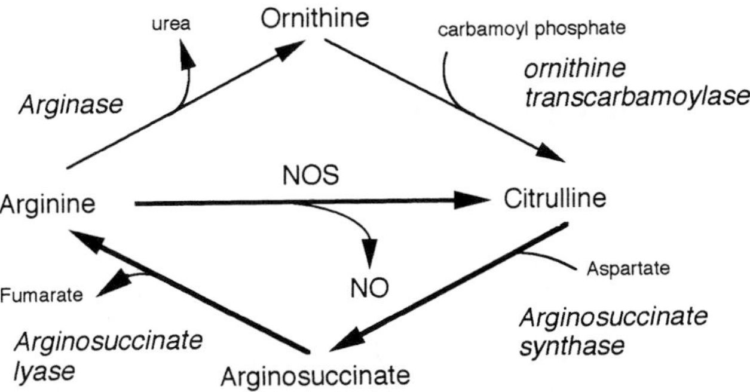

Figure 55–2. Arginine-citrulline cycle. L-Citrulline, the by-product of nitric oxide (NO) synthesis, is recycled to L-arginine by the formation of arginosuccinate (modified urea cycle, *thick arrows*). The formation of L-citrulline by the urea cycle *(thin arrows)* is restricted to the liver and kidney, which possess carbamoyl-phosphate and ornithine transcarbamoylase. However, other tissues rich in NO synthase (NOS), such as the endothelium and the brain, contain the enzymes arginosuccinate synthase and arginosuccinate lyase, allowing the formation of L-arginine from L-citrulline. The determination of [^{3}H]citrulline from [^{3}H]arginine is a means to assess NO formation, provided that there is no urea cycle.

which can form in the body when oxidized NO reacts with highly reactive thiol (-SH) groups. Indeed, some authors[9] have concluded that endothelium-derived relaxing factor behaves more like RSNO than NO on interaction with vascular smooth muscle in a system replete with physiologic thiols. Moreover, RSNOs have been identified in vivo[10] and appear to be more potent smooth muscle relaxants than is NO itself.[11] The majority of endogenously produced NO circulates in plasma as RSNOs, which stabilize NO bioactivity and probably play roles in transporting and targeting NO to specific effector sites.

Formation of nitrosylhemoglobin has been observed in animals and humans given endotoxin and nitroglycerin, respectively. It has been demonstrated that incubation of RSNOs with hemoglobin, instead of giving rise to a reaction between NO and oxygenated heme groups, inactivating the NO, originated the formation of hemoglobin-SNO. Exposure to NO, however, produced mainly methemoglobin.[8] Thus, hemoglobin has the newly discovered dual function of inactivating NO at the heme group and transporting NO by forming hemoglobin-SNO at the cysteine residues. Furthermore, the finding of higher levels of hemoglobin-SNO in arterial than in mixed venous blood of rats suggests that hemoglobin takes on NO in the lungs and delivers it to the tissues.[8] This new function of hemoglobin could have a role in the regulation of blood pressure, because injection of hemoglobin (lacking SNO) in rats caused the blood pressure to rise, but blood pressure did not change when hemoglobin-SNO was administered.[8]

PHYSIOLOGIC ROLES OF NITRIC OXIDE

Shear stress and different agonists, such as bradykinin, adenosine, histamine, thrombin, or acetylcholine, induce an increase

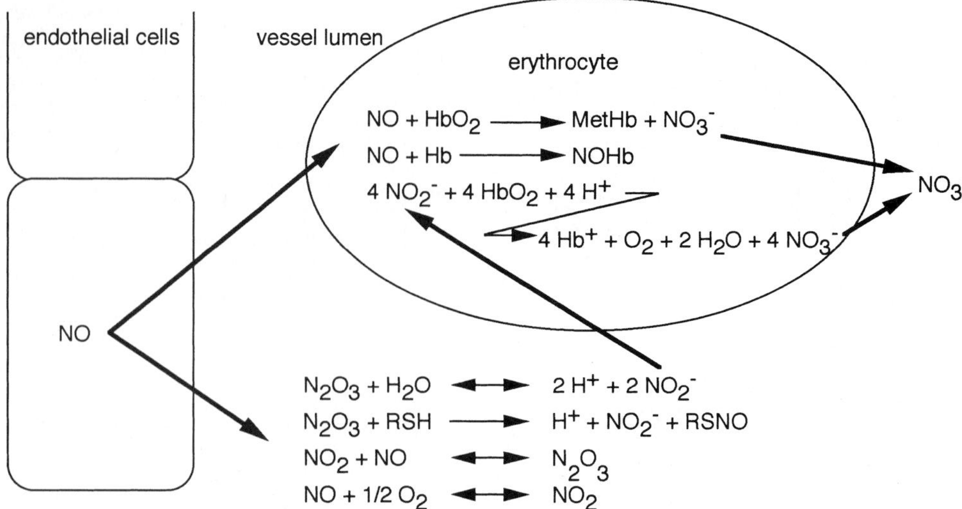

Figure 55–3. Metabolism of nitric oxide (NO) in blood. Released from the endothelial cell into the blood, NO is rapidly oxidized to nitrite (NO_2^-), which reacts with hemoglobin, forming nitrate (NO_3^-). NO reaching the erythrocyte directly forms nitrosylhemoglobin (NOHb), for the heme group in deoxy-Hb has a high affinity for NO, or methemoglobin (metHb) and NO_3^-. Alternatively (not shown), nitrosohemoglobin (SNO-Hb) may be formed in arterial blood, for the thiol groups in the cys residues of oxy-Hb have a very high affinity for NO to form nitrosothiols. The end products of these reaction are NO_3^-, NOHb, MetHb, and nitrosothiols (RSNOs). NO_2 = nitrogen dioxide; N_2O_3 = dinitrogen trioxide.

in intracellular calcium concentration, activating cNOS to produce small amounts of NO (see Fig. 55–1). Given its short half-life, NO must induce biologic effects at locations close to its site of production (paracrine action). NO diffuses to adjacent cells, where because of its affinity for heme iron, it reacts with soluble guanylate cyclase (sGC), resulting in the formation of cyclic guanosine monophosphate (cGMP), subsequent stimulation of cGMP-dependent protein kinase, decrease in intracellular calcium concentration, and vascular smooth muscle relaxation. Pulsatile flow-induced NO release maintains the cardiovascular system in a constant state of vasodilation. Nitrovasodilators in clinical use (nitroglycerin, sodium nitroprusside) act by being metabolized to NO and thereby causing sGC activation. NO also exerts effects on the endothelial cell (autocrine action), most notably a feedback inhibition of its own synthesis.

Other cGMP-mediated effects include (1) inhibition of fibrinogen binding to the IIb/IIIa receptor, (2) inhibition of phosphorylation of myosin light chains and of protein kinase C, (3) stimulation of phosphorylation of the beta subunit of glycoprotein I, and (4) modulation of response mediated by phospholipases A_2 and C.

NO also has a physiologic role as an anti-inflammatory molecule. Indeed, conditions associated with diminished NO are associated with changes consistent with an acute inflammatory response,[12] such as increased leukocyte-endothelial cell adhesion, platelet-leukocyte aggregation, albumin leakage, and increased formation of oxygen free radicals. NOS inhibitors, by increasing superoxide availability, destabilize mast cells and cause platelet-activating factor (PAF) and leukotriene B_4 release, expression of P-selectin on the endothelial surface, and subsequent increased leukocyte adhesivity.[13-15] Physiologically produced NO destroys superoxide anion, because inhibition of NOS results in an increased oxidative stress,[15] and superoxide is known to increase leukocyte recruitment.

NO helps maintain a low microvascular permeability.[16] The increased vascular permeability associated with NOS inhibitors occurs in two phases, one leukocyte-independent phase and a subsequent leukocyte-dependent phase, which is probably mediated by the release of PAF. It has been suggested that cGMP has a role in maintaining normal cytoskeletal integrity and that the effects of NOS inhibitors on vascular permeability are due to a destructuration of the normal cytoskeleton and endothelial cell retraction.[17]

Other physiologic actions of NO include its antiproliferative effects (which may have importance in vascular smooth muscle cell hyperplasia at sites of endothelial damage or arteriosclerosis) and its effects on hormone (growth hormone, corticotropin, thyroid-stimulating hormone, oxytocin, vasopressin) release.

Thus, under physiologic conditions, NO plays important roles as a tonic vasodilator, antiadhesive and antiaggregatory molecule for platelets and neutrophils, and superoxide scavenger. In this context, it is expected that conditions associated with decreased NO production (i.e., ischemia-reperfusion injury) or increased destruction (i.e., increased superoxide availability) may result in the abrogation of these normal functions, leading to increased leukocyte adhesivity to the endothelium, increased platelet aggregability, and vascular hyperpermeability.

PATHOPHYSIOLOGIC ROLES OF NITRIC OXIDE

The increased amounts of NO generated in inflammatory conditions are toxic for cell function.[18] A number of mechanisms outlined here are involved in NO-mediated cytotoxicity.

The interaction of NO with Fe-S-containing enzymes involved in adenosine triphosphate (ATP) generation, such as aconitase (Krebs cycle), NADH ubiquinone oxidoreductase and succinate ubiquinone oxidoreductase (electron transport chain), and enzymes of the deoxyribonucleic acid (DNA) synthesis pathway, results in inhibition of these enzymes and consequent decreased cellular respiration and intracellular ATP depletion.[19] Interaction of NO with thiol-containing enzymes can cause adenosine diphosphate (ADP) ribosylation and subsequent inactivation of glyceraldehyde-phosphate dehydrogenase, an enzyme involved in glycolysis.[20] NO may cause DNA damage resulting in activation of the enzyme poly-adenosine 5′-diphosphate (ADP)-ribose-synthetase (PARS) (see later). Moreover, NO modulates expression of numerous genes[21] and decreases the activity of sGC by decreasing the expression of genes encoding normal alpha and beta subunits of the enzyme,[21] which may be an important homeostatic mechanism for sGC desensitization to attenuate NO-mediated cytotoxicity or hemodynamic compromise in conditions of increased NO production. At high concentrations, NO not only binds to iron in proteins but also functionally inactivates protein-associated iron, thereby damaging protein and cell function.

NO reacts with superoxide (O_2^-) to form peroxynitrite ($ONOO^-$), a powerful oxidant. The high concentration of superoxide dismutase (SOD) normally present in cells keeps superoxide at low levels under physiologic conditions. However, superoxide reacts with NO three times faster than with SOD, and large amounts of NO out-compete SOD for superoxide.

The effects of peroxynitrite are critically dependent on the environmental conditions. For instance, both peroxynitrite and superoxide inactivate aconitase, but superoxide does so about 100 times faster than peroxynitrite does. NO production will slow the rate of superoxide-induced aconitase inactivation by forming peroxynitrite. Glutathione, normally present at high levels in mitochondria, reacts faster with peroxynitrite than with superoxide, forming thiols. Under these conditions, NO confers resistance to superoxide. However, if glutathione is depleted by oxidant stress, all formed peroxynitrite is free to react with and damage aconitase because peroxynitrite is a more powerful oxidant than superoxide.[22]

A second example is that the oxidant potential of peroxynitrite is determined not by the amount of its precursors NO and superoxide but by the ratio between the two. In fact, excess NO (by the administration of an NO donor) reduced the peroxynitrite-induced depression of mitochondrial respiration in endothelial cells.[23] These considerations are relevant because they may help explain findings in which both NOS inhibitors and NO donors seem to be beneficial.

Peroxynitrite is toxic through several mechanisms:

1. Oxidation of iron sulfur centers, sulfhydryl groups, lipids, and zinc fingers occurs in various important molecules.
2. At a slower rate, peroxynitrite spontaneously decomposes to form hydroxyl radicals.
3. In the presence of the metal catalyst Fe^{3+}, superoxide nitrates tyrosine residues in proteins, blocking critical phosphorylation reactions in signal transduction cascades, and can make proteins antigenic. The detection of nitrotyrosine in tissues is indicative of NO-related oxidative stress.
4. Induction of single-strand DNA breaks and subsequent PARS activation lead to intracellular ATP depletion. It has been shown that peroxynitrite causes depression of mitochondrial respiration, vasodilation, and impaired endothelium-dependent vasodilation by a PARS-dependent mechanism.[2, 23, 24]

By these mechanisms, iNOS seems to be beneficial for the host in certain infections and inflammatory conditions, playing an important role in mediating the destruction of intracellular organisms and tumor cells. However, iNOS may also be detrimental, causing cytotoxic effects to the host's own cells. For example, iNOS expression may benefit the host because it is required for wound closure, for normal angiogenesis to sustain survival of a skin flap, and to attenuate pulmonary leukocyte recruitment in lipopolysaccharide (LPS)–challenged mice.[2] On the other hand, iNOS may be related to lethality and lung damage in LPS-challenged mice and to lung damage in hemorrhagic shock.[2]

The role of iNOS in sepsis has been studied in mice rendered genetically deficient in iNOS. In one study, iNOS-deficient mice[25] showed no differences in survival compared with wild-type and homozygous knockout mice treated with LPS at doses of 5 and 15 mg/kg, but survival improved with 30 mg/kg of LPS. Mice deficient in iNOS failed to restrain the replication of *Listeria monocytogenes* in vivo and lymphoma cells in vitro and showed less marked LPS-induced hypotension. LPS-induced liver damage was similar in normal and iNOS-deficient mice. In another study, iNOS deficiency in mice completely prevented death after treatment with 12.5 mg/kg of LPS.[26] In a third study, iNOS-deficient mice treated with 12.5 or 25 mg/kg of LPS showed no increase in NOx levels and had the same mortality rate as that of wild-type mice.[27] The cause of these discrepancies is unknown and may be related to differences in the genetic backgrounds of the mutant and control mice used in these experiments.

ROLE OF NITRIC OXIDE IN THE HEMODYNAMIC CHANGES OF SEPSIS

A large body of evidence supports the concept that an excessive release of NO contributes to cardiovascular dysfunction in sepsis,[28-34] not only in models of gram-negative bacteremia or endotoxemia but also in gram-positive septic shock.[35] An excessive release of NO has been implicated in sepsis-induced hypotension, vascular hyporeactivity to pressor agents, decreased tissue oxygen extraction, decreased myocardial contractility, and decreased skeletal muscle contractility. NO also appears to be responsible for interleukin-2 (IL-2)–induced cardiovascular changes in patients with renal carcinoma as well as in vasodilation associated with cirrhosis.

The acute NO release induced by LPS in vivo[31, 36, 37] is caused by the activation of cNOS, possibly by LPS-induced bradykinin[38] or PAF[39] release, which are known activators of cNOS. The acute (within 60 minutes) vascular hyporeactivity to vasoconstrictor agents in LPS-treated rats was prevented by the NOS inhibitor *N*-monomethyl-L-arginine (L-NMMA) but not by dexamethasone, an inhibitor of iNOS expression,[39] whereas dexamethasone pretreatment prevented the vascular hyporeactivity and hypotension at 180 minutes. A significant increase in measurable NOS activity was noted in tissues only at 180 minutes after endotoxin. These results suggested that the immediate vascular hyporeactivity in septic shock is caused by an enhanced formation of NO due to activation of cNOS, and the delayed hypotension and vascular hyporeactivity are due to enhanced NO formation by endotoxin-induced iNOS.

The depressed vascular response to pressor agents characteristic of septic shock is compounded by a decreased response to endothelium-dependent vasodilators.[30, 33] The cause of this reduced release of stimulated NO is not totally understood but may involve several mechanisms, such as an alteration in signal transduction for NO release, a down-regulation of cNOS messenger ribonucleic acid (mRNA) by tumor necrosis factor-α (TNF-α), cytotoxicity of NO in high concentrations for the endothelium itself, a negative feedback mechanism by which NO may inhibit its own production, decreased L-arginine availability, and NO inactivation by an increase in oxygen-derived free radicals induced by the septic stimulus. Recent evidence indicates that peroxynitrite has a determinant role in sepsis-induced endothelial dysfunction.[23, 40]

Effects of Nitric Oxide Synthase Inhibitors

In view of the role of NO in modulating the vascular changes of sepsis, several therapeutic approaches to inhibit the actions of NO can be envisioned (Fig. 55–4), including:

1. Inhibition of NOS activity (i.e., by L-arginine analogs).
2. Inhibition of its induction process (i.e., by glucocorticoids).

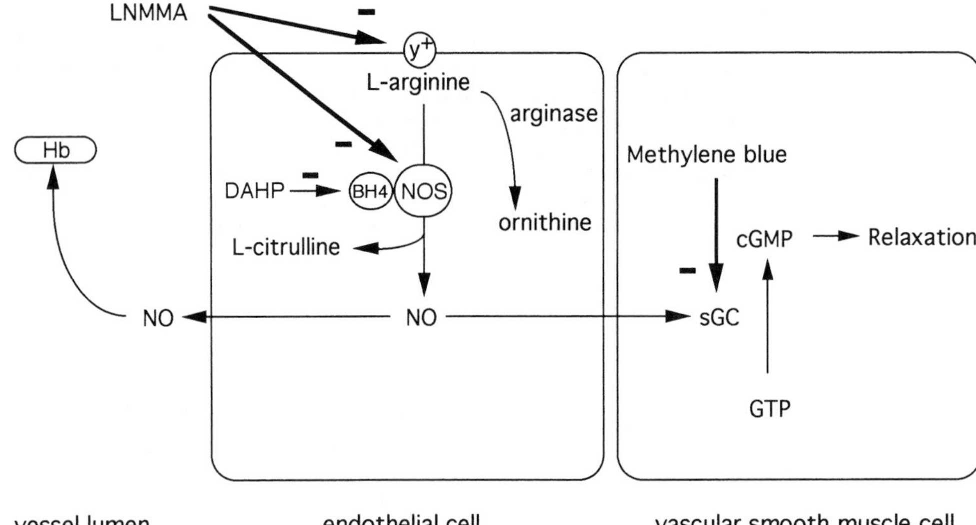

Figure 55–4. Schematic representation of the nitric oxide (NO) formation from L-arginine and the different steps where NO synthesis or action can be inhibited. NO synthesis can be blocked by different L-arginine analogs, such as L-*N*-monomethyl-arginine (L-NMMA). NO action can be blocked by hemoglobin (Hb), which rapidly scavenges circulating NO. Activation of soluble guanylate cyclase (sGC) can be inhibited by methylene blue. Nitric oxide synthase (NOS) activity can also be diminished by inhibition of cofactor supply by 2,4-diamino-6-hydroxypyrimidine (DAHP), which inhibits tetrahydrobiopterin (BH4) synthesis, or by limiting L-arginine availability by arginase. GTP = guanosine triphosphate; cGMP = cyclic guanosine monophosphate.

3. Scavenging of circulating NO (i.e., by hemoglobin).
4. Inactivation of sGC (with methylene blue).

The activity of iNOS can also be modulated by regulation of cofactor supply, such as through the inhibition of the synthesis of tetrahydrobiopterin, an essential cofactor for NOS, and by regulation of arginine availability through the exogenous administration of arginase.

L-Arginine analogs may show some selectivity for one NOS isoform. For instance, N^G-cyclopropyl-L-arginine, N^G-nitro-L-arginine, and N^G-nitro-L-arginine methyl ester (L-NAME) are more selective for cNOS. N^G-Amino-L-homoarginine, N^G-amino-L-arginine, and L-NMMA are approximately equipotent on cNOS and iNOS. Aminoguanidine and some related guanidines, as well as substituted isothiourea compounds, such as *S*-methylisothiourea, show selectivity toward iNOS.

Nonselective NOS inhibitors lead to less marked hypotension and improve vascular reactivity in sepsis.[31–34] However, they can also be associated with the abrogation of the physiologic functions normally served by NO. Pretreatment with different nonselective NOS inhibitors increased LPS-induced mortality in rats,[41–43] and plasma levels of TNF and IL-6 were higher.[43] L-NMMA increased LPS-induced liver injury[44] and intestinal damage in endotoxemic rats.[45] The protective effects of NO in endotoxemia are probably due to the reduction of oxygen radical–mediated injury and to the prevention of intravascular thrombosis.[46]

The vasoconstrictor effect of NOS inhibitors was associated with an increase in right and left cardiac filling pressures and a decreased cardiac output.[33] In endotoxemic dogs, NOS inhibition decreased cardiac index and oxygen delivery,[47, 48] and N^ω-amino-L-arginine caused seizure-like activity in normal dogs and increased lactic acidosis, liver damage, and mortality rate in dogs infused with endotoxin.[48] NOS inhibition also decreased regional (splanchnic, renal) blood flow[49–51] when it was administered before or early after the septic challenge.

Therefore, a number of studies have indicated that nonselective NOS inhibition can lead to an increased inflammatory response, reduced systemic and regional blood flow, more marked organ dysfunction, and a higher mortality rate in experimental models of sepsis. The causes of these deleterious effects associated with NOS inhibition can be due to

- Excessive vasoconstriction and decreased blood flow
- Use of an excessive dose of the NOS inhibitor
- Enhanced thrombi formation and increased platelet and leukocyte adhesivity to the endothelium
- Increase in proinflammatory cytokines
- Inhibition of NO-mediated antibacterial effects
- Use of nonselective NOS inhibitors, leading to inhibition of cNOS

Selective Versus Nonselective Nitric Oxide Synthase Inhibition

The use of selective NOS inhibitors (inhibitors of iNOS rather than cNOS) is supported by the concept that NO from cNOS is necessary for certain physiologic functions, and its inhibition may compromise several important functions normally regulated by NO, leading to decreased organ perfusion, thrombi formation, and increased leukocyte adhesivity. This concept is supported by two pieces of evidence: (1) the reported adverse effects of nonselective NOS inhibitors in models of sepsis outlined before, and (2) the finding that the administration of L-NMMA at high doses in septic rabbits and rats is associated with more severe organ failure and an increased mortality rate, whereas the administration of high-dose L-NMMA plus an NO donor, or of lower doses of L-NMMA, is beneficial.[52, 53]

Thus, it has been proposed that selective NOS inhibition would be an appropriate strategy for blocking excessive NO production in sepsis. Aminoguanidine is a selective iNOS inhibitor. Studies in a rat model of endotoxic shock have shown that pretreatment with aminoguanidine (1) ameliorated the delayed (after 60 minutes of the septic challenge) endotoxin-induced hypotension and vascular hyporeactivity, (2) attenuated renal, liver, and pancreatic dysfunction, and (3) improved survival.[54] *S*-Methylisothiourea, another selective iNOS inhibitor, reversed LPS-induced hypotension and vascular hyporeactivity in rats, ameliorated liver and renal dysfunction, and improved survival.[55-57]

Therefore, selective inhibition of inducible but not of endothelial NOS attenuates circulatory failure and multiple organ failure caused by endotoxemia. Despite the rationale of using selective NOS, however, in all studies in which detrimental effects of nonselective NOS inhibitors have been shown, the agent under study was administered either before or shortly after the septic challenge, well before the expression of iNOS could have taken place, and the dose was not titrated against any physiologic parameter, such as blood pressure. The negative results of those studies indicate the importance of NO generation by cNOS in the early phase of sepsis. Once sepsis has been established, it is possible that NOS inhibition by use of a nonselective inhibitor, carefully titrated against a physiologic parameter (i.e., blood pressure), does not totally suppress NO production and functions necessary for normal physiology of the cardiovascular, hematologic, and immune systems. This point is highlighted by the finding that NOS inhibitors given before or shortly after endotoxin increased mortality, whereas the same intervention given at a later time improved survival.[58]

On the other hand, sepsis is associated with a marked decrease in endothelium-dependent vasodilation, suggesting deficient endothelial NO production. Furthermore, TNF-α down-regulates cNOS mRNA. Therefore, whether there is significant production of endothelial NO to be spared (i.e., with the use of selective NOS inhibitors) in sepsis is debatable.

Regulation of Inducible Nitric Oxide Synthase Expression

Pretreatment with glucocorticoids inhibits iNOS expression,[59] leading to attenuation of delayed hypotension and vascular hyporeactivity in rat models of septic and hemorrhagic shock.[39, 60] Adrenalectomized rats showed a greater degree of iNOS induction and more severe cardiovascular failure after endotoxin. This effect was prevented by the administration of small doses of exogenous glucocorticoids.[61] Endogenous glucocorticoids suppress iNOS induction and are involved in endotoxin tolerance in vivo.[62] At least some of the anti-inflammatory effects of glucocorticoids are due to inhibition of iNOS expression.

Other inhibitors of iNOS expression include:

- Cyclosporine
- Nifedipine
- Dithiocarbamates (which suppress the action of transcription factor NF-κB in stimulated cells, a required step for iNOS induction)
- Anticytokine treatments (i.e., anti-TNF monoclonal antibodies, IL-1 receptor antagonist, and the PAF receptor antagonist WEB2086)
- Endogenous polyamines

Stroma-Free Hemoglobin as a Treatment for Septic Shock

Hemoglobin causes vasoconstriction by its NO-scavenging effect. Other proposed mechanisms of action include enhancement of endothelin release and inhibition of the enzyme NOS.[63] Cross-linked stroma-free hemoglobin increases arterial pressure in normal rats[64] as well as in bacteremic dogs[65] and endotoxemic pigs.[66] The pressor effect of diaspirin cross-linked hemoglobin (DCLH) is accompanied by indirect evidence of improved tissue perfusion.[66] The administration of hemoglobin is not without potential adverse effects in experimental models of sepsis, and there are reports of the induction of pulmonary damage, exacerbation of pulmonary hypertension and hypoxemia, LPS binding that augments the activity of endotoxin, stimulation of the production of cytokines by mononuclear cells, activation of complement, induction of liver and kidney injury, and an increased mortality rate.

An interesting pilot study in 14 patients with septic shock who received boluses of 10 g of DCLH has indicated that vasopressor support could be substantially reduced without signs of tissue hypoperfusion, although cardiac output decreased.[67] Future studies should determine whether this intervention is safe and effective for the treatment of patients with septic shock.

ROLE OF NITRIC OXIDE IN ORGAN DYSFUNCTION IN SEPTIC SHOCK

Nitric Oxide and Intestinal Dysfunction in Sepsis

NO has been implicated both in the maintenance of normal intestinal physiology and in mediating disease-related changes in intestinal function. The origin of NO in the gut may be nNOS, eNOS, or iNOS as well as a nonenzymatic source. The release of NO from nonadrenergic, noncholinergic neurons plays a role in the coordinated propagation of intestinal contents and sphincter relaxation and in gastric dilatation after food ingestion. NO is the major inhibitory factor of gut wall smooth muscle.

NO in the intestine may also have a nonenzymatic origin, by reduction of swallowed nitrate to nitrite and then to NO in acidic conditions and from anaerobic organisms that use nitrite and nitrate for respiration. Intraluminal NO may have an important role in inhibiting the growth of luminal flora. Of note, swallowing, gastric acidity, and luminal anaerobic microorganisms are all reduced in critically ill patients, possibly leading to a reduced amount of luminal NO. It has been speculated that reduced intraluminal NO could be involved in the relationship between loss of gastric acidity (i.e., by anti-H_2 treatment) and the development of nosocomial pneumonia.

In the endothelium, NO plays a role in the regulation of mucosal blood flow.[68] The protective effects in several models of mucosal injury, including endotoxemia and ischemia-reperfusion injury, may be associated with NO-mediated (1) maintenance of blood flow, (2) antiadhesive neutrophil properties, (3) increase in mucous secretion, and (4) mast cell stabilization.

NO exerts a tonic effect in the maintenance of low permeability to middle-range hydrophilic macromolecules, and NOS inhibition exacerbates LPS-induced mucosal damage in animal models of sepsis.[16, 69] On the other hand, it has been proposed that NO also has a causative role in intestinal injury in sepsis. LPS-injected rats show up-regulation of iNOS enzymatic activity in small intestinal and colonic epithelial cells and loss of cellular viability.[70] Aminoguanidine decreased bacterial translocation in LPS-treated rats and ameliorated endotoxin-induced bacterial translocation.[71] NO can promote translocation in a variety of ways, such as by inducing ileus and subsequent bacterial overgrowth and translocation or by altering epithelial permeability. Therefore, endotoxin-induced gut barrier dysfunction is dependent on the induction of iNOS.

In summary, NO is both protective and detrimental for the intestinal epithelium. NO from cNOS is protective during the early phase of sepsis, probably by helping maintain mucosal blood flow and by inhibiting PAF and histamine release from mast cells.[72] During later phases of sepsis, NO is cytotoxic, and inhibition of its synthesis results in attenuation of LPS-induced barrier dysfunction.

NO-induced mucosal epithelial hyperpermeability is related

to intracellular ATP depletion[73] and derangement in the distribution of F-actin.[74] Acidic conditions exacerbate the effects of NO on mucosal permeability and favor the formation of the potent oxidizing agent peroxinitrous acid (ONOOH) from peroxynitrite. It is these species ($ONOO^-$/ONOOH) that probably mediate the cytotoxic effects of NO by inactivation of mitochondrial aconitase, activation of PARS, and subsequent intracellular ATP depletion. Peroxynitrite increased the permeability and depleted the ATP content of cultured epithelial monolayers through a PARS-dependent mechanism[75] (see earlier). ATP depletion may be causally linked to intestinal epithelial barrier dysfunction, because a slight decrease in intracellular ATP content led to epithelial hyperpermeability in human intestinal epithelial cell monolayers,[76] probably by increasing intracellular calcium concentration.[77] Interestingly, NO donors not only increased permeability and depleted ATP but also increased intracellular calcium concentration.[78]

Nitric Oxide and Liver Dysfunction in Sepsis

The finding that nonselective NOS inhibitors administered to rats increased LPS-induced liver damage[46, 79] has led to the concept that NO has a protective role for liver function during sepsis. *S*-Methylisothiourea either did not change LPS-induced liver dysfunction[80] or, in rats treated with a higher dose of LPS, prevented hepatic damage.[55] Interestingly, iNOS does not seem to have a role in LPS-induced liver damage.[2, 25, 81]

The beneficial effects of selective NOS inhibitors could be related to an attenuation of the harmful effects associated with excessive NO production from iNOS in the liver, such as inhibition of mitochondrial respiration and gluconeogenesis, inhibition of total protein synthesis in cultured hepatocytes, and inhibition of bile canalicular contraction.

Nitric Oxide and Heart and Muscle Dysfunction in Sepsis

NO has also been implicated in the sepsis-induced decrease in skeletal muscle contractility because NOS inhibitors reversed in vitro the decreased contractility of diaphragmatic muscle.[82] NO also has a negative inotropic effect on the heart, as has been shown in papillary muscle and rat myocytes.[83] Whether these in vitro effects are relevant for cardiac function in vivo is unknown because the increase in afterload after NOS inhibition may determine a decrease in cardiac output regardless of any improvement in myocardial contractility. Moreover, it is unclear whether the amounts of NO generated during sepsis are sufficient to achieve the effects observed in vitro.

NITRIC OXIDE SYNTHASE INHIBITION IN HUMAN SEPTIC SHOCK

The idea that increased release of NO is involved in systemic hypotension and decreased vascular resistance of human septic shock is based on studies showing that:

1. Plasma concentrations of NOx are increased in patients with septic shock and are related to organ failure and prognosis.
2. NOx levels are related to some hemodynamic alterations.
3. NOS inhibitors in patients with septic shock are associated with beneficial effects.

The hypothesis that NOS inhibition may be beneficial in human septic shock is based not only on the possibility of improving vascular hyporeactivity and its sequelae (i.e., blood flow maldistribution, tissue hypoxia) but also on the hope that blocking NO could improve organ function because of the suppression of NO-mediated cytotoxic effects. However, although NOS inhibition improves vascular reactivity in humans with septic shock, the relationship between excessive NO release and the development of organ failure or death has not been confirmed at present.

Increased NOx plasma concentrations have been detected in adults[84] and children with sepsis[85, 86] and correlated with the Acute Physiology and Chronic Health Evaluation (APACHE) III score in postoperative patients[87] as well as with the magnitude of the inflammatory response (as measured by IL-6 plasma levels) in children with sepsis syndrome.[88] NOx levels also correlate negatively with blood pressure or systemic vascular resistance[84, 89] and positively with endotoxemia.[89]

Preliminary studies showed that inhibitors of NO synthesis are associated with vasoconstrictive properties in patients with septic shock[90, 91] that were reversed by L-arginine.[91] More recently, phase I and phase II clinical trials have been completed. The administration of fixed-dose rates of L-NMMA (from 1.0 to 20.0 mg/kg/hour) to different cohorts of patients with septic shock enabled norepinephrine therapy to be reduced or removed, with a tendency for cardiac index to fall, without impairment in left ventricular performance (measured as the left ventricular stroke work index).[92-94]

In a subsequent phase II clinical trial in which L-NMMA was titrated to maintain a mean arterial pressure of 70 mm Hg or higher in 312 patients with septic shock while withdrawal of concurrent vasopressors was attempted, resolution of shock (ROS) at 72 hours was attained in 39.1% of patients receiving L-NMMA and in 23.7% of those receiving placebo ($P < .005$).[95] No significant effect on 28-day mortality was observed (47% in the treatment group versus 48% in the placebo group). However, ROS at 72 hours was associated with a better 28-day survival rate (74% survival rate of patients with ROS versus 55% of patients with no ROS). The study groups did not differ in the incidence of reported adverse experiences.[96] Pulmonary hypertension was reported more often in the treatment group than in the placebo group. Pulmonary hypertension or right-sided heart dysfunction was reported overall in 10 of 156 (6%) in the treatment group and in four of 156 (3%) in the placebo group[97] and, among those with a mean pulmonary arterial pressure of 35 mm Hg or higher, in five of 17 (29%) in the treatment group and in one of 14 (7%) in the placebo group.

Thus, it seems that acute administration of NOS inhibitors in humans with septic shock leads to an increase in blood pressure accompanied by a fall in cardiac output and a rise in systemic and pulmonary vascular resistance. Prospective controlled clinical trials in patients with septic shock treated with L-NMMA for 72 hours after a rigorous algorithm aimed at decreasing conventional vasopressor support have shown that treatment with L-NMMA is associated with an increased incidence of ROS without untoward effects. Because ROS was associated with a better 28-day survival rate, it has been suggested that L-NMMA may significantly improve survival. Therefore, a phase III study has been designed to test this hypothesis and is now under way. Only this large, well-designed, prospective clinical trial will answer the question of whether NOS inhibition with L-NMMA in patients with septic shock improves survival in this deadly condition.

ROLE OF NITRIC OXIDE IN OTHER FORMS OF SHOCK

Hemorrhagic Shock

Like other forms of shock, hemorrhagic shock induces a state of vascular hyporeactivity and abnormal endothelium-dependent vasodilation.[98] Hemorrhagic shock in rats is associated with early (first 120 minutes) and late vascular hyporeactivity, probably caused by activation of cNOS and induction of iNOS, respectively.[60] The mechanism for the activation of cNOS is unclear but may be related to release of bradykinin, ATP, and serotonin. The mechanism for the induction of iNOS in hemorrhagic shock is unknown, but hemorrhage-induced release of TNF may be involved.

The role of NO in organ failure in hemorrhagic shock is controversial. Inhibition of NOS in rats subjected to hemorrhagic shock improved blood pressure,[99] decreased shock-induced gastric lesions, prolonged survival time,[100] and improved renal function and glomerular filtration rate.[101] Others have shown that nonselective NOS inhibition in hemorrhagic shock increased liver damage.[102] On the contrary, other studies in a model of hemorrhagic and traumatic shock in rats have shown that NO donors improved blood pressure, mesenteric artery endothelial function, and survival.[103, 104]

Trauma patients had lower than normal nitrate levels, whereas nontrauma surgical patients with sepsis had nitrate levels above normal.[84] The low capacity of trauma patients to generate nitrate persisted if sepsis occurred. On the basis of these results, it was hypothesized that iNOS expression was suppressed in trauma patients and that this deficit could be related to immunosuppression in these patients.

Ischemia-Reperfusion Injury

Ischemia-reperfusion is associated with leukocyte adherence and emigration, platelet-leukocyte aggregation, increased albumin leakage, mast cell degranulation, and epithelial hyperpermeability. All these findings feature the results of NOS inhibition, leading to the hypothesis that a lack of NO could be responsible for the ischemia-reperfusion–induced vascular dysfunction. There is evidence to support the concept that there is both a decrease in NO production and an increase in NO inactivation due to superoxide formation during the reperfusion phase.[105, 106] NO donors provided protection against ischemia-reperfusion injury, reducing albumin leakage, mast cell degranulation, and leukocyte recruitment, preventing epithelial hyperpermeability, and improving endothelium-dependent vasodilation and survival rate.[107] These effects may be due to the superoxide-scavenging effects and antiadhesive neutrophil properties of NO.

Other studies, however, have demonstrated that NO is damaging in ischemia-reperfusion injury. NOS inhibition limits leukocyte recruitment and protein leakage in postischemic lung and skeletal muscle[108] as well as reduces contractile dysfunction associated with ischemia-reperfusion.[109] In these models, protection was also achieved by oxygen free radical scavengers, suggesting that it is the interaction between oxygen free radicals and NO, possibly to form peroxynitrite, that is responsible for tissue injury.

Shock Due to Low Cardiac Output

Under normal conditions, there is a balance between vasoconstrictive adrenergic stimuli and NO-mediated vasodilator tone.[110, 111] In sheep subjected to a low cardiac output state, blood pressure and systemic vascular resistance are much better maintained if N^G-nitro-L-arginine is infused.[112] The released NO interacts with the sympathetic nervous system and prevents effective compensation of cardiovascular responses to the low-output state.

It appears that shock caused by low cardiac output is associated with alterations in both basal and stimulated release of NO. Stimulated release of NO is decreased in this condition,[113] leading to an impaired endothelial control of vascular tone. In vascular rings from dogs with heart failure, it has been reported that L-NMMA induced a greater increase in resting vascular tension compared with that of control subjects.[114] In a chronic model of pacing-induced heart failure in dogs,[115] L-arginine induced a decrease in vascular resistance. Thus, heart failure may be accompanied by induced (substrate-dependent) NOS and increased basal release of NO. Whether basal NO production is enhanced or decreased in patients with chronic low-output state is controversial.[116]

ACKNOWLEDGMENT

This manuscript was supported in part by FIS No. 98/0196.

References

1. Kelm M, Yoshida K: Metabolic fate of NO and related N-oxides. *In:* Methods in Nitric Oxide Research. M Feelisch, JS Stamler (Eds). Chichester, England, John Wiley & Sons Ltd, 1996, pp 47–58.
2. Nathan C: Inducible nitric oxide synthase: What difference does it make? J Clin Invest 1997; 100:2417–2423.
3. Hecker M, Sessa WC, Harris HJ, Angaard EE, Vane JR: The metabolism of L-arginine and its significance for the biosynthesis of endothelium-derived relaxing factor. Cultured endothelial cells recycle L-citrulline to L-arginine. Proc Natl Acad Sci USA 1990; 87:8612–8616.
4. Sessa WC, Hecker M, Mitchell JA, Vane JR: The metabolism of L-arginine and its significance for the biosynthesis of endothelium-derived relaxing factor: L-Glutamine inhibits the generation of L-arginine by cultured endothelial cells. Proc Natl Acad Sci USA 1990; 87:8607–8611.
5. Wu G, Meininger CJ: Regulation of L-arginine synthesis from L-citrulline by L-glutamine in endothelial cells. Am J Physiol 1993; 265:H1965–H1971.
6. Ralevic V, Khalil Z, Helme RD, Dusting GJ: Role of nitric oxide in the actions of substance P and other mediators of inflammation in rat skin microvasculature. Eur J Pharmacol 1995; 284:231–239.
7. Xu H, Pearl RG: Effect of L-glutamine on pulmonary hypertension in the perfused rabbit lung. Pharmacology 1994; 48:260–264.
8. Li J, Bonaventura C, Bonaventura J, Stamler JS: *S*-Nitrosohaemoglobin: A dynamic activity of blood involved in vascular control. Nature 1996; 380:221–226.
9. Wei EP, Kontos HA: H_2O_2 and endothelium-dependent cerebral arteriolar dilation. Hypertension 1990; 16:162–169.
10. Stamler JS, Jaraki O, Osborne J, Simon D, Keaney J, Vita J, Singel D, Valeri CR, Loscalzo J: Nitric oxide circulates in mammalian plasma as an *S*-nitroso adduct of serum albumin. Proc Natl Acad Sci USA 1992; 89:7674–7677.
11. Gaston B, Drazen J, Jansen A, Sugarbaker DA, Loscalzo J, Richards W, Stamler JS: The relaxation of human bronchial smooth muscle by *S*-nitrosothiols in vitro. J Pharmacol Exp Ther 1994; 268:978–984.
12. Gaboury JP, Kubes P: Endogenous antiadhesive molecules. *In:* Physiology and Pathophysiology of Leukocyte Adhesion. Granger DN, Schmid-Schoenbein G (Eds). New York, Oxford University Press, 1994, pp 241–260.
13. Kubes P, Kanwar S, Niu XF, Gaboury JP: Nitric oxide synthesis inhibition induces leukocyte adhesion via superoxide and mast cells. FASEB J 1993; 7:1293–1299.
14. Davenpeck KL, Gauthier TW, Lefer AM: Inhibition of endothelial-derived nitric oxide promotes P-selectin expression and actions in the rat microcirculation. Gastroenterology 1994; 107:1050–1058.
15. Niu XF, Smith CW, Kubes P: Intracellular oxidative stress induced by nitric oxide synthesis inhibition increases endothelial cell adhesion to neutrophils. Circ Res 1994; 74:1133–1140.
16. Kubes P, Granger DN: Nitric oxide modulates microvascular permeability. Am J Physiol 1992; 262:H611–H615.
17. Kubes P: Nitric oxide–induced microvascular permeability alterations: A regulatory role for cGMP. Am J Physiol 1993; 265:H1910–H1915.
18. Thomae KR, Joshi PC, Davies P, Pitt BR, Billiar TR, Simmons

RL, Nakayama DK: Nitric oxide produced by cytokine-activated pulmonary artery smooth muscle cells is cytotoxic to cocultured endothelium. Surgery 1996; 119:61-66.
19. Stadler J, Curran RD, Ochoa JB, et al: Effect of endogenous nitric oxide on mitochondrial respiration of rat hepatocytes in vitro and in vivo. Arch Surg 1994; 126:186-191.
20. Zhang J, Snyder SH: Nitric oxide stimulates auto-ADP-ribosylation and inhibition of glyceraldehyde-3-phosphate dehydrogenase. J Biol Chem 1992; 267:16771-16774.
21. Filipov G, Bloch DB, Block KD: Nitric oxide decreases stability on mRNA encoding soluble guanylate cyclase subunits in rat pulmonary artery smooth muscle cells. J Clin Invest 1997; 100:942-948.
22. Stamler J, Piantadosi CA: O=ONO: It is CO. J Clin Invest 1996; 97:2165.
23. Szabó C, Cuzzocrea S, Zingarelli B, O'Connor M, Salzman AL: Endothelial dysfunction in a rat model of endotoxic shock. J Clin Invest 1997; 100:723-735.
24. Szabó C, Zingarelli B, Salzman AL: Role of poly-ADP ribosyltransferase activation in the nitric oxide- and peroxynitrite-induced vascular failure. Circ Res 1996; 78:1051-1063.
25. MacMicking JD, Nathan C, Hom G, et al: Altered responses to bacterial infection and endotoxic shock in mice lacking inducible nitric oxide synthase. Cell 1995; 81:641-650.
26. Wei XQ, Charles IG, Smith A, et al: Altered immune responses in mice lacking inducible nitric oxide synthase. Nature 1995; 375:408-411.
27. Laubach VE, Shesely EG, Smithies O, Sherman PA: Mice lacking inducible nitric oxide synthase are not resistant to lipopolysaccharide-induced death. Proc Natl Acad Sci USA 1995; 92:10688-10692.
28. Salvemini D, Korbut R, Anggard E, Vane J: Immediate release of nitric oxide-like factor from bovine aortic endothelial cells by *E. coli* lipopolysaccharide. Proc Natl Acad Sci USA 1990; 87:2593-2597.
29. Lorente JA, Landín L, Esteban A: Role of nitric oxide in the regulation of vascular tone in septic shock. *In:* Update in Intensive Care and Emergency Medicine. Vincent JL (Ed). Berlin, Springer-Verlag, 1994, pp 75-89.
30. Julou-Schaeffer G, Gray GA, Fleming I, Schott CC, Parratt JR, Stoclet JC: Loss of vascular responsiveness induced by endotoxin involves L-arginine pathway. Am J Physiol 1990; 259:H1038-H1043.
31. Thiemermann C, Vane JR: Inhibition of nitric oxide synthesis reduces the hypotension induced by bacterial lipopolysaccharide in the rat in vivo. Eur J Pharmacol 1990; 182:591-594.
32. Meyer J, Traber LD, Nelson S, Lentz CW, Nakazawa H, Herndon D, Noda H, Traber DL: Reversal of hyperdynamic response to continuous endotoxin administration by inhibition of NO synthesis. J Clin Invest 1992; 73:324-328.
33. Lorente JA, Landín L, Renes E, et al: Role of nitric oxide in the hemodynamic changes of sepsis. Crit Care Med 1993; 21:759-767.
34. Landín L, Lorente JA, Renes E, Canas P, Jorge P, Liste D: Inhibition of nitric oxide synthesis improves the vasoconstrictive effect of noradrenaline in sepsis. Chest 1994; 106:250-256.
35. De Kimpe SJ, Hunter ML, Bryant CE, Thiemermann C, Vane JR: Delayed circulatory failure due to the induction of nitric oxide synthase by lipoteichoic acid from *Staphylococcus aureus* in anaesthetized rats. Br J Pharmacol 1995; 114:1317-1323.
36. Kilbourn RG, Jubran A, Gross SS, et al: Reversal of endotoxin-mediated shock by N^G-methyl-L-arginine, an inhibitor of nitric oxide synthesis. Biochem Biophys Res Commun 1990; 172:1132-1138.
37. Kilbourn RG, Gross SS, Jubran A, Adams A, Griffith OW, Levi R, Lodato RF: N^G-methyl-L-arginine inhibits tumor necrosis factor-induced hypotension: Implications for the involvement of nitric oxide. Proc Natl Acad Sci USA 1990; 87:3629-3632.
38. Fleming I, Dambacher T, Busse R: Endothelium-derived kinins account for the immediate response of endothelial cells to bacterial lipopolysaccharide. J Cardiovasc Pharmacol 1992; 20(Suppl 12):S135-S138.
39. Szabó C, Mitchell JA, Thiemermann C, Vane JR: Nitric oxide-induced hyporeactivity to noradrenaline precedes the induction of nitric oxide synthase in endotoxin shock. Br J Pharmacol 1993; 108:786-792.
40. Szabó C: The role of peroxynitrite in the pathophysiology of shock, inflammation and ischemia-reperfusion injury. Shock 1996; 6:79-88.
41. Cohen J, Silva A: NO inhibitors and septic shock (Letter). Lancet 1992; 339:751.
42. Minnard EA, Shou J, Naama H, Cech A, Gallagher H, Daly J: Inhibition of nitric oxide synthesis is detrimental during endotoxemia. Arch Surg 1994; 129:142-148.
43. Tiao G, Rafferty J, Ogle C, Fischer JE, Hasselgren PO: Detrimental effect of nitric oxide synthase inhibition during endotoxemia may be caused by high levels of tumor necrosis factor and interleukin-6. Surgery 1994; 116:332-338.
44. Billiar TR, Curran RD, Harbrecht BG: Modulation of nitrogen oxide synthesis in vivo: N^G-Monomethyl-L-arginine inhibits endotoxin-induced nitrite/nitrate biosynthesis while promoting hepatic damage. J Leukoc Biol 1990; 48:565-569.
45. Hutcheson IR, Whittle BJR, Boughton-Smith NK: Role of nitric oxide in maintaining vascular integrity in endotoxin-induced acute intestinal damage in the rat. Br J Pharmacol 1990; 101:815-820.
46. Harbrecht BG, Billiar TR, Stadler J, Demetris AJ, Ochoa J, Curran RD, Simmons RL: Inhibition of nitric oxide synthesis during endotoxemia promotes intrahepatic thrombosis and an oxygen radical-mediated hepatic injury. J Leukoc Biol 1992; 52:390-394.
47. Klabunde RE, Ritger RC: N^G-Monomethyl-L-arginine restores arterial blood pressure but reduces cardiac output in a canine model of endotoxic shock. Biochem Biophys Res Commun 1991; 178:1135-1140.
48. Cobb JP, Natanson C, Hoffman WD, et al: N^ω-Amino-L-arginine, an inhibitor of nitric oxide synthesis, raises vascular resistance but increases mortality rates in awake canines challenged with endotoxin. J Exp Med 1992; 176:1175-1182.
49. Spain DA, Wilson MA, Garrison RN: Nitric oxide synthase inhibition exacerbates sepsis-induced renal hypoperfusion. Surgery 1994; 116:322-331.
50. Mulder MF, van Lambalgen AA, Huisman E, et al: Protective role of NO in the regional hemodynamic changes during acute endotoxemia in rats. Am J Physiol 1994; 266:H1558-H1564.
51. Pastor CM, Payen DM: Effects of modifying nitric oxide pathway on liver circulation in a rabbit endotoxin shock model. Shock 1994; 2:196-202.
52. Nava E, Palmer RMJ, Moncada S: Inhibition of nitric oxide synthesis in septic shock: How much is beneficial? Lancet 1991; 338:1555-1557.
53. Wright CE, Rees DD, Moncada S: The protective and pathological roles of nitric oxide in endotoxin shock. Cardiovasc Res 1992; 26:48-57.
54. Wu CC, Chen SJ, Szabó C, Thiemermann C, Vane JR: Aminoguanidine attenuates the delayed circulatory failure and improves survival in rodent models of endotoxic shock. Br J Pharmacol 1995; 114:1666-1672.
55. Szabó C, Southan GJ, Thiemermann C: Beneficial effects and improved survival in rodent models of septic shock with *S*-methylisothiourea sulfate, a potent and selective inhibitor of inducible nitric oxide synthase. Proc Natl Acad Sci USA 1994; 91:12472-12476.
56. Aranow JS, Zhuang J, Wang H, Larkin V, Smith M, Fink MP: A selective inhibitor of inducible nitric oxide synthase prolongs survival time in a rat model of bacterial peritonitis: Comparison with two nonselective strategies. Shock 1996; 5:116-121.
57. Wu CC, Ruetten H, Thiemermann C: Comparison of the effects of aminoguanidine and N^ω-nitro-L-arginine methyl ester on the multiple organ dysfunction caused by endotoxaemia in the rat. Eur J Pharmacol 1996; 300:99-104.
58. Rees D, Monkhouse J, Moncada S: N^G-Monomethyl-L-arginine HCl (L-NMMA: 546C88) improves survival in a conscious instrumented mouse model of endotoxic shock. Endothelium 1995; 3(Suppl):S116.
59. Radomski MW, Palmer RMJ, Moncada S: Glucocorticoids inhibit the expression of an inducible, but not the constitutive, nitric oxide synthase in vascular endothelial cells. Proc Natl Acad Sci USA 1990; 87:10043-10047.
60. Thiemermann C, Szabó C, Mitchell JA, Vane JR: Vascular hyporeactivity to vasoconstrictor agents and hemodynamic decompensation in hemorrhagic shock is mediated by nitric oxide. Proc Natl Acad Sci USA 1993; 90:267-271.

61. Szabó C, Thiemermann C, Vane JR: Inhibition of the production of nitric oxide and vasodilator prostaglandins attenuates the cardiovascular response to bacterial endotoxin in adrenalectomized rats. Proc R Soc Lond B Biol Sci 1993; 253:233–238.
62. Szabó C, Thiemermann C, Wu CC, Perreti M, Vane JR: Attenuation of the induction of nitric oxide synthase by endogenous glucocorticoids accounts for endotoxin tolerance in vivo. Proc Natl Acad Sci USA 1994; 91:271–275.
63. Bone HG, Schnarts PJ, Booke M, McGuire R, Harper D, Traber LD, Traber DL: Oxalated pyridoxalated hemoglobin polyoxyethylene conjugate normalizes the hyperdynamic circulation in septic sheep. Crit Care Med 1997; 25:1010–1018.
64. Sharma AC, Gulati A: Effect of diaspirin cross-linked hemoglobin and norepinephrine on systemic hemodynamics and regional circulation in rats. J Lab Clin Med 1994; 123:299–308.
65. Crowley JP, Metzger J, Gray J, et al: Infusion of stroma-free cross-linked hemoglobin during acute gram-negative bacteremia. Circ Shock 1993; 41:144–149.
66. Aranow JS, Wang H, Zhuang J, Fink MP: Effect of human hemoglobin on systemic and regional hemodynamics in a porcine model of endotoxemic shock. Crit Care Med 1996; 24:807–814.
67. Reah G, Bodenham AR, Mallik A, Daily EK, Przybelski RJ: Initial evaluation of diaspirin cross-linked hemoglobin (DCLHb) as a vasopressor in critically ill patients. Crit Care Med 1997; 25:1480–1488.
68. Spain DA, Wilson MA, Bar-Natan MF, Garrison RN: Role of nitric oxide in small intestinal microcirculation during bacteremia. Shock 1994; 2:41–46.
69. Boughton-Smith NK, Hucheson IR, Deakin AM, et al: Protective effect of *S*-nitro-*N*-acetyl-penicillamine in endotoxin-induced acute intestinal damage in the rat. Eur J Pharmacol 1994; 191:485–488.
70. Tepperman BL, Brown JF, Korolkiewicz R, Whittle BJR: Nitric oxide synthase activity, viability and cyclic GMP levels in rat colonic and epithelial cells: Effects of endotoxin challenge. J Pharmacol Exp Ther 1994; 271:1477–1482.
71. Unno N, Wang H, Menconi MJ, Tytgat SHAJ, Larkin V, Smith M, Morin MJ, Chavez A, Hodin RA, Fink MP: Inhibition of inducible nitric oxide synthase ameliorates endotoxin-induced gut mucosal barrier dysfunction in rats. Gastroenterology 1997; 113:1246–1257.
72. Kanwar S, Wallance JL, Befus D, et al: Nitric oxide synthesis inhibition increases epithelial permeability via mast cells. Am J Physiol 1994; 266:G222–G229.
73. Salzman AL, Menconi MJ, Unno N, Ezzell RM, Gasey DM, Gonzalez PK, Fink MP: Nitric oxide dilates tight junctions and depletes ATP in cultured Caco-2BBe intestinal epithelial monolayers. Am J Physiol 1995; 193:G923–G933.
74. Hinshaw DB, Armstrong BC, Burger JM, Beals TF, Hyslop PA: ATP and microfilaments in cellular oxidant injury. Am J Pathol 1988; 132:479–488.
75. Szabó C, Saunders C, O'Connor M, Salzman AL: Peroxynitrite causes energy depletion and increases permeability via activation of poly(ADP-ribose) synthetase in pulmonary epithelial cells. Am J Respir Cell Mol Biol 1997; 16:105–109.
76. Unno N, Menconi MJ, Salzman AL, Smith M, Hagen S, Ge Y, Ezzell RM, Fink MP: Hyperpermeability and ATP depletion induced by chronic hypoxia or glycolytic inhibition in Caco-2BBe monolayers. Am J Physiol 1996; 270:G1010–G1021.
77. Unno N, Fink MP: BAPTA inhibits elevation of cytosolic free Ca^{2+} ($[Ca^{2+}]i$) during chemical hypoxia and ameliorates junctional hyperpermeability in human intestinal epithelial monolayers. Surg Forum 1996; 47:197–199.
78. Tsuji Y, Unno N, Menconi MJ, Smith M, Fink MP: Nitric oxide donors increase cytosolic ionized calcium in cultured human intestinal epithelial cells. Shock 1996; 6:19–24.
79. Billiar TR, Harbrecht BG: Resolving the nitric oxide paradox in acute tissue damage. Gastroenterology 1997; 113:1405–1407.
80. Harbrecht BG, Billiar TR, Stadler J, Demetris AJ, Ochoa J, Curran RD, Simmons RL: Inhibition of nitric oxide synthesis during endotoxemia promotes intrahepatic thrombosis and an oxygen radical-mediated hepatic injury. J Leukoc Biol 1992; 52:390–394.
81. Vos TA, Gouw ASH, Klok PA, et al: Differential effects of nitric oxide synthase inhibitors on endotoxin-induced liver damage in rats. Gastroenterology 1997; 113:1323–1333.
82. Boczkowski J, Lanone S, Ungureanu-Longrois D, Danialou G, Fournier T, Aubier M: Induction of diaphragmatic nitric oxide synthase after endotoxin administration in rats. J Clin Invest 1996; 98:1550–1559.
83. Brady AJ, Poole-Wilson PA, Harding SE, Warren JB: Nitric oxide production within cardiac myocytes reduces their contractility in endotoxemia. Am J Physiol 1992; 263:H1963–H1966.
84. Ochoa JB, Udekwu AO, Billiar TR, et al: Nitrogen oxide levels in patients after trauma and during sepsis. Ann Surg 1991; 214:621–626.
85. Shi Y, Li HQ, Shen CK, et al: Plasma nitric oxide levels in newborn infants with sepsis. J Pediatr 1993; 123:435–438.
86. Wong HR, Carcillo JA, Burckart G, et al: Increased serum nitrite and nitrate levels in children with the sepsis syndrome. Crit Care Med 1995; 23:835–842.
87. van Dissel JT, Groeneveld PHP, Maes B, van Furht R, Frolich M, Feuth HDM: Nitric oxide: A predictor of morbidity in postoperative patients? Lancet 1994; 344:1579–1580.
88. Doughty LA, Kaplan SS, Carcillo JA: Inflammatory cytokine and nitric oxide reponses in pediatric sepsis and organ failure. Crit Care Med 1996; 24:1137–1143.
89. Gómez-Jiménez J, Salgado A, Mourelle M, Martín MC, Segura RM, Peracaula R, Moncada S: L-Arginine:nitric oxide pathway in endotoxemia and human septic shock. Crit Care Med 1995; 23:253–258.
90. Petros A, Lamb G, Leone A, Moncada S, Bennett D, Vallance P: Effects of a nitric oxide inhibitor in humans with septic shock. Cardiovasc Res 1994; 28:34–39.
91. Lorente JA, Landín L, de Pablo R, Renes E, Liste D: The L-arginine pathway in the sepsis syndrome. Crit Care Med 1993; 21:1287–1295.
92. Vincent JL, Colice G, Grover R, Zacardelli D, Guntupalli K, Watson D, for the Wellcome International Septic Shock Study Group: The effects of 546C88 in left ventricular performance in patients with septic shock. Intensive Care Med 1995; 21:S20.
93. Anzueto A, Lodato R, Lorente J, Holzapfel L, Grover R, Takala J, for the Wellcome International Septic Shock Study Group: Multicenter placebo-controlled, double-blind trial of the nitric oxide synthase inhibitor 546C88 in patients with septic shock: Acute hemodynamic effects. Am J Respir Crit Care Med 1997; 155:A263.
94. Guntupalli K, Grover R, Jeffs R, Colice G, Watson D, Vincent JL, for the Wellcome International Septic Shock Study Group: Effects of 546C88 on selected indices of organ function in patients with septic shock. Intensive Care Med 1995; 21:S21.
95. Anzueto A, Beale R, Holzapfel L, Arneson C, Rover R, for the Glaxo Wellcome International Septic Shock Study Group: Multicentre, placebo-controlled, double-blind study of the nitric oxide synthase inhibitor 546C88 in patients with septic shock: Effect on resolution of shock and survival. Intensive Care Med 1997; 23:S57.
96. Takala J, Guntupalli K, Donaldson J, Watson D, for the Glaxo Wellcome International Septic Shock Study Group: Multicentre, placebo-controlled, double-blind study of the nitric oxide synthase inhibitor 546C88 in patients with septic shock: Effect on early non-cardiovascular organ function. Intensive Care Med 1997; 23:S51.
97. Lodato RF, Bakker J, Balk R, Grossman S, for the Glaxo Wellcome International Septic Shock Study Group: Multicentre, placebo-controlled, double-blind study of the nitric oxide synthase inhibitor 546C88 in patients with septic shock: Effect in those with pulmonary hypertension. Intensive Care Med 1997; 23:S55.
98. Szabó C, Csaki C, Benyo Z, Reivich M, Kovach AGB: Role of the L-arginine–nitric oxide pathway in the changes in cerebrovascular reactivity following hemorrhagic hypotension and retransfusion. Circ Shock 1991; 37:307–316.
99. Klabunde RE, Slayton KJ, Ritger RC: N^G-Methyl-L-arginine restores arterial pressure in hemorrhaged rats. Circ Shock 1993; 40:47–52.
100. Zingarelli B, Squadrito F, Altavilla D, Calapai G, Campo GM, Calo M, Saitta A, Caputi AP: Evidence for a role of nitric oxide in hypovolemic hemorrhagic shock. J Cardiovasc Pharmacol 1992; 19:982–986.
101. Lieberthal W, McGarry AE, Sheils J, Valeri CR: Nitric oxide inhibition in rats improves blood pressure and renal function during hypovolemic shock. Am J Physiol 1991; 261:F868–F872.

102. Harbrecht BG, Wu B, Watkins SC, Marshall SC, Keefer LK: Targeting nitric oxide (NO) delivery in vivo. Design of a liver-selective NO donor prodrug that blocks tumor necrosis factor-α-induced apoptosis and toxicity in the liver. J Med Chem 1997; 40:1947–1954.
103. Symington PA, Ma X-L, Lefer AM: Protective actions of *S*-nitroso-*N*-acetylpenicillamine (SNAP) in a rat model of hemorrhagic shock. Methods Find Exp Clin Pharmacol 1992; 14:789–797.
104. Cristopher TA, Ma X-L, Lefer AM: Beneficial action of *S*-nitroso-*N*-acetylpenicillamine, a nitric oxide donor, in murine traumatic shock. Shock 1994; 1:19–24.
105. Kurose I, Wolf R, Grisham MB, Granger DN: Modulation of I/R-induced microvascular dysfunction by nitric oxide. Circ Res 1994; 74:376–382.
106. Kanwar S, Tepperman BL, Payne D, Sutherland LR, Kubes P: Time course of nitric oxide production and epithelial dysfunction during I/R of the feline small intestine. Circ Shock 1994; 42:135–140.
107. Carey C, Siegfried MR, Ma XL, Weyrich AS, Lefer AM: Antishock and endothelial protective actions of a NO donor in mesenteric ischemia and reperfusion. Circ Shock 1992; 38:209–216.
108. Seekamp A, Mulligan MS, Till GO, Ward PA: Requirements for neutrophil products and L-arginine ischemia-reperfusion injury. Am J Pathol 1993; 142:1–10.
109. Matheis G, Sherman MP, Buckberg GD, Haybron DM, Young HH, Ignarro LJ: Role of L-arginine–nitric oxide pathway in myocardial reoxygenation injury. Am J Physiol 1992; 262:H616–H620.
110. Gonzalez C, Fernandez A, Martin C, Moncada S, Estrada C: Nitric oxide from endothelium and smooth muscle modulates responses to sympathetic nerve stimulation: Implications for endotoxin shock. Biochem Biophys Res Commun 1992; 86:150–156.
111. Navarro J, Sánchez A, Diz J, et al: Hormonal, renal and metabolic alterations during hypertension induced by chronic inhibition of NO in rats. Am J Physiol 1994; 267:R1516–R1521.
112. Lorente JA, Landín L, Canas P, Albaya A, Delgado MA, Albaya A, Renes E, Jorge P, Liste D: Effects of nitric oxide synthesis inhibition in the cardiovascular response to low output shock. Crit Care Med 1996; 24:482–487.
113. Wang J, Seyedi N, Xu X-B, Wolin MS, Hintza TH: Defective endothelium-mediated control of coronary circulation in conscious dogs after heart failure. Am J Physiol 1994; 266:H670–H680.
114. O'Murchu B, Miller VM, Perella MA, Burntett JC: Increased production of nitric oxide in coronary arteries during congestive heart failure. J Clin Invest 1994; 93:165–171.
115. Elsner D, Muntze A, Kromer E, Riegger GA: Systemic vasoconstriction induced by inhibition of nitric oxide synthesis is attenuated in conscious dogs with heart failure. Cardiovasc Res 1991; 25:438–440.
116. Webb DJ, McMurray JJV: Enhanced basal nitric oxide production in heart failure (Letter). Lancet 1994; 344:887.

56

Apoptosis in Critical Illness

Yuchi Li, PhD • Jeffrey A. Kazzaz, PhD
Stuart Horowitz, PhD

APOPTOSIS AND NECROSIS

Cell death is often thought to occur via one of two distinct modes: apoptosis or necrosis. However, it may be best to think of necrosis as a consequence rather than a mode of cell death, because even apoptosis can eventually result in "secondary" necrosis. It is conceivable that there are other modes of programmed cell death in addition to apoptosis, all of which currently fall under the heading of necrosis.

Apoptosis, a form of programmed cell death, is the process of cellular self-destruction and involves a specific series of events.[1] It can be a scheduled and physiologically regulated event, occurring during normal cell turnover and development and in response to viral infection. For the most part, *necrosis* is the result of unscheduled, acute injury and in vivo can result in or from an inflammatory response, which can be local or systemic.[2] On the other hand, when cells in tissue die via apoptosis, they are removed through phagocytosis by neighboring healthy cells.[1] Thus, the observation that inflammation can be circumvented has given rise to the current notion that apoptosis is a protective mode of cell death.[1]

Apoptosis was originally defined morphologically by cell shrinkage and chromatin condensation. These are relatively late manifestations of apoptosis, however, and a great deal of attention has been focused on the biochemical and molecular events that constitute intermediate steps along the apoptotic pathway. It is unclear whether intervention along these steps will result in cell survival, necrosis, or some intermediate form of cell death. In addition, the early signal transduction events leading to apoptosis are subjects of intense study. It is known that apoptosis can be regulated at a growing number of checkpoints, depending on the cell type and the initial trigger.

Apoptosis in Development and Homeostasis

Apoptosis is a form of programmed cell death that occurs during development and, in many cases, under normal physiologic conditions. For example, the process of morphogenesis in the embryo occurs, in part, through the elimination of cells that are necessary for only a limited time span. Such elimination generally takes place through apoptosis.

One of best examples of apoptosis during embryogenesis is in limb development. Separation of the digits from the limb bud occurs by precise patterns of massive mesodermal cell death through apoptosis.[3] In all normal tissues, the homeostatic balance between cell proliferation and cell death depends, in part, on apoptosis and its regulation. In hematopoietic homeostasis, stem cell renewal is continuously counterbalanced by apoptosis. In early B cell and T cell development, apoptosis is required to eliminate cells with nonfunctional antigen receptors and is critical for removing self-reactive cells at the immature lymphocyte stage before they reach maturity.

The consequences of unregulated apoptosis can be severe. The inappropriate induction of apoptosis in lymphocyte populations plays a major role in the pathogenesis of acquired immunodeficiency syndrome (AIDS), whereas ineffective apoptosis has been associated with autoimmunity, inflammation, and the development of hematologic malignancies.[4] Deregulated apoptosis might also be involved in cancer, neurodegenerative disorders, viral and bacterial infections, and even the aging process itself.[5–7] Although extensive reviews of apoptosis and diseases have been published,[2, 8] this chapter focuses on several systems related to critical illness and describes apoptosis in lung injury.

Cancer

Cancer growth represents an imbalance between cell proliferation and cell death. Cells in a wide variety of human malignancies have a decreased ability to undergo apoptosis in response to at least some physiologic stimuli.[9] This is most apparent in metastatic tumors. The molecular bases for the increased resistance of tumor cells to undergo apoptosis and several genes that are critical in the regulation of apoptosis have been defined. The p53 gene product is required for cells to initiate apoptosis in response to genotoxic damage.[10–12] It is also fundamental in the pathway that leads from the sensing of DNA damage to the initiation of apoptosis. At least 50% of all malignant tumors have mutations or rearrangements of both copies of the *p53* gene on human chromosome 17. Included in this group are 80% of colon cancers, 50% of lung cancers, and 40% of breast cancers.

A wide variety of chemotherapeutic agents and irradiation work by initiating DNA damage. The inability of cells to undergo apoptosis in response to DNA damage may underlie the enhanced resistance to chemotherapeutic agents and radiation in those *p53*-deficient tumors. On the other hand, tumors can arise if the antiapoptosis gene *bcl-2* becomes dysregulated, resulting in cells that live much longer than normal.[8] Overexpression of *bcl-2* specifically prevents cells from initiating apoptosis in response to a number of stimuli, and the induction of genes that inhibit *bcl-2* can induce apoptosis in a wide variety of tumor types.[13–15] Abnormal expression of *bcl-2* has been found in prostate cancer, colon cancer, and neuroblastoma.[16–18]

Inflammation

Acute inflammation is characterized by the recruitment of neutrophils, which are loaded with potent proteolytic enzymes, toxic cationic proteins, and chemotactic factors that have proven roles in amplifying the inflammatory response. Rather than being programmed to die by necrosis, allowing uncontrolled escape of proinflammatory contents, the short-lived neutrophils appear to be constitutively programmed to undergo apoptosis. This limits their proinflammatory potential and results in rapid and specific recognition and clearance by macrophages and phagocytes.[19] Moreover, even the uptake of large numbers of apoptotic neutrophils by macrophages fails to elicit phagocyte secretion of proinflammatory mediators, such as granule enzymes, thromboxane, and chemokines, emphasizing the injury-limiting potential of neutrophil clearance by apoptosis.

Not only neutrophils but also eosinophil granulocytes are programmed to undergo apoptosis, followed by phagocyte uptake. Furthermore, apoptosis can mediate clearance of another major player in the inflammation-repair response, the myofibroblast. Although recruitment of large numbers of myofibroblasts is an important event in repair of skin wounds, proper healing requires the apoptotic destruction of many of these cells, probably preventing the formation of hypertrophic scars.[20]

Finally, apoptosis is likely to play an important role in vascular remodeling during angiogenesis and revascularization of injured tissue. Failure to undergo apoptosis has been implicated as a key pathogenic event in eosinophilia, which is associated with a variety of chronic inflammatory diseases, particularly allergic manifestations, such as bronchial asthma and atopic dermatitis.[21, 22] Failure to remove myofibroblasts may be an important risk factor for proinflammatory scarring.

Neurodegenerative Disorders

Loss of specific sets of neurons characterizes a wide variety of neurologic diseases, such as Alzheimer's disease, Parkinson's disease, amyotrophic lateral sclerosis, retinitis pigmentosa, spinal muscular atrophy, and various forms of cerebellar degeneration.[23] The cell loss in these diseases does not induce an inflammatory response, and apoptosis appears to be the mode of cell death.

Although the exact triggers for apoptosis are not known, oxidative stress, calcium toxicity, mitochondrial defects, excitatory toxicity, and deficiency of survival factors have been surmised to contribute to the pathogenesis of these disorders.[24] Each of these pathways is involved in neuronal apoptosis. For example, Alzheimer's disease is associated with the progressive accumulation of β-amyloid peptide in plaques, and β-amyloid peptide can induce death of cultured central nervous system neurons.[25] Mutations in β-amyloid precursor protein are associated with some forms of familial Alzheimer's disease.

Acute Lung Injury

Acute lung injury (ALI), the rapid disruption of the gas exchange apparatus in response to noxious environmental or endogenous agents, is a common and deadly condition. Each year, more than 150,000 patients are treated nationwide and more than 50% of afflicted patients die.[26] The disease process begins with an explosive inflammatory response in the alveolar wall. In the aftermath of the resultant tissue destruction, extensive fibroproliferation in the alveolar airspace can ensue, involving fibroblasts, capillaries, and their connective tissue products.[27] Although necrosis is the descriptor typically used to characterize pulmonary cell death during active lung injury, studies have revealed that apoptosis also plays an important role.[28–30] Our laboratory has been studying apoptosis in acute lung injury using three distinct models:

- Hyperoxia
- Oleic acid
- Bacterial pneumonia

Some of this work and other studies have been reviewed.[31]

Therapy with supraphysiologic concentrations of oxygen (O_2) is required in a number of clinical situations, but this use of O_2 may be accompanied by tissue damage.[32, 33] For example, hyperoxia plays a role in the etiology of bronchopulmonary dysplasia in premature infants.[34, 35] The general problem of O_2 toxicity involves several organs, most notably the lungs.[36] The pathology of O_2-induced acute lung injury includes inflammation and permeability changes of the alveolar-capillary membrane, causing extensive pulmonary edema and severe decreases in respiratory function.[37]

The observation that inflammation can be circumvented by apoptosis (versus necrosis) in tissues has given rise to the popular notion that apoptosis is a protective mode of cell death.[1] Despite this paradigm, the question of whether apoptosis occurs during acute tissue injury in complex organs has not been addressed. We therefore studied acute injury in the lung.[29] Lung injury is known to be multifaceted, involving cascades of events that can be initiated by a wide variety of primary insults.[38] Acute lung injury is usually accompanied and exacerbated by pulmonary inflammation. Because of the complex nature of this injury, we hypothesized that cell death might be multimodal, involving not only necrosis but also apoptosis.[38]

Severe pneumonitis is a prominent feature of hyperoxic acute lung injury. To study apoptosis during the development of hyperoxic acute lung injury, we used the in situ terminal deoxynucleotidyl transferase–mediated dUTP nick end labeling (TUNEL) assay.[39] In a mouse model of hyperoxic lung injury, TUNEL-positive, apoptotic nuclei were clearly evident at a time when lung injury was severe compared with that in control unexposed mice. To confirm independently that the TUNEL assay was an accurate reflection of apoptosis in acutely injured tissue, isolated genomic DNA from exposed and control lungs was studied. DNA isolated from apoptotic cells is visualized by agarose gel electrophoresis as 200-bp (base pair) ladders, a hallmark of apoptosis in nucleated cells.[40] Acutely injured hyperoxic lungs exhibited nucleosomal DNA ladders, typical of apoptosis, and these ladders were not detected in control lung. Moreover, this response was not generalized to other organs that were not injured because ladders were not evident in the liver DNA of the same animals.

Interleukin-1β (IL-1β)-converting enzyme (ICE) and other members of the caspase family of proteases are activated in apoptosis. To determine whether ICE up-regulation occurs in hyperoxia-induced acute lung injury, we examined the expression of ICE in untreated and hyperoxic mouse lungs. ICE expression was induced compared with control lungs. In particular, the activated form of ICE, p20, was present exclusively in nuclei of injured lung cells.

Barazzone and colleagues[30] have examined several other aspects of apoptosis-related gene expression in mouse lungs. Individual members of the Bcl-2 gene family can either inhibit or promote apoptosis, depending on the relative abundance of the proteins and the timing of their expression. To begin to understand the role of the *Bcl-2* family in hyperoxic cell death, northern blots were probed for Bcl-x and Bax, two members whose increased expression is associated with promotion of cell death. Prolonged hyperoxic exposure was associated with an eightfold increase in the relative abundance of Bax messenger ribonucleic acid (mRNA) and a 12-fold increase in Bcl-x. These data provide the rationale for further investigation of the *Bcl-2* family in hyperoxic acute lung injury. *Fas* and *p53* (other apoptosis-related proteins) were also up-regulated in this study; however, neither *Fas*-null nor *p53*-null mice showed any changes in susceptibility to O_2 toxicity (as measured by wet-to-dry lung weight ratios or pulmonary edema), suggesting that these pathways are not of central importance in hyperoxic lung death.[30]

Apoptosis and Tolerance to Hyperoxia

The presence of apoptosis in the acutely injured lung may be part of a protective mechanism to limit the extent of injury or inflammation, as has been proposed during resolution of acute respiratory distress syndrome (ARDS).[41, 42] If apoptosis is also protective during acute lung injury, animals that are relatively resistant to such injury can be predicted to exhibit apoptosis sooner than sensitive animals. To examine this possibility, we studied two models of differential sensitivity to hyperoxia: inbred mice[43] and adult versus newborn rabbits.[44] The results of these quantitative studies indicate that the extent of apoptosis was well correlated with the severity of hyperoxic acute lung injury and inversely correlated with resistance.[29]

In a study of cell death in hyperoxic adult rats, animals showed more apoptosis in their lungs with advancing exposure to hyperoxia.[45] These observations indicate that lung apoptosis during pulmonary O_2 toxicity is conserved among mammals and suggest that this response is of fundamental importance. However, we have also found that the percentage of cells undergoing apoptosis is highly variable among these species, with mice exposed to 100% O_2 having the most intense response. Moreover, quantitative studies of models of acquired (versus inbred) resistance to hyperoxia in rats suggest that there is no simple relationship between the extent of apoptosis and resistance or sensitivity to hyperoxia.[45] It may be necessary to identify the pulmonary cell types undergoing apoptosis in order to shed further light on the connection between programmed cell death and tolerance to acute lung injury.

Apoptosis in Other Models of Acute Lung Injury

Although apoptosis during hyperoxia is widespread and appears to involve many cell types in lung, the timing of the onset and persistence of apoptosis is concurrent with the influx of neutrophils, which themselves are likely to undergo apoptosis during pulmonary inflammation. A commonly used model of acute lung injury with a much more rapid onset involves the intravenous administration of oleic acid, which causes severe lung injury characterized by pulmonary edema, decreased pulmonary function, and fulminant inflammation.[46] Oleic acid injury in the rabbit is severe after only 1 hour.[47] In rabbits, apoptosis was evident in oleic acid–induced acute lung injury but was not observed in control animals given the vehicle alone. Oleic acid injury was distinct from hyperoxia in that the pattern of apoptosis was focal, correlating with patchy foci of injury known to occur in lung tissue in this model.[46] Thus, in a different model of acute lung injury, in which the insult is primary vascular, apoptosis was also well correlated with severe lung injury. In this model, the timing of injury is too rapid to be attributable to dying neutrophils.

To test whether apoptosis occurs during acute lung injury of bacterial origin, we used a model of streptococcal pneumonia. In rats infected with a bolus of *Streptococcus sanguis*, acute and severe pneumonia developed over the course of 1 day.[48, 49] Apoptosis was evident in infected lungs as soon as 8 hours after infection. This early time point was clearly in the acute pneumonitic phase, well before the onset of resolution of the infection. Apoptosis occurred during a time of severe pulmonary inflammation, as evident by 4′,6-diamidino-2-phenylindole (DAPI) fluorescence, which showed a large neutrophil infiltrate. In contrast, apoptosis in nearby airway epithelial cells was prominent. A more detailed discussion of these data may be found in Mantell and coworkers.[29] Apoptosis is also a prominent feature of the repair phase in bacterial pneumonia, as described in detail by Kazzaz[28] and Rhodes,[48, 49] and their colleagues and by us (unpublished observations). During repair, however, the cell types that undergo apoptosis change, depending on whether the repair is successful or whether it leads to fibrosis.

In Vivo Lung Injury Experiments

It has generally been thought that a distinguishing feature of apoptosis is that it occurs without eliciting an inflammatory response, whereas necrosis causes inflammation. Our data suggest that this paradigm should be reevaluated because it does not adequately account for our observations. Using three different models, we found that apoptosis is clearly a feature of acute lung injury. We call this "unscheduled" apoptosis because acute lung injury does not follow a schedule and is not a programmed event. Moreover, the onset of acute lung injury caused by oleic acid (1 hour) is too short to allow significant apoptosis of infiltrating neutrophils or macrophages, indicating that apoptosis occurred in lung cells. Yet, except for the obvious apoptosis in airway epithelium, it is difficult to identify definitively the cell types involved, especially in the gas exchange regions. Such identification requires electron microscopy or dual-label methods.[44]

Resolution of Acute Lung Injury

In patients who survive acute lung injury, granulation tissue resolves in concert with repopulation of the air-liquid interface by type II epithelial cells. Effective repair is completed when the epithelium assumes its physiologic conformation. A key event associated with resolution of acute lung injury is the removal of intra-alveolar cells resulting from fibroproliferation. Excess hyperplastic type II cells must also be removed. Thus, an important aspect of tissue remodeling is apoptosis, which may be part of a protective mechanism to limit the extent of injury or inflammation. This has been proposed in resolution of ARDS.[41, 42]

Polunovsky and coworkers[41] showed that bronchoalveolar lavage fluids from patients undergoing resolution of ARDS contained substances that could induce apoptosis in cultured pulmonary artery endothelial cells and fibroblasts, whereas lavage fluids from patients in earlier stages of ARDS or from normal individuals did not. Moreover, histologic examination of resolving lung tissue revealed apoptotic cells.

In a study of patients with acute lung injury and patients with chronic interstitial pneumonia, the presence of apoptosis in type II cells and the presence of proliferation in a variety of lung cells were examined.[50] In general, there was an inverse relationship between proliferation of type II cells (which was common in chronic interstitial pneumonia and unresolved acute lung injury) and type II cell apoptosis. In patients with resolving acute lung injury, type II cell apoptosis was common and cellular proliferation at the alveolar level was generally absent. However, patients with chronic pneumonia had ongoing type II cell proliferation and minimal apoptosis. These experiments suggest that apoptosis is also part of the repair process, and when it occurs appropriately, fibrosis is prevented.

In an attempt to understand what role apoptosis has in the outcome of pneumonia, our laboratory studied two models of bacterial pneumonia in experimental animals that result in either resolution or fibrosis.[48, 49] Infection with either *S. sanguis* or *Streptococcus pneumoniae* type 25 results in acute pneumonitis within 8 hours of infection; however, whereas the *S. sanguis* infection becomes mostly resolved over the time course of 1 week, the *S. pneumoniae* infection does not and the lungs become fibrotic.[48, 49] TUNEL assays demonstrated that at 8 hours after infection, during the acute stage of infection, apoptotic activity was evident in both models involving predominantly bronchiolar and alveolar epithelial cells[28] (Kazzaz et al, unpublished observations). The resolving lungs formed an abscess at the base of the lung after days. Within these abscesses, apoptotic nuclei were predominantly neutrophils. By 4 days in the resolving model, little edema was evident, the abscesses became more organized, and few if any TUNEL-positive cells were seen in the portions of the lung that had clearly resolved. However, apoptotic cells were still found in the abscess and the area immediately adjacent to it, particularly in the alveolar epithelium. At 8 days after infection, the resolving lung was mostly repaired, except for an abscess that persisted at the base. Few apoptotic cells were seen outside or adjacent to the abscess by TUNEL assay, but apoptosis was still clearly evident in the abscess. At this time point in the fibrosing model, widespread apoptosis persisted.

Overall, in the resolving model, apoptosis was limited in the abscess during resolution. In contrast, apoptosis persisted and became more widespread in the fibrosing model. This study demonstrates that apoptosis is a feature of both the acute and resolving stages of pneumonia. It is a component of resolution and fibrosis in the lung, and the difference between normal and abnormal resolution of pneumonia may depend on the ability to limit apoptosis. It seems that the cell types undergoing apoptosis may be crucial in determining outcome. Although fibrosis is a proliferative disease, cell death is a prominent factor (as in cancer). The cell types involved in the ratio of cell death and cell proliferation might be a key factor in determining whether injury resolves or the lungs become fibrotic.

Nonapoptotic Programmed Cell Death in Lung

Although unscheduled apoptosis is a prominent component of acute lung injury resulting from hyperoxia and other causes, apoptosis is not the only mode of cell death occurring in such lungs.[28, 29] Direct exposure of cultured human alveolar epithelial (A549) cells to hyperoxia does not result in apoptosis.[28] We have made virtually identical observations on other lung epithelial cell lines, including mouse lung epithelial (MLE-12) cells and rat epithelial (SV-40T2) cells, which are type II cell derived. Similarly, HeLa cells (from cervical carcinoma) do not undergo apoptosis in response to hyperoxia. We have also exposed two different primary cell types of human lung to hyperoxia in culture: vascular endothelial cells (HVEC-L) and bronchial epithelial cells (NHBE). Neither cell line underwent apoptosis in response to hyperoxia. Like the transformed cells, these primary cells swelled and died over a period of days of exposure to hyperoxia. These data indicate that many epithelial cell lines (as well as endothelial HVEC-L cells) do not die via apoptosis when cultured in conditions of hyperoxia. However, Jyonouchi and colleagues[51] reported that a few Madin-Darby canine kidney (MDCK) epithelial cells in culture died via apoptosis after 2 days in hyperoxia, but only when first grown to near-confluence; this suggests that the mode of cell death triggered by a particular stimulus may differ among cell types.

Nonapoptotic cell death in hyperoxia occurs over several days—sufficient time for the elaboration of a program of gene expression. We therefore sought to understand transcription factor activity and signal transduction during hyperoxia compared with cell death triggered by apoptotic stimuli. Apoptotic cell death can be prevented by the activation of nuclear factor κB (NF-κB),[52-55] a multisubunit transcription factor that regulates genes involved in inflammation, infection, and stress.[56] NF-κB activation may be part of a survival program used to escape other forms of cell death. We examined NF-κB in A549 cells exposed to concentrations of H_2O_2 that cause apoptosis or hyperoxia. Despite the activation and induction of NF-κB by molecular O_2, the cells do not escape death.[57] These observations are summarized next.

After release from the inhibitory binding protein I-κB, NF-κB translocates to the nucleus, regulating transcription. NF-κB activation was studied during hyperoxia by immunolocalization of the p65 subunit of NF-κB. In control A549 cells grown in room air, immunofluorescence was weak, and p65 was evident primarily in the cytoplasm. Nuclear fluorescence was clearly evident by 30 minutes of hyperoxia, and it increased over the course of 1 day. The cells became slightly swollen by 24 hours, and fluorescence became more intense not only in the nuclei but also in the cytoplasm of many cells.

In contrast, cells undergoing H_2O_2-induced apoptosis showed a nuclear evacuation of NF-κB. The translocation of p65 to the nucleus is consistent with NF-kB activation. Increased immunofluorescence suggested that the level of p65 protein also increased. Western blots showed that, indeed, NF-κB levels were increased as soon as 30 minutes of exposure to 95% O_2 and peaked by 24 hours. However, H_2O_2-induced apoptosis caused no increased NF-κB protein. Northern blots showed that by 30 minutes of O_2 exposure there was a slight increase in steady-state levels of p65 mRNA and that message levels increased over the course of 1 day and remained elevated for 2 days. In contrast, there was no increase in NF-κB expression during H_2O_2-induced apoptosis.

The differential activation and expression of NF-κB during different modes of cell death suggest the existence of different signaling pathways. We have therefore begun to decipher the transcriptional regulatory events that occur in the early phases of oxidant-induced death. One early response to stress involves the transient expression of the c-Fos and c-Jun proto-oncogenes. The transcription complex known as AP-1 includes the Fos-Jun dimer and not only is reported to be redox-sensitive but also is activated in lungs of hyperoxic rats.[58]

To study AP-1 regulation during hyperoxia, we exposed mouse lung epithelial (MLE-12) cells to 95% O_2 for up to 24 hours. Cells were harvested at various time points and mRNA assayed by northern blots for Fos and Jun expression. Compared with those in control cells (transferred and replated at the same time in fresh medium), both c-Fos and c-Jun transcript levels were elevated transiently (at 30 minutes) and then returned rapidly to baseline. Interestingly, both mRNAs were again increased in abundance at 16 to 24 hours (unpublished observations).

The c-Fos promoter is sometimes regulated by the p42 and p44 mitogen-activated protein kinase (MAP kinase) cascade.[59] To investigate whether p42 and p44 MAP kinases are activated by hyperoxia, we used antibodies raised against the activated form of the proteins. We detected no changes in the levels of activated p42 or p44 during exposure to hyperoxia. In contrast, within 10 minutes of incubation in an apoptosis-inducing concentration of H_2O_2, there was a significant increase in phosphorylated p42 and p44, indicating that signaling events are different in these two modes of oxidant-induced lung epithelial cell death.

Increased abundance of c-Fos and c-Jun transcripts can be associated with activation of their corresponding proteins. Jun phosphorylation, necessary for activation, was thus assayed. Western blots were incubated with an antibody specific for phosphorylated c-Jun. A rise in the level of phosphorylated c-Jun was observed within 0.5 hour. The appearance of a second, higher-migrating band suggested the presence of additional phosphorylation. Similar to the mRNA, phosphorylated c-Jun levels decreased after this brief rise but increased again at 16 to 24 hours. Jun phosphorylation can be mediated by Jun kinase (JNK). To examining a possible role for JNK, we performed a JNK "pull-down" experiment. In this assay, cell lysates were incubated with affinity beads bound to glutathione-S-transferase (GST)-Jun fusion protein to "pull down" JNK. In this case, an increase in phosphorylated Jun was evident only at the late phase, at 16 to 24 hours, suggesting that early signaling and late signaling of Jun activation may be different (unpublished results).

These preliminary data on hyperoxic signaling indicate that NF-κB translocation (and presumptive activation) is not a result of the p42-p44 MAP kinase pathway but a likely downstream consequence of activation of the JNK pathway. Moreover, c-Jun and its phosphorylation are increased in a biphasic fashion, the first phase occurring within 30 minutes and the second after 16 hours. On the basis of these observations and the fact that the Fos-Jun transcription complex AP-1 has been shown to have a role not only in the immediate-early response to stress but also in cell death,[60] we postulate the existence of multiple signal transduction pathways in hyperoxia-induced cell death.

SUMMARY

Acute lung injury is associated with multimodal cell death, including apoptosis. In the acute phase of injury, the extent of apoptosis is often correlated with the severity of the injury—the more apoptosis, the worse the injury. However, apoptosis is also associated with the resolution of acute lung injury and with fibrosis. It is therefore likely that the extent of apoptosis may not be as important to the final outcome as the cell types that undergo apoptosis, the timing of cell death, and the relative rates of death versus proliferation.

Other forms of programmed cell death may be operative during acute lung injury, especially during hyperoxia. More work is needed to understand the regulation of nonapoptotic cell death. Taken together, it appears that reducing the extent of cell death sometimes can mitigate acute lung injury (e.g., during the acute phase) and that at other times augmenting the extent of cell death hastens recovery (e.g., during resolution). We recommend further investigation before one proceeds with simplistic approaches to either increase or decrease the extent of cell death in acute lung injury.

References

1. Steller H: Mechanism and genes of cellular suicide. Science 1995; 267:1445.
2. Thompson CB: Apoptosis in the pathogenesis and treatment of disease. Science 1995; 267:1456.
3. Hammar SP, Mottet NK: Tetrazolium salt and electron-microscopic studies of cellular degeneration and necrosis in the interdigital areas of the developing chick limb. J Cell Sci 1971; 8:229.
4. McKenna SL, Cotter TG: Functional aspects of apoptosis in hematopoiesis and consequences of failure. Adv Cancer Res 1997; 71:121.
5. Vaux DL, Haecker G, Strasser A: An evolutionary perspective on apoptosis. Cell 1994; 76:777.
6. Bursch W, Oberhammer F, Schulte-Hermann R: Cell death by apoptosis and its protective role against disease. Trends Pharmacol Sci 1992; 13:245.
7. Warner HR, Hodes RJ, Pocinki K: What does cell death have to do with aging? J Am Geriatr Soc 1997; 45:1140.
8. Savill J: Apoptosis in disease. Eur J Clin Invest 1994; 24:715.
9. Hoffman B, Liebermann DA: Molecular controls of apoptosis: Differentiation/growth arrest primary response genes, proto-oncogenes, and tumor suppressor genes as positive and negative modulators. Oncogene 1994; 9:1807.
10. Lowe SW, Schmitt EM, Smith SW, et al: p53 is required for radiation-induced apoptosis in mouse thymocytes. Nature 1993; 362:847.
11. Clarke AR, Purdie CA, Harrison DJ, et al: Thymocyte apoptosis induced by p53-dependent and independent pathways. Nature 1993; 362:849.
12. Lee JM, Bernstein A: p53 mutations increase resistance to ionizing radiation. Proc Natl Acad Sci U S A 1993; 90:5742.
13. Hockenbery DM, Nunez G, Milliman C, et al: Bcl-2 is an inner mitochondrial membrane protein that blocks programmed cell death. Nature 1990; 348:334.
14. Vaux DL, Cory S, Adams JM: *Bcl-2* gene promotes haemopoietic cell survival and cooperates with c-*myc* to immortalize pre-B cells. Nature 1988; 335:440.
15. Hockenbery DM, Oltvai ZN, Yin X-M, et al: Bcl-2 functions in an antioxidant pathway to prevent apoptosis. Cell 1993; 75:241.
16. McDonnell TJ, Troncoso P, Brisbay SM, et al: Expression of the protooncogene *bcl-2* in the prostate and its association with emergence of androgen-independent prostate cancer. Cancer Res 1992; 52:6940.
17. Hague A, Moorghen M, Hicks D, et al: BCL-2 expression in human colorectal adenomas and carcinomas. Oncogene 1994; 9:3367.
18. Castle VP, Heidelberger KP, Bromberg J, et al: Expression of the apoptosis-suppressing protein bcl-2′ in neuroblastoma is associated with unfavorable histology and N-myc amplification. Am J Pathol 1993; 143:1543.
19. Savill J: Apoptosis in resolution of inflammation. J Leukoc Biol 1997; 61:375.
20. Darby I, Skalli O, Gabbiani G: Alpha-smooth muscle actin is transiently expressed by myofibroblasts during experimental wound healing. Lab Invest 1990; 63:21.
21. Holgate ST: The 1992 Cournand Lecture. Asthma: Past, present and future. Eur Respir J 1993; 6:1507.
22. Kroegel C, Virchow JC Jr, Luttmann W, et al: Pulmonary immune cells in health and disease: The eosinophil leucocyte (part I). Eur Respir J 1994; 7:519.
23. Isacson O: On neuronal health. Trends Neurosci 1993; 16:306.
24. Choi DW: Excitotoxic cell death. J Neurobiol 1992; 23:1261.
25. Loo DT, Copani A, Pike CJ, et al: Apoptosis is induced by beta-amyloid in cultured central nervous system neurons. Proc Natl Acad Sci U S A 1993; 90:7951.
26. Rinaldo JE, Rogers RM: Adult respiratory distress syndrome. N Engl J Med 1982; 306:900.

27. Fukuda Y, Ishizaki M, Masuda Y, et al: The role of intraalveolar fibrosis in the process of pulmonary structural remodeling in patients with diffuse alveolar damage. Am J Pathol 1987; 126:171.
28. Kazzaz JA, Xu J, Palaia TA, et al: Cellular oxygen toxicity—oxidant injury without apoptosis. J Biol Chem 1996; 271:15182.
29. Mantell LL, Kazzaz JA, Xu J, et al: Unscheduled apoptosis during acute inflammatory lung injury. Cell Death Differ 1997; 4:600.
30. Barazzone C, Horowitz S, Rodriguez I, et al: Oxygen toxicity in mouse lung: Pathways to cell death. Am J Respir Cell Mol Biol 1998; 19:573.
31. Niederman M: Respiratory infection in the critically ill: Mechanisms and the role of apoptosis in the response to infection. Sepsis 1998; 1:153.
32. Northway WH Jr, Rosam RC, Porter DY: Pulmonary disease following respirator therapy of hyaline-membrane disease. Bronchopulmonary dysplasia. N Engl J Med 1967; 276:357.
33. Horowitz S, Davis JM: Lung injury when development is interrupted by premature birth. *In:* Growth and Development of the Lung. McDonald JA (Ed). New York, Marcel Dekker, 1997, p 577.
34. Pappas CT, Obara H, Bensch KG, et al: Effect of prolonged exposure to 80% oxygen on the lung of the new born mouse. Lab Invest 1983; 48:735.
35. Frank L, Roberts RJ: Endotoxin protection against oxygen-induced acute and chronic lung injury. J Appl Physiol 1979; 45:699.
36. Wispe JR, Roberts RJ: Molecular basis of pulmonary oxygen toxicity. Clin Perinatol 1987; 14:651.
37. Freeman BA, Mason RJ, Williams MC, et al: Antioxidant enzyme activity in alveolar type II cells after exposure of rats to hyperoxia. Exp Lung Res 1986; 10:203.
38. Spragg RG: DNA strand break formation following exposure of bovine pulmonary artery and aortic endothelial cells to reactive oxygen products. Am J Respir Cell Mol Biol 1991; 4:4.
39. Gavrieli Y, Sherman Y, Ben-Sasson SA: Identification of programmed cell death in situ via specific labeling of nuclear DNA fragmentation. J Cell Biol 1992; 119:493.
40. Leist M, Gantner F, Bohlinger I, et al: Murine hepatocyte apoptosis induced in vitro and in vivo by TNF-alpha requires transcriptional arrest. J Immunol 1994; 153:1778.
41. Polunovsky VA, Chen B, Henke C, et al: Role of mesenchymal cell death in lung remodeling after injury. J Clin Invest 1993; 92:388.
42. Uhal BD, Joshi I, True AL, et al: Fibroblasts isolated after fibrotic lung injury induce apoptosis of alveolar epithelial cells in vitro. Am J Physiol 1995; 269:L819.
43. Piedboeuf B, Johnston CJ, Watkins RH, et al: Increased expression of tissue inhibitor of metalloproteinases (TIMP-I) and metallothionein in murine lungs after hyperoxic exposure. Am J Respir Cell Mol Biol 1994; 10:123.
44. Veness-Meehan KA, Cheng ER, Mercier CE, et al: Cell-specific alterations in expression of hyperoxia-induced mRNAs of lung. Am J Respir Cell Mol Biol 1991; 5:516.
45. Otterbein L, Chin BY, Mantell L, et al: Hyperoxia induces apoptosis in the rat lung: Marker of injury or tolerance? Am J Physiol 1998; 275:L14.
46. Schuster DP: ARDS: Clinical lessons from the oleic acid model of acute lung injury. Am J Respir Crit Care Med 1994; 149:245.
47. Hall SB, Lu RZ, Venkitaraman AR, et al: Inhibition of pulmonary surfactant by oleic acid: Mechanisms and characteristics. J Appl Physiol 1992; 72:1708.
48. Rhodes GC, Tapsall JW, Lykke AW: Alveolar epithelial responses in experimental streptococcal pneumonia. J Pathol 1989; 157:347.
49. Rhodes GC, Lykke AW, Tapsall JW, et al: Abnormal alveolar epithelial repair associated with failure of resolution in experimental streptococcal pneumonia. J Pathol 1989; 159:245.
50. Bardales RH, Xie SS, Schaefer RF, et al: Apoptosis is a major pathway responsible for the resolution of type II pneumocytes in acute lung injury. Am J Pathol 1996; 149:845.
51. Jyonouchi H, Sun S, Mizokami M, et al: Cell density and antioxidant vitamins determine the effects of hyperoxia on proliferation and death of MDCK epithelial cells. Nutr Cancer 1997; 28:115.
52. Barinaga M: Life-death balance within the cell. Science 1996; 274:724.
53. Beg AA, Baltimore D: An essential role for NF-κB in preventing TNF-alpha-induced cell death. Science 1996; 274:782.
54. Van Antwerp DJ, Martin SJ, Kafri T, et al: Suppression of TNF-alpha-induced apoptosis by NF-κB. Science 1996; 274:787.
55. Wang CY, Mayo MW, Baldwin AS: TNF- and cancer therapy-induced apoptosis: Potentiation by inhibition of NF-kappaB. Science 1996; 274:784.
56. Schreck R, Rieber P, Baeuerle PA: Reactive oxygen intermediates as apparently widely used messengers in the activation of the NF-kappa B transcription factor and HIV-1. EMBO J 1991; 10:2247.
57. Li Y, Kazzaz JA, Mantell LL, et al: NFκB is activated by hyperoxia but does not protect from cell death. J Biol Chem 1997; 272:20646.
58. Choi AM, Sylvester S, Otterbein L, et al: Molecular responses to hyperoxia in vivo: Relationship to increased tolerance in aged rats. Am J Respir Cell Mol Biol 1995; 13:74.
59. Treisman R: Ternary complex factors: Growth factor regulated transcriptional activators. Curr Opin Genet Dev 1994; 4:96.
60. Preston GA, Lyon TT, Yin Y, et al: Induction of apoptosis by c-Fos protein. Mol Cell Biol 1996; 16:211.

57

Infections in the Surgical Critical Care Unit

Steven M. Steinberg, MD, FACS
Ronald Lee Nichols, MD, MS, FACS

Postoperative infectious complications are a common cause of morbidity and mortality in the surgical intensive care unit (ICU). These infections most commonly involve the urinary or respiratory tract, invasive catheters, or the operative wound. Patients in ICUs are, by the nature of their clinical status, much more likely to have nosocomial infections than the general hospital population. Although the rate of hospital-acquired infection in the general hospital population is approximately 5%,[1] the rate of nosocomial infection in surgical ICU patients is estimated to be twofold to fivefold higher.[2] Many factors that seem to be associated with this higher risk of infection have been described. Craven and colleagues[3] found that ICU confinement of longer than 3 days, the presence of shock, the use of arterial catheters, and the use of urinary catheterization for longer than 10 days were all linked to significant increases in the incidence of nosocomial infection. Many clinical characteristics seem to be related to the development of infection in ICU patients (Table 57–1).

Although the straight-line logic that infections led to sepsis, which led to multiple organ failure, which led to death was operational in the past (as evidenced by the work of Fry and others,[4, 5] who reported that infection is related to the development of the multiple system organ failure syndrome and to higher mortality), more recently those concepts have come into question. For example, Poole and colleagues[6] reported on 749 patients admitted to the ICU, 73 of whom experienced multiple organ failure. Although infection was very common in this subset of patients, there was no statistical relationship between any infection and death. Death was strongly associated with severe sepsis syndrome.

The evaluation of the critically ill patient in the ICU to determine the focus of infection is often difficult and commonly provides conflicting data. Furthermore, we have come to realize that clinical signs of sepsis, such as fever, leukocytosis, high cardiac output, and low peripheral vascular resistance, may result from other, noninfectious causes. Shock resulting from any cause, severe multiple trauma, acute pancreatitis, the presence of nonviable tissue, and reperfusion injury may all result in the clinical picture of sepsis. Such underlying conditions should be vigorously sought and treated. Patients with these conditions should be supported by all hemodynamic, ventilatory, nutritional, and other means available.

We often search, however, for a "treatable" source of a patient's sepsis, which is most commonly a nosocomial infection. We have found that a systematic, head-to-toe search for the site of infection in the critically ill surgical patient with sepsis is of utmost importance. Nevertheless, first and foremost, any search for infection in a surgical patient must address the prior condition of the patient. This includes not only the patient's preexisting diseases but also any history of invasive procedures that have been performed.

Frequently, the occurrence of infectious complications or organ failure in a surgical ICU patient is closely associated with complications of the operations previously performed. Any investigation for the site of infection in a critically ill patient must start at that patient's known site of disease or operation. For example, in the patient who has undergone a gastrointestinal (GI) tract operative procedure, the clinician's index of suspicion must be extremely high for complications of that operation, including anastomotic dehiscence, peritonitis, and intra-abdominal abscess. Before the sepsis can be attributed to an infection at a distant site, the patient must be evaluated for complications of the original disease process or operation that may have resulted in infection. Investigation for other hospital-acquired infections should be carried out either concomitantly or after the original disease site has been examined.

This chapter reviews those infections acquired in the hospital setting that may result in sepsis in the critically ill surgical patient (Table 57–2).

WOUND INFECTION

In a frequently cited national study published in 1964, the overall incidence of postoperative wound infection was reported to be 7.5%.[7] The incidence varied from surgeon to surgeon, from hospital to hospital, and from one surgical procedure to another. The lowest infection rate (2%) followed "clean" operations, such as elective orthopedic procedures and herniorrhaphy, in which the possible sources of wound contamination were solely airborne or exogenous. "Clean-

TABLE 57–1. Risk Factors for the Development of Intensive Care Unit (ICU) Infections

Risk Factors
Age > 70 yr
Shock
Coma
Steroids
Chemotherapy
ICU stay > 3 days
Previous antibiotic therapy
Mechanical ventilation
Invasive monitoring
Urinary catheter use > 10 days
Acute renal failure
Head or multiple trauma
Surgical rather than medical patient

TABLE 57–2. Nosocomial Infections Common to the Intensive Care Unit Patient

Surgical Site	***Abdomen***
Wound infection	Peritonitis
	Abscess
Head and Neck	*Clostridium difficile* enterocolitis
Sinusitis	Urinary tract infection
Meningitis	
Ventriculitis	***Catheter-Related Infections***
Parotitis	Arterial catheters
	Central venous catheters
Chest	Swan-Ganz catheters
Pneumonia	
Lung abscess	
Empyema	

contaminated" operations that resulted in the additional exposure of the operative site to the endogenous microflora had higher rates of infection (>5%). In 1977, Green and Wenzel[8] reported that the average hospital stay doubled and that hospitalization costs were thus increased when postoperative wound infection developed after any of six common elective operations were performed.

The economic, physical, and psychologic impact of postoperative wound sepsis and other serious infections mandates the use of preventive methods. The most critical of these are proper surgical technique and sound judgment (i.e., in the choice of operation, on the part of a responsible surgeon and surgical team). In addition, well-controlled prospective, blinded clinical studies have defined the circumstances in which antibiotic prophylaxis is of benefit as well as the situations in which the risks of prophylaxis outweigh the expected benefits.

Classification of Surgical Wounds

Surgical wounds are generally classified as (1) clean, (2) clean-contaminated, (3) contaminated, or (4) dirty.[9]

Clean wounds are those from operations in the course of which the GI, genitourinary, or respiratory tract has not been entered. The usual causes of postoperative infections in this case are the aerobic exogenous bacteria, such as staphylococci, that enter the wound during the operation. The overall infection rate in clean surgical procedures is often quoted to be in the range of 2% to 3%.

Clean-contaminated wounds are those from elective operations in the course of which the GI, genitourinary, or respiratory tract has been entered. The risk of infection in this case is higher than in clean surgical procedures, generally between 5% and 10%. The primary cause of infection is the endogenous microflora of the organ that has been surgically resected.

Contaminated wounds are those from operations during which acute inflammation (without pus formation) or gross spillage of GI contents has been encountered. Infections in this case are primarily due to endogenous bacteria, and the infection rate is about 20%.

Dirty wounds are those from operations in which gross pus is encountered. As with the other types of wounds, infections in this case are primarily related to the involved organ's endogenous microflora. The infection rate approaches 40%.

Non–Antibiotic-Associated Factors That Influence Wound Infection Rates

Many factors have been regarded, without convincing evidence, as influencing the incidence of postoperative wound infection in clean operations, such as preoperative scrub technique, surgical glove damage, barrier materials, and "laminar flow" air systems in the operating room (Table 57–3).[9] Several factors, however, are clearly associated with higher risk of wound infection.

The longer the period of *preoperative hospitalization*, the greater the infection rate.[9] Northey[10] observed that virtually every patient is colonized with nosocomial bacteria within 2 weeks of admission to a critical care unit. The colonizations are usually by hospital-acquired, antibiotic-resistant organisms.

Having the patient use *hexachlorophene*-containing antiseptics for the *preoperative shower* on the evening before surgery is associated with a significantly lower postoperative wound infection rate.[9] The decrease in infection rate has not been observed when regular soap is used in the preoperative shower. *Razor shaving* of the operative site on the day before surgery appears to increase the postoperative infection rate.[9] The increase results from the growth and multiplication of skin microorganisms in the damaged epithelium after the razor shave. For this reason, when razor shaving is to be employed, it should be confined to the immediate preoperative period. Studies have shown, however, that the lowest postoperative infection rate occurs if no shaving is performed; clipping with a barber's shears or using a depilatory cream before surgery has been associated with a low wound infection rate.[9, 11]

TABLE 57–3. Factors Influencing the Development of Postoperative Wound Infections in Clean Surgical Procedures According to Level of Importance

Very Important (Infection Rate Doubled)
Period of preoperative hospitalization prolonged
Shaving of the operative site on the day before surgery
Duration of operation prolonged
Use of prophylactic abdominal drains
Operation performed in the presence of an active remote infection
Important (Infection Rate Less Than Doubled but Significantly Increased)
Preoperative showering with antiseptic not performed
Probably Not Important (No Significant Increase in Infection Rate)
Surgeon's hand scrub: iodophor instead of hexachlorophene
Patient skin preparation: iodophor instead of hexachlorophene
Use of plastic skin drapes
Use of "laminar flow" air systems

Generally, each hour added to the *duration of operation* results in a doubling of the infection rate.[9] Shapiro and coworkers[12] have reported on a prospective study of risk factors for infection after hysterectomy. They observed that the statistically significant benefit of antibiotic prophylaxis in decreasing wound sepsis after operations lasting 1 hour was lost for operations lasting more than 3.3 hours. This finding undoubtedly relates to the pharmacokinetics of antibiotic prophylaxis as well as to greater bacterial wound colonization in lengthy, complicated operative procedures. Repeated doses of prophylactic antibiotics given during the operation may be necessary for procedures lasting more than 3 hours, especially when agents with short half-lives are used.

Nora and colleagues[13] reported on the dangers of the *prophylactic use of drains* after abdominal surgery. On the basis of their common detection of skin bacteria at the interior of the abdominal drains, these researchers have stressed the "two-way street" concept (i.e., that bacteria may just as easily enter the body along the drain tract as be removed by the drain). Magee[14] demonstrated that the presence of either Silastic or latex Penrose drains in an experimental wound dramatically enhanced the wound's infection rate, even in the presence of subinfective doses of bacteria. From these experimental and clinical studies, it appears that the prophylactic use of abdominal drains is unwarranted and may indeed be a dangerous practice. When drains are required to empty localized collections, they should be placed through sites other than the primary surgical incision to decrease the incidence of subsequent wound infection.

Significant increases in postoperative wound infection occur when an elective procedure is done in the presence of an *active remote infection*.[9] It is thus prudent to initiate treatment for urinary, pulmonary, or skin infections at least 48 hours before elective operative procedures are attempted.

Types of Clinical Wound Sepsis

Most postoperative wound infections are uncomplicated, involving only the skin and subcutaneous tissues. Infrequently, they progress to become necrotizing infections, which may involve the fascia and muscle. The usual clinical presentation of uncomplicated wound infection consists of the following symptoms, which often begin between the fourth and eighth postoperative days:

- Local incisional pain (dolor)
- Tenderness
- Swelling (tumor)
- Redness (rubor)
- Increased warmth (calor)
- Elevated body temperature

When infection occurs during the first 48 hours after operation, it is characteristically caused by either clostridia or β-hemolytic streptococci. In such a case, the dramatic clinical presentation of gangrenous infections may include profound systemic toxicity and rapid local advance of the infection, which often involves all layers of the body wall. A high mortality rate (60% to 80%) can be expected unless a rapid diagnosis is made on the basis of clinical presentation and the results of a Gram stain of wound fluid.

Treatment consists of parenteral administration of antimicrobial agents (usually penicillin G alone) and aggressive, prompt surgical debridement of all infected tissue. Additionally, hyperbaric oxygen therapy should be employed if it is locally available.

In clean operations in which the GI, genitourinary, and respiratory tracts have not been entered, exogenous *Staphylococcus aureus* is the usual cause of infection; in contrast, infection by a polymicrobial aerobic-anaerobic flora that closely resembles the normal endogenous microflora of the surgically resected organ occurs in clean-contaminated operations. The cardinal features of treatment of an uncomplicated wound infection are operative drainage and local wound care.

Prevention of Wound Infection

Much progress has been made since the mid-1980s in the appropriate use of antibiotic prophylaxis in the patient undergoing surgery. Well-controlled, prospective, blinded studies have identified many areas in which antibiotic prophylaxis is of benefit as well as those clinical settings in which the risks of antibiotic prophylaxis outweighed the expected value.[15]

Historically, the most common errors included the widespread use of antibiotic prophylaxis in clean surgical procedures as well as faulty timing of the initial administration of the selected agents. Currently, the most common error is the practice of continuing use of the antibiotic agents beyond the time necessary for maximum benefit (>72 hours).[16]

In order to obtain the greatest effect from the use of prophylactic antibiotics, one must be aware of the following factors:

1. The timing of administration should offer maximum benefit while minimizing adverse effects.
2. The route of administration must be appropriate.
3. The choice of antibiotic agent should be based on the types of organisms that usually cause infection.
4. A dosage necessary to attain efficacious tissue or serum levels must be administered.

Timing of Antibiotic Prophylaxis

The effective use of prophylactic antibiotics depends to a great extent on the appropriate timing of their administration.[17] Intravenously administered antibiotics in effective doses should first be given within 30 minutes of the operative incision. This is accomplished if the anesthesiologist starts the antibiotic infusion when he or she establishes intravenous access in the operating room just before the induction of anesthesia.

Such timing of antibiotic administration results in the presence of therapeutic drug levels in the wound and related tissues during the operation but does not allow for the development of bacterial resistance. Administration of the drugs should be continued for less than 24 hours, a period during which the concentration of bacteria in the wound may exceed the capacity of the tissues to destroy them. Continuation of prophylactic drug therapy beyond 24 hours increases the risk of drug toxicity or bacterial superinfection and does not reduce the incidence of subsequent infection. One to three doses of antimicrobial agents, with the first dose given just before operative incision as just described, are sufficient for prophylaxis.

When prophylaxis is accomplished with orally administered antibiotics, as is common for elective colon resection, the agents should be given only during the 24 hours before operation. Longer periods of preoperative preparation are not necessary and have been associated with the isolation of resistant organisms within the colonic lumen at the time of resection.[18]

Route of Administration

Intravenous administration is preferred in most surgical patients. Administering antibiotics intravenously in a relatively small volume of diluent over a short time results in high serum concentrations that are reflected in more rapid entry of antibiotics into, and higher early concentrations of antibiotics in, wound fluid. Administration of equivalent doses of antibiotics by either continuous intravenous infusion or intermittent intramuscular injection produces lower blood concentrations and later entry of the drugs into wound fluid. Oral administration of poorly absorbed antibiotics has a major role only in the elective preparation of patients undergoing colon operations.[19]

Choice of Antibiotics

No single antibiotic agent or combination of agents can be relied on for effective prophylaxis in the various clinical settings of the surgical critical care unit. The agent or agents employed should be chosen primarily on the basis of efficacy against the microorganisms that usually cause the infectious complications in each clinical setting.[9] For example, in uncomplicated cardiovascular or orthopedic operations, the usual cause of postoperative infections is aerobic streptococci or staphylococci. The organisms responsible for infection after GI or gynecologic surgery are more complex, and selecting appropriate prophylactic antibiotics in this situation requires an understanding of the polymicrobial nature of the endogenous microflora at each site. The microorganisms usually responsible for infection in different surgical disciplines are listed in Table 57-4.

Antibiotic Prophylaxis in Clean Surgical Procedures

In the past, the use of prophylactic antibiotics in clean surgical procedures has been limited to procedures in which a prosthetic foreign body has been implanted.[15] The general attitude has been that any benefit from the use of antibiotic prophylaxis in clean surgical cases is outweighed by its potentially harmful effects, which include toxic and allergic drug reactions as well as bacterial or fungal superinfections. Low infection rates in clean procedures are best obtained through strict adherence to the principles of good surgical technique.

The presence of any foreign body, however, disables wound healing. Even a single suture in a wound is sufficient to cause suppuration with a bacterial inoculum that by itself does not result in infection.[20] Foreign material interferes with normal wound defense mechanisms, so fewer bacteria are necessary

TABLE 57–4. Microorganisms Most Commonly Isolated from Sites of Postoperative Infection

Surgical Discipline/ Infection Site	Aerobes	Anaerobes
Gastrointestinal		
Mouth	Streptococci	*Bacteroides* (other than *Bacteroides fragilis*), peptostreptococci, fusobacteria
Esophagus	Same as for mouth	Same as for mouth
Stomach	Enteric gram-negative bacilli, streptococci	Same as for mouth
Biliary	Enteric gram-negative bacilli, group D streptococci	Clostridia
Distal ileum	Enteric gram-negative bacilli	*B. fragilis,* peptostreptococci, clostridia
Colon	Same as for distal ileum	Same as for distal ileum
Gynecologic	Same as for distal ileum	Same as for distal ileum
Orthopedic	Staphylococci, streptococci	
Thoracic	Streptococci, pneumococci	Bacteroides (other than *B. fragilis*), peptostreptococci
Cardiovascular	Staphylococci, streptococci	
Urologic	Enteric gram-negative bacilli, group D streptococci	

to cause infection. A large, multicenter, prospective randomized study of antibiotic prophylaxis in clean surgical procedures, such as inguinal hernia repair and breast procedures, has demonstrated the apparent value of antibiotic prophylaxis in reducing wound infection.[21]

The risk of infections in patients undergoing clean surgical procedures with prosthetic devices, such as total hip replacement and implantation of cardiac valves or vascular grafts, is low. When infection does occur in these patients, however, the result most often is catastrophic. Prophylaxis with antistaphylococcal drugs may reduce the incidence of postoperative infection in such cases and is therefore recommended.[15] Penicillinase-resistant penicillins, such as methicillin, oxacillin, and nafcillin, have commonly been employed for prophylaxis in this clinical setting. Higher numbers of infections in this setting, however, have been reported to be due to *Staphylococcus epidermidis,* an organism that has a degree of resistance to this group of semisynthetic penicillins. It is for this reason that first-generation cephalosporins, which usually exhibit good activity against many of the organisms that commonly cause postoperative sepsis, continue to be the drugs of choice. If significant antibiotic resistance is suspected or proven, the use of vancomycin may be desirable.

PERITONITIS AND INTRA-ABDOMINAL ABSCESS

Significant improvement in the survival of patients with intra-abdominal infection was observed early in the 20th century; mortality rates fell from 90% to 40% to 50% primarily because of the realization that surgical intervention was necessary to cure most intra-abdominal infections. The mortality rate has decreased only minimally over the last 50 years, however, despite the discovery and use of effective antibiotics and the advent of modern critical care. Secondary bacterial peritonitis primarily occurs following the leakage of the endogenous microflora from a diseased or traumatized intraperitoneal hollow viscus. The extent of dissemination and the severity of the infection within the peritoneal cavity depend on a number of factors, including:

- Source of contamination
- Duration of contamination
- Presence of adjuvant substances
- Bacterial synergy
- Adequacy of the host defense response

Hemoglobin, ascitic fluid, fibrin clots, necrotic tissue, bile, and barium sulfate have all been demonstrated to promote the establishment of intra-abdominal bacterial infection.[22]

The polymicrobial nature of intra-abdominal infections and the pathogenic characteristics of anaerobes were first recognized by Altemeier[23, 24] in patients with perforated appendicitis. The conclusions of his studies, published in 1938 and 1942, were as follows:

1. The majority of the bacteria do not produce a fatal peritonitis when injected in pure culture.
2. Many avirulent strains of bacteria, particularly *Escherichia coli,* become highly virulent in the presence of dead tissue.
3. In mixed culture, these bacteria show a synergistic action, producing a high level of pathogenicity.
4. Peritonitis appears to be an infection resulting from the synergistic activities of the various bacterial symbionts present.

These studies were not elaborated on for nearly three decades, until modern anaerobic microbiologic techniques were introduced, allowing for the better classification of the organisms in both normal flora and postoperative infection studies.[25]

Experimental models of intra-abdominal sepsis have provided much insight with regard to bacterial synergy and also the need to treat such infection with antibiotics active against both aerobes and anaerobes. Intra-abdominal sepsis is, at times, a two-phase disease process, with acute peritonitis and bacteremia occurring early, and intra-abdominal abscesses developing later on in the survivors of the first phase. Aerobes seem to be responsible for the high mortality in acute peritonitis, whereas anaerobes are necessary for the development of intra-abdominal abscesses in the survivors. The use of antibiotics directed against both aerobes and anaerobes is significant in decreasing the mortality rate associated with early peritonitis and late abscess formation in experimental intra-abdominal sepsis.[26, 27] Subsequent studies have demonstrated that the most important virulence factor for *Bacteroides fragilis* is its polysaccharide capsule.

Clinical Presentation

The diagnosis of intra-abdominal infection is usually suggested by the patient's history and the typical physical findings. Abdominal pain is present in almost all patients with peritonitis or abscess. The physical findings—involuntary guarding and tenderness—are localized in patients with abscess but diffuse in patients with generalized peritonitis. The pain and tenderness are worsened by any movement, including coughing and jarring of the hospital bed. Absence of bowel sounds and abdominal distention occur owing to paralytic ileus. Patients with intra-abdominal infection also have fever, and they may have other symptoms and signs related to hypovolemia due to fluid sequestration within the peritoneal cavity. With adequate fluid resuscitation, the patients manifest the typical hyperdynamic state associated with sepsis. Increases in the peripheral polymorphonuclear leukocyte count commonly exceed 15,000 cells per mm^3, with a shift to the left often observed.

Plain or contrast radiologic examinations of the abdomen and chest may be helpful in demonstrating perforations, ileus, space-occupying lesions, and free fluid. Specialized radiologic tests, such as ultrasound and computed tomography, are most helpful in searching for localized intra-abdominal fluid collections. In patients with ascites, paracentesis may be helpful.

In patients without ascites and with borderline findings on physical examination, peritoneal lavage may be extremely helpful in diagnosis. The technique was first described in this clinical setting by Richardson and colleagues[30] in 1983. It requires the intraperitoneal placement of a catheter, either by cutdown or by the percutaneous route, followed by the instillation of 1 L of saline. The fluid is then drained off, and an aliquot is examined. The diagnosis of peritonitis is made if (1) gross pus, bile, or feces is present in the fluid, (2) the leukocyte count is higher than 500 polymorphonuclear leukocytes per mm^3, or (3) bacteria or food fibers are seen on microscopic examination. It is important to obtain samples of the fluid from peritoneal lavage as well as the fluid from paracentesis for both aerobes and anaerobes.

Therapy

The most critical aspects of the treatment of secondary peritonitis are early diagnosis and prompt intervention. Pitcher and Musher[31] found a strong correlation between the interval from presentation to treatment and the subsequent perioperative morbidity and mortality. Antibiotic use, ICU care, and other adjunctive modalities do not compensate for delays in definitive treatment.

Frequently, the exact cause of the peritonitis is not ascertained until abdominal exploration is performed. For therapeutic purposes, it is helpful to classify intra-abdominal infections as either diffuse or localized. *Localized* infections are more commonly amenable to operative resection, surgical drainage, or percutaneous catheter drainage. *Diffuse* suppurative peritonitis is not particularly responsive to these types of treatment alone; other approaches, such as open abdominal packing, radical peritoneal debridement, peritoneal lavage, and planned repeated abdominal explorations, have been recommended as additional therapeutic options.

Treatment of Localized Infection

Resection

Resectional therapy for disease such as gangrenous appendicitis, cholecystitis, bowel infarction, or perforated diverticulitis is the standard of care. In the past, the operative treatment of perforated diverticulitis was conducted in three stages: (1) drainage of abscess with diverting colostomy, (2) resection of the involved colon, and finally (3) closure of the colostomy. Most surgeons today combine the first and second stages.

With the ability to drain abscesses percutaneously, however, another potential approach is as follows:

1. Percutaneous drainage of the peridiverticular abscess to allow the patient's symptoms and signs of infection to resolve.
2. Mechanical and antibiotic preparation of the colon.
3. Resection of the involved portion of colon with primary anastomosis.

It remains to be seen whether this approach will become widely applicable.

Drainage

The optimal method of treating abscesses continues to be incision and drainage, and many techniques are available. Percutaneous drainage of intra-abdominal abscesses was first reported by Grønvall and colleagues[32] in 1977. Comparisons of percutaneous drainage with surgical drainage of abdominal abscesses are extremely variable and suffer from the lack of evidence from prospective, randomized studies.

On the basis of currently available data, we believe that percutaneous drainage of intra-abdominal abscesses is not advisable in the presence of the following factors:

1. Complex abscesses, which are defined as those that (a) have more than two septations, (b) are in continuity with the gastrointestinal tract, (c) are filled with thick debris, or (d) contain primarily fungi.
2. More than two abscesses.
3. Pancreatic abscesses.
4. Drainage pathways that would necessitate traversing bowel or uncontaminated body cavities.

The success rate for percutaneous drainage of abscesses in favorable circumstances should range from 80% to 90%.

Treatment of Diffuse Intra-abdominal Infections

Although the overriding principle in the management of localized purulent collections (incision and drainage) is accepted and the major controversies concerning management are over differences in technique, the same cannot be said about the treatment principles for diffuse suppurative peritonitis. Several approaches to this condition are available.

Simple Drainage

Simple drainage of the peritoneal cavity in the setting of diffuse suppurative peritonitis is totally ineffective, possibly because drains are rapidly walled off by fibrin deposition along the drain tract.

Continuous Postoperative Peritoneal Lavage

Continuous peritoneal lavage refers to the placement of irrigation catheters in the peritoneal cavity *at the time of operation* to irrigate the peritoneal cavity with fluid in an effort to dilute or wash away bacteria and other toxic substances during the postoperative period. It is extremely important to note that (1) the use of this technique has been proposed only as a therapeutic adjunct after exploratory laparotomy has been used to control the inciting factors in the development of peritonitis and (2) the technique is of no use by itself.

The technique usually involves instilling 1 L of fluid over 5 to 10 minutes, allowing it to remain in the peritoneal cavity for approximately 30 minutes, and then draining it out over 20 to 25 minutes.[33] This process is repeated until either the effluent becomes totally clear or an arbitrary point in time has been reached. The choice of fluid and of any additives to it, such as antibiotics and heparin, varies widely among the proponents of the technique.

Many nonrandomized studies have shown a survival advantage with the use of continuous postoperative peritoneal lavage; however, five of the six prospective published studies show no improvement with lavage.[34] Because this technique has not convincingly been demonstrated to improve survival, we believe that it should be used only in highly selected patients, such as those with peritonitis and renal failure who require peritoneal dialysis for the renal failure.

Intraoperative Irrigation

Although intraoperative irrigation with crystalloid solutions has not been shown to decrease either mortality or the rate of recurrence of abscesses, virtually all studies have supported the use of intraoperative peritoneal irrigation with or without antibiotic-containing solutions in patients with diffuse bacterial peritonitis. Schumer and colleagues[35] demonstrated that crystalloid irrigation reduced the number of bacteria remaining in the peritoneal cavity. Although Rosato and coworkers[36] also showed a reduction in the concentration of adjuvant substances following irrigation, they were unable to show any reduction in either mortality or rate of subsequent abscess formation.

Various antibiotics, including cephalothin (1 g/L), kanamycin (1 g/L), bacitracin (50,000 U/L), chloramphenicol, and other aminoglycosides, have all been used enthusiastically but have rarely been shown to decrease the incidence of recurrent intra-abdominal infection. When intraoperative irrigation is used, attention should be devoted to possible antibiotic toxicities that may occur as a result of rapid absorption and the presence of high systemic serum levels of the drugs.

Radical Peritoneal Debridement

In 1975, Hudspeth[37] introduced the concept of radical peritoneal debridement for the treatment of generalized peritonitis. The technique involves the complete exposure of the entire peritoneal cavity. Initially, all free peritoneal fluid and pus are suctioned out of the abdomen. Then, the entire peritoneal cavity is meticulously debrided. All fibrin peels are removed from the serosal surfaces of the bowel. In the only study comparing radical peritoneal debridement with standard therapy, Polk and Fry[38] reported no difference in outcome.

Leaving the Peritoneal Cavity Open

The concept of treating the peritoneal cavity as a large abscess cavity and of managing generalized peritonitis by packing it open was revived in 1979.[39] Since that time, several reports on the use of this technique or modifications of it have been published.

The combination of the use of polypropylene mesh to avoid evisceration and of planned repeated returns to the operating room has been widely adopted and practiced in the specific group of patients who have severe generalized bacterial peritonitis. The decision is made at the initial operation, on the basis of operative findings, to return the patient to the operating room daily to break up loculations and debride dead tissue. The abdomen is closed when no further fluid collections or necrotic debris can be found. No prospective, randomized clinical studies comparing the packing of the abdomen open or any of its variations with any other form of treatment has been published.

This open type of treatment has been proposed to have the following advantages over standard therapy:

1. A decrease in intra-abdominal pressure, which improves blood flow to the abdominal viscera.
2. Daily elimination of purulent and necrotic material to maintain control over infection by lessening the bacterial burden.
3. The prompt recognition of intra-abdominal complications. The risks of bowel perforation and fistula formation may be higher with this procedure.

Antibiotic Selection

Unlike patients with superficial wound abscesses, in whom surgical drainage alone suffices, patients with intra-abdominal infections are best managed with a combination of surgical repair, excision, diversion, or drainage and therapy with appropriately chosen, parenterally administered antibiotics.

The antibiotic therapy should be initiated as soon as the diagnosis is made preoperatively and should be continued during the operation and into the postoperative period. The choice of ideal agent or agents and the necessary duration of therapy remain controversial. On the basis of experimental and clinical studies, the chosen antibiotics must have activity against both colonic aerobes and anaerobes, including *B. fragilis*.[27, 40] Conventional antibiotic regimens for peritonitis have consisted of an aminoglycoside and either clindamycin or metronidazole; however, the use of single-antibiotic therapy effective against both aerobic and anaerobic organisms has been espoused. The antibiotics that are commonly used singly or in combination are listed in Table 57–5.

The appropriate duration of antibiotic therapy in patients with established peritonitis is controversial. The data of Lennard and coworkers[41] indicate that if a patient is afebrile but still has leukocytosis at the conclusion of the antibiotic course, the risk that the patient has ongoing or recurrent intra-abdominal infection is 33%. In this study, 79% of patients who were still febrile at the conclusion of their antibiotic course had recurrent infection. No patient who was afebrile and whose white blood cell count was normal had recurrent intra-abdominal infection. One must realize, however, that no randomized, prospective study comparing different durations of antibiotic therapy has ever been performed in secondary peritonitis. Solomkin and colleagues[42] showed that the mean duration of therapy in patients with peritonitis in whom the endpoints of therapy—normal white blood cell count and absence of fever—were achieved was approximately 9 days.

These studies and others have led the Surgical Infection Society[43] to make the following recommendations:

1. Plan a 5- to 7-day course of antibiotics directed at aerobic gram-negative bacilli and anaerobic bacteria for diffuse peritonitis or localized intra-abdominal abscess.
2. If there is no clinical improvement within 4 to 5 days, strongly consider the possibility that (a) source control has been inadequate, (b) there is further undrained localized pus,

TABLE 57–5. Parenteral Antibiotic Agents Currently Used for Therapy of Intra-abdominal Infection

Combination Therapy
AEROBIC COVERAGE*
Amikacin
Aztreonam
Cefotaxime
Ceftriaxone
Ciprofloxacin
Gentamicin
Tobramycin
ANAEROBIC COVERAGE†
Chloramphenicol
Clindamycin
Metronidazole
Single-Drug Therapy
AEROBIC/ANAEROBIC COVERAGE WITH SINGLE AGENT
Ampicillin/sulbactam
Cefotetan
Cefoxitin
Ceftizoxime
Imipenem/cilastatin
Pipericillin/tazobactam
Ticarcillin/clavulanic acid

*To be combined with a drug having anaerobic activity.
†To be combined with a drug having aerobic activity.

or (c) an inadequately treated extra-abdominal infection exists and should be vigorously sought.

Conclusion

Control of the source of peritoneal soilage, cleanup of the peritoneal cavity, and antibiotics are all important in the treatment of established intra-abdominal infection. Failure in any one of the three areas results in a less than optimum outcome.

The antibiotic regimen should include coverage for both aerobic gram-negative rods and anaerobic organisms. Duration of antibiotic treatment should range from 5 to 10 days and possibly up to 14 days. If there has not been a significant clinical response by day 4 or 5 of therapy, one must consider the presence of either ongoing intraperitoneal infection or extra-abdominal infection that is being inadequately treated with the chosen antibiotic regimen. If the patient still shows signs of sepsis at the conclusion of the antibiotic course, a vigorous search for ongoing intra-abdominal and extra-abdominal infections should begin.

HEAD AND NECK INFECTIONS

The most common hospital-acquired infections of the head and neck are sinusitis and central nervous system infections, including meningitis and ventriculitis.

Sinusitis

Sinusitis is a commonly overlooked source of sepsis and should be suspected in patients who have sustained facial trauma or who have any type of tube passing through the nares. Since Arens and coworkers[44] first described this problem and reported a 2% incidence in an ICU population, several other reports have appeared that indicate that sinusitis is an even more common occurrence in ICU patients than was previously thought. O'Reilly and colleagues[45] reported a 27% incidence of sinusitis; reviews of the subject describe occurrence rates that range between the two values just cited.

Sinusitis is most commonly associated with nasotracheal intubation, but its occurrence with the use of nasogastric tubes has also been reported. Facial trauma is also a predisposing factor. The maxillary sinuses are involved in 50% to 75% of all cases of sinusitis in facial trauma, and the involved sinus is almost always on the same side as the nasal tube. The mechanism by which sinusitis occurs is assumed to be obstruction of the sinus ostia, which results in the accumulation of fluid in the sinus and then in secondary infection.

Diagnosis is difficult because most patients do not exhibit the typical symptoms of sinusitis or, because of depressed mental status, cannot relate their symptoms to their physicians. The diagnosis is most easily made with computed tomography of the face and sinuses. Plain sinus radiographs are not particularly helpful, probably because of the difficulty in properly positioning these critically ill patients to obtain adequate radiographic images.

Unlike the situation with primary sinusitis, the bacteria involved in sinusitis secondary to intubation are usually gram-negative bacilli, *S. aureus,* or anaerobes. Treatment consists of removal of the nasal tube, use of decongestant sprays and antibiotics appropriate for the implicated organism, and, most important, drainage of the sinus.

Parotitis

Parotitis is rarely seen in the critically ill surgical patient. This infection is probably caused by inspissation of saliva in Stensen's duct in dehydrated patients, which results in ductal obstruction. With a better understanding of fluid therapy in surgical patients, postoperative parotitis seems to have become a disease of the past. Early reports of the disease tended to stress the importance of *S. aureus*; however, several reports of parotitis due to gram-negative bacilli have appeared in the literature.

THORACIC INFECTIONS

The intrathoracic infections most commonly seen in the ICU are pneumonia, lung abscess, and empyema. Additionally, because of the great number of cardiac surgical procedures performed in the United States, mediastinitis is not infrequently seen in surgical ICUs.

Pneumonia

The incidence of pneumonia is related to underlying lung injury (e.g., that caused by adult respiratory distress syndrome [ARDS] or pulmonary contusion), mechanical ventilation for longer than 48 hours, prolonged preoperative hospitalization, thoracic or upper abdominal incision, and, possibly, the use of certain types of stress ulcer prophylactic agents.[46]

The mechanism by which pneumonia occurs in ICU patients is thought to be aspiration, inhalation, or hematogenous spread. Aspiration of upper airway and oropharyngeal secretions seems to be the most common mode. The bacteriology of ICU-acquired pneumonias tends to confirm this assertion. Approximately 70% to 75% of ICU-related pneumonias are caused by aerobic gram-negative bacilli, whereas 15% to 20% are caused by *S. aureus,* and 5% to 15% by *Candida* species.[47] In only 2% to 15% of normal humans do gram-negative bacilli colonize the upper airways; however, in 55% to 75% of critically ill patients, colonization of the upper airway occurs within the first few days of the ICU stay. Driks and colleagues[48] have demonstrated an association between colonization of the stomach by gram-negative bacilli and the subsequent development of pneumonia in the presence of the same organisms.

A number of factors, both related to the primary illness and iatrogenic in nature, contribute to the higher risk of pneumonia in ICU patients (Table 57–6). Normal barriers to infection are breached, including the mucociliary clearance mechanism in the tracheobronchial tree and the normally acidic nature of the stomach. Endotracheal tubes prevent the normal mucociliary mechanism from functioning and from clearing secretions. To minimize the risk of stress-related GI ulceration, we alkalize the stomach; this measure allows for overgrowth of lower GI tract bacteria in the stomach, which then colonize the upper aerodigestive tract. Another risk factor for pneumonia is that the ICU patient's mental status may be depressed because of head trauma, narcotics, sedatives, or central nervous system failure from sepsis, decreasing the ability to cough.

TABLE 57–6. Risk Factors for Intensive Care Unit–Related Pneumonia

Age
Aspiration
Head trauma
History of smoking
Lung injury—adult respiratory distress syndrome, pulmonary contusion
Prior use of antibiotics
Prolonged preoperative hospitalization
Pulmonary edema
Stress ulcer prophylaxis with antacids
Upper abdominal or thoracic incision

Diagnosis

The diagnosis of pneumonia in otherwise critically ill patients can be very difficult to establish. Other factors are often present that may account for the patient's fever and leukocytosis. Chest radiography is frequently not helpful because many patients with pneumonia already have infiltrates secondary to other pulmonary disease, such as adult respiratory distress syndrome or pulmonary contusion.

Because of these difficulties, a number of diagnostic techniques involving sputum analysis have been developed. Determination of the quantity and quality of sputum, Gram's stain of the sputum, and sputum culture can suggest a diagnosis but are not diagnostic tests. We have found examination of the quantity and quality of sputum to be a good guide, however, to the diagnosis of pneumonia. The presence of copious amounts of purulent sputum is consistent with the pneumonia process, and the diagnosis can usually be confirmed by Gram's stain of the sputum. The absence of white blood cells in a sputum sample obtained through an endotracheal tube almost completely precludes the diagnosis of pneumonia, whereas the presence of white blood cells in combination with intracellular bacteria ensures the diagnosis. Many times, the Gram stain of the sputum demonstrates white blood cells and one or more morphologic types of bacteria, none of which is intracellular. In this instance, the findings of sputum analysis should guide the choice of antibiotics; once the sputum culture and sensitivity results are known, the antibiotic may be changed if necessary. In patients without endotracheal tubes, however, 25% to 50% of sputum cultures show a discrepancy with respect to the organisms they contain compared with sputum samples collected more distally in the tracheobronchial tree. This finding almost certainly represents either colonization of the upper airways with organisms different from those causing the pneumonia or contamination by the oral flora. Various techniques have been described to improve the specificity of sputum culture in these cases, including (1) transtracheal aspiration and (2) bronchoscopic protected sampling of the lower respiratory tract.

With *transtracheal aspiration,* a small angiocatheter is passed through the cricothyroid membrane and a sputum sample is obtained via the angiocatheter. This collection method has the advantage of bypassing the mouth and thus avoiding contamination by oral flora. Analysis of a sample obtained in this manner to identify the true pathogen is much more reliable than analysis of an expectorated sputum sample. However, this technique cannot be performed when an endotracheal tube is in place, and it is associated with a small risk of pneumothorax, subcutaneous emphysema, and hemorrhage.

Bronchoscopy has also been used to obtain sputum samples. Some contamination by oral flora always occurs because the bronchoscope must pass through the upper aerodigestive tract. In *protected brush sampling,* a sterile brush protected within a plastic tube is passed through the bronchoscope. When the area to be sampled is reached, the brush is pushed out of the end of the plastic tube, the sample is obtained, and the brush is withdrawn back into the plastic tubing. The brush is then removed from the patient and cut off into culture media. In *protected specimen bronchoalveolar lavage,* sterile saline is introduced through the sterile plastic tubing, is aspirated, and is then cultured. Both methods of sputum sampling have significantly better accuracy than other techniques of sputum sampling. We suggest using a bronchoscopic sampling technique for a case of pneumonia that does not seem to respond clinically to treatment directed by standard sputum sampling techniques.

Most ICU-acquired pneumonias reflect the bacterial flora within the ICU. Within a short time of arriving in an ICU, a patient's own normal bacterial flora is replaced by the ICU flora. This process is exacerbated by the use of broad-spectrum antibiotics, which decimate the patient's more antibiotic-sensitive normal bacterial flora and allow for overgrowth of the resistant ICU bacteria.

Prevention of ICU-Acquired Pneumonia

Several concepts and techniques developed since the mid-1980s seem to decrease the incidence of ICU-related pneumonia: (1) the use of enteral (not parenteral) nutrition, (2) alteration of the type of stress ulcer prophylaxis, (3) early fixation of pelvic and long bone fractures, and (4) selective gut decontamination.

Enteral versus Parenteral Nutrition

Since the initial discovery that a patient's nutrition can be maintained with total parenteral nutrition (TPN), it has become clear that this modality represents a great advance and that it has saved many lives. The use of TPN in critically ill patients has not met with total success, however. With the popularity of the concept of the "gut origin septic state" and the role of the gastrointestinal tract in sepsis and multiple organ failure, studies comparing TPN and enteral nutrition have repeatedly demonstrated the superiority of enteral feedings in decreasing infectious complications as well as the intensity of the sepsis syndrome.[49]

Several prospective studies comparing enteral nutrition with parenteral nutrition in critically ill trauma patients have now shown a lower incidence of ICU-related pneumonia in patients who receive enteral nutrition.

In a study by Moore and coworkers,[50] 59 patients who sustained severe abdominal trauma were randomly grouped to receive equal amounts of calories and protein by either the enteral ($n = 29$) or parenteral ($n = 30$) route. No patients who received enteral nutrition had pneumonia, whereas pneumonia did develop in 20% (six of 30) of the group receiving TPN ($P < .03$ between groups).

In another study by Kudsk and colleagues,[51] 68 patients who sustained blunt or penetrating abdominal trauma were randomly grouped to receive either enteral nutrition or TPN. Only 6% of patients who received enteral feedings had pneumonia, whereas 29% of patients who received TPN did so.

Furthermore, Bower and associates[52] demonstrated fewer nosocomial infections and shorter hospital stay in patients receiving an enteral formula supplemented with arginine, nucleotides, and fish oil than in patients receiving a standard enteral formula. Battistella and coworkers[53] also showed that the use of lipid emulsion in a TPN regimen is associated with a significantly higher risk of infection and prolonged pulmonary failure.

We rarely use TPN in our surgical patients, and we generally begin enteral feedings on the first postoperative day, as soon as a patient is hemodynamically stable.

Stress Ulcer Prophylaxis

One of the great advances in modern critical care has been the recognition that the incidence of significant GI stress hemorrhage can be decreased from approximately 15% to 5% through the use of antacids, histamine$_2$ (H_2) blockers (e.g., cimetidine, ranitidine, famotidine), sucralfate, or misoprostol. Because of the association of increased gastric pH, gastric colonization with enteric organisms, and the development of ICU-related pneumonia with these same organisms, the relationship between the type of stress ulcer prophylaxis and pneumonia has been the subject of several investigations.

In 1987, Driks and associates[48] and Tryba[54] both reported that the use of sucralfate rather than antacids seemed to be related to a lower incidence of ICU-acquired pneumonia.

Kappstein and coworkers[55] found the same to be true when they compared sucralfate and cimetidine; they reported a 46% incidence of nosocomial pneumonia in the cimetidine group and a 27% incidence of nosocomial pneumonia in the sucralfate group. All of these researchers suggested that the increase in gastric pH—which is associated with the use of antacids or H_2 blockers and with the subsequent colonization of the stomach with enteric organisms—is the primary factor related to the higher incidence of pneumonia.

Several reports, however, have concluded that no relationship exists between stress ulcer prophylaxis regimen and ICU-acquired pneumonia. Simms and colleagues[56] found no difference in incidence of pneumonia among their groups of subjects who received antacids (30%), cimetidine (28%), or sucralfate (27%). Cook and associates,[57] using meta-analysis techniques, found no compelling evidence to support the concept that one form of stress ulcer prophylaxis is superior to any other form in minimizing the risk of nosocomial pneumonia. They concluded that most of the prior studies suffered from methodologic deficiencies, such as small sample size and the failure to separate antacids and H_2 blockers in the study groups.

Early Fracture Fixation

In the past, fractures in patients with multiple trauma were fixed almost as an afterthought: The other serious injuries were dealt with at the time of presentation, and the patient was then taken to the ICU, where the fractures would be treated with bed rest and traction. Through the insight of such traumatologists as John Border and Thomas Rüedi, the recognition that patients with multiple trauma "did better" with early fracture fixation piqued the interest of a number of trauma groups. Seibel and coworkers[58] demonstrated a lower rate of acute respiratory failure in patients with early fixation (within 24 to 48 hours of injury) of femur fractures than in patients with late fixation.

Bone and coworkers[59] and Behrman and associates[60] demonstrated a decrease in the incidence of pneumonia and also noted (1) shorter time requirements for mechanical ventilation, (2) lower incidence of adult respiratory distress syndrome, (3) fewer ICU and hospital days, (4) lower mortality rate, and (5) lower care costs in the groups that underwent immediate stabilization of femur fractures compared with the groups treated initially with traction followed by late fixation. These researchers have theorized early fracture fixation has the following benefits:

- Allows for the early mobilization of the patient, so that he or she may be transferred from the bed and into the upright position early postoperatively
- Decreases ongoing blood loss with the resultant possibility of shock
- Helps to minimize ongoing soft tissue injury

Selective Gut Decontamination

The concept of selective gut decontamination grew out of the belief that some pneumonias are due to the aspiration of gastric contents colonized by enteric organisms. The thinking was that if the cycle could be interrupted before the aspiration stage, the incidence of ICU-acquired pneumonia might decrease. This technique—in which nonabsorbable antibiotics effective against aerobic gram-negative bacteria and *Candida* species were swabbed into the oropharynx and given via a nasogastric tube—was noted to be effective in preventing infections in patients with leukemia.[61]

Stoutenbeek and colleagues[62] were the first to demonstrate the efficacy of selective gut decontamination in trauma patients. They used a regimen consisting of (1) the application in the oropharynx of a sticky paste containing 2% each of polymyxin E, tobramycin, and amphotericin B four times daily along with (2) the administration of the same antibiotics via the nasogastric tube and (3) the intravenous administration of a third-generation cephalosporin. In a nonrandomized trial of this approach in comparison with historical controls from their own ICU, they found that selective gut decontamination decreased the incidences of pneumonia, urinary tract infection, bacteremia, and wound infection.

Three other prospective, randomized studies have confirmed the findings of Stoutenbeek's group. Kerver and coworkers[63] used the same antibiotic regimen as used by the Stoutenbeek group, but in a patient population comprising both trauma and nontrauma surgical patients; they found a significant decrease in pneumonia and intra-abdominal infections but no alteration in the mortality rate of the group receiving the selective gut decontamination regimen. Using only polymyxin E, tobramycin, and amphotericin B administered by capsule or nasogastric tube (no oropharyngeal paste or systemic antibiotics), Godard and associates[64] were also able to verify the previous findings: a reduction in the overall number of gram-negative infections and a lower incidence of ICU-acquired pneumonia. A 12% mortality rate was found in the group receiving selective gut decontamination, compared with an 18% rate in the control group (not a significant difference). The study by Godard's group had the advantage of including all patients admitted to the ICU—trauma, nontrauma surgical, and medical patients.

Flaherty and coworkers[65] found that selective gut decontamination (with polymyxin, gentamicin, and nystatin) and stress ulcer prophylaxis with antacids or H_2 blockers, or both, significantly decreased the incidence of all infections, including pneumonia, compared with sucralfate therapy for stress ulcer prophylaxis and no selective gut decontamination. Overall, the rate of all infections was 12% in the group undergoing selective gut decontamination, compared with 27% in the group given sucralfate; the incidence of pneumonia was similarly less in the former group (2% and 9%, respectively).

A study by Cerra and colleagues,[66] who used nystatin and norfloxacin in 94 critically ill patients via nasogastric tube (no oropharyngeal application), demonstrated a decrease in the incidence of pneumonia and other nosocomial infections in the group receiving selective gut decontamination. They did not, however, report a reduction in mortality or in the incidences of multiple organ failure or adult respiratory distress syndrome. Similarly, Gastinne and coworkers[67] were not able to demonstrate any difference in either incidence of pneumonia or mortality between selective gut decontamination and placebo.

Although the use of nonabsorbable antibiotics in the oropharynx and GI tract may reduce the incidence of nosocomial pneumonia, the intravenous use of antibiotics to prevent ICU-related pneumonia has not been successful. In a large, multicenter study carried out in Europe, approximately 1300 patients were randomly grouped to receive either cefoxitin, penicillin G, or no antibiotic.[68] The incidence of pneumonia was 6% in both the cefoxitin and penicillin groups, and 7% in the patients receiving no prophylactic antibiotics.

We do not recommend the use of selective gut decontamination because of the lack of evidence that it improves survival and because of the expense it adds to the patient's care.

Empyema

Empyema is a complication of pneumonia, trauma, or chest tube placement. After trauma, empyema most commonly occurs from the incomplete evacuation of blood from the pleural space. We recommend that any hemothorax that is not completely drained by tube thoracostomy should be operatively evacuated within 3 to 7 days of injury.

Controversy surrounds the use of prophylactic antibiotics for the duration of chest tube placement.[15] Since the mid-1980s, several retrospective and prospective reviews on this subject have appeared in the literature. The reporting researchers' conclusions are divided with regard to whether antibiotics are helpful in preventing empyema in patients with chest trauma who require tube thoracostomy. In these reports, the risk of empyema ranged from 1.2% to 7%. The researchers who reported the higher rate of empyema found that antibiotics lowered the empyema rate, whereas those who observed a lower rate of empyema found no benefit attributable to prophylactic antibiotics. It seems likely that factors such as emergency placement of a chest tube, hemothorax (as opposed to pneumothorax), and manipulation of the chest tube are all associated with a higher incidence of empyema.

Lung Abscess

Lung abscess most commonly is a complication of pneumonia, and its bacteriology depends on the cause and microbiology of the pneumonia. For example, pneumonias secondary to aspiration cause abscesses that harbor anaerobes.

Regardless of the pathogen, the treatment of lung abscesses involves their drainage. In the majority of patients, repeated bronchoscopy is needed to break into the abscess cavity and to drain the abscess internally into the tracheobronchial tree. We recommend at least daily bedside flexible bronchoscopic drainage until the amount of purulence is significantly decreased and the systemic signs of infection begin to resolve. External drainage or resection of pulmonary abscesses is uncommonly necessary and fraught with complications, the most common and most devastating of which is bronchopleural fistula.

CATHETER-RELATED INFECTIONS

(see also Chapter 59)

It is estimated that 2.5 million central venous catheters and 100,000 arterial catheters are placed in patients in the United States each year. Because catheter-related sepsis occurs in 3% to 5% of all intravascular catheter placements, the magnitude of the problem is clear.

Catheter-related sepsis has been defined as either bacteremia associated with intravascular catheters or sepsis (fever, leukocytosis) that resolves with removal of the catheter. The diagnosis is strengthened when the organism cultured from the blood is the same as that obtained from the catheter tip. Catheter contamination from the skin is the most common mode of infection, followed by seeding of the catheter from a remote site, catheter or tubing contamination at the connecting hub, and infusate colonization. The most commonly encountered organisms associated with catheter-related infection are staphylococci (*S. aureus* and *S. epidermidis*), *Candida albicans,* and gram-negative bacilli. Each accounts for approximately 25% of catheter-related infections.

Risk factors related to the development of catheter-related infection are as follows:

- Nature of the underlying disease
- Duration of catheterization
- Location of the catheter
- Expertise of the physician who places the catheter
- Use of multi-lumen catheters
- Catheter care
- Material of which the catheter is constructed

Catheter-related sepsis is more likely to develop in patients in critical care units than in patients on hospital wards. It is not clear, however, whether this finding is a result of patients' underlying illnesses or of the fact that intravascular catheters used in ICU patients tend to be manipulated more, are in place longer, and are more often placed under emergency circumstances than catheters used in hospital ward patients.

A duration of catheterization of longer than 3 days has been shown to be linked with a higher rate of catheter sepsis.[69] The site of cannulation is an important determinant, in that femoral venous cannulas are the most likely to be colonized, followed by internal jugular catheters, with subclavian catheters having the lowest risk.

Single-lumen and multiple-lumen catheters seem to carry approximately the same risk of catheter-related infection, and changing central venous catheters over a guide wire or moving them to a new site does not seem to result in a lower incidence of infection.[70, 71] Although results of studies comparing single-lumen and multiple-lumen catheters are mixed, triple-lumen catheters tend to present a slightly higher risk of colonization than single-lumen catheters.

The development of catheter-related bacteremia is closely related to the number of colony-forming units (CFUs) cultured off the catheter tip on semiquantitative culture.[72] When fewer than 15 CFUs are cultured from the catheter tip, catheter-related bacteremia is rare. This fact is the basis for many of the suggested plans of catheter maintenance. The most controversial aspect of catheter maintenance concerns the routine changing of catheters in the nonseptic patient. Recommendations to change the catheter to a different site every 3 to 7 days, to change the catheter-over-guide wire every 3 to 7 days, and to leave the catheter in place without routine replacement have all been made.

Eyer and associates[73] reported a study in which 112 consecutive surgical ICU patients were randomly assigned to three catheter management protocols: (1) changing the catheter to an entirely new site every 7 days, (2) changing the catheter-over-guide wire every 7 days, or (3) no weekly change at all. The study evaluated central venous, pulmonary artery, and arterial catheters. All catheters were changed if a positive blood culture result was obtained since the most recent catheter change; if evidence of exit site infection was present; or if the patient manifested sepsis without any other obvious source. The incidences of catheter-related sepsis episodes per patient were similar for all groups (0.17 for guide-wire changes, 0.22 for complete changes, and 0.16 for no changes).

The algorithm for catheter changes that we follow is detailed in Figure 57–1.

Treatment

The treatment of catheter-related infection involves removal of the catheter and the administration of antibiotics. The appropriate duration of antibiotic therapy is a subject of controversy. Most clinicians continue antibiotic therapy only as long as a patient manifests systemic signs of infection (e.g., fever, leukocytosis). Longer courses of antibiotic therapy (up to 10 to 14 days) may be necessary, however, to prevent complications of staphylococci-related bacteremias. In retrospective studies, both Raad and Sabbagh[74] and Mylotte and McDermott[75] suggested that continuing antibiotic therapy for 10 to 14 days is associated with a lower incidence of recurrent bacteremia or of endocarditis.

Prevention

The most important means of decreasing the incidence of catheter-related sepsis is strict adherence to aseptic technique during catheter placement and care. Caps, masks, gowns, and gloves should certainly be used during placement of pulmo-

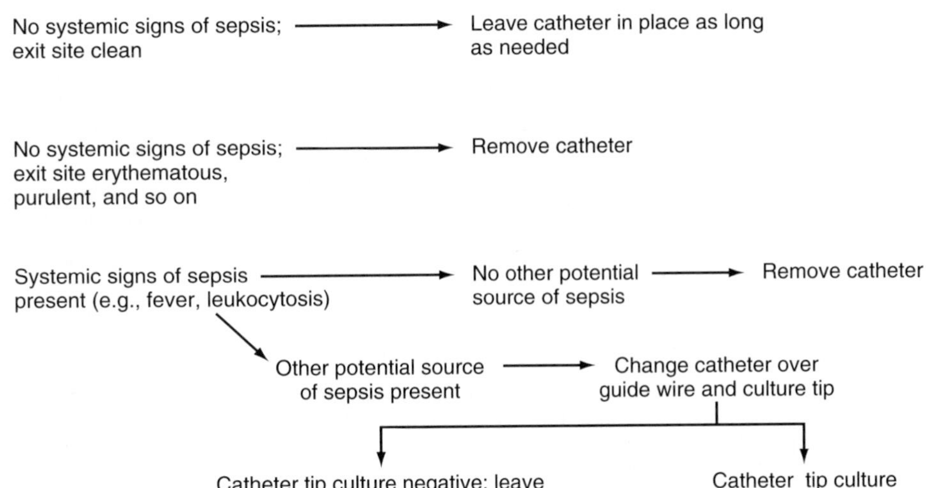

Figure 57–1. Algorithm for managing arterial, central venous, and pulmonary artery catheters.

nary artery and central venous catheters and possibly even for placement of arterial catheters.

A number of other adjunctive techniques have been developed to minimize the incidence of catheter-related sepsis. They include the bonding of antibiotics and silver compounds to the catheter, the use of a sterile, protective plastic sleeve over pulmonary artery catheters, and utilization of a silver ion–impregnated cuff. The silver ion–impregnated cuff fits over the catheter at the time of placement. It is made of collagen and allows for a firm anchoring of the catheter in the subcutaneous tissue. It acts as both a mechanical and a chemical barrier to bacteria and has been shown to minimize the incidence of skin site infections as well as catheter-related sepsis.

Complications

The occurrence of subacute bacterial endocarditis and suppurative thrombophlebitis of the great veins is an uncommon but deadly complication of the placement of central venous and pulmonary artery catheters and of transvenous pacemakers. It has been demonstrated that, within 1 to 2 days after placement of a central venous or pulmonary artery catheter, damage to the endothelium occurs; this damage is hypothesized to be responsible for the higher risk of endocarditis and phlebitis.

ABDOMINAL INFECTIONS

Most intra-abdominal infections that occur in critically ill surgical patients are secondary to the patients' underlying disease or represent a complication of a surgical procedure. Several "abdominal" infections do not, however, belong in these categories. They are discussed here.

Clostridium difficile–Related Enterocolitis

Clostridium difficile–related enterocolitis is not uncommon in the critically ill patient treated with antibiotics. It tends to cluster in "mini-epidemics" and almost always follows the use of antibiotics. There may be a substantial lag between the withdrawal of antibiotics and the development of colitis. It is our experience that *C. difficile*–related enterocolitis can manifest a full spectrum of features, from mild diarrhea and other nonspecific symptoms to a necrotizing enterocolitis with bowel perforation.

Diagnosis is made on the basis of results from assay of a stool specimen for *C. difficile* toxin. The disease commonly (but not always) affects the distal sigmoid colon and rectum and can be diagnosed on sigmoidoscopic examination by detection of the classic pseudomembranes. Presence of the disease cannot be excluded, however, if pseudomembranes are not seen.

Although oral vancomycin is slightly more effective than either orally or intravenously administered metronidazole, metronidazole is the agent of choice because of growing concern about the development of vancomycin-resistant bacteria. Occasionally, a patient has a fulminant form of enterocolitis, and systemic signs of sepsis result from the *C. difficile* infection. If bowel perforation occurs, if signs of peritoneal irritation are present, or if sepsis becomes increasingly more severe, the patient should undergo exploratory laparotomy and resection of the involved colon.

Urinary Tract Infection

Urinary tract infection is the most common hospital-acquired infection; however, it seems to be a less important problem in critically ill patients than in hospital ward patients. The development of urinary tract infection is directly related to the duration of urinary bladder catheterization. In one study, only 2.6% of urine specimens cultured were positive in patients whose catheters had been in place for fewer than 4 days.[76] The rate of positive urine culture results increases dramatically after 5 days of catheterization.

The diagnosis is usually easily made on the basis of urinalysis and culture results. The combination of white blood cells on microscopic examination or leukocyte esterase in the urine and the growth of an organism (usually > 100,000 CFUs/mL) confirms the diagnosis. The organisms most commonly isolated are gram-negative aerobes and *Candida* species.

Urinary tract infection seems to be declining in incidence. This may be because of the use of closed drainage systems and improvement in nursing protocols for catheter care. Performance of routine catheter culture in patients without sepsis, use of prophylactic antibiotics, and frequent catheter changes are not necessary and do not seem to reduce the incidence of urinary tract infection.

SUMMARY

A multitude of infections can result in sepsis in critically ill patients. We believe that the best way to evaluate these patients is to develop a list of diagnostic possibilities based on whether they have risk factors for specific infections, and not to simply perform "pan-culturing." Our approach to evaluation yields useful diagnostic information and avoids inadequate, ineffective, and unnecessary treatment, whether with antibiotics or with any other therapeutic modalities.

References

1. Pories SE, Gamelli RL, Mead PB, et al: The epidemiologic features of nosocomial infections in patients with trauma. Arch Surg 1991; 126:97.
2. Maki DG: Risk factors for nosocomial infection in intensive care. Arch Intern Med 1989; 149:30.
3. Craven DE, Kunches LM, Lichtenberg DA, et al: Nosocomial infection and fatality in medical surgical intensive care unit patients. Arch Intern Med 1988; 148:1161.
4. Fry DE, Pearlstein L, Fulton RL, et al: Multiple system organ failure: The role of uncontrolled infection. Arch Surg 1980; 115:136.
5. Pin RW, Wertz MJ, Lennard ES, et al: Determinants of organ malfunction or death in patients with intra-abdominal sepsis: A discriminant analysis. Arch Surg 1983; 118:242.
6. Poole GV, Muakkassa FF, Griswold JA: The role of infection in outcome of multiple organ failure. Am Surg 1993; 59:727.
7. Ad Hoc Committee of the Committee on Trauma, National Research Council Division of Medical Sciences: Factors influencing the incidence of wound infection. Ann Surg 1964; 160(Suppl):32.
8. Green JW, Wenzel RP: Postoperative wound infection: A controlled study of the increased duration of hospital stay and direct cost of hospitalization. Ann Surg 1977; 185:264.
9. Nichols RL: Surgical wound infection. Am J Med 1991; 91(Suppl 3B):54S.
10. Northey D: Microbial surveillance in a surgical intensive care unit. Surg Gynecol Obstet 1974; 139:321.
11. Balthazar ER, Colt J, Nichols RL: Preoperative hair removal: A random, prospective study. South Med J 1982; 75:799.
12. Shapiro M, Munoz A, Tager IB, et al: Risk factors for infection at the operative site after abdominal or vaginal hysterectomy. N Engl J Med 1982; 307:1661.
13. Nora PF, Vanecko RM, Bransfield JJ: Prophylactic abdominal drains. Arch Surg 1972; 105:173.
14. Magee C: Potentiation of wound infection by surgical drains. Am J Surg 1976; 131:547.
15. Antimicrobial prophylaxis for surgery. Med Lett 1993; 35:91.
16. Shapiro M, Townsend TR, Rosner B, et al: Use of antimicrobial drugs in general hospitals: Patterns of prophylaxis. N Engl J Med 1979; 301:351.
17. Burke JF: The effective period of preventive antibiotic action in experimental incisions and dermal lesions. Surgery 1961; 50:161.
18. Nichols RL: Bowel preparation. *In*: Surgical Infections: Diagnosis and Treatment. Meakins JL (Ed). New York, Scientific American, 1994, p 151.
19. Nichols RL, Condon RE, Grobach SL, et al: Efficacy of preoperative antimicrobial preparation of the bowel. Ann Surg 1972; 176:227.
20. Howe CW: Experimental studies on determinants of wound infection. Surg Gynecol Obstet 1966; 123:507.
21. Platt R, Zaleznik DF, Hopkins CC, et al: Perioperative antibiotic prophylaxis for herniorrhaphy and breast surgery. N Engl J Med 1990; 322:153.
22. Dunn D, Rotstein O, Simmons R: Fibrin in peritonitis: IV. Synergistic intraperitoneal infection caused by *Escherichia coli* and *Bacteroides fragilis* within fibrin clots. Arch Surg 1984; 119:139.
23. Altemeier W: The bacterial flora of acute perforated appendicitis: A bacteriologic study based upon one hundred cases. Ann Surg 1938; 107:517.
24. Altemeier W: The pathogenicity of the bacteria of appendicitis peritonitis: An experimental study. Surgery 1942; 11:374.
25. Nichols RL, Smith JW: Wound and intra-abdominal infections: Microbiological considerations and approaches to treatment. Clin Infect Dis 1993; 16(Suppl 4):266.
26. Weinstein WM, Onderdonk AB, Bartlett JG, et al: Experimental intra-abdominal abscesses in rats: Development of an experimental model. Infect Immun 1974; 10:1250.
27. Nichols RL, Smith JW, Fossedal EN, et al: Efficacy of parenteral antibiotics in the treatment of experimentally induced intra-abdominal sepsis. Rev Infect Dis 1979; 1:302.
28. Kasper DL: The polysaccharide capsule of *Bacteroides fragilis* subspecies *fragilis*: Immunochemical and morphologic definition. J Infect Dis 1976; 133:79.
29. Onderdonk AB, Kasper DL, Cisneros RL, et al: The capsular polysaccharide of *Bacteroides fragilis* as a virulence factor: Comparison of the pathogenic potential of encapsulated and unencapsulated strains. J Infect Dis 1977; 136:82.
30. Richardson J, Flint L, Polk H: Peritoneal lavage: A useful diagnostic adjunct for peritonitis. Surgery 1983; 94:826.
31. Pitcher W, Musher D: Critical importance of early diagnosis and treatment of intra-abdominal infection. Arch Surg 1982; 117:328.
32. Grønvall J, Grønvall S, Hegedüs V: Ultrasound-guided drainage of fluid-containing masses using angiographic catheterization techniques. AJR 1977; 131:323.
33. Stephen M, Loewenthal J: Continuing peritoneal lavage in high-risk peritonitis. Surgery 1979; 85:603.
34. Leiboff AR, Soroff HS: The treatment of generalized peritonitis by closed postoperative peritoneal lavage: A critical review of the literature. Arch Surg 1987; 122:1005.
35. Schumer W, Lee D, Jones B: Peritoneal lavage in postoperative therapy of late peritoneal sepsis. Surgery 1964; 55:841.
36. Rosato E, Oram-Smith J, Mullis W, et al: Peritoneal lavage treatment in experimental peritonitis. Ann Surg 1972; 175:384.
37. Hudspeth A: Radical surgical debridement in the treatment of advanced generalized bacterial peritonitis. Arch Surg 1975; 110:1233.
38. Polk H, Fry D: Radical peritoneal debridement for established peritonitis: The results of a prospective randomized clinical trial. Ann Surg 1980; 192:350.
39. Steinberg D: On leaving the peritoneal cavity open in acute generalized suppurative peritonitis. Am J Surg 1970; 137:216.
40. Walker AP, Nichols RL, Wilson RF, et al: Efficacy of a β-lactamase inhibitor combination for serious intra-abdominal infections. Ann Surg 1993; 217:115.
41. Lennard E, Dellinger E, Wertz M, et al: Implications of leukocytosis and fever at conclusion of antibiotic therapy for intra-abdominal sepsis. Ann Surg 1982; 195:19.
42. Solomkin JS, Reinhart HH, Dellinger EP, et al: Results of a randomized trial comparing sequential intravenous/oral treatment with ciprofloxacin plus metronidazole to imipenem/cilastatin for intra-abdominal infections. Ann Surg 1996; 223:303.
43. Bohnen JM, Solomkin JS, Dellinger EP, et al: Guidelines for clinical care: Anti-infective agents for intra-abdominal infection: A Surgical Infection Society Policy Statement. Arch Surg 1992; 127:83.
44. Arens JF, LeJeune FE, Webre DR: Maxillary sinusitis, a complication of nasotracheal intubation. Anesthesiology 1974; 40:415.
45. O'Reilly MJ, Reddick EJ, Black W, et al: Sepsis from sinusitis in nasotracheally intubated patients: A diagnostic dilemma. Am J Surg 1984; 147:601.
46. Craven DE, Kunches LM, Kilinsky V, et al: Risk factors for pneumonia and fatality in patients receiving continuous mechanical ventilation. Am Rev Respir Dis 1986; 133:729.
47. Burchard K: Diagnosis and treatment of pneumonia in the surgical intensive care unit. Surg Gynecol Obstet 1989; 171(Suppl):35.
48. Driks MR, Craven DE, Celli BR, et al: Nosocomial pneumonia in intubated patients given sucralfate as compared with antacids or histamine type 2 blockers. N Engl J Med 1987; 317:1376.
49. Border JR, Hassett J, LaDuca J, et al: The gut origin septic states in blunt multiple trauma (ISS = 40) in the ICU. Ann Surg 1987; 206:427.
50. Moore FA, Moore EE, Jones TN, et al: TEN versus TPN following major abdominal trauma: Reduced septic morbidity. J Trauma 1989; 29:916.
51. Kudsk KA, Croce MA, Fabian TC, et al: Enteral vs. parenteral feeding: Effects on septic morbidity following blunt and penetrating abdominal trauma. Ann Surg 1992; 215:503.
52. Bower RH, Cerra FB, Bershadsky B, et al: Early enteral administration of a formula (Impact) supplemented with arginine, nucleotides, and fish oil in intensive care unit patients: Results of a multicenter, prospective, randomized clinical trial. Crit Care Med 1995; 23:436.
53. Battistella FD, Widergren JT, Anderson JT, et al: A prospective,

randomized trial of intravenous fat emulsion administration in trauma victims requiring total parenteral nutrition. J Trauma 1997; 43:52.
54. Tryba M: Risk of acute stress bleeding and nosocomial pneumonia in ventilated intensive care unit patients: Sucralfate versus antacids. Am J Med 1987; 83(Suppl 3B):117.
55. Kappstein I, Schulgen G, Friedrich T, et al: Incidence of pneumonia in mechanically ventilated patients treated with sucralfate or cimetidine as prophylaxis for stress bleeding: Bacterial colonization of the stomach. Am J Med 1991; 91(Suppl 2A):125S.
56. Simms HH, DeMaria E, McDonald L, et al: Role of gastric colonization in the development of pneumonia in critically ill trauma patients: Results of a prospective randomized trial. J Trauma 1991; 31:531.
57. Cook DJ, Laine LA, Guyatt GH, et al: Nosocomial pneumonia and the role of gastric pH: A meta-analysis. Chest 1991; 100:7.
58. Seibel R, LaDuca J, Hassett J, et al: Blunt multiple trauma (ISS 36), femur traction, and the pulmonary failure-septic state. Ann Surg 1985; 202:283.
59. Bone LB, Johnson KD, Weigelt J, et al: Early versus delayed stabilization of femoral fractures: A prospective randomized study. J Bone Joint Surg [Am] 1989; 71:336.
60. Behrman SW, Fabian TC, Kudsk KA, et al: Improved outcome with femur fractures: Early vs. delayed fixation. J Trauma 1990; 30:792.
61. Sleyfer DT, Mulder NH, de Vries-Hospers HG, et al: Infection prevention in granulocytopenic patients by selective decontamination of the digestive tract. Eur J Cancer 1980; 16:859.
62. Stoutenbeek CP, van Saene HK, Miranda DR, et al: The effect of selective decontamination of the digestive tract on colonization and infection rate in multiple trauma patients. Intensive Care Med 1984; 10:185.
63. Kerver AJ, Rommes JH, Mevissen-Verhage EA, et al: Prevention of colonization and infection in critically ill patients: A prospective randomized study. Crit Care Med 1988; 16:1087.
64. Godard J, Guillaume C, Reverdy ME, et al: Intestinal decontamination in a polyvalent ICU: A double-blind study. Intensive Care Med 1990; 16:307.
65. Flaherty J, Nathan C, Kabins S, et al: Pilot trial of selective decontamination for prevention of bacterial infection in an intensive care unit. J Infect Dis 1990; 162:1393.
66. Cerra FB, Maddaus MA, Dunn DL, et al: Selective gut decontamination reduces nosocomial infections and length of stay but not mortality or organ failure in surgical intensive care unit patients. Arch Surg 1992; 127:163.
67. Gastinne H, Wolff M, Delatour F, et al: A controlled trial in intensive care units of selective decontamination of the digestive tract with nonabsorbable antibiotics. N Engl J Med 1992; 326:594.
68. Mandelli M, Mosconi P, Langer M, et al: Prevention of pneumonia in an intensive care unit: A randomized multicenter clinical trial. Crit Care Med 1989; 17:501.
69. Gil RT, Kruse JA, Thill-Baharozian MC, et al: Triple- vs. single-lumen central venous catheters: A prospective study in a critically ill population. Arch Intern Med 1989; 149:1139.
70. Farkas JC, Liu N, Bleriot JP, et al: Single- versus triple-lumen central catheter-related sepsis: A prospective randomized study in a critically ill population. Am J Med 1992; 93:277.
71. Badley AD, Steckelberg JM, Woolan PC, et al: Infectious rates of central venous pressure catheters: Comparison between newly placed catheters and those that have been changed. Mayo Clin Proc 1996; 71:838.
72. Maki DG, Weise CE, Sarafin HW: A semiquantitative method for identifying intravenous catheter-related infection. N Engl J Med 1977; 296:1305.
73. Eyer S, Brummitt C, Crossley K, et al: Catheter-related sepsis: Prospective, randomized study of three methods of long-term catheter maintenance. Crit Care Med 1990; 18:1073.
74. Raad II, Sabbagh MF: Optimal duration of therapy for catheter-related *Staphylococcus aureus* bacteremia: A study of 55 cases and review. Clin Infect Dis 1992; 14:75.
75. Mylotte JM, McDermott C: *Staphylococcus aureus* bacteremia caused by infected intravenous catheters. Am J Infect Control 1987; 15:1.
76. Martinez OV, Civetta JM, Anderson K, et al: Bacteriuria in the catheterized surgical intensive care patient: A prospective survey of 100 patients. Crit Care Med 1986; 14:188.

58

Antimicrobial Therapy in the Critical Care Setting

Joan E. Kapusnik-Uner, PharmD
Marjorie Robinson, PharmD • Merle A. Sande, MD

The diagnosis of and therapy for infections represent a major function of the critical care physician. Intensive care unit (ICU) infections are often severe and are encountered either as a cause of admission to an ICU or as a complication of other severe illnesses. Also, bacterial sepsis remains a common cause of late death in trauma victims.[1] The diagnosis of infection in the ICU patient may be obvious or extremely difficult. Infection may have a dramatic presentation with high temperature, leukocytosis with left shift, hypotension, disseminated intravascular coagulopathy, renal insufficiency, and respiratory failure. On the other hand, patients admitted to the ICU for presumed shock, respiratory insufficiency, or coma may ultimately not have infection as an underlying diagnosis despite the presence of classic signs and symptoms.[2] The patient presenting with respiratory insufficiency is an excellent example of the dilemma faced by the ICU physician, who must try to distinguish between infectious and noninfectious causes.

The scope of fungal infections in the ICU setting has changed, in that endemic mycoses are continuing to be a problem in cancer patients and in those individuals with underlying human immunodeficiency virus infection. Also, in the United States, nosocomial opportunistic fungal infections have increased in hospitals during the 1990s.[3]

This chapter reviews a rational approach to the diagnosis and treatment of bacterial infections encountered by the ICU physician. Diagnostic tests and a general approach to selecting empirical antibiotic treatments are described. A summary of the pertinent pharmacology data for the individual antibiotics is given, with an emphasis on spectrum of activity, pharmacokinetics including the threshold creatinine clearance used for dose adjustment, toxicities, and dosing guidelines.[4] Infections commonly found in the ICU patient along with a rationale to their antimicrobial treatment are also described.

DIAGNOSIS OF INFECTION

Once infection is suspected in the ICU patient, the physician's goal is to identify the infecting pathogen. Usually, a specific bacteriologic diagnosis is made through isolation of the pathogen by culture or identification by staining techniques.

Before the availability of culture data in a particular patient, one can usually obtain clues as to the identity of the pathogen by performing a Gram stain of "material" from the suspected site of infection. When the Gram stain reveals only a single morphologic type of bacteria, such as gram-positive cocci or gram-negative bacilli, this organism should be treated empirically as the etiologic pathogen. Morphologic characteristics cannot indicate whether the pathogen is anaerobic or aerobic, but certain clues can help to identify the organism. For example, gram-positive cocci in clusters are likely to be staphylococci, encapsulated gram-positive diplococci are probably *Streptococcus pneumoniae*, small gram-negative cocci are *Neisseria* species, and coccobacillary organisms are consistent with *Haemophilus* species.

When the Gram stain reveals multiple morphologic types of bacteria, this may represent contamination during the process of obtaining the specimen (e.g., contamination of a wound swab specimen by the normal skin flora), or the presence of multiple morphologic types of bacteria can be an accurate reflection of a polymicrobial, or mixed, infection. The specificity and usefulness of the Gram stain or culture specimens are related directly to the care with which the specimen is obtained.[5] Compulsive care must be used to minimize contamination. This is obviously difficult in obtaining samples from nonsterile body sites (e.g., respiratory secretions obtained from a patient on a ventilator, because the endotracheal tube or upper airway is colonized by large numbers of bacteria).

SELECTION OF ANTIBIOTICS

A number of patient-specific historical and clinical factors must be taken into account before an empirical antibiotic regimen is selected.[6] For example, several aspects of the patient's history must be considered:

1. Is the infection community-acquired or hospital-acquired? Community-acquired infections are, in general, caused by bacteria that are more susceptible to a wide range of antimicrobial agents and may be treated with "standard," less toxic, and less expensive agents. Hospital-acquired (nosocomial) infections, however, may be caused by pathogens with complex antimicrobial resistance patterns and may require potentially more toxic and expensive drugs.

2. What is the patient's underlying illness? Certain diseases predispose patients to infections caused by specific pathogens. For example, multiple myeloma is associated with infections caused by encapsulated bacteria, such as *S. pneumoniae* and *Haemophilus influenzae;* patients with leukemia and leukopenia and burn victims are predisposed to infections with *Pseudomonas aeruginosa;* and diabetes mellitus is associated with polymicrobial infections caused by *Staphylococcus aureus* and anaerobic organisms. Thus, if a patient with such an underlying illness is thought to have an infection, the empirical antibiotic regimen is tailored to cover these organisms.

3. What is the suspected primary focus of infection? Different anatomic sites are characteristically infected by specific microorganisms. For example, the urinary tract and biliary tree are usually infected by enteric (aerobic) gram-negative bacilli, whereas endocarditis is caused by aerobic gram-positive cocci, such as *S. aureus* and viridans group streptococci, and meningitis is caused by encapsulated organisms, such as *S. pneumoniae, Neisseria meningitidis,* and *H. influenzae*.

4. Has the patient been treated with antibiotics recently? If the patient has acquired a new infection during or shortly after treatment with antibiotics, the new infection or superinfection is likely to be caused by a more resistant pathogen.

5. In patients already receiving antibiotics, bacterial growth obtained may be suppressed in cultures owing to the presence of antibiotic in the actual culture specimen. Thus, culture results may be less helpful for pathogen identification.

The appropriate selection of antimicrobial agents for empirical therapy also requires a reasonable understanding of drug pharmacology, including the mechanism of action (bactericidal versus bacteriostatic), antimicrobial spectrum of activity, pharmacokinetics, potential toxicities, and appropriate dose and dosing interval for a given clinical scenario. There are several important considerations:

1. When should a bactericidal versus a bacteriostatic antibiotic be selected? Bactericidal antibiotics kill bacteria without the assistance of host defenses and thus are important for the cure of infections when the host immune response is not adequate. Three clinical settings require bactericidal therapy for cure: (a) meningitis, because there are decreased antibodies and complement (C3b) in cerebrospinal fluid (CSF) as well as the lack of surface phagocytosis; (b) infectious endocarditis, in which a dense fibrin-platelet meshwork encases a large bacterial inoculum (vegetation) and is impermeable to the effects of circulating white blood cells (WBCs); and (c) infections in neutropenic patients. Bacteriostatic drugs, in contrast, inhibit the normal growth cycle of bacteria but do not lyse or kill the organisms. Bacteriostatic agents, such as tetracyclines, macrolides, and clindamycin, generally provide adequate therapy when host defenses are intact.

2. The general spectrum of activity for an antimicrobial agent must be understood. The usefulness of a specific agent in an institution may be monitored by the microbiology, infectious diseases, and infection control departments. An antibiogram, which outlines an institution's susceptibility pattern to specific microorganisms, is helpful for the empirical antimicrobial selection process. The ICU physician must be informed of susceptibilities of common ICU pathogens because they may vary among institutions and also within a given institution (e.g., *Enterobacter* species, *Acinetobacter* species, and *Pseudomonas* species).

3. Pharmacokinetics is important because the physician must understand the distribution and elimination characteristics of an antimicrobial agent. For example, infections occurring in the CSF (i.e., meningitis), biliary tract, or urinary tract may be difficult to treat because certain drugs may not adequately distribute to those sites. The routes of elimination for each agent are important for the drug selection process to ensure adequate urine and bile concentrations for the treatment of infection at these sites. Also, toxicities may occur when elimination routes are impaired.

4. The dose and dosing intervals are selected with the following factors in mind: the pathogen's minimum inhibitory concentration (MIC), the severity of infection, the body size of the patient (affecting the drug's volume of distribution), and the route of drug elimination relative to the patient's organ function. Inadequate drug regimens can result in treatment failure and the emergence of antimicrobial resistance, whereas excessive drug administration may result in toxicity and unnecessary expense.

5. The toxicity profile of antimicrobial agents is important for the overall clinical outcome. Factors that contribute to potential toxicities may be avoided or carefully monitored (i.e., excessive serum drug concentrations, renal dysfunction, concomitant administration of drugs with similar toxicities).

During the first 48 to 72 hours of empirical antimicrobial therapy, the patient must be watched closely for signs of clinical deterioration or improvement. If the patient's status deteriorates, the following possibilities should be considered:

- Presence of an undrained or undebrided focus of infection
- A too-narrow spectrum of antimicrobial coverage
- Inadequate penetration of drug to the focus of infection
- Subtherapeutic dose or interval for the severity of infection or for the patient's body size

When culture and sensitivity results are available, the antimicrobial regimen should be reassessed and tailored to the narrowest spectrum, least toxic, and least expensive agents. It is crucial to tailor antimicrobial agents, even when patients have "responded" to therapy. This is done to minimize the alterations in the patient's bacterial flora, which occur with prolonged use of broad-spectrum antibiotics. Shortened courses of therapy and narrow-spectrum coverage to both help minimize the "antibiotic pressure" that promotes antimicrobial resistance[7] and reduce the incidence of bacterial superinfections caused by resistant pathogens (e.g., fungi and *Enterococcus* species). Drug toxicities and expense may also be reduced by decreasing the duration of therapy.

ANTIMICROBIAL AGENTS

β-Lactam Antimicrobial Agents

Penicillin G

Penicillin G remains clinically useful for a variety of serious infections. Penicillin G potassium is acid-labile and, therefore, is not used widely as an oral agent for systemic infections. Phenoxypenicillin, penicillin VK, is more acid-stable and is the preferred oral penicillin salt formulation. Aqueous crystalline penicillin G potassium is administered parenterally (intramuscularly or intravenously). The procaine and benzathine salts are for intramuscular injection only; these preparations are less useful for infections in the ICU because relatively low serum concentrations result after drug administration.

The mechanism of action of β-lactam antimicrobial agents (penicillins, cephalosporins, monobactams, and carbapenems) is related to their ability to inhibit bacterial cell wall synthesis and in some organisms trigger lysis of the cell wall. β-Lactams bind to various intracellular proteins called penicillin-binding proteins (PBPs) and exert their effects at several stages of cell wall synthesis. The affinity and specificity of different β-lactams for different PBPs may help to explain why the various agents have differing spectrums of activity. Alterations in binding to certain PBPs have also been associated with antimicrobial resistance.

Bacteria may become resistant to the penicillins by several mechanisms. The most important mechanism is through the production of enzymes called β-lactamases. These enzymes act irreversibly on the β-lactam drug molecule itself, causing hydrolysis of the β-lactam ring. Gram-positive bacteria produce, for the most part, plasmid-mediated β-lactamases, which are secreted extracellularly (i.e., out of the bacteria) into the host infection site. Conversely, gram-negative organisms uniformly produce β-lactamases (chromosome mediated or plasmid mediated; constitutive or inducible) but concentrate these enzymes intracellularly in the periplasmic space. Other mechanisms of resistance include decreased antibiotic penetration through the outer cell wall membrane and altered PBPs, resulting in decreased antibiotic binding.

Gram-positive cocci, for the most part, have remained highly sensitive to penicillin G. The susceptible aerobic organisms include *Enterococcus* species (not *Enterococcus faecium)*, group A streptococci *(Streptococcus pyogenes)*, group B streptococci *(Streptococcus agalactiae)*, group C streptococci, viridans group streptococci, *Streptococcus bovis,* and the anaerobic gram-positive cocci, including *Peptostreptococcus* species and *Peptococcus* species. Notably, the incidence of intermediate-level or high-level penicillin resistance in *S. pneumoniae* has risen significantly in the late 1990s. *Listeria monocytogenes, Neisseria meningitidis,* and *Clostridium* species *(C. perfringens* and *C. tetani)* are also susceptible. Routine sensitivity testing may not be performed for some of these organisms because resistance is rare. However, report of *S. pneumoniae* resistance to penicillin makes screening of these organisms necessary.[8]

Most strains of *S. aureus* and *Staphylococcus epidermidis* do produce β-lactamases and are, therefore, resistant to penicillin G and ampicillin. In addition, most strains of *S. epidermidis* are methicillin-resistant (MRSE), a resistance mechanism mediated by elaboration of a unique enzyme, PBP-2A.[9] There is an increasing incidence of methicillin-resistant *S. aureus* (MRSA), such that ICU physicians should be aware of the MRSA incidence in their institutions. The susceptibility testing of cephalosporins against MRSE and MRSA may give misleading information (falsely susceptible) because standard sensitivity tests do not detect small numbers of these resistant organisms. *Therefore, no cephalosporin is recommended in the treatment of infection caused by MRSE or MRSA.*

Penicillin G is eliminated from the body primarily by renal tubular secretion and glomerular filtration. Therefore, dosage adjustments must be made in patients with significant renal insufficiency (<40 mL/min). The serum elimination half-life of penicillin is approximately 30 minutes in patients with normal renal function. Penicillin distributes widely into body fluids, except for CSF, although in patients with meningitis (inflamed meninges), penicillin enters the CSF more easily and achieves therapeutic concentrations against susceptible bacteria when high-dose penicillin is administered (a total of 12 to 20 million units per day). Intravenous aqueous crystalline penicillin G is usually administered by intermittent infusion. Moderate-to-severe infections caused by susceptible organisms are adequately treated by 1 to 3 million units every 2 to 6 hours (Table 58–1). For meningitis and endocarditis, the higher doses (a total of 12 to 20 million units per day) are usually recommended.

The major adverse reactions from penicillin G are hypersensitivity reactions. Several chemical entities have been implicated as the cause. Antigenic determinants (metabolites) of penicillin hypersensitivity are formed by in vivo hydrolysis of the β-lactam ring and are classified as major and minor determinants, depending on how frequently they are involved in hypersensitivity reactions. The major antigenic determinant, the penicilloyl metabolite, elicits an immunoglobulin E (IgE) antibody response but results in accelerated urticarial reactions and maculopapular rashes.[10] The various minor determinants elicit an IgE antibody response, which mediates most of the anaphylactic reactions. Skin testing with the single, commercially available preparation penicilloyl polylysine (Pre-Pen) does not routinely predict which patient will have the more important anaphylactic reaction. It is, therefore, inadequate and is not routinely recommended. Skin testing with extemporaneously prepared penicillin solutions is also inadequate.

Other than hypersensitivity reactions, penicillin G rarely causes toxicity. Drug accumulation in renal failure may predispose patients to generalized seizures, which are less responsive to anticonvulsant therapy. Central nervous system (CNS) toxicity may also appear as lethargy, confusion, and multifocal myoclonus. Cation intoxication may occur during high-dose penicillin therapy because of the large potassium load and also because of excessive obligate anion excretion of the penicillin molecules. In patients with renal failure, serum potassium concentration should be monitored during high-dose therapy with the potassium penicillin salt preparation; alternatively, penicillin G sodium may be specially ordered.

Clinically, penicillin G is still the single agent of choice for treatment of most streptococcal infections. Because *Enterococcus* species are uniquely "tolerant" of penicillin's action (i.e., antimicrobial action results in only a bacteriostatic effect), penicillin should be combined with gentamicin to achieve bactericidal activity for treatment of life-threatening infections such as enterococcal endocarditis and meningitis. This so-called synergistic effect achieved with penicillin and gentamicin against *Enterococcus* species is also produced by the combination of penicillin and gentamicin against viridans streptococci, a combination again used only in special circumstances (i.e., short-course therapy for endocarditis).

Ampicillin

Ampicillin, a semisynthetic derivative of penicillin, is active against most strains of bacteria sensitive to penicillin G and

TABLE 58–1. Miscellaneous Penicillins

Variable	Aqueous Penicillin G (Potassium Salt)	Ampicillin	Nafcillin
Route of elimination	Renal	Renal and biliary	Hepatic, biliary, and renal
Dose adjustment creatinine clearance threshold	<40 mL/min	<10 mL/min	No change
Adult dosage regimen	1–3 MU every 2–6 hr	1–2 g every 4–6 hr	1–2 g every 4–6 hr
Average peak concentration (dose)	10 mg/L (1 MU)	47 mg/L (2 g)	40 mg/L (1 g)
Sodium content	0.3 mEq/MU	3.0 mEq/g	2.9 mEq/g

MU = million units.

against some aerobic gram-negative bacilli. Susceptible Enterobacteriaceae include some strains of *Escherichia coli, Proteus* species, and *Salmonella* species. Ampicillin distributes throughout body tissues and fluids and is eliminated by renal and biliary mechanisms. The normal serum elimination half-life in adults is 1.1 to 1.3 hours, and dosage adjustments may be necessary only in severe renal impairment (e.g., creatinine clearance below 10 mL/min). Ampicillin cannot be detected in CSF with uninflamed meninges, but therapeutic concentrations for susceptible organisms are achieved in meningitis with large doses of drug. Dosages range from 1 to 2 g every 4 to 6 hours (see Table 58–1).

Amoxicillin, a close chemical and pharmacologic relative of ampicillin, is more acid-stable and is, therefore, more effectively absorbed from the gastrointestinal tract. Amoxicillin is available only as an oral preparation in the United States. Its spectrum of activity is identical to that of ampicillin, although it is not recommended in the treatment of infectious diarrhea because of low concentrations achieved in bile and stool. Ampicillin and amoxicillin are more likely to cause rashes than do other penicillins, but these are usually benign, macular rashes and are *unrelated* to "true penicillin allergy."

Nafcillin

The emergence of staphylococcal resistance to penicillin G made necessary the development of a class of drugs called the β-lactamase–stable penicillins. Nafcillin, methicillin, and oxacillin, also called penicillinase-resistant penicillins, are parenteral semisynthetic agents. The use of nafcillin is restricted appropriately to the treatment of suspected or documented *S. aureus* infections. Nafcillin is less active than penicillin G against the other "penicillin-sensitive" organisms, such as streptococci, and is not an acceptable alternative in the treatment of enterococcal infections. Nafcillin is excreted unchanged in the urine (30%) to a lesser extent than other penicillins. Most of the drug is metabolized in the liver or eliminated in bile. The serum elimination half-life of nafcillin is approximately 1 hour, and penetration into CSF is usually adequate for the treatment of staphylococcal meningitis. The dose ranges from 1 to 2 g every 4 to 6 hours (see Table 58–1).

Adverse reactions associated with nafcillin are similar to those observed with other penicillins. In addition, dose-related neutropenia is reported to occur with high-dose (>10 g/d), long-term (>10 days) therapy. Interstitial nephritis associated with methicillin and hepatotoxicity associated with oxacillin have somewhat reduced the clinical usefulness of these two drugs, making nafcillin the parenteral penicillinase-resistant penicillin of choice.

Antipseudomonal Penicillins

Ticarcillin, Mezlocillin, and Piperacillin

Carbenicillin, introduced in 1967, was the first β-lactam antibiotic with reliable antipseudomonal activity and represented a dramatic improvement in the prognosis of pseudomonal infections. Unfortunately, large carbenicillin dosages needed to be given (30 g/day), which meant a large sodium salt load as well. Ticarcillin has a spectrum of activity similar to that of carbenicillin but is more active by weight and is active against more strains of *Pseudomonas* species. This increased activity by weight meant that smaller dosages and, therefore, a lower salt load could be administered. The main mechanism of resistance against these drugs is inactivation by β-lactamases, although decreased cell wall permeability has also been documented. Mezlocillin and piperacillin have greater activity against gram-negative anaerobes, anaerobic and aerobic streptococci, and *Enterococcus* species compared with ticarcillin. Mezlocillin has activity that is equal to that of ticarcillin against *P. aeruginosa,* whereas piperacillin's activity is somewhat better than ticarcillin's. These three agents owe their increased activity against *Pseudomonas* species to enhanced cell wall permeability and increased binding to PBP-3 (responsible for bacterial septation).

The elimination half-life of these agents varies from approximately 1 hour for ticarcillin to 1.3 hours for both piperacillin and mezlocillin. These last two agents have an even longer half-life when larger doses are administered. These higher doses have dose-dependent rates of elimination (i.e., the higher the dose, 4 g versus 3 g, the longer the elimination half-life). Thus, higher doses (4 g) that are given less frequently (every 6 to 8 hours) are used to take advantage of this pharmacokinetic feature. The dosing schedule for ticarcillin is usually 3 g every 4 to 6 hours for a serious infection (every 4 hours for pseudomonal infections).

Because the distribution and penetration of these penicillins into CSF, even with inflamed meninges, are negligible, they are not reliable for the treatment of meningitis. The primary route of elimination for ticarcillin is the kidney, and dosage adjustment is recommended for patients when the creatinine clearance falls below 60 mL/min. Combined renal and biliary routes of elimination are important for mezlocillin (dose adjustment at below 30 mL/min) and piperacillin (dose adjustment at below 40 mL/min) (Table 58–2).

Adverse reactions include those seen with other penicillins. In addition, antipseudomonal penicillins can cause a qualitative platelet defect in which the antibiotic blocks platelet aggregation. Another problem resulting from large daily doses of these penicillins is the concomitant salt load. Each antibiotic molecule is dibasic and, if excreted, acts as an obligate anion when it is eliminated, leading to potassium wasting and hypokalemia. The large amount of sodium administered with these antibiotics may also lead to fluid retention and electrolyte imbalances.

β-Lactamase Inhibitor Combinations

Ampicillin plus Sulbactam (Unasyn), Ticarcillin plus Clavulanate (Timentin), and Piperacillin plus Tazobactam (Zosyn)

Sulbactam, clavulanate (clavulanic acid), and tazobactam are unique compounds that irreversibly bind to and inactivate β-lactamase enzymes. When combined with ampicillin, ticarcil-

TABLE 58–2. Extended-Spectrum Antipseudomonal Penicillins

Variable	Ticarcillin	Mezlocillin	Piperacillin
Route of elimination	Renal	Renal and biliary	Renal and biliary
Dose adjustment creatinine clearance threshold	<60 mL/min	<30 mL/min	<40 mL/min
Adult dosage regimen	3 g every 4–6 hr	2–4 g every 6 hr	4 g every 6 hr
Average peak concentration (dose)	218 mg/L (3 g)	217 mg/L (3 g)	227 mg/L (4 g)
Sodium content	5.2–6.5 mEq/g	1.75–1.85 mEq/g	1.85 mEq/g

lin, and piperacillin, respectively, they prevent destruction by β-lactamases and have increased our utilization of these "older" drugs. These combination drugs are active against previously susceptible organisms but have an expanded spectrum of activity, which notably includes *S. aureus* (but not MRSA) and *Bacteroides fragilis*. Some aerobic gram-negative bacilli are also included in the expanded spectrum, although the chromosome-mediated β-lactamases found in *Citrobacter* species, *Enterobacter* species, indole-positive *Proteus* species, *Providencia* species, and *Serratia* species may not be uniformly inhibited.

The development of ampicillin plus sulbactam became of interest because β-lactamase enzymes elaborated from gram-positive and gram-negative bacteria had diminished the usefulness of ampicillin monotherapy. Sulbactam, when combined with ampicillin in the commercially available 2:1 ratio, inhibits important plasmid-mediated β-lactamases, thus increasing the spectrum of activity of ampicillin to include β-lactamase-producing strains of *Neisseria* species (mostly *N. gonorrhoeae), Moraxella catarrhalis, S. aureus, E. coli, Proteus* species, *Klebsiella* species, *Acinetobacter* species, and *Bacteroides* species, including *B. fragilis*. Organisms that are ampicillin susceptible remain so with the combination and include *Enterococcus* species, aerobic and anaerobic streptococci, and *L. monocytogenes*. *P. aeruginosa* and other nosocomial gram-negative bacilli remain resistant to ampicillin plus sulbactam, as do MRSA and MRSE. Because the spectrum of activity is so broad for this combination agent, it has been effective monotherapy for many community-acquired mixed infections, such as pelvic inflammatory disease and other intra-abdominal infections as well as in polymicrobial skin and soft-tissue infections, including diabetes-related infections.

The addition of sulbactam to ampicillin does not change the pharmacokinetic profile of ampicillin. Usual ampicillin/sulbactam dosages range from 1.5 to 3.0 g every 6 hours. Both drugs have a serum elimination half-life of approximately 1 hour; renal elimination is the primary route, and dose adjustment is recommended when the creatinine clearance falls below 30 mL/min (Table 58–3).

Biliary excretion of sulbactam appears to be less than that of ampicillin, which may have an impact on the adequate treatment of hepatobiliary infections caused by β-lactamase–producing organisms. Although ampicillin and sulbactam do penetrate into CSF in patients with meningitis, there is a lack of adequate clinical efficacy studies for this indication. The toxicity profile of ampicillin plus sulbactam is essentially the same as that observed for ampicillin; the most common adverse reactions are diarrhea, skin reactions, and nausea and vomiting.

The addition of clavulanic acid to ticarcillin has broadened its spectrum of activity in the same way as that of sulbactam to ampicillin. Organisms that were susceptible to ticarcillin remain so with the combination; however, *S. aureus* and *B. fragilis* (major producers of β-lactamases) are now also susceptible. Elimination is not altered with the clavulanic acid–ticarcillin product. Ticarcillin, 3 g, is combined with clavulanic acid, 100 mg, in the commercially available preparation. Dosages of 3.1 g every 4 to 6 hours are recommended, and dose adjustment is necessary when the creatinine clearance falls below 60 mL/min. Piperacillin-tazobactam is given in a dose of 3.375 g every 6 hours (3 g of piperacillin with 375 mg of tazobactam). Dose adjustments are recommended for a creatinine clearance below 40 mL/min (see Table 58–3). Adverse reactions to these β-lactamase inhibitor combinations are similar to those observed with the individual antibiotics; however, the incidence of diarrhea is reported to be higher.

First-Generation and Second-Generation Cephalosporins

Cefazolin

Cephalosporium is a fungus that produces cephalosporin C. Most of the presently available cephalosporin antibiotics are semisynthetic derivatives of this compound. The cephalosporin nucleus is similar to that of the penicillins with the same β-lactam ring, and their mechanism of action is similar. Cefazolin is a first-generation cephalosporin that has proved to be safe and effective against many pathogenic aerobic gram-positive cocci and gram-negative bacilli. It became a popular substitute in patients with a history of penicillin allergy. It has been reported that approximately 5% to 10% of patients who demonstrate allergy to penicillin also appear to experience a cross-reaction to the cephalosporins. Although this may be an acceptable risk in patients reporting a "non-life-threatening" reaction from penicillin (e.g., hives, rash), *it is not an acceptable risk* in the patient who gives a history of immediate reactions or anaphylaxis. There is no skin test that will definitively predict which penicillin-allergic patient will experience a cephalosporin cross-reaction. Therefore, when antimicrobial therapy is indicated in a patient with a history of penicillin

TABLE 58–3. β-Lactamase Inhibitor Combination Antimicrobials

Variable	Ampicillin plus Sulbactam	Ticarcillin plus Clavulanate	Piperacillin plus Tazobactam
Route of elimination	Renal and biliary	Renal	Renal and biliary
Dose adjustment creatinine clearance threshold	<30 mL/min	<60 mL/min	<40 mL/min
Adult dosage regimen	1.5–3 g every 6 hr	3.1 g every 4–6 hr	3.375 g every 6 hr
Average peak concentration (dose)	47 mg/L (2 g)	325 mg/L (3.1 g)	250 mg/L (3.375 g)
Sodium content	5 mEq/1.5 g	4.75 mEq/g	N/A

anaphylaxis, most authorities recommend not using a β-lactam antibiotic when possible.[11]

Gram-positive cocci that are cefazolin-resistant (and also other cephalosporins) include *Enterococcus* species, MRSE, and MRSA, even though in vitro tests may sometimes give contrary data. The aerobic gram-negative bacilli that are usually cefazolin sensitive include *E. coli, Klebsiella* species, and *Proteus mirabilis*, although nosocomial strains are often resistant. Oral gram-positive anaerobic streptococci are sensitive, but gram-negative anaerobes are resistant (e.g., *Bacteroides* species).

Cefazolin offers advantages over cephalothin, which was the first available parenteral cephalosporin. It has the same spectrum of activity, although in vitro cephalothin may be more stable against β-lactamase enzymes. However, cefazolin is used more often because of its favorable pharmacokinetic profile, with a more prolonged serum half-life (0.5 hour for cephalothin versus 1.5 to 2 hours for cefazolin), thus allowing less frequent administration. Cefazolin is also better tolerated as an intramuscular injection. Since cefazolin is excreted primarily by glomerular filtration, dosage adjustments must be made in patients with decreased renal function (creatinine clearance below 55 mL/min). The therapeutic dose range is 1 to 2 g every 6 to 8 hours. Only small quantities of the drug are excreted into the bile, and unreliable drug concentrations are found in CSF, even with inflamed meninges (Table 58–4).

Local reactions (e.g., phlebitis) related to intravenous administration of cefazolin are the most frequently observed adverse effects. Hypersensitivity (allergic) reactions may occur but to a lesser degree than with penicillins. They may appear as anaphylaxis, immediate reaction with shortness of breath and urticarial rash, serum sickness, a positive Coombs' reaction with or without hemolytic anemia, morbilliform rash, fever, pruritus, and eosinophilia. There is a significant rate of cross-reaction in patients allergic to penicillin who will then have an allergic reaction to cephalosporins. This is why a complete allergy history is important, in that if anaphylaxis is reported from the penicillin, cephalosporins should be avoided when possible.[11]

Cefuroxime

Cefuroxime is active against cefazolin-sensitive organisms, but it is also active against *H. influenzae*, even β-lactamase–producing strains. Nosocomial strains of *E. coli, Proteus* species, and *Klebsiella* species may be more sensitive to cefuroxime than to cefazolin. However, *S. aureus* is less susceptible. Drug distribution occurs widely throughout the body, including penetration into CSF. Cefuroxime, however, has been shown to be less effective than ceftriaxone in the treatment of *H. influenzae* meningitis and is, therefore, not routinely recommended.[12]

The main route of elimination is the kidneys, and dose adjustment is recommended at a creatinine clearance below 20 mL/min. A serum elimination half-life of approximately 80 minutes allows dosing of 750 mg or 1.5 g every 8 hours. Most patients who have an infection require only the 750-mg dose. Side effects of cefuroxime include those described for cefazolin.

Cefoxitin and Cefotetan

Cefoxitin and cefotetan are predominantly active against the same bacteria as cefuroxime is. Important additions to their spectrum of activity are anaerobic gram-negative organisms, especially *B. fragilis*, as well as *N. gonorrhoeae* and aerobic gram-negative bacilli, such as *Serratia* species. A unique characteristic of cefoxitin is its increased resistance to hydrolysis by various β-lactamases. Cefoxitin and cefotetan, however, are less active against some gram-positive organisms, including staphylococci and streptococci.

These drugs are eliminated mainly by the kidneys; therefore, dosage adjustments must be made in patients with decreased renal function (<50 mL/min and <30 mL/min, respectively). A peak serum concentration of 75 mg/L is achieved after a 1-g intravenous dose of cefoxitin, and the elimination half-life is approximately 45 minutes, compared with cefotetan with a half-life of 3 to 4.6 hours and a peak serum concentration of 140 mg/L. Dosage regimens for cefoxitin in the treatment of infections (as opposed to lower doses for surgical prophylaxis) range from 1 to 2 g every 4 to 8 hours; the regimen for cefotetan is 1 to 2 g every 12 hours (see Table 58–4).

Potential adverse reactions from these agents are similar to those from other cephalosporins, although cefotetan can cause a "disulfiram reaction" as well as bleeding from inhibition of the synthesis of vitamin K–dependent coagulation factors. These reactions have rarely been reported at the currently recommended dosing range of 1 to 2 g every 12 hours.

Third-Generation and Fourth-Generation Cephalosporins

The third-generation cephalosporins represented a significant advance in spectrum of activity and pharmacokinetics over older cephalosporins. Important features include the following:

- Greater β-lactamase stability
- Increased affinity for gram-negative bacilli PBP-1 and PBP-3
- Longer serum elimination half-lives
- Better penetration into CSF

These compounds show enhanced activity against *H. influenzae* and *Neisseria* species as well as most strains of Enterobacteriaceae, including nosocomial strains. Like other cephalosporins, they are not active against *Enterococcus* species, *L. monocytogenes*, MRSA, and MRSE and have variable activity against *B. fragilis* and *P. aeruginosa*. The chromosome-mediated β-lactamases of aerobic gram-negative bacilli hydrolyze most third-generation cephalosporins to some degree. In general, higher, more predictable CSF concentrations, greater than 10% of the simultaneous serum concentrations, are achievable with these cephalosporins, making them useful for the treatment of meningitis caused by susceptible organisms.

Cefotaxime

Cefotaxime and its desacetylcefotaxime metabolite are active against most Enterobacteriaceae except for *Enterobacter*

TABLE 58–4. First-Generation and Second-Generation Cephalosporins

Variable	Cefazolin	Cefuroxime	Cefoxitin	Cefotetan
Route of elimination	Renal	Renal	Renal	Renal and biliary
Dose adjustment creatinine clearance threshold	<55 mL/min	<20 mL/min	<50 mL/min	<30 mL/min
Adult dosage regimen	1–2 g every 6–8 hr	0.75–1.5 g every 8 hr	1–2 g every 4–8 hr	1–2 g every 12 hr
Average peak concentration (dose)	140 mg/L (1 g)	50 mg/L (750 mg)	75 mg/L (1 g)	140 mg/L (1 g)
Sodium content	2 mEq/g	2.4 mEq/g	2.3 mEq/g	3.5 mEq/g

species. The metabolite may be less active by weight than is cefotaxime. Some evidence suggests that cefotaxime and desacetylcefotaxime may act synergistically against some bacteria. A significant inoculum effect is seen with the chromosome-mediated β-lactamases of *Serratia* species, indicating that for certain infections, a high concentration of β-lactamase enzymes may destroy the drug's activity. Unfortunately, cefotaxime is readily hydrolyzed by the plasmid-mediated β-lactamases of *Pseudomonas* species and *B. fragilis*. The gram-positive activity of cefotaxime is comparable to that of cefuroxime. Cefotaxime has been useful in the treatment of serious infections (e.g., meningitis) due to penicillin-resistant *S. pneumoniae.*

The pharmacokinetics of both cefotaxime parent compound and its active metabolite should be considered when one is making decisions concerning dosing. Cefotaxime is eliminated by liver metabolism to desacetylcefotaxime as well as by the kidneys and bile. After a 2-g intravenous dose of cefotaxime, serum levels of 80 to 90 mg/L are achieved, but cefotaxime has a relatively short half-life of 0.9 to 1.7 hours. The desacetyl metabolite, on the other hand, is eliminated more slowly (half-life of 1.4 to 1.9 hours), mainly by further liver metabolism and renal excretion. In renal failure, the clearance of cefotaxime and metabolite is minimally affected, and thus dosage adjustments do not need to be made, except in cases of severe insufficiency (<20 mL/min). The "usual" dosing schedule varies widely for cefotaxime, from 1 to 2 g every 4 to 8 hours. Complications of cefotaxime therapy are similar to those of other β-lactam antibiotics (Table 58–5).

Ceftizoxime

The spectrum of antimicrobial activity for ceftizoxime is similar to that of cefotaxime. The drug is hydrolyzed by chromosomal β-lactamase of *Enterobacter* species and is not usually active against *P. aeruginosa*. A potential difference between this third-generation cephalosporin and the others is its improved activity against *B. fragilis*, which is comparable to that of cefoxitin and cefotetan. The gram-positive spectrum of activity and patterns of resistance are similar to those of cefotaxime.

Approximately 85% to 88% of the drug is excreted by the kidneys, with a serum elimination half-life ranging between 1.4 and 1.9 hours, thus allowing a dosing interval of 6 to 8 hours. Ceftizoxime is concentrated in the bile in the absence of biliary obstruction. A normal dosage of 1 to 2 g every 8 hours must be adjusted for patients with renal failure (see Table 58–5).

Ceftazidime

The aerobic gram-negative spectrum for ceftazidime is exceptionally broad. Ceftazidime appears to be the most β-lactamase stable of the third-generation cephalosporins. It alone is stable with respect to the chromosomal β-lactamase of *Serratia* species and is the most stable against the β-lactamase of *Pseudomonas* species. Ceftazidime is also the most active against *Proteus* species because of its stability with respect to its chromosomal β-lactamases. However, ceftazidime is readily hydrolyzed by β-lactamases from *B. fragilis* and, therefore, should not be used as a single agent when infection with this organism is suspected. Gram-positive activity is adequate for nonenterococcal streptococci but is marginal for most nafcillin-sensitive *S. aureus*.

A peak serum concentration of 200 mg/L is obtained from a 2-g intravenous dose with a serum elimination half-life of approximately 1.4 to 2 hours. The dosing range is 1 to 2 g every 6 to 12 hours. Ceftazidime is cleared predominantly by the kidneys and some in the bile; thus, in renal insufficiency, dosage adjustments should be made (see Table 58–5).

Ceftazidime has been used as a single agent and in combination with an aminoglycoside to treat a variety of infections including pneumonia, osteomyelitis, sepsis, abscesses, cellulitis, urinary tract infections, and especially infection caused by *P. aeruginosa*, including those infections complicating cystic fibrosis. Febrile neutropenic cancer patients (white blood cell count < 500/mm^3) are often empirically given ceftazidime monotherapy.[13] Adverse reactions reported with ceftazidime include those ordinarily found with other β-lactam antibiotics.

Ceftriaxone

Ceftriaxone has a number of unique properties. The drug is active against gram-negative bacteria and is stable against their chromosomal and plasmid-mediated β-lactamases. The gram-negative antibacterial spectrum for ceftriaxone is similar to that of cefotaxime and ceftizoxime, except for *P. mirabilis* and *Morganella morganii*, which are more sensitive to ceftriaxone, and it is less active against *Pseudomonas* species. The gram-positive antibacterial spectrum is also similar to that of cefotaxime. Like ceftazidime, ceftriaxone is not reliable for coverage of *B. fragilis*.

Ceftriaxone's pharmacokinetic profile is unique among the third-generation cephalosporins, with both high serum drug concentrations and a long serum elimination half-life. This is in part due to the high protein binding of this agent. A 1-g intravenous dose yields a peak serum concentration of approximately 150 mg/L, and the serum elimination half-life ranges from 5.4 to 10.9 hours. Thus, ceftriaxone may be given once every 24 hours for most infections. Penetration into the CSF is impressive in patients with inflamed meninges with concentrations of 7% to 11% of the simultaneous serum levels. Dosing in meningitis should be more frequent (1 to 2 g every 12 hours) to maintain an adequate CSF drug concentration. Sixty per cent of drug is excreted by the kidneys, and 40% is metabolized by the liver or excreted in bile; therefore, dosage adjustments are not necessary in patients with renal insufficiency (see Table 58–5).

Adverse reactions reported are similar to those of other β-lactam agents. In addition, ceftriaxone has been reported to cause biliary sludging, stone formation, and biliary obstruction thought to be due to drug chelation with calcium.[14]

TABLE 58–5. Third-Generation and Fourth-Generation Cephalosporins

Variable	Cefotaxime	Ceftizoxime	Ceftazidime	Ceftriaxone	Cefepime
Route of elimination	Hepatic, renal, and biliary	Renal	Renal	Renal and biliary	Renal
Dose adjustment creatinine clearance threshold	<20 mL/min	<80 mL/min	<50 mL/min	No change	<60 mL/min
Adult dosage regimen	1–2 g every 4–8 hr	1–2 g every 8 hr	1–2 g every 6–12 hr	1–2 g every 12–24 hr	1–2 g every 12 hr
Average peak concentration (dose)	45 mg/L (1 g)	85 mg/L (1 g)	70 mg/L (1 g)	150 mg/L (1 g)	80 mg/L (1 g)
Sodium content	2.2 mEq/g	2.6 mEq/g	2.3 mEq/g	3.6 mEq/g	N/A

Cefepime

Cefepime is a fourth-generation cephalosporin with a broader spectrum of activity against both gram-positive and gram-negative aerobic bacteria than the third-generation cephalosporins. Cefepime is active against all *Streptococcus* species. Cefepime is highly active against *S. pneumoniae* (MIC ≤ 0.05 mg/L). However, it demonstrates variable activity against intermediate penicillin-resistant (MIC 0.1 to 1.0 mg/L) and high-level penicillin-resistant (MIC > 2.0 mg/L) strains. Cefepime demonstrates activity greater than that of ceftazidime and similar to that of cefotaxime against most *Streptococcus* species. Methicillin-sensitive *S. aureus* and *S. epidermidis* are susceptible to cefepime. Like all other cephalosporins, cefepime does not have clinically significant inhibitory activity against methicillin-resistant *S. epidermidis* and *S. aureus* and has no activity against *Enterococcus* species. Cefepime has greater inhibitory activity than ceftazidime and cefotaxime against the Enterobacteriaceae family.

Unlike third-generation cephalosporins, cefepime is stable to hydrolysis by many plasmid-mediated and chromosome-mediated β-lactamases and is a poor inducer of type 1 β-lactamases. The drug thus demonstrates excellent in vitro activity against cefotaxime-resistant and ceftazidime-resistant isolates of *Enterobacter aerogenes, Enterobacter cloacae,* and *Citrobacter freundii.* Cefepime has activity similar to that of ceftazidime against *P. aeruginosa, Stenotrophomonas maltophilia,* and *Acinetobacter calcoaceticus* and activity similar to that of ceftazidime and cefotaxime against *H. influenzae*. Compared with ceftizoxime, cefepime has minimal activity against *B. fragilis* species.

The average peak serum drug concentration after a 1-g intravenous infusion is approximately 80 mg/L. Cefepime has a half-life of 1.3 to 2.3 hours and is primarily excreted by the kidney. Dosage adjustment is recommended in patients with renal failure with a threshold creatinine clearance of 60 mL/min (see Table 58–5). The usual dose ranges from 1 to 2 g given every 12 hours, but it can be increased to a maximum of 6 g/day in severely ill patients. Cefepime is well tolerated (e.g., side effects in fewer than 5% of patients); headache is the most common adverse event, followed by rash, nausea, diarrhea, vomiting, and constipation.[15]

Monobactam and Carbapenem Agents

Aztreonam

Aztreonam is a synthetic monobactam antibiotic that is truly a "narrow-spectrum" antimicrobial agent with activity only against aerobic gram-negative bacilli (e.g., Enterobacteriaceae). Although stable with respect to most of the plasmid-mediated and chromosome-mediated β-lactamases produced by these organisms, an inoculum effect (see cefotaxime for explanation of inoculum effect) is seen with *Serratia marcescens, Enterobacter* species, *Klebsiella* species, and *Pseudomonas* species. This compound is hydrolyzed by the β-lactamase of *B. fragilis. H. influenzae, Neisseria* species, many Enterobacteriaceae (*E. coli, E. aerogenes, Klebsiella* species, *Proteus* species), *Salmonella*, and *Shigella* have low MICs, ranging from 0.05 to 0.25 mg/L. The nosocomial gram-negative bacteria such as *E. cloacae, C. freundii*, and *Serratia* species have higher MICs from 2 to 4 mg/L, whereas *Acinetobacter* species have an MIC of 6 mg/L and *P. aeruginosa* has an MIC of 8 mg/L or higher.

The average peak serum aztreonam concentration after a 1-g intravenous infusion ranges from 90 to 164 mg/L. The half-life is reported to be 1.3 to 2.2 hours, with the kidney being the primary excretion route. Dose adjustment is warranted for a creatinine clearance less than 30 mL/min (Table 58–6). The usual dose ranges from 1 to 2 g every 8 hours. Significant CSF penetration has been reported in patients with inflamed meninges, although this drug is not routinely recommended in meningitis. Aztreonam penetrates into other tissues, fluids, and urine at concentrations many times the MIC of most sensitive pathogens.

Adverse reactions to aztreonam are similar to those reported for other β-lactam antimicrobials. Aztreonam appears to display low immunologic cross-reactivity with other β-lactam antibiotics and may be useful in patients with non-life-threatening allergies to β-lactams.[16] Its safety in patients with a history of anaphylaxis due to β-lactam antibiotics is not clear. A potential benefit of aztreonam's narrow spectrum of activity (i.e., not active against anaerobic bacteria or gram-positive aerobes) is that it may have minimal effect on normal gastrointestinal flora, thus decreasing the incidence of diarrhea and superinfections.

Imipenem-Cilastatin and Meropenem

Imipenem and meropenem are parenteral carbapenems that are highly resistant to degradation by the β-lactamase enzymes produced by gram-negative and gram-positive organisms, particularly those that are plasmid-mediated. These broad-spectrum drugs are potent against community-acquired gram-positive organisms as well as the more resistant nosocomial gram-negative bacilli. Meropenem demonstrated less inhibitory activity against methicillin-susceptible *S. aureus* than that of imipenem. Both are inactive against MRSA and have unreliable activity against *Enterococcus* species, *Mycoplasma pneumoniae, Chlamydia* species, *Legionella* species, and *L. monocytogenes.*

Imipenem and meropenem inhibited the growth of all strains of *B. fragilis* and *Fusobacterium* species. Meropenem is more active than imipenem in vitro against Enterobacteriaceae, *H. influenzae,* and *N. gonorrhoeae* and had an MIC of 4 mg/L for 90% of *P. aeruginosa* isolates.

An intravenous infusion of 500 mg of imipenem results in a peak serum concentration of 33 mg/L and has a serum elimination half-life of approximately 0.85 to 1.3 hours. This serum concentration is relatively low; however, imipenem is a potent drug, and most Enterobacteriaceae have low MICs (see Table 58–6). A 1-g intravenous infusion of meropenem resulted in a peak serum concentration ranging between 53 and 61 mg/L. Both imipenem and meropenem are primarily excreted by the kidneys (70% to 80% and 54% to 79%, respectively). Meropenem, like imipenem, requires dose adjustment in patients with renal impairment (creatinine clearance, <50 mL/min for meropenem, <70 mL/min for imipenem).

High urine concentrations are not observed after imipenem administration because of significant drug hydrolysis (metabolism) by proximal tubule brush border dehydropeptidase enzymes. Unfortunately, the resulting metabolites are nephrotoxic. Therefore, the currently marketed imipenem product also contains cilastatin, a dipeptidase inhibitor. The addition of cilastatin results in higher urine imipenem concentrations and decreased formation of the potentially nephrotoxic metabolites. Imipenem dosages must be adjusted in renal failure because drug accumulation may lead to neurotoxicity (e.g., seizures). Meropenem is stable to inactivation by human renal dehydropeptidase and unlike imipenem does not require the additional administration of cilastatin.

CSF penetration of these agents is excellent (20% to 30%); however, because of the potential for CNS toxicity, imipenem is used rarely in the treatment of meningitis. Meropenem has excellent CSF penetration, and unlike imipenem, it does not appear, to date, to increase the risk of seizures.

Adverse reactions for imipenem and meropenem are similar to those reported for other β-lactam antimicrobials (i.e., hypersensitivity reactions). However, because of the broad spec-

TABLE 58–6. Monobactam and Carbapenem Agents

Variable	Aztreonam	Imipenem	Meropenem
Route of elimination	Renal and hepatic	Renal and metabolic?	Renal
Dose adjustment creatinine clearance threshold	<30 mL/min	<70 mL/min	<50 mL/min
Adult dosage regimen	1–2 g every 8 hr	0.5–1.0 g every 6–8 hr	1.0–2.0 g every 8 hr
Average peak concentration (dose)	90–164 mg/L (1 g)	33 mg/L (500 mg)	53–61 mg/L (1 g)
Sodium content	None	2.8–3.2 mEq/g	3.92 mEq/g

trum of activity, superinfections are reported to occur with enterococci and fungi. Mild renal failure has been seen along with elevated liver enzymes for imipenem. Of some concern is the association of imipenem with seizures. The reported incidence is less than 1% and occurs in patients with renal failure or with preexisting seizure disorders.[17] Imipenem and meropenem may cause allergic reactions in patients known to have a history of penicillin or cephalosporin allergy. Thus, imipenem and meropenem should be avoided if possible in patients with a history of anaphylaxis from other β-lactams.[18]

Aminoglycoside Antibiotics

The most commonly used parenteral aminoglycoside antibiotics are gentamicin, tobramycin, and amikacin. Streptomycin's usefulness has declined for the treatment of bacterial infections but has increased in the therapy for infections with *Mycobacterium tuberculosis*, especially for multidrug-resistant strains.

Aminoglycosides are rapidly bactericidal against aerobic gram-negative bacilli, although their exact mechanism of action is not completely understood. Drug easily passes by aqueous porin channels through the outer cell wall membranes of gram-negative bacilli, entering into the periplasmic space. Aminoglycosides cannot easily pass through the thicker outer cell wall membrane of gram-positive bacteria and thus have higher MICs to these organisms. Drug molecules are then transported across the cytoplasmic membrane, which appears to be an active process closely linked to electron transport, oxidative phosphorylation, and cellular respiration. This transport mechanism is impaired under conditions of low pH, high osmolality, and reduced oxygen tension. Thus, in certain clinical settings, aminoglycoside antimicrobials may not be maximally effective (e.g., acidic fluids, such as ascites; anaerobic environments, such as poorly perfused tissue or abscesses). Aminoglycosides are known to bind irreversibly to the 30S ribosomal subunit and to alter protein synthesis.

There are three well-described mechanisms by which bacteria develop resistance to the aminoglycosides. First, ribosomal mutation alters the site of aminoglycoside attachment. This phenomenon has been rare except for some strains of enterococci. Second, bacteria may become resistant to aminoglycosides by preventing penetration of the drug through the outer bacterial cell membrane or by preventing active transport through the cytoplasmic membrane. Anaerobic organisms are thought to be resistant because of the latter mechanism (the absence of the oxygen-dependent active transport system). Finally, the most important mechanism of bacterial resistance for aerobic gram-negative bacilli is plasmid-mediated enzyme production, which occurs within the periplasmic space.

Aminoglycosides have exposed hydroxyl and amino groups that are the potential sites of enzymatic modification. These enzymes inactivate aminoglycosides by adenylation, acetylation, or phosphorylation. Amikacin is the aminoglycoside most stable to these enzymatic effects because it has fewer sites for enzymatic attack. The antibacterial activity of aminoglycosides is directed primarily against aerobic gram-negative bacilli. Most are active against strains of Enterobacteriaceae, such as *E. coli*, *Klebsiella* species, *Enterobacter* species, *Proteus* species, and *Serratia* species. Strains of *P. aeruginosa*, *Citrobacter* species, *Acinetobacter* species, and *Providencia stuartii* are usually more resistant. When in vitro testing is performed, tobramycin appears to be the aminoglycoside most active against the various *Pseudomonas* species, including *P. aeruginosa*. Other pseudomonal strains, such as *Burkholderia cepacia*, are more resistant to all aminoglycosides. Their synergistic activity with penicillins or vancomycin against aerobic gram-positive bacteria is primarily limited to viridans streptococci, *Enterococcus* species, and *Staphylococcus* species.

Aminoglycoside concentrations are generally low in various infected secretions and tissues, such as respiratory secretions, pleural fluid, CSF, and aqueous humor. These low concentrations are predictable because of the simultaneously low serum concentrations, the high molecular polarity, and the relatively short serum elimination half-life. However, high drug concentrations are found in the proximal tubular cells of the renal cortex, which is thought to correlate with the nephrotoxic potential of aminoglycosides.[19]

Traditionally, it has been thought that careful drug dose titration was needed for aminoglycosides because of their narrow therapeutic window. An aminoglycoside loading dose was usually given to achieve the desired peak serum concentration for Enterobacteriaceae of 5 to 10 mg/L for gentamicin and tobramycin and 15 to 30 mg/L for amikacin (Table 58–7). Maintenance doses and dosing intervals are adjusted on the basis of the patient's estimated creatinine clearance because glomerular filtration is the major route of elimination. Empirical maintenance doses for gentamicin and tobramycin range from 1.2 to 1.5 mg/kg every 8 hours and for amikacin are 7.5 mg/kg every 8 to 12 hours. Clinical scenarios when dosage reductions may be necessary include advanced age, decreased renal blood flow, intrinsic renal disease, and azotemia. Higher drug dosages may be required in neonates, in burn patients, with serious pseudomonal infections, or in patients with cystic fibrosis.

Serum drug concentration monitoring is necessary for all patients with life-threatening gram-negative infections.[20] Peak serum concentrations (30 minutes after a 30-minute infusion) are measured to ensure the adequacy of antimicrobial activity against a specific pathogen. Therefore, the desired peak concentration may be different among patients, ranging from 5 to 10 mg/L. Measuring the trough serum concentration (just before receiving a dose) allows assessment of whether drug accumulation is occurring, which is a risk factor for nephrotoxicity and ototoxicity. Most clinicians adjust dosing to achieve a trough concentration of less than 2 mg/L. The frequency of monitoring of serum drug concentrations will vary among patients (usually once weekly throughout therapy) but should be more frequent in patients with changing renal function or in those with more resistant pathogens (see Table 58–7).

Life-threatening adverse reactions from aminoglycosides are rare but may include neuromuscular blockade, similar to that seen with *d*-tubocurarine, which may result in muscle weakness and respiratory depression with apnea, especially with administration by rapid intravenous bolus dosing. Patients at increased risk include those who have myasthenia gravis and severe hypocalcemia and patients who have been concurrently receiving a neuromuscular blocking agent. All aminoglycosides can cause irreversible or reversible damage to the hair cells of the inner ear. Auditory and vestibular toxicity has been reported with equal frequency for amikacin, tobramycin, and gentamicin, whereas streptomycin appears to cause predominantly vestibular toxicity. The ototoxic effects of aminoglycosides may be potentiated by concurrent administration of other ototoxic agents (e.g., loop diuretics). It is postulated that all persons receiving an aminoglycoside will incur some damage to the hair cells, an effect that will accumulate over time with subsequent use of aminoglycosides, other ototoxic drugs, or auditory insults.

Nephrotoxicity is the most common complication of aminoglycoside therapy. It appears to be most common in older, debilitated patients and in those with preexisting renal disease. In addition, ICU patients with hypotension or contracted intravascular volume from volume depletion, diuretic therapy, or contrast dyes are at specific risk. Nephrotoxicity is also incurred in patients who have had previous aminoglycoside therapy or who are receiving concurrent drugs known to be nephrotoxic (e.g., amphotericin). Nephrotoxicity is usually mild and reversible. Because aminoglycosides are useful in the treatment of serious infections, their use should not be avoided just because of the potential risk of nephrotoxicity. Close monitoring of serum drug concentrations will help to minimize this toxicity.

A new strategy for dosing aminoglycosides is being used by many clinicians. A single large daily dose of aminoglycosides or "once-daily" aminoglycosides may be more effective than (or at least as effective as) and less toxic than the traditional divided daily doses.[21-23] This new regimen takes advantage of the concentration-dependent killing power of aminoglycosides (i.e., the higher the drug serum concentration, the faster the rate of bacterial killing).[22] This new dosing regimen additionally provides a prolonged period at the end of the dosing interval when the serum drug concentration is low (or undetectable by assay methods employed by clinical laboratories). This method of drug administration allows the aminoglycoside molecules the time they need to efflux out of the end-organ cells (hair cells of the ear and proximal tubular cells of the kidney), which results in reduced ototoxicity and nephrotoxicity. A recommended empirical dose in adults with serious aerobic gram-negative infections and normal renal function is 5 to 7 mg/kg given once daily for gentamicin and tobramycin and 20 mg/kg per day for amikacin. The threshold creatinine clearance in these patients when dose reduction (or a more prolonged dosing interval) is necessary is 60 mL/min for this once-daily regimen (see Table 58–7). It is still advisable to monitor serum drug concentrations when the once-daily regimen for treatment of infection is continued for more than a few days, especially in patients with high creatinine clearance estimates (i.e., >100 mL/min), when the dosing interval may need to be shortened to every 12 hours.

Anti-anaerobe Antimicrobial Agents

Clindamycin

Clindamycin, a semisynthetic derivative of lincomycin, is a bacteriostatic antimicrobial agent. The exact mechanism by which clindamycin inhibits bacterial protein synthesis is not known, but the inhibition is eventually accomplished by binding to the 50S ribosomal subunit. Aerobic gram-positive organisms other than enterococci are susceptible, whereas aerobic gram-negative bacilli are completely resistant. Clindamycin is effective against most clinically important anaerobes (gram-positive cocci and gram-negative bacilli), including *B. fragilis*, although rates of resistance for *B. fragilis* of 15% and higher have been reported in specific institutions.

Clindamycin is available as oral and intravenous-intramuscular formulations. After a 600-mg intravenous infusion, the peak serum concentration achieved is approximately 10 mg/L, many times the MICs of susceptible organisms. The drug is well distributed into most body tissues and fluids but does not penetrate the blood-brain barrier to any reliable extent. Therefore, this drug would not be appropriate for the treatment of meningitis. In addition, it exerts only a bacteriostatic effect. Adequate parenteral therapy ranges from 600 to 900 mg every 6 to 12 hours. Clindamycin is predominantly metabolized by the liver to inactive compounds (90%), but a small amount of unchanged drug is also eliminated by the kidneys. Thus, no adjustments need to be made for renal insufficiency, but they may be necessary in severe liver disease (e.g., cirrhosis). The normal serum elimination half-life is 2 to 4 hours (Table 58–8).

Pseudomembranous colitis (diarrhea, abdominal pain, fever, mucus and blood in the stool), a highly publicized complication of clindamycin therapy, is due to the production of exotoxin by resistant strains of *Clostridium difficile*. Treatment consists of first discontinuing clindamycin and then administering oral metronidazole or oral vancomycin if symptoms persist.[24] This adverse effect has also been associated with most other antibiotics and is not specific for clindamycin. Other reported adverse effects from clindamycin include nausea, vomiting, diarrhea, rash, local thrombophlebitis, and increased liver enzymes.

Metronidazole

Metronidazole is a nitroimidazole drug that is highly active against obligate anaerobes, but it does not have clinically significant activity against facultative anaerobic and aerobic organisms. Its mechanism of action has not been fully eluci-

TABLE 58–7. Aminoglycosides

Variable	Gentamicin	Tobramycin	Amikacin
Route of elimination	Renal	Renal	Renal
Traditional target peak concentration for Enterobacteriaceae	5-10 mg/L	5-10 mg/L	15-30 mg/L
Traditional target trough concentration for Enterobacteriaceae	<2.0 mg/L	<2.0 mg/L	5-10 mg/L
Traditional dosage regimen for Enterobacteriaceae	1.2-1.5 mg/kg every 8 hr	1.2-1.5 mg/kg every 8 hr	7.5 mg/kg every 8-12 hr
Dose adjustment creatinine clearance threshold for "once-daily" regimen	<60 mL/min	<60 mL/min	<60 mL/min
"Once-daily" regimen (only for *select* adult patients)	5-7 mg/kg every 24 hr	5-7 mg/kg every 24 hr	20 mg/kg every 24 hr

TABLE 58–8. Antianaerobe Antimicrobials

Variable	Clindamycin	Metronidazole
Route of elimination	Hepatic	Hepatic and renal
Dose adjustment creatinine clearance threshold	Adjustment in hepatic cirrhosis	Adjustment in hepatic cirrhosis only
Adult dosage regimen	600 or 900 mg every 6–12 hr	500 or 750 mg every 8–12 hr
Average peak concentration (dose)	10 mg/L (600 mg)	26 mg/L (7.5 mg/kg)

dated but probably has to do with its nitro group being reduced within anaerobes by low-redox-potential electron transport proteins. It is also effective in the treatment of trichomoniasis, amebiasis, and giardiasis.

Metronidazole is a rapidly bactericidal agent that is active against gram-negative anaerobic bacilli such as the various *Bacteroides* species, including *B. fragilis*. Gram-positive bacilli, such as *Clostridium* species, are nearly all sensitive as well. Unfortunately, anaerobic gram-positive cocci are less susceptible (*Peptococcus* and *Peptostreptococcus*) but are inhibited, whereas other anaerobic streptococci are resistant. Until recently, acquired resistance to metronidazole was not described; however, resistant *B. fragilis* isolates and treatment failures of trichomonal infections have now been reported.

The peak serum concentration achieved after a 7.5 mg/kg intravenous dose of metronidazole is approximately 26 mg/L, and the serum elimination half-life is 6 to 8 hours (see Table 58–8). Usual dosing varies widely depending on the site and severity of infection. The most frequently administered dose of metronidazole for bacterial infections is 500 mg because it is available in a premixed minibag. Higher dosages (7.5 mg/kg) may be necessary in large patients or for the treatment of CNS infections. A dosing interval of every 8 to 12 hours should be used because this agent has a long half-life. Most of an intravenous dose of metronidazole is metabolized by the liver to inactive metabolites, which are then eliminated by the kidney. No dosage adjustments need be made in renal failure. However, with significant hepatic dysfunction, therapy should be monitored for toxicities and dosage reductions should be made. Metronidazole penetrates well into body tissues and fluids, including penetration into CSF, in which concentrations have been reported to be 43% of simultaneous serum concentrations in patients with meningitis.

Adverse reactions specific to metronidazole have been reported to include metallic taste, anorexia, and nausea. The urine may turn dark or reddish brown, causing some unnecessary concern. Neurologic side effects include peripheral neuropathy, manifesting as tingling and paresthesias, as well as CNS effects including vertigo, seizures, and ataxia. A disulfiram-like reaction may also occur during concurrent drug therapy with an alcohol-containing product or ingestion of alcoholic beverages. Symptoms of a disulfiram reaction are hypotension, nausea, flushing, and tachycardia. Metronidazole may be responsible for clinically significant drug-drug interactions with warfarin. Metronidazole is thought to decrease warfarin metabolic clearance (increasing the half-life) and thus increase or prolong warfarin's hypoprothrombinemic effects.

Quinolones

Ciprofloxacin, Ofloxacin, and Levofloxacin

These are the currently available parenteral quinolone antimicrobials. The bactericidal mechanism of action for these agents is unique and involves inhibition of deoxyribonucleic acid (DNA) gyrase (topoisomerase) enzymes. Their spectrum of activity is similar; most aerobic gram-negative bacilli are susceptible, including *P. aeruginosa*. All anaerobic organisms are resistant, whereas aerobic gram-positive cocci have variable susceptibility. Because these drugs are used specifically for respiratory tract infections, great care should be taken to rule out the possibility of *S. pneumoniae* infection before one of these three quinolones is selected; these antimicrobials are not recommended, even though in vitro test results may show this organism to be marginally susceptible.[25] *S. aureus* and *S. epidermidis*, including MRSA and MRSE, have been susceptible. Unfortunately, the emergence of resistance occurs rapidly in patients who receive quinolones as monotherapy for severe infections from previously susceptible MRSA and MRSE.

With regard to most gram-positive bacteria, quinolones have a "narrow therapeutic window"; that is, the achievable (nontoxic) peak concentrations are close to the MICs of the organisms. However, the uncontrolled use of ciprofloxacin has quickly promoted the rapid emergence of ciprofloxacin resistance both for *S. aureus* and for *P. aeruginosa* (with cross-resistance conferred to other quinolones).[26] The addition of rifampin to a ciprofloxacin regimen is believed to help prevent this emergence of resistance. Quinolones also have activity against atypical organisms, including *Chlamydia* species and *Legionella* species, as well as various strains of *Mycobacterium*, including *M. tuberculosis*. Levofloxacin is the L-isomer of ofloxacin and has demonstrated an antibacterial activity twice that of ofloxacin.

Ciprofloxacin is eliminated by the kidneys and by liver metabolism, whereas ofloxacin and levofloxacin are mostly excreted by the kidney. Their approximate serum elimination half-lives are 3 to 5 hours, 4 to 8 hours, and 6 to 8 hours, respectively. Drug accumulation occurs to a significant extent in renal insufficiency; thus, dosage adjustment is necessary when creatinine clearance falls below 30 mL/min (Table 58–9). Drug distribution occurs widely throughout body tissues and fluids, with concentrations in many fluids exceeding serum drug concentrations. Penetration into CSF (11% to 46%) is reported to occur in patients with meningitis. However, because these drugs have a narrow therapeutic window, they are not routinely recommended in the treatment of meningitis.

Dosing recommendations for ciprofloxacin and ofloxacin are 200 to 400 mg every 12 hours; however, every 8 hours has been used in severe infections or with *P. aeruginosa* infections. The dose recommended for levofloxacin is 250 to 500 mg every 24 hours. Ciprofloxacin has the best microbiologic activity against *P. aeruginosa*. Levofloxacin has excellent in vitro activity against common community-acquired organisms; in vitro, it demonstrates lower MICs compared with ofloxacin; in addition, it has pharmacokinetic advantages resulting in once-daily dosing for most infections.

Quinolone dose amounts are somewhat limited by adverse reactions that occur more commonly when serum drug concentrations exceed 6.0 mg/L because of the risks of CNS toxicities. Headache and restlessness as well as seizures and psychosis have been reported in 1% to 2% of patients. Other adverse reactions include gastrointestinal side effects, rash, arthralgias, and increased liver enzymes. The arthropathy observed in children is severe enough that the drugs are contraindicated except in life-threatening infections (e.g., resistant pseudomonal infection in cystic fibrosis patients). A clinically significant drug-drug interaction is reported with ciprofloxacin

TABLE 58–9. Quinolones

Variable	Ciprofloxacin	Ofloxacin	Levofloxacin	Trovafloxacin
Route of elimination	Renal and hepatic	Renal	Renal	Hepatic, biliary, and renal
Dose adjustment creatinine clearance threshold	≤30 mL/min	≤50 mL/min	<50 mL/min	No adjustment in renal insufficiency (adjustment in hepatic cirrhosis)
Adult dosage regimen	200–400 mg every 8–12 hr	200–400 mg every 12 hr	250–500 mg every 24 hr	100–300 mg every 24 hr
Average peak concentration (dose)	4 mg/L (400 mg)	4 mg/L (400 mg)	5.7 mg/L (500 mg)	3.1 mg/L (200 mg)

and warfarin, which results in increased prothrombin time and possible bleeding.[27, 28]

Trovafloxacin

Trovafloxacin is a fluoroquinolone that is a broad-spectrum antibacterial agent with activity against many gram-positive, gram-negative, and anaerobic bacteria. Trovafloxacin has activity against *Streptococcus* and *Staphylococcus* species; it has activity similar to that of ciprofloxacin against *H. influenzae* and *M. catarrhalis* and similar or less activity against Enterobacteriaceae and *P. aeruginosa. N. gonorrhoeae, Chlamydia trachomatis, M. pneumoniae, Legionella pneumoniae,* and *B. fragilis* are organisms for which trovafloxacin has demonstrated inhibitory activity.

Trovafloxacin is 75% bound by plasma proteins and is rapidly distributed into most target tissues. A 200-mg oral dose of trovafloxacin is conjugated (metabolism) and is 23% and 63% recovered in the urine and stool, respectively. Intravenous trovafloxacin is administered as the pro-drug alatrofloxacin. Dosing recommendations for trovafloxacin are 100 to 300 mg given once every 24 hours with no adjustments needed for renal insufficiency (see Table 58–9), but dose adjustment is required in patients with significant liver dysfunction. The adverse effect profile is similar to that of other quinolones; dizziness is the most common adverse event reported.[29]

Miscellaneous Agents

Vancomycin

In the 1950s, vancomycin was the agent of choice for penicillin-resistant staphylococcal infection; however, after the introduction of penicillinase-resistant penicillins (e.g., nafcillin) and later cephalosporins, this status was altered. When first introduced in 1956, preparations contained approximately 80% vancomycin and 20% impurities with unknown microbiologic activity and toxicity. A high incidence of adverse reactions including nephrotoxicity, ototoxicity, fever, and phlebitis was initially reported. Today, preparations are more pure and thus cause fewer reactions.

Vancomycin is a narrow-spectrum drug that exerts its bactericidal effect by irreversibly binding to the cell wall of susceptible gram-positive bacteria and inhibits cell wall synthesis. This drug has unique antimicrobial activity against MRSA and MRSE.[30] It is also active against gram-positive bacilli, streptococci, and *Enterococcus* species. However, resistance to vancomycin has increased dramatically, particularly in nosocomial strains of *E. faecium*.

Like the penicillins, vancomycin is not bactericidal against enterococci. When a bactericidal effect is necessary to treat specific infections like enterococcal endocarditis, it may be achieved with the synergistic combination of vancomycin plus an aminoglycoside (usually gentamicin). *Clostridium* species and *Corynebacterium* species are gram-positive bacilli and are usually susceptible to vancomycin; however, gram-negative aerobes and anaerobes are all resistant.

Vancomycin is not absorbed from the gastrointestinal tract; thus, the oral route of administration has been reserved for the treatment of pseudomembranous colitis. Intramuscular administration of vancomycin is contraindicated because of adverse reactions (i.e., pain, tenderness, or muscle necrosis). Intravenous drug should be administered only during a period of at least 60 minutes because rapid infusions may cause the "red neck" or "red man" syndrome with nausea, chills, hypotension, urticaria, and macular rashes.[31] Also, thrombophlebitis can be minimized by administering vancomycin in at least 200 mL of fluid and by reducing the infusion rate.

There is conflict in the literature regarding appropriate monitoring of peak and trough vancomycin concentrations.[32] The peak concentration should be monitored in patients if there is concern about drug accumulation (e.g., in acute renal failure) and should be kept below 60 mg/L to minimize ototoxicity. The trough concentration should be monitored for efficacy and should remain in the range of 5 to 10 mg/L (above the MIC of the pathogen being treated). To achieve these desired steady-state serum concentrations quickly, an initial loading dose of approximately 17.5 mg/kg (using total body weight in the calculation) is recommended. The maintenance dose regimen is based on the patient's renal function. Patients with normal renal function may require a total daily maintenance dose of 10 to 15 mg/kg given every 12 hours. Adjustments for decreased renal function can be estimated by monitoring serum drug concentrations (Table 58–10). Vancomycin penetrates well into various body fluids except the CSF. Penetration of vancomycin, even in patients with meningitis, may be erratic, and thus intrathecal drug administration may be required. Vancomycin is not significantly concentrated, specifically in the bile or aqueous humor.

Erythromycin

Erythromycin belongs to the macrolide class and demonstrates bacteriostatic activity against gram-positive organisms such as streptococci. Other macrolide antibiotics have a broader spectrum of activity. *S. aureus* may also be susceptible, but resistance may develop to erythromycin during therapy. Acquired resistance may be exclusively erythromycin resistance or may also include resistance to clindamycin. Erythromycin is also clinically useful for the treatment of infections resulting from *Treponema pallidum* (syphilis) as well as atypical organisms such as *M. pneumoniae, Chlamydia* species, and *Legionella pneumophila*. Erythromycin inhibits bacterial protein synthesis by reversibly binding to the 50S ribosomal subunit. Erythromycin more rapidly penetrates bacterial cell walls in the non-ionic drug state (pK_a 8.8) and thus is most effective in an alkaline environment; activity decreases in acidic surroundings, such as in an abscess or in urine.

Erythromycin lactobionate and erythromycin gluceptate are the available intravenous preparations. Intramuscular injection is avoided because of pain. These two erythromycin esters are inactive, and in vivo hydrolysis must occur to free active erythromycin base. Peak serum concentrations after 500 mg of the lactobionate salt are approximately 10 mg/L. Erythromycin is mostly metabolized by the liver but is eliminated to a

TABLE 58–10. Miscellaneous Agents

Variable	Vancomycin	Erythromycin (Lactobionate)	Trimethoprim-Sulfamethoxazole
Route of elimination	Renal	Hepatic and biliary	Hepatic and renal
Dose adjustment creatinine clearance threshold	≤30 mL/min	No adjustment	<50 mL/min
Adult dosage regimen	10–15 mg/kg every 12 hr (adjust for volume of distribution and renal function)	0.5–1.0 g every 6 hr	5–15 mg/kg/day divided every 6–12 hr (of trimethoprim component) and 15 mg/kg/day for PCP specifically
Average peak concentration (dose)	20 mg/L (1 g)	10 mg/L (500 mg)	9.0/105 mg/L (160/800 mg)

PCP = *Pneumocystis carinii* pneumonia.

small degree as unchanged drug in the urine and bile. The serum elimination half-life of erythromycin ranges from 0.8 to 3.0 hours. Erythromycin penetrates fairly well into body tissues and fluids, except CSF, even in patients with inflamed meninges. For serious infections, 0.5 to 1.0 g should be administered every 6 hours (see Table 58–10).

Thrombophlebitis associated with drug infusion is a frequent problem; however, severe adverse reactions (i.e., tinnitus and transient deafness) have rarely been reported with intravenous administration. The oral formulations have all been known to cause an exceptionally high incidence of gastrointestinal side effects, and erythromycin estolate has been associated with reversible jaundice.

Trimethoprim-Sulfamethoxazole

Trimethoprim-sulfamethoxazole (TMP-SMZ) is a broad-spectrum combination product available as a fixed 1:5 ratio. Both drugs are folate synthesis antagonists and act synergistically to inhibit or kill susceptible bacteria. Aerobic streptococci and staphylococci are susceptible, as are aerobic enteric gram-negative bacilli. *Enterococcus* species and anaerobic gram-negative bacilli, such as *B. fragilis*, are resistant. Most strains of *P. aeruginosa* are resistant; however, *Stenotrophomonas maltophilia*, a multiresistant nosocomial pathogen, is usually susceptible.

TMP-SMZ is well absorbed from the gastrointestinal tract and is also tolerated after intravenous infusion (except for some thrombophlebitis). Therapeutic ratio concentrations of 1:20 are observed in most body fluids, which appears to be an optimal ratio for synergistic activity. Both drugs are metabolized by the liver and are eliminated by the kidney. Serum elimination half-lives are 8 to 11 hours and 10 to 13 hours, respectively. Drug accumulation as well as toxic metabolite accumulation can occur in severe renal insufficiency, such that dosage reduction is recommended. TMP-SMZ does penetrate into CSF (40% to 50%) in meningitis; however, this drug is mostly bacteriostatic and is, therefore, not acceptable for the routine treatment of bacterial meningitis.

Drug dosages are calculated as total daily dose of TMP component, 5 to 15 mg/kg/day; serious gram-negative bacillary infections require the higher dosage, and 15 mg/kg/day is recommended for *Pneumocystis carinii* pneumonia. The total daily dose is divided every 6 to 12 hours so that no more than 400 mg of TMP is given at one time because of toxicities. The dose-limiting toxicity of intravenous TMP-SMZ is usually gastrointestinal intolerance (see Table 58–10).

Other adverse reactions to TMP-SMZ include, most notably, hypersensitivity reactions such as rash, fever, epidermal necrolysis, and Stevens-Johnson syndrome. Hematologic toxicities (anemia, neutropenia, and thrombocytopenia) may be treatable with concomitant administration of folinic acid. Hepatitis and CNS reactions are also reported, but most patients tolerate this drug well. The incidence, however, of adverse reactions has been reported to be extremely high in patients with acquired immunodeficiency syndrome (AIDS). The mechanism of this increased risk of toxicity is not well understood but is thought to be related to altered drug metabolism. A clinically significant drug-drug interaction is reported with TMP-SMZ and warfarin, which results in increased prothrombin time and possible bleeding.

COMMONLY ENCOUNTERED INTENSIVE CARE UNIT INFECTIONS

Pneumonias

Community-Acquired Pneumonias

Community-acquired pneumonias in relatively healthy people rarely result in illness severe enough to require ICU admission. In persons with significant underlying medical disease (alcoholism, malignant neoplasms, malnutrition, diabetes, sickle cell disease, congestive heart failure, or chronic obstructive lung disease), however, pneumonia can have severe consequences.

S. pneumoniae is a common cause of adult pneumonia in the community, whereas pneumonia in younger adults and children may be caused by viruses, *Mycoplasma pneumoniae*, *Chlamydia pneumoniae*, and *Legionella* species as well. Community-acquired bacterial pneumonia is usually characterized by respiratory symptoms, cough, shortness of breath, purulent sputum, and occasionally pleuritic chest pain. The diagnosis depends on signs of infection, such as fever, chills, leukocytosis, and abnormal findings on chest radiography. The sputum Gram stain should show polymorphonuclear cells and a predominant microorganism with rare epithelial cells. The diagnosis may be confirmed by sputum culture and occasionally by positive blood cultures.

Because *S. pneumoniae* is the most common cause of community-acquired pneumonia, a penicillin is the treatment of choice in most cases. However, because the respiratory tract of patients with chronic obstructive pulmonary disease or of smokers is frequently colonized by *H. influenzae*, multiple organisms may be seen on sputum Gram stain or culture. Consequently, the true pneumonic pathogen may not be distinguishable, so that empirical treatment with ampicillin, which covers both organisms, may be initiated. Unfortunately, in many communities, the prevalence of penicillin-resistant pneumococcus (MIC > 0.1 mg/L) and β-lactamase–producing *H. influenzae* may be significant; thus, third-generation cephalosporins serve as alternatives.

Atypical pneumonias must be treated with erythromycin; in the rare case of *Klebsiella pneumoniae*, which is reported to occur in older, debilitated, and alcoholic patients, an extended-spectrum penicillin or cephalosporin plus gentamicin should be added. When aspiration is believed to be a contributing factor in the pathogenesis of pneumonia, oral anaerobe coverage including *Bacteroides* species must be added. This can be achieved by administration of clindamycin, cefoxitin, or β-lactamase inhibitor combination agents. *P. carinii* pneumonia must always be considered in a patient with human immunodeficiency virus (HIV) infection and is treated with TMP-SMZ.

Hospital-Acquired Pneumonias

Hospitalized patients, especially those with endotracheal tubes or tracheostomies undergoing mechanical ventilation, are at increased risk for pneumonia. Hospital-acquired pneumonia develops in five to 10 patients per 1000 hospital admissions and has a mortality rate of 20% to 50%.[33] These pneumonias are most commonly caused by aerobic gram-negative bacilli including *K. pneumoniae, Proteus* species, *Serratia marcescens, E. coli, Enterobacter cloacae*, and *P. aeruginosa*. In addition, *S. aureus* is reported to be responsible for some nosocomial pneumonias and appears to be more common in patients on ventilators. Other organisms, such as anaerobes and fungi, are infrequently responsible for nosocomial pneumonias. Fungal pneumonia may especially occur in immunocompromised patients (e.g., transplant recipients) or in patients who have been taking broad-spectrum antibiotics for prolonged periods.

The gram-negative bacilli encountered in nosocomial pneumonias may be resistant to many standard antibiotics such as ampicillin, cefazolin, gentamicin, and TMP-SMZ. Consequently, the extended-spectrum penicillins, penicillin and β-lactamase inhibitor combinations, or third-generation cephalosporins are required. If the extended-spectrum penicillins are selected, the addition of gentamicin or tobramycin is recommended because of the lack of stability in the former against some β-lactamases and for synergy. Because of the high morbidity and mortality associated with gram-negative pneumonia, particularly *Pseudomonas* pneumonia, synergistic combination therapy is frequently recommended, especially in the septic patient. The specific choice of drugs may depend on the unique sensitivity pattern of an ICU.

If gram-positive cocci are seen on the Gram stain, *S. aureus* must be considered a potential pathogen. Vancomycin is the drug of choice for MRSA, which may be common in the ICU setting. As previously described, cephalosporins should not be considered a substitute for vancomycin in the treatment of infections resulting from MRSA or MRSE, even if in vitro test results show the organism to be susceptible.

Urinary Tract Infections

Community-acquired urinary tract infections rarely cause urosepsis unless there is a structural abnormality of the genitourinary tract. Patients may occasionally appear with sepsis from pyelonephritis and have normal genitourinary anatomy; however, usually the patients may have ignored symptoms for prolonged periods or are debilitated. In hospitalized patients, instrumentation or the presence of a urinary catheter predisposes the patient to urinary tract infection.

Community-acquired urinary tract infections are usually caused by enteric gram-negative bacilli, which are increasingly resistant to ampicillin and TMP-SMZ but remain susceptible to most first-generation cephalosporins, quinolones, and aminoglycosides. The organisms causing hospital-acquired urinary tract infections are those nosocomial gram-negative bacilli that colonize the patient and may include more resistant organisms, such as *P. aeruginosa*. Vancomycin-resistant *Enterococcus* has also been described as a urinary tract pathogen, and thus susceptibility testing for *Enterococcus* under these circumstances of nosocomial infection may be recommended. Extended-spectrum penicillins, third-generation cephalosporins, or β-lactamase inhibitor combination agents may be used empirically as monotherapy. Alternatively, in cases of septic shock, the addition of an aminoglycoside is recommended. There are theoretical reasons why aminoglycosides may be less effective when they are used alone in the treatment of complicated urosepsis. Within renal abscess cavities or the renal medulla, aminoglycosides may be relatively inactive owing to low pH or anaerobic environment.

Urosepsis should be suspected in the patient who has signs of systemic infection (e.g., chills, fever, leukocytosis, and hypotension) in addition to flank pain and lower abdominal pain. Confirmatory laboratory findings include pyuria with or without WBC casts and Gram stain of urine with many bacteria of a single morphologic type. The diagnosis is confirmed by isolation of the infecting organism from blood or urine cultures.

Treatment must include assessment (with sonogram, intravenous pyelogram, or computed tomographic scan) and removal of the urinary tract obstruction because antibiotic therapy alone is not adequate. Nevertheless, antibiotics are essential for treating bacteria in the bloodstream and the genitourinary tract.

Meningitis

Patients with bacterial meningitis may be admitted to an ICU because of lethargy, obtundation and need for airway protection, treatment of seizures and hemodynamic instability, or other systemic consequences of infection (see Chapter 60). Cure of meningitis requires the administration of adequate doses of bactericidal antibiotics. Early institution of adjuvant steroid therapy (dexamethasone) has been shown to reduce morbidity in *H. influenzae* meningitis in children.[34] *S. pneumoniae* is the most common cause of community-acquired meningitis in adults, followed by *Neisseria meningitidis, Listeria monocytogenes*, and rarely *H. influenzae*. Postneurosurgical meningitis may be caused by a variety of pathogens, including nosocomial gram-negative bacilli as well as staphylococci.

The diagnosis should be suspected on the basis of the appropriate clinical syndrome but is established by Gram stain and culture of CSF and blood. When a primary site of pneumococcal or *H. influenzae* infection, such as the lung or sinus, is identified, meningitis is probably due to the same organism. Meningitis associated with CSF leaks or rhinorrhea (post-traumatic) is usually caused by *S. pneumoniae*. The CSF findings characteristic of bacterial meningitis are high WBC count with a predominance of polymorphonuclear cells, a decrease in CSF glucose concentration (less than 50% that of serum glucose), and elevated protein level. If the infecting agent is not isolated by cultures, a bacteriologic diagnosis can sometimes be made by detection of the capsular antigens in the CSF or blood by counterimmunoelectrophoresis.

Thus, empirical therapy for bacterial meningitis in most patients consists of ampicillin or high-dose penicillin G (20 million units per day adjusted for renal insufficiency). Ceftriaxone has replaced this regimen in regions where penicillin-resistant *S. pneumoniae* has been found. Patients at risk for enteric gram-negative bacilli or *H. influenzae* infection should receive ceftriaxone. Because no one cephalosporin is active against *L. monocytogenes*, penicillin or ampicillin should be included in a patient's regimen if this organism is suspected (i.e., the elderly, immunocompromised patients, neonates).

Vancomycin should be administered if MRSA or MRSE is suspected in postneurosurgical patients. It is recommended for the treatment of pneumococcal meningitis because of the rising incidence of penicillin-resistant *S. pneumoniae*.

Adjuvant therapy with dexamethasone is important for children with *H. influenzae* meningitis. Its use in adults is controversial, but it may be used to reduce cerebral edema in patients with increased intracranial pressure or CNS dysfunction, such as an altered mental status or a focal neurologic deficit.

Endocarditis and Endovascular Infections

Endocarditis is an infection in which the host defense has limited ability to control bacterial growth. Vegetations on heart valves are avascular masses of fibrin, platelets, and bacteria that do not contain WBCs. Consequently, the choice of bactericidal antibiotics is crucial for cure.

Left-sided native valve endocarditis may have a wide variety of presentations that require ICU admission or complicate a patient's hospital course. Patients may be admitted with a stroke, cerebral hemorrhage, bowel infarct, myocardial infarction, limb ischemia, or renal failure. These manifestations are consequences of systemic embolization or congestive heart failure resulting from valve dysfunction. Patients with right-sided endocarditis (particularly common in intravenous drug users) may have septic pulmonary emboli.

The diagnosis is based on recognition of the appropriate clinical syndrome, as described previously, and documentation of sustained bacteremia. At least two blood specimens obtained 30 minutes apart should be positive for a single organism; an echocardiogram may be helpful if valve vegetations are seen, but it is normal in a significant number of the cases.

Left-sided native valve endocarditis is most commonly caused by streptococci (viridans streptococci, 30% to 40%; *Enterococcus* species, 5% to 18%; others, 15% to 25%); staphylococci cause 20% to 35% of cases mostly from *S. aureus*, with few cases of *S. epidermidis*; and aerobic gram-negative bacilli cause 1.5% to 13%. Intravenous drug users are particularly susceptible to *S. aureus* infection of the tricuspid valve.

Empirical therapy for community-acquired native valve endocarditis must include an antimicrobial agent that is active against viridans streptococci; therefore, penicillin plus gentamicin (low-dose 1 mg/kg every 8 hours) is administered. Coverage for *S. aureus* with nafcillin may be added, depending on the clinical presentation and risk factors. Vancomycin should be reserved for MRSA and for patients who have anaphylactic hypersensitivity reactions to β-lactams. The duration of therapy is usually 4 to 6 weeks. The addition of low-dose gentamicin is to achieve synergy with nafcillin against *S. aureus* and may decrease the duration of fever and positive blood cultures. The synergistic combination of nafcillin and gentamicin may also decrease the total duration of therapy in selected patients with right-sided endocarditis from 4 weeks to 2 weeks.

For streptococcal (nonenterococcal) endocarditis, penicillin plus gentamicin is the regimen of choice. The addition of gentamicin may decrease the required treatment duration to 2 weeks, whereas enterococcal endocarditis treatment is always prolonged (4 to 6 weeks) because it is difficult to cure. Therapy must continue with the combination of penicillin or ampicillin (or vancomycin in penicillin-allergic patients) plus gentamicin because the penicillin alone is not bactericidal against the enterococcus. Gentamicin is the aminoglycoside of choice; however, increasing resistance to gentamicin is being observed, such that all enterococcal strains causing endocarditis should have susceptibility testing.

Prosthetic valve endocarditis is usually subdivided into two stages: *early* (<2 months after operation) and *late*. Staging of this infection is important because the bacteriology is different in these two groups.

In early prosthetic valve endocarditis, *S. epidermidis* (27%), *S. aureus* (20%), aerobic gram-negative bacilli (19%), and fungi (13%) are the most common organisms. Empirical therapy must include vancomycin for MRSA and MRSE as well as an aminoglycoside. If *S. epidermidis* is isolated, rifampin, 300 mg orally twice a day, may be added. Unfortunately, valve replacement is frequently required, with streptococcal infections having the best prognosis.

Late endocarditis is usually caused by streptococci, but staphylococci and gram-negative bacilli are not uncommon. Therefore, empirical therapy for late prosthetic valve endocarditis must include coverage for all of these organisms.

References

1. Polk HC Jr: Factors influencing the risk of infection after trauma. Am J Surg 1993; 165(Suppl 2A):2S.
2. Bates DW, Sands K, Miller E, et al: Predicting bacteremia in patients with sepsis syndrome. J Infect Dis 1997; 176:1538.
3. Fridkin SK, Jarvis WR: Epidemiology of nosocomial fungal infections. Clin Microbiol Rev 1996; 9:499.
4. MedAxon: The American Hospital Formulary Service: Drug Information plus First DataBank CD ROM Product. McEvoy GK (Ed). Bethesda, Md, American Society of Health System Pharmacists, July 1998.
5. Wilson ML: General principles of specimen collection and transport. Clin Infect Dis 1996; 22:766.
6. Chambers HF, Sande MA: Antimicrobial agents: General considerations. *In:* Goodman and Gilman's The Pharmacological Basis of Therapeutics. 9th ed. Molinoff PB, Ruddon RW (Eds). New York, McGraw-Hill, 1996, p 1029.
7. Shlaes DM, Gerding DN, John JF JR, et al: Society for Healthcare Epidemiology of America and Infectious Diseases Society of America joint committee on the prevention of antimicrobial resistance: Guidelines for the prevention of antimicrobial resistance in hospitals. Clin Infect Dis 1997; 25:584.
8. Appelbaum PC: Antimicrobial resistance in *Streptococcus pneumoniae*: An overview. Clin Infect Dis 1992; 15:77.
9. Chambers HF: Methicillin resistance and staphylococci: Molecular and biochemical basis and clinical implications. Clin Microbiol Rev 1997; 10:781.
10. Padovan E, Bauer T, Tongio MM, et al: Penicilloyl peptides are recognized as T cell antigenic determinants in penicillin allergy. Eur J Immunol 1997; 27:1303.
11. Mandell GL, Petri WA Jr: Antimicrobial agents: Penicillins, cephalosporins, and other beta-lactam antibiotics. *In:* Goodman and Gilman's The Pharmacological Basis of Therapeutics. 9th ed. Molinoff PB, Ruddon RW (Eds). New York, McGraw-Hill, 1996, p 1088.
12. Lebel MH, Hoyt MJ, McCracken GH Jr: Comparative efficacy of ceftriaxone and cefuroxime for treatment of bacterial meningitis. J Pediatr 1989; 114:1049.
13. Pizzo PA, Hathorn JW, Hiemenz J, et al: A randomized trial comparing ceftazidime alone with combination antibiotic therapy in cancer patients with fever and neutropenia. N Engl J Med 1986; 315:552.
14. Park HZ, Lee SP, Schy AL: Ceftriaxone-associated gallbladder sludge. Gastroenterology 1991; 100:1665.
15. Barradell LB, Bryson HM: Cefepime: A review of its antibacterial activity, pharmacokinetic properties and therapeutic use. Drugs 1994; 47:471.
16. Mandell GL, Petri WA Jr: Antimicrobial agents: Penicillins, cephalosporins, and other beta-lactam antibiotics. *In:* Goodman and Gilman's The Pharmacological Basis of Therapeutics. 9th ed. Molinoff PB, Ruddon RW (Eds). New York, McGraw-Hill, 1996, p 1097.
17. Pestotnik SL, Classen DC, Evans RS, et al: Prospective surveillance of imipenem/cilastatin use and associated seizures using a hospital information system. Ann Pharmacother 1993; 27:497.
18. Wiseman LR, Wagstaff AJ, Brogden RN, et al: Meropenem. A review of its antibacterial activity, pharmacokinetic properties and clinical efficacy. Drug 1995; 50:73.
19. Aronoff GR, Pottratz ST, Brier ME, et al: Aminoglycoside accumulation kinetics in rat renal parenchyma. Antimicrob Agents Chemother 1983; 23:74.
20. Watling SM, Dasta JF: Aminoglycoside dosing considerations in intensive care unit patients. Ann Pharmacother 1993; 27:351.
21. Prins JM, Buller HR, Kuiijpeer EJ, et al: Once versus thrice daily gentamicin in patients with serious infections. Lancet 1993; 341:335.
22. Kapusnik JE, Hackbarth CJ, Chambers HF, et al: Single, large, daily dosing versus intermittent dosing of tobramycin for treating experimental *Pseudomonas* pneumonia. J Infect Dis 1988; 158:7.

23. Nicolau DP, Freeman CD, Belliveau PP, et al: Experience with a once-daily aminoglycoside program administered to 2184 adult patients. Antimicrob Agents Chemother 1994; 39:650.
24. Fekety R, Shah AB: Diagnosis and treatment of *Clostridium difficile* colitis. JAMA 1993; 269:71.
25. Lee BL, Padula AM, Kimbrough RC, et al: Infectious complications with respiratory pathogens despite ciprofloxacin therapy. N Engl J Med 1991; 325:520.
26. Ball P: Emergent resistance to ciprofloxacin amongst *Pseudomonas aeruginosa* and *Staphylococcus aureus*. Clinical significance and therapeutic approaches. J Antimicrob Chemother 1990; 26(Suppl F):165.
27. Marchbanks CR: Drug-drug interactions with fluoroquinolones. Pharmacotherapy 1993; 13:23S.
28. Fuchs PC, Barry AL, Brown SD, et al: Prevalence of resistance to three fluoroquinolones: Assessment of levofloxacin disk test error rates and surrogate predictors of levofloxacin susceptibility. Antimicrob Agents Chemother 1996; 40:1633.
29. Haria M, Lamb HM: Trovafloxacin. Drugs 1997; 54:435.
30. Hackbarth CJ, Chambers HF: Methicillin-resistant staphylococci: Detection methods and treatment of infections. Antimicrob Agents Chemother 1989; 33:995.
31. Newfield P, Roizen MF: Hazards of rapid administration of vancomycin. Ann Intern Med 1979; 91:581.
32. Freeman CD, Quintiliani R, Nightingale CH: Vancomycin therapeutic drug monitoring: Is it necessary? Ann Pharmacother 1993; 27:594.
33. Scheld WM, Mandell GL: Nosocomial pneumonia: Pathogenesis and recent advances in diagnosis and therapy. Rev Infect Dis 1991; 9:743S.
34. Schaad UB, Lips U, Gnehm HE, et al: Dexamethasone therapy for bacterial meningitis in children: Swiss Meningitis Study Group. Lancet 1993; 342:457.

59

Catheter Colonization and Catheter-Related Bacteremia

Scott Norwood, MD, FACS, FCCM

It is estimated that nosocomial bloodstream infections occur at a rate of 1.3 to 14.5 per 1000 hospital admissions, resulting in 62,500 deaths per year.[1] The proportion of primary bloodstream infections from nosocomial sources increased from 51% in 1981 to 71% in 1992, and at least 20% of the infections were due to intravascular devices. Primary bloodstream infection is the fourth most common nosocomial infection, preceded only by urinary tract infections, pneumonia, and surgical site infections.[2] Intravascular devices are the source of most primary bloodstream infections, and 90% of these infections are secondary to central venous catheters.[3]

Catheter-related bloodstream infection (CR-BSI) is important because it contributes to significant morbidity, prolonged hospitalization, and excess hospital costs. The incidence and risk of death from all sources of nosocomial bloodstream infections and CR-BSI have progressively increased since the mid-1980s.[2]

Although multiple studies of risk factors and preventive strategies have been published, a 1995 survey of physicians' central venous catheter practices documented a high percentage of potentially detrimental protocols and site care practices.[4] This may explain the observed increase of CR-BSI since the mid-1980s. Such practices may contribute to the dramatic increase in primary bloodstream infections identified in patients with central venous catheters.[2]

This chapter clarifies some of the commonly used terms associated with CR-BSI, discusses theories of pathogenesis, risk factors, and available diagnostic techniques, and reviews the existing data on infections associated with the most common types of vascular catheters.

DEFINITIONS

Most studies provide no consensus on precise definitions or terms for describing catheter bacterial or fungal colonization and CR-BSI, leading to diversity in the reported incidence of these problems.[5] Guidelines from the Hospital Infection Control Practices Advisory Committee (HICPAC) of the Centers for Disease Control and Prevention (CDC)[6] and a separate Roundtable Consensus Conference on short-term central venous catheter access[7] clarify some of these definitions. Although it is clear that inanimate objects do not become "infected," there is strong evidence to suggest that bacteria may be able to live and multiply on catheter surfaces, deriving nutrients from catheter polymers, the deposited glycocalyx of certain bacterial species, and other nonviable bacteria.[8] Erroneous delineations of contamination, colonization, and actual infection have led to confusion and incorrect interpretation of many clinical investigations.[9] The following definitions are derived from the current publication from HICPAC[6] and from personal communication with members of the Roundtable Consensus Conference[7]:

Device-related bloodstream infection: A bacteremia or fungemia that is the direct consequence of colonization of some aspect of the implanted device and is not related to infection at another site. The intravascular portion of the device is contaminated to sufficiently high levels that organisms have gained access to the bloodstream.[7]

Colonized catheter: A positive catheter culture result (a positive result from culture of the catheter tip or intracutaneous segment) without evidence of systemic infection. (This definition has commonly been used in earlier studies as the definition for "catheter-related infection.") Semiquantitative (rolled catheter segment) or quantitative (sonication) techniques can be used to determine whether a catheter is considered colonized ($\geq$ 15 colony-forming units [CFUs] or $\leq$ 1000 [10^3] CFUs by semiquantitative or quantitative technique, respectively). Values of less than 15 CFUs by semiquantitative culture and less than 10^3 CFUs by quantitative culture are regarded as a negative culture, a contamination, or an insignificant infection requiring no therapy.[7]

Catheter-related bloodstream infection (CR-BSI): A positive catheter culture with concomitant isolation of the same organism (species, strain, subtype) from the blood. There should be no other identifiable source of infection.[7] Subtyping is an invaluable aid in diagnosing a suspected CR-BSI, especially during periods of active surveillance. CR-BSI has often been a "diagnosis of exclusion," that is, isolation of an organism without identification of a distant site of infection and without isolation of the organism from the catheter (previously termed "suspected CR-BSI"). Diagnosing CR-BSI without obtaining the appropriate catheter culture should be avoided because a diagnosis of CR-BSI requires strict adherence to the definition stated.[7]

Infusate-related bloodstream infection: Isolation of the same organism from the infusate and from separate percutaneous peripheral blood cultures with no other identifiable source of infection.[7]

Local catheter-related infection: Growth of 15 or more CFUs from a catheter specimen by semiquantitative culture or 10^3 or more CFUs from a catheter by quantitative culture with accompanying signs of inflammation (e.g., erythema, warmth, swelling, or tenderness) at the skin exit site.[6] Local signs of inflammation do not necessarily indicate significant infection or mandate immediate catheter removal in every situation.

Septic thrombosis: A relatively rare complication occurring when a cannulated vein is thrombosed and the clot is infected with microorganisms.[7]

In addition to these definitions, other investigators have defined "exit site infection" as the presence of an obvious exudate or inflammation (erythema, tenderness, or induration) within 2 cm of the catheter exit site.[10, 11] This definition should be used with caution, however, because some catheters in place for prolonged periods may cause a local inflammatory response without the presence of bacteria. In this situation, a diagnosis of "infection" should not be made, and removal of the catheter may not be necessary. Culture of the drainage or of the skin around the insertion site may be helpful, in that a positive bacterial culture result assists in confirming the presence of an exit site infection. Cultures of the skin around the insertion site have good negative predictive value.[10, 12, 13]

PATHOGENESIS

Investigators have shown that microbial colonization and biofilm formation are universal, occurring as early as 1 day after catheter insertion.[8, 14] The presence of colonization or biofilm formation, however, does not necessarily represent the presence of infection. The final determinant whether such colonization causes clinical infection is multifactorial. A multitude of host factors, catheter composition, and the interaction between microorganisms and the catheter surface may all contribute to the pathogenesis of CR-BSI.[15] Multiple sites are incriminated as potential sources for microbial entry into an intravenous or intra-arterial delivery system (Fig. 59-1).

Four pathogenic theories for CR-BSI have been proposed. The prevailing hypothesis is that bacterial colonization and subsequent CR-BSI begin at the interface of the catheter and the skin insertion site.[10, 16] The patient's skin bacteria are the most common source of organisms causing CR-BSI.[17] Host proteins such as fibronectin rapidly coat the catheter following insertion and provide a substrate for *Staphylococcus aureus*.[10] Multiple species of *Staphylococcus epidermidis* (also referred to as coagulase-negative staphylococci) are responsible for the majority of catheter colonizations causing CR-BSI.[17, 18] These bacteria produce a glycocalyx or "slime" composed of a specific polysaccharide adhesive that mediates attachment of the bacteria to the catheter surface.[10, 19] In vitro electron microscopy identifies coagulase-negative staphylococci adherent to irregularities in catheter surfaces within 30 minutes following inoculation.[8] Microcolonies may develop within 1 hour, and heavy colonization occurs within 6 to 12 hours.[20] The glycocalyx coating can serve as a barrier against antibiotics, phagocytic neutrophils, and macrophages.[8, 20] In vitro studies also show that bacteria are able to grow on catheter surfaces even when externally supplied nutrients are absent.[8, 21, 22] This seems possible only if bacteria are capable of using catheter components or other bacterial cells as nutrient sources. Catheter surface erosion does occur, suggesting that catheter components, added antithrombogenic layers, or endogenous proteins coating the catheter surface are possible nutritional sources.

A second theory suggests that the catheter hub may be the primary source for CR-BSI.[23] Bacteria may be introduced via one or more hubs from frequent manipulations, migrating down the inner luminal surface and gaining access to the venous circulation. A study by Segura and colleagues[23] identified a 10% rate of CR-BSI associated with hub contamination. The majority of patients in this study were not ICU patients, however, and the mean duration of catheterization was longer than 2 weeks. This mode of infection is probably more commonly seen in patients with long-term catheterization.[23, 24]

One study evaluating the pathogenesis and epidemiology of pulmonary artery (PA) CR-BSI showed that approximately 17% of colonizations or CR-BSIs occurred from hub contamination.[25] However, species antibiograms and plasmid profiles of bacterial isolates confirmed that 80% of catheter colonizations and CR-BSIs still developed from skin entry sites.[25]

According to the third theory, remote infections may produce catheter seeding from bacteremia. Although this scenario is possible, hematogenous catheter seeding is probably uncommon as a source of ongoing CR-BSI.[14, 26] It has been suggested that many catheter infections from fungal and enteric organisms, such as enterococci, *Escherichia coli*, and *Klebsiella,* may infect catheters by hematogenous spread.[27] In vitro catheter experiments with gram-negative bacteria indicate that most gram-negative organisms show extensive bacterial adherence to catheter surfaces.[28] Antimicrobial-treated *Pseudomonas* species also develop a bacterial slime that is similar to that of *S. epidermidis* and is capable of coating catheter surfaces. In these in vitro experiments, antibiotics did not eliminate gram-negative bacteria from the catheters. These data substantiate the clinical impression that it is very difficult, if not impossible, to eliminate colonization of long-term central venous catheters by gram-negative organisms with the use of antibiotics alone.[28]

Infusate contamination has been implicated as a possible fourth mechanism.[29-31] Parenteral nutrition solutions[32] and lipid emulsions[33] can support bacterial and fungal growth,[26] but the present risk from infusate contamination is considered very low.

RISK FACTORS

Risk factors for catheter colonization and CR-BSI can be grouped into *patient-related* and *hospital-related* factors.[26] The following features may be considered patient-related risk factors:

- Age (i.e., <1 year or >60 years)
- Alteration of host defense mechanisms
- Severity of underlying disease
- Remote sources of infection
- Heavy bacterial skin colonization
- Changes in skin integrity from disease (psoriasis)[7] or trauma (burns)[26]

Patient-related factors usually cannot be altered but must be considered in the development of catheter maintenance protocols.

Many hospital-related factors can be altered, and prevention protocols should focus on these risks. Although the number of catheter manipulations and the experience of the individual performing the catheter insertion are considered risk factors, they commonly cannot be changed or controlled. Cutdowns should be avoided if possible because the incidence of catheter-related complications is higher than with the percutaneous technique.[34] The most common risk factors that can be altered or controlled are discussed separately.

Anatomic Site of Insertion

A number of studies strongly suggest that the internal jugular site is a risk factor.[25, 35-37] Possible explanations include the close proximity to oropharyngeal secretions, greater catheter motion from neck movement, and difficulty with maintaining a sterile occlusive dressing.[25]

The femoral site is also more likely to become heavily

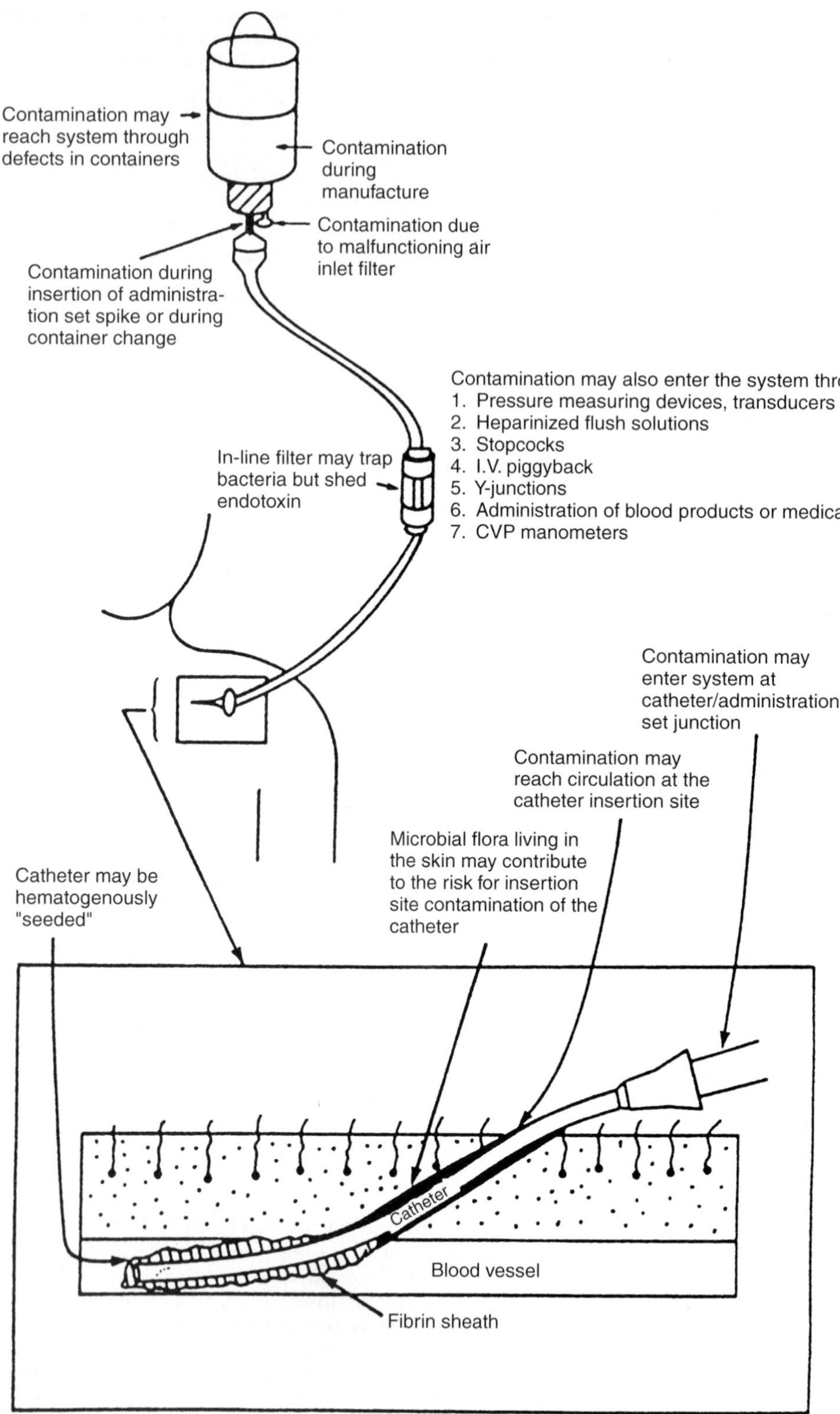
Contamination may reach system through defects in containers
Contamination during manufacture
Contamination due to malfunctioning air inlet filter
Contamination during insertion of administration set spike or during container change
Contamination may also enter the system through:
1. Pressure measuring devices, transducers
2. Heparinized flush solutions
3. Stopcocks
4. I.V. piggyback
5. Y-junctions
6. Administration of blood products or medications
7. CVP manometers
In-line filter may trap bacteria but shed endotoxin
Contamination may enter system at catheter/administration set junction
Contamination may reach circulation at the catheter insertion site
Microbial flora living in the skin may contribute to the risk for insertion site contamination of the catheter
Catheter may be hematogenously "seeded"
Catheter
Blood vessel
Fibrin sheath

Figure 59–1. Potential sites of microbial entry, colonization, and catheter-related bloodstream infection for intravenous delivery systems. (From Henderson DK: Intravascular device–associated infection: Current concepts and controversies. Infect Surg 1988; 7:366.)

colonized, with greater risk for CR-BSI. A study by Kemp and associates[37] in patients receiving total parenteral nutrition found the overall incidences of catheter colonization to be 36% for femoral, 17% for internal jugular, and 5% for subclavian sites. The incidence of CR-BSI was not provided. "Catheter infection" was defined as 15 or more CFUs in catheter tip cultures by semiquantitative culture.

Although earlier studies reported the successful use of the femoral site for long-term parenteral therapy,[38, 39] these studies incorporated a subcutaneous tunneling process into the femoral vein, by which the catheter tip was located in the inferior vena cava. Femoral vein cannulation is considered safe when the catheter site is used for no longer than 3 days and when dressing changes are made frequently.[40] Data that my colleagues and I have collected suggest that colonization of femoral sites, even with the use of chlorhexidine and silver sulfadiazine–bonded catheters, is significantly higher than colonization of subclavian or internal jugular catheter sites.[41]

Duration of Catheter Use

The incidence of significant catheter colonization and CR-BSI is directly proportional to the length of time a catheter is used. The optimal time for catheter removal, however, is unknown. The risk that any catheter may cause CR-BSI is low if the catheter is removed within 3 days. Critically ill patients usually need venous access for prolonged periods, and it is not clear when a catheter should be removed to prevent complications and yet optimize time of catheter use. Two studies suggest that central venous and pulmonary artery catheters should not have predetermined life spans.[42, 43] Another study in cancer patients provides evidence that peripheral arterial catheters should be removed within 4 to 6 days and PA catheters within 4 to 7 days of insertion.[44]

Because risk factors are multifactorial, global recommendations for catheter removal may not be applicable to all patients. Generally, catheters should be removed (1) when they are no longer needed or (2) if CR-BSI is suspected on the basis of examination of the entry site and appropriate cultures to confirm clinical suspicions (see diagnostic techniques later). Individual hospitals, individual intensive care units, and, in certain situations, individual practitioners should study their catheter infection rates to develop guidelines appropriate for their practice and environment. Rates of CR-BSIs per 1000 catheter-days may then be calculated for comparison with published standards.[6, 7] Recommendations and guidelines for catheter exchange may be used to optimize prevention of CR-BSI and to prolong site use on the basis of existing published data.

Critically Ill versus Noncritically Ill Patients

A review of all prospective studies using quantitative culture techniques reported data varying from a low risk of 0.7% per day in catheters used for total parenteral nutrition to 3.3% per day for central venous catheters.[45] Many of these studies did not distinguish critically ill patients from other hospitalized patients or septic from nonseptic patients. One study examining multiple-lumen central venous catheter infection rates in critically ill patients reported no infections or significant catheter colonization in critically ill nonseptic patients, compared with a 26.3% incidence of catheter colonization (previously termed "catheter-related infection") and a 9.6% incidence of CR-BSI in critically ill septic patients.[46] This study also suggested that the number of days a patient is hospitalized prior to catheter insertion may contribute to a higher incidence of catheter colonization leading to CR-BSI.[46]

Catheter Composition

Earlier, stiffer catheters were associated with a higher risk of thrombosis and infection.[47, 48] Although more flexible silicone and polyurethane catheters may be less thrombogenic with less in vitro bacterial adherence,[49] later studies question this premise. Gilsdorf and colleagues,[50] after studying four different intravenous catheter materials, concluded that the decreases in in vitro bacterial adherence and thrombogenicity conferred by newer catheter materials did not improve resistance to catheter colonization and subsequent bacteremia. Their study demonstrated that *S. epidermidis* was adherent to polymeric silicone (Silastic), polytetrafluoroethylene (Teflon), and two types of polyurethane. These researchers speculated that bacterial adherence to these catheter materials in the absence of nutrients probably reflects one of the following[50]:

- Organism resistance to nutritional inadequacy
- The organism's ability to use catheter materials as nutrients
- Expression of adherence factors that do not depend on either growth or nutrition

DIAGNOSTIC TECHNIQUES

Investigators still do not agree on a diagnostic standard for catheter infections. Significant problems exist with both clinical and microbiologic criteria.[2] The clinical diagnosis of a significant catheter infection that requires treatment by either catheter removal, antibiotics, or both is insensitive and nonspecific. Assuming that reasonable sterile technique during insertion and appropriate site care have been utilized, even the presence of erythema and purulent drainage is considered an unreliable indicator in some situations.[51, 52] Routine qualitative broth cultures are too sensitive for diagnosing CR-BSI,[45] giving false-positive rates up to 50%.[53] Routine swab sampling and culture of the catheter exit site in the absence of local or systemic signs of infection may also be too sensitive, although some investigators suggest that periodic semiquantitative swab sampling and culture of central venous catheter skin exit sites have a negative predictive value of at least 95%.[54]

The inaccuracy of clinical diagnosis has led to a variety of microbiologic diagnostic techniques. Because each method has advantages and disadvantages, some investigators have suggested that simply performing peripheral blood cultures and clinical evaluation may be all that is necessary and cost effective.[55] Both quantitative and semiquantitative catheter cultures require catheter removal to make the diagnosis, prompting some investigators to infer that such cultures have minimal impact on the treatment of most hospitalized patients.[56]

The inappropriate removal of both long-term and short-term central venous catheters has created a variety of catheter exit site and quantitative blood culture techniques. Heavy colonization of the skin exit site is considered the most common precursor to CR-BSI. Catheter colonization and CR-BSI are associated with positive skin site culture results, especially quantitative cultures yielding 50 or more CFUs.[57] In a study of cancer patients with long-term nontunneled Silastic catheters, surveillance, quantitative skin cultures and quantitative catheter cultures were nonspecific and insensitive in determining CR-BSI. When quantitative skin cultures were performed only in those patients with clinical findings suspicious for CR-BSI, however, this modality was highly sensitive, specific, and predictive.[58] The technique of obtaining specimens for quantitative skin cultures has been described in detail by Bjornson and colleagues.[27]

Quantitative Blood Cultures

The paired quantitative blood culture is another technique used for diagnosis of CR-BSI without the need to remove the catheter. This technique, first described by Wing and associates,[59] involves obtaining blood culture specimens simultaneously through the catheter and peripherally and then performing quantitative comparisons of the bacterial concentrations in the two specimens. In the original study, a diagnosis of CR-BSI was made if blood removed through the catheter had more CFUs per millimeter than blood taken from a peripheral vein. Since then, other studies have shown that a fivefold to 10-fold increase in the number of microorganisms grown from the catheter-drawn specimen is necessary to make the diagnosis.[60–62] Although the ideal ratio has not been determined, it is believed that the diagnosis of CR-BSI can be confirmed if the catheter blood quantitative culture colony count is fivefold higher than the peripheral blood culture colony count. If, however, the catheter blood quantitative culture value is more than 0 but the peripheral blood culture value is 0, a diagnosis of CR-BSI cannot be made[2] and the catheter may merely be colonized.

Paired quantitative blood cultures have not gained widespread clinical use because many microbiology laboratories do not perform them and because the results have not always been considered useful. Moonens and associates[63] showed that Gram's stains of blood removed through total parenteral nutrition catheters for paired quantitative blood cultures had a 100% positive predictive value and a 42% negative predictive value for diagnosing CR-BSI. Thus, Gram's stain enabled the rapid presumptive diagnosis of CR-BSI and earlier initiation of antimicrobial therapy.[63]

Catheter Culture Techniques

Various quantitative catheter culture techniques have been developed to separate true infection from colonization.[45] The semiquantitative (roll-plate) technique developed by Maki and colleagues[53] is the best-studied and most commonly utilized method for surveillance cultures. A 5-cm catheter segment (tip or intracutaneous) is rolled across a blood-agar plate in a reproducible, defined manner. In the original study, a positive result was defined as 15 or more CFUs per plate, although most of the culture-positive catheters yielded confluent growth.[53] A positive catheter segment culture result (≥ 15 CFUs, now defined as catheter colonization) resulted in a 16% risk of subsequent CR-BSI.

Members of the Roundtable Consensus Conference have recommended that both the catheter tip and the intracutaneous segment be cultured when CR-BSI is suspected.[7] One study of infections in PA catheters showed that only 61% of semiquantitative tip cultures were positive in catheters known to be infected.[64] Intracutaneous segment cultures were positive in 83%, however, and culturing both the tip and the intracutaneous segment (of the PA catheter introducer) resulted in a 94% positive rate.[64]

Other, more complex techniques have been used to distinguish true infection from colonization, including Gram's stain,[65] broth quantitative cultures,[66] and "sonicated" quantitative catheter cultures.[67] Moyer and associates[68] compared various culture techniques for diagnosis of catheter colonization and CR-BSI. They considered semiquantitative culture the best test for making the diagnosis of "catheter-related infection" but regarded paired quantitative blood culture of specimens simultaneously withdrawn through the catheter and peripherally as an acceptable approach in patients with very difficult venous access or long-term indwelling catheters.[59, 68, 69]

Culture Recommendations

One study has suggested that central venous catheters removed within 5 days of placement may not require culture because the information usually has no clinical impact on therapy.[56] Although surveillance cultures and culture of catheters used less than 5 days may not be routinely indicated, this suggestion does not imply that catheters in place for longer periods should not be cultured, especially when CR-BSI is suspected. It is generally recognized that the risk of infection is very low if catheters are placed under sterile conditions, cared for appropriately, and removed in 3 to 5 days. Therefore, routine culture of such catheters is not indicated except during surveillance periods for quality improvement purposes.

Sherertz[1] has provided the following recommendations for catheter cultures, which are both clinically useful and cost effective:

1. Unless conducting clinical research or investigating a problem, one should perform catheter cultures only when they are clinically indicated.
2. The roll-plate method for peripheral cultures should be used (semiquantitative culture method).
3. For removable central venous catheters, either the roll-plate technique (semiquantitative culture), vortex method, or sonication may be used.
4. Paired quantitative blood culture specimens obtained through the catheter and from a peripheral vein may be helpful in deciding whether to remove an implanted central venous catheter.

Although Sherertz[1] recommends that only the tip of the central venous catheter be sampled for culture, others recommend culturing both the tip and the intracutaneous segment simultaneously.[7, 64] These latter recommendations should also be used for surveillance purposes if an institution identifies a CR-BSI rate higher than 2% to 3% (number of catheter infections per 100 catheters) or a catheter colonization rate greater than 15%.[7]

A recurring question concerns the value of qualitative broth blood cultures of samples obtained through the central catheter (TTC) to diagnose CR-BSI or catheter colonization. Qualitative broth cultures have been advocated for confirming the diagnosis of bacteremia from all causes (e.g., pneumonia, abscess) but not specifically for CR-BSI.[69] This practice should be considered only when short-term catheters have been in place for relatively short periods (<4 days). Strict antiseptic preparation of the hub is mandatory to prevent false-positive culture results.[69] Catheter microbial colonization may contaminate TTC blood specimens, and unless paired quantitative blood cultures are being performed, the TTC results should not be used to diagnose CR-BSI. Generally, qualitative TTC cultures should be avoided unless the physician knows precisely how the specimens are obtained and how long the short-term catheter has been in place. Qualitative TTC cultures are indicated only if it is impossible to obtain blood culture specimens from peripheral venipuncture.

CATHETER AND SITE MAINTENANCE

Skin preparation prior to insertion and appropriate site maintenance are crucial factors in preventing CR-BSI. Long-term maintenance of catheters and insertion sites has been studied extensively, including the type and frequency of dressing changes, intravenous tubing changes, skin antiseptics, topical ointments, and guide-wire exchange to diagnose or prevent infection. Great care should be taken in preparing the site for catheter insertion, including the use of careful antiseptic skin preparation and large, sterile drapes. Ideally, sterile gowns, gloves, surgical head covers, and masks are also used during nonurgent situations when time permits.

Antiseptics, Ointments, and Dressing Materials

A study assessing the efficacy of cutaneous antiseptics evaluated 668 catheterizations randomly grouped for skin preparation with 10% povidone-iodine, 70% alcohol, or 2% aqueous chlorhexidine.[70] Chlorhexidine provided the best protection against catheter colonization, with an incidence of 2.3% versus 7.1% and 9.3% for alcohol and povidone-iodine, respectively (P = .02). The rate of CR-BSI was also lower: 0.5%

versus 2.3% and 2.6%, respectively.[70] Another study evaluating epidural catheter colonization also strongly supported the use of chlorhexidine as the first-line skin antiseptic.[71]

Chlorhexidine, a cationic biguanide, is a potent germicide against nearly all nosocomial bacteria and yeasts.[70] Unlike povidone-iodine or alcohol, chlorhexidine provides residual cutaneous antibacterial activity that persists for several hours after application, and its germicidal activity is not neutralized by blood, serum, or other protein-rich biomaterials.[70] Another study compared a 4% alcohol-based solution of 0.25% chlorhexidine gluconate and 0.025% benzalkonium chloride with 10% povidone-iodine for care of central venous and arterial catheter insertion sites.[72] The rate of "catheter-related sepsis" in this study was 12 per 1000 catheter-days in the chlorhexidine-treated sites versus 21 per 1000 catheter-days for the povidone-iodine sites.[72]

Various ointments are also routinely used. In a large prospective study, Maki and Band[73] concluded that topical antimicrobial ointments conferred only modest protection, primarily for peripheral venous catheters remaining in place for more than 4 days. If ointments are used at all, these researchers recommended topical polymyxin-neomycin-bacitracin ointment for peripheral catheters and iodophor ointment for central venous and arterial catheters.[74] The Hospital Infection Control Practices Advisory Committee for the CDC now recommends that topical antimicrobial ointments not be used on the insertion sites of peripheral venous catheters or short-term nontunneled central venous catheters.[6]

The frequency and type of dressing changes have also been extensively studied. It is recommended that sterilely inserted peripheral intravenous catheters be removed at 48 to 72 hours to minimize the risk of phlebitis.[6] Peripheral catheters that were inserted under emergency conditions should be removed within 24 hours and replaced at a new site.[6] The dressing should be replaced when the catheter is replaced (i.e., at 48 or 72 hours) or when the dressing becomes damp, loosened, or soiled. It is important that the peripheral venous catheter site be inspected daily. Therefore, transparent dressings are almost universally used for peripheral catheters.[6]

In a large study of dressing regimens for more than 2000 polytetrafluoroethylene peripheral venous catheters, Maki and Ringer[74] found no difference in skin site colonization, catheter colonization, or CR-BSI among dry gauze, transparent polyurethane, and iodophor-transparent dressings. They recommended that for a peripheral catheter placed under sterile conditions, either sterile dry gauze or a transparent dressing could be left in place until the catheter was removed at 48 to 72 hours. Other studies suggest that bacterial colonization of peripheral venous catheters increases under transparent dressings, raising catheter colonization rates and hospital costs.[75]

Two studies have implicated transparent dressings for central venous catheters as being associated with a higher incidence of catheter colonization and associated CR-BSI.[76, 77] An analysis of previously published studies in the English literature demonstrated a statistically significant higher risk of catheter colonization for catheter sites with transparent dressings than for those with dressings of dry cotton gauze and tape, and a trend toward increased CR-BSI.[78] The study reported a 53% higher risk of catheter colonization (previously defined as catheter-related infection) for peripheral catheters and a 63% to 78% higher risk of significant colonization for central venous catheters.

It is important to understand that most of these earlier studies and the subsequent meta-analysis looked at conventional nonpermeable polyurethane dressings. A later study by Maki and associates[79] compared conventional (nonpermeable) polyurethane, highly permeable polyurethane, and sterile gauze and tape dressings for pulmonary artery catheters. In this study, cutaneous bacterial colonization under the dressing at the time of catheter removal was lowest with gauze and tape ($10^{1.3}$ CFUs); intermediate with the highly permeable polyurethane dressing ($10^{1.8}$ CFUs; $P < .01$); and highest with the conventional (nonpermeable) polyurethane dressing ($10^{2.1}$ CFUs; $P < .001$). There were no significant differences in catheter segment colonization or CR-BSI among the three groups.[79] These researchers concluded that polyurethane dressings appear to be safe for use with pulmonary artery catheters and may be left in place for up to 5 days between dressing changes.[79]

Conventional nonpermeable transparent dressings probably impede moisture evaporation from the insertion site and may, therefore, enhance bacterial colonization, especially in critically ill or diaphoretic patients.[75-77] Disadvantages of transparent dressings include poor adhesion in diaphoretic patients or with use of topical ointments and, depending on frequency of use, greater expense.[4] If central venous or pulmonary artery catheters are used for prolonged periods, nonpermeable transparent dressings should be avoided. Further studies with semipermeable transparent dressings are needed to ensure that these newer, more expensive dressings are as safe as tape and gauze for short-term catheterization.[4]

Replacement Schedules and Guide-Wire Exchange

Two schools of thought exist regarding guide-wire exchange for prevention of catheter colonization and CR-BSI. The first suggests that routine exchange of a catheter to a new site or by guide wire at a predetermined interval confers protection. The second allows for central venous catheters to be left in place until the development of clinical suspicion or signs of catheter colonization or CR-BSI. Both practices have inherent risks. With routine catheter exchange, the patient is exposed to the potential risk of pneumothorax or injury to major vessels.[9] Recontamination and subcutaneous tract infection may occur during an improperly performed guide-wire exchange.[9] It is also well known that the risk of infection increases with time if catheters remain in place indefinitely.

Most studies evaluating guide-wire exchange show that the technique is safe and effective for diagnosing CR-BSI and for prolonging use of a catheter site.[46, 80-82] Guide-wire exchange is effective in diagnosing catheter colonization and CR-BSI as long as every attempt is made to "sterilize" the entire external portion of the in situ catheter and the surrounding skin before the exchange. This practice not only prevents contamination of the new catheter during exchange but also yields more accurate semiquantitative culture results, because the catheters are removed through a "sterile field."[30] If bacteria are truly capable of growing and multiplying on catheter surfaces without external nutrient sources, as suggested by in vitro studies,[8, 20, 50, 83] guide-wire exchange may help prevent infection by removing significant numbers of externally and internally adherent bacteria before the development of a colony number sufficient to cause bacteremia or local infection.

One criticism of guide-wire exchange is that intracutaneous tract colonization or contamination during the exchange may perpetuate local infection and allow for subsequent infection of the new catheter. One study proved this possibility to be unlikely; 12 culture-positive catheters were replaced with new catheters by guide-wire exchange, and subsequent catheters removed from the same sites showed no growth in eight catheters (67%), probable contamination in one (8%), and positive cultures in only three (25%).[42] An observational cohort study of 2470 patients receiving central venous catheters showed that subsequent catheters exchanged over guide wires were at no higher risk for CR-BSI than a second catheter placed at a new anatomic site.[82] These studies suggest, as previously hypothesized by Bozzetti and colleagues,[84] that guide-wire exchange may confer some protection against CR-BSI. Because there is an increased risk of bacteremia, however, when culture results for removed catheters are positive,[53] it is therefore recommended that the new catheter be removed from the colonized site and another catheter be inserted at a different anatomic site when semiquantitative (≥ 15 CFUs) or quantitative (>10^3 CFUs) culture results for the removed catheter are positive. If the culture results for the catheter segment initially removed by guide-wire exchange are not positive (<15 CFUs semiquantitative; <10^3 CFUs quantitative), the new catheter placed via guide wire into the old site may be left in place.

Two studies investigated the infection risk of different methods of managing long-term vascular catheters in critically ill patients.[42, 43] Cobb and associates[43] studied four different methods of replacing central venous and PA catheters. Patients were randomly grouped to receive (1) a new catheter at a new site every 3 days, (2) a guide-wire exchange at the existing site every 3 days, (3) a new catheter and new site only when clinically indicated, or (4) a guide-wire exchange only when infection was suspected. Of the 160 patients studied, 5% had CR-BSI, 16% had catheter colonization, and 9% had major mechanical complications. Insertions at new sites were associated with more mechanical complications when compared to the guide-wire exchanged catheters (5% versus 1%; P = .005).[43] Although the results were not statistically significant, patients who were randomly assigned to guide-wire exchanges were considered more likely to have bacteremia after the first 3 days of catheterization when compared to patients who received catheters at a new site (6% versus 0%; P = .06). The researchers concluded that routine replacement of central vascular catheters every 3 days does not prevent infection and that guide-wire exchange may increase the risk of bacteremia.[43]

Eyer and colleagues[42] evaluated three different methods of site management for multiple-lumen, single-lumen, central, PA, and arterial catheters used for 7 or more days: (1) catheter exchange to a new site every 7 days, (2) no scheduled catheter change at any particular time but exchange to a new site when clinically indicated, and (3) guide-wire exchange every 7 days. In all groups, a catheter change was mandatory for a positive blood culture, exit site infection (defined as purulent drainage, expanding erythema or cellulitis, or a positive qualitative swab culture result for the exit site specimen), or clinical signs of sepsis without a definite source. These workers found no difference in infection risk among the three methods of long-term catheter care, recommending that the method with the fewest complications and least expense be used.

These two studies support the following general guidelines:

1. Central, PA, and arterial catheters should not be routinely changed at specific intervals.
2. Guide-wire exchange is appropriate when a new catheter is needed or when CR-BSI is suspected, because the method is safer.[42]
3. If there is evidence of a skin exit site infection, however, removing the old catheter and placing a new catheter at a new site would be most appropriate.[42]

Suggested Method for Guide-Wire Exchange

The following procedure of guide-wire exchange is recommended:

1. Guide-wire exchange begins with a complete sterilization of the external portion of the existing catheter before the guide wire is placed: All intravenous tubing, including parenteral nutrition tubing, is carefully separated from the catheter hubs and replaced with sterile caps or plugs. The separated intravenous tubing tips are also sterilely protected until they are reconnected to the new catheter.
2. Sterile, disposable gowns and gloves are worn by personnel performing the procedure, along with surgical hats and masks, and a sterile field for the necessary equipment is prepared on a bedside table.
3. The distal ports of the catheter to be exchanged are placed on a sterile paper barrier (usually provided in the new catheter kit), and the insertion site, along with a 10-cm circumferential area of skin and the entire external portion of the catheter from insertion site to capped hubs, is scrubbed for 5 minutes with 10 cm × 10 cm gauze pads soaked in 4% chlorhexidine skin cleanser. The important aspect of this preparation is that the chlorhexidine be allowed to remain in contact with the skin and the external portion of the catheter for at least 5 minutes.
4. After this scrub, the excess soap is carefully removed from the area with dry 10 cm × 10 cm gauze pads, and the skin sutures securing the catheter are removed with a No. 11 disposable scalpel.
5. The operator then exchanges sterile surgical gloves, and the entire area is draped with six sterile cloth surgical towels, or other large sterile barriers, with the distal catheter hubs being carefully removed from the now contaminated sterile paper barrier to the new sterile cloth barrier.
6. A sterile guide wire is carefully inserted through the distal port of the catheter after removal of the cap, with care taken that the wire does not touch the external portion of the hub.
7. The old catheter is carefully removed, with care taken to avoid contact with the surrounding skin.
8. Appropriate culture specimens are then obtained by amputating the 5-cm intracutaneous segment and the 5-cm distal tip of the catheter. This can be done with a sterile disposable suture removal kit (Johnson & Johnson Products, Inc., Skillman, N.J.). The segments are placed into two separate culturettes (Baxter Healthcare Corporation, McGaw Park, Ill.) and transported immediately to the microbiology laboratory for semiquantitative cultures.
9. The portion of the guide wire protruding from the skin is then cleaned with 4% chlorhexidine. Prior to handling the new catheter, it is best to change gloves for a third time. A new catheter is then placed over the guide wire into the proper anatomic position.
10. The catheter is sutured into place after the guide wire is removed.

A chest roentgenogram is generally not required after guide-wire exchange.

For central venous catheters (16 to 30 cm in length), both the tip and the intracutaneous 5-cm segments from the removed catheter are sent for semiquantitative culture. For pulmonary artery catheters and introducers, the 5-cm tip of the pulmonary artery catheter and the 5-cm intracutaneous segment of the catheter introducer are sent in separate culturettes for semiquantitative culture.

INFECTION RISKS OF SPECIFIC CATHETER TYPES

Pulmonary Artery Catheters

Several studies have shown that the risk of infection from PA catheters has decreased substantially over the past decade.[25, 79, 85, 86] Mermel and colleagues,[25] in an extensive study of the pathogenesis and epidemiology of PA catheter infections, found a 22% incidence of colonization and a 0.7% incidence of CR-BSI.

Another study of 69 PA catheters reported a 21.7% incidence of catheter colonization (≥ 15 CFUs by semiquantitative culture).[64] Catheterization for longer than 5 days was associated with a higher risk of colonization and a 13.3% risk of CR-BSI if catheter colonization developed.[64] The risk of catheter colonization was 41.2% if the catheter remained in place longer than 5 days, but only 15.4% if the catheter was used for 5 days or less.[64] In a later study, all episodes of CR-BSI occurred with catheters that had been in place for 5 or more days.[79] These two studies and others[87-89] demonstrate that the risk of CR-BSI from PA catheters is relatively low when the catheters are used for 5 days or less and when reasonable insertion site care is given. Clearly, the risk for CR-BSI increases when PA catheters are used for prolonged periods.

Multiple-Lumen Central Venous Catheters

Multiple-lumen central venous catheters were first introduced into clinical practice in the early 1980s and have rapidly increased in popularity, especially for use in critically ill patients.[5] These catheters have been implicated as a potential risk factor for CR-BSI. The risk of catheter colonization of multiple-lumen central venous catheters ranges from 6.9% to 11.5%, with an associated CR-BSI rate of 1.3% to 13.1%.[90-93] Kruse and Shah[5] reviewed all of the studies on CR-BSI in multiple-lumen central venous catheters from 1984 through 1992[5]; these researchers concluded that although a few trials suggest that the risk of infection is higher with multiple-lumen catheters, most have not.[5] Many of these studies used total parenteral nutrition as the entry criterion for patient selection; others combined PA catheter data. Such criteria and comparisons may bias results of these studies, because patients with multiple-lumen or PA catheters are usually more critically ill than patients with single-lumen catheters. Therefore, the perceived higher infection rate may be related not to the type of catheter but rather to difficulty in maintaining sterility, more frequent catheter manipulations, and the patients' immune status.

In one such study, Clark-Christoff and associates[92] examined the rate of CR-BSI in 78 patients with single-lumen catheters and 99 patients with triple-lumen catheters. All of the patients were considered to be at high risk for catheter colonization and associated CR-BSI. The researchers concluded that more frequent catheter manipulations with triple-lumen catheters caused a higher rate of infection and that, therefore, these catheters should not be used routinely for total parenteral nutrition. Eyer and colleagues[42] reported a 3.4% incidence of catheter colonization with an associated 2.1% incidence of CR-BSI in triple-lumen catheters used for an average of 22.6 days. Several other studies also found no higher risk of CR-BSI associated with triple-lumen catheters.[37, 46, 80, 90, 91, 93]

Another study separated multiple-lumen catheter infections in critically ill surgical patients according to whether the patients were septic (with other sources of infection) or nonseptic (no source of infection identified).[46] There were no episodes of significant catheter colonization (defined as ≥ 15 CFUs by semiquantitative culture) or CR-BSI in the nonseptic critically ill patients; the incidence of catheter colonization in the septic group was 26.3%, and the incidence of CR-BSI was 9.6%.[46] The rate of catheter colonization (previously termed catheter-related infection) per 100 days was only 0.9 for both septic and nonseptic patients combined, which is very similar to rates previously published for single-lumen catheters.[46] This study concluded that the risk of infection for multiple-lumen catheters is no higher than for single-lumen catheters, but septic patients are probably at higher risk regardless of the type of catheter used.[46]

Despite these findings, many experts in the field of device-associated infection believe that multiple-lumen central venous catheters are a probable risk factor compared with single-lumen catheters.[6, 7] They believe that multiple ports increase the frequency of catheter manipulation and that, possibly because of the larger diameter of some of these catheters, the insertion sites may be more prone to infection.[6] In the critically ill patient, the benefits of multiple-lumen catheters must be individually weighed against the potential higher risk of infection.

Arterial Catheters

In 1979, Band and Maki[94] studied arterial catheter-related infections and determined that the predominant variables for infection risk at that time were percutaneous versus cutdown insertion (ninefold increase in CR-BSI with cutdowns) and extended arterial cannulation time (>4 days). The overall incidence of catheter-related infection (now considered significant catheter colonization) was 18%, with 70% of the infections occurring in catheters used longer than 96 hours.[94] All five episodes of CR-BSI in this study occurred in patients with catheter sites used for more than 96 hours.[94]

A later study also suggested that extended cannulation time is an important factor and reemphasized that the risk of infection for arterial catheter sites used less than 96 hours is virtually nonexistent.[95] In this later study, 27% of sites used for more than 96 hours became colonized, as evidenced by positive swab cultures of the entry sites. Significant catheter colonization (defined as ≥ 15 CFUs on semiquantitative culture) developed in 9.5% of radial and femoral artery sites used for up to 14 days (mean, 6.4 days), although there were no documented episodes of CR-BSI. Significant colonization (≥ 15 CFUs by semiquantitative culture) developed in 44% of axillary sites after 96 hours of use.[95] The researchers concluded that (1) radial and femoral artery sites could be used for prolonged periods if skin site colonization were controlled with strict local site care and (2) guide-wire exchange could also be used to confirm the presence of catheter colonization for arterial catheters.[95] This relatively low risk of significant arterial catheter colonization and CR-BSI has been confirmed in other studies.[96]

Long-Term Central Venous Catheters

Although seldom used in the acute critically ill patient, catheters for long-term central venous access in both the inpatient and outpatient setting are becoming more common for patients requiring total parenteral nutrition and chemotherapy. In cancer patients, the catheters most frequently used have been long-dwelling tunneled catheters (Hickman, Broviac, Groshong[97]). These catheters provide life-prolonging therapy over extended periods by allowing for nutritional support, antibiotics, and chemotherapy without the need for frequent intravenous line changes.[97]

The incidence of significant catheter colonization with tunneled central venous catheters is approximately 2 per 1000 catheter-days.[98] Historically, the importance of tunneling long-dwelling catheters has been emphasized. This practice has been the principal strategy for preventing infection in these catheters, especially in cancer patients over the past two decades.[97] Two studies have questioned this practice, however, showing no difference in infection rates between tunneled and nontunneled long-dwelling subclavian catheters.[99, 100]

For long-dwelling catheters, four more definitions of infection (in addition to those given at the beginning of the chapter) must be considered, as follows:

Catheter exit site infection: Presence of inflammation or purulent exudate at the catheter exit site.[101]

Tunnel infection: Inflammation extending along the tract of a subcutaneously tunneled catheter more than 2 cm from the skin exit site.[101]

Septic thrombophlebitis: Thrombosis of a cannulated vein with inflammation and microbial invasion of the vein wall.[97]

Suppurative thrombophlebitis: A more severe case of septic thrombophlebitis in which the vein lumen is filled with pus.[97]

Peripherally Inserted Central Venous Catheters

Since 1990, peripherally inserted central venous catheters (PICCs) for long-term venous access have become more popular. These catheters may be used as a bridge between short-term venous access (<2 to 3 weeks) and long-term access (≥ 3 months). One review reported the average duration of PICC use to be in the range of 20 to 50 days.[102] These catheters are inserted through the basilic or cephalic vein and are used primarily in outpatients. The majority of studies indicate a low rate of infection.[102, 103] One study, however, showed a higher rate of infection with PICCs than with nontunneled silicone catheters placed directly into the subclavian vein.[99] PICCs are not very useful in patients with acute critical illness.

NOVEL TECHNIQUES

Attachable Silver-Impregnated Cuffs

An attachable subcutaneous cuff made of an inner silicone sleeve and an outer layer of bovine collagen impregnated with silver ion (Vitacuff, Vitaphore Corporation, Plainsboro, N.J.) was the first significant technologic advance specifically designed for preventing CR-BSI from short-term central venous catheterization. The results of two prospective randomized studies suggest that the cuff may substantially reduce the risk of catheter colonization (defined as ≥ 15 CFUs on semiquantitative culture).[51, 104] These studies reported reductions in rates of catheter colonization from 28.9% to 9.1% (P = .002)[51] and 34.5% to 7.7%.[104] No significant differences in the rates of CR-BSI were identified with the use of the cuff in either study.[51, 104]

Other studies have failed to demonstrate any benefit of the cuff in critically ill and septic patients.[9, 80] One observational study showed a higher rate of catheter colonization (31%) and fungemia (20%) by *Candida* species.[80] Dahlberg and colleagues[105] were also unable to show any short-term or long-term benefits of the attachable silver-impregnated cuff in a prospective randomized study of hemodialysis patients.

Antiseptic-Impregnated and Antibiotic-Impregnated Catheters

Central venous catheters impregnated with various antiseptic and antibiotic agents have been developed in an attempt to reduce the frequency of CR-BSI.

A multiple-lumen catheter coated with silver silvadiazine and chlorhexidine antiseptics has been commercially available for several years (Arrowgard, Arrow Corporation, Reading, Pa.). A prospective, randomized study compared this new catheter with a standard polyurethane multiple-lumen central venous catheter.[106] The results in 405 catheters studied showed that the antiseptic-coated catheters were twofold less likely to be colonized with bacteria than standard catheters (24.6% versus 1.0%; P = .02).[106]

In a prospective randomized study, Collin[107] observed a ninefold reduction in catheter colonization (termed catheter-related infection, and defined as 15 or more CFUs on semiquantitative culture) with the use of the antiseptic-bonded multiple-lumen catheter (18% versus 2%; P = .001). These data translated to rates of catheter-related infections per 1000 catheter-days of 2.27 for antiseptic-coated catheters and 24.68 for standard catheters (P = .001). Collin[107] concluded that the use of antiseptic-impregnated catheters significantly reduced the rate of "catheter-related infections." In addition, the low infection rate over time permitted less frequent guidewire exchanges and catheter removals, thereby reducing patient risk and hospital costs.[107]

Another study of 244 antiseptic-bonded catheters used for prolonged periods (mean, 11.7 ± 8.74 days; range, 1 to 51 days) identified a rate of CR-BSI per 1000 days as 1.57,[41] which compares favorably with that for long-term tunneled central catheters.[98] The CR-BSI rate per 1000 days was even lower (0.98) when subclavian sites were analyzed separately.[41]

Silver sulfadiazine and chlorhexidine are antiseptics possessing broad-spectrum antimicrobial properties, and the combination of these two antiseptics exhibits synergistic activity while preventing the emergence of resistant strains of bacteria.[108] Laboratory studies in different animal models have shown a significant reduction in skin and catheter bacterial colonization,[109] bacterial adherence,[108] and biofilm formation[108] with the use of catheters impregnated with silver sulfadiazine and chlorhexidine. Additionally, there was no clinical, pathologic, or microbiologic evidence of local or systemic toxicity from these antiseptics.[108] Both chlorhexidine and silver sulfadiazine are more protective against the most virulent organisms that cause CR-BSI (*S. aureus* and *Candida* species).[106] Despite these laboratory findings and clinical studies showing benefits, however, other studies have failed to show a benefit from antiseptic-impregnated catheters.[110, 111] Given the additional cost of these catheters, their use has not been universally accepted.

Trooskin and coworkers[112] first demonstrated the feasibility of antibiotic bonding to catheter surfaces.[108] Cefazolin,[112, 113] rifampin and minocycline,[114-116] and teicoplanin[117] have all been used to impregnate central venous catheters to reduce infection. Currently, such technology is commercially available. There is concern, however, that the general use of surface antibiotics for preventing CR-BSI may potentially select for resistance and contribute to the emergence of more antibiotic-resistant organisms.[7] The successful strategy for future reduction in CR-BSI clearly is in developing catheter surfaces that are resistant to colonization, either by developing new catheter materials or by impregnating catheter surfaces with antiseptics or antibiotics. Currently, impregnating catheter surfaces seems to be the area of greater promise.[115, 118]

RECOMMENDATIONS

The following recommendations are based on the studies reviewed in this chapter, published HICPAC CDC guidelines,[6] and the Roundtable Consensus Conference on the use of short-term central venous catheters.[7]

Physicians in critical care units are encouraged to study their own patient populations to determine the incidence of significant catheter colonization and CR-BSI and to develop appropriate guidelines for catheter exchange and site maintenance. On the basis of currently available information, peripheral arterial, central venous, and PA catheters do not require "routine" exchange either to a different site or over a guide wire. Although the risk of colonization and bacteremia increases with time, the optimal time for catheter removal is not known for peripheral arterial, central venous, and PA

TABLE 59–1. Recommendations for Short-Term Catheter Placement

Catheter Type	Preferred Anatomic Site(s) (in Order of Preference)	Frequency of Catheter Exchange	Guide-Wire Exchange an Option?
Peripheral venous catheter	Upper extremity[b]	48–72 hr[b]	No
Emergency peripheral venous catheter[a]	Upper extremity[b]	24 hr[b]	No
CVC (single-lumen or multiple-lumen)	Subclavian[b–d]	Routine replacement not recommended[b–d]	Yes
	Internal jugular	Routine replacement not recommended[b–d]	Yes
	Femoral	5 days[d]	Yes
Peripherally inserted CVC	Upper extremity	No recommendation[b]	Yes
PA catheter and PA catheter introducer	No recommendation[b]	5 days[b]	Yes
Short-term hemodialysis	No recommendation[b]	No recommendation[b]	No recommendation[b]
Peripheral arterial catheters	Radial[d]	No more than every 4 days[b] (routine replacement not recommended[d])	Yes[d]
	Femoral		
	Axillary		

[a]Catheter inserted under emergency conditions, in which sterile preparation may have been less than optimal.
[b]Hospital Infection Control Practices Advisory Committee guidelines. (Data from Pearson ML, et al: Infect Control Hosp Epidemiol 1996; 17:438.[6])
[c]Consensus Conference recommendations. (Civetta JM, personal communication, November 21, 1997.[7])
[d]Author's recommendation.
CVC = central venous catheter; PA = pulmonary artery.

catheters. Routine catheter exchange in critically ill patients does not alter infection risks.

Recommendations for short-term catheter placement are outlined in Table 59–1.

Any catheter (peripheral or central) that is placed under less than ideal conditions should be treated as a potential source of infection. Generally, such a catheter should be removed and a new catheter inserted at a different site if catheterization is needed for longer than 48 hours. Ideal conditions for catheter insertion include:

- Use of sterile, disposable surgical gowns, masks, hats, and gloves
- Careful preparation of the skin site with an appropriate antiseptic solution
- Wide draping of the area to create an adequate sterile field

The subclavian site is preferred over the internal jugular or femoral site for long-term (>72 hours) catheter use because of the higher colonization rates associated with neck and groin insertion sites.

The absolute indication for either removal or guide-wire exchange of a catheter is the presence of an unexplained bacteremia. In the critical care setting, fever is an unreliable indicator of CR-BSI. Guide-wire exchange using the strict protocol described in this chapter is an acceptable alternative to placing a catheter at a different site, because only about 20% to 25% of catheters removed for suspected infection actually yield positive semiquantitative culture results, and less than 10% are associated with CR-BSI.

In my experience, antiseptic-impregnated central venous and PA catheter introducers allow for prolonged catheter use without significantly increasing the risk of CR-BSI over time.[41] Individual institutions and critical care units should review their infection rates and catheter insertion practices to determine whether this readily available technology is cost effective for their patients. I prefer daily site cleansing with 4% chlorhexidine and alcohol, followed by placement of a dry dressing consisting of sterile gauze and occlusive tape. Antibiotic ointments do not seem to provide an added benefit, and there is insufficient evidence to strongly recommend the use of clear plastic dressings over tape and gauze, in terms of preventing infection and reducing costs. Adherence to strict protocols for site preparation at the time of insertion and for maintenance during the life of the catheter is crucial in critically ill patients if catheters are to remain in place for prolonged periods without increasing the risk for infection.

References

1. Sherertz R: Surveillance for infections associated with vascular catheters. Infect Control Hosp Epidemiol 1996; 17:746.
2. Pittet D, Wenzel R: Nosocomial bloodstream infections. Arch Intern Med 1995; 155:1177.
3. Maki DG: Infections due to infusion therapy. *In:* Hospital Infections. Bennett JV, Brachman PS (Eds). Boston, Little, Brown & Co, 1992, p 849.
4. Clemence M, Walker D, Farr B: Central venous catheter practices: Results of a survey. Am J Infect Control 1995; 23:5.
5. Kruse J, Shah N: Detection and prevention of central venous catheter-related infections. Nutr Clin Pract 1993; 8:163.
6. Pearson ML, Hierholzer WJ, Garner JS, et al: Guideline for prevention of intravascular device-related infections. Infect Control Hosp Epidemiol 1996; 17:438.
7. Civetta JM: Personal communication at Roundtable Consensus Conference: Short-Term Central Venous Catheter (CVC) Access: Controlling Infectious Complications, Chicago, November 21, 1997.
8. Peters G, Loui R, Pulverer G: Adherence and growth of coagulase-negative staphylococci on surfaces of intravenous catheters. J Infect Dis 1982; 146:479.
9. Bonawitz SC, Hammel EJ, Kirkpatrick JR: Prevention of central venous catheter sepsis: A prospective randomized trial. Am Surg 1991; 47:618.
10. Adal K, Farr B: Central venous catheter-related infections: A review. Nutrition 1996; 12:208.
11. Press OW, Ramsey PG, Larson EB, et al: Hickman catheter infections in patients with malignancies. Medicine 1984; 63:189.
12. Cercenado E, Ena J, Rodriguez-Creixems M, et al: A conservative procedure for the diagnosis of catheter-related infections. Arch Intern Med 1990; 150:1417.
13. Armstrong CW, Mayhall CG, Miller KB, et al: Clinical predictors

of infection of central venous catheters used for total parenteral nutrition. Infect Control Hosp Epidemiol 1986; 11:71.
14. Anaissie E, Samonis G, Kontoyiannis D, et al: Role of catheter colonization and infrequent hematogenous seeding in catheter-related infections. Eur J Clin Microbiol Infect Dis 1995; 14:134.
15. Goldman DA, Pier GB: Pathogenesis of infections related to intravascular catheterization. Clin Microbiol Rev 1993; 6:176.
16. Bjornson HS: Pathogenesis, prevention, and management of catheter-associated infections. New Horiz 1993; 1:271.
17. Wijngaerden E, Bobbaers H: Intravascular catheter related bloodstream infection: Epidemiology, pathogenesis and prevention. Acta Clin Belg 1997; 52:9.
18. Martin MA, Pfaller MA, Wenzel RP: Coagulase-negative staphylococcal bacteremia. Ann Intern Med 1989; 110:9.
19. Muller E, Takeda S, Shiro H, et al: Blood proteins do not promote adherence of coagulase-negative staphylococci to biomaterials. Infect Immun 1991; 59:3323.
20. Passerini L, Lam K, Costerton JW, et al: Biofilms on indwelling vascular catheters. Crit Care Med 1992; 20:665.
21. Herrman M, Lai QJ, Albrecht RM, et al: Adhesion of *Staphylococcus aureus* to surface-bound platelets: Role of fibrinogen, fibrin, and platelet integrins. J Infect Dis 1993; 167:312.
22. Wang I-W, Anderson JM, Marchant RE: *Staphylococcus epidermidis* adhesion to hydrophobic biomedical polymer is mediated by platelets. J Infect Dis 1993; 167:329.
23. Segura M, Alvarez-Lerma F, MaTellado J, et al: A clinical trial on the prevention of catheter-related sepsis using a new hub model. Ann Surg 1996; 223:363.
24. Raad I, Costerton W, Sabharwal U, et al: Ultrastructural analysis of indwelling vascular catheters: A quantitative relationship between luminal colonization and duration of placement. J Infect Dis 1993; 18:400.
25. Mermel LA, McCormick RD, Springman SR, et al: The pathogenesis and epidemiology of catheter-related infection with pulmonary artery Swan-Ganz catheters: A prospective study using molecular subtyping. Am J Med 1991; 91(Suppl 3B):1975.
26. Henderson DK: Intravascular device–associated infection: Current concepts and controversies. Infect Surg 1988; 7:365.
27. Bjornson HS, Colley R, Bower RH, et al: Association between microorganism growth at the catheter insertion site and colonization of the catheter in patients receiving total parenteral nutrition. Surgery 1982; 92:720.
28. Penner J, Allerberger F, Dierich M, et al: In vitro experiments on catheter-related infections due to gram-negative rods. Chemotherapy 1993; 39:336.
29. Kovacevich DS, Faubion WC, Bender JM, et al: Association of parenteral nutrition catheter sepsis with urinary tract infections. JPEN J Parenter Enteral Nutr 1986; 10:639.
30. Pettigrew RA, Lang SDR, Haydock DA, et al: Catheter-related sepsis in patients on intravenous nutrition: A prospective study of quantitative catheter cultures and guidewire changes for suspected sepsis. Br J Surg 1985; 72:52.
31. Maki DG, Rhame FS, Mackel DC, et al: Nationwide epidemic of septicemia caused by contaminated intravenous products: I. Epidemiologic and clinical features. Am J Med 1976; 60:471.
32. Goldman DG, Martin WT, Worthington JW: Growth of bacteria and fungi in total parenteral nutrition solutions. Am J Surg 1973; 126:314.
33. Crocket KS, Noga R, Filibeck DG, et al: Microbial growth comparisons of five commercial parenteral lipid emulsions. JPEN J Parenter Enteral Nutr 1984; 8:391.
34. Moran JM, Atwood RP, Rowe MI: A clinical and bacteriologic study of infections associated with venous cutdowns. N Engl J Med 1965; 272:554.
35. Richet H, Hubert B, Nitemberg G, et al: Prospective multicenter study of vascular-catheter-related complications and risk factors for positive central-catheter cultures in intensive care unit patients. J Clin Microbiol 1990; 28:2520.
36. Hagley MT, Martin B, Gast P, et al: Infections and mechanical complications of central venous catheters placed by percutaneous venipuncture and over guidewires. Crit Care Med 1992; 20:1426.
37. Kemp L, Burge J, Choban P, et al: The effect of catheter type and site on infection rates in total parenteral nutrition patients. JPEN J Parenteral Enteral Nutr 1994; 18:71.
38. LaSala RA, Starker PM, Askanazi J: The saphenous system for long-term parenteral nutrition. JPEN J Parenteral Enteral Nutr 1987; 11:259.
39. Curtas S, Bonaventura M, Meguid MM: Cannulation of inferior vena cava for long-term central venous access. Surg Gynecol Obstet 1989; 186:121.
40. Purdue GF, Hunt JL: Vascular access through the femoral vessels: Indications and complications. J Burn Care Rehabil 1986; 7:498.
41. Norwood S, Wilkins H, Fernandez L, et al: A prospective analysis of infection rates using antiseptic-bonded central venous catheters. Crit Care Med 1998; 26(Suppl):A44.
42. Eyer S, Brummitt C, Crossley K, et al: Catheter-related sepsis: Prospective, randomized study of three methods of long-term catheter maintenance. Crit Care Med 1990; 18:1073.
43. Cobb DK, High KP, Sawyer RG, et al: A controlled trial of scheduled replacement of central venous and pulmonary-artery catheters. N Engl J Med 1992; 327:1062.
44. Raad I, Umphrey J, Khan A, et al: The duration of placement as a predictor of peripheral and pulmonary arterial catheter infections. J Hosp Infect 1993; 23:17.
45. Hampton AA, Sheretz RJ: Vascular access infections in hospitalized patients. Surg Clin North Am 1988; 68:47.
46. Norwood SH, Jenkins G: An evaluation of triple-lumen catheter infections using a guidewire exchange technique. J Trauma 1990; 30:706.
47. Welch GW, McKeel DW, Silverstein P, et al: The role of catheter composition in the development of thrombophlebitis. Surg Gynecol Obstet 1974; 138:421.
48. Stillman RM, Soliman F, Garcia L, et al: Etiology of catheter-associated sepsis. Arch Surg 1977; 112:1497.
49. Linder LE, Curelaru I, Gustavsson B, et al: Material thrombogenicity in central venous catheterization: A comparison between soft, antebrachial catheters of silicone elastomer and polyurethane. JPEN J Parenter Enteral Nutr 1984; 8:399.
50. Gilsdorf JR, Wilson K, Beals TF: Bacterial colonization of intravenous catheter materials in vitro and in vivo. Surgery 1989; 106:37.
51. Maki DG, Cobb I, Carman JK, et al: An attachable silver-impregnated cuff for prevention of infection with central venous catheters: A prospective, randomized multi-center trial. Am J Med 1988; 85:307.
52. Sherertz RJ, Raad II, Belani A, et al: Three year experience with sonicated vascular catheter cultures in a clinical microbiology laboratory. J Clin Microbiol 1990; 28:76.
53. Maki DG, Weise CE, Sarafin HW: A semiquantitative culture method for identifying intravenous catheter–related infection. N Engl J Med 1977; 296:1305.
54. Cercenado E, Ena J, Rodriguez-Creixems M, et al: A conservative procedure for the diagnosis of catheter-related infections. Arch Intern Med 1990; 150:1417.
55. Reimer L: Catheter-related infections and blood cultures. Clin Lab Med 1994; 14:51.
56. Widmer AF, Nettleman M, Flint K, Wenzel RP: The clinical impact of culturing central venous catheters: A prospective study. Arch Intern Med 1992; 152:1299.
57. Armstrong CW, Mayhall CG, Miller KB, et al: Clinical predictors of infection of central venous catheters used for total parenteral nutrition. Infect Control Hosp Epidemiol 1990; 11:71.
58. Raad I, Baba M, Bodey G: Diagnosis of catheter-related infections: The role of surveillance and targeted quantitative skin cultures. Clin Infect Dis 1995; 20:593.
59. Wing EJ, Norden CW, Shadduck RK, Winkelstein A: Use of quantitative bacteriologic techniques to diagnose catheter-related sepsis. Arch Intern Med 1979; 139:482.
60. Flynn PM, Shenep JL, Barrett FF: Differential quantitation with a commercial blood culture tube for diagnosis of catheter-related infection. J Clin Microbiol 1988; 26:1045.
61. Mosca R, Curta S, Forbes B, et al: The benefits of isolator cultures in the management of suspected catheter sepsis. Surgery 1987; 102:718.
62. Raucher HS, Hyatt AC, Barzilai A, et al: Quantitative blood cultures in the evaluation of septicemia in children with Broviac catheters. J Pediatr 1984; 104:29.
63. Moonens F, Alami S, Gossum A: Usefulness of gram staining of blood collected from total parenteral nutrition catheter for rapid

diagnosis of catheter-related sepsis. J Clin Microbiol 1994; 32:1578.
64. Rello J, Coll P, Net A, et al: Infection of pulmonary artery catheters: Epidemiologic characteristics and multivariate analysis of risk factors. Chest 1993; 103:132.
65. Cooper GL, Hopkins GC: Rapid diagnosis of intravascular catheter-associated infection by direct gram staining of catheter segments. N Engl J Med 1985; 312:1142.
66. Cleri DJ, Corrado ML, Seligman SJ: Quantitative culture of intravenous catheters and other intravascular inserts. J Infect Dis 1980; 141:781.
67. Raad II, Sabbagh MF, Rand KH, et al: Quantitative tip culture methods and the diagnosis of central venous catheter-related infections. Diagn Microbiol Infect Dis 1992; 15:13.
68. Moyer MA, Edwards LD, Farley L: Comparative culture methods on 101 intravenous catheters. Arch Intern Med 1983; 143:66.
69. Wormser GP, Onorato IM, Preminger TJ, et al: Sensitivity and specificity of blood cultures obtained through intravascular catheters. Crit Care Med 1990; 18:152.
70. Maki DG, Ringer M, Alvarado CJ: Prospective randomized trial of povidone-iodine, alcohol, and chlorhexidine for prevention of infection associated with central venous and arterial catheters. Lancet 1991; 338:339.
71. Shapiro JM, Bond EL, Garman JK: Use of a chlorhexidine dressing to reduce microbial colonization of epidural catheters. Anesthesiology 1990; 73:625.
72. Mimoz O, Pieroni L, Lawrence C, et al: Prospective, randomized trial of two antiseptic solutions for prevention of central venous or arterial catheter colonization and infection in intensive care unit patients. Crit Care Med 1996; 24:1818.
73. Maki DG, Band JD: A comparative study of polyantibiotic and iodophor ointments in prevention of vascular catheter-related infection. Am J Med 1981; 70:739.
74. Maki DG, Ringer M: Evaluation of dressing regimens for prevention of infection with peripheral intravenous catheters. JAMA 1987; 258:2396.
75. Craven DE, Lichtenberg DA, Kunches LM, et al: A randomized study comparing a transparent polyurethane dressing to a dry gauze dressing for peripheral intravenous catheter sites. Infect Control 1985; 6:361.
76. Conly JM, Grieves K, Peters B: A prospective randomized study comparing transparent and dry gauze dressings for central venous catheters. J Infect Dis 1989; 159:310.
77. Dickerson N, Horton P, Smith S, et al: Clinically significant central venous catheter infections in a community hospital: Association with type of dressing. J Infect Dis 1989; 169:720.
78. Hoffman KK, Weber DJ, Samsa GP, et al: Transparent polyurethane film as an intravenous catheter dressing: A meta-analysis of the infection risks. JAMA 1992; 267:2072.
79. Maki DG, Stolz SS, Wheeler S, Mermel LA: A prospective, randomized trial of gauze and two polyurethane dressings for site care of pulmonary artery catheters: Implications for catheter management. Crit Care Med 1994; 22:1729.
80. Norwood S, Hajjar G, Jenkins L: The influence of an attachable subcutaneous cuff for preventing catheter infections in critically ill surgical and trauma patients. Surg Gynecol Obstet 1992; 175:33.
81. Civetta JM, Hudson-Civetta JA, Nelson LD, et al: Utility and efficacy of guidewire changes (Abstract). Crit Care Med 1987; 15:380.
82. Badley AD, Steckelberg JM, Wollani PC, Thompson RL: Infectious rates of central venous pressure catheters: Comparison between newly placed catheters and those that have been changed. Mayo Clin Proc 1996; 71:838.
83. Gristina AG: Biomaterial-centered infection: Microbial adhesion versus tissue integration. Science 1987; 237:1588.
84. Bozzetti F, Terno G, Bonfanti G, et al: Prevention and treatment of central venous catheter sepsis by exchange via a guidewire. Ann Surg 1983; 198:48.
85. Ricard P, Martin R, Marcous JA: Protection of indwelling vascular catheters: Incidence of bacterial contamination and catheter-related sepsis. Crit Care Med 1985; 13:541.
86. Damen J, Bolton D: A prospective analysis of 1400 pulmonary artery catheterizations in patients undergoing cardiac surgery. Acta Anaesthesiol Scand 1986; 30:386.
87. Myers ML, Austin TW, Sibbald WJ: Pulmonary artery catheter infections. Ann Surg 1985; 201:237.
88. Hudson-Civetta JA, Civetta JM, Martinez OV, et al: Risk and detection of pulmonary artery catheter-related infection in septic surgical patients. Crit Care Med 1987; 15:29.
89. Civetta JM, Hudson-Civetta JA, Dion L: Duration of illness affects catheter-related infection and bacteremia (Abstract). Presented at the 27th Interscience Conference on Antimicrobial Agents and Chemotherapy, Atlanta, October 11-12, 1988.
90. Manglano R, Martin M: Safety of triple lumen catheters in the critically-ill. Am Surg 1991; 57:370.
91. Farkas JC, Liu N, Bleriot JP, et al: Single- versus triple-lumen central catheter-related sepsis: A prospective randomized study in a critically-ill population. Am J Med 1992; 93:277.
92. Clark-Christoff N, Watters VA, Sparks W, et al: Use of triple-lumen subclavian catheters for administration of total parenteral nutrition. JPEN J Parenter Enteral Nutr 1992; 16:403.
93. Lee RB, Buckner M, Sharp KW: Do multi-lumen catheters increase central venous catheter sepsis compared to single-lumen catheters? J Trauma 1988; 28:1472.
94. Band JD, Maki DG: Infections caused by arterial catheters used for hemodynamic monitoring. Am J Med 1979; 67:735.
95. Norwood SH, Cormier B, McMahan NG, et al: Prospective study of catheter-related infection during prolonged arterial catheterization. Crit Care Med 1988; 16:836.
96. Leroy O, Beuscart C, Santre C, et al: Nosocomial infections associated with long-term artery cannulation. Intensive Care Med 1989; 15:241.
97. Farr BM: Vascular catheter related infections in cancer patients. Surg Oncol Clin North Am 1995; 4:493.
98. Howell PB, Walters PE, Donowitz GR, et al: Risk factors for infection of tunneled central venous catheters in adult cancer patients. Cancer 1995; 75:1367.
99. Raad I, Davis S, Becker M, et al: Low infection rate and long durability of nontunneled Silastic catheters. Arch Intern Med 1993; 153:1791.
100. Andrivet P, Bacquer A, VuNgoc C, et al: Lack of clinical benefit from subcutaneous tunnel insertion of central venous catheters in immunocompromised patients. Clin Infect Dis 1994; 18:199.
101. Press OW, Ramsey PG, Larson EB, et al: Hickman catheter infections in patients with malignancies. Medicine 1984; 63:189.
102. Merrell S, Peatross B, Grossman M, et al: Peripherally inserted central venous catheters. West J Med 1994; 160:25.
103. Graham DR, Keldermans MM, Klemm LW, et al: Infectious complications among patients receiving home intravenous therapy with peripheral, central, or peripherally placed central venous catheters. Am J Med 1991; 91:3.
104. Flowers RH, Schwenzer KJ, Kopel RF, et al: Efficacy of an attachable subcutaneous cuff for the prevention of intravascular catheter-related infection. JAMA 1989; 261:878.
105. Dahlberg PJ, Agger WA, Singer JR, et al: Subclavian hemodialysis catheter infections: A prospective, randomized trial of an attachable silver-impregnated cuff for prevention of catheter-related infections. Infect Control Hosp Epidemiol 1995; 16:506.
106. Carlson R: Antiseptic-releasing catheter reduces infections: An interview with Dennis Maki, M.D. Oncology Times 1992; 14:23.
107. Collin GR: Use of an antiseptic-impregnated central venous catheter for the prevention of catheter-related infections: Results of a prospective, randomized trial. Crit Care Med 1997; 25(Suppl):A84.
108. Greenfield JI, Sampath L, Popilskis SJ, et al: Decreased bacterial adherence and biofilm formation on chlorhexidine and silver sulfadiazine-impregnated central venous catheters implanted in swine. Crit Care Med 1995; 23(5):894.
109. Modak SM, Sampath L: Development and evaluation of a new polyurethane central venous antiseptic catheter: Reducing central venous catheter infections. Complications Surg 1992; 11:23.
110. Ciresi DL, Albrecht RM, Volkers PA, Scholten DJ: Failure of antiseptic bonding to prevent central venous catheter-related infection and sepsis. Am Surgeon 1996; 62:641.
111. Pemberton LB, Ross V, Cuddy P, et al: No difference in catheter sepsis between standard and antiseptic central venous catheters. Arch Surg 1996; 131:986.
112. Trooskin SZ, Donetz AP, Harvey RA, et al: Prevention of catheter sepsis by antibiotic bonding. Surgery 1985; 97:546.

113. Kamal GD, Pfaller MA, Rempe LE, et al: Reduced intravascular catheter infection by antibiotic bonding. JAMA 1991; 265:2364.
114. Raad I, Darouiche R, Hachem R, et al: Antibiotics and prevention of microbial colonization of catheters. Antimicrob Agents Chemother 1995; 39:2397.
115. Darouiche R, Raad I, Bodey G, Musher D: Antibiotic susceptibility of staphylococci isolated from patients with vascular catheter-related bacteremia: Potential role of the combination of minocycline and rifampin. Int J Antimicrob Agents 1995; 6:31.
116. Raad I, Darouiche R, Hauhem R, et al: The broad-spectrum activity and efficacy of catheters coated with minocycline and rifampin. J Infect Dis 1996; 173:418.
117. Bach A, Darby D, Bottiger B, et al: Retention of the antibiotic teicoplanin on a hydromer-coated central venous catheter to prevent bacterial colonization in postoperative surgical patients. Intensive Care Med 1996; 22:1066.
118. Sherertz RJ, Carruth WA, Hampton AA, et al: Efficacy of antibiotic-coated catheters in preventing subcutaneous *Staphylococcus aureus* infection in rabbits. J Infect Dis 1993; 167:98.

60

Central Nervous System Infections

David W. Haas, MD • Allen B. Kaiser, MD

Physiologic and anatomic barriers make direct medical and surgical intervention difficult in the critically ill patient with central nervous system (CNS) infection. Physiologically, the blood-brain barrier impairs delivery of many antimicrobials, and anatomic barriers are created by the bony calvarium and the central location of the ventricular system.

In addition, noninfectious conditions may mimic CNS infection. For example, a necrotic brain tumor may be clinically indistinguishable from a brain abscess. In general, it is prudent to address the infectious possibilities immediately in such situations.

A final problem is that many pathogens produce identical clinical syndromes. Timely identification of the specific etiologic agent is crucial. Fortunately, most pathogens can be identified from early laboratory tests, such as Gram stains of cerebrospinal fluid (CSF) or of pus aspirated from a brain abscess. Epidemiologic clues may also suggest specific microorganisms; pathogens associated with community-acquired infections differ from those acquired in a hospital. In short, proper therapy for CNS infection demands an understanding of the anatomy and physiology of the CNS, the pharmacokinetics of antimicrobial agents, and the epidemiology of infecting pathogens.

BACTERIAL MENINGITIS

Anatomy

Bacterial meningitis is a pyogenic infection of the cerebral ventricles and the subarachnoid space, with bacteria usually confined to the nutrient-rich CSF. Most CSF is formed by the choroid plexus of the ventricles, enters the subarachnoid space at the cisterna magna, flows around the cerebral hemispheres, and is reabsorbed by the arachnoid villi (Fig. 60–1). In the adult, CSF is produced at approximately 500 mL/day whereas the CSF space averages 140 mL in volume. The cerebral subarachnoid space joins the spinal subarachnoid space at the cisterna magna. Flow through the spinal subarachnoid space is of variable velocity and direction.

There are numerous potential and actual spaces among the layers of the meninges (Fig. 60–2). Meningitis involves the actual space (i.e., the subarachnoid space). The brain parenchyma is usually not infected in uncomplicated bacterial meningitis, even when the illness follows a fulminant course. Exceptions occur in neonates, in whom *Citrobacter freundii* and *Haemophilus influenzae* may cause focal cerebritis or microabscesses adjacent to the pia. In adults, *Listeria monocytogenes* meningitis may be complicated by cerebritis, brain abscess, or both.

How does bacterial meningitis cause such profound CNS dysfunction when neural tissues are not directly infected or involved in the associated inflammatory response? Likely factors may include (1) bacterial toxins that affect underlying neural structures; (2) occlusion of cortical blood vessels that traverse the subarachnoid space (see Fig. 60–2); (3) damage to nerve roots that traverse the subarachnoid space, causing cranial or spinal nerve dysfunction; (4) impairment of CSF flow (see Fig. 60–1), which leads to hydrocephalus; and (5) bacterial products that stimulate release of cytokines, which cause capillary leakage, cerebral edema, and possibly direct neuronal injury.

The CSF-filled space should not be viewed as a single compartment. The small size of the foramina of Luschka and Magendie probably ensures unidirectional caudal flow. This flow, the cephalad flow within the cerebral subarachnoid space, and the imprecise flow within the lumbar area suggest three distinct compartments. This compartmentalization has implications for therapy because movement of medications and infectious agents between compartments depends on rates and directions of CSF flow.

Infectious agents may invade the CSF by at least three routes (Table 60–1). First, the vascular structures of the choroid

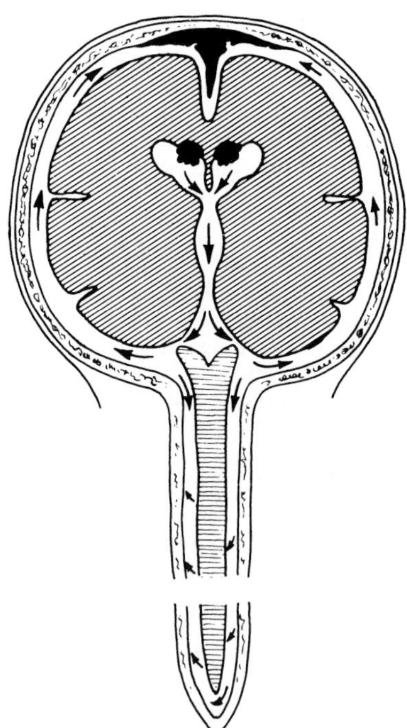

Figure 60–1. Cerebrospinal fluid (CSF) flow within the central nervous system. CSF formed at the choroid plexus of the cerebral ventricles rapidly enters the subarachnoid space at the foramina of Luschka and Magendie. From the cisterna magna, an organized flow of CSF occurs around the convexities of the brain to the arachnoid villi. There are multiple pathways of bidirectional flow around the spinal cord.

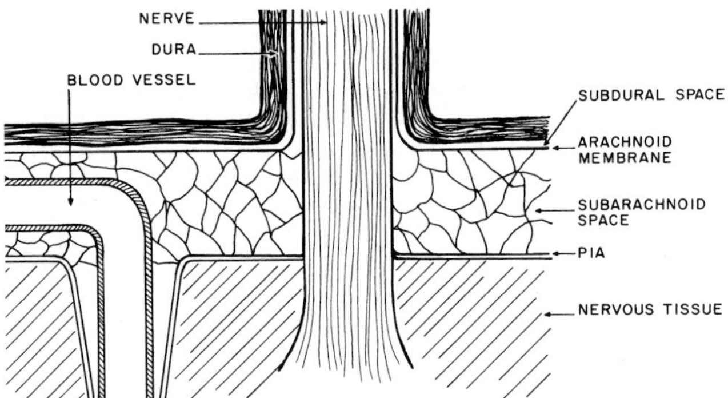

Figure 60–2. This diagram of the potential and actual spaces between the layers of the meninges shows the relationship of blood vessels and nerve roots to the subarachnoid space.

plexus and pia and the vessels that traverse the subarachnoid space may serve as conduits during systemic bacteremia. The frequency of ventriculitis during meningitis suggests that the choroid plexus is an important route.

A second, less common route is direct invasion across the protective meninges. Disruption of the dura by trauma or surgery may allow direct invasion of the CSF, and CSF drainage from sites of surgery and trauma indicates a break in dural continuity. Emissary veins provide another pathway for bacteria to spread from contiguous foci into the subarachnoid space. These veins traverse the skull and dura, directly connecting the soft tissues of the head and neck with the venous system of brain and meninges, including the arachnoid villi. Although blood in the emissary veins usually flows away from the brain, the CNS veins and dural sinuses do not contain valves, and retrograde flow of bacteria is possible. Congenital defects may occur at any point from the glabrata to the cauda equina, offering additional direct communication with the subarachnoid space.[1]

Finally, organisms rarely may reach the ventricles or subarachnoid space from within the neural tissue (e.g., rupture of a brain abscess into the CSF).

TABLE 60–1. Routes by Which Bacteria May Enter the Subarachnoid Space

Bloodstream

Most likely pathogens: pneumococci, meningococci, *Haemophilus influenzae, Escherichia coli* (neonates), group B streptococci (neonates)
- *Choroid plexus:* may be most common site of invasion
- *Meningeal blood vessels:* located throughout the subarachnoid space
- *Arachnoid villi:* a possible route of invasion, located between the sagittal sinus and subarachnoid space

Transdural Route

Most likely pathogens: pneumococci, gram-negative enteric bacilli, staphylococci (especially coagulase-negative), *H. influenzae*
- *Surgery:* including ventriculoatrial and ventriculoperitoneal shunts
- *Trauma:* especially when cribriform plate or petrous bone is fractured
- *Parameningeal infective focus:* including sinusitis, otitis, osteomyelitis; emissary veins may serve as conduit
- *Congenital defects:* including myelomeningocele and spinal dermal sinus

Transparenchymal Route

Most likely pathogens: anaerobic bacteria

Occurs when brain abscess ruptures into ventricles or subarachnoid space

Pathophysiology

The unique anatomy and composition of the CSF-filled compartments create an environment that, relative to other tissues, encourages persistence of microorganisms. Phagocytosis is most effective when a polymorphonuclear leukocyte can trap a bacterium against a host tissue surface; the large fluid-filled spaces of the ventricles and subarachnoid space deny such phagocytic surfaces. Mobilization of polymorphonuclear leukocytes is delayed during the early stages of infection. In addition, CSF contains little immunoglobulin.[2] Most important, complement, which rapidly kills many bacteria and assists in chemotaxis, phagocytosis, and intracellular killing, is absent from normal CSF. These features dictate that once the CSF is inoculated with pathogens, a self-limited illness is virtually impossible.[3]

These limited local defense mechanisms may explain the importance of the use of bactericidal antibiotics in bacterial meningitis. Lepper and Dowling[4] showed that treatment of pneumococcal meningitis with penicillin was associated with lower mortality than the combination of penicillin and tetracycline. Tetracycline, a bacteriostatic antibiotic, effectively "neutralizes" the bactericidal activity of penicillin. Although tetracycline may be as effective as penicillin for many extra-CNS infections and produces acceptable CSF levels, its inferior performance suggests that host defenses cannot compensate for its lack of bacterial killing. Chloramphenicol, which is bactericidal against most *H. influenzae* and pneumococci, may be as effective as ampicillin for meningitis caused by susceptible strains of these organisms. (Chloramphenicol is not optimal therapy for many penicillin-resistant pneumococci, as discussed later.) However, it is rarely bactericidal against gram-negative enteric bacilli, and failures are common when gram-negative bacillary meningitis is treated with chloramphenicol.[5]

CLINICAL COURSE OF PYOGENIC MENINGITIS

Most patients with bacterial meningitis exhibit only modest impairment of higher integrative functions on presentation. Several days of malaise, fever, and headache are typical, and meningismus is usually present.[6] The CSF indices are almost always abnormal, and a Gram stain or culture of the fluid usually reveals the infecting pathogen unless antibiotics were administered beforehand. Despite the availability of antibiotics active against all common causes of acute bacterial meningitis in adults, the overall mortality remains approximately 25%.[7]

For unclear reasons, in some patients pyogenic meningitis follows a different course. Such patients experience a fulminant illness that rapidly (<48 hours) produces signs and symptoms of both systemic and CNS infections. In addition to having fever, headache, and meningismus, such patients exhibit early impairment of sensorium, ranging from lethargy to coma. Despite appropriate antimicrobial therapy, mortality rates of approximately 50% have been reported for such patients.[8]

A successful outcome is inversely related to the degree of impairment of higher integrative functions when therapy is initiated. At some point, progression to morbidity or mortality becomes irreversible. A parallel exists in herpes simplex encephalitis, in which mortality is 50% to 65% in patients who present with severe cognitive impairment versus 10% to 30% without such impairment.[9, 10] Adults who are obtunded on admission with community-acquired bacterial meningitis may be three times more likely than more alert patients to die of the infection.[7]

Syndromes of Central Nervous System Infection

Definitive diagnosis of bacterial meningitis requires laboratory confirmation. Involvement of the CNS by other pathogens (e.g., viruses, fungi, mycobacteria) and noninfectious processes (e.g., subarachnoid hemorrhage) may produce identical syndromes. In practice, infection of the CNS usually presents as a subacute illness characterized by fever, headache, and meningismus (i.e., the *subacute CNS infection syndrome*). A smaller percentage of patients with CNS infection present with a rapidly progressing illness (<24 to 48 hours) with early impairment of higher integrative functions and represent the *acute meningitis syndrome* (Table 60–2).

The following topics include approaches to acute meningitis and subacute CNS infection syndromes. These approaches prioritize the competing needs of obtaining a precise etiologic diagnosis and instituting early antimicrobial therapy.

Acute Meningitis Syndrome

Early recognition of and therapy for acute meningitis syndrome are essential to prevent mortality and excessive morbidity. The initial manifestation may be subtle, with a low-grade headache or upper respiratory tract infection. Once meningeal symptoms (vomiting, severe headache, and stiff neck) develop, however, the clinical course is dramatic. Patients appear "toxic," and higher integrative functions may deteriorate rapidly. In older patients, the signs and symptoms may be indistinct, consisting only of fever, irritability, confusion, poor appetite, or seizures. Nonetheless, such cases may progress to coma within hours.

The physician should initiate antimicrobial therapy within 30 minutes of encountering the patient with acute meningitis syndrome and should not withhold therapy while awaiting the CSF Gram stain results (Fig. 60–3). A brief history should elicit antibiotic (especially penicillin) allergy and identify risk factors such as immunosuppression, recent surgery, or trauma. A brief physical examination should exclude papilledema or focal neurologic defects. Papilledema and focal defects (excluding Todd's paralysis) are rare in acute meningitis and are indications for immediate empirical antimicrobial therapy with a third-generation cephalosporin (cefotaxime or ceftriaxone) plus vancomycin combined with either metronidazole or chloramphenicol because of the possibility of a brain abscess caused by anaerobic organisms. A computed tomography (CT) or magnetic resonance imaging (MRI) scan should follow immediately to rule out a mass lesion, which might produce uncal herniation if a lumbar puncture were performed.

TABLE 60–2. Etiology of Acute and Subacute Syndromes of Central Nervous System (CNS) Infection

Acute Meningitis Syndrome

Rapid onset (<24–48 hr) of fever, headache, or meningismus, with early impairment of higher integrative functions
- *Common:* pyogenic meningitis (pneumococcal, meningococcal, *Haemophilus*, other)
- *Uncommon:* viral encephalitis (especially herpes simplex), subarachnoid bleed, and brain tumor (with rupture)
- *Rare:* viral meningitis, granulomatous meningitis (cryptococcal, mycobacterial), carcinomatous meningitis, and brain tumor

Subacute CNS Infection Syndrome:

Subacute onset (>24–48 hr) of fever, headache, or meningismus, with no or gradual impairment of higher integrative functions
- *Common:* viral meningitis, viral encephalitis, pyogenic meningitis
- *Uncommon:* brain abscess, brain tumor, granulomatous meningitis
- *Rare:* cerebrovascular accident, carcinomatous meningitis

Antibiotics should be administered within the first 30 minutes to patients with acute meningitis syndrome even if diagnostic results are incomplete (see text on therapy later). Therapy is often delayed in practice because physicians make the mistake of waiting for the results of a scan or lumbar puncture before starting therapy.[11] The importance of administering antibiotics to patients with the acute meningitis syndrome within 30 minutes, *regardless of how far the diagnostic process has progressed*, cannot be overemphasized. Therapy can be modified later on the basis of the Gram stain or culture results. Rarely does a noninfectious process, such as subarachnoid hemorrhage, produce this syndrome.

Subacute Central Nervous System Infection Syndrome

Febrile illness associated with a somewhat more gradual progression of signs and symptoms of CNS involvement defines the subacute CNS infection syndrome. Headache can be mild or severe, and neck stiffness can be minimal or marked. However, patients should be oriented and clinically stable, as evidenced by a gradual (>24 to 48 hour) progression of symptoms. Although pyogenic organisms are frequently implicated, many cases are caused by nonpyogenic pathogens and noninfectious factors.

Herpes simplex encephalitis, brain abscess, and meningitis due to fungi, mycobacteria, or viruses may all produce moderate fever, worsening headache, and progressive impairment of higher integrative functions. On occasion, carcinomatous meningitis, brain tumor, and subarachnoid bleeding cause similar findings (see Table 60–2). To avoid inappropriate therapy and unnecessary hospitalization, one should carefully weigh the decision to institute antimicrobial agents. If pyogenic meningitis is still a possibility after evaluation, however, antimicrobial therapy should be given (see later).

The first priority in managing subacute CNS infection syndrome is "rapid diagnosis" versus the "rapid therapy" approach to acute meningitis syndrome. A physician should take 1 to 2 hours to carefully evaluate a patient and relevant laboratory data (Fig. 60–4). Peripheral blood granulocytosis (>10,000/mm^3), CSF pleocytosis (cell counts > 1000/mm^3), elevated CSF protein (>100 mg/dL), or decreased CSF glucose (<40 mg/dL) favor a bacterial etiology.

If the history and examination findings suggest a space-occupying lesion, lumbar puncture and even antimicrobial therapy can be safely delayed for 1 to 2 hours pending results of emergency CT or MRI scan. If longer delays are likely, empirical therapy before lumbar puncture may be preferred if a space-occupying lesion is a possibility. Other causes of subacute CNS infection syndrome are discussed later (see Brain Abscess and Viral Infections of the Central Nervous System).

Therapy of Pyogenic Meningitis

Pneumococci, meningococci, and rarely *H. influenzae* cause most cases of community-acquired bacterial meningitis in previously healthy adults.[12] Intravenous penicillin (18 to 24 million units/day) had traditionally been the treatment of choice. However, β-lactamase–positive *H. influenzae* and, more important, pneumococci that are intermediately (minimal inhibitory concentration ≥ 0.1 μg/mL) or highly (minimal inhibitory concentration > 1 μg/mL) resistant to penicillin have altered this approach. At least 15% to 20% of clinical isolates of *Streptococcus pneumoniae* in the United States are resistant to penicillin.[13] The extent to which penicillin-resistant pneumococci are resistant to cephalosporins, chloramphenicol, sulfonamides, and tetracyclines is highly variable. To date, vancomycin is active against virtually all pneumococci.

Initial therapy for most patients with bacterial meningitis

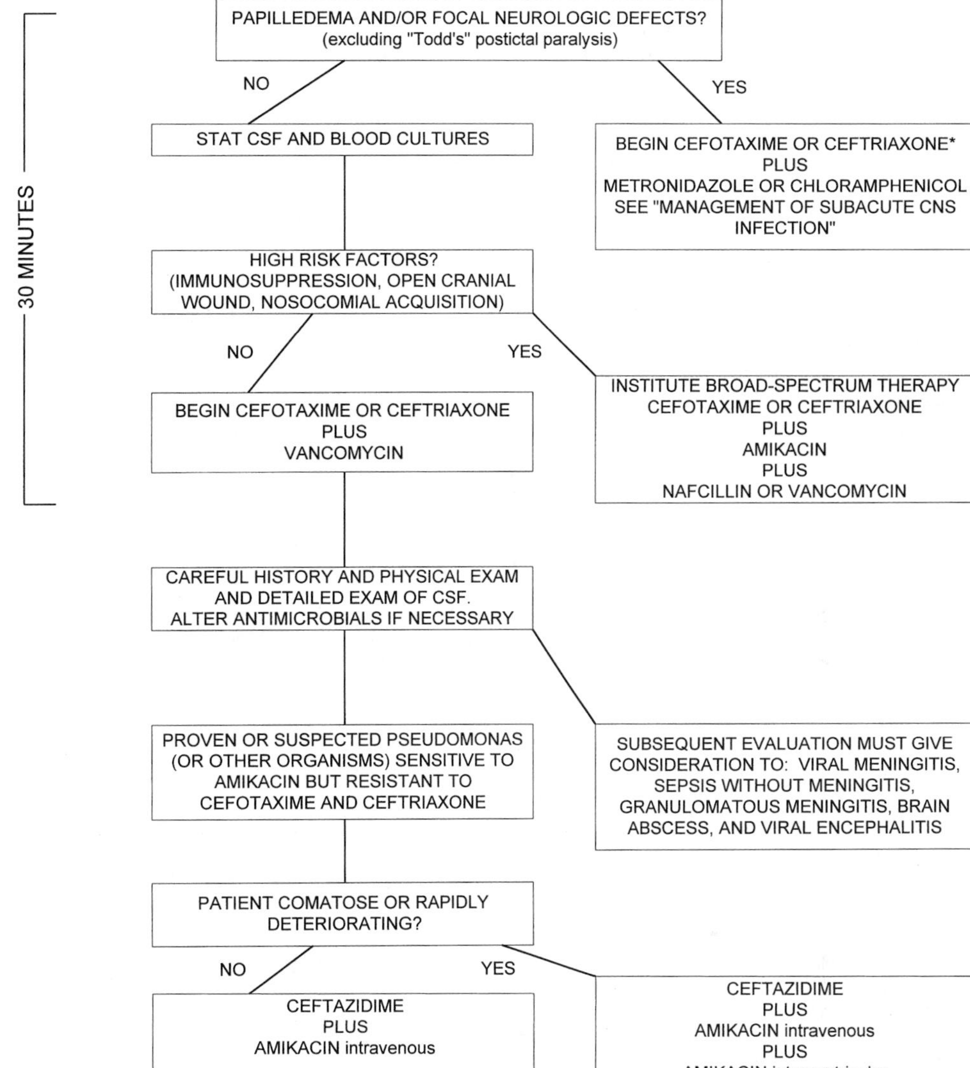

(Fulminant course, <48 hr, with fever, headache, usually with impaired sensorium and stiff neck)
30 MINUTES
PAPILLEDEMA AND/OR FOCAL NEUROLOGIC DEFECTS? (excluding "Todd's" postictal paralysis)
NO
YES
STAT CSF AND BLOOD CULTURES
BEGIN CEFOTAXIME OR CEFTRIAXONE* PLUS METRONIDAZOLE OR CHLORAMPHENICOL SEE "MANAGEMENT OF SUBACUTE CNS INFECTION"
HIGH RISK FACTORS? (IMMUNOSUPPRESSION, OPEN CRANIAL WOUND, NOSOCOMIAL ACQUISITION)
NO
YES
BEGIN CEFOTAXIME OR CEFTRIAXONE PLUS VANCOMYCIN
INSTITUTE BROAD-SPECTRUM THERAPY CEFOTAXIME OR CEFTRIAXONE PLUS AMIKACIN PLUS NAFCILLIN OR VANCOMYCIN
CAREFUL HISTORY AND PHYSICAL EXAM AND DETAILED EXAM OF CSF. ALTER ANTIMICROBIALS IF NECESSARY
PROVEN OR SUSPECTED PSEUDOMONAS (OR OTHER ORGANISMS) SENSITIVE TO AMIKACIN BUT RESISTANT TO CEFOTAXIME AND CEFTRIAXONE
SUBSEQUENT EVALUATION MUST GIVE CONSIDERATION TO: VIRAL MENINGITIS, SEPSIS WITHOUT MENINGITIS, GRANULOMATOUS MENINGITIS, BRAIN ABSCESS, AND VIRAL ENCEPHALITIS
PATIENT COMATOSE OR RAPIDLY DETERIORATING?
NO
YES
CEFTAZIDIME PLUS AMIKACIN intravenous (Consider AMIKACIN intralumbar)
CEFTAZIDIME PLUS AMIKACIN intravenous PLUS AMIKACIN intraventricular

Figure 60–3. Algorithm for the management of patients with the acute meningitis syndrome. See Table 60-3 for specific antimicrobial doses *(asterisk)*.

should include a third-generation cephalosporin, such as cefotaxime or ceftriaxone. These drugs are bactericidal against the common pathogens of acute meningitis and are adequate for most penicillin-resistant pneumococci. However, because some penicillin-resistant pneumococci are also resistant to cephalosporins, vancomycin should be administered concomitantly.[14] Vancomycin should not be used alone as initial therapy because of its marginal CNS penetration and poor activity against *H. influenzae* and meningococci.

Chloramphenicol, when used for high-level penicillin-resistant pneumococcal meningitis, has been associated with a high failure rate, even when the organisms appear to be susceptible to chloramphenicol in vitro.[15] Pneumococci are the most common cause of bacterial meningitis in the elderly, and these same considerations apply. However, gram-negative bacilli and *L. monocytogenes* are commonly implicated in elderly patients.[12] A wide spectrum of pathogens cause meningitis in immunosuppressed patients. On rare occasion, in patients with no immunologic defects, fungi, protozoa, and unusual bacteria may cause acute or subacute meningitis. After initiation of therapy, every effort should be made to identify the infecting pathogen.

Large systemic doses of third-generation cephalosporins (e.g., cefotaxime and ceftriaxone) are bactericidal against the common pathogens of bacterial meningitis (most pneumococci, meningococci, and all *H. influenzae*).[16] The third-generation cephalosporins are also effective in enteric gram-negative meningitis. *Escherichia coli, Klebsiella*, and other susceptible bacilli can be treated with these agents. A third-generation cephalosporin is indicated for patients who are relatively stable and infected with an enteric gram-negative organism presumed to be sensitive to the cephalosporins (see Fig. 60–3). Successful treatment of enteric gram-negative meningitis is associated with trough CSF antibiotic levels five to 10 times the minimal inhibitory concentration of the organism.[17] A third-generation cephalosporin plus vancomycin is not indicated for every case of bacterial meningitis. Moribund patients, patients with resistant organisms, or patients who do not respond to such therapy may require intraventricular aminoglycoside therapy (see Fig. 60–3).

The doses of antimicrobial agents used for CNS infections are presented in Table 60–3. Some CNS pathogens cannot be reliably treated with cefotaxime or ceftriaxone, and alternative therapy is presented in Table 60–4.

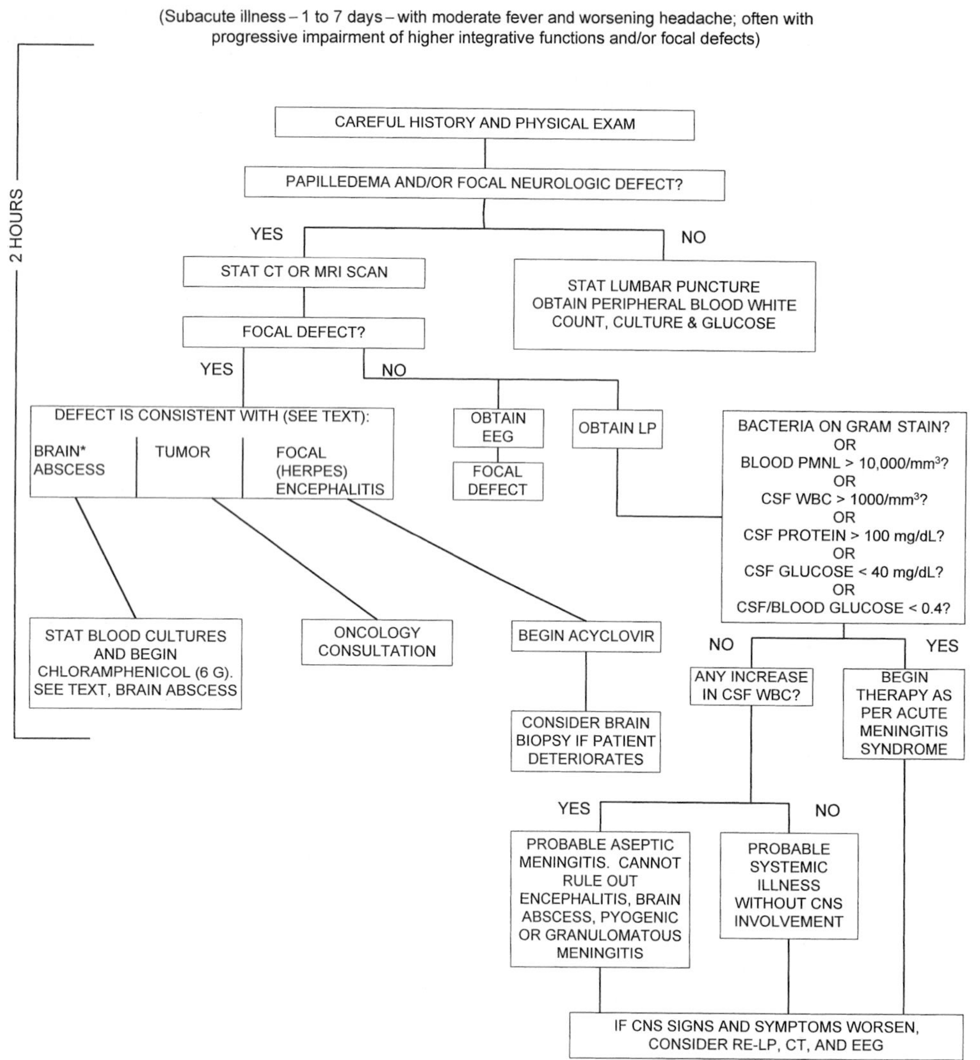

Figure 60–4. Algorithm for the management of patients with the subacute central nervous system (CNS) infection syndrome. If CT is not diagnostic for brain abscess, multiple antimicrobial therapy may be indicated pending further evaluation *(asterisk)*. CT = computed tomography; EEG = electroencephalogram; MRI = magnetic resonance imaging; PMNL = polymorphonuclear leukocyte; WBC = white blood cell; CSF = cerebrospinal fluid; RE-LP = repeat lumbar puncture.

The duration of therapy in bacterial meningitis varies with the pathogen and the clinical response. A normal host with pneumococcal or meningococcal meningitis is unlikely to experience relapse after clinical improvement, and appropriate antibiotics should be given for 7 days.[18] For pneumococcal and *H. influenzae* meningitis, 10 to 14 days of therapy are recommended.[14] Because antibiotic penetration into CSF falls as meningeal inflammation subsides, parenteral antibiotics are recommended for the entire course.

Abnormalities of the CSF (high protein level, high white blood cell count, and low glucose concentration) persist for days to weeks. Resolution of symptoms should serve as adequate evidence of success. In the patient who responds poorly to 48 hours of therapy, repeated lumbar puncture and head CT or MRI are indicated. Neither a scan nor repeated lumbar puncture is indicated for patients with pneumococcal or meningococcal meningitis who steadily improve with therapy. In contrast, the response to therapy in gram-negative enteric meningitis is less consistent. CSF cultures and Gram's stain should be monitored daily. After the CSF becomes sterile, an additional 7 days of aggressive antimicrobial therapy is warranted.

Adults with acute bacterial meningitis commonly have predisposing infections, including pneumonia, sinusitis, otitis, or endocarditis.[7] Therapy for meningitis usually treats the primary cause. Exceptions include endocarditis, which requires prolonged therapy with bactericidal antibiotics, and brain abscess, which may require surgical drainage or prolonged antimicrobial therapy.

Use of Corticosteroids

Much of the morbidity of bacterial meningitis is caused by the vigorous inflammatory response. Corticosteroids block inflammation, and animal studies clearly show that the addition of corticosteroids to antibacterial regimens improves survival. However, the role of corticosteroids for patients with pyogenic meningitis is controversial.

Four double-blind placebo-controlled studies of dexamethasone adjuvant therapy for children with acute bacterial meningitis showed benefits, including decreased neurologic sequelae (mostly in terms of hearing loss) and, in one study, improved survival.[19–21] However, most patients were infected with *H. influenzae*, now an unusual cause of meningitis in developed countries. In addition, corticosteroids may impair penetration of vancomycin into the CSF and the rate of killing of penicillin-resistant pneumococci.[22] Nevertheless, dexamethasone administration with the first dose of antibiotic (0.6 mg/kg/day intravenously in four divided doses for the first 4 days of antibiotic treatment) is occasionally used to treat children age 2 months and older who are at risk for *H. influenzae* meningitis (i.e., those not previously vaccinated against *H.*

TABLE 60–3. Dosages of Antimicrobial Drugs for Treatment of Central Nervous System Infection

Drug	Dosage (by Total Body Weight)	Usual Dosage (for 70-kg Adult)
Acyclovir	10 mg/kg IV every 8 hr	700 mg IV every 8 hr
Amikacin	15 mg/kg IV load, then 7.5 mg/kg every 12 hr*	1050 mg IV load, then 525 mg IV every 12 hr*
Intrathecal	0.1 mg · lb^{-1} · day^{-1}	15 mg/day
Intraventricular	0.1 mg · lb^{-1} · day^{-1}	15 mg/day
Ampicillin	30 mg/kg IV every 4 hr	2 g IV every 4 hr
Cefotaxime	30 mg/kg IV every 4 hr	2 g IV every 4 hr
Ceftazidime	30 mg/kg IV every 6 hr	2 g IV every 6 hr
Ceftriaxone	30 mg/kg IV every 12 hr	2 g IV every 12 hr
Chloramphenicol	15 mg/kg IV every 6 hr	1 g IV every 6 hr
Metronidazole	7.5 mg/kg IV every 6 hr	500 mg IV every 6 hr
Nafcillin	30 mg/kg IV every 4 hr	2 g IV every 4 hr
Penicillin G	60,000–70,000 units/kg IV every 4 hr	4–5 million units IV every 4 hr
Trimethoprim-sulfamethoxazole	5 mg/kg IV every 6 hr	350 mg IV every 6 hr†
Vancomycin	15–30 mg/kg IV every 12 hr	1–2 g IV every 12 hr*

*Adjust dose on the basis of serum levels.
†Dose indicates trimethoprim component.

influenzae), although this practice in becoming less common. Routine corticosteroid use for adults is not advised.[23]

Complications

Systemic complications may dominate the clinical course of acute bacterial meningitis. Forty per cent of patients with pneumococcal meningitis have concomitant sepsis. The sepsis is usually from an extra-CNS focus, such as pneumonia. Less commonly, sepsis represents seeding of the bloodstream from the infected meninges. Whether bacteremia precedes or follows meningeal infection, the sepsis demands immediate attention. General supportive measures are crucial. Other complications, such as aspiration of gastric contents, seizures, and gastrointestinal bleeding, must be monitored and prevented if possible.

When *Neisseria meningitidis* is causative, rhinorrhea or sore throat is often antecedent, followed by fever, chills, and a petechial rash. Failure to recognize a febrile rash as meningococcemia may allow evolution to necrotizing vasculitis with loss of extremities (Fig. 60–5) or death. Progression to acute meningitis syndrome is not inevitable, but patients often have CSF cultures positive for *N. meningitidis* even when signs and symptoms of direct CNS involvement are lacking. Physiologic doses of steroids may be necessary when fulminant meningococcemia is complicated by hypotension due to adrenal insufficiency.[24]

As inflammatory exudate fills the ventricles and subarachnoid space, impairment of cranial and spinal nerve roots, cerebral infarction and edema, hydrocephalus, and subdural effusion may occur. As many as 15% of patients experience impaired ocular movement, and 11% have hemiparesis or quadriparesis.[25] Fortunately, focal defects may resolve during recovery (Table 60–5).

Hydrocephalus can cause morbidity long after the infection has resolved. The availability of CT and MRI has improved management of this complication. Subdural effusions have been associated with *H. influenzae* meningitis in children; however, the importance of this complication and the need to aspirate such effusions are debatable. Cerebral infarction and edema have developed in the course of aggressive infection or delayed therapy.[26] Anecdotal reports suggest that high-dose steroids, specifically dexamethasone, may be lifesaving when intracranial pressure is markedly elevated.

Focal Central Nervous System Defects

Focal neurologic abnormalities and papilledema are unusual at presentation in pyogenic meningitis and suggest a focal lesion (see Figs. 60–3 and 60–4). Interpretation of CT, MRI, or electroencephalographic findings is central to treating such patients. Brain abscess, tumor, or herpetic encephalitis is best detected with this information (Table 60–6). The absence of papilledema or focal neurologic defects in a patient with headache, fever, and progressive impairment of higher integrative functions suggests that meningitis is more likely and that lumbar puncture is needed. Uncal herniation is extremely unlikely in such a patient, and it is hazardous to delay a diagnostic lumbar puncture should pyogenic meningitis be present.

TABLE 60–4. Bacterial Meningitis Pathogens Not Adequately Treated with Cefotaxime or Ceftriaxone

Organism	Antimicrobial Agent
Pseudomonas aeruginosa	Ceftazidime plus amikacin
Listeria monocytogenes	Trimethoprim-sulfamethoxazole or ampicillin
Staphylococcus aureus (methicillin susceptible)	Nafcillin
S. aureus (methicillin resistant)	Vancomycin
Enterobacter species (β-lactam–resistant strains)	Trimethoprim-sulfamethoxazole
Pneumococci (some high-level penicillin-resistant strains)	Vancomycin or imipenem

TABLE 60–5. Focal Neurologic Signs in Bacterial Meningitis

Early onset (defect is present at or shortly after presentation)
- Often accompanied by focal or generalized seizures
- Possibly related to meningeal vasculitis or cortical ischemia
- Usually reversible

Late onset (defect develops late in course, often as patient is otherwise recovering)
- Probably related to cortical vein thrombosis
- May be reversible

Persisting (present on presentation and worsens during therapy)
- Usually represents a major complication or mistaken diagnosis: brain abscess, herpes encephalitis, subdural empyema
- Often requires a major change in therapy

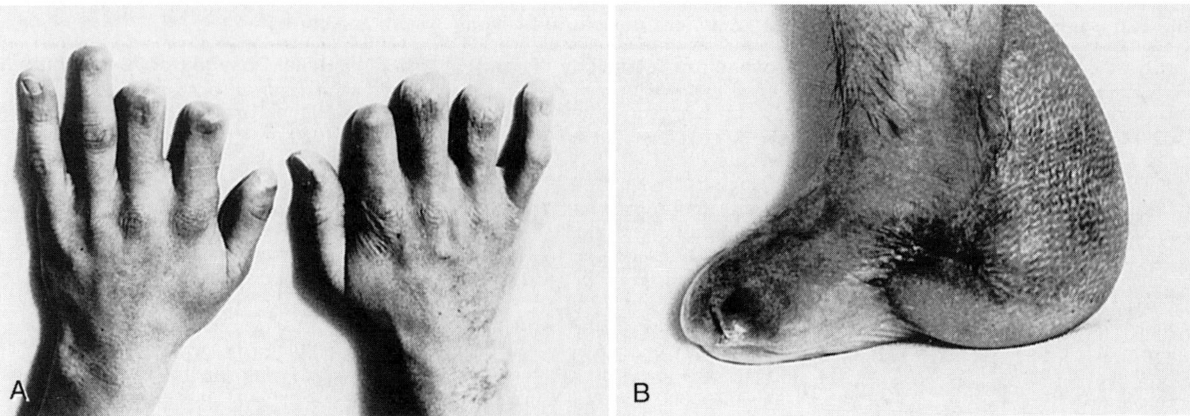

Figure 60–5. Extremities of the hands *(A)* and foot *(B)* in a 14-year-old boy who was observed by two physicians as his petechial rash progressed to "bruises" (purpura fulminans); the lesions were not recognized as the hallmarks of *Neisseria meningitidis*-induced sepsis. In addition to the loss of extremities caused by the necrotizing vasculitis of meningococcemia, signs and symptoms characteristic of the acute meningitis syndrome rapidly developed.

BRAIN ABSCESS

Pyogenic brain abscess, a localized suppurative infection of parenchymal CNS tissue, may involve any region from the cerebral cortex to the conus medullaris. Despite modern antibiotic therapy and refined surgical and radiographic techniques, mortality rates are approximately 15% to 25%. This poor prognosis is related to its relative infrequency and the technical difficulty of surgical intervention. Patients with altered sensoria on presentation clearly have a worse prognosis.[27] In most cases, CT or MRI provides sufficient information for optimal management. MRI is more sensitive for small or early lesions and better visualizes the cerebellum and brain stem.

Pathophysiology

A brain abscess begins as a localized area of parenchymal cellulitis (cerebritis) that evolves to necrosis and frank suppuration. The initial stage, characterized by vascular congestion, petechial hemorrhage, cerebral edema, and tissue softening, is demonstrable by MRI. As cerebritis progresses, CT findings become abnormal, revealing a capsule-like hyperemic zone surrounding the area of inflammation. In time, liquefaction results in frank abscess formation.

As the abscess matures, a dense capsule is formed. In relatively avascular areas of the brain, collagen formation is delayed. Once formed, however, the capsule resolves slowly. When necrosis is rapid and capsule formation delayed, as in the relatively avascular cerebral white matter, abscess rupture is more likely. In some cases, edema is the dominant process.

In the preantibiotic era, contiguous foci (middle ear, mastoids, and sinuses) caused most brain abscess. With the availability of antibiotics, however, such complications have become less common. An increasing proportion of cases is due to distant foci of infection, or they originate from unknown sites. With hematogenous seeding, abscesses tend to develop in the middle cerebral artery distribution. The etiologic pathogen relates to the route of infection (Table 60–7). The bacteria most often isolated from brain abscess are aerobic and anaerobic streptococci, although enteric gram-negative rods, staphylococci, pneumococci, and *Nocardia asteroides* may be pres-

TABLE 60–6. Differential Diagnosis of Central Nervous System Infection and Tumor

	Brain Abscess	Bacterial Meningitis	Herpetic Encephalitis	Brain Tumor
History				
Headache	Severe, often focal	Severe, generalized	Mild to severe	Absent to severe
Focal defect	Often	Occasional	Occasional	Usual
Progression	Days to weeks	Hours to days	Days	Days to months
Physical Examination				
Fever/degree	Usual/low-grade	Always/high	Usual/variable	Rare
Early focal signs	Often	Occasional	Occasional	Usual
Pressure signs	Often	Rare	Occasional	Often
Distal infection	Often	Often	Unrelated	Unrelated
CT or MRI Scan				
Focal	Always*	No	Occasional	Always
Ring effect/onset	Often/late†	—	No	Often/early

*May be negative or nonspecific during first 48 hours of illness.
†Development of abscess wall will be delayed by steroid therapy.
CT = computed tomography; MRI = magnetic resonance imaging.

TABLE 60–7. Brain Abscess

	Origin	Organism*	Incidence (% of Total)	Location
Contiguous foci (70%)	Middle ear	ANA and A streptococci, *Bacteroides fragilis,* A GNR	35%	Temporal lobe
	Mastoids	A GNR, *B. fragilis,* ANA and A streptococci	15%	Cerebellum
	Sinuses	ANA streptococci, *Bacteroides,* staphylococci, *Haemophilus,* pneumococcus	15%	Frontal lobe
	Trauma	Staphylococci, ANA bacteria	5%	Site of trauma
	Lungs	ANA streptococci, A GNR, *Nocardia*	10%	Occur at cortical junction along distribution of middle cerebral artery, involving frontal, parietal, and temporal lobes.
	Right-to-left shunts	Staphylococci, ANA and A streptococci	5%	
Distal foci (30%)	Abdominal infections	A and ANA GNR	5%	Abscesses are often multiple.
	Unknown sites	A and ANA streptococci	10%	

*Mixed infections are common.
ANA = anaerobic; A = aerobic; GNR = gram-negative rods.

ent. Fungi such as *Aspergillus* and protozoa such as amoebae can also be etiologic agents.[28-32]

Clinical Course

The variable signs and symptoms of brain abscess relate to variations in location, size, and rapidity of development. At one extreme, the course may span weeks, with few constitutional symptoms. In this setting, signs and symptoms of a space-occupying lesion predominate and neoplasm is the primary diagnostic concern. In contrast, a previously asymptomatic brain abscess may rupture into the subarachnoid space, causing death within hours. The differential diagnosis in this setting includes an acute cerebral vascular event and pyogenic meningitis. However, brain abscess usually progresses subacutely for 7 to 14 days.

Classic symptoms include excruciating headache, low-grade fever, and focal neurologic signs. Occasionally, a patient may have no symptoms referable to the CNS, and the absence of fever does not preclude the diagnosis.

Lumbar puncture may demonstrate increased cells and protein level and normal or decreased glucose concentration. However, organisms are identified in only 10% of cases. Because lumbar puncture may be life-threatening in the presence of an expanding brain abscess, this procedure should be avoided when a focal lesion is likely. This is particularly important because CSF parameters are nonspecific and CSF culture is rarely positive in the patient with brain abscess.

Parameningeal foci cause brain abscess as the inflammatory process erodes through bone and meningeal tissues (see Table 60–7). Chronic otitis, sinusitis, or postsurgical and post-traumatic dural defects in a patient with progressive neurologic deterioration strongly suggest brain abscess.

Bacterial pathogens also invade neural tissues via hematogenous spread. The presence of chronic extrameningeal suppurative foci or illicit intravenous drug use predisposes to brain abscess. Pulmonary filtration helps protect the host from hematogenous seeding of the brain. However, when cyanotic heart disease or pulmonary arteriovenous fistulas are present, brain abscesses may occur.[33] About one fifth of patients have no recognized source of infection, and delayed diagnosis in these cases may increase mortality. Brain abscesses associated with endocarditis are rare but, when present, are often multiple and small. Rarely, bacterial meningitis causes intracerebral abscess.

The CNS complications of brain abscess relate to both the inflammation and the space-occupying lesion. Nonspecific complications include aspiration, gastrointestinal bleeding, and general inanition. The specific signs and symptoms of brain abscess relate to the space-occupying effect and may offer the most easily recognizable clues; however, even these findings may be absent or impossible to differentiate clinically from other causes of space-occupying lesions. When surrounding edema is excessive, aggressive therapy with corticosteroids is warranted. If a brain abscess ruptures into the subarachnoid space or into a cerebral ventricle, the patient's condition will rapidly deteriorate.

Computed Tomography and Magnetic Resonance Imaging

CT and MRI techniques are particularly valuable in assessing brain abscesses. Changes in lesion size can be accurately followed from week to week. Neurosurgical intervention can be guided by assessment of proximity to vital neural structures. An expanding abscess may be aggressively drained; conversely, a stable or shrinking abscess can be assiduously observed.

CT scanning has some limitations, particularly in the early cerebritis stage. In addition, the cerebellum, brain stem, and spinal cord may not be well visualized, and CT may not detect lesions of 1.5 cm or smaller. For such lesions, MRI scan enhanced with intravenous gadolinium is more sensitive. However, most symptomatic brain abscesses are detectable by CT except for multiple, small abscesses associated with endocarditis. Persons thus affected may have major functional impairment but only nonspecific changes on CT.

Although CT and MRI may assess the maturity of the abscess and associated capsule, misinterpretation can occur. Because the vascularity of the cerebral white matter is modest in comparison to that of the gray matter, CT may erroneously suggest that capsule formation is lagging behind the inflammatory process in lesions involving the white matter. Steroid therapy may delay or even reverse CT findings by delaying true capsule formation.

Therapy

Combined antimicrobial therapy and surgical drainage constitute the classic management of pyogenic brain abscesses. The antimicrobial agents must cross the blood-brain barrier and should be administered for prolonged periods. Aspiration of the abscess is usually required to isolate the pathogens and to guide therapy. Positive cultures from blood or suppurative foci occasionally establish a presumptive etiologic diagnosis, allowing a preliminary therapeutic regimen to be instituted. Because neurologic status may change rapidly, frequent evaluation of patients is crucial.

Brain abscess can resolve with antimicrobial therapy alone, and the use of CT has encouraged continuation of medical therapy without surgery in patients who are stable and in whom the cause has been determined by appropriate cultures.[34] However, neurosurgical intervention is indicated (1) in patients who deteriorate because of the space-occupying effect, (2) for aspiration and culture to define specific antimicrobial therapies, and (3) for abscesses that do not respond to medical therapy.

Steroids should not be routinely employed. In patients with edema and neurologic deterioration, however, high-dose steroids are indicated.

VIRAL INFECTIONS OF THE CENTRAL NERVOUS SYSTEM

All components of the CNS are vulnerable to viral infection. The resultant clinical syndrome may be meningitis, encephalitis, or myelitis. Acute viral meningitis is manifested by meningeal irritation, CSF pleocytosis, and an uncomplicated clinical course. Impairment of higher integrative functions dominates viral encephalitis. Personality changes may occur, with irritability and inability to concentrate. Patients may also experience fever, persisting headache, nausea, and vomiting. As a result of parenchymal involvement, CNS function may deteriorate over several days through confusion, lethargy, somnolence, and coma. Systemic symptoms become more prominent as CNS dysfunction worsens. Meningismus may develop at any point during viral encephalitis or may remain absent.

Pathophysiology

Viruses most commonly enter the CNS hematogenously. Virus may initially traverse mucous membranes (e.g., enteroviruses) or be inoculated into subcutaneous tissues (e.g., arthropod-borne viruses). After local replication within extraneural tissues, sustained viremia occurs. Alternatively, virus may gain access to the CNS by neuronal spread, as when rabies virus spreads along peripheral nerves into the CNS. The olfactory tracts may provide a route of entry for herpes simplex virus.[35]

Individual viruses demonstrate affinities for different areas of the CNS. Enteroviruses and mumps viruses usually involve the ependyma and tissues of the subarachnoid space, producing meningeal irritation. In contrast, arthropod-borne and rabies viruses almost always involve the parenchyma and cause encephalitis. In older children and adults, herpes simplex virus type 1 characteristically causes temporal lobe encephalitis, whereas herpes simplex virus type 2 more typically causes meningitis.[35] Such affinities are not absolute. For example, enteroviruses may on rare occasions cause encephalitis.

Acute Viral Meningitis

Many viruses cause meningitis. A pathogen usually cannot be isolated from adults with presumed viral meningitis, and the term *aseptic meningitis* describes this syndrome. Acute viral meningitis is common in neonates and young adults but is unusual after age 40 years.

Non-neonatal acute viral meningitis typically develops during the summer or fall in otherwise healthy young adults. Several days of chills, myalgias, and malaise are followed by excruciating headache, photophobia, stiff neck, nausea, and vomiting. Lumbar puncture reveals clear fluid with normal glucose concentration, mildly elevated protein level, and lymphocytic pleocytosis. The illness resolves without sequela. The meningeal symptoms last 7 to 10 days, with malaise persisting for as long as 6 weeks. Differentiation from bacterial or fungal infection is the primary goal of management (Fig. 60–6). In children, a CSF lactate level above 30 mg/dL, although not specific for bacterial meningitis, is unusual during viral meningitis and may be of some diagnostic use.[36, 37] Therapy is entirely symptomatic.

Viral Encephalitis

A host of viral agents infect the parenchyma of the brain or spinal cord to produce encephalitis or myelitis, respectively. Both diseases impair neurologic function and may cause irreversible neuronal injury. Viral encephalitis is typically an acute febrile illness associated with headache, an altered level of consciousness disproportionate to systemic illness, behavioral or speech disturbances, and often neurologic signs such as seizures or hemiparesis. In contrast, viral myelitis spares higher integrative functions.

Noninfectious syndromes may mimic viral encephalitis and myelitis, and virtually any component of the CNS may be involved. Specific antiviral therapy is available for few causes of encephalitis. When cerebral or spinal cord edema compromises CNS function, high-dose corticosteroids are indicated.

Herpes Encephalitis

Unlike most viral infections, herpes simplex encephalitis is amenable to antiviral therapy. This illness may occur at any age and tends to produce a rapidly devastating course. Successful treatment requires prompt administration of intravenous acyclovir. The mortality of documented untreated infections may exceed 70%, although mild or asymptomatic cases may occur. The morbidity from surrounding cerebral edema may be considerable.

Herpes simplex encephalitis involves the temporal lobes in the majority of cases. This localization causes aphasia, anosmia, temporal lobe seizures, and focal neurologic defects. Such findings, often with a severe prodromal headache and progressing to confusion, lethargy, or coma, suggest the diagnosis. Electroencephalography is superior to CT in detecting localization of the infection.[9] In some cases, MRI findings are abnormal when electroencephalographic and CT findings are not diagnostic. Unfortunately, a wide range of signs and symptoms may occur. A CSF polymerase chain reaction test for herpes simplex virus is positive in most cases and strongly suggests the diagnosis.[38] Serology alone is not diagnostic, and CSF may be normal or nonspecifically abnormal. A rising titer of antibodies in the CSF may confirm the diagnosis but does not appear until 1 week or more into the illness. Empirical therapy with acyclovir is often used in critically ill patients with encephalitis and evidence of focal CNS involvement. Brain biopsy with culture is rarely indicated except when response to acyclovir is not prompt. A full 10-day course of antiviral therapy should be administered if herpes simplex encephalitis is suspected.[39]

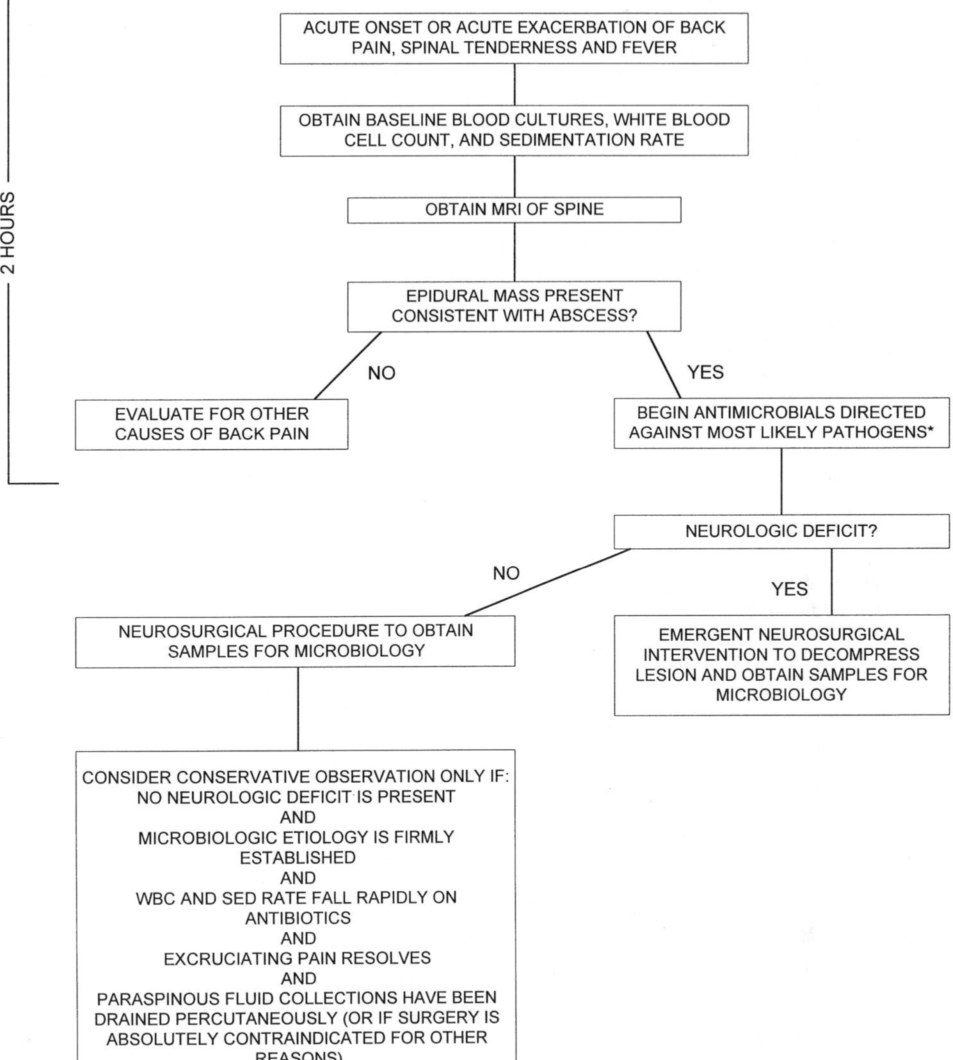

Figure 60–6. Algorithm for the management of patients with the spinal cord epidural abscess syndrome. If MRI cannot be performed, myelogram (the lateral cervical approach may be required), high-contrast CT, or CT-myelography may be an acceptable alternative to localize an epidural abscess. If abscess drainage can be performed promptly, antimicrobial drugs may be withheld until specimens for microbiologic analysis are obtained; they can then be immediately administered in the operating room or radiology suite *(asterisk)*.

Central Nervous System Infection and the AIDS Patient

CNS dysfunction is common in patients with the acquired immunodeficiency syndrome (AIDS). Neurologic disease may be a result of direct CNS involvement by many pathogens. CT or MRI and lumbar puncture are indicated for any patient with AIDS with significant headache or altered mental status, even when CNS symptoms do not dominate the picture. Because mass lesions are prevalent, lumbar puncture should generally be deferred until after CT or MRI. Common mass lesions in AIDS are toxoplasmosis, lymphoma, and progressive multifocal leukoencephalopathy. Enhancement after the administration of an intravenous contrast agent favors toxoplasmosis or lymphoma and makes progressive multifocal leukoencephalopathy, at present untreatable, unlikely.

Most patients with toxoplasmosis have detectable serum antibodies to *Toxoplasma gondii*, sometimes at low titer, and a negative test response for serum antibody makes the diagnosis much less likely. Laboratories that assay *Toxoplasma* antibody by serial dilution should use an initial serum dilution of 1:2 or less. Toxoplasmosis usually responds dramatically to appropriate antimicrobials, although lifelong therapy may be necessary to prevent relapse. For contrast-enhancing CNS mass lesions, positron emission tomography often differentiates CNS lymphoma from toxoplasmosis and other lesions in patients with advanced AIDS.[40]

Cryptococcal meningitis is also common in AIDS. Almost all patients with AIDS with cryptococcal meningitis have detectable cryptococcal antigen in both serum and CSF, often at high titer (e.g., >1:100,000). The optimal therapy for cryptococcal meningitis in AIDS is evolving. In most cases, initial therapy should include both amphotericin B and 5-flucytosine.

PARADURAL ABSCESS

The epidural space is between the dura and the bony structures of the skull and vertebral column; the subdural space is between the subarachnoid membrane and the dura (see Fig. 60–2). Unlike the subarachnoid space, the paradural tissues are only potential spaces, with the arachnoid membrane and the dura resisting the spread of infection across their surfaces.

Although subdural abscesses are more common within the cranium and epidural abscesses within the vertebral column, the causes, pathophysiology, and therapies are similar. These abscesses usually develop from a contiguous infection, surgery, or trauma.

In the skull, the epidural tissues are dense and epidural abscess is unusual. The subarachnoid membrane is less adherent to the dura, making the subdural space the more likely site of infection. The reverse is true in the vertebral column, where a thin layer of fat and blood vessels separate the dura from the vertebral bony structures. Infection here is more likely to involve the epidural space. Once established, infection may dissect within the epidural space for considerable distances.

Cranial subdural empyema may be clinically indistinguishable from a brain abscess. Subdural abscess is usually related to infection of the paranasal sinuses and, less commonly, to the ears or mastoids.[41] Trauma, surgical intervention, or hematogenous sources cause the remaining cases. Organisms common to sinusitis, including nonhemolytic streptococci, pneumococci, *Haemophilus*, anaerobes, and staphylococci, cause most infections. Gram-negative enteric bacilli may be associated with middle ear and mastoid infection.

An epidural abscess of the vertebral column classically progresses rapidly from spinal ache to paralysis.[42] Although most such abscesses are caused by *Staphylococcus aureus*, unusual pathogens such as *Pseudomonas* have been frequently recognized in immunosuppressed patients and illicit drug users. Trauma or surgery of the vertebral column is a recognized cause of epidural abscess, and various organisms have been noted in this setting. Although most cases are community acquired, approximately one sixth occur postoperatively.

Paradural abscesses tend to evolve rapidly, often producing irreversible damage to underlying neural structures. Antibiotics alone are rarely an option, and immediate neurosurgical drainage remains the mainstay of therapy. CT has greatly aided the management of subdural cranial abscess.

Spinal Epidural Abscess Syndrome

The spinal epidural abscess syndrome usually begins with localized severe spinal pain. Higher integrative functions generally remain intact; systemic manifestations are rarely severe enough to cause cortical dysfunction. Symptoms usually progress through four clinical phases: spinal ache, nerve root pain, radicular weakness, and paralysis. Back pain with fever, focal tenderness, and sensory or motor deficits strongly suggests this disease. The neck may be stiff, and a source of hematogenous seeding may be identified in three fourths of patients.

The rapidity of diagnosis depends on the severity of the signs and symptoms (see Fig. 60–6). The diagnostic study of choice is MRI, which defines cord compression and the presence and extent of abscess, identifies drainable paraspinal fluid collections, and diagnoses concomitant vertebral osteomyelitis. Other procedures, such as myelography and CT scanning, may be used if MRI cannot be done. Emergency neurosurgical intervention is generally considered mandatory for this infection, both to obtain tissue for microbiology and for decompression. Some patients have been successfully treated with antibiotics alone, without surgical intervention. Nonsurgical management might be considered if, on frequent examination, weakness does not develop in the patient receiving antibiotic therapy; if severe pain does not persist; and if fever, peripheral white blood cell count, and sedimentation rate all decline on therapy.[43, 44] Unfortunately, sudden neurologic impairment develops in some patients even weeks into conservative therapy, presumably because of vascular compromise of the cord.

Patients with neurologic defects require a more aggressive approach to management. Frequent neurologic examinations are mandatory for a patient with fever and recent severe back pain. The neurologic deficit may initially be limited to a loss of pain sensation in the perianal region (second sacral dermatome). Weakness indicates the need for immediate neurosurgical consultation and MRI. If myelography is performed, CSF should be obtained for examination.

Degenerative disease and metastatic tumor may mimic epidural abscess, especially if fever is present. A metastatic tumor of the spinal cord can rapidly produce severe neurologic deficits, and a history of malignant disease may be suggestive. Metastatic tumors are often best treated with steroids and radiotherapy. If fever cannot be easily attributed to another site of infection or inflammation, MRI will usually distinguish among degenerative spinal disease, metastatic tumor, and epidural abscess. In some cases, exploratory surgery may be necessary for diagnosis. Other considerations include transverse myelitis or hematoma.

Spinal epidural abscess demands prompt antimicrobial therapy to minimize residual weakness or paralysis. Community-acquired abscesses are usually due to *S. aureus* and should be treated with nafcillin. If methicillin-resistant staphylococci are prevalent, vancomycin should be substituted. Recent urinary tract infection, decubitus ulcers, or vertebral surgery suggests the presence of gram-negative bacilli, and a third-generation cephalosporin, with or without an aminoglycoside, should be added. Treatment may be modified when culture results are available.

SEPSIS SYNDROME

Acutely ill patients with the sepsis syndrome experience CNS dysfunction late in the course of illness. Gram-negative sepsis frequently produces this syndrome, and multiple organ failure may occur. Patients are not always observed early in the illness, and at presentation, signs and symptoms of CNS disease may dominate the illness (Fig. 60–7).

During treatment, general supportive measures take precedence over CNS concerns. After a brief assessment, general

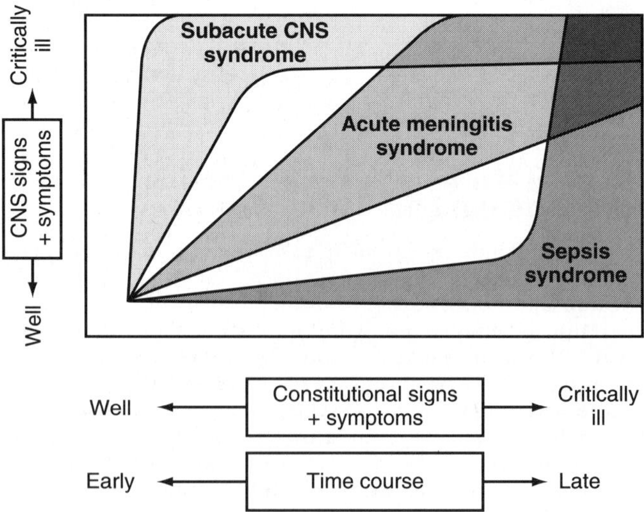

Figure 60–7. Graphic representation of the clinical presentations of the subacute central nervous system (CNS) infection syndrome, the acute meningitis syndrome, and the sepsis syndrome. On the vertical axis is the spectrum of CNS signs and symptoms (e.g., loss of higher integrative functions or of focal sensory or motor deficits). On the horizontal axis are the spectrum of constitutional symptoms (e.g., fever and malaise) and the time course of the different syndromes. SED = sedimentation; WBC = white blood cell; MRI = magnetic resonance imaging.

life-support measures should correct hypotension, hypoxia, and anuria. As soon as easily accessible body fluid specimens are obtained for culture, broad-spectrum antimicrobial agents should be administered. At this point, a history should be carefully taken and physical examination performed and the patient treated as outlined for subacute CNS infection syndrome (see Fig. 60-4). Delays in directly assessing the CNS are justifiable only when the history has been adequate to document that a clear-cut systemic illness preceded the onset of CNS symptoms and signs. Otherwise, a more aggressive use of lumbar puncture and CT or MRI is warranted (see Figs. 60-3 and 60-4).

SUMMARY

Acute infection of the CNS may warrant drastic therapeutic maneuvers. Because the four major syndromes of CNS infection (i.e., acute meningitis syndrome, subacute CNS infection syndrome, spinal epidural abscess syndrome, and sepsis syndrome) differ in signs and symptoms as well as in approaches to definitive diagnosis and therapy, it is important to distinguish among them. Moreover, diverse infectious and noninfectious causes may produce similar syndromes in the CNS. For therapy to be effective, it must be instituted within minutes to hours of the initial evaluation. Thus, in the practice of critical care medicine involving CNS disease, the physician must carefully coordinate therapy and diagnosis to offer the earliest possible therapy for all likely disease processes while efficiently working to identify the specific disease process.

References

1. Mount LA: Congenital dermal sinuses. JAMA 1949; 139:1263.
2. Simberkoff MS, Moldover NH, Rahal JJ Jr: Absence of detectable bactericidal and opsonic activities in normal and infected human cerebrospinal fluids. J Lab Clin Med 1980; 95:362.
3. Tunkel AR, Scheld WM: Pathogenesis and pathophysiology of bacterial meningitis. Clin Microbiol Rev 1993; 6:118.
4. Lepper MH, Dowling HF: Treatment of pneumococcal meningitis with penicillin compared with penicillin plus aureomycin. Arch Intern Med 1951; 88:489.
5. Rahal JJ Jr, Simberkoff MS: Bactericidal and bacteriostatic action of chloramphenicol against meningeal pathogens. Antimicrob Agents Chemother 1976; 10:322.
6. Baldwin LN, Henderson A, Thomas P, et al: Acute bacterial meningitis in young adults mistaken for substance abuse. Br Med J 1993; 306:775.
7. Durand ML, Calderwood SB, Weber DJ, et al: Acute bacterial meningitis: A review of 493 episodes. N Engl J Med 1993; 328:21.
8. Carpenter RR, Petersdorf RG: The clinical spectrum of bacterial meningitis. Am J Med 1962; 33:262.
9. Whitley RJ, Soong S, Linneman C Jr, et al: Herpes simplex encephalitis. JAMA 1982; 247:317.
10. Whitley RJ, Alford CA, Hirsch MS, et al: Vidarabine versus acyclovir therapy in herpes simplex encephalitis. N Engl J Med 1986; 314:144.
11. Talan DA, Guterman JJ, Overturf GD, et al: Analysis of emergency department management of suspected bacterial meningitis. Ann Emerg Med 1989; 18:856.
12. Wenger JD, Hightower AW, Facklam RR, et al: Bacterial meningitis in the United States, 1986: Report of a multistate surveillance study. J Infect Dis 1990; 162:1316.
13. Bradley JS, Scheld WM: The challenge of penicillin-resistant *Streptococcus pneumoniae* meningitis: Current antibiotic therapy in the 1990s. Clin Infect Dis 1997; 24:S213.
14. Quagliarello VJ, Scheld WM: Treatment of bacterial meningitis. N Engl J Med 1997; 336:708.
15. Friedland IR, Klugman KP: Failure of chloramphenicol therapy in penicillin-resistant pneumococcal meningitis. Lancet 1992; 339:405.
16. Congeni BL: Comparison of ceftriaxone and traditional therapy of bacterial meningitis. Antimicrob Agents Chemother 1984; 25:40.
17. Wright PF, Kaiser AB, Bowman CM, et al: The pharmacokinetics and efficacy of an aminoglycoside administered into the cerebral ventricles in neonates: Implications for further evaluation of this route of therapy in meningitis. J Infect Dis 1981; 143:141.
18. Lin T-Y, Chrane DF, Nelson JD, McCracken GH: Seven days of ceftriaxone therapy is as effective as ten days' treatment for bacterial meningitis. JAMA 1985; 253:3559.
19. Lebel MH, Freij BJ, Syrogiannopoulos GA, et al: Dexamethasone therapy for bacterial meningitis—results of two double-blind, placebo-controlled trials. N Engl J Med 1998; 319:964.
20. Girgis NI, Farid Z, Mikhail IA, et al: Dexamethasone treatment for bacterial meningitis in children and adults. Pediatr Infect Dis J 1989; 8:848.
21. Odio CM, Faingezicht I, Paris M, et al: The beneficial effects of early dexamethasone administration in infants and children with bacterial meningitis. N Engl J Med 1991; 324:1525.
22. Paris MM, Hickey SM, Uscher MI, Shelton S, Olsen KD, McCracken GH: Effect of dexamethasone on therapy of experimental penicillin- and cephalosporin-resistant pneumococcal meningitis. Antimicrob Agents Chemother 1994; 38:1320.
23. Townsend GC, Scheld WM: The use of corticosteroids in the management of bacterial meningitis in adults. J Antimicrob Chemother 1996; 37:1051.
24. Boswirth DC: Reversible adrenocortical insufficiency in fulminant meningococcemia. Arch Intern Med 1979; 139:823.
25. Dodge PR, Swartz MN: Bacterial meningitis—a review of selected aspects. N Engl J Med 1961; 272:954.
26. Pfister HW, Feiden W, Einhaupl KM: Spectrum of complications during bacterial meningitis in adults. Results of a prospective clinical study. Arch Neurol 1993; 50:575.
27. Seydoux C, Francioli P: Bacterial brain abscesses: Factors influencing mortality and sequelae. Clin Infect Dis 1992; 15:394.
28. Garfield J: Management of supratentorial intracranial abscess: A review of 200 cases. Br Med J 1969; 2:7.
29. Brewer NS, MacCarty CS, Wellman WE: Brain abscess: A review of recent experience. Ann Intern Med 1975; 82:571.
30. Dreissen JJR, van Alphen HAM: Brain abscess and subdural empyema. J Neurol Neurosurg Psychiatry 1976; 39:481.
31. Jefferson AA, Keogh AJ: Intracranial abscesses: A review of treated patients over 20 years. Q J Med 1977; 46:389.
32. Fischbein CA, Rosenthal A, Fischer EG, et al: Risk factors for brain abscess in patients with congenital heart disease. Am J Cardiol 1974; 34:97.
33. Press OW, Ramsey PG: Central nervous system infections associated with hereditary hemorrhagic telangectasia. Am J Med 1984; 77:86.
34. Boom WH, Tuazon CU: Successful treatment of multiple brain abscesses with antibiotics alone. Rev Infect Dis 1985; 7:189.
35. Whitley RJ: Viral encephalitis. N Engl J Med 1990; 323:242.
36. Bland RD, Lister RC, Ries JP: Cerebrospinal fluid lactic acid level and pH in meningitis. Dis Child 1974; 128:151.
37. Jordan GW, Statland B, Halsted C: CSF lactate in diseases of the CNS. Arch Intern Med 1983; 143:85.
38. Anderson NE, Powell KF, Croxson MC: A polymerase chain reaction assay of cerebrospinal fluid in patients with suspected herpes simplex encephalitis. J Neurol Neurosurg Psychiatry 1993; 56:520.
39. Landry ML, Booss J, Hsiung GD: Duration of vidarabine therapy in biopsy-negative herpes simplex encephalitis. JAMA 1982; 247:332.
40. Pierce MA, Johnson MDJ, Maciunas RJ, et al: Evaluating contrast-enhancing brain lesions in patients with AIDS by using positron emission tomography. Ann Intern Med 1995; 123:594.
41. Kaufman DM, Miller MH, Steigbigel NH: Subdural empyema: Analysis of 17 recent cases and review of the literature. Medicine (Baltimore) 1975; 54:485.
42. Baker AS, Ojemann RG, Swartz MN, et al: Spinal epidural abscess. N Engl J Med 1975; 293:463.
43. Wheeler D, Keiser P, Rigamonti D, Keay S: Medical management of spinal epidural abscesses—case report and review. Clin Infect Dis 1992; 15:22.
44. Baker AS, Ojemann RG, Baker RA: Editorial response to Wheeler et al. To decompress or not to decompress—spinal epidural abscess. Clin Infect Dis 1992; 15:28.

61

Pneumonia in the Immunosuppressed Patient

David L. Paterson, MBBS, FRACP • Nina Singh, MD

Pneumonia is a significant cause of morbidity and mortality in immunosuppressed patients. It is the most common reason for immunosuppressed patients to be managed in intensive care units (ICUs). The incidence of pneumonia in immunosuppressed populations varies, from 15% in solid-organ transplant recipients to greater than 50% in patients with advanced human immunodeficiency virus (HIV) infection.[1] Mortality exceeds 90% for specific infections in some groups; however, early diagnosis and institution of appropriate antimicrobial therapy, especially when immunosuppression can be reduced, can improve outcome significantly.

This chapter outlines the normal host defenses against pneumonia and how they are reduced in immunosuppressive conditions. The epidemiology, diagnostic approach, and management of common presentations of pneumonia in immunosuppressed patients is also discussed.

NORMAL HOST DEFENSES AGAINST PNEUMONIA

The lungs have an immense and intense interaction with the outside environment. A vast array of defenses protect the lungs from invading pathogens in the course of this exposure. At a most basic level, mechanical defenses remove the bulk of potentially harmful agents from the lungs. Aerodynamic filtration and impaction of large particulates (>10 μm) by the nasopharynx, mucociliary clearance, and coughing are the principal means of mechanical defense. Only particles smaller than 3 μm are deposited on the alveolar surface. In the alveoli, defenses take three forms.

First, resident alveolar defense mechanisms are the primary line of defense against alveolar invasion. Extracellular surfactant has antibacterial activity against staphylococci and some gram-negative bacilli and fungi.[2] Alveolar macrophages are the resident cellular defenders of the lung. Derived from monocyte precursor cells and differentiated in the lungs, they are involved in the clearance of particulates, macromolecular debris, and organisms from the lung's epithelial surfaces. To do this, the macrophage must recognize the foreign material and then destroy it. The recognition process can be nonspecific, but more often it is related to a specific antibody or complement fraction. Phagocytosis follows recognition of the material. If it is an organism that is engulfed, killing takes place within a phagolysosome by way of oxidative and nonoxidative mechanisms. Oxidative mechanisms in alveolar macrophages can kill staphylococci but not gram-negative bacilli or *Cryptococcus* or *Toxoplasma* organisms. Nonoxidative mechanisms include use of proteases, lysozyme, and defensins (broad-spectrum cytotoxic peptides), among other agents.

Second, an inflammatory response is necessary for effective clearance of most organisms. Although alveolar macrophages are important, if the microbial burden is large or the microbes are particularly virulent, a dual phagocytic system involving polymorphonuclear neutrophils (PMNs) from the systemic vasculature is crucial. Important chemotaxins involved in attracting PMNs include the complement 5 molecule and its fragments, leukotriene B_4 and numerous chemotactic cytokines, including interleukin-8 (IL-8). Directed migration of the PMNs into the alveolar space is the end result of a complex cytokine-mediated process involving endothelial cells, cell adhesion molecules, alveolar epithelial cells, and mononuclear phagocytes.

Third, specific pulmonary immune responses are essential for defending the lung against pathogens such as virulent encapsulated bacteria, viruses, and intracellular organisms that survive inside alveolar macrophages, such as mycobacteria and fungi. Antigen-specific T and B lymphocytes need to proliferate and differentiate to hold in check such organisms. An early event in this process is activation of T lymphocytes,[3] which requires interaction between the T cell and an antigen-presenting cell (APC), a cell that can present the antigen on its surface in association with the major histocompatibility complex (MHC). Alveolar macrophages are ineffective antigen-presenting cells; dendritic cells in the interstitium, alveolar septum, and throughout the columnar epithelium of the bronchi are the major antigen-presenting cells of the lung. Activated CD4 and CD8 T lymphocytes have key roles in pulmonary defenses against pathogens, particularly mycobacteria, fungi, and viruses. They produce high levels of interferon-gamma, granulocyte-macrophage colony stimulating factor, and tumor necrosis factor, which recruit and activate monocytes from the circulation. Activated CD8 cytotoxic T lymphocytes can lyse virus-infected cells. CD4 T lymphocytes contribute to the regulation of B cell expansion and differentiation. After migrating from the bone marrow, B lymphocytes differentiate in the lung to mature antibody-producing plasma cells. Antibody gains access to the alveoli, where it activates complement, neutralizes pathogens and their toxins, and functions as opsonins to enhance macrophage recognition and ingestion of extracellular pathogens.

Before leaving the topic of host defenses, we must point out that in some instances pneumonia is an immune-mediated condition. For example, evidence from animal and limited human studies suggest that replication of cytomegalovirus (CMV) *per se* in the lung is unrelated to the development of pathologic effects. Rather, a host immune response is required for induction of pneumonia. CMV may be harbored in the lungs of patients with advanced HIV infection without producing pneumonitis, possibly because these patients cannot mount a pathogenic T cell response. In contrast, in allogeneic-bone marrow transplant recipients, the pneumonia may be due to uncontrolled accumulation and recruitment of host T cells in the lungs.[4]

IMMUNOSUPPRESSIVE CONDITIONS AS THEY AFFECT HOST DEFENSES

Immunosuppression can be broadly defined as a state in which the response of the host to a foreign antigen is subnormal. Numerically the most common groups with immunosuppression include (1) patients with HIV infection, (2) patients with a hematologic malignancy or solid tumor receiving chemotherapy, (3) transplant recipients, and (4) patients with an autoimmune disorder receiving corticosteroids, methotrexate, or other immunosuppressive drugs. Each of these immunosuppressive states has an adverse effect on the host defenses against pneumonia described earlier (Table 61–1).

Rare causes of immunosuppression include the congenital (primary) immunodeficiencies. These conditions usually produce specific defects in the host's defenses against pneumonia (Table 61–2). Such defects are relatively "pure," and as a result, limited classes of organisms are susceptible. For example, Bruton's X-linked agammaglobulinemia is associated with a block in the normal maturation of immunoglobulin-producing

TABLE 61–1. Host Defenses Against Pneumonia and Examples of Their Compromise by Immunosuppressive Conditions

Host Defense	Defect	Consequence of Defect
Mechanical Defense		
Nasopharyngeal filtration	Intubation of the trachea	Aspiration and subsequent infection with mouth or stomach flora
Mucociliary clearance	Poor nutrition leading to impaired integrity of mucosal epithelial cells	Bacterial and fungal colonization of lower respiratory tract
Cough reflex	Altered neurologic function leading to diminished cough	Bacterial and fungal colonization of lower respiratory tract; *Legionella* infection
Epithelial barriers	Mechanical disruption by invasive procedures	Bacterial and fungal colonization of lower respiratory tract and skin
Alveolar Defense		
Alveolar macrophages	Disrupted function induced by corticosteroids and other immunosuppressive drugs	Propensity for intracellular microbes; poor containment of mycobacteria
Inflammatory Response		
Polymorphonuclear neutrophils	Diminished number because of cytotoxic chemotherapy or marrow aplasia/ invasion	Infection with gram-negative bacilli or *Aspergillus*
Specific T and B Cell Immune Responses		
CD4+ T lymphocytes	Diminished number due to HIV infection	Infection with *Pneumocystis carinii,* mycobacteria, fungi, herpesviruses
B lymphocytes	Diminished function due to multiple myeloma, CLL, or hypogammaglobulinemia	Infection with *Streptococcus pneumoniae,* or *Haemophilus influenzae*

HIV = human immunodeficiency virus; CLL = chronic lymphocytic leukemia.

B cells that results in the absence of circulating mature B cells, plasma cells, and serum immunoglobulin. It is not surprising, therefore, that organisms that are normally dealt with by immunoglobulin, such as *Streptococcus pneumoniae* and *Haemophilus influenzae,* are common in patients with agammaglobulinemia.

The etiology of pneumonia in patients with acquired immunosuppression may also be predicted because of well-described patterns observed with known defects induced in the host defense. For example, patients with recent-onset neutropenia are likely to be infected with gram-negative bacilli (typically *Pseudomonas aeruginosa*), and patients with HIV and a CD4 count just under 200 cells/mm^3 are likely to have *Pneumocystis carinii* pneumonia. The risk of infection in immunosuppressed patients depends not only on the type of immunosuppression but also on its intensity and duration. The incidence and severity of infection in neutropenic patients are inversely proportional to the absolute neutrophil count.[5] Gram-negative bacterial infections are uncommon when the absolute neutrophil count is above 500 cells/mm^3 then begin to rise in frequency when the neutrophil count falls below 500 cells; and they are most prevalent as the absolute neutrophil count approaches zero. The duration of neutropenia is also important; patients with prolonged neutropenia are more likely to have invasive aspergillosis. With HIV infection, the likelihood of opportunistic infection is inversely proportional to CD4 lymphocyte counts. It is now known that plasma viral load measurements independently predict outcome of HIV infection.[6–8]

A specific time line for pulmonary infection can be constructed for each type of transplant recipient. A similar plot can be constructed for patients with HIV infection, based on the CD4 cell count. Such illustrations can be extraordinarily useful for determining the likelihood of various causes of pneumonia in the immunosuppressed host (Tables 61-3 to 61-5).

Unfortunately, it would be simplistic to believe that acquired immunosuppression always results in a predictable narrow spectrum of disease. Many immunosuppressed patients have multiple types of immunosuppression. For example, patients with advanced HIV infection may have T lymphocyte depletion and B lymphocyte dysfunction. In addition, they may be neutropenic as a result of zidovudine and have poor nutritional status as a result of *Cryptosporidium* diarrhea. All of these factors can change the spectrum of possible causes of pneumonia. In contrast, an allogeneic bone marrow transplant recipient may (1) be neutropenic from pre-transplantation conditioning with cyclophosphamide, (2) be receiving corticosteroids and cyclosporine for prophylaxis against graft-versus-host disease, and (3) have mucosal breaches from longstanding central venous lines.

Finally, liver transplant recipients may be receiving corticosteroids and tacrolimus to prevent rejection, may have an endotracheal tube disrupting the mechanical barriers provided by the upper respiratory tract, and may be infected with immunomodulating viruses such as CMV and hepatitis C virus.

For patients with acquired immunosuppression, the risk of pneumonia is therefore related to the cumulative defects produced by different treatments and underlying disease processes. Thus, many patients have defects in all host defenses—disrupted mechanical barriers to pulmonary infection, decreased alveolar macrophage function, decreased neutrophil number or function, and reduced T and B cell function. It is also important to consider not only the current state of immunosuppression but episodes of immunosuppression that may have occurred in the past. For example, corticosteroid boluses given for graft rejection do not immediately increase the risk of infection; this comes 3 to 4 weeks later. Although protease inhibitors can dramatically diminish the circulating load of HIV, it is unlikely that patients who previously had low CD4 lymphocyte counts will experience total restoration of immunocompetence.

TABLE 61–2. Primary Immunodeficiencies and Their Relationship to Different Causes of Pneumonia

Condition	Defect	Description of Pneumonia
B Lymphocyte Deficiencies		
X-linked agammaglobulinemia (Bruton's)	Absence of B cells, plasma cells, and antibody	Recurrent *Haemophilus influenzae, Streptococcus pneumoniae, Staphylococcus aureus, Pseudomonas aeruginosa, Mycobacterium pneumoniae,* or *Pneumocystis carinii* pneumonia after maternal antibody is consumed (i.e., after first 4–6 mo of life)
Selective IgG subclass deficiencies	Selective deficiencies of IgG	Wide spectrum, from recurrent severe bacterial pneumonias to few abnormalities to normal
Selective IgA deficiency	Serum IgA <5 mg/dL (severe deficiency)	Wide spectrum, from recurrent *S. pneumoniae* and *H. influenzae* pneumonia to few abnormalities
Hyper-IgM immunodeficiency	Elevated IgM but reduced IgG, IgA	Recurrent bacterial pneumonia (usually not overwhelming); sometimes *P. carinii*
T Lymphocyte Deficiencies		
DiGeorge's syndrome	Thymic aplasia with reduced CD4 and CD3 cells (CD8 cells normal)	Severe viral pneumonia (herpes, measles), sometimes *P. carinii,* fungal, or gram-negative bacterial
Purine nucleoside phosphorylase deficiency	Marked T cell depletion (CD4:CD8 ratio normal)	*P. carinii* and viral pneumonia
Mixed T and B Cell Deficiencies		
Common variable immunodeficiency	Various B cell activation or differentiation defects plus gradual deterioration of T cell number and function	Recurrent pneumonia or chronic bronchiectasis presenting in childhood or adulthood. Organisms include *P. carinii,* cytomegalovirus, varicella-zoster virus, *S. pneumoniae, H. influenzae*
Severe combined immunodeficiency	Severely reduced IgG and absent T cells	*P. carinii* within first 9 months of life; subsequent viral or *Legionella* pneumonia
Wiskott-Aldrich syndrome	Decreased T cell number and function; low IgM; sometimes low IgG	*S. pneumoniae, H. influenzae,* herpesvirus, *P. carinii* pneumonia, usually by age 6 yr
Ataxia-telangiectasia	Decreased T cell number and function; IgA, IgE, IgG_2 and IgG_4 deficiency	*S. aureus, S. pneumoniae, H. influenzae* recurrent pneumonia, leading to bronchiectasis
Complement Disorders		
C3 deficiency	Congenital absence of C3 or consumption of C3 due to deficiency of C3b inactivator	Recurrent pneumonia due to *S. pneumoniae, H. influenzae,* or Enterobacteriaceae
Phagocyte Defects		
Kostmann's syndrome, Shwachman-Diamond syndrome, and cyclic neutropenia	Low polymorphonuclear leukocyte count	Pneumonia due to *S. aureus, P. aeruginosa,* or Enterobacteriaceae
Chronic granulomatous disease	Defect in NADPH oxidase in phagocytic cells	Pneumonia and pulmonary abscess due to *S. aureus, Escherichia coli, Klebsiella, Enterobacter, Serratia, Pseudomonas,* or *Aspergillus* species
Chediak-Higashi syndrome	Impaired microbicidal activity of phagocytes	*S. aureus* or *H. influenzae* (less commonly *Aspergillus*) pneumonia

Ig = immunoglobulin; NADPH = nicotinamide adenine dinucleotide phosphate, reduced form.

THE ROLE OF THE ENVIRONMENT IN PNEUMONIA

The likelihood that a particular pathogen will cause pneumonia in an immunosuppressed patient depends not only on the level and type of immunosuppression but also on environmental pathogens. Although some organisms that produce pneumonia in immunosuppressed patients (e.g., enteric gram-negative bacilli) are endogenous, are harbored by most people, and cause disease only when host defenses are breached, others are acquired from the environment, usually through the air (Table 61-6).

Aspergillus is a classic example. The organism is ubiquitous in the environment and is easily acquired by inhalation. Immunocompetent persons who have functional alveolar macrophages and neutrophils are protected from vascular invasion by the organism. In immunosuppressed patients, however, outbreaks of invasive aspergillosis have been linked to construction activity in or near a transplantation or a hematology unit, *Aspergillus* proliferation on poorly maintained air conditioning units, and exposure to large amounts of dust produced by emptying vacuum cleaner bags.[9-11]

Much debate attends the modes of acquisition of *P. carinii* and of *Legionella* species. Some investigators hypothesize that *P. carinii* infection is acquired in childhood, becomes part of the host's resident microbial flora, and remains quiescent until immunosuppression allows replication of the organisms. Others believe that *P. carinii* infections are transient and repeated but can be held in check by an intact immune system. Although rare, some clusters of infection have occurred in immunosuppressed hosts, suggesting exposure to a common source patient.[12] A number of reports have linked outbreaks

TABLE 61–3. Occurrence of Causes of Pneumonia in Solid-Organ Transplant Recipients in Various Time Periods After Transplantation

	Months After Transplantation				
Pathogen	*<1*	*1–2*	*2–6*	*6–12*	*>12*
MRSA	XXX	X			
Gram-negative bacilli	XXX	X			
Legionella	X	X	X		
Aspergillus	X	XXX	X		
Cytomegalovirus	X	XXX	XXX		
Nocardia			X	X	X
Mycobacterium			X	X	X
Cryptococcus			X	XX	XX
Coccidioides	X	X	XX	X	X

MRSA = methicillin-resistant *Staphylococcus aureus*.
Key: XXX = very common; XX = occasional; X = rare but does occur.

TABLE 61–5. Relation Between Likely Agents of Pneumonia in HIV-Infected Patients and CD4 Count

	CD4 Cell Count (cells/mm³)			
Agent	*>500*	*200–500*	*50–200*	*<50*
Streptococcus pneumoniae	XXX	XXX	X	
Haemophilus influenzae	XX	XX	X	
Mycobacterium tuberculosis	X	XXX	XX	X
Cryptococcus		X	XX	XX
Pneumocystis carinii			XXX	XXX
Cytomegalovirus				XXX
Mycobacterium avium				XXX
Aspergillus				XX

Key: XXX = very common; XX = occasional; X = rare but does occur.

of *Legionella* infection to hospital cooling towers; however, more evidence supports aspiration of contaminated tap water as an important mode of transmission.[13] Hospital outbreaks of *Legionella* can be curtailed by disinfecting tap water distribution systems. In our unit, transplant recipients are prohibited from consuming tap water.

Earlier we discussed timelines for the occurrence of pneumonia in immunosuppressed patients (see Tables 61-3 to 61-5). The occurrence of infection outside these timelines indicates that environmental contamination may be the source of the infection. For example, invasive pulmonary aspergillosis in a patient who has been neutropenic for only a few days heightens suspicion of increased amounts of *Aspergillus* in the environment from construction work or another source. Clusters of infection are another indication of potential common environmental sources of pathogens. In some circumstances (e.g., occurrence of methicillin-resistant *Staphylococcus aureus,* vancomycin-resistant enterococci, or extended-spectrum β-lactamase–producing *Klebsiella pneumoniae*), "multiresistant" bacteria may be spread from unsuspected colonized patients on the hands of hospital staff.

The hospital environment is a more likely source of infection than the community; however a number of causes of pneumonia in immunosuppressed hosts can be acquired in the community. These include tuberculosis, the geographically restricted dimorphic fungi (*Histoplasma, Coccidioides,* and *Blastomyces*), cryptococcosis, and infection with the intestinal nematode *Strongyloides stercoralis.* Each of these infections may occur in a transplant recipient by way of reactivation of previous infection, primary infection, or reinfection. Primary community-acquired pneumonia in the immunosuppressed host can be due to respiratory viruses such as respiratory syncytial virus, adenovirus, and influenza virus.

APPROACH TO DIAGNOSIS

Diagnosis of pneumonia in immunosuppressed patients should follow the usual steps: history taking, physical examination, noninvasive tests, and invasive procedures. The simple combination of history taking, physical examination, and chest radiography can often dramatically narrow the differential diagnosis, but an important caveat needs to be mentioned. Caution must be exercised in use of the principle of Ockham's razor: *Entities are not to be multiplied without necessity.* In other branches of internal medicine, given all the patient's symptoms, signs, and noninvasive laboratory test results, a physician finds that one unifying diagnosis can explain the illness. Pneumonia in the immunosuppressed patient may be due to several intercurrent infections (or noninfectious conditions) in a single patient. For example, an HIV patient can have simultaneous *P. carinii* pneumonia and pulmonary infiltrates due to pulmonary Kaposi's sarcoma, or a neutropenic

TABLE 61–4. Occurrence of Causes of Pneumonia in Bone Marrow Transplant Recipients in Various Time Periods After Transplantation

	Months After Transplantation				
Pathogen	*<1*	*1–2*	*2–6*	*6–12*	*>12*
MRSA	XX	X	X		
Gram-negative bacilli	XXX	X			
Streptococcus pneumoniae		X	X	X	X
*Aspergillus**	XX	XX	XXX		
Cytomegalovirus		XXX	XXX		
HSV	XX				
HHV-6	X	XX	XX		
Adenovirus	XX	XX	XX	X	X
RSV	XXX	XX	XX	X	X
VZV			X	X	X

*Early infections with *Aspergillus* occur when patients are neutropenic. Late infections occur when patients are receiving corticosteroids for graft-versus-host disease or when persistently neutropenic.

MRSA = methicillin-resistant *Staphylococcus aureus;* HSV = herpes simplex virus; HHV-6 = human herpesvirus-6; RSV = respiratory syncytial virus; VZV = varicella-zoster virus

Key: XXX = very common; XX = occasional; X = rare but does occur.

TABLE 61–6. Environmental Sources of Organisms That Produce Pneumonia in Immunosuppressed Patients

Organism	Source
MRSA, VRE	Other patients, via hands of hospital staff
Multiresistant gram-negative bacilli	Other patients, via hands of hospital staff
Legionella	Cooling towers, tap water
Mycobacterium	Usually from person-to-person spread; rarely from milk (*Mycobacterium bovis*)
Histoplasma, Coccidioides, Blastomyces	Inhalation of organisms from soil
Aspergillus	Construction area, dusty air conditioners, etc. (airborne)
Cryptococci	Soil or pigeon feces (airborne)
Cytomegalovirus	Often endogenous (HIV-infected patients); can come from donor organ or blood transfusion (transplant setting)

MRSA = Methicillin-resistant *Staphylococcus aureus;* VRE = vancomycin-resistant enterococci; HIV = human immunodeficiency virus.

patient can have bacterial pneumonia and invasive pulmonary aspergillosis.

In many cases, an invasive procedure is necessary for an accurate diagnosis to be made. Unfortunately, even after the most intensive investigation, only nonspecific information may be forthcoming; empirical treatment must then be based on relevant epidemiologic information.

History and Physical Examination

History Taking

The overall level, duration, and type of immunosuppression can incline suspicion toward certain clinical entities. For example, an antiretroviral drug-naive, HIV-infected patient with a CD4 count between 50 and 200 cells/mm^3 is highly likely to have pneumonia caused by *P. carinii.* Unfortunately, the diagnostic possibilities increase with increasing immunosuppression and duration of immunocompromise.

The tempo and mode of onset of pneumonia are also important. Rapidly progressive pneumonia of less than 24 hours' duration in a neutropenic or "ventilated" patient usually suggests a bacterial (often gram-negative) cause. In contrast, viral, *P. carinii,* and *Aspergillus* pneumonias have a subacute onset over several days to a week.

A chronic course is more likely to suggest tuberculosis or infection with *Nocardia* or *Cryptococcus* organisms, or one of the geographically restricted fungi. A history of travel or residence in a Third World country or the Southwestern United States may further heighten clinical suspicion of particular causes of chronic pneumonia—tuberculosis and coccidioidomycosis, respectively. Occupational and recreational history is sometimes important; *Rhodococcus equi* is sometimes (but not always) associated with exposure to horses.

Finally, since pneumonia in the immunosuppressed patient may have noninfectious causes (e.g., drug-induced pneumonitis), full knowledge of the patient's drug history is essential. The nature of the patient's symptoms can be important. As many as 50% of patients with legionellosis have gastrointestinal symptoms, especially watery diarrhea. Invasive pulmonary aspergillosis may present with symptoms that mimic pulmonary thromboembolism (pleuritic chest pain, dyspnea, hemoptysis) and occasionally with massive hemoptysis.

Physical Examination

Physical examination may also help narrow the "infectious differential diagnosis." Patients with bacterial pneumonia are likely to be febrile, tachycardiac, and tachypneic, whereas patients with nocardiosis or cryptococcosis are often afebrile and have normal pulse and respiratory rates. Careful examination of the patient's skin for signs of cutaneous infection with *Nocardia* or *Cryptococcus* organisms is also essential. Rarely, patients with invasive pulmonary aspergillosis have an coexisting cutaneous infection around the insertion sites of long-standing central venous catheters.

Radiology

Chest Radiography

Virtually all modern definitions of pneumonia include the necessity that pulmonary infiltrate be visualized by radiologic assessment (Figs. 61-1 to 61-3). In some circumstances, findings from the history (particularly type and intensity of immunosuppression, and tempo of onset of the pneumonia) combined with the radiographic appearance can virtually clinch the diagnosis. For example, an HIV-infected patient with CD4 count less than 200 cells/mm^3 who is not taking prophylaxis against *P. carinii* and whose subacute pneumonic process is visualized radiographically as an interstitial alveolar butterfly pattern spreading from the hilar region should be given high-dose trimethoprim-sulfamethoxazole, since *P. carinii* pneumonia is highly likely. Many times, however, radiologic examination may simply narrow the diagnostic possibilities and guide empirical treatment before an invasive investigation can be performed (Tables 61-7 and 61-8).

Radiologic assessment is also necessary to guide the choice of invasive investigation. If a pulmonary nodule is shown to be peripheral in location, percutaneous needle aspiration may be feasible. In contrast, radiologic evidence of a peribronchovascular (interstitial) infiltrate may best be investigated by flexible fiberoptic bronchoscopy, allowing bronchoalveolar lavage (BAL) or bronchoscopic biopsy.

Pneumonia in immunosuppressed patients exhibits certain typical patterns demonstrable by chest radiography. Unfortunately, although the patterns to be described are frequently seen, organisms can produce atypical patterns, especially if the patient is profoundly immunosuppressed. Alveolar pneumonia (airspace or lobar pneumonia) typically is caused by *Pneumococcus* organisms and is characterized by an inflammatory exudate in peripheral alveoli. Air bronchograms are frequently present on radiography. While the process is typified by complete lobar involvement, often the involvement is not extensive. In immunosuppressed patients, this form of consolidation is frequently multilobar, like that caused by *Legionella* species. Advanced infection with *Aspergillus* or *Nocardia* organisms or *Mycobacterium tuberculosis* may also produce this radiographic pattern, although discrete nodular infiltrates are more usual. Bronchopneumonia occurs when the inflammatory response occurs in the bronchi and surrounding parenchyma. Radiographically, this produces a more patchy appearance than that of alveolar pneumonia. Segmental bronchopneumonia is commonly observed with viral pneumonia, and with pneumonias caused by *S. aureus, H. influenzae, Chlamydia pneumoniae, Mycoplasma pneumoniae,* and occasionally *Pneumococcus* organisms.

Peribronchovascular infiltrates (interstitial pneumonia) are manifested radiographically as a reticular or reticulonodular pattern. Early *P. carinii* infection characteristically has this appearance, as do CMV, varicella-zoster virus (VZV), and herpes simplex virus infections. Nodular infiltrates are characteristic of subacute or chronic fungal, mycobacterial, and nocardial infections. Nodular infiltrates of more rapid onset can be the

TABLE 61–7. Possible Causes of Acute-Onset Pneumonia* in Immunosuppressed Patients by Chest Radiographic Abnormality

Consolidation	NONINFECTIOUS
INFECTIOUS	Pulmonary edema
Gram-negative bacilli	Leukoagglutinin reaction
Staphylococcus aureus	***Nodular Infiltrate***
Legionella	INFECTIOUS
Anerobes (aspiration)	*S. aureus*
NONINFECTIOUS	*Legionella*
Pulmonary hemorrhage	NONINFECTIOUS
Pulmonary thromboembolism	Pulmonary calcification
Peribronchovascular Infiltrate	***Cavitary Lesions***
INFECTIOUS	INFECTIOUS
Gram-negative bacilli	*S. aureus*
S. aureus	*Pseudomonas aeruginosa*
Legionella	

*Acute onset is defined as development of significant pneumonia within 24 hours.

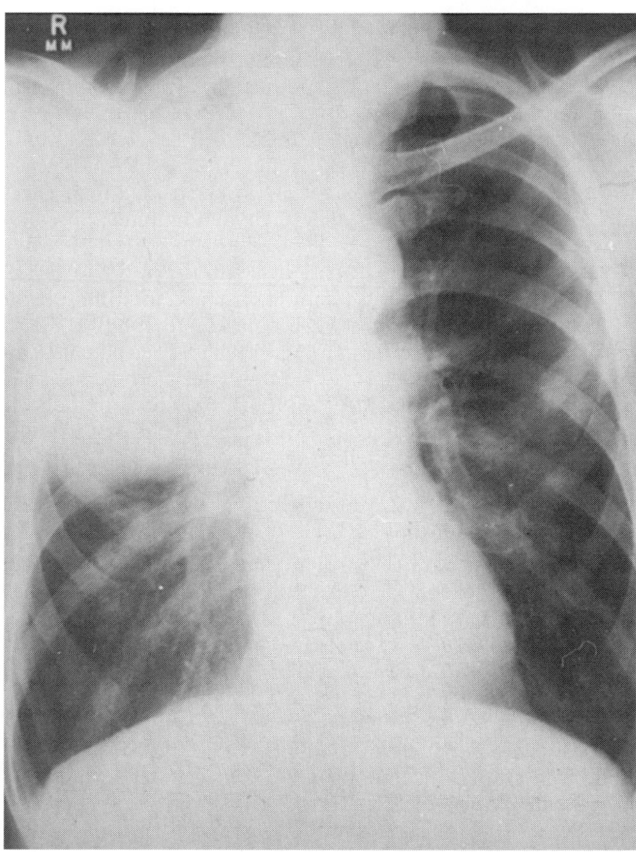

Figure 61–1. Chest roentgenogram of patient with B cell deficiency and overwhelming *Streptococcus pneumoniae* pneumonia.

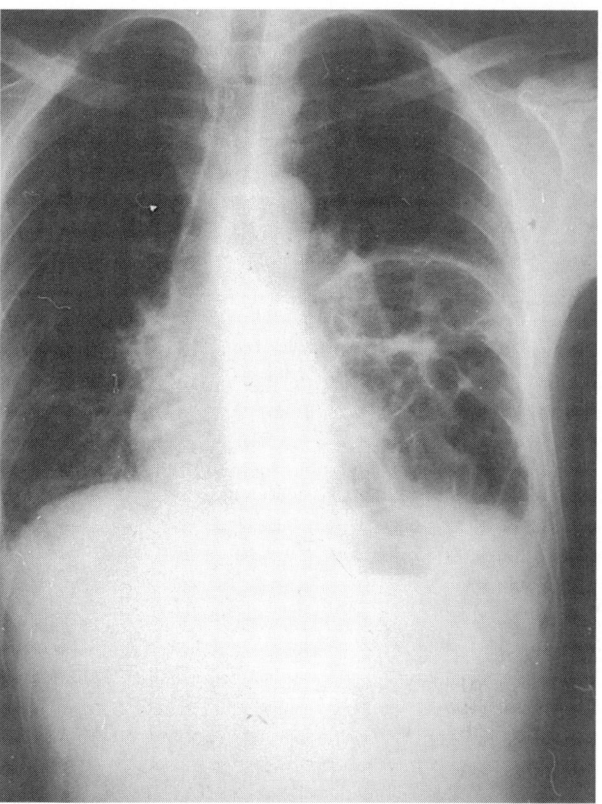

Figure 61–2. Chest roentgenogram of HIV-infected patient receiving pentamidine as prophylaxis against *Pneumocystis carinii* who presented with cough, dyspnea, and pleuritic chest pain. Unusual cystic lesion on left side was due to *P. carinii.*

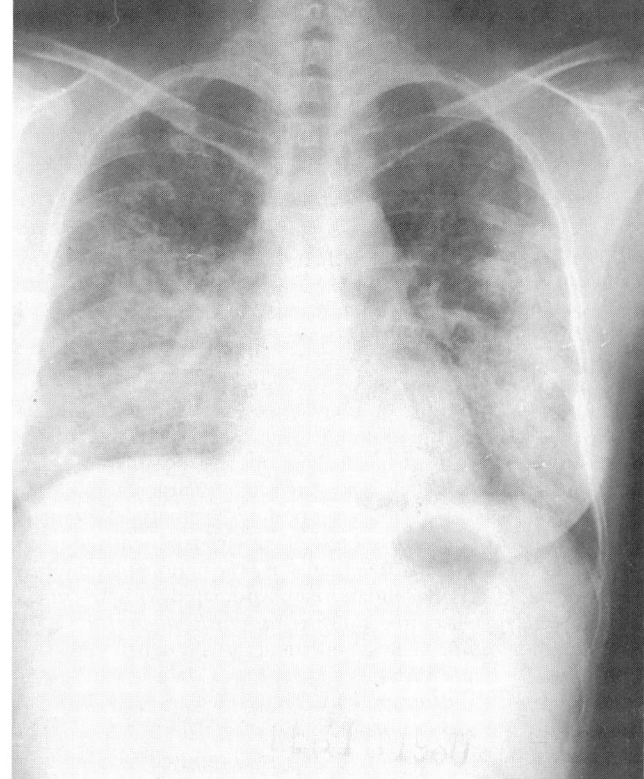

Figure 61–3. Chest roentgenogram of immunosuppressed patient with diffuse viral pneumonia, most likely respiratory syncytial virus.

TABLE 61–8. Common Differential Diagnoses of Subacute or Chronic Onset Pneumonia* in Immunosuppressed Patients by Chest Radiographic Abnormality

Consolidation

INFECTIOUS

- Fungi, especially *Aspergillus fumigatus*
- *Nocardia*
- Tuberculosis

NONINFECTIOUS

- Drug-induced
- Radiation-induced
- Pulmonary thromboembolism

Peribronchovascular Infiltrate

INFECTIOUS

- *Pneumocystis carinii*
- Viruses (cytomegalovirus, human herpesvirus 6, respiratory syncytial virus, influenza virus, adenovirus)

NONINFECTIOUS

- Drug-induced
- Radiation-induced

Nodular

INFECTIOUS

- Fungi, especially *Cryptococcus neoformans, Coccidioides immitis, Aspergillus* organisms
- *Nocardia*
- Tuberculosis
- *Rhodococcus equi*
- *Bartonella* species

NONINFECTIOUS

- Adenocarcinoma
- Squamous cell carcinoma
- Post-transplantation lymphoproliferative disorder

Cavitation

INFECTIOUS

- *Legionella,* especially *Legionella micdadei*
- *R. equi*
- *Mycobacterium tuberculosis*
- *Aspergillus*

NONINFECTIOUS

- Bronchogenic carcinoma

*Subacute-chronic onset is defined as a process developing over several days to weeks.

result of *S. aureus* or *P. aeruginosa* infection, either as a primary event or sometimes as a result of infected emboli originating from an infected intravascular catheter.

Radiographically, nodules can be described as spherical or oval intrapulmonary opacities that are well enough circumscribed to permit measurement of their diameter.[14] Sometimes, multiple very small nodules can be seen. These may be caused by miliary infection due to tuberculosis, histoplasmosis, or blastomycosis, or if they are slightly larger, to VZV or CMV infection. *Masses* are large nodules (sometimes defined as larger than 6 cm in diameter). They are frequently due to *Cryptococcus* or *Nocardia* organisms. Cavitation of nodules, masses, or areas of consolidation are associated with *M. tuberculosis, R. equi, Legionella micdadei, P. aeruginosa, S. aureus, Aspergillus* species, and sometimes other fungi.

Computed Tomography

Although plain chest films are usually all that is necessary to establish a radiographic pattern, chest computed tomography (CT) plays an important role in diagnosis of pneumonia in immunosuppressed patients. CT of the chest can determine whether pneumonia is necrotizing, whether mediastinal lymphadenopathy is present, whether (and how many) small granulomatous lesions or nodules are present, and whether a pleural effusion or empyema accounts for part of the pulmonary density observed on chest films. There is increasing evidence that high-resolution CT is more sensitive than chest radiography in detecting pneumonia in immunosuppressed patients.[14–16]

In a study of neutropenic patients who had fever for more than 2 days despite empirical antibiotic treatment, thin-section CT showed findings suggestive of pneumonia about 5 days earlier than did chest radiography.[15] This was particularly important for fungal pneumonia, because delay in diagnosis is associated with high risk of death. Furthermore, a number of highly typical CT appearances can be associated with fungal (especially *Aspergillus*) pneumonia, especially in neutropenic patients.

Nuclear Medicine Scans

Nuclear medicine scans are generally nonspecific but may occasionally be useful for excluding certain infectious causes of pneumonia in immunosuppressed patients. For example, a normal gallium 67 (^{67}Ga) scan may exclude *P. carinii* infection. Similarly, radiolabeled indium 111 (^{111}In) human immunoglobulin may occasionally be useful in excluding invasive pulmonary aspergillosis in immunosuppressed patients with negative or nonspecific radiographic findings.[17] This scan may also be useful in assessing resolution of *P. carinii* infection, which is not possible with ^{67}Ga scans.

Simple Noninvasive Tests

Simple noninvasive tests sometimes support the clinical impression gained by history taking, physical examination, and chest radiography, and they may even obviate the need for an

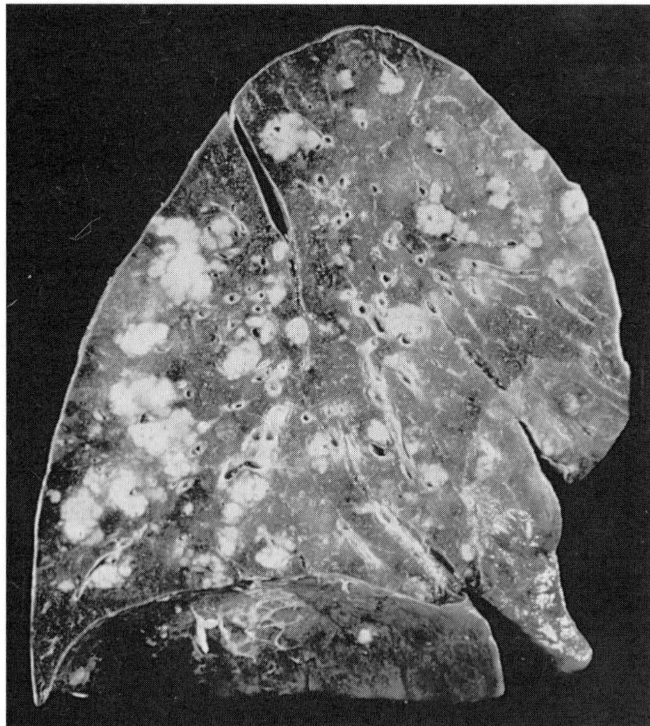

Figure 61–4. Autopsy specimen of lung shows widespread infection with *Mycobacterium tuberculosis.*

invasive procedure to establish the diagnosis. The cautions mentioned earlier against assuming that only one disease process is present in the immunosuppressed patient at any given time must nevertheless be remembered.

Arterial Blood Gas Analysis

Arterial blood gas analysis should be performed on any immunosuppressed patient with significant pneumonia unless the patient has a bleeding diathesis. Pulse oximetry is a reasonable noninvasive alternative for selected patients, but it may be inaccurate in patients with acute respiratory failure owing to peripheral vasoconstriction from shock or the use of vasopressors. Severe anemia, onychomycosis, fingernail polish, and carboxyhemoglobin or methemoglobin may all cause falsely depressed measures of oxygen saturation on pulse oximetry. Significant hypoxemia is an indication to use corticosteroids in addition to antimicrobials in the treatment of *P. carinii* pneumonia. Good oxygenation is almost always maintained with chronic processes such as tuberculosis, nocardiosis, and many fungal infections, whereas hypoxemia is typical of acute bacterial and viral pneumonias.

Sputum and Secretions

Examination of sputum or respiratory tract secretions obtained via endotracheal suction can be valuable and should be attempted when an immunosuppressed patient is thought to have pneumonia. A high-quality sample is required. For sputum, this is lower respiratory tract secretions produced by cough. Saliva is useless. Microscopically, a good sample contains numerous PMNs and few squamous cells. Laboratories that reject unsatisfactory specimens should be contacted if the patient is neutropenic. The value of Gram staining and routine bacteriologic culture is lower for sputum from immunosuppressed patients than for that from immunocompetent ones. The finding of *S. pneumoniae, H. influenzae,* or Enterobacteriaceae bacilli may represent bacterial pneumonia, but just as likely represents colonization and masks another infectious process. In contrast, the finding of a fungus such as *Aspergillus fumigatus* is much more significant than it is in an immunocompetent host: predictive values of positive sputum culture for subsequent development of invasive aspergillosis are as high as 82% for bone marrow recipients and 72% for liver transplant recipients.[10, 18] Specialized media should be set up for culture of fungi, *Legionella* organisms, or mycobacteria from sputum. Culture of *Legionella, Cryptococcus neoformans,* or *M. tuberculosis* (but not necessarily other mycobacteria) is diagnostic and is an indication to commence appropriate therapy.

Induced sputum samples are obtained by administration of aerosolized hypertonic saline. The applicability of the test is limited to alert, cooperative patients, but the test provides a better alveolar sample than regular expectorated sputum does. The test is of greatest use in diagnosis of *P. carinii* pneumonia (diagnostic yield up to 75%). The specimen can be stained with immunofluorescent monoclonal antibodies or Giemsa or silver stain. Induced sputum can also be used as samples for mycobacterial smears and cultures from patients who do not have a cough, and can be examined for fungi and cells with viral inclusions. While a positive result from induced sputum is an indication for specific antimicrobial treatment, a negative result does not rule out any of the infections listed earlier.

Serologic and Other Blood Tests

Blood for culture should be taken from all patients. Culture findings are most useful for detecting bacterial pathogens. Detection of CMV or human herpesvirus-6 (HHV-6) in peripheral blood can be accomplished by cell culture of buffy coat, direct fluorescent antibody examination of buffy coat using the shell vial method, antigenemia assays (e.g., PP65 antigen), and polymerase chain reaction (PCR) of peripheral blood. Antigenemia assays and PCR are becoming increasingly popular for detection of CMV infection as they are rapid and accurate. Invasive CMV disease, however, still needs to be verified by lung biopsy.

Detection of serum cryptococcal antigen is a very specific test that should be used to evaluate pneumonia in HIV-infected patients and transplant recipients. Surveillance serologic tests for the *Aspergillus* antigen galactomannan may also be useful in high-risk transplant recipients and neutropenic patients. Serologic tests for antibody against *Histoplasma capsulatum, Coccidioides immitis, Legionella* species, *M. pneumoniae, C. pneumoniae,* and respiratory viruses (influenza A and B, respiratory syncytial virus, adenoviruses, and parainfluenza virus) can also be performed in selected patients but a convalescent sample may be necessary to demonstrate a diagnostic rise in titer.

Miscellaneous Noninvasive Tests

The diagnosis of *Legionella pneumophila* serogroup 1 infection can be made by detection of antigen in urine.[19] Although this serogroup is responsible for as many as 80% of cases of *Legionella* pneumonia, other species and serogroups cannot be detected by this method. The tuberculin skin test is often performed to assess pneumonia, but a negative result should never supersede culture in excluding the diagnosis of tuberculosis, since many immunosuppressed patients are anergic. Fungal skin tests are compromised for the same reason.

Flexible Fiberoptic Bronchoscopy

Fiberoptic bronchoscopy has become the cornerstone of assessment of pneumonia in immunosuppressed patients and has a diagnostic yield of 60% to 90% in patients with HIV infection and about 50% in those with other forms of immunosuppression. Although all of the diagnostic techniques mentioned earlier can heighten one's suspicion of certain clinical entities, the requirement for tissue, or at the very least a lower respiratory tract sample, taken from the area likely involved by disease, is best approached by fiberoptic bronchoscopy. BAL is almost always performed; bronchoscopic biopsy improves the yield but can be risky for patients who have bleeding disorders not reversible with blood product support or who are severely hypoxemic. Fiberoptic bronchoscopy also affords an opportunity to visually inspect the anatomy of the tracheobronchial tree (e.g., for infectious processes such as tracheobronchial aspergillosis) and to collect bronchial washings and brushings, although these modalities have been largely replaced by BAL.

Bronchoalveolar Lavage

BAL has proved to be of greatest use in the diagnosis of diffuse pulmonary infiltrates, particularly those due to *P. carinii* infection in HIV-infected patients and to pulmonary hemorrhage in other immunosuppressed patients. In such cases, it is diagnostic in as many as 95% of cases. In part, because of its success with *P. carinii* pneumonia, BAL has become such a popular mode of investigating pulmonary infiltrates in immunosuppressed patients that its limitations are forgotten. For example, the significance of CMV identified by BAL in HIV-infected patients is unclear.[20] At least 50% of all severely immunosuppressed HIV-infected patients shed CMV in respiratory secretions. In one study, 72% of BAL samples from HIV-infected patients with pulmonary symptoms contained CMV, but pathologic evidence of CMV pneumonia was demonstrated in only 3% of them.[21] In contrast, the yield of all infectious diagnoses for BAL in patients with hematologic malignancies is low:

a "microbiologic diagnosis" in only 28% of patients whose symptoms are consistent with pulmonary infection.[22] The diagnostic yield for BAL with invasive pulmonary aspergillosis is only 45% to 62%. BAL has limited use in evaluating nodular infiltrates and for detecting noninfectious processes such as drug toxicity, metastatic malignancy, and the adult respiratory distress syndrome (ARDS).

BAL is also criticized because of the high associated rate of false-positive bacterial isolations due to contamination from the upper airway. Protected BAL is a variation of conventional BAL in which sealed probes or distally protected catheters are used to avoid contact between the fluid used in BAL and oral and upper airway organisms that could contaminate the suction channel of the bronchoscope.[23] This technique has been used to discriminate between upper airway colonizers and lower respiratory tract pathogens, particularly in ventilator-associated pneumonia. Protected brushings can also be used. Quantitative culture has added another level of sophistication to the procedure. Although such techniques are widely used in some centers, their role remains controversial because of questions about accuracy and about what constitutes the threshold concentration of bacteria that is defined as significant.

Transbronchial Lung Biopsy

Transbronchial lung biopsy, although limited by the contraindications mentioned earlier, is particularly useful in definitive diagnosis of viral pneumonia and noninfectious causes of pulmonary infiltrates in immunosuppressed populations. Transbronchial biopsy has found an important place in lung transplantation. It provides specimens for histologic diagnosis of acute graft rejection and CMV pneumonia.[24, 25] In patients with hematologic malignancies, the technique can distinguish leukemic infiltrates and radiation and drug-induced pneumonitis from pneumonia of infectious causes. Unfortunately, the nonspecific or negative findings in a sizable proportion of patients probably reflect sampling errors and the operator dependence of the procedure. Complications include hemorrhage, pneumothorax, and transient hypoxemia.

Nonbronchoscopic Lung Biopsy

Alternatives to bronchoscopic biopsy may be useful when a diagnosis cannot be made by bronchoscopic techniques or when peripheral nodules or cavities are present (Table 61-9).

Thoracoscopy

Thoracoscopic transpleural lung biopsy is a useful and well-tolerated procedure for some patients. Excellent results have been obtained in patients with diffuse interstitial pulmonary disease.[26] The procedure is also useful in focal, pleura-based disease in the periphery of the lung. The procedure can be carried out with local analgesia, but because a pneumothorax is created by virtue of the approach, a chest tube is needed for several days after the procedure.

Percutaneous Needle Biopsy

Percutaneous needle biopsy of the lung is often the diagnostic procedure of choice for peripherally located nodules or cavities. The procedure is not appropriate for diffuse lung disease. CT guidance much improves the diagnostic yield of the needle biopsy. Microscopy and culture for fungi, *Nocardia* organisms, and mycobacteria can be performed, as can cytologic examination for malignant cells. The specimen is usually insufficient for histopathologic examination. Pneumothorax is the major complication, although its frequency has been reduced by using small-gauge needles.

A combination of CT-guided needle localization of small nodules and simultaneous injection of methylene blue to improve recognition of the nodule, followed by thoracoscopic resection of the localized nodule has been used successfully in transplant recipients.[27]

Open Lung Biopsy

Open lung biopsy is regarded as the definitive procedure for diagnosis of pneumonia in immunosuppressed patients because a large tissue sample (potentially from several different sites) can be obtained. Open lung biopsy provides a specific diagnosis for 60% to 90% of immunosuppressed patients so investigated. It is most often used when previous diagnostic maneuvers have been unsuccessful, pulmonary infiltrates are spreading rapidly, hypoxemia is worsening, and the patient has a potentially treatable underlying condition. Thus, it is rarely used in patients with advanced HIV infection or relapsing acute myelogenous leukemia, but it is quite applicable to transplant recipients and those with collagen vascular disease.

Like other diagnostic procedures, open lung biopsy is less successful in patients with hematologic malignancy than in those with immunosuppression of other causes. It may, however, identify noninfectious causes of pulmonary infiltrate (e.g., antineoplastic drug toxicity or lymphocytic interstitial pneumonia) that other diagnostic methods cannot. An advantage is that it offers control over complications of the biopsy, including bleeding and air leaks. Its disadvantages include intubation and general anesthesia. Procedure-related mortality is 1%.

TABLE 61–9. Evaluation of Immunosuppressed Patients with Nodular Pneumonia of Subacute or Chronic* Onset

1. Contrast-enhanced chest CT scan to confirm radiographic diagnosis
2. History
   a. Type of immunosuppression: transplant (PTLD), human immunodeficiency virus (Kaposi's sarcoma)
   b. Underlying disease: history of carcinoma (metastatic hepatocellular carcinoma)
   c. Geographic location: southwest United States (coccidioidomycosis), developing nations (tuberculosis)
   d. Previous positive purified protein derivative (PPD) test (tuberculosis)
   e. Headache or neurologic symptoms (cerebral aspergillosis or nocardiosis)
   f. Exposure to animals (horses, *Rhodococcus equi;* cats, *Bartonella;* dogs, *Echinococcus*)
3. Physical examination
   a. Skin lesions (nocardiosis, cryptococcosis, Kaposi's sarcoma)
4. Noninvasive laboratory evaluation
   a. Blood cultures (*Cryptococcus, R. equi*)
   b. PPD (tuberculosis)
   c. Serology (*Cryptococcus, Aspergillus, Bartonella, Echinococcus,* Epstein-Barr virus)
   d. Tumor markers: alpha-fetoprotein (adenocarcinoma)
5. Tissue and microbiologic diagnosis
   a. Punch biopsy of skin lesions
   b. Thoracoscopic excision or percutaneous fine-needle biopsy
      (1) Histology (all diagnoses)
      (2) Special stains (*Nocardia,* fungi, mycobacteria)
      (3) Culture, including specialized media (*Legionella, Nocardia, Bartonella,* mycobacteria, fungi, viruses)

Modified from Paterson DL, Singh N, Gayowski T, Marino R: Pulmonary nodules in liver transplant recipients. Medicine 1998; 77:50-58.

*Subacute-chronic onset is defined as a process that develops over several days to weeks.

PPD = purified protein derivative; CT = computed tomography; PTLD = post-transplantation lymphoproliferative disorder.

EPIDEMIOLOGY AND IDENTIFICATION OF SPECIFIC AGENTS OF PNEUMONIA

Gram-Positive cocci

Streptococcus pneumoniae

Pneumococci are the most common cause of pneumonia in patients with normally functioning immune systems; however, all immunosuppressed patients are also at risk, some at higher risk than others. For example, serious pneumococcal infection is 200 times more common in persons with HIV infection than in age-matched "healthy" persons.[28] Pneumococcus is the most common bacterial pathogen in nonhospitalized patients with multiple myeloma, lymphoma, or chronic lymphocytic leukemia. Patients who undergo splenectomy for hematologic disease or other causes are at increased risk, as are bone marrow transplant recipients with graft-versus-host disease and functional asplenia. Recurrent pneumococcal pneumonia is often the presentation of congenital immunodeficiencies. In all groups of immunosuppressed patients, *S. pneumoniae* can produce nosocomial pneumonia.

Diagnosis of pneumococcal pneumonia rests on culture from blood, sputum, or other respiratory tract specimens. Segmental or lobar consolidation, as seen on radiographic examination, is present only in the minority of cases in immunosuppressed hosts.

Staphylococcus aureus

S. aureus pneumonia usually occurs as a result of intubation and aspiration, although septic pulmonary emboli sometimes develop from infected thrombotic material in the venous system (related to central venous catheters). In isolates from immunosuppressed patients in tertiary referral centers methicillin-resistant *S. aureus* (MRSA) now far exceeds in prevalence more susceptible strains. MRSA strains with reduced susceptibility to vancomycin and teicoplanin have now been recorded.[29, 30] Like other forms of bacterial pneumonia, *S. aureus* pneumonia is identified by culture of blood or respiratory tract specimens. A variety of patterns are seen on chest radiography, although rapid cavitation of bronchopneumonia should increase suspicion of staphylococcal disease.

Coagulase-negative staphylococci, although often cultured from respiratory tract specimens from immunosuppressed patients, are rarely a cause of significant pneumonia. Other diagnostic possibilities should be entertained for such findings.

Enterococci and Nonpneumococcal Streptococci

Enterococcal pneumonia is exceedingly unusual, although enterococci (including vancomycin-resistant *Enterococcus faecium*[31] is sometimes found in endotracheal aspirates or "unprotected BAL" specimens. Viridans streptococci are also much more likely to be a contaminant of mouth flora than the true cause of pneumonia.

Gram-Positive Bacilli

Rhodococcus equi

R. equi has long been recognized to be a cause of pneumonia in horses. It is now better known as a cause of pneumonia in HIV-infected patients, though transplant recipients are also at risk.[32, 33] Although the patient often recalls exposure to horses, the long persistence of these organisms in macrophages may account for exceptions to this rule. The clinical presentation tends to be insidious: fever, fatigue, and nonproductive cough. Cavitary lesions (particularly in the upper lobes) with air-fluid levels are seen on chest radiographs. The organism can be grown from blood cultures, but biopsy and culture of the chest lesions can also differentiate this infection from tuberculosis (which it resembles clinically). Sometimes the organism is partially acid-fast, but culture reveals highly mucoid, salmon pink–colored colonies that grow well on ordinary media.

Nocardia

Nocardia species are an important cause of pulmonary nodules in immunosuppressed patients. Infections occur particularly in patients who have lymphoreticular neoplasms or are receiving long-term corticosteroid therapy. Solid organ transplant recipients and patients with HIV infection are also at risk.[34] Onset of infection tends to be subacute or chronic. Sometimes subcutaneous abscesses coexist with pneumonia. Unfortunately, in immunosuppressed hosts, dissemination can occur from the lungs, via the blood, to the brain.

The classic radiographic appearance is single or scattered nodules or masses. Cavitation may occur, but confluent bronchopneumonia, complete lobar consolidation, empyema, and reticulonodular infiltrates can all be seen. Isolation of *Nocardia* organisms from skin lesions greatly increases the likelihood that pulmonary lesions are due to the organism. Culture of specimens from percutaneous needle biopsy of lung nodules is a common mode of diagnosis, although sputum and bronchoscopic specimens occasionally yield the organism. Blood cultures are rarely positive. The laboratory should be alerted to the possibility of *Nocardia,* as a modified Ziehl-Neelson stain that decolorizes with 1% sulfuric acid instead of acid alcohol is best for directly demonstrating the organism in clinical specimens. The organism is only weakly gram-positive, so routine Gram stains may not be adequate. Culture can be performed on routine blood agar, although growth is not rapid.

Gram-Negative Bacilli

Haemophilus influenzae

Splenectomized patients are at increased risk for serious *H. influenzae* type B infections, as are patients with Hodgkin's disease and multiple myeloma. Congenital B cell deficiencies also place the patient at increased risk for recurrent *H. influenzae* pneumonia. The significance of *H. influenzae* in sputum is sometimes doubtful, as the organism may be colonizing only the airways. Occasionally, serious *H. influenzae* pneumonia occurs in patients with advanced HIV infection and produces an interstitial pneumonia resembling that produced by *P. carinii.* The clinical picture also resembles that of *P. carinii* pneumonia: subacute onset, nonproductive cough, hypoxemia, and increased lactate dehydrogenase levels.[35, 36]

Enterobacteriaceae

Bacteria of the family Enterobacteriaceae include *Escherichia coli, K. pneumoniae, Serratia marcescens,* and *Enterobacter cloacae.* These organisms of gut origin frequently colonize the mouths and upper respiratory tracts of hospitalized patients. Most pneumonias caused by these organisms result from microaspiration of upper airway secretions that have been colonized with these bacteria. The classic lobar pneumonia of community-acquired *K. pneumoniae* infection is rarely seen in immunosuppressed patients, who typically have hospital-acquired bronchopneumonia (including ventilator-associated pneumonia). Neutropenic patients may have rapidly progressive pneumonia associated with shock. Immunosuppressed patients are becoming increasingly likely to be colonized with strains of Enterobacteriaceae possessing extended-spectrum β-lactamases, a fact that complicates treatment of pneumonia due to these organisms.[37]

Acinetobacter Species

Like the Enterobacteriaceae, *Acinetobacter* species colonize the respiratory tracts of hospitalized patients. Endotracheal intubation appears to carry significant risk. *Acinetobacter* pneumonia is frequently a multilobar bronchopneumonia.

Pseudomonas aeruginosa and Other Related Organisms

Bacteremic *P. aeruginosa* pneumonia occurs principally in neutropenic patients after cancer chemotherapy but may also be seen in patients with HIV infection. This is a fulminant disease associated with rapid onset of sepsis and respiratory failure. Radiographic appearance varies with the interval since onset; early signs are pulmonary vascular congestion, interstitial edema, and early pulmonary edema, whereas after 2 to 3 days a more extensive mixture of alveolar and interstitial infiltrates is seen. On pathologic examination, necrotic nodules are observed, often with hemorrhage.[38] Cavitation may result from the necrosis. Ventilator-associated pneumonia due to *P. aeruginosa* may be less aggressive than primary bacteremic pneumonia but is still associated with significant mortality.

Burkholderia cepacia is a frequent colonizer of patients with cystic fibrosis and can cause pneumonia in lung transplant recipients. Bacteremia is common and is associated with high fever and severe progressive respiratory failure.

Stenotrophomonas maltophilia behaves in a similar manner to *P. aeruginosa.* It can cause bacteremic pneumonia in neutropenic patients or ventilator-associated pneumonia in other immunosuppressed populations.

Legionella

Legionella pneumonia occurs with increased frequency in transplant recipients,[39, 40] but only sporadic cases of it have been reported in other profoundly immunosuppressed populations. The incubation period for Legionnaires' disease is 2 to 10 days, so most cases in transplant recipients are actually acquired in hospital. Early in the illness, the patient experiences only nonspecific symptoms and a mild cough. Diarrhea is present in as many as 50%, changes in mental status may occur, and hyponatremia (serum sodium <130 mEq/L) may be noted on blood chemistry studies. Although the chest radiograph may be normal early on, most cases have abnormal radiographic appearances when first assessed. The initial changes are often unilateral and tend to affect the lower lobe, but they soon progress to multilobar disease. Cavitation and apparent abscess formation are not uncommon in immunosuppressed hosts receiving corticosteroids.[41]

Legionella pneumonia is almost certainly underdiagnosed, as the organism does not grow on standard bacterial culture media. Microbiology laboratories should be asked to use specialized media (e.g., buffered charcoal yeast extract agar [BCYE]) on BAL and sputum samples when this organism is suspected. Direct fluorescent antibody (DFA) tests have been used on respiratory specimens but are probably less sensitive than culture. A urine test for *L. pneumophila* serogroup 1 antigen is available whose sensitivity is comparable to those of other methods. Serologic detection of antibodies is widely performed, but, as it often takes 4 to 12 weeks for an antibody response to *Legionella* infection to develop, it provides a diagnosis only in retrospect.

Chlamydia pneumoniae and *Mycoplasma pneumoniae*

C. pneumoniae and *M. pneumoniae* are common causes of community-acquired pneumonia in the normal healthy population. Their epidemiologies in immunosuppressed persons have not been firmly established. Pneumonia usually has a subacute course. Initially, radiographs demonstrate unilateral interstitial or reticulonodular infiltrates, but they may become bilateral with more advanced disease.

Mycobacteria

Mycobacterium tuberculosis

Tuberculosis occurs with increased frequency in patients with T cell deficiencies (especially HIV infection), transplant recipients, patients with neoplastic disease (especially Hodgkin's disease), and patients receiving prolonged corticosteroid therapy. Manifestations of tuberculosis vary with the degree of immunosuppression. For example, HIV-infected patients with well-preserved CD4 lymphocyte counts have positive tuberculin skin reactions, predisposition to upper lobe involvement, and frequently, cavitation. In contrast, HIV-infected patients with CD4 cell counts less than 50/mm^3, are usually anergic, may have lower and middle lobe involvement on chest radiography, and rarely have cavitation. Disseminated extrapulmonary disease is also more common in those who are more profoundly immunosuppressed.

Sputum induction should be considered when a patient does not cough. Ziehl-Neelson or fluorochrome staining and culture of sputum or other respiratory secretions remain the cornerstones of diagnosis. Given the diversity of presentations of tuberculosis in immunosuppressed patients, these tests should be considered routine for the evaluation of pneumonia in this patient population.

Nontuberculous Mycobacteria

Mycobacterium avium complex (MAC) frequently produces disseminated disease in HIV-infected patients with CD4 counts less than 50/mm^3 who are not protected by azithromycin, clarithromycin, or rifabutin prophylaxis. Actually, the lung is an unusual site of disease in HIV-infected patients. MAC isolated from the sputum of HIV-infected patients is usually a colonizer. Diagnostic confusion arises when acid-fast organisms are seen in sputum or BAL fluid and culture results are not available. *M. tuberculosis* cannot be distinguished accurately from MAC on the basis of stained smears. The BACTEC radiometric system for culturing mycobacteria, in combination with highly specific DNA probes to differentiate *M. tuberculosis* from MAC, can reduce the time for a definitive diagnosis to little more than 10 to 14 days. Depending on the relative local prevalences of *M. tuberculosis* and MAC, many clinicians opt to treat for tuberculosis on the basis of positive smears rather than waiting for definitive speciation to initiate therapy.

Other mycobacterial species occasionally cause pneumonia in immunosuppressed hosts, including *Mycobacterium kansasii, M. malmoense, M. haemophilum,* and *M. fortuitum.* Treatment regimens vary so accurate speciation needs to be performed.

Fungi

Pneumocystis carinii

P. carinii produces pneumonia in patients with a wide variety of immunosuppressive conditions but most notably those who have T lymphocyte deficiencies like those associated with HIV infection. The risk of *P. carinii* pneumonia increases when the CD4 cell count falls below 200/mm^3. The infection is now rare in HIV-infected patients taking protease inhibitors, which significantly reduce the HIV load, even when pretherapy CD4 counts were less than 200 cells/mm^3. For solid-organ transplant recipients, the risk of infection is greatest in the first 6 months after transplantation, although some risk probably persists as long as the patient receives immunosuppressive therapy. The risk increases when bolus corticosteroids or OKT3 is used to treat rejection. Failure to use prophylaxis (especially trimethoprim-sulfamethoxazole) for either advanced HIV infection or during the early months after solid-organ transplantation, increases the risk of *P. carinii* pneumonia. Other immunosuppressed groups at risk for *P. carinii* pneumonia include those with collagen vascular diseases such as Wegener's granulomatosis[42] and, less often, cancer patients treated with chemotherapy or radiotherapy.[43]

Occasionally, the chest radiograph is normal even in the presence of overt pulmonary symptoms due to *P. carinii.* In this circumstance, gallium scans are often positive. More often, the chest film is abnormal by the time the patient presents for medical attention. An interstitial alveolar butterfly pattern is most characteristic, but in the early stages of infection diffuse, fine, bilateral perihilar infiltrates are seen. Unusual patterns of infection (nodules, cysts, pneumothoraces, unilateral infiltrates, lobar consolidations) may be seen, depending on variables such as use of aerosolized pentamidine for prophylaxis, previous episodes of the disease, and time until presentation. Cystic changes and upper lobe involvement appear to be more common when aerosolized pentamidine is used as prophylaxis.

Although an abnormal chest film is sufficient to prompt further investigation to definitively diagnose *P. carinii* pneumonia, CT may show interstitial and micronodular changes not visible by chest radiography. Radiolabeled ^{111}In human immunoglobulin imaging may be useful in detecting superimposed focal infection with other organisms and the diffuse changes typical of *P. carinii.*

The diagnosis of *P. carinii* pneumonia depends on identifying the organisms by a direct staining technique—immunofluorescence staining using monoclonal antibodies to *P. carinii,* or the less specific toluidine blue O or silver stain (both of which stain the cyst wall) or Giemsa or Diff-Quik stains (for sporozoites, trophozoites, or intracystic bodies). PCR, used in some centers, has high specificity and sensitivity.

The choice of specimen is important. Routine sputum examinations have poor yield, but using hypertonic saline to induce sputum improves diagnostic capability considerably (30% to 75% of cases positive by more invasive methods will be positive). BAL, alone or combined with transbronchial lung biopsy and coupled with immunofluorescence staining, is "positive" in more than 95% of cases. Resorting to open lung biopsy is rarely necessary. Patients often harbor dead organisms in respiratory secretions for many weeks after successful treatment of *P. carinii* pneumonia. This may confuse the diagnostic picture when new respiratory tract findings have developed.

In all cases of presumed or confirmed *P. carinii* pneumonia, arterial blood gases should be measured, because corticosteroid therapy is indicated for patients with marked hypoxemia. Finally, it must be remembered that infection with other organisms may be intercurrent with *P. carinii* pneumonia and may account for a delayed or poor response to anti-*Pneumocystis* therapy.

Aspergillus

Invasive aspergillosis is an important cause of pneumonia in the immunosuppressed host by virtue of its high mortality rate. It occurs in all immunosuppressed populations, including transplant recipients, patients rendered neutropenic by treatment for hematologic malignancy, patients with advanced HIV infection, and children with chronic granulomatous disease. The rates of *Aspergillus* pneumonia in the first year after transplantation are as follows: for kidney transplantation, 0.7%; pancreas, 1.3%; liver, 1.7%; autologous hematopoietic stem cells, 2.6%; heart, 6.2%; related-donor allogeneic bone marrow, 6.7%; lung, 8.4%; and unrelated-donor allogeneic bone marrow, 10.3%.

Risk factors for invasive pulmonary aspergillosis include (1) delayed recovery from neutropenia, (2) severe graft-versus-host disease necessitating large doses of steroids for bone marrow recipients, and (3) poor graft function, CMV infection, renal failure requiring hemodialysis and OKT3 use in solid-organ transplant recipients. Construction activity in or near a unit where immunosuppressed patients are housed is also a risk factor for infection.[10]

Onset of invasive pulmonary aspergillosis may be insidious, but unsuspected dissemination of infection can increase the mortality rate to 92% for bone marrow recipients, 87% for liver recipients, and approximately 75% for other immunosuppressed populations. In neutropenic patients this form of pneumonia may present as fever that is unresponsive to empirical antibiotic therapy, or, much less often, as acute, rapidly progressive pneumonia. Sometimes the clinical picture resembles that of pulmonary embolism and infarction, with dyspnea, cough, pleuritic chest pain, and hemoptysis. Massive hemoptysis due to invasion of the infection into major vessels may occur.

Pulmonary nodules or wedge-shaped areas of consolidation are typical on chest radiography.[44, 45] Chest CT is more sensitive than chest radiography, and characteristically shows a halo of "ground-glass" attenuation around focal nodules. This corresponds pathologically to hemorrhage around a focus of pulmonary infarction. Particularly on resolution of neutropenia, cavitation occurs, being evident radiographically as an air crescent around a focal region of consolidation.[44, 45] *Aspergillus* tracheobronchitis can occur (typically in lung transplant recipients but sometimes in other populations); chest radiographs are normal or unchanged from baseline films.

The finding of *Aspergillus* organisms in culture of respiratory tract specimens from immunosuppressed patients is a powerful predictor of invasive pulmonary aspergillosis and an indication for institution of antifungal therapy. Unfortunately, *Aspergillus* organisms are cultured from sputum in only 8% to 34% of patients with invasive pulmonary aspergillosis and from the BAL fluid of 45% to 62%.[16, 46, 47] Although PCR of BAL fluid is potentially more sensitive than culture, in practice the risk of contaminating reaction buffers or patient samples with *Aspergillus* conidia is great, and contamination reduces the positive predictive value of the test.

Bronchoscopic or open lung biopsy is the "gold standard" of diagnosis, but waiting for this proof of infection to initiate therapy frequently risks treatment failure owing to unsuspected disseminated disease. There is clearly a need for diagnostic tests that detect *Aspergillus* infection before significant vascular invasion occurs. Surveillance serologic tests performed twice a week during the "at-risk period" are emerging as a useful tool for early diagnosis. Enzyme-linked immunosorbent assay (ELISA) to detect an *Aspergillus* antigen, galactomannan, in serum has sensitivity of 76% and specificity of 85%. ELISA results can be available within 4 hours of collecting the sample and in some patients are positive as long as 28 days before symptoms or radiographic signs of invasive pulmonary aspergillosis become evident.[48] Although detection of immunoglobulin G antibodies to *A. fumigatus* in serum has not been studied as extensively, it may also predate radiographic signs of aspergillosis by several weeks.[49]

Cryptococcus neoformans

Although pulmonary cryptococcal infection can affect persons with intact immune systems, it is more often found in immunosuppressed patients. More than 50% of cases now occur in HIV-infected patients, and solid-organ transplant recipients, patients with Hodgkin's disease, and those who require long-term corticosteroid therapy are sometimes infected. Two varieties of *C. neoformans* can be cultured. *C. neoformans* var. *neoformans* grows best in composted bird droppings and affects both immunocompetent and immunosuppressed persons, whereas *C. neoformans* var. *gattii* is associated with certain eucalyptus trees, almost always affects immunocompetent persons, and has a tendency to produce focal pulmonary or cerebral lesions (cryptococcomas).

Most immunosuppressed patients with pulmonary cryptococcosis have fever and cough, although the fever tends to be mild. Transplant recipients, other patients receiving corticosteroid therapy, HIV-infected patients with relatively well-preserved CD4 counts, and patients with Hodgkin's disease have nodular or patchy alveolar infiltrates. Sometimes masses (nodules > 6 cm in diameter) are seen. Cavitation is rare. In contrast, patients with HIV infection and low CD4 counts may have diffuse interstitial infiltrates or alveolar consolidation.

The serum cryptococcal antigen is a useful, easy, noninvasive test that rapidly provides diagnostic information on immunosuppressed patients with pneumonia. Several caveats bear mention. In patients with cryptococcal pneumonia whose disease is not disseminated beyond the lung, the serum cryptococcal antigen assay may be negative. In rare cases, infection with a nonencapsulated strain of *C. neoformans* is accompanied by a false-negative test result. Infection with *Trichosporon beigelii* is a rare cause of a false-positive serum cryptococcal antigen.

Sputum cultures are positive for *C. neoformans* in as many as 50% of patients with cryptococcal pneumonia. Cultures of BAL fluid are positive in 50% to 90% of cases. Staining BAL fluid with India ink can provide rapid diagnosis of infection. Cryptococcal antigen testing of BAL fluid can also be performed,[50] although many laboratories do not regard this test as routine. Biopsy of nodules or mass lesions can provide definitive diagnosis; culture and pathologic examination of tissue can be performed. Cryptococci may be somewhat difficult to visualize on routine hematoxylin-eosin staining, so Mayers' mucicarmine stain (which stains the fungal capsule) should be requested.

Whenever an immunosuppressed patient is determined to have cryptococcal pneumonia, a search should be mounted for extrapulmonary sites of infection. In about 80% of cases in immunosuppressed patients, intercurrent meningitis is uncovered by cerebrospinal fluid (CSF) examination. Cutaneous cryptococcosis is also sometimes observed, and it can be clinically indistinguishable from bacterial cellulitis.[51] Patients who also have meningitis may need more intensive and prolonged therapy than those who have pneumonia only.

Histoplasma capsulatum, *Coccidioides immitis*, and *Blastomyces dermatitidis*

HIV-infected patients and solid-organ transplant recipients are more likely to present with *H. capsulatum, C. immitis,* or *B. dermatitidis* infection compared with other immunosuppressed patients. These fungal infections are geographically restricted. Importantly, cases are often identified outside endemic areas in immunosuppressed patients who travel to or lived in endemic regions, sometimes years earlier. Their previously dormant infections are reactivated in response to immunosuppression. New exogenous infections are also common in those who are living in endemic regions.

Histoplasmosis is disseminated in more than 60% of immunosuppressed patients with the infection. Miliary or diffuse infiltrates may be seen on chest films. Occasionally, a syndrome resembling septic shock is observed that is marked by rapid development of respiratory failure and widespread pulmonary infiltrates. Rapid diagnostic methods include antigen detection in blood, urine, or BAL fluid and methenamine-silver staining of peripheral blood or bone marrow. Results of these tests can be available within 24 hours. Fungal cultures provide the definitive diagnosis, but results take 2 to 4 weeks to develop. Serologic test results can be false negative with acute infection or when the immunosuppressed host is not producing antibody, or they can be false positive owing to previous episodes of the disease. Histoplasmin skin tests are not recommended.

Coccidioidomycosis also is characterized by disseminated infection in immunosuppressed hosts.[52] Spherules in respiratory secretions or tissues are characteristic. Cultures from sputum or other respiratory specimens can be positive within 3 to 5 days. Although serologic testing has limitations in immunosuppressed patients, antibodies are detected in more than 80% of HIV-infected persons with the fungal infection. Skin tests are usually negative.

Blastomycosis is the least common of the endemic mycoses. Upper lobe nodular infiltrates are characteristic, but miliary or diffuse infiltrates can be associated with disseminated disease. Fungal stains of respiratory tract secretions are usually positive, and they are the most accessible means of rapid diagnosis. Blastomycosis antigen, which cross-reacts with *H. capsulatum,* may be detected in urine or blood. Culture is the only means for definitive diagnosis.

Mucormycosis, Pulmonary Candidiasis, and Unusual Fungal Infections

Mucormycosis is seen in as many as 8% of patients with leukemia examined at autopsy, and occasionally in solid-organ transplant recipients. Clinically, pulmonary mucormycosis resembles invasive pulmonary aspergillosis. The fungi have a distinctive appearance on tissue biopsy, but no other rapid diagnostic tests exist. Sputum and BAL specimens are rarely helpful. Definitive diagnosis relies on culture from biopsy specimens.

Candida albicans is often a colonizer in sputum or BAL specimens, but in lung transplant recipients, it can cause a fulminant pneumonia within the first 2 weeks after transplantation. The donor lungs are the most likely source of infection. Septic pulmonary emboli due to *Candida* organisms may occur in immunosuppressed patients with infected central venous catheters. In neutropenic patients or liver transplant recipients, disseminated candidiasis may also involve the lungs and will be diagnosed by culturing *Candida* at other sites.

Many other fungi can produce pneumonia in immunosuppressed patients, including *Pseudallescheria boydii,* which produces a clinical appearance like that of invasive pulmonary aspergillosis, especially in neutropenic patients; *Penicillium marneffei,* which produces a patchy pneumonic process as part of disseminated infection in HIV-infected patients; and *Sporothrix schenckii,* which produces cavitary lesions in patients taking long-term corticosteroid therapy.

Viruses

Cytomegalovirus

CMV pneumonia in immunosuppressed patients has traditionally been associated with a high mortality rate. For example, in bone marrow transplant recipients, biopsy-proven CMV pneumonia was an inexorable process that progressed rapidly to death in at least 80% of patients. However, modern methods of preemptive treatment (particularly those based on antigen detection or PCR of peripheral blood) and, in selected situations, prophylaxis, have markedly reduced the impact of this infection on immunosuppressed persons.

The clinical presentation of CMV pneumonia is not vastly different from that of other infectious diffuse pneumonias. Gradual onset of nonproductive cough, dyspnea, and fever is typical. Physical examination of the chest may be unrevealing. Chest radiography shows bilateral infiltrates, although sometimes in early stages of the infection unilateral, focal, or nodular infiltrates are observed. As the infection progresses, diffuse consolidation and marked hypoxemia develop. Timing of the infection may give some clue to its presence. In bone marrow transplant recipients the median time of onset is 60 days after transplant, and the disease is rare more than 150 days after transplantation. Exceptions do exist; occasionally CMV pneumonia occurs before engraftment,[53] and in patients with chronic graft-versus-host disease the infection may occur 6 to 12 months after transplantation.

Diagnosis from BAL fluid is considerably more reliable than in HIV-infected patients (see earlier section on Flexible Fiberoptic Bronchoscopy). Most cases of CMV pneumonia in bone marrow transplant recipients occur in patients who were seropositive for CMV before transplantation. In contrast, in solid-organ transplant recipients, CMV pneumonia is most likely to occur in seronegative recipients of an organ from a CMV-positive donor.[54] In such patients, pneumonia is generally part of a clinical syndrome characterized by fever, constitutional symptoms, and atypical lymphocytosis that develop 1 to 4 months after transplantation. Primary CMV pneumonia in lung transplant recipients can be particularly severe and has been linked to acute graft rejection, invasive aspergillosis, and bronchiolitis obliterans. True CMV pneumonia in HIV-infected patients occurs only when the CD4 cell count is less than $50/mm^3$.

Definitive diagnosis of CMV pneumonia requires demonstration of Cowdry type A intracytoplasmic inclusion bodies in areas of inflammation. Sometimes, even with infection, the inclusion bodies cannot be detected. Immunohistochemical markers may detect CMV-specific antigen in tissue in these cases of so-called histologically occult pneumonia.

Other Herpesviruses

The exact role of ***human herpesvirus 6*** in producing pneumonia in immunosuppressed patients remains to be determined.[55] It appears to be responsible for some cases of pneumonia in bone marrow transplant recipients.[56] Its role in HIV infection is controversial. Diagnosis is made by PCR or culture from BAL fluid, although the breakpoint value for true infection, as opposed to asymptomatic shedding, is not known. Growth from a peripheral blood sample probably indicates active systemic infection. Serologic tests are not helpful in attributing pneumonia to this organism.

Pneumonia due to ***herpes simplex viruses*** (HSVs) undoubtedly occurs, although results from BAL specimens can be misleading owing to contamination from the oropharynx. Hematogenous dissemination of HSV can produce severe diffuse interstitial pneumonitis.

The lung is the major visceral target of chickenpox, and *VZV pneumonia* usually occurs 3 to 7 days after onset of the skin lesions. Pneumonitis can be rapidly progressive over a few days. Disseminated zoster, involving the lung, can develop in persons previously infected with VZV. During VZV pneumonia, the virus can be cultured from sputum or BAL fluid. Cytologic examination of sputum may show multinucleate giant cells with intranuclear inclusions. Not uncommonly, other causes of pneumonia coexist with VZV; then diagnosis and therapy are complicated.

Recent evidence suggests a new herpesvirus, HHV-8, may be associated with development of ***Kaposi's sarcoma***.[57] Kaposi's sarcoma involves the lungs in as many as 25% of those with skin involvement. Typical lesions can be visualized on bronchoscopy. Detection of HHV-8 deoxyribonucleic acid in the BAL fluid has been described,[58] but it is not yet known how specific this test is for pulmonary Kaposi's sarcoma.

Respiratory Viruses (Influenza virus, Respiratory Syncytial Virus, Adenovirus)

Over the last decade it has become increasingly clear that common respiratory viruses frequently cause pneumonia in immunosuppressed patients. The pneumonia can be severe, and mortality is as high as 50% for bone marrow transplant recipients.[59] In solid-organ transplant recipients, these infections mainly affect children. Neutropenic patients with hematologic malignancies are also infected. Severely immunosuppressed patients with upper respiratory tract symptoms should have nasopharyngeal aspiration or washing for viral detection by direct fluorescence antibody tests and viral culture. In more advanced cases, BAL fluid can also be subjected to these tests and lung biopsy specimens can be examined for typical viral changes, such as multinucleate syncytial cells with intracytoplasmic viral inclusions, as seen in respiratory syncytial virus pneumonia. Accurate serologic assessment usually requires acute-phase and convalescent serum samples.

Respiratory syncytial virus is the most common community respiratory tract virus to cause pneumonia. The initial presentation is rhinorrhea and nasal and sinus congestion, but the infection quickly progresses to pneumonia, especially in the first month after transplantation.[59] Unless treatment is initiated rapidly the death rate is close to 100%.[59]

Influenza virus pneumonia in immunosuppressed patients also commences with upper respiratory tract symptoms. In both bone marrow transplant recipients and patients with hematologic malignancies, it can progress to life-threatening disease, particularly if they are neutropenic.[59, 60] Mortality is highest among patients who remain neutropenic for a long time. Secondary bacterial pneumonia is common.

Parainfluenza virus pneumonia in adult bone marrow transplant recipients has a 37% mortality rate.[61] In most patients, it develops within 100 days after transplantation. *Picornavirus pneumonia* also follows the typical pattern of upper respiratory tract symptoms followed by diffuse pneumonia, and has a mortality rate of 25% in bone marrow transplant recipients. *Adenoviruses* are associated with hepatitis in transplant recipients, but they can also cause pneumonia (independently or in conjunction with hepatitis). In contrast to the pulmonary infection due to other respiratory viruses mentioned earlier, pneumonia due to adenovirus is not usually preceded by upper respiratory tract symptoms. Usually, the pneumonia is a bilateral, interstitial process, but pleural effusions occur in 20% of cases.

Helminths

Strongyloides stercoralis

S. stercoralis is an intestinal nematode (roundworm) that can infect humans for years. Most cases are acquired in tropical regions (including southern parts of the United States) through skin contact with soil contaminated with the infective filariform larvae. Infection with *S. stercoralis* is potentially lethal, because massive larval invasion of the lungs can occur in immunosuppressed hosts (hyperinfection syndrome). This has been described in patients with HIV infections and hematologic malignancies, transplant recipients, and others taking corticosteroids. A cycle of autoinfection occurs when rhabditiform larvae penetrate into the vascular tree via the bowel wall or the perianal skin. The larvae follow the venous circulation to the right side of the heart and then to the pulmonary alveolar capillary bed, whence they penetrate into the alveolar space.

Diffuse pulmonary infiltrates occur that can cavitate. The pneumonia is frequently accompanied by severe abdominal pain. Passenger bacteria that accompany the migrating nematodes into the blood can cause polymicrobial bacteremia.

Peripheral eosinophilia is often observed but is not universal. The diagnosis is based on demonstration of filariform larvae in sputum, BAL fluid, or stool. Formal-ether concentrates of sputum should be requested if the diagnosis is suspected. Serum antibody tests are available, but in immunosuppressed patients their sensitivity is diminished. However, serologic and stool examinations should be performed in patients with a "relevant geographical history" before immunosuppressive therapy is commenced, because treatment of uncomplicated gastrointestinal infection is far easier than treatment of the hyperinfection syndrome.

Protozoa

Microsporidia have emerged as significant pathogens in patients with advanced HIV infection. Although these organisms usually produce diarrhea, disseminated infection can occur. Pulmonary involvement presents with small interstitial infiltrates. The laboratory should be alerted to the possibility of microsporidial pulmonary involvement in patients with advanced HIV infection in whose stool microsporidia have been detected. Sputum or BAL fluid can then be examined with Giemsa or modified trichrome stains to detect these tiny organisms. *Cryptosporidium,* an organism that also usually produces diarrhea, can occasionally produce respiratory infection and is detected with modified acid-fast stains.

Toxoplasma pneumonia is rare, but it can affect HIV-infected patients and solid-organ transplant recipients. Amebiasis, leishmaniasis, and babesiosis can all have pulmonary manifestations when they are disseminated infections in immunosuppressed hosts. Relevant exposure history should be sought.

NONINFECTIOUS CAUSES OF PNEUMONIA

To complicate the diagnosis of pneumonia in immunosuppressed patients, there are many non-infectious causes of pulmonary infiltrates (Table 61–10). Suspicion of these entities is aroused by relevant exposure history (chemotherapeutic agents, radiotherapy), history of malignancy (Kaposi's sarcoma, hematologic malignancy, hepatocellular carcinoma), and nonspecific or negative findings on microbiologic evaluation. Early diagnosis by biopsy can allow effective therapy, whether it be withdrawal of the inducing agent or corticosteroid or chemotherapy. Of all the noninfectious causes of pulmonary infiltrates, pulmonary edema, pulmonary embolism, adult respiratory distress syndrome, and pulmonary hemorrhage are most common. Septic shock, without lung infection, may produce diffuse pulmonary infiltrates. Aggressive therapy of pulmonary edema or septic shock is sometimes required before further assessment of infectious causes of pneumonia can be pursued.

TABLE 61–10. Noninfectious Differential Diagnoses of Pneumonia in Immunosuppressed Hosts

Transplant Recipients
Pulmonary edema
Adult respiratory distress syndrome
Pulmonary calcification
Metastatic carcinoma
Post-transplantation lymphoproliferative disorder
OKT3 administration
Drugs (e.g., azathioprine)
Human Immunodeficiency Virus Infection
Kaposi's sarcoma
Lymphoma
Bleomycin sulfate
Pulmonary alveolar proteinosis
Pulmonary emboli
Hematologic Malignancies
Pulmonary edema
Radiation pneumonitis
Chemotherapeutic agents (bleomycin, busulfan, chlorambucil, cyclophosphamide, cytosine arabinoside, hydroxyurea, melphalan, methotrexate, mitomycin, nitrosurea, procarbazine)
Recurrent leukemia or lymphoma
Leukemic cell lysis pneumopathy
Pulmonary emboli
Pulmonary alveolar proteinosis

EMPIRICAL AND SPECIFIC THERAPY

With many presentations of pneumonia in immunosuppressed patients, antimicrobial therapy must commence empirically because of the risk of rapid disease progress and worsening hypoxemia. The chronic progression of pulmonary nodules is one exception. To a large extent, the decision to commence empirical therapy rests on assessment of the patient's clinical status. A frequent concern about empirical institution of antimicrobial agents is that they will preclude making a precise microbiologic diagnosis. Certainly, before antimicrobial agents are given, simple but potentially very useful tests such as blood cultures should be performed.

The choice of empirical therapy depends on the stage of the immunosuppression process, the use of prophylactic antimicrobial therapy, and the radiologic and epidemiologic findings. For example, patients with granulocytopenia whose pneumonia develops with their initial fever usually require only antibacterial therapy. This should cover principally gram-negative bacilli, including *P. aeruginosa.* Traditionally, an anti-*Pseudomonas* β-lactam antibiotic plus an aminoglycoside are chosen, although some physicians recommend monotherapy with ceftazidime or a carbapenem. Local resistance patterns (e.g., a high incidence of extended-spectrum β-lactamase–producing Enterobacteriaceae) may call for modification of this approach. Only when no response occurs within 48 to 72 hours is broader-spectrum coverage added or bronchoscopy performed.

In contrast, persistently neutropenic patients who develop a new focal pulmonary infiltrate while receiving antibiotic therapy have a much broader differential diagnosis. Such patients are at such high risk for fungal infection that we recommend aggressive empirical antifungal therapy, including amphotericin deoxycholate in large doses (1 to 1.5 mg/kg per day) or a lipid formulation of amphotericin. Empirical addition of itraconazole or 5-flucytosine should be seriously considered. Traditionally, much smaller doses of amphotericin (e.g., 0.5 mg/kg per day) are used empirically, because many believe that renal toxicity associated with larger doses can be justified only when fungal infection has been proven by microbiologic or histopathologic studies. We believe, however, that the mortality associated with invasive fungal pneumonia in neutropenic patients is so great as to override such concerns. Empirical therapy with lipid preparations of amphotericin, when compared to amphotericin deoxycholate in a randomized controlled trial in neutropenic patients, was rarely associated with significant nephrotoxicity.[62] Invasive diagnostic procedures can be arranged, but only after aggressive empirical antifungal therapy has been instituted.

The choice of empirical treatment of severe pneumonia with diffuse or interstitial infiltrates in nonneutropenic patients depends on whether prophylaxis has been used against *P. carinii,* time since transplantation, or CD4 lymphocyte count. Trimethoprim-sulfamethoxazole should be included in the empirical regimen if no *P. carinii* prophylaxis was being given. A macrolide or quinolone active against *Legionella* organisms (e.g., azithromycin, erythromycin, ciprofloxacin) should be included, especially if *Legionella* samples have been cultured from the hospital's water system. Ganciclovir may be used empirically in transplant recipients at high risk.

When specific organisms are known, targeted therapy should be initiated (Table 61-11). Antimicrobial agents alone, however, may not suffice to treat pneumonia in immunosuppressed patients. Supportive therapy, possibly including mechanical ventilation, may need to be considered. Decreasing or eliminating immunosuppressive therapy and improving neutrophil number and function with granulocyte colony-stimulating factor is essential. Surgery may be useful, particularly for focal fungal infections such as aspergillosis and mucormycosis. Identification and appropriate treatment of infection in extrapulmonary sites is also important. Many antimicrobial agents interact with cyclosporine or tacrolimus; such interactions can be avoided by careful choice of antibiotic or by dose adjustment.[63] Particular attention must be paid to the duration of therapy, especially for organisms such as *M. tuberculosis, R. equi,* and most of the fungi. HIV-infected patients may need to continue maintenance therapy all their lives after the initial intensive therapy is completed.

PREVENTION OF PNEUMONIA

Much can be done to prevent pneumonia in immunosuppressed populations: prevention of colonization, antimicrobial prophylaxis, surveillance with preemptive therapy, and immunomodulation or immunoprophylaxis.

Prevention of colonization is probably the most important measure for preventing pneumonia. Its principles are relatively simple, but in practice are rarely implemented properly. Horizontal transmission of resistant bacteria from other patients via the hands of health care workers is a major problem that can easily be prevented by handwashing. Drinking water contaminated with *Legionella* organisms can be prevented by disinfecting the hospital water distribution system. Risk of *P. aeruginosa* infection in neutropenic patients may be reduced

TABLE 61–11. Treatment Regimens for Selected Infectious Pneumonias in Immunosuppressed Patients

Pathogen	Treatment of Choice	Comment
Bacteria		
Streptococcus pneumoniae	Penicillin	High-level (but not intermediate) penicillin resistance may require cefotaxime or vancomycin.
Methicillin-resistant *Staphylococcus aureus*	Vancomycin	Removal of infected central venous lines may be important.
Rhodococcus equi	Azithromycin plus rifampin	Optimal regimen not yet determined. Other possibilities include combinations with erythromycin, vancomycin, aminoglycosides, or imipenem.
Nocardia	TMP-SMZ	Ceftriaxone and imipenem are also useful in some species.
Haemophilus influenzae	Ampicillin	Ampicillin plus β-lactamase inhibitor appropriate if organism produces β-lactamase.
Enterobacteriaceae	Ciprofloxacin or third-generation cephalosporin	Extended-spectrum β-lactamase are producers best treated with a carbapenem.
Acinetobacter	Imipenem or ceftazidime	Ampicillin-sulbactam may be useful for resistant strains.
Pseudomonas aeruginosa	Ceftazidime, piperacillin, or carbapenem plus tobramycin	High peaks of aminoglycoside are required
Burkholderia cepacia	TMP-SMZ	Imipenem, ciprofloxacin, minocycline, or chloramphenicol may be alternative.
Stenotrophomonas maltophilia	TMP-SMZ	Ticarcillin/clavulanate may be alternative.
Legionella	Azithromycin or ciprofloxacin	Add rifampin in severe cases.
Cryptococcus pneumoniae	Azithromycin or doxycycline	β-Lactams are not effective.
Mycobacterium pneumoniae	Azithromycin or erythromycin	Doxycycline is an alternative.
Mycobacterium tuberculosis	Isoniazid, rifampin, ethambutol, and pyrazinamide	Susceptibilities must be tested.
Fungi		
Pneumocystis carinii	TMP-SMZ	Add corticosteroids with hypoxemia.
Aspergillus	Lipid preparation of amphotericin or high-dose amphotericin deoxycholate (1-1.5 mg/kg)	Combination with G-CSF, GM-CSF, itraconazole, or 5-flucytosine is recommended.
Cryptococcus neoformans	Amphotericin or fluconazole	Surgery should be considered for focal disease.
Mucormycetes	Lipid preparation of amphotericin or high-dose amphotericin deoxycholate (1-1.5 mg/kg)	Surgery is almost always needed.
Viruses		
Cytomegalovirus	Ganciclovir	G-CSF may be needed to prevent neutropenia.
Respiratory syncytial virus	Ribavirin	Some use immunoglobulin in addition.
Influenza virus	Amantadine or rimantidine	Resistance may emerge during treatment.
Human herpesvirus 6	Ganciclovir	G-CSF may be needed to prevent neutropenia.
Herpes simplex virus	Acyclovir	Famciclovir is an alternative.
Varicella-zoster virus	Acyclovir	Famciclovir is an alternative.

TMP-SMZ = trimethoprim-sulfamethoxazole; G-CSF = granulocyte colony-stimulating factor; GM-CSF = granulocyte-monophage colony-stimulating factor.

by withholding fresh leafy vegetables. Respiratory transmission of mycobacteria, viruses, and fungi in hospitals has been conclusively demonstrated. In many institutions, it is necessary to accommodate all HIV-infected patients with pneumonia in respiratory isolation until three smears of sputum samples are shown to be negative. Patients with VZV, influenza, or respiratory syncytial virus should also be accommodated in respiratory isolation. Accommodation of neutropenic bone marrow transplant recipients in rooms with laminar airflow and high-efficiency particulate air (HEPA) filtration reduces their risk for invasive aspergillosis.[10] Construction activity in the hospital is also a risk factor for invasive pulmonary aspergillosis and should be appropriately contained.

In recent years, clinicians have embraced widespread antimicrobial prophylaxis as a means of preventing pneumonia and other infections in immunosuppressed patients. While strategies such as use of trimethoprim-sulfamethoxazole to prevent *P. carinii* pneumonia in HIV-infected patients and transplant recipients is clearly of benefit, prophylaxis against other fungi, bacteria, and viruses is not definitively of benefit. Vancomycin resistance in enterococci and staphylococci, fluconazole resistance in yeasts, and ganciclovir resistance in CMV are becoming major concerns. Alternatives to widespread prophylaxis include selective use in identified high-risk groups or preemptive use of antimicrobials.[64] The preemptive strategy consists of regular surveillance testing (usually by way of PCR or antigen detection in blood) and, when results are positive, short-term therapy for asymptomatic or minimally symptomatic patients. Preemptive treatment has been most used to manage CMV and *Aspergillus* infections.

Immunomodulation and immunoprophylaxis are widely used. Inactivated vaccines (e.g., against influenza virus and pneumococcus) are indicated for virtually all immunosuppressed patients. In general, live vaccines should not be used. Intravenous pooled immunoglobulin is indicated for patients with immunoglobulin deficiencies. Finally, reducing the duration of neutropenia by using granulocyte colony–stimulating factor is appropriate for selected neutropenic patients.

References

1. Singh N, Gayowski T, Wagener M, Marino IR, Yu VL: Pulmonary infections in liver transplant recipients receiving tacrolimus. Transplantation 1996; 61:396.
2. Coonrod JD, Lester RL, Hsu LC: Characterization of the extracellular bactericidal factors of rat alveolar lung material. J Clin Invest 1984; 74:1269.
3. Croft M: Activation of naive, memory and effector T cells. Curr Opin Immunol 1994; 5:431.
4. Grundy JE, Shanley JD, Griffiths PD: Is cytomegalovirus interstitial pneumonitis in transplant recipients an immunopathological condition? Lancet 1987; 2:996.
5. Bodey GP, Buckley M, Sathe YS, et al: Quantitative relationships between circulating leukocytes and infection in patients with acute leukemia. Ann Intern Med 1996; 64:328.
6. Hughes MD, Johnson VA, Hirch MS, et al: Monitoring plasma HIV-1 RNA levels in addition to CD4 lymphocytes improves assessment of antiretroviral therapeutic response. Ann Intern Med 1997; 126:929.
7. O'Brien WA, Hartigan PM, Daar ES, et al: Changes in plasma HIV RNA levels and CD4+ lymphocyte count predicts both response to antiretroviral therapy and therapeutic failure. Ann Intern Med 1997; 126:939.
8. Mellors JW, Munoz A, Giorgi J, et al: Plasma viral load and CD4+ lymphocytes as prognostic markers of HIV-1 infection. Ann Intern Med 1997; 126:946.
9. Weems JJ, Davis BJ, Tablan OC, Kaufman L, Martone WJ: Construction activity: An independent risk factor for invasive aspergillosis and zygomycosis in patients with hematologic malignancy. Infect Control 1987; 8:71.
10. Wald A, Leisenring W, van Burik J, Bowden RA: Epidemiology of *Aspergillus* infections in a large cohort of patients undergoing bone marrow transplantation. J Infect Dis 1997; 175:1459.
11. Anderson K, Morris G, Kennedy H, et al: Aspergillosis in immunocompromised paediatric patients: Associations with building hygiene, design, and indoor air. Thorax 1996; 51:256.
12. Chave J, David S, Wauters J, et al: Transmission of *Pneumocystis carinii* from AIDS patients to other immunosuppressed patients: A cluster of *Pneumocystis carinii* pneumonia in renal transplant recipients. AIDS 1991; 5:927.
13. Yu VL: Could aspiration be the major mode of transmission for *Legionella*? Am J Med 1993; 95:13.
14. Paterson DL, Singh N, Gayowski T, Marino IR: Pulmonary nodules in liver transplant recipients. Medicine 1998; 77:50–58.
15. Heussel CP, Kauczor HU, Heussel G, Fischer B, Mildenberger P, Thelen M: Early detection of pneumonia in febrile neutropenic patients: Use of thin-section CT. AJR Am J Roentgenol 1997; 169:1347.
16. Caillot D, Casasnovas O, Bernard A, et al: Improved management of invasive pulmonary aspergillosis in neutropenic patients using early thoracic computed tomographic scan and surgery. J Clin Oncol 1997; 15:139–147.
17. Oyen WJG, Claessens RAMJ, Raemaekers JMM, et al: Diagnosing infection in febrile granulocytopenic patients with indium 111–labeled human immunoglobulin G. J Clin Oncol 1992; 10:61.
18. Kusne S, Torre CJ, Manez R, et al: Factors associated with invasive lung aspergillosis and the significance of positive *Aspergillus* culture after liver transplantation. J Infect Dis 1992; 166:1379.
19. Stout JE, Yu VL: Legionellosis. N Engl J Med 1997; 337:682.
20. Baughman RP: Cytomegalovirus: The monster in the closet? Am J Respir Crit Care Med 1997; 156:1.
21. Mann M, Shelhamer JH, Masur H, et al: Lack of clinical utility of bronchoalveolar lavage cultures for cytomegalovirus in HIV infection. Am J Respir Crit Care Med 1997; 155:1723.
22. Eriksson B-M, Dahl H, Wang F-Z, et al: Diagnosis of pulmonary infections in immunocompromised patients by fiber-optic bronchoscopy with bronchoalveolar lavage and serology. Scand J Infect Dis 1996; 28:479.
23. Nieto JMS, Alcarez AC: The role of bronchoalveolar lavage in the diagnosis of bacterial pneumonia. Eur J Clin Microbiol Infect Dis 1995; 14:839.
24. Chan CC, Abi-Saleh WJ, Arroliga AC, et al: Diagnostic yield and therapeutic impact of flexible bronchoscopy in lung transplant recipients. J Heart Lung Transplant 1996; 15:196.
25. Boehler A, Vogt P, Zollinger A, Weder W, Speich R: Prospective study of the value of transbronchial lung biopsy after lung transplantation. Eur Respir J 1996; 9:658.
26. Dijkman JH, van der Meer JWM, Bakker W, et al: Transpleural lung biopsy by the thoracoscopic route in patients with diffuse interstitial pulmonary disease. Chest 1982; 82:76.
27. Schwarz RE, Posner MC, Plunkett MB, Selby RR, Landreneau RJ: Needle-localized thoracoscopic resections of small indeterminate pulmonary nodules in transplant patients. Clin Transplant 1994; 8:378.
28. Redd SC, Rutherford GW, Sande MA, et al: The role of human immunodeficiency virus infection in pneumococcal bacteremia in San Francisco residents. J Infect Dis 1990; 162:1012.
29. Hiramatsu K, Hanaki H, Ino T, et al: Methicillin-resistant *Staphylococcus aureus* clinical strains with reduced vancomycin susceptibility. J Antimicrob Chemother 1997; 40:135–136.
30. CDC Update. *Staphylococcus aureus* with reduced susceptibility to vancomycin—United States, 1997. MMWR Morb Mortal Wkly Rep 1997; 46:813.
31. Linden PK, Pasculle AW, Manez R, et al: Differences in outcomes for patients with bacteremia due to vancomycin-resistant *Enterococcus faecium* or vancomycin-susceptible *E. faecium*. Clin Infect Dis 1996; 22:663.
32. Sane DC, Durack DT: Infection with *Rhodococcus equi* in AIDS. N Engl J Med 1986; 314:56.
33. Le Lay G, Martin F, Leroyer C, Abalain ML, Credoz L, Chastel C: *Rhodococcus equi* causing bacteraemia and pneumonia in a pulmonary transplant patient. J Infect 1996; 33:239.
34. Forbes GM, Harvey FAH, Philpott-Howard JN, et al: Nocardiosis in liver transplantation: Variation in presentation, diagnosis and therapy. J Infect 1990; 20:11.
35. Moreno S, Martinez R, Barros C, et al: Latent *Haemophilus influenzae* pneumonia in patients infected with HIV. AIDS 1991; 5:967.

36. Schlamm HT, Yancovitz SR: *Haemophilus influenzae* pneumonia in young adults with AIDS, ARC or risk of AIDS. Am J Med 1989; 86:11.
37. Paterson DL, Ko W, Von Gottenberg A, et al: In vitro susceptibility and clinical outcome of bacteremia due to extended-spectrum beta-lactamase (ESBL) producing *Klebsiella pneumoniae.* Clin Infect Dis 1998; 27:956.
38. Fetzer AE, Werner AS, Hagstrom JWC: Pathologic features of pseudomonal pneumonia. Am Rev Respir Dis 1967; 96:1121.
39. Singh N, Muder RR, Yu VL, Gayowski T: *Legionella* infection in liver transplant recipients: Implications for management. Transplantation 1993; 56:1549–1551.
40. Harrington RD, Woolfrey AE, Bowden R, McDowell MG, Hackman RC: Legionellosis in a bone marrow transplant center. Bone Marrow Transplant 1996; 18:361.
41. Ebright JR, Tarakji E, Brown WJ, et al: Multiple bilateral lung cavities caused by *Legionella pneumophila:* A case report and review of the literature. Infect Dis Clin Pract 1993; 2:195.
42. Ognibene FP, Shelhamer JH, Hoffman GS, et al: *Pneumocystis carinii* pneumonia: A major complication of immunosuppressive therapy in patients with Wegener's granulomatosis. Am J Respir Crit Care Med 1995; 151:795.
43. Arend SM, Kroon FP, van't Wout JW: *Pneumocystis carinii* pneumonia in patients without AIDS, 1980 through 1993. Arch Intern Med 1995; 155:2436.
44. Mori M, Galvin JR, Barloon TJ, Gingrich RD, Stanford W: Fungal pulmonary infections after bone marrow transplantation: Evaluation with radiography and CT. Radiology 1991; 178:721.
45. Logan PM, Muller NL: High-resolution computed tomography and pathologic findings in pulmonary aspergillosis: A pictorial essay. Can Assoc Radiol J 1996; 47:444.
46. Hopwood V, Johnson EM, Cornish JM, et al: Use of the Pastorex *Aspergillus* antigen latex agglutination test for the diagnosis of invasive aspergillosis. J Clin Pathol 1995; 48:210.
47. Guillemain R, Lavarde V, Amrein C, et al: Invasive aspergillosis after transplantation. Transplant Proc 1995; 41:1307.
48. Verweij PE, Stynen D, Rijs AJMM, et al: Sandwich enzyme-linked immunosorbent assay compared with Pastorex latex agglutination test for diagnosing invasive aspergillosis in immunocompromised patients. J Clin Microbiol 1995; 33:1912.
49. Tomee JFC, Mannes PM, van der Bij W, et al: Serodiagnosis and monitoring of *Aspergillus* infections after lung transplantation. Ann Intern Med 1996; 125:197.
50. Baughman RP, Rhodes JC, Dohn MN, et al: Detection of cryptococcal antigen in bronchoalveolar lavage fluid: A prospective study of diagnostic utility. Am Rev Respir Dis 1992; 145:1226.
51. Singh N, Gayowski T, Wagener MM, Marino IR: Clinical spectrum of invasive cryptococcosis in liver transplant recipients receiving tacrolimus immunosuppression: Prospective study with ecologic and pathogenic implications. Clin Transplant 1997; 11:66.
52. Holt CD, Winston DJ, Kubak B, et al: Coccidioidomycosis in liver transplant patients. Clin Infect Dis 1997; 24:216.
53. Limaye AP, Bowden RA, Myerson D, Boeckh M: Cytomegalovirus disease occurring before engraftment in marrow transplant recipients. Clin Infect Dis 1997; 24:830.
54. Falagas ME, Snydman DR, George MJ, et al: Incidence and predictors of cytomegalovirus pneumonia in orthotopic liver transplant recipients. Transplantation 1996; 61:1716.
55. Singh N, Carrigan DR: Human herpesvirus-6 in transplantation: An emerging pathogen. Ann Intern Med 1996; 124:1065.
56. Cone RW, Hackman RC, Huang M-L, et al: Human herpesvirus 6 in lung tissue from patients with pneumonitis after bone marrow transplantation. N Engl J Med 1993; 329:156.
57. Chang Y, Cesarman E, Pessin MS, et al: Identification of herpesvirus-like DNA sequences in AIDS-associated Kaposi's sarcoma. Science 1994; 266:1865.
58. Cathomas G, Tamm M, McGandy CE, Perruchoud AP, Mihatsch MJ, Dalquen P: Detection of herpesvirus-like DNA in the bronchoalveolar lavage fluid of patients with pulmonary Kaposi's sarcoma. Eur Respir J 1996; 9:1743.
59. Whimbey E, Champlin RE, Couch RB, et al: Community respiratory virus infections among hospitalized adult bone marrow transplant recipients. Clin Infect Dis 1996; 22:778.
60. Yousef HM, Englund J, Couch R, et al: Influenza among hospitalized adults with leukemia. Clin Infect Dis 1997; 24:1095.
61. Lewis VA, Champlin R, Englund J, et al: Respiratory disease due to parainfluenza virus in adult bone marrow transplant recipients. Clin Infect Dis 1996; 23:1033.
62. Walsh T, Bodensteiner D, Hiemenz J, et al: A randomized, double-blind trial of AmBisome (liposomal amphotericin B) versus amphotericin B in the empirical treatment of persistently febrile neutropenic patients (Abstract LM-90). *In:* Abstracts of the 37th Interscience Conference on Antimicrobial Agents and Chemotherapy, Toronto, 1997. N Engl J Med 1999; 340:764.
63. Paterson DL, Singh N: Interactions between tacrolimus and antimicrobial agents. Clin Infect Dis 1997; 25:1430.
64. Singh N, Yu VL, Mieles L, et al: Failure of high-dose acyclovir and success of short-course preemptive ganciclovir therapy in preventing cytomegalovirus disease in liver transplant recipients: A prospective randomized trial. Ann Intern Med 1994; 120:375.

62

Infections in Patients with Neoplastic Disease

Amar Safdar, MD • Donald Armstrong, MD

Patients with neoplastic diseases have a greater tendency to acquire infections than the general population. The causes of infections range from agents in the community such as seasonal influenza virus or respiratory syncytial virus (RSV) to perennial organisms like *Streptococcus pneumoniae.* In patients with nosocomial alterations in normal microflora, invasion with organisms such as *Pseudomonas* and *Enterobacter* species may be promoted.[1] Resistant bacterial species such as methicillin-resistant *Staphylococcus aureus* (MRSA) and vancomycin-resistant enterococcis (VREF) also may be encountered.

Agents that usually have low virulence potential can cause serious, invasive infections in patients with altered immune function, whether due to an underlying neoplasm or antineoplastic therapy. The organisms in this setting can range from normal skin flora such as *Candida* species, the normally nonpathogenic saprophyte *Pneumocystis carinii* (PC), or commensal organisms like dematiaceous fungi, which can function as virulent pathogens.[2]

Even with the current advances in medicine, it remains a daunting task to establish timely diagnoses of infectious diseases in critically ill patients with neoplasms. Often, prompt institution of appropriate therapy is crucial.

Fever has been described as the most frequent clinical presentation of infection. Nonspecific contributory signs may occur, like the relative bradycardia associated with *Salmonella* septicemia or *Brucella* infection or the tachycardia with hypotension that may appear early in the course of clostridial sepsis in patients with a rapidly decompensating febrile state. Pyrexia, even though it is the most common sign of infections in general, may be absent from the clinical presentation. A study of cancer patients at the Memorial Sloan-Kettering Cancer Center (MSKCC) in New York, from 1950 to 1971, found that 20% of the subjects had no documented febrile response during disseminated *Mycobacterium tuberculosis* infection.[3]

Therapy with adrenocorticoid hormones may effectively suppress fever. To complicate the issue further, fever due to an underlying lymphoproliferative disease or to certain solid tumors can mimic an infectious syndrome.

This chapter is divided into three sections. The first section describes prevalent infections due to specific immune deficits and the epidemiology of infectious agents. The second focuses on infections relative to an underlying neoplasm and certain organisms and clinical syndromes peculiar to neoplastic disease. Finally, we address the infectious complications seen in the increasing population of bone marrow transplant recipients.

TABLE 62–2. Effect of Leukocyte Count on Outcome of Bacteremia

Absolute Neutrophil Count	Lymphoma and Leukemia	Solid Tumor
≥500/mm³ mortality rate	29.0%	26.0%
≤500/mm³ mortality rate	46.0%	36.0%

I OVERVIEW

CLASSIFICATION

Infections in cancer patients are categorized by the nature of the underlying immunosuppression and may result from the antineoplastic therapy or the neoplastic disease itself (Table 62–1). The predisposing immune defects can be divided into three broad categories:

1. Granulocytopenia.
2. Cell-mediated immunity: T lymphocyte–dependent immune defect or monocyte-macrophage–dependent immune defect.
3. Humoral immunity: B lymphocyte–dependent immune defect, hypogammaglobinemia, splenic dysfunction.

Granulocytopenia

Granulocytopenia (see Table 62–1) secondary to cytotoxic antineoplastic therapy may be profound and prolonged with the prevalent use of highly potent cytotoxic agents. The low neutrophil counts can result from hematopoietic neoplasms or myelophthisis due to extensive bone marrow infiltration by solid tumor cells or advanced-stage lymphoreticular neoplasms and "empty marrows" in patients suffering from aplastic anemia or myelodysplastic syndrome. Besides the decreased absolute neutrophil count, persons with acute leukemia have dysfunctional polymorphonuclear leukocytes. The cytotoxic agents used to treat cancer, such as methotrexate, 6-mercaptopurine, daunorubicin, vincristine, asparaginase, and prednisone, can disrupt chemotaxis, phagocytosis, and even intracellular microbial killing.[4] Prolonged corticosteroid therapy or poorly managed hyperglycemia, irradiation, and, in situations of prolonged hypoxemia, acidosis or hypovolemia, can either predispose to infections with the pyogenic bacteria or hamper recovery because of dysfunctional granulocytes. The risk of infections in patients with low neutrophil counts is directly related to the degree of neutropenia (Table 62–2). The potential for infection increases rapidly with the drop in granulocyte count below 500 cells/µL, and the likelihood of severe infections appears to correlate directly with the absolute neutrophil count (ANC) in the peripheral blood below 100 cells/µL.[5, 6, 6a] The duration of granulocytopenia and rapidity of decline in granulocyte counts are independent predictors not only of the risk of infections but also of the clinical outcome.

The principal role of polymorphonuclear leukocytes is to orchestrate the acute inflammatory reaction to microbial invasion. Thus, the absence or mildness of symptoms or signs can be misleading, and empirical antimicrobial therapy must be started at the earliest suspicion of infection. The overall incidence of documented infections in granulocytopenic cancer patients ranges from 40% to 60%, although some centers have reported rates as low as 20%.[5, 6a]

The factors contributing to the development of infections during neutropenia are summarized in Table 62–3. The mucositis involving the gastrointestinal tract presents clinically as ulceration of the buccal mucosa, malabsorption states, or, in severe cases, gastrointestinal bleeding. It is frequently observed with the use of larger doses of potent myelosuppressive cytotoxic antineoplastic agents such as paclitaxel or etoposide (VP16).

TABLE 62–1. Microorganisms Associated with Neutropenia

Bacteria	Fungi	Viruses
Common	***Common***	***Common***
AEROBIC	*Candida* spp.	HSV
CNS	*Aspergillus* spp.	***Uncommon***
Staphylococcus aureus	***Uncommon***	VZV
Streptococcus spp.	*Trichosporon* spp.	CMV
Enterococcus spp.	*Fusarium* spp.	
Enterobacteriaceae	*Pseudoallescheria boydii*	
Pseudomonas aeruginosa	*Malassezia furfur*	
Less Common	Zygomycetes	
AEROBIC		
Corynebacterium jeikeium		
Bacillus spp.		
Enterobacter spp.		
Acinetobacter spp.		
Serratia spp.		
Pseudomonas organisms not *P. aeruginosa*		
Aeromonas spp.		
Stenotrophomonas maltophilia		
ANAEROBIC		
Clostridium perfringens		
Clostridium septicum		
Bacteroides fragilis		

CNS = coagulase-negative streptococci; HSV = herpes simplex virus; VZV = varicella zoster virus; CMV = cytomegalovirus.

TABLE 62–3. Factors Contributing to Infection in Neutropenia

1. Mucositis
   a. Altered ciliary function and clearing
2. Venous access
   a. Indwelling central venous catheter
   b. Hickman, Broviac
   c. Mediport devices
3. Infusion ports
   a. Peritoneal
   b. Hepatic artery pumps
   c. Ommaya and epidural catheters
4. Urinary catheters
5. Mechanical obstruction
   a. Colon carcinoma
   b. Endobronchial cancers
6. Altered mental status
   a. Loss of gag reflex

Bacterial Infections

Cancer patients are at higher risk for septicemia from oral commensal microorganisms such as alpha-hemolytic streptococci (e.g., *Streptococcus mitis*) or the enteric aerobic gram-negative bacteria (e.g., *Escherichia coli, Klebsiella* or *Enterobacter* species, or *Pseudomonas aeruginosa).*[6, 6b] On occasion, enterococci, diphtheroids, and anaerobic bacteria such as *Clostridium* species or *Bacteroides* species can gain access to the bloodstream, and, less frequently *Capnocytophaga* (DF-1) species may invade and disseminate in profoundly neutropenic patients.[2, 9]

Intravenous Device–Related Infections

The universal use of long-term central venous access catheters (CVCs) has played a key role in the re-emergence of bacteremia due to the gram-positive bacteria in neutropenic hosts. Coagulase-negative staphylococci are the most frequent cause of bacteremia, followed by *S. aureus.*[9a–9c] Less often, *Corynebacterium jeikeum* (CDC-JK), enterococci, and *Bacillus* species can lead to bloodstream infections.

Fungal Infections

The death rate in neutropenic patients at MSKCC with *Candida* septicemia has been considerably reduced from 84% in 1966 to 35% to 45% in more recent years.[9a, 10, 11] Despite aggressive antibacterial and antifungal therapy, however, the mortality rate has not significantly improved since 1990. The incidence of fungal infection in neutropenic patients is dependent on multiple endogenous and external influences (Table 62–4) and appears to differ among institutions.[12] Data from the National Nosocomial Infections Surveillance (NNIS) system collected during 1980 to 1990 shows an increase in the hospital-acquired fungal infection rate from 2.0 to 3.8 per 1000 patient discharges. The overall incidence of infection caused by fungal pathogens reported in 1980 was 6.0%, and at the end of the study period had increased to 10.2%.[13] The increasing rate of candidemia among febrile neutropenic patients has been evident.

The incidence of candidemia in the United States rose from 1.0 per 1000 discharges in 1980 to 4.9 per 1000 in 1990, making *Candida* species the fourth most prevalent cause of positive blood cultures.[13] A species shift, from *Candida albicans* to the less triazole-responsive *Candida tropicalis,* has been observed. The increase in *Candida glabrata* and *Candida krusei* infections in this population is probably due to selection of intrinsically azole resistant strains by increased azole use.[14–16]

The overall mortality rate for invasive *Candida* infections associated with relapse of hematologic malignancies that require cytotoxic chemotherapy has remained between 70% and 90%.[10, 17] However, the mortality rate for patients with candidemia (all species) without evidence of tissue invasion ranges from 39% to 50% among a comparable patient population.[9a] Candidemia is a poor indicator of invasive candidiasis, as 40% to 60% of patients with hematogenous disseminated candidiasis have negative blood cultures.

Like the factors that contribute to bacterial infections, fungemia is related to the degree (less than 150 cells/μL) and the duration (more than 5 to 7 days) of neutropenia. It also bears a relationship to the presence of an indwelling central venous access catheter.[9, 9a, 10, 11] Candidemia associated with CVCs can progress to systemic dissemination and to solid organ infections, especially in the heart and kidneys. Alternatively, with candidemia from gastrointestinal sources such as severe mucositis, the dissemination is more likely to involve the viscera in the portal circulation, such as the liver and spleen. Skin lesions due to fungal emboli are far more common with *C. tropicalis* fungemia. In one study fungal emboli were responsible for more than 70% of all such lesions.[10]

Fever is the most common presentation of *Aspergillus* infections in granulocytopenic cancer patients. The incidence of systemic aspergillosis is disproportionately high in patients with leukemia, about seven times greater than in patients with a lymphoreticular malignancy.[18, 19] Most often involved are the lungs (Table 62–5), and owing to the propensity of the organism to invade blood vessels and cause intravascular thrombosis, pulmonary infarctions and hemorrhages can lead to a dramatic clinical presentation of massive hemoptysis. On occasion patients with reduced pulmonary reserves and those receiving large doses of adrenocorticoid hormone therapy may present with respiratory symptoms of acute onset leading to acute respiratory distress as an initial manifestation of pulmonary *Aspergillus* infection.

Extrapulmonary *Aspergillus* infections frequently involve the paranasal sinuses. Less commonly, brain abscess or cerebritis may occur, and only rarely fatal heart infection. Cutaneous infections can be either primary (appearing at intravenous access sites) or can produce indurated lesions along pressure points on the body. The classic multiple ecthmyic lesions with

TABLE 62–4. Risk Factors for Candidemia

Neutropenia
≤150 Neutrophils
≥1 wk duration
Central venous catheter (Hickman, Brovaic, Mediport)
Broad-spectrum antibiotics
Chemotherapy
Total parenteral nutrition
Candida colonization
Abdominal surgery
Mucositis
Corticosteroids
Prolonged hospitalization (~20–30 days)
Relapse of neoplasm
Diabetes mellitus
Radiation therapy
Extremes of age
Bone marrow transplantation
Graft-versus-host disease (acute and chronic)
Donor mismatch

TABLE 62–5. Organ Involvement with Aspergillosis in Cancer Patients*

	No. of Cases	
Organ Involved	***Meyer et al.***	***Young and Bennett***
Lung	90	92
Brain	9	13
Heart	9	7
Gastrointestinal tract	9	21
Kidney	7	12
Liver	5	12
Thyroid	4	9
Spleen	3	—
Diaphragm	1	5
Bladder	1	0
Disseminated infection (≥2 organs)	23/93	34/98

Data from Meyer RD, Young LS, Armstrong D: Am J Med, 1973; 54:6–15; and Young RC, Bennett JE: Aspergillosis: The spectrum of disease in 98 patients. Medicine 1970; 49:147–173.

*Incidence of aspergillosis in patients with leukemia was seven times greater than in patients with lymphoma.

TABLE 62–6. Predominant Types of Lung Involvement with Pulmonary Aspergillosis

Type of Involvement	No. of Cases	
	*Meyer et al.**	*Young and Bennett†*
Bronchopneumonia	37	32
Hemorrhagic infarction	34	32
Focal necrosis	5	3
Aspergilloma (cavitating)	5	1
Bronchitis	4	9
Microabscesses	2	10
Interstitial	2	0
Lobular pneumonia	2	0
Lobar pneumonia	1	9
Solitary granuloma	0	1
Solitary lung abscess	0	3

*Data from Meyer RD, Young LS, Armstrong D: Am J Med 1973; 54:6–15.
†Data from Young RC, Bennett JE: Aspergillosis: The spectrum of disease in 98 patients. Medicine 1970; 49:147–173.

a large area of central gangrenous necrosis signal disseminated disease. Early skin biopsy is the fastest and most reliable way of making a diagnosis of persistent dermal lesions in this population; however, therapy must not be withheld while pursuing the diagnosis. The most important prognostic indicator of favorable outcome is resolution of neutropenia and early antifungal therapy. In most instances prompt antifungal therapy[2, 6b, 20] is started empirically.

In the earlier literature the most frequent pulmonary presentation of invasive *Aspergillus* infection was bronchopneumonia and hemorrhagic infarctions.[18, 21] Focal necrosis and invasive cavitary lesions were less common (Table 62–6). With the wider availability of more sensitive radiographic techniques, such as high-resolution computed tomography (Fig. 62–1), early focal infections are being diagnosed more frequently and treated earlier. This should contribute to a more favorable outcome in neutropenic patients. Infections caused by *Fusarium* species are hard to distinguish on clinical grounds from those of *Aspergillus. Fusarium* has a tendency to cause bloodstream and cutaneous infection. A similar pattern is observed with *Trichosporon beigelli* infections. Both fungi have exhibited less than optimal response to amphotericin B.

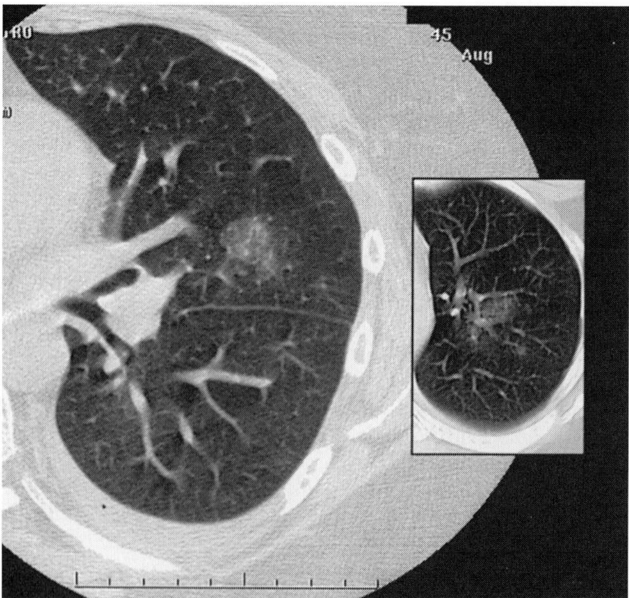

Figure 62–1. High-resolution CT scan image. Midlung field focal nodular opacity seen with early *Aspergillus flavus* infection. *Inset,* Standard (non–contrast-enhanced) CT shows focal opacities with *A. flavus.*

Viral Infections

Patients with neutropenia are at higher risk for recrudescence of herpes simplex virus (HSV) infection. These most often involve the oropharynx and may extend to the esophagus, leading to severe odynophagia and dysphagia. Perianal or genital HSV-2 or HSV-1 reactivation causes morbidity, as the very painful lesions heal slowly and provide portals of entry for perianal bacterial or fungal superinfections. A high index of suspicion for HSV infection in neutropenic patients with fever of an obscure source may help to lower the potential risk of superinfection and prompt early initiation of antiviral therapy.

Very rarely, HSV infection is disseminated. Systemic HSV infection often involves the lungs, central nervous system, gastrointestinal tract, and the liver. Patients with chemotherapy-induced granulocytopenia and an underlying T lymphocyte defect may be at a higher risk of reactivation of Varicella-zoster virus (VZV). It may present as single or multidermatomal involvement, and rarely results in systemic dissemination, but when it does the organs usually affected are lungs, liver, and the gastrointestinal tract. An infrequent but potentially fatal VZV nondermatomal infection of the autonomic nervous system supplying the bowel presents as an acute abdomen mimicking a perforated viscus. Unless treated early, it is nearly always fatal.

Cell-Mediated Immune Deficits

(Table 62–7)

The immune response mediated by thymus-derived lymphocytes plays a central role in the type IV hypersensitivity response. This component of the immune system controls monocyte-macrophage antigen handling and intracellular microbial elimination via various cytokines and lymphokines. Immunocompromised patients are highly susceptible to infections with intracellular microorganisms, and the extent of the immune deficit is proportional to the stages of the underlying neoplasm—lymphocytic leukemia,[22] Hodgkin's disease, or uncommon ones such as hairy cell leukemia and adult T cell leukemia and lymphoma (ATL). Certain antineoplastic agents may potentiate or be the primary cause of defects in the cell-mediated immune response. Examples include fludarabine, cladribine, and agents used to induce T lymphocyte suppression such as cyclosporine, tacrolimus, plus corticosteroids, which have independent potential to cause a wide range of immune dysfunctions.

There is also a cancer-related predilection for certain infections. Patients with relapsed Hodgkin's disease, while receiving antineoplastic agents and radiation therapy, have a 25% or better chance for VZV reactivation,[23] and a higher risk than the general population for disseminated infection. Incidences of *P. carinii* pneumonia as high as 20% have been observed in children receiving maintenance chemotherapy for acute lymphocytic leukemia (ALL).[24] They develop *P. carinii* pneumonia (PCP) with the classic features of dry cough, progressive dyspnea, and interstitial infiltrates on radiography. Those with hairy cell leukemia (independent of chemotherapy) have a higher rate of PCP, owing both to the profound underlying cell-mediated immune compromise and to suboptimal macrophage handling of intracellular microorganisms. These patients also have a higher incidence of mycobacterial infections, especially *Mycobacterium kansasii* and *Mycobacterium avium* complex.

TABLE 62–7. Pathogens Associated with Cell-Mediated Immune Deficits

Bacteria	Fungi	Parasite	Viruses
Listeria monocytogenes	*Cryptococcus neoformans*	*Toxoplasma gondii*	Varicella-zoster
Salmonella spp.	*Candida* spp. (local)	*Strongyloides stercoralis*	Herpes simplex
Nocardia asteroides	*Histoplasma capsulatum*	*Cryptosporidium*	Cytomegalovirus
Mycobacterium tuberculosis and other mycobacteria	*Coccidioides immitis*	*Cyclospora*	***Less Common***
Legionella spp.	*Pneumocystis carinii*	*Microsporidium*	Influenza
Rhodococcus equi			Parainfluenza
Less Common			Respiratory syncytial virus
Brucella spp.			Adenovirus
			Measles virus
			Epstein-Barr virus
			Human herpesvirus

Patients with lymphomas, especially those suffering from Hodgkin's disease, tend to develop reactivation of pulmonary infections with *Mycobacterium tuberculosis.*[3]

Certain viruses stand out as common pathogens in this group of cancer patients. HSV (types I and II) carry increased risk for dissemination, depending on the degree of cell-mediated immune compromise, which correlates with the stage of the malignancy. Cytomegalovirus (CMV) usually presents as reactivation of an infection acquired in the remote past but can also be an acute infection acquired in a transfusion of blood products. The end organ affected most often in these patients is the lungs, and one must bear in mind that the presentation may not always be the classic bilateral interstitial infiltrates and non-productive cough, as focal pulmonary infections can also occur. The gastrointestinal tract is the next most commonly affected organ; however, unlike in patients with acquired immunodeficiency syndrome (AIDS), retinitis is a rare complication of CMV viremia in patients with hematopoietic neoplasms.[25]

Humoral Immunity and Splenic Dysfunction (Table 62–8)

Hypogammaglobinemia may appear as an important immune defect in patients suffering from chronic lymphocytic leukemia and in patients with advance stages of multiple myeloma, both due to increased immunoglobulin catabolism and reduced immunoglobulin synthesis secondary to B cell dysfunction. Both result in reduction in normally functioning immunoglobulins. In addition, there is a relative deficiency of opsonization of selected bacteria. The same type of deficient B cell response without hypogammaglobinemia may appear in bone marrow recipients. Patients who undergo splenectomy for an underlying neoplastic disease also become infected with the same type of bacteria, which may be opsonized but are not cleared owing to the absence of the spleen. These patients are very susceptible to a widely disseminated and rapidly fatal infection with *Streptococcus pneumoniae.* Septicemia caused by *Haemophilus influenzae, Neisseria meningitidis,* or certain intra- and extraerythrocytic parasites such as *Plasmodium* and *Babesia* species pose serious threats to this group of patients. Vaccination against these bacteria does not produce an effective antibody response in patients who have been splenectomized or who have a B cell defect. Splenectomized patients and bone marrow transplant recipients should be considered for long-term or even life long prophylaxis with an appropriate antibiotic and strict screening of blood products for *Plasmodium* and *Babesia* species.

Occasionally, patients with chronic lymphocytic leukemia have an underlying cellular immune defect that makes them vulnerable to infection by pathogens such as *P. carinii* and *Giardia lamblia.* The latter can mimic a chronic malabsorption disorder.

EPIDEMIOLOGY

The epidemiology of infections in cancer patients is associated with changes in the microflora that may result from the home or hospital environment and with factors such as travel, occupation, hobbies, pets, or other animals.

Hospital Environment

The microflora and macroflora (e.g., in ventilation and water supply systems and fomites) associated with hospitals and other chronic care facilities such as nursing homes and dialysis centers can cause a change in the patient's normal flora. Antibiotics have become the single most prominent promoter of resistant microorganisms that can colonize these patients. Among other factors that appear to play a role are degree and duration of immunosuppression, invasive procedures, and duration of hospital stay.

TABLE 62–8. Pathogens Associated with Humoral Immune Deficits

Disease	Bacterium	Fungus	Parasite	Virus
Spleen				
Splenectomy	*Streptococcus pneumoniae*		*Babesia* spp.	Varicella-zoster virus (?)
Hyposplenism	*Haemophilus influenzae*		*Plasmodium* spp.	
	Neisseria meningitidis			
B Cell Defect				
Multiple myelomoa	*S. pneumoniae*	*Pneumocystis carinii*	*Giardia lamblia* (?)	Echovirus
Chronic lymphocytic leukemia	*H. influenzae*			
Post–marrow transplant	*N. meningitidis*			

TABLE 62–9. Transfusion-Related Infections

Bacterium	Fungus	Virus	Parasite
Pseudomonas fluorescens	*Candida* spp.	Hepatitis B	*Plasmodium* spp.
Yersinia spp.		Hepatitis C	*Toxoplasma gondii*
Brucella spp.		Hepatitis non-A, non-B, or non-C	*Babesia* spp.
Salmonella spp.		Cytomegalovirus	*Trypanosoma cruzi*
Enterobacter agglomerans		Epstein-Barr virus	
Enterobacter cloacae		Human immunodeficiency virus	
		Human T lymphotropic virus 1	
		Human T lymphotropic virus 2	

The gastrointestinal tract of the patient may become colonized with resistant *Escherichia coli, Klebsiella* or *Enterobacter* species, or *P. aeruginosa* as a result of antibiotic-related selection pressure or by plasmid-mediated transfer of resistant genes from hospital-acquired microorganisms. Waterborne pseudomonads or *Serratia marcescens* may colonize the lower urinary tract and intravenous catheter sites. Hospital-acquired *S. aureus* and MRSA may colonize the upper respiratory passages, usually the nasopharynx. CDC-JK colonizes the skin around the axilla and groin regions. Use of topical povidone baths may help reduce colonization, and consequently, the risk for bacteremia and CVC-related infections.[46]

Candida species tend to infect certain types of hospitalized patients. *C. albicans* or *C. tropicalis* can cause mucous membrane infections, which in the presence of mucositis and neutropenia can become invasive. Fungemia can result from a gastrointestinal or a CVC source. On the other hand, *Candida parapsilosis* tends to cause fungemia arising from CVC's in patients who require total parenteral nutrition.

P. carinii infection has been observed in clusters reported from several institutions. We recommend respiratory isolation for suspected or proven *P. carinii* infections. Scabies may be troublesome—and severe in immunocompromised patients. Transmission occurs via person-to-person spread and inadequately disinfected fomites.

Seasonal respiratory viruses such as RSV, influenza virus, and parainfluenza virus spread by droplet transmissions or direct contact are hazards to severely immunodeficient patients. These infections can cause serious morbidity and mortality. RSV lower respiratory tract infection can be severe and even fatal for leukemia and bone marrow transplantation patients. VZV may cause a life-threatening infection in susceptible patients including healthy seronegative health care workers and cancer patients with cellular immune deficits. VZV infection can be transmitted during the prevesicular (prodromal) phase via the respiratory route and subsequently from viral shedding from noncrusted cutaneous lesions. The infections associated with transfusion of blood products (Table 62–9) in the hospital can further complicate the evaluation of febrile patients with cancer.

Geographic Considerations

It is essential to know where a patient has lived or traveled. Latent infections with endemic pathogens can be reactivated months to years later in severely immunocompromised patients. These organisms include endemic mycoses, such as *Histoplasma* capsulation and *Coccidioides immitis,* and parasites, such as *Strongyloides stercoralis.*

Home Environment

Close contacts with family or friends can result in transmission of organisms such as RSV, influenza viruses, *Mycobacterium tuberculosis,* and resistant bacteria from a chronic care facility. Cytomegalovirus, scabies, or hepatitis A virus can be brought home from a day-care center or from school. Children in a household with an immunocompromised cancer patient should not be vaccinated with live attenuated vaccines lest viral shedding pose a transmission risk for the immunocompromised household contact.

Work, Habits, and Hobbies

Working with farm animals and exposure and contact with wild animals and household pets can expose us to a variety of pathogens. Some common infections, such as those with *Campylobacter* species, have been attributed to contact with dogs, and infection with *Capnocytophaga canimorsus* (DF-II) can be life-threatening in neutropenic or splenectomized patients exposed to canine saliva. Cats can transmit oocysts of *Toxoplasma gondii,* which can cause severe disease.

II

INFECTIONS RELATED TO AN UNDERLYING NEOPLASM

ADULT T CELL LEUKEMIA AND LYMPHOMA

Adult T cell leukemia and lymphoma (ATL) was first described by Takatsuki in 1977. It was subsequently attributed to the newly discovered human T lymphotropic virus type I (HTLV-I). An associated immune defect of T cells was a feature of the disease, and as many as 80% developed opportunistic viral infections. The lungs are a common site of infection, which may lead to progressive respiratory insufficiency early in the course of the disease. The well-recognized noninfectious complication in patients suffering from ATL is hypercalcemia induced by parathyroid hormone–related protein, which is thought to be secreted by the ATL cells. Cytomegalovirus accounts for 70% of the infections involving the lungs, and in half of cases it is responsible for adrenal necrosis.[26] The second most common pathogen group is fungi. Invasive aspergillosis involving the lung, and occasionally candidemia, can cause fever and sepsis. Infections with *Cryptococcus neoformans,* and rarely *Mucor* species, have also been observed. Like patients with other hematologic neoplasms associated with an underlying defect in the type IV hypersensitivity reaction, more than 10% of these patients are at risk for *P. carinii* pneumonia.[26] Patients with ATL from the Caribbean are especially prone to the hyperinfection syndrome with *S. stercoralis.*

Infections and immunomodulation develop not only in acute ATL but also in the chronic, smoldering type, and it has been observed as early as the HTLV-I carrier state, before malignant transformation.[27] The hyperinfection syndrome due to *S. stercoralis* can also be seen at this time and heralds the onset of the disease.

HAIRY CELL LEUKEMIA

Hairy cell leukemia is a rare lymphoproliferative malignancy of B cell origin. The underlying immune deficit includes profound T lymphocyte dysfunction plus granulocytopenia, monocytopenia, and leukocyte functional abnormalities. Splenectomy to enhance neutrophil counts carries increased risk of serious pyogenic infections by encapsulated bacteria. Owing to cellular immune and monocyte function defects, mycobacterial infections are common. Most frequently encountered are *M. kansasii* and *M. avium* pulmonary infections, which at the time of diagnosis are usually disseminated. Occasionally hairy cell leukemia patients present with infections caused by HSV, CMV, *Candida, Listeria, Salmonella,* or *Cryptococcus* organisms or *P. carinii.*

CHRONIC LYMPHOCYTIC LEUKEMIA

Hypogammaglobinemia is the principal immunologic deficit in patients with advanced chronic lymphocytic leukemia. (CLL).[19] The risk of severe infection by encapsulated pyogenic bacteria does not decrease with antineoplastic chemotherapy. Splenectomy increases the risk for life-threatening pneumococcal infection. As pneumococcal vaccination is apparently of little benefit to these patients, lifelong antibiotic prophylaxis with penicillin or erythromycin or long-acting macrolides may be of benefit, but the question requires further investigation. The prophylactic antibiotic of choice for penicillin-resistant pneumococci is not known, and some investigators would continue to use penicillin.

NEUTROPENIC ENTEROCOLITIS

The incidence of acute necrotizing enterocolitis is around 10% in children with leukemia. Neutropenic enterocolitis is growing more prevalent but is now less common as a terminal illness.[28] It is most frequently associated with the profound and longstanding neutropenia and increasing potency of cytotoxic chemotherapeutic agents.[28, 29] The agents that promote gastrointestinal tract ulceration (i.e., cytosine arabinoside [Ara-C], etoposide [VP-16], and occasionally daunomycin) exhibit statistically significant associations with this syndrome. At one center, 90% of typhlitis cases occurred within 30 days of chemotherapy, and risk was inversely related to recovery of the neutrophil counts.[28, 29] Patients with severe ulcers and necrosis are likely to suffer perforation during the granulocyte recovery phase.

Common clinical symptoms are fever, abdominal pain and distention, and nearly one third of patients present with acute lower gastrointestinal tract bleeding. Microorganisms most often isolated in children with typhlitis are *Pseudomonas* species, *E. coli, S. aureus,* and *Clostridium* species, especially *C. septicum.* Cultures grow a fungus such as a *Candida* or less commonly, *Aspergillus* species, from the affected sites in a few living patients and in half of those examined post mortem.

In the majority of patients, conservative medical treatment and aggressive antibiotic and antifungal therapy have been keys to drastically reducing deaths associated with neutropenic enterocolitis, which some two decades ago was thought to be uniformly fatal. Hollow viscus perforation or imminent perforation (as in patients with advanced pneumatosis intestinalis) may be an indication for surgical intervention.[29]

LISTERIOSIS

Since the 1950s, *Listeria monocytogenes* infection has emerged as an uncommon but serious illness in patients with T lymphocyte dysfunctions.[30] Historically, *L. monocytogenes* infection of the gravid uterus of animals and humans has been recognized as a cause of chorioamnionitis. More recently, self-limited foodborne outbreaks have been connected to *L. monocytogenes* contamination of cheeses and processed foods.

In cancer patients the infection may present as septicemia, with or without central nervous system (CNS) involvement. Rarely, it presents as a complicated CNS infection such as intracranial abscess and hydrocephalus. The heart, liver, spleen, and pancreas occasionally are involved. Serous body cavity infections presenting as peritonitis or pleurisy have been reported.

Patients with Hodgkin's disease, acute or chronic leukemia, and multiple myeloma have a greater predilection for *L. monocytogenes* infection. When, occasionally, solid tumor patients with widespread metastatic disease, as from breast or female genitourinary tract cancer, develop serious life-threatening *Listeria* infection, the prognosis is grave.[31]

Listeriosis has a high relapse rate in patients treated less than 2 weeks for bacteremia or less than 6 weeks for meningitis. Even with modern medical care this infection carries a high mortality rate—30% to 35% according to one study.[31]

TUBERCULOSIS

Reactivation of a latent infection is responsible for most cases of tuberculosis in immunocompromised patients with a T cell defect. Lymphoproliferative disorders[23] and patients with metastatic breast cancer and locally spreading gynecologic malignancy appear to have more frequent reactivation of infection with *M. tuberculosis.* In a study of 201 cancer patients at a cancer center, the overall mortality rate was 17%.[3]

Patients with nonresectable lung cancer undergoing chemotherapy and those with head and neck neoplasms treated with radiation therapy stand out as populations at high risk for reactivation of previously acquired tuberculous infection. These two patient groups have mortality rates of 7% and 13% from *M. tuberculosis* infection, respectively.[3]

Disseminated infections usually follow cytotoxic chemotherapy, with or without corticosteroid use. Most of these patients, however, do not exhibit a miliary pattern on chest roentgenography. Unless aggressively pursued for a microbiologic or histopathologic diagnosis, the mortality rate may approach 90%, and the diagnosis is often established on the post mortem examination.[3]

NOCARDIOSIS

Infection by *Nocardia asteroides* in patients with neoplastic diseases usually presents as bronchopneumonia or lobar pneumonia. CNS involvement may be an indolent process or a fulminant necrotizing infection leading to single or multiple abscess formation.[30] Predisposing neoplasms are as described for *M. tuberculosis*. The common denominator is a T lymphocyte defect.[32]

There is an association of nocardiosis and large doses of prednisone administered for more than 2 to 4 weeks. Nocardiosis even with appropriate antibiotic therapy (sulfonamides, trimethoprim-sulfamethoxazole [TMP-SMZ] for 4 to 6 months) has a mortality rate greater than 50%, although this may be related to the advanced underlying disease.

FEVER AND SEPSIS

Patients with granulocytopenia and those with profound T lymphocyte suppression (e.g., due to fludarabine therapy) may present with clinical sepsis with no evident source of infection. The microorganisms listed in Table 62-1 are microflora associated with the integument or the gastrointestinal or genitourinary tract. In neutropenic patients, after obtaining adequate cultures, empirical antibiotics, antifungal, or antiviral therapy must be instituted promptly to reduce morbidity and the high mortality associated with sepsis.[20]

Most regimens in neutropenic patients include an anti-*Pseudomonas* beta lactam plus an aminoglycoside.[6] Third-generation cephalosporins such as ceftazidime and newer agents such as cefepime, with or without an aminoglycoside, are acceptable regimens. The aminoglycoside offers synergy against some gram-negative bacilli and may have some activity against *S. aureus.* If MRSA is a common hospital pathogen, vancomycin should be added. Additionally, vancomycin should be included if *S. viridans* organisms resistant to beta lactams are prevalent. The increasing incidence of coagulase-negative staphylococci in cancer patients is related to the use of indwelling central venous catheters.[9b, 9c]

In patients with reduced renal function a combination of two anti-*Pseudomonas* beta-lactam antibiotics can be used instead of an aminoglycoside. The role of fluoroquinolones is evolving in combination therapy with an anti-*Pseudomonas* penicillin or third-generation cephalosporins. In cases of documented penicillin or cephalosporin allergy, monobactams (e.g., aztreonam) should be considered. For febrile granulocytopenic patients who cannot tolerate aminoglycosides, or when *P. aeruginosa* infections are not likely, monotherapy with a "non–anti-*Pseudomonas*" third-generation cephalosporin, such as ceftriaxone, or combination therapies using second-generation cephalosporins remain reasonable alternative regimens. These regimens have also been used when the duration of neutropenia is estimated to be only a week to 10 days and *P. aeruginosa* infection is highly unlikely.

In centers with an increase in infections with *Stenotrophomonas maltophilia,* empirical use of TMP-SMZ in combination with an aminoglycoside has been found to be reasonably effective. Similarly, in centers with a high incidence of bacteremia due to highly resistant species such as *Enterobacter,* empirical use of imipenem and an aminoglycoside (e.g., amikacin) may be justified as first-line empirical therapy for critically ill neutropenic patients. For persons with unexplained fever and a history of splenectomy, empirical therapy against encapsulated bacteria, especially *S. pneumoniae,* with either ampicillin, 150 mg/kg daily, or penicillin, 300,000 units/kg daily, plus ceftriaxone, 1 to 2 g IV every 12 to 14 hours daily, should be considered for treatment of ampicillin-resistant *H. influenzae.* In addition, vancomycin use must be considered because of the emergence of penicillin-resistant *S. pneumoniae* in certain geographic areas and hospitals and chronic care facilities.

In the treatment of patients with cell-mediated immune defects, *P. carinii* pneumonia must be suspected with progressive respiratory distress of unclear cause, and empiric therapy must be considered with TMP-SMZ in doses of 15 to 20 mg/kg per day in four divided doses. In patients with a history of tuberculosis exposure, empiric treatment with isoniazid, 300 mg daily, rifampin, 600 mg daily, pyrazinamide, 25 to 30 mg/kg per day, and ethambutol, 15 mg/kg per day, must be considered while diagnostic measures are undertaken.

Antibiotic therapy is usually continued until the fever has resolved and the neutrophil count has been restored. In cases of prolonged neutropenia, when the temperature has returned to normal for 3 to 5 days, antibiotics can be stopped, one at a time, at 48-hour intervals.

In clinically stable patients who remain febrile, changes of antibiotics and addition of antifungal agents may not always be necessary, as infection in these patients might be suppressed and not eliminated; however, the possibility of super-

TABLE 62–10. Preferred Therapies for Life-Threatening Opportunistic Fungal Infections

Infection	Initial Therapy	Completion or Maintenance
Aspergillosis	Amphotericin B (IV) 1.0–1.5 mg/kg/day	Itraconazole (PO) 5 mg/kg/day
Candidiasis	Amphotericin B (IV) 1.0 mg/kg/day	Fluconazole (PO or IV) 200–400 mg/day
Zygomycosis	Amphotericin B (IV) 1.0–1.5 mg/kg/day	Amphotericin B 1.0 mg/kg/day
Cryptococcosis	Amphotericin B (IV) 1 mg/kg/day *plus* Flucytosine (PO) 100 mg/day in four doses	Fluconazole (PO or IV) 200–400 mg/day
Histoplasmosis	Amphotericin B (IV) 1.0 mg/kg/day	Itraconazole (PO) 5 mg/kg/day
Coccidioidomycosis	Amphotericin B (IV) 1.0 mg/kg/day	Fluconazole (PO or IV) 200–400 mg/day

PO = by mouth; IV = intravenous.

infection by a resistant pathogen or of a recrudescent viral infection must always be kept in mind.

In the persistently febrile neutropenic patient receiving broad-spectrum antibacterial treatment for 3 to 7 days without response, antifungal therapy (Table 62-10) should be started with amphotericin B at 0.7 to 1 mg/kg per day.[10] We prefer 1 mg/kg per day and, instead of a test dose, the initial full dose can be administered at first very slowly to avoid acute reactions, and then, if tolerated, the rate of infusion can be increased. We prefer amphotericin B over fluconazole as initial treatment of suspected acute fungal infections, although the choice of agents may vary between centers.[33] Combined therapy with other agents such as rifampin or 5-flucytosine for candidiasis or aspergillosis has not been proven to be superior to amphotericin B alone. The addition of flucytosine at 100 mg/kg per day in four divided doses to amphotericin B results in earlier sterilization of CSF in patients with cryptococcosis.[30] Blood levels of flucytosine should be maintained at 25 to 50 μg/mL.

Catheter-related infections can be treated with antibiotics administered via all catheter ports for a period of 2 weeks, for infections due to coagulase-negative staphylococci and CDC-JK. When endovascular infection is suspected more prolonged therapy (4 to 6 weeks) may be necessary. Fungemia due to *C. albicans* or *C. tropicalis* may also require a longer course of therapy, but bloodstream infections due to *C. parapsilosis* and *C. glabrata* may respond to therapy of shorter duration. Most would remove catheters, if possible, for fungal or resistant bacterial infections.

III

INFECTIONS IN BONE MARROW RECIPIENTS

In this section we briefly discuss the conventional infectious diseases (also discussed elsewhere) and elaborate on a few less common infections in the population of allogeneic bone marrow transplant recipients. The immune defects have a temporal relationship to the various stages of marrow transplantation (Fig. 62-2). Immediately after transplantation, mu-

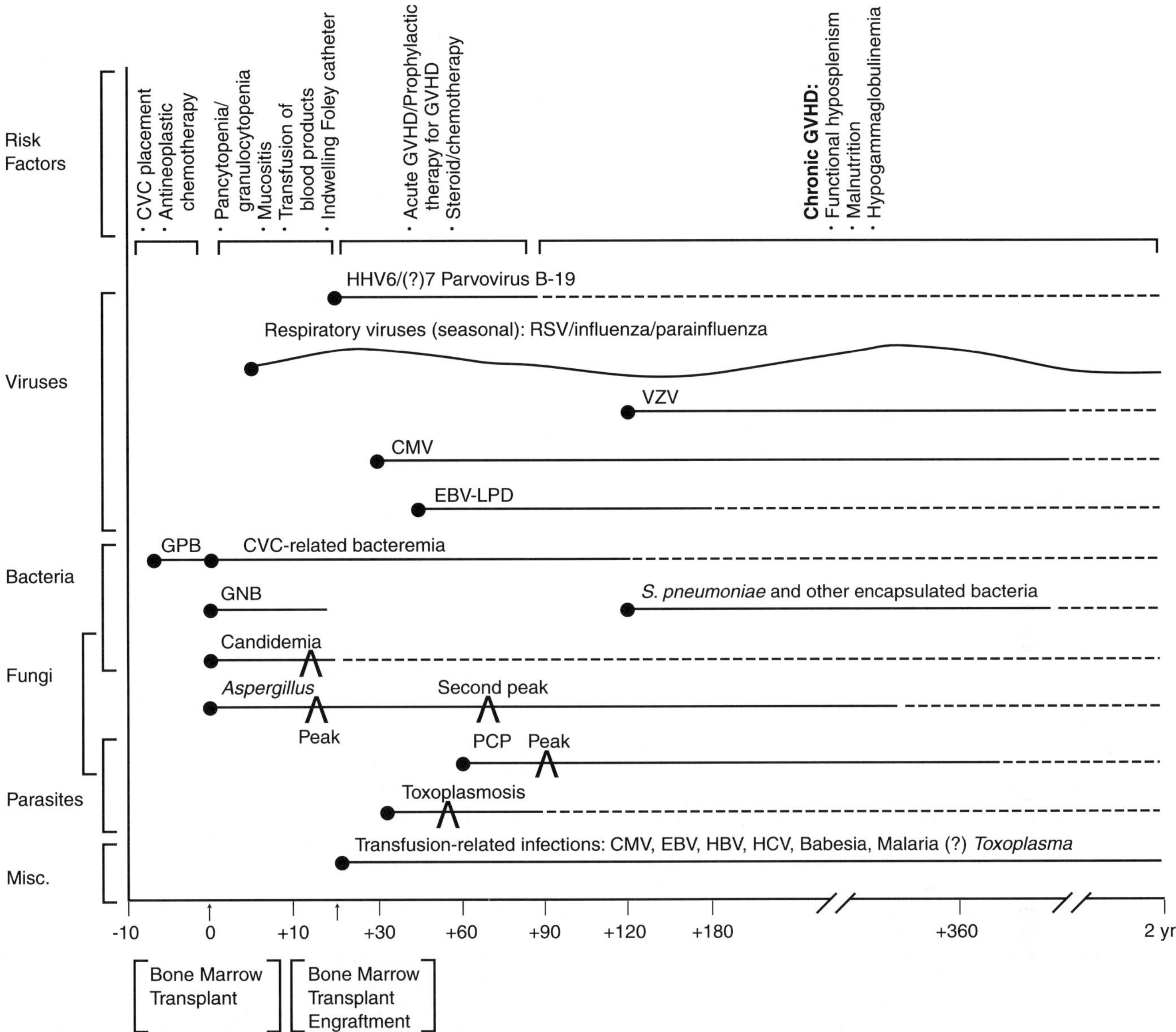

Figure 62–2. Infections in patients with allogeneic bone marrow transplant. RSV = respiratory syncytial virus; VZV = varicella zoster virus; CMV = cytomegalovirus; EBV = Epstein-Barr virus; LPD = lymphoproliferative disorder; GNB = gram-negative bacteria; GPB = gram-positive bacteria; CVC = central venous catheter; PCP = *Pneumocystis carinii* pneumonia; HBV = hepatitis B virus; HCV = hepatitis C virus; HHV = human herpesvirus; GVHD = graft-versus-host disease.

cositis, neutropenia, and CVCs are the main predisposing factors to infections. The organisms include gram-positive cocci such as coagulase-negative staphylococci and *S. aureus* and less commonly other *Streptococcus* species.

The Enterobacteriaceae (*E. coli, Klebsiella* species) and *Enterobacter* species are associated with ulceration in the gastrointestinal tract and mucositis during neutropenia. The duration and the degree of neutropenia remain universal indicators for the incidence of infection. Neutrophil counts less than 150 cell/μL for longer than 3 or 4 weeks have an independent relationship with survival, despite prophylactic and preemptive therapeutic measures. Fungemia becomes a concern with low neutrophil counts beyond 5 to 7 days. Recently, an increase in candidemia earlier in the course of neutropenia has been noted in patients following bone marrow transplantation and a shift toward non-*C. albicans Candida* bloodstream infection.[34] The difficulty in establishing an early diagnosis of fungal infection has led to the widespread use of empiric therapy with amphotericin B as the standard of care in these patients.

Invasive infections by *Aspergillus* species usually involve the lungs, and less frequently the paranasal sinuses. Solid visceral infections such as hepatosplenic abscesses and brain lesions are less common.[35] Prolonged severe neutropenia and large doses of systemic adrenocorticoid hormone predispose to these infections.

Hepatosplenic mycotic abscesses are most frequently seen in the second and the third month after marrow allograft following an extended period of neutropenia. These usually become clinically evident during the granulocyte recovery phase. In addition to *Candida* and *Aspergillus* species, other fungi can cause invasive disease, including *Trichosporon beigelli, Fusarium* species, *Pseudallescheria boydii,* and the *Zygomycetes.*

The most important predictor of outcome is the recovery of a stable functional neutrophil count. The therapy of choice is amphotericin B in doses of 1 mg/kg body weight per day. The therapeutic role of triazoles like fluconazole for *Candida* and *Trichosporon* and itraconazole for *Aspergillus* and *Fusarium* infections is uncertain at the present time. *P. boydii* infections are especially resistant to antifungals, and miconazole may be the only effective agent. With the availability of lipid formulations of amphotericin with relatively less nephrotoxicity, the management of patients with markedly reduced renal function, drug-induced acute tubular necrosis, or unmanageable electrolytes and acid-base disturbances may be facilitated.

The introduction of laminar air flow rooms on transplantation units has helped in reducing clusters of *Aspergillus* infections, especially during periods of construction. Special respiratory precautions during seasonal community respiratory virus outbreaks may help to prevent life-threatening complications in this vulnerable population; however, the practice of reverse isolation has not consistently provided benefit to marrow allograft patients. On the contrary, this practice exacerbates the social isolation experienced by these psychologically stressed subjects.

Thanks to the universal use of acyclovir prophylaxis for HSV in HSV-seropositive patients the potential for local HSV recurrence and disseminated infections, such as encephalitis and occasionally pneumonitis, has been markedly reduced.[36] Secondary bacterial and fungal infections due to portal or systemic entry from either skin or mucous membrane disruption as a result of HSV ulcerative lesions are uncommon.

T lymphocyte dysfunction, along with $CD4^+$ and $CD8^+$ lymphocytopenia, is worst around 45 to 60 days after conventional allogeneic marrow transplantation. The most common infection during this period is reactivation of CMV. The infection may be seen even earlier in patients who require large doses of systemic corticosteroids for early-onset acute graft-versus-host disease seen most commonly in "non–T cell depleted" transplant recipients.[37] The lungs appear most often to be affected by CMV, and owing to the severity of lymphopenia the untreated infection can rapidly progress to respiratory failure and death. The radiographic presentation may lead to the diagnosis, but a high degree of suspicion and early detection of CMV viremia with the blood neutrophil (PP65), antigenemia, or early detection of viral replication in the cell cultures by direct immunofluorescence assays (e.g., shell vial test) has helped to institute timely anti-CMV therapy. Therapy with ganciclovir and anti-CMV immunoglobulin has significantly reduced mortality in transplant patients, from 80% to less than 50% associated with CMV pneumonia.[25] Preemptive ganciclovir therapy has decreased the overall incidence of CMV disease. The utility of other anti-viral agents, such as foscarnet, in the absence of documented CMV ganciclovir resistance has not been evaluated in prospective controlled trials. Additionally, the use of combinations of foscarnet and ganciclovir needs further clinical evaluation.

CMV-seronegative recipients of bone marrow from a CMV-seropositive donor are at high risk for severe CMV disease after transplantation. The introduction of preemptive ganciclovir therapy for the first 100 days after BMT has significantly improved survival in these patients.[38]

The incidence of VZV reactivation has decreased since the introduction of prophylactic acyclovir to prevent HSV recrudescence.[39] For the patient with multidermatomal or disseminated VZV infection, large intravenous doses of acyclovir (10 mg/kg every 8 hours) or ganciclovir are the treatments of choice.[40] PCP[24] is not a common complication in the bone marrow transplant population, as TMP-SMZ prophylaxis has become the standard of care. Rare instances of breakthrough PCP have been reported in sulfa-allergic patients receiving aerosolized pentamidine prophylaxis.

Toxoplasmosis may occur from reactivation of previously acquired infection or, uncommonly, as an acute primary infection transmitted via transfusion of blood products or bone marrow *source* from a seropositive donor. Common presentations are fever of uncertain origin with progressive pulmonary disease and respiratory compromise, and occasionally neurologic symptoms due to brain abscesses.[41, 42] The diagnosis requires a high degree of suspicion and the demonstration of *T. gondii* tachyzoites in bronchoalveolar lavage fluid or biopsy specimens. The present availability of polymerase chain reaction methods for the demonstration of tachyzoite DNA has facilitated early diagnosis and treatment. Sulfadiazine and pyrimethamine are the drugs of choice. For subjects with sulfa intolerance, clindamycin can be substituted without significantly altering the treatment outcome.

Rare infections due to the polyoma virus (CJK-BK) may cause hemorrhagic cystitis and or progressive multifocal leukoencephalopathy which can lead to high morbidity and mortality in this population. Unremitting diarrhea caused by gastrointestinal tract infection due to rotavirus, is not a management problem only in the pediatric transplant population; adult patients can also have a protracted course. Community respiratory viral infections can be life threatening. The early course of infection can appear as a non-specific febrile rhinorrhea, but failure to diagnose promptly and to intervene can result in rapidly progressive lower respiratory tract compromise.

On occasion patients receiving Epstein-Barr virus (EBV)–seropositive-donor derived bone marrow develop EBV-induced lymphoproliferative disorder (EBV-LPD). EBV-infected B lymphocytes undergo immortalization, which may result in a progressive lymphocytic infiltrative disease or lymphoma. The mean time of onset for EBV-LPD, as for other infections (such as CMV, PCP, and VZV) associated with the T lymphocyte "nadir," is 1½ to 6 months following marrow transplant. The time of onset can be delayed beyond 180 days in patients who receive large doses of systemic corticosteroids for chronic graft-versus-host disease. The incidence of EBV-LPD is less than 1% in the unmodified BMT procedure, but the recipients of marrow from HLA antigen–mismatched unrelated donors have a severalfold higher risk of EBV-LPD. There is an independent risk of EBV-LPD associated with the degree and the type of T cell depletion process employed. T cell–specific monoclonal antibodies carry an LPD incidence as high as 26%, whereas processes that deplete both T and B lymphocytes by using antibodies (i.e., compth-1) have no reported cases of EBV-LPD.[43]

The organs involved in EBV-LPD disease appear to be related to the specific immunosuppressive agents. For example, patients receiving azathioprine have a twofold higher risk of central nervous system involvement, whereas in individuals receiving prophylactic or therapeutic cyclosporine the primary organ involved is the gastrointestinal tract. The most frequent clinical presentation is nontender cervical lymphadenopathy. About a third of patients present with exudative tonsilitis, and 25% with pulmonary symptoms. Fever was found in 80% of patients.[44]

EBV monoclonal B-cell lymphoma tumors are refractory to conventional antiviral and antineoplastic agents. The therapy reported from the allogeneic transplantation group at MSKCC has emerged as the standard treatment for EBV-LPD. It is based on the principle of an adaptive transfer of donor-derived EBV-specific cytotoxic T cells that can induce a durable and complete remission of EBV-LPD in severely CD3 and CD4 lymphocytopenic marrow allograft recipients.[44]

In patients with chronic graft-versus-host disease the invading microorganisms are associated with the primary organ involved—skin, gastrointestinal tract, liver, and occasionally lungs. The underlying immune defect, apart from the secondary myelosuppression, is altered type IV hypersensitivity either due to prolonged T lymphocyte dysfunction or as the result of transplant rejection therapy. Both hypogammaglobulinemia and hyposplenism make these patients prone to disseminated infections by the encapsulated bacteria, most frequently *S. pneumoniae,* occasionally *H. influenzae,* and *N. meningitidis.* The lack of opsonization and ineffective bloodstream clearance by the dysfunctional spleen can lead to fatal *S. pneumoniae* septicemia in cases of delayed diagnosis and late institution of effective therapy. Owing to the decrease in secretory antibodies there is an increased risk of sinopulmonary infections that can become chronic. This is probably due to the sicca syndrome and associated reduced primary defenses such as absence of salivary lysozyme.

Human herpesvirus 6 and 7 and human parvovirus B-19 infections can occur during the immediate or late phase following the marrow allograft. With human herpesvirus 6 primary infection, the classic triad of primary infection, including fever, skin rash, and lymphadenopathy, is uncommon or often self-limiting. The three clinical syndromes requiring anti-herpesvirus 6 therapy with foscarnet in BMT recipients are myelosuppression (i.e., secondary granulocytopenia, anemia, thrombocytopenia), encephalitis, and pneumonitis.[45] Bone marrow suppression and even secondary marrow graft failure can result from reactivation of parvovirus B-19 infection; however, the role of this infection in secondary graft failure is controversial.

Late-onset invasive fungal infections (e.g., *Aspergillus*) are increasingly recognized complications, especially in patients on therapy for chronic graft-versus-host disease. Some transplant services are maintaining their patients on long-term antifungal prophylaxis. Clinical efficacy of this measure needs further evaluation.

The profound impairment of humoral immunity and cellular immune responses involving a decline in helper T cells ($CD3^{+}4^{+}$), impairment of natural killer cell functions, and recovery of these responses in various combination are delayed up to 12 to 24 months after allogenic marrow transplantation. The factors complicating the processes of total immune reconstitution following BMT are still obscure.

References

1. Armstrong D, Young LS, Meyer RD, Blevins AH: Infectious complications of neoplastic disease (Review). Med Clin North Am 1971; 55:729–745.
2. Bodey GP: Infections in cancer patients. Cancer Treat Rev 1975; 2:89–128.
3. Kaplan MH, Armstrong D, Rosen P: Tuberculosis complicating neoplastic disease: A review of 201 cases. Cancer 1974; 33:850–858.
4. Pickering LK, Ericsson CD, Kohl S: Effect of chemotherapeutic agents on metabolic and bactericidal activity of polymorphonuclear leukocytes. Cancer 1978; 42:1741–1746.
5. Bodey GP, Buckley M, Sathe YS, Freireich EJ: Quantitative relationships between circulating leukocytes and infection in patients with acute leukemia. Ann Intern Med 1966; 64:328–340.
6. Pizzo PA, Armstrong D, Bodey G, et al: The design, analysis and reporting of clinical trials on the empirical antibiotic management of the neutropenic patient. Report of a consensus panel. J Infect Dis 1990; 161:397–401.

6a. Schimpff SC: Empiric antibiotic therapy for granulocytopenic cancer patients. Am J Med 1986; 80(Suppl 5C):13–20.

6b. Pizzo PA, Walsh TJ: Fungal infections in the pediatric cancer patient. Semin Oncol 1990; 17(Suppl 6):6–9.

7. Wynne JW, Armstrong D: Clostridial septicemia. Cancer 1972; 29:215–221.
8. Kagnoff MF, Armstrong D, Blevins A: *Bacteroides* bacteremia. Experience in a hospital for neoplastic diseases. Cancer 1972; 29:245–251.
9. Singer C, Kaplan MH, Armstrong D: Bacteremia and fungemia complicating neoplastic diseases: A study of 364 cases. Am J Med 1977; 62:732–742.

9a. White MH: Epidemiology of invasive candidiasis: Recent progress and current controversies. Int J Infect Dis 1997; 1(suppl 1):7–10.

9b. Wade JC, Schimpff SC, Newman KA, Wiernik PH: *Staphylococcus epidermidis:* An increasing cause of infection in patients with granulocytopenia. Ann Intern Med 1982; 97:503–508.

9c. EORTC International Antimicrobial Therapy Cooperative Group, and the National Cancer Institute of Canada–Clinical Trials Group: Vancomycin added to empirical combination antibiotic therapy for fever in granulocytopenic cancer patients. J Infect Dis 1991; 163:951–958.

10. Horn R, Wong B, Kiehn TE, Armstrong D: Fungemia in a cancer hospital: Changing frequency, earlier onset, and results of therapy. Rev Infect Dis 1985; 7:646–655.
11. Whimbey E, Kiehn TE, Brannon P, Blevins A, Armstrong D: Bacteremia and fungemia in patients with neoplastic disease. Am J Med 1987; 82:723–730.
12. Wey SB, Mori M, Pfaller MA, Woolson RF, Wenzel RP: Risk factors for hospital-acquired candidemia: A matched case-control study. Arch Intern Med 1989; 149:2349–2353.
13. Beck-Sague C, Jarvis WR: Secular trends in the epidemiology of nosocomial fungal infections in the United States, 1980–1990. National Nosocomial Infections Survallence System: J Infect Dis 1993; 167:1247–1251.
14. Jarvis WR: Epidemiology of nosocomial fungal infections with emphasis on *Candida* species. Clin Infect Dis 1995; 20:1526–1530.
15. Maksymiuk AW, Thongprasert S, Hopfler R, Luna M, Fainstein V, Bodey GP: Systemic candidiasis in cancer patients. Am J Med 1984; 77:20–27.
16. Abi-Said D, Anaissie E, Uzun O, Raad I, Pinzcowski H, Vartivarian S: The epidemiology of hematogenous candidiasis caused by different *Candida* species. Clin Infect Dis 1997; 24:1122–1128.
17. Meunier-Carpentier F, Kiehn TE, Armstrong D: Fungemia in the immunocompromised host. Changing patterns, antigenemia, high mortality. Am J Med 1981; 71:363–370.
18. Meyer RD, Young LS, Armstrong D, Yu B: Aspergillosis complicating neoplastic diseases. Am J Med 1973; 54:6–15.
19. Salonen J, Nikoskelainen J: Lethal infections in patients with hematological malignancies. Eur J Haematol 1993; 51:102–108.
20. Hughes WT, Armstrong D, Bodey GP, Feld R, Mandell GL, Meyers JD, Pizzo PA, Schimpff SC, Shenep JL, Wade JC, et al: Guidelines for use of antimicrobial agents in neutropenic patients with unexplained fever. J Infect Dis 1990; 161:381–396.
21. Young RC, Bennett JE, Vogel CL, Carbone PP, DeVita VT: Aspergillosis: The spectrum of the disease in 98 patients. Medicine (USA) 1970; 49:147–173.
22. Salonen J, Nikoskelainen J: Lethal infections in patients with hematological malignancies. Eur J Hematol 1993; 51:102–108.
23. Armstrong D, Minamoto G: Infectious complications of Hodgkin's disease. *In* Hodgkin's disease: The Consequences of Survival. Lacher MJ, Redman JR: Philadelphia, Lea & Febiger, 1989, p 151–167.
24. Sepkowitz KA, Brown AE, Telzak EE, Gottlieb S, Armstrong D: *Pneumocystis carinii* pneumonia among patients without AIDS at a cancer hospital. JAMA 1992; 267:832–837.
25. Wingard JR: Viral infections in leukemia and bone marrow transplant patients. Leuk Lymphoma 1993; 11(S2):115–125.
26. Suzumiya J, Marutsuka K, Nabeshima K, Nawa Y, Koono M, Tamura K, Kimura N, Hisano S, et al: Autopsy findings in 47 cases of adult T-cell leukemia/lymphoma in Miyazaki Prefecture, Japan. Leuk Lymphoma 1993; 11:281–286.
27. Hanada S, Uematsu T, Iwahashi M, Nomura K, Utsunomiya A, Kodama M, Ishibashi K, Terada A, et al: The prevalence of human T-cell leukemia virus Type 1 infection in patients with hematologic and non-hematologic diseases in an adult T-cell leukemia-endemic area of Japan. Cancer 1989; 64:1290–1295.
28. Katz JA, Wagner ML, Gresik MV, Mahoney DH Jr, Fernbach DJ: Typhilitis: A 18-year experience and postmortem review. Cancer 1990; 65:1041–1047.
29. Sloas MM, Flynn PM, Kaste SC, Patrick CC: Typhilitis in children with cancer: A 30-year experience. Clin Infect Dis 1993; 17:484–490.
30. Armstrong D, Wong B: Central nervous system infections in immunocompromised hosts. Ann Rev Med 1982; 33:293–308.

31. Louria DB, Hensle T, Armstrong D, Colliins HS, Blevins A, Krugman D, Buse M: Listeriosis complicating malignant diseases: A new association. Ann Intern Med 1967; 67:260–281.
32. Young LS, Armstrong D, Blevins A, Lieberman P: *Nocardia asteroides* infection complicating neoplastic disease. Am J Med 1971; 50:356–367.
33. Bernard EM, Armstrong D: Treatment of opportunistic fungal infections: Clinical overview and protective. Int J Infect Dis 1997; 1(suppl 1):28–31.
34. Goodrich JM, Reed EC, Mori M, Fisher LD, Skerrett S, Dandliker PS, Klis B, Counts GW, et al: Clinical features and analysis of risk factors for invasive candidal infection after marrow transplantation. J Infect Dis 1991; 164:731–740.
35. Wald A, Leisenring W, Van Burik JA, Bowden RA: Epidemiology of *Aspergillus* infections in a large cohort of patients undergoing bone marrow transplantation. J Infect Dis 1997; 175:1459–1466.
36. Saral R, Burns WH, Laskin OL, Santos GW, Lietman PS: Acyclovir prophylaxis of herpes-simplex virus infections: A randomized double-blind, controlled trial in bone marrow transplant recipients. N Engl J Med 1981; 305:63–67.
37. Wingard JR, Piantadosi S, Burns WH, Zahurah ML, Santos GW, Saral R: Cytomegalovirus infections in bone marrow transplant recipients given intensive cytoreduction therapy. Rev Infect Dis 1990; 12(S7):S793–S804.
38. Goodrich JM, Bowden RA, Fisher L, Keller C, Schoch G, Meyers JD: Ganciclovir prophylaxis to prevent cytomegalovirus disease after allogeneic marrow transplant. Ann Intern Med 1993; 118:173–178.
39. Saral R, Ambinder RF, Burns WH, Angelopulos CM, Griffin DE, Burke PJ, Lietman PS: Acyclovir prophylaxis against herpes simplex virus infections in patients with leukemia: A randomized double-blind placebo-controlled study. Ann Intern Med 1983; 99:773–776.
40. Locksley RM, Flournoy N, Sullivan KM, Meyers JD: Infection with varicella-zoster virus after marrow transplantation. J Infect Dis 1985; 152:1172–1181.
41. Slavin MA, Meyres JD, Remington JS, Hackman RC: *Toxoplasma gondii* infection in marrow transplant recipients: A 20 year experience. Bone Marrow Transplant 1994; 13:549–557.
42. Derouin F, Gluckman E, Beauvais B, Devergie A, Melo R, Monny M, Lariviere M: *Toxoplasma* infection after human allogeneic bone marrow transplantation: Clinical and serologic study of 80 patients. Bone Marrow Transplant 1986; 1:67–73.
43. O'Reilly RJ, Small TN, Papadopoulos E, Lucas K, Lacerda J, Koulova L: Biology and adoptive cell therapy of Epstein-Barr virus–associated lymphoproliferative disorder in recipients of marrow allografts. Immunol Rev 1997; 157:195–216.
44. Papadopoulos EB, Ladanyi M, Emanuel D, Mackinnon S, Boulad F, Carabasi MH, Castro-Malaspina H, Childs BH, Gillio AP, Small TN, et al: Infusions of donor leukocytes to treat Epstein-Barr virus–associated lymphoproliferative disorders after allogenenic bone marrow transplantation. N Engl J Med 1994; 330:1185–1191.
45. Yoshiikawa T, Suga Y, Asano Y, Nakashima T, Yazaki T, Sobue R, Hirano M, Fukuda M, Kojima S, Matsuyama T: Human herpes virus-6 infection in bone marrow transplantation. Blood 1991; 78:1381–1384.
46. Armstrong D, Schmitt HJ: *Corynebacterium jeikeium. In:* Infections in Immunocompromised Infants and Children. Patrick CC (Ed). New York, Churchill Livingstone, 1992, pp 511–516.

63

Management of HIV and AIDS-Related Infection in the Intensive Care Unit

John M. Luce, MD • Robert M. Wachter, MD

Many changes have occurred in the overall management of patients with human immunodeficiency virus (HIV) infection and the acquired immunodeficiency syndrome (AIDS) since such patients were first identified in the United States in the early 1980s. Inspired by increased understanding of the natural history of HIV infection, these changes have profoundly influenced the critical care of HIV-infected patients. Because this influence is so important, this chapter begins with a discussion of insights into the biology and epidemiology of HIV infection and general changes in the prevention, treatment, and outcome of HIV-related disease. We then describe the respiratory diseases, including *Pneumocystis carinii* pneumonia (PCP), that frequently cause respiratory failure in patients with HIV infection and thereby prompt their admission to the intensive care unit (ICU). Next, we outline current diagnostic approaches and therapy for PCP, which remains the most common respiratory reason for ICU admission. Finally, we consider studies of the outcome of ICU admission for HIV-related diseases, including respiratory failure caused by PCP, and try to answer the crucial question of which patients with such diseases benefit from admission to the ICU.

INSIGHTS INTO THE BIOLOGY AND EPIDEMIOLOGY OF HIV INFECTION

For many years, HIV infection has been viewed as a process of progressive cellular immune dysfunction leading inexorably to death. Such infection was thought to include an initial viremia, followed by a latent period in which HIV was contained within $CD4^+$ lymphocytes and other cells and replicated minimally. Eventually, the virus proliferated and killed the cells that contained it, at which point a second viremia occurred. At the same time, opportunistic infections and neoplasms occurred in the presence of the severe HIV-induced immune deficiency.

This traditional view has been challenged by the development of quantitative HIV assays and the demonstration that HIV and $CD4^+$ lymphocyte replication and destruction rates during infection are as high as 10 billion virions per day.[1, 2] Use of such assays has also led to the discovery that, after HIV transmission, most patients manifest rapid HIV replication with high serum levels, followed by a cellular immune response and an abrupt reduction in viral load in blood but with persistent viral activity in lymphoid tissue.[3] The amount of virus at the point of initial replication provides important prognostic information. For example, high initial concentrations of virus (>30,000 copies/mm^3) presage rapid progression in terms of the slope of $CD4^+$ cell decline, time to an AIDS-defining diagnosis, and length of survival, whereas low concentrations (<5000 copies/mm^3) predict a more favorable prognosis.[4]

On average, 8 to 10 years pass before patients experience the opportunistic infections and neoplasms that characterize

AIDS. The infections that occur are influenced by many host factors, most of which are unknown. Nevertheless, it is clear that the types of infections suffered by HIV-infected patients are related in part to differences in their environment. This presumably accounts for the finding that, other than bacteria, *Mycobacterium tuberculosis* is the organism that most commonly causes lower respiratory tract infection among AIDS patients in Africa, whereas *P. carinii* remains the dominant organism in the United States.[5, 6]

The first American patients with what came to be known as HIV infection and AIDS were white homosexual and bisexual men in Los Angeles and New York.[7, 8] Infection with HIV was largely confined to the gay community in the United States through the early 1980s, although a heterosexual form of the disease was noted to be predominant in Africa and other areas. Subsequently, HIV has increasingly been spread through injection drug use and heterosexual contact, and AIDS is now clearly a disease of women and children as well as men in the United States.[9] It has also become a disease of poverty, as HIV infection is increasingly prevalent in blacks, Latinos, and other minority groups. Metropolitan areas with the highest AIDS rates per 100,000 population in the United States in 1996 were New York (120.1), Miami (99.4), Jersey City, New Jersey (97.7), San Francisco (95.0), and West Palm Beach, Florida (85.4).[10] All of these areas have large homosexual or minority communities in which HIV infection is increasingly widespread.

CHANGES IN THE PREVENTION, TREATMENT, AND GENERAL OUTCOME OF HIV-RELATED DISEASE

Management of HIV-infected patients early in the AIDS epidemic was based largely on the diagnosis and treatment of opportunistic infection and neoplasms. These disorders were usually diagnosed late in the course of HIV infection, and their treatment too often yielded poor results. However, as the natural history of HIV infection was better understood, a test for the presence of the virus became available, and monitoring of CD4 cell levels became common, clinicians began to offer secondary and then primary prophylaxis for opportunistic infections.[11] In 1987, antiretroviral therapy in the form of zidovudine was shown to be effective, and soon other nucleoside analogs became available.[12, 13] In concert with chemoprophylaxis for opportunistic infections, these agents offered the first real hope that HIV infection and its immunologic sequelae could be arrested, if not cured.

Hope has increased manyfold with the introduction of protease inhibitors, a new class of drugs active against HIV. By March 1996, the U.S. Food and Drug Administration (FDA) had approved three such agents: saquinavir mesylate, ritonavir, and indinavir.[14] Results of studies presented at the Eleventh International AIDS Conference suggested that more than half of patients taking protease inhibitors in addition to nucleoside analogs demonstrated a significant decrease in viral load and an increase in $CD4^+$ lymphocyte levels.[15] Increasingly, clinicians have advocated the administration of what has come to be called highly active antiretroviral therapy (HAART) as outlined in annually updated recommendations from the United States Panel of the International AIDS Society.[16] Although HAART is not effective in all patients, and although resistance to protease inhibitors may become problematic, it appears at this writing that many treated patients with HIV infection may avoid hospitalization and enjoy a longer life expectancy. The cost for this therapeutic success ranges from $12,000 to $15,000 per patient per year.[16]

Because adherence to treatment is essential for HAART to be successful, because poor adherence may cause drug resistance in addition to low effectiveness, and because the money spent on protease inhibitors may be better used for other interventions, debate exists over whether the new drugs should be made available to the homeless and marginally housed members of American society. Between 9% and 20% of this population is HIV infected, and the prevalence of alcoholism, drug abuse, and mental illness within it is high.[17] The authors of a review[18] of protease inhibitors among the homeless recommended that these agents be offered to all patients whose living situation and clinical management can be stabilized but that less aggressive antiretroviral therapy using only reverse transcriptase inhibitors be recommended for unstable patients.

RESPIRATORY DISEASE TRENDS AMONG HIV-INFECTED PATIENTS

Previous reports describing the respiratory manifestations of HIV infection were limited, for the most part, to small series of patients and cross-sectional studies. However, the Pulmonary Complications of HIV Study, in which a cohort of over 1130 HIV-infected patients without AIDS at study entry were followed at six United States centers from 1988 until 1994, has identified the broad spectrum of respiratory disorders that occur in such patients over time. Upper respiratory tract infections were the most common respiratory infections among HIV-infected patients in this study, as they were among patients not infected by HIV. However, lower respiratory tract infections increased as CD4 cell levels decreased among the HIV-infected patients and, presumably, as viral load increased. Acute bronchitis was the predominant lower respiratory tract infection among HIV-infected cohort members with CD4 cell counts greater than or equal to 500 cells/mm^3.[19]

Among the cohort members with CD4 cell counts of 200 to 499 cells/mm^3, the incidences of bacterial pneumonia and PCP each increased an average of 40% per year. Among cohort members with entry CD4 cell levels of less than 200 cells/mm^3, acute bronchitis, bacterial pneumonia, and PCP occurred at high rates without discernible time trends and despite chemoprophylaxis in more than 80% of patients, the rate of lower respiratory tract infections increased as the CD4 cell levels declined. Throughout the 6 years of the study, injection drug users experienced a higher incidence of bacterial pneumonia than did homosexual and bisexual men.[19]

Regarding PCP in particular, multivariate analysis revealed that recurrent undiagnosed fevers, night sweats, oropharyngeal thrush, and unexplained weight loss were associated with increased risk among cohort members with CD4 cell levels greater than 200/mm^3. A decline in the diffusing capacity for carbon monoxide on pulmonary function testing was also seen among patients who later had PCP. Although PCP occurred in patients despite prophylaxis, subjects whose CD4 cell counts declined below 200 cells/mm^3 and who were not receiving preventive therapy were nine times more likely to have PCP within 6 months than subjects who received such therapy. Men were more likely to have PCP than women, and white subjects had three times the risk of incurring PCP of black subjects. There were no significant differences in risk by HIV transmission category, age, education, or the use of zidovudine or other nucleoside analogs.[20]

The Pulmonary Complications of HIV Study also showed the following:

1. Many patients with HIV disease are admitted to the ICU with nonrespiratory problems.
2. Not all those admitted with respiratory problems have PCP.
3. Admission for respiratory infections requiring mechanical ventilation is associated with a high mortality rate.

4. Mechanical ventilation for nonrespiratory disorders carries a more favorable prognosis.

Of the 1130 adults with HIV infection who did not have AIDS at the time of enrollment in the study, 510 patients had a total of 1320 hospital admissions, and 63 patients had a total of 68 admissions to the ICU. Twenty-five (40%) of the patients admitted to the ICU died during that admission.[21]

Only 24 patients were admitted to the ICU with a principal diagnosis of lung disease: 11 had PCP, and six of them (55%) died. Four had bacterial pneumonia, two had pulmonary edema caused by renal failure, and one each had pulmonary tuberculosis, pulmonary Kaposi's sarcoma, pneumothorax, acute respiratory distress syndrome (ARDS), pulmonary fibrosis, cytomegalovirus pneumonia, and adenocarcinoma metastatic to the lungs. Eleven (79%) of these 13 patients died. Thirty-nine patients had 47 ICU admissions for nonrespiratory problems, such as gastrointestinal disorders, cardiovascular disorders, sepsis syndrome, and neurologic disorders. Nine (23%) of these patients died. Of the 28 patients who received mechanical ventilation, seven (25%) had PCP (five died), seven had other lung infections (six died), and 14 received ventilation for nonrespiratory disorders (only five died).[21]

CURRENT DIAGNOSTIC APPROACHES AND THERAPY FOR *PNEUMOCYSTIS CARINII* PNEUMONIA

The Pulmonary Complications of HIV Study and earlier investigations[22–25] indicate that PCP remains the most frequent cause of respiratory failure prompting admission of HIV-infected patients to the ICU in the United States. The clinical presentation of PCP can range from the subtle to the fulminant. Most patients have most or all of the following symptoms or signs: fever, tachypnea, dyspnea with a nonproductive or scant productive cough, and a chest that is either clear to auscultation or has dry rales.[26] Symptoms have generally been present for days to weeks before the diagnosis is made. It has been uncommon for patients to be in respiratory failure at the time they present for medical attention. At San Francisco General Hospital, for example, only six of 77 patients (8%) who received intensive care for PCP and respiratory failure were taken directly to the ICU at the time of hospital admission.[23] Unfortunately, because a lack of current studies, whether this pattern remains today is unclear.

Severe pneumonia caused by *P. carinii* is similar in presentation and pathogenesis to ARDS. As in ARDS, the organism appears to cause a widespread capillary leak.[27] The chest roentgenogram, therefore, usually resembles that in ARDS: a diffuse, bilateral interstitial infiltration. Less commonly, PCP results in diffuse and focal airspace consolidation, cysts and pneumatoceles, and pneumothorax. Finally, about 5% to 10% of patients who prove to have PCP initially have normal chest roentgenograms.[26]

The diagnosis of PCP is made when the organism is identified in the pulmonary secretions of a patient with a compatible clinical presentation. In patients suspected of having PCP, the least invasive diagnostic test is an examination of a sputum specimen induced by inhalation of a hypertonic saline aerosol. In experienced hands, this test has 79% sensitivity and a negative predictive value of 61%.[26] This yield may be increased when fluorescein-conjugated monoclonal antibodies are used.[28] Despite vigorous attempts at sputum induction, however, the diagnosis is not made by this method in at least 20% to 40% of patients with PCP. Moreover, sputum induction is generally not possible in patients who have marked respiratory distress or who are intubated.

When the sputum examination is negative or when sputum cannot be induced, fiberoptic bronchoscopy with bronchoalveolar lavage (BAL) is the procedure of choice, with a sensitivity for PCP above 90%.[29] Early bronchoscopy with BAL should be performed as soon as possible in patients with suspected PCP and a negative induced sputum examination.[30] Although the addition of transbronchial biopsy generally adds little to the yield of lavage in the diagnosis of PCP, it is helpful in HIV-infected patients with other pulmonary infections.[31] It is thus a reasonable initial invasive study when the probability of PCP is low and a useful follow-up test when the BAL fails to demonstrate PCP.

The mainstays of therapy for moderate to severe PCP are intravenous trimethoprim-sulfamethoxazole (TMP-SMX) and pentamidine isethionate.[32] Unfortunately, both drugs are poorly tolerated by AIDS patients, with the frequency of adverse drug reactions often exceeding 50%. Toxic effects of TMP-SMX include nausea, rash, leukemia, thrombocytopenia, hyponatremia, and renal dysfunction. Toxic effects of pentamidine include nausea, orthostatic hypotension, pancreatitis, hypoglycemia or hyperglycemia, leukopenia, thrombocytopenia, and renal dysfunction. Notably, some patients destined to respond to either drug experience transient clinical deterioration during the first 3 to 5 days of treatment, possibly because of an inflammatory response to dead or dying organisms that may increase capillary permeability and pulmonary edema formation. This edema formation may be worsened if patients are given overly large amounts of intravenous fluids.

The potential toxicity of TMP-SMX and pentamidine has led to a search for other less toxic agents and routes of drug delivery. Although in one study aerosolized pentamidine was as efficacious as and less toxic than intravenous TMP-SMX in the treatment of acute PCP, intubated patients were excluded from this protocol.[32] Furthermore, because deposition of aerosolized pentamidine in the endotracheal tube may depress lung levels of the drug, this therapy cannot be recommended for intubated patients with PCP.[33] Intravenous trimetrexate and oral atovaquone have also been shown to be efficacious in patients with mild to moderate PCP, but their use in critically ill patients is limited.[34, 35] As a result, these agents cannot be recommended at the present time.

The high frequency of toxic reactions and worsened respiratory failure after standard antimicrobial treatment of PCP, as well as observations of dramatic improvement with the use of corticosteroids, motivated intense interest in the adjuvant use of these drugs several years ago. This interest prompted several controlled trials[36, 37] demonstrating that the adjuvant use of corticosteroids, along with standard anti-*Pneumocystis* therapy, decreases the risk of respiratory failure and death in patients with AIDS and moderate to severe PCP.

On the basis of a review of published and unpublished studies, a National Institutes of Health–University of California Expert Panel recommended that the equivalent of 40 mg of oral prednisone be given twice daily to patients with AIDS, PCP, and arterial oxygen tension (PO_2) levels in room air of less than 70 mm Hg or arterial-alveolar PO_2 gradients of more than 35 mm Hg.[38] The expert panel recommended that the initial dose be maintained during days 1 through 5 of therapy and then tapered gradually over 3 weeks. Although the panel recommended further study of whether patients already in respiratory failure from PCP benefit from adjuvant corticosteroids, most clinicians use these drugs in this setting.

Because severe PCP is a form of ARDS, positive end-expiratory pressure (PEEP) often increases the arterial PO_2 and decreases shunt fraction. However, these increases may be relatively modest, and therefore this benefit of PEEP must be weighed against its known risks, including barotrauma and decreased cardiac output. Because PEEP can be administered to spontaneously breathing patients via continuous positive airway pressure through a tightly fitting face mask or endotracheal tube, not all PCP patients with respiratory failure require mechanical ventilation. Nevertheless, most such patients have a greatly increased work of breathing and generally require ventilatory support as their pulmonary disease progresses. Most patients are ventilated either with the assist-control mode or with intermittent mandatory ventilation at a high ventilator rate. At San Francisco General Hospital, pressure control ventilation is used frequently to reduce the risk of barotrauma by lowering peak and mean airway pressures. The pressure support mode or continuous positive airway pressure may be helpful during weaning.[33]

OUTCOME AND UTILIZATION OF INTENSIVE CARE FOR HIV-RELATED DISEASES

The previously mentioned Pulmonary Complications of HIV Study[21] demonstrated that the majority of HIV-infected patients who received intensive care in six centers in the United States from 1988 until 1994 did so for nonrespiratory problems and that only a minority of these patients died. The same point was made in a study[39] of the course of 120 consecutive AIDS patients admitted to the ICU in a hospital in Paris, France, between 1990 and 1993. Of these patients, 60 had acute respiratory failure, 27 manifested central nervous system dysfunction, 15 had pneumothorax, 13 were in shock, and 3 had other conditions. Overall, 34 patients (35%) died and 86 (65%) survived. Sixteen of the 60 patients (27%) with acute respiratory failure died, but only eight of 27 (30%) with central nervous system dysfunction, one of 15 (6%) with pneumothorax, six of 13 (46%) of those with shock, and three of five (60%) with other conditions. Multivariate analysis identified three factors predicting poor ICU outcome: poor performance on a physiologic score on admission, time between AIDS diagnosis and ICU admission of more than 1 year, and a low albumin level. Long-term survival after ICU discharge depended only on the severity of AIDS and not on the particulars of the opportunistic infection. The investigators concluded that AIDS patients should be admitted to the ICU on the same basis as other patients.

Despite this conclusion, the mortality rate of mechanically ventilated patients was 61% in this study from Paris, compared with 9% in patients who did not undergo ventilation, and mortality exceeded 80% for ventilated patients with acute respiratory failure. Similarly, in the Pulmonary Complications of HIV Study,[21] 84% of patients ventilated for acute respiratory failure died, versus 36% of patients ventilated for nonrespiratory disorders. Thus, although patients with nonrespiratory disorders seem to benefit from provision of aggressive care even if they require mechanical ventilation, benefit is less apparent among patients who require mechanical ventilation for acute respiratory failure.

Because PCP remains the most common cause of respiratory failure in AIDS patients and the most common reason for ICU admission, more is known about the outcome of intensive care for AIDS patients with PCP than for any other group. All studies to date of ICU outcome for AIDS patients with PCP indicate that such patients have a poor short-term prognosis, especially if they require mechanical ventilation. For example, an investigation conducted in a Paris hospital between 1987 and 1992 revealed that 27 (82%) of 33 mechanically ventilated AIDS patients with PCP died.[40] The mortality rate was 50% among patients for whom mechanical ventilation was started early in the course of acute respiratory failure but rose to almost 100% when mechanical ventilation was started after 5 days of treatment with TMP-SMX and corticosteroids.

Similarly, investigators at a hospital in Vancouver, British Columbia, have demonstrated that the proportion of patients with PCP who required hospitalization at their institution decreased from 100% in 1981 to 1987 to 78% in 1987 to 1991. The proportion of these hospitalizations associated with acute respiratory failure decreased from 21% in 1981 to 1987 to 9% in 1987 to 1991. Although the proportion of AIDS patients with acute respiratory failure resulting from PCP who received mechanical ventilation in their ICU decreased from 89% in 1981 to 1987 to 64% in 1987 to 1991, the case fatality rate among those ventilated patients increased from 50% in 1981 to 1987 to 89% in 1987 to 1991. These changes were associated with a significant increase in the early administration of corticosteroid for AIDS-related PCP, suggesting to the investigators that patients who require mechanical ventilation despite maximal treatment have a dismal prognosis.[41]

We completed a study[42] of the outcome, cost, and cost-effectiveness of critical care for patients with AIDS, PCP, and severe respiratory failure requiring mechanical ventilation at San Francisco General Hospital over a 10-year period, 1981 to 1991. This cohort of patients was divided into three groups for analysis: patients admitted to the ICU in 1981 to 1985 (era I), those admitted from 1986 to 1988 (era II), and those admitted from 1989 to 1991 (era III). Twenty-eight (25%) of these 113 patients survived to hospital discharge: 6 (19%) of 43 in era I, 13 (39%) of 33 in era II, and 9 (25%) of 37 in era III. In era I, only a low albumin level correlated with ICU mortality; in era III, a low $CD4^+$ lymphocyte level on admission and the development of pneumothorax were predictive of death before hospital discharge. Indeed, nine of the 10 patients who had pneumothoraces during this period left the ICU alive.

The mean ICU length of stay for all patients during era I was 10.6 days, compared with 6.9 days in era II and 10.6 days in era III. These differences could be explained by the improved survival during era II. Reflecting the reduced length of stay during era II, mean ICU charges were $43,125, $25,614, and $47,083 during the three periods. The post-ICU hospital charges for the 28 patients who survived the hospital discharge in all three eras averaged $92,903, whereas the charges for patients who died averaged $46,334.

Assuming that ventilated patients would have died that day had they not received mechanical ventilation, the cost of ICU care and subsequent hospitalization was $124,781 per year of life saved during the 10 years of this study. In era I, ICU admission and hospitalization cost $305,795 per year of life saved. This figure fell to $94,528 for patients in era II but rose to $215,233 for patients in era III. The improvement in cost-effectiveness in era II was due to shortened ICU length of stay and improved survival rates, whereas the worsening cost-effectiveness in era III was due to a falling survival rate and a longer length of stay. The cost-effectiveness of critical care for patients in era III, $215,233, was considerably more than that of ICU care for patients with solid tumors ($82,845) and ICU care for patients with hematologic malignancies (189,339) during the same period, not to mention general interventions such as chemoprophylaxis for PCP ($14,000).

Unfortunately, follow-up studies of the outcome, cost, and cost-effectiveness of critical care for AIDS patients requiring mechanical ventilation for PCP have not been reported from San Francisco General Hospital or other institutions in recent years. Nevertheless, investigations to date have suggested that the prognosis of such patients is poor, particularly if they have not responded to anti-*Pneumocystis* agents and corticosteroids. The same can probably be said for AIDS patients with respiratory failure with pneumonia caused by bacteria, *M. tuberculosis*, or other microorganisms, although outcome data for these patients are more limited than for patients with PCP. Given the high cost and limited cost-effectiveness of critical care of patients who have failed a reasonable course (e.g., at least 5 days) of treatment, it seems ethically appropriate to discourage ICU admission of such patients or offer them only a short therapeutic trial.

The prognosis remains uncertain for patients who have not received antimicrobial therapy before ICU admission, including patients for whom PCP, tuberculosis, or other pulmonary infections are the first manifestations of advanced infection with HIV. This part is particularly relevant in light of the advances in antiretroviral therapy and chemoprophylaxis discussed earlier. Presumably, patients with acute respiratory failure who have not responded to nucleoside analogs, protease inhibitors, chemoprophylactic agents, and antimicrobial therapy for pneumonia are highly unlikely to benefit from admission to the ICU. Admission of such patients, therefore, should be discouraged. However, patients who have not had access to or have not availed themselves of highly active antiretroviral therapy cannot be thought of as having failed treatment. We believe that patients such as these deserve to be offered a therapeutic trial in the ICU.

References

1. Wei X, Ghosh SK, Taylor ME, et al: Viral dynamics in human immunodeficiency virus type I infection. Nature 1995; 373:117-122.
2. Ho DD, Neumann AV, Perelson KS, Chen W, Leonard VM, Markowitz M: Rapid turnover of plasma virions and CD4 lymphocytes in HIV-1 infection. Nature 119; 373:123-126.
3. Pantaleo G, Graziosi C, Demarest JF, et al: HIV infection is active and progressive in lymphoid tissue during the clinically latent stage of disease. Nature 1993; 362:355-358.
4. Mellors JW, Rinaldo CR Jr, Gupta P, White RM, Todd JA, Kingsley LA: Prognosis in HIV-1 infection predicted by the quantity of virus in plasma. Science 1996; 272:1167-1170.
5. Murray JF, Mills J: Pulmonary infectious complications of human immunodeficiency virus infection: Part I. Am Rev Respir Dis 1990; 141:1356-1372.
6. Murray JF, Mills J: Pulmonary infectious complications of human immunodeficiency virus infection: Part II. Am Rev Respir Dis 1990; 141:1582-1598.
7. Gottlieb MS, Schroff R, Schanker HM, et al: *Pneumocystis carinii* pneumonia and mucosal candidiasis in previously healthy homosexual men. Evidence of a new acquired cellular immunodeficiency. N Engl J Med 1981; 305:1425-1431.
8. Masur H, Michelis MA, Greene JB, et al: An outbreak of community-acquired *Pneumocystis carinii* pneumonia: Initial manifestation of cellular immune dysfunction. N Engl J Med 1981; 305:1431-1438.
9. Khabbaz RF, Onorato IM, Cannon RO, et al: Seroprevalence of HTLV-I and HTLV-II among intravenous drug users and persons in clinics for sexually transmitted diseases. N Engl J Med 1992; 326:375-380.
10. Centers for Disease Control: AIDS annual rates per 100,000 population United States, January-December 1996. JAMA 1997; 277:1510.
11. Fischl MA, Dickinson GM, La Voie L: Safety and efficacy of sulfamethoxazole-trimethoprim chemoprophylaxis for *Pneumocystis carinii* pneumonia in AIDS. JAMA 1988; 259:1185-1189.
12. Fischl MA, Richmann DD, Greico MH, et al: The efficacy of azidothymidine (AZT) in the treatment of patients with AIDS and AIDS-related complex: A double-blind, placebo-controlled trial. N Engl J Med 1987; 317:185-191.
13. Kahn JO, Lagakos SW, Richman DD, et al: A controlled trial comparing continued zidovudine with didanosine in human immunodeficiency virus infection. N Engl J Med 1992; 327:581-587.
14. Bartlett JG: Protease inhibitors, a new class of drugs against human immunodeficiency virus. JAMA 1997; 277:1865-1866.
15. Ermini EK: Maintenance of long-term virus suppression in patients treated with the protease inhibitors Crixivan (indinavir) (Abstract MDB 170). *In*: Programme and Abstracts of the XI International Conference on AIDS, Vancouver, July 7-12, 1996.
16. Carpenter CCJ, Fischl MA, Hammer SM, et al: Antiretroviral therapy for HIV infection in 1997: Updated recommendations of the International AIDS Society USA panel. JAMA 1997; 277:1962-1969.
17. Zolopa AR, Hahn JA, Gorter R, et al: HIV and tuberculosis infection in San Francisco's homeless adults: Prevalence and risk factors in a representative sample. JAMA 1994; 272:455-461.
18. Bangsberg D, Tulsky JP, Hecht FM, Moss AR: Protease inhibitors in the homeless. JAMA 1997; 278:63-65.
19. Wallace JM, Hansen NI, Lavange L, et al: Respiratory disease trends in the pulmonary complications of HIV infection study cohort. Am J Respir Crit Care Med 1997; 155:72-80.
20. Stansell JD, Osmond DH, Charlebois E, et al: Predictors of *Pneumocystis carinii* pneumonia in HIV-infected persons. Am J Respir Crit Care Med 1997; 155:60-66.
21. Rosen MJ, Clayton K, Schneider RF, et al: Intensive care of patients with HIV infection: Utilization, critical illnesses, and outcomes. Am J Respir Crit Care Med 1997; 155:67-71.
22. Wachter RM, Luce JM, Turner J, Volberding P, Hopewell PC: Intensive care of patients with the acquired immunodeficiency syndrome: Outcome and changing patterns of utilization. Am Rev Respir Dis 1986; 134:891-896.
23. Wachter RM, Russi MB, Bloch DA, Hopewell PC, Luce JM: *Pneumocystis carinii* pneumonia and respiratory failure in AIDS: Improved outcomes and increased use of intensive care units. Am Rev Respir Dis 1991; 143:251-256.
24. Rogers PL, Lane HC, Henderson DK, Parrillo J, Masur H: Admission of AIDS patients to a medical intensive care unit: Causes and outcome. Crit Care Med 1989; 17:113-117.
25. Friedman Y, Franklin C, Rackow EC, Weil MH: Improved survival in patients with AIDS, *Pneumocystis carinii* pneumonia, and severe respiratory failure. Chest 1989; 96:862-866.
26. Hopewell PC: *Pneumocystis carinii* pneumonia: Diagnosis. J Infect Dis 1988; 157:1115-1119.
27. Sankary RM, Turner J, Lipavsky A, Howes EL Jr, Murray JF: Alveolar-capillary block in patients with AIDS and *Pneumocystis carinii* pneumonia. Am Rev Respir Dis 1988; 137:443-449.
28. Kovacs JA, Ng VL, Masur H, et al: Diagnosis of *Pneumocystis carinii* pneumonia: Improved detection in sputum with use of monoclonal antibodies. N Engl J Med 1988; 318:589-593.
29. Golden JA, Hollander H, Stulbarg MS, Gamsu G: Bronchoalveolar lavage as the exclusive diagnostic modality for *Pneumocystis carinii* pneumonia: A prospective study among patients with the acquired immunodeficiency syndrome. Chest 1986; 90:18-22.
30. Huang L, Hecht FM, Stansell JD, Montanti R, Hadley WK, Hopewell PC: Suspected *Pneumocystis carinii* pneumonia with a negative induced sputum examination: Is early bronchoscopy useful? Am J Respir Crit Care Med 1995; 151:1866-1871.
31. Cadranel J, Gillet-Juvin K, Antoine M, et al: Site-directed bronchoalveolar lavage and transbronchial biopsy in HIV-infected patients with pneumonia. Am J Respir Crit Care Med 1995; 152:1103-1106.
32. Masur H: Prevention and treatment of *Pneumocystis* pneumonia. N Engl J Med 1992; 327:1853-1860.
33. Wachter RM, Luce JM, Hopewell PC: Critical care of patients with AIDS. JAMA 1992; 267:541-547.
34. Allegra CJ, Chabner BA, Tuazon CU, et al: Trimetrexate for the treatment of *Pneumocystis carinii* pneumonia in patients with the acquired immunodeficiency syndrome. N Engl J Med 1987; 317:978-985.
35. Dohn MN, Weinberg WG, Torres RA, et al: Oral atovaquone compared with intravenous pentamidine for *Pneumocystis carinii* pneumonia in patients with AIDS. Ann Intern Med 1994; 121:174-180.
36. Montaner JSG, Lawson LM, Levitt N, Belzberg A, Schechter MT, Ruedy J: Corticosteroids prevent early deterioration in patients with moderately severe *Pneumocystis carinii* pneumonia and the acquired immunodeficiency syndrome (AIDS). Ann Intern Med 1990; 113:14-20.
37. Gagnon S, Boota AM, Fischl MA, Baier H, Kirksey OW, La Voie L: Corticosteroids as adjunctive therapy for severe *Pneumocystis carinii* pneumonia in the acquired immunodeficiency syndrome: A double-blind, placebo-controlled trial. N Engl J Med 1990; 323:1444-1450.
38. The National Institutes of Health University of California Expert Panel for Corticosteroids and Adjunctive Therapy for *Pneumo-*

cystis carinii Pneumonia: Consensus statement on the use of corticosteroids as adjunctive therapy for *Pneumocystis* pneumonia in the acquired immunodeficiency syndrome. N Engl J Med 1990; 323:1500–1504.
39. Lazard T, Retel O, Guidet B, Maury E, Valleron A-J, Offenstadt G: AIDS in a medical intensive care unit: Immediate prognosis and long-term survival. JAMA 1996; 276:1240–1245.
40. Staikowsky F, Lafon B, Guidet B, Denis M, Mayaud C, Offenstadt G: Mechanical ventilation for *Pneumocystis carinii* pneumonia in patients with the acquired immunodeficiency syndrome: Is the prognosis really improved? Chest 1993; 104:756–762.
41. Hawley PH, Ronco JJ, Guillemi SA, et al: Decreasing frequency but worsening mortality of acute respiratory failure secondary to AIDS-related *Pneumocystis carinii* pneumonia. Chest 1994; 106:1456–1459.
42. Wachter RM, Luce JM, Safrin S, Berrios DC, Charlebois E, Scitovsky AA: Cost and outcome of intensive care for patients with AIDS, *Pneumocystis carinii* pneumonia, and severe respiratory failure. JAMA 1995; 273:230–235.

64

Infections After Solid Organ Transplantation

Peter K. Linden, MD, DMD

Infections occurring after allograft transplantation are still generally acknowledged to be a major variable in organ recipient morbidity and mortality.[1, 2] A reciprocal relationship between allograft viability and infection is often apparent; allograft dysfunction caused by technical errors often manifests as infection (e.g., cholangitis resulting from hepatic allograft vascular compromise; urosepsis complicating a ureteral anastomosis leak in a kidney recipient). Alternatively, infectious complications may adversely affect the allograft, either directly (e.g., cytomegalovirus [CMV] hepatitis in hepatic grafts) or indirectly, as in the case of rejection that ensues after the withdrawal or tapering of immunosuppression in the face of overwhelming infection. Superimposed on a 20-year trend of decreasing overall 1- and 5-year post-transplantation mortality rates, infection remains the leading primary or associated cause of mortality for all categories of organ transplantation.[1] Nevertheless, enormous advances have been made over the past 20 years that have created a more favorable standard of care and better graft and patient survival. These have included, in part, the chemoprophylaxis of opportunistic infections (herpes simplex virus [HSV], CMV, *Pneumocystis carinii*), improved surgical techniques, and the more refined application of conventional cyclosporine-based immunosuppression plus the introduction of alternative agents, including FK-506.[3]

Since the last edition of this textbook, noteworthy clinical advances have been made in the management of post-transplantation infection and serious new challenges have arisen. A special concern has been the rapid evolution of drug-resistant pathogens, which have disproportionately threatened immunocompromised patients, new and unique pathogens, and the relative shortage of donor organs, which has lengthened candidate waiting periods. New strategies for prophylaxis or preemptive therapy and novel anti-infective agents are some important recent developments. This chapter updates for intensive care (ICU) clinicians these recent advances and challenges in a dynamic and important field.

EPIDEMIOLOGY

The incidence of post-transplantation infection from several recent major series of solid organ recipients is illustrated in Table 64–1.[4–12] The frequency and severity of infections vary much, depending on the transplanted organ and the transplant center. The extensive nature of liver and small intestinal transplantation procedures contribute significantly to the higher rates of serious infection, as compared with kidney transplants. Similarly, kidney-pancreas transplantation has a higher incidence of infection than solitary kidney transplantation, owing to the greater prevalence of underlying diabetes and to complications associated with either alkaline pancreatic drainage into the bladder or pancreatic-enteric anastomosis complications.[13] Variance among medical centers is, in part, secondary to both candidate selection policies (high-risk or low-risk) and the intensity and quality of immunosuppression regimens.

TEMPORAL PATTERNS OF INFECTION

The time course of infections in the post-transplantation period is conveniently grouped into three consecutive but overlapping periods:

- Early infections, within the first month
- A middle period, between the 2nd and 6th months
- Late infections, which can occur sporadically throughout life.

This stereotypical pattern was conveniently set forth as a timetable for kidney recipients in the early 1980s.[14] New prophylactic and preemptive strategies have partially modified both the timing and the composition of post-transplantation infection today. Infections in the early, middle, and late post-transplantation periods are summarized in Table 64–2.

Early Infections

The most severe and life-threatening infections tend to cluster in the first month after transplantation. Both biologic and iatrogenic factors are responsible for the high rates of early serious infection. The disruption of anatomic barriers, establishment of artificial vascular and excretory (urine, bile) anastomoses, and the sheer duration of surgery are major predisposing factors for early postoperative infection.[1, 2] Pretransplant host conditions (diabetes, uremia, alcoholism, liver failure, malnutrition, immunosuppression) whose effects are carried over into the postoperative period can impair wound healing and further compromise local host defenses.

Infections present or incubating before the transplantation

TABLE 64–1. Rates of Serious Infection Based on the Category of Solid-Organ Transplant

Transplant	Institution	Years	Infections (%)	Associated Mortality (%)
Liver	Pittsburgh	1985–1987	83	23
Liver	Mayo Clinic	1984–1985	53	9
Liver	Baylor	1988–1989	47	8
Kidney	Minnesota	1987–1990	65	8
Kidney	Netherlands	1985–1986	26	NA
Heart	Loyola	1986–1986	67	0
Heart	Multicenter	1980–1987	57	5
Pancreas	Mayo	1987–1991	79	18
Intestinal	Pittsburgh	1991–1993	92	NA

NA = not available.

TABLE 64–2. Common Infections After Solid-Organ Transplantation Based on the Time of Presentation

Early (Weeks 1–4)
All Solid-Organ Recipients
Superficial wound infection
Bacterial pneumonia
Urinary tract infection
Catheter infection
Kidney Recipients
Pyelonephritis
Perinephric/parenchymal abscess
Liver Recipients
Cholangitis
Intra-abdominal abscess
Peritonitis
Hepatic abscess
Heart and Heart-Lung Recipients
Sternal wound infection
Mediastinitis
Empyema
Middle (Months 2–6)
CMV
Epstein-Barr virus (PTLD)
Legionellosis
Tuberculosis
Nocardia
Aspergillus
Pneumocystis carinii
Late (After 6 Months)
P. carinii
Cryptococcosis
Herpes zoster virus
CMV retinitis
Community-acquired pathogens
Streptococcus pneumoniae
Influenza

PTLD = post-transplantation lymphoproliferative disorder; CMV = cytomegalovirus.

may be manifested clinically only shortly after the transplantation procedure. Allograft immunotolerance is lowest during the early months, so larger doses of both baseline and supplemental immunosuppression are required to prevent and treat rejection. Early primary dysfunction of the allograft, especially in liver and heart-lung recipients, may culminate in single or multiple system organ failure and enhance the risk for infection. Finally, exposure to virulent or "multiresistant" nosocomial pathogens may enhance the risk for serious infection in the weeks after the transplant procedure.

Early infections—within the first month—are most often postoperative superficial or deep wound infections. Bacterial pathogens derived from the host's endogenous or antibiotic-modified flora predominate; however, fungal infections, particularly *Candida* species, also pose a serious threat. Reactivated mucocutaneous HSV infections are classically associated with this early period as well; however, acyclovir prophylaxis has dramatically reduced the frequency of this complication.

Intermediate Infections

Several major categories of infection classically present during the intermediate post-transplantation period (months 2 to 6). Despite significant advances in prophylactic and preemptive strategies, CMV remains the dominant pathogen during this period and has a wide range of presentations, including a febrile syndrome, focal invasive disease (pneumonia, hepatitis, or enteritis), and disseminated disease. Serious short-term sequelae of CMV disease include allograft rejection mediated either by CMV-induced up-regulation of allograft class II human lymphocyte antigen (HLA) expression compounded by the iatrogenic tapering of immunosuppression and higher risks for bacterial or fungal superinfection due to virus-enhanced, cell-mediated immunosuppression.[15, 16] The cumulative effects of iatrogenic immunosuppression coupled with nosocomial exposure or reactivation of a dormant infection may culminate in serious, life-threatening infection due to certain bacteria (*Mycobacterium tuberculosis* or *Legionella, Listeria*, or *Nocardia* species), fungi (*Aspergillus, Cryptococcus*, endemic mycoses, *P. carinii)*, and protozoa (*Strongyloides stercoralis, Toxoplasma gondii)*, and other opportunistic pathogens.

Late Infections

Late post-transplantation infections are secondary to a diverse spectrum of pathogens. The frequency and severity of infection in this period may be partially related to the intensity and duration of antecedent immunosuppressive therapy. Thus, patients with chronic rejection and a high immunosuppressant requirement are at higher risk for late infections. Relapsing forms of infection—bronchitis in lung recipients, cholangitis in patients undergoing liver grafts with biliary duct disease, and chronic urinary tract infections in kidney recipients—are not uncommon.[17]

Endogenous reactivation of viruses (varicella-zoster virus [VZV], hepatitis B or C, Epstein-Barr virus [EBV]), and bacteria (*M. tuberculosis*) is most common in this category. CMV chorioretinitis is well described in this late period,[18] as is a more recent trend of late CMV infection in graft recipients treated with an intensive CMV prophylaxis regimen.[19] Infections with community-acquired pathogens (influenza, *Streptococcus pneumoniae, Staphylococcus aureus*) also occur, but potentially with a more fulminant course or atypical clinical presentation. *P. carinii*, now taxonomically classified as a fungus, was responsible for moderate to severe pneumonitis in as many as 15% of solid organ recipients prior to the use of chemoprophylaxis. Trimethoprim-sulfamethoxazole (TMP-SMZ) prophylaxis has dramatically diminished this threat, but pneumocystosis occurs sporadically as a result of either physician withdrawal of TMP-SMZ or patient noncompliance. Occasionally, late technical allograft complications, such as hepatic artery thrombosis in a liver recipient, may also occur and present as sepsis with enteric bacteremia or candidemia.

SOURCES OF PATHOGENS IN ORGAN RECIPIENTS

The organ recipient is susceptible to an enormously broad range of potential pathogens, in large part because of the compromise of anatomic barriers and iatrogenic immunosuppression directed principally toward cell-mediated immunity. Placed in simple perspective, these pathogens are either endogenous (i.e., originating within the host) or exogenous (i.e., newly acquired from the physical environment [human contacts or inanimate objects], allograft, or transfused blood products). A more subtle distinction is required, however, because certain organisms may be acquired either exogenously and cause early clinical disease (primary tuberculosis, CMV-positive allograft causing infection in a CMV-seronegative recipient) or endogenously as a tissue-latent phase that is reactivated in the setting of host immunosuppression (reactivated pulmonary tuberculosis or CMV disease in a CMV-seropositive recipient).

Endogenous bacterial flora colonize the mucosal surfaces of the upper respiratory, gastrointestinal, and genitourinary tracts as well as the skin surface (predominantly gram-positive flora).

The composition of this "normal" flora is usually modified by exposure to the animate nosocomial environment (other patients via the health care worker vector) and the inanimate environment (air, water, medical equipment). In addition, prior antibiotic use favors the proliferation of multiresistant bacterial flora and the overgrowth of *Candida* species. This "modified endogenous flora" is a common concern because many allograft recipients have had an extended period of ICU or non-ICU nosocomial exposure during the donor search before the transplantation procedure. Such potential pathogens may be resistant to the "protocolized" antibiotic prophylaxis administered to all transplant recipients at a particular transplant center with a high prevalence of resistant bacteria.

Several nosocomial multiresistant bacterial species have become quite problematic in some transplant categories during the past decade. Strains of enterococci very resistant to vancomycin and all other appropriate antimicrobials have produced significant morbidity and mortality in liver recipients, given the propensity for this organism to cause hepatobiliary and intra-abdominal infection.[20-22] Moreover, candidates who become colonized with vancomycin-resistant enterococci (VRE) have been shown to have a high rate of early post-transplantation VRE infection, owing in part to the lack of effective chemoprophylaxis. Nosocomial acquisition of methicillin-resistant *S. aureus* in the candidate period has been shown to increase the risk for post-transplantation staphylococcal infection, for which therapy remains limited to parenteral vancomycin.[23] Multiresistant or panresistant *Pseudomonas aeruginosa* is especially problematic in cystic fibrosis patients undergoing lung transplantation.[24]

Latent endogenous organisms are characteristically contained within certain organ tissues by an intact host cell-mediated immune system. After a variable period of cell-mediated immunosuppression, these organisms may reactivate to cause clinical disease in the allograft recipient. Organisms with reactivation potential include bacteria *(M. tuberculosis)*, the herpesviruses (HSV, VZV, CMV, and EBV), fungi *(Histoplasma capsulatum, Coccidioides immitis)*, protozoa *(T. gondii)*, and parasites *(S. stercoralis)*. The probability of one's harboring these organisms depends on specific variables for each. For instance, geographic origin is the major determinant for developing latent infection with *C. immitis* (southwestern United States) or *Strongyloides* (southeastern United States, Caribbean); however, seroprevalence studies demonstrate a uniformly high rate of latent infection for type 1 human herpes simplex virus (HHV1), VZV, and EBV: more than 95% of adults demonstrate seropositivity.

CMV is an important exception. A wide range (40% to 100%) of adults possess serum immunoglobulin G antibodies indicative of prior primary CMV infection.[25] Laboratory evidence that confirms the presence of a tissue-latent phase for a particular organism before transplantation is crucial because it can prospectively guide prophylactic and diagnostic management in the post-transplantation period. These measures may include isoniazid prophylaxis for candidates with positive purified protein derivative of tuberculin (PPD) skin tests and intensified antiviral prophylaxis in CMV-seronegative recipients of CMV-seropositive allografts. In contrast to bone marrow transplantation, the shortage of donor solid organs prevents prospective matching of CMV-seronegative allografts exclusively for CMV-seronegative recipients. Many transplantation centers have also discontinued preferential administration of CMV-seronegative blood products to CMV-seronegative recipients, owing to the prevailing importance of the allograft as the CMV source and to cost issues.[26]

Exogenous organisms may be transmitted to the organ recipient (1) from the physical environment (air, water, bed linens, food), (2) by direct contact with health care personnel, and (3) from the donor allograft or transfused blood products. Outbreaks of infections of certain exogenous organisms among cohorted transplant patients can be the alert to a contaminated environmental source.[27] Airborne spread of *Aspergillus* spores from hospital construction and recirculated ventilation patterns has been associated with well-documented cluster epidemics of invasive aspergillosis.[28, 29] *Cryptococcus, Mucorales, Histoplasma*, and many other less common fungi *(Dactylaria, Fusaria, Pseudoallescheria boydii)* invade via air in the lungs; however, the precise environmental contact source is usually unknown.

Exogenous bacterial pathogens to which transplant recipients are particularly vulnerable include *Legionella, Listeria monocytogenes*, and *Nocardia* species. Best described are nosocomial outbreaks of pneumonia caused by *Legionella pneumophila, Legionella micdadei*, and several other species from a contaminated hospital hot water supply.[30-32] However, because *Legionella* bacteria are fairly ubiquitous community pathogens, sporadic cases of legionellosis may affect nonhospitalized organ recipients any time in the post-transplantation period. Nocardiasis remains an uncommon infection, although earlier series reported a somewhat higher incidence among heart and kidney recipients.[1] *Listeria* is most often transmitted via contaminated food sources and is still the most common bacterial central nervous system (CNS) pathogen among organ recipients. It has been speculated that the common use of TMP-SMZ for prophylaxis of pneumocystosis may serendipitously provide protection from other sulfa-susceptible pathogens (e.g., *Nocardia, Listeria*, and *Toxoplasma* species).[2, 33]

The donor allograft represents a proven source of potential pathogens that is unique to the organ recipient population. Over the past 30 years, this route of transmission has generally been narrowed to either undetectable organisms or pathogens for which there is no prospective indication by which to eliminate the potential donor from consideration. Clinician knowledge of organisms in this latter group may still be significant for guiding subsequent prophylaxis in the recipient. Examples include CMV, hepatitis B and C viruses, *Toxoplasma*, and the tracheal bacterial cultures of lung donors.

Before the availability of screening methods, there were numerous reports of transmission of hepatitis B and C and human immunodeficiency virus 1 (HIV-1), with serious or fatal sequelae. Before HIV-1 antibody screening in 1985, cases of donor-to-recipient HIV-1 transmission with rapid progression to full-blown acquired immunodeficiency syndrome (AIDS) were reported for all major solid organ transplant groups.[34, 35] HIV transmission has also been rare since the use of systematic HIV antibody screening as a result of false-negative determinations in the "window" period of HIV seroconversion.[36] Further sophistication of HIV screening has largely eliminated HIV as a transmissible agent in the transplant setting. Serologic screening has drastically diminished the threat of donor transmission of this agent; however, hepatitis C transmission may still occur because of the significant window period when there is no detectable antibody. Some transplant centers utilize organs from donors who are positive for hepatitis B core antibody or hepatitis C antibody for those patients who already have chronic hepatitis B or C infection or for desperately ill candidates.[37] Post-transplantation prophylaxis for the viral hepatitides are discussed later in this chapter. Rare but well-documented cases of proven donor-recipient transmission are reported for HSV, *Aspergillus*, and *M. tuberculosis*.[38-40]

ROLE OF IATROGENIC IMMUNOSUPPRESSION

The multicomponent immunosuppressive regimens required by all solid-organ recipients for the prevention and treatment of allograft rejection are a key determinant for the development of post-transplantation infection. The major immunosuppressants can be categorized as corticosteroids, cytotoxic or antiproliferative drugs (including azathioprine, mycophenolate, and cyclophosphamide), and agents directed either at the CD4 lymphocyte (OKT3, antilymphocyte globulin or rabbit antithymocyte globulin) or at its lymphokine production (cyclosporine, FK-506). The "infection-potentiating" effect of any immunosuppressive drug has some specificity based on its targets. It is difficult, however, to attribute any given infection to one specific immunosuppressive agent because most post-transplantation regimens contain multiple immunosuppressants and there are many other immunosuppressive and non-immunosuppressive risk factors for infection.

Corticosteroids cause broad impairment of host defenses, having effects on the neutrophil inflammatory response, macrophage antigen processing, antibody production, and cell-mediated immunity. These effects are, to some extent, both dose- and duration-dependent. This association is best illustrated by the drop in the incidence of both infections and infection-related mortality in kidney, liver, and heart recipients coincident with the introduction of cyclosporine, which allowed a relative reduction of corticosteroid doses.[41–43] Notably, steroids are not potent inducers of CMV disease or other invasive viral illnesses. Other adverse effects of steroid therapy in organ recipients include impairment of wound healing and an altered clinical presentation that may result in delayed diagnosis of a serious infection.

Both cyclosporine and FK-506 appear to improve the risk-benefit ratio as it pertains to infectious complications, owing to the diminished need for other immunosuppressants to prevent or treat rejection. Both agents selectively depress helper T lymphocyte interleukin-2 (IL-2) synthesis without depressing neutrophil, macrophage, or antibody-mediated defense.[44, 45] Moreover, the low rates of infection in cyclosporine-treated, non-organ recipients (i.e., autoimmune disease) are additional evidence of its favorable infection risk profile.[46] After the introduction of cyclosporine in 1980, multiple prospective or historically controlled trials consistently demonstrated reduced rates of serious bacterial and viral (but not fungal) infection, as compared with steroid-azathioprine-antilymphocyte regimen–treated recipient groups.[47] Daily monitoring of serum blood cyclosporine levels in the early post-transplantation period has decreased the chance for underimmunosuppression or overimmunosuppression and has allowed individualization of cyclosporine dosing. The recent addition of cyclosporine microemulsion (Neoral) has facilitated the dosing of cyclosporine compared to the conventional cyclosporine preparation.[48] Two prospective trials comparing cyclosporine to FK-506 (tacrolimus) in liver recipients demonstrated equivalent rates of patient or graft survival and the incidence of infection and lymphoproliferative disease.[49, 50]

Antilymphocyte therapy with either polyclonal (antilymphocyte globulin [ALG]) or monoclonal (murine OKT3) antibody is used at many transplant centers for either induction in the early post-transplantation period or for treatment of steroid-refractory acute rejection. Several reports suggested higher rates of invasive CMV disease in kidney, liver, and heart recipients as compared with either historic or contemporary controls.[51, 52] EBV-mediated post-transplantation lymphoproliferative disorder (PTLD) was also strongly associated with a previous course of OKT3 or sequential use of Minnesota ALG and OKT3 in kidney recipients.[53, 54]

Immunosuppression may be radically tapered or completely withdrawn without excessive allograft rejection in the setting of life-threatening infection or electively in the late post-transplantation period in carefully selected organ recipients.[55–57] Recent observations of a possible host-donor immunologic "chimerism" may explain allograft tolerance in some recipients.[58] Finally, renal transplant recipients are unique in that allograft nephrectomy and conversion to hemodialysis, allowing withdrawal of all immunosuppression, may improve clinical outcomes.[59]

INFECTIONS RELATED TO THE TRANSPLANTATION PROCEDURE

The category of organ transplantation is a major determinant for the sites of infection, particularly in the early post-transplantation period. Both the allograft organ and contiguous tissue structures are especially vulnerable to infection, for a variety of reasons relating to retained fluid collections, foreign bodies, and technical complications. Such infections merit separate discussion based on the type of transplant. In contrast, certain opportunistic infections occur in all types of transplant recipients because all are exposed to exogenous organisms from similar sources (donor graft, blood products, and nosocomial and community physical environments), and all uniformly require varying degrees of T cell–directed immunosuppression. Therefore, a separate pathogen-based discussion for these infections, with an emphasis on notable differences between organ transplant types, is presented subsequently.

Kidney Transplantation

The most common infectious problems are urinary tract infections (UTIs): some series demonstrate rates exceeding 40% within the first year of transplantation. Independent risk factors include prolonged bladder catheterization, degree of organ mismatch, patient age, and history of urologic complications. Simultaneous pancreas-kidney transplantation with bladder drainage is associated with a higher rate of UTI than enteric pancreatic drainage.[60] The spectrum of infecting organisms is no different from those that cause native UTIs, aerobic gram-negative bacilli and enterococci predominating. Among immunocompromised hosts kidney recipients are exquisitely susceptible to the adverse effects of UTI.[61] Early UTI is characteristically more refractory to conventional therapy and is associated with more severe sequelae (pyelonephritis, bacteremia, sepsis) than UTIs occurring after the third post-transplantation month. Both symptomatic and asymptomatic infections merit aggressive therapy. Appropriate management includes 4 to 6 weeks of antibiotic therapy, removal of the bladder drainage catheter, if possible, and post-therapy follow-up urine cultures. Tapering of immunosuppression is rarely indicated, except in the setting of superimposed sepsis. Recurrent infections or relapse with the same organism should prompt a search for structural sources (parenchymal abscess) and functional abnormalities (ureterovesical reflux, urethral stricture, neurogenic bladder). Rarely, graft nephrectomy is indicated for complicated upper UTI. Prophylaxis with TMP-SMZ or ciprofloxacin has shown clear reductions in the rate of early UTIs.[62]

Wound infection rates in most series are generally within the expected range for clean-contaminated surgery (5% to 10%) conducted with appropriate antibiotic prophylaxis. Preoperative host risk factors include poorly controlled uremia, diabetes, and malnutrition. The majority of wound infections are superficial and are easily treated with antibiotics and drainage. Postoperative hematomas, lymphoceles, and urinomas resulting from technical errors much potentiate the risk of deep perinephric wound infection. These complications can have devastating consequences, including mycotic aneurysm formation in the vascular pedicle, sepsis, and graft failure. Transplant nephrectomy is often the only lifesaving measure for deep perinephric space infections. Rare causes of early infections in kidney recipients are also described, including direct transmission of infectious agents via the donor kidney (e.g., *M. tuberculosis*, HSV[38, 39]), primary or reactivated papovavirus infection manifesting as a ureteral stenosis or interstitial nephritis,[63, 64] hemorrhagic pyelonephritis or acute tubular necrosis caused by adenovirus,[65, 66] and deep wound infection with *Mycoplasma hominis*.[67]

Liver Transplantation

Serious infectious complications are most likely to occur within 4 weeks after liver transplantation. Liver recipients have the highest rates of bloodstream infection among all solid organ recipients.[68] Pretransplant risk factors for infection include chronic hepatitis C infection, a recent episode of spontaneous bacterial peritonitis, and pretransplant immunosuppression.[5, 69] Surgical entry into the biliary tree and proximal gastrointestinal tract is a necessary but predisposing cause of the high postoperative infection rates. A recent study has shown a close relationship of the enteric organism in bile or the jejunum and operative site infections.[70] Such infections are principally intra-abdominal and are closely related to a number of factors, including duration of surgery, type and viability of the biliary anastomosis, and adequacy of vascular supply via a reconstructed recipient-to-host hepatic arterial system.

Duration of Surgery

A prospective analysis from the University of Pittsburgh demonstrated a significant correlation between the number of operative hours (composed of the transplant operation alone or subsequent surgery, or both) and the number of episodes of infection and the probability of deep-seated fungal infection.[5] Such a relationship probably captures multiple inherent risk factors for which operative time is an easily measurable marker, including hemorrhage, technical difficulties, and the risk of intra-abdominal contamination with endogenous flora via intestinal or biliary spillage or translocation.

Type and Viability of the Biliary Anastomosis

A second operation (retransplantation or duct revision) requiring a choledochojejunostomy anastomosis is also associated with a significantly higher infection rate than choledochocholedochostomy.[5] Serious intra-abdominal infection may occur secondary to a bile leak or biliary obstruction. Leakage of bile can manifest as fever or sepsis, with or without enteric bacteremia, and it usually presents within the first 2 weeks after transplantation. An elevated serum bilirubin value is characteristic and occasionally is mistaken for acute rejection. Underlying reasons for a bile leak are usually either vascular insufficiency or are purely technical in nature. Management includes early surgical correction or temporary external biliary drainage along with appropriate antibiotic therapy.[71] Biliary obstruction usually presents later and is most often due to anastomotic stenosis or intrahepatic strictures.

Adequacy of Vascular Supply Via a Reconstructed Recipient-to-Host Hepatic Arterial System

Thrombosis of the hepatic artery may present as relapsing enteric bacteremias, hepatic abscess, fulminant hepatic necrosis, or indolent breakdown of the extrahepatic biliary anastomosis or intrahepatic biliary tree.[72] The quality and intensity of immunosuppression probably are not major inciting risk factors for these infections; however, continued immunosuppression may contribute to poor healing and impair recovery from a serious pyogenic infection.

Heart and Lung Transplantation

The most significant sites of infection after heart, lung, or heart-lung transplantation are the lung parenchyma and other compartments of the chest cavity (pleural space, mediastinum). Independent risk factors for early infection include prolonged cardiopulmonary bypass time, an implanted artificial heart device, and oral flora in the tracheal cultures of lung donors.[73] Mediastinitis is an uncommon but potentially devastating complication. Its incidence was 2.5% and 2.8% in two recent series.[74, 75] Risk factors include prior sternotomy, early post-transplantation hemorrhage, staphylococcal pneumonitis, diabetes, and early rejection. Inciting events are primary contamination at transplantation, a sternal wound infection, or leakage of secretions from the tracheal anastomosis into the peritracheal tissue in lung recipients. *S. aureus* or *Staphylococcus epidermidis* organisms are predominant; however, gram-negative bacteria and other less common pathogens, including *M. hominis*[76] and *Nocardia*,[77] have been reported. Presenting local signs include incisional erythema, purulent drainage, and an unstable sternum. Computed tomography (CT) provides confirmatory evidence in most cases. Successful management can be achieved in most cases with a combination of systemic antibiotics and open debridement with irrigation or closure using muscle flaps.

Lung and heart-lung recipients are at high risk for bacterial pneumonia as a result of, for example, compromised secretion clearance secondary to airway denervation, anastomosis breakdown, loss of lymphatic drainage, donor inoculum of organisms, or pretransplant conditions that predispose to chronic lung infection, such as cystic fibrosis or obstructive lung disease.[1] Pneumonia may occur as early as the second post-transplantation day. Diagnostic confusion with early acute graft rejection is not uncommon; however, the distinction is best made by careful clinical and laboratory examination. Early therapy is guided by knowledge of donor tracheal cultures and recipient native lung flora. Bronchoscopic lavage or brushing is the most common technique for obtaining culture material to guide definitive antimicrobial therapy.

Pancreas Transplantation

Cumulative early experience with pancreatic transplantation has shown a high rate of serious intra-abdominal infections and significant associated mortality.[11] Lumbreras and colleagues found a 53% incidence of bacterial infection within the first 3 months, related principally to the surgical procedure.[11] The majority were deep wound infections, such as pelvic or intra-abdominal abscesses or peritonitis. Allograft pancreatitis secondary to ischemic preservation injury or operative trauma and bowel contamination are the principal mechanisms. Controversy persists as to whether the optimal approach to pancreatic exocrine drainage is an enteric anastomosis or the more orthodox technique of bladder drainage.

Bowel and Multivisceral Transplantation

Transplantation of the small intestine, with or without other intra-abdominal viscera, is associated with a very high rate of early infection, owing to the extensive and prolonged nature of the surgery and the intensive immunosuppression required to control the strong tendency for early allograft rejection. In a series of 16 intestinal recipients, 15 experienced two or more episodes of bacterial or fungal infection.[12] There is a high incidence of apparent intestinal translocation of enteric bacteria and fungi as a result of intraluminal overgrowth and loss of mucosal integrity caused by concomitant graft rejection. Paradoxically, immunosuppression must be intensified during these episodes to restore intestinal mucosal integrity.[78]

OPPORTUNISTIC INFECTIONS

Opportunistic Bacteria

Infections with opportunistic bacteria can be either epidemic, usually in the nosocomial setting, or sporadic, usually in the late post-transplantation period. Many opportunistic bacteria are pathogenic, even in persons with entirely normal host defenses. Immunocompromised organ recipients are notable for several reasons, including higher attack rates after exposure, more fulminant or therapy-refractory disease, and clinical presentations different from those of immunocompetent hosts. These features are partly attributable to the facilitation of intracellular growth and persistence of certain pathogens secondary to compromise of cell-mediated immunity.

Legionellosis

Within several years after the 1976 Philadelphia Legionnaires' disease epidemic came several reports of nosocomial legionellosis in renal transplant units that were associated with significant morbidity and mortality figures.[31, 79] Since that time, there has been a rapid growth of knowledge pertaining to the prevention of legionellosis by hyperchlorination of hospital water supplies, better diagnostic techniques, and emphasis on early, effective treatment. Nevertheless, *Legionella* remains a low-frequency pathogen that is more often a late community-acquired infection, although nosocomial epidemics resulting from undetected failure of the water eradication system are still described. Thus, any case of legionellosis in a transplant unit should prompt a search for nosocomial sources. *L. pneumophila*, serogroup 1, causes the vast majority (80% to 90%) of cases; other *L. pneumophila* serogroups and *L. micdadei* accounting for most others.

Direct aerosolization into the distal airways and aspiration of contaminated water are believed to be the principal modes of acquisition.[80] Early reports emphasized a high prevalence of nonspecific clinical and laboratory signs (nonproduction of sputum, diarrhea, hyponatremia, elevated transaminase levels, and de novo renal insufficiency); however, current opinion derived from aggregate experience has diminished their prospective diagnostic value.[80] The majority of transplant recipients with legionellosis still manifest high-grade fever, even when they are given corticosteroids. Chest radiographic findings in the transplant recipient are typically uni- or multilobar alveolar infiltrates that do not much differ from those of "normal" hosts, although early cavitation appears to be described more frequently among immunosuppressed patients.[81] Extrapulmonary legionellosis described in solid organ recipients includes hepatitis in a liver recipient, peritonitis in a kidney recipient, and a pericardial effusion in a heart recipient.[82-84] Such evidence demonstrates that hematogenous dissemination of this organism may occur with or without clinically evident pulmonary disease.

Early diagnosis necessitates a high index of suspicion because special microbiologic stains and culture methods are required. Rapidly available tests are most valuable because they may prompt early therapeutic intervention. Direct fluorescent antibody examination of respiratory secretions was the most frequently used rapid method, but it has only 50% sensitivity. Both the *Legionella* gene probe, which detects all *Legionella* species with excellent sensitivity and specificity, and the urine radioimmunoassay for antigenuria have superior sensitivity and remain positive even during early therapy. *Legionella* culture remains the "gold standard"; however, growth requires special media (buffered charcoal yeast agar) and may not produce results until the fifth day. *Legionella* bacteremia is detectable in as many as 20% of documented pneumonia cases but also requires specific communication with the microbiology laboratory because special subplating methods are required.

Treatment delay is ill tolerated by transplant recipients and should be started on an empirical basis for clinically suspected cases. Intravenous erythromycin (4 g/day) has the longest cumulative record of success, although no prospective comparative trials against other agents effective in vitro are available. Coadministration of rifampin is recommended for severe cases or refractory disease. Interference with cyclosporine or FK-506 metabolism is well described for both erythromycin and rifampin, which presents a unique problem for the organ recipient. Close monitoring of drug levels is recommended for guiding appropriate immunosuppressive dosing. Agents with less or no drug interference that appear promising for the treatment of *Legionella* include the quinolones (ciprofloxacin, ofloxacin) and the new-generation macrolide antibiotic, clarithromycin.[85, 86] Duration of treatment should be, at minimum, 21 days, because relapses are associated with shorter courses. Cavitary disease or slow responders may require longer periods of therapy.

Tuberculosis

The incidence of *M. tuberculosis* disease among solid-organ recipients is higher than that in the general population but still relatively low. Two large series of kidney recipients from Denver and Minnesota showed occurrences of only three cases each from recipient populations of 400 and 845, respectively.[87, 88] A 9-year study of liver transplantation at the University of Pittsburgh documented only five cases from a total of 2380 recipients.[89]

In a large retrospective series of kidney, liver, and heart transplant recipients the incidence was only 0.8% (51 cases), the predominant presentation being pulmonary (63%), followed by extrapulmonary (12%) and disseminated (25%).[90] The consistently low incidence of tuberculosis (TB) is somewhat unexpected because of the number of risk factors that favor a higher incidence of reactivated TB. These include pretransplantation chronic conditions associated with TB (alcoholism, uremia, cirrhosis, steroid therapy), organ recipients from endemic countries, and post-transplantation immunosuppression. The actual incidence is probably higher, owing to missed antemortem diagnosis and fewer postmortem examinations at many transplant centers. Moreover, the rising incidence of TB since the late 1980s, in both the general population and immunocompromised groups such as those with HIV, may in the future favor higher rates of TB in the organ recipient population. Most TB in transplant recipients is due to reactivation of latent endogenous foci; however, systematic cohorting of hospitalized transplant patients and a poor primary T cell containment response (resulting from immunosuppression) render organ recipients extremely susceptible to primary disease after exposure to an active case of pulmonary disease.

Nosocomial outbreaks are characterized by fulminant progressive primary disease and high mortality rates.[91] The spectrum of clinical presentation is more diverse, the incidence of disseminated disease in one study of kidney recipients[92] being as high as 38.7% with a 59.8% rate of extrapulmonary disease, as compared with 17.5% of cases in the overall United States population.[93] Other atypical features in transplant recipients include middle and lower lobe reactivated pulmonary disease, poorly visible or absent tissue granulomas, a high rate of bone and joint disease, and transmission to the recipient via reactivation in the donor organ.[39] Diagnostic methods are no different than those for TB in the general population; however, the value of the purified protein derivative (PPD) skin test is significantly diminished because of the high prevalence of cutaneous anergy. Prior bacille Calmette-Guérin vaccination may cause a PPD reaction; however, this does not necessarily confer immunity to adult organ recipients. Preliminary data from two new diagnostic modalities, gene probe and polymerase chain reaction (PCR) appear promising.

No data are available from prospective trials of antituberculous therapy among organ recipients. Standard treatment with a minimum of three first-line agents (isoniazid, rifampin, ethambutol, pyrazinamide) for at least 12 months is usually recommended, with excellent treatment success even with continued immunosuppression. Shorter courses of therapy have been reported to be successful, but there is only limited available experience.[94] Recipients with risk factors for isoniazid resistance or multidrug resistance such as isoniazid prophylaxis failure, prior incomplete therapy, and foreign natives will require broader empirical regimens until definitive susceptibility results are available. It is imperative to implement full respiratory isolation measures (negative-pressure, closed room, and proper masking) for suspected or documented pulmonary disease with positive acid-fast bacilli smears. Infectivity should rapidly wane within 1 to 2 weeks of initiating appropriate antituberculosis therapy.

Isoniazid hepatotoxicity is a major concern, particularly for liver recipients. In a series of 13 who received isoniazid after liver transplantation, five who were receiving a multidrug regimen demonstrated biochemical and histologic findings of hepatotoxicity, whereas none of the patients receiving prophylaxis with only isoniazid developed toxicity.[95] Rifampin may also augment the hepatic metabolism of both cyclosporine and FK-506.

Atypical mycobacteria are less common opportunistic bacterial pathogens in solid-organ recipients. The most common organism in this category is *Mycobacterium kansasii*, for which there are numerous reports of both focal and disseminated invasive disease. Others include *Mycobacterium haemophilum, Mycobacterium chelonei, Mycobacterium marinum*, and *Mycobacterium avium-intracellulare*. In contrast to *M. tuberculosis*, these organisms are not capable of person-to-person spread, and thus cases with pulmonic involvement do not require respiratory isolation measures. Treatment is multifaceted with both multidrug chemotherapy directed by susceptibility testing and surgical debridement in some instances.

Nocardiosis

Nocardia asteroides is a gram-positive or modified acid-fast–positive, rod-shaped organism with characteristic beading and branching morphology. Despite its environmental pervasiveness, the documented incidence of infection in the transplant population has always been low. Over the past decade, some speculate that the widespread use of sulfa prophylaxis for *P. carinii* may have further diminished the incidence of nocardiosis; however, this remains unproven.[2] Qualitative improvements in immunosuppression may also be instrumental, because a series of nocardiosis in renal transplant recipients demonstrated a 0.7% incidence in the post-cyclosporine era compared with a rate of 2.6% in pre-cyclosporine era controls.[96]

Nocardia bacteria usually gain entry via inhalation of aerosolized organisms with secondary hematogenous spread, most often to the central nervous system (CNS), skin, and subcutaneous tissues, although involvement of all viscera has been described. Initial clinical presentation is most frequently a subacute febrile illness with clinical and radiographic pulmonic disease. In the minority of patients, the pulmonary focus is silent and only a skin, CNS, or other visceral manifestation is present. *Nocardia* species grow aerobically on routine blood agar, but their growth properties are slower than most bacterias.[1] Thus, early notification of the microbiology laboratory of clinical suspicion of nocardiosis may be instrumental in detecting the organism. Because of its low rate of occurrence, no prospective trials have compared the therapeutic efficacy of agents with activity in vitro against species of *Nocardia*.

Sulfa drugs (TMP-SMZ, sulfisoxazole, sulfadiazine) have the longest track record of success when used for an optimal period, at least 3 to 6 months.[97, 98] Sulfa-intolerant persons have responded to alternative agents, including minocycline and amoxicillin-clavulanic acid.

Opportunistic Fungal Infections

Infection secondary to opportunistic fungi continues to have the highest associated case fatality rates among all categories of infectious agents in the solid-organ recipient. Despite improved survival in the cyclosporine era, there was no measured decrease in the incidence of fungal infection in a combined series of kidney and heart recipients.[46] The incidence of fungal infections is highest among liver recipients and is progressively lower among heart-lung, heart, and kidney recipients, respectively.[99] *Candida, Aspergillus*, and *Cryptococcus* organisms constitute more than 90% of all fungal infection.

Candida species are the predominant cause in all organ transplant groups with the exception of heart recipients, who may have a higher incidence of *Aspergillus* infection.[100] Other less common fungal species that have become increasingly recognized pathogens include *Mucorales* and other filamentous, nonpigmented fungi *(Fusarium, Curvularia, Trichosporon beigelii)* and pigmented fungi *(Dactylaria)*. Finally, fungi with a strong geographic concentration, termed endemic, such as *Coccidioides, Histoplasma*, and *Blastomyces*, may occasionally cause either reactivated disease in organ recipients native to these regions or progressive primary infection after initial exposure. The discussion is limited to post-transplant infections resulting from the major fungal pathogens *Candida, Aspergillus*, and *Cryptococcus*.

Candida Infections

Invasive disease secondary to *Candida* species remains the most common type of fungal infection in the organ transplant population. Such infection is most often confirmed within the first 2 to 3 post-transplant months, when recent surgery and other fungal selection factors have their strongest influence. Most *Candida* infections are believed to arise from the host's endogenous intestinal flora; however, cluster outbreaks of non–*Candida albicans* infections suggest that transmission from exogenous sources may occur as well.

Risk factors for candidiasis have been studied most extensively in the liver transplant population. A multivariate analysis of 91 fungal infections among 355 liver recipients[101] demonstrated the following statistically significant risk factors:

- Retransplantation
- Reintubation, severe illness at time of transplantation
- Higher intraoperative transfusion requirements
- Choledochojejunostomy biliary reconstruction
- Post-transplant course complicated by bacterial infection, antibiotic therapy, and vascular problems related to the graft

The spectrum of infectious disease caused by *Candida* species ranges from mucosal involvement only (stomatitis, esophagitis, cystitis) to bloodstream infection indicative, usually, of either a catheter-related source or true multivisceral invasion. The crude mortality rates associated with candidemia in immunocompromised patients still range upward from 50%.[102, 103] However, the sensitivity of candidemia as an indicator of deep-seated disease is notoriously poor: only 30% to 40% of patients with postmortem invasive disease have antemortem candidemia. Conversely, candidemia in solid-organ recipients should never be assumed to be a blood culture contaminant, transient event, or a catheter-related source (for which simple catheter removal is adequate).

There are few other specific signs of candidiasis in the organ recipient population; nodular skin lesions and retinal infiltrates are occasionally seen in the oncologic population but only rarely observed in transplant recipients. The presence of *Candida* at multiple sites (urinary or respiratory tract, gut) has poor positive predictive value for the presence of a deep-seated *Candida* infection, because many organ recipients have either preexisting colonization or experience colonization de novo in the post-transplant period.[104] However, the predictive value of non–*C. albicans* species *(Candida tropicalis)* in surveillance cultures for invasive disease has been shown to be higher than *C. albicans* in bone marrow recipients.[105] Reliable criteria that necessitate antifungal therapy include histopathologic demonstration of yeast or pseudohyphae in deep tissue specimens or positive cultures from a sterile body site.[106] Unfortunately, there has been little progress toward the development of a sensitive and specific serologic assay for significant *Candida* infection.

Some studies have demonstrated an ecologic shift from a predominance of *C. albicans* species to other *Candida* species.[107] In particular, the emergence of *Candida glabrata* and *Candida krusei* infections has been attributed, in part, to the increased use of fluconazole, for either prophylaxis or therapy, as these species are azole-resistant.[108]

Superficial *Candida* infections (stomatitis, esophagitis) are usually responsive to enteral nystatin or fluconazole, whereas severe cases may be treated with systemic amphotericin. The prognosis of invasive candidiasis infection remains poor, even in the setting of aggressive therapy. Amphotericin B at dose ranges of 0.5 to 1.0 mg/kg/day remains the primary treatment modality. Improved outcome with the addition of 5-flucytosine has been reported. A clinical trial comparing fluconazole to amphotericin B for candidemia demonstrated equivalent efficacy, but this study excluded organ recipients and other immunocompromised patients.[109] Fluconazole may cause a dramatic increase in cyclosporine or FK-506 levels because of its interference with hepatic cytochrome P-450 metabolism. Recently approved lipid formulations of amphotericin B preparations have shown similar or improved rates of efficacy for a variety of mycoses and are clearly less nephrotoxic than conventional amphotericin B.[110]

Aspergillus Infection

Aspergillus are filamentous fungi that are ubiquitous in the environment (soil, dust) and are capable of causing contamination of laboratory specimens, true colonization, or invasive disease. Conditions that favor the airborne release and spread of spores (hospital construction or heavy dust contamination in air conduits) clearly enhance the risk of aspergillosis in the post-transplantation period. Most infections are secondary to two species: *Aspergillus fumigatus* and *Aspergillus flavus*. The primary host defense against aspergillosis is alveolar macrophages, which contain the spore phase, and neutrophils, which have activity against the hyphal form.[111]

Organ recipients are rendered vulnerable to invasive disease principally because of the depression of the pulmonary mononuclear cell line (alveolar macrophage) and perhaps qualitative suppression of the neutrophil. The first three post-transplantation months show the highest incidence because of the combined effects of profound immunosuppression, antibiotic pressure, and nosocomial exposure. Invasive disease most often begins in the lungs as a febrile focal pneumonitis. The radiographic picture may also include solitary or multiple nodules with or without cavitation. Hemoptysis, although nonspecific, may be a clinical manifestation of angioinvasive pulmonary disease. Less common sites of primary inoculation include the sinuses, open surgical wounds, and the skin. Not uncommonly, the primary site of infection is either subclinical or undiagnosed, the subsequent diagnosis being established in distant organs as endocarditis, cerebral abscess, or disseminated disease.

Establishing a definitive diagnosis of invasive aspergillosis can be difficult. The histopathologic demonstration of tissue-invasive hyphal forms with dichotomous 45°-angle branching remains the gold standard. Because less common pathogenic fungi, however, may have a similar morphologic appearance on tissue stains (e.g., *P. boydii, Dactylaria, Alternaria, Fusarium*), concomitant growth of an *Aspergillus* species in the specimen confirms the diagnosis. The significance of an *Aspergillus* isolate in a respiratory specimen from a solid-organ recipient is variable and thus is best interpreted in association with the clinical and radiographic findings.[112, 113]

Lung transplant recipients are a unique class owing to their high rate of asymptomatic lung colonization with *Aspergillus* in the candidate period secondary to chronic lung disease.[114] Conversely, invasive aspergillosis evolved without antecedent positive cultures in at least 20% of cases in one series.[115] Despite their well-known ability for hematogenous dissemination, *Aspergillus* organisms rarely grow in routine or fungal blood cultures. Innovative methods for detecting them, including tests for metabolites and polymerase chain reaction, are promising but still not widely available.

The prognosis for invasive aspergillosis in all organ recipient groups has remained poor, with mortality ranges from 50% to 93%.[116] Responsible factors include difficulties in establishing an early diagnosis when disease is localized, a poor response in vivo to amphotericin B, and fatal relapse after the completion of amphotericin B therapy. The standard of therapy remains large doses of amphotericin B (1 to 1.5 mg/kg/day). Some reports demonstrate favorable experience with oral itraconazole and lipid formulations of amphotericin; however, the overall numbers are small.[117-119] Surgical resection of discrete pulmonary, cutaneous, or other visceral lesions may be an effective form of therapy in selected patients.[120-122]

Preventive measures should be comprehensive and include sealing off hospital construction sites, high-efficiency particulate air (HEPA) filtration, and nosocomial air surveillance cultures. Localized prophylaxis with nebulized or intranasal amphotericin B appears promising in bone marrow and cancer patients but has not been tested in organ recipients. Itraconazole may provide systemic chemoprophylaxis during nosocomial outbreaks or in recipients with colonization in the candidate period.

Cryptococcus Infection

Cryptococcus neoformans is a ubiquitous yeast pathogen that causes a sporadic low frequency of infection in all categories of solid-organ recipients.[1, 123] Unlike *Candida* and *Aspergillus* infections, cryptococcosis may occur in the very late post-transplantation period. No specific environmental or host risk factors have been discovered that favor the development of cryptococcal disease. Pretransplant harboring of the organism has rarely been demonstrated; however, routine screening with cryptococcal serologic tests is not regarded as either cost effective or clinically efficacious. The organism usually gains entry via inhalation of airborne yeast forms. Pulmonary manifestations are usually subclinical; however, on occasion a febrile pneumonitis is evident. Early diagnosis and treatment of the infection at this stage may obviate the two most common sequelae, meningitis and disseminated disease. Other uncommon primary manifestations have included skin nodules, cellulitis, and retinitis. The meningeal syndrome is usually characterized by a subacute (lasting weeks) progressive fever, headache, and visual disturbances, with or without true meningismus.

Cerebrospinal fluid (CSF) findings include mononuclear pleocytosis of fewer than 500 cells, moderate elevation in protein, and a normal or mildly depressed glucose level. CSF cryptococcal antigen (latex agglutination) testing is invariably positive, whereas positive India ink staining is present in 40% to 50% of patients. Head computed tomographic (CT) findings are variable. They may include noncommunicating hydrocephalus, meningeal enhancement, and discrete lesions (cryptococcoma) only rarely. Poor prognostic factors include a positive blood culture, high CSF cryptococcal antigen titer, and an attenuated CSF inflammatory response.[124] Combination therapy with amphotericin B (0.5 mg/kg/day) and flucytosine (150 mg/kg/day), divided every 6 hours) for a minimum of 6 weeks is recommended.[125] Intrathecal or intraventricular amphotericin B (0.1 to 0.5 mg/day) has been reported to enhance the clinical response in severe cases[126]; however, its independent contribution has not been rigorously studied. Fluconazole has shown equivalent efficacy in the AIDS population, and early noncomparative results in transplant patients are promising.[127, 128] Despite in vitro susceptibility of *Cryptococcus* to either amphotericin or fluconazole, clinical failure is not infrequent, principally because of late presentation, mechanical CNS complications such as hydrocephalus, and late clinical relapse.

Viral Infections

The herpesvirus family constitutes the dominant group of viral pathogens in solid-organ recipients, largely because of their widespread prevalence as latent organisms in the general population and their capability for reactivation. Thus, both the donor organ and certain recipient tissues can harbor these potentially pathogenic viruses. All viruses in this family are implicated as important causes of post-transplantation morbidity and mortality. These include HSV, CMV, VZV, and EBV, and the recently identified virus, human herpesvirus 6 (HHV-6). Other significant viral pathogens include hepatitis B, hepatitis C, adenovirus, polyomaviruses, and parvovirus B19.

Herpes Simplex Virus

Reactivated HSV infections may occur in HSV-seropositive recipients, usually during the early post-transplantation period. Common sites include the oropharynx (HSV-1) and genital lesions in recipients who are seropositive for HSV-2. Classically, lesions are painful vesicles; however, traumatized or unroofed lesions may appear as coalesced ulcers. Localized mucocutaneous HSV usually is responsive to intravenous or oral acyclovir therapy, which hastens healing, shortens the period of viral shedding, and may prevent progression to more serious disease.[129] Less commonly, disseminated cutaneous infection or visceral involvement (esophagitis, hepatitis, pneumonitis) may cause life-threatening sequelae.[130]

The spectrum of more severe HSV disease may represent a true primary infection in a seronegative recipient via HSV transmission from the donor organ. These infections may have a fulminant course with high mortality despite intravenous acyclovir therapy. Definitive diagnosis for any HSV infection requires the demonstration of typical multinucleate giant cells on either cytologic or histologic specimens, cytopathologic effect in viral cell culture, or immunofluorescence staining for HSV antigens. Low-dose oral acyclovir (200 to 400 mg three or four times a day) may prevent or modify both mucocutaneous and visceral HSV infection.[131] Although acyclovir-resistant HSV strains have been increasingly reported in HIV-infected patients receiving long-term acyclovir prophylaxis, so far these strains have not been prevalent in organ recipients. Clinical experience with famciclovir and valacyclovir, two recently approved antiviral agents with efficacy against HSV, has been limited in solid-organ recipients.

Varicella-Zoster Virus

The vast majority (90%) of adult solid-organ recipients are VZV-seropositive as a result of childhood chickenpox and are thus considered immune to exogenous reinfection with VZV. Rare instances of primary varicella may occur in VZV-seronegative recipients after exposure to an incubating case of chickenpox. Such cases can be severe, with interstitial pneumonitis–induced respiratory failure and multiple organ dissemination. Postexposure prophylaxis with varicella-zoster immune globulin, administered within 72 hours of exposure, may abort or modify the primary varicella syndrome. Reactivated disease, commonly termed *herpes zoster* or *shingles*, occurs in organ recipients at a constant low frequency of 10% to 15%. The time of occurrence may be months or even years after transplantation. Single or multidermatomal, unilateral, painful vesicular eruption is the most common clinical manifestation. Although usually self-limited, some cases progress from cutaneous disease to visceral dissemination.

Early intervention with large doses of intravenous acyclovir (30 mg/kg/day) may shorten the clinical syndrome, promote healing, and prevent progression to visceral dissemination in immunosuppressed patients.[132] Varicella vaccination is projected to have clinical and economic benefit in pediatric solid-organ recipients; however, experience with this recently approved vaccine remains limited in immunocompromised patients.[133]

Cytomegalovirus

In recent years, CMV has been the most intensively investigated pathogen in solid-organ recipients. Thus, fatal or life-threatening invasive disease is less commonly manifested now, owing to significant developments in techniques and strategies for the early detection, treatment, and prevention of CMV infection and disease.

CMV remains the most common single infectious agent in all categories of organ transplantation.[1, 2] CMV infection and disease occur in most organ recipients within the first three post-transplantation months; however, delayed adverse effects in the allograft may be seen months to years later. Symptomatic CMV infection has been associated with fungal and other opportunistic infections in kidney, heart, and liver transplant recipients.[134–136] This effect may be mediated by CMV-induced depression of helper T lymphocyte subsets and expansion of suppressor T lymphocyte subsets with impairment of cellular immunity.[134, 137]

CMV also activates a variety of proinflammatory cytokines (i.e., vascular cell adhesion molecule, intercellular adhesion molecule-1) that enhance the presentation of major histocompatibility complex (MHC) class II surface allograft antigens, which appear to enhance both acute and chronic allograft rejection.[138] Late graft dysfunction in each respective allograft category (vanishing bile duct syndrome in liver recipients, glomerulotubular damage and renal artery stenosis in kidney recipients, and atherosclerotic disease in cardiac grafts) are sequelae associated with significant prior CMV disease.[139–142]

Either the virus is transmitted to the recipient via the donor organ (less frequently blood products), or the recipient CMV strain may reactivate from a state of latency. Thus, seropositive recipients may have either reactivation of the latent strain or superinfection with the donor strain. CMV infection is defined as either *asymptomatic*, which only denotes evidence of either prior acquisition of the virus (positive CMV serology) or viral shedding without symptoms, or *symptomatic* (also termed *disease*), in which the host has clinical, biochemical, virologic, or histopathologic findings of an active CMV process. The status of the recipient's native CMV immunity is a major determinant of the frequency and severity of CMV disease after transplantation[143, 144]; CMV-seronegative recipients who sustain a primary CMV infection have a rate of symptomatic CMV infection as high as 70% in some series, more serious morbidity, and more frequent relapses than seropositive recipients with either reactivation or superinfection.

Immunosuppression with antilymphocyte therapy also potentiates the risk of CMV disease.[145] Symptomatic CMV disease tends to cluster between the second and sixth post-transplantation months, with or without CMV-directed chemoprophylaxis. Clinical presentation is diverse, ranging from a simple CMV syndrome of fever, malaise, and atypical lymphocytosis to serious focal or disseminated invasive disease. Thus, CMV pneumonitis in heart-lung and lung recipients tends to dominate the clinical picture, whereas CMV hepatitis is a more frequent problem in liver recipients. The attributable mortality is variable in many series because of differences in the definition of disease and organ transplant category. CMV pneumonia has a mortality as high as 64% among solid-organ recipients, even with antiviral therapy.[146]

The common and rare acute manifestations of CMV disease are shown in Table 64–3. Diagnosis of invasive disease requires at least the demonstration of typical CMV inclusions in tissue or cytology (e.g., pneumonitis) or virologic evidence of CMV along with a compatible clinical picture. The rapid shell vial centrifugation method allows fast detection (24 to 48 hours) of CMV early antigens in buffy coat, urine, respiratory tract, and tissue specimens[147]; however, the latest-generation tests for CMV, such as the pp65 assay for leukocyte antigenemia or quantitative PCR are becoming the most rapid and accurate methods for establishing the presence of CMV disease.[148, 149]

Intravenous ganciclovir for 2 to 3 weeks remains the primary therapeutic option for invasive CMV disease in solid-organ recipients. Numerous noncomparative series in solid-organ recipients have shown a clinical benefit with ganciclovir therapy, but no placebo-controlled trials are available.[150, 151] Ganciclovir therapy may, however, permit continued immunosuppression for concomitant graft rejection and thus reduce the risk of worsening the CMV disease.[152] The principal limiting toxicity is bone marrow suppression, usually manifesting as leukopenia during the second week of therapy. Ganciclovir must be carefully dosed according to measured or estimated creatinine clearance, since inappropriately large doses may cause severe myelosuppression. CMV strains with ganciclovir resistance were usually confined to HIV-infected patients receiving long-term ganciclovir; however, a recent report of clinical failure in a ganciclovir-treated lung transplant recipient indicates that this phenomenon may threaten solid-organ recipients.[153] Ganciclovir resistance should be considered when patients show a poor clinical response or evidence of persistent CMV excretion.

Foscarnet has a more serious side effect profile than ganciclovir, and there is less clinical experience in solid-organ recipients as a primary treatment modality for CMV disease. It continues to be used most often for patients intolerant of ganciclovir or in refractory cases. Finally, CMV-specific hyperimmune globulin has demonstrated clear survival benefit in bone marrow recipients with CMV pneumonia; however, its adjunctive therapeutic benefit in solid-organ recipients has not convincingly been shown in clinical trials.[154]

Strategies to prevent CMV disease have proliferated since the late 1980s, yet the optimal clinical-effective and cost effective methods remain unknown. A meta-analysis of 13 prospective, controlled CMV prophylaxis trials in solid-organ patients showed protection from CMV disease (RR = 0.50; $P < .001$), but no decrease in graft loss, rejection, or death in the prophylaxis groups.[155] A second approach to CMV prevention that has gained popularity, termed *preemptive*, couples a course of antiviral therapy with either early signs of CMV replication using a sensitive monitoring assay or with a high-risk post-transplantation event (i.e., antilymphocyte therapy). Preemptive strategies have the advantage of targeting organ recipients with incubating CMV disease and avoiding antiviral-related toxicity and costs in lower-risk patients. Some prophylactic and preemptive strategies are summarized in Table 64–4.[156–165]

TABLE 64–3. Acute and Delayed Manifestations of Cytomegalovirus Disease

Organ Invasive Disease
- Mononucleosis syndrome
- Hepatitis
- Pneumonitis
- Gastroesophagitis
- Enteritis
- Colitis
- Encephalitis
- Retinitis
- Adrenalitis
- Cutaneous vasculitis

Immune-Mediated Disease
- Allograft rejection (acute and chronic)
- Superinfection with nonviral pathogens
- Allograft dysfunction
- Glomerulonephritis (renal recipients)
- Vanishing bile duct syndrome (liver recipients)
- Accelerated coronary atherosclerosis (cardiac recipients)
- Bronchiolitis obliterans (lung recipients)

Epstein-Barr Virus

Serologic evidence of prior EBV infection is present in more than 95% of adult solid-organ recipients; however, only 1% to 2% of these recipients have EBV-related post-transplantation lymphoproliferative disease (PTLD). However, EBV-seronegative adults exposed to EBV via the allograft or transfused blood products had a PTLD incidence of 33%.[166] Antirejection therapy with OKT3 also increases the risk for PTLD.[53, 54] Strong evidence linking EBV with the PTLD includes the isolation of EBV deoxyribonucleic acid (DNA) sequences and viral proteins in both hyperplastic and frank lymphatic and visceral tumor tissue.[167] High EBV immune globulin viral capsid antibody titer may be present. The histologic appearance of such tumors ranges from polymorphous hyperplasia to frank lymphoma with monomorphic cells.[168] The median time from transplantation to presentation is 3 to 5 months in most solid-organ groups, the highest incidences being in heart, lung, and intestinal transplant recipients.

Recipients with unexplained fever, adenopathy, atypical lymphocytosis or leukopenia, pulmonary, gastrointestinal or CNS lesions, or splenomegaly should undergo aggressive work-up for PTLD. A favorable clinical response may occur with judicious tapering of immunosuppression alone.[169] Antiviral therapy with acyclovir is often added; however, its true clinical benefit is not known.

Occasionally, both surgical excision and antineoplastic che-

TABLE 64–4. Prophylaxis and Preemptive Regimens for Cytomegalovirus (CMV) in Solid-Organ Recipients

Solid Organ	Regimen Comparison	CMV Disease Rates	
		Regimen (%)	*Comparator (%)*
Prophylaxis			
Kidney[155]	AC 3200 mg/day × 12 wk vs. PL	7.5	29.0
Liver[156]	IV GA/PO AC × 12 wk vs. PO AC	28.0	9.0
Liver[157]	PO GA (days 10–98) vs. PL	4.8	18.9
Liver[158]	CMVIG × 16 wk vs. PL	4.8	19.0
Lung[159]	IV GA × 6 wk	81.0	—
Preemptive			
Kidney[160]	IV GA with (+) PCR vs. IV GA for sx	40.0	60.0
Liver[161]	IV GA with (+) pp65*	12.0	—
Liver[162]	IV GA with CMV shedding vs. PO AC × 24 wk	4.0	29.0
Liver[163]	IV GA started with OKT3 × ≥ 4 wk vs. ≤ IV GA × 2 wk	2.2	50.0
Lung[164]	IV GA × 21 days with antigenemia vs. IV GA with sx	0	27.7

*Only in CMV-positive donors to CMV-negative recipients.
GA = ganciclovir; AC = acyclovir; PL = placebo; CMVIG = hyperimmune anti-CMV globulin; sx = CMV symptoms; PO = oral dosing; IV = intravenous dosing.

motherapy are required for aggressive visceral disease with monoclonal cell surface markers and autonomous tumor behavior that is unresponsive to recovery of the host's immune system. Some reports have shown benefit with allogeneic (donor) HLA-compatible leukocyte infusion for refractory PTLD.[170] The prophylactic efficacy of anti-CMV globulin in EBV-seronegative pediatric organ recipients is under investigation.

Human Herpesvirus 6

Human herpesvirus 6 (HHV-6) is a recently characterized herpesvirus closely related to CMV. Post-transplantation HHV-6 infection has been described in renal and liver recipients manifesting anything from asymptomatic viral shedding and seroconversion to a variable syndrome of fever, rash, blood dyscrasias (leukopenia, anemia), and invasive visceral disease (pneumonitis, hepatitis) at a median time of 50 days after transplantation.[171-173] A close association with CMV disease has also been seen. Treatment with ganciclovir may shorten the clinical course, but ganciclovir-resistant variants have been isolated.

Parvovirus B19

Parvovirus B19 has been shown to cause fever, rash, and a variety of blood dyscrasias, including aplastic anemia, leukopenia, and pure red blood cell aplasia in a variety of organ recipients.[174, 175] Detection of parvovirus B19 DNA by PCR can be performed in blood, bone marrow, and other tissues. Large doses of intravenous immunoglobulin, with or without erythropoietin, may be an effective treatment, although spontaneous remission has also been observed.[175]

CHEMOPROPHYLAXIS AND OTHER PREVENTIVE MEASURES

Measures to prevent certain types of infectious complications in organ recipients may vary, depending on the transplant category or transplant center. There is poor consensus on many of these interventions because of inherent difficulties in performing comparative prospective trials. Some are well supported in nontransplant populations, such as AIDS and cancer patients, and have been adapted for use in the solid organ recipients. Currently, most organ recipients all receive prophylaxis directed against perioperative wound infection, *P. carinii*, HSV, and some type of antifungal prophylaxis regimen. Table 64–5 summarizes some preventive and chemoprophylaxis strategies.

TABLE 64–5. Chemoprophylaxis and Other Preventive Measures After Solid-Organ Transplantation

Pathogen	Chemoprophylaxis	Dosage/Comments
Candida spp.	Mycostatin	2–4 million units/day
	Fluconazole	400 mg/day × 10 wk
	Amphotericin B	10–20 mg/day
Aspergillus	Itraconazole	100–200 mg/day
	Aerosolized amphotericin	
Herpes simplex virus	Acyclovir	200 mg q.i.d.
Varicella-zoster virus	VZIG	Postexposure prophylaxis
Pneumocystis carinii	Trimethoprim-sulfamethoxazole	160/800 every other day
	Aerosolized pentamidine	300 mg/mo
	Dapsone	50–100 mg/day
Toxoplasma gondii	Pyrimethamine	50 mg/day
Mycobacterium tuberculosis	Isoniazid	100 mg/day × 12 mo
Streptococcus pneumoniae	Pneumovax	1–2 months pretransplantation
Haemophilus influenzae	Influenza vaccination	Annually
	Amantadine	
Hepatitis B	HBIG ± lamivudine	6–12 mo* lifelong

*In liver recipients with chronic hepatitis B infection or recipients of hepatitis B core IgG-positive donor livers.
VZIG = varicella zoster immune globulin; HBIG = hepatitis B immune globulin; q.i.d. = four times daily.

References

1. Patel R, Paya CV: Infections in solid-organ transplant recipients. Clin Microbiol Rev 1997; 10:86–124.
2. Fishman JA, Rubin RH: Infections in solid organ transplant recipients. N Engl J Med 1998; 338:1741–1751.
3. Kusne S, Fung J, Alessiana M, et al: Infections during a randomized trial comparing cyclosporine to FK 506 immunosuppression in liver transplantation. Transplant Proc 1992; 24:429–430.
4. Mora NP, Gonwa TA, Goldstein RM, et al: Risk of postoperative infection after liver transplantation: A univariate and stepwise logistic regression analysis of risk factors in 150 consecutive patients. Clin Transplant 1992; 46:443–449.
5. Kusne S, Dummer JS, Ho M, et al: Infections after liver transplantation: An analysis of 101 consecutive cases. Medicine 1988; 67:132–143.
6. Paya CV, Hermans PE, Washington JA, et al: Incidence, distribution, and outcome of episodes of infection in 100 orthotopic liver transplantations. Mayo Clin Proc 1989; 64:555–564.
7. O'Connell JB, Pirarre R, Sullivan HJ, et al: Heart transplantation at Loyola University Medical Center: The first two years. J Heart Transplant 1986; 5:54.
8. Linder J: Infection as a complication of heart transplantation. J Heart Transplant 1988; 7:390–394.
9. van Dorp WT, Kootte AM, van Gemerrt GW, et al: Infections in renal transplant patients treated with cyclosporine or azathioprine. Scand J Infect Dis 1989; 21:75–80.
10. Brayman KL, Stephanian E, Matas A, et al: Analysis of infectious complications occurring after solid organ transplantation. Arch Surg 1992; 127:38–47.
11. Lumbreras C, Fernandez I, Velosa J, Munn S, Sterioff S, Paya CV: Infectious complications following pancreatic transplantation: Incidence, microbiological and clinical characteristics, and outcome. Clin Infect Dis 1995; 20:512–520.
12. Todo S, Tzakis A, Reyes J, et al: Small intestinal transplantation in humans with or without the colon. Transplantation 1994; 57:840–848.
13. Smets YF, van der Pijl JW, van Dissel JT, Ringers J, de Fijter JW, Lemkes HH: Infectious disease complications of simultaneous pancreas kidney transplantation. Nephrol Dial Transplant 1997; 12:764–771.
14. Rubin RH, Wolfson JS, Cosimi AB, et al: Infection in the renal transplant recipient. Am J Med 1981; 70:405–411.
15. Rubin RH: The indirect effects of cytomegalovirus infection on the outcome of organ transplantation. JAMA 1989; 261:3607–3609.
16. Rand KH, Pollard RB, Merigan TC, et al: Increased pulmonary superinfection in cardiac transplant patients undergoing primary cytomegalovirus infection. N Engl J Med 1978; 298:951–953.
17. Goya N, Tanabe K, Iguchi Y, et al: Prevalence of urinary tract infection during outpatient follow-up after renal transplantation. Infection 1997; 25:101–105.
18. Egbert PR, Pillard RB, Gallagher JB, et al: Cytomegalovirus retinitis in immunosuppressed hosts. Ann Intern Med 1980; 93:664–670.
19. Martin M, Manez R, Linden PK, et al: A prospective randomized trial comparing sequential ganciclovir–high dose acyclovir to high dose acyclovir for the prevention of cytomegalovirus disease in adult liver transplant recipients. Transplantation 1994; 58:779–785.
20. Linden PK, Pasculle AW, Manez R, Kramer DJ, Fung JJ, Pinna AD, Kusne S: Differences in outcomes for patients with bacteremia due to vancomycin-resistant *Enterococcus faecium* or vancomycin-susceptible *E. faecium*. Clin Infect Dis 1996; 22:663–670.
21. Papanicolaou GA, Meyers BR, Meyers J, Mendelson MH, Lou W, Emre S, Sheiner P, Miller C: Nosocomial infections with vancomycin-resistant *Enterococcus faecium* in liver recipients: Risk factors for acquisition and mortality. Clin Infect Dis 1996; 23:760–766.
22. Newell KA, Millis JM, Arow PM, Bruce DS, Woodle ES, Cronin DC, et al: Incidence and outcome of infection by vancomycin-resistant *Enterococcus* following orthotopic liver transplantation. Transplantation 1998; 63:439–442.
23. Chang FY, Singh N, Gayowski T, Drenning SD, Wagener MM, Marion IR: *Staphylococcus aureus* nasal colonization and association with infections in liver transplant recipients. Transplantation 1998; 65:1169–1172.
24. Aris RM, Gilligan PH, Neuringer IP, Gott KK, Rea J, Yankaskas JR: The effects of panresistant bacteria in cystic fibrosis patients on lung transplant outcome. Am J Respir Crit Care Med 1997; 155:1699–1704.
25. Krech U: Complement-fixing antibodies against cytomegalovirus in different parts of the world. Bull WHO 1973; 49:103–106.
26. Falagas ME, Snydman DR, Ruthazer R, et al: Primary cytomegalovirus infection in liver transplant recipients: Comparison of infections transmitted via donor organs and via transfusions. Clin Infect Dis 1996; 23:292–297.
27. Rubin RH: The compromised host as sentinel chicken (Editorial). N Engl J Med 1987; 317:1151–1153.
28. Sarubbi FA, Kopt HB, Wilson MB, et al: Increased recovery of *Aspergillus* from respiratory specimens during hospital construction. Am Rev Respir Dis 1982; 125:33–38.
29. Lentino JR, Rosenkranz MA, Michaels JA, et al: Nosocomial aspergillosis: A retrospective review of airborne disease secondary to road construction and contaminated air conditioners. Am J Epidemiol 1982; 116:430–437.
30. Doebbeling BN, Ishak MA, Wade BH, et al: Nosocomial *Legionella micdadei* pneumonia: 10 years experience and a case-control study. J Hosp Infect 1989; 13:289–298.
31. Tobin JO, Beare J, Dunnill MS, et al: Legionnaire's disease in a transplant unit: Isolation of the causative agent from shower baths. Lancet 1980; 2:118–121.
32. Prodinger WM, Bonatti H, Allerberger F, et al. *Legionella* pneumonia in transplant recipients: A cluster of cases of eight years' duration. J Hosp Infect 1994; 26:191–202.
33. Andreone PA, Olivari MT, Elick B, et al: Reduction of infectious complications following heart transplantation with triple-drug immunotherapy. J Heart Transplant 1986; 5:13–19.
34. Prompt CA, Reiss MM, Grillo FM, et al: Transmission of AIDS virus at renal transplantation. Lancet 1985; 2:672.
35. Rubin RH, Jenkins RL, Shaw BW, et al: The acquired immunodeficiency syndrome and transplantation. Transplantation 1987; 44:1–4.
36. Simonds RJ, Holmberg SD, Hurwitz RL, et al: Transmission of human immunodeficiency virus type 1 from a seronegative organ and tissue donor. N Engl J Med 1992; 326:726–732.
37. Dodson SF, Issa S, Araya V, et al: Infectivity of hepatic allografts with antibodies to hepatitis B virus. Transplantation 1997; 64:1582–1584.
38. Dummer JS, Armstrong J, Ho M, et al: Transmission of infection with herpes simplex virus by renal transplantation. J Infect Dis 1987; 155:202–206.
39. Peters TG, Reiter CG, Boswell RL: Transmission of tuberculosis by kidney transplantation. Transplantation 1984; 38:514–516.
40. Keating MR, Guerrero MA, Daly RC, Walker RC, Davies SF: Transmission of invasive aspergillosis from a subclinically infected donor to three different organ transplant recipients. Chest 1996; 109:1119–1124.
41. Dummer JS, Hardy A, Poorsattar A, et al: Early infections in kidney, heart, and liver transplant recipients on cyclosporine. Transplantation 1983; 36:259–267.
42. Hofflin JM, Potasman I, Baldwin JC, et al: Infectious complications in heart transplant recipients receiving cyclosporine and corticosteroids. Ann Intern Med 1987; 106:209–216.
43. The Canadian Multicentre Transplant Study Group: A randomized clinical trial of cyclosporine in cadaveric renal transplantation. N Engl J Med 1986; 314:1219–1225.
44. Borel JF, Feurer C, Gubler GU, et al: Biological effects of cyclosporine A: A new antilymphocytic agent. Agents Actions 1976; 6:468–475.
45. Sawada S, Suzuki G, Kawase Y, et al: Novel immunosuppression agent, FK 506 in vitro effects on the cloned T cell activation. J Immunol 1987; 139:1797–1803.
46. Kim JH, Perfect JR: Infection and cyclosporine. Rev Infect Dis 1989; 11:677–690.
47. Palestine AG, Nussenblatt RB, Chan CC: Side effects of systemic cyclosporine in patients not undergoing transplantation. Am J Med 1984; 77:652–656.
48. Frei UA, Neumayer HH, Buchholz B, et al: Randomized, double-blind, one-year study of the safety and tolerability of

cyclosporine microemulsion compared with conventional cyclosporine in renal transplant patients. Transplantation 1998; 65:1455–1460.
49. Wiesner RH: A long-term comparison of tacrolimus (FK506) versus cyclosporine in liver transplantation: A report of the United States FK506 Study Group. Transplantation 1998; 66:493–499.
50. The US Multicenter FK 506 Liver Study Group: A comparison of tacrolimus (FK 506) and cyclosporine for immunosuppression in liver transplantation. N Engl J Med 1994; 331:1110–1115.
51. Singh N, Dummer JS, Ho M, et al: Infections with cytomegalovirus and other herpes viruses in 121 liver transplant recipients: Transmission by donated organ and the effect of OKT3 antibodies. J Infect Dis 1988; 154:124–131.
52. Nicol DL, MacDonald AS, Beliltsky P, et al: Reduction by combination prophylactic therapy with CMV hyperimmune globulin and acyclovir of the risk of primary CMV disease in renal transplant recipients. Transplantation 1993; 55:841–846.
53. Swinnen LJ, Costanzo-Nordin MR, Fisher SG, et al: Increased incidence of lymphoproliferative disorder after immunosuppression with the monoclonal antibody OKT3 in cardiac transplant recipients. N Engl J Med 1990; 323:1723–1728.
54. Cockfield SM, Preiksaitis J, Harvey E, et al: Is sequential use of ALG and OKT3 in renal transplants associated with an increased incidence of fulminant post-transplant lymphoproliferative disorder? Transplant Proc 1991; 23:1106–1107.
55. Padbury RT, Gunson BK, Dousset B, et al: Steroid withdrawal from long term immunosuppression in liver allograft recipients. Transplantation 1993; 55:789–794.
56. O'Connell JB, Bristow MR, Rasmussen LG, et al: Cardiac allograft function with corticosteroid-free maintenance immunosuppression. Circulation 1990; 82(Suppl IV):318–321.
57. Mazariegos GV, Reyes J, Marino IR, et al: Weaning of immunosuppression in liver transplant recipients. Transplantation 1997; 63:253–249.
58. Starzl TE, Demetris AJ, Trucco M, et al: Systemic chimerism in human female recipients of male livers. Lancet 1992; 340:876–877.
59. Gregoor PJ, Kramer P, Weimar W, van Saase JL: Infections after renal allograft failure in patients with or without low-dose maintenance immunosuppression. Transplantation 1997; 63:1528–1530.
60. Kuo PC, Johnson LB, Schweitzer EJ, Bartlett ST: Simultaneous pancreas/kidney transplantation—a comparison of enteric and bladder drainage of exocrine pancreatic secretions. Transplantation 1997; 63:238–243.
61. Tolkoff-Rubin NE, Rubin RH: Urinary tract infection in the immunocompromised host. Lessons from kidney transplantation and the AIDS epidemic. Infect Dis Clin North Am 1997; 11:707–717.
62. Fox BC, Sollinger HW, Belzer FO, et al: A prospective, randomized, double-blind study of trimethoprim-sulfamethoxazole for prophylaxis of infection in renal transplantation: Clinical efficacy, absorption of trimethoprim-sulfamethoxazole, effects on the microflora, and the cost-benefit of prophylaxis. Am J Med 1990; 89:255–274.
63. Gardner SD, Mackenzie EFD, Smith C, et al: Prospective study of the human polyomaviruses BK and JC and cytomegalovirus in renal transplant recipients. J Clin Pathol 1984; 37:578–586.
64. Mathur VS, Olson JL, Darragh TM, Yen TS: Polyomavirus-induced interstitial nephritis in two renal transplant recipients: Case reports and review of the literature. Am J Kidney Dis 1997; 29:754–758.
65. Shinohara Y, Hashimoto K, Ikegami M, et al: Hemorrhagic kidney graft pyelonephritis caused by type 37 adenovirus infection. Transplant Proc 1992; 24:1565–1566.
66. Mathur SC, Squiers EC, Tatum AH, et al: Adenovirus infection of the renal allograft with sparing of pancreas graft function in the recipients of a combined kidney-pancreas transplant. Transplantation 1998; 65:138–141.
67. Miranda C, Carazo C, Banon R, et al: *Mycoplasma hominis* infection in three renal transplant recipients. Diagn Microbiol Infect Dis 1990; 13:329–331.
68. Wagener MM, Yu VL: Bacteremia in transplant recipients: A prospective study of demographics, etiologic agents, risk factors, and outcomes. Am J Infect Control 1992; 20:239–247.
69. Singh N, Gayowski T, Wagener MM, Marion IR: Increased infections in liver transplant recipients with recurrent hepatitis C virus hepatitis. Transplantation 1996; 61:402–406.
70. Arnow PM, Zachary KC, Thistlethwaite JR, et al: Pathogenesis of early operative site infections after orthotopic liver transplantation. Transplantation 1998; 65:1500–1503.
71. Lerut J, Gordon RD, Iwatsuki S, et al: Biliary tract complications in human orthotopic liver transplantation. Transplantation 1987; 43:47–50.
72. Tzakis AG, Gordon RD, Shaw BW, et al: Clinical presentation of hepatic artery thrombosis after liver transplantation in the cyclosporine era. Transplantation 1987; 40:667–671.
73. Zenati M, Dowling RD, Dummer JS, et al: Influence of the donor lung on development of early infections in lung transplant recipients. J Heart Transplant 1990; 9:508–509.
74. Baldwin RT, Radovanevic B, Sweeny MS, et al: Bacterial mediastinitis after heart transplantation. J Heart Lung Transplant 1992; 1:545–549.
75. Karwande SV, Renlund DG, Olsen SL, et al: Mediastinitis in heart transplantation. Ann Thorac Surg 1992; 54:1039–1045.
76. Boyle EM, Burdine J, Bolman RM: Successful treatment of *Mycoplasma* mediastinitis after heart-lung transplantation. J Heart Lung Transplant 1993; 12:508–512.
77. Thaler F, Gotainer B, Teodori G, et al: Mediastinitis due to *Nocardia asteroides* after cardiac transplantation. Intensive Care Med 1992; 18:127–128.
78. Starzl TE, Todo S, Tzakis A, et al: Multivisceral and intestinal transplantation. Transplant Proc 1992; 24:1217–1223.
79. Haley CE, Cohen ML, Halter J, et al: Nosocomial Legionnaire's disease: A continuing common-source epidemic at Wadsworth Medical Center. Ann Intern Med 1979; 90:583–586.
80. Edelstien PH: Legionnaire's disease. Clin Infect Dis 1993; 16:741–749.
81. Gombert ME, Josephson A, Goldstein EJC, et al: Cavitary Legionnaire's pneumonia: Nosocomial infection in renal transplant recipients. Am J Surg 1984; 147:402–405.
82. Arnouts PJ, Ramael MR, Ysebaert DK, et al: *Legionella pneumophila* peritonitis in a kidney transplant patient. Scand J Infect Dis 1991; 23:19–122.
83. Tokunaga Y, Concepcion W, Berquist WE, et al: Graft involvement by *Legionella* in a liver transplant recipient. Arch Surg 1992; 127:475–477.
84. Valentina HA, Hunt SA, Gibbons R, et al: Increasing pericardial effusion in cardiac transplant recipients. Circulation 1989; 79:603–609.
85. Meyer RD: Role of the quinolones in the treatment of legionellosis. J Antimicrob Chemother 1991; 28:623–625.
86. Hamedani P, Juzar A, Hafeez S, et al: The safety and efficacy of clarithromycin in patients with *Legionella* pneumonia. Chest 1991; 100:1503–1506.
87. Neff TA, Hudgel DW: Miliary tuberculosis in a renal transplant recipient. Am Rev Respir Dis 1973; 108:677–678.
88. Ascher NL, Simmons RL, Marker S, et al: Tuberculous joint disease in transplant patients. Am J Surg 1978; 135:853.
89. Higgins RD, Kusne S, Reyes J, et al: *Mycobacterium tuberculosis* after liver transplantation: Management and guidelines for prevention. Clin Transplant 1992; 6:81–90.
90. Aguado JM, Herrero JA, Gavalda J, et al: Clinical presentation and outcome of tuberculosis in kidney, liver and heart transplant recipients in Spain. Spanish Transplantation Infection Study Group, GESITRA. Transplantation 1997; 63:1278–1286.
91. Sundberg R, Shapiro RR, Darras F, et al: A tuberculosis outbreak in a renal transplant program. Transplant Proc 1991; 23:3091–3092.
92. Quinibi WY, Al-Sibai B, Taher S, et al: Mycobacterial infection after renal transplantation: Report of 14 cases and review of the literature. Q J Med 1990; 77:1039–1060.
93. Rieder HL, Snider DE, Cauthen GM: Extrapulmonary tuberculosis in the United States. Am Rev Respir Dis 1990; 141:347–351.
94. Grauhan O, Lohmann R, Lemmens P, et al: Mycobacterial infections after liver transplantation. Langenbecks Arch Chir 1995; 380:171–175.
95. Schluger LK, Sheiner PA, Jonas M, et al: Isoniazid hepatotoxicity after orthotopic liver transplantation. Mt Sinai J Med 1996; 63:364–369.

96. Arduino RC, Johnson PC, Miranda AG: Nocardiosis in renal transplant recipients undergoing immunosuppression with cyclosporine. Clin Infect Dis 1993; 16:505–512.
97. Simpson GL, Stinson EB, Egger MJ, et al: Nocardial infections in the immunocompromised host: A detailed study in a defined population. Rev Infect Dis 1981; 3:492–507.
98. Wallace RJ, Septimus EJ, Williams TW, et al: Use of trimethoprim-sulfamethoxazole for treatment of infections due to *Nocardia*. Rev Infect Dis 1982; 4:312–325.
99. Paya CV: Fungal infections in solid-organ transplantation. Clin Infect Dis 1993; 16:677–689.
100. Linder J: Infection as a complication of heart transplantation. J Heart Transplant 1988; 7:390–394.
101. Castaldo P, Stratta RJ, Wood RP, et al: Clinical spectrum of fungal infections after orthotopic liver transplantation. Arch Surg 1991; 126:149–156.
102. Rantala A, Niinikoski J, Lehtonen O-P: Yeasts in blood cultures: Impact of early therapy. Scand J Infect Dis 1989; 21:557–561.
103. Komshian SV, Uwaydah AK, Sobel JD, et al: Fungemia caused by *Candida* species and *Torulopsis glabrata* in the hospitalized patient: Frequency, characteristics, and evaluation of factors influencing outcome. Rev Infect Dis 1989; 11:379–390.
104. Tollemar J, Ericzon BG, Holmberg K, et al: The incidence and diagnosis of invasive fungal infections in liver transplant recipients. Transplant Proc 1990; 22:242–244.
105. Tollemar JU, Holmberg K, Ringden O, et al: Surveillance tests for the diagnosis of invasive fungal infections in bone marrow transplant recipients. Scand J Infect Dis 1989; 21:205–212.
106. Edwards JE, Bodey GP, Bowden RA, et al: International conference for the development of a consensus in the management and prevention of severe candidal infections. Clin Infect Dis 1997; 25:43–59.
107. Pfaller MA, Jones RN, Messer SA, Edmond MB, Wenzel RP and the SCOPE Participant Group: National surveillance of nosocomial bloodstream infection due to species of *Candida* other than *Candida albicans*: Frequency of occurrence and antifungal susceptibility in the SCOPE program. Diagn Microbiol Infect Dis 1998; 30:121–129.
108. Fortun J, Lopez-San Roman A, Velasco JJ, et al: Selection of *Candida glabrata* strains with reduced susceptibility to azoles in four liver transplant patients with invasive candidiasis. Eur J Clin Microbiol Infect Dis 1997; 16:314–318.
109. Rex JH, Bennett JE, Sugar AM, et al: A randomized trial comparing fluconazole with amphotericin B for the treatment of candidemia in patients without neutropenia. N Engl J Med 1994; 331:1325–1330.
110. Walsh TJ, Hiemenz JW, Seibel NL, et al: Amphotericin B lipid complex for invasive fungal infections: Analysis of safety and efficacy in 556 cases. Clin Infect Dis 1998; 26:1383–1396.
111. Khardori N: Host-parasite interaction in fungal infections. Eur J Clin Microbiol Infect Dis 1989; 8:331–351.
112. Yu VL, Muder RR, Poorsatar A: Significance of isolation of *Aspergillus* from the respiratory tract in diagnosis of invasive pulmonary aspergillosis. Am J Med 1986; 81:249–254.
113. Horvath JA, Dummer S: The use of respiratory tract cultures in the diagnosis of invasive pulmonary aspergillosis. Am J Med 1996; 100:171–178.
114. Paradowski LJ. Saprophytic fungal infections and lung transplantation—revisited. J Heart Lung Transplant 1997; 16:524–531.
115. Kusne S, Torre-Cisneros J, Manez R, et al: Factors associated with invasive lung aspergillosis and the significance of positive *Aspergillus* culture after liver transplantation. J Infect Dis 1992; 166:1379–1383.
116. Denning DW: Therapeutic outcome in invasive aspergillosis. Clin Infect Dis 1996; 23:608–615.
117. Denning DW, Tucker RM, Hanson LH, et al: Treatment of invasive aspergillosis with itraconazole. Am J Med 1989; 86:791–800.
118. Denning DW, Lee JY, Hostetler JS, et al: NIAID Mycoses Study Group multicenter trial of oral itraconazole therapy for invasive aspergillosis. Am J Med 1994; 97:135–144.
119. Merhav H, Mieles L: Amphotericin B lipid complex in the treatment of invasive fungal infections in liver transplant patients. Transplant Proc 1997; 29:2670–2674.
120. Mayer JM, Nimer L, Carroll K: Isolated pulmonary *Aspergillus* infection in cardiac transplant recipient: Case report and review. Clin Infect Dis 1992; 15:698–700.
121. Loria KM, Salinger MH, Frohlich TG, et al: Primary cutaneous aspergillosis in a heart transplant recipient treated with surgical excision and oral itraconazole. J Heart Lung Transplant 1992; 11:156–159.
122. Salerno CT, Ouyand GW, Pederson TS, et al: Surgical therapy for pulmonary aspergillosis in immunocompromised patients. Ann Thorac Surg 1998; 65:1415–1419.
123. Jabbour N, Reyes J, Kusne S, Martin M, Fung J: Cryptococcal meningitis after liver transplantation. Transplantation 1996; 61:146–149.
124. Diamond RD, Bennett JE: Prognostic factors in cryptococcal meningitis: A study of 111 cases. Ann Intern Med 1974; 80:181.
125. Bennett JE, Dismukes WE, Duma RJ, et al: A comparison of amphotericin B alone and combined with flucytosine in the treatment of cryptococcal meningitis. N Engl J Med 1979; 301:126–131.
126. Polsky B, Depman MR, Gold JWM, et al: Intraventricular therapy of cryptococcal meningitis via a subcutaneous reservoir. Am J Med 1986; 81:24–28.
127. Robinson PA, Knirsch AK, Joseph JA: Fluconazole for life-threatening fungal infections in patients who cannot be treated with conventional antifungal agents. Rev Infect Dis 1990; 12(Suppl 3):S349–S363.
128. Conti DJ, Tolkoff-Rubin NE, Baker GP Jr, et al: Successful treatment of invasive fungal infection with fluconazole in organ transplant recipients. Transplantation 1989; 48:692–695.
129. Chou S, Gallagher JC, Merigan TC: Controlled clinical trial of intravenous acyclovir to treat mucocutaneous herpes simplex after marrow transplantation. Lancet 1981; 1:1392–1394.
130. Kusne S, Schwartz M, Berinig MK, et al: Herpes simplex virus hepatitis after solid organ transplantation in adults. J Infect Dis 1991; 163:1001–1007.
131. Pettersson E, Hovi T, Ahonen T, et al: Prophylactic oral acyclovir after renal transplantation. Transplantation 1985; 39:279–281.
132. Shepp DH, Dandliker PS, Meyers JD: Treatment of varicella-zoster virus infection in severely immunocompromised patients. N Engl J Med 1986; 314:208–212.
133. Kitai IC, King S, Gafni A: An economic evaluation of varicella vaccine for pediatric liver and kidney transplant recipients. Clin Infect Dis 1993; 17:441–447.
134. George MJ, Snydman DR, Werner BG, et al: The independent role of cytomegalovirus as a risk factor for invasive fungal disease in orthotopic liver transplant recipients. Am J Med 1997; 103:106–113.
135. Gorensek MJ, Stewart RW, Keys TF, et al: Symptomatic cytomegalovirus infection as a significant risk factor for major infections after cardiac transplantation. J Infect Dis 1988; 158:884–887.
136. Schooley RT, Hirsch MS, Colvin RB, et al: Association of herpes group virus infections with T-lymphocyte subset alterations, glomerulopathy and opportunistic infections following renal transplantation. N Engl J Med 1983; 308:307–313.
137. Maher P, O'Toole CM, Wreghitt TG, et al: Cytomegalovirus infection in cardiac transplant recipients is associated with chronic T cell subset ratio inversion with expansion of a Leu7+ TS-C+ subset. Clin Exp Immunol 1985; 62:515–524.
138. von Willebrand E, Pettersson E, Ahonen J, Hayry P: CMV infection class II antigen expression, and human kidney allograft rejection. Transplantation 1986; 42:374–367.
139. O'Grady JG, Alexander GJM, Sutherland S, et al: Cytomegalovirus infection and donor/recipient HLA antigens: Interdependent cofactors in pathogenesis of vanishing bile duct syndrome after liver transplantation. Lancet 1988; 2:302–305.
140. Richardson WP, Colvin RB, Cheeseman SH, et al: Glomerulopathy associated with cytomegalovirus viremia in renal allografts. N Engl J Med 1981; 305:57–63.
141. Pouria S, State OI, Wong W, Hendry BM: CMV infection is associated with transplant renal artery stenosis. Q J Med 1998; 91:185–189.
142. Grattan MT, Moreno-Cabral CE, Stames VA, et al: Cytomegalovirus infection is associated with cardiac allograft rejection and atherosclerosis. JAMA 1989; 261:3561–3566.
143. Weir MR, Irwin BC, Maters AW, et al: Incidence of cytomegalovirus disease in cyclosporine-treated renal transplant recipients based on donor/recipient pretransplant immunity. Transplantation 1987; 43:187–193.

144. Rubin RH: Infection in the organ transplant recipient. *In*: Clinical Approach to Infection in the Compromised Host. 3rd ed. Rubin RH, Young LS (Eds). New York, Plenum, 1994, pp 629–705.
145. Snydman DR: Treatment of cytomegalovirus pneumonia in solid organ recipients. *In*: Ganciclovir Therapy for Cytomegalovirus Infection. Spector S (Ed). New York, Marcel Dekker, 1991, p 145.
146. Paya CV, Smith TF, Ludwig J, et al: Rapid shell viral culture and tissue histology compared with serology for the rapid diagnosis of cytomegalovirus infection in liver transplantation. Mayo Clin Proc 1989; 64:670–675.
147. Niubo J, Perez JL, Martinez-Lacasa JT, et al: Association of quantitative cytomegalovirus antigenemia with symptomatic infection in solid organ transplant patients. Diagn Microbiol Infect Dis 1996; 24:19–24.
148. Abecassis MM, Koffron AJ, Kaplan B, et al: The role of PCR in the diagnosis and management of CMV in solid organ recipients: What is the predictive value for the development of disease and should PCR be used to guide antiviral therapy? Transplantation 1997; 63:275–279.
149. Erice A, Chou S, Biron KK, et al: Progressive disease due to ganciclovir-resistant cytomegalovirus in immunocompromised patients. N Engl J Med 1989; 320:289–293.
150. Dunn DL, Mayoral JL, Gillingham KT, et al: Treatment of invasive cytomegalovirus disease in solid organ transplant recipients with ganciclovir. Transplantation 1991; 51:98–106.
151. Snydman DR: Ganciclovir therapy for cytomegalovirus disease associated with renal transplants. Rev Infect Dis 1988; 10:S554.
152. Dunn DL, Mayoral JL, Gillingham KT, et al: Simultaneous treatment of concurrent rejection and tissue invasive cytomegalovirus disease without detrimental effects upon patient or allograft survival. Clin Transplant 1992; 46:413–420.
153. Alain S, Honderlick P, Grenet D, et al: Failure of ganciclovir treatment associated with selection of a ganciclovir-resistant cytomegalovirus strain in a lung transplant recipient. Transplantation 1997; 63:1533–1536.
154. Zaia JA: Prevention and treatment of cytomegalovirus pneumonia in transplant recipients. Clin Infect Dis 1993; 17(Suppl 2):S392–S399.
155. Couchoud C, Cucherat M, Haugh M, Pouteil-Noble C: Cytomegalovirus prophylaxis with antiviral agents in solid organ transplantation. Transplantation 1997; 65:641–647.
156. Balfour HH Jr, Chace BA, Stapleton JT, et al: A randomized placebo-controlled trial of oral acyclovir for the prevention of cytomegalovirus disease in recipients of renal allografts. N Engl J Med 1989; 320:1381–1387.
157. Martin M, Manez R, Linden PK, et al: A prospective randomized trial comparing sequential ganciclovir–high dose acyclovir to high dose acyclovir for prevention of CMV disease. Transplantation 1994; 58:779–785.
158. Gane E, Saliba F, Valdecasas GJ, et al: Randomised trial of efficacy and safety of oral ganciclovir in the prevention of cytomegalovirus disease in liver-transplant recipients. The Oral Ganciclovir International Transplantation Study Group. Lancet 1997; 350:1729–1733.
159. Snydman DR, Werner BG, Dougherty NN, et al: Cytomegalovirus immune globulin prophylaxis in liver transplantation: A randomized double-blind, placebo-controlled trial. Ann Intern Med 1993; 119:984–991.
160. Kelly JL, Albert RK, Wood DE, Raghy G: Efficacy of a 6-week prophylactic ganciclovir regimen and the role of serial cytomegalovirus antibody testing in lung transplant recipients. Transplantation 1995; 59:1144–1147.
161. Brennan DC, Garlock KA, Lippmann BA, et al: Control of cytomegalovirus-associated morbidity in renal transplant patients using intensive monitoring and either preemptive or deferred therapy. J Am Soc Nephrol 1997; 8:118–125.
162. Grossi P, Kusne S, Rinaldo C, et al: Guidance of ganciclovir therapy with pp65 antigenemia in cytomegalovirus-free recipients of livers from seropositive donors. Transplantation 1996; 61:1659–1660.
163. Singh N, Yu VL, Mieles L, Wagener MM, Miner RC, Gayowski T: High dose acyclovir compared with short-course preemptive ganciclovir therapy to prevent cytomegalovirus disease in liver transplant recipients: A randomized trial. Ann Intern Med 1994; 120:375–381.
164. Winston DJ, Imagawa DK, Holt CD, Kaldas F, Shaked A, Bussutil RW: Long term ganciclovir prophylaxis eliminates serious cytomegalovirus disease in liver transplants receiving OKT3 therapy for rejection. Transplantation 1995; 60:1357–1360.
165. Egan JJ, Lomaz J, Barber L, et al: Preemptive treatment for the prevention of cytomegalovirus disease in lung and heart transplant recipients. Transplantation 1998; 65:747–752.
166. Manez R, Breinig MC, Linden P, et al: Posttransplant lymphoproliferative disease in primary Epstein-Barr virus infection after liver transplantation: The role of cytomegalovirus disease. Clin Infect Dis 1997; 176:1462–1467.
167. Ho M, Jaffe R, Miller G, et al: The frequency of Epstein-Barr virus infection and associated lymphoproliferative syndrome after transplantation and its manifestations in children. Transplantation 1988; 45:719–727.
168. Starzl T: The diagnosis and treatment of posttransplant proliferative disorders. Curr Probl Surg 1988; 25:371–465.
169. Starzl TE, Nalesnik MA, Porter KA, et al: Reversibility of lymphomas and lymphoproliferative lesions developing under cyclosporine-steroid therapy. Lancet 1984; 1:583–587.
170. Emanuel DJ, Lucas KG, Mallory GB, et al: Treatment of posttransplant lymphoproliferative disease in the central nervous system of a lung transplant recipient using allogeneic leukocytes. Transplantation 1997; 63:1691–1694.
171. Lautenschlager I, Hockerstedt K, Linavuori K, Taskinen E: Human herpesvirus-6 infection after liver transplantation. Clin Infect Dis 1998; 26:702–707.
172. Singh N, Carrigan DR, Gayowski T, Marino IR: Human herpesvirus-6 infection in liver transplant recipients: Documentation of pathogenicity. Transplantation 1997; 64:674–678.
173. Morris DJ, Littler E, Arrand JR, et al: Human herpesvirus 6 infection in renal transplant recipients. N Engl J Med 1989; 320:1560–1561.
174. Chang FY, Singh N, Gayowski T, Marino IR: Parvovirus B19 infection in a liver transplant recipient: Case report and review in organ transplant recipients. Clin Transplant 1996; 10:243–247.
175. Wicki J, Samii K, Cassinotti P, et al: Parvovirus B19-induced red cell aplasia in solid-organ transplant recipients: Two case reports and review of the literature. Hematol Cell Ther 1997; 39:199–204.

65

Bacterial Pneumonia in Adult Respiratory Distress Syndrome

Jay I. Peters, MD • Jacqueline J. Coalson, PhD

Adult respiratory distress syndrome (ARDS) occurs with a spectrum of severity and is clinically defined by bilateral infiltrates, a ratio of $Pa{O_2}$ to $FI{O_2} \leq 200$, and either a pulmonary artery occlusive pressure of 18 mm Hg or less or no clinical evidence of elevated left arterial pressure.[1] When the injury is less severe ($Pa{O_2}$ ratio > 200 mm Hg but ≤ 300 mm Hg), the syndrome is termed "acute lung injury." The acute changes in the lung function, typically in gas exchange, result from structural changes in the alveolar-capillary membrane leading to the development of noncardiogenic pulmonary edema through increased vascular permeability. The histologic lesion, termed "diffuse alveolar damage" (DAD), evolves through uniform stages despite the wide differences in the clinical cause of ARDS.[2]

The histologic appearances of the lung can generally be divided into three histologic overlapping stages that correlate with the clinical evolution of the disease[3] (see Chapter 125).

The *exudative stage* occurs during the first week after the onset of respiratory failure. Light microscopy reveals hyaline membranes along the alveolar ducts, capillary congestion, interstitial and alveolar edema, and hemorrhage with neutrophil aggregation. By 7 to 14 days, the *proliferative-reparative stage* predominates and is characterized by proliferation of type II alveolar epithelial cells and fibroblasts. Fibroblasts migrate into the alveolar exudate and convert it to cellular granulation tissue and subsequently into dense fibrous tissue *(fibrotic phase).*

Until the early 1970s, it was generally believed that patients with ARDS died of hypoxemic respiratory failure with underlying proliferative lung lesions as a consequence of the DAD process. In 1986, however, a pathologic review of 77 postmortem examinations in a study population with ARDS documented that more than 70% of the patients had evidence of bronchopneumonia at autopsy, and in 21% it was the only lung finding. Only nine patients had severe pulmonary fibrosis (reparative DAD).[4] In this same ARDS study population, multiple organ failure, death, and infection were highly interrelated, the most common cause of death being multiple organ failure rather than uncorrectable hypoxemia, of which only 2 of 141 patients died.[5, 6] Other studies confirmed these findings.

In a prospective study by Montgomery and coworkers, only 16% of deaths from ARDS were from irreversible hypoxemia and 80% of these patients had ongoing *sepsis syndrome* at the time of death.[7] Although early deaths (within 72 hours) could be attributed to the underlying illness or injury, most late deaths were related to sepsis syndrome and multiple organ failure. In this study, a pulmonary source was implicated in 75% of patients who acquired the sepsis syndrome after the onset of ARDS.[7] Sepsis syndrome continues to be a common complication among ARDS patients. In a recent prospective study of more than 200 patients, Suchyta and coworker found sepsis as a complication in 60% of patients.[8] Pneumonia was the cause of ARDS in 40% of the patients, and 23% of these patients died of progressive respiratory failure. The authors speculated that perhaps the inflammation associated with pneumonia altered the lungs' reparative process.

Lung infection not only is a common complication and a frequent cause of death in patients with acute lung injury but also is a common initiating event of ARDS. Pneumonia and aspiration accounted for nearly 37% of the 741 patients with acute respiratory failure enrolled by the multiple centers in the extracorporeal membrane oxygenation (ECMO) trial.[9] These same two categories accounted for 66% of the 90 patients selected from this larger group of patients for randomization to ECMO or control treatment. In studies of ARDS, the percentage of patients with pneumonia has varied widely, probably dependent on how the patient populations were selected by the investigators.[10, 11]

Bacterial infection in nonpulmonary sites is significantly related to the problem of adult respiratory failure and nosocomial pneumonia. Sepsis was thought to be the causative factor in approximately 15% of the patients with acute respiratory failure in the ECMO trial.[9] In surgical patients, especially after trauma, sepsis has been reported to account for as many as 90% of fatal cases of ARDS, clearly documenting that it is the most common cause of severe and ultimately fatal lung injury.[12] The pathogenesis of sepsis with its numerous cascading mediators not only is increasingly complex but its definition also continues to undergo refinement. In 1991, the American College of Chest Physicians/Society of Critical Care Medicine developed a refined set of terms and definitions to describe the *systemic inflammatory response syndrome* (SIRS), sepsis, sepsis syndrome, and septic shock.[13] This conference extended the concept that inflammatory mediators may be initiated by infection or noninfectious insults like pancreatitis, multiple trauma, and tissue injury or ischemia. During a systemic inflammatory response, the lungs become prone to infection and augmentation of the lungs' defense mechanisms during critical periods may prove to be beneficial in the treatment of patients with ARDS.

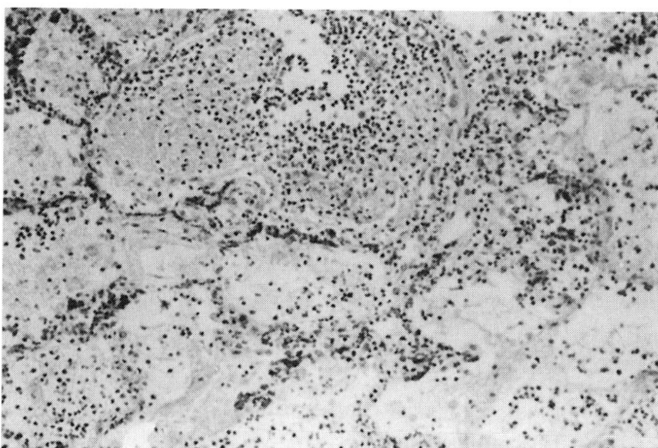

Figure 65–1. Lung specimen from a patient with documented sepsis who died 7 days after onset of acute respiratory distress syndrome. Alveolar walls are engorged with red blood cells. The alveolar spaces contain edema, fibrin strands, and numerous polymorphonuclear neutrophils (PMNs). (Hematoxylin and eosin, ×150.)

The term SIRS has been applied to patients who manifest signs of infection or inflammation in the absence of a definitive site.[14] One theory to explain the process is the translocation of bacteria or endotoxin across the gastrointestinal mucosa in severely ill patients.[15] Another hypothesis may be that the development of nosocomial pneumonia may escape clinical detection and trigger systemic inflammation. The lungs in septic patients can be the recipients of a metastatic bloodborne infection from another organ, the source of a clinically silent focus of pneumonia that "feeds" the septic process,[5] or the septic process via its widespread permeability defect can simply inactivate the lungs' local defenses and allow the lungs to acquire nosocomial pneumonia via aspiration of oropharyngeal flora. All result in histologic evidence of pneumonia in the lungs of patients (Figs. 65–1 and 65–2).

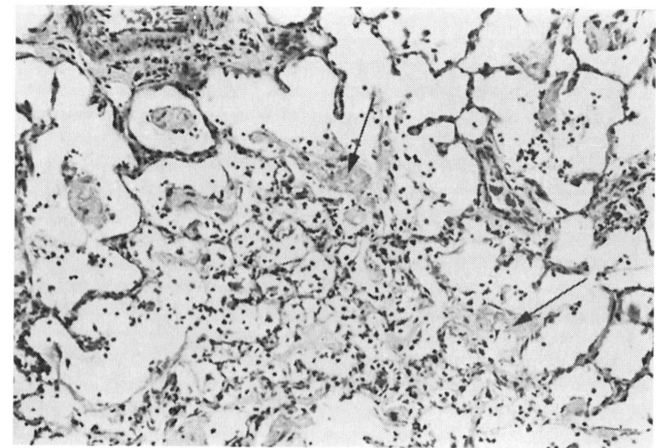

Figure 65–2. Baboon lung exposed to 80% oxygen for 11 days. Fibrin aggregates *(arrows)*, the result of exudative diffuse alveolar damage, are intermixed with an "alveolitis" of alveolar macrophages and fewer polymorphonuclear neutrophils. This is the most severe lesion manifested in this model. (Hematoxylin and eosin, ×150.)

It is now clear that nosocomial pneumonia in patients with ARDS is frequently characterized by the sepsis syndrome and accompanied by multiple organ failure.[7, 16] Bacterial infection, either of the lung itself or at nonpulmonary sites, is a major contributor to the poor prognosis of ARDS.[17] The events that allow us to understand how pulmonary infection is manifested in a patient with ARDS mandate an understanding of the normal defense mechanisms in the lungs and how their disruption can result in patients' increased vulnerability to infection in the intensive care unit (ICU).

DEFENSE MECHANISMS OF THE LUNG

The lung represents the largest epithelial surface of the body with a surface area of 70 m^2. During respiration, the upper and lower airways are exposed to a multitude of microorganisms and airborne particles. The respiratory system has developed extraordinary defense mechanisms to prevent infections of the respiratory tract (Table 65–1). The mucociliary apparatus, along with the important gag and cough reflexes, has a pivotal role in removing inhaled microbes. Bacterial *adherence* (binding of bacteria) to epithelial cells and interbacterial *inhibition* (receptor sites occupied by gram-positive organisms in normalcy) prevent colonization of the oropharynx and tracheobronchial tree with gram-negative organisms, an important but incompletely understood defense mechanism. The lungs complement these defense mechanisms with several immunoglobulins, IgA at the airway level and IgG at the alveolar level, and other secretions, including lysozyme, lactoferrin, surfactant, and fibronectin. The interrelated activities of these factors allow for entrapment and neutralization of microbes and their subsequent removal on the mucociliary blanket. Bronchus-associated lymphoid tissue and lymphocytes add needed immunologically competent cells. At the alveolar level, the alveolar macrophages function effectively in a normal host to remove those microbes smaller than 0.2 mm, which may bypass all of the airway physical and mechanical barriers in the airways.

The alveolar macrophage is the primary cell that serves to maintain the sterility of the terminal airways and alveoli. The alveolar macrophage can eliminate challenges of 10^5–10^6 organisms without recruiting polymorphic neutrophils (PMNs) into the airspace.[18] If, however, the challenge is too great or the virulence of the organisms high, the macrophage, through cell-to-cell signaling, can recruit PMNs from the pulmonary microvasculature. An increasing body of evidence shows that cytokines secreted by alveolar macrophages and other lung cells, especially tumor necrosis factor (TNF), interleukin-1 (IL-1), and IL-8, are capable of attracting PMNs into the terminal airway as well as activating PMNs for enhanced respiratory burst and phagocytosis.[18–20] Recent clinical investigations showed that the cytokine functions of alveolar macrophages are down-regulated after sepsis.[21] This phenomenon of down-regulation may, under most circumstances, protect the host from continual activation and inflammatory injury; however, this protective mechanism may render the host vulnerable to subsequent infection at an adjacent or distant site, such as the lung. These findings of down-regulation in the pulmonary immune system have led to studies of augmenting the lungs' defense mechanisms with exogenous interferon gamma (IFN-γ) or granulocyte–colony-stimulating factor (G-CSF).[22, 23]

Although conventional wisdom suggests that increasing the number of PMNs would worsen acute lung injury, G-CSF has been shown to attenuate endotoxin-induced lung injury in both a guinea pig and a sheep model.[24, 25] Clinical studies are ongoing to evaluate the role of G-CSF in non-neutropenic patients with severe pneumonia. Inflammatory mediators, such as TNF, interleukins, eicosanoids, interferons, and CSFs, may play a pivotal role in the inflammatory response to both infectious and noninfectious insults. Whether the pathogenesis of these infectious and noninfectious inflammatory states are the same remains controversial. However, most physicians do accept that some "clinically septic" patients never experience bacteremia and others lack a source of documented infection even at autopsy.

TABLE 65–1. Defense Mechanisms of the Respiratory System

Normal oropharyngeal bacterial flora
Aerodynamic filtration
Airway reflexes
Cough
Gag
Bronchoconstriction
Mucociliary escalator
Oropharyngeal and airway secretions: saliva, mucus
Lactoferrin
Complement
Surfactant
Fibronectin
Alpha$_1$-antitrypsin
Lysozyme
Immunoglobulins IgA and IgG
Bronchus-associated lymphoid tissue lymphocytes
Alveolar macrophages

COLONIZATION OF THE RESPIRATORY TRACT

Nosocomial bacterial pneumonias develop in hospitalized patients and are due to a shift of flora that can be documented when patients become progressively sicker.[26] The endogenous microflora in the oropharynx of a healthy individual usually consists of nonpathogenic, gram-positive (*Streptococcus salivarius*, lactobacilli), and anaerobic bacteria. When exposed to large quantities of pathogenic bacteria, a normal host will clear the organisms within 6 hours of exposure.[27] Colonization of the oropharynx in healthy individuals with gram-negative bacilli is very uncommon, occurring in only 1% to 6% of subjects. The same low incidence of gram-negative bacilli colonization is found among personnel caring for patients in ICUs.

Colonization of the upper respiratory tract by gram-negative bacilli is mediated by alterations in the surface properties of the epithelial cells.[28, 29] Experimentally, it is known that after exposure to malnutrition, general surgery, or renal dysfunction, buccal cell adherence increases significantly. The organisms most likely to spread during infections have specialized surfaces that enable them to adhere to cell surfaces (e.g., pili, fibrillae, lipotichoic acid, and so on). The risk factors responsible for oropharyngeal colonization with gram-negative bacilli include neutropenia, prior antibiotic therapy, alcoholism, azotemia, coma, diabetes, serious illness, hypotension, intubation, smoking, surgery, and neutralization of gastric acid.[28, 29]

In a prospective study of patients hospitalized in a medical ICU, Johanson and coworkers demonstrated that in those who had nosocomial pneumonia, gram-negative bacilli were cultured from the oropharynx in 85%.[30] Critically ill patients also can exhibit colonization of the tracheobronchial tree. Tillotson and Finland[31] examined 149 antibiotic-treated patients with primary pneumonia. Lower airway colonization with pathogenic bacteria (e.g., *Staphylococcus aureus, Klebsiella pneumoniae, Escherichia coli, Haemophilus influenzae, Pseudomonas aeruginosa,* and others) developed in 59% of these patients.[31] In 48 patients treated with mechanical ventilation and endotracheal intubation, Schwartz and colleagues determined that by day 8 of illness, more than two thirds of the patients had gram-negative bacilli in tracheal aspirates.[32] Several investigators have shown that polyvinylchloride endotracheal tubes provided a surface to which pathogenic bacteria adhere in great numbers[18] and that intubation significantly increased the risk of gram-negative pneumonia.

One hypothesis to explain colonization of the upper respiratory tract suggested that during times of illness, an elaboration of proteases took place that removed fibronectin from the surface of epithelial cells.[28, 33] Removal of fibronectin increased the exposure of binding sites and allowed adherence by gram-negative organisms.[30] Another group of investigators have demonstrated changes in the binding properties of the buccal epithelium for various lectins (large glycoproteins) at the time of gram-negative colonization.[34] Their data suggested that an alteration of the glycoprotein content of the epithelial cells rather than an increased exposure of the binding sites may be the underlying mechanism for colonization of gram-negative organisms.

Niederman and associates, examining patients with tracheostomies, showed that in about half of the study group persistent colonization of the lower airways developed. In these colonized subjects, pneumonia occurred at a threefold greater frequency.[35] Although some of the non-Enterobacteriaceae (*Pseudomonas* and *Acinetobacter*) may be from an exogenous environmental source, the gram-negative bacilli that colonize the oropharynx and tracheobronchial tree of patients with ARDS are usually not acquired from an environmental source but are acquisitions from the gram-negative organisms that reside in a patient's gastrointestinal tract or are acquired from another patient's bacterial flora. These organisms are transmitted from patient to patient on the hands of personnel.[36]

PATHOGENESIS OF PNEUMONIA

The mechanisms by which microorganisms enter the lower respiratory tract include inhalation, aspiration, hematogenous spread, and inoculation from contiguous sites of infection. Clinically, inhalation and aspiration are the predominant routes of delivery of microbes into the airways. The manner by which bacteria are presented to the lungs is the primary determinant of whether or not infection will develop. Berendt showed in a primate model that deposition of 10^7 *K. pneumoniae* in an aerosol failed to produce pneumonia, whereas 10^4 organisms delivered as a fluid bolus into the trachea consistently produced pneumonia.[37] In humans, infection by inhalation of microbes probably occurs in only a few particular instances, such as infection caused by viruses, *Legionella*, mycobacteria, and fungi.

Microaspiration of bacteria from a colonized oropharynx or tracheobronchial tree is the primary route of acquisition of microbes into the lung. Organisms that colonize the upper respiratory tract may be abundantly present in secretions. Concentrations of organisms may be as high as 10^8/mL,[36] so that aspiration of even small quantities of secretions are sufficient to deliver a massive bacterial inoculum into the lungs. Aspiration of oropharyngeal secretions occurs in at least 45% of healthy individuals during sleep and in 70% of patients with depressed levels of consciousness.[38] Cuffed endotracheal tubes do not protect against aspiration of small volumes of secretions from the oropharynx because of the milking of small quantities around the endotracheal cuff during cycles of the ventilator.[32] The endotracheal tube can also serve as a conduit of microbes from health care givers and equipment used in respiratory therapy. In fact, the risk of pneumonia is six to 21 times greater in intubated patients than in other hospitalized patients.[39] Finally, retrograde migration to the oropharynx from a stomach colonized with microbes can occur, after which aspiration into the lungs can result.[40, 41] Acid-neutralizing therapy with antacids and H_2 blockers allows gastric pH to rise, permitting gram-negative organisms in the stomach to increase exponentially.

The probability of producing pneumonia using a bolus delivery is enhanced by an increase in either the number of bacteria instilled or the volume of the inoculum. If a bolus is delivered in a mucin suspension and is not removed, multiplication with persistence of bacteria occurs in the distal portion of lung and results in edema, inflammation, and accumulation of bacterial products. Experimentally, in normal animals, 10^7 and greater bacterial concentrations delivered as a bolus routinely induce clinical pneumonia and can cause death of the animal.[37, 42] However, diffuse alveolar damage reduces the host's level defenses and allows the induction of pneumonia by aspirated secretions containing smaller quantities of microbes.

Experimental settings that more closely mimic the compromised host in an ICU environment have been developed to assess how infection augments lung injury. Johanson and colleagues examined the effects of bacterial superinfection on injured hamster lungs pretreated with 100% oxygen. Inocula of both 10^3 and 10^6 organisms elicited pneumonias.[43] In an oleic acid–induced lung injury model in the baboon, animals that sustained a superimposed pneumonia and bacteremia had a precipitous clinical course when compared with baboons treated with oleic acid only.[44] Likewise, lung injury induced by 80% oxygen produces a mild DAD lesion in baboons during an 11-day period. However, if infection is induced by an intrabronchial inoculation of *P. aeruginosa* organisms on day 6, the animals sustain a severe lung injury, clearly documenting the detrimental effect of infection on a predamaged lung[45] (Fig. 65–3; see also Fig. 65–2). Recent research revealed that the bronchoalveolar and serum levels of pro-inflammatory cytokines do not differentiate between ARDS in the absence of lung infections and states of severe primary or secondary pneumonia.[46] In contrast to cardiogenic pulmonary edema, ARDS and pneumonia present with comparable and systemic inflammatory sequelae. Other investigators performed serial lavages between day 3 and day 21 in patients with persistence

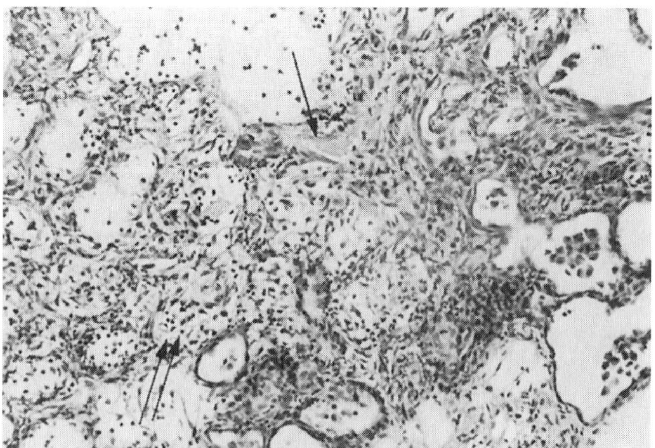

Figure 65–3. Baboon lung exposed to 80% oxygen for 6 days, followed by intrabronchial instillation of *Pseudomonas* organisms. A residual fibrin aggregate is identified *(arrow)*, but the alveoli are filled with organizing fibrous connective tissue *(double arrow)* that is infiltrated with both polymorphonuclear neutrophils and mononuclear cells. (Hematoxylin and eosin, ×150.)

of ARDS.[47] This group found a persistence of cytokines (IL-8, IL-1β) even as late as 2 to 3 weeks after the onset of ARDS.

It is assumed that the antibacterial defense mechanisms are impaired in patients with ARDS (Table 65–2). The presence of endotracheal tubes that markedly reduce mucociliary transport and the presence of pulmonary edema and alveolar hypoxia that impair the bactericidal capacity of the lungs are among suggested mechanisms. Edema fluid can interfere with the bactericidal function of alveolar macrophages and the antibacterial function of surfactant by reducing its quantity and changing its functional characteristics.[27, 48] The interaction of bacilli with the alveolar macrophages and PMNs within the alveolar space has been studied by a number of investigators.[36] Deposition of 10^9 organisms by aerosolization results in a rapid clearance and no infection with *S. aureus* and other gram-positive organisms.[49] Low-virulence organisms, such as those found in normal oropharyngeal flora, do not require PMNs or circulating antibody; however, inhalation of gram-negative bacilli is associated with a longer clearance time and a rapid recruitment of PMNs in distal airways.[50] Neutropenia is associated with a more impaired clearance of gram-negative bacilli than macrophage depletion.[51]

Nosocomial pneumonias in patients with ARDS are usually polymicrobial because the organisms are selected from a larger group of colonizing pathogens in the tracheobronchial and oropharyngeal secretions.[6, 52] Why only certain organisms subsequently elicit pneumonia is not well understood. Enteric gram-negative bacilli are the predominant pathogens in patients with ARDS. Gram-negative organisms were found in 75% of the cases in a study by Fagon and colleagues[52] and in 56% of patients in a study by Seidenfeld and associates.[6] In both studies, the most common gram-negative pathogen was *P. aeruginosa*.[6, 52] The specific risk factors identified with the causation of *P. aeruginosa*-induced pneumonia in patients with ARDS are leukopenia, corticosteroid therapy, intravascular monitoring devices, and respiratory therapy equipment.[28] Gram-positive isolates accounted for 52% and 32%, respectively, of the bacteria cultured from the patients in these two studies.[6, 52]

Calibration of the histologic findings of pneumonia with quantitative bacterial cultures of the lung has been experimentally carried out. In baboons and hamsters with either normal lungs or lungs damaged by oleic acid or oxygen, a correlation was found between the appearance of histologic pneumonia and greater than 10^4 colony-forming units (CFUs) per gram of lung tissue.[43, 53] Lungs demonstrating fewer bacteria did not contain characteristic histologic foci of infection. In a patient study, bacterial infections of the lung that had been manifested clinically also contained at least 10^4 CFUs/g of tissue.[54] The presence of more than 10^5 CFUs/mL of exudate has been used by Bartlett to document the presence of lung pneumonia.[55] Bacterial infections of the lung that had been manifested clinically also contained at least 10^4 CFUs/g of tissue.[54] Another study, using postmortem lung examination within 3 days of bronchoscopy, found histologic pneumonia associated with 10^3 CFUs/mL with protected sterile brush, 10^4 CFUs/mL with bronchoalveolar lavage fluid, and 10^5–10^6 with quantitative endotracheal aspirations.[56]

TABLE 65–2. Pathogenetic Steps in Nosocomial Pneumonia Caused by Gram-Negative Bacilli

Onset of predisposing factors
Serious illness, surgery, antibiotics, and so on; initiate proteases
Colonization (acquisition)
Adherence properties of the oropharyngeal and tracheobronchial airway epithelium altered; gram-negative bacilli acquired
Entry into lungs
Aspiration of colonized upper-airway secretions or neutralized gastric secretions
Interaction with defense mechanisms
Host's inadequate local and systemic defenses allow bacterial multiplication
Formation of pneumonitic inflammatory exudate
Edema, inflammatory cell infiltrates, and bacterial products collect in airspaces
Egress from lungs
Spread can occur via lymphatics and/or bloodstream

CLINICAL ASPECTS OF PNEUMONIA

Nosocomial pneumonia frequently occurs in critically ill patients whose lungs are being mechanically ventilated. Because the clinical diagnosis is difficult, the true incidence is still subject to controversy. In fact, no prospective human study has ever been performed evaluating the diagnosis of pneumonia exclusively in ARDS patients. Most of the literature relates to ventilator-associated pneumonia in critically ill patients, some of whom have ARDS. Among all the patients admitted to hospitals, infections of the respiratory tract represent one of the most common nosocomial infections along with urinary tract and surgical wound infections.[57] The risk of respiratory tract infection, however, varies among different patient groups. Johanson and coworkers determined that the risk of nosocomial pneumonia in 213 patients admitted to medical ICUs was approximately 12%, including 24% of patients with acute respiratory failure.[30] Fagon and colleagues[52] documented that the risk of infection increases with the duration of mechanical ventilation. In 567 patients treated with mechanical ventilation, the overall rate of infection was 9%, but the risk was 6.5% after 10 days, 19% after 20 days, and 28% after 30 days of ventilation.[52]

The most comprehensive study, by Rouby and coworkers, evaluated the histologic and bacteriologic aspects of 83 mechanically ventilated, critically ill ICU patients in the immediate postmortem period.[58] Of these patients, 84% developed acute diffuse lung injury with clinical sepsis during hospitalization and 52% demonstrated definite bronchopneumonia on histologic examination. The majority of these pneumonias were severe, confluent bronchopneumonias, and some were associated with abscess formation.

Extensive data that define the risk or frequency of nosocomial pneumonia in specific patient populations (such as those with ARDS) are lacking, but several studies have come from various populations, including medical/surgical, surgical, medical, or respiratory ICU populations. Only a few of these studies, however, have distinguished between pneumonia as a cause of ARDS and pneumonia that arises as a complication of ARDS. In 1975, Fulton and Jones observed that 45% of their patients had primary pneumonia and 50% had nosocomial pneumonias.[59] In the study by Seidenfeld and associates, 21% of the patients had pneumonia that initiated ARDS and 53% had pneumonia as a complication during their hospital course.[6] Pneumonia was the cause in 33% and a complication in 34% of 583 patients with ARDS enrolled in the European collaborative study.[60]

However, estimates of the frequency of lower respiratory tract infection in patients with ARDS are questionable because of inadequacy of current diagnostic techniques. The usual clinical criteria for diagnosis of nosocomial pneumonia include fever, leukocytosis, and purulent tracheobronchial secretions, and a new or changing infiltrate on chest x-ray. However, each of these criteria is commonly encountered whether or not bacterial infection is present in patients with ARDS.

This problem is further complicated by the fact that nearly all patients with ARDS are colonized with gram-negative bacilli with a reservoir of secretions pooled above the endotracheal tube. Secretions in the lower airway may originate from aspiration of tracheal secretions or from tracheobronchitis or a pneumonia. The presence of purulent secretions, even at bronchoscopy, is neither sensitive nor specific for pneumonia.[61]

When Andrews and associates examined the accuracy of these criteria in an overall assessment in the diagnosis of nosocomial pneumonia among 30 patients who died with acute respiratory failure, the presence or the absence of bacterial pneumonia was misdiagnosed in 30% of the cases.[62] Pneumonias in the study were definitively diagnosed for purposes of comparison at autopsy by examining multiple sections of the lungs of patients who died with acute respiratory failure. The diagnosis of histologic pneumonias was diagnosed by the presence of an intense PMN inflammatory exudate that centers on terminal or respiratory bronchioles and extends into subjacent and surrounding alveoli. Of the 58% of patients with histologically diagnosed pneumonia, one third were judged clinically not to have pneumonia. Of the 42% without histologically proven pneumonia, one fifth were judged to have clinical evidence of pneumonia. Chastre and coworkers[63] also found that nosocomial pneumonias are underdiagnosed clinically when compared with histologic findings at autopsy.

Other investigators have since offered criteria to allow a definite diagnosis of pneumonia to be made clinically.[41] Salata and coworkers confirm a nosocomial pneumonia diagnosis when a new or progressive pulmonary infiltrate develops with (1) positive pleural fluid or blood cultures for the same organism as in a tracheal aspirate, (2) radiographic cavitation, (3) histopathologic demonstration of pneumonia or necrosis, or (4) new fever, leukocytosis, and purulent tracheal aspirate.[64] While a new or progressive pulmonary density, fever, leukocytosis, and purulent secretions invariably indicate pneumonia in a previously healthy individual, they lack specificity (31% to 40%) in the setting of mechanical ventilation and ARDS.[65] Alternative causes of pulmonary densities include progressive ARDS or cardiogenic pulmonary edema, aspiration of blood or gastric contents, infarction or hemorrhage, neoplastic infiltration, fibroproliferation seen with ARDS, pleural fluid, and volume loss (i.e., atelectasis).

Meduri and coauthors undertook a prospective study to identify the relative frequency of conditions causing fever and pulmonary densities in 50 patients receiving mechanical ventilation with clinical features of pneumonia.[66] A comprehensive protocol was initiated to diagnose infections and noninfectious inflammatory processes, thromboembolic disease, atelectasis, congestive heart failure, pulmonary fibroproliferation, and drug fever. Fever originated from an infection in 37 of 45 patients; however, infectious were less common in patients with ARDS. In patients with ARDS, 11 of 20 were confirmed to have infection. Pneumonia (in five) and catheter-related infection (in four) were most common, whereas sinusitis and urinary tract infection were seen less often (in two each). Noninfectious causes of fever included pulmonary fibroproliferation, pancreatitis, and venous thrombosis. Even in the setting of clinical pneumonia with bacteremia, several studies have found extrapulmonary sources of the bacteremia in 57% to 64% of patients receiving mechanical ventilation.[67, 68]

Because of the lack of sensitivity and specificity in a pneumonia diagnosis, invasive procedures have been developed to collect secretions directly from the involved lower respiratory tract while minimizing contamination from bacteria colonizing the airways. The original work by Higuchi and Johanson[28] and Chastre and colleagues,[54] correlating protected specimen brush (PSB) with lung histology and tissue culture, has promoted the growth of clinical investigation in the field. Among bronchoscopic techniques, the PSB is the modality that has been used by most clinical investigators.

Using 10^3 CFU/mL as a breakpoint to define a positive PSB culture has proved useful in animal and human studies.[53, 67, 69] The PSB, which samples as little as 0.001 mL of lung secretions, is diluted in 1 mL of holding medium for processing, and a growth of 10^3 CFU/mL represents 10^5 to 10^6 bacteria per milliliter. When properly used, the PSB collects respiratory secretions with a minimum degree of contamination. The area to be sampled is sometimes problematic, but most clinicians sample areas of new infiltrate on radiograph, areas with subsegmental purulence, or dependent areas. Autopsy studies have shown that nosocomial pneumonia predominantly involves the posterior portions of the lower lobes but that the pneumonias are frequently disseminated into each lobe.[53, 70] Clinical studies supporting this observation have varied, however; several have reported sterility of different sample sites in lungs,[71, 72] whereas others have shown close correlation between culture samples when obtained from different lobes.[73, 74]

Quantitative cultures of the PSB have an overall sensitivity between 64% to 100% (mean, 82%) and specificity from 69% to 100% (mean, 92%). Quantitative cultures, however, show a significant quantitative discordance in as many as 17% of patients.[65] Dreyfuss and associates reexamined the significance of borderline growth (at least 10^2 but less than 10^3 CFU/mL) in patients with ventilator-associated pneumonia.[75] A second PSB showed significant organisms (at least 10^3 CFU/mL) in 35% of patients. Therefore, the consensus conference on standardization of bronchoscopic techniques in diagnosis of pneumonia recommended cultures within 1 $\log_{10}$ of the cutoff values should be interpreted with caution (Table 65–3).[61]

Bronchoalveolar lavage (BAL) is the sequential instillation and aspiration of a physiologic solution into a subsegment of the lung. BAL samples a larger portion of the lung parenchyma than PSB and is estimated to recover five to 10 times the number of organisms obtained by PSB. The initial infusion of 20 mL is discarded to reduce contamination; however, some studies show upper airway contamination in up to 30% of patients.[76] Sensitivity and specificity of quantitative BAL in diagnosis of nosocomial pneumonia has ranged from 72% to

TABLE 65–3. Bronchoscopic Techniques in the Diagnosis of Pneumonia

High-risk patients
Respiratory: $Pao_2 < 70$ mm Hg on $FIO_2 > 70\%$; PEEP ≥ 15 cm H_2O; bronchospasm
Cardiac: recent myocardial infarction (≤ 48 hr), unstable angina; mean blood pressure < 75 mm Hg on vasopressors
Hematologic: platelet count < 20,000 mm^3;* PT or PTT 1.5 × control
Ventilator settings
FIO_2 at 100%; respiratory rate: 15–20/min; peak inspiratory flow $\leq$ 60 L/min
Set alarms to allow adequate ventilation
Designate thresholds of pneumonia
PSB $\geq 10^3$ CFUs/mL
BAL $\geq 10^4$ CFUs/mL
ICOs > 2%
Borderline values = within 1 $\log_{10}$ of threshold for PSB or BAL

*Risk of bleeding with PSB.
ICOs = intracellular organisms; PT = prothrombin time; PTT = partial thromboplastin time; PSB = protected specimen brush; BAL = bronchoalveolar lavage; CFUs = colony-forming units; PEEP = positive end-expiratory pressure.

100% and from 69% to 100%, respectively.[61] A recent modification of the catheter with a distal sterile plug has allowed for lower rates of contamination.

Two groups of investigators have studied the efficacy of protected bronchoalveolar lavage (PBAL). PBAL sensitivity and specificity were 82% to 85% and 83% to 86%, respectively.[77, 78] Recovery of larger quantities of secretions allows for microscopic analysis of the specimen before the quantitative cultures are available. Patients with ventilator-associated pneumonia show an increase in the total neutrophil count, with a mean percentage ranging from 77% to 82%, and elastin fibers have been identified in about 50% of the patients. These findings are nondiagnostic, since similar findings have been noted in noninfectious inflammatory processes, like ARDS. Identification of intracellular organisms in more than 2% of phagocytic cells is considered specific for pneumonia (95% to 100%) and has a reported sensitivity above 75%.[61]

The influence of antibiotic therapy on PSB and BAL is considerable, and efforts to obtain bronchoscopic specimens before initiation of antibiotic therapy are strongly recommended. The culture results of PSB and BAL in patients receiving antibiotic therapy can be difficult to interpret either by precluding the recovery of organisms at a significant concentration in respiratory secretions or by causing results to be falsely positive.[79, 80] False-positive cultures are believed to occur because antibiotics predispose to colonization of the upper airway associated with aspiration of secretions containing high bacterial loads. Antibiotics have been associated with a false-positive culture rate of 41% to 60% for PSB and 35% for BAL.[79, 80] Specimens obtained within 12 hours of starting antibiotics are still useful in identifying a causative pathogen (sensitivity, 70%); however, it is preferable to obtain specimens for culture prior to antibiotic administration or 48 hours after discontinuing antibiotics.[61]

Despite the extensive literature regarding the invasive techniques for diagnosis of nosocomial pneumonia in patients, bronchoscopic evaluation (PSB or BAL) should not be considered the standard of care in evaluating patients with ARDS. These procedures are invasive and expensive and have never been studied in a randomized, prospective fashion. There are no data showing a reduction in mortality or a reduction in the time on mechanical ventilation or in the ICU when such protocols are applied to patients with ventilator-associated pneumonia. Two recent studies have given encouraging results in utilizing quantitative cultures of the endotracheal aspirate in evaluation of pneumonia in mechanically ventilated patients.[81, 82] Using a diagnostic threshold of 10^5 CFU/mL, sensitivity and specificity approaching PSB and BAL may be achieved. Further studies will be necessary to establish if this technique is clinically useful.

OUTCOMES AND CONCLUSIONS

The outcome of patients with ARDS and nosocomial pneumonia has been reported to be extremely poor. The mortality rate of nosocomial pneumonia alone has been reported to be between 55% and 75% in mechanically ventilated patients.[16, 39, 83, 84] In ARDS study populations, the presence of infection of any source has been associated with a poor outcome and with multiple organ failure. Seidenfeld and colleagues demonstrated a survival rate of 67% in patients with no infection versus 21% when infection of any type was present; the mortality rate was 88% when pneumonia complicated ARDS in this study series.[6] In the ARDS patient population of Montgomery and coworkers, pulmonary sources of infection predominated when ARDS developed, followed by sepsis. Of late sepsis, 75% of cases were secondary to pneumonia and were considered to be the direct or contributing cause of death in 54% of these patients.[7]

Investigators have found that the mortality of nosocomial pneumonias of various causes differs. For example, Fagon and coworkers showed that the mortality of *Pseudomonas* and of *Acinetobacter* and *S. aureus* was greater than that of other types of gram-negative pneumonias.[52] Prior antiobotic therapy was more common in patients who developed *P. aeruginosa* and *Acinetobacter* species than other gram-negative pneumonias.[52] Celis and coworkers showed a higher mortality rate in a group of patients with gram-negative pneumonias due to high-risk causes than in patients with gram-negative pneumonias attributed to other causes.[39]

In general, regimens that provide coverage for enteric gram-negative bacilli (i.e., *P. aeruginosa, Klebsiella* species, and *E. coli*) and against *S. aureus* should be selected for patients with ARDS and pneumonia, and vancomycin is administered if the potential pathogen is methicillin-resistant. The European experience of selective digestive decontamination has successfully reduced the incidence of pneumonia, but the mortality rates due to multiple organ failure have not been altered. In baboon models of ARDS, Johanson and colleagues prevented pneumonia with the use of topical respiratory antibiotics.[53] The use of intravenous penicillin, along with topical polymyxin B, gentamicin, or both, reduced the severity of histologic pneumonia and the bacterial loads (characterized by a bacterial index). Concern remains, however, that the use of these approaches on a widespread basis might cause emergence of antibiotic-resistant strains in the ICU environment.

A recent prospective study attempted to determine the incidence of pulmonary infection in patients with ARDS and the impact of nosocomial pneumonia on survival.[85] Patients underwent serial bronchoscopy and quantitative BAL and PSB between day 3 to day 21 after the onset of ARDS. Pneumonia was confirmed in only 16% of patients, and the mortality rate of 43% was lower than previous reports by this same group. Interpretation of this data is difficult because almost all patients were receiving broad-spectrum antibiotics and bronchoscopy was not performed for a clinical suspicion of pneumonia. Over the past few years, several reports have documented a significant and long-awaited improvement in ARDS.[86] Because most of these studies use historic controls, the studies should be interpreted with caution. Many authors propose a slow, but definite, improvement in survival of patients with ARDS through small but additive effects: (1) pressure control or reverse I/E ratio ventilation, (2) better control of fluid balance, (3) use of corticosteroids in the late phases of the syndrome, and (4) earlier diagnosis and better antibiotic therapy for nosocomial pneumonia.

Prophylactic antibiotics are not recommended, since administering antibiotics to patients without infection may lead to antibiotic-resistant bacteria that have been associated with a higher mortality.[87, 88] Although it has never been studied specifically in ARDS, some experts recommend a trial of early empirical antibiotic therapy in the early phase of the disease when sepsis is presumed to be the cause.[89] When clinical manifestations of pneumonia develop in patients with ARDS, the physician must understand the complexity of this clinical presentation and should proceed with a diagnostic evaluation to rule out pneumonia and other potential causes of fever and pulmonary densities. The use of invasive procedures should be based on the risk of the procedure in a specific patient; the potential utility of the data obtained (i.e., significantly less useful in patients on antibiotics); and the physiologic response of the patient to the inflammatory insult (i.e., progressive hypoxemia, sepsis syndrome). Once specimens are obtained for culture, empirical antibiotics should be administered in unstable patients or patients with minimal pulmonary reserve.

Bassin and Niederman have presented an excellent review on strategies for the prevention of pneumonia.[90] Future studies must address means to reduce bacterial adherence of gram-negative bacilli to airway cells. Development of antibodies against gram-negative bacteria would be helpful to use in patients with pneumonia. An important advance that would make a major impact on the emergence of the sepsis syndrome would be a means to enhance the integrity and intactness of the intestinal mucosa to prevent translocation of bacteria or bacterial products from the intestine. Early augmentation of host defenses and subsequent use of immunomodulators may be necessary to prevent systemic infection from leading to multiple organ failure. Because of the complexity of the various clinical situations that can predispose patients to the development of nosocomial pneumonia, a multipronged approach undoubtedly must be created for successful treatment of ARDS in the ICU setting.

References

1. Bernard GR, Artigas A, Brigham KL, et al: The American-European Consensus Conference on ARDS: Definitions, mechanisms, relevant outcomes, and clinical trial coordination. Am J Respir Crit Care Med 1994; 149:818.
2. Katzenstein AA, Askin FB: Surgical pathology of non-neoplastic lung disease. *In:* Major Problems in Pathology. 2nd ed. Bennington JL (Ed). Vol 13. Philadelphia, WB Saunders, 1990, pp 9–57.
3. Tomashefski JF: Pulmonary pathology of the adult respiratory distress syndrome. Clin Chest Med 1990; 11:593.
4. Coalson JJ: Pathology of sepsis, septic shock and multiple organ failure. *In:* Sibbald WJ, Sprung CL (Eds). New Horizons: Perspectives on Sepsis and Septic Shock. Fullerton, Calif, Society of Critical Care Medicine, 1986, pp 27–59.
5. Bell RC, Coalson JJ, Smith JD, et al: Multiple organ failure and infection in adult respiratory distress syndrome. Ann Intern Med 1983; 99:293.
6. Seidenfeld JJ, Pohl DF, Bell RC, et al: Incidence, site, and outcome of infections in patients with the adult respiratory distress syndrome. Am Rev Respir Dis 1986; 134:12.
7. Montgomery AB, Stager MA, Carrico C, et al: Causes of mortality in patients with the adult respiratory distress syndrome. Am Rev Respir Dis 1985; 132:485.
8. Suchyta MR, Clemmer TP, Elliott CC, et al: The adult respiratory distress syndrome: A report of survival and modifying factors. Chest 1992; 101:1074.
9. Extracorporeal support for respiratory insufficiency: Collaborative study (December 1979). Washington, DC, National Heart, Lung, and Blood Institute, U.S. Department of Health, Education, and Welfare, Public Health Division, 1979.
10. Baumann WR, Jung RC, Koss M, et al: Incidence and mortality of adult respiratory distress syndrome: A prospective analysis from a large metropolitan hospital. Crit Care Med 1986; 14:1.
11. Fowler AA, Hamman RF, Good JT, et al: Adult respiratory distress syndrome: Risk with common predispositions. Ann Intern Med 1983; 98:593.
12. Walker L, Eiseman B: The changing pattern of post-traumatic respiratory distress syndrome. Ann Surg 1975; 181:693.
13. Bone RC, Balk RA, Cerra FB, et al: American College of Chest Physicians/Society of Critical Care Medicine Consensus Conference: Definitions for sepsis and multiple-organ failure and guidelines for the use of innovative therapies in sepsis. Chest 1992; 101:1644.
14. Bone RC: Toward an epidemiology and natural history of SIRS (systemic inflammatory response syndrome). JAMA 1992; 268:3452.
15. Deitch EA: The role of intestinal barrier failure and bacterial translocation in the development of systemic infection and multiple organ failure. Arch Surg 1990; 125:403.
16. Craven DE, Kunches LM, Kilinsky V, et al: Risk factors for pneumonia and fatality in patients receiving continuous mechanical ventilation. Am Rev Respir Dis 1986; 133:792.
17. Sessler CN, Bloomfield GL, Fowler AA III: Current concepts of sepsis and acute lung injury. Clin Chest Med 1996; 17:213.
18. Nelson S, Mason CM, Kolls J, et al: Pathophysiology of pneumonia. Clin Chest Med 1995; 16:1.
19. Nelson S, Bagby GJ, Summer W: Anti-tumor necrosis factor-alpha antibody suppresses pulmonary antibacterial defenses. Am Rev Respir Dis 1991; 143S:393.
20. Ulich TR, Yin S, Guo K, et al: The intratracheal administration of endotoxin and cytokines: The interleukin-1 (IL-1) receptor antagonist inhibits endotoxin- and IL-1–induced acute inflammation. Am J Pathol 1991; 138:521.
21. Simpson SQ, Modi HN, Balk RA, et al: Reduced alveolar macrophage production of tumor necrosis factor during sepsis in mice and men. Crit Care Med 1991; 19:1060.
22. Jaffe HA, Buhl R, Mastrangeli A, et al: Organ specific cytokine therapy. J Clin Invest 1991; 88:2.
23. Yasuda H, Ajiki Y, Shimozato T, et al: Therapeutic efficacy of granulocyte colony-stimulating factor alone and in combination with antibiotics against *Pseudomonas aeruginosa* infections in mice. Infect Immun 1990; 58:2502.
24. Kanazawa M, Ishizaka A, Hasegawa N, et al: Granulocyte colony-stimulating factor does not enhance endotoxin-induced acute lung injury in guinea pigs. Am Rev Respir Dis 1992; 145:1030.
25. Koizumi T, Kubo KJ, Shinozaki S, et al: Granulocyte colony-stimulating factor does not exacerbate endotoxin-induced lung injury in sheep. Am Rev Respir Dis 1993; 148:132.
26. Johanson WG, Pierce AK, Sanford TP: Changing pharyngeal flora of hospitalized patients: Emergence of gram-negative bacilli. N Engl J Med 1969; 281:1137.
27. LaForce FM: Effects of alveolar lining material on phagocytic and bacterial activity of lung macrophages against *Staphylococcus aureus.* J Lab Clin Med 1976; 88:691.
28. Higuchi JH, Johanson WG: The relationship between adherence of *Pseudomonas aeruginosa* to upper respiratory cells in vitro and susceptibility to colonization in vivo. J Lab Clin Med 1980; 95:698.
29. Palmer LB: Bacterial colonization: Pathogenesis and clinical significance. Clin Chest Med 1987; 8:455.
30. Johanson WG Jr, Pierce AK, Sanford JP, et al: Nosocomial respiratory infections with gram-negative bacilli: The significance of colonization of the respiratory tract. Ann Intern Med 1972; 77:701.
31. Tillotson JR, Finland M: Bacterial colonization and clinical superinfection of the respiratory tract complicating antibiotic treatment of pneumonia. J Infect Dis 1969; 119:597.
32. Schwartz DB, Olson DE, Kauffman CA: Influence of aspiration on tracheal colonization following endotracheal intubation. Am Rev Respir Dis 1984; 129:A182.
33. Woods DE, Straus DC, Johanson WG, et al: Role of salivary protease activity in adherence of gram-negative bacilli to mammalian buccal epithelial cells in vivo. J Clin Invest 1981; 68:1435.
34. Mason CM, Summer WR, Dal Nogare AR: Lectin binding characteristics of buccal and tracheal epithelium in rats with gram-negative bacillary colonization. Am Rev Respir Dis 1991; 143:A291.
35. Niederman MS, Ferranti RD, Ziegler A, et al: Respiratory infection complicating long-term tracheostomy: The implication of persistent gram-negative tracheobronchial colonization. Chest 1984; 85:39.
36. Johanson WG Jr: Bacterial infection in ARDS: Pathogenetic mechanisms and consequences. In: Textbook of Critical Care. 2nd ed. Shoemaker WC, Ayres S, Grenvik A (Eds): Philadelphia, WB Saunders, 1989, pp 845–853.
37. Berendt RF: Relationship of method of administration to respiratory virulence of *Klebsiella pneumoniae* for mice and squirrel monkeys. Infect Immun 1978; 20:581.
38. Huxley EJ, Viroslav J, Gray WR, et al: Pharyngeal aspiration in normal subjects and patients with depressed consciousness. Am J Med 1978; 64:564.
39. Celis R, Torres A, Gatell J, et al: Nosocomial pneumonia: A multivariable analysis of risk and prognosis. Chest 1988; 93:318.
40. Atherton ST, White DJ: Stomach as source of bacteria colonizing respiratory tract during artificial ventilation. Lancet 1978; 2:968.
41. Pingleton SK, Fagon JV, Leeper KV: Patient selection for clinical investigation of ventilator-associated pneumonia: Criteria for evaluating diagnostic techniques. Chest 1992; 102(Suppl 1):553S.
42. Onofrio JM, Toews GB, Lipscomb MF, et al: Granulocyte-alveolar macrophage interaction in the pulmonary clearance of *Staphylococcus aureus.* Am Rev Respir Dis 1983; 127:335.

43. Johanson WG Jr, Higuchi JH, Woods DE, et al: Dissemination of *Pseudomonas aeruginosa* during lung infection: Role of oxygen-induced lung injury. Am Rev Respir Dis 1985; 132:358.
44. Campbell DG, Coalson JJ, Johanson WG Jr: The effect of bacterial superinfection on lung function after diffuse alveolar damage. Am Rev Respir Dis 1984; 129:974.
45. Coalson JJ, King RJ, Winter VT, et al: Oxygen and pneumonia-induced lung injury: I. Pathological and morphometric studies. J Appl Physiol 1989; 67:346.
46. Schutte H, Lohmeyer J, Rosseau S, Ziegler S, Siebert C, Kielisch H, Pralle H, Grimminger F, Morr H, Seeger W: Bronchoalveolar and systemic cytokine profiles in patients with ARDS, severe pneumonia and cardiogenic pulmonary edema. Eur Respir J 1996, 9:1858.
47. Goodman RB, Strieter RM, Martin DP, et al: Inflammatory cytokines in patients with persistence of the acute respiratory distress syndrome. Am J Respir Crit Care Med 1996; 154:602.
48. Juers J, Rogers RM, McCurdy JB: Enhancement of bactericidal capacity of alveolar macrophages by human "alveolar lining material." Clin Res 1975; 23:348.
49. Huber GL, LaForce FM, Johanson WG Jr: Experimental models in pulmonary antimicrobial defenses. *In:* Respiratory Defense Mechanisms. Brain JD, Proctor DF, Reid L (Eds): New York, Marcel Dekker, 1977, pp 983–1022.
50. Pierce AK, Reynolds RC, Harris GD: Leukocytic response to inhaled bacteria. Am Rev Respir Dis 1977; 116:679.
51. Rehm SR, Gross GN, Pierce AK: Early bacterial clearance from murine lungs. Species-dependent phagocyte response. J Clin Invest 1980; 66:194.
52. Fagon JY, Chastre J, Domart Y, et al: Nosocomial pneumonia in patients receiving continuous mechanical ventilation: Prospective analysis of 52 episodes with use of a protected specimen brush and quantitative culture techniques. Am Rev Respir Dis 1989; 139:877.
53. Johanson WG Jr, Seidenfeld JJ, Gomez P, et al: Bacteriologic diagnosis of nosocomial pneumonia following prolonged mechanical ventilation. Am Rev Respir Dis 1988; 137:259.
54. Chastre J, Viau F, Brun P, et al: Prospective evaluation of the protected specimen brush for the diagnosis of pulmonary infections in ventilated patients. Am Rev Respir Dis 1984; 130:924.
55. Bartlett JG: Invasive diagnostic techniques in pulmonary infections. *In:* Respiratory Infections: Diagnosis and Management. 2nd ed. Pennington JE (Ed): New York, Raven Press, 1989, pp 52–68.
56. Marquette CH, Copin MC, Wallet F, et al: Diagnostic tests for pneumonia in ventilated patients: Prospective evaluation of diagnostic accuracy using histology as a diagnostic gold standard. Am J Respir Crit Care Med 1995; 151:1878.
57. Centers for Disease Control: National nosocomial infections study report: Annual summary, 1984. MMWR 1986; 35:17S.
58. Rouby J, de Lassale EM, Poette P, et al: Nosocomial bronchopneumonia in the critically ill: Histology and bacteriologic aspects. Am Rev Respir Dis 1992; 146:1059.
59. Fulton RL, Jones CE: The cause of post-traumatic respiratory insufficiency in man. Surg Gynecol Obstet 1975; 140:179.
60. Carlet J, Hemmer M, Flandre P, et al: Infection and ARDS: A complex interaction: A prospective study of 583 patients. Am Rev Respir Dis 1989; 139:A270.
61. Meduri GU, Chastre J: The standardization of bronchoscopic techniques for ventilator-associated pneumonia. Chest 1992; 102:557S.
62. Andrews CP, Coalson JJ, Smith JD, et al: Diagnosis of nosocomial bacterial pneumonia in acute, diffuse lung injury. Chest 1981; 80:254.
63. Chastre J, Fagon JT, Soler P, et al: Diagnosis of nosocomial bacterial pneumonia in intubated patients undergoing ventilation: Comparison of the usefulness of bronchoalveolar lavage and the protected specimen brush. Am J Med 1988; 85:499.
64. Salata RA, Lederman MM, Shales DM, et al: Diagnosis of nosocomial pneumonia in intubated, intensive care unit patients. Am Rev Respir Dis 1987; 135:426.
65. Meduri GU: Diagnosis and differential diagnosis of ventilator-associated pneumonia. Clin Chest Med 1995; 16:61.
66. Meduri GU, Mauldin GL, Wunderink RG, et al: Causes of fever and pulmonary densities in patients with clinical manifestations of ventilator-associated pneumonia. Chest 1994; 106:221.
67. Fagon JY, Chastre J, Hance AJ, et al: Detection of nosocomial lung infection in ventilated patients: Use of a protected specimen brush and quantitative culture techniques in 147 patients. Am Rev Respir Dis 1988; 138:110.
68. Bryan CS, Reynolds KL: Bacteremic nosocomial pneumonia: Analysis of 172 episodes from a single metropolitan area. Am Rev Respir Dis 1984; 128:668.
69. Meduri GU, Beals D, Maijub G, et al: Protected bronchoalveolar lavage: A new bronchoscopic technique to retrieve uncontaminated distal airway secretions. Am Rev Respir Dis 1991; 143:855.
70. Dever LL, Johanson WG Jr: Pneumonia complicating adult respiratory distress syndrome. Clin Chest Med 1995; 16:147.
71. Baughman RP, Thorpe JE, Staneck J, et al: Use of the protected specimen brush in patients with endotracheal or tracheostomy tubes. Chest 1987; 91:233.
72. Belenchia JM, Wunderink RG, Meduri GU, et al: Alternative causes of fever in ARDS patients suspected of having pneumonia. Am Rev Respir Dis 1991; 143:A683.
73. Pham LH, Brun-Buisson C, Legrand P, et al: Diagnosis of nosocomial pneumonia in mechanically ventilated patients: Comparison of a plugged telescoping catheter with the protected specimen brush. Am Rev Respir Dis 1991; 143:1055.
74. Pugin J, Auckenthaler R, Mili N, et al: Diagnosis of ventilator-associated pneumonia by bacteriologic analysis of bronchoscopic and nonbronchoscopic blind bronchoalveolar lavage fluid. Am Rev Respir Dis 1991; 143:1121.
75. Dreyfuss D, Mier L, Le Bourdelles G, et al: Clinical significance of borderline quantitative protected brush specimen culture results. Am Rev Respir Dis 1993; 147:946.
76. Torres A, de la Bellacasa JP, Xaubet A, et al: Diagnostic value of quantitative cultures of broncho-alveolar lavage and telescoping plugged catheters in mechanically ventilated patients with bacterial pneumonia. Am Rev Respir Dis 1989; 140:306.
77. Barreiro B, Dorca J, Catala I: Protected bronchoalveolar lavage with balloon-tipped catheter in the diagnosis of ventilator-associated pneumonia. Am Rev Respir Dis 1993; 147:A39.
78. Castella J, Puzo C, Ausina V, et al: Diagnosis of pneumonia with a method of protected bronchoalveolar lavage. Eur Respir J 1991; 4:407S.
79. Marquette CH, Herengt F, Saulnier F, et al: Protected specimen brush in the assessment of ventilator-associated pneumonia: Selection of a certain lung segment for bronchoscopic sampling is unnecessary. Chest 1993; 103:243.
80. Torres A, Martos A, de la Bellacasa JP, et al: Specificity of endotracheal aspiration, protected specimen brush, and bronchoalveolar lavage in mechanically ventilated patients. Am Rev Respir Dis 1993; 147:952.
81. El-Ebiary M, Torres A, Gonzalez J, Puig de la Bellacasa J, Garcia C, Jimenez de Anta M, Ferrer M, Rodriquez-Roisin R: Quantitative cultures of endotracheal aspirates for the diagnosis of ventilator-associated pneumonia. Am Rev Respir Dis 1993; 148:1552.
82. Marquette CH, Copin M-C, Wallet F, et al: Diagnostic tests for pneumonia in ventilated patients: Prospective evaluation of diagnostic accuracy using histology as a diagnostic gold standard. Am J Respir Crit Care Med 1995; 151:1878.
83. DuMoulin GC, Hedley-Whyte J, Paterson DG, et al: Aspiration of gastric bacteria in antacid-treated patients: A frequent cause of postoperative colonization of the airway. Lancet 1982; 1:242.
84. Stevens RM, Teres D, Skillman JJ, et al: Pneumonia in an intensive care unit: A thirty-month experience. Arch Intern Med 1974; 134:106.
85. Sutherland KR, Steinberg KP, Maunder RJ, et al: Pulmonary infection during the acute respiratory distress syndrome. Am J Respir Crit Care Med 1995; 152:550.
86. Lemaire F: The prognosis of ARDS: Appropriate optimism? Intensive Care Med 1996; 22:371.
87. Kollef MH: Ventilator-associated pneumonias: A multivariate analysis. JAMA 1993; 270:1965.
88. Leeper KV Jr: Diagnosis and treatment of pulmonary infections in adult respiratory distress syndrome. New Horiz 1993; 1:550.
89. Kollef MH, Schuster DP: The acute respiratory distress syndrome. N Engl J Med 1995; 332:27.
90. Bassin AS, Niederman MS: Prevention of ventilator-associated pneumonia. Clin Chest Med 1995; 16:195.

66

Intra-abdominal Sepsis

John M. Kellum, MD, FACS

Postoperative or post-traumatic infection has supplanted hemorrhage as the leading cause of death on general surgical and trauma services. The average cost of a postoperative infection in 1992 was about $28,000, whereas that of an average intensive care unit (ICU) stay for infection complicated by organ system failure was $150,000.[1]

Since the last edition of this textbook, numerous studies of monoclonal antibodies against endotoxin-lipopolysaccharide, leukotrienes, and tumor necrosis factor (TNF) have failed to demonstrate an improvement in the prevention or therapy of intra-abdominal sepsis. Selective decontamination of the digestive tract with oral antibiotics has been studied in Germany. Results show some improvement in pulmonary and urinary tract infections but no improvement in overall survival. Enteral feeding has been superior to parenteral feeding in preventing nosocomial infections in critcally ill patients.[2] More recently, an enteral diet containing constituents, thought to be immune-enhancing, was shown to reduce overall septic complications, hospital stay, and the development of intra-abdominal abscess in victims of severe trauma.[3]

HISTORICAL PERSPECTIVE

19th Century War Surgery

The history of surgical infection is really the history of war surgery. During the American Civil War, a gunshot wound to an extremity was tantamount to an amputation or to death from gas gangrene; a gunshot wound to the abdomen was almost uniformly fatal. Surgeons were not generally prepared to undertake celiotomy under such circumstances. Although Joseph Lister had described his antiseptic technique in the 1860s,[4] it was not widely accepted at military field hospitals of the day and, in fact, remained controversial well into the 1880s.[5]

20th Century War Surgery

In the 1880s, Billroth founded his famous surgical school in Vienna and demonstrated that gastrectomy was feasible using Listerian technique. At the time of World War I, however, the military war wound still had a ghastly rate of fatal infection. On the Western Front alone, it was estimated that 50,000 German soldiers died of gas gangrene.[6]

Prior to World War I, Landsteiner had described the elements of the ABO blood compatibility system.[7] During this war, however, surgeons had poor supplies of blood for transfusion and were ignorant of the volumes of blood needed to combat hemorrhagic shock. Blalock,[8] working at the Vanderbilt School of Medicine's surgical research laboratories in the 1930s, did pioneering work in the understanding of shock and blood replacement. Thus, by World War II a much improved management of hemorrhagic problems prevailed; yet the prevention and treatment of sepsis remained relatively primitive.

Sulfa antibiotics and penicillin had been discovered before the beginning of World War II, but their limited availability caused them to be of marginal benefit to the overall military medical effort. When penicillin became available in May 1944, a reduction in case fatality rates for abdominal wounds and in the incidence of postoperative bacterial peritonitis was observed with its use, in contrast to previous treatment of soldiers with sulfonamides alone.[9] During World War II, however, important policies were established with regard to the treatment of war wounds. Standardized methods of wide debridement of soft tissue wounds were developed, and those had a more profound effect on the reduction of cases of gas gangrene than did the availability of penicillin. Just as important was the directive by the Surgeon General in 1943, mandating that all colonic injuries be handled by colostomy[10]; this policy is credited with greatly reducing the death rate from intra-abdominal sepsis following this injury.

During the Korean and Vietnam conflicts, great improvements were made in expediting the evacuation of the wounded from the battlefield into appropriate field hospitals with well-trained surgeons, nurses, and corpsmen.[11] The importance of massive intravenous therapy with crystalloid early in the resuscitative effort to avoid acute renal failure was first appreciated during the Korean conflict.[1] As antibiotics were widely used for the first time to prevent infection, a change in the character of wound pathogens became apparent. Instead of β-hemolytic *Streptococcus* and *Clostridium perfringens,* surgeons encountered the scourge of the early 1950s, *Staphylococcus aureus.*

With the development of semisynthetic antibiotics with good staphylococcal coverage, the gram-negative aerobes (e.g., *Escherichia coli, Klebsiella pneumoniae,* and other Enterobacteriaciae) emerged as important pathogens around the time of the Vietnam War, in both military and civilian hospitals. With the progressive development of more powerful antibiotics, the aerobic pathogens gradually changed; the havoc wreaked by *Pseudomonas aeuruginosa* is a good example. On the other hand, the anaerobic pathogens remained the same with *Bacteroides fragilis* (whose virulence had been originally described by Meleney and colleagues[12] in the 1930s), still the important pathogen with regard to intra-abdominal sepsis.

Relationship Between Aerobic and Anaerobic Bacteria

Although many surgeons questioned the pathogenicity of anaerobic organisms, the experimental work of Weinstein and coworkers[13] demonstrated that the presence of *B. fragilis* was necessary to produce an experimental intra-abdominal abscess in rats, which developed about the 7th day after mixed peritoneal contamination. On the other hand, gram-negative aerobes were more important in the early bacteremic, septic phase, which resulted in a 43% mortality in the first 3 days in this model. Thus, it appears that a synergistic relationship exists between aerobic and anaerobic bacterial species of the type usually encountered with mixed bacterial contamination from bowel injury or perforation. Gram-negative aerobes, such as *E. coli,* caused the early septic phase with the elaboration of *endotoxin.* Endotoxin is generally credited for the massive peripheral vasodilatation observed in septic shock with consequent subnormal peripheral vascular resistance and arterial hypotension. To the contrary, obligate anaerobes, like *B. fragilis,* do not elaborate endotoxin but are required for the establishment and maintenance of an intra-abdominal abscess.[13]

Antibiotic Prophylaxis of Colon Surgery

A major landmark in the successful prevention of intra-abdominal sepsis following elective surgery was the randomized, prospective multicenter trial of an oral antibiotic combination in addition to a mechanical bowel preparation versus a mechanical bowel preparation *alone* prior to colon surgery.[14] Carried out at Veterans Administration Hospitals, this study demonstrated a highly significant reduction in the incidence of wound infections ($P < .001$), intra-abdominal abscesses ($P < .02$), and anastomotic leaks ($P < .05$) in the group receiving oral antibiotics. The antibiotics used were neomycin (aerobic microbe coverage) and erythromycin (anaerobic coverage) in three 1-gram doses each.

Theory of Translocation of Bacteria Across the Bowel Wall

In 1985, Deitch and colleagues,[15] extending a theme of prior investigation going back over 100 years, reported that certain stressful clinical circumstances were accompanied by the overgrowth of luminal bacteria in the distal small intestine or colon with actual movement of bacteria or bacterial by-products across the basement membrane with localization in the mesenteric lymph nodes and in the portal circulation in the rat. The circumstances included burns,[15] endotoxemia,[16] hemorrhagic shock,[17] intestinal ischemia,[18] obstructive jaundice,[19] malnutrition,[20] withdrawal of oral diet with substitution of oral total parenteral nutrition,[21] or a low-fiber diet.[22]

This model was proposed as a possible explanation for the persistence of septic signs and the development of multiple organ dysfunction (MOD) in some severely ill patients recovering from severe trauma or peritonitis with no other apparent source of infection. Earlier, Polk and Shields[23] had recommended routine laparotomy for abdominal surgery patients who manifested signs of organ dysfunction with no other apparent source of infection. Norton,[24] however, reported that such laparotomies frequently yielded negative findings and that once sequential, multiple organ system dysfunction was established, draining persistent abdominal collections rarely was associated with survival.

Although the clinical relevance of bacterial translocation as a source of persistent sepsis and organ dysfunction is far from proven, the theory has opened up a renewed interest in the subject of what nutrients or humoral factors are important in the maintenance of gut integrity. From the experimental work of Windmueller,[25] Souba,[26] and Wilmore[27] and their colleagues, there is clinical evidence that both glutamine (either enterally or parenterally administered) and enteral fiber are necessary to prevent the transduction of luminal bacteria in humans. This idea had arisen from the laboratory finding that enterocytes in tissue culture appear to prefer glutamine, oxaloacetic acid, and other ketone bodies to glucose as a nutrient.[25]

DEMOGRAPHICS

As reported by Saini and colleagues[28] 100 consecutive patients with intra-abdominal abscesses were treated at a Boston teaching hospital; 61% of the abscesses resulted from spontaneous intra-abdominal disease, 10% were the result of trauma, and 29% were complications of abdominal surgery. Of the 61 patients with spontaneous intra-abdominal causes, appendicitis occurred in 16 (26%), diverticulitis in 12 (20%), primary liver abscess in seven (11%), perforated colon cancer in six (10%), Crohn's disease, perforated peptic ulcer, and pancreatitis in three each (5%), and miscellaneous causes in 11 (18%). The mean age of patients with intra-abdominal infections was 56 years (range, 12 to 82). There was a slight predominance of males over females (57% versus 43%, respectively).

In patients whose intra-abdominal sepsis is a complication of abdominal surgery, the overwhelming majority have had surgery of the alimentary tract. In the series of Saini and colleagues,[28] for example, 73% of patients with intra-abdominal abscesses had undergone gastrointestinal or biliary surgery; of this group, 73% had colonic operations. Given the normal flora of the gastrointestinal tract (Fig. 66–1), this preponderance of postoperative infections is not surprising. Whereas most infections in "clean" surgical procedures arise from exogenous bacterial contamination, most infections complicating "clean-contaminated" gastrointestinal operations are from endogenous contamination.

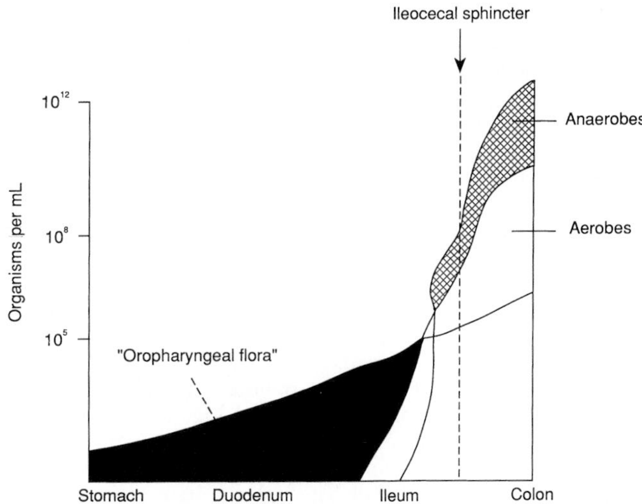

Figure 66–1. The normal bacterial flora of the human alimentary tract. While an exponential rise for both aerobic and anaerobic microorganisms was observed in the distal half on the ileum, the anaerobic exceeded the aerobic density by 10^3 organisms/mL of luminal fluid in the distal colon. (Modified with permission from a drawing by Sherwood A. Gorbach, MD, Division of Infectious Diseases, Tufts New England Medical Center, Boston.)

The distribution of abscesses is shown in Figure 66–2. The subphrenic collection remained the most common intra-abdominal abscess, followed by pelvic localization.[28]

RISK OF SEPSIS AND ANTIBIOTIC PROPHYLAXIS IN SURGICAL PATIENTS

Classification of Surgical Procedures

Both elective and emergency surgery can be stratified into four categories that help predict the likelihood of postoperative infection.

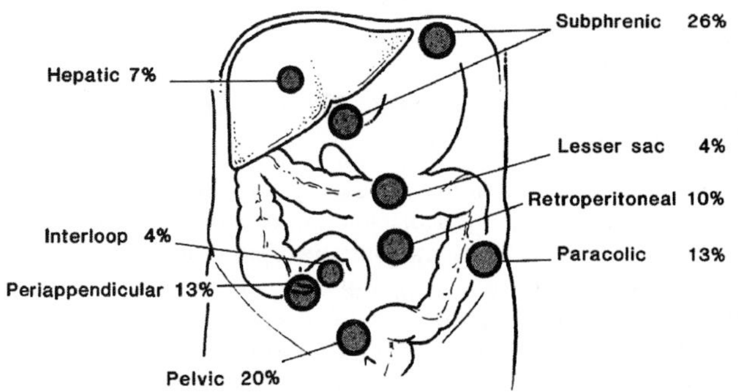

Figure 66–2. Peritoneal location of 130 intra-abdominal abscesses in 100 consecutive patients treated at Tufts New England Medical Center Hospital. From Saini S, Kellum JM, O'Leary MP, et al: Improved localization and survival in patients with intra-abdominal abscesses. Am J Surg 1983; 145:136–142.

1. *Clean.* An incision is made through antiseptically prepared integument but does not cross mucous membranes. These procedures are associated with a wound infection rate of less than 2%.[29] Inguinal hernia repair is a common example.

2. *Clean-contaminated.* A mucous membrane is crossed in a manner whereby contamination is controlled. Most elective alimentary tract operations fall under this category, including cholecystectomy, pancreatectomy, hepatectomy, and intestinal procedures. Figure 66–2 demonstrates the wide variation in the intestinal flora under normal, nondiseased conditions between the various regions of the gastrointestinal tract.[30] Because of the large variation in potential inocula, there is a wide range of predicted infection rates (5% to 15%), depending on whether the surgeon is opening the pylorus or the colon.

3. *Contaminated.* Penetrating trauma of the abdomen may cause contamination not only by crossing a mucous membrane in an uncontrolled fashion but also by passing through unprepared integument and causing devascularization of soft tissue of the abdominal wall. The infection rate averages 20%.

4. *Dirty.* This category includes massive contamination or the crossing of prepared integument when the surgeon must operate on a grossly infected process, such as a large diverticular abscess or osteomyelitis. If skin is closed in these cases, the infection rate exceeds 35%.

An appreciation of these principles allows the surgeon to prepare patients and to conduct operations in such a way as to lower the infection rates. The principles of prophylactic antibiotics are as follows:

1. The risk of infection of an operation should exceed the risk of side effects of antibiotics (~ 5%) except when one is placing vascular prosthetic grafts, for example, in which the implications of an infection are life-threatening.

2. Antibiotics must be given prior to the expected time of contamination so that antibiotic tissue levels in the wound and peritoneum are maximum at the time of contamination.

3. Antibiotic therapy should be tailored to cover the anticipated pathogens contaminating the wound or peritoneum.

4. A narrow-spectrum antibiotic should be chosen, if possible, to prevent the emergence of resistant strains which may lead to the development of nosocomial infections in the hospital environment. For example, a first- generation cephalosporin is usually preferable to a second- or third-generation cephalosporin in elective gallbladder surgery, since it can be expected to provide coverage against common bile pathogens and both streptococci and staphylococci. A first-generation drug is also significantly less expensive.

5. When the entrance in the distal half of the ileum or the colon must be surgically entered, oral antibiotics effective against both aerobic and anaerobic organisms should be employed with a brief preoperative course to reduce the inoculum of contamination.

Selective Decontamination of the Digestive Tract

The selective decontamination theory is based on the susceptibility of critically ill surgical patients to bacterial colonization of the gastrointestinal tract, aspiration pneumonia, and hospital-acquired infections.[31, 32] Stoutenbeek[33] and Hartenauer[34] and their colleagues have studied the theory of suppression of gut flora to prevent nosocomial infection and persistent sepsis from translocation of bacteria. Hartenauer's group used a combination of oral polymyxin E, tobramycin, and amphotericin B in ICU patients at risk for nosocomial infections and multiple organ dysfunction. In a prospective, consecutive crossover controlled study, they found a significantly lower rate of nosocomial bronchopulmonary and urinary tract infections in the antibiotic group than in the placebo group; however, there was no reduction in mortality between the two treatment groups. While still attracting interest in selected centers, this technique has not become widely accepted in the United States.

BIOCHEMISTRY

Endotoxin

Many of the gram-negative aerobic organisms, such as *E. coli*, liberate endotoxin, which is rapidly absorbed through the peritoneum into the circulation. Later, after the formation of an abscess, these same organisms can elaborate endotoxin, which is absorbed into the venous drainage of the abscess wall. In either case, the lipopolysaccharide component of endotoxin is thought to initiate the release of a cascade of mediators of the inflammatory process. Endotoxin itself appears to cause a profound collapse of vascular tone and systemic hypotension.

The most common form of endotoxin-induced hypotension is so-called "warm shock." The cardiac index is elevated, and the patient's skin feels warm as a result of a combination of fever and peripheral vasodilatation. Much less commonly, the cardiac index is depressed; this latter form is associated with a high early mortality.

Leukocyte and Platelet Mediators

After endotoxin invades the circulation, it activates macrophages, which in turn release TNF and interleukins.[1] It also activates platelets to release platelet-activating factor (PAF), which causes platelets to aggregate and causes localized vasoconstriction by release of vasoactive substances, such as serotonin.

Prostanoids

Through activation of leukocytes and platelets, inflammatory mediators (e.g., prostacyclin, thromboxane) are released.[1] These can give rise to pulmonary lesions that culminate in the development of adult respiratory distress syndrome (ARDS). Sielaff and coauthors,[35] studying experimental septic shock in the pig, demonstrated that prior administration of ibuprofen, a prostaglandin synthetase inhibitor, largely blocks the characteristic pulmonary lesion seen in that model. The eicasanoids are also thought to be partly responsible for the microcirculatory damage of gastrointestinal mucosa seen in endotoxin-induced shock.[24]

Oxygen-Derived Free Radicals

Leukocytes contain vesicles that are rich in precursors of oxygen radicals. In clinical situations in which tissue ischemia followed by reperfusion occurs (such as hemorrhagic or septic shock), xanthine oxidase catalyzes the conversion of hyoxanthine—itself a product of the effect of ischemia on tissue adenosine triphosphate—to oxidants and nonoxidative toxins. In addition, leukocytes adhere to vascular endothelial cells, resulting in neutrophil activation with elaboration of oxygen radicals and other toxins that cause a microcirculatory injury, leading to increased capillary permeability and interstitial edema. This theory is supported by the morphologic findings of ARDS, which is associated with interstial edema and platelet, neutrophil, and fibrin debris in the pulmonary microcirculation.[1]

None of these mechanisms is mutually exclusive. Certainly, the elaboration of cytokines from activated macrophages and leukocytes is complementary to the microcirculatory theory of multiple organ dysfunction. Furthermore, it is possible that bacterial translocation can initiate some of the macrophage activation and leukocyte adherence to endothelium, which lead to organ dysfunction. The cellular and humoral mediators of multiple organ dysfunction and bacterial translocation are detailed in other chapters (see Sections III, VIII, and X).

DIAGNOSIS

Clinical Features

Patients with intra-abdominal abscesses from spontaneous abdominal disease frequently present with an acute abdomen. Examples are perforated appendicitis, acute diverticulitis, and perforated peptic ulcer. Classical clinical findings of intra-abdominal abscess include fever (usually > 102°F), leukocytosis, and localized abdominal tenderness. Postoperative abscesses are more difficult to detect because these signs are often present after abdominal surgery in patients without abscesses. In the series of Saini and colleagues,[28] clinical findings were the indication for operative drainage in 41% of patients with intra-abdominal abscesses.

Radiologic Features

Classical plain x-ray films of the abdomen may be helpful in the diagnosis. Such films may demonstrate abnormal collections of gas or fluid. Fig. 66–3 demonstrates an air-fluid level in a large left subphrenic abscess that was a complication of a perforated peptic ulcer.

Contrast gastrointestinal radiography may also be used to detect and localize intra-abdominal abscesses. Figure 66–4 demonstrates how a barium enema can localize a pericolic abscess in a patient with acute diverticulitis.

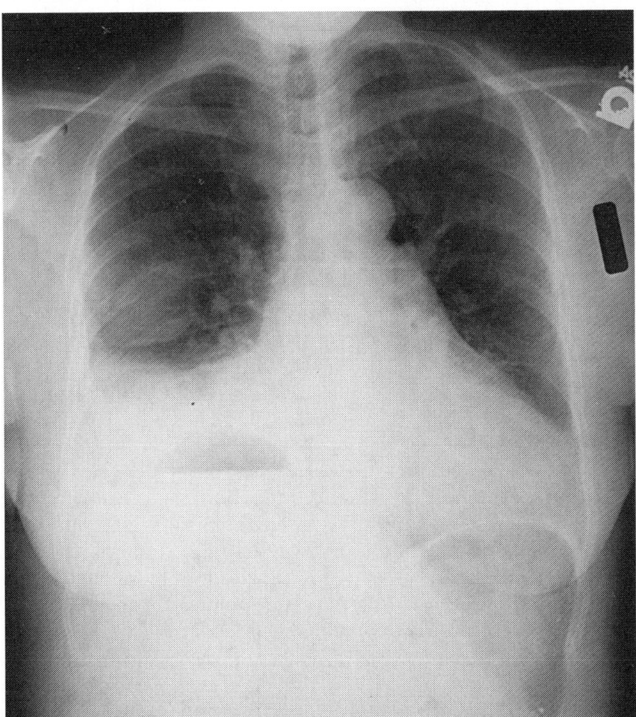

Figure 66–3. Plain radiograph of the chest and upper abdomen demonstrates a right subdiaphragmatic abscess with an air-fluid level. This patient presented with right upper quadrant abdominal pain, right shoulder pain, and fever. At operation, a chronic, sealed-off duodenal ulcer perforation was discovered to be the cause of the abscess.

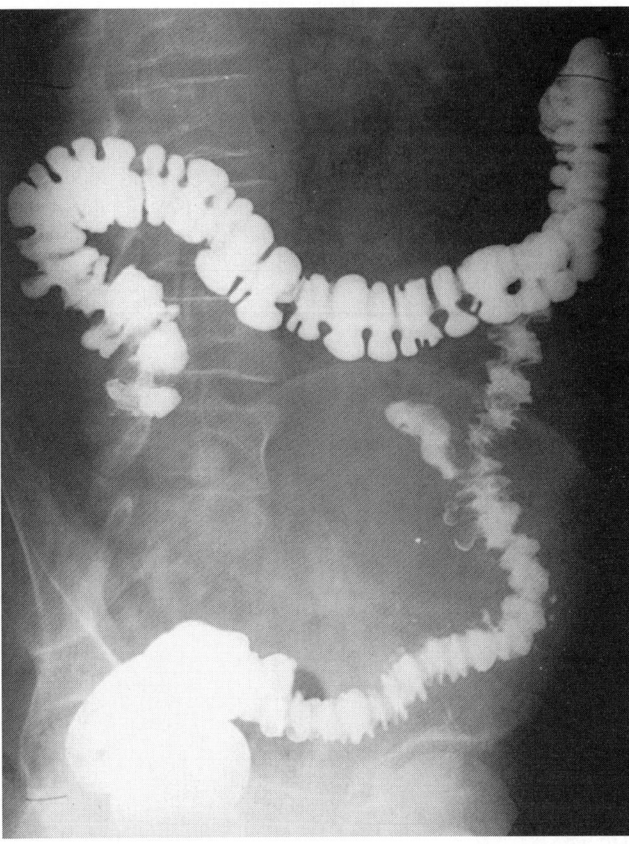

Figure 66–4. A contrast radiograph of the colon (barium enema) demonstrates diverticulitis of the sigmoid colon with perforation into a pericolic abscess.

Modern imaging techniques, however, have revolutionized the diagnosis of intra-abdominal abscess. Saini[28] reported that computed tomography was diagnostically superior to both gallium scintigraphy and ultrasonography. Figure 66–5 demonstrates an abscess associated with sigmoid colonic diverticuli-

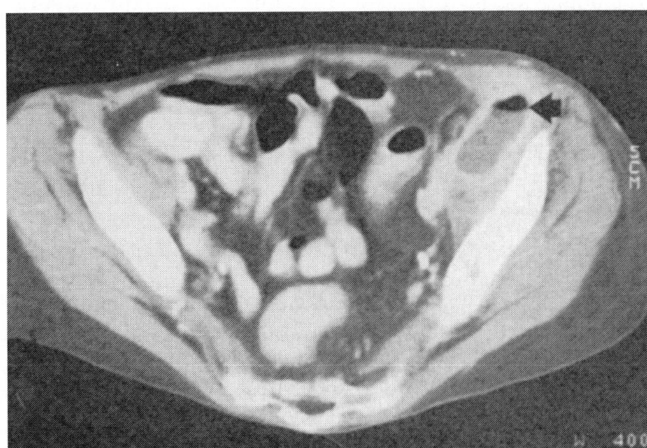

Figure 66–5. Diverticular abscess with drainage A 57-year-old woman with Crohn's disease and breast cancer presented with left lower quadrant pain, fever, and leukocytosis. A collection with an air-fluid level (*arrow*) was located anterior to the left iliac muscle. Note the enhancing rind.

tis. The advantages of CT include the ability to differentiate fluid and gas within an abscess from that inside the gastrointestinal lumen. CT was superior to ultrasound examination when the localization of an abscess was not previously suspected by clinical evidence, when a pelvic or interloop abscess was present and, most important, when multiple intra-abdominal collections were involved.[28] In cases of generalized peritoneal contamination, a fever occurring 5 or more days postoperatively and not explainable by other causes (e.g., pulmonary atelectasis or pneumonia, urinary tract infection, wound infection, thrombophlebitis, intravenous catheter infection, or drug reaction) is an indication for CT of the entire abdomen and pelvis. The reduced mortality for intra-abdominal abscess patients reported by Saini's group.[28] was attributed to earlier diagnosis, largely as a result of the availability of CT scans rather than any improvement in the therapy for multiple organ dysfunction. Goris and van Dalen[32] have noted that the mortality for multiple organ dysfunction has remained stubbornly constant at 60%.

THERAPY

Fluid/Pressor Therapy of Septic Shock

In septic shock related to intra-abdominal sepsis, the diagnosis is frequently established after the placement of a Swan-Ganz catheter for monitoring pulmonary capillary wedge pressure and cardiac output. The hypotension of septic shock, in contrast to that seen with hemorrhagic shock or cardiac failure, is usually associated with elevated cardiac index and a markedly decreased systemic vascular resistance. Mixed venous oxygen content is usually high or normal, reflecting the presence of significant arteriovenous shunting associated with the septic state. (See also Chapters 5 and 8.)

Antibiotics

In the early stages of intra-abdominal sepsis antibiotic therapy should be broad-spectrum, aimed at covering potential aerobic gram-negative and anaerobic microorganisms. When a patient has been in the hospital, especially in the ICU, for several days, the antibiotics should offer coverage for *P. aeruginosa.*

If aminoglycosides are used, it is important to measure peak and trough levels after early doses to avoid ototoxicity and nephrotoxicity. Prolonged dosing intervals can be calculated from readily available tables in the case of reduced renal function. A detailed discussion of antibiotic therapy for surgical infection is included in Chapter 57.

Nutrition

One of the more promising advances in preventing septic complications in susceptible surgical and trauma patients involves the early institution of enteral feeding. While this idea could be related to the theory of bacterial translocation, this association has not been proven in clinical studies. Moore and colleagues,[2] in a multicenter, prospective trial, compared early institution of an elemental diet via tube jejunostomies with total parenteral nutrition in victims of severe trauma. A meta-analysis demonstrated that the enterally fed patients had a significantly lower incidence of bronchopulmonary, urinary tract, and overall infections.

Kudsk and colleagues randomized trauma patients to an enteral diet containing glutamine, arginine, ribonucleotides, and omega-3 fatty acids (immune-enhancing diet) or to an isonitrogenous, isocaloric diet. A third group with no early enteral access but with comparable injury severity scores served as a control group. Significantly fewer major infectious complications developed in patients randomized to the immune-enhancing diet (6%; n = 17) than in those in the isonitrogenous group (41%; P = .02, n = 18) or the control group (58%, P = .002, n = 19). The duration of hospital stay, regimen of therapeutic antibiotics, and development of intra-abdominal abscess were significantly lower in patients receiving the enhanced enteral diet than in the two other groups.

Drainage of Intra-abdominal Abscesses

Although most abscesses necessitate drainage, certain intra-abdominal abscesses can sometimes be cured with antibiotic therapy alone. For example, multiple small hepatic abscesses secondary to cholangitis sometimes resolve with just antibiotics. The explanation is that liver abscesses, like some lung and brain abscesses, may communicate with the ductile system draining the organ and thus may be partially drained. Small pericolic abscesses associated with acute diverticulitis often resolve with antibiotic therapy alone. Kellum and coworkers[36] reported that nearly 90% of patients with acute diverticulitis—all of whom are thought to have colonic microperforations and pericolic collections—will respond to antibiotics alone, equally well if treated with cefoxitin alone, or a combination of gentamicin and clindamycin. Again, the communication of a pericolic abscess with a perforated diverticulum affords at least partial drainage. Because most intra-abdominal abscesses do not communicate with drainage conduits, they do not resolve without some form of drainage.

Percutaneous Catheter Drainage of Abscesses

Gerzof and associates[37] reported a highly successful series of patients treated with CT-guided or ultrasound-guided placement of drainage catheters in intra-abdominal abscesses. In this report, the authors emphasized the importance of the following factors in the success of the technique:

1. Complete drainage of all abscesses or loculations.
2. Broad-spectrum antibiotic coverage prior to manipulation.
3. Follow-up imaging or contrast studies to document complete resolution of the abscess.
4. Availability of a safe route for percutaneous catheter drainage.
5. Availability of surgical backup.

In this series,[37] 61 (86%) of 71 abscesses in 67 patients were successfully drained. There were 11 complications (15%); six deaths were attributable to sepsis, three of which were related to inadequate drainage. Only one abscess recurred during the follow-up from 2 to 5 years.

Percutaneous drainage is particularly valuable in patients with unilocular, solitary abscesses and in those with organ failure or coagulopathy, when conventional surgical drainage carries a high risk of mortality. Contraindications include patients with a surgical abdomen in whom intestinal perforation or gangrene is likely or patients in whom the drainage route would violate a hollow viscus or the pleural space.

Surgical Drainage and Drains

Saini's group[28] reported that since the availability of CT, the mortality for open surgical drainage had fallen from 30% to 12%. The complication rate was high (28% in this series of 100 consecutive patients), including recurrent abscesses, enterocutaneous fistulas, and superinfection with resistant organisms. The authors noted that imaging tests made extraserous or regional surgical drainage more accurate and recommended this approach over transperitoneal drainage (through a vertical midline incision) because of a lower observed morbidity. Open drainage was preferable for multiple abscesses, for CT-localized interloop abscesses, and for most pelvic abscesses.

The use of various types of drains are largely the personal preference of the surgeon. *Active suction drains* have the advantage that negative pressure is used to continuously evacuate the contents of an abscess cavity, and there is less contamination from the drain itself. Disadvantages include the tendency of suction drains to become plugged and the greater likelihood of some of the stiffer suction drains to erode into intestines or blood vessels.

Passive drains, such as the redoubtable Penrose drain, are less likely to become plugged, especially if they are placed through a large opening in the abdominal wall; they are also less likely to erode into vital structures. On the other hand, they require more active management from the surgeon in that they must be moved frequently to avoid being walled off from the target collection. Another disadvantage is the greater potential for external contamination.

Ancillary Therapies

Monoclonal antibodies against the lipopolysaccharide component of endotoxin have been developed and tested in humans. Unfortunately, because early promising data have not been substantiated in larger clinical trials, these therapies have not been approved for widespread clinical usage. Despite this setback, various biotechnology companies are developing these promising techniques. Antibodies to TNF, interleukins, and PAF have been developed and are beginning to be used in clinical trials involving septic patients.

In addition, non-antibodies are being developed by means of monoclonal techniques to replace various deficient elements found in the patient with sepsis. For example, a monoclonally synthesized surfactant is being clinically tested in surgical patients with sepsis who are thought to be at high risk for ARDS.

Additional Therapies

Another strategy, still in the investigative phase, includes the use of triiodothyronine to improve the inotropic action of the heart under the stress of septicemia. A second is the use of allopurinol to block the action of xanthine oxidase in catalyzing the production of oxygen radicals in the ischemia-reperfusion model of septic shock.

SUMMARY

At present, aggressive diagnosis and therapies, which are aimed at the prevention of sequential multiple organ system failure, should be the main goal of the surgeon treating peritonitis and intra-abdominal sepsis. Even if successful strategies are developed to combat the ravages of multiple organ failure, they will be extravagantly expensive not only in terms of financial costs, but also, more importantly, in terms of patient morbidity.

References

1. Deitch EA: Multiple organ failure, pathophysiology and potential future therapy. Ann Surg 1992; 216:117–134.
2. Moore, FA, Feliciano, DV, Andrassy, RJ, et al: Early enteral feeding, compared with parenteral, reduces postoperative septic complications: The results of a meta-analysis. Ann Surg 1992; 216:172–183.
3. Kudsk KA, Minard G, Croce MA, et al: A randomized trial of isonitrogenous enteral diets after severe trauma: An immune-enhancing diet reduces septic complications. Ann Surg 1996; 224:531–540.
4. Haagensen CD, Lloyd WEB: A Hundred Years of Medicine. New York, Sheridan House, 1943, pp 239–248.
5. Ravitch M: A Century of Surgery 1880-1980. Philadelphia, JB Lippincott, 1981.
6. Garrison FH: Notes on the History of Military Medicine. Washington, DC, Association of Military Surgeons, 1922, pp 188–206.
7. Landsteiner K: Individual differences in human blood. Science 1931; 73:403.
8. Blalock A: Acute circulatory failure as exemplified by shock and hemorrhage. Surg Gynecol Obstet 1934; 58:551–561.
9. Drye JC: Penicillin and sulfonamide therapy (2410 casualties). *In:* Surgery in World War II. Vol II. General Surgery. Coates JB, DeBakey ME (Eds). Washington DC, Office of the Surgeon General, Department of the Army, 1947, pp 197–201.
10. Hays SB: Policy on Large Bowel Injuries. Circular Letter No. 178. Washington, DC, Office of the Surgeon General, Department of the Army, October 23, 1943.
11. Barrett O: U.S. medicine in Vietnam: The early years. *In:* Internal Medicine in Vietnam. Vol II. General Medicine and Infectious Diseases. Ognibene AJ, Barrett O (Eds). Washington, DC, Office of the Surgeon General, Department of the Army, 1982, pp 21–38.
12. Meleney FL, Opps S, Harvey HD, et al: Peritonitis: II. Synergism of bacteria commonly found in peritoneal exudates. Arch Surg 1932; 25:709–721.
13. Weinstein WM, Onderdonk AH, Bartlett JG, et al: Experimental intra-abdominal abscesses in rats: Development of an experimental model. Infect Immun 1974; 10:1250–1255.
14. Clarke JS, Condon RE, Bentley DW, et al: Preoperative oral antibiotics reduce septic complications of colon operations: Results of a prospective, randomized double-blind clinical study. Am J Surg 1977; 186:251–259.
15. Deitch EA, Maejima K, Berg R: Effect of oral antibiotics and bacterial overgrowth on the translocation of the GI tract microflora in burned rats. J Trauma 1985; 25:385–392.
16. Deitch EA, Berg R, Specian R: Endotoxin promotes the translocation of bacteria from the gut. Arch Surg 1987; 122:185–190.
17. Baker JW, Deitch EA, Berg RD, et al: Hemorrhagic shock induces bacterial translocation from the gut. J Trauma 1988; 28:896–906.
18. Bennion RS, Wilson SE, Williams RA: Early portal anaerobic bacteremia in mesenteric ischemia. Arch Surg 1984; 119:151–155.
19. Deitch EA, Sittig K, Li M, et al: Obstructive jaundice promotes bacterial translocation from the gut. Am J Surg 1990; 159:79–84.
20. Deitch EA, Xu DZ, Qi L, et al: Protein malnutrition alone and in combination with endotoxin impairs systemic and gut-associated immunity. JPEN J Parenter Enteral Nutr 1992; 16:25–31.
21. Mainous M, Xu DZ, Lu Q, et al: Oral-TPN–induced bacterial translocation and impaired immune defences are reversed by refeeding. Surgery 1991; 110:277–283.
22. Spaeth G, Berg RD, Specian RD, et al: Food without fiber promotes bacterial translocation from the gut. Surgery 1990; 108:240–246.
23. Polk HC, Shields CL: Remote organ failure: a valid sign of occult intra-abdominal infection. Surgery 1977; 81:310–313.
24. Norton LW: Does drainage of intra-abdominal pus reverse multiple organ failure? Am J Surg 1985; 149:347–350.
25. Windmueller HG: Glutamine utilization by the small intestine. Adv Enzymol 1982; 53:202–231.
26. Souba WW, Scott TE, Wilmore DW: Intestinal consumption of intravenously administered fuels. JPEN J Parenter Enter Nutr 1985; 9:18–22.
27. Wilmore DW, Goodwin CW, Aulick LH, et al: Effect of injury and infection on visceral metabolism and circulation. Ann Surg 1980; 192:491–504.
28. Saini S, Kellum JM, O'Leary MP, et al: Improved localization and survival in patients with intra-abdominal abscesses. Am J Surg 1983; 145:136–142.
29. Nichols RL: Classification of surgical wounds and nonoperative factors influencing surgical wound infection. *In:* Decision Making in Surgical Sepsis. Nichols RL, Hyslop NE, Bartlett JG (Eds). Philadelphia, BC Decker, 1991, pp 20–22.
30. Bartlett JG: The normal flora. *In:* Surgical Infections, Selective Antibiotic Therapy. Condon RE, Gorbach SL (Eds): Baltimore, Williams & Wilkins, 1981, pp 1–6.

31. Van der Waaij D, Berghuis-de Vries JM, Lekkerkerk-van der Wees JEC: Colonization resistance of the digestive tract in conventional and antibiotic-treated mice. J Hyg (Camb) 1971; 69:405–411.
32. Goris RJA, van Dalen R: Selective decontamination in the intensive care unit. *In:* Advances in Trauma and Critical Care. Vol 7. Maull KI (Ed): St. Louis, Mosby-Year Book, 1992, pp 61–78.
33. Stoutenbeek CP, Van Saene HKF, Miranda DR, et al: The effect of selective decontamination of the digestive tract on colonization and infection rate in multiple trauma patients. Intensive Care Med 1984; 10:185–192.
34. Hartenauer U, Thulig B, Diemer W, et al: Effect of selective flora suppression on colonization, infection, and mortality in critically ill patients: A one-year, prospective consecutive study. Crit Care Med 1991; 19:463–473.
35. Sielaff TD, Sugerman HJ, Tatum JL, et al: Successful treatment of adult respiratory distress syndrome by histamine and prostaglandin blockade in a porcine pseudomonas model. Surgery 1987; 102:350–357.
36. Kellum JM, Coppa GF, Way LR, et al: Randomized, prospective comparison of cefoxitin with gentamicin-clindamycin in the treatment of acute colonic diverticulitis. Clin Ther 1992; 14:376–384.
37. Gerzof SG, Robbins AH, Johnson WC, et al: Percutaneous catheter drainage of abdominal abscesses: A five year experience. N Engl J Med 1981; 305:653–657.

67

Laboratory Diagnosis of Infection

Michael R. Jacobs, MB, BCh, PhD, MRCPath

Infections in critically ill patients, either as primary diseases or as complications of other conditions, carry a high mortality and require prompt and appropriate diagnosis and therapy. The laboratory diagnosis of infection in critical care medicine consists of (1) collection and direct examination of specimens, (2) culture for bacterial, viral, and fungal pathogens, (3) antimicrobial susceptibility testing, and (4) serologic diagnosis of infection.

SPECIMEN COLLECTION

Collection of adequate, appropriate, and representative samples is crucial to successful laboratory examination,[1] particularly in critical care medicine. Basic antiseptic precautions can easily be omitted in the flurry of activity surrounding a critically ill patient, and diagnostic material may be unavailable or may be obtained only after institution of antimicrobial therapy. Results of investigations performed on a specimen are valid only if the specimen is correctly collected, transported, and processed.

Ideal specimens are collected from normally sterile body sites and should not be contaminated by indigenous organisms of the skin or mucous membranes.[2, 3] The quantity should be adequate, particularly if the specimen is to be examined for low numbers of multiple groups of organisms. Tissue rather than swabs should be submitted whenever possible.

Specimens should be promptly transported to the laboratory under conditions designed to protect fastidious organisms and prevent overgrowth of any contaminants. Each specimen is accompanied by relevant information about the patient, including clinical diagnosis and examinations required, and each should be promptly examined and cultured on appropriate media.

If possible, specimens are collected before the institution of antimicrobial therapy, and use of topical anesthetics or preservative-containing solutions should be avoided.[2] Procedure guides for collecting and transporting specimens and information about facilities available, routine laboratory practices, and interpretation of results should be obtained from laboratory staff. Many institutions have developed policies for limiting the extent and frequency of microbiologic investigations on the basis of patient population, prevalence of pathogens, and length of hospitalization.[4, 5]

Respiratory Specimens

Important respiratory tract infections in critically ill patients include acute primary pneumonias as well as pneumonias secondary to endotracheal intubation, impaired host defenses (resulting from malignancies, immunosuppressive drugs, or chemotherapy), diabetes, alcoholism, and congestive heart failure. Because expectorated sputum is often difficult or impossible to obtain from these patients, material for examination can be sampled by bronchoscopy, transtracheal aspiration, or open lung biopsy.[6] Bronchoscopy with double-lumen catheters minimizes oropharyngeal contamination of specimens; however, the local anesthetic agents that are used during bronchoscopy possess antibacterial properties, and results of bronchoscopically obtained specimens should be interpreted with caution. Protected brush bronchoscopic or alveolar lavage sampling permits the use of quantitative culture techniques.

Transtracheal aspiration is indicated when sputum cannot be obtained, when Gram's stain or culture of sputum does not yield a clear pathogen, when a respiratory infection has responded poorly to antimicrobial therapy, and when there is a possibility of superinfection.[6] The technique is used less commonly than before because of the ease of bronchoscopic sampling. Transtracheal aspiration is carried out as follows:

1. The patient's neck is extended, a local anesthetic agent is injected over the cricothyroid membrane, and the trachea is entered through the membrane with a large-bore needle containing an indwelling catheter. The needle is angled downward, toward the patient's coccyx.
2. After the needle has entered the trachea, the catheter is advanced several inches, and the needle is withdrawn.
3. Sputum is aspirated from the catheter with a syringe; if no material is obtained, 1 to 2 mL of preservative-free sterile saline can be injected and aspirated.

Transtracheal aspirates bypass the oropharynx and can, therefore, be cultured in both anaerobic and aerobic media. Significant complications of transtracheal aspiration are hemoptysis, subcutaneous emphysema, aspiration, and cellulitis. The procedure can have false-positive results because of oropharyngeal aspiration or tracheal colonization and false-negative results because of prior antimicrobial therapy or bronchial obstruction.

Open lung biopsy is an alternative to bronchoscopy but is usually necessary only in immunocompromised hosts. Although the procedure is associated with low mortality and morbidity, it is contraindicated in patients with hypoxia and thrombocytopenia.[6]

Blood Specimens

Patients with sepsis are often in septic shock and, therefore, critically ill. Prompt, adequate, and aseptic collection of blood for culture before antimicrobial therapy is started is essential to confirm the diagnosis and identify the causative pathogen and its antimicrobial susceptibility.[2]

Blood is best collected by direct venipuncture with a needle and syringe or a sterile transfer set; to avoid contamination, vacuum tubes should be used with sterile, prepackaged needle holders. Additional specimens can be collected from arterial or venous access catheters, but such specimens may demonstrate only colonization of the line rather than sepsis and should not be the only blood specimens submitted for culture.

Venipuncture is performed as follows:

1. The venipuncture site is first disinfected with 70% alcohol, followed by 2% iodine or an iodophor, which should remain in contact with the skin for at least a minute.
2. Residual iodine is then removed with an alcohol pad.
3. Ten to 20 mL of blood is collected in a syringe by venipuncture.
4. The syringe needle is changed, and the blood is injected into two broth bottles, one aerobic and one anaerobic. The optimal volume ratio of blood to broth is 1:10; commercial broth bottles usually contain 30 to 100 mL of broth, requiring 3 to 10 mL of blood per bottle.[1]

Bacteremia is best demonstrated by detection of the same organism in multiple blood cultures collected over several hours from different venipuncture sites. In critical care medicine, it is often not possible to delay the start of antimicrobial therapy later than immediately after the initial set of culture specimens are obtained. The alternative is to collect two culture sets from different venipuncture sites with a delay as short as a few minutes or to collect a second set of cultures in commercially available resin-containing antimicrobial removal systems shortly after antimicrobial therapy has begun. Because multiple specimens should be collected in all patients with suspected sepsis, the collection time should be clearly noted on each requisition so that the relationship among clinical condition, antimicrobial therapy, procedures performed, and culture results can be assessed.

Vascular catheter tips should be submitted for culture when removed.[2] Blood required for culture for viruses and *Leptospira* can be collected in sterile, heparinized tubes.[3]

Urine Specimens

Urine is best collected as a clean-catch, midstream specimen after appropriate cleansing of the external genitalia.[1] This is usually not possible in critically ill patients, and the laboratory should be notified about specimens not optimally collected. If urine culture is particularly important, suprapubic aspiration can be used to obtain a specimen. Suprapubic aspirates should be clearly identified because any growth from these specimens is significant.

In catheterized patients, urine should be collected with a needle and syringe directly from the clamped catheter. Such specimens should be clearly identified because they are not evaluated with conventional quantitation. Urinary catheter tips should not be submitted for culture because they reflect only what is colonizing the catheter, not necessarily the patient.

Urine specimens should be transported to the laboratory as soon as possible and submitted for culture within an hour of collection. Specimens can be refrigerated if any delay is anticipated.

Other Specimens

Body fluids and exudates, pus, and swabs of mucous membranes should be submitted to the laboratory as rapidly as possible.[1, 2] If anaerobic culture is required, anaerobic transport media should be used.

DIRECT EXAMINATION OF SPECIMENS

Direct microscopic examination of specimens, as either wet mounts or stained smears, is extremely important in the diagnosis of many infections.[1, 2] Specimens can be examined for various microbial antigens and other products as well as for inflammatory cells and chemical composition.

Wet Mounts

Direct examination of a fluid specimen on a slide and under a coverslip can be extremely useful for demonstrating protozoa and inflammatory cells. Dark-ground or phase-contrast illumination reveals bacteria, including spirochetes, and other organisms. *Cryptococcus neoformans* can be demonstrated by mixing a drop of India ink with a drop of cerebrospinal fluid (CSF) or other body fluid; the India ink is a negative stain that outlines the capsule of the organism. Potassium hydroxide wet mounts are useful for detecting fungi, particularly in sputum.

Stained Smears

Gram's Stains

Stained smears are commonly performed on a wide variety of specimens and often provide diagnostic information in infectious conditions. Gram-stained smears of body fluids and exudates can show inflammatory cells as well as bacteria. Clumps of gram-positive cocci suggest staphylococci or peptococci; chains of gram-positive cocci suggest streptococci or peptostreptococci; large gram-positive bacilli suggest clostridia; large gram-negative bacilli suggest Enterobacteriaceae; and small gram-negative bacilli suggest *Pseudomonas, Haemophilus*, or *Bacteroides* species. Bacterial morphology can be highly variable, however, particularly in material from abscesses or from patients on antimicrobial therapy, and overinterpretation of smears must be avoided.

Gram's stains of sputum are helpful when the presence of inflammatory cells suggests pneumonia; however, if oral squamous epithelial cells and a wide variety of organisms are observed, the specimen includes saliva and should be discarded.[1] Pneumonia caused by *Streptococcus pneumoniae, Haemophilus influenzae, Staphylococcus aureus*, and Enterobacteriaceae can often be identified with a high level of accuracy from a Gram-stained sputum sample.[6]

Gram's stains of urine are highly suggestive of significant bacteriuria if two or more bacteria are seen per oil-immersion field of well-mixed, uncentrifuged urine.[1] Gram-negative bacilli suggest Enterobacteriaceae, and gram-positive cocci suggest enterococci or staphylococci.

Gram's stain can be easily and rapidly performed by the physician attending the patient. Good results, however, require considerable experience and expertise, because decolorization time depends on the nature of the material being stained. As already mentioned, overinterpretation of smears should be avoided. Because many organisms have similar appearances, those in Gram-stained smears should be described according to their morphology as well as their degree of staining. Finally, the preparation of Gram's stain reagents should be checked, and a supply of smears containing a mixture of gram-positive cocci and gram-negative bacilli should be provided as quality control slides to be stained by anyone using the reagents.

Acid-Fast and Fluorescent Stains

Mycobacteria do not stain readily with Gram's method, but they resist acid decolorization and thus can be identified through the use of various acid-fast stains on sputum and other specimens.[2] Both Ziehl-Neelsen stain, which uses hot carbolfuchsin, and Kinyoun's stain, which uses cold, concentrated carbolfuchsin, stain mycobacteria red. Auramine stains mycobacteria a bright yellow under suitable fluorescent illumination.

Fluorescein-tagged fluorescent antibody stains are useful in demonstrating various pathogens, such as *Legionella pneumophila, Pneumocystis carinii, Francisella tularensis*, and common respiratory viruses.[1, 7] Fluorescein appears bright green under suitable fluorescent illumination. Other staining methods are silver stains of biopsy specimens for fungi and *P. carinii*, and Giemsa's stains of blood smears for malarial parasites. All staining procedures, particularly fluorescent stains, require adequate controls.

DETECTION OF MICROBIAL PRODUCTS

The only commonly available techniques for detecting microbial products directly in specimens are various immunologic methods used to identify microbial antigens and direct gene probes to detect *Neisseria gonorrhoeae* and *Chlamydia trachomatis*.[7, 8] Considerable advances have been made in the development of amplified gene probes, for example by the polymerase chain reaction (PCR).[9] Availability of commercial products has improved.[10]

In patients with meningitis, capsular polysaccharide antigens of *H. influenzae, S. pneumoniae, Neisseria meningitidis*, or *C. neoformans* can be detected in CSF and sometimes in serum, sputum, urine, and effusion fluids. Antigens can be demonstrated by counterimmunoelectrophoresis (CIE), latex agglutination, or staphylococcal coagglutination,[7] but false-positive and false-negative results limit the application of these procedures. CIE of CSF is best for the diagnosis of bacterial meningitis, and latex agglutination of CSF or serum is best for the diagnosis of cryptococcal infection. CIE of serum, sputum, or urine detects up to 75% of bacteremic pneumococcal agents in pneumonia but only 45% of nonbacteremic agents. Moreover, antigen can persist in urine for up to 6 weeks after onset of illness and may not accurately reflect a patient's current disease.[7]

Enzyme-linked immunosorbent assays (ELISAs) are being developed for the detection of bacterial and viral antigens using enzyme-labeled antibodies. Examples of infections that can be identified by the ELISA technique are rotavirus infection, gonorrhea, and legionnaires' disease.

Molecular diagnostic techniques, such as PCR-based methods, are currently in routine use in many institutions (1) to detect infectious agents rapidly, (2) to detect agents that are not readily cultured, (3) to quantitate viral load, and (4) to detect genes or gene mutations responsible for antimicrobial resistance.[9] Another useful application is genetic fingerprinting of organisms to identify and characterize strains associated with outbreaks of disease or colonization.[10, 11] Availability, cost, and turnaround time remain major limiting factors in the universal use of such methods.[11]

CULTURE METHODS

The wide variety of bacteria, fungi, viruses, and protozoa that can cause infections requires different isolation techniques. Most laboratories choose techniques on the basis of ease of use, local prevalence of various infectious diseases, clinical usefulness, and availability of equipment and facilities.[1] Physicians should be aware which procedures are routine and which are available on request, either on site or at a referral laboratory. To ensure its optimal laboratory handling, each specimen should be identified by the patient's age, clinical presentation and diagnosis, travel history, known exposure to specific pathogens, and any antimicrobial therapy.[1, 2] Laboratory tests should be specifically requested, particularly when unusual infections are suspected.

Specimens are usually processed for groups of organisms, such as rapidly growing bacteria (aerobic and anaerobic), mycobacteria, fungi, chlamydiae, and viruses. Rapidly growing bacteria are generally isolated from specimens that are streaked onto a variety of agar media and incubated aerobically (supplemented with 5% to 10% carbon dioxide [CO_2], if necessary) or anaerobically. Selective and enrichment media are used to select pathogens from normal flora. Blood agar allows the growth of many common bacteria in 24 to 48 hours, whereas chocolate agar encourages the growth of more fastidious organisms, such as *Haemophilus* and *Neisseria* species. MacConkey's agar is specific for growth and differentiation of enteric gram-negative bacilli.

Mycobacteria can be isolated on various solid media, such as Löwenstein-Jensen agar, in 2 to 3 weeks. Detection within a week is possible through the use of liquid media containing carbon 14–labeled substrates.[12]

Fungi can be readily isolated on most bacteriologic media after prolonged incubation if antibacterial agents are added to inhibit bacterial growth. Incubation for several weeks at 30°C and 37°C may be required for growth of systemic fungi.[1] Special techniques are required for the isolation of molds from blood, such as the lysis-centrifugation method.

Viruses and chlamydiae can be isolated by animal inoculation or by inoculation of hens' eggs or mammalian cell cultures.[3] Cell cultures are commonly used but do not grow all viruses.

Respiratory Specimens

Diagnosis of bacterial pneumonia can be confirmed by culture of sputum, transtracheal aspirates, or biopsy material (1) on blood agar under CO_2 for pneumococci and staphylococci; (2) on chocolate agar under CO_2 for *Haemophilus*; (3) on MacConkey's agar for enteric gram-negative bacilli; or (4) on enriched blood agar incubated anaerobically for anaerobes (only for suitable specimens, such as transtracheal aspirates or material from open lung biopsy).[1, 2] *Mycoplasma pneumoniae* can be isolated on special media, but its isolation is rarely attempted owing to its slow growth and to inadequate material for culture.[13] Mycobacteria and many fungi require prolonged aerobic incubation. *Legionella pneumophila* and other *Legionella* species can be cultured from respiratory specimens on charcoal–yeast extract agar under CO_2; sputum is the least suitable specimen for isolating these organisms. Viral isolation can be attempted from all respiratory specimens.[3]

Blood Specimens

The diagnosis of sepsis is best made by the presence of sustained bacteremia. After direct inoculation of blood into liquid culture media, culture broths are incubated at 35°C and are examined several times daily. Growth is detected by observation of macroscopic turbidity, blind subculture, measurement of CO_2 released from ^{14}C-labeled substrates, or other indicators of bacterial metabolic activity.[1, 2]

Most bacteria and yeasts grow in common commercial blood culture media, but prolonged incubation is often required to isolate yeasts and *Brucella* species. Biphasic broth-agar media can also be used for prolonged incubation. Antimicrobial-removing resin media or lysis-centrifugation systems may be used in addition to these media for specimens from patients who are receiving antimicrobial therapy or in whom fungal infection is suspected.

Predominant bloodstream pathogens in the 1990s have been *Escherichia coli*, *Klebsiella pneumoniae*, *S. aureus*, coagulase-negative staphylococci, and *Enterococcus* species, particularly vancomycin-resistant *Enterococcus faecium*.[14] Leading sources of bacteremia are intravenous catheters, the respiratory and genitourinary tracts, and intra-abdominal foci. Other notable pathogens currently seen in bloodstream infections are fungi and *Mycobacterium avium*; the frequency of anaerobes has declined.

Urine Specimens

Quantitation of organisms in voided urine is used to differentiate infection (>100,000 organisms per milliliter) from urethral and perineal contamination (<10,000 mixed organisms per milliliter).[1] Urine is cultured quantitatively on blood and MacConkey's agar with a calibrated 1-mL loop. Any growth may be significant in catheter and suprapubic specimens of urine, and specimens obtained from patients receiving antimicrobial therapy need to be interpreted with caution.

Other Specimens

Specimens from normally sterile sites are usually cultured for bacteria aerobically and anaerobically on blood agar; chocolate agar is used if fastidious organisms are suspected.[1, 2] Specimens from mucous membranes or the gastrointestinal tract often require selective and enrichment media to allow isolation of specific pathogens (e.g., *Salmonella* species from feces and *N. gonorrhoeae* from the cervix, urethra, throat, or rectum).[1, 2]

Identification of Isolates

Most common bacteria, fungi, and mycobacteria are identified from the following features:

- Ability to grow on cell-free media
- Colonial morphology on solid media
- Rate of growth
- Temperature requirements
- Stained microscopic morphology
- Biochemical or antigenic properties

Atypical isolates, unusual organisms, and differentiation of phage types or serotypes of an organism are generally referred to a reference laboratory for investigation. Identification of epidemic strains can be achieved by many molecular methods, such as deoxyribonucleic (DNA) fingerprinting, plasmid profiles, and multilocus enzyme electrophoresis.[15]

Growth of viruses and chlamydiae can be detected in cell cultures from cytopathic effects, such as cell rounding, cell clustering, syncytial formation, and intranuclear or intracytoplasmic inclusions.[13] Hemadsorption, direct immunofluorescence, and interference can also indicate viral growth. Final identification of a virus requires specific neutralization of viral activity by homologous antiserum.

ANTIMICROBIAL SUSCEPTIBILITY TESTS

Determining the susceptibility of isolated pathogens to appropriate antimicrobial agents is an important function of clinical microbiology laboratories. The development and spread of resistant nosocomial pathogens, as well as the increasing numbers of immunocompromised patients and new antimicrobial agents, emphasize the importance of rapid and accurate susceptibility testing of isolates from critically ill patients.

In vivo susceptibility is influenced by the following factors:

- Host defense mechanisms
- Concentrations of antimicrobial agents at the site of infection
- Natural course, nature, and severity of the infection
- Any delay in starting therapy
- Effects of other therapeutic measures, such as surgery

In vitro susceptibility depends on the following:

- The organism
- Growth medium
- Atmosphere
- Inoculum size
- Length and temperature of incubation

Because these factors have been standardized for common rapidly growing bacteria,[16] the outcome of infection is affected mainly by in vivo factors.

Organisms are regarded as *susceptible* to an antimicrobial agent if they are inhibited in vitro by a concentration of the agent that is lower than serum concentrations achievable with the usual drug dosage.[17] *Resistant* organisms are not inhibited or are inhibited only at concentrations above those attainable. Susceptibility and resistance are expressed as the *minimal inhibitory concentration* (MIC) of an antimicrobial agent required to inhibit growth of a defined population of organisms or as categories based on antimicrobial levels in various body sites. Most susceptibility tests are based directly or indirectly on MIC determination[18] and require strict standardization and quality control.

Surveillance of antimicrobial resistance patterns is important for developing guidelines for antimicrobial therapy and for controlling spread of resistant strains.[18] In addition, the use of processes to integrate antimicrobial susceptibility results from individual patients into hospital information systems has been shown to improve patient management by monitoring the differences between antimicrobial susceptibility of pathogens and antibiotic therapy being used.[19]

Determination of Minimal Inhibitory Concentration

For determination of MIC, serial twofold dilutions of antimicrobial agents in a suitable growth medium, such as Mueller-Hinton broth, are prepared in test tubes (macrodilution method) or in microdilution wells (microdilution method), with an inoculum of 10^5 to 10^6 organisms per milliliter.[16, 17] MICs can also be performed by the agar dilution method; multiple inocula of 10^4 organisms per spot are placed on antimicrobial agent–containing plates with a replicating device. After overnight incubation at 35°C, the lowest antimicrobial concentration that completely inhibits growth is the MIC.

Minimal bactericidal concentrations (MBCs) can be determined by quantitative subculture; the MBC is the lowest concentration of antimicrobial agent that produces at least a 99.9% reduction in the original inoculum.[16] MBCs are now rarely determined, however, because of a lack of reproducibility of results and the absence of quality-control strains.

The macrodilution method produces reproducible MIC results, but it is time-consuming and expensive. The microdilution method produces results identical to those obtained with macrodilution for gram-positive bacteria and results one dilution lower for enteric gram-negative bacteria[20]; this method is commercially available in the form of frozen or lyophilized trays. Agar dilution, the most reproducible MIC determination method, allows testing of up to 36 organisms simultaneously on a standard agar plate.[16]

A new method for MIC determination is the E test, which is performed with a plastic carrier strip that releases an antimicrobial gradient when placed on an agar plate. It combines the simplicity of disk diffusion with the accuracy of MIC determination. The E test is particularly useful for susceptibility testing of fastidious organisms, such as *S. pneumoniae, H. influenzae*, and anaerobes.[18]

MICs are expressed in micrograms per milliliter and should be at least twofold to fourfold lower than mean achievable drug levels to produce an adequate therapeutic response. MICs can also be qualitatively expressed by predetermined resistance categories based on achievable serum drug concentrations, as follows[16] (Table 67–1):

1. A *susceptible* organism is inhibited by levels of antimicrobial agents readily attained in the blood on usual dosage, including oral when applicable.
2. An *intermediate* organism is inhibited only by drug blood levels achieved with fairly high dosage or when the drug is concentrated (e.g., in urine).
3. A *resistant* organism is resistant to commonly achievable drug levels.

These general categories are influenced by the patient's condition, drug pharmacokinetics, renal and hepatic disease, age, the presence of shock, and effects of other drugs. These categories may need to be modified for infections in sites of poor drug penetration, such as CSF.

Disk-Diffusion Tests

The zone of growth inhibition around a disk containing an antimicrobial agent is inversely proportional to the MIC of the antimicrobial agent.[21, 22] Up to 12 different disks can be placed on a Petri dish, 15 cm in diameter, containing Mueller-Hinton agar seeded with a test organism. Zones of inhibition are recorded after overnight incubation at 35°C. The organism is categorized as (1) susceptible, (2) intermediate (moderately susceptible), or (3) resistant to the antimicrobial agent on each disk according to the diameter of the zone of inhibition around the disk. The disk-diffusion method usually used is the Kirby-Bauer procedure, which is limited by the range of drugs and organisms that can be tested. Anaerobes should not be tested by disk diffusion.[21]

Automated Tests

The MIC and disk-diffusion methods require overnight incubation in addition to the 24 hours usually required to isolate the

TABLE 67–1. Minimum Inhibitory Concentrations (MICs): Interpretative Standards for Enteric Gram-Negative Staphylococci and Enterococci

	MIC (μ/mL)		
Antimicrobial Agent	***Susceptible***	***Intermediate****	***Resistant***
β-Lactams			
PENICILLINS			
Ampicillin, ampicillin-sulbactam, amoxicillin-clavulanate			
When testing Enterobacteriaceae	≤8.00	16	≥32.00
When testing staphylococci	≤0.25	—	≥0.5
When testing enterococci	≤8.00	—	≥16.00
When testing other streptococci	≤0.25	0.5–4	≥8.00
Penicillin G			
When testing staphylococci	≤0.12	—	≥0.25
When testing enterococci	≤8.00	—	≥16.00
When testing pneumococci	≤0.06	0.12–1	≥2.00
When testing other streptococci	≤0.12	0.25–2	≥4.00
Oxacillin and nafcillin†			
When testing staphylococci	≤2.00	—	≥4.00
Mezlocillin, ticarcillin, ticarcillin-clavulanate, piperacillin			
When testing Enterobacteriaceae	≤16.00	32–64	≥128.00
When testing *Pseudomonas aeruginosa*	≤64.00	—	≥128.00
CEPHALOSPORINS			
Cephalothin, cefazolin, cefoxitin, cefuroxime, ceftazidime, cefepime	≤8.00	16	≥32.00
Cefotaxime, ceftriaxone, ceftizoxime	≤8.00	16–32	≥64.00
Cefotetan, cefoperazone	≤16.00	32	≥64.00
CARBAPENEMS			
Imipenem, meropenem	≤4.00	8	≥16.00
MONOBACTAMS			
Aztreonam	≤8.00	16	≥32.00
Aminoglycosides			
Gentamicin, tobramycin	≤4.00	8	≥16.00
Amikacin	≤16.00	32	≥64.00
Glycopeptides			
Vancomycin	≤4.00	8–16	≥32.00
Macrolides			
Erythromycin, clindamycin	≤0.50	1–4	≥8.00
Azithromycin, clarithromycin	≤2.00	4	≥8.00
Quinolones			
Ciprofloxacin	≤1.00	2	≥4.00
Levofloxacin	≤2.00	4	≥8.00

*Intermediate MICs approach achievable blood and tissue levels, and response rates may be lower than for strains with susceptible MICs. Strains with intermediate MICs can be treated in body sites where drugs are concentrated, such as urine, or when high dosages of drugs, such as β-lactams, are used. This category also indicates a buffer zone to allow for minor technical errors with toxic agents.

†Oxacillin-resistant and nafcillin-resistant staphylococci are resistant to all β-lactams.

organism. The obvious need for faster turnaround times in the care of critically ill patients has led to the development of commercial systems that produce susceptibility results in 3 to 7 hours.[23] Staphylococci, enterococci, and enteric gram-negative bacilli can be tested by any of several commercially available systems that read and interpret results photometrically.[24] These automated systems perform adequately in comparison with MIC results and can test between nine and 20 drugs at one time. They should be used with caution, however, and results for important isolates should be confirmed by conventional methods. Manufacturers' recommendations must be strictly followed with these systems to avoid erroneous results.

Beta-lactamase Production

Penicillin and ampicillin-resistant strains of *H. influenzae* and *S. aureus* produce β-lactamases that can be demonstrated by various methods. Beta-lactamase production by *H. influenzae* can be rapidly detected by the acidimetric or chromogenic cephalosporin methods.[25] Demonstration of β-lactamase production by *S. aureus* is more difficult and may require induction by oxacillin or methicillin.

Choosing Susceptibility Tests and Agents

The choice of susceptibility testing method depends on (1) the organism to be tested, (2) the techniques available, and (3) the need for speed or accuracy. The choice of antimicrobial agents to be tested is determined by (1) the organism to be tested, (2) its site of isolation, and (3) local patterns of susceptibility and antimicrobial use.[26]

Some antimicrobial agents, such as amikacin and the newer β-lactams, are tested or reported only if resistance to older aminoglycosides or β-lactams is detected. Susceptibility to groups of antimicrobial agents can be determined by testing against one member of the group (Table 67–2).

Because critically ill patients are often treated with combinations of antimicrobial agents, the interaction of these agents is important.[25, 27] Effective antimicrobial combinations are either synergistic or additive. These effects can be assessed in vitro by testing the rate of killing of an organism with drugs alone and in combined drugs in a checkerboard titration. Many drug combinations are known to be synergistic in vivo, particularly β-lactams with aminoglycosides, and do not need to be tested in combination.[27] Combinations known to be antagonistic in vivo include penicillin G with tetracycline in pneumococcal meningitis and chloramphenicol with a β-lactam agent in meningitis caused by enteric gram-negative bacilli.

Severe mycobacterial infections, such as miliary tuberculosis, are rare but are increasingly being encountered in critically ill patients. Conventional mycobacterial susceptibility tests take 2 to 3 weeks. Such testing can be performed within a week, however, on isolates of *Mycobacterium tuberculosis* with the use of a radiometric method.[12, 28]

Susceptibility of yeasts and molds to amphotericin B and imidazoles can be determined through the use of techniques similar to MIC determinations for bacteria.[29] These techniques, however, are difficult to perform and are best done by specialist reference laboratories.

DETERMINING BACTERICIDAL ACTIVITY OF BODY FLUIDS

The bactericidal activity of serum and other body fluids reflects the adequacy of antimicrobial therapy.[25, 30] The best assessment is made by drawing peak and trough serum samples; peak samples are drawn 15 to 30 minutes after intravenous infusion or 1 hour after intramuscular injection of the antimicrobial agent; trough samples are drawn just before the next drug dose.

Determination of serum bactericidal activity, often referred to as the *Schlichter test*, is performed by preparing serial twofold dilutions of the patient's serum in tubes of Mueller-Hinton broth and inoculating each tube with a suspension of 5×10^5 organisms per milliliter.[25] After overnight incubation, bacteriostatic levels are read and tubes are subcultured to determine bactericidal dilutions. Results are expressed as end-point serum dilutions.

Criteria for acceptable bactericidal levels have not been clearly defined except in endocarditis, in which peak serum bactericidal dilutions of 1:8 or greater correlate with a favorable outcome. These tests are rarely performed.

MONITORING ANTIMICROBIAL LEVELS

Measurement of concentrations of antimicrobial agents in serum and other body fluids can confirm that therapeutic drug levels (i.e., above in vitro MIC values) have been attained but levels approaching toxicity have been avoided.[31, 32] Although most drugs do not usually require monitoring, aminoglycosides,[31, 32] chloramphenicol,[33, 34] and vancomycin[31] produce dose-related toxicity. Gentamicin and tobramycin trough values greater than 2 mg/mL and amikacin trough values greater than 10 mg/mL are associated with nephrotoxicity.[31, 35] Reversible hematopoietic toxicity of chloramphenicol occurs with serum concentrations greater than 25 mg/mL, particularly in patients with liver or renal disease.[33, 34] Renal disease, obesity, dehydration, edema, major burns, and fever can all alter aminoglycoside distribution, resulting in potentially toxic drug levels.[32]

Peak and trough serum samples for antimicrobial assay should be drawn as discussed previously. All specimens must be labeled with sampling time, times of drug administration, drug dosage and route of administration, and other drugs being administered, particularly antimicrobial agents. This labeling is necessary to minimize drug interactions, such as the inactivation of aminoglycosides by high concentrations of carbenicillin, and to ensure that the assay procedure is appropriate.[36, 37]

Drugs can be assayed by microbiologic, biochemical, and chromatographic methods.[1] Microbiologic methods require at least 24 hours and are difficult to perform if patients are receiving multiple antimicrobial agents. Biochemical methods using antibodies with radioactive, enzyme, or fluorescent labels are widely used for aminoglycosides. Chloramphenicol, which is now rarely used, is best assayed by high-pressure liquid chromatography.[38] The utility of monitoring vancomycin levels is controversial because there is a poor correlation of serum levels to either toxicity or efficacy.[39, 40]

SEROLOGIC DIAGNOSIS OF INFECTIONS

Although antibody detection is rarely useful for the management of critically ill patients, serologic evaluation can be important in providing a diagnosis during convalescence.[40] Acute-phase sera should be collected, if possible, in patients with febrile illnesses, and convalescent samples should be drawn 1 to 6 weeks later. There are many techniques to detect antibodies, and commercial reagents are increasingly available. Examples of infections causing severe illness that can be diagnosed serologically are typhoid fever, brucellosis, tularemia, legionnaires' disease, all acute viral diseases, histoplasmosis,

TABLE 67–2. Recommended Antimicrobial Agents to be Tested According to Organism and Site of Isolation*

Enteric Gram-Negative Isolates from Urine	***Staphylococci***
Ampicillin†	Penicillin G
Amoxicillin-clavulanate	Amoxicillin-clavulanate
Ampicillin-sulbactam	Ampicillin-sulbactam
Trimethoprim	Oxacillin or nafcillin
Tetracycline†	Cephalothin
Nitrofurantoin	Erythromycin
Sulfisoxazole†	Clindamycin
Nalidixic acid	Imipenem or meropenem
Mezlocillin, piperacillin, or ticarcillin	Vancomycin
Gentamicin	Gentamicin
Tobramycin	Amikacin
Amikacin	Clarithromycin or azithromycin
Cephalothin†	Ciprofloxacin or levofloxacin
Cefoxitin	Trimethoprim-sulfamethoxazole
Cefuroxime	***Enterococci***
Third-generation cephalosporins‡	Ampicillin†
Imipenem or meropenem	Pencillin G
Ciprofloxacin or levofloxacin	Ciprofloxacin or levofloxacin
Enteric Gram-Negative Isolates from Other Sites	Gentamicin (high-level resistance)
Ampicillin†	Nitrofurantoin§
Amoxicillin-clavulanate	Vancomycin
Ampicillin-sulbactam	***Nonenterococcal Streptococci***
Trimethoprim	Penicillin G
Chloramphenicol	Erythromycin
Aztreonam	Clindamycin
Gentamicin	Clarithromycin or azithromycin
Tobramycin	Vancomycin
Amikacin	**Streptococcus pneumoniae**
Imipenem or meropenem	Penicillin G‖
Cephalothin†	Cefotaxime or ceftriaxone
Cefoxitin	Erythromycin
Cefuroxime	Vancomycin
Mezlocillin, piperacillin, or ticarcillin	**Haemophilus influenzae**
Third-generation cephalosporins‡	Ampicillin†
Ciprofloxacin or levofloxacin	Amoxicillin-clavulanate or ampicillin-sulbactam
Pseudomonas, Xanthomonas, *and* Acinetobacter	Cefotaxime or ceftriaxone
Piperacillin	Tetracycline
Aztreonam	Trimethoprim
Mezlocillin or ticarcillin	Sulfisoxazole†
Ceftazidime or cefepime	Ciprofloxacin or levofloxacin
Trimethoprim-sulfamethoxazole	***Anaerobes***
Gentamicin	Penicillin G
Tobramycin	Ampicillin
Netilmicin	Ampicillin-clavulanate or ampicillin-sulbactam
Amikacin	Ticarcillin, mezlocillin, or piperacillin
Imipenem or meropenem	Ticarcillin-clavulanate
	Clindamycin
	Imipenem or meropenem
	Metronidazole
	Cefoxitin

* The most appropriate antimicrobials to test are best determined by the clinical laboratory in consultation with medical staff, infectious disease practitioners, and the pharmacy. Antimicrobials in each list have proven clinical efficacy for the listed organism group and acceptable in vitro test performance.

† These agents represent similar agents (e.g., ampicillin represents amoxicillin; cephalothin represents cephaloridine, cephalexin, cefazolin, and cephradine).

‡ Cefotaxime, ceftazidime, ceftizoxime, ceftriaxone, or moxalactam.

§ For urinary isolates only.

‖ For disk-diffusion testing, oxacillin or methicillin disks reflect penicillin G susceptibility more accurately than penicillin G disks.

rickettsial typhus and spotted fevers, toxoplasmosis, and amebiasis.[41]

VALUE OF DIAGNOSTIC MICROBIOLOGY IN CRITICAL CARE MEDICINE

Diagnostic microbiologic procedures can identify the infectious cause of a disease and determine its optimal therapy. Rapid determination of these results is vital in critical care medicine, particularly for patients with sepsis, pneumonia, meningitis, or neutropenia. Faster bacterial isolation, identification, and susceptibility tests now allow results to be obtained on the day after specimen collection rather than 2 days after. For results to be of value for the initial management of critically ill patients, however, this time delay needs to be shortened to 1 or 2 hours; only antigen-detection procedures currently fulfill this requirement, and their usefulness is limited. Direct microscopic examination of specimens remains the only rapid diagnostic procedure that is always available and can be performed with simple reagents and microscopes.

In critically ill patients with suspected infections, broad-spectrum therapy can be guided by Gram's stain results until culture and susceptibility results are known. Adequate collection of appropriate specimens is crucial for the generation of meaningful laboratory results and should not be neglected in the rush to initiate antimicrobial therapy in a critically ill patient.

Microbiology laboratories can provide valuable information about the antimicrobial susceptibility of pathogens, serum bactericidal activity, serum drug levels, and activity of drugs in combination. Antimicrobial therapy may still fail, however, for the following reasons[26]:

- Failure of drug absorption or distribution
- Accelerated drug inactivation
- Inadequate dosage
- Inactivation of drugs when mixed in infusion fluids before administration
- Failure of drugs to reach organisms in abscesses or the central nervous system
- Development of pathogen resistance during therapy
- Drug antagonism
- Superinfection
- Impairment of local or general host defenses

Consultation among physicians and clinical microbiology personnel does much to identify many of these factors and to optimize patient care. Improvements in rapid diagnostic procedures will be a major advance in the diagnosis and management of the critically ill patient.

References

1. Washington JA (Ed): Laboratory Procedures in Clinical Microbiology. 2nd ed. New York, Springer-Verlag, 1985.
2. Isenberg HD, Washington JA, Doern GV, et al: Specimen collection and handling. *In*: Manual of Clinical Microbiology. 5th ed. Balows A, Hausler JR, Herrmann KL, et al (Eds). Washington, DC, American Society for Microbiology, 1991, p 15.
3. Lennette DA: Preparation of specimens for virological examination. *In*: Manual of Clinical Microbiology. 5th ed. Balows A, Hausler JR, Herrmann KL, et al (Eds). Washington, DC, American Society for Microbiology, 1991, p 818.
4. Wilson ML: Clinically relevant, cost-effective clinical microbiology: Strategies to decrease unnecessary testing. Am J Clin Pathol 1997; 107:154.
5. Christenson JC, Overall JC: Proper use of the clinical microbiology laboratory. Pediatr Rev 1995; 16:62.
6. Donowitz GR, Mandell GL: Acute pneumonia. *In*: Principles and Practices of Infectious Diseases. 2nd ed. Mandell GL, Douglas RG, Bennett JE (Eds). New York, John Wiley & Sons, 1985, p 394.
7. Fung JC, Tilton RC: Detection of bacterial antigens by counterimmunoelectrophoresis, coagglutination and latex agglutination. *In*: Manual of Clinical Microbiology. 4th ed. Lennette EH, Balows A, Hausler JR, et al (Eds). Washington, DC, American Society for Microbiology, 1985, p 883.
8. Tenover FC: Molecular methods for the clinical microbiology laboratory. *In*: Manual of Clinical Microbiology. 5th ed. Balows A, Hausler JR, Herrmann KL, et al (Eds). Washington, DC, American Society for Microbiology, 1991, p 119.
9. Tang YW, Procop GW, Persing DH: Molecular diagnosis of infectious disease. Clin Chem 1997; 43:2021.
10. Sandin RL, Rinaldi M: Special considerations for the clinical microbiology laboratory in the diagnosis of infections in the cancer patient. Infect Dis Clin North Am 1996; 10:413.
11. Pfaller MA, Herwaldt LA: The clinical microbiology laboratory and infection control: Emerging pathogens, antimicrobial resistance, and new technology. Clin Infect Dis 1997; 25:858.
12. Horstmeier CD, DeYoung DR, Doerr KA, et al: A comparison of a radiometric method and conventional media for recovery of mycobacteria in clinical specimens (Abstract No. C187). *In*: Abstracts of the 82nd Annual Meeting of the American Society for Microbiology, Washington, DC, 1982.
13. Menegus MA, Douglas RG: Viruses, rickettsia, chlamydia and mycoplasmas. *In*: Principles and Practices of Infectious Diseases. 2nd ed. Mandell GL, Douglas RG, Bennett JE (Eds). New York, John Wiley & Sons, 1985, p 138.
14. Weinstein MP, Towns ML, Quartey SM, et al: The clinical significance of positive blood cultures in the 1990s: A prospective comprehensive evaluation of the microbiology, epidemiology, and outcome of bacteremia and fungemia in adults. Clin Infect Dis 1997; 24:584.
15. Pfaller MA: Typing methods for epidemiological investigation. *In*: Manual of Clinical Microbiology. 5th ed. Balows A, Hausler JR, Herrmann KL, et al (Eds). Washington, DC, American Society for Microbiology, 1991, p 171.
16. National Committee for Clinical Laboratory Standards: Performance Standards for Antimicrobial Susceptibility Testing; Eighth Informational Supplement M100-S8. Wayne, Pa, National Committee for Clinical Laboratory Standards, 1998.
17. Barry AL: The Antimicrobial Susceptibility Test: Principles and Practices. Philadelphia, Lea & Febiger, 1976.
18. Sahm DF, Tenover FC: Surveillance for the emergence and dissemination of antimicrobial resistance in bacteria. Infect Dis Clin North Am 1997; 11:767.
19. Schifman RB, Pindur A, Bryan JA: Laboratory practices for reporting bacterial susceptibility tests that affect antibiotic therapy. Arch Pathol Lab Med 1997; 121:1168.
20. Barry AL, Jones RN, Gavan TL: Evaluation of the Micro-Media system for quantitative antimicrobial susceptibility testing: A collaborative study. Antimicrob Agents Chemother 1978; 13:61.
21. National Committee for Clinical Laboratory Standards: Performance Standards for Antimicrobic Disk Susceptibility Tests. 5th ed. Villanova, Pa, National Committee for Clinical Laboratory Standards, 1993.
22. National Committee for Clinical Laboratory Standards: Performance Standards for Antimicrobial Susceptibility Testing: Fourth Informational Supplement. Villanova, Pa, National Committee for Clinical Laboratory Standards, 1992.
23. Randall EL: State of the art susceptibility testing with the Autobac MTS. *In*: Rapid Methods and Automation in Microbiology. Tilton RC (Ed). Washington, DC, American Society for Microbiology, 1982, p 295.
24. Kelly MT, Latimer JM, Balfour LC: Comparison of three automated systems for antimicrobial susceptibility testing of gram-negative bacilli. *In*: Rapid Methods and Automation in Microbiology. Tilton RC (Ed). Washington, DC, American Society for Microbiology, 1982, p 302.
25. Schoenknecht FD, Sabath LD, Thornsberry C: Special tests. *In*: Manual of Clinical Microbiology. 4th ed. Lenette EH, Balows A, Hausler JR, et al (Eds). Washington, DC, American Society for Microbiology, 1985, p 1.
26. Sanders WG, Sanders CC: Significance of *in vitro* antimicrobial susceptibility tests in care of the infected patient. *In*: Significance of Medical Microbiology in the Care of Patients. Lorain V (Ed). Baltimore, Williams & Wilkins, 1977, p 186.
27. Krogstad DJ, Moellering RC: Antimicrobial combinations. *In*: Antibiotics in Laboratory Medicine. 2nd ed. Lorain V (Ed). Baltimore, Williams & Wilkins, 1986, p 537.
28. McClatchy JK: Antimycobacterial drugs: Mechanisms of action, drug resistance, susceptibility testing, and assays of activity in biological fluids. *In*: Antibiotics in Laboratory Medicine. 2nd ed. Lorain V (Ed). Baltimore, Williams & Wilkins, 1986, p 181.
29. Shadomy S, Pfaller MA; Laboratory studies with antifungal agents: Susceptibility tests and quantitation in body fluids. *In*: Manual of Clinical Microbiology. 5th ed. Balows A, Hausler JR, Herrmann KL, et al (Eds). Washington, DC, American Society for Microbiology, 1991, p 1173.
30. Stratton CW, Weinstein MP, Reller LB: Correlation of serum bactericidal activity with antimicrobial agent level and minimal bactericidal concentration. J Infect Dis 1982; 145:160.
31. Appel GB, Neu HC: The nephrotoxicity of antimicrobial agents. N Engl J Med 1977; 296:722.
32. Pechere JC, Dugal R: Clinical pharmacokinetics of aminoglycoside antibiotics. Clin Pharmacokinet 1979; 4:170.
33. Scott JL, Finegold SM, Belkin GA, et al: A controlled double-blind study of the hematologic toxicity of chloramphenicol. N Engl J Med 1965; 272:1137.
34. Suhrland LG, Weisberger AS: Chloramphenicol toxicity in liver and renal disease. Arch Intern Med 1963; 112:747.

35. Dahlgren JG, Anderson ET, Hewitt WL: Gentamicin blood levels: A guide to nephrotoxicity. Antimicrob Agents Chemother 1975; 8:58.
36. Henderson JL, Polk RE, Kline BJ: *In vitro* inactivation of gentamicin, tobramycin, and netilmicin by carbenicillin, azlocillin, or mezlocillin. Am J Hosp Pharm 1981; 38:1167.
37. Pickering LK, Gearhart P: Effect of time and concentration upon interaction between gentamicin, tobramycin, netilmicin, or amikacin and carbenicillin or ticarcillin. Antimicrob Agents Chemother 1979; 15:592.
38. Pickering LK, Hoecker JL, Kramer WG, et al: Assays for chloramphenicol compared: Radioenzymatic, gas chromatographic with electron capture and gas chromatographic-mass spectrophotometric. Clin Chem 1979; 25:300.
39. Cantu TC, Yamanaka-Yeun NA, Lietman PS: Serum vancomycin concentrations: Reappraisal of their clinical value. Clin Infect Dis 1994; 18:533.
40. Moellering RC: Monitoring serum vancomycin levels: Climbing the mountain because it is there? (Editorial). Clin Infect Dis 1994; 18:544.
41. White A: Serologic diagnosis. *In*: Principles and Practices of Infectious Diseases. Mandell GL, Douglas RG, Bennett JE (Eds). New York, John Wiley & Sons, 1979, p 192.

68

Malaria and Other Tropical Infections in the Intensive Care Unit

Daniel G. Bausch, MD, MPH

Although the spectrum of possible "tropical" infections in a patient with exposures overseas may initially seem daunting, a detailed history of the travel itinerary, activities, and exposures can often significantly narrow the differential diagnosis. This must include more than simply recording the countries to which the patient traveled. Exposures of a business traveler staying at hotels and eating at restaurants in a major city may be drastically different from those of a student backpacking through rural areas of the same country. Knowledge of the endemic area of given diseases, drug resistance patterns, and incubation periods is vital (Table 68-1 and Fig. 68-1). In addition, most "nontropical" infections are also common in developing countries. Thus, although the differential diagnosis must be expanded to include tropical pathogens, common illnesses seen in both developing and industrialized countries must still be considered.

Patients prone to tropical infections can be divided into three groups:

1. Returning travelers who have little or no immunity to tropical pathogens.
2. Persons residing in areas endemic for tropical illnesses who are often immune to disease, if not infection.
3. Individuals originally from endemic areas but now residing elsewhere who have, in the absence of exposure, experienced a waning of their immunity and may again be susceptible.

The degree of immunity may exert profound effects on the presentation and severity of illness. For example, a returning traveler may develop severe malaria at a relatively low parasitemic load, whereas a resident of sub-Saharan Africa with an equal degree of parasitemia may be asymptomatic. Young children, regardless of geographic origin, represent an immunologically naive and thus susceptible group once maternal antibody has waned (past 6 months of age). Genetic differences in susceptibility may also exist, such as resistance to *Plasmodium vivax* in blacks resulting from the absence of Duffy group antigens or the relative protection against all malaria species afforded to those carrying the sickle cell trait.[1]

For returning travelers, knowledge of pretravel vaccinations and prescribed and administered chemoprophylaxis (which often turn out not to be the same) is imperative, although these do not confer 100% protection and should not be used to discard a given entity from the differential diagnosis. Patients as well as physicians frequently err in the adherence to and the prescribing of appropriate prophylactic regimens.[2] Chemotherapy, complete or partial, may prolong the incubation period or may alter the presentation of the illness. Individuals initially from endemic areas are usually less likely to seek pretravel medical advice before making a visit home and also often have considerably more exposures to tropical pathogens during their visit than do short-term travelers from industrialized countries.[3]

Although both returning travelers and travelers hailing from endemic areas may have complicating underlying health conditions, these problems may be less likely to be previously diagnosed in the latter group. Underlying diabetes, hypertension, malnutrition, chronic anemia, intestinal parasites, tuberculosis, and human immunodeficiency virus (HIV) or hepatitis B infection may be discovered at the time of the acute illness.[4] Infection with multiple tropical pathogens is common in those living in endemic areas. Thus, the finding of a given pathogen cannot automatically be assumed to be the cause of the patient's current illness.

MALARIA

Epidemiology and Etiology

Malaria is the most common serious infection in tropical countries as well as in returning travelers and therefore should be considered in any patient reporting travel in endemic areas or with exposure to unscreened blood products ("transfusion malaria") or blood-contaminated needles. Increasing travel and immigration over the past few decades have resulted in increases in imported malaria in the United States and Canada.[5, 6] The risk of acquiring severe *P. falciparum* malaria is highest for those traveling to sub-Saharan Africa and New Guinea, moderate in India, and comparatively low in Southeast Asia and Latin America.[7, 8] In addition, malaria is occasionally reported in individuals without reported travel.[9] This exposure may result from the carriage of malaria-infected passengers (who may be asymptomatic) or anopheline mosquitoes on aircraft arriving from endemic areas. The parasite may then be secondarily transmitted by anopheline mosquitoes endemic in some industrialized countries.

Four *Plasmodium* species cause malaria in humans: *P. falciparum*, *P. vivax*, *P. ovale*, and *P. malariae* (Table 68-2). Although all may produce severe consequences in a debilitated patient, potentially fatal malaria that merits attention in an intensive care unit can be grouped into three categories:

1. Severe complications of *P. falciparum*, most notably cerebral malaria in children and, less commonly, in nonimmune adults (Table 68-3). These account for the vast majority of deaths and chronic sequelae associated with malaria.
2. Splenic rupture, which occurs most frequently with *P. vivax*.
3. Chronic nephrotic syndrome caused by immune complex

Text continued on page 774

TABLE 68–1. Some Tropical Diseases that May Cause Severe Illness Meriting Admission to an Intensive Care Unit

Disease and Organism	Usual Clinical Presentation	Usual Incubation Period	Geographic Distribution	Mode of Transmission and Typical Risk Factors
Protozoa and Helminths				
African trypanosomiasis (*Trypanosoma brucei gambiense* and *T. b. rhodesiense*)*			Sub-Saharan Africa	Tsetse fly bite, camping, safari
Hemolymphatic stage	Systemic febrile illness, lymphadenopathy, hepatosplenomegaly, 30% have history of chancre, rarely DIC and thrombocytopenia	3–21 days		
Meningoencephalitic stage	Headache, somnolence, change in mental status, extrapyramidal and cerebellar signs	Months to years		
Babesiosis (*Babesia* spp.)	Systemic febrile illness, occasionally hepatosplenomegaly	3–28 days	North America, Europe	Tick bite, rarely via blood transfusion; especially severe when splenectomized
Cerebral cysticercosis (*Taenia solium*)	Seizures, headache, change in mental status, muscle pain	Years	Worldwide, especially Latin America and India	Ingestion of cysticerci in contaminated pork (taeniasis), ingestion of *T. solium* eggs in human feces (cysticercosis); areas where pigs allowed to roam free
Cerebral toxoplasmosis (*Toxoplasma gondii*)	Fever, meningoencephalitis, focal neurologic deficits, seizures, change in mental status	Reactivation disease often occurring many years after exposure	Worldwide	Ingestion of cysts in under-cooked meat or oocysts from exposure to cat feces; immunocompromised host
CNS schistosomiasis (*Schistosoma* spp., especially *S. japonicum*)	Encephalopathy, meningoencephalitis, transverse myelitis, seizures	Weeks to months	Africa, Asia, Caribbean, Middle East, South America	Skin penetration of cercaria when swimming or bathing in contaminated water
Eosinophilic meningitis (*Angiostrongylus cantonensis*)	Headache, meningitis, sometimes cranial nerve involvement, fever minimal	1–7 days	Southeast Asia, South Pacific	Ingestion of larvae in undercooked mollusks, crustaceans, or frogs
Fulminant necrotizing colitis or appendicitis caused by *Entamoeba histolytica*	Fever, abdominal pain, bloody diarrhea in colitis, may have perforation	3–21 days	Worldwide	Fecal-oral; most often in malnourished, elderly, or immunocompromised
Leak of rupture of echinococcal cyst (*Echinococcus* spp.)	Allergic symptoms: urticaria, pruritus, anaphylaxis	Years	Worldwide	Ingestion of eggs in feces of infected carnivores such as dogs and wolves; raising of domestic livestock
Malaria				
Plasmodium falciparum	Systemic febrile illness (see text for complications)	8–25 days	Tropics, worldwide	Mosquito bite, transfusion
Plasmodium vivax†	Systemic febrile illness	8–27 days	Tropics, worldwide	Mosquito bite, transfusion
Plasmodium ovale†	Systemic febrile illness	9–17 days	Tropics, worldwide	Mosquito bite, transfusion
Plasmodium malariae	Systemic febrile illness	15–30 days	Tropics, worldwide	Mosquito bite, transfusion
Overwhelming strongyloidiasis (*Strongyloides stercoralis*)	Fever, abdominal pain and distention, shock, pulmonary and CNS involvement common	2–3 wk for initial infection, may be maintained via autoinfection for decades	Worldwide	Skin contact with contaminated soil; miliary training exercises. Dissemination may occur in immunocompromised patients.
Primary amebic meningoencephalitis (*Naegleria fowleri* and *Acanthamoeba* spp.)	Fever, meningoencephalitis	3–7 days	Sporadic areas worldwide	Entry of trophozoite through the nose; swimming in contaminated fresh warm water; hot springs
Visceral leishmaniasis (*Leishmania* spp.)	Systemic febrile illness, weight loss, hepatosplenomegaly, lymphadenopathy, sometimes changes in skin pigmentation	2–21 wk	Tropics, worldwide	Sandfly bite

Table continued on following page

TABLE 68–1. Some Tropical Diseases that May Cause Severe Illness Meriting Admission to an Intensive Care Unit *Continued*

Disease and Organism	Usual Clinical Presentation	Usual Incubation Period	Geographic Distribution	Mode of Transmission and Typical Risk Factors
Viral				
Dengue hemorrhagic fever and dengue shock syndrome	Systemic febrile illness; retro-orbital, joint, and bone pain; petechial rash, bleeding complications, shock	2–7 days	Tropics, worldwide	Mosquito bite
Eastern equine encephalitis	Fever, encephalitis, change in mental status, seizures	4–21 days	Eastern United States, Caribbean, South America	Mosquito bite
Hepatitis A	Systemic febrile illness, light-colored stools, dark urine, jaundice	2–7 wk	Worldwide	Fecal-oral, ingestion of seafood from contaminated seabeds
Hepatitis B	As for hepatitis A	1–5 mo	Worldwide	Sexual transmission, exposure to blood, vertical transmission (mother to child)
Hepatitis D	As for hepatitis A	1–3 mo	Worldwide	Requires coinfection with hepatitis B virus; predominantly blood-borne transmission
Japanese encephalitis	Fever, encephalitis, focal neurologic deficits, seizures	4–21 days	Asia	Mosquito bite, seasonal
Measles	Fever, conjunctivitis, coryza, conjunctivitis, cough, rash, Koplik's spots	5–14 days	Worldwide	Person to person via aerosolized virus
Monkeypox	Fever, diffuse vesicular rash resembling chickenpox but involving palms and soles	3–21 days (?)	Central and West Africa	Person to person as well as exposure to infected squirrels and monkeys
Poliomyelitis	Fever, acute flaccid paralysis, meningeal signs, muscle pain	9–12 days	Worldwide except Western Hemisphere	Person to person
Rabies	Fever, change in mental status, autonomic instability, photophobia, aerophobia, paralysis	20–90 days	Worldwide	Animal bite or bat exposure; spelunking
Tick-borne encephalitis	Fever, encephalitis, focal neurologic deficits, seizures	7–14 days	Central and East Asia, Europe, North Africa, North America	Tick bite
Venezuelan equine encephalitis	Most often system febrile illness, encephalitis in only 1%–4%	4–21 days	Latin America, southern United States	Mosquito bite; areas where equines raised (natural reservoir)
Viral hemorrhagic fevers (Ebola, Marburg, Lassa, Junin, Machupo, Congo-Crimean, Rift Valley, hantaviruses, others)	Variable: usually systemic febrile illness with capillary leak syndrome, may or may not exhibit frank hemorrhage, low cardiac output, shock, ARDS	3–28 days	Select areas worldwide	Exposure to rodent excreta, person to person, tick or mosquito bite, some unknown
Yellow fever	Systemic febrile illness, jaundice, gastrointestinal hemorrhage, delirium, shock	3–6 days	South America, Africa	Mosquito bite
Bacterial				
Anthrax (*Bacillus anthracis*)	Systemic febrile illness with pulmonary involvement (inhalation), abdominal pain and bloody diarrhea (ingestion) and shock, cutaneous ulcer or eschar (skin exposure)	2–10 days	Worldwide	Inhalation, ingestion, or skin exposure to spores; exposure to domestic animals or animal by-products

Botulism (*Clostridium botulinum*)	Bilateral cranial nerve deficits with symmetric descending weakness, fever absent	1–3 days	Worldwide	Toxin ingestion or wound contamination; home-canned foods, soil contamination
Brucellosis (*Brucella* spp.)	Systemic febrile illness, may involve large bones and joints, spine	2–8 wk	Worldwide	Ingestion of contaminated milk; inhalation, skin or conjunctival inoculation from contact with farm animals
Campylobacter (*Campylobacter* spp.)	Fever, abdominal pain and diarrhea, sometimes bloody	1–7 days	Worldwide	Fecal-oral
Typhoid fever (*Salmonella typhi*)	Systemic febrile illness, abdominal pain, rash, intestinal perforation and bleeding	8–28 days	Worldwide	Fecal-oral
Cholera (*Vibrio cholerae*)	Copious "rice water" diarrhea, abdominal pain, severe hypovolemia, fever minimal or absent	1–3 days	Tropics, worldwide	Fecal-oral, ingestion of seafood from contaminated seabeds
Diphtheria (*Clostridium diphtheriae*)	Low-grade fever, cough, pharyngitis, oropharyngeal membrane, neck swelling, mucosal bleeding, myocarditis, polyneuritis	3–7 days	Worldwide, especially temperate areas	Person to person, respiratory transmission as well as through breaks in the skin
Hemolytic uremic syndrome and other virulent *Escherichia coli*	Fever and bloody diarrhea followed by hemolysis and renal failure (HUS); other virulent *E. coli:* systemic febrile illness with abdominal pain and diarrhea, usually not bloody	2–5 days for diarrheal illness with hemolysis and uremia occurring within the following 10 days	Worldwide	Ingestion of poorly cooked meat, fecal-oral
Melioidosis (*Pseudomonas pseudomallei*)	Systemic febrile illness, often with pneumonia or local suppurative infection, shock (especially if immunosuppressed)	2–21 days	Asia, especially Thailand	Exposure to infected animals, person to person (?), often immunocompromised host (usually AIDS)
Oroya fever (*Bartonella bacilliformis*)	Systemic febrile illness, acute anemia, jaundice	2–3 wk	Peru, Ecuador, and Colombia	Sandfly bite; hiking, camping
Pertussis (*Bordetella pertussis*)	Low-grade fever, coryza, rhinorrhea, paroxysmal dry cough	5–21 days	Worldwide	Person to person, adults vaccinated as children again susceptible for milder disease
Plague (*Yersinia pestis*)	Fever, localized tender lymphadenitis ("bubo"), pneumonia in pneumonic plague, shock	2–8 days	Worldwide	Flea bite or person to person; areas of high rat densities
Shigellosis (*Shigella* spp.)	Fever, abdominal pain, dysentery	1–5 days	Worldwide	Fecal-oral
Tetanus (*Clostridium tetani*)	Diffuse muscle spasms, opisthotonos, trismus, autonomic dysfunction	3–21 days	Worldwide	Soil contamination of wound, commonly involves umbilical stump in neonates
Trench fever (*Bartonella quintana*)	Systemic febrile illness, sometimes with skin rash and hepatosplenomegaly	3–38 days	Worldwide	Louse bite; areas of crowding or poor sanitation, more severe in immunocompromised

Table continued on following page

TABLE 68–1. Some Tropical Diseases that May Cause Severe Illness Meriting Admission to an Intensive Care Unit *Continued*

Disease and Organism	Usual Clinical Presentation	Usual Incubation Period	Geographic Distribution	Mode of Transmission and Typical Risk Factors
Rickettsia and Spirochetes				
Boutonneuse fever (*Rickettsia conorii*)	Systemic febrile illness, peripheral rash, eschar at site of tick bite ("tache noire")	7–14 days	Africa, Europe, Middle East, India	Tick bite; camping, safari
Endemic typhus (*Rickettsia typhi*)	Systemic febrile illness, rash in approximately 50%, sometimes seizures or change in mental status	7–14 days	Worldwide	Infected flea feces rubbed into broken skin; situations of high rat densities, can also be transmitted by fleas from cats
Epidemic typhus (*Rickettsia prowazekii*)	Systemic febrile illness, centripetal rash, no eschar	7–14 days	Worldwide, especially cold climates	Infected louse feces rubbed into broken skin; situations of crowding and poor sanitation, refugee camps
Leptospirosis (*Leptospira interrogans*)	Systemic febrile illness, meningitis, rash, minority show hepatorenal syndrome or encephalitis, sometimes pulmonary infiltration and hemorrhage	2–20 days	Worldwide	Exposure to urine or standing water contaminated by urine of many types of mammals; hunting, military exercises
Q fever (*Coxiella burnetti*)	Systemic febrile illness, may manifest pneumonia, endocarditis, hepatitis, osteomyelitis, neurologic abnormalities	14–39 days	Worldwide	Inhalation of organism from products of infected livestock or pets, including milk, urine, feces, and especially birth products; farmers, ranchers
Rat bite fever (*Spirillum minor* or *Streptobacillus moniliformis*)‡	Systemic febrile illness, peripheral rash, sometimes with desquamation, polyarthritis in *S. moniliformis,* eschar or ulcer at site of bite in *S. minor*	2–28 days	Worldwide, especially Asia and North America	Bite of rat or other animal that preys on rats, ingestion of food contaminated by rat
Relapsing fever (*Borrelia* spp.)	Systemic febrile illnesses with recrudescence, rash, neurologic abnormalities	4–18 days	Worldwide	Louse (*Borrelia recurrentis*) or tick bite (various *Borrelia* spp.)
Scrub typhus (*Rickettsia tsutsugamushi*)	Systemic febrile illness, centripetal rash, often lymphadenopathy and eschar at site of tick bite	6–18 days	Asia, Australia, Pacific islands	Mite bite
Fungi				
Aspergillosis (*Aspergillus* spp.)	Fever with pulmonary infiltrates, pulmonary "fungus ball" (aspergilloma), transient infiltrates and allergic symptoms in allergic bronchopulmonary aspergillosis	1–4 wk	Worldwide	Inhalation of spores from soil
Blastomycosis (*Blastomyces dermatitidis*)	Systemic febrile illness, pneumonia; bone, skin, and GU tract involvement	1–4 wk, reactivation may occur	North America, sub-Saharan Africa	Inhalation of spores from soil
Candidiasis (*Candida* spp.)	Mucosal and skin colonization, systemic febrile illness with solid organ involvement in immunosuppressed or those with long-term antibiotic use	1–4 wk	Worldwide	Direct inoculation into skin or mucous membranes, colonization of catheters

Coccidioidomycosis (*Coccidioides immitis*)	Systemic febrile illness, pneumonia, pulmonary cavities, meningeal, skin, and bone involvement	1–4 wk, reactivation may occur in immunocompromised	Dry, desert areas of the Americas	Inhalation of spores from soil; immunocompromised host (usually AIDS)
Chromoblastomycosis (various fungi)	Nodular, hyperkeratotic skin lesions	1–4 wk	Tropics, worldwide	Traumatic implantation of fungus in skin, soil exposure
Cryptococcosis (*Cryptococcus neoformans*)	Often mild meningitis, low-grade fever, nonfocal neurologic examination, sometimes seizures or pulmonary involvement	1–4 wk, reactivation may occur in immunocompromised	Worldwide	Inhalation of spores from soil and bird excreta, especially pigeons; usually immunocompromised host (usually AIDS)
Histoplasmosis (*Histoplasma capsulatum*)	Fever, peumonia, may involve lymph nodes, mediastinum, skin and bone marrow	1–4 wk, reactivation may occur	Tropics, worldwide	Inhalation of spores from soil
Mycetoma (various fungi and bacteria)	Chronic swollen limb with nodules, sinus tracts, drainage of pus and "grains"	Weeks to months	Semidesert areas of Latin America, Africa, and India	Traumatic implantation of fungus in skin, soil exposure
Mucormycosis (various fungi from the order Mucorales)	Fever, CNS infiltration with loss of consciousness, black exudate around mucous membranes of face, pulmonary infiltrates	1–7 days	Worldwide	Inhalation of spores from soil, traumatic inoculation of wound; usually immunocompromised host (diabetes mellitus or steroid use)
Paracoccidioidomycosis (*Paracoccidioides brasiliensis*)	Systemic febrile illness with lung, bone, skin, lymph node, mucous membrane, and adrenal gland involvement	1–4 wk, reactivation may occur	Latin America	Inhalation of spores from soil
Pneumocystosis (*Pneumocystis carinii*)§	Fever, dyspnea, dry cough, hypoxemia, often only mild findings on pulmonary auscultation and CXR	Reactivation disease occurring in immunocompromised host years after infection	Worldwide	Inhalation; immunocompromised host (usually AIDS)
Mycobacteria				
Mycobacterium leprae	Wide range of presentations: hypopigmented skin rash, neurasthenic spots (tuberculoid), multiple nodular lesions (lepromatous)	Months to years??	Worldwide	Unknown
Mycobacterium tuberculosis	Fever, productive cough with pulmonary infiltrates, most commonly upper lobes, often cavities; miliary tuberculosis, meningitis, and GU involvement all also common	Usually reactivation years after infection	Worldwide	Person to person via inhalation
Scrofula (*Mycobacterium scrofulaceum*)	Fever, lymphadenitis	Weeks to months	Worldwide	Soil exposure
Prions				
Creutzfeldt-Jacob disease	Change in mental status, myoclonus, spasticity, rigidity, extrapyramidal and cerebellar signs and symptoms, occasionally seizures	Months to years	Worldwide?	Recipients of cadaveric transplants or injections of biomedical products derived from infected patients, contaminated surgical apparatuses, person to person(?), ingestion of contaminated beef or lamb(?)

**T. b. rhodesiense* typically progresses much faster than *T. b. gambiense*.
†Relapses may appear months to years after initial infection.
‡This disease can be caused by both the spirochete *Spirillum minor* and gram-negative bacteria *Streptobacillus moniliformis*.
§The taxonomy of this organism remains in question. Variably classified among fungi and protozoa.
DIC = disseminated intravascular coagulation; CNS = central nervous system; HUS = hemolytic-uremic syndrome; AIDS = acquired immunodeficiency syndrome; GU = genitourinary; CXR = chest x-ray.

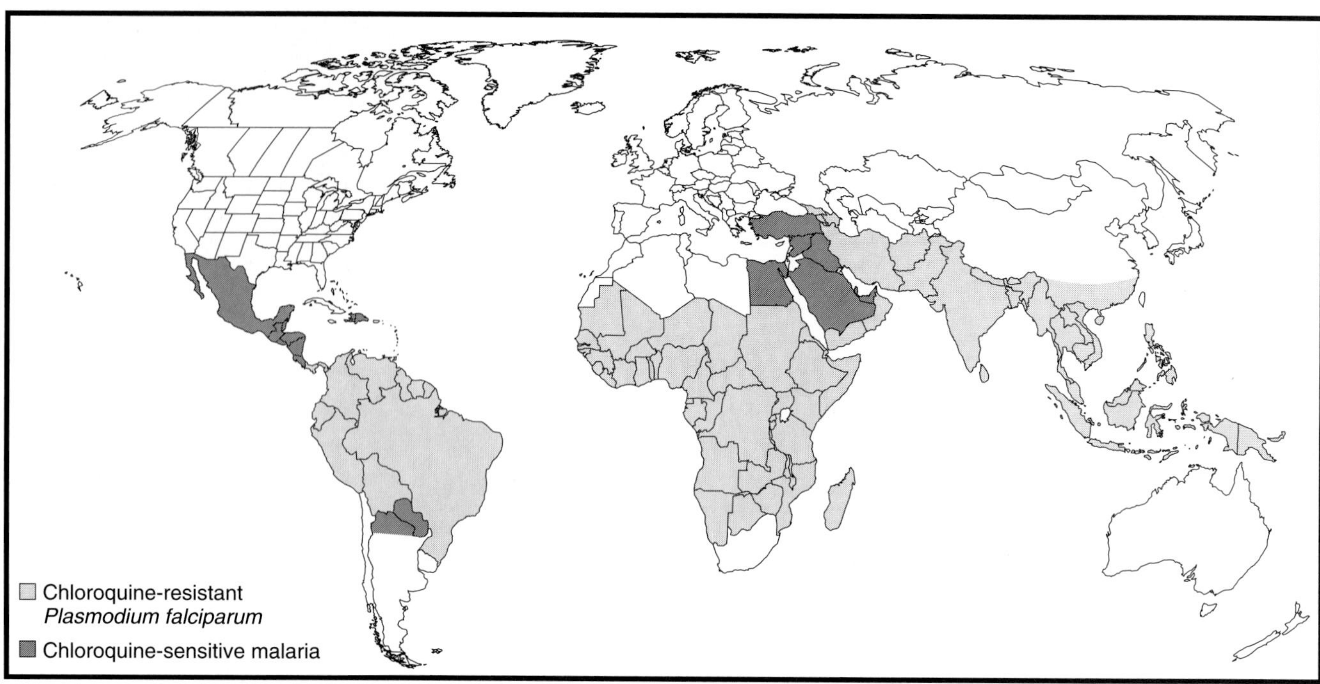

Figure 68–1. Distribution of malaria and chloriquine-resistant *Plasmodium falciparum*, 1997. (Modified from Centers for Disease Control and Prevention [CDC]: Health Information for International Travel 1996–1997. Atlanta, 1997.)

nephritis associated with *P. malariae*, usually seen in children and often complicated by overwhelming bacterial infection.

Uncomplicated Malaria

Malaria is classically described as producing stages of symptoms that progress over an 8- to 12-hour period, constituting a "paroxysm." These correspond to the period of schizont rupture and appearance of ring forms (merozoites) in the blood, which are accompanied by the release of a number of host inflammatory mediators.

The paroxysm classically begins suddenly with a "cold stage" in which the patient experiences rigors and chills, often accompanied by headache, nausea, and vomiting. Intense peripheral vasoconstriction may result in pale, goose-pimpled skin and cyanosis of the lips and nail beds. Within a few hours the "hot stage" ensues, with high fever, flushed skin, throbbing headache, and palpitations. Febrile convulsions may occur in young children. This proceeds to the "defervescent stage" in which a drenching sweat and resolution of the fever occur. The exhausted patient often then sleeps.

Although a classic periodicity is described for the different malaria species (see Table 68–3), this occurs only when the infection has persisted untreated long enough to allow synchronization of schizont rupture. Furthermore, schizont rupture tends to be asynchronous in primary infections, usually the case in returning travelers. Therefore, malaria may often result in persistently spiking fevers difficult to distinguish from fever produced by many other infectious organisms. Thus, the absence of a classic paroxysm and periodicity should not be used to exclude the diagnosis of malaria. The classic paroxysm may be accompanied by cough, myalgias, back pain, postural hypotension, abdominal pain, diarrhea, and weakness. Rash and lymphadenopathy are not typical of malaria and suggest another diagnosis.

Severe Malaria

Most cases of severe malaria are due to *P. falciparum*, which, unlike the other malaria parasites, infects erythrocytes of all

TABLE 68–2. Features of the Four Plasmodial Species of Malaria

Feature	*P. falciparum*	*P. vivax*	*P. ovale*	*P. malariae*
Chloroquine resistance	Yes	No*	No	No
Asexual cycle (hr)	48 (tertian)	48 (tertian)	48 (tertian)	72 (quartan)
Relapse	No	Yes	Yes	No
Characteristic on thin blood film	Rings predominate, multiply infected RBCs, high parasitemia, rings with thread-like cytoplasm, double nuclei, banana-shaped gametocytes	Enlarged RBCs, Schüffner's dots, trophozoite cytoplasm ameboid, 12–24 merozoites in mature schizont	Oval RBCs with fringed edges, Schüffner's dots, trophozoite cytoplasm compact, 6–16 merozoites in mature schizont	Trophozoite cytoplasm compact (band forms), 6–12 merozoites in mature schizont, RBC unchanged

Modified from Miller LH, Warrell DA: Malaria. *In:* Tropical and Geographical Medicine. 2nd ed. Warren KS, Mahmoud AA (Eds). New York, McGraw-Hill, 1990, p 246.
**P. vivax* resistance to chloroquine now reported in some areas of Southeast Asia, Oceania, and South America.
RBC = red blood cell.

TABLE 68–3. Frequent Complications of *Plasmodium falciparum* Malaria

Cerebral malaria
Acute renal failure
Anemia
Pulmonary edema and acute respiratory distress syndrome
Bacterial superinfection and shock
Hypoglycemia
Splenic rupture or tear
Premature labor, abortion, and low birth weight

ages, allowing high levels of parasitemia that often correlate with morbidity and mortality (see Table 68–3). *P. falciparum* causes decreased erythrocyte deformability and the production of small protrusions or "knobs" on erythrocyte membranes that mediate the adhesion of parasitized red blood cells (RBCs) to the venular endothelium. A host of inflammatory mediators, such as tumor necrosis factor-α (TNF-α), interleukin-1, kinins, and reactive nitrogen intermediates, are also produced.[10] These may up-regulate and activate endothelial adhesion molecules, such as intracellular adhesion molecule 1 (ICAM-1) and E-selectin, again promoting vascular adhesion of parasitized cells. The sum total of this cascade is sequestration of parasitized erythrocytes in the microvasculature with resultant sluggish flow, obstruction, impaired oxygen delivery, and organ dysfunction.[10, 11]

The most profound effects are usually on the cerebral capillaries, although a host of tissues may be effected, including the kidney, liver, spleen, placenta, intestine, lung, bone marrow, heart, and retina. Ring hemorrhages may develop at the sites of obstructed vessels, perhaps facilitated by thrombocytopenia resulting from splenic sequestration of platelets. The inflammatory cytokines may also mediate such pathologic processes as hypoglycemia, lactic acidemia, shock, gut mucosal damage, and increased permeability and neutrophil aggregation in the lung. Host genetic as well as parasite strain differences probably play a role in the ultimate course of the disease.

Cerebral Malaria

This is the most frequent severe complication of plasmodium infection, accounting for most fatalities as well as chronic sequelae. Strictly defined, cerebral malaria implies unrousable coma caused by *P. falciparum*.[12] High fevers and febrile convulsions may produce transiently altered mental status without true involvement of the cerebral microvasculature and thus technically do not constitute cerebral malaria. However, in clinical practice, persistent changes in sensorium that cannot be attributed to other processes such as bacterial meningitis or viral encephalitis should be considered cerebral malaria until proved otherwise.

The altered sensorium of cerebral malaria may develop gradually within a few days of onset of illness or manifest as persistent coma after a generalized convulsion. The most common neurologic picture is that of a symmetric upper motor neuron lesion with hypertonia, hyperreflexia, clonus, absent abdominal reflexes, and extensor Babinski's responses. Hypotonia and acute cerebellar ataxia are sometimes seen as well, especially in India and Sri Lanka. There is usually a diffuse, symmetric encephalopathy, sometimes with signs of frontal lobe release such as a pout reflex and bruxism, although there is usually no grasp reflex and the gag reflex is normally maintained. Both decorticate and decerebrate posturing may occur. Meningismus, opisthotonos, and a disconjugate gaze are frequently seen. Nystagmus and a sixth-nerve palsy are more rare. Pupils are usually symmetric with intact pupillary, corneal, oculocephalic, and oculovestibular reflexes. Photophobia, severe neck rigidity, and papilledema are almost never seen.

Seizures may occur in up to 50% of cases of cerebral malaria. Although generalized seizures are classically reported, partial motor seizures, with or without secondary generalization, may occur. Although often showing only diffuse cortical dysfunction, electroencephalographic (EEG) studies may sometimes reveal underlying status epilepticus even when it is not clinically noted.[13]

Acute Renal Failure

Acute renal failure (ARF) is seen in about 30% of adult patients with cerebral malaria but is less common in children. It is usually due to acute tubular necrosis and is most often reversible. Renal ischemia caused by hypovolemia, renal vasoconstriction, microvascular obstruction, and pigment nephropathy related to hemolysis may all contribute. Electrolyte abnormalities such as hyponatremia, hypocalcemia (usually related to albumin loss), hypophosphatemia, and metabolic acidemia as well as fluid overload threatening pulmonary edema may result. "Blackwater fever" refers to a syndrome of high mortality in which ARF occurs in those manifesting low or absent parasitemia. It was classically seen in people of northern European descent working in Africa or South America and thought to be related to immune hemolysis induced by the antimalarial drug quinine.

Anemia

Anemia occurs in virtually all cases of severe *P. falciparum* malaria and is particularly profound in young children.[14] Destruction of parasitized erythrocytes occurs via hemolysis. In addition, erythrocytes may be lost from the circulation because of increased antibody sensitivity, phagocytosis, and removal by the reticuloendothelial system. Furthermore, bone marrow production is inhibited.[15] The degree of anemia generally correlates with the bilirubin level and level of parasitemia. It may be exacerbated by underlying glucose-6-phosphate dehydrogenase deficiency in the setting of administration of oxidant antimalarial drugs and iron deficiency anemia caused by malnutrition. Significant jaundice and hemoglobinuria may result.

Pulmonary Edema and Acute Respiratory Distress Syndrome

Pulmonary complications are typically the most lethal of the complications of malaria, usually occurring late in the course of the illness. Edematous lungs showing interstitial edema and inflammatory cell infiltrates are seen at autopsy in most fatal cases.

Shock

So-called algid malaria, referring to hypotension and shock, may resemble and indeed sometimes be due to secondary gram-negative sepsis. This is often seen in the setting of hyperparasitemia with concomitant hypoglycemia and lactic acidemia and may progress to multiple organ system failure and death. Whether or not bacteria are isolated, a classic septic shock picture is typical, with elevated cardiac index and decreased systemic vascular resistance.[16] Splenic rupture may occasionally be a cause (see later).

Hypoglycemia

This is a frequently seen and sometimes major complication, especially in pregnant women and young children. Although sometimes asymptomatic in pregnancy, this is often manifested by convulsions, impaired consciousness, and extensor posturing. Serum insulin levels are low and lactate, alanine, and counterregulatory hormones appropriately elevated. The administration of quinoline antimalarials can contribute to this hypoglycemia (see later).

Splenic Complications

Splenomegaly is common in infection with all four malaria parasites. Unlike virtually all the other complications of malaria, however, which are more associated with *P. falciparum*, splenic complications are more commonly noted with *P. vivax* infection. Nonimmune patients are at greater risk. Although the term with catastrophic implications "spontaneous splenic rupture" has traditionally been used, in reality a range of hematomas or tears of varying severity may occur. Overeager examiners have been suggested to play a role in the pathogenesis, although no cases of clear palpation-induced rupture have been reported. Fever, tachycardia, vomiting, prostration, abdominal pain or guarding, tender splenomegaly, hypovolemia, and rapidly worsening anemia are common presenting features. Abdominal pain may be localized or diffuse, mild or severe. Shock may ensue. Diaphragmatic irritation after rupture may cause referred pain to the left shoulder, supraclavicular, or scapular regions (Kehr's sign). This is present in about one half of cases and is said to have good specificity for rupture.

Tropical splenomegaly syndrome, also sometimes termed hyperreactive malarial syndrome (HMS), refers to a condition of massive splenomegaly, high titers of total serum immunoglobulin M (IgM) and malaria-specific antibodies, scant or absent parasitemia, and response to antimalarial agents. It is seen in individuals with a history of residence in an endemic area and can be associated with any malaria species. Host genetic factors appear to play a role.[17]

Malaria in Pregnant Women and Children

In addition to being more susceptible to infection, pregnant women and their fetuses are particularly in danger with malaria, with increased risk of maternal and fetal death, premature delivery, and low birth weight. Malaria parasites can often be found in the placenta and may impair oxygen and nutrient transport to the fetus. Disease is most severe in primiparae, especially from nonendemic areas. In contrast, women from endemic areas are usually asymptomatic with the exception of the effects of anemia, again more severe in primiparae. Congenital malaria is rare except in infants born to nonimmune mothers.[18]

Febrile convulsions are common, especially in younger children. As a child becomes older than 3 to 4 years, convulsions become more likely to represent cerebral malaria.[19] As compared with adults with cerebral malaria, children have a shorter history of fever before progressing to coma (average about 2 days). Cough, nausea, vomiting, and diarrhea may be present and falsely suggest a diagnosis other than malaria. Jaundice, pulmonary edema, and ARF are uncommon in children. Conversely, anemia is common and often severe, as are hypoglycemia and its sequelae.

Other Complications

Mild hepatocellular damage may occur and be manifested by elevated liver function tests. This is rarely clinically significant, however. At least theoretically, metabolic clearance of antimalarial medications and lactate could be impaired, and there could be deficits in the production of coagulation factors and albumin. In addition, an association between severe malaria infection and hepatitis B surface antigen carriage has been noted.[20]

Impaired flow in intestinal capillaries with resultant mucosal erosion may explain the gram-negative sepsis occasionally seen. Although subendocardial and epicardial hemorrhages have been noted at autopsy, myocarditis does not occur and primary cardiac events are relatively rare in malaria. In addition to febrile convulsions, hyperpyrexia can cause central nervous system (CNS) damage and, in pregnant women, fetal distress. Disseminated intravascular coagulation (DIC) is seen in less than 10% of severe cases. A host of secondary complications, including aspiration pneumonia, gram-negative septicemia (especially with nontyphoid salmonella), parvovirus infection, and endemic Burkitt's lymphoma may be related to falciparum malaria. Unlike the situation with many other tropical illnesses, there does not appear to be a significant interaction between malaria and HIV infection.[21] Thrombocytopenia, although frequent, is not usually associated with bleeding or correlated with disease severity.

Laboratory and Ancillary Studies

Uncomplicated cases may manifest mild hemolytic anemia, thrombocytopenia, leukopenia (of both neutrophils and lymphocytes), and albuminuria. In severe malaria more profound laboratory abnormalities may be noted, including profound anemia and thrombocytopenia; leukocytosis with a left shift; prolonged coagulation factors sometimes with increased fibrin split products and diminished fibrinogen reflecting DIC; hyponatremia; hypoalbuminemia; hypophosphatemia; lactic acidemia; and elevation of hepatic enzymes, lactate dehydrogenase (LDH), bilirubin, blood urea nitrogen (BUN), and creatinine. Urinalysis may reveal proteinuria, RBCs and RBC casts, and hemoglobinuria. Coagulation defects and thrombocytopenia often correlate with the degree of parasitemia.[21]

Although findings such as increased brain volume and occasionally brain swelling have been noted in computed tomographic (CT) and magnetic resonance imaging (MRI) studies in cerebral malaria, these tests are generally not helpful clinically and are indicated only to rule out suspected mass lesions when the diagnosis of cerebral malaria is not certain.[22]

Diagnosis

Because malaria often presents with nonspecific signs and symptoms, making a clinical diagnosis may be difficult. Although almost all patients have a history of fever, they may frequently be afebrile at the time of examination.[23] Physicians in industrialized countries who are unfamiliar with the disease may not initially include malaria in the differential diagnosis. Delayed diagnosis is frequent and associated with a poor outcome.[3, 24] Although patients with other species of malaria parasite may not present for months or even years after infection, most of those with *P. falciparum* present within 6 months of exposure.[2]

The differential diagnosis includes most febrile illnesses found in the tropics, including typhoid fever, bacterial pneumonia, leptospirosis, relapsing fever, enteropathogenic *Escherichia coli* and other enteric pathogens, influenza, hepatitis, meningococcal infection, rickettsial infections, viral hemorrhagic fevers, and arboviral infections (see Table 68–1). Babesiosis may present both clinically and microscopically similarly to malaria in patients without travel to malaria-endemic areas. Cerebral malaria must be distinguished from bacteria meningitis, the viral meningoencephalitides, metabolic coma, and intoxications.

Specific laboratory diagnosis is made via the examination of thick and thin Giemsa-stained smears. Thick smears are more sensitive in generally diagnosing malaria, and thin smears allow identification of the specific parasite as well as a quantitative assessment of the level of parasitemia. Smears should be taken as soon as the diagnosis of malaria is considered, without waiting for manifestation of a classic paroxysm. Parasitemia may be undetectable in the early stages of the illness, in those from endemic areas who are semi-immune, and in those who have previously self-administered antimalarials, a common practice in malaria-endemic areas.[25] In addition, levels of parasitemia may fluctuate. Thus, repeated smears may be necessary for diagnosis. However, a blood film is unlikely to be falsely negative in a patient with severe disease.[8] Despite this, negative smears should not prevent the prompt administration of antimalarial therapy if the diagnosis is strongly suspected. Conversely, asymptomatic parasitemia is common in children from endemic areas and thus a positive smear does not necessarily signify a clinical case under these circumstances.

Considerable expertise at reading malaria smears may be necessary to distinguish the parasites. Infection with more than one species of malaria parasite is common. The most important point is to distinguish *P. falciparum*, with its concomitant risk of severe complications, from the other plasmodium species (see Table 68-3). Superimposed platelets, particles of stain, pits in the slide, RBC inclusions such as Howell-Jolly bodies and those seen in siderocytes, and other intracellular pathogens such as *Bartonella* and *Babesia* must be distinguished from malaria parasites.

Newer diagnostic modalities, such as the quantitative buffy coat technique, acridine orange staining of blood smears, and the ParaSight-F dipstick test, may be more sensitive than microscopy and aid in the diagnosis of difficult cases.[26] A retrospective diagnosis in nonimmune patients can be made via immunofluorescent antibody testing on acute and convalescent sera.

As cerebral malaria is often indistinguishable from bacterial meningitis, lumbar puncture must be performed in all suspected cases.[27] In cerebral malaria the cerebrospinal fluid (CSF) opening pressure is usually normal. A few lymphocytes and moderate elevation of protein may be seen. High CSF lactate and low glucose indicate a poor prognosis.

CT or MRI scanning of the abdomen is the usual diagnostic modality when splenic rupture is considered, although ultrasonography, arteriography, bleeding scans, or exploratory laparotomy may sometimes be needed.

Management

As delay of therapy is associated with increased mortality, empirical treatment should be implemented immediately in all suspected cases after appropriate blood specimens are obtained.[24] Features that indicate severe disease meriting admission to the intensive care unit (ICU) and urgent intravenous therapy include change in mental status, seizures or other neurologic findings suggestive of cerebral malaria, acute renal failure, pulmonary edema, shock, hypoglycemia, spontaneous bleeding or DIC, acidemia, hyperparasitemia (>250,000 parasitized RBCs per μL or >5% of RBCs), jaundice, hyperpyrexia, and severe anemia. In these critically ill patients, chloroquine-resistant *P. falciparum* should be assumed until proven otherwise. Furthermore, chloroquine-resistant *P. vivax* has now been reported from areas of Southeast Asia, Oceania, and South America.[28, 29]

The quinoline derivatives, quinine and quinidine, administered intravenously every 8 hours, are the drugs of choice in severe malaria. Quinine therapy should be initiated with a loading dose of 16.7 mg base/kg followed by a maintenance dose of 8.3 mg/kg. All doses should be infused over 4 hours. If quinine or mefloquine has been taken within the previous 12 hours, the loading dose is omitted. In the United States, where intravenous quinine is no longer available, quinidine gluconate can be substituted at a loading dose of 10 mg/kg over 1 hour (the maximum is 600 mg for both children and adults), followed by a continuous infusion of 0.02 mg/kg/min.[30] Intravenous therapy should be maintained until the patient can swallow quinine sulfate capsules (600 mg every 8 hours in adults, 25 mg/kg/day divided every 8 hours in children) to complete a total treatment course of 7 days. If the patient requires more than 72 hours of intravenous treatment, the dose should be reduced by 30% to 40% because of decreased renal clearance and volume of distribution. Doses must also be diminished in patients with renal insufficiency.

Commonly occurring side effects of the quinolines are those of "cinchonism": nausea, vomiting, headache, dysphoria, vasodilation, tinnitus, and changes in auditory and visual acuity. These are usually mild at standard doses. Irreversible or severe side effects such as seizures and coma are extremely rare and are usually associated with overdosing or an underlying CNS disorder. The simultaneous use of two quinoline compounds (i.e., mefloquine and quinine) or re-treatment with the same quinoline within a short period of time may predispose to severe side effects.[31] It may be difficult to distinguish possible CNS drug toxicities from the effects of cerebral malaria. Quinidine has, on rare occasions, been associated with psychiatric disorders.[32] In addition to the hypoglycemia often produced by the plasmodium infection itself, hypoglycemia may be due to quinine-induced stimulation of insulin, especially in pregnancy.[33] Hypophosphatemia may be precipitated by intravenous glucose administration and/or quinoline-induced hyperinsulinemia and may disturb CNS function.[23] Levels of digoxin, mefloquine, neuromuscular blocking agents, and oral anticoagulants may all be increased with quinoline administration.

Severe side effects consisting of cardiac conduction abnormalities (prolonged Q-T interval), hypotension, blindness, deafness, and coma may occur when serum quinoline levels exceed 20 mg/L. In addition, bolus injections can cause fatal hypotension and cardiac dysrhythmias. Cardiac monitoring should be performed with intravenous quinoline use, especially with quinidine, which, although more potent against the malaria parasite, is also generally more toxic. Infusion rates of quinidine should be decreased if the Q-T interval increases by more than 25% of its baseline level. Quinine metabolism appears to be decreased in children with kwashiorkor but increased in those with marasmus.[34] Despite the potential cardiac toxicity of various antimalarials and the presence of shock in severe cases, the heart appears remarkably resilient in malaria infection and the mode of death is rarely primary cardiac failure or dysrhythmia.[35]

The level of parasitemia should be monitored via examination of a thin blood smear every 12 hours. A decrease of 75% should be noted within 48 hours of initiating therapy. If this does not occur, a resistant parasite should be considered. Low-level quinine resistance has now been reported in parts of Southeast Asia and sub-Saharan Africa.[36, 37] If resistance is suspected, doxycycline, 100 mg IV every 12 hours, should be added except in pregnant women and young children.[38]

A variety of newer compounds, presently unavailable in the United States, may also be effective: artemisinin and its derivatives appear as efficacious as quinine.[39] The addition of iron chelators such as desferrioxamine has been demonstrated to hasten clearance of the parasite and shorten the duration of cerebral malaria coma, perhaps through depriving the malaria parasite of necessary iron as well as enhancing the T helper immune response and protecting against iron-mediated peroxidant cerebral tissue damage.[40] The newer macrolides, atovaquone, and the antioxidant pentoxifylline may also have therapeutic roles.[41-43] Some of the beneficial effects of antimalarial compounds may be exerted by modification of the host response to malaria infection in addition to their direct effect on the parasite.

Although few controlled data exist, exchange transfusion has been employed in cases of severe disease with high parasitemia with apparent benefit.[44] Beneficial effects may include the reduction of both parasite load and cytokine mediators of inflammation as well as improved oxygen transport.

Careful attention to fluid balance is imperative, especially considering the poor prognosis once acute respiratory distress syndrome or pulmonary edema develops. Measurements of urine output and daily weight should be routinely performed. Monitoring of central venous pressure should be considered in delicate cases, such as those with respiratory distress or compromised renal function. Considering that the prognosis associated with pulmonary failure is considerably poorer than that of ARF, some authors recommend the early use of inotropes rather than excessive fluids in the setting of hypotension.[23] Dialysis is indicated for ARF and may aid not only through improved fluid balance and control of acidemia but also via the removal of circulating cytokine mediators of inflammation. Although observations are limited, the quinolines appear not to be dialyzed.[45] Cautious transfusion of packed RBCs is usually indicated when the hematocrit falls below 20%.[23] Concurrent administration of diuretics or low-dose dopamine may be warranted to avoid fluid overload. Metabolic acidosis should be treated by improving pulmonary gas exchange, correcting hypovolemia, and treating associated septicemia. In patients with profound shock, blood should be drawn for cultures and broad-spectrum antibiotics begun because of the risk of concomitant bacterial septicemia.

Blood glucose should be checked frequently, especially in pregnant patients, and 50% glucose administered when needed. Results of studies on the efficacy of continuous intravenous infusion of 5% dextrose in controlling hypoglycemia have been mixed.[46, 47] Quinoline-induced hypoglycemia may be prevented by the administration of somatostatin analogs followed by glucagon.[48]

Seizures can be prevented with a single intramuscular injection of phenobarbital, 3.5 mg/kg.[49] Trials of the routine administration of iron have not shown efficacy despite the frequent finding of anemia.[50] Although the risk of bleeding is low, aspirin should be avoided in the presence of thrombocytopenia. Steroids are detrimental in severe malaria and should not be used.[51] Although splenectomy may be necessary in those with splenic rupture, many patients can be managed conservatively with supportive therapy.[17]

Malaria therapy in pregnancy raises several special concerns. Although few prospective studies exist, it appears that the quinolines can be given in standard doses in the pregnant patient. Despite theoretical concerns about their abortifacient properties, this has not been shown to be a practical problem even with extensive use.[52] In resistant or refractory cases, intravenous clindamycin, 150 to 900 mg every 8 hours, should be added to the quinoline.[18] Few data are available for the newer antimalarial agents. In late pregnancy fetal monitoring should be begun before the initiation of quinoline therapy so that the effects of the disease can be distinguished from those of drug toxicity. Although fetal distress is usually the result of placental insufficiency, it may sometimes be related to high maternal temperature and hypoglycemia. Thus, these should be carefully monitored and treated accordingly. Fluid balance is particularly crucial in pregnant patients, as the sudden increase in peripheral vascular resistance post partum may precipitate pulmonary edema. Exchange transfusion may be useful. Early obstetric intervention should be considered for the benefit of both mother and fetus.

The principles of management for children are the same as for adults, although doxycycline is contraindicated in those younger than 8 years of age. As febrile convulsions are common and may complicate the presentation by suggesting cerebral malaria, fever should be controlled by the use of acetaminophen, cooling blankets, and baths.

Prognosis

Reported case fatality rates in severe malaria range from 2% to 50%.[53-56] Findings that correlate with a poor prognosis in most studies include respiratory distress or acute respiratory distress syndrome, depth and duration of coma, hypoglycemia, hyperlactemia, biochemical evidence of hepatic or renal dysfunction, multiple seizures, younger age, severe anemia, and treatment in a rural health facility as opposed to an ICU.[21, 23, 57-60] There is a semiquantitative relationship between level of parasitemia and risk of death, especially in nonimmune patients.

Although fewer than 10% of adults with cerebral malaria have persistent neurologic sequelae, this number may be as high as 40% in children, especially if hypoglycemia occurred.[46, 53] Commonly seen sequelae include hemiparesis, cerebellar ataxia, and extrapyramidal rigidity.[55] Children who survive without obvious neurologic sequelae appear to develop normally neuropsychologically.[61]

OTHER TROPICAL INFECTIONS

Although fevers occurring in individuals with exposures in the tropics should be considered to be malaria until proven otherwise, the differential diagnosis is broad. Table 68–1 gives an overview of nonmalarial illnesses that may be considered.

References

1. Frideman MJ: Erythrocytic mechanism of sickle-cell resistance to malaria. Proc Natl Acad Sci U S A 1978; 75:1994–1997.
2. Svenson JE, MacLean JD, Gyorkos TW, et al: Imported malaria. Arch Intern Med 1995; 155:861–868.
3. Moore TA, Tomayko JF, Wierman AM, et al: Imported malaria in the 1990s. Arch Fam Med 1994; 3:130–136.
4. Adebajo AO, Smith DJ, Hazleman BL, et al: Seroepidemiological associations between tuberculosis, malaria, hepatitis B, and AIDS in West Africa. J Med Virol 1994; 42:366–368.
5. Lackritz EM, Lobel HO, Howell BJ, et al: Imported *Plasmodium falciparum* malaria in American travelers to Africa. JAMA 1991; 265:383–385.
6. Yechouron A, Nguyen C, MacLean JD, et al: The changing pattern of imported malaria. Can Dis Wkly Rep 1988; 14:133–136.
7. Lewis SJ, Davidson RN, Ross EJ, et al: Severity of imported falciparum malaria: Effect of taking anti-malarial prophylaxis. Br Med J 1992; 305:741–743.
8. Centers for Disease Control: Recommendations for the prevention of malaria among travelers. MMWR Morb Mortal Wkly Rep 1990; 47:1–10.
9. Centers for Disease Control: Probable locally acquired mosquito-transmitted *Plasmodium vivox* infection—Georgia, 1996. MMWR Morb Mortal Wkly Rep 1997; 46:264–267.
10. Miller LH, Good MF, Milon G: Malaria pathogenesis. Science 1994; 264:1878–1883.
11. Turner G: Cerebral malaria. Brain Pathol 1997; 7:569–582.
12. Warrell DA, Molyneux ME, Beales PF: Severe and complicated malaria. Trans R Soc Med Hyg 1990; 84(Suppl 2):1–65.
13. Crawley J, Smith S, Kirkham F, et al: Seizures and status epilepticus in childhood cerebral malaria. Q J Med 1996; 89:591–597.
14. Allen SJ, O'Donnell, Alexander ND, et al: Severe malaria in children in Papua New Guinea. Q J Med 1996; 89:779–788.
15. Phillips RE, Pasvol G: Anaemia of *Plasmodium falciparum* malaria. Baillieres Clin Haematol 1993; 5:315–330.
16. Bruneel F, Gachot B, Timsit JF, et al: Shock complicating severe falciparum malaria in European adults. Intensive Care Med 1997; 23:698–701.
17. Zingmand BS, Viner BL: Splenic complications in malaria: Case report and review. Clin Infect Dis 1993; 16:223–232.

18. Silver HM: Malarial infection during pregnancy. Infect Dis Clin North Am 1997; 11(1):99-107.
19. Wattanagoon Y, Srivilairit S, Looareesuwan S, et al: Convulsions in childhood malaria. Trans R Soc Trop Med Hyg 1994; 88:426-428.
20. Thuraz MR, Kwiatkowski D, Torok ME, et al: Association of hepatitis B surface antigen carriage with severe malaria in Gambian children. Nat Med 1995; 1:374-375.
21. Niyongabo T, Deloron P, Aubry P, et al: Prognostic indicators in adult cerebral malaria: A study in Burundi, an area of high prevalence of HIV infection. Act Trop 1994; 56:299-305.
22. Looareesuwan S, Wilairatana P, Krishna S, et al: Magnetic resonance imaging of the brain in patients with cerebral malaria. Clin Infect Dis 1995; 21:300-309.
23. Blumberg L, Lee RP, Lipman J, et al: Predictors of mortality in severe malaria: A two year experience in a non-endemic area. Anaesth Intensive Care 1996; 24:217-223.
24. Greenberg AE, Lobel HO: Mortality from *Plasmodium falciparum* malaria in travelers from the United States, 1959-1987. Ann Intern Med 1990; 113:326-327.
25. Snow RW, Peshu N, Forster D, et al: The role of shops in the treatment and prevention of childhood malaria on the coast of Kenya. Trans R Soc Trop Med Hyg 1992; 86:237-239.
26. Craig MH, Sharp BL: Comparative evaluation of four techniques for the diagnosis of *Plasmodium falciparum* infections. Trans R Soc Trop Med Hyg 1997; 91:279-282.
27. Wright PW, Avery WG, Ardill WD, et al: Initial clinical assessment of the comatose patient: Cerebral malaria vs. meningitis. Pediatr Infect Dis J 1993; 12(1):37-41.
28. Phillips EJ, Keystone JS, Kain KC: Failure of combined chloroquine and high dose primaquine therapy for *Plasmodium vivax* malaria acquired in Guyana, South America. Clin Infect Dis 1996; 23:1171-1173.
29. Longworth MD: Drug-resistant malaria in children and travelers. Pediatr Clin North Am 1995; 42:649-654.
30. Centers for Disease Control: Intravenous quinidine gluconate in the treatment of severe *Plasmodium falciparum* infections. MMWR 1985; 34:371.
31. Phillips-Howard PA, ter Kuile FO: CNS adverse events associated with antimalarial agents. Drug Saf 1995; 12:370-383.
32. Deleu D, Schmedding E: Acute psychosis as idiosyncratic reaction to quinidine: Report of two cases. BMJ 1987; 294:1001-1002.
33. Davis TM, Suputtamongkol Y, Spencer JL, et al: Glucose turnover in pregnant women with acute malaria. Clin Sci (Colch) 1994; 86:83-90.
34. Treluyer JM, Roux A, Mugnier C, et al: Metabolism of quinine in children with global malnutrition. Pediatr Res 1996; 40:558-563.
35. Bethell DB, Phuong PT, Phuong CX et al: Electrocardiographic monitoring in severe falciparum malaria. Trans R Soc Trop Med Hyg 1996; 90:266-269.
36. Pukrittayakamee S, Supanaranond W, Looareesuwan S, et al: Quinine in severe falciparum malaria: Evidence of declining efficacy in Thailand. Trans R Soc Trop Med Hyg 1994; 88:324-327.
37. Jelinek T, Schelbert P, Loscher T, et al: Quinine resistant falciparum malaria acquired in east Africa. Trop Med Parasitol 1995; 46(1):38-40.
38. Waiz A, Hossain MR, Chakraborty B, et al: Triple drug therapy with quinine, cotrimoxazole and tetracycline in the management of cerebral malaria—a review of 254 cases. Bangladesh Med Res Counc Bull 1995; 21(2):77-80.
39. Van Hensbroek MB, Onyiorah E, Jaffar S, et al: A trial of artemether or quinine in children with cerebral malaria. N Engl J Med 1996; 335:69-75.
40. Mabeza GF, Biemba G, Gordeuk VR: Clinical studies of iron chelators in malaria. Act Haematol 1996; 95(1):78-86.
41. Tarlow MJ, Block SL, Harris J, et al: Future indications for macrolides. Pediatr Infect Dis J 1997; 16:457-462.
42. De Alencar FE, Cerutti C Jr, Durlacher RR, et al: Atovaquone and proguanil for the treatment of malaria in Brazil. J Infect Dis 1997; 175:1544-1547.
43. Di Perri G, Di Perri IG, Monteiro GB, et al: Pentoxifylline as a supportive agent in the treatment of cerebral malaria in children. J Infect Dis 1995; 171:1317-1322.
44. Vachon F, Wolff M, Lebras J, et al: Exchange transfusion as an adjunct to the treatment of severe falciparum malaria. Clin Infect Dis 1992; 14:1269-1270.
45. Sukontason K, Karbwang J, Rimchala W, et al: Plasma quinine concentrations in falciparum malaria with acute renal failure. Trop Med Int Health 1996; 1:236-242.
46. Taylor TE, Molyneux ME, Wirima JJ, et al: Blood glucose levels in Malawian children before and during the administration of intravenous quinine for severe falciparum malaria. N Engl J Med 1988; 319:1040-1047.
47. White NG, Warrell DA, Chantahvanich P, et al: Severe hypoglycemia and hyperinsulinemia in falciparum malaria. N Engl J Med 1983; 309:61-66.
48. Phillips RE, Warrell DA, Looareesuwan S, et al: Effectiveness of SMS 201-995, a synthetic, long-acting somatostatin analogue, in treatment of quinine-induced hyperinsulinaemia. Lancet 1986; 1:713-716.
49. White NJ, Looareesuwan S, Philips RE, et al: Single dose phenobarbitone prevents convulsions in cerebral malaria. Lancet 1988; ii:64-66.
50. Van den Hombergh J, Dalderop E, Smit Y: Does iron therapy benefit children with severe malaria-associated anaemia? A clinical trial with 12 weeks supplementation of oral iron in young children from the Turiani Division, Tanzania. J Trop Pediatr 1996; 42:220-227.
51. Hoffman SL, Rustama D, Pnujabi NH, et al: High-dose dexamethasone in quinine-treated patients with cerebral malaria: A double-blind, placebo-controlled trial. J Infect Dis 1988; 158:325-331.
52. Phillips-Howard PA, Wood D: The safety of antimalarial drugs in pregnancy. Drug Saf 1996; 14:131-145.
53. Genton B, al-Yaman F, Alpers MP, et al: Indicators of fatal outcome in paediatric cerebral malaria: A study of 134 comatose Papua New Guinean children. Int J Epidemiol 1997; 26:670-676.
54. Van Hensbroek MB, Palmer A, Jaffar S, et al: Residual neurologic sequelae after childhood cerebral malaria. J Pediatr 1997; 131:125-129.
55. Bajiya HN, Kochar DK: Incidence and outcome of neurological sequelae in survivors of cerebral malaria. J Assoc Physicians India 1996; 44:679-681.
56. Jaffar S, Van Hensbroek MB, Palmer A, et al: Predictors of a fatal outcome following childhood cerebral malaria. Am J Trop Med Hyg 1997; 57:20-24.
57. Olumese PE, Sodeinde O, Gbadegesin RA, et al: Respiratory distress adversely affects the outcome of childhood cerebral malaria. Trans R Soc Trop Med Hyg 1995; 89:634.
58. Mabeza GF, Moyo VM, Thuma PE, et al: Predictors of severity of illness on presentation in children with cerebral malaria. Ann Trop Med Parasitol 1995; 89:221-228.
59. Marsh K, Forster D, Waruiru C, et al: Indicators of life-threatening malaria in African children. N Engl J Med 1995; 332:1399-1404.
60. Zucker JR, Lackritz EM, Ruebush TK 2nd, et al: Childhood mortality during and after hospitalization in western Kenya: Effect of malaria treatment regimens. Am J Trop Med Hyg 1996; 55:655-660.
61. Muntendam AH, Jaffar S, Bleichrodt N, et al: Absence of neuropsychological sequelae following cerebral malaria in Gambian children. Trans R Soc Trop Med Hyg 1996; 90:391-394.

69

Antimicrobial Resistance and Other Epidemiologic Considerations in the Intensive Care Unit

Michael Edmond, MD, MPH

Each year in the United States, nosocomial infections develop in 5% to 10% of hospitalized patients and cause the death of 80,000 patients.[1] The Centers for Disease Control and Prevention (CDC) report that the incidence of nosocomial infections is increasing, and nosocomial infections are now the fourth leading cause of death in the United States.[1]

During the 1990s, both the number of critical care beds and the proportion of hospital beds in intensive care units (ICUs) have risen as an expanding proportion of patients are managed in the outpatient setting. As technology has advanced, it has also for the most part become more invasive, leaving the body's normal defensive barriers damaged and the potential for development of infection greatly increased. Moreover, we have witnessed a growing proportion of immunosuppressed patients in the ICU setting, and there is no other area in the hospital where the usage of antimicrobial agents is as dense. Last, the poor compliance of health care workers with hand washing and other infection control measures enables nosocomial pathogens to travel from patient to patient. Thus, the ICU is an epicenter for nosocomial infections and the development of antibiotic resistance.

This chapter focuses on the problems of antimicrobial resistance and the prevention of nosocomial infections in the ICU.

ANTIMICROBIAL RESISTANCE

In a 1997 CDC-sponsored surveillance study at eight hospitals, antimicrobial resistance was more commonly encountered in ICU patients than in ward patients and outpatients.[2] Specifically, rates of methicillin resistance in *Staphylococcus aureus* and coagulase-negative staphylococci, ceftazidime resistance in *Enterobacter cloacae* and in *Pseudomonas aeruginosa*, and vancomycin resistance in enterococci were significantly higher in the ICU setting. On the basis of this study, epidemiologists at the CDC have recommended that resources directed toward control of antimicrobial resistance should be particularly focused on the ICU setting.[2]

During the 1980s and 1990s, a shift in nosocomial pathogens has resulted in the emergence of pathogens of relatively low intrinsic virulence. These organisms proliferated with the ability to support bodily functions by mechanical means, the use of invasive devices for diagnosis and therapy, and the introduction of intensely broad-spectrum antimicrobial agents. These "new" pathogens included the coagulase-negative staphylococci, enterococci, and *Candida*. All three groups have become increasingly antibiotic-resistant in recent years. Thus, there has been a trend toward nosocomial infections caused by organisms that are relatively nonvirulent but antibiotic-resistant, although virulent organisms, such as *S. aureus* and gram-negative bacilli, remain problematic in the critical care setting. Three groups of pathogens, *S. aureus*, enterococci, and the Enterobacteriaceae, are examined in further detail.

Staphylococcus aureus

Staphylococcus aureus has played an important role in American hospitals for several decades. Within a few years after the introduction of penicillin, the first reports of penicillinase-producing strains were reported. These strains became increasingly common in the 1950s, and today, very few strains of *S. aureus* are susceptible to penicillin G. In the early 1960s, the penicillinase-resistant penicillins were introduced; however, within a year of the introduction of methicillin, methicillin-resistant strains of *S. aureus* (MRSA) were detected.

Until the 1970s, methicillin resistance remained uncommon in the United States. Since that time, resistant strains have become increasingly prevalent. In 1975, only 2% of *S. aureus* strains causing nosocomial infections were methicillin-resistant; by 1996, 35% of strains were.[3] Most MRSA strains currently exhibit resistance to other antibiotics, including erythromycin, clindamycin, and tetracycline. The rate of methicillin resistance in parts of Europe is even worse. In a very large point prevalence study conducted in 1992 and involving more than 1400 European ICUs and 10,000 patients, 60% of *S. aureus* isolates causing nosocomial infections were found to be resistant to methicillin.[4]

In 1996, Hiramatsu and colleagues[5] isolated the first strain of *S. aureus* from a clinical specimen that did not display full susceptibility to vancomycin. The organism was isolated from a sternal wound infection of a child and displayed a vancomycin minimum inhibitory concentration (MIC) of 8 μg/mL. Soon thereafter, it was determined that 20% of *S. aureus* isolates in the index hospital displayed the same resistance pattern, and many other Japanese hospitals were also detecting such isolates.[6] One year later, two patients in the United States were found to be infected with strains of methicillin-resistant *S. aureus* that had reduced susceptibility to vancomycin (MIC = 8 μg/mL).[7]

In the three patients described in these studies, prolonged courses of vancomycin had been administered prior to detection of the strains with reduced vancomycin susceptibility. Moreover, high-level vancomycin resistance has been experimentally transferred from *Enterococcus faecalis* to *S. aureus* in both in vitro and in vivo models.[8] Thus, strains of *S. aureus* with intermediate resistance to vancomycin have emerged, and the specter of fully resistant strains looms on the horizon. Given the virulent nature of *S. aureus*, high-level resistance to vancomycin will likely portend high rates of mortality in infected patients.

All clinical isolates of *S. aureus* should be tested for vancomycin susceptibility.[9] Because initial identification of vancomycin-resistant *S. aureus* may be laboratory error stemming from culture of *S. aureus* mixed with other organisms, cultures should be repeated to obtain a pure *S. aureus* strain.

The primary site of colonization by MRSA is the anterior nares. From there, other parts of the body may become colonized, most notably the axillae, groin, and perineal area. Colonization with *S. aureus* is intermittent in 50% of the population and prolonged in 30%; 20% of people never become colonized.[10] The estimated half-life of nasal colonization is 40 months.[11] From the epidemiologic standpoint, the colonized but uninfected patient is important, because such a patient may serve as a reservoir for transmission of MRSA to other patients in the hospital, usually via transient hand contamination of health care workers. Health care workers may themselves become colonized and serve as a reservoir for transmission to patients.

Contact precautions (described later) should be instituted for patients found to be colonized or infected with MRSA.

Enterococci

The enterococci are well-designed to function as important nosocomial pathogens. Because they are part of the normal gut flora in most humans, they are ubiquitous organisms. They exhibit intrinsic resistance to numerous antimicrobials and have acquired resistance to essentially all antibiotics to which they have been exposed. Hardy physical characteristics allow them to survive in the environment for prolonged periods. Lastly, contamination of the hands of health care workers who are noncompliant with hand-washing protocols provide the potential for spread from patient to patient in the hospital setting.

Overall, enterococci account for 10% of all infections occurring in the hospital.[12] Currently, the enterococci are the third most common cause of nosocomial bloodstream infections, accounting for 11% of these infections (SCOPE* Project, 1998, unpublished data). In a study of 110 severe enterococcal infections, Patterson and associates[13] found that nearly half the cases occurred in the ICU.

Enterococci are intrinsically resistant to penicillin (relative resistance), pencillinase-resistant penicillins, cephalosporins, clindamycin, trimethoprim-sulfamethoxazole, and low levels of aminoglycosides. Acquired high-level resistance of enterococci to aminoglycosides was reported in 1970 for streptomycin and in 1979 for gentamicin. Vancomycin resistance for these organisms was first reported in 1986 in Europe[14] and soon spread to the United States. By the early 1990s, many hospitals in the eastern United States were isolating enterococcal strains resistant to all available antimicrobials. These strains are now endemic in many institutions.

Vancomycin-resistant enterococci (VRE) play a pathogenic role in intra-abdominal infections, surgical wound infections, bloodstream infections, and urinary tract infections. Numerous case-control studies have evaluated risk factors for the development of VRE colonization and infection. The antimicrobial agents that have been identified as risk factors are vancomycin,[15-22] third-generation cephalosporins,[19, 21, 23-25] ciprofloxacin,[18] and antianaerobic agents (metronidazole, imipenem, and clindamycin).[26, 27]

The other risk factors for colonization and infection by VRE in a hospitalized patient are as follows:

- Prolonged hospital stay[15, 16, 28, 29]
- ICU stay[22, 23, 27]
- Proximity to other patients with VRE[30]
- Care from a nurse caring for patients with VRE[30]
- Neutropenia[25]
- Intestinal colonization with VRE[26]
- Hematologic malignancy[20]
- Severe illness[18, 20]
- Bone marrow transplantation[20]
- Liver transplantation[21]

Thus, patients in the ICU setting may have multiple risk factors for colonization and infection by VRE.

Enterobacteriaceae

The family Enterobacteriaceae contains numerous genera, many of which are part of the normal human intestinal flora. Some of these organisms, however, are also important causes of nosocomial infections, including *Escherichia coli*, *Citrobacter* species, *Enterobacter* species, *Klebsiella* species, *Proteus* species, and *Serratia* species. Typical sites of infection are the urinary tract, the respiratory tract, surgical wounds, and the bloodstream.

*SCOPE = Surveillance and Control of Pathogens of Epidemiologic Importance.

Resistance in these organisms occurs via numerous mechanisms, a complete discussion of which is beyond the scope of this chapter. The important classes of antimicrobials to which the enteric organisms have acquired resistance are the aminoglycosides, quinolones, and β-lactams.

Studies from ICUs have shown that rates of resistance to the aminoglycosides vary according to the individual drug, bacterial species, site of infection, and prior exposure to this class of drugs.[31, 32] Rates of susceptibility correlate with achievable drug concentrations at that site (i.e., isolates from sites with the highest concentrations of aminoglycosides exhibit the highest rates of aminoglycoside susceptibility). Analysis of susceptibility rates by body site shows the following pattern[31]:

Urine > Blood > Wound > Respiratory tract

In studies from critical care units, amikacin retains the greatest activity (>90% of isolates susceptible),[31] followed by tobramycin (69% to 88% susceptible),[31-33] with gentamicin as the least active (40% to 72% susceptible).[31-33]

Ciprofloxacin activity against the enteric gram-negative organisms varies by pathogen and by geographic area.[31-34] In the United States, these organisms are generally susceptible.[31, 34] It should be noted, however, that one gram-negative pathogen common in the ICU but not of the Enterobacteriaceae family, *P. aeruginosa*, has become increasingly resistant to ciprofloxacin.[34]

Although resistance to the β-lactams can occur via several mechanisms, the most prevalent mechanism of resistance is the production of β-lactamases. Numerous β-lactamases have been described. In the Enterobacteriaceae, extended-spectrum β-lactamases have become increasingly prevalent since their first description in the early 1980s. These enzymes inactivate the expanded-spectrum cephalosporins (e.g., cefotaxime, ceftazidime, ceftriaxone) and aztreonam. In a national surveillance study conducted from 1987 to 1991, 40% of nosocomial *Enterobacter* infections were found to be resistant to ceftazidime. Moreover, ICU stay was identified as an independent predictor of ceftazidime resistance in *Enterobacter* and *Klebsiella pneumoniae* nosocomial infections.[35] In another large study of antimicrobial resistance in U.S. ICUs, one third of *Enterobacter* isolates were resistant to ceftazidime.[31] Repeated cultures of *Enterobacter* from ICU patients show an increase in resistance (13% to 28%).[32, 36]

PREVENTION AND CONTROL OF NOSOCOMIAL INFECTIONS AND ANTIBIOTIC RESISTANCE IN THE CRITICAL CARE UNIT

A multifaceted approach is required to prevent the development and transmission of nosocomial infections as well as the development of antibiotic resistance. Four concurrent processes are essential: hand washing, isolation techniques, prudent use of antimicrobials, and surveillance for nosocomial infections.

Hand Washing

Because the majority of nosocomial infections are transmitted via the contact route, primarily via the hands of health care workers,[37] it seems intuitively obvious that hand washing is vital to prevent hospital-acquired infections. In fact, hand washing remains the single most important means of preventing the transmission of nosocomial pathogens. Nonetheless, observational studies in ICUs have found that hand-washing compliance by health care workers is generally less than

50% and in some units may be less than 20%.[38–43] Most of these studies have also shown that hand-washing compliance by physicians lags behind that of other members of the health care team.[38, 39, 41, 42] It has been estimated that a 1.5-fold to twofold increase in hand-washing compliance would result in a 25% to 50% decrease in the incidence of nosocomial infections.[40] Unfortunately, most studies designed to improve hand-washing compliance have not demonstrated a lasting positive effect on the behavior of health care workers.

The microorganisms on the hand can be divided into transient flora and resident flora.[44] The *resident* flora comprises coagulase-negative staphylococci, *Micrococcus*, and *Corynebacterium*. These organisms are generally of low virulence and are rarely transmitted to patients except when introduced via invasive procedures.[45] They are not easily removed through hand washing. The *transient* flora, however, are important causes of nosocomial infections. These organisms are acquired primarily by contact, are loosely attached to the skin, and are easily washed off. The purpose of hand washing in the hospital is to remove the transient flora recently acquired through contact with patients or environmental surfaces.[45]

Health care workers should wash their hands thoroughly before and after each patient contact. In critical care units in hospitals with high rates of antibiotic-resistant organisms, medicated hand-washing agents should be used instead of bland soap. Studies have shown that chlorhexidine and isopropyl alcohol are superior to bland soap and water in the removal of vancomycin-resistant enterococci and multiply-resistant gram-negative organisms from the hands.[46] However, chlorhexidine has the advantage of producing a residual antibacterial effect (i.e., a previous hand wash may kill organisms newly introduced onto the hands of health care workers before the next hand wash occurs).[47] Moreover, in a large trial comparing chlorhexidine with 60% isopropyl alcohol as a hand-washing agent in three ICUs at the University of Iowa, Doebbeling and colleagues[40] demonstrated that use of chlorhexidine resulted in a significantly lower nosocomial infection rate. Thus, chlorhexidine appears to be the agent of choice in the ICU.

To encourage compliance with hand washing, sinks in the ICU should be readily accessible and optimally in the immediate vicinity of each bed. In areas where sinks are not close by, wall-mounted dispensers with medicated, alcohol-based waterless agents should be installed. When the hands are visibly soiled, however, waterless agents alone are not adequate.

Gloves

Gloves should be worn by health care workers to prevent contamination of the hands with microorganisms, to prevent exposure of the health care worker to blood-borne pathogens, and to reduce the risk of transmission of microorganisms from the hands of the health care worker to the patient. Unfortunately, some health care workers mistakenly believe that the use of gloves reduces the need for hand washing. Contamination of the hands may occur, however, with organisms on the surface of the gloves as they are removed,[48] and some gloves have small tears that may allow organisms to contaminate the hands. Thus, gloves should be viewed as a protective barrier but not as a substitute for hand washing.

Isolation in the Intensive Care Unit

The latest version of isolation guidelines from the CDC is much easier to understand and implement than previous iterations. In this system, two tiers of isolation are utilized: (1) *standard* precautions for all patients and (2) *transmission-based* precautions for patients who have certain confirmed or suspected infectious processes.

Standard Precautions

Standard precautions, which have replaced "universal precautions," are designed to (1) protect the health care worker from blood-borne pathogens and (2) reduce the potential for transmission of pathogens. Standard precautions apply to the following[49]:

- Blood
- All body secretions and excretions (except sweat)
- Nonintact skin
- Mucous membranes

Essential elements of standard precautions are outlined in Table 69–1.

Transmission-Based Precautions

Three categories of transmission-based precautions have been developed:

- Airborne
- Droplet
- Contact

Essential elements of transmission-based precautions are shown in Table 69–1. Clinical scenarios and pathogens that warrant these precautions are delineated in Table 69–2.

Airborne Precautions

Airborne precautions are designed to prevent the transmission of organisms by droplet nuclei or dust particles; these agents are limited to *Mycobacterium tuberculosis*, varicella-zoster virus, and measles virus. Thus, airborne precautions should be used for patients with confirmed or suspected active pulmonary or laryngeal tuberculosis, varicella, measles, or disseminated zoster, and for immunosuppressed patients with localized zoster.[49]

Airborne precautions require special engineering considerations with regard to air handling. Specifically, the isolation room must be maintained at negative pressure in comparison with air in the areas outside the room to prevent droplet nuclei from wafting out of the room and into adjacent areas. In addition, air in the isolation room should ideally be exhausted to the outdoors; when this cannot be accomplished, the air should be passed through high-efficiency filters.[50]

Federal regulations require that respiratory protection be worn by all persons entering the isolation room. Masks approved by the National Institute for Occupational Safety and Health for such use must be able to filter 1-μm particles with an efficiency of 95% (N-95 masks). Health care workers who are to wear these masks must be fit-tested for them and taught to check their masks for fit each time they are used.[50]

Although every ICU does not need the ability to provide airborne isolation, medium-sized and large hospitals should have the capability to provide airborne isolation in the critical care setting. For hospitals with multiple critical care units considering the retrofitting of existing rooms to provide airborne isolation, it may be more economical to put multiple isolation rooms in one ICU to serve all critical care settings rather than putting an airborne isolation room in each unit.

Droplet Precautions

Droplet precautions are implemented to prevent the transmission of organisms via droplets generated when the infected patient coughs, sneezes, or talks or when procedures are performed in such a patient that may induce coughing (e.g., suctioning, bronchoscopy). A health care worker who approaches within 3 feet of patients infected with droplet-transmissible agents should wear a mask to prevent contact of

TABLE 69–1. Essential Elements of Standard and Transmission-Based Isolation Precautions*

		Transmission-Based Precautions		
Element	**Standard Precautions**	***Airborne Precautions***	***Droplet Precautions***	***Contact Precautions***
Room	Private room for patients who contaminate the environment or cannot maintain appropriate hygiene	Negative-pressure, private room with air exhausted to outdoors or through high-efficiency filtration Keep door closed	Private room Door may remain open	Private room Dedicate use of noncritical patient-care items to a single patient
Masks	For procedures or activities likely to generate splashes or sprays of blood, body fluids, secretions, or excretions	N-95 mask or portable respirator for those entering room Surgical mask should be placed on patient's face for transport outside isolation room	For entering room Surgical mask should be placed on patient's face for transport outside isolation room	
Face shield and eye protection	For procedures or activities likely to generate splashes or sprays of blood, body fluids, secretions, or excretions			
Gowns	For procedures or activities likely to generate splashes or sprays of blood, body fluids, secretions, or excretions			If clothing will contact patient, surfaces, items in room If patient has diarrhea, ileostomy, colostomy, or uncontained wound drainage Remove gown before leaving room
Gloves	When touching blood, body fluids, secretions, excretions, contaminated items, mucous membranes, nonintact skin Remove promptly after use, before touching noncontaminated items, and before touching next patient			When entering room
Hand washing	After touching blood, body fluids, secretions, excretions, contaminated items Immediately after glove removal Between patients			Use medicated hand-washing agent

Modified from Garner JS: Hospital Infection Control Practices Advisory Committee: Guideline for isolation precautions in hospitals. Infect Control Hosp Epidemiol 1996; 17:53.

*Based on guidelines published by Centers for Disease Control and Prevention (CDC).

TABLE 69–2. Indications for Transmission-Based Isolation Precautions

	Airborne Precautions	Droplet Precautions	Contact Precautions
Known or suspected diseases or pathogens	Measles Tuberculosis, pulmonary or laryngeal Varicella* Zoster (disseminated or in immunocompromised patient)*	Adenovirus (infants, children)* Diphtheria, pharyngeal *Haemophilus influenzae* meningitis, epiglottitis *H. influenzae* pneumonia (infants, children) Influenza Meningococcal infections Mumps *Mycoplasma* pneumonia Parvovirus B19 Pertussis Plague, pneumonic Rubella Streptococcal (group A) pharyngitis, pneumonia, scarlet fever (infants, young children)	Abscess, not covered or drainage not contained Adenovirus (infants, children)* Cellulitis, uncontrolled drainage Decubitus ulcer, infected and drainage not contained *Clostridium difficile* enterocolitis Conjunctivitis, acute viral Diphtheria, cutaneous *Escherichia coli* O157:H7 colitis (diapered or incontinent patients) Enteroviral infections (infants, young children) Furunculosis (infants, young children) Group A streptococcal major skin, burn or wound infection) Hemorrhagic fevers (Lassa, Marburg, Ebola) Hepatitis A (diapered or incontinent patients) Herpes simplex virus (neonatal; disseminated; severe primary mucocutaneous) Impetigo Lice Major (noncontained) abscess, cellulitis, or decubitus MDR bacteria (e.g., MRSA, VRE, GISA, GRSA) infection or colonization Parainfluenza infection (infants, children) Pediculosis, scabies Rotavirus (diapered or incontinent patients) Respiratory syncytial virus infection (infants, children, immunocompromised) Rubella, congenital Scabies Streptococcal (group A) major skin, wound, or burn infection *Staphylococcus aureus* major skin, wound, or burn infection *Shigella* (diapered or incontinent patients) Varicella* *Yersinia enterocolitica* enteritis, disseminated, or in immunocompromised patient Zoster (disseminated or in immunocompromised patient)*
Scenarios requiring empiric implementation of precautions	Vesicular rash* Maculopapular rash with coryza and fever Cough, fever, and upper lobe pulmonary infiltrate Cough, fever, and any pulmonary infiltrate in HIV-infected patient or patient at high risk for HIV infection	Meningitis Petechial or ecchymotic rash with fever Paroxysmal or severe persistent cough during periods of pertussis activity	Abscess or draining wound that cannot be covered Acute diarrhea with likely infectious cause in incontinent or diapered patient Diarrhea in an adult with history of recent antibiotic use History of infection or colonization with MDR organisms Respiratory infections in infants and young children Skin, wound, or urinary tract infection in a patient with a recent hospital or nursing home stay in a facility where MDR organisms are prevalent Vesicular rash

*Condition requires two types of precautions.
MDR = multidrug-resistant; MRSA = methicillin-resistantS. *aureus*; VRE = vancomycin-resistant enterococci; GISA = *S. aureus* with intermediate resistance to glycopeptides; GRSA = glycopeptide-resistant *S. aureus*; HIV = human immunodeficiency virus.

droplets with mucous membranes.[49] Most droplet-transmitted infections are seen in the pediatric setting; important droplet-transmitted infections seen in the adult critical care setting are invasive *Haemophilus influenzae* infections, invasive meningococcal infections, and influenza.

Droplet precautions are generally easy to implement in the critical care setting, particularly in units with one patient per room. Open bays with multiple patients should be avoided when possible for patients requiring droplet precautions.

Contact Precautions

Owing to the high rate at which patients are colonized or infected with multidrug-resistant organisms in the critical care setting, contact precautions are the form of isolation most commonly needed in this setting. Some experts advocate using contact precautions empirically for all intensive care patients, because most such patients not already infected or colonized with epidemiologically important organisms are at high risk for infection or colonization with these organisms.

Contact precautions are indicated for patients colonized or infected with methicillin-resistant *S. aureus*, vancomycin-resistant enterococci, and multidrug-resistant gram-negative bacilli.[49] Another group of patients requiring this type of isolation is patients with diarrheal illnesses that are presumed or confirmed to be of an infectious origin. In the critical care setting, *Clostridium difficile* enteritis is an important indication.[49]

New Pathogens, New Guidelines

Are the established CDC isolation guidelines sufficient to deal with new pathogens? Although contact precautions should prevent the transmission of staphylococci with reduced susceptibility to vancomycin, the implications of dissemination of these organisms are significant. This issue prompted some experts to propose more stringent guidelines to control these organisms prior to reports of their emergence.[51]

The CDC published interim guidelines for infection control in 1997 but has not issued final guidelines.[3] In addition to implementation of contact precautions, the CDC recommended that (1) the number of persons with access to colonized or infected patients be limited, (2) infection control personnel monitor and strictly enforce compliance with infection control practices, and (3) surveillance cultures be performed on health care workers to monitor for potential colonization with the resistant strain.[3] If a health care worker becomes colonized, decolonization with mupirocin should be attempted.[51]

When a patient is reported to be infected by a *S. aureus* strain with reduced susceptibility to vancomycin, the clinician should ensure that the laboratory has confirmed the finding, because the most common reason for detection of reduced vancomycin susceptibility is an erroneous result due to testing of a mixed rather than pure culture. While the laboratory is confirming the finding, at a minimum contact precautions should be instituted for the patient.

Surveillance for Nosocomial Infections

The purpose of surveillance is to monitor for the development of nosocomial infections. When surveillance is performed over an extended time (at least 1 year), endemic infection rates can be established, allowing ICU personnel to know how many infections can be expected in any give period. When infection rates significantly exceed the baseline (endemic) rate, an *outbreak* exists; this finding should prompt infection control personnel to work with ICU personnel to determine the cause of the outbreak.

To be most effective, surveillance should be concurrent (i.e., performed while patients are hospitalized rather than through retrospective chart review after their discharge). Also, surveillance should be *active;* that is, trained professionals should systematically review each patient's chart and detect infections on the basis of standardized definitions.

In *passive surveillance*, ICU personnel are asked to report infections to the infection control department. This latter approach is problematic, in that (1) standardized definitions for infections may not be used appropriately or at all, depending on the individual health care worker's level of understanding, and (2) unit personnel may forget or may have a disincentive to report infections. Thus, accurate rates of infection are unlikely to be determined by passive surveillance. Nevertheless, *sentinel surveillance* (the ICU physician or nurse reports an unusual observation to infection control personnel) remains useful in early identification of epidemics.

The ICU and infection control personnel should meet to discuss the type of surveillance to be performed in the ICU. At a minimum, surveillance for bloodstream, urinary tract, respiratory tract, and surgical wound infections should be conducted for all patients in the ICU. In addition, periodic meetings are essential to review trends in nosocomial infections. Cooperation between these two groups is of utmost importance. To provide the most meaningful feedback to ICU personnel, the surveillance personnel should report infection rates with device-day denominators when appropriate (e.g., ventilator-associated pneumonias per ventilator-day, bloodstream infections per central line–days). Expressing infection rates with device-day denominators also facilitates interhospital comparison of infection rates.

In addition to surveillance for nosocomial infections, laboratory-based surveillance should be implemented. This procedure involves monitoring culture results and antimicrobial susceptibility results, including isolates representing colonization. Although most hospital microbiology laboratories publish yearly antibiograms, it may be useful also to review unit-based antibiograms, because important trends in the development of antibiotic resistance in the critical care unit may be hidden in the antibiogram of the entire hospital.

It is also useful to separate microbiologic data according to body site. Koontz[52] observed that antibiotic-resistant, gram-negative strains were isolated from respiratory tract, urinary tract, and wound specimens 3 years before organisms with the same antibiogram were isolated from blood specimens. Thus, monitoring the antimicrobial susceptibility patterns of non-bloodstream isolates may detect emerging resistance patterns sooner.

Engineering and Design Considerations

Ideally, each patient in the ICU should be placed in a separate room. Unfortunately, many older hospitals still contain open bays and lack sufficient space to construct individual patient rooms. Separate clean and dirty utility areas help to prevent environmental contamination.

As mentioned previously, adequate numbers and placement of sinks are imperative to encourage compliance with hand washing.

Sharps containers should be placed near each bedside. Containers should be constructed of puncture-resistant material and should be emptied when three-fourths full to prevent sharps from protruding from the container.

Containers for biohazardous waste and regular waste should be conveniently placed throughout the environment.

Antibiotic Control

Over the past several years, many hospitals have developed and implemented antibiotic control programs. These range from limiting the number of antimicrobial agents on the formulary to more restrictive programs, such as automatic "stop" orders and the requirement of infectious diseases consultation for approval to prescribe certain agents. Interestingly, the driving force behind many of these programs has been not concerns about worsening antimicrobial resistance but rather cost savings. One particularly problematic issue in the critical care unit is treatment based on culture results that represent colonization and not true infection. This inappropriate use of antibiotics poses additional selective pressure for increasingly resistant organisms.

Other Considerations

In addition to surveillance, infection control personnel should interact with the ICU to help develop infection control policies as well as to aid in educational programs for infection control. Infection control personnel also can provide important assistance in the evaluation of new products that may have implications for infection control.

References

1. Nosocomial infections. Infect Control Today 1998; 2:10.
2. Archibald L, Phillips L, Monnet D, et al: Antimicrobial resistance in isolates from inpatients and outpatients in the United States: Increasing importance of the intensive care unit. Clin Infect Dis 1997; 24:211.
3. Centers for Disease Control and Prevention: Interim guidelines for prevention and control of staphylococcal infection associated with reduced susceptibility to vancomycin. MMWR Morb Mortal Wkly Rep 1997; 46:626.
4. Vincent J-L, Bihari DJ, Suter PM, et al: The prevalence of nosocomial infection in intensive care units in Europe: Results of the European Prevalence of Infection in Intensive Care (EPIC) Study. JAMA 1995; 274:639.
5. Hiramatsu K, Aritaka N, Hanaki H, et al: Dissemination in Japanese hospitals of strains of *Staphylococcus aureus* heterogeneously resistant to vancomycin. Lancet 1997; 350:1670.
6. Centers for Disease Control and Prevention: Reduced susceptibility of *Staphylococcus aureus* to vancomycin—Japan 1996. MMWR Morb Mortal Wkly Rep 1997; 46:624.
7. Centers for Disease Control and Prevention: Update: *Staphylococcus aureus* with reduced susceptibility to vancomycin—United States, 1997. MMWR Morb Mortal Wkly Rep 1997; 46:813.
8. Noble WC, Virani Z, Cree RGA: Co-transfer of vancomycin and other resistance genes from *Enterococcus faecalis* NCTC 12201 to *Staphylococcus aureus*. FEMS Microbiol Lett 1992; 93:195.
9. Hospital Infection Control Practices Advisory Committee: Recommendations for preventing the spread of vancomycin resistance. Infect Control Hosp Epidemiol 1995; 16:105.
10. Fekety FR Jr: The epidemiology and prevention of staphylococcal infection. Medicine 1964; 43:593.
11. Sanford MD, Widmer AF, Bale MJ, et al: Efficient detection and long-term persistence of the carriage of methicillin-resistant *Staphylococcus aureus*. Clin Infect Dis 1994; 19:1123.
12. Emori TG, Gaynes RP: An overview of nosocomial infections, including the role of the microbiology laboratory. Clin Microbiol Rev 1993; 6:428.
13. Patterson JE, Sweeney AH, Simms M, et al: An analysis of 110 serious enterococcal infections: Epidemiology, antibiotic susceptibility, and outcome. Medicine 1995; 74:191.
14. Leclercq R, Derlot E, Duval J, et al: Plasmid-mediated resistance to vancomycin and teicoplanin in *Enterococcus faecium*. N Engl J Med 1988; 319:157.
15. Rubin LG, Tucci V, Cercenado E, et al: Vancomycin-resistant *Enterococcus faecium* in hospitalized children. Infect Control Hosp Epidemiol 1992; 13:700.
16. Karanil LV, Murphy M, Josephson A, et al: A cluster of vancomycin-resistant *Enterococcus faecium* in an intensive care unit. Infect Control Hosp Epidemiol 1992; 13:195.
17. Boyle JF, Soumakis SA, Rendo A, et al: Epidemiologic analysis and genotypic characterization of a nosocomial outbreak of vancomycin-resistant enterococci. J Clin Microbiol 1993; 31:1280.
18. Morris JG Jr, Shay DK, Hebden JN, et al: Enterococci resistant to multiple antimicrobial agents, including vancomycin: Establishment of endemicity in a university medical center. Ann Intern Med 1995; 123:250.
19. Moreno F, Grota P, Crisp C, et al: Clinical and molecular epidemiology of vancomycin-resistant *Enterococcus faecium* during its emergence in a city in southern Texas. Clin Infect Dis 1995; 21:1234.
20. Shay DK, Goldmann DA, Jarvis WR: Reducing the spread of antimicrobial-resistant microorganisms: Control of vancomycin-resistant enterococci. Pediatr Clin North Am 1995; 42:703.
21. Tornieporth NG, Roberts RB, John J, et al: Risk factors associated with vancomycin-resistant *Enterococcus faecium* infection or colonization in 145 matched case patients and control patients. Clin Infect Dis 1996; 23:767.
22. Papanicolaou GA, Meyers BR, Meyers J, et al: Nosocomial infections with vancomycin-resistant *Enterococcus faecium* in liver transplant recipients: Risk factors for acquisition and mortality. Clin Infect Dis 1996; 23:760.
23. Livornese LL Jr, Dias S, Samel C, et al: Hospital-acquired infection with vancomycin-resistant *Enterococcus faecium* transmitted by electronic thermometers. Ann Intern Med 1992; 117:112.
24. Handwerger S, Raucher B, Altarac D, et al: Nosocomial outbreak due to *Enterococcus faecium* highly resistant to vancomycin, penicillin, and gentamicin. Clin Infect Dis 1993; 16:750.
25. Montecalvo MA, Horowitz H, Gedris C, et al: Outbreak of vancomycin-, ampicillin-, and aminoglycoside-resistant *Enterococcus faecium* bacteremia in an adult oncology unit. Antimicrob Agents Chemother 1994; 38:1363.
26. Edmond MB, Ober JF, Weinbaum DL, et al: Vancomycin-resistant *Enterococcus faecium* bacteremia: Risk factors for infection. Clin Infect Dis 1995; 20:1126.
27. Dever LL, China C, Eng RHK, et al: Vancomycin-resistant *Enterococcus faecium* in a Veterans Affairs medical center: Association with antibiotic usage. Am J Infect Control 1998; 26:40.
28. Gordts B, Van Landuyt H, Leven M, et al: Vancomycin-resistant enterococci colonizing the intestinal tracts of hospitalized patients. J Clin Microbiol 1995; 33:2842.
29. Wade JJ: The emergence of *Enterococcus faecium* resistant to glycopeptides and other standard agents: A preliminary report. J Hosp Infect 1995; 30:483.
30. Boyce JM, Opal SM, Chow JW, et al: Outbreak of multidrug-resistant *Enterococcus faecium* with transferable vanB class vancomycin resistance. J Clin Microbiol 1994; 32:1148.
31. Itokazu GS, Quinn JP, Bell-Dixon C, et al: Antimicrobial resistance rates among aerobic gram-negative bacilli recovered from patients in intensive care units: Evaluation of a national postmarketing surveillance program. Clin Infect Dis 1996; 23:779.
32. Jarlier V, Fosse T, Philippon A, and the ICU Study Group: Antibiotic susceptibility in aerobic gram-negative bacilli isolated in intensive care units in 39 French teaching hospitals (ICU study). Intensive Care Med 1996; 22:1057.
33. Khurana CM, Wojack BR: Prevalence of ciprofloxacin resistance in multiresistant gram-negative intensive care isolates. Infection 1994; 22(Suppl 2):S99.
34. Tillotson GS, Dorrian I, Bloneau J: Fluoroquinolone resistance: Mechanisms and epidemiology. J Med Microbiol 1997; 46:457.
35. Burwen DR, Banerjee SN, Gaynes RP, et al: Ceftazidime resistance among selected nosocomial gram-negative bacilli in the United States. J Infect Dis 1994; 170:1622.
36. Manian F, Meyer L, Jenne J, et al: Loss of antimicrobial susceptibility in aerobic gram-negative bacilli repeatedly isolated from patients in intensive-care units. Infect Control Hosp Epidemiol 1996; 17:222.
37. Bauer TM, Ofner E, Just HM, et al: An epidemiological study assessing the relative importance of airborne and direct contact transmission of microorganisms in a medical intensive care unit. J Hosp Infect 1990; 15:301.
38. Sproat LJ, Inglis TJJ: A multicentre survey of hand hygiene practice in intensive care units. J Hosp Infect 1994; 26:137.
39. Conley JM, Hill S, Ross J, et al: Handwashing practices in an intensive care unit: The effects of an educational program and its relationship to infection rates. Am J Infect Control 1989; 17:330.

40. Doebbeling BN, Stanley GL, Sheetz CT, et al: Comparative efficacy of alternative hand-washing agents in reducing nosocomial infections in intensive care units. N Engl J Med 1992; 327:88.
41. Kaplan LM, McGuckin M: Increasing handwashing compliance with more accessible sinks. Infect Control 1986; 7:408.
42. Albert RK, Condie F: Hand-washing patterns in medical intensive-care units. N Engl J Med 1981; 304:1465.
43. Graham M: Frequency and duration of handwashing in an intensive care unit. Am J Infect Control 1990; 18:77.
44. Price PB: The bacteriology of normal skin: A new quantitative test applied to a study of the bacterial flora and the disinfectant action of mechanical cleaning. J Infect Dis 1938; 63:301.
45. Steere AC, Mallison GF: Handwashing practices for the prevention of nosocomial infections. Ann Intern Med 1975; 83:683.
46. Wade JJ, Desai N, Casewell MW: Hygienic hand disinfection for the removal of epidemic vancomycin-resistant *Enterococcus faecium* and gentamicin-resistant *Enterobacter cloacae*. J Hosp Infect 1991; 18:211.
47. Wade JJ, Casewell MW: The evaluation of residual antimicrobial activity on hands and its clinical relevance. J Hosp Infect 1991; 18(Suppl B):23.
48. Doebbeling BN, Pfaller MA, Houston AK, et al: Removal of nosocomial pathogens from the contaminated glove: Implications for glove reuse and handwashing. Ann Intern Med 1988; 109:394.
49. Garner JS: Hospital Infection Control Practices Advisory Committee: Guideline for isolation precautions in hospitals. Infect Control Hosp Epidemiol 1996; 17:53.
50. Centers for Disease Control and Prevention: Guidelines for preventing the transmission of *Mycobacterium tuberculosis* in health-care facilities, 1994. MMWR Morb Mortal Wkly Rep 1994; 43:1.
51. Edmond MB, Wenzel RP, Pasculle AW: Vancomycin-resistant *Staphylococcus aureus*: Perspectives on measures needed for control. Ann Intern Med 1996; 124:329.
52. Koontz FP: Microbial resistance surveillance techniques: Blood culture versus multiple body site monitoring. Diagn Microbiol Infect Dis 1992; 15(Suppl 2):31S.

A. ENDOCRINOLOGY

70

Thyroid Emergencies

Robert C. Smallridge, MD, FACP

Patients with hyperthyroidism and hypothyroidism are usually treated as outpatients. However, when hyperthyroidism is severe, is associated with other medical illnesses, or reaches a state of decompensation *(thyroid storm)*, intensive inpatient management is indicated. Similarly, patients who have profound hypothyroidism or myxedema coma should be treated in the critical care environment. Furthermore, patients may be euthyroid but need specialized care because they have an anatomic enlargement of the thyroid gland that has created an emergency.

Aside from the bona fide conditions of thyroid hormone excess and deficiency, a common problem encountered in acutely ill patients is a constellation of thyroid blood test abnormalities. This condition is referred to as *nonthyroidal illness* or *euthyroid sick syndrome*,[1, 2] and hormone replacement therapy for it is not generally recommended. However, the literature suggests that in certain circumstances thyroid hormone therapy may be beneficial; the current status of this controversy is described in this chapter.

THYROID PHYSIOLOGY

An overview of the brain-hypothalamic-pituitary-thyroid axis is depicted in Figure 70–1. The dominant influence controlling thyroid hormone secretion is the pituitary hormone thyrotropin (TSH), a glycoprotein that is under both positive and negative feedback regulation. Thyrotropin-releasing hormone is principally responsible for stimulating the secretion of TSH, whereas estrogen has a minor positive effect, enhancing the TSH response to thyrotropin-releasing hormone (TRH). The thyroid hormones thyroxine (T_4) and triiodothyronine (T_3) play an essential role in the negative feedback inhibition of TSH secretion. In addition, several other hormones, including cortisol (and other glucocorticoids), dopamine, and somatostatin, all inhibit TSH release.

TSH, by acting through a plasma membrane receptor on thyroid follicular cells, stimulates iodide uptake and thyroid hormone synthesis and secretion. Under certain conditions, patients with autoimmune thyroid disease develop circulating immunoglobulins that can affect thyroid function by binding to the TSH receptor. These proteins (TSH-receptor antibodies) can produce hyperthyroidism (Graves' disease). Alternatively, some antibodies bind to the TSH receptor without causing stimulation, and these may produce hypothyroidism.

Under normal circumstances, TSH maintains circulating levels of T_4 and T_3 within a narrow physiologic range. All of the T_4 is produced and secreted by the thyroid gland. This amounts to about 90 μg/day. However, only approximately 20% of circulating T_3 is manufactured by the thyroid gland; the rest is derived from deiodination by the enzyme 5′-deiodinase. This process occurs in many peripheral tissues, especially those of the liver and kidney. Other pathways of metabolic degradation of thyroxine exist,[3] and it has been suggested that sulfation may play a prominent role in critically ill individuals.[4]

Thyroid hormones circulate bound to three proteins: T_4-binding globulin, transthyretin, and albumin. The amount of T_4 circulating in its unbound form is only 0.03%, and that of T_3 is but 0.3%. Nevertheless, it is only this extremely small fraction of hormone (especially of T_3) that is transported into cells and is responsible for the myriad biologic responses influenced by thyroid hormones.

THYROID FUNCTION TESTS

Thyroid hormones affect virtually every tissue and organ system in the body, and the symptoms and signs elicited by their excess or deficiency are numerous. Unfortunately, none of the symptoms or signs is specific for thyroid disease; thus, clinical examination, although an important element of any evaluation, is not diagnostic of thyroid dysfunction. In the setting of severe illness, the accurate diagnosis of thyroid disease can be difficult. Thyroid function tests, especially measurements of serum hormones, are an essential element in the decision-making process.

The selection of appropriate tests, in conjunction with an

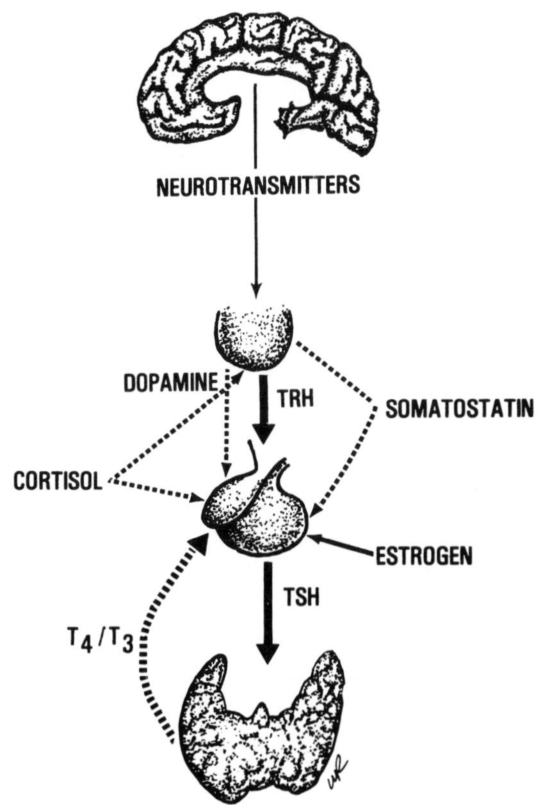

Figure 70–1. Schematic drawing of the hypothalamic-pituitary-thyroid axis and its hormonal control. *Solid lines* indicate a positive influence, and *dashed lines* represent a negative influence. The width of a line represents the relative importance of the effect. TRH = thyrotropin (TSH)-releasing hormone; T_4 = thyroxine; T_3 = triiodothyronine. (From Smallridge RC: Thyrotropin-secreting pituitary tumors. Endocrinol Metab Clin North Am 1987; 16:766.)

appreciation of the variables that can confound their interpretation in hospitalized patients, can simplify the testing procedure. Even so, pitfalls await the skilled clinician. An overview of commonly ordered tests and of the directional changes observed in various diseases is given in Table 70–1. The total T_4 level has been used for more than 2 decades. Since almost all of the T_4 measured in this assay is bound to several proteins, factors altering the quantity, affinity, or capacity of these proteins elevate or lower the T_4 value and may mislead the physician into thinking that a patient is either hyperthyroid or hypothyroid. This difficulty has been avoided by simultaneously performing an in vitro test (the T_3 uptake test) and then by deriving a free T_4 index. The free T_4 index correlates well with the "gold standard" thyroid test, serum free T_4 (measured by equilibrium dialysis). Measurement of free T_4 traditionally has not been readily available because of its involved cost and time factors. Unfortunately, the free T_4 index is not always reliable in the setting of critical illness, and in response diagnostic products companies have produced many kit assays designed to measure free T_4 levels. Several assays that appear to be reliable in measuring thyroid function in critically ill patients have been reported in the literature.[5]

A serum T_3 determination is not helpful in evaluating hospitalized patients suspected of being hypothyroid, because inhibition of 5′-deiodinase activity results in low T_3 levels in euthyroid persons afflicted with a variety of medical or surgical disorders.[1, 2] Documentation of an increased total or free T_4 level is usually sufficient to support a diagnosis of hyperthyroidism. In some cases, the T_4 level is normal, and one must demonstrate a high T_3 level (a condition known as T_3 *toxicosis*). A reverse T_3 (rT_3) level may be helpful; this hormone level is low in patients with hypothyroidism but elevated in those with nonthyroidal illness. The reason for the increase in rT_3 is that the enzyme that converts T_4 to T_3 also is responsible for the degradation of rT_3.

Measurements of serum TSH also are valuable. TSH is suppressed in all patients with hyperthyroidism except for those with the rare disorders of thyroid hormone resistance and TSH-secreting pituitary tumors.[6–8] When serum free T_4 is low, elevation of TSH is diagnostic of primary hypothyroidism. In critically ill patients, however, TSH levels may be partially suppressed, and some patients with hypothyroidism have values within the normal range. The mechanism may include the effects of increased endogenous cortisol or of the administration of steroids or dopamine, or both, to such patients.

THYROTOXICOSIS AND THYROID STORM

Thyrotoxicosis is present whenever excess amounts of thyroid hormones, either endogenous or exogenous in origin, are circulating in the bloodstream. When the underlying process is overproduction and secretion of hormone by the thyroid gland, hyperthyroidism exists.

Pathophysiology

Numerous organ systems are affected. The cardiovascular system is subject to many changes, including an increase in heart rate, stroke volume, cardiac output, and cardiac contractility. Peripheral vascular resistance is reduced.[9, 10] Changes in the respiratory system include tachypnea, a reduction in vital capacity, diffusing capacity, and lung compliance in combination with an increase in the ventilatory responses to hypercapnia and hypoxia.[11] Muscle weakness accounts at least in part for these disturbances.[12] Gastrointestinal function is enhanced,[13] with a shortening of intestinal transit time, an increase in duodenal basal electrical activity, and, at times, a secretory diarrhea. The central nervous system is subject to an increase in catecholamine turnover and an increase in receptor sensitivity to neurotransmitters.

Clinical Presentation

The symptoms and signs of the typical case of hyperthyroidism reflect the enhancing influence of excessive amounts of thyroid hormone on the function of many organs (Table 70–2). At times, one system may predominate; that is, a patient may be referred to a cardiologist because of tachyarrhythmias, to a pulmonologist because of dyspnea, to a rheumatologist because of myopathy, to a gastroenterologist because of diarrhea, or to a dermatologist because of severe pruritus. Older patients may have a paucity of symptoms and signs, with thyroid enlargement frequently being absent.[14, 15]

A patient may require hospitalization because of complications arising from his or her hyperthyroid state. Older patients frequently experience atrial fibrillation, with incidences of approximately 30% to 40%.[14, 15] Significant cardiovascular events include congestive heart failure, unstable angina, and myocardial infarction (even in patients with normal coronary arteries). Other less common arrhythmias include complete heart block and ventricular arrhythmias, which can be lethal. A variety of neurologic conditions such as stroke, myasthenia gravis, periodic paralysis, seizures, and myopathies may also prompt hospital admission.[16] Pregnant women with hyperemesis gravidarum may demonstrate increases of both total and free T_4 and T_3 levels; interestingly, these abnormalities usually resolve spontaneously. The cause of hyperthyroidism in hyperemesis may be chorionic gonadotropin (CG), as serum CG levels correlate with free T_4, and CG has thyrotrophic activity in cultured cells.[17]

The most dangerous complication of hyperthyroidism is a state of systemic decompensation known as *thyroid storm*.[18, 19] The hallmarks of this life-threatening disorder in-

TABLE 70–1. Serum Thyroid Hormone Tests in Health and Disease

	Total T_4	T_3U	FT_4 Index	Free T_4	T_3	rT_3	TSH
Euthyroid	N	N	N	N	N	N	N
Hyperthyroid	↑	↑	↑	↑	↑	↑	↓
Hypothyroid	↓	↓	↓	↓	N, ↓	↓	↑
TBG excess	↑	↓	N	N	↑	↑	N
TBG deficiency	↓	↑	N	N, ↓	↓	↓	N
Nonthyroidal illness	N, ↓	↑	N, ↓	↑, N, ↓	↓	↑	N, ↓
FDH	↑	N	↑	N	N	N	N

From Smallridge RC: Metabolic and anatomic thyroid emergencies: A review. Crit Care Med 1992; 20:276. © Williams & Wilkins, 1992.

TBG = thyroxine-binding globulin; FDH = familial dysalbuminemic hyperthyroxinemia; T_3 = triiodothyronine; T_4 = thyroxine; T_3U = T_3 uptake; FT_4 = free T_4; rT_3 = reverse T_3; N = normal; ↑ = increased; ↓ = decreased.

TABLE 70–2. Symptoms and Signs of Thyrotoxicosis and Thyrotoxic Crisis

Thyrotoxicosis	Crisis
Neuromuscular	***Neuromuscular***
Emotional lability	Agitation
Short attention span	Emotional lability
Tremor	Apathy
Weakness	Delirium
Periodic paralysis	Seizures
	Coma
Cardiovascular	***Cardiovascular***
Tachycardia	Congestive heart failure
Systolic hypertension	Arrhythmias
Atrial fibrillation	
Thermoregulation	***Thermoregulation***
Warm, moist skin	Fever
Heat intolerance	
Gastrointestinal	***Gastrointestinal***
Hyperdefecation	Vomiting
	Diarrhea
	Jaundice
Nutritional	***Nutritional***
Increased appetite	Severe weight loss
Weight loss	Vitamin deficiencies

clude fever, cardiac dysfunction (arrhythmias, congestive heart failure), and neurologic changes ranging from agitation and restlessness to confusion, disorientation, delirium, seizures, and coma. Thyroid storm develops in the setting of untreated or undertreated hyperthyroidism and is associated with some precipitating event. Situations known to trigger this critical condition include surgery, infections and other acute medical illnesses, trauma, labor and delivery, and emotional stress. It is imperative that an initiating factor be carefully sought for and corrected.

Differential Diagnosis

Thyrotoxicosis is suspected when blood tests show an elevated free T_4 index or free T_4. An assortment of conditions collectively referred to as *euthyroid hyperthyroxinemia*[20] must be distinguished from thyrotoxicosis (Table 70–3). Individuals with euthyroid hyperthyroxinemia are clinically euthyroid, and a carefully taken history and observations on physical examination should suggest the correct diagnosis. Occasionally, thyrotoxicosis is suspected clinically but the serum T_4 level is normal. When this scenario arises, a determination of serum T_3 level should be ordered because T_3 toxicosis may be present.

The most reliable test for distinguishing between hyperthyroidism and other causes of thyrotoxicosis is the radioactive iodine uptake test. Table 70–4 indicates how this test can help one to narrow the differential diagnosis. Graves' disease is the most common cause of hyperthyroidism and is associated with an undetectable serum TSH level. Toxic multinodular goiter is less common in the United States than in other countries. Although symptoms are often less pronounced than in Graves' disease, older patients are susceptible to the development of complications, especially if they receive an iodine load, as may occur when diagnostic radiographic dye studies are performed. Inappropriate TSH secreting disorders,[6–8] although uncommon, are being recognized much more often than in the past owing to the advent of sensitive TSH assays.

TABLE 70–3. Differential Diagnosis of Euthyroid Hyperthyroxinemia

Alterations in thyroid hormone/plasma protein binding
- Inherited
  - TBG excess
  - TBPA excess
  - Familial dysalbuminemic hyperthyroxinemia
- Acquired
  - Nonthyroidal illness
    - Liver disease
    - Acute intermittent porphyria
    - Estrogen secreting tumors
  - Drugs
    - Narcotics (e.g., methadone, heroin)
    - Oral contraceptives
    - Perphenazine
    - 5-Fluorouracil
    - Clofibrate
  - Physiologic (pregnancy)
  - T_4 autoantibodies

Transient hyperthyroxinemia
- Acute medical illness
- Acute psychiatric disease
- Hyperemesis gravidarum

Drug-induced hyperthyroxinemia
- Amiodarone
- Iodinated contrast agents (e.g., ipodate, iopanoate)
- Heparin

Thyroid hormone resistance (generalized)

From Smallridge RC: Metabolic and anatomic thyroid emergencies: A review. Crit Care Med 1992; 20:276. © Williams & Wilkins, 1992.

T_4 = thyroxine; TBPA = thyroxine-binding prealbumin; TBG = thyroxine-binding globulin.

Patients with these disorders usually do not present with such acute disease that hospitalization is likely.

Neonatal thyrotoxicosis, due to transplacental transfer of maternal thyroid-stimulating immunoglobulins, occurs in the offspring of fewer than 1% of women with a history of Graves' disease. It should be suspected in any pregnant woman with such a history, even if her hyperthyroidism had been treated years previously. Newborns with this illness may develop heart failure and thus require careful observation until the condition resolves over several weeks to months after birth.

TABLE 70–4. Differential Diagnosis of Thyrotoxicosis

Increased Radioactive Iodine Uptake
- Diffuse hyperplasia (Graves' disease)
- Toxic multinodular goiter
- Solitary autonomous nodule
- Neonatal thyrotoxicosis
- Syndromes of inappropriate TSH secretion
  - TSH tumors
  - Thyroid hormone resistance (central)
- Trophoblastic tumor

Decreased Radioactive Iodine Uptake
- Destructive thyroiditis
  - Subacute (viral)
  - Postpartum (autoimmune)
  - Painless, nonpostpartum
- Iodine-induced (e.g., amiodarone)
- Thyrotoxicosis factitia
- Metastatic thyroid carcinoma
- Struma ovarii

Modified from Smallridge RC: Metabolic and anatomic thyroid emergencies: A review. Crit Care Med 1992; 20:276. © Williams & Wilkins, 1992.

TSH = thyroid-stimulating hormone.

Most causes of low radioactive iodine uptake thyrotoxicosis do not produce illness of such severity that hospitalization is necessary. However, accidental or suicidal ingestion of large amounts of thyroid hormone can be quite serious.[21] Similarly, patients who have drug-induced thyrotoxicosis (e.g., that caused by iodine or amiodarone) may have life-threatening disease.[22]

Therapy

Management of patients with uncomplicated hyperthyroidism of mild to moderate severity can be accomplished on an outpatient basis. Patients are usually rendered euthyroid with antithyroid drugs (either methimazole or propylthiouracil). Adrenergic symptoms can be controlled initially with β-blocker therapy. Approximately one third of patients with Graves' disease may go into long-term remission after a year of antithyroid drug treatment. Individuals with small goiters (<40 g) and a short duration of symptoms (<6 months) are more likely to respond. Thyroid ablation, preferably with iodine 131 (^{131}I) but occasionally with surgical thyroidectomy, is quite effective not only for patients with Graves' disease but also for those with nodular diseases. Thyroid ablation is *not* recommended for the syndromes of TSH secretion; proper therapy should focus on decreasing TSH secretion.

Patients with severe hyperthyroidism may benefit from a period of hospitalization. Restricted activity, ensurance of compliance with medications, and education may promote recovery. Certainly, anyone who manifests confounding medical problems may need to be admitted to a hospital. It is important to remember that the metabolism of some drugs is enhanced by hyperthyroidism. Specifically, digoxin[23] and adrenergic blockers[24] may be required in larger than usual doses, and patients should be carefully monitored for side effects.

Once euthyroidism is attained, atrial fibrillation often spontaneously converts to sinus rhythm. Nakazawa and coworkers[25] found this to be true in 62% of 163 patients. In most individuals, conversion occurred within 3 weeks of euthyroidism and never after 4 months. Therefore, elective cardioversion is recommended if atrial fibrillation persists for more than 16 weeks. The question of whether patients with atrial fibrillation should receive anticoagulation drugs while hyperthyroid has not been addressed prospectively. Petersen and Hansen[26] retrospectively evaluated 610 patients with untreated thyrotoxicosis, of whom 91 had atrial fibrillation; they found that age, but not atrial fibrillation, was a significant risk factor for the development of stroke. However, others[27] have recommended anticoagulation for patients with thyrotoxic atrial fibrillation to reduce the likelihood of a cerebrovascular accident.

The most severe form of hyperthyroidism, thyroid storm, should always be managed in the intensive care unit (ICU). Table 70–5 outlines the recommended approach. General supportive measures are essential in the overall scheme. Fever reduction decreases metabolic demands and also the percentage of free T_4. Because salicylates may affect the binding of thyroid hormones to plasma proteins, acetaminophen is the preferred antipyretic agent.[18, 19]

Large fluid losses due to sweating, vomiting, and diarrhea need to be aggressively replaced with fluids and electrolyte solutions. Glucose and vitamins are also important, as these patients have been catabolic for a prolonged period of time. Hemodynamic monitoring may be required because heart failure (including high output) may be present. As noted earlier, higher doses of digoxin may be needed; β-blockers should be used with caution.

Pharmacologic intervention is essential and should be approached in several ways. Antithyroid drugs should be given initially and frequently to prevent further thyroid hormone synthesis. Either propylthiouracil or methimazole can be given orally or crushed and delivered by nasogastric tube. Rectal delivery of antithyroid drugs has also been reported.[28, 29]

Inhibition of the release of T_4 and T_3 acutely from the thyroid gland is of utmost importance and can be accomplished with either a saturated solution of potassium iodide or Lugol's solution. This therapy works immediately and is effective for several weeks. An initial dose of antithyroid drug must be given *before* the first dose of iodide because administration of iodide to an unblocked thyroid gland can worsen a patient's status. Lithium can also be used, but this drug's side effects limit its popularity. If lithium is used, blood levels must be monitored and maintained within a range of 0.5 to 1.5 mmol/L.

A third means of improving the clinical condition in thyroid storm is to inhibit conversion of T_4 to T_3. The most effective agent, and one which has been studied extensively, is ipodate sodium (Oragrafin). In one study, patients' serum T_3 levels fell by 73% within 1 day and remained at this level for almost 6 months with continued daily ipodate sodium therapy.[30] Caution in its long-term use is advised, since escape from its beneficial effects has been reported.[31] An additional acute effect of this drug is inhibition of hormone secretion, since it contains large amounts of iodide. Propylthiouracil and glucocorticoids may block conversion of T_4 to T_3 and have an additive effect when combined.[32]

Reduction of the hyperadrenergic state is desired, and β-blocker therapy is effective in this regard. Propranolol has been favored for many years, in part because it has been shown to inhibit conversion of T_4 to T_3 in hyperthyroid patients. It should be noted that some severely hyperthyroid individuals with cardiac disease maintain cardiac output by increasing their heart rate. Injudicious use of a β-blocker could precipitate heart failure.[33] The short-acting β_1-blocker esmolol has been used in several patients with thyrotoxic crisis[34] and may offer some advantage over propranolol for two reasons: (1) it is a more cardioselective antagonist and (2) its biologic effects dissipate more rapidly. Two loading doses may be needed, and maintenance doses of up to 350 $\mu g \cdot kg^{-1} \cdot min^{-1}$ have been used.

The last management option involves T_4 removal. Occasional reports have demonstrated the efficacy of plasmapheresis and hemoperfusion.[18, 19, 35] In a few Graves' disease patients who manifested thyrotoxic crisis while receiving medical therapy, immediate surgical thyroidectomy has been successful.[36] With aggressive management as outlined here, these latter approaches should need to be entertained only rarely.

Most forms of thyrotoxicosis associated with a low radioactive iodine uptake do not pose a medical emergency. Two that do are *thyrotoxicosis factitia* and *iodine-induced thyrotoxicosis*. Factitious disease is usually brought on accidentally in children and as the result of suicide attempt in adults. Emesis and gastric lavage should be instituted acutely. β-Blockers and barbiturates have been recommended for management of tachycardia and for sedation. Other reported therapies have included plasmapheresis, steroid therapy, and treatment with iopanoic acid.[21] Bile acid sequestrants have also been employed.[37]

Patients receiving large doses of iodine-containing compounds chronically, such as asthmatic or cardiac patients (of the latter, those taking amiodarone), may experience severe hyperthyroidism up to the point of thyroid storm. This event can pose difficult management problems because the body stores of iodine may remain elevated for months. Surgery has been used successfully when medical therapy does not control the disease.[38] Amiodarone-induced thyrotoxicosis (AIT) type 1

TABLE 70–5. Management of Decompensated Hyperthyroidism (Thyroid Crisis)

Management	Route of Administration
General Measures	
Antipyresis	
Acetaminophen	PO
Cooling blankets	
Blockade of central nervous system thermoregulatory centers	IV
Hydration: fluids, electrolytes	IV
Nutrition: glucose, vitamins	IV
Antibiotics	IV
Cardiac therapy	IV, PO
Specific Measures	
Inhibition of T_4 synthesis	
PTU: 200–400 mg PO q6h	PO, NG, rectal
MMI: 20–40 mg PO q6h	PO, NG, rectal
Inhibition of T_4 release	
Iodides	
SSKI: 5 drops q6h	PO, rectal
Lugol's solution: 10 gtt q8h	PO
Lithium: 300–900 mg/day	PO
Sodium ipodate (see below)	PO
Inhibition of conversion of T_4 to T_3	
PTU	PO, NG, rectal
Sodium ipodate: 0.5–1.0 g/day	PO
Glucocorticoids (dexamethasone, 2 mg q6h)	IV, PO
Propranolol (see below)	IV, PO
Inhibition of adrenergic effects	
Propranolol: 1.0 mg (IV); 40–120 mg q6h (PO)	IV, PO
Esmolol: 500-μg/kg loading dose over 1 min; then 50–200 μg/kg per minute	IV
T_4 removal	
Plasmapheresis	
Dialysis	
Hemoperfusion	
Bile salt-binding resins	

From Smallridge RC: Metabolic and anatomic thyroid emergencies: A review. Crit Care Med 1992; 20:276. © Williams & Wilkins, 1992.
PO = oral; IV = intravenous; q = every; NG = nasogastric; PTU = propylthiouracil; T_4 = thyroxine; MMI = methimazole; SSKI = saturated solution of potassium iodide.

may respond to methimazole and potassium perchlorate, whereas thyroid-destructive AIT (type 2) responds to glucocorticoids.[39]

HYPOTHYROIDISM AND MYXEDEMA COMA

Hypothyroidism can be either primary (thyroid gland failure) or secondary (due to pituitary insufficiency). Primary hypothyroidism is most commonly the result of an autoimmune destruction of the thyroid gland (autoimmune thyroiditis, or Hashimoto's disease). Thyroid disease is fivefold to 10-fold more common in women than in men, and the incidence of symptomatic disease increases with age. Above the age of 60 years, approximately 5% of women become hypothyroid. Because hypothyroidism develops gradually and because many of the symptoms are attributed to advancing age, the diagnosis is frequently delayed. Other causes of primary thyroid insufficiency include ablation (with ^{131}I or surgery) and the use of certain drugs (e.g., lithium and diphenylhydantoin). Amiodarone can produce hypothyroidism as well as hyperthyroidism.

Secondary hypothyroidism is much less common than primary hypothyroidism. The most likely cause would be a pituitary tumor, but hypothalamic injury (meningiomas, infiltrative diseases such as sarcoidosis or tuberculosis) or carotid artery aneurysms occasionally produce hypothyroidism. In all of these situations, careful attention should be devoted to determination of the possible existence of other pituitary hormone deficiencies.

Pathophysiology

Hypothyroidism alters the function of many organs, generally in a fashion opposite to that of hyperthyroidism.[16] The cardiovascular system responds with bradycardia and a reduction in stroke volume, cardiac index and contractility, and oxygen consumption as well as with an increase in peripheral vascular resistance.[10] Pulmonary changes include hypoventilation and an impaired hypoxemic and hypercapnic ventilatory drive as well as muscle weakness and obstructive sleep apnea.[40, 41] These abnormalities may lead to acute hypercapnic respiratory failure. Central nervous system changes involve a decrease in oxygen and glucose utilization, a reduction in cerebral blood flow, and an increase in cerebrovascular resistance. The kidneys may demonstrate impaired renal water excretion, and the intestinal tract may manifest impaired motility. Anemia—both physiologic (from reduced oxygen demands) and secondary (both iron deficiency and megaloblastic)—is common. Myopathic changes are frequent, and peripheral and cranial nerve neuropathies have been reported.

Clinical Presentation

Symptoms and signs commonly observed in hypothyroidism are listed in Table 70–6. Additionally, hypothyroidism may

TABLE 70–6. Symptoms and Signs of Hypothyroidism and Myxedema Coma

Hypothyroidism	Myxedema (Coma)
Neuromuscular	***Neuromuscular***
Fatigue	Psychosis
Weakness	Obtundation/coma
Slowed mentation	
Delayed deep tendon reflexes	
Muscle cramps	
Cardiovascular	***Cardiovascular***
Bradycardia	Bradycardia
Hypertension	Pericardial effusion
Gastrointestinal	***Gastrointestinal***
Constipation	Ileus
	Megacolon
Thermoregulation	***Thermoregulation***
Cold intolerance	Hypothermia
Cool dry skin	

present as other common illnesses such as heart failure, intestinal pseudo-obstruction, bleeding disorder (an acquired von Willebrand's abnormality), anemia, or cerebrovascular disease.[42, 43]

The most severe presentation of hypothyroidism is myxedema coma, with or without respiratory failure.[44, 45] This condition usually follows exposure to an external stress. Precipitating events include infections, surgery, trauma, injudicious use of oxygen, or a variety of acute medical illnesses. Use of medications, especially sedative and hypnotic agents, can produce a decompensated state in older hypothyroid patients. The condition is more likely to occur in the winter because hypothermia is also a triggering factor.

Differential Diagnosis

The diagnosis of primary hypothyroidism is readily made when a patient's serum TSH concentration is elevated and the T_4 level is low or low normal. Difficulty arises when a total T_4 value is below normal but the TSH is within the normal range. In the outpatient setting, the possibilities include a protein-binding abnormality and secondary or central hypothyroidism. A normal free T_4 index or free T_4 concentration would be expected with the former possibility. If pituitary or hypothalamic disease is suspected, a careful history and physical examination should be performed to seek evidence of the presence of other hormone deficiencies. Measurement of other anterior pituitary hormones confirms the diagnosis and characterizes the extent of pituitary insufficiency.

When a hospitalized patient with a systemic illness is found to have a low T_4 level and a normal TSH concentration, one must consider several possibilities. Most commonly, nonthyroidal illness is responsible. Although one would expect the free T_4 level to be normal, when measured with some commercial assays it is found to be either increased or reduced. The results of several commercial assays have compared well with equilibrium dialysis measurements in hospitalized patients.[5] Confounding the situation is the occurrence of normal TSH levels in some ill patients with primary hypothyroidism; once the acute illness resolves, TSH increases. Finally, secondary hypothyroidism must also be entertained. Although not readily available, a serum rT_3 assay may clarify the problem because the level of this hormone is low in hypothyroidism but elevated in nonthyroidal illness. A more readily available test—measurement of the resin T_3 uptake—may provide similar information: resin T_3 uptake is low in hypothyroidism and increased (often markedly) in nonthyroidal illness.

Management

Uncomplicated hypothyroidism is treated on an outpatient basis.[46] Young patients with mild to moderate disease can be started on L-thyroxine (L-T_4), 50 to 100 μg/day, and their serum TSH levels measured at 4 to 6 weeks later. Upward adjustment of hormone dosage should be performed until the TSH value is suppressed to within the normal range. The full replacement dose is approximately 1.7 $\mu g \cdot kg^{-1} \cdot day^{-1}$.[47] Older individuals or any patients with known coronary artery disease should be managed more conservatively. L-T_4 can initiate or exacerbate angina,[10, 48] so treatment should proceed slowly. An initial dose of L-T_4 should be no greater than 12.5 to 25 μg/day. Patients should be questioned about the development of any cardiac symptoms, and serum TSH level should be measured before any increase in dosage is made. Changes in dosage should be small (12.5 to 25 μg) and made no more frequently than every 6 weeks.

Although central hypothyroidism is much less common than primary disease, it is important to recognize. Patients with concomitant secondary adrenal insufficiency should receive replacement hydrocortisone therapy before initiation of thyroid hormone treatment, since an increase in metabolic rate caused by the latter might induce acute adrenal insufficiency.

Profound hypothyroidism/myxedema coma is an endocrine emergency with a high mortality rate. The diagnosis should be considered in any obtunded or comatose patient for whom no obvious cause can be identified. Hypothermia or the absence of fever in a patient with a known infection is possible.

Management of myxedema coma should be conducted in the ICU. A variety of general supportive measures are essential (Table 70–7). If hypothermia is present, covering the patient with blankets is helpful. Active warming with heating devices should be avoided, however, because doing so may produce vasodilation and a lowering of blood pressure. An adequate blood volume should be restored. Hypothyroidism impairs

TABLE 70–7. Management of Decompensated Hypothyroidism (Myxedema Crisis)

General Measures
Hypothermia
Use blankets only—no heating devices
Hydration
Maintain adequate blood volume
Avoid water intoxication
Nutrition: glucose, vitamins
Antibiotics
Cardiac therapy
Correct hypotension
Glucocorticoids (stress doses)
Anticipate and treat heart failure
Correct anemia
Pulmonary therapy
Monitor arterial blood gases
Ventilatory support
Treat infection
Intestinal atony
Specific Measures
Thyroid hormone
Initial dose: 200–300 μg L-T_4 IV
Maintenance: 50–100 μg L-T_4 per day IV

From Smallridge RC: Metabolic and anatomic thyroid emergencies: A review. Crit Care Med 1992; 20:276.

free water clearance; monitoring of electrolytes is important to avoid hyponatremia. Adequate glucose maintenance is required to prevent the development of hypoglycemia. Dilated cardiomyopathy has been reported;[49] thus, careful hemodynamic monitoring is essential. Drug metabolism is prolonged, so care must be taken to avoid toxicity if digoxin is used.[50] Stress doses of steroids are recommended because the integrity of the pituitary-adrenal axis is usually unknown. Formal testing can be done at a later time. A careful search for an underlying infection is a must, and broad-spectrum antibiotic coverage is advised pending the receipt of culture results.

Close monitoring of pulmonary status is vital. Patients with hypothyroidism may hypoventilate, and they are sensitive to drugs that can depress respiration. They may require therapy for acute respiratory failure. Gastrointestinal tract abnormalities may also complicate the management plan, as hypotonia, ileus, or megacolon may occur.

Ideally, therapy for hypothyroidism in comatose patients should be restricted to only those persons identified as unequivocally hypothyroid. Unfortunately, this is not always possible, because laboratory values available at the time of decision making do not always distinguish between this disorder and nonthyroidal illness. Since delay in therapy can be fatal, early treatment with thyroid hormone has been advocated,[44] even though this approach may mean that some individuals may be treated unnecessarily. Thyroid therapy can be discontinued as a patient's situation becomes more clear.

Because absorption may be impaired, thyroid hormone should be given intravenously. A loading dose of L-T_4 (300 to 500 μg IV) followed by daily doses of 50 to 100 μg has been recommended.[44, 45] The rationale for a large initial dose is that endogenous stores of thyroid hormone are depleted. Kaptein and coworkers[51] have reported that large doses of L-T_4 may not cause cardiovascular complications in critically ill patients. However, Hylander and Rosenqvist[52] reported a greater mortality rate in patients who had high serum T_3 levels when treated for myxedema coma. In the absence of definitive guidelines for management of this disorder, an intermediate approach of giving 300 μg L-T_4 followed by daily doses of 50 to 100 μg might lessen the possibility of the occurrence of cardiac complications.

Therapy in Surgical Patients

Some patients are recognized to be hypothyroid shortly before surgery is needed. In the past, it was believed that anesthetic and surgical complications were more common in such patients.[53] Three studies performed in the 1980s have provided more complete information on this subject. In two of the reports,[54, 55] mild to moderate hypothyroidism had little influence on surgical complications. Ladenson and associates[56] reported the occurrence of intraoperative hypotension, heart failure, and some postoperative gastrointestinal and neuropsychiatric problems that were managed without sequelae. Importantly, the investigators observed no increased occurrence of cardiopulmonary difficulties, infections, impaired wound healing, or blood loss or any increase in the number of days spent in the hospital or in the incidence of death. Whether these observations can be extrapolated to all patients with hypothyroidism, including those with longstanding and severe disease, is unknown.

When surgery is elective, it seems reasonable to delay the procedure until the hypothyroid state has been reversed. However, these studies suggest that if surgery is more urgent, a patient has a reasonably good chance of tolerating the operation successfully. One special situation is surgery for the cardiac patient who presents with severe angina pectoris.[53] In individuals undergoing cardiac bypass, surgery was found to be more successful if thyroid replacement was begun after the operation (presumably because of the impact of thyroid hormone on myocardial oxygen consumption). Cardiac patients should now be at even less risk because the introduction of better antianginal drugs and balloon angioplasty has eliminated the potential risk of general anesthesia in the hypothyroid patient.

Neurosurgeons must be familiar with the issues involved in managing hypothyroidism, particularly as it relates to hypothalamic and pituitary disorders. Before surgery, patients must be screened for the possibility of deficiencies of multiple pituitary hormones. Most critical is the recognition of adrenocorticotropic hormone (ACTH) deficiency because administration of stress doses of glucocorticoids are required perioperatively. Should surgery be indicated for a benign tumor, such as a pituitary adenoma, the decision to correct the hypothyroidism before surgery depends on whether resection is urgent because the tumor impinges on vital structures, such as the optic chiasm. In hypothyroid patients, not all pituitary masses warrant surgery. In some persons with primary hypothyroidism, generalized compensatory pituitary enlargement develops from prolonged TSH production. These individuals may present with visual field changes, and computed tomography and magnetic resonance imaging scans show a pituitary mass with suprasellar extension. Surgery is *not* the appropriate treatment; thyroid hormone use decreases the size of the pituitary gland back to normal.[6, 8] Thus, it is essential to measure serum TSH concentration in any patient before surgical exploration is performed.

THYROID HORMONE AND CRITICAL ILLNESS

Numerous studies have shown that serum T_3 and (in some patients) T_4 levels are reduced in critical illness. Serum free T_4 levels, measured by equilibrium dialysis, are usually normal or elevated, and TSH levels are not increased. This reduction in T_3 level is reproduced in fasted subjects. In the latter, physiologic supplements of oral T_3 have increased skeletal muscle breakdown, and it is believed that the impairment of conversion of T_4 to T_3 in such situations protects a patient from excessive catabolism. Therefore, administering thyroid hormone to patients with nonthyroidal illness has been discouraged.[1, 2] Two controlled studies have addressed this issue. Becker and colleagues[57] gave L-T_3 to patients with extensive burns and found neither beneficial nor detrimental effect. Brent and Hershman[58] gave L-T_4 to a small group of patients with severe medical or surgical disease and also found no benefit. The tissue concentrations of thyroid hormones in patients with nonthyroidal illness have not been well studied.

Arem and coworkers[59] measured cell contents of T_4 and T_3 in 12 patients dying of nonthyroidal illness and in another 10 healthy persons killed suddenly by trauma. Tissue concentrations of T_3 were reduced in the liver, lung, kidney, pituitary, hypothalamus, and cerebral cortex of patients with nonthyroidal illness; T_4 levels were lower in the liver. The crucial question raised by these findings is whether they indicate the presence of tissue hypothyroidism.

Since the mid-1980s, several bodies of literature have provided evidence—albeit preliminary or controversial—for a beneficial role of thyroid hormone in selected circumstances related to critical illness. The most numerous works are found in the literature on organ transplantation. Several investigators have claimed that giving small doses of thyroid hormone to donors before organ removal improves organ survival[60] and, when given to recipients, reduces the need for inotropic support and the number of days spent in the ICU.[61] Animal studies indicate that the effect may be due to improvement in cellular metabolic function. Not all reports are favorable, and worsening of metabolic acidosis with T_3 therapy has been reported.[62]

T_3, when given in sufficient quantity to raise serum free T_3 levels to normal, acts as an inotropic agent in patients undergoing myocardial revascularization, a condition of nonthyroidal illness.[1, 2] Finally, evidence from studies in experimental animals demonstrates that pharmacologic doses of T_4 protect against the development of acute renal failure. This result may be because of an effect of the hormone on plasma membrane functions or epidermal growth factor action.[63] The possible benefit of this therapy in human acute renal failure is unknown.

At this time, thyroid hormone use cannot be recommended in any of the conditions described in this section. The results do raise the possibility that thyroid hormone use may be warranted under specific circumstances but that its clinical application, if any, requires additional carefully designed clinical trials.

OBSTRUCTIVE THYROID EMERGENCIES

Thyroid enlargement, in the absence of biochemical abnormalities, can create a surgical emergency.[16, 64, 65] Although the thyroid gland usually can expand when it is in its normal cervical location, a substernally located thyroid gland can cause obstruction within the thoracic inlet. Frequent symptoms include dyspnea, dysphagia, and a sense of fullness or choking. Less common but more serious is the occurrence of acute respiratory failure, respiratory arrest, or the superior vena cava syndrome. The most useful diagnostic tool for detecting upper airway obstruction is the flow-volume loop,[66] which should be obtained for every patient with a substernal or intrathoracic goiter. Although the superior vena cava syndrome is most often caused by a malignancy, this disorder occasionally may be due to a benign goiter.[16, 64, 65] It can be cured by surgery.

Rarely, massive upper gastrointestinal hemorrhage that results from downhill varices produced by goiter has been reported.[16, 65] Although most goiters are benign, sudden thyroid enlargement should suggest the presence of malignancy, such as a thyroid lymphoma or an anaplastic carcinoma. The former is amenable to therapy,[67] whereas the latter carries a dismal prognosis.[68]

Surgery is the preferred treatment for compressive goiters, although endoscopic insertion of a tracheal endoprosthesis has been used in inoperable patients.[69] Radioiodine also can substantially reduce the size of nontoxic goiters by an average of 40% after a year. It is of no value for acute emergencies but may be considered in older patients with significant comorbid diseases who have no significant airway obstruction.[70]

SUMMARY

Thyroid emergencies are not common. When they do occur, they may be attributed to either biochemical or anatomic abnormalities. The management of patients with these disorders is multidisciplinary and may require the expertise of a critical care physician and nurse, an endocrinologist, a pulmonologist, a cardiologist, and a surgeon.

References

1. Chopra IJ: Euthyroid sick syndrome: Is it a misnomer? J Clin Endocrinol Metab 1997; 82:329.
2. McIver B, Gorman CA: Euthyroid sick syndrome: An overview. Thyroid 1997; 7:125.
3. Engler D, Burger AG: The deiodination of the iodothyronines and of their derivatives in man. Endocr Rev 1984; 5:151.
4. LoPresti JS, Mizuno L, Nimalysuria A, et al: Characteristics of 3,5,3′-triiodothyronine sulfate metabolism in euthyroid man. J Clin Endocrinol Metab 1991; 73:703.
5. Wong TK, Pekary AE, Hoo GS, et al: Comparison of methods for measuring free thyroxin in nonthyroidal illness. Clin Chem 1992; 38:720.
6. Smallridge RC: Thyrotropin-secreting pituitary tumors. Endocrinol Metab Clin North Am 1987; 16:765.
7. Refetoff S, Weiss RE, Usala SJ: The syndromes of resistance to thyroid hormone. Endocr Rev 1993; 14:348.
8. Beck-Peccoz P, Brucker-Davis F, Persani, L, et al: Thyrotropin-secreting pituitary tumors. Endocr Rev 1996; 17:610.
9. Woeber KA: Thyrotoxicosis and the heart. N Engl J Med 1992; 327:94.
10. Dillmann WH: Cardiac function in thyroid disease: Clinical features and management considerations. Ann Thorac Surg 1993; 56:S9.
11. Kendrick AH, O'Reilly JF, Laszlo G: Lung function and exercise performance in hyperthyroidism before and after treatment. Q J Med 1988; 256:615.
12. Siafakas NM, Milona I, Salesiotou V, et al: Respiratory muscle strength in hyperthyroidism before and after treatment. Am Rev Respir Dis 1992; 146:1025.
13. Wegener M, Wedmann B, Langhoff T, et al: Effect of hyperthyroidism on the transit of a caloric solid-liquid meal through the stomach, the small intestine, and the colon in man. J Clin Endocrinol Metab 1992; 75:745.
14. Davis PJ, Davis FB: Hyperthyroidism in patients over the age of 60 years. Medicine 1974; 53:161.
15. Tibaldi JM, Barzel US, Albin J, et al: Thyrotoxicosis in the very old. Am J Med 1986; 81:619.
16. Smallridge RC: Metabolic and anatomic thyroid emergencies: A review. Crit Care Med 1992; 20:276.
17. Goodwin TM, Montoro M, Mestman JH, et al: The role of chorionic gonadotropin in transient hyperthyroidism of hyperemesis gravidarum. J Clin Endocrinol Metab 1992; 75:1333.
18. Burch HB, Wartofsky L: Life-threatening thyrotoxicosis: Thyroid storm. Endocrinol Metab Clin North Am 1993; 22:263.
19. Tietgens ST, Leinung MC: Thyroid storm. Med Clin North Am 1995; 79:169.
20. Borst GC, Eil C, Burman KD: Euthyroid hyperthyroxinemia. Ann Intern Med 1983; 98:366.
21. Cohen JH III, Ingbar SH, Braverman LE: Thyrotoxicosis due to ingestion of excess thyroid hormone. Endocr Rev 1989; 10:113.
22. Georges J-L, Normand J-P, Lenormand M-E, et al: Life-threatening thyrotoxicosis induced by amiodarone in patients with benign heart disease. Eur Heart J 1992; 13:129.
23. Bonelli J, Haydl H, Hruby K, et al: The pharmacokinetics of digoxin in patients with manifest hyperthyroidism and after normalization of thyroid function. Int J Clin Pharmacol 1978; 16:302.
24. Feely J, Stevenson IH, Crooks J: Increased clearance of propranolol in thyrotoxicosis. Ann Intern Med 1981; 94:472.
25. Nakazawa HK, Sakurai K, Hamada N, et al: Management of atrial fibrillation in the post-thyrotoxic state. Am J Med 1982; 72:903.
26. Petersen P, Hansen JM: Stroke in thyrotoxicosis with atrial fibrillation. Stroke 1988; 19:15.
27. Atwood JE, Albers GW: Anticoagulation and atrial fibrillation. Herz 1993; 18:27.
28. Nabil N, Miner DJ, Amatruda JM: Methimazole: An alternative route of administration. J Clin Endocrinol Metab 1982; 54:180.
29. Yeung S-CJ, Go R, Balasubramanyam A: Rectal administration of iodide and propylthiouracil in the treatment of thyroid storm. Thyroid 1995; 5:403.
30. Shen D-C, Wu S-Y, Chopra IJ, et al: Long-term treatment of Graves' hyperthyroidism with sodium ipodate. J Clin Endocrinol Metab 1985; 61:723.
31. Roti E, Gardini E, Minelli R, et al: Sodium ipodate and methimazole in the long-term treatment of hyperthyroid Graves' disease. Metabolism 1993; 42:403.
32. Croxson MS, Hall TD, Nicoloff JT: Combination drug therapy for treatment of hyperthyroid Graves' disease. J Clin Endocrinol Metab 1977; 45:623.
33. Ikram H: The nature and prognosis of thyrotoxic heart disease. Q J Med 1985; 213:19.

34. Brunette DD, Rothong C: Emergency department management of thyrotoxic crisis with esmolol. Am J Emerg Med 1991; 9:232.
35. Preuschof L, Keller F, Bogner U, et al: Plasma exchange and hemoperfusion in iodine-induced thyrotoxicosis. Blood Purif 1991; 9:164.
36. Schaaf L, Greschner M, Paschke R, et al: Thyrotoxic crisis in Graves' disease: Indication for immediate surgery. Klin Wochenschr 1990; 68:1037.
37. Shakir KMM, Michaels RD, Hays JH, et al: The use of bile acid sequestrants to lower serum thyroid hormones in iatrogenic hyperthyroidism. Ann Intern Med 1993; 118:112.
38. Köbberling J, Hintze G, Becker H-D: Iodine-induced thyrotoxicosis—A case for subtotal thyroidectomy in severely ill patients. Klin Wochenschr 1985; 63:1.
39. Bartalena L, Brogioni S, Grasso L, et al: Treatment of amiodarone-induced thyrotoxicosis, a difficult challenge: Results of a prospective study. J Clin Endocrinol Metab 1996; 81:2930.
40. Ambrosino N, Pacini F, Paggiaro PL, et al: Impaired ventilatory drive in short-term primary hypothyroidism and its reversal by 1-triiodothyronine. J Endocrinol Invest 1985; 8:533.
41. Rajagopal KR, Abbrecht PH, Derderian SS, et al: Obstructive sleep apnea in hypothyroidism. Ann Intern Med 1984; 101:491.
42. Robuschi G, Safran M, Braverman LE, et al: Hypothyroidism in the elderly. Endocr Rev 1987; 8:142.
43. Tachman ML, Guthrie GP Jr: Hypothyroidism: Diversity of presentation. Endocr Rev 1984; 5:456.
44. Nicoloff JT, LoPresti JS: Myxedema coma: A form of decompensated hypothyroidism. Endocrinol Metab Clin North Am 1993; 22:279.
45. Jordan RM: Myxedema coma: Pathophysiology, therapy, and factors affecting prognosis. Med Clin North Am 1995; 79:185.
46. Mandel SJ, Brent GA, Larsen PR: Levothyroxine therapy in patients with thyroid disease. Ann Intern Med 1993; 119:492.
47. Hennessey JV, Evaul JE, Tseng Y-C, et al: L-Thyroxine dosage: A reevaluation of therapy with contemporary preparations. Ann Intern Med 1986; 105:11.
48. Levine HD: Compromise therapy in the patient with angina pectoris and hypothyroidism. Am J Med 1980; 69:411.
49. Ladenson PW, Sherman SI, Baughman KL, et al: Reversible alterations in myocardial gene expression in a young man with dilated cardiomyopathy and hypothyroidism. Proc Natl Acad Sci U S A 1992; 89:5251.
50. Croxson MS, Ibbertson HK: Serum digoxin in patients with thyroid disease. Br Med J 1975; 3:566.
51. Kaptein EM, Quion-Verde H, Swinney RS, et al: Acute hemodynamic effects of levothyroxine loading in critically ill hypothyroid patients. Arch Intern Med 1986; 146:662.
52. Hylander B, Rosenqvist U: Treatment of myxoedema coma-factors associated with fatal outcome. Acta Endocrinol 1985; 108:65.
53. Becker C: Hypothyroidism and atherosclerotic heart disease: Pathogenesis, medical management, and the role of coronary artery bypass surgery. Endocr Rev 1985; 6:432.
54. Weinberg AD, Brennan MD, Gorman CA, et al: Outcome of anesthesia and surgery in hypothyroid patients. Arch Intern Med 1983; 143:893.
55. Drucker DJ, Burrow GN: Cardiovascular surgery in the hypothyroid patient. Arch Intern Med 1985; 145:1585.
56. Ladenson PW, Levin AA, Ridgway EC, et al: Complications of surgery in hypothyroid patients. Am J Med 1984; 77:261.
57. Becker RA, Vaughan GM, Ziegler MG, et al: Hypermetabolic low triiodothyronine syndrome of burn injury. Crit Care Med 1982; 10:870.
58. Brent GA, Hershman JM: Thyroxine therapy in patients with severe nonthyroidal illnesses and low serum thyroxine concentration. J Clin Endocrinol Metab 1986; 63:1.
59. Arem R, Wiener GJ, Kaplan SG, et al: Reduced tissue thyroid hormone levels in fatal illness. Metabolism 1993; 42:1102.
60. Novitzky D: Novel actions of thyroid hormone: The role of triiodothyronine in cardiac transplantation. Thyroid 1996; 6:531.
61. Jeevanandam V: Triiodothyronine: Spectrum of use in heart transplantation. Thyroid 1997; 7:139.
62. Randell TT, Höckerstedt KAV: Triiodothyronine treatment is not indicated in brain-dead multiorgan donors: A controlled study. Transplantation Proc 1993; 25:1552.
63. Wagener OE, Lieske JC, Toback FG: Molecular and cell biology of acute renal failure: New therapeutic strategies. New Horiz 1995; 3:634.
64. Newman E, Shaha AR: Substernal goiter. J Surg Oncol 1995; 60:207.
65. Mack E: Management of patients with substernal goiters. Surg Clin North Am 1995; 75:377.
66. Miller MR, Pincock AC, Oates GD, et al: Upper airway obstruction due to goitre: Detection, prevalence and results of surgical management. Q J Med 1990; 274:177.
67. Butler JS Jr, Brady LW, Amendola BE: Lymphoma of the thyroid: Report of five cases and review. Am J Clin Oncol 1990; 13:64.
68. Nel CJC, van Heerden JA, Goellner JR, et al: Anaplastic carcinoma of the thyroid: A clinicopathologic study of 82 cases. Mayo Clin Proc 1985; 60:51.
69. Noppen M, Meysman M, Dhondt E, et al: Upper airway obstruction due to inoperable intrathoracic goitre treated by tracheal endoprosthesis. Thorax 1994; 49:1034.
70. Huysmans D, Hermus A, Edelbroek M, et al: Radioiodine for nontoxic multinodular goiter. Thyroid 1997; 7:235.

71

Diabetic Emergencies

Guillermo E. Umpierrez, MD, FACP
Thomas R. Ziegler, MD

A balance between hepatic glucose production and glucose utilization in peripheral tissues tightly regulates plasma glucose concentration. A complex interplay of glucose-lowering and glucose-raising factors maintains the plasma glucose concentration within a narrow range, roughly 4.0 to 7.0 mmol/L (72 to 126 mg/dL), and prevents the devastating consequences of hyperglycemia and hypoglycemia. Life-threatening complications of diabetes mellitus are diabetic ketoacidosis (DKA), hyperglycemic hyperosmolar syndrome (HHS), and hypoglycemic crises. DKA and HHS are related to insulin deficiency. Hypoglycemia is a major problem for many patients with diabetes, especially those with drug-treated diabetes. This chapter reviews the pathogenesis, diagnosis, and management of these major complications of diabetes mellitus.

DIABETIC KETOACIDOSIS

Diabetic ketoacidosis is a complex metabolic disturbance of carbohydrate, lipid, and protein metabolism characterized by hyperglycemia, hyperketonemia, and metabolic acidosis. DKA occurs in the presence of absolute or near-absolute insulin deficiency, such as in patients with insulin-dependent (type 1) diabetes mellitus. However, patients with non-insulin-dependent (type 2) diabetes are also at risk during the catabolic stress of acute illness.

In contrast to popular belief, DKA is more common in adults than in children.[1] In community-based studies, more than 40% of patients with DKA are older than 40 years, and more than 20% are older than 55 years.[1, 2] Many of these adult patients with DKA had type 2 diabetes, because 29% of the patients were obese, had measurable insulin secretion, and had a low prevalence of autoimmune markers of beta cell destruction.[3]

Because most cases of DKA occur in patients with a known history of diabetes mellitus (~80%), this acute metabolic complication should be largely preventable through early detection, patient education, and outpatient management. DKA

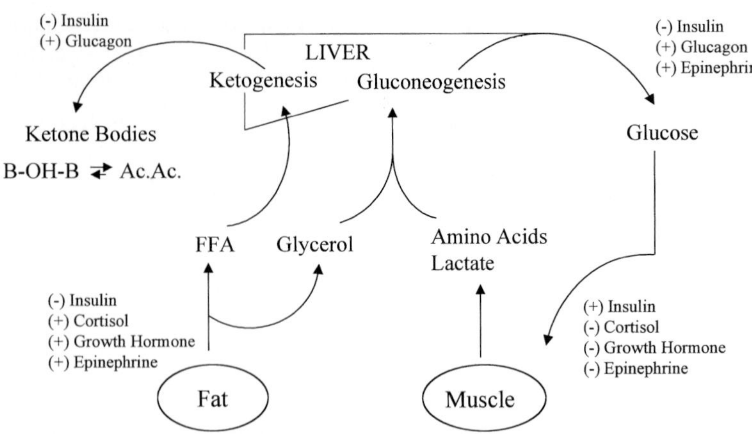

Figure 71–1. Role of insulin and counterregulatory hormones in the pathogenesis of diabetic ketoacidosis (DKA) and hyperglycemic hyperosmolar nonketotic syndrome (HHS). FFA = free fatty acids.

continues, however, to be an important cause of morbidity and mortality among patients with diabetes.[4, 5] It is estimated that DKA accounts for 9% to 28% of all diabetes-related hospital admissions,[6, 7] and epidemiologic studies in the United States indicate that hospitalizations for DKA are increasing.[5] In community-based studies, the incidence varied from 8 episodes per 1000 person-years for DKA at all ages to 13.4 per 1000 person-years among diabetic persons in whom the diagnosis of diabetes was made before age 30 years.[4, 8] Data for DKA from hospital discharge surveys in the United states during 1989 to 1991[4] indicated an annual average of 100,000 cases, with discharge rates higher for black males than for black females, white females, and white males.

Despite advances in the treatment of DKA, it remains a serious event, with mortality rates as high as 5% to 10%.[4, 7, 9] Mortality of this disease increases substantially with aging; mortality rates for patients aged 65 to 75 years reach 20% to 40%.[9, 10] Death in patients with DKA rarely results from the metabolic complications of hyperglycemia or metabolic acidosis, but rather relates to the underlying medical illness (i.e., trauma, infection) that precipitated the ketoacidosis.

Pathogenesis

Diabetic ketoacidosis is characterized by uncontrolled hyperglycemia, metabolic acidosis, and increased circulating total body ketone concentration. Ketoacidosis results from the lack or ineffectiveness of insulin with concomitant elevation of counterregulatory hormones (glucagon, catecholamines, cortisol, and growth hormone).[11, 12]

The physiologic effects of insulin and counterregulatory hormones are shown in Figure 71–1. Insulin controls hepatic glucose production by suppressing hepatic gluconeogenesis and glycogenolysis. In insulin-sensitive tissues, such as muscle, insulin promotes protein anabolism, glucose uptake, and glycogen synthesis, and inhibits glycogenolysis and protein breakdown. In addition, insulin is a powerful inhibitor of lipolysis, free fatty acid (FFA) oxidation, and ketogenesis. The counterregulatory hormones promote metabolic pathways opposite to insulin action, in both the liver and peripheral tissues.[12–14] During metabolic decompensation, the association of insulin deficiency and insulin resistance alters glucose production and disposal and increases lipolysis and production of ketone bodies.

The pathophysiologic basis for hyperglycemia and ketoacidosis in DKA is shown in Figure 71–2. Hyperglycemia results from increased hepatic glucose production and impaired glucose utilization in peripheral tissues. Increased gluconeogenesis results from the high availability of gluconeogenic precursors (alanine, lactate, and glycerol) and from the greater activity of gluconeogenic enzymes (phosphoenolpyruvate carboxykinase [PEPCK], fructose-1,6-bisphosphatase, and pyruvate carboxylase).[12, 15] In addition, both hyperglycemia and high ketone levels cause an osmotic diuresis, which leads to hypovolemia and decreased glomerular filtration rate; the latter further aggravates hyperglycemia.[13, 15]

The mechanisms underlying the higher production of ketones have been discussed in a number of reviews.[12, 16, 17] The association of insulin deficiency with higher concentrations of catecholamines, cortisol, and growth hormone activates hormone-sensitive lipase in adipose tissue. This enzyme causes endogenous triglyceride breakdown with subsequent release of large amounts of fatty acids into the circulation.[13, 16] Elevated FFAs are transported into the hepatic mitochondria, where they are oxidized to ketone bodies, a process stimulated predominantly by glucagon.[14] Glucagon lowers the hepatic levels of malonyl coenzyme A (CoA), the first-committed intermediate in the synthesis of long-chain fatty acids (lipogenesis) and a potent inhibitor of fatty acid oxidation.[17] Malonyl CoA inhibits carnitine palmitoyl transferase I (CPT I), an enzyme that regulates movement of FFA into the mitochondria. Therefore, reduction in malonyl CoA leads to stimulation of

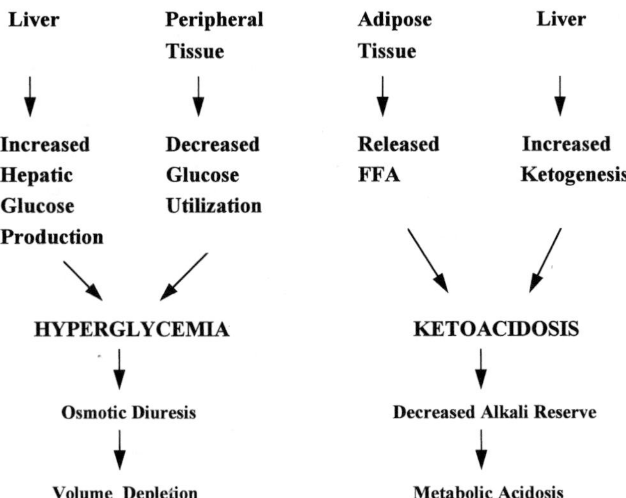

Figure 71–2. Pathogenesis of acute metabolic decompensation in diabetes mellitus. (From Umpierrez GE, Khajavi M, Kitabchi AE: Diabetic ketoacidosis and hyperglycemic hyperosmolar nonketotic syndrome. Am J Med Sci 1996; 311:225–233.)

CPT I and effectively increases ketoacid production. In addition to increased ketone body production, there is evidence that decreased clearance of ketoacids contributes to the development of DKA.

Precipitating Causes

DKA is the initial manifestation of diabetes in 20% to 30% of patients with type 1 diabetes. In known diabetic patients, precipitating factors for DKA include infections, intercurrent illnesses, psychologic stress, and noncompliance with therapy (Table 71-1). Infection is the most common precipitating factor for DKA, occurring in 30% to 50% of cases.[1, 6, 7] Urinary tract infection and pneumonia account for the majority of infections. Other acute conditions that may precipitate DKA are cerebrovascular accident, alcohol abuse, pancreatitis, pulmonary embolism, myocardial infarction, and trauma. Drugs that affect carbohydrate metabolism, such as corticosteroids, thiazides, sympathomimetic agents (e.g., dobutamine and terbutaline), and pentamidine, may also precipitate the development of DKA.

Noncompliance and psychologic factors have also been emphasized as contributors to the incidence of DKA. In a survey of 341 female patients with type 1 diabetes, Polonsky and associates[18] reported that psychologic problems complicated by eating disorders were a contributing factor in 20% of recurrent ketoacidosis episodes in young women. Rydall and coworkers[19] reported that up to one third of young women with type 1 diabetes had eating disturbances that affected the management of their diabetes and increased the risk of microvascular complications. Factors that may lead young subjects to omit taking their insulin include (1) fear of gaining weight if their disease is under good metabolic control, (2) fear of hypoglycemia, (3) rebellion against authority, and (4) diabetes-related stress.

Noncompliance with therapy has also been reported to be a major precipitating cause of DKA in urban black and medically indigent patients. Both Musey and colleagues[20] and Umpierrez and associates[2] reported that in urban black patients, poor compliance with insulin accounted for more than 50% of cases of DKA in patients admitted to a major urban hospital. Similarly, another study reported that rates of hospitalization for DKA in diabetic patients without health insurance or with Medicaid insurance alone was two to three times higher than comparable rates among diabetic persons with private health insurance.[21]

Although the use of continuous subcutaneous insulin infusion by an insulin pump was associated with a higher risk of DKA,[22] mechanical improvements in such devices and the use of frequent home glucose monitoring have reduced this complication considerably. In one of the largest prospective studies of therapy and follow-up for type 1 diabetes, the Diabetes Control and Complications Trial,[23] the incidence of DKA was quite low in patients treated with continuous insulin infusion devices.

TABLE 71–1. Causes of Diabetic Ketoacidosis (DKA) and Hypoglycemic Hyperosmolar Syndrome (HHS)

Precipitating Cause	Admissions (%)	
	DKA*	HHS†
Infection	30–35	40–60
Failure to take insulin	15–40	0–35
New-onset diabetes	20–25	20–25
Medical illnesses	10–20	10–15
Unknown	2–10	—

* Data from Umpierrez GE, et al: Arch Intern Med 1997; 157:669[2]; Kitabchi AE, et al: *In* Joslin's Diabetes Mellitus. 13th ed. Kahn CR, et al (Eds). Philadelphia, Lea & Febiger, 1994, pp 738–770[7]; and Morris LR, et al: Ann Intern Med 1986; 105:836.[35]

† Data from Umpierrez GE, et al: Arch Intern Med 1997; 157:669[2]; Kitabchi AE, et al: *In* Joslin's Diabetes Mellitus. 13th ed. Kahn CR, et al (Eds). Philadelphia, Lea & Febiger, 1994, pp 738–770[7]; and Gerich JE, et al: J Clin Invest 1976; 57:875.[12]

Diagnosis

Symptoms and Signs

The clinical presentation of DKA usually develops rapidly, over a span of less than 24 hours. Polyuria, polydipsia, and weight loss may be present for several days prior to the development of ketoacidosis, whereas vomiting and abdominal pain are commonly the presenting symptoms. Abdominal pain sometimes mimicking an acute abdomen is especially common in children; although the cause has not been elucidated, delayed gastric emptying and ileus induced by electrolyte disturbances and metabolic acidosis have been implicated as possible causes of the abdominal pain in DKA.

Physical examination reveals signs of dehydration, including loss of skin turgor, dry mucous membranes, tachycardia, and hypotension. Mental status can vary from full alertness to profound lethargy; however, fewer than 20% of patients are hospitalized with loss of consciousness.[2, 7] Acetone odor on the breath and labored Kussmaul's respiration may also be present on admission, particularly in patients with severe metabolic acidosis. Although the most common precipitating event in DKA is infection, most patients are normothermic or even hypothermic at presentation. If a patient with DKA becomes febrile, a vigorous search for an underlying infection must be undertaken.

Laboratory Findings

Although the diagnosis of DKA can be suspected on clinical grounds, the confirmation is based on laboratory tests. The syndrome of DKA consists of the triad of hyperglycemia, ketosis, and acidemia. Diagnostic criteria for DKA accepted by most experts in the field are as follows[6, 7, 13]:

- Blood glucose level higher than 250 mg/dL
- pH lower than 7.3
- Serum bicarbonate concentration lower than 15 mEq/L
- Moderate ketonemia (β-hydroxybutyrate and acetoacetic acid levels higher than 3 mmol/L)

The key diagnostic feature is the elevation in circulating total blood ketone concentration. In clinical practice, assessment of augmented ketonemia is usually made with the nitroprusside reaction, which provides a semiquantitative estimation of acetoacetate and acetone levels. This reagent test can underestimate the severity of ketoacidosis, however, because the assay does not recognize the presence of β-hydroxybutyrate. Rapid and specific enzymatic tests that measure β-hydroxybutyrate and acetoacetate in small samples have become available[24, 25] and are preferable in establishing the diagnosis of ketoacidosis.

Accumulation of ketoacids usually results in a high anion gap metabolic acidosis. The anion gap is calculated by subtracting the sum of chloride (Cl) and bicarbonate (HCO_3) concentrations from the sodium (Na) concentration [$Na - (Cl + HCO_3)$]. The normal anion gap is 12 ± 2 mEq/L.

Clinicians should be aware that the diagnosis of DKA can be confounded by the coexistence of other acid-base disorders. The arterial pH may be normal or even high, depending on the level of respiratory compensation as well as by the presence of metabolic alkalosis from frequent vomiting, diuretic use, or volume contraction. Similarly, the blood glucose concentration may be normal or only minimally elevated in 15% of patients with DKA (<300 mg/dL), such as in alcoholic subjects or in patients receiving insulin. In addition, a wide variability in the type of metabolic acidosis has been reported. Androgue and coworkers[26] reported that 46% of patients admitted for DKA had a high anion gap acidosis, 43% had mixed anion gap acidosis and hyperchloremic metabolic acidosis, and 11% had only hyperchloremic metabolic acidosis.

In clinical practice, determination of the anion gap and calculation of the delta gap (Δ gap) are useful clinical tools for detecting mixed acid-base disturbances, which may not be evident from measurement of pH or bicarbonate.[27, 28] In an uncomplicated high anion gap metabolic acidosis (i.e., DKA), for every 1-mmol/L rise in the anion gap, there should be a concomitant fall of 1 mmol/L in the bicarbonate concentration. In a patient with DKA, any significant deviation from this rule implies the existence of mixed acid-base disorder.[27, 29] If the rise in calculated anion gap is greater than the fall in serum bicarbonate, a superimposed metabolic alkalosis is usually present. Conversely, if the rise in anion gap is lower than the fall in bicarbonate, a concomitant non–anion gap hyperchloremic metabolic acidosis is usually present.

Not all patients who present with ketoacidosis have DKA. Patients with chronic ethanol abuse and a recent binge culminating in nausea, vomiting, and acute starvation may present with alcoholic ketoacidosis. The key diagnostic feature that differentiates diabetic from alcohol-induced ketoacidosis is the concentration of blood glucose. DKA is characterized by severe hyperglycemia, but the presence of ketoacidosis without hyperglycemia in an alcoholic patient is virtually diagnostic of alcoholic ketoacidosis. In addition, some patients whose food intake has been low (less than 500 calories/day) for several days may present with starvation ketosis. A healthy subject, however, is able to adapt to prolonged fasting by (1) increasing the clearance of ketones by the peripheral tissues (brain and muscle) and (2) enhancing the kidney's ability to excrete ammonia to compensate for the higher acid production.[30] Therefore, a patient with starvation ketosis rarely presents with a serum bicarbonate concentration less than 18 mEq/L.[30]

Most patients with DKA present with leukocytosis; however, a leukocyte count greater than 25,000/mm^3 or the presence of more than 10% neutrophil bands is seldom seen in the absence of bacterial infection.[15] The admission serum sodium level is usually low because of the osmotic flux of water from the intracellular to the extracellular space in the presence of hyperglycemia. An increase in serum sodium concentration in the presence of hyperglycemia indicates a rather profound water loss.

The severity of the sodium and water deficit may be assessed as follows: The serum sodium level can be corrected by the addition of 1.6 mEq/L to the measured serum sodium level for every 100 mg/dL by which the glucose level exceeds 100 mg/dL.[13] Extreme hypertriglyceridemia, which may be present during the DKA as a result of impaired lipoprotein lipase activity, may cause lipemic serum with spurious lowering of serum sodium (pseudohyponatremia).

The admission serum potassium concentration is usually elevated in patients with DKA. These high levels occur because of a shift of potassium from the intracellular to the extracellular space as a result of acidemia, insulin deficiency, and hypertonicity. Similarly, the admission serum phosphate level may be normal or elevated because of metabolic acidosis. Dehydration also can lead to increases in total serum protein, albumin, amylase, and creatine phosphokinase concentrations in patients with acute diabetic decompensation.

Treatment

Successful treatment of DKA requires frequent monitoring of patients, correction of hypovolemia and metabolic disorders, and careful search for the precipitating cause of DKA. A flow sheet is invaluable for recording vital signs, volume and rate of fluid administration, insulin dosage, and urine output and to assess the efficacy of medical therapy.

Fluid Therapy

Because patients with DKA are invariably volume-depleted (fluid deficit of 4 to 6 L), priority should be given to fluid resuscitation and electrolyte replacement.

Initial fluid therapy is directed toward expansion of intravascular volume and restoration of renal perfusion. Isotonic saline (0.9% NaCl), infused at a rate of 500 to 1000 mL/hour during the first 2 hours, is usually adequate, but in patients with hypovolemic shock, a third or fourth liter of isotonic saline may be needed to restore normal blood pressure and tissue perfusion. For children, intravenous fluid should be given at 20 mL/kg/hour, or 500 mL/m^2/hour, in the initial phase.

After intravascular volume depletion has been corrected, the normal saline infusion should be reduced to 250 mL/hour or changed to 0.45% saline, depending on the serum sodium concentration. The free water deficit can be estimated, on the basis of the corrected serum sodium concentration, with the following equation[31]:

$$\text{water balance} = 0.6\,(\text{body weight in kg}) \times \left(1 - \frac{[\text{corrected sodium}]}{140}\right)$$

The goal is to replace half the estimated water deficit over a period of 12 to 24 hours. The fluid requirement of children with DKA must be carefully calculated, and replacement should be carried out slowly over a period of 36 to 48 hours to avoid rapid shifts of fluids into the brain and the development of cerebral edema.[32] For young children, the average recommended rate of intravenous fluid administration is 5 to 8 mL/kg/hr, with a maximum of 4 L/m^2/24 hours.[33]

Once the plasma glucose concentration reaches 250 mg/dL, replacement fluids should contain 5% to 10% dextrose, to (1) allow continued administration of insulin until ketonemia is controlled and (2) avoid hypoglycemia.[2, 28] An additional important aspect of fluid management in hyperglycemic states is to replace the volume of urinary losses. Failure to adjust fluid replacement for urinary losses may delay correction of electrolyte levels and water deficit.

Insulin Therapy

The cornerstone of management of diabetic ketoacidosis is insulin administration. Insulin therapy increases peripheral glucose utilization and decreases hepatic glucose production, thereby lowering blood glucose concentration. In addition, it inhibits the release of free fatty acids from adipose tissue and decreases ketogenesis, leading to the reversal of ketogenesis.

Regular insulin given intravenously by continuous infusion remains the drug of choice. Intermittent infusion or hourly boluses of low-dose intravenous insulin should be avoided because of regular insulin's short half-life. We recommend an initial intravenous bolus of regular insulin of 0.1 U/kg, followed by a continuous infusion of regular insulin at a dose of 0.1 U/kg/hour until blood glucose levels reach 250 mg/dL.[2, 28] At this time, dextrose should be added to intravenous fluids, and the insulin infusion rate reduced to 0.05 U/kg/hour. Thereafter, the rate of insulin administration is adjusted to maintain glucose levels at approximately 200 mg/dL and is continued until ketoacidosis is resolved.

During insulin therapy, capillary blood glucose levels should be determined every 1 to 2 hours at the bedside with the use of a glucose oxidase reagent strip, and blood should be drawn every 4 hours for determinations of serum electrolytes, glucose, blood urea nitrogen (BUN), creatinine, magnesium, phosphorus, and venous pH.

In 1997, Umpierrez and associates[2] reported the results of an insulin adjustment protocol designed to keep plasma glucose levels between 160 and 220 mg/dL during treatment of patients with hyperglycemic emergencies. In 144 patients with DKA and 23 patients with hyperglycemic hyperosmolar nonketotic syndrome treated with this protocol, serum glucose levels came into target range within 8 hours, and the mean duration of treatment to clear ketoacidosis was 18 hours. Compared with treatment of patients without a predefined protocol, this insulin adjustment protocol resulted in a fourfold lower incidence of hypoglycemic events (5% versus 23%).[2]

Potassium

Despite a total body potassium deficit of 3 to 5 mEq/kg, the serum potassium level in most patients with DKA is at or above the upper limits of normal.[34] With initiation of therapy, the extracellular potassium concentration invariably falls. Rehydration lowers the serum potassium level by exerting a dilutional effect and by increasing urinary potassium excretion. Both insulin therapy and correction of acidosis decrease serum potassium levels by stimulating cellular potassium uptake in peripheral tissues.[7, 34] Therefore, to prevent hypokalemia, most patients should be given intravenous potassium during the course of DKA therapy.

We recommend potassium replacement with intravenous potassium chloride (20 to 30 mEq/L) as soon as the serum potassium concentration is below 5.5 mEq/L. The treatment goal is to maintain serum potassium levels within the normal range (i.e., 4 to 5 mEq/L). In some hyperglycemic patients with severe potassium deficiency, insulin administration may precipitate profound hypokalemia,[35] which can induce life-threatening arrhythmias and respiratory muscle weakness. Thus, if the initial serum potassium is equal to or lower than 3.0 mEq/L, potassium replacement should begin immediately using an infusion of potassium chloride at a rate of 10 to 20 mEq/hour, and one may consider withholding insulin therapy until sufficient intravenous potassium replacement is given (1 to 2 hours).

Bicarbonate

Bicarbonate administration in patients with DKA remains controversial. Severe metabolic acidosis can lead to impaired myocardial contractility, cerebral vasodilation and coma, and several gastrointestinal complications.[13, 17] Rapid alkalinization, however, may result in hypokalemia, paradoxic central nervous system acidosis, and worsened intracellular acidosis (as a result of increased carbon dioxide production) with overshoot alkalosis.[13, 17] Controlled studies have failed to show any benefit from bicarbonate therapy in patients with DKA and arterial pH between 6.9 and 7.1.[36] Nevertheless, most experts in the field recommend that in patients with severe metabolic acidosis (pH $<$ 6.9 to 7.0), 44.6 mEq of sodium bicarbonate should be added to 1 L of hypotonic saline until pH rises to at least 7.0. If the arterial pH is 7.0 or higher, no bicarbonate therapy is necessary.

Phosphate

Total body phosphate deficiency is universally present in patients with DKA, but its clinical relevance and the benefits of replacement therapy remain uncertain. Several studies have failed to show any beneficial effect of phosphate replacement on clinical outcome.[7] Furthermore, aggressive phosphate therapy is potentially hazardous, as indicated in case reports of children with DKA in whom hypocalcemia and tetany developed secondary to intravenous administration of phosphate.[33] Theoretic advantages of phosphate therapy include prevention of respiratory depression and generation of erythrocyte 2,3-diphosphoglycerate.

Because of these potential benefits, careful phosphate replacement may be indicated in patients with cardiac dysfunction, anemia, or respiratory depression, and in those with serum phosphate concentrations lower than 1.0 to 1.5 mg/dL.[7, 28] If phosphate replacement is needed, it should be administered as a potassium salt, by giving half as potassium phosphate and half as potassium chloride. In such patients, because of the risk of hypocalcemia, serum calcium and phosphate levels must be monitored during phosphate infusion.

Transition to Subcutaneous Insulin

Patients with DKA should be treated with continuous intravenous insulin until ketoacidosis is resolved. Criteria for resolution of ketoacidosis are as follows:

- Blood glucose level lower than 200 mg/dL
- Serum bicarbonate level 18 mEq/L or higher
- Venous pH greater than 7.3
- Calculated anion gap 14 mEq/L or less

When these criteria are achieved, subcutaneous insulin therapy can be started.

If the patient is able to eat, split-dose therapy with both regular (short-acting) insulin and intermediate-acting insulin may be given. Patients with known diabetes may be given insulin at the dosage they were receiving before the onset of DKA. In patients with newly diagnosed diabetes, an initial total insulin dose of 0.6 U/kg/day is usually sufficient to achieve and maintain metabolic control. Two thirds of this total daily dose should be given in the morning and one third in the evening as a split-mixed dose.

If the patient is not able to eat, we prefer to continue the intravenous insulin infusion protocol. However, the patient could receive subcutaneous regular insulin every 4 hours according to a sliding scale while an infusion of 5% dextrose in half-normal saline is given at a rate of 100 to 200 mL/hour.

Although serum β-hydroxybutyrate levels are usually lower than 1.5 mmol/L at resolution of DKA,[25] we do not recommend routine measurements of ketone levels during therapy. In some patients, however, such as those with prolonged metabolic acidosis, with combined diabetic and lactic acidosis, or with other mixed acid-base disorders, direct measurement of β-hydroxybutrate levels may be indicated. During treatment of DKA, the use of the nitroprusside test, which measures acetoacetate and acetone levels but fails to determine β-hydroxybutyrate concentration, should be avoided, because the fall in acetoacetate lags behind the resolution of DKA.[25, 36]

HYPERGLYCEMIC HYPEROSMOLAR SYNDROME

Hyperglycemic hyperosmolar syndrome (HHS) was first described by Dreschfeld[37] more than a century ago. The condition received little attention, however, until 1957, when Sament and Schwartz[38] reported their experience with a diabetic syndrome characterized by marked stupor without ketosis (diabetic hyperosmolar syndrome). During the past few decades, this syndrome has been the focus of several excellent reviews.[6, 7, 39]

Although HHS and DKA often are discussed as distinct entities, most diabetologists agree that they represent two extremes in a spectrum of emergencies caused by poorly controlled diabetes. Indeed, many patients have features of HHS and DKA. In a retrospective review of a large number of patients with decompensated diabetes, Wachtel and associates[40] reported that 22% of patients with hyperglycemic crises had DKA, 45% had HHS, and 32% had features of both disorders.

Most patients with HHS have type 2 diabetes mellitus. The typical patient with HHS has undiagnosed diabetes, is between 55 and 70 years of age, and commonly is a nursing home resident. The incidence of HHS is difficult to determine because of the lack of population-based studies, the absence of a universally accepted definition, and the multiple combined illnesses often found in these patients. The incidence of HHS as the primary diagnosis at the Memphis Regional Medical Center from 1981 to 1989 was 0.05% of all diabetes-related admissions.[7] In a prospective study of urban African-Americans, we found that of a total of 4991 adult patients admitted with the primary diagnosis of diabetes mellitus, 439 patients (9%) met biochemical criteria for DKA, and 23 patients (0.5%) for HHS.[2] Mortality attributed to HHS is considerably higher than for DKA, reported rates being 5% to 35%. Mortality in HHS is most likely dependent on underlying illness or comorbidities.[4, 7, 8]

Pathogenesis

Hyperglycemic hyperosmolar syndrome is defined as a state of severe metabolic decompensation characterized by severe hyperglycemia, hyperosmolality, and dehydration in the absence of significant ketoacidosis.[4, 8, 39] Although the pathogenesis of HHS has not been completely elucidated, relative insulin deficiency and increased concentrations of counterregulatory hormones characterize this syndrome. The absence or minimal presence of ketosis, the key difference from DKA, has been speculatively explained by a higher plasma level of endogenous insulin secretion and lower levels of counterregulatory hormones in patients with HHS.

Insulin secretion in patients with HHS is higher than in patients with DKA.[41] Serum concentrations of C peptide (an indicator of endogenous insulin secretion) in HHS are sometimes several times higher than those found in patients with DKA. In patients with HHS, the higher insulin concentration is sufficient to suppress lipolysis and ketogenesis but inadequate to regulate hepatic glucose production and promote glucose utilization. Lower levels of counterregulatory hormones also could be responsible for reduced FFA levels in HHS. Gerich and colleagues[12] reported that circulating levels of FFA, glucagon, cortisol, and growth hormone are lower in individuals with HHS than in patients with DKA. Later studies, however, found that circulating levels of glucagon and catecholamines are comparably elevated in HHS and DKA.[42] Thus, owing to these conflicting results, the role of counterregulatory hormones in the pathogenesis of ketogenesis in HHS has not been well established. Another potential mechanism for the lack of ketosis in HHS involves the inhibitory effect of hyperosmolality on lipolysis, insulin secretion, and glucose uptake.[22]

Disturbances in hydration and electrolyte balance are of great importance in the pathogenesis of HHS. The osmotic diuresis due to hyperglycemia is characterized by urinary concentrations of solutes roughly similar to half-normal saline, with combined urinary sodium and potassium concentrations of approximately 70 to 80 mEq/L.[13] Because HHS evolves over several days, continued osmotic diuresis leads to hypernatremia, particularly in elderly patients with compromised renal function or inability to drink water to keep up with urinary losses. The resulting hypernatremia and hyperglycemia, coupled with inadequate water intake and excess water loss, result in profound volume contraction. Hypovolemia leads to progressive decline in glomerular filtration rate and aggravation of the hyperglycemic state.

Precipitating Causes

Precipitating causes of HHS are shown in Table 71-1. HHS is the initial manifestation of diabetes in 7% to 17% of patients.[2, 3, 9] Infection is the major precipitating factor, occurring in 30% to 60% of patients; urinary tract infections and pneumonia are the most common infections.[39, 40] In many instances, an acute illness, such as cerebrovascular accident or myocardial infarction, provokes the release of counterregulatory hormones or compromises the access to water. Certain medications that cause DKA may also precipitate the development of HHS. These include glucocorticoids, thiazide diuretics, phenytoin, and β-blockers.[43]

Diagnosis

The diagnostic criteria for HHS are as follows:

- Plasma glucose concentration higher than 600 mg/dL
- Serum osmolality greater than 320 mOsm/kg
- The absence of ketoacidosis

Although by definition, patients with HHS have a serum pH greater than 7.3, a serum bicarbonate greater than 18 mEq/L, and negative ketone bodies in urine and plasma, mild ketonemia may be present.[22]

The importance of increased serum osmolality in the clinical presentation and outcome of patients with hyperglycemic crises has been well established.[2, 39, 40] Altered sensorium (lethargy, stupor, coma) correlates better with hyperosmolality than with the patient's age or the severity of acid-base disturbance. In a report of 23 patients with HHS, we found that the mean serum osmolality in patients who presented in coma was greater than 340 mOsm/Kg, higher than in noncomatose patients.[2] Some other researchers have advocated use of "effective" serum osmolality rather than total plasma osmolality to define the hyperosmolar state.[39, 44] Because urea is distributed equally in all body compartments, and because its accumulation does not induce an osmotic gradient across the cell membrane, it may be more appropriate to consider "effective" osmolality (Eosm), which excludes the concentration of urea. Formulas for calculation of serum osmolality (Sosm) and effective osmolality are as follows:

$$\text{Sosm} = 2\ \text{Na (mEq/L)} + \frac{\text{glucose (mg/dL)}}{18} + \frac{\text{BUN (mg/dL)}}{2.8}$$

$$\text{Eosm} = 2\ \text{Na (mEq/L)} + \frac{\text{glucose (mg/dL)}}{18}$$

The most common clinical presentation for patients with HHS is altered sensorium.[2, 39] Physical examination reveals signs of volume depletion with loss of skin turgor, weakness, tachycardia, and hypotension. Fever due to underlying infection is common, and signs of acidosis (Kussmaul's respiration, acetone breath odor, and warm skin) are usually absent. In some patients, focal neurologic signs (hemiparesis, hemianopsia) and seizures (partial motor seizures more common than generalized) may be the dominant clinical features, resulting in a common misdiagnosis of stroke. Despite the focal nature of neurolgic findings, the neurologic manifestations of HHS often reverse completely after correction of the metabolic disorder.

In addition to hyperglycemia and hyperosmolality, the laboratory profile of HHS on admission consists of normal to elevated serum sodium and potassium concentrations. Serum bicarbonate concentration may be slightly decreased but is usually higher than 15 to 18 mEq/L. Approximately 50% of patients with HHS have an increased anion gap metabolic acidosis as the result of concomitant ketoacidosis or an increase in serum lactate levels. Blood urea nitrogen and creatinine levels are commonly elevated, and initial azotemia may have both prerenal and renal causes. Leukocytosis, with cell counts in the range of 10,000/mm^3 to 15,000/mm^3, is common, and values greater than 20,000/mm^3 are suggestive of an underlying bacterial infection. Elevation of creatine phosphokinase may be observed and is often due to rhabdomyolysis.

Treatment

General therapeutic measures for HHS are similar to those recommended for patients with DKA. In general, the treatment of HHS should be directed at replacing the volume deficit, correcting hyperosmolality and electrolyte disturbances, and managing the underlying illness that may have precipitated metabolic decompensation. These goals are best achieved by managing the patient in an intensive care unit.

Fluid Therapy

Most patients with HHS are severely dehydrated on admission, with fluid deficits often ranging from 8 to 12 L in adults.[7, 39] Most investigators recommend initial fluid therapy with normal saline at a rate of 500 to 1000 mL/hour for 1 to 2 hours, directed toward expansion of intravascular volume and restoration of renal perfusion. Subsequent fluid therapy is administered as 0.45% saline at a rate of 200 to 500 mL/hour and aimed at replacing half of the estimated volume deficit during the first 12 to 24 hours.

Fluid administration may also significantly improve hyperglycemia and hypertonicity through a decline in counterregulatory hormone levels[7, 39, 40] and improvement in renal perfusion that leads to enhanced glucose excretion. Hydration alone has been shown to reduce the glucose concentration by 17% to 80% during a period of 12 to 14 hours,[39] representing an average plasma glucose reduction rate of 25 to 50 mg/dL/hour.

Insulin Therapy

Continuous infusion of a low-dose insulin regimen is the treatment of choice for patients with HHS. Subcutaneous administration of regular insulin should be avoided, because absorption of insulin from subcutaneous sites may be unpredictable in the presence of dehydration. Figure 71–3 presents an algorithm for the treatment of hyperglycemic crises (DKA and HHS).

In brief, insulin is administered as an initial bolus of 0.1 U/kg followed by a continuous infusion calculated to deliver 0.1 U/kg/hour and continued at this rate until blood glucose decreases to approximately 250 mg/dL.[27] At this time, intravenous fluids should be changed to dextrose-containing solutions, and the insulin dose should be decreased by 50% (0.05 U/kg/hour), or to 2 to 3 U/hour.[27] Thereafter, the rate of insulin administration is adjusted to maintain a blood glucose level of approximately 200 mg/dL.

Intravenous insulin infusion is usually continued until the patient is hemodynamically stable, the level of consciousness has improved, and the patient is able to tolerate food intake. Although most patients require insulin therapy after recovery from HHS, some patients may not require insulin; their diabetes may be controlled with diet alone or with diet plus an oral hypoglycemic agent.[39, 43]

Potassium

Mild to moderate hyperkalemia is commonly found in patients with HHS despite severe total body potassium depletion. Hyperglycemia and hyperosmolality cause a shift of potassium from the intracellular compartment into plasma[12] and may contribute to a false estimate of total body potassium. The serum potassium deficit in patients with HHS is 3 to 5 mEq/kg of body weight.[39]

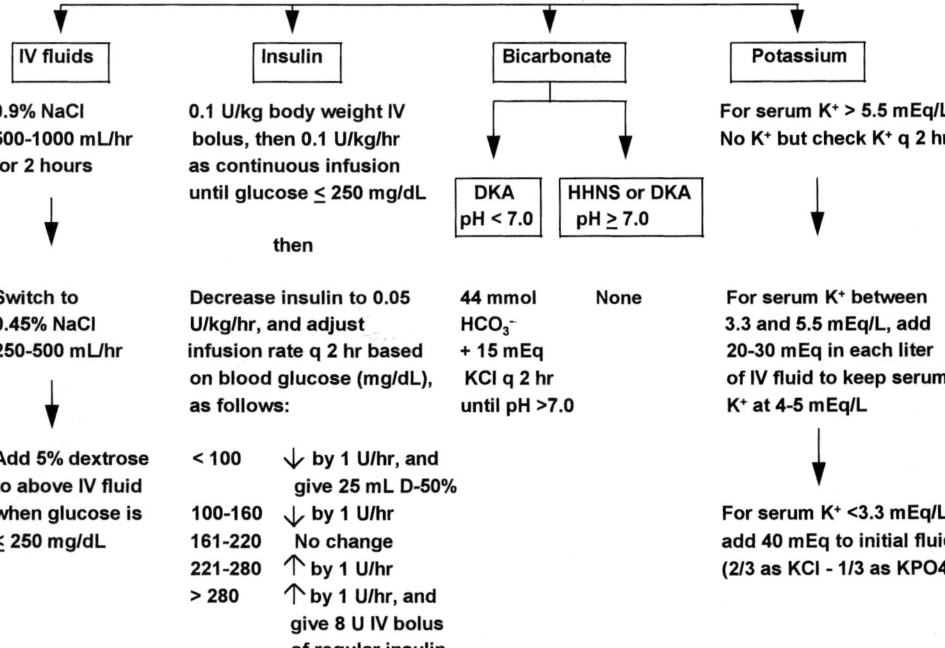
After history and physical examination, obtain complete blood count, chemistry profile, and blood gases STAT, then:
IV fluids
Insulin
Bicarbonate
Potassium
0.9% NaCl
500-1000 mL/hr
for 2 hours
0.1 U/kg body weight IV bolus, then 0.1 U/kg/hr as continuous infusion until glucose ≤ 250 mg/dL
then
DKA pH < 7.0
HHNS or DKA pH ≥ 7.0
For serum K^+ > 5.5 mEq/L
No K^+ but check K^+ q 2 hr
Switch to
0.45% NaCl
250-500 mL/hr
Decrease insulin to 0.05 U/kg/hr, and adjust infusion rate q 2 hr based on blood glucose (mg/dL), as follows:
44 mmol HCO_3^- + 15 mEq KCl q 2 hr until pH >7.0
None
For serum K^+ between 3.3 and 5.5 mEq/L, add 20-30 mEq in each liter of IV fluid to keep serum K^+ at 4-5 mEq/L
Add 5% dextrose to above IV fluid when glucose is ≤ 250 mg/dL
< 100 ↓ by 1 U/hr, and give 25 mL D-50%
100-160 ↓ by 1 U/hr
161-220 No change
221-280 ↑ by 1 U/hr
> 280 ↑ by 1 U/hr, and give 8 U IV bolus of regular insulin
For serum K^+ <3.3 mEq/L, add 40 mEq to initial fluid (2/3 as KCl - 1/3 as KPO4)
Lab follow-up: Measure glucose by finger stick q 2 hr and serum glucose, electrolytes, Mg^{++}, PO_4^-, and venous pH q 4 hr until resolution of ketoacidosis

Figure 71–3. Algorithm for treatment of diabetic ketoacidosis (DKA) and hyperglycemic hyperosmolar nonketotic syndrome (HHNS) at Grady Memorial Hospital. (From Umpierrez GE, Kelly JP, Navarrete JE, et al: Hyperglycemic crises in urban blacks. Arch Intern Med 1997; 157:669.)

The principles of potassium replacement in HHS are the same as those in DKA. We recommend that potassium replacement be initiated after serum levels fall below 5.5 mEq/L in the presence of adequate urine output. Generally, potassium replacement at a rate of 20 to 30 mEq/hour is appropriate[7, 39, 43]; the goal is to maintain a serum potassium concentration within the normal range, 4 to 5 mEq/L.

Phosphate

The average deficit of phosphate in HHS is 1 mmol/kg. Although severe phosphate deficiency may be associated with substantial morbidity and mortality, there is little evidence that phosphate replacement in HHS improves clinical outcome. In patients with severe hypophosphatemia, 20 to 30 mEq/L of potassium phosphate can be added to replacement fluids. Because phosphate therapy may be associated with lowering of serum calcium concentration,[32] serum phosphate levels should be carefully monitored throughout the course of treatment.

HYPOGLYCEMIA

Hypoglycemia is the most common complication of treatment of diabetes mellitus. The vast majority of episodes occur in insulin-treated subjects, but hypoglycemia also occurs in patients treated with oral hypoglycemic agents.[45, 46] In major prospective clinical trials, 65% of patients with insulin-dependent (type 1) diabetes[23] and 11% of patients with non–insulin-dependent (type 2) diabetes being treated with insulin[47] suffered episodes of severe hypoglycemia over approximately 6 years of intensive therapy for their diabetes. Results from the Diabetes Control and Complications Trial indicate that patients with type 1 diabetes treated with conventional insulin therapy suffered an average of one episode of symptomatic hypoglycemia per week, and those receiving intensive insulin therapy had an average of two such episodes per week.[23]

Biochemically, *hypoglycemia* can be defined as a plasma glucose level below 50 mg/dL. In clinical practice, hypoglycemia is defined as a state of abnormally low plasma (blood) glucose level that is typically, but not invariably, associated with adrenergic (autonomic) symptoms, neuroglycopenic symptoms, or both.[48] Hypoglycemia may range from a very mild lowering of blood glucose concentration (60 to 70 mg/dL) with minimal or no symptoms to severe hypoglycemia with glucose levels below 40 mg/dL and severe neurologic symptoms, such as seizures, disorientation, and loss of consciousness.

The differential diagnosis of hypoglycemia is shown in Table 71–2. In adults, hypoglycemia can be divided into *fasting* (unrelated to food and usually occurring more than 4 hours after a meal) and *postprandial* (within 4 hours of a meal). Fasting hypoglycemia can be the result of drugs, critical illnesses, certain hormonal deficiency states, non–islet cell tumors, and beta cell tumors. Postprandial or alimentary hypoglycemia is usually reported after gastric surgery and rarely as an idiopathic disorder. In addition to all causes of adult hypoglycemia, several causes of hypoglycemia are unique to children[49, 50]; they include neonatal hypoglycemia, specific enzyme deficiencies, and ketogenic hypoglycemia of childhood.

In patients with diabetes, the vast majority of hypoglycemic events result from drugs, particularly insulin and oral agents. Hypoglycemia associated with insulin therapy is usually related to errors in dosage, delaying or skipping of meals, exercise, and intensity of metabolic control. The risk of hypoglycemia is increased by the development of renal failure, impairment of counterregulation, *hypoglycemia unawareness* (loss of the perception of warning symptoms of developing hypoglycemia), and autonomic neuropathy (gastroparesis). Diabetic patients in whom hypoglycemia develops while they are taking sulfonylureas are usually older than 60 years of age and have renal insufficiency.[4] Oral hypoglycemic agents, such as metformin, troglitazone, and acarbose, are not expected to cause hypoglycemia because they do not stimulate insulin secretion.

TABLE 71–2. Causes of Hypoglycemia

Fasting Hypoglycemia
Drugs
Insulin, sulfonylurea
Ethanol
Pentamidine, salicylates, β-blockers
Critical illness
Liver failure
Renal failure
Congestive heart failure
Sepsis
Hormone deficiency states
Adrenal insufficiency
Hypopituitarism
Hypothyroidism
Non–islet cell tumors
Mesenchymal tumors
Hepatoma
Adenocarcinoma
Carcinoid tumors
Endogenous hyperinsulinism
Insulinoma
Nesidioblastosis
Postprandial Hypoglycemia
Alimentary hypoglycemia
Idiopathic

In children, as well as in adults, ethanol consumption has been shown to be an important cause of hypoglycemia in both diabetic and nondiabetic subjects.[51, 52] Severe ethanol consumption depletes nicotinamide adenosine dinucleotide (NAD), a cofactor critical for the utilization of gluconeogenic precursors (lactate, amino acids, glycerol). Other drugs associated with hypoglycemia are pentamidine, salicylates, and nonselective β-blockers.

Critical illnesses, such as severe liver disease, renal insufficiency, congestive heart failure, and sepsis, may be associated with a higher risk of hypoglycemia in diabetic patients. In such patients, hypoglycemia may result from diminished glycogen stores, reduced hepatic glucose production, or both. Hypoglycemia is common in children, in whom (1) glucose demands are accelerated by medical or surgical stress, (2) glycogen stores are depleted by chronic disease, and (3) caloric supply is inadequate because of fasting and insufficient dextrose administration.[50, 53] In addition, hypopituitarism, adrenal insufficiency, and hypothyroidism may cause hypoglycemia in nondiabetic subjects. Hypoglycemia may require reduction of insulin dosage in diabetic subjects, especially during a period of caloric deprivation or under the stress of an intercurrent illness.[54, 55] Other causes of hypoglycemia are rare in diabetes.

Diagnosis

The symptoms of hypoglycemia have been classified into two major groups, those due to activation of the autonomic nervous system and those due to neuroglycopenia. Increased catecholamine secretion causes adrenergic manifestations such as sweating, nervousness, fatigue, hunger, and tachycardia. Neuroglycopenic symptoms consist of dizziness, confusion, difficulty in speaking and thinking, and behavioral changes as well as seizures and coma. Recurrent episodes of severe hypoglycemia, ethanol abuse, β-blocking agents, and defective counterregulation may be associated with a state of *hypoglycemia unawareness.*[56, 57] Patients with hypoglycemia unawareness have been found, in a prospective study, to have a nearly sevenfold increase in the frequency of severe iatrogenic hypoglycemia.[56]

Documentation of hypoglycemia requires demonstration of a below-normal blood glucose concentration, preferably coupled with symptoms that are rapidly reversed by measures that raise blood glucose levels (Whipple's triad). In patients with diabetes who are receiving pharmacologic therapy, the diagnosis of hypoglycemia may be rapidly established with a blood glucose self-monitoring device; however, if measurement of blood glucose is not possible, one should assume that hypoglycemia is present on the basis of symptoms and treat it empirically.[49]

In patients with suspected hypoglycemia but without an apparent precipitating cause, blood samples should be drawn before therapeutic intervention, for determination of glucose, cortisol, insulin, C peptide, and sulfonylurea levels. The diagnosis of insulin-mediated hypoglycemia depends on the presence of inappropriately high insulin levels relative to a low plasma glucose concentration. Patients with endogenous hyperinsulinism (insulinoma) have measured plasma insulin levels equal to or greater than 6 μU/mL (36 pmol/L) and serum C peptide levels equal to or greater than 0.6 ng/mL (0.2 nmol/L).[58] In contrast, elevated insulin levels in association with suppressed C peptide levels suggest exogenous (surreptitious) insulin administration. Ingestion of sulfonylurea stimulates endogenous insulin secretion and may result in concentrations of glucose, insulin, and C peptide levels identical to those of patients with insulinoma; its occult use may be detected by measurement of sulfonylurea in blood or urine.[59]

Treatment

The urgent treatment of symptomatic hypoglycemia requires restoration of normoglycemia by administration of carbohydrates or glucose. Most patients (i.e., insulin-treated diabetics) do not require hospitalization unless hypoglycemia is extremely severe or they become unresponsive.[4, 49]

Mild to moderate hypoglycemia in alert patients can be treated with 20 g oral glucose (dextrose tablets, candy, fruit juices) or glucagon therapy. In severe cases, adult patients should receive 25 g glucose intravenously (50 mL 50% dextrose), with re-treatment in 15 to 20 minutes if necessary.

Intravenous glucose infusion may be necessary (5% to 10% dextrose in water) at a rate sufficient to maintain the blood glucose level above 100 mg/dL. A bolus of 25% dextrose (0.5 g/kg) is administered, followed by a constant infusion of 5% to 10% dextrose to maintain adequate blood glucose levels. When the patient awakens, a high-carbohydrate diet, consisting of more than 300 g carbohydrates per day, is started, followed by slow tapering of the intravenous glucose infusion over a period of 24 hours. Glucagon (1 mg) in adults can be given IV or IM when it is not feasible to give intravenous glucose. Comparable therapeutic measures are recommended in children.[60]

The prevention of recurrent episodes of hypoglycemia requires correction of the underlying cause. Insulin dose should be adjusted, and offending drugs should be discontinued. Patients with hormonal deficiencies, such as hypopituitarism, adrenal insufficiency, and hypothyroidism, should be treated appropriately.

References

1. Faich GA, Fishbein HA, Ellis SE: The epidemiology of diabetic acidosis: A population-based study. Am J Epidemiol 1983; 117:551.
2. Umpierrez GE, Kelly JP, Navarrete JE, Casals MMC, Kitabchi AE: Hyperglycemic crises in urban Blacks. Arch Intern Med 1997; 157:669.
3. Umpierrez GE, Casals MMC, Gebhart SSP, Mixon PS, Clark WS, Phillips LS: Diabetic ketoacidosis in obese African Americans. Diabetes 1995; 44:790.
4. Fishbein HA, Palumbo PJ: Acute Metabolic Complications in Diabetes: Diabetes in America (National Diabetes Data Group). (NIH Publication No. 95-1468.) Bethesda, Md, National Institutes of Health, 1995, pp 283–291.
5. Centers for Disease Control, Division of Diabetes Translations: Diabetes Surveillance, 1991. Washington, DC, U.S. Government Printing Office, 1992, pp 635–1150.
6. Marshall SM, Walker M, Alberti KGGM: Diabetic ketoacidosis and hyperglycemic nonketotic coma. *In*: International Textbook of Diabetes Mellitus. Alberti KGGM, DeFronzo RA, Keen H, Zimmel P (Eds). London, John Wiley & Sons, 1992, pp 1151–1164.
7. Kitabchi AE, Fisher JN, Murphy MB, Rumbak MJ: Diabetic ketoacidosis and the hyperglycemic hyperosmolar nonketotic state. *In*: Joslin's Diabetes Mellitus. 13th ed. Kahn CR, Weir GC (Eds). Philadelphia, Lea & Febiger, 1994, pp 738–770.
8. Johnson DD, Palumbo PJ, Chu C: Diabetic ketoacidosis in a community-based population. Mayo Clin Proc 1980; 55:83.
9. Sheppard MC, Wright AD: The effect on mortality of low-dose insulin therapy for diabetic ketoacidosis. Diabetes Care 1982; 5:111.
10. Snorgaard O, Eskilder PC, Vadstrup S, Nerup J: Diabetic ketoacidosis in Denmark: Epidemiology, incidence rates, precipitating factors and mortality rates. J Intern Med 1989; 226:223.
11. McGarry JD, Foster DW: Hormonal control of ketogenesis: Biochemical considerations. Arch Intern Med 1977; 137:495.
12. Gerich JE, Lorenzi M, Bier DM, et al: Effects of physiologic levels of glucagon and growth hormone on human carbohydrate and lipid metabolism: Studies involving administration of exogenous hormone during suppression of endogenous hormone secretion with somatostatin. J Clin Invest 1976; 57:875.
13. DeFronzo RA, Matsuda M, Barret E: Diabetic ketoacidosis: A combined metabolic-nephrologic approach to therapy. Diabetes Rev 1994; 2:209.
14. DelPrato S, Castellino P, Simonson DC, DeFronzo RA: Hyperglucagonemia and insulin-mediated glucose metabolism. J Clin Invest 1987; 79:547.
15. Waldhaush W, Kleinberger G, Korn A, et al: Severe hyperglycemia: Effects of rehydration on endocrine derangements and blood glucose concentration. Diabetes 1979; 28:577.
16. Schreiber M, Kamel KS, Cheema-Dhadly S, Halpein Ml: Ketoacidosis. Diabetes Rev 1994; 2:98.
17. Foster DW, McGarry JD: The metabolic derangements and treatment of diabetic ketoacidosis. N Engl J Med 1983; 309:159.
18. Polonsky WH, Anderson BJ, Lohrer PA, et al: Insulin omission in women with IDDM. Diabetes Care 1994; 17:1178.
19. Rydall AC, Rodin GM, Olmsted MP, et al: Disordered eating behavior and microvascular complications in young women with insulin-dependent diabetes mellitus. N Engl J Med 1997; 336:1849.
20. Musey VC, Lee JK, Crawford R, Klatka MA, McAdams D, Phillips LS: Diabetes in urban African Americans: I. Cessation of insulin therapy is the major precipitating cause of diabetic ketoacidosis. Diabetes Care 1995; 18:483.
21. Weissman JS, Gatsonis C, Epstein AM, et al: Rates of avoidable hospitalization by insurance status in Massachusetts and Maryland. JAMA 1992; 268:2388.
22. Kitabchi AE, Rumbak MJ: Diabetic ketoacidosis: Diagnosis; diabetic ketoacidosis: treatment; hyperosmolar nonketotic coma; and maintenance treatment after hyperglycemic crisis. *In*: Decision Making in Emergency Medicine. Callahan MI, Barton CW, Schumaker HM (Eds). Philadelphia, BC Decker, 1990, pp 178–185.
23. DCCT Research Group: The effect of intensive treatment of diabetes on the development and progression of long-term complications in insulin-dependent diabetes mellitus. N Engl J Med 1993; 329:977.
24. Koch DD, Feldbruegge DH: Optimized kinetic method for automated determination of β-hydroxybutyrate. Clin Res 1987; 33:1761.
25. Androgue HJ, Wilson H, Boyd AE, et al: Plasma acid-base patterns in diabetic acidosis. N Engl J Med 1982; 307:1603.

26. Salem MM, Mujais SK: Gaps in the anion gap. Arch Intern Med 1992; 152:1625.
27. Umpierrez GE, Khajavi M, Kitabchi AE:. Diabetic ketoacidosis and hyperglycemic hyperosmolar nonketotic syndrome. Am J Med Sci 1996; 311:225.
28. Wrenn K: The delta (Δ) gap: An approach to mixed acid-base disorders. Ann Intern Med 1990; 19:123.
29. Cahill GF: Starvation in man. N Engl J Med 1970; 282:675.
30. Feig PU, McCurdy DK: The hypertonic state. N Engl J Med 1977; 297:1444.
31. Rosenbloon AL: Intracerebral crises during treatment of diabetic ketoacidosis. Diabetes Care 1990; 13:22.
32. Rosenbloom AL, Hannas R: Diabetic ketoacidosis: Treatment guidelines. Clin Pediatr 1996; 261:266.
33. Androgue HJ, Lederer ED, Suki WN: Determinants of plasma potassium levels in diabetic ketoacidosis. Medicine 1986; 65:163.
34. Abranson E, Anky R: Diabetic acidosis with initial hypokalemia: Therapeutic implications. JAMA 1966; 196:401.
35. Morris LR, Murphy MB, Kitabchi AE: Bicarbonate therapy in severe diabetic ketoacidosis. Ann Intern Med 1986; 105:836.
36. Umpierrez GE, Watts NB, Phillips LS: Clinical utility of β-hydroxybutyrate determined by reflectance meter in the management of diabetic ketoacidosis. Diabetes Care 1995; 18:137.
37. Dreschfeld J: The Bradshawe Lecture on diabetic coma. Br Med J 1886; 2:358.
38. Sament S, Schwartz MB: Severe diabetic stupor without ketosis. S Afr Med J 1957; 31:893.
39. Ennis ED, Stahl EJVB, Kreisberg RA: The hyperosmolar hyperglycemic syndrome. Diabetes Rev 1994; 2:115.
40. Wachtel TJ, Tetu-Mouradjain LM, Goldman DL, et al: Hyperosmolality and acidosis in diabetes mellitus: A three-year experience in Rhode Island. J Gen Intern Med 1991; 6:495.
41. Cowle CC, Port FK, Wolfe RA, et al: Disparities in incidence of diabetic end-stage renal disease according to race and type of diabetes. N Engl J Med 1989; 321:1074.
42. Turpin BP, Duckworth WC, Solomon SS: Simulated hyperglycemic hyperosmolar syndrome: Impaired insulin and epinephrine effects upon lipolysis in the isolated rat fat cell. J Clin Invest 1979; 63:403.
43. Cruz-Caudillo JC, Sabatini S: Diabetic hyperosmolar syndrome. Nephron 1995; 69:201.
44. Lorber D: Nonketotic hypertonicity in diabetes mellitus. Med Clin North Am 1993; 79:39.
45. Cryer PE: Hypoglycemia: The limiting factor in the management of IDDM. Diabetes 1994; 43:1378.
46. Fisher KF, Lees JA, Newman JH: Hypoglycemia in hospitalized patients: Causes and outcomes. N Engl J Med 1986; 315:12145.
47. UK Prospective Diabetes Study Group: Overview of 6 years' therapy of type II diabetes: A progressive disease. Diabetes 1995; 44:1249.
48. Cryer PE: Hypoglycemia. *In*: Medicine for the Practicing Physician. 4th ed. Hurst JW (Ed). Stanford, Conn, Appleton & Lange, 1996, pp 646–651.
49. Cryer PE: Hypoglycemic disorders. *In*: Hypoglycemia: Pathophysiology, Diagnosis and Treatment. Cryer PE (Ed). New York, Oxford University Press, 1997, pp 127–168.
50. Haymond MW: Hypoglycemia in infants and children. Endocrinol Metab Clin North Am 1989; 18:211.
51. Malouf R, Brust JCM: Hypoglycemia: Causes, neurological manifestations, and outcome. Ann Neurol 1985; 17:421.
52. Devenyi P: Alcoholic hypoglycemia and alcoholic ketoacidosis: Sequential events of the same process? Can Med Assoc J 1982; 127:513.
53. Haymond MW, Karl IE, Clarke WL, et al: Differences in circulating substrates during short term fasting in men, women and children. Metabolism 1982; 18:211.
54. Daughaday WH: The pathophysiology of IGF-II hypersecretion in non-islet tumor hypoglycemia. Diabetes Rev 1995; 3:62.
55. Cryer PE, Fisher JN, Shamoon H: Hypoglycemia. Diabetes Care 1994; 17:734.
56. Gold AE, MacLeod KM, Frier BM: Frequency of severe hypoglycemia in patients with type I diabetes with impaired awareness of hypoglycemia. Diabetes Care 1994; 17:697.
57. Frier BM: Hypoglycemia unawareness. *In*: Hypoglycemia and Diabetes: Clinical and Physiological Aspects. Frier BM, Fisher BM (Eds). London, Edward Arnold, 1993, pp 284–301.
58. Service FJ: Hypoglycemic disorders. N Engl J Med 1995.
59. Seltzer HS: Drug-induced hypoglycemia. Endocrinol Metab Clin North Am 1989; 18:163.
60. Weigle CGM: Metabolic and endocrine diseases in pediatric intensive care. *In*: Textbook of Pediatric Intensive Care. Rogers MC (Ed). Baltimore, Williams & Wilkins, 1987, pp 1057–1109.

72

Adrenal Insufficiency

Elizabeth Beale, MD
Howard Belzberg, MD, FCCM, FCCP, FACP

Adrenal insufficiency is gaining importance in the intensive care unit (ICU). It is becoming apparent that in certain subgroups of critically ill patients, the incidence is higher than was previously suspected. It is essential to make the diagnosis because untreated adrenal insufficiency has a mortality rate approaching 100% and treatment is simple and may be lifesaving. Diagnosis, however, is difficult for several reasons:

1. The clinical features are nonspecific.
2. Typical features may be masked by coexisting illnesses or therapy.
3. Currently used diagnostic criteria may not be valid in the critically ill patient.

The etiology of adrenal insufficiency in the critically ill patient has not been well studied, but recent work suggests that it is often multifactorial, de novo in onset, and transient.

Despite treatment, the mortality rate is still approximately 50% in critically ill patients with adrenal insufficiency. Although this is undoubtedly partly due to coexistent disease, it may also be due to delayed diagnosis and treatment. It is recommended that when adrenal insufficiency is suspected, the patient be treated emergently with glucocorticoids before laboratory results are obtained; if a beneficial response is seen, treatment is continued.

INCIDENCE

Estimates of the incidence of adrenal insufficiency in critically ill patients vary widely and depend on the population studied as well as on the diagnostic criteria used (Table 72–1). Estimates range from less than 1% to 20%.[1-3] Few large prospective studies have been performed in the ICU setting, and different criteria have been used for making the diagnosis in the studies.[1-6] Most published reports of adrenal insufficiency in the ICU involve case reports.[7-15]

In the general population, adrenal insufficiency occurs in 40 to 60 per million.[16] By contrast, recent reports suggest that the frequency of occurrence is much higher in certain critically ill patients. For example, in a subgroup of hypotensive or failed-to-wean ICU patients older than 55 years who had been in the ICU for more than 14 days, the incidence of adrenal insufficiency was 11%.[6] In end-stage acquired immunodeficiency syndrome (AIDS), the incidence of adrenal insufficiency may be as high as 5%.[16] Overall, the incidence in critically ill patients in the ICU has been estimated to range from about 0.7% to 1.4%,[2, 5, 6] but the incidence of adrenal insufficiency, especially that developing de novo during the ICU stay, has not been well studied.[6]

Trauma patients are at lower risk than nontrauma surgical

TABLE 72–1. Reported Incidence of Adrenal Insufficiency

Population	Incidence	Reference
General	40–60/million population	7, 16
ICU patients	<1%–20%	1–3
SICU	0.66% (7/1054)	6
SICU trauma patients	0.23% (1/442)	6
SICU nontrauma patients	0.98% (6/612)	6
SICU stay > 14 days	6% (6/99)	6
SICU > age 55 yr	1.7% (7/417)	6
SICU stay > 14 days *and* age > 55 yr	11% (6/54)	6
General trauma and surgery	0.005% (3/60,000)	40
Blunt abdominal trauma	0.08% (1/1200)	41
Adrenal injury diagnosis on CT scan after blunt abdominal trauma	5% (1/20)	41
Children suspected of having intra-abdominal injury after blunt abdominal trauma	0% (0/1155)	42
Post-traumatic adrenal hemorrhage in children thought to have intra-abdominal injury after blunt abdominal trauma	0% (0/34)	42
Urologic surgery	0.01% (1/8109)	43
Cardiac surgery	0.11% (1/4364)	34
Liver transplant recipients requiring ICU admission	6% (2/36)	7
Unexplained hypotension within 48 hr of abdominal surgery in patients > 65 yr	5% (5/105)	17
AIDS	5%	16
Eosinophilia in ICU patients	23% (7/31)	5

AIDS = acquired immunodeficiency syndrome; CT = computed tomography; ICU = intensive care unit; SICU = surgical intensive care unit.

ICU patients,[6] and this has been attributed to their younger age and generally better health before hospitalization. Blunt trauma to the abdomen may cause bilateral adrenal hemorrhage, but this is unusual and unlikely to be associated with adrenal insufficiency.[9]

An abnormally low random or stimulated serum cortisol level is the most common diagnostic feature of adrenal insufficiency, and the incidence of adrenal insufficiency depends on the diagnostic test and the reference range used. Thus, Span and coworkers[1] found a relatively low incidence of adrenal insufficiency in their study of ICU patients when the cutoff level for adrenal insufficiency was a random cortisol level below 11 μg/dL. Later investigators noted a higher incidence when a lower limit of normal of 15 μg/dL was used in critically ill patients.[6] The role of stress in critically ill patients makes it difficult to establish "normal" levels of cortisol and to identify when patients have relatively insufficient levels. Use of the standard cosyntropin test may lead to underestimation of the incidence of adrenal insufficiency, and the low-dose cosyntropin test may be a more appropriate test in the ICU setting.[17]

ETIOLOGY

Adrenal insufficiency results when there are inadequate amounts of adrenal hormones to meet the body's physiologic requirements (Table 72–2). Cortisol deficiency is the major cause of morbidity and mortality, but aldosterone deficiency that occurs with primary adrenal insufficiency may also play a pathogenetic role. Adrenal insufficiency may be due to disruption of the hypothalamic-pituitary-adrenal axis, increased glucocorticoid metabolism, resistance to adrenal hormone actions, increase in the requirements for glucocorticoids, or any combination of these factors. In contrast to adrenal insufficiency in the noncritically ill patient, the etiology and pathogenesis of adrenal insufficiency in the critically ill patient are often obscure and the presentation is typically nonspecific.

Primary Adrenal Insufficiency

Primary adrenal insufficiency arises from a pathologic process in the adrenal gland itself. At least 90% of the gland must be destroyed for adrenal insufficiency to occur in otherwise healthy patients. In noncritically ill patients, 65% to 80% of primary adrenal insufficiency is due to autoimmune adrenalitis. This is a chronic condition occurring in 39 to 60 per million population. The mean age at diagnosis is 40 years, and women are more commonly affected than men.[16, 18] The disease is due to destruction of the adrenal gland by antibodies and cytotoxic lymphocytes and may be associated with other autoimmune endocrinopathies (type I and type II polyglandular syndromes).

Infection is a major cause of primary adrenal insufficiency. Tuberculosis is responsible for about 30% of adrenal insufficiency in the general population, and this rate may rise because resistance to therapy is increasing. Fungal infections, in particular disseminated histoplasmosis, may also cause adrenal insufficiency.[19] In the late stages of AIDS, 5% of patients have been reported to have overt adrenal insufficiency caused by destruction of the adrenal glands by opportunistic infection,[16] thus making it a common cause of primary adrenal insufficiency. Ten per cent of patients with advanced AIDS may have subclinical abnormalities of adrenal function.[18]

Acute bilateral adrenal hemorrhage usually occurs in hospitalized patients and may be due to a variety of causes, including sepsis, coagulopathy, ischemia, hypotension, and trauma. The onset of adrenal insufficiency is usually abrupt. Rao and colleagues[20] reported that adrenal hemorrhage occurred in patients who were critically ill from other causes, especially heart disease and infection. The three major risk factors were thromboembolic disease, coagulopathy, and the postoperative state. Coagulopathy causing adrenal insufficiency may be either iatrogenic (e.g., warfarin or heparin therapy) or pathologic. The usual tests for anticoagulation (activated partial thromboplastin time, partial thromboplastin time) need not be abnormal for bilateral adrenal hemorrhage to occur. Dahlberg and associates[21] described 19 patients with acute bilateral adrenal hemorrhage who were taking anticoagulants; all had clotting parameters in the therapeutic range. Adrenal hemorrhage has also been associated with heparin-induced thrombocytopenia. Adrenal insufficiency may occur with thromboembolic disorders, such as the antiphospholipid syndrome, and

TABLE 72–2. Causes of Adrenal Insufficiency

Primary	***Central***
Autoimmune	Long-term glucocorticoid therapy with
Isolated Addison's adrenalitis	Rapid tapering or withdrawal
Part of type I or type II polyglandular autoimmune syndrome	Failure to increase dose during stress
Infection	Transient ACTH deficiency postoperatively
Meningococcal septicemia	Pituitary or metastatic carcinoma
Tuberculosis	Hypothalamic tumor
Systemic fungal infection, including histoplasmosis, cryptococcosis, blastomycosis, and coccidioidomycosis	Craniopharyngioma
Acquired immunodeficiency syndrome (AIDS)	Pituitary surgery or irradiation
Opportunistic infection	Infiltrative disorders
Viral, e.g., human immunodeficiency virus, *Cytomegalovirus*	Lymphocytic hypophysitis
Bacterial, e.g., tuberculosis, *Mycobacterium avium-intracellulare*	Sarcoidosis
Fungal, e.g., histoplasmosis	Histiocytosis X
Protozoal, e.g., toxoplasmosis	Empty sella syndrome
Kaposi's sarcoma	Postpartum pituitary necrosis (Sheehan's syndrome)
Adrenomyeloneuropathy	Necrosis or bleeding into a pituitary macroadenoma
Adrenoleukodystrophy	Head trauma, including lesions of the pituitary stalk
Metastatic carcinoma	Isolated ACTH deficiency
Extensive bilateral metastases	Chronic alcoholism
Withdrawal of glucocorticoid therapy	***Increased Degradation of Glucocorticoid***
Lymphoma	Treatment of hypothyroidism
Isolated glucocorticoid deficiency	Rifampin
Infiltrating diseases	Most anticonvulsants (phenytoin, barbiturates, carbamazepine; less so, valproic acid)
Sarcoidosis	***Resistance to Glucocorticoid Action or Increased Demand***
Amyloidosis	Acquired immunodeficiency syndrome (AIDS)
Hemochromatosis	Functional hypoadrenalism
Acute bilateral adrenal hemorrhage, necrosis, or thrombosis due to	***Limited Adrenal Reserve***
Sepsis (especially meningococcal septicemia)	Age (>55 yr)
Anticoagulant therapy	Malnutrition
Antiphospholipid syndrome	Prolonged hospital and ICU stay
Idiopathic thrombocytopenic purpura	Chronic alcoholism
Thromboemboli	High APACHE II score
Heparin-induced thrombocytopenia	High TISS score
Surgical removal of functioning adrenal adenoma	Stress in the form of trauma, surgery, infection, dehydration
Trauma	***Multifactorial***
Medications: etomidate, ketoconazole, aminoglutethimide, mitotane, metyrapone	

ACTH = adrenocorticotropic hormone; APACHE = Acute Physiology and Chronic Health Evaluation; ICU = intensive care unit; TISS = Therapeutic Intervention Scoring System.

with idiopathic thrombocytopenic purpura. Acute bilateral adrenal hemorrhage may occur after blunt abdominal trauma as a result of increased abdominal pressure causing retrograde venous blood flow into the adrenal glands. Of 269 patients who died after a motor vehicle accident or blunt force, 7% had adrenal injury or hemorrhage, but the number who had adrenal insufficiency is not known.[22] The classic infective cause of acute bilateral adrenal hemorrhage is meningococcal septicemia, but it may also occur with streptococcal pneumonia and with other gram-negative infections, including those due to streptococcus and *Haemophilus influenza* type b, and certain bacillus infections.[18]

Adrenomyeloneuropathy is increasingly being recognized as a cause of adrenal insufficiency in young men. It is an X-linked recessive disorder associated with spastic paralysis. Adrenal insufficiency may occur before or after the onset of the neurologic disease.[16]

Isolated glucocorticoid deficiency may result from adrenal unresponsiveness to adrenocorticotropic hormone (ACTH).[16] It is a rare familial condition with clinical features of cutaneous pigmentation, weakness, hypoglycemia, and seizures. ACTH levels are elevated, and aldosterone levels are normal.[23] Although the adrenal gland is a frequent site of tumor metastases, these rarely cause clinical adrenal insufficiency.[24] This may partly be due to the frequent chemotherapeutic use of corticosteroids. Certain pharmacologic agents, including etomidate and ketoconazole, interfere with adrenal mitochondrial enzymes and may precipitate acute adrenal insufficiency. Similarly, aminoglutethimide and other chemotherapeutic agents may cause or precipitate acute adrenal insufficiency by inhibiting the conversion of cholesterol to corticosteroids.[25-27] Removal of a supposed nonfunctioning adrenal "incidentaloma" may precipitate an adrenal crisis if it is in fact functional and causing suppression of the hypothalamic-pituitary-adrenal axis.[28]

Central Adrenal Insufficiency

Central adrenal insufficiency is due to dysfunction of the pituitary gland or the hypothalamus (see Table 72–2). If the adrenal insufficiency is due to an abnormality in the pituitary gland, it may be referred to as *secondary*; if the abnormality is in the hypothalamus, the adrenal insufficiency is termed *tertiary*.

Long-term glucocorticoid therapy is the most common cause of central adrenal insufficiency, which usually results from suppression of corticotropin-releasing hormone release.[16] It is estimated that 6 million people in the United States have subclinical central adrenal insufficiency secondary to exogenous glucocorticoid use and that this may become overt under stress.[29] Suppression of the hypothalamic-pituitary axis has been reported to occur within 5 to 7 days of starting therapy with a dose of 60 mg daily of prednisone and may persist for up to 9 months after withdrawal of exogenous glucocorticoids.[30] However, the exact dose and duration of administration of glucocorticoids required to suppress the hypothalamic-pituitary axis have not been established, and few cases of acute adrenal insufficiency due purely to withdrawal of exogenous glucocorticoids have been reported.[18] Adrenal insufficiency may occur after administration of glucocorticoids by any route, including inhaled and topical administration.[31] Rapid tapering or withdrawal of glucocorticoids or failure to increase doses during stress, such as may occur inadvertently during critical illness or injury when no history is available from the patient, may also precipitate adrenal insufficiency. The underlying disease for which the treatment was prescribed may also recur after glucocorticoid withdrawal, further increasing the glucocorticoid requirements and complicating management.

Merry and colleagues[17] described several cases in which they noted postoperative adrenal insufficiency due to transient ACTH deficiency. They found that 5% of 105 patients older than 65 years within 48 hours of abdominal surgery had glucocorticoid-responsive hypotension and a low random serum cortisol level (<15 μg/dL), a normal response to the standard (250 μg) cosyntropin stimulation test, and an abnormally low cortisol level after a low-dose (1 μg) cosyntropin stimulation test. The cause of the adrenal insufficiency was not clear. None of the patients received previous glucocorticoid treatment or had a chronic pituitary disorder. Chronic alcoholism may have contributed in two of the four patients, and etomidate was used in three of the four.

Postpartum pituitary necrosis or bleeding (*Sheehan's syndrome*), necrosis or infarction of a pituitary macroadenoma, head trauma, lesions of the pituitary stalk, and pituitary surgery for Cushing's disease or other pituitary surgery may cause abrupt or delayed onset of central adrenal insufficiency. Adrenal insufficiency may occur 5 to 10 years after pituitary fossa radiation for a pituitary tumor. Infiltrative and malignant conditions, such as pituitary carcinoma or metastatic carcinoma to the hypothalamic-pituitary area, craniopharyngioma, sarcoidosis, histiocytosis X, and the empty sella syndrome, may cause central adrenal insufficiency and are usually associated with other pituitary hormonal disorders, including diabetes insipidus. Lymphocytic hypophysitis may be associated with pure ACTH deficiency. Chronic alcohol ingestion inhibits the ACTH response to insulin hypoglycemia and may play a role in adrenal insufficiency in the stressed, critically ill patient.

Relative Insufficiency

In addition to the classic causes of glucocorticoid deficiency, it is possible that adrenal insufficiency may arise from a relative insufficiency of glucocorticoids (see Table 72-2). This relative insufficiency may be secondary to (1) increased degradation of glucocorticoids, (2) resistance to glucocorticoid action, or (3) increased demand.

Adrenal insufficiency may be unmasked by various medications that increase the hepatic metabolism of cortisol. These include rifampin and most anticonvulsants (phenytoin, phenobarbitone, carbamazepine, and, less so, valproic acid).[5] Treatment of hypothyroidism (which may be associated with autoimmune adrenalitis) may unmask occult adrenal insufficiency by increasing the metabolism of corticosteroids by hepatic enzymes.[16]

Although it is not widely viewed as a cause of adrenal insufficiency, resistance to cortisol action may play a role in the pathogenesis of adrenal insufficiency. In patients with AIDS, adrenal insufficiency has been described despite normal circulating levels of cortisol, and resistance to glucocorticoid action has been demonstrated in lymphocytes.[32] Baldwin and Allo[12] described four patients who had clinical features of an adrenal crisis and who had levels of cortisol after standard (250 μg) cosyntropin stimulation testing that would generally rule out adrenal insufficiency yet who responded to physiologic doses of glucocorticoid. The authors hypothesized a syndrome of functional hypoadrenalism. The incidence of this disorder has not been prospectively studied in the ICU.

Multifactorial Causes

In several studies,[5-7, 12, 17] it is apparent that adrenal insufficiency develops because of cumulative demands on and insults to the adrenal gland. Patients may be predisposed to the development of acute adrenal insufficiency by having poor adrenal reserve. The following factors appear to contribute to the development of adrenal insufficiency in the critically ill patient:

- Increasing age (>55 years)
- Malnutrition
- Prolonged hospital and ICU stay
- Chronic alcoholism
- High Acute Physiology and Chronic Health Evaluation (APACHE) II score;
- High Therapeutic Intervention Scoring System (TISS) score
- Stress in the form of trauma, surgery, infection, and dehydration

Medications listed before, including prior glucocorticoid use, have frequently been associated with adrenal insufficiency in the ICU.[6, 7]

CLINICAL PRESENTATION

In the non-ICU setting, adrenal insufficiency is usually insidious in onset and typically presents with nonspecific features, such as weakness, weight loss, lethargy, depression, and gastrointestinal symptoms. By contrast, in virtually all cases of adrenal insufficiency reported in the ICU setting, the diagnosis has been made when the patient is in an acute adrenal crisis.[5, 6, 12, 17] Furthermore, in the critically ill patient, the presenting picture may be altered by coexisting disease and ongoing supportive therapy, and features of chronicity, such as hyperpigmentation and loss of axillary hair, are infrequent.[5] Even subacute findings, such as electrolyte imbalances, may be absent.

The typical ICU patient with adrenal insufficiency is older than age 55 years and has had a prolonged (>14 days) ICU stay. Adrenal insufficiency occurs more frequently in patients with a high TISS or APACHE score and is more likely to occur in a nontrauma patient than in a trauma patient.[6] Predisposing factors include malnutrition and chronic alcoholism. There may be a history of drug use that predisposes to adrenal insufficiency, such as prior or inadequate glucocorticoid use, etomidate, anticonvulsant therapy, or rifampin.

The acute presentation may be precipitated by a physical stressor, such as surgery, trauma, infection, or dehydration. Features of the etiologic mechanism, such as tuberculosis, AIDS, or a pituitary tumor, may be present. Refractory shock (i.e., hypotension not responding to fluids or inotropes) is the main clinical feature in the critically ill patient. Patients with adrenal insufficiency may have high-output circulatory failure (cardiac index > 4 L/min/m^2) with tachycardia, hypotension, and a low systemic vascular resistance (<500 dyne · sec/cm^5 · m^2)[12, 18] and a normal-to-high pulmonary capillary wedge pressure.[18, 33]

The differential diagnosis includes sepsis, neurogenic shock, overdose of a vasodilator drug, arteriovenous shunt, severe anemia, thyrotoxicosis, cirrhosis, beriberi, and pregnancy. This condition is due to loss of vascular tone because of cortisol deficiency, both directly and through its permissive actions on catecholamines and vasoactive peptides.[33]

Many features of adrenal insufficiency are nonspecific and may be difficult to identify in a noncommunicating patient with multiple problems (Table 72–3). Possible presenting features are fever (temperature higher than 39°C, especially with negative cultures and no other evidence of sepsis) and mental status changes (weakness, fatigue, lethargy, agitation, confusion, psychosis, and coma). These may occur without hemodynamic instability. A conscious patient may complain of arthralgias or myalgias. Dehydration is common. Gastrointestinal alterations, such as anorexia, nausea, vomiting, diarrhea, abdominal pain, and weight loss, may also occur.

Two features specific to primary adrenal insufficiency are hyperpigmentation and hyperkalemia. Hyperpigmentation is due to the melanocyte-stimulating effect of elevated ACTH. It is especially marked over extensor surfaces and on the lips, dental gingival margin, buccal mucosa, and scars.[18] Hyperkalemia is due to damage to the zona glomerulosa with loss of production of mineralocorticoids; however, like other features of adrenal insufficiency in critically ill patients, hyperkalemia may be masked by therapy or other pathologic processes.

Other presenting features may help identify the adrenal insufficiency as primary. Vitiligo is sometimes seen and is thought to be due to autoimmune destruction of melanocytes; it is associated with primary autoimmune adrenalitis. Abdominal or flank pain and abdominal rigidity may be seen in conscious patients with adrenal hemorrhage or thrombosis.[18, 34] Women with primary or central adrenal insufficiency have scanty axillary and pubic hair because of adrenal androgen deficiency, whereas men have scanty body hair with adrenal insufficiency only when gonadotropin levels are affected. Hypoparathyroidism, mucocutaneous candidiasis, autoimmune thyroid disease, or insulin-dependent diabetes mellitus may be present with adrenal insufficiency if it is longstanding and part of an autoimmune polyglandular endocrinopathy.[16]

A pale skin without anemia is reported with central adrenal insufficiency. Amenorrhea, small testicles, secondary hypothy-

TABLE 72–3. Clinical Presentation of Adrenal Insufficiency

Primary and Central Adrenal Insufficiency

CARDIOVASCULAR

- Hypotension
- Tachycardia
- High-output circulatory failure
- Low systemic vascular resistance
- Impaired hemodynamic response to catecholamines and fluid therapy

NEUROLOGIC

- Confusion
- Fatigue
- Agitation
- Coma
- Psychosis

MUSCULAR

- Myalgia
- Arthralgia
- Weakness

GASTROINTESTINAL AND ABDOMINAL

- Anorexia
- Nausea
- Vomiting
- Diarrhea
- Constipation
- Weight loss
- Abdominal or flank pain, abdominal rigidity with adrenal hemorrhage or thrombosis

METABOLIC

- Hyponatremia
- Hypoglycemia
- Mild metabolic acidosis
- Slightly elevated creatinine concentration
- Hypercalcemia

HEMATOLOGIC

- Eosinophilia
- Lymphocytosis
- Neutropenia
- Mild normocytic, normochromic anemia

MISCELLANEOUS

- Fever

Primary Adrenal Insufficiency

- Hyperpigmentation of extensor surfaces, scars, mucous membranes
- Vitiligo
- Hyperkalemia
- Scanty axillary and pubic hair (female patients only)
- Autoimmune thyroid disease
- Type I autoimmune polyglandular syndrome (adrenal insufficiency, hypoparathyroidism, mucocutaneous candidiasis)
- Type II autoimmune polyglandular syndrome (adrenal insufficiency, autoimmune thyroid disease, and insulin-dependent diabetes mellitus)
- Neurologic signs with adrenomyeloneuropathy

Central Adrenal Insufficiency

- Pallor without anemia
- Headache
- Visual symptoms

May Be Associated with Pituitary Insufficiency

- Gonadotropin deficiency
  - Scanty axillary and pubic hair
  - Amenorrhea
  - Small testes
  - Delayed puberty
- Thyrotropin deficiency
  - Secondary hypothyroidism
  - Prepubertal growth deficit
- Diabetes insipidus

roidism, delayed puberty, headache, and visual symptoms may also be present.

Possible biochemical alterations that should suggest adrenal insufficiency are hyponatremia, hyperkalemia, acidosis, slightly elevated creatinine concentration, hypoglycemia, and rarely hypercalcemia. Fluid and electrolyte alterations may be masked by concomitant therapy with these agents. Alkaline phosphatase activity was reported to be elevated in four of 16 patients with Addison's disease and corrected after 1 week of glucocorticoid therapy.[18]

Eosinophilia was present in 3% of ICU patients, of whom 23% had adrenal insufficiency, and 82% of these responded to hydrocortisone.[5] Eosinophilia is found in 20% of patients with chronic adrenal insufficiency. Lymphocytosis, neutropenia, and a mild normocytic, normochromic anemia may also be seen.

DIAGNOSIS

Clinical Diagnosis

The diagnosis of adrenal insufficiency is usually confirmed by the use of biochemical criteria. In the critically ill patient, however, a clinical diagnosis is sufficient for commencement of treatment.[5, 6, 12, 16] This is so for two reasons:

1. The criteria for diagnosis of adrenal insufficiency that are currently used in the ICU may not always be valid in the critically ill patient because they were derived from studies in the non-ICU population. In particular, the normal cortisol range in critically ill patients is uncertain, and the standard cosyntropin stimulation test is unreliable in new-onset central adrenal insufficiency.
2. In a critically ill patient, untreated adrenal insufficiency carries a mortality of almost 100%, and patients usually present in a crisis. Immediate treatment, before biochemical confirmation is obtained, may be lifesaving.

Thus, clinical features as described in the preceding section may, in critically ill patients, be adequate grounds for a therapeutic trial of glucocorticoids.

Laboratory Assessment

The indications for and interpretation of laboratory tests of adrenal insufficiency in the critically ill patient are described in Table 72–4.

Random Cortisol Testing

A blood sample should be drawn for evaluation of the plasma cortisol level as soon as the diagnosis of adrenal insufficiency is considered. It is preferable to draw baseline samples before initiation of therapy with glucocorticoids, because most glucocorticoids cross-react with cortisol during the assay. Dexamethasone is generally considered not to cross-react and thus is often the first therapeutic glucocorticoid used if diagnostic testing is not complete.

An ACTH level should be determined at the same time as the initial cortisol level. The normal reference range for cortisol in critically ill patients is still being determined, and a cortisol level in the standard "normal range" (6 to 18 μg/dL) does not exclude adrenal insufficiency in the critically ill patient.[2] Many authors consider that a level of more than 20 μg/dL is adequate in critically ill patients, but others are more cautious, raising the level to 25 μg/dL, and it has been stated that "there is no upper limit above which the diagnosis can safely be excluded."[16] A serum cortisol level of less than 10 μg/dL[16] or even 15 μg/dL[6] in a critically ill patient has been considered to be diagnostic of adrenal insufficiency. By contrast, in the noncritically ill patient, a level as low as 6 μg/dL may be considered normal.[16]

Because the random cortisol level is often in the indeterminate range of 10 to 20 μg/dL, further testing is frequently required (i.e., cosyntropin stimulation testing). In practice, determination of the baseline cortisol level and the cosyntropin stimulation test can easily be done simultaneously.

In the nonstressed, noncritically ill patient, peak cortisol production occurs in the morning, and a blood sample drawn between 6 AM and 8 AM is often the first screening test of cortisol done for adrenal insufficiency. In the critically ill patient, however, pharmacologic and physiologic factors can override the normal diurnal pattern, making the morning cortisol determination of no particular value.

Cosyntropin Stimulation Testing

Cosyntropin stimulation tests are the most widely used provocative tests of adrenal function in the ICU. Unlike the "gold standard" insulin hypoglycemia and metyrapone tests, which activate the entire hypothalamic-pituitary-adrenal axis, cosyntropin directly stimulates the adrenal gland. Cosyntropin stimulation tests are simple, quick, and safe to perform, however, and most study results are comparable to the insulin hypoglycemia and metyrapone test results in chronic adrenal insufficiency.

Standard Short Cosyntropin Test

The standard short cosyntropin test is the most widely used test for the diagnosis of adrenal insufficiency in the critically ill patient. After a blood sample is drawn for determination of baseline cortisol and ACTH levels, 250 μg of cosyntropin is injected intravenously (preferred in critically ill patients) or intramuscularly; further samples for cortisol levels are drawn at 30 minutes and 60 minutes. Because there is no significant difference between 30- and 60-minute cortisol levels, one of these two samples may be omitted.

Interpretation of this test is controversial. The most widely accepted criteria for normality are a peak level above 20 μg/dL[16] in a critically ill patient and a rise of 7 μg/dL[5] above the baseline value. A doubling of the baseline value of cortisol has also been used to indicate normal adrenal function. Other authors, however, have reported clinical improvement after giving corticosteroids to patients with stimulated levels as high as 36 μg/dL.[12] These studies lend support to the concept that biochemical criteria may be misleading.

A major concern is that the test does not accurately detect recent-onset central adrenal insufficiency, which may constitute a large proportion of adrenal insufficiency in the ICU.[16] The 250 μg of cosyntropin used in the standard cosyntropin test is supraphysiologic; that is, the serum levels of the synthetic ACTH used in this test exceed the ACTH levels found during stress.

Low-Dose Short Cosyntropin Test

The low-dose short cosyntropin test is gaining acceptance as a more accurate and physiologic test for diagnosing adrenal insufficiency in the ICU. This test is used to detect all cases of adrenal insufficiency that the standard short test detects as well as recent-onset secondary adrenal insufficiency,[6] and it may become the test of choice for adrenal insufficiency in the ICU. It is performed in the same manner as the standard short test, except that only 1 μg of cosyntropin is injected. Because a much smaller dose of cosyntropin is being used, care must be taken that it is all injected intravenously. The cosyntropin can be diluted before injection to ensure complete administration.

Long Cosyntropin Test

The long cosyntropin test (3 days) is helpful for differentiating primary from central adrenal insufficiency. It has been largely replaced by ACTH measurement.

TABLE 72–4. Laboratory Assessment of Adrenal Insufficiency in the Critically Ill Patient

Test	Indication	Interpretation	Method	Reference
Random plasma cortisol	Initial screening test for all patients with suspected adrenal insufficiency	Plasma cortisol level <10 μg/dL confirms adrenal insufficiency; 10–15 μg/dL suggests adrenal insufficiency. Plasma cortisol level >25 μg/dL usually excludes adrenal insufficiency in an adequately stressed patient. Plasma cortisol between 10 and 20–25 μg/dL is an indeterminate result, and a cosyntropin stimulation test should be done.		2, 6, 16, 17, 44, 45
Standard short cosyntropin test	Initial test for all critically ill patients and for all patients with a random plasma cortisol level between 10 and 20 μg/dL Not for suspected recent-onset central adrenal insufficiency or mild secondary adrenal insufficiency	Peak plasma cortisol level of >20–25 μg/dL is generally considered to exclude adrenal insufficiency; similarly, a rise in plasma cortisol of >7 μg/dL is generally considered normal. The rise in cortisol may be less in an already stressed patient.	Inject 250 μg cosyntropin intravenously or intramuscularly. Measure plasma cortisol level at 0 minutes, 30 minutes, and 60 minutes.	5, 16, 17, 46, 47
Low-dose short cosyntropin test	Suspected recent-onset central adrenal insufficiency or mild secondary adrenal insufficiency Suspected adrenal insufficiency with normal result on standard short cosyntropin test	As for the standard short cosyntropin test	Inject 1 μg-cosyntropin intravenously. Measure plasma cortisol level at 0 minutes, 30 minutes, and 60 minutes. Cosyntropin may be diluted to facilitate complete intravenous injection.	6, 17
Adrenocorticotropic hormone (ACTH)	Differentiation of primary from central adrenal insufficiency	Normal plasma ACTH level: 5–45 pg/mL In primary adrenal insufficiency, plasma ACTH level is usually >100 pg/mL. In central adrenal insufficiency, plasma ACTH level is usually low but may be in the normal range.		16, 45
Corticotropin-releasing hormone (CRH) test	Differentiation of hypothalamic and pituitary adrenal insufficiency This test is also used to rule out primary adrenal insufficiency. Some prefer it to the cosyntropin test because it evaluates the pituitary-adrenal axis.	Inadequate rise in plasma ACTH and cortisol	1 μg/kg or 100 μg CRH intravenously Measure plasma ACTH and plasma cortisol levels every 15 minutes for 60–90 minutes.	16
Plasma renin activity (PRA) and plasma aldosterone	Suspected mineralocorticoid deficiency with primary adrenal insufficiency May help differentiate primary from central adrenal insufficiency	Primary adrenal insufficiency: PRA > 3 ng/dL Plasma aldosterone <5 ng/mL with no rise after cosyntropin stimulation test		45

ACTH Testing

In the critically ill patient, an ACTH level should be determined simultaneously with the random cortisol level. Levels are decreased within a few hours of exogenous glucocorticoid administration. A high level is generally found with primary adrenal insufficiency, and a low level with central adrenal insufficiency. ACTH levels alone cannot be relied on for making the diagnosis of adrenal insufficiency; pulsatility of ACTH may lead to an incorrect diagnosis, and ACTH levels vary widely in critically ill patients and tend to correlate poorly with levels of cortisol. It has been suggested that other factors (such as endothelin) play a role in glucocorticoid release, accounting for this dissociation between pituitary ACTH and glucocorticoid secretion.

Corticotropin-Releasing Hormone Testing

Corticotropin-releasing hormone (CRH) may become a valuable diagnostic aid in differentiating pituitary, hypothalamic, and primary adrenal insufficiency. Studies so far show it to be highly sensitive in the diagnosis of adrenal insufficiency. Reference ranges are still being determined. ACTH usually peaks at 15 to 30 minutes after CRH is given; cortisol peaks at 30 to 45 minutes.

Other Localization Tests

The insulin hypoglycemia and the metyrapone tests used to differentiate primary and central adrenal insufficiency are not generally indicated for use in critically ill patients because they are potentially hazardous and time-consuming, and alternative tests are available. Adrenal autoantibodies are highly sensitive and specific for autoimmune adrenalitis. Plasma aldosterone levels are low and renin levels are high with primary adrenal insufficiency, whereas levels are usually normal with central adrenal insufficiency.[16]

Computed Tomography of the Adrenals

Computed tomography (CT) of the adrenal glands is useful in determining the cause of primary adrenal insufficiency. CT should be deferred until the patient is in a hemodynamically stable condition. Marked enlargement of the adrenal glands in patients with adrenal insufficiency is usually a sign of active tuberculosis. Enlargement also occurs with fungal infection, metastatic carcinoma, lymphoma, and AIDS. Blunt trauma typically causes a rounded enlargement of the adrenal gland on abdominal CT scan. There is often a central hematoma in the medulla surrounded by an enhanced cortex. The periadrenal fat may be stranded by hemorrhage, and blood may also track along the ipsilateral hemidiaphragm. Calcification of the adrenal glands may be seen with tuberculosis. Chronic autoimmune adrenalitis causes adrenal gland atrophy.[18] CT-guided fine-needle biopsy may be helpful in the differential diagnosis of an adrenal mass. Adrenal incidentalomas are adrenal masses noted incidentally on 1% to 2% of adrenal imaging studies. They are usually benign and biochemically inactive, but evaluation for activity and follow-up is recommended.[35]

Magnetic resonance imaging of the head is usually superior to CT scan for diagnosis of central adrenal insufficiency caused by lesions of the hypothalamus or pituitary and should be ordered in patients with visual disturbances or headaches who are thought to have a tumor. CT scan of the head is recommended if bony invasion or calcification by a craniopharyngioma is suspected.

TREATMENT

The mainstay of therapy for adrenal insufficiency is glucocorticoid replacement. Fluids, electrolytes, and glucose may also be required. The underlying pathologic process and other precipitating factors should be evaluated and treated appropriately (Table 72-5).

TABLE 72–5. Management of Adrenal Insufficiency

Situation	Management
Hemodynamically unstable patient with suspected adrenal insufficiency	1. Draw blood sample for determination of baseline cortisol and ACTH levels. 2. Immediately give hydrocortisone sodium succinate (Solu-Cortef) 100 mg bolus IV, then either hydrocortisone sodium succinate 100–200 mg q 24 hr by continuous IV infusion or 100 mg IV q 8 hr; *or* If a cosyntropin test is to be performed immediately, give dexamethasone 2 mg IV bolus in place of bolus hydrocortisone. Once cosyntropin testing has been completed, change to hydrocortisone sodium succinate 100–200 mg q 24 hr by continuous IV infusion, or 100 mg IV q 8 hr. 3. Give isotonic saline with 5% glucose intravenously for hypovolemia and hyponatremia. 4. Treat underlying cause and precipitating factors.
Suspected adrenal insufficiency in a stable patient	1. Draw blood sample for determination of baseline cortisol and ACTH levels and perform cosyntropin stimulation test. 2. Once the diagnosis is established, or on the basis of clinical suspicion, give hydrocortisone sodium succinate (Solu-Cortef), 100–200 mg every 24 hours by continuous infusion or, alternatively, 100 mg intravenously every 8 hours. 3. Give isotonic saline with 5% glucose intravenously for hypovolemia and hyponatremia. 4. Treat underlying cause and precipitating factors.
Maintenance	1. Taper stress doses of hydrocortisone as patient's condition improves. Usual maintenance doses of hydrocortisone are 25 mg daily: 15 mg in the morning and 10 mg in the evening. 2. Mineralocorticoid may be necessary for primary adrenal insufficiency. Usual dose is fludrocortisone, 0.05 mg–0.2 mg daily. 3. The hydrocortisone dose should be doubled or tripled with stress. 4. The patient should carry identification and be educated regarding condition.

Indications for Treatment

Because untreated adrenal insufficiency carries a mortality of almost 100%, treatment is essential and should be given on clinical suspicion alone in an emergency situation.[18] In a critically ill patient, treatment can be initiated with dexamethasone without affecting either the results of the tests or the quality of the treatment. In less urgent cases, treatment may be withheld until the results of the random cortisol and cosyntropin stimulation tests have been obtained. Beneficial results have been documented with glucocorticoid administration to patients with plasma cortisol values within the "normal" range. A normal test result should thus not preclude treatment if there is a strong clinical suspicion that the patient has adrenal insufficiency.[5, 12, 16]

Glucocorticoids

The usual recommended stress dose of hydrocortisone is 50 to 100 mg intravenously every 6 to 8 hours. An initial bolus of 100 mg intravenously followed by a continuous 24-hour infusion of 100 to 200 mg of hydrocortisone has been recommended.[16] Improvement in the patient's condition is often dramatic and seen within hours of initiation of therapy. Stress doses of hydrocortisone provide adequate glucocorticoid and mineralocorticoid activity.

Because dexamethasone does not cross-react with cortisol in current assays, it has been used to treat critically ill patients while diagnostic tests are being completed. Dexamethasone, however, has no mineralocorticoid activity and thus is not the treatment of choice in these patients. Furthermore, because diagnostic testing for adrenal insufficiency can be completed within half an hour, it should seldom be necessary to use dexamethasone in a case of suspected adrenal insufficiency.

In the stable patient, a blood sample for determination of the baseline cortisol and ACTH levels should be drawn and a cosyntropin simulation test performed. Depending on the urgency of the situation, hydrocortisone may be started on clinical suspicion while test results are pending.

The dose of glucocorticoid should be tapered as the patient improves. In cases of transient adrenal insufficiency that has been noted in critically ill patients,[17] therapy can eventually be discontinued. For persistent adrenal insufficiency, maintenance therapy is necessary (usually 20 to 25 mg of hydrocortisone daily). Additional mineralocorticoid may be necessary in the long-term management of primary adrenal insufficiency; a single daily dose of fludrocortisone (0.05 to 0.2 mg) is usually given.[16]

The usual maintenance dose of glucocorticoids is 25 mg hydrocortisone, 15 mg in the morning and 10 mg in the evening.[16] The maintenance dose of glucocorticoids should be doubled or tripled with fever, surgery, or other major stress. The dose should be titrated to avoid overmedication resulting in features of glucocorticoid (Cushing's syndrome) or mineralocorticoid (hypertension, heart failure, hypokalemia) excess. During treatment of acute adrenal insufficiency, cortisol's mineralocorticoid actions are generally considered adequate for physiologic needs. However, some authorities have recommended the addition of a mineralocorticoid (e.g., deoxycorticosterone, 10 mg intramuscularly) in any case with severe hypotension or shock.

Fluids and Electrolytes

The fluid of choice in hypovolemic patients is isotonic saline with 5% glucose. Large volumes may be required, and the patient's hemodynamic response should be monitored. Hyponatremia usually responds to glucocorticoid therapy and saline administration.[16]

Treatment of Associated Pathologic Conditions

Patients with etiologic processes, such as tuberculosis, or related conditions, such as autoimmune hypothyroidism, will require treatment for these conditions. Rifampin and thyroxine therapy both increase cortisol degradation, and the physician should take care that adequate replacement glucocorticoid doses are provided in order to avoid precipitating a crisis. Patients should carry identification documenting that they have adrenal insufficiency and should be educated regarding their condition.

PREVENTION OF ADRENAL INSUFFICIENCY

The clinician should anticipate the development of adrenal insufficiency, especially in a high-risk individual. A patient with a cushingoid appearance may have recently been taking glucocorticoids, as may patients with medical conditions in which glucocorticoids are used, such as asthma. There is individual susceptibility to hypothalamic-pituitary-adrenal axis suppression by exogenous glucocorticoids, and a crisis may be precipitated by a relatively mild stress, such as a minor infection in patients receiving low doses of glucocorticoids or in patients previously taking glucocorticoids. Patients who are within 1 to 2 years of treatment with high-dose glucocorticoids should be given 50 to 100 mg of hydrocortisone daily in two to three divided doses for minor illnesses or procedures. For a major illness or procedure, 300 mg of hydrocortisone should be given intravenously during 24 hours.

The low-dose short cosyntropin test is reported to be more sensitive than the standard cosyntropin test in detecting mild central adrenal insufficiency and may be used preoperatively to assess adrenal function.[36] Presurgical screening is recommended in the following situations:

- Elderly patients
- Patients who have been hospitalized for a prolonged time
- Malnourished or alcoholic individuals
- Patients who have other risk factors for adrenal insufficiency

Patients currently receiving high-dose glucocorticoid therapy should continue with their usual regimen for minor illnesses or procedures. If vomiting occurs, the equivalent of the maintenance dose can be given intravenously. For a major illness or procedure, 300 mg of hydrocortisone should be given intravenously during 24 hours. The intravenous glucocorticoid is usually started 6 hours before surgery.

Tapering of glucocorticoids is started once the patient's condition improves. The rate of tapering depends on the dose of glucocorticoids given and the duration for which they were received.[29]

OUTCOME

The mortality of untreated adrenal insufficiency is reported to be 100%.[5, 6, 16] Even with treatment, the mortality rate in critically ill patients is approximately 50%. Many patients, even those who eventually die, who have a diagnosis of adrenal insufficiency show a dramatic response to glucocorticoids within hours of its administration. Death is frequently due to coexisting diseases but in some cases may be due to glucocorticoid therapy started too late.

A correlation has been found between the baseline cortisol level and survival. In patients with severe illness, cortisol levels are positively correlated with the degree of illness and negatively correlated with survival. Rothwell and Lawler[37] have derived an endocrine index using cortisol, thyroxine, and thyroid-stimulating hormone that is reported to be a better predictor than the APACHE II score of outcome in the ICU.

ALDOSTERONE DEFICIENCY

Aldosterone is a mineralocorticoid secreted from the zona glomerulosa of the adrenal cortex. Secretion is primarily under the influence of the renin-angiotensin system, with ACTH and serum potassium playing lesser roles. Production is increased by a decrease in sodium intake, and mild cases of aldosterone deficiency may become apparent only during periods of sodium restriction. Aldosterone deficiency leads to an inability to retain sodium and excrete potassium, causing volume depletion and hyperkalemia.

Etiology and Pathogenesis

Aldosterone deficiency may occur as an isolated entity or as part of global adrenal insufficiency (Table 72–6). Aldosterone deficiency occurs with cortisol deficiency in primary adrenal insufficiency. It is usually not found with secondary adrenal insufficiency because its production is not directly ACTH-dependent. With marked atrophy of the adrenal gland, however, aldosterone deficiency may occur.

Isolated hypoaldosteronism is usually divided into two groups: *hyporeninemic* hypoaldosteronism (the more common form) and *hyperreninemic* hypoaldosteronism (see Table 72–6).

Hyporeninemic Hypoaldosteronism

Hyporeninemic hypoaldosteronism is usually a result of diabetic nephropathy and mild renal failure and is probably due to decreased renin production by the nephropathic kidney. It may also occur with nephropathy in chronic renal failure, AIDS, interstitial nephritis (including drug-induced interstitial nephritis), and congenital renin deficiency.

TABLE 72–6. Causes of Hypoaldosteronism

I. **Part of global adrenal insufficiency**
II. **Secondary to defects of the renin-angiotensin system**
   A. Hyporeninemic hypoaldosteronism (low renin production)
      1. Renal disease with secondary decreased renin production
         a. Diabetic nephropathy
         b. Chronic renal failure
         c. Systemic lupus erythematosus
         d. Acquired immunodeficiency syndrome (AIDS)
         e. Interstitial nephritis
      2. Congenital familial defect in renin production
      3. Drugs that suppress renin-angiotensin system
         a. β-Adrenergic receptor blockers
         b. Prostaglandin-synthesis inhibitors
         c. Potassium-sparing diuretics
   B. Low angiotensin
   C. Low angiotensin-converting enzyme
   D. Low angiotensin receptors
III. **Isolated hypoaldosteronism**
   A. Hyperreninemic hypoaldosteronism
      1. Severe illness
      2. Congenital corticosterone methyl oxidase deficiency
      3. Postoperative after removal of aldosterone-secreting tumor
      4. Autoimmune disease
      5. Heparin
      6. Hemochromatosis
      7. Hypoparathyroidism
      8. Pretectal disease of the nervous system
      9. Severe postural hypotension

Hyperreninemic Hypoaldosteronism

Hyperreninemic hypoaldosteronism occurs secondary to the inability of the adrenal gland to synthesize aldosterone, usually because of a defect in corticosterone methyl oxidase. Prolonged heparin use may cause hyperreninemic hypoaldosteronism by a direct suppressive effect on the zona glomerulosa. Hyperreninemic hypoaldosteronism has been found to occur in severely ill patients, especially after prolonged hypotension. The mortality in these patients is 80%, and the syndrome may be due to adrenal insufficiency or a shift in steroid biosynthesis from mineralocorticoids to glucocorticoids, possibly related to prolonged ACTH stimulation. Unlike other forms of isolated hypoaldosteronism, this illness is not associated with significant hyperkalemia.

Isolated hypoaldosteronism may also occur after removal of an aldosterone-secreting tumor, in patients with hemochromatosis, pretectal disease of the nervous system, and in severe postural hypotension.

Clinical Presentation

Isolated aldosterone deficiency typically presents with unexplained hyperkalemia in an older patient with mild renal failure. Related complications include arrhythmias, weakness, or even sudden death. The hyperkalemia is disproportionately high for the degree of renal failure, a complication that usually occurs only with a glomerular filtration rate of less than 10 mL/min. Hyperkalemia occurs with normal sodium intake in severe cases, but in mild cases, the hyperkalemia may be present only with sodium restriction. Sodium wasting is not usually clinically apparent. Impaired ammonia excretion may lead to a mild hyperchloremic metabolic acidosis. Features of glucocorticoid deficiency are present if the hypoaldosteronism is part of global adrenal insufficiency.

Diagnosis

Accurate diagnosis of isolated aldosterone deficiency usually requires demonstration of the inability of aldosterone to increase after stimulation (sodium restriction, upright posture). The first step in the diagnosis is to exclude other causes of hyperkalemia and then to demonstrate normal glucocorticoid production (i.e., normal cortisol levels). Once global adrenal insufficiency has been excluded, renin and aldosterone should be measured in the baseline, supine state and then again after the patient has been upright for several hours and sodium restricted. Low renin and low aldosterone levels that fail to rise with stimulation confirm hyporeninemic hypoaldosteronism, whereas a high renin level and low aldosterone level are found with hyperreninemic hypoaldosteronism. If both renin and aldosterone levels are high, the diagnosis is *pseudohypoaldosteronism*. These stimulation tests are rarely performed in the critically ill patient.

Treatment

Mild hypoaldosteronism frequently does not warrant treatment other than addressing the cause and avoiding aggravating factors. If the patient is hypertensive or in mild heart or renal failure, furosemide may be used. More severe hypoaldosteronism with hypotension is treated with fludrocortisone, starting with 0.05 mg/day. The final dose of fludrocortisone is frequently higher in patients with isolated hypoaldosteronism than that required for treatment of global adrenal insufficiency (i.e., 0.2 mg daily). The dose is adjusted until there is no postural or supine hypotension, a normal serum potassium concentration, and no edema. The plasma renin level may be measured to aid dosing and should be maintained in the high-normal range.[38, 39] Patients should maintain an adequate fluid and salt intake, especially during stress periods.

References

1. Span LFR, Hermus ARMM, Bartelink AKM, et al: Adrenocortical function: An indicator of severity of disease and survival in chronic critically ill patients. Intensive Care Med 1992; 18:93–96.
2. Lamberts SW, Bruining HA, deJong FH: Corticosteroid therapy in severe illness. N Engl J Med 337:1285–1292.
3. Sibbald WJ, Short A, Cohen MP, Wilson RF: Variations in adrenocortical responsiveness during severe bacterial infections. Ann Surg 1977; 186:29–33.
4. Jurney TH, Cockrell JL, Lindberg JS, et al: Spectrum of serum cortisol response to ACTH in ICU patients. Chest 1987; 92:292–295.
5. Angelis M, Yu M, Takanishi D, et al: Eosinophilia as a marker of adrenal insufficiency in the surgical intensive care unit. J Am Coll Surg 1996; 183:589–596.
6. Barquist E, Kirton O: Adrenal insufficiency in the surgical intensive care unit patient. J Trauma 1997; 42:27–31.
7. Singh N, Gayowski T, Marino IR, et al: Acute adrenal insufficiency in critically ill liver transplant recipients: Implications for diagnosis. Transplantation 1995; 59:1744–1745.
8. Crump JA, Beard MEJ, Angus HB, et al: Acute adrenal insufficiency: A new presentation of Castleman's disease. J Intern Med 1995; 238:81–84.
9. Lewis JV: Bilateral adrenal hemorrhage after blunt trauma: Diagnosis by computed tomography. South Med J 1994; 87:1269–1271.
10. Blake DP, Bessey PQ: Adrenocortical neoplasm disguised as a post-traumatic perinephric hematoma. Milit Med 1996; 161:173–175.
11. Szalados JE, Vukmir RB: Acute adrenal insufficiency resulting from adrenal hemorrhage as indicated by post-operative hypotension. Intensive Care Med 1994; 20:216–218.
12. Baldwin WA, Allo M: Occult hypoadrenalism in critically ill patients. Arch Surg 1993; 128:673–676.
13. Sutherland FWH, Naik SK: Acute adrenal insufficiency after coronary artery bypass grafting. Ann Thorac Surg 1996; 62:1516–1517.
14. Lefevre N, Delauney L, Hingot JL, et al: Bilateral massive adrenal haemorrhage complicating anaphylactic shock: A case report. Intensive Care Med 1996; 22:447–449.
15. Claussen MS, Landercasper J, Cogbill TH: Acute adrenal insufficiency presenting as shock after trauma and surgery: Three cases and review of the literature. J Trauma 1992; 32:94–100.
16. Oelkers W: Adrenal insufficiency. N Engl J Med 1996; 355:1206–1211.
17. Merry WH, Caplan RH, Wickus GG, et al: Postoperative acute adrenal failure caused by transient corticotropin deficiency. Surgery 1994; 116:1095–1100.
18. Werbel SS, Ober KP: Acute adrenal insufficiency. Endocrinol Metab Clin North Am 1993; 22:303–328.
19. Kannan CR: Diseases of the adrenal cortex. Dis Mon 1988; 34:627–638.
20. Rao RH, Vagnucci AH, Amico JA: Bilateral massive adrenal hemorrhage: Early recognition and treatment. Ann Intern Med 1989; 110:227–235.
21. Dahlberg PJ, Goellner MH, Pehling GB: Adrenal insufficiency secondary to adrenal hemorrhage. Two case reports and a review of cases confirmed by computed tomography. Arch Intern Med 1990; 150:905–909.
22. Porter JM, Muscato K, Patrick JR: Adrenal hemorrhage: A comparison of traumatic and nontraumatic deaths. J Natl Med Assoc 1995; 87:569–571.
23. Spark RJ, Etzkorn JR: Absent aldosterone response to ACTH in familial glucocorticoid deficiency. N Engl J Med 1977; 297:917–920.
24. Kung AW, Pun KK, Lam K, et al: Addisonian crisis as presenting feature in malignancies. Cancer 1990; 65:177–179.
25. Wagner RL, White PF, Kan PB, et al: Inhibition of adrenal steroidogenesis by the anesthetic etomidate. N Engl J Med 1984; 310:1415–1421.
26. Sonino N: The use of ketoconazole as an inhibitor of steroid production. N Engl J Med 1987; 317:812–818.
27. Chin R: Adrenal crisis. Crit Care Clin 1991; 7:23–42.
28. Huiras CM, Pehling GB, Caplan RH: Adrenal insufficiency after operative removal of apparently nonfunctional adrenal adenomas. JAMA 1989; 261:894–898.
29. Boulanger BR, Gann DS: Management of the trauma victim with pre-existing endocrine disease. Crit Care Clin 1994; 10:537–554.
30. Graber AL, Ney RL, Nicholson WE, et al: Natural history of pituitary-adrenal recovery following long-term suppression with corticosteroids. J Clin Endocrinol Metab 1965; 25:11–16.
31. Passmore JM Jr: Adrenal cortex. *In:* Endocrine Aspects of Acute Illness. Geethood GW, Chernow B (Eds). New York, Churchill Livingstone, 1986, pp 97–134.
32. Norbiato G, Bevilacqua M, Vago T, et al: Cortisol resistance in acquired immune deficiency syndrome. J Clin Endocrinol Metab 1992; 74:608–613.
33. Dorin RI, Kearns PJ: High output circulatory failure in acute adrenal insufficiency. Crit Care Med 1988; 16:296–297.
34. Alford WC Jr, Meador CK, Mihalevich J, et al: Acute adrenal insufficiency following cardiac surgical procedures. J Thorac Cardiovasc Surg 1979; 78:489–493.
35. Staren ED, Prinz RA: Selection of patients with adrenal incidentalomas for operation. Surg Clin North Am 1995; 75:499–509.
36. Dickstein G, Shechner C, Nicholson WE, et al: Adrenocorticotropin stimulation test: Effects of basal cortisol level, time of day, and suggested new sensitive low dose test. J Clin Endocrinol Metab 1991; 72:773–778.
37. Rothwell PM, Lawler PG: Prediction of outcome in intensive care patients using endocrine parameters. Crit Care Med 1995; 23:78–83.
38. Oelkers W, Lage M: Control of mineralocorticoid substitution in Addison's disease by plasma renin measurement. Klin Wochenschr 1976; 54:607–612.
39. Oelkers W, Diederich S, Bähr V: Diagnosis and therapy surveillance in Addison's disease: Rapid adrenocorticotropin (ACTH) test and measurement of plasma ACTH, renin activity, and aldosterone. J Clin Endocrinol Metab 1992; 75:259–264.
40. Vandam LD, Moore FD: Adrenocortical mechanisms related to anesthesia. Anesthesiology 1960; 21:531–552.
41. Burks DW, Mirvis SE, Shanmuganathan K: Acute adrenal injury after blunt abdominal trauma: CT findings. AJR Am J Roentgenol 1992; 158:503–507.
42. Sivit CJ, Ingram DJ, Taylor GA, et al: Posttraumatic adrenal hemorrhage in children: CT findings in 34 patients. AJR Am J Roentgenol 1992; 158:1299–1302.
43. Mohler JL, Flueck JA, McRoberts JW: Adrenal insufficiency following unilateral adrenalectomy: A case report. J Urol 1986; 135:554–556.
44. Swingle WW, Brannick LJ, Osborn M, et al: Effect of gluco- and mineralocorticoid adrenal steroids on fluid and electrolytes of fasted adrenalectomized dogs. Proc Soc Exp Biol Med 1957; 96:446–452.
45. Grinspoon SK, Biller BMK: Clinical review 62: Laboratory assessment of adrenal insufficiency. J Clin Endocrinol Metab 1994; 79:923–931.
46. May ME, Vaughn ED, Carey RM: Adrenocortical insufficiency—clinical aspects. *In:* Adrenal Disorders. Vaughn ED Jr, Carey RM (Eds). New York, Thieme Medical, 1989, pp 171–189.
47. Oelkers W, Diederich S, Bähr V: Recent advances in diagnosis and therapy of Addison's disease. *In:* Bhatt HR, James VHT, Besser GM, et al (Eds). Advances in Thomas Addison's Diseases. Vol 1. London, Journal of Endocrinology, Thomas Addison Society, 1994, pp 69–80.

73

Endocrine Emergencies

K. Patrick Ober, MD

Of the many endocrine emergencies that are encountered in the practice of medicine, hypoglycemia, diabetes insipidus, pheochromocytoma, and carcinoid crisis are emphasized in this chapter. Each of these complex endocrine disorders is potentially life-threatening if it is not recognized promptly and managed effectively.

HYPOGLYCEMIA

Glucose has an essential function as the fundamental energy source for the brain. This critical fuel requirement creates a need for a consistently available and uninterrupted supply of glucose. An intricate homeostatic system has evolved to ensure adequate availability of glucose at all times; postabsorptive (fasting) levels of plasma glucose are generally kept within the fairly narrow range of 60 to 100 mg/dL (3.3 to 5.6 mmol/L). This stability is maintained even under the disruptive circumstances of calorie deprivation and increased energy requirements that occur with severe trauma, febrile illnesses, and other catabolic states. The maintenance of adequate serum glucose levels is a crucial function of the stress response, and the increased secretion of "stress hormones," such as cortisol, catecholamines, and growth hormone contributes to the provision of consistent glucose availability. A failure in the life-sustaining system for maintaining serum glucose levels can lead to severe dysfunction of many organs and ultimately death.[1]

The central nervous system (CNS) is the major site of glucose utilization. The brain uses 85% to 90% of the glucose that is produced in the infant and about 50% in the adult. Glucose moves down a concentration gradient across the blood-brain barrier; this movement is facilitated by glucose transport proteins.

Clinical Features

The clinical effects of hypoglycemia are variable and are related to duration and severity of the hypoglycemia. Although most symptoms are short-lived, with reversal occurring promptly after restoration of blood glucose levels, some neurologic deficits can persist for days or even weeks if the hypoglycemia has been particularly severe or prolonged; in rare cases, the neurologic damage may be irreversible. The neurologic effects of hypoglycemia include confusion, disorientation, combativeness, and seizures. Ataxia, hemiparesis, coma, decortication, decerebration, choreoathetosis, and "locked-in" syndrome have all been reported. There has been concern about possible long-term intellectual impairment after hypoglycemia, although this is not fully established. Hypoglycemia may be responsible for up to 5% of the deaths in young patients with diabetes.

Hypothermia is a well-recognized accompaniment of hypoglycemia; the degree of hypothermia is related to the severity of the hypoglycemia. After an early increase in metabolic heat production due to increased sympathoadrenal activity, heat dissipation at the skin surface causes a subsequent fall in core temperature by evaporative heat loss from sweating and conduction of heat to the periphery. The hypothermia of hypoglycemia may be a protective response, because lower brain temperature during hypoglycemia has been shown to limit neuronal loss.

Four major counterregulatory hormones are involved in the defense against hypoglycemia, with a hierarchy of response. Decreases in the plasma glucose concentration to the threshold of 65 mg/dL (3.6 mmol/L) provoke the secretion of glucagon and epinephrine, the hormones of greatest counterregulatory importance.

The single most important counterregulatory hormone is *glucagon*, which enhances hepatic glycogenolysis and gluconeogenesis and is necessary for full recovery from hypoglycemia.

Epinephrine becomes essential in the absence of glucagon (common in the patient with insulin-dependent diabetes due to autoimmune islet cell loss).

Growth hormone and *cortisol* are slower to act as counterregulatory agents, do not make any substantial contribution to glucose counterregulation during acute hypoglycemia, and cannot compensate effectively for hypoglycemia in the absence of glucagon and epinephrine; thus, they are of secondary importance in the counterregulation of hypoglycemia. Cortisol levels do not increase until the blood glucose level falls below 55 mg/dL.[2]

As the major user of glucose, the brain is a primary organ for recognizing and directing the counterregulatory response to hypoglycemia. However, the counterregulatory hormones are activated before the development of CNS symptoms or cognitive dysfunction. As plasma glucose levels fall to the range of 60 to 65 mg/dL, the triggering of catecholamine release causes the adrenergic symptoms of tachycardia, palpitation, tremor, and pallor, and these symptoms become even more severe with further declines in glucose concentrations. Decrease in plasma glucose concentration to the level of 55 mg/dL (3.1 mmol/L) initiates autonomic symptoms (anxiety, hunger, irritability, trembling, and sweating), mediated by specific glucose-sensing centers in the ventromedian hypothalamic nuclei of the brain. Further lowering of glucose concentration leads to development of neuroglycopenic symptoms (weakness, confusion, faintness, headache, impaired concentration, cognitive impairment, behavioral abnormalities, and even coma and seizures). The specific sites in the CNS that detect glucopenia and initiate the counterregulatory response are not clearly identified; redundant glucose-sensing neurons are located in widespread brain regions.[1]

Diagnosis

The definition of hypoglycemia is problematic and somewhat arbitrary. The finding of a low plasma glucose level is not sufficient by itself. Remarkable nadirs of blood sugar, to the range of 20 to 30 mg/dL, can occur in perfectly healthy people under varying physiologic conditions (e.g., intense exercise by athletes and fasting in healthy women). For the diagnosis of hypoglycemia to be established, a patient must exhibit all three features of "Whipple's triad":

1. CNS manifestations of low glucose concentration ("neuroglycopenic symptoms"): confusion, disorientation, unusual behavior, seizures, and coma.

"β-Adrenergic" manifestations alone are not sufficient to define hypoglycemia—tachycardia, tremor, palpitation, and diaphoresis are nonspecific and are commonly associated with anxiety, fear, and a multitude of other nonhypoglycemic stresses.

2. A simultaneous blood glucose level less than 40 mg/dL (2.2 mmol/L).

3. Recovery from the symptoms after glucose administration.

Methodology-related aspects of glucose measurement can be a potential problem in the assessment of glucose levels in some critically ill patients. Finger-stick glucose measurements in hypotensive patients can be misleadingly lower than the simultaneous measurement in venous blood, perhaps because of peripheral vasoconstriction with continuous tissue glucose consumption.

When the presence of hypoglycemia has been determined on the basis of Whipple's triad, it is essential to establish the specific cause (Table 73–1). Approximately 1.2% of adults who are hospitalized in a tertiary care hospital have hypoglycemia. About half of the hypoglycemic episodes are attributable to insulin administration; decreased calorie intake due to illness or hospital procedures is an important cofactor. Chronic renal failure in the nondiabetic patient is the second most common cause of hypoglycemia. Chronic malnutrition, acute calorie deprivation, and liver disease are other contributors. The overall hospital mortality in this group of hypoglycemic patients is around 27%; mortality is related to the number of risk factors for hypoglycemia and the degree of hypoglycemia, even though hypoglycemia per se is rarely the cause of death.[3]

Treatment

The immediate therapy for hypoglycemia consists of glucose administration. Before glucose treatment, a blood sample for determination of insulin and C peptide levels should be drawn in the patient who does not have an obvious cause of hypoglycemia. In the hypoglycemic patient who is still alert and oriented, 20 g of oral glucose or 40 g of carbohydrate as orange juice corrects hypoglycemia; a smaller amount of orange juice (20 g of carbohydrate) and milk (20 g of carbohydrate) provides partial correction. Patients who are confused, combative, or comatose should receive 25 g of glucose intravenously; oral glucose therapy in such patients may cause aspiration and therefore should be avoided. The use of 1 mg of intravenous glucagon is equally effective in restoring serum glucose levels in patients with insulin-induced hypoglycemia,[4] but glucagon has no effect in patients whose hepatic glycogen stores are depleted (e.g., calorie-deprived alcoholic patients).

TABLE 73–1. Causes of Hypoglycemia

1. Insulin excess
   a. Insulinoma
   b. Insulin administration
   c. Sulfonylureas
   d. Insulin autoimmune hypoglycemia
   e. Autoantibodies to the insulin receptor
2. Non-islet cell tumors: typically large tumors of mesenchymal, hepatocellular, hematologic, or neuroendocrine origin that produce insulin-like growth factor II (IGF-II)
3. End-stage renal disease
4. Liver diseases
5. Congestive heart failure
6. Endocrine deficiencies
   a. Growth hormone deficiency
   b. Cortisol deficiency
7. Ketotic hypoglycemia
8. Enzyme deficiencies
9. Infectious diseases
   a. *Plasmodium falciparum* malaria
   b. Sepsis
10. Medications and toxins
   a. Sulfonylureas
   b. Ethanol
   c. Salicylate poisoning
   d. β-Blocking drugs
   e. Other drugs
      (1) Pentamidine, disopyramide, ritodrine, quinine, haloperidol
      (2) In renal failure: trimethoprim-sulfamethoxazole, propoxyphene
   f. Pyriminil (Vacor)—rodenticide
   g. Unripened Caribbean akee fruit ("Jamaican vomiting illness")

DIABETES INSIPIDUS

Clinical Features

Diabetes insipidus is manifested by an inability to conserve water. *Polyuria* (defined as urine volumes above 30 mL/kg/day) and *polydipsia* are the most common clinical features; patients usually become aware of the polyuria at volumes above 3 to 4 L/day. Hypertonicity (hypernatremia) can also be seen, but this occurs only when the patient has an impaired thirst mechanism, is not fully responsive, or has no access to water.

Diagnosis

Before therapy is initiated, it is imperative to exclude other processes that may resemble diabetes insipidus. Osmotic diuresis should always be considered a possible etiologic factor of polyuria and polydipsia; it can be caused by infusion of mannitol or elevated levels of glucose or urea (as in postobstructive diuresis). As soon as an osmotic diuresis is ruled out, the next step is to confirm that the patient has a *hypotonic polyuria*, which is defined as increased urine volume with decreased urine osmolality (<300 mOsm/kg). The three causes of hypo-osmolar polyuria are:

1. Inadequate secretion of antidiuretic hormone (ADH): *central or neurogenic diabetes insipidus.*
2. Impaired renal responsiveness to ADH: *nephrogenic diabetes insipidus.*
3. Increased water intake: *primary polydipsia.*

The diagnosis of diabetes insipidus requires the simultaneous documentation of serum hypertonicity (>295 mOsm/kg) and hypernatremia (>145 mEq/L) in the setting of hypo-osmolar polyuria. Because even a slight increase in serum osmolality triggers an increase in free water intake in patients who have an intact thirst mechanism and ready access to free water, serum hypertonicity and hypernatremia rarely occur spontaneously. On occasion, a water deprivation test may be required to establish the diagnosis of diabetes insipidus. Several versions of this test have been advocated, but the goal is the same for each—documentation of urinary hypo-osmolality in the context of serum hyperosmolality. A positive test result rules out primary polydipsia and establishes diabetes insipidus as the underlying disorder.

Subsequently, central diabetes insipidus should be differentiated from nephrogenic diabetes insipidus by the injection of vasopressin or one of its analogs. With central diabetes insipidus, vasopressin decreases urine volume and increases urine concentration; with nephrogenic diabetes insipidus, there is no response to the exogenous hormone. Some patients may have indeterminate responses, and a blunted response can occur in patients with primary polydipsia due to a "washed-out" renal concentration gradient.[5] Once the diagnosis of central diabetes insipidus is made, appropriate imaging studies are required to define the anatomic basis of the process (possibilities include primary CNS lesions, metastatic disease, infiltrative processes, and trauma).

Treatment

The most straightforward, safe, and inexpensive treatment of central diabetes insipidus is the simple replacement of the free water that is being "wasted" by the kidneys. This can be accomplished by the patients themselves, assuming an intact thirst mechanism (which in some cases may be injured by the same pathologic process that caused the diabetes insipidus) and ready access to water. However, severe polyuria and polydipsia are often intolerable to the patient, and use of pharmacologic vasopressin replacement is commonly employed. The situation is even more complicated in the patient who has no thirst awareness or who cannot voluntarily obtain water (such as the patient who is not fully responsive because of surgery, trauma, or other medical problems). In most patients with well-established central diabetes insipidus, hormone replacement should be employed.

In alert patients, DDAVP (1-desamino-8-D-arginine vasopressin) is the preferred vasopressin replacement because of its quick onset of action (1 hour), relatively long duration of action (6 to 24 hours), and high level of antidiuretic activity with slight vasopressor effect. Used as a nasal aerosol, a single bedtime dose may be sufficient to control overnight symptoms, which are usually the most bothersome. At times, a divided regimen is used if daytime symptoms are a problem. The dosage can be adjusted by 10-μg increments until an effective dose is reached. An oral form is also available.

In the critically ill patient, careful monitoring of weight, electrolyte values, and intake and output is essential. Parenteral DDAVP (intravenously, subcutaneously, or intramuscularly) is the preferred vasopressin replacement, using a starting dose of 1 μg.[6] Hourly monitoring of urine output and osmolality guides further dosing. Thoughtful intravenous fluid replacement is a crucial component of management and should be in the form of dextrose-containing water solutions—the patient's predominant fluid loss is that of free water, and use of saline solutions presents an unnecessary solute load that further increases renal water loss.

In patients with postoperative diabetes insipidus, control is usually achieved with doses of 1 to 4 μg DDAVP subcutaneously every 12 hours. Careful monitoring of fluid balance is essential because of the possibility of "breakthrough" polyuria at the lower dose and risk of hyponatremia and fluid overload at the higher dose range.[5] The risk of profound hyponatremia is considerable if excess hypotonic fluid is administered in the setting of DDAVP-driven antidiuresis. Thus, an increase of urine output (hypotonic polyuria) should be allowed before the next DDAVP dose is given. Extreme care is required so as not to "get ahead" on fluid input. Maintenance hypotonic fluid replacement therapy should be switched from intravenous to oral as soon as the patient is able to sense thirst and drink adequate amounts of water (the patient's thirst mechanism, if intact, is an excellent guide to adequacy of water replacement and will avoid overreplacement).

Post-traumatic diabetes insipidus is occasionally seen after head trauma and usually resolves within 3 to 5 days. Recovery is not recognized unless the patient is periodically allowed to be a little "behind" on fluids; persistent aggressive free water infusion results in a continued hypotonic polyuria resembling ongoing diabetes insipidus. Periodic lowering of the rate of fluid administration aids in identification of recovery and limits the risk of hyponatremia. However, some patients may have permanent diabetes insipidus.

The most treacherous pattern of post-traumatic diabetes insipidus is *triphasic diabetes insipidus*. The patient presents with diabetes insipidus starting hours to days after injury (reflecting the impairment of vasopressin secretion due to "shock" of the magnocellular neurons). Release of stored vasopressin from the injured neurons creates a second phase of "inappropriate" vasopressin release that may develop within several days and persist for up to 2 weeks after injury. During the second phase, the patient is at risk for severe hyponatremia if large quantities of free water are infused. The third phase consists of recurrent and permanent diabetes insipidus due to the progressive death of the magnocellular neurons by retrograde axonal degeneration. At this stage, patients should be treated with lifelong replacement therapy.

PHEOCHROMOCYTOMA

Clinical Features

Pheochromocytomas are relatively rare tumors that arise from chromaffin tissues of the sympathetic nervous system. Clinical manifestations of the tumors can be attributed to increased catecholamine production.[7] The clinical features are protean; the most important manifestations are hypertension (either sustained or paroxysmal, frequently labile and difficult to control), headache, diaphoresis, palpitations, hyperglycemia, and clinical features of a hypermetabolic state. The differential diagnosis is broad, as noted in Table 73–2.

Diagnosis

The diagnosis of pheochromocytoma is confirmed by elevated levels of catecholamines or catecholamine metabolites in plasma or in urine. There is probably no single "best" test. Plasma catecholamines, urine catecholamines, and urine catecholamine metabolites (e.g., metanephrine and vanillylmandelic acid) are elevated in most patients with pheochromocytomas. Tradeoffs between test sensitivity and specificity are recurrent problems in diagnosis[8]; tests that are touted for their high sensitivity (such as tests of plasma catecholamines) suffer from having a relatively low specificity and can give misleadingly elevated results in many disorders in which excessive catecholamine secretion is a secondary response to stress.[9] Provocative tests are risky and should be avoided.

TABLE 73–2. Differential Diagnosis of Pheochromocytoma

- Acute mercury poisoning (acrodynia)
- β-Adrenergic hyperresponsive state
- Alcohol withdrawal
- Anxiety or panic disorder
- Autonomic dysfunction
- Baroreflex failure
- Carcinoid syndrome
- Catecholamine conjugation defects
- Drugs
  - Amphetamines
  - Ephedrine
  - Isoproterenol
  - Phenylephrine
  - Pseudoephedrine
- Eclampsia
- Endocrine secretory tumors
- Hypertension
- Hyperthyroidism
- Hypoglycemia
- Monoamine oxidase inhibitor and hypertensive crisis
- Mitral valve prolapse
- Myocarditis
- Paroxysmal hypertension after clonidine withdrawal
- Post-traumatic stress disorder exacerbation
- Surreptitious self-injection of epinephrine

Modified from Werbel SS, Ober KP: Pheochromocytoma: Update on diagnosis, localization and management. Med Clin North Am 1995; 79:131–153.

Once a pheochromocytoma is confirmed by biochemical measurements, localization of the tumor is necessary. Computed tomography detects the majority of pheochromocytomas, but in some circumstances magnetic resonance imaging or nuclear medicine scans can provide additional information.

Treatment

Surgical removal is the only definitive treatment of pheochromocytomas. Preoperative medical management is essential to a good outcome. Without adequate medical control of blood pressure, the patient is at high risk for hypertensive crisis with the induction of anesthesia, surgical manipulation of the tumor, or other stress. Postoperatively, the patient with poorly controlled blood pressure may have severe problems with hypotension, possibly reflecting a state of functional volume depletion due to chronic vasoconstriction.

Preoperative therapy should be aimed at controlling the blood pressure and overcoming chronic vasoconstriction, allowing reestablishment of effective circulating volume. Establishment of good α-adrenergic control is the critical first step.[7] β-Adrenergic blockade should never be started before α-blockade is established. In the absence of an α-blocking agent, β-blockade alone can result in unopposed α-adrenergic stimulation (producing a state of vasoconstriction that is not offset by the vasodilatory effects of the β_2-receptors), creating the potential for resultant hypertensive crisis, pulmonary edema, and shock. Effective α-adrenergic blockers include phenoxybenzamine, 10 mg twice daily (increasing to 0.5 to 1.0 mg/kg daily), or prazosin hydrochloride, 2 to 5 mg three to four times daily; there has been less experience with terazosin, 1 to 20 mg daily, or doxazosin, 1 to 16 mg daily.

β-Adrenergic blocking drugs should be employed as needed to control or prevent severe tachycardia and tachyarrhythmias, but only after α-blockade has been well established (as defined by normalization of blood pressure).

An alternative approach to adrenergic receptor blockade, but one that is less commonly used, is the inhibition of catecholamine synthesis. Metyrosine, a competitive inhibitor of tyrosine hydroxylase (the rate-limiting step in catecholamine synthesis) can be started at 250 mg every 6 hours and titrated upward by 250 to 500 mg daily, to a total dose of 4 g every day if needed.

During surgery, or with an acute hypertensive crisis in a nonsurgical setting, blood pressure elevations respond well to intravenous phentolamine, nitroglycerin, or sodium nitroprusside. Esmolol can be used to manage tachyarrhythmias. After tumor removal, hypotension becomes the most common blood pressure problem, but hypotension is less likely to occur if there has been good blood pressure control for at least a week before surgery. Postoperative hypotension usually responds well to volume replacement. Pressor agents should be used only if there is failure to respond to volume repletion. Other postoperative problems include hypoglycemia; patients should have glucose monitoring within the first 3 hours of tumor removal. If a patient has bilateral pheochromocytomas and undergoes bilateral adrenalectomies, glucocorticoid replacement is essential.

CARCINOID CRISIS

Carcinoid Syndrome

Carcinoid tumors are derived from the enterochromaffin cells found throughout the gastrointestinal tract and bronchi. Most carcinoid tumors are biochemically silent and present only with mass effects, such as obstruction. However, carcinoids are capable of producing a variety of peptides and amines, and the "carcinoid syndrome" occurs when clinical symptoms are caused by these substances. Because of hepatic metabolism of the products of carcinoid tumors that are predominantly secreted into the portal circulation, systemic symptoms do not occur unless there are hepatic metastases from a gastrointestinal carcinoid tumor (or, less commonly, direct secretion of tumor products into the systemic circulation by ovarian or bronchial carcinoids). Flushing, diarrhea, and heart disease are the major features of the carcinoid syndrome.

The flushing is erythematous, usually affects the upper body, and can be of variable duration and severity. Compared with the carcinoids of gastrointestinal origin, bronchial carcinoids are notable for severe and prolonged flushes that may last for many hours and are associated with increased tear formation, sweating, salivation, facial edema, diarrhea, and hypotension. Carcinoid flushing is frequently spontaneous but can be precipitated by alcohol ingestion, meals, or anxiety. The flushing is probably related to the release of kinins; kallikrein is released by carcinoids either spontaneously or after stimulation by alcohol or catecholamines and generates bradykinin from plasma kininogens. In milder cases, flushing can be prevented simply by the avoidance of known precipitants. With gastric carcinoids, the distinctive flush is mediated by histamine, and a combination of H_1 and H_2 antagonists (such as diphenhydramine, 50 mg every 6 hours, and cimetidine, 300 mg every 6 hours) has been helpful. For most patients, however, the use of the long-acting somatostatin analog octreotide (100 to 500 μg subcutaneously every 8 to 12 hours) is the most effective agent for management of flushes; interferon-α, which is used to reduce tumor mass, can also alleviate flushing in some patients.

Diarrhea is common and frequently (but not consistently) related to episodes of flushing. The diarrhea, usually watery, is related to increased motility and possibly to intestinal secretion; serotonin is the likely stimulus. Loperamide is effective treatment. Serotonin antagonists, such as cyproheptadine and methysergide, are also effective, but octreotide is the most effective agent for patients who are refractory to other approaches.[10]

The heart disease of carcinoid syndrome is predominantly right-sided, related to fibrosis of the endocardium and valves (tricuspid regurgitation or stenosis is the most common lesion, but pulmonic stenosis can also occur). The fibrosis is attributed to the effects of serotonin. Serotonin also contributes to the asthma that occurs in some patients with carcinoid syndrome. Measurement of the principal serotonin metabolite (5-hydroxyindoleacetic acid) is the cornerstone of diagnosis for carcinoid.

Carcinoid Crisis

Carcinoid crisis is essentially an exaggerated and extreme flushing episode associated with severe hypotension triggered by the outpouring of vasoactive substances from the carcinoid tumor. The crisis may be manifested by hypotension, prolonged flushing, confusion, and even coma. Carcinoid crisis may occur without an obvious precipitant but can also be triggered by a number of stimuli, which include induction of anesthesia, surgery, chemotherapy, or abdominal palpation. Because of the severe fall in blood pressure that may be refractory to traditional therapies, such as fluids, crystalloid replacement, and vasopressors, carcinoid crisis is potentially life-threatening. The risk of carcinoid crisis can be lowered by avoidance of flush-provoking agents, such as catecholamines.

If a crisis occurs, hypotension responds to octreotide acetate, 100 μg intravenously, and this agent should be available when patients with carcinoid syndrome are undergoing surgery or starting chemotherapy.[11] In acute situations, octreotide has been effective in patients who have not responded to intravenous fluids, calcium, and epinephrine.[12] Intravenous doses of 100 to 500 μg have been safely administered. Methoxamine, 3 to 5 mg, can be used if octreotide is not available, but other pressor agents should be avoided. Prophylactic use of octreotide is recommended in patients who have severe carcinoid symptoms (or who have had a previous hypotensive episode) and are to undergo induction of anesthesia or start chemotherapy. Therapeutic levels sufficient to minimize the likelihood of carcinoid storm can be achieved by the subcutaneous administration of 250 to 500 μg octreotide 1 to 2 hours before the induction of anesthesia.[13]

References

1. Ober KP: Alterations in fuel metabolism in critical illness: Hypoglycemia. *In:* Endocrinology of Critical Disease. Ober KP (Ed). Totowa, NJ, Humana Press, 1997, pp 211-231.
2. Service FJ: Hypoglycemic disorders. N Engl J Med 1995; 332:1144-1152.
3. Fischer KF, Lees JA, Newman JH: Hypoglycemia in hospitalized patients: Causes and outcomes. N Engl J Med 1986; 315:1245-1250.
4. Collier A, Steedman DJ, Patrick AW: Comparison of intravenous glucagon and dextrose in treatment of severe hypoglycemia in an accident and emergency department. Diabetes Care 1987; 10:712-715.
5. Ober KP: Diabetes insipidus. Crit Care Clin 1991; 7:109-125.
6. Buonocore CM, Robinson AG: The diagnosis and management of diabetes insipidus during medical emergencies. Endocrinol Metab Clin North Am 1993; 22:411-423.
7. Werbel SS, Ober KP: Pheochromocytoma: Update on diagnosis, localization and management. Med Clin North Am 1995; 79:131-153.
8. Ober KP: Uncle Remus and the cascade effect in clinical medicine: Brer Rabbit kicks the Tar-Baby. Am J Med 1987; 82:1009-1013.
9. Rolih CA, Ober KP: The endocrine response to critical illness. Med Clin North Am 1995; 79:211-224.
10. Feldman JR: The carcinoid syndrome. Endocrinologist 1993; 3:129-135.
11. Marsh HM, Martin JK Jr, Kvols LK, et al: Carcinoid crisis during anesthesia: Successful treatment with somatostatin analog. Anesthesiology 1987; 66:89-91.
12. Kvols LK, Martin JK, Marsh HM, Moertel CG: Rapid reversal of carcinoid crisis with a somatostatin analog (Letter). N Engl J Med 1985; 313:1229-1230.
13. Kvols LK: Therapy of the malignant carcinoid syndrome. Endocrinol Metab Clin North Am 1989; 18:557-568.

74

Neuroendocrine Immunology in the Critically Ill Patient

Edwin Lee, MD • Gary P. Zaloga, MD, FCCM

Neuroendocrine immunology represents an emerging area of critical care that deals with bidirectional interactions between the immune and neuroendocrine systems.[1] Cells of the immune system secrete substances that modulate function of the nervous and endocrine systems. In return, cells of the endocrine and nervous systems secrete substances that modulate immune function.

Anterior pituitary hormones are important for the regulation of cellular metabolism and immunologic homeostasis.[2] For example, prolactin, estrogens, dehydroepiandrosterone sulfate (DHEAS), growth hormone, and insulin-like growth factor 1 (IGF-1) possess immunostimulatory effects, whereas adrenocorticotropin (ACTH), glucocorticoids, progesterone, and testosterone have immunosuppressive actions.[1-4]

Researchers have recently discovered that leukocytes and endocrine glands synthesize and secrete similar hormones.[1, 4-6] For example, T lymphocytes secrete ACTH, enkephalins, endorphins, thyroid-stimulating hormone (TSH), gonadotropins, growth hormone, prolactin, parathyroid hormone-related peptide, and IGF-1. Macrophages secrete ACTH, endorphins, growth hormone, substance P, IGF-1, and atrial natriuretic peptide. Receptors for hormones have also been found on leukocytes (i.e., prolactin, ACTH, TSH, growth hormone, β-endorphin). Moreover, leukocytes secrete releasing hormones that can stimulate various endocrine glands (i.e., corticotropin-releasing hormone, luteinizing hormone-releasing hormone, thyrotropin-releasing hormone (TRH), and gonadotropin-releasing hormone). Interestingly, leukocyte hormonal responses vary with the stimulus.[1, 4] Endotoxin primarily stimulates release of ACTH, staphylococcal endotoxin A releases TSH, and mixed lymphocyte reactions release chorionic gonadotropin. Although leukocytes release less hormone per cell than endocrine cells do, total leukocytes outnumber pituitary cells and can produce more total hormone. These findings indicate that paracrine and autocrine mechanisms may be involved in regulating interactions between the endocrine and immune systems. They also suggest that hormones are intricate components of both the neuroendocrine and immune systems.

Neuroendocrine hormone secretion and action are exquisitely sensitive to stress and especially to critical illness. Illness depresses triiodothyronine (T_3), thyroxine (T_4), TSH, luteinizing hormone (LH), follicle-stimulating hormone (FSH), testosterone, prolactin, estradiol, and IGF-1 levels. On the other hand, illness increases epinephrine, norepinephrine, dopamine, cortisol, growth hormone, and glucagon levels. Interestingly, some studies suggest that endocrine hormone profiles are better predictors of outcome than is the Acute Physiology and Chronic Health Evaluation (APACHE) score.[7, 8] Alterations in endocrine function may represent both adaptive and maladaptive responses to critical illness. This chapter discusses the effects of hormones on immune function in critically ill patients.

GROWTH HORMONE

Loss of cell protein is a natural consequence of critical illness and impairs organ function (including the immune system). Negative nitrogen balance occurs when protein loss (catabolism) is greater than synthesis (anabolism). Persistent hypercatabolism has many adverse effects on the body. It impairs protein synthesis, depletes cells of vital proteins, and increases morbidity and mortality.[9] Unfortunately, body loss of protein continues during critical illness despite use of aggressive nutritional support.[10, 11] This has caused many to administer anabolic hormones to critically ill patients in an attempt to improve protein homeostasis.

Human growth hormone is a 191-amino acid protein that is secreted from the anterior pituitary gland. Growth hormone release is stimulated by growth hormone-releasing hormone (GHRH) produced in the hypothalamus and is inhibited by somatostatin. In healthy adults, growth hormone secretion is pulsatile; the highest levels occur in the early evening, the lowest levels during rapid eye movement sleep. Pulsatile and diurnal secretion of growth hormone is important for optimal response to growth hormone but is lost during critical illness.

Growth hormone produces many of its metabolic effects by stimulating production of IGF-1 in the tissues. Circulating IGF-1 is primarily of liver origin. IGF-1 and growth hormone (through IGF-1-independent mechanisms) stimulate protein anabolism and lipolysis.[9] Growth hormone also causes insulin resistance and hyperglycemia. However, these effects are offset by the hypoglycemic actions of IGF-1.

Interest in the ability of growth hormone to stimulate protein synthesis and improve nitrogen balance began in the 1940s when Cuthbertson and coworkers[12] demonstrated an attenuation of protein loss in rats with femoral fractures when these animals were administered an extract from bovine pituitary glands. In 1961, Liljedahl and colleagues[13] administered growth hormone to severely burned patients and demonstrated improved nitrogen retention. Recombinant human growth hormone (rhGH) has been available for clinical use since 1985. Subsequent studies in burn patients have demonstrated the ability of rhGH to increase the rate of wound healing in skin graft donor sites, reduce donor site healing times, increase nitrogen retention, and decrease hospital stay.[14-17] Growth hormone has been found to increase the production of important proteins, such as laminin, collagen types IV and VII, and cytokeratin, in burn patients.[18]

The use of growth hormone in patients who have sepsis and who have sustained trauma has not demonstrated any clinically significant improvement in outcome. Some studies demonstrate decreased nitrogen losses associated with increased fatty acid oxidation and improved protein synthesis.[19-22] For example, Ziegler and associates[22] reported an attenuation in nitrogen excretion when growth hormone was used up to 41 days after injury in trauma and burn patients; other studies, however, did not confirm an improvement in nitrogen balance, increase in IGF-1 levels, or improved septic score with administration of growth hormone.[23, 24] Dahn and coworkers[24] compared the results of growth hormone administration to normal volunteers and septic patients. Growth hormone did not decrease nitrogen loss, increase splanchnic amino acid uptake, or increase IGF-1 levels in the septic patients. The lack of an anabolic effect from growth hormone in critically ill patients may be secondary to acquired growth hormone resistance during severe illness.

Two large phase III clinical trials of recombinant growth hormone in critically ill intensive care unit patients were concluded in 1997. These two prospective, randomized, and placebo-controlled trials were conducted in Europe and included catabolic patients undergoing open heart and abdominal surgery or patients suffering from multiple trauma or acute respiratory failure. The patients were given a dose of growth hormone of 16 IU (5.3 mg) or 24 IU (8 mg) per day according to body weight. The maximum treatment time was 21 days. A total of 532 patients were included in the two studies. Two hundred fifty-nine patients received growth hormone, 264 received placebo, and nine were not treated. The results of the two studies were similar and showed a significantly higher mortality in growth hormone–treated patients. The mortality rate was 18.2% in placebo-treated patients (48/264) and 41.7% (108/259) in the growth hormone–treated group. The reasons for the increased mortality remain unclear. However, on the basis of the results of these trials, the use of growth hormone for the treatment of acute catabolism in critically ill patients is not recommended.

The anabolic effects of growth hormone are primarily mediated by IGF-1, a peptide whose synthesis is largely controlled by growth hormone, thyroid hormone, insulin, and nutritional status. Thus, poor nutritional status, low thyroid hormone levels (i.e., euthyroid sick syndrome), and insulin resistance may blunt the actions of growth hormone and may be responsible for its diminished effectiveness in some studies. The activity of IGF-1 is also modulated by insulin-like growth factor–binding proteins (IGFBPs). Six different IGFBPs have been identified. The most abundant is IGFBP-3, which serves as the major carrier protein or intravascular store of IGF-1.[9] Thus, low levels of IGFBP-3 in critically ill patients may impair the anabolic actions of IGF-1.

Acquired growth hormone resistance is common during critical illness (i.e., trauma, sepsis, surgery).[25, 26] Patients have elevated growth hormone levels associated with low IGF-1 levels.[25] In addition, critically ill patients have low levels of IGFBP-3, high levels of the inhibitory binding protein IGFBP-1, and increased serum protease activity that reduces the affinity of IGFBP-3 for IGF-1.[27] The net effect of these changes is diminished anabolic action of IGF-1. Dopamine is an inhibitor of growth hormone release, and studies demonstrate that dopamine infusion (even at low levels of 2 μg/kg/min) inhibits growth hormone secretion in critically ill patients.[28] Dopamine also suppresses the thyroidal axis.[3] Thus, use of dopamine in critically ill patients may contribute to the catabolic state by reducing secretion of the body's major anabolic hormones.

Growth hormone improves cardiac performance in dilated cardiomyopathies associated with growth hormone deficiency.[29, 30] On the basis of these findings, Fazio and coworkers[31] administered growth hormone (4 IU every other day subcutaneously) for 3 months to patients with idiopathic dilated cardiomyopathies (non–growth hormone–deficient). There was improvement in hemodynamics, myocardial energy metabolism, myocardial mass, left ventricular chamber size, and clinical status. The beneficial effects diminished 3 months after discontinuation of growth hormone treatment. Thus, growth hormone may have potential beneficial effects in the treatment of nonischemic myocardial contractile failure.

Growth hormone has been evaluated as a means of improving respiratory strength and decreasing weaning time from mechanical ventilation in patients with respiratory failure. Pape and colleagues[32] administered growth hormone to patients with stable uncomplicated chronic obstructive pulmonary disease (COPD) and reported a 27% improvement in inspiratory force. In a noncontrolled pilot study of 53 patients with prolonged ventilator dependency, growth hormone (0.04 to 0.14 mg/kg/day) was thought to improve weaning from mechanical ventilation.[33] In a subsequent prospective randomized controlled clinical trial, however, growth hormone did not improve muscle strength or decrease ventilatory time despite improving nitrogen balance.[34]

Growth hormone and IGF-1 are required for optimal cellular and humoral immune responses, and both molecules are synthesized and secreted by immunocompetent cells.[35-38] Both agents are required for growth of the thymus and synthesis of thymulin, an important immune hormone. They are important for production of immunoglobulins, cytolytic activity of T lymphocytes, natural killer (NK) cell activity, differentiation of neutrophils, and production of tumor necrosis factor (TNF)-α. Growth hormone augments the production of superoxide anions by macrophages and neutrophils, similar to interferon-γ. Growth hormone and IGF-1 promote survival of granulocytes and monocytes by inhibiting apoptosis.[2, 35, 38] Despite these findings, patients with growth hormone deficiency or defects in the growth hormone receptor (i.e., Laron's syndrome) lack clinically significant immunodepression.

On the other hand, postsurgical patients with low growth hormone levels demonstrate depressed immune function compared with postsurgical patients with higher growth hormone levels.[39] There is a reduction in the T lymphocyte helper (CD4) to suppressor (CD8) cell ratio. Growth hormone administration (0.1 IU/kg subcutaneously daily) to patients receiving chronic steroid therapy associated with a diminished growth hormone response to GHRH also improved CD4:CD8 ratios.[40]

Vara-Thorbeck and associates[41] randomized 180 patients undergoing elective open cholecystectomy with and without choledochoduodenostomy to control or growth hormone treatment (8 IU/day subcutaneously for 1 week). Serum immunoglobulin levels and skin antigen testing responses improved significantly in the group receiving growth hormone compared with the control subjects. The treatment group experienced significantly lower wound infection rates (3.4% versus 17%) and a shorter hospital stay (9.6 versus 12.5 days). Further studies are needed to confirm these interesting findings.

Growth hormone administration has been shown to improve nitrogen balance in many but not all studies.[18–22] Despite apparent improvement in protein synthesis in various groups of patients, data regarding clinical cost-effectiveness of this expensive therapy are lacking. Growth hormone administration does not appear to decrease the patient's stay in the hospital or intensive care unit, to improve weaning from mechanical ventilation, to improve healing of surgical wounds, or to lower infection rates in most studies. Current data suggest that growth hormone administration may increase mortality in acutely catabolic patients. The hormone is not recommended for use in critically ill patients. Further studies regarding efficacy in selected subsets of patients who may benefit from this therapy are required.

INSULIN-LIKE GROWTH FACTOR 1

IGF-1 stimulates glucose uptake and oxidation, lipid synthesis, bone formation, protein synthesis, and myelin synthesis. It also improves renal blood flow, myocardial contractility, function of immune cells, and neuronal survival.[37, 42–47] Because of these effects and the low levels of IGF-1 in many critically ill patients, administration of IGF-1 may be beneficial in critically ill patients. Unfortunately, few studies of IGF-1 administration have been performed in critically ill patients. IGF-1 has been shown to improve glucose control in patients with chronic diabetes with insulin resistance but has not been studied in diabetic ketoacidosis. IGF-1 can improve cardiac function in experimental models of cardiomyopathy.[44, 45] Its effects in humans with cardiomyopathy are unknown.

IGF-1 inhibits lysine oxidation, decreases protein breakdown, and improves glucose uptake in burn patients.[48] It also improves nitrogen balance in patients with traumatic head injuries.[49] Unfortunately, IGF-1 infusion decreases growth hormone levels (by negative feedback) and IGFBP-3 levels. Interestingly, in a small study of head-injured patients, those who achieved higher IGF-1 levels with IGF-1 administration (>350 ng/mL) had improved survival.[49] In contrast, infusion of IGF-1 did not improve nitrogen balance in other studies.[50–52]

IGF-1 improves renal blood flow,[53] glomerular filtration rate,[53] and recovery from experimental ischemia-induced acute renal failure in rats.[54, 55] However, IGF-1 did not improve recovery in a prospective randomized clinical trial of critically ill patients with ischemia-induced acute renal failure. Kudsk and associates[46] studied the effect on immune function of IGF-1 infusion (0.01 mg/kg/hr for 14 days). IGF-1 improved CD4:CD8 ratios compared with the control group. However, this study was small, there were almost twice as many patients in the study than in the control group, and the study group had higher baseline CD4:CD8 ratios. In addition, IGF-1 failed to significantly bring about increased CD4 or decrease CD8 counts. Thus, IGF-1 is not recommended for routine use in critically ill patients.

Because growth hormone produces metabolic effects that are independent of IGF-1, many have proposed that combined growth hormone and IGF-1 administration would produce superior effects compared with either agent alone. Kupfer and colleagues[56] administered combined therapy (0.05 mg/kg growth hormone subcutaneously once daily plus IGF-1 at a rate of 12 μg/kg/hr) to seven calorically restricted volunteers and demonstrated improved nitrogen balance. Combined therapy was more effective than single-agent therapy; however, these patients were not critically ill and no physiologic benefit was demonstrated.

Alternatively, one might administer GHRH or growth hormone–releasing peptide-2 (GHRP-2) in an attempt to increase levels of both growth hormone and IGF-1. Van den Berghe and coworkers[57] administered GHRH plus GHRP-2 or GHRP-2 to critically ill patients and reported increases in growth hormone and IGF-1 levels. The clinical benefit of such therapy in critically ill patients requires further study.

PROLACTIN

Prolactin is secreted from the anterior pituitary gland in a pulsatile and circadian fashion. It is also secreted by lymphocytes. Prolactin secretion is tonically inhibited by dopamine (dopamine-2 receptors), opiates, and glucocorticoids. Release can be increased by dopamine antagonists, such as haloperidol and metoclopramide. Importantly, exogenous administration of dopamine (even at low doses) also attenuates prolactin release.[3, 58]

In addition to its effects on lactation, prolactin possesses important actions on the immune system (i.e., B and T cells, macrophages).[36] Hypoprolactinemia (from hypophysectomy or use of dopamine agonists) suppresses antibody formation and inhibits delayed cutaneous hypersensitivity responses.[59] Suppression of prolactin secretion with dopamine agonists decreases T cell–dependent activation of macrophages and B cell and T cell proliferation.[58, 60, 61] Dopamine agonists suppress splenocyte and lymphocyte synthesis of interferon-γ. Immunocompetence is restored by administration of prolactin or use of a dopamine antagonist. Dopamine agonists also increase mortality from *Listeria* in mice.[61, 62] This effect is antagonized by prolactin administration. Prolactin administration to animals with hemorrhagic shock improves cytokine release and decreases mortality from subsequent sepsis.[63, 64] Bromocriptine, a dopamine agonist, is being used as adjuvant immunosuppressive treatment of autoimmune disease and organ transplantation.[65] Dopamine agonists have also been effective immunosuppressive agents in the treatment of experimental allergic encephalitis and adjuvant-induced arthritis.

Devins and coworkers[58] administered dopamine to critically ill patients (5 μg/kg/min). Dopamine suppressed prolactin levels by more than 90%. In addition, in vitro T cell proliferative responses to concanavalin A (ConA) were significantly lower in the dopamine-treated group than in the control group. Whether hypoprolactinemia increases the risk of infection in critically ill patients remains unclear.

SEX HORMONES

The three major sex hormones in the body are (1) estrogens, (2) testosterone, and (3) dehydroepiandrosterone (DHEA). DHEA also exists in the sulfated form (DHEAS). During critical illness, there is a suppression of the gonadal axis. The result is a decrease in levels of LH, FSH, estrogen, testosterone, and DHEAS.[66–68] Dopamine infusion also suppresses release of the sex hormones.[69] Hypogonadism induced by critical illness may have evolved as an adaptive mechanism. There is a decrease in sexual drive and a shift in hormonal synthesis away from sex hormones to glucocorticoids.[67]

DHEAS modulates immune function. In humans, DHEAS enhances interleukin-2 (IL-2) production and increases T cell cytotoxicity.[70, 71] DHEA stimulates Th1 cell function and enhances T lymphocyte function. DHEAS also antagonizes the suppressive effects of glucocorticoids on lymphocyte proliferation. Low levels of DHEAS during critical illness accentuate the immunosuppressive effects of elevated cortisol levels.[72] DHEA modulates immune function in postmenopausal women by increasing the cytotoxicity of NK cells.[73] DHEA also preserved immunocompetence in burned mice.[71] Studies are needed to determine whether DHEA or DHEAS can improve immune function and decrease infections in critically ill patients.

Testosterone and estrogens also modulate immune function. In general, androgens and progesterone attenuate the immune response whereas estrogens increase immune responses. Androgens interfere with maturation of B cells and increase T suppressor function.[74] Estrogens augment the function of B lymphocytes, inhibit T suppressor cells, facilitate T helper maturation, and increase macrophage maturation and function. Interestingly, autoimmune disease is higher in female patients than in male patients,[74] an effect that may relate to differences in levels of sex hormones. The effect of androgens and estrogens on immune function and infectious risk in critically ill patients is unknown.

THYROID HORMONES

Thyroid hormones modulate gene expression and regulate the activity of immune cells. TSH increases the proliferative response of B and T lymphocytes to mitogens and increases antibody production.[75] Thus, alterations in levels of thyroid hormones during critical illness may impair immune function.

Nonthyroidal illness (such as critical illness) and dopamine administration suppress the thyroidal axis and result in a decrease in TRH, TSH, T_4, and T_3 levels.[3, 76-79] Release of tissue factors within the brain and peripheral tissues during critical illness suppresses the secretion of releasing hormones and impairs the conversion of T_4 to T_3. Interestingly, IL-1, IL-6, TNF, and interferon-γ also inhibit the release of TSH and lower thyroid hormone levels, whereas IL-2 stimulates TSH release.[75] These changes in thyroid hormone levels associated with illness are known as the euthyroid sick syndrome.[80] Low levels of T_4 and T_3 during critical illness are associated with a poor outcome.[81, 82] However, the effects of T_3 or T_4 administration on the morbidity and mortality of critically ill patients have been variable; some studies suggest improvement,[83-90] whereas others could find no benefits.[91-93]

Thyroid hormones regulate the respiratory centers and modulate the ventilatory response to hypoxia and hypercapnia. They are also important for contractile function and endurance of the respiratory muscles. Although thyroid hormone replacement improves respiratory function in hypothyroid patients, it does not appear to improve respiratory function in euthyroid sick patients with respiratory failure. To date, there is no conclusive evidence to suggest that administration of thyroid hormone to critically ill patients decreases infections or improves respiratory muscle function, cardiovascular function, or outcome.

GLUCOCORTICOIDS

Adrenocorticotropin (ACTH) and cortisol are elevated during critical illness and are part of the stress response. Higher cortisol levels occur in patients with more severe illnesses and negatively correlate with survival.[94] Glucocorticoids depress immune function[95-97] by inhibiting B and T lymphocytes, macrophages, and neutrophils. These agents decrease IL-1 and TNF release by macrophages, decrease interferon-γ and IL-2 release by T lymphocytes, and block the inflammatory actions of IL-1. They suppress IL-2 production and lymphocyte proliferation. These agents are frequently used to induce immune suppression in patients with immune-mediated diseases or inflammatory disorders.

Glucocorticoids improve outcome in patients with adrenal insufficiency. However, the majority of studies indicate that they do not improve outcome in patients with intact adrenal function and sepsis[98, 99] or the adult respiratory distress syndrome (ARDS). Some benefit on respiratory function is reported in patients with fibroproliferative late-stage ARDS.[100, 101] Glucocorticoids are beneficial as immunosuppressive agents in the treatment of a variety of inflammatory disorders, such as asthma and vasculitis.[97]

ADRENOMEDULLARY-IMMUNE INTERACTIONS

Critical illness stimulates the release of catecholamines from the adrenal medulla and nerve terminals. These agents play critical roles in the cardiovascular and metabolic response to illness. Recent evidence indicates that immune cells can influence the secretion of catecholamines from the adrenal medulla. Adrenal denervated rats increase their plasma epinephrine levels after infection. In addition, leukocytes secrete a small peptide that promotes catecholamine secretion from adrenal chromaffin cells.[102-104] Thus, immune cell activation of the sympathoadrenal system may contribute to catecholamine secretion during inflammatory states. Interestingly, epinephrine inhibits but β-adrenergic blockade enhances release of the peptide. The immune-mediated release of epinephrine may have evolved as a redundancy to neural-mediated epinephrine release to ensure adequate energy supply (i.e., glucose, fatty acids) and cardiovascular function during stress and infection. In this regard, leukocytes are obligate glucose users.

Cytokines released from leukocytes modulate activity of the hypothalamic-pituitary-adrenal axis.[105, 106] In addition, increases in adrenal catecholamine secretion have an impact on the function of the immune system by direct effects on leukocytes and indirect effects on the hypothalamic-pituitary axis.[107-109] Dopamine, epinephrine, norepinephrine, and phosphodiesterase inhibitors alter activity of lymphocytes, macrophages, neutrophils, and NK cells and alter cytokine production and antigen-induced leukocyte proliferative responses. These effects are discussed in the next sections.

DOPAMINE

Low-dose dopamine infusion (2 to 5 μg/kg/min) produces plasma dopamine levels of approximately 10^{-7} mmol/L, nearly 100-fold to 1000-fold higher than concentrations generated by endogenous secretion. Although circulating dopamine does not cross the mature blood-brain barrier, dopamine-2 receptors are accessible to circulating dopamine within the anterior pituitary and hypothalamic median eminence (outside the blood-brain barrier). Dopamine receptors are also accessible on human B and T lymphocytes.[110]

The anterior pituitary gland plays a crucial role in metabolic and immunologic homeostasis. Hormones regulated by the anterior pituitary are both immunostimulatory (i.e., prolactin, DHEAS, growth hormone, estrogens) and immunosuppressive (i.e., glucocorticoids, testosterone). Receptors for growth hormone and prolactin are of the same class as interleukin receptors. Dopamine is a normal regulator of pituitary function, and infusion of dopamine (even at levels of 0.5 to 2.0 μg/kg/min) suppresses the secretion of most anterior pituitary hormones (i.e., prolactin, growth hormone, LH, FSH, TSH) except for ACTH (which stimulates the production of cortisol).[3, 58, 111] Suppression of TSH and T_4 and T_3 levels can further reduce thyroid hormone levels in patients with the euthyroid sick syndrome.[112] The net result of dopamine administration is an increase in the ratio of immunosuppressive to immunostimulating hormones and immune suppression.

Dopamine can produce immunosuppressive effects by acting directly on leukocytes. Dopamine-2 receptors are present on both B and T lymphocytes.[110] Dopamine decreases intracellular cyclic adenosine monophosphate (cAMP) levels in lymphocytes through dopamine-2 receptors coupled to inhibitory G proteins. It inhibits *N*-formyl-methionyl-leucyl-phenylalanine (FMLP)–induced superoxide anion generation (respiratory burst) in polymorphonuclear leukocytes, interferon-γ synthesis in macrophages, and mitogen-induced lymphocyte proliferation.[113-115] When it is administered to critically ill patients, dopamine (5 μg/kg/min) decreases mitogen (i.e., concanavalin A) stimulation of T lymphocyte proliferation.[58] Dopamine also suppresses delayed cutaneous hypersensitivity responses, mixed lymphocyte culture responses, generation of cytotoxic T cells, and antibody responses (see discussion of prolactin).

Although dopamine suppresses immune function in critically ill patients, its effects on infection are less clear. Because a lack of evidence confirms beneficial effects of dopamine for the protection of renal function and maintenance of intestinal perfusion and because the effects of dopamine on the neuroendocrine axis are unlikely to be beneficial, we caution against the long-term use of dopamine in critically ill patients.

α-ADRENERGIC AND β-ADRENERGIC AGONISTS

Immune cells contain β-adrenergic receptors that regulate immune function.[116-124] β-Adrenergic receptor activation on lymphocytes decreases antibody synthesis, mitogen-induced lymphocyte transformation, T lymphocyte–mediated cytolytic activity, synthesis of complement, and total lymphocyte and T cell subset numbers. Increasing intracellular cAMP concentrations with β-adrenergic agonists (primarily β_2 effect) also inhibits neutrophil adhesiveness, chemotaxis, phagocytosis, and lysosomal enzyme release. These agents inhibit oxygen free radical production[118] and FMLP-induced chemoluminescence by neutrophils.[120] The immunosuppressive effects of β-adrenergic agonists may help reduce tissue injury but may also diminish immune defenses.

Epinephrine and norepinephrine inhibit production of TNF (a proinflammatory cytokine) by mononuclear cells, microglial cells, and human blood cells stimulated with endotoxin.[121-123] This effect has been demonstrated with epinephrine administration both in vitro and in vivo (30 ng/kg/min). Epinephrine also augments release of IL-10, an anti-inflammatory cytokine. Pretreatment of mice with α_2- and β-adrenergic agonists modulates endotoxin-induced TNF secretion. Norepinephrine, the major neurotransmitter of the sympathetic nervous system, and isoproterenol decrease endotoxin-induced release of TNF in mice (a β_1-adrenergic effect).

On the other hand, propranolol increases the TNF response, whereas prazosin (an α-adrenergic antagonist) reduces the TNF response. Prazosin's inhibitory response results from increased sympathetic output induced by blocking presynaptic α_2-inhibitory receptors. Adrenalectomy does not abolish the effect of α_2 antagonists, confirming that their effect is not mediated through increased secretion of adrenal steroids. However, ganglionic blockade of sympathetic outflow does inhibit the effects of α_2-adrenergic agonists.

Thus, α_2-adrenergic agonists augment release of TNF by inhibiting sympathetic output; β-adrenergic agonists decrease TNF release through β_1 receptors on leukocytes. In vivo, there is an equilibrium between stimulatory and inhibitory effects of catecholamines on TNF-secreting cells. These actions are regulated through α_2 and β_1 adrenoceptors located on these cells. The effect of up-regulation and down-regulation of adrenergic receptors on immune function during critical illness requires further study. Lymphocytes also appear capable of synthesizing catecholamines.[125] Thus, an autocrine loop exists whereby lymphocytes synthesize catecholamines and the catecholamines inhibit lymphocyte proliferation and differentiation. This mechanism may allow lymphocytes to down-regulate their own activity.

PHOSPHODIESTERASE INHIBITORS

Phosphodiesterase inhibitors increase levels of cAMP in leukocytes and produce effects similar to those of β-adrenergic agonists.[126-132] Inflammatory cells contain predominantly phosphodiesterase types III and IV. Physiologic levels of methylxanthines (nonselective phosphodiesterase inhibitors) and amrinone (phosphodiesterase inhibitor type III) suppress the release of TNF-α from blood monocytes and alveolar macrophages, decrease the release of interferon-γ and IL-1 during endotoxic shock, up-regulate production of IL-10 and IL-6 (anti-inflammatory cytokines), reduce phagocytic and bactericidal capabilities of polymorphonuclear leukocytes and macrophages, decrease release of reactive oxygen species by macrophages, diminish the proliferative response of T lymphocytes to mitogens, and decrease the cytotoxic activity of NK cells.[126-132] The effect on infection rates and the possible synergistic immune depression between β agonists and phosphodiesterase inhibitors have not been studied in critically ill patients.

Leukocyte-endothelial cell interactions play important roles in the pathophysiologic processes of sepsis, acute lung injury, and multiple organ failure. Cytokines such as IL-1 stimulate endothelial cells to express surface adhesion molecules that bind with neutrophils and monocytes. The net effect can be either inflammatory cell injury or enhanced bactericidal defenses. Increased levels of cAMP inhibit expression of cytokine-mediated endothelial cell adhesion molecules, such a E-selectin and vascular cell adhesion molecule 1 (VCAM-1). Amrinone (at clinically relevant doses) inhibits IL-1β–induced increases in endothelial cell expression of E-selectin, intercellular adhesion molecule 1 (ICAM-1), and VCAM-1.[133, 134] Dopamine also decreases expression of E-selectin.

SUMMARY

It is now clear that an intricate bidirectional signaling system exists between neurons, endocrine glands, and immune cells. Each component of the system can synthesize compounds with hormonal properties and can influence the activity of the other components. There are major alterations in cell function and secretory products from these cells (i.e., cytokines, hormones, catecholamines) during critical illness. In addition, many of the agents used to treat critically ill patients alter function of these cells (i.e., dopamine, epinephrine, norepinephrine, amrinone). The net effect of these changes favors immunosuppression. Immunosuppression may have evolved to protect the host from immune-mediated organ injury. However, prolonged immunosuppression undoubtedly predisposes the critically ill patient to infection. Clearly, further investigation is needed into the use of hormone replacement and the effects of catecholamine and phosphodiesterase inhibitor administration on immune function and infection rates in critically ill patients.

References

1. Reichlin S: Neuroendocrine-immune interactions. N Engl J Med 1993; 329:1246–1253.
2. Kooijman R, Hooghe-Peters EL, Hooghe R: Prolactin, growth

hormone, and insulin-like growth factor-I in the immune system. Adv Immunol 1996; 63:377-454.
3. Van den Berghe G, de Zegher F: Anterior pituitary function during critical illness and dopamine treatment. Crit Care Med 1996; 24:1580-1590.
4. Weigent DA, Carr DJ, Blalock JE: Bidirectional communication between the neuroendocrine and immune systems. Ann N Y Acad Science 1989; 579:17-27.
5. Weigent DA, Blalock JE: Interactions between the neuroendocrine and immune systems: Common hormones and receptors. Immunol Rev 1987; 100:79-108.
6. Blalock JE, Smith EM: A complete regulatory loop between the immune and neuroendocrine systems. Fed Proc 1985; 44:108-111.
7. Jarek MJ, Legare EJ, McDermott MT, et al: Endocrine profiles for outcome prediction from the intensive care unit. Crit Care Med 1993; 21:543-550.
8. Rothwell PM, Lawler PG: Prediction of outcome in intensive care patients using endocrine parameters. Crit Care Med 1995; 23:78-83.
9. Wolf SE, Barrow RE, Herndon DN: Growth hormone and IGF-I therapy in the hypercatabolic patient. Baillieres Clin Endocrinol Metab 1996; 10:447-463.
10. Streat SJ, Beddoe AH, Hill GL: Aggressive nutritional support does not prevent protein loss despite fat gain in septic intensive care patients. J Trauma 1987; 27:262-266.
11. Loder PB, Smith RC, Kee AJ, et al: What rate of infusion of intravenous nutrition solution is required to stimulate uptake of amino acids by peripheral tissues in depleted patients? Ann Surg 1990; 211:360-368.
12. Cuthbertson DP, Shaw GB, Young FG: The anterior pituitary gland and protein metabolism: III. The influence of anterior pituitary extract on the rate of wound healing. J Endocrinol 1941; 2:475-478.
13. Liljedahl SO, Gemzell CA, Plantin LO, et al: Effect of human growth hormone in patients with severe burns. Acta Chir Scand 1961; 22:1-14.
14. Herndon DN, Barrow RE, Kunkel KR, et al: Effects of recombinant human growth hormone on donor-site healing in severely burned children. Ann Surg 1990; 212:424-431.
15. Gilpin DA, Barrow RE, Rutan RL, et al: Recombinant human growth hormone accelerates wound healing in children with large cutaneous burns. Ann Surg 1994; 220:19-24.
16. Sherman SK, Demling RH, LaLonde C, et al: Growth hormone enhances re-epithelialization of human split graft donor sites. Surg Forum 1988; 40:37-39.
17. Gore DC, Honeycutt D, Jahoor F, et al: Effect of exogenous growth hormone on whole-body and isolated-limb protein kinetics in burned patients. Arch Surg 1991; 126:38-43.
18. Herndon DH, Hawkins HK, Nguyen TT, et al: Characterization of growth hormone enhanced donor site healing in patients with large cutaneous burns. Ann Surg 1995; 221:649-659.
19. Douglas RG, Humberstone DA, Haystead A, et al: Metabolic effects of recombinant human growth hormone: Isotopic studies in the postabsorptive state and during total parenteral nutrition. Br J Surg 1990; 77:785-790.
20. Petersen SR, Holaday NJ, Jeevanandam M: Enhancement of protein synthesis efficiency in parenterally fed trauma victims by adjuvant recombinant human growth hormone. J Trauma 1994; 36:726-733.
21. Voerman HJ, Strack van Schijndel RJM, Groeneveld ABJ, et al: Effects of recombinant human growth hormone in patients with severe sepsis. Ann Surg 1992; 216:648-655.
22. Ziegler TR, Young LS, Ferrari-Baliviera E, et al: Use of human growth hormone combined with nutritional support in a critical care unit. JPEN J Parenter Enteral Nutr 1990; 14:574-581.
23. Gottardis M, Benzer A, Koller W, et al: Improvement of septic syndrome after administration of recombinant human growth hormone (rhGH)? J Trauma 1991; 31:81-86.
24. Dahn MS, Lange MP, Jacobs LA: Insulin-like growth factor I production is inhibited in human sepsis. Arch Surg 1988; 123:1409-1414.
25. Ross R, Miell J, Freeman E, et al: Critically ill patients have high basal growth hormone levels with attenuated oscillatory activity associated with low levels of insulin-like growth factor-I. Clin Endocrinol 1991; 35:47-54.
26. Bentham J, Rodriguez-Arnao J, Ross RJM: Acquired growth hormone resistance in patients with hypercatabolism. Horm Res 1993; 40:87-91.
27. Donaghy AJ, Baxter RC: Insulin-like growth factor bioactivity in its modification in growth hormone resistant states. Baillieres Clin Endocrinol Metab 1996; 10:421-446.
28. Van den Berghe G, Zegher F, Lauwers P, et al: Growth hormone secretion in critical illness: Effect of dopamine. J Clin Endocrinol Metab 1994; 79:1141-1146.
29. Cuneo RC, Wilmshurst P, Lowy C, et al: Cardiac failure responding to growth hormone (Letter). Lancet 1989; 1:838-839.
30. Frustaci A, Perrone GA, Gentiloni N, et al: Reversible dilated cardiomyopathy due to growth hormone deficiency. Anat Pathol 1992; 97:503-511.
31. Fazio S, Sabatini D, Capaldo B, et al: A preliminary study of growth hormone in the treatment of dilated cardiomyopathy. N Engl J Med 1996; 334:809-814.
32. Pape GS, Friedman M, Underwood LE, et al: The effect of growth hormone on weight gain and pulmonary function in patients with chronic obstructive lung disease. Chest 1991; 99:1495-1500.
33. Knox JB, Wilmore DW, Demling RH, et al: Use of growth hormone for postoperative respiratory failure. Am J Surg 1996; 171:576-580.
34. Pichard C, Kyle U, Chevrolet J, et al: Lack of effects of recombinant growth hormone on muscle function in patients requiring prolonged mechanical ventilation: A prospective, randomized, controlled study. Crit Care Med 1996; 24:403-413.
35. Auernhammer CJ, Strasburger CJ: Effects of growth hormone and insulin-like growth factor I on the immune system. Eur J Endocrinol 1995; 133:635-645.
36. Murphy WJ, Rui H, Longo DL: Minireview: Effects of growth hormone and prolactin; immune development and function. Life Sci 1995; 57:1-14.
37. Bjerknes R, Aarskog D: Priming of human polymorphonuclear neutrophilic leukocytes by insulin-like growth factor I: Increased phagocytic capacity, complement receptor expression, degranulation, and oxidative burst. J Clin Endocrinol Metab 1995; 80:1948-1955.
38. Kelley KW: The role of growth hormone in modulation of the immune response. Ann N Y Acad Sci 1990; 594:95-103.
39. Dahn MS, Mitchell RA, Smith S, et al: Altered immunologic function and nitrogen metabolism associated with depression of plasma growth hormone. JPEN J Parenter Enteral Nutr 1984; 8:690-694.
40. Giustina A, Bussi AR, Jacobello C, et al: Effects of recombinant human growth hormone (GH) on bone and intermediary metabolism in patients receiving chronic glucocorticoid treatment with suppressed endogenous GH response to GH-releasing hormone. J Clin Endocrinol Metab 1995; 80:122-129.
41. Vara-Thorbeck R, Guerrero JA, Rosell J, et al: Exogenous growth hormone: Effects on the catabolic response to surgically produced acute stress and on postoperative immune function. World J Surg 1993; 17:530-538.
42. Quin JD: The insulin-like growth factors. Q J Med 1992; 82:81-90.
43. Le Roith D: Insulin-like growth factors. N Engl J Med 1997; 336:633-640.
44. Ambler GR, Johnston BM, Maxwell L, et al: Improvement of doxorubicin induced cardiomyopathy in rats treated with insulin-like growth factor I. Cardiovasc Res 1993; 27:1368-1373.
45. Duerr RL, Huang S, Miraliakbar HE, et al: Insulin-like growth factor-I enhances ventricular hypertrophy and function during the onset of experimental cardiac failure. J Clin Invest 1995; 95:619-627.
46. Kudsk KA, Mowatt-Larssen C, Bukar J, et al: Effect of recombinant human insulin-like growth factor I and early total parenteral nutrition on immune depression following severe head injury. Arch Surg 1994; 129:66-71.
47. Tapson VF, Boni-Schnetzler M, Pilch PF, et al: Structural and functional characterization of the human T lymphocyte receptor for insulin-like growth factor I in vitro. J Clin Invest 1988; 82:950-957.
48. Cioffi WG, Gore DC, Rue LW III, et al: Insulin-like growth factor-I lowers protein oxidation in patients with thermal injury. Ann Surg 1994; 220:310-319.

49. Hatton J, Rapp RP, Kudsk KA, et al: Intravenous insulin-like growth factor-I (IGF-I) in moderate-to-severe head injury: A phase II safety and efficacy trial. J Neurosurg 1997; 86:779–786.
50. Goeters C, Mertes N, Tacke J, et al: Repeated administration of recombinant human insulin-like growth factor-I in patients after gastric surgery. Ann Surg 1995; 222:646–653.
51. Mauras N, Horber FF, Haymond MW: Low dose recombinant human insulin-like growth factor-I fails to affect protein anabolism but inhibits islet cell secretion in humans. J Clin Endocrinol Metab 1992; 75:1192–1197.
52. Guler HP, Schmid C, Zapf J, et al: Effects of recombinant insulin-like growth factor I on insulin secretion and renal function in normal human subjects. Proc Natl Acad Sci USA 1989; 86:2868–2872.
53. Hirschberg R, Kopple JD: Evidence that insulin-like growth factor I increases renal plasma flow and glomerular filtration rate in fasted rats. J Clin Invest 1989; 83:326–330.
54. Feld S, Hirschberg R: Growth hormone, the insulin-like growth factor system, and the kidney. Endocr Rev 1996; 17:423–480.
55. Ding H, Kopple JD, Cohen A, Hirschberg R: Recombinant human insulin-like growth factor-I accelerates recovery and reduces catabolism in rats with ischemic acute renal failure. J Clin Invest 1993; 91:2281–2287.
56. Kupfer SR, Underwood LE, Baxter RC, et al: Enhancement of the anabolic effects of growth hormone and insulin-like growth factor I by use of both agents simultaneously. J Clin Invest 1993; 91:391–396.
57. Van den Berghe G, Zegher F, Veldhuis JD, et al: The somatotropic axis in critical illness: Effect of continuous growth hormone (GH)–releasing hormone and GH-releasing peptide-2 infusion. J Clin Endocrinol Metab 1997; 82:590–599.
58. Devins SS, Miller A, Herndon BL, et al: Effects of dopamine on T-lymphocyte proliferative responses and serum prolactin concentrations in critically ill patients. Crit Care Med 1992; 20:1644–1649.
59. Nagy E, Berczi I, Wren GE, et al: Immunomodulation by bromocriptine. Immunopharmacology 1983; 6:231–243.
60. Russell DH, Kibler R, Matrisian L, et al: Prolactin receptors on human T and B lymphocytes: Antagonism of prolactin binding by cyclosporin. J Immunol 1985; 134:3027–3031.
61. Bernton EW, Meltzer MS, Holaday JW: Suppression of macrophage activation and T-lymphocyte function in hypoprolactinemic mice. Science 1988; 239:401–404.
62. Holaday JW: Neuroendocrine-immune interactions and their relevance to the pharmacology of critical care medicine. Klin Wochenschr 1991; 69:13–19.
63. Zellweger R, Zhu X, Wichmann MW, et al: Prolactin administration following hemorrhagic shock improves macrophage cytokine release capacity and decreases mortality from subsequent sepsis. J Immunol 1996; 157:5748–5754.
64. Zellweger R, Wichmann MW, Ayala A, et al: Prolactin: A novel and safe immunomodulating hormone for the treatment of immunodepression following severe hemorrhage. J Surg Res 1996; 63:53–58.
65. Carrier M, Wild J, Pelletier C, et al: Bromocriptine as an adjuvant to cyclosporine immunosuppression after heart transplantation. Ann Thorac Surg 1990; 49:129–132.
66. Fourrier F, Jallot A, Leclerc L, et al: Sex steroid hormones in circulatory shock, sepsis syndrome, and septic shock. Circ Shock 1994; 43:171–178.
67. Lephart ED, Baxter CR, Parker CR Jr: Effect of burn trauma on adrenal and testicular steroid hormone production. J Clin Endocrinol Metab 1987; 64:842–848.
68. Spratt DI, Cox P, Orav J, et al: Reproductive axis suppression in acute illness is related to disease severity. J Clin Endocrinol Metab 1993; 76:1548–1554.
69. Van den Berghe G, de Zegher F, Wouters P, et al: Dehydroepiandrosterone sulphate in critical illness: Effect of dopamine. Clin Endocrinol 1995; 43:457–463.
70. Suzuki T, Suzuki N, Daynes RA, et al: Dehydroepiandrosterone enhances IL-2 production and cytotoxic effector function of human T cells. Clin Immunol Immunopathol 1991; 61:202–211.
71. Araneo BA, Shelby J, Li GZ, et al: Administration of DHEA to burned mice preserves normal immunological competence. Arch Surg 1993; 128:318–325.
72. Blauer KL, Poth M, Rogers WM, et al: Dehydroepiandrosterone antagonizes the suppressive effects of dexamethasone on lymphocyte proliferation. Endocrinology 1991; 129:3174–3179.
73. Casson PR, Andersen RN, Herrod HG, et al: Oral dehydroepiandrosterone in physiologic doses modulates immune function in postmenopausal women. Am J Obstet Gynecol 1993; 169:1536–1539.
74. Schuurs AHWM, Verheul HAM: Effects of gender and sex steroids on the immune response. J Steroid Biochem 1990; 35:157–172.
75. Weigent DA, Blalock JE: Associations between neuroendocrine and immune systems. J Leukoc Biol 1995; 58:137–150.
76. Chopra IJ: Euthyroid sick syndrome: Is it a misnomer? J Clin Endocrinol Metab 1997; 82:329–334.
77. Burmeister LA: Reverse T_3 does not reliably differentiate hypothyroid sick syndrome from euthyroid sick syndrome. Thyroid 1995; 5:435–441.
78. Van den Berghe G, de Zegher F, Vlasselaers D, et al: Thyrotropin-releasing hormone in critical illness: From a dopamine-dependent test to a strategy for increasing low serum triiodothyronine, prolactin, and growth hormone concentrations. Crit Care Med 1996; 24:590–595.
79. Zaloga GP, Chernow B, Smallridge RC, et al: A longitudinal evaluation of thyroid function in critically ill surgical patients. Ann Surg 1985; 201:456–464.
80. Zaloga GP, Smallridge RC: Thyroidal alterations in acute illness. Semin Respir Med 1985; 7:95–107.
81. Kaptein EM, Weiner JM, Robinson WJ, et al: Relationship of altered thyroid hormone indices to survival in nonthyroid illness. Clin Endocrinol 1982; 16:565–574.
82. Slag MF, Morley JE, Elson MK, et al: Hypothyroxinemia in critically ill patients as a predictor of high mortality. JAMA 1981; 245:43–45.
83. Hesch RD, Husch M, Kodding R, et al: Treatment of dopamine-dependent shock with triiodothyronine. Endocr Res Commun 1981; 8:229–237.
84. Novitzky D, Cooper DKC, Reichart B: Hemodynamic and metabolic responses to hormonal therapy in brain-dead potential organ donors. Transplantation 1987; 43:852–854.
85. Dulchavsky SA, Hendrick SR, Dutta S: Pulmonary biophysical effects of triiodothyronine augmentation during sepsis-induced hypothyroidism. J Trauma 1993; 35:104–109.
86. Dulchavsky SA, Kennedy PR, Geller ER, et al: T_3 preserves respiratory function in sepsis. J Trauma 1991; 31:753–759.
87. Klemperer JD, Klein I, Gomez M, et al: Thyroid hormone treatment after coronary-artery bypass surgery. N Engl J Med 1995; 333:1522–1527.
88. Novitzky D, Cooper DKC, Swanepoel A: Inotropic effect of triiodothyronine (T_3) in low cardiac output following cardioplegic arrest and cardiopulmonary bypass: An initial experience in patients undergoing open heart surgery. Eur J Cardiothorac Surg 1989; 3:140–145.
89. Klemperer JD, Klein IL, Ojamaa K, et al: Triiodothyronine therapy lowers the incidence of atrial fibrillation after cardiac operations. Ann Thorac Surg 1996; 61:1323–1329.
90. Jeevanandam V: Triiodothyronine: Spectrum of use in heart transplantation. Thyroid 1997; 7:139–145.
91. Brent GA, Hershman JM: Thyroxine therapy in patients with severe nonthyroidal illnesses and low serum thyroxine concentration. J Clin Endocrinol Metab 1986; 63:1–8.
92. Becker RA, Vaughan GM, Ziegler MG, et al: Hypermetabolic low triiodothyronine syndrome of burn injury. Crit Care Med 1982; 10:870–875.
93. Bennett-Guerrero E, Jimenez JL, White WD, et al: Cardiovascular effects of intravenous triiodothyronine in patients undergoing coronary artery bypass graft surgery. JAMA 1996; 275:687–692.
94. Jurney TH, Cockrell JL, Lindberg JS, et al: Spectrum of serum cortisol response to ACTH in ICU patients: Correlation with degree of illness and mortality. Chest 1987; 92:292–295.
95. Gillis S, Crabtree GR, Smith KA: Glucocorticoid-induced inhibition of T cell growth factor production. J Immunol 1979; 123:1624–1631.
96. Larsson EL: Cyclosporin A and dexamethasone suppress T cell responses by selectively acting at distinct sites of the triggering process. J Immunol 1980; 124:2828–2833.
97. Chin R, Eagerton DC, Salem M: Corticosteroids. *In:* The Pharma-

cologic Approach to the Critically-Ill Patient. 3rd ed. Chernow B (Ed). Baltimore, Williams & Wilkins, 1994, pp 715–740.
98. Bone RC, Fisher CJ Jr, Clemmer TP, et al: A controlled clinical trial of high-dose methylprednisolone in the treatment of severe sepsis and septic shock. N Engl J Med 1987; 317:653–658.
99. Bernard GR, Luce JM, Sprung CL, et al: High-dose corticosteroids in patients with the adult respiratory distress syndrome. N Engl J Med 1987; 317:1565–1570.
100. Meduri GU, Chinn AJ, Leeper KV, et al: Corticosteroid rescue treatment of progressive fibroproliferation in late ARDS. Chest 1994; 105:1517–1527.
101. Biffl WL, Moore FA, Moore EE, et al: Are corticosteroids salvage therapy for refractory acute respiratory distress syndrome? Am J Surg 1995; 170:591–596.
102. Roberts JC, Jones SB: Chromaffin cell epinephrine secretion mediated by a macrophage peptide: The role of endotoxin. Shock 1997; 7:211–216.
103. Roberts JC, Mathews HL, De Poter W, et al: Mononuclear-cell peptide mediation of chromaffin-cell epinephrine secretion. Neuroimmunomodulation 1996; 3:119–130.
104. Jones SB, Wang Z, Wang X, et al: Immune cells mediate epinephrine secretion from bovine chromaffin cells in vitro. Life Sci 1993; 53:447–451.
105. Besedovsky HO, del Rey A, Klusman I, et al: Cytokines as modulators of the hypothalamic-pituitary-adrenal axis. J Steroid Biochem Mol Biol 1991; 40:613–618.
106. Zhou ZZ, Jones SB: Involvement of central vs peripheral mechanisms in mediating sympathoadrenal activation in endotoxic rats. Am J Physiol 1993; 265:683–688.
107. Madden KS, Sanders VM, Felten DL: Catecholamine influences and sympathetic neural modulation of immune responsiveness. Annu Rev Pharmacol Toxicol 1995; 35:417–448.
108. Hatfield SM, Petersen BH, Di Micco JA: Beta-adrenoceptor modulation of the generation of murine cytotoxic T-lymphocytes in vitro. J Pharmacol Exp Ther 1986; 239:460–466.
109. Felten DL, Felten SY, Berlinger DL, et al: Noradrenergic sympathetic neural interaction with the immune system: Structure and function. Immunol Rev 1987; 100:225–260.
110. Santambrogio L, Lipartiti M, Bruni A, et al: Dopamine receptors on human T and B lymphocytes. J Neuroimmunol 1993; 45:113–120.
111. Van den Berghe G, de Zegher F, Lauwers P: Dopamine suppresses pituitary function in infants and children. Crit Care Med 1994; 22:1747–1753.
112. Van den Berghe G, de Zegher F, Lauwers P: Dopamine and sick euthyroid syndrome in critical illness. Clin Endocrinol 1994; 41:731–737.
113. Yamazaki M, Matsuoka T, Yasui K, et al: Dopamine inhibition of superoxide anion production by polymorphonuclear leukocytes. J Allergy Clin Immunol 1989; 83:967–972.
114. Sternberg EM, Wedner HJ, Leung MK, et al: Effect of serotonin (5-HT) and other monoamines on murine macrophages: Modulation of interferon-gamma induced phagocytosis. J Immunol 1987; 138:4360–4365.
115. Kouassi E, Bowkhris W, Descotes J, et al: Selective T-cell defects by dopamine administration in mice. Immunopharmacol Immunotoxicol 1987; 9:477–488.
116. Hadden JW, Hadden EM, Middleton E: Lymphocyte blast transformation-I: Demonstration of adrenergic receptors in human peripheral lymphocytes. Cell Immunol 1970; 1:583–595.
117. Besedovsky HO, Del Rey A, Sorkin E, et al: Immunoregulation mediated by the sympathetic nervous system. Cell Immunol 1979; 48:346–355.
118. Weiss M, Schneider EM, Tarnow J, et al: Is inhibition of oxygen radical production of neutrophils by sympathomimetics mediated via beta-2 adrenoceptors? J Pharmacol Exp Ther 1996; 278:1105–1113.
119. Galant SP, Underwood S, Duriseti L, et al: Characterization of high affinity beta-2 adrenergic receptor binding of (-)[^{3}H]dihydroalprenolol to human polymorphonuclear cell particulates. J Lab Clin Med 1978; 92:613–618.
120. Opdahl H, Benestad HB, Nicolaysen G: Effect of beta-adrenergic agents on human neutrophil granulocyte activation with *N*-formyl-methionyl-leucyl-phenylalanine and phorbol myristate acetate. Pharmacol Toxicol 1993; 72:221–228.
121. Van der Poll T, Coyle SM, Barbosa K, et al: Epinephrine inhibits tumor necrosis factor-alpha and potentiates interleukin-10 production during human endotoxemia. J Clin Invest 1996; 97:713–719.
122. Sekut L, Champion BR, Page K, et al: Anti-inflammatory activity of salmeterol: Down-regulation of cytokine production. Clin Exp Immunol 1995; 99:461–466.
123. Elenkov IJ, Hasko G, Kovacs KJ, et al: Modulation of lipopolysaccharide-induced tumor necrosis factor-alpha production by selective alpha- and beta-adrenergic drugs in mice. J Neuroimmunol 1995; 61:123–131.
124. Del Rey A, Besedovsky HO, Sorkin E, et al: Immunoregulation mediated by the sympathetic nervous system: II. Cell Immunol 1981; 63:329–334.
125. Bergquist J, Tarkowski A, Ekman R, et al: Discovery of endogenous catecholamines in lymphocytes and evidence for catecholamine regulation of lymphocyte function via an autocrine loop. Proc Natl Acad Sci USA 1994; 91:12912–12916.
126. Spatafora M, Chiappara G, Merendino AM, et al: Theophylline suppresses the release of tumor necrosis factor-alpha by blood monocytes and alveolar macrophages. Eur Respir J 1994; 7:223–228.
127. Nelson S, Summer WR, Jakob GJ: Aminophylline-induced suppression of pulmonary antibacterial defenses. Am Rev Respir Dis 1985; 131:923–927.
128. Scordamaglia A, Ciprandi G, Ruffoni S, et al: Theophylline and the immune response: In vitro and in vivo effects. Clin Immunol Immunopathol 1988; 48:238–246.
129. Jilg S, Barsig J, Leist M, et al: Enhanced release of interleukin-10 and soluble tumor necrosis factor as novel principles of methylxanthine action in murine models of endotoxic shock. J Pharmacol Exp Ther 1996; 278:421–431.
130. Leist M, Auer-Barth S, Wendel A: Tumor necrosis factor production in the perfused mouse liver and its pharmacologic modulation of methylxanthines. J Pharmacol Exp Ther 1996; 276:968–976.
131. Nemeth ZH, Hasko G, Szabo C, et al: Amrinone and theophylline differentially regulate cytokine and nitric oxide production in endotoxemic mice. Shock 1997; 7:371–375.
132. Giroir BP, Beutler B: Effect of amrinone on tumor necrosis factor production in endotoxemic shock. Circ Shock 1992; 36:200–207.
133. Fortenberry JD, Huber AR, Owens ML: Inotropes inhibit endothelial cell surface adhesion molecules induced by interleukin-1B. Crit Care Med 1997; 25:303–308.
134. Pober JS, Slowik MR, de Luca LG, et al: Elevated cyclic AMP inhibits endothelial cell synthesis and expression of endothelial adhesion molecule-1 but not intercellular adhesion molecule-1. J Immunol 1993; 150:5114–5123.

B. METABOLISM

75

Acid-Base Balance (Quantitation)

Robert Schlichtig, MD

Abnormal arterial acid-base balance is among the best predictors of mortality in critical care[1-3] and an early detector of serious conditions. Its quantitation facilitates recognition (Table 75-1) and expedites treatment of the underlying disease.

There are two general causes of abnormal acid-base balance in clinical medicine: respiratory and metabolic. Both produce changes in pH, carbon dioxide partial pressure (P_{CO_2}), and

TABLE 75–1. Examples of Serious Conditions That Can Be Detected by Blood Gas Analysis

Acute Respiratory Acidosis

Central nervous system depression (e.g., drugs, brain stem injury)
Near-terminal respiratory muscle fatigue (e.g., status asthmaticus, pulmonary edema, Guillain-Barré syndrome)

Acute Respiratory Alkalosis

Sepsis
Pulmonary embolus
Acute hepatic failure

Metabolic Acidosis

Hyperchloremic acidosis (e.g., diarrhea, renal tubular acidosis)
Lactic acidosis (dysoxia, sepsis)
Ketosis (diabetic ketoacidosis, alcoholic ketoacidosis)
Sulfuric acidosis (renal failure)
Ingested poisons

Metabolic Alkalosis

Nasogastric suction
Intravascular volume contraction

Compensated Respiratory Acidosis

Chronic obstructive pulmonary disease

Compensated Respiratory Alkalosis

Chronic liver disease

bicarbonate (HCO_3^-). For practical purposes, CO_2 is an acid. When it is excreted by cells, it liberates H^+ from water. It returns the H^+ back to water when the CO_2 is exhaled. Thus, abnormal arterial PCO_2 ($PaCO_2$) means that there is a respiratory (i.e., lung ventilatory) abnormality. Abnormal $PaCO_2$ is also typical of metabolic abnormalities, because they stimulate a (partial) respiratory compensation. Hence, abnormal $PaCO_2$ might represent either a primary respiratory or a primary metabolic problem. Discriminating between respiratory and metabolic components of acid-base abnormalities has long been a major stumbling block for clinicians, particularly when they try to make urgent decisions.

To assist in the recognition of acid-base disorders, some have devised a scheme similar to the one depicted in Figure 75-1. Patients with primary respiratory disturbances (of either sudden or long duration) have abnormal arterial pH that is opposite in direction to the abnormal $PaCO_2$. Primary metabolic disturbances have the opposite effect (i.e., changes in pH and $PaCO_2$ that are the same in direction). Underlying this behavior is an apparent attempt of the body to maintain pH close to normal,[4] with respiratory and metabolic abnormalities tending to balance each other out. Unfortunately, this simple scheme captures only part of the information obtainable and can lead to wrong clinical decisions in many important instances. One reason is that the compensators are sometimes impaired; that is, there may be more than one disturbance. For example, a patient with a lactic (metabolic) acidosis may develop respiratory failure, retain CO_2, and have decreased pH and increased $PaCO_2$. Thus, the blood gas interpretation suggested by Figure 75-1 is unreliable.

In an effort to distinguish metabolic from respiratory acid-base abnormalities, many schemes have been introduced over the better part of the 20th century. These schemes have seemed at odds with each other because one counted weak ions *(buffer base)*, another strong ions (strong ion difference), and yet another some strong and some weak ions (anion gap). Some use plasma (PCO_2 versus HCO_3^-), some whole blood *(base excess)*, and others all of the fluid surrounding cells *(standard base excess)*. It should come as no surprise that these schemes do not really produce different conclusions—they are all conceptually and quantitatively consistent with each other.[5-7]

Standard base excess (SBE) is an old and simple concept for assessing acid-base status. It is as reliable as any other concept and deconvolutes the interpretation of "arterial blood gases." It quantifies the metabolic component of the acid-base abnormality, just as $PaCO_2$ quantifies respiratory abnormalities. This permits clinicians to recognize the primary disturbance as well as normal and abnormal compensation. Most commercial blood gas analyzers calculate SBE and can optionally print it together with the pH, PCO_2, and HCO_3^-. Although SBE is not a new concept, the idea that SBE is qualitatively and quantitatively consistent with all the other acid-base schemes has been demonstrated only in the 1990s.[5-7]

Introductory sections of this chapter outline the basic physicochemistry and physiology of acid-base disorders and the derivation of SBE. The material is largely superfluous as far as clinical decision making is concerned, but it provides the rationale for using the SBE method in place of more cumbersome schemes. The material is provided for readers who might be attracted to the simplicity of the SBE approach but are not comfortable that SBE is consistent with the other methods. Others may wish to refer directly to "Clinical Quantitations of Primary, Compensatory, and Mixed Disturbances" later to see how SBE together with the anion gap can be used to make clinical diagnoses.

PHYSICOCHEMISTRY OF ACID-BASE BALANCE

An acid is an H^+ donor. Hydrochloric acid (HCl) gives up H^+ when added to blood. A base is an H^+ acceptor. Sodium bicarbonate ($NaHCO_3$) removes H^+ when added to blood. CO_2 behaves like an acid because most of it combines with H_2O to form carbonic acid (H_2CO_3), which dissociates almost completely to HCO_3^- and H^+ as defined by the Henderson-Hasselbalch equation.

The concentration of H^+ in tissue is extremely small, only about one-millionth that of HCO_3^-, and is thus usually expressed as the negative logarithm of H^+, the pH. From a

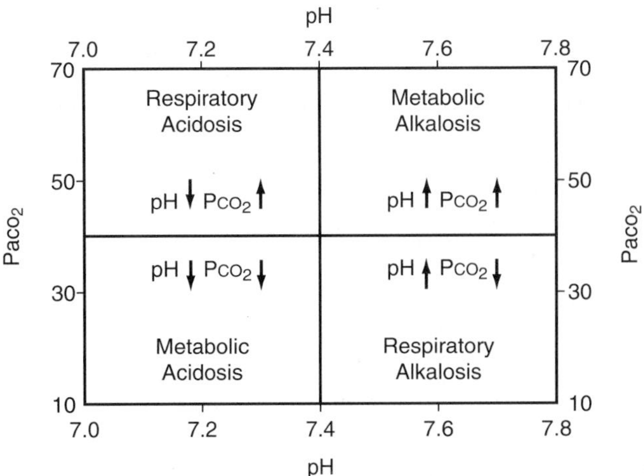

Figure 75–1. Unreliable method for interpreting blood gases. A primary respiratory disturbance normally causes changes in pH (*x*-axis) and $PaCO_2$ (*y*-axis) that are opposite in direction (*upper left* and *lower right*). A primary metabolic abnormality normally causes changes in pH and $PaCO_2$ that are in the same direction (*lower left* and *upper right*). Because important exceptions to this scheme are common, however, this method should not be employed alone.

physicochemical perspective, the H^+ concentration is entirely passive, being determined by P_{CO_2} and metabolic acids and bases.[8-11] From a physiologic perspective, the H^+ concentration is a potent stimulator of lung ventilation and tissue metabolism. This necessary juxtaposition of physicochemical and physiologic reasoning has created much confusion.

Neutral pH simply means that $H^+ = OH^-$. At normal mammalian temperature, neutral pH is 6.8; at 0°C, neutral pH is 8.0, however, because less H_2O dissociates to H^+ and OH^- at lower temperatures. The pH is normally 0.6 pH unit larger than neutral in arterial plasma of all species, regardless of normal body temperature. Inside cells the pH is closer to neutral, as in the seawater from which we evolved.

The chemistry of pH, P_{CO_2}, bicarbonate, and buffers was firmly established in the early years of the 20th century and codified later by several groups. Current reviews are available.[5, 6]

Electroneutrality, Strong Versus Weak Ions, and Strong Ion Difference

Electroneutrality means that the net ionic charge in a given solution is zero.[8-11] In pure 0.9% saline, for example, the concentration of sodium cation, Na^+, equals that of chloride anion, Cl^-. If pure potassium bicarbonate is added, $Na^+ + K^+ = Cl^- + HCO_3^-$. To be precise, ions of minuscule concentration such as H^+ and OH^- should be included too, that is, $H^+ + Na^+ + K^+ = OH^- + Cl^- + HCO_3^- + CO_3^-$; however, for most purposes, these minuscule ions create unnecessary clutter in descriptions of an electrical balance sheet.

Of the four major ions in the preceding solutions, Na^+, K^+, and Cl^- are called "strong" because they are always free, that is, cannot combine with other ions and so lose their charge. HCO_3^- is weak because it can be forced to combine with another weak ion, H^+, to form H_2CO_3, CO_2, and H_2O and so lose its electrical charge.

A simple example illustrates the important differences between strong and weak ions. Suppose 10 millimoles (mM) of pure HCl is added to 1 L of solution with 140 mM Na^+, 105 mM Cl^-, and 25 mM HCO_3^- (Fig. 75-2). Cl^- dissociates from H^+, because Cl^- is a strong ion in solution, so the Cl^- concentration increases to 115 mM. The Na^+ concentration remains 140 mM, because Na^+ is also a strong ion and cannot be forced to combine with Cl^-. The HCO_3^- concentration does not remain at its original value of 25 mM, and the 10 mM of H added to the solution does not remain free. Instead, almost all of the H^+ combines with HCO_3^- to form CO_2 and H_2O. H^+ has been forced to combine with HCO_3^- because electroneutrality must be preserved. Hence, HCO_3^- decreases by slightly less than 10 mM, and the very small increase of H^+ makes up the difference, with the H^+ concentration ending up greater than it was before (Fig. 75-2). The strong ions are all ionized because they are strong, whereas most of the weak ions no longer are, because they are weak.

This simple example illustrates the usefulness of electroneutrality in estimating unknown quantities; that is, the net ionic charge difference between the strong cations and anions, called the *strong ion difference* (SID), dictates the net ionic charge of weak anions, such as HCO_3^- and H^+. In this instance,

$$Na^+ - Cl^- = SID = HCO_3^-$$

This understanding is helpful in quantitation, because it would be easier and more accurate to estimate SID by measuring HCO_3^- than by measuring Na^+ and Cl^-. Analyzers cannot determine the $Na^+ - Cl^-$ difference with as much precision as they can the HCO_3^- concentration. Later we show that it is easier to estimate SID in an analogous manner in physiology (as buffer base) than it is to measure SID directly.

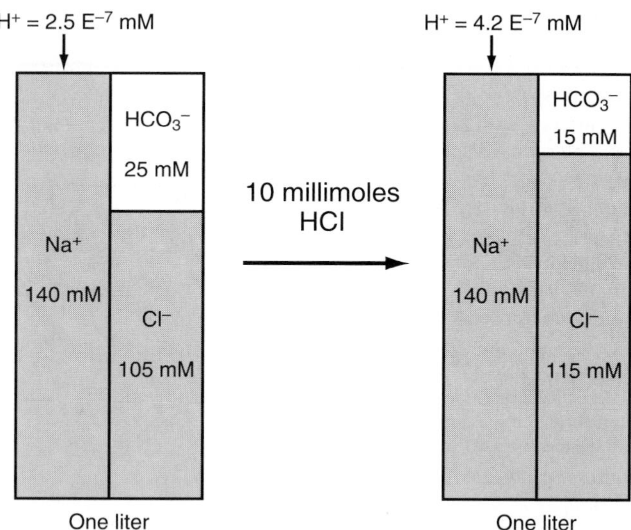

Figure 75–2. Electroneutrality, strong versus weak ions, and strong ion difference. If you can remember the following three facts simultaneously, you will understand a major portion of acid-base theory. First, the sum of the positives (including Na^+ and H^+) must equal the sum of the negatives (Cl^-, La^-, HCO_3^-). Second, the strong ions (Na^+, Cl^-, La^-) are always dissociated, no matter what else happens *(shaded boxes)*, whereas the weak ions (HCO_3^- and H^+) can lose their charge *(clear boxes)*. Third, the concentration difference between the strong ions or strong ion difference therefore determines the concentrations of the weak ions. In this example, addition of 10 millimoles of hydrochloric acid to 1 liter of solution forces a decrease in HCO_3^- and increase in H^+ because Cl^- is strong, whereas HCO_3^- and H^+ are weak.

Chemical Equilibrium

What distinguishes a strong ion from a weak one is the unique pattern by which each establishes chemical equilibrium. An important example is lactic acid (LaH), which, like any acid, dissociates to its conjugate base, lactate (La^-):

$$LaH \leftrightarrow La^- + H^+$$

The proportion associated (LaH) or dissociated (La^-) is characterized by a constant, k, where

$$LaH \times k = La^- \times H^+$$

This equation makes intuitive sense when one notices that if lactic acid is half (50%) dissociated, then $LaH = La^-$ and k must equal H^+. The k for lactic acid is 0.000138, giving pk = 3.86.[12] Half of lactic acid is dissociated at a pH of 3.86. At any pH greater than 6.0, more than 99.9% of lactic acid is ionized, making La^- a strong anion in physiology (Fig. 75-3) and a determinant of SID.

Three Independent Determinants of Acid-Base Status

Electroneutrality and chemical equilibrium are forces governing acid-base balance. Another, the Gibbs-Donnan equilibrium, governs ion exchanges across membranes (see later) and is also important in quantitation. There are also three independent variables that affect acid-base balance[8-11]:

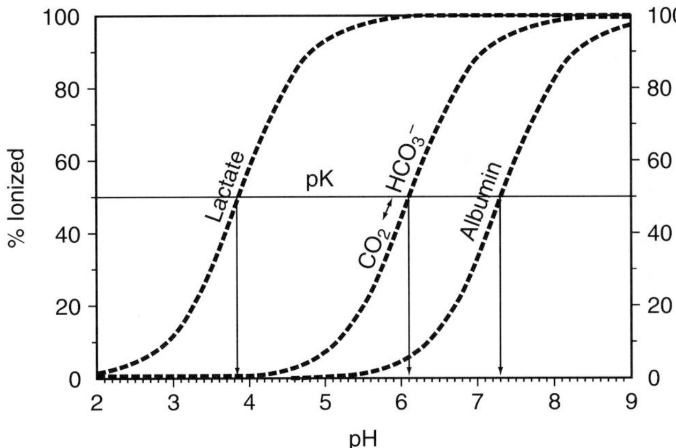

Figure 75–3. Chemical equilibrium. Whether an ion is "strong" or "weak" depends on its pK (i.e., the pH at which half of the substance is ionized, the other half not). The pK of lactate is 3.9 (i.e., more than 99% of it is ionized at pH greater than 6). Carbonic acid and albumin are weak acids because substantial portions of them are neutral in the physiologic range, requiring that their ionized concentrations be computed.

- P_{CO_2} (respiratory)
- SID (metabolic)
- Nonvolatile weak acid (buffer)

The first two (P_{CO_2} and SID) are clinically relevant because they can change sufficiently to produce large changes in pH. The last (nonvolatile buffer) can be an equally important variable in theory but does not vary enough to cause pH changes of clinical relevance,[13] as shown later.

Carbon Dioxide

The most familiar independent variable is P_{CO_2}. In arterial blood, P_{CO_2} varies with ventilation and is normally about 40 mm Hg. It is quantified clinically as partial pressure of the gas (P_{CO_2}). Alternatively, P_{CO_2} can be multiplied by its solubility coefficient (α) to give concentration in millimoles per liter (mM). The coefficient α is a function of temperature, and is 0.0306 at 37°C.[14, 15] In water,

$$CO_2 + H_2O \leftrightarrow H_2CO_3 \leftrightarrow HCO_3^- + H^+$$

The mathematical translation of this equation into numbers is often presented in a somewhat convoluted manner but is really no more complex than the equation describing chemical equilibrium for lactate presented earlier. The H_2CO_3 (middle of the reaction) intermediate can be ignored, as can the H_2O concentration (left-hand side of the reaction), which is large and practically constant. Hence, bicarbonate ion can be predicted in the same manner as lactate ion:

$$CO_2 \times K = HCO_3^- \times H^+$$

where K is the dissociation constant of CO_2. The K, α, and partial pressure of CO_2 can be lumped together to give

$$40 \text{ mm Hg} \times 24 = 24 \text{ mM} \times 40 \text{ mM}$$

More popular is the same equation expressed by taking the negative logarithm of both sides and rearranging, giving the Henderson-Hasselbalch equation:

$$pH = pK + \log[HCO_3^-/(\alpha \times P_{CO_2})]$$

pK is 6.1, so $CO_2 = HCO_3^-$ at a pH of 6.1, just as LaH = La^- at a pH of 3.86 (see Fig. 75–3).

The only independent variable in these equations is P_{CO_2}: pH and HCO_3^- depend on it. However, pH and P_{CO_2} can both be measured accurately, and no matter what else happens, either of the last two equations can be used to calculate HCO_3^-, a useful number. For example, it was simpler to estimate SID from HCO_3^- than it was to measure it directly in the solution containing Na^+, Cl^-, and HCO_3^-.

Nonvolatile Weak Acid Buffer

A buffer is a molecule that takes up or releases substantive (i.e., millimolar) quantities of H^+ in the physiologic range as pH changes. For example, HCO_3^- took up nearly 10 mM of H^+ in the preceding example. However, HCO_3^- cannot buffer its own progenitor (CO_2) and so cannot prevent acid-base changes produced by changing CO_2, which is volatile. Thus, HCO_3^- is not an independent variable, and the term nonvolatile buffer is used to distinguish the second independent determinant of acid-base status. Nonvolatile weak acid buffers in blood are mainly hemoglobin (Hb), albumin, and inorganic phosphate (P_i). The abbreviation for ionized weak acid buffer is A^-, for unionized weak acid buffer is AH, and for total weak acid buffer is ATOT. Hence

$$ATOT = A^- + HA$$

The dissociation of any given HA (e.g., albumin or Hb) is just like that for lactate and carbonic acid:

$$HA \leftrightarrow A^- + H^+$$

and can be described mathematically in the same way as for lactic acid and carbonic acid:

$$HA \times k = A^- \times H^+$$

Hence, A^- can be calculated from pH and ATOT, just as HCO_3^- can be calculated from pH and P_{CO_2} using the last two equations. Because K values for ATOT (e.g., albumin) are close to the physiologic range, buffering of respiratory and metabolic acids is quite good, even at the extremes of albumin and Hb concentration. Hb and albumin do not have true pK values because they are large molecules composed of so many amino acid buffers. For practical purposes,[10] however, each behaves as if it were a buffer with a single pK value (see Fig. 75–3). Both buffer metabolic and respiratory acids best in the physiologic range.

Strong Ion Difference and Buffer Base

The third independent variable determining acid-base balance in a fluid is SID, the concentration difference between the strong anions and strong cations. SID is the newest name for the "metabolic" variable, although the same concept was clearly evident long before the 1940s.[8, 18] It may be the purest physicochemical expression of "metabolic" but proved long ago to be unnecessarily cumbersome in physiology.[10]

Potentially life-threatening disease states ultimately produce changes in strong ions such as La^- (dysoxia or sepsis), β-hydroxybutyrate$^-$ (βOHB^-; diabetic ketoacidosis), and SO_4^- (renal failure) that produce large enough changes in SID to force noticeable changes in pH. The pure metabolic variable (SID) in a patient with lactic acidosis, diabetic ketoacidosis, or uremic acidosis would be

$$SID = Na^+ + K^+ - Cl^- - La^- - \beta OHB^- - AcAc^- - SO_4^{2-}$$

To measure SID directly from the concentrations of all these strong ions would be difficult and impractical. SID determines and equals the net charge of weak ions (HCO_3^- and A^-). Hence, it is quite a bit easier to estimate SID as

$$SID = HCO_3^- + A^-$$

where A^- is Hb^- with or without $albumin^-$ and P_i^-.

It turns out to be more accurate to estimate SID as the sum of HCO_3^- (calculated from PCO_2 and pH) and A^- (calculated from ATOT and pH), just as it was more accurate to calculate SID from HCO_3^- in the solution of NaCl, $NaHCO_3$, and HCl described earlier.[8, 10, 11, 16] This best choice method for estimating the pure metabolic SID component of acid-base status has been employed since the 1950s, although the sum of $HCO_3^- + A^-$ was then referred to as *buffer base* (BB).[8, 10] Even at this turn of the millennium, estimation of SID as BB (i.e., $HCO_3^- + A^-$) remains the most practical method for quantifying accurately the metabolic component of an acid-base disturbance, although the name buffer base is now used mainly by a few surviving original investigators. The term remains appropriate, because BB is what typically is actually computed, for determining SID accurately. Few laboratories can measure all of the potential strong ions, and BB calculation is needed to determine the quantity of unmeasured strong ion.

Base Excess or Strong Ion Difference Excess

The metabolic variable is SID. It is measured as its metabolic mirror image, BB, which is $HCO_3^- + A^-$. What matters in physiology and clinical medicine, however, is the magnitude of deviation from normal metabolic balance.[10] This physiologic quantity is called base excess (BE), short for buffer base excess. No accuracy is sacrificed in the transition from BB to BE. BE is almost, but not quite, the same as the deviation from normal SID or BB. Normal BE is 0 mM, a nice round number. The precise definition of BE is the change in concentration of added strong acid or base needed to restore pH to normal (7.4) at normal PCO_2 (40 mm Hg). The BE definition is easy to grasp when one realizes that if PCO_2 is 40 mm Hg, the abnormality in pH is purely metabolic. BE rendered practical the juxtaposition of physicochemical and physiologic reasoning. It was thoroughly validated conceptually and quantitatively during the polio epidemics of the 1950s by Siggaard-Andersen and colleagues.

The strict definition of BE involves adding strong acid or base to the sample, but the actual practice does not. BE is estimated from HCO_3^- and A^- (see earlier). HCO_3^- is estimated from pH and PCO_2, and A^- is estimated from pH and hemoglobin in whole blood or from albumin and phosphate in plasma. The A^- and HCO_3^- are added together to give BB. BE is computed as the difference between the actual BB and that expected at pH 7.4, $PaCO_2$ is 40 mm Hg for a particular patient.[17] Positive BE means metabolic alkalosis; negative BE means metabolic acidosis. BE could just as well be called *SID excess* (SIDex) because one could not add a strong acid (e.g., HCl) or a strong base (e.g., NaOH) to a solution without changing the SID and because SID is BB. It has been shown that the independently derived BE[10, 17] and SID[9, 10, 12] equations provide nearly identical numerical values when SID is properly translated to SIDex in this manner.[7]

BE can be expressed for plasma alone, erythrocytes alone, whole blood (erythrocytes in plasma), or the entire extracellular fluid.[17] In each instance, the definition remains the same, that is, the change in metabolic balance that would be needed to restore normal metabolic homeostasis at normal PCO_2. BE of whole blood is more complicated than BE of plasma or erythrocytes, because acid-base conditions are so different in red blood cells and plasma. For example, the normal erythrocyte pH is 7.19, whereas the normal plasma pH is 7.40. The SID and ATOT values of the two compartments differ as well.[11] Nevertheless, it has been widely appreciated since the 1940s that the whole-blood BE or BB or SID can be calculated using just plasma pH and PCO_2.[8, 10] Hemoglobin measurement, which was once common practice, is no longer needed (see later). In any event, BE of whole blood or extracellular fluid (ECF) can be estimated using the pH and PCO_2 of plasma because red blood cell and plasma fluids are predictably related to each other by the Gibbs-Donnan equilibrium, a law that is just as important as electroneutrality and chemical equilibrium. The Gibbs-Donnan equilibrium[10, 17, 19] becomes a dominant force whenever a membrane (e.g., the erythrocyte membrane) prevents permeation of ATOT buffer (e.g., Hb) while permitting free passage of other ions (e.g., Cl^- and HCO_3^-). Its end result, for quantitative purposes, is that the plasma pH resulting from addition of metabolic or respiratory acid to whole blood (or even to interstitial fluid) can always be predicted, even though the resulting SIDs in the individual compartments can differ.[17, 20, 21]

The importance of Gibbs-Donnan interactions between plasma and red blood cell buffers has sometimes been neglected,[22] resulting in incorrect conclusions with regard to cause and effect.[13, 20] It has been pointed out that the plasma SID correlates reasonably well with the whole-blood BE.[23] However, they are numerically far different, and this direct comparison is substantively incorrect,[20] explaining why the BE of whole blood has been used in preference to the SID or BB of plasma since the inception of these concepts in the early 1900s.[8, 10]

PHYSIOLOGY AND STANDARD BASE EXCESS

The body regulates two kinds of acids. Respiratory acid (CO_2) is generated mainly by combustion in the mitochondria, where cells use the energy of available food by combining it with O_2. Between 70% and 100% of the O_2 is normally excreted as CO_2, depending on the fuel. CO_2 generates H^+ by combining with H_2O, producing HCO_3^- at the same time. Metabolic acid generates H^+ by decreasing SID, forcing a millimeter decrease in the weak ions HCO_3^- and A^- and a nanomolar increase in the weak ion H^+. Metabolic acid can be ingested (Cl^-, SO_4^{2-}) or synthesized de novo (La^-, β-hydroxybutyrate$^-$).

Respiratory Acid-Base Balance Regulation

The respiratory center normally regulates arterial plasma pH on a minute-to-minute basis, retaining or excreting CO_2 "acid," by regulating the frequency and volume of lung ventilation. The respiratory center responds mainly to signals from PO_2, pH, and PCO_2, with PO_2 being the strongest stimulus to ventilation and PCO_2 the weakest.[4] The CO_2 excretion rate eventually equals the CO_2 production rate, whether the $PaCO_2$ is 30 mm Hg (pregnancy) or 70 mm Hg, as in chronic obstructive pulmonary disease (COPD). CO_2 coming from tissues simply "pours" down its gradient between pulmonary capillary blood and pulmonary alveolar gas, like water falling over a dam. Eventually, the flow over the dam is the same, regardless of its height. The "height" of the dam (and so PCO_2 of the body) is determined by lung ventilation, permitting pH regulation.

Metabolic Acid-Base Balance Regulation

Whereas lungs can correct blood pH rapidly, kidneys can do so only slowly. Mole for mole, strong anions and CO_2 are similar in their ability to change pH. However, strong anions are excreted mainly in urine, which flows at only a fraction of the lung ventilation rate, and strong anions are also more difficult to export than CO_2. This explains why lungs can respond nearly instantaneously to a change in metabolic acid-base balance, whereas kidneys require several days to respond fully to a change in lung ventilation.

Kidney regulation of the metabolic acid-base balance is typically described in terms of the HCO_3^- or H^+ balance. Alternatively, the same processes can be understood in terms of the strong ion balance. This SID reasoning is a conceptual mirror of the conventional HCO_3^- or H^+ reasoning with regard to cause and effect. For example, infusion of sodium bicarbonate into a normal subject stimulates the kidney to excrete "HCO_3^-." The dynamics of this perturbation was described many years ago in terms of urinary SID,[9] although that term was not then in use. The response of the kidney in that circumstance was retention of Cl^- relative to Na^+ and K^+, lowering the net whole-body SID. Although HCO_3^- was indeed excreted, it was renal strong cation (Na^+ and K^+) excretion relative to anion excretion that caused it. The resulting increase in urine SID forced HCO_3^- excretion so as to preserve electroneutrality in urine. Thus, HCO_3^- is indeed excreted but only because urinary SID increases.

Gastrointestinal acid-base dynamics can also be viewed from the SID perspective. Gastric parietal cells can raise gastric juice H^+ simply by secreting Cl^- in excess of strong cation. The large increase in H^+ is maintained in the stomach lumen because gastric mucosa together with its mucous layer can support a large pH gradient between lumen and cells. The resulting gastric acidity minimizes bacterial growth in the stomach and facilitates early digestion. When these gastric juices pass into the duodenum, the acidifying Cl^- (low SID) is neutralized by alkalinizing Na^+ (as $NaHCO_3$), secreted by pancreas and other distal enteric cells, so that there is no change in the balance of strong ions in the body as a whole. The Na^+ is eventually reabsorbed with the Cl^-. If the patient vomits, however, or if his or her gastric secretions are emptied by a nasogastric tube, Cl^- exits the body, causing alkalosis (by raising SID). The colon normally reabsorbs K^+ and Na^+, maintaining a normal body SID when it does so successfully. During diarrhea, the SID is smaller, resulting in body acidosis.

Normal Patterns of Response to Abnormal Respiration or Metabolism

The normal or expected compensations of respiratory for metabolic acid-base abnormalities and of metabolic for respiratory ones have been charted by many investigators over many years using arterial blood gases. Pooled data of these investigators are shown in Figure 75-4, expressed in terms of the acid-base variables directly regulated by the body, H^+ and Pa_{CO_2}.[4] Populations of patients with only one primary disturbance were selected by these investigators on clinical grounds.

The data of Figure 75-4 are consistent with the scheme displayed in Figure 75-1. Primary disturbances in Pa_{CO_2} regulation (see top two panels) produce changes in H^+ that are in the same direction as the disturbance in Pa_{CO_2}, because CO_2 splits water to form H^+ when added to solution or returns H^+ to water when it leaves. The H^+ deviation from normal is larger acutely (see top panel) than it is in the chronic condition (see middle panel), after the kidneys have compensated by removing or retaining metabolic acid (Cl^-) or base (Na^+, K^+). Primary metabolic disturbances (see bottom panel) produce changes in H^+ that are compensated almost immediately by changes in Pa_{CO_2}, which are in the opposite direction. Because lungs can normally compensate for pH much more quickly than the kidneys can, the response is more or less

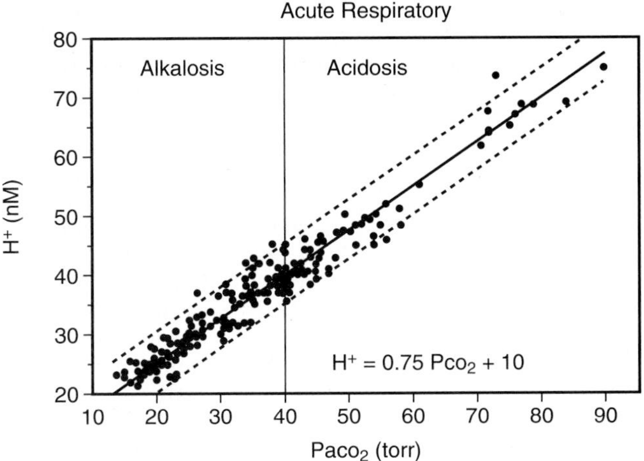

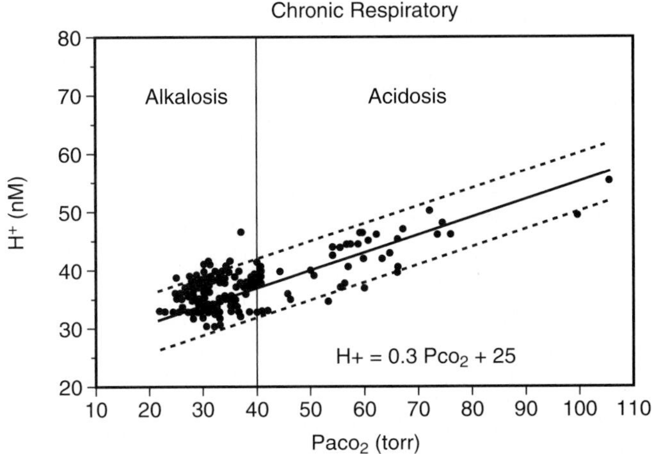

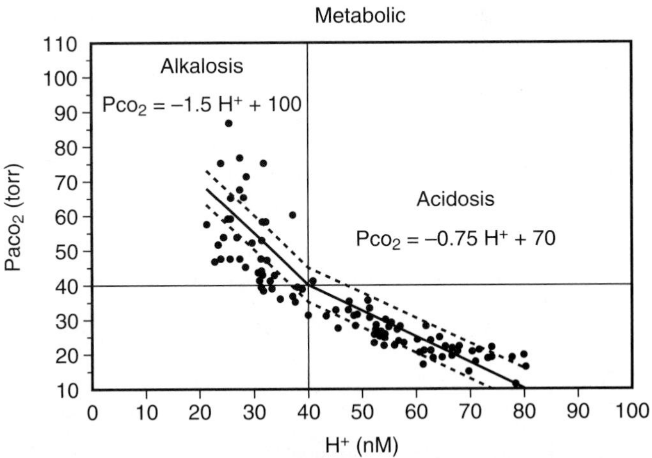

Figure 75–4. Half a century's worth of published clinical data for patients considered on clinical grounds to have acute respiratory disturbances *(top)*, chronic respiratory disturbances *(middle)*, and metabolic disturbances *(bottom)*. Data are displayed in terms of the acid-base variables that are ultimately regulated—H^+ and Pa_{CO_2}.

immediate. Compensation for a primary respiratory or metabolic abnormality is never complete at steady state, so the pH is at least partly abnormal in the original direction.

Although H^+ and $Paco_2$ are the variables to which regulatory receptors in brain and kidney respond (see Fig. 75-4), the expected interactions of respiratory and metabolic alterations are usually expressed, for clinical purposes, in terms of plasma HCO_3^- and $Paco_2$ (Fig. 75-5). Plasma HCO_3^- is not a variable that is directly regulated by the body, but equations describing expected relations between HCO_3^- and $Paco_2$ are somewhat easier to deal with clinically than equations relating H^+ and $Paco_2$.[24] Figure 75-5 is therefore an improvement on Figure 75-4, as far as care providers are concerned. Nevertheless, clinicians tend to neglect even the conventional HCO_3^- versus $Paco_2$ diagram (Fig. 75-5) because the equations are difficult to remember, the diagram is tedious to use, and the distinction between respiratory and metabolic alterations is indirect.

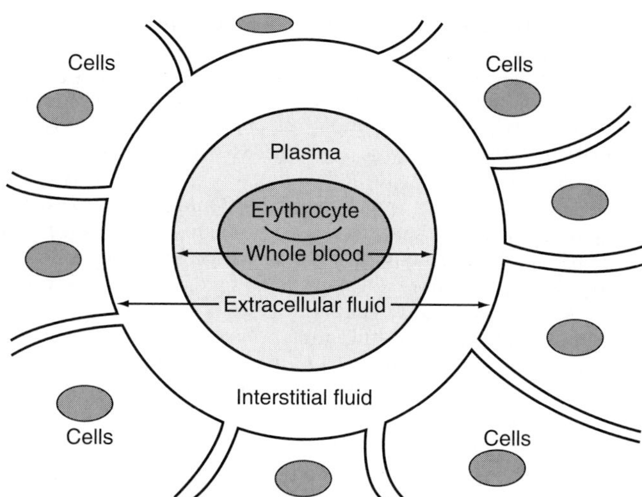

Figure 75–6. The extracellular fluid (ECF) is composed of plasma (~3 L), red blood cells (~2 L), and interstitial fluid (~10 L). ECF is the common reservoir for delivery of nutrients and clearance of wastes for all the tissues in the body, making it sensitive to major acid-base changes in the tissues.

Standard Base Excess

SBE quantifies the metabolic abnormality of the ECF in mM. It is not the same as the whole-blood BE but is the BE of whole blood together with its surrounding interstitial fluid. ECF (Fig. 75-6) is the mobile fluid reservoir trapped between cells (e.g., hepatocytes, myocytes, enterocytes, neurons); it serves as the conduit between cells and the outside environment from which nutrients (O_2, food) are taken and into which wastes (CO_2, urea, solid waste) are excreted. ECF includes plasma (~3 L), red blood cells (~2 L), and interstitial fluid (~10 L). ECF flows through arteries, veins, and lymphatics, mixing constantly. The acid-base status of the ECF (not just plasma or just whole blood) is therefore the vehicle through which acid-base regulation is accomplished. SBE is computed from the same variables that the body regulates, plasma H^+ and $Paco_2$ (see Fig. 75-4); predicts expected compensation just as well[5,6]; and is as good a predictor of compensation as the more conventional HCO_3^- versus $Paco_2$ approach (see Fig. 75-5). A diagram of SBE versus $Paco_2$ is shown in Figure 75-7. The SBE approach (see Fig. 75-7) deconvolutes the distinction between respiratory and metabolic alterations. Blood gas analyzers compute SBE as

$$SBE = 0.9287[HCO_3^- - 24.4 + 14.83\ (pH - 7.4)]$$

The first term in the equation (i.e., $0.9 \times HCO_3^- - 24.4$) derives the change in HCO_3^- from the normal value in ECF. The second term (i.e., $0.9 \times 15 \times pH - 7.4$) gives the deviation of A^- from the normal value in ECF. The sum of the two gives the change in BB (or in SID) needed to restore the metabolic acid-base status to normal in the entire ECF. The equation is written in terms of arterial plasma, which is a thoroughly mixed, oxygenated sample of blood that was in equilibrium with ECF when it was flowing through capillaries

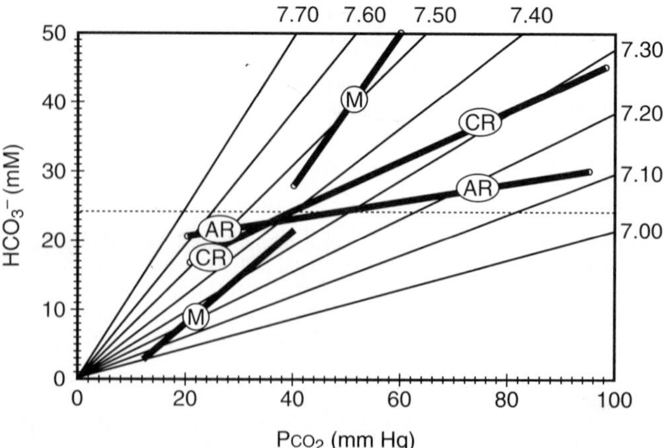

Figure 75–5. A plasma bicarbonate versus $Paco_2$ diagram, conventionally used to express the data shown in Figure 75-4. AR = acute respiratory; CR = chronic respiratory; M = metabolic.

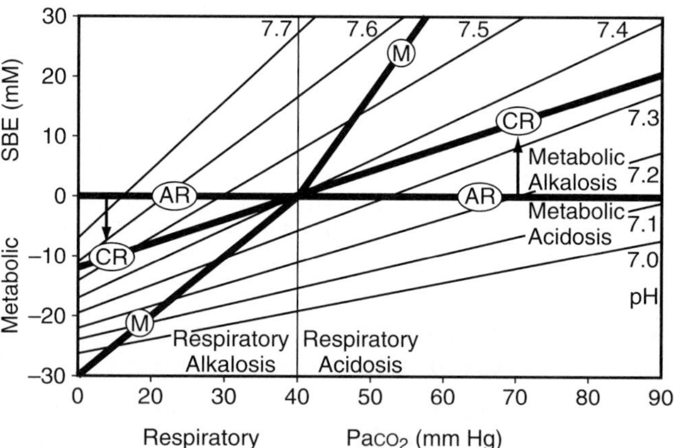

Figure 75–7. Grogogram for recognizing the major categories of acid-base disturbance. Derived from the same data as Figure 75-4, with the same confidence limits. Metabolic (standard base excess [SBE]) is on the *y*-axis; respiratory ($Paco_2$) is on the *x*-axis. Respiratory acidosis versus alkalosis is divided by the vertical $Paco_2$ = 40 mm Hg line; metabolic acidosis versus alkalosis is divided by the horizontal SBE = 0 line. SBE is zero during acute respiratory (AR) disturbances because there is no metabolic disturbance. During chronic respiratory (CR) disturbances, a change in metabolic (SBE) counteracts the change in respiratory ($Paco_2$) such that the change in SBE equals the change in $Paco_2$ times 0.4. Metabolic disturbances (M) stimulate or depress ventilation differently. During acute metabolic acidosis, the diaphragms are stimulated to change $Paco_2$ by a value that equals the change in SBE. During acute metabolic alkalosis, the diaphragms are depressed, changing $Paco_2$ by only 0.6 times the change in SBE.

and remains representative of ECF conditions when it flows from central veins into arteries, where it can be sampled.

The SBE calculation assumes that ATOT of the ECF is equivalent to blood with an Hb concentration of 5 g/dL. Even if the true average Hb concentration of the ECF were as low as 1 g/dL, however, the maximum error in the calculation would be only 3 mM.[5] The error would be zero mM at a Pa_{CO_2} of 40 mm Hg and 3 mM at a Pa_{CO_2} well in excess of 100 mm Hg. This explains why patients with widely varying protein buffer concentrations (Hb and albumin) respond so similarly to abnormalities in respiratory and metabolic acid-base status (see Fig. 75-4). Nonvolatile weak acid buffer (ATOT) is indeed an important determinant of acid-base status from the physicochemical perspective, but clinical ECF variations in ATOT are too small and too slow to cause acid-base perturbations in physiology.[13, 20]

CLINICAL QUANTITATION OF PRIMARY, COMPENSATORY, AND MIXED DISTURBANCES

Respiratory and metabolic acid-base abnormalities are quantified as

$$\text{respiratory disturbance} = \Delta P_{CO_2}$$

where ΔP_{CO_2} is $P_{CO_2} - 40$ in mm Hg, and

$$\text{metabolic disturbance} = \text{SBE}$$

where SBE is in mM.[5, 6] Most commercial blood gas analyzers calculate SBE and print it if programmed to do so. Arterial blood is needed to distinguish metabolic from respiratory changes, because the acid-base status of venous blood reflects a number of factors other than just lung ventilation.[21, 25]

Acute Respiratory Disturbances

In a patient with a purely respiratory acid-base abnormality,

$$\text{SBE} = 0$$

where confidence limits are ± 5 mM. SBE is zero because there is no metabolic disturbance, just a respiratory one (Fig. 75-8). The same equation applies to both acute respiratory acidosis (e.g., oversedation, acute respiratory failure) and acute respiratory alkalosis (e.g., sepsis, acute liver failure).

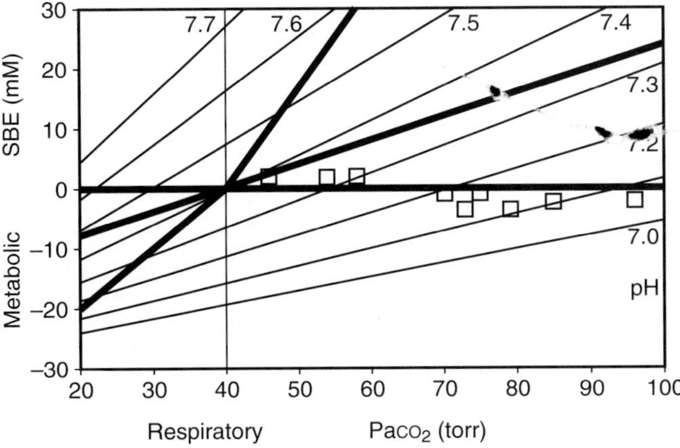

Figure 75–8. Data for a patient with primary alveolar hypoventilation, superimposed on a grogogram. Standard base excess (SBE) remains 0 ± 5 mM because the disturbance is almost entirely respiratory.

CASE HISTORY

A 67-year-old woman with severe COPD was admitted to the hospital for dyspnea. Optimal medical management failed to improve her symptoms. She was transferred first for observation to the intermediate care unit, where she became unresponsive, and then to the intensive care unit, where arterial blood gases (ABGs) showed pH 7.19, Pa_{CO_2} 70 mm Hg, P_{O_2} 249 mm Hg. She was given mechanical ventilation. Within 48 hours, she was rested and able to breathe on her own and was extubated. She ate a small lunch, drank a little, ate a mouthful or two of dinner, talked sparingly with a number of family members, but gradually became sleepy and difficult to arouse. She breathed at a constant rate of 25 breaths/min, but her breathing seemed progressively more shallow. Her pulse oximeter showed arterial oxygen saturation (Sa_{O_2}) between 88% and 92%. Around 9 PM ABG values were obtained because she was no longer arousable. They showed pH 7.10, P_{CO_2} 85 mm Hg, P_{O_2} 50 mm Hg. She was intubated again and extubated again. She was offered no resuscitation or, alternatively, tracheostomy with a goal of nighttime ventilation. Her family was large (multiple generations), local, and caring, and was able and willing to take care of her with home ventilation. She wanted neither, because she believed that she could breathe on her own without medical assistance. Finally, after a third course of mechanical ventilation, she realized that she could not remember any of the intubations and decided to have a tracheostomy.

Commentary

SBE was 0 ± 5 mM throughout because the problem was purely respiratory. There was no metabolic abnormality. She had "primary alveolar hypoventilation" caused by generalized weakness. There did not appear to be any other serious problem. Her data are shown in Figure 75-8.

Metabolic Acidosis

Primary metabolic disorders stimulate or depress ventilation to compensate for the abnormal pH, just as the primary respiratory disorders do. However, the compensation occurs much more quickly, because the respiratory muscles can quickly change P_{CO_2}. To see whether ventilation is compensating normally for the pH imbalance, one can use the following equation:

$$\Delta Pa_{CO_2} = \text{SBE}$$

CASE HISTORY

A 21-year-old man was admitted to the surgical ward one evening because of suspicion of an acute abdomen. He had been nauseated for 6 days, complaining of severe dull epigastric pain. Several years earlier, a diagnosis of congestive cardiomyopathy had been confirmed, but his father stated that his son had no exercise limitation and that he could play basketball with his friends when he wanted to. Abdominal ultrasonography was normal, and there was no free air on an obstructive series. Electrolytes were normal, with a normal anion gap (see later). "Liver enzymes" were minimally elevated. The afternoon of the next day, the patient appeared cyanotic to the nursing staff, who provided 100% O_2. The patient's lips and nail beds were blue, he was curled in a fetal position, and he was moaning. His blood pressure was 90/60. A pulse oximeter provided no reading. ABG values were obtained and revealed pH 7.13, P_{CO_2} 19 mm Hg, P_{O_2} 109 mm Hg, SBE −20 mM. A central line was inserted, yielding a central venous oxygen saturation of 53%. An echocardiogram demonstrated severe global hypokinesis and an ejection fraction of about 10%. Dobutamine was started at 3 μg/kg/min and advanced gradually to 10 μg/kg/min while arrhythmias were sought. Plasma electrolyte determinations were repeated, and revealed an anion gap of 19 mM. The young man's abdominal pain improved markedly, and he was no longer curled in a fetal position, although he was still obviously ill. Liver function tests (LFTs) were repeated, and transaminases were in the 200s (IUs)

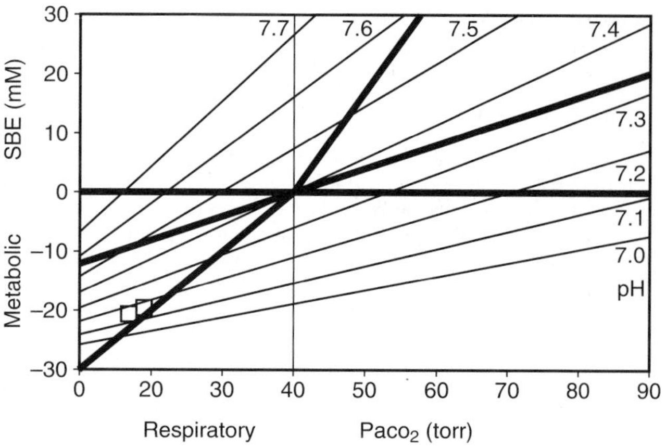

Figure 75–9. Data for a patient with metabolic acidosis, superimposed on a grogogram. $Paco_2$ is 0 ± 5 mm Hg of that expected for a patient with a standard base excess (SBE) of -20 mM.

because of liver ischemia. He was transferred by helicopter to a cardiac transplantation center.

Commentary

This patient was suffering from cardiogenic shock resulting from myocarditis. The O_2 supply was inadequate to support O_2 demand (dysoxia), resulting in anaerobic metabolism with lactic acidosis. Initially, it appeared on clinical grounds (cyanosis) as though his arterial blood was hypoxic, suggesting a lung problem. However, ABG determinations revealed a normal arterial Po_2 with a markedly decreased SBE (severe metabolic acidosis) and normal respiratory compensation ($Paco_2$ -19 within $\pm$ 5 mM of the SBE) (Fig. 75–9). His lungs were responding appropriately, maintaining normal arterial Po_2 as well as a Pco_2 adequate to maintain plasma pH near the expected range.

Metabolic Alkalosis

Metabolic alkalosis normally depresses ventilation, allowing Pco_2 to rise and correct pH toward normal; however, the degree of respiratory depression is less marked:

$$\Delta Paco_2 = 0.6 \times SBE$$

Familiar to most intensivists is the patient who has received massive intravascular volume resuscitation during the nadir of illness, with most of this fluid leaking into the interstitial space, but who then mobilizes this fluid into the circulation during early convalescence. Particularly when furosemide is used to expedite the fluid mobilization, a contraction alkalosis typically develops in these patients. If, for example, SBE increases to $+10$ mM as a consequence of the contraction alkalosis, $Paco_2$ should be $40 + 0.6 \times 10$ or 46 mM. If Pco_2 in the same patient were 30 mm Hg, the clinician might consider, for example, fear, anxiety, or new onset of sepsis.

Chronic Respiratory Disturbances

If the patient's $Paco_2$ remains constantly elevated for several days, the kidneys are stimulated to restore pH toward normal. Hence, whereas acute respiratory disturbance results in an SBE near zero, a chronic respiratory disturbance results in an SBE different from zero, namely

$$SBE = 0.4 \times \Delta Paco_2$$

The direction of change in SBE (up or down) is in the same direction as that in Pco_2 (up or down) that stimulated it.

ANION GAP AND DETECTION OF SERIOUS METABOLIC ACIDOSES

SBE and $Paco_2$ provide the only available quantitation of respiratory and metabolic acidosis and alkalosis. The main limitation of SBE is that it does not discriminate between *non-anion gap acidoses*, which tend to be less urgent, and the *positive anion gap acidoses*, which tend to be more serious. Examples of the latter conditions are lactic acidosis (dysoxia and/or sepsis), ketosis (diabetic ketoacidosis), and poisoning. When the type of acidosis cannot be distinguished with certainty on clinical grounds, plasma electrolyte (i.e., Na^+, K^+, Cl^-, HCO_3^-) analysis is needed. Anion gap determination is also needed to detect metabolic acidosis when it is counterbalanced by metabolic alkalosis (see the clinical example later).

Anion gap is usually measured in venous plasma. Here, we can estimate HCO_3^- as total CO_2 by adding strong acid to the plasma sample. The strong acid (usually sulfuric acid) converts all the HCO_3^- to CO_2; the Pco_2 is measured as partial pressure and then converted to mM. This total CO_2 is a reasonable estimate of HCO_3^- in plasma. By itself, however, the plasma HCO_3^-, is not helpful for determining the cause of its abnormality without additional information. As shown in Figure 75–5, decreased HCO_3^- might be due to acute metabolic acidosis, to acute respiratory alkalosis, or to chronic respiratory alkalosis. Increased HCO_3^- may be due to metabolic alkalosis, acute respiratory acidosis, or chronic respiratory acidosis. In venous plasma, it can also be due to low venous O_2 saturation.[21, 25]

Approximate Anion Gap

The anion gap is based on the electroneutrality principle (see earlier), according to which the main positive ionic charges in plasma (Na^+ and K^+) have to be approximately equal to the main negative ionic charges (Cl^-, HCO_3^-, and A^-), where A^- is negatively charged nonvolatile buffer. Normally $Na^+ + K^+ = Cl^- + HCO_3^- + A^-$, and normally the anion gap (AG) equals A^-:

$$AG = Na^+ + K^+ - Cl^- - HCO_3^- = A^-$$

The anion gap, or A^-, is normally 3 to 11 mM in plasma, if K^+ is included. It represents ionized albumin and P_i.[16] If the anion gap is abnormally large, there are more negatively charged substances than can be accounted for by just A^-. The extra negatives may be lactate (La^-) or ketone bodies ($AcAc^-$ or β-OHB^-). Anion gap is measured in plasma, usually venous, because that is the most convenient place to measure it. If there are abnormal quantities of La^-, $AcAc^-$, β-OHB^- in venous plasma, there are abnormal quantities of La^-, $AcAc^-$, or β-OHB^- in whole blood and ECF.

The plasma anion gap supplements information provided by ABG analysis (SBE or abnormal position on a diagram of HCO_3^- versus $Paco_2$). For example, the finding of a positive anion gap in the 21-year-old patient with cardiogenic shock provided strong supporting evidence for the presence of a lactic acidosis. The anion gap is also a reasonable screening tool. Had this patient's plasma electrolytes on admission shown a positive anion gap, the diagnosis of lactic acidosis related to cardiogenic shock might have been made earlier.

The main problem with the anion gap is that the normal range is so large, partly because albumin and P_i concentrations can vary so greatly. For example, a hypoalbuminemic patient can have a normal anion gap despite significant lactic acidosis.

The anion gap also increases with alkalosis because it equals A^-, which becomes plentiful when H^+ is scarce.

Toward a More Precise Anion Gap

Some authors have proposed adjusting the normal range for anion gap by the patent's albumin[26] and phosphate,[27] thereby avoiding the problem of insensitivity. Each g/dL of albumin has a charge of 2.8 mM at pH 7.4 and each mg/dL of phosphate has a charge of 0.59 mM at pH 7.4. At a typical venous pH (which is not 7.4), the "normal" anion gap for a given patient can be estimated as

$$AG = 2(\text{albumin}) + 0.5(\text{phosphate})$$

The following method should be precise[20]:

$$AG = A^- = pH\,[(1.16 \times \text{albumin}) + (0.42 \times P_i)] - 5.83 \times \text{albumin} - 1.28 \times P_i$$

The latter equation requires measurement of plasma pH in the sample in addition to the measurement of albumin and phosphate. This equation seems to be accurate[28] and is entirely consistent with the former one, but it is new and relatively untried. The main limitation of both is the accuracy of the measurement of $Na^+ + K^+ - Cl^-$ as well as the accuracy of pH, albumin, and P_i. Further work is needed to determine confidence limits and values in routine care of patients. The general concept of measuring anion gap more precisely has led to what is now often referred to as the *strong ion gap* (SIG).[29] It may also be referred to as the BB − SID gap.

MIXED DISORDERS

If the compensation for a given acid-base disturbance is appropriate (see Fig. 75–5 or Fig. 75–7), there is only one disorder. For example, the acid-base disorder of the 21-year-old man with cardiogenic shock was acute metabolic acidosis with respiratory compensation. If acute respiratory distress syndrome had developed after reperfusion of his ischemic intestine, however, his lungs might have become so stiff and noncompliant that he would be unable to lower Pa_{CO_2} to the level expected for his metabolic acidosis. Hence, even if the Pa_{CO_2} were then 40 mm Hg, the patient could be said to have metabolic acidosis and respiratory acidosis, because respiratory compensation would be less than expected (Fig. 75–10).

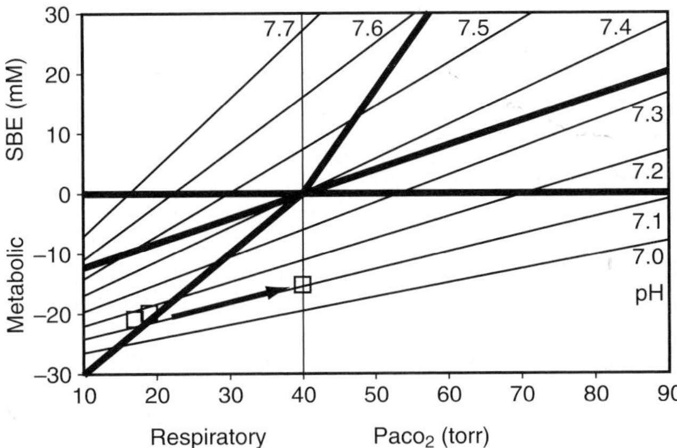

Figure 75–10. Hypothetical data. If the patient whose data are shown in Figure 75–9 had a normal Pa_{CO_2}, he could be considered to have a mixed disturbance—metabolic acidosis with inappropriate ventilation (i.e., with respiratory acidosis).

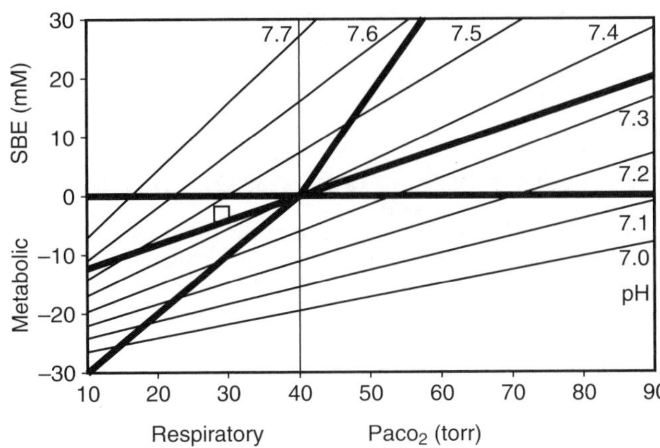

Figure 75–11. Data for a patient with severe metabolic acidosis resulting from renal failure as well as severe metabolic alkalosis from nasogastric suction. The standard base excess (SBE) is nearly zero because the two disturbances cancel each other out.

Most mixed disorders are easy to recognize with an acid-base map, because the patient's data do not fall within ± 5 mM or mm Hg of the dark lines. Others, however, can be missed. Strict attention to the anion gap can usually prevent a misdiagnosis.

CASE HISTORY

A 78-year-old woman experienced severe "abdominal angina" for 2 months with postprandial nausea and vomiting. An angiogram revealed celiac artery stenosis, a 5-cm abdominal aortic aneurysm, and right renal artery stenosis. Intraoperatively, exposure of the celiac artery origin required that her diaphragm and two ribs be divided. A fibrous band about the celiac origin was divided, and the aortic aneurysm was repaired. Renal failure occurred even though there was no intraoperative hypotension, there was minimal blood loss, and 9 L of isotonic fluid had been administered. She required a total of 25 L of resuscitation fluid in the first 4 days to replace that which seemed to have escaped into the interstitial space as a consequence of necessary operative trauma. By postoperative day 9, she was no longer edematous because combined nasogastric and chest tube drainage had been nearly 5 L/day. She was extubated. With room air, her ABG determinations revealed pH 7.46, Pa_{CO_2} 29 mm Hg, P_{O_2} 94 mm Hg, HCO_3^- 20.3 mM, and SBE −3 mM. Blood urea nitrogen was 75, and serum creatinine was 4.5. Plasma Na^+ was 126, K^+ 4.0, Cl^- 79, and HCO_3^- 25 mM. Anion gap was 26 mM. Her data are shown in Figure 75–11.

Commentary

Analysis of SBE versus Pa_{CO_2} (see Fig. 75–11) or of HCO_3^- versus Pa_{CO_2} (see Fig. 75–5) would lead the unwary clinician to conclude that this patient had acute or chronic respiratory alkalosis, because the data lie within ± 5 mM of either. The SBE of -3 mM (within ±5 mM of zero) is inconsistent with the anion gap of 26 mM, suggesting another interpretation of the results. SBE is the quantity of strong acid or base that would be needed to restore the pH of the ECF to 7.4 if Pa_{CO_2} were 40 mm Hg. The progressive buildup of SO_4^{2-} (a strong anion) in renal failure has been largely counterbalanced by the gastric loss of the strong anion Cl^-. This patient could be said to have a triple disorder—hypochloremic metabolic alkalosis, metabolic acidosis of renal failure, and acute respiratory alkalosis.

An example with more urgent implications would be a patient with chronic respiratory acidosis, Pa_{CO_2} 70 mm Hg, pH 7.35, HCO_3^- 38 mM, and SBE 12 mM, in whom lactic acidosis develops as a result of septic shock. The rise in lactate could counterbalance the SBE of 12 mM, lowering it to zero, giving the mistaken appearance of an acute respiratory acidosis. The same incorrect diagnosis would be apparent using either a diagram of HCO_3^- versus $Paco_2$ (see Fig. 75-5) or a diagram of SBE versus $Paco_2$ (see Fig.75-7). Anion gap would typically be positive in such a case, although an astute clinician should already have guessed the correct diagnosis before the plasma electrolytes became available.

ACID-BASE QUANTITATION IN TISSUE

The same acid-base principles that apply to flowing blood also apply to tissue. The acid-base question in tissue currently of greatest interest to intensivists is whether or not the O_2 supply is adequate. The quest by intensivists for a reliable parameter for detecting dysoxia has often been referred to as their "holy grail." The use of tissue acid-base status seems to be a step in the right direction. An inadequate O_2 supply stimulates anaerobic glycolysis and the formation of lactic acid, which at human pH levels is a strong acid, equipotent with HCl. When tissue lactate increases, HCO_3^- is forced to lose its charge to preserve electroneutrality and so becomes CO_2 and H_2O. The result is tissue hypercarbia and acidemia.

Acid-base balance in stomach tissue of patients, as it relates to the adequacy of O_2 supply, is being explored in clinical practice. Most publications have reported gastric tissue pH, "pHi" or "pHim," that was calculated by measuring Pco_2 in a silicone (Silastic) balloon (tonometer) at the tip of a nasogastric tube. ABG values must also be obtained, arterial HCO_3^- calculated from them using the Henderson-Hasselbalch equation, and then tissue pH calculated by a second use of the same equation, this time using the balloon Pco_2 and arterial HCO_3^-. Tissue pH calculated in this manner seems to be reasonably accurate when blood flow is adequate.[30]

An important misconception regarding gastric tissue pH is that there is a single critical value for it.[31] In actuality (i.e., in nature), tissue pH closely parallels arterial pH as the pH of the ECF changes.[32] For example, the tissue pH of a patient with severe diabetic ketoacidosis is acidic, simply because the blood perfusing the tissue is acidic. If the clinician further wishes to know whether the tissue is dysoxic, what matters is not the absolute tissue pH but, rather, the difference between tissue pH and arterial pH. Gastric tissue pH is not easily measured directly.

A simpler approach is to look at the tissue-arterial Pco_2 difference, avoiding the need for the Henderson-Hasselbalch equation. Two separate attempts[28, 33] to define it yielded different values, partly because of differences in the methods used to measure tissue Pco_2. In any event, efforts so far suggest that the tissue-arterial Pco_2 difference is a sensitive indicator of tissue dysoxia. The definition of critical arterial-tissue Pco_2 difference ought to be possible using multiple independent methods.

SUMMARY

Primary respiratory and primary metabolic disturbances both produce abnormal arterial Pco_2. To quantify the metabolic abnormality, the only additional number needed is the arterial plasma pH, from which SBE (standard base excess) can be computed. During an acute respiratory disturbance, SBE is zero, because there is no metabolic compensation. During chronic respiratory disturbance, SBE changes by 0.4 times the change in $Paco_2$ to compensate (partially) for the change in pH. During metabolic alkalosis, the compensatory increase in respiratory acid ($Paco_2$) is 0.6 times the decrease in metabolic acid. During metabolic acidosis, the compensatory decrease in $Paco_2$ equals the increase in SBE. The anion gap (in arterial or venous plasma) detects the most worrisome metabolic acidoses, whereas SBE does not discriminate between anion gap and non-anion gap acidoses.

Further refinements of the anion gap may prove helpful in care of patients. Use of the tissue acid-base balance seems the best current prospect for detecting inadequate O_2 supply to individual organs, but this approach is not yet sufficiently developed to be used routinely in clinical practice.

ACKNOWLEDGMENT

The author thanks Professor John W. Severinghaus for editorial assistance.

References

1. Knaus WA, Wagner DP, Draper EA, et al: The APACHE III prognostic system: Risk prediction of hospital mortality for critically ill hospitalized adults. Chest 1991; 100:1619–1636.
2. Cloutier CT, Lowery BD, Carey LC: Acid-base disturbances in hemorrhagic shock in 66 severely wounded patients prior to treatment. Arch Surg 1969; 98:551–557
3. Maynard N, Bihari D, Beale R, et al: Assessment of splanchnic oxygenation by gastric tonometry in patients with acute circulatory failure. JAMA 1993; 270:1203–1210.
4. Berger AJ: Control of breathing. *In*: Textbook of Respiratory Medicine. Murray JF, Nadel JA (Eds). Philadelphia, WB Saunders, 1994, pp 199–218.
5. Schlichtig R, Grogono AW, Severinghaus JW: Human $Paco_2$ and standard base excess compensation for acid-base imbalance. Crit Care Med 1998; 26:1173–1179.
6. Schlichtig R, Grogono AW, Severinghaus JW: Current status of acid-base quantitation in physiology and medicine. Anesthesiol Clin North Am 1998; 16:211–233.
7. Schlichtig R: Base excess vs. strong ion difference: Are they really different? Physiologist 1996; 39:146.
8. Singer RB, Hastings AB: An improved clinical method for the estimation of disturbances of the acid-base balance of human blood. Medicine (Baltimore) 1948; 27:223–242.
9. Singer RB, Clark JK, Barker ES, Crosley AP, Elkinton JR: The acute effects in man of rapid intravenous infusion of hypertonic sodium bicarbonate solution. I. Changes in acid-base balance and distribution of the excess buffer base. Medicine (Baltimore) 1955; 34:51–95.
10. Siggaard-Andersen O: The Acid-Base Status of Blood. 4th ed. Copenhagen, Munksgaard, 1974.
11. Stewart PA: How to Understand Acid-Base: A Quantitative Acid-Base Primer for Biology and Medicine. New York, Elsevier/North-Holland, 1981, p 136.
12. Lehninger AL: Biochemistry. *In*: The Molecular Basis of Cell Structure and Function. New York, Worth Publishers, 1970, p 47.
13. Wilkes P: Hypoproteinemia, strong-ion difference, and acid-base status in critically ill patients. J Appl Physiol 1998; 84:1740–1748.
14. Severinghaus JW, Stupfel M, Bradley AF: Accuracy of blood pH and Pco_2 determinations. J Appl Physiol 1956; 9:189–196.
15. Severinghaus JW, Stupfel M, Bradley AF: Variations of serum carbonic acid pK′ with pH and temperature. J Appl Physiol 1956; 9:197–203.
16. Figge J, Mydosh T, Fencl V: Serum proteins and acid-base equilibria: A follow-up. J Lab Clin Med 1992; 120:713–719.
17. Siggaard-Andersen O: The Van Slyke equation. Scand J Clin Lab Invest 1977; 37(Suppl 146):15–20.
18. Stewart PA: Modern quantitative acid-base chemistry. Can J Physiol Pharmacol 1983; 61:1444–1461.
19. Funder J, Wieth JD: Chloride and hydrogen ion distribution between human red cells and plasma. Acta Physiol Scand 1966; 68:234–245.
20. Schlichtig R: [Base excess] vs [strong ion difference]: Which is more helpful? Ad Exp Med Biol 1997; 411:91–96.
21. Schlichtig R: [Base excess] and [strong ion difference] during O_2-CO_2 exchange. Ad Exp Med Biol 1997; 411:97–102.
22. McAuliff JJ, Lind LJ, Leith DE, Fencl V: Hypoproteinemic alkalosis. Am J Med 1986; 81:86–90.
23. Kellum JA, Bellomo R, Kramer DJ, Pinsky MR: Splanchnic buffering of metabolic acid during early endotoxemia. J Crit Care 1997; 12:7-12.

24. Narins RG, Emmett M: Simple and mixed acid-base disorders: A practical approach. Medicine (Baltimore) 1980; 59:161–187.
25. Schlichtig R: Simulation of maximum respiratory venous P_{CO_2} in vitro. Acta Anaesthesiol Scand 1995; 39(Suppl 107):143–149.
26. Gabow PA: Disorders associated with an altered anion gap. Kidney Int 1985; 27:472–483.
27. Kellum JA: Recent advances in acid-base physiology applied in critical care. *In*: Yearbook of Intensive Care and Emergency Medicine. Vincent JL (Ed). Heidelberg, Springer-Verlag, (in press).
28. Rozenfeld RA, Dishart MK, Tønnessen TI, Schlichtig R: Methods for detecting intestinal ischemic anaerobic metabolic acidosis by local P_{CO_2}. J Appl Physiol 1996; 81:1834–1842.
29. Kellum JA, Kramer DJ, Pinsky MR: Strong ion gap: A methodology for exploring unexplained anions. J Crit Care 1995; 10:51–55.
30. Antonsson JB, Boyle CC, Kruithoff KL, et al: Validation of tonometric measurement of gut intramural pH during endotoxemia and mesenteric occlusion in pigs. Am J Physiol 1990; 259:G519–G523.
31. Schlichtig R, Mehta N, Gayowski TJP: Tissue-arterial P_{CO_2} difference is a better marker of ischemia than intramural pH (pHi) or arterial pH-pHi difference. J Crit Care 1996; 11:51–56.
32. Adler S: The simultaneous determination of muscle cell pH using a weak acid and weak base. J Clin Invest 1972; 51:256–265.
33. Schlichtig R, Bowles SA: Distinguishing between aerobic and anaerobic appearance of P_{CO_2} in intestine during low flow. J Appl Physiol 1994; 76:2443–2451.

76

Diagnosis and Treatment of Acid-Base Disorders

John A. Kellum, MD

In general, acid-base disorders are more important for what they tell the clinician than for any harm they pose to the patient. Most acid-base disorders are mild and well tolerated, but they allow the astute clinician to recognize underlying disorders that otherwise might be difficult to diagnose or even suspect. For example, salicylate intoxication is one of only a few disorders that routinely produce both a primary respiratory alkalosis and a primary positive–anion gap metabolic acidosis. Correctly interpreting this mixed acid-base disorder allows one to quickly arrive at a short differential diagnosis and to obtain salicylate levels to confirm the exact diagnosis. Thus, even though this acid-base disorder itself is usually benign, the disorder that causes it can be life-threatening.

Under certain circumstances, however, acid-base derangements are themselves dangerous. Such is the case when the disorders are extreme (e.g., pH < 7.0 or pH > 7.7) or when they develop quickly. Severe abnormalities may cause organ dysfunction, which may have a broad range of clinical manifestations (e.g., cerebral edema, seizures, decreased myocardial contractility, pulmonary vasoconstriction, systemic vasodilation). Furthermore, even less extreme derangements may produce harm because of the patient's response to the abnormality. For example, a spontaneously breathing patient with metabolic acidosis attempts to compensate by increasing minute ventilation. This may lead to respiratory muscle fatigue with respiratory failure or diversion of blood flow from vital organs to the respiratory muscles, resulting in organ injury. The increased catecholamine levels associated with acidemia may lead to cardiac arrhythmias in critically ill patients or increase myocardial oxygen demand in patients with acute myocardial infarction. In such cases, it may be prudent not only to treat the underlying disorder but also to provide symptomatic treatment for the acid-base disorder itself. Accordingly, it is important to understand both the causes of acid-base disorders and the limitations of various treatment strategies.

In Chapter 75, the basic mechanisms of acid-base balance were reviewed, focusing on the physicochemical determinants of pH in the blood and tissues. These determinants are the difference between strong cations (e.g., Na^+, K^+) and strong anions (e.g., Cl^-, lactate) known as the *strong ion difference* (SID); the total weak acid "buffers" (A_{TOT}), which include mainly albumin and phosphate; and the partial pressure of carbon dioxide (P_{CO_2}). These three variables (SID, A_{TOT}, and P_{CO_2})—and only these three—can independently affect plasma pH. Dependent variables are H^+ and HCO_3^-, whose concentrations in plasma are determined by SID, A_{TOT}, and P_{CO_2}. Changes in H^+ concentration in plasma occur as a result of changes in the dissociation of water and A_{TOT} brought about by the electrochemical forces produced by changes in SID and P_{CO_2}. The *standard base excess* (SBE) is mathematically equivalent to the change in SID required to restore pH to 7.4 given a P_{CO_2} of 40 mm Hg and the prevailing A_{TOT}. Thus, an SBE of -10 mEq/L means that the SID is 10 mEq less than that required to achieve pH 7.4.

The main difference between this physical-chemical approach and other approaches is the emphasis on independent and dependent variables. Only changes in the independent variables (SID, A_{TOT}, and P_{CO_2}) can bring about changes in the dependent variables (H^+ and HCO_3^-). Movements of H^+ or HCO_3^- per se cannot affect their concentrations in plasma unless changes in SID, A_{TOT}, or P_{CO_2} also occur. Several other reviews of this approach are also available in the literature.[1-4] In this chapter, these principles are applied to the clinical arena and the diagnosis and treatment of individual disorders are reviewed. At the end, a unified approach to the patient with acid-base imbalance is presented along with some brief examples.

METABOLIC ACID-BASE DISORDERS

Metabolic acid-base derangements are produced by a significantly greater number of underlying disorders and are almost always more difficult to treat than respiratory disorders. Traditionally, metabolic acidoses and alkaloses have been categorized according to the ions that are responsible for the disorder. Examples include lactic acidosis and chloride-responsive alkalosis. It is important to recognize that metabolic acidosis is produced by a decrease in the SID, which produces an electrochemical force that results in an increase in the free H^+ concentration (see Chapter 75). A decrease in SID may be brought about by generation of organic anions (e.g., lactate, ketones), loss of cations (e.g., diarrhea), mishandling of ions (e.g., renal tubular acidosis) or addition of exogenous anions (e.g., iatrogenic acidosis, poisonings). By contrast, metabolic alkaloses occur as a result of an inappropriately large SID, although the SID need not be greater than the "normal" 40 to 42 mEq/L. This alkalosis may be brought about by loss of anions in excess of cations (e.g., vomiting, diuretics) or rarely by administration of strong cations in excess of strong anions (e.g., transfusion of large volumes of banked blood).

Similarly, the treatment of metabolic acid-base disorders requires a change in the SID. Metabolic acidoses are repaired by increasing the plasma Na^+ concentration more than the plasma Cl^- concentration (e.g., by sodium bicarbonate [$NaHCO_3$] administration), and metabolic alkaloses are repaired by replacing Cl^- either as sodium chloride (NaCl) in large volumes, potassium chloride (KCl), or even hydrogen chloride (HCl). So-called chloride-resistant metabolic alkaloses are resistant to chloride only because of ongoing renal losses that increase in response to increased Cl^- replacement (e.g., hyperaldosteronism).

Pathophysiology

It follows that disorders in metabolic acid-base balance occur in one of three ways: (1) as a result of dysfunction of the primary regulating organs, (2) as a result of exogenous administration of drugs or fluids that alter the body's ability to maintain normal acid-base balance, or (3) as a result of abnormal metabolism that overwhelms the ability of the normal defense mechanisms to work. The organs responsible for regulating SID in both health and disease are the kidneys and, to a lesser extent, the gastrointestinal (GI) tract.

The Kidney

Plasma flows to the kidneys at a rate of approximately 600 mL/min. The glomeruli filter this plasma to yield filtrate at 120 mL/min, and the filtrate is in turn processed by reabsorption and secretion mechanisms in the tubule cells along which the filtrate passes on its way to the ureters. More than 99% of the filtrate is normally reabsorbed and returned to the plasma. Thus, the kidney can excrete only a small amount of strong ion into the urine each minute, and several minutes to hours are therefore required to affect the SID significantly.

The handling of strong ions by the kidney is extremely important because every Cl^- filtered but not reabsorbed decreases the SID. Because most of the human diet contains similar ratios of strong cations to strong anions, sufficient Cl^- is usually available for this to be the primary regulating mechanism. This mechanism is particularly apparent when we consider that renal Na^+ and K^+ handling is influenced by other priorities (e.g., intravascular volume and plasma K^+ homeostasis). Accordingly, "acid handling" by the kidney is generally mediated through Cl^- balance. How the kidney handles Cl^- is obviously important. Traditional approaches to this problem have focused on H^+ excretion and emphasized the importance of NH_3 (ammonia) and its add-on cation NH_4^+. However, H^+ excretion per se is irrelevant, as water provides an essentially infinite source of free H^+. Indeed, the kidney does not excrete H^+ any more as NH_4^+ than it does as H_2O. The purpose of renal ammoniagenesis is to allow the excretion of Cl^- without Na^+ or K^+, and this is achieved by supplying a weak cation (NH_4^+) to excrete with Cl^-.

Occasionally, urine pH is used incorrectly to interpret changes in plasma pH as produced by the action of the kidneys. It is important to realize that urine pH tells us nothing about plasma pH and little about renal "acid" excretion. The urine contains a number of low-molecular-weight substances that are at such low levels in plasma as to be negligible but are concentrated in the urine. For example, ionized phosphates exist in plasma at very low concentrations (<2 mEq/L). These ions constitute a small part of A_{TOT} but have minimum effects on plasma pH. The kidney, however, concentrates these ions to the point that they have a significant effect on urine pH. The presence of phosphate ions in the urine has no effect on plasma SID, PCO_2, or A_{TOT} and, therefore, no effect on plasma pH.

Renal-Hepatic Interaction

As we can see from the preceding discussion, NH_4^+ is important to systemic acid-base balance not because of its carriage of H^+ or because of its direct action in the plasma (normal plasma NH_4^+ concentration is <0.01 mEq/L) but because of its "co-excretion" with Cl^-. Of course, NH_4^+ is produced not only in the kidney. Hepatic ammoniagenesis (and, as we shall see, glutaminogenesis) is also important for systemic acid-base balance and, as expected, is tightly controlled by mechanisms sensitive to plasma pH.[5] Indeed, this reinterpretation of the role of NH_4^+ in acid-base balance is supported by the evidence that hepatic glutaminogenesis is stimulated by acidosis.[6] Nitrogen metabolism by the liver can result in either urea, glutamine, or NH_4^+. Normally, the liver does not release more than a small amount of NH_4^+; rather, it incorporates the nitrogen into either urea or glutamine. Hepatocytes have enzymes that enable them to produce either of these end products, and both allow for the regulation of plasma NH_4^+ at suitably low levels. Urea and glutamine, however, have significantly different effects at the level of the kidney. Glutamine is used by the kidney to generate NH_4^+ and facilitate the excretion of Cl^-. Thus, the production of glutamine can be seen as having an alkalinizing effect on plasma pH because of the way in which the kidney utilizes it.

Further support for this scenario comes from the discovery of an anatomic organization of hepatocytes according to their enzyme content.[7] Hepatocytes with a propensity to produce urea are positioned closer to the portal venule and thus have the first chance at the NH_4^+ delivered. Acidosis inhibits ureagenesis, and under these conditions more NH_4^+ is available for the downstream hepatocytes, which are predisposed to produce glutamine. Thus, the leftover NH_4^+ is "packaged" as glutamine for export to the kidney, where it is used to facilitate Cl^- excretion.

The Gastrointestinal Tract

The GI tract is an important cause of metabolic acid-base imbalance. Along its length, the GI tract handles strong ions quite differently. In the stomach, Cl^- is pumped out of the plasma and into the lumen, reducing the SID of the gastric juice and thus reducing the pH. On the plasma side, the SID is increased by the loss of Cl^- and the pH is increased, producing the so-called alkaline tide, which occurs at the beginning of a meal when gastric acid secretion is maximum.[8] In the duodenum, Cl^- is reabsorbed and the plasma pH is restored. Normally, only slight changes in plasma pH are evident because Cl^- is returned to the circulation almost as soon as it is removed. If gastric secretions are removed from the patient, however, either by suction catheter or by vomiting, Cl^- is progressively lost and the SID steadily increases. It is the Cl^- loss, not the H^+, that is the determinant of plasma pH. Although H^+ is "lost" as HCl, it is also lost with every molecule of water removed from the body. When Cl^- (a strong anion) is lost without loss of a strong cation, the SID is increased and therefore the plasma H^+ concentration is decreased. When H^+ is "lost" as water (HOH) rather than HCl, there is no change in the SID and hence no change in the plasma H^+ concentration.

In contrast to the stomach, the pancreas secretes fluid into the small intestine that has an SID much higher than that of plasma and is low in Cl^-. Thus, the plasma perfusing the pancreas has its SID decreased, a phenomenon that peaks about an hour after a meal and helps counteract the alkaline tide. If large amounts of pancreatic fluid are lost (e.g., from surgical drainage), an acidosis results as a consequence of the decreased plasma SID.

In the large intestine, fluid also has a high SID because most of the Cl^- has been removed in the small intestine and the remaining electrolytes are mostly Na^+ and K^+. The body normally reabsorbs much of the water and electrolytes from this fluid, but when severe diarrhea exists, large amounts of cations can be lost. If this loss is persistent, the plasma SID decreases and acidosis results.

In addition to the acid-base effects of abnormal loss of strong ions from the lumen of the GI tract, the small intestine, in particular, may contribute strong ions to the plasma. This

TABLE 76–1. Causes of an Increased Anion Gap

Common Causes	*Rare Causes*
Renal failure	Dehydration
Ketoacidosis	Sodium salts
Diabetic	Sodium lactate
Alcoholic	Sodium citrate
Starvation	Sodium acetate
Metabolic errors	Sodium penicillin (>50 million units/day)
Lactic acidosis	
Toxins	Carbenicillin (>30 g/day)
Methanol	Decreased unmeasured cation
Ethylene glycol	Hypomagnesemia
Salicylates	Hypokalemia
Paraldehyde	Hypocalcemia
	Alkalosis

contribution is most apparent when mesenteric blood flow is compromised and lactate is produced, sometimes in large quantities. Although global hypoperfusion may compromise the mesentery, the intestine does not appear to be a source of lactic acid in resuscitated sepsis[9] (see later section on lactic acidosis). Moreover, whether the GI tract is capable of regulating strong ion uptake in a compensatory fashion has not been well studied. There is some evidence that the gut may modulate systemic acidosis in experimental endotoxemia by removing anions from the plasma.[10] The full capacity of this organ to affect acid-base balance is unknown, however.

Metabolic Acidosis

Traditionally, metabolic acidoses have been categorized according to the presence or absence of unmeasured anions. We can routinely detect these unmeasured anions by examining the plasma electrolytes and calculating the anion gap (AG) as described in the following. The differential diagnosis for a positive-AG acidosis is shown in Table 76–1. Non-AG acidoses can be divided into three types: (1) renal, (2) gastrointestinal, and (3) iatrogenic (Fig. 76–1). In the intensive care unit (ICU), the most common types of metabolic acidosis include lactic acidosis, ketoacidosis, iatrogenic acidosis, and toxin-produced acidosis.

Even extreme acidosis appears to be well tolerated by healthy individuals, particularly when the exposure is brief. For example, healthy individuals may achieve an arterial pH less than 7.15 and a lactate concentration above 20 mEq/L during maximum exercise.[11] Chronically, however, even mild acidemia (pH < 7.35) may produce metabolic bone disease and protein catabolism. Furthermore, critically ill patients may not tolerate even brief episodes of acidemia.[12] The potential effects of metabolic acidosis and alkalosis on vital organ function are shown in Table 76–2. There appear to be significant

TABLE 76–2. Potential Clinical Effects of Metabolic Acid-Base Disorders

Metabolic Acidosis	Metabolic Alkalosis
Cardiovascular	***Cardiovascular***
Decreased inotropy	↑ Inotropy (Ca^{2+} entry)
Conduction defects	Altered coronary blood flow*
Arterial vasodilatation	Digoxin toxicity
Venous vasoconstriction	***Neuromuscular***
Oxygen Delivery	Neuromuscular excitability
Decreased oxyhemoglobin binding	Encephalopathy
Decreased 2,3-DPG (late)	Seizures
Neuromuscular	***Metabolic Effect***
Respiratory depression	Hypokalemia
Decreased sensorium	Hypocalcemia
Metabolism	Hypophosphatemia
Protein wasting	Impaired enzyme function
Bone demineralization	***Oxygen Delivery***
Catecholamine, PTH, and aldosterone stimulation	Increased oxyhemoglobin affinity
Insulin resistance	Increased 2,3-DPG (delayed)
Gastrointestinal Effect	
Emesis	
Electrolytes	
Hyperkalemia	
Hypercalcemia	
Hyperuricemia	

*Animal studies have shown both increased and decreased coronary artery blood flow.
2,3-DPG = 2,3-diphosphoglycerate; PTH = parathyroid hormone.

differences between metabolic acidosis and respiratory acidosis in terms of the outcome of patients, and this suggests that the underlying disorder is perhaps more important than the absolute degree of acidemia.[13]

If prudence dictates that symptomatic therapy is to be provided, consideration should be given to the likely duration of the disorder. If the disorder is expected to be short-lived (e.g., diabetic ketoacidosis), maximizing respiratory compensation is usually the safest approach. When the disorder resolves, ventilation can be quickly reduced to normal and there are no lingering effects of therapy. By contrast, if the SID is increased (e.g., by using $NaHCO_3$), there is a risk of alkalosis when the underlying disorder resolves. If the disorder is likely to be more chronic (e.g., renal failure), therapy aimed at restoring the SID is indicated. In all cases, the therapeutic target can be determined from the SBE quite accurately. As discussed in Chapter 75, the SBE corresponds to the amount by which the SID must change in order to restore the pH to

URINE STRONG ION DIFFERENCE (NA + K – Cl)

(+) **Renal Tubular Acidosis**	(–) **Nonrenal**
Urine pH > 5.5	Gastrointestinal
Distal (type I)	Diarrhea
	Small-bowel/pancreatic drainage
Urine pH < 5.5	
Low serum K^+	Iatrogenic
Proximal (type II)	Parenteral nutrition
	Saline
High serum K^+	Carbonic anhydrase inhibitors
Aldosterone deficiency (type IV)	Anion exchange resins

Figure 76–1. Differential diagnosis of a hyperchloremic metabolic acidosis.

7.4 if we assume a P_{CO_2} of 40 mm Hg. Thus, if the SID is 30 mEq/L and the SBE is −10 mEq/L, the target SID is 40 mEq/L. Accordingly, the plasma Na^+ concentration would have to increase by 10 mEq/L for $NaHCO_3$ administration to repair the acidosis completely. If increasing the plasma Na^+ concentration is inadvisable for other reasons (e.g., hypernatremia), $NaHCO_3$ administration is also inadvisable.

In addition, $NaHCO_3$ administration is associated with certain disadvantages. Large (hypertonic) doses given rapidly may actually decrease the blood pressure[14] and have the potential to cause sudden, severe increases in P_{CO_2}.[15] Accordingly, it is important to assess patients' ventilatory status before $NaHCO_3$ is administered, particularly patients who are not mechanically ventilated. $NaHCO_3$ infusion also affects the serum K^+ and Ca^+ concentrations, and these need to be monitored closely.

Alternative therapies for metabolic acidosis have been developed in order to avoid some of these disadvantages. Carbicarb is an equimolar mixture of sodium carbonate (Na_2CO_3) and $NaHCO_3$.[16] Carbicarb works by increasing the plasma Na^+ concentration in the same way that $NaHCO_3$ works, but Carbicarb does not increase P_{CO_2}. Animal studies have shown mixed results with Carbicarb,[17] and human experience is extremely limited.

Tromethamine (Tris buffer or Tham) is a synthetic buffer that consumes CO_2 and readily penetrates cells.[18] Tromethamine is a weak base (dissociation constant pK = 7.9) and, as such, is unlike other plasma constituents. The major advantage of this agent is that it does not alter the SID, and thus there is no concern about having to increase the plasma Na^+ concentration in order to achieve an effect. Accordingly, it is often used in situations in which $NaHCO_3$ cannot be used because of hypernatremia. Even though this agent has been available since the 1960s, data are surprisingly limited in humans with acid-base disorders. In small uncontrolled studies, tromethamine appeared to be effective in reversing metabolic acidosis secondary to ketoacidosis or renal failure without obvious toxicity.[19] When concentrations exceeding 0.3 M were used, however, adverse reactions were reported, including hypoglycemia, respiratory depression, and even fatal hepatic necrosis. In Europe, a mixture of tromethamine, acetate, $NaHCO_3$, and disodium phosphate is available (Tribonate). This mixture seems to have fewer side effects than tromethamine alone, but experience is still limited.

The Anion Gap and the Strong Ion Gap

For more than 30 years, the AG has been used by clinicians and has evolved into a major tool for evaluating acid-base disorders.[20] The AG is calculated, or rather estimated, from the differences between the routinely measured concentrations of serum cations (Na^+ and K^+) and anions (Cl^- and HCO_3^-). Normally, this difference or "gap" is made up by albumin and, to a lesser extent, by phosphate. Sulfate and lactate also contribute a small amount, normally less than 2 mEq/L. There are also unmeasured cations such as Ca^{2+} and Mg^{2+}, and these tend to offset the effects of sulfate and lactate except when either is abnormally increased (Fig. 76–2). Plasma proteins other than albumin can be either positively or negatively charged but in the aggregate tend to be neutral,[21] except in rare cases of abnormal paraproteins such as those in multiple myeloma. In practice, the AG is calculated as follows:

$$AG = (Na^+ + K^+) - (Cl^- + HCO_3^-)$$

Because of its low and narrow extracellular concentration, K^+ is often omitted from the calculation. Normal values with relatively wide ranges reported by most laboratories are 12 ± 4 mEq/L (if K^+ is considered) and 8 ± 4 mEq/L (if K^+ is not considered). The value of a "normal AG" has decreased since the introduction of more accurate methods for measuring the Cl^- concentration.[22, 23] However, the various measurement techniques available mandate that each institution reports its own expected normal AG.

The utility of the AG derives primarily from its ability to quickly and easily limit the differential diagnosis for a patient with metabolic acidosis. If an increased AG is present, the explanation is almost invariably found among four disorders: ketosis, lactic acidosis, poisoning, and renal failure.[24] Besides these, several conditions can alter the accuracy of AG estimation, and they are frequently seen in critical illness.[25, 26]

Dehydration may induce a parallel increment in the apparent AG by increasing the concentration of all the ions. Severe hypoalbuminemia causes a decrease in the AG, and it has been recommended that the AG be corrected for the prevailing albumin concentration because each gram-per-deciliter (g/dL) decline in serum albumin reduces the apparent AG by 2.5 to 3 mEq/L.[27] Respiratory and metabolic alkaloses are associated with an increase of up to 3 to 10 mEq/L in the apparent AG after enhanced lactate production (resulting from stimulated phosphofructokinase enzymatic activity), the reduction in the ionized weak acids (A^-), and possibly the additional effect of dehydration (with its own impact on AG calculation). A low Mg^{2+} concentration with associated low K^+ and Ca^{2+} concentrations and the administration of sodium salts of poorly reabsorbable anions (such as β-lactam antibiotics) are known causes of an increased AG.[28] Certain parenteral nutrition formulations, such as those containing acetate, may increase the AG, and citrate may rarely have the same effect in the setting of multiple blood transfusions, particularly if massive doses of banked blood are used, such as during liver transplantation.[29] None of these rare causes, however, increases the AG significantly,[30] and each is usually easily identified.

Some additional cases of an increased AG of unknown cause have been reported. In the nonketotic hyperosmolar state of diabetes, an AG has been found that remains unexplained.[31] Unmeasured anions have been reported in the blood of patients with sepsis[32, 33] and liver disease[34, 35] and in experimental animals given endotoxin.[36] These anions may be the source of much of the unexplained acidosis seen in patients with critical illness.[37]

Additional doubt has been cast on the diagnostic value of the AG in certain situations.[25, 33] Salem and Mujais[25] found routine reliance on the AG to be "fraught with numerous pitfalls." The primary problem with the AG is its reliance on the use of a "normal" range produced by albumin and to a lesser extent phosphate as discussed earlier. These constituents may be grossly abnormal in patients with critical illness, leading to a change in the normal range for these patients. Moreover, because these anions are not strong anions, their charge is altered by changes in pH. This has prompted some authors to adjust the normal range for the AG by the patient's albumin[27] or even phosphate[38] concentration. Each g/dL of albumin has a charge of 2.8 mEq/L at pH 7.4 (2.3 mEq/L at 7.0 and 3.0 mEq/L at 7.6), and each mg/dL of phosphate has a charge of 0.59 mEq/L at pH 7.4 (0.55 mEq/L at 7.0 and 0.61 mEq/L at 7.6).

Thus, a convenient way to estimate the normal AG for a given patient is by use of the following formula[38]:

$$\text{"normal" AG} = 2(\text{albumin g/dL}) + 0.5(\text{phosphate mg/dL})$$

or in international units (IU):

$$\text{"normal" AG} = 0.2(\text{albumin g/L}) + 1.5(\text{phosphate mmol/L})$$

When this patient-specific normal range was used to examine the presence of unmeasured anions in the blood of critically

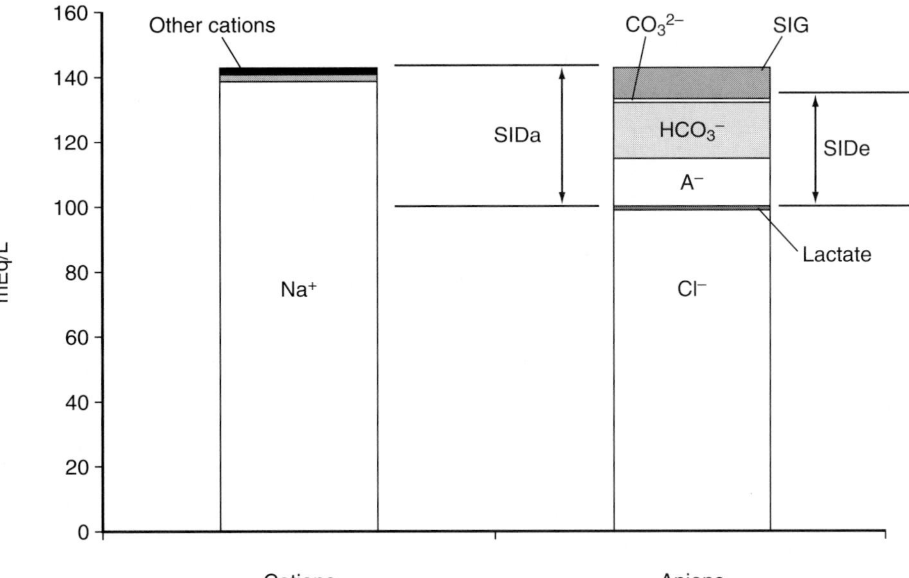

Figure 76–2. Charge balance in blood plasma. "Other cations" include Ca^{2+} and Mg^{2+}. The strong ion difference (SID) is always positive (in plasma) and SID − SIDe (effective) must equal zero. Any difference between SID apparent (SIDa) and SIDe is the strong ion gap (SIG) and must represent unmeasured anions. (From Kellum JA: Metabolic acidosis in the critically ill: Lessons from physical chemistry. Kidney Int 1998; 153:S81–S86.)

ill patients, the accuracy of this method improved from 33% with the routine AG (normal range = 12 mEq/L) to 96%.[38] This technique should be used only when the pH is less than 7.35, and even then it is accurate only within 5 mEq/L. When more accuracy is needed, the reader is referred to slightly more complicated methods of estimating A^-.[34, 39]

Another alternative to the traditional AG is the SID. By definition, the SID must be equal and opposite to the negative charges contributed by A^- and total CO_2 (see Chapter 75). The latter value, the sum of charges from A^- and total CO_2, has been termed "SID-effective" (SIDe).[21] The apparent SID (SIDa) is obtained by measurement of each individual ion. The SIDa and the SIDe should both equal the true SID. If SIDa and SIDe differ, unmeasured ions must exist. If SIDa is greater than SIDe these ions are anions, and if SIDa is less than SIDe they are cations. This difference has been termed the *strong ion gap* (SIG) to distinguish it from the AG.[34] Unlike the AG, the SIG is normally zero and does not change with changes in pH or albumin concentration, as does the AG.

Positive Anion Gap Acidoses

Lactic Acidosis

In many forms of critical illness, lactate is the most important cause of metabolic acidosis.[40] Lactate has been shown to correlate with outcome in patients with hemorrhagic[41] and septic shock.[42] Lactic acid is traditionally viewed as the predominant source of metabolic acidosis occurring in sepsis.[43] In this view, lactic acid is released primarily from the musculature and the gut as a consequence of tissue hypoxia. Moreover, the amount of lactate produced is thought to correlate with the total oxygen debt, the magnitude of the hypoperfusion, and the severity of shock.[40]

This view has been challenged by the observations that during sepsis, even with profound shock, resting muscle does not produce lactate. Indeed, studies by various investigators have shown that the musculature may actually consume lactate during endotoxemia.[9, 44, 45] Data concerning the gut are less clear. There is little question that underperfused gut can release lactate; however, it does not appear that the gut releases lactate during sepsis if its perfusion is maintained. Under such conditions, the mesentery is either neutral to or even takes up lactate.[9, 44] Perfusion is probably a major determinant of mesenteric lactate metabolism. In a canine model of sepsis in which endotoxin was used, gut lactate production could not be shown when flow was maintained with dopexamine hydrochloride.[45]

It is interesting that studies in animals as well as humans have shown that the lung may be a prominent source of lactate in the setting of acute lung injury.[9, 46–48] Although studies such as these do not address the underlying pathophysiologic mechanisms of hyperlactatemia in sepsis, they do suggest that the conventional wisdom regarding lactate as evidence of tissue dysoxia is an oversimplification at best. Indeed, many investigators have begun to offer alternative interpretations of hyperlactatemia in this setting.[47–51]

Table 76–3 lists several alternative sources of hyperlactatemia. These include metabolic dysfunction resulting from mitochondrial enzymatic derangements, which can and do lead to lactic acidosis. In particular, pyruvate dehydrogenase (PDH), the enzyme responsible for moving pyruvate into the Krebs cycle (Fig. 76–3), is inhibited by endotoxin.[52] Data from other studies, however, suggest that increased aerobic metabolism may be more important than metabolic defects or anaerobic metabolism. Gore and colleagues[53] observed increased glucose and pyruvate production and oxidation in

TABLE 76–3. Mechanisms Associated with Increased Serum Lactate Concentration

Tissue Hypoxia
Hypodynamic shock
Organ ischemia
Hypermetabolism
Increased aerobic glycolysis
Increased protein catabolism
Hematologic malignancies
Decreased Clearance of Lactate
Liver failure
Shock
Inhibition of Pyruvate Dehydrogenase
Thiamine deficiency
Endotoxin?
Activation of Inflammatory Cells?

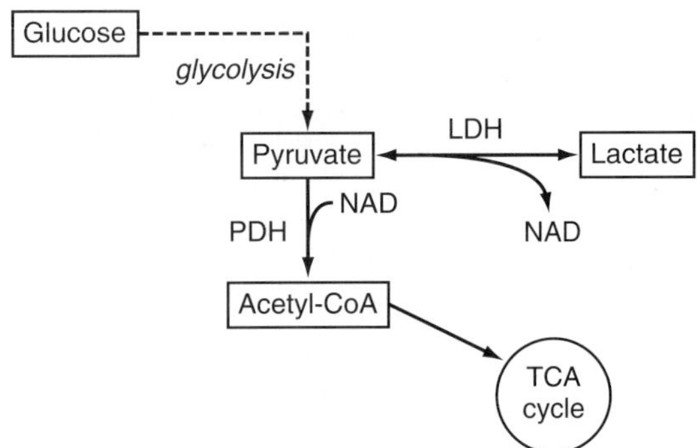

Figure 76–3. Simplified metabolic pathway for lactate. Note that lactate production generates nicotinamide-adenine dinucleotide (NAD), which is essential for metabolism of pyruvate. LDH = lactate dehydrogenase; PDH = pyruvate dehydrogenase; TCA = trichloroacetic acid.

patients with sepsis. Furthermore, when PDH was stimulated by dichloroacetate, there was an additional increase in oxygen consumption but a decrease in glucose and pyruvate production. These results suggest that hyperlactatemia in sepsis occurs as a consequence of increased aerobic metabolism rather than tissue hypoxia or PDH inhibition.

Such findings are consistent with known metabolic effects of lactate production on cellular bioenergetics.[54] Lactate production alters the cytosolic and hence mitochondrial redox state such that the increased ratio of reduced nicotinamide-adenine dinucleotide (NADH) to NAD supports oxidative phosphorylation as the dominant source of ATP production. Finally, use of catecholamines, especially epinephrine, also results in lactic acidosis, presumably by stimulating cellular metabolism (e.g., increased hepatic glycolysis), and may be a common source of lactic acidosis in the ICU.[55, 56] Interestingly, this phenomenon does not appear to occur with either dobutamine or norepinephrine[56] and does not appear to be related to decreased tissue perfusion.

Although controversy exists about the source and interpretation of lactic acidosis in critically ill patients, there is no question about the ability of lactate accumulation to produce acidemia. Lactate is a strong ion by virtue of the fact that at a pH within the physiologic range, it is almost completely dissociated (i.e., the pK of lactate is 3.9; at a pH of 7.4, 3162 ions are dissociated for every one that is not). Because the body can produce and dispose of lactate rapidly, it functions as one of the most dynamic components of the SID. Lactic acid, therefore, can produce significant acidemia.

Just as often, however, critically ill patients have hyperlactatemia that is much greater than the amount of acidosis seen. In fact, hyperlactatemia may exist without any metabolic acidosis at all. This is not because acid "generation" is separate from lactate production, such as through "unreversed ATP hydrolysis."[57] Phosphate is a weak acid and does not contribute substantially to metabolic acidosis even under extreme circumstances. Furthermore, the H^+ concentration is determined not by how much H^+ is produced or removed from the plasma but rather by changes in the dissociation of water and weak ions. Virtually anywhere in the body, pH is above 6.0 and lactate behaves as a strong ion. Its generation decreases the SID and results in an increased H^+ concentration.

There are two possible explanations for increased lactate without increased H^+. First, if lactate is added to the plasma not as lactic acid but rather as the salt of a strong acid (e.g., sodium lactate), there is little change in the SID because a strong cation (Na^+) is being added along with a strong anion. In fact, as lactate is removed by metabolism, the remaining Na^+ increases the SID, resulting in metabolic alkalosis. Hence, it would be possible to give enough lactate to increase the plasma lactate concentration without increasing the H^+ concentration. The amount of exogenous lactate required would be quite large, because normal metabolism results in the turnover of approximately 1500 to 4500 millimoles of lactic acid per day. Thus, only large amounts of lactate infused rapidly would result in appreciable increases in the plasma lactate concentration. For example, the use of lactate-based hemofiltration fluid may result in hyperlactatemia with an *increased* plasma HCO_3^- concentration and pH.

The second and more important mechanism whereby hyperlactatemia exists without acidemia (or with less acidemia than expected) is correction of the SID by the elimination of another strong anion from the plasma. This was demonstrated by Madias and colleagues.[58] In the setting of sustained lactic acidosis induced by lactic acid infusion, these investigators found that Cl^- moves out of the plasma space, thus normalizing pH. Under these conditions, hyperlactatemia may persist but base excess may be normalized by compensatory mechanisms to restore the SID.

Traditionally, lactic acidosis is subdivided into *type A*, in which the mechanism is tissue hypoxia, and *type B*, in which there is no hypoxia.[59] This distinction may be artificial, however. Disorders such as sepsis may be associated with lactic acidosis caused by a variety of mechanisms (see Table 76–3), some type A and others type B. A potentially useful method of distinguishing anaerobically produced lactate from lactate from other sources is to measure the serum pyruvate concentration. The normal ratio of lactate to pyruvate is 10:1,[60] with ratios greater than 25:1 considered to be evidence of anaerobic metabolism.[51] This approach makes biochemical sense because, as shown in Figure 76–3, pyruvate is shunted into lactate during anaerobic metabolism, dramatically increasing the lactate-to-pyruvate ratio. The precise test characteristics, including normal ranges and sensitivity and specificity data, have not yet been defined for patients. Accordingly, this method remains investigational.

Treatment of lactic acidosis remains controversial. The only noncontroversial approach is to treat the underlying cause. This assumes that the underlying cause can be identified with a significant degree of certainty, which is not always possible. The assumption that hypoperfusion is always the most likely cause has been seriously challenged, especially in the case of well-resuscitated patients (as discussed earlier). Thus, therapy aimed at increasing oxygen delivery may not be effective. Indeed, if epinephrine is used, lactic acidosis may worsen.

The use of $NaHCO_3$ is equally controversial. In perhaps the most widely cited study on this topic, hypoxic lactic acidosis was induced in anesthetized dogs by ventilating them with gas containing little oxygen.[61] These animals were then treated with $NaHCO_3$ or with placebo, and, surprisingly, the group receiving $NaHCO_3$ actually exhibited an increase in both plasma lactate and H^+ concentrations compared with control animals. Furthermore, the $NaHCO_3$-treated animals experienced a decrease in cardiac output and blood pressure not seen in the control animals. A potential explanation for these findings is that the HCO_3^- was converted to CO_2, which increased the $Pa{CO_2}$ not only in the blood but also inside the cells of these animals with a fixed minute ventilation. The resulting intracellular acidosis might have been detrimental to myocardial function. However, these hypotheses have not been supported by subsequent studies, which have not demonstrated paradoxical intracellular acidosis or even detrimental hemodynamic effects after $NaHCO_3$ treatment in experimental hypoxic lactic acidosis.[62] Furthermore, it is not clear how this type of hypoxic lactic acidosis in well-perfused animals is related to the clinical conditions in which lactic acidosis occurs.

Two clinical trials have been conducted to determine the effectiveness of $NaHCO_3$ therapy in reversing acidosis and improving hemodynamics in patients with lactic acidosis.[63, 64] The results of both studies were the same; $NaHCO_3$ neither improved nor worsened systemic hemodynamics despite improving arterial pH. There was also no evidence that $NaHCO_3$ treatment worsened tissue hypoxia.

In summary, although there is little evidence that $NaHCO_3$ administration is helpful in lactic acidosis, there is also no strong evidence that it is harmful. Given the potentially serious effects of severe acidemia in critically ill patients discussed earlier and the fact that lactate metabolism by the liver is impaired during severe acidemia,[65] I recommend that treatment be instituted to maintain a pH above 7.20. The form of treatment that is best depends on the patient's underlying problem. $NaHCO_3$ is effective only to the extent that the plasma Na^+ concentration can be increased.

An alternative treatment would be to increase pyruvate metabolism to acetyl coenzyme A (CoA) rather than to lactate (see Fig. 76-3). This can be done by stimulating the enzyme pyruvate dehydrogenase, which catalyzes this reaction. This is the mechanism of action of dichloroacetate, which is effective in lowering lactate levels and improving pH (to a small degree) in patients with lactic acidosis.[66] However, dichloroacetate does not appear to improve outcome.[67]

Ketoacidosis

Another common cause of a metabolic acidosis with a positive AG is ketoacidosis. Ketones are formed by β-oxidation of fatty acids, a process inhibited by insulin. In insulin-deficient states (e.g., diabetes), ketone formation may quickly become out of control because severely elevated blood glucose concentrations produce an osmotic diuresis, which may lead to volume contraction. This state is associated with elevated cortisol and catecholamine secretion, which further stimulates free fatty acid production.[68] In addition, an increase in glucagon relative to insulin leads to decreased malonyl CoA and increased carnitine palmitoyl transferase levels, the combination of which increases ketogenesis.

Ketone bodies include acetone, acetoacetate, and β-hydroxybutyrate. Both acetoacetate and β-hydroxybutyrate are strong anions (pK 3.8 and 4.8, respectively).[69] Thus, like lactate, they decrease the SID and increase the H^+ concentration. Ketoacidosis may result from diabetes (DKA) or alcohol (AKA). The diagnosis is established by measuring serum ketones. It is important to understand, however, that the nitroprusside reaction measures only acetone and acetoacetate and not β-hydroxybutyrate. Thus, the state of measured ketosis is dependent on the ratio of acetoacetate to β-hydroxybutyrate. This ratio is low when lactic acidosis coexists with ketoacidosis because the reduced redox state of lactic acidosis favors production of β-hydroxybutyrate.[70] In such circumstances, the apparent level of ketosis is small compared with the amount of acidosis and the elevation of the AG. There is also a risk of confusion during treatment of ketoacidosis, because ketones as measured by the nitroprusside reaction may increase despite resolution of the acidosis. This increase occurs as a result of the rapid clearance of β-hydroxybutyrate with improvement in acid-base balance without change in the measured level of ketosis. Furthermore, ketones may even appear to increase as β-hydroxybutyrate is converted to acetoacetate. Hence, it is better to monitor the success of therapy by measuring pH and AG than by assaying serum ketones.

The treatment of DKA includes insulin and large amounts of fluid; 0.9% saline is usually recommended. Potassium replacement is often required as well. Fluid resuscitation reverses the hormonal stimuli for ketone body formation, and insulin allows the metabolism of ketones and glucose. Administration of $NaHCO_3$ may produce a more rapid rise in the pH by increasing the SID, but there is little evidence that this is desirable. Furthermore, to the extent that the SID is increased by increasing the plasma Na^+ concentration, the SID will be too high once the ketosis is cleared, resulting in "overshoot" alkalosis. In any case, such measures are rarely necessary and should probably be avoided except in extreme cases.[71]

A more common problem in the treatment of DKA is persistence of acidemia after resolution of the ketosis. This hyperchloremic metabolic acidosis occurs as Cl^- replaces ketoacids, thus maintaining a decreased SID and pH. This appears to occur for two reasons. First, exogenous Cl^- is often provided in the form of 0.9% saline, which, if given in large enough quantities, results in a so-called dilutional acidosis (see later). Second, it appears that some amount of increased Cl^- reabsorption occurs as ketones are excreted in the urine. It has also been suggested that the increased tubular Na^+ load produces electrical-chemical forces that favor Cl^- reabsorption.[72]

The acidosis seen in AKA is usually less severe. The treatment consists of fluids and glucose instead of the insulin used in DKA.[73] Indeed, insulin is contraindicated because it may cause precipitous hypoglycemia.[74] Thiamine must also be given to avoid precipitating Wernicke's encephalopathy.

Renal Failure

Although renal failure may produce a hyperchloremic metabolic acidosis, especially when chronic, the buildup of sulfates and other acids frequently increases the AG. However, the increase is usually not large.[75] Similarly, uncomplicated renal failure rarely produces severe acidosis except when it is accompanied by high rates of acid generation such as with hypermetabolism.[76] In all cases, the SID is decreased and is expected to remain so unless some therapy is provided. Hemodialysis permits removal of sulfate and other ions and allows normal Na^+ and Cl^- balance to be restored, thus returning the SID to normal (or near normal). However, patients who do not yet require dialysis and those who are between treatments often require some other therapy to increase the SID. $NaHCO_3$ is used as long as the plasma Na^+ concentration is not already elevated. Other options include Ca^{2+}, which usually requires replacement anyway. Replacement of Ca^{2+} cannot increase the SID much because of the rather narrow range of free Ca^{2+} (0.975–1.125 mmol/L). Even though Ca^{2+} is a divalent cation, it is unreasonable to expect its administration to have much effect on the SID.

Poisons

Metabolic acidosis with an increased AG is a major feature of various types of drug and substance intoxications (see Table 76-1). Again, it is generally more important to recognize these disorders so that specific therapy can be provided than to treat the acid-base disorder that they produce. For a more detailed discussion of management of these disorders, see Chapter 12.

Other and Unknown Causes

As discussed earlier, some cases of an increased AG of unknown cause have been reported. In the nonketotic hyperosmolar state of diabetes, an AG has been found that remains unexplained.[31] Even when careful methods have been applied using the SIG or similar strategies, unmeasured anions have been reported in the blood of patients with sepsis[32, 33] and liver disease[34] and in experimental animals given endotoxin.[35] Furthermore, unknown cations also appear in the blood of some critically ill patients.[33] The significance of these findings remains to be determined.

Non–Anion Gap (Hyperchloremic) Acidoses

Hyperchloremic metabolic acidosis occurs as a result of either increased Cl^- relative to strong cations, especially Na^+, or loss of cations with retention of Cl^-. As seen in Figure 76–1, these disorders can be separated by history and by examination of the urinary Cl^- concentration. When acidosis occurs, the normal response of the kidney is to increase Cl^- excretion. Failure to do so identifies the kidney as the source of acidosis. Extrarenal hyperchloremic acidoses occur as a result of exogenous Cl^- loads (iatrogenic acidosis) or loss of cations from the lower gastrointestinal tract without proportional loss of Cl^-.

Renal Tubular Acidosis

Examination of the urine and plasma electrolytes and pH and calculation of the urine SIDa allows one to diagnose most cases of renal tubular acidosis (RTA) correctly (see Fig. 76–1).[77] Caution must be exercised when the plasma pH is greater than 7.35 because this may turn off urinary Cl^- excretion. In such circumstances, it may be necessary to infuse sodium sulfate or furosemide. These agents stimulate Cl^- and K^+ excretion and may be used to unmask the defect and to probe K^+ secretory capacity.

The mechanisms of RTA are not well established. It is likely that much of the confusion has occurred as a result of attempting to understand the physiology from the point of view of regulating H^+ and HCO_3^- concentrations. As we have discussed, this is simply inconsistent with the principles of physical chemistry. The kidney does not excrete H^+ any more as NH_4^+ than it does as H_2O. The purpose of renal ammoniagenesis is to allow the excretion of Cl^-, which balances the charge of NH_4^+. The defect in all types of RTA is inability to excrete Cl^- in proportion to Na^+, although the reasons vary by type. Treatment is largely dependent on whether the kidney responds to mineralocorticoid replacement or whether there is loss of Na^+ that can be replaced as $NaHCO_3$.

Classic distal (type I) RTA responds to $NaHCO_3$ replacement, and generally 50 to 100 mEq/day is required. In this type of RTA, K^+ defects are also common and K^+ replacement is also required. A variant of the classic distal RTA is a hyperkalemic form, which is actually more common than the classic type. The central defect here appears to be impaired Na^+ transport in the cortical collecting duct. These patients also respond to $NaHCO_3$ replacement. Proximal (type II) RTA is characterized by both Na^+ and K^+ reabsorption defects. The disorder is uncommon and is usually part of the Fanconi syndrome, in which reabsorption of glucose, phosphate, urate, and amino acids is also impaired. Treatment of this disorder with $NaHCO_3$ is ineffective, as increased ion delivery merely results in increased excretion. Thiazide diuretics have been used to treat this disorder with varying success.

Type IV RTA is caused by aldosterone deficiency or resistance. Diagnosis of these disorders is confirmed by the high serum K^+ and low urine pH (<5.5). Treatment is usually most effective if one can remove the cause, which is most commonly drugs such as nonsteroidal anti-inflammatory agents, heparin, or potassium-sparing diuretics. Occasionally, mineralocorticoid replacement is required.

Gastrointestinal Acidosis

Diarrhea significant enough to produce a hyperchloremic metabolic acidosis is usually difficult to miss. Fluid secreted into the gut lumen contains higher amounts of Na^+ than Cl^-, similar to the differences in plasma. Extremely large losses of these fluids, particularly if volume is replaced with fluids containing equal amounts of Na^+ and Cl^-, results in a decrease in the plasma Na^+ concentration relative to the Cl^- concentration and a decrease in the SID. Such a scenario can be avoided if fluids such as lactated Ringer's solution are used instead of water or saline. Ringer's solution has a more physiologic SID and therefore does not produce acidosis except in rare circumstances (see section on lactic acidosis).

Iatrogenic Acidosis

Two of the most common causes of a hyperchloremic metabolic acidosis are iatrogenic and both involve administration of chloride. Modern parenteral nutrition formulas contain weak anions such as acetate in addition to Cl^-, and the balance of the anions can be adjusted depending on the acid-base status of the patient. If sufficient amounts of weak anions are not provided the plasma Cl^- concentration increases, decreasing the SID and resulting in acidosis. A similar condition may arise when saline is used for fluid resuscitation, resulting in a *dilutional acidosis*.

Dilutional acidosis was first described more than 50 years ago,[78, 79] although some have argued that it is only a minor issue at best.[80] In healthy animals, large doses of NaCl have been demonstrated to produce only a minor hyperchloremic acidosis.[81] These studies have been interpreted as showing that if dilutional acidosis occurs, it is only in the extreme case and even then it is only mild. This line of reasoning cannot be applied to critically ill patients for two reasons. First, large-volume resuscitation is commonly required for patients with sepsis and trauma, and these patients may receive crystalloid infusions of 5 to 10 times their plasma volumes in a single day. Second, the reasoning fails to consider the fact that critically ill patients are frequently not in normal acid-base balance to begin with. These patients may have lactic acidosis or renal insufficiency. Furthermore, critically ill patients may not be able to compensate normally by increasing ventilation and may have abnormal buffer capacity because of hypoalbuminemia. In ICU patients[82] as well as in animals with experimental sepsis,[83] dilutional acidosis does occur and can produce significant acid-base derangements.

From Chapter 75, the mechanism of dilutional acidosis should be clear. Solutions containing equal amounts of Na^+ and Cl^- affect the plasma concentrations of Na^+ and Cl^- differently because the normal Na^+ concentration is 35 to 45 mEq/L greater than the normal Cl^- concentration. Adding 154 mEq/L of both ions in, for example, 0.9% saline increases the Cl^- concentration more than the Na^+ concentration. It may be less obvious why critically ill patients are more susceptible to this disorder than healthy subjects. Apparently, many critically ill patients have a significantly lower SID than healthy individuals even when these patients have no evidence of a metabolic acid-base derangement.[84] This is not surprising when one considers that the positive charge of the SID is balanced by the negative charges of A^- and total CO_2 and that many critically ill patients are hypoalbuminemic and tend to have reduced A^-. Because the body defends P_{CO_2} for other reasons, a reduction in A^- leads to a reduction in SID by the body in order to maintain normal pH. Thus, a typical ICU patient might have an SID of 30 mEq/L rather than 40 to 42 mEq/L. If the same patient develops a metabolic acidosis (e.g., lactic acidosis), the SID decreases further. If the patient is resuscitated with large volumes of 0.9% saline, it produces a significant metabolic acidosis. These effects are demonstrated by the example in Table 76–4. Note that as the SID decreases, so does the pH despite the "compensatory" hyperventilation. Also note that the fall in pH is greater when the SID changes from 22 to 16 mEq/L than when it changes from 32 to 22 mEq/L. This relationship is further illustrated in Figure 76–4 and demonstrates that a patient with a lower baseline SID is more susceptible to a subsequent acid load.

The clinical implication for management of patients in the ICU is that when large volumes of fluid are used for resuscitation they should be more physiologic than saline. One alterna-

TABLE 76–4. Effects of Lactic Acidosis and Resuscitation with Saline*

Condition	SID (mEq/L)	pH	P_{CO_2} (mm Hg)	SBE (mEq/L)
Baseline	32	7.41	40	0.5
Lactic acidosis	22	7.32	30	−9.8
10 liters of 0.9% saline	16	7.19	26	−17.1

*Results for a 70-kg man with lactic acidosis (arterial whole blood lactate 10 mmol/L), subsequent resuscitation with 10 liters of 0.9% saline, no urine output, and as yet no change in lactate concentration. Baseline Na^+ and Cl^- concentrations are 130 mEq/L and 102 mEq/L, respectively.

P_{CO_2} = partial pressure of carbon dioxide; SBE = standard base excess; SID = strong ion difference.

tive is lactated Ringer's solution. In this fluid the difference between Na^+ and Cl^- concentrations is more physiologic and thus the SID is closer to normal (~28 mEq/L, whereas the SID of saline is 0 mEq/L). Of course, this assumes that the lactate in lactated Ringer's solution is metabolized, which, as discussed earlier, is almost always the case.

Unexplained Hyperchloremic Acidosis

Critically ill patients sometimes manifest hyperchloremic metabolic acidosis for reasons that are not clear. Often, these patients have other coexisting types of metabolic acidosis, making the precise diagnosis difficult. For example, some patients with lactic acidosis have more acidosis than can be explained by the increase in lactate concentration[32] and patients with sepsis and acidosis frequently have normal lactate levels.[85] Unexplained anions are often the cause,[32-34] but there may also be a hyperchloremic acidosis. Saline resuscitation may be responsible for much of this acidosis, as discussed previously, but evidence from experiments with endotoxemic animals suggests that as much as a third of the acidosis is still unexplained.[83]

A potential explanation for this finding is the partial loss of a Donnan equilibrium between plasma and interstitial fluid. The severe accompanying capillary leak results in loss of albumin from the vascular space, necessitating the movement of another ion to maintain charge balance between the two compartments. If Cl^- moved into the plasma space to restore charge balance, a strong anion would be replacing a weak anion and a hyperchloremic metabolic acidosis would result. At present, this hypothesis remains unproven.

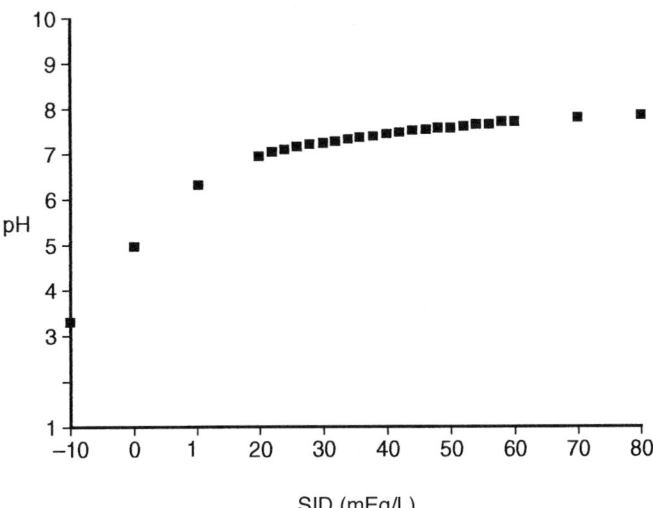

Figure 76–4. Plot of pH versus strong ion difference (SID). For this plot, ATOT and P_{CO_2} were held constant at 18 mEq/L and 40 mm Hg, respectively. A water dissociation constant for blood of 4.4×10^{-14} (mEq/L) is assumed. Note how steep the pH curve becomes at SID less than 20 mEq/L. (Adapted from Kellum JA: Metabolic acidosis in the critically ill: Lessons from physical chemistry. Kidney Int 1998; 53:S81–S86.)

Metabolic Alkalosis

Metabolic alkalosis occurs as a result of an increased SID. This may be secondary to losses of anions (e.g., Cl^- from the stomach) or increases in cations (rare). Metabolic alkaloses can be divided into those in which Cl^- losses are *temporary* and Cl^- can be effectively replaced (chloride responsive) and those in which hormonal mechanisms produce *ongoing* losses that can, at best, be temporarily offset by Cl^- administration (chloride-resistant) (Table 76–5). As with hyperchloremic acidosis, these disorders can be distinguished by examination of the urinary Cl^- concentration.

Chloride-Responsive Disorders

Chloride-responsive disorders usually occur as a result of Cl^- losses from the stomach such as with vomiting or gastric drainage. The treatment is to replace the Cl^-. This can be done slowly with NaCl or more rapidly with KCl or even HCl. Saline plus KCl is usually the treatment of choice because volume depletion usually coexists with these disorders. Dehydration in turn stimulates aldosterone secretion, which results in Na^+ reabsorption and loss of K^+ (and Cl^-). Saline is effective, even though it contains Na^+, because the administration of equal amounts of Na^+ and Cl^- results in larger relative increases in Cl^- concentration than Na^+ concentration (see iatrogenic acidosis). In rare circumstances, when neither K^+ nor volume depletion is a problem, it may be desirable to give back Cl^- as HCl.

Diuretics and other forms of volume contraction produce

TABLE 76–5. Differential Diagnosis of Metabolic Alkalosis (Increased Strong Ion Difference)

Chloride Loss < Sodium

- Chloride responsive (urine Cl^- concentration < 10 mmol/L)
  - Gastrointestinal losses
    - Vomiting
    - Gastric drainage
    - Chloride-wasting diarrhea (villous adenoma)
  - After diuretic use
  - After hypercapnea
- Chloride unresponsive (urine Cl^- concentration > 20 mmol/L)
  - Mineralocorticoid excess
    - Primary hyperaldosteronism (Conn's syndrome)
    - Secondary hyperaldosteronism
    - Cushing's syndrome
    - Liddle's syndrome
    - Bartter's syndrome
    - Exogenous corticoids
    - Excessive licorice intake
  - Ongoing diuretic use

Exogenous Sodium Load > Chloride

- Sodium salt administration (acetate, citrate)
  - Massive blood transfusions
  - Parenteral nutrition
  - Plasma volume expanders
  - Sodium lactate (Ringer's solution)

Other

- Severe deficiency of intracellular cations
  - Magnesium, potassium

metabolic alkalosis predominantly by stimulating aldosterone, as discussed earlier. However, diuretics also induce K^+ and Cl^- excretion directly, further complicating the problem and inducing metabolic alkalosis more rapidly.

Chloride-Resistant Disorders

Chloride-resistant disorders are characterized by an increased urinary Cl^- concentration (>20 mmol/L) (see Table 76–5). They are said to be "chloride-resistant" because of ongoing Cl^- losses. Most commonly, the losses are a result of increased mineralocorticoid activity. Treatment requires that the underlying disorder be addressed (Table 76–6).

Other Causes of Metabolic Alkalosis

In rare instances, an increased SID and, therefore, metabolic alkalosis occur as a result of cation administration rather than anion depletion. This disorder arises, for example, in milk-alkali syndrome and with intravenous administration of strong cations without strong anions. The latter occurs with massive blood transfusion because Na^+ is given with citrate (a weak anion) instead of Cl^-. Similar results are observed when parenteral nutrition formulations contain too much acetate and not enough Cl^- to balance the Na^+ load.

RESPIRATORY ACID-BASE DISORDERS

Respiratory disorders are far easier to diagnose and treat than metabolic disorders because the mechanism is always the same, although the underlying disease process may vary. CO_2 is produced by cellular metabolism or by the titration of HCO_3^- by metabolic acids. Normally, alveolar ventilation is adjusted to maintain the arterial P_{CO_2} between 35 and 45 mm Hg. When alveolar ventilation is increased or decreased out of proportion to P_{CO_2} production, a respiratory acid-base disorder exists.

Pathophysiology

CO_2 production by the body (at 220 mL/min) is equal to 15,000 mmol/day of carbonic acid.[86] This compares to less than 500 mmol/day for all nonrespiratory acids that are managed by the kidney and gut. Pulmonary ventilation is adjusted by the respiratory center in response to signals from Pa_{CO_2}, pH, and P_{O_2}, as well as some signals from exercise, anxiety, wakefulness, and others. The normal Pa_{CO_2} of 40 mm Hg is attained by a precise match of alveolar ventilation to metabolic CO_2 production. Pa_{CO_2} changes in a "compensatory" ventilatory response to altered arterial pH produced by metabolic acidosis or alkalosis in predictable ways that are detailed in the preceding chapter.

Respiratory Acidosis

When CO_2 elimination is inadequate compared with the rate of tissue production, Pa_{CO_2} increases to a new steady state determined by the new relationship between alveolar ventilation and CO_2 production. Acutely, this increase in P_{CO_2} increases both the H^+ and HCO_3^- concentrations according to the carbonic acid equilibrium equation (see Chapter 75). Thus, this change in HCO_3^- concentration is mediated by chemical equilibrium, not by any systemic adaptation. Similarly, this increased HCO_3^- concentration does not "buffer" the H^+ concentration. There is no change in the SID and hence no change in SBE. Tissue acidosis always occurs in respiratory acidosis because CO_2 builds up in the tissue. If the Pa_{CO_2} remains increased, compensation occurs and the SID increases to restore the H^+ concentration toward normal. This is accomplished primarily by Cl^- removal from the plasma space.

Because movement of Cl^- into the tissues or the red blood cells results in intracellular acidosis (complicated by the existence of an increased tissue P_{CO_2}), Cl^- must be removed from the body to achieve a lasting effect on SID. The kidney is designed to do this, as discussed already, and the GI tract is not (although the adaptive capacity of this route of Cl^- elimination has not been fully explored). Accordingly, patients with renal disease have a difficult time adapting to chronic respiratory acidosis. When renal function is intact, Cl^- is eliminated in the urine, and after a few days the SID is in-

TABLE 76–6. Treatment of Metabolic Alkalosis

Condition	Treatment
Primary aldosteronism	Spironolactone or other agents that block distal tubular sodium reabsorption improve alkalosis, hypokalemia, and hypertension. Large doses may be necessary. Restriction of sodium intake and potassium supplementation may be necessary. When an adenoma can be identified, surgery is curative. When the cause is bilateral adrenal cortical hyperplasia, therapy is medical. Dexamethasone is effective in long-term therapy of familial dexamethasone-responsive aldosteronism.
Secondary aldosteronism	Angiotensin-converting enzyme inhibitors are usually effective. Repair of the underlying lesion, if feasible, may be required.
Cushing's syndrome	Caused by pituitary oversecretion of ACTH: surgery or radiation Caused by adrenal adenoma or carcinoma: adrenalectomy Caused by secondary or ectopic ACTH production: address the underlying malignancy.
Liddle's syndrome	Triamterene may be effective.
Bartter's syndrome	Treatment often unsatisfactory in the long term. Potassium-sparing diuretics, potassium and magnesium supplementation, angiotensin-converting enzyme inhibitors, and cyclooxygenase inhibitors are partially effective.
Exogenous corticoids	Discontinuation of the offending agent or agents and vigorous initial potassium replacement.
Severe potassium or magnesium depletion	Replacement of these electrolytes (may require very large amounts).

From Spital A, Garella S: Correction of acid-base derangements. *In:* Critical Care Nephrology. Ronco C, Bellomo R (Eds). Dordrecht, The Netherlands, Kluwer Academic Publishers, 1998, pp 311–328.
ACTH = adrenocorticotropic hormone.

creased to a level necessary to return the pH toward 7.35. It is unclear whether this amount of time is required by the physiologic constraints of the system or to avoid being overly sensitive to transient changes in alveolar ventilation. In any case, this adaptation results in an increased pH for any degree of hypercarbia. According to the Henderson-Hasselbalch equation, the increased pH results in an increased HCO_3^- concentration for a given PCO_2. Thus, the "adaptive" increase in HCO_3^- concentration *results from* rather than being the *cause of* the increased pH. Although the HCO_3^- concentration is a convenient and reliable marker of metabolic compensation, it is not the mechanism. This point is more than semantic because only changes in the independent variables of acid-base balance (PCO_2, ATOT, SID) can affect the plasma H^+ concentration and HCO_3^- is not an independent variable.

Diseases of Ventilatory Impairment

As with virtually all acid-base disorders, treatment begins with addressing the underlying disorder. Acute respiratory acidosis can be caused by central nervous system (CNS) suppression, neuromuscular disease or impairment (e.g., myasthenia gravis, hypophosphatemia, hypokalemia), or airway and parenchymal lung disease (e.g., asthma, acute respiratory distress syndrome [ARDS]). This last category of conditions also produces primary hypoxia, not just alveolar hypoventilation. The two can be distinguished by using the alveolar gas equation:

$$PAO_2 = PIO_2 - PaCO_2/R$$

where R is the respiratory exchange coefficient (generally taken as 0.8) and PIO_2 is the inspired oxygen tension (room air is approximately 150 mm Hg). Thus, as $PaCO_2$ increases, PAO_2 decreases in a predictable fashion. If the PAO_2 is reduced further, there is a defect in gas exchange.

Chronic respiratory acidosis is most often caused by chronic lung disease (e.g., chronic obstructive pulmonary disease [COPD]) or chest wall disease (e.g., kyphoscoliosis). Rarely, its cause is central hypoventilation or chronic neuromuscular disease.

When and How to Treat

Another aspect of respiratory acidosis apparent from the alveolar gas equation is that the primary threat to life comes not from acidosis but from hypoxemia. With room air, the $PaCO_2$ cannot exceed 80 mm Hg before life-threatening hypoxemia results. Accordingly, supplemental oxygen is required in the treatment of these patients. Unfortunately, oxygen administration alone is almost never sufficient treatment and the defect in ventilation must be addressed directly. When the underlying cause can be addressed quickly (e.g., reversal of narcotics with naloxone), it may be possible to avoid endotracheal intubation. More often this is not the case and mechanical ventilation must be initiated. Mechanical support is indicated when the patient is unstable or at risk for instability or when CNS function deteriorates. Furthermore, for patients who are exhibiting signs of respiratory muscle fatigue, mechanical ventilation should be instituted before respiratory failure occurs. Thus, it is not the absolute $PaCO_2$ value that is important but, rather, the clinical condition of the patient.

Chronic hypercapnia requires treatment when there is an acute deterioration. In this setting, it is important not to try to restore the $PaCO_2$ to 35 to 45 mm Hg; instead treatment should be tailored to the patient's baseline $PaCO_2$ if it is known. If the baseline $PaCO_2$ is not known, a target $PaCO_2$ of 60 mm Hg may be reasonable. Overventilation has two undesirable consequences. First, life-threatening alkalemia may occur if the $PaCO_2$ is rapidly normalized in a patient with chronic respiratory acidosis and an appropriately large SID. Second, even if the $PaCO_2$ is corrected slowly, the patient's plasma SID decreases over time, making it impossible to wean the patient from mechanical ventilation.

Other options for treatment of hypercarbia include noninvasive ventilation using a Bi-PAP system. This technique can be useful in the management of some patients, particularly when their sensorium is not impaired.[87] Rapid infusion of $NaHCO_3$ in respiratory acidosis can induce acute respiratory failure if alveolar ventilation is not increased to account for the increased CO_2. Thus, if $NaHCO_3$ is to be used, it must be administered slowly and alveolar ventilation adjusted appropriately. Furthermore, as discussed previously, $NaHCO_3$ works by increasing the plasma Na^+ concentration. If this is not possible or not desirable, $NaHCO_3$ should be avoided.

Occasionally, it is useful to reduce CO_2 production. This can be accomplished by reduction of carbohydrate in nutritional support, control of temperature in the febrile patient, and sedation of the anxious or combative patient. Treatment of shivering in the postoperative period can reduce CO_2 production. However, it is unusual to control hypercarbia with these techniques alone.

Permissive Hypercapnia

There has been considerable interest in ventilator-associated lung injury. Overdistention of alveoli can result in tissue injury and microvascular permeability leading to interstitial and alveolar edema. Compared with ventilatory strategies that employ lower pressures and volumes, prolonged exposure to increased airway pressure and lung volumes has been shown to result in lung pathology and decreased survival of animals.[88, 89] For these reasons, it is often necessary to tolerate a reduced minute ventilation and hence an elevated $PaCO_2$. This practice is often referred to as permissive hypercapnia or controlled hypoventilation. Uncontrolled studies suggest that this method may reduce mortality in patients with severe ARDS.[13]

Permissive hypercapnia, however, is not without risks. Sedation is mandatory, and even neuromuscular blocking agents are frequently required. Intracranial pressure increases, as does transpulmonary pressure, making this technique unusable for patients with brain injury and right ventricular dysfunction. There is controversy about how low the pH can be. Whereas some have reported good results even with pH less than 7.0,[13] most authors have advocated more modest pH reductions (pH above 7.25).

Respiratory Alkalosis

Respiratory alkalosis may be the most frequently encountered acid-base disorder. It occurs in those who reside at high altitude and in a number of pathologic conditions, the most important of which include salicylate intoxication, early sepsis, hepatic failure, and hypoxic respiratory disorders. Respiratory alkalosis also occurs with pregnancy and with pain or anxiety.

Hypocapnia appears to be a particularly bad prognostic indicator in patients with critical illness.[90] Like acute respiratory acidosis, acute respiratory alkalosis results in a small change in HCO_3^- concentration as dictated by the Henderson-Hasselbach equation. If hypocapnia persists, the SID begins to decrease as a result of renal Cl^- reabsorption. After 2 to 3 days, the SID assumes a new, lower, steady state.[91] Severe alkalemia is unusual in respiratory alkalosis, and management is therefore directed at the underlying cause. Typically, these mild acid-base changes are clinically more important for what they can alert the clinician to, in terms of underlying disease, than for any threat they pose to the patient. In rare cases, respiratory depression with narcotics is necessary.

Pseudorespiratory Alkalosis

The presence of arterial hypocapnia in profound circulatory shock has been termed pseudorespiratory alkalosis.[92] This condition can be seen when alveolar ventilation is supported but the circulation is grossly inadequate. In such conditions, the mixed venous P_{CO_2} is significantly elevated but the arterial P_{CO_2} is normal or even decreased as a result of decreased CO_2 delivery to the lung and increased pulmonary transit time. Overall CO_2 clearance is thus markedly decreased, and patients have profound tissue acidosis, usually both metabolic and respiratory. The metabolic component comes from tissue hypoperfusion and hyperlactatemia. Arterial oxygen saturation may also appear adequate despite tissue hypoxemia. This condition is rapidly fatal unless systemic hemodynamics can be normalized.

UNIFIED APPROACH TO THE PATIENT WITH ACID-BASE IMBALANCE

We now outline an approach to the patient with an acid-base disorder, focusing in particular on mixed disorders. As in much of medicine, there are numerous ways to arrive at the correct answer, and the approach outlined here is not necessarily any better than other approaches available. The method described here, however, focuses on the readily available clinical information and in these times of cost containment may be more "user friendly" than some of the more traditional approaches. In addition, this approach is consistent with the physicochemical principles of acid-base balance outlined in this chapter and in Chapter 75, both of which the reader is advised to consult when reading the following text.

Characterizing the Disorder

The first step in the approach to a patient with an acid-base imbalance is to characterize the disorder. Since acid-base imbalances are usually recognized by abnormalities in the venous plasma electrolyte concentrations, it is appropriate to start there. Although HCO_3^- is a dependent variable, using the venous HCO_3^- concentration is the easiest way to screen for acid-base disorders. A normal HCO_3^- concentration, however, in no way excludes the presence of even serious acid-base derangements. Therefore, if the history and physical examination lead one to suspect a disease process that results in an acid-base imbalance, more investigation is required. Still, the venous plasma electrolytes provide useful information.

The HCO_3^- concentration is normally 22 to 26 mEq/L. Increases in HCO_3^- concentration occur with primary and compensatory metabolic alkaloses and decreases occur with primary or compensatory metabolic acidoses. Regrettably, in mixed disorders, the HCO_3^- concentration may be misleading and the presence of any abnormality in HCO_3^- concentration requires further investigation. In addition to examining the HCO_3^- concentration, venous blood can be used to calculate the anion gap ($Na^+ + K^+ - Cl^- - HCO_3^-$). If the HCO_3^- concentration or AG is abnormal or if there is clinical suspicion of a mixed disorder, arterial blood should be sampled for blood gas analysis. This test provides information on the pH, Pa_{CO_2}, and SBE. Simple disorders conform to the equations presented in Chapter 75, but "mixed" disorders are also quite common. A summary of this information is present in Table 76-7. These methods are successful in characterizing simple acid-base disorders and mixed disorders (see the following).

In patients with acidemia, the next step is to examine the AG. This is not done when there is alkalemia because results may often be misleading. Alkalemia increases the charge on albumin and stimulates nonanaerobic hyperlactatemia, both of which increase the AG. Furthermore, the presence of unexplained anions in the absence of acidosis is of uncertain clinical significance. If the AG is calculated from an alkalemic blood sample, only significant abnormalities (>22 mEq/L) should be considered important. More often, however, it is not oversensitivity but rather undersensitivity that plagues the AG calculation. As outlined earlier, the accuracy of the AG can easily be improved by using a patient-specific normal range rather than a standard one. If unmeasured anions are detected, it is a good idea to compare their amounts with the abnormality in SBE. For example, if the calculated AG is 5 mEq/L greater than expected and the SBE is −15 mEq/L, a mixed metabolic acidosis is present. The unmeasured anions (e.g., ketones) account for an SBE of −5 mEq/L, and some other process is responsible for another 10 mEq/L. Such a condition might occur, for example, if large amounts of 0.9% saline were used to treat a patient with DKA. As the ketosis resolves, the acidosis persists because the SID is kept low by exogenous Cl^- administration.

TABLE 76–7. Acid-Base Patterns in Simple Disorders

pH	$PaCO_2$	SBE	Disorder
<7.35	<35	< −5	Metabolic acidosis
>7.45	>45	> +5	Metabolic alkalosis
<7.35	>45	0 ± 5	Acute respiratory acidosis
<7.35	>45	> +5*	Chronic respiratory acidosis
>7.45	<35	0 ± 5	Acute respiratory alkalosis
>7.45	<35	< +5*	Chronic respiratory alkalosis

*For chronic disorders, SBE should be defined by the following equation: $SBE = 0.4(Pa_{CO_2} - 40) \pm 5$.

Pa_{CO_2} = arterial carbon dioxide pressure; SBE = standard base excess.

Determining the Cause

Once the disorder has been characterized, the clinician must integrate the information obtained from the history and physical examination in order to arrive at an accurate diagnosis. The differential diagnoses for various disorders are listed in Tables 76-1, 76-3, and 76-5.

Case Histories

The following cases provide an illustration of the foregoing approach. Although these may represent "extreme" cases, they are not unusual in the ICU, and they serve to illustrate the need to appreciate the basic principles of acid-base balance outlined in Chapter 75 and the present chapter.

CASE HISTORY 1

The patient was a 65-year-old white man with a history of rheumatoid arthritis, non-insulin-dependent diabetes mellitus (diet-controlled), hypertension, COPD, and a remote history of cholecystectomy for acute cholecystitis. Outpatient medications include ibuprofen, nifedipine, albuterol, and ipratropium bromide (Atrovent) inhalers. He was often noncompliant with medical appointments. He was involved in a motor vehicle accident and sustained injuries to his right anterior chest and upper abdomen.

The diagnosis included rib fractures, pulmonary contusion, and a grade III liver laceration. He underwent surgery for liver laceration. The surgical team found extensive adhesions, and a large amount of blood was lost during the operation. The patient was resuscitated with lactated Ringer's solution and blood products in the trauma bay as well as in the operating room. Analysis of arterial blood obtained in the operating room revealed a pH of 7.10, a Pa_{CO_2} of 30 mm Hg, and an SBE of −19 mEq/L. The plasma lactate concentration was 11.5 mEq/L, and additional blood products and 120 mEq of $NaHCO_3$

were given for resuscitation. When the patient arrived in the ICU, his blood gas analysis revealed a pH of 7.35, a $Paco_2$ of 35 mm Hg, an SBE of −5 mEq/L, and a lactate concentration of 8.0 mEq/L. His hematocrit was 29%, and he was given more blood and colloid. After 6 hours in the ICU, his pH had increased to 7.60, the $Paco_2$ was 33 mm Hg, the SBE was +10 mEq/L, and the lactate concentration was 2.0 mEq/L. At this point, the patient had a fairly straightforward metabolic alkalosis as evidenced by an increased SBE and a mild respiratory alkalosis shown by the $Paco_2$ of 33 mm Hg. The metabolic component was due to a combination of lactate clearance, massive blood transfusion (citrate), and $NaHCO_3$ administration. The respiratory component was due to ventilator settings, ordered to adjust for a metabolic acidosis that had now cleared. The ventilator setting was reduced, allowing the $Paco_2$ to increase to 55 mm Hg to normalize the pH to 7.40.

On the fifth postoperative day, the patient could not be weaned from mechanical ventilation and a routine set of electrolytes revealed a progressive evolving metabolic acidosis. The plasma HCO_3^- concentration had been decreasing at a rate of approximately 2 mEq/L/day and was now 20 mEq/L. The AG was calculated as 12 mEq/L and the phosphate and albumin concentrations were within normal limits (making this a normal AG value). An arterial blood gas analysis revealed a pH of 7.28, Pco_2 of 40 mm Hg, and SBE of −7.5 mEq/L. Accordingly, the diagnoses were a primary hyperchloremic metabolic acidosis and also a respiratory acidosis, because there should have been an element of respiratory compensation and there was not.

The patient was returned to assist-control ventilation and the $Paco_2$ decreased to 30 mm Hg, suggesting that the patient was unable to progress with weaning because of mechanical insufficiency, probably related to his chest wall injury. At this point, evaluation of the hyperchloremic metabolic acidosis focused on the urine electrolytes. The patient had not received diuretics, and the arterial pH was less than 7.35. In this case, urine electrolyte analysis should have been reliable. The results of the urine analysis were as follows: Na^+ 50 mEq/L, K^+ 30 mEq/L (plasma K^+ was 5.0 mEq/L), Cl^- 40 mEq/L, and pH 5.0. Thus, the patient's urine SIDa was 40 mEq/L, and from Figure 76–1 we see that he had a renal tubular acidosis (RTA). The urine pH was also low (5.0), indicating that this was not a distal RTA, and on the basis of his plasma K^+ of 5.0 mEq/L the diagnosis was type IV RTA. This diagnosis was consistent with the patient's history of diabetes mellitus and use of ibuprofen. The type IV RTA was likely to have been the cause of some of the acidosis seen in the first blood gas analysis, because the SBE of −19 mEq/L was only partly explained by the lactate concentration of 11.5 mEq/L. The management of this type of RTA primarily involves removing the inciting agents (nonsteroidal anti-inflammatory agents), and most cases resolve without further treatment.

The preceding case history also demonstrates that acid-base disorders in critically ill patients are often dynamic and multifactorial. Frequent reassessment is often necessary, particularly in the early stages of illness.

CASE HISTORY 2

This patient was a 55-year-old woman who had returned from the operating room 6 hours previously after having undergone orthotopic liver transplantation. The allograft was slow to function, and there was evidence of significant preservation injury. The arterial lactate concentration was 16 mEq/L and rising. An arterial blood gas analysis revealed a pH of 7.16, Pco_2 of 32 mm Hg, and SBE of −16 mEq/L. Thus, the patient had a pure metabolic acidosis secondary to lactic acid. The ventilation was also inadequate, and because the patient was heavily sedated, she was not able to compensate normally. The respiratory rate on the mechanical ventilator was increased from 14 to 18 breaths/min in an effort to decrease the Pco_2 to 25 to 28 mm Hg.

The lactic acid was entirely responsible for the acidosis because the negative SBE value was exactly equal to the lactate concentration (i.e., no mixed acidosis was present). The source of the lactic acidosis was almost certainly delayed hepatic function with little or no uptake of lactate by the liver. In such situations, the liver may actually produce additional lactate. However, the pulmonary capillary wedge pressure was 14 mm Hg and the right ventricular end-diastolic volume 120 mL. Additional fluids were given to reduce the likelihood that anaerobic lactate production was also present. Colloids were chosen for this indication because the patient's albumin was 2.0 g/dL (secondary to the underlying liver disease) and because saline might worsen the acidosis by further decreasing the SID. Even lactated Ringer's solution might transiently worsen the SID in this case because of the severe hepatic dysfunction. A liter of 5% albumin solution was given intravenously. In addition, the patient's urine output was poor and the serum Na^+ and Cl^- concentrations were 130 and 105 mEq/L, respectively. Accordingly, she was also given 120 mEq of $NaHCO_3$.

After these treatments a repeated arterial blood gas analysis revealed the following: pH 7.32, Pco_2 25 mm Hg, and SBE −12 mEq/L. The lactate concentration was still 16 mEq/L. Over the next 12 hours, the lactate concentration decreased to 10 mEq/L, the liver was making bile, the patient was waking up, and the urine output improved considerably. The mechanical ventilator was adjusted multiple times to keep the Pco_2 in the appropriate range for the resolving acidosis and was now set at 12 breaths per minute. Repeated arterial blood gas analysis revealed a pH of 7.40, Pco_2 of 35 mm Hg, and SBE of −1 mEq/L. At first glance, the complete correction of the acidosis seemed to contrast with the persisting hyperlacticemia. Indeed, the lactate concentration of 10 mEq/L should produce an SBE in a corresponding range. The lactic acid still in the bloodstream was no less "acidic" than it had been 12 hours earlier.

Examination of the patient's electrolytes revealed what has changed. Serum Na^+ and Cl^- concentrations were now 132 and 102 mEq/L, respectively. These seemingly small changes from 130 and 105 mEq/L earlier have enormous importance. Twelve hours before, the patient's SID had been 18 mEq/L. Increasing the serum Na^+ concentration by 2 mEq/L and decreasing the serum Cl^- by 3 mEq/L and lactate by 6 mEq/L resulted in an increase in the SID of 11 mEq/L, and the SID was now 29 mEq/L. The patient's intact renal function as well as intercompartmental shifts allowed the decrease in serum Cl^- concentration. The serum Na^+ concentration increased as a result of exogenous Na^+ administration (both as $NaHCO_3$ and as 5% albumin solution), and the lactate decreased as the allograft function improved. The "baseline" SID was low (30 mEq/L) because the ATOT was low (albumin was 2 g/dL and phosphate 3 mg/dL).

As the remaining lactate cleared over the next few hours, the SID would increase to nearly 40 mEq/L and the patient would become alkalemic unless steps were taken to reduce minute ventilation further. Allowing the Pco_2 to increase to 45 mm Hg resulted in the pH remaining less than 7.50, and over the next several hours the kidneys restored the SID to the baseline concentration by retaining Cl^-. Over the next few weeks to months, the new liver increased the albumin concentration, and as the ATOT improved the kidneys slowly adjusted the SID upward until a new steady state was reached.

References

1. Kellum JA: Metabolic acidosis in the critically ill: Lessons from physical chemistry. Kidney Int 1998; 53:S81–S86.
2. Stewart PA: Modern quantitative acid-base chemistry. Can J Physiol Pharmacol 1983; 61:1444–1461.
3. Jones NL: A quantitative physciochemical approach to acid-base physiology. Clin Biochem 1990; 23:89–195.
4. Leblanc M, Kellum JA: Biochemical and biophysical principles of hydrogen ion regulation. *In*: Critical Care Nephrology. Ronco C, Bellomo R (Eds). Dordrecht, The Netherlands, Kluwer Academic Publishers, 1998, pp 261–277.
5. Bourke E, Haussinger D: pH homeostasis: The conceptual change. Contrib Nephrol 1992; 100:58–88.
6. Oliver J, Bourke E: Adaptations in urea and ammonium excretion in metabolic acidosis in the rat: A reinterpretation. Clin Sci Mol Med 1975; 48:515–520.
7. Atkinson DE, Bourke E: pH Homeostasis in terrestrial vertebrates: Ammonium ion as a proton source. *In*: Comparative and Environmental Physiology. Mechanisms of Systemic Regulation, Acid-Base Regulation, Ion Transfer and Metabolism. Vol 22. Heisler N (Ed). Berlin, Springer, 1995, pp 1–26.
8. Moore EW: The alkaline tide. Gastroenterology 1967; 52:1052–1054.
9. Bellomo R, Kellum JA, Pinsky MR: Visceral lactate fluxes during early endotoxemia in the dog. Chest 1996; 110:198–204.
10. Kellum JA, Bellomo R, Kramer DJ, Pinsky MR: Splanchnic Buff-

ering of Metabolic Acid During Early Endotoxemia. J Crit Care 1997; 12:7–12.
11. Lindinger MI, Heigenhauser GJF, McKelvie RS, Jones NL: Blood ion regulation during repeated maximal exercise and recovery in humans. Am J Physiol 1992; 262:R126–R136.
12. Forrest DM, Walley KR, Russel JA: Impact of acid-base disorders on individual organ systems. *In*: Critical Care Nephrology. Ronco C, Bellomo R (Eds). Dordrecht, The Netherlands, Kluwer Academic Publishers, 1998, pp 297–310.
13. Hickling KG, Walsh J, Henderson S, Jackson R: Low mortality rate in adult respiratory distress syndrome using low-volume, pressure-limited ventilation with permissive hypercapnia: A prospective study. Crit Care Med 1994; 22:1568–1578.
14. Kette F, Weil MH, Gazmuri RJ: Buffer solutions may compromise cardiac resuscitation by reducing coronary perfusion pressure. JAMA 1991; 266:2121–2126.
15. Hindman BJ: Sodium bicarbonate in the treatment of subtypes of lactic acidosis: Physiologic considerations. Anesthesiology 1990; 72:1064–1076.
16. Bersin RM, Arieff AI: Improved hemodynamic function during hypoxia with Carbicarb, a new agent for the management of acidosis. Circulation 1988; 77:227–233.
17. Spital A, Garella S: Correction of acid-base derangements. *In*: Critical Care Nephrology. Ronco C, Bellomo R (Eds). Dordrecht, The Netherlands, Kluwer Academic Publishers, 1998, pp 311–328.
18. Bleich HL, Swartz WB: Tris buffer (THAM): An appraisal of its physiologic effects and clinical usefulness. N Engl J Med 1966; 274:782–787.
19. Arieff AI: Bicarbonate therapy in the treatment of metabolic acidosis. *In*: The Pharmacologic Approach to the Critically Ill Patient. Chernow B (Ed). Baltimore, Williams & Wilkins, 1994, p 973.
20. Narins RG, Emmett M: Simple and mixed acid-base disorders: A practical approach. Medicine (Baltimore) 1980; 59:161–187.
21. Figge J, Mydosh T, Fencl V: Serum proteins and acid-base equilibria: A follow-up. J Lab Clin Med 1992; 120:713–719.
22. Sadjadi SA: A new range for the anion gap. Ann Intern Med 1995; 123:807.
23. Winter SD, Pearson R, Gabow PG, Schultz AL, Lepoff RB: The fall of the serum anion gap. Arch Intern Med 1990; 150:311–313.
24. Levinsky NG: Acidosis and alkalosis. *In*: Harrison's Principles of Internal Medicine. 11th ed. Brauwald E, Isselbacher KJ, Petersdorf RG, et al (Eds). New York, McGraw-Hill, 1987.
25. Salem MM, Mujais SK: Gaps in the anion gap. Arch Intern Med 1992; 152:1625–1629.
26. Oster JR, Perez GO, Materson BJ: Use of the anion gap in clinical medicine. South Med J 1988; 81:229–237.
27. Gabow PA: Disorders associated with an altered anion gap. Kidney Int 1985; 27:472–483.
28. Whelton A, Carter GG, Garth M, et al: Carbenicillin-induced acidosis and seizures. JAMA 1971; 218:1942–1943.
29. Kang Y, Aggarwal S, Virji M, et al: Clinical evaluation of autotransfusion during liver transplantation. Anesth Analg 1991; 72(1):94–100.
30. Narins RG, Jones ER, Townsend R, et al: Metabolic acid-base disorders: Pathophysiology, classification and treatment. *In*: Fluid Electrolyte and Acid-Base Disorders. Arieff AI and DeFronzo RA (Eds). New York, Churchill Livingston, 1985, pp 269–385.
31. Arieff AI, Carroll HJ: Nonketotic hyperosmolar coma with hyperglycemia: Clinical features, pathophysiology, renal function, acid-base balance, plasma-cerebrospinal fluid equilibria and the effects of therapy in 37 cases. Medicine (Baltimore) 1972; 51:73–94.
32. Mecher C, Rackow EC, Astiz ME, Weil MH: Unaccounted for anion in metabolic acidosis during severe sepsis in humans. Crit Care Med 1991; 19:705–711.
33. Gilfix BM, Bique M, Magder S: A physical chemical approach to the analysis of acid-base balance in the clinical setting. J Crit Care 1993; 8:187–197.
34. Kellum JA, Kramer DJ, Pinsky MR: Strong ion gap: A methodology for exploring unexplained anions. J Crit Care 1995; 10:51–55.
35. Kirschbaum B: Increased anion gap after liver transplantation. Am J Med Sci 1997; 313:107–110.
36. Kellum JA, Bellomo R, Kramer DJ, Pinksy MR: Hepatic anion flux during acute endotoxemia. J Appl Physiol 1995; 78:2212–2217.
37. Mehta K, Kruse JA, Carlson RW: The relationship between anion gap and elevated lactate. Crit Care Med 1986; 14:405–414.
38. Kellum JA, Kramer DJ, Pinsky MR: Closing the GAP: A simple method of improving the accuracy of the anion gap (Abstract). Chest 1996; 110:18S.
39. Schlichtig R: [Base excess] vs [strong ion difference]: Which is more helpful? Adv Exp Med Biol 1997; 411:91–96.
40. Mizock BA, Falk JL: Lactic acidosis in critical illness. Crit Care Med 1992; 20:80–93.
41. Weil MH, Afifi AA: Experimental and clinical studies on lacate and pyruvate as indicators of the severity of acute circulatory failure (shock). Circulation 1970; 41:989–1001.
42. Blair E: Acid-base balance in bacteremic shock. Arch Intern Med 1971; 127:731–739.
43. Madias NE: Lactic acidosis. Kidney Int 1986; 29:752–774.
44. van Lambalgen AA, Runge HC, van den Bos GC, Thijs LG: Regional lactate production in early canine endotoxin shock. Am J Physiol 1988; 254:E45–E51.
45. Cain SM, Curtis SE: Systemic and regional oxygen uptake and delivery and lactate flux in endotoxic dogs infused with dopexamine. Crit Care Med 1991; 19:1552–1560.
46. Brown S, Gutierrez G, Clark C, Nelson C, Tiu A: The lung as a source of lactate in sepsis and ARDS. J Crit Care 1996; 11:2–8.
47. Kellum JA, Kramer DJ, Lee KH, Mankad S, Bellomo R, Pinsky MR: Release of lactate by the lung in acute lung injury. Chest 1997; 111:1301–1305.
48. De Backer D, Creteur J, Zhang H, Norrenberg M, Vincent J-L: Lactate production by the lungs in acute lung injury. Am J Respir Crit Care Med 1997; 156:1099–1104.
49. Stacpoole PW: Lactic acidosis and other mitochondrial disorders. Metab Clin Exp 1997; 46:306–321.
50. Fink MP: Does tissue acidosis in sepsis indicate tissue hypoperfusion? Intensive Care Med 1996; 22:1144–1146.
51. Gutierrez G, Wolf ME: Lactic acidosis in sepsis: A commentary. Intensive Care Med 1996; 22:6–16.
52. Kilpatrick-Smith L, Dean J, Erecinska M, Silver IA: Cellular effects of endotoxin in vitro. II. Reversibility of endotoxic damage. Circ Shock 1983; 11:101–111.
53. Gore DC, Jahoor F, Hibbert JM, DeMaria EJ: Lactic acidosis during sepsis is related to increased pyruvate production, not deficits in tissue oxygen availability. Ann Surg 1996; 224:97–102.
54. Connett RJ, Honig CR, Gyeski TEJ, Brooks GA: Defining hypoxia: A systems view of V_{O_2}, glycolysis, energetics, and intracellular P_{O_2}. J Appl Physiol 1990; 68:833–842.
55. Bearn AG, Billing B, Sherlock S: The effect of adrenaline and noradrenaline on hepatic blood flow and splanchnic carbohydrate metabolism in man. J Physiol (Lond) 1951; 115:430–441.
56. Levy B, Bollaert P-E, Charpentier C, et al: Comparison of norepinephrine and dobutamine to epinephrine for hemodynamics, lactate metabolism, and gastric tonometric variables in septic shock: A prospective randomized study. Intensive Care Med 1997; 23:282–287.
57. Zilva JF: The origin of acidosis in hyperlactatemia. Ann Clin Biochem 1978; 15:40–43.
58. Madias NE, Homer SM, Johns CA, Cohen JJ: Hypochloremia as a consequence of anion gap metabolic acidosis. J Lab Clin Med 1984; 104:15–23.
59. Cohen RD, Woods HF: Lactic acidosis revisited. Diabetes 1983; 32:181–191.
60. Kreisberg RA: Lactate homeostasis and lactic acidosis. Ann Intern Med 1980; 92:227–237.
61. Graf H, Leach W, Arieff AI: Evidence for a detrimental effect of bicarbonate therapy in hypoxic lactic acidosis. Science 1985; 227:754–756.
62. Rhee KH, Toro LO, McDonald GG, Nunnally RL, Levin DL: Carbicarb, sodium bicarbonate, and sodium chloride in hypoxic lactic acidosis. Chest 1993; 104:913–918.
63. Cooper DJ, Walley KR, Wiggs BR, Russell JA: Bicarbonate does not improve hemodynamics in critically ill patients who have lactic acidosis: A prospective, controlled clinical study. Ann Intern Med 1990; 112:492–498.
64. Mathieu D, Neviere R, Billard V, Fleyfel M, Wattel F: Effects of bicarbonate therapy on hemodynamics and tissue oxygenation in patients with lactic acidosis: A prospective, controlled clinical study. Crit Care Med 1991; 19:1352–1356.
65. Cohen RD: The production and removal of lactate: Lactate in acute conditions. *In*: International Symposium on Lactate in Acute

Conditions. Bossart H, Perret C (Eds). Basel, Karger, 1979, pp 10-19.
66. Stacpoole PW, Lorenz AC, Thomas RG, Harman EM: Dichloroacetate in the treatment of lactic acidosis. Ann Intern Med 1988; 108:58-63.
67. Stacpoole PW, Wright EC, Baumgartner TG, et al: A controlled clinical trial of dichloroacetate for treatment of lactic acidosis in adults. N Engl J Med 1992; 327:1564-1569.
68. Alberti KGMM: Diabetic emergencies. Br Med J 1989; 45:242-263.
69. Magder S: Pathophysiology of metabolic acid-base disturbances in patients with critical illness. *In*: Critical Care Nephrology. Ronco C, Bellomo R (Eds). Dordrecht, The Netherlands, Kluwer Academic Publishers, 1998, pp 279-296.
70. Bakerman S: ABC's of Interpretive Laboratory Data. Greenville, NC, Interpretive Laboratory Data, 1984, p 3.
71. Androque HJ, Tannen RL: Ketoacidosis, hyperosmolar states, and lactic acidosis. *In*: Fluids and Electrolytes. Kokko JP, Tannen RL (Eds). Philadelphia, WB Saunders, 1996, pp 643-674.
72. Good DG: Regulation of bicarbonate and ammonium absorption in the thick ascending limb of the rat. Kidney Int 1991; 40:S36-S42.
73. Fulop M: Alcoholic ketoacidosis. Endocrinol Metab Clin North Am 1993; 22:209-219.
74. Wrenn KD, Slovis CM, Minion GE, Rutkowski R: The syndrome of alcoholic ketoacidosis. Am J Med 1991; 91:119-128.
75. Widmer B, Gerhardt RE, Harrington JT, Cohen JJ: Serum electrolyte and acid base composition: The influence of graded degrees of chronic renal failure. Arch Intern Med 1979; 139:1099-1102.
76. Harrington JT, Cohen JJ: Metabolic acidosis. *In*: Acid-base. Cohen JJ, Kassirer JP (Eds). Boston, Little, Brown & Co, 1982, pp 121-225.
77. Batlle DC, Hizon M, Cohen E, Gutterman C, Gupta R: The use of the urine anion gap in the diagnosis of hyperchloremic metabolic acidosis. N Engl J Med 1988; 318:594-599.
78. Cheek DB: Changes in total chloride and acid-base balance in gastroenteritis following treatment with large and small loads of sodium chloride. Pediatrics 1956; 17:839-847.
79. Shires GT, Tolman J: Dilutional acidosis. Ann Intern Med 1948; 28:557-559.
80. Garella S, Chang BS, Kahn SI: Dilution acidosis and contraction alkalosis: Review of a concept. Kidney Int 1975; 8:279-283.
81. Garella S, Tzamaloukas AH, Chazan JA: Effect of isotonic volume expansion on extracellular bicarbonate stores in normal dogs. Am J Physiol 1973; 225:628-636.
82. Mathes DD, Morell RC, Rohr MS: Dilutional acidosis: Is it a real clinical entity? Anesthesiology 1997; 86:501-503.
83. Kellum JA, Bellomo R, Kramer DJ, Pinsky MR: Etiology of metabolic acidosis during saline resuscitation in endotoxemia. Shock 1998; 9:364-368.
84. Kellum JA: Recent advances in acid-base physiology applied to critical care. *In*: Yearbook of Intensive Care and Emergency Medicine. Vincent JL (Ed). New York, Springer-Verlag, 1998, pp 577-587.
85. Gilbert EM, Haupt MT, Mandanas RY, Huaringa AJ, Carlson RW: The effect of fluid loading, blood transfusion, and catecholamine infusion on oxygen delivery and consumption in patients with sepsis. Am Rev Respir Dis 1986; 134:873-878.
86. Gattinoni L, Lissoni A: Respiratory acid-base disturbances in patients with critical illness. *In*: Critical Care Nephrology. Ronco C, Bellomo R (Eds). Dordrecht, The Netherlands, Kluwer Academic Publishers, 1998, pp 297-312.
87. Brochard L, Mancebo J, Wysocki M, et al: Noninvasive ventilation for acute exacerbations of chronic obstructive pulmonary disease. N Engl J Med 1995; 333:817-822.
88. Tsuno K, Miura K, Takeya M, Kolobow T, Morioka T: Histopathologic pulmonary changes from mechanical ventilation at high peak airway pressures. Am Rev Respir Dis 1991; 143:1115-1120.
89. Sugiura M, McCulloch PR, Wren S, Dawson RH, Froese AB: Ventilator pattern influences neutrophil influx and activation in atelectasis-prone rabbit lung. J Appl Physiol 1994; 77:1355-1365.
90. Gennari FJ, Kassirer JP. Respiratory alkalosis. *In*: Acid-Base. Cohen JJ, Kassirer JP (Eds). Boston, Little, Brown & Co, 1982, pp 349-376.
91. Cohen JJ, Madias NE, Wolf CJ, Schwartz WB: Regulation of acid-base equilibrium in chronic hypocapnia: Evidence that the response of the kidney is not geared to the defense of extracellular [H^+]. J Clin Invest 1976; 57:1483-1489.
92. Adrogue HJ, Madias NE: Management of life-threatening acid-base disorders: Part II. N Engl J Med 1998; 338:107-111.

77

Sodium and Potassium Disorders

Juan Carlos Ayus, MD, FACP • Carlos Caramelo, MD

Sodium and potassium disorders are common in critically ill patients and frequently result in increased morbidity and mortality. Early recognition and appropriate treatment of these disorders can limit their adverse effects. Appropriate treatment requires a basic understanding of sodium and potassium pathophysiology. This chapter reviews water equilibrium and hyponatremic, hypernatremic, hypokalemic, and hyperkalemic states. Disorders of divalent ions are discussed elsewhere in this book.

PHYSIOLOGY OF WATER EQUILIBRIUM

Balance of Body Water, Dimensions, Composition, and Exchange

In healthy individuals and in normal conditions, approximately 50% of the lean body mass in females and 60% in males is water. This amount of water is distributed in the intracellular compartment (two thirds of the total body water) and extracellular compartment (one third of the total body water). The extracellular water is distributed between plasma and interstitial fluid in one-fourth and three-fourths proportions, respectively.[1]

Water metabolism is regulated by complex mechanisms that involve diverse levels of integration and control (i.e., the central nervous system, the cardiovascular and renal systems, and a host of endo-, para-, and autocrine mediators). The objective of the whole system is to maintain constant water content of the organism and constant water distribution between the different compartments. In general, the body's water conservation system is not maximally stressed, because daily exchanges with the outside environment are not more than 5% of the total body content of water.

Cell membranes can be considered maximally permeable to water, and accordingly there is an osmotic equilibrium between intra- and extracellular compartments. The extracellular osmolarity, which depends on the plasma sodium concentration, is equivalent to intracellular osmolality, which depends on the intracellular concentration of potassium. The necessity to maintain this equivalence determines all cellular adaptations to osmotic changes, through either the gain or the release of osmotically active solutes. Other solutes such as urea or glucose are necessary, albeit in a less important fashion, for the maintenance of plasma osmolality. Urea is, however, not relevant in terms of generating an osmotic gradient, because of its free transmembrane permeability.[1]

The water content of the organism is regulated by input and output systems. Output occurs via urine formation, fecal excretion, and cutaneous and respiratory evaporation. The physiologic priority is the elimination of the daily solute load, which mandates an obligatory loss of water as the solvent for excreted solutes. These minimum obligatory losses are a function of the magnitude of the solute load and of the ability to concentrate urine and need to be replaced by the ingestion of an equivalent quantity of water.[1]

Main Mechanisms of Control

Thirst and urine concentration are the main defenses against hyperosmolarity, whereas water excretion is the principal defense against hypo-osmolality caused by excessive ingestion. The maintenance of water equilibrium also requires the hormone arginine vasopressin (AVP), also called antidiuretic hormone (ADH). AVP binds to specific receptors on the collecting ducts (V_2 receptors), which are coupled to cyclic adenosine monophosphate (cAMP) formation. The activation of these receptors by AVP promotes the recruitment and membrane attachment of water channels formed by a specific protein, aquaporin 2, which allow water reabsorption to the interstitium. AVP results in decreased urine flow and increased urine osmolality. There is a wide range of values for normal urinary osmolality, from a minimum of 50 to 80 mOsm/kg H_2O to a maximum of approximately 1200 mOsm/kg H_2O. The osmotic threshold for AVP secretion is about 280 mOsm/kg H_2O. Thirst starts to be stimulated at approximately 290 mOsm/kg H_2O. Both the thirst center and AVP production are located in the hypothalamus. AVP is transported by neurosecretion from the hypothalamus to the neurohypophysis.

AVP production is regulated by several factors, including plasma osmolality, effective circulating volume, and stimuli such as nausea, stress, temperature, and other hormonal mediators. The fact that the extracellular fluid is an NaCl-water solution implies that sodium and water alterations are related. Therefore, most hypernatremic and hyponatremic situations are actually due to changes in water content, and although the kidney is the organ that generates these water abnormalities, it is the brain that suffers the consequences of cellular volume alterations (Fig. 77–1).

Renal Water Handling

The diluting segment of the nephron needs adequate water and solute delivery in order to generate free water. A decrease in solute ingestion (as seen in malnutrition or malabsorption) or glomerular filtration rate (GFR) or an increase in proximal tubular reabsorption may diminish the amount of fluid delivered to the distal nephron and thus limit the renal capacity to excrete water. Furthermore, tubulointerstitial nephropathies or administration of diuretics may depress free water excretion by disturbing the normal structure or function of the diluting segment. Finally, the dilute tubular fluid present in the late portion of the thick ascending limb of Henle's loop must be allowed to traverse the remaining portions of the nephron without substantial water reabsorption taking place. The water permeability of the most distal nephron sites is determined in large part by the amount of circulating antidiuretic hormone, AVP. The role of AVP in the distal nephron is to increase water permeability in responsive segments, thus permitting reabsorption of water generated in the diluting segment. Suppression of AVP synthesis and/or release is required for the elaboration of a maximally dilute urine. In normal circumstances, very small decreases in plasma osmolality are sufficient to suppress maximally the release of AVP from the posterior pituitary.[1]

HYPONATREMIC STATES

In clinical practice, hypo-osmolar states are usually suspected when the plasma sodium is found to be low. Although hyponatremia usually implies hypo-osmolality, actual measured osmolality may be low, normal, or even elevated in patients with hyponatremia.[1] Before an aggressive therapeutic regimen is begun, however, it is vital to prove that the plasma osmolality is indeed low.

Symptomatic Hyponatremia

Most cases of symptomatic hyponatremia occur in a small subset of clinical settings. The situations of postoperative hyponatremia, hypotonic states complicating treatment with oxytocin, hyponatremia caused by decompensated psychosis, compulsive water drinking, and diuretic-associated hyponatremia are described next.

Water retention out of proportion to sodium retention is noted in surgical patients. This is accompanied by decreases in urine output and plasma sodium and an increase in urine salt excretion.[2, 3] The factors responsible for this can be broadly classified into alterations in AVP secretion, changes in intrarenal water handling, excessive hypotonic fluid administration, and drug effects. In postsurgical patients, it has been

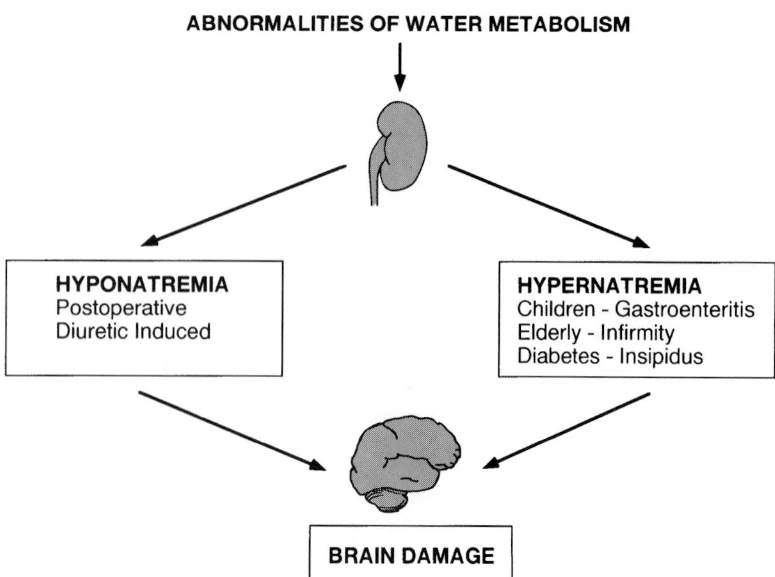

Figure 77–1. Abnormal handling of electrolytes and water by the kidney results in changes in brain volume regulation that lead to brain damage.

found that AVP levels are increased compared with preoperative values.[3] Only a small minority of surgical patients, about 1%, develop hyponatremia, and symptomatic hyponatremia occurs in about 10% of these subjects.[3] Excessive hypotonic fluid absorption contributes to hyponatremia in men undergoing transurethral resection of the prostate (TURP) and women undergoing hysteroscopic endometrial ablation.[4, 5] Because of the routine use of electrocautery during TURP and endometrial ablation, electrolyte solutions cannot be used as irrigating fluids. Instead, mannitol, glycine, and sorbitol are the favored fluids. In a procedure lasting 2 hours, upward of 2.4 L of these sodium-free solutions might be absorbed. This amount is often sufficient to decrease plasma sodium to levels that may induce symptoms (<120 mmol/L). When glycine is the irrigating fluid, another possible cause of altered mental status is acute ammonia toxicity, which can theoretically result from the metabolism of absorbed glycine.[5]

The most important step to be taken in the prevention of postoperative hyponatremia is careful consideration of the choice of intravenous fluids. *Hypotonic solutions are seldom, if ever, appropriate in postoperative patients.*[2, 3] These patients have limited capabilities to excrete water. Unless there is a definite reason to suspect the existence of a deficit of free water, isotonic sodium chloride (154 mM NaCl) is the preferred fluid.

Oxytocin is a drug that is used commonly to hasten labor and in the treatment of gastrointestinal (GI) hemorrhage. At relatively low doses (<20 mU/min) oxytocin has little antidiuretic potency. However, at doses of 50 mU/min or greater, urine flow can be inhibited in a dose-dependent fashion to less than 10% of preinfusion rates.[1] The antidiuretic actions of oxytocin can cause hyponatremia.

Patients with psychiatric disorders and psychogenic polydipsia are also at risk for severe hyponatremia. Although many neuroleptic agents are said to stimulate the release of AVP, the number of reports in which this has been well documented is surprisingly small. Water clearance in a hyponatremic psychotic patient was abnormal when he received haloperidol but not during a drug-free interval.[1]

Hyponatremia ultimately develops in a sizable number of patients receiving diuretics. Although this process is frequently mild and asymptomatic, it can be severe and quite acute.[6] The negative sodium balance induced by the diuretic agent represents an additional stimulus for the nonosmotic release of AVP. Agents with a preferential site of action in the cortical diluting segment (such as thiazides) further impair the ability to excrete a water load. Host factors also predispose to the development of diuretic-induced hyponatremia. These include malnutrition, advanced age, and female gender.[6] In some patients, marked stimulation of thirst is a probable predisposing factor.[7]

Brain Adaptation to Hyponatremia

Briefly, adaptation of the brain to hyponatremia occurs as a consequence of the following sequence of events. Hyponatremia leads to the movement of water into brain cells. Vasopressin and perhaps other hormones also lead to direct movement of water into brain cells independent of the effects of hyponatremia. The early adaptation of brain to hyponatremia-mediated edema is through loss of blood and cerebrospinal fluid, followed by extrusion of sodium from brain cells by several pathways.[2] Loss of potassium and amino acids follows later, in an attempt to decrease brain cell osmolality without a gain of water.[2]

Hyponatremic encephalopathy occurs when a hyponatremic patient exhibits symptoms that are secondary to increased intracranial pressure associated with brain edema.[2] Because the brain is encased within a rigid compartment, little parenchymal swelling can occur before intracranial pressure increases and central nervous system (CNS) symptoms develop. When hyponatremic encephalopathy occurs, the initial symptoms may be dramatic, including such severe manifestations as seizures and respiratory arrest. Hypoxemia is a prominent feature in this condition.[3, 8] *Noncardiogenic pulmonary edema* can also be the clinical presentation of hyponatremia. Furthermore, hypoxemia impairs brain adaptation and worsens cerebral edema.[9] Thus, awareness of the situations in which an unrecognized symptomatic hypotonic state is possible is the first and most important step in management. The most common situation in which this occurs is in the *postoperative* patient. As discussed earlier, multiple factors conspire against the ability of the kidney to excrete a water load in postsurgical subjects. Every postoperative patient should be considered at risk for the development of hyponatremia and appropriate prophylactic measures taken.[2, 3]

Although postoperative hyponatremic encephalopathy can occur in anyone, younger female patients demonstrate a clear predisposition for the occurrence of brain damage or death. Studies have demonstrated that the age and gender of the patient are major determinants of brain damage caused by hyponatremia.[3, 10] In general, most adult patients with symptomatic hyponatremia (serum sodium of 128 mmol/L or less) who do not suffer permanent neurologic damage are older women or men of any age, whereas those who die or incur permanent brain injury are younger women (Fig. 77–2).

Treatment of Hypotonic States

Early treatment of symptomatic hyponatremia is required in order to prevent long-term neurologic sequelae. If respiratory arrest or coma develops before therapy is initiated, the prognosis is usually grave even if hyponatremia is ultimately corrected. When symptoms are present, rapid treatment is required with hypertonic NaCl with a loop diuretic.[11, 12] The guidelines for treatment are to raise the plasma sodium by no more than 20 to 25 mmol/L over the first 48 hours[11] (Table 77–1; Fig. 77–3). However, the possibility that these patients may undergo a significant water diuresis during treatment should always be considered. In this situation, the use of a vasopressin analog, desmopressin (deamino-D-arginine-vasopressin [DDAVP]), is indicated to curtail the water diuresis and thus prevent correction of serum sodium by more than 25 mmol/L in the initial 48 hours.[11] This treatment may also apply to other situations in which a spontaneous diuresis occurs during correction of hyponatremia, such as in patients who are compulsive water drinkers.

HYPERNATREMIC STATES

Because sodium with its accompanying anions constitutes the great majority of osmoles in the plasma, hypertonicity is always present if hypernatremia is present.[13] The plasma osmolality should be determined early during the clinical evaluation of patients with hypertonic conditions. The major solutes that contribute to plasma osmolality in normal subjects are sodium with its accompanying anions, urea, and glucose. An estimate of osmolality that is useful clinically is obtained from the formula:

$$\text{plasma osmolality} = 2(\text{Na}) + \text{BUN (mg/dL)}/2.8 + \text{glucose (mg/dL)}/18$$

where BUN is blood urea nitrogen.

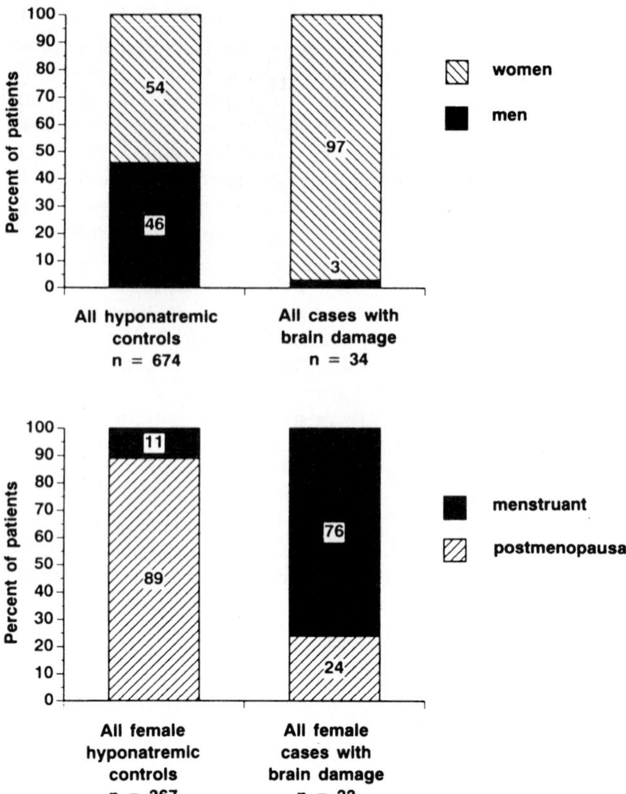

Figure 77–2. Effects of gender and menstruant status on brain damage from hyponatremic encephalopathy. *Top panel,* The proportions of men and women who did (cases) and did not (controls) have permanent brain damage are compared. The relative risk for death or permanent brain damage is 28 times greater in women than in men (95% confidence interval [CI], 5 to 141). *Bottom panel,* The proportion of women with hyponatremia who were or were not menstruant, who did (cases) or did not (controls) have permanent brain damage. The relative risk for dying or brain damage from postoperative hyponatremia is 26 times greater for menstruant women than for postmenopausal women (95% CI, 11 to 62). (From Ayus JC, Wheeler JM, Arieff AI: Postoperative hyponatremic encephalopathy in menstruant women. Ann Intern Med 1992; 117:891-897.)

Causes of Hypernatremia

In infants, gastroenteritis with diarrhea is the most common cause of hypernatremia. Small children may also become hypernatremic after accidental administration of a high solute load, particularly accidental substitution of NaCl for sugar in preparation of formula or improper dilution of concentrated formulas.[13]

In adults, causes of hypernatremia include nasogastric hyperalimentation, nonketotic hyperosmolar coma, acute renal failure, renal tubular damage, improper mixture of dialysis fluid, dehydration secondary to either fever or elevated ambient temperature, pituitary or renal diabetes insipidus (DI), seawater ingestion, and hyperadrenocorticoid states. Excessive administration of hypertonic solutions of $NaHCO_3$ to critically ill patients suffering cardiac arrest has also been associated with a dangerously elevated plasma osmolality.[13]

DI is most commonly central or neurogenic and is characterized by total or partial failure to synthesize or secrete ADH (vasopressin). Most causes for central DI involve destruction of the hypothalamic-hypophyseal structures responsible for producing ADH; for DI to be present, the lesions must decrease ADH secretion by at least 75%.[13]

Nephrogenic DI (NDI) is characterized by inability of the renal tubules to respond to ADH in the presence of normal hormone concentrations. The pathogenesis involves disruption of the countercurrent mechanism that generates a hypertonic medullar and papillary interstitial space or from disruption of the capacity for ADH to increase the osmolality of the collecting duct. Although NDI may be congenital, acquired (i.e., drug-induced) NDI is much more common.[13]

A group of adult patients in whom the entity of hypernatremia with its attendant sequelae is not appreciated are chronic alcoholic subjects with end-stage liver disease who present with fulminant liver failure and hepatic encephalopathy.[13] Such patients are often treated with oral lactulose as therapy for their hepatic encephalopathy. Hypernatremia may complicate such therapy.[13] Patients with lactulose-associated hypernatremia have a mortality of 87%; for patients without hypernatremia, the mortality rate is 60%.

Clinical Manifestations of Hypernatremia

The signs and symptoms of hypernatremia are variable. In experimental hyperosmolality, findings include nystagmus, myoclonic jerking of the extremities, severe weight loss, decreased food intake, and ultimately respiratory failure and death.[14] Seizures are commonly present and roughly correlate with the degree of hypernatremia. Associated laboratory abnormalities include metabolic acidosis and hyperglycemia.[14] The abnormalities in glucose metabolism are important therapeutically and are addressed further later.

Initially, brain cells shrink because of osmotic water abstraction, but ultimately the cells nearly regain the water content they had in the control state by virtue of a combination of net solute uptake and generation of solute de novo. Studies of hypernatremia have shown that over the course of 7 days, water content of the brain decreases by approximately 10% but eventually recovers to within 98 to 99% of the control value.[14] This is largely accompanied by an increase in brain solute content. The increase in solute serves to protect brain

TABLE 77–1. Treatment of Hypotonic States

High-risk groups: *Younger females and children.* Most important step is prevention: avoidance of hypotonic fluid administration in *surgical patients.* Measure plasma osmolality to confirm hypo-osmolality.

Symptomatic Hyponatremia (Headache, Nausea, Emesis, Weakness)

ACUTE TREATMENT

1. Start treatment with hypertonic (515 mM) NaCl infusion; use an infusion pump in an intensive care unit setting.
2. Monitor serum sodium every 2 hr until the patient is stable and symptom-free.
3. Stop hypertonic NaCl when the patient is symptom-free or serum sodium is increased by 20–25 mmol/L *in the initial 48 hours* of therapy to avoid cerebral demyelinating lesions.
4. Avoid hypernatremia or normonatremia during the initial 5 days of therapy, particularly in patients with alcoholism or liver disease.

CHRONIC TREATMENT

1. Fluid restriction
2. Demeclocycline
3. Oral urea
4. Lithium
5. Vasopressin V_2 receptor antagonists

Asymptomatic Hyponatremia

1. Fluid restriction
2. Treatment of underlying disease

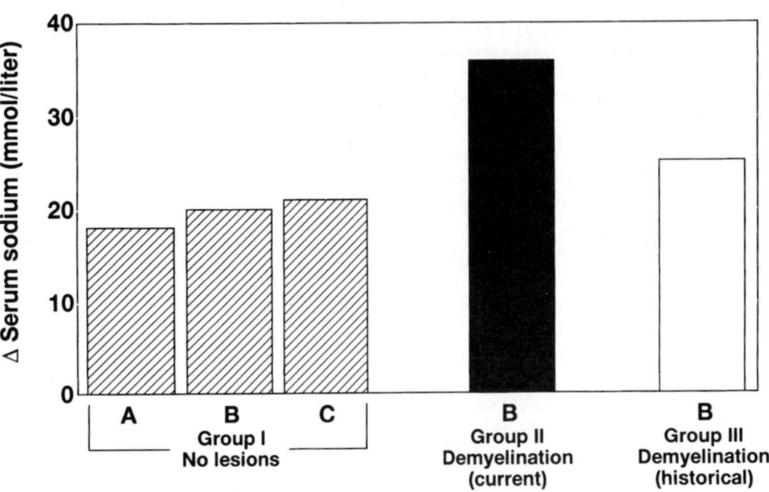

Figure 77–3. Absolute change in serum sodium concentration in the three groups of patients. In group I, concentrations were measured at the end of treatment with hypertonic saline (A), 24 hours after initiation of treatment (B), and 48 hours after initiation of treatment (C). In groups II and III, concentrations were measured at the end of treatment with hypertonic saline. (From Ayus JC, Krothapalli RK, Arieff AI: Treatment of symptomatic hyponatremia and its relation to brain damage. N Engl J Med 1987; 317:1190–1195.)

cell volume from further dehydration, which could lead to structural damage.[14] However, this initial protective effect may eventually become deleterious during correction of hypernatremia if the plasma sodium is somehow decreased more rapidly than the brain is able to dissipate the idiogenic osmoles[14] (Fig. 77–4).

Hypernatremia is associated with considerable long-term morbidity and mortality in both children and adults. The mortality of elderly patients with hypernatremia was found to be 42% in one study, and neurologic morbidity was present in 38% of the survivors.[13] One especially noteworthy finding in this series was the fact that mortality was higher in patients with hypernatremia that developed in the hospital. The authors attributed this finding to a more complicated clinical setting and delayed recognition of hypertonicity in the hospitalized subjects.[13]

Treatment of Hyperosmolar States

The goal of therapy for hypernatremia is the reduction of plasma osmolality toward normal by the administration of free water in excess of solute. When water administration is planned, the major therapeutic questions are the type of fluid to be given and its rate and route of administration. In adult patients with hypernatremia, 280 mM dextrose in water (5% dextrose in water [D_5W]) has commonly been administered. Later information suggests that therapy for hypernatremia with glucose-containing solutions (280 mM glucose in H_2O) may lead to cerebral intracellular lactic acidosis, with increased mortality.[13] In addition, an osmotic diuresis caused by glucose hastens renal water losses and slows correction of the hypertonic state. Furthermore, the metabolism of glucose is seldom if ever normal in patients with hypernatremia.[13] Rec-

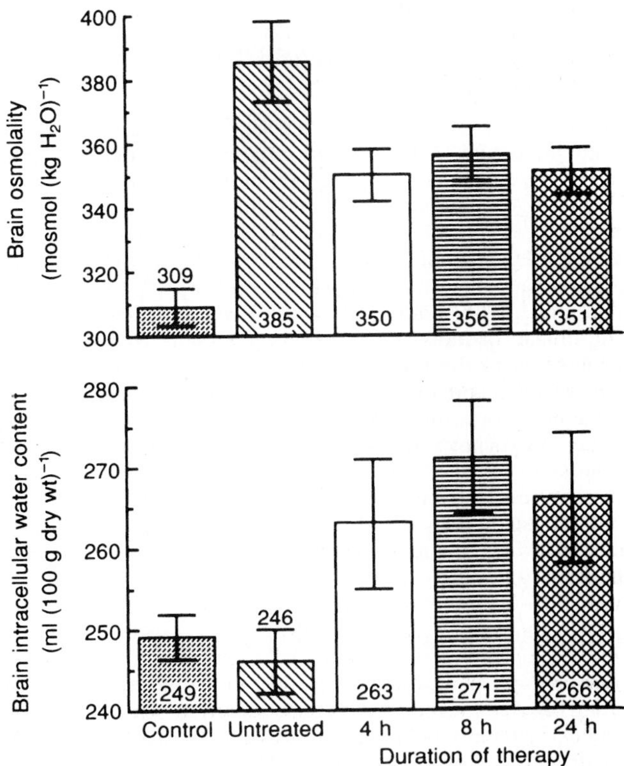

Figure 77–4. Brain osmolality and intracellular water content in rabbits before and after treatment for hypernatremia. *Upper panel:* Brain osmolality in control rabbits, rabbits with untreated chronic (1 week) hypernatremia, and rabbits in which hypernatremia was lowered to normal values over 4, 8, or 24 hours. All values in rabbits with treated hypernatremia are significantly less than the value in rabbits with chronic hypernatremia ($P < .01$) and significantly greater than control ($P < .01$). *Lower panel:* Corresponding values for brain intracellular water content. Values after therapy over 4, 8, or 24 hours are significantly greater than both the control and 1 week hypernatremia values ($P < .01$). (From Ayus JC, Armstrong DL: Central nervous system effects of hyponatremia and its therapy in rats and rabbits. J Physiol (Lond) 1996; 421:243–255.)

TABLE 77–2. Treatment of Hyperosmolar States

1. The patient should initially receive colloid, such as plasma or a plasma substitute or isotonic saline, to replete intravascular volume.
2. Fluid deficit should be estimated on the basis of serum sodium, body weight, and total body water. The deficit should be given over 48–72 hr, aiming for a decrement in serum osmolality of approximately 1 mOsm per liter/hr. In severe hypernatremia (>170 mEq/L) serum sodium should *not* be corrected to below 150 mEq/L in the first 48–72 hr. Maintenance fluids, which include replacement of urine volume with hypotonic fluid, are given in addition to the deficit.
3. Hypotonic fluid should be administered. The usual replacement fluid is 77 mEq/L NaCl (0.5 N saline). In general, solutions containing glucose should be *avoided* and an oral route of administration should be used.
4. Plasma electrolytes should be monitored every 2 hr until the patient is neurologically stable.

ommendations for treatment of chronic hypernatremia in adults, when the hypernatremia is due primarily to water loss, are listed in Table 77–2.

Treatment of central DI consists of administering a synthetic analog of ADH, desmopressin or DDAVP. Some clinicians are still using injectable forms of vasopressin, but this is not the treatment of choice. Other treatments, which include the use of substances such as chlorpropamide, clofibrate and its derivatives, and thiazide diuretics, are of only secondary value in the treatment of DI. During the puerperal period there may be a rare form of DI caused by excessive vasopressinase activity; it is necessary to identify it, because it does not respond to vasopressin but does respond to desmopressin. Nephrogenic DI is difficult to treat. Drugs contributing to NDI should be discontinued, if possible. The only treatment available for NDI is administration of thiazidic diuretics, which stimulate an ADH-independent increase in proximal tubular resorption and a decrease in polyuria.[13]

REGULATION OF POTASSIUM HOMEOSTASIS

Potassium is primarily an intracellular cation, with 98% of total body potassium (3000 to 4000 mEq) being located intracellularly. The cell potassium concentration is approximately 120 to 140 mEq/L, whereas the extracellular potassium concentration is between 3.5 and 4.5 mEq/L. This intercompartmental gradient is maintained by the activity of Na^+K^+-ATPase, which pumps Na^+ out of and K^+ into the cell in a 3:2 ratio.[15] Oral ingestion or IV administration of potassium leads initially to the uptake of most of the excess potassium by the cells, in proportion to the relative distribution of potassium between extracellular and intracellular spaces (1:35 to 1:40). Plasma potassium concentration is a function of the relationship between potassium entry, the intercompartmental distribution of potassium, and potassium excretion. Alterations in potassium concentration have marked effects on membrane polarity, with consequences for all cells in which polarization-depolarization cycles are functionally relevant (e.g., cardiac, neuromuscular cells).[15]

Renal Management of Potassium

The kidney has a principal role in the maintenance of potassium balance, varying potassium secretion with changes in dietary or parenteral intake (up to 120 to 140 mEq/day). Only small amounts of potassium are lost each day in stool and sweat (<15 mEq). Almost all of the filtered potassium is reabsorbed in the proximal tubule and the loop of Henle, so that less than 10% of the filtered load is delivered to the early distal tubule. In comparison with these reabsorptive processes, potassium is secreted by the collecting tubules. Secretion and reabsorption in these segments are responsible for urinary potassium excretion and are regulated by physiologic needs.[15] Aldosterone increases potassium secretion and is critical for renal tubular adaptation to changes in potassium. An increase in plasma potassium or extracellular volume (ECV) depletion stimulates aldosterone secretion, thereby promoting the excretion of potassium in the urine. The contrary occurs during potassium depletion and ECV expansion.

Measurement of aldosterone levels is of little clinical utility in the intensive care setting. Instead, the effect of aldosterone can be examined by estimating the transtubular potassium gradient (TTKG) at the end of the cortical collecting tubule:

$$\text{TTKG} = \frac{\text{urine K/(urine osm/plasma osm)}}{\text{plasma K}}$$

The TTKG in normal conditions is approximately 8 to 9, and a value below 7 in a hyperkalemic patient is suggestive of a decreased effect of aldosterone. In ECV depletion, the high potassium luminal concentration and the low urine flow lead to a reduction in the absolute rate of potassium secretion. The combination of increased aldosterone release and reduced distal flow allows sodium to be conserved without substantially affecting potassium balance. On the other hand, the presence of nonsuppressible aldosterone secretion in a euvolemic or hypervolemic patient, as occurs in primary hyperaldosteronism, enhances urinary potassium excretion and hypokalemia occurs.[15]

Elements of Diagnosis and Factors Regulating Potassium Levels

Several coexisting factors influence potassium entry into the cells:

Catecholamines

Stimulation or suppression of receptors favors or impairs, respectively, the cellular entry of potassium. These actions have practical consequences for patients in the intensive care unit (ICU). The increment in the plasma potassium concentration after a potassium load is enhanced in the presence of β_2-adrenergic blockade, the release of epinephrine and insulin during a stress response can acutely lower the plasma potassium concentration, and the administration of β-receptor agonists can lower the plasma potassium level.

Insulin Deficiency, Hyperglycemia, and Hyperosmolality

Insulin promotes potassium entry into cells.[15] On the other hand, the ability to handle a potassium load is impaired with insulin deficiency. Hyperosmolality induced by either hyperglycemia or solutes such as mannitol induces translocation-dependent hyperkalemia. This is caused by osmotic water movement from the cells into the extracellular fluid, which drags potassium out of the cells. The plasma potassium concentration may rise by as much as 0.4 to 0.8 mEq/L for every 10 mOsm/kg elevation in the effective plasma osmolality.

Acid-Base Alterations

Changes in the extracellular pH produce reciprocal H^+ and potassium shifts between cells and the extracellular fluid (ECF).[15] As a result, potassium tends to move into cells with alkalemia and out of cells with acidemia.[15] On the average, the plasma potassium concentration rises by 0.6 mEq/L (range, 0.2 to 1.7 mEq/L) for every 0.1 unit reduction in extracellular pH. However, a fall in pH is less likely to raise the plasma potassium concentration in patients with lactic acidosis or ketoacidosis.[15] Moreover, respiratory acidosis and alkalosis induce relatively small changes in potassium balance.[15]

Cell Breakdown and Catabolism

Any cause of increased tissue breakdown results in release of potassium into the extracellular fluid; hyperkalemia may occur in this setting, particularly in patients with some degree of renal failure. Clinical examples include trauma, the administration of cytotoxic or radiation therapy to patients with hematologic malignancies, and rhabdomyolysis.[15]

Hyperaldosteronism

The presence of one of the forms of primary mineralocorticoid excess should be suspected in any patient with the triad of hypertension, unexplained hypokalemia, and metabolic alkalosis. Screening should be performed in all patients with otherwise unexplained hypokalemia and in those with severe or resistant hypertension.[15]

Hypoaldosteronism

Any cause of decreased aldosterone release or effect, such as that induced by hyporeninemic hypoaldosteronism or certain drugs, can diminish the efficiency of potassium secretion and lead to hyperkalemia. The rise in the plasma potassium concentration is generally small in patients with normal renal function but can be clinically important in the presence of underlying renal insufficiency; this aspect should be taken into account in the ICU setting, because hyporeninemic hypoaldosteronism may be responsible for some cases of unexplained hyperkalemia (e.g., increased potassium load resulting from gastrointestinal blood loss in a patient with hypoaldosteronism). Hyporeninemic hypoaldosteronism most often occurs in patients 50 to 70 years of age with diabetic nephropathy or chronic interstitial nephritis of any origin, such as gouty nephropathy, nephrolithiasis, analgesic nephropathy, sickle cell renal disease, and urinary tract disease, who have mild to moderate renal insufficiency. Patients with primary adrenal insufficiency have low aldosterone and cortisol levels but a high plasma renin activity because of the commonly associated volume depletion and hypotension.[15]

Renal Failure

In contrast to acute renal failure, significant hyperkalemia (potassium above 5.5 mmol/L) is uncommon in patients with chronic renal disease, as the ability to maintain potassium excretion at near-normal levels is maintained until a decrease of about 80% in glomerular filtration rate is reached. Some patients have hyperkalemia and impaired potassium excretion despite normal aldosterone release and normal sodium handling. This seemingly selective impairment in potassium handling, which does not respond to exogenous mineralocorticoid, has been described with acute renal transplant rejection, cyclosporine treatment, and lupus nephritis.[15]

Drug Intoxication and Poisoning

In different types of poisoning, potassium alterations are important factors in determining the patient's outcome. Unless renal function is impaired or rhabdomyolysis is severe, hyperkalemia is a relatively uncommon metabolic complication of poisoning. In contrast, marked hypokalemia is a more common problem and may have serious sequelae. Most potassium disturbances in acute poisoning are due to disruption of extrarenal control mechanisms, notably the activity of Na^+,K^+-adenosine triphosphatase (Na^+,K^+-ATPase) and K^+ channels.[15] Hypokalemia occurs because of increased Na^+,K^+-ATPase activity (e.g., $beta_2$ agonist, theophylline, or insulin poisoning), competitive blockade of potassium channels (e.g., barium or chloroquine poisoning), gastrointestinal losses, and/or alkalosis. Hyperkalemia follows inhibition of Na^+,K^+-ATPase activity (e.g., by digoxin), increased uptake of potassium salts, disruption of intermediary metabolism (e.g., cyanide poisoning), activation of potassium channels (e.g., fluoride poisoning), and the presence of acidosis and rhabdomyolysis, particularly if the latter is complicated by renal failure.[15]

TABLE 77–3. Guidelines for Examining the Hyperkalemic Patient

Assess Increased Potassium Intake
Assess a Shift of Potassium from Intracellular to Extracellular Fluid
Metabolic acidosis
β_2-Adrenergic blockade
Insulin deficiency
Necrosis or depolarization
Assess Cause of Reduced Potassium Loss in Urine
Renal failure
Low aldosterone action
Decreased distal nephron flow rate

HYPERKALEMIA

The major causes of hyperkalemia are shown in Table 77–3. The primary symptoms of hyperkalemia are related to impaired neuromuscular transmission and depression of cardiac function. Membrane excitability is dependent on the resting membrane potential, which depends on the ratio of intracellular to extracellular potassium concentration. The level of potassium in the blood is correlated with mortality. In one study, mortality was 14% with a potassium level of 7 mmol/L, 42% with a potassium level of 8 mmol/L, and 100% with a potassium level of more than 8 mmol/L. Mortality and electrocardiographic studies support the contention that 7 mmol/L levels is a critical value for potassium. There is, however, substantial individual variability in the level of potassium at which symptoms develop, mostly dependent on concomitant factors such as Ca^{2+} and H^+ concentrations and, more important, with the time it takes to reach hyperkalemic values. Monitoring of hyperkalemia should be done by electrocardiogram (Table 77–4); however, a marked decrease in skeletal muscle strength is a harbinger of impending myocardial alterations.

Treatment of Hyperkalemia

Specific treatment of hyperkalemia is directed at antagonizing the membrane effects of potassium, driving extracellular potassium into the cells, and/or removing excess potassium from the body. The first step in the treatment of hyperkalemia is to eliminate sources of potassium entry, such as dietary sources,

TABLE 77–4. Summary of Electrocardiographic Changes During Hyperkalemia

1. Increased T-wave amplitude
2. Decreased R-wave amplitude
3. ST segment depression
4. Decreased P-wave amplitude
5. Prolonged PR, QRS, and QT intervals
6. Absent P waves
7. Ventricular arrhythmias

TABLE 77–5. Drug-Related Hyperkalemia

Drugs Containing Potassium
Example:
Potassium chloride, salt substitutes

Drugs That Cause a Potassium Shift from Intracellular to Extracellular Fluid
Hormone antagonists
β_2-Adrenergic blockers
Drugs that impair insulin release from cells (e.g., diazoxide)
Cell depolarizers (digitalis)

Drugs That Interfere with Potassium Excretion in the Urine
Drugs that interfere with renin-angiotensin-aldosterone axis
Release from adrenal gland (e.g., heparin)
Decreased renin release (β_2-adrenergic blockers)
Converting enzyme inhibitors (e.g., captopril)
Angiotensin II antagonists
Drugs that block aldosterone binding to its receptors
Spironolactone
Drugs that cause interstitial nephritis
Sodium channel blockers (amiloride, triamterene, trimethoprim)
Most common: combinations of more than one of the preceding drugs

salt substitutes, or potassium supplements, and to discontinue drugs that may potentiate hyperkalemia, such as nonsteroidal anti-inflammatories or angiotensin-converting enzyme inhibitors (Table 77–5).

Calcium directly antagonizes the membrane effects of hyperkalemia through still incompletely identified mechanisms. The protective effect of calcium begins within minutes but does not last. As a result, calcium infusions are indicated, mostly when electrocardiographic (ECG) changes are severe. The usual dose is 1 ampule (10 mL) of 10% calcium gluconate. This dose is infused over a 3-minute period. ECG changes should be monitored, and another dose can be given after 5 minutes if ECG changes fail to improve.

Potassium can be shifted intracellularly by administering insulin-glucose, sodium bicarbonate, or β_2-adrenergic agonists. Effective insulin therapy usually leads to a 0.5 to 1.5 mEq/L fall in the plasma potassium concentration. Insulin is given as 10 units of regular insulin, together with 40 to 50 g of glucose to avoid hypoglycemia. Sodium bicarbonate administration produces a metabolic alkalosis, stimulating potassium movement into cells. It can be added to glucose or saline solution, although spectacular effects on potassium concentration cannot be expected. Data do not support the efficacy of the common practice of administering $NaHCO_3$ for the emergency treatment of hyperkalemia in patients receiving maintenance dialysis.[15] The β_2-adrenergic agonists drive potassium into cells by increasing Na^+,K^+-ATPase activity and are a readily available adjuvant treatment for rapidly reducing plasma potassium concentration. Albuterol is the adrenergic agent of choice for severe hyperkalemia. Side effects are tachycardia and possible induction of angina and arrhythmias in susceptible subjects. Thus, these agents are basically contraindicated for patients with heart disease.[15]

Potassium can be removed from the body with diuretics and cation exchange resins. Either thiazide or loop diuretics can be used, and the major cation exchange resin available is sodium polystyrene sulfonate (Kayexalate; 1 g binds approximately 1 mEq of potassium). Hemodialysis is also effective for decreasing plasma potassium levels, as 30 to 40 mEq of potassium can be extracted in a regular dialysis session.[15]

HYPOKALEMIA

The main signs and symptoms of hypokalemia are the characteristic electrocardiographic changes with dysrhythmias, hypoperistalsis, paralytic ileus, and lack of muscular tone and strength. The development of hypokalemia is of greatest concern in patients with underlying heart disease, hypertension, or hepatic cirrhosis. Hypokalemia can precipitate hepatic coma in some patients with advanced hepatic cirrhosis, at least in part because of increased renal ammonium synthesis. Subjects with concurrent digitalis therapy or a plasma potassium concentration less than 3.0 mEq/L are particularly prone to cardiac arrhythmias.[15] In addition, hypokalemia may contribute to an increased incidence of sudden death in patients with hypertension and left ventricular hypertrophy and is a risk factor for multifocal atrial tachycardia, especially in patients with chronic obstructive lung disease. Potassium depletion by itself can induce a variety of relatively rapid, frequently overlooked changes in renal function. These include ADH resistance with impaired urinary concentration, increased ammonia production, and altered renal bicarbonate and sodium reabsorption.[15]

Hypokalemia results from three primary causes (Table 77–6):

- Decreased potassium intake
- Increased entry of potassium into cells
- Increased potassium losses

Decreased dietary intake or decreased parenteral administration causes hypokalemia only in rare cases or after considerably long periods of insufficient potassium input. However, decreased intake exacerbates hypokalemia in patients with increased potassium losses. Either metabolic or respiratory alkalosis can promote potassium entry into cells, albeit in small amounts (<0.4 mEq/L decrease of plasma potassium for every 0.1-unit rise in pH).[15] A major reason for the association of hypokalemia with alkalemia is that the underlying cause of alkalemia (e.g., diuretics, vomiting, or hyperaldosteronism) causes both H^+ and K^+ losses. Transient catecholamine-related hypokalemia can be seen during stress-induced release of epinephrine or administration of β_2-adrenergic agonists to treat asthma, heart failure, hypotension, or premature labor.[16]

In a series of patients with severe asthma, the mean basal plasma potassium level at the beginning of an untreated severe crisis was 3.54 mmol/L; the value decreased to 2.9 mmol/L in a short period of time after intensive β_2-agonist treatment.[16] An association between hypothermia and hypokalemia, related

TABLE 77–6. Causes of Hypokalemia

Decreased Potassium Intake

Potassium Shift into Cells
Acid-base disorders
Alkalosis
Hormones
Insulin
β_2-Adrenergic agonists
Anabolism
Growth
Recovery from diabetic ketoacidosis
Total parenteral nutrition

Increased Potassium Losses
Vomiting or nasogastric aspiration
Diarrhea
Diuretics
Hyperaldosteronism
Hypomagnesemia
Antibiotics and other drugs (penicillin derivatives, amphotericin B, cisplatin, and toluene)

Rare Disorders
Hereditary hypokalemic periodic paralysis
Hyperthyroidism

to potassium redistribution to the cells, appears in a number of postoperative patients. On the basis of this observation, administration of $NaHCO_3$, insulin, digitalis, and calcium to patients suffering from hypothermia must be done with caution because hypokalemia may coexist with low body temperature and predispose patients to lethal dysrhythmias.[15]

Loss of gastric or intestinal secretions for any cause (vomiting, diarrhea, laxatives, or tube drainage) is associated with potassium depletion primarily related to increased urinary losses.[15] Use of agents that limit gastric acid production is a preventive method in patients with prolonged gastroduodenal drainage.[15]

Diuretics that act proximal to the potassium secretory site (e.g., acetazolamide, loop diuretics, and thiazide-type diuretics) increase potassium excretion by increasing distal delivery and stimulating aldosterone synthesis.[15] Moreover, nonreabsorbable anions such as β-hydroxybutyrate or some antibiotics (penicillin, carbenicillin) can lead to marked increases in potassium excretion.

Treatment of Hypokalemia

Although hypokalemia can be transiently induced by the entry of potassium into cells, most cases result from unreplaced losses. The total potassium deficit in patients with potassium loss can only be approximated, because there is no strict correlation between the plasma potassium concentration and total body potassium stores. A plasma potassium level of 3.0 mEq/L suggests a deficit of 200 to 300 mmol of potassium. Levels below 2.0 mEq/L are frequently accompanied by a deficit of more than 500 mmol.[15] However, these estimates of body potassium depletion apply only when the depletion is chronic. Acute decreases in plasma potassium are associated with much lower levels of depletion.

Potassium chloride is the first-choice preparation for potassium repletion, especially in the setting of chloride-responsive metabolic alkalosis.[15] Patients with severe hypokalemia are given intravenous KCl at a concentration of 20 to 40 mEq/L and at a rate of 10 mEq/hr. Occasionally, patients with severe hypokalemia may require potassium repletion at rates of 20 to 30 mEq/hr. Saline- rather than dextrose-containing intravenous fluids are indicated at the beginning of the therapy to avoid stimulation of insulin secretion, which might lead to further hypokalemia. Hypomagnesemia is frequently associated with hypokalemia.[17] It is important to remember that magnesium is required for potassium entry into cells. Thus, magnesium administration is frequently necessary for potassium retention in hypokalemic, critically ill patients. In a controlled study of hypokalemic patients in the ICU, individuals receiving magnesium sulfate required less potassium replacement.[17] Defective normalization of potassium content might be responsible in part for the increased mortality related to hypomagnesemia in critically ill patients.[15]

It must be emphasized that rapid intravenous administration of potassium is potentially dangerous (e.g., causes arrhythmias) even in potassium-depleted patients. Even though a central vein catheter is preferable for potassium administration, the top of the catheter should not enter the heart, to avoid bathing the cardiac pacemaker cells with a concentrated potassium solution. Monitoring the physiologic effects of hypokalemia is essential, as when these problems are no longer severe, the rate of potassium repletion should be decreased.[18] Major risks of potassium administration are cardiac arrhythmias and rebound hyperkalemia. However, studies report that potassium chloride infusions at a high concentration (200 mmol/L) and high rate (20 mmol/hr) are well tolerated, decrease the frequency of ventricular arrhythmias, and do not cause transient hyperkalemia.[16] It is important to estimate and replace potassium losses during repletion, especially continued urinary losses related to diuretic therapy or aldosterone effect. The use of potassium-sparing diuretics (amiloride, triamterene, and spironolactone) for these patients can limit further urinary losses of both potassium and magnesium.[16]

References

1. Berl T, Schrier RW: Clinical disorders of water metabolism. *In:* Renal and Electrolyte Disorders. Schrier RW (Ed). Philadelphia, Lippincott-Raven, 1997, pp 1–71.
2. Ayus JC, Varon J, Fraser C: Pathogenesis and management of hyponatremic encephalopathy. Curr Opin Crit Care 1995; 1:452–459.
3. Ayus JC, Wheeler JM, Arieff AI: Postoperative hyponatremic encephalopathy in menstruant women. Ann Intern Med 1992; 117:891–897.
4. Arieff AL, Ayus JC: Endometrial ablation complicated by fatal hyponatremic encephalopathy. JAMA 1993; 270:1230–1232.
5. Ayus JC, Arief AI: Glycine-induced hypo-osmolar hyponatremia. Arch Intern Med 1997; 157:223–226.
6. Ayus JC: Diuretic induced hyponatemia. Arch Intern Med 1986; 146:1295–1296.
7. Friedman E, Shadel M, Halkin H, Farfel Z: Thiazide-induced hyponatremia: Reproducibility by single dose rechallenge and analysis of pathogenesis. Ann Intern Med 1989; 110:24–30.
8. Ayus JC, Arieff AI: Pulmonary complications of hyponatremic encephalopathy: Noncardiogenic pulmonary edema and hypercapnic respiratory failure. Chest 1995; 107:517–521.
9. Wexler ZS, Ayus JC: Hypoxic and ischemic hypoxia exacerbates brain injury associated with metabolic encephalopathy in laboratory animals. J Clin Invest 1994; 93:256–264.
10. Arieff AI, Ayus JC, Fraser CL: Hyponatremia and death or permanent brain damage in healthy children. Br Med J 1992; 304:1218–1222.
11. Ayus JC, Krothapalli RK, Arieff AI: Treatment of symptomatic hyponatremia and its relation to brain damage: A prospective study. N Engl J Med 1987; 317:1190–1195.
12. Sarnaik AP, Meert K, Hackbarth R, Fleischmann L: Management of hyponatremic seizures in children with hypertonic saline: A safe and effective strategy. Crit Care Med 1991; 19:758–762.
13. Arieff AI, Ayus JC: Pathogenesis and management of hypernatremia. Curr Opin Crit Care 1996; 2:418–423.
14. Ayus JC, Armstrong DL, Arieff AI: Effects of hypernatremia in the central nervous system and its therapy in rats and rabbits. J Physiol (Lond) 1996; 492:243–255.
15. Peterson LN, Levi M: Disorders of potassium metabolism. *In:* Renal and Electrolyte Disorders. Schrier RW (Ed). Philadelphia, Lippincott-Raven, 1997, pp 192–240.
16. Khan MA: Plasma potassium in acute severe asthma before and after treatment. Br J Clin Pract 1989; 43:363–365.
17. Whang R, Whang DD, Ryan MP: Refractory potassium depletion: A consequence of magnesium deficiency. Arch Intern Med 1992; 152:40–45.
18. Siegel D, Hulley SB, Black DM, et al: Diuretics, serum and intracellular electrolyte levels, and arrhythmias in hypersensitive men. JAMA 1992; 267:1083–1089.

78

Calcium, Magnesium, and Phosphorus Disorders

Gary P. Zaloga, MD, FCCM • Pamela R. Roberts, MD

Calcium, magnesium, and phosphorus are divalent ions that are essential for normal cell and organ function. These ions play key roles in many metabolic, physiologic, and structural processes. They are important regulators of enzyme activity, protein synthesis and degradation, cell messenger systems, and energy metabolism. Alterations in the extracellular or intracellular levels of these ions are common in critically ill patients. Optimal treatment of critically ill patients requires a knowledge of the pathophysiology and treatment of disorders of these ions.[1]

PHYSIOLOGIC FUNCTION

Calcium

Calcium is the primary regulator of movement in the body. Thus, it is essential for normal excitation-contraction coupling in cardiac, smooth, and skeletal muscle. Calcium also regulates contractile elements involved in the processes of ciliary motion, opening of intercellular channels (i.e., permeability), endocytosis, exocytosis, diapedesis, mitosis, meiosis, neurotransmission, and secretion (i.e., hormones, enzymes). Calcium is an important cell messenger that couples extracellular events (i.e., receptor activation) to intracellular enzyme and metabolic alterations. For example, it is important for the cardiovascular actions of β-adrenergic and α-adrenergic agonists. Calcium ions are responsible for pacemaker activity and the plateau phase of the action potential. They are also important activators of enzymes, such as the proteases, lipases, and nucleases, and are required for blood coagulation.

Although many calcium-activated processes are essential for normal cell integrity, calcium also activates processes that are detrimental to cell function and may even result in cell death.[2-4] These include catecholamine resistance, digestive enzyme activation (proteases, lipases, nucleases), free radical production, cytokine release, vasoconstriction, and programmed cell death (apoptosis). Thus, normal cell function requires controlled regulation of cytoplasmic calcium levels.

Magnesium

Magnesium is an essential cofactor for more than 300 enzymatic reactions in the body. These enzymes include the adenosine triphosphatases (ATPases, both Na^+, K^+-ATPase and Ca^{2+}-ATPase); cyclases (e.g., adenylate cyclase); and enzymes involved in deoxyribonucleic acid (DNA) synthesis, oxidation reactions, fatty acid synthesis, and glycolytic pathways.[5] Magnesium is important for membrane stability and ion channel function,[5] and it helps maintain the electrical membrane potential (through effects on potassium flux). Magnesium is also an important regulator of calcium channels and parathyroid hormone (PTH) secretion and action.[6-10] Magnesium is a component of Mg^{2+}-adenosine triphosphate (ATP), the primary energy source for the cell. It is also required for protein synthesis (along with potassium and phosphorus). Most intracellular magnesium is associated with organic compounds.

Phosphorus

Phosphorus bonds are used for cell energy (e.g., ATP, creatine phosphate). Phosphorus is also an essential component of 2,3,-diphosphoglycerate (2,3-DPG, important for offloading of oxygen from hemoglobin), cyclic adenosine monophosphate (cAMP), cyclic guanosine monophosphate (cGMP), ribonucleic acid (RNA), DNA, and inositol polyphosphates. In addition, it is involved in acid-base balance, regulation of the glycolytic pathway, and regulation of renal synthesis of 1,25-dihydroxyvitamin D, and it is required for protein synthesis. Phosphorus is an essential structural component of bone (required for mineralization) and cell membranes (e.g., phospholipids).

MEASUREMENT

In contrast to univalent ions, such as sodium and potassium, divalent ions are carried on circulating proteins (primarily albumin) in the blood. Thus, calcium, magnesium, and phosphorus circulate in the blood in ionized (physiologically active), chelated, and protein-bound forms[1, 11-13] (Table 78-1). The quantity of calcium and magnesium that is protein bound is clinically significant; direct measurement of the ionized forms is required for accurate assessment of physiologically active quantities. In fact, most patients with low total calcium and magnesium levels (usually from low albumin levels) have normal ionized calcium and magnesium concentrations. Numerous studies in critically ill patients indicate that total and calculated ionized calcium and magnesium levels are poor indicators of true circulating ionized calcium and magnesium status.[14-18] This is especially true in severely ill patients and postsurgical patients with low albumin levels.

The primary location of the ion is also important in interpreting blood, plasma, or serum levels. Magnesium and phosphorus are primarily intracellular ions (similar to potassium). Thus, circulating (extracellular) levels may not reflect intracellular status. On the other hand, calcium is primarily extracellular. Extracellular free calcium levels are 10,000 times higher than intracellular free calcium levels, and the ionized calcium level is a good indicator of the extracellular calcium status. The movement of the divalent ions into and out of cells and cellular compartments (where they exert biologic effects) is regulated by various pumps, exchangers, and channels and is influenced by hormones and intracellular messengers.

Technology (ionized ion electrodes) is available for assessment of ionized calcium and magnesium concentrations. Binding of these ions to albumin is pH-dependent. Acidosis decreases protein binding whereas alkalosis increases protein binding.[1] Thus, acute changes in blood pH (hyperventilation, administration of bicarbonate) can alter ionized levels of the ions. However, excess circulating ion is excreted by the kidneys in patients with intact renal function. Lowered circulating ionized calcium levels are normalized by PTH-induced release of calcium from bone.

The physiologically active levels (ionized) of calcium, magnesium, and phosphorus can be altered by the presence of circulating chelators (such as citrate and albumin). Chelators bind the ions, decreasing their ionized levels while at the same time elevating total levels. Thus, total levels of these ions can be deceptive in patients receiving chelators. Although citrate is an excellent chelator of calcium, levels of calcium can be maintained by the parathyroid–vitamin D axis in most patients receiving blood transfusions. Clinically significant ionized hypocalcemia is seen only in patients receiving rapid blood transfusion during resuscitation and in patients with hypothermia, hepatic failure, or renal failure.[1] Citrate is metabolized by temperature-dependent hepatic enzymes in the liver and excreted through the kidneys.

TABLE 78–1. Circulating Forms of Divalent Ions

Ion	Total	Ionized	Chelated	Protein Bound
Calcium	8.5–10.5 mg/dL 2.1–2.6 mmol/L	4.2–5.2 mg/dL 1.0–1.3 mmol/L 50%	1.3–1.6 mg/dL 0.3–0.4 mmol/L 10%–15%	3.4–4.2 mg/dL 0.8–1.0 mmol/L 35%–40%
Magnesium	1.7–2.4 mg/dL 1.4–2.0 mEq/L 0.7–1.0 mmol/L	0.9–1.3 mg/dL 0.8–1.1 mEq/L 0.4–0.55 mmol/L 55%	0.26–0.36 mg/dL 0.2–0.3 mEq/L 0.1–0.15 mmol/L 15%	0.5–0.72 mg/dL 0.4–0.6 mEq/L 0.2–0.3 mmol/L 30%
Phosphorus	2.5–4.5 mg/dL 0.8–1.45 mmol/L	1.4–2.5 mg/dL* 0.4–0.8 mmol/L 55%	0.8–1.4 mg/dL 0.24–0.44 mmol/L 30%	0.4–0.7 mg/dL 0.1–0.2 mmol/L 15%

*Circulates as HPO_4; H_2PO_4; sodium, calcium, and magnesium salts; and PO_4.

REGULATION

Calcium is primarily stored in the skeleton (~1000 g), and circulating levels are maintained within narrow limits by the parathyroid-vitamin D-bone axis.[1, 11] PTH secretion is stimulated by ionized hypocalcemia and suppressed by ionized hypercalcemia and elevated 1,25-dihydroxyvitamin D levels. PTH fluctuates on a minute-per-minute basis and is the primary regulator of circulating calcium levels. PTH secretion is stimulated by mild ionized hypomagnesemia but suppressed by severe ionized hypomagnesemia and hypermagnesemia.[6, 7, 9] In addition, normal magnesium levels are required for normal actions of PTH on bone.[8, 10, 19] Thus, extreme alterations in circulating magnesium levels are common causes of ionized hypocalcemia.[6–10, 19, 20]

PTH stimulates the release of calcium from bone, absorption from the gastrointestinal tract (through vitamin D), and reabsorption from the renal tubules. Vitamin D is also an important regulator of ionized calcium status. Vitamin D is synthesized in the skin, a reaction requiring ultraviolet light, and absorbed from the diet (fat-soluble vitamin). It is 25-hydroxylated in the liver and 1-hydroxylated in the kidney. Renal 1-hydroxylase activity is regulated by PTH (increases activity), inorganic phosphorus (low phosphorus level increases activity), growth hormone, hydrogen ions, and calcitonin levels. 1,25-Dihydroxyvitamin D is the active form of the hormone. It increases the resorption of calcium from bone and absorption of calcium from the gastrointestinal tract. Calcitonin plays a lesser role in the normal regulation of circulating calcium levels. Declines in plasma calcium concentration decrease calcitonin secretion, leading to increased bone resorption and decreased renal calcium excretion. During acute hypercalcemia, calcitonin levels increase, resulting in a decrease in bone resorption and renal synthesis of 1,25-dihydroxyvitamin D. In addition, acute elevations in calcitonin have been associated with ionized hypocalcemia (e.g., during infection).

Phosphorus and magnesium balance is maintained by the intestinal tract (absorption), kidneys (excretion), and bone (mineralization versus resorption).[1, 12, 13] However, the kidneys are the primary regulators of circulating levels. These ions are freely filtered at the glomerulus and reabsorbed along the renal tubules through sodium-dependent cotransport. Renal phosphorus excretion is increased by PTH, PTH-related peptide, calcitonin, vasopressin, atrial natriuretic peptide, dopamine, metabolic acidosis, volume expansion, glucose, amino acids, saline, sodium bicarbonate, and ketones. It is decreased by vitamin D, growth hormone, insulin-like growth factor 1, glucocorticoids, thyroid hormone, and metabolic alkalosis.

The principal mechanism for long-term adaptation to phosphorus supply is adaptation of the renal transport mechanisms. During dietary phosphorus restriction, phosphorus transport is high and urinary phosphorus excretion is low. The reverse occurs with high phosphorus intake. The mechanisms for signal transduction within the kidneys are unknown but appear to reside within the renal tubular cell.

Magnesium is absorbed primarily in the loop of Henle (50%); lesser amounts are absorbed in the proximal (25%) and distal (5%) convoluted tubules.[13] Magnesium reabsorption is increased by PTH, vitamin D, metabolic alkalosis, hypocalcemia, intravascular volume depletion, and magnesium depletion; it is decreased by calcium (hypercalcemia), diuretics, phosphorus depletion, metabolic acidosis, hypermagnesemia, and intravascular volume expansion. However, the primary factors regulating magnesium reabsorption in the kidneys reside within the renal tubular cells and are influenced directly by circulating magnesium levels.

Thus, patients with renal disease are at risk for hypermagnesemia and hyperphosphatemia. In addition, there is an obligate loss of these ions in stool, through the skin, and in the urine. Dysfunction of the renal tubules that results in the inability to reclaim these ions (i.e., renal wasting) can lead to low circulating levels when losses exceed intake.

ION BALANCE

Calcium, magnesium, and phosphorus balance is maintained through both intake and output (through urine, feces, and skin) (Table 78-2). Poor dietary intake of magnesium and phosphorus can result in body depletion of these ions because of obligate losses in urine, in stool, and through the skin. Calcium levels in the blood are well maintained despite lack of dietary intake of calcium because of mobilization of calcium from bone. However, persistent negative calcium balance will result in osteoporosis. Thus, maintenance of dietary intake of these ions is important for maintenance of normal body mineral homeostasis.

TABLE 78–2. Ion Balance (Daily)

	Calcium	Magnesium	Phosphorus
Dietary intake	1000 mg	300 mg	1000 mg
Intestinal absorption	400 mg	150 mg	600 mg
Feces	800 mg	150 mg	550 mg
Filtered by kidneys	10000 mg	3500 mg	4500 mg
Urine	180 mg	125 mg	400 mg
Total body stores	1000 g	24 g	800 g

ETIOLOGY

Hypocalcemia

Ionized hypocalcemia (ionized calcium level below 1.0 mmol/L)[1, 21] results from one of four basic disorders (Table 78-3): inadequate PTH secretion or action, inadequate vitamin D secretion or action, bone resistance to PTH or vitamin D, and circulating chelators. Ionized hypocalcemia does not result from inadequate calcium intake because release of bone calcium is adequate for maintenance of normal circulating calcium levels (provided the PTH-vitamin D axis is intact). Inadequate PTH secretion or action may result from underlying hypoparathyroidism, severe hypomagnesemia,[8, 16] hypermagnesemia,[7] and other acquired defects in PTH secretion or action.[8, 10, 19, 22] Acquired defects in PTH secretion have been reported in patients with sepsis,[22] pancreatitis, rhabdomyolysis, and systemic inflammatory states. Cytokines and other circulating factors released during these disease states are believed to suppress the parathyroid glands. Such a process may have evolved to be protective because slight lowering of calcium levels is protective in animal models of sepsis and ischemia-reperfusion injury. In some patients, ionized hypocalcemia develops in association with a low PTH level after a prolonged period of hypercalcemia. These patients with posthypercalcemic hypocalcemia are believed to have parathyroid gland suppression from their hypercalcemia. The syndrome is rarely severe and usually resolves during a few days.

Vitamin D deficiency may result from inadequate vitamin intake in the diet or lack of synthesis in the skin (i.e., no ultraviolet light exposure). Vitamin D is a fat-soluble vitamin, and absorption from the gastrointestinal tract requires pancreatic enzymes, bile, and an intact mucosa. Thus, absorption of vitamin D is impaired in patients with pancreatic insufficiency (e.g., pancreatitis), biliary obstruction (e.g., biliary cirrhosis), inadequate bile production (e.g., cirrhosis), short-gut syndromes, and severe inflammatory bowel disease. Vitamin D is hydroxylated in the liver (25-hydroxylation) and kidney (1-hydroxylation) to the active form of vitamin D, 1,25-dihy-

TABLE 78–3. Causes of Hypocalcemia, Hypomagnesemia, and Hypophosphatemia

Hypocalcemia	Hypomagnesemia	Hypophosphatemia
Impaired PTH Action Primary hypoparathyroidism Pseudohypoparathyroidism Acquired hypoparathyroidism Neck surgery Radioiodine Infiltrative disease (e.g., cancer) Hypomagnesemia Sepsis Burns Pancreatitis Rhabdomyolysis Posthypercalcemic ***Impaired Vitamin D Action*** Poor dietary intake Malabsorption Liver disease Renal disease Hypomagnesemia Sepsis Rhabdomyolysis Pseudohypoparathyroidism Phenytoin, phenobarbital Rifampin, isoniazid Ketoconazole ***Calcium Chelation or Precipitation*** Phosphate (e.g., tumor lysis) Citrate EDTA Albumin Hungry bone syndromes Osteoblastic malignant neoplasms Fat embolism Pancreatitis Rhabdomyolysis Ethylene glycol (oxalate) Protamine Sodium sulfate Sodium fluoride ***Decreased Bone Resorption*** Calcitonin (e.g., toxic shock) Cisplatin Bisphosphonates Plicamycin Gallium nitrate	***Gastrointestinal Losses*** Reduced absorption Malabsorption (e.g., short bowel) Laxative abuse Fistulas or nasogastric suction Reduced intake Malnutrition Hyperalimentation Intravenous fluids ***Renal Losses*** Renal disease Glomerulonephritis Tubular disorders Interstitial nephritis Diuretic phase of acute tubular necrosis Hypercalcemia Hyperaldosteronism Hyperthyroidism Phosphorus deficiency Diabetic ketoacidosis ***Drug-Induced Renal Losses*** Diuretics Aminoglycosides, amphotericin B Cisplatin Carbenicillin, pentamidine Cyclosporine Thyroid hormone Digoxin Calcium, cellulose phosphate Ethanol Saline Citrate Catecholamines ***Miscellaneous Losses*** Pregnancy and lactation Severe sweating Burns (skin) Hungry bone syndrome Sepsis Hypothermia Cardiopulmonary bypass Dialysis Refeeding syndrome Glucose, insulin	***Gastrointestinal Losses*** Malabsorption Emesis, diarrhea Nasogastric suction Phosphorus-binding antacids Alcohol, vitamin D deficiency ***Renal Losses*** Renal tubular defects Hyperparathyroidism Hypercalcemia of malignancy Hypomagnesemia, hypokalemia Acidosis Vitamin D deficiency Diuretics, volume expansion Recovery from acute tubular necrosis After renal transplantation Alcohol abuse, diabetes mellitus ***Transcellular Shift*** Refeeding syndrome Carbohydrate loading Recovery from hypothermia Recovery from burns Alkalosis Alcoholism Diabetic ketoacidosis (insulin) Sepsis Salicylate poisoning Hungry bone syndrome Anabolic steroids ***Drug-Induced Losses*** Anabolic steroids Antacids Calcitonin Diuretics Theophylline Epinephrine (beta agonists) Glucagon Insulin Sodium bicarbonate Salicylates Alcohol Glucocorticoids ***Miscellaneous Losses*** Dialysis Inadequate phosphorus intake

EDTA = ethylenediaminetetraacetic acid; PTH = parathyroid hormone.

droxyvitamin D. Activation of vitamin D is impaired in patients with renal disease, severe liver disease, and sepsis. These patients are at risk for the development of ionized hypocalcemia.

Bone resistance to calcium-mobilizing hormones such as PTH and 1,25-dihydroxyvitamin D can cause ionized hypocalcemia. Bone resistance may be caused by hypomagnesemia and drug administration. Examples of drugs associated with ionized hypocalcemia include bisphosphonates, plicamycin, cisplatin, and calcitonin. Patients with severe skeletal loss from osteoporosis can usually mobilize adequate calcium to prevent the development of ionized hypocalcemia.

The final major cause of ionized hypocalcemia is *chelation*. Chelators bind calcium faster than it can be released from bone. The net result is ionized hypocalcemia with a normal or elevated total blood calcium level. Chelation is common after administration of citrate,[23-25] phosphate, albumin, ethylene glycol,[26] fluoride, and noncalcified radiocontrast dyes. Citrate is used as a preservative in blood and is metabolized by temperature-dependent enzymes in the liver and excreted by the kidneys. Thus, citrate clearance is impaired in patients with hypothermia, liver insufficiency, and renal insufficiency. These patients are at risk for hypocalcemia. On the other hand, normothermic patients with relatively normal liver and renal function and an intact parathyroid–vitamin D axis can usually tolerate 3 to 4 units of citrated blood per hour. Phosphate is a potent chelator of calcium but also causes calcium precipitation, inhibition of bone resorption, and suppression of renal synthesis of 1,25-dihydroxyvitamin D. Thus, hyperphosphatemia is a common cause of ionized hypocalcemia. Causes of hyperphosphatemia include phosphate administration, tumor lysis, renal failure, and rhabdomyolysis. Ethylene glycol is metabolized to oxalate, a calcium chelator.[26] The hypocalcemia of pancreatitis was at one time believed to result from chelation of calcium in tissues due to fat necrosis. However, the amount of calcium deposited in tissue beds is unlikely to be the primary cause of hypocalcemia. Defects in the PTH–vitamin D axis are thought to be the primary cause of hypocalcemia.[1]

Hypocalcemia rarely occurs as part of a syndrome characterized by accelerated bone formation (i.e., "hungry bone syndromes"). These syndromes may occur in patients after parathyroidectomy or thyroidectomy for hyperactive glands. These patients have accelerated bone resorption because of excess production of PTH or thyroid hormones. When the stimulus for bone resorption is acutely removed by surgery, bone formation may exceed mineral supply, and hypocalcemia results. The hypocalcemia is usually accompanied by hypophosphatemia and hypomagnesemia. Increased bone formation and hypocalcemia may also occur in patients with osteoblastic metastasis from malignant neoplasms of prostate, breast, and lung.

Hypocalcemia may occur in patients with fat embolism. The hypocalcemia probably results from a combination of chelation, increased protein binding of calcium, and reduced calcium mobilization. Hypocalcemia is associated with the toxic shock syndrome. The exact pathogenesis of the syndrome is undefined, but increased release of calcitonin is believed to contribute to the hypocalcemia. In addition, hypocalcemia after thyroidectomy may result from calcitonin release.[27] Ionized hypocalcemia is common in patients undergoing cardiopulmonary bypass surgery.[28] Hypocalcemia results from dilution and chelation of calcium. Parathyroid gland secretion is normal in most patients, and ionized calcium levels return to normal after bypass.

Hypercalcemia

Ionized hypercalcemia (ionized calcium level above 1.3 mmol/L)[1, 29] occurs when calcium enters the vascular space faster than it can be removed (primarily through renal excretion). Thus, renal insufficiency predisposes patients to ionized hypercalcemia. The major causes of ionized hypercalcemia (Table 78–4) are calcium release from the bone and increased calcium intake (e.g., calcium supplements, milk-alkali syndrome). Excess release of bone calcium may be due to (1) erosion of bone from malignant neoplasms, (2) release of calcium from bone due to immobilization, or (3) humoral stimulation of calcium release as a result of excess PTH, PTH-related peptide, thyroid hormone, catecholamines (e.g., pheochromocytoma), vitamin D, vitamin A, transforming growth factor-α, or interleukin-1. Few tumors secrete PTH.

The most common malignant neoplasms associated with hypercalcemia are lung, breast, hematologic, head and neck, renal, and prostate cancers.[30, 31] Most humoral hypercalcemia of malignancy results from tumor secretion of PTH-related peptides,[30-33] many of which can be detected by available assays. Interestingly, most PTH-related peptides stimulate the release of calcium from bone but fail to stimulate the 1-hydroxylase enzyme in the kidney. The result is an elevated PTH level (due to cross-reaction in PTH assays) but a low 1,25-dihydroxyvitamin D level. Some malignant neoplasms (e.g., lymphoma, Hodgkin's disease) and granulomas (e.g., sarcoid, tuberculosis, histoplasmosis, coccidioidomycosis, berylliosis, silicosis) express 1-hydroxylase activity and can cause hypercalcemia because of excess synthesis of 1,25-dihydroxyvitamin D.[34-38] We have also seen a few patients who have hypercalcemia after a period of hypocalcemia. The hypercalcemia most likely results from increased production of PTH and 1,25-dihydroxyvitamin D, stimulated by the period of hypocalcemia. The cause for the ionized hypocalcemia resolves faster than the calcium-mobilizing hormones can readjust (perhaps owing to parathyroid gland hyperplasia). The mild hypercalcemia in these patients resolves without treatment.

A number of syndromes of hypercalcemia are also associated with hypocalciuria. The hypercalcemia results from decreased renal calcium excretion with or without altered synthesis or action of PTH. Hypocalciuric hypercalcemia may occur as an inherited syndrome (familial hypocalciuric hypercalcemia)[39, 40] or in patients with hypothyroidism,[41] with lithium toxicity, after thiazide administration, and with adrenal insufficiency. The familial syndrome is benign and does not require treatment.

Hypomagnesemia

Hypomagnesemia (magnesium level below 1.4 mEq/L, 0.7 mmol/L, or 1.7 mg/dL)[1, 18, 42-45] is common in critically ill patients, occurring in 25% to 70% of patients (depending on the type of illness or injury). A decrease in total magnesium level is common in patients with low albumin levels (because of a decrease in the protein-bound fraction; see Table 78–1). Many of these patients have normal ionized magnesium levels. Ionized hypomagnesemia occurs when magnesium losses from the body (from urine, stool, secretions, or skin) exceed intake from the diet (see Table 78–3). In contrast to calcium, maintenance of circulating magnesium levels is dependent on dietary intake.

Despite the presence of magnesium in bone, no regulatory system exists to mobilize the magnesium. Because there is an obligatory loss of magnesium from the body, inadequate intake (e.g., malnutrition) can cause ionized hypomagnesemia. Ionized hypomagnesemia may also occur from increased losses (e.g., diuretics, diarrhea) despite maintenance of normal intake. Many critically ill patients with previously normal magnesium status can experience clinically significant ionized hypomagnesemia within 3 to 4 days of their illness.

Ionized hypomagnesemia may result from decreased gastro-

TABLE 78–4. Causes of Hypercalcemia, Hypermagnesemia, and Hyperphosphatemia

Hypercalcemia	Hypermagnesemia	Hyperphosphatemia
Malignant neoplasia	Renal failure	Reduced renal excretion
Hyperparathyroidism	Excess magnesium intake	Renal insufficiency
Immobilization	Antacids	Hypoparathyroidism
Calcium administration	Supplements	PTH resistance
Renal causes	Diet	Hyperthyroidism
Chronic renal failure	Enemas	Acromegaly
Recovery from acute renal failure	Parenteral nutrition	Bisphosphonates
After renal transplantation	Eclampsia	Tumoral calcinosis
Posthypocalcemic hypercalcemia	Preterm labor	Children
Hypocalciuric hypercalcemias	Hypothyroidism	Increased phosphorus intake
Familial	Adrenal insufficiency	Laxatives
Hypothyroidism	Lithium toxicity	Diet
Lithium	Hypocalciuric hypercalcemia	Supplements
Thiazides		Potassium phosphate
Adrenal insufficiency		Enemas
Bartter's syndrome		Vitamin D
Granulomatous disease		Release from tissues
Sarcoidosis		Hemolysis
Histoplasmosis		Tumor lysis
Coccidioidomycosis		Rhabdomyolysis
Tuberculosis		Sepsis
Hyperthyroidism		Malignant hyperpyrexia
AIDS		Fulminant hepatitis
Phosphorus depletion		Severe hypothermia
Pheochromocytoma		Acidosis
Acromegaly		
Drug-induced		
Calcium		
Lithium		
Milk-alkali syndrome		
Theophylline		
Thiazides		
Vitamin D or A toxicity		

AIDS = acquired immunodeficiency syndrome; PTH = parathyroid hormone.

intestinal absorption or increased stool losses of magnesium, increased loss of magnesium through the urine, and internal redistribution of magnesium (see Table 78–3). Decreased gut absorption of magnesium is frequently coupled with increased secretion and is seen in patients with inflammatory bowel disease, gastroenteritis, pancreatic insufficiency, fistulas, short-bowel syndromes, ileal bypass, and other bowel diseases associated with diarrhea. Unabsorbed fat can form complexes with magnesium and also decrease its absorption. Lower-tract secretions are higher in magnesium (10 to 14 mEq/L) than upper tract secretions (1 to 2 mEq/L).

A large number of diseases and medications disrupt renal conservation of magnesium and result in hypomagnesemia (see Table 78–3).[44] Renal magnesium wasting is present when urinary magnesium losses exceed 12 mg (0.5 mmol) per day in the presence of ionized hypomagnesemia. Renal causes of hypomagnesemia include glomerulonephritis, tubular disorders, interstitial nephritis, diabetes mellitus, diuretics, aminoglycosides,[45] amphotericin B, cyclosporine, cisplatin, cardiac glycosides, ethanol, calcium, and sodium chloride.

Occasional patients may have ionized hypomagnesemia as a result of an acute shift of magnesium into the cell (i.e., redistribution; see Table 78–3). Such shifts occur in patients with refeeding syndromes, after administration of glucose or amino acids, and after insulin or catecholamine administration.

Hypomagnesemia may not reflect total body magnesium depletion because only a small fraction of total body magnesium is found in extracellular fluids. Most of the ion is found in the intracellular space and bone. In addition, serious magnesium depletion may exist in the presence of normal or elevated blood magnesium concentrations. Despite these concerns, long-term hypomagnesemia is almost always associated with decreased intracellular ion levels.

Hypermagnesemia

Hypermagnesemia (magnesium level above 2.0 mEq/L, 1 mmol/L, or 2.4 mg/dL) results when intake of magnesium exceeds excretion.[33, 44] Normal kidneys can excrete large amounts of magnesium. Thus, hypermagnesemia (see Table 78–4) usually results from excess administration of magnesium in patients with renal insufficiency. The most common causes are the administration of magnesium-containing antacids, enemas, intravenous fluids, or nutrition. Serum magnesium levels are well maintained in patients with chronic renal diseases until creatinine clearance declines below 10 mL/min in patients with normal dietary intake. Administration of magnesium to patients with eclampsia or preterm labor also causes hypermagnesemia. Hypermagnesemia may result in patients with normal magnesium intake in whom renal excretion of magnesium is diminished as a result of hypothyroidism, adrenal insufficiency, lithium intoxication, and familial hypocalciuric hypercalcemia.

Hypophosphatemia

Hypophosphatemia (phosphorus level below 2.5 mg/dL)[1, 46–49] results from three primary mechanisms (see Table 78–3):

- Intracellular shift of phosphorus (redistribution)
- Increased loss of phosphorus through the kidneys
- Decreased gastrointestinal absorption (increased loss) of phosphorus

Phosphorus shifts intracellularly during carbohydrate administration and nutritional support (e.g., refeeding, intravenous administration of dextrose). Phosphorus is also used for protein synthesis and cell replication, and intracellular uptake occurs during anabolic responses. Acute respiratory and metabolic alkalosis stimulates glycolysis, consuming phosphorus in the process. In addition, drugs such as insulin and catecholamines stimulate the transcellular movement of phosphorus.

Phosphorus is lost in the urine as a result of tubular defects in phosphorus reabsorption. In addition, increased levels of PTH, acidosis, diuretics, vitamin D deficiency, and recovery from acute renal failure (diuretic phase) cause phosphaturia and hypophosphatemia. Inadequate phosphorus intake alone rarely causes hypophosphatemia because of the wide availability of phosphorus in foods. However, marginal phosphorus intake coupled with another cause for hypophosphatemia is frequently associated with hypophosphatemia. Gastrointestinal loss of phosphorus may result from decreased absorption or increased phosphorus secretion. Common causes include malabsorption states, diarrhea, fistula drainage, and phosphorus-binding antacids (aluminum or magnesium hydroxide).

Many factors contribute to phosphorus depletion in the alcoholic patient. These include poor dietary intake, use of phosphorus-binding antacids, vomiting, magnesium deficiency, refeeding syndrome, and renal phosphorus wasting. Diabetes mellitus is a common cause of phosphorus depletion. Phosphorus is lost in the urine because of glycosuria, ketonuria, polyuria, and acidosis. There is also a shift of phosphorus out of cells and into the plasma during insulin deficiency. Much of this phosphorus is lost in the urine, contributing to total body phosphorus depletion. After insulin administration, phosphorus shifts into cells, and blood levels fall. Severe phosphorus depletion in these patients can contribute to insulin resistance. Respiratory alkalosis depresses blood phosphorus levels to a greater extent than does metabolic alkalosis (because of more pronounced intracellular alkalosis). Intracellular alkalosis causes a shift of phosphorus into cells owing to increased utilization of phosphorus by the cell (especially if glucose is present) by a number of metabolic processes (e.g., glycolysis).

Hypophosphatemia may not reflect total body phosphorus depletion because only a small fraction of total body phosphorus is found in extracellular fluids. Most of the ion is found in the intracellular space and bone. In addition, serious phosphorus depletion may exist in the presence of normal or elevated serum phosphorus concentrations. Despite these concerns, long-term hypophosphatemia is almost always associated with decreased intracellular ion levels.

Hyperphosphatemia

Hyperphosphatemia (phosphorus level above 4.5 mg/dL) results from three basic mechanisms[1, 47, 50, 51] (see Table 78-4):

- Reduced renal excretion
- Increased entrance of phosphorus into the extracellular space from the intracellular space
- Increased phosphorus or vitamin D intake

Phosphorus is removed from the body primarily by renal excretion. Thus, as glomerular filtration decreases, so does phosphorus clearance. Phosphorus levels may increase before there is a clear elevation of blood urea nitrogen or creatinine. In patients with chronic renal insufficiency, phosphorus excretion is usually maintained until glomerular filtration rates decrease below 25 mL/min. In acute renal insufficiency, however, hyperphosphatemia occurs at higher glomerular filtration rates because there is less time for the remaining tubules to compensate, and acute renal failure is frequently associated with higher entry of phosphorus into the vascular space. Elevated levels of phosphorus are also seen in patients with hypoparathyroidism, hyperthyroidism, or acromegaly and after use of bisphosphonates. Higher phosphorus levels are found in children because of increased concentrations of growth hormone and insulin-like growth factor 1.

Hyperphosphatemia may occur when cells are damaged, releasing their intracellular store of phosphorus. Examples include cancer chemotherapy (e.g., leukemia, lymphoma), rhabdomyolysis, malignant hyperpyrexia, fulminant hepatitis, sepsis, hemolysis, and severe hypothermia. Finally, excess intake of phosphorus (e.g., enemas, laxatives), especially in patients with renal insufficiency, can result in hyperphosphatemia.

CLINICAL FEATURES

Hypocalcemia

Ionized hypocalcemia affects all tissues in the body. However, the primary organs affected clinically are the neuromuscular and cardiovascular systems[1, 21] (Table 78-5). Symptoms of hypocalcemia are most prominent when the blood calcium level falls rapidly. There is considerable variability in the level of ionized calcium at which symptoms occur.

Ionized hypocalcemia results in neuromuscular irritability and includes hyperactive reflexes, muscle spasms, paresthesias, seizures, and tetany. The seizures seen in patients with hypocalcemia represent generalized tetanic responses and are not usually associated with aura, unconsciousness, or incontinence. Although neuromuscular weakness has been reported in some animal models, weakness in humans usually reflects the underlying disease causing the hypocalcemia rather than the hypocalcemia itself.

Cardiovascular alterations are uncommon until ionized calcium levels decrease below 0.7 to 0.8 mmol/L (normal, 1.0 to 1.3 mmol/L). Patients may have hypotension, bradycardia, arrhythmias, and impaired cardiac contractility.[52-56] Hypocalcemia may also impair the action of digitalis.[53] However, catecholamine action is not impaired.[57] Electrocardiographic changes induced by hypocalcemia include sinus bradycardia, QT interval prolongation, and ST interval lengthening. These changes are not reliable indicators of the presence of or degree of hypocalcemia. Hypocalcemia may also precipitate life-threatening laryngospasm or bronchospasm and can contribute to respiratory muscle weakness.

Calcium levels in the blood decrease in patients with sepsis, ischemia-reperfusion injuries, and other states associated with systemic inflammation. However, most of these states are associated with elevated levels of intracellular calcium.[2, 58] Because elevated intracellular calcium levels impair cell function (e.g., uncouple oxidative phosphorylation, decrease receptor–intracellular messenger coupling), increase the activation of digestive enzymes (e.g., lipases, proteases, nucleases), and increase the production of free radicals, calcium administration to these patients is thought to be detrimental. The lowering of circulating calcium levels in these patients is believed to be protective.[2-4] Thus, we do not advocate administering calcium to patients unless the ionized calcium level is below 0.8 mmol/L (decreased by at least 20% from normal). Although there are no prospective randomized trials of calcium therapy in humans with ionized hypocalcemia, experimental studies support the detrimental effects of calcium administration to animals with ischemia and sepsis.

Hypercalcemia

Clinical features of hypercalcemia[1, 29] reflect the underlying disease (e.g., malignant neoplasia) as well as organ dysfunction

TABLE 78–5. Clinical Features of Hypocalcemia, Hypomagnesemia, and Hypophosphatemia

Hypocalcemia	Hypomagnesemia	Hypophosphatemia
Cardiovascular	Cardiovascular	General
Hypotension	Arrhythmias	Weakness, malaise
Cardiac insufficiency	Heart failure	Myocardial insufficiency
Bradycardia, heart block	Coronary artery spasm	Impaired pressor responses
Arrhythmias	Hypertension	Myopathy, muscle weakness
Cardiac arrest	Digitalis sensitivity	Respiratory insufficiency
Insensitivity to digitalis	PR and QT prolongation	Renal dysfunction
QT and ST prolongation	Neuromuscular	Rhabdomyolysis
Neuromuscular	Muscle weakness	Hematologic
Tetany	Spasm, tremor	Hemolysis
Spasm	Seizures	Platelet dysfunction
Paresthesias	Tetany	Leukocyte dysfunction
Seizures	Paresthesias	Impaired immune function
Weakness	Confusion, disorientation	Skeletal
Chvostek's and Trousseau's signs	Obtundation, coma	Osteomalacia, rickets
Basal ganglia and extrapyramidal calcification	Ataxia, nystagmus	Fractures
Papilledema	Depression	Increased bone resorption
Respiratory	Irritability	Metabolic
Laryngeal spasm	Psychosis	Impaired glucose tolerance
Apnea	Personality change	Insulin resistance
Bronchospasm	Gastrointestinal	Hypermagnesemia
Psychiatric	Anorexia	Hypercalciuria
Anxiety	Nausea, vomiting	Acidosis
Dementia	Ileus	Neurologic
Depression	Abdominal cramps	Ataxia
Irritability	Metabolic	Altered mentation
Psychosis	Hypocalcemia	Confusion, delirium
Confusion	Hypokalemia	Obtundation, coma
Neurosis	Hypophosphatemia	Irritability
Cataracts	Nephrolithiasis (calcium oxalate)	Paresthesias
Dry skin, brittle nails		Seizures
Coarse hair		Tremor
		Peripheral neuropathy
		Gastrointestinal
		Anorexia
		Nausea, vomiting
		Hepatic failure or necrosis

(Table 78-6). Symptoms are more likely when blood calcium concentration increases rapidly and in patients with higher calcium levels. The primary organ systems affected by hypercalcemia are neuromuscular, cardiovascular, gastrointestinal, and renal.

Neuromuscular manifestations include muscle weakness, hyporeflexia, memory impairment, disorientation, lethargy, coma, headache, and seizures. Hypercalcemia increases vascular resistance and blood pressure, depresses the response to β-adrenergic agonists,[59-61] impairs cardiac contractility, and may cause arrhythmias. QT interval shortening may be detected on the electrocardiogram but is not a reliable indicator of the presence of hypercalcemia.[62] Hypercalcemia also increases the action of digitalis and predisposes to toxicity.

Renal manifestations include the development of calculi (nephrolithiasis), calcium precipitation (nephrocalcinosis), disruption of renal tubular function, and interstitial nephritis. Calcium impairs sodium and water reabsorption and may result in nephrogenic diabetes insipidus. The result can be polyuria, dehydration, impairment in renal perfusion, and renal failure. Intravascular volume depletion coupled with reduced renal perfusion exacerbates hypercalcemia, and circulating calcium levels can reach high values (>20 mg/dL). Hypercalcemia may also cause anorexia, pancreatitis, and vasculitis.

Hypomagnesemia

The clinical features of hypomagnesemia,[1, 42] like those of hypocalcemia, relate to increased neuronal irritability and cardiovascular alterations (see Table 78-5). Neuromuscular symptoms and signs include muscle weakness, spasms, paresthesias, lethargy, disorientation, coma, apathy, seizures, and tetany. Hypomagnesemia may present as respiratory failure or failure to wean from the ventilator.[63] Neuromuscular symptoms are rare unless the total serum magnesium level is less than 1.0 to 1.2 mg/dL. Magnesium is required for PTH secretion, and PTH and vitamin D action and hypomagnesemia may cause hypocalcemia.[6, 10, 19] Magnesium is also a cofactor for the Na^+,K^+-ATPase enzyme and can result in renal potassium wasting and intracellular potassium depletion.[64-67] Potassium depletion, in addition to magnesium depletion, can cause muscle weakness and cardiac arrhythmias.

Some studies report an inverse relationship between magnesium intake and coronary artery disease, myocardial infarction, arrhythmias, and sudden death. There are also reports of low blood magnesium levels in patients with heart disease admitted to the hospital.[68-71] Meta-analysis of numerous reports suggests that intravenous magnesium therapy given early after myocardial infarction reduces arrhythmias and mortality.[72, 73] The Second Leicester Intravenous Magnesium Intervention Trial (LIMIT-2), a prospective randomized double-blind placebo-controlled study, demonstrated a significant reduction in mortality from coronary artery disease in the magnesium-treated group.[74] There was also a decrease in heart failure. In contrast, the Fourth International Study of Infarct Survival (ISIS-4) failed to confirm these findings.[75] Magnesium administration has been shown to reduce arrhythmias in patients with myocardial ischemia, after myocardial infarction, and after cardiac surgery. In addition to cardiac arrhythmias, magnesium depletion may result in heart failure, coronary artery spasm, and hypertension. There is increased sensitivity to digitalis and vasoconstrictors.

Hypomagnesemia is associated with increased release of endothelin and proinflammatory cytokines. Cytokine-induced injury is increased and outcome from sepsis is diminished in hypomagnesemic animals.

Hypermagnesemia

Hypermagnesemia[1] is well tolerated until circulating magnesium levels exceed 4 to 6 mg/dL. These high levels of magnesium can impair neuromuscular transmission and cause loss of deep tendon reflexes, muscle weakness, and respiratory failure (see Table 78–6). Severe hypermagnesemia may also cause vasodilation,[76] hypotension, heart block, and cardiac arrest. Magnesium may cause vasodilation by blocking calcium entry[77] or causing the release of prostacyclin.[78] Other features of severe hypermagnesemia are hypocalcemia (suppression of parathyroid glands)[7, 20] and increased neuromuscular sensitivity to the effects of muscle relaxants.

Hypophosphatemia

Cellular phosphorus depletion affects all cells in the body by depleting energy stores (e.g., ATP, creatine phosphate), diminishing membrane phospholipids, limiting second-messenger generation (e.g., cAMP and cGMP, phosphoinositides), reducing levels of 2,3-DPG (modulates hemoglobin-oxygen affinity), and reducing substrate for the synthesis of DNA and RNA. Symptoms and signs are unusual unless the circulating phosphorus level is less than 2 mg/dL. Most patients with levels below 1 mg/dL manifest cellular dysfunction. Clinical features (see Table 78–5) include muscle weakness, respiratory insufficiency, impaired weaning from mechanical ventilation, tremor, paresthesia, encephalopathy, ataxia, lethargy, coma, seizures, anorexia, rhabdomyolysis, hemolysis, renal dysfunction, hepatic insufficiency, impaired immune function, insulin resistance, impaired gluconeogenesis, impaired vasopressor responses, and cardiac insufficiency.[1, 46, 79–91]

Severe hypophosphatemia has a variety of effects on renal function. There is a fall in glomerular filtration rate; diminished tubular uptake of glucose, calcium, magnesium, and bicarbonate; increased synthesis of 1,25-dihydroxyvitamin D; and diminished excretion of hydrogen ions. Prolonged and severe phosphorus depletion can cause a metabolic acidosis.

Hyperphosphatemia

Hyperphosphatemia produces clinical manifestations (see Table 78–6) primarily by decreasing circulating calcium levels and causing calcium precipitation.[1, 50] Soft-tissue calcium phos-

TABLE 78–6. Clinical Features of Hypercalcemia, Hypermagnesemia, and Hyperphosphatemia

Hypercalcemia	Hypermagnesemia	Hyperphosphatemia
Cardiovascular	Decreased deep tendon reflexes	Hypocalcemia
Hypertension	Muscle weakness	Ectopic calcification (e.g., renal, periarticular, skin, blood vessels, corneal)
Arrhythmias	Respiratory failure	Neurologic
Digitalis sensitivity	Paralysis	Lethargy
Catecholamine resistance	Cardiovascular	Somnolence
QT shortening	Bradycardia	Coma
Urinary system	Hypotension	Secondary hyperparathyroidism and renal osteodystrophy
Nephrocalcinosis	Heart block	
Nephrolithiasis	Cardiac arrest	
Tubular dysfunction (e.g., free water loss)	PR, QRS, ST prolongation	
Polyuria (nephrogenic diabetes insipidus)	Neurologic	
Glomerular disorders	Lethargy	
Interstitial nephritis	Somnolence	
Gastrointestinal	Coma	
Peptic ulcers	Nausea, vomiting	
Pancreatitis	Urinary retention	
Constipation		
Anorexia		
Nausea, vomiting		
Neuromuscular		
Weakness, hypotonia		
Hyporeflexia		
Neuropsychiatric		
Depression, lethargy		
Obtundation, coma		
Memory impairment		
Psychosis		
Disorientation, confusion		
Headache		
Seizures		
Skeletal		
Osteopenia		
Fractures		
Miscellaneous		
Skin necrosis		
Pruritus		
Conjunctivitis		
Hypomagnesemia		
Ectopic calcification		
Vasculitis		

phate precipitation usually occurs when the calcium × phosphate product exceeds 70. In addition, alkalosis favors precipitation. Soft-tissue calcification can result in an inflammatory response, vasculitis, organ injury, and organ failure. The kidney is one of the most commonly injured organs.

TREATMENT

Hypocalcemia

In patients with suspected hypocalcemia (usually on the basis of a low total calcium level), an ionized calcium level should be measured to confirm the diagnosis. Most patients with a low total circulating calcium level do not have ionized hypocalcemia. Magnesium and phosphorus levels should also be checked and levels of these ions corrected if they are abnormal. Administration of calcium to hyperphosphatemic patients can be deleterious (inducing calcium precipitation) and may cause death. In addition, it is difficult to normalize calcium levels in patients with hypomagnesemia until the magnesium level is corrected. If it is clinically indicated, blood samples should be sent for assessment of PTH and vitamin D levels.

A large body of evidence indicates that cellular calcium overload is a primary mechanism for cellular dysfunction and cell death after ischemia and shock (including sepsis).[2, 58] Current data suggest that mild ionized hypocalcemia is protective during states of systemic inflammation, ischemia, and sepsis.[2-4] Because hypocalcemic symptoms are unusual unless the ionized calcium level is less than 0.8 mmol/L (normal, 1.0 to 1.3 mmol/L), we do not routinely recommend treatment in critically ill patients unless levels are below 0.8 mmol/L.

Symptomatic ionized hypocalcemia and ionized calcium levels below 0.7 to 0.8 mmol/L should be treated with intravenous calcium[1, 21] (Table 78–7). Initial therapy in adults consists of the administration of a calcium bolus (100 mg elemental calcium during 5 to 10 minutes) followed by an infusion of 0.5 to 1.0 mg/kg/hr of elemental calcium. Bolus administration of intravenous calcium produces only a transient rise in circulating calcium, with levels returning toward baseline during 0.5 to 2.0 hours. Although the form of intravenous calcium administered is not important, because the small differences in their ionization have little clinical significance, the clinician must be aware that various preparations (e.g., calcium chloride, calcium gluceptate, calcium gluconate) contain different amounts of elemental calcium per gram of calcium salt. Response to calcium therapy varies with each individual, depending on renal function and the status of the parathyroid–vitamin D axis. Thus, ionized calcium levels should be followed and the dose adjusted to keep the level above 0.8 mmol/L (mild hypocalcemic range) or within the low-normal range (1.0 to 1.1 mmol/L).

It is important that one treat the underlying disease responsible for the hypocalcemia (e.g., sepsis, hypomagnesemia). Drugs that are aggravating the hypocalcemia should be discontinued and another drug substituted if possible (e.g., loop diuretics). Calcium is irritating to veins and should be diluted before administration. Calcium is best administered through a central vein. Calcium chloride should not be injected intramuscularly; however, when intravenous access is not available, calcium gluceptate can be administered intramuscularly. Calcium salts should not be administered with bicarbonate because the two precipitate. Calcium should be administered cautiously to patients receiving digitalis because increased calcium levels predispose to digitalis toxicity.

Response to calcium therapy should be monitored by following clinical symptoms and signs, vital signs, the electrocardiogram, and ionized calcium levels. One should also check

TABLE 78–7. Treatment of Hypocalcemia, Hypomagnesemia, and Hypophosphatemia

Hypocalcemia	Hypomagnesemia	Hypophosphatemia
Evaluate and treat underlying disease Remove offending drugs Treat hypomagnesemia Treat hyperphosphatemia Treat hypokalemia Administer calcium *Parenteral:* 100 mg elemental calcium IV during 5–10 min, followed by 0.5–1.0 mg/kg/hr; taper to effect *Oral:* 0.5–1 g every 6 hr ***Calcium Preparations*** INTRAVENOUS Calcium chloride (10%): 272 mg calcium (13.6 mEq) per 10 mL Calcium gluconate (10%): 93 mg calcium (4.6 mEq) per 10 mL ORAL Calcium carbonate: 500 mg; 40% elemental calcium Calcium gluconate: 500 mg; 9% elemental calcium Calcium lactate: 650 mg; 13% elemental calcium Calcium citrate: 1000 mg; 24% elemental calcium Calcium glubionate: 115 mg calcium per 5 mL ***Vitamin D Metabolites***	Evaluate and treat underlying disease Remove offending drugs Treat other electrolyte disturbances Administer magnesium *Intravenous:* magnesium chloride (1 g = 118 mg magnesium = 9 mEq magnesium) or sulfate (1 g = 98 mg magnesium = 8 mEq magnesium; give 1 g magnesium as bolus during 5 minutes followed by 0.5–1 g/hr; reduce dose for renal failure *Oral:* give magnesium oxide (1 tablet = 241 mg magnesium = 20 mEq magnesium) or magnesium gluconate (500-mg tablet = 27 mg magnesium = 2.3 mEq magnesium); 20–80 mEq/day in divided doses (≈1 g magnesium per day); reduce dose for renal failure; give additional magnesium for excess losses ***Conversion of Units for Magnesium*** 1 mEq = 0.5 mmol = 12.3 mg	Evaluate and treat underlying disease Remove offending drugs Treat other electrolyte disorders Administer phosphorus *Intravenous* (try to avoid this route because it may lead to calcium phosphate precipitation): give potassium phosphate (93 mg/mL PO_4; 4 mEq/mL potassium) or sodium phosphate (93 mg/mL PO_4; 4 mEq/mL Na); if depletion is recent and uncomplicated, give 0.6 mg (0.02 mmol)/kg/hr; if depletion is prolonged or multifactorial, give 0.9 mg (0.03 mmol)/kg/hr; reduce dose for renal failure *Oral:* 1000–1200 mg elemental phosphorus per day in divided doses (every 6–12 hr); give additional quantity for excess losses; reduce dose for renal failure. ***Oral Preparations*** Neutra-Phos: 250 mg PO_4 Potassium-PO_4: 125, 250 mg PO_4 per tablet Whole milk: 1 mg/mL PO_4 Skim milk: 0.9 mg/mL PO_4

TABLE 78–8. Treatment of Hypercalcemia, Hypermagnesemia, and Hyperphosphatemia

Hypercalcemia	Hypermagnesemia	Hyperphosphatemia
Evaluate and treat underlying disease; consider surgery for hyperparathyroidism and chemotherapy for malignant disease	Evaluate and treat underlying disease	Evaluate and treat underlying disease
General measures Mobilization Remove offending drugs Restrict calcium intake Correct electrolyte disorders; monitor electrolyte levels	Antagonize neuromuscular and cardiac effects: administer 1 g calcium chloride (10%) IV during 5–10 min	Decrease phosphorus intake
Replete intravascular volume with intravenous normal saline	Reduce magnesium intake and intestinal absorption Phosphate Cellulose phosphate	Increase renal phosphorus excretion Saline plus furosemide Dialysis for renal failure
Increase urinary calcium excretion with saline plus furosemide; maintain urine output at 200–300 mL/hr; consider dialysis for patients with renal failure	Increase renal excretion Administer intravenous saline and furosemide Dialysis for renal failure	Reduce gastrointestinal absorption of phosphorus Aluminum hydroxide (30–60 mL every 6 hr) Calcium carbonate (1–2 g every 6 hr)
Decrease bone resorption Pamidronate, 15–45 mg in 250 mL saline IV during 2–4 hr for up to 10 days Calcitonin, 4–8 IU/kg every 6–12 hr IV, SC, or IM Plicamycin, 15–25 μg/kg IV in 1 L saline during 4–24 hr every 2–7 days Gallium nitrate, 200 mg/m² in 1 L saline daily by continuous infusion for 5 days	Shift magnesium into cells with glucose and insulin	Administer calcium cautiously for symptomatic hypocalcemia (hyperphosphatemia may cause calcium precipitation in the blood)
Calcium chelators Phosphate, 500–1000 mg orally every 6 hr; 50 mmol/L PO_4 by continuous infusion every 8–12 hr Phospho-Soda, 5 mL rectally every 6 hr		
Glucocorticoids, 40–100 mg prednisone or methylprednisolone/day		

levels of magnesium, phosphorus, potassium, and creatinine at periodic intervals (every 6 to 12 hours during initial therapy). Once ionized calcium levels are at the desired level, patients may be switched to enteral calcium (see Table 78-7). Most patients with persistent hypocalcemia require 2 to 4 g of elemental calcium per day (in divided doses every 6 hours). When enteral calcium alone is insufficient for maintenance of ionized calcium levels, vitamin D should be added. Vitamin D is rarely required during the period of critical illness because calcium levels can be easily maintained with use of the intravenous route. If the clinician is unfamiliar with the use of vitamin D for managing hypocalcemia, endocrine consultation should be sought.

Adverse effects from calcium administration are similar to the effects of hypercalcemia (see Table 78-6). Hypercalciuria is common and may result in renal calculi or nephrocalcinosis. Urinary calcium excretion should be monitored and kept below 350 mg per gram creatinine. When calcium excretion is high, administration of a thiazide diuretic (25 to 50 mg orally twice daily) may help reduce urinary calcium excretion. Other common effects of calcium administration include increased systemic vascular resistance, hypertension, flushing, nausea, and vomiting.

Hypercalcemia

The definitive treatment of hypercalcemia[1, 29, 92, 93] involves eliminating the cause of the hypercalcemia (e.g., hyperparathyroidism, malignant neoplasm, excess calcium intake). Most causes of hypercalcemia require specific treatment aimed at the underlying disease. For example, surgery is the preferred treatment of hyperparathyroidism; however, while investigation of the etiology of the hypercalcemia is under way, it may be necessary to lower the circulating calcium level to prevent organ injury and death.

The goal of therapy for hypercalcemia (Table 78-8) is to minimize calcium entry into the circulation while maximizing exit from the circulation.[1, 29] General measures include the following:

- Hydration to restore intravascular volume and tissue perfusion
- Correction of electrolyte abnormalities (e.g., potassium, magnesium)
- Removal of offending drugs (e.g., thiazides, vitamins A and D, calcium)
- Restriction of calcium intake (both enteral and parenteral)
- Mobilization of the patient (to reduce calcium release from bone)

First-line therapy involves increasing renal excretion of calcium through the use of saline and furosemide (20 to 40 mg intravenously as needed). Saline restores intravascular volume and renal perfusion, increasing glomerular filtration of calcium. Saline also inhibits calcium reabsorption in the renal tubule. Furosemide inhibits calcium and sodium reabsorption, increasing calcium excretion in the urine. Saline and furosemide are adjusted to maintain a urine output of 200 to 300 mL/hr. Close monitoring of the patient is essential to prevent volume overload, pulmonary edema, hypokalemia, and hypomagnesemia. If the patient has renal failure, calcium may be removed by use of dialysis or hemofiltration.

Second-line therapy is aimed at reducing calcium release from bone (the primary cause of most hypercalcemias). The drugs of choice for reducing bone resorption are the bisphosphonates (see Table 78-8). These agents are chemical analogs of pyrophosphate that are resistant to hydrolysis by phosphatases. Bisphosphonates are absorbed to hydroxyapatite crystals on the bone surface and inhibit bone resorption and formation. They also inhibit osteoclast activity. These agents are poorly absorbed from the gastrointestinal tract and should be given intravenously for the treatment of hypercalcemia. Pamidronate and etidronate disodium are approved for treatment of hypercalcemia in the United States. Clodronate and alendronate are also available in other countries. In the United States, pamidronate is the drug of choice for treating hypercalcemia.[94] It may be given as a daily infusion of 15 to 45 mg (in 250 mL normal saline during 2 to 4 hours) for up to 10 days or as a single infusion of 30 to 90 mg (in saline during 4 to 24 hours). Onset of action is usually within 24 to 48 hours, and the duration of action can be up to several weeks. Seventy per cent to 100% of hypercalcemic patients will become eucalcemic after a single intravenous infusion of 60 to 90 mg. These drugs are excreted by the kidneys, and the dosage should be adjusted in patients with renal failure. Adverse effects include transient temperature elevations, transient leukopenia, hypophosphatemia, hypokalemia, hypomagnesemia, and myalgias.

Third-line therapy is rarely required. Third-line agents (see Table 78-8) are less effective or associated with more side effects compared with first-line and second-line agents. Calcitonin binds to receptors on the osteoclast and inhibits its activity. Calcitonin also increases renal excretion of calcium. Despite safety and few side effects (e.g,, nausea, vomiting, abdominal cramps, rash, flushing, diarrhea), calcitonin lacks potency for the treatment of hypercalcemia (approximately 25% of patients do not respond and 80% remain hypercalcemic) and is associated with tachyphylaxis (within 48 to 72 hours). It may be given by the subcutaneous, intramuscular, or intravenous routes at a dose of 4 to 8 IU/kg every 6 to 12 hours. Calcitonin has a rapid onset of action, typically within 6 to 24 hours. Calcitonin may be useful when it is added to a bisphosphonate to allow faster reduction of the calcium level.

Plicamycin (previously mithramycin) is an inhibitor of RNA synthesis and is cytotoxic to osteoclasts. Associated toxicities limit its usefulness for treating hypercalcemia. It is reserved for patients who fail to respond to bisphosphonates. Plicamycin is administered in a dosage of 15 to 25 μg/kg in 1 L of normal saline intravenously during 4 to 24 hours. The dose is repeated every 2 to 7 days, as needed. Onset of action is within 12 hours of drug administration, with the maximal effect seen within 24 to 48 hours. Calcium levels become normalized in 75% to 80% of patients. Side effects include nausea, vomiting, cellulitis at the infusion site (especially if there is extravasation), cytopenias (bone marrow toxicity), hepatic toxicity, renal toxicity, and platelet inhibition.

Gallium nitrate adsorbs to hydroxyapatite crystals and inhibits bone resorption.[95] It is administered as a continuous infusion (200 mg per square meter body surface area in 1 L normal saline) daily for 5 days. Onset of action is 48 to 72 hours, and the maximal response is seen at 5 to 6 days. Eucalcemia is achieved in 75% to 85% of patients. Adverse effects include nephrotoxicity, hypophosphatemia, anemia, nausea, vomiting, and hypotension.

Inorganic phosphate is also effective for the treatment of hypercalcemia but is associated with potentially lethal side effects. These characteristics restrict its use to patients with life-threatening hypercalcemia in whom other therapies have failed. Phosphate decreases calcium levels by inhibiting osteoclast-mediated bone resorption, decreasing gut calcium absorption, inhibiting renal synthesis of 1,25-dihydroxyvitamin D, and precipitating calcium in tissues. Calcium precipitation in tissues (e.g., lungs, heart, kidneys, blood vessels) can lead to organ damage, hypotension, and death. Orally and rectally administered phosphates are safer than intravenously administered phosphates.

Glucocorticoids (e.g., prednisone, 40 to 100 mg daily) are effective in treating hypercalcemia associated with excess intake of vitamin D or vitamin A or excess production of vitamin D by tumors and granulomatous disease processes. These agents are also effective in treating hypercalcemia associated with hematologic cancers, such as multiple myeloma, lymphoma, and leukemia (because of direct tumoricidal effects).

Hypomagnesemia

Magnesium deficiency is treated by eliminating the cause for the hypomagnesemia (usually increased loss from the body) and administration of magnesium[1, 42] (see Table 78-7). The amount, route, and duration of magnesium administration depend on the etiology and severity of depletion. Drugs that are increasing magnesium loss (e.g., diuretics, aminoglycosides) should be discontinued or switched to alternative agents if possible. Mild asymptomatic hypomagnesemia can be treated with diet alone. However, patients with moderate (<1.4 mg/dL) or severe (<1.0 mg/dL) hypomagnesemia or symptoms should receive enteral or parenteral supplements.

Severe or life-threatening hypomagnesemia (e.g., cardiac arrhythmias) should be treated with intravenous magnesium. We recommend giving 1 to 2 g of magnesium sulfate (8 to 16 mEq) during 5 to 10 minutes followed by 0.5 to 1.0 g/hr as an infusion. The dosage should be reduced for patients with renal insufficiency. Levels should be monitored at appropriate intervals (every 4 hours during initial therapy) and dosage adjusted to maintain a high-normal circulating magnesium level. Potassium levels should also be monitored and replacement given if necessary. Treatment is usually carried out for 3 to 5 days to allow time for repletion of intracellular stores.

Once circulating levels have been maintained in the normal range, patients can be switched to maintenance dosages of magnesium through the enteral or parenteral routes. Most adult patients with normal renal function require 0.4 mEq/kg/day orally or 0.1 to 0.2 mEq/kg/day intravenously plus excess losses (e.g., from urine, stool, fistulas, or skin). Bolus doses of magnesium (2 to 4 g intravenously) are excreted quickly by the kidneys. Thus, it is better to administer magnesium as a continuous infusion or smaller intermittent doses. Magnesium may also be administered intramuscularly (4 g IM every 4 to 6 hours). Magnesium oxide is the preferred agent for enteral administration. Magnesium-containing antacids are poorly absorbed. The major side effect of enteral magnesium is diarrhea or loose stools.

During magnesium repletion, it is important to monitor circulating magnesium (to avoid severe hypermagnesemia), potassium, and calcium levels. We also monitor blood pressure, heart rate, clinical status (e.g., neurologic, respiratory), and occasionally the electrocardiogram (especially if the patient has arrhythmias).

There has been debate in the literature regarding the value of magnesium in patients with underlying ischemic cardiac disease. Despite this debate, most studies indicate that magnesium has antiarrhythmic, anti-ischemic, antioxidant, cytoprotective, and antiatherosclerotic effects. The majority of studies indicate that magnesium decreases arrhythmias after myocardial infarction[72-74] and coronary artery bypass surgery. Magnesium also improves outcome after myocardial ischemia.[72-74] The only major study that failed to confirm these findings was ISIS-4.[75] However, ISIS-4 was primarily designed to evaluate the effects of thrombolytic agents. In addition, magnesium was given after thrombolytic administration (after reperfusion). One would expect magnesium to be most beneficial when it is given before reperfusion. Overall, we believe that magnesium is useful and safe for the treatment of ischemic cardiac disease and highly recommend it. Magnesium has been effective in treating arrhythmias even in patients with normal circulating magnesium levels. Magnesium is one of the preferred treatments of digitalis-induced arrhythmias and torsades de pointes.

Hypermagnesemia

Hypermagnesemia rarely causes problems unless the circulating magnesium level is above 4 to 5 mg/dL. Levels below this value can be treated conservatively by decreasing intake of magnesium. Obligate losses of magnesium in stool, secretions, and urine usually lower the magnesium level during a few days. Neuromuscular and cardiac toxicity of hypermagnesemia can be antagonized by administering intravenous calcium (5 to 10 mEq during 5 to 10 minutes) (see Table 78-8). The antagonistic effect of calcium is only transient and allows time for removal of magnesium from the body. Saline plus furosemide is effective for enhancing renal excretion in patients with adequate renal function. Dialysis can be used in patients with renal failure. One can also attempt to shift magnesium intracellularly with glucose and insulin.

Hypophosphatemia

Serious life-threatening consequences from hypophosphatemia are common when the circulating phosphorus level decreases below 1 mg/dL, and these patients should receive aggressive phosphorus repletion (usually by the intravenous route).[1, 46] Cell dysfunction also occurs when phosphorus levels are below 2 mg/dL, and these patients should receive phosphorus supplementation. All drugs contributing to hypophosphatemia should be discontinued if possible (e.g., phosphorus-binding antacids, diuretics).

For immediate correction of profound or symptomatic hypophosphatemia, intravenous therapy is preferred (see Table 78-7). Oral phosphorus requires time for absorption and may cause diarrhea. Intravenous phosphorus should be administered cautiously because it may cause hypocalcemia and calcium phosphate precipitation in the blood. Hypocalcemia is more likely in patients with hypomagnesemia (suppressed PTH release), and calcium phosphate formation is potentiated by alkalosis. If phosphorus depletion is recent (total body stores are only mildly depleted), we administer 0.6 mg (0.02 mmol)/kg/hr; if depletion is prolonged and multifactorial, we administer 0.9 mg (0.03 mmol)/kg/hr. Circulating phosphorus levels should be checked every 6 to 12 hours and replacement adjusted accordingly. Hyperkalemia may occur if phosphorus is administered as potassium phosphate. Phosphorus administration may need to be decreased in patients with renal failure.

Once phosphorus levels are stable or in patients with lesser degrees of hypophosphatemia, phosphorus may be administered as enteral therapy. Maintenance therapy consists of administering 1000 to 1200 mg elemental phosphorus per day in divided doses plus excess losses (see Table 78-7). It usually takes 5 to 7 days to replete body stores of phosphorus after a period of severe depletion. The most common side effect of enteral phosphorus is diarrhea. We recommend monitoring circulating phosphorus, calcium, potassium, and creatinine levels during repletion therapy. The best form of therapy for hypophosphatemia is prevention, which can be easily achieved if circulating phosphorus levels are checked on a daily basis in critically ill patients.

Hyperphosphatemia

Therapy for hyperphosphatemia (see Table 78-8) is aimed at the following[1, 50]:

- Treatment of the underlying disorder
- Elimination of the phosphorus source (e.g., diet, laxatives, cell lysis)
- Removal of phosphorus from the circulation
- Correction of associated hypocalcemia

Phosphorus intake should be restricted and phosphorus excretion in the urine increased by use of a combination of saline plus furosemide. Phosphorus absorption can be diminished and phosphorus removed from the body through the gut by use of binders such as aluminum hydroxide and calcium carbonate. Gut phosphorus binders are beneficial even if no oral phosphorus is given (by binding secreted phosphorus). When calcium carbonate is administered, close monitoring is essential to prevent hypercalcemia. In addition, calcium should not be used in patients with serum phosphorus levels greater than 7 to 8 mg/dL to avoid calcium phosphate precipitation. Phosphorus levels should be lowered by other means before calcium is administered. Dialysis can be used to remove phosphorus in patients with renal failure. One may also choose to shift phosphorus intracellularly by use of glucose and insulin.

SUMMARY

Calcium, magnesium, and phosphorus are essential ions for normal physiologic function. They are vital to the body's response to critical illness. Abnormalities in divalent ion homeostasis are common during critical illness and frequently contribute to organ dysfunction. It is important to recognize the clinical features of altered ion homeostasis, to understand how to assess these abnormalities, and to be capable of appropriately treating disorders of divalent ion homeostasis.

References

1. Zaloga GP, Chernow B: Divalent ions: Calcium, magnesium, and phosphorus. *In:* The Pharmacologic Approach to the Critically Ill Patient. 3rd ed. Chernow B (Ed). Baltimore, Williams & Wilkins, 1994, pp 777-804.
2. Zaloga GP, Malcolm D: Calcium as a mediator in septic shock. *In:* Handbook of Mediators in Septic Shock. Neugebauer E, Holaday J (Eds). Boca Raton, Fla, CRC Press, 1993, pp 475-485.
3. Malcolm DS, Zaloga GP, Holaday JW: Calcium administration increases the mortality of endotoxic shock in rats. Crit Care Med 1989; 17:900-903.
4. Zaloga GP, Sager A, Prielipp R, Ward K: Low dose calcium administration increases mortality during septic peritonitis. Circ Shock 1992; 37:226-229.
5. White RE, Hartzell HC: Magnesium ions in cardiac function: Regulation of ion channels and second messengers. Biochem Pharmacol 1989; 38:859-867.
6. Anast CS, Winnacker JL, Forte LR, Burns TW: Impaired release of parathyroid hormone in magnesium deficiency. J Clin Endocrinol Metab 1976; 42:707-717.
7. Cholst IN, Steinberg SF, Tropper PJ, Fox HE, Segre GV, Bilezikian JP: The influence of hypermagnesemia on serum calcium and parathyroid hormone levels in human subjects. N Engl J Med 1984; 310:1221-1225.

8. Rude RK, Oldham SB, Singer FR: Functional hypoparathyroidism and parathyroid hormone end-organ resistance in human magnesium deficiency. Clin Endocrinol 1976; 5:209–224.
9. Brown EM, Chen CJ: Calcium, magnesium and the control of PTH secretion. Bone Miner 1989; 5:249–257.
10. Freitag JJ, Martin KJ, Conrades MB, et al: Evidence for skeletal resistance to parathyroid hormone in magnesium deficiency. Studies in isolated perfused bone. J Clin Invest 1979; 64:1238–1244.
11. Kumar R: Calcium metabolism. *In:* The Principles and Practice of Nephrology. Jacobson HR, Striker GE, Klahr S (Eds). St. Louis, Mosby-Year Book, 1995, pp 964–971.
12. Hruska KA, Kovach KL: Phosphate balance and metabolism. *In:* The Principles and Practice of Nephrology. Jacobson HR, Striker GE, Klahr S (Eds). St. Louis, Mosby-Year Book, 1995, pp 986–992.
13. Sutton RAL, Sakhaee K: Magnesium balance and metabolism. *In:* The Principles and Practice of Nephrology. Jacobson HR, Striker GE, Klahr S (Eds). St. Louis, Mosby-Year Book, 1995, pp 1005–1008.
14. Moore EW: Ionized calcium in normal serum, ultrafiltrates and whole blood determined by ion exchange electrodes. J Clin Invest 1970; 49:318–334.
15. Zaloga GP, Chernow B: Hypocalcemia in critical illness. JAMA 1986; 256:1924–1929.
16. Zaloga GP, Chernow B, Cook D, Snyder R, Clapper M, O'Brian JT: Assessment of calcium homeostasis in the critically ill surgical patient. The diagnostic pitfalls of the McLean-Hastings nomogram. Ann Surg 1985; 202:587–594.
17. Ladenson JH, Lewis JW, Botd JC: Failure of total calcium corrected for protein, albumin, and pH to correctly assess free calcium status. J Clin Endocrinol Metab 1978; 46:986–993.
18. Zaloga GP, Wilkens R, Tourville J, Wood D, Klymer DM: A simple method for determining physiologically active calcium and magnesium concentrations in critically ill patients. Crit Care Med 1987; 15:813–816.
19. Johannesson AJ, Raisz LG: Effects of low medium magnesium concentration on bone resorption in response to parathyroid hormone and 1,25-dihydroxyvitamin D in organ culture. Endocrinology 1983; 113:2294–2298.
20. Eisenbud E, LoBue CL: Hypocalcemia after therapeutic use of magnesium sulfate. Arch Intern Med 1976; 136:688–691.
21. Mundy GR, Reasner CA: Hypocalcemia. *In:* The Principles and Practice of Nephrology. Jacobson HR, Striker GE, Klahr S (Eds). St. Louis, Mosby-Year Book, 1995, pp 971–977.
22. Zaloga GP, Chernow B: The multifactorial basis for hypocalcemia during sepsis. Studies of the parathyroid hormone–vitamin D axis. Ann Intern Med 1987; 107:36–41.
23. Howland WS, Schweizer O, Jascott D, Ragasa J: Factors influencing the ionization of calcium during major surgical procedures. Surg Gynecol Obstet 1976; 143:895–900.
24. Kahn RC, Jascott D, Carlon GC, Schweizer O, Howland WS, Goldiner PL: Massive blood replacement: Correlation of ionized calcium, citrate, and hydrogen ion concentration. Anesth Analg 1979; 58:274–278.
25. Denlinger JK, Nahrwold ML, Gibbs PS, Lecky JH: Hypocalcemia during rapid blood transfusion in anaesthetized man. Br J Anaesth 1976; 48:995–1000.
26. Turk J, Morell L: Ethylene glycol intoxication. Arch Intern Med 1986; 146:1601–1603.
27. Watson CG, Steed DL, Robinson AG, Deftos LJ: The role of calcitonin and parathyroid hormone in the pathogenesis of post-thyroidectomy hypocalcemia. Metabolism 1981; 30:588–589.
28. Robertie PG, Butterworth JF, Royster RL, et al: Normal parathyroid hormone responses to hypocalcemia during cardiopulmonary bypass. Anesthesiology 1991; 75:43–48.
29. Mundy GR, Reasner CA: Hypercalcemia. *In:* The Principles and Practice of Nephrology. Jacobson HR, Striker GE, Klahr S (Eds). St. Louis, Mosby-Year Book, 1995, pp 977–986.
30. Mundy GR: Hypercalcemia of malignancy. Kidney Int 1987; 31:142–155.
31. Mundy GR, Ibbotson KJ, D'Souza SM, et al: The hypercalcemia of cancer: Clinical implications and pathogenic mechanisms. N Engl J Med 1984; 310:1718–1727.
32. Insogna KL: Humoral hypercalcemia of malignancy. The role of parathyroid hormone–related protein. Endocrinol Metab Clin North Am 1989; 18:779–794.
33. Stewart AF, Horst R, Deftos LJ, Cadman EC, Lang R, Broadus PE: Biochemical evaluation of patients with cancer-associated hypercalcemia: Evidence for humoral and nonhumoral groups. N Engl J Med 1980; 303:1377–1383.
34. Breslau NA, McGuire JL, Zerwekh JE, Frenkel EP, Pak CY: Hypercalcemia associated with increased serum calcitriol levels in three patients with lymphoma. Ann Intern Med 1984; 100:1–6.
35. Zaloga GP, Eil C, Medberry CA: Humoral hypercalcemia in Hodgkin's disease. Association with elevated 1,25-dihydroxycholecalciferol levels and subperiosteal bone resorption. Arch Intern Med 1985; 145:155–157.
36. Adams JS: Vitamin D metabolite-mediated hypercalcemia. Endocrinol Metab Clin North Am 1989; 18:765–778.
37. Bell NH, Stern PH, Pantzer E, Sinha TK, DuLuca HF: Evidence that increased circulatory 1,25-dihydroxyvitamin D is the probable cause for abnormal calcium metabolism in sarcoidosis. J Clin Invest 1979; 64:218–225.
38. Mason RS, Frankel T, Chan YL, Lissner D, Posen S: Vitamin D conversion by sarcoid lymph node homogenate. Ann Intern Med 1984; 100:59–61.
39. Marx SJ, Attie MF, Levine MA, Spiegel AM, Downs RW, Lasker RD: The hypocalciuric or benign variant of familial hypercalcemia: Clinical and biochemical features in fifteen kindreds. Medicine (Baltimore) 1981; 60:397–412.
40. Heath H: Familial benign (hypocalciuric) hypercalcemia. A troublesome mimic of mild primary hyperparathyroidism. Endocrinol Metab Clin North Am 1989; 18:723–740.
41. Zaloga GP, Eil C, O'Brian JT: Reversible hypocalciuric hypercalcemia associated with hypothyroidism. Am J Med 1984; 77:1101–1104.
42. Sutton RAL, Sakhaee K: Hypomagnesemia. *In:* The Principles and Practice of Nephrology. Jacobson HR, Striker GE, Klahr S (Eds). St. Louis, Mosby-Year Book, 1995, pp 1008–1012.
43. Chernow B, Barmberger S, Stoiko M, et al: Hypomagnesemia in patients in postoperative intensive care. Chest 1989; 95:391–397.
44. Zaloga GP, Roberts JE: Magnesium disorders. *In:* Endocrine Emergencies. Zaloga GP (Ed). Probl Crit Care 1990; 4:425–436.
45. Zaloga GP, Chernow B, Pock A, Wood B, Zaritsky A, Zucker A: Hypomagnesemia is a common complication of aminoglycoside therapy. Surg Gynecol Obstet 1984; 158:561–565.
46. Kovach KL, Hruska KA: Hypophosphatemia. *In:* The Principles and Practice of Nephrology. Jacobson HR, Striker GE, Klahr S (Eds). St. Louis, Mosby-Year Book, 1995, pp 993–999.
47. Zaloga GP: Phosphate disorders. *In:* Endocrine Emergencies. Zaloga GP (Ed). Probl Crit Care 1990; 4:416–424.
48. Knochel JP: The pathophysiology and clinical characteristics of severe hypophosphatemia. Arch Intern Med 1977; 137:203–220.
49. Knochel JP: The clinical status of hypophosphatemia: An update. N Engl J Med 1985; 313:447–449.
50. Kovach KL, Hruska KA: Hyperphosphatemia. *In:* The Principles and Practice of Nephrology. Jacobson HR, Striker GE, Klahr S (Eds). St. Louis, Mosby-Year Book, 1995, pp 1000–1005.
51. Peppers MP, Geheb M, Desai T: Endocrine crisis. Hypophosphatemia and hyperphosphatemia. Crit Care Clin 1991; 7:201–214.
52. Chaimovitz C, Abinader E, Benderly A, Better OS: Hypocalcemic hypotension. JAMA 1972; 222:86–87.
53. Chopra D, Janson P, Sawin CT: Insensitivity to digoxin associated with hypocalcemia. N Engl J Med 1977; 296:917–918.
54. Connor TB, Rosen BL, Blaustein MP, Applefeld MM, Doyle LA: Hypocalcemia precipitating congestive heart failure. N Engl J Med 1982; 307:869–872.
55. Drop LJ: Ionized calcium, the heart and hemodynamic function. Anesth Analg 1985; 64:432–451.
56. Ginsburg R, Esserman LJ, Bristow MR: Myocardial performance and extracellular calcium in a severely failing human heart. Ann Intern Med 1983; 98:603–606.
57. Butterworth JF, Strickland RA, Zaloga GP: Hemodynamic actions and drug interactions of calcium and magnesium. *In:* Endocrine Emergencies. Zaloga GP (Ed). Probl Crit Care 1990; 4:402–415.
58. Zaloga GP, Washburn D: Multiorgan failure is associated with elevated free intracellular calcium in human sepsis. Chest 1988; 94(Suppl):6S.
59. Zaloga GP, Willey S, Malcolm D, Chernow B, Holaday JW: Hypercalcemia attenuates blood pressure response to epinephrine. J Pharmacol Exp Ther 1988; 247:949–952.

60. Zaloga GP, Strickland RA, Butterworth JF, Mark LJ, Mills SA, Lake CR: Calcium attenuates epinephrine's beta-adrenergic effects in postoperative heart surgery patients. Circulation 1990; 81:196–200.
61. Butterworth JF, Zaloga GP, Prielipp RC, Tucker WY, Royster RL: Calcium inhibits the cardiac stimulating properties of dobutamine but not amrinone. Chest 1992; 101:174–180.
62. Ellman H, Dembin H, Seriff N: The rarity of shortening of the QT interval in patients with hypercalcemia. Crit Care Med 1982; 10:320–322.
63. Molloy DW, Dhingra S, Solven FR, Wilson A, McCarthy DS: Hypomagnesemia and respiratory muscle power. Am Rev Respir Dis 1984; 129:497–498.
64. Whang R, Flink EB, Dyckner T, Wester PO, Aikawa JK, Ryan MP: Magnesium depletion as a cause of refractory potassium repletion. Arch Intern Med 1985; 145:1686–1689.
65. Whang R, Morosi HJ, Rodgers D, Reyes R: The influence of sustained magnesium deficiency on muscle potassium repletion. J Lab Clin Med 1967; 70:895–902.
66. Ryan MP, Whang R, Yamalis W, Aikawa JK: Effect of magnesium deficiency on cardiac and skeletal muscle potassium during dietary potassium restriction. Proc Soc Exp Biol Med 1973; 143:1045–1047.
67. Webb S, Schade DS: Hypomagnesemia as a cause of persistent hypokalemia. JAMA 1975; 233:23–24.
68. Rector WG, DeWood MA, Williams RV, et al: Serum magnesium and copper levels in myocardial infarction. Am J Med Sci 1981; 281:25–29.
69. Dyckner T: Serum magnesium in acute myocardial infarction: Relation to arrhythmias. Acta Med Scand 1960; 207:59–66.
70. Flink EB, Brick JE, Shane SR: Alterations of long-chain free fatty acids and magnesium concentrations in acute myocardial infarction. Arch Intern Med 1981; 141:441–443.
71. Abraham AS, Shaoril R, Shimonovitz E, et al: Serum magnesium levels in acute medical and surgical conditions. Biochem Med 1980; 24:21–26.
72. Teo KK, Yusuf S, Collins R, et al: Effects of intravenous magnesium in suspected acute myocardial infarction: Overview of randomized trials. Br Med J 1991; 303:1499–1503.
73. Lau J, Antman EM, Jimenez-Silva J, et al: Cumulative meta-analysis of therapeutic trials for myocardial infarction. N Engl J Med 1992; 327:248–254.
74. Woods KL, Fletcher S, Roffe C, et al: Intravenous magnesium sulphate in suspected acute myocardial infarction: Results of the second Leicester Intravenous Magnesium Intervention Trial (LIMIT-2). Lancet 1992; 339:1553–1558.
75. Collins R, Peto R, Flather M, et al: ISIS-4: A randomized factorial trial assessing early oral captopril, oral mononitrate, and intravenous magnesium sulphate in 58,050 patients with suspected acute myocardial infarction. Lancet 1995; 345:669–685.
76. Altura BM, Altura BT: Magnesium ions and contraction of vascular smooth muscles: Relationship to some vascular diseases. Fed Proc 1981; 40:2672–2679.
77. Levine BS, Coburn JW: Magnesium, the mimic/antagonist of calcium. N Engl J Med 1984; 310:1253–1254.
78. Rude R, Manoogian C, Ehrlick P, et al: Mechanisms of blood pressure regulation by magnesium in man. Magnesium 1989; 8:266–273.
79. Berner YN, Shike M: Consequences of phosphate imbalance. Annu Rev Nutr 1988; 8:121–148.
80. Gravelyn TR, Brothy N, Siegert C, Peters-Golden M: Hypophosphatemia-associated respiratory muscle weakness in a general inpatient population. Am J Med 1988; 84:870–876.
81. Darsee JR, Nutter DO: Reversible severe congestive cardiomyopathy in three cases of hypophosphatemia. Ann Intern Med 1978; 89:867–870.
82. Fuller TJ, Nichols WW, Brenner BJ, Peterson JC: Reversible depression in myocardial performance in dogs with experimental phosphorus deficiency. J Clin Invest 1978; 62:1194–1200.
83. O'Connor LR, Wheeler WS, Bethune JE: Effect of hypophosphatemia on myocardial performance in man. N Engl J Med 1977; 297:901–903.
84. Kreusser W, Vetter HO, Mittmann U, Horl WH, Ritz E: Haemodynamics and myocardial metabolism of phosphorus depleted dogs: Effects of catecholamines and angiotensin II. Eur J Clin Invest 1982; 12:219–228.
85. Aubier M, Murciano D, Lecocguic Y, et al: Effect of hypophosphatemia on diaphragmatic contractility in patients with acute respiratory failure. N Engl J Med 1985; 313:420–424.
86. Newman JH, Neff TA, Ziporin P: Acute respiratory failure associated with hypophosphatemia. N Engl J Med 1977; 296:1101–1103.
87. Varsano S, Shapiro M, Taragan R, Bruderman I: Hypophosphatemia as a reversible cause of refractory ventilatory failure. Crit Care Med 1983; 11:908–909.
88. Zaloga GP: Hypophosphatemia in patients with chronic obstructive pulmonary disease. J Crit Ill 1992; 7:364–375.
89. Agusti AG, Torres A, Estopa R, Agustividal A: Hypophosphatemia as a cause of failed weaning. Crit Care Med 1984; 12:142–143.
90. Craddock PR, Yawata Y, VanSanten L, Gilberstadt S, Silvis S, Jacob HS: Acquired phagocyte dysfunction: A complication of the hypophosphatemia of parenteral hyperalimentation. N Engl J Med 1974; 290:1403–1407.
91. DeFronzo RA, Lang R: Hypophosphatemia and glucose intolerance: Evidence for tissue insensitivity to insulin. N Engl J Med 1980; 303:1259–1263.
92. Bilezikian JP: Management of acute hypercalcemia. N Engl J Med 1992; 326:1196–1203.
93. Edelson GW, Kleerekoper M: Hypercalcemic crisis. Med Clin North Am 1995; 79:79–92.
94. Sawyer N, Newstead C, Drummond A, Cunningham J: Fast (4-h) and slow (24-h) infusion of pamidronate disodium (aminohydroxypropylidene diphosphate [APD]) as single shot treatment of hypercalcemia. Bone Miner 1990; 9:122–128.
95. Warrell RP, Bockman RS, Coonley CJ, Isaacs M, Staszewski H: Gallium nitrate inhibits calcium resorption from bone and is effective treatment for cancer-related hypercalcemia. J Clin Invest 1984; 73:1487–1490.

C. NUTRITION

79

Enteral Nutrition

Pamela R. Roberts, MD • Gary P. Zaloga, MD, FCCM

ENTERAL NUTRITION

Cellular and organ function depends on an adequate supply of nutrients. Cells require nutrients for (1) growth and division; (2) enzyme production and activity; (3) carbohydrate, fat, and protein synthesis; (4) muscle contraction and relaxation; and (5) numerous other cellular functions. Nutrients are also needed for more complex physiologic processes, such as wound repair, neurohumoral secretion, immune function, and gut integrity. Protein catabolism and malnutrition can decrease organ mass and impair function of organ systems (i.e., cardiac, pulmonary, immune, renal, gastrointestinal, and hepatic) when nutrients are not available in sufficient amounts. Numerous studies show that malnutrition is associated with increased morbidity and mortality in critically ill patients.[1-5]

We believe that outcome after injury is related to both adequate metabolic and hemodynamic resuscitation of the patient. In this chapter, we review roles of specific nutrients, optimal delivery and timing of nutritional support, techniques of early enteral feeding, complications of enteral nutrition, nutrition for specific diseases, and our approach to feeding critically ill patients.

TIMING OF NUTRITIONAL SUPPORT

The question of when to initiate nutritional support in seriously ill patients, especially previously well-nourished ones, is under intense study. Many patients can tolerate short periods of starvation after severe stress (e.g., cardiopulmonary bypass surgery); however, prolonged starvation impairs organ function, predisposes to infection, increases morbidity, and can result in death. Optimal timing of nutritional support is most likely disease-specific. For example, it may be beneficial to initiate nutritional support within hours of certain injuries (e.g., burns, severe trauma). In contrast, deferring nutritional support in some patients (e.g., those who undergo elective cholecystectomy) may be of little consequence. The preinjury nutritional status of a patient is another important determinant of the appropriate time to begin nutritional support.

The neuroendocrine-immune response to illness is characterized by the breakdown of skeletal muscle, gastrointestinal mucosa, and other tissues (presumably to provide nutrients for more vital organs, such as those of the immune and cardiovascular systems). Although this system of tissue breakdown may provide adequate nutrients for maintenance of organ integrity during moderate and short-lived stress states, severe and prolonged stress erodes visceral proteins, impairs organ function, compromises immune defenses, and delays wound healing.

The concept of nutritional support has evolved over the past decade from the idea of simple delivery of calories and protein to metabolic resuscitation of organs. Recent research has shown that administration of specific nutrients can support gut integrity, minimize liver injury, improve gut and liver blood flow, hasten wound healing, improve immune function, lower infection rates, and improve outcome. Some patients may "tolerate" periods of starvation; however, their outcome may be improved by nutritional support. The human body is capable of storing nutrients and mobilizing them during times of exogenous nutrient deprivation. Most cells are dependent on constant delivery of nutrients for maintenance of optimal cell function, but it is clear that nutrient delivery to cells during starvation is not as effective as postprandial nutrient delivery. In addition, critical illness interferes with storage and mobilization of nutrients and interconversion of nutrient substrates (owing to organ dysfunction). The net result is that substrates may become limited during illness and compromise organ function. For example, critical illness can outstrip the supply of some nonessential amino acids, causing them to become essential during critical illness (i.e., "conditionally essential nutrients"). There may also be an increased demand for amino acids and antioxidant substances, which results in depletion states and organ injury.

Investigations of the effects of fasting on organ function and injury have been performed in cell, organ, and animal models. These findings indicate that fasting can compromise gut function, the gut barrier, mesenteric blood flow, immune function, protein synthesis, wound healing, liver function, and renal function. Studies of gut integrity in thermally injured guinea pigs indicate that the bowel becomes edematous, loses mucosal integrity, and permits bacterial translocation within 24 to 72 hours of injury. The gut is protected from such injury by immediate institution of enteral feeding.[6]

Both animal and human studies demonstrate that early enteral feeding blunts the hypermetabolic or hypercatabolic response to injury.[7-11] Our group[12] found that in rats enteral feeding protected the liver from damage after hemorrhage. We believe the enteral nutrients improved blood flow to the gut and liver following hemorrhage. We[13] investigated the effects of enteral nutrients on renal blood flow in fasting rats and discovered better renal blood flow with administration of enteral nutrients than with enteral fluids. In other studies of early feeding,[14] we randomized rats to receive nutrients or water enterally in a model of glycerol-induced rhabdomyolysis and acute renal failure. Animals receiving enteral nutrients had significantly better renal blood flow and glomerular filtration rates (GFRs) after injury and better survival 72 hours after injury (78% versus 35%).

Effects of timing of enteral nutritional support on wound healing have been investigated in animal studies. Moss and colleagues[15, 16] evaluated the effect of early enteral feeding on colonic anastomotic healing in dogs. Dogs fed enterally immediately after surgery had better colonic anastomotic bursting pressure and wound collagen synthesis when compared with unfed controls. In rats fed early after surgery, Zaloga and coworkers[17] reported twice the abdominal wound strength at 1 week with early feeding compared to animals not fed until day 3 after surgery. These investigations indicate that wound healing is enhanced by early administration of enteral nutrients.

Tanigawa and colleagues[18] isolated livers from fed and fasted rats and exposed the livers to 2½ hours of normothermic ischemia. They assessed liver injury by measuring products of lipid peroxidation. Lipid peroxidation was significantly (sixfold to 10-fold) greater in the fasted ischemic group. The results indicate that fasting enhances lipid peroxidation after ischemia and that nutrient delivery prior to ischemia may protect from oxidative damage. The mechanisms for the protective effects of feeding are believed to result from augmentation of cellular antioxidant systems. Lipid peroxidative injury is also a component of other organ injuries frequently encountered in the critical care setting (e.g., sepsis, acute respiratory distress syndrome [ARDS]).

We have reviewed the published literature of 19 prospective controlled clinical studies that compared early and delayed enteral nutritional support,[19-37] and key aspects of these studies are summarized in Table 79–1. Eighteen of the studies were randomized. A study by Kudsk and coauthors[30] used a nonrandomized control group for delayed feeding. In most of the studies, the early-fed group received enteral feeding within 24 hours of hospital admission, whereas the delayed feeding groups were not fed until 3 to 5 days after admission. In some of the studies,[20, 33, 35, 36] patients in the early- fed group received nutrient supplementation via the oral route. We defined outcome in terms of complications, infections, length of stay, hospitalization cost, or survival. Seven studies involved abdominal surgery patients, seven evaluated patients with trauma or burn injury, four involved patients with hip fractures, and one study evaluated patients with liver transplants. Four studies demonstrated improvement in survival with early feeding.[20, 35-37] However, 16 of 19 studies demonstrated an improvement in at least one of the outcome criteria with early nutrient administration.

Thus, most of the prospective controlled trials in seriously ill or injured patients indicate that early enteral nutritional support improves outcomes in seriously ill patients. We conclude that available data support use of early enteral nutrition. No studies indicate an advantage to delaying nutritional support in seriously ill patients.

ROUTE OF NUTRITIONAL SUPPORT

Nutritional support may be administered by enteral or parenteral routes. Although nutrition support experts agree that "If the gut works, use it," many seriously ill patients with a functional gut continue to receive total parenteral nutrition (TPN). Reasons for widespread use of TPN include (1) ease and reliability of administration and (2) problems with delivery of nutrients to patients with gastrointestinal dysfunction. The gastrointestinal tract evolved to process nutrients via complex mechanisms. Results from numerous animal and human studies indicate that enteral nutrition is superior to parenteral nutrition.[38-40]

TABLE 79–1. Early Versus Delayed Feeding of Critically Ill Patients: Summary of 19 Prospective Controlled Trials

Author	Condition	Result
Sagar et al.[19]	Major gastrointestinal surgery; n = 30	E group had significant reduction in weight loss and LOS.
Alexander et al.[20]	Burn injury; n = 18	High-protein group had significant increase in survival as compared with control group.
Moore and Jones[21]	Abdominal trauma; n = 63	E group had significant reduction in septic morbidity and nonsignificant reductions in LOS and cost.
Grahm et al.[22]	Head injury (Glasgow Coma Scale <10); n = 32	E group had significantly fewer infections and days in the ICU.
Chiarelli et al.[23]	Burn injury; n = 20	E feeding was associated with significant reduction of hypermetabolic state and incidence of bacteremias and with nonsignificant decrease in hospital stay.
Schroeder et al.[24]	Elective bowel resection; n = 32	E group demonstrated significantly improved wound healing, but no difference in total complications. E group showed a trend toward shorter hospital stays.
Eyer et al.[25]	Blunt trauma; n = 38	No difference in LOS, ventilator days, organ system failure, or mortality. E group had more infections.
Jenkins et al.[26]	Burn injury; n = 80; E group received enteral feeding during and after operative procedures; D group had enteral feeding withheld perioperatively.	Despite greater % third-degree burns, E group had significantly fewer wound infections. E group showed trend toward shorter LOS per % third-degree burn.
Hasse et al.[27]	Liver transplantation; n = 31	E group had lower incidence of viral and bacterial infections.
Beier-Holgersen and Boesby[28]	Major abdominal surgery (bowel resection); n = 60	E group had significant reduction in infections and complications, regained colon function faster, had a nonsignificant decrease in LOS. More patients in the D group required ICU. Hospital cost was 25% lower for E group.
Carr et al.[29]	Gastrointestinal resection; n = 28	E group had fewer complications.
Kudsk et al.[30]	Trauma; nonrandomized controlled study of early feeding with immunity-enhancing formula as compared with nonfed control group; n = 35	E group had significant decrease in infections, complications, and hospital stay and nonsignificant reduction in hospital charges.
Watters et al.[31]	Esophagectomy and pancreatoduodenectomy; n = 28	E group had lower postoperative vital capacity and FEV_1, lower postoperative mobility; LOS was similar.
Heslin et al.[32]	Gastrointestinal cancer surgery; n = 195	No difference in complications, infections, LOS, or mortality.
Schilder et al.[33]	Major abdominal gynecologic surgery; n = 96	E group had shorter LOS.
Bastow et al.[34]	Femur fracture; n = 122	E group had shorter LOS.
Delmi et al.[35]	Femur fracture; n = 59	E group had fewer complications and mortality, and significantly shorter hospital stay.
Tkatch et al.[36]	Femur fracture; n = 62	E group had fewer complications and deaths, and significantly shorter hospital stay.
Sullivan et al.[37]	Hip fracture requiring surgery; n = 17	E group had significantly better survival.

E = early fed or supplemented group; D = delayed feeding or unsupplemented group; LOS = length of stay; ICU = intensive care unit; FEV_1 = functional expiratory volume in 1 second.

Using an animal model of abdominal sepsis, Kudsk and coworkers[41, 42] compared effects of enteral and parenteral nutrition. Survival was better with enteral nutrition in both malnourished (70% versus 30%) and well-nourished (60% versus 20%) animals. Studies by the authors[43] and others[44] also demonstrated improved survival in enterally fed animals with endogenous infection induced by methotrexate. Petersen and colleagues[45] reported better survival in protein-depleted animals with peritonitis receiving enteral nutrients. Similarly, Zaloga's group[46] reported better survival rates with enteral than with parenteral nutrient delivery in animals after hemorrhagic hypotension.

Animal experiments have assessed effects of enteral nutrition and TPN on organ function. Many studies indicate that TPN is poor at maintaining gut integrity. The presence of enteral nutrients is a potent trophic stimulus for the gastrointestinal tract. These nutrients directly stimulate gut growth and indirectly stimulate gut growth via production of gut trophic hormones such as enteroglucagon. Enteral nutrients also increase gut blood flow.[47–52] Other studies demonstrate that gut atrophy occurs in the absence of luminal nutrients.[47–56] The gut atrophy includes loss of mucosal mass, increased permeability, loss of gut-associated lymphoid tissue (GALT), and loss of secretory immunoglobulin A (IgA).[55, 56] The net result is increased viability of translocating bacteria.[55] TPN results in loss of liver function in comparison to enteral nutrition.[57–60] It is postulated that the diminished liver function results from decreased secretion of gastrointestinal trophic factors. In animal studies, enteral nutrition supported better body weight maintenance and gain compared with TPN,[50, 51, 61, 62] increased organ mass,[50, 51, 53] and improved protein synthesis in the postoperative period.[63]

In human studies, Fong and colleagues[64] examined the systemic response to endotoxin in individuals pretreated for one week with either TPN or enteral nutrition. Endotoxin injection resulted in higher body temperature, lower blood pressure, increased circulating lactate levels, and greater tumor necrosis factor (TNF) secretion in the TPN-pretreated subjects. The authors postulated that the TPN "primed" the host to mount an exaggerated response to endotoxin. The clinical relevance of this study to the treatment of human sepsis is unclear.

Prospective, randomized clinical trials have compared enteral and parenteral nutrition after surgery, trauma, and chemotherapy. Routine use of perioperative TPN for patients undergoing major surgery was evaluated in 18 controlled studies and analyzed by meta-analysis.[65, 66] Routine perioperative use of TPN was not beneficial compared to oral feeding. In the Veterans Administration Cooperative Study,[67] enteral nutrition and TPN were compared in malnourished elective surgical patients. The TPN group received one week of preoperative TPN in an effort to improve nutritional status before surgery. Data revealed a significantly higher rate of sepsis in the TPN group (14% versus 6%). Overall, complications and mortality were similar for both study groups. The study indicated that enteral feeding was superior to TPN in malnourished patients undergoing elective surgical procedures.

Route of nutrient administration has been studied most extensively in trauma patients. Adams and colleagues[68] randomized trauma patients to TPN or enteral nutrition. They reported no significant differences in intensive care unit (ICU) stay, hospital stay, ventilator time, infection rate, or nutritional response between groups. In this study, cost of TPN was threefold higher than that of enteral nutrition. Moore and associates[69] randomized abdominal trauma patients to TPN or enteral nutrition. The enteral nutrition group had a significantly lower rate of infection and improved visceral protein responses. Meta-analysis[70] of enteral nutrition and TPN studies of trauma patients also reported significantly fewer infections in the enteral nutrition patients (18% versus 35%). Kudsk and colleagues[71] randomized 98 patients with severe abdominal trauma to receive enteral nutrition or TPN. The infection rate was significantly lower in the enteral nutrition group (15.7% versus 40%), and, notably, the incidence of pneumonia and intra-abdominal abscess was also significantly lower.

Young and colleagues[72] randomized neurosurgical patients to TPN or enteral nutrition. Despite significantly lower protein and calorie intakes in the enteral nutrition group over the first 10 days of nutrition, outcomes were similar in the two groups. Additionally, Hadley's group[73] found no differences in outcomes for head-injured patients randomized to TPN or enteral nutrition.

Route of nutritional support has been evaluated in cancer chemotherapy patients. Koretz[74] reviewed 17 studies and found no significant benefit for TPN over enteral nutrition, in terms of tumor response, outcome, complication rate, or cost. Klein and coworkers[75] analyzed 28 prospective randomized trials and reported that TPN may reduce complications when administered preoperatively to malnourished gastrointestinal cancer patients; however, they found no significant improvements with TPN in survival, treatment tolerance, or outcome of other cancer patients receiving radiotherapy or chemotherapy. Significantly higher infection rates were reported in chemotherapy patients who received TPN. The American College of Physicians[76] published a position paper after reviewing 12 prospective, randomized, controlled trials that compared TPN and enteral nutrition in cancer chemotherapy patients. In this meta-analysis, TPN was associated with a significantly higher infection rate, lower survival rate, and decreased tumor responses.

In general, then, enteral nutrition appears to be superior to TPN. Benefits range from direct effects on gastrointestinal integrity to indirect effects on hormones and immune function. Most patients have adequate small intestine function and should receive their nutritional support by the enteral route. It is clear that delivery of nutrients via the gastrointestinal route improves outcomes for critically ill patients.

GUT FUNCTION

The gastrointestinal tract is divided into sections: esophagus, stomach, small intestine, and large intestine. Gastric emptying and colonic motility are decreased in critically ill patients. In constrast, small-intestinal motility, digestion, and absorption remain functional during critical illness and are adequate for enteral nutrition. The entity termed *ileus* (a dilated and non-functioning small intestine) is rare. Adequacy of small-intestine function has been documented in studies utilizing barium or radiolabeled compound movement, absorption of vitamin B_{12} or D-xylose, and measurement of small-bowel myoelectrical activity. Thus, the key issue *for* early enteral feeding is the ability to deliver nutrients directly into the small intestine in patients with impaired gastric and colonic motility. Over the past 15 years, small-bowel feeding has become routine after burn injury, multiple trauma, abdominal surgery, major vascular surgery, severe head injury, cardiopulmonary arrest, respiratory failure, and other critical illnesses.

Historically, physicians used the presence or absence of bowel sounds as criteria to determine when to initiate enteral feeding. Bowel sounds result from air moving through the small intestine. The presence of bowel sounds requires gastric emptying and gastric air. Many seriously ill patients have gastroparesis and are treated with nasogastric suctioning. These patients have little movement of air from the stomach to small intestine and, therefore, decreased bowel sounds. To declare absence of bowel sounds, one should listen for 2 to 4 minutes in each of the four abdominal quadrants. In practice, few clinicians listen for more than a few seconds. In addition, the quantity of bowel sounds does not correlate directly with gut motility. Thus, bowel sounds are a poor indicator of small-intestine function. The presence of bowel sounds is a better indicator of active gastric emptying. Injection of air into the small intestine almost always results in auscultatable bowel sounds.

True ileus is detected by clinical examination (i.e., abdominal distention) and radiologic evidence of dilated, air-filled loops of small intestine. Patients with true ileus need evaluation of the specific causes (e.g., narcotics, pancreatitis). Passage of flatus or stool indicates return of colonic motility, which may not occur until a week or more after injury. Patients with impaired colonic motility can be fed with fiber-free enteral formulations.

SPECIFIC NUTRIENTS

The number and variety of nutritional formulas available are increasing rapidly. Review of specific formulas is beyond the scope of this chapter, and extensive reviews are found elsewhere.[77] We briefly review the major nutrient classes and their roles in metabolism. Understanding these basic concepts should help the physician choose an appropriate formula for each patient.

Protein

Intact Protein, Peptides, Amino Acids

Both the quantity and quality of protein vary in enteral formulas. Protein content of formula varies between 19 and 94 g/L.

Protein forms include intact protein (e.g., casein, soy, whey), peptides, and free amino acids. In the normal diet, protein is consumed in the intact form and is then utilized via a complex process of digestion and absorption. Protein digestion begins in the stomach by hydrolysis secondary to pepsin and hydrochloric acid. After leaving the stomach, protein digestion continues in the small bowel by pancreatic enzymes (i.e., chymotrypsin, trypsin) and mucosal peptidases. A combination of small peptides (70%) and amino acids is produced. Free amino acids, dipeptides, and tripeptides may enter the enterocyte via specific transporters. In addition, however, small quantities of larger peptides (>3 amino acids) enter the circulation from the intestine by processes yet undefined, which may include pinocytosis. This transport system does not maintain nitrogen balance but is capable of transporting small amounts of physiologically active peptides.[78-82] The authors believe that absorbed bioactive peptides may have physiologic consequences such as stimulation of growth factors and regulation of blood flow.[79] Data suggest that approximately 30% to 70% of the nitrogen absorbed and in the portal circulation may take the form of small peptides.[83, 84]

In normal digestion, proteins are degraded to peptides and amino acids. When a patient's digestion is intact, it is best to feed an intact protein diet. When digestion is impaired (e.g., by pancreatic insufficiency, sepsis, multiple trauma, shock, and severe malnutrition), a diet containing large amounts of small peptides (<10 amino acids in length) is advantageous.

Few data support the use of amino acid–based diets instead of intact protein- or peptide-based formulas.[85-87] Reported disadvantages of amino acid–based diets include:

- Gut atrophy[88-92]
- Bacterial translocation[89, 93]
- Decreased liver function[94-96]
- Poorer growth and wound healing[88, 97-99]
- Decreased visceral protein synthesis[90]
- Increased diarrhea[90, 100]
- Poorer nitrogen balance[87, 99]
- Higher mortality, compared with intact protein and peptide diets[89, 90, 94, 95, 101-106]

Peptide-based formulas are associated with numerous advantages, as compared with intact protein formulations. Benefits of peptide-based diets include:

- Improved nitrogen absorption[86, 87, 107-109]
- Decreased stool output and diarrhea[110, 111]
- Improved protein synthesis[112]
- Better growth and wound repair[97, 98, 110, 111, 113, 114]
- Increased insulin growth factor 1 (somatomedin C) levels[88]
- Better gut maintenance[113, 114]
- Enhanced hepatic protein synthesis[95, 109, 111, 115]

Hepatic function can be assessed by measuring (1) changes in levels of circulating hepatic proteins (e.g., prealbumin, transferrin, retinol-binding protein) or (2) clearance of bilirubin. Brinson and Kolts[110] reported better absorption and improved transferrin and albumin levels in patients receiving a peptide diet, as compared with an intact protein diet.

Meredith and associates[111] compared an intact protein diet with a peptide-based diet in patients with multiple trauma. Patients receiving the peptide-based diet had less diarrhea, greater increases in hepatic proteins (prealbumin, transferrin, albumin), and shorter hospital stays. Ziegler's group[109] reported better nitrogen absorption and visceral protein levels in ICU patients fed a peptide-based diet than in those given an intact protein diet.

We[115] compared a peptide diet with an intact protein diet in trauma patients. Patients fed the peptide diet maintained higher levels of prealbumin, transferrin, and retinol-binding protein. Similarly, visceral protein levels were higher in geriatric patients[116] and patients with inflammatory bowel disease[117] who took peptide diets than in those fed amino acid and conventional (food) diets. Conversely, Mowatt-Larsen and colleagues[118] found no difference in visceral protein levels when trauma patients were randomized to a peptide diet or an intact protein diet. Collectively, most studies suggest that peptide diets support better liver function in critical illness.

As the concentration of peptides in the formula increases, net nutrient absorption is improved[107, 108] and diarrhea is decreased.[100] The specific protein used may be important. We[119] evaluated growth in rats fed diets containing different intact proteins (i.e., casein, soy, whey) and found more growth in animals fed soy.[119] Bounous and Kongshavn[120] reported increased immune responsiveness in the animals that received lactoalbumin protein hydrolysates compared with those fed casein protein hydrolysates. Sitren and associates[121] assessed mortality after methotrexate in mice fed diets of different protein sources (casein or soy). Loose stools were observed in 60% of the casein group but in none of the soy group. The soy group maintained better body weight and had higher survival rates (60% versus 20%). The difference in outcome may have resulted from differences in peptide products generated during protein digestion. This group[121] also compared outcomes for methotrexate-treated mice fed diets containing free amino acids, hydrolyzed casein, whole casein, or soy protein. Mortality was 100% with amino acids, 60% with intact casein, 0% with hydrolyzed casein, and 0% with soy protein.

Numerous peptides that possess biologic actions have been identified.[79] Carnosine (β-alanyl-histidine) is found in meat and is absorbed intact in the gastrointestinal tract. Roberts' group[98] observed improved wound healing in rats given carnosine supplement in an amino acid–based formula. Cyclo-histidine-proline (c-his-pro) and β-casomorphin are peptides found in currently available peptide formulations.

C-his-pro, an active component of thyrotropin-releasing hormone (TRH), is absorbed through the intestinal tract.[78] It is capable of stimulating release of thyroid-stimulating hormone (TSH), regulating blood flow, affecting neurotransmission, and improving blood pressure in shock models; it is also an opiate antagonist.

β-Casomorphin, a peptide derived by trypsin and chymotrypsin hydrolysis of casein, has opiate activity and is thought to regulate gut motility, permeability,[122] secretion, and absorption. Other investigators[123, 124] have demonstrated that peptides generated during protein digestion possess immune-modulating properties.

Arginine

Arginine is an important amino acid for protein synthesis, creatine synthesis, production of nitric oxide, and the urea cycle.[125] It is synthesized by the body and previously was considered nonessential. It is believed now that cellular demand for arginine may exceed the body's synthesizing capability during growth and critical illness.[125, 126] Arginine deficiency can impair function of the urea cycle, can cause hyperammonemia and increased orotate excretion, and limits synthesis of nitric oxide, an important regulator of vascular tone, immune function, cardiac contractility, and neuroendocrine secretion. Therefore, arginine is now considered a "conditionally essential" amino acid. Arginine is also a secretagogue and in pharmacologic doses can stimulate secretion of growth hormone, prolactin, glucagon, and adrenal catecholamines. Most of the recent nutritional interest in arginine is based on its effects on immune function and wound healing.

When fed diets deficient in arginine,[125, 127] traumatized animals exhibit impaired growth and healing. Supplementation with arginine (1% to 3%) improves nitrogen balance and lessens weight loss in animals after injury.[125, 127-130] Arginine improves wound healing in rats when supplemented in chow (1%)[127, 130] or intravenous nutrition (7.5 g/L).[131] Failure of arginine to improve wound healing in hypophysectomized rats suggests that its effects were dependent on the hypothalamic-pituitary axis.[130] Alternatively, studies indicate that arginine's effects on wound healing are not associated with increases in growth hormone.[125, 132]

Hepatic protein synthesis was studied in control and septic rats during TPN with arginine and with glycine supplementation.[133] The animals "supplemented" with arginine had increased liver protein synthesis (i.e., histone, fibrinogen, albumin, total liver protein).

Arginine supplementation (15 g/day intravenous or 25 g/day enteral) was evaluated in humans and was found to improve nitrogen balance only minimally.[134, 135] In other studies,[136, 137] arginine was supplemented at 30 g/day for 2 weeks, and its effects on wound healing were determined in healthy human volunteers by implantation of subcutaneous polytetrafluoroethylene tubing. Arginine supplementation improved wound healing by increasing collagen deposition.

Supplementation with arginine enhances lymphocyte blastogenic responses to mitogens in animals[125, 131, 136, 138, 139] and humans.[126, 135, 140] Barbul and colleagues[138] demonstrated that 1% arginine-supplemented chow increased thymic weight and cellularity in both healthy and injured (femoral fracture) rats. Arginine supplementation also increased mitogen stimulation of thymic lymphocytes in healthy and injured animals. Notably, arginine prevented the decrease in mitogen stimulation that follows injury. In other studies, arginine enhanced skin allograft rejection, decreased tumor induction, and produced antitumor effects in animals.[125, 127]

Barbul and colleagues[136, 141] found improved lymphocyte responses to mitogens in healthy humans after oral arginine supplementation (30 g/day). Daly and colleagues[135] reported that arginine supplementation improved T lymphocyte responses to concanavalin A (Con-A) and phytohemagglutinin (PHA) in postoperative cancer patients; however, no differences were found in infections or outcome between control and arginine-supplemented patients. In contrast, Sigal and colleagues[142] reported that parenteral arginine alone (no nutritional support) did not increase mitogen-related lymphocyte proliferation in postoperative patients. The net effects of these studies indicate that arginine can stimulate the activity of a variety of immune cells (i.e., is immunity-enhancing).

Saito and coworkers[143] studied burned guinea pigs (30% total body burn) fed an intact protein diet supplemented with different quantities of arginine (1% to 4% of total calories). There were no differences between arginine and control groups in weight loss, urinary vanillylmandelic acid (VMA) levels, plasma cortisol or glucagon levels, nitrogen balance, transferrin levels, C3, or carcass or gastrocnemius muscle weights. Resting energy expenditure was greater in the groups fed arginine. Delayed cutaneous hypersensitivity responses were improved in the 1% to 2% arginine-supplemented group. After injection of *Staphylococcus aureus*, skin lesions (abscesses) were smaller in the arginine-supplemented groups. Mortality was 56% in the control and the 4% arginine-supplemented groups, 29% in the 1% arginine-supplemented group, and 22% in the 2% arginine-supplemented group. These mortality data suggest a dose effect, with 1% and 2% arginine improving survival and 4% arginine increasing mortality in the control group. Results of this study (i.e., worse outcomes with more arginine) support the need for studies in humans aimed at optimizing the arginine dose and limiting adverse side effects.

Studies by Madden and colleagues[144] evaluated survival when arginine was given via different routes or at different intervals from induction of peritonitis caused by cecal ligation and puncture (CLP) in rats. When arginine was administered enterally starting immediately after CLP, arginine had no effect on survival. Arginine improved survival in animals given arginine enterally 3 days before CLP and continued after CLP. Arginine also improved survival in animals given arginine intravenously after CLP. Impaired intestinal absorption, or perhaps increased arginine utilization, may explain why the post-CLP enteral arginine group did not exhibit improved survival.

Efficacy of arginine supplementation in guinea pig peritonitis induced by *Escherichia coli* and *S. aureus* infusion was examined by Gonce and associates.[145] In contrast to other studies, survival was 54% for animals in the control group (0% arginine), 41% in the 2% and 4% arginine groups, and 9% in the 6% arginine group. No differences in albumin, transferrin, or C3 levels were seen between groups. The arginine-supplemented groups exhibited lower nitrogen balances.

Synthesis of nitric oxide (i.e., endothelium-derived relaxant factor) is arginine-dependent.[146] Rat aortic rings incubated with endotoxin have decreased reactivity to norepinephrine.[147, 148] L-arginine potentiates this effect, whereas the L-arginine antagonist N-monomethyl-L-arginine (NMMA) restores the contractile response to norepinephrine. L-Arginine administration reverses this effect and results in a depressed contractile response. In vivo, endotoxin infusion depresses the pressor response to norepinephrine.[148] This effect is inhibited by NMMA. L-Arginine reverses the effect in vivo of NMMA, causing norepinephrine resistance. In vivo and in vitro endotoxin acts on vascular tissue to induce resistance to norepinephrine secondary to the activation of the L-arginine pathway.[147] Similarly, TNF causes hypotension when administered intravenously. TNF is believed to be important in the hypotension and decreased organ perfusion in sepsis and other forms of shock. TNF infusion decreases blood pressure in dogs[149]; this effect is reversed with NMMA. The effect of NMMA is antagonized and hypotension is restored by infusion of L-arginine. Therefore, it appears that nitric oxide production from arginine mediates the hypotension caused by TNF.

It remains unclear whether arginine supplementation predisposes to hypotension in human sepsis. As a vasodilator, arginine may improve organ perfusion and wound healing by enhancing blood flow. Thus, the effects of arginine supplementation or arginine antagonism need further evaluation, especially in shock states. Importantly, however, arginine supplementation combined with ω-3 long-chain fatty acids in a complete nutritional formula has not caused hypotension in patients after sepsis, trauma, burns, or surgery.

Glutamine

Glutamine is the most abundant free amino acid in body tissues and plasma. An important component of proteins, it functions as a nitrogen carrier and energy source.[150, 151] It is an important regulator of protein synthesis and gluconeogenesis. It is synthesized in most tissues of the body and has been considered a "nonessential" amino acid. Recent data suggest that, during critical illness, tissue needs for glutamine can outstrip endogenous synthesis. In these situations, supplementation of exogenous glutamine can be beneficial. Therefore, many consider glutamine to be "conditionally essential." Glutamine is synthesized at the fastest rate in muscle, but the greatest rate of glutamine metabolism occurs in the intestine. Glutamine is also a precursor for the neurotransmitters glutamate and γ-aminobutyric acid.

Glutamine is consumed by replicating cells and is an important fuel for gastrointestinal tract maintenance and repair.[151-156] Glutamine deficiency is associated with gut atrophy during stress. Maintaining the integrity of the gastrointestinal tract is a major goal in the treatment of critically ill patients because translocation of bacteria and toxins via the gastrointestinal tract is thought to be a cause of multiple organ failure. Large doses of glutamine have been shown to prevent gut atrophy, maintain bowel integrity, and prevent bacterial translocation after various insults, which include methotrexate toxicity[157] and radiation injury.[158] A number of animal studies report that glutamine-supplemented TPN improves gut mass.[159-161] However, glutamine-supplemented TPN is less effective than standard enteral nutrition for maintenance of gut integrity and function.[160]

Current TPN solutions contain no glutamine because of its instability in solution over long storage periods. This absence of glutamine contributes to gut atrophy during TPN therapy. Glutamine amino acids can be added to TPN formula immediately before infusion. They are stable in solution over short periods (24 hours). Glutamine peptides are stable in solution over long periods (months) and are being evaluated in clinical trials; these trials are reviewed elsewhere.[150, 152, 162]

Most studies of enteral glutamine supplementation have compared a glutamine-supplemented amino acid diet with a glutamine-deficient amino acid diet.[161, 163-165] These investigations show that glutamine supplementation increases gut mass, barrier function, and survival in animals. The clinical relevance of these studies, however, is questionable, since none of the commercially available enteral formulations is glutamine-deficient, and most formulas utilize intact proteins instead of amino acids.

Fox and colleagues[157, 164] studied the effect of glutamine-supplemented enteral feeding on survival after methotrexate in rats. They reported 100% mortality in animals fed a glutamine-deficient amino acid diet and 80% mortality in animals fed a glutamine-supplemented amino acid diet. Using the same experimental design, McAnena and associates[94] studied the effect of polypeptide feeding on survival after methotrexate in rats. Animals receiving an amino acid diet had 100% mortality, and those fed the polypeptide diet had 30% mortality. Mortality increased as the quantity of amino acids in the diet increased.

Shou's group[89, 103] also utilized methotrexate-treated rats to study the effect of diet on gut mass, bacterial translocation, and survival. A glutamine-supplemented amino acid diet increased gut mass more than a glutamine-deficient amino acid diet; however, gut mass was even greater in animals fed intact protein diets. Bacterial translocation was 100% with the glutamine-deficient amino acid diet, 70% with the glutamine-supplemented amino acid diet, and 0% with the intact protein diet. Mortality was 100% with the glutamine-deficient amino acid diet, 75% with the glutamine-supplemented amino acid diet, and 0% with the intact protein diet.

The effect of glutamine on gut adaptation after massive small-bowel resection in rats was evaluated by Vanderhoff and colleagues.[166] A chow diet was supplemented with glutamine, glycine, or glucose. No differences in gut mass were reported among the 3 groups. Wells and coworkers[167] evaluated a chow diet, an intact protein diet, and a glutamine-supplemented intact protein diet in rats inoculated with endotoxin and given metronidazole. They found no differences in gut histology or bacterial translocation between groups. Barber and colleagues,[168] supplementing a peptide diet with glutamine, found no significant effect of glutamine on gut mass, bacterial translocation, or survival after endotoxin challenge.

The effects of glutamine on immune function have been evaluated in numerous studies in vitro. Glutamine enhances murine peritoneal macrophage function in vitro.[169] Furukawa and associates[170] reported that rats with bacterial peritonitis fed diets supplemented with either free glutamine or glutamine in oligopeptide form exhibited enhanced peritoneal and hepatic bacterial clearance compared with animals fed a glutamine-deficient diet. Similarly, glutamine augments the bactericidal activity in vitro of neutrophils from burn patients.[171]

O'Riordain and colleagues[172] studied the effects of glutamine (glycyl-glutamine dipeptide)-supplemented TPN on immune function in surgical patients. They found increased T cell mitogenic responses in patients receiving glutamine, but no differences between patient groups in the proinflammatory cytokines interleukin-6 (IL-6) and TNF.

Ziegler and colleagues[173] reported that humans tolerated oral and intravenous supplemental glutamine well. In a randomized, double-blind, controlled trial in bone marrow transplant recipients, patients treated with glutamine-supplemented TPN had improved nitrogen balance, fewer infections, and shorter lengths of hospital stay than patients who received standard TPN.[174] Others[175, 176] also reported improved nitrogen balance in surgical patients given glutamine-supplemented TPN.

Houdijk's group[177] randomized patients with severe multiple trauma to a glutamine-supplemented enteral formula or an isocaloric, isonitrogenous enteral feeding regimen. Patients who received the glutamine-supplemented enteral formula had a significant decrease in incidences of pneumonia, bacteremia, and sepsis, as compared with the control group.

All commercial enteral formulas contain glutamine in the free form or as a component of peptides or intact proteins. The optimal amount and form of glutamine (i.e., free amino acid, peptides, or protein) for gut maintenance and immune function is not known; however, it is clear that glutamine is important for gut maintenance and that glutamine requirements outstrip the body's synthetic capabilities in severe stress. Feeding glutamine-deficient diets results in gut atrophy and bacterial translocation in animal models of critical illness, but there is little evidence that glutamine supplementation improves the physiologic effects of complex diets containing peptides or intact proteins. An enteral formula containing supplemental glutamine has now been marketed. A recent randomized clinical trial[177] reported benefits (i.e., fewer infections) with its use in trauma patients. More conclusive evidence of its benefits in critically ill patients is lacking.

Cysteine and Glycine

Decreased levels of several amino acids, including cysteine and glycine, have been reported in patients after severe trauma.[178, 179] In vitro, hepatocytes require these amino acids for the production of secretory proteins.[180] Cysteine, glycine, and glutamate are precursors for the synthesis of glutathione (an antioxidant). Glutathione production is thought to be important during the inflammatory response.[181] Grimble and coworkers[182] reported that rats fed diets supplemented with glycine or cysteine had higher glutathione levels and lower ceruloplasmin levels after injection with TNF-α than did animals fed diets supplemented with alanine. These data suggest roles for glycine and cysteine in the response to inflammation and the possibility of optimizing glutathione levels with diet in stressed patients. For example, whey protein contains more cysteine than other intact proteins, and whey (intact or hydrolyzed) diets may offer a means of increasing glutathione levels.

Histidine

We evaluated the effects of histidine on organ function. In rats, intravenous infusion of histidine increased urine output and free water clearance.[183] Histidine also caused decreased renal cell production of cyclic adenosine monophosphate (cAMP) in vitro and decreased urinary cAMP levels in vivo.[184, 185]

Conclusion

We conclude that there is little absorptive advantage for peptide-based diets over intact protein-based diets in patients with intact digestive and absorptive functions. Patients with intact digestion can generate physiologically active peptides from intact protein in the gut. We believe that there are advantages to feeding peptide-based formulas to patients with impaired digestion or amino acid transport; however, few data are available to support the superiority of amino acid–based formulas over intact protein or peptide formulas. Different protein sources (i.e., casein, whey, soy, meat) can cause different physiologic responses; however, the optimal source or mixture of sources remains to be evaluated in future studies. Numerous studies suggest that amino acids possess specific biogenic actions. Both arginine and glutamine possess specific biologic activity beyond their "nutrient" value. The optimal dose and optimal form (i.e., amino acid, peptide) for delivery of specific amino acids (i.e., arginine, glutamine, cysteine, glycine, histidine) remain to be determined. In addition, diseases that might respond to administration of these amines need to be identified.

Fat

Lipids have many diverse functions in cells, but their primary roles are as energy sources and as membrane components. They provide energy at the rate of 9.3 kcal/kg body weight. Besides providing energy, lipids participate in the regulation of cardiovascular tone (i.e., prostaglandins), are components of cell membranes (i.e., phospholipids), and act as cellular messengers (i.e., phosphoinositides). Lipids in the diet differ in the number of carbon atoms, the number of double bonds, and the position of the double bonds. Structural differences result in unique physiologic properties of the lipid molecules. Short-chain fatty acids contain two to four carbon atoms, medium-chain fatty acids have six to 10 carbons, and long-chain fatty acids have 12 to 28 carbons. The ω-terminus is the carbon atom farthest from the carboxy terminal. Linoleic acid (18:2ω-6) has 18 carbon atoms and two double bonds. The first double bond is at the sixth carbon from the ω-terminus.

Linoleic acid is essential for normal growth and development and must be provided in the diet; that is, it is an essential fatty acid. It is the precursor of arachidonic acid (20:4ω-6), which is metabolized to prostaglandins and leukotrienes. Approximately 3% of the diet is required as linoleic acid; however, most nutritional formulations provide 10% to 20% of calories as linoleic acid.

Fatty acid composition of cell membranes is affected by lipid content of the diet.[186–191] Dietary modification of fatty acids alters lymphocyte function,[186, 187] enzyme activity,[192] and cellular receptor responsiveness.[193] These physiologic effects may result from dietary fatty acid–induced alterations in membrane structure and function.

Dietary lipids have potent effects on immune function.[186–188, 190, 191] These lipids may alter immune function by affecting energy supply, essential fatty acid availability, cell membrane fluidity, fat-soluble vitamin supply, membrane receptor coupling, eicosanoid synthesis, and cytokine release. Fatty acids may also alter expression of genes involved in inflammation and other cell functions.[194]

Diets rich in linoleic acid (i.e., corn oil, safflower oil, soybean oil, sunflower oil, parenteral lipids) or exogenous administration of linoleic acid suppresses mitogen-induced (PHA, Con-A) lymphocyte proliferation.[186, 189, 195–197] For instance, diets containing 30% corn oil suppressed mitogenic responses of isolated monkey lymphocytes to Con-A, PHA, and pokeweed mitogen.[197]

Monounsaturated fats, saturated fats, and medium-chain triglycerides have negligible effects on mitogen-induced lymphocyte stimulation. In contrast, diets rich in saturated fats inhibit chemotaxis, phagocytosis, and bactericidal activity of isolated neutrophils.[186] Diets high in saturated fats also reduce macrophage adherence and phagocytosis.

Normal immune function requires small quantities of dietary linoleic acid; however, large amounts suppress components of the immune system.[186, 187] This suppressive effect may also be useful for preventing organ rejection. For example, administration of linoleic acid prolongs allograft survival in animals, whereas diets low in linoleic acid hasten allograft rejection.[186, 187, 195] On the other hand, a high intake of linoleic acid may predispose to infection. Alternatively, essential fatty acid deficiency suppresses antibody production and delayed cutaneous hypersensitivity responses,[186] and may result in immunosuppression.

Diets high in ω-6 long-chain polyunsaturated fatty acids (PUFAs) depress mitogenic responses of T lymphocytes and splenocytes, promote tumorigenesis, and decrease B lymphocyte antibody production. Suppressive effects may be mediated through release of cellular factors (i.e., prostaglandins and cytokines). Immunosuppressive effects may be beneficial in certain situations. They may help to minimize tissue damage early after injury.

Eicosanoids derived from PUFAs are important factors in the immune response. When antigens stimulate immune cells, arachidonic acid is released from the cells by action of phospholipase. The amount of arachidonic acid released is proportional to the quantity in the cell membranes, which is affected by dietary lipid intake (primarily linoleic acid). Arachidonic acid is then metabolized to a variety of eicosanoids via the cyclooxygenase and lipoxygenase pathways. Linoleic acid is the precursor of monoenoic and dienoic prostaglandins, which can be immunosuppressive. Alternatively, ω-3 PUFAs are precursors of trienoic prostaglandins, which are less immunosuppressive (i.e., less platelet aggregation from thromboxane A_3 [TxA_3], less immunosuppression from prostaglandin E_3 [PGE_3]).

Low concentrations of PGE_2 are permissive to portions of the immune system (i.e., promote lymphocyte proliferation). In contrast, high concentrations of PGE_2 are suppressive to macrophages and lymphocytes. High levels are produced in patients with sepsis, burns or traumatic injury, or ARDS, and after major surgery or blood transfusion.[186] Increased dietary ω-6 PUFA favors production of PGE_2. For example, Johnston and Marshall[198] fed animals with corn oil (high linoleic acid), linseed oil (high in ω-3 fat linolenic acid), or coconut oil (rich in medium-chain triglycerides). Mononuclear cell production of PGE_2 was highest in animals fed corn oil and lowest in those fed linseed oil.

The physiologic role of high levels of PGE_2 is uncertain. It may be part of a negative feedback system "designed" to minimize the immune response and reduce cytokine production after injury. High levels of PGE_2 have anti-inflammatory actions and suppress mitogen responses, clonal proliferation, antigenic stimulation, cytokine production by lymphocytes, generation of cytotoxic cells, lymphocyte migration, and antibody production.[186] PGE_2 also inhibits neutrophil lysosomal release, suppresses mast cell degranulation, and dilates vessels. Long-term overproduction of PGE_2 may predispose to infection.

Leukotrienes (LTs) are metabolites of the ω-3 and ω-6 PUFAs and are important inflammatory mediators in sepsis, shock, trauma, and hypermetabolic states. They are produced by numerous immune cells, including lymphocytes, macrophages, mast cells, neutrophils, and other cells. LTs have a variety of physiologic effects. LTB_4 is a chemoattractant for activation of neutrophils and a stimulator of killer cell activity.[186, 190, 191] It is also chemotactic for lymphocytes and monocytes, enhances lymphocyte adherence, inhibits antibody production, and can stimulate IL-2 production. LTC_4, LTD_4, and

LTE_4 are bronchial constrictors. LTC_4 and LTD_4 also increase vascular permeability. In general, LTs are immune stimulators at physiologic levels.

Fish oils contain high concentrations of the ω-3 long-chain fatty acids eicosapentaenoic acid (EPA) and docosahexaenoic acid (DHA). These fatty acids compete with arachidonic acid for cyclooxygenase. Animals fed diets rich in EPA and DHA produce less PGE_2, LTB_4, LTC_4, and 6-keto-PGF_{1a}.[186, 187, 190, 191, 199] Supplementation with dietary ω-3 PUFAs (i.e., linolenic acid) decreases endotoxin-induced production of TxA_2, prostacyclin, and TNF in equine peritoneal macrophages.[200, 201] The clinical significance of these effects is unclear.

The total fat content of the diet can alter LT synthesis. LTE_4 synthesis was greater with a 5% ω-6 PUFA diet than with a 20% diet.[187] In addition, ω-3 PUFAs were more effective in decreasing synthesis of eicosanoids and LTs in low-fat diets (5%) than in high-fat ones (20%).[187]

The immune system is extremely complex. The first stages of defense involve nonspecific immunity—macrophages, neutrophils, complement, and the acute-phase response. Specific immunity recognizes, remembers, and destroys invading organisms. Mechanisms of specific immunity include cell-mediated immunity and humoral immunity. Effects of different lipids and combinations of lipids on all elements of the immune system have not been determined. It is possible that a lipid that enhances one component may suppress another. Overall effects are difficult to predict from isolated studies and clinical trials using altered lipid sources in combination with other nutrients. Specific trials of different dietary lipid combinations would be helpful in determining effects.

ANIMAL AND HUMAN STUDIES. Cytokines produced by various organs are believed to contribute to organ failure in critically ill patients. Feeding diets enriched in ω-3 PUFAs may diminish cytokine production. These diets decreased TNF and IL-1 secretion from endotoxin-stimulated monocytes. Kuppfer cells from rats fed ω-3 PUFAs for 6 weeks exhibited decreased production of TNF.[187] Cerra and coworkers[202] evaluated rat Kuppfer cell secretion of PGE_2 and TxB_2 in response to endotoxin stimulation. Animals fed menhaden oil (ω-3 PUFA) produced less PGE_2 and TxB_2 than animals fed corn oil or safflower oil.

Mochizuki and colleagues[203] performed studies in burned guinea pigs to determine the optimal total fat content for enteral diets following thermal injury. They reported that 5% to 15% safflower oil was optimal for protein synthesis and preservation of muscle mass. Higher concentrations (30% to 50%) were associated with adverse effects on muscle mass, nitrogen balance, and transferrin levels.

Other investigators studied the effects of lipid composition on outcome in models of critical illness. Intravenous and oral administration of fish oils increased survival in guinea pigs following endotoxin administration.[186] Similar effects were observed with prostaglandin synthesis inhibitors (i.e., ibuprofen, indomethacin). In other studies, mortality was increased in rats after cecal ligation and puncture as dietary ω-6/ω-3 PUFA increased.[202] Alexander and associates[204] reported higher mortality in animals fed linoleic acid diets (10% lipid diet) than in those fed fish oil or safflower oil diets.[204] The fish oil group also had lower resting metabolic energy expenditure, less weight loss, higher transferrin levels, and better opsonic indices.

Trocki and colleagues[205] also administered fish oil to burned guinea pigs. Animals fed 5%, 15%, 30%, or 50% of nonprotein calories as fish oil had similar mortality rates, resting metabolic expenditures, transferrin levels, macrophage bactericidal indices, and opsonic indices. Thermally injured rats fed a structured, lipid-containing, medium-chain triglyceride (60%) and fish oil (40%) diet had better nitrogen balances, lower energy expenditures, and decreased net protein catabolism than animals fed safflower oil diets.[206]

Peck and associates[207] fed mice diets containing different fats for two to three weeks. The animals then were subjected to a 20% burn and to infection with *Pseudomonas aeruginosa*. More animals fed a fish oil–supplemented diet died than did animals fed a safflower-supplemented diet (78% versus 27%). Mortality was intermediate in animals fed oleic acid– (44%) or coconut oil (58%)–supplemented diets. PGE_2 production was less profuse in the fish oil group. Peck's group found no differences in T and B lymphocyte functions. Interestingly, these results contrast with those observed in burned but not infected animals. Thus, it is possible that nonlymphocyte functions of the immune system (i.e., macrophages, neutrophils) were responsible for improved survival in the safflower group compared with the fish oil group. Different lipids may have varying effects at various times after injury. For example, immunosuppression from PGE_2 may be beneficial early after injury to minimize the inflammatory response and limit organ injury; however, prolonged immunosuppression may predispose to infection and worse outcomes.

Clouva-Molyvdas and colleagues[208] investigated the role of different lipid sources (coconut oil, fish oil, oleic acid, safflower oil) on survival from peritonitis in mice (*P. aeruginosa* and *Salmonella typhimurium*). Animals received 5% or 40% of total calories from fat for two to three weeks. Mortality was not significantly different between groups. Peck and colleagues[209] randomized guinea pigs to diets with varying fat contents (3.5% to 56% of calories) and fat compositions (fish oil, safflower oil, 50/50 mixture). The amount of fat did not affect survival in experimental peritonitis; however, the lipid composition significantly affected survival. The 50/50 mixture group had 39% survival; the safflower group, 20% survival; and the fish oil group, 9% survival. Delayed cutaneous hypersensitivity response was greatest in the fish oil group, intermediate in the 50/50 mixture group, and lowest in the safflower oil group. PGE_2 production by splenic macrophages was greatest in the safflower oil group, intermediate in the 50/50 mixture group, and least in the fish oil group. In this study, delayed cutaneous hypersensitivity response and PGE_2 production did not predict survival in this infection model. Results of this study suggest that outcomes from infections are best with fat mixtures, but the optimal fat mixture has not been determined.

Use of intravenous lipids in parenteral nutrition has caused concern because these preparations contain large amounts of linoleic acid (ω-6 PUFA). Hamawy and colleagues[210] administered TPN with 50% and 0% lipid to animals with leg fracture and infection. Lipid was given as long-chain triglycerides (LCT) or 75% medium-chain triglycerides (MCT) plus 25% LCT. Reticuloendothelial function was better in the animals fed the MCT-LCT mixture. Similarly, reticuloendothelial dysfunction was described in normal and burned guinea pigs when LCT preparations were administered.[211] Intraperitoneal "intralipid" slowed clearance of *S. aureus* from the peritoneal cavities of mice and increased its dissemination to other organs.[212] It increased death rates in animals infected with *Streptococcus* species.[213] Intravenous linoleic acid–supplemented nutrition prolongs graft survival and potentiates blood transfusion–induced immunosuppression.[214] Linoleic acid also prolongs graft survival and has additive effects when combined with cyclosporine.[215] Other studies determined that intravenous lipid supplementation had no effect on Kuppfer cell phagocytosis in septic rats.[216] In vitro, human leukocytes incubated with lipid emulsions rich in linoleic acid have impaired chemotaxis and diminished bactericidal activity.[213, 217, 218] Mitogen-stimulated and IL-2–activated human lymphocyte proliferation are both inhibited by lipid emulsions.[219] These lipids also diminish production of cytotoxic lymphokine-activated killer cells.

Cheney and colleagues[220] noted an association between the quantity of intravenous lipid administered to bone marrow transplant recipients and the incidence of infection. Freeman and associates[221] reported a significant association between use of intravenous lipid and staphylococcal bacteremia in neonates. These studies indicate that linoleic acid possesses immunosuppressive effects.

In healthy subjects, dietary supplementation with EPA and DHA alters cytokine and prostaglandin production. After 6 weeks (but not 3 weeks) of supplementation, LTB_4 generation is reduced.[222] LTB_4-induced chemotaxis is also decreased. Endres and colleagues[223] fed ω-3 PUFA to healthy subjects for 6 weeks and measured mononuclear cell cytokine release secondary to stimulation in vitro with endotoxin, *S. aureus*, and PHA. TNF, IL-1, and PGE_2 production were lowered by the diet. Similarly, LTB_4-induced chemotaxis was diminished; thus, in healthy subjects, ω-3 PUFA attenuates release of inflammatory mediators.

Luostarinen and Saldeen[224] supplemented healthy volunteers with fish oil (5.4 g EPA and 3.2 g DHA) for 4 weeks. They reported that dietary fish oil decreased superoxide generation by neutrophils without altering neutrophil lysosomal enzyme release.

Clinical studies report that fish oil supplementation has beneficial effects on acute inflammatory conditions, rheumatoid arthritis, multiple sclerosis, and lupus, and that it prolongs graft survival. Meydani and coworkers[225] supplemented diets of healthy young and older women with ω-3 PUFA (2.4 g/day) for 12 weeks and found decreased mitogenic response in the older women after 12 weeks' supplementation.

Effects of fish oil supplementation on critically ill patients are unclear. Morlion and associates[226] randomized postsurgical patients to TPN with either soybean oil emulsion or fish oil plus soybean oil emulsion for 5 days after surgery. They evaluated plasma and membrane fatty acid composition and LT-synthesizing capacity of lymphocytes. At the end of the study period, EPA concentration was increased (2.5-fold), and LTB_5 and LTC_5 synthesis were increased in the patients who received fish oil in the lipid emulsion. Production rates of LTB_4 and LTC_4 were similar in both groups.

Gadek's group[227] randomized patients with ARDS to a standard enteral formula or an isocaloric, isonitrogenous formula supplemented with ω-3 long-chain fatty acids (i.e., γ-linolenic acid, EPA) and antioxidants. Patients receiving the ω-3 long-chain fatty acid–enriched diet demonstrated reduced lung inflammation, a lower incidence of new organ failures, decreased ventilator time, and shorter ICU and hospital stays.

In conclusion, lipid content of the diet affects cellular and metabolic activity. Lipids alter membrane composition and function, generation of cytokines and prostaglandins, immune cell function, and the body's response to infection. Diets high in linoleic acid appear to be immunosuppressive. Decreasing linoleic acid in the diet improves immune function. The ω-6 PUFA linoleic acid and the ω-3 PUFA linolenic acid are essential fatty acids and must be supplied in the diet. The optimal fat blend for critically ill patients remains unclear, but many recommend an ω-6 PUFA–ω-3 PUFA ratio of 1:1. Optimal fat intake is thought to range from 20% to 40% of total calories, given as a mixture of MCTs, ω-6 PUFA, and ω-3 PUFA. The authors favor balanced fat formulas that contain the required amounts of linoleic acid (i.e., 5% to 10% of nonprotein calories) mixed with other lipids (i.e., MCTs, ω-3 PUFA, and saturated fats).

Carbohydrate

Carbohydrate may be provided as simple sugars or complex polysaccharides, such as starch and fiber. Some fibers (i.e., pectin) escape digestion in the upper gastrointestinal tract and reach the colon, where bacteria metabolize them into short-chain fatty acids (acetate, propionate, butyrate).[228] Short-chain fatty acids stimulate electrolyte and water absorption, increase colonic blood flow, stimulate colonic proliferation, and are preferential fuels for the colon. They are also metabolized to glutamine and ketones and can be used as fuel by the small intestine. Short-chain fatty acids are easily absorbed and metabolized by both large and small bowels. Clearance of short-chain fatty acids is primarily via the liver. In humans, short-chain fatty acids are derived from fermentation of fiber in the large bowel, and they contribute to energy of the body. Colonic absorption of short-chain fatty acids is estimated to provide 5% to 10% of daily energy requirements.[229] Acetate and butyrate are converted to acetylcoenzyme A; propionate is converted to succinylcoenzyme A. Some fibers (e.g., cellulose, lignin) are not digested in the gastrointestinal tract and add bulk to the stool. These fibers are stool softeners and stimulate bowel mobility. Most liquid nutritional formulas do not contain these fibers, but patients may benefit from supplementation. The fibers must be administered enterally and must remain in the colon long enough to undergo bacterial fermentation. During antibiotic therapy, bacterial fermentation may be limited owing to changes in intestinal microflora. Altered fermentation may lead to gut atrophy and decreased gut barrier integrity.

Dietary fibers have many effects on gastrointestinal integrity.[230] Pectin and guar (digestible fibers) stimulate proliferation and maturation of intestinal cells.[230-233] Metabolizable fibers increase gastrointestinal mucosal enzyme activity and gut absorption.[230-234] Infusion of short-chain fatty acids into the colon of animals improves colon anastomosis healing[235] and increases gut mucosal deoxyribonucleic acid (DNA) content.[236] Koruda and colleagues[237] reported that supplementation of parenteral nutrition with short-chain fatty acids decreased the gut atrophy associated with TPN. Harig and coworkers[238] found that infusion of short-chain fatty acids into the colon of patients with diversion colitis reduced bowel inflammation. Pectin supplementation of elemental diets improves intestinal adaptation after small-bowel resection.[237] In another study, pectin supplementation decreased colonic inflammation in experimental colitis[239] and improved healing of colonic anastomoses in rats.[240]

Although some fibers accelerate gastrointestinal transit, pectin delays gastric emptying[241] and prolongs transit time.[242] Pectin supplementation decreases the incidence of liquid stools in patients receiving tube feeding,[230, 243] and may help to decrease diarrhea. "Unmetabolizable," or bulk, fibers have minimal effects on these parameters, as they enhance colonic transit and produce larger and softer stools.[242] They are thus used to treat constipation. These fibers may increase stool viscosity in patients with diarrhea. Bulk fibers do not decrease the incidence of diarrhea.[244]

Glucose synthesis is increased in critically ill patients and is not fully suppressed by administration of exogenous glucose. Hyperglycemia is a result of accelerated gluconeogenesis, glycogenolysis, and insulin resistance. Lactate, glycerol, alanine, and other amino acids are substrates for glucose production. Both glucose and fat metabolism are enhanced in critical illness. This suggests that the body can use both fuel sources efficiently. Glucose cannot totally suppress lipid oxidation, and lipid cannot fully suppress glucose oxidation. There is no metabolic advantage to giving patients only one fuel source as there is no absolute preference for either glucose or lipid.

Glucose or lipid administration has nitrogen-sparing effects,[245-250] but these effects "plateau."[251] After the plateau is reached, increasing the amounts does not further reduce protein breakdown. Supplemental insulin to prevent hyperglycemia may help to suppress protein catabolism.[252, 253]

Carbohydrate feeding has the undesirable side effect of excessive carbon dioxide production (V_{CO_2}). Increased V_{CO_2} increases minute ventilation and work of breathing. Hypercarbia and respiratory failure can develop in patients with diminished respiratory function. Askanazi and associates[254] reported that septic patients overfed glucose (i.e., 1.5 to 2 times the resting energy expenditure) demonstrated elevated oxygen consumption, V_{CO_2}, and minute ventilation.

Lipid has been substituted for carbohydrate as a calorie source to avoid hypercapnia and respiratory acidosis and failure. Studies reveal that lipid-glucose combinations cause less carbon dioxide production and lower minute ventilation than glucose alone[255-257]; however, studies that report clinically significant increases in V_{CO_2} with high-carbohydrate formulas administered calories in excess of requirements. When carbohydrate or carbohydrate plus lipid was provided in amounts that matched energy expenditure, few significant differences were observed in V_{CO_2} between treatment groups. Some enteral formulas are designed to increase the lipid:glucose ratio. No significant differences in V_{CO_2} were found when glucose-lipid diets containing 30% to 50% lipid (administered at rates that matched energy needs) were compared.[258] Yet, high-fat enteral diets increase the incidence of gastrointestinal side effects (i.e., abdominal distention, bloating, diarrhea).

Nucleic Acids

Because the body can synthesize nucleic acids, they are not considered essential dietary components. Their importance as nutrients remains unclear. They are not present in parenteral nutrition or in most enteral formulations.

Some studies suggest that nucleic acids play a role in the immune response. Diets deficient in nucleic acids suppress mixed lymphocyte responses, mitogen-stimulated lymphocyte proliferation, cardiac allograft rejection, graft-versus-host disease, and delayed cutaneous hypersensitivity.[259-264] Nucleotide supplementation reverses these effects. Nucleotide-deficient diets enhance cyclosporine immunosuppression,[262, 263] decrease activity of natural killer cells in vitro, and are associated with decreased synthesis of IL-2.[261] In contrast, these diets are associated with increased macrophage activation. The dietary effects of nucleotides are both time- and dose-dependent. Uracil appears to be of major importance in nucleotide preparations.[262, 264]

Animals given *Candida albicans*[259, 265] or *S. aureus*[266, 267] have increased mortality when fed nucleotide-free diets. Because the role of nucleotide supplementation in treatment of human diseases has not been adequately evaluated, support for its use is lacking. Some of the immunity-enhancing enteral formulas, however, do contain nucleotides (i.e, yeast ribonucleic acid [RNA]).

Nutrient Combinations

Randomized, controlled trials have not been performed to evaluate the individual effects or various doses of specific nutrients (e.g., arginine, glutamine, ω-3 PUFAs, peptides, and nucleotides) on infection rates or outcomes for critically ill patients. Recent analyses[268-270] of prospective controlled trials[227, 271-285] of immunity-enhancing formulas (containing combinations of immune nutrients) concluded that these formulas were associated with better outcomes for critically ill patients.

Most of the early studies of immunity-enhancing diets were criticized, because they did not compare isonitrogenous or isocaloric regimens. In 1990, Gottschlich and associates[271] reported significant decreases in wound infections and ICU stays for burn patients fed a diet enriched with arginine and ω-3 PUFAs. This diet was also associated with a trend toward lower rates of pneumonia and death.

Cerra's group[272] randomized 20 trauma patients to an immunity-enhancing diet or an intact protein diet. Although there were no differences in infection rates or mortality between these small groups, patients who received the "immune" diet exhibited increased mononuclear cell mitogenic responses.

Daly and coworkers[273] randomized patients undergoing gastrointestinal surgery for malignancy to an immunity-enhancing diet or an intact protein formula. The intact protein group received significantly less protein and their nitrogen balance was more negative. Lengths of stay were similar; however, the incidence of infections plus wound-healing complications was lower in the "immune" diet group.

Bower and colleagues[274] performed a large multicenter, double-blind, randomized trial that compared an immunity-enhancing diet to an intact protein formula in critically ill patients. Patients fed the "immune" diet received more protein. The "immune formula" significantly decreased lengths of stay (21 versus 29 days) in the sepsis subgroup. The "immune" diet group tended to have fewer infections and shorter lengths of stay than the control group.

A study by Brown and coworkers[275] evaluated trauma patients randomized to an "immune" diet or a standard diet, and reported 71% fewer infections ($P < .05$) in the former group.

In a study by Moore and associates,[276] trauma patients fed an immune formula had significantly fewer abdominal abscesses and organ failures. In that trial, the immune-formula group tended to need fewer days on the ventilator, in the ICU, and in the hospital.

More recent studies compared isonitrogenous and isocaloric dietary regimens. Daly's group[277] compared post–gastrointestinal surgery patients fed either an immune formula or a standard formula (isocaloric and isonitrogenous) and found fewer infections and wound complications and shorter lengths of stay (16 versus 22 days) in the immune group. Kudsk and associates[278] reported similar observations—fewer major infections and shorter lengths of stay—for trauma patients randomized to an immune diet as compared with those fed a standard diet.

Two additional studies of gastrointestinal surgery patients[279, 280] reported fewer infections and shorter lengths of stay for the patients fed an immune formula. One study that evaluated septic patients randomized to an immune formula or a standard diet reported fewer new infections in the immune group.[281] This study by Galban and associates[281] is the only trial of immune-enhancing enteral formulas that reported a significant decrease in mortality.

Weimann and colleagues[282] conducted a trial in a small number of severely injured patients. The investigators found significantly fewer systemic inflammatory response syndrome (SIRS) days per patient and lower multi-organ failure scores per patient among those fed an immune formula. Atkinson and coworkers[283] randomized mixed medical and surgical patients to an immune formula or a standard formula and reported that successful early enteral feeding with an immune formula decreased lengths of stay in the ICU and the hospital, reduced time on mechanical ventilation, and lowered the incidence of SIRS.

Houdijk's group[177] randomized trauma patients to receive a glutamine-enriched enteral formula and reported significantly lower incidences of pneumonia, bacteremia, and sepsis in the glutamine-supplemented group as compared with the control group. In contrast, Mendez and colleagues[284] found no better outcomes in trauma patients fed an immune diet.

Gadek's group[227] evaluated an enteral formula enhanced

TABLE 79–2. Mineral Requirements

Mineral	Recommended Daily Intake: Enteral	Recommended Daily Intake: Parenteral
Sodium	90–150 mEq	90–150 mEq
Potassium	60–90 mEq	60–90 mEq
Magnesium	350 mg	10–30 mEq
Calcium	1000 mg	10–20 mEq
Phosphorus	1000 mg	10–35 mmol

with EPA, γ-linolenic acid, and antioxidants. This nutrient mixture was compared to a control diet in a randomized, double-blind, multicenter trial of patients with ARDS.[227] The investigators reported significantly reduced pulmonary neutrophil recruitment and inflammation, lower incidence of new organ failures, and shorter lengths of stay in ARDS patients fed the enriched diet.

Currently, few data exist to indicate which of the current enteral immune-enhancing formulas is superior to the others. Only one published clinical trial compared 2 immune formulas.[286] They found no differences in outcomes between groups. These are the first generation of immune-enhancing enteral formulations, and we anticipate improvements. In conclusion, extensive review of prospective, randomized, clinical trials comparing early enteral feeding with immune-enhancing and standard enteral diets indicates that the immune formulas are highly likely to improve outcome and reduce hospitalization costs.

Water

Water requirements depend on the body water content and ongoing water losses (in urine, stool, skin, respiratory tract). It is difficult to predict specific body water needs, which can vary from 1.5 to 6 L/day. Clinical assessment is helpful in determining water requirements (e.g., decreased skin turgor suggests a need for more water). A rising blood urea nitrogen (BUN)/creatinine ratio, concentrated urine, and hypernatremia also suggest an increased need for fluids or water. On the other hand, hyponatremia usually results from an excess of body water that "dilutes" sodium. Most adult patients require approximately 1 mL of water per kilocalorie consumed (1.5 mL/kcal for infants).

Micronutrients

Human requirements for vitamins, minerals, and trace elements in critical illness have not been determined. Provision of at least the recommended daily allowance (RDA) of each vitamin is advocated to prevent complications of deficiency. Minerals should be provided in doses that maintain adequate serum levels. Trace elements, such as zinc and copper, should be supplied to avoid deficiency states. Levels of vitamins and trace elements are not clinically useful indicators of deficiency.

TABLE 79–3. Vitamin Requirements

Vitamin	Deficiency	Recommended Daily Intake: Enteral	Recommended Daily Intake: Parenteral
Vitamin A	Night blindness, impaired wound healing, male sterility	1000–2000 μg (3300–6600 IU)	1000 μg (3300 IU)
Vitamin D	Rickets, osteomalacia, hypocalcemia	400 IU (10 μg)	200 IU (5 μg)
Vitamin E	Edema, hemolysis, oxidant damage	400–800 IU	400–800 IU
Vitamin K	Bleeding, prolonged clotting times	65–80 μg	10 mg/wk
Vitamin C	Scurvy, delayed wound healing, perifollicular hemorrhage, petechiae, ecchymoses, bleeding gums, oxidant injury	100–500 mg	100 mg
Thiamine (B_1)	Beriberi, Wernicke-Korsakoff syndrome	1.0–3.0 mg	3 mg
Riboflavin (B_2)	Angular stomatitis, cheilosis, glossitis	1.1–1.8 mg	3.6 mg
Niacin	Pellagra, raw tongue, atrophic papillae, tongue fissuring, dementia, diarrhea	10–20 mg	40 mg
Folate	Macrocytic anemia, stomatitis, glossitis, diarrhea, malabsorption	0.2–0.4 mg	0.4 mg
Pyridoxine (B_6)	Oxalate stones, polyneuritis, seborrhea, glossitis, seizures, microcytic anemia	1.6–2.0 mg	4 mg
Vitamin B_{12}	Megaloblastic anemia, neuropathy, stomatitis, glossitis	3 μg	5 μg
Pantothenic acid	Lethargy, nausea, vomiting, abdominal pain, paresthesias	5–10 mg	15 mg
Biotin	Skin rash, alopecia, lethargy, depression, paresthesias	150–300 μg	60 μg

Minerals

Minerals are required for normal body function (see chapters on divalent ions and sodium and potassium). The major minerals in the human body are sodium, potassium, magnesium, calcium, and phosphorus. Most formulas supply the normal recommended dietary amounts (Table 79-2) of these minerals when total calorie expenditure is met. Many patients lose excessive amounts of these minerals and require supplementation. In contrast, with renal insufficiency, potassium, magnesium, and phosphorus accumulate, and dietary restriction may be warranted. Increasing magnesium intake may also improve cardiovascular function, decrease arrhythmias, and protect from organ injury.

Vitamins

Vitamins (Table 79-3) are necessary for metabolism of carbohydrates, fats, and protein. They are important cofactors for enzyme activity. The following vitamins are essential for humans:

- Vitamins A, D, E, and K (fat-soluble)
- Vitamins C, B_1 (thiamine), B_2 (riboflavin), B_6 (pyridoxine), B_{12}, folate, niacin, pantothenic acid, and biotin (water-soluble)

For an extensive review of vitamin biochemistry and requirements, the reader is referred elsewhere.[287]

Most enteral formulas supply the normal recommended dietary amounts of essential vitamins (see Table 79-3) when total calorie expenditure is met. Little is known of the changes in vitamin requirements associated with critical illness, trauma, and surgery. Vitamin deficiencies impair cell and organ function and recovery from illness. Because the biologic half-life of fat-soluble vitamins is usually long, significant deficiencies of fat-soluble vitamins are rare. Provision of adequate calories and protein with TPN reduces mobilization of body fat and minimizes release of fat-soluble vitamins. Patients receiving TPN are at risk for fat-soluble vitamin deficiencies when supplementation is inadequate. Because tissue stores of water-soluble vitamins are small, deficiencies can develop soon after onset of malnutrition. Supplementation of water-soluble vitamins during TPN is mandatory (see Table 79-3).

Supplements may be needed during enteral nutrition if losses or needs are expected to increase. Some advocate the administration of larger quantities of vitamins C and E for their antioxidant functions. Others recommend giving large amounts of vitamin A (10,000 to 25,000 IU/day) to improve wound healing in critically ill patients (particularly those receiving corticosteroids) and in patients with diabetes.[288]

Trace Elements

Trace minerals are inorganic elements that regulate many metabolic processes in the body. Many function as constituents of enzyme complexes. Eight trace minerals (Table 79-4) are essential for humans: iron, iodine, cobalt, zinc, copper, chro-

TABLE 79–4. Trace Mineral Requirements

Trace Element	Deficiency	Recommended Daily Intake: Enteral	Recommended Daily Intake: Parenteral
Iron	Microcytic anemia, sore tongue, angular stomatitis	10–15 mg	2.5 mg
Iodine	Goiter, hypothyroidism	150 μg	—
Cobalt		Given as vitamin B_{12}	Given as vitamin B_{12}
Zinc	Dermatitis, hypogonadism, cellular immune deficiency, impaired taste, impaired wound healing	15 mg	2.5–4.0 mg
Copper	Microcytic anemia, neutropenia, hypotonia, depigmentation, cerebral degeneration	1.5–3 mg	0.5–1.5 mg
Chromium	Glucose intolerance, peripheral neuropathy, weight loss	50–200 μg	10–15 μg
Manganese	Encephalitis-like syndrome, extrapyramidal syndrome	2.0–5.0 mg	0.15–0.8 mg
Selenium	Myalgias, heart failure	50–70 μg	20–40 μg

mium, manganese, and selenium. Most formulas supply the normal recommended dietary amounts (see Table 79-4) of these minerals when total calorie expenditure is met by administration of the formula. It is not clear how the RDA values should be applied to critically ill patients. Some recommend increasing administration of some of the trace elements for a variety of specific purposes (e.g., increased zinc intake to enhance wound healing).[288] No data from clinical trials are available to support or dispute such recommendations.

TECHNIQUES OF ENTERAL FEEDING

Enteral nutritional support can be delivered by the oral, gastric, or small-intestinal route.[289-299] Physiologic responses (e.g., anabolism) are optimal when the oral route is used, followed by the gastric and then the small-intestinal route.[289] Thus, we believe that the oral route is the preferred one for nutritional support. Unfortunately, this route may not be an option in some patients because of depressed mental status, anorexia, or problems with swallowing that increase the risk of aspiration. These patients may be fed via the gastric or small-intestinal route. For patients with intact gastric emptying who are not at significant risk of aspiration, the gastric route is preferred. Alternatively, when gastric emptying is delayed or aspiration is a concern, small-intestinal feeding is the best option.

Gastric feeding is delivered via nasogastric tubes, small-bore feeding tubes, or gastrostomy tubes. We prefer larger-bore nasogastric tubes or gastrostomy tubes when gastric residual monitoring is necessary. Nasogastric or orogastric tubes are generally easily placed via the nose or mouth. Confirmation of gastric placement (e.g., aspiration of gastric contents or bile) is mandatory prior to gastric feeding. Gastrostomy tubes can be placed using the percutaneous endoscopic gastrostomy method[292-294, 296] or surgically.[294, 295, 297, 298]

Feeding into the small bowel is accomplished through small-bore feeding tubes inserted through the nose or oral cavity. Such tubes are passed through the stomach and pylorus and into the small intestine. We prefer to place the tip of the tube into the distal duodenum or proximal jejunum. In 92% of critically ill patients, we have been successful in passing feeding tubes into the small intestine using a bedside "corkscrew" method.[291] Other techniques for effectively placing these tubes into the small intestine include fluoroscopic or endoscopic guidance and surgery.[295, 296, 298, 299] With a combination of these methods, successful placement is possible in more than 99% of critically ill patients.

Some clinicians place feeding tubes into the stomach and wait until they migrate into the small intestine. This approach may be reasonably effective (30% to 70%) in ward patients, but it has little efficacy (<5%) in most critically ill patients with impaired gastric emptying. One study[300] indicated efficacy of a one-time dose of intravenous erythromycin in improving migration of feeding tubes from the stomach into the small intestine. Metoclopramide has not proved reliable in promoting migration of feeding tubes into the small intestine of a critically ill patient, although it may help to decrease gastric reflux. Cisapride may also be effective as a promotility agent.

Jejunal feeding tubes may be used to provide enteral nutrition.[294-299] Typically, these are placed at the time of abdominal surgery. Small-diameter needle catheter jejunostomy tubes are problematic owing to their tendency to be clogged by some nutritional formulations. Therefore, we prefer larger-diameter jejunal catheters.

An aggressive approach to ensuring placement of small-bowel feeding tubes is necessary for administration of early enteral nutrition. When oral nutrition is not feasible, gastric or small bowel options should be considered. We believe that the choice of (1) duodenal tube or jejunal tube, (2) "blind" bedside or fluoroscopic or endoscopic guidance, or (3) surgical techniques is best made according to individual patient characteristics and local resources.

APPROACH TO ENTERAL FEEDING

Enteral feeding should be initiated within 12 to 48 hours of admission to the ICU. Therefore, when oral feeding is not feasible, a gastric feeding tube should be placed in most patients and feeding should be attempted before placement of a small-bowel feeding tube. Alternatively, when a patient is at high risk for poor gastric emptying (because of severe multiple trauma, history of gastric paresis) or for aspiration, a small-bowel tube can be placed. The head of the bed should be elevated 30 degrees to decrease the risk of aspiration.

In adults, feeding may be administered in boluses of 100 to 250 mL every 2 to 4 hours or by continuous infusion starting at 25 to 30 mL/hr and increased by 10 to 25 mL/hr every 1 to 4 hours, as tolerated (i.e., gastric residual volumes <150 mL) until the calorie goal (25 to 30 kcal/kg/day) is delivered. If the protein goal is not achieved, a formula with a higher protein-calorie ratio is in order or protein can be added to the formula. Gastric residual volumes should be monitored every 4 hours, before giving the next bolus. If an adult's gastric residuum is more than 150 mL, feedings should be withheld for 2 hours and then resumed.

Some clinicians prefer to increase feedings (for adults) more slowly (i.e., ~10 mL/hr every 6 to 12 hours), but often this is not necessary. The goal rate of infusion should be met by the third day of therapy, or frequently earlier. When gastric emptying is impaired and nutritional goals are not achievable via gastric delivery, small-bowel feeding should be instituted and advanced to goal rates. Feeding formulas should not be diluted. Formula osmolality is typically 300 to 600 mOsm/kg of water, and this rarely causes diarrhea.

NUTRITION FOR SPECIFIC DISEASE STATES

Systemic Inflammatory Response Syndrome

In patients with SIRS from trauma, burn injury, or sepsis, enteral nutrition is associated with decreases in infectious complications (see Route of Nutritional Support earlier). Enteral formulations enriched with specific nutrients, such as arginine, ω-3 long-chain fatty acids, and RNA, have been associated with shorter hospital stays and fewer infectious complications. Many clinical trials demonstrate improved outcomes when patients are fed enteral formulations containing nutrient combinations designed to enhance immune function. These trials are detailed elsewhere (see Nutrient Combinations).

Acute Pancreatitis

Of all patients with pancreatitis admitted to the hospital 20% are estimated to have severe pancreatitis and are at high risk for development of medical complications. Oral nutrition is typically prohibited by many factors, such as abdominal pain, nausea and vomiting, gastric atony, paralytic ileus, and partial duodenal obstruction secondary to pancreatic enlargement, among others. Decreases in luminal pancreatic enzymes and in absorption of ingested substrates produce maldigestion. Excessive protein loss may occur as a result of inflammation of peritoneal and retroperitoneal surfaces, diarrhea, or fistula.

Many metabolic and nutritional alterations are induced by pancreatitis. Energy expenditure is widely variable. About 50%

of severely ill patients exhibit dramatic increases in energy expenditure; studies report that resting energy expenditure may be increased 149% above predicted levels.[301] These studies report that about 40% of patients are normometabolic and about 10% hypometabolic (as low as 77% of predicted value). Carbohydrate metabolism is altered by an increase in the glucagon:insulin ratio, impaired beta cell function, insulin resistance, and increased gluconeogenesis. Fat metabolism is altered by increased lipolysis and lipid oxidation and by impaired clearance of lipids from the blood resulting in hyperlipidemia and hypertriglyceridemia. Changes in protein metabolism are manifested by accentuation of net protein catabolism, increased ureagenesis, and net nitrogen losses as great as 20 to 40 g/day. Micronutrient and vitamin deficiencies are common and include calcium, magnesium, zinc, thiamine, and folate. Negative energy balance frequently results from reduced nutrient intake and increased metabolic demands. Persistently negative nitrogen balance is associated with higher mortality.

"Pancreatic rest" (i.e., no enteral nutrients) has been a common therapy for pancreatitis, but its benefit in acute or chronic pancreatitis has never been proven. The general goal of pancreatic rest is to decrease exocrine pancreatic secretions (i.e., protein enzymes, fluids, and bicarbonate). Oral feeding often leads to recurrence of symptoms and elevation of amylase and lipase levels. Indeed, the site of enteral nutrient delivery affects pancreatic secretion. Gastric infusion of nutrients produces more profuse pancreatic secretions than does duodenal infusion. Jejunal infusion causes even less pancreatic stimulation. Animal studies by Ragins and colleagues[302] showed little or no pancreatic stimulation when an elemental diet was infused into the jejunum at neutral pH.

The traditional approach to nutritional support of a patient with pancreatitis consists of restricting oral feeding and, if the patient cannot eat within a week, administering parenteral nutrition. Others begin parenteral feeding immediately on hospital admission if the patient is malnourished or is not expected to eat within 3 to 5 days. Interestingly, results from prospective randomized trials indicate that early enteral feeding into the small bowel is tolerated well by patients with pancreatitis and is associated with improved outcome.[303, 304]

Sax and colleagues[305] compared TPN to no nutrition support in 54 patients with pancreatitis. There was no benefit from TPN, and patients who received TPN had more infections and longer hospital stays. McClave's group[306] compared TPN to small-bowel feeding in 30 patients with acute pancreatitis. Enterally fed patients "normalized" their amylase earlier, were eating earlier, and stayed in the hospital fewer days. Although these findings were not statistically significant, there was a trend in the direction of improved outcomes in the enteral-feeding group. Costs of nutritional support were significantly lower for the "enteral group."

Kalfarentzos and associates[307] compared TPN to enteral feeding in 38 patients with acute, severe pancreatitis. They tolerated enteral feeding well. Patients fed enterally experienced fewer complications and episodes of sepsis than those who received TPN. The cost of nutritional support was lower for the enteral group. Windsor and coworkers[308] reported the results of a prospective randomized study of TPN and enteral nutrition in 34 patients with severe, acute pancreatitis (amylase value >1000, computed tomographic evidence of necrosis). Enteral feeding was associated with faster resolution of inflammatory markers, decreased evidence of endotoxin translocation, greater total antioxidant capacity, and reduced rates of SIRS, sepsis, and organ failure. ICU stays were significantly shorter in the enteral group, as were total hospital stays.

These trials suggest that early enteral nutrition should be the preferred route of nutritional support for patients with pancreatitis.

Inflammatory Bowel Disease

Patients with inflammatory bowel disease typically have decreased nutrient intake and malabsorption and higher rates of protein-losing enteropathy and drug-nutrient interactions. Protein-calorie malnutrition and specific nutrient deficiencies result. Many prospective randomized clinical trials have evaluated the clinical efficacy of enteral nutrition in patients with Crohn's disease. Unfortunately, most of the studies are limited by small sample size, heterogeneity of patients, a large number of withdrawals from the diet groups, and variations in diet composition. These trials were evaluated by meta-analysis,[309-311] which determined that overall remission rates were lower in enteral nutrition–treated than in steroid-treated patients and that there was no advantage demonstrated for use of elemental formulas over nonelemental ones. Studies using ω-3 fatty acids from fish oil to treat inflammatory bowel disease report conflicting results in treating Crohn's disease[312, 313] and decreases in disease activity in patients with ulcerative colitis.[314-317] Effects of enteral formulas designed to enhance immune function have not been evaluated in inflammatory bowel disease.

In general, bowel rest is not necessary to produce clinical remission of inflammatory bowel disease. Enteral nutrition should be attempted first and TPN used only when patients cannot tolerate enteral nutrition.[318, 319] Studies suggest that steroid therapy is more effective than enteral nutritional therapy in inducing remission in patients with Crohn's disease. Further studies of enteral nutrition for inflammatory bowel disease are needed before conclusions can be drawn about optimal nutrient-pharmacologic combination therapies.

Acute Renal Failure

Most patients with renal failure should be fed via the enteral route. No prospective randomized clinical trials have assessed the efficacy of enteral nutrition in critically ill patients with acute renal failure. Many of these patients are hypercatabolic, secondary to comorbid conditions, and they also lose excessive amounts of nutrients through dialysis. Additionally, the stress of hemodialysis or continuous renal replacement procedures themselves can increase nutritional demands. Thus, patients with acute renal failure who are receiving dialysis or ultrafiltration therapy may need larger quantities of nutrients (i.e., amino acids). Patients with acute renal failure should receive a minimum of 1.0 g/kg/day of protein. Protein needs are expected to be greater for patients with acute renal failure who have sustained polytrauma, burn injury, or significant surgical wounds, and for these patients we recommend administration of 1.2 to 1.5 g/kg/day of protein. Protein intake for critically ill patients should not be limited to less than 1.0 g/kg/day in an attempt to obviate dialysis therapy. In anticipation of losses via dialysis, critically ill patients receiving hemodialysis (i.e., amino acid losses of 3 to 5 g/hour) should be given 1.2 to 1.5 g/kg/day of protein.

Specific nutritional considerations of peritoneal dialysis relate primarily to glucose and amino acids.[318] Peritoneal dialysis fluid contains glucose, and one should consider this when determining the total calories to be administered. Because peritoneal dialysis removes an estimated 40 to 60 g amino acid per day, amino acid requirements are increased.

Oliguric and anuric renal failure are associated with fluid intolerance. Increased plasma levels of potassium, magnesium, and phosphorus can also result. Enteral formulas with relatively smaller amounts of fluid and electrolytes may be useful in these patients. Dialysis therapy may be necessary to achieve adequate nutritional support. Clinical benefits of enteral nutrition and optimal formulations and timing of therapy have not been specifically established in critically ill patients with acute renal failure.

Liver Disease

Patients having liver failure as a single-organ failure may be hypermetabolic. Most exhibit increased losses of potassium, magnesium, and zinc. Fluid restriction is often instituted for treatment of significant ascites. Patients require careful fluid and electrolyte management. Several prospective randomized controlled trials found that patients hospitalized for complications of cirrhosis tolerated enteral nutrition well and that it improved hepatic function, hepatic encephalopathy, and Child's score.[320-322]

Encephalopathy often complicates liver failure, but these patients require protein for recovery from organ failure. Some protein (1.0 to 1.3 g/kg/day) should be provided in these cases.[318] When encephalopathy persists or worsens or when nutritional needs are not met, one should consider use of enteral products designed for isolated liver failure (e.g., increased branched-chain amino acids and decreased aromatic and sulfur-containing amino acids). These special formulations may not improve outcome in these patients, but they may benefit individual patients by improving mental function. No trials of enteral nutrition in fulminant liver failure resulting from viral hepatitis or drugs have been conducted.

COMPLICATIONS OF ENTERAL NUTRITION

Enteral nutrition may be associated with complications, including malpositioned feeding tubes, aspiration of gastric contents, and diarrhea. Patients may experience complications secondary to the feeding access device. Feeding tubes inserted through the nose are associated with sinusitis, dysphagia, gastroesophageal reflux, and irritation of the nasal, pharyngeal, esophageal, or gastric regions. Percutaneous tubes are associated with tube exit site infections and dislodgment of the stomach or small intestine from the abdominal wall with resultant spillage of gastrointestinal contents into the peritoneal cavity. Tube blockage can occur with any type of feeding access, but it becomes more likely as the internal diameter of the tube decreases. Despite the variety of complications that can occur, with the exception of pulmonary aspiration, life-threatening complications are rare.

Malpositioned Feeding Tubes

Malpositioned feeding tubes are most often associated with blind bedside methods of tube placement. Critically ill patients are believed to be at increased risk for misplacement into the endobronchial tree or pleural space, secondary to alterations of mental status induced by injury or sedation, absence of the gag reflex, inability to cough, dysphagia, or endotracheal intubation. To avoid pulmonary damage and pneumothorax, the tube position in the gastrointestinal tract should be confirmed before the tube is inserted all the way. Acceptable methods include radiographic confirmation, assessment of myoelectrical activity, aspiration of gastric contents (which typically have a pH of 2 to 4), or aspiration of bile.[323] Alternatively, direct laryngoscopy may be used to visualize the tube passing into the esophagus.

Auscultation findings can be misleading. A feeding tube placed into the base of the left lung can produce sounds similar to those heard in tubes placed into the stomach. Pneumothorax is more frequent with central line placement than with feeding tube placement (1.7% versus 0.3%).[324, 325]

Aspiration of Gastric Contents

Pulmonary aspiration is one of the most serious complications of enteral feeding.[326-331] Large gastric volume is believed to predispose to gastric reflux and aspiration, but the amount of gastric residual volume that predisposes to aspiration is not known and depends on the patient's position, competence of the lower esophageal sphincter, and stomach size.[326-328, 332]

Saliva and gastric secretions contribute to gastric residuum. Most healthy fasting adults have gastric residual volumes of 100 mL or less.[333] Large gastric residual volume may result from gastroparesis. The literature frequently quotes a wide range of incidences of aspiration and associated high mortality; however, a study that assessed the risk of pulmonary aspiration in enterally fed patients found the incidence of aspiration to be about 5%, with little or no associated mortality.[328]

Delivery of nutrients to the small intestine minimizes the risk of pulmonary aspiration.[329, 330] A nasogastric tube is often needed to decompress the stomach and prevent large gastric residual volumes. Addition of dye to the feeding formula is a convenient and inexpensive method for detecting reflux of formula into the stomach from the small bowel or dislodgment of a small bowel tube into the stomach. Elevating the head of the bed 30 to 45 degrees also minimizes gastric reflux and aspiration.[326, 327] Treating gastroparesis with promotility agents (i.e., erythromycin, metoclopramide, or cisapride) may be useful in decreasing gastric volume and the risk of aspiration.

Diarrhea

Diarrhea may occur in patients receiving enteral nutrition.[334-338] Diarrhea can result from drug therapy, gut atrophy, impaired digestion and absorption, hypersecretory states, gut infection (e.g., *Clostridium difficile*, *Vibrio cholerae*, *Salmonella* species), hypoalbuminemia, or fecal impaction. Drugs commonly associated with diarrhea include magnesium (i.e., antacids), sorbitol (a vehicle for many elixir drugs), and antibiotics (which induce bacterial overgrowth). Digestion and absorption are altered in patients with malnutrition, after severe injury (trauma or burns), and by diseases that decrease bile production or enzyme secretion (i.e., pancreatitis, cystic fibrosis). Diarrhea can also be a manifestation of gut failure in patients with multiple organ failure.

Definitions of diarrhea vary in the literature, and this has led to wide variations in reported incidences. We and others[336] prefer to define "diarrhea" as production of excessive stool, specifically more than 250 g/day. Many critically ill patients have rectal incontinence, which may result in numerous bowel movements but not true diarrhea. The stools of many tube-fed patients are often of liquid or pasty consistency owing to lack of fiber.

Formula osmolality is still unfairly blamed for much "tube-feeding diarrhea." Keohane and colleagues[337] performed a definitive study indicating that osmolality is not responsible for the diarrhea associated with enteral feeding. Therapeutic regimens that recommend decreasing the volume or concentration of enteral formulas should be avoided because they only deprive patients of needed nutrients.

Most diarrhea can be successfully managed with enteral nutrition. Prescribed medications should be reviewed and any that could be causing the diarrhea should be discontinued when possible. Substitutes should be found for drugs containing sorbitol (e.g., crushed pills in water). Prokinetic agents given for gastroparesis may cause diarrhea once gastrointestinal motility has improved. The cause of the diarrhea should be determined and specific treatment instituted, as appropriate, especially with infectious diarrhea. Frequently, diarrhea can be decreased by altering dietary intake (i.e., reducing long-chain fatty acids, using peptide-based diets) or by giving opiates. Fiber supplementation may result in more solid stools. Stool output can be managed with diapers, fecal incontinence bags, or rectal Foley catheters. Fluids and electrolytes must be monitored in patients with diarrhea, and adequate replacement provided. Most diarrhea resolves as the patient's condition improves. Persistence of diarrhea often indicates gut failure and the multiple organ dysfunction syndrome, with its associated high mortality rate.

Other Complications

Sinusitis and otitis media may occur secondary to use of nasal feeding tubes. Erosions at insertion sites are another possible complication. Dislodgment of a gastrostomy or jejunostomy tube is a rare complication. Metabolic complications, such as hyperglycemia in diabetic patients should be managed with insulin therapy. Rare but potentially life-threatening complications, such as severe hypophosphatemia or hypokalemia, may occur in the hypermetabolic or severely malnourished patient being refed after a period of starvation (i.e., refeeding syndrome). These electrolytes should be monitored for derangements and treatment given, as needed, to avoid adverse consequences. Overfeeding is associated with metabolic complications, poor gastrointestinal tolerance, and worse outcomes[339] and should be avoided.

SUMMARY

Enteral feeding is the preferred route of nutritional support in critically ill patients. Nutrient administration should be initiated as soon as possible after admission to the hospital. Oral nutrition is best, but when patients cannot eat an adequate amount of nutrients safely, feeding via a gastric or small-bowel feeding tube is in order. Recent advances in nutrition research have produced enteral formulas using specific nutrients that can modulate immune responses and improve outcomes in critically ill patients. Successful enteral feeding requires skill and close attention to feeding tube position, possible complications, and nutritional responses.

References

1. Hill GL: Body composition research: Implications for the practice of clinical nutrition. JPEN J Parenter Enteral Nutr 1992; 16:197-218.
2. Windsor JA, Hill GL: Weight loss with physiologic impairment: A basic indicator of surgical risk. Ann Surg 1988; 207:290-296.
3. Windsor JA, Hill GL: Risk factors for postoperative pneumonia: The importance of protein depletion. Ann Surg 1988; 208:209-214.
4. Haydock DA, Hill GL: Impaired wound healing in surgical patients with varying degrees of malnutrition. JPEN J Parenter Enteral Nutr 1986; 10:550-554.
5. Windsor JA, Hill GL: Protein depletion and surgical risk. Aust N Z J Surg 1988; 58:711-715.
6. Saito H, Trocki O, Alexander JW, Kopcha R, Heyd T, Joffe SN: The effect of route of nutrient administration on the nutritional state, catabolic hormone secretion, and gut mucosal integrity after burn injury. JPEN J Parenter Enteral Nutr 1987; 11:1-7.
7. Dominioni L, Trocki O, Mochizuki H, Fang CH, Alexander JW: Prevention of severe postburn hypermetabolism and catabolism by immediate intragastric feeding. J Burn Care Rehabil 1984; 5:106-112.
8. Mochizuki H, Trocki O, Dominioni L, Brackett KA, Joffe SN, Alexander JW: Mechanism of prevention of postburn hypermetabolism and catabolism by early enteral feeding. Ann Surg 1984; 200:297-310.
9. McArdle AH, Palmason C, Brown RA, Brown HC, Williams HB: Early enteral feeding of patients with major burns: Prevention of catabolism. Ann Plast Surg 1984; 13:396-401.
10. Jenkins M, Gottschlich M, Alexander JW, Warden GD: Effect of immediate enteral feeding on the hypermetabolic response following severe burn injury (Abstract). JPEN J Parenter Enteral Nutr 1989; 13:12.
11. Mochizuki H, Trocki O, Dominioni L, Alexander JW: Reduction of postburn hypermetabolism by early enteral feeding. Curr Surg 1985; 42:121-125.
12. Bortenschlager L, Roberts PR, Black KW, Zaloga GP: Enteral feeding minimizes liver injury during hemorrhagic shock. Shock 1994; 2:351-354.
13. Roberts PR, Black KW, Zaloga GP: Effect of fasting and refeeding on renal blood flow: Implications for perioperative management (Abstract). Anesthesiology 1997; 87:A228.
14. Roberts PR, Black KW, Zaloga GP: Enteral feeding improves outcome and protects against glycerol-induced acute renal failure in the rat. Am J Respir Crit Care Med 1997; 156:1265-1269.
15. Greenstein A, Rogers P, Moss G: Doubled fourth day colorectal anastomotic strength with complete retention of intestinal mature wound collagen and accelerated deposition following immediate full enteral nutrition. Surg Forum 1978; 29:78-81.
16. Moss G, Greenstein A, Levy S, Bierenbaum A: Maintenance of GI function after bowel surgery and immediate enteral full nutrition: I. Doubling of canine colorectal anastomotic bursting pressure and intestinal wound mature collagen content. J Parenter Enteral Nutr 1980; 4:535-538.
17. Zaloga GP, Bortenschlager L, Black KW, Prielipp R: Immediate postoperative enteral feeding decreases weight loss and improves wound healing after abdominal surgery in rats. Crit Care Med 1992; 20:115-118.
18. Tanigawa K, Kim YM, Lancaster JR, Zar HA: Fasting augments lipid peroxidation during reperfusion after ischemia in the perfused rat liver. Crit Care Med 1999; 27:401-406.
19. Sagar S, Harland P, Shields R: Early postoperative feeding with elemental diet. BMJ 1979; 1:293-295.
20. Alexander W, MacMillan BG, Stinnett JD, et al: Beneficial effects of aggressive protein feeding in severely burned children. Ann Surg 1980; 192:505-517.
21. Moore EE, Jones TN: Benefits of immediate jejunostomy feeding after major abdominal trauma—a prospective, randomized study. J Trauma 1986; 26:874-880.
22. Grahm TW, Zadrozny DB, Harrington T: The benefits of early jejunal hyperalimentation in the head-injured patient. Neurosurgery 1989; 25:729-735.
23. Chiarelli A, Enzi G, Casadei A, Baggio B, Valeno A, Mazzoleni F: Very early nutrition supplementation in burned patients. Am J Clin Nutr 1990; 51:1035-1039.
24. Schroeder D, Gillanders L, Mahr K, Hill GL: Effects of immediate postoperative enteral nutrition on body composition, muscle function, and wound healing. JPEN J Parenter Enteral Nutr 1991; 15:376-383.
25. Eyer SD, Micon LT, Konstantinides FN, et al: Early enteral feeding does not attenuate metabolic response after blunt trauma. J Trauma 1993; 34:639-643.
26. Jenkins ME, Gottschlich MM, Warden GD: Enteral feeding during operative procedures in thermal injuries. J Burn Care Rehab 1994; 15:199-205.
27. Hasse JM, Blue LS, Goldstein RM, et al: Early enteral nutrition support in patients undergoing liver transplantation. JPEN J Parenter Enteral Nutr 1995; 19:437-443.
28. Beier-Holgersen R, Boesby S: Influence of postoperative enteral nutrition on postsurgical infections. Gut 1996; 39:833-835.
29. Carr CS, Ling KDE, Boulos P, Singer M: Randomised trial of safety and efficacy of immediate postoperative enteral feeding in patients undergoing gastrointestinal resection. BMJ 1996; 312:869-871.
30. Kudsk KA, Minard G, Croce MA, et al: A randomized trial of isonitrogenous enteral diets after severe trauma. Ann Surg 1996; 224:531-543.
31. Watters JM, Kirkpatrick SM, Norris SB, et al: Immediate postoperative enteral feeding results in impaired respiratory mechanics and decreased mobility. Ann Surg 1997; 226:369-380.

32. Heslin MJ, Latkany L, Brooks AD, et al: A prospective, randomized trial of early enteral feeding after resection of upper gastrointestinal malignancy. Ann Surg 1997; 226:567–577.
33. Schilder JM, Hurteau JA, Look KY, et al: A prospective controlled trial of early postoperative oral intake following major abdominal gynecologic surgery. Gynecol Oncol 1997; 67:235–240.
34. Bastow MD, Rawlings J, Allison SP: Benefits of supplementary tube feeding after fractured neck of femur: A randomised controlled trial. Br Med J 1983; 287:1589–1592.
35. Delmi M, Rapin CH, Bengoa JM, et al: Dietary supplementation in elderly patients with fractured neck of the femur. Lancet 1990; 335:1013–1016.
36. Tkatch L, Rapin CH, Rizzoli R, et al: Benefits of oral protein supplementation in elderly patients with fracture of the proximal femur. J Am Coll Nutr 1992; 11:519–525.
37. Sullivan DH, Nelson CL, Bopp MM, Puskarich-May CL, Walls RC: Nightly enteral nutrition support of elderly hip fracture patients: A phase I trial. J Am Coll Nutr 1998; 17:155–161.
38. Kudsk KA, Minard G: Enteral nutrition. *In*: Nutrition in Critical Care. Zaloga GP (Ed). St. Louis, Mosby-Year Book, 1994, pp 331–360.
39. Zaloga GP: Nutrition and prevention of systemic infection. *In*: Critical Care: State of the Art, Vol 12. Fullerton, Calif, Society of Critical Care Medicine, 1991, pp 31–79.
40. Zaloga GP, MacGregor DA: What to consider when choosing enteral or parenteral nutrition. J Crit Ill 1990; 5:1180–1200.
41. Kudsk KA, Carpenter G, Petersen S, Sheldon GF: Effect of enteral and parenteral feeding in malnourished rats with *E. coli*-hemoglobin adjuvant peritonitis. J Surg Res 1981; 31:105–110.
42. Kudsk KA, Stone JM, Carpenter G, Sheldon GF: Enteral and parenteral feeding influences mortality after hemoglobin-*E. coli* peritonitis in normal rats. J Trauma 1983; 23:605–609.
43. Zaloga GP, Prielipp RC, Ward KA: Total parenteral nutrition (TPN) increases mortality following methotrexate-induced endogenous sepsis (Abstract). Anesthesiology 1990; 73:A1232.
44. Alverdy JC, Aoys F, Moss BS: Parenteral nutrition results in bacterial translocation from the gut and death following chemotherapy. JPEN J Parenter Enteral Nutr 1990; 14:8S.
45. Petersen ST, Kudsk KA, Carpenter G, Sheldon GF: Malnutrition and immunocompetence: Increased mortality following an infectious challenge during hyperalimentation. J Trauma 1981; 21:528–533.
46. Zaloga GP, Knowles R, Black KW, Prielipp R: Total parenteral nutrition increases mortality after hemorrhage. Crit Care Med 1991; 19:54–59.
47. Ryan GP, Dudrick SJ, Copeland EM, Johnson LR: Effects of various diets on colonic growth in rats. Gastroenterology 1979; 77:658–663.
48. Johnson LR, Copeland DM, Dudrick SJ, Lichtenberger LM, Castro GA: Structural and hormonal alterations in the gastrointestinal tract of parenterally fed rats. Gastroenterology 1975; 68:1177–1183.
49. Levine GM, Deren JJ, Steiger E, Sinno R: Role of oral intake in maintenance of gut mass and disaccharide activity. Gastroenterology 1974; 67:975–982.
50. Johnson LR, Copeland EM, Dudrick SJ, Lichtenberger LM, Castro GA: Structural and hormonal alterations in the gastrointestinal tract of parenterally fed rats. Gastroenterology 1975; 68:1177–1183.
51. Thompson JS, Vaughan WP, Forst CF, Jacobs DL, Weekly JS, Rikkers LF: The effect of the route of nutrient delivery on gut structure and diamine oxidase levels. JPEN J Parenter Enteral Nutr 1987; 11:28–32.
52. Lickley HL, Track NS, Vranic M, Bury KD: Metabolic responses to enteral and parenteral nutrition. Am J Surg 1978; 135:172–176.
53. Kudsk KA, Stone JM, Carpenter G, Sheldon GF: Effects of enteral and parenteral feeding of malnourished rats on body composition. J Trauma 1982; 22:904–906.
54. Czernichow B, Galluser M, Hasselmann M, Doffoel M, Raul F: Effects of amino acids in mixtures given by enteral or parenteral route on intestinal morphology and hydrolases in rats. JPEN J Parenter Enteral Nutr 1991; 16:259–263.
55. Alverdy JC, Aoys E, Moss GS: Total parenteral nutrition promotes bacterial translocation from the gut. Surgery 1988; 104:185–190.
56. Alverdy J, Chi HS, Sheldon GF: The effect of parenteral nutrition on gastrointestinal immunity: The importance of enteral stimulation. Ann Surg 1985; 202:681–684.
57. Lindor KD, Fleming CR, Abrams A, Hirschkorn MA: Liver function values in adults receiving total parenteral nutrition. JAMA 1979; 241:2398–2400.
58. Riely CA, Fine PL, Boyer JL: Progressively rising serum bile acids—a common effect of parenteral nutrition (Abstract). Gastroenterology 1979; 77:A34.
59. Knodell RG, Spector MH, Brooks DA, Keller FX, Kyner WT: Alterations in pentobarbital pharmacokinetics in response to parenteral and enteral alimentation in the rat. Gastroenterology 1980; 79:1211–1216.
60. Knodell RG, Steele NM, Cerra FB, Gross JB, Solomon TE: Effects of parenteral and enteral hyperalimentation on hepatic drug metabolism in the rat. J Pharmacol Exp Ther 1984; 229:589–597.
61. Saito H, Trocki O, Alexander JW, Kopcha R, Heyd T, Joffe SN: The effect of route of nutrient administration on the nutritional state, catabolic hormone secretion, and gut mucosal integrity after burn injury. JPEN J Parenter Enteral Nutr 1987; 11:1–7.
62. Rivera A Jr, Bhatia J, Rassin DK, Gourley WK, Catarau E: In vivo biliary function in the adult rat: The effect of parenteral glucose and amino acids. JPEN J Parenter Enteral Nutr 1989; 13:240–245.
63. Hiramatu T, Saito S, Taniwka K, Gukushima R, Moriaka Y: The beneficial effects of postoperative enteral nutrition on protein metabolism and immunocompetence in rats with gastrectomy (Abstract). JPEN J Parenter Enteral Nutr 1990; 14:10S.
64. Fong Y, Marano MA, Barber A, He W, Moldawer LL, Bushman ED, Coyle SM, Shires GT, Lowry SF: Total parenteral nutrition and bowel rest modify the metabolic response to endotoxin in humans. Ann Surg 1989; 210:449–457.
65. Detsky AS, Baker JP, O'Rourke K, Goel V: Perioperative parenteral nutrition: A meta-analysis. Ann Intern Med 1987; 107:195–203.
66. American College of Physicians: Perioperative parenteral nutrition. Ann Intern Med 1987; 107:252–253.
67. Veterans Affairs Total Parenteral Nutrition Cooperative Study Group: Perioperative total parenteral nutrition in surgical patients. N Engl J Med 1991; 325:525–532.
68. Adams S, Dellinger EP, Wertz JM, Oreskovisch MR, Simonowitz D, Johansen K: Enteral versus parenteral nutritional support following laparotomy for trauma: A randomized prospective trial. J Trauma 1986; 26:882–892.
69. Moore FA, Moore EE, Jones TN, McCroskey BL, Peterson VM: TEN versus TPN following major abdominal trauma—reduced septic morbidity. J Trauma 1989; 29:916–923.
70. Moore FA, Feliciano DV, Andrassy RJ, MeArdles AH, Booth FV, Morgenstein-Wagner TB, Kellum JM Jr, Welling RE, Moore EE: Early enteral feeding, compared with parenteral, reduces postoperative complications. The results of a meta-analysis. Ann Surg 1992; 216:172–183.
71. Kudsk KA, Croce MA, Fabian TC, Minard G, Tollety EA, Poret HA, Kuhl MR, Brown RO: Enteral versus parenteral feeding: Effects on septic morbidity after blunt and penetrating abdominal trauma. Ann Surg 1992; 215:503–513.
72. Young B, Ott L, Twyman D, Norton J, Rapp R, Tibbs P, Haack D, Brivins B, Dempsey R: The effect of nutritional support on outcome from severe head injury. J Neurosurg 1987; 67:668–676.
73. Hadley MN, Grahm TW, Harrington T, Schiller WR, McDermott MK, Posillico DB: Nutritional support and neurotrauma: A critical review of early nutrition in forty-five acute head injury patients. Neurosurgery 1986; 19:367–373.
74. Koretz RL: Parenteral nutrition: Is it oncologically logical? J Clin Oncol 1984; 2:534–538.
75. Klein S, Simes J, Blackburn GL: Total parenteral nutrition and cancer clinical trials. Cancer 1986; 58:1378–1386.
76. American College of Physicians: Parenteral nutrition in patients receiving cancer chemotherapy. Ann Intern Med 1989; 110:734–736.
77. Hopkins B: Enteral nutrition products. *In*: Nutrition in Critical Care. Zaloga GP (Ed). St. Louis, Mosby-Year Book, 1995, pp 439–467.
78. Roberts PR, Black KW, Zaloga GP: Small bowel absorption of bioactive peptides in rats: Implications for nutritional therapeutics (Abstract). Crit Care Med 1995; 23:A98.

79. Roberts PR, Zaloga GP: Dietary bioactive peptides. New Horiz 1994; 2:237–243.
80. Amoss M, Rivier J, Guillemin R: Release of gonadotropins by oral administration of synthetic LRF or a tripeptide fragment of LRF. J Clin Endocrinol Metab 1972; 35:175–177.
81. Gardner MG: Intestinal assimilation of intact peptides and proteins from the diet—a neglected field? Biol Rev 1984; 59:289–301.
82. Danforth F, Moore RO: Intestinal absorption of insulin in the rat. Endocrinology 1959; 65:118–123.
83. Gardner ML: Absorption of intact peptides: Studies on transport of protein digests and dipeptides across rat small intestine in vitro. Q J Exp Physiol 1982; 67:629–637.
84. Webb KE Jr: Amino acid and peptide absorption from the gastrointestinal tract. Fed Proc 1986; 45:2268–2271.
85. Zaloga GP: Nutrition and prevention of systemic infection. *In*: Critical Care: State of the Art. Vol 12. Fullerton, Calif, Society of Critical Care Medicine, 1991, pp 31–79.
86. Zaloga GP: Studies comparing intact protein, peptide, and amino acid formulas. *In:* Uses of Elemental Diets in Clinical Situations. Bounos G (Ed). Boca Raton, Fla, CRC Press, 1993, pp 201–217.
87. Zaloga GP: Physiologic effects of peptide-based formulas. Nutr Clin Practice 1990; 5:231–237.
88. Zaloga GP, Ward KA, Prielipp RC: Effect of enteral diets on whole body and gut growth in unstressed rats. JPEN J Parenter Enteral Nutr 1991; 15:42–47.
89. Shou J, Lieberman MD, Hoffman K, Leon P, Redmond HP, Davies H, Daly JM: Dietary manipulation of methotrexate-induced enterocolitis. JPEN J Parenter Enteral Nutr 1991; 15:307–312.
90. Trocki O, Mochizuki H, Dominioni L, Alexander JW: Intact protein versus free amino acids in the nutritional support of thermally injured animals. J Parenter Enteral Nutr 1986; 10:139–145.
91. Janne P, Carpenter Y, Williams G: Colonic mucosal atrophy induced by a liquid elemental diet in rats. Am J Dig Dis 1977; 22:808–812.
92. Birke H, Thorlacius-Ussing O, Hessov I: Trophic effect of dietary peptides on mucosa in the rat small bowel. JPEN J Parenter Enteral Nutr 1990; 14:16S.
93. Alverdy JC, Aoys E, Moss GS: Total parenteral nutrition promotes bacterial translocation from the gut. Surgery 1988; 104:185–190.
94. McAnena OJ, Harvey LP, Bonau RA, Daly JM: Alteration of methotrexate toxicity in rats by manipulation of dietary components. Gastroenterology 1987; 92:354–360.
95. Zaloga GP, Knowles R, Black KW, Prielipp RC: Total parenteral nutrition increases mortality after hemorrhage. Crit Care Med 1991; 19:54–59.
96. Knodell RG: Effects of formula composition on hepatic and intestinal drug metabolism during enteral nutrition. JPEN J Parenter Enteral Nutr 1990; 14:34–38.
97. Imondi AR, Stradley RP: Utilization of enzymatically hydrolyzed soybean protein and crystalline amino acid diets by rats with exocrine pancreatic insufficiency. J Nutr 1974; 104:793–801.
98. Roberts PR, Black KW, Santamauro JT, Zaloga GP: Dietary peptides improve wound healing following surgery. Nutrition 1997; 14:266–269.
99. Poullain MG, Cezard JP, Roger L, Mendy F: Effect of whey proteins, their oligopeptide hydrolysates and free amino acid mixtures on growth and nitrogen retention in fed and starved rats. JPEN J Parenter Enteral Nutr 1974; 13:382–386.
100. Plumb JA, Gardner GL: Can elemental diets reduce the intestinal toxicity of 5-fluorouracil? JPEN J Parenter Enteral Nutr 1983; 7:351–357.
101. Zaloga GP, Prielipp RC, Ward KA: Total parenteral nutrition (TPN) increases mortality following methotrexate-induced endogenous sepsis (Abstract). Anesthesiology 1990; 73:A1232.
102. Jones BJ, Lees R, Andrews J, Frost P, Silk DB: Comparison of an elemental and polymeric enteral diet in patients with normal gastrointestinal function. Gut 1983; 24:78–84.
103. Shou J, Lieberman MD, Hoffman K, Redmond HP, Leon P, Davies H, Daly JM: Dietary manipulation of methotrexate (MTX)-induced enterocolitis. JPEN J Parenter Enteral Nutr 1990; 14:12S.
104. Fox AD, Kripke SA, DePaula J, Berman JM, Settle RG, Rombeau JL: Effect of a glutamine-supplemented enteral diet on methotrexate-induced enterocolitis. JPEN J Parenter Enteral Nutr 1988; 12:325–331.
105. Harvey LP, McAnena OJ, Mehta BM, Daly JM: Reversibility of elemental liquid diet-induced methotrexate toxicity by refeeding with chow. JPEN J Parenter Enteral Nutr 1987; 11:119–123.
106. Stanford JR, King D, Carey L, Anderson G: The adverse effects of elemental diets on tolerance for 5-FU toxicity in the rat. J Surg Oncol 1977; 9:493–501.
107. Granger DN, Brinson RR: Intestinal absorption of elemental and standard enteral formulas in hypoproteinemic (volume expanded) rats. JPEN J Parenter Enteral Nutr 1988; 12:278–281.
108. Brinson RR, Pitts VL, Taylor AE: Intestinal absorption of peptide enteral formulas in hypoproteinemic (volume expanded) rats: A paired analysis. Crit Care Med 1989; 17:657–660.
109. Ziegler F, Ollivier JM, Cynober L, Masini JP, Coudray-Lucas C, Levy E, Giboudeau J: Efficacy of enteral nitrogen support in surgical patients: Small peptides vs non-degraded proteins. Gut 1990; 31:1277–1283.
110. Brinson RR, Kolts BE: Diarrhea associated with severe hypoalbuminemia: A comparison of a peptide-based chemically defined diet and standard enteral alimentation. Crit Care Med 1988; 16:130–136.
111. Meredith JW, Ditesheim JA, Zaloga GP: Visceral protein levels in trauma patients are greater with peptide diet than intact protein diet. J Trauma 1990; 30:825–829.
112. Monchi M, Vaugelade P, Vaissade P, Rerat A: Net protein utilization after duodenal infusion of small peptides or free amino acids in growing rats. JPEN J Parenter Enteral Nutr 1991; 15:29S.
113. Bounous G, Hugon J, Gentile JM: Elemental diet in the management of the intestinal lesion produced by 5-fluorouracil in the rat. Can J Surg 1971; 14:298–311.
114. Bounous G, Maestracci D: Use of an elemental diet in animals during treatment with 5-fluorouracil (NSC-19893). Cancer Treat Rev 1976; 60:17–22.
115. Zaloga GP, Meredith JW, Roberts P, Bortenschlager L, Black K, Henningfield M: Improved hepatic protein responses with hydrolyzed protein versus intact protein diets after trauma. Crit Care Med 1991; 20:S94.
116. Feller A, Rudman D, Caindec N: Comparison of nutritional efficacy of Peptamin and Vivonex TEN elemental diets in elderly tube fed subjects. JPEN J Parenter Enteral Nutr 1989; 13:12S.
117. Smith JL, Arteaga C, Heymsfield SB: Increased ureagenesis and impaired nitrogen use during infusion of a synthetic amino acid formula: A controlled trial. N Engl J Med 1982; 306:1013–1018.
118. Mowatt-Larsen CA, Brown RO, Wojtysiak SL, Kudsk KA: Enteral nutrition efficacy and tolerance: Comparison of peptide with standard formulas. JPEN J Parenter Enteral Nutr 1991; 15:32S.
119. Zaloga SJ, Black KW, Roberts PR, Zaloga GP: Dietary peptide profile modulates body nitrogen utilization: Implications for nutritional support (Abstract). Anesthesiology 1995; 83:A242.
120. Bounous G, Kongshavn PA: Influence of dietary proteins on the immune system of mice. J Nutr 1982; 112:1747–1755.
121. Sitren HS, Johns LG, Solomon PL: Modulation of methotrexate (MTX) toxicity by protein source in solid diets and in enteral formulas. JPEN J Parenter Enteral Nutr 1993; 17:32S.
122. Brinson RR, Pitts WM, Benoit J: Effect of β-casomorphin, a casein hydrolysate derivative, on intestinal permeability in volume expanded hypoproteinemic rats. JPEN J Parenter Enteral Nutr 1990; 14:10S.
123. Yoshikawa M, Kishi K, Takahashi M, Watanabe A, Miyamura T, Yamazaki M, Chiba H: Immunostimulating peptide derived from soybean protein. Ann N Y Acad Sci 1993; 685:375–376.
124. Jaziri M, Migliore-Samour D, Casabianca-Pignede MR, Keddad K, Morgat JL, Jolles P: Specific binding sites on human phagocytic blood cells for Gly-Leu-Phe and Val-Glu-Pro-Ile-Pro-Tyr, immunostimulating peptides from human milk proteins. Biochim Biophys Acta 1992; 1160:251–261.
125. Barbul A: Arginine: Biochemistry, physiology, and therapeutic implications. JPEN J Parenter Enteral Nutr 1986; 10:227–238.
126. Barbul A: Arginine and immune function. Nutrition 1990; 6:53–62.
127. Seifter E, Rettura G, Barbul A, Levenson SM: Arginine: An essential amino acid for injured rats. Surgery 1978; 84:224–230.
128. Chyun JH, Griminger P: Improvement of nitrogen retention by arginine and glycine supplementation and its relation to collagen synthesis in traumatized mature and aged rats. J Nutr 1984; 114:1697–1704.

129. Sitren HS, Fisher H: Nitrogen retention in rats fed on diets enriched with arginine and glycine: I. Improved N retention after trauma. Br J Nutr 1977; 37:195–208.
130. Barbul A, Rettura G, Levenson SM, Seifter E: Wound healing and thymotropic effects of arginine: A pituitary mechanism of action. Am J Clin Nutr 1983; 37:786–794.
131. Barbul A, Fishel RS, Shimazu S, Wasserkrug HL, Yoshimura NN, Tao RC, Efron G: Intravenous hyperalimentation with high arginine levels improves wound healing and immune function. J Surg Res 1985; 31:328–334.
132. Barbul A, Wasserkrug HL, Yoshimura NN, Tao RC, Efron G: High arginine levels in intravenous hyperalimentation abrogate post-traumatic immune suppression. J Surg Res 1984; 36:620–624.
133. Leon P, Redmond HP, Stein TP, Shou J, Schluter MD, Kelly C, Lanza-Jacoby S, Daly JM: Arginine supplementation improves histone and acute phase protein synthesis during gram-negative sepsis in the rat. JPEN J Parenter Enteral Nutr 1991; 15:503–508.
134. Elsair J, Poey J, Issad H, et al: Effect of arginine chlorhydrate on nitrogen balance during the three days following routine surgery in man. Biomedicine 1978; 29:312–317.
135. Daly JM, Reynolds J, Thom A, Kinsley L, Dietrick-Gallagher M, Shou J, Ruggieri B: Immune and metabolic effects of arginine in the surgical patient. Ann Surg 1988; 208:512–523.
136. Barbul A, Lazarou SA, Efron DT, Wasserkrug HL, Efron G: Arginine enhances wound healing and lymphocyte immune responses in humans. Surgery 1990; 108:331–337.
137. Kirk SJ, Hurson M, Regan MC, Holt DR, Wasserkrug HL, Barbul A: Arginine stimulates wound healing and immune function in elderly human beings. Surgery 1993; 114:155–160.
138. Barbul A, Wasserkrug HL, Seifter E, Rettura G, Levenson SM, Efron G: Immunostimulatory effects of arginine in normal and injured rats. J Surg Res 1980; 29:228–235.
139. Barbul A, Wasserkrug HL, Sisto DA, Seifter E, Rettura G, Levenson SM, Efron G: Thymic stimulatory actions of arginine. JPEN J Parenter Enteral Nutr 1980; 4:446–449.
140. Kirk SJ, Regan MC, Wasserkrug HL, Sodeyama M, Barbul A: Arginine enhances T-cell responses in athymic nude mice. JPEN J Parenter Enteral Nutr 1992; 16:429–432.
141. Barbul A, Sisto DA, Wasserkrug HL, Efron G: Arginine stimulates lymphocyte immune response in healthy human beings. Surgery 1981; 90:244–251.
142. Sigal RK, Shou J, Daly JM: Parenteral arginine infusion in humans: Nutrient substrate or pharmacologic agent? JPEN J Parenter Enteral Nutr 1992; 16: 423–428.
143. Saito H, Trocki O, Wang SL, Gonce SJ, Joffe SN, Alexander JW: Metabolic and immune effects of dietary arginine supplementation after burn. Arch Surg 1987; 122:784–789.
144. Madden HP, Breslin RJ, Wasserkrug HL, Efron G, Barbul A: Stimulation of T-cell immunity by arginine enhances survival in peritonitis. J Surg Res 1988; 44:658–663.
145. Gonce SJ, Peck MD, Alexander JW, Miskell PW: Arginine supplementation and its effect on established peritonitis in guinea pigs. JPEN J Parenter Enteral Nutr 1990; 14:237–244.
146. Palmer RM, Rees DD, Ashton DS, Moncada S: L-Arginine is the physiological precursor for the formation of nitric oxide in endothelium-dependent relaxation. Biochem Biophys Res Commun 1988; 153:1251–1256.
147. Fleming I, Gray GA, Julou-Schaeffer G, Parratt JR, Stoclet JC: Incubation with endotoxin activates the L-arginine pathway in vascular tissue. Biochem Biophys Res Commun 1990; 171:562–568.
148. Julou-Schaeffer G, Gray GA, Fleming I, Schott C, Parratt JR, Stoclet JC: Loss of vascular responsiveness induced by endotoxin involves L-arginine pathway. Am J Physiol 1990; 259:H1038–H1043.
149. Kilbourn RG, Gross SS, Jubran A, Adams J, Griffith OW, Levi R, Lodato RF: NG-methyl-L-arginine inhibits tumor necrosis factor-induced hypotension: Implications for the involvement of nitric oxide. Proc Natl Acad Sci U S A 1990; 87:3629–3632.
150. Souba WW: Glutamine: Physiology, Biochemistry, and Nutrition in Critical Illness. Austin, Texas, R. G. Landes, 1995, pp 93–105.
151. Souba WW, Smith RJ, Wilmore DW: Glutamine metabolism by the intestinal tract. JPEN J Parenter Enteral Nutr 1985; 9:608–617.
152. Proceedings of an international glutamine symposium—glutamine metabolism in health and disease: Basic science and clinical aspects. JPEN J Parenter Enteral Nutr 1990; 14(Suppl):39S–146S.
153. Wilmore DW, Smith RJ, O'Dwyer ST, Jacobs DO, Ziegler TR, Wang XD: The gut: A central organ after surgical stress. Surgery 1988; 104:917–923.
154. Windmueller HG, Spaeth AE: Uptake and metabolism of plasma glutamine by the small intestine. J Biol Chem 1974; 249:5070–5079.
155. Windmueller HG, Spaeth AE: Identification of ketone bodies and glutamine as the major respiratory fuels in vivo for postabsorptive rat small intestine. J Biol Chem 1978; 253:69–76.
156. Windmueller HG, Spaeth AE: Intestinal metabolism of glutamine and glutamate from the lumen as compared to glutamine from the blood. Arch Biochem Biophys 1975; 171:662–674.
157. Fox AD, Kripke SA, De Paula J, Berman JM, Settle RG, Rombeau JL: Effect of a glutamine-supplemented enteral diet on methotrexate-induced enterocolitis. JPEN J Parenter Enteral Nutr 1988; 12:325–331.
158. Klimberg VS, Souba WW, Dolson DJ, et al: Prophylactic glutamine protects the intestinal mucosa from radiation injury. Cancer 1990; 66:62–68.
159. Klimberg VS, Souba WW, Sitren H, Plumley DA, Salloum RM, Hautamaki RD, Bland KI, Copeland EM III: Glutamine-enriched total parenteral nutrition supports gut metabolism. Surg Forum 1989; 15:175–177.
160. Hwang TL, O'Dwyer ST, Smith RJ, et al: Preservation of small bowel mucosa using glutamine-enriched parenteral nutrition (Abstract). Surg Forum 1987; 38:56.
161. O'Dwyer ST, Smith RJ, Kripke SA, et al: New fuels for the gut. *In:* Clinical Nutrition: Enteral and Tube Feeding. 2nd ed. Rombeau JL, Caldwell MD (Eds). Philadelphia, WB Saunders, 1990, pp 540–555.
162. Karner J, Roth E, Ollenschlager G, et al: Glutamine-containing dipeptides as infusion substrates in the septic state. Surgery 1989; 106:893–900.
163. Jacobs DO, Evans A, O'Dwyer ST, Smith RJ, Wilmore DW: Disparate effects of 5-fluorouracil on the ileum and colon of enterally fed rats with protection by dietary glutamine. Surg Forum 1987; 38:45–47.
164. Fox AD, Kripke SA, Berman JR, Settle RG, Rombeau JL: Reduction of the severity of enterocolitis by glutamine-supplemented enteral diets. Surg Forum 1987; 38:43–44.
165. Klimberg VS, Dolson DJ, Salloum RM, Bland KI, Copeland EM III, Souba WW: Radioprotection with a glutamine-enriched elemental diet. JPEN J Parenter Enteral Nutr 1990; 14:9S.
166. Vanderhoff JA, Park JHY, Mohammadpour H, Blackwood D: Absence of trophic effect of glutamine on intestinal adaptation following massive bowel resection. JPEN J Parenter Enteral Nutr 1990; 14:8S.
167. Wells CL, Jechorek RP, Erlandsen SL, Lavin PT, Cerra FB: The effect of dietary glutamine and dietary RNA on ileal flora, ileal histology, and bacterial translocation in mice. Nutrition 1990; 6:70–83.
168. Barber AE, Jones WG III, Minei JP, Fahey TJ III, Moldawer LL, Rayburn JL, Fischer E, Keogh CV, Shires GT, Lowry SF: Glutamine or fiber supplementation of a defined formula diet: Impact on bacterial translocation, tissue composition, and response to endotoxin. JPEN J Parenter Enteral Nutr 1990; 14:335–343.
169. Parry-Billings M, Evans J, Calder PC, et al: Does glutamine contribute to immunosuppression after major burns? Lancet 1990; 336:523–525.
170. Furukawa S, Saito H, Inaba T, Lin MT, Inoue T, Naka S, Fukatsu K, et al: Glutamine-enriched enteral diet enhances bacterial clearance in protracted bacterial peritonitis, regardless of glutamine form. JPEN J Parenter Enteral Nutr 1997; 21:208–214.
171. Ogle CK, Ogle JD, Mao JX, et al: Effect of glutamine on phagocytosis and bacterial killing by normal and pediatric burn patient neutrophils. JPEN J Parenter Enteral Nutr 1994: 18:128–133.
172. O'Riordain MG, De Beaux A, Fearon KCH: Effect of glutamine on immune function in the surgical patient. Nutrition 1996; 12:S82–S84.
173. Ziegler TR, Benfell K, Smith RJ, Young LS, Brown E, Ferrari-Baliviera E, et al: Safety and metabolic effects of L-glutamine administration in humans. JPEN J Parenter Enteral Nutr 1990; 14:137S–146S.

174. Ziegler TR, Young LS, Benfell K, Scheltinga M, Hortos K, Bye R, et al: Clinical and metabolic efficacy of glutamine-supplemented parenteral nutrition after bone marrow transplantation. Ann Intern Med 1992; 116:821–828.
175. Stehle P, Zander J, Mertes N, Albers S, Puchstein C, Lawin P, Furst P: Effect of parenteral glutamine peptide supplements on muscle glutamine loss and nitrogen balance after major surgery. Lancet 1989; 1:231–233.
176. Hammarqvist F, Wernerman J, Ali R, von der Decken A, Vinnars E: Addition of glutamine to total parenteral nutrition after elective abdominal surgery spares free glutamine in muscle, counteracts the fall in muscle protein synthesis, and improves nitrogen balance. Ann Surg 1989; 209:455–461.
177. Houdijk AP, Rijnsburger ER, Jansen J, Wesdorp RIC, Weiss JK, McCamish MA, Teerlink T, Meuwissen SGM, Haarman HJ, Thijs LG, Van Leeuwen PAM: Randomised trial of glutamine enriched enteral nutrition on infectious morbidity in patients with multiple trauma. Lancet 1998; 352:772–776.
178. Jeevanadam M, Young DH, Ramais L, Schiller WR: Amino aciduria of severe trauma. Am J Clin Nutr 1989; 49:814–822.
179. Wannamacher RW: Key role of various individual amino acids in host response to infection. Am J Clin Nutr 1977; 30:1269–1280.
180. Hutson SM, Stinson-Fisher C, Shiman R, Jefferson LS: Regulation of albumin synthesis by hormones and amino acids in primary cultures of rat hepatocytes. Am J Physiol 1987; 252:E291–E298.
181. Meister A: New aspects of glutathione biochemistry and transport-selective alteration of glutathione metabolism. Nutr Rev 1984; 42:397–410.
182. Grimble RF, Jackson AA, Persaud C, Wride MJ, Delers F, Engler R: Cysteine and glycine supplementation modulate the metabolic response to tumor necrosis factor-α in rats fed a low protein diet. J Nutr 1992; 122:2066–2073.
183. Roberts P, Black K, Zaloga G: Histidine infusion enhances free water clearance (Abstract). Chest 1993; 104(Suppl):2S.
184. Roberts P, Zaloga G, Black K: Histidine infusion enhances free water excretion by inhibiting cAMP generation in the kidney. Anesthesiology 1993; 79(Suppl 3A): A278.
185. Roberts P, Black K, Zaloga G: Histidine enhances free water clearance and decreases urinary cAMP excretion. Crit Care Med 1994; 22:A210.
186. Kinsella JE, Lokesh B: Dietary lipids, eicosanoids, and the immune system. Crit Care Med 1990; 18:S94–S113.
187. Johnston PV: Dietary fat, eicosanoids and immunity. Adv Lipid Res 1985; 21:103–141.
188. Kinsella JE, Lokesh B, Broughton S, Whelan J: Dietary polyunsaturated fatty acids and eicosanoids: Potential effects on the modulation of inflammatory and immune cells: An overview. Nutrition 1990; 6:24–62.
189. Wan JM, Teo TC, Babayan VK, Blackburn GL: Lipids and the development of immune dysfunction and infection. JPEN J Parenter Enteral Nutr 1988; 12:43S–52S.
190. Calder PC: Dietary fatty acids and the immune system 1998; 56:S70–S83.
191. Calder PC: Effects of fatty acids and dietary lipids on cells of the immune system. Proc Nutr Soc 1996; 55: 127–150.
192. Swanson JE, Lokesh BR, Kinsella JE: Ca^{2+}-Mg^{2+} ATPase of mouse cardiac sarcoplasmic reticulum is affected by membrane n-6 and n-3 polyunsaturated fatty acid content. J Nutr 1989; 119:364–372.
193. Alam SQ, Ren YF, Alam BS: [^{3}H]Forskolin- and [^{3}H]dihydroalprenolol-binding sites and adenylate cyclase activity in hearts of rats fed diets containing different oils. Lipids 1988; 23:207–213.
194. Simopoulos AP: The role of fatty acids in gene expression: Health implications. Ann Nutr Metab 1996; 40:303–311.
195. Meade CJ, Mertin J: Fatty acids and immunity. Adv Lipid Res 1978; 16:127–165.
196. Locniskar M, Nauss KM, Newberne PM: The effect of quality and quantity of dietary fat on the immune system. J Nutr 1983; 113:951–961.
197. Meydani SN, Nicolosi RJ, Hayes KC: Effect of long-term feeding of corn oil or coconut oil diets on immune response and prostaglandin E_2 synthesis on squirrel and cebus monkeys. Nutr Res 1985; 5:993–1002.
198. Johnston DV, Marshall LA: Dietary fat, prostaglandins, and the immune response. Prog Food Nutr Sci 1984; 8:3–25.
199. Yoshino S, Ellis EF: Effects of a fish oil-supplemented diet on inflammation and immunological processes in rats. Int Arch Allerg Appl Immunol 1987; 84:233–240.
200. Morris DD, Henry MM, Moore JN, Fischer K: Effect of dietary linolenic acid on endotoxin-induced thromboxane and prostacyclin production by equine peritoneal macrophage. Circ Shock 1989; 29:311–318.
201. Morris DD, Henry MM, Moore JN: Dietary alpha linolenic acid reduces endotoxin-induced tumor necrosis factor activity production by equine macrophage (Abstract). Circ Shock 1990; 31:82.
202. Cerra FB, Alden PA, Negro F, Billiar T, Svingen BA, Licari J, Johnson SB, Holman RT: Sepsis and exogenous lipid modulation. JPEN J Parenter Enteral Nutr 1988; 12:63S–68S.
203. Mochizuki H, Trocki O, Dominioni L, Ray MB, Alexander JW: Optimal lipid content for enteral diets following thermal injury. JPEN J Parenter Enteral Nutr 1984; 8:638–646.
204. Alexander JW, Saito H, Trocki O, Ogle CK: The importance of lipid type in the diet after burn injury. Ann Surg 1986; 204:1–8.
205. Trocki O, Heyd TJ, Waymack JP, Alexander JW: Effects of fish oil on postburn metabolism and immunity. JPEN J Parenter Enteral Nutr 1987; 11:521–528.
206. Teo TC, DeMichele SJ, Selleck KM, Babayan VK, Blackburn GL, Bistrian BR: Administration of structured lipid composed of MCT and fish oil reduces net protein catabolism in enterally fed burned rats. Ann Surg 1989; 210:100–107.
207. Peck MD, Alexander JW, Ogle CK, Babcock GF: The effect of dietary fatty acids on response to *Pseudomonas* infection in burned mice. J Trauma 1990; 30:445–452.
208. Clouva-Molyvdas P, Peck MD, Alexander JW: Short-term dietary lipid manipulation does not affect survival in two models of murine sepsis. JPEN J Parenter Enteral Nutr 1992; 16:343–347.
209. Peck MD, Ogle CK, Alexander JW: Composition of fat in enteral diets can influence outcome in experimental peritonitis. Ann Surg 1991; 214:74–82.
210. Hamawy KJ, Moldawer LL, Georgieff M, Valicenti AJ, Babayan VK, Bistrian BR, Blackburn GL: The effect of lipid emulsions on the reticuloendothelial system function in the injured animal. JPEN J Parenter Enteral Nutr 1985; 9:559–565.
211. Sobrado J, Moldawer LL, Pomposelli JJ, Mascioli EA, Babayan VK, Bistrian BR, Blackburn GL: Lipid emulsions and reticuloendothelial system function in healthy and burned guinea pigs. Am J Clin Nutr 1985; 42:855–863.
212. Nugent KM: Intralipid effects on reticuloendothelial function. J Leukoc Biol 1984; 36:123–132.
213. Fischer GW, Hunter KW, Wilson SR, Mease AD: Diminished bacterial defenses with intralipid. Lancet 1980; 2:819–820.
214. Perez RV, Munda R, Alexander JW: Dietary immunoregulation of transfusion-induced immunosuppression. Transplantation 1988; 45:614–617.
215. Perez RV, Munda R, Alexander JW: Augmentation of donor-specific transfusion and cyclosporin effects with dietary linoleic acid. Transplantation 1989; 47:937–940.
216. Nishiwaki H, Iriyama K, Asami H, Kihata M, Hioki T, Asakawa T, Suzuki H: Influences of an infusion of lipid emulsion on phagocytotic activity of cultured Kupffer's cells in septic rats. JPEN J Parenter Enteral Nutr 1986; 10:614–616.
217. Nordenstrom J, Jarstrand C, Wiernik A: Decreased chemotactic and random migration of leukocytes during intralipid infusion. Am J Clin Nutr 1979; 32:2416–2422.
218. Jarstrand C, Berghem L, Lahnborg G: Human granulocyte and reticuloendothelial system function during intralipid infusions. JPEN J Parenter Enteral Nutr 1978; 2:663–670.
219. Sedman PC, Ramsden CW, Brenan TG, Guillou PJ: Pharmacological concentrations of lipid emulsions inhibit interleukin-2-dependent lymphocyte responses in vitro. JPEN J Parenter Enteral Nutr 1990; 14:12–17.
220. Cheney CL, Lenssen P, Aker SN: Association of intravenous lipid emulsion with risk of infection (Abstract). J Am Coll Nutr 1990; 9:532.
221. Freeman J, Goldmann DA, Smith NE, Sidebottom DG, Epstein MF, Platt R: Association of intravenous lipid emulsion and coagulase-negative staphylococcal bacteremia in neonatal intensive care units. N Engl J Med 1990; 323:301–308.
222. Lee TH, Hoover RL, Williams JD, Sperling RI, Ravalese J III, Spur

BW, Robinson DR, Corey EJ, Lewis RA, Austen KF: Effect of dietary enrichment with eicosapentaenoic and docosahexaenoic acids on in vitro neutrophil and monocyte leukotriene generation and neutrophil function. N Engl J Med 1985; 312:1217-1224.
223. Endres S, Ghorbani R, Kelley VE, Georgilis K, Lonnemann G, van der Meer JW, Cannon JG, Rogers TS, Klempner MS, Weber PC, et al: The effect of dietary supplementation with n-3 polyunsaturated fatty acids on the synthesis of interleukin-1 and tumor necrosis factor by mononuclear cells. N Engl J Med 1989; 320:265-271.
224. Luostarinen R, Saldeen T: Dietary fish oil decreases superoxide generation by human neutrophils: Relation to cyclooxygenase pathway and lysosomal enzyme release. Prostaglandins Leukot Essent Fatty Acids 1996; 55:167-172.
225. Meydani SN, Endres S, Woods MM, Goldin BR, Soo C, et al: Oral (*n*-3) fatty acid supplementation suppresses cytokine production and lymphocyte proliferation: Comparison between young and older women. J Nutr 1991; 121:547-555.
226. Morlion BJ, Torwesten E, Lessire H, Sturm G, Peskar BM, Furst P, Puchstein C: The effect of parenteral fish oil on leukocyte membrane fatty acid composition and leukotriene-synthesizing capacity in patients with postoperative trauma. Metabolism 1996; 45:1208-1213.
227. Gadek JF, DeMichele S, Karlstad M, Murray M, Pacht E, Donahoe M, Albertson T, Van Hoozen C, Wennberg A, Nelson J, Noursalehi M: Enteral nutrition with eicosapentaenoic acid (EPA), γ-linoleic acid (GLA) and antioxidants reduces pulmonary inflammation and new organ failures in patients with acute respiratory distress syndrome (ARDS). Chest 1998; 114: 277S.
228. Mortensen PB, Clausen MR, Bonnen H, Hove H, Holtug K: Colonic fermentation of ispaghula, wheat bran, glucose, and albumin to short-chain fatty acids and ammonia evaluated in vitro in 50 subjects. JPEN J Parenter Enteral Nutr 1992; 16:433-439.
229. McNeil NI: The contribution of the large intestine to energy supplies in man. Am J Clin Nutr 1984; 39:338-342.
230. Palaccio JC, Rolandelli RH, Settle RG, et al: Dietary fiber's physiologic effects and potential applications to enteral nutrition. *In:* Clinical Nutrition: Enteral and Tube Feeding. 2nd ed. Rombeau JL, Caldwell MD (Eds). Philadelphia: WB Saunders, 1990, pp 556-574.
231. Tasman-Jones C, Jones AL, Owen RL: Jejunal morphological consequences of dietary fiber in rats (Abstract). Gastroenterology 1978; 74:1102.
232. Jacobs LR: Effect of dietary fiber on mucosal growth and cell proliferation in the small intestine of the rat: A comparison of oat bran, pectin, and guar with total fiber deprivation. Am J Clin Nutr 1983: 37:954-960.
233. Koruda MJ, Rolandelli RH, Settle RG, Saul SH, Rombeau JL: The effect of a pectin-supplemented elemental diet on intestinal adaptation to massive small bowel resection. JPEN J Parenter Enteral Nutr 1986; 10:343-350.
234. Brown RC, Kelleher J, Losowsky MS: The effect of pectin on the structure and function of the rat small intestine. Br J Nutr 1979; 42:357-365.
235. Rolandelli RH, Koruda MJ, Settle RG, Rombeau JL: Effects of intraluminal infusion of short-chain fatty acids on the healing of colonic anastomosis in the rat. Surgery 1986; 100:198-204.
236. Kripke SA, Fox AD, Berman JM, Settle RG, Rombeau JL: Stimulation of intestinal mucosal growth with intracolonic infusion of short-chain fatty acids. JPEN J Parenter Enteral Nutr 1989; 3:109-116.
237. Koruda MJ, Rolandelli RH, Settle RG, Zimmaro DM, Rombeau JL: Effect of parenteral nutrition supplemented with short-chain fatty acids on intestinal adaptation to massive small bowel resection. Gastroenterology 1988; 95:715-720.
238. Harig JM, Soergel KH, Komorowski RA, Wood CM: Treatment of diversion colitis with short-chain fatty acid irrigation. N Engl J Med 1986; 320:23-28.
239. Rolandelli RH, Saul SH, Settle RG, Jacobs DO, Trerotola SO, Rombeau JL: Comparison of parenteral nutrition and enteral feeding with pectin in experimental colitis in the rat. Am J Clin Nutr 1988; 47:715-721.
240. Rolandelli RH, Koruda MJ, Settle RG, Rombeau JL: The effect of enteral feedings supplemented with pectin on the healing of colonic anastomoses in the rat. Surgery 1986; 99:703-707.
241. DiLorenzo C, Williams CM, Hajnal F, Valenzuela JE: Pectin delays gastric emptying and increases satiety in obese subjects. Gastroenterology 1988; 95:1211-1215.
242. Spiller GA, Chernoff MC, Hill RA, Gates JE, Nassar JJ, Shipley EA: Effect of purified cellulose, pectin and a low-residue diet on fecal volatile fatty acids, transit time and fecal weight in humans. Am J Clin Nutr 1980; 33:754-759.
243. Zimmaro DM, Rolandelli RH, Koruda MJ, Settle RG, Stein TP, Rombeau JL: Isotonic tube feeding formula induces liquid stool in normal subjects: Reversal by pectin. JPEN J Parenter Enteral Nutr 1989; 13:117-123.
244. Hart GK, Dobb GJ: Effect of a fecal bulking agent on diarrhea during enteral feeding in the critically ill. JPEN J Parenter Enteral Nutr 1988; 12:465-468.
245. Shaw JH, Wolfe RR: An integrated analysis of glucose, fat, and protein metabolism in severely traumatized patients: Studies in the basal state and the response to total parenteral nutrition. Ann Surg 1989; 209:63-72.
246. Bark S, Holm I, Hakansson I, Wretlind A: Nitrogen-sparing effect of fat emulsion compared with glucose in the postoperative period. Acta Chir Scand 1976; 142:423-427.
247. Nordenstrom J, Askanazi J, Elwyn DH, Martin P, Carpentier YA, Robin AP, Kinney JM: Nitrogen balance during total parenteral nutrition—glucose vs fat. Ann Surg 1983; 197:27-33.
248. Baker JP, Detsky AS, Stewart S, Whitwell J, Marliss EB, Jeejeebhoy KN: Randomized trial of total parenteral nutrition in critically ill patients: Metabolic effects of varying glucose-lipid ratios as the energy source. Gastroenterology 1984; 87:53-59.
249. Shaw JH, Holdaway CM: Protein-sparing effect of substrate infusion in surgical patients is governed by the clinical state, and not by the individual substrate infused. JPEN J Parenter Enteral Nutr 1988; 12:433-440.
250. deChalain TM, Michell WL, O'Keefe SJ, Ogden JM: The effect of fuel source on amino acid metabolism in critically ill patients. J Surg Res 1992; 52:167-176.
251. Iapichino G, Gattinoni L, Solca M, Radrizzani D, Zucchetti M, Langer M, Vesconi S: Protein sparing and protein replacement in acutely injured patients during TPN with and without amino acid supply. Intensive Care Med 1982; 8:25-31.
252. Brooks DC, Sessey PQ, Black PR, Aoki TT, Wilmore DW: Insulin stimulates branched chain amino acid uptake and diminishes nitrogen flux from skeletal muscle of injured patients. J Surg Res 1986; 40:395-405.
253. Jahoor F, Shangraw RE, Miyoshi H, Wallfish H, Herndon DN, Wolfe RR: Role of insulin and glucose oxidation in mediating the protein catabolism of burns and sepsis. Am J Physiol 1989; 257:E323-E331.
254. Askanazi J, Rosenbaum SH, Hyman AI, Silverberg PA, Milic-Emili J, Kinney JM: Respiratory changes induced by the large glucose loads of total parenteral nutrition. JAMA 1980; 243:1444-1447.
255. Askanazi J, Nordenstrom J, Rosenbaum SH, Elwyn DH, Hyman AI, Carpentier YA, Kinney JM: Nutrition for the patient with respiratory failure: Glucose vs. fat. Anesthesiology 1981; 54:373-377.
256. Herve P, Simmonneau G, Girard P, Cerrina J, Mathieu M, Duroux P: Hypercapnic acidosis induced by nutrition in mechanically ventilated patients: Glucose vs. fat. Crit Care Med 1985; 13:537-540.
257. Heymsfield SB, Head CA, McManus CB III, Seitz S, Staton GW, Grossman GD: Respiratory, cardiovascular, and metabolic effects of enteral hyperalimentation: Influence of formula dose and composition. Am J Clin Nutr 1984; 40:116-130.
258. Talpers SS, Romberger DJ, Bunce SB, Pingleton SK: Nutritionally associated increased carbon dioxide production. Excess total calories vs. high proportion of carbohydrate calories. Chest 1992; 102:551-555.
259. VanBuren CT, Kulkarni AD, Fanslow WC, Rudolph FB: Dietary nucleotides, a requirement for helper/inducer T-lymphocytes. Transplantation 1985; 40:694-697.
260. Van Buren CT, Kulkarni AD, Schandle VB, Rudolph FB: The influence of dietary nucleotides on cell-mediated immunity. Transplantation 1983; 36:350-352.
261. Carver JD, Cox WI, Barness LA: Dietary nucleotide effects upon

murine natural killer cell activity and macrophage activation. JPEN J Parenter Enteral Nutr 1980; 14:18–22.
262. Rudolph FB, Kulkarni AD, Fanslow WC, Pizzini RP, Kumar S, VanBuren CT: Role of RNA as a dietary source of pyrimidines and purines in immune function. Nutrition 1990; 6:45–62.
263. VanBuren CT, Kim E, Kulkarni AD, Fanslow WC, Rudolph FB: Nucleotide-free diet and suppression of the immune response. Transplant Proc 1987; 19:57–59.
264. VanBuren CT, Rudolph FB, Kulkarni AD, Pizzini RP, Fanslow WC, Kumar S: Reversal of immunosuppression induced by a protein-free diet: Comparison of nucleotides, fish oil, and arginine. Crit Care Med 1990; 18:S114–S117.
265. Fanslow WC, Kulkarni AD, VanBuren CT, Rudolph FB: Effect of nucleotide restriction and supplementation on resistance to experimental murine candidiasis. JPEN J Parenter Enteral Nutr 1988; 12:49–52.
266. Kulkarni AD, Fanslow WC, Drath DB, Rudolph FB, VanBuren CT: Influence of dietary nucleotide restriction on bacterial sepsis and phagocyte cell function in mice. Arch Surg 1986; 121:169–172.
267. Kulkarni AD, Fanslow WC, Rudolph FB, VanBuren CT: Effect of dietary nucleotides on response to bacterial infections. JPEN J Parenter Enteral Nutr 1986; 10:169–171.
268. Zaloga GP: Immune-enhancing enteral diets: Where's the beef? Crit Care Med 1998; 26:1143–1146.
269. Zaloga GP, Roberts PR: Early enteral feeding improves outcome. *In*: Yearbook of Intensive Care and Emergency Medicine. Vincent JL (Ed). Berlin, Springer-Verlag, 1997, pp 701–714.
270. King BK, Kudsk KA: Can an enteral diet decrease sepsis after trauma? Adv Surg 1998; 31:53–78.
271. Gottschlich MM, Jenkins M, Warden GD, et al: Differential effects of three dietary regimens on selected outcome variables in burn patients. JPEN J Parenter Enteral Nutr 1990; 14:225–236.
272. Cerra FB, Lehmann S, Konstantinides N, et al: Improvement in immune function in ICU patients by enteral nutrition supplemented with arginine, RNA, and menhaden oil is independent of nitrogen balance. Nutrition 1991; 7:193–199.
273. Daly JM, Lieberman MD, Goldfine J, et al: Enteral nutrition with supplemental arginine, RNS, and ω-3 fatty acids in patients after operation: Immunologic, metabolic and clinical outcome. Surgery 1992; 112:56–67.
274. Bower RH, Cerra FB, Bershadsky B, et al: Early enteral administration of a formula (Impact) supplemented with arginine, nucleotides, and fish oil in intensive care unit patients: Results of a multicenter, prospective, randomized clinical trial. Crit Care Med 1995; 23:436–449.
275. Brown RO, Hunt H, Mowatt-Larssen CA, Wojtysiak SL, Henningfield MF, Kudsk KA: Comparison of specialized and standard enteral formulas in trauma patients. Pharmacotherapy 1994; 14:314–320.
276. Moore FA, Moore EE, Kudsk KA, et al: Clinical benefits of an immune-enhancing diet for early postinjury enteral feeding. J Trauma 1994; 37:607–615.
277. Daly JM, Weintraub FN, Shou J, Rosato EF, Lucia M: Enteral nutrition during multimodality therapy in upper gastrointestinal cancer patients. Ann Surg 1995; 221:327–338.
278. Kudsk KA, Minard G, Croce MA, et al: A randomized trial of isonitrogenous enteral diets after severe trauma: An immune-enhancing diet reduces septic complications. Ann Surg 1996; 224:531–543.
279. Senkal M, Mumme A, Eickhoff U, et al: Early postoperative enteral immunonutrition: Clinical outcome and cost-comparison analysis in surgical patients. Crit Care Med 1997: 25:1489–1496.
280. Braga M, Gianotti L, Vignali A, Cestari A, Bisagni P, Di Carlo V: Artificial nutrition after major abdominal surgery: Impact of route of administration and composition of the diet. Crit Care Med 1998; 26:24–30.
281. Galban C, Celaya S, Marco P, et al: An immune-enhancing enteral diet reduces mortality and episodes of bacteremia in septic ICU patients (Abstract). JPEN J Parenter Enteral Nutr 1998; 22:S13.
282. Weimann A, Bastian L, Werner EB, Grotz M, Hansel M, Lotx J, Truatwein C, Tusch G, Schlitt HJ, Regel G: Influence of arginine, omega-3 fatty acids and nucleotide-supplemented enteral support on systemic inflammatory response syndrome and multiple organ failure in patients after severe trauma. Nutrition 1998; 14:165–172.
283. Atkinson S, Sieffert E, Bihari D: A prospective randomized double-blind controlled clinical trial of enteral immunonutrition in the critically ill. Crit Care Med 1998; 26:1164–1172.
284. Mendez C, Jurkovich GJ, Garcia I, Davis D, Parker A, Maier RV: Effects of an immune-enhancing diet in critically injured patients. J Trauma 1997; 42:933–941.
285. Chlebowski RT, Beall G, Grosvenor M, et al: Long-term effects of early nutritional support with new enterotropic peptide-based formula vs standard enteral formula in HIV-infected patients: Randomized prospective trial. Nutrition 1993; 9:507–512.
286. Saffle JR, Wiebke G, Jennings K, Morris SE, Barton RG: Randomized trial of immune-enhancing enteral nutrition in burn patients. J Trauma 1997; 42:793–802.
287. Zaloga GP, Bortenschlager LW: Vitamins. *In:* Nutrition in Critical Care. Zaloga GP (Ed). St. Louis, Mosby-Year Book, 1994, pp 217–241.
288. Roberts PR: Nutrition and wound healing. *In:* Nutrition in Critical Care. Zaloga GP (Ed). St. Louis, Mosby-Year Book, 1994, pp 525–544.
289. Young EA, Cioletti LA, Traylor JB, Balderas V: Gastrointestinal response to oral versus gastric feeding of defined formula diets. Am J Clin Nutr 1982; 35:715–726.
290. Zaloga GP, Roberts PR: Bedside placement of enteral feeding tubes in the intensive care unit. Crit Care Med 1998; 26:987–988.
291. Zaloga GP: Bedside method for placing small bowel feeding tubes in critically ill patients: A prospective study. Chest 1991; 100:1643–1646.
292. Ponsky JL, Cauderer MW: Percutaneous endoscopic gastrostomy: A nonoperative technique for feeding gastrostomy. Gastrointest Endosc 1981: 27:9–11.
293. Mellinger JD, Ponsky JL: Percutaneous endoscopic gastrostomy: State of the art, 1998. Endoscopy 1998; 30:126–132.
294. Baskin WN: Advances in enteral nutrition techniques. Am J Gastroenterol 1992; 87:1547–1553.
295. Marks JM, Ponsky JL: Access routes for enteral nutrition. Gastroenterologist 1995; 3:130–140.
296. Ponsky JL, Gauderer MW, Stellato TA, Aszodi A: Percutaneous approaches to enteral alimentation. Am J Surg 1985; 1499:102–105.
297. Kirby DF, Dellege MH, Fleming CR: American Gastroenterological Association technical review on tube feeding for enteral nutrition. Gastroenterology 1995; 108:1282–1301.
298. Minard G: Enteral access. Nutr Clin Pract 1994; 9:172–182.
299. Baskin W: PEJ placement: A new steerable catheter technique. Am J Gastroenterol 1989; 84:63.
300. Kalliafas S, Choban PS, Ziegler D, Drago S, Flancbaum L: Erythromycin facilitates postpyloric placement of nasoduodenal feeding tubes in intensive care unit patients: Randomized double-blinded, placebo-controlled trial. JPEN J Parenter Enteral Nutr 1996; 20:385–388.
301. Dickerson RN, Vehe KL, Mullen JL, Feurer ID: Resting energy expenditure in patients with pancreatitis. Crit Care Med 1991;19:484–490.
302. Ragins H, Levenson SM, Signer R, et al: Intrajejunal administration of an elemental diet at neutral pH avoids pancreatic stimulation. Am J Surg 1973; 126:606–614.
303. Klein S, Kinney J, Jeejeebhoy K, Alpers D, Hellerstein M, Murray M, Twomey P, et al: Nutrition support in clinical practice: Review of published data and recommendations for future research directions. JPEN J Parenter Enteral Nutr 1998; 21:133–156.
304. McClave SA, Snider H, Owens N, Sexton LK: Clinical nutrition in pancreatitis. Dig Dis Sci 1997; 42:2035–2044.
305. Sax HC, Warner BW, Talamini MA, Hamilton FN, Bell RH, Fischer JE, Bower RH: Early total parenteral nutrition in acute pancreatitis: Lack of beneficial effects. Am J Surg 1987; 153:117–124.
306. McClave SA, Greene LM, Snider HL, Makk JK, Cheadle WG, Owens NA, et al: Comparison of the safety of early enteral vs parenteral nutrition in mild acute pancreatitis. J Parenter Enteral Nutr 1997; 21:14–20.
307. Kalfarentzos F, Kehagias J, Kokkinis K, Gogos CA: Enteral nutrition is superior to parenteral nutrition in severe acute pancreatitis: Results of a randomized prospective trial. Br J Surg 1997; 84:1665–1669.
308. Windsor ACJ, Kanwar S, Li AGK, et al: Compared to parenteral nutrition, enteral feeding attenuates the acute phase response

and improves disease severity in acute pancreatitis. Gut 1998; 42:431-435.
309. Griffiths AM, Ohlsson A, Sherman PM, et al: Meta-analysis of enteral nutrition as a primary treatment of active Crohn's disease. Gastroenterology 1995; 108:1056-1067.
310. Trallori MA, D'Albasio GD, Milla M, et al: Defined-formula diets versus steroids in the treatment of active Crohn's disease. Scand J Gastroenterol 1996; 31:267-272.
311. Fernandez-Banares F, Cabre E, Esteve-Comas M, et al: How effective is enteral nutrition in inducing clinical remission in active Crohn's disease? A meta-analysis of the randomized clinical trials. JPEN J Parenter Enteral Nutr 1995; 19:356-369.
312. Belluzi A, Brignola C, Campieri M, et al: Effect of an enteric-coated fish oil preparation on relapses in Crohn's disease. N Engl J Med 1996; 334:1557-1560.
313. Lorenz-Meyer H, Bauer P, Nicolay C, et al: Omega-3 fatty acids and low carbohydrate diet for maintenance of remission of Crohn's disease. Scand J Gastroenterol 1996; 31:778-785.
314. Aslan A, Tridafilopoulos G: Fish oil fatty acid supplementation in active ulcerative colitis: A double-blind, placebo-controlled, cross-over study. Am J Gastroenterol 1992; 87:432-437.
315. Lorenz R, Weber PC, Szimnau P, et al: Supplementation with n-3 fatty acids from fish oil in chronic inflammatory bowel disease: A randomized, placebo-controlled, double-blind cross-over trial. J Intern Med 1989; 225:225-232.
316. Hawthorne AB, Daneshmend TK, Hawkey CJ, et al: Treatment of ulcerative colitis with fish oil supplementation: A prospective 12 month randomized controlled trial. Gut 1992; 33:922-928.
317. Stenson WF, Cort D, Rodgers J, et al: Dietary supplementation with fish oils in ulcerative colitis. Ann Intern Med 1992; 116:609-614.
318. Cerra FB, Benitez MR, Blackburn GL, Irwin RS, Jeejeebhoy K, Katz DP, Pingleton SK, et al: Applied nutrition in ICU patients: A consensus statement of the American College of Chest Physicians. Chest 1997; 111:769-778.
319. Duerksen DR, Nehra V, Bistrian BR, Blackburn GL: Appropriate nutritional support in acute and complicated Crohn's disease. Nutrition 1998; 14:462-465.
320. Kearns PJ, Young H, Garcia G, et al: Accelerated improvement of alcoholic liver disease with enteral nutrition. Gastroenterology 1992; 102:200-205.
321. Hirsch S, Bunout D, de la Maza R, et al: Controlled trial of nutrition supplementation in outpatients with symptomatic alcoholic cirrhosis. JPEN J Parenter Enteral Nutr 1993; 17:119-124.
322. Coare E, Gonzalez-Huix FG, Abad-Lacruz A, et al: Effect of total enteral nutrition on the short-term outcome of severely malnourished cirrhotics. Gastroenterology 1990; 98:715-720.
323. Metheny N, Wehrle MA, Wiersema L, Clark J: Testing feeding tube placement: Auscultation vs pH method. Am J Nurs 1998; 98:37-42.
324. Roundtable Conference: Enteral Nutritional Support for the 1990's: Innovations in Nutrition, Technology, and Techniques. Columbus, Ohio, Ross Laboratories, 1992, pp 1-51.
325. Roubenoff R, Ravich WJ: Pneumothorax due to nasogastric feeding tubes: Report of four cases, review of the literature, and recommendations for prevention. Arch Intern Med 1989; 149:184-188.
326. Torres A, Serr-Batlles J, Ros E, Piera C, Puig de la Bellacasa J, Cobos A, Lomena F, Rodriguez-Roisin R: Pulmonary aspiration of gastric contents in patients receiving mechanical ventilation: The effect of body position. Ann Intern Med 1992; 116:540-543.
327. Ibanez J, Panafiel A, Raurich JM, Marse P, Jorda R, Mata F: Gastroesophageal reflux in intubated patients receiving enteral nutrition: Effect of supine and semirecumbent positions. JPEN J Parenter Enteral Nutr 1992; 16:419-422.
328. Mullan H, Roubenoff RA, Roubenoff R: Risk of pulmonary aspiration among patients receiving enteral nutrition support. JPEN J Parenter Enteral Nutr 1992; 16:160-164.
329. Lazarus BA, Murphy JB, Culpepper L: Aspiration associated with long-term gastric versus jejunal feeding: A critical analysis of the literature. Arch Phys Med Rehabil 1990; 71:46-53.
330. Burtch GD, Shatney CH: Feeding jejunostomy (versus gastrostomy) passes the test of time. Am Surg 1987; 53:54-57.
331. Elpern EH: Pulmonary aspiration in hospitalized patients. Nutr Clin Pract 1997; 12:5-13.
332. Mobarhan S, Kazi N: Enteral feeding associated gastroesophageal reflux and aspiration pneumonia. Nutr Rev 1996; 54:324-328.
333. McClave SA, Snider HL, Lowen CC, McLaughlin AJ, Greene LM, McCombs RJ, Rodgers L, Wright RA, Roy TM, Schumer MP, et al: Use of residual volume as a marker for enteral feeding intolerance: Prospective blinded comparison with physical examination and radiographic findings. JPEN J Parenter Enteral Nutr 1992; 16:99-105.
334. Edes TE, Walk BE, Austin JL: Diarrhea in tube-fed patients: Feeding formula not necessarily the cause. Am J Med 1990; 88:91-93.
335. Guenter PA, Settle RG, Perlmutter S, Marino PL, DeSimone GA, Rolandelli RH: Tube feeding-related diarrhea in acutely ill patients. JPEN J Parenter Enteral Nutr 1991; 15:277-280.
336. Mobarhan S, DeMeo M: Diarrhea induced by enteral feeding. Nutr Rev 1995; 53:67-70.
337. Keohane PP, Attrill H, Love M, Frost P, Silk DBA: Relation between osmolality and gastrointestinal side effects in enteral nutrition. Br Med J 1984; 288:678-680.
338. Ringel AF, Jameson GL, Foster ES: Diarrhea in the intensive care unit. Crit Care Clin 1995; 11:465-477.
339. Zaloga GP, Roberts P: Permissive underfeeding. New Horiz 1994; 2:257-263.

80

Total Parenteral Nutrition for the Critically Ill Patient

Jeffrey A. Sternberg, MD • Stephanie A. Rohovsky, MD
George L. Blackburn, MD, PhD
Timothy J. Babineau, MD

Total parenteral nutrition (TPN) is a pharmacologic therapy whereby nutrients, vitamins, electrolytes, and medications are delivered via the central venous route to patients who are unable to tolerate enteral nutrition. Prior to the development of parenteral nutrition in the 1960s, critically ill patients often died of malnutrition-associated complications. Severe illnesses requiring an intensive care unit (ICU) stay place a patient's restorative forces in direct competition with the relentless progression of nutritional depletion. In the pre-nutrition support era, patients either recovered rapidly and resumed eating or succumbed to the weakening effects of malnutrition, such as infection, impaired wound healing (dehiscence or anastomotic leak), and multisystem organ dysfunction.

In conjunction with this clinical observation was the new appreciation that premorbid nutritional status and nutrient administration greatly influence the body's response to trauma and sepsis.[1] Parenteral alimentation was thus developed during the late 1960s in an attempt to positively influence these factors. Unfortunately, early enthusiasm for parenteral nutrition lead to the administration of excessive calories in order to promote a "positive" nitrogen balance in critically ill patients. Instead of improving outcome, such "hyperalimentation" led to major metabolic complications that mitigated against many of the beneficial effects of nutrition support. The dangers of overfeeding are now well appreciated, however, and we have progressed from an era of hyperalimentation to one in which calories approximating a patient's basal energy requirements are delivered. In addition, the indications for parenteral nutrition have been more clearly defined, and, as this is a potent pharmacologic therapy, it should be applied selectively rather than routinely.

The use of parenteral nutrition, while controversial in some settings, has been accepted as an effective means of sustaining life and promoting recovery in critically ill patients incapable of ingesting, absorbing, or assimilating nutrients. TPN has also proved appropriate for similar non–critically ill patients who have preexisting malnutrition and for nonstressed but hospitalized persons who can take nothing by mouth (NPO status) for 5 to 7 days. The goals of parenteral nutrition remain supportive:

1. Improving wound healing.
2. Bolstering immune function.
3. Influencing acid-base and mineral homeostasis.
4. Minimizing obligate nitrogen loss in the catabolic postinjury state.

In this chapter we present an overview of parenteral nutrition and a guide to its appropriate use in the ICU setting.

STARVATION, MALNUTRITION, AND THE METABOLIC RESPONSE TO INJURY

To effectively administer nutrition support in the ICU, one must have a rudimentary understanding of the exchange of labile nutrients between the major body compartments during states of fasting and stress. The body is divided into *lean* and *adipose* components (Fig. 80–1). The lean portion is further divided into *extracellular mass* (extracellular fluid, plasma proteins, and skeleton) and *body cell mass* (skeletal muscle, viscera).

During a protracted fast in a nonstressed patient, a fall in serum insulin enables mobilization of metabolic fuels. Glucose is initially derived from hepatic glycogen stores (muscle is unable to release glucose from glycogen into the systemic circulation) for the first 24 to 48 hours, after which hepatic gluconeogenesis using peripherally released amino acids and glycerol (the latter is released during lipolysis) continue to supply the body's glucose-dependent tissues (immune system, brain, renal medulla) with fuel. With continued fasting, ketogenesis occurs and free fatty acids become the body's primary fuel, thus decreasing the need for amino acid mobilization and preserving skeletal muscle. The body exists in a state of maximal resource conservation, sustaining itself on energy-rich fat, minimizing the loss of lean tissue (nitrogen losses, a measure of protein breakdown, approach 4 to 5 g/day), and reducing basal energy expenditure. Interestingly, serum albumin concentrations are usually not depressed in this state of pure *protein-calorie malnutrition* (PCM), or *marasmus*. Immune function typically remains intact in such subjects, but reserves are limited and these patients are incapable of resisting severe or prolonged systemic stress, such as major surgery or acute pancreatitis (Table 80–1). Patients with marasmic PCM appear obviously malnourished and wasted as, for example, are those with esophageal obstruction or anorexia nervosa. This "pure" form of unstressed starvation is not typically seen in the ICU setting.

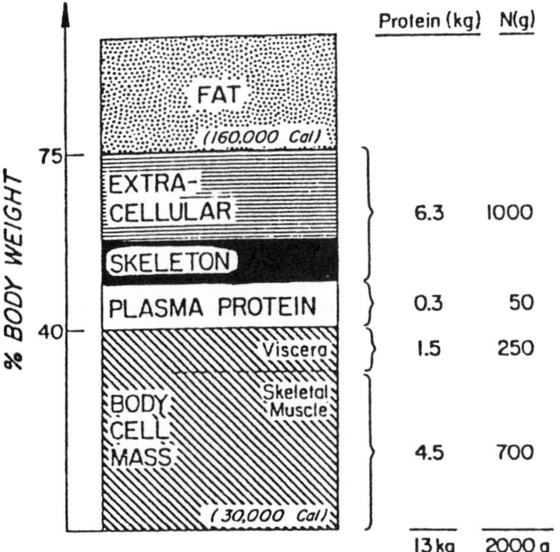

Figure 80–1. Relative size and protein content of the four major body compartments. (Adapted with permission from Blackburn GL, Bistrian BR, Maini BS: Nutritional and metabolic assessment of the hospitalized patient. J Parenter Enteral Nutr 1977; 1:11–22.)

TABLE 80–1. Protein-Calorie Malnutrition (PCM) and Surgical Risk

PCM	Serum Albumin	Surgical Risk
Marasmus	→ or ↑	↑
End-stage disease, cachexia	↓ ↓	↑ ↑
Kwashiorkor, hypoalbuminemic PCM	↓ ↓ ↓	↑ ↑ ↑

Another form of malnutrition commonly seen in hospitalized patients is the *cachexia syndrome* associated with end-stage illnesses such as the wasting syndrome of acquired immunodeficiency syndrome (AIDS), cancer cachexia syndrome, and end-stage liver disease. Decreased oral intake and a mild systemic inflammatory response contribute to a modest increase in peripheral protein catabolism and cause a mild elevation of acute phase reactant proteins, a slight depression of serum albumin, and an increased surgical risk proportional to the degree of weight loss.[2] This form of malnutrition increasingly is contributing to morbidity in ICU patients.

The more commonly encountered clinical form of PCM in critical illness is *hypoalbuminemic malnutrition*, a kwashiorkor-like disorder. After significant injury, the body's metabolic processes are reprioritized by a group of endogenous mediators, including the counterregulatory hormones cortisol, glucagon, catecholamines, and growth hormone in addition to aldosterone, antidiuretic hormone, eicosanoid derivatives, and cytokines such as tumor necrosis factor (TNF), interleukin-1 (IL-1), and IL-6 (Table 80–2). Consequent to the ensuing systemic inflammatory process is an increase in basal metabolic rate, the development of insulin resistance, trace metal redistribution, and water and salt retention. Gluconeogenesis, normally an insulin-sensitive process, becomes decoupled from hormonal control, which can lead to hyperglycemia in nondiabetic patients when glucose is provided in modest amounts. As a result, insulin levels are mildly elevated and ketoadaptation does not occur.[2] This exaggerated metabolic response is orchestrated primarily by the liver and the immune system. Large quantities of metabolic fuels are mobilized from their storage depots in the periphery (skeletal muscle and adipose tissue) to meet the demands of the metabolically more active viscera (particularly the liver, the immune system, and the injury site) (Fig. 80–2). Rapid substrate cycling occurs to maintain an available circulating pool of glucose, amino acids, and fatty acids for essential organ function and repair; however, some authors have suggested that this cycling may in part be a wasteful process that contributes to a futile increase in visceral metabolic rate and thermogenesis.[3]

Critical illness triggers a survival response in the host, whereby lean tissue is systematically catabolized in order for the organism as a whole to survive. In contrast to uncomplicated starvation, whereby fat losses are greater than lean

TABLE 80–2. Physiologic Impacts of Starvation and of Stress

	Starvation	Stress
Protein		
Catabolism	+	+ + +
Carbohydrate		
Glycogenolysis	+	+ + +
Gluconeogenesis	+	+ + +
Lipid		
Lipolysis	+ + +	+ +
Ketosis	+ + +	− − −
Metabolic Alterations		
Mobilization of protein, glucose, lipid	Passive	Active
Energy expenditure	Decreases	Increases
Serum albumin	Stable	Drops precipitously
Urine urea nitrogen (assuming adequate protein-energy stores)	<5 g/day	>10 g/day

Adapted from Daley B, Cahill S, Driscoll D, et al: Parenteral and enteral nutrition. *In:* Gastrointestinal Pharmacotherapy. Wolfe M (Ed). Philadelphia, WB Saunders, 1993, pp 293–316.

Key: Plus and minus signs indicate the degree of activation or suppression.

TABLE 80–3. Composition of Weight Loss in Starvation and Stress

Condition	Fat (%)	Lean Tissue (%)
Simple starvation, first wk	60	40
Simple starvation, second wk	67–75	25–33
Cachexia	50	50
Acute injury	25	75

Unpublished data courtesy of B. R. Bistrian, MD, PhD.

tissue losses, severe catabolic stress utilizes skeletal muscle breakdown preferentially as metabolic fuel (Table 80–3). Patient inactivity further contributes to skeletal muscle wasting by encouraging amino acid mobilization due to disuse, and the resultant profound muscle weakness contributes to respiratory dysfunction and generalized morbidity. The serum albumin concentration rapidly falls after injury, regardless of the premorbid nutritional status, owing to a combination of factors, including decreased production by the liver, increased degradation, and extravascular sequestration. Serum albumin is thus useful as a gauge of systemic inflammation rather than as a nutritional marker. Patients with stress-induced hypoalbuminemic malnutrition may not appear grossly malnourished and may be difficult for the untrained eye to recognize because of the fluid overload that often accompanies the critically ill state. These patients are at increased risk for infectious complications, sepsis, and multisystem organ failure and death, despite their noncachectic appearance.[4]

Severe catabolic stress, such as that associated with trauma, burns, severe sepsis, or pancreatitis, can lead to the loss of 20 to 30 g of urinary nitrogen (UN) a day. Each gram of nitrogen represents approximately 6.25 g of protein, each gram of which in turn accounts for approximately 5 g of lean tissue. Therefore, a patient with 25 to 30 g of UN will loose up to 800 to 900 g of lean tissue a day, representing more than a kilogram of actual body weight (males, 75% to 85% lean tissue; females, 70% to 75% lean tissue). Patient water and salt avidity during acute illness, however, may mask this functional tissue loss.

Death is known to occur after the loss of approximately 50% of one's lean tissue mass, or approximately 1000 g of nitrogen for a 70-kg male. (Each gram of nitrogen represents approximately 30 g of lean tissue.) Patients expressing a severe stress response are incapable of adequately sustaining this process without rapidly depleting their substrate reserves, resulting in organ dysfunction and immunosuppression. For a nonstressed individual of normal body composition, death typically occurs after a 3-month fast. For critically ill patients, this time period is compressed to 1 month; for severely catabolic patients who entered the hospital with some degree of preexisting malnutrition (the majority of critically ill patients), this period may be as short as 14 days. Functional deficits ensue before death. The goal is to intervene before nutritional deficiencies occur, thus underscoring the importance of initiating *early* nutritional support in critically ill patients.

Malnutrition is a common component of many disease processes and is most broadly defined as a substantial lean tissue loss due to illness or prolonged inadequate dietary intake.[1] As many as 50% of all hospitalized patients are malnourished.[5, 6] Risk factors for PCM include:

1. Protracted inflammatory conditions (inflammatory bowel disease, rheumatic disease).

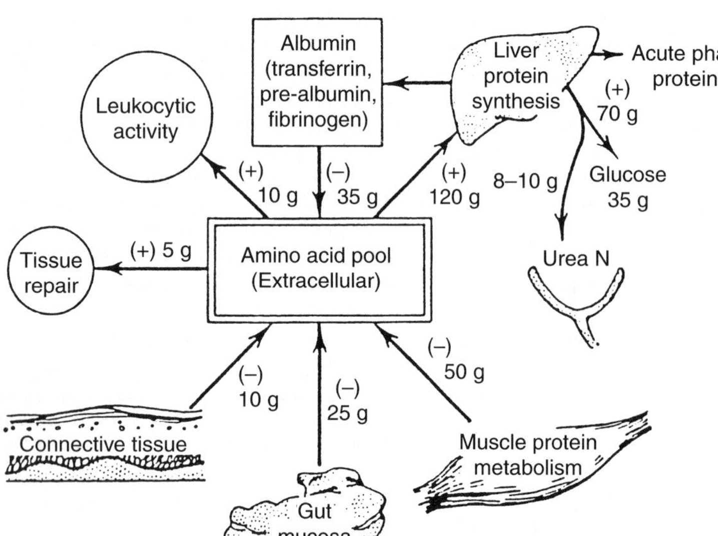

Figure 80–2. Functional redistribution of body cell mass after acute stress provides nitrogen for protein synthesis by the liver and immune system. *Arrows* reflect the net release (−) or uptake (+) of amino acids by various tissues. (From Blackburn GL: Nutrition in surgical patients. *In*: Hardy's Textbook of Surgery. Hardy JD, Kukora JS, Pass HI [Eds]. Philadelphia, JB Lippincott, 1988, pp 86–105.)

2. Preexisting organ dysfunction (congestive heart failure or cirrhosis).
3. Malignancy.

Other patients may be well nourished and healthy before becoming critically ill (acute pancreatitis or multitrauma), but they become rapidly debilitated and nutritionally depleted from their amplified injury response. Consequently, efforts to recognize malnutrition, prevent its progression, or abate its development are of paramount importance in the ICU.

GOALS OF NUTRITION SUPPORT IN THE INTENSIVE CARE UNIT

Parenteral nutrition serves as a primary therapy for pure PCM. In such unstressed subjects, TPN increases net protein synthesis and increases body cell mass (BCM) when combined with physical activity. The role of parental nutrition in critically ill patients, however, is mainly supportive. TPN administration slows the deterioration of nutritional status, which is rapid in unsupported severely catabolic patients. In this stressed population, parenteral nutrition is capable of promoting visceral protein synthesis to a greater degree than it is able to decrease the breakdown of skeletal muscle. The overall effect is the net diminution, but not complete inhibition, of protein catabolism.[7]

With today's available means of nutrition support, positive nitrogen balance and skeletal muscle anabolism are not possible in critically ill patients owing to their heightened metabolic response and inactivity.[8-11] There is no evidence to suggest that energy balance is beneficial for stressed patients. In fact, even if it were possible, evidence exists that aggressive attempts to reverse catabolism by providing excessive calories are potentially harmful.[12, 13] Nitrogen and calorie balance have never been convincingly demonstrated to correlate with outcome and should each be viewed as surrogate markers of illness severity. Lean tissue accretion through the administration of nutrition support becomes possible only after the metabolic response to injury subsides and the patient begins to convalesce.

In severely stressed patients, four factors directly promote the development of malnutrition:

- Immobility
- Anorexia
- Anabolic inefficiency
- Increased catabolism

Of these consequences of illness, nutrition support (both enteral and parenteral) can remove the anorectic component from the equation but has only a limited effect on the others.[2] In critical illness, the principal goals of nutrition support are to:

1. Provide substrate (protein, carbohydrate, lipid, electrolytes, minerals, and vitamins) for ongoing metabolic functions.
2. Maximize protein synthesis and limit protein catabolism.
3. Bolster immune function and improve wound healing.
4. Improve cardiac and respiratory function by restoring glycogen stores in cardiac and diaphragmatic muscle.
5. Correct acid-base and electrolyte disturbances.
6. Potentially modify the systemic inflammatory response.

The eventual goal for any patient receiving TPN or enteral nutrition via a feeding tube is the resumption of enteral nutrition via the oral route.

WHO SHOULD RECEIVE NUTRITION SUPPORT?

All critically ill patients require a thorough nutritional assessment to determine who is likely to benefit from nutrition support and whether nutrition is to be provided via an enteral route, parenteral route, or a combination. In addition, the decision to administer parenteral nutrition may be influenced by the presence of metabolic or acid-base disturbances that are best addressed by this therapy. Three principal factors predict the need for nutrition support: current nutritional status (i.e., body composition), the anticipated duration of inadequate nutrient intake, and the presence and degree of the stress response.[14] Because a majority of critically ill patients are malnourished, are unable to eat for long periods, and have a heightened systemic inflammatory response, most will require some form of nutrition support. Nonetheless, a thorough nutritional assessment is useful for establishing the likelihood of a critically ill patient developing malnutrition-related complications, since nutrition support has inherent risks and should be used discriminately.

A nutritional assessment begins with a thorough history and physical examination. A history of comorbid illnesses with components of nausea, vomiting, diarrhea, or weight loss is important. The finding of recent (within 6 months) unintentional weight loss is often the easiest and most important clinical indicator that correlates closely with the degree of risk (Table 80–4). Functional deficits begin to develop with weight loss in excess of 10%, even in obese patients. When weight loss reaches 20%, the ability to combat stress is severely diminished and nutritional intervention is mandated. Many patients are unable to relate an accurate history, and other assessment methods are commonly employed. Moderate to severe malnutrition is usually present in individuals whose current weight is less than 85% of the ideal body weight for height. The body mass index (BMI) is often a more useful indicator. Defined as weight in kilograms divided by the square of height in meters, it normalizes body weight for height and is independent of sex. A value less than 18 is consistent with significant malnutrition.[2]

For many critically ill patients, weight alone may be a poor indicator of nutrition status, as short-term fluctuations in total body water may account for changes in weight. Physical examination can help place a patient's weight in the proper clinical context. Fluid overload can be signified by peripheral edema, ascites, or anasarca. Temporal and peripheral muscle wasting may occur, signifying probable PCM even in the face of weight gain. Other nutritional indicators may be more useful in these fluid-expanded subjects.

Upper arm anthropometry is a useful tool for assessing malnutrition. This technique reveals information about lean body mass and fat reserves that is based on standard values and correlates with nutrition status.[15, 16] Measurements of mid-arm circumference and triceps skinfold thickness are used to calculate the mid-arm muscle circumference. A value below the 5th percentile is consistent with a loss of approximately 30% of normal lean body mass and is an absolute indication for nutritional intervention.

Serum levels of visceral protein markers such as albumin, prealbumin, retinol-binding protein, transferrin, and insulin-like growth factor I (somatomedin C) have commonly been used as indicators of nutritional status. Low serum levels of these proteins, however, loosely correlate with nutritional

Table 80–4. Evaluation of Weight Loss in Critically Ill Patients

Time (mo)	Clinically Significant Weight Loss (%)	Severe Weight Loss (%)
1	5	10
3	5–10	15
6	10	20

depletion, as they can be relatively normal in cases of pure PCM, such as anorexia nervosa; instead, they should be viewed as markers of the severity of the systemic inflammatory response. These markers are depressed in acute and chronic processes that activate inflammatory cascades (e.g., infection, pancreatitis, active rheumatoid conditions, cirrhosis, congestive heart failure). Serum protein marker levels fall rapidly in well-nourished patients with severe, acute inflammatory processes and remain depressed until that condition has subsided, whether or not they have received adequate nutritional support. Although the levels of the different serum protein markers change at different rates owing to their variable serum half-lives and volumes of distribution, they "trend" in the same direction. Because the serum albumin level tracks with the degree and duration of ongoing systemic inflammation, it is a good predictor of patient outcome and remains the prototypical serum marker (Fig. 80–3).[7]

Because most critically ill patients have severe inflammatory processes and require nutritional support, it follows that hypoalbuminemia in the ICU is associated with the need for nutritional intervention. Exogenous albumin administration may raise serum albumin levels in hypoalbuminemic patients but does not decrease morbidity or mortality.[17] Its addition to the TPN admixture is not useful but potentially harmful. Albumin can become glycosylated when mixed with hypertonic dextrose solutions, thereby losing many of its functional characteristics.[18] When used to increase intravascular oncotic pressure transiently to aid in diuresis, albumin is best administered in bolus fashion, followed immediately by diuretic therapy.

Hypoalbuminemia in sick patients is due to the conglomerate effect of three separate forces[2]:

1. Extravasation of albumin into the extravascular compartment owing to an increase in capillary permeability to form a new equilibrium. (This shift in the equilibrium between intravascular and extravascular albumin has the most rapid and largest effect on serum albumin levels.)
2. Down-regulation of hepatic albumin synthesis by the actions of the cytokines TNF, IL-1, and IL-6. (Albumin is thus termed a *negative acute-phase reactant.*)
3. Increased albumin catabolic rate.

Additional techniques for measuring nutritional status or following catabolic rate are commonly employed in the ICU and are useful academic tools. A 24-hour urine collection is such a method of obtaining information about lean body mass. The amount of creatinine excreted in the urine over 24 hours is proportional to skeletal muscle mass. The creatinine height index (CHI) is the ratio of measured creatinine excreted to the expected excreted creatinine based on that of control subjects matched by age, sex, and ideal body weight.[7] Values below 85% indicate moderate PCM, and values less than 60% signify severe loss of lean body mass.[19] Urinary creatinine measurements in patients with fluctuating serum creatinine levels may yield less useful data. A 24-hour urine collection for urea nitrogen provides an indirect measurement of the severity of the stress response and can emphasize the need for early nutritional intervention in patients.

The use of techniques such as delayed cutaneous hypersensitivity and total lymphocyte count as predictors of the need for nutritional intervention are too insensitive to yield useful information in the ICU. Many additional assessment methods have been formulated and have a role in clinical research. Even with all these tools, however, there is no single gold standard.[20] Clinical acumen remains the most important factor when one is determining the presence of malnutrition and the need for nutritional intervention.

INITIATING NUTRITION SUPPORT

Deciding when to initiate nutrition support for an ICU patient depends on the nutritional assessment and the severity of illness. For moderately malnourished patients with a modest systemic inflammatory response, nutrition support should be started after a period without food of no more than 5 to 7 days. In critically ill patients, however, nutrition support should be instituted within the first 48 to 72 hours of arrival in the ICU, provided that they have been adequately resuscitated.

Choosing the appropriate route of nutrition support for a critically ill patient is an important decision predicated on a patient's clinical situation. Although enteral feeding is always the preferred route for patients with a functional gastrointestinal tract, many critically ill patients have relative or absolute contraindications to enteral feedings. Patients with severe diarrhea, abdominal distention, high nasogastric tube output, pancreatitis, or unobtainable safe access to the gastrointestinal tract are poor candidates for enteral nutrition. The complications of enteral nutrition include pulmonary aspiration, diarrhea, and intestinal ischemia or infarction.[21] Owing to the seriousness of the last complication, hemodynamically unstable patients with low cardiac outputs and patients on moderate to large doses of alpha agonists should not be fed by the enteral route.[2] In addition, many critically ill patients are difficult to feed safely enterally, because of either feeding intolerance or respiratory failure with aspiration risk.[22] Such prob-

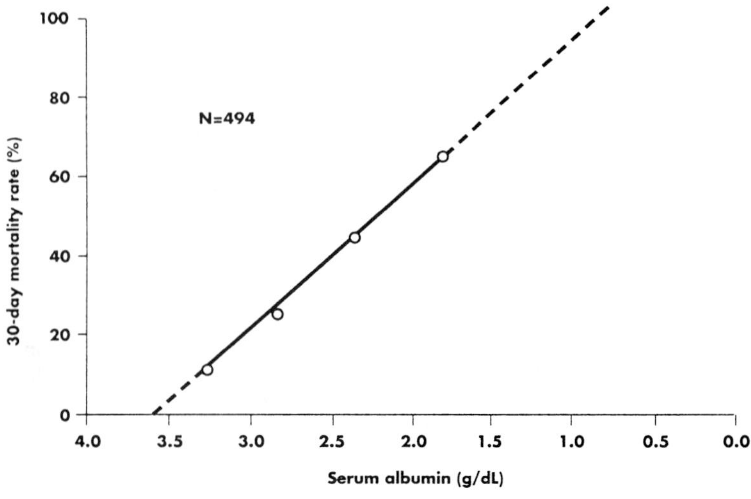

Figure 80–3. Correlation of serum albumin concentration and 30-day mortality in hospitalized subjects. (Adapted from Reinhardt GF, Myskofsky JW, Wilkens DB, et al: Incidence and mortality of hypoalbuminemic patients in hospitalized veterans. JPEN J Parenter Enteral Nutr 1980; 4:357–359.)

lems in administering enteral feeding need to be anticipated early in the ICU course of a patient so as not to delay the provision of nutrition support.

Parenteral nutrition offers some potential advantages over enteral nutrition for critically ill patients, such as improved metabolic, electrolyte, and micronutrient management; better acid-base manipulation; drug delivery capabilities (histamine H_2 blockers, metoclopramide, insulin, heparin); and ensured nutrient delivery without the concerns of gastrointestinal intolerance, compliance with transnasal feeding tubes, or absorption. Additionally, as most critically ill patients will already have central venous access, parenteral nutrition can be started without the added risk of central line insertion.

Concerns over the use of parenteral nutrition in the ICU have included mucosal atrophy of the bowel and bacterial translocation. Although these effects have been demonstrated in rodents, they have not been shown to occur in humans.[23-26] Although commonly asserted in the literature, the increase in septic complications often associated with use of TPN can usually be correlated with the prevalence of hyperglycemia in study populations. There is no direct evidence that TPN alone is immunosuppressive in human subjects. Another potential metabolic complication of TPN is hepatic steatosis, which is avoidable with careful calorie administration. To date, the route of feeding has never been shown conclusively to be an independent predictor of infection or poor outcome.

THE PARENTERAL FORMULA

Parenteral formulas contain both nutrient and non-nutrient elements; thus, TPN not only delivers nutrition but also regulates fluid, electrolyte, and acid-base homeostasis. In prescribing TPN for an ICU patient, one must take into account changes in the patient's volume status, ability to tolerate extra intravenous fluid, glycemic control, arterial pH, and serum electrolyte concentrations. For these reasons, patient-specific parenteral formulas are preferential for critically ill patients. An overriding consideration in the administration of TPN is to do no harm. Corrective measures made with the parenteral formula should err on the conservative side, taking into account the anticipated metabolic changes over a 24-hour period.

The volume of the parenteral formula is an important factor to consider in critically ill patients. In the ICU, patient volume requirements can vary unpredictably. For volume-restricted patients, nutrition support should be limited to 1 L of solution.[27] Although this necessitates a period of permissive underfeeding, energy balance is not a short-term goal of nutrition support and the additional volume required to fully feed such patients may be detrimental.[12, 13] Because many unstable patients require large volumes of resuscitation fluids, additional volume should be provided as extra dextrose-free intravenous fluid.

ENERGY REQUIREMENTS

Ideally, calories should be provided by the parenteral formula in amounts similar to those utilized by the patient. Therefore, the energy requirement of a patient is derived from an estimation of basal energy expenditure (BEE). The BEE is expressed in terms of kilocalories (kcal) burned during a 24-hour period and includes the energy used for vital processes in the resting state (metabolism, circulation, breathing, and thermoregulation[7]). The energy expenditure of most critically ill patients is less than that of nonhospitalized subjects, owing to the former group's inactivity, preexisting PCM, and age. (The elderly have less lean tissue per unit height and weight.[28]). Exceptions to this rule do exist; young polytrauma patients or burn patients can have a BEE of 35 to 40 kcal/kg of body weight.[29]

Numerous methods exist for calculating or measuring BEE. The simplest and most accurate method of estimating a patient's energy requirements is as follows (with the above noted exceptions):

$$\text{energy requirement} = 25 \text{ kcal/kg/day}$$

This formula is based on studies demonstrating that critically ill patients generally have energy expenditures of 22 to 24 kcal/kg.[28] The weight used for calculating energy expenditure (and other substrate requirements in this chapter) is the ideal body weight (IBW).[30] For obese individuals (>130% of IBW), the IBW plus 25% of the obese weight (actual weight − IBW) should be used for the calculation. This upward adjustment accounts for the extra visceral and supportive tissue that accompanies adiposity.[31]

The Harris-Benedict equation has been traditionally employed to calculate BEE.[32] These values along with the accompanying stress factors generally overestimate the true energy expenditure of critically ill patients as they were derived before the development of modern ICU practices, which have reduced the intensity of the systemic response to injury. Strict use of the Harris-Benedict equation multiplied by stress factors can lead to overfeeding, one of the principal errors made in TPN support.[2] Clinical and experimental evidence indicates that this practice is potentially harmful for the following reasons:

1. Overfeeding often leads to hyperglycemia, especially in stressed subjects, and is known to decrease neutrophil and macrophage function as well as immunoglobulin opsonization.[33, 34] Hyperglycemia increases the incidence of nosocomial infection, including catheter-related infections and candidemia.[35] The risk of infection may be five times as high when serum glucose rises above 220 mg/dL.[36] Hyperglycemia also can precipitate hypermetabolism through insulin-induced catecholamine secretion, leading to increased protein catabolism.[2]
2. Overfeeding can lead to hepatic steatosis as excessive dextrose calories are increasingly disposed of by nonoxidative pathways, including de novo *lipogensis*, whereby the liver directly converts glucose to lipid. This process, besides leading to hepatic dysfunction, has an energy cost that further promotes hypermetabolism.
3. Overfeeding leads to an increase in the respiratory quotient and lipogenesis, which can compromise patient respiratory function.[7]

Avoidance of overfeeding and attempts to aggressively maintain euglycemia during TPN administration are imperative to realize benefit from this therapy and decrease the infectious risk. To date, no study has ever demonstrated a clinical benefit to feeding at a patient's BEE as compared with feeding below this value. Because of the potential risks of even moderate hyperglycemia, "permissive underfeeding" has a theoretical appeal.[13]

The most accurate method for determining the energy expenditure of a patient is through the use of the *metabolic cart* with *indirect calorimetry*. The cart measures oxygen consumption and carbon dioxide production. These values can in turn be used to calculate a patient's respiratory quotient (moles of carbon dioxide produced ÷ moles of oxygen consumed) and the BEE using the modified Weir equation.[32] The metabolic cart is becoming a standard piece of equipment in most academic ICUs. When available, it is most helpful for determining the BEE of patients to whom standard methods of energy estimation are not easily applied, such as those who are morbidly obese, are elderly, weigh less than 50 kg, or are edematous. Additionally, the metabolic cart should be used for burn and trauma patients and for those requiring prolonged nutrition support.

PROTEIN REQUIREMENTS

Corporeal protein exists in one of three forms: (1) structural, (2) functional (e.g., enzymes), or (3) a portion of a small, tightly regulated circulating pool of free amino acids. Parenterally administered amino acids can be incorporated into one of these compartments or oxidized to yield glucose and urea.

Optimal protein intake (calorie value of 4 kcal/g) for critically ill patients is approximately 1.5 g/kg/day.[37] This amount of protein intake can decrease the degree of nitrogen loss in catabolic patients, mostly by enhancing visceral protein synthesis and to a lesser degree by diminishing peripheral protein catabolism.[7] Delivering additional amounts of protein does not further reverse this trend and does not yield a positive nitrogen balance.[8, 9] Nutrition support during acute injury, therefore, is able to lessen nitrogen losses but does not build lean tissue. Only when the systemic response to injury has subsided are patients capable of becoming anabolic.

Protein calories count in the total calorie calculations of a parenteral formula, since delivered amino acids do not yield net protein synthesis. Even when the inflammatory response subsides, only a small portion of the delivered protein is utilized for protein synthesis. Providing amounts of protein in excess of 1.7 g/kg/day results in excessive ureagenesis rather than contributing to protein anabolism.[9] When the recommended amount of protein is provided, its contribution to increases in patient blood urea nitrogen (BUN) is small (only 5 to 15 g/dL) as compared with the same from a hypercatabolic patient's endogenous protein turnover (as high as 200 g of protein a day). Uremia in such settings is an indication for dialysis rather than for a decrease in the amount of protein delivered. For the protein-sparing effects of parenterally administered glucose and lipid to be realized, adequate amounts of protein must be provided.[7]

All available parenteral amino acid formulas contain adequate amounts of both essential amino acids (EAAs) and nonessential amino acids for most critically ill patients, and providing additional amounts of EAAs has not proved beneficial. Parenteral solutions enriched in branched chain amino acids (BCAAs = valine, leucine, isoleucine) have potential use in the treatment of patients with acute renal failure or hepatic encephalopathy. Compared with non-BCAAs, which are hepatically metabolized, BCAAs are metabolized by skeletal muscle and, therefore, do not directly contribute to hepatic urea production. In addition, BCAAs compete with aromatic amino acids (thought to contribute to hepatic encephalopathy) for the carrier, which is responsible for their transport into the brain, thus potentially decreasing the latter's passage across the blood-brain barrier. BCAAs may also improve the efficiency with which protein is utilized.

So far, BCAA-enriched parenteral formulas have not reduced mortality in acute renal failure.[38] Studies of their use in patients with significant hepatic encephalopathy, too, have yielded mixed results. BCAAs appear to benefit by reducing encephalopathy grade and possibly improving survival when used in very protein-intolerant patients suffering from chronic (not acute) hepatic encephalopathy.[20] In such patients, protein administration should be reduced to 1.0 g/kg/day. Because of their increased cost and arguable efficacy, BCAAs should not be used as first-line treatment for hepatic encephalopathy. There is no proof that BCAA-enriched parenteral formulas are beneficial for critically ill patients with sepsis or trauma.[20]

The use of glutamine in parenteral formulas has received considerable attention. Formerly limited by its instability in standard parenteral formulas, glutamine is now available as a soluble dipeptide (alanyl-glutamine). Glutamine's theoretical utility in critical illness is inferred from its need as a fuel by rapidly dividing tissues (enterocytes, colonocytes, and immune tissues), as a nitrogen donor for purine and pyrimidine synthesis, and by the kidney to excrete an acid load. Furthermore, the rapid decline in serum glutamine concentrations in sepsis has been used as an argument for empirically administering pharmacologic doses of this amino acid to critically ill patients.

Initial studies of glutamine-enriched TPN demonstrated a reduction in length of hospital stay for patients undergoing bone marrow transplantation.[39] This effect, however, has not been reproduced in subsequent studies. In a trial utilizing glutamine-enriched TPN in critically ill patients, there was a decrease in 6-month mortality in the study group compared with the control group, despite identical early survival rates.[38] This finding needs to be tested in subsequent studies before glutamine-enriched parenteral solutions can be recommended for critically ill patients.

GLUCOSE

Parenteral carbohydrate is supplied as dextrose (3.4 kcal/g) and constitutes the primary source of calories in the TPN admixture. Glucose is required for phagocytosis and is an excellent cardiac fuel, capable of increasing cardiac output when administered in conjunction with insulin and potassium. Parenterally administered glucose has one of four metabolic fates:

1. Burning, or oxidization.
2. Becoming part of a tightly regulated serum pool.
3. Nonoxidative disposal by being converted to glycogen in the liver, cardiac muscle, or skeletal muscle.
4. Nonoxidative disposal by being directly converted to fat in the liver.*

Central, or hepatic, insulin resistance is common in severely stressed patients and is characterized by the reduced capacity of insulin to inhibit hepatic gluconeogenesis. Peripheral insulin resistance reduces the ability of skeletal muscle from participating fully in the uptake of metabolic fuels. Owing to these factors, the dextrose content of the initial TPN solution should be minimal, 50 to 150 g of dextrose per day, depending on whether or not hyperglycemia is present. TPN should not be initiated until hyperglycemia has been adequately controlled (<220 mg/dL) with either a subcutaneously administered insulin sliding scale or a continuous insulin drip.

Once euglycemia has been achieved (insulin added to the TPN formula or an insulin drip run if necessary), the dextrose load can be increased by 50 g/day. Optimal glycemia control is a serum glucose value of 150 to 180 mg/dL. Insulin can be added to the parenteral formula as the dextrose content is advanced to maintain glycemia control. For metabolically labile patients, patients with unpredictable subcutaneous absorption, or patients who require excessive doses of insulin, an accessory insulin infusion is appropriate.

The route of insulin administration should follow the route of dextrose delivery; parenterally administered dextrose is best managed with intravenous regular insulin (as a drip or as part of the nutrient admixture), whereas enterally administered dextrose is best managed with a subcutaneous, long-acting

*A minor glucose disposal pathway in normal humans (<1% of daily energy expenditure), de novo lipogenesis becomes an increasingly important pathway with excessive administration of parenteral glucose calories (glucose calories > BEE) and in disease states, including critical illness, cirrhosis, and AIDS.[40]

Table 80–5. Incidence of Hyperglycemia in Nondiabetic Patients Receiving Total Parenteral Nutrition

Rate of Dextrose Infusion	Incidence (%)
<4 (mg/kg/min), 24 kcal/kg	0
4.1–5, >24–30 kcal/kg	11
>5, >30 kcal/kg	49

Data from Rosemarin D, Wardlow G, Mirtallo J: Hyperglycemia with high continuous infusion rates of total parenteral nutrition glucose. Nutr Clin Pract 1996; 11:151.

variety. When one is advancing the dextrose content of TPN, the insulin-dextrose ratio of the previous bag should serve as a guide. Diabetic patients who require TPN require more than 100% of their usual insulin needs once they receive their calorie goal.

Most critically ill patients do not tolerate, nor do they require, more than 400 g of dextrose per day. Rates of dextrose infusion of 4 mg/kg/min (~ 400 g/day for a 70-kg man) should be considered the upper limit of parenteral dextrose infusion; however, most patients require considerably fewer calories than this.[41] Increasing the rate of infusion can lead to hyperglycemia and de novo lipogenesis with its ensuing metabolic complications (hepatic steatosis, early hypertransaminemia, late hyperbilirubinemia, elevation of the respiratory quotient above 1, and increased work of breathing (Table 80–5).[33] With the current practice of modest calorie provision and the use of mixed fuels (lipid-containing TPN admixtures) to decrease hepatic lipogenesis, this process is becoming more rare. Intrahepatic cholestasis and shock liver are two conditions commonly encountered in critically ill patients. These processes can mimic de novo lipogenesis. Clinical acumen should suggest the correct diagnosis in such situations, avoiding inappropriate discontinuation of TPN in such patients, who typically are unstable and difficult to feed enterally.

When one is calculating the total dextrose calories supplied to a patient, medications and drips using 5% dextrose in water (D_5W) as a vehicle, which can amount to substantial volume and dextrose loads in some ICU patients, should be carefully evaluated and included in the calorie calculations.

LIPID

Lipid metabolism during stress is a complex and incompletely understood process. Consequently, lipid administration as part of the parenteral formula remains controversial. Currently available lipid emulsions in the United States are composed solely of long-chain triglycerides (LCTs) and provide 9 kcal/g. Because they are supplied as 20% emulsions, parenteral lipids are actually less calorie-dense than parenteral dextrose solutions. When administered improperly, lipid emulsions:

1. Inhibit the reticuloendothelial system and impair phagocyte function, particularly that of Kupffer cells.[42]
2. Worsen oxygenation in the adult respiratory distress syndrome (ARDS).[43]
3. Carry an infectious risk when administered separately over a prolonged time (lipid emulsions by themselves serve as an excellent culture medium but are bactericidal once mixed with hypertonic dextrose solutions).
4. Promote production of immunosuppressive eicosanoid derivatives.

To avoid these untoward effects, the rate of lipid administration for a severely stressed patient should never exceed 0.11 g/kg/hour and should remain below 20% of the total calories delivered.[7] For an ICU patient, 20 to 40 g of lipid per day is typical.

The potential beneficial effects of parenteral lipid administration are:

1. A decrease in de novo lipogenesis.
2. A decrease in the dextrose administered to diabetic patients and potentially better glycemia control.
3. Enhanced protein sparing if coadministered with sufficient protein.
4. Prevention of essential fatty acid deficiency.*
5. A reduction of the parenteral admixture's osmolarity and, consequently, its phlebitic potential.
6. A decrease in carbon dioxide production and thus reduction of the respiratory quotient.

Total nutrient admixtures (3-in-1 formulations) should be used whenever possible because continuous lipid administration avoids many of the immunosuppressive associations of bolus lipid infusions and may reduce the incidence of glucose-associated complications. Serum triglyceride levels should be checked periodically after administration of parenteral lipid emulsions and the lipid component of the TPN discontinued if this level rises above 400 to 500 mg/dL. Although not available in the United States, alternative forms of lipids, including medium-chain triglycerides (MCTs) and omega-3 fatty acids (fish oil), are under investigation for parenteral use.

ELECTROLYTES

Electrolytes are administered as components of the parenteral formula on the basis of need, and there are no "standard" doses. Electrolytes are given to replenish deficits, make up for ongoing losses, and effect a change in the patient's electrochemical milieu (i.e., influence acid-base homeostasis or elevate a cation concentration to influence cardiac function). A thorough daily accounting of fluid losses and an understanding of fluid composition is imperative (Table 80–6).

In addition to the guidelines for administration already mentioned, sodium is given to influence intravascular volume status. Sodium is given liberally when volume expansion is desired and is restricted for intravascularly overexpanded patients (those in congestive heart failure or renal failure).

Chloride, while a dependent anion that follows sodium and potassium shifts and losses, is very important in relation to a patient's acid-base homeostasis. Large chloride losses, as in nasogastric tube output or large bowel diarrhea, can lead to the development of metabolic alkalosis. If patients are kept in chloride balance (losses = replacement), this disturbance does not occur. Mild metabolic alkalosis may respond to chloride repletion with either the sodium or potassium salt (as long as serum sodium and potassium concentrations permit). Once the serum pH rises above 7.50 in a patient with metabolic alkalosis, when a patient has a chloride-unresponsive alkalosis (e.g., secondary to steroid administration), or when the serum sodium or potassium concentration does not permit administration of moderate amounts of sodium or potassium chloride, use of 0.1 M hydrochloric acid (HCl) is required. HCl is a safe and effective method of treating metabolic alkaloses. Usually 50 to 100 mEq/L is delivered per day, and venous or arterial blood gases are followed to monitor effect. HCl should not be utilized to treat pure respiratory alkalosis. Concentrations of HCl greater than 0.1 M should not be used, as they can cause central venous catheter damage. HCl is absolutely contraindi-

*This rare entity is difficult to produce in stressed patients owing to their elevated catechol levels, which promote lipolysis (adipose stores contain EFAs).

TABLE 80–6. Composition of Gastrointestinal Secretions*

Source	Approximate Volume (mL/24 hr)	Secretion (mEq/L)			
		Sodium	Potassium	Chloride	Bicarbonate
Saliva	1500 (500–2000)	8 (2–10)	26 (20–30)	10 (8–20)	30
Stomach	1500 (500–4000)	60 (10–116)	7 (0–30)	120 (8–150)	0
Gallbladder	400 (50–800)	145 (135–155)	5 (3–10)	100 (83–110)	35 (20–45)
Pancreas	1500 (200–2000)	140 (110–185)	5 (3–10)	25 (55–95)	70 (50–110)
Ileum	3000	140	5	104	50 (40–140)
Colon	250 (100–400)	60	30	40	—

*Numbers in parentheses are ranges.

cated in lipid-containing nutrient admixtures, owing to its ability to "crack" the emulsion and produce potentially lethal fat emboli.

Metabolic acidosis is similarly treated with the addition of sodium and potassium acetate to the parenteral formula. Sodium bicarbonate is incompatible for use in TPN, as it forms insoluble coprecipitates. Bicarbonate salts should never be infused through a common intravenous line with TPN.

MICRONUTRIENTS

Calcium, magnesium, phosphate, and trace elements are typically added to the TPN admixture daily, although the exact parenteral requirements have not been clearly elucidated. Typical doses of calcium (administered as calcium gluconate) and magnesium (administered as magnesium sulfate) supplementation are approximately 10 mEq/day for each, which should maintain normal serum concentrations in the absence of excessive losses. Approximately half of serum calcium is bound to albumin, and stressed, hypoalbuminemic patients have falsely depressed serum calcium concentrations. The ionized (physiologically active) calcium measurement is more useful in this setting.

The usual parenteral daily supplement of phosphorus is 30 to 40 mmol/day. It is administered as the sodium or potassium salt, and its maximal rate of delivery should not exceed 1 mmol/kg/day. Phosphorus is essential for building lean tissue and for forming the energy-rich phosphates that fuel metabolism. Omission of phosphorus from the parenteral formula can lead to cardiac dysfunction and even death. Phosphorus should be excluded only when the measured serum concentration is high (as in renal failure). An inverse relationship exists between calcium and phosphorus, and administration of one can depress the serum concentration of the other. Many clinical states (e.g., renal failure) and medications (e.g., steroids and diuretics) affect serum calcium, magnesium, and phosphorus concentrations. Daily administration should be based on serum concentrations.

While many micronutrient disorders can be treated appropriately with the TPN admixture, when large doses of minerals are required to correct a disturbance a secondary infusion should be used to supplement the TPN additives. In such cases, overcorrection of the disorder can be avoided by discontinuing the piggyback infusion instead of discarding the entire TPN bag.

Trace elements are added daily. Replacement is largely empirical. Serum zinc and iron levels can be decreased during stress as part of the metabolic response to injury. Zinc is an important cofactor in numerous enzymatic reactions and plays an important role in wound healing. Large zinc losses can be expected with high gastrointestinal output (e.g., those resulting from ileostomy or fistula). Approximately 10 mg of zinc is lost per liter of diarrhea. Each day 5 to 20 mg of zinc can be added to the TPN admixture. Supplemental iron, on the other hand, is added to the TPN admixture only when iron deficiency anemia is detected. Parenteral iron should not be used to treat the hypoferremia of stress, as it can increase oxidative injury, promote bacterial growth, and worsen sepsis.

Finally, although rarely seen in stressed hospitalized patients, vitamin deficiencies do occur when supplementation is not provided. Perhaps the most striking example of such a deficiency is the lactic acidosis seen when thiamine has been omitted from the parenteral admixture.[44] This has occasionally resulted in death. A multivitamin containing the 12 essential vitamins is added daily to the TPN admixture. Vitamin K (10 mg) is given separately, once a week by subcutaneous injection, to avoid deficiency of this fat-soluble vitamin (unless contraindicated). Critically ill patients who are receiving antibiotics are especially at risk for coagulopathy secondary to vitamin K deficiency owing to alterations in the normal gastrointestinal flora.

CENTRAL VENOUS LINES: INSERTION, MAINTENANCE, AND COMPLICATIONS

TPN delivery requires central venous access, most often in the subclavian or internal jugular vein. The subclavian vein is the preferred site of central access because of improved dressing care that may reduce infectious complications. ICU patients often already have central venous lines (CVLs); thus, catheter insertion and its attendant risks are obviated. Although a new, dedicated noncontaminated catheter is preferred, TPN may be infused through any available central line, including the venous infusion port (VIP) of a pulmonary artery catheter.

The two most common problems related to CVLs that arise once access has been established are catheter-related infection and central venous thrombosis. The incidence of CVL infection is usually reduced by a nutrition support service whose dedicated nurses provide improved dressing and line care.[45] Appropriate administration of TPN by itself does not increase the incidence of line infections. Line infections are prevented by strict aseptic insertion technique and proper line care. Patients receiving TPN who demonstrate fever, increased white blood cell count, or hyperglycemia may have a CVL infection. Blood for culture should be obtained, peripherally and centrally, and the catheter should be exchanged over a guide wire and its tip sent for culture. Finally, routine catheter exchange is not performed unless for specific clinical indications.

A second major complication associated with CVLs is catheter-related thrombosis. Unless otherwise contraindicated, heparin is added daily to the parenteral admixture in doses ranging from 3000 to 12,000 units/day, to reduce this risk.[46] The primary goal is to raise the partial thromboplastin time to the high normal range (28 to 30 seconds). This dose should be reduced to 3000 units per day in patients with 50,000 to 100,000 platelets per deciliter and is discontinued when platelet counts fall below 50,000.[47] Doses larger than 12,000 units have been associated with partial thromboplastin time prolongation and may cause bleeding. Patients with a partial thromboplastin time of less than 25 seconds are at especially high risk for catheter-related central venous thrombosis. Patients with inflammatory bowel disease, obesity, pancreatitis, or cancer; women receiving estrogen replacement therapy; and smokers fit into this category and often require larger than usual doses of heparin.

TOTAL PARENTERAL NUTRITION ADDITIVES

Use of the TPN admixture for drug delivery has its advantages. First, this practice is cost effective because materials and personnel time can be eliminated when drugs are added to the TPN admixture. Second, the addition of drugs to the TPN solution eliminates volume that the patient would typically receive from piggybacked intravenous solutions. Third, violations of the CVL ports are minimized, which likely decreases the incidence of catheter-related infections. Last, the continuous infusion of certain medications (e.g., histamine H_2 antagonists) produces steady-state drug levels that may enhance drug efficacy and reduce drug interactions.[48]

Histamine H_2 receptor antagonists are routinely used in the care of critically ill ICU patients and can be added directly to the TPN admixture. Benefits include prevention and treatment of stress-related gastritis, reduction of nasogastric tube losses, and decreases in small-bowel and ostomy losses. Finally, regular insulin, metoclopramide, aminophylline, and steroids are occasionally added to the TPN admixture.

OBESITY AND CRITICAL ILLNESS

Obesity in a critically ill patient deserves special discussion. Obesity (weight 30% > ideal body weight or BMI > 30) and morbid obesity (weight 100 pounds > ideal body weight or BMI > 40) significantly increase morbidity and mortality from critical illness.[49] Stressed obese patients lose lean body mass and fat stores just as do nonobese patients, leading to PCM. For nonstressed obese patients, a protein-sparing modified diet has been employed for weight loss. A modification of this approach (moderately hypocaloric TPN) has been developed for obese critically ill patients: protein supplied in normal "stress" amounts (1.5 g/kg of adjusted ideal body weight/day), and total calories are provided at approximately 500 kcal less than the expected resting energy expenditure.[50] Obese patients have large depots of adipose tissue (which also contain EFAs) that are easily mobilized during times of stress. An optimal protein synthetic response can thus be achieved with about 1500 kcals.[1] The lower carbohydrate intake is less likely to precipitate hyperglycemia, and endogenous fatty acids are released to make up the calorie gap. Finally, lipids are not usually administered unless hyperglycemia supervenes.

SUMMARY

TPN can provide nutritional and metabolic support for critically ill patients. Through the provision of total nutrient admixtures, the net protein breakdown that accompanies the stress response can be reduced by promoting synthesis. Furthermore, TPN helps to preserve host defenses, lean body mass, and visceral organ function and can maintain the proper metabolic and electrochemical milieu in critically ill patients. Despite the appeal of the adage "more is better," parenteral calorie delivery should not exceed energy expenditure. Appropriate nutritional support as part of the overall ICU schema for critically ill patients may shorten length of stay in the ICU and decrease morbidity, the ultimate goal being improved survival.[51]

References

1. Daley B, Cahill S, Driscoll D, et al: Parenteral and enteral nutrition. *In:* Gastrointestinal Pharmacotherapy. Wolfe M (Ed). Philadelphia, WB Saunders, 1993, pp 293–316.
2. Sternberg J, Bistrian BR: Nutrition support in the patient with gastrointestinal disease. *In*: Therapy of Digestive Disorders. Wolfe M (Ed). Philadelphia, WB Saunders. (in press).
3. Wolfe RR, Herndon DN, Jahoor F, et al: Effect of severe burn injury on substrate cycling by glucose an fatty acids. N Engl J Med 1987; 317:403.
4. McClave SA, Mitoraj TE, Thielmeier KA, et al: Differentiating subtypes (hypoalbuminemic vs. marasmic) of protein-calorie malnutrition: Incidence and clinical significance in a university hospital setting. J Parenter Enteral Nutr 1992; 4:337.
5. Bistrian B, Blackburn G, Hallowell E, et al: Protein nutritional status of general surgical patients. JAMA 1974; 230:858.
6. Bistrian B, Blackburn G, Vitale J, et al: Prevalence of malnutrition in general medical patients. JAMA 1976; 235:1567.
7. APEX: The preceptorship for excellence in parenteral nutritional support. *In*: Health Management Solutions. Bristan BR (Ed). Norwalk, Conn, 1996.
8. Streat S, Beddoe A, Hill G: Aggressive nutritional support does not prevent protein loss despite fat gain in septic intensive care patients. J Trauma 1987; 27:262.
9. Wolfe RR, Goodenough RD, Burke JF: Response of protein and urea kinetics in burn patients to different levels of protein intake. Ann Surg 1983; 197:163.
10. Rodriguez DJ, Clevenger FW, Osler TM, et al: Obligatory negative nitrogen balance following spinal cord injury. JPEN J Parenter Enteral Nutr 1991; 15:319.
11. Shikora S: Nutrition support for the critically ill. *In*: Nutrition Support: Theory & Therapeutics. Shikora S, Blackburn GL (Eds). New York, Chapman and Hall, 1997, pp 464–485.
12. Pomposelli J, Bistrian B: Is TPN immunosuppressive? New Horiz 1994; 2:224.
13. Zaloga G, Roberts P: Permissive underfeeding. New Horiz 1994; 2:257.
14. Stack J, Babineau T, Bistrian B: Assessment of nutritional status in clinical practice. Gastroenterologist 1996; 4:S8.
15. Frisancho AR: Triceps skinfold and upper arm muscle size norms for assessment of nutritional status. Am J Clin Nutr 1974; 27:1052.
16. Frisancho AR: New norms of upper limb fat and muscle areas for assessment of nutritional status. Am J Clin Nutr 1981; 34:2540.
17. Foley EF, Borlase BC, Benotti PN, et al: Albumin therapy in the critically ill. Arch Surg 1990; 125:739.
18. Doweiko JP, Bistrian BR: The effect of glycosylated albumin on platelet aggregation. JPEN J Parenter Enteral Nutr 1994; 18:516.
19. Eisenstein C, Van Way CW III: Nutritional assessment. *In*: Handbook of Surgical Nutrition. Van Way CW III (Ed). Philadelphia, JB Lippincott, 1992, pp 107–118.
20. Klein S, Kinney J, Jeejeebhoy K, et al: Nutrition support in clinical practice: Review of published data and recommendations for future research directives. JPEN J Parenter Enteral Nutr 1997; 21:133.
21. Smith-Choban P, Max MH: Feeding jejunostomy: A small bowel stress test? Am J Surg 1988; 155:112.
22. Babineau TJ, Hernandez E, Forse RA, et al: Symptomatic hyperlipasemia after cardiopulmonary bypass: Implications for enteral nutritional support. Nutrition 1993; 9:237.
23. Sedman P, Macfie J, Palmer M, et al: Preoperative parenteral nutrition is not associated with mucosal atrophy or bacterial translocation in humans. Br J Surg 1991; 82:1663.
24. Sedman P, Macfie J, Sagar P, et al: The prevalence of gut translocation in humans. Gastroenterology 1994; 107:643.
25. Buchman AL, Mestecky J, Moukarzel A, et al: Intestinal immune function is unaffected by parenteral nutrition in man. J Am Coll Nutr 1995; 14:656.
26. Alpers DH, Stenson WF: Does total parenteral nutrition–induced intestinal mucosal atrophy occur in humans and can it be affected

by enteral supplements? Curr Opin Gastroenterol 1996; 12:169-173.
27. Babineau TJ, Swails W, Stewart S, et al: Nutritional support of patients following cardiopulmonary bypass: Required modifications of the TPN solution. Crit Care Med 1995; 23:A101.
28. Hunter D, Jaksic T, Lewis D, et al: Resting energy expenditure in the critically ill: Estimations versus measurement. Br J Surg 1988; 75:875.
29. Frankenfield D, Omert L, Badellino M, et al: Correlation between measured energy expenditure and clinically obtained variables in trauma and sepsis patients. JPEN J Parenter Enteral Nutr 1994; 18:398.
30. Blackburn GL, Bistrian BR, Maini BS: Nutritional and metabolic assessment of the hospitalized patient. J Parenter Enteral Nutr 1977; 1:11.
31. McMahon M, Bistrian B: The physiology of nutritional assessment and therapy in protein-calorie malnutrition. Disease A Month 1990; 7:375.
32. Van Way CW III: Nutritional support in the injured patient. Surg Clin North Am 1991; 71:537.
33. Rosemarin D, Wardlow G, Mirtallo J: Hyperglycemia with high continuous infusion rates of total parenteral nutrition glucose. Nutr Clin Pract 1996; 11:151.
34. Kwuon M, Ling P, Lyndon E, et al: Immunologic effects of acute hyperglycemia in non-diabetic rats. JPEN J Parenter Enteral Nutr 1997; 21:91.
35. Hostetter M: Handicaps to host defense: Effects of hyperglycemia on C_3 and *Candida albicans*. Diabetes 1990; 39:271.
36. Pomposelli J, Baxter J, Babineau T, et al: Early postoperative glucose control predicts nosocomial infection rate in diabetic patients. JPEN J Parenter Enteral Nutr 1998; 22:77.
37. Shaw JHF, Wildbore M, Wolfe RR: Whole body protein kinetics in severely septic patients: The response to glucose infusion and total parenteral nutrition. Ann Surg 1987; 205:288.
38. McCowen KC, Chan S, Bistrian BR: Total parenteral support. Curr Opin Gastroenterol 1998; 14:157.
39. Ziegler TR, Young LS, Benfell K, et al: Clinical and metabolic efficacy of glutamine-supplemented parenteral nutrition after bone marrow transplantation: A randomized, double blind, controlled study. Ann Intern Med 1992; 116:821.
40. Hellerstein M, Schwarz J, Neese R: Regulation of de novo lipogenesis in humans. Annu Rev Nutr 1996; 16:523.
41. Wolfe R, O'Donnell T, Stone M, et al: Investigation of factors determining the optimal glucose infusion rate in total parenteral nutrition. Metabolism 1980; 29:892.
42. Seidner DL, Mascioli EA, Istan NW, et al: The effects of long chain triglyceride emulsions on reticuloendothelial system function in humans. JPEN J Parenter Enteral Nutr 1989; 13:614.
43. Bistrian BR: Novel lipid sources in parenteral and enteral nutrition. Proc Nutr Soc 1997; 56:1.
44. Centers for Disease Control and Prevention (CDC): Lactic acidosis traced to thiamine deficiency related to nationwide shortages of multivitamins for total parenteral nutrition. JAMA 1997; 278:109.
45. Nelson DB, Kien CL, Mohr B, et al: Dressing changes by specialized personnel reduce infection rates in patients receiving central venous parenteral nutrition. JPEN J Parenter Enteral Nutr 1986; 10:220.
46. Imperial J, Bistrian BR, Bothe A, et al: Limitation of central vein thrombosis in parenteral nutrition by continuous infusion of low dose heparin. J Am Coll Nutr 1983; 2:263.
47. Driscoll DF, Blackburn GL: Total parenteral nutrition 1990: A review of its current status in hospitalized patients, and the need for patient-specific feedings. Drugs 1990; 40:346.
48. Driscoll DF, Lowell JA, Nompleggi D, et al: Continuous versus intermittent cimetidine infusion in critically ill hospitalized patients: Role of TPN admixture as drug vehicle. Nutrition 1990; 6:383.
49. Hubert HB, Feinleib M, McNamara PM, et al: Obesity as an independent risk factor for cardiovascular disease: 26 year follow-up of participants in the Framingham Heart Study. Circulation 1983; 67:968.
50. Baxter J, Bistrian B: Moderately hypocaloric parenteral nutrition in the critically ill obese patient. Nutr Clin Pract 1989; 4:133.
51. Heyland DK, MacDonald S, Keefe L, et al: Total parenteral nutrition in the critically ill patient. JAMA 1998; 280:2008.

81

Pediatric Enteral and Parenteral Surgical Nutrition

Walter J. Chwals, MD

Practitioners have long recognized the crucial role of nutrition in the proper growth and development of the healthy child. In recent years, research in this area has focused more on the special needs of the premature infant as technological advances in neonatal support have made possible the survival of neonates much earlier in gestation. Furthermore, an improved understanding of the particular needs of the metabolically stressed infant, which, in many respects, are different from those of the older child or adult, has led to altered strategies in the nutritional resuscitation of these children. Because injury itself, as well as the disease processes that frequently necessitate intensive care, visits a metabolic insult, a thorough understanding of the unique features of the injury response in infants and children and the therapeutic considerations that may best support the child during this period are an important responsibility of the pediatric practitioner. Improvement in mortality and morbidity in this population of patients certainly rests, in large part, on the better understanding of these principles.

This chapter addresses the special considerations that should be taken into account in treating critically ill infants and children after acute injury in contrast to the metabolic and nutritional needs of the healthy child. Specific attention is also directed to the particular needs of the premature infant.

BODY COMPOSITION, FLUID, AND ELECTROLYTE HOMEOSTASIS

Perinatal Body Composition Alterations

During gestation, total body water (TBW) decreases and extracellular fluid (ECF)/intracellular fluid (ICF) compartment ratios increase as a proportion of total body weight (i.e., TBW decreases from 90% to 80% during gestation, equals about 73% in the 10-day-old neonate, and decreases to 60% in the adult). During the first week of life, the newborn infant loses about 5% TBW (78% decreases to 73% TBW) as a result of diuresis, which accounts for an overall weight loss during this period, even as the child is growing. TBW losses continue gradually, decreasing to 60% of total body weight by 18 months of life. These changes are accompanied by a relative increase in ICF (20% at 20 weeks of gestation, 35% at birth, and 40% at 18 months relative to total body weight) and a concomitant decrease in ECF (60% at 20 weeks of gestation, 45% at birth, and 20% at 18 months relative to total body weight.

Preterm infants are born with relatively high percentages of TBW and ECF compared with term infants. The process of eliminating this excess water and solute, which would normally occur during weeks to months in utero, is accelerated and occurs within a matter of days to weeks postnatally. Infants with earlier gestational age require a greater amount of postnatal time to achieve the equivalent fluid compartment ratios of term infants. Both premature and term infants require an initial period of physiologic diuresis and weight loss to remove excess TBW and solute. Replacing fluid lost during this physiologic diuresis can lead to volume excess, especially in premature infants. Even in the face of excess fluid administration, however, preterm infants can regulate renal water and sodium excretion to complete this elimination process (up to 140 mL/kg/day).[2]

Studies show that excess intravenous fluids in premature infants may alter the clinical outcome by increasing the incidence of patent ductus arteriosus, left ventricular failure and congestive heart failure, respiratory distress syndrome, bronchopulmonary dysplasia, and necrotizing enterocolitis. In infants who weigh less than 1500 g, the period of diuresis-associated weight loss extends through the first 2 weeks of life and primarily involves volume decrease within the ECF compartment (plasma volume remains constant). Preterm infants may tolerate fluid restriction better than fluid excess owing to changes that appear to affect primarily the interstitial fluid space. The clinical strategy is toward more conservative fluid management.

The total body content of the major extracellular electrolytes (especially sodium and chloride) decreases in proportion to the changes in the ECF/ICF compartment ratio during the first week of life. Increased urinary sodium excretion results in a negative sodium balance and may be the physiologic mechanism involved in initiating postnatal diuresis. Increasing the sodium content of intravenous fluids does not reduce this fluid contraction but instead results in increased sodium excretion.[3] In addition, infants of older gestational age but with intrauterine growth retardation have compartmental water volumes similar to those of less mature infants of the same birth weight.[4] They also undergo a mandatory physiologic diuresis, and replacement of this volume should not be calculated into their fluid requirements.

Perinatal Fluid and Sodium Regulation

Most of the regulatory mechanisms for volume status change respond to the plasma compartment and are a function of developmental maturation. A sensitive, low-pressure cardiopulmonary reflex exists during the first week of life. This mechanism leads to increased sodium excretion during periods of hypervolemia, and its sensitivity diminishes with postnatal development.[5] The immature juxtaglomerular apparatus responds to decreased perfusion by releasing renin; as the infant matures, the trigger pressure increases.[6]

The immature kidney has an elevated fractional excretion of sodium (FE_{Na}). This can be seen in the differences between preterm and term neonatal kidneys and between term neonatal kidneys and those of older children.[7] As the kidney matures, the ratio of glomeruli to distal tubules decreases, leading to a decrease in FE_{Na}. Sympathetic nervous input to the kidney, which would normally decrease sodium excretion, is attenuated in the immediate postnatal period. Despite the increased excretion of sodium, the immature kidney has a lower capacity to excrete a sodium load owing to a decrease in tubular Na^+, K^+-ATPase activity and functional immaturity of the tubular basolateral cell membranes.[8] Dopamine infusion increases glomerular filtration rate and sodium excretion to a similar degree in adults and neonates. The renin-angiotensin system is active and well developed in the neonate; however, the immature kidney is less responsive to exogenous aldosterone.

The difficulty involved in managing postnatal fluids, especially in premature neonates, relates to the balance between the physiologic need for diuresis and the functional immaturity of the kidney, which primarily regulates this process. Premature infants have a decreased glomerular filtration rate and concentrating capacity. In contrast to the volume-loaded preterm infant kidney, which can adequately clear free water, the inefficient concentrating capability of the immature kidney necessitates adequate volume replacement during periods of dehydration, and a delicate balance must be maintained.

Insensible Water Loss

Water loss in neonates and infants can be divided into insensible water loss, excretion of renal solute, water loss in stool, and water and electrolytes lost during normal homeostasis. Insensible losses are free water losses that occur through the skin and respiratory tract. The rate of loss through the respiratory tract is dependent on tidal volume, respiratory rate, temperature, and the humidity of inspired and expired air. In term and near-term infants (more than 32 weeks of gestation), respiratory losses can account for up to one third of insensible losses. Although infants have greater insensible losses at earlier gestational ages, respiratory losses in this population are proportionally less owing to increased loss through the skin.

In all infants, regardless of age, transepithelial water loss (TEWL) makes up most insensible losses. The degree of TEWL varies inversely with body weight and age. Younger infants have a higher ratio of body surface area to body weight. Environmental factors also play a significant role. Use of radiant warmers and phototherapy can increase temperature and decrease humidity, exacerbating evaporative losses. Extremely low birth weight infants have a poorly developed insulating white fat layer and skin that is not yet keratinized, allowing increased cutaneous loss of free water. In infants, TEWL can be reduced significantly during transport by use of an impermeable plastic cover. Fever can increase insensible losses by about 7 mL/kg/day for each degree above 37.2°C (99°F). In very low birth weight infants, TEWL can exceed the volume of fluid excreted by the kidneys, but transcutaneous losses decrease steadily as postnatal age increases. Free water should be used to replace insensible losses. Complications of fluid loss include hyperosmolality, which can lead to an increased risk of intracerebral hemorrhage.

Tables are available to aid in estimating TEWL in neonatal patients. These use either weight or postnatal and gestational age to compare the amount of TEWL in the respective groups. The simplest of these tables estimates TEWL at 30 to 60 mL/kg/day for neonates who weigh less than 1500 g, and 15 to 35 mL/kg/day in neonates who weigh more than 1500 g.[9]

Body Fat

The body fat compartment is generated during the last 2 months of gestation and reaches about 10% of total body weight at term. Most body fat is contained in *white adipose tissue,* which serves as an insulating blanket against energy loss and for the storage of caloric energy. A second type of fat is stored as *brown adipose tissue* (BAT), which can compose up to 10% of total body fat at term. Infants with intrauterine growth retardation have markedly reduced total body fat, exhibited by decreased skinfold thickness and ponderal index, defined as birth weight in grams times 100, divided by body length in centimeters.[10] Ponderal index and skinfold thickness correlate with lean body mass in premature and neonatal infants. As gestational age increases in both small-for-gestational age (SGA) and appropriate-for-gestational age (AGA) infants, there is a significant decrease in percentage of lean body mass relative to total body weight, indicating increased adipose tissue stores.

Infants undergo a tremendous temperature shock at birth, coming from a protected thermoneutral environment into the cool surroundings of the external world. To survive, evolution has provided a means by which infants can generate heat and maintain their temperature. Two mechanisms exist by which an infant can generate heat. These are shivering thermogenesis, in which muscle contraction generates heat, and nonshivering thermogenesis, which is due to the presence of BAT.

BAT can generate large amounts of heat and can convert thyroxine to triiodothyronine (T_3). Biochemically, BAT is identical to white fat, except for the presence of thermogenin, an uncoupling protein that allows BAT to generate heat.[11] In infants, BAT makes up 1% to 2% of birth weight and is concentrated in the axillary and perirenal areas. During periods of cooling, there is a rapid redistribution of cardiac output, resulting in increased blood flow to the BAT. Excess energy used to generate heat can rapidly lead to a depletion of energy stores needed for homeostasis, and BAT is strongly dependent on an adequate supply of lipids. Even routine nursing procedures performed on the premature infant in an incubator can lead to a temperature drop as great as 2 to 3°C, requiring up to 2 hours for restoration of thermoneutrality.[12]

At birth, human infants are completely dependent on nonshivering thermogenesis for maintaining body temperature. The onset of nonshivering thermogenesis is delayed by a placental factor that is thought to inhibit thermogenin. As this factor disappears during the first few days of neonatal life, there is a gradual increase in BAT thermogenin activity. As the BAT is slowly replaced by white adipose tissue, the infant becomes dependent on shivering thermogenesis.

Very premature infants carry out nonshivering thermogenesis poorly because of inadequate BAT stores (which develop during the last 3 months of gestation). Full-term infants can keep their body temperature at a level much higher than that of the environment, whereas premature infants tend to be more poikilothermic. The rate of lipid depletion in BAT and the loss of nonshivering thermogenesis capability are accelerated in malnourished and sick infants.

Maintenance Fluids and Electrolytes

Maintenance intravenous fluids and electrolytes are the amounts of fluids and solutes required for basal needs and to replace the usual daily losses from the respiratory, integumentary, gastrointestinal, and genitourinary systems.

Maintenance fluid volume replacement can be estimated by the use of data in Table 81-1. The infant liver, especially in the premature baby, is low in glycogen reserves, and replacement with 10% dextrose in quarter-normal saline is recommended to provide some carbohydrate calorie supplement for the brain. In infants older than 1 year of age, 5% dextrose in half-normal saline is an appropriate choice for maintenance. Both neonates and older infants should have about 2 mEq/kg/day of potassium added to their maintenance fluids to replace daily potassium losses. These maintenance fluid estimates should be reduced in the first 2 to 5 days of life owing to the neonate's physiologic need for diuresis. This principle is countered by the increase in TEWL in the very premature neonate. Although there is some controversy, a general fluid-replacement guideline would be to deliver 70 to 80 mL/kg/day for near-term and term newborns during the first week of life.

With earlier gestational age, increases in maintenance fluid needs are appropriate in the first several days of life. After this initial period of physiologic diuresis, maintenance should be calculated on the basis of Table 81-1. The loss of water and electrolytes in stool is usually negligible unless diarrhea is present. The presence of significant emesis or daily nasogastric tube losses should be accounted for in calculating replacement fluids. Daily fistula losses and other surgical drainage also need to be calculated into maintenance requirements. These losses should be accurately measured and replaced on a volume-to-volume basis with appropriate fluids. Electrolyte losses may be calculated after results are obtained from the analysis of electrolytes of an aliquot from the drainage site multiplied by 24-hour output.

TABLE 81–1. Estimation of Maintenance Fluid Requirements

Body Weight	Fluid
First 10 kg	100 (mL/kg/day)
Second 10 kg	50 (mL/kg/day)
Each additional kg	20 (mL/kg/day)

TABLE 81–2. Electrolyte Composition of Gastrointestinal Fluids

Fluid	Na^+ (mEq/L)	K^+ (mEq/L)	Cl^- (mEq/L)	HCO_3^- (mEq/L)
Saliva	10	26	10	30
Stomach	60	10	130	—
Duodenum	140	5	80	—
Bile	145	5	100	35
Pancreas	140	5	75	115
Ileum	140	5	104	30
Colon	60	30	40	—

Table 81-2 provides the electrolyte composition of the commonly encountered gastrointestinal fluids. Gastric losses proximal to the pylorus contain sodium, chloride, potassium, and hydrogen ion. The hydrogen ion concentration [H^+] is 100 mEq/L at a pH of 1.0, 10 mEq/L at a pH of 2.0, and so on, in a logarithmic fashion. Because an infant's gastric pH is usually 3.0 to 4.0, gastric electrolyte losses can be replaced readily with half-normal to normal saline containing 10 mEq of potassium chloride per liter. Intestinal losses distal to the pylorus are ultrafiltrates of plasma and are readily replaced with a balanced salt solution such as lactated Ringer's. Urinary loss of sodium is about 2 to 3 mEq/kg/day, with a loss of potassium of 1 to 2 mEq/kg/day. Usual daily maintenance replacement should include 3 to 4 mEq of sodium and 2 mEq of potassium per kilogram in the form of the chloride salts.

NUTRITIONAL REQUIREMENTS AND DELIVERY IN THE HEALTHY CHILD

Nutritional needs can be divided into the general categories of energy, protein, nonprotein, and noncalorie substrate delivery. Amounts in children differ from those in adults, primarily because of increased requirements for growth and activity in children. This is especially true during early infancy when visceral organ growth is rapid and extensive relative to muscle and fat growth.

Energy Requirements

Energy can be partitioned into (1) maintenance metabolic needs (basal metabolic rate, activity, and heat loss to the environment) and (2) growth needs. Energy requirements are age-related and are three to four times higher for infants than for adults (Table 81-3). In healthy, metabolically nonstressed neonates, weight gain occurs when absorbed energy (metabolizable energy) exceeds energy expenditure. Growth increases proportional to the amount of energy delivery greater than 55 to 60 kcal/kg/day (basal metabolic rate).[13] For every 5 kcal excess absorbed, approximately 1 g of new tissue is generated.[14] In term neonates, a goal growth rate of approximately 15 g/kg/day can be achieved with energy delivery of 110 to 120 kcal/kg/day. In low-birth-weight (<1500 g) infants,

TABLE 81–3. Age-Adjusted Nutritional Requirements

Age (yr)	Energy* (kcal/kg/day)	Protein* (g/kg/day)
0–1	120–90	2.5–2.0
1–7	90–75	2.0–1.5
8–12	75–60	1.5
12–18	60–30	1.5–1.0
>18	30–25	1.0

Modified from Wretlind A: Complete intravenous nutrition: Theoretical and experimental background. Nutr Metab 1972; 14(Suppl):1–57; and Fomon SJ: Requirements and recommended dietary intakes of protein during infancy. Pediatr Res 1991; 30:391–395.

*Values on the left in each column indicate requirements at the lowest age interval for healthy, nonstressed subjects.

approximately 150 kcal/kg/day is needed to achieve this weight gain.[14] Normal healthy infants use about 35% to 40% of their daily calorie intake for growth (energy cost of tissue synthesis and energy stored in new tissue) during the first 6 months of life. At 2 years of age, only about 2% to 5% of energy intake is used for this purpose (Fig. 81–1). The basal metabolic rate is about 50 to 55 kcal/kg/day in infancy and gradually declines to about 20 to 25 kcal/kg/day during adolescence.[15]

Protein Requirements

Growth can be expressed in terms of protein accretion, which is the amount of protein generated as new tissue. Nitrogen accounts for approximately 2% of total body weight at birth in contrast to just above 3% in the adult. Most of this difference is made up in the first year of life because of rapid somatic growth. During this first year, the infant increases its body length by twofold and body weight by threefold. Parenchymal growth is particularly accelerated during this period. For instance, the brain mass increases to 60% of its normal adult size during the first year of life. However, energy needs take metabolic precedence, so that protein will be preferentially used as an energy source (even if protein delivery is low) if nonprotein substrate delivery is inadequate to meet energy needs.

In the healthy infant, protein accretion as a function of body weight is highest in the neonate (0.93 g/kg/day) and decreases progressively from that point. Protein accretion is 0.5 g/kg/day during the second and third months of life, 0.26 g/kg/day during the fifth and sixth months of life, 0.18 g/kg/day from 9 to 12 months of age, and 0.08 g/kg/day between 2 and 3 years of age.[16] Protein accretion is dependent on the amount of protein actually absorbed (metabolizable protein), the efficiency of conversion of various dietary proteins into tissue protein (estimated at 90% for breast milk but only 70% for soy protein found in infant formula), and the protein lost during breakdown.

Protein lost because of incomplete enteral absorption and breakdown can be estimated by measuring stool, urine, and skin nitrogen content and is calculated to be approximately 0.95 g/kg/day of protein during the first year of life. Taking these factors into account and allowing for the interpatient variability, the estimated enteral protein requirement is approximately 2.6 g/kg/day during the neonatal period, 2.0 g/kg/day at 2 to 3 months of age, and 1.3 g/kg/day at 1 year of life. Values may be somewhat less for parenteral delivery because of decreased absorptive losses.

In the premature or SGA child, protein needs are proportionately higher (ranging to 3.5 g/kg/day) owing to substantially increased urinary nitrogen losses and increased catch-up growth requirements (~20% higher than the 3.0 g/kg/day needed to support intrauterine growth rates).[17]

Nonprotein Requirements

Most infant formulas provide a relatively balanced delivery of nonprotein calories, in the range of 45% of total calorie intake each for carbohydrate and fat. In the postnatal period, infant metabolism is characterized by a greater dependence on lipid substrate in addition to carbohydrate substrate for energy needs.[18] There is substantial evidence that premature infants, because of impaired fat absorption by immature gut, may benefit from increased concentrations of medium-chain triglycerides (MCTs) in enteral formulas.[19] Carbohydrates remain important as a source of energy for children and are optimally provided in the form of starches, such as those found in cereals, vegetables, and flour.

Noncalorie Requirements

Trace elements are found in relatively small amounts in the diet but are essential for human metabolism. They include iron, zinc, iodine, selenium, copper, manganese, chromium, molybdenum, and cobalt (Table 81–4).

Iron is present in hemoglobin and iron-binding proteins such as myoglobin, transferrin, ferritin, and hemosiderin. It is essential for several important enzymes, including cytochromes and leukocyte myeloperoxidase.[20] The principal function of iron involves oxygen transport.

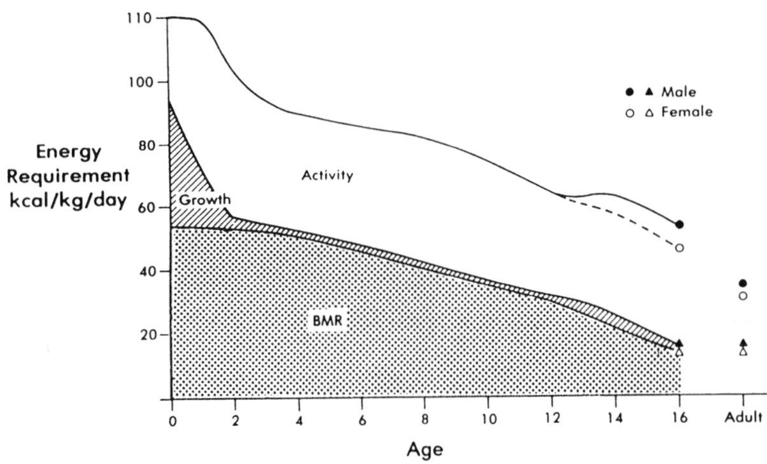

Figure 81–1. Change in energy requirement per kilogram of body weight during growth. BMR = basal metabolic rate. (From Holliday MA: Body composition and energy needs during growth. *In:* Human Growth: A Comprehensive Treatise, 2nd ed. Vol 2: Postnatal Growth Neurobiology. Falkner F, Tanner JM [Eds]. New York, Plenum Publishing, 1986, p 102.)

TABLE 81–4. Recommended Daily Dietary Allowances

		Infants		Children			11–18 yr	
	Nutrient	*<6 mo*	*>6 mo*	*1–3 yr*	*4–6 yr*	*7–10 yr*	*Male*	*Female*
Fat-Soluble	Vitamin A (μg)	375	375	400	500	700	1000	800
	Vitamin D (μg)	7.5	10	10	10	10	10	10
	Vitamin E (μg)	3.0	4.0	6	7	7	10	8
	Vitamin K (μg)	5.0	10	15	20	30	65	55
Water-Soluble	Vitamin C (mg)	30	35	40	45	45	50–60	50–60
	Thiamin (mg)	0.3	0.4	0.7	0.9	1.0	1.5	1.1
	Riboflavin (mg)	0.4	0.5	0.8	1.1	1.2	1.8	1.3
	Niacin (mg)	6.0	6.6	9.0	12	13	20	15
	Vitamin B_6 (mg)	0.3	0.6	1.0	1.1	1.4	2.0	1.4
	Folate (μg)	25	35	50	75	100	200	180
	Vitamin B_{12} (μg)	0.3	0.5	0.7	1.0	1.4	2.0	2.0
	Biotin (μg)	10	15	50	65	120	200	150
Minerals	Calcium (mg)	400	600	800	800	800	1200	1200
	Phosphorus (mg)	300	500	800	800	800	1200	1200
	Magnesium (mg)	40	60	80	120	170	350	280
Trace Elements	Iron (mg)	6	10	10	10	10	12	15
	Zinc (mg)	5	5	10	10	10	15	12
	Iodine (μg)	40	50	70	90	120	150	150
	Selenium (μg)	10	15	20	20	30	70	55
	Copper (mg)	0.5	1.0	1.0	2.0	2.5	2.5	2.5
	Manganese (mg)	0.5	1.0	1.0	2.0	3.0	3.5	3.5
	Chromium (μg)	10	60	60	100	200	200	200
	Molybdenum (μg)	30	80	80	150	300	350	350

Modified from Recommended Dietary Allowances. 10th ed. Washington, DC, National Academy Press, 1989, pp 85–258.

Zinc is an essential cofactor in more than 200 mammalian enzymes. It plays an important role in cell division, growth, wound healing, and immunity.[21] Zinc-dependent enzymes include deoxyribonucleic acid (DNA) and ribonucleic acid (RNA) polymerases, carbonic anhydrase, and alkaline phosphatase. Zinc is transported principally by albumin. Increased supplementation should be considered when gastrointestinal losses are high (e.g., diarrhea, high ostomy output).

Iodine is essential for thyroxine and triiodothyronine function. Deficiency syndromes have not been reported during short-term total parenteral nutrition (TPN), but supplementation is important over the longer term (short-bowel syndrome).

Selenium is essential for glutathione peroxidase function.[22] Deficiencies in children can result in cardiomyopathy. Additional supplementation should be considered if gastrointestinal losses are high. Selenium delivery should be reduced in infants with renal failure.

Copper is an important component of several oxidative enzymes, including ceruloplasmin, cytochrome oxidase, and copper-zinc superoxide dismutase (important antioxidant). Copper requirements increase in association with high jejunal losses. In addition to neutropenia and iron-resistant hypochromic microcytic anemia, copper deficiency in infants results in osteoporosis and retarded bone growth.[23]

Manganese is an important function component of a number of enzymes, such as manganese superoxide dismutase (antioxidant) and pyruvate decarboxylase (important in energy metabolism). Manganese deficiency can impair production of hyaluronic acid, chondroitin sulfate, and other mucopolysaccharides essential for growth and maintenance of connective tissue, cartilage, and bone.[20] Manganese requirements increase in association with high jejunal losses. Because more than 90% is excreted in the bile, patients with cholestatic liver disease should not receive supplementation. Hypermanganesemia has been associated with basal ganglia alterations in infants receiving long-term TPN.[24]

Chromium (trivalent form) is important in the maintenance of adequate glucose tolerance.[25] Although deficiencies have not occurred with short-term TPN, insulin-resistant hyperglycemia has been associated with the use of chromium-free TPN for more than 5 months. Chromium delivery should be reduced in infants with renal failure.

Molybdenum is essential for xanthine oxidase and sulfite oxidase (antioxidants) function.[26] Molybdenum delivery should be reduced in infants with renal failure. Cobalt is an important component of vitamin B_{12}.

Vitamin requirements are listed in Table 81–4. They may be categorized, on the basis of affinity, into fat-soluble (vitamins A, D, E, and K) and water-soluble (vitamins B_1, B_6, B_{12}, C, riboflavin, niacin, folate, and biotin) classes. Vitamin A is important in maintaining vision (retinoic acid metabolism), and deficiencies can result in night blindness, growth retardation, and impaired resistance to infection. Vitamin A intoxication has been associated with increased intracranial pressure in infants.[27] Vitamin D is necessary for normal bone growth and development, and deficiencies have been associated with idiopathic hypocalcemia. Vitamin C and vitamin D requirements are reported to be greater for infants than for older children.[28] In critically ill infants, vitamin C and particularly vitamin E may be beneficial in reducing oxidative stress by facilitating removal of superoxide radicals. These putative benefits have yet to be established clinically; however, one study suggests that vitamin E may reduce the incidence of intraventricular hemorrhage in high-risk neonates.[29] Vitamin K is routinely administered at birth to prevent neonatal coagulopathy.[30] Infants also require increased supplements of calcium, phosphorus, and folate.

Special Considerations in Low-Birth-Weight Infants

The principal goal of protein-calorie nutritional support in low-birth-weight infants is to generate postnatal growth rates that match intrauterine growth. Preterm infants are developmentally immature and have low energy stores in the form of hepatic glycogen content and subcutaneous adipose tissue. Calorie reserves in the 1000-g infant are about 100 kcal/kg/day, in contrast to those of the term baby, which measure 1500 to 1800 kcal/kg/day. It is particularly important to recognize these low energy reserves, especially with early prematurity or SGA infants, because they exist in the fat mass, not as glycogen. There are no glycogen reserves in the neonatal liver. Furthermore, brain tissue is exclusively dependent on glucose as a fuel source, and the neonatal brain represents 10% of total body weight, in contrast to the adult brain, which represents 2% of total body weight. Premature and SGA infants, therefore, are at extraordinary risk for development of hypoglycemia if adequate exogenous glucose is not provided because they have little compensatory endogenous reserves to mobilize. In addition, functional immaturity of fatty acid oxidative enzymes may impede mobilization of the small fat reserves they do have.[31] For this reason, it is critically important to provide approximately 6 mg/kg/min of dextrose (10 g/kg/day) to meet the metabolic needs of the brain.[32]

Because of accelerated organ growth rates, protein requirements may reach 3 to 4 g/kg/day in otherwise healthy low-birth-weight infants to achieve the desired weight gain of 15 g/kg/day.[17] Cysteine, proline, taurine, and histidine are viewed as conditionally essential amino acids in these infants owing to decreased endogenous synthesis rates stemming from immature development of enzyme systems.[33]

Physiologic jaundice is increased and prolonged in low-birth-weight infants as a result of an inability to conjugate bilirubin. Because fatty acids compete with bilirubin for albumin-bonding sites, parenteral lipid administration should be reduced to decrease the risk of kernicterus. As a guideline, lipid delivery is reduced to 1 g/kg/day if albumin is less than 2.5 g/dL, in association with serum bilirubin concentrations of greater than 12 mg/dL during the first 2 postnatal weeks of life. Moreover, increased carnitine administration may be helpful to improve fatty acid use (improved transmitochondrial membrane transport) in these infants.[34]

Requirements for elemental calcium (5 to 7.5 mEq/kg/day) and phosphate (1 to 2 mEq/kg/day) in low-birth-weight infants are generally impossible to achieve, either enterally or parenterally, because they precipitate out of solution at these concentrations owing to the lower pH of infant amino acid formulas. The use of calcium glycerophosphate or monobasic phosphate, however, allows greater quantities of calcium and phosphate delivery.

Increased magnesium administration is also required, especially with hepatic dysfunction due to diseases such as neonatal hepatitis and biliary atresia. Vitamin requirements for low-birth-weight infants are controversial. There is growing concern that these needs, particularly of the lipid-soluble vitamins, may be overestimated, although conclusive data are lacking. Trace elements are essential for growth and development, and requirements are increased in low-birth-weight infants.[35]

ROUTE OF DELIVERY

Enteral Delivery

A large body of literature now exists to establish the substantial advantages of enteral, compared with parenteral, nutritional delivery. These advantages include the following[36]:

- Better maintenance of the structural and functional integrity of the gastrointestinal tract
- Decreased risk of bacterial translocation
- Greater ease and safety of administration
- More physiologic and efficient use of nutrient substrates
- Decreased risk of hepatobiliary complications
- Improved outcome
- Improved cost effectiveness

Breast-feeding remains the optimal method for nutritional support of the healthy neonate. In addition to fostering bonding between mother and child, breast milk provides optimal nutrient content to support growth and provides immunoactive substrates. These advantages may be particularly important in the premature child who can tolerate enteral nutrition because breast milk, especially when it is fortified, can result in faster catch-up growth in this population of infants.[37] Breast milk can be fortified with commercially available protein and calcium supplements. Supplemental iron and vitamin D are suggested if breast milk is continued after 4 months. Primarily because of inadequate calcium deposition, fortified breast milk is recommended for premature infants.

During gestation, the fetus relies on maternal endocrine function and nutrient substrate delivery through the placenta to support growth and development. Although the fetus is able to swallow amniotic fluid at 16 to 17 weeks of gestation, efficient sucking and swallowing capability do not occur until the 33rd and 35th weeks of gestation. Furthermore, adequate gastric emptying and lower esophageal sphincter function do not occur until the 34th week of gestation. Adequate sucrose and maltose activity is present after the 32nd week, and adequate lactose activity occurs at about 36 to 38 weeks of gestation. In addition, adequate levels of bile salt production and secretion are not present until later in the third trimester of gestation. These developmental features become increasingly important as the gestational age at birth decreases, especially with SGA infants.

Infant enteral formulas generally mimic breast milk in calorie density but provide more protein, calcium, phosphorus, and iron. Most formulas are within an iso-osmolar range. Products designed for premature infants contain even higher concentrations of these constituents, and many include a substantial portion of fat substrate as MCT. Formulas designed to meet the specific protein-calorie and noncalorie nutrient requirements of low-birth-weight infants are available in concentrations of 24 and 27 kcal per ounce. However, these hyperosmolar preparations should be administered slowly at first because they may overtax the immature gut and result in feeding intolerance. Whey protein is used to reduce curd formation and promote gastric emptying. Because gastric emptying is inversely proportional to calorie density and osmolarity, concentrated preparations must be used with caution because they can predispose to gastroesophageal reflux and aspiration.

In premature infants, the initial use of a carefully placed soft gastric or transpyloric feeding tube for continuous drip feedings may be beneficial until gastric function improves and swallow coordination matures. These feeding tubes should be placed beyond the pyloric sphincter, and preferably beyond the ligament of Treitz, to prevent aspiration until gastric emptying mechanisms mature sufficiently to accommodate intragastric feeding. Only continuous drip feedings may be used beyond the pylorus. Such feeding should be initiated at rates of 1 mL/hr and advanced cautiously, but even this relatively small amount of nutrition is probably adequate to stimulate gut functional development and maintain the integrity of the gut barrier.[38]

In children who have prolonged tube-feeding needs, placement of a gastrostomy tube may be performed. When gastric or nasogastric tube feeding is initiated or increased, residual gastric volumes should be checked every 4 hours to determine that residual volumes do not exceed 50% of the volume delivered.

Although enteral feeding is generally safer than parenteral feeding, complications can occur from improper use, poor gastric emptying, tube migration, bacterial contamination of the formula, underlying illness, or medications.[39] The most frequent serious complication is the pulmonary aspiration of formula. This risk can be reduced by elevating the upper torso to a 30-degree angle or by keeping the child in a prone position and by advancing the nasogastric tube to a transpyloric position, preferably beyond the ligament of Treitz.

Inadequate absorption can result in poor growth or diarrhea. Measuring the biochemical products of malabsorption is better than measuring the volume of diarrhea to evaluate feeding intolerance.[40] Carbohydrate malabsorption can be documented by a fecal pH of less than 5.5 and the presence of greater than 0.25 g/dL of reducing substances in the stool. Fat malabsorption is assessed by measuring the fat content of a 72-hour stool collection. After 6 months of age, healthy infants should absorb 90% of ingested fat.

Parenteral Delivery

Parenteral nutrition is necessary in patients who cannot tolerate adequate enteral nutritional delivery for an extended period (usually 5 days or more) owing to prolonged gastrointestinal dysfunction. Historically, the clinical feasibility of TPN was first successfully established in the nutrition of babies with gastroschisis and short-bowel syndrome. In addition, parenteral nutrition is frequently used to supplement protein-calorie needs in critically ill patients who can tolerate only limited enteral nutritional delivery. Because highly concentrated (>12.5 g/dL) carbohydrate solutions quickly induce thrombophlebitis in peripheral veins, TPN must be administered through a central venous catheter. The catheter tip is usually advanced to the junction of the superior vena cava with the right atrium to facilitate rapid dilution of the infused hyperosmolar solution with blood in a large, high-flow chamber. The development of small-caliber, soft polyurethane catheters has reduced complications associated with erosion of the catheter tip through the vessel wall. The addition of heparin (1 U/mL) to solution may reduce the risk of central vein thrombosis.

Peripheral vein parenteral nutrition (PPN) may be useful for periods of 1 to 2 weeks, either as the sole source of nutritional support or to supplement enteral nutrient delivery.[41] For a reduced risk of thrombophlebitis, solution osmolality should not exceed 600 mOsm/L, and dextrose concentrations should not exceed 12.5 g/dL. The addition of lipid emulsions, either in combination with protein and carbohydrate (three-in-one compounded solutions) or piggybacked into polyurethane catheters with protein-carbohydrate solutions, can decrease the irritative effects of hypertonic carbohydrate infusion. This enables the safe nutrient delivery of up to 85 kcal/kg/day (about 850 mOsm).

The use of PPN prevents the complication of central vein thrombosis as well as the technical and mechanical complications (pneumothorax, catheter tip–induced central vein and right atrial erosion or perforation) associated with the placement of central catheters. The short-term use of femoral venous catheters is a safe alternative for PPN delivery, associated in one study with a low catheter sepsis rate (2%).[42] Percutaneously placed central venous catheters also appear to offer substantial advantage over surgically placed central venous catheters in significantly reducing sepsis rates in neonatal and pediatric intensive care patients.[43]

In infants requiring long-term TPN, cyclic delivery has been shown to be safe and effective.[44] The cyclic administration of carbohydrate mimics, to some extent, the intermittent nature of oral feeding. When TPN is cycled off, serum glucose and insulin concentrations fall, lipid oxidation increases, and lipid storage decreases. All these factors have putative benefit in reducing liver dysfunction, a complication frequently observed in infants receiving long-term TPN.

The complications associated with parenteral feeding, some of which are discussed earlier, may be:

- Mechanical or technical (related to the catheter, pump, or placement)
- Metabolic (related to fluid, electrolyte, and organ function)
- Nutritional (related to excessive or inadequate nutrient delivery)
- Infectious

In one study, the overall infection rate associated with TPN administration was 5%, with considerable variability based on site of placement and lumen number.[45] The risk of many of these complications is substantially reduced if a complete nutritional support team, including well-trained physicians, nurses, dietitians, and pharmacists, takes part in nutritional delivery.

Drawbacks of Total Parenteral Nutrition

A substantial number of randomized, prospective trials have compared TPN with enteral nutritional delivery in acutely stressed high-risk patients (including children). Meta-analysis of eight of these trials (involving high-risk surgical patients) shows a significant reduction in septic complications (18% versus 35%) in the enterally fed group of patients.[46] A study of burn patients demonstrated significantly increased mortality (63% versus 26%) in the group randomized to receive TPN supplementation of enteral calories versus enteral calories alone.[47] A study of adult trauma patients has shown that the enteral group infection rate is significantly lower than that of the parenteral group, as determined by fewer cases of pneumonia and intra-abdominal abscesses.[48]

These data support the preferential use of enteral nutritional delivery to the degree clinically feasible. Parenteral nutrition remains an important clinical modality until the gut can accommodate full nutritional delivery to meet the needs of the child. However, some enteral nutrition should be initiated, even in small amounts, as early as possible to maintain the integrity of the intestinal barrier. As gut function improves, parenteral nutrition should be weaned as enteral nutrition is increased.

NUTRITIONAL ASSESSMENT

Accurate nutritional and metabolic assessment is particularly difficult in the neonatal and pediatric intensive care settings. The metabolic events that accompany acute injury states are incompletely understood and frequently cause changes that render standard techniques based on assumptions derived from nonstressed subjects invalid.

Anthropometry

The standard for assessing the adequacy of nutritional delivery in the healthy nonstressed child is growth. Growth may be assessed by body weight norms for age and sex,[49] which norms have been revised for premature infants. Body length, head circumference, and body weight are commonly used in infants, as is height in older children. Malnutrition in nonstressed children more accurately can be determined by weight-for-height and height-for-age evaluation.[50] Acute and chronic malnutrition can approach 15% to 50%, respectively, in hospitalized children.[51]

An accurate and detailed history is the crucial first step in the nutritional assessment of the pediatric patient. A complete dietary history should be obtained, including the nature and duration of any symptoms or signs related to compromised dietary intake. Primary among these is any history of recent weight loss or retardation of growth (in infancy through adolescence). The presence and duration of nausea, vomiting, food aversion, anorexia, early satiety, fatigue, weakness, diarrhea, abdominal pain, fever, and frequency of infections are all important potential indicators of malnutrition with potential for outcome significance.[52]

Anthropometric measurements should always include accurate weight and height data, which should be recorded on a growth chart appropriate for age. In infants, a head circumference measurement should also be obtained. Comparison with previous growth chart recordings should be carried out to establish growth velocity. Of these various measurements, weight for height, or weight/height percentile, is the best indicator of nutritional status (better than weight for age).[53] Weight/height percentile can be calculated from published National Center for Health Statistics data.[54]

Arm circumference and triceps skinfold measurements can be used to calculate muscle and fat compartments but are operator-dependent and can provide misleading data if the measurement is carried out incorrectly. It is important to measure with nonstretchable tape and to employ the same anatomic landmarks in measuring.[55] For instance, mid-upper arm circumference (AC) should be measured exactly halfway between the acromion and the olecranon. Triceps skinfold thickness (TSF) should be measured at this same point with skinfold calipers.[56] Arm muscle circumference (AMC), which is representative of the muscle compartment, can then be calculated as follows:

$$AMC = AC - TSF$$

TSF assesses the thickness of the subcutaneous adipose layer. In contrast to adults, fat stores in children are almost exclusively confined to the subcutaneous fat compartment. This compartment constitutes the major body energy reserve and diminishes as a function of malnutrition severity. In children, a significant correlation exists between weight/height percentile and both TSF and AMC.[57] Caveats, in addition to operator-associated variability, include compartment fluid shifts induced during acute metabolic stress states (caused, for instance, by inflammation, infection, surgery, intensive chemotherapy, and so on) and malignant neoplasia-related fluid accumulations (ascites). All can lead to gross inaccuracies in the interpretation of anthropometric data.

Biochemical assessment includes evaluation of visceral proteins. Although serious hypoalbuminemia (<3.0 g/dL) is not observed in most nonstressed malnourished pediatric patients, it is sometimes present and has been associated with compromise of muscle function.[52] Shorter half-life visceral proteins, such as prealbumin and transferrin, also accurately reflect protein compartment losses resulting from malnutrition-related catabolism (see section on visceral protein status).

Two nonspecific markers of protein nutrition that may reflect immunologic competence can be assessed clinically by calculating the total lymphocyte count (TLC) and delayed cutaneous hypersensitivity (DCH). Data suggesting that TLC is a marker of malnutrition stem from studies that have documented malnutrition-related pediatric thymic atrophy[58] and reduced TLC (<2500/mm^3) in about 20% of malnourished children (versus no reduction below this number in well-nourished children).[59] Low TLC (<1500/mm^3 versus >2000/mm^3 for nutritionally replete patients) has been documented in hospitalized adult patients[60] but does not correlate well with outcome parameters such as mortality and morbidity.[61] Reasons for lack of correlation may be related to the wide range of normal TLC (1000 to 4000/mm^3) and the fact that TLC does not reflect ratios of helper T cells to suppressor T cells.

Calculations of TLC may be performed by multiplying the total white blood cell count by the percentage of lymphocytes. During acute metabolic stress and oncologic therapy, TLC is valueless as a measure of malnutrition, but increasing counts after therapy may be related to accelerated bone marrow recovery made possible by nutritional support.[62]

DCH is a measure of impaired antibody reactivity to a series of skin test antigens.[63] The synthesis of antibodies may be impaired by malnutrition and the resulting decreased protein synthesis.[64] In addition to T cell dysfunction, DCH is another possible factor associated with the anergy-related immunocompromise observed during cancer cachexia.

Anergy established on the basis of DCH has been associated with a reduced lymphocyte proliferative response in malnourished children.[59] In a large population of adult surgical patients, anergy has been associated with a significantly increased incidence of sepsis and mortality compared with immunocompetent patients. These immunologic assessment modalities assume previous exposure of the child to the antigens tested and are valueless during periods of acute metabolic stress and after chemotherapy.

Indications for Supplemental Nutrition

Criteria for identifying children who are malnourished differ somewhat in various published reports. In general, the following surveillance criteria can be used to identify children who are malnourished or likely to require supplemental nutritional support:

1. Interval or total weight loss of greater than 5% during the past 3 to 6 months in older children.
2. Weight-to-height ratio less than or equal to 90% or weight/height percentile less than or equal to the 10th percentile.
3. Serum albumin concentration less than or equal to 3.2 g/dL (in the absence of acute metabolic stress within the past 14 days).
4. Adipose energy reserves as determined by TSF less than or equal to the 5th percentile for age and gender.
5. A decrease in the current percentile for weight (or height) of at least two percentile channels during the past 3 to 6 months in older children (for instance, weight of the 75th to 90th percentile might decrease to the 25th to 50th percentile for age and gender).
6. Voluntary food intake less than 70% of estimated requirements for 5 days for well-nourished patients.
7. Anticipated gut dysfunction for more than 5 days for well-nourished patients.
8. DCH-established anergy in any nonstressed child older than 2 years of age before treatment.

METABOLIC ASSESSMENT

Acute Metabolic Stress Response

In response to a variety of local or systemic injury stimuli (such as trauma, sepsis, and acute inflammatory conditions), a series of metabolic changes occur that characterize the acute stress state. Among the early features of the injury response is the release of cytokines, followed rapidly by important alterations in the hormonal environment. Increased counterregulatory hormone concentrations are associated with insulin and growth hormone resistance. As a result of this response, a sequence of metabolic events is initiated that includes the catabolism of endogenous stores of protein, carbohydrate, and fat to provide essential substrate intermediates and energy necessary to fuel the ongoing response process. Amino acids from catabolized proteins flow to the liver, where they provide substrate for the synthesis of acute-phase proteins and glucose (gluconeogenesis). Therefore, acute metabolic stress response represents a hypermetabolic, hypercatabolic state that results in the loss of endogenous tissue (Fig. 81–2). Growth, which is an anabolic process, is inhibited during periods of acute metabolic stress. As the acute metabolic stress response resolves, adaptive anabolic metabolism ensues to restore catabolic losses. In children, this phase is characterized by the resumption of somatic growth.

Insulin is a potent anabolic hormone responsible for glycogen synthesis and the storage of carbohydrate, lipogenesis and the storage of fat, and new protein synthesis. Insulin and insulin-like growth factor 1 (IGF-1) are essential hormones for somatic growth in infants and children. Acute metabolic stress is characterized by substantial increases in serum concentrations of catecholamines, glucagon, and cortisol, which are referred to as counterregulatory hormones because they oppose the anabolic effects of insulin. Serum concentrations of these metabolic stress–related hormones increase as a result of cytokine release.[65]

Glucagon induces glycolysis and gluconeogenesis. These effects counteract the anabolic effects of insulin. Increased glycolysis results in increased serum lactate and alanine concentrations. These amino acids provide the substrate necessary for the endogenous regeneration of glucose (the Cori cycle and alanine cycle). These cycles are major contributors to altered carbohydrate metabolism during acute metabolic stress.

Cortisol induces muscle proteolysis and promotes gluconeogenesis. Glucocorticoids cause the muscle proteolysis associated with cytokine release, and they have been shown to be a predictor of protein breakdown and hypermetabolism in acutely stressed adults. The major amino acid sources for gluconeogenesis are alanine and glutamine from skeletal muscle and gut, respectively. Hepatic uptake of these amino acids is accelerated during acute metabolic stress.[66] Like glucagon, cortisol also causes insulin resistance. Although insulin concentrations may be increased during acute metabolic stress, its anabolic effects are inhibited.

Catecholamines cause hyperglycemia by promoting hepatic

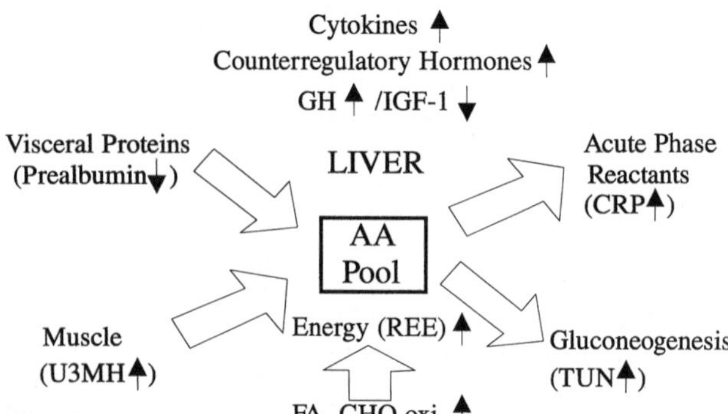

Figure 81–2. Metabolic response to acute injury. GH = growth hormone; IGF-I = insulin-like growth factor I; AA = amino acid; CRP = C-reactive protein; TUN = total urinary nitrogen; FA, CHO oxi = fatty acid and carbohydrate oxidation; U3MH = urinary 3-methylhistidine; REE = resting energy expenditure.

glycogenolysis, by causing conversion of skeletal muscle glycogen to lactate (which is then transported to the liver for conversion to glucose through the Cori cycle), and by suppressing the pancreatic secretion of insulin. Catecholamines also induce lipolysis, which results in the mobilization of free fatty acids. Finally, catecholamines, in addition to glucagon and cortisol, induce hypermetabolism, which is associated with an increase in the basal metabolic rate.

In health, the major actions of growth hormone are to decrease protein catabolism and promote protein synthesis, to promote fat mobilization and the conversion of free fatty acids to acetylcoenzyme A, and to decrease glucose oxidation while increasing glycogen deposition. However, the anabolic effects of growth hormone, particularly as they relate to protein metabolism, are mediated principally by IGF-1. During acute metabolic stress, IGF-1 concentrations decrease and IGF-1 inhibitory binding concentrations increase. In this state, the substrate-mobilizing effects of growth hormone prevail and result in increased lipolysis and free fatty acid oxidation.

Both term and premature neonatal infants are capable of generating a counterregulatory response to surgically induced injury.[67, 68] The response is relatively short-lived (24 hours) and can be dampened by fentanyl anesthesia. However, this response may differ according to the age and physiologic maturity of the subject. For instance, children from 2 to 20 years of age do not appear to have significant differences in cortisol production immediately after surgery, despite considerable age differences and variable durations of surgically induced stress.[69] In contrast, neonatal infants immediately after open heart surgery (without substantive fentanyl anesthesia) can generate only approximately 50% of the average 2-year-old child's surgically induced cortisol response.[68] Furthermore, neonatal infants clearly can generate a graded response based on the degree of severity of surgical stress.[70] Moreover, work in preterm baboons also demonstrates a graded counterregulatory hormone response based on injury severity.[68] However, the onset of the response appears to be delayed and of longer duration than the hormonal response reported in more mature, stressed infants, thus suggesting the possibility that functional immaturity associated with earlier gestational development may play a role in this process.

As previously mentioned, surgical trauma per se may not visit a particularly severe injury insult.[71] Stable infants undergoing elective surgical intervention do not generally have an appreciable energy response to operative trauma.[72] However, if surgical procedures are classified on the basis of the magnitude of the procedure, a small, but significant, increase in energy response can be observed in association with major versus minor operative trauma.[73] In general, though, the predominant stimulus of the energy response to injury in infants requiring surgery depends on the insult of the underlying disease process that necessitates the surgery rather than the operative procedure itself.[74]

Anabolic Hormone Resistance During Acute Metabolic Stress

Since the dawn of human existence, the metabolic response to acute injury and disease has been characterized by an associated decrease or absence of exogenous nutrient intake (*anorexia*). A predominant clinical feature of serious illness in neonates is feeding intolerance or a decreased willingness to feed. This phenomenon causes the sick infant to rely on the mobilization of endogenous fuel stores for the provision of substrates and energy required during the period of acute metabolic stress. Because normal anabolic metabolism, which essentially results in the removal of substrates from the circulation and their deposition in tissue stores, would appear to be counterproductive in the face of increased demands for substrate mobilization, and because the advent of exogenous nutritional support has occurred extremely recently within the time frame of human development, the attenuation of anabolic hormone effects in response to acute injury states teleologically represents an important evolutional compensatory mechanism. This mechanism is characterized by the suppression of, or resistance to, the anabolic effects of at least two key hormones, insulin and growth hormone.

Because the anabolic effects of these hormones are various and depend on a multitude of associated conditions, it is important to define which of these effects and associated conditions are altered in regard to "resistance," for example:

- Nature of the injury insult (i.e., sepsis versus burn)
- Substrate pool affected (i.e., glucose versus protein)
- Region of the body sampled (i.e., splanchnic, hepatic, peripheral muscle, or systemic circulatory beds)
- Absence or presence and type of exogenous substrate support
- Timing of samples taken relative to the injury event
- Use of exogenous hormonal supplementation

Lack of attention to these details has led to considerable controversy, especially in relation to the nature of insulin resistance.[75-80]

Insulin resistance is defined as increased glucose production, lipolysis, fatty acid oxidation, and proteolysis as well as decreased glucose uptake and storage associated with high serum glucose, amino acid, and insulin concentrations. Septic and acute injury states in adults are characterized by an inability to use glucose despite increased serum glucose, amino acid, and lipid concentrations.

Early studies in these populations of patients demonstrated hyperglycemia in association with elevated serum insulin concentrations,[76, 77] and this hyperglycemia could not be reversed by the administration of substantial pharmacologic insulin doses. Later studies in septic adults report failure of exogenous insulin to suppress hepatic glucose production despite concomitant provision of exogenous glucose.[79] Data obtained by use of various limb clamp techniques, criticized because they are nonphysiologic, conflict to some degree with total-body study results. When patients with sepsis were studied with use of a hyperglycemic glucose clamp, no significant reductions in glucose storage or oxidation were observed, and total glucose disposal was decreased.[78] However, when such patients were compared with healthy adults by use of a euglycemic hyperinsulinemic clamp with increasing insulin doses, there was a suppressed insulin effect in the septic group, suggesting a possible insulin receptor defect.[80]

In another study of severely septic adults, increases in both glucose production and clearance were demonstrated in association with a decreased glucose-stimulated insulin secretion, which raises the possibility that glucose uptake may be insulin-independent in sepsis.[81] Conflicting data relative to whether glucose oxidation is appropriate to circulating insulin levels may be at least in part explained by the fact that pyruvate dehydrogenase activity is dependent on the nature of the injury insult. For instance, the activity of this enzyme is depressed in septic adults (thus reducing aerobic metabolism and glucose oxidation),[82] whereas there is a 40-fold increase in activity in burned adults.[83]

Because insulin is known to promote protein anabolism, primarily by decreasing proteolysis, the protein breakdown observed in acute metabolic stress states has been ascribed to insulin resistance.[84] However, despite the presence of proteolysis, the protein anabolic effect of insulin has been reported to be intact.[85] Furthermore, decreased leucine oxidation and improved nitrogen retention have been observed in hyperinsulinemic burned patients.[86]

In one study, the exogenous provision of extremely large insulin doses during a 7-day period in severely burned adults was shown to increase muscle protein synthesis (approximately 350% relative to that of controls subjects), and this effect was associated with a sixfold increase in amino acid transport from the circulating to the muscle pool.[87] Although this report suggests that exogenous insulin may be useful in promoting protein synthesis in severely catabolic patients, to achieve this effect, insulin was infused at rates that resulted in serum concentrations of 900 μU/mL, which are more than 10 times higher than the range generally observed (55 to 70 μU/mL) in injured patients. In addition, although all study groups were fed enterally (protein intake of approximately 2.1 g/kg/day and 60 kcal/kg/day), the insulin group received an additional 80 kcal/kg/day as intravenous 50% dextrose to prevent insulin-induced hypoglycemia, raising serious questions about the negative impact of this excessive glucose load on the liver. Also, although muscle protein synthesis was increased, there was no improvement in the rate of burn or wound healing compared with that of the control group (R.R. Wolfe, personal communication).

The use of exogenous insulin at much lower infusion rates has been reported to improve nitrogen secretion in moderately stressed adult patients after abdominal surgery.[88] When protein intake was increased from 1.5 to 3.0 g/kg/day, however, there was no significant difference in improved nitrogen retention between the insulin and control groups.

In health, the major actions of growth hormone are to decrease protein catabolism and promote protein synthesis, to promote fat mobilization and the conversion of free fatty acids to acetylcoenzyme A, and to decrease glucose oxidation while increasing glycogen deposition. However, the anabolic effects of growth hormone, particularly as they relate to protein metabolism, are mediated principally by IGF-1. During acute metabolic stress, IGF-1 levels fall, and IGF-1 inhibitory binding protein concentrations rise.[89] In this state, the substrate-mobilizing effects of growth hormone prevail and result in increased lipolysis and fatty acid oxidation. These findings demonstrate an anabolic growth hormone resistance during acute metabolic stress states.

Although exogenous growth hormone administration reverses the catabolic effects of acute injury in moderately stressed adults and severely burned children,[90] in a completed study, exogenous infusions of this hormone (0.2 mg/kg/day × 7 days) did not elicit an anabolic response in critically ill neonates with necrotizing enterocolitis or gastroschisis.[91] In this same population of patients, however, exogenous growth hormone significantly improved lipid substrate utilization in both term and premature infants.[92]

Protein Metabolism During Acute Metabolic Stress

Visceral Proteins

Normally, the liver synthesizes a number of proteins that constitute labile pools within the serum compartment. Among others, these proteins include albumin, transferrin, prealbumin, and retinol-binding protein. These proteins account for early nitrogen losses resulting from catabolism induced by injury. Compared with albumin (half-life [$t_{1/2}$], 20 days), both prealbumin ($t_{1/2}$ = 2 days) and retinol-binding protein ($t_{1/2}$ = 10 hours) have shorter serum half-lives and constitute smaller protein pools. Visceral proteins with shorter half-lives correlate better with other variables of malnutrition. For instance, prealbumin concentrations decrease rapidly in response to

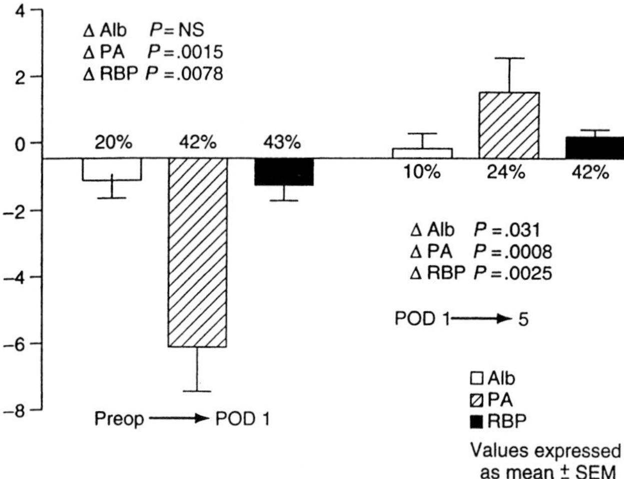

Figure 81–3. Mean percentage change (Δ) of visceral proteins during acute metabolic stress. Statistical analysis used the paired Student's *t*-test. Alb-serum albumin (g/dL); PA-serum prealbumin (mg/dL); RBP-serum retinol-binding protein (mg/dL); Preop-within 24 hours before surgery; POD-postoperative day.

acute injury and are more significantly depressed than albumin[93] (Fig. 81-3). Infant studies also demonstrate a precipitous decrease in visceral protein concentrations in response to acute metabolic stress that return to normal as the insult resolves.[94] Prealbumin is a better marker than albumin for assessment of nutritional repletion and the recovery of visceral protein synthesis in critically ill infants.[95]

A study of metabolically stressed neonates shows a significantly increased ability to recover anabolic metabolism (as established by serum prealbumin levels) in premature versus near-term babies after injury, perhaps related to accelerated growth capacity of the fetus during the third trimester of gestation versus the term infant.[96]

Total Urinary Nitrogen

Protein and fat catabolism during acute metabolic stress results in increased urinary nitrogen losses. Protein catabolism increases the size of the hepatic free amino acid pool. The liver dominates a substantial portion of these amino acids to synthesize glucose (gluconeogenesis); this results in increased nitrogen that is excreted in the urine as urea. Fat catabolism (*lipolysis*) yields increased free fatty acids, which, when oxidized, result in ketone body formation. These keto acids are buffered by ammonia and excreted in the urine.[97]

Because urea nitrogen losses correlate poorly with ammonia nitrogen losses in the urine during injury states, it is preferable to measure 24-hour total urinary nitrogen (TUN).[98] Because serial urinary nitrogen measurements reflect the degree and duration of catabolism resulting from various categories of injury and correlate grossly with hypermetabolism (increased stress-related energy expenditure),[71] this technique can be used to monitor the acute metabolic stress response and may also be valuable in determining injury severity.[99] I have noted a small (0.2 to 0.5 g of N_2) but significant increment in TUN during the first 2 to 4 days after major surgery in infants. These values return to normal levels by postoperative days 7 to 10 (Fig. 81-4). Similar changes have been noted by others[100] and may also reflect nutritional repletion as the acute stress response resolves. I have observed higher TUN in septic infants, but interpatient variability precludes estimating these losses from clinical impression alone.

Acute-Phase Proteins

In response to acute injury stimuli, the hepatic synthesis of certain specialized proteins, called acute-phase proteins, is dramatically increased. This process is mediated by cytokines (principally interleukin-6[101]) that selectively redirect hepatic protein synthesis, such that the synthesis of acute-phase proteins is increased while the synthesis of visceral protein is retarded.[102] These proteins carry out a number of important immunologic and repair functions during the acute stress period. C-reactive protein (CRP) is one such acute-phase reactant that in general reaches peak serum levels at 24 to 48 hours after injury. Because its serum half-life is 4 to 6 hours, decreases in the hepatic synthesis of CRP as the acute metabolic stress response resolves are promptly reflected in decreased serum levels of this acute-phase protein.

In children, marked increases in serum CRP concentrations have been observed after a variety of metabolic stress stimuli, even in immunosuppressed hosts. In infants, this same effect has been noted in response to bacterial causes. Investigations of the perioperative acute-phase response in infants and neonates have demonstrated significant increases in serum CRP concentrations within 24 hours after injury insult that later return toward normal values as the child recovers.[94] These changes in serum acute-phase protein levels appear to coincide with urinary nitrogen excretion, thus demonstrating two important aspects of altered protein metabolism during acute metabolic stress (see Fig. 81-4).

Energy Expenditure

Energy expenditure is a characteristic feature of metabolism that can be measured by the amount of heat released. This is the principle of *direct calorimetry,* in which energy release is quantified by the amount of heat required to raise the temperature of 1 mL of water by 1°C from to 15.5° to 16.5° (1 calorie). Because this method involves confining the subject in a closed calorimeter for extended periods, it is impractical for clinical use. In contrast, *indirect calorimetry* can be carried out at the patient's bedside and involves the measurement of the differences in oxygen and carbon dioxide concentrations between a known volume (minute ventilation) of inspired and expired gas. In this way, oxygen consumption (Vo_2) and carbon dioxide production (Vco_2) may be calculated on the basis of known and constant relationships between Vo_2, Vco_2, and heat produced (energy expenditure) for many metabolic processes. These include, among others, the oxidation of various carbohydrates, fats, and proteins as well as lipogenesis. The respiratory quotient (RQ), which may be expressed as Vco_2/Vo_2, is also specific and constant for each of these processes, for instance, the total oxidation of carbohydrate (RQ = 1.0) or fat (RQ = 0.7). For lipogenesis (the synthesis of fat from carbohydrate), the RQ equals 2.75.[103]

The value of indirect calorimetry in the intensive care setting lies in the fact that estimations of energy expenditure based on other clinical criteria are notoriously inaccurate. The actual measured energy expenditure (MEE) is frequently much less than predicted values based on clinical grounds. Although average MEE values in large series of patients tend to differentiate various degrees of injury,[71] individual subjects can respond to similar injury states with widely diverse MEE values. A study of critically ill infants found a 3.5-fold difference in MEE (adjusted for age and weight) between the lowest and highest interpatient values.[104]

Serial Metabolic Monitoring and Clinical Outcome

The value of establishing injury severity lies in the metabolic response to such injury and the ability to predict clinical

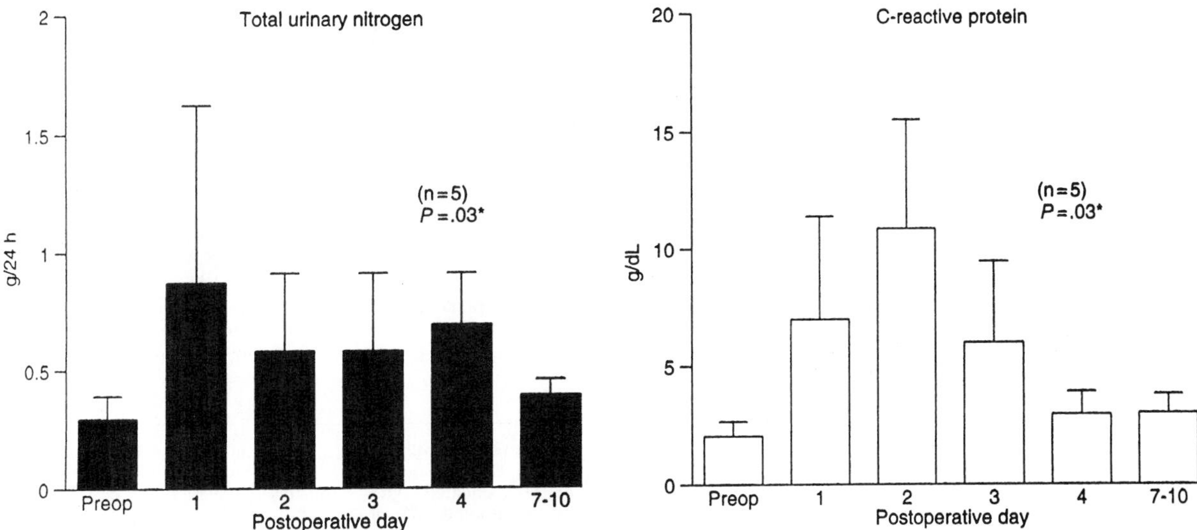

Figure 81–4. Infant metabolic response to surgical stress. Preoperative values were obtained within 24 hours before surgery.

outcome from that response. This allows the evaluation of treatment programs on the basis of comparable severity scores. The implication is that when injury response is stratified, severity-related therapeutic strategies can be developed to supplement or enhance the response and improve the outcome. A scoring system relating injury severity (based on multiple physiologic variables) to mortality has been devised for pediatric patients. This Pediatric Risk of Mortality (PRISM) scoring system is difficult to use because of the numerous variables required for assessment.[105]

As previously discussed, surgically induced changes in serum counterregulatory hormone concentrations have been shown to correlate well with a severity score of operative trauma in infants.[70] Another study has suggested that metabolic response parameters (energy expenditure and nitrogen excretion) may be useful in predicting mortality in the pediatric intensive care setting. This system has been shown to correlate favorably with PRISM mortality risk predictions but offers the advantage of easier implementation.[106]

Because of the necessity of serial evaluation to establish the pattern of the injury response, the ease of application is an important feature of any scoring system. This fact is significant because injury severity is a function not only of intensity but also of duration of the insult. In support of this concept is a study of critically ill surgical infants in which daily serum protein indices, including CRP and prealbumin, were measured throughout the perioperative period in critically ill infants stratified to high-stress and low-stress groups.[94] Serum prealbumin levels were lower and remained depressed for a significantly longer time in the high-stress than in the low-stress group (Fig. 81–5). When infants were grouped according to postoperative mortality (within 30 days of surgery), significant decreases in preoperative serum prealbumin levels and increases in peak CRP levels were observed in nonsurvivors, thus suggesting the potential predictive value of these metabolic indices for serial perioperative evaluation in this population of patients (Fig. 81–6). The strongest potential mortality predictor was found to be ongoing depression in day 5 prealbumin levels. Failure of the liver to resume visceral protein synthesis by this time (indicating continued acute metabolic stress) was associated with the most significant increase in infant mortality seen in this critical care population of infants (Fig. 81–7).

Serial monitoring of the acute metabolic stress response may also be useful in detecting postoperative complications. The normal postoperative stress response pattern is characterized by a gradual decrease in acute metabolic parameters as a function of recovery from the initial injury insult. When postoperative complications occur, such as wound infection, anastomotic leak, or sepsis, an abrupt increase in acute injury response parameters results, usually within 12 hours of the new metabolic insult. This concept is supported by an investigation involving surgical infants in which subjects who suffered infectious complications postoperatively were compared with those whose postoperative course was complication free.[107] Results showed that serial protein metabolic stress response monitoring with CRP and prealbumin was superior to conventional indices of infection (body temperature and leukocyte count and differential) in predicting postoperative bacterial infection in early infancy. Guidelines for infant metabolic monitoring during acute metabolic stress are listed in Table 81–5.

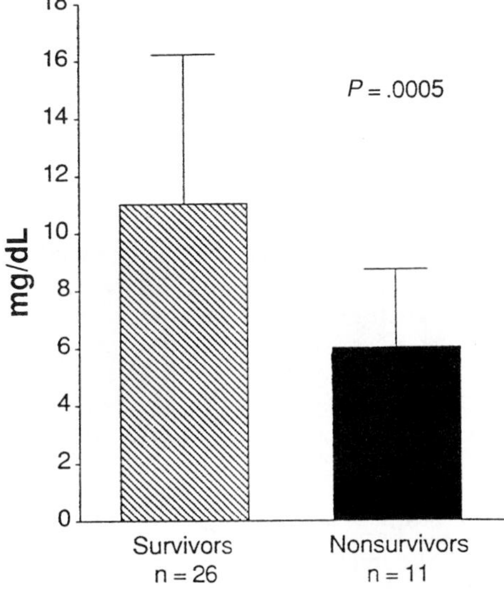

Figure 81–5. Serum prealbumin concentrations obtained within 24 hours before surgery. n = number of patient data points obtained during this time interval.

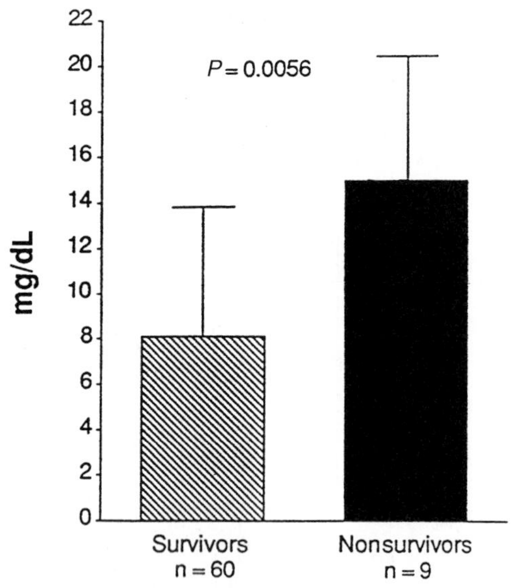

Figure 81–6. Peak serum C-reactive protein (CRP) concentrations obtained within 48 hours following surgery. n = the number of patient data points obtained during this time interval.

TABLE 81–5. Guidelines for Infant Metabolic Monitoring During Acute Stress

Parameter	Stress Characteristics Evaluated
Prealbumin	Visceral protein catabolism Hepatic synthesis
Total urinary nitrogen	Protein and fat catabolism Gluconeogenesis $NB = N_I - [TUN + 75 mg/kg/day]$
C-reactive protein	Acute-phase response
Indirect calorimetry	Energy expenditure and RQ $EB = E_I - MEE$ $RQ = V\text{CO}_2/V\text{O}_2$

NB = nitrogen balance; N_I = 24-hour nitrogen intake; TUN = total urinary nitrogen; EB = energy balance; E_I = 24-hour energy intake; MEE = measured energy expenditure, RQ = respiratory quotient; $V\text{O}_2$ = oxygen consumption; $V\text{CO}_2$ = carbon dioxide production.

OVERFEEDING

Overfeeding occurs when the administration of calories or specific substrate exceeds the requirements to maintain metabolic homeostasis. These requirements, which vary according to the patient's age, state of health, and underlying nutritional status, are substantially altered during periods of injury-induced acute metabolic stress. Excess nutritional delivery during this period can further increase the metabolic demands of an acute injury and place an added burden on the lungs and liver. The result is not only to exacerbate pulmonary and hepatic pathophysiologic processes but also to increase the risk of mortality. It is important, therefore, to ensure that calorie intake not exceed demand during the period of acute metabolic response in critically ill infants and children.

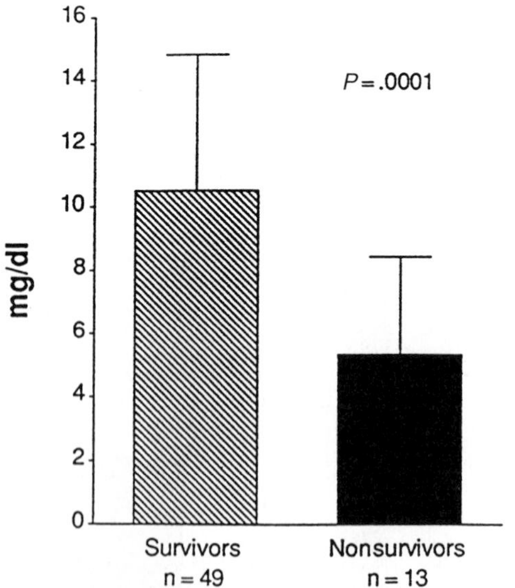

Figure 81–7. Late postoperative serum prealbumin concentrations obtained from postoperative days (POD) 4 to 7 (average values). These prealbumin concentrations in surviving infants represent a substantial increase from POD 1 levels that was not observed in the nonsurvivors, thus indicating ongoing acute metabolic stress in the latter (nonsurvivor) group. n = the number of patient data points obtained during this time interval.

Effect on Respiration

Carbohydrate overfeeding, either with or without excessive calorie delivery, can have a significant negative effect on respiration. *Lipogenesis* (the biosynthesis of fat from carbohydrate) is an energy-requiring process characterized by an increase in $V\text{CO}_2$ relative to $V\text{O}_2$. The RQ for pure lipogenesis is 2.75.[103] Lipogenesis represents the only metabolic process with an RQ consequence of greater than 1. Because other metabolic processes with RQs of 1 or less also occur simultaneously in vivo (i.e., lipid oxidation, RQ = 0.7; carbohydrate oxidation, RQ = 1; and protein oxidation, RQ = 0.8), and the measured RQ represents the net effect of all of these processes, RQ values in excess of 1 represent high lipogenic activity and are usually associated with overfeeding. In infants, increased carbon dioxide production, resulting from excess carbohydrate administration, can cause an increase in respiratory rate necessary to remove excess carbon dioxide.[108] Excess protein delivery has been shown to exacerbate this effect in adults by increasing respiratory sensitivity to carbon dioxide.[109] Substituting lipid for some of the carbohydrate administered, usually 25% to 35%, is effective (in both infant and adult studies) in reducing carbon dioxide production and lipogenesis, thus resulting in decreased RQ.[108, 110–113]

In acute injury states, particularly with severe metabolic stress, hypermetabolism (increased MEE) resulting from increased $V\text{O}_2$ accompanies the increases in $V\text{CO}_2$ due to overfeeding. Overfeeding in these stressed patients can result in increased respiratory requirements caused by increased carbon dioxide production,[114–116] even though these changes may not be accurately reflected in total RQ.[117] Maximum glucose oxidation rates exist for metabolically stressed as well as for nonstressed subjects. Glucose administered in excess of maximum oxidation rates undergoes fat biosynthesis (lipogenesis), resulting in substantial increases in carbon dioxide production.[115] The importance of avoiding excessive nutritional delivery is confirmed by studies that demonstrate that overfeeding can result in ventilatory dependency in patients with decreased pulmonary reserve.[109, 118, 119] This ventilatory dependency is due to the inability of patients with limited pulmonary function to adequately eliminate increased carbon dioxide produced when excessive total calorie and, particularly, carbohydrate intake is metabolized. Preterm infants are especially vulnerable to the respiratory effects of overfeeding because of their immature pulmonary development and limited respiratory reserve.

Effect on Hepatic Morphology and Function

A number of metabolic alterations are the result of total calorie overfeeding and carbohydrate overfeeding. In healthy subjects and clinically stable patients, excessive glucose intake induces increased insulin levels, resulting in decreased fatty acid oxidation, reduced ketogenesis, increased glucose oxidation, and increased lipogenesis. In addition, the insulin-glucagon ratio increases in the portal vein, in association with increased hepatic deposition of fat (steatosis) and increased serum levels of hepatic enzymes, indicating hepatic cellular injury.[120]

In one study of stable adult patients overfed (average, 177% of predicted energy expenditure) with glucose-based TPN, liver biopsy results showed fatty infiltration and incipient intrahepatic cholestasis within 5 days of the initiation of intravenous nutrition.[121] After 21 days, biopsy results showed bile duct proliferation, canalicular bile plugs, centrilobular cholestasis with the bile pigment in hepatocytes, and periportal inflammation. Liver function test results were elevated in 83% of the subjects by a mean of 14 days, and the number of liver function test abnormalities increased in proportion to the increased amount of carbohydrate calories infused. These changes are typical of a number of similar studies involving overfed subjects.[115, 120, 122, 123]

Similar alterations have been documented in several studies involving clinically stable infants receiving glucose-based TPN; however, the onset of these changes is more rapid, particularly in preterm neonates. This phenomenon may be due to hepatic functional immaturity.[124]

Acute metabolic stress increases lipolysis and free fatty acid oxidation relative to glucose oxidation, owing to conterregulatory hormone–induced insulin resistance. These endocrine effects reduce the efficiency with which exogenous carbohydrate is metabolized. With excessive carbohydrate delivery, serum insulin, glucose, glucose oxidation, and fatty acid oxidation increase, and lipogenesis remains high.[125] These metabolic events further predispose the liver to hepatic cellular injury, resulting in hepatic dysfunction. Furthermore, glucose oxidation is dependent on pyruvate dehydrogenase for entry of pyruvate into the tricarboxylic acid cycle. During acute injury due to sepsis, increased serum concentrations of lactate and alanine suggest that pyruvate dehydrogenase activity may be inhibited as part of the metabolic stress response.[82] Excess glucose administration increases the hepatic work demand to metabolize increased amounts of these substrate intermediates.[125]

Lipid overfeeding with long-chain triglyceride (LCT) formulations can inhibit the ability of the reticuloendothelial system of the liver to clear bacteria during acute injury states.[126] Decreased hepatic clearance is associated with increased bacterial sequestration in the lung, resulting in increased pulmonary neutrophil activation and the release of inflammatory mediators. LCT contains high concentrations of linoleic acid, an arachidonic acid precursor, which increases substrate availability for prostaglandin synthesis. Replacing LCT with MCT, which is absorbed directly into the blood from the gut and does not pass through the liver, restores liver reticuloendothelial system function and reduces lung bacterial sequestration.

Stress metabolism cannot be reversed by overfeeding during critical illness. Instead, overfeeding further increases the negative impact of stress by increasing the hypermetabolic demands associated with it and by augmenting the hepatic workload.[116] Finally, hepatic compromise due to overfeeding during nonstress periods may decrease hepatic metabolic function in response to subsequent acute injury, especially sepsis. Cecal ligation and puncture in rats previously overfed enterally for 6 days resulted in marked decreases in hepatic (and whole-body) protein synthesis relative to the normal-intake group.[127] Hepatomegaly was 67% greater in the overfed group, but liver protein per gram of tissue was significantly less relative to normally fed animals. It is particularly noteworthy that hepatic dysfunction and pathomorphologic changes due to carbohydrate-based TPN nutritional delivery not only are observed earlier in infants than in adults but also, among this population of infants, evolve most rapidly in patients who are severely stressed, especially those who are septic.[122]

Effect on Survival

It is logical to assume that the damaging aspects of overfeeding during acute metabolic stress would have a negative impact on survival, but proof of this hypothesis remains elusive in many human studies owing to the different nature of various injury stimuli and the diverse responses they induce in individual patients. Also, the limitations in the design of experimental human protocols preclude the more definitive methods of evaluation available in more rigidly controlled animal studies.

As previously discussed, the increased metabolic demands imposed by overfeeding result in increased glucose production, glucose and lipid oxidation, carbon dioxide production associated with lipogenesis, insulin/glucagon ratio, and lactate and alanine cycling. Although whole-body protein synthesis rates increase in some stressed populations, protein breakdown is not substantially decreased in response to overfeeding.[128] These alterations result in increased respiratory work required to remove excess carbon dioxide and increased hepatic work required to metabolize the excess substrates created. Excessive substrate calorie administration augments energy requirements to process the increased substrate load, resulting in further hypermetabolism due to diet-induced thermogenesis. Overfeeding has been documented to increase hypermetabolism (MEE) by 34% in acutely stressed adult subjects after the initiation of excess protein-calorie delivery.[116]

The effects of calorie overfeeding with high-carbohydrate delivery were evaluated in postoperative adults retrospectively grouped on the basis of RQ higher than 0.95 (high-calorie) versus RQ of less than 0.95 (low-calorie) values.[129] The high-calorie group received 150% MEE, and the low-calorie group received 100% MEE. Glucose calories were 77% of the total calorie intake in the high-calorie group (yielding an average RQ of 1.12), compared with glucose calories of 60.6% (yielding an RQ of 0.73) in the low-calorie group. Mortality was significantly greater in the overfed group than in the group delivered calories equal of MEE (40% versus 29%; $P < .05$).

In a prospective study of septic guinea pigs grouped by calorie intake (100, 125, 150, or 175 kcal/kg/day), there was a significant increase in mortality and decrease in survival time in the animals fed 150 and 175 kcal/kg/day (the mortality rate was 100% in both groups).[130] On the other hand, 175 kcal/kg/day was optimal for guinea pigs subjected to thermal injury.[131] This underscores the differing nutritional requirements based on the nature of the injury insult and the metabolic stress response that it induces. As discussed previously, data on septic stress suggest that pyruvate dehydrogenase activity is inhibited as part of the metabolic stress response.[82] In contrast, data generated in burned children show that pyruvate dehydrogenase activity is not decreased but, rather, is amplified during this type of acute injury.[83] In sepsis, glucose infusion results in increased levels of lactate and alanine; whereas in thermal stress, increased glucose oxidation occurs, and less lactate and alanine are generated. This may help to explain why the increased nutritional delivery appropriate for burn injury might constitute overfeeding during sepsis in the same animal model.

Another consideration involves the impact of prestress overfeeding on the subsequent metabolic stress response. When acute bacterial peritonitis was induced in rats after 6 days of enteral overfeeding (175% of normal intake), the mortality rate increased to 53%, in contrast to the 14% mortality rate observed in normal-intake animals. These changes were associated with decreased hepatic and whole-body protein synthesis, which may reflect a reduced metabolic capability to meet the demands of acute injury in the overfed group.

Precise calorie delivery is best determined during acute injury states by measuring energy expenditure. Owing to substantial interpatient variability, estimates of energy needs on the basis of disease categories, subject age, or body composition can be misleading and usually result in overfeeding. Overfeeding cannot reverse tissue catabolism until the acute metabolic stress response has resolved. In acutely stressed children, MEE constitutes the total energy requirement, and calorie delivery in excess of this amount should be avoided until metabolic stress parameters indicate resolution of the acute injury state.[89]

Nutritional Repletion During Metabolic Stress and Growth Recovery

As previously discussed, the acute metabolic stress response represents a predominantly catabolic state. Endogenous tissue stores of protein, carbohydrate, and fat are invariably decreased during this period, and growth is impeded. Approximately 30% to 35% of predicted energy requirements for healthy infants are needed for growth (Fig. 81-8). In addition,

TABLE 81–6. Guidelines for Infant Nutritional Support During Acute Stress

Post-injury Nutrition (Enteral or Parenteral)
Protein, 2.5 g/kg/day
Fat, 1 g/kg/day
Carbohydrate, 10 g/kg/day
Increase Nutrition Intake (Enteral Route Preferred)
Respiratory quotient (<1.05 or decreased × 48 hr)

because of the reductions in activity and insensible losses typically observed in sedated infants in a thermoneutral intensive care environment, calorie requirements during acute metabolic stress are reduced to amounts necessary to meet *basal* metabolic needs alone (Table 81-6). Therefore, if calorie repletion based on the predicted requirements for healthy infants is administered during the acute phase of metabolic stress in critically ill infants, when the energy required for growth is negligible, substantial overfeeding is likely.[104]

Infant energy expenditure after complication-free surgical procedures does not increase substantially above measured baseline values.[72, 73] The characteristics of injury metabolism will be present only during the acute stress response period. For surgical stress alone, this period is relatively short, generally less that 48 hours.[67] For this reason, studies that attempt to evaluate surgically related acute stress changes during later postoperative periods are potentially flawed[132] and may introduce misleading conclusions. The magnitude of the stress response becomes much more difficult to predict if a substantial portion of the injury insult results from an additional, nonsurgical factor, such as burn trauma or sepsis. In a study of infants with a wide variety of stress insults, there was substantial interpatient variability in MEE relative to the predicted basal metabolic rate.[104] This variability, in large part, may be attributable to substantial differences in the acute

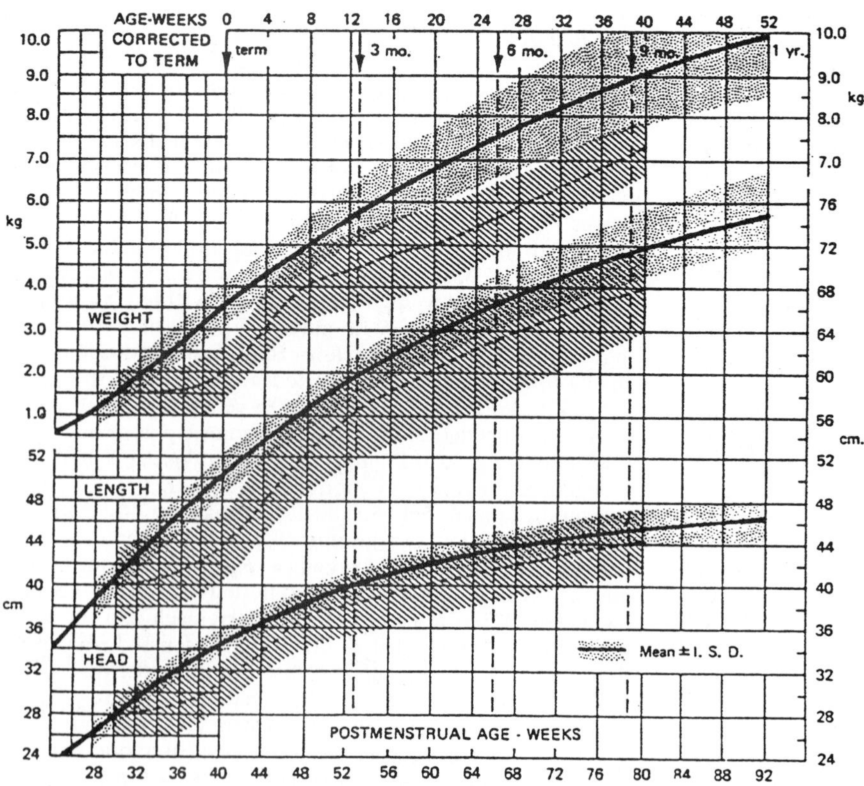

Figure 81–8. The *diagonal shading* represents longitudinal growth of sick preterm infants, 28 to 32 weeks' gestation (mean ± 1 SD) superimposed on Babson's curve for postnatal growth in well infants. Note the growth cessation during acute illness. (From Maisels MJ, Marks KH: Growth chart for sick premature infants [Letter]. J Pediatr 1981; 98:663–664.)

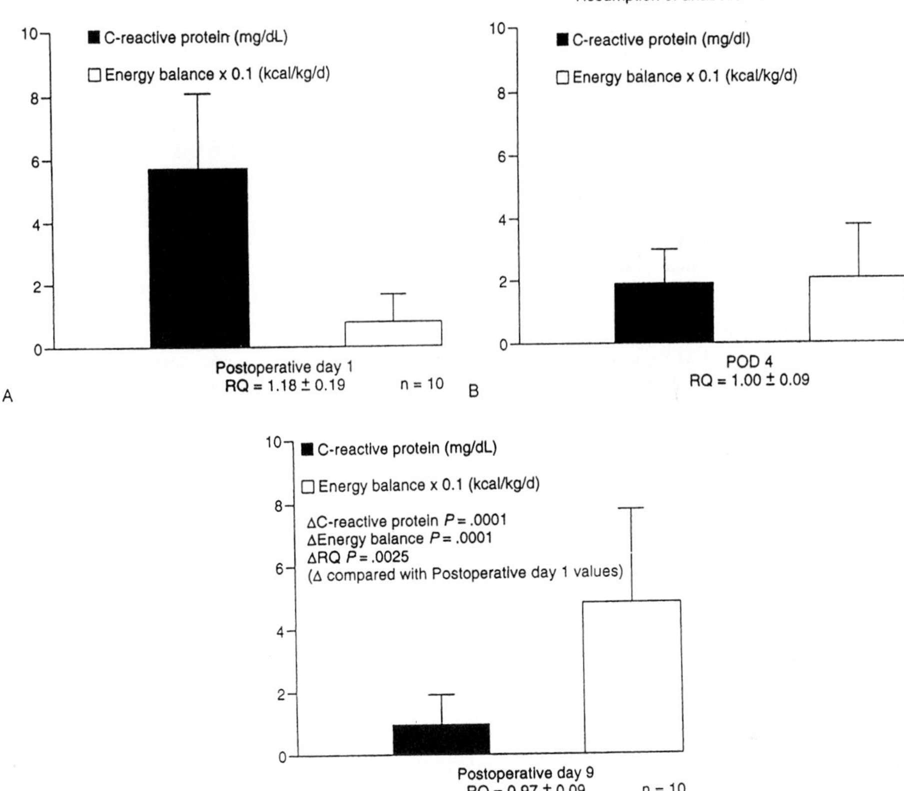

Figure 81–9. *A, Top,* Initial postoperative catabolism. Despite predictably low energy balance associated with basal energy delivery, the respiratory quotient (RQ) is greater than 1.0 during acute metabolic stress, with C-reactive protein (CRP) high, suggesting substantial lipogenesis at caloric intake that is moderately in excess of energy expenditure on postoperative day (POD) 1. *B, Middle,* Resumption of anabolic metabolism. Twofold increase in energy balance at constant basal energy intake associated with decreasing respiratory quotient and return of CRP toward normal serum concentrations suggests increasing use of caloric intake for anabolic metabolism as acute stress response resolves. *C, Bottom,* Normal growth recovery following acute injury. After increase in energy delivery to normal, nonstress calorie intake levels, energy balance reaches values appropriate for adequate growth, associated with a respiratory quotient below 1.0 and low CRP concentrations. Changes (Δ) in POD 9 CRP, energy balance, and respiratory quotient values are statistically significant relative to POD 1 values.

metabolic demands imposed by the underlying disease process.[74]

As the acute phase of metabolic stress resolves, the adaptive anabolic phase ensues, resulting in resumption of somatic growth. Recovery is characterized by decreasing concentrations of CRP and TUN values in association with increasing prealbumin. This trend can be established by the serial post-injury monitoring of these parameters[133] (Fig. 81–9).

To avoid premature increments in calorie delivery, daily indirect calorimetric measurements are carried out to assess RQ. Because RQ equals V_{CO_2}/V_{O_2} and because overfeeding causes increased lipogenesis (and increased V_{CO_2} relative to V_{O_2}) excessive calorie intake (especially excessive carbohydrate intake) generally results in an RQ of greater than 1.0.

For reasons previously discussed, metabolically stressed neonates appear to be particularly susceptible to overfeeding. Indirect calorimetric measurements in this population of infants reveal RQ well in excess of 1 when calorie delivery exceeds energy expenditure. For this reason, calories should be administered to match MEE needs only until acute metabolic stress has subsided (CRP < 2 mg/dL),[134] at which time calories can be advanced to promote growth recovery.[133] If indirect calorimetry is unavailable, only *basal* metabolic needs[15] should be delivered until CRP falls below stress levels. Because it has been shown that infant growth can be inhibited in association with acute illness,[134] this method provides a potentially useful guide to advance calorie delivery and optimize growth recovery without overfeeding infants during the acute phase of the metabolic response to injury.

References

1. Friis-Hansen B: Body water compartments in children: Changes during growth and related changes in body composition. Pediatrics 1961; 28:169–181.
2. Lorenz JM, Kleinman LI, Kotgol UR: Water balance in very low birth weight infants: Relationships to water and sodium intake and effect on outcome. J Pediatr 1982; 101:423–432.
3. Bidiwala KS, Lorenz JM, Kleinman LI: Renal function correlates of postnatal diuresis in preterm infants. Pediatrics 1988; 82:50–58.
4. Peterson S, Gotfredsen A, Knudsen FU: Lean body mass in small for gestational age and appropriate for gestational age infants. J Pediatr 1988; 113:886–889.
5. Smith FG, Klinkefus JM, Robillard JE: Effects of volume expansion on renal sympathetic nerve activity and cardiovascular and renal function in lambs. Am J Physiol 1992; 262:R651–R658.
6. Anderson DF, Parks CM, Faber JJ: Arterial pressure after chronic reductions in suprarenal aortic flow in fetal lambs. Am J Physiol 1987; 253:H838–H844.
7. Engelke SC, Shah BL, Vasan U: Sodium balance in very low birthweight infants. J Physiol 1978; 93:837–841.
8. Fukuda Y, Bertorello A, Aperia A: Ontogeny of the regulation of Na/K-ATPase activity on the renal proximal convoluted tubule cell. Pediatr Res 1991; 30:131–134.
9. Roy RN, Sinclair JC: Hydration of the low birth-weight infant. Clin Perinatol 1975; 2:393–417.
10. Forbes GB: Methods for determining composition of the human body. Pediatrics 1962; 29:477–494.
11. Cannon B, Nedergaard J: The biochemistry of an inefficient tissue: Brown adipose tissue. Essays Biochem 1985; 20:110–164.
12. Nedergaard J, Cannon B: Brown adipose tissue: Development and function. *In:* Fetal and Neonatal Physiology. Polin RA, Fox WW (Eds). Philadelphia, WB Saunders, 1992, p 314.
13. Catzeflis C, Schutz Y, Micheli JL, et al: Whole body protein synthesis and energy expenditure in very low birth weight infants. Pediatr Res 1985; 19:679–687.
14. Reichman BL, Chessex P, Putet G: Partition of energy metabolism and energy cost of growth in the very low-birth weight infant. Pediatrics 1982; 69:446–451.
15. Talbot FB: Basal metabolism standards for children. Am J Dis Child 1938; 55:455–459.
16. Fomon SJ: Requirements and recommended dietary intakes of protein during infancy. Pediatr Res 1991; 30:391–395.

17. Zlotkin SH, Bryan MH, Anderson GH: Intravenous nitrogen and energy intakes required to duplicate in utero nitrogen accretion in prematurely born human infants. J Pediatr 1981; 99:115–120.
18. Carlson SE, Barness LA: Macronutrient requirements for growth. *In:* Nutrition in Pediatrics. Walker WA, Watkins JB (Eds). Boston, Little, Brown, & Co, 1985, pp 3–15.
19. Dupont C, Rocchiccioli F, Bougneres PF: Urinary excretion of dicarboxylic acids in term newborns fed with 5% medium-chain triglycerides-enriched formula. J Pediatr Gastroenterol Nutr 1987; 6:313–314.
20. Linder MC: Nutrition and metabolism of the trace element. *In:* Nutritional Biochemistry and Metabolism: With Clinical Applications. Linder MC (Ed). New York, Elsevier, 1991, pp 215–276.
21. Patrick J. Zinc. *In:* CRC Handbook of Clinical Chemistry. Werner M (Ed). Boca Raton, Fla, CRC Press, 1989, pp 275–278.
22. Rotruck JT, Pope AL, Ganther HE, Swanson AB, Hafeman DG, Hoekstra WG: Selenium: Biochemical role as a component of glutathione peroxidase. Science 1973; 179:588–590.
23. Karpel JT, Peden VH: Copper deficiency in long-term parenteral nutrition. J Pediatr 1972; 80:32–36.
24. Reynolds AP, Kiely E, Meadows N: Manganese in long term paediatric parenteral nutrition. Arch Dis Child 1994; 71:527–528.
25. Mertz W: Chromium in human nutrition: A review. J Nutr 1993; 123:626–633.
26. Johnson JL, Rajagopalan KV, Cohen HJ: Molecular basis of the biologic function of molybdenum: Effect of tungsten on xanthine oxidase and sulfite oxidase in the rat. J Biol Chem 1974; 249:859–866.
27. Mahoney C, Mangolis M, Knauss TA, Labbe RF: Chronic vitamin A intoxication in infants fed chicken liver. Pediatrics 1980; 65:893–896.
28. American Academy of Pediatrics Committee on Nutrition: Nutritional needs of low birth weight infants. Pediatrics 1985; 75:976–1086.
29. Phelps DL: The role of vitamin E therapy in high-risk neonates. Clin Perinatol 1988; 15:955–963.
30. Suttie J: Vitamin K responsive hemorrhagic disease of infancy. J Pediatr Gastroenterol Nutr 1990; 11:4–6.
31. Letton RW, Chwals WJ: Endotoxin-induced hepatocyte energy status and metabolic compensation in adult versus neonatal rabbits. Surg Forum 1996; 47:683–686.
32. Battaglia FC: Chronic intrauterine deprivation. *In:* Intrauterine Asphyxia and the Developing Fetal Brain. Gluck L (Ed). Chicago, Year Book Medical Publishers, 1977, pp 331–338.
33. Miller RG, Jahoor F, Jaksic T: Decreased cysteine and proline synthesis in parenterally fed, premature infants. J Pediatr Surg 1995; 30:953–957.
34. Brasseur D, Johansson A, Goyens P, et al: Carnitine (C) balance in the parenterally fed premature neonate receiving a new C-containing fat emulsion. JPEN J Parenter Enteral Nutr 1991; 15(Suppl):25S.
35. Greene HL, Hambidge KM, Schanler R, et al: Guidelines for the use of vitamins, trace elements, calcium, magnesium, and phosphorus in infants and children receiving total parenteral nutrition: Report of subcommittee on pediatric parenteral nutrient requirements from the Committee on Clinical Practice Issues of the American Society of Clinical Nutrition. Am J Clin Nutr 1988; 48:1324–1342.
36. Chellis MJ, Sander SV, Webster H, Dean JM, and Jackson D: Early enteral feeding in the pediatric intensive care unit. JPEN J Parenter Enteral Nutr 1996; 20:71–73.
37. Nutrition Committee, Canadian Paediatric Society: Nutrient needs and feeding of premature infants. Can Med Assoc J 1995; 152:1765–1785.
38. Lucas A, Bloom SR, Aynsley-Green A: Gut hormones and minimal enteral feeding. Acta Paediatr Scand 1986; 75:719–723.
39. Brown RO, Carlson SD, Cowan GSM, et al: Enteral nutritional support management in a university teaching hospital: Team versus non-team. JPEN J Parenter Enteral Nutr 1987; 11:52–56.
40. Roberts P, Meredith JW, Black K, Zaloga G: Diarrhea does not alter impaired small bowel absorption following trauma. JPEN J Parenter Enteral Nutr 1993; 17:34S.
41. Payne-James JJ, Khawaja HT: First choice for total parenteral nutrition: The peripheral route. JPEN J Parenter Enteral Nutr 1993; 17:468–478.
42. Friedman B, Kanter G, Titus D: Femoral venous catheters: A safe alternative for delivering parenteral alimentation. Nutr Clin Pract 1994; 9:69–72.
43. Chatas MK, Paton JB: Sepsis outcomes in infants and children with central venous catheters: Percutaneous versus surgical insertion. J Obstet Gynecol Neonatal Nurs 1996; 6:500–506.
44. Collier S, Crouch J, Hendricks K, Caballero B: Use of cyclic parenteral nutrition in infants less than 6 months of age. Nutr Clin Pract 1994; 9:65–68.
45. Kemp L, Burge J, Choban P, Harden J, Mirtallo J, Flancbaum L: The effect of catheter type and site on infection rates in total parenteral nutrition patients. JPEN J Parenter Enteral Nutr 1994; 18:71–74.
46. Moore FA, Feliciano DV, Andrassy RJ, et al: Early enteral feeding, compared with parenteral, reduces postoperative septic complications. Ann Surg 1992; 216:172–183.
47. Herndon DN, Barrow RE, Stein M, et al: Increased mortality with intravenous supplemental feeding in severely burned patients. J Burn Care Rehabil 1989; 10:309–313.
48. Kudsk KA, Groce MA, Favian TC, Minard G, Tolley EA, Poret HA, Kuhl MR, Brown RO: Enteral versus parenteral feeding. Ann Surg 1992; 215:503–513.
49. Hamill PVV, Drizd TA, Johnson CL: Physical growth: National Center for Health Statistics percentiles. Am J Clin Nutr 1993; 32:607–629.
50. Waterlow JR: Classification and definition of protein-calorie malnutrition. Br Med J 1972; 3:566–569.
51. Merritt RJ, Suskind RM: Nutritional survey of hospitalized pediatric patients. Am J Clin Nutr 1979; 32:1320–1325.
52. Donaldson SS, Wesley MN, DeWys W, Suskind RM, Jaffe N, van Eys J: A study of the nutritional status of pediatric cancer patients. Am J Dis Child 1981; 135:1107–1112.
53. Trowbridge FL: Clinical and biochemical characteristics associated with anthropometric nutritional categories. Am J Clin Nutr 1979; 32:758–766.
54. Rao KV, Singh D: An evaluation of the relationship between nutritional status and anthropometric measurements. Am J Clin Nutr 1970; 23:83–93.
55. Grant A: Nutritional Assessment Guidelines. Seattle, Cutter Laboratories, 1979, pp 11–22.
56. Hamill PVV, Drizd TA, Johnson C, Reed RB, Roche AF, Moore WM: Physical growth: National Center for Health Statistics percentiles. Am J Clin Nutr 1979; 32:607–629.
57. Carter P, Carr D, van Eys J, Coody D: Nutritional parameters in children with cancer. J Am Diet Assoc 1983; 82:616–622.
58. Smythe PM, Brereton-Stiles GG, Grace JH, et al: Thymolymphatic deficiency and depression of cell-mediated immunity in protein-calorie malnutrition. Lancet 1971; 28:939–944.
59. Chandra RK: Immunocompetence in undernutrition. J Pediatr 1972; 81:1194–1200.
60. Bistrian BR, Blackburn GL, Scrimshaw N, Flatt JP: Cellular immunity in semistarved states in hospitalized adults. Am J Clin Nutr 1975; 28:1148–1155.
61. Mullen JL, Buzby GP, Matthews DC, Smale BF, Rosato EF: Reduction of operative morbidity and mortality by combined preoperative and postoperative nutritional support. Ann Surg 1980; 192:604–613.
62. Hays DM, Merritt RJ, White L, et al: Effect of total parenteral nutrition on marrow recovery during induction therapy for acute nonlymphocytic leukemia in childhood. Med Pediatr Oncol 1983; 11:134–140.
63. Neumann CG, Lawlor GJ, Stiehm ER, Swenseid ME, Newton C, Herbert J, Ammann AJ, Jacob M: Immunological responses in malnourished children. Am J Clin Nutr 1975; 28:89–104.
64. Law DK, Dudrick SJ, Abdou NI: The effect of dietary protein depletion on immunocompetence. Ann Surg 1974; 179:168–173.
65. Michie HR, Spriggs DR, Manogue KR, Sherman MD, Revhaug A, O'Dwyer ST, Arthur K, Dinarello CA, Cerami A, Wolff SW: Tumor necrosis factor and endotoxin induce similar metabolic responses in human beings. Surgery 1988; 104:280–286.
66. Pacitti AJ, Austgen TR, Souba WW: Adaptive regulation of alanine transport in hepatic plasma membrane vesicles from the endotoxin-treated rat. J Surg Res 1991; 51:46–53.
67. Anand KJS, Hanson DD, Hickey PR: Hormonal-metabolic stress responses in neonates undergoing cardiac surgery. Anesthesiology 1990; 73:661–670.

68. Taylor AF, Lally KP, Chwals WJ, McCurnin DC, Gerstmann DR, Shade RA, deLemos RA: Hormonal response of the premature primate to operative stress. J Pediatr Surg 1993; 28:844–846.
69. Khilnani P, Munoz R, Salem M, Gelb C, Todres ID, Chernow B: Hormonal responses to surgical stress in children. J Pediatr Surg 1993; 28:1–4.
70. Anand KJS, Aynsley-Green A: Measuring the severity of surgical stress in newborn infants. J Pediatr Surg 1988; 23:297–305.
71. Long CL, Schaffel N, Geiger JW, Schiller WR, Blakemore WS: Metabolic response to injury and illness: Estimation of energy and protein needs from indirect calorimetry and nitrogen balance. JPEN J Parenter Enteral Nutr 1979; 3:452–456.
72. Shanbhogue RL, Lloyd DA: Absence of hypermetabolism after operation in the newborn infant. JPEN J Parenter Enteral Nutr 1992; 16:333–336.
73. Jones MO, Pierro A, Hammond P, Lloyd DA: The metabolic response to operative stress in infants. J Pediatr Surg 1993; 28:1258–1263.
74. Chwals WJ, Letton RW, Jamie A, Charles B: Stratification of injury severity using energy expenditure response in surgical infants. J Pediatr Surg 1995; 30:1161–1164.
75. Gump FE, Long C, Killian P, Kinney JM: Studies of glucose intolerance in septic injured patients. J Trauma 1974; 14:378–388.
76. Evans EI, Butterfield WJH: The stress response in the severely burned. Ann Surg 1951; 134:588–613.
77. Howard JM: Studies of the absorption and metabolism of glucose following injury. The systemic response to injury. Ann Surg 1955; 141:321–326.
78. White RH, Frayn KN, Little RA, et al: Hormonal and metabolic responses to glucose infusion in sepsis by the hyperglycaemic glucose clamp technique. JPEN J Parenter Enteral Nutr 1987; 11:345–353.
79. Long CL, Kinney JM, Geiger JW: Nonsuppressability of gluconeogenesis by glucose in septic patients. Metabolism 1976; 25:193–201.
80. Henderson AA, Frayn KN, Galasko CS, Little RA: Dose-response relationships for the effects of insulin on glucose and fat metabolism in injured patients and control subjects. Clin Sci (Colch) 1991; 80:25–32.
81. Dahn MS, Jacobs LA, Smith S, et al: The relationship of insulin production to glucose metabolism in severe sepsis. Arch Surg 1985; 120:166–172.
82. Vary TC, Siegel JH, Nakatani T, et al: Effects of sepsis on activity of pyruvate dehydrogenase complex in skeletal muscle and liver. Am J Physiol 1986; 250:E634–E640.
83. Wolfe RR, Jahoor F, Herndon DN, et al: Isotopic evaluation of the metabolism of pyruvate and related substrates in normal adult volunteers and severely burned children: Effect of dichloroacetate and glucose infusion. Surgery 1991; 110:54–67.
84. Frayn KN, Little RA, Stoner HB, Galasko CS: Metabolic control in non-septic patients with musculoskeletal injuries. Injury 1984; 16:73–79.
85. Brooks DC, Bessey PQ, Black PR, et al: Insulin stimulates branched chain amino acid uptake and diminished nitrogen flux from skeletal muscle of injured patients. J Surg Res 1986; 40:395–405.
86. Jahoor F, Shangraw RE, Miyoshi H, et al: Role of insulin and glucose oxidation in mediating the protein catabolism of burns and sepsis. Am J Physiol 1989; 257:E323–E331.
87. Sakurai Y, Aarsland A, Herndon DN, et al: Stimulation of muscle protein synthesis by long-term insulin infusion in severely burned patients. Ann Surg 1995; 222:283–297.
88. Valarini R, Sousa MF, Kalil R, et al: Anabolic effects of insulin and amino acids in promoting nitrogen accretion in postoperative patients. J Parenter Enteral Nutr 1994; 18:214–218.
89. Chwals WJ, Bistrian BR: Role of exogenous growth hormone and insulin-like growth factor I in malnutrition and acute metabolic stress: A hypothesis. Crit Care Med 1991; 19:1317–1322.
90. Herndon DN, Barrow RE, Kunkel KR, et al: Effects of recombinant human growth hormone on donor-site healing in severely burned children. Ann Surg 1990; 12:424–431.
91. Chwals WJ: Adjunctive growth hormone during acute metabolic stress in neonates. 4th International Congress on the Immune Consequences of Trauma, Shock and Sepsis. Munich, March 4–8, 1997, p 27.
92. Letton RW, Chwals WJ, Jamie A, et al: Neonatal lipid utilization increases with injury severity: Recombinant human growth hormone versus placebo. J Pediatr Surg 1996; 31:1068–1074.
93. Fletcher JP, Little JM, Guest PK: A comparison of serum transferrin and serum prealbumin as nutritional parameters. JPEN J Parenter Enteral Nutr 1987; 11:144–147.
94. Chwals WJ, Fernandez ME, Jamie AC, Charles BJ: Relationship of metabolic indices to postoperative mortality in surgical infants. J Pediatr Surg 1993; 28:819–822.
95. Chwals WJ, Fernandez ME, Charles BJ, et al: Serum visceral protein levels reflect protein-calorie repletion in neonates recovering from major surgery. J Pediatr Surg 1992; 27:317–321.
96. Tueting JL, Chwals WJ, Byerley LO: Anabolic recovery relative to degree of prematurity following acute injury in neonates. J Pediatr Surg 1999; 34:13–17.
97. Felig P, Marliss EB, Cahill GF Jr: Metabolic response to human growth hormone during prolonged starvation. J Clin Invest 1971; 50:411–421.
98. Loder PB, Kee AJ, Horsburgh R, et al: Validity of urinary urea nitrogen as a measure of total urinary nitrogen in adult patients requiring parenteral nutrition. Crit Care Med 1989; 17:309–312.
99. Bistrian BR: A simple technique to estimate severity of stress. Surg Gynecol Obstet 1979; 148:675–678.
100. Rickham PP: The Metabolic Response to Neonatal Surgery. Cambridge, Mass, Harvard University Press, 1957, pp 7–93.
101. Ohzato H, Yoshizaki K, Nishimoto N, Ogata A, Tagoh H, Monden M, Gotoh M, Kishimoto T, Mori T: Interleukin-6 as a new indicator of inflammatory status: Detection of serum levels of interleukin-6 and C-reactive protein after surgery. Surgery 1992; 111:201–209.
102. Dickson PW, Bannister D, Schreiber G: Minor burns lead to major changes in synthesis rates of plasma proteins in the liver. J Trauma 1987; 27:283–286.
103. McGilvery RW: Biochemistry: A Functional Approach. Philadelphia, WB Saunders, 1979, p 532.
104. Chwals WJ, Lally KP, Woolley MM, et al: Measured energy expenditure in critically ill infants and young children. J Surg Res 1988; 44:467–472.
105. Pollack MM, Ruttimann UE, Getson PR: Pediatric risk of mortality (PRISM) score. Crit Care Med 1988; 16:1110–1116.
106. Steinhorn DM, Green TP: Severity of illness correlates with alterations in energy metabolism in the pediatric intensive care unit. Crit Care Med 1991; 19:1503–1509.
107. Chwals WJ, Fernandez ME, Jamie AC, Charles BJ, Rushing JT: Detection of postoperative sepsis in infants with the use of metabolic stress monitoring. Arch Surg 1994; 129:437–442.
108. Piedboeuf B, Chessex P, Hazan J, et al: Total parenteral nutrition in the newborn infant: Energy substrates and respiratory gas exchange. J Pediatr 1991; 118:97–102.
109. Askanazi J, Weissman C. LaSala P, et al: Effect of protein intake on ventilatory drive. Anesthesiology 1984; 60:106–110.
110. Bresson JL, Bader B, Rocchiccioli F, et al: Protein-metabolism kinetics and energy-substrate utilization in infants fed parenteral solutions with different glucose-fat ratios. Am J Clin Nutr 1991; 54:370–376.
111. Van Aerde JEE, Sauer PJJ, Pencharz PB, et al: Effect of replacing glucose with lipid on the energy metabolism of newborn infants. Clin Sci 1989; 76:581–588.
112. Salas-Salvado J, Molina J, Figueras J, et al: Effect of the quality of infused energy on substrate utilization in the newborn receiving total parenteral nutrition. Pediatr Res 1993; 33:112–117.
113. Delafosse B, Bouffard Y, Viale JP, et al: Respiratory changes induced by parenteral nutrition in postoperative patients undergoing inspiratory pressure support ventilation. Anesthesiology 1987; 66:393–396.
114. Elwyn DH, Kinney JM, Jeevanandam M, et al: Influence of increasing carbohydrate intake on glucose kinetics in injured patients. Ann Surg 1979; 190:117–127.
115. Burke JF, Wolfe RR, Mullany CJ: Glucose requirements following burn injury. Ann Surg 1979; 190:274–285.
116. Askanazi J, Carpentier YA, Elwyn DH, et al: Influence of total parenteral nutrition on fuel utilization in injury and sepsis. Ann Surg 1980; 191:40–46.
117. Askanazi J, Rosenbaum S, Hyman R: Respiratory changes induced by the large glucose loads of total parenteral nutrition. JAMA 1980; 243:1444–1447.

118. Van den Berg B, Stam H: Metabolic and respiratory effects of enteral nutrition in patients during mechanical ventilation. Intensive Care Med 1988; 14:14:206–211.
119. Askanazi J, Nordenstrom J, Rosenbaum SH, et al: Nutrition for the patient with respiratory failure: Glucose versus fat. Anesthesiology 1990; 54:373–377.
120. Nussbaum MS, Fischer JE: Pathogenesis of hepatic steatosis during total parenteral nutrition. *In:* Nyhus LM (Ed). Surgery Annual. Norwalk, Conne, Appleton & Lange, 1991, pp 1–11.
121. Lowry SF, Brennan MF: Abnormal liver function during parenteral nutrition: Relation to infusion excess. J Surg Res 1979; 26:300–306.
122. Payne-James JJ, Silk DB: Heptobiliary dysfunction associated with total parenteral nutrition. Dig Dis 1992; 9:106–124.
123. Freund HR: Abnormalities of liver function and hepatic damage associated with total parenteral nutrition. Nutrition 1991; 7:1–6.
124. Das JB, Cosentino CM, Levy MF, et al: Early hepatobiliary dysfunction during total parenteral nutrition: An experimental study. J Pediatr Surg 1993; 28:14–18.
125. Bursztein S, Elwyn DH, Askanazi J: Energy metabolism and indirect calorimetry in critically ill and injured patients. Acute Care 1988; 14–15:91–110.
126. Sobrado J, Moldawer LL, Pomposelli JJ, et al: Lipid emulsions and reticuloendothelial system function in healthy and burned guinea pigs. Am J Clin Nutr 1985; 42:855–863.
127. Yamazaki K, Maiz A, Moldawer LL, et al: Complications associated with the overfeeding of infected animals. J Surg Res 1986; 40:152–158.
128. Koea JB, Shaw JHF: Total parenteral nutrition in surgical illness: How much? How good? Nutrition 1992; 8:275–281.
129. Vo NM, Waycaster M, Acuff RV, et al: Effects of postoperative carbohydrate overfeeding. Am Surg 1987; 53:632–635.
130. Alexander JW, Gonce SJ, Miskell PW, et al: A new model for studying nutrition in peritonitis. Ann Surg 1989; 209:334–340.
131. Dominioni L, Trocki O, Fang CH, et al: Enteral feeding in burn hypermetabolism: Nutritional and metabolic effects of different levels of calorie and protein intake. JPEN J Parenter Enteral Nutr 1985; 9:269–279.
132. Billeaud C, Piedboeuf B, Chessex P: Respiratory gas exchange in response to fat-free parenteral nutrition: A comparison after thoracic or abdominal surgery in newborn infants. J Pediatr Surg 1993; 28:11–13.
133. Chwals WJ: Overfeeding the critically ill child: Fact or fantasy? New Horiz 1994; 2:147–155.
134. Letton RW, Chwals WJ, Jamie A, Charles B: Early postoperative alterations in infant energy use increase the risk of overfeeding. J Pediatr Surg 1995; 30:988–993.

82

Micronutrient Deficiencies

Khursheed N. Jeejeebhoy, MBBS, PhD, FRCPC

The major part of our dietary intake is composed of water, proteins, carbohydrates, fats, and electrolytes. However, for the utilization of these nutrients it is essential to absorb other substances, called micronutrients, in relatively smaller and in some instances minute amounts. These micronutrients belong to two main groups of substances called *trace elements* and *vitamins*. The former are inorganic elements, and the latter are complex organic compounds. Both are essential because they regulate metabolic processes as constituents of enzyme complexes required for the utilization of carbohydrates, proteins, and fats.

TRACE ELEMENTS

General Aspects

Cotzias[1] defined an *essential* trace element as one that has the following characteristics:

1. It is present in the healthy tissues of all living things.
2. The tissue concentration is constant from one animal to the next.
3. Withdrawal leads to a reproducible functional and/or structural abnormality.
4. Addition of the element prevents the abnormality.
5. The abnormality is associated with a specific biochemical change.
6. The biochemical change is prevented or cured along with the observed clinical abnormality when the nutrient is given.

In animal studies, 15 elements have been found to be essential for health. They are iron, zinc, copper, chromium, selenium, iodine, cobalt, manganese, nickel, molybdenum, fluorine, tin, silicon, vanadium, and arsenic. However, according to the strict criteria suggested by Cotzias, only the first seven have been shown to be necessary for health in humans. Of these, cobalt is essential only as part of the corrin ring in vitamin B_{12}.

Trace elements are absorbed as inorganic substances and as organic compounds. In natural foods, the latter often predominate. Because the absorption of the two forms may differ, results of studies with inorganic test substances cannot be equated with the availability of the same elements in organic form in food. For example, heme iron is absorbed efficiently, and the availability of this form of iron cannot be judged from studies with elemental iron. Similarly, chromium as an inorganic salt is poorly absorbed, but the organic form in yeast is well absorbed.

Absorbed trace elements circulate as protein-bound complexes that are not always in free equilibrium with tissue stores. For example, the exchangeable plasma copper is present in small amounts bound to albumin. In contrast, the major form of circulating copper, ceruloplasmin, is not freely exchangeable. For this and other reasons, total circulating levels may not reflect the availability of an element for nutritional needs.

Tissue stores of a trace element may not be available to meet needs during a period of deficient supply for two reasons. First, they may be incorporated in enzyme proteins that do not exchange with the free pool; second, during anabolism there is net flow of trace elements into cells, so that cellular stores cannot be mobilized.

The converse applies in catabolism. For example, in hypercatabolic states, even though zinc is being lost and the patient is in negative zinc balance, plasma zinc is normal because of net outflow from tissue stores.[2] When nutritional support is given, resulting in protein synthesis, a positive zinc balance occurs, but plasma levels fall and deficiency results unless exogenous zinc is given. Because the action of trace elements depends on other factors such as age, metabolic and nutritional states (anabolic or catabolic), and availability of agonists and antagonists, clinical deficiency cannot be predicted by simple demonstration of a low blood level of the element. As an example of this complexity, it has been found that at least some degree of selenium deficiency can be overcome by giving vitamin E. Also, children with selenium-responsive Keshan disease have levels of plasma selenium no lower than those of children with phenylketonuria receiving artificial diets, yet the latter do not show a clinical deficiency.

These findings make it imperative to look for subclinical functional changes to enable us to define needs. For example, even in patients who did not have an overt clinical deficiency of zinc, Wolman and colleagues[2] showed that a negative zinc balance was associated with reduced nitrogen retention and carbohydrate tolerance, justifying the need for maintaining balance. Finally, the route of excretion of most trace elements, except chromium, is mainly through the gastrointestinal tract. This raises the possibility that abnormal gastrointestinal losses may increase requirements in patients with disease of the gastrointestinal tract. Another consequence of the gastrointestinal route of excretion is that renal disease does not reduce the need to give these elements.

Iron

Iron Requirements in the Intensive Care Unit

There are no data on the needs for iron in the intensive care unit (ICU). Concern has been expressed that increased levels of circulating iron are associated with an increased incidence of infections.[3] However, these data have shown an increased incidence of malaria, neonatal *Escherichia coli* infection, and infections related to *Vibrio vulnificus* in patients with hemochromatosis.[4] On the other hand in nonmalarious countries iron supplementation has been beneficial and reduced sepsis rates.[3]

Recommendations for Intravenous Iron

A dilute solution of iron dextran can be used to provide 1 to 2 mg of iron per day to replace physiologic losses.[5]

Zinc

Zinc is a widely distributed element in foodstuffs (shellfish, liver, milk, and wheat bran) and in the human body. It has been identified as a part of about 120 enzymes.[6] Among them are carbonic anhydrase, carboxypeptidase, alkaline phosphatase, oxidoreductases, transferases, ligases, hydrolases, lyases, and isomerases. Although the syndrome of zinc deficiency cannot be identified with the dearth of any one enzyme, zinc deficiency does have a pronounced effect on nucleic acid metabolism, thus influencing protein and amino acid metabolism.

Zinc is an integral constituent of deoxyribonucleic acid (DNA) polymerase, reverse transcriptase, ribonucleic acid (RNA) polymerase, transfer RNA (tRNA) synthetase, and the protein chain elongation factor.[6] Thus, zinc deficiency can alter protein synthesis at a number of different points, and it is not surprising that in the absence of zinc, growth arrest occurs. Furthermore, zinc deficiency is teratogenic as determined by animal studies and observations of patients with untreated acrodermatitis enteropathica. This finding suggests that zinc deficiency may affect gene expression. In experimental studies of unicellular organisms, it has been shown that zinc deficiency changes the nature of RNA polymerase and the base composition of messenger RNA (mRNA). The translated peptides contain a preponderance of arginine-rich peptides that can bind to anions such as phosphate groups in nucleic acids and alter their action. Such an alteration may affect the synthesis of histones, proteins that are known to reduce the activity of DNA as a template.[6]

The preceding experimental findings about zinc and nucleic acids are interesting, in view of the clinical observation that a number of functions dependent on protein synthesis are suppressed by zinc deficiency. These include growth, cellular immunity,[7,8] fertility, hair growth, wound healing,[9] and plasma protein levels. Thus, it is obvious that zinc deficiency leads to profound disturbances of protein synthesis. In addition, in volunteer studies, experimental mild zinc deficiency reduced thymulin levels and the CD4/CD8 ratio.[10]

Zinc Requirements and Recommendations

It is recommended that zinc be taken at 15 mg/day in the diet of adults. On the basis of a mean absorption of 20%, this amounts to about 3 mg of absorbed zinc per day. Zinc intake during pregnancy does not need to be increased, but during lactation the intake should be increased by 7 mg/day for the first month of lactation and by 4 mg/day subsequently. Wolman and colleagues[2] found that patients receiving parenteral nutrition who did not have diarrhea required about 2.5 mg/day for balance. Requirements increased with increased catabolism and gastrointestinal losses (by 12 mg per liter of small intestinal fluid and 17 mg per liter of stool).

In addition to replacing losses, infants need zinc for growth. This is especially true of preterm infants, because two thirds of the infant's zinc is transferred from the mother during the last 10 to 12 weeks of normal gestation. It has been estimated that 0.5 to 0.75 mg of zinc is taken up per day during the last 3 weeks of gestation and the first 3 weeks of postnatal life in babies who gain 1.5 kg, making the requirements about 300 to 500 μg/kg/day. James and MacMahon[11] found that infants required 300 μg/kg/day to maintain balance. In older children, 50 μg/kg/day maintained normal serum levels, and it was recommended that 100 μg/kg/day be given as a safe intake for growth.[12] In addition, supplementation is required for abnormal gastrointestinal losses, but these doses have not been determined experimentally.

Zinc Requirements in the Intensive Care Unit

In the ICU, zinc status can be difficult to evaluate because of many factors. Sepsis reduces plasma levels. Increased losses result from intestinal drainage. In addition, with raw wounds and burns, zinc losses amount to a mean of 27 mg/day.[13] The ratio of zinc to nitrogen in these exudates was found to be 2.8 mg Zn/g N, which is as high as that in muscle tissue (i.e., 2.0 mg Zn/g N[13]). Increased zinc losses in urine amounting to 3 to 7 mg/day occur after head injury[14] and burns.[15] Whereas the urinary zinc peaked at a week in head-injured patients, that in patients with burns peaked 2 to 5 weeks after injury, which appeared to be due to a tubular defect in the kidney. After coronary bypass surgery, prolonged low plasma zinc levels also suggest zinc deficiency.[16] These findings suggest that zinc losses in injured and burned patients are increased to a variable extent.

Copper

Copper is found in many foods, including organ meats, shellfish, legumes, and cocoa. It is widely distributed in human tissues and is a part of enzymes such as cytochrome-*c* oxidase, superoxide dismutase, dopamine β-hydroxylase, monoamine oxidase, and lysyl oxidase. In addition, 90% of the plasma copper is in the form of ceruloplasmin. The major effects of copper deficiency are expressed through the consequences of ceruloplasmin and lysyl oxidase deficiencies.

Ceruloplasmin is an iron oxidase. Iron released by red blood cell breakdown is taken up by macrophages. It is then released from macrophages and bound to transferrin for transport to iron-storing and iron-requiring tissues. Similarly, storage iron in the liver is in equilibrium with transferrin. Ceruloplasmin oxidizes ferrous iron and aids in transfer of iron from stores to transferrin. It is believed that iron in cells is reduced by riboflavin to the ferrous form to cross the cell membrane and that after crossing it has to be reoxidized to the ferric form to bind to transferrin. Therefore, copper deficiency results in conditioned iron deficiency.

Mature collagen and elastin are characterized by the presence of cross-links formed from precursor peptides such as α-aminoadipic acid δ-semialdehyde, or allysine, and δ-hydroxy-α-aminoadipic acid δ-semialdehyde, or hydroxyallysine. These substances are formed by the oxidative deamination of peptidyl lysine or hydroxylysine residues. This process depends on the copper-containing enzyme lysyl oxidase.

In addition to the effects of copper deficiency on iron and collagen, another result is leukopenia.

Copper Requirements and Recommendations

The normal diet supplies 2 to 4 mg/day and with this intake deficiency has never been observed in adults. In utero, a major part of body copper is gained during the last 10 weeks of gestation, and it is estimated that a premature or neonatal infant retains 100 to 130 μg/kg/day over a 3-week period. In malnourished infants, between 40 and 135 μg/kg/day is required.

In adult patients receiving a parenteral nutrition regimen, Shike and coworkers[17] found that 0.3 mg/day was sufficient to meet the needs of patients without diarrhea. The requirement rose to 0.5 mg/day in those with diarrhea. In contrast, the requirement fell to 0.1 mg/day in patients with abnormal liver function.[23] These figures compare well with those of Jacobson and Western,[18] who obtained a positive balance with all patients but one by giving 0.24 to 0.29 mg of copper per day. In infants, the need, based on balance, is for 50 μg/kg/day. However, the range varies between 10 and 50 μg/kg/day.[11] Hence, caution should be exercised in order to avoid overload, and the lower figure of 20 μg/kg/day has been suggested. For older children, 20 μg/kg/day has been found sufficient to meet needs.[12]

Copper Requirements in the Intensive Care Unit

Copper excretion from burn wounds can amount to 4 mg/day[13] and is associated with depressed serum copper levels as well as increased urinary copper.[19] These findings suggest increased requirements in these patients. Gastrointestinal losses from diarrhea and fistulas can also increase needs.

Chromium

Good dietary sources of chromium are brewer's yeast, corn oil, vegetables, and whole grains. Chromium deficiency in animals has been found to cause a syndrome of glucose intolerance similar to that of clinical diabetes. The abnormalities found were corrected by giving chromium.[20] This element is also important in promoting insulin action in peripheral tissues. In vitro, chromium enhances insulin stimulation of glucose oxidation and lipogenesis in adipose tissue. In muscle it also increases insulin-induced glycogenesis. Insulin-stimulated amino acid transport is also positively influenced by chromium.

This set of observations in animals is supported by the finding that the intravenous administration of chromium increased glucose utilization in a patient with chromium deficiency.[21] Chromium administration to this patient also increased the fall in circulating leucine levels in response to a glucose load. Because the insulin response to the glucose load was normal, this observation suggests that chromium enhances insulin-stimulated tissue uptake of leucine. The respiratory quotient (RQ) was low and the plasma free fatty acid (FFA) levels were high before the administration of chromium. The low RQ and high FFA levels show that fat mobilization and oxidation were continuing despite normal insulin levels. Administration of chromium reduced free fatty acid levels, increased the RQ, and promoted glucose oxidation for energy. Thus, chromium is one of the factors that influence insulin sensitivity.

Chromium Requirements and Recommendations

For the adult, oral chromium requirements have not been determined. Deficiency in patients receiving total parenteral nutrition may be due to continuous glucose loading resulting in higher urinary excretion, which in turn increases requirements. It was estimated that in one such patient the needs might have been increased to 10 to 20 μg/day. For infants, balance studies by James and MacMahon[11] indicated a requirement of 0.14 to 0.2 μg/kg/day. However, balance studies in more patients with a spectrum of clinical conditions need to be done to obtain the required information.

Chromium Requirements in the Intensive Care Unit

In view of glucose intolerance with a metabolic diabetic state, chromium requirements are likely to be increased in septic patients. However, there are no data at present to support this concept. Studies showing high plasma chromium levels in patients receiving long-term total parenteral nutrition (TPN) have appeared and have been interpreted as showing chromium overload. However, glucose-based TPN increases chromium losses, and these levels are likely to be the result of glucose loading.[21]

Selenium

Selenium is interrelated with other antioxidants, such as vitamin E. Deficiency of one can be partially corrected by giving the other. To understand the need for these two micronutrients, it is necessary to examine the alternative means by which oxygen is reduced in biologic systems. Normally, the enzyme cytochrome oxidase accepts electrons from cytochrome *c* at the end exposed to the cytosol and discharges them by reacting with $4H^+$ to form water. The alternative path involves the monovalent addition of electrons to form superoxide. The superoxide, if left unaltered, disproportionates to hydrogen peroxide (H_2O_2) and oxygen. The H_2O_2 can also react by the Haber-Weiss[22] reaction with superoxide to form hydroxyl ions. Thus, in the absence of appropriate controls, a number of reactive peroxide and hydroxyl radicals can form and damage the cell. In well-nourished cells, superoxide dismutase (SOD) disproportionates superoxide to H_2O_2 and the peroxide so formed is reduced by glutathione peroxidase (GSHpx) to water.

$$O_2 \xrightarrow{e^-} O_2^- \xrightarrow{e^-} O_2^{2-}$$

$$O_2^- + H_2O_2 \rightarrow O_2 + OH^- + OH$$

$$O_2^- + H^+ \xrightarrow{SOD} H_2O_2 \xrightarrow{GSHpx} H_2O$$

Glutathione peroxidase is an enzyme made up of four subunits, each containing selenocysteine as an integral part of the molecule. In association with superoxide dismutase, it controls the levels of superoxide and peroxide in the cell. This in turn affects lipid peroxidation of polyunsaturated fatty acids in cell membranes. Vitamin E is another line of defense and controls the formation of hydroperoxides in the fatty acid residues of phospholipids, a process that depends on the antioxidant role of the vitamin and also involves its entering into a structural relation with membrane phospholipids. Finally, lipid hydroperoxides may be reduced by GSHpx to hydroxy acids.

Biologic reactions that produce superoxide are (1) enzyme reactions, such as those involving xanthine oxidase; (2) metabolic pathways, such as the hexose monophosphate shunt and oxidative reactions mediated by cytochrome P_{450}; (3) interaction of dioxygen with the electron transport chain in the mitochondria; and (4) phagocytosis, in which a burst of oxidative metabolism is associated with generation by the hexose monophosphate shunt of reduced nicotinamide-adenine dinucleotide phosphate (NADPH), which in turn is used by NADPH oxidase to generate superoxide. The excess superoxide is controlled by SOD and GSHpx. Hence, it is not surprising that bacterial killing is affected by selenium deficiency. In addition, some antineoplastic agents such as bleomycin produce superoxide.

Thus, a number of different pathophysiologic situations and metabolic states can increase superoxide evolution and the need for protection by vitamin E and GSHpx.

Selenium is incorporated into tissue proteins as selenocysteine. The incorporation of selenium into an amino acid occurs via a unique tRNA and into protein through specific codons in the mRNA. Protein catabolism releases toxic selenocysteine, which is rapidly hydrolyzed by selenocysteine β-lyase with release of free selenium.

Selenium Requirements and Recommendations

Human metabolic studies suggest a minimum selenium intake of 0.25 μmol/day,[23] and in studies from China the minimum intake was 0.38 μmol/day. In North American volunteers, the requirement has been estimated to be 0.68 μmol/day.[24] The recommended daily allowance (RDA) is defined as 0.011 μmol/kg/day. This allowance should be increased by 0.12 and 0.24 μmol/day, respectively, in pregnant and lactating women.

Patients receiving parenteral nutrition without added selenium may have selenium deficiency with associated muscle weakness,[25] and in two patients receiving long-term TNP cardiomyopathy has also been described.[26, 27] Selenite has been given at 60 to 120 μg/day without toxic effects to patients receiving home parenteral nutrition (HPN) and has succeeded in maintaining levels of plasma selenium.

Selenium Requirements in the Intensive Care Unit

Selenium levels were reduced in ICU patients and continued to fall with increasing length of stay.[28] In this study, selenium excretion was inversely related to nitrogen balance, suggesting that increased protein catabolism resulted in selenium loss. In another series, burn patients had reduced plasma and erythrocyte selenium levels, reduced glutathione peroxidase levels, and reduced renal excretion of selenium.[29] These data suggest increased selenium requirements in ICU patients, but the exact requirements are not known.

VITAMINS

Vitamins are essential nutrients that are active in minute quantities. Although it seems obvious that these substances have to be included in any regimen of TPN in order to avoid deficiency, their optimal dose and frequency of administration have not been studied in detail in patients receiving TPN. The recommendations derived from available studies have been based upon simple observations of plasma or blood levels during a given regimen.[30–32]

Fat-Soluble Vitamins

Vitamin A

Vitamin A occurs in nature in three forms. All-*trans*-retinol or A_1 and 3-dehydroretinol or A_2 are the forms found in mammals. In vegetables, vitamin A occurs as the precursor β-carotene.

REQUIREMENTS IN THE ICU. Because vitamin A is required for epithelial differentiation and cell multiplication, its requirement is likely to be increased in patients with injury. In burn patients vitamin A levels fell rapidly,[33] but unlike levels of retinol binding protein, they did not recover for weeks in patients with a burn surface area greater than 20%, suggesting deficiency. The requirements are clearly not known.

Vitamin D

REQUIREMENTS IN THE ICU. The RDA for vitamin D is difficult to judge because the skin synthesizes a great deal of vitamin D. The RDA of 200 IU/day is quite generous considering the variable amount synthesized by the skin. The RDA for pregnant and lactating women has been set at 400 IU/day. In states of malabsorption, intake should be raised. In patients receiving TPN, hypercalcemia may develop when intravenous vitamin D_2 is given,[34, 35] and hypercalcemia in this situation appears to be associated with pancreatitis.[36] We therefore do not routinely add vitamin D to TPN. If vitamin D is added, the patient should be monitored for development of hypercalcemia and pancreatitis. In this context, it should be remembered that when the serum albumin is reduced, the presence of a normal serum calcium level indicates hypercalcemia.

Vitamin E

There are seven forms of vitamin E. Three of these, α-tocopherol, β-tocopherol, and γ-tocopherol, are found in the diet. In addition, the molecule of α-tocopherol has several asymmetric centers that give rise to stereoisomers. Natural α-tocopherol is biologically the most potent and is composed of only one isomer. It is called RRR-α-tocopherol. The synthetic compound has eight isomers and is only 74% as potent as the natural compound. It is called all-rac-α-tocopherol. Dietary tocopherol is expressed as RRR-α-tocopherol equivalents (α-TEs). One α-TE is equal to the activity of 1 mg of RRR-α-tocopherol. β-Tocopherol is 50% and γ-tocopherol 10% as active as RRR-α-tocopherol.

REQUIREMENTS IN THE ICU. There is increasing evidence that free radical injury and peroxidation are responsible for many conditions seen in the ICU. They include heart failure, reperfusion injury, cytokine-induced injury, and effects of drugs. Vitamin E at 100 mg/day has been shown to reduce circulating lipid peroxide levels in burn patients.[37] Cytokine-induced muscle proteolysis was prevented by giving vitamin E,[38] and the locomotor dysfunction of neutrophils after blunt trauma was improved by vitamin E.[39] These findings suggest that vitamin E requirements are increased and are likely to be of special importance in critically ill patients. The exact dose remains to be determined.

Vitamin K

There are several chemical forms of vitamin K, but all are characterized by a quinone ring connected to a side chain that varies with the compound. Three main forms—K_1 (synthesized by plants), K_2 (of microbial origin), and the synthetic parent compound K_3 or menadione (2-methyl-1,4-naphthoquinone)—are important in human nutrition. K_2 is formed in the gut by bacteria by the removal of the side chain from longer chain analogs.

REQUIREMENTS IN THE ICU. In malnourished patients, subnormal levels of vitamin K_1 were identified and when such patients received broad-spectrum antibiotics, prolonged prothrombin times and reduced levels of factor VII occurred. These complications were not observed in patients who had normal vitamin K_1 levels on admission.[40] This study suggests that vitamin K should be given to malnourished patients in the ICU.

Water-Soluble Vitamins

These vitamins are distinguished by the fact that most contain nitrogen (unlike fat-soluble vitamins) and are components of coenzymes that catalyze biochemical reactions. Five of these vitamins are especially concerned with energy metabolism: thiamine, riboflavin, niacin, biotin, and pantothenate.

Thiamine (Vitamin B_1)

REQUIREMENTS IN THE ICU. The optimal dose of thiamine for critically ill patients has not been determined. In one study of patients with major trauma who were fed enterally or parenterally with 1.24 to 2.1 mg of thiamine, all developed evidence of severe biochemical thiamine deficiency.[41] Using the same biochemical criteria, 5.0 mg/day avoids deficiency.[42]

Riboflavin (Vitamin B_2)

REQUIREMENTS. The oral intake should be 0.6 mg per 1000 kcal. Hence, in an average adult the intake should be 1.2 to 1.6 mg/day. During pregnancy and lactation an additional 0.3 to 0.5 mg/day should be given. For adult patients receiving TPN, the American Medical Association (AMA) recommends 3.6 mg/day. In other studies, 1.8 to 10 mg has been used and shown to be adequate biochemically.[43, 44]

Pantothenic Acid

REQUIREMENTS. There is insufficient evidence regarding oral requirements for humans, but 4 to 7 mg/day is suggested. For patients receiving TPN, the AMA recommends 15 mg/day in adults.

Niacin

REQUIREMENTS. The recommended oral intake is 6.6 mg of niacin equivalents (NEs) per 1000 kcal. Thus, about 13 to 18 mg/day should be taken by adults. During pregnancy and lactation, respectively, an additional 2 and 5 NE/day is recommended. For TPN, the AMA recommends 40 mg/day in adults.

Pyridoxine (Vitamin B_6)

REQUIREMENTS. The oral intake in adults should be 1.6 to 2.0 mg/day based on the fact that the requirement is related to protein intake in the proportion of 0.016 mg/g protein. During pregnancy and lactation, intake should be increased to 2.5 to 2.6 mg/day. Kishi and colleagues[42] found that 3 mg/day during TPN was adequate on the basis of transaminase activity. By contrast, 5.5 mg/day was not sufficient for all patients receiving TPN at home.[45] In acutely sick patients, 15 mg caused serum levels to rise.[44] The AMA recommends 4 mg/day for adults receiving TPN.

Biotin

REQUIREMENTS. About 30 to 100 μg/day is the recommended oral intake. Pregnancy does not increase requirements, and data for lactation are insufficient. However, the dietary intake is only an approximation, especially in the case of TPN, because a significant amount of biotin is synthesized in the intestine and the availability of synthesized biotin has been questioned. For patients receiving TPN, the AMA recommends an intake of 60 μg/day.

Folic Acid and Folates

REQUIREMENTS. The requirement for adults is 3 μg/kg/day. This is increased to 500 μg/day during pregnancy. An additional 100 μg/day of folate should be given during lactation. The use of drugs such as phenytoin and sulfasalazine inhibits absorption of folate. For such patients receiving such drugs, supplemental folate should be given by mouth. Alcoholism interferes with the metabolism of folate and increases requirements. For patients receiving TPN, the current vitamin preparations given intravenously provide more than enough folate.

Vitamin B_{12}

REQUIREMENTS. The RDA for vitamin B_{12} is 2.0 μg/day. During pregnancy and lactation, an additional 0.2 and 0.6 μg/day, respectively, are recommended. In patients with pernicious anemia and those with an ileal resection or ileal lesions, malabsorption occurs. These patients should be given 100 μg/mo by intramuscular injection. High-dose oral therapy with 1 mg/day has been used successfully for patients with malabsorption. However, oral high-dose therapy is not recommended. For patients receiving TPN, 3 μg/day is given.

Ascorbic Acid

REQUIREMENTS IN THE ICU. Critical illness is associated with evidence of free radical injury (see vitamin E). Among the free radical scavengers is vitamin C, and it has been shown that vitamin C in high doses reduces microvascular protein flux and permeability after burn injury.[46] In addition, it improves leukocyte dysfunction after blunt trauma.[39]

Requirements for a number of these vitamins are known for the normal state, but the effects of sepsis and trauma on the requirements for vitamins given intravenously and in enteral feedings are still not clear.

References

1. Cotzias GC: Role and importance of trace substances in environmental health. *In:* Proceedings of the First Annual Conference on Trace Substances in Environmental Health. Vol 1. DD Hemphill (Ed). Columbia, Mo, University of Missouri, 1967, pp 5–19.
2. Wolman SL, Anderson GH, Marliss EB, Jeejeebhoy KN: Zinc in total parenteral nutrition: Requirements and metabolic effects. Gastroenterology 1979; 73:458–467.
3. Oppenheimer SJ: Iron and infection: The clinical evidence. Acta Paediatr Scand Suppl 1989; 361:53–62.
4. Muench KH: Hemochromatosis and infection: Alcohol and iron, oysters and sepsis. 1989; Am J Med 87:40N–43N.
5. Wan KK, Tsallas G: Dilute iron dextran formulation for addition to parenteral nutrient solutions. Am J Hosp Pharm 1980; 37:206–210.
6. Vallee BL, Falchuk KH: Zinc and gene expression. Philos Trans R Soc Lond B Biol Sci 1981; 294:185–197.
7. Golden MHN, Golden BE, Harland PSEG, et al: Zinc and immunocompetence in protein-energy malnutrition. Lancet 1978; 1:1226–1227.
8. Fernandes G, Nair M, Onoe K, et al: Impairment of cell-mediated immunity functions by dietary zinc deficiency in mice. Proc Natl Acad Sci U S A 1979; 76:457–461.
9. Golden MHN, Golden BE, Jackson AA: Skin breakdown in kwashiorkor responds to zinc (Letter). Lancet 1980; 1:1256.
10. Prasad AS, Meftah S, Abdallah J, Kaplan J, Brewer GJ, Bach JF, Dardenne M: Serum thymulin in human zinc deficiency. J Clin Invest 1988; 82:1202–1210.
11. James BE, MacMahon RA: Balance studies of 9 elements during complete intravenous feeding of small premature infants. Aust Paediatr J 1976; 12:154–162.
12. Ricour C, Duhamel J-F, Gros J, et al: Estimates of trace element requirements of children receiving total parenteral nutrition. Arch Fr Pediatr 1977; 34(Suppl 7):92–100.
13. Berger MM, Cavadini C, Bart A, Mansourian R, Guinchard S, Bartholdi I, Vandervale A, Krupp S, Chioléro R, Freeman J, Dirren H: Cutaneous copper and zinc losses in burns. Burns 1992; 18:373–380.
14. McClain CJ, Twyman DL, Ott LG, Rapp RP, Tibbs PA, Norton JA, Kasarskis EJ, Dempsey RJ, Young B: Serum and urine zinc response in head-injured patients. J Neurosurg 1986; 64:224–230.
15. Boosalis MG, Solem LD, Cerra FA, Konstantinides F, Ahrenholz DH, McCall JT, McClain CJ: Increased urinary zinc excretion after thermal injury. J Lab Clin Med 1991; 118:538–545.
16. Antila H, Salo M, Näntö V, Irjala K, Brenner R, Vapaavuori M:

Serum iron, zinc, copper, selenium and bromide concentrations after coronary bypass operation. JPEN J Parenter Enteral Nutr 1990; 14:85–89.
17. Shike M, Roulet M, Kurian R, et al: Copper metabolism and requirements in total parenteral nutrition. Gastroenterology 1981; 81:290–297.
18. Jacobson S, Western P-O: Balance study of twenty trace elements during total parenteral nutrition in man. Br J Nutr 1977; 37:107–126.
19. Boosalis MG, McCall JT, Solem LD, Arnholz DH, McClain CJ: Serum copper and ceruloplasmin levels and urinary copper excretion in thermal injury. Am J Clin Nutr 1986; 44:899–906.
20. Anderson RA: Chromium metabolism and its role in disease processes in man. Clin Physiol Biochem 1986; 4:31–41.
21. Jeejeebhoy KN, Chu RC, Marliss EB, et al: Chromium deficiency, glucose intolerance and neuropathy reversed by chromium supplementation in a patient receiving long-term total parenteral nutrition. Am J Clin Nutr 1977; 30:531–538.
22. Haber F, Weiss J: The catalytic decomposition of hydrogen peroxide by iron salts. Philos Trans R Soc Lond A 1934; 147:332–351.
23. Stewart RDH, Griffiths NM, Thomson CD, et al: Quantitative selenium metabolism in normal New Zealand women. Br J Nutr 1978; 40:45–54.
24. Levander OA, Sutherland B, Morris VC, et al: Selenium balance in young men during selenium depletion and repletion. Am J Clin Nutr 1981; 34:2662–2669.
25. Brown MR, Cohen HJ, Lyons JM, Curtis TW, Thunberg B, Cochran WJ, Klish WJ: Proximal muscle weakness and selenium deficiency associated with long term parenteral nutrition. Am J Clin Nutr 1986; 43:549–554.
26. Lane HW, Dudrick S, Warren DC: Blood selenium levels and glutathione peroxidase activities in university students and chronic intravenous hyperalimentation subjects. Proc Soc Exp Biol Med 1981; 167:383–390.
27. Fleming CR, Fleming JT, McCall JT, et al: Selenium deficiency and fatal cardiomyopathy in a patient on home parenteral nutrition. Gastroenterology 1982; 83:689–693.
28. Hawker FH, Stewart PM, Snitch PJ: Effects of acute illness on selenium homeostasis. Crit Care Med 1990; 18:442–446.
29. Hunt DR, Lane HW, Beesinger D, Gallagher K, Halligan R, Johnston D, Rowlands BJ: Selenium depletion in burn patients. JPEN J Parenter Enteral Nutr 1984; 8:695–699.
30. Lowry SF, Goodgame JT, Maher MM, et al: Parenteral vitamin requirements during feeding. Am J Clin Nutr 1978; 31:2149–2158.
31. Nichoalds GE, Meng HC, Caldwell MD: Vitamin requirements in patients receiving total parenteral nutrition. Arch Surg 1977; 112:1061–1064.
32. Vanamee P, Shils ME, Burke AW, et al: Multivitamin preparations for parenteral use: A statement by the nutrition advisory group. JPEN J Parenter Enteral Nutr 1979; 3:258–261.
33. Cynober L, Desmoulins D, Lioret N, Aussel C, Hirsch-Marie H, Saizy R: Significance of vitamin A and retinol binding protein serum levels after burn injury. Clin Chim Acta 148:247–253, 1985.
34. Shike M, Harrison JE, Sturtridge WC, Tam CS, Bobechko PE, Jones G, Murray TM, Jeejeebhoy KN: Metabolic bone disease in patients receiving long-term total parenteral nutrition. Ann Intern Med 1980; 92:343–350.
35. Shike M, Sturtridge WC, Tam CS, Harrison JE, Jones G, Murray TM, Husdan H, Whitwell J, Wilson DR, Jeejeebhoy KN: A possible role of vitamin D in the genesis of parenteral-nutrition-induced metabolic bone disease. Ann Intern Med 1981; 95:560–568.
36. Izsak EM, Shike M, Roulet M, Jeejeebhoy KN: Pancreatitis in association with hypercalcemia in patients receiving total parenteral nutrition. Gastroenterology 1980; 79:555–558.
37. Mingjian Z, Qifang W, Laxing G, Hong J, Zongyin W: Comparative observation of changes in serum lipid peroxides influenced by supplementation of vitamin E in burn patients and healthy controls. Burns 1992; 18:19–21.
38. Cannon JG, Meydani SN, Fielding RA, Fiatarone MA, Meydani M, Farhangmehr M, Orencole SF, Blumberg JB, Evans WJ: Acute phase response in exercise. II. Association between vitamin E, cytokines and muscle proteolysis. Am J Physiol 1991; 260:R1235–R1240.
39. Maderazo EG, Woronick CL, Hickingbotham N, Jacobs L, Bhagavan HN: A randomized trial of replacement antioxidant vitamin therapy for neutrophil locomotory dysfunction in blunt trauma. J Trauma 1991; 31:1142–1150.
40. Cohen H, Scott D, Mackie J, Shearer M, Bax R, Karran SJ, Machin SJ: The development of hypoprothrombinaemia following antibiotic therapy in malnourished patients with low serum vitamin K_1 levels. Br J Haematol 1988; 68:63–66.
41. McChonachie I, Haskew A: Thiamine status after major trauma. Intensive Care Med 1988; 14:628–631.
42. Kishi H, Nishii S, Ono T, et al: Thiamin and pyridoxine requirements during intravenous hyperalimentation. Am J Clin Nutr 1979; 32:332–338.
43. Stromberg P, Shenkin A, Campbell RA, et al: Vitamin status during total parenteral nutrition. JPEN J Parenter Enteral Nutr 1981; 5:295–299.
44. Bradley JA, King RFJC, Schorah CJ: Vitamins in intravenous feeding: A study of water-soluble vitamins and folate in critically ill patients receiving intravenous nutrition. Br J Surg 1978; 65:492–494.
45. Jeejeebhoy KN, Langer B, Tsallas G, et al: Total parenteral nutrition at home: Studies in patients surviving 4 months to 5 years. Gastroenterology 1976; 71:943–953.
46. Matsuda T, Tanaka H, Hanumadass M, Gayle R, Yuasa H, Abcarian H, Matsuda H, Reyes H: Effects of high-dose vitamin C administration on postburn microvascular fluid and protein flux. J Burn Care Rehabil 1992; 13:560–566.

83

Nutrition for the Critically Ill Geriatric Patient

Thomas G. Baumgartner, PharmD, MEd, FASHP, BCNSP

If I had my way I'd make health catching instead of disease.

— Robert Green Ingersall

The geriatric patient, not unlike other patients, must receive sustenance to meet basic needs. The critically ill geriatric patient, not unlike other geriatric patients, must also receive nourishment to accommodate unusual states of stress. Today, it is a clinical challenge to provide nutrition since the choice of nutritional precursors needed to address healthy or disease states remains unclear. The aging process further compounds the challenge. This chapter highlights the aging process as it relates to the critically ill geriatric population and their nutritional management in the intensive care setting.

THE AGING PROCESS

Aging theories include population, organ, and cellular classifications. The population classification is based on either metabolic rate or collagen cross-linking. Organ demise is proposed to be associated with immune compromise, hormonal changes, or a central nervous system (CNS) pacemaker. Cellular mechanisms have the most scientific support and include (1) recessive or dominant mutations in somatic cells, (2) physiological err frequency increases, (3) glycation, (4) genetic code alterations, and (5) free radical aberrations. Interestingly, in animals, caloric restriction has been shown to decelerate the rate of aging through glycation reductions, oxidative damage, and gene expression alterations.

The effects of aging have been defined through measurements of muscle mass and body fat ratios, aerobic capacity, bone density, tactile response time, forced expiratory volume, and visual and auditory tests. At the cellular level, aging has been followed by serial changes in basement membrane, epidermal turnover rates, collagen ratios, sebaceous gland architecture, microvascular changes, elastic fiber content, and hormonal and cytokine concentrations. On the chromosomal level, gene length, teleomere position, and deoxyribonucleic acid (DNA) strand breakage rates have been studied.

Of key interest are the longitudinal studies that are beginning to show that number, type, and function of T cells may be associated with longevity, morbidity, and mortality in free-living elderly humans. Multifaceted alterations in the ability of T cells from older donors to respond to stimulation are being dissected, and pathways that are compromised in the elderly, compared with the young, are being defined.[1]

Functional capabilities appear to be the mainstay for appraisal of well-being, but they are poorly predicted by chronologic age. Physical, behavioral, and cognitive functions of the aged, with or without disease, span a broad spectrum. Although signs and symptoms in the geriatric population should not be readily attributed to old age, a decreasing efficiency of organ function in the aged is likely to be part of the aging process. For example, the kidney is composed of approximately 1 million nephrons that gradually, particularly after chronolgic age 30, trickle away, decade by decade, a process that is directly reflected in marked decline of organ efficiency. Similarly, other organ systems contribute to an overall apoptotic demise. Human aging is likely best characterized as the progressive constriction of each organ system's homeostatic reserve. Each organ system's decline appears to be independent of changes in other organ systems and is influenced by diet, environment, and personal habits. Because of a lack of physiologic reserve, a functional older person may maintain health into old age but may become increasingly vulnerable to stress and illness (i.e., may be unable to maintain homeostasis).[2]

Age-related physiologic changes are important to consider when one is making diagnostic and therapeutic decisions. Clinicians need to be aware of the ramifications of the aging process, especially with regard to decreased functional reserve and tolerance to therapeutic interventions. Thoughtful clinical application of this concept improves medical outcomes and enhances patients' quality of life in their later years.[3] General mortality has been shown to conform to Gompertz' dynamics through age 96 years for both men and women.[4]

The most vulnerable organ system is the first to be compromised with the onset of disease in the elderly. Many ailments plague the aged (Table 83–1).

The elderly (with chronic diseases) are at high risk for nutritional abnormalities. Insufficient nutritional intake has been associated with old age, loneliness, physical and mental handicaps, immobility, and chronic illness. On the other hand, obesity is also common in the United States, so that excess nutritional intake is closely associated with the expression of many diseases. Nonetheless, independent of dietary deficiency, dietary excess or disease, there is progressive loss of lean body mass in aging. Men can lose twice as much lean body mass as women. In addition to weight loss, there is a decrease in basal metabolic rate and skeletal mass (and height) and an increase in mean body fat (up to twice as much in women). A reduction in physical activity, with the above compositional changes, results in decreased energy and protein requirements in the aging patient. Therefore, it is particularly imperative to avoid overfeeding. Providing too much amino acid or protein can increase respiratory drive (although not reflected in hypercapnea in arterial gas) and renal solute load. Excessive carbohydrate intake can cause fatty liver infiltration, hypercapnea, increased work of breathing, dehydration, hyperglycemia, and complement fixation compromise.

TABLE 83–1. Common Diseases of the Aged Population

Anemia
Coronary artery disease
Basal cell carcinoma
Chronic lymphatic leukemia
Chronic pain
Chronic renal failure
Cognitive impairment
Decubitus ulcers
Degenerative osteoarthritis
Dementia
Depression
Diabetes mellitus
Diabetic hyperosmolar nonketotic coma
Fecal issues (increased transit, decreased transit, dysmotility)
Gout
Heart failure
Herpes zoster
Hip fracture
Lymphoma
Metabolic bone disease
Monoclonal gammopathies
Osteoarthritis
Osteoporosis
Parkinsonism
Polymyalgia rheumatica
Prostatic carcinoma
Sleep disturbances
Stroke
Tuberculous infections
Urinary incontinence
Urinary precipitancy
Vascular (venous and arterial) insufficiency

Increased lipid supplementation has been associated with immunocompromise.

These considerations must be balanced, however, with the provision of enough of these macronutrients to provide the following:

1. Sufficient nitrogen-containing macronutrients as precursors for catecholamines, hormones, cytokines, and other proteins.
2. Enough carbohydrate, as dextrose or (glycerin), to drive nutrients into the cell under the control of insulin.
3. Adequate lipid to normalize hepatic function; as much as one third of phase I hepatic metabolism can fall off without daily intravenous lipid.

Patients receiving postoperative 2000 kcal total parenteral nutrition (TPN) regimens providing all nonprotein calories as dextrose ($n = 16$) showed a 34% reduction of mean antipyrine clearance after 7 days of TPN compared with controls ($n = 13$, $P < .05$). This effect was seen also in patients receiving a 1600 kcal dextrose-based regimen ($n = 8$). In patients receiving a 2000 kcal TPN regimen in which 500 kcal were provided as lipid ($n = 10$), mean antipyrine clearance was not significantly different from that of the control group.[5] Lipids are also needed, of course, to prevent and treat essential fatty acid deficiency. The least invasive feeding route should be used, and careful monitoring of the regimen instituted to avoid deficiencies or excesses.

Older individuals will continue to make up a major portion of patients requiring critical care, particularly those undergoing surgery. Age and chronic disease-related factors blunt the reserves with which the elderly can meet the demands of critical illness.

Resumption of normal functional abilities should be the primary target of nutritional support in the geriatric population. Grip strength monitoring may be useful for detecting skeletal (respiratory) muscle weakness. Without adequate nutrition and tissue perfusion, skeletal muscle strength can decline significantly in just a few days. Simple grip strength may be a useful alternative to complex nutritional markers.[6] Skeletal muscle weakness may precede and predict the development of insulin resistance.[7]

Immobility and malnutrition place the elderly at high risk for muscle atrophy and pressure ulcers. Exercise should be encouraged not only because of its beneficial effects on blood pressure, cardiovascular conditioning, glucose homeostasis, bone density, and even longevity but also for its influence in improving mood and sleep and in preventing constipation and falls. Increased (up to 30 times) movement of nutrients to target sites occurs during and following exercise.

In further support of exercise and physical therapy, immobility predisposes to muscle atrophy, deep venous thrombosis, atelectasis, hypostatic pneumonia, constipation, functional urinary incontinence, and loss of motivation. Of course, the systemic inflammatory response syndrome (SIRS) or sepsis is the most serious extended complication of immobility.

Immune competency decreases with aging, and T cell-dependent functions are most compromised, most likely a result of involution of the thymus gland. Defects in T cell proliferative capacity and responsiveness, interleukin-2 (IL-2) production and receptor expression, signal transduction, and cytotoxicity are frequently cited problems associated with immunosenescence.

Wound healing may be impaired in the elderly and may contribute to the development of pressure sores. Nutrients are important for wound healing, and intake should be optimized in these patients. Adequate protein and energy are required for each gram of collagen synthesized, but anabolism cannot take place without sufficient micronutrients.

Constipation is common in the elderly.[8] It can be a symptom of organic disease, or it may represent a colonic or anorectal functional disorder of unknown etiology called *chronic idiopathic constipation*. The untoward effects that may result from laxative abuse can be greater than those of constipation.[9] Insufficient dietary fiber, fluid deprivation, and immobility all lend to constipation. Moreover, complications of constipation, such as fecal impaction, fecal incontinence, ulceration, and obstruction can be catastrophic in the debilitated elderly patient.

AGING PHYSIOLOGY AND NUTRITION

The nutritional management of the critically ill geriatric patient must be carefully balanced, with consideration given to (1) the sensitivity and specificity of diagnostic and treatment tools, (2) organ dysfunction or failure, (3) CNS impairments (cognitive, sensory, delirium), (4) age-related changes in physiology and pharmacodynamics, (5) increased vulnerability to delirium, (6) immobility complications, and (7) multiple concurrent illnesses. Gut integrity, particularly in association with the organ that consumes the most oxygen, the liver, is important. In fact, gut perfusion is now being related to overall prognosis with the use of intramucosal carbon dioxide partial pressure (P_{CO_2}) measurement or calculated intramucosal pH (pHi) of gastric tonometry. Continual gastric P_{CO_2} measurement (P_{iCO_2}) is a monitoring technique with high sensitivity in detecting gastrointestinal hypoperfusion based on an intramucosal CO_2 accumulation. The clinical significance of the primary parameter P_{iCO_2} as well as the suitability of this technique as a monitoring tool for the daily routine must continue to be assessed.[10]

It is interesting, however, that changes in gastric motility or blood flow to the aged gut do not appear to alter the efficiency with which moieties move from the gut to the systemic circulation.[11, 11a]

Despite the widespread belief that *enteral* nutrition is superior to *parenteral* nutrition in humans, there may be little difference between the two. That is, enteral nutrition is not safer; has no demonstrable benefit with respect to either measured physiologic parameters or intestinal morphology, permeability or function; has no demonstrable benefit with respect to bacterial translocation; and carries a better outcome only in abdominal trauma, cancer chemotherapy, and ulcerative colitis. Associated costs of each route also need to be reappraised based on more invasive enteral access and decreasing parenteral nutrition prices.[12]

Once a preferred route is selected, specific organ status must be evaluated to determine the nature of the formulation and how to tailor it to the patient. The particular concerns relative to nutrition and organ function (heart, lung, kidney, liver, gastrointestinal route) are described next.

Nutrition and the Aging Heart

Cardiac cachexia is associated with cellular hypoxia, decreased caloric intake and assimilation, increased caloric expenditure, and anorexia from medications used to treat the patient with heart disease. Digoxin and diuretic medications must be carefully monitored. These medications can result in excessive urinary losses of micronutrients, especially potassium, magnesium, and calcium. Micronutrient, particularly electrolyte, imbalance contributes to arrhythmias and impaired cardiac contractibility. Malnutrition resulting from chronic low cardiac output states (i.e., cardiac cachexia) is not uncommon and contributes to mortality and morbidity, especially in older people. Impaired absorption of fat has been related to the clinical severity of heart failure. Lipid is a preferred substrate for myocardial function.[13] Decreased lipid intake can alter membrane structure and contribute to arrhythmias.

Comprehensive hemodynamic, metabolic, and clinical studies indicate that acceptable levels of nutrition support can be provided to malnourished patients with severe congestive heart failure resulting in improvement of their clinical status without adversely influencing cardiac function.[14] The mechanisms for alterations in body composition as a consequence of cardiac cachexia are multifactorial, but major causes may be cytokine-mediated host responses to the underlying disease.[15] Hypermetabolism increases energy expenditure, resulting in weight loss and chronic heart failure.[16]

Mesenteric ischemia may develop owing to advanced atherosclerosis combined with low cardiac output states. Cardiac atrophy impairs cardiac contractibility and leads to a low cardiac output state. This effect is accentuated in patients with a history of myocardial disease who have lost tissue due to infarction.

Nutrition and the Aging Lung

Malnutrition is both a cause and a result of pulmonary failure. A successful outcome to the treatment of pulmonary failure often hinges on appropriate and aggressive nutritional therapy. Metabolic stresses caused by nutritional therapeutic intervention in the patient with pulmonary failure must be anticipated.[17] Undernutrition is associated with important alterations in respiratory muscle structure and function. Undernutrition-related effects on respiratory muscles, by inducing respiratory muscle weakness through derangements in muscle energy production, transport, and utilization, may represent important "metabolic" factors in the pathogenesis of ventilatory failure.[18]

Patients with chronic obstructive pulmonary disease (COPD) are frequently malnourished. These patients are predisposed to infection and a subsequent increase in mortality. Nutritional support is mandatory to prevent visceral deterioration, but adverse effects of nutrition support can be harmful to patients with COPD. Excessive calories (especially glucose) increases CO_2 production and can precipitate respiratory failure.[19] Low body weight, a potentially modifiable factor, is associated with increased respiratory mortality, but whether it is a casual factor or a marker of declining health remains unclear.[20]

Carbohydrate is likely the most injurious macrosubstrate to the lung when overdosed because it has a respiratory quotient (RQ) = $\dot{V}CO_2/\dot{V}O_2$ of 1; that is, the CO_2 produced, divided by the oxygen (O_2) that is required to consume 1 mole of dextrose, is the same. Therefore, excessive carbohydrate can increase respiratory demands and can fatigue the respiratory muscles. The effects of excessive amino acid or protein (on pulmonary drive and immunocompromise) and lipid intake (immunocompromise) are less clear. The infectious implications are founded in burned guinea pig work describing increased sepsis secondary to excess protein supplementation and immunocompromise secondary to proposed deleterious cytokine shower.

Human studies have shown that low-fat nutrition support decreases infectious morbidity and shortens length of stay in burn patients. Fish oil does not seem to add clinical benefit to low-fat solutions. Of key importance, low-fat feeding nutrition regimens modulate cortisol-binding globulin and the concentration of free circulating cortisol after severe stress.[21] Investigation describing no increase in the incidence of bacteremia or fungemia in bone marrow transplant patients receiving low-dose and high-dose lipid supplementation supports the use of lipid in SIRS or sepsis patients.

Experimental data have implicated intravenous lipids as being immunosuppressive, yet evidence that lipids are associated with an increase in clinically documented infections is sparse. A prospective trial conducted in patients with hematologic malignancies who were undergoing bone marrow transplantation compared the incidence of bacteremia and fungemia during the first month after the transplant. Patients (n = 512) were randomly assigned to receive 6% to 8% (a low dose) or 25% to 30% (the standard dose) of total daily energy as a 20% lipid emulsion. These data indicate that moderate amounts of intravenous lipid-rich in linoleic acid are not associated with an increased incidence of bacterial or fungal infections in patients undergoing bone marrow transplantation and receiving TPN.[22] This study has challenged earlier suggestions of cytokine shower secondary to lipids and suggest that lipids appear to be less of a problem on infectious status.

Ventilatory control is also affected by age. The ventilatory response to hypoxia and CO_2 (that generally occurs postoperatively) is significantly reduced in healthy older men. Decreases in cough effectiveness, mucociliary clearance, altered gag reflex, swallowing problems, positional impact, CNS depression, and immunocompromise associated with aging predispose the critically ill geriatric patient to pulmonary infections. These effects are worsened by the adverse effects of malnutrition on lung function; these include decreased respiratory muscle function, decreased ventilatory drive, and altered lung defense mechanisms.[23]

Malnutrition is common in patients receiving mechanical ventilation. Poor nutritional status contributes to impaired respiratory muscle function, altered lung structure, diminished ventilatory response, and resistance to infection.[24] An associated increased work of breathing as well as an increased respiratory muscle oxygen expenditure also takes place. Delayed decision making lends to prolonged periods of no nutrition, and diagnostic testing often leads to insufficient periods of feeding.

Oxygen consumption and energy expenditure can be estimated in patients with a pulmonary artery catheter in place (cardiac output × arterial-venous oxygen difference). This result is then multiplied by 10 to accommodate denominations if the Fick equation is derived. Once O_2 consumption (250 mL/min, within normal limits) has been determined, the Weir equation provides an approximate energy expenditure.

Alternatively, energy expenditures can be assessed by indirect calorimetry. Energy expenditure and oxygen consumption are affected by many factors (Table 83–2). CO_2 in arterial gases does not reflect protein or amino acid dosing but, of course, increases with increasing carbohydrate or lipid supplementation. There may be a reduction in $Paco_2$ with increasing nitrogen intake (increased ventilatory response).

Patients with emphysema demonstrate an increase in protein and carbohydrate oxidation in fasting and fed states.[25]

Malnutrition reduces respiratory muscle mass and contractile force through atrophy of type II fibers and impaired energy metabolism. Nutritional repletion restores respiratory muscle function but may add to ventilatory work. Nutritional repletion also enhances weaning from mechanical ventilation.[26]

In cachectic subjects, the diaphragm muscle mass and thickness are reduced in proportion to the reduction in body weight. In addition, respiratory muscle strength and endurance are reduced more dramatically than the weight loss. This finding suggests that malnutrition induces a reduction in muscular mass that is associated with a decrease in contractility. Diaphragmatic weakness may increase the risk of respiratory failure in patients with COPD.[27]

Energy goal estimations for the critically ill geriatric patients can be derived by several means. A total of 25 to 30 kcal/kg per day is commonly used. Others calculate basal energy expenditure (BEE) and add a factor for work of breathing secondary to nutrients and the ventilator. Still others use a metabolic cart to determine O_2 consumption, CO_2 production, and energy needs. If a pulmonary artery catheter is in place, the Fick and Weir equations provide a calculated O_2 consumption and BEE, respectively.

TABLE 83–2. Factors That Cause Decreases or Increases in Oxygen Consumption

Decreases
Age
Hypothermia (without shivering)
Mechanical ventilation (i.e., decreased work of breathing)
Medications (i.e., analgesics, sedatives)
Paralysis
Sleep
Increases
Alkalosis
Bath
Chest physical therapy
Chest x-ray studies
Dressing change
Hyperthermia
Major surgery
Medications (i.e., catecholamines)
Nutrition
Physical examination
Respiratory failure
Sepsis
Suctioning
Turning
Visitors

Fluid overload can result from increased retention of sodium and, subsequently, water. Careful assessment of volume status is important to ensure adequate intravascular volume while minimizing pulmonary edema.[28]

Antioxidants in the lung have a protective role against oxidative damage. Therefore, maintenance of sufficient antioxidant status, especially with trace elements and vitamins, may protect lungs from oxidative injuries.[29]

Nutrition and the Aging Kidney

Individualizing dietary replacement for the critically ill geriatric patient with renal disease has become increasingly important.

There is a steady decline in glomerular filtration rate (GFR) (i.e., creatinine clearance) with age. Creatine in muscle also decreases at about the same rate as the GFR. However, the decline of renal function with age is highly variable among individuals. Approximately half of renal plasma flow and perhaps one third of the creatinine clearance or GFR falls off with aging. Longitudinal studies on the rate of decline in renal function with age show that in one third there is no change in creatinine clearance with advancing age, another subgroup showed a linear decrease with age, and still others actually showed improvement in renal function as they got older.[30] Dosage adjustments of medications excreted primarily by the kidneys should not be based on serum creatinine values but, rather, on measured or at least estimated creatinine clearance. Urine concentration and dilution, tubular secretion and reabsorption, and hydrogen ion secretion are all reduced in the geriatric patient, thereby predisposing these patients to fluid retention, electrolyte disorders, and acid-base imbalance.

The critically ill patient with acute renal failure (ARF) should receive enteral nutrition if the gut is functional and parenteral nutrition if it is not. It may be necessary to curtail enteral nutrition during dialytic procedures to avoid shunting of blood to the mesentery and the subsequent effect on blood pressure. Although mesenteric ischemia is uncommon in the general population, it is frequently encountered in patients undergoing long-term hemodialysis. In such patients, excessive ultrafiltration or a too rapid filtration rate can favor ischemia. Prophylactic measures must be taken at the first sign of ischemia, especially since clinical and biologic features of mesenteric ischemia remain largely nonspecific.[31]

Specialized renal amino acid formulas with higher essential (and thus branched-chain) amino acid content have not been more advantageous than standard formulas containing mixed amino acids.[32]

Protein intake should match metabolic demands and should not be restricted in patients with renal disease unless severe renal solute load becomes problemic. If creatinine clearances are less than than 30 mL/min, sodium, potassium, chloride, and protein create additive renal solute loads that may further injure the kidney. The critically ill patient generally requires 1 to 1.3 g of amino acids/kg per day parenterally, while the parenteral needs of the unstressed patient are met by providing approximately the oral recommended daily (dietary) allowance (RDA) of 0.8 g of amino acids/kg per day. Geriatric patients, however, may have protein needs that are 20% higher than previously determined.

Serum albumin concentrations decrease with age, and values below 38 g/L are associated with increased morbidity, mortality, and disability in older patients. The extent to which the decreases are associated independently with changes in metabolism, dietary intake, physical activity, morbidity, or body composition is not clear. Decreases with age in serum albumin concentrations are associated with muscle loss (sarcopenia). This association is independent of other factors that may affect muscle mass and albumin concentration. The increased risk of disability with low serum albumin concentrations observed in these patients may actually reflect an association with sarcopenia.[33] Protein removal by continuous dialytic methods may eliminate increasingly more amino acids than by intermittent or peritoneal dialysis.

Protein losses during continuous renal replacement therapy (CRRT) have been reported to be as high as 1.3 g/L. With CRRT outputs of up to 50 L/day, these values would amount to protein losses of up to 65 g/day. Protein losses during CRRT are substantially lower than previously reported and depend on the serum protein concentration and the predominant nature of solute removal (convection or diffusion). These losses can vary between 12 and 75 g/day.[34] CRRT has found widespread use and acceptance during the 1990s. The various modalities differ in the following:

- Type of access (arteriovenous or venovenous)
- Application of convective clearance (continuous hemofiltration), diffusive clearance (continuous hemodialysis), or a combination of both (continuous hemodiafiltration)
- Site where the replacement fluid enters the circuit (predilution or postdilution)

Continuous therapies incorporate several advantages, such as:

- Improved hemodynamic stability
- The possibility of unlimited alimentation
- Optimal fluid balance
- Gradual urea removal without fluctuations

Major disadvantages include:

- The ongoing necessity of continuous anticoagulation
- Immobilization of the patient
- Possible side effects from lactate-containing replacement fluid or dialysate.

CRRT has certainly made the management of critically ill patients easier. In particular, oligoanuric patients with diuretic-resistant volume overload and hemodynamically unstable patients with ARF and concomitant sepsis or multiorgan failure appear to benefit most from continuous treatment. The role of continuous hemofiltration as a method of removing serum cytokines in patients with sepsis but without ARF is still controversial and needs further clinical assessment. Furthermore, intermittent hemodialysis is preferable in patients with hemorrhagic diathesis because it can be easily performed without anticoagulants.[35]

The hallmark of the metabolic alterations in ARF is accelerated protein breakdown that cannot be effectively suppressed by provision of exogenous nutritional substrates. Specific uremic toxic effects, insulin resistance, hormonal derangements, metabolic acidosis, circulating proteases, inflammatory mediators (i.e., cytokines) and dialysis-related losses of nutritional substrates all contribute to the activation of protein degradation.[36]

Metabolism in ARF is also affected by an impairment of the multiple metabolic and endocrine functions of the kidney. Various amino acids are synthesized or interconverted by the kidneys and may become conditionally indispensable. The kidney is also an important organ in the degradation of peptides, such as peptide hormones. As a consequence of these metabolic aberrations, imbalances in amino acid pools in plasma and in the intracellular compartment occur in ARF and elimination and utilization of infused amino acids is altered. Protein or amino acid requirements are influenced more by (1) the nature of the illness causing ARF, (2) the extent of hypercatabolism, (3) by associated complications, and (4) the type and frequency of renal replacement therapy than by renal dysfunction per se.[37, 38]

Intradialytic parenteral nutrition (IDPN) has been advocated for the management of malnutrition in hemodialysis patients. The rationale for its use is that patients are unable to increase oral intake to meet their nutritional needs or that the oral route is not effective in managing malnutrition in this group of patients. However, numerous studies using IDPN have failed to demonstrate efficacy with this costly mode of treatment.[39]

Prealbumin (transthyretin, thyroid-binding prealbumin) is a visceral protein and serves as an anabolic marker because it has a half-life of about 1½ days. Since prealbumin transports retinoids and since the geriatric patient in renal failure generally has elevated serum concentrations of vitamin A, serum prealbumin concentrations in these patients can be spuriously higher. Nonetheless the baseline concentration and a demonstrated rise in prealbumin define *anabolism*.

Markers of iron homeostasis are also affected in patients with renal failure. Serum ferritin, hemoglobin, serum iron, and total body iron stores were studied in 20 patients with chronic renal failure treated conservatively and in 20 patients undergoing regular hemodialysis. There was no relationship between serum iron or transferrin and bone marrow iron deposits, but serum ferritin concentration was a good indicator of increased marrow iron stores. All patients with serum ferritin levels above 300 μg/L had increased iron stores. Serum ferritin assay is a useful noninvasive technique for detecting iron overload in uremic and hemodialyzed patients,[40] but increased serum ferritin concentrations may be associated with other conditions (e.g., inflammatory states, sepsis).[41, 42]

Selenium deficiency may occur in chronic uremic patients and may alter thyroid gland function.[43] Thyroid hormone levels are reduced in patients with ARF despite normal thyroid-stimulating hormone (TSH) serum concentrations. An increase in thyroxine (T_4) concentrations is apparent during treatment with selenium and may be related to a favorable outcome in ARF. Thyroid hormone concentrations paralleled plasma selenium levels, indicating a possible influence of selenium on thyroid function in ARF.[44]

Creatine is the precursor of serum creatinine (both also appear as urine non-urea nitrogen). Because lean body mass decreases with aging, serum creatinine levels may appear lower in older patients for a given glomerular filtration rate (GFR). However, doubling the serum creatinine level is still related to halving of the GFR. Cellular water and basal metabolic rate in a 90-year-old person are about 80% those in a 30-year-old, whereas cardiac index falls to 70% in the 90-year-old. The GFR, as measured by inulin, is about 60%, whereas renal blood flow (diodrast and para-amino hippurate), vital capacity and maximum breathing capacity decrease by approximately 50%. It is important that we be aware of the decreased renal function and subsequent fluid as well as solute (paticularly sodium, potassium, chloride, and protein) restrictions.

Acid-base balance is far more important than solute load corrections in stabilizing renal function and should be addressed aggressively.

Nutrition and the Aging Liver

Branched Chain Amino Acids

Although hepatic mass decreases with aging, hepatic function remains at normal levels. In patients with hepatic failure, branched chain–enriched amino acid (BCAA) formulas improve encephalopathy. A meta-analysis of six large studies demonstrated an improvement in overall survival when patients with liver disease were fed a TPN formula containing increased amounts of BCAAs.[45] Pooled analysis of five randomized controlled studies showed a highly significant improvement in mental recovery ($P < .001$) from high-grade encephalopathy over follow-up times varying from 5 to 14 days. Two studies reported an increased risk of death in the treatment group. Two others showed a clear benefit from administration of parenteral nutrition: The aggregate relative risk (for encephalopathy) reduction was 0.59 (95% confidence interval, 0.23 to 0.80; $P = .002$). Addition of unpublished data from a third positive study increased the relative risk reduction to 0.82 ($P < .0001$), and even the most conservative interpretation of the published data still yielded a significant reduction in mortality ($P = .023$).[46]

Based on the results of the two largest, long-term studies, the use of oral BCAAs in the prevention and treatment of chronic encephalopathy is recommended for patients with advanced cirrhosis who are intolerant to alimentary proteins.[47] Other studies have shown that BCAA administration reduces serum concentrations of aromatic amino acids but fails to improve cerebral function and to decrease mortality in patients with hepatic encephalopathy. In contrast to the potential beneficial effects noted in hepatic encephalopathy, there is no solid evidence that BCAA-enriched nutritional regimens reduce the mortality rate in patients with trauma or sepsis.[48] Higher concentrations of BCAA formulas (45% versus 35% renal or hepatic solutions) have not shown beneficial effects in septic patients.[49]

Albumin

Hepatic albumin synthesis does not decline until about 75% to 90% of liver function is lost. The liver synthesizes about 200 mg/kg per day. However, synthesis can be increased to as much as 400 mg/kg per day. One must appreciate the distribution of total body albumin to understand the pharmacodynamics associated with the provision of colloidal agents. The intravascular albumin half-life is 2 to 3 weeks, whereas extravascular (two thirds total body albumin) has short half-lives (i.e., hours). Each gram of colloidal agent, whether carbohydrate-based (e.g., hydroxyethylstarch, dextran) or protein-based (e.g., albumin, plasma protein fraction) draws about 20 to 25 mL of extravascular fluid into the intravascular compartment. In addition to their primary oncotic pressure role, protein-based agents bind and transport a variety of moieties, that include electrolytes, trace elements, vitamins, hormones, and medications.

Normal serum albumin levels have been associated with a shorter inflammatory phase of wound healing and normal angiogenesis, collagen synthesis, and wound remodeling. Albumin levels below 2.5 g/dL represent a 50% loss of the normal plasma colloid oncotic pressure and may contribute to gastrointestinal tract mucosal edema and diarrhea. A serum albumin level of 2.5 g/dL can be used to predict those patients who will experience diarrhea when fed by mouth. In fact, several authors have found that up to 100% of patients with a serum albumin below 1.5 g/dL have diarrhea with enteral feeding. Hypoalbuminemic patients receiving TPN have markedly shortened plasma albumin half-lives.[50]

Although hypoalbuminemia is associated with increased severity of illness, capillary leak, greater inflammatory responses, mucosal edema, poorer wound healing, and diarrhea, there are no data to indicate that these parameters are reversed by albumin administration. Albumin may have detrimental effects by causing transcapillary leak into tissues and subsequently increasing extravascular fluid through oncotic draw. Rapid infusion may result in pulmonary edema. Albumin solutions contain about 15.4 mEq sodium/dL that can contribute to sodium overload ("salt-poor" albumin is a misnomer). Prolonged albumin infusion has been associated with hypofibrinogenemia. Reduced coagulation activity following albumin supplementation seems partly caused by a decrease of coagulation protein content; increased fibrinolysis in the albumin patients is not the cause. Decreased coagulation protein content parallels the decrease in coagulation activity and the need for postresuscitation blood transfusions.[51]

In large, heathy, aging populations, clinically meaningful decreases in serum albumin have not been found, although there is a very modest reduction with advancing age.[52] Serum albumin levels may be markedly decreased in older patients suffering from malnutrition or severe chronic disease and such changes may alter medication binding.[53, 54]

In one small study,[55] each patient with a serum albumin level less than 2.6 g/dL experienced diarrhea. No patient with a serum albumin level of 2.6 g/dL or greater developed diarrhea, regardless of the type of nutritional support received. Four of the 12 patients with hypoalbuminemia and diarrhea were placed on a peptide-based, chemically defined diet, after which the diarrhea resolved and serum albumin concentrations increased. Others have concluded that hypoalbuminemia-related diarrhea during tube feeding is significantly higher in patients with albumin levels less than 2 g/dL, and patients with hypoalbuminemia due to chronic malnutrition have a significantly higher incidence of diarrhea than those with acute malnutrition, such as burned patients.[56]

Nutrition and the Aging Gastrointestinal Tract

In critically ill geriatric patients, the gastrointestinal tract must be carefully assessed before the introduction of enteral nutrition. Many chronic diseases or iatrogenic reasons (i.e., devices, stents, medications) may place the aged, friable gut at risk if it is used for feeding. As with other patients, the type of feeding (i.e., clear, full liquid, soft, or regular) should be appreciated. If adequate intake is not possible, supplemental or full enteral formula feeding should be considered within 3 to 5 days (to include preadmission dietary history). The location of the feeding tube should be distal to lesions and obstructions. Thrombocytopenia may predispose the geriatric patient to bleeding, and tubes may be undesirable mediators of bleeding. SIRS or sepsis may increase risk of translocation in critically ill geriatric patients.[57]

Intestinal absorption is generally not affected by aging, although organ dysfunction (i.e., hepatic, pancreatitic) may contribute to decreased bioavailability of medications and nutrients. The effect of renal failure on intestinal absorption of dietary fatty acids is not known. In animal models, however, the rates of amino acid transport, determined both in vivo and in vitro, were significantly lower in short-term than in long-term renal failure.[58]

Choline and inositol have been promoted as effective digestants, but convincing information is lacking. Choline is crucial for sustaining life. It modulates the basic signaling processes within cells, is a structural element in membranes, and is vital during critical periods in brain development. Choline metabolism is also closely interrelated with the metabolism of methionine and folate. The patient who is fed intravenously is part of a vulnerable population.[59, 60]

Pancreatic enzymes[61] may be lacking and may predispose to malabsorption. Intestinal dysmotility may also present problems in the geriatric patient. Small-intestinal overgrowth with colonic-type bacterial should be considered in subjects aged 75 years of age or older with chronic diarrhea, anorexia, or nausea, even in the absence of clues such as clinically apparent predisposition or vitamin B_{12} deficiency. Small-intestinal dysmotility, rather than fasting hypochlorhydria or mucosal immunosenescence, probably is responsible for the prevalence of bacterial overgrowth in this group.[62]

Nutrition and Other Conditions

Neurologic injury initiates a cascade of local and systemic metabolic responses. Patients become hypermetabolic, hypercatabolic, and hyperglycemic demonstrating decreased immunocompetency and altered gastrointestinal tract function. Provision of an adequate supply of nutrients is associated with improved outcome. Because of the high incidence of gastroparesis, enteral nutritional support of patients with acute head injury has traditionally been difficult and has led to frequent use of small-bowel feedings or TPN. Evidence indicates that early small-bowel feeding of patients with acute head injury results in a decreased incidence of infections and shorter stay in the intensive care unit (ICU).[63]

The effects of TPN versus enteral nutrition were studied in patients following major neurosurgery. Enteral nutrition after neurosurgical procedures is associated with an accelerated normalization of nutritional status and an improved substrate tolerance. Enteral nutrition was thought to oppose early postoperative absorption disturbances of the small intestine.[64]

Pancreatitis

TPN is commonly used to treat ICU patients who have pancreatitis. Although rapid infusions of fat have been shown to cause a reduction in gallbladder volume, studies of longer infusion time have shown no associated cholecystokinin stimulation. Subjects who received 10% fat emulsion (Intralipid, Kabivitrum, Stockholm) over 3 hours demonstrated reduced gallbladder volume. This effect was statistically significant at about 80 minutes of lipid influsion and became progressively more marked as the infusion progressed, reaching a reduction of approximately 30% during the third hour of infusion.[65]

Continuous intravenous (IV) insulin infusion, although a national standard, may be associated with insulin resistance compared with pulsed infusions of insulin for hyperglycemic control. The greater efficacy of pulsed insulin administration in suppressing hepatic glucose production is accompanied by an equipotent effect on glucose utilization.[66] When IV insulin is administered, half of the previous day's sliding scale given subcutaneously, is placed in the TPN solution and delivered intravenously (usually over 24 hours) to keep the blood glucose level below 220 mg/dL. The dose is adjusted according to blood glucose values.

Two possible mechanisms for glucose mediated organ damage are glycation of proteins (complement fixation compromise) and the polyol pathway. Tight control of blood glucose concentrations has been shown to decrease the risk of microvascular complications.[67, 68] Diabetic patients also manifest increased vascular permeability. The use of increasing amounts of exogenous insulin may increase the transcapillary escape rate of albumin.[69] On the other hand, physiologic hyperinsulinemia does not affect systemic albumin permeability in healthy subjects or normoalbuminuric, non–insulin-dependent diabetes mellitis (NIDDM) patients. In contrast, in NIDDM patients, but not in healthy subjects, insulin increases the urinary excretion of albumin and protein markers of proximal tubular function.[70]

The American Diabetes Association recommendations for nutrient intake in the unstressed diabetic patient include 0.8 to 1 g of protein/kg per day (less with renal failure), 55% to 60% of calories from carbohydrates (unrefined carbohydrate with fiber), and less than 30% of calories from fat. Because optimal protein, carbohydrate, and lipid intake for the critically ill diabetic patient are unknown, current recommendations are similar to those for critically ill patients. Vitamin C has been of benefit in both type I and type II diabetes in terms of increased hydroxylation of collagen during synthesis.[71] Decreased ascorbic acid levels in leukocytes of type II diabetic patients suggest that supplementation may be beneficial.[72]

Patients with diabetes also have alterations in neutrophil function, putting them at an increased risk for infection, including decreased adhesiveness, poor chemotaxis, decreased opsonization, decreased phagocytosis, and reduced intracellular killing. They also have decreased cell-mediated immunity with decreased lymphocyte transformation, reduced macrophage-lymphocyte interaction, and an impaired delayed-type hypersensitivity. Transient hyperglycemia in patients receiving TPN may be associated with impaired immune function. The effects of short-term hyperglycemia on one aspect of antimicrobial immune function (i.e., the ability of immunoglobulin G [IgG] to fix complement) have been investigated. A significant reduction in complement fixation by immunoglobulin occurred with elevated glucose concentrations, and this effect may play a clinically significant immunosuppressive role in transiently hyperglycemic patients.[73] One may be able to improve leukocyte dysfunction by maintaining excellent glucose control in diabetic patients with blood glucose below 200 mg/dL. A blood glucose level below 220 mg/dL is necessary to avoid complement fixation compromise.

In the diabetic patient, parenteral or enteral nutrition should be initiated with only 150 g of dextrose (enough to supply the brain and erythrocyte with preferred substrate) over the first 24 hours. Approximately one third to one half of the patient's usual total daily subcutaneous insulin dose is generally added to the TPN solution. Additional subcutaneous insulin should be administered using a sliding scale regimen written as a standing order with the dose of insulin based on bedside glucose measurements. After the first 24 hours, approximately half of the additional regular subcutaneous insulin administered over the 24-hour period is added to the TPN solution prior to increasing the rate or concentration of dextrose. Evidence suggests that continuous infusion, rather than bolus administration, of insulin may be associated with insulin resistance. It must also be remembered that IV insulin has a very short half-life (a couple of minutes) with a relatively short biologic half-life (½ hr). Although IV insulin availability is decreased by binding to IV containers, tubing, and in-line filters,[74-77] the addition of amino acid to TPN solutions virtually eliminates the adsorption to containers or tubing.

Anabolic Hormones

Nutrition plays a pivotal role in the regulation of both growth hormone (GH) and insulin-like growth factor-1 (IGF-1) secretions; GH and IGF-1 in turn significantly influence the use of nutrients in humans and animals. Fasting and caloric or protein restriction increase circulating values of GH and decrease those of IGF-1. In humans, both hormones seem to enhance protein anabolism but only for short periods. Secondary effects are mainly hypoglycemia with IGF-1 and hyperglycemic with GH.[78, 79] Secretion of GH declines by 14% with each decade in normal adults after 20 years of age; IGF-1 also decreases with aging.

Administration of GH may attenuate several important decrements in body composition (i.e., lean body mass) and in function associated with aging. Short-term side effects of GH therapy include edema, carpal tunnel syndrome, and arthralgia. Further studies of GH replacement are needed to examine issues such as dosage, tolerance, and efficacy before the widespread use of GH is advocated for older populations.[80] No adverse effects (e.g., hypoglycemia) that might be attributed to recombinant human IGF-1 therapy were observed in ICU patients with SIRS.[81] Circulating epinephrine at plasma concentrations, similar to those reached during physical stress, stimulates the production of binding protein (IGFBP-1) in humans.[82] The IGFs mediate the anabolic effects of GH on protein synthesis in muscle and skeletal tissues.

Administration of GH to normal volunteers who have been made catabolic by caloric restriction improves nitrogen balance. Administration of somatomedin-C (IGF-1) to catabolic normal volunteers also results in improved nitrogen balance and, unlike GH, does not induce insulin resistance. GH was anabolic in patients with severe chronic obstructive lung disease (COPD) and resulted in improved chest wall muscle strength. Both IGF-1 and GH have the potential to improve muscle mass and function in patients who are catabolic as a result of the severity of their underlying disease state.[83] Although IGF-1 is regulated by nutritional intake independently of growth hormone,[84] its use in critically-ill patients, at this time, is unclear.

Although extended studies are required, preliminary findings suggest potential therapeutic benefits of dehydroepiandrosterone (DHEA) in immunodeficient states,[85] such as complement fixation compromise in diabetic patients. It is particularly important to control blood glucose levels during steroid administration, sepsis, or surgical stress.

The clinical effect of perioperative nutrition from 28 controlled clinical trials has been reported. Preoperative nutritional support is indicated in patients with high-grade malnutrition.[86]

Glucose administration during severe stress does not suppress enhanced hepatic glucose production or lipolysis. This phenomenon, related to tissue insulin resistance and elevated protein catabolism, produces a progressive loss of body cell mass and fosters development of malnutrition.[87]

Cytokines, notably TNF and IL-1, suppress synthesis of lipoprotein lipase, which decreases the rate of triglyceride fatty acid (TGFA) clearance. Hypertriglyceridemia, then, can develop in the absence of elevated plasma free fatty acid levels.[88]

Early nutritional supplementation decreases the incidence of septic complications by improving overall nutritional status and by maintaining immune competence and wound healing.[89] It is widely appreciated that substantial losses of body protein do occur in critically ill patients with sepsis despite aggressive nutritional support.[90, 91]

Aging is associated with a number of changes in circulating hormone concentrations (Table 83-3). These changes are superimposed on the effects of critical illness.

Thyroid Hormones

As a normal response to injury, the body's ability to convert the stored form of thyroid hormone (T_4) into the active form

TABLE 83–3. Circulating Hormones in Older People

Decreased
1,25-Dihydroxyvitamin D
Aldosterone
Calcitonin
Dehydroepiandrosterone
Estradiol (females)
Growth hormone
Insulin-like growth factor-1
Renin
Testosterone
Triiodothyronine (T_3)
Increased
Follicle-stimulating hormone
Insulin
Norepinephrine
Parathyroid hormone
Prolactin (no change in females)
Vasopressin (daytime only; decreased levels at night)

(triiodothyronine [T_3]) becomes impaired. There is increased conversion of T_4 to an inactive thyroid hormone known as *reverse T_3* (rT_3) rather than T_3. The syndrome of low T_3 (*sick euthyroid syndrome*), seen in acute illness, is an adaptive strategy to reduce the normal effects of T_3 on resting energy expenditure. Selenium plays a role in the conversion of T_4 to T_3. Iodothyronine 5′-deiodinase, which is mainly responsible for peripheral T_3 production, has been demonstrated to be a selenium-containing enzyme. In older patients, reduced peripheral conversion of T_4 to T_3 and overt hypothyroidism are frequently observed. Repletion of selenium may improve thyroid hormone activation in the elderly.[92]

In critically ill patients, however, normalization of T_3 values by replacement of thyroid hormone has had no beneficial effect on clinical outcome. Although thyroid hormones stimulate appetite, the effect is primarily related to an increase in metabolic rate. Overuse of thyroid hormone can result in weight loss (increased metabolism) and can aggravate underlying cardiorespiratory disease. Depression is the most common cause of weight loss and anorexia in older persons. Cytokine release has also been associated with the wasting effects of cancer and rheumatoid arthritis. Numerous medications have been used to treat the anorexia of aging:

- GH
- Megestrol
- Cyproheptadine
- Tetrahydrocannabinol
- Anabolic steroids
- Prokinetic agents
- Antidepressants

All critically ill patients should receive an individualized anorexia assessment that may include treatment with several agents.

NUTRITIONAL ASSESSMENT

Nutritional support of the critically ill geriatric patient is based on the ability to treat the underlying disease and accommodate the desires of the patient and family. There is no requirement to administer nutritional support when death is imminent. A clinical technique called "subjective global assessment" (SGA) that evaluates nutritional status based on features of the history and physical examination has been a reliable, easily used tool for patient nutritional assessment.[93] The subjective global assessment is a good tool for assessing nutritional status prior to an acute illness (Table 83–4). Of primary importance to nutritional goal setting is an appreciation of lean body mass (i.e., mass of the thigh relative to the longest bone in the body, the femur).

Older patients are particularly vulnerable to malnutrition. Contributing factors include:

- Cognitive impairment
- Poor dentition
- Drug-nutrient interactions
- Poor sight
- Poor hand-to-mouth coordination
- Need for assistance at meals
- Presence of depression
- Respiratory dysfunction
- Altered sense of taste and smell
- Swallowing difficulties.

As the duration of hospital stay increases, the likelihood of malnutrition generally rises.

Of course, providing either tube feeding or TPN to hospitalized patients is not a benign procedure and can be associated with appreciable risks,[94] including the development of septic, mechanical, or metabolic complications. In the critically ill older patient, the risks are heightened owing to the effects of aging on vital organ function as well as on the body's ability to respond to injury and infection. In addition, the existence of comorbid disease increases the rate of complications.[95] Critical illness often creates a vigorous metabolic response to permit the repair of injured tissues.[96]

TABLE 83–4. Abbreviated Nutrition Assessment

Subjective Global Assessment

I. ***History***

Weight Change
  Loss over past 6 months:
  Change in past two weeks:
Dietary intake changes:
GI Sx:
Functional Capacity:
Disease relation to nutritional requirements:
    Stress (none, moderate, high)

II. ***Physical (0 = nl, 1+ = mild, 2+ = moderate, 3+ = severe)***

Subcutaneous fat:
Muscle wasting:
Ankle edema:
Sacral edema:
Ascites:

III. ***SGA rating***

A = Well nourished
B = Moderately malnourished
C = Severely malnourished

From Detsky AS, McLaughlin JR, Baker JP, Johnston N, Whittaker S, Mendelson RA, Jeejeebhoy KN: What is subjective global assessment of nutritional status? J Parenter Enteral Nutr 1987; 11:8–13.

GI = gastrointestinal; Sx = symptoms; SGA = subjective assessment.

Fluid Balance

Changes in routine nutrition assessment parameters (i.e., visceral proteins) and body composition are affected by fluid balance; thus, they are not specific indicators of the adequacy of nutritional support in ICU patients.[97] Because of changes in total body water and intracellular water, IV fluid management must be dynamically adjusted for the older patient. During periods of fever and stress (e.g., postoperatively), daily water requirements may be more than doubled.

On the other hand, fluid-restricted formulas may be required in the volume-overloaded critically ill patient. Fluid restriction can be accomplished using 1.5 to 2 kcal/mL enteral or TPN formulas made with more concentrated constituents (i.e., 15% amino acids, 70% dextrose, and 20% lipid). Because fluid-restricted patients are at risk for development of protein-calorie and micronutrient deficiencies,[98] nutrient intake should be closely monitored.

IV catheters are composed of a variety of materials (polyvinylchloride, polyethylene, silicon, hydromer-coated polyurethane, standard polyurethane, fluoroethylene, propylene, or polytef). The hydromer-coated polyurethane carries with it the lowest rate of thrombogenicity.[99] Measures that decrease bacterial adherence reduce the incidence of infections.[100] Bacterial attachment has been found to be lower on glycerophosphorylcholine-containing polyurethanes, both in the absence of and after preadsorption with plasma proteins.[101] The use of central venous catheters coated with antibiotics (e.g., minocycline, rifampin) has been shown to significantly reduce the incidence of catheter-related infection.

Coating catheters with minocycline and rifampin inhibits ultrastructural colonization of indwelling catheters and maintains effective antimicrobial activity for at least 2 weeks.[102]

Catheter-related infection (CRI) accounts for a large percentage of nosocomial infections, and related bacteremia is a common complication. Bacteremia arises in approximately one of 15 episodes of catheter-related infection and causes considerable morbidity and occasional mortality as well as increased medical costs. Semiquantitative tip culture by the roll-plate method is the cornerstone for diagnosis of catheter-related infection in routine practice. However, there is a great deal of interest in alternative methods for diagnosis without catheter withdrawal, since treatment of the patient can be successfully completed with the infected device maintained in place. Conservative management includes perfusion of antibiotics through the infected catheter and the antibiotic-lock technique.[103] A significant decrease in staphylococcal, gram-negative, and fungal intraluminal colonization after instillation of appropriate antimicrobial has been achieved.[104, 105]

Filters are presently used within IV administration sets or add-ons to existing administration sets. They are designed primarily to remove bacteria and fungus, but they also remove particles (tens of thousands in a typical parenteral nutrition solution) and trap air emboli. The 0.22-μm filter is used for most IV solutions that must be filtered. The 0.45-μm filter does not filter out several organisms, such as *Haemophilus* or *Pseudomonas* species. Still larger sizes (1 to 5 μm) are used to filter primarily fungus and particulates in lipid-containing solutions. IV filters are composed of many different types of materials and include cellulose ester, polyacrylate, polypropylene, polyethylene, or posidyne nylon.[66] The posidyne nylon filter is also pyrogen-retentive.[106]

Route of Nutrient Delivery

Critically ill patients are susceptible to injury of the intestinal mucosa, changes in gut permeability, and failure of intestinal defense mechanisms. These conditions put patients at risk for infection and multiple organ dysfunction syndrome. Specific therapies are needed to prevent gut failure during critical illness. Translocation of bacteria, mediators of the inflammatory response, and the microcirculation play a role in the response to critical illness. Enteral nutrition that includes glutamine and arginine may enhance gut function and may improve outcomes.[107]

Interruptions in enteral feeding may lead to inadequate nutritional support, highlighting the importance of performing daily nutritional monitoring (intakes, outputs, calorie counts) so as to prevent malnutrition.[108] The most common ICU feeding complication in enterally fed critically ill patients has been interruption in continuous tube feedings.[109] Inactive patients and patients with fecal incontinence are at risk for fecal impaction. Dehydration or fluid restriction may lead to constipation or impaction. Early enteral nutrition investigations in critically ill patients promise to better address these kinds of problems.[110]

Septic patients in the ICU have increased lactulose and L-rhamnose urine excretion ratios (0.23 ± 0.19) compared with control subjects (0.03 ± 0.01; $P < .001$), consistent with increased gastrointestinal permeability in sepsis. Septic patients had decreased L-rhamnose/3-*O*-methyl-D-glucose urine excretion ratios (0.14 ± 0.07) compared with normal controls (0.28 ± 0.08; $P < .001$), consistent with decreased gastrointestinal functional absorptive capacity in sepsis. In sum, ICU patients with acute sepsis exhibited increased gastrointestinal permeability and decreased gastrointestinal functional absorptive capacity in comparison with healthy control subjects. These abnormalities may contribute to the pathophysiology of sepsis.[111]

Failure of the gut barrier remains central to the hypothesis that toxins escaping from the gut lumen contribute to activation of the host's immune inflammatory defense mechanisms, subsequently leading to the autointoxication and tissue destruction seen in the septic response characteristic of multiorgan failure. A "vicious circle" of increased intestinal permeability, leading to toxic mediator release, resulting in a further increase in gut permeability is generated. Additionally, the systemic and local inflammatory cells that become activated in the gut contribute to the systemic response characteristic of the sepsis syndrome and multiorgan failure.[112] A randomized controlled trial of enteral versus parenteral nutrition after major upper gastrointestinal tract surgery showed no clinical benefit of the enteral route. Enteral nutrition did not modulate gut barrier function postoperatively.[113] On the other hand, a number of prospective randomized trials in trauma and postoperative patients demonstrated a decreased incidence of infection in enteral versus parenterally fed patients.

In contrast to what is commonly stated, nearly 90% of older people are capable of acidifying gastric contents, even in the basal, unstimulated state. Of those patients who were consistent hyposecretors of acid, most had serum markers of atrophic gastritis.[114] Patients with hypochlorhydria are at increased risk for bacterial colonization of the stomach and for pneumonia.

The gastrointestinal tract entry point (i.e., nasogastric, nasojejunal, percutaneous endoscopic gastrostomy, nasoduodenal, oral-duodenal, oral-jejunal, jejunostomy) is decided by the type of trauma or location of the lesion. Once an access plan is developed, the motility and function of the bowel leads to formula type selection (i.e., elemental, polymeric, organ-specific, and immune-modulating). The formula volume is a balance between hourly tolerance and approximated daily needs. Ultimately, delivery may be intermittent, continuous, or cyclic and is individualized to the patient. *Cyclic* (part of the day) versus *continuous* enteral or parenteral nutrition has been useful in terms of clearing lipid from tissues (especially in the liver), however, concentrating nutrients in smaller time frames of administration has also been associated with hypercapnea. In patients with inflammatory bowel disease treated by parenteral nutrition, the incidence of TPN-induced cholestasis may be reduced by discontinuous (cyclic) TPN.[115] Critical illness frequently leads to organ dysfunction and is an evolving area of nutritional support.[116]

The timing of the feeding appears to be of paramount importance because early enteral nutrition may maintain muscle mass by blunting the cytokine-mediated hypermetabolic response.[117] Humoral immunity parameters, particularly IgA and IgM, do not appear to be statistically different between enteral and parenteral routes.[118]

The infusion of enteral products into the small bowel reduces the incidence of formula aspiration if the infusion is beyond the pylorus. To minimize aspiration pneumonitis on tube insertion, one must take care not to lubricate the tube with an ointment having an external phase that is oil-based.

Most nutritional experts favor the use of the enteral over the parenteral route whenever possible, with some studies documenting a decreased incidence of infection and reduced cost. Because enteral feeding better supports gut function and the immune response, parenteral nutrition is reserved for the patient with gastrointestinal tract dysfunction who cannot tolerate enteral feeding. A multidisciplinary team approach to patient selection, assessment, and monitoring is recommended.[119]

NUTRITION FORMULAS

Many critically ill patients are malnourished, and *refeeding syndrome* can develop if nutritional repletion is too aggressive (i.e., hypophosphatemia, hypokalemia and hypomagnesemia, hyperglycemia). Therefore, feeding should be initiated with complete formulas at half the calculated needs and advanced to full feeding over 2 to 3 days.

In addition to concurrent medical illness, factors contributing to malnutrition in the elderly include inadequate income, problems with shopping or preparing meals, poor eating habits, and difficulties with dentures. Excess or megadosing of nutrients, especially micronutrients, may also be present.

Protein Macrosubstrate

Up to 65% of elderly hospitalized patients are said to be protein-energy undernourished at admission, or they acquire nutritional deficits while hospitalized.[120] Loss of lean body mass (LBM) is a hallmark of aging and of acute and chronic illness. Loss of more than 40% of LBM is incompatible with life. The causes in aging remain obscure, although changes in GH production, physical activity, and cytokines IL-1β and TNF-α may play a role.[121]

Cytokines such as IL-1, TNF-α, and IL-6 mediate a variety of host responses to trauma and infection, including skeletal muscle proteolysis.[122] Host responses to infectious and inflammatory stimuli are altered with aging antagonists, such as IL-1 receptor antagonist. These cytokine antagonists reduce IL-2 production and the capability of T cells to proliferate, thereby inhibiting responses in the elderly.[123]

The oral RDA of protein for an unstressed healthy adult is about 0.8 g/kg of body weight, and for a stressed healthy adult it is about 1.2 to 1.5 g/kg. Of this dietary protein, about 20% of the constituent amino acids should be essential amino acids, since these cannot be synthesized in adequate amounts by the body and must be present in the diet. Most parenteral amino acid formulas are approximately 50% essential amino acids. The essential amino acid content of enteral formulas varies with the protein source but generally contains greater than 20% essential amino acids.

Protein needs of critically ill patients are not constant. They change with the degree of catabolism, degree of injury, phase of illness, and renal function. In one study, monitoring of an individualized program of nutritional support provided a greater mean daily weight gain, allowed greater amounts of nutrients to be provided, and was cost effective compared with the use of a standardized solution without individualized monitoring.[124]

The acute-phase response to injury or infection is associated with alterations in dynamics of many trace elements, particularly iron, zinc, and copper. The decline in serum iron and zinc levels with a concominant rise in the serum copper level is brought about by changes in the concentration of specific tissue proteins controlled by cytokines, especially IL-1, TNF, and IL-6.[125] Globulins and acute-phase reactants rise, and visceral proteins, such as albumin and prealbumin, decline for approximately 1 week after injury. At that time, visceral proteins begin to rise and acute-phase reactants normalize. Thus, visceral proteins are not specific markers of nutritional status.

Protein supplementation is an important substrate for proteins that are synthesized and secreted as part of the acute phase response to illness or injury (Table 83–5).

Protein breakdown (i.e., catabolism) is part of the response to illness and injury. Critically ill patients may lose extraordinary amounts of nitrogen. Quantitation of nitrogen losses is difficult, and large amounts may be lost in urine, stool, and other secretions. Urinary losses are also difficult to detect because of inaccuracies of measurement techniques, interference by hematuria, medication metabolites, and circadian rhythm of urea excretion.

Serum albumin concentration is frequently used to define nutritional status. The data indicate that serum albumin is a valid measure of nutritional state for epidemiologic surveys (i.e., lack of acute illness, presence of chronicity). However, as a result of the low sensitivity and specificity, it is a poor parameter for evaluating the individual patient's nutritional state because serum concentration interpretation is limited by state of health and fluid status.[126]

TABLE 83–5. Cytokine and Hormonal Acute-Phase Response

Aldosterone	C-reactive protein
Tumor necrosis factor-α	Glucagon/insulin
α_1-Antichymotrypsin	Growth hormone
α_2-Macroglobulin	Interleukin-1
Catecholamines	Interleukin-2
Cortisol	

Serum albumin serves better as a predictor of survival or as an epidemiologic tool rather than a reliable nutrition monitoring parameter. In addition, other reasons that cast doubt on the validity of albumin as a nutritional tool include:

1. Intravascular concentration (due to circadian rhythm) is as much as 0.75 g/day.
2. Intravascular albumin represents only 30% to 40% of total body albumin.
3. The half-life of intravascular albumin is 2 to 3 weeks (extravascular half-lives are in hours).
4. Positional impact is 10% to 15% (greater hemoconcentration with sitting or standing).

Prealbumin (transthyretin, thyroid binding prealbumin) is a short-acting (36-hour) visceral protein (unrelated to albumin). Because of its shorter half-life, it is frequently used as a nutritional marker in critically ill patients. Increasing concentrations in critically ill patients usually suggest control of the underlying disease process plus adequate nutritional support. Prealbumin concentrations are affected by underlying diseases (particularly those associated with thyroid or renal function) and volume status.[127]

Skin tests to assess delayed hypersensitivity or T-cell function are difficult to interpret in aged patients, who show declining cellular immunity. Waning of tuberculin sensitivity appears to be an integral part of the aging process.[128] Steroid administration, stress, critical illness, and sepsis also depress responses. In addition, vitamin deficiency is likely to be associated with anergy.[129] Therefore, skin testing is of little value as an aid to nutrition support in the critically ill patient.

Glutamine is an amino acid that has many metabolic roles in the body, including protection of tissue integrity and enhancement of the immune response. Low plasma and tissue levels of glutamine in the critically ill suggest that demand may exceed endogenous supply, and with the profound muscle wasting that occurs, the supply of glutamine may become critical to survival. Patients who cannot tolerate enteral feeding are solely dependent on conventional TPN that does not contain glutamine. Continuing work in this area suggests a role for supplemental glutamine during TPN.[130]

Energy Macrosubstrates

Carbohydrate

Glucose is a preferred substrate for a variety of tissues, but the brain and erythrocyte, in particular, require about 150 g/day. The maximal rate of glucose oxidation is 5 to 7 mg of glucose/kg per minute. This rate may be lower in the critically ill geriatric patient, who is compromised secondary t› stress, sepsis, or medications that are associated with abnormal glucose metabolism. Exceeding a glucose renal threshold of about 180 mg/dL glucose (interindividual variations) may be associated with an osmotic diuresis and dehydration. Exceeding a blood glucose level of 220 mg/dL for more than 16 hours results in complement fixation compromise (glycation of immunoglobulins) and immune depression. Increased morbidity secondary to carbohydrate overload includes fatty liver infiltration and hypercapnea. Fructose is an alternative carbohydrate source that does not require insulin for metabolism.[131]

Hemoglobin A_{1c} and, more recently, fructosamine are useful in management of older diabetic patients. Serum fructosamine provides an estimation of the glycemic state during the preceding 10 to 20 days. The turnover of serum proteins is, in general, faster than that of hemoglobin. Therefore, fructosamine is faster responding than Hb A_{1c} to recompensation or fluctuations in glycemic control, as observed in labile metabolic situations. On the other hand, under conditions of stable metabolic control, fructosamine values correlate closely to those of Hb A_{1c}.[132] The fasting blood glucose level is not significantly altered by age, but the 2- and 3-hour postprandial blood glucose is higher in the aged.

The presence of bacteria or their products (e.g., endotoxin) either directly or indirectly (via stimulation of mononuclear phagocytes to release cytokines) activates the immune response. The use of glucose by these tissues, which are predominantly glycolytic, is stimulated, resulting in increased lactate production. Simultaneous glucose uptake by skeletal muscle also contributes to hyperlactacidemia. The excess CO_2 from this anaerobic imbalance can drive respiratory quotients toward lipogenic levels of 1.3. Sepsis and stress are associated with insulin insensitivity and resistance; resolution is frequently associated with reduced insulin requirements.

Aging and severity of illness interact to exaggerate the increases in blood glucose levels that accompany TPN with hypertonic glucose. Serum insulin responses to TPN decline with aging, likely reflecting reduced insulin secretion. Diminished insulin responses may contribute to hyperglycemia and represent a diminished anabolic signal in such patients. The acutely ill elderly patient is predisposed to hyperglycemia and should be monitored carefully even when pre-TPN blood glucose values are normal.[133]

Lipid

IV fat emulsion products are derived from soybeans or a mixture of soybean and safflower oil. The products contain about 15 mM phosphate per liter, in addition to selenium, and about 60 μg of vitamin K per 100 mL (30 μg in the 10%). Both hyperphosphatemia and warfarin interaction secondary to lipid infusion have been reported.[134] If warfarin is given, the International Normalized Ratio (INR) should be monitored daily to ensure adequate anticoagulation.[135] In patients receiving IV lipids, a normal vitamin K_1 status can be maintained during long-term TPN without vitamin K_1 supplementation. However, vitamin K supplementation cannot be abandoned until the vitamin K content of emulsions is standardized by manufacturers. A weekly supply of 250 to 400 μg of vitamin K_1 is enough to maintain and even restore a normal vitamin K_1 status in TPN.[136]

IV lipid for patient use is available in 10% and 20% concentrations, but the use of the 20% product has been advocated to avoid the lipoprotein-X (LP-X) problems associated with the 10%. Hyperlipidemia during IV Intralipid 10% is induced almost exclusively by the increased LP-X.[137] The role of LP-X is unclear.[138–142]

Metabolites of arachidonic acid (i.e., proinflammatory compounds) formed from omega-6 essential fatty acids (n-6), play a pathologic role in mortality from sepsis. Metabolites of eicosapentaenoic acid, formed from omega-3 essential fatty acids (n-3), are less potent inflammatory mediators. Dietary restriction of n-6 fatty acids or supplementation with n-3 fatty acids in the form of fish oil has been shown to decrease the production of n-6 metabolites and to improve survival in a rat peritonitis model.[143] Omega-3 fatty acids can be found in a variety of enteral formulas. Their effects in humans remain to be clarified. Since the compositional ratio of n-6 to n-3 is approximately 4:1 in the human and 2.5:1 in other animal models, structured IV lipids of both of these long-chain lipids as well as medium-chain lipid combinations will likely be available in the future. The IV lipid injectables are about 50% linoleic acid (n-6), with only very small concentrations of linolenic acid (n-3).

Increased unsaturation of cell membrane fatty acids is said to have a major impact on membrane fluidity. Intralipid contains triglycerides composed of polysaturated fatty acids and lecithin as an emulsifier. Circulating lipoproteins interact with lymphocyte-specific membrane receptors (that inhibit antigen- and mitogen-induced blastogenesis). However, Intralipid alters neither the lipid composition of lymphocyte membrane nor membrane fluidity. Furthermore, if modulation of membrane lipid composition by Intralipid does occur, cellular self-regulation (by fatty acid synthesis to keep the membrane fluidity stable) is likely.[144]

Long-term omega-3 fatty acid supplementation reduces cytokine production and T cell mitogenesis. This reduction may be greater in older individuals. Although (n-3) fatty acid–induced reduction in cytokine production may have beneficial anti-inflammatory effects, its suppression of IL-2 production and lymphocyte proliferation may not be desirable.[145] Supplemental omega-3 fatty acids have been used to treat inflammation in patients with inflammatory bowel disease, arthritis, and autoimmune disorders. However, their effectiveness in treating inflammatory disorders in critically ill patients is unproven.

Essential fatty acid requirements (for prevention of deficiency) are estimated to be approximately 1% to 4% of total energy requirements and should be in the form of linoleic acid. Patients with chronic intestinal disease should be evaluated for deficiencies and imbalances and treated with substantial amounts of supplements rich in essential fatty acids, such as oral vegetable and fish oils or IV lipids.[146] Alpha-linolenic acid deficiency was described in five adults receiving long-term gastric tube feeding with a commercially available powdered formula mixed with water, fat-free milk, or both. Scaly dermatitis and skin atrophy developed. Three patients receiving the same powder mixed with whole milk showed no signs of essential fatty acid deficiency. In four patients, supplementation with cod liver oil and soya oil for 4 weeks normalized n-3 acids in plasma and red blood cells, whereas n-6 acid levels remained unchanged or decreased slightly. At the same time, skin changes were reversed.

Minimal daily requirement of alpha-linolenic acid and of long-chain omega-3 (n-3) fatty acids are estimated to be 0.2% to 0.4% and 0.1% to 0.2% of calories, respectively.[147] Omega-6 lipids (linoleic acid), such as soybean (parenteral amino acids and IV lipid), safflower, sunflower, and corn oils, are approximately 60% linoleic acid. These precurse even-numbered icosanoids (i.e., prostaglandin E_2 [PGE_2], prostacyclin [PGI_2], thromboxane [TXA_2]), but odd-numbered icosanoids (i.e., PGE_3, leukotriene E_3 [LTE_3], TXA_3) are precursed by omega-3 lipids (linolenic acid), such as peanut and canola oils. The plasma lipid alterations characteristic of essential fatty acid deficiency generally appear 1 to 2 weeks after the initiation of fat-free parenteral nutrition and may be associated with a reduction in prostaglandin formation.

The relationship between exclusion of fat from the diet and changes in intraocular pressure (IOP) and PGE_2 plasma levels has been studied. The results indicated that 3 weeks after the omission of dietary fat, a significant reduction in IOP levels occurred and persisted throughout the follow-up period of 7 weeks. Plasma PGE_2 levels were also significantly reduced in patients receiving fat-free parenteral nutrition for 3 weeks compared with levels measured while patients were on a fat-containing diet.[148]

TPN, either lipid-based or glucose-based, has been shown to be a safe and effective therapy for reversing the malnutrition of acute pancreatitis.[149] Others have also shown no adverse effects on the pancreas with the provision of IV fat in parenteral regimens.[150]

The diagnosis of carnitine deficiency is based on a determination of free carnitine and acylcarnitine levels in serum, urine, or tissues. Carnitine in the human body is derived from the intake of preformed dietary carnitine and biosynthesized carnitine, stemming from the metabolism of lysine and methionine. Carnitine is synthesized in liver and kidney, stored in skeletal muscle, and excreted mainly in urine. Carnitine has two main functions: (1) transporting long-chain fatty acids into the mitochondrial matrix for beta-oxidation to provide cellular energy and (2) modulating the rise in intramitochondrial acyl-CoA/CoA ratio, which relieves the inhibition of many intramitochondrial enzymes involving glucose and amino acid catabolism. Thus, the main consequence of carnitine deficiency is impaired energy metabolism.[151] Older patients are at risk for carnitine deficiency.

Micronutrients

Micronutrients play key roles in many of the metabolic processes that promote survival from critical illness. For vitamins, these processes include oxidative phosphorylation, which is altered in the patient with systemic inflammation, and protection against oxidative mediators. Trace elements are essential for direct antioxidant activity, and they function as cofactors for a variety of antioxidant enzymes. Wound healing and immune function also depend on adequate levels of vitamins and minerals. Of extreme importance is the ease with which a deficiency state can develop in the critically ill because of decreased nutrient intakes and increased requirements.[152]

Electrolytes

Approximately a dozen electrolytes, as well as vitamins, and half a dozen trace elements are used in enteral and parenteral formulas. Commonly assessed micronutrients include major minerals (sodium, potassium, calcium, phosphate, magnesium, chloride, bicarbonate), trace elements (iron, zinc) and vitamins (B_{12}, folic acid). Although biochemical assessment of other micronutrients is possible, the clinical appreciation of mineral and vitamin deficiencies usually requires recognition of corresponding signs and symptoms.

Hypocalcemia is common in critically ill patients. The aging patient is predisposed to decreased concentrations of 1,25-dihydroxyvitamin D (a hormone that aids in calcium absorption). Hypocalcemia is associated with a prolonged QT interval and cardiovascular insufficiency. Dietary sodium excess contributes to urinary calcium losses.[153] Ionized calcium concentrations have also been found to be useful because many ICU patients have alterations in both arterial pH and serum albumin levels.[154] Free fatty acids increase calcium binding to the albumin molecule. Alterations in free fatty acid concentrations during critical illness may contribute to the poor correlation between corrected total serum calcium and ionized calcium concentrations in critically ill patients. In addition, acute elevations in circulating free fatty acid concentrations may contribute to hypocalcemia in patients with defects in bone calcium mobilization.[155]

The effect of aging on the relationship between the concentrations of blood ionized calcium and of serum parathyroid hormone (PTH) have been explored. Serum concentrations of PTH in elderly men were twice those in younger men, whereas blood ionized calcium did not differ between the two groups. With IV infusion of calcium gluconate, the minimum PTH concentration was two-fold to three-fold higher in elderly men. These findings suggest that, with aging, the relationship between calcium and PTH is altered such that at any given level of calcium, the concentration of PTH is higher.[156] The higher PTH concentrations may contribute to osteopenia. Optimal oral calcium intakes of 37.5 mmol (1500 mg)/day have been proposed for older people. However, high-calcium diets may reduce net zinc absorption and balance and may increase the zinc requirement in adults.[157]

The aging critically ill patient is also susceptible to alterations in magnesium and phosphorus homeostasis. Renal insufficiency predisposes to elevated concentrations. On the other hand, poor dietary intake, use of various medications, and underlying disease can lead to deficiency states. Levels of these ions should be monitored in the critically ill geriatric patient. Compensatory metabolic alterations secondary to chronic starvation predispose malnourished patients to refeeding syndrome. Providing nutritional support, either from a no-feeding to a feeding situation or from a lower feeding regimen to a more aggressive feeding level, initiates an intracellular shift of potassium, magnesium, and phosphate that results in many adverse effects.[158, 159] The most imporant of these is a shift to the left of the hemoglobin:oxygen dissociation curve. This becomes quite problematic if there are additive factors that may also tighten the hemoglobin:oxygen affinity (i.e., alkalemia, hypocapnia, hypothermia). Aggressive TPN support has been followed by acute cardiopulmonary decompensation associated with severe hypophosphatemia and other metabolic abnormalities. Despite attempts at phosphate correction, progressive failure of multiple organ systems can lead to death.[160]

Hypocalcemia cannot be normalized without correcting hypomagnesemia. Magnesuria secondary to catecholamine shower, intestinal losses, various medications, and the unreliability of serum concentrations (even ionized) lend to the true difficulty in defining magnesium deficiency.[161]

Trace Elements

Enteral nutrition, whether by mouth or by tube, is fraught with problems that may influence kinetics. Even parenteral nutrition, although delivered to the intravascular milieu, carries with it no guarantee that trace minerals will indeed reach their target sites. Trace elements should always be included in the nutritional regimen. We should not assume that there are stores of micronutrients that permit delay in supplementation, since the patient may be seriously depleted on entry into the intensive care arena.[162] The elderly are predisposed to trace element deficiencies because of poor diet, use of various medications, and underlying disease.

Trace elements that are included in enteral formulations include the ones with RDAs (i.e., iodine, iron, selenium, zinc) and estimated safe and adequate daily dietary intakes (i.e., chromium, copper, fluoride, manganese, molybdenum). The American Medical Association trace element recommendations for parenteral administration include chromium, copper, manganese, and zinc. In addition, selenium, molybdenum, iron, and iodide are available.

Chromium

Chromium, as previously discussed, is a part of glucose tolerance factor associated with the activity of insulin, and hyperglycemia may signal its deficiency. Significant concentrations of chromium and zinc contaminations, however, have been found in a variety of parenteral nutrition components that exceed even current dosing recommendations.[163]

Selenium

Selenium status influences thyroid hormones in the critically ill geriatric patient, mainly by modulating T_4 levels.[164, 165] The relationship between selenium and T_4/T_3 indicates that reduced T_4 to T_3 deiodination might also be related to decreases in serum selenium concentrations,[166] which have been reported to be decreased in critically ill patients. As with many micronutrients, however, redistribution into tissues contributes to the decrease and makes serum concentrations difficult to interpret. Platelet, erythrocyte, and urinary assessments of selenium and glutathione peroxidase further define the need for supplemental selenium. Both selenium and vitamin E provide similar antoxidant activity.[167]

Zinc

Serum zinc levels fall as an early response to inflammation, infection, and injury. Zinc, too, is redistributed (to liver, bone marrow, thymus, and the site of injury or inflammation) in the critically ill patient. This redistribution is mediated by IL-1 and other cytokines secreted from macrophages.[168] Large losses of zinc can occur via intestinal losses (i.e., 12 mg/L fistula fluid and 17 mg/kg of stool). When supplemented orally, the clinician must be aware that about 25% of zinc sulfate is elemental zinc and approximately 20% is bioavailable, so that only about 11 mg elemental zinc of a 220-mg zinc sulfate dosage will reach target sites. Since 15 mg of elemental zinc is the RDA or oral requirement, multiple doses may need to be given.[169] Critically ill (particularly postsurgical) patients have higher requirements. Zinc deficiency can have marked effects on virtually all components of the immune system. Strong epidemiologic data support the belief that Zinc deficiency is a major factor underlying immune dysfunction in select human populations. Zinc may also be essential for the activity and binding of protein kinase C in lymphocyte membranes, a critical factor in the activation and inactivation of immunoregulatory genes.[170]

It is interesting that when serum zinc concentrations fall, as with severe injury or sepsis, serum copper and ceruloplasmin levels increase. On the other hand, long-term zinc use can be associated with copper deficiency.[171, 172] In addition to zinc excess, reports indicate that copper deficiency also occurs secondary to gastric resection, unsupplemented total parenteral nutrition, or general malnutrition. The microcytic, hypochromic anemia secondary to copper deficit is almost always heralded by a neutropenia. Both anemia and neutropenia caused by copper deficiency are well-known consequences of long-term TPN[173, 174] and has also been reported in long-term enteral nutrition.[175]

Iron

As with zinc, serum iron levels fall as a result of the cytokine-mediated response to infection or injury. Iron is sequestered in Kuppfer cells of the liver during inflammation. Iron deficiency needs to be confirmed before iron supplementation is given to patients, particularly over long periods. Oversupplementation of iron can lead to organ injury secondary to cellular iron overload. Genetic hemochromatosis is a metabolic autosomal recessive disease characterized by excessive iron absorption; accumulation of iron in the liver, heart, pancreas, and endocrine glands gives rise to organ damage and dysfunction. Some studies indicate that hemachromatosis, once thought to be rare and fatal, is quite frequent (up to two to five homozygotes for 1000 inhabitants). When subjects are recognized and treated before onset of cirrhosis, they have a normal life expectancy.[176]

Aluminum

The use of modern analytic methods has demonstrated that aluminum salts can be absorbed from the gut and concentrated in various human tissues, including bone, parathyroid glands, and brain. High concentrations of aluminum have been detected in the brain tissue of patients with Alzheimer's disease. Various reports have suggested that high aluminum intakes may be harmful to some patients with bone disease or renal impairment.

The most common foods with substantial amounts of aluminum-containing additives include some processed cheeses, baking powders, cake mixes, frozen doughs, pancake mixes, self-rising flours, and pickled vegetables. The aluminum-containing nonprescription drugs include some antacids, buffered aspirins, antidiarrheal products, douches, and hemorrhoidal medications.[177] Additives to TPN solutions that are contaminated with aluminum include albumin, calcium, and phosphate salts. In addition, Shohl's solution and other citrate-containing solutions (blood components or alkalinizing agents) contain much aluminum.

Vitamins

The oldest age category in the 1989 edition of the Recommended Dietary Allowances was 51 years and above. A review of past and newer data suggests that the current oral RDAs for older people are too low for riboflavin, vitamin B_6, folic acid, vitamin B_{12}, vitamin D, and calcium and are probably too high for vitamin A.

Parenteral vitamins include the fat-soluble (vitamins A, D, E, K), the semi–water-soluble (cyanocobalamin, folic acid) and the water-soluble vitamins (thiamine, riboflavin, niacin, pyridoxine, and vitamin C). Biotin, another semi–water-soluble vitamin, and pantothenic acid, a water-soluble vitamin, are included in the estimated safe and adequate daily dietary intakes recommendations.

Aging is associated with impaired immune responses and increased infection-related morbidity. Healthy older subjects who received vitamin supplements had higher numbers of certain T-cell subsets and natural killer (NK) cells, enhanced proliferation response to mitogen, increased IL-2 production, higher antibody response, and higher NK cell activity. These subjects were also less likely to have illness due to infections. Therefore, supplementation with a modest physiologic amount of micronutrients may improve immunity and may decrease the risk of infection in old age.[178]

The effects of vitamin supplementation on grip strength and immune function was studied in a group of institutionalized geriatric patients with a relatively higher prevalence of low, and below acceptable, biochemical parameters of vitamin C, pyridoxine, folic acid, riboflavin, iron, and zinc nutriture. The improved vitamin status had a positive and statistically significant effect on delayed cutaneous hypersensitivity, one of the parameters of cellular immunity.[179] Decreased serum concentrations of 25-hydroxyvitamin D has also been related to impaired immune competence. Results from population-based sample of elderly individuals suggest that inadequate vitamin D status is, indeed, an important public health problem that may be readily addressed by adequate vitamin D intake or sunlight exposure.[180] Fortified liquid milk and vitamin supplements have been associated with significantly higher serum 25-hydroxyvitamin D levels. These results emphasize the need for foodstuff fortification and supplement use in healthy older people as well as "high-risk" housebound and institutionalized older people.[181]

If the critically ill geriatric patient can tolerate partial feeding, oral vitamins should be included. The oral dietary recom-

TABLE 83–6. Oral Vitamin Requirements: Dietary Recommended Intake (DRI)

Biotin	300 μg
Folate	400 μg
Niacin (B_3)	20 mg
Pantothenic acid (B_5)	10 mg
Riboflavin (B_2)	1.7 mg
Thiamin (B_1)	1.5 mg
Pyridoxine (B_6)	2 mg
Vitamin A	5000 IU
Vitamin B_{12}	6 μg
Vitamin C	60 mg
Vitamin D	400 IU
Vitamin E	30 IU
Vitamin K	80 μg

IU = International Units; mg = milligrams; μg = micrograms.

mended intake and parenteral vitamin products are listed in Tables 83-6 and 83-7, respectively.

Thiamin, folic acid, vitamin B_{12} injections, ascorbic acid (vitamin C), phytonadione (vitamin K), riboflavin (vitamin B_2), niacin (vitamin B_3), calcitriol (1,25 dihydroxycholecalciferol) and pyridoxine (vitamin B_6) are available for parenteral use. With the exception of IV calcitriol, all can be added to TPN solutions. Vitamin A is also available for intramuscular (IM) use only.

Supplementation with vitamins C, E, and A or beta carotene increases the activation of cells involved in tumor immunity in the elderly. Supplementation with vitamin A, a relatively weak antioxidant, has also been shown to decrease morbidity and mortality associated with measles infections in children.[182]

In a double-blind, placebo-controlled trial, healthy older adults (60 years or above) in a metabolic research unit received either a placebo or oral vitamin E supplements (800 mg/dL of α-tocopherol acetate) for 30 days. Supplementation improved several parameters of immune function in vivo and in vitro.[183]

In a few instances, thrombocytopenia may actually be due to isolated deficiency of folate.[184, 185] Risk factors for acute folate deficiency are extensive tissue damage due to sepsis, trauma or surgery, and ARF requiring renal replacement therapy. The diagnosis is based on bone marrow examination showing marked megaloblastic changes because serum folate levels and red blood cell folate levels may be normal.[186] Folate values have been shown to be lower postoperatively, increasing the risk of hematologic toxicity in patients given folate-free parenteral nutrition after a surgical operation.[187]

In the setting of renal failure (acute or chronic), vitamin A serum concentrations are increased. Vitamin A is osteolytic and may increase serum calcium concentrations.[188]

Elevated plasma levels of homocysteine and disulfide adducts of homocysteine, collectively termed "homocyst(e)ine," are associated with increased risk of thrombotic and atherosclerotic vascular disease. Dietary interventions to lower plasma homocysteine (e.g., folate, vitamin B_{12}, and pyridoxine supplementation) have been proposed as a global strategy to decrease the prevalence of vascular disease.[189] It is apparent that elevated homocysteine status, in the absence of vitamin deficiency and low, but not deficient, vitamin B_{12} status are important risk factors for increased chromosome damage in lymphocytes.[190, 191] A serum cobalamin level lower than 250 pmol/L, combined with high values of plasma homocysteine and serum methylmalonic acid, confirms the diagnosis of vitamin B_{12} deficiency. A low serum and erythrocyte folate level and high plasma homocysteine confirm folate deficiency.[192] Hyperhomocysteinemia has been described in patients deficient in folate and in vitamins B_{12} and B_6.

Deficiency of pyridoxine has been associated with immunologic changes observed in older persons infected with human immunodeficiency virus (HIV) and those with uremia or rheumatoid arthritis.[193] Vitamin B_6 deficiency impairs in vitro indices of cell-mediated immunity in healthy elderly adults. IL-2 production and lymphocyte proliferation impairment may be reversible by vitamin B_6 repletion.[194] Infection and trauma cause inflammatory stress in patients. Tissue damage, enhanced inflammatory mediator production, and suppressed lymphocyte function may occur as a consequence. The antioxidative vitamins, ascorbic acid, and the tocopherols are important not only for limiting tissue damage but also in preventing increased cytokine production, a consequence of excessive activation of nuclear factor-κB (NF-κB). In humans, dietary supplementation with ascorbic acid (vitamin C), tocopherols, and vitamin B_6 enhances a number of aspects of lymphocyte function. The effect is most apparent in older people.[195]

Vitamin C can also exhibit pro-oxidant effects, however, and may undesirably increase the mobilization of iron. Humans have two circulating iron-binding proteins to soak up free iron to prevent it from generating toxic quantities of free radicals:

- Transferrin, a high-affinity, low-capacity protein (2 atoms of iron per molecule of transferrin) for which there are receptors on the surface of every iron-requiring cell
- Ferritin, a lower-affinity, high-capacity protein (maximum of 4500 atoms of iron per molecule of ferritin) for which there are receptors only on the surface of iron-storage cells, such as reticuloendothelial cells.

Ferritin protein is an acute-phase reactant that sharply rises in the presence of inflammation, whereas transferrin is a reverse acute-phase reactant that falls in the presence of inflammation.[196] Iron is a double-edged sword. National Health and Nutrition Examination Survey (NHANES) I data indicate that high body iron stores, manifested by increased transferrin saturation, are associated with an increased cancer risk. Other data show increased heart attack risk.[197]

Many critically ill patients receive histamine-H_2 antagonists, and concerns about diminishing the protective acid barrier abound (i.e., microorganism permeability, nutrient assimilation, medication needs, delayed gastric emptying, vitamin B_{12} deficiency).[198] Oral ranitidine (150 mg twice a day) resulted in a nonsignificant decrease of intrinsic factor concentration and intrinsic factor output but was responsible for malabsorption of protein-bound cobalamin. This malabsorption was reversible on discontinuation of ranitidine.[199]

The response rate to vitamin supplements suggests that

TABLE 83–7. Adult Parenteral Multivitamin Products

	A (IU)	D (IU)	E (IU)	B_1 (mg)	B_2 (mg)	B_3 (mg)	B_5 (mg)	B_6 (mg)	B_{12} (μg)	C (mg)	Biotin (mg)	Folic Acid (mg)
Astra (MVI-12)	3,300	200	10	3	3.6	40	15	4	5	100	0.06	0.4
Fujisawa (MVC)	10,000	1000	5	50	10	100	25	15		500		

metabolic evidence of vitamin deficiency is common in the elderly, even in the presence of normal serum vitamin levels. Metabolite assays permit identification of older subjects who may benefit from vitamin supplements.[200]

MEDICATION-NUTRIENT INTERACTIONS

No review of nutritional support in the critically ill geriatric patient would be complete without mentioning the role of nutritional status in the pharmacodynamics of medicinals. Disease states and nutritional conditions affect nutrient status and a drug's therapeutic efficacy. While a medication's pharmacokinetic profile can usually be predicted, it can also be dramatically modified by nutrients and by certain pathophysiologic conditions, including aging, disease, and genetics.[201] Nutritional status, sex, hormonal status, and circadian rhythm also affect the pharmacodynamics of a drug. Food-drug interactions can lead to a loss of therapeutic efficacy or toxic effects of drug therapy. Generally, the effect of food on drugs results from a reduction in the drug's bioavailability;[202] however, an alteration in drug clearance can occur owing to the effect of certain foods on medication metabolism[203] or on excretory functions.

Medications that cause xerostomia may affect the ability to chew and swallow. This leads to avoidance of certain foods, which raises the possibility that xerostomia may contribute to undernutrition in older persons.[204] Gastric emptying is delayed with oral fat, IV lipid, and many medications. As a rule, the longer the time in the stomach, the better the absorption in the small intestine (if the drug is not acid-labile). The less the ionization, the better the absorption. Medications or foods with pKa* of 3 to 8 will be affected by the pH of the gastrointestinal tract (gastric pH = 1 to 2; colonic pH = 6 to 8). The extent to which drugs exhibiting weakly acid or basic properties are ionized depends on their ionization potential (pKa) and the pH of their milieu. Weakly acidic drugs that are lipid-soluble in their nonionized state diffuse freely across the cell membrane and on entering a relatively basic intracellular compartment become trapped and accumulate within the cell.[205] Other effects of nutrients on the absorption phenomenon include stimulation of enzymatic metabolism and presystemic metabolism (first-pass effect), which are useful for prodrugs when hydrolysis can take place before absorption from the bowel (i.e., clorazepate, erythromycin ethyl succinate). Specific amino acids at the absorption sites may be needed to absorb the medication in an optimal manner. Active transport moieties can be affected by agents that disrupt normal cell metabolism (i.e., sodium fluoride, which inhibits energy to the active transport system). Drug absorption can also be influenced by villous atrophy (i.e., isoniazid, aspirin, chloramphenicol), radiation (i.e., digoxin), celiac disease (i.e., propranolol), and complexation.[206]

SUMMARY

Dysregulation of apoptosis *(a genetically controlled process that removes unwanted or damaged cells) may underlie the pathogenesis of autoimmune diseases and aging.*[207] *Accompanying this state of programmed cell death in the aged is the metabolic response to injury that is associated with hypermetabolism. This process induces a redistribution of body nitrogen away from the skeletal mass and toward the viscera and areas of increased metabolic activity, such as the surgical wound, the zone of inflammation, and toward cells producing mediators. Exogenously administered nitrogen increases the rate of protein synthesis, but it does not affect the catabolic process. Carefully balancing macronutrients can achieve caloric (energy) equilibrium.*[208]

The clinician must be ever vigilant in the choice of the right route, in the avoidance of underfeeding as well as overfeeding, and in the relationship of the disease state and its treatment to the nutritional regimen. Diligently selecting the right mix of kilocalories to nitrogen in concert with an understanding of micronutrient (electrolytes, trace elements, and vitamins) supplementation will lend to more optimal nutrition support for the critically ill geriatric patient in the intensive care arena.

ACKNOWLEDGMENT

I would like to acknowledge T. James Gallagher, MD, FCCM, and Andrea Gabrielli, MD, for their generous review of this work and for their continuing collegiality in the nutritional care of the critically ill geriatric patient.

References

1. Pawelec G, Adibzadeh M, Solana R, Beckman I: The T cell in the ageing individual. Mech Ageing Dev 1997; 93:35–45.
2. Troncale JA: The aging process: Physiologic changes and pharmacologic implications. Postgrad Med 1996; 99:111–114, 120–122.
3. Troncale JA: The aging process. Physiologic changes and pharmacologic implications. Postgrad Med 1996; 99:111–114.
4. Riggs JE, Millecchia RJ: Mortality among the elderly in the U.S., 1956–1987: Demonstration of the upper boundary to Gompertzian mortality. Mech Ageing Dev 1992; 62:191–199.
5. Burgess P, Hall RI, Bateman DN, Johnston ID: The effect of total parenteral nutrition on hepatic drug oxidation. J Parenter Enteral Nutr 1987; 11:540–543.
6. Gough DB, White M, Morrin M, Joyce W, Phelan D, Fitzpatrick JM, Gorey TF: The relationship between a nutritional index and acute physiology score in critical illness. Ir J Med Sci 1992; 161:565–568.
7. Lazarus R, Sparrow D, Weiss ST: Handgrip strength and insulin levels: Cross-sectional and prospective associations in the Normative Aging Study. Metabolism 1997; 46:1266–1269.
8. Lux G, Orth KH, Bozkurt T: Constipation is not a disease but a symptom. Ther Umsch 1994; 51:177–189.
9. Shafik A: Constipation: Pathogenesis and management. Drugs 1993; 45:528–540.
10. Knichwitz G, Brussel T: [Intramucosal P_{CO_2} measurement as gastrointestinal monitoring]. Anaesthesiol Intensivmed Notfallmed Schmerzther 1997; 32:479–487.
11. Schmucker DL: Aging and drug disposition: An update. Pharmacol Rev 1985; 37:133–148.
11a. Castleden CM, Volans CN, Raymond K: The effect of aging on drug absorption from the gut. Age Aging 1977; 6:138–143.
12. Lipman TO: Grains or veins: Is enteral nutrition really better than parenteral? A look at the evidence. JPEN J Parenter Enteral Nutr 1988; 22:167–182.
13. King D, Smith ML, Chapman TJ, Stockdale HR, Lye M: Fat malabsorption in elderly patients with cardiac cachexia. Age Ageing 1996; 25:144–149.
14. Paccagnella A, Calo MA, Caenaro G, Salandin V, Jus P, Simini G, Heymsfield SB: Cardiac cachexia: Preoperative and postoperative nutrition management. JPEN J Parenter Enteral Nutr 1994; 18:409–416.
15. Freeman LM, Roubenoff R: The nutrition implications of cardiac cachexia. Nutr Rev 1994; 52:340–347.
16. Shiihara H: [Pre- and postoperative nutritional assessment of cardiac cachexia]. Nippon Kyobu Geka Gakkai Zasshi 1991; 39:183–191.
17. Pinard B, Geller E: Nutritional support during pulmonary failure. Crit Care Clin 1995; 11:705–715.
18. Fiaccadori E, Zambrelli P, Tortorella G: [Physiopathology of respiratory muscles in malnutrition]. Minerva Anestesiol 1995; 61:93–99.

*pKa = pH at which 50% of a compound is ionized.

19. Rose W: Total parenteral nutrition and the patient with chronic obstructive pulmonary disease. J Intraven Nurs 1992; 15:18-23.
20. Gray DK, Gibbons L, Shapiro SH, Macklem PT, Martin JG: Nutritional status and mortality in chronic obstructive pulmonary disease. Am J Respir Crit Care Med 1996; 153:961-966.
21. Garrel DR, Razi M, Lariviere F, Jobin N, Naman N, Emptoz-Bonneton A, Pugeat MM: Improved clinical status and length of care with low-fat nutrition support in burn patients. J Parenter Enteral Nutr 1995; 19:482-491.
22. Lenssen P, Bruemmer BA, Bowden RA, Gooley T, Aker SN, Mattson D: Intravenous lipid dose and incidence of bacteremia and fungemia in patients undergoing bone marrow transplantation. Am J Clin Nutr 1998; 67:927-933.
23. Pingleton SK, Harmon GS: Nutritional management in acute respiratory failure. JAMA 1987; 257:3094-3099.
24. Keithley JK: Nutritional needs and support of mechanically ventilated patients. Medsurg Nurs 1997; 6:74-75.
25. Verbeken EK, Cauberghs M, Mertens I, Clement J, Lauweryns JM, Van de Woestijne KP: The senile lung: Comparison with normal and emphysematous lungs. 2. Functional aspects. Chest 1992; 101:800-809.
26. Rochester DF: Malnutrition and the respiratory muscles. Clin Chest Med 1986; 7:91-99.
27. Dureuil B, Matuszczak Y: Alteration in nutritional status and diaphragm muscle function. Nutr Dev 1998; 38:175-180.
28. Rosado M, Banner MJ: Ascites and its effects upon respiratory muscle loading and work of breathing. Crit Care Med 1996; 24:538-540.
29. Dow L, Tracey M, Villar A, Coggon D, Margetts BM, Campbell MJ, Holgate ST: Does dietary intake of vitamins C and E influence lung function in older people? Am J Respir Crit Care Med 1996; 154:1401-1404.
30. Lindeman RD, Tobin JD, Shock NW: Longitudinal studies on the rate of decline in renal function with age. J Am Geriatr Soc 1985; 33:278-285.
31. Hachache T, Milongo R, Kuentz F, Guergour M, Maynard C, Meftahi H, Foret M, Maurizi J, Cordonnier DJ: [Mesenteric ischemia in hemodialyzed patients]. Presse Med 1997; 26:410-413.
32. Mirtallo JM, Schneider PJ, Mavko K, Ruberg RL, Fabri PJ: A comparison of essential and general amino acid infusions in the nutritional support of patients with compromised renal function. J Parenter Enteral Nutr 1982; 6:109-113.
33. Baumgartner RN, Koehler KM, Romero L, Garry PJ: Serum albumin is associated with skeletal muscle in elderly men and women. Am J Clin Nutr 1996; 64:552-558.
34. Mokrzycki MH, Kaplan AA: Protein losses in continuous renal replacement therapies. J Am Soc Nephrol 1996; 7:2259-2263.
35. Manns M, Sigler MH, Teehan BP: Continuous renal replacement therapies: An update. Am J Kidney Dis 1998; 32:185-207.
36. Mege JL, Sanguedolce MV, Purgus R, Moulin B, Bongrand P, Capo C, Olmer M: Chronic and intradialytic effects of high-flux hemodialysis on tumor necrosis factor-alpha production: Relationship to endotoxins. Am J Kidney Dis 1992; 20:482-488.
37. Druml W: Protein metabolism in acute renal failure. Miner Electrolyte Metab 1998; 24:47-54.
38. van Bommel EF, Ponssen HH: Intermittent versus continuous treatment for acute renal failure: Where do we stand? Am J Kidney Dis 1997; 30(5 Suppl 4):S72-S79.
39. Wolfson M: The cost and bother of intradialytic parenteral nutrition are not justified by available scientific studies. ASAIO J 1993; 39:864-867.
40. Aljama P, Ward MK, Pierides AM, Eastham EJ, Ellis HA, Feest TG, Conceicao S, Kerr DN: Serum ferritin concentration: A reliable guide to iron overload in uremic and hemodialyzed patients. Clin Nephrol 1978; 10:101-104.
41. Herbert V, Jayatilleke E, Shaw S, Rosman AS, Giardina P, Grady RW, Bowman B, Gunter EW: Serum ferritin iron, a new test, measures human body iron stores unconfounded by inflammation. Stem Cells 1997; 15:291-296.
42. Soboleva MK, Gavalov SM: [The iron overload syndrome in patients with severe bacterial inflammatory diseases and convalescents]. Gematol Transfuziol 1993; 38:21-24.
43. Napolitano G, Bonomini M, Bomba G, Bucci I, Todisco V, Albertazzi A: Thyroid function and plasma selenium in chronic uremic patients on hemodialysis treatment. Biol Trace Elem Res 1996; 55:221-230.
44. Makropoulos W, Heintz B, Stefanidis I: Selenium deficiency and thyroid function in acute renal failure. Ren Fail 1997; 19:129-136.
45. Naylor CD, O'Rourke K, Detsky AS, Baker JP: Parenteral nutrition with branched-chain amino acids in hepatic encephalopathy: A meta-analysis. Gastroenterology 1989; 97:1033-1042.
46. DerSimonian R: Parenteral nutrition with branched-chain amino acids in hepatic encephalopathy: Meta-analysis. Hepatology 1990; 11:1083-1084.
47. Fabbri A, Magrini N, Bianchi G, Zoli M, Marchesini G: Overview of randomized clinical trials of oral branched-chain amino acid treatment in chronic hepatic encephalopathy. J Parenter Enteral Nutr 1996; 20:159-164.
48. Wahren J, Denis J, Desurmont P, Eriksson LS, Escoffier JM, Gauthier AP, Hagenfeldt L, Michel H, Opolon P, Paris JC, Veyrac M: Is intravenous administration of branched chain amino acids effective in the treatment of hepatic encephalopathy? A multicenter study. Hepatology 1983; 3:475-480.
49. Garcia-de-Lorenzo A, Ortiz-Leyba C, Planas M, Montejo JC, Nunez R, Ordonez FJ, Aragon C, Jimenez FJ: Parenteral administration of different amounts of branched-chain amino acids in septic patients: Clinical and metabolic aspects. Crit Care Med 1997; 25:418-424.
50. Spiess A, Mikalunas V, Carlson S, Zimmer M, Craig RM: Albumin kinetics in hypoalbuminemic patients receiving total parenteral nutrition. JPEN J Parenter Enteral Nutr 1996; 20:424-428.
51. Lucas CE, Ledgerwood AM, Mammen EF: Altered coagulation protein content after albumin resuscitation. Ann Surg 1982; 196:198-202.
52. Campion EW, deLabry LO, Glynn RJ: The effect of age on serum albumin in healthy males: Report from the Normative Aging Study. J Gerontol 1988; 43:M18-M20.
53. MacLennan WJ, Martin P, Mason BJ: Protein intake and serum albumin levels in the elderly. Gerontology 1977; 23:360-367.
54. Conti MC, Goralnik JH, Salive ME, et al: Serum albumin level and physical disability as predictors of mortality in older persons. JAMA 1994; 272:1036-1042.
55. Brinson RR, Kolts BE: Hypoalbuminemia as an indicator of diarrheal incidence in critically-ill patients. Crit Care Med 1987; 15:506-509.
56. Hwang TL, Lue MC, Nee YJ, Jan YY, Chen MF: The incidence of diarrhea in patients with hypoalbuminemia due to acute or chronic malnutrition during enteral feeding. Am J Gastroenterol 1994; 89:376-378.
57. Baue AE, Durham R, Faist E: Systemic inflammatory response syndrome (SIRS), multiple organ dysfunction syndrome (MODS), multiple organ failure (MOF): Are we winning the battle? Shock 1998; 10:79-89.
58. Pahl MV, Barbari A, Vaziri ND, Hollander D, Sanchez M, Oveisi F, Patel N: Intestinal absorption of arachidonic acid in experimental azotemia. Life Sci 1990; 46:1649-1656.
59. Blusztajn JK: Choline, a vital amine. Science 1998; 281:794-795.
60. Zeisel SH, Blusztajn JK: Choline and human nutrition. Annu Rev Nutr 1994; 14:269-296.
61. Toskes PP: Medical management of chronic pancreatitis. Scand J Gastroenterol Suppl 1995; 208:74-80.
62. Riordan SM, McIver CJ, Wakefield D, Bolin TD, Duncombe VM, Thomas MC: Small intestinal bacterial overgrowth in the symptomatic elderly. Am J Gastroenterol 1997; 92:47-51.
63. Roberts PR: Nutrition in the head-injured patient. New Horiz 1995; 3:506-517.
64. Suchner U, Senftleben U, Eckart T, Scholz MR, Beck K, Murr R, Enzenbach R, Peter K: Enteral versus parenteral nutrition: Effects on gastrointestinal function and metabolism. Nutrition 1996; 12:13-22.
65. Priori P, Pezzilli R, Panuccio D, Nardi R, Gullo L: Stimulation of gallbladder emptying by intravenous lipids. JPEN J Parenter Enteral Nutr 1997; 21:350-352.
66. Bratusch-Marrain PR, Komjati M, Waldhausl WK: Efficacy of pulsatile versus continuous insulin administration on hepatic glucose production and glucose utilization in type I diabetic humans. Diabetes 1986; 35:922-926.
67. Sypniewski E Jr, Mirtallo JM, Schneider PJ: Hyperosmolar, hyperglycemic, nonketotic coma in a patient receiving home total parenteral nutrient therapy. Clin Pharm 1987; 6:69-73.

68. Swidan SZ, Montgomery PA: Effect of blood glucose concentrations on the development of chronic complications of diabetes mellitus. Pharmacotherapy 1998; 18:961–972.
69. Nestler JE, Barlascini CO, Tetrault GA, Fratkin MJ, Clore JN, Blackard WG: Increased transcapillary escape rate of albumin in nondiabetic men in response to hyperinsulinemia. Diabetes 1990; 39:1212–1217.
70. Catalano C, Muscelli E, Quinones Galvan A, Baldi S, Masoni A, Gibb I, Torffvit O, Seghieri G, Ferrannini E: Effect of insulin on systemic and renal handling of albumin in nondiabetic and NIDDM subjects. Diabetes 1997; 46:868–875.
71. Schneir M, Ramamurthy N, Golub L: Dietary ascorbic acid normalizes diabetes-induced underhydroxylation of nascent type I collagen molecules. Coll Relat Res 1985; 5:415–422.
72. Akkus I, Kalak S, Vural H, Caglayan O, Menekse E, Can G, Durmus B: Leukocyte lipid peroxidation, superoxide dismutase, glutathione peroxidase and serum and leukocyte vitamin C levels of patients with type II diabetes mellitus. Clin Chim Acta 1996; 244:221–227.
73. Hennessey PJ, Black CT, Andrassy RJ: Nonenzymatic glycosylation of immunoglobulin G impairs complement fixation. J Parenter Enteral Nutr 1991; 15:60–64.
74. Weber SS, Wood WA, Jackson EA: Availability of insulin from parenteral nutrient solutions. Am J Hosp Pharm 1977; 34:353–357.
75. Doglietto GB, Bellantone R, Bossola M, Perri V, Ratto C, Pacelli F, Sofo L, Migliore A, Manna R, Crucitti F: Insulin adsorption to three-liter ethylene vinyl acetate bags during 24-hour infusion. JPEN J Parenter Enteral Nutr 1989; 13:539–541.
76. Marcuard SP, Dunham B, Hobbs A, Caro JF: Availability of insulin from total parenteral nutrition solutions. JPEN J Parenter Enteral Nutr 1990; 14:262–264.
77. Overett TK, Bistrian BR, Lowry SF; Hopkins BS, Miller D, Blackburn GL: Total parenteral nutrition in patients with insulin-requiring diabetes mellitus. J Am Coll Nutr 1986; 5:79–89.
78. Jeevanandam M, Holaday NJ, Petersen SR: Integrated nutritional, hormonal, and metabolic effects of recombinant human growth hormone (rhGH) supplementation in trauma patients. Nutrition 1996; 12:777–787.
79. Yarwood GD, Ross RJ, Medbak S, Coakley J, Hinds CJ: Administration of human recombinant insulin-like growth factor–I in critically ill patients. Crit Care Med 1997; 25:1352–1361.
80. Bouillanne O, Rainfray M, Tissandier O, Nasr A, Lahlou A, Cnockaert X, Piette F: Growth hormone therapy in elderly people: An age-delaying drug? Fundam Clin Pharmacol 1996; 10:416–430.
81. Yarwood GD, Ross RJ, Medbak S, Coakley J, Hinds CJ: Administration of human recombinant insulin-like growth factor–I in critically ill patients. Crit Care Med 1997; 25:1352–1361.
82. Fernqvist-Forbes E, Hilding A, Ekberg K, Brismar K: Influence of circulating epinephrine and norepinephrine on insulin-like growth factor binding protein–1 in humans. J Clin Endocrinol Metab 1997; 82:2677–2680.
83. Clemmons DR, Underwood LE: Role of insulin-like growth factors and growth hormone in reversing catabolic states. Horm Res 1992; 38 (Suppl 2):37–40.
84. Burgess EJ: Insulin-like growth factor 1: A valid nutritional indicator during parenteral feeding of patients suffering an acute phase response. Part 2. Ann Clin Biochem 1992; 29:137–144.
85. Khorram O, Vu L, Yen SS: Activation of immune function by dehydroepiandrosterone (DHEA) in age-advanced men. J Gerontol A Biol Sci Med Sci 1997; 52:M1–M7.
86. Muller JM, Thul P, Ablassmaier B: [Perioperative nutritional therapy and its relevance for postoperative outcome]. Chirurg 1997; 68:574–582.
87. Chiolero R, Revelly JP, Tappy L: Energy metabolism in sepsis and injury. Nutrition 1997; 13 (9 Suppl):45S–51S.
88. Spitzer JJ, Bagby GJ, Meszaros K, Lang CH: Alterations in lipid and carbohydrate metabolism in sepsis. J Parenter Enteral Nutr 1988; 12(6 Suppl):53S–58S.
89. Kuhn MM: Nutritional support for the shock patient. Crit Care Nurs Clin North Am 1990; 2:201–220.
90. Streat SJ, Beddoe AH, Hill GL: Aggressive nutritional support does not prevent protein loss despite fat gain in septic intensive care patients. J Trauma 1987; 27:262–266.
91. Jeevanandam M, Holaday NJ, Petersen SR: Posttraumatic hormonal environment during total parenteral nutrition. Nutrition 1993; 9:333–338.
92. Olivieri O, Girelli D, Azzini M, Stanzial AM, Russo C, Ferroni M, Corrocher R: Low selenium status in the elderly influences thyroid hormones. Clin Sci Colch 1995; 89:637–642.
93. Morley JE: Anorexia in older persons: Epidemiology and optimal treatment. Drug Aging 1996; 8:134–155.
94. American Society for Parenteral and Enteral Nutrition. JPEN J Parenter Enteral Nutr 1993; 17(4 Suppl):1SA–52SA.
95. Driscoll DF; Bistrian BR: Special considerations required for the formulation and administration of total parenteral nutrition therapy in the elderly patient. Drugs Aging 1992; 2:395–405.
96. Mirtallo JM: Assessing the nutritional needs of the critically-ill patient. Drug Intell Clin Pharm 1990; 24(11 Suppl):S20–S23.
97. Phang PT, Aeberhardt LE: Effect of nutritional support on routine nutrition assessment parameters and body composition in intensive care unit patients. Can J Surg 1996; 39:212–219.
98. Opper FH, Burakoff R: Nutritional support of the elderly patient in an intensive care unit. Clin Geriatr Med 1994; 10:31–49.
99. Dunkirk SG, Gregg SL, Duran LW, Monfils JD, Haapala JE, Marcy JA, Clapper DL, Amos RA, Guire PE: Photochemical coatings for the prevention of bacterial colonization. J Biomater Appl 1991; 6:131–156.
100. Merritt K, Chang CC: Factors influencing bacterial adherence to biomaterials. J Biomater Appl 1991; 5:185–203.
101. Baumgartner JN, Yang CZ, Cooper SL: Physical property analysis and bacterial adhesion on a series of phosphonated polyurethanes. Biomaterials 1997; 18:831–837.
102. The Texas Medical Center Catheter Study Group, Raad II, Darouiche RO, Dupuis J, Abi-Said D, Gabrielli A, Hachem R, Wall M, Harris R, Jones J, Buzaid A, Robertson C, Shenaq S, Curling P, Burke T, Ericsson C: Central venous catheters coated with minocycline and rifampin for the prevention of catheter-related colonization and bloodstream infections: A randomized, double-blind trial. Crit Care Med 1998; 26:219–224. Ann Intern Med 1997; 127:267–274.
103. Capdevila JA: Catheter-related infection: An update on diagnosis, treatment, and prevention. Int J Infect Dis 1998; 2:230–236.
104. Andris DA, Krzywda EA, Edmiston CE, Krepel CJ, Gohr CM: Elimination of intraluminal colonization by antibiotic lock in silicone vascular catheters. Nutrition 1998; 14:427–432.
105. Krzywda EA, Andris DA, Edmiston CE Jr, Quebbeman EJ: Treatment of Hickman catheter sepsis using antibiotic lock technique. Infect Control Hosp Epidemiol 1995; 16:596–598.
106. Baumgartner TG, Schmidt GL, Thakker KM, Sitren HS, Cerda JJ, Mahaffey SM, Copeland EM 3d: Bacterial endotoxin retention by inline intravenous filters. Am J Hosp Pharm 1986; 43:681–684.
107. Stechmiller JK, Treloar D, Allen N: Gut dysfunction in critically ill patients: A review of the literature. Am J Crit Care 1997; 6:204–209.
108. Stechmiller J, Treloar DM, Derrico D, Yarandi H, Guin P: Interruption of enteral feedings in head injured patients. J Neurosci Nurs 1994; 26:224–229.
109. Medley F, Stechmiller J, Field A: Complications of enteral nutrition in hospitalized patients with artificial airways. Clin Nurs Res 1993; 2:212–223.
110. Frost P, Bihari D: The route of nutritional support in the critically-ill: Physiological and economical considerations. Nutrition 1997; 13(9 Suppl):58S–63S.
111. Johnston JD, Harvey CJ, Menzies IS, Treacher DF: Gastrointestinal permeability and absorptive capacity in sepsis. Crit Care Med 1996; 24:1144–1149.
112. Swank GM, Deitch EA: Role of the gut in multiple organ failure: bacterial translocation and permeability changes. World J Surg 1996; 20:411–417.
113. Reynolds JV, Kanwar S, Welsh FK, Windsor AC, Murchan P, Barclay GR, Guillou PJ. 1997 Harry M: Vars Research Award: Does the route of feeding modify gut barrier function and clinical outcome in patients after major upper gastrointestinal surgery? JPEN J Parenter Enteral Nutr 1997; 21:196–201.
114. Aryeh H, Brady DA, Schaal SE, Samloff M, Dedon J, Ruhl CE: Gastric acidity in older adults. JAMA 1997; 278:659–662.
115. Zazzo JF, Millat B: [Postoperative continuous or cyclic total parenteral nutrition]. Ann Fr Anesth Reanim 1984; 3:111–115.
116. Zaloga G, Ackerman MH: A review of disease-specific formulas. AACN Clin Issues Crit Care Nurs 1994; 5:421–435.

117. Sax HC: Early nutritional support in critical illness is important. Crit Care Clin 1996; 12:661-666.
118. Buchman AL, Mestecky J, Moukarzel A, Ament ME: Intestinal immune function is unaffected by parenteral nutrition in man. J Am Coll Nutr 1995; 14:656-661.
119. Reilly H: Parenteral nutrition: An overview of current practice. Br J Nurs 1998; 7:461-467.
120. Sullivan D, Lipschitz D: Evaluating and treating nutritional problems in older patients. Clin Geriatr Med 1997; 13:753-768.
121. Roubenoff R: Hormones, cytokines and body composition: Can lessons from illness be applied to aging? J Nutr 1993; 123(2 Suppl):469-473.
122. Cannon JG, Meydani SN, Fielding RA, Fiatarone MA, Meydani M, Farhangmehr M, Orencole SF, Blumberg JB, Evans WJ: Acute phase response in exercise: II. Associations between vitamin E, cytokines, and muscle proteolysis. Am J Physiol 1991; 260(6 Pt 2):R1235-R1240.
123. Catania A, Airaghi L, Motta P, Manfredi MG, Annoni G, Pettenati C, Brambilla F, Lipton JM: Cytokine antagonists in aged subjects and their relation with cellular immunity. J Gerontol A Biol Sci Med Sci 1997; 52:B93-B97.
124. Dice JE, Burckart GJ, Woo JT, Helms RA: Standardized versus pharmacist-monitored individualized parenteral nutrition in low-birth-weight infants. Am J Hosp Pharm 1981; 38:1487-1489.
125. Shenkin A: Trace elements and inflammatory response: Implications for nutritional support. Nutrition 1995; 11(1 Suppl):100-105.
126. Forse RA, Shizgal HM: Serum albumin and nutritional status. J Parenter Enteral Nutr 1980; 4:450-454.
127. Measurement of visceral protein status in assessing protein and energy malnutrition: Standard of care. Prealbumin in Nutritional Care Consensus Group. Nutrition 1995; 11:169-171.
128. Dorken E, Grzybowski S, Allen EA: Significance of the tuberculin test in the elderly. Chest 1987; 92:237-240.
129. Toss G, Symreng T: Delayed hypersensitivity response and vitamin D deficiency. Int J Vitam Nutr Res 1983; 53:27-31.
130. Griffiths RD, Palmer TE, Jones C: Parenteral glutamine supply in intensive care patients. Nutrition 1996; 12(11-12 Suppl):S73-S75.
131. Adolph M, Eckart A, Eckart J: [Fructose vs. glucose in total parenteral nutrition in critically ill patients]. Anaesthesist 1995; 44:770-781.
132. Henrichs HR: [Diagnosis of the diabetic metabolic status using fructosamine (and HbA1c) determination: The glycation quotient Glyc-Q, the glycation nomogram]. Wien Klin Wochensch Suppl 1990; 180:64-69; discussion 78-81.
133. Kahn SE, Larson VG, Beard JC, et al: Effect of exercise on insulin action, glucose tolerance, and insulin secretion in aging. Am J Physiol 1990; 258(6 Pt 1):E937-E943.
134. Vernon WB, Atkins JM, Stewart RD: Hyperphosphatemia from lipid emulsion in a patient on total parenteral nutrition. J Parenter Enteral Nutr 1988; 12:84-87.
135. MacLaren R, Wachsman BA, Swift DK, Kuhl DA: Warfarin resistance associated with intravenous lipid administration: Discussion of propofol and review of the literature. Pharmacotherapy 1997; 17:1331-1337.
136. Chambrier C, Leclercq M, Saudin F, Vignal B, Bryssine S, Guillaumont M, Bouletreau P: Is vitamin K_1 supplementation necessary in long-term parenteral nutrition? JPEN J Parenter Enteral Nutr 1998; 22:87-90.
137. Tashiro T, Mashima Y, Yamamori H, Horibe K, Nishizawa M, Sanada M, Okui K: Increased lipoprotein X causes hyperlipidemia during intravenous administration of 10% fat emulsion in man. JPEN J Parenter Enteral Nutr 1991; 15:546-550.
138. Tashiro T, Mashima Y, Yamamori H, Sanada M, Nishizawa M, Okui K: Intravenous Intralipid 10% vs. 20%, hyperlipidemia, and increase in lipoprotein X in humans. Nutrition 1992; 8:155-160.
139. Narayanan S: Biochemistry and clinical relevance of lipoprotein X. Ann Clin Lab Sci 1984; 14:371-374.
140. Haumont D, Richelle M, Deckelbaum RJ, Coussaert E, Carpentier YA: Effect of liposomal content of lipid emulsions on plasma lipid concentrations in low birth weight infants receiving parenteral nutrition. Part 1. J Pediatr 1992; 121:759-763.
141. Miyahara T, Fujiwara H, Yae Y, Okano H, Okochi K, Torisu M: Abnormal lipoprotein appearing in plasma of patients who received a ten percent soybean oil emulsion infusion. Surgery 1979; 85:566-574.
142. Abe M, Kawano M, Tashiro T, Yamamori H, Takagi K, Morishima Y, Shirai K, Saitou Y, Nakajima N: Catabolism of lipoprotein-X induced by infusion of 10% fat emulsion. Nutrition 1997; 13:417-421.
143. Johnson JA 3d, Griswold JA, Muakkassa FF: Essential fatty acids influence survival in sepsis. J Trauma 1993; 35:128-131.
144. Zhang D, Li T, Wang W: [The effect of Intralipid on the membrane fluidity of lymphocytes from human blood]. Chung Hua Wai Ko Tsa Chih 1995; 33:273-275.
145. Meydani SN, Endres S, Woods MM, Goldin BR, Soo C, Morrill-Labrode A, Dinarello CA, Gorbach SL: Oral (n-3) fatty acid supplementation suppresses cytokine production and lymphocyte proliferation: Comparison between young and older women. J Nutr 1991; 121:547-555.
146. Siguel EN, Lerman RH: Prevalence of essential fatty acid deficiency in patients with chronic gastrointestinal disorders. Metabolism 1996; 45:12-23.
147. Bjerve KS, Thoresen L, Mostad IL, Alme K: Alpha-linolenic acid deficiency in man: Effect of essential fatty acids on fatty acid composition. Adv Prostaglandin Thromboxane Leukot Res 1987;17B:862-865.
148. Naveh-Floman N, Belkin M: Prostaglandin metabolism and intraocular pressure. Br J Ophthalmol 1987; 71:254-256.
149. Sitzmann JV, Steinborn PA, Zinner MJ, Cameron JL: Total parenteral nutrition and alternate energy substrates in treatment of severe acute pancreatitis. Surg Gynecol Obstet 1989; 168:311-317.
150. Grant JP, James S, Grabowski V, Trexler KM: Total parenteral nutrition in pancreatic disease. Ann Surg 1984; 200:627-631.
151. Tanphaichitr V, Leelahagul P: Carnitine metabolism and human carnitine deficiency. Nutrition 1993; 9:246-254.
152. Demling RH, DeBiasse MA: Micronutrients in critical illness. Crit Care Clin 1995; 11:651-673.
153. Bennett WM: Drug interactions and consequences of sodium restriction. Am J Clin Nutr 1997; 65(2 Suppl):678S-681S.
154. Chernow B, Zaloga G, McFadden E, Clapper M, Kotler M, Barton M, Rainey TG: Hypocalcemia in critically-ill patients. Crit Care Med 1982; 10:848-851.
155. Zaloga GP, Willey S, Tomasic P, Chernow B: Free fatty acids alter calcium binding: A cause for misinterpretation of serum calcium values and hypocalcemia in critical illness. J Clin Endocrinol Metab 1987; 64:1010-1014.
156. Portale AA, Lonergan ET, Tanney DM, Halloran BP: Aging alters calcium regulation of serum concentration of parathyroid hormone in healthy men. Part 1. Am J Physiol 1997; 272:E139-E146.
157. Wood RJ, Zheng JJ: High dietary calcium intakes reduce zinc absorption and balance in humans. Am J Clin Nutr 1997; 65:1803-1809.
158. Brooks MJ, Melnik G: The refeeding syndrome: An approach to understanding its complications and preventing its occurrence. Pharmacotherapy 1995; 15:713-726.
159. Solomon SM, Kirby DF: The refeeding syndrome: A review. JPEN J Parenter Enteral Nutr 1990; 14:90-97.
160. Weinsier RL, Krumdieck CL: Death resulting from overzealous total parenteral nutrition: The refeeding syndrome revisited. Am J Clin Nutr 1981; 34:393-399.
161. Baumgartner TG: Magnesium assessment: Is it worth the work? Adv Gastroenterol Hepatol Clin Nutr 1997; 2:213-216.
162. Baumgartner TG: Trace elements in clinical nutrition. Nutr Clin Pract 1993; 8:251-263.
163. Hak EB, Storm MC, Helms RA: Chromium and zinc contamination of parenteral nutrient solution components commonly used in infants and children. Am J Health Syst Pharm 1998; 55:150-154.
164. Olivieri O, Girelli D, Azzini M, Stanzial AM, Russo C, Ferroni M, Corrocher R: Low selenium status in the elderly influences thyroid hormones. Clin Sci (Colch) 1995; 89:637-642.
165. Berger MM, Lemarchand-Beraud T, Cavadini C, Chiolero R: Relations between the selenium status and the low T_3 syndrome after major trauma. Intensive Care Med 1996; 22:575-581.
166. Olivieri O, Girelli D, Stanzial AM, Rossi L, Bassi A, Corrocher R: Selenium, zinc, and thyroid hormones in healthy subjects: Low T_3/T_4 ratio in the elderly is related to impaired selenium status. Biol Trace Elem Res 1996; 51:31-41.

167. Sanders DE: Vitamin E/selenium. J Am Vet Med Assoc 1986; 188:227.
168. Giles L, Smiciklas-Wright H, Fosmire G, Derr J: Variations in plasma zinc in older men and women. Biol Trace Elem Res 1994; 41:235–243.
169. Ripa S, Ripa R: Zinc and the elderly. Minerva Med 1995; 86:275–278.
170. Keen CL, Gershwin ME: Zinc deficiency and immune function. Annu Rev Nutr 1990; 10:415–431.
171. Broun ER, Greist A, Tricot G, Hoffman R: Excessive zinc ingestion: A reversible cause of sideroblastic anemia and bone marrow depression. JAMA 1990; 264:1441–1443.
172. Simon SR, Branda RF, Tindle BF, Burns SL: Copper deficiency and sideroblastic anemia associated with zinc ingestion. Am J Hematol 1988; 28:181–183.
173. Banno S, Niita M, Kikuchi M, Wakita A, Takada K, Mitomo Y, Niimi T, Yamamoto T: [Anemia and neutropenia in elderly patients caused by copper deficiency for long-term enteral nutrition]. Rinsho Ketsueki 1994; 35:1276–1281.
174. Tamura H, Hirose S, Watanabe O, Arai K, Murakawa M, Matsumura O, Isoda K: Anemia and neutropenia due to copper deficiency in enteral nutrition. JPEN J Parenter Enteral Nutr 1994 Mar-Apr; 18:185–189.
175. Percival SS: Neutropenia caused by copper deficiency: Possible mechanisms of action. Nutr Rev 1995; 53:59–66.
176. Cartabellotta A, Montalto G: [Genetic hemochromatosis: Importance of population screening?]. Recenti Prog Med 1996; 87:118–123.
177. Lione A: The prophylactic reduction of aluminium intake. Food Chem Toxicol 1983; 21:103–109.
178. Chandra RK: Effect of vitamin and trace-element supplementation on immune responses and infection in elderly subjects. Lancet 1992; 340:1124–1127.
179. Suboticanec K, Stavljenic A, Bilic-Pesic L, Gorajscan M, Gorajscan D, Brubacher G, Buzina R: Nutritional status, grip strength, and immune function in institutionalized elderly. Int J Vitam Nutr Res 1989; 59:20–28.
180. Jacques PF, Felson DT, Tucker KL, Mahnken B, Wilson PW, Rosenberg IH, Rush D: Plasma 25-hydroxyvitamin D and its determinants in an elderly population sample. Am J Clin Nutr 1997; 66:929–936.
181. Keane EM, Healy M, O'Moore R, Coakley D, Walsh JB: Hypovitaminosis D in the healthy elderly. Br J Clin Pract 1995; 49:301–303.
182. Bendich A: Physiological role of antioxidants in the immune system. J Dairy Sci 1993; 76:2789–2794.
183. Vitamin E supplementation enhances immune response in the elderly. Nutr Rev 1992; 50:85–87.
184. Watson AJ, Lawlor E, Temperley IJ, Keogh JA: Severe thrombocytopenia secondary to acute folate deficiency. Ir J Med Sci 1981; 150:125.
185. Mant MJ, Connolly T, Gordon PA, King EG: Severe thrombocytopenia probably due to acute folic acid deficiency. Crit Care Med 1979; 7:297–300.
186. Geerlings SE, Rommes JH, van-Toorn DW, Bakker: Acute folate deficiency in a critically ill patient. Neth J Med 1997; 51:36–38.
187. Tennant GB, Smith RC, Leinster SJ, O'Donnell JE, Wardrop CA: Amino acid infusion induced depression of serum folate after cholecystectomy. Scand J Haematol 1981; 27:333–338.
188. Russell RM: The impact of disease states as a modifying factor for nutrition toxicity. Nutr Rev 1997; 55:50–53.
189. Lentz SR: Homocysteine and vascular dysfunction. Life Sci 1997; 61:1205–1215.
190. Refsum H, Fiskerstrand T, Guttormsen AB, Ueland PM: Assessment of homocysteine status. J Inherit Metab Dis 1997; 20:286–294.
191. Fenech MF, Dreosti IE, Rinaldi JR: Folate, vitamin B_{12}, homocysteine status and chromosome damage rate in lymphocytes of older men. Carcinogenesis 1997; 18:1329–1336.
192. Berentsen S, Talstad I: [Homocysteine and methylmalonic acid. New tests—for what benefit?]. Tidsskr Nor Laegeforen 1996; 116:2677–2679.
193. Rall LC, Meydani SN: Vitamin B_6 and immune competence. Nutr Rev 1993; 51:217–225.
194. Meydani SN, Ribaya-Mercado JD, Russell RM, Sahyoun N, Morrow FD, Gershoff SN: Vitamin B-6 deficiency impairs interleukin 2 production and lymphocyte proliferation in elderly adults. Am J Clin Nutr 1991; 53:1275–1280.
195. Grimble RF: Effect of antioxidative vitamins on immune function with clinical applications. Int J Vitam Nutr Res 1997; 67:312–320.
196. Herbert V, Shaw S, Jayatilleke E: Vitamin C–driven free radical generation from iron. J Nutr 1996; 126(4 Suppl):1213S–1220S.
197. Herbert V, Shaw S, Jayatilleke E, Stopler-Kasdan T: Most free-radical injury is non-related: It is promoted by iron, hemin, holoferritin and vitamin C, and inhibited by desferoxamine and apoferritin. Stem Cells (Dayt) 1994; 12:289–303.
198. Force RW, Nahata MC: Effect of histamine H_2-receptor antagonists on vitamin B_{12} absorption. Ann Pharmacother 1992; 26:1283–1286.
199. Belaiche J, Zittoun J, Marquet J, Nurit Y, Yvart J: [Effect of ranitidine on secretion of gastric intrinsic factor and absorption of vitamin B_{12}]. Gastroenterol Clin Biol 1983; 7:381–384.
200. Naurath HJ, Joosten E, Riezler R, Stabler SP, Allen RH, Lindenbaum J: Effects of vitamin B_{12}, folate, and vitamin B_6 supplements in elderly people with normal serum vitamin concentrations. Lancet 1995; 346:85–89.
201. Thomas JA: Drug nutrient interactions. Nutr Rev 1995; 53:271–282.
202. Williams L, Davis JA, Lowenthal DT: The influence of food on the absorption and metabolism of drugs. Med Clin North Am. 1993; 77:815–829.
203. Bailey K: Physiological factors affecting drug toxicity. Regul Toxicol Pharmacol 1983; 3:389–398.
204. Loesche WI, Bromberg I, Terpenning MS, Bretz WA, Dominguez BL, Grossman NS, Langmore SE: Xerostomia, xerogenic medications and food avoidances in selected geriatric groups. J Am Geriatr Soc 1995; 43:401–407.
205. Gerweck LE: Tumor pH: Implications for treatment and novel drug design. Semin Radiat Oncol 1998; 8:176–182.
206. Dressman JB, Berardi RR: Dermentzoglou LC: Upper gastrointestinal (GI) pH in young, healthy men and women. Pharm Res 1990; 7:756–761.
207. Thatte U, Dahanukar S: Apoptosis: Clinical relevance and pharmacological manipulation. Drugs 1997; 54:511–532.
208. Negro F, Cerra FB: Nutritional monitoring in the ICU: Rational and practical application. Crit Care Clin 1988; 4:559–572.

84

Obesity in the Critically Ill Patient

Larry Bortenschlager, MD • Gary P. Zaloga, MD, FCCM

Obesity is the most common and costly nutritional problem in the United States. This chronic disease affects 33% of adults[1–4] and the incidence appears to be increasing. Health care costs are approximately $68 billion per year; an additional $30 billion per year are spent on weight reduction programs and special foods.[4, 5] Total health care costs for obesity represent approximately 8% of total health care costs.[6] Obesity is also a common cause of disability and death.[4] Obesity-related conditions are estimated to contribute to 300,000 deaths yearly, ranking second only to smoking as a cause of preventable death.[4] Treatment directed toward long-term reduction of body weight is largely ineffective, and 90% to 95% of persons who lose weight subsequently regain it.[7]

Accurate measurement of body fat requires specialized techniques (e.g., isotopic methods, dual-photon absorptiometry). Because these techniques are expensive and not readily available, careful measurements of height and weight are usually

TABLE 84–1. Health Hazards of Obesity

Organ or System	Disease
Cardiac	Coronary artery disease Angina pectoris, myocardial infarction Cardiomyopathy, heart failure Arrhythmias
Vascular	Hypertension Deep venous thrombosis Stroke
Pulmonary	Sleep apnea, obesity-hypoventilation syndrome Pulmonary hypertension Pulmonary embolism Aspiration pneumonia
Metabolic	Dyslipidemias Diabetes mellitus
Hepatobiliary	Cholelithiasis, cholecystitis Hepatic steatosis
Rectum, colon, prostate	Cancer
Female reproductive tract, breast	Cancer
Miscellaneous	Osteoarthritis, gout Fractures

used clinically to assess overweight patients. "Obesity" represents an excess of fat for height, and "overweight" represents excess body weight for height. One can be overweight as a result of obesity or as a result of excess muscle mass (as occurs in body builders). Overweight not resulting from fat does not carry the same increased health risks as obesity. Thus, when one is confirming a diagnosis of obesity, it is important to distinguish between obesity and overweight. Overweight is defined as a body mass index (BMI), or weight in kilograms divided by the square of the height in meters, greater than 25 to 28. A BMI greater than 28 is associated with increased morbidity and mortality[8] and is almost always associated with an increase in body fat. A central distribution of body fat (ratio of waist circumference to hip circumference greater than 0.9 for females and 1.0 for males) is associated with higher morbidity and mortality than a peripheral distribution of fat.[9] Risks of obesity are also greater in patients with increased abdominal fat compared with gluteal fat. In addition, morbidity and mortality are higher in patients who have been obese since childhood.

The prevalence of obesity varies with the population (i.e., country, age, sex, race). It is higher in Mexican Americans and blacks than in whites. It is also higher in the poor and women. In the United States, approximately 33% of the adult population has a BMI greater than 27. Of the obese population, 42% (35 million Americans) are severely obese (BMI greater than 31).

Obesity predisposes to a large variety of diseases that increase both morbidity and mortality[9–11] (Table 84–1). These conditions include coronary artery disease, myocardial infarction, cardiomyopathy, heart failure, hypertension, hypercholesterolemia, hypertriglyceridemia, diabetes mellitus, obstructive sleep apnea, obesity hypoventilation syndrome, pulmonary hypertension, cholelithiasis, hepatic steatosis, cancer (i.e., rectum, colon, prostate, female reproductive tract, gallbladder, breast), osteoarthritis, gout, fractures, deep venous thrombosis, and pulmonary embolism. Severe obesity (BMI $>$ 40) is associated with an increased risk of sudden death.

Thus, it is clear that obesity contributes to many diseases that result in admission to an intensive care unit (ICU). In a review of surgical patients, Choban and colleagues[12] found that 37% of adults undergoing elective surgery were overweight (BMI $>$ 27) and 17% were severely obese (BMI $>$ 31). In a review of trauma patients,[13] 24% were overweight and 10% severely obese. Because of the high prevalence of obesity, these patients are frequent users of critical care. In addition, obese patients have more complications and consume more resources than their lean counterparts. This chapter describes the pathophysiology, organ effects, and medical and surgical treatment of obesity.

PATHOPHYSIOLOGY OF OBESITY

Obesity results from nutrient imbalance as more foodstuffs are stored as fat than are used for energy and metabolism. The control of food intake and energy expenditure is mediated via numerous endocrine and neural signals (Table 84–2) from adipose tissue, endocrine glands, the neurologic system, and gastrointestinal systems, and these signals are integrated by the central nervous system.[1] Interactions between mediators are complex (as in sepsis). There are many redundancies and interactions between mediators. Thus, it is unlikely that a single pharmacologic manipulation can control obesity.

Eating is affected by both biochemical factors and psychologic factors. The primary areas of the brain that control eating are the arcuate and paraventricular nuclei in the ventro-

TABLE 84–2. Mediators of Obesity

Organ or System	Decrease Appetite or Increase Energy Expenditure	Increase Appetite or Decrease Energy Expenditure
Gastrointestinal	Glucagon, cholecystokinin, glucagon-like peptides, bombesin, glucose	Opioid peptides, neurotensin, growth hormone-releasing hormone, somatostatin
Endocrine	Epinephrine (β receptor), estrogens, thyroid hormone	Epinephrine (α receptor), androgens, glucocorticoids, insulin, peptide YY, progesterone, thyroid hormone
Adipose	Leptin	
Peripheral nervous system	Norepinephrine (β receptor)	Norepinephrine (α receptor)
Central nervous system	Dopamine, serotonin, γ-aminobutyric acid, cholecystokinin	Galanin, opioid peptides, growth hormone-releasing hormone, somatostatin
Hypothalamus	Norepinephrine, serotonin, neuropeptide Y, glucagon-like peptide-1, corticotropin-releasing hormone	Norepinephrine, serotonin, neuropeptide Y, glucagon-like peptide-1, corticotropin-releasing hormone

medial hypothalamus. Afferent neural and hormonal signals modulate the release of peptides that affect food intake and efferent signals to the hypothalamic-pituitary axis and autonomic nervous system that alter energy expenditure. Lesions in these areas of the brain result in hyperphagia, increased insulin release, hypometabolism, and obesity.

The control of food intake involves positive and negative sensory feedback, gastric and intestinal distention, the effects of nutrients, nutrient reserves, and metabolism.[14] Hunger and satiety are controlled by both positive and negative sensory signals related to the appearance, smell, color, taste, texture, and temperature of food. Hunger is also affected by stimulation of oropharyngeal receptors and blood glucose level.

Distention of the gastrointestinal tract negatively affects food intake. In addition, chemoreceptors in the gastrointestinal tract, liver, and brain respond to carbohydrate (i.e., glucose), free fatty acids, peptides, and hormones stimulated by these nutrients to modulate food intake. Satiety receptors are found along the entire gastrointestinal tract. The satiety effects of diet are mediated by hydrolytic products, not polymeric nutrients. Suppression of food intake is achieved by sugars that utilize the glucose transporter, fatty acids 12 carbons in length or longer, and the amino acids L-phenylalanine and L-tryptophan. Drugs such as acarbose (an inhibitor of α-1,4-glucosidases) and orlistat (a lipase inhibitor) reduce the satiety effects of food. Nutrients also inhibit gastric emptying, stimulate pancreatic secretion, and increase intestinal motility (all of which decrease appetite). Feedback regulation from food is probably mediated by a combination of neural and hormonal signals arising in the gastrointestinal tract. The intensity of feedback inhibition of intake depends on the number of sensors that are activated (i.e., length of intestine exposed to the nutrients).

Hormones and peptides that increase food intake include opioid peptides (e.g., endorphin, dynorphin, β-casomorphin), neuropeptide Y, galanin, aldosterone, corticosterone, growth hormone–releasing hormone, insulin, and peptide YY. Agents that inhibit intake of food include cholecystokinin, bombesin, neurotensin, anorectin, calcitonin, enterostatin, corticotropin-releasing hormone (CRH), glucagon, vasopressin, somatostatin, insulin, and thyrotropin-releasing hormone (TRH). Finally, leptin (secreted by adipocytes) inhibits food intake and increases energy expenditure.

Of the many hormones that control food intake (see Table 84–2), insulin, cholecystokinin, leptin, and neuropeptide Y are major regulators[1]:

Insulin decreases food intake by inhibiting expression of neuropeptide Y in the brain, enhancing the anorectic effects of cholecystokinin, and inhibiting neuronal reuptake of norepinephrine. Insulin may also affect food intake by modulating the effect of leptin.

Cholecystokinin is secreted by the duodenum in response to food and decreases food intake. It is also synthesized by the brain, and intracranial cholecystokinin also decreases food intake. Although cholecystokinin does not penetrate the blood-brain barrier, gastrointestinal cholecystokinin may modulate food intake via afferent neuronal signals from the intestines to the brain.

Leptin[1, 15–17] is synthesized and secreted by adipose tissue and represents an afferent satiety signal from fat stores. Leptin administration reduces food intake and increases energy expenditure, resulting in reduced body fat. Leptin expression is increased by insulin, glucocorticoids, and estrogens and decreased by beta agonists and androgens. The mechanism of action of leptin remains unclear, but some of its actions appear to be mediated by decreasing or blocking the actions of neuropeptide Y. Thus, decreased leptin action (decreased levels, abnormal peptide) or leptin resistance could cause obesity. Most obese patients do not have an abnormal leptin; however, leptin resistance probably contributes to obesity in many patients.

Neuropeptide Y links various afferent signals from the endocrine, gastrointestinal, and nervous systems to effectors of energy intake and expenditure. Neuropeptide Y is synthesized in the arcuate nucleus of the hypothalamus and transported axonally to the paraventricular nucleus of the hypothalamus, its major site of action. It is also synthesized by the adrenal glands and sympathetic nervous system but does not penetrate the blood-brain barrier. Neuropeptide Y is a potent appetite stimulant. Its synthesis is increased by insulin and glucocorticoids and decreased by leptin and estrogens.

Genetic factors contribute greatly to the development of obesity. More than 70 different genes have been identified that contribute to obesity.[18] It is estimated that 80% of the variance in BMI is attributable to genetic factors. Genetic factors affect tissue fat distribution, physical activity, resting metabolic rate, changes in energy expenditure in response to eating, eating behavior, food preference, and rates of lipolysis. Given the importance of energy stores for survival and reproductive capacity, the ability to conserve energy in the form of adipose tissue would at one time have offered a survival advantage. Humans are enriched with genes that favor energy intake and storage and diminish energy expenditure. However, easy access to calorically dense foods and sedentary lifestyle have made the metabolic consequences of these genes maladaptive.

Environmental factors also contribute to the development of obesity. Such factors include the abundance of food, cost of food, characteristics of food (e.g., high fat content), availability of food, and activity factors (e.g., exercise).

The body regulates energy expenditure[19] via neural and endocrine systems. Energy expenditure is the sum of resting energy expenditure plus energy consumed by physical activity (e.g., exercise, excess respiratory work) and the thermogenic effect of food. A reduction in any one of the three can lead to obesity. The sympathetic nervous system, parasympathetic nervous system, adrenal glands, gastrointestinal tract, and thyroid gland modulate body energy expenditure. In addition, many cytokines (e.g., tumor necrosis factor, interleukin-1) are now recognized to increase body energy expenditure and are responsible for the increased resting energy expenditure seen during critical illness.

EFFECTS OF OBESITY ON ORGAN FUNCTION

Obesity affects the function of many organ systems in the body and predisposes to a variety of diseases. These include coronary artery disease, myocardial infarction, heart failure, hypertension, dyslipidemias (lower high-density lipoprotein [HDL], elevated low-density lipoprotein [LDL] and very-low-density lipoprotein [VLDL], elevated triglycerides), diabetes mellitus, sleep apnea, obesity hypoventilation syndrome, pulmonary hypertension, gallbladder disease, arthritis, deep vein thrombosis, pulmonary emboli, and cancer (see Table 84–1). Patients with many of these diseases improve with weight loss.

Obesity is characterized by an increase in total blood volume and resting cardiac output.[20–23] The increase in cardiac output is primarily the result of an increase in stroke volume rather than heart rate. Left ventricular preload is increased and systemic vascular resistance is reduced in normotensive individuals. However, systemic vascular resistance is raised in hypertensive patients. Resting oxygen consumption is increased and correlated with body weight.[22] The net result can be left ventricular dilation and/or hypertrophy.[24] Cardiac weight is frequently increased as a result of hypertrophy. Chronic hypertension in the obese patient contributes to the hypertrophy. Left ventricular filling pressures may be elevated because of increased preload and reduced ventricular compliance.[20-23] Both ventricular diastolic dysfunction[25] and systolic dysfunction are common in severely obese patients and contribute to heart failure.

Coronary artery disease is common in obese patients. The likelihood of myocardial ischemia or infarction increases as left ventricular mass and metabolic demands increase. All of these factors predispose to cardiac arrhythmias and sudden death. Fluid loading is poorly tolerated by obese patients with cardiac dysfunction.

Obesity predisposes to coronary artery disease and its consequences (angina pectoris, myocardial infarction, arrhythmias, heart failure).[26] Coronary artery disease is more common in obese patients with central versus peripheral obesity. Other predisposing factors for coronary artery disease in the obese patient are hyperlipidemia (decreased HDL, elevated LDL and VLDL), diabetes mellitus, hypertension, and tobacco use.

Obesity may be associated with a cardiomyopathy that is independent of the presence of other risk factors such as hypertension, diabetes mellitus, and hyperlipidemia (the cardiomyopathy of obesity). Despite an elevated resting cardiac output, obese patients frequently demonstrate impaired left ventricular contractility, both at rest and with exercise.[22, 27-31] Decreased myocardial β-adrenergic receptors in the heart may contribute to decreased contractility.[30, 31] Diastolic dysfunction usually develops before systolic dysfunction. Many patients remain asymptomatic despite cardiac dysfunction. Others manifest cardiac dysfunction with dyspnea on exertion, orthopnea, shortness of breath at rest, and peripheral edema. Many obese patients decrease their activity level because of shortness of breath, an effect that masks symptoms of heart failure and contributes to additional weight gain. Cardiomyopathy can be worsened by the development of pulmonary hypertension, valvular heart disease, and hypoxia in patients with sleep apnea and hypoventilation syndromes. It is important to note that some of the oral appetite suppressants have been associated with the development of pulmonary hypertension and valvular disease (see section on treatment of obesity).

Cardiomyopathy and cardiac ischemia in obese patients predispose to a variety of atrial and ventricular arrhythmias as well as sudden death. Atrial tachydysrhythmias such as atrial fibrillation and multifocal atrial tachycardia are common. Left and right axis deviation, P pulmonale, low voltage, and left-right ventricular hypertrophy may be seen on the electrocardiogram.

The treatment of cardiomyopathy in obese patients is similar to that in other patients. Important considerations include (1) reduction of preload, (2) use of agents that decrease afterload, (3) heart rate control in patients with atrial tachyarrhythmias, and (4) use of agents that improve both systolic and diastolic function. Weight loss can improve symptoms and cardiac function in some patients.

Obesity predisposes to hypertension.[26] Sixty per cent of obese individuals who are 20% or more overweight have hypertension. Ten per cent exhibit severe forms of the disease and have end-organ involvement (heart, kidneys, eyes). Hypertension is a major risk factor for stroke in the obese patient.[32] Weight gain is an important risk factor for the development of or exacerbation of hypertension in both the young and old. Blood pressure decreases and may become normal with weight loss in overweight persons.[32] When blood pressure is measured in the obese patient, it is important to use the proper blood pressure cuff size. Cuffs that are too small may result in artificially high blood pressure values.

The exact cause of hypertension in obese individuals is unclear. Most likely, it results from the additive effects of several organ derangements. As total body fat mass increases, so does blood flow to the expanding adipose tissue. Body metabolic rate and oxygen consumption increase, stimulating an increase in cardiac output. Normally, the rise in cardiac output occurs with a reduction in systemic vascular resistance and maintenance of a normal blood pressure. However, as obesity becomes more severe, systemic vascular resistance and blood pressure increase. Insulin resistance occurs and is associated with hyperinsulinemia. Hyperinsulinemia and a decreased renal filtration surface result in renal tubule sodium reabsorption, intravascular volume expansion, and sympathetic hyperactivity. Plasma levels of renin and aldosterone may also be elevated.

Pulmonary function is adversely affected by obesity.[33-36] Function of the respiratory muscles and diaphragmatic excursion are impaired in the severely obese. There is restriction of the ability of the chest wall to expand. Vital capacity, total lung capacity, functional residual capacity, forced expiratory volume in 1 second, and expiratory reserve volume are all reduced in the morbidly obese. These parameters are usually normal in those with mild to moderate obesity.

The fall in expiratory reserve volume is presumably due to small-airway closure.[37] Lung compliance is reduced secondary to low lung volumes and elevated hemidiaphragms (especially during recumbency). Thus, the obese patient is predisposed to atelectasis and ineffective clearing of mucus. Work of breathing and body energy expenditure are increased because of abnormal chest elasticity, increased chest wall resistance, increased airway resistance, abnormal diaphragmatic position, upper airway resistance, and higher production of carbon dioxide.[33-35] To help minimize the work of breathing, obese individuals take more frequent but smaller breaths. The ability to increase minute ventilation is limited. Ventilation-perfusion mismatch is common (especially in the supine position) and may cause hypoxemia.[34, 38] Severe hypoxemia contributes to an increased risk of sudden death. Most hypoxemic patients have normal or low carbon dioxide levels. However, abnormalities in the control of ventilation are common in obese patients.

Obese patients may have sleep apnea and the obesity-hypoventilation syndrome. Sleep apnea is usually of the obstructive type.[39] Pure central sleep apnea is uncommon. An increase in the circumference of the head, as well as BMI, increases the risk of sleep apnea. Fat deposition, redundant soft tissue in the airway, and relaxation of the pharyngeal and glossus muscles during sleep contribute to sleep apnea. The obesity-hypoventilation syndrome develops in a small percentage of patients with sleep apnea (~5%). This syndrome is characterized by a depressed respiratory response to hypoxia and hypercapnia, frequent episodes of apnea resulting in hypoxemia, daytime somnolence, irregular breathing, and an increased work of breathing. Hypoxemia and hypercapnea can cause pulmonary hypertension and cor pulmonale. Right ventricular failure may eventually result in left ventricular failure, further compromising oxygenation. Respiratory failure can also occur. Hypercapnea can be severe enough to cause lethargy, somnolence, and coma.

Patients with hypoxemia and sleep apnea can improve quickly with weight reduction.[40, 41] Pulmonary hypertension and heart failure also improve with weight reduction; the degree of improvement depends on the length of time the condition has been present and the degree of underlying heart disease. The cornerstone of treatment of patients with obesity-hypoventilation syndrome is administration of oxygen and reversal of hypoxemia. It is also important to minimize hypercapnea and reverse acidosis. Overadministration of oxygen can suppress respiratory drive and lead to further hypercapnia and acidosis. Thus, oxygen therapy must be closely monitored and carefully titrated. We aim for a Po_2 of 55 to 60 torr and/or an oxygen saturation of 88% to 90%. Most patients can be managed without intubation through use of nasal oxygen or noninvasive ventilation (i.e., bilevel positive-pressure ventilation). When respiratory failure is severe, mentation is depressed, and other organ failures occur (e.g., cardiac failure), intubation and mechanical ventilation are required. Polycythemia may be present as a result of chronic hypoxemia and may require specific treatment (i.e., phlebotomy). Heart failure is usually treated with diuretics and inotropic agents. Patients with pulmonary hypertension and heart failure are at high risk for hypotension when vasodilators are administered. Vasodilators may also exacerbate hypoxemia by inhibiting hypoxic pulmonary vasoconstriction. The use of inhaled nitric oxide and other pulmonary vasodilators for these patients requires further study. Medroxyprogesterone has been used to improve ventilatory drive and blood gases in patients with obesity-hypoventilation syndrome. Its use in treating acute ventilatory failure is less clear.

Although patients may be obese, they are frequently malnourished and may suffer from protein, vitamin, and mineral deficiencies. Deficiencies of potassium, magnesium, and phosphorus may predispose to respiratory muscle weakness and respiratory failure. Thus, nutritional support is an important adjuvant to therapy in these patients. Respiratory drives and respiratory muscle strength are also influenced by thyroid hormone. Obese patients with respiratory failure should be evaluated for hypothyroidism and treated accordingly. Acetazolamide has been used to decrease serum bicarbonate levels in patients with obesity-hypoventilation syndrome. This agent should be used cautiously and patients monitored closely during treatment. Although metabolic alkalosis can induce hypoventilation, bicarbonate levels may have increased in response to rising carbon dioxide levels. Lowering of bicarbonate with acetazolamide may exacerbate acidosis, pulmonary hypertension, and heart failure.

Endotracheal intubation is frequently difficult in the obese patient.[42] Contributing factors include limited neck mobility, a large tongue, increased upper airway soft tissue, and limited mouth opening.

Weaning from mechanical ventilation is difficult in the obese patient with hypoventilation. These patients may live with lower Po_2 and higher Pco_2 values than lean individuals. Measures of vital capacity, tidal volume, minute ventilation, maximum minute ventilation, maximum negative inspiratory pressure, and respiratory rate are usually abnormal and do not necessarily contraindicate weaning. Atelectasis is common during weaning, and the ability to clear secretions (via cough) is frequently impaired. No ventilator mode or weaning protocol has proved to be superior to others in weaning the obese patient. Respiratory mechanics are better in the upright than in the supine position. We favor the use of intermittent T-piece trials and extubation when the patient tolerates a 2-hour trial. Respiratory muscle fatigue can develop quickly in obese patients during weaning because of small endotracheal tubes, supine positioning, requirement to open valves in the ventilatory circuit, agitation or anxiety, and increased work of breathing superimposed on underlying respiratory and cardiac insufficiency. Obese patients with hypoventilation are also extremely sensitive to sedative drugs (perhaps because of an abnormal respiratory center).

The risk of aspiration is increased in the obese patient. Factors contributing to pneumonia include higher volumes of gastric fluid, higher gastric pH, increased intra-abdominal pressure, and greater incidence of gastroesophageal reflux. These patients are best managed in the semi-upright position.

Pulmonary complications are increased in obese patients after surgery compared with their lean counterparts.[20, 33, 43–45] Pulmonary dysfunction is accentuated by thoracic and upper abdominal incisions. Pain control strategies with minimal respiratory depression, such as epidural analgesia, can improve postoperative respiratory function in these patients. Early physical mobilization and aggressive chest physiotherapy are also recommended.

Obesity is one of the major risks factors for pulmonary embolism.[46] Postoperative obese patients also have a higher incidence of pulmonary embolism.[47, 48] Decreased mobility, venous stasis, and altered coagulation contribute to thrombosis. Diminished levels of antithrombin III and fibrinolytic activity have been reported.[49, 50] Immobilized obese patients should receive prophylaxis against deep venous thrombosis.

Weight gain is associated with increased insulin concentrations, enhanced insulin resistance, hyperglycemia, and diabetes mellitus.[26] Even modest weight loss significantly improves glycemic control.[32, 51, 52] Both energy restriction and weight reduction improve glycemic control in patients with diabetes mellitus. Correction of weight excess can reverse the abnormalities of insulin secretion, clearance, and action on glucose metabolism in markedly obese patients and may allow discontinuation of insulin treatment and antidiabetic drugs.[53, 54]

As body weight increases, the size of fat cells increases. The deposition of triacylglycerol in subcutaneous and visceral depots is associated with an increase in the production of cholesterol. Increased cholesterol production in turn is associated with increased cholesterol secretion in bile and an increased risk (threefold to fourfold) of gallstone formation and gallbladder disease.[26]

Patients with obesity have an increased risk of cancer.[55] Overweight men with colorectal and prostate cancers have higher mortality rates. Overweight women have higher rates of endometrial, cervical, ovarian, breast, and gallbladder cancers.

The prevalence of osteoarthritis and gout is also increased in obese patients. Arthritis contributes to immobility and exacerbates weight gain.

TREATMENT OF OBESITY

The goal of treatment is to reduce weight to such an extent that the excess morbidity and mortality rates of obesity revert to baseline values.[32] Unfortunately, many patients cannot adhere to programs designed to achieve these optimal goals. Lesser degrees of weight reduction also have beneficial health effects. It is important to establish reasonable and attainable goals for weight reduction, yet weight reduction alone does not necessarily improve health, and drug therapies and surgery for obesity may be detrimental to health. Because treatments may entail health risks for the patient, it is important to grade the risk-benefit ratio of any proposed therapy for obesity (Table 84–3).

Medical Management

Energy Expenditure

The bases of weight loss are reduced caloric intake and increased energy expenditure. Both protein and carbohydrate can be converted to fat. Thus, altering the relative proportions of protein, carbohydrate, and fat in the diet without reducing calories is not effective for weight loss.[56] Fat has a high caloric content, and reducing fat intake may be one mechanism for

TABLE 84–3. Obesity Treatments from Low to High Risk

Reduced Caloric Intake	Increased Energy Expenditure
Low Risk	
Behavior modification	Increased activity (exercise)
Decreased dietary intake	Thermogenic drugs
Anorexic drugs	Agents that inhibit nutrient absorption
Gastric reduction surgery	
Intestinal bypass surgery	
High Risk	

decreasing total caloric intake. In addition, decreased fat intake and increased protein intake suppress voluntary energy intake. Thus, there may be an advantage to the use of low-fat, high-protein diets for the management of obesity.

Diet composition does not directly influence resting energy expenditure. The main determinant of resting metabolic rate is fat-free mass (with fat having a lesser effect). Thus, diet composition may indirectly affect energy expenditure via effects on body composition. Energy expenditure is affected by the thermic effect of food, which represents the energy expended in digesting, absorbing, interconverting, and storing ingested nutrients. Overall, the thermic effect of food is small, accounting for 6% to 10% of total energy expenditure. Both the amount and composition of food can affect the thermic effect of food. However, varying the fat and carbohydrate content of food over normal ranges of 20% to 60% of total calories has little significant effect on energy expenditure.

When negative energy balance is achieved through reduced energy intake, there is a reduction in energy expenditure because of a reduction in the thermic effect of food. As weight reduction occurs, the resulting decrease in body mass is accompanied by a reduction in resting energy expenditure. In addition, the energy required for physical activity decreases because the energy cost of movement is less at lower body mass. Thus, as weight is lost, there is a reduction in energy expenditure that makes further weight loss more difficult.

Diets with drastically altered proportions of nutrients may be dangerous. There are minimum body requirements for proteins, essential fatty acids, vitamins, and minerals. Depletion of these nutrients can increase morbidity and mortality. It is far better to establish long-term weight control by using a diet containing a modest restriction of calories. Very-low-calorie diets (i.e., 400 to 800 calories per day) should be used only under supervision by a trained physician and only when there is medical urgency for weight reduction. These patients require mineral and vitamin supplementation to avoid deficiencies of these nutrients. Adverse metabolic effects (e.g., dehydration, electrolyte imbalance, orthostatic hypotension, hyperuricemia, ventricular arrhythmias) are common with these diets. It is also important to note that dieting can decrease morbidity and mortality without reducing weight. For example, decreasing fat (and cholesterol) intake can reduce cardiovascular morbidity without causing weight reduction. Energy expenditure varies greatly between individuals. Thus, one should estimate or measure energy expenditure in an obese patient so that one can prescribe an appropriate reducing diet for the patient; a deficit of approximately 3500 kcal results in 1 pound of weight loss.

Daily energy expenditure per unit of lean body mass is similar in lean and obese subjects at their usual body weight. However, small (i.e., 10%) decreases in body weight result in declines in energy expenditure. Thus, a formerly obese patient requires approximately 15% fewer calories to maintain normal body weight than a person of the same body composition who has never been obese. This decrease in energy expenditure results from decreases in both resting and nonresting energy expenditure and reflects a state of increased metabolic efficiency.

Initial evaluation of the obese patient should rule out underlying metabolic disease that requires specific treatment. Such diseases include hypothyroidism, Cushing's syndrome, insulinomas, leptin deficiency (rare), hypothalamic-pituitary disease, pseudohypoparathyroidism, and hypogonadal syndromes. Rarely has obesity been reported to develop after central nervous system injury resulting from head trauma, brain surgery, or central nervous system infection. Interestingly, obesity may develop in animals after infection with various viruses that damage the hypothalamus (i.e., canine distemper virus, Borna disease virus, avian and human adenoviruses, and Rous-associated virus type 7).

Lifestyle

The *first line* of treatment for obesity involves lifestyle alterations, which must be continued indefinitely. These include increased activity (exercise) and reduced caloric intake. Increased activity helps promote dietary compliance. Lifestyle changes for maintenance of weight loss are difficult. Caloric restriction is effective for reducing weight,[57] and most patients can reduce their weight in the short term. Adherence to caloric restriction is partly a function of the intensity of supervision of the weight loss program. Behavior modification has been beneficial as an adjunct to caloric restriction and exercise programs. Average weight loss is 8.5 kg over 21 weeks.[4] Thus, the efficacy of drug treatment must be judged against the efficacy of nondrug treatment regimens (which are safer).

Unfortunately, few patients are able to reduce their weight to ideal body weight levels with caloric restriction or behavioral modification alone. Two thirds of patients who lose weight regain it within 1 year, and almost all patients regain weight within 5 years.[4, 57] It is likely that this inability to lose weight and sustain weight loss results from biochemical factors. Numerous drugs may contribute to obesity by stimulating appetite or improving nutrient storage. These drugs include glucocorticoids, insulin, oral hypoglycemics, phenothiazines, tricyclic antidepressants, cyproheptadine, and valproic acid. Obesity should be treated as a chronic disease requiring long-term treatment, similar to diabetes mellitus or hypertension.

The *second line* of treatment for obesity is reduction of other risk factors. These include smoking, hypertension, elevated cholesterol, and diabetes mellitus. Weight reduction is effective in treating hypertension and diabetes mellitus. However, if weight reduction cannot be achieved or risk factors persist, aggressive treatment is required.

Drugs

Drug therapy represents *third-line therapy* for obesity.[4, 51, 58–61] To date, none of the available drugs have proved to be effective for long-term weight loss that improves the overall health of the obese population, and drug therapy cannot be recommended for treatment of most obese patients. A variety of drugs are available for the treatment of obesity (Table 84–4). Antiobesity drugs can be classified into three categories on the basis of their mechanisms of action: (1) those that reduce food intake, (2) those that alter metabolism either before or after absorption, and (3) those that increase energy expenditure. Although some of these agents are effective in promoting weight loss, weight is quickly regained when the drugs are stopped. The vast majority of drugs used to treat obesity are

TABLE 84–4. Drug Therapy of Obesity

Drug	Mechanism of Action	Adverse Effects and Comments
Sympathomimetic agents Phentermine Phenmetrazine Phendimetrazine Benzphetamine Diethylpropion Mazindol Phenylpropanolamine	Stimulate brain catecholamine pathways, decreasing appetite or increasing energy expenditure	Hypertension Cardiac ischemia or infarction Cardiac arrhythmias Palpitations, tachycardia Cardiac arrest Stroke Seizures Psychosis, agitation, euphoria Anxiety Central nervous system vasculitis Dry mouth Constipation Disturbed sleep Headache
Serotonin reuptake inhibitors Fenfluramine Fluoxetine Dexfenfluramine Sertraline	Increase brain serotonin, decreasing appetite	Pulmonary hypertension Cardiac valve defects Dry mouth Urinary urgency, polyuria Diarrhea Dizziness Disturbed sleep, vivid dreams Memory loss Depression
Combined effects on brain catecholaminergic and serotoninergic pathways Sibutramine Phentermine + fenfluramine	Stimulate brain catecholaminergic and serotoninergic pathways	Combines adverse effects of sympathomimetic agents and serotonin reuptake inhibitors
β_3-Adrenergic agonists	Increase energy expenditure	Drugs under development Tremor
Lipase inhibitors Tetrahydrolipostatin	Decrease digestion and absorption of fat	Diarrhea, flatus, oily stools Deficiency of fat-soluble vitamins
Leptin	Decreases appetite and increases energy expenditure; decreases neuropeptide Y	Agent undergoing clinical studies
Neuropeptide Y antagonists	Decrease appetite	Agents under development
Tumor necrosis factor	Decreases appetite	Agent under study
Cholecystokin agonists	Suppress appetite	Drugs under development
Thyroid hormone	Increases energy expenditure	Hypertension Tachycardia Cardiac arrhythmias Cardiac ischemia or infarction Osteoporosis Anxiety, agitation Psychosis Many others

central appetite suppressants that act on brain catecholamine and serotonin pathways. These include:

- Sympathomimetic drugs
- Serotonin reuptake inhibitors
- Agents that affect both catecholaminergic and serotoninergic pathways.

Sympathomimetic Agents

Amphetamine and methamphetamine were two of the first sympathetic agents used to suppress appetite in the treatment of obesity. These agents mimic the effects of the sympathetic transmitters epinephrine, norepinephrine, and dopamine. However, because of numerous adverse cardiovascular and central nervous system effects and their abuse potential, the amphetamines were abandoned for the treatment of obesity. Newer sympathomimetic agents with less abuse potential were subsequently developed and include phentermine, phenmetrazine, phendimetrazine, benzphetamine, diethylpropion, mazindol, and phenylpropanolamine. Phenylpropanolamine is found in most of the over-the-counter diet pills. These agents increase brain concentrations of catecholamines or act directly on catechol receptors to decrease appetite and/or increase energy expenditure.

A review of the effectiveness of these agents for weight loss[59] indicated that the drug-treated group lost approximately 0.5 pound more per week than the placebo-treated group. However, most of these studies were short term (usually 4–6 weeks), and the long-term effectiveness and medical benefits (reduced morbidity and mortality) of these drugs remain unproved. These agents act as stimulants and have many cardiovascular and central nervous system side effects. They have been reported to increase blood pressure and are associated with cardiac arrhythmias, cardiac ischemia, myocardial infarction, cardiac arrest, stroke, and bowel infarction. These effects are more likely to occur in patients with underlying cardiovascular disease (e.g., atherosclerosis), common in many obese patients. They also stimulate the brain and may result in anxiety, agitation, psychosis, and seizures.

The effects of these agents vary between individuals, and the risk of adverse consequences increases as the dose is increased. However, a significant body of medical evidence indicates that severe life-threatening central nervous system and cardiovascular events may occur with doses of the drugs that are used routinely to treat obesity. Thus, any potential benefits of these agents in promoting weight loss seem to be outweighed by their medical risks.

Serotonin Reuptake Inhibitors

Serotonin reuptake inhibitors increase serotonin levels in the brain and suppress appetite.[59] The serotonin reuptake inhibitors include fenfluramine,[62] dexfenfluramine (the dextro stereoisomer of *dl*-fenfluramine),[51, 63–65] and fluoxetine.[66–68] Fenfluramine also acts to release serotonin at nerve endings.[59] These drugs have fewer stimulant effects on the heart and brain than sympathomimetic agents.

Serotonin reuptake inhibitors have been more effective than placebo in producing weight loss. They also sustain weight loss over 1 to 4 years (provided patients continue to take the drugs).[69–71] Weight is quickly regained when the drugs are discontinued. Unfortunately, fenfluramine and dexfenfluramine have been associated with the development of pulmonary hypertension,[72–75] cardiac valve lesions (primarily aortic insufficiency and mitral regurgitation),[76–78] and depression. Some patients develop valvular lesions without murmurs or symptoms. These lesions can be detected by echocardiography. Patients with valvular lesions are at risk for endocarditis. Pulmonary hypertension may result from the vasoconstrictive effects of serotonin. Elevated serotonin levels may also cause cardiac valvular lesions, which appear morphologically similar to those found in the carcinoid syndrome.

Serotonin induces arterial spasm and has been implicated in Raynaud's phenomenon. In this regard, the serotonin reuptake inhibitor dexfenfluramine has been implicated as a cause of digital necrosis,[79] lower extremity arterial ischemia,[80] and coronary artery spasm.[81] Interestingly, fenfluramine[72, 82, 83] and dexfenfluramine[84] improve insulin sensitivity. Fenfluramine and dexfenfluramine have been withdrawn from the market at the request of the Food and Drug Administration (FDA).

Fluoxetine (marketed as an antidepressant) has been associated with weight loss in a number of clinical studies. The drug was more effective than placebo when used for 8 weeks. Most patients treated for longer periods of time (16 to 20 weeks) regained weight.[4] The drug may be useful for long-term weight loss in the subset of patients who do not regain weight while taking the drug.

Combination Drugs

A third group of agents has both catecholaminergic and serotoninergic agonist effects and includes sibutramine[85] (an inhibitor of both norepinephrine and serotonin reuptake) and the combination of phentermine and fenfluramine.[4] Weintraub and coworkers[71] combined two agents with different mechanisms of action (phentermine and fenfluramine), used in smaller doses, and were able to obtain long-term weight loss. However, weight was quickly regained upon discontinuation of the drugs. This combination of drugs has been associated with valvular heart disease.[76, 77] There is limited long-term experience with sibutramine. To date, pulmonary hypertension and cardiac valve lesions have not been reported with the drug, but substantial increases in blood pressure can occur. Other common adverse effects include headache, dry mouth, constipation, and insomnia. Sibutramine was approved for the treatment of morbid obesity, but the combination pill (phentermine and fenfluramine) has the undesirable side effects of both its constituent agents and has been removed from the market.

Studies indicate that the β_3-adrenergic receptor is involved in the regulation of energy expenditure.[86, 87] Thermogenic agents aimed at activating this receptor are under development. Thyroid extract, the first drug used to treat obesity, was used in the late 1800s. Thyroid hormone administration increases energy expenditure and can be effective in causing weight reduction. Certainly, hypothyroid patients can benefit from thyroid hormone administration. In general, obese patients do not have a low metabolic rate and are not hypothyroid. The administration of thyroid hormone to euthyroid individuals can be associated with numerous adverse cardiovascular and metabolic effects and is not recommended.

Lipase inhibitors (e.g., tetrahydrolipstatin) prevent the digestion and absorption of ingested fats.[88, 89] These agents increase fat content in the stool and may cause flatus, oily stools, diarrhea, and deficiencies of fat-soluble vitamins. Their use for the treatment of obesity awaits clinical trials.

A number of experimental agents are under evaluation for the treatment of obesity. These include leptin.[90] Initial results suggest that leptin administration can decrease body weight, but its long-term efficacy for the control of obesity requires further study. Other agents under evaluation include neuropeptide Y antagonists, cholecystokinin agonists, and tumor necrosis factor.

Surgical Management

Surgery can be dramatically effective in the treatment of obesity and may cure obesity-associated diabetes mellitus and hypertension. Because of the morbidity and mortality associated with surgery, it is recommended only for the severely obese (BMI > 40). The procedures most commonly used to treat obesity are gastric reduction surgery and jejunoileal bypass. Gastric banding to reduce gastric volume is rarely performed today because of late weight gain and risk of gastric perforation.

Gastric restrictive surgery with gastric bypass (bypassing most of the stomach and duodenum) offers the best treatment for patients with intractable morbid obesity. The success rate of the surgery approaches 75%. Most patients lose more than 50% of their excess weight.[91, 92] Major morbidity is seen in fewer than 10% of these high-risk patients and mortality is approximately 1%. Vertical banded gastroplasty is also performed in some centers.[93] Weight loss results are not as good with this procedure.

After gastric restrictive surgery, long-term nutritional deficiencies can develop.[94–96] The most common deficiencies are vitamin and mineral deficiencies, dehydration, and protein-calorie malnutrition as a result of reduced intake and/or absorption. Vomiting may occur with overeating. Common nutrient abnormalities include deficiencies of vitamins B_{12}, A, K, and D; folate; and thiamine. Deficient minerals include iron, calcium, magnesium, and potassium. These deficiencies should be treated with oral vitamin and mineral supplements. Vitamin B_{12} deficiency may result from inadequate dietary intake, inadequate release of the vitamin from its food source because of decreased acid or pepsin production in the remaining stomach pouch, inadequate mixing of vitamin B_{12} with R protein in the stomach, decreased availability of intrinsic factor, and decreased formation of vitamin B_{12}–intrinsic factor complex. Most patients with gastric bypass procedures cannot maintain adequate levels of vitamin B_{12} from diet alone and require oral or parenteral supplementation (500 to 600 μg/day orally). Untreated vitamin B_{12} deficiency can cause macrocytic anemia, leukopenia, thrombocytopenia, glossitis, and neurologic derangements. Folate deficiency is usually due to decreased intake and may result in macrocytic anemia, leukopenia, thrombocytopenia, and glossitis. It can be prevented by oral vitamin supplementation (1 mg/day). Iron deficiency results from decreased intake and malabsorption (bypass of duodenum) and causes a microcytic anemia. Iron supplementation is helpful. Dehydration results from decreased fluid intake (gastric restriction) and fluid losses in diarrhea and vomiting. Deficiencies may develop many years after gastric or bowel surgery, and long-term monitoring may be required.

Other complications of gastric restrictive surgery include stomal stenosis and ulceration, intussusception, gallstones, gallbladder sludge, dumping syndrome, and rarely liver failure. Many patients require cholecystectomy because of symptomatic gallbladder disease.

The jejunoileal bypass was the standard surgical treatment for obesity until it was replaced by gastric restrictive surgery in the 1980s. Although it is infrequently performed today, the clinician may still encounter patients who have undergone this surgical procedure. The operative mortality of the procedure is less than 1% in experienced hands, and most patients lose nearly one third of their preoperative weight. The operation involves connecting approximately 35 cm of proximal jejunum to 10 cm of distal ileum with an end-to-end or end-to-side anastamosis.[97] The jejunoileal bypass causes weight loss via malabsorption and reduced intake. The cause of the reduced intake remains unknown, but it may be related to the bacteria present in the blind loop of intestine created by the procedure.

Complications of this procedure include hepatic steatosis, cirrhosis, and liver failure.[97] Hepatic fibrosis occurs in 50% of patients by 6 years after surgery. Hepatic failure, arthritis, skin lesions, and renal failure are believed to be caused by bacterial overgrowth in the blind loop. These complications are associated with a vasculitis accompanied by tissue and circulating immune complexes that contain antibodies to colonic bacteria. Improvement of the immune complex disease occurs after treatment with corticosteroids and antibiotics that reduce colonic bacteria.

Other complications include itching, gallstones, enteritis, pneumatosis cystoides intestinalis, bowel obstruction, fluid loss, electrolyte abnormalities, and a non–anion gap acidosis (bicarbonate loss). Bypass enteritis is characterized by constipation, bloating, and fever. This condition usually responds to antibiotics such as metronidazole. The most common electrolyte abnormalities involve potassium, calcium, and magnesium deficiencies (largely caused by malabsorption).

Deficiency of vitamin D (a fat-soluble vitamin) and decreased calcium absorption may lead to osteomalacia and hypocalcemia. Most patients improve with calcium and vitamin D supplementation. Treatment with metronidazole may also improve calcium homeostasis (implicating bacteria overgrowth as a cause of hypocalcemia). A non–anion gap acidosis may develop as a result of bile acid irritation of the colonic mucosa, causing bicarbonate secretion along with malabsorption of bicarbonate.

Renal disease can develop in patients after jejunoileal bypass. Etiologic mechanisms include immune complex disease, nephrocalcinosis, and calcium oxalate stone disease. Increased oxalate absorption and hyperoxaluria are common. These patients are best managed with low-oxalate diets and oral oxalate binders (e.g., calcium).

Malabsorption contributes to low levels of vitamin A, β-carotene, and vitamin B_{12}. Some patients require parenteral vitamin B_{12} supplementation. Malabsorption of medications is also common and may necessitate much larger drug doses. Monitoring of drug blood levels, clinical response, or both is the best means of adjusting drug dosages.

Intestinal adaptation (increased length and thickness of jejunum and ileum) takes place after surgery and may explain regain of weight in some patients. Other complications of jejunoileal bypass include a 60-fold increased risk of tuberculosis and an increased risk of systemic fungal infections, such as coccidioidomycosis. Intestinal bypasses are rarely performed today because of the unacceptable long-term nutritional and medical consequences.[98]

ADVERSE EFFECTS OF WEIGHT LOSS

Weight loss, especially rapid weight loss, has been associated with a number of adverse effects.[32] Most of the effects result from nutrient deficiencies related to decreased food intake. Rapid weight loss in obese patients increases the risk for gallstone formation and cholecystitis. Interestingly, the lithogenicity of bile, which is elevated in obesity, is increased further during weight loss. Once weight loss is achieved, the risk diminishes. Other adverse effects of weight loss include loss of lean body mass, cardiac arrhythmias, water loss (diuresis), disturbances of electrolytes (potassium, magnesium, phosphorus, calcium, sodium), liver dysfunction, elevated uric acid levels, constipation, hypotension, hair loss, cold intolerance, and immune compromise.

NUTRITIONAL SUPPORT

Despite the presence of excess body fat and preserved lean body mass, obese patients are similar to other critically ill patients when it comes to nutritional support. Protein-calorie malnutrition and mineral-vitamin deficiencies can develop quickly after critical illness. It is not advisable for these patients to lose weight during critical illness (unless weight loss is part of their therapy). Priorities of the underlying illness and healing take precedence over weight loss. In addition, underlying malnutrition is common in obese patients despite their increased weight and predisposes to increased morbidity and mortality.

Although there are no clinical trials of early feeding in obese critically ill patients alone, it is reasonable to extrapolate from early feeding trials in critically ill patients because many of the patients were obese. These trials indicate that outcome is improved with early nutritional support (see Chapter 79).

Equations for the calculation of energy and protein requirements are unreliable for obese patients.[99] Indirect calorimetry can be useful for the estimation of energy intake. If calorimetry is not available, we recommend giving 25 to 30 kcal/kg ideal body weight (IBW) per day and 1.2 to 1.5 g protein/kg IBW per day. Enteral nutrition should be the primary route of nutritional support for the obese patient.

If weight loss is desirable (e.g., in a patient with obesity-hypoventilation syndrome), hypocaloric nutrition can be used to treat obese patients. Dickerson and colleagues[100] demonstrated that nitrogen balance could be achieved in mild to moderately stressed obese patients receiving hypocaloric nutritional support (average intake 15 kcal/kg IBW per day and 2.1 g protein/kg IBW per day). Over 48 days, patients lost 10 kg of body weight. Burge and coworkers[101] performed a prospective randomized double-blind study of hypocaloric nutritional support in obese hospitalized patients (50% energy expenditure; 2 g protein/kg IBW per day). More than 90% of patients achieved positive nitrogen balance without adverse effects. Hypocaloric feeding also improves glucose control in diabetic patients.

The aim of hypocaloric feeding is to allow patients to mobilize fat for energy while sparing protein. Administration of exogenous protein or growth hormone attenuates tissue protein losses. Hypocaloric nutrition and growth hormone administration have been shown to diminish protein loss in patients after surgery and trauma. However, the effect of hypocaloric nutrition[100-102] with or without growth hormone on outcome in critically ill patients has not been studied. Hormonal alterations during critical illness impair the body's response to growth hormone. Thus, we use only hypocaloric nutrition (with added protein) for patients whose illness (e.g., obesity-hypoventilation syndrome) would be ameliorated by weight reduction.

DRUG DOSING

The distribution, metabolism, protein binding, and clearance of drugs may be altered in the obese patient, independent of underlying disease.[103-109] Certainly, administering drugs (e.g., digoxin, aminophylline, aminoglycosides, cyclosporine) on the basis of actual body weight can result in overdosing and toxic effects. The enteral absorption of drugs is usually normal in the obese patient. However, plasma factors (e.g., lipoproteins, triglycerides, cholesterol, free fatty acids) that bind to plasma transport proteins can alter protein binding of drugs.[110, 111] The volume of distribution (V_d) of drugs is clearly altered in obesity, especially that of lipophilic agents. The V_d of weakly lipophilic drugs (e.g., aminoglycosides, quinolones) is moderately increased in obesity, but the V_d of highly lipophilic agents (e.g., benzodiazepines, verapamil, sufentanil) is significantly increased. The clearance of most hepatically metabolized drugs is not reduced in obesity. Hepatic clearance of methylprednisolone and propranolol, however, is reduced in obesity.[104-112] The clearance of renally cleared drugs depends on the glomerular filtration rate, which is frequently increased in obese patients. Because of underlying disease, however, glomerular filtration may be decreased in obesity. Because of the complex nature of altered drug pharmacokinetics in obesity, we recommend close monitoring of drug levels and clinical endpoints of drug action in these patients.

SUMMARY

The impact of obesity on outcome and resource utilization in the ICU has not been studied. However, on the basis of limited studies[113-115] and clinical experience, it is generally believed that obesity contributes to increased morbidity and mortality, increased length of stay, and increased costs of critical illness.

References

1. Rosenbaum M, Leibel RL, Hirsch J: Obesity. N Engl J Med 1997; 337:396-407.
2. Kuczmarski RJ, Flegal KM, Campbell SM, Johnson CL: Increasing prevalence of overweight among US adults. JAMA 1994; 272:205-211.
3. Van Itallie TB: Prevalence of obesity. Endocrinol Metab Clin North Am 1996; 25:887-905.
4. National Task Force on the Prevention and Treatment of Obesity: Long term pharmacotherapy in the management of obesity. JAMA 1996; 276:1907-1915.
5. Wolf AM, Colditz GA: The cost of obesity: The US perspective. Pharmacoeconomics 1994; 5(Suppl):34-37.
6. Colditz GA: Economic costs of obesity. Am J Clin Nutr 1992; 55(Suppl):503-507.
7. Wadden TA: Treatment of obesity by moderate and severe caloric restriction: Results of clinical trials. Ann Intern Med 1993; 229:688-693.
8. Van Itallie T: Health implications of overweight and obesity in the United States. Ann Intern Med 1985; 103:983-988.
9. Sjostrom L: Morbidity and mortality of severely obese subjects. Am J Clin Nutr 1992; 55(Suppl):508-515.
10. Bray GA: Health hazards of obesity. Endocrinol Metab Clin North Am 1996; 25:907-919.
11. National Institutes of Health Consensus Development Panel on the Health Implications of Obesity: Health implications of obesity: National Institues of Health Consensus Development Conference Statement. Ann Intern Med 1985; 103:1073-1078.
12. Choban PS, Heckler R, Burge J, et al: Nosocomial infections in obese surgical patients. Am Surg 1995; 61:1001-1005.
13. Choban PS, Maynes C, Weireter LJ: Obesity and increased mortality in blunt trauma. J Trauma 1991; 31:1253-1257.
14. Geiselman PJ: Control of food intake. Endocrinol Metab Clin North Am 1996; 25:815-829.
15. Halaas JL, Gajiwala KS, Maffei M, et al: Weight-reducing effects of the plasma protein encoded by the obese gene. Science 1995; 269:543-546.
16. Collins S, Kuhn CM, Petro AE, Swick AG, Chrunyk BA, Surwit RS: Role of leptin in fat regulation. Nature 1996; 380:677.
17. Pelleymounter MA, Cullen M, Baker MJ, et al: Effects of the obese gene product on body weight regulation in *ob/ob* mice. Science 1995; 269:540-543.
18. Perusse L, Changon YC, Bouchard C: The human obesity gene map: The 1996 update. Obes Res 1997; 5:49-61.
19. DeLany JP, Lovejoy JC: Energy expenditure. Endocrinol Metab Clin North Am 1996; 25:831-846.
20. Vaughan RW, Conaham TJI: Part I: Cardiopulmonary consequences of morbid obesity. Life Sci 1980; 26:2119-2127.
21. Backman L, Freyschuss U, Hallbert D, et al: Cardiovascular function in extreme obesity. Acta Med Scand 1983; 149:437-439.
22. DeDivitus O, Fazio S, Pateto M, et al: Obesity and cardiac function. Circulation 1981; 64:477-480.
23. Rexrode KM, Manson JE, Hennekens CH: Obesity and cardiovascular disease. Curr Opin Cardiol 1996; 11:490-495.
24. Lauer MS, Anderson KM, Kannel WB, et al: The impact of obesity on left ventricular mass and geometry: The Framingham Heart Study. JAMA 1991; 266:231-236.
25. Berkalp B, Cesur V, Corapcioglu D, et al: Obesity and left ventricular diastolic dysfunction. Int J Cardiol 1995; 52:23-26.
26. Pi-Sunyer FX: Medical hazards of obesity. Ann Intern Med 1993; 119(Suppl):655-660.
27. Nakajma T, Fujioka S, Tokunaga K, et al: Noninvasive study of left ventricular performance in obese patients: Influence of duration of obesity. Circulation 1985; 7:481-486.
28. Alpert MA, Singh A, Terry BE, et al: Effect of exercise on left ventricular systolic function and reserve in morbid obesity. Am J Cardiol 1989; 63:1478-1482.
29. Licata G, Scaglione R, Barbagallo M: Effect of obesity on left ventricular function studied by radionuclide angiocardiography. Int J Obes 1991; 15:295-302.
30. Merlino G, Scaglione R, Carrao S, et al: Association between reduced lymphocyte beta-adrenergic receptors and left ventricular dysfunction in young obese subjects. Int J Obes Relat Metab Disord 1994; 18:699-703.
31. Merlino G, Scaglione R, Paterna S, et al: Lymphocyte beta-adrenergic receptors in young subjects with peripheral or central obesity: Relationship with central haemodynamics and left ventricular function. Eur Heart J 1994; 15:786-792.
32. Pi-Sunyer FX: Short-term medical benefits and adverse effects of weight loss. Ann Intern Med 1993; 119(Suppl):722-726.
33. Marik P, Varon J: The obese patient in the ICU. Chest 1998; 113:492-498.
34. Ray C, Sue D, Bray G, et al: Effects of obesity on respiratory function. Am Rev Respir Dis 1983; 128:501-506.
35. Thomas PS, Cowen ERT, Hulands G, et al: Respiratory function in the morbidly obese before and after weight loss. Thorax 1989; 44:382-386.
36. Collins LC, Hoberty PD, Walker JF, et al: The effect of body fat distribution on pulmonary function tests. Chest 1995; 107:1298-1302.
37. Douglas FG, Chong PY: Influence of obesity on peripheral airway patency. J Appl Physiol 1972; 33:559-563.
38. Holley HS, Milic-Emili J, Becklake MR, et al: Regional distribution of pulmonary ventilation and perfusion in obesity. J Clin Invest 1967; 46:475-481.
39. Vgontzas AN, Tan TL, Bixler EO, et al: Sleep apnea and sleep disruption in obese patients. Arch Intern Med 1994; 154:1705-1711.

40. Garay SM, Rapoport D, Sorkin B, Epstein H, Feinberg I, Goldring RM: Regulation of ventilation in the obstructive sleep apnea syndrome. Am Rev Respir Dis 1981; 124:451–457.
41. Sugerman HJ, Baron PL, Fairman RP, Evans CR, Vetrovec GW: Hemodynamic dysfunction in obesity hypoventilation syndrome and the effects of treatment with surgically induced weight loss. Ann Surg 1988; 207:604–613.
42. Williamson JA, Webb RK, Szekely S, et al: The Australian Incident Monitoring Study: Difficult intubation—an analysis of 2,000 incident reports. Anaesth Intensive Care 1993; 21:602–607.
43. Rose DK, Cohen MM, Wigglesworth DF, et al: Critical respiratory events in the postanesthesia care unit: Patient, surgical, and anesthetic factors. Anesthesiology 1994; 81:410–418.
44. Agarwal N, Shibutani K, San Filippo JA: Hemodynamic and respiratory changes in surgery of the morbidly obese. Surgery 1982; 92:226–233.
45. Pasulka PS, Bistrian BR, Benotti PN: The risks of surgery in obese patients. Ann Intern Med 1986; 104:540–546.
46. Goldhaber SZ, Goldstein E, Stampfer ML, et al: A prospective study of risk factors for pulmonary embolism in women. JAMA 1997; 227:642–645.
47. Clayton JK, Anderson JR, McNicol GP: Post-operative prediction of postoperative deep vein thrombosis. Br Med J 1976; 2:910–912.
48. Kakkar VV, Howe CT, Nicolaides AN, et al: Deep vein thrombosis of the leg: Is there a "high-risk" group? Am J Surg 1970; 120:527–530.
49. Bern MM, Bothe AJ, Bistrian B, et al: Effects of low-dose warfarin on antithrombin III levels in morbidly obese patients. Surgery 1983; 94:78–83.
50. Almer L, Janzon L: Low vascular fibrinolytic activity in obesity. Thromb Res 1975; 6:171–175.
51. Scheen AJ: Antiobesity drugs in the management of diabetes. Int Diabetes Monit 1997; 9:1–8.
52. Wing RR, Blair EH, Bonomi P, et al: Caloric restriction per se is a significant factor in improvement in glycemic control and insulin sensitivity during weight loss in obese NIDDM patients. Diabetes Care 1994; 17:30–36.
53. Letiexhe MR, Scheen AJ, Gerard PL, et al: Post-gastroplasty recovery of ideal body weight normalizes glucose and insulin metabolism in obese women. J Clin Endocrinol Metab 1995; 80:364–369.
54. Pories WJ, MacDonald KG, Flickinger EG, et al: Is type II diabetes (NIDDM) a surgical disease? Ann Surg 1992; 215:633–643.
55. Garfinkel L: Overweight and cancer. Ann Intern Med 1985; 103:1034–1036.
56. Leibel RL, Hirsch J, Appel BE, Checani GC: Energy intake required to maintain body weight is not affected by wide variation in diet composition. Am J Clin Nutr 1992; 55:350–355.
57. Wadden TA: Treatment of obesity by moderate and severe caloric restriction. Ann Intern Med 1993; 119(Suppl):688–693.
58. Silverstone T: Appetite suppressants—a review. Drugs 1992; 43:820–836.
59. Bray GA: Use and abuse of appetite-suppressant drugs in the treatment of obesity. Ann Intern Med 1993; 119(Suppl):707–713.
60. Bray GA, Ryan DH: Drugs used in the treatment of obesity. Diabetes Rev 1997; 5:83–103.
61. Atkinson RL: Use of drugs in the treatment of obesity. Annu Rev Nutr 1997; 17:383–403.
62. Salmela PI, Sotaniemi EA, Viikari J, et al: Fenfluramine therapy in non-insulin-dependent diabetic patients: Effects on body weight, glucose homeostasis, serum lipoproteins and antipyrine metabolism. Diabetes Care 1981; 4:535–540.
63. Davis R, Faulds D: Dexfenfluramine: An updated review of its therapeutic use in the management of obesity. Drugs 1996; 52:696–724.
64. Guy-Grand B, Crepaldi G, Lefebvre P, et al: International trial of long-term dexfenfluramine in obesity. Lancet 1989; 2:1142–1145.
65. Guy-Grand B: Clinical studies with dexfenfluramine: From past to future. Obes Res 1995; 3(Suppl):491–496.
66. Fuller RW, Wong DT: Fluoxetine: A serotonergic appetite suppressant drug. Drug Dev Res 1988; 17:1–15.
67. Wise SD: Clinical studies with fluoxetine in obesity. Am J Clin Nutr 1992; 55(Suppl):181–184.
68. Darga LL, Carroll-Michals L, Botsford SJ, Lucas CP: Fluoxetine's effect on weight loss in obese subjects. Am J Clin Nutr 1991; 54:321–325.
69. Douglas JG, Gough J, Preston PG, et al: Long term efficacy of fenfluramine in treatment of obesity. Lancet 1983; 1:384–386.
70. Guy-Grand B, Apfelbaum M, Crepaldi G, Gries A, Lefebvre P, Turner P: International trial of long-term dexfenfluramine in obesity. Lancet 1989; 2:1142–1145.
71. Weintraub M, Sundaresan PR, Schuster B, et al: Long term weight control study: I–VII. Clin Pharmacol Ther 1992; 51:581–646.
72. Abenhaim L, Moride Y, Brenot F, et al: Appetite-suppressant drugs and the risk of primary pulmonary hypertension. N Engl J Med 1996; 335:609–616.
73. McMurray J, Bloomfield P, Miller HC: Irreversible pulmonary hypertension after treatment with fenfluramine. Br Med J 1986; 292:239–240.
74. Atanassoff PG, Weiss BM, Schmid ER, Tornic M: Pulmonary hypertension and dexfenfluramine (Letter). Lancet 1992; 339:436.
75. Mark ES, Patalas ED, Chang HT, Evan RJ, Kessler SC: Fatal pulmonary hypertension associated with short term use of fenfluramine and phentermine. N Engl J Med 1997; 337:602–606.
76. Connolly HM, Crary JL, McGoon MD, et al: Valvular heart disease associated with fenfluramine-phentermine. N Engl J Med 1997; 337:581–588.
77. Rasmussen S, Corya BC, Glassman RD: Valvular heart disease associated with dexfenfluramine (Letter). N Engl J Med 1997; 337:636.
78. Cannistra LB, Davis SM, Bauman AG: Valvular heart disease associated with dexfenfluramine. N Engl J Med 1997; 337:636.
79. Marinella MA, Berrettoni BA: Digital necrosis associated with dexfenfluramine. N Engl J Med 1997; 337:1776.
80. Prate B, Spreux A, Chichmanian RM, et al: Ischémie subaigue distale du membre inférieur gauche au cours d'un traitement associant dexfenfluramine et minocycline. Therapie 1992; 47:438–439.
81. Evrard P: Myocardial infarction associated with dextrofenfluramine. BMJ 1990; 301:1050.
82. Turtle JR, Burgess JA: Hypoglycemic action of fenfluramine in diabetes mellitus. Diabetes 1973; 22:858–867.
83. Verdy M, Charbonneau L, Verdy I, et al: Fenfluramine in the treatment of non-insulin-dependent diabetics: Hypoglycemic versus anorectic effect. Int J Obes 1983; 7:289–297.
84. Scheen AJ, Paolisso G, Salvatore T, Lefebvre PJ: Improvement of insulin-induced glucose disposal in obese patients with NIDDM after 1-wk treatment with *d*-fenfluramine. Diabetes Care 1991; 14:325–332.
85. Bray GA, Ryan DH, Gordon D, et al: A double-blind randomized placebo-controlled trial of sibutramine. Obes Res 1996; 4:263–270.
86. Himms-Hagen J, Danforth E: The potential role of B_3-adrenoceptor agonists in the treatment of obesity and diabetes. Curr Opin Endocrinol Diabetes 1996; 3:59–65.
87. Arch JRS, Wilson S: Prospects for β_3-adrenoceptor agonists in the treatment of obesity and diabetes. Int J Obes 1996; 20:191–199.
88. Drent ML, Van der Veen EA: Lipase inhibition. A novel concept in the treatment of obesity. Int J Obes 1993; 7:241–244.
89. Drent ML, Larsson I, William-Olsson T, et al: Orlistat (RO1-8-0647), a lipase inhibitor, in the treatment of human obesity: A multiple dose study. Int J Obes Relat Metab Disord 1995; 19:221–226.
90. Caro JF, Sinha MK, Kolaczynski JW, et al: Leptin—the tale of an obesity gene. Diabetes 1996; 45:1455–1462.
91. Sugarman HJ, Londrey GL, Kellum JM, et al: Weight loss with vertical banded gastroplasty and Roux-Y gastric bypass for morbid obesity with selective versus random assignment. Am J Surg 1989; 157:93–102.
92. Pories WJ, Swanson MS, MacDonald KG, et al: Who would have thought it? An operation proves to be the most effective therapy for adult-onset diabetes mellitus. Ann Surg 1995; 222:339–352.
93. Printen KJ, Halverson JD: Hemic micronutrients following vertical banded gastroplasty. Am Surg 1988; 54:267–268.
94. Halverson JD: Metabolic risk of obesity surgery and long term follow up. Am J Clin Nutr 1992; 55:602S–605S.
95. Halverson JD: Micronutrient deficiencies after gastric bypass for morbid obesity. Am Surg 1986; 52:594–598.

96. Avinoah E, Ovnat A, Charuzi I: Nutritional status seven years after Roux-en-Y gastric bypass surgery. Surgery 1992; 111:137–142.
97. Greenway FL: Surgery for obesity. Endocrinol Metab Clin North Am 1996; 25:1005–1027.
98. Kirkpatrik JR: Jejunoileal bypass: A legacy of late complications. Arch Surg 1987; 122:610–614.
99. Choban PS, Burge JC, Flancbaum L: Nutrition support of obese hospitalized patients. Nutr Clin Pract 1997; 12:149–154.
100. Dickerson RN, Rosato EF, Mullen JL: Net protein anabolism with hypocaloric parenteral nutrition in obese stressed patients. Am J Clin Nutr 1986; 44:747–755.
101. Burge JC, Goon A, Choban PS, et al: Efficacy of hypocaloric total parenteral nutrition in hospitalized obese patients: A prospective, double-blind randomized trial. JPEN J Parenter Enteral Nutr 1994; 18:203–207.
102. Baxter JK, Bistrian BR: Moderate hypocaloric parenteral nutrition in the critically ill obese patient. Nutr Clin Pract 1989; 4:133–135.
103. Abernethy DR, Greenblatt DL: Drug disposition in obese humans: An update. Clin Pharmacokinet 1986; 11:199–213.
104. Cheymol G: Clinical pharmacokinetics of drugs in obesity: An update. Clin Pharmacokinet 1993; 25:103–114.
105. Blouin RA, Kolpek JH, Mann HJ: Influence of obesity on drug disposition. Clin Pharm 1987; 6:706–714.
106. Li L, Miles MV, Lakkis H, et al: Vancomycin-binding characteristics in patients with serious infections. Pharmacotherapy 1996; 16:1024–1029.
107. Zahorska-Markiewicz B, Waluga M, Zielinski M, et al: Pharmacokinetics of theophylline in obesity. Int J Clin Pharmacol Ther 1996; 34:393–395.
108. Flechner SM, Kolbeinsson ME, Tam J, et al: The impact of body weight on cyclosporine pharmacokinetics in renal transplant recipients. Transplantation 1989; 47:806–810.
109. Traynor AM, Nafziger AN: Aminoglycoside dosing weight correction factors for patients of various body sizes. Antimicrob Agents Chemother 1995; 39:545–548.
110. Wasan KM, Lopex-Berestein G: The influence of serum lipoproteins on the pharmacokinetics and pharmacodynamics of lipophilic drugs and drug carriers. Arch Med Res 1993; 24:395–401.
111. Suh B, Craig WA, England AC, et al: Effect of free fatty acids on the protein binding of antimicrobial agents. J Infect Dis 1981; 143:986–997.
112. Morgan DJ, Bray M: Lean body mass as a predictor of drug dosage: Implications for drug therapy. Clin Pharmacokinet 1994; 26:292–307.
113. Smith-Choban P, Weireter LJ, Maynes C: Obesity and increased mortality in blunt trauma. J Trauma 1991; 31:1253–1257.
114. Rose DK, Cohen MM, Wigglesworth DF, et al: Critical respiratory events in the postanesthesia care unit: Patient, surgical and anesthetic factors. Anesthesiology 1994; 81:410–418.
115. Goldhaber SZ, Goldstein E, Stampfer ML, et al: A prospective study of risk factors for pulmonary embolism. JAMA 1997; 277:642–645.

D. Pharmacology

85

Sedatives and Analgesics in Critical Care

Angela M. Hadbavny, MS, PharmD • John W. Hoyt, MD

RATIONALE FOR USE OF SEDATION AND ANALGESIA IN THE INTENSIVE CARE UNIT

The typical intensive care unit (ICU) is not a calm, restful place. Even in the most modern ICU constructed to provide a more humane environment, patients are immersed in a whirlwind of noise, equipment, people, and activity. Personal space and autonomy are violated. Patients are often restrained in bed because they are attached to equipment and intravascular lines. Severe illness, pain, anxiety, fear, inability to communicate adequately with ICU personnel, and possible psychiatric problems may be present in the critically ill and may result in the development of delirium.[1] Besides improvement of the environment, other nonpharmacologic measures to minimize the development of agitation and delirium include frequent communication with and orientation of patients and maintenance of a normal wake-sleep cycle. Simple massage and back rubs have been shown to promote sleep and to provide some pain relief.[2, 3]

Despite nonpharmacologic measures, most ICU patients require some form of sedation and often pain medication to make their hospital stay more comfortable and to promote safety and compliance with therapeutic measures, such as mechanical ventilation. Perhaps the most important part of managing agitation, anxiety, delirium, and pain in the critically ill patient is to try to identify and treat the underlying cause. Metabolic derangements, hypoxia, infections, combinations of drugs, withdrawal from drugs, and severe pain can make a patient agitated, delirious, and uncooperative. Administering sedatives may only make a patient with persistent pain more confused, less able to communicate, and more difficult to treat. If possible, one should address the underlying cause of the pain or discomfort rather than just treat the symptoms. For adequate assessment and treatment of a patient, sedatives and analgesics must often be given before complete information about a patient's condition is available. As soon as possible, however, the physiologic problems should be addressed. This may remove the need for sedatives and analgesics. The classic example is the elderly patient who is perfectly functional under normal circumstances but who gets an infection and becomes confused and delirious. When the fever and infection are gone, the patient's behavior returns to normal.

In terminally ill patients, although the disease may not be curable, pain, delirium, and dyspnea should be treated and patients made comfortable until their death.[4] Unfortunately, reports of inadequate sedation of patients therapeutically paralyzed with neuromuscular blocking agents, which have no effect on central nervous system (CNS) sensory or cognitive function, demonstrate that the need for adequate sedation, preferably with amnesic and analgesic properties, cannot be overemphasized.[5] One way to ensure adequate sedation in paralyzed patients is to use bedside-processed electroencephalographic monitoring. This type of electroencephalogram (EEG) cannot be used to show seizure activity but can indicate whether a patient is awake or asleep and has been in use in the operating room by anesthesiologists for years.[6, 7]

The choice of which sedatives and analgesics to use in ICU patients has in recent years become controversial. Good randomized clinical studies elucidating and comparing the pharmacokinetics and pharmacodynamics of these drugs in critically ill patients are scarce. Much of the published literature on sedation and analgesia is more applicable to the non-ICU patient or the nonhospitalized patient. For example, respiratory depression is a major concern with these drugs in spontaneously breathing patients but is much less important in the ICU. Pain is a subjective problem best explained by the person having it. The critical care health professional must anticipate and treat pain, anxiety, and delirium in patients who often cannot communicate the reason for their agitation. The desired endpoints of therapy are difficult to quantitate and vary according to the population of patient's and the practices of the health care institution.

Several evaluation tools or scales are available for assessing the depth of sedation or pain intensity that permit titration of drug therapy according to some measurable endpoint.[2, 6, 8] The choice of sedative agent or analgesic is usually a function of the physician's prior training and clinical experience and the guidelines and formulary of the health system in which he or she practices. In this age of managed care and cost containment, the cost of individual agents along with the overall clinical status of the patient should be considered. The Society of Critical Care Medicine has published an excellent set of practice parameters for intravenous (IV) analgesia and sedation for adult ICU patients.[9] However, because critically ill patients and their continually changing conditions may respond differently to similar treatments, the clinician should learn about several sedative and analgesic agents and be aware of possible adverse events associated with their use. Doses should be titrated to adequately manage the patient's problems but avoid toxicities due to impaired drug elimination. The intensivist should also be aware that there are adjunctive therapeutic agents that may not be part of the usual ICU armamentarium of agents but may be efficacious and even necessary for adequate management of agitation, delirium, and especially pain.[10] The most commonly used sedatives and analgesics are discussed with emphasis on indications for their use, contraindications, and adverse effects common to critically ill patients.

ANALGESICS

General Concepts About Pain and Its Assessment

Pain is an unpleasant and emotional sensory experience associated with potential or actual tissue damage. Pain and suffering are private, subjective, and internal experiences that are not directly observable or measurable. It is difficult to objectively assess or measure pain. Whenever possible, pain assessment should involve the patient's own report describing the type, location, and severity of the pain. Instruments such as the visual analog scale (VAS) numerical rating scales, behavioral rating scales, and other questionnaires may be used to quantitate the severity of pain and the response to analgesic therapy.[8] In a critically ill patient, communication may be hampered; therefore, physiologic signs of pain, such as increased heart rate, blood pressure, palmar sweating, or tears (crying), must often be used as indicators of pain. The injury, pathologic process, or disease causing the pain should obviously be identified and treated if possible. Analgesics are used to provide symptomatic relief.

There are three types of pain:

1. *Somatic* pain results from activation of somatic afferent nerves without injury to peripheral nerves or the CNS. Somatic pain is typically well localized.
2. *Visceral* pain results from activation of visceral nociceptors and is a deep, aching, cramping sensation.
3. *Neuropathic* pain results from direct injury to peripheral receptors, nerves, or the CNS. Neuropathic pain tends to be severe, burning, shooting, lancinating, or dysesthetic in character and is difficult to control with standard opioid analgesics.[11]

The initial pain sensation resulting from tissue injury is amplified and prolonged by the release of inflammatory mediators, such as prostaglandins, cytokines, histamine, serotonin, and substance P, and by resetting of the sensitivity of nerves involved in pain sensation.[12] The actions of some analgesics, for example, nonsteroidal anti-inflammatory drugs (NSAIDs) and steroids, involve decreasing the effects of inflammatory mediators. Other analgesics, such as opioids, anticonvulsants, local anesthetics, antidepressants, and alpha$_2$ agonists, act through receptors in the CNS or by modulation of neuronal transmission of pain or its perception.

Standard Routes of Administration for Analgesia

In the ICU, analgesia is generally provided by the IV route; however, some analgesia may be administered epidurally, intrathecally, through feeding tubes, or orally. Rectal administration is sometimes used in outpatients who cannot take oral medications, with bioavailability similar to that with oral administration. The intramuscular (IM) route is generally not used for administering any medications in the ICU. IM injections are painful, cause muscle damage, and most importantly result in unpredictable drug absorption in critically ill patients. Continuous subcutaneous infusions are used outside the hospital usually for patients with no IV access.[13]

Alternative Routes

Transdermal and Intranasal Analgesia

The transdermal and intranasal routes of analgesic administration are a more recent development. Only one analgesic, *fentanyl,* is available in the United States for transdermal administration. The patches deliver 25 μg/hr per 10 cm^2 and come in doses of 25, 50, 75, and 100 μg/hr that deliver fentanyl for up to 72 hours.[11] Transdermal fentanyl is effective for outpatient maintenance therapy; however, problems with using the patches include high cost and the dose is not easily titratable with slow onset and offset of effect. Patients require supplemental doses of analgesics for the 12 to 24 hours required for the patch to take effect. There is also a prolongation of fentanyl elimination after removal of the patch because of a subcutaneous depot of drug.[14]

Butorphanol, a partial opioid agonist pharmacologically similar to pentazocine and nalbuphine, is available in a nasal spray. Transnasal butorphanol has been used to relieve migraine headaches in outpatients and occasionally used postoperatively for moderate to severe pain in patients with fractures.[14] Butorphanol and other partial agonists and mixed agonist-antagonist opioids are generally not recommended for use in ICU patients because these medications may precipitate opioid withdrawal in patients who have been receiving chronic opioid therapy and may also cause psychotomimetic effects.[9, 13] Transnasal butorphanol at a dose of 1 or 2 mg (2 mg given as a 1 mg puff in each nostril) every 4 to 6 hours may be useful in treating opioid-induced persistent pruritus that does not respond to administration of antihistamines.[15] There is one report of apraxia, reversible with naloxone, after a single dose of intranasal butorphanol that rendered the patient unable to speak or move.[16]

Patient-Controlled Analgesia

Patient-controlled analgesia (PCA) may be used for administration of the analgesic agent by either the IV or epidural route. PCA requires an alert, cooperative patient who can press the button to deliver a demand dose of medication from a preprogrammed, securely locked pump. PCA pumps have limited utility in critically ill patients except perhaps in treating postoperative pain. The patient should be given a loading dose of the analgesic agent to provide pain relief, and then the pump is set to deliver subsequent boluses of medication on demand. There is a time lockout interval programmed to prevent dosing prematurely. Typical PCA pump IV morphine doses range from 0.5 to 3 mg with a lockout period of 5 to 20 minutes. A typical PCA fentanyl IV dosing regimen would be boluses of 15 to 50 μg with a lockout period of 3 to 10 minutes.[17] Some PCA pumps are capable of giving a background continuous infusion of analgesic. The infusion lowers the safety factor in using PCA to prevent overdose; however, patients with high opioid requirements due to chronic pain or those with frequently interrupted sleep may benefit.[18]

With *patient-controlled epidural analgesia* (PCEA), less opioid analgesia is necessary to give pain relief. An opioid, such as morphine sulfate or fentanyl alone or combined with the local anesthetic bupivacaine, have been administered by PCEA.[19] The satisfaction of patients with PCA is high because control over analgesia is maintained by the patient to match pain intensity.

Epidural and Intrathecal Methods for Delivery of Analgesia

Spinal Anatomy

A brief clarification of the *neuraxial* routes of delivery of analgesia is warranted. The spinal cord is covered by three membranes and the outermost bony structure and ligaments of the vertebral column. The innermost membrane covering the spinal cord is the pia mater, which is rich in vascular supply. Moving outward, one finds the next membrane, the arachnoid mater. In between the pia mater and arachnoid mater is the *subarachnoid space* or *intrathecal space,* which contains cerebrospinal fluid (CSF) and is the site of intrathecal injection.

The next layer above the arachnoid mater is the dura mater, a tough membrane. The narrow space between the dura mater and the arachnoid mater is filled with lymph. The arachnoid is so close to the dura that when the dura is punctured, the arachnoid is also punctured and the subarachnoid space is entered. The *epidural,* peridural, or extradural space is located between the bony and ligamentous walls of the spinal canal and outer surface of the dura mater. The epidural space contains nerve roots, fat tissue with a rich capillary supply, and a valveless venous system that connects with the intracranial venous sinuses and pelvic venous supply. The epidural space narrows as it ascends; therefore, a given volume of injected agent will affect a greater number of segments when it is injected into the cervical and thoracic spinal regions compared with the lumber regions.

When a drug is injected into the epidural space, usually only a small amount (~4% for morphine) penetrates the dura and gets into the CSF to affect the spinal cord and nerve roots. Drugs distribute into epidural fat and epidural veins and are absorbed systemically.[20] In general, the epidural route of administration is less likely than the intrathecal route to cause serious adverse effects; however, the intrathecal route provides more potent analgesia with smaller doses of drug.

Complications

Some complications of epidural catheter placement and injection[20] include:

- Inadvertent dural puncture
- Infection
- Bleeding
- Catheter migration
- Inappropriate drug injection

Inadvertent dural puncture can result in administration of drug intrathecally, causing unexpected hemodynamic changes or respiratory arrest. If a catheter is inadvertently placed through the dura, it may be used as an intrathecal catheter provided all drug doses are adjusted appropriately and personnel are aware of the catheter's actual location. Inadvertent dural puncture may result in headache, which should be treated with increased oral or IV fluid intake, supine position, analgesics, and placement of a blood patch (injecting autologous blood at the site of the puncture injury). If the dural puncture occurs above the L-2 level, spinal injury may result.

Strict aseptic technique for placement and maintenance of epidural and intrathecal catheters is extremely important to prevent meningitis and epidural abscess. Bleeding during placement or after removal of an epidural catheter may result in an epidural or subarachnoid hematoma. Symptoms of hematoma include sensory and motor deficits, paralysis, or bladder and bowel incontinence.[20] Back pain is not always present with subarachnoid or epidural hematoma. Hemorrhage is more likely if anticoagulants such as low-molecular-weight heparins have been administered or the patient has a bleeding diathesis.[14, 21]

Migration of an epidural catheter can result in loss of analgesia, unilateral analgesia, decreased dermatomal spread (local anesthetic agents), or increased toxicity if the catheter has gone intravascular. Intravascular injections of local anesthetic agents can cause seizures, cardiac arrhythmias, and cardiac arrest.

Inadvertent injection of drugs intended for IV injection into epidural or intrathecal catheters can result in serious problems, including paralysis. Only preservative-free products intended for epidural injection should be used. Injection ports should be covered and properly labeled.[20]

Neuraxial Analgesic Pharmacology

Lipid solubility of a drug is directly related to its speed of onset, extent of dermatomal spread, and duration of analgesia when it is given epidurally. Morphine, which is highly hydrophilic, spreads rostrally and has a long onset of action: fentanyl, which is lipophilic, is exactly the opposite in its activity. Morphine tends to provide a wider area of analgesia and can cause more centrally mediated adverse effects, such as delayed respiratory depression. Fentanyl, because of its high lipid solubility, tends to have a rapid onset of analgesia, a more localized action, and a better safety profile when it is administered epidurally.[14] The onset of action of epidurally administered local anesthetics can be accelerated by prior injection of sodium bicarbonate, which raises pH and causes local anesthetic molecules to become unionized and able to rapidly diffuse across the dura to the site of action.[20]

Analgesic agents may be injected epidurally or intrathecally by either (1) *bolus injection* or (2) *continuous infusion.*

Bolus injection eliminates the need for an infusion pump; however, the risk of adverse events is higher than with continuous infusion because of rapid attainment of high peak drug concentrations. Continuous infusions tend to provide a constant level of analgesia with lower incidence of respiratory depression.[20]

Important risk factors for development of respiratory depression after epidural injection of analgesics[22] include:

- Older age
- Concomitant administration of other oral or parenteral sedatives or opioids
- Thoracic surgery or prolonged surgery
- Unintentional subarachnoid injection

Epidural administration of bupivacaine has resulted in respiratory arrest and death in opioid-tolerant patients. The mechanism appears to be removal of the pain stimulus that normally drives respiration and prevents respiratory depression.[23] Monitoring of respiratory rate (<10 breaths/min) and level of consciousness is usually adequate to detect respiratory depression. Ongoing respiratory monitoring is recommended for 12 hours after bolus injection of morphine and for the duration of a continuous infusion of opioid. Continuous monitoring may be discontinued after discontinuation of the continuous infusion.[22]

Opioid Analgesics

Analgesic Effects

Opioids, particularly morphine and fentanyl, are the most widely used class of analgesic agents in the ICU. Opioids bind to specific receptors located in the spinal cord and brain and alter nociceptive transmission and modulate pain. Opiate receptors are classified into five types: mu_1 and mu_2, kappa, delta, epsilon, and sigma. Binding of opiate agonists to CNS mu receptors results in analgesia and sedation plus the side effects of respiratory depression, constipation, urinary retention, confusion, miosis, bradycardia, euphoria, and nausea.[9, 20] Opioid receptors have been demonstrated in peripheral tissues, such as inflamed knee joints. *Intra-articular* injection of small doses of opioids (e.g., 5 to 6 mg morphine), provides long-lasting pain relief that is reversible by naloxone.[18] Opioid analgesics should generally be given on a continuous or scheduled intermittent basis, with as-needed supplemental or bolus doses. A loading or bolus dose to attain therapeutic blood levels should be administered IV before a continuous infusion is started.[9]

Unfortunately, critically ill patients (and pain patients in general) often receive inadequate pain control because of unwarranted fears of narcotic addiction or side effects.[9, 11, 14] Previous exposure to opioids, either illicit or prescribed for chronic pain, can lead to physical *tolerance.*[24] Tolerance in ICU patients may also be manifested by the requirement for increasing doses of opioids to maintain analgesia and accommodation to side effects such as sedation.[25] Opioid-tolerant ICU patients should be given sufficient oral or IV opioids to prevent withdrawal and additional opioids or other analgesics to provide adequate analgesia.[26, 27] Epidural analgesia alone may relieve pain but is often insufficient to prevent withdrawal in opioid-tolerant patients; consequently, additional systemic opioid may be needed.[14]

Because analgesia produced by opioids generally does not have a ceiling effect, increasing doses produce increased analgesia.[13] In some patients with chronic pain, especially patients with neuropathic pain that is treated with morphine, *hyperalgesia* may occur. Hyperalgesia is a centrally mediated phenomenon in which pain increases when morphine is given through a reversal of postsynaptic inhibition. Hyperalgesia does not appear to occur with opioids that are not conjugated in the liver, such as fentanyl, sufentanil, alfentanil, and methadone.[28, 29] *Myoclonus* may also occur in patients receiving morphine and is treatable by changing to alternative opioid therapy or by adding clonazepam.[27–29]

Patients with neuropathic pain due to terminal illness or nonmalignant pain who no longer obtain adequate analgesia from epidural or intrathecal opioids alone may obtain pain relief from the addition of epidural or intrathecal administration of the $alpha_2$ agonist clonidine or a local anesthetic such as bupivacaine.[30–32] Epidural *clonidine* is infused at rates of 12.5 to 70 μg/hr or intrathecally at 8 to 400 μg/day.[30, 31] Limited data in patients with terminal cancer who have lost their response to morphine indicate that addition of subanesthetic doses of *ketamine* dramatically relieves pain. Ketamine acts at the NMDA (*N*-methyl-D-aspartate) receptor, which promotes development of hyperalgesia.[10, 33] Ketamine is similar to phencyclidine (PCP) and may cause terrifying hallucinations, necessitating coadministration of haloperidol, droperidol, or benzodiazepines. It is thus recommended for use only when other analgesic options are ineffective.[9, 10, 33, 34]

Side Effects

Opioids cause a number of troublesome side effects that may sometimes be lessened by changing to an opioid of a different structural class. True allergic reactions to opioids are rare; however, some opioids, especially morphine, meperidine, and codeine, may cause histamine release with accompanying flushing, itching, and urticaria.[14] Pruritus that is caused by opioids is usually not a histamine-mediated problem. Pruritus is due to direct effects of opioids at the medulla and trigeminal nerve.[29] Antihistamines may give some relief because of sedative effects. Itching not relieved by antihistamines, especially in patients receiving spinal or epidural opioids, can be treated by administering small doses of *naloxone* or a continuous low-dose IV naloxone infusion. Injection of small doses of a mixed opiate agonist-antagonist, such as 2.5 mg IV or 10 mg subcutaneous *nalbuphine* or intranasal *butorphanol,* has been used to relieve itching.[14, 15, 20, 29]

Respiratory depression, airway obstruction, and loss of airway protective reflexes should be monitored in ICU patients treated with opioids by observance of arterial oxygen saturation with pulse oximetry and by close attention to respiratory rate.[9] Respiratory depression can be reversed by the opiate antagonist naloxone.[14, 29] Clinicians should be aware that the stimulant drugs *methylphenidate* (Ritalin) and *dextroamphetamine* are sometimes used for patients with chronic pain or cancer-related pain to counteract excessive sedation and possible respiratory depression while also providing enhanced analgesia.[11, 13]

Gastrointestinal symptoms, including nausea, vomiting, gastric retention, ileus, and constipation, are common and may respond to standard pharmacologic treatments (e.g., antiemetics, metoclopramide, cisapride, laxatives); however, ileus is usually unresponsive to treatment in ICU patients. Severe nausea and vomiting can be relieved by small doses of naloxone or nalbuphine if other therapies fail.[13, 14, 29] A new peripherally acting agent, *methylnaltrexone,* should be available shortly to safely relieve some gastrointestinal adverse effects of opioids, such as delayed gastric emptying and constipation.[35] With use of naloxone, only small injections of 0.1 to 0.2 mg should be administered to prevent precipitation of withdrawal or loss of pain control.[14]

Morphine and Hydromorphone

Morphine is the naturally occurring prototype opiate that is widely used for pain control in the United States. It is inexpensive and is available in a variety of dosage forms. Morphine is metabolized in the liver and conjugated to produce *morphine-6-glucuronide,* an active metabolite with potent sedative and analgesic activity that is eliminated through the kidneys. Morphine and its metabolite accumulate in patients with hepatic or renal impairment, causing prolonged sedation.[36, 37] The onset of action of a single IV dose of morphine is relatively slow, about 5 to 10 minutes, because of low lipid solubility.[17] The duration of action is 2 to 7 hours. Morphine can cause vasodilation and hypotension, especially if it is injected rapidly in a patient with insufficient intravascular volume.[37]

Morphine is known to cause spasm of the sphincter of Oddi, and many physicians do not use it in patients with pancreatic or biliary tract disease. *Meperidine* has been the preferred analgesic in these patients because it has little effect on smooth muscle, but this has not been demonstrated in clinical studies.[13, 38] It has been suggested that patients suffering from pain due to pancreatitis may be treated with mixed agonist-antagonist opioids. These agents do not cause spasm,[38]; however, agonist-antagonist opioids may precipitate withdrawal or reverse pain control in patients previously treated with opioid agonists, such as meperidine and morphine.[9, 13, 27]

Starting doses of morphine in opioid-naieve patients are 1 to 15 mg IV bolus, and starting continuous IV infusion rates are 1 to 20 mg/hour.[17, 37] Because of extreme pain and the development of tolerance, patients have been known to require 7 g of morphine per day.[39] Epidural morphine continuous infusion rates start at 0.1 to 1.5 mg/hr.[20] Because of its analgesic, sedative, and euphoric effects, morphine is often administered to dying patients to relieve pain and dyspnea.[4] Dying patients not already receiving morphine can be administered small bolus doses of IV morphine, 1 to 2 mg, every 10 minutes until they are comfortable. A continuous infusion may then be started at an hourly rate equal to 50% of the cumulative bolus dose.[40]

Hydromorphone is a semisynthetic derivative of morphine that is more lipophilic with five to six times the analgesic potency of morphine when given intravenously but with less euphoria and lower incidence of nausea and pruritus when given epidurally.[17, 18, 41] It is available in a wide variety of dosage forms, including highly concentrated solutions for injection, which may be more useful for patients with high analgesic requirements, subcutaneous administration, or use in portable or implantable infusion pumps with small reservoirs.[13] When a patient is switched from one opioid to another (e.g., from morphine to hydromorphone), cross-tolerance among opioids is not complete. Therefore, the equianalgesic dose should be calculated on the basis of potency, and the patient should then be started on 50% of the calculated dose to avoid overdosage.[42] Hydromorphone is hepatically converted into inactive metabolites that are renally eliminated. IV bolus doses start at 0.5 to 2 mg, infusion rates at 0.2 to 0.5 mg/hour.[9, 17] Epidural continuous infusion doses start at 0.15 to 0.3 mg/hour.[20, 41]

Fentanyl and Its Derivatives

Fentanyl is the other frequently used opioid in ICU patients. It is a synthetic opioid agonist that is about 100 times more potent than morphine. It has fever sedative and euphoric effects than morphine. Fentanyl does not cause histamine release or hypotension when it is injected and is safer to use in hemodynamically unstable patients.[9, 37] Because fentanyl is lipophilic, onset of effect after IV injection is rapid, within 1 minute. Its short duration of action of 30 to 60 minutes for a single dose is due to redistribution into peripheral tissues.[9, 36, 37] Fentanyl is metabolized by the liver to inactive metabolites,[36, 42] but, patients with renal insufficiency may display prolonged sedation if they are maintained on continuous fentanyl therapy.[43] After prolonged use, even in patients with normal renal and hepatic function, fentanyl tends to accumulate in fat, which can prolong its effects.[9, 36, 37]

IV bolus doses of fentanyl range from 1 to 2 μg/kg or 50 to 150 μg and should be injected over 1 to 2 minutes. More rapid injection can cause chest rigidity, which may need to be treated with a neuromuscular blocking agent and mechanical ventilation.[9, 42] Respiratory depression is more likely if fentanyl is administered with benzodiazepines.[42] Continuous IV infusions of fentanyl start at 30 to 100 μg/hour and are titrated to achieve adequate analgesia.[9, 42] In one report, a terminally ill cancer patient required a continuous fentanyl IV infusion of 4250 μg/hour to obtain adequate pain relief. An ICU patient who had tolerance to fentanyl infusion required 6000 μg/hour.[25, 39] Fentanyl transdermal patches are used to provide continuous pain control in outpatients.[11, 13, 14, 44] Epidural continuous infusion rates are 20 to 150 μg/hour.[20]

The fentanyl derivatives alfentanil and sufentanil do not seem to offer any advantage over fentanyl for analgesia in ICU patients and are expensive.[9, 45] *Alfentanil* is faster in onset than fentanyl and has one third the duration of action but is only one fourth to one tenth as potent.[44] Alfentanil has a prolonged duration of action in patients with hepatic failure owing to accumulation.[45] *Sufentanil* is five to 10 times more potent than fentanyl, is more lipophilic, and has a shorter duration of action than that of fentanyl.[44] Sufentanil has less potent metabolites, accumulates in renal failure, and can cause prolonged respiratory depression.[36]

Remifentanil is a new fentanyl derivative that has rapid onset and offset of action. It is rapidly eliminated by plasma and tissue esterases. Because of this, patients who have received remifentanil require initiation of another analgesic agent soon after remifentanil is discontinued. In contrast to the other fentanyl derivatives, remifentanil cannot be administered epidurally or intrathecally because the current formulation contains glycine, which causes motor dysfunction. Continuous IV infusion rates for remifentanil range from 0.025 to 0.2 μg/kg/min.[46]

Meperidine (Pethidine)

Meperidine, also called pethidine, is a synthetic opioid with analgesic activity similar to that of morphine but with one tenth the potency. Meperidine is converted into a neurotoxic metabolite, *normeperidine,* which accumulates with impaired renal function.[9, 36, 47, 48] The metabolite causes CNS excitation, tremors, myoclonus, and seizures even in patients with normal renal function or hepatic dysfunction.[9, 47–49] The administration of meperidine should also be avoided in patients treated with monoamine oxidase inhibitors (within the past 21 days) or amphetamines because this can precipitate a fatal syndrome of excitation, hyperpyrexia, and seizures.[27, 42] In patients who have taken phenobarbital or hepatic enzyme inducers, production of normeperidine is increased, leading to greater accumulation.[27, 48] The Agency for Health Care Policy and Research has recommended that meperidine be used only for brief courses in healthy patients who have shown an unusual reaction or allergy to morphine.[9, 47]

Nonsteroidal Anti-inflammatory Drugs

NSAIDs have a limited role in analgesia in the ICU. They are efficacious for pain due to inflammatory processes or malignant disease involving bone. There is a ceiling effect to analgesia produced by NSAIDs. Increasing the dose above a maximum level increases the risk of adverse effects but not analgesia. NSAIDs have the potential risk of gastrointestinal bleeding, bleeding secondary to platelet dysfunction, and development of renal insufficiency. Renal complications are more likely in older patients and in those with hypovolemia, cardiac disease, or preexisting renal impairment.[9, 11]

Only one NSAID, *ketorolac,* is available for parenteral use in the United States. Ketorolac administration may be oral (PO), IM, or IV. Parenteral administration of ketorolac is limited to a maximum dose of 120 mg/day, 30 mg every 6 hours, in patients younger than 65 years who weigh at least 50 kg and have normal renal function. Patients 65 years old or older, with renal failure, or who weigh less than 50 kg should receive a maximum of 60 mg/day given as 15 mg every 6 hours. Ketorolac has caused an increased risk of gastrointestinal bleeding and acute renal failure in patients dependent on prostaglandins to maintain renal blood flow.[14] There are scattered reports of ketorolac given as a continuous infusion or intermittent IV doses in cancer patients for periods of 14 days to 11 months.[50-52] Misoprostol given at a dose of 100 or 200 μg four times a day helps prevent gastrointestinal toxicity due to NSAID therapy.[42, 50, 51]

Local Anesthetic Agents

Local anesthetics, such as bupivacaine, lidocaine, and ropivacaine, relieve pain by blocking nociceptive transmission. Increasing concentrations of local anesthetics increase the depth of nerve penetration and produce *analgesia, sympathetic block,* then *sensory block,* and finally *motor block.* When local anesthetics are given epidurally, there is always some degree of autonomic blockade. If administered in the lumbar area, they cause vasodilation in the lower extremities, which increases perfusion and decreases the likelihood of thromboembolic disease but can also cause hypotension. Adequate hydration and maintenance of the supine position prevent hypotension. Administration of epidural local anesthetics at the thoracic level causes sympathetic blockade, which may decrease the risk of postoperative ileus.[26] Coadministration of a local anesthetic agent with an opioid epidurally—usually bupivacaine with fentanyl or its derivatives—tends to lower the dose of both agents required for good analgesia and minimizes the occurrence of adverse effects.[18, 20, 41] Sometimes an epidural catheter is inserted to provide anesthesia during surgery and is then used in the ICU to provide continued analgesia. This is especially true in orthopedic surgery because epidural analgesia permits early ambulation and better tolerance of physical therapy.[18] Epidural analgesia is also used successfully postsurgically to control pain after thoracic, abdominal, and genitourinary surgery.[14]

The most widely used local anesthetic agent is *bupivacaine,* which is lipid-soluble. It has a long duration of action, tends to accumulate in epidural fat, and does not attain meaningful systemic concentrations, which minimizes the occurrence of serious adverse effects. Adverse effects, (e.g., CNS toxicity with generalized seizures, cardiac toxicity with arrhythmias, cardiac arrest refractory to resuscitation) can be minimized by administration of epidural local anesthetics by continuous infusion rather than by large bolus injections that may result in high serum concentrations.[20] Local anesthetics can cause urinary retention by parasympathetic blockade of the sacral nerves.[20] Bupivacaine and a new agent, *ropivacaine,* are less likely to cause motor blockade that inhibits voluntary movement.[19] Transient or permanent paralysis has occurred when large amounts of a local anesthetic were accidentally injected subdurally.[20] Patients with chronic neuropathic pain have been successfully managed with intrathecal continuous coadministration of bupivacaine and opioids for as long as 11 months.[32] When analgesia is initiated with bupivacaine in opioid-tolerant patients, close monitoring is required to decrease the dose of opioid because of the real danger of respiratory arrest.[23]

Local anesthetics are also used in peripheral nerve blocks either as anesthesia during surgery or for pain control. Peripheral nerve blocks with local anesthetics are effective in treating unrelenting neuropathic or *sympathetically maintained pain* (SMP).[3, 10, 14, 53] Intrapleural injection of these agents is used after surgery to control incisional pain and chest wall pain.[14] The oral calcium channel blocker *nifedipine* is sometimes a useful adjunct in treating SMP, perhaps by causing vasodilation.[53] Nerve blocks are sometimes used as temporary blocks, which if successful, are followed by longer-lasting neurolytic injections of alcohol or phenol.[3, 27, 53] Local anesthetics, combined with epinephrine, are used to prolong the action of the local anesthetic as a "chemical tourniquet"; however, this combination should be avoided in areas at risk for ischemia or necrosis, such as the digits.[14, 54] Nerve blocks may be maintained by administering repeated doses of a local anesthetic agent into catheters placed directly into a nerve plexus.[18]

Systemic infusions of lidocaine have been used on a limited basis for control of rapidly progressive neuropathic pain. The dose is 1 to 5 mg/kg given IV over 20 to 60 minutes.[10, 54] Patients may also be given the oral local anesthetic *mexiletine* at a starting dose of 150 mg/day, which is gradually increased until good analgesia is achieved or a maximum of 900 mg/day is reached. The electrocardiogram (ECG) should be monitored, and patients with cardiac disease are at increased risk for adverse effects.[10]

Other Adjunctive Analgesics

A number of adjuvant analgesics are useful for cancer pain and for various difficult to control pain syndromes, such as neuropathic pain and *central post-stroke pain* (CPSP).

Clonidine

Clonidine, the $alpha_2$ agonist, was previously mentioned in the discussion of opioids because it is effective in treating neuropathic or central pain that is refractory to opioids. Clonidine acts by inhibiting norepinephrine release at presynaptic adrenergic fibers, which lessens pain transmission. It is administered by the epidural or intrathecal routes.[30, 31] The use of oral, IV, peripheral block injection, and transdermal clonidine for pain control is being investigated.[10, 30, 53] Treatment should begin with low doses with gradual dose escalation. Sedation, hypotension, and bradycardia are the major side effects.[30, 31]

Corticosteroids

Corticosteroids are useful adjuncts for treatment of cancer pain of bone, visceral, neuropathic, or sympathetic origin.[53, 55] The corticosteroids are hormones that affect many organ systems in the body, they have anti-inflammatory effects and antiedema and analgesic activity through effects on nerve depolarization. Corticosteroids are useful in syndromes of spinal cord compression and brain metastases, and they tend to counteract nausea and anorexia and stimulate appetite. Epidural steroids are useful for both malignant and nonmalignant pain.[10, 55] The preferred oral agent is *dexamethasone* because of its high potency, long duration of action, and minimum mineralocorticoid effect. A reasonable starting dose is 10 mg daily.[55] The dose of steroid should be gradually tapered down to the lowest effective dose during a period of weeks.[10, 13] Corticosteroids are associated with a number of toxicities, including immune suppression and infections, gastritis, hypertension, fluid retention, hyperglycemia, osteoporosis, aseptic necrosis of bone, proximal muscle weakness, Cushing's habitus, and psychiatric disorders.[13, 55] The benefits of corticosteroids to patients with a limited life expectancy generally outweigh these risks.[10]

Tricyclic Antidepressants and Anticonvulsant Agents

Tricyclic antidepressants and anticonvulsants have been used with some success for the treatment of diabetic peripheral neuropathy and trigeminal neuralgia. Both of these drug classes also have some utility as analgesics in patients with severe neuropathic pain due to cancer and other causes. The antidepressant with the most clinical experience is *amitriptyline;* however, most of the older tricyclic antidepressants that inhibit norepinephrine reuptake are efficacious as analgesics. The newer serotonin reuptake inhibitors have not shown analgesic efficacy. The anticonvulsants used for pain control are phenytoin, carbamazepine, clonazepam, gabapentin, and valproate. In general, the initial dose of antidepressant is low. The dose is increased to an effective level that may be lower than the dose used to treat depression. Doses are also increased for anticonvulsants until standard anticonvulsant doses are attained.[10, 13, 53]

Central post-stroke pain affects up to 6% of stroke patients and is not limited to involvement of the thalamus as was previously thought. It is common in younger patients with mild motor affliction and is characterized by a partial or total deficit of temperature sense and/or sharpness sensation.[58] Pain intensity varies from mild to severe and can affect the hemibody, an entire limb, the upper extremities and face, or small spots on the face or body. Even the light touch of a cotton sheet can exacerbate the pain.[57]

The mainstay of therapy for CPSP is administration of adrenergically acting antidepressants. If these are not effective, mexiletine may be added.[56, 57] Phenytoin, carbamazepine, and clonazepam have also been efficacious for treating patients with sudden paroxysmal bouts of lancinating pain; the antidepressants are more effective for the background, burning type of pain.[57] The earlier antidepressant therapy is initiated, the more likely it is to be effective. Conventional analgesics are generally ineffective for CPSP.[58]

SEDATIVES

General Concepts

Assuming that the clinician is attempting to identify and treat the underlying reasons for agitation and has provided adequate pain control, sedation may still be required by many ICU patients.[1, 2, 58] The ideal sedative should cause drowsiness, anxiolysis, amnesia, muscle relaxation (antispasmodic), and reduced agitation (motor restlessness). It may be helpful for this agent to possess anticonvulsant properties. Sedation reduces the risk of complications associated with the stress response and helps patients tolerate routine ICU care.[2, 9, 58]

It is now common to adjust the dose of sedative drugs according to some form of sedation scale. The most common scales are similar to the Ramsay scale, which rates sedation numerically, with 1 indicating a wide awake and agitated patient and 6 denoting a totally unresponsive patient.[2, 6, 8, 34] Ideally, the patient should be calm, slightly sleepy, but easily awakened and responsive to commands, a 2 or 3 on the Ramsay scale. Deeper levels of sedation are sometimes necessary in life-threatening hemodynamic instability, severe pulmonary disease, or increased oxygen demand. Sometimes the dose of sedative is high enough to cause cardiovascular problems, such as hypotension. In this case, paralysis with a neuromuscular blocking agent may be required. Sedation scales permit titration to the level ordered by the physician and permit more uniform documentation of the response to medication, which is useful for clinical research as well as for improved patient care.[2, 6, 8] The bedside EEG can be used to monitor brain function and sedation in patients receiving neuromuscular blockers or when normal assessment is impossible.[6, 7, 59]

Sedatives are generally administered by the IV or oral routes in critical care units. Oral administration of sedative and analgesic agents is less expensive than the IV route and works well in patients who are being enterally fed, who are expected to need prolonged sedation (e.g., receiving mechanical ventilation), and who have fairly stable sedative requirements.[60] The extremely high cost of sedative agents, particularly midazolam and propofol, has encouraged health professionals to seek ways to provide adequate sedation and minimize drug treatment costs.[9, 45, 60–62]

The pharmacology of the commonly used sedative agents in the critical care setting—benzodiazepines, propofol, butyrophenones, chlorpromazine, and alpha$_2$ agonists—is presented. Except for the alpha$_2$ agonists, the common sedative agents used in the ICU have no analgesic activity. Opioid analgesics and sedatives are synergistic and are commonly used in combination regimens, particularly opioids and benzodiazepines.[9, 63] The pharmacodynamics and pharmacokinetics of the sedative agents are as variable as the critically ill patient and are not always predictable. Factors such as changing renal function, hepatic dysfunction, heart failure, age, and length and method of administration (single bolus versus prolonged infusion) may drastically alter the results of treatment with sedative agents.

Benzodiazepines

The benzodiazepines are the most frequently used sedative agents in the ICU. This class of drugs causes hypnosis, anxiolysis, amnesia, relaxation of muscle spasms, and reduced convulsant activity.[42] Benzodiazepines are widely used because of their ability to blunt the patient's recall. Benzodiazepines act at the gamma-aminobutyric acid (GABA) receptor complex in the CNS. They bind to a specific site on the GABA receptor complex to cause movement of chloride ions into the nerve cell, resulting in hyperpolarization.[34, 59]

Benzodiazepines may not be suitable for some delirious or psychiatrically ill patients who may become more confused and agitated. These patients may need antipsychotic medications, such as the butyrophenones.[59] In the elderly, benzodiazepines may cause a paradoxical excitation and agitation that worsens with escalating doses.[34, 58] Benzodiazepines do cause a dose-dependent respiratory depression, although it is less profound than that seen with opioids. Synergism with opioids, alcohol, and other depressant drugs may make respiratory depression more likely. Cardiovascular adverse effects due to benzodiazepines are rare and consist mainly of hypotension, which generally occurs with rapid IV injection, particularly of products containing propylene glycol in the formulations, such as lorzepam and diazepam. Benzodiazepine administration can also cause hypotension in hypovolemic patients.[34] Benzodiazepines are contraindicated in patients with narrow-angle glaucoma.[42]

With the exception of lorazepam and oxazepam, the benzodiazepines are metabolized by the liver into pharmacologically active compounds that significantly prolong the duration of action. Lorazepam and oxazepam are conjugated in the liver to form inactive glucuronide compounds.[34, 58] The pharmacodynamic effects of benzodiazepines, such as sedation, do not correlate with the pharmacokinetic half-life clearance of the drugs measured in blood samples. This is because the benzodiazepines are lipid-soluble and move in and out of the CNS rapidly (redistribution), allowing the patient to wake up, even though the drug may persist in the blood or peripheral tissues for many hours.[2, 45, 64]

Patients in alcohol withdrawal are often managed with a benzodiazepine regimen. The choice of benzodiazepine depends on which of the pharmacokinetic properties the clinician wants to use. Some physicians believe that the benzodiazepines with longer half-lives, such as diazepam and chlordiazepoxide, provide a smoother, self-tapering treatment of alcohol withdrawal.[64] Others are concerned about drug accumulation, particularly in the elderly and in hepatic disease, and favor oxazepam and lorazepam.[65] More easily titratable regimens using midazolam or propofol are better suited for managing the unpredictable fluctuating symptoms of delirium tremens (DTs).[66] Alcoholic patients often require high doses of benzodiazepines because of cross-tolerance.[59]

Flumazenil

Flumazenil is a benzodiazepine receptor antagonist that is administered by IV injection. It reverses many of the clinical effects of benzodiazepines. Routine use of flumazenil in the ICU to reverse sedation is generally not recommended because the drug may precipitate seizures or cardiac arrhythmias in predisposed individuals (history of seizures, post–cardiac arrest, head injury, cerebral hypoxia, chronic benzodiazepine use) or in cases of mixed drug overdose with drugs that lower the seizure threshold, particularly cyclic antidepressants and cocaine.[34, 67] To reverse benzodiazepine sedation, 0.2 mg is given IV over 15 seconds, followed by additional doses at 1 minute intervals until the desired level of consciousness is achieved. The maximum dose is 1 mg. In a benzodiazepine overdose, 0.2 mg flumazenil is given during 30 seconds followed by 0.5 mg over 30 seconds at 1-minute intervals to a maximum of 5 mg.[42, 67]

The half-life of elimination of flumazenil is shorter than that of all the benzodiazepines; therefore, re-sedation is likely when flumazenil is given to reverse sedation, necessitating repeated IV bolus doses or administration of a continuous infusion. Flumazenil is not always a replacement for intubation and mechanical ventilation, and the cost of a continuous flumazenil infusion may be higher than the cost of mechanical ventilation.[34, 67] However, flumazenil is of diagnostic value in patients who do not awaken after known benzodiazepine administration.[59]

Diazepam

Diazepam is an extremely lipophilic benzodiazepine that has a rapid onset of action, 0.5 to 5 minutes after IV injection, because it easily enters the CNS.[9, 34, 58, 68] Diazepam was the first benzodiazepine and is inexpensive.[45] The original propylene glycol and alcohol injectable formulation causes burning and phlebitis when it is given IV.[9, 68] This problem has been lessened by production of a sterile preparation of diazepam in fat emulsion (Dizac, Diazemuls).[42, 69] The duration of action of a single IV dose is short, 30 to 100 minutes, because the drug rapidly leaves the CNS and distributes peripherally.[9, 70]

A typical adult dose is 0.1 to 0.2 mg/kg or 2 to 15 mg every 3 to 4 hours. In the elderly patient, 2 mg may be appropriate; others may require up to 15 mg cardioversion.[42, 58] The drug should be injected at rates less than or equal to 5 mg/min.[58, 69] Diazepam is rarely given as a continuous infusion or by repeated injections to critically ill patients, since it becomes a long-acting sedative. This is because of accumulation in peripheral tissues, especially with hepatic dysfunction. Diazepam is converted into *desmethyldiazepam,* which, like the parent drug, has an extremely long half-life (200 hours) and is pharmacologically active.[9, 34, 58, 65] Diazepam is generally administered undiluted as intermittent IV injections because large volumes of fluid are required to dissolve the drug. Also, the drug should not be administered through IV tubing containing polyvinyl chloride because it is lost by adsorption to the plastic.[9]

Some clinicians switch to diazepam if a patient is receiving mechanical ventilation and requires sedation for longer than 5 days.[60] With its rapid onset and offset as a single IV dose and low cost, diazepam is suitable for short-term, rapid-onset sedation during a procedure or before the start of continuous sedation with lorazepam, as discussed next.

Lorazepam

Lorazepam is an "intermediate-acting" benzodiazepine that is less lipophilic than diazepam and midazolam. After an IV injection, the onset of action is within 5 to 20 minutes, peaking at about 30 minutes.[9, 34, 58] The decreased lipophilicity results in a smaller distribution volume and less potential for drug accumulation in peripheral tissues. Further, lorazepam is hepatically converted to an inactive compound by glucuronidation. This process is less affected by liver disease.[2, 9] Elimination of lorazepam is generally not altered by hepatic or renal disease.[9, 58, 65] All of these properties result in the interesting phenomenon that patients receiving lorazepam for extended periods may demonstrate more rapid awakening than those receiving midazolam for extended periods. Doses of up to 10 mg/hour have been demonstrated to be safe and effective in critically ill patients.[9, 58]

Lorazepam is formulated with polyethylene glycol and propylene glycol, which, administered in large quantities, can cause possible toxicities, such as hyperosmolality, metabolic acidosis, and acute tubular necrosis, unrelated to the drug itself.[71–73] Therefore, the maximum dose of, 10 mg/hour should not be exceeded. If sedation with lorazepam at that dose is inadequate, a different sedative agent should be added or substituted in the sedation regimen.

Lorazepam may be administered by either intermittent IV injections or continuous IV infusion. Lorazepam is poorly soluble in aqueous solution, making it more difficult to prepare a diluted solution for continuous infusion. A lorazepam solution can be prepared at certain concentrations (e.g., 0.1, 0.16, 0.2, or 1 mg/mL), preferably in glass bottles of 5% dextrose solution. The admixture should not be refrigerated, exposed to heat, or infused by a roller or volumetric pump infusion device because those tend to agitate the solution, causing the drug to precipitate out of solution.[61, 62, 74, 75] Others infuse the undiluted 2-mg/mL product by syringe pump through a central line. Continuous infusion doses generally range from 0.25 to 6 mg/hour, with usual doses of 1 to 3 mg/hour.[61] The recommended starting IV bolus dose of lorazepam is 0.44 mg/kg or 2 to 4 mg administered every 2 to 4 hours.[9, 58] In elderly or debilitated patients, a lower dose of 0.5 or 1 mg is appropriate.[42] Lorazepam should be diluted with an equal volume of sterile water, normal saline, or 5% dextrose in water before injection and should be administered at a maximum rate of 2 mg/min to avoid hypotension from the other ingredients in the formulation.[58]

Because of lorazepam's slow onset of action, sedation should be initiated with a bolus injection of either diazepam or midazolam, which take effect rapidly.[61] Many institutions have chosen lorazepam as their sedative of choice for critically ill patients requiring sedation for longer than 24 or 48 hours.[9, 45, 60–62] Lorazepam is safe, effective, and inexpensive, resulting in decreased drug costs and no difference in time for weaning from mechanical ventilation after tapering or stopping sedation.

Midazolam

Midazolam is traditionally considered to be a short-acting benzodiazepine, which is true when it is given for a short time in patients with normal hepatic, renal, and cardiac function. Midazolam is metabolized in the liver to *1-hydroxymidazolam,* which is pharmacologically active and has a half-life similar to that of the parent drug. Midazolam and its metabolite may accumulate after continued administration in the critically ill patient, causing prolongation of sedative effects, especially in the elderly and in patients with renal, hepatic, or congestive heart failure or decreased plasma albumin levels. The half-life of elimination of midazolam in ICU patients is 3.8 to 7.7 hours and may be as long as 26 hours in these patients, who may remain sedated for hours to days after the drug is discontinued.[9, 45] Tolerance to midazolam has occurred in younger patients who demonstrate violent withdrawal reactions hours to days after the drug is discontinued. After prolonged midazolam therapy, it is suggested that the drug be tapered rather than abruptly discontinued or a longer-acting benzodiazepine substituted.[2, 9]

Midazolam is easily prepared for IV infusions because of its high water solubility. Once injected into the patient, it undergoes a pH-dependent ring closure that renders it highly lipophilic and permits it to rapidly enter the CNS.[9, 34] Onset of sedation occurs within 0.7 to 2.5 minutes, similar to onset of diazepam.[9, 68] Single IV doses of the drug have a short duration of action owing to rapid redistribution out of the CNS into peripheral tissues.[9, 68] Continuous IV infusions, which are easily titrated, are used to maintain sedation in the critically ill patient after an initial bolus injection.

ICU patients generally require 1 to 20 mg/hour of midazolam for adequate sedation, but higher doses have been reported.[9, 58] The usual IV bolus dose is 1 to 2.5 mg of midazolam, but higher doses may be used in extremely agitated patients.[42, 59] Patients recover from the sedative effects of a single IV dose of midazolam in 30 to 100 minutes, as with diazepam.[70]

Midazolam is a convenient, titratable, effective sedative in the ICU setting. However, its high cost compared with that of other benzodiazepines has led to recommendations that midazolam be used for short-term sedation for less than 24 to 48 hours and for IV bolus dosing before initiation of a sedative regimen using lorazepam.[9, 45, 60–62]

Propofol

Propofol, or di-isopropylphenol, is an anesthetic agent that at subanesthetic doses possesses sedative, anxiolytic, and hypnotic activity; at high doses, it can cause amnesia. Patients should generally be monitored closely and intubated and mechanically ventilated if necessary because of the risk of respiratory depression, hypoxia, and apnea. Propofol is not an analgesic, so adequate analgesia must be given to patients in pain or to those patients undergoing painful procedures.[2, 9, 34, 76] Propofol has antiemetic activity and controls both postoperative and chemotherapy-induced vomiting. It also seems to possess anticonvulsant properties.[76]

Propofol is extremely lipophilic, causing it to have a rapid onset and offset of effect. Onset is within 0.7 to 5 minutes, and duration of action of a single dose is brief, 2 to 30 minutes, because of rapid CNS penetration and subsequent redistribution into peripheral tissues.[34, 37, 45] With continued administration, propofol does accumulate in peripheral fat tissues, but this does not have any significant effect on the recovery time.[9, 34, 37] Because of its pharmacokinetic and pharmacodynamic properties, sedation with propofol is appropriate in patients with neurologic disorders, such as head trauma, because they may be easily awakened for assessment.[2, 37]

The drug is generally administered by continuous infusion, with bolus doses of 1 to 2.5 mg/kg given only for extreme agitation or for a brief procedure, such as cardioversion. Bolus administration is discouraged in critically ill or hypovolemic patients because of the risk of hypotension; propofol can cause venodilation, bradycardia, and negative inotropic effects.[2, 34] If hypotension occurs, administration of dopamine or other pressor agent, 6% hetastarch, and a temporary decrease or discontinuation of vasodilators may be required.[34, 37, 59]

Propofol infusions may be rapidly titrated to achieve the desired level of sedation, which makes it particularly suitable for managing life-threatening agitation or delirium tremens.[59, 66] Infusions are usually started at 0.5 or 1 mg/kg/hour and increased every 5 to 10 minutes until the patient is adequately sedated or the manufacturer's recommended maximum dose of 6 mg/kg/hour is reached. Higher infusion rates are considered anesthetic doses.[59] Continuous infusions of propofol and midazolam are equally effective for sedation of ICU patients. A shorter time to weaning and extubation has been reported with propofol. Economic advantages are less clear because of the high cost and may be seen only with short-term use (less than 24 hours) of propofol.[2, 45, 62] It is recommended that propofol be used for short-term sedation for a maximum of 24 to 48 hours or until other less costly agents may be substituted.[9]

Propofol is formulated in a sterile 10% soybean oil-in-water emulsion that decreases burning and pain when it is injected into peripheral veins. Preferably, propofol should be administered by central vein.[9] It is available in a 1% or 10 mg/mL emulsion; however, a 2% product is being tested as a means of decreasing the fat load that is infused during propofol therapy.[9, 77] Propofol 1% provides 1.1 kcal/mL, which must be considered in the design and monitoring of the patient's nutritional regimens to avoid hypertriglyceridemia, hyperlipemia, calorie overload with elevated $Paco_2$ and respiratory acidosis, or lactic acidosis.[2, 9, 34, 37, 77, 78] Other adverse effects are tolerance and physical dependence, withdrawal seizures, and infection due to improper handling of the propofol.[2, 34] Propofol should be handled with strict aseptic technique as for total parenteral nutrition solutions, which are a good growth medium for microorganisms. The solution should not be hung for longer than 12 hours after the bottle is spiked. If propofol is removed from its original container, it should be discarded after 6 hours. Propofol should be administered through a dedicated line with tubing changes every 12 hours to prevent sepsis.[2, 9, 34] The manufacturer of propofol emulsion has now added ethylenediaminetetraacetic acid (EDTA) as a bacteriostatic agent.[2]

Haloperidol and Other Neuroleptics

Delirium is characterized by disorganized thought and speech, decreased level of consciousness, and altered sensory perception usually from organic causes. It is often difficult to distinguish delirium from anxiety-induced agitation. Delirious patients often remove catheters, extubate themselves, or injure themselves. All possible causes of delirium, including other drugs, should be eliminated before pharmacotherapy is tried.[1, 2, 9, 58] *Haloperidol* is a high-potency butyrophenone neuroleptic drug that is effective in the treatment of delirium in the critically ill.

Haloperidol is a dopamine receptor antagonist that has a calming effect manifested by reduced interest in the environment, reduced emotion and affect, and reduced initiative. Patients become less agitated, less aggressive, and less anxious but retain intellectual function. Haloperidol does not possess significant sedative effects, but it often decreases the need for other sedatives. Haloperidol does not cause respiratory depression. It is usually administered to ICU patients by either bolus or continuous IV injection, which seems to cause less frequent extrapyramidal reactions; however, some acute dystonic reactions, such as laryngospasm, may occur.[2, 9, 58, 79]

Haloperidol is an α-adrenergic blocker and can cause hypotension in patients who are volume-depleted or receiving antihypertensive therapy.[58] Haloperidol can cause prolongation of the QT interval and torsades de pointes, particularly in patients who are receiving large doses (>50 mg/day) or who have abnormal serum calcium, potassium, or magnesium levels. Other drugs affecting the QT interval or cardiac disease can be synergistic with haloperidol in causing cardiac conduction problems. Patients should be on a cardiac monitor, and the ECG should be checked for prolongation of the corrected QT interval to greater than 440 msec or a 25% lengthening of the QT interval above baseline.[2, 9, 79, 80] Droperidol is a neuroleptic with antiemetic activity that causes a higher incidence of sedation and hypotension than haloperidol does and also causes QT prolongation. *Droperidol* is not recommended for use in ICU patients as a sedative.[9, 58, 80]

The usual starting IV bolus dose of haloperidol is 0.5 to 10 mg, depending on the severity of the agitation. It should be administered over 1 minute, then repeated, and sometimes doubled, every 30 minutes until delirium is controlled or a maximum of 40 mg has been given. A benzodiazepine such as lorazepam may be added. Fifty percent to 100% of the total dose can then be given in divided doses during 24 hours or administered as a continuous infusion at doses up to 40 mg/hour. The dose is then gradually tapered, depending on the patient's condition.[9, 58, 59, 63, 79, 80]

Chlorpromazine, a low-potency phenothiazine neuroleptic, shares the increased risk of excess sedation and hypotension, which makes it a less useful sedative in ICU patients.[9, 58] However, chlorpromazine has been shown to be effective when it is administered to dying cancer patients along with morphine to control symptoms of restlessness and dyspnea.[4, 81] Chlorpromazine may be given IV, but it is usually given orally, rectally, or IM. Doses are 12.5 mg or 25 mg given IV or 25 mg given rectally every 4 to 12 hours.[4, 81]

Alpha$_2$ Agonists

This class of agents represents the future of sedative and analgesic research. Alpha$_2$ agonists possess both sedative and analgesic activities. *Clonidine* has been investigated for use as a sedative and is used in the treatment of alcohol withdrawal through the oral and transdermal routes. It is not yet available for IV administration in the United States. A highly selective injectable alpha$_2$ agonist available in Europe, *dexmedetomidine,* has anxiolytic activity similar to that of the benzodiazepines and is currently being investigated in this country. Clonidine and dexmedetomidine both can lower blood pressure and cause bradycardia.[2, 59, 64, 66]

SUMMARY

For the past 30 years of critical care, the primary objective of ICU practitioners has been the development of monitoring and life-support technology to treat the patient with life-threatening disease. Attention to the alleviation of symptoms has been uncommon. Palliation has been rare and in the minds of many clinicians refers only to the management of pain and suffering in patients dying of a malignant disease. Palliation *comes from the Latin word for "cloak" and means to make less severe or mitigate or shield against. We believe that palliation is an essential part of the practice of critical care not only for patients who are likely to die of their illness in the ICU but also for that 90% of patients who usually survive admission to the ICU. Sedatives and analgesics are two of the primary tools of palliation. High-quality analgesia should be a high priority for all critical care practitioners. If that is not enough to palliate against the symptoms of the patient, sedatives should be added to the treatment regimen. Palliation reduces the stress response of critical illness and is as important to good critical care practice as any of the life-support and monitoring practices that are so important to state-of-the-art critical care.*

References

1. Inaba-Roland KE, Maricle RA: Assessing delirium in the acute care setting. Heart Lung 1992; 21:48–55.
2. Hassan E, Fontaine DK, Nearman HS: Therapeutic considerations in management of agitated or delirious critically ill patients. Pharmacotherapy 1998; 18:113–129.
3. Urba SG: Nonpharmacologic pain management in the terminally ill. Clin Geriatr Med 1996; 12:301–311.
4. National Institutes of Health: Symptoms in terminal illness: A research workshop. Rockville, Md, National Institutes of Health, 1997; http://www.nih.gov./ninr/end-of-life.htm.
5. Wagner BKJ, Zavotsky KE, Sweeney JB, Palmeri BA, Hammond JS: Patient recall of therapeutic paralysis in a surgical critical care unit. Pharmacotherapy 1998; 18:358–363.
6. Crippen DW: Neurological monitoring in the intensive care unit. New Horiz 1994; 2:107–120.
7. Crippen DW: Using bedside EEGs to monitor sedation during neuromuscular blockade. J Crit Ill 1997; 12:519–524.
8. Habibi S, Coursin D: Assessment of sedation, analgesia, and neuromuscular blockade in the perioperative period. Int Anesthesiol Clin 1996; 34:215–241.
9. Society of Critical Care Medicine: Practice parameters for systemic intravenous analgesia and sedation for adult patients in the intensive care unit. Practice parameters for sustained neuromuscular blockade in the adult critically ill patient. Anaheim, Calif, Society of Critical Care Medicine, 1995. Abridged version in Crit Care Med 1995; 23:1596–1600.
10. Portenoy RK: Adjuvant analgesic agents. Hematol Oncol Clin North Am 1996; 10:103–119.
11. Rigas M: Economic considerations in the pharmacologic management of pain. Pharmacol Ther 1997; 22:454–468.
12. Yaksh TL, Malmberg AB: Central pharmacology of nociceptive transmission. *In* Textbook of Pain. 3rd ed. Melzack R, Wall P (Eds). Edinburgh, Churchill Livingstone, 1994, pp 165–200.
13. Levy MH: Pharmacologic management of cancer pain. Semin Oncol 1994; 21:718–739.
14. Follin S, Charland S: Acute pain management: Operative or medical procedures. Ann Pharmacother 1997; 31:1068–1076.
15. Dunteman E, Karanikolas M: Transnasal butorphanol for the treatment of opioid-induced pruritus. J Pain Symptom Manage 1996; 12:255–260.
16. Gora-Harper ML, Sunahara JF, Gray MS: Intranasal butorphanol-induced apraxia. Ann Pharmacother 1995; 15:798–800.
17. Lubenow TR, McCarthy RJ: Management of acute postoperative pain. *In:* Clinical Anesthesia. 2nd ed. Barash PG, Cullen BF, Stoelting RK (Eds). Philadelphia, JB Lippincott, 1992, pp 1547–1577.
18. D'Amours RH, Ferrante M: Postoperative pain management. J Orthop Sports Phys Ther 1996; 24:227–236.
19. Mulroy MF: Epidural opioid delivery methods: Bolus, continuous infusion, and patient-controlled epidural analgesia. Reg Anesth 1996; 21(Suppl 6S):100–104.
20. Shafer AL, Donnelly AJ: Management of postoperative pain by continuous epidural infusion of analgesics. Clin Pharm 1991; 10:745–764.
21. Food and Drug Administration: Q and A's: Low molecular weight heparins/heparinoids and spinal/epidural anesthesia. U.S. Food and Drug Administration, May 6, 1998: http//www.fda.gov/medwatch/safety/1998/lovq&a.htm.
22. Mulroy MF: Monitoring opioids. Reg Anesth 1996; 21 (Suppl 6S):89–83.
23. Piquet CY, Malleret MP, Lemoigne AH, Barjhoux CE, Danel VC, Vincent FH: Respiratory depression following administration of intrathecal bupivacaine to an opioid dependent patient. Ann Pharmacother 1998; 32:653–655.
24. Portenoy RK: Tolerance to opioid analgesics: Clinical aspects. Cancer Surv 1994; 21:49–65.
25. Shafer A, White PF, Schuttler J, Rosenthal MH: Use of a fentanyl infusion in the intensive care unit: Tolerance to its anesthetic effects? Anesthesiology 1983; 59:245–248.

26. De Leon-Casasola OA: Postoperative pain management in opioid-tolerant patients. Reg Anesth 1996; 21 (Suppl 6S):114–116.
27. Caraceni A, Portenoy RK: Pain management in patients with pancreatic carcinoma. Cancer Suppl 1996; 78:639–653.
28. Sjogren P, Jonsson T, Jensen NH, Drenck NE, Jensen TS: Hyperalgesia and myoclonus in terminal cancer patients treated with continuous intravenous morphine. Pain 1993; 55:93–97.
29. Chaney MA: Side effects of intrathecal and epidural opioids. Can J Anaesth 1995; 42:891–903.
30. Eisenach JC, De Kock M, Klimscha W: α-Adrenergic agonists for regional anesthesia: A clinical review of clonidine (1984–1995). Anesthesiology 1996; 85:655–674.
31. Duraclon (clonidine hydrochloride injection) formulary kit and package inset. Roxane Laboratories, Inc., Columbus, Ohis, September 1996.
32. Krames ES, Lanning RM: Intrathecal infusional analgesia for non-malignant pain: Analgesic efficacy. J Pain Symptom Manage 1993; 8:539–548.
33. Mercadante S: Ketamine in cancer pain: An update. Palliat Med 1995; 10:225–230.
34. Kress JP, O'Connor MF, Pohlman AS, Hall JB: Sedating critically ill ventilated patients: A pharmacologic primer. J Crit Ill 1997; 12:287–299.
35. Murphy DB, Sutton JA, Prescott LF, Murphy MB: Opioid-induced delay in gastric emptying. A peripheral mechanism in humans. Anesthesiology 1997; 87:765–770.
36. Davies, G, Kingswood C, Street M: Pharmacokinetics of opioids in renal dysfunction. Clin Pharmacokinet 1996; 31:410–422.
37. Birmingham MC: Use of sedatives and hypnotics in the intensive care unit. Pharmaguide to Hospital Medicine (Bayer Corp Pharmaceuticals) 1998; 10:1–4, 9–11.
38. Isenhower HL, Mueller BA: Selection of narcotic analgesics for pain associated with pancreatitis. Am J Health Syst Pharm 1998; 55:480–486.
39. Lenz K, Dunlop DS: Continuous fentanyl infusion in severe cancer pain. Ann Pharmacother 1998; 32:316–319.
40. Cohen MH, Anderson AJ, Krasnow SH, Spagnolo SV, Citron ML, Payne M, Fossieck BE: Continuous intravenous infusion of morphine for severe dyspnea. South Med J 1991; 84:229–234.
41. De Leon-Casasola OA, Lema MJ: Postoperative epidural opioid analgesia: What are the choices? Anesth Analg 1996; 83:867–875.
42. USP DI Drug Information for the Health Care Professional. 18th ed. Vol 1. Rockville, Md, The United States Pharmacopeial Convention, Inc, 1998.
43. Koehntop DE, Rodman JH: Fentanyl pharmacokinetics in patients undergoing renal transplantation. Pharmacotherapy 1997; 17: 746–752.
44. Clotz MA, Nahata MC: Clinical uses of fentanyl, sufentanil, and alfentanil. Clin Pharm 1991; 10:581–593.
45. Armstrong DK, Crisp CB: Pharmacoeconomic issues of sedation, analgesia, and neuromuscular blockade in critical care. New Horiz 1994; 2:85–93.
46. Burkle H, Dunbar S, Van Aken H: Remifentanil: A novel, short-acting mu-opioid. Anesth Analg 1996; 83:646–651.
47. Agency for Health Care Policy and Research: Acute pain management: Operative or medical procedures and trauma, part 1 and part 2. Clin Pharm 1992; 11:309–331, 391–414.
48. Danziger LH, Martin SJ, Blum RA: Central nervous system toxicity associated with meperidine use in hepatic disease. Pharmacotherapy 1994; 14:235–238.
49. Hagmeyer KO, Mauro LS, Mauro VF: Meperidine-related seizures associated with patient-controlled analgesia pumps. Ann Pharmacother 1993; 27:29–32.
50. Miller LJ, Kramer MA: Pain management with intravenous ketorolac. Ann Pharmacother 1993; 27:307–308.
51. Middleton RK, Lyle JA: Ketorolac continuous infusion: A case report and review of the literature. J Pain Symptom Manage 1996; 12:190–194.
52. Gordon RL: Prolonged central intravenous ketorolac continuous infusion in a cancer patient with intractable pain. Ann Pharmacother 1998; 32:193–196.
53. Lipman AG: Analgesic drugs for neuropathic and sympathetically maintained pain. Clin Geriatr Med 1996; 12:501–515.
54. Backonja MM: Local anesthetics as adjuvant analgesics. J Pain Symptom Manage 1994; 9:491–499.
55. Watanabe S, Brurera E: Corticosteroids as adjuvant analgesics. J Pain Symptom Manage 1994; 9:442–445.
56. Segatore M: Understanding central post-stroke pain. J Neurosci Nurs 1995; 27:28–35.
57. Bowhser D: The management of central post-stroke pain. Postgrad Med J 1995; 71:598–604.
58. Fish DN: Treatment of delirium in the critically ill patient. Clin Pharm 1991; 10:456–466.
59. Crippen DW: Pharmacologic treatment of brain failure and delirium. Crit Care Clin 1994; 10:733–766.
60. Watling SM, Johnson M, Yanos J: A method to produce sedation in critically ill patients. Ann Pharmacother 1996; 30:1227–1231.
61. Hadbavny AM, Hoyt JW: Promotion of cost-effective benzodiazepine sedation. Am J Hosp Pharm 1993; 50:660–661.
62. Devlin JW, Holbrook AM, Fuller HD: The effect of ICU sedation guidelines and pharmacist intervention on clinical outcomes and drug cost. Ann Pharmacother 1997; 31:689–695.
63. Watling SM, Dasta JF, Seidl EC: Sedatives, analgesics, and paralytics in the ICU. Ann Pharmacother 1997; 31:148–153.
64. Erstad BL, Cotugno CL: Management of alcohol withdrawal. Am J Health Syst Pharm 1995; 52:697–709.
65. Peppers MP: Benzodiazepines for alcohol withdrawal in the elderly, and in patients with liver disease. Pharmacotherapy 1996; 16:49–58.
66. Crippen DW: Strategies for managing delirium tremens in the ICU: How to control fluctuating symptoms and minimize the risk of organ damage. J Crit Ill 1997; 12:140–149.
67. Kantor GSA: Flumazenil: A review for clinicians. Am J Anesthesiol 1997; 24:84–88.
68. Buhrer M, Maitre PO, Crevoisier C, Stanski DR: Electroencephalographic effects of benzodiazepines. II. Pharmacodynamic modeling of the electroencephalographic effects of midazolam and diazepam. J Clin Pharmacol Ther 1990; 48:555–567.
69. Dizac package insert. Ohmeda PPD, Inc., Pharmacia AB, Liberty Corner, N J, September 1994.
70. Ariano RE, Kassum DA, Aronson KJ: Comparison of sedative recovery time after midazolam versus diazepam administration. Crit Care Med 1994; 22:1492–1496.
71. Nolen JG, Cerra FB: Propylene glycol–induced lactic acidosis secondary to a continuous infusion of lorazepam. Pharmacotherapy 1993; 13:abstract 43.
72. Laine GA, Hossain SMH, Solis RT, Adams SC: Polyethylene glycol nephrotoxicity secondary to prolonged high-dose intravenous lorazepam. Ann Pharmacother 1995; 29:1110–1114.
73. Seay RE, Graves PJ, Wilkin MK: Comment: Possible toxicity from propylene glycol in lorazepam infusion. Ann Pharmacother 1997; 31:647–648.
74. Grillo JA, Barie PS: Precipitation of lorazepam during infusion by volumetric pump. Am J Health Syst Pharm 1996; 53:1850–1851.
75. Volles DF, Boullata JI, Gelone SP, Grillo JA: More on usability of lorazepam admixtures for continuous infusion. Am J Health Syst Pharm 1996; 53:2753–2755.
76. Borgeat A, Wilder-Smith OHG, Suter PM: The nonhypnotic therapeutic applications of propofol. Anesthesiology 1994; 80:642–656.
77. McLeod G, Dick J, Wallis C, Patterson A, Cox C, Colvin J: Propofol 2% in critically ill patients: Effect on lipids. Crit Care Med 1997; 25:1976–1981.
78. Marinella MA: Lactic acidosis associated with propofol (Letter). Chest 1996; 109:292.
79. Riker RR, Fraser GL, Cox PM: Continuous infusion of haloperidol controls agitation in critically ill patients. Crit Care Med 1994; 22:433–440.
80. Lawrence KR, Nasraway SA: Conduction disturbances associated with administration of butyrophenone antipsychotics in the critically ill: A review of the literature. Pharmacotherapy 1997; 17:531–537.
81. McIver B, Walsh D, Nelson K: The use of chlorpromazine for symptom control in dying cancer patients. J Pain Symptom Manage 1994; 9:341–345.

86

Neuromuscular Blocking Drugs in Patients in the Intensive Care Unit

Richard C. Prielipp, MD

Neuromuscular blocking (NMB) drugs were introduced to clinical practice in the operating room by anesthesiologists in 1942. Use of NMB drugs in the intensive care unit (ICU) soon followed, and as many as 5% of ICU patients received continuous administration of NMB drugs for 24 hours or more.[1] Lately, use of NMB drugs in the ICU has decreased[2] because of untoward side effects such as prolonged motor weakness, myopathy, accumulation of toxic drug metabolites, and drug tachyphylaxis.[3-12] These problems may be diminished by appropriate NMB drug selection and administration, identification of drug-drug interactions, optimization of drug delivery, monitoring of NMB drug effects, and understanding of the pathophysiology of NMB-associated neuromuscular injury. NMB drugs also vary in acquisition costs and may constitute a significant fraction of the ICU pharmacy budget.[13, 14] Pharmacoeconomic evaluation of ICU drugs must also take into account secondary costs such as personnel time, use of infusion devices and twitch monitors, long-term effects of drug and active metabolites, and potential morbidity or mortality secondary to prolonged weakness, myopathy, or neuropathy syndromes.[14]

GENERAL CONSIDERATIONS

Relationship of Structure to Activity

The neuromuscular junction expresses nicotinic acetylcholine receptors (nAChRs) on *presynaptic* nerve endings (which act in a positive feedback to mobilize more transmitter for subsequent release), as well as several million postsynaptic cholinergic receptors concentrated in the junctional folds of the muscle membrane opposite the nerve ending (Fig. 86-1). The neurotransmitter acetylcholine (ACh) has a positively charged quaternary ammonium ($[N\text{-}C_4]^+$) group that binds the negatively charged alpha subunit of the cholinergic receptor.[15, 16] When activated by two ACh molecules, the receptor opens a channel for the flow of positively charged ions (sodium and calcium) into and potassium out of the muscle cell, inducing sufficient current to depolarize the muscle end plate and trigger muscle contraction.

All nondepolarizing NMB drugs competitively antagonize postjunctional ACh receptors.[15-17] NMB drugs also vary in their prejunctional effects. The remarkable specificity of NMB drugs is related to the molecular structure of the acetylcholine molecule being functionally duplicated within the structure of NMB drugs such as pancuronium (Fig. 86-2). Nondepolarizing NMB drugs are large, bulky structures that are chemically categorized in two classes[18]: the benzylisoquinolinium[19] and the aminosteroid[20] compounds. The depolarizing NMB succinylcholine is a linear molecule composed of two acetylcholine molecules attached end to end via acetate groups.[21]

Quaternary ammonium drugs, in addition to their NMB effect, vary in their potential to activate or antagonize other receptors. Effects at muscarinic receptors may result in bradycardia or tachycardia, and blockade of nicotinic autonomic ganglia may produce significant hypotension. Endogenous release of vasoactive amines such as norepinephrine and histamine may lead to sympathomimetic effects of hypotension.[15, 17] Structural differences appear to play a major role in the development of these side effects.[19, 20, 22]

Drug dose is inversely related to NMB potency.[15] The most potent drugs are used in smaller doses (i.e., fewer drug molecules), generally resulting in fewer side effects. Thus, drugs such as doxacurium and pipecuronium are noteworthy for their lack of hemodynamic or autonomic interactions.[19, 20, 22, 23] But administration of smaller quantities of these potent compounds also means that there are fewer molecules circulating to antagonize neuromuscular junctional ACh receptors, resulting in a slower onset of action. In practice, the speed of NMB drug onset has few clinical implications in most ICU situations compared with use in the operating theater.

Indications for and Interactions of Neuromuscular Blocking Drugs in the Intensive Care Unit

Because all NMB drugs are totally devoid of sedative and analgesic activity, their use must be accompanied by the administration of narcotics and sedative drugs. In fact, many patients may have adequate ventilation and management without NMB drugs if appropriate quantities of analgesics and sedatives are administered. The common and generally recognized uses of NMB drugs in the ICU are summarized in Table 86-1. Optimization of mechanical ventilation is the most frequent indication, especially in patients with acute lung injury requiring newer, more sophisticated modes of ventilation. Pharmacokinetic and pharmacodynamic properties of NMB drugs are summarized in Table 86-2, and adverse effects are outlined in Table 86-3. The interactions of NMB agents with other drugs are summarized in Table 86-4.

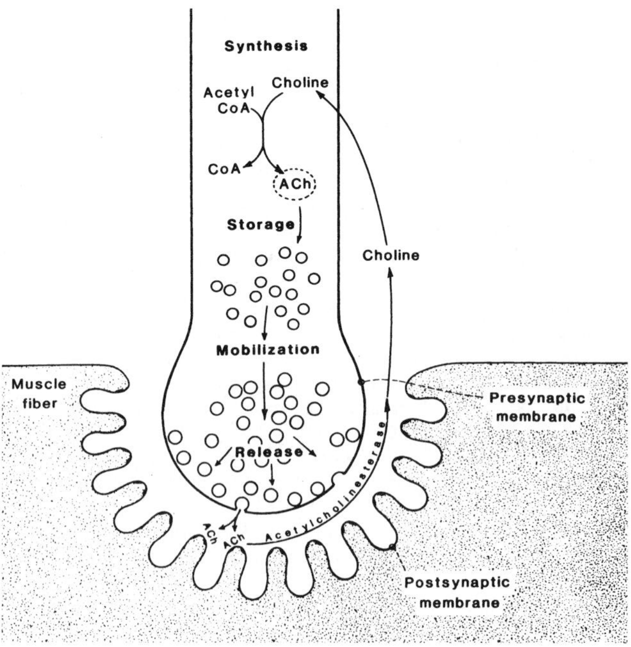

Figure 86–1. Diagram of the neuromuscular junction, site of 1 to 10 million nicotinic acetylcholine receptors (nAChR) concentrated in the junctional folds of the muscle end plate. The neurotransmitter acetylcholine is released from axonal vesicles in response to neuronal action potentials. (From Lebowitz PW, Ramsey FM: Muscle relaxants. *In:* Barash PG, Cullen BF, Stoelting RK [Eds]. Clinical Anesthesia. Philadelphia, JB Lippincott, 1989, p 341.)

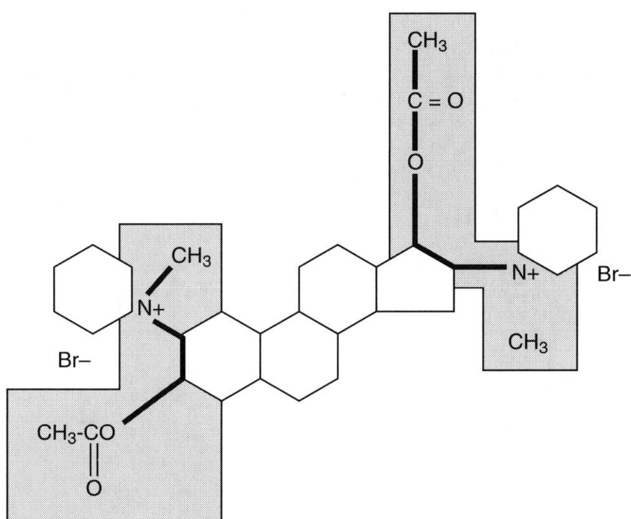

Figure 86–2. Receptor specificity is imparted by the incorporation of the basic acetylcholine (ACh) molecule (highlighted, bold) within the basic structure of the aminosteroid neuromuscular blocking (NMB) drugs, such as pancuronium. NMB drug binding occurs at the alpha subunit of the nAChR. The presence of the bulky, steroid backbone of the NMB drug (pancuronium) assists in effectively blocking the cation channel. (From Prielipp RC, Coursin DB: Applied pharmacology of common neuromuscular blocking agents in critical care. New Horiz 1994; 2:34.)

NEUROMUSCULAR BLOCKING DRUGS

Classification

The ideal NMB drug would be rapid in onset, have a predictable offset, be nontoxic, lack deleterious cardiovascular or autonomic effects, undergo a defined means of metabolism and excretion preferably independent of end-organ function, and be inexpensive.[15, 18, 22, 24] Although many of these characteristics are found in clinically available drugs, no approved drug meets all criteria. Several drugs, however, approach the ideal.[15, 18, 22, 25]

NMB drugs are traditionally classified by mode of action, structure, and duration of action. Mechanistically, neuromuscular blockade occurs via one of two different pharmacologic modes. Drugs that act as prolonged agonists at the nACh receptor are called depolarizing agents (e.g., succinylcholine). A second group of agents (nondepolarizers, e.g., pancuronium) bind noncovalently and competitively to nACh receptors, thereby inhibiting neuromuscular transmission. Clinically available nondepolarizing drugs can be grouped into two basic structural categories. The benzylisoquinolinium drugs tend to be potent (and therefore slower in onset) NMB drugs that are eliminated by the kidneys or Hofmann elimination and may trigger histamine release. Conversely, the aminosteroid compounds are less potent, have a faster onset of action, are eliminated by the liver with active metabolites, and lack significant histamine release or autonomic interactions. Last, NMB drugs may be classified as short-, intermediate-, or long-acting on the basis of their duration of action.

TABLE 86–1. Uses of Neuromuscular Blocking Drugs in Patients in the Intensive Care Unit

Common Indications

- Facilitating synchrony between mechanical ventilator and patient (e.g., with status asthmaticus)
- Facilitating endotracheal intubation
- Selected patients with intracranial hypertension
- Eliminating shivering
- Decreasing O_2 consumption
- Optimizing conditions for imaging or diagnostic studies
- Immobility of patient during invasive procedures or transport
- Emergent control of agitated or combative patient

Less Frequent Indications

- Supportive therapy for tetanus or status epilepticus (with electroencephalographic monitoring)
- Selected patients with severe cardiovascular instability

Short-Acting Drugs

Succinylcholine

Succinylcholine is the only ultrashort-acting, depolarizing NMB drug in current clinical use in the United States. Muscle fasciculations, followed by flaccid muscle paralysis, characterize depolarizing neuromuscular blockade. Succinylcholine, structurally consisting of two ACh molecules "back to back," mimics the pharmacologic action of acetylcholine at the nAChR. However, because succinylcholine is metabolized more slowly than acetylcholine, the motor end plate is subjected to a sustained depolarizing stimulation, rendering the end plate region electrically refractory and functionally unexcitable (receptor desensitization). The muscle loses its ability to contract in response to subsequent stimuli for a period of 5 to 10 minutes. This prolonged stimulation of the nAChR channel by succinylcholine also results in a large influx of sodium and calcium ions (down their concentration gradients) and a simultaneous efflux of potassium ions (briefly increasing the serum potassium concentration [K^+] 0.5–1.0 mEq/L).

The typical succinylcholine neuromuscular block occurs within 60 seconds of an intubating dose (1.0 to 1.5 mg/kg) and is clinically heralded by muscle fasciculations, particularly in the hands, feet, and face. Succinylcholine undergoes rapid redistribution and ester hydrolysis by plasma pseudocholinesterase at a maximum rate of 100 μg/kg/min. This limits the clinical duration of action to 5 to 7 minutes. Various disease states (such as severe liver disease, myxedema, protein-calorie malnutrition, and malignancy), as well as pregnancy, may result in a quantitative decrease in plasma pseudocholinesterase levels, which prolongs the duration of action of succinylcholine by 50% to 100%. In addition, a plasma pseudocholinesterase enzyme variant may be inherited as a homozygous recessive trait with a frequency of 1:2500, and these individuals are noteworthy for ultraslow metabolism of succinylcholine. Afflicted patients are paralyzed for 1 to 3 hours or longer after a single intubating dose of succinylcholine.

Adverse effects of succinylcholine limit its widespread application. These include cardiac arrhythmias (junctional rhythms, sinus arrest, bradycardia, or tachycardia); diffuse myalgia; myoglobinuria (especially in children); malignant hyperthermia; increases in intraocular, intragastric, or intracranial pressure; and increases in serum potassium. Most noteworthy is lethal hyperkalemia triggered in patients with acute neurologic, crush, or burn injuries.[21] Succinylcholine is therefore contraindicated for patients with major thermal burns, significant crush injuries, spinal cord transection, malignant hyperthermia, acute upper or lower motor neuron lesions, certain muscular dystrophies (i.e., myotonia congenita or dystrophica), and severe, prolonged infections such as uncontrolled peritonitis.

In summary, succinylcholine still occupies a unique niche in the family of NMB drugs. It remains the drug of choice in situations in which speed of onset and short duration of action are priorities. However, its side effects and potential complications limit widespread utilization in the ICU popula-

TABLE 86–2. Selected Drugs for Intensive Care Unit Use

	Benzylisoquinolinium Drugs				
	Tubocurarine (Curare)	*Cisatracurium (Nimbex)*	*Atracurium (Tracrium)*	*Doxacurium (Nuromax)*	*Mivacurium (Mivacron)*
Introduced (yr)	1942	1995	1983	1991	1992
ED_{95} dose (mg/kg)	0.51	0.05	0.25	0.025–0.030	0.075
Initial dose (mg/kg)	0.2–0.3	0.20	0.4–0.5	Up to 0.1	0.15–0.25
Duration (min)	80	45–60	25–35	120–150	10–20
Infusion described	?	Yes	Yes	Yes	Yes
Infusion dose (μg/kg/min)	—	2.5–3.0	4–12	0.3–0.5	9–10
Recovery (min)	80–180	90	40–60	120–180	10–20
% Renal excretion	40–45	Hofmann elimination	5–10 (uses Hofmann elimination)	70	Inactive metabolites
Renal failure	Increased effect	No change	No change	Increased effect	Increased duration
% Biliary excretion	10–40	Hofmann	Minimal (uses Hofmann elimination)	Unclear	—
Hepatic failure	Minimal change to mild increased effect	Minimal to no change	Minimal to no change	?	Increased duration
Active metabolites	No	No	No, but can accumulate laudanosine	?	No
Histamine release hypotension	Marked	No	Minimal but dose dependent	None	Minimal but dose dependent
Vagal block tachycardia	Minimal	No	No	No	No
Ganglionic blockade hypotension	Marked	No	Minimal to none	No	No
Prolonged ICU block	?	Rare	Rare	Too early to tell	Too early to tell
Estimated U.S. ICU use	NR	Increasing	Minimal	Infrequent	Rare-NR
Cost ($) (24-hr estimate)	NR	$200–225	$500	$100–150	$700

	Aminosteroids			
	Pancuronium (Pavulon)	*Vecuronium (Norcuron)*	*Pipecuronium (Arduan)*	*Rocuronium (Zemuron)*
Introduced (yr)	1972	1984	1991	1994
ED_{95} dose (mg/kg)	0.07	0.05	0.05	0.3
Initial dose (mg/kg)	0.1	0.1	0.085–0.1	0.6–1.0
Duration (min)	90–100	35–45	90–100	30
Infusion described	Yes	Yes	No	Yes
Infusion dose (μg/kg/min)	1–2	1–2	0.5–2.0	10–12
Recovery (min)	120–180	45–60	55–160	20–30
% Renal excretion	45–70	50	50+	33
Renal failure	Increased effect	Increased effect, especially metabolites	Increased duration	Minimal
% Biliary excretion	10–15	35–50	Minimal	<75
Hepatic failure	Mild increased effect	Variable, mild	Minimal	Moderate
Active metabolites	Yes: 3-OH and 17-OH-pancuronium	Yes: 3-desacetylvecuronium	Not reported	No
Histamine release hypotension	None	None	None	None
Vagal block tachycardia	Modest to marked	No	No	Some at higher doses
Ganglionic blockade hypotension	No	No	No	No
Prolonged ICU block	Yes	Yes	No reports	No reports
Estimated U.S. ICU use	Variable	Decreasing	Uncommon	Variable
Cost (%) (24-hr estimate)	$10	$185–200	No data	$300

Modified from Prielipp RC, Coursin DB: Applied pharmacology of common neuromuscular blocking agents in critical care. New Horiz 1994; 2:34.
ED_{95} = 95% effective dose; ICU = intensive care unit; NR = not recommended.

tion. These limitations of succinylcholine may be circumvented by the Food and Drug Administration (FDA) approval of ORG 9487, an investigational low-potency, steroid-based, rapid-onset NMB drug. ORG 9487 is unique as a nondepolarizing NMB drug because it can be reversed by neostigmine 2 minutes after its administration, resulting in a recovery profile similar to that of succinylcholine.[26]

Mivacurium

Mivacurium (see Table 86–2) is currently the shortest acting nondepolarizing (benzylisoquinolinium) NMB drug.[19] It is associated with histamine release and has a duration of action of 15 to 25 minutes when administered as a bolus. Mivacurium is metabolized by plasma cholinesterase, the same enzyme that degrades succinylcholine. Therefore, prolonged neuromuscular blockade can occur in the same clinical situations as with succinylcholine. The drug's short duration of action requires that it be administered as a continuous infusion in the ICU; however, the cost of such an infusion would be prohibitive (see Table 86–2). Thus, mivacurium is used primarily for intubation in the ICU in patients for whom succinylcholine is contraindicated. Major metabolites of mivacurium are renally excreted.

Intermediate-Acting Drugs

Atracurium

Atracurium (see Table 86–2) is an intermediate-acting, benzylisoquinolinium NMB drug marketed as a racemic mixture of 10 stereoisomers.[15, 17, 19, 22, 27] Neuromuscular blockade occurs over 3 to 4 minutes after injection of 0.3 to 0.6 mg/kg. Rapid administration may trigger histamine release with secondary hypotension. A unique aspect of atracurium is its degradation via the *Hofmann reaction,* a nonenzymatic, spontaneous breakdown that occurs at normal body temperature and pH and is independent of renal or hepatic function.[18, 19, 28] However, accumulation of one major metabolite, laudanosine, may produce excitatory central nervous system (CNS) toxicity, such as seizures. The threshold for laudanosine CNS stimulation in humans remains unknown, but because laudanosine is renally excreted, it may accumulate to a greater degree when prolonged infusions are used in critically ill patients with renal failure.

Cisatracurium

Cisatracurium (see Table 86–2) is the R-*cis,* R′-*cis* isomer that normally constitutes about 15% of the commercial NMB drug mixture marketed as atracurium (Fig. 86–3). The features that distinguish it from atracurium are greater potency, no dose-related histamine release, less interaction with autonomic ganglia, and generation of threefold less laudanosine. Like atracurium, it undergoes Hofmann elimination, so drug elimination occurs independent of end-organ function. Intravenous doses of 0.2 mg/kg (four times the 95% effective dose [ED_{95}]) provide good conditions for endotracheal intubation in 90 seconds and last 45 to 60 minutes. Continuous infusions titrated from 2.5 to 3.0 μg/kg/min may be utilized for ICU patients.[29]

Vecuronium

Vecuronium (see Table 86–2) is an aminosteroid that differs in structure from pancuronium by the deletion of a methyl group at the 2*N*-piperidino position of the steroid molecule.[15, 17, 20] This substitution eliminates the vagolytic effects such as tachycardia and hypertension associated with pancuronium injections. Vecuronium is administered in the ICU as an intermittent bolus or continuous infusion. It undergoes hepatic hydrolysis to three different desacetyl metabolites: 3-, 17-, and 3,17-desacetylvecuronium, which vary in NMB activity. The 3-desacetyl metabolite is estimated to be 80% as potent as the parent compound; the others are far less potent.[11, 30] Metabolites such as 3-desacetylvecuronium accumulate in renal failure, especially when complicated by uremia, and are one of the causes of prolonged weakness in this group of patients.[11, 30]

Rocuronium

Rocuronium, introduced in 1994, is also an aminosteroid NMB drug (see Table 86–2) chemically related to vecuronium. Intravenous doses of 0.6 to 1.2 mg/kg produce good to excellent intubating conditions within 60 seconds,[31] rivaling succinylcholine for speed of onset. Rocuronium has an intermediate duration of action (30 to 45 minutes), no cardiovascular side effects, and elimination primarily via the hepatobiliary system

TABLE 86–3. Potential Adverse Effects of Neuromuscular Blocking Drugs in the Intensive Care Unit

Anxiety or stress in the awake patient
Risk of ventilator disconnection or airway mishap
Autonomic and cardiovascular interactions
Tachycardia or bradycardia
Hypotension or hypertension
Accumulation of parent drug or drug metabolites (e.g., laudanosine, 3-desacetylvecuronium)
Decreased lymphatic flow, respiratory clearance
Risk of generalized deconditioning, skin breakdown, peripheral nerve injury
Unpredictable risk of prolonged muscle weakness and postparalytic syndrome (myopathy)
Drug cost
Central nervous system toxicity with prolonged administration
Interactions with leukocytes (immune suppression)

TABLE 86–4. Drug Interactions with Neuromuscular Blocking (NMB) Drugs

Drugs That Potentiate the Action of Nondepolarizing NMB Drugs
Halogenated anesthetics
Local anesthetics
Lidocaine
Antibiotics
Aminoglycosides (gentamicin, tobramycin, amikacin)
Polypeptides (polymyxin B)
Other antibiotics (clindamycin, tetracycline)
Antiarrhythmics
Procainamide
Quinidine
Magnesium
Calcium channel blockers
β-Adrenergic blockers
Chemotherapeutic agents
Cyclophosphamide
Dantrolene
Diuretics
Furosemide (biphasic response)
Thiazides
Lithium carbonate
Cyclosporine
Drugs That Antagonize the Actions of Nondepolarizing NMB Drugs
Phenytoin
Carbamazepine
Theophylline
Sympathomimetic agents
Chronic exposure to nondepolarizing NMB drugs

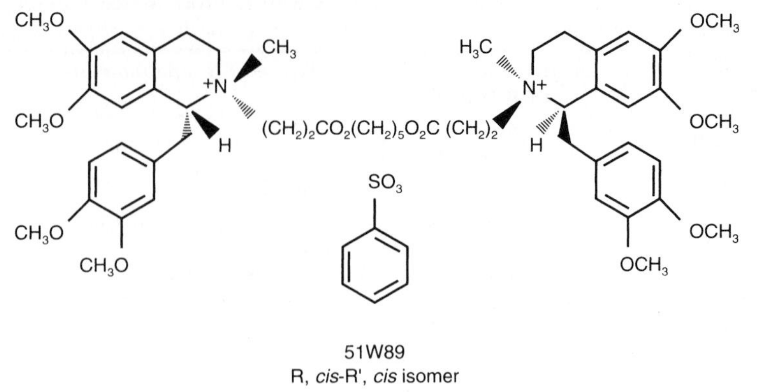

Figure 86–3. Structure of cisatracurium (51W89), the R, cis-R′, *cis* isomer of atracurium, with four chiral centers (highlighted with bold atomic bond markings). This structure is representative of the benzylisoquinolinium class of neuromuscular blocking drugs.

(but with minimum liver metabolism). Either intermittent bolus (mean dose = 14 to 68 mg/hr) or continuous infusion (30 to 50 mg/hr) may be utilized in adult and pediatric ICU patients.[32, 33] However, the $t\frac{1}{2}^{\beta}$ (terminal half-life) at least triples in ICU patients when the drug is given for prolonged periods, because the volume of distribution at steady state increases threefold.[32]

Long-Acting Drugs

d-Tubocurarine

d-Tubocurarine (curare) (see Table 86–2) is the prototypic benzylisoquinolinium NMB drug.[19] Although the first NMB used in the ICU (for the treatment of tetanus), it is rarely used now because of associated histamine release and ganglionic blockade resulting in hypotension. It undergoes predominantly renal excretion with some minor biliary excretion. The $t\frac{1}{2}^{\beta}$ of curare is markedly prolonged in patients with renal and hepatic dysfunction. The degree of biliary excretion, however, does increase in patients with renal failure.

Metocurine

Metocurine is a trimethylated derivative of *d*-tubocurare. It is twice as potent as the parent compound and associated with far less histamine release and less ganglionic blockade.[19] It is minimally metabolized, undergoes predominantly renal excretion, and has an extended half-life in patients with renal failure because it does not undergo hepatic or biliary elimination.

Pancuronium

Pancuronium (see Table 86–2) is a synthetic, bisquaternary aminosteroid NMB drug[20] that is vagolytic and sympathomimetic. These changes in autonomic tone may result in tachycardia, hypertension, and increased cardiac output[34] and are likely to occur despite the timing and method of drug delivery in ICU patients. Pancuronium is metabolized to hydroxylated derivatives such as 3-OH-pancuronium, which is 50% as potent as the parent drug.[20] Thus, the NMB effects of pancuronium accumulate with repeated dosing. Both pancuronium and its metabolites are mainly excreted by the kidney, but the duration of action may be prolonged in patients with either hepatic or renal insufficiency. The long duration of action permits administration in the ICU as either intermittent boluses or continuous infusion.[34, 35]

Pipecuronium

Pipecuronium (see Table 86–2) is also a long-acting aminosteroid NMB drug,[20, 22, 23] which facilitates its ICU administration via intermittent boluses.[35] It is longer acting than pancuronium but is not associated with cardiovascular side effects or autonomic interactions. It is metabolized by the liver to 3-desacetylpipecuronium and then renally excreted.

Doxacurium Chloride

Doxacurium chloride (see Table 86–2), a benzylisoquinolinium NMB drug introduced in 1991, is noted for its potency ($ED_{95} \approx 0.025$ mg/kg) and lack of hemodynamic or autonomic interactions.[19, 23, 36, 37] Repeated doxacurium dosing of patients in the operating room (OR) and ICU[34] has not been associated with tachycardia or accumulation. The drug is primarily excreted unchanged by the kidneys and minimally metabolized. There may be modest prolongation of doxacurium blockade in patients with renal or hepatic insufficiency.

TWITCH MONITORING IN THE INTENSIVE CARE UNIT

Traditionally, the degree of neuromuscular blockade in the operating room is routinely monitored by qualitative grading of a motor response to transcutaneous peripheral nerve stimulation.[38–41] In this way, neuromuscular function can be assessed independently of confounding variables such as sedation, alterations in mental status, or the patient's cooperation. Most authorities now recommend routine use of a hand-held peripheral nerve stimulator in the ICU to titrate the depth of neuromuscular blockade and prevent significant and unnecessary NMB drug overdose. Indeed, routine use of neuromuscular function monitoring with a peripheral nerve stimulator has been advocated to limit, if not eliminate, prolonged weakness after use of NMB drugs in the ICU.[8]

Although it is theoretically desirable, avoiding periods of profound (or complete) neuromuscular block with twitch monitoring in ICU patients cannot guarantee return of normal neuromuscular function once the NMB drug is discontinued. Traditionally, the ulnar nerve at the wrist is stimulated while evaluating the motor response of the adductor pollicis brevis muscle of the thumb.[41] Use of other peripheral nerve sites (such as facial nerve stimulation while grading the orbicularis oculi muscle or stimulation of the peroneal nerve of the upper leg while grading foot dorsiflexion) is also feasible. Patients with strokes, paraplegia, or dense peripheral neuropathies should be monitored on unaffected limbs, because affected extremities exhibit altered responses (resistance) to neuromuscular blockade.

The train-of-four (TOF) is the most reliable and convenient method for clinical monitoring of neuromuscular blockade, particularly in awake patients, for whom more vigorous tetanic stimulation is both uncomfortable and stressful.[38, 39] With the TOF, four supramaximal stimuli (40 to 60 mA current) are delivered at 2 Hz (i.e., one stimulus every 0.5 second) and the motor twitch response to the fourth stimulus (T4) is compared with the twitch response to the first stimulus (T1). Nondepolarizing blockade is characterized by a progressive decrement in successive motor twitch responses (a TOF response < 0.7) (Fig. 86–4), the presence of fade during tetanic stimulation, and the presence of post-tetanic facilitation.[38, 39, 41] The number of motor responses after TOF stimulation closely correlates with the percentage of receptors occupied by NMB drugs at the neuromuscular junction.[39] Visual or tactile evaluation of the TOF response is clinically adequate for most applications in the ICU. More precise characterization of the motor response is possible with commercially available force transducer-recorders.

The main shortcoming of peripheral nerve stimulation is that global muscle function is inferred from the response of a single peripheral muscle group.[40] For instance, the diaphragm and laryngeal muscles are more resistant to neuromuscular blockade than the adductor pollicis brevis muscle and also recover more quickly after cessation of NMB drugs. In some patients, a TOF count of zero at the adductor pollicis muscle may not correlate with a level of neuromuscular blockade sufficient to manage adequately clinical endpoints such as elimination of coughing during suctioning, elimination of peripheral motor movements, or dyssynchrony ("triggering") of the ventilator. Thus, a TOF count of zero does not necessarily represent a failure of monitoring or drug titration but may reflect both the difficulty of administering NMB drugs in the ICU and the need for clinical endpoints discrepant with the monitored twitch at the adductor pollicis. It is important, therefore, to utilize a combination of both peripheral nerve stimulation and clinical assessment to evaluate neuromuscular function and degree of neuromuscular blockade.

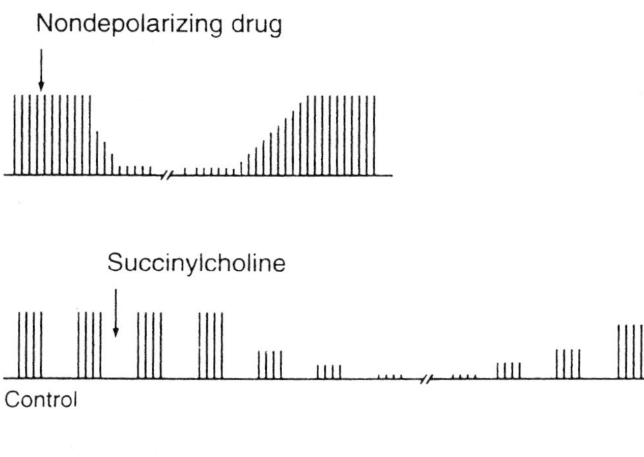

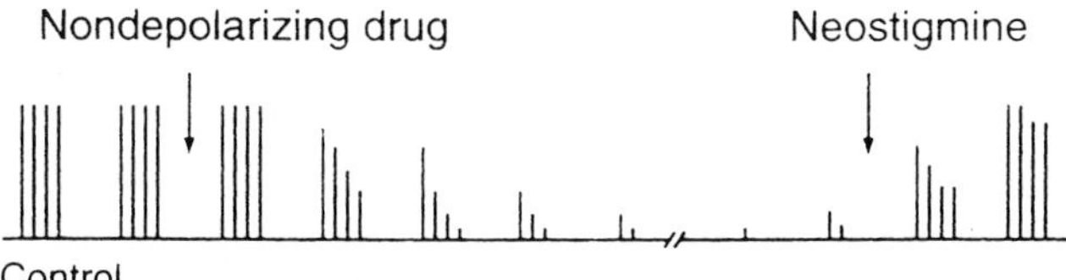

Figure 86–4. *Top panel:* Effect of a nondepolarizing neuromuscular blocking (NMB) drug (pancuronium) on the single-twitch response at 1 Hz. *Middle panel:* Effect of succinylcholine (a depolarizing NMB drug) on the train-of-four (TOF) response applied at 2 Hz after a baseline period is established. All four twitches are depressed equally, and there is no fade of the response during either onset or recovery from this type of neuromuscular block. *Bottom panel:* The more common effect of a nondepolarizing NMB drug producing a decrement in the TOF response ("fade"). The TOF response can be advantageous, in that no baseline period is required for effective monitoring. In this case, recovery was hastened by use of the anticholinesterase drug, neostigmine. (From Hunter JM: New neuromuscular blocking drugs. N Engl J Med 1995; 332:1691.)

Critically ill patients rarely require dense (e.g., 100%) receptor blockade. NMB drugs should be titrated to the minimally effective dose, maintaining the smallest degree of neuromuscular blockade that provides optimal care of the patient. A fixed level of neuromuscular blockade is difficult to maintain in ICU patients because of factors such as changing body temperature; alterations of muscle blood flow; altered electrolytes; and use of concomitant medications such as aminoglycosides, magnesium, and calcium channel blockers (see Table 86–4).

SIDE EFFECTS AND COMPLICATIONS OF NEUROMUSCULAR BLOCKING DRUGS IN THE INTENSIVE CARE UNIT

Caution must be exercised in order to limit potential adverse effects associated with use of NMB drugs in the ICU (see Table 86–3). Precautions include:

- A secured, patent, mechanical airway
- Adequate ventilation
- Appropriate inspired oxygen concentration
- Concurrent sedation and analgesia
- Precautions with pressure points on the eyes or skin
- Prophylaxis for deep venous thrombosis
- Intermittent neurologic assessment

Unexpected complications after NMB use in the ICU include prolonged recovery and even myopathy after discontinuation of NMB drug administration. These events may be related to the unrestricted use of NMB drugs in the ICU, variable modes of administration, excessive depth of neuromuscular blockade, the specific drug administered, and NMB drug interactions. Other unresolved issues include the possible benefit of routine monitoring of neuromuscular function (see earlier), lack of familiarity with newer NMB drugs, the effects of prolonged immobility, and the severity of systemic illness with associated neuromuscular pathology. It is helpful to characterize these adverse effects into *pharmacologic, physiologic,* and *toxic* mechanisms. In addition, "prolonged weakness" in the ICU may be defined as neuromuscular recovery that requires significantly longer than expected on the basis of accepted pharmacokinetic parameters generally recognized for the NMB drugs (e.g., > 120 minutes after discontinuation of intermediate-acting NMB drugs such as atracurium or vecuronium). "Myopathy" is defined as the clinical triad of persistent clinical paresis, increased serum creatine kinase (CK) concentrations, and abnormal motor unit electromyography (EMG) but normal sensory nerve conduction studies (NCSs) after administration of NMB drugs in the ICU.

Pharmacologic Adverse Effects

The steroid-based NMB drugs pancuronium and vecuronium are used frequently in the ICU.[42, 43] Not surprisingly, most case reports of ICU patients with prolonged weakness and myopathy concern patients who receive steroid-based NMB drugs.[12] The association between steroid-based NMB agents and muscle weakness must be examined carefully, because many ICU patients display altered NMB drug pharmacokinetics.[28] For instance, vecuronium undergoes hepatic hydrolysis to three metabolites, excreted primarily in the bile, that vary in NMB activity.[11] The 3-desacetyl metabolite is estimated to be 80% as potent as the parent compound; the 17- and 3,17-desacetylvecuronium metabolites are far less potent.[30] The 3-desacetylvecuronium metabolite accumulates in normal volun-

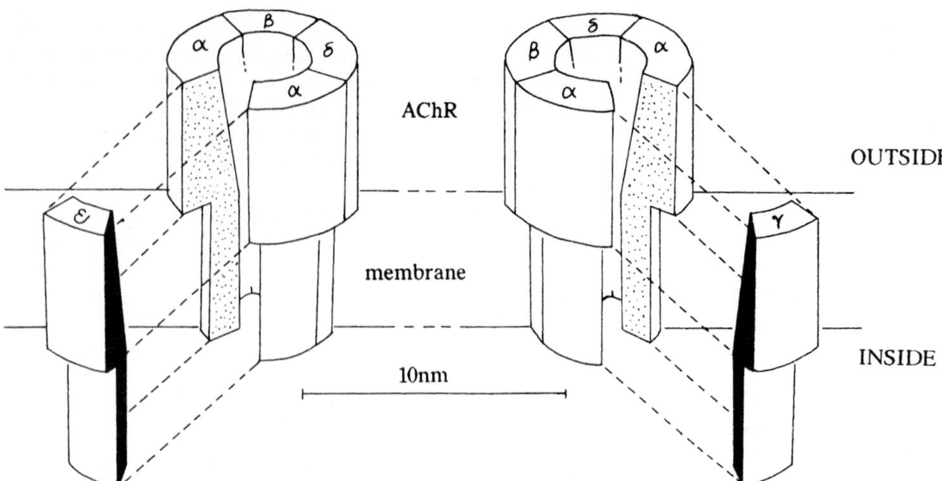

Figure 86–5. The mature, adult nicotinic acetylcholine receptor *(left)* and the immature, or fetal variant receptor *(right)*. These receptors differ by a single subunit substitution, which produces immature receptors characterized by 10-fold greater ionic activity, rapid metabolic turnover, and extrajunctional proliferation. (From Martyn JA, White DA, Gronert GA, et al: Up- and down-regulation of skeletal muscle acetylcholine receptors. Anesthesiology 1992; 76:822.)

teers[44] and patients in renal failure[11] and is poorly dialyzed and minimally ultrafiltered. In addition, Segredo and colleagues[11, 30] found a threefold increase in the elimination half-life for vecuronium because of an increased volume of distribution in patients receiving prolonged administration. The hepatic elimination of 3-desacetylvecuronium is decreased in patients who are uremic for 36 hours or more.[30] Thus, the accumulation of both 3-desacetylvecuronium and vecuronium[44] in renal failure probably contributes to prolonged weakness in this subset of ICU patients.[11, 30]

Pancuronium is a similar bisquaternary NMB drug that is desacetylated at the C3 position of the steroid nucleus to 3-desacetylpancuronium. The 3-OH metabolite is lipophilic, 90% bound to plasma proteins, approximately 50% as active as the parent pancuronium,[45] and may accumulate in patients with renal insufficiency. The combination of decreased clearance, increased volume of distribution, and accumulation of active 3-OH metabolites in renal failure may be a pharmacologic mechanism for prolonged weakness in many ICU patients.[11, 44]

A wide range of drugs interact with NMB drugs. These drug-drug interactions may either antagonize or potentiate the effect of NMB drugs (see Table 86–4). There is also concern that increased toxicity may occur when NMB drugs are administered with corticosteroids.[7, 10, 12, 46] The long-term effects and potential toxicities of many of these interactions are under investigation, especially those not secondary to altered pharmacokinetics or dynamics.

Pathophysiologic Adverse Effects

Pathophysiologic changes occur at the nerve, neuromuscular junction, and muscle in critically ill patients. These changes are enhanced when patients are immobilized or denervated secondary to CNS or spinal cord injury as well as during NMB drug–induced paralysis. The nAChR may be triggered to revert to a fetal variant structure (Fig. 86–5), characterized by an increase in total number, extrajunctional proliferation, and "resistance" to nondepolarizing NMB drugs.[47] This change may account for the observation that some ICU patients develop tachyphylaxis with NMB drugs.[48] The proliferation and distribution of these altered receptors across the myomembrane can, however, simultaneously sensitize patients to depolarizing drugs such as succinylcholine (Table 86–5). Succinylcholine stimulation of the immature, fetal receptors increases cation transport, which may be manifest clinically as life-threatening hyperkalemia.[21]

Additional investigations of the effects of critical illness and prolonged NMB exposure on nerves, neuromuscular junctions, and muscle are ongoing. For instance, there is increasing recognition of an entity termed *critical illness polyneuropathy* (CIP).[49, 50] The sensory and motor polyneuropathy of CIP differentiates this process from other neurologic and myopathic processes encountered in the critically ill (Table 86–6). CIP is a sensory-motor polyneuropathy that is manifest as distal extremity motor weakness with atrophy, reduced reflexes, and preserved cranial nerve function. CIP occurs most

TABLE 86–5. Up- and Down-regulation of Nicotinic Acetylcholine Receptors

Physiologic Stress	Change in Nicotinic Acetylcholine Receptor	Clinical Consequences
Major body burns Motor neurologic deficits Denervation syndromes Muscle crush injury Prolonged immobilization Muscle atrophy Severe infections Prolonged exposure to NMB drugs	Increased	1. Resistance to usual doses of NMB drugs (tachyphylaxis) 2. Marked sensitivity to agonists (i.e., hyperkalemic response to succinylcholine)
Myasthenia gravis Exercise conditioning Organophosphorus poisoning?	Decreased	1. Sensitivity to usual doses of NMB drugs 2. Resistance to succinylcholine

Data from Yentis SM: Suxamethonium and hyperkalemia. Anaesth Intensive Care 1990; 18:92; and Martyn JA, White DA, Gronert GA, et al: Up-and-down regulation of skeletal muscle acetylcholine receptors: Effects on neuromuscular blockers. Anesthesiology 1992; 76:822.

NMB = neuromuscular blocking.

TABLE 86–6. Diagnostic Characteristics of Intensive Care Unit Patients with Prolonged Weakness After Neuromuscular Blocking Drugs

Diagnosis	History	Physical Examination and Laboratory	Muscle or Nerve Biopsy	EMG, NCS	Course
Postparalysis syndrome	NMB drug use (aminosteroid more common) May occur with NMB drug alone Consider drug interactions (especially concurrent steroids)	Diffuse weakness Sparing of sensory function Potential for elevation of CK	Early change: selective thick-filament degeneration (EM) or local loss of ATPase activity (LM) Late change: muscle fiber necrosis	Small cMAP NL snAP NL or near NL NCV Myopathic change (only in patient with steroids and NMB drugs) With NMB drugs alone see type II atrophy (disuse)	Favorable for the most part, but patient may have prolonged recovery period
Critical illness polyneuropathy	Commonly occurs with sepsis More frequent in elderly, severely ill patients	Sensory and motor involvement	Predominantly axonal degeneration	Consistent with distal axonal sensorimotor polyneuropathy	May have protracted process with unfavorable outcome Outcome mainly related to underlying pathology
Steroid-induced myopathy	Acute or chronic process Occurs more commonly in proximal muscles	Systemic sequelae of steroid use (skin changes, diabetes, body habitus, hypertension)	Type II muscle fiber atrophy	NL or, if severe, mild myopathic change	Tends to be favorable
Deconditioning syndrome	Occurs with immobile, highly catabolic patients in the ICU May be exacerbated by deafferentation associated with dense neuromuscular blockade	Diffuse weakness and loss of muscle mass and skin	Muscle biopsy not indicated but if done shows type II fiber atrophy	Essentially NL	Dependent on underlying pathology
Guillain-Barré syndrome	Associated with underlying viral infection and ascending polyneuropathy	Diffuse motor weakness Potential involvement of cranial nerves Possible autonomic lability	Not indicated	Compatible with demyelinating sensorimotor polyneuropathy	Favorable, appears to improve with immunoglobulin or plasmapheresis
Myasthenia gravis	Variable but frequently progressive fatigue and bulbar signs	Muscle fatiguability	Not indicated	Decremental response on repetitive stimulation at 2 Hz MUP variability on EMG	Dependent on aggressiveness of disease; favorable with cholinesterase inhibitors, steroids, and thymectomy as needed
Acute rhabdomyolysis	Associated with crush injuries, drug overdose, or toxic ingestions	Increased CK Check [HPO_4^{2-}] Urine myoglobin	Diffuse muscle fiber necrosis	Spontaneous activity with myopathic changes	Favorable, depends on associated pathology and injury
Central pontine myelinolysis	Rapid electrolyte alterations	Locked-in syndrome	Not indicated	NL	Poor

From Prielipp RC, Coursin DB, Wood KE, Murray MJ: Complications associated with sedative and neuromuscular blocking drugs in critically ill patients. Crit Care Clin 1995; 11:983–1003.

ATPase = adenosine triphosphatase; CK = creatine kinase; cMAP = compound motor action potential; EM = electron microscopy; EMG = electromyography; ICU = intensive care unit; LM = light microscopy; MUP = motor unit potential; NCV = nerve conduction velocity; NL = normal; NMB = neuromuscular blocking; snAP = sensory action potential.

commonly in elderly patients with sepsis who are severely ill for prolonged periods. Up to 70% of ICU patients with sepsis are reported to experience some elements of CIP. The process is associated with high mortality, but if patients survive the underlying disease, they may make a full recovery. However, recovery requires a protracted period (3 to 6 months) of hospitalization and supportive care. CIP is a diagnosis of exclusion that is made after examination of the clinical setting, determination that the patient has a diffuse sensory-motor deficit, and appropriate findings on EMG and nerve conduction studies. CIP is thought to be the result of primary axonal degeneration, perhaps related to microvascular ischemia of the nerve during the systemic inflammatory response syndrome.[49, 51] It does not appear to be directly related to the use of NMB drugs. It is differentiated from Guillain-Barré syndrome by the absence of inflammatory changes in nerve fibers and the presence of normal cerebrospinal fluid.

TABLE 86–7. Differential Diagnosis in Patients with Prolonged Weakness After Neuromuscular Blocking (NMB) Drugs

Residual NMB drug effect secondary to parent drug, drug metabolite, or drug-drug interaction
Myasthenia gravis
Eaton-Lambert syndrome
Muscular dystrophies
Guillain-Barré syndrome
Central nervous system injury or lesion
Spinal cord injury
Steroid myopathy
Critical illness polyneuropathy
Disuse atrophy
Severe electrolyte toxicity (e.g., magnesium)
Severe electrolyte deficiency (e.g., hypophosphatemia)

Toxic Adverse Effects

The incidence of weakness after prolonged use of NMB drugs in the ICU remains unknown, although Op de Coul and colleagues[10] reported muscle weakness (of unknown and variable etiology) in 20% of consecutive patients who received long-term administration of pancuronium. Murray and coworkers[1] monitored prospectively patients in the ICU at the Mayo Clinic and estimated the risk of clinically significant prolonged neuromuscular block as 5%. The actual incidence is probably dependent on numerous factors, including the administration of various antibiotics (aminoglycosides), corticosteroids,[46] anticonvulsants, magnesium, calcium channel blocking drugs, and other medications that may interact with NMB drugs (see Table 86–4).[52] The incidence of true myopathy is less than that of prolonged weakness in the ICU, but it is difficult to quantitate precisely.

The direct toxicity of NMB drugs is poorly characterized but may be additive to alterations of NMB drug pharmacology and changes in the nAChR discussed previously. In addition, alterations in nerve, muscle, and the neurojunction may increase the toxicity of normally nontoxic drugs or drug metabolites.[12, 53] Concerns about untoward effects of NMB drugs in the ICU have even led some to advocate elimination of prolonged use of NMB drugs for critically ill patients. Others have suggested that certain NMB drugs may be better suited than others in the ICU setting, in which renal failure, hepatic failure, NMB drug tachyphylaxis, and concurrent use of parenteral corticosteroids (e.g., for status asthmaticus, acute lung injury, connective tissue disease) are common.[50–54] Unfortunately, much of the evidence for direct toxicity remains anecdotal.

Acute myopathy, often referred to as *postparalytic quadriparesis* or *tetraparesis,* is an infrequent but major complication of prolonged NMB administration in the critically ill.[4, 8, 53, 55–57] This entity must be differentiated from other causes of weakness in ICU patients (Table 86–7; see Table 86–6). Afflicted patients demonstrate diffuse weakness that persists long after the NMB drug is discontinued. Neurologic examination reveals a global motor deficit that tends to afflict proximal and distal muscles equally.

Zochodne and coworkers[57] reviewed the electrophysiologic changes associated with acute myopathy in seven ICU patients, all of whom demonstrated preservation of sensory neural pathways. Barohn and colleagues[53] described three patients with myopathy that was characterized by low-amplitude compound motor action potentials, normal sensory studies, and fibrillations. Muscle biopsy showed loss of thick myosin filaments. Variable increases in CK may be detected, depending on the timing of laboratory determinations and the initiation of the myopathic process. Thus, there may be justification for routinely screening high-risk ICU patients with serial CK determinations during the infusion of NMB drugs. It is not clear whether drug combinations such as aminosteroid NMB drugs and corticosteroids increase the risk of myopathy.

There have been some reports of a myopathy development after ICU administration of the benzylisoquinolinium NMB drugs (e.g., atracurium).[27, 54] One was a report of myopathy occurring in two patients after ICU administration of atracurium and corticosteroids, confirmed by either increased serum CK or EMG and NCS evaluations.[54] Myopathy occurred in both of these ICU patients despite the routine use of a peripheral nerve twitch monitor and frequent titration of the NMB drug infusion.

The evaluation of a patient with prolonged weakness, paresis, and possible myopathy after discontinuation of NMB drugs requires a systematic approach (Fig. 86–6; see Table 86–7). This approach should include a thorough history and physical examination combined with review of recent medications and identification of related nerve or muscle pathology. Potential residual neuromuscular blockade should be investigated with a peripheral nerve stimulator.[38–40] In addition, early neurologic consultation with appropriate diagnostic examination, including EMG and NCS, CK analysis, and muscle biopsy, should be performed. Characteristics of clinical findings in some of the processes considered in the differential diagnosis of prolonged weakness after NMB administration are noted in Table 86–6. Patients with postparalysis myopathy require ongoing reassurance and aggressive supportive care. The long-term prognosis is dependent on underlying pathology but, for the most part, is favorable. However, the recovery period may be protracted.

PROSPECTIVE STUDIES OF NEUROMUSCULAR BLOCKING DRUGS USE IN THE INTENSIVE CARE UNIT

Rocuronium

Sparr and colleagues[32] reported rocuronium drug requirements for bolus administration (median dose = 0.34 mg/kg/hr) and continuous infusion (0.54 mg/kg/hr) in 32 adult ICU patients. NMB drug requirements decreased during the first 6 to 9 hours, because the $t_{1/2}^{\beta}$ and the volume of distribution at steady state increased threefold.[32] Median time for recovery to the fourth twitch in the TOF stimulation was 100 minutes after bolus administration and 60 minutes after rocuronium drug infusion. Pediatric patients may require significantly larger doses (0.76 mg/kg/hr) initially and during maintenance infusion (0.95 mg/kg/hr).[33]

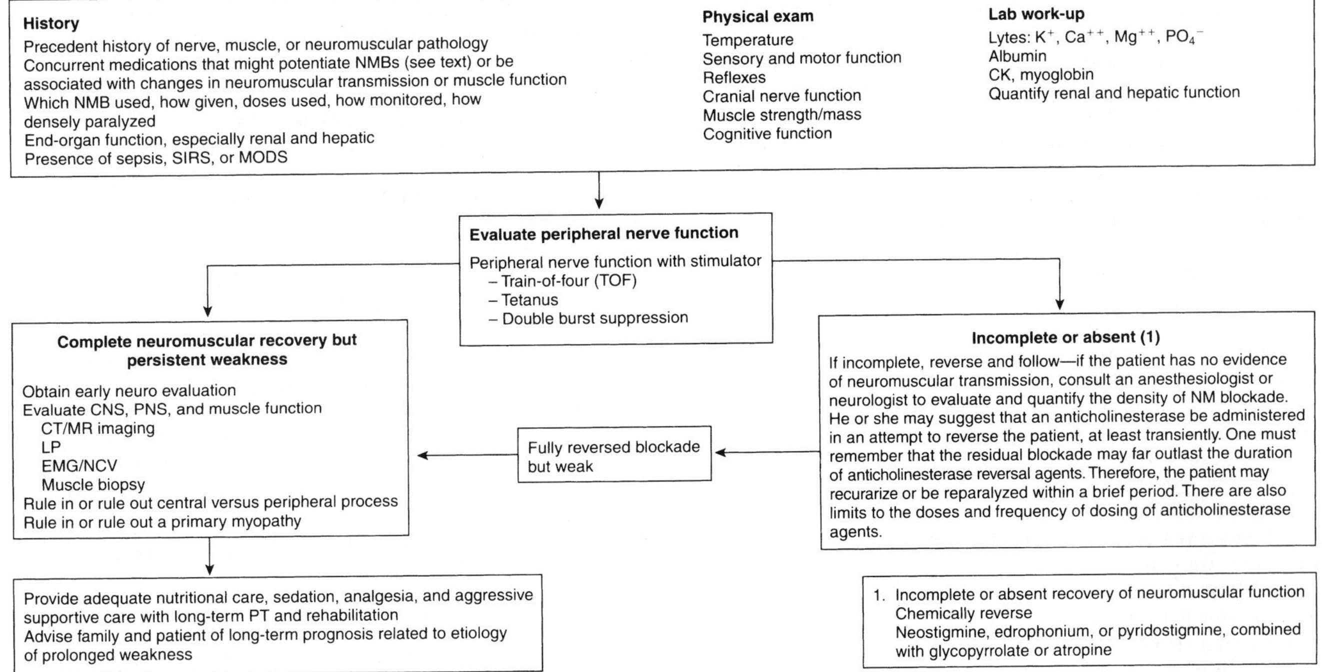

History
Precedent history of nerve, muscle, or neuromuscular pathology
Concurrent medications that might potentiate NMBs (see text) or be associated with changes in neuromuscular transmission or muscle function
Which NMB used, how given, doses used, how monitored, how densely paralyzed
End-organ function, especially renal and hepatic
Presence of sepsis, SIRS, or MODS
Physical exam
Temperature
Sensory and motor function
Reflexes
Cranial nerve function
Muscle strength/mass
Cognitive function
Lab work-up
Lytes: K^+, Ca^{++}, Mg^{++}, PO_4^-
Albumin
CK, myoglobin
Quantify renal and hepatic function
Evaluate peripheral nerve function
Peripheral nerve function with stimulator
– Train-of-four (TOF)
– Tetanus
– Double burst suppression
Complete neuromuscular recovery but persistent weakness
Obtain early neuro evaluation
Evaluate CNS, PNS, and muscle function
CT/MR imaging
LP
EMG/NCV
Muscle biopsy
Rule in or rule out central versus peripheral process
Rule in or rule out a primary myopathy
Fully reversed blockade but weak
Incomplete or absent (1)
If incomplete, reverse and follow—if the patient has no evidence of neuromuscular transmission, consult an anesthesiologist or neurologist to evaluate and quantify the density of NM blockade. He or she may suggest that an anticholinesterase be administered in an attempt to reverse the patient, at least transiently. One must remember that the residual blockade may far outlast the duration of anticholinesterase reversal agents. Therefore, the patient may recurarize or be reparalyzed within a brief period. There are also limits to the doses and frequency of dosing of anticholinesterase agents.
Provide adequate nutritional care, sedation, analgesia, and aggressive supportive care with long-term PT and rehabilitation
Advise family and patient of long-term prognosis related to etiology of prolonged weakness
1. Incomplete or absent recovery of neuromuscular function
Chemically reverse
Neostigmine, edrophonium, or pyridostigmine, combined with glycopyrrolate or atropine

Figure 86–6. One strategy for a systematic approach to the ICU patient with prolonged weakness, paresis, and possible myopathy. The history, physical examination, and laboratory studies are important elements for securing a diagnosis. CT = computed tomography; MR = magnetic resonance; EMG = electromyelography; PNS = peripheral nervous system; LP = lumbar puncture; NCV = nerve conduction velocity; CK = creatine kinase; PT = physical therapy; NMB = neuromuscular blocker; SIRS = systemic inflammatory response syndrome; MODS = multiorgan dysfunction syndrome. (From Prielipp RC, Coursin DB, Wood KE, Murray MJ: Crit Care Clin 1995; 11:1983.)

Doxacurium and Pancuronium

Murray and coworkers[34] compared bolus injection of pancuronium (0.05 mg/kg) and doxacurium (0.025 mg/kg) in a double-blind, randomized study of 40 severely ill adult patients paralyzed for 2 to 3 days in the ICU. Neuromuscular blockade was monitored with a peripheral nerve stimulator and additional boluses were given as clinically indicated. Pancuronium significantly increased heart rate by 11 beats per minute, but there was no change after doxacurium. Furthermore, neuromuscular recovery (to appearance of T4 in the TOF) was more variable and prolonged (279 ± 229 minutes) after pancuronium than after doxacurium (138 ± 46 minutes).[34] Patients with renal insufficiency (creatinine clearance < 50 mL/min) had prolonged recovery if they received pancuronium.

The dose requirements and neuromuscular recovery after doxacurium administered as a continuous infusion have been defined in adult ICU patients with head injuries.[37] Patients were paralyzed for 66 ± 12 hours (range 20 to 109.5 hours). The doxacurium infusion rate was similar at the beginning (1.0 ± 0.1 mg/hr) and end (1.3 ± 0.4 mg/hr) of the study. Doxacurium bolus had no effect on heart rate, mean arterial pressure, or intracranial pressure. After discontinuation of doxacurium infusion, neuromuscular recovery required 118 ± 19 minutes (similar to that reported by Murray and coworkers). There were no complications, prolonged weakness, or myopathies in these neurosurgical patients.

Cisatracurium and Vecuronium

The dose-response and recovery pharmacodynamics of two intermediate-acting NMB drugs, cisatracurium and vecuronium, were compared in a prospective, randomized, double-blind multicenter study of 58 critically ill adults.[29] These NMB drugs were administered as an infusion for 1 to 5 days, titrated by peripheral nerve stimulation and twitch monitoring. Cisatracurium infusion averaged 2.6 ± 0.2 mg/kg/min for a mean duration of 80 ± 7 hours. Neuromuscular recovery to a 70% TOF ratio took 63 ± 12 minutes. Vecuronium infusion averaged 0.9 ± 0.1 μg/kg/min for a mean duration of 66 ± 12 hours. By contrast, neuromuscular recovery after vecuronium required a significantly longer time, averaging 387 ± 163 minutes. In addition, prolonged recovery of neuromuscular function occurred more commonly after vecuronium drug infusion (13 of 30 patients) than after cisatracurium (two of 28 patients).

Cisatracurium and Atracurium

The pharmacodynamics and pharmacokinetics of the two benzylisoquinolinium intermediate-acting NMB drugs cisatracurium and atracurium were examined in a prospective, randomized, double-blind study of 12 mechanically ventilated ICU patients paralyzed for 1 to 2 days.[58] Neuromuscular recovery to a 70% TOF ratio required 60 minutes after the cisatracurium infusion and 62 minutes after atracurium. Cisatracurium was 2.5 times more potent than atracurium in these ICU patients, which translated to significantly lower plasma laudanosine concentrations after cisatracurium (peak value = 1.3 μg/mL) than after atracurium (maximum concentration = 4.4 μg/mL).[58]

OTHER CONTROVERSIES ABOUT LONG-TERM NEUROMUSCULAR BLOCKING DRUG USE IN THE INTENSIVE CARE UNIT

Patients with Head Trauma

Head injury and brain trauma may increase intracranial pressure (ICP). At least 50% of patients with severe head injury manifest an ICP greater than 20 mm Hg. Although the specific pathologic effects of increased ICP are yet to be defined, the outcome of patients after head injury is worse when ICP remains elevated. However, there is no agreement about optimal therapy for increased ICP associated with head trauma. Traditional management utilizes controlled hyperventilation, fluid restriction, head elevation, diuretics, cerebrospinal fluid (CSF) drainage, and routine use of NMB drugs. Paralysis with NMB drugs can effectively prevent or blunt the potent sympathetic and other reflex responses to tracheal suctioning that would otherwise result in rapid increases in ICP.[59] In addition, NMB drugs facilitate the use of controlled hyperventilation. Despite the efficacy of NMB drugs in facilitating control of intracranial hypertension in patients with head injury, administration of NMB drugs (as part of a routine protocol for ICU patients with trauma) has not been shown to improve patients' outcome.[60]

Hsiang and colleagues[61] reviewed 514 patients with severe head trauma (Glasgow Coma Scale score ≤ 8) collated in the Traumatic Coma Data Bank from 1984 to 1987. Approximately half of these patients received early and routine use of NMB drugs; the other half did not. Patients receiving early, routine use of NMB drugs (group 1) were characterized by significantly longer ICU stay (8 versus 5 days), more frequent pneumonia, and a trend toward a higher rate of sepsis.[61] Although the mortality was lower in group 1 patients who received early NMB drugs (24% versus 39%, $P < .001$), this group also had significantly more vegetative and severely disabled survivors. Significant limitations are inherent in this study, but it raises important questions regarding use of NMB drugs and a prospective study is warranted. Currently, the use of NMB drugs for control of ICP in patients with head trauma remains controversial.

Central Nervous System Effects of Long-Term Administration

Curare (*d*-tubocurarine) causes marked CNS excitation in animals when applied directly to the cerebral cortex. Szenohradszky and coworkers[62] determined the seizure threshold (in rats) after intrathecal administration of various NMB drugs. The potency for inducing seizures (atracurium > pancuronium > vecuronium) was not related to peripheral potency as a muscle relaxant (pancuronium > vecuronium > atracurium). It is unknown what drug concentration develops in the CSF of patients receiving prolonged administration of NMB drugs in the ICU, especially if they suffer head trauma with disruption of the blood-brain barrier.

Cardone and colleagues[63] suggested that the CNS toxicity may be due to accumulation of intracellular calcium secondary to sustained activation of acetylcholine receptor ion channels by NMB drugs. Interestingly, neither atracurium or laudanosine increased intracellular calcium in experimental brain slices. Further investigation of CNS toxicities is warranted, especially in patients with head trauma or encephalopathy who receive prolonged NMB infusions.[64]

Tachyphylaxis

The pharmacologic development of tachyphylaxis (i.e., rapid acquisition of clinical hyporeactivity as a result of frequent or continuous exposure to a NMB drug) may be seen in both pediatric and adult ICU patients within 24 to 72 hours of the onset of neuromuscular blockade.[65, 66] True tachyphylaxis is denoted by a tripling or quadrupling of the starting NMB dose,[66] and infusion rates of vecuronium as high as 32 mg/hr have been recorded.[48] Multiple factors may account for tachyphylaxis in ICU patients. These include improper storage of certain labile NMB drugs, alterations in plasma protein binding or volume of NMB drug distribution, alterations in body temperature or acid-base balance, and proliferation of immature (or "fetal") nACh receptors at the neuromuscular junction and across the myomembrane.[47, 65] Chronic, partial neuromuscular blockade, like partial or complete deafferentation injury, may trigger proliferation of these abnormal, "fetal variant" nACh receptors[67] (see Fig. 86-5). These receptors are characterized by greater ionic activity, rapid metabolic turnover, and extrajunctional proliferation (see Table 86-5).

Hogue and coworkers[47] showed that the development of these extrajunctional receptors could be stimulated in rats by chronic subclinical infusion of curare. Autopsy data for ICU patients confirmed that an increased density of skeletal muscle nACh receptors was associated with an increased requirement for NMB drugs. Thus, some patients with increased nACh receptors may develop tachyphylaxis with NMB drugs in the ICU setting and perhaps become more susceptible to developing prolonged weakness or myopathy as a consequence.

Neuromuscular Blocking Drugs in the Elderly

Because of decreased cardiac output to skeletal muscle, the onset of paralysis is delayed in elderly patients after NMB drug administration. In addition, the half-life of many NMB drugs, such as vecuronium, rocuronium, and pancuronium, is increased, probably as a result of reduced renal and hepatic function. However, plasma clearance of atracurium and cisatracurium is not altered in the elderly, because of Hofmann elimination.

Leukocyte Activity and Neuromuscular Blocking Drugs

Limited information is available on interactions of the immune system and NMB drugs. Anecdotal evidence, such as that reported by Hsiang and colleagues,[61] shows a higher rate of pneumonia (29% versus 15%) and sepsis (11% versus 7%) in head-injured patients managed with early use of NMB drugs than in patients not routinely receiving NMB drugs. Others have noted a significantly increased rate of postsurgical pneumonias with the long-acting NMB drug pancuronium (12.7%) compared with the intermediate-acting drug atracurium (5.1%). The mechanism is not clear, but pancuronium has been reported to inhibit polymorphonuclear neutrophil adherence and migration[68] in high concentrations (1.3 μg/mL blood) as well as alter leukocyte membrane fluidity.[69] Although the clinical significance of these findings is not clear, it is speculated that NMB drugs directly interact with the immune system, and this biochemical effect potentiates infectious problems associated with immobility (e.g., decreased clearance of respiratory secretions).

SUMMARY

NMB drugs are administered in large doses over prolonged periods to severely ill patients with one or more organ failures in the ICU. These drugs may have potential untoward effects. Some of these are readily predictable, whereas others are not. Major concerns are appropriate drug selection and delivery, monitoring, and neuromuscular recovery of patients who receive NMB drugs for 24 hours or more. Myopathy and paresis have been reported after prolonged use of NMB drugs in the ICU. Further investigation needs to characterize this process fully, identify those at risk, and outline mechanisms for preventing or limiting the injury. Prolonged weakness may occur secondary to changes in the basic pharmacology or elimination of NMB drugs in ICU patients. Pathophysiologic changes in the nerve, muscle, or neuromuscular junction may also play a role in the development of some cases of prolonged weakness or myopathy. Concerns about the potential for direct or indirect toxicity of NMB drugs to skeletal muscle and the central nervous system remain. Resolution of these issues will improve the selection and optimal administration of NMB drugs to ICU patients.

References

1. Murray MJ, Strickland RA, Weiler C: The use of neuromuscular blocking drugs in the intensive care unit: A US perspective. Intensive Care Med 1993; 19(Suppl 2):S40.
2. Elliot JM, Bion JF: The use of neuromuscular blocking drugs in intensive care practice. Acta Anaesthesiol Scand Suppl 1995; 106:70.
3. Coursin DB: Neuromuscular blockade: Should patients be relaxed in the ICU? Chest 1992; 102:988.
4. Douglass JA, Tuxen DV, Horne M, et al: Myopathy in severe asthma. Am Rev Respir Dis 1992; 146:517.
5. Giostra E, Magistris MR, Pizzolato G, et al: Neuromuscular disorder in intensive care unit patients treated with pancuronium bromide: Occurrence in a cluster group of seven patients and two sporadic cases, with electrophysiologic and histologic examination. Chest 1994; 106:210.
6. Gooch JL, Suchyta MR, Balbierz JM, et al: Prolonged paralysis after treatment with neuromuscular junction blocking agents. Crit Care Med 1991; 19:1125.
7. Hansen-Flaschen J, Cowan J: Neuromuscular blockade in the intensive care unit: More than we bargained for. Am Rev Respir Dis 1993; 147:234.
8. Hoyt JW: Persistent paralysis in critically ill patients after the use of neuromuscular blocking agents. New Horiz 1994; 2:48.
9. Kupfer Y, Namba T, Kaldawi E, et al: Prolonged weakness after long-term infusion of vecuronium bromide. Ann Intern Med 1992; 117:484.
10. Op de Coul AA, Lambregts PC, Koeman J, et al: Neuromuscular complications in patients given Pavulon® (pancuronium bromide) during artificial ventilation. Clin Neurol Neurosurg 1985; 87:17.
11. Segredo V, Caldwell JE, Matthay MA, et al: Persistent paralysis in critically ill patients after long-term administration of vecuronium. N Engl J Med 1992; 327:524.
12. Watling SM, Dasta JF: Prolonged paralysis in intensive care unit patients after the use of neuromuscular blocking agents: A review of the literature. Crit Care Med 1994; 22:884.
13. Armstrong DK, Crisp CB: Pharmacoeconomic issues of sedation, analgesia, and neuromuscular blockade in critical care. New Horiz 1994; 2:85.
14. Rudis MI, Guslits BJ, Peterson EL, et al: Economic impact of prolonged motor weakness complicating neuromuscular blockade in the intensive care unit. Crit Care Med 1996; 24:1749.
15. Ramsey FM: Basic pharmacology of neuromuscular blocking agents. Anesthesiol Clin North Am 1993; 11:219.
16. Dreyer F: Acetylcholine receptor. Br J Anaesth 1982; 54:115.
17. Bevan DR, Donati F: Muscle relaxants. *In:* Clinical Anesthesia. 2nd ed. Barash PG, Cullen BF, Stoelting RK (Eds). Philadelphia, JB Lippincott, 1992, p 481.
18. Hunter JM: New neuromuscular blocking drugs. N Engl J Med 1995; 332:1691.
19. Belmont MR, Maehr RB, Wastila WB, et al: Pharmacodynamics and pharmacokinetics of benzylisoquinolinium (curare-like) neuromuscular blocking drugs. Anesthesiol Clin North Am 1993; 11:251.
20. Ducharme J, Donati F: Pharmacokinetics and pharmacodynamics of steroidal muscle relaxants. Anesthesiol Clin North Am 1993; 11:283.
21. Yentis SM: Suxamethonium and hyperkalaemia. Anaesth Intensive Care 1990; 18:92.
22. Mirakhur RK: Newer neuromuscular blocking drugs: An overview of their clinical pharmacology and therapeutic use. Drugs 1992; 44:182.
23. Rathmell JP, Brooker RF, Prielipp RC, et al: Hemodynamic and pharmacodynamic comparison of doxacurium and pipecuronium with pancuronium during induction of cardiac anesthesia: Does the benefit justify the cost? Anesth Analg 1993; 76:513.
24. Harper NJ: Neuromuscular blocking drugs: Practical aspects of research in the intensive care unit. Intensive Care Med 1993; 19(Suppl 2):S80.
25. Prielipp RC, Coursin DB: Applied pharmacology of common neuromuscular blocking agents in critical care. New Horiz 1994; 2:34.
26. Wierda JM, van den Broek L, Proost JH, et al: Time course of action and endotracheal intubating conditions of Org 9487, a new short-acting steroidal muscle relaxant: A comparison with succinylcholine. Anesth Analg 1993; 77:579.
27. Werner MU, Nielsen HK, Jensen AG, et al: Atracurium in the intensive care unit. Acta Anaesthesiol Scand 1987; 31(Suppl 86):200.
28. Prielipp RC, Jackson MJ, Coursin DB: Comparison of the neuromuscular recovery after paralysis with atracurium versus vecuronium in an ICU patient with renal insufficiency. Anesth Analg 1994; 78:775.
29. Prielipp RC, Coursin DB, Scuderi PE, et al: Comparison of the infusion requirements and recovery profiles of vecuronium and cisatracurium 51W89 in intensive care unit patients. Anesth Analg 1995; 81:3.
30. Caldwell JE, Szenohradszky J, Segredo V, et al: The pharmacodynamics and pharmacokinetics of the metabolite 3-desacetylvecuronium (ORG 7268) and its parent compound, vecuronium, in human volunteers. J Pharmacol Exp Ther 1994; 270:1216.
31. Puhringer FK, Khuenl-Brady KS, Koller J, et al: Evaluation of endotracheal intubating conditions of rocuronium (ORG 9426) and succinylcholine in outpatient surgery. Anesth Analg 1992; 75:37.
32. Sparr HJ, Wierda JM, Proost JH, et al: Pharmacodynamics and pharmacokinetics of rocuronium in intensive care patients. Br J Anaesth 1997; 78:267.
33. Tobias JD: Continuous infusion of rocuronium in a paediatric intensive care unit. Can J Anaesth 1996; 43:353.
34. Murray MJ, Coursin DB, Scuderi PE, et al: Double-blind, randomized, multicenter study of doxacurium vs. pancuronium in intensive care unit patients who require neuromuscular-blocking agents. Crit Care Med 1995; 23:450.
35. Khuenl-Brady KS, Reitstätter B, Schlager A, et al: Long-term administration of pancuronium and pipecuronium in the intensive care unit. Anesth Analg 1994; 78:1082.
36. van Miert MM, Hunter JM: Neuromuscular blocking agents in critically ill patients. Curr Opin Anaesthesiol 1994; 7:375.
37. Prielipp RC, Robinson JC, Wilson JA, et al: Dose response, recovery, and cost of doxacurium as a continuous infusion in neurosurgical intensive care unit patients. Crit Care Med 1997; 25:1236.
38. Hudes E, Lee KC: Clinical use of peripheral nerve stimulators in anaesthesia. Can J Anaesth 1987; 34:525.
39. Brull SJ: An update on monitoring of neuromuscular function. Curr Opin Anaesthesiol 1992; 5:577.
40. Donati F, Bejan DR: Not all muscles are the same (Editorial). Br J Anaesth 1992; 68:235.
41. Davidson JE: Neuromuscular blockade: Indications, peripheral nerve stimulation, and other concurrent interventions. New Horiz 1994; 2:75.
42. Hansen-Flaschen JH, Brazinsky S, Basile C, et al: Use of sedating drugs and neuromuscular blocking agents in patients requiring mechanical ventilation for respiratory failure. JAMA 1991; 266:2870.
43. Klessig HT, Geiger HJ, Murray MJ, et al: A national survey on the practice patterns of anesthesiologist intensivists in the use of muscle relaxants. Crit Care Med 1992; 20:1341.
44. Wright PM, Hart P, Lau M, et al: Cumulative characteristics of atracurium and vecuronium: A simultaneous clinical and pharmacokinetic study. Anesthesiology 1994; 81:59.
45. Miller RD, Agoston S, Booij LH, et al: The comparative potency and pharmacokinetics of pancuronium and its metabolites in anesthetized man. J Pharmacol Exp Ther 1978; 207:539.
46. Danon MJ, Carpenter S: Myopathy with thick filament (myosin) loss following prolonged paralysis with vecuronium during steroid treatment. Muscle Nerve 1991; 14:1131.
47. Hogue CW Jr, Itani MS, Martyn JA: Resistance to *d*-tubocurarine in lower motor neuron injury is related to increased acetylcholine

receptors at the neuromuscular junction. Anesthesiology 1990; 73:703.
48. Coursin DB, Klasek G, Goelzer SL: Increased requirements for continuously infused vecuronium in critically ill patients. Anesth Analg 1989; 69:518.
49. Bolton CF, Young GB, Zochodne DW: The neurologic complications of sepsis. Ann Neurol 1993; 33:94.
50. Bolton CF: Muscle weakness and difficulty in weaning from the ventilator in the critical care unit. Chest 1994; 106:1.
51. Witt NJ, Zochodne DW, Bolton CF, et al: Peripheral nerve function in sepsis and multiple organ failure. Chest 1991; 99:176.
52. Erkola O: Complications of neuromuscular blockers: Interaction with concurrent medications and other neuromuscular blockers. Anesthesiol Clin North Am 1993; 11:427.
53. Barohn RJ, Jackson CE, Rogers SJ, et al: Prolonged paralysis due to nondepolarizing neuromuscular blocking agents and corticosteroids. Muscle Nerve 1994; 17:647.
54. Meyer KC, Prielipp RC, Grossman JE, et al: Prolonged weakness after infusion of atracurium in two intensive care unit patients. Anesth Analg 1994; 78:772.
55. Margolis BD, Khachikian D, Friedman Y, et al: Prolonged reversible quadriparesis in mechanically ventilated patients who received long-term infusions of vecuronium. Chest 1991; 100:877.
56. Partridge BL, Abrams JH, Bazemore C, et al: Prolonged neuromuscular blockade after long-term infusion of vecuronium bromide in the intensive care unit. Crit Care Med 1990; 18:1177.
57. Zochodne DW, Ramsay DA, Saly V, et al: Acute necrotizing myopathy of intensive care: Electrophysiological studies. Muscle Nerve 1994; 17:285.
58. Boyd AH, Eastwood NB, Parker CJ, et al: Comparison of the pharmacodynamics and pharmacokinetics of an infusion of cis-atracurium (51W89) or atracurium in critically ill patients undergoing mechanical ventilation in an intensive therapy unit. Br J Anaesth 1996; 76:382.
59. Werba A, Weinstabl C, Petricek W, et al: Vecuronium prevents increases in intracranial pressure during routine tracheobronchial suctioning in neurosurgical patients. Anaesthesist 1991; 40:328.
60. Prough DS, Joshi S: Does early neuromuscular blockade contribute to adverse outcome after acute head injury? Crit Care Med 1994; 22:1349.
61. Hsiang JK, Chestnut RM, Crisp CB, et al: Early, routine paralysis for intracranial pressure control in severe head injury: Is it necessary? Crit Care Med 1994; 22:1471.
62. Szenohradszky J, Trevor AJ, Bickler P, et al: Central nervous system effects of intrathecal muscle relaxants in rats. Anesth Analg 1993; 76:1304.
63. Cardone C, Szenohradszky J, Yost S, et al: Activation of brain acetylcholine receptors by neuromuscular blocking drugs: A possible mechanism of neurotoxicity. Anesthesiology 1994; 80:1155.
64. Werba A, Gilly H, Weindlmayr-Goettel M, et al: Porcine model for studying the passage of non-depolarizing neuromuscular blockers through the blood-brain barrier. Br J Anaesth 1992; 69:382.
65. Hunter JM: Resistance to non-depolarizing neuromuscular blocking agents. Br J Anaesth 1991; 67:511.
66. Coursin DB, Meyer DA, Prielipp RC: Doxacurium infusion in critically ill patients with atracurium tachyphylaxis. Am J Health Syst Pharm 1995; 52:635.
67. Martyn JA, White DA, Gronert GA, et al: Up-and-down regulation of skeletal muscle acetylcholine receptors: Effects on neuromuscular blockers. Anesthesiology 1992; 76:822.
68. Smith CJ, Edwards AE, Gower DE, et al: Leucocyte migration: Effects of in vitro exposure to anaesthetic agents: Possible potentiation of effects by adrenaline. Eur J Anaesthesiol 1992; 9:463.
69. Aloui R, Gallet H, Biot N, et al: Behavior of leukocyte membrane fluidity in presence of anaesthetic drugs: Comparison between allergic patients and control subjects. Gen Pharmacol 1993; 24:419.

87

Basic Pharmacologic Principles and Drug Monitoring

Drew A. MacGregor, MD • Tom A. Martin, PharmD, BCPS

The clinical pharmacist has become an integral member of the critical care health care team, providing vital information concerning drug effects, drug-drug interactions, therapeutic drug monitoring (TDM), and numerous other pharmacologic details commonly overlooked by physicians and nurses. As patients with more complex multiple organ system dysfunction are cared for in the intensive care unit (ICU), the necessity to better understand pharmacologic principles continues to increase. This chapter reviews some of the basic pharmacologic principles and supplies examples of pharmacodynamics and pharmacokinetics to demonstrate the usefulness of these principles when applied to critically ill patients. The chapter also demonstrates the importance and benefit of TDM, again providing specific examples pertaining to the ICU.

PHARMACODYNAMICS

In the broad sense, pharmacodynamics is the study of how individual drugs affect specific organs, receptors, or the body in whole and of the mechanisms by which drugs exert these effects. Since the mid-1980s, there has been an explosion of information pertaining to the receptor sites of drugs, the interactions of drugs with these receptors, and the physiologic effects of these interactions. This in turn has allowed physicians to make more appropriate use of medications that are designed for very specific physiologic effects.

One of the finest examples of pharmacodynamics was the isolation, elucidation, and specification of the β-adrenergic receptor (β-AR) and β-adrenergic receptor agonists. The β-AR is a complex assimilation of numerous subunits, including the membrane-bound cellular receptor, regulatory proteins located within the membrane (G proteins), and the enzyme adenylyl cyclase.[1] Activation of the β-AR initiates molecular interactions with the G proteins, which in turn increase the activity of adenylyl cyclase, increasing the production of intracellular cyclic adenosine monophosphate (cAMP). The cAMP stimulates intracellular protein kinase reactions, which in turn activate phosphorylase enzymes, including the class of phosphorylases that induce conformational changes in the voltage-regulated cellular membrane calcium channels, allowing for an influx of ionized calcium into the myocardial cell. As a result of the change in intracellular calcium, calcium channels associated with the sarcoplasmic reticulum open, release large concentrations of calcium, and stimulate interactions between actin and myosin in muscle.

The research into the pharmacodynamics of the β-AR and the agonists for these receptors has allowed for improved pharmacologic support of the failing heart.[2] For example, experimental data indicate that epinephrine and isoproterenol are more efficacious and potent β-AR agonists than are dobutamine, dopamine, and dopexamine.[3] Although numerous theories explain this fact, one pharmacodynamic explanation is that epinephrine and isoproterenol possess higher "binding frequency" than do the less potent agonists; that is, a single molecule of epinephrine or isoproterenol can bind to a β-AR, activate the cascade of events just described, and get released from the receptor, being free in the plasma to circulate and activate more β-AR. Dobutamine and the other less potent β-AR agonists bind to the cellular receptor for a much longer time and are less capable of activating additional receptor complexes. Thus, in the time it takes for a weak β-AR agonist to stimulate a small number of receptors, epinephrine may have stimulated hundreds or even thousands of β-ARs. This has been demonstrated clinically by an increased inotropic effect for epinephrine for a given degree of chronotropic effect in comparison with that for dobutamine in patients recovering from coronary bypass surgery.[4]

Improved understanding of β-AR pharmacodynamics has also helped explain the changes in β-AR density associated with the failing heart.[1, 5-7] In normal people, there are approximately 10 β_1 receptors for every β_2 receptor in the heart. In chronic congestive heart failure, however, the number of β_1 receptors decreases to a far greater extent than does the number of β_2 receptors, and the ratio can reach approximately 5:3. Thus, in healthy human volunteers and/or animal models, β_1 agonists are better cardiac stimulants than are β_2 agonists. In contrast, stimulation of the β_2-AR becomes a much more efficacious therapy in patients with congestive heart failure.[8, 9]

Additional terms used to describe the pharmacodynamics of various drug combinations include *additive effects*, which refers to two drugs that have pharmacologic effects within the body that are greater than the effects of either drug alone and can usually be expressed as the algebraic summation of the effects. Two drugs whose effect is greater than the expected summation of both drugs are said to have *synergistic effects*. *Antagonistic effects* occur when drugs combine to produce effects that are less than the sum of the individual effects of the drugs.

In the same β-AR example, the cAMP produced by β-adrenergic stimulation is rapidly hydrolyzed by enzymes known as phosphodiesterases. Thus, the addition of a phosphodiesterase inhibitor (e.g., amrinone, milrinone) results in increases in myocardial contractility that are more pronounced than the maximal effect produced by a β-AR agonist alone; the drugs demonstrate an additive effect.[10-12] On the other hand, combining two different β-AR agonists may result in no additive effect or in a partially antagonistic effect. An antagonistic interaction may result from the weaker agonist's acting as a competitive inhibitor for binding sites on the β-AR.[13] Antibiotics are commonly used together for their synergistic effects. For example, ampicillin and an aminoglycoside are commonly used in combination for the treatment of *Enterococcus faecalis* infection. The combined effect of cell wall synthesis (the penicillins) and ribosomal activity (aminoglycosides) results in much greater bacterial killing than would be achieved by either drug alone or from the additive effect of both drugs in isolation. It is extremely important to recognize which drugs may offer additive or synergistic effects and those that may yield antagonistic results when combined.

Pharmacodynamics also play important roles in the toxicity or side effects of numerous drugs used in critical care. Medications that are metabolized through the hepatic microsomal enzyme system, specifically by the cytochrome P_{450} enzyme system, markedly alter the pharmacodynamics of other drugs that are also metabolized through this pathway. A common example in organ transplantation is the addition of the antibiotic erythromycin to a transplant recipient.[14, 15] This drug dramatically increases the plasma levels of the antirejection drug cyclosporine, allowing for lower dosages of this very expensive agent. Conversely, failure to recognize this interaction can lead to cyclosporine toxicity. Such drug-drug interactions are of vital importance in the ICU, in which multiple medications are frequently required for the simultaneous treatment of multiple concurrent illnesses.

PHARMACOKINETICS

Pharmacokinetics is the quantitative study of how drugs enter the body, are distributed within the various organ systems, and are eliminated from the body. Kinetics become quite complicated in view of the absorption of an orally administered pro-drug, which must be adequately absorbed from the gastrointestinal (GI) tract, transported to the liver for partial metabolism to the active drug, further transported to the site(s) or organ(s) of action, metabolized, and eliminated from the body. In critically ill patients, we routinely avoid some of the complicating factors of pharmacokinetics by directly injecting drugs into the vascular system rather than worrying about the absorption characteristics and first-pass effects through the enteral circulation and the liver.

Classic descriptions of pharmacokinetics use the "fluid-in-a-bucket" analogy: A measured amount of drug distributed within a given volume of fluid results in very precise estimation of drug concentration. The single drug in a single bucket is the one-*compartment* model, and although the simplicity of this analogy does not apply directly to most physiologic systems, it does allow for better comprehension of more complex systems. For example, if a bolus of drug is injected into the vascular system and is neither absorbed nor distributed to any other tissues (i.e., remains in the vascular system), the initial concentration of the drug can be calculated as follows:

$$\text{bolus dose} = X_0$$
$$\text{volume of distribution} = V_d$$
$$\text{initial concentration} = C = X_0/V_d$$

Similarly, we can reverse this formula and measure the concentration of drug (C) in plasma after a bolus dose (X_0) and calculate the volume of distribution (V_d) of that drug. With this volume of distribution, a more precise dose of drug required to achieve a desired plasma concentration can be calculated. This model also allows for precise determination of half-life ($t_{1/2}$), which is the time required for drug concentration to fall by 50%, which can be easily measured and calculated.

As any drug is removed from a compartment (vascular space or other), there is a *rate constant (k)* that describes the rate at which drug is eliminated from that compartment. The clearance (Fig. 87-1) of a drug can then be calculated as follows:

$$\text{clearance} = Q = kV$$

Unfortunately, few drugs administered adhere to this one-compartment model. In fact, most drugs appear to be best described by two- or three-compartment models, with rate constants and clearances described for each compartment.[16, 17] Rate constants can be determined for drug distribution from one compartment (e.g., vascular) to another (e.g., soft tissues) or for excretion from the body (elimination rate constant, k_e).

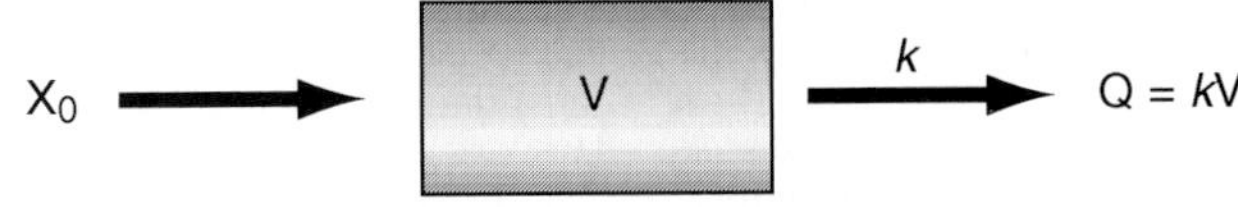

Figure 87–1. A bolus dose of drug (X_0) given into volume (V) is removed at a specific clearance (Q), according to the rate constant *k*.

Figure 87–2 helps demonstrate pharmacokinetics in a two-compartment model. Injectable drugs immediately enter the circulating blood volume, and the central compartment (plasma) demonstrates a peak rise in drug concentration after administration. Some portion of the drug, however, is distributed into a second (and perhaps even a third) compartment. These peripheral compartments may be the reticuloendothelial system, intracellular fluid volume, or any other isolated physiologic space, but rarely are these "compartments" directly attributable to an anatomic structure. In addition to the amount of drug that is terminally eliminated by the body (again represented by the elimination constant, k_e), drug is also being removed from the central compartment and redistributed back into the central compartment from the peripheral or secondary compartment; the rate constants k_{12} and k_{21} characterize the intercompartmental transfer of drug.

One example of the importance of multicompartment models is the tricyclic class of antidepressants. After the drug is absorbed into the bloodstream, these highly lipophilic drugs are distributed into tissues separate from the plasma, which results in very low plasma levels despite potentially large amounts of drug within the body. Whereas k_{12} (the distribution from the plasma to the tissues) is very large, k_{21} (the release of drug from the tissues back to the central, or plasma compartment) is very small. In addition, the plasma volume of distribution (V_1) is small, but the volume of distribution in the tissues (V_2) is huge. Because of these facts, drug elimination is very slow, and toxic effects can last for a considerable length of time. Thus, treatment of tricyclic overdose is difficult because enhancing elimination is not very effective and because complete removal of drug from the plasma by means of hemodialysis or charcoal hemofiltration (equivalent to maximizing k_e) does very little to eliminate the bulk of the drug that is in the body.[18]

This multicompartment understanding of pharmacokinetics is redefining the concept of half-life as well. In a one-compartment model, the half-life is the time required for drug concentration in the plasma (the single compartment) to fall by 50%.

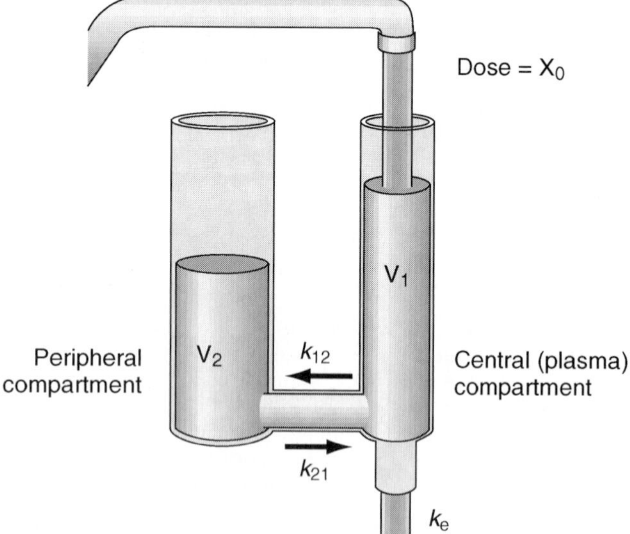

Figure 87–2. Model of pharmacokinetics in a two-compartment model. Drug administered to the central (plasma) compartment is distributed to a peripheral (tissue) compartment according to the rate constant, k_{12} and is redistributed back to the central compartment according to the rate constant, k_{21}. Terminal elimination from the body is determined by the clearance (Q), which is dependent upon the elimination rate constant, k_e.

In the multicompartment model, it is possible to consider the plasma half-life, the tissue half-life, the elimination half-life, and the therapeutic half-life, each of which has a slightly different focus for the theoretical and/or mathematical representation of elimination and metabolism for each compartment. A number of studies have demonstrated how mathematical models can be used to more precisely calculate the half-life and other pharmacokinetic variables of multicompartment drugs.[16, 17, 19, 20]

The complexity of multicompartment models is important in order to fully understand the potential benefits and risks of drugs, especially as new drugs are brought onto the market to replace older medications. Figure 87–3 demonstrates a three-compartment model for four different opioid agonist analgesics. In each model, a central (plasma) compartment receives the drug via injection and has a rapid rise in concentration, with a corresponding rate of terminal elimination. The second, or peripheral, compartment (shown on the left) corresponds to the central nervous system (CNS), on which the drug has its therapeutic benefit. The CNS compartment has a very rapid exchange with the central compartment for all of the opioids, but each agonist demonstrates a different volume of distribution for this compartment. Similarly, each agonist redistributes within a third compartment (shown on the right of each figure) but at a much slower rate (i.e., smaller k_{13}).

With these illustrations, some facts about each of the opioid agonists can be demonstrated. For example, if drug is continuously added to the central (plasma) compartment in a concentration that exceeds the elimination of the drug, the drug will be redistributed quickly into the compartment on the left (e.g., the CNS) *and* will be slowly but continuously redistributed into the larger peripheral compartment on the right. The dose given to the central compartment can be adjusted to maintain a certain level of effect, primarily as a result of levels in the CNS compartment. Because this compartment has a rapid equilibration with the central compartment, drug dose and CNS effect are closely linked. When the drug is discontinued, however, the levels fall from both the central and the CNS compartments according to the elimination constants for each drug (e.g., the size of the drainage hole in the bucket). However, drug in the tissue compartment is redistributed back to the central compartment (which rapidly redistributes it into the CNS compartment). As a result, drugs with large tissue compartments (e.g., sufentanil, fentanyl) have the potential for significant accumulation in the tissues and, as a result of redistribution from this tissue compartment, a prolonged effect after drug discontinuance. Drugs such as remifentanil and alfentanil have much smaller volumes of distribution for both the CNS and the tissue compartments and thus are less likely to demonstrate prolonged effect, even when the drug has been given for a long time.

THERAPEUTIC DRUG MONITORING

Despite the implied precision of predicting drug levels and clearances using multiple-compartment pharmacokinetics, TDM in the critical care setting is still analogous to raking leaves in a hurricane. Constant change in patient dynamics makes for difficult interpretation of static measurements of drug concentration data. The lack of strong data to support the concept that achieving target drug concentrations affects outcomes in critically ill patients causes many physicians and pharmacists to question the role that repeated serum concentration measurements play in optimal patient care. Critically ill patients are, however, at an increased risk for development of adverse therapy outcomes as a result of alterations in drug pharmacokinetics and pharmacodynamics. The absorption,

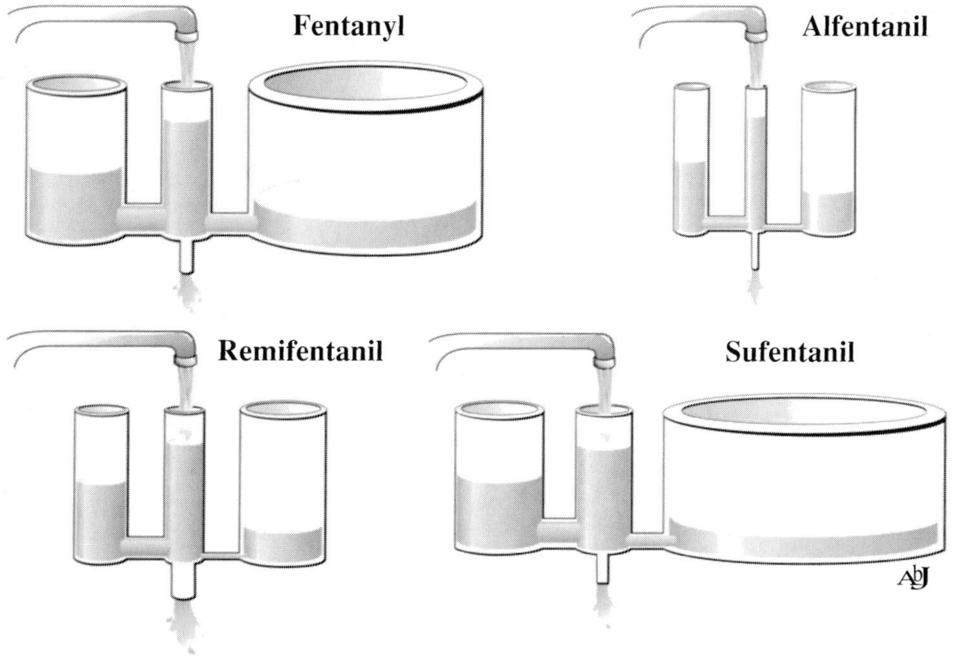

Figure 87–3. Pharmacokinetic models for four opioid agonists. Each agonist has volumes of distribution for the central (plasma) compartment, a central nervous system (CNS) compartment *(left)* and a separate peripheral (tissue) compartment *(right)*. Each compartment has different rate constants as well, which lead to the differences in duration of effect for each of the drugs. (Courtesy of P. E. Scuderi MD, Department of Anesthesiology, Wake Forest University School of Medicine.)

distribution, metabolism, and elimination of drugs administered to the critically ill patient are affected by a multitude of host-specific factors, ranging from hemodynamic and nutritional status to concurrent disease states and related pharmacotherapy. The pharmacodynamics of drug therapy are altered as a result of acute changes in the affinity and number of binding sites, as has been described for β-ARs. The lack of direct assessment parameters for many drugs necessitates use of surrogate markers, which further contributes to the difficulty of assessing drug therapy in these patients.

Thus, the art of the science of TDM is the ability to use multiple static data to assess an ever-changing clinical situation. Patient-specific pharmacokinetic parameters derived from strategically obtained serum drug concentrations can be used to individualize doses for patients with variable distribution volumes and elimination characteristics. The goal of TDM in the ICU is to help ensure cost-effective drug therapy that maximizes outcomes while minimizing complications. In the subsequent sections of this chapter, we analyze the use of TDM for different classes of medications used in the critical care environment.

Table 87–1 lists seven criteria developed by Spector and associates that would ideally be met in order to justify the use of TDM.[21] No single agent "currently satisfies" all seven of these criteria, but the goal of TDM is to meet as many of these standards as possible. Table 87–2 lists many of the drugs for which plasma or blood levels can be measured and which of the Spector criteria each drug fulfills. The final criterion for any drug monitoring program should be that determination of drug levels alters patient care in an evidence-based manner. The criteria listed in Table 87–1 help the physician to determine whether such evidence exists.

Aminoglycosides

The aminoglycoside antibiotics are the prototypical drugs for which TDM is employed to individualize therapy. They exhibit first-order, one-compartment elimination characteristics, which makes for easy bedside interpretation of serum concentrations. Aminoglycosides are distributed primarily into body water, so clinical conditions associated with changes in fluid status warrant closer monitoring. The tenuous fluid status that accompanies critical illness predisposes affected patients to variable aminoglycoside volumes of distribution, which in turn can lead to wide fluctuations in serum concentrations across the standard dose range. As a result, alternative dosing strategies are often necessary to achieve the desired goals of therapy.[22]

Studies have supported the premises that higher serum concentrations produce better outcomes (both in terms of bacterial killing and in resolution of infections) and that elevated trough concentrations for prolonged periods of time increase the likelihood of developing adverse effects.[23] Thus, the basic goal with aminoglycoside therapy is to achieve high peak concentrations and very low trough concentrations in the plasma. Traditional dosing methods attempt to achieve target concentrations on the basis of the specific site of infection. Peak concentrations of gentamicin and tobramycin for uncomplicated urinary tract infections and for synergy with gram-positive organisms are generally considered to be 3 to 5 μg/mL, whereas the target range for bacteremia and other

TABLE 87–1. Seven Criteria for the Use of Therapeutic Drug Monitoring

I. An appropriate drug assay is available (satisfactory accuracy and precision, small sample volume requirements, short analysis time, minimal cost, and high assay specificity).
II. There is documented and significant interindividual variability in drug absorption, elimination, and distribution.
III. Adequate pharmacokinetic data concerning the drug are available.
IV. The pharmacologic effect is proportional to the plasma drug concentration.
V. A narrow range exists between the efficacious and toxic drug concentrations.
VI. A constant pharmacologic effect over an extended period of time exists.
VII. Clinical studies exist that define the therapeutic and toxic ranges of the drug.

Adapted from Spector R, Park GD, Johnson GF, Vesell EF: Therapeutic drug monitoring. Clin Pharmacol Ther 1988; 43:345–353.

TABLE 87–2. Medications Fulfilling Criteria for Effective Therapeutic Drug Monitoring

Drug	I	II	III	IV	V	VI	VII	Comments
Amikacin	×	×	×	×	×		×	Trough only if dosing once daily to document clearance
Digoxin	×	×	×				×	Accumulates in renal failure; monitor potassium and magnesium
Gentamicin	×	×	×	×	×		×	Trough only if dosing once daily to document clearance; nomogram available for 7 mg/kg doses
Lidocaine	×	×	×		×			Dose to effect; monitor concentrations to avoid toxicity
Phenytoin	×	×			×			Free phenytoin concentrations are technically difficult to determine; nonlinear kinetics are exhibited at therapeutic serum concentrations; dose to effect; monitor concentrations to avoid toxicity
Procainamide	×	×		×	×			Dose to effect; monitor concentrations to avoid toxicity
Quinidine	×	×		×	×			Dose to effect; monitor concentrations to avoid toxicity; nonlinear kinetics may be exhibited
Theophylline	×	×	×		×			Multiple disease states and drug interactions alter kinetics; monitor concentrations to avoid toxicity; nonlinear kinetics may be exhibited
Tobramycin	×	×	×	×	×		×	Trough only if dosing once daily to document clearance; nomogram available for 7 mg/kg doses
Vancomycin	×	×	×					Trough only in renal insufficiency to document clearance

serious gram-negative infection is 6 to 8 μg/mL. Because the aminoglycosides do not penetrate pulmonary tissue as well, peak plasma levels between 8 and 10 μg/mL are considered desirable for treating pneumonia.[24] Peak concentrations should be measured 30 minutes after a 30-minute infusion or 15 minutes after a 60-minute infusion. All gentamicin and tobramycin troughs should be measured immediately before the next dose and should be less than 2 μg/mL. Amikacin peak concentrations for most infections should be 20 to 30 μg/mL, and troughs should be less than 10 μg/mL. These values represent steady-state concentrations, so the common practice is to wait until at least the third or fourth dose before measuring concentrations.

The fact that most critically ill patients never achieve the elusive steady-state condition adds to the difficulty in interpretation of blood concentrations. Some clinicians advocate obtaining first-dose peak and trough concentrations in order to make necessary dosage adjustments more rapidly. One underlying assumption with this method is that obtaining higher peak concentrations early in therapy produces better outcomes. This concept has been substantiated by in vitro data and at least supported by in vivo data and is the basis of once-daily dosing of aminoglycosides. This dosing method takes advantage of the finding that microbiologic and clinical efficacy seem to be related to the ratio of peak concentrations to the minimum inhibitory concentration (peak:MIC) for concentration-dependent antibiotics, such as the aminoglycosides. Thus higher peaks result in more efficient bacterial killing, and the longer interval between doses allows for complete drug clearance from the renal cortex, which has been shown to reduce the risk of toxicity.

Controversy also exists as to the optimal dose and concentration sampling time for aminoglycosides. Nicolau and associates[25] developed a nomogram to achieve a target peak concentration of 20 μg/mL (10 times the MIC of the most troublesome pathogen) and a 4-hour drug-free period (<0.5 μg/mL). This group has advocated giving an initial 7 mg/kg dose of gentamicin or tobramycin and adjusting the dosing interval on the basis of a blood concentration measurement taken approximately 8 hours (range, 6 to 14 hours) later. This nomogram should not be used with doses other than 7 mg/kg. One alternative sampling method for doses less than 7 mg/kg in patients with questionable renal function is to check a trough value before the second dose to document that the patient is able to clear the drug. This value should ideally be less than 0.5 μg/mL to allow for a drug-free period. The drawback with this strategy is that one cannot know how long the concentration is below the MIC or the lower limit of the assay. In each instance, the ultimate goal is to define the dose-response curve for each given patient; it is desirable to reach peak blood levels approximately 10 times the MIC for the cultured pathogen, and drug levels should be nearly undetectable 2 to 4 hours before the next dose, to help minimize toxicity.

One additional note of caution is that there is a difference between once-daily dosing and traditional once-a-day dosing. In the former case, the goal is to maximize the peak:MIC ratio and provide a drug-free period. The latter method describes the fact that the clearance of aminoglycosides for a given patient can be markedly reduced by renal dysfunction or other causes, and thus the drug remains in higher concentrations for more prolonged periods of time, increasing the risks of toxicity. Therefore, patients with renal impairment need a longer interval between drug doses to achieve trough concentrations of less than 2 μg/mL for gentamicin and tobramycin. The administered dose of aminoglycoside must also be lower (1 to 2 mg/kg) to prevent such high peak concentrations that will not be cleared from the body during the 24-hour period. The concern in using these antibiotics when clearance is markedly decreased is compromising efficacy (peak concentrations) versus increasing risk of toxicity (trough concentrations).

Vancomycin

The routine monitoring of serum vancomycin concentrations continues to be debated.[26-30] In contrast to the aminoglycosides, no direct relationship has been shown between serum concentration and patient outcome. In vitro data suggest that vancomycin exhibits non–concentration-dependent initial killing action against gram-positive organisms such as *Staphylococcus aureus, E. faecalis, Streptococcus pyogenes,* and *Strep-*

tococcus pneumoniae and that vancomycin appears to inhibit regrowth of these organisms for 0.5 to 3.5 hours *after* the concentration falls below the MIC.[31-34] These characteristics suggest that the ideal dosing strategy for vancomycin, like that for the β-lactams, would be one that maintains serum concentrations above the MIC of the organism for the entire dosing interval. One option for dosing antibiotics with this type of sustained in vitro activity is to administer the antibiotic via continuous infusion so as to optimize the antimicrobial killing patterns.[35, 36] However, although this practice has been used with some β-lactams, the applicability of the data to clinical practice for vancomycin has yet to be determined.[37]

Vancomycin in doses to maintain trough concentrations of at least 5 to 10 μg/mL may be appropriate because the vancomycin MIC for most organisms is 1 μg/mL, and thus serum concentrations would be 5 to 10 times the MIC for the entire dosing interval. Organism location must also be considered in assessment of therapy. The vancomycin molecule is too large to penetrate body cavities very well. Vancomycin distribution into the pulmonary epithelial lining fluid of critically ill patients has been shown to be approximately 20%.[38] Therefore, serum trough concentrations of 5 to 10 μg/mL would keep the pulmonary lining fluid concentration above the MIC for the dosing interval for organisms with MICs of 1 μg/mL. Patients with organisms with MICs of 2 μg/mL or higher require more aggressive dosing, with a target trough concentration of 20 μg/mL. Vancomycin penetration into cerebrospinal fluid is very poor, so patients with penicillin-resistant gram-positive meningitis or shunt infections often require intrathecal or intrashunt administration.

Documentation of toxicity related to vancomycin concentration is also lacking. The nephrotoxicity and ototoxicity historically associated with vancomycin are now believed to have been secondary to impurities in the early formulation of the drug, rather than to serum vancomycin concentrations. There does, however, appear to be an increased risk for these adverse effects when vancomycin is combined with an aminoglycoside.

The fact that vancomycin exhibits multicompartmental pharmacokinetic properties serves to further confuse the issue of whether monitoring concentrations is practical. The lack of a consensus on the optimal time to obtain peak concentrations results from an uncertainty as to which "peak" concentration is important. A concentration obtained immediately after the end of the infusion represents the maximum serum concentration achieved during that dosing interval (i.e., peak concentration in the central [vascular] compartment). However, if efficacy and toxicity are indeed related to concentration, the greatest concern would be with the maximum concentration achieved in the tissue compartment, rather than in the serum. This concentration occurs at the end of the distributional phase, which displays considerable interpatient variability. Vancomycin also does not fit consistently into either a two- or three-compartment model. This is because of variable volumes of distribution, variable rate constants, and variations in terminal clearance, determined partly by renal function. The result is a less than ideal estimation of distributional half-life, which ranges from 0.5 to more than 3 hours, making dosage adjustments on a proportional basis impractical. Serum concentrations obtained 1 to 2 hours after the end of the infusion to allow for the intercompartmental distribution process create confusion because the resulting serum concentration typically falls outside the accepted "therapeutic" range of 30 to 40 μg/mL. This often results in numerous unnecessary dosage adjustments. Because of these considerations, routine monitoring of serum vancomycin levels has been eliminated from many clinical practices.

Moellering described some clinical scenarios in which monitoring vancomycin concentrations may be prudent: (1) patients receiving vancomycin/aminoglycoside combinations; (2) anephric patients undergoing hemodialysis and receiving infrequent doses of vancomycin for serious systemic infections (especially if the newer high-flux dialysis membranes are being used); (3) patients receiving higher-than-usual doses of vancomycin; and (4) patients with rapidly changing renal function.[30] Critically ill patients often meet one or all of these criteria because of the nature of their disease states; however, it remains to be proven that monitoring vancomycin levels actually influences outcome, and thus each patient's condition should dictate whether monitoring vancomycin concentrations is practical.

Phenytoin

Anticonvulsants, in contrast to aminoglycoside antibiotics, generally exert their therapeutic benefit by maintaining plasma levels, whereas their toxicity is generally attributable to excessive peak concentrations; thus monitoring anticonvulsant therapy in critically ill patients typically involves trying to achieve the lowest effective dose. Also in contrast to antibiotics, anticonvulsants have a definite, more easily monitored therapeutic endpoint; therefore, serum concentrations play a lesser role in the designing of drug dosing regimens. However, phenytoin may be the exception to this rule.

Phenytoin does not exhibit standard pharmacokinetics, in that at blood concentrations above approximately 4 μg/mL, the drug exhibits Michaelis-Menten (capacity-limited or saturable) kinetics; that is, alterations in the administered dose do not produce proportional changes in serum concentrations, and small dosage increases may result in phenytoin levels in excess of the generally accepted therapeutic range of 10 to 20 μg/mL. The fact that phenytoin is highly protein-bound (more than 90%) also makes for difficulties in dosing in patients with reduced albumin and/or elevated blood urea nitrogen (BUN) concentrations. The free (unbound) phenytoin concentration is the more important concentration because only free drug is able to exert a pharmacologic effect.

Unfortunately, because free phenytoin concentrations are technically difficult to determine, most hospital laboratories send these samples out to other facilities. The typical 2-day turnaround time makes this process impractical in the critically ill patient. Many equations have been proposed to estimate free phenytoin concentrations on the basis of measured total concentrations; however, the correlation between the measured free concentrations and the calculated free concentrations has not been strong enough to warrant routine use of these formulas.

Anderson and colleagues proposed a revised Winter-Tozer equation that appears to be more accurate in trauma victims and elderly patients with hypoalbuminemia.[39] In general, the clinician should be aware that patients with clinical situations associated with higher free fractions of phenytoin (i.e., decreased binding sites or displacement) require total serum trough concentrations lower than the accepted range of 10 to 20 μg/mL. Clinicians should avoid the tendency to chase serum concentrations in lieu of clinical assessment.

Antiarrhythmics

Despite the increasing number of drugs for which serum concentrations can be measured, monitoring antiarrhythmic drug therapy follows the same basic premise as with phenytoin. Most drugs are dosed to effect, the acceptable concentration being whatever suppresses the arrhythmia without causing side effects. Antiarrhythmics for which serum concentration monitoring is common are digoxin, procainamide (and

N-acetylated procainamide [NAPA]), quinidine, and lidocaine. Of these agents, digoxin and procainamide are the two most commonly used in the ICU.

Digoxin represents a difficult problem for TDM because of its large volume of distribution (~7 L/kg) and long half-life, resulting from its multicompartment distribution. Despite these pharmacokinetic considerations, therapeutic benefit does appear to correlate with serum levels of the drug. Loading doses should be given to rapidly achieve therapeutic concentrations of 1.5 to 2.4 ng/mL for atrial fibrillation and 0.5 to 1.2 ng/mL for inotropic effects. Maintenance regimens should be designed to achieve the lowest effective trough concentration. Studies have shown that the risk for adverse effects dramatically increases once the steady-state serum concentration exceeds 2 ng/mL; thus, monitoring drug levels in patients who are prone to changes in digoxin clearance (e.g., those with renal dysfunction or hypoperfusion states) appears warranted. In addition to elevated drug levels, hypokalemia, hypomagnesemia, and hypercalcemia have all been reported to potentiate digoxin toxicity.

Therapeutic drug monitoring for procainamide presents additional challenges. Procainamide itself exerts antiarrhythmic effects and is metabolized initially in the liver, where it is acetylated to NAPA. This metabolite has class III antiarrhythmic activity, and both compounds produce toxicity when the drug levels exceed approximately 10 μg/mL. This relatively narrow therapeutic index, the lack of correlation between dosage changes and proportional changes in serum concentrations, and the correlation of serum concentrations with antiarrhythmic effects makes monitoring procainamide and NAPA serum concentrations an acceptable practice. Most critically ill patients require a continuous infusion to maintain concentrations of each compound between approximately 4 and 10 μg/mL, with a combined level (procainamide plus NAPA) of between 10 and 15 μg/mL. Once the patient's condition has stabilized and medications can be administered by mouth or through a nasogastric or an orogastric tube, patients may be switched to the instant-release product at doses starting at 500 mg every 3 to 6 hours to maintain trough procainamide concentrations in the range of 4 to 10 μg/mL.

Theophylline

Theophylline's role in treating acute asthmatic and bronchospastic episodes continues to be questioned. As such, theophylline use in critical care is generally limited to patients on stable maintenance regimens before admission to the ICU. These patients are commonly started on continuous theophylline infusions until they are able to take the oral, immediate-release product. The sustained-release products are reserved for ward patients who are preparing for discharge. The definition of optimal theophylline therapy continues to evolve as new discoveries are made into its pharmacokinetics and pharmacodynamics. There has been interest in changing the accepted therapeutic range from 10 to 20 μg/mL to 5 to 15 μg/mL to help reduce the occurrence of adverse effects, especially tachydysrhythmias.[40] However, data supporting efficacy at lower concentrations are lacking. Central to this argument is the discovery that theophylline may also exhibit Michaelis-Menten kinetics (similar to those of phenytoin) in some patients at therapeutic serum concentrations. As a result, dosage changes do not always produce proportional changes in serum concentrations. This situation may expose these patients to a higher risk of adverse effects with small changes in dose. The fact that serious adverse effects, including seizures and cardiovascular toxicity, may occur at near-normal concentrations further serves to confuse the risk-benefit analysis of monitoring theophylline levels. As a general rule, dose increases greater than 25% are not recommended once the serum concentration exceeds 10 μg/mL.

Theophylline clearance is affected by numerous medications and disease states. It is metabolized by the cytochrome P_{450} system in the microsomal fraction of the hepatocyte into four primary metabolites, one of which is caffeine. Drugs such as cimetidine, ciprofloxacin, erythromycin, propranolol, and verapamil have been shown to reduce theophylline clearance. Phenobarbital, phenytoin, and rifampin each enhance theophylline clearance. Diseases such as chronic obstructive pulmonary disease, cirrhosis, heart failure, hypothyroidism, hyperthyroidism, and cystic fibrosis have been shown to variably affect theophylline clearance. In view of the significant pathophysiologic changes and the number of medications that accompany the treatment of critical illness, it seems prudent to recommend monitoring theophylline concentrations along with the clinical signs and symptoms of toxicity, such as tachycardia, nausea, vomiting, agitation, arrhythmias, and seizures.

SUMMARY

Even though the concentrations of more and more drugs are able to be measured in serum, the data to support specific therapeutic ranges for most drugs in the critical care setting remain arguably weak. However, most clinicians agree that there are many drugs for which the therapeutic index is narrow enough to support the concept that too much or not enough of these drugs puts the patient at undue risk for therapy failure or toxic complications. Although TDM is certainly not an exact science, it does help make an even more inexact science (critical care medicine) more individualized than giving "standard" doses to patients with abnormal homeostasis. The key to making TDM practical is realizing its proper role in patient care and learning how to interpret the serum concentration data within the context of the patient's clinical condition.

References

1. Bristow MR, Hershberger RE, Port JD, Gilbert EM, Sandoval A, Rasmussen R, Cates AE, Feldman AM: β-adrenergic pathways in nonfailing and failing human ventricular myocardium. Circulation 1990; 82(Suppl I):I12–I25.
2. Bristow MR, Ginsburg R, Minobe W, Cubicciotti RS, Sageman WS, Lurie K, Billingham ME, Harrison DC, Stinson EB: Decreased catecholamine sensitivity and β-adrenergic-receptor density in failing human hearts. N Engl J Med 1982; 307:205–211.
3. MacGregor DA, Prielipp RC, Butterworth JF IV, James RL, Royster RL: Relative efficacy and potency of β-adrenoceptor agonists for generating cAMP in human lymphocytes. Chest 1996; 109:194–200.
4. Butterworth JF IV, Prielipp RC, Royster RL, Spray BJ, Kon ND, Wallenhaupt SL, Zaloga GP: Dobutamine increases heart rate more than epinephrine in patients recovering from aortocoronary bypass surgery. J Cardiothorac Vasc Anesth 1992; 6:535–541.
5. Summers RJ, Molnaar P, Russell F, Elnatan J, Jones CR, Buxton BF, Chang V, Hambley J: Coexistence and localization of beta 1- and beta 2-adrenoceptors in the human heart. Eur Heart J 1989; 10(Suppl B):11–21.
6. Heitz A, Schwartz J, Velly J: β-Adrenoceptors of the human myocardium: Determination of β1 and β2 subtypes by radioligand binding. Br J Pharmacol 1983; 80:711–717.
7. Buxton BF, Jones CR, Molenaar P, Summers RJ: Characterization and autoradiographic localization of beta-adrenoceptor subtypes in human cardiac tissues. Br J Pharmacol 1987; 92:299–310.
8. Fowler MB, Laser JA, Hopkins GL, Minobe E, Bristow MR: Assessment of the β-adrenergic receptor pathway in the intact failing human heart: Progressive receptor down-regulation and subsensitivity to agonist response. Circulation 1986; 74:1290–1302.
9. Brodde OE, Zerkowski HR, Borst HG, Maier W, Michel MC: Drug-

and disease-induced changes of human cardiac beta-1 and beta-2 adrenoceptors. Eur Heart J 1989; 10(Suppl B):38–44.
10. Jones JL, Gengo PJ, Dodam JR, Hellyer PW: Amrinone combined with dobutamine improves hemodynamics and oxygen delivery without down-regulation of cardiac β-adrenergic receptor density in porcine endotoxemia. Shock 1995; 3:224–234.
11. Vincent JL, Leon M, Berre J, Melot C, Kahn RJ: Addition of enoximone to adrenergic agents in the management of severe heart failure. Crit Care Med 1992; 20:1102–1106.
12. Prielipp RC, Butterworth JF IV, Zaloga GP, Robertie PG, Royster RL: Effects of amrinone on cardiac index, venous oxygen saturation and venous admixture in patients recovering from cardiac surgery. Chest 1991; 99:820–825.
13. Prielipp RC, Butterworth JF IV, Royster RL, Pang J, Zaloga GP: Dobutamine antagonizes cAMP production by epinephrine in human lymphocytes. Anesth Analg 1993; 76:S334.
14. Hughes CM, Swanton JG, Collier PS: Cyclosporin A and erythromycin: A study of a drug interaction in the in situ perfused rat liver model. Biopharm Drug Dispos 1993; 14:615–625.
15. Turgeon DK, Leichtman AB, Lown KS, Normolle DP, Deeb GM, Merion RM, Watkins PB: P_{450} 3A activity and cyclosporine dosing in kidney and heart transplant recipients. Clin Pharmacol Ther 1994; 56:253–260.
16. Prielipp RC, MacGregor DA, Butterworth JF IV, Meredith JW, Levy JH, Wood KE, Coursin DB: Pharmacodynamics and pharmacokinetics of milrinone administration to increase oxygen delivery in critically ill patients. Chest 1996; 109:1291–1301.
17. Shafer A, Sung ML, White PF: Pharmacokinetics and pharmacodynamics of alfentanil infusions during general anesthesia. Anesth Analg 1986; 65:1021–1028.
18. Frommer DA, Kulig KW, Marx JA, Rumack B: Tricyclic antidepressant overdose: A review. JAMA 1987; 257:521–526.
19. Hughes MA, Glass PS, Jacobs JR: Context-sensitive half-time in multicompartment pharmacokinetic models for intravenous anesthetic drugs. Anesthesiology 1992; 76:334–341.
20. Katz R, Kelly HW: Pharmacokinetics of continuous infusions of fentanyl in critically ill children. Crit Care Med 1993; 21:995–1000.
21. Spector R, Park GD, Johnson GF, Vesell ES: Therapeutic drug monitoring. Clin Pharmacol Ther 1988; 43:345–353.
22. Watling SM, Dasta JF: Aminoglycoside dosing considerations in intensive care unit patients. Ann Pharmacother 1993; 27:351–357.
23. Moore RD, Lietman PS, Smith CR: Clinical response to aminoglycoside therapy: Importance of the ratio of peak concentration to minimal inhibitory concentration. J Infect Dis 1987; 155:93–99.
24. Moore RD, Smith CR, Lietman PS: Association of aminoglycoside plasma levels with therapeutic outcome in gram-negative pneumonia. Am J Med 1984; 77:657–662.
25. Nicolau DP, Freeman CD, Belliveau PP, Nightingale CH, Ross JW, Quintiliani R: Experience with a once-daily aminoglycoside program administered to 2,184 adult patients. Antimicrob Agents Chemother 1995; 39:650–655.
26. Edwards DJ, Pancorbo S: Routine monitoring of vancomycin concentrations: Waiting for proof of its value. Clin Pharmacokinet 1987; 6:652–654.
27. Rodvold KA, Zokufa H, Rotschafer JC: Routine monitoring of serum vancomycin concentrations: Can waiting be justified? Clin Pharm 1987; 6:655–658.
28. Sayers JF, Shimasaki R: Routine monitoring of serum vancomycin concentrations: The answer lies in the middle (letter). Clin Pharmacokinet 1988; 7:18.
29. Cantu TG, Yamanaka-Yuen NA, Lietman PS: Serum vancomycin concentrations: Reappraisal of their clinical value. Clin Infect Dis 1994; 18:533–543.
30. Moellering RC Jr: Monitoring serum vancomycin levels: Climbing the mountain because it is there? Clin Infect Dis 1994; 18:544–546.
31. Flandrois JP, Fardel G, Carret G: Early stages of in vitro killing curve of LY146032 and vancomycin for *Staphylococcus aureus*. Antimicrob Agents Chemother 1988; 32:454–457.
32. Garrison MW, Vance-Bryan K, Larson TA, Toscano JP, Rotschafer JC: Assessment of effects of protein binding on daptomycin and vancomycin killing of *Staphylococcus aureus* by using an in vitro pharmacodynamic model. Antimicrob Agents Chemother 1990; 34:1925–1931.
33. Hanberger H, Nilsson LE, Maller R, Isaksson B: Pharmacodynamics of daptomycin and vancomycin on *Enterococcus faecalis* and *Staphylococcus aureus* demonstrated by studies of initial killing and postantibiotic effect and influence of Ca^{2+} and albumin on these drugs. Antimicrob Agents Chemother 1991; 35:1710–1716.
34. Odenholt-Tornqvist I, Lowdin E, Cars O: Postantibiotic sub-MIC effects of vancomycin, roxithromycin, sparfloxacin, and amikacin. Antimicrob Agents Chemother 1992; 36:1852–1858.
35. Benko AS, Cappelletty DM, Kruse JA, Rybak MJ: Continuous infusion versus intermittent administration of ceftazidime in critically ill patients with suspected gram-negative infections. Antimicrob Agents Chemother 1996; 40:691–695.
36. Nicolau DP, Nightingale CH, Banevicius MA, Fu Q, Quintiliani R: Serum bactericidal activity of ceftazidime: Continuous infusion versus intermittent injections. Antimicrob Agents Chemother 1996; 40:61–64.
37. James JK, Palmer SM, Levine DP, Rybak MJ: Comparison of conventional dosing versus continuous-infusion vancomycin therapy for patients with suspected or documented gram-positive infections. Antimicrob Agents Chemother 1996; 40:696–700.
38. Lamer C, de Beco V, Soler P, Calvat S, Fagon JY, Dombret MC, Farinotti R, Chastre J, Gibert C: Analysis of vancomycin entry into pulmonary lining fluid by bronchoalveolar lavage in critically ill patients. Antimicrob Agents Chemother 1993; 37:281–286.
39. Anderson GD, Pak C, Doane KW, Griffy KG, Temkin NR, Wilensky AJ, Winn HR: Revised Winter-Tozer equation for normalized phenytoin concentrations in trauma and elderly patients with hypoalbuminemia. Ann Pharmacother 1997; 31:279–284.
40. Self TH, Heilker GM, Alloway RR, Kelso TM, Abou-Shala N: Reassessing the therapeutic range for theophylline on laboratory report forms: The importance of 5–15 mcg/mL. Pharmacotherapy 1993; 13:590–594.

88

Alterations in Drug Disposition in the Elderly

John W. Devlin, PharmD
Barbara J. Zarowitz, PharmD, FCCM

In the United States, the population older than 65 years (the elderly) will double and the population older than 80 years (the old elderly) will nearly triple by the year 2040.[1] The elderly currently make up more than half of all intensive care unit (ICU) admissions. This proportion is likely to increase over time. Although younger patients admitted to the ICU might be expected to do better than elderly patients, age itself is a poor predictor of critical illness-related outcomes, such as mortality and quality of life.[2]

Older patients consume nearly three times as many prescription drugs as younger patients and therefore are at risk for experiencing significantly more drug-drug interactions and adverse drug reactions (ADRs).[3] Factors that contribute to adverse reactions in the critically ill elderly patient include (1) polypharmacy, (2) low body mass, (3) excessive length of therapy, (4) preexisting chronic disease, (5) organ dysfunction, (6) a history of prior drug reactions, and (7) prescription errors[4] (Table 88-1). An analysis of prescribing errors in a large hospitalized cohort found advanced age to be the most common pathophysiologic factor not appropriately accounted for when the initial selection of drug dosage was made.[5] Because of the high incidence of adverse drug reactions in this population, an adverse reaction should be included in the differential diagnosis of any new sign or symptom. An

TABLE 88–1. Possible Reasons for Increases in Drug Reactions in the Elderly

Reason	Comment
1. Taking multiple medications	Important cause of drug interactions
2. Delayed absorption	Unimportant
3. Decreased first-pass effect	Of rare importance
4. Altered hepatic metabolism	Common, important
5. Impaired metabolic adaptability	Probably important
6. Low serum albumin levels, altered protein binding	Increases glomerular filtration and tissue drug concentrations
7. Impaired renal function	Very important
8. More body fat, less water	Occasionally important
9. Substantial malnutrition	Important
10. Changed organ susceptibility to adverse effects with aging	Probably important, inadequately studied
11. Underlying confusion or dementia	Masks adverse effects; decreases ability to assess patient
12. Reduced movement (immobility)	Decreased basal metabolic rate, creatinine production, and muscle mass
13. Enhanced central nervous system penetration	Important
14. Exaggerated or minimized response	Important

Adapted from Iber FL, Murphy PA, Connor ES: Age-related changes in the gastrointestinal system: Effects on drug therapy. Drugs Aging 1994; 5:34–48.

unrecognized adverse drug reaction, if left undiagnosed, may lead to the prescribing of additional medications, each having its own potential for adverse effects.[6]

This chapter reviews important age-related pharmacokinetic and pharmacodynamic changes that occur in critically ill elderly patients and provides recommendations for optimizing the pharmacologic aspects of care in this population. Although common trends and changes that have been observed in the elderly are identified throughout this chapter, a great degree of heterogeneity exists among elderly critically ill patients (i.e., biologic age is not synonymous with chronologic age). Little information exists about drug use in the old elderly, yet this is probably the population most at risk for adverse events. For elderly critically ill patients, drug therapy should be individualized and each patient should be carefully monitored for adverse effects.

AGE-RELATED PHARMACOKINETIC CHANGES IN CRITICAL ILLNESS

Familiarity with pharmacokinetic parameters such as bioavailability, volume of distribution, elimination half-life, and clearance greatly enhances the clinician's ability to optimize drug therapy. Pharmacokinetic knowledge helps the clinician select the appropriate drug and dosage regimen to achieve the desired therapeutic goal while minimizing adverse effects. Older patients have many age-related physiologic changes, including impairment of baseline organ function. These age-related changes are further complicated by superimposed critical illness, leading to large interindividual variability in drug disposition.

Absorption

The pharmacokinetic term that describes the extent of drug absorption is *bioavailability.* When a drug is administered intravenously, it is completely available systemically and is therefore 100% bioavailable (bioavailablity [F] = 1). Factors such as reduced gastric acidity and impaired gastrointestinal motility in the older patient may slow the rate of dissolution and absorption after oral or nasogastric tube drug administration. The clinical significance of these changes, however, is minor, since the total amount of drug absorbed (i.e., area under the curve) usually remains unchanged.[3]

Common alterations that affect absorption in critically ill patients in all age groups include:

- Incomplete oral disintegration or dissolution
- Gut wall edema or stasis
- Alterations in gastric or intestinal blood flow
- Concurrent therapy with anticholinergic agents, narcotic analgesics, antacids, or enteral feeds

Bioavailability may be decreased by as much as 50% to 80% when drugs such as phenytoin or sucralfate are administered concomitantly with enteral nutriments. Individual absorption characteristics of each drug should be examined before one relies on the adequacy of the oral route of administration.[7]

Subcutaneous, intramuscular, and rectal routes of administration (except for subcutaneous heparin) are not recommended for elderly ICU patients, because alterations in blood flow to the injection site and rectal mucosa and decreased muscle mass and subcutaneous tissue may impair absorption. Consequently, the intravenous route is the primary route of medication administration in the ICU.[7]

Distribution

The relationship between the amount of drug in the body and the plasma concentration after absorption and distribution is expressed by a proportionality constant called the apparent *volume of distribution* (V_d). It reflects a nonphysiologic compartment into which drug disperses and may be affected by body size, physicochemical characteristics of the drug, tissue binding, plasma protein binding, and regional blood flow. In general, drugs that remain within the plasma have a small V_d (<0.3 L/kg), whereas agents that are more lipophilic and sequestered outside the circulation usually have a much greater V_d (>1 L/kg).[7]

In the elderly, lean body mass decreases by 10% to 20% but total body mass changes little because of increases in adipose tissue[8] (Fig. 88–1). Because of these changes, hydrophilic drugs have a lower V_d and lipophilic drugs a higher V_d. The larger V_d for lipophilic agents such as anesthetics, barbiturates, and benzodiazepines may result in a longer half-life ($t\frac{1}{2}$), because the drug is more slowly redistributed from fat back to the bloodstream before being cleared from the body. Whereas the V_d of some drugs such as digoxin and cimetidine is reduced in the elderly, the V_d for other agents such as tobramycin and pancuronium is similar across all age groups.[9]

Critical illness itself may be a more important determinant of V_d than the patient's age. Most critically ill patients have an increase in total body water (e.g., after resuscitation) that may lead to lower plasma concentrations of low-V_d hydrophilic drugs. Critical illness–induced increases in free water dramatically increase the volume of distribution for aminoglycosides and may lead to lower than expected peak concentrations unless the dose is increased.[10] Increased extracellular and total body water and decreased body cell mass can occur, even in the presence of central volume contraction in hypoalbuminemic patients.[7] Continual assessment of fluid distribution by monitoring fluid inputs and outputs, pulmonary capillary wedge pressure, serum albumin, and subcutaneous edema is essential when establishing loading doses of medications.

Baseline plasma protein concentrations, already altered in older people, may change dramatically in the presence of

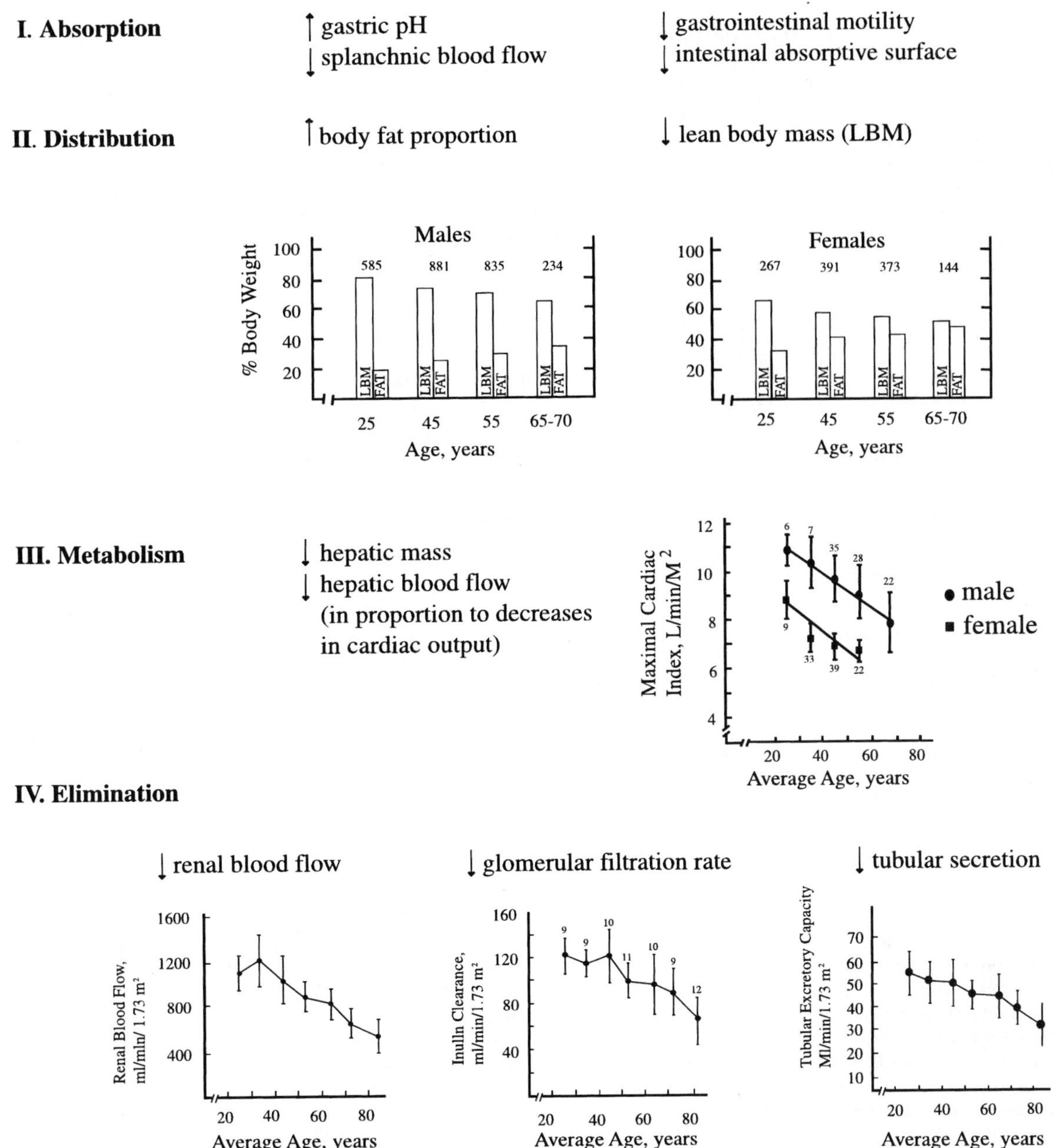

Figure 88–1. Physiologic changes with aging that may affect drug disposition are reflected. (From Evans WE, Schentag JJ [Eds]: Applied Pharmacokinetics: Principles of Therapeutic Drug Monitoring. 3rd ed. Vancouver, Wash, Applied Therapeutics, 1992, pp 9-1–9-43.)

critical illness and affect the amount of unbound or free drug in the body. Decreases in albumin, prealbumin, and transferrin observed in patients with burns, heart failure, liver disease, sepsis, uremia, and trauma may lead to transient increases in the free fraction of acidic drugs such as phenytoin, theophylline, and warfarin.[11]

The concentrations of acute-phase reactants such as α1-acid glycoprotein, already increased in elderly patients with a concomitant chronic inflammatory disease such as rheumatoid arthritis, may dramatically increase in patients with burns, infections, myocardial infarctions, and surgery. In these situations, increased binding of basic drugs (e.g., lidocaine) may lead to decreased effects, necessitating an increase in dose.[7]

Clearance

Whereas the initial loading dose is usually based on the estimated volume of distribution, the maintenance dose, once steady state is reached, is dependent on clearance. "Clearance" is a term based on the concept of the whole body acting as a drug-eliminating system. Hepatic and renal drug excretions, which together form the major clearance pathways, can be affected by both critical illness and age.

Critical illness has variable effects on drugs cleared primarily by the liver. The clearance of high intrinsic clearance drugs (e.g., labetalol, morphine, lidocaine), whose elimination is dependent primarily on liver blood flow, is reduced in states of hepatic hypoperfusion.[7] As hepatic blood flow decreases by about 30% between ages 30 and 75 years (see Fig. 88–1), older patients are particularly sensitive to the impairments in hepatic perfusion and hepatocellular function commonly seen in critically ill patients with shock, congestive heart failure, and sepsis[12] (Fig. 88–2).

Drugs dependent primarily on enzymatic function rather than liver blood flow for their clearance are considered low-

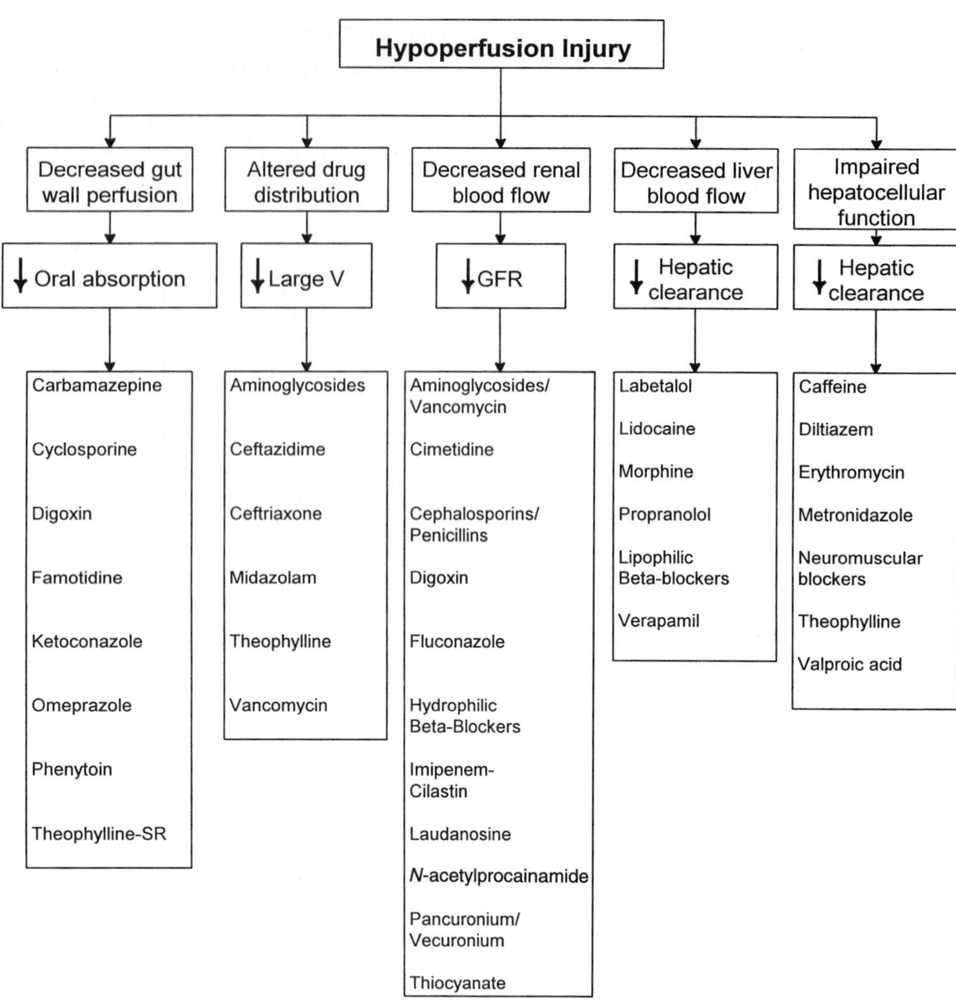

Figure 88–2. Hypoperfusion-induced changes in blood flow and organ system function may result in decreased absorption, altered distribution, impaired renal excretion, and decreased hepatic metabolism of clinically important drugs. GFR = glomerular filtration rate.

extraction drugs and may require dosage adjustment in patients with liver dysfunction. Animal models of traumatic injury have demonstrated differential decreases in both *phase I* (*nonsynthetic* functionalization reactions: oxidation, reduction, hydrolysis) and phase II (*synthetic* conjugation reactions: glucuronidation, sulfation, acetylation, and methylation) biotransformations. *Phase II* reactions are less affected by acuity of illness and age than phase I reactions.[7] The elimination of diazepam, which is oxidatively metabolized to active metabolites, is prolonged in the elderly. Lorazepam, in contrast, is eliminated by conjugation, a pathway not significantly affected by age[13] (Table 88–2).

The overall metabolic activity of the liver declines with advancing age as a result of decreases in both hepatic mass and blood flow[12] (see Fig. 88–1). Age-related changes in microsomal and cytoplasmic enzyme activity occur in animals but have never been conclusively demonstrated in humans.[14] It is likely that genetic and environmental factors, such as concomitant illness, baseline nutrition, alcohol use, and prescription drug use, are more important determinants of metabolic function than age alone. Genetic polymorphism, which may alter hepatic biotransformation by a factor of 5 and hepatic clearance by a factor of 30, persists in the elderly.[15] Therefore, an older patient who is a poor metabolizer of a substrate clears it from the body much more slowly than an elderly rapid metabolizer. Stereoselective drug metabolism, in which one enantiomer of a racemic drug (e.g., verapamil, warfarin, cimetidine) is preferentially metabolized, occurs more frequently in older people than in the young.[16]

Enzyme functional capacity is altered by concurrent drug therapy with enzyme-inducing agents (phenobarbital, phenytoin, rifampin, carbamazepine) or enzyme-inhibiting agents (cimetidine, omeprazole, erythromycin, quinolone antibiotics).[17] The overall clinical significance of the observed effect depends on the following:

- Potency of the offending agent
- Fraction of total clearance accounted for by metabolism
- Isoenzyme family affected
- Route of administration
- Selected dose

Compared with induction, direct metabolic inhibition occurs faster and usually produces more clinically important effects. Hepatic enzyme induction, the onset of which ranges from 2 to 10 days, is often reduced in the elderly.[18] Specific recommendations for dosage adjustment for hepatically cleared drugs are available.[19]

Drug-induced hepatotoxicity appears to be more prevalent in the elderly. Intrinsic hepatotoxicity (dose related) is usually the result of decreased elimination (e.g., in the elderly patient with multiple organ failure). Idiosyncratic hepatotoxicity (dose unrelated) is more common in elderly patients receiving isoniazid, halothane, or sulindac and may be related to dysfunctional antioxidant mechanisms.[20]

Reduced renal elimination of medications is a factor that complicates pharmacotherapy in the elderly critically ill patient. After the age of 25, the glomerular filtration rate (GFR) progressively declines at a rate of approximately 0.5 to 1 mL/

TABLE 88–2. Effects of Aging on the Clearance of Some Oxidized and Conjugated Drugs

Drug	Effect	Reference
Oxidized		
Chlordiazepoxide	↓↓	Am J Psychiatry 1977; 134:559
Desmethyldiazepam	↓↓	Br J Clin Pharmacol 1979; 7:119
Erythromycin	↓↓	Eur J Clin Pharmacol 1990; 39:161
Haloperidol	↓↓	Neuropsychobiology 1996; 33:12
Midazolam	↓↓	Biochem Pharmacol 1992; 44:275
Nicardipine	↓↓	Am Heart J 1989; 117:256
Nifedipine	↓↓	Br J Clin Pharmacol 1988; 25:297
Phenytoin (free)	↓↓	Clin Pharmacokinet 1981; 6:389
Propranolol	↔	Br J Clin Pharmacol 1979; 7:49
Theophylline	↓↓	Eur J Clin Pharmacol 1989; 36:29
Verapamil	↓↓	Acta Med Scand 1984; 681(Suppl):25
Conjugated		
Acetaminophen	↓	Br J Clin Pharmacol 1990; 30:634
Lamotrigine	↓	J Pharm Med 1991; 1:121
Lidocaine	↓↓	J Cardiovasc Pharmacol 1983; 5:1093
Lorazepam	↓	Clin Pharmacol Ther 1979; 26:103
Metronidazole	↔	Hum Exp Toxicol 1990; 9:155
Morphine	↓	Age Ageing 1989; 18:258
Oxazepam	↔	Clin Pharmacol Ther 1981; 30:805

Modified from Woodhouse K, Wynne HA: Age-related changes in hepatic function: Implications for drug therapy. Drugs Aging 1992; 2:243.
↔ = none; ↓ = minor; ↓↓ = significant.

min per 70 kg/year. By age 80, GFR has decreased by about 40%.[21] These changes are secondary to age-related decreases in renal mass, loss of functional nephrons, and diminished renal artery perfusion. Critical illness may further impair renal function in the elderly because of reduced perfusion (e.g., with shock); intrinsic renal damage secondary to ischemia, drugs, and toxins; or immunologic injury (see Fig. 88–2). Decreasing renal function increases the half-life of renally cleared drugs, leading to parent drug and metabolite accumulation, and may increase the potential for toxicity, particularly with drugs that have a narrow therapeutic index (Table 88–3).

Generally, a linear relationship exists between renal drug clearance and creatinine clearance (Cl_{CR}). Elderly patients, many of whom are immobile and malnourished, frequently have low serum creatinine concentrations that mask the ability to detect a reduction in the GFR via serial serum creatinine concentrations. The age-adjusted Cockcroft and Gault equation, used to estimate the GFR by calculating a creatinine clearance, has poor validity for critically ill patients, especially those with poor baseline renal function.[22, 23] A further complicating factor, applicable to critically ill patients of any age, is the fact that renal function may change rapidly and, therefore, increased plasma creatinine values may lag behind a diminished GFR.[23] Dosage regimens for many of the drugs used in the elderly ICU population may be modified using linear regression equations and empirical recommendations.[24]

TABLE 88–3. Drugs That Commonly Induce Acute Renal Failure or Complicate Chronic Renal Failure in Critically Ill Elderly Patients

Aminoglycosides
Amphotericin B
Angiotensin-converting enzyme inhibitors
Diuretics
Nonsteroidal anti-inflammatory drugs
Radiocontrast media
Vasopressors

AGE-RELATED PHARMACODYNAMIC CHANGES IN CRITICAL ILLNESS

The term *pharmacodynamics* refers to effects resulting from the interaction between drugs and biologic systems. Whereas the term *pharmacokinetics* describes drug disposition, pharmacodynamics pertains to drug effects. Elderly critically ill patients, because of multiple organ dysfunction and impaired homeostatic responses, may have an increased sensitivity to drug effects.[25] This increased sensitivity is usually manifest as either an increased therapeutic response or a dose-related adverse effect. Pharmacologic intensity of effect can be altered by the pharmacokinetic factors previously reviewed (i.e., inadequate drug concentration at the receptor site secondary to altered absorption, distribution, or elimination) and receptor-related factors (e.g., number, occupancy, and translocation of the receptor within the membrane) (Fig. 88–3).

In clinical practice, increased responsiveness or excess effect is frequently demonstrated in the elderly for drugs having neurologic, cardiovascular, gastrointestinal, and anti-infective effects, but age-related pharmacodynamic changes have been demonstrated in controlled, clinical studies for only a handful of drugs, including metoclopramide, opioid analgesics, and warfarin.[25] It should be emphasized that elderly patients, as a group, are heterogeneous (e.g., the healthy 65-year-old versus the frail 90-year-old) and thus it is difficult to make generalizations about pharmacodynamics in this population.

SPECIFIC PHARMACOTHERAPY PROBLEMS RELATED TO ORGAN SYSTEMS

Although it is important for the clinician to recognize potential age-related pharmacokinetic and pharmacodynamic changes when prescribing drug therapy for the elderly ICU population, little can usually be done to alter these parameters. When designing a pharmacotherapeutic regimen for the elderly ICU patient, it is more important that the clinician utilize the best available evidence in the literature to support therapeutic efficacy and to prevent or identify potential drug-induced adverse effects.

A major limitation to predicting an elderly patient's response to drug therapy is the paucity of comparative drug trials that include elderly patients. Only since 1990 has the Food and Drug Administration (FDA) required drugs intended for use in the elderly to undergo testing in this population and to be labeled with prescribing information for patients older than 65 years.[26] At present, prescribing decisions are often made through the extrapolation of drug study results involving younger, healthier patients who may respond differently to therapy. For example, even though 80% of deaths from acute myocardial infarction occur in patients older than 65 years, a review found that 60% of 214 randomized trials studying therapies for acute myocardial infarction excluded patients older than age 75.[27] Well-designed postmarketing surveillance studies may be one method by which to increase information about drug use in this population.[6]

Central Nervous System

Elderly patients frequently have baseline neurologic deficits resulting from previous strokes, underlying dementia, or parkinsonism. Visual and hearing impairments coupled with an increased sensitivity to sedative agents, such as the benzodiazepines, often make drug-induced neurologic adverse effects difficult to detect.[9] Drugs with anticholinergic effects (e.g., antihistamines, phenothiazines) can be problematic and have been associated with confusion. Delirium and confusion have

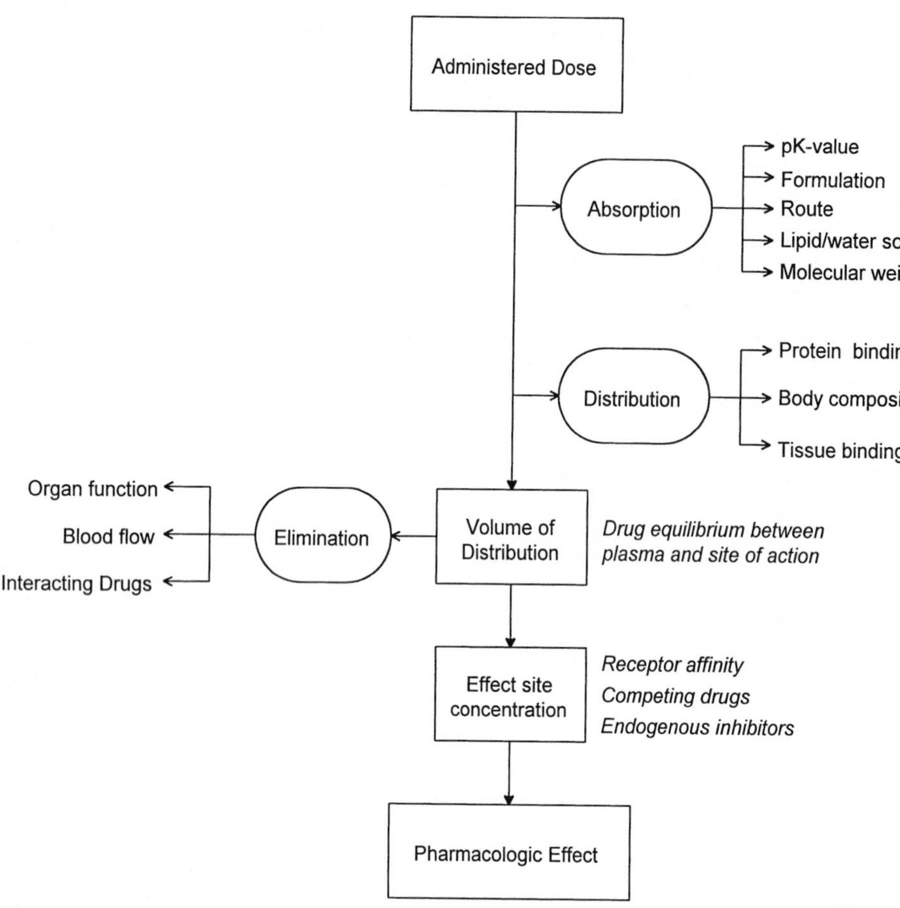

Figure 88–3. Drug pharmacokinetic and pharmacodynamic factors can alter the intensity of the pharmacologic effect. Factors that affect absorption, distribution, effect site concentration, and elimination are schematically represented.

also been caused by histamine (H_2) receptor antagonists (e.g., cimetidine), tricyclic antidepressants, long-half-life benzodiazepines, and corticosteroids and by withdrawal reactions to short-half-life benzodiazepines such triazolam or midazolam. Drug-induced delirium and confusion are amplified in the setting of critical illness through a variety of concomitant, underlying physiologic, psychosocial, and environmental factors.

Metabolism of phenytoin (Vmax) is decreased in older patients. Because of the saturable metabolism of phenytoin, small increases in dose may lead to large increases in plasma concentration. Elderly patients generally require only 80% of the total daily phenytoin dose needed by younger patients, although some critically ill subpopulations (e.g., patients with neurotrauma) may require higher than normal doses.[11, 28] No clinically significant changes have been reported for carbamazepine or valproate in elderly patients. Phenobarbital is not routinely recommended for use in the elderly, except as a third-line agent for status epilepticus, because of the increased incidence of oversedation and paradoxical central nervous system (CNS) excitation seen in this population.

Elderly patients are more sensitive to benzodiazepines because of a combination of pharmacokinetic and pharmacodynamic factors. Of the benzodiazepines, lorazepam is less likely to accumulate in the elderly because it is cleared primarily by glucuronidation and, unlike midazolam and diazepam, is not oxidatively metabolized to active metabolites.[13] The elderly may be more sensitive to the sedative and hypotensive effects of propofol. Butyrophenones such as haloperidol, sometimes required to manage delirium-related agitation, should be started at a low dose to avoid hypotension as well as prolonged corrected QT interval–related effects.

Older patients are at increased risk for nondepolarizing, neuromuscular blocker–related prolonged motor weakness. Other concomitant factors, besides age, that increase the risk of prolonged motor weakness include (1) gender (female), (2) length of paralytic use, (3) underlying hepatic and renal insufficiency, and (4) concomitant therapy with aminoglycosides or corticosteroids.[29]

A study comparing patients who experienced prolonged motor weakness related to paralytics (the majority being elderly) with matched control subjects estimated that the median length of ICU stay increased from 4 to 42 days and the median charges increased from $22,191 to $91,476 for the patients with prolonged weakness.[30] Train-of-four monitoring decreases the amount of neuromuscular blocker administered and leads to faster recovery from paralysis.[31] Baseline changes (e.g., electrolyte disturbances, preexisting neuromuscular disease, obesity, peripheral edema) are often present in elderly critically ill patients and may result in interpretive problems when train-of-four monitoring is used.[32] To avoid prolonged motor weakness, clinicians should regularly reassess the need for continued paralysis and discontinue therapy when it is no longer indicated.

Elderly patients often require lower doses of narcotics, in part because of their higher threshold for pain and atypical pain presentation (e.g., nausea and vomiting). The use of meperidine should be avoided because of its low potency and increased incidence of CNS-related adverse effects such as seizures—particularly for patients with renal insufficiency, in whom the active metabolite (normeperidine) is more likely to accumulate.[9]

The half-life of morphine is unchanged in the elderly because both the volume of distribution and clearance are reduced.[33] Although morphine is generally considered the analgesic of choice in the ICU, it must be used cautiously for patients with renal insufficiency because of the potential risk for accumulation of its active 6-glucuronide metabolite.[33]

Opiates with partial agonist-antagonist activity, such as pentazocine and butorphanol, should not be used in the elderly because their analgesic effectiveness is low and the occurrence of delirium is frequent.

Elderly patients are at a particularly high risk for nonsteroidal anti-inflammatory agent (NSAID)–induced adverse effects, such as gastrointestinal hemorrhage and renal insufficiency. Agents such as ketorolac and indomethacin are not recommended in this population.[34]

Cardiovascular

Age-related cardiovascular changes are often difficult to distinguish from underlying cardiac disease because nearly 50% of the elderly population have abnormal cardiac pathology. By age 75 years, approximately 90% of the normal pacemaker cells and as many as 50% of the bundle of His cells are lost, resulting in a greater incidence of chronic atrioventricular blocks. Other age-related changes include bradycardia resulting from excessive vagal tone, a decreased heart rate response to stress, and a lower cardiac index. Altered blood pressure homeostasis may lead to increased responsiveness to vasodilators and calcium channel blockers.[35]

Age-related declines in β-adrenoreceptor (βAR) function may be associated with decreased responsiveness to β-adrenergic agonists and higher circulating plasma norepinephrine concentrations. Although it is well established that the chronotropic and inotropic responses to isoproterenol (a nonselective beta agonist) and exercise (a β_1AR-mediated response) are impaired in the elderly, the effect of age on β_2AR responsiveness is unclear. Studies to date suggest that β_2AR-mediated chronotropic cardiac responsiveness is reduced in the elderly but that β_2AR-mediated metabolic responsiveness is unaltered.[36] The effects of aging on β_2AR-mediated cardiac inotropic and vascular responsiveness are equivocal. The magnitude of and likelihood of experiencing withdrawal effects from β-blockers are similar in both young and old patients.[36] The clinical relevance of altered β-adrenergic function, however, may be minor, as most agents used in the ICU that act on β receptors (e.g., albuterol, dopamine) are titrated to clinical effect. In contrast, in a population of patients with decompensated congestive heart failure, dobutamine was shown to augment cardiac output and stroke volume significantly less in elderly patients and to provide no hemodynamic benefits at infusion rates above 5 μg/kg/min.[37]

Several drugs with cardiovascular mechanisms should be prescribed and monitored carefully when used in the elderly ICU patient. Because the distribution volume of digoxin is dependent on lean body mass, loading doses usually need to be reduced for the elderly. In addition, maintenance doses should be reduced for patients with concomitant renal insufficiency and for patients taking drugs that inhibit digoxin clearance (e.g., verapamil, amiodarone).[38] The electrocardiogram (ECG) is a more sensitive predictor of the efficacy and toxicity of digoxin than serum concentrations. β-blockers need to be used with caution in the elderly, since bradyarrhythmic and blood pressure–related effects may be exaggerated because of underlying age-related changes (e.g., decreased baroreceptor responsiveness, a lower baseline heart rate, and β-adrenoreceptor functional impairment).[39]

Calcium channel blockers are commonly used for the treatment of tachyarrhythmias, hypertension, and angina. Verapamil induces sinus node depression and bradyarrhythmias more often in the elderly.[35] Older patients receiving nifedipine have a greater decrease in blood pressure and less compensatory reflex tachycardia than younger patients because of increased nifedipine bioavailability and decreased clearance.[9] The safety of short-acting nifedipine for blood pressure control has been questioned.[40] Diminished clearance of the angiotensin-converting enzyme (ACE) inhibitor (ACEI) lisinopril may lead to greater blood pressure–lowering effects.[9] Patients who require an ACEI for afterload reduction or blood pressure control, particularly if they are also receiving a diuretic, should be started on a small dose of a short-acting ACEI, such as captopril, and both blood pressure and renal function should be regularly monitored.

Diuretic agents frequently induce electrolyte abnormalities, including hypokalemia and hypomagnesemia, that predispose patients to tachyarrhythmias and impair respiratory muscle strength.[41] Care must be taken not to induce hypovolemia by overdiuresis because older patients are less able to decrease urine flow, increase urine osmolality, and conserve sodium than younger patients. The elderly may experience a higher incidence of loop diuretic–induced ototoxicity, particularly after the rapid infusion of large doses.[42]

Antiarrhythmic drugs are being used less frequently in the ICU, particularly for patients with asymptomatic tachyarrhythmias, because of the accumulating evidence that they affect outcome detrimentally.[35] If antiarrhythmic therapy is started, it is important to consider age-related decreases in drug clearance that may increase the risk of adverse effects such as arrhythmias. The clearance of quinidine, procainamide, and lidocaine is decreased in the elderly. A higher incidence of lidocaine-related adverse effects, such as bradyarrhythmias, confusion, and seizures, has been documented.[43] Reversible, medication-related causes of tachyarrhythmias should always be considered in the elderly. Examples of such medications are beta agonists (e.g., albuterol, dobutamine), theophylline, erythromycin, and haloperidol. The Advanced Cardiac Life Support (ACLS) guidelines for elderly adults recommend a decrease in the dose of lidocaine maintenance infusions by 50% and avoidance of high-dose epinephrine boluses, as they have been demonstrated to worsen the outcome of patients in this population.[44]

Although there is no evidence to suggest that heparin dose requirements are affected by age, bleeding complications and heparin-induced thrombocytopenia have been reported to occur more frequently in the elderly.[45] Critically ill elderly patients tend to have lower warfarin dosage requirements. This may result from decreased hepatic function, reduced vitamin K intake, and concomitant administration of drugs that inhibit warfarin metabolism (e.g., amiodarone) or induce hypoprothrombinemia (e.g., cefotetan).[46] Although the incidence of warfarin-related bleeding is higher in the old elderly, other factors besides age, such as anticoagulation intensity, are stronger predictors of bleeding risk.[46]

Because most trials of thrombolytic agents after myocardial infarction have excluded patients older than age 75 years, data are insufficient to establish a firm risk-benefit assessment of thrombolytic therapy for this population. Although elderly patients are at greater risk for thrombolytic-related adverse effects, the much greater beneficial effects of these agents on absolute mortality have led to recommendations that their use be increased.[47]

Gastrointestinal

The high incidence of constipation and ileus observed in elderly critically ill patients is usually due not to physiologic age-related changes but to inadequate fluid and nutritional intake or drugs (e.g., narcotic analgesics). Gastrointestinal motility is often further compromised in these patients by concomitant mesenteric hypoperfusion and sepsis.[18]

To optimize the enteral route for nutrition and drug administration, prokinetic agents, such as metoclopramide, cisapride, and erythromycin, are utilized. Metoclopramide has been associated with both increased arginine vasopressin release in elderly patients, an effect that may exacerbate hyponatremia, and a higher incidence of extrapyramidal effects, such as akathisia.[9] Increasing age places patients at higher risk for both cisapride-induced and erythromycin-induced corrected QT interval prolongation.[48]

Although age older than 65 years has been reported to be a risk factor for stress-related hemorrhage, a large cohort study reported that patients' ages were similar in both bleeding and nonbleeding groups.[49] Elderly patients may be particularly susceptible to CNS-related toxicity of H_2-receptor antagonists. Clearance of both cimetidine and ranitidine is reduced in elderly patients, with concomitant end-organ failure further compromising elimination.[18]

Elderly, mechanically ventilated patients may be at greater risk for development of tracheal colonization and nosocomial pneumonia. Drug therapy may exacerbate ventilator-associated pneumonia risk factors; these include:

- Gastroesophageal reflux secondary to theophylline
- Calcium channel blocker–induced lowering of esophageal sphincter tone
- H_2-blocker–related increases in bowel pH leading to small-bowel bacterial overgrowth[50]

Pulmonary

Pulmonary function tests in the elderly reveal decreased vital capacity and forced expiratory volume but unchanged total lung capacity and tidal volume. Baseline PaO_2 usually decreases (<80 mm Hg) with age, whereas pH and $PaCO_2$ remain unchanged. Patients are less able to protect their airway, and their responses to hypoxia and hypercarbia are diminished. Furthermore, the effects of sedatives and analgesics persist because of decreased clearance and may further blunt respiratory response and function.

No age-related differences in response have been shown for the inhaled bronchodilators albuterol and ipratropium.[51] A placebo-controlled trial demonstrated an increase in asymptomatic simple and complex tachyarrhythmias during $beta_2$ agonist treatment potentially related to $beta_2$ agonist–induced hypokalemia.[52] In the elderly, a reduced bronchodilator response to theophylline, coupled with a markedly increased incidence of seizures and tachyarrhythmias, suggests that there is little indication for the use of theophylline in this population.[53]

Anti-infectives

The emergence of resistance to many common antibiotics has emphasized the need to achieve optimal antibiotic tissue levels over the dosage interval, especially for agents that demonstrate concentration-dependent killing. Age-related and critical illness–related decreases in renal function require appropriate dose reductions for renally excreted anti-infective agents, such as β-lactams, vancomycin, aminoglycosides, co-trimoxazole, and fluconazole. One retrospective review of ceftazidime therapy in the elderly concluded that 75 of the 111 patients (68%) were prescribed an excessive ceftazidime dose in relation to renal function. The excessive doses were estimated to cost $13,800.[54]

Once-daily aminoglycoside dosing, utilizing the postantibiotic and concentration-dependent killing properties of aminoglycosides, is as safe and as effective as multiple daily dosing in a population of non–critically ill, elderly patients.[55] Although few studies have evaluated this dosing strategy in critically ill elderly patients, its use would seem advantageous, particularly for fluid-resuscitated patients with an increased aminoglycoside V_d.

Clearance of erythromycin is decreased in elderly patients.[9] In addition, age has been reported to be a major risk factor for the development of erythromycin-induced torsades de pointes.[48] Serum quinolone levels have been reported to increase with age.[56] Of the quinolones, ofloxacin has been associated with a higher incidence of adverse drug-related events, presumably because of its longer serum half-life.[56] Elderly patients are at an increased risk for co-trimoxazole–induced hyperkalemia.[57] Elderly, institutionalized patients have a significantly higher carriage rate of *Clostridium difficile*, particularly with prior stool softener and antacid use, and are at an increased risk for antibiotic-associated pseudomembranous colitis.[58]

Few elderly critically ill patients have been included in comparative studies examining the various liposomal amphotericin B products. The liposomal products may be advantageous in patients with disseminated fungal infections and concomitant acute renal failure.

SUMMARY

A thorough understanding of the physiologic changes that occur in the elderly critically ill patient, coupled with an awareness of the pharmacokinetic and pharmacodynamic profiles of drugs commonly used in this population, allows the ICU clinician to optimize therapeutic efficacy and to avoid adverse drug reactions. Table 88–4 contains strategies that may aid the clinician in reaching these goals.

Although age-related changes in drug disposition are usually aligned with known age-related physiologic changes, many questions remain regarding the role of altered plasma proteins in drug distribution, the cause of altered drug me-

TABLE 88–4. Principles of Appropriate Prescribing for the Elderly Patient in the Intensive Care Unit

Obtain a complete history from the patient, family members, nursing home, primary care physician, and/or community pharmacist of present prescription and OTC medications, allergies, and alcohol intake as well as previous drug-related adverse effects.
Avoid prescribing medications empirically when the benefit of the medication is questionable.
Review medication lists daily. Discontinue any medications that are no longer indicated.
Monitor the frequency of use of PRN medications, in particular, narcotics and other CNS depressants.
Know the drugs you are using. Know the pharmacologic profile of the medications you prescribe and the potential adverse effects and toxicities. Monitor patients closely for deterioration of functional parameters that could be drug-related.
Start low, and increase doses slowly when possible. Always use the minimum dose necessary for efficacy. Use drug monitoring when available and appropriate.
Treat adequately. Use doses sufficient to achieve the therapeutic goal, as tolerated. Do not withhold therapy for treatable diseases.
Use new agents with particular caution. Most new compounds have not been thoroughly evaluated in the elderly population and the risk-benefit ratio is often unclear.

Adapted from Parker BM, Cusack BJ, Vestal RE: Pharmacokinetic optimization of drug therapy in elderly patients. Drugs Aging 1995; 7:10–18.

CNS = central nervous system; OTC = over the counter; PRN = pro re nata (as necessary).

tabolism, and quantification of the temporal relationship between drugs entering body organs and the subsequent pharmacologic response.[59] *There is an urgent need for more pharmacokinetic and pharmacodynamic studies in elderly patients of drugs commonly used in the ICU. For drug compounds in development, these studies should be completed while drugs are still in phase II and phase III of development.*

Most adverse drug reactions observed in the elderly are pharmacologically predictable side effects of commonly used drugs and therefore can be prevented. Drugs with the best risk-benefit profile and those likely to induce the fewest adverse effects should be considered first-line options. Therapy should be initiated at a low dose and then carefully titrated until the lowest effective dose is achieved, especially in patients known to have compromised organ function, concomitant disease, or altered homeostasis. Drug therapy that does not result in a beneficial effect or that is suspected of inducing an adverse effect should be stopped.

Last, the ICU clinician should be careful not to withhold potentially lifesaving drug therapy on the grounds of age alone.[60]

References

1. Schneider E, Guralnik J: The aging of America. JAMA 1990; 263:2335.
2. Chelluri L, Grenvik A: Intensive care for critically ill elderly: Mortality, costs, and quality of life. Arch Intern Med 1995; 155:1013.
3. Montamat S, Cusack B, Vestal R: Management of drug therapy in the elderly. N Engl J Med 1989; 321:303.
4. Jue SG, Vestal RE: Adverse drug reactions in the elderly: A critical review. *In*: Medicine in Old Age: Clinical Pharmacology and Drug Therapy. O'Malley K (Ed). London, Churchill Livingstone, 1985, p 52.
5. Lesar TS, Briceland L, Stein DS: Factors related to errors in medication prescribing. JAMA 1997; 277:312.
6. Rochon PA, Gurwitz JH: Geriatrics septet: Drug therapy. Lancet 1995; 326:32.
7. Zarowitz BJ: Pharmacologic principles. *In*: Textbook of Critical Care. 3rd ed. Ayres SM, Grenvik A, Holbrook PR, et al (Eds). Philadelphia, WB Saunders, 1995, pp 1141–1154.
8. Novak LP: Aging, total body potassium, fat-free mass, and cell mass in males and females between the ages of 18 and 85 years. J Gerontol 1972; 27:438.
9. Nielson C: Pharmacologic considerations in critical care of the elderly. Clin Geriatr Med 1994; 10:71–89.
10. Dasta JF, Armstrong DK: Variability in aminoglycoside pharmacokinetics in critically ill surgical patients. Crit Care Med 1988; 16:327.
11. Boucher BA, Kuhl DA, Fabina TC, et al: Effect of neurotrauma on hepatic drug clearance. Clin Pharmacol Ther 1991; 50:487.
12. Wynn HA, Goudevenos J, Rawlins MD, et al: Hepatic drug clearance: The effect of age using indocyanine green as a model compound. Br J Clin Pharmacol 1990; 30:634.
13. Greenblatt DJ, Harmatz JS, Shader RI: Clinical pharmacokinetics of anxiolytics and hypnotics in the elderly: I. Therapeutic considerations. Clin Pharmacokinet 1991; 21:165.
14. Schmucker DL, Woodhouse KW, Wang RK, et al: Effects of age and gender on in vitro properties of human liver microsomal monooxygenases. Clin Pharmacol Ther 1990; 48:365.
15. Hunt CM, Westerkam WR, Stave GM, et al: Hepatic cytochrome P-4503A activity in the elderly. Mech Ageing Dev 1992; 64:189.
16. Chandler MHH, Scott SR, Blouin RA: Age-associated stereoselective alterations in hexobarbital metabolism. Clin Pharmacol Ther 1988; 43:436.
17. Brouwer KCR, Dukes GE, Powell JR: Influence of liver function on drug disposition. *In*: Applied Pharmacokinetics: Principles of Therapeutic Drug Monitoring. 3rd ed. Evans WE, Schentag JJ, Jusko J (Eds). Vancouver, Wash, Applied Therapeutics, 1992, pp 6-1–6-59.
18. Iber FL, Murphy PA, Connor ES: Age-related changes in the gastrointestinal system: Effects on drug therapy. Drugs Aging 1994; 5:34.
19. Kubisty Ca, Arns PA, Wedland PJ, Branch RA: Adjustment of medications in liver failure. *In*: Pharmacologic Approach to the Critically Ill Patient. 3rd ed. Chernow B (Ed). Baltimore, Williams & Wilkins, 1994, pp 95–113.
20. Schenker S, Bay M: Drug disposition and hepatotoxicity in the elderly. J Clin Gastroenterol 1994; 18:232–237.
21. Sokoll LJ, Russell RM, Sadowski JA: Establishment of creatinine clearance reference values for older women. Clin Chem 1994; 40:2276.
22. Cockcroft DW, Gault MH: Prediction of creatinine clearance from serum creatinine. Nephron 1976; 16:31.
23. Robert S, Zarowitz BJ: Is there a reliable index of glomerular filtration rate in critically ill patients? Ann Pharmacother 1991; 25:169.
24. Bennet WM, Aronoff GR, Golper TA, et al: Drug Prescribing in Renal Failure. 3rd ed. Philadelphia, American College of Physicians, 1994.
25. Feely J, Coakley D: Altered pharmacodynamics in the elderly. Clin Geriatr Med 1990; 6:269.
26. FDA: Guideline for the Study of Drugs Likely to Be Used in the Elderly. Rockville, Md, Food and Drug Administration, Center for Drug Evaluation and Research, 1989, p 16.
27. Gurwitz JH, Col NF, Avorn J: The exclusion of the elderly and women from clinical trials in acute myocardial infraction. JAMA 1992; 268:1417.
28. Bauer LA, Blouin RA: Age and phenytoin kinetics in adult epileptics. Clin Pharmacol Ther 1982; 31:301.
29. Watling SM, Dasta JF: Prolonged paralysis in intensive care unit patients after the use of neuromuscular blocking agents: A review of the literature. Crit Care Med 1994; 22:884.
30. Rudis MI, Guslits BJ, Peterson EL, et al: Economic impact of prolonged motor weakness complicating neuromuscular blockade in the intensive care unit. Crit Care Med 1996; 24:1749.
31. Rudis MI, Sikora CA, Angus E, et al: A prospective, randomized, controlled evaluation of peripheral nerve stimulation versus standard clinical dosing of neuromuscular blocking agents in critically ill patients. Crit Care Med 1997; 25:575.
32. Rudis MI, Guslits BJ, Zarowitz BJ: Technical and interpretive problems of peripheral nerve stimulation in monitoring neuromuscular blockade in the intensive care unit. Ann Pharmacother 1996; 30:165.
33. Baillie SP, Bateman DN, Coates PE, et al: Age and the pharmacokinetics of morphine. Age Ageing 1989; 28:258.
34. Griffin MR, Ray WA, Schaffner W: Nonsteroidal anti-inflammatory drug use and death from peptic ulcer in elderly persons. Ann Intern Med 1988; 109:359.
35. Duncan AK, Vittone J, Fleming KC: Cardiovascular disease in elderly patients. Mayo Clin Proc 1996; 71:184–196.
36. Scarpace PJ, Tumer N, Mader SL: Beta-adrenergic function in aging: Basic mechanisms and clinical implications. Drugs Aging 1991; 1:116.
37. Rich MW, Imburgia M: Inotropic response to dobutamine in elderly patients with decompensated congestive heart failure. Am J Cardiol 1990; 65:519.
38. Passmore AP, Johnston GD: Digoxin toxicity in the aged: Characterizing and avoiding the problem. Drugs Aging 1991; 1:364.
39. Stolarek I, Scott PJ, Caird FI: Physiological changes due to age: Implications for cardiovascular therapy. Drugs Aging 1991; 1:467.
40. Grossman E, Messerli FH, Grodzicki T, et al: Should a moratorium be placed on sublingual nifedipine capsules given for hypertensive emergencies and pseudoemergencies? JAMA 1996; 276:1328.
41. Isaac G, Holland OB: Drug-induced hypokalemia: A cause for concern. Drugs Aging 1992; 2:35.
42. Rybal LP: Ototoxicity of loop diuretics. Otolaryngol Clin North Am 1993; 26:829.
43. Cusack B, O'Malley K, Lavan J, et al: Protein binding and disposition of lignocaine in the elderly. Eur J Clin Pharmacol 1985; 29:323.
44. American Heart Association: Advanced cardiac life support. JAMA 1992; 268:2199.
45. Campbell NRC, Hull RD, Brant R, et al: Aging and heparin-related bleeding. Arch Intern Med 1996; 156:857.
46. Redwood M, Taylor C, Bain BJ, et al: The association of age with dosage requirements for warfarin. Age Ageing 1991; 20:217.
47. Krumholz HM, Pasternak RC, Weinstein MC, et al: Cost effective-

ness of thrombolytic therapy with streptokinase in elderly patients with suspected acute myocardial infarction. N Engl J Med 1992; 327:7.
48. Tschida SJ, Guay DRP, Straka RJ, et al: QTc-interval prolongation associated with slow intravenous erythromycin lactobionate infusions in critically ill patients: A prospective evaluation and review of the literature. Pharmacotherapy 1996; 16:663.
49. Cook DJ, Fuller HD, Guyatt GH, et al: Risk factors for gastrointestinal bleeding in critically ill patients. N Engl J Med 1994; 330:377.
50. Haboubi NY, Montgomery RD: Small-bowel bacterial overgrowth in elderly people: Clinical significance and response to treatment. Age Ageing 1992; 13:21.
51. Kradjan WA, Driesner NK, Abuan TH, et al: Effect of age on bronchodilator response. Chest 1992; 101:1545.
52. Higgins RM, Cookson WOCM, Lane DJ, et al: Cardiac arrhythmias caused by nebulized beta-agonist therapy. Lancet 1987; 2:863.
53. Shannon M, Lovejoy FH Jr: The influence of age vs peak serum concentration on life-threatening events after chronic theophylline intoxication. Arch Intern Med 1990; 150:2045.
54. Vlasses PH, Bastion WA, Behal R, et al: Ceftazidime dosing in the elderly: Economic implications. Ann Pharmacother 1993; 27:967.
55. Koo J, Tight R, Rajkumar V, et al: Comparison of once daily versus pharmacokinetic dosing of aminoglycosides in elderly patients. Am J Med 1996; 101:177.
56. Fihn SD, Callahan CM, Martin DC, et al: Quinolones in the elderly. Drugs 1995; 49(Suppl 2):112.
57. Modest GA, Price B, Mascoli N: Hyperkalemia in elderly patients receiving standard doses of trimethoprim-sulfamethoxazole. Ann Intern Med 1994; 120:437.
58. McFarland LV, Surawicz CM, Stamm WE: Risk factors for *Clostridium difficile* carriage and *C. difficile*-associated diarrhea in a cohort of hospitalized patients. J Infect Dis 1990; 162:678.
59. Crome P, Flanagan RJ: Pharmacokinetic studies in elderly people: Are they necessary? Clin Pharmacokinet 1994; 26:243.
60. Montague TJ, Wong RY, Burton JR, et al: Changes in acute myocardial infarction risk and patterns of practice for patients older and younger than 70 years, 1987–1990. Can J Cardiol 1992; 8:596.

89

Applied Cardiovascular Physiology in the Critically Ill

Michael L. Hess, MD, FACC
William S. Sibbald, MD, FRCP(C)

A detailed appreciation of factors responsible for the alteration of cardiac function in critical illness requires knowledge of both the molecular basis of cardiac function and its influence on cardiac mechanics as it relates to both normal and pathologic conditions. Only then can therapeutics be rationally applied to the cardiovascular support of critically ill patients. This chapter reviews both systolic and diastolic abnormalities at the cell and organ level and explains how these are assessed at the bedside. Pressure-volume (P-V) loops are used in a theoretic sense to relate cellular mechanisms to abnormalities of cardiovascular function and the effects of various therapies in the critically ill patient.

CELLULAR PHYSIOLOGY OF MYOCARDIAL FUNCTION

Cellular Determinants of Contractility

The interaction of the proteins actin, myosin, and the troponin complex results in contractile activity of the myocardial muscle fibers. Engagement of actin and myosin occurs when calcium (Ca^{2+}) levels in the cytosol increase in the presence of adequate adenosine triphosphate (ATP). This process is regulated by a complex that consists of troponin C and other proteins. Troponin C contains a Ca^{2+}-specific binding site with variable affinity for Ca^{2+}.[1] When Ca^{2+} is bound to troponin C, *tropomyosin* (a protein bound to the troponin complex, which inhibits actin-myosin interaction in the absence of troponin C) undergoes a conformational change, allowing for actin-myosin interaction and contraction.

Removal of Ca^{2+} from the cytosol results in dissociation from troponin C, with subsequent cessation of actin-myosin cross-linkage. This event signals the end of contractile activity and the start of relaxation. This process is known as inactivation.[2]

Calcium and Cyclic Adenosine Monophosphate

Alterations in the delivery, use, and myofibrillar sensitivity to and removal of Ca^{2+} from the myofibril and the myocyte cytosol constitute the biologic basis for the vast majority of the abnormalities in both contractility and relaxation. Ca^{2+}, stored in the sarcoplasmic reticulum (SR), is released from storage sites. In addition, Ca^{2+} entry from extracellular locations participate in the contractile process.

Entry of Ca^{2+} from extracellular locations occurs through voltage-dependent gated "slow channels," activated by membrane depolarization, or via sodium-calcium (Na-Ca^{2+}) exchange across the sarcolemma. This Ca^{2+}, rather than participating directly in activation of contraction, causes release of Ca^{2+} from the SR,[3] so-called Ca^{2+}-dependent Ca^{2+} release. The Ca^{2+} released from the SR binds to troponin, with subsequent contractile activity.

In addition, elevated levels of cyclic adenosine monophosphate (cAMP), the major intracellular second messenger, cause increased Ca^{2+} influx by recruitment of additional voltage-dependent channels, previously dormant. This is accomplished by cAMP-mediated transfer of phosphates to *phospholamban,* a protein linked to the voltage-gated channels. Phospholamban, a protein within the SR, when phosphorylated by cAMP-dependent mechanisms, results in increased SR uptake of Ca^{2+}.[4] This is noted to occur primarily after adrenergic stimuli. All of these mechanisms result in increased contraction.[5]

Altered Ca^{2+} kinetics are responsible for the increases in contractility. The increased contractility of postextrasystolic beats,[6,7] increased heart rate (HR)[8,9] and—during pharmacologic manipulation with cardiac glycosides—phosphodiesterase inhibitors,[10] sympathomimetic amines,[9] and caffeine[4] are dependent on changes in intracellular Ca^{2+} or cAMP levels.

Individual muscle units in the failing and hypertrophied ventricle have depressed function.[11] The myocardial depression accompanying anoxia,[12] acidosis,[13] hypothyroidism, barbiturate use, administration of local and general anesthetic agents, use of Ca^{2+} antagonists,[14] and ischemia[15] all result from abnormalities in the Ca^{2+}-dependent mechanisms described here.

Mediators of Contractility

Various mediators act independently by linking stimulated acetylcholine receptors to intracytoplasmic enzyme systems that alter the contractile state of the myocardium. The most well-characterized of these systems, the *guanine nucleotide regulatory proteins,*[16] are coupled to acetylcholine receptors and possibly to receptors for nitric oxide and endothelins.

Beta Receptors and Guanine Nucleotide Regulatory Proteins

Adrenergic stimulation of cardiac myocytes is a very important regulator of both Ca^{2+} influx and cAMP levels within the cell (Fig. 89–1). The predominant beta receptor of myocytes, when stimulated, increases the manufacture of cAMP. This in turn, results in increased Ca^{2+} influx. Ca^{2+} channels that are under the influence of beta receptor–mediated increases in cAMP are known as *receptor-operated channels.*[17,18]

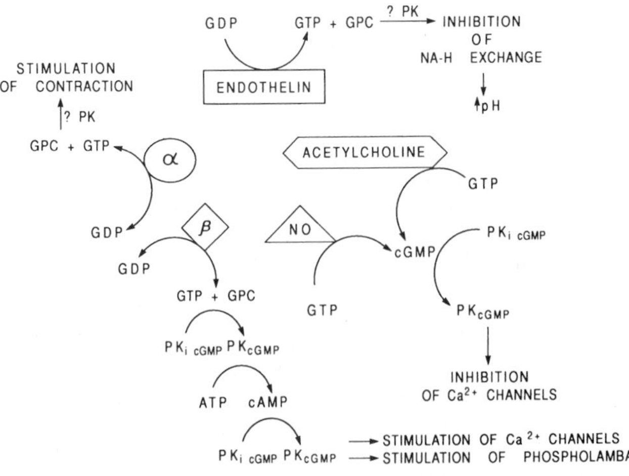

Figure 89–1. Receptors and intracellular signaling via G proteins (see text). GDP = guanosine diphosphate; GTP = guanosine triphosphate; GPC = G protein complex; PK = active protein kinase; PK_i = inactive protein kinase; α = alpha receptor; β = beta receptor; NO = nitrous oxide receptor.

Stimulation of beta receptors on the cell surface results in activation of adenylate cyclase (AC) and subsequent increases in cAMP levels. This results in increased Ca^{2+} influx with resultant increases in contractile force. The coupling between beta receptors and AC occurs through guanine cyclic nucleotides, also known as *G proteins.*[19] G proteins have both stimulatory and inhibitory influences on AC. The G protein complex in its active form contains guanosine triphosphate (GTP). When present, this protein "couples" the beta receptor to AC, and when beta receptor adrenergic stimulation occurs, results in the formation of cAMP and subsequent increases in intracellular calcium. The G protein complex is capable of degrading its bound GTP to guanosine diphosphate (GDP) when beta receptor stimulation ceases, thereby no longer stimulating AC. G proteins also have a pivotal role in stimulation of cardiac contractility by a receptor stimulation through a *cAMP-independent* mechanism[20] which results in increased contractility within a single heartbeat (see Fig. 89–1). Cyclic AMP-dependent mechanisms have demonstrated delays in response of 2 to 20 seconds, as opposed to G protein pathway delays in response of 150 msec. This allows alterations in Ca^{2+} flux within a single heart beat, an explanation of the observed phenomenon of increased contractility immediately after increased stimulation.

Inhibitory G proteins, when activated by stimulated acetylcholine receptors, inhibit Ca^{2+} influx.[21] This phenomenon occurs via a cyclic guanosine monophosphate (cGMP)-mediated mechanism. A cGMP system, similar to the cAMP system, activates cGMP protein kinase (cGMP-PK), which inhibits calcium inward currents previously stimulated by cAMP.[22] Additionally, cGMP-mediated inhibition of Ca^{2+} channels has been demonstrated *not* to be a result of cAMP hydrolysis or a result of inhibition of cAMP-PK but a direct effect of cGMP-PK.

In addition to changes in receptor function, molecular alterations in receptor production in various disease states occur. In dilated cardiomyopathies, both beta receptor messenger ribonucleic acid (mRNA) and absolute receptor levels were found to be depressed.[23] At the same time, $beta_1$ receptor kinase levels were elevated. Beta receptor kinase, the molecule responsible for phosphorylation of beta-adrenergic receptors, is elevated when beta receptors are dysfunctional (uncoupled). This may provide an explanation for the catecholamine insensitivity observed in failing hearts as well as after cardiopulmonary bypass.[24]

Nitric Oxide

Nitric oxide has been shown to affect cardiac contractility. It has been found in many tissue types, including ventricular myocytes, where its physiologic effects are mediated via cGMP. Cholinergic myocardial depressant effects, as evidenced by inhibition of the effect of the muscarinic agonist carbachol, are inhibited by antagonists of nitric oxide (methylene blue and oxyhemoglobin) as well as by L-arginine (the natural substrate of nitric oxide synthesis analogs), which inhibit nitric oxide. In addition, the positive inotropic action of the beta agonist isoproterenol is enhanced by nitric oxide inhibition. These data indicate that the effect of nitric oxide is to activate the inhibitory receptor cyclic nucleotide interaction through cGMP mechanisms (see Fig. 89–1).

Nitric oxide has been implicated in the myocardial response to sepsis. It has been well documented that myocardial depression in septic shock occurs secondary to a yet undefined substance. One potential substance, tumor necrosis factor (TNF), has been shown in vitro to depress the activity of spontaneously beating rat cardiomyocytes in tissue culture. Inhibition of nitric oxide synthesis by *N*-methyl-arginine blocked TNF-induced cardiomyocyte depression.[25] Additionally, methylene blue, an inhibitor of guanylate cyclase,[26] prevented TNF-induced cardiomyocyte depression.

Although the cellular mechanism of the depression noted in septic myocardium has not yet been well characterized, it may be due to alterations in Ca^{2+} handling. Abnormalities of beta receptor function, as measured by decreased levels of cAMP in peripheral lymphocytes in septic patients, as well as possible abnormalities in patients with sepsis have been elicited.[27] The exact cellular level of this defect, whether this abnormality of beta receptor function is receptor downregulation or reduced transcription of beta receptor genes, has not been determined.

Endothelin

Endothelin-1, a 21-amino acid vasoconstrictor peptide released from the vascular endothelium, was isolated by Yangisawa and colleagues.[28] Since that time, four additional isoforms and a closely related substance, *vasoactive intestinal contractor*, have been isolated. These substances have been found ubiquitously in mammalian tissues. Their intracardiac site of genesis is unknown but is believed to be the endothelium of the coronary arteries and microvasculature. Various vasodilator and vasoconstrictor substances released from the vascular endothelium alter blood flow and, in this way, indirectly affect cardiac contractility.[29] Of these locally elaborated paracrine substances, the endothelins have been most extensively studied.

High-affinity receptors for endothelins in mammalian atria and ventricles have been isolated. In vitro, these substances are potent vasoconstrictors and positive inotropes, acting via a yet incompletely defined mechanism. Kelly and colleagues[30] demonstrated that at constant cytosolic Ca^{2+} levels, using the Ca^{2+}-specific intracellular probe Fura-2, endothelins cause marked increases in the contractility of isolated rat ventricular myocytes. This observation suggests that endothelins may sensitize the myofibrils to calcium.

As previously discussed, an increase in intracellular pH results in increased myofibrillar sensitivity for Ca^{2+}, thereby increasing contractility. Endothelin causes an increase in intracellular pH with a subsequent increase in contraction when studied in rat ventricular myocytes. This effect is completely inhibited by pretreatment with amiloride, which inhibits sodium-hydrogen ion exchange across the sarcolemmal membrane and, hence, prevents increases in intracellular pH.[31] Furthermore, the effect of endothelin appears to be mediated via G proteins participating in signal transduction after binding of endothelin to its sarcolemmal receptor (see Fig. 89–1).

Cellular Determinants of Relaxation

Just as abnormalities of contraction have as their cellular basis derangements of Ca^{2+} handling, so does relaxation. Cessation of the inward Ca^{2+} current (or inactivation) by closure of voltage-limited channels begins the period of relaxation at the myocyte level, with the rate and extent of Ca^{2+} removal affecting the rate and extent of relaxation. Inactivation signals the end of actin-myosin interaction. However, this single term does not adequately describe the interplay of processes that are occurring at the cellular level to facilitate relaxation. An SR Ca^{2+} pump, in the presence of adequate ATP, pumps Ca^{2+} into the SR from the cytosol. In addition, the Na-Ca^{2+} exchange pump (also ATP requiring), which allows influx of Ca^{2+} during contraction, also participates in the transport of Ca^{2+} out of the cell across the sarcolemma. The affinity of myofibril for Ca^{2+} also affects relaxation. As the myofibril shortens, its affinity for Ca^{2+} decreases, limiting Ca^{2+} effects. All of these mechanisms are facilitated or inhibited by drugs or neurohumoral factors.

Few researchers have focused on critically ill patients to assess the cellular basis of relaxation in critical illness; however, these processes have been extensively studied in dilated cardiomyopathies, left ventricular (LV) hypertrophy, ischemia, and hypertrophic cardiomyopathy. Impairment of relaxation in these patients occurs secondary to increased levels of Ca^{2+} within the myocyte in diastole[32] owing to diminished function of the SR pump, decreased expression at the genetic level for this pump (as evidenced by decreased mRNA levels),[33] decreased phospholamban activity[34] or levels of phospholamban mRNA,[35] down-regulation or uncoupling of beta receptors,[36] or inhibition of function by G protein.

MECHANICS OF SYSTOLIC FUNCTION

Determinants of Stroke Volume

Systemic blood pressure is the product of cardiac output and total peripheral resistance; an increase in either results in an increase in blood pressure unless, of course, a compensatory depression occurs in the opposite variable. Disordered autoregulation of blood flow to microvascular beds disturbs the normal relationship of cardiac output, total peripheral resistance, and blood pressure. Therefore, determinants of central flow (cardiac output) assume greater importance. In addition, these same systemic illnesses can influence the cardiac output directly by altering the determinants of cardiac output (i.e., heart rate and stroke volume [SV]).

Definition

Stroke volume is defined as that portion of blood that is ejected from the ventricle by a single heart beat. The magnitude of SV is determined by the following influences:

- Ventricular preload
- Ventricular afterload
- Ventricular contractility
- Heart rate

Preload

Studies of isolated heart muscle preparations provided the basis for an understanding of both ventricular preload and afterload. From these studies, ventricular *preload* was initially related to the degree of myocardial fiber length at the onset of a contraction. Because a change in muscle length was accompanied by changes in sarcomere length, the sarcomere was thereby recognized as the fundamental unit that defined contraction of cardiac muscle. The sarcomere, therefore, represents the ultrastructural basis for *Starling's law of the heart,* which states that the force of muscle contraction is dependent on initial muscle length.

In this context, Gordon and associates[37] first showed that the force of contraction developed in myocardial muscle was proportional to sarcomere length. The clinical expression of this relationship between muscle length and the force of a subsequent contraction is the observation that cardiac work increases as end-diastolic ventricular size or preload increases. Ventricular preload, therefore, may be assessed as (1) end-diastolic stress, (2) end-diastolic volume (EDV), or (3) end-diastolic dimension (EDD). End-diastolic stress and EDD are clinically measured with echocardiography. EDV can be measured by either echocardiography or nuclear scientigraphic measurements. However, repeated measurements are time-consuming. The most common and earliest measure of ventricular preload is the measurement of end-diastolic filling pressures. Early clinical studies reported ventricular preload as measured by end-diastolic filling pressures, such as the central venous pressure for the right ventricle (RV) and the pulmonary capillary wedge pressure (PCWP) for the left ventricle (LV).[38] Because end-diastolic pressure (EDP) relates to EDV not by any linear function but exponentially,[39] an EDP cannot be adequately substituted as a measure of ventricular preload.[40]

Afterload

Pertinent concepts that initially defined ventricular afterload also originated from studies of isolated heart muscle. In these studies, *afterload* was defined as the weight the muscle fiber had to lift once contraction had been initiated. Clinically, however, the ventricle does not lift a weight, it ejects a viscous fluid load into a viscoelastic system. Therefore, the definition of afterload, described by experiments using isolated muscle preparations, does not adequately account for the load the ventricle must eject against in vivo. In fact, any ideal definition of ventricular afterload should acknowledge several elements, including ventricular intracavitary pressure, wall thickness, chamber radius, and geometry. Although difficult to assess clinically, the afterload faced by either ventricle during ejection is probably best represented by systolic wall tension, or stress.[41] Wall stress reflects an integration of the effects of two major loads: a *vascular load* and the load imposed by the ventricle itself. The vascular load is determined by the cross-sectional area of the vascular bed, the elasticity of the vascular wall, and the viscosity of the blood; all can be isolated in the laboratory by measurement of vascular input impedance spectral.[42]

The ventricular load represents the combined effects of the physiologic properties of cardiac muscle cells as well as ventricular shape and size.[43] However, ventricular afterload cannot be easily measured if this strict physiologic definition is used; it is therefore clinically approximated if one measures the mean pressure that the ventricle is exposed to during ejection or if one calculates the appropriate vascular resistance (i.e., systemic or pulmonary vascular resistance).[44] Independent ventricular afterload changes may profoundly influence ventricular muscle shortening and, hence, cardiac output and systemic oxygen transport.[45]

Contractility

The inotropic state of the heart refers to the vigor of ventricular contraction when both preload and afterload are known and held constant. Contractility is the most difficult determinant to measure accurately because almost every known index of contractility proposed is dependent, to various degrees, on ventricular preload or afterload.

Pressure-Volume Loops

The interaction of the three determinants of SV (preload, afterload, and contractility) may be conceptualized by analysis of P-V loops for isolated cardiac beats.[46] Understanding this approach to describing ventricular function further clarifies the interaction of the physiologic determinants of SV. Pressure-volume relations are particularly useful for describing the pathophysiology of clinical disorders encountered in the critically ill as well as mechanisms by which different therapeutic interventions might affect the ventricular stroke output in this patient population.

A ventricular P-V loop can be inscribed by continuous measurement of ventricular volume and pressure (Fig. 89-2). At the end of ventricular contraction, the pressure within the ventricle falls. Ventricular filling is initiated when ventricular pressure has decreased below the atrial pressure (point A in Fig. 89-2); with ventricular filling, diastole begins. Subsequently, activation of cardiac muscle by an action potential initiates isovolumic contraction at end-diastole (point B); isovolumic contraction continues until ventricular pressure exceeds aortic diastolic pressure when ejection begins (point C); at end-systole (point D), isovolumic relaxation is initiated. Joined together, points A, B, C, and D inscribe a single P-V loop, and the area within this loop reflects the stroke work

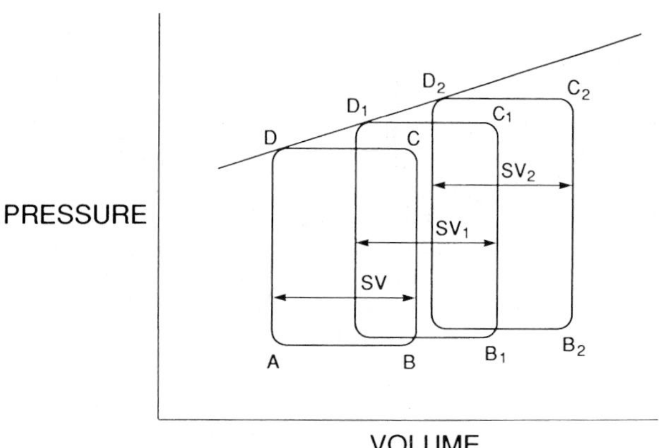

Figure 89–2. Ventricular pressure-volume loops. The loop bounded by points A, B, C, and D represents the resting pressure-volume relationship for an entire cardiac cycle. Diastole occurs between points A and B. Isovolumic contraction occurs between points B and C. At point C, the ventricular pressure exceeds the aortic pressure, and ejection commences. Ejection continues until the energy substrate is utilized by end-systolic (point D). Isovolumic relaxation then occurs, and diastole starts when ventricular pressure drops below the atrial pressure. Increasing afterload (C_1, C_2) is compensated by increases in end-diastolic volume and pressure, as noted by points B_1 and B_2. The end-systolic points (D, D_1, D_2) for each of these loops all fall on a single line, which is called the *isovolumic pressure line* and which reflects the inotropic state. SV = stroke volume.

performed by the ventricle during this one cardiac cycle. In this context, it is thereby intuitive that stroke work is made up of both volume and pressure work.

When ventricular afterload is increased at a constant inotropic state, as hypothetically represented by points C_1 and C_2 in Figure 89–2, new P-V loops are constructed because stroke work now increases proportional to the increase in afterload. Flow work or SV is maintained by a compensatory increase in EDV (B_1 and B_2). The end-systolic point of each loop (upper left corner of each loop, points D, D_1, D_2) falls along a single line, an *isovolumic pressure line,* the slope of which reflects the resting contractile or inotropic state.

This activity is further illustrated in Figure 89–3. The ventricle with depressed contractility is indicated by the P-V loop bounding stroke volume (SV_1). An inotrope given to this depressed ventricle would shift the isovolumic pressure line upward and to the left, resulting in larger SV for any given level of preload (SV_2 and SV_3).

The *Frank-Starling mechanism,* or preload recruitable stroke work, can now be described by these concepts. At a constant inotropic and afterload state, increases in preload as represented by points B_1 and B_2 in Figure 89–4 result in increased SV_1 to SV_2).

Clinical Methods of Measuring Contractility

Traditionally, contractility was a measure of the overall vigor with which the ventricular geometry changed or by a rise in pressure over time (dp/dt) within the cavity of the LV. The most common measurement, the *ejection fraction,* measures a percentage change in the size of LV in two dimensions by planimetry or by the difference in radionuclide counts between systole and diastole in the case of gated blood pool scanning. These methods, although convenient, do not control variables that affect contractility, such as preload, heart rate, and afterload, making independent estimates of contractility impossible. The dp/dt also varies with heart rate, preload, and afterload.

Clinically, contractility may be most easily conceptualized as an increase in SV when preload, afterload, and heart rate are unchanged. This situation is the ideal, however, and more precise measurement of contractility is often needed for clinical decision making and for research application.

An excellent load-independent measure of contractility, both in vivo and ex vivo isolated heart preparations, is that of end-systolic P-V relations.[47] This is the point of P-V curve at end-systole. Alterations in afterload and preload without a change in contractility result in formation of a straight line with a constant volume intercept (the isovolumic pressure line). This slope of this line reflects the intrinsic contractility of the ventricle (see Figs. 89–2 and 89–3), and because the volume intercept does not change with alterations in preload and afterload, it is considered to be load-independent. More recent studies, however, have shown that these relationships can be curvilinear with changes in load and inotropy. Furthermore, the isovolumic pressure line can be constructed only by pharmacologic intervention, nuclear or angiographic as-

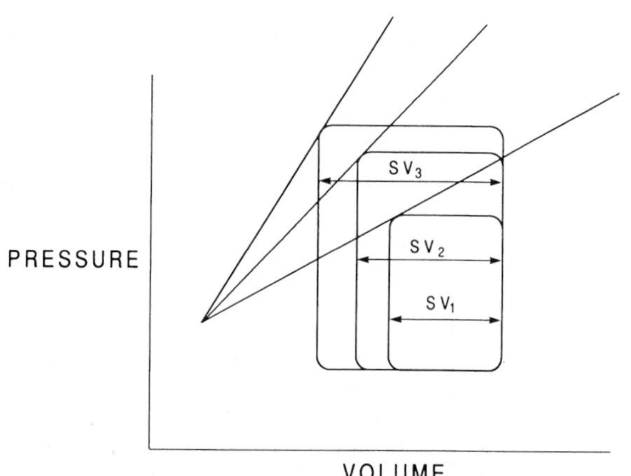

Figure 89–3. Ventricular pressure-volume loops at varying levels of contractility depicted by three different isovolumic lines. End-diastolic pressure does not change, but stroke volume (SV) increases with increasing contractility ($SV_1<SV_2<SV_3$).

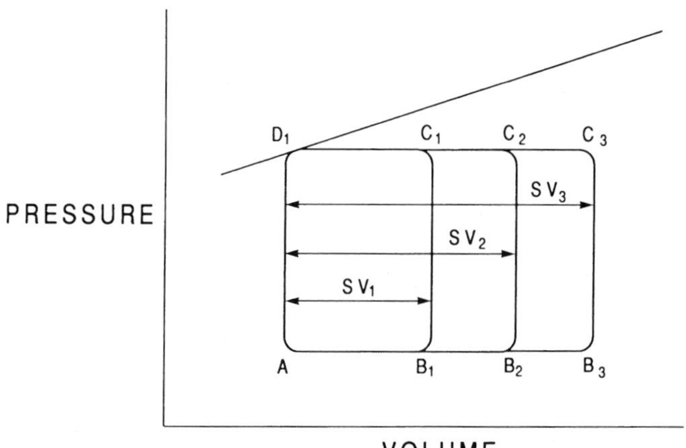

Figure 89–4. Ventricular pressure-volume loops at different preloads. Contractility and afterload are held constant. Increases in preload increase stroke volume (SV) and stroke work as a function of the Frank-Starling mechanism.

sessment of volume, and invasive pressure monitoring, thus limiting its use in clinical practice.

A method of contractility evaluation that is independent of both preload, afterload, and heart rate has been described by Colan and colleagues.[48] The rate-corrected velocity of circumferential fiber shortening (Fig. 89-5) is a powerful measure of contractility with both research and clinical application. This measure describes the fractional shortening of the LV as measured by echocardiography from the parasternal short axis dimension (see Fig. 89-5, *left upper panel* and *lower panel*).

$$\frac{\dfrac{EDD - ESD}{EDD}}{ET_c}$$

where EDD is end-diastolic dimension, ESA is end-systolic dimension, and ET_c, (the rate-corrected ejection time) is the ejection time (taken from external carotid pulse tracings) divided by the square root of the R-R interval.

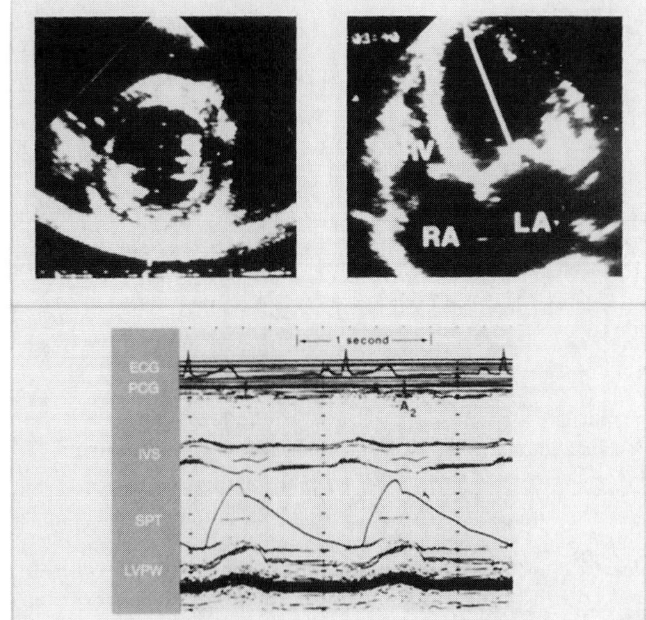

Figure 89–5. Noninvasively acquired data for determination of left ventricular (LV) force-velocity relations. The *upper left-hand panel* shows the two-dimensional short axis image through which the M-mode recording *(lower panel)* was obtained and the minor axis dimensions were measured. The *upper right-hand panel* shows an apical four-chamber, two-dimensional image from which long-axis measurements are made. The externally calibrated subclavian pulse tracing (SPT) is used to acquire simultaneous pressure data *(lower panel)*. End-systole is identified by aortic valve closure (A_2) on the phonocardiogram (PCG). End-diastole is defined as the peak of the R wave on the electrocardiogram (ECG). IVS = interventricular septum; LVPW = left ventricular posterior wall; RV = right ventricle; RA = right atrium; LA = left atrium. (From Borow KM, Marcus RH, Neuman A, et al: Modern noninvasive techniques for the assessment of left ventricular systolic performance. *In:* Heart Disease: A Textbook of Cardiovascular Medicine. 4th ed. Braunwald E [Ed]. Philadelphia, WB Saunders, 1982, p 31.)

MECHANICS OF DIASTOLE

Left Ventricular Compliance and the Diastolic Left Ventricular Pressure-Volume Relationship

The nonlinear relationship between pressure and volume during ventricular diastole is depicted in Figure 89-2. The diastolic phase of the cardiac cycle extends from points A to B. A shift to the right in this diastolic pressure relationship is depicted by points B to B_1 and B_1 to B_2. These shifts reflect either a change in the operating chamber stiffness of the LV, as is normally noted with increased filling[49] or these changes may occur as a result of various disease states (Fig. 89-6).[50]

Abnormal shifts in ventricular pressure at a given volume, reflecting a change in ventricular compliance outside of the norm (Fig. 89-7) where contractility is held constant[49] is represented by a shift from the loop bounded by the broken line to that bounded by the solid line. The result of increased chamber stiffness (decreased compliance) is a decreased EDV for a given EDP. This nonlinear relationship of EDP and EDV is critically important in the clinical treatment of patients and is a source of significant error in hemodynamic manipulations.[40] Assessment of EDV as EDP results in incorrect assumptions of the cause of decreased stroke work (see area bounded by loops in Fig. 89-7). The contractile state has not changed, as evidenced by the slope of the isovolumic pressure line, which reflects the intrinsic contractile state of the myocardium. Instead, the cause of the decrease in stroke work has been the decrease in preload (EDV), which is not evident by measurement of EDP alone.

Factors That Affect the Diastolic Pressure-Volume Relationship

Left ventricular diastolic function depends on many factors, some intrinsic to the heart itself (e.g., the active energy-dependent process of relaxation and material properties of the myocardium) and some extrinsic to the LV (e.g., pericardial constraining forces and ventricular interaction). Furthermore, Gilbert and Glantz[50] suggest the subdivisions of *extent of relaxation* (i.e., the completeness of relaxation) and the *rate of relaxation*. Alterations in the extent, rate, or both characterize the abnormalities of relaxation and result in characteristic hemodynamic patterns (Fig. 89-8).[50]

Extent of Relaxation

The extent of relaxation is the major determinant of EDV and EDP because these are measurements made at the end of the relaxation process. Abnormalities in extent of relaxation affect the end-diastolic P-V relationship in the greatest manner. Abnormalities in the rate of relaxation, however, tend to have minimum effect on the end-diastolic P-V relationship, because they occur early in diastole and therefore do not alter EDP and EDV to any appreciable extent.

The extent of relaxation may be viewed as the compliance properties of the LV at the point where relaxation is complete (i.e., end diastole). Alterations in the determinants of this relationship that are *intrinsic* to the myocardium result in shifts of the diastolic pressure volume curve. *LV geometry* (i.e., thickness, size, and chamber dimension) in large part determines the LV end-diastolic P-V relationship, as determined by mathematic approximations based on Laplace's law.[50] Alterations in the LV end-diastolic P-V relationship may occur secondary to the change in elastic properties as the ventricle stretches during filling. Changes in the diastolic P-V relationship that depend on the rate at which the LV deforms are known as *viscoelasticity*, a property that the myocardium shares with most biomaterials. This property is manifested when filling rates are highest, occurring during the first half of diastole or after atrial contraction. *Stress relaxation* (a

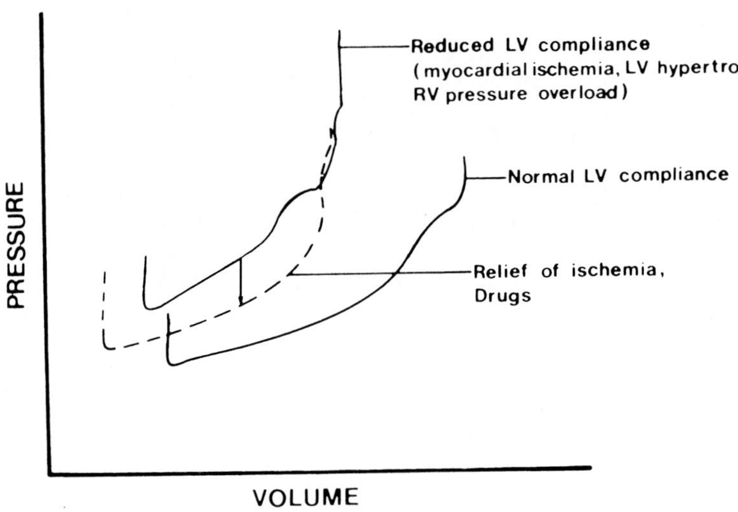

Figure 89–6. Causes of shifts in the left ventricular (LV) diastolic pressure-volume relationship. Various factors can either increase or reduce compliance and shift the curve either upward and to the left or downward and to the right.

decrease in the distending pressure of the ventricle over time) and *creep* (a rightward shift in the diastolic P-V relationship) are two experimental manifestations of viscosity. The clinical importance of viscoelasticity has been disputed.

Other dynamic changes in relaxation that occur during ventricular filling are due to alterations in the elastic properties and the rate of relaxation of the myocardium mediated by changes in the load sensed by the LV during relaxation. These *load-dependent relaxation* phenomena cause instantaneous changes in LV compliance as well as in the rate of relaxation that are independent of heart rate when LV muscle is abruptly stretched.

An additional determinant of the diastolic P-V relationship is *coronary vascular turgor.* The effect of this on the extent of relaxation is primarily through its erectile effect on LV stiffness.[51] This decreases LV diastolic compliance by increasing LV wall volume, resulting in a higher EDP for a given volume. This effect seems to be independent of pericardial influences and predominates in the late diastolic filling period, thereby influencing the extent of relaxation, albeit to a small degree. In addition, the constraining effect of the pericardium and the degree of ventricular interaction affect the extent of relaxation.

Alterations in Extent of Relaxation Secondary to Intrinsic Myocardial Disorders

Left ventricular hypertrophy results in abnormalities of relaxation that are characteristic of the manner in which the hypertrophy developed and of the type of hypertrophy formed.[52] Chronic volume overload, as in mitral or aortic insufficiency or due to physical conditioning, results in *eccentric hypertrophy,* characterized by increased ventricular volume but little or no change in elasticity. This results in little increase in pressure at increased volumes. In contrast, chronic pressure overload, as in aortic stenosis or chronic untreated hypertension, results in *concentric hypertrophy,* with increased elastic stiffness and an elevated EDP for a given volume. Geometrically, pressure overload or hypertrophy is characterized by additional myocytes in parallel with existing cells; volume overload (eccentric hypertrophy) results in increased length of existing myocytes. Alterations in Ca^{2+} metabolism result in elevated myocyte diastolic Ca^{2+} levels. These factors

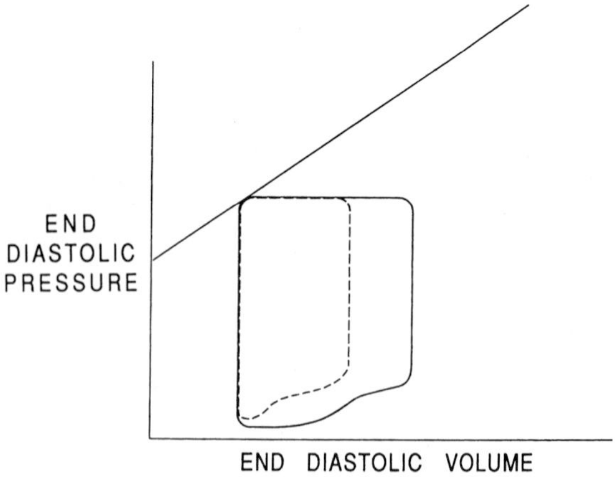

END DIASTOLIC PRESSURE

END DIASTOLIC VOLUME

Figure 89–7. Effect of changes in compliance on stroke volume. Ventricular pressure-volume loops are constructed for two different conditions in the same heart. Contractility and ejection pressure do not change. The only change has been an upward shift to the left in the left ventricular diastolic pressure-volume relationship of the loop bounded by the *broken line* caused by a decrease in the compliant properties of the myocardium. This results in a reduction both in end-diastolic volume at a given end-diastolic pressure and in the area enclosed by the loop (decreased stroke volume).

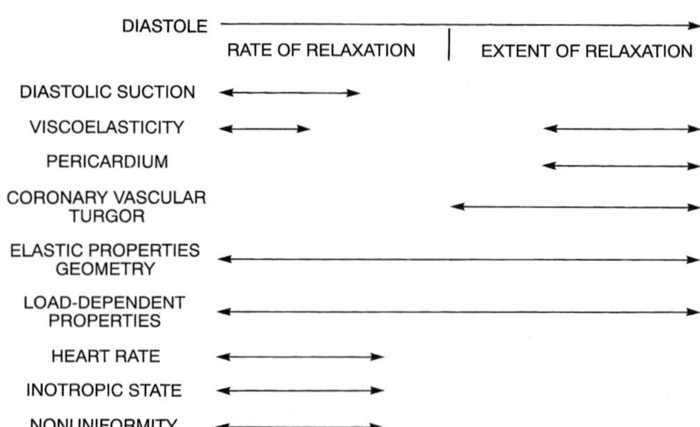

Figure 89–8. Factors affecting the diastolic pressure-volume relationship and their time-course of effect during diastole. The duration of effect (distances bounded by *arrows*) and the mechanism of action of each factor (i.e., rate of relaxation or extent of relaxation, or both) are diagrammed. (Modified from Gilbert JC, Glantz SA: Determinants of left ventricular filling and of the diastolic pressure-volume relation. Circ Res 1989; 64:827. Reproduced with permission. Copyright 1989, American Heart Association.)

account for the elevated EDP in chronic pressure overload hypertrophy.

Ischemia affects the extent of relaxation, as evidenced by upward shift in end-diastolic P-V relationship when myocardial oxygen demand outstrips supply.[53] Pacing-induced ischemia after the creation of a coronary stenosis in dogs results in such a shift in the pressure volume relationship at end diastole (Fig. 89–9). These effects are independent of pericardial, right ventricular, or lung interactions, implying a change in the intrinsic myocardial elastic properties. Changes in diastolic properties secondary to changes in myocardial Ca^{2+} handling,[37] as well as in hydrogen ion accumulation[54] and repeated systolic stretch of the ischemia segment,[55] interact to produce the observed changes.

The changes in ventricular compliance seem to be restricted to the region of active ischemia.[55] Furthermore, uninvolved areas show evidence of a proportional increase in regional size and pressure (with a resultant constant diastolic P-V relation) to maintain stroke volume by the Starling mechanism. Hence, during acute ischemia, the remaining normal areas of myocardium appear to use the Frank-Starling mechanism to maintain stroke volume in compensation for the effects of abnormal contractility or an upward shift of the regional diastolic P-V relationship within the ischemic areas.

Rate of Relaxation

The rate of relaxation, results primarily in changes in the rate of diastolic early filling.[50] The determinants of relaxation rate are many, and their interactions complicated (see Fig. 89–9). Increases in heart rate and inotropy result in increased rates of relaxation. Alterations in end-diastolic loading conditions result in changes in the rate of relaxation during experimental conditions. *Nonuniformity* of relaxation,[2] which describes a nonuniform distribution of load and electric inactivation during diastole in space and time, results in alterations in the rate of relaxation. *Ventricular suction,* or the ability of the ventricle to generate pressures below equilibrium diastolic pressures, may alter the rate and extent of LV filling. Finally, ischemia can alter the rate as well as the extent of relaxation. Resolution of ischemia results in reversal of these changes.

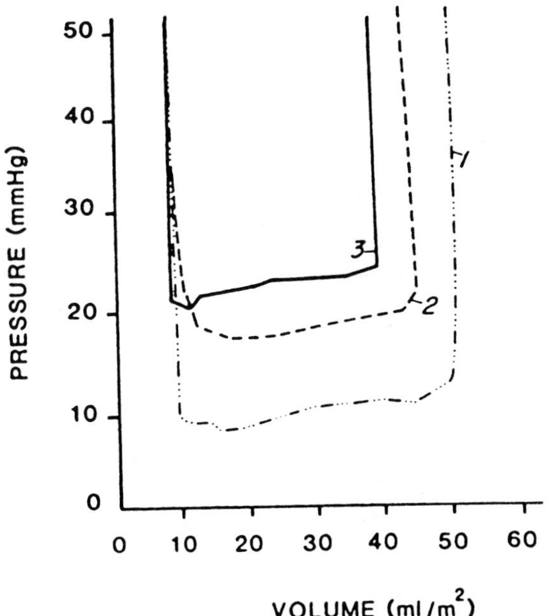

Figure 89–9. Pressure-volume loops that illustrate the ischemic response to pacing in dogs with coronary stenosis. Note the shift upward and to the left during progressive pacing; this shift represents predominant diastolic dysfunction (line 1 = 84 beats/min; line 2 = 110 beats/min; line 3 = 135 beats/min). (From Aroesty JM, McKay RG, Heller GV, et al: Simultaneous assessment of left ventricular systolic and diastolic function during pacing-induced ischemia. Circulation 1985; 71:889.)

Extrinsic Influences on the Diastolic Pressure-Volume Relationship

It is now apparent that external loads profoundly influence ventricular compliance properties. Specifically, the right ventricle (RV),[56] the pericardium[57] and the lungs[58] all may acutely induce shifts of the LV diastolic P-V relationship.

Pericardial Influences

The influence of the pericardium in the diastolic P-V relationship is a function of both its stiffness and its ability to constrain the entire heart.[59] An increase in size of one ventricle therefore causes an increase in the EDP for a given volume (i.e., a shift upward in the P-V relationship) (Fig. 89–10). The constraining effect of normal pericardium is dependent on its intrinsic compliance and how it affects LV pressures. Just as dilation of the RV affects the LV diastolic P-V relation, dilation of the LV (i.e., high LV filling pressure) amplifies the pericardium's influence. This has been demonstrated by measurement of the diastolic P-V relation before and after removal of the pericardium.[57] Little normal pericardial effect is observed at normal filling pressures.

In addition, the intact pericardium allows interaction between the atria and the LV as well as between RV and LV. The effect of left atrial (LA) pressure is approximately one-quarter that of the RV pressure in determining the LV diastolic pressure.[60]

Assessment of pericardial constraint in patients is difficult. Experimental systems are overly invasive, and measurement artifacts influence pressure measurements.[50] RV or right atrial (RA) pressure under normal conditions serves as a useful measurement of pericardial influence but may be of limited use in patients with RV hypertrophy, cor pulmonale, and pulmonary hypertension as well as after drainage of chronic pericardial tamponade.

Right Ventricular Influences

Studies of RV influence on LV compliance[58, 61] have demonstrated that an upward shift of the LV diastolic P-V curve (i.e., reduced compliance) accompanies RV volume increases at end diastole (Fig. 89–11); although this effect is present with the pericardium open, the coupling is much stronger when it is closed.[57] Ventricular interaction is thus an important mechanism underlying acute reductions in LV compliance whether the RV is enlarged as a result of pressure or volume overload. Ventricular interaction may also be responsible for some of the improved LV compliance properties observed with the administration of vasoactive medications that reduce volume return to the RV (e.g., nitrates).[62]

The importance of appreciating the influence of RV pressure and volume overload, as well as the use of cardiotonic medications, on the LV diastolic P-V relationship is apparent from clinical studies of patients with adult respiratory distress syndrome (ARDS). This work, summarized in Table 89–1, describes changes in pulmonary capillary wedge pressure (PCWP) and LV preload in two clinical circumstances:

1. At three levels of pulmonary pressures, which thereby represented a progressive increase in RV afterload.[63]
2. In patients in whom an inotrope was required to maintain adequate systemic oxygen transport.[64]

In patients with acute pulmonary hypertension, an increase in the PCWP was found to be reflected by a constant LV EDV

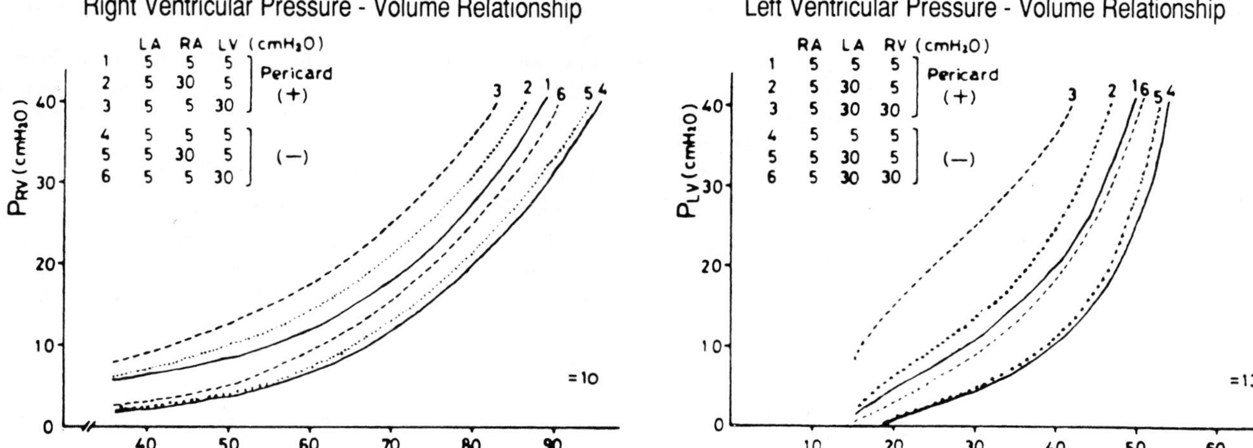

Figure 89–10. Effect of the pericardium on chamber pressure-volume relations. The ventricular pressure-volume relation of one ventricle is shifted upward when the pressure in one or more of the other chambers is increased. The pericardium causes this interaction to be more forceful. In addition, the direct interaction effect of the right ventricle on the left is greater than that of the left ventricle on the right, particularly with the pericardium intact. The representative right *(A)* and left *(B)* ventricular pressure-volume curves from isolated, perfused dog hearts were obtained while the other three chambers were held at various pressures from 5 to 30 cm H_2O (4–22 mm Hg) with and without the pericardium. Curves 1, 2, and 3 in each situation were with the pericardium (pericard [+]). Curves 4, 5, and 6 were without the pericardium (pericard [−]). PRV = right ventricular pressure; PLV = left ventricular pressure; VRV = right ventricular volume; VLV = left ventricular volume. (From Maruyama Y, Ashikawa K, Isoyama S, et al: Mechanical interactions between four heart chambers with and without the pericardium in canine hearts. Circ Res 1982; 50:86. Copyright 1982, American Heart Association.)

(preload), thereby demonstrating the effect of a pressure-overloaded RV to induce a depression in LV compliance properties. That is, LV chamber stiffness was altered with pulmonary hypertension, so that the LV end-diastolic P-V curve was progressively shifted left with each successive increase in pulmonary artery pressure. Alterations in LV geometry were also noted with increasing pulmonary hypertension. The LV septal/free wall axis appears disproportionately reduced compared with either the base-to-apex or the anteroposterior axis.[56, 58] Acute pulmonary hypertension induced by glass bead embolization confirms that (1) upward shifts in the LV diastolic P-V relationship occur with changes in RV afterload (i.e., a reduction in LV compliance) and (2) this effect is largely mediated by a reduction in the dimension of the LV septum to the free wall and an increase in intrapericardial pressure.[58] Similarly, during administration of inotropes, patients with ARDS demonstrated a higher mean PCWP than those without, although LV preload was again similar within the two groups (see Table 89–1). Hence, LV compliance was reduced in patients receiving inotropic support of systemic oxygen transport compared with patients in whom inotropes were not used.

Reduced LV preload with RV dilation due to acute pulmonary hypertension may be the result of either the direct ventricular interaction described earlier resulting in reduced LV distensibility and a series interaction in which LV output falls because of reduced RV output in both steady-state and transient conditions, especially with the pericardium in place. It has been determined that this series interaction is responsible for approximately one half of the RV-LV interaction with an intact pericardium. After removal of the pericardium, the dependence on series interaction of the RV and LV rises to four fifths.

Other investigators have found conflicting results in this area[65] but have not considered the delay in RV input to LV input. Calvin and Ascah[66] have demonstrated a significant series interaction occurring in an open pericardial model of pulmonary hypertension. Furthermore, LV hypertrophy results in far less dependence on direct ventricular interaction but on a greater series interaction either with or without the pericardium in place.[67]

TABLE 89–1. Effect of Pulmonary Hypertension and the Administration of Inotropes on Left Ventricular Compliance Properties (Mean ± SD Values)

	Mean Blood Pressure (mm Hg)	PCWP (mm Hg)	LV End-Diastolic Volume (mL/m²)
Pulmonary hypertension			
Mean pulmonary artery pressure (mm Hg)			
Less than 20		5.0 ± 2*	87 ± 32
21–30		12.7 ± 4*	87 ± 31
Greater than 30		18.4 ± 4*	91 ± 27
Inotropes			
No inotropes	92 ± 15	12 ± 5	97 ± 31
Inotropes	78 ± 16†	15 ± 4†	96 ± 38

* $P < .05$, by analysis of variance between the three groups.
† $P < .05$, no inotropes vs. inotropes.
PCWP = pulmonary capillary wedge pressure; LV = left ventricular.

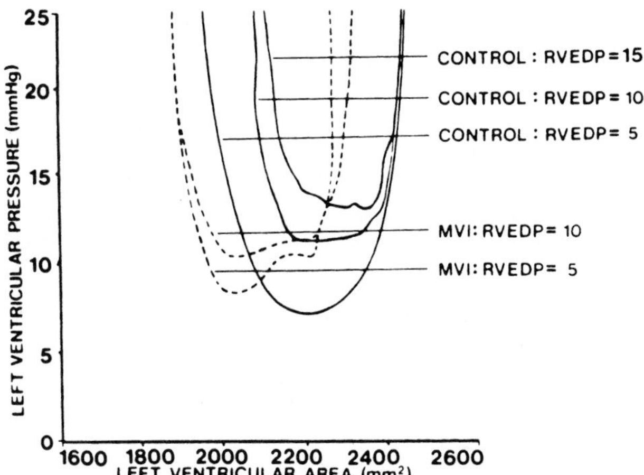

Figure 89–11. Effect of volume loading of the right ventricle on the left ventricular diastolic pressure-volume (measured as area in square millimeters) relationship during control and with pulmonary hypertension induced by microvascular lung injury. Volume loading shifts the pressure-area relationship upward during both control *(solid lines)* and microvascular injury *(dashed lines)*. RVEDP = right ventricular end-diastolic pressure. (From Calvin JE, Baer RW, Glantz SA: Pulmonary injury depresses cardiac systolic function through Starling mechanism. Am J Physiol 1986; 251:H722.)

The effects of RV pressure overload induced by glass bead embolization on the LV P-V relationship are diagrammatically illustrated in Figure 89–12.[61] This figure demonstrates an upward shift in the LV diastolic P-V relationship after the induction of acute pulmonary hypertension as well as a decrease in LV end-diastolic size. Stroke work is depressed because of the Frank-Starling relationship (Fig. 89–13).[58] Both direct and series interactions are likely present in this case. However, volume loading can restore LV preload to its baseline state. This observation suggests a dominance of the series interaction over the direct interaction in RV pressure overload.

The fall in preload-mediated LV stroke output that accompanies right heart failure[68] and acute RV overload[69] reduces cardiac output and oxygen transport. Because blood pressure also eventually decreases, RV subendocardial ischemia[68] develops further, contributing to the failure of the RV and exacerbating all of the events just described.

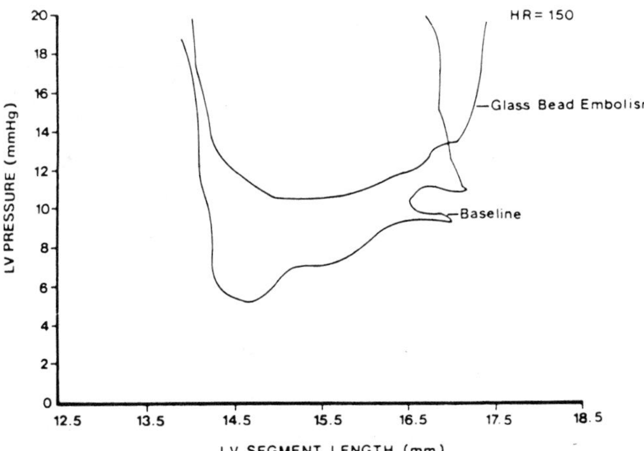

Figure 89–12. The left ventricular (LV) diastolic pressure–segment length relationship during acute pulmonary hypertension at similar preloads and heart rate (HR). Acute pulmonary hypertension shifts the relationship upward. (From Calvin JE Jr, Langlois S, Garneys G: Ventricular interaction in a canine model of acute pulmonary hypertension and its modulation by vasoactive drugs. J Crit Care 1988; 3:43.)

Patients with lung disease may, by a different mechanism than RV-LV interaction, experience a rise in the LV end-diastolic P-V relationship. Gomez and colleagues[70] have described global LV hypertrophic changes occurring as a result of chronic pulmonary hypertension secondary to experimentally induced chronic obstructive pulmonary disease (COPD) in dogs. Previous investigators have also noted LV hypertrophy associated with RV pressure afterload secondary to pulmonary artery banding. It is postulated that sustained stress of the RV may lead to LV hypertrophy if the RV and LV myocardium act as a single structure. Alternatively, substance released by the RV as it hypertrophies may induce LV hypertrophy. Other investigators have postulated that increased RV wall tension, when sustained, results in LV hypertrophy.

The practical clinical significance of these two examples of ventricular interaction may then be summarized as follows: If the PCWP is used to define LV preload, volume resuscitation to support preload-dependent ventricular stroke output might be limited in patients with severe pulmonary hypertension or those receiving inotropes before a normal LV preload is attained. That is, a normal LV preload in patients with severe pulmonary hypertension or in those concurrently receiving inotropic agents is likely reflected by a substantially higher PCWP than is found in those without these considerations. A depression in LV compliance that is observed with pulmonary hypertension or the use of the inotropic agents evokes a substantial increase in the hydrostatic pressure (i.e., PCWP) responsible for determining fluid flux across the pulmonary microvascular membrane at a constant LV preload. Therefore, the critical hydrostatic pressure within the pulmonary microvasculature, which if exceeded results in abnormal accumulation of extravascular lung water (i.e., pulmonary edema), is at

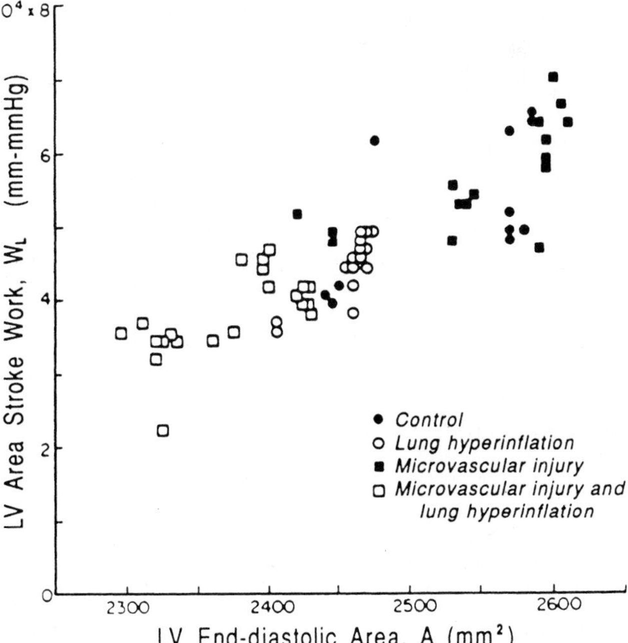

Figure 89–13. Relationship of left ventricular (LV) area stroke work to LV end-diastolic area in an experimental model of dog. The acute pulmonary hypertension produced by a glass microvascular injury relationship is linear. Neither microvascular injury nor lung hyperinflation changed LV performance beyond the effect associated with the changes in end-diastolic LV size. (From Calvin JE, Baer RW, Glantz SA: Pulmonary injury depresses cardiac systolic function through Starling mechanism. Am J Physiol 1986; 251:H722.)

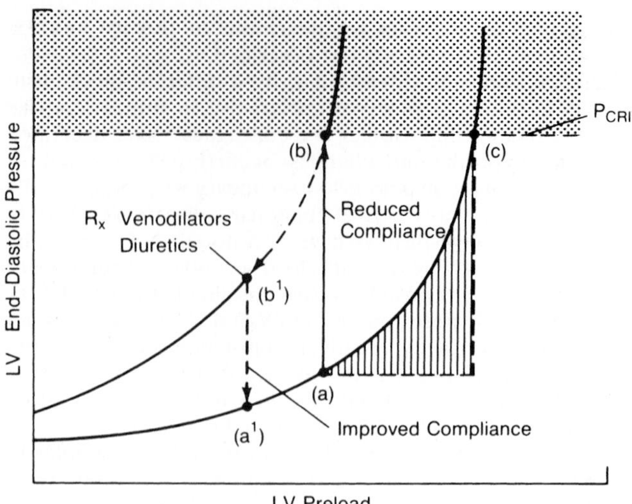

Figure 89–14. Left ventricular (LV) end-diastolic pressure-volume relationships. The critical hydrostatic pressure (P_{CRIT}) in the pulmonary microvascular membrane is exceeded at a lower preload when LV compliance is reduced by inotropes or by pulmonary hypertension. Treatment (Rx) aimed at reducing pulmonary capillary hydrostatic pressure usually improves LV compliance.

a lower LV preload (hence, a lower preload-mediated stroke output) both in patients receiving inotropes and in those with pulmonary hypertension (Fig. 89-14, point b versus c).

Interactions between the LV and both the RV and PA are also extremely important in explaining the hemodynamics of low cardiac output states complicating RV wall infarction. Previous researchers have characterized the decrease in LV distensibility with RV ischemia and infarction.[71] Calvin[60] has demonstrated that upward shifts in the LV diastolic P-V relationships and decreased LV filling observed during RV infarction are related to both RV and PA interaction with the LV (Fig. 89-15).

Effect of Positive End-Expiratory Pressure on the Left Ventricular End-Diastolic Pressure-Volume Relationship

A reduction in LV compliance has been observed with the institution of positive end-expiratory pressure (PEEP), further

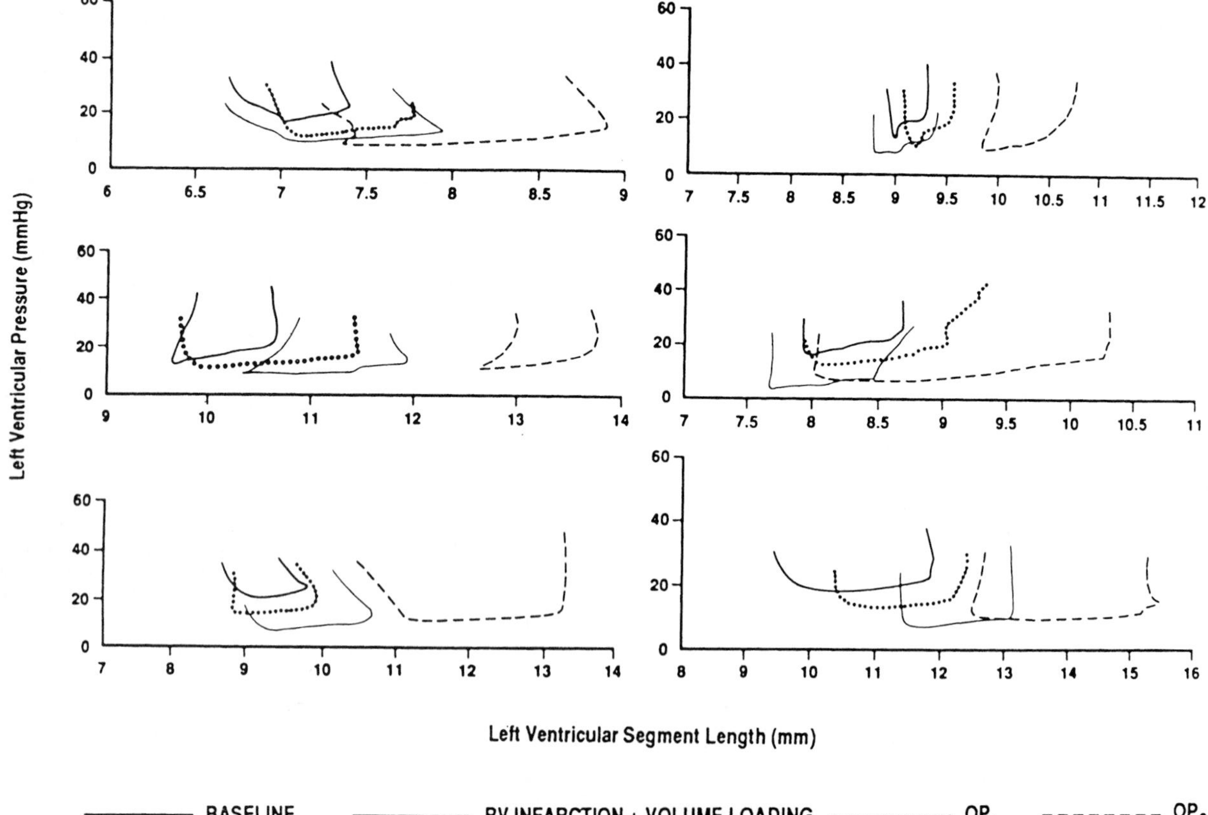

Figure 89–15. Plots of left ventricular (LV) diastolic pressure-segment length relations in an experimental model of right ventricular (RV) infarction. Volume loading after RV infarction shifted the relation further upward in all experiments. Partial opening of the pericardium (OP_1) shifted it downward, and complete opening of the pericardium (OP_2) returned it to baseline levels of pressure (although lengths increased). (From Calvin JE: Optimal right ventricular filling pressures and the role of pericardial constraint in right ventricular infarction in dogs. Circulation 1991; 84:852.)

depressing ventricular preload beyond the decrease produced by the reduction in venous return. Jardin and associates[72] suggested that the cause of a depression in LV compliance with the use of PEEP was a leftward septal shift consequent to RV pressure overload (i.e., the concept of direct ventricular interaction due to a PEEP afterloading effect on the right ventricle, resulting in increased right-sided volume).

Others[58] have, however, concluded that PEEP alters LV distensibility by increasing intrapericardial pressures through the external force it applies to the surface of the heart (Fig. 89–16). In one study, Calvin and colleagues[58] simulated PEEP by hyperinflation of the lung in an open-chest animal model. Although such a model would be expected to underestimate the PEEP effects, end-expiratory airway pressures of 15 mm Hg were maintained. A reduction in both RV and LV size resulted with this amount of positive airway pressure, primarily through a reduction in both RV and LV septal to free wall dimensions. Despite the reduction in ventricular size, intracavitary pressures were unchanged from control. This observation defined that a primary effect of lung hyperinflation was to reduce ventricular compliance by the lungs physically compressing both ventricles from the outside; there was no evidence that the RV dilated under the effects of the increased RV afterload. Hence, RV dilation could not be responsible for a leftward septal shift.

It has been also been noted that PEEP restricted outward expansion of the LV lateral wall during diastole; the position of the septum was not displaced by PEEP. It would therefore appear that PEEP is capable of causing a leftward shift in LV PV relationships (i.e., reduced compliance) by altering biventricular geometry because of direct compressive forces exerted on the heart surface with its use.

Clinical Measurement of Diastolic Abnormalities

The rate of relaxation is described by the time constant of relaxation, which is exponentially related to the fall in LV

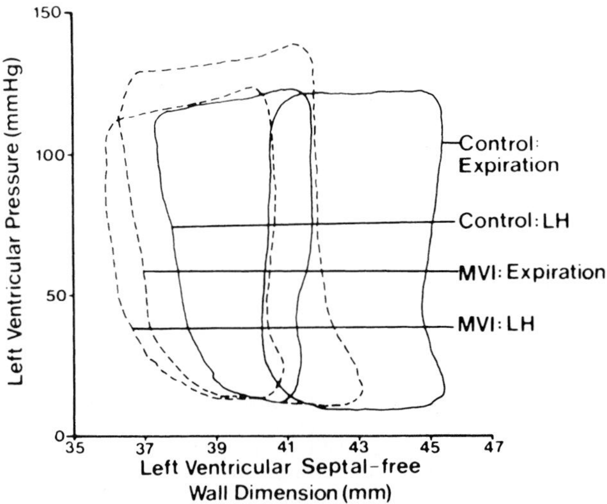

Figure 89–16. The ventricular septal free-wall pressure-dimension relationship during lung hyperinflation. End-expiratory loops during both a control period and a microvascular injury (MVI) are compared with loops taken during a lung hyperinflation, which is equivalent to an end-expiratory pressure of 15 mm Hg. Note the leftward shift of the end-diastolic points, which confirms a reduction in end-diastolic size or volume. However, this shift occurs with very little decrease in end-diastolic pressure, which suggests that the lungs exerted an external force on the heart. (From Calvin JE, Baer RW, Glantz SA: Pulmonary injury depresses cardiac systolic function through Starling mechanism. Am J Physiol 1986; 251:H722.)

pressure over time and can be measured by invasive experimental and clinical systems.[50] The time of isovolumic pressure decrease, beginning with the end of mechanical systole and lasting through mitral valve opening, is used to calculate the time constant of relaxation. The required cumbersome equations cannot be easily applied at the bedside but can be used to measure relaxation rates during coronary arteriography.[73]

Doppler filling velocity patterns provide an excellent noninvasive measurement of changes in the rate and extent of relaxation,[74] provided certain caveats are kept in mind. Alterations in chamber stiffness (e.g., a decrease in compliance seen in various disease states) without alteration in relaxation rate result in changes in the pattern of Doppler filling time-velocity integrals, which have gained wide acceptance as indicators of diastolic compliance abnormalities. These changes are characterized by a decreased velocity of rapid filling (E wave) and augmented atrial contribution to filling (A wave) as the atrium contracts into a noncompliant ventricular chamber (Fig. 89–17, top panel).

This pattern has been noted in concentric LV hypertrophy,[75] in hypertrophic cardiomyopathy,[76] and with acute ischemia during angioplasty[77] as well as in normal patients with increasing age and heart rate and with inspiration.[77]

These disease states result in abnormalities in the Doppler filling pattern that characterize both the extent and rate of relaxation. The foregoing description represents the complex interaction of both early and late diastolic relaxation abnormalities, with early diastolic abnormalities predominating.[78] In patients with unimpaired rates of relaxation and primary alterations in ventricular compliance, late diastolic filling, a reflection of the extent of relaxation, is primarily affected. The result is a decrease in atrial filling velocities, represented by a diminution in the A wave, which was seen in a subgroup of patients with coronary artery disease studied by Stoddard and coworkers (see Fig. 89–17).[78] Conversely, alteration in the rate of relaxation (an early diastolic phenomenon) while chamber stiffness does not vary results in a diminution of the early filling of the ventricle and a larger atrial contribution (see Fig. 89–14). However, patients with elevated LA pressures secondary to significant mitral regurgitation exhibit maintained or exaggerated peak filling velocities, a manifestation of the increased driving force of the elevated LA pressure to ventricular early diastolic filling.[79] Even in patients with hypertrophic cardiomyopathy, this is not a reflection of impairment to late diastolic filling atrial contraction, as might first be surmised (Fig. 89–18). Therefore, one should make assumptions based on Doppler-derived ventricular filling patterns in light of the overall hemodynamic picture, taking into account atrial pressure, valvular lesions, and age-adjusted normal values.

Nishimura and colleagues[79] reported their experience with noninvasive determination of measuring continuous-wave Doppler velocities of mitral regurgitation. Correlation between measured invasively and LV pressure curves derived from Doppler velocity curves through application of a modification of the Bernoulli equation was obtained. This, however, required knowledge of the LV EDP, an invasively derived variable. A calculation approximation could be made with the addition of 20 mm Hg to the Doppler-derived atrioventricular pressure gradient, but according to the researchers, it is less accurate but acceptable.

SUMMARY

This chapter has presented a comprehensive review of current concepts put forth by many talented investigators in the field of ventricular performance. An understanding of the basic tenets of their detailed studies should allow a more rational treatment plan to be devised for the critically ill

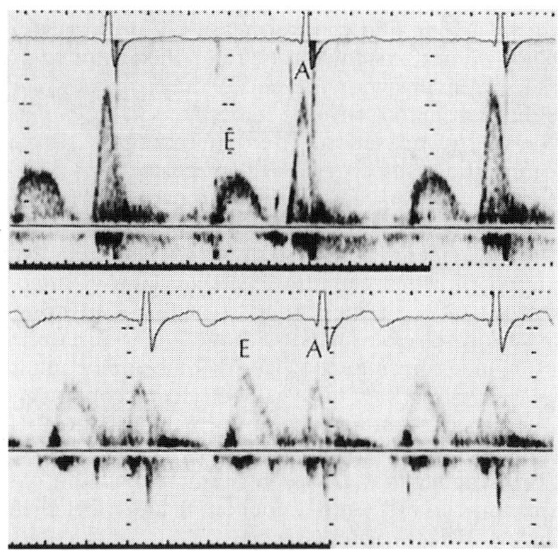

Figure 89–17. Pulsed Doppler mitral inflow velocities illustrating a diminished early filling velocity (E) and augmentation of atrial filling velocities (A) *(top panel)* compared with normal mitral inflow velocity patterns *(bottom panel)*.

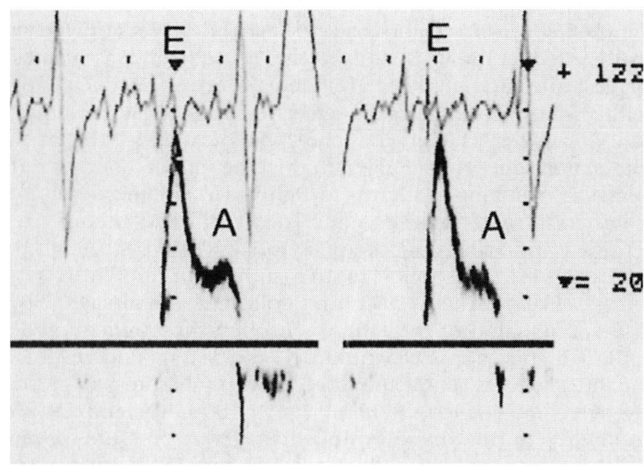

Figure 89–18. Pulsed Doppler mitral flow velocities demonstrating augmented early filling velocities (E) with blunted atrial filling patterns (A) that are characteristic of alterations in relaxation extent.

patient. Although many of the subjects addressed cannot be directly measured or observed, their complex interaction in the production of such measured variables as heart rate, blood pressure, SV, systemic vascular resistance, pulmonary vascular resistance, cardiac output, and PCWP can be better inferred if a good grasp of the material is achieved.

As a continued source of clinical "head scratching," the PCWP and its relationship to stroke output deserve special attention. The PCWP itself is not always indicative of optimal ventricular filling. Both the LV and RV are characterized by inherent stiffness properties, which in turn may be altered by various diseases affecting the ventricles themselves. The pulmonary circulation that joins them as well as drugs and positive-pressure ventilation establishes the well-appreciated difficulty in assessment of ventricular preload by measuring end-diastolic filling pressure, such as the PCWP in the LV and the central venous pressure in the RV.

It is possible, however, to use information gained by following the trend in a measured PCWP or central venous pressure to make inferences with regard to ventricular compliance properties and to thereby appropriately define goal-directed therapy. When the goal of therapy is to match systemic oxygen with peripheral oxygen needs, the options to accomplish this are defined in the oxygen transport equation. To increase flow, fluid administration to enhance SV by augmenting preload is usually preferred if the PCWP is not so high that any further increase would risk a decrease in arterial oxygen content with the development or worsening of pulmonary edema. With a PCWP less than 10 to 12 mm Hg, a fluid challenge may be instituted; an increase in the PCWP of equal to or less than 5 mm Hg with a 250- to 500-mL fluid bolus implies that the LV is operating on the relatively flat portion of its diastolic P-V curve, and another fluid challenge may very well be attempted if further augmentation in SV is believed necessary to increase oxygen transport (Fig. 89–19). This process may be continued until the PCWP increases by an amount equal to or greater than 5 mm Hg, which implies that the LV is now operating on the relatively steep ascending portion of the P-V curve. At

FLUID CHALLENGE

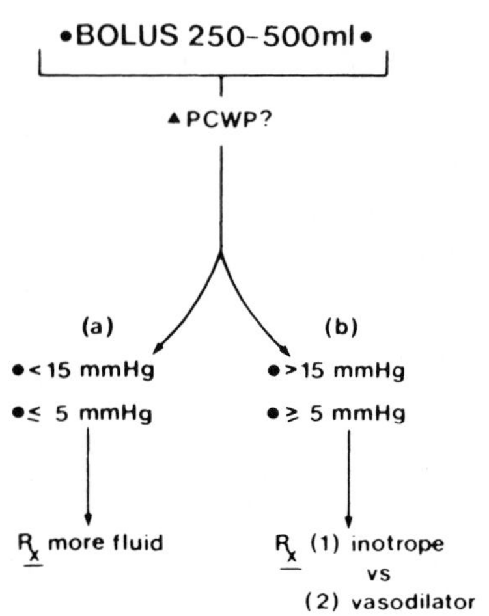

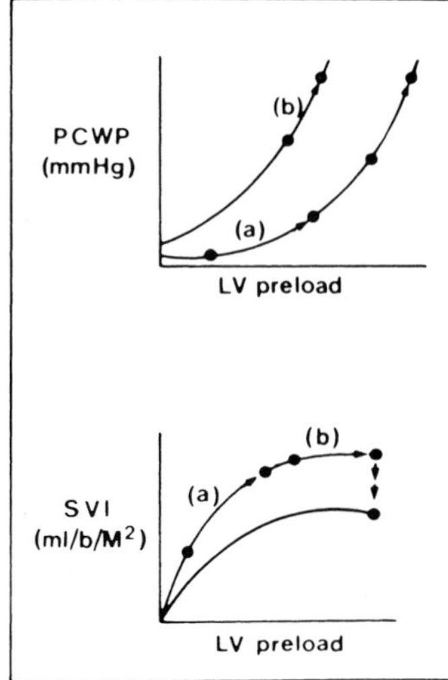

Figure 89–19. A clinical algorithm for volume loading in a critically ill patient. The absolute value of the pulmonary capillary wedge pressure (PCWP) and the magnitude of its change after a moderate volume load help dictate further therapy (see text). SVI = stroke volume index.

TABLE 89–2. Effect of Systemic Vasodilators in Cardiac Disease and Adult Respiratory Distress Syndrome

	Cardiac Disease		Adult Respiratory Distress Syndrome
	Phentolamine	***Nitroprusside***	***Nitroprusside***
Mean BP (mm Hg)	92 ± 14 → 82 ± 11†	92 ± 13 → 82 ± 14†	102 ± 16 → 84 ± 15†
Cardiac index	3.2 ± 0.8 → 3.7 ± 1.2†	3.7 ± 1.2 → 4.3 ± 1.3†	4.0 ± 1.1 → 4.1 ± 0.6
SV	38 ± 11 → 44 ± 10†	42 ± 15 → 47 ± 19†	38 ± 8 → 40 ± 5
PCWP	16 ± 6 → 11 ± 6†	17.5 ± 15 → 15 ± 4†	14 ± 5 → 14 ± 6
LV EDV	102 ± 39 → 124 ± 70	103 ± 40 → 110 ± 41	84 ± 29 → 78 ± 29

† $P > .05$ by Student's *t*-test.
SV = stroke volume; PCWP = pulmonary capillary wedge pressure; LV EDP = left ventricular end-diastolic pressure; BP = blood pressure.

this point, further fluid administration may simply increase the PCWP to approach the capillary hydrostatic pressure limit without any significant effect on preload mediated SV. If an increase in oxygen transport is still required, the choice is now restricted to using inotropic or vasodilating agents to augment SV. If blood pressure is sufficiently stable to allow cautions titration of a vasodilator, the effect of this therapy may be to increase SV primarily as well as to improve LV compliance. The latter effect, a decrease in PCWP at a constant or slightly reduced preload, may then allow further fluid administration and, hence, an even greater increase in preload-mediated SV.

Without stability of systemic pressures sufficient to allow confidence in administration of a vasodilator, inotropes are the final alternative when the need is to increase SV and, hence, oxygen transport. By increasing contractility, inotropes do increase SV but potentially at the expense of reducing LV compliance (Table 89–2).

With the development of invasive techniques to measure ventricular diastolic filling as volume versus pressure, these interrelationships may become more clear in the day-to-day bedside practice of medicine. A volume-detecting catheter with the ability to measure both EDV and end-systolic volume as well as PCWP is now being used clinically and may be helpful in evaluations of difficult hemodynamic situations. It has been found to be of greatest use in those patients with RV disorders that traditionally have presented difficult hemodynamic assessments.

Echocardiographic measures of cardiac output have been highly accurate when properly applied, but they are often difficult to perform in critically ill patients and do not allow frequent sampling. Gated nuclear imaging, especially in patients with RV disorders and sepsis, when combined with thermodilution cardiac output monitoring or with continuous cardiac output monitoring, has allowed us to quantitate the cause of many hemodynamic derangements that are not obvious with conventional methods.

Finally, noninvasive measurement of contractility, by characterization of the fractional velocity of shortening corrected for heart rate, has proved useful in treating critically ill patients. However, success again depends on technical factors in image acquisition and the need for reproducibility requiring skilled personnel and interpretation of these images.

References

1. Housmans PR, Lee NKM, Blinks JR: Active shortening retards the decline of the intracellular calcium transient in mammalian heart muscle. Science 1983; 221:159.
2. Brutsaert DL, Rademakers FE, Sys SU: Triple control of relaxation: Implications in cardiac disease. Circulation 1984; 69:190.
3. Kohmoto O, Spitzer KW, Movsesian MA, et al: Effects of intracellular acidosis on [Ca^{2+}]; transients, transsarcolemmal Ca^{2+} fluxes, and contraction in ventricular myocytes. Circ Res 1990; 66:622.
4. Lee HC, Smith N, Mohabir R, et al: Cytosolic calcium transients from the beating mammalian heart. Physiol Sci 1987; 94:7792.
5. Hicks MJ, Shigekawa M, Katz AM: Mechanism by which cyclic adenosine 3′:5′-monophosphate-dependent protein kinase stimulates calcium transport in cardiac sarcoplasmic reticulum. Circ Res 1979; 44:384.
6. Hoffman BF, Bindler E, Suckling EE: Postextrasystolic potentiation of contraction in cardiac muscle. Am J Physiol 1956; 185:95.
7. Ross J, Sonnenblick EH, Kaiser GA, et al: Electroaugmentation of ventricular performance and oxygen consumption by repetitive application of paired electrical stimuli. Circ Res 1965; 16:332.
8. Higgins CB, Vatner SF, Franklin D, et al: Extent of regulation of the heart's contractile site in the conscious dog by alteration in the frequency of contraction. J Clin Invest 1973; 53:1187.
9. Katz AM: Regulation of myocardial contractility 1958–1983: An odyssey. J Am Coll Cardiol 1983; 1:52.
10. Colluci WS, Wright RF, Braunwald E: New positive inotropic agents in the treatment of congestive heart failure: Part 2. N Engl J Med 1986; 314:349.
11. Braunwald E, Sommenblick EH, Ross J Jr: Mechanisms of cardiac contraction and relaxation in heart disease. *In:* Heart Disease: A Textbook of Cardiovascular Medicine, 4th ed. Braunwald E (Ed). Philadelphia, WB Saunders, 1992, p 351.
12. Beirholm EA, Grantham RN, O'Keefe DD, et al: Effects of acid-base changes, hypoxia and catecholamines on ventricular performance. Am J Physiol 1975; 228:1555.
13. Williamson JR, Schaffer SW, Ford C, et al: Contribution of tissue acidosis to ischemic injury in the perfused rat heart. Circulation 1976; 53:I-3.
14. Braunwald E: Mechanism of action of calcium-channel–blocking agents. N Engl J Med 1982; 307:1618.
15. Levine MJ, Harada K, Meuse AJ, et al: Excitation contraction upcoupling during ischemia in blood perfused dog heart. Biochem Biophys Res Comm 1991; 179:502.
16. Gilman AG: G proteins: Transducers of receptor-generated signals. Ann Rev Biochem 1987; 56:615.
17. Katz AM: Cyclic adenosine monophosphate effects on the myocardium: A man who blows hot and cold with one breath. J Am Coll Cardiol 1983; 2:143.
18. Homey CJ, Graham RM: Molecular characterization of adrenergic receptors. Circ Res 1985; 56:635.
19. Neer EJ, Clapham DE: Role of G protein subunits in transmembrane signalling. Nature 1988; 333:129.
20. Yatani A, Brown AM: Rapid β-adrenergic modulation of cardiac calcium channel currents by a fast G protein pathway. Science 1989; 245:71.
21. Mery PF, Lohmann SM, Walter U, et al: Ca^{2+} current is regulated by cyclic GMP-dependent protein kinase in mammalian cardiac myocytes. Proc Natl Acad Sci USA 1991; 88:1197.
22. Nawrath H: Cyclic AMP and cyclic GMP may play opposing roles in influencing force of contraction mammalian myocardium. Nature 1986; 262:509.
23. Ungerer M, Bohm M, Elce JS, et al: Altered expression of β adrenergic receptors in the failing human heart. Circulation 1993; 87:454.
24. Schranz D, Droege A, Broede A, et al: Uncoupling of human

cardiac β-adrenoreceptors during cardiopulmonary bypass with cardioplegic cardiac arrest. Circulation 1993; 87:422.
25. Kumar A, Kosuri R, Kandula P, et al: Tumor necrosis factor–induced myocardial cell depression is mediated by nitric oxide and cyclic GMP generation. Crit Care Med 1994; 22:A191.
26. Schneider F, Lutaun P, Hasselmann M, et al: Methylene blue increases systemic vascular resistance in human septic shock. Intensive Care Med 1992; 18:309.
27. Silverman HJ, Penaranda R, Orens JB, et al: Impaired β-adrenergic receptor stimulation of cyclic adenosine monophosphate in human septic shock: Association with myocardial hyporesponsiveness to catecholamines. Crit Care Med 1993; 21:31.
28. Yangisawa M, Kurihara H, Kimura S, et al: A novel potent vasoconstrictor peptide produced by vascular endothelial cells. Nature 1988; 332:411.
29. Kramer BK, Nishida M, Kelly RA, et al: Myocardial actions of a new class of cytokines. Circulation 1992; 85:350.
30. Kelly RA, Eid H, Kramer BK, et al: Endothelin enhances the contractile responsiveness of adult rat ventricular myocytes to calcium by a pertussive toxin–sensitive pathway. J Clin Invest 1990; 86:1164.
31. Kramer BK, Smith TW, Kelly RA: Endothelin and increased contractility in adult rat ventricular myocytes: Role of intracellular alkalosis induced by activation of the protein kinase C–dependent Na^+-H^+. Circ Res 1991; 68:260.
32. Limas CJ, Olivari M, Goldenberg IF, et al: Calcium uptake by cardiac sarcoplasmic reticulum in human dilated cardiomyoathy. Cardiovasc Res 1987; 21:601.
33. Mercadier J, Lompr A, Duc P, et al: Altered sarcoplasmic reticulum Ca^{2+}-ATPase gene expression in the human ventricle during end-stage heart failure. J Clin Invest 1990; 85:305.
34. Feldman MD, Copelas L, Gwathmey JK, et al: Deficient production of cyclic AMP: Pharmacologic evidence of an important cause of contractile dysfunction in patients with end-stage heart failure. Circulation 1987; 75:331.
35. Feldman AM, Ray PE, Silan CM, et al: Selective gene expression in failing human heart. Circulation 1991; 83:1866.
36. Bristow MR, Hershberger RE, Port JD, et al: β-Adrenergic pathways in nonfailing and failing human ventricular myocardium. Circulation 1990; 82:112.
37. Gordon AM, Huxley AF, Julian FJ: The variation in isometric tension with sarcomere length in vertebrate fibers. J Physiol 1966; 184:170.
38. Diamond G, Forrester JS: Effect of coronary artery disease and acute myocardial infarction on left ventricular compliance in man. Circulation 1992; 45:11.
39. Glanta SA, Parmley WW: Factors which affect the diastolic pressure-volume curve. Circ Res 1978; 43:171.
40. Calvin JE, Diredger AA, Sibbald WJ: Does the pulmonary capillary wedge pressure predict left ventricular preload in critically ill patients? Crit Care Med 1981; 9:437.
41. Regan DM: Calculation of left ventricular wall stress. Circ Res 1990; 67:245.
42. Lloyd TR, Donnerstein RL: Afterload dependence of echocardiographic left ventricular ejection force determination. Am J Cardiol 1991; 67:901.
43. Grossman W, Jones D, McLaurin LP: Wall stress and patterns of hypertrophy in the human left ventricle. J Clin Invest 1975; 56:56.
44. Yin FCP, Liu Z: Estimating arterial resistance and compliance during transient conditions in humans. Am J Physiol 1989; 257:H19.
45. Takoka H, Takeuchi M, Odake M, et al: Comparison of hemodynamic determinants for myocardial oxygen consumption under different contractile states in human ventricle. Circulation 1993; 87:59.
46. Chatterjee K, Parmley WW: The role of vasodilator therapy in heart failure. Prog Cardiovasc Dis 1977; 19:301.
47. Sagawa K: The end-systolic pressure-volume relation of the ventricle: Definition, modifications and clinical use. Circulation 1981; 3:1223.
48. Colan SD, Borow KM, Neumann A: Left ventricular end-systolic wall stress-velocity of fiber shortening relation: A load-independent index of myocardial contractility. J Am Coll Cardiol 1984; 4:715.
49. Gaasch WH, Levine HJ, Quinones MA, et al: Left ventricular compliance: Mechanisms and clinical implications. Am J Cardiol 1976; 38:645.
50. Gilbert JC, Glantz SA: Determinants of left ventricular filling and of the diastolic pressure-volume reaction. Circ Res 1989; 64:827.
51. Momomura S, Ingwall JS, Parker JA, et al: The relationship of high energy phosphates, tissue pH, and regional blood flow to diastolic distensibility in the ischemic dog myocardium. Circ Res 1985; 57:822.
52. Lorell BH, Grossman W: Cardiac hypertrophy: The consequences for diastole. J Am Coll Cardiol 1987; 9:1189.
53. Apstein CS, Grossman W: Opposite initial effects of supply and demand ischemia on left ventricular diastolic compliance: The ischemia-diastolic paradox. J Mol Cell Cardiol 1987; 19:119.
54. Ikenouchi H, Kohmoto O, McMillan M, et al: Contributions of $[Ca^{2+}]i$, [Pi] and pH to altered diastolic myocyte tone during partial metabolic inhibition. J Clin Invest 1991; 88:55.
55. Sasyama S, Nonogi H, Miyazaki S, et al: Changes in diastolic properties of the regional myocardium during pacing-induced ischemia in human subjects. J Am Coll Cardiol 1985; 5:599.
56. Stool EW, Mulins CB, Leshin SJ, et al: Dimensional changes of the left ventricle during acute pulmonary arterial hypertension in dogs. Am J Cardiol 1974; 33:868.
57. Glantz SA, Misback GA, Moores WY, et al: The pericardium substantially affects the left ventricular diastolic pressure-volume relationship in the dog. Circ Res 1978; 42:433.
58. Calvin JE, Baer RW, Glantz SA: Pulmonary injury depresses cardiac systolic function through Starling mechanism. Am J Physiol 1986; 251:H722.
59. Tyson GS, Maier GW, Olsen CO, et al: Pericardial influences on ventricular filling in the conscious dog. Circ Res 1984; 54:173.
60. Calvin JE: Optimal right ventricular filling pressures and the role of pericardial constraint in right ventricular infarction in dogs. Circulation 1991; 84:852.
61. Calvin JE Jr, Langlois S, Garneys G: Ventricular interaction in a canine model of acute pulmonary hypertension and its modulation by vasoconstrictive drugs. J Crit Care 1988; 3:42.
62. Ludbrook PA, Byrne JD, McKnight RC: Influence of right ventricular hemodynamics on left ventricular diastolic pressure-volume relations in man. Circulation 1979; 59:21.
63. Sibbald WJ, Driedger AA: Right ventricular function in acute disease states: Pathophysiologic considerations. Crit Care Med 1984; 11:339.
64. Raper R, Cunningham D, Sibbald W: The influence of CAD on diastolic biventricular function in sepsis. Clin Invest Med 1985; 8:A69.
65. Olson CO, Tyson GS, Maiter GW, et al: Dynamic ventricular interaction in the conscious dog. Circ Res 1983; 52:85.
66. Calvin JE, Ascah KJ: Impact of leftward septal shift and potential role of ischemia in its production during experimental right ventricular pressure overload. J Crit Care 1992; 7:106.
67. Slinker BK, Chagas ACP, Glantz SA: Chronic pressure overload hypertrophy decreases direct ventricular interaction. Am J Physiol 1987; 253:H347.
68. Calvin JE, Quinn B: Right ventricular pressure overload during acute lung injury: Cardiac mechanics and the pathophysiology of right ventricular systolic dysfunction. J Crit Care 1989; 4:251.
69. Calvin JE: Right ventricular afterload mismatch during acute pulmonary hypertension and its treatment with dobutamine: A pressure segment length analysis in a canine model. J Crit Care 1989; 4:239.
70. Gomez A, Unruh H, Mink SN: Altered left ventricular chamber stiffness and isovolumic relaxation in dogs with chronic pulmonary hypertension caused by emphysema. Circulation 1993; 87:247.
71. Goto Y, Yamoto J, Saito M, et al: Effects of right ventricular ischemia on left ventricular geometry and the end-diastolic pressure-volume relationship in the dog. Circulation 1985; 72:1104.
72. Jardin F, Farcot J, Boisante L, et al: Influence of positive end-expiratory pressure on left ventricular performance. N Engl J Med 1981; 304:387.
73. Kass DA, Midei M, Brinker J, et al: Influence of coronary occlusion during PTCA on end-systolic and end-diastolic and pressure-volume relations in humans. Circulation 1990; 81:447.
74. Rokey R, Kuc LC, Zoghbi WA, et al: Determination of parameters of left ventricular diastolic filling with pulsed Doppler echocardi-

ography: Comparison with cineangiography. Circulation 1985; 71:543.
75. Pearson AC, Labovitz AJ, Mrosek D, et al: Assessment of diastolic function in normal and hypertrophied hearts: Comparison of Doppler echocardiography and M-mode echocardiography. Am Heart J 1987; 113:1417.
76. Maron BJ, Spirito P, Green KJ, et al: Noninvasive assessment of left ventricular diastolic function by pulsed Doppler echocardiography in patients with hypertrophic cardiomyopathy. J Am Coll Cardiol 1987; 10:733.
77. Labovita AJ, Lewen MK, Kern M, et al: Evaluation of left ventricular systolic and diastolic dysfunctioning during transient myocardial ischemia produced by angioplasty. J Am Coll Cardiol 1987; 10:748.
78. Stoddard MF, Pearson AC, Kern MJ, et al: Left ventricular diastolic function: Comparison of pulsed Doppler echocardiographic and hemodynamic indexes in subjects with and without coronary artery disease. J Am Coll Cardiol 1989; 13:327.
79. Nishimura RA, Schwartz RS, Tajik AJ, et al: Noninvasive measurement of rate of left ventricular relaxation by Doppler echocardiography: Validation with simultaneous cardiac catheterization. Circulation 1993; 88:146.

90

The Coronary Arteries in Unstable Angina Pectoris, Acute Myocardial Infarction, and Sudden Coronary Death

William C. Roberts, MD

This chapter reviews and compares coronary arterial findings in patients with fatal unstable angina pectoris (UAP), acute myocardial infarction (AMI), and sudden coronary death (SCD).

AMOUNTS OF CORONARY ARTERIAL LUMINAL NARROWING IN THE THREE CORONARY SUBSETS

The amounts of coronary arterial narrowing observed at necropsy in patients with UAP, AMI, and SCD are generally enormous.[1] As shown in Table 90–1, from a necropsy study of 80 patients with these three coronary events (SCD in 31, AMI in 27, and UAP in 22), an average of 2.9 of the four major (right, left main, left anterior descending, and left circumflex) coronary arteries were severely (>75% decrease in cross-sectional area) narrowed at some points, and no significant differences were observed among the three coronary subsets.[1] The patients with UAP had a much higher frequency of severe narrowing of the left main coronary artery (10 of 22 patients [45%]) than did the AMI (3 of 27 patients [11%]) and SCD (3 of 31 patients [10%]) groups.

A more sophisticated approach to determining degrees of luminal narrowing is to examine the entire lengths of the four major epicardial coronary arteries. One technique involves incising each of the four major coronary arteries transversely at 5-mm intervals and then preparing a histologic section from each 5-mm segment. Normally, the total length of the four major arteries is about 27 cm (right, 10 cm; left main, 1 cm; left anterior descending, 10 cm; and left circumflex, 6 cm); thus, about 55 5-mm-long segments from each heart are available for examination.

Studies using this approach in the patients with UAP, AMI, and SCD are summarized in Table 90–2.[1] Of the 4016 5-mm segments studied in the 80 patients, 38% were narrowed 76% to 100% in cross-sectional area by plaque alone (controls, 3%); 34% were narrowed 51% to 75% (controls, 22%); 20% were narrowed 26% to 50% (controls, 44%); and only 7% were narrowed 25% or less (controls, 31%). Similar degrees of narrowing by plaque alone in all four categories of narrowing were observed in the groups with AMI and SCD; the patients with UAP had significantly more severe coronary narrowing than did the other two groups.

In general, therefore, patients with fatal UAP have more extensive severe narrowing by plaque alone of the four major epicardial coronary arteries than do patients with either AMI or SCD, and the patients with UAP, compared with the other two groups, have a significantly higher frequency of severe narrowing of the left main coronary artery.

COMPOSITION OF CORONARY ATHEROSCLEROTIC PLAQUES IN THE THREE CORONARY SUBSETS

Until the late 1980s,[2, 6] no detailed information was available concerning the composition of atherosclerotic plaques in the epicardial coronary arteries of patients with fatal coronary events. Kragel and associates,[2, 3] using a computerized morphometry system, traced the various components of atherosclerotic plaques in histologic sections prepared from 1438 5-mm segments of the four major epicardial coronary arteries in 37 patients with fatal coronary artery disease (UAP in 10, AMI in 15, and SCD in 12 patients). The results are summarized in Table 90–3. The dominant component of the coronary atherosclerotic plaques in all three subsets of patients was fibrous tissue, accounting for about 80% of the plaques in each subset; extracellular lipid (pultaceous debris) and calcium each made up about 5% of the plaques, and several miscellaneous components formed the remainder of the plaques. The cellular component of the fibrous tissue occu-

TABLE 90–1. Number of Major (Right, Left Main, Left Anterior Descending, and Left Circumflex) Coronary Arteries Narrowed More Than 75% in Cross-Sectional Area by Atherosclerotic Plaque in Fatal Coronary Artery Disease

Coronary Event	Patients (n)	Mean Age (Years)	Number of Four Arteries per Patient >75% Narrowed in Cross-Sectional Area by Plaque				
			4	*3*	*2*	*1*	*Mean*
Sudden coronary death	31	47	3	20	6	2	2.8
Acute myocardial infarction	27	59	3	14	10	0	2.7
Unstable angina pectoris	22	48	10	8	3	1	3.2
Totals	80	51	16 (20%)	42 (52%)	19 (24%)	3 (4%)	2.9
Controls	40	52	0 (0)	5 (5%)	12 (13%)	21 (23%)	0.7

TABLE 90–2. Amounts of Cross-Sectional Area Narrowing of Each 5-mm Segment of the Four Major (Right, Left Main, Left Anterior Descending, and Left Circumflex) Epicardial Coronary Arteries by Atherosclerotic Plaques in Subjects with Fatal Coronary Artery Disease

Subgroup	Patients (n)	Mean Age (Years)	Number of 5-mm Segments	Per Cent Segments Narrowed				
				0–25%	*25%–50%*	*51%–75%*	*76%–100%*	*Mean Score*
Sudden coronary death	31	47	1564	7%	23%	34%	36%	2.98
Acute myocardial infarction	27	59	1403	5%	23%	38%	34%	3.01
Unstable angina pectoris	22	48	1049	11%	12%	29%	48%	3.12
Totals	80	51	4016	7%	20%	34%	38%	3.02
Controls	40	52	1849	31%	44%	22%	3%	1.97

pied a larger portion of plaque in the patients with UAP and SCD, and the acellular (dense) component of fibrous tissue occupied a larger portion of the plaque in the AMI group. In all three subsets, the amount of dense fibrous tissue increased as plaque size increased (or as lumen size decreased) and the amount of cellular fibrous tissue decreased as plaque size increased.

FREQUENCY AND TYPES OF ACUTE LESIONS IN THE MAJOR CORONARY ARTERIES IN THE THREE CORONARY SUBSETS

Considerable effort has been directed toward understanding the acute coronary events that may be responsible for the development of UAP, AMI, and SCD. From angiographic, angioscopic, and necropsy studies, it has been speculated that plaque rupture and hemorrhage with overlying intraluminal thrombus, which are the acute lesions usually responsible for AMI, are also responsible for UAP and maybe SCD.

Kragel and associates[4] examined 3101 5-mm segments of 268 epicardial coronary arteries of 67 patients with fatal coronary events (UAP in 14, AMI in 31, and SCD in 21 patients). The results of these detailed studies are summarized in Table 90–4. The frequency of *intraluminal thrombus* was similar in the UAP and SCD groups (29% in each) and significantly lower than that in the AMI group (69%). The thrombus was nonocclusive in the patients with UAP and in five of six patients with SCD but was nonocclusive in only four of the 22 patients with AMI. The composition of the nonocclusive and occlusive thrombi also was different: The nonocclusive thrombus consisted mainly of platelets, and the occlusive thrombus mainly of fibrin. Of the 32 patients with thrombus, plaque rupture was found in association with the thrombus in 17 patients (53%): in none of the four patients with UAP, in two of the six patients with SCD, and in 15 (83%) of the 22 patients with AMI. In the 15 patients with thrombus unassociated with plaque rupture, hemorrhage into the plaque at the site of thrombus was found in seven: in three of the four patients with UAP, in two of the six patients with SCD, and in two of the 32 patients with AMI.

Plaque rupture was found in 33 (49%) of the 67 patients. Its frequency was insignificantly different in the groups with UAP (36% [5 of 14] and SCD (19% [4 of 21]): In both groups the frequency was significantly less than in the group with AMI (75% [24 of 32]).

Plaque hemorrhage was observed in 27 (40%) of the 67 patients, and its frequency was significantly lower in the groups with UAP (21% [3 of 14]) and SCD (19% [4 of 21]) than in the group with AMI (63% [20 of 32]). Plaque hemorrhage was associated with plaque rupture or intraluminal thrombus in 20 (74%) of the 27 patients with plaque hemorrhage: in four of the 14 patients with unstable angina, in four of 21 with sudden death, and in 13 of the 32 with acute infarction.

Multiple small vascular channels were present in 60 (90%) of the 67 patients and with an insignificantly different frequency in each of the three patient groups (see Table 90–1). The frequency of multiluminal channels in each 5-mm-long segment of coronary artery was significantly higher in the group with UAP (12% [66 of 572]) than in either the SCD (7% [72 of 999]) or AMI groups (7% [107 of 1530]).

Thus, comparison of findings from examination of a histologic section from each of 3101 5-mm segments of 268 major epicardial coronary arteries from 67 patients with fatal coronary artery disease disclosed that the frequency of three acute coronary lesions (intraluminal thrombus, plaque rupture, and plaque hemorrhage) was similar in patients with UAP and SCD and that the frequency of each of these acute lesions was significantly higher in patients with a fatal first transmural AMI. Furthermore, although multiluminal channels (not acute lesions) within plaques were frequent in all three patient groups, these lesions were found significantly more often in 5-mm segments of coronary arteries in the group with UAP than in the groups with SCD and AMI, where their frequency was similar.

Several angiographic studies[5-9] have identified either intraluminal filling defects consistent with thrombus or specific morphologic lesions (eccentric narrowings with irregular borders) in patients with UAP, and these defects have been used to distinguish such patients from those with stable angina.

TABLE 90–3. Mean Composition of Coronary Arterial Atherosclerotic Plaques in the Four Major Epicardial Coronary Arteries

Components of Plaque	Mean Per Cent of Plaque Containing Various Components in the Four Major Coronary Arteries (1438 Segments)		
	Unstable Angina Pectoris (n = 10)	*Acute Myocardial Infarction (n = 15)*	*Sudden Coronary Death (n = 12)*
Dense fibrous tissue	35	46	29
Loose fibrous tissue	1	3	3
Cellular fibrous tissue	52	32	50
Calcium	4	4	8
Pultaceous debris	4	8	4
Foam cells	0	1	0
Foam cells and lymphocytes	3	4	6
Inflammatory infiltrates without significant numbers of foam cells	1	2	1

TABLE 90–4. Frequency of Acute Coronary Lesions and Multiluminal Channels at Necropsy in Patients with Unstable Angina Pectoris, Sudden Coronary Death, and Acute Myocardial Infarction

Coronary Subset	No. of Patients	Coronary Arteries			
		Thrombus	*Plaque Rupture*	*Plaque Hemorrhage*	*Multiluminal Channels*
Unstable angina pectoris	14	4 (29%)*	5 (36%)*	3 (21%)*	14 (100%)
Sudden coronary death	21	6 (29%)*	4 (19%)*	4 (19%)*	17 (81%)
Acute myocardial infarction	32	22 (69%)†	24 (75%)†	20 (63%)†	29 (90%)
Totals	67	32 (48%)	33 (49%)	27 (40%)	60 (90%)

Statistical significance of acute coronary lesions (*) in unstable angina and sudden coronary death versus those lesions (†) found in acute myocardial infarction.

Comparison of postmortem angiographic and histologic findings[10] in patients with coronary artery disease (not necessarily UAP), however, has shown that these irregular eccentric lesions may represent not only sites of intraluminal thrombus but also plaque rupture, plaque hemorrhage, or organized thrombus. In addition, three angioscopic studies[11-13] have identified intraluminal thrombus and ulceration or rupture of plaque in patients with UAP. On the basis of these studies, it has been widely speculated that the lesion responsible for the development of UAP is an ulcerated plaque over which nonocclusive intraluminal thrombus develops.

Before accepting that this hypothesis is indeed true for all or most patients with UAP, we must consider the limitations of the previous studies.[5-13] Interpretation of the significance of the eccentric irregular lesions seen angiographically in patients with UAP is based largely on the work of Levin and Fallon,[10] who compared postmortem coronary arteriograms and histologic sections of coronary artery narrowings in 39 patients who died either after coronary artery bypass surgery or of consequences of AMI. (Because the trauma of bypass surgery may be associated with plaque rupture or plaque hemorrhage or both, patients who had undergone this procedure were excluded from the study by Kragel and colleagues.[4]

Levin and Fallon identified 38 narrowings that had irregular borders or intraluminal lucencies on angiography. Of these, 8 (21%) were acute or organizing nonocclusive thrombi overlying atherosclerotic plaque, six (16%) were nonocclusive thrombi overlying sites of plaque rupture or hemorrhage, 10 (26%) were sites of plaque hemorrhage or rupture without thrombus, six (16%) contained recanalized thrombus (presumably multiluminal channels), and 21% showed narrowing of the segment by plaque without any complicating acute lesion. More than a third of the irregular eccentric lesions studied, therefore, showed no acute lesion that would account for the abrupt change in symptoms in the setting of UAP. In the study by Kragel and coworkers, plaques containing multiluminal channels, although common to all three groups of patients, were most frequent in the group with UAP.

When interpreting reports of angiographic or angioscopic studies in patients with UAP, one presumes that the patients did not have left ventricular necrosis (AMI) at the time of study, an assumption that may or may not be true. Guthrie and associates[14] studied 12 patients with UAP who died shortly after coronary artery bypass surgery. At autopsy, four of the 12 patients had AMI that histologically appeared to have occurred before the operation, and AMI was not suspected clinically in any of the four patients. Therefore, in studies of living patients, it may be difficult to determine whether the patients have pure UAP or have combined UAP and AMI.

Information about coronary artery morphology in patients with UAP is scant and difficult to interpret for several reasons. UAP is rarely fatal, and those patients who do die during the period of UAP usually have undergone a coronary angioplasty or bypass procedure or have experienced an AMI shortly before death. In patients with AMI preceded by UAP, intracoronary lesions may not be representative of those occurring in patients with UAP not complicated by AMI.

Information about the acute coronary lesions in patients who died shortly after coronary artery bypass surgery has been provided in several studies. Guthrie and colleagues[14] described 12 patients and Roberts and Virmani[15] described 19 patients with UAP who died shortly after coronary bypass surgery. In both studies, the frequency of intraluminal thrombus was low (8% and 12%, respectively) when patients with AMI were excluded. In a separate report, Virmani and Roberts[16] described the frequency of extravasated erythrocytes and fibrin in the plaque of 17 of the 22 patients with UAP. Plaque hemorrhage (erythrocytes with or without fibrin) was identified in 94% of their patients. It is likely that surgical manipulation of the epicardial coronary arteries was responsible for the plaque hemorrhage in many of these cases.

In a study of UAP with fatal outcome, Falk[17] provided information about the frequency of acute lesions in the epicardial coronary arteries of patients with SCD, UAP, and AMI. He described necropsy findings in "25 patients, all of whom died of acute coronary thrombosis within 24 hours after the onset of acute symptoms." Of the 24 patients for whom clinical information was available, 15 clearly had UAP, two had an equivocal history of UAP, and seven did not have UAP. Of these 25 patients, 15 had coagulative necrosis (AMI) that, as determined histologically, was compatible with an age of less than 24 hours. In these patients, he described lamellar thrombi (21 of 25 patients, including 14 of 15 with UAP), 81% of which were associated with plaque rupture and hemorrhage. Neither the frequency of plaque rupture nor the number of thrombotic episodes differed between the patients with and without UAP. Because all of these patients died suddenly (some with UAP and some with UAP complicated by AMI), the three ischemic syndromes cannot be analyzed individually.

Davies and associates[18] studied 90 patients who died suddenly outside the hospital within 6 hours of the onset of pain "or other symptoms." The data were presented in a report entitled "Intramyocardial platelet aggregation in patients with unstable angina suffering sudden ischemic cardiac death." Of their 90 patients, 36 (40%) had chest or arm pain at some time in the 2 weeks preceding death. The history of chest pain was obtained by a coroner's police officer from the next of kin who had been living with the patient. Thus, the history was not obtained from the patient or a physician. None of the 90 patients had been admitted to a hospital with increasing chest pain. No information about the presence or absence of chest pain at rest was available for any patient. Thus, in none of the 90 patients was the type, location, or severity of the pain known. Nevertheless, these patients were considered to have had UAP. Necropsy in the 90 patients disclosed the following: 31 (30%) had nonocclusive intracoronary thrombus, 22 (24%) had SCD associated with "regional coagulative necrosis" (AMI), and 23 (25%) had nontransmural necrosis. Of the

36 patients with chest or arm pain at some time in the 2 weeks before death, 35 had plaque rupture identified in one of the major epicardial coronary arteries. Of the 54 without chest pain in the 2 weeks before death, 51 had plaque rupture.

Thus, it remains unknown whether the patients in that study had UAP. Some probably did have UAP, but some clearly had AMI, and most would fulfill most investigators' definition of SCD. Diagnosis of UAP in persons not admitted to the hospital and with a history obtained by a nonphysician is difficult, to say the least.

Multiluminal vascular channels were present in 90% of the 67 patients studied by Kragel and colleagues.[4] These channels most likely represented organized thrombus (the consequence of a previous nonfatal thrombotic event) and were usually at a site where the lumen was severely narrowed by plaque. Multiluminal channels were observed in a significantly higher percentage of the 5-mm coronary segments in the patients with UAP than in those with either SCD or AMI.

The lower frequency of plaque rupture and occlusive thrombus in the groups with UAP and SCD than in the group with AMI may be a reflection of differences in plaque composition between these groups. Likewise, the similarity in the frequency of these acute coronary lesions in patients with UAP and SCD may reflect the similarity in plaque composition in these two groups. As described earlier, in all three types of patients, the mean percentage of dense fibrous tissue, calcific deposits, and pultaceous debris increases with increasing degrees of luminal narrowing and the mean percentage of cellular fibrous tissue decreases. Severely narrowed segments in the AMI group (those narrowed more than 75% in cross-sectional area) contained significantly more pultaceous debris and significantly less calcium and cellular fibrous tissue than did similarly narrowed segments in the UAP and SCD groups. Because occlusive thrombus is almost exclusively found in association with rupture of a lipid-rich plaque, the greater the amount of pultaceous debris, the greater is the frequency of plaque rupture and occlusive thrombus.

The characteristic lesion in patients with a fatal first AMI, then, is an occlusive thrombus overlying a ruptured plaque rich in pultaceous debris; in patients with UAP, it is a severely narrowed segment frequently containing multiluminal channels with or without a small nonocclusive thrombus; in patients with SCD without left ventricular necrosis, it is a segment of coronary artery with significant luminal narrowing by atherosclerotic plaque with or without platelet-rich nonocclusive thrombus. Thus, the frequency of acute coronary lesions (intraluminal thrombus, plaque rupture, and plaque hemorrhage) in patients with UAP (not complicated by AMI) and SCD (not complicated by AMI) is similar, and the frequency of these lesions is significantly lower than that observed in patients with AMI.

References

1. Roberts WC: Qualitative and quantitative comparison of amounts of narrowing by atherosclerotic plaques in the major epicardial coronary arteries at necropsy in sudden death, transmural acute myocardial infarction, transmural healed myocardial infarction and unstable angina pectoris. Am J Cardiol 1989; 64:324–328.
2. Kragel AH, Reddy SG, Wittes JT, et al: Morphometric analysis of the composition of atherosclerotic plaques in the four major epicardial coronary arteries in acute myocardial infarction and in sudden coronary death. Circulation 1989;80:1747–1756.
3. Kragel AH, Reddy SG, Wittes JT, et al: Morphometric analysis of the composition of coronary arterial plaques in isolated unstable angina pectoris with pain at rest. Am J Cardiol 1990; 66:562–567.
4. Kragel AH, Gertz SD, Roberts WC, et al: Morphologic comparison of frequency and types of acute lesions in the major epicardial coronary arteries in unstable angina pectoris, sudden coronary death and acute myocardial infarction. J Am Coll Cardiol 1991;18:801–808.
5. Cowley JM, DiSciasco G, Rehr RB, et al: Angiographic observations and clinical relevance of coronary thrombus in unstable angina pectoris. Am J Cardiol 1989; 63:108E–113E.
6. Gotoh K, Minamino T, Katoh O, et al: The role of intracoronary thrombus in unstable angina: Angiographic assessment and thrombolytic therapy during ongoing anginal attacks. Circulation 1988;77:526–534.
7. Ambrose JA, Winters SL, Stern A, et al: Angiographic morphology and the pathogenesis of unstable angina pectoris. J Am Coll Cardiol 1985;5:609–616.
8. Vetrovec GW, Leinbach RC, Gold HK, et al: Intracoronary thrombolysis in syndromes of unstable ischemia: Angiographic and clinical results. Am Heart J 1982;104:946–952.
9. Holmes DR, Hartzler GO, Smith HC, et al: Coronary artery thrombosis in patients with unstable angina. Br Heart J 1981;45:411–416.
10. Levin DC, Fallon JT: Significance of the angiographic morphology of localized coronary stenoses: Histopathologic correlations. Circulation 1982;66:316–320.
11. Hombach V, Hoher M, Kochs M, et al: Pathophysiology of unstable angina pectoris: Correlations with angioscopic imaging. Eur Heart J 1988;9 (Suppl N):40–45.
12. Forrester JS, Litvack F, Grundfest W: A perspective of coronary disease seen through the arteries of living man. Circulation 1987;75:505–513.
13. Sherman CT, Litvack F, Grundfest W, et al: Coronary angioscopy in patients with unstable angina pectoris. N Engl J Med 1986;315:913–919.
14. Guthrie RB, Vlodaver Z, Nicoloff DM, et al: Pathology of stable and unstable angina pectoris. Circulation 1975;51:1059–1063.
15. Roberts WC, Virmani R: Quantification of coronary arterial narrowing in clinically-isolated unstable angina pectoris: An analysis of 22 necropsy patients. Am J Med 1979;67:792–799.
16. Virmani R, Roberts WC: Extravasated erythrocytes, iron, and fibrin in atherosclerotic plaques in coronary arteries in fatal coronary heart disease and their relation to intraluminal thrombus: frequency and significance in 57 necropsy patients and in 2958 five-mm segments of 224 major epicardial coronary arteries. Am Heart J 1983;105:788–797.
17. Falk E: Unstable angina with fatal outcome: Dynamic coronary thrombosis leading to infarction and/or sudden death. Circulation 1985;71:699–708.
18. Davies MJ, Thomas AC, Knapman PA, et al: Intramyocardial platelet aggregation in patients with unstable angina suffering sudden ischemic cardiac death. Circulation 1986;73:418–427.

91

Treatment of Myocardial Infarction

Thomas Killip, MD

ETIOLOGY AND PATHOLOGY

In the overwhelming majority of cases, myocardial infarction (MI) is caused by coronary artery disease secondary to coronary atherosclerosis. Other causes occurring in less than 5% of cases are coronary spasm induced by drugs (especially cocaine) or of unknown cause; coronary embolization, as in the presence of aortic valve disease or bacterial endocarditis; and paradoxical embolization in the presence of a patent foramen ovale. In rare instances, massive blunt trauma to the chest may sever the left anterior descending coronary artery, inducing acute symptoms. Myocardial infarction also occurs uncommonly in certain congenital heart diseases, such as anomalous origin of a coronary artery from the pulmonary artery.

The clinical consequences of coronary artery disease are depicted in Figure 91–1. If the extent of intimal swelling due to atheroma is modest (generally less than 50% reduction of the internal diameter of the blood vessel) so that coronary blood flow is unimpeded, remaining normal at rest and during exertion, ischemia is unlikely and symptoms are absent. When coronary blood flow to one or more myocardial regions is significantly reduced, at rest or during exercise, below the threshold required for adequate oxygenation or nutrition (a reduction in the internal diameter of the culprit vessel of 50% to 70% or more), ischemic syndromes generally accompanied by characteristic chest discomfort develop. Four ischemic syndromes are recognized clinically (see Fig. 91–1). Although they are classified as distinct entities, it may be difficult to identify the ischemic syndrome in a particular patient when first seen, because the syndromes may merge. MI is the major threat in the unstable patient, for example, and the clinical situation may rapidly change.

Many patients with angina remain stable, having relatively few episodes characteristically reproduced by a similar level of exertion, for many months or years. In other patients, however, the angina becomes more severe, often with a crescendo character, or occurs at rest, requiring more frequent nitroglycerin therapy. Occurrence of angina at rest suggests ischemia despite the reduced cardiac demand and generally demands urgent medical attention. Whether patients have unstable angina, non–Q-wave myocardial infarction, or Q-wave myocardial infarction is generally determined initially from an analysis of the history and the electrocardiogram (ECG) obtained during initial evaluation.

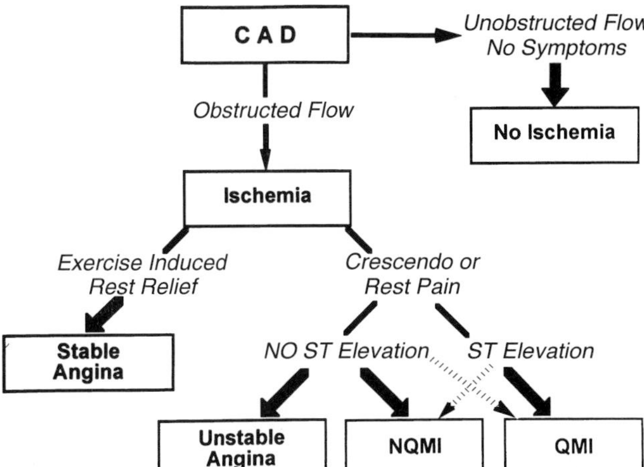

Figure 91–1. Myocardial ischemic syndromes. Swelling of the coronary artery intima by the atherosclerotic process may be insufficient to interfere with normal flow patterns; ischemia is absent and the patient has no symptoms. When coronary blood flow is decreased sufficiently by a reduction in the internal diameter of the coronary artery of at least 50% to 70%, ischemic chest pain may develop. In stable angina, discomfort is typically associated with exertion and relieved by rest or sustained-release (SL) nitroglycerin, generally in a reproducible pattern. Crescendo or rest precordial ischemic pain usually implies unstable angina, non–Q-wave myocardial infarction (MI), or Q-wave MI. Unstable angina and non–Q-wave MI are frequently associated with acute development of a partially obstructive thrombus adherent to the atherosclerotic plaque and ST-segment depression on the electrocardiogram. Q-wave MI is characterized by ST-segment elevation and occlusive thrombi acutely complicating coronary artery disease (CAD). NQMI = non–Q-wave MI; QMI = Q-wave MI. (Modified from Heart Disease: A Textbook of Cardiovascular Medicine. 5th ed. Braunwald E [Ed]. Philadelphia, WB Saunders, 1997, p 1187.)

PATHOGENESIS

According to current understanding, the atherosclerotic process evolves initially from a fatty streak, a raised, yellowish, lipid-containing streak readily visible on the inner surface of involved arteries when viewed at postmortem examination.[1] That the streak is a response to injury was first proposed in the 1970s. The battleground for coronary artery disease is the intima. The media and adventitia do not appear to be primarily involved.

Injury to the intima, such as flow stress, stimulates local expression of vascular cell adhesion molecules, leading to local binding of circulating monocytes. It is known that elevated blood lipids and, possibly, some viruses and bacteria also induce the gene controlling this molecule. Some of the adherent monocytes enter the subendothelial space, moving between the endothelial cells. A major component of the fatty streak also is smooth muscle. Smooth muscle is not normally found in the intima but migrates from the media to the areas of infiltrated monocytes in response to a variety of stimuli, including platelet-derived growth factor.

The pathology of coronary artery disease has a major inflammatory component. In addition to characteristic pathologic findings, C-reactive protein, or acute-phase reactor, is elevated in patients with ischemic syndromes. Reports suggest that elevated C-reactive protein as a marker for coronary artery disease predicts a poor prognosis.[2] Whether this substance is a marker for atherosclerosis or is related to its cause is not known.

The monocytes in the fatty streak or infiltrating the subendothelial space become transformed into macrophages and develop receptors for engulfing lipid, especially oxidized low-density lipoprotein (LDL). Over time, they become converted to the characteristic foam cells found in atheroma. As the atheroma builds up in the subintimal space, bulging into the lumen of the coronary artery, connective tissue forms over the surface, gradually being transformed into fibrotic cap. Ischemic syndromes develop when the atheroma with its fibrous cap reduces the internal diameter of the coronary vessel to 50% to 70% (a 75% to 90% obstruction of the cross-sectional area). The acute unstable coronary syndromes—unstable angina, non–Q-wave myocardial infarction, Q-wave myocardial infarction—are generally precipitated by the development of an occlusive or partially occlusive thrombus that abruptly or progressively further narrows the lumen, reduces coronary blood flow, and causes profound ischemic symptoms.

According to our current understanding, a coronary thrombus is initiated after rupture of a vulnerable atherosclerotic plaque. Rupture of the plaque exposes humoral elements and platelets to tissue factors ordinarily protected in the subendothelial space. These tissue factors initiate a coagulation cascade with the initiation of thrombin production and the conversion of fibrinogen to fibrin as well as alteration in platelet structure and function, leading to aggregation and the platelet plug[3] (Fig. 91–2). Coronary artery thrombi have both red (humoral clotting cascade) and white (platelet) components, which have been recognized on pathologic examination and seen directly during angioscopy in patients with myocardial infarction or unstable angina.[4]

The mechanisms by which these two components of the clot develop are briefly reviewed, because the management, especially of acute myocardial infarction, is undergoing rapid change on the basis of an understanding of the molecular

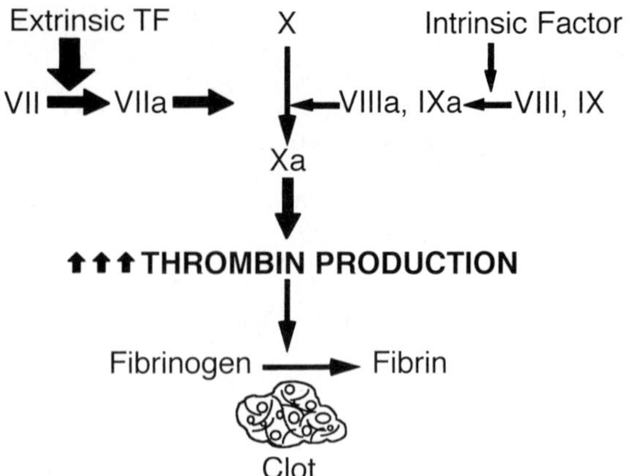

Figure 91–2. Current concepts of activation of the coagulation cascade following plaque rupture in coronary thrombosis. Tissue factor (TF), not normally exposed to blood elements, is activated by disruption of the atherosclerotic plaque activating factor VII. Intrinsic factor in the circulating blood is not thought to play as large a role as TF. Activated factor Xa participates in the prothrombinase complex; a single molecule generates many molecules of thrombin. The end product of coagulation, the clot, is a complex conglomeration of fibrin and platelets with both red fibrin and white platelet components visible on a direct angioscopy of human coronary arteries. (After Antman EM: *In* Cardiology Rounds. Vol 1. No 2. Boston, Brigham and Women's Hospital, 1997, pp 1–7.)

biology of the coronary thrombus and the development of drugs to retard or prevent key components in the thrombotic sequence. An understanding of both the clotting sequence and the platelet aggregation sequence assists the emergency physician and the cardiologist in making wise therapeutic choices for the management of the coronary thrombotic syndromes, especially with the development of new pharmacologic approaches.

Clotting

Following rupture of the plaque, exposure to tissue factor (factor VII) is activated (factor VIIa) (see Fig. 91–2). Activation of extrinsic tissue factor, factor VIIIa, and factor IXa is thought to be less important. Factor VIIa activates factor X. Activated factor Xa is a critical component in the clotting cascade, because it engenders multiple molecules of thrombin. Thrombin, in turn, activates the conversion of fibrinogen to fibrin, which precipitates as strands, developing multiple cross-linkages with aggregated platelets and forming the physical clot.

Platelets

When platelets are exposed to the subendothelial matrix, proteins such as collagen and von Willebrand's factor bind to receptors (glycoprotein Ia/IIa and Ib receptors), causing *adhesion* of the platelets to the site of injury.[5] The platelets then become *activated,* their shape changes, and degranulation releases thromboxane A_2, serotonin, and other highly reactive molecules. The glycoprotein IIb/IIIa receptors, of which there are many thousands on each platelet, are activated and bind with von Willebrand's factor and fibrinogen, which is converted to fibrin strands. Simultaneously, the platelets *aggregate* with one another. The end result is a rapidly accumulating thrombus compromising coronary blood flow and producing ischemic symptoms.[6] Thus, the sequence of platelet change is *adhesion, activation, aggregation.*

CLINICAL FEATURES

Approximately 50% of patients presenting with first MI have only single-vessel disease. In acute Q-wave infarction, characterized by new onset of ST-segment elevation, angiographic study has shown complete occlusion of the culprit coronary artery by thrombus in more than 80% of instances.[7] In non–Q-wave infarction, generally characterized by ST-segment depression in two or more continuous leads, similar studies have revealed the culprit coronary artery partially occluded by thrombus in the majority of cases. Unstable angina is also characterized by partially occluding thrombi in the culprit coronary artery. Although patients presenting to the emergency room with ischemic chest pain can usually retrospectively be classified as having one of the four ischemic syndrome categories defined in Figure 91–1, such accuracy is usually not possible at the time of presentation.

Q-wave infarcts, manifesting in the classic mode as ST-segment elevation, can usually be readily recognized from analysis of the initial ECG, and appropriate therapy initiated. The evidence that fibrinolytic therapy is effective in Q-wave infarction is unequivocal, and treatment with an appropriate agent should be initiated as rapidly as possible. Mortality reduction after thrombolysis is greatest with anterior infarcts; inferior infarcts and infarcts in other locations also respond favorably, but their mortality is low; hence the salvage is not as large. Current evidence does not support the use of thrombolytic agents in the treatment of unstable angina or non–Q-wave MI, although generally, other treatment measures as described here are applied.

THE OPEN ARTERY HYPOTHESIS

Beginning more than two decades ago, the experimental work of Reimer and coworkers[8] in dogs demonstrated that the duration of coronary occlusion directly influenced the mass of left ventricle infarcted. Interestingly, electron microscopic change in myocardial mitochondria was observed within 2 minutes of coronary occlusion. Myocardial salvage was greatest when treatment (i.e., restoration of coronary blood flow) was begun within 1 hour. A variety of clinical and experimental observations document a direct relationship between survival or preservation of left ventricular function and time to good physiologic reperfusion following onset of myocardial infarction. Thus the GUSTO (Global Utilization of Streptokinase and Tissue Plasminogen Activator to Treat Occluded Arteries) investigators[9, 10] showed that survival could be directly related to the time from onset of symptoms to beginning of definitive treatment. However, there was only minor improvement in left ventricular ejection fraction with earlier treatment and maximal restoration of coronary flow. Jeremy and associates[11] demonstrated in an observational study that spontaneous patency following myocardial infarction prevented extensive ventricular remodeling. Despite the emphasis in many studies on the importance of earliest possible thrombolytic treatment for Q-wave infarction, other data suggest that treatment up to 12 hours, and possible even up to 24 hours after onset of symptoms may be beneficial.[12] Although the benefit is much reduced with late treatment, there is evidence that ventricular function may be preserved and that ventricular remodeling, with its adverse consequences, may be prevented or retarded. In addition, a careful experimental study in rats suggested that reperfusion at a time that did not limit infarct size still had a major effect on improving ventricular remodeling.[13]

The concept in Q-wave infarction (the consequence of total occlusion of a coronary artery secondary to a recent thrombus and a ruptured atherosclerotic plaque) that reopening of the culprit artery spontaneously or by therapeutic intervention as quickly as possible, but perhaps even as late as 24 hours, reduces initial mortality, preserves ventricular function, and hence influences late mortality is termed the "open artery hypothesis." Recognition of the clinical truth of this hypothesis motivates the drive to reopen the occluded artery and maintain its patency over the long term as well as the intense effort from basic scientists and clinical investigators to improve current treatment of Q-wave infarction and the other ischemic syndromes.

During the acute phase and after recovery, the prognosis of MI is directly related to the volume of left ventricular myocardium infarcted. Studies in the pre-revascularization era documented that survival with 50% or more of infarcted left ventricular mass was unusual, whether the damage occurred as one massive insult or as a series of small events over time.[14] In the current era, successful revascularization reduces the mass of left ventricular myocardium in jeopardy, but it is likely that the relationship between mass of infarcted left ventricle and prognosis will stand the test of time.

DIAGNOSIS

Heart disease is the leading cause of mortality in the western world, among both men and women, accounting for about one in every four deaths in patients older than 35 years. A high index of suspicion must be maintained when any patient older than about 35 years complains of persistent chest pain that lasts more than 20 minutes, suggesting the possibility of myocardial ischemia. After age 50 years, women have an increasing incidence of coronary heart disease, yet the significance of the complaint of chest pain may not be recognized as readily in a woman as in a man. Women are more reticent about seeking medical attention for chest pain, and on average, they delay seeking medical attention by several hours compared with men.

Rapid triage, diagnosis, and treatment of patients with suspected ischemic chest pain are imperative. In a patient in whom Q-wave infarction is likely, the goal of recording the first ECG in 10 minutes and beginning administration of the first dose of a fibrinolytic agent within 20 to 30 minutes of initial contact should be maintained as a continual challenge to the treatment team. The success of fibrinolytic therapy in reducing mortality is in an inverse linear relationship, hour by hour, with time from onset of symptoms. Although retrospective analysis of the GISSI-1 (Gruppo Italiano iper lo Studio della Streptochinasi nell'Infarto Micordico)[15] data suggested that salvage was greatly increased if treatment (in this study, streptokinase) was initiated within the first hour of symptoms ("the golden hour"),[15] combined analysis from many studies totaling several thousands of patients does not suggest evidence of a sharp increase in salvage during the first hour.[12] Nevertheless, the sooner definitive therapy is applied, the sooner coronary perfusion in the affected area may be restored, the more likely that myocardium is salvaged, and the better the prognosis.

Following a rapid history and a focused physical examination, the most important initial diagnostic test is the 12-lead electrocardiogram. If a patient's previous ECG was normal, sensitivity and specificity of this test are approximately 80% to 85% for detection of myocardial infarction; if the previous ECG was abnormal, the accuracy is much reduced. In the first 1 to 3 hours after onset of myocardial infarction, the electrocardiogram in Q-wave infarction is usually diagnostic, with marked ST-segment elevation in two or more contiguous leads. A strictly posterior Q-wave infarct may be overlooked, because the pattern of Q-wave and ST-segment elevation from a posterior surface is reversed in leads V_1 and V_2, presenting as small or modest R waves with ST-segment depression.

The diagnosis of Q-wave infarction is generally not obscured by right bundle branch block, but it may be difficult to recognize in the presence of left bundle branch block (LBBB). Sgarbossa and colleagues[16] have reviewed the criteria for diagnosis of Q-wave infarction in the presence of LBBB. Non-Q-wave infarctions may manifest as alterations in the direction and amplitude of the T-wave vector with ST segment depression. When the diagnosis of Q-wave infarct is evident from the initial ECG, appropriate therapy must be undertaken immediately.

Diagnosis of MI is confirmed by a rise in serum activity of specific myocardial enzymes several hours after the acute event. Creatine kinase (CK) with measurement of the MB fraction (isoenzyme with muscle and brain subunits [CKMB]) has stood the test of time and remains the most widely available and reliable diagnostic tool. The usual routine is to obtain blood samples for serum myocardial enzyme assay at the time of first encounter and then at 8, 16, and 24 hours. CKMB begins to rise 4 to 6 hours after the onset of myocardial infarction, reaching a peak at about 30 hours and subsiding by 72 hours.[17] For greatest usefulness, it is important to have a responsive laboratory system that can provide a result within 1 to 2 hours of receipt of a specimen.

Other enzymes, such as tropinin and myoglobin, have also been evaluated. The tropinins have about the same time course for onset of serum activity as CKMB but are elevated for as much as 120 hours. Tropinins are much more sensitive to myocardial damage, showing increased levels of serum activity with so-called micro-infarcts. Myoglobin response has an earlier onset, with the first rise detected at 1 to 2 hours and peak activity at about 10 hours after onset of infarction.

Chest Pain; Rule Out Myocardial Infarction

A diagnostic dilemma commonly encountered, especially in the emergency departments of urban hospitals, is "Chest pain; rule out myocardial infarction."[18, 18a] The patient is middle-aged, often female, complaining of chest pain with atypical features. Because some individuals with MI present with atypical features—even, sometimes, without pain—the complaints must be taken seriously. The patient should be carefully evaluated for the presence of ischemic heart disease despite the fact that the majority of patients, especially premenopausal women presenting with atypical complaints, prove not to have significant coronary artery disease. If the initial ECG is normal, the probability of acute MI is exceedingly low (about 3%) and the prognosis is excellent.

A number of emergency systems have developed chest pain diagnostic units, generally nearby but conveying a more restful ambience than the standard emergency department environment. Patients are monitored, serial enzymes are evaluated, and further diagnostic evaluation is arranged on an outpatient basis if ischemia or myocardial infarction appears to be absent or of low probability. In such instances, the patient is discharged in 24 to 36 hours.

ACUTE PHASE

Age is the single most important prognostic factor in MI. In patients aged 70 years or younger, a hospital mortality from MI of 3% to 6% has been reported, whereas in patients 85 years or older, the risk is 35% or higher. Although various other prognostic factors have been identified, outcome depends on the amount of left ventricle damage, the combination of acute infarction and scar, and the extent of coronary artery disease. A large infarct with single-vessel coronary disease may be relatively well tolerated, yet smaller infarctions in the presence of old scar and extensive coronary atherosclerosis may be poorly tolerated.[19]

A generation ago, Killip and Kimball[20] described a simple system for bedside evaluation of left ventricular function based on the presence or absence of pulmonary rales, advanced left ventricular failure, or cardiogenic shock. Despite the crudity of the physiologic evaluation, the classification remains accurate. The classification is as follows:

- *Class I:* No evidence of heart failure
- *Class II:* Pulmonary rales suggestive of early left ventricular failure
- *Class III:* Pulmonary edema
- *Class IV:* Cardiogenic shock

Patients in class I have an excellent prognosis. Those in class II have a somewhat reduced prognosis. Patients in class III or class IV have a sharply higher mortality. Indeed, cardiogenic shock remains a difficult therapeutic problem, with minimal evidence of progress in treatment, until perhaps the last few years. Evaluating patients with MI on a daily basis according to our simple scheme provides useful prognostic information.

TREATMENT

Treatment of myocardial infarction is designed to (1) relieve symptoms, (2) limit the extent of myocardial damage, (3) reduce cardiac work and hence reverse ischemia, and (4) manage complications. About half of the deaths from acute MI occur within the first 4 to 6 hours. Thus, management in an acute care setting during the first few hours is critical. The most common factor limiting early treatment is denial. Although there is widespread public awareness of the significance of chest pain as a symptom of heart attack, delay in seeking medical aid is all too common, especially among women. Studies have shown that older women who live alone or are the functioning heads of their households often delay seeking medical help, with potentially severe consequences.[21] Because the major cause of early mortality is primary ventricular fibrillation (ventricular fibrillation occurring without significant prodromal ventricular ectopic beats), access to a monitoring unit as early as possible is essential.

Pain

The initial discomfort of MI may be agonizingly severe. Morphine, 2 to 4 mg IV, repeated as needed, is often highly effective in treating the pain of MI. Morphine has adverse effects, including respiratory depression, some decrease in myocardial contractility, bradycardia, and vasodilatation, so the response of the patient must be closely watched. The hypotensive effect of morphine often responds to simple elevation of the lower extremities. The ischemic pain of MI may also be relieved by nitroglycerin, which may be administered sublingually (0.4 mg repeated once or twice as necessary), followed by continuous intravenous drip if required. Rapid and effective use of IV nitroglycerin may sharply reduce the need for morphine.

Oxygen

Increased left ventricular filling pressure consequent to myocardial dysfunction of acute MI raises pulmonary venous pressure, increases the work of breathing, and reduces pulmonary capillary oxygen tension and partial pressure of arterial oxygen. Hence, treatment with oxygen administered via nasal prongs at a rate of 4 to 6 L/min is reasonable for the first 36 to 48 hours in uncomplicated MI. More profound left ventricular dysfunction with pulmonary congestion may require more efficient means of oxygen delivery. Evidence is lacking that continued use of oxygen after the first 1 to 2 days in a good-risk patient provides therapeutic benefit.

Aspirin and Platelet Dysfunction

Increased platelet aggregability is intimately associated with coronary atherosclerosis.[6] Phasic alterations in platelet function correlate with the circadian rhythm for occurrence of MI in the waking hours and have been used to identify patients at high risk for recurrent ischemia or extension of infarction. The acute phase of myocardial infarction initiates platelet activation and aggregation. This action is further increased by fibrinolytic therapy, raising the risk of coronary artery reocclusion and further myocardial damage.

The Second International Study of Infarct Survival (ISIS-2)[22] conclusively demonstrated that 162.5 mg of enteric-coated aspirin administered immediately to patients with MI reduced hospital mortality by 23% compared with placebo. These initial results have been repeatedly confirmed and extended by other studies of the use of aspirin in combination with various thrombolytic agents. Hence, all patients with suspected MI should receive aspirin in at least this dose immediately, chewed and swallowed for rapid effect, on first encounter and daily thereafter.

Aspirin acetylates platelet cyclooxygenase for the life of the platelet, blocking synthesis of certain prostacyclines, especially thromboxane A_2, and thus inhibiting aggregation in vivo. A dose of 162.5 mg produces virtual complete inhibition of cyclooxygenase in less than 1 hour for the life of the platelet, which is 8 to 10 days. Lower doses may take several hours to accomplish intermission. Doses higher than 325 mg may produce adverse effects. Hence, the initial dose upon recognition of MI should be ½ or 1 full tablet (325 mg) of aspirin.

Restoration of Coronary Flow

Thrombolytics

It is now recognized that the acute ischemic syndromes unstable angina, non–Q-wave infarction, and Q-wave infarction are characterized by the development of thrombi at the site of a nonocclusive atherosclerotic plaque (see Fig. 91-1). Thrombi do not appear to play a role in the development of stable, exercise-induced angina pectoris. In Q-wave myocardial infarction, the culprit coronary artery generally is totally occluded by the combination of plaque and recent thrombus. In non–Q-wave infarctions and in unstable angina, the blood vessels remain patent although narrowed by plaque and thrombus. Fibrinolytic therapy has not proved useful in altering the natural history of unstable angina or non–Q-wave infarction.[23] Catastrophic herniation of the plaque into the lumen to completely obstruct the coronary artery is uncommon, occurring in 5% or less of Q-wave MI.[24]

The report of the Fibrinolytic Therapy Trialists' Collaborative Group (FTTCG)[12] illustrated that mortality in Q-wave infarcts is substantially reduced (25% to 30%) by treatment with fibrinolytic therapy of patients with either ST segment elevation or bundle branch block up to 12 hours and possibly as much as 18 to 20 hours after the onset of symptoms. The absolute benefits are greatest in patients with anterior ST-segment elevation, but patients with inferior ST-segment elevation, who have a lower risk, also benefit. Patients with Q-wave infarcts have the highest risk and the greatest benefit from fibrinolysis. The sooner the treatment, the greater the salvage.

Too few patients receiving treatment 12 hours or more after onset of symptoms have been studied for firm judgments to be made about the efficacy of fibrinolysis when treatment is delayed. Nonrandomized studies of small groups of patients and some animal experiments suggest that ventricular function may still be preserved secondary to reduced left ventricular remodeling despite little effect on mortality.[11, 13] The FTTCG overview suggested that age is no bar to fibrinolysis, and that the benefit is greater than the risk even in patients 75 years or older.[12] Many authorities believe that age alone should not be a bar to fibrinolytic treatment in the absence of clear-cut contraindications.

The FTTCG overview of all large trials found that in patients with ST-segment elevation and bundle branch block treated within 12 hours of onset of symptoms, fibrinolytic therapy prevents 20 to 30 deaths per 1000 patients treated. In a large trial, this advantage was accompanied by about four extra strokes per 1000 patients, two of which were associated with early death. Generally, the risk of stroke with fibrinolytic treatment has been found to be between 0.8% and 2%.

Debate has focused on the choice of fibrinolytic agent and whether heparin should be utilized as a routine adjunct therapy. Three large clinical trials—GISSI-2,[25] ISIS-3,[22, 22a] and GUSTO-1[9]—have compared the effectiveness of different thrombolytic agents.

In GISSI-2 and its international study extension, 20,891 patients with acute MI were randomly assigned within 6 hours of onset of symptoms to receive either streptokinase (1.5 million units over 30 to 60 min) or tissue plasminogen activator (t-PA) (alteplase, 100 mg over 3 hours). All patients received 325 mg of aspirin daily and were randomized to receive heparin (12,500 units SC twice daily) or no heparin. No significant differences were noted in total mortality between t-PA and streptokinase and between heparin and no heparin.

ISIS-3 compared t-PA, streptokinase, and anisoylated plasminogen-streptokinase activator complex (APSAC). More than 41,000 patients were randomly assigned to receive the three agents. All patients received 162.5 mg of aspirin daily and were also randomly assigned to receive subcutaneous heparin (12,500 units SC twice daily) or no heparin. No advantage for heparin was observed. No mortality differences were noted among the three thrombolytic agents, and aside from a slight decrease in the reinfarction rate with patients receiving t-PA, no differences were found in the complication rates. Results of both GISSI-2 and ISIS-3 suggested that the relatively inexpensive streptokinase is as effective as t-PA, which costs six to seven times more.

The GUSTO trial was designed to determine whether the rapidity of return to coronary artery patency influenced mortality.[9] Patients with anterior MI who were receiving "front-loaded" doses of t-PA and intravenous heparin had a 20% reduction in mortality compared with those receiving streptokinase. The GUSTO trial also noted that intravenous heparin was not more effective than subcutaneous heparin in the streptokinase arm of the trial. An angiographic substudy of GUSTO reported that patency of the culprit artery 90 minutes after therapy was highest in patients treated with t-PA and intravenous heparin. Patients with open arteries had greater improvement in left ventricular function and a somewhat lower mortality at 30 days. Interestingly, although the patency rate at 90 minutes was highest in the subsets of patients receiving t-PA and heparin, patency in all groups was similar at 180 minutes, suggesting that the earlier the artery is opened, the better the prognosis.

GUSTO has been interpreted by its participants and the majority of North American cardiologists as demonstrating a therapeutic advantage for fibrinolysis with so-called front-loaded t-PA combined with heparin therapy. This is not the universal view, however. Collins and associates,[26] a group of distinguished British clinical scientists and biostatisticians, have criticized the "selective emphasis" on subsection analysis as leading to a false emphasis on a significant difference among the therapies studied. These researches agree that the t-PA–based regimens probably opened occluded arteries about 30 to 60 minutes earlier than did the streptokinase regimen. They argue, however, that this modest shortening of delay is likely to decrease the immediate mortality by only about 1 to 2 deaths per 1000 subjects studied, and they note that this putative advantage is associated with the hazard of additional cerebral hemorrhage (trials have established a slightly higher risk of cerebral hemorrhage from t-PA than from streptokinase). According to these authors,[26] the advantage of using t-PA, if any, is slight indeed.

Results of the various trials of thrombolytics can be summarized as follows:

1. Effective fibrinolysis reduces mortality and salvages myocardium in both anterior and inferior Q-wave MI by restoring coronary flow, at least over the short term. Fibrinolysis is not effective in non–Q-wave MI or in unstable angina.
2. The sooner a patient is treated, the better, for up to at least 12 hours and possibly as long as 18 to 24 hours after onset.
3. A front-loaded dose of t-PA combined with closely monitored intravenous heparin may be slightly more effective than streptokinase with subcutaneous or intravenous heparin.
4. Bleeding, both intracranial and at puncture sites, is the main complication of fibrinolysis.
5. The risk of intracranial bleeding is slightly higher with t-PA than with other agents. The overall risk appears to be 0.8% to 2%.

Percutaneous Transluminal Coronary Angioplasty

Fibrinolytic therapy of acute myocardial infarction has a number of disadvantages. As mentioned, it carries a risk of intracerebral bleed. Almost all intracerebral bleeds engender serious ongoing morbidity, and about half are fatal. Full restoration of coronary flow, so-called TIMI-3 flow, is achieved in only about 50% of cases. Furthermore, the flow may be of short duration, because reocclusion occurs in a significant percentage of cases.[27] Additionally, although the thrombus may be lysed, the atherosclerotic plaque remains, protruding into the lumen and possibly generating new thrombotic obstructions. Since the first comparison of percutaneous transluminal coronary angioplasty (PTCA) and thrombolysis in patients with acute myocardial infarction, there has been increasing enthusiasm to intervene mechanically to destroy the thrombus and dilate the culprit artery in acute MI.

Weaver and coworkers[28] have reviewed the seven randomized trials comparing PTCA and thrombolysis with a meta-analysis comparing the effects on death, reinfarction, major bleeding, total stroke, and hemorrhagic stroke. The studies were small, with combined totals of 1290 patients subjected to PTCA and 1316 patients undergoing lytic therapy, but the results were consistent and impressive. Duration of symptoms varied from less than 6 hours in several trials to less than 12 hours in others. Duration of follow-up was to discharge in some studies, and to 30 days in others. The mean time to treatment was 26 minutes longer for PTCA than with lytic therapy. There was a significant reduction in the odds of death favoring primary PTCA. The risk of mortality was 4.4% with PTCA and 6.5% with thrombolysis, representing 21 more lives saved per 1000 patients treated with PTCA. The risk of death or nonfatal infarction was lower in patients treated with primary PTCA, as were the rates of total stroke and hemorrhagic stroke. Although the total number of patients studied was small, weaver and coworkers[28] conclude that "there is good evidence of significant reductions in the risk of death, myocardial infarction and stroke attributable to PTCA" compared with lytic therapy in myocardial infarction.

The results of the Weaver analysis are dramatic and may influence our approach to treatment of myocardial infarction; however, several caveats are in order: The reports involve small numbers of patients in several trials, the protocols varied, and meta-analysis may underemphasize differences and falsely assume a commonality among patients and protocols. Less than 10% of the hospitals in the United States have cardiac catheterization laboratories, so rapid access to this high-technology care is limited. Furthermore, and most important, the studies were carried out by highly experienced, highly motivated, expert invasive cardiologists. If PTCA is to become more widespread in the treatment of myocardial infarction in the community, it will have to be demonstrated that the technical skills applied to the patients with acute MI meet the standards of the academic medical centers that carried out the clinical trials.

Heparin

In North America, patients with myocardial infarction or unstable angina are commonly treated with intravenous heparin for 48 hours or longer, commencing when the diagnosis is entertained. The GUSTO trial compared various combinations of streptokinase, t-PA, subcutaneous heparin, and intravenous heparin in myocardial infarction, and all patients received concomitant aspirin. The investigators concluded from an angiographic substudy that "front-loaded" t-PA (100 mg in 90 minutes IV as a 15-mg bolus initially; then 0.75mg/kg over the next 30 minutes to a maximum of 50 mg; then 0.5 mg/kg over the next 60 minutes to a maximum of 35mg) and IV heparin produce the highest rate of culprit artery patency at 90 minutes. On the basis of this study, the majority of patients treated in the United States currently receive the front-loaded t-PA dosage plus IV heparin as previously described.

That heparin is indicated and useful in treatment of myocardial infarction is not a universal opinion. Collins and associates,[26] in an exhaustive analysis of clinical trials in the treatment of acute MI involving a total of more than 68,000 patients receiving various combinations of heparin, aspirin, and fibrinolytics, concluded that there is little added benefit from the use of heparin. Most of the trials evaluating the effectiveness of heparin took place in the pre-aspirin era. Heparin adds little to the effect of aspirin. According to the Collins review, heparin has a modest effect in reducing mortality during hospitalization, but no gain can be demonstrated after 35 days, or 6 months post-MI.[26] Heparin is clearly associated with an increase in major bleeds, although careful adjustment of dose according to weight does reduce this risk. High doses engender higher rates of intracranial hemorrhage. Collins and associates conclude, "Available evidence with respect to heparin . . . does not provide any clear justification for routine heparin therapy in patients with suspected acute myocardial infarction (or unstable angina)."[26]

The Future

Since the mid-1980s, the results of clinical trials and the introduction of aspirin, β-adrenergic blockers, fibrinolytic agents, and, possibly, heparin as well as other drugs have revolutionized the treatment of impending myocardial infarction, reducing mortality and preserving ventricular function.

A look back a few years from now, however, will no doubt reveal our current pharmacologic approach as crude. Patency of the culprit artery is achieved in only about 50% of cases. The nonocclusive thrombus associated with unstable angina and non–Q-wave infarction is not readily susceptible to current treatment. Aspirin has only a modest antiaggregatory effect on platelets. In vitro, aspirin blocks about 20% of the antiaggregatory effect of adenosine diphosphate (ADP) on platelets, compared with 30% for the thienopyridines (ticlopidine and clopidogrel), and about an 80% effect for the glycoprotein IIb/IIIa receptor blocking agents. Furthermore, the fibrinolytics have a paradoxical effect on clot formation. Lysis of fibrin exposes thrombin, which not only greatly enhances thrombin activity through an autocatalytic process but also is a potent platelet activator.

Current therapy for MI is good, better than it was, but far from perfect. Thus, despite the putative advantage of PTCA in selected (and lucky) patients with acute MI, there is an intense pharmacologic effort to identify newer agents or combinations of agents to more definitively attack the heart of the ischemic problem: thrombus adherent to altered atherosclerotic plaque in the culprit coronary artery.

New Pharmacologic Approaches

Although the thienopyridines, as mentioned, are more potent platelet antiaggregators than aspirin, unfortunately their full therapeutic effect requires 2 to 4 days of oral therapy.

Heparin may or may not be advantageous in treatment of acute MI, but it is a drug with many problems. Standard unfractionated heparin, a heterogeneous mixture of polysaccharide chains, acts by activating antithrombin III, thus accelerating its ability to inhibit thrombin and factor Xa by about a thousandfold. However, it has a variable anticoagulant effect, requires frequent serum activated partial thromboplastin time (aPTT) analyses for proper dosing, and is prone to cause thrombocytopenia or, occasionally, the heparin-induced thrombocytopenia syndrome.

To date, the newer direct antithrombin drugs, such as hirudin and bivalirudin (Hirulog), which inhibit thrombin directly without requiring antithrombin III, have not been shown to have a clinical advantage regarding outcome compared with standard undifferentiated heparin.[29-32] Low-molecular-weight heparins, which have a more predictable anticoagulant effect, less sensitivity to platelet factor IV, and a lower rate of inducing thrombocytopenia, have also undergone trial in ischemic syndromes, with promising results.[33-36] The low-molecular-weight heparin preparations need to be evaluated on an individual basis because of important chemical differences, but studies suggest the possibility of their therapeutic effectiveness in unstable angina and non–Q-wave MI.

A new class of drugs, the glycoprotein IIb/IIIa inhibitors, which bind to the glycoprotein IIb/IIIa receptor, thus blocking the final common pathway for platelet aggregation, are being evaluated in a variety of clinical situations. The EPILOG,[37] PRISM,[38, 38a] and other studies have demonstrated the effectiveness of abciximab, a Fab antibody fragment directed against the glycoprotein IIb/IIIa receptor, in reducing ischemic complications and reocclusion following PTCA and in unstable angina. Other molecular glycoprotein IIb/IIIa receptor inhibitors, such as Integrelin (a peptide) and tirofiban (lamifiban), also being evaluated in a variety of thrombus-induced ischemic conditions. The possibility that these new drugs, when used in imaginative and sequential combinations, may further enhance treatment will no doubt be very much in the forefront of clinical trials for the next few years.

For example, could early treatment, perhaps in the ambulance or at home, with a reduced dose of a fibrinolytic drug, a more potent antiplatelet aggregatory drug with rapid action, in association with low-molecular-weight heparin, possibly together with an antithrombin or a glycoprotein IIA/IIIB receptor inhibitor for early effective thrombolysis, be followed by transportation to a medical center for PTCA with or without stenting? In what sequence? Which drugs? What dosage? It seems highly likely that our current treatment of impending MI, both Q-wave and non–Q-wave infarctions, and perhaps also unstable angina will change progressively and incrementally as new outcome data accumulate.

β-Adrenergic Blockers

β-Adrenergic blocking agents (β-blockers) decrease heart rate, blood pressure, and cardiac work with a consequent reduction in myocardial oxygen consumption. They also lower blood free fatty acids, possibly having a beneficial effect on cardiac arrhythmia. Randomized trials have demonstrated that β-blockers reduce morbidity and mortality not only in the first few hours or days after onset of acute MI, but also in the following months and years.[23] In the absence of contraindications, intravenous β-blockers may be administered during the first few hours of MI. Contraindications include heart rate less than 60 beats/min, hypotension, moderate or severe left ventricular failure, evidence of peripheral hypoperfusion, varying degrees of atrioventricular block, chronic obstructive pulmonary disease or asthma, severe peripheral vascular disease, and insulin-dependent diabetes mellitus.

Either of the following regimens may be used:

1. Atenolol: 5 mg IV over 5 minutes, repeat in 10 minutes; if well tolerated, 50 mg PO 10 minutes later and 12 hours later, followed by 50 or 100 mg daily thereafter
2. Metoprolol: 5 mg IV over 2 to 5 minutes, repeated three times; if well tolerated, 50 mg every 12 hours beginning 15 minutes after last IV dose

Heart rate and blood pressure should be carefully monitored during the IV dosage of a β-blocker and thereafter. Dosage is reduced if bradycardia or hypotension develops. Untoward effects may be reversed with isoproterenol, 1 to 5 μg/min IV.

Nitrates

Nitrates have a major role in the management of ischemic symptoms, especially pain.[23] Their effective use may sharply reduce the need for opiate therapy. Nitrates are vasodilators, having a major effect on the capacitance system, but also dilating arteries and arterioles, and even effecting some vasodilation of the atherosclerotic vessels. Nitrates are pro-drugs that must be converted by mechanisms not fully understood to nitric oxide, which stimulates guanylyl cyclase, converting guanosine triphosphate to cyclic guanosine monophosphate, which effects the vasodilation. Nitrates also reduce platelet adhesion and aggregation.

All nitrates induce tolerance with loss of hemodynamic effect, although the mechanism is poorly understood. Putative explanatory factors have included the persistence of plasma volume expansion, sulfhydryl depletion, and increased production of superoxide anion. Vitamin E has been reported to prevent the development of some aspects of nitrate tolerance, lending credence to the superoxide theory.[39]

For the treatment of ischemia, nitroglycerin may be administered initially in the emergency room sublingually, one to three times in sequence in the standard dose of 0.3 or 0.4 mg per tablet. Intravenous nitroglycerin is often highly effective in relieving ischemic symptoms. Generally, the aim is to reduce systemic blood pressure by 10 to 20 mm Hg but not to less than 80 to 90 mm Hg systolic. Infusion is started at a rate of 5–10 μg/min, and the dose is increased by 5–10 μg every few minutes until the desired response is achieved.

Calcium Antagonists

Although useful in the management of hypertension, calcium antagonists have not been shown to reduce morbidity or mortality in the early treatment or secondary prevention of acute MI. They do not appear to offer any additional advantage when beta-adrenergic blockers and aspirin are given. Diltiazem appears to have modest long-term beneficial effects in some patients in the absence of heart failure but is associated with higher mortality in the presence of left ventricular failure.[23]

Glucose, Potassium, and Insulin

Exogenous glucose is a more efficient fuel than free fatty acids or glycogen, and it is more likely to prevent ischemic injury, according to experimental data. Glycolysis-derived adenosine triphosphate (ATP) preferentially supports cell membrane ion transport and hence preserves cell wall integrity. A published overview of nine clinical randomized trials suggested improved outcome in the treatment of acute MI with glucose-potassium-insulin mixtures. However, because of the small number of patients evaluated, the statistical power of the individual trials was low. Despite more than 30 years of discussion, a large randomized clinical trial designed to definitively determine the efficacy of this form of treatment has yet to be carried out.

Angiotensin-Converting Enzyme Inhibitors

In Q-wave MI, ventricular remodeling with thinning and ballooning of the infarct segment, producing progressive ventricular enlargement and ultimately reduced ventricular function, occurs in as many as 40% of patients. A number of large, randomized clinical trials have demonstrated a benefit, in terms of mortality and preservation of ventricular function, when oral angiotensin-converting enzyme (ACE) inhibitors have been administered. Thus, it is recommended that ACE inhibitors should generally be started orally within the first 24 hours after thrombolytic therapy has been completed if blood pressure is stable.[23] If there is little or no evidence of ventricular dysfunction after 6 weeks, the ACE inhibitors can be discontinued. In the presence of reduced ventricular function, the drugs should generally be continued. Therapy should be initiated with a low dose, ½ to ¼ of the usual starting dose; the dose should be gradually increased over the next 2 to 4 days.

Magnesium

The value of supplemental magnesium in MI remains controversial. The second most abundant intracellular cation, magnesium has a number of physiologic effects, including systemic and coronary vasodilation, antiplatelet activity, suppression of automaticity, and protection of myocytes against calcium overload during ischemia. Although one meta-analysis suggested a significant effect of magnesium on mortality in MI, the results of a subsequent large, randomized clinical trial were negative.[40] The American College of Cardiology/American Heart Association guidelines for the management of acute MI conclude that a reduction in mortality may be seen in high-risk patients provided that magnesium therapy is administered soon after the onset of symptoms (preferably less than 6 hours).[23] The guidelines suggest a bolus of 2 g over 5 to 15 minutes followed by an infusion of 18 g over 24 hours, but they indicate that the optimum dose has not been established.

MYOCARDIAL STUNNING AND HIBERNATION

Two possible consequences of prolonged ventricular dysfunction, myocardial stunning and myocardial hibernation, have attracted considerable attention. In *myocardial stunning,* a contraction abnormality persists for a time after an episode of ischemia despite restoration of flow.[41] The hypocontractile state responds to positive inotropic drugs and is thought to be secondary to excess cytosolic calcium released from sarcoplasmic reticulum damaged by oxygen-derived free radicals. Stunning has been extensively investigated in experimental animals and probably occurs in humans in a number of situations, such as after thrombolysis following MI, after cardiopulmonary bypass, and possibly after exercise-induced ischemia.

Hibernating myocardium is defined as "persistent contractile dysfunction that is associated with reduced coronary flow but preserved myocardial viability."[41] The dysfunction is reversed when coronary flow is restored. Improved ventricular function has been observed after coronary bypass surgery and angioplasty in the apparent absence of recent ischemia, suggesting that the hibernating myocardium had responded to revascularization. Clearly, unrecognized recurrent ischemia could induce changes in left ventricular function, stimulating hibernation.

Documenting the presence of stunned or hibernating myocardium or differentiating between the two conditions may be difficult clinically. These concepts imply, however, that not all ventricular dysfunction in patients with coronary artery disease is necessarily irreversible. Positron emission tomography scanning has been advanced as a diagnostic modality that can identify poorly functioning but viable myocardium to assist a clinician in evaluating whether revascularization in the presence of apparent chronic ventricular dysfunction might lead to significant contractile improvement.[42]

COMPLICATIONS

Arrhythmia

During the first few days after MI, the presence of some arrhythmia is almost universal. Supraventricular arrhythmia, including atrial tachycardia, atrial flutter, and atrial fibrillation, occurs in about 5% of cases, similar to the incidence in the normal population. Patients with a previous history of heart failure and dilated left atrium are somewhat more likely to have a bout of fibrillation or flutter. The incidence of atrial fibrillation increases with age, in large anterior infarcts, and with the development of heart failure. Fibrinolytic therapy reduces the incidence of atrial fibrillation. Atrial fibrillation increases the likelihood of systemic embolization; about half of the embolic events occur during the first day.[23]

Initial treatment is generally focused on controlling heart rate. An intravenous β-blocker, such as atenolol, esmolol, or metoprolol, may be given. Intravenous metoprolol may be administered in doses of 5mg every 3 to 5 minutes for three doses to slow the rate to an acceptable level, followed by oral doses as described earlier. If the heart rate is rapid and there is evidence of hemodynamic compromise, immediate direct-current cardioversion is indicated. Direct-current conversion is not applied routinely, however, because the atrial arrhythmia usually recurs in the first day or two. Spontaneous conversion to sinus rhythm after a few days is the rule.

First-degree heart block and Wenckebach's phenomenon commonly accompany inferior and posterior infarction in the first few hours after onset. These abnormalities are generally self-limited and subside within a few hours. If the ventricular rate slows because of excessive block, atropine in doses of 0.5 mg IV may be cautiously administered to a total dose of 1 to 2 mg. Administration of atropine in doses less than 0.5 mg may paradoxically produce severe bradycardia, presumably owing to transient central nervous system stimulation. Complete heart block in an anterior MI with a slow ventricular response usually denotes massive MI and is an ominous sign. Treatment with an intravenous pacemaker should be initiated, but technical problems not uncommonly occur, related in part to the difficulty of placing the pacemaker catheter in uninvolved ventricular muscle.[23]

Ventricular arrhythmias are extremely common in the first 48 to 72 hours after MI. Within the first few hours of infarction, primary ventricular fibrillation may occur. Although the incidence of *primary fibrillation* (fibrillation in the absence of prodromal ventricular premature beats) appears to have declined during the past decade, this rhythm is the major immediate cause of the high early mortality in the first few hours after the onset of symptoms. The decreased occurrence may relate to changes in lifestyle, especially the decline in cigarette smoking among men, the widespread use of β-blockers in patients with ischemic heart disease, the use of aspirin, and perhaps other measures.

Almost all patients with MI have some ventricular arrhythmia during the first 72 hours of monitoring. Many authorities have advocated the prophylactic use of intravenous lidocaine to prevent serious arrhythmia during the first 2 or 3 days of hospitalization. Clinical trials, however, fail to demonstrate an advantage of prophylactic lidocaine or any other prophylactic antiarrhythmic. Thus, treatment of ventricular arrhythmia on demand rather than prophylactic therapy is currently recommended.[23]

Ventricular tachycardia complicating MI may be *sustained* (>30 seconds and/or with hemodynamic compromise), *nonsustained* (<30 seconds), monomorphic, or polymorphic. Short bursts of ventricular tachycardia are common in the first 48 hours of MI but do not appear to predict more sustained arrhythmia. Sustained episodes of ventricular tachycardia that are well tolerated hemodynamically may be treated with lidocaine, procainamide, or amiodarone, as follows:

1. *Lidocaine:* 1.0 to 1.5 mg/kg as initial bolus, followed by additional doses of 0.5 to 0.75 mg/kg every 5 to 10 minutes to a maximum dose of 3 mg/kg. Following loading, an infusion of 2 to 4 mg/min may be added. Infusion rates should be reduced in older patients or in the presence of heart failure or hepatic dysfunction to avoid lidocaine toxicity.
2. *Procainamide:* Loading infusion of 10 to 15 mg/kg (500 to 1250 mg), given at a rate of 20 mg/min over 30 to 60 minutes, followed by maintenance infusion of 1 to 4 mg/min.[23] Infusion rates should be reduced in the presence of renal dysfunction.[23]
3. *Amiodarone:* 150 mg infused over 10 minutes followed by constant infusion of 1.0 mg/min for 6 hours and then a maintenance infusion of 0.5 mg/min.[23]

Rapid *polymorphic* ventricular tachycardia is the equivalent of ventricular fibrillation and should be treated with immediate direct-current precordial shock. Immediate cardioversion is generally not needed for ventricular rates less than 150 beats/min. Recurrent refractory ventricular arrhythmia in the hemodynamically unstable patient may reflect (1) electrolyte imbalance, especially severe hypokalemia or hypomagnesemia; (2) severe and persistent ischemia or infarction; or (3) cardiogenic shock.[23]

Right Ventricular Infarction

Involvement of the right ventricle occurs in 30% to 50% of posterior-inferior infarcts, carries a high risk of mortality, and identifies candidates for urgent consideration for revascularization.[43] Loss of right ventricular propulsion is characterized by hypotension, low pulmonary capillary wedge pressure reflecting inadequate left ventricular filling, and intolerance of hypotensive agents such as nitroglycerin. The triad of hypotension, clear lung fields, and elevated jugular venous pressure is an important clinical clue to the diagnosis.

The diagnosis of right ventricular infarct may be made with a high level of certainty by examination of the QRS complex in lead V_{4R}. One non–ST-segment elevation is the most helpful ECG finding.[44] In patients who present with inferior infarction and hypotension, measurement of pulmonary artery and pulmonary capillary wedge pressure with the Swan-Ganz technique may be required to distinguish left ventricular forward failure or incipient cardiogenic shock, hypovolemia, or right ventricular infarction.

In the presence of low capillary wedge pressure, administration of a volume load is helpful. In hypovolemia, volume administration should increase systemic pressure with maintenance of normal right ventricular hemodynamics. In right ventricular infarction, a high right ventricular filling pressure must be supported by administration of excess volume to maintain adequate left ventricular filling pressures.

Hemodynamic Instability and Cardiogenic Shock

Cardiogenic shock may be present at the initial encounter or may develop during the first day of treatment or even later. Early recognition of the pre-shock state has a major influence on effective treatment. High systemic vascular resistance may maintain systolic pressure despite a profound reduction in stroke volume. Such patients may be pale, cool, and restless, and palpation of a major peripheral artery (carotid, axillary, femoral) reveals markedly diminished pulse volume. A rising heart rate with persistent tachycardia is an important clue to the pre-shock state. It is important to rule out other causes of hypotension, such as extensive right ventricular infarction, rupture of the ventricular septum, rupture of the papillary muscle producing mitral regurgitation, and cardiac tamponade. A bedside transthoracic or transesophageal echocardiogram may be helpful in establishing the diagnosis.

Aggressive circulatory support is generally required in the treatment. Historically, the mortality has been 75% or greater. Some reports have suggested that revascularization may improve prognosis; if confirmed by clinical trials, these findings would represent the first reduction in the mortality of cardiogenic shock in decades.[45, 46] Pharmacologic therapy may be temporarily effective. Dopamine, an alpha-beta agonist, is administered IV at 0.5 to 1 μg/kg/min. The dose is increased until a satisfactory response is achieved. High doses induce vasoconstriction. Dobutamine, a beta agonist, is given IV at rates of 2.5 to 10 μg/kg/min and sometimes in higher doses. Combinations of inotropes and vasodilators, such as dobutamine, milrinone, nitroprusside, and nitroglycerin, may also be used in low-output states.

An intra-aortic counterpulsating balloon, which increases mean arterial pressure and augments diastolic coronary perfusion, may provide temporary support. Several left ventricular assist devices are being evaluated in the treatment of cardiogenic shock. There is no evidence that the counterpulsating balloon or other assist devices improve prognosis, but they may temporarily support the circulation until definitive treatment can be initiated.

Patients with cardiogenic shock should be promptly treated with fibrinolytic agents in the absence of contraindications. Anecdotal reports have suggested an occasional dramatic response, presumably due to effective reopening of the occluded culprit artery. The most exciting new approach to the treatment of cardiogenic shock is the application of PTCA or emergency bypass surgery for revascularization of the involved myocardium. The pooled hospital mortality rate obtained from a series of reports on PTCA was 46%,[47] although the overall success rate of the procedure in terms of restoring satisfactory coronary flow was only 73%. Similarly, the pooled mortality rate from a series of surgical reports was 32%.[47] Both these mortality rates are significantly below historical mortality, but the possibility of marked selection bias is ever-present. The open artery hypothesis can be well tested in patients with cardiogenic shock; greatest risk = greatest gain. The need for clinical trials of revascularization therapy that are carefully designed and meticulously carried out is paramount.

Mural Thrombus

Ventricular thrombus develops in about 30% of patients with apical-anterior transmural MI. In patients at risk, it is reasonable to obtain an echocardiogram between the third and fifth days. If thrombus is present, intravenous heparin is given for several days, followed by warfarin (Coumadin) therapy for 3 months. Serial echocardiography is used to monitor the status of the thrombus and guide the discontinuance of anticoagulants.

Pericarditis

A transient friction rub is not uncommon in the first few days after transmural MI. Surprisingly, thrombolytic therapy does not increase the incidence of hemorrhagic pericardial effusion, a rare complication of MI in the pre-anticoagulant era. The pericarditis is generally self-limited, although the symptoms may be confused with those of recurrent ischemia or peptic ulcer disease. If rub and pericardial pain are persistent, treatment with a nonsteroidal anti-inflammatory agent such as indomethacin may be useful.

RECOVERY PHASE

Patients with uncomplicated MI may generally be discharged from the hospital in 5 to 7 days. Long-term prognosis is influenced by the extent of coronary artery disease, preservation of left ventricular function, age, and coexisting morbid factors, such as diabetes and the potential for malignant arrhythmia. Many authorities recommend either a submaximal exercise test prior to discharge or a symptom-limited exercise test 2 weeks or more after onset of acute MI to determine the patient's functional capacity and to identify, on the basis of poor response, patients who may be candidates for revascularization.[23] In the United States, patients treated in academic centers commonly undergo angiography and angioplasty prior to discharge, but this is not the practice in Canada.

After discharge, aspirin (81, 162.5, or 325 mg daily) should be continued to reduce mortality and the risk of subsequent reinfarction. Prophylactic administration of β-blockers reduces postinfarct mortality by 20% to 30%, although the possible benefit in low-risk patients is controversial. Maximum benefit occurs during the first year. Calcium channel blockers have not been shown to reduce postinfarct mortality in randomized clinical trials, although diltiazem may be of benefit in some low-risk groups with preserved left ventricular function. Patients with ventricular extrasystoles do not benefit from treatment with class I antiarrhythmias; indeed, randomized trials suggest that these agents actually increase mortality. Episodes of sustained ventricular tachycardia or recurrent cardiac arrest may need electrophysiologic testing. Treatment with amiodarone or an implantable defibrillator may be required.

Identification and modification of risk factors constitute a major component of postinfarct treatment. Cessation of smoking, management of hypertension, and normalization of cholesterol abnormality improve outcome. Growing evidence that successful cholesterol reduction retards progression and, to some extent, influences regression of atherosclerotic obstructive lesions should motivate both patients and doctors to maintain effective lipid-lowering therapy after infarction. As mentioned earlier, angiotensin-converting enzyme inhibitors reduce ventricular modeling, especially in patients with large anterior transmural MI, and should be initiated routinely within the first 24 hours in the absence of contraindications. ACE inhibitors may be discontinued after 6 to 8 weeks in patients who have normal ventricular function after MI but are continued, perhaps indefinitely, in the patient in whom the infarct has altered ventricular shape or reduced function.

References

1. Hajjar DP, Nicholson AC: Atherosclerosis. Am Sci 1995; 83:459-467.
2. Garfinkel E, Duronto E, Cerda M, et al: Patients with unstable angina related with C-reactive protein and *Chlamydia pneumoniae* infection (Abstract). Eur Heart J 1996; 17(Suppl):578.
3. Loscalzo J, Schafer AI: Overview of hemostasis and fibrinolysis. *In:* New Therapeutic Agents in Thrombosis and Thrombolysis. Sasahara AA, Loscalzo J (Ed). New York, NY: Marcel Dekker, 1997, pp 1-7.
4. Thieme T, Wernecke KD, Meyer R, et al: Angioscopic evaluation of atherosclerotic plaques: Validation by histomorphologic analysis and association with stable and unstable coronary syndromes. J Allergy Clin Immunol 1996; 28:1-6.
5. Willerson JT, Golino P, Eidt J, et al: Platelet mediators and unstable coronary artery disease. Circulation 1989; 80:198-205.
6. Fuster V, Badimon L, Badimon JJ, Chesebro JH: The pathophysiology of coronary artery disease and the acute coronary syndromes. N Engl J Med 1992; 326:242-250, 310-318.
7. Davies MJ, Woolf N, Robertson WB: Pathology of acute myocardial infarction with particular reference to occlusive coronary thrombi. Br Heart J 1976; 38:659-664.
8. Reimer KA, Lowe JE, Rasmussen MM, Jennings RB: The wave front phenomenon of ischemic cell death: Myocardial infarct size vs. duration of coronary occlusion in dogs. Circulation 1977; 56:786-794.
9. The GUSTO Investigators: An international randomized trial comparing four thrombolytic strategies for acute myocardial infarction. N Engl J Med 1993; 329:673-682.
10. The GUSTO Angiographic Investigators: The effects of tissue plasminogen activator, streptokinase, or both on coronary-artery patency, ventricular function, and survival after acute myocardial infarction. N Engl J Med 1993; 329:1615-1622.
11. Jeremy RW, Hackworthy RA, Bautovich G, et al: Infarct artery perfusion and changes in left ventricular volume in the month after acute myocardial infarction. J Am Coll Cardiol 1987; 9:989-995.
12. Fibrinolytic Therapy Trialists' (FTT) Collaborative Group: Indications for fibrinolytic therapy in suspected acute myocardial infarction: Collaborative overview of early mortality and major morbidity results from all randomized trials of more than 1,000 patients. Lancet 1994; 343:311-322. [Erratum, Lancet 1994; 343:742.]
13. Hochman JS, Choo H: Limitation of myocardial infarct expansion by reperfusion independent of myocardial salvage. Circulation 1987; 75:299-306.
14. Alonso DR, Scheidt S, Post M, et al: Pathophysiology of cardiogenic shock: Quantification of myocardial necrosis, clinical, pathologic and electrocardiographic correlation. Circulation 1973; 48:588-596.
15. GISSI (Gruppo Italiano per lo Studio della Streptochinasi nell'Infarto miocardico): Effectiveness of intravenous thrombolytic treatment in acute myocardial infarction. Lancet 1986; 1:397-401.
16. Sgarbossa EB, Pinski SL, Barbagelata A, et al: Electrocardiographic diagnosis of acute myocardial infarction in the presence of left bundle-branch block. Engl J Med 1996; 334:481-487.
17. Lee TH, Goldman L: Serum enzyme assays in the diagnosis of acute myocardial infarction: Recommendations based on a quantitative analysis. Ann Intern Med 1986; 105:221.
18. Gomez MA, Anderson JL, Karagounis LA, et al: An emergency department-based protocol for rapidly ruling out myocardial ischemia reduces hospital time and expense: Results of a randomized study (ROMIO). J Am Coll Cardiol 1996; 28:25-33.

18a. Roberts RR, Zalenski RJ, Menash EK, et al: Costs of an emergency department-based accelerated diagnostic protocol vs. hospitalization in patients with chest pain: A randomized controlled trial. JAMA 1997; 278:1670-1676.

19. Norris RM, Barnaby PF, Brandt PWT, et al: Prognosis after recovery from first acute myocardial infarction: Determinants of reinfarction and sudden death. Am J Cardiol 1984; 53:408.
20. Killip T, Kimball JT: Treatment of myocardial infarction in a coronary care unit: A two year experience with 250 patients. Am J Cardiol 1967; 20:457.
21. Alonzo AA: The impact of the family and lay others on care-seeking during life-threatening episodes of suspected coronary artery disease. Soc Sci Med 1986; 22:1297-1311.
22. ISIS-2 (Second International Study of Infarct Survival) Collaborative Group: Randomized trial of intravenous streptokinase, oral aspirin, both, or neither among 17, 187 cases of suspected acute myocardial infarction: ISIS-2. Lancet 1988; 2:349-360.

22a. Third International Study of Infarct Survival Collaborative Group (ISIS-3): A randomised comparison of streptokinase vs. tissue plasminogen activator vs. antistreplase and of aspirin plus heparin vs. aspirin alone among 41,299 cases of suspected acute myocardial infarction. Lancet 1992; 339:753-770.

23. Ryan T, Anderson J, Antman E, et al: ACC/AHA guidelines for the management of patients with acute myocardial infarction: A report of the American College of Cardiology/American Heart Association Task Force on Practice Guidelines (Committee on Management of Acute Myocardial Infarction). J Am Coll Cardiol 1996; 28:1328-1428.
24. Falk E, Shah PK, Fuster V: Coronary plaque disruption. Circulation 1995; 92:657-671.
25. Gruppo Italiano per lo Studio della Sopravvivenza nell'Infarto Miocardico: GISSIS: A factorial randomised trial of alteplase versus streptokinase and heparin versus no heparin among 12,490 patients with acute myocardial infarction. Lancet 1990; 336:65-71.
26. Collins R, Peto R, Baigent C, Sleight P: Aspirin, heparin, and fibrinolytic therapy in suspected myocardial infarction. N Engl J Med 1997; 336:847-860.
27. Topol EJ: Toward a new frontier in myocardial reperfusion therapy: Emerging platelet preeminence. Circulation 1998; 97:211-218.
28. Weaver WD, Simes JR, Betriu A, et al: Comparison of primary coronary angioplasty and intravenous thrombolytic therapy for acute myocardial infarction: A quantitative review. JAMA 1997; 278:2093-2098.
29. Cannon CP, Maraganore JM, Loscalzo J, et al: Anticoagulant effects of Hirulog, a novel thrombin inhibitor, in patients with coronary artery disease. Am J Cardiol 1993; 71:778-782.
30. Ohman EM, Slovak JP, Anderson RL, et al: Potent inhibition of thrombin with efegatran in combination with t-PA in acute myocardial infarction: Results of a multicenter randomized dose ranging trial (Abstract). Circulation 1996; 94:I-430.
31. Weaver WD, Fung A, Lorch G, et al: Efegatran and streptokinase vs. T-PA and heparin for treatment of acute MI (Abstract). Circulation 1996; 94:I-430.
32. Vermeer F, Vahanian A, Fels PW, et al: Intravenous argatroban versus heparin as co-medication to alteplase in the treatment of acute myocardial infarction: Preliminary results of the ARGAMI pilot study (Abstract). J Am Coll Cardiol 1997; 29:185A.
33. Fragmin during Instability in Coronary Artery Disease (FRISC) Study Group: Low-molecular-weight heparin during instability in coronary artery disease. Lancet 1996; 347:561-568.
34. Swahn E, Wallentin L, FRISC Study Group: Low-molecular-weight heparin (Fragmin) during instability in coronary artery disease (FRISC). Am J Cardiol 1977; 80(5A):25E-29E.
35. Cohen M, Demers C, Gurfinkel EP, et al: A comparison of low-molecular-weight heparin with unfractionated heparin for unstable coronary artery disease. N Engl J Med 1997; 337:447-452.
36. The Thrombolysis in Myocardial Infarction (TIMI) IIA Trial Investi-

gators: Dose-ranging trial of enoxaparin for unstable angina: Results of TIMI 11A. J Am Coll Cardiol 1997; 29:1474-1482.
37. The EPILOG Investigators: Platelet glycoprotein IIb/IIIa receptor blockade and low-dose heparin during percutaneous coronary revascularization. N Engl J Med 1997; 336:1689-1696.
38. The Platelet Receptor Inhibition in Ischemic Syndrome Management (PRISM) Study Investigators: A comparison of aspirin plus tirofiban with aspirin plus heparin for unstable angina. N Engl J Med 1998; 338:1498-1505.
38a. The Platelet Receptor Inhibition in Ischemic Syndrome Management in Patients Limited by Unstable Signs and Symptoms (PRISM-PLUS) Study Investigators: Inhibition of the platelet glycoprotein IIb/IIIa receptor with tirofiban in unstable angina and non-Q-wave myocardial infarction. N Engl J Med 1998; 338:1488-1497.
39. Parker JD, Parker JO: Nitrate therapy for stable angina pectoris. N Engl J Med 1998; 338:520-531.
40. ISIS-4: A randomized factorial trial assessing early captopril, oral mononitrate and intravenous magnesium sulphate in 58,050 patients with suspected myocardial infarction. Lancet 1995; 345:669-685.
41. Bolli R: Myocardial stunning in man. Circulation 1992; 86:1671-1690.
42. Tillisch J, Brunken R, Marschall R, et al: Reversibility of cardiac wall motion abnormalities predicted by positron tomography. N Engl J Med 1986; 314:884-888.
43. Zehender M, Kasper W, Kander E, et al: Right ventricular infarction as an independent predictor of prognosis after acute inferior infarction. N Engl J Med 1993; 328:982-988.
44. Robalino BD, Whitlow PL, Underwood DA, Salcedo EE: Electrocardiographic manifestations of right ventricular infarction. Am Heart J 1989; 118:138-144.
45. Goldberg RJ, Gore JM, Alpert JS, et al: Cardiogenic shock after acute myocardial infarction: Incidence and mortality from a community-wide perspective, 1975-1988. N Engl J Med 1991; 325:1117-1122.
46. Hochman JS, Boland J, Sleeper LA, et al, and the SHOCK Registry Investigators: Current spectrum of cardiogenic shock and effect of early revascularization on mortality: Results of an international registry. Circulation 1995; 91:873-881.
47. Hochman JS: Cardiogenic shock: Can we save the patient? Am Coll Cardiol Ed Highlights 1996; 12:1-5.

92

Contemporary Thrombolytic Therapy in Acute Myocardial Infarction

Yves Janin, MD • Michael L. Hess, MD, FACC

Disruption of an atherosclerotic plaque allows blood to enter and expand the plaque and exposes its highly thrombogenic lipid and collagen core, resulting in activation of the thrombotic cascade and in platelet adhesion and activation. Endothelial dysfunction, vasospasm, low endogenous fibrinolytic activity, increased catecholamine levels, high shear flow rates across the site of plaque disruption, increasing thrombus burden, obstruction to coronary arterial flow, and decreasing coronary perfusion pressure with resultant stasis in the vicinity of the plaque result in total coronary arterial occlusion and an acute myocardial infarction (MI). The recognition that thrombotic coronary artery occlusion is invariably present in the early stages of acute myocardial infarction[1] and the observation that the infusion of thrombolytic agents within the infarct-related artery early after the onset of symptoms result in recanalization of the occluded coronary artery[2] have led to the development of thrombolytic therapy for the acute management of MI.

HUMAN TISSUE-TYPE PLASMINOGEN ACTIVATOR

Human tissue-type plasminogen activator (t-PA), a 68-kD_a serine protease, is a 527 amino acid glycoprotein, organized by 17 disulfide bridges into a series of five discrete, essentially autonomous, independently folded, structural domains that are strikingly homologous to domains found in other secreted and cell surface proteins.[3] Approximately 10% of its molecular mass is due to carbohydrate.[4]

Residues 4 to 50 of the t-PA molecule form a "Finger" domain (F), which is closely related to the fibrin-binding Finger structure of fibronectin and is extremely stable.[4]

Residues 51 to 87 form a domain that is homologous with the epidermal growth factor (EGF) domain and with urokinase (u-PA), another plasminogen activator.

Residues 88 to 175 (Kringle 1) and 176 to 263 (Kringle 2) form two contiguous domains, each built around three intradomain disulfide bridges. They have thermodynamic properties similar to those of the kringles in plasminogen.[4] The determinants of clearance are located within the Kringle 1 domain.[5]

Residues 277 to 527, the serine protease domain, constitute the catalytic domain, which is homologous with members of the chymotrypsin family of serine proteases. It contains two modules that interact cooperatively with each other at neutral pH and are "de-cooperated" at low pH or by removal of the Finger/EGF region.[4]

The five domains of t-PA are encoded by a total of 12 exons, of which only the fibronectin-like Finger domain and the EGF-like domain, which mediate the high-affinity binding of t-PA to fibrin, are each entirely coded by unique single exons that have been incorporated into a large number of genes coding for multidomain extracellular proteins, including t-PA, u-PA, protein C, and factors IX and X.[6]

t-PA consists of a single-chain polypeptide that, on activation via hydrolysis of the Arg^{275}-Ile^{276} peptide bond, assumes a two-chain form.[7] t-PA is unusual in the family of serine proteases because it is active in both the single-chain and the two-chain forms, whereas most of the others exist as zymogens and require proteolytic cleavage to a two-chain form in order to release full enzymatic activity. Provided that they are bound to fibrin, both the single-chain and double-chain t-PA have equal potency.[8]

t-PA has only one substrate in vivo: the zymogen plasminogen. By cleaving a single peptide bond, Arg^{560}-Val^{561}, t-PA converts inactive plasminogen into the voracious protease; plasmin, which solubilizes the cross-linked fibrin that forms the meshwork of blood clots.[8]

Deletion of the Kringle 2 domain results in a threefold decrease in affinity of t-PA for fibrin and a twofold increase in the number of Finger domain-specific binding sites. Thus, the presence of both the Finger domain and Kringle 2 prevents the utilization of one binding site on a fibrin monomer.[8] The Finger domain is essential for the efficient initiation of fibrinolysis.

t-PA binds to fibrin by simultaneously using the Finger domain and Kringle 2, via a Finger domain-specific binding site and an internal lysine residue in the vicinity of that binding site.[8] Once bound, the t-PA molecule becomes fixed on the fibrin polymer in a specific correct orientation to yield a high-affinity binding site for Glu-plasminogen, which binds exclusively and with high affinity to the t-PA-fibrin complex at the end-to-end junction between two fibrin or fragment X molecules in the protofibril, resulting in a ternary complex that converts plasminogen to plasmin. The digestion of fibrin by plasmin releases carboxyl-terminal lysine residues to which plasminogen binds, resulting in a conformational change that is more readily activated by t-PA than solution-phase Glu-plasminogen. These lysine residues also bind to t-PA, via the lysine binding site of Kringle 2, and increase ternary complex formation.[8]

t-PA is a poor enzyme in the absence of fibrin, but the presence of fibrin strikingly enhances the activation rate of plasminogen by a factor of 1000.[9] Plasmin formed on the fibrin surface has both its lysine binding site and its active site occupied, and it is only slowly inactivated by α_2-antiplasmin; free plasmin, when formed, is rapidly inhibited by α_2-antiplasmin. Extremely high plasminogen concentrations of 15 μM (10 times the physiologic concentration in plasma) have been demonstrated in the superficial layer of a partially degraded fibrin clot.[10]

The specific activity of Alteplase is 550,000 to 667,000 IU/mg.[11] The therapeutic dose of t-PA in the accelerated t-PA regimen used for intravenous administration in acute myocardial infarction is 100 mg.

Large quantities of t-PA (48 million to 60 million units) are necessary to dissolve occlusive thrombi because t-PA is cleared extremely quickly from the circulation. The elimination of t-PA from the plasma is biphasic, with the half-life of the initial faster phase being 3 to 6 minutes in humans.[3] t-PA variants in which the Finger or EGF-like domains are deleted are ineffective plasminogen activators at physiologic concentrations, but they behave similarly to wild type t-PA at the steady-state plasma concentrations required for coronary reperfusion in acute myocardial infarction.[12, 13] Platelets contain large amounts of plasminogen activator inhibitor-1 (PAI-1), which is the principal endogenous inhibitor of t-PA. The second-order rate constant for association of PAI-1 with t-PA is extremely high and accounts for the initial, fast phase, inhibition of t-PA by human plasma. Residues 296 to 302 and 304 are not involved in the catalytic functions of t-PA, but they play an important role in the interaction of t-PA with its cognate serpin PAI-1.[14]

The major site of removal and catabolism of t-PA is the liver, where parenterally administered t-PA accumulates rapidly and is then degraded over several hours. Two types of hepatic cells are involved in this process. The *endothelial cells*, which clear 40% of wild-type t-PA, carry mannose receptors that recognize asparagine-linked mannose-rich oligosaccharides on circulating glycoproteins and the mannose-rich oligosaccharide of t-PA attached to [117]asparagine in Kringle 1.[3] The hepatic *parenchymal cells* have a specific t-PA receptor, the low-density lipoprotein receptor-related protein that is identical to the α_2-macroglobulin receptor and that recognizes the tyrosine[67] residue of the EGF-like domain of t-PA. This receptor binds free t-PA with moderate efficiency and complexes it with very high affinity to PAI-1.

GOAL OF REPERFUSION THERAPY

In patients with acute MI, rapid restoration of unrestricted antegrade flow in the infarct-related artery has been established as the primary determinant of an improved clinical outcome.[15] A meta-analysis of TEAM-2,[16] TEAM-3,[17] four German multicenter studies,[18] the GUSTO* angiographic substudy,[19, 20] and the TAMI† trials,[21] and five prospective, controlled thrombolytic therapy studies of acute MI of adequate size, requiring ST-segment elevation at entry and using early (< 24 hours) angiography, revealed that optimal outcome was only achieved with the restoration of TIMI* perfusion grade 3 flow in the infarct-related artery.[22] For the combined study,[22] there was a significantly lower mortality (in-hospital or 30-day) in patients with TIMI grade 3 flow (3.7%) compared with both: patients with TIMI grade 2 flow (7.0%) and with TIMI grade 0/1 flow (8.8%). Times to enzymatic peaks from initiation of thrombolytic therapy were significantly reduced in patients who achieved TIMI grade 3 flow compared with those with TIMI grades below 3. The left ventricular ejection fraction was significantly higher with TIMI grade 3 (TIMI-3) flow than with TIMI grade 2 flow (a difference of 4 to 5 percentage points), and there was a significant improvement in regional wall motion in patients with TIMI grade 3 compared with TIMI grade 2 flow.[22] Thus, early and complete restoration of flow in the infarct-related artery is associated with a significantly improved survival and clinical outcome.

*GUSTO = Global Utilization of Streptokinase and Tissue Plasminogen Activator for Occluded Arteries trial.

†TAMI = Thrombolysis and Angioplasty in Myocardial Infarction trial.

Once the clinical diagnosis of acute MI has been established, a question needs to be resolved: Is the patient a candidate for thrombolytic therapy?

SPECIAL CONSIDERATIONS

Time to Treatment

Because the evolution of myocardial necrosis in acute MI and the myocardial salvage following restoration of coronary blood flow are time-dependent, thrombolytic therapy should be administered as soon as possible if there are no contraindications (Table 92–1).[23, 24]

In the TIMI-2 trial,[24] each hour gained in the administration of the thrombolytic agent resulted in a 1% decrease in the absolute mortality and in 10 lives saved per 1000 patients treated. In GUSTO-I,[25, 26] irrespective of the thrombolytic randomization, a delay in the time to thrombolysis from the time of symptom onset adversely affected mortality and the development of heart failure and cardiogenic shock. Similarly, in the Late Assessment of Thrombolytic Efficacy (LATE) study,[26] patients with acute MI and ST-segment elevation who were treated with recombinant t-PA (rt-PA) less than 3 hours after hospital admission had a significantly lower mortality rate at 1 year than did those treated after 3 hours (Table 92–2).

In a systematic overview of nine major trials that randomized more than 1000 patients between fibrinolytic therapy and control, the Fibrinolytic Therapy Trialists' (FTT) Collaborative Group[27] reported that among the 45,000 patients presenting with ST-segment elevation or left bundle branch block, the relation between benefit and delay from symptom onset indicated a highly significant mortality reduction (1.6 additional

*TIMI = Thrombolysis in Myocardial Infarction.

TABLE 92–1. Indications for Thrombolytic Therapy

1. Chest pain lasting longer than 20 min
   and
2. ST-segment elevations ≧1 mm in two contiguous leads
   or
   ST-segment depressions in leads V_1 and V_2 consistent with a posterior myocardial infarction
   and
3. *Time:* Onset of the pain to diagnosis of acute myocardial infarction
   Less than 12 hours: all patients
   12–24 hours: patients with persistent chest pain and patients at high risk

TABLE 92–2. Key Points in the Use of Thrombolytic Therapy in Acute Myocardial Infarction

1. Time to administration is critical. Each hour gained to administration results in a 1% decrease in mortality.
2. Age is not a contraindication. Elderly patients (>75 yr) demonstrate an improvement in survival but with an *increased* incidence of stroke.
3. Suspected occlusion of saphenous vein grafts: angioplasty preferred. If angioplasty is unavailable, administer thrombolytic therapy.
4. Mortality rates tend to be higher in women with comorbidity, but successful thrombolytic therapy produces equivalent benefits.
5. Although thrombolytic therapy can prevent cardiogenic shock, it is not the preferred treatment. Primary angioplasty is preferred.

lives saved per 1000 patients treated, for each hour earlier that treatment began) of about 30 per 1000 for those presenting within 0 to 6 hours and of about 20 per 1000 for those presenting 7 to 12 hours from onset and a statistically uncertain benefit of about 10 per 1000 for those presenting at 13 to 18 hours. Although later treatment was associated with a larger excess of deaths on days 0 to 1, mortality reduction during days 2 to 35 was little affected by the time patients were treated.[28] The LATE study[26] evaluated the effect of t-PA in a double-blind randomized fashion in 5711 patients with acute MI presenting 6 to 24 hours after onset of symptoms. Patients who were treated within 12 hours of symptom onset had a significant 25.6% reduction in mortality at 35 days of follow-up.

In the TAMI-6 Study, patients with ST-segment elevation on electrocardiography, presenting 6 to 24 hours after the onset of symptoms, who were randomly assigned to t-PA had a significantly higher infarct-related artery patency at 24 hours, but in-hospital and 6-month mortality rates were similar as the patients were randomly assigned to placebo.[29, 30] Although there was no difference in ejection fraction at the 6-month follow-up in the two groups, only the placebo group exhibited a significant increase in median end-diastolic volume as compared with the acute phase.[30]

During the evolution of an acute MI, a variable combination of coronary arterial thrombosis and vasoconstriction frequently result in spontaneous intermittent coronary artery recanalization and reocclusion.[31] Spontaneous reperfusion of the occluded infarct-related artery occurs in 13% to 20% of patients and contributes to the limitation of infarct size.[1, 30, 32, 33] The stress of the clinical condition itself results in an increase in epinephrine levels, which in turn activates platelets.[34] These patients present with a longer duration of stuttering chest pain and may still have viable myocardium in the territory of the infarct-related artery.

In the presence of collateral vessels to the infarct-related artery, viability of the acutely ischemic myocardium may be preserved, especially at the periphery of the jeopardized territory.[35–37] In these patients, late administration of thrombolytics may salvage this ischemic but viable water-shed zone.

Late restoration of the patency of the infarct-related artery is better than persistent occlusion. An open artery following MI is the most significant predictor of long-term survival in patients with single-vessel disease.[38–41] Late administration of thrombolytics in patients with acute MI that involves a large territory in the presence of continuing chest pain, by opening the infarct related artery, (1) reduces the extent of left ventricular remodeling, cavity dilatation, and wall stress[30, 42]; (2) decreases the electrical instability of the myocardium[43]; and (3) provides a possible source of collateral flow to other coronary arterial territories.

Elderly Patients

In older patients, the in-hospital mortality rate is much greater than in the overall group of patients with MI, with almost a fourfold increased risk in the "oldest" compared to the "youngest" subgroups in three large major trials.[44–46] In ISIS-2,* the mortality rate of patients older than age 80 years, who were treated with streptokinase and aspirin, decreased from 37% to 20%, a 46% reduction.[44] In the GUSTO trial,[46] the 30-day mortality rate of patients older than age 75 years, treated with accelerated t-PA and intravenous heparin, was 19.1% but a rate of 20.2% in those who received streptokinase and intravenous heparin; the respective 30-day mortality rates for patients age 75 years or younger were 4.4% and 5.5%. Thus, although the relative mortality reduction following therapy with accelerated t-PA and intravenous heparin was smaller (6% versus 20%) in patients older than 75 years, the absolute reduction was similar to that of patients 75 years or younger.

When older patients receive thrombolytic therapy, the incidence of intracerebral hemorrhage and infarction is higher than in younger patients. In the accelerated t-PA with intravenous heparin branch of the GUSTO trial,[46] patients older than age 75 had a 4% incidence of all strokes and a 2% incidence of hemorrhagic strokes; in patients 75 years or younger treated in the same manner, the respective incidences were 1.2% and 0.5%, respectively.

In the GUSTO trial,[46] the incidence of the combined 30-day mortality or nonfatal stroke in patients older than 75 years was 20.6% for those treated with accelerated t-PA and intravenous heparin and 21.5% for those treated with streptokinase and intravenous heparin, a 0.9% reduction. Among patients aged 75 years or younger, the combined incidence of death or nonfatal stroke was 5.2% for those treated with accelerated t-PA and intravenous heparin and 6.3% for those who received streptokinase and intravenous heparin, a 1.1% reduction. Thus, although the incidence of intracerebral hemorrhage and infarction is increased in patients older than 75 years who are treated with accelerated t-PA and intravenous heparin, there is a clear-cut favorable net clinical benefit, with nine fewer deaths or nonfatal strokes per 1000 patients compared with 11 fewer deaths or nonfatal strokes in patients aged 75 years or younger.

Right Ventricular Infarction

The right ventricle, compared with the left, is less prone to infarction and better able to tolerate prolonged ischemia without necrosis, thus making these patients attractive candidates for reperfusion.[29] Patients with right ventricular infarction have a stiff, noncompliant ventricle that is dependent on high filling pressures and that may not tolerate the reduction in preload induced by nitroglycerin. Cardiogenic shock associated with right ventricular infarction is characterized by high right atrial pressures and normal or low left ventricular filling pressures.

Treatment involves the rapid administration of large volumes of fluid in order to achieve a pulmonary capillary wedge pressure of 18 to 20 mm Hg. Patients who remain hypotensive after volume loading may be treated with the infusion of the inotropic agent dobutamine, the insertion of an intra-aortic balloon pump, and primary coronary angioplasty.

*Second International Study of Infarct Survival.

Prior Coronary Artery Bypass Graft Surgery

In the GUSTO trial, patients with acute MI who have had a previous coronary artery bypass graft surgery (CABG) procedure had a significantly higher 24-hour, 30-day, and 1-year mortality rate than patients without prior CABG surgery.[47] These patients also had a significantly higher incidence of complications, including cardiogenic shock, pulmonary edema, recurrent ischemia, and reinfarction.

In about two thirds of the patients with prior CABG who later have an acute MI, the culprit vessel is a vein graft that is frequently occluded by a large thrombus. Grines and coworkers[47] reported that after intravenous thrombolytic therapy, successful reperfusion occurred in only two of eight grafts (25%) but intragraft thrombolysis or angioplasty restored flow in eight of 10 grafts (80%) (see Chapter 93). In a series of 130 patients with prior CABG and MI, O'Keefe and colleagues[48] reported that primary angioplasty was associated with an 86% success rate in vein grafts and a similar in-hospital mortality rate in patients with or without previous CABG (see Chapter 93). If a cardiac catheterization laboratory is rapidly available, acute MI patients with prior CABG should undergo primary angioplasty. If there are no catheterization facilities, the patient should receive thrombolytic therapy.

Gender

The GUSTO-I trial[30] has shown that even though women were significantly older; had more hypertension, diabetes, hypercholesterolemia, heart failure, and shock; and had a significantly higher 30-day mortality than men, they demonstrated a similar 90-minute patency rate (TIMI-3 flow) of the infarct-related artery, a similar 90-minute ejection fraction, and regional ventricular function in the presence of TIMI-2 or TIMI-3 flow and no significant difference in left ventricular function at 5- to 7-day follow-up (see Table 92–2).

Cardiogenic Shock

Cardiogenic shock is an uncommon complication of acute MI. It was associated with a mortality rate of about 80% in the prethrombolytic era and still carries a grave prognosis, with an in-hospital mortality of 56%.[49, 50] In the GUSTO-I trial,[50] cardiogenic shock was present in 0.77% of the enrolled patients on arrival and developed in 6.5% of the patients after hospital admission. In patients treated with accelerated rt-PA, cardiogenic shock was much less likely to develop than in patients treated with the other thrombolytic regimens, thus making rt-PA the preferred thrombolytic agent for prevention of cardiogenic shock.[49] However, rt-PA was less effective in patients presenting in cardiogenic shock, possibly because when coronary perfusion pressure is low, the efficacy of the thrombolysis is limited by the diffusion constraints of the thrombolytic agent[51] and by the passive collapse of the compliant zones of the infarct-related artery.[52]

An aggressive strategy of early angiography and revascularization in the GUSTO-I patients with acute MI and cardiogenic shock who received thrombolytic therapy was associated with a significant reduction in 30-day and 1-year mortality.[50] Early institution of an intra-aortic balloon pump was associated with a trend toward a lower 30-day and 1-year all-cause mortality despite an increased risk of bleeding and adverse events.[53]

Therefore, if an experienced cardiac catherization laboratory is immediately available, patients in cardiogenic shock should undergo emergency coronary angiography and revascularization as indicated. If an experienced cardiac catheterization laboratory is not available, or if there is going to be a delay before angiography, thrombolytic therapy should be administered and insertion of an intra-aortic balloon pump in the presence of refractory cardiogenic shock should be considered.

Hypertension

Patients with acute MI who present with hypertension should not be routinely excluded from thrombolytic therapy. Indeed, in ISIS-II, among the 1141 patients who presented with a systolic blood pressure greater than 175 mm Hg, streptokinase therapy resulted in a mortality rate of 5.7% in contrast to a rate of 8.7% in the placebo group[54] (Table 92–3).

Hypertensive patients whose systolic blood pressure drops to below 180 mm Hg and whose diastolic blood pressure decreases below 105 mm Hg after therapy with morphine, nitrates, and β blockers should be considered for thrombolytic therapy. Patients who remain severely hypertensive (systolic blood pressure > 200 mm Hg, diastolic blood pressure > 110 mm Hg) should be referred for cardiac catheterization and primary angioplasty.

Cardiopulmonary Resuscitation

Patients who have sustained a cardiac arrest and require less than 10 minutes of cardiopulmonary resuscitation (CPR) should not be excluded from receiving thrombolytic therapy.[55] In a review of 59 patients from the first three TAMI trials, who required less than 10 minutes of CPR before receiving thrombolytic therapy or within 6 hours of treatment, Tenaglia and coauthors found no bleeding complications directly attributable to CPR. In the 60-Minutes Myocardial Infarction Project from Germany,[18] thrombolysis in nonrandomized CPR patients with acute MI and without a left bundle branch block was independently associated with a significantly lower hospital mortality despite an increased incidence of bleeding complications. However, patients who undergo prolonged CPR or who have an altered mental state after CPR should be referred for primary angioplasty (see Table 92–3).

Peptic Ulcer Disease

A history of gastrointestinal bleeding in the preceding 2 months is a relative contraindication to thrombolytic therapy. However, since a well-treated peptic ulcer should heal within

TABLE 92–3. Contraindications to Thrombolytic Therapy

Absolute
Active internal bleeding
Previous intracranial bleeding, cerebral neoplasm, or major intracranial pathology
Stroke or head trauma within 6 months
Known allergy to the thrombolytic agent
Aortic dissection
Acute pericarditis
History of serious bleeding tendency
Relative
Surgery or gastrointestinal bleeding within 2 months
Pregnancy or within 1 month post partum
Severe, persistent hypertension (diastolic blood pressure > 100 mm Hg)
Trauma including cardiopulmonary resuscitation with rib fractures within 2 weeks
Hemorrhagic retinopathy
Bleeding diathesis or concurrent use of oral anticoagulants
Active peptic ulcer disease

1 month, patients with a treated peptic ulcer may be considered for thrombolytic therapy if they have had no evidence of bleeding in the preceding month (see Table 92–3).

Diabetic Retinopathy

Patients with diabetes mellitus have an increased incidence of coronary artery disease and have a worse clinical outcome following an acute MI.[56] In the GUSTO-I trial, none of the 6011 diabetic patients had a clinically recognized intraocular hemorrhage, and the upper 95% confidence interval (CI) for the incidence of intraocular hemorrhage in these patients was 0.05%.[56] Diabetic retinopathy, therefore, should not be considered a contraindication to thrombolysis in patients with acute MI.

Menstruation

Menstruation is not a contraindication to thrombolytic therapy and is not associated with an increase in risk of severe bleeding.[57] However, there may be a clinically significant increase in the risk of moderate vaginal bleeding not linked with any adverse outcome in GUSTO-I (Table 92–4).[57]

Other Relative Contraindications

Puncture of a subclavian or jugular vein is not an absolute contraindication to thrombolysis, but it can result in noncompressible bleeding and airway compromise.[58] Patients who have been taking warfarin may be at increased risk for bleeding.[54, 59] In the presence of a left ventricular thrombus, thrombolytic therapy may result in partial lysis and embolization of thrombus fragments.

DOSING AND ADMINISTRATION

If there are contraindications for thrombolytic therapy, the patient should be immediately referred for emergency primary cardiac catheterization and angioplasty (see Table 92–3 and Chapter 93). In the absence of contraindications to thrombolytic therapy, the accelerated t-PA regimen[60, 61] should be ordered and immediately administered. Accelerated t-PA is administered as an intravenous bolus of 15 mg, followed by an infusion of 50 mg or 0.75 mg/kg over the next 30 minutes, then by an infusion of 35 mg or 50 mg/kg administered over 60 minutes, for a total of up to 100 mg given over 90 minutes (see Table 92–5).

To ensure delivery of the thrombolytic agent to the thrombus in the infarct-related artery, an adequate coronary perfusion pressure must be ensured and hypotension aggressively treated. All patients should receive aspirin in the absence of major contraindications (Table 92–5).

TABLE 92–4. Special Considerations in Regard to Thrombolytic Therapy in the Presence of Comorbidity

1. Hypertension is *not* a contraindication. Treated blood pressure < 180/105 mm Hg: safe to proceed. Blood pressure > 180/105 mm Hg: refer for primary angioplasty.
2. CPR: If < 10 minutes in duration, proceed with thrombolysis: > 10 minutes or altered mental status, refer for primary angioplasty.
3. Active peptic ulcer disease within the previous 2 months: a relative contraindication.
4. Diabetic retinopathy and menstruation are *not* contraindications.
5. For patients taking warfarin (Coumadin), for patients who have undergone subclavian or jugular vein puncture, or in known thrombus, be very *careful.*

TABLE 92–5. Dosing and Administration

1. Accelerated t-PA: IV bolus of 15 mg followed by 50 mg or 0.75 mg/kg over 30 minutes; then 35–50 mg/kg over the next 60 minutes, for a total of up to 1000 mg over 90 minutes.
2. All patients should receive aspirin (e.g., 325 mg).
3. Coadministration of heparin 5000-unit bolus followed by 1000 units/hr IV. Target a PTT = 50–70 sec at 12 hr from initiation of therapy.

t-PA = tissue plasminogen activator; PTT = partial thromboplastin time.

Attempts have been made to modify the rt-PA dosing protocol in order to facilitate its administration and to improve its reperfusion success rate.[62, 63]

In the continuous infusion versus double-bolus administration of alteplase trial,[62] 7169 patients with acute MI were randomly assigned to weight-adjusted, accelerated infusion of 100 mg of alteplase or to a bolus of 50 mg of alteplase over 1 to 3 minutes, followed 30 minutes later by a second bolus of 50 mg. The trial was stopped because of the poorer clinical outcomes in the double-bolus group. Mortality at 30 days, the primary end point, was higher with two bolus doses of alteplase (7.98%) than with an accelerated infusion of alteplase (7.53%), resulting in an absolute difference of 0.44%, with a one-sided 95% upper boundary of 1.49%, which was not significant. There was, however, no significant difference in the rate of stroke, bleeding complications, and major cardiac events and procedures at 30 days between the two groups.

Gulba and coworkers[62] used computer simulation models of the plasma rt-PA levels to develop a new 60-minute alteplase dosing regimen designed to produce a high rt-PA plasma concentration that is maintained over 60 minutes, an initially high peak rt-PA plasma level, and maintenance below the rt-PA threshold, beyond which "plasminogen steal" occurs.[63] This new protocol involved administration of rt-PA as an intravenous bolus of 20 mg, followed immediately by a continuous infusion of an additional 80 mg of rt-PA over 60 minutes, together with a concomitant infusion of heparin designed to maintain the activated partial thromboplastin time (aPTT) between 50 and 80 seconds. The dose was administered to 254 patients presenting within 6 hours of the onset of symptoms. At coronary angiography performed 90 minutes after the start of therapy, TIMI grade 3 flow and total patency (TIMI grades 2 and 3 flow) of the infarct-related artery were found in 81.1% and 87% of the patients, respectively. This new dosing protocol awaits further study in larger, double-blind multicenter trials.

Antithrombotic Therapy: Heparin

Administration of a thrombolytic agent results in lysis of the thrombus and exposure of the various thrombogenic portions of the ruptured plaque, including its highly thrombogenic lipid core. Furthermore, thrombolytic therapy results in a marked activation of thrombin.[64, 66] Thrombin bound to fibrin remains active[67] and is released during fibrinolysis as thrombin-bound fibrin degradation products which retain the capacity to convert fibrinogen to fibrin and activate platelets.[67, 68] As successive layers of fibrin are removed, inaccessible molecules of thrombin are exposed at the surface of the residual clot and contribute to the occurrence of coagulation during thrombolytic therapy.

In a study of 55 patients with acute MI who were treated with urokinase or t-PA and underwent coronary angiography at 90 minutes and 24 to 36 hours, Gulba and colleagues[69] found that although thrombin-antithrombin III complex levels decreased in patients with persistent patency, they increased in the patients undergoing unsuccessful thrombolysis and in those with early reocclusion. Thus, the use of intravenous heparin is of paramount importance in inactivating the free thrombin formed in the vicinity of the lysing thrombus and, thus, in decreasing the incidence of reocclusion.

Heparin should be administered as a 5000-unit bolus, followed by a 1000 unit/hour intravenous infusion. In patients who weigh less than 80 kg, the initial heparin infusion rate should be 800-units/kg. The aPTT should be determined 6 hours later. The heparin infusion rate should be adjusted to achieve a target aPTT of 60 to 70 seconds, since in the GUSTO-I trial an aPTT that ranged from 50 to 70 seconds at 12 hours from initiation of therapy was associated with the lowest rates for 30-day mortality, stroke, and bleeding.[70] In patients who receive thrombolytics, the lytic state can produce a transient coagulation defect that can prolong the aPTT for up to 24 hours. Therefore, the dose of heparin should be adjusted upward only in the first 12 hours if it is below the therapeutic range. The heparin infusion should be discontinued after 48 hours unless other indications, such as post-MI angina, atrial fibrillation, left ventricular mural thrombus, severely depressed left ventricular systolic function, large anterior MI, or deep venous thrombosis dictate a more prolonged course of heparinization.

Results

Accelerated t-PA with immediate intravenous heparin in the GUSTO-I trial[25] was associated with a small but significant decrease of 9 per 1000 in mortality, a decrease of 7 per 1000 of borderline significance in the prespecified combined clinical end point of death and nonfatal stroke, and a significant excess of cerebral hemorrhage of 2.3 per 1000. The 24-hour mortality in group receiving activated t-PA with intravenous heparin was 2.4%, which was significantly lower than in either of the streptokinase treatment arms of the trial. The 30-day mortality rate with accelerated t-PA with intravenous heparin was 6.3%, which was significantly lower than in either of the two streptokinase regimens. Patients aged 75 years or younger had a 30-day mortality of 4.4% compared with a 30-day mortality of 19.1% in those older than 75 years.

Multivariate analysis of the predictors of mortality in the GUSTO-I patients[71] identified five baseline characteristics that were significantly associated with an increased 30-day mortality:

- Age
- Lower systolic blood pressure
- Higher Killip class
- Elevated heart rate
- Anterior infarction

Of these, age was the most significant factor influencing 30-day mortality with rates of 1.1% in patients younger than 45 years and 20.5% in patients older than 75 years.

The 90-minute angiographic coronary patency rate (TIMI grade 3 or 2) in the GUSTO angiographic study[19] was 81% with accelerated t-PA and heparin, with more than two thirds of the patent infarct-related arteries having TIMI grade 3 flow (normal flow) but with only a 54% total incidence of TIMI grade 3 flow reperfusion. The 30-day mortality rate for patients with a completely open (TIMI grade 3) infarct-related artery at 90 minutes was 4.2% in contrast to 8.2% for patients with a closed artery (TIMI grade 0/1). In addition, patients who had normal coronary flow at 90 minutes had a significantly lower mortality rate than those who had TIMI grade 0, 1, or 2 flow at 90 minutes.[19] The accelerated t-PA with heparin GUSTO group included a significantly higher percentage of patients with preserved regional wall motion at 90 minutes and at 5 to 7 days compared with the streptokinase groups. However, there was no statistically significant difference in left ventricular ejection fraction in all three treatment groups at each time interval. The ventricular function at 90 minutes was strongly related to survival. In patients with an ejection fraction less or equal to 45%, 30-day survival rate was 85.3%; in patients with an ejection fraction greater than 45%, 30-day survival rate was 96.1%.[19]

COMPLICATIONS

Failure to Recanalize the Infarct-Related Artery

Exposure of the ruptured atherosclerotic plaque, with its highly thrombogenic portions, high-grade coronary artery stenosis, large thrombus burden, marked thrombin activation, platelet activation with release of vasoactive amines and procoagulant substances, platelet thrombi, vasospasm, and decreased coronary perfusion pressure, contributes to decreasing the efficiency of thrombolysis, thus leading to a failure to recanalize the infarct-related artery.

In the TIMI trials,[72] 179 (25%) of 723 patients with acute MI who were treated within 6 hours of the onset of symptoms with either t-PA, urokinase, or a combination, failed to achieve patency of the infarct-related artery at 90 minutes after thrombolytic therapy. In the GUSTO trial,[19] 52 (19%) of the 272 patients who received an accelerated infusion of rt-PA with heparin had an occluded (TIMI grade 0/1 flow) infarct-related artery at 90 minutes.

Persistence or reccurrence of the chest pain and of the electrocardiographic manifestations of acute MI, after the administration of the thrombolytic and implementation of the adjunctive therapy, is an indication for rescue angioplasty. The occurrence at any time of hemodynamic instability, cardiogenic shock, or acute pulmonary edema is an indication for emergency primary or rescue angioplasty.

Bleeding

The main complication of thrombolytic therapy is bleeding, and the most dreaded and disastrous one is intracerebral hemorrhage. From a combined analysis of five studies, Simoons and colleagues[71] collected 150 patients with documented intracranial hemorrhage. By multivariate analysis, they found that age over 65 years, body weight below 70 kg, hypertension on hospital admission, and administration of t-PA were the four independent predictors of risk for intracranial bleeding. In the GUSTO trial[25], the combined incidence of intracerebral hemorrhage and infarction among the 10,376 patients treated with accelerated t-PA and intravenous heparin was 1.6%, with a 4% incidence in patients older than 75 years and a 1.2% incidence in those aged 75 years or younger. Stroke was associated with a high mortality rate. In the total GUSTO study, 41% of all strokes were fatal and 31% were disabling. The incidence of severe or life-threatening bleeding was significantly lower (0.9%) with the accelerated t-PA with intravenous heparin regimen compared with the two streptokinase regimens.[25]

The combined 30-day mortality or nonfatal stroke in the accelerated t-PA with intravenous heparin arm of the GUSTO trial was 7.2%. This figure was significantly reduced in contrast to a combined 30-day mortality or nonfatal stroke incidence of 8.2% in the streptokinase with intravenous heparin group and an incidence of 8% in the streptokinase with subcutaneous heparin group.

Univariate analysis in patients treated with 100 mg of rt-PA in the TIMI-II trial revealed increased frequencies of major and of major or minor hemorrhagic events with weight below 70 kg, female gender, a history of hypertension, a 5-hour fibrinogen level below 100 mg/dL, a 50-minute rt-PA plasma level above 1500 mg/dL, and physical signs of cardiac decompensation. Of these characteristics, a history of hypertension was the most prevalent one associated with major bleeding.[72]

In the GUSTO-I trial,[73] multivariate analysis revealed that the four independent and most powerful predictors of bleeding after thrombolytic therapy were, in order, older age, lighter body weight, female sex, and African ancestry. Worsening in Killip class was related to a significant increase in the incidence of bleeding complications for patients in the United States but not for patients elsewhere. The most common sources of moderate and severe bleeding were procedure-related, and the most common site of spontaneous bleeding was the gastrointestinal tract. By multivariate analysis, adjusting for the baseline characteristics of the patients, hypertension was not a significant independent predictor of the risk of bleeding.

Reocclusion

The following factors contribute to reocclusion of an infarct-related artery:

- Incomplete thrombolysis
- Persistence of a highly thrombogenic focus in the arterial wall
- High shear rates across a significant residual stenosis
- Plasminogen and platelet activation
- Inadequate antithrombin therapy

A meta-analysis of 28 studies of thrombolytic therapy for acute MI with three angiograms (one with an occluded artery, one with a reperfused artery, and a third for the assessment of reocclusion) found an incidence of reocclusion of 16 ± 10%.[74] In the TIMI trials,[75] reocclusion of the infarct-related artery at a median of 7 days occurred in 9% of the 419 patients by t-PA, urokinase, or a combination. Compared with the patients with a patent infarct-related artery, these patients had a significantly higher in-hospital mortality (12.8% versus 4%) and complication rate and a significantly lower left ventricular ejection fraction.[75]

Among the patients treated with accelerated t-PA and heparin, the GUSTO angiographic substudy[19] noted a reocclusion rate of 7.4% at 5 to 7 days of follow-up angiography. In the patients with TIMI grade 3 flow at 90 minutes, an overall reocclusion rate of 5.9% was found. However, the rate of reinfarction (4.1%) was relatively low in the activated t-PA with heparin treatment group.[26]

In spite of these limitations, rapid and effective administration of thrombolysis to appropriate patients early in the course of MI reduces mortality, prevents shock, preserves myocardial function, and ultimately prolongs life.

SUMMARY

Thrombolytic therapy for acute MI saves lives.

The thrombolytic agents now available for clinical use have a number of limitations, including:

- *Administration by continuous infusion*
- *Inability to restore patency of the infarct-related artery*
- *Prolonged time to reperfusion*
- *Acute reocclusion of the infarct-related artery*
- *Systemic fibrinogenolysis*
- *Significant bleeding*
- *Hemorrhagic strokes*

Even with these limitations, rapid and effective administration of thrombolytic agents to appropriate patients early in the course of MI reduces mortality and improves quality of life.

ACKNOWLEDGMENTS

This work was performed during the tenure of Dr. Janin as a National Institutes of Health fellow (HL 07537). The authors thank Ms. Sylvia Converse for her preparation of this manuscript.

References

1. DeWood MA, Spores J, Notske R, Mouser LT, Borroughs R, Golden MS, Lang HT: Prevalence of total coronary occlusion during the early hours of transmural myocardial infarction. N Engl J Med 1980; 303:897–902.
2. Rentrop KP, Blanke H, Karsch KR, Wiegand V, Kostering K, Oster H, Leitz K: Acute myocardial infarction: Intracoronary application of nitroglycerin and streptokinase. Clin Cardiol 1979; 2:354–363.
3. Bassell-Dupuy R, Jiang NY, Bittick T, Madison E, McGookey D, Orth K, Shohet R, Sambrook J, Gething MJ: Tyrosine 67 in the epidermal growth factor–like domain of tissue-type plasminogen activator is important for clearance by a specific hepatic receptor. J Biol Chem 1992; 267:9968–9977.
4. Novokhanty VV, Ingham KC, Medved LV: Domain structure and domain-domain interactions of recombinant tissue plasminogen activator. J Biol Chem 1991; 266:12994–13001.
5. Keyt BA, Paoni NF, Refino CJ, Berleau L, Nguyen H, Chow A, Lai J, Pena L, Pater C, Ogez J, Etchevery T, Botstein D, Bennett WF: A faster-acting and more potent form of tissue plasminogen activator. Proc Natl Acad Sci USA 1994; 91:3670–3674.
6. Larsen GR, Henson K, Blue Y: Variants of human tissue-type plasminogen activator: Fibrin binding, fibrinolytic, and fibrinogenolytic characterization of genetic variants lacking the fibronectin finger-like and/or the epidermal growth factor domains. J Biol Chem 1988; 263:1023–1029.
7. Hu, CK, Kohnert U, Wilhelm O, Fischer S, Llinas M: Tissue-type plasminogen activator domain-deletion mutant BM 06.022: Modular stability, inhibitor binding and activation cleavage. Biochemistry 1994; 33:11760–11766.
8. Horrevoets AJF, Smilde A, deVries C, Pannekoek H: The specific roles of finger and kringle 2 domains of tissue-type plasminogen activator during in vitro fibrinolysis. J Biol Chem 1994; 269:12639–12644.
9. Rijken D, Hoylaerts M, Collen D: Fibrinolytic properties of one-chain and two-chain human extrinsic (tissue-type) plasminogen activator. J Biol Chem 1982; 257:2920–2925.
10. Sakharov DV, Rijken DC: Superficial accumulation of plasminogen during clot lysis. Fibrinolysis 1994; 8(Suppl I):83-87.
11. Loscalzo J, Braunwald E: Tissue plasminogen activator. N Engl J Med 1988; 319:925–931.
12. Collen D, Lijnen HR, Vanlinthout I, Kieckens, Nelles L, Stassen JM: Thrombolytic and pharmacokinetic properties of human tissue-type plasminogen activator variants, obtained by deletion and/or duplication of structural/functional domains, in a hamster pulmonary embolism model. Thromb Haemost 1991; 65:174–180.
13. Collen D, Stassen JM, Larsen G: Pharmacokinetics and thrombolytic properties of deletion mutants of human tissue-type plasminogen activator in rabbits. Blood 1988; 71:216–219.
14. Madison EL, Goldsmith EJ, Gerard RD, Gething M-JH, Sambrook JF: Serpin-resistant mutants of human tissue-type plasminogen activator. Nature 1989; 339:721–723.
15. Rentrop PK: Restoration of antegrade flow in acute myocardial infarction: The first 15 years. J Am Coll Cardiol 1995; 25:1S–2S.
16. Karagounis L, Sorensen LG, Menlove RL, Moreno F, Anderson JL: Does thrombolysis in myocardial infarction (TIMI) perfusion grade 2 represent a most patent or a most occluded artery? Enzymatic and electrocardiographic evidence from the TEAM-2 study. J Am Coll Cardiol 1992; 19:1–10.

17. Anderson JL, Karagounis LA, Becker LC Sorensen SG, Menlove RL: TIMI perfusion grade 3 but not grade 2 results in improved outcome after thrombolysis for myocardial infarction. Circulation 1993; 87:1829–1839.
18. Vogt A, von Essen R, Tebbe U, Feurerer W, Appel, KF, Neuhaus KL: Impact of early perfusion status of the infarct-related artery on short term mortality after thrombolysis for acute myocardial infarction: Retrospective analysis of four German multicenter studies. J Am Coll Cardiol 1993; 21:1391–1395.
19. The GUSTO Angiographic Investigators: The effects of tissue plasminogen activator, streptokinase or both on coronary artery patency, ventricular function, and survival after acute myocardial infarction. N Engl J Med 1993; 329:1615–1622.
20. Simes RJ, Topol EJ, Holmes DR, White HD, Rutsch WR, Vahanian A, Simoons ML, Morris D, Betriu A, Califf RM, Ross AM: Link between the angiographic substudy and mortality outcomes in a large randomized trial of myocardial reperfusion. Circulation 1995; 91:1923–1928.
21. Lincoff AM, Topol EJ, Califf RM, Sigmon KN, Lee KL, Ohman EM, Rosenchein U, Ellis SG: Significance of a coronary artery with Thrombolysis in Myocardial Infarction grade 2 flow “patency” (outcome in the Thrombolysis and Angioplasty in Myocardial Infarction Trials). Am J Cardiol 1995; 75:871–876.
22. The TIMI Study Group: Comparison of invasive and conservative strategies after treatment with intravenous tissue plasminogen activator in acute myocardial infarction: Results of the Thrombolysis in Myocardial Infarction (TIMI) Phase II trial. N Engl J Med 1989; 320:618–627.
23. Cannon CP, Antman EM, Walls R, Braunwald E: Time as an adjunct agent to thrombolytic therapy. J Thromb Thrombol 1994; 1:27–34.
24. Newby KL, Rutsch WR, Califf RM, Simoons ML, Aylward PE, Armstrong PW, Woodlief LH, Lee KL, Topol EJ, van de Werf F: Time from symptom onset to treatment and outcomes after thrombolytic therapy. J Am Coll Cardiol 1996; 27:1646–1655.
25. The GUSTO Investigators: An international randomized trial comparing four thrombolytic strategies for acute myocardial infarction. N Engl J Med 1993; 329:673–682.
26. Langer A, Goodman SG, Topol EJ, Charlesworth A, Skene AM, Wilcox RG, Armstrong PW: Late Assessment of Thrombolytic Efficacy (LATE) study: Prognosis in patients with non–Q wave myocardial infarction. J Am Coll Cardiol 1996; 27:1327–1332.
27. Fibrinolytic Therapy Trialists' (FTT) Collaborative Group: Indications for fibrinolytic therapy in suspected acute myocardial infarction: Collaborative review of early mortality and major morbidity results from all randomized trials of more than 1000 patients. Lancet 1994; 343:311–322.
28. Bates ER: Revisiting reperfusion therapy in inferior myocardial infarction. J Am Coll Cardiol 1997; 30:334–342.
29. Woodfield SL, Lundergan CF, Reiner JS, Thompson MA, Rohrbeck SC, Deychak Y, Smith JO, Burton JR, McCarthy WF, Califf RM, White HD, Weaver WD, Topol EJ, Ross AM: Gender and acute myocardial infarction: Is there a different response to thrombolysis? J Am Coll Cardiol 1997; 29:35–52.
30. Hackett D, Davies G, Chierchia S, Maseri A: Intermittent coronary occlusion in acute myocardial infarction: Value of combined thrombolytic and vasodilator therapy. N Engl J Med 1987; 317:1055–1059.
31. Chesebro JH, Knatterud G, Roberts R, Borer J, Cohen LS, Dalen J: Thrombolysis in Myocardial Infarction (TIMI) trial, Phase I: A comparison between intravenous tissue plasminogen activator and intravenous streptokinase. Clinical findings through hospital discharge. Circulation 1987; 76:142–154.
32. Wharton TP, Marsalese D, Brodie BR: How often do infarct-related arteries show early perfusion without prior thrombolytic therapy, and should these vessels be dilated acutely? Results from TAMI-2. Circulation 1995; 92:1530–1537.
33. Becker RC: Seminars in thrombosis, thrombolysis and vascular biology: 3. Platelet activity in cardiovascular disease. Cardiology 1991; 79:49–63.
34. Clements IP, Christian TF, Higano ST, Gibbons RJ, Gersh BJ: Residual flow to the infarct zones as determinant of infarct size after direct angioplasty. Circulation 1993; 88:1527–1533.
35. Mizuno K, Koriuchi K, Matui H, Miyamoto A, Arakawa K, Shibuya T, Kuitia A, Nakamura H: Role of coronary collateral vessels during transient coronary occlusion during angioplasty assessed by hemodynamic, electrocardiographic and metabolic changes. J Am Coll Cardiol 1988; 12:624–528.
36. Habib GB, Heibig J, Forman SA, Brown BG, Roberts R, Terin ML, Bolli R: Influence of coronary collateral vessels on myocardial infarct size in humans: Results of Phase I Thrombolysis in Myocardal Infarction (TIMI) trial. Circulation 1991; 83:739–746.
37. Califf RM, Topol EJ, Gersh BJ: From myocardial salvage in acute myocardial infarction: The role of reperfusion therapy. J Am Coll Cardiol 1989; 14:1382–1488.
38. Braunwald E: Myocardial reperfusion, limitation of infarct size, reduction of left ventricular dysfunction, and improved survival: Should the paradigm be expanded? Circulation 1989; 79:441–444.
39. Braunwald E: The open-artery theory is alive and well—again. N Engl J Med 1992; 329:1650–1652.
40. Cigarroa RG, Lang RA, Hillis LD: Prognosis after acute myocardial infarction in patients with and without residual antegrade coronary blood flow. Am J Cardiol 1989; 64:155–160.
41. Fortin DF, Califf RM: Long-term survival from acute myocardial infarction: Salutary effect of an open coronary vessel. Am J Med 1990; 88:9N–15N.
42. Goldman L: Electrophysiological testing after myocardial infarction: A paradigm for assessing the incremental value of a diagnostic test. Circulation 1991; 83:1090–1092.
43. Wilcox RG, von der Lippe G, Olsson CG, Jensen G, Skene AM, Hampton JR: Effects of alteplase in acute myocardial infarction: 6-month results from the ASSET study. Lancet 1990; 335:1175–1178.
44. ISIS-2 (Second International Study of Infarct Survival) Collaborative Group: Randomized trial of intravenous streptokinase, oral aspirin, or neither among 17, 187 cases of suspected acute myocardial infarction: ISIS-2. Lancet 1988; 2:349–369.
45. Gruppo Italiano per lo Studio Streptochinasi nell' Infarto Miocrdico (GISSI): Long-term effects on intravenous thrombolysis in acute myocardial infarction: Final report of the GISSI study. Lancet 1987; 2:871–874.
46. White HD, Barbash GI, Califf RM, Simes RJ, Granger CB, Weaver D, Kleiman NS, Aylward PE, Gore JM, Vehanian A, Lee KL, Ross AM, Topol EJ: Age and outcome with contemporary thrombolytic therapy: Results from the GUSTO-I trial. Circulation 1996; 94:1826–1833.
47. Grines CL, Booth DC, Nissen SE, Gurley JC, Bennett KA, O'Connor WN, DeMaria AN: Mechanism of acute myocardial infarction in patients with prior coronary artery bypass grafting and therapeutic implications. Am J Cardiol 1990; 65:1292–1296.
48. O'Keefe JH Jr, Bailey WL, Rutherford BD, Hartzler GO: Primary angiolasty for acute myocardial infarction in 1,000 consecutive patients: Results in an unselected population and high-risk subgroups. Am J Cardiol 1993; 72:107G–115G.
49. Holmes DR, Bates ER, Kleiman NS, Sadowski Z, Horgan JHS, Morris DC, Califf RM, Berger PB, Topol EJ: Contemporary reperfusion therapy for cardogenic shock: The GUSTO-I trial experience. J Am Cardiol 1995; 26:668–674.
50. Berger PB, Holmes DR, Stebbins AL, Bates ER, Califf RM, Topol EJ: Impact of an aggressive invasive catheterization and revascularization strategy on mortality in patients with cardiogenic shock in the Global Utilization of Streptokinase and Tissue Plamsminogen Activator for Occluded Arteries (GUSTO-I) trial. Circulation 1997; 96:122–127.
51. Zidansek A, Blinc A: The influence of transport parameters and enzyme kinetics of the fibrinolytic system on thrombolysis: Mathematical modeling of two idealized cases. Thromb Haemost 1991; 65:553–559.
52. Li KA, Santamore WP, Morley DL, Tulenko TN: Stenotic amplication of vasoconstriction responses. Am J Physiol 1989; 256:H1044–H1051.
53. Anderson RD, Ohman M, Holmes DR Jr, Col J, Stebbins Al, Bates ER, Stomel RJ, Granger CB, Topol EJ, Califf RM: Use of intraaortic balloon counterpulsation in patients presenting with cardiogenic shock: Observations from the GUSTO-I study. J Am Coll Cardiol 1997; 30:708–715.
54. Simoons ML, Maggioni AP, Knatterud G, Leimberger JD, deJaegere P, van Domburg R, Boersma E, Frazosi MG, Califf R, Schroder R, Braunwald E: Individual risk assessment for intracranial hemorrhage during thrombolytic therapy. Lancet 1993; 342:1523–1528.

55. Tenaglia AN, Califf RM, Candela RJ, Kereiakes DJ, Berrios E, Young SY, Stack RS, Topol EJ: Thrombolytic therapy in patients requiring cardiopulmonary resuscitation. Am J Cardiol 1991; 68:1015–1019.
56. Mahaffey KW, Granger CB, Toth CA, White HD, Stebbins AL, Barbas GI, Vahanian A, Topol EJ, Califf RM: Diabetic retinopathy should not be a contraindication to thrombolytic therapy for acute myocardial infarction: Review of occular hemorrhage incidence and location in the GUSTO-I trial. J Am Coll Cardiol 1997; 30:1606–1610.
57. Karnash SL, Granger CB, White HD, Woodlief LH, Topol EJ, Califf RM: Treating menstruating women with thrombolytic therapy: Insights from the global utilization of streptokinase and tissue plasminogen activator for occluded coronary arteries (GUSTO-I) trial. J Am Coll Cardiol 1995; 26:1651–1656.
58. Chapman GD, Ohman EM, Topol EJ, Candela RJ, Kereiakes DJ, Samaha J, Berrios E, Pieper KS, Young SY, Califf RM: Minimizing the risk of inappropriately administering thrombolytic therapy (Thrombolysis and Angioplasty in Myocardial Infarction [TAMI] study group). Am J Cardiol 1993; 71:783–787.
59. De Jaegere PP, Arnold AA, Balk AH, Simoons ML: Intracranial hemorrhage in association with thrombolytic therapy: Incidence and clinical predictive factors. J Am Coll Cardiol 1992; 19:289–294.
60. Neuhaus KL, Feurerer W, Jeep-Tebbe S, Niederer W, Vogt A, Tebbe U: Improved thrombolysis with a modified dose regimen of recombinant tissue-type plasminogen activator. J Am Coll Cardiol 1989; 14:1566–1569.
61. The Continuous Infusion Versus Double-Bolus Administration of Alteplase (COBALT) Investigators. A comparison infusion of alteplase with double-bolus administration for acute myocardial infarction. N Engl J Med: 1997; 337:1124–1130.
62. Gulba DC, Tanswell P, Dechend R, Sosada M, Weis A, Waigand J, Uhlich F, Hauck S, Jost S, Raffenbeul W, Lichtlen PR, Dietz R: Sixty minute alteplase protocol: A new accelerated recombinant tissue-type plasminogen activator regimen for thrombolysis in acute myocardial infarction. J Am Coll Cardiol 1997; 30:1611–1617.
63. Torr SR, Nachowiak DA, Fujii S, Sobel BE: "Plasminogen steal" and clot lysis. Am J Cardiol 1992; 19:1085–1090.
64. Rapold HJ: Promotion of thrombin activity by thrombolytic therapy without simultaneous anticoagulation. Lancet 1990; 1:481–482.
65. Eisenberg PR, Miletich JP: Induction of marked thrombin activity by pharmacologic concentrations of plasminogen activators in non-anticoagulated whole blood. Thromb Res 1989; 55:636–643.
66. Schiele R, Rustige J, Burczk U, Koch A Harmjanz D, Tebbe U, Senges J: Thrombolysis after resuscitation in acute myocardial infarction. J Am Coll Cardiol February 1966:297A.
67. Eisenberg PR, Miletich JP: Induction of marked thrombin activity by thrombolytic therapy without simultaneous anticoagulation. Lancet 1990; 1:481–482.
68. Mirshahi M, Soria J, Faivre R, Lu H, Courtney M, Roitsch C, Tripier D, Caen P: Evaluation of the inhibition by heparin and hirudin of coagulation activation during rt-A-induced thrombolysis. Blood 1989; 74:1025–1030.
69. Gulba DC, Barthels M, Westhoff-Bleck M, Jost S, Raffenbeul W, Daniel WG, Hecker H, Lichtlen PR: Increased thrombin levels during thrombolytic therapy in acute myocardial infarction relevance for the success of therapy. Circulation 1991; 83:937–944.
70. Lee KL, Woodlief LH, Topol EJ, Weaver D, Betriu A, Col J, Simoons M, Alward P, van de Werf F, Califf RM: Predictors of 30-day mortality in the era of reperfusion for acute myocardial infarction: Results of an international trial of 41201 patients. Circulation 1995; 91:1659–1668.
71. Simoons ML, Maggioni AP, Knatterud G, Leimberger JD, de Jaegere P, van Domburg R, Boersma E, Franzosi MG, Califf R, Schrooder R, Braunwald E: Individual risk assessment for intracranial hemorrhage during thrombolytic therapy. Lancet 1993; 342:1523–1528.
72. Bovill EG, Terrin ML, Stump DC, Berke AD, Frederick M, Collin D, Feit F, Gore JM, Hillis LD, Lambrew CT, Leiboff R, Mann KG, Markis JE, Pratt CM, Sharkey SW, Tracy RP, Chesbro JH: Hemorrhagic events during therapy with recombinant tissue-type plasminogen activator, heparin, and aspirin for acute infarction: Results of the thrombolysis in myocardial infarction (TIMI), phase II trial. Ann Int Med 1991; 115:256–265.
73. Berkowitz SD, Granger CB, Pieper KS, Lee KL, Gore JM, Simoons M, Armstrong PW, Topol EJ, Califf RM: Incidence and predictors of bleeding after contemporary thrombolytic therapy for myocardial infarction. Circulation 1997; 95:2508–2516.
74. Verheugt FWA, Meijer A, Lagrand WK, van Eenige MJ: Reocclusion: The flip side of coronary thrombolysis. J Am Coll Cardiol 1996; 27:766–773.
75. Ohman ME, Califf RM, Topol EJ, Candela R, Abbottsmith C, Ellis S, Sigmon KN, Kereiakes D, George B, Stack R: Consequences of reocclusion after successful reperfusion therapy in acute myocardial infarction. Circulation 1990; 82:781–791.

93

Interventional Therapies for Cardiogenic Shock

Yves Janin, MD • George Vetrovec, MD, FACC
Michael L. Hess, MD, FACC

BACKGROUND

Definition

The cardinal signs of cardiogenic shock are tissue perfusion inadequate to meet metabolic demands and resulting in end-organ dysfunction manifested by altered mental status, confusion, agitation, hypotension, acute pulmonary edema, hypoxemia, oliguria, and cyanosis.

Cardiogenic shock is defined as:

- Systolic blood pressure below 90 mm Hg for at least 1 hour that is not responsive to fluid administration alone and that is secondary to cardiac dysfunction

associated with

- Signs of tissue hypoperfusion or a cardiac index below 2.2 L/min/m^2 or systolic blood pressure that is less than 90 mm Hg within 1 hour after the administration of positive inotropic agents.

Cardiogenic shock develops when more than 40% of the left ventricle is nonfunctional.[1-3] A significant portion of the left ventricle does not have to be acutely infarcted; it just has to be nonfunctioning. Thus, cardiogenic shock can develop in (1) a patient who had at least one prior myocardial infarction that resulted in a large scar, (2) a patient with balanced chronic heart failure in whom ischemia or infarction of a previously unaffected myocardial territory suddenly develops, and (3) a patient with a nonischemic cardiomyopathy secondary to chronic hypertension or valvular disease, resulting in significant impairment of left ventricular systolic function who has acute myocardial ischemia resulting from either coronary artery disease or a coronary artery embolization secondary to atrial fibrillation. It is also evident that the development of acute ischemia in a relatively small myocardial territory, in a patient with a large amount of hibernating or stunned myocardium, can rapidly precipitate cardiogenic shock. Therefore, the consequences of an acute myocardial ischemic event depend on (1) the size of the myocardial territory involved and (2) the "substrate" (i.e., status of the remainder of the left ventricular myocardium and any associated disease of the coronary arteries not involved by infarction).[4, 5]

Etiology of Cardiogenic Shock

Complications of Myocardial Infarction

It is critical to realize that not all shock states occurring in the context of acute myocardial ischemia are cardiogenic in nature. Acute myocardial infarction is usually accompanied by diaphoresis, which can be profuse and accompanied by nausea and vomiting, resulting in dehydration—and, sometimes, significant contraction of the intravascular volume. In these patients, shock is readily reversible with rapid fluid administration. In other patients, acute myocardial ischemia can be accompanied by a severe vasovagal reaction of the cardioinhibitory and/or vasodepressor type, which respond to atropine, fluid administration, and, if necessary, vasopressors and external cardiac pacing. Patients with an inferior myocardial infarction can present with a variety of heart blocks, which can result in shock and which can be rapidly treated with atropine and external cardiac pacing. New-onset atrial fibrillation, even with a controlled heart rate, or an accelerated junctional rhythm in the setting of an acute myocardial ischemic event, can result in shock. In patients with diastolic dysfunction and a stiff left ventricle, shock can develop secondary to hypertension, hypertrophy, or chronic ischemia, since atrial contraction contributes as much as 20% to 30% of left ventricular filling.

Patients can present with acute myocardial infarction in the setting of other serious conditions that can be obscured by the ischemic chest pain and the electrocardiographic (ECG) pattern. For example, acute gastrointestinal bleeding in a patient with coronary artery disease or an acute pulmonary embolus can result in acute myocardial ischemia and infarction and should be suspected. It is also critical to always remember that acute aortic dissection can involve the aortic root and result in acute myocardial infarction. Equally important is to consider acute cardiac tamponade secondary to Dressler's syndrome, as the cause of shock in a patient with a recent myocardial infarction who now presents with shock and an ECG pattern that could be consistent with acute myocardial ischemia. A patient with steroid dependence, a malignancy, opportunistic infection, or the acquired immunodeficiency syndrome or a transplant recipient may have unrecognized adrenocortical insufficiency, which may be manifested by shock induced by the stress of a cardiac catheterization or an acute myocardial infarction.

Post Intervention

Shock in patients who have undergone any type of cardiac catheterization or percutaneous transluminal coronary angioplasty (PTCA), especially with the use of atherectomy devices or lasers, can be particularly ominous. Acute closure secondary to intracoronary thrombosis and occlusion can be diagnosed immediately by electrocardiography and by the clinical presentation. This should be treated very aggressively with fluids, vasopressors, positive inotropic agents, intra-aortic balloon pump (IABP) counterpulsation, and appropriate intravenous anticoagulation with heparin while one is awaiting emergency transport of the patient to the cardiac catheterization laboratory for immediate angiography and restoration of antegrade flow in the occluded coronary artery. The treatment of acute closure is prompt restoration of antegrade Thrombolysis in Myocardial Infarction (TIMI) grade 3 coronary flow, and no time should be lost in unnecessary diagnostic maneuvers. Since the shock state is not reversed until the coronary artery has been reopened, this dramatic complication is treated in the catheterization laboratory.

In the interventional setting, one should not forget that cardiac tamponade can occur after an apparently uneventful right heart catheterization (Swan-Ganz catheterization) or so-called routine coronary angiography or coronary intervention. Temporary pacemaker wires can perforate the right ventricle, especially in the setting of an acute right ventricular infarction, and produce delayed cardiac tamponade. Distended jugular veins in the setting of shock, Kussmaul's sign, and electrical alternans on electrocardiography, although not specific, should prompt suspicion of cardiac tamponade. Echocardiography should be performed promptly at the bedside to evaluate this possibility and to direct the pericardiocentesis, which reverses the shock state. While echocardiography is awaited, fluids should be administered in an attempt to increase left ventricular preload.

Shock subsequent to cardiac catheterization or another coronary intervention can also be secondary to (1) profuse osmotic diuresis from the contrast agent, or to (2) overzealous diuresis, in the catheterization laboratory, of a patient with diastolic dysfunction and left ventricular hypertrophy who is preload-dependent (a condition that may be exacebated by excessive bleeding during the coronary intervention, especially if large coronary-guiding catheters and devices are used). Bleeding in the femoral area with subsequent hypovolemic shock at the vascular access site, with or without subcutaneous rupture of a femoral arterial pseudoaneurysm and retroperitoneal bleeding, can be quite extensive in "anticoagulated" patients. In these patients, it is crucial to promptly reverse the hypovolemia in order to restore the coronary perfusion pressure, since decreased perfusion of a recently dilated coronary artery results in stasis in the area of the iatrogenically ruptured plaque, which, together with the dysfunctional endothelium of these arteries and the increased cathecholamine levels, results in intense activation of the coagulation cascade, platelet activation, and vasospasm, leading to acute closure.

Shock can also develop after coronary angiography in a patient with severe disease of the left main coronary artery, especially in the presence of left ventricular systolic dysfunction. This can be a sequela to mechanical trauma to the left main coronary artery induced by catheter engagement in its lumen, which can result in spasm or plaque disruption and thrombosis. Management consists of immediate insertion of an IABP, institution of vasopressor and inotropic support, intravenous anticoagulation, and prompt surgical consultation and referral.

Because cardiac catheterizations are frequently performed in anticipation of peripheral vascular surgery in patients who have multiple risk factors for coronary artery disease, rupture of a previously undiagnosed abdominal aortic aneurysm should also be considered in the presence of other unexplained shock in such patients.

Left ventriculography performed in a patient with a recent anterior myocardial infarction and a previously unrecognized left ventricular thrombus or aortography in a patient with floating aortic wall atherosclerotic debris can lead to dislodgment and embolization. If the mesenteric arteries are involved, bowel ischemia and massive extravasation of fluid in the bowel wall and mesentery can result and lead to shock.

Initial Treatment

When shock develops in a cardiac patient, the most probable cause should always be considered and promptly and aggressively treated while the most life-threatening causes are ruled out or confirmed by a history of the clinical event, physical examination, and readily available diagnostic techniques such as electrocardiography and echocardiography.

A cardiologist should be consulted immediately. An arterial line should be placed in all patients because noninvasive blood pressure measurements correlate poorly with the actual blood pressure. Central lines should be used preferentially. When a large-gauge intravenous line is desired, the femoral vein in the groin or the external jugular vein high in the neck should be used. Puncture of noncompressible vessels should be avoided if possible, in the eventuality that the patient will need thrombolytic therapy. Therapy should not be delayed while preparations are being made for central line or Swan-Ganz catheter insertion and monitoring. In these critically sick and unstable patients, aggressive therapy should be instituted immediately with vasopressors, positive inotropic agents, fluids as indicated, and maintenance of adequate oxygenation. External transcutaneous pacemakers are preferred, since they are not time-consuming in their application and do not have the risk of myocardial perforation that accompanies transvenous pacemakers, especially when these are placed in agitated patients.

Although Swan-Ganz catheters can be inserted at the bedside via a femoral vein with fluoroscopic guidance, they may not remain in position in agitated patients or those who "fight the ventilator." If the tip falls back into the right ventricle, ventricular tachycardia can result. This condition should be promptly considered and the catheter be withdrawn immediately to the inferior vena cava, without confirmation by fluoroscopy, instead of risking continuing ventricular tachycardia. Advanced Cardiac Life Support (ACLS) protocols are ineffective in this setting. Swan-Ganz catheters should preferentially be inserted under fluroscopic guidance.

ACUTE MYOCARDIAL INFARCTION

The Global Utilization of Streptokinase and Tissue Plasminogen Activator for Occluded Coronary Arteries (GUSTO-I) trial,[6] which studied a total of 41,201 patients with acute myocardial infarction who presented within 6 hours of onset of symptoms, reported its findings on the largest cohort of cardiogenic shock patients prospectively identified in a randomized trial.[7–9] Cardiogenic shock was identified in 7.2% of the patients.[7] It was present on arrival in 0.7% of the patients, and it developed after the initial admission to the hospital in 6.5% of the patients in the setting of recurrent ischemia or reinfarction. Of the patients with cardiogenic shock, 11% presented with shock, and the remaining 89% developed shock after admission. The majority who developed cardiogenic shock did so in the first 48 hours after randomization. Older age, female sex, hypertension, diabetes mellitus, previous myocardial infarction, and anterior myocardial infarction were significantly more common in patients with cardiogenic shock as compared with those without shock. Patients with cardiogenic shock had a longer delay time prior to the administration of thrombolysis than those who did not.[7]

In the GUSTO-I trial, in-hospital complications were significantly more common in patients with cardiogenic shock than in the others.[7] Asystole, the most frequent arrhythmia, occurred in 40% of the patients with cardiogenic shock and in 3% of those without shock. Reinfarction and recurrent ischemia were significantly increased in patients with cardiogenic shock (10% and 26%, respectively) as compared with those without shock (3% and 19%, respectively).[4] Fifty-seven per cent of the 315 patients who were in cardiogenic shock on arrival and 56% of the 2657 patients who had shock after the initial admission died in the hospital compared with in-hospital mortality of only 3% for the 37,764 patients who did not develop shock. All patients in cardiogenic shock have the same high mortality risk, regardless of whether shock is present on arrival or whether it develops after the implementation of thrombolysis and other medical therapeutics. Whether cardiogenic shock was present on arrival or developed after admission, there was no significant difference in the incidence of major clinical events and in the in-hospital and 30-day mortality rates, with respect to the four different thrombolytic strategies.[7]

PRIMARY CORONARY ANGIOPLASTY

The development of cardiogenic shock in the setting of acute myocardial infarction is ominous, as shock is the most common cause of death in hospitalized patients with acute myocardial infarction.[7–13] Prompt reestablishment of antegrade flow in the infarct-related artery is crucial to the survival of these critically sick patients.[8–15]

In patients with acute myocardial infarction, rapid restoration of unrestricted antegrade TIMI grade 3 flow in the infarct-related artery has been established as the principal determinant of an improved clinical outcome.[16] A meta-analysis of TEAM-2,[17] TEAM-3,[18] four German multicenter studies,[19] the GUSTO angiographic substudy,[20, 21] and the TIMI trials,[22] five prospective, controlled thrombolytic therapy studies of acute myocardial infarction requiring ST-segment elevation at entry and using early (<24 hours) angiography, revealed that optimal outcome was achieved only with restoration of TIMI grade 3 flow in the involved artery.[23] For the combined study, mortality (in-hospital or 30-day) was significantly lower in patients with TIMI-3 flow (3.7%) as compared with both patients with TIMI-2 flow (7.0%) and those with TIMI-0/1 flow (8.8%). Times to enzymatic peaks from initiation of thrombolytic therapy were significantly reduced in patients who achieved TIMI-3 flow, compared with those with TIMI grades below 3.[23] The left ventricular ejection fraction was significantly higher with TIMI-3 flow as compared with TIMI-2 flow: the difference averaged 4 to 5 percentage points, and there was significantly better regional wall motion in patients with TIMI-3 as compared with those who had TIMI-2 flow.[23] Thus, early and complete restoration of flow in the infarct-related artery is associated with significantly improved survival and clinical outcome in patients with acute myocardial infarction.

This finding is particularly true for critically ill patients whose acute myocardial infarction is complicated by cardiogenic shock.[2, 8, 11–15] Although thrombolytic therapy of patients with acute myocardial infarction and cardiogenic shock is associated with a significant reduction in the 30-day mortality as compared with no thrombolysis, the magnitude of its impact is small, as shown in the multicenter randomized How Effective Are Revascularization Options in Cardiogenic Shock trial (HEROICS),[24] which reported a 30-day mortality of 80% in patients who received thrombolytic therapy and of 100% in those who received conventional nonrevascularization therapy.

In a nonrandomized study[12] of 50 patients with acute myocardial infarction, with no mechanical complications or cardiogenic shock, receiving medical therapy including IABP counterpulsation, vasopressors and thrombolytic therapy the in-hospital and 1-year survival rates were significantly better in the PTCA group (64% and 52%, respectively) in contrast to the nonrevascularized group (24% and 12%). A retrospective review of the experience of four centers, from 1982 to 1985[13] with emergency PTCA in patients with cardiogenic shock complicating an acute myocardial infarction, found that in-hospital survival was significantly better for those who underwent successful PTCA than those for whom the PTCA was unsuccessful (69% versus 20%).

The SHOCK trial registry,[11] an international multicenter registry of patients in cardiogenic shock in the United States and Belgium that was initiated in January 1992 and completed in April 1993, reported on a very heterogeneous group of 214 patients who had cardiogenic shock complicating acute myocardial infarction. This group included patients with ST-segment elevation, new Q waves, or new left bundle branch block (LBBB) and another group of patients with ST depression and/or T-wave inversion or old LBBB. Only 47% of the patients in the former group received thrombolytic therapy. The in-hospital mortality rate of the patients who underwent coronary angiography was significantly lower than that of those who were not catheterized (51.3% versus 85.2%). There was, however, no difference in the in-hospital mortality of the patients who underwent early revascularization (24 hours after the diagnosis of shock) and those not undergoing revascularization (51% versus 58%). After adjustment for cardiac catheterization status, the use of an IABP did not affect in-hospital mortality of this extremely heterogenous group of patients. Excluding patients with concomitant conditions that would preclude emergency revascularization for cardiogenic shock, patients with causes of cardiogenic shock other than left ventricular dysfunction and those with ST-segment depressions, "old" LBBB, or nonspecific ECG changes, the SHOCK registry investigators found that, among the 150 trial-eligible patients, in-hospital mortality was significantly lower for those selected to undergo early revascularization (50%) than for those given either late revascularization or none (67%).[13]

A report on patients from the same registry with cardiogenic shock and a history of coronartery bypass graft (CABG)[25] found that, compared with patients who never had CABG, these patients had a higher in-hospital mortality rate (75% versus 63.9%) and that only a minority (7.4%) were referred for "redo" CABG. The in-hospital mortality rates for the patients with cardiogenic shock and prior CABG who underwent revascularization by either PTCA or CABG were significantly lower than that for those who were not revascularized (56.5% versus 84.4%). These findings support aggressive revascularization for this high-risk group of patients.

Although the success rate of primary PTCA for acute myocardial infarction can be as high as 97.1%, as reported by the Primary Angioplasty in Myocardial Infarction (PAMI) Study group,[25] primary PTCA in patients with cardiogenic shock complicating acute myocardial infarction has a significantly lower success rate.[8, 14, 15] In the Society for Cardiac Angiography and Interventions registry of primary PTCA performed within 24 hours of onset of acute myocardial infarction in 4366 patients, for the years 1990 through 1994,[14] the success rate for PTCA was 91.5%. Emergency CABG was performed in 3.4% of the patients, and the in-hospital mortality rate was 2.6%, although in that registry late mortality may have been incompletely reported. The predictors of an unsuccessful PTCA were older age, lower laboratory PTCA volume, an IABP in place, cardiogenic shock, and moribund status.[14] PTCA was successful in 77.6% of the 313 patients with cardiogenic shock, a significantly lower rate than the 90.4% success rate in the 4053 patients without shock.

In the Mid-America Heart Institute's experience with 1000 consecutive, unselected patients whose acute myocardial infarction was treated with primary PTCA,[15] the success rate of PTCA in the 79 patients in cardiogenic shock was 82%, which was significantly less than the success rate of 95% in the absence of shock. In this series, the in-hospital mortality rate of the patients in cardiogenic shock treated with primary PTCA was 44%, in contrast to a rate of 5% in the patients without shock.[15] In comparison to the patients in cardiogenic shock who had an unsuccessful primary PTCA, a successful primary PTCA significantly reduced in-hospital mortality from 79% to 37%:

- Patency of the infarct-related artery is one of the most important predictors of in-hospital mortality. In the GUSTO-I trial,[7] cardiac catheterization was performed in 1351 (45%) of the 2972 patients who were in cardiogenic shock. Of these catheterized patients 907 (67%) were "revascularized"; 340 (25%) were referred for coronary artery bypass; and of the remaining 1011 patients 567 (56%) underwent coronary angioplasty.[7]
- The 30-day mortality for the 1621 patients in cardiogenic shock who did not undergo cardiac catheterization was 74% (1200 patients). The 30-day mortality for the 2065 patients in shock not undergoing revascularization was 66% (1370 patients). Among the 907 patients in shock undergoing revascularization with either PTCA or CABG, the 30-day mortality was significantly reduced to 29% (263 patients) in the entire revascularization group and in each subgroup (165 patients with PTCA and 98 patients with CABG).

TABLE 93–1. Cardiogenic Shock and Myocardial Infarction: Key Points

1. Cardiogenic shock is the most common cause of death in hospitalized patients with acute myocardial infarction.
2. *Prompt* reestablishment of coronary flow is crucial.
3. Thrombolytic therapy generally *prevents* the development of shock. It is *not* the preferred modality for established cardiogenic shock.
4. Primary percutaneous transluminal coronary angioplasty (PTCA) is the preferred first and urgent form of therapy. This procedure can increase survival.
5. Intra-aortic balloon pumps have *not* been associated with increased survival. Early insertion may be of benefit as a "bridge" to emergent PTCA.

As a comparison, among the patients in whom shock did not develop in the GUSTO-I, the 30-day mortality of the 16,563 patients who did not undergo cardiac catheterization, was 5.6% (934 patients), and that of the 11,466 patients undergoing revascularization was 0.9% (107 patients).[7]

In a subgroup analysis of these 2200 patients from GUSTO-I who developed cardiogenic shock and underwent cardiac catheterization, coronary angiography was performed within 24 hours of the onset of shock in 406 (18%). Patients who underwent early angiography were significantly younger, had had significantly fewer earlier angina episodes and myocardial infarction, and were significantly more likely to have a family history of coronary artery disease and of hyperlipidemia. For the patients who underwent angiography within 24 hours of onset of shock, the 30-day mortality was 38% (155 patients), which is significantly lower than the mortality rate of 61% (1100 patients) in the patients who had delayed angiography.[8] The mortality difference between these two groups of patients remained significant 1 year after enrollment in the trial: 44.2% versus 66.4%.

Early angioplasty was performed in 197 patients. It was successful in 148 (75%), whose 30-day mortality was 35%—significantly lower than that of 55% for the 49 patients (25%) whose angioplasty was unsuccessful.[5] By multivariate analysis, the aggressive strategy of early coronary angiography and revascularization was independently associated with a reduction in 30-day mortality (odds ratio, 0.43). Interestingly, the 173 patients who underwent early angiography but no revascularization procedure within 24 hours, had a significantly lower 30-day mortality: 35% as compared with 62% for the group in whom early angiography was not performed. A review of 100 of these former patients for whom angiographic data were available revealed that the infarct-related artery was patent (TIMI grade 2 or 3 flow) in 52 and that it had normal (TIMI grade 3) flow in 30.[8]

Thus, an aggressive strategy of early coronary angiography and revascularization in patients with acute myocardial infarction complicated by cardiogenic shock and treated with thrombolytic therapy is associated with a significant reduction in 30-day mortality that is independent of the baseline clinical characteristics (Table 93–1).[7, 8]

INTRA-AORTIC BALLOON PUMP

Since its first clinical insertion for cardiogenic shock complicating an acute myocardial infarction in 1968,[26] the use of

IABP counterpulsation for the control of ongoing myocardial ischemia has become steadily more prevalent, whereas its use for support of hemodynamic decompensation (including cardiogenic shock) has remained relatively constant.[27] Furthermore, percutaneous insertion of an IABP is associated with a high rate of vascular complications, ranging from 10.2% in a general cardiac surgery population to 60% in a series of 80 patients with cardiogenic shock complicating acute myocardial infarction who underwent emergency surgical revascularization.[10]

In cardiac surgical series, the mortality associated with IABP insertion to stabilize medically refractory ischemia in the preoperative period was significantly lower than when it was placed intraoperatively or postoperatively.[28] IABP counterpulsation is still infrequently used for acute myocardial infarction complicated by cardiogenic shock, owing to the inherent reluctance to use this large-bore catheter in association with thrombolytic therapy and in part, to the lack of definitive data about its efficacy.

In the GUSTO-I trial the decision to insert an IABP in patients with acute myocardial infarction and cardiogenic shock who received thrombolytic therapy was made by the treating physician.[7, 8, 29] Of the 310 patients who on arrival had cardiogenic shock, an IABP was inserted within 1 calendar day of admission ("early-IABP group") in 62 (20%) and after day 1 or not at all ("no-IABP group") in 248 (80%).[29] The median time to death was 67 hours in the early-IABP group and 7.2 hours in the no-IABP group. Surviving longer, the early-IABP group had more ischemic events and underwent more procedures. There was significantly greater use of inotropic agents, hemodynamic monitoring, intubation, and pacemaker support in the early-IABP group. Recurrent ischemia (20% versus 9%) and reinfarction (5% versus 0.8%) were significantly more common in the early-IABP group.

Cardiac catheterization was performed in 84% of the patients in the early-IABP group and in 28% of the patients in the no-IABP group. In the 51 patients who underwent coronary angiography in the early-IABP group, the median time to catheterization was 5.5 hours. In the early-IABP group, coronary angioplasty was performed in 42% of the patients and in 20% of the patients who underwent CABG. In contrast, in the no-IABP group only 9% of the patients underwent PTCA, and only 4% CABG. As expected, the early-IABP group had significantly more bleeding, with patients receiving a mean of 4 units of packed red blood cells.[29]

There was no significant difference in the in-hospital mortality between the early-IABP and no-IABP groups (48% and 59%, respectively). There was a trend toward a lower 30-day mortality in the early-IABP group (47% versus 60%), which became insignificant after adjustment for the baseline clinical predictors of mortality. In addition, there was no significant difference in the 30-day mortality between the patients who underwent revascularization in both groups; however, the unadjusted 1-year mortality was significantly lower in the early-IABP group (57% versus 67%).[29]

Among the patients with acute myocardial infarction who presented in cardiogenic shock, more than 50% of the overall 30-day deaths occurred within the first 8 hours in those who were critically ill and in whom the initiation of IABP counterpulsation did not affect survival. The 30-day mortality continued to be higher, however, in the no-IABP group, which suggests the possibility that the earlier use of IABP might have improved survival.[29]

In a retrospective review of 46 patients with acute myocardial infarction and cardiogenic shock who received thrombolytic therapy within 12 hours of onset of symptoms in a community hospital, Kovack and coworkers found that the community hospital survival for both those who were transferred to a tertiary care center and those who were not was 93% for the patients who were also treated with an IABP (inserted an average of 5.7 hours from the onset of chest pain) and 37% for those without IABP.[28] This observation suggests that early insertion of an IABP in patients with acute myocardial infarction complicated by cardiogenic shock and treated with thrombolytics may increase their survival and allow transfer to a tertiary care facility for revascularization (see Table 93-1).

One practical note: To minimize bleeding and/or vascular complications, an experienced angiographer should obtain access. If feasible, a single anterior arterial puncture should be made to minimize bleeding risk. Furthermore, femoral access should be cephalic, to avoid accessing the superficial femoral artery. Ischemic complications are fewer when arterial access is obtained in the common femoral artery.

EMERGENCY SURGICAL REVASCULARIZATION

In general, surgical revascularization performed early after acute myocardial infarction is associated with an excessive death rate, which reflects the fact that patients referred for CABG have significantly more extensive coronary artery disease, more multivessel disease, and lower left ventricular systolic function.[30-32] The Myocardial Infarction Triage and Intervention (MITI) registry reviewed the records of 1299 patients who underwent CABG in the setting of acute myocardial infarction.[32] Thrombolytic therapy was administered to only 23.6%. There was no significant difference in the hospital mortality for the patients "operated" within 24 hours of admission and those who underwent later surgery. In the Thrombolysis and Angioplasty in Myocardial Infarction I (TIMI-I) trial of intravenous tissue plasminogen activator (t-PA) and PTCA for acute myocardial infarction,[33] there was no in-hospital mortality in the absence of preoperative cardiogenic shock among the 16 patients who underwent CABG within 7.3 ± 1.9 hours of the onset of chest pain.

These results are not in accordance with those of the randomized, double-blind, GUSTO trial,[6] in which 3526 (8.6%) of the 41,021 patients with acute myocardial infarction who received thrombolytic therapy within 6 hours of onset of symptoms underwent surgical revascularization during the initial hospital period.[31] This included 130 of the 2972 patients in cardiogenic shock who underwent cardiac catheterization.[8, 30] For the entire group, the 30-day mortality was substantial in patients undergoing CABG within the first 2 days of the acute myocardial infarction but rapidly decreased thereafter. CABG performed on day 1 was associated with a 30-day mortality rate of 21%.[30] The risk of death after CABG and within 30 days of enrollment was directly related to the development of a mechanical complication and inversely related to the left ventricular ejection fraction and the time from enrollment until surgery.[30] Thus cardiogenic shock may be treated successfully with emergency cardiac surgical revascularization.[10]

In the MITI registry,[32] cardiogenic shock at the time of admission was not significantly associated with hospital mortality. This group, however, included only 22 (1.7%) of the 1299 patients with acute myocardial infarction who underwent CABG. In the TAMI-I trial,[33] CABG performed within 7.3 ± 1.9 hours of the onset of chest pain in eight patients who developed cardiogenic shock after initiation of tissue plasminogen activator (t-PA) was associated with in-hospital mortality of 37.5% (three patients).

Allen and colleagues[10] reported a remarkable series of 80 consecutive patients in cardiogenic shock complicating an acute myocardial infarction and not due to mechanical compli-

TABLE 93–2. Surgical Considerations in the Management of Cardiogenic Shock and Myocardial Infarction: Key Points

1. Emergency coronary artery bypass surgery is a viable alternative for patients with cardiogenic shock.
2. With appearance of a new systolic murmur after myocardial infarction, think acute ventricular septal defect and/or mitral regurgitation. Emergent echocardiography, followed by cardiac catheterization and surgical consultation, is a must.
3. Postinfarction ventricular septal defect carries a high mortality rate. Acute mitral regurgitation is usually due to involvement of the posterior medial papillary muscle. Emergent insertion of an intra-aortic balloon pump is a necessity. Do not delay surgery.

cations, who were dependent on inotropic support and IABP conterpulsation at the time of surgery and who did not receive thrombolytics. Ninety-four per cent (75) of these patients were able to be weaned postoperatively from both inotropic and IABP support, and 83% (66) survived the 30-day postoperative period. Delay of surgical revascularization longer than 18 hours after onset of cardiogenic shock was associated with significant prolongation in the duration of postoperative inotropic and IABP support and significantly higher 30-day mortality as compared with operation within 18 hours of onset of shock (31% versus 7%, respectively). Early and late mortality were related to (1) time from myocardial infarction to surgery, (2) time from shock to surgery, (3) history of myocardial infarction, and (4) preoperative organ failure.[10] Previous myocardial infarction had occurred in eight of 11 patients (73%) who died perioperatively after undergoing delayed (>18 hours) revascularization. (Table 93–2).

Therefore, patients in cardiogenic shock who are found, on coronary angiography, to have more than 50% stenosis of the left main coronary artery with either a left anterior descending or a circumflex infarct–related vessel, 75% stenosis of the left main artery with a right coronary infarct-related vessel, severe disease of all three coronary arteries, or coronary anatomy unsuitable for PTCA should be considered for emergency surgical revascularization. Immediate consultation with a cardiac surgeon should also be sought while the patient is still in the catheterization laboratory so that if urgent surgery were to be rejected, selected angioplasty might be beneficial.

MECHANICAL COMPLICATIONS OF ACUTE MYOCARDIAL INFARCTION

The sudden occurrence of electromechanical dissociation and profound shock during or after thrombolytic therapy in a previously hemodynamically stable patient should immediately prompt suspicion of acute aortic dissection with rupture into the pericardial sac, acute cardiac free wall rupture, and inappropriate thrombolysis of a patient with unrecognized acute pericarditis that is now complicated by acute pericardial tamponade. Because there is no appropriate medical therapy for these conditions, cardiac surgical consultation should be immediate. Acute attempts to stabilize such patients include volume replacement, pressure support, and pericardiocentesis.

Postinfarct Ventricular Septal Rupture and Acute Mitral Regurgitation

All patients with acute myocardial infarction should be thoroughly examined on admission and frequently thereafter. Any new systolic murmur should immediately lead to suspicion of a mechanical complication, especially in the presence of hemodynamic compromise, heart failure of new onset, or recurrence of chest pain. In addition, a mechanical complication should be suspected when any hemodynamic instability is observed, regardless of the physical findings. A murmur of severe acute mitral regurgitation may be very short in duration and may not be detected in an agitated patient who suddenly develops pulmonary edema.

Mortality remains high when ventricular septal rupture or acute mitral regurgitation complicates acute myocardial infarction and causes cardiogenic shock.[34-36] A high index of suspicion, together with timely diagnosis, prompt implementation of therapy, and surgical consultation, is thus necessary to improve the chances of survival.

A definitive differential diagnosis between these two conditions cannot be made by physical examination. Both conditions present with a systolic murmur, which can be apical, radiating to the axilla, and associated with a thrill. Once the diagnosis is confirmed, aggressive therapy should be immediately instituted. Arrangements should be made immediately for emergency echocardiography followed by cardiac catheterization and cardiac surgical consultation. If the patient has a Swan-Ganz catheter, right atrial, pulmonary arterial, and radial arterial oxygen saturation values should be obtained, to document the presence of a left-to-right shunt. Transthoracic echocardiography should be performed together with color Doppler flow mapping of the entire interventricular septum, from base to apex. Echocardiography[16] can visualize and assess the size of most ventricular septal ruptures and determine right and left ventricular function, estimate pulmonary artery pressures, evaluate the mitral and tricuspid valves, assess the need for valve repair or replacement, and rule out a second mechanical complication of myocardial infarction or an associated free wall rupture. The sensitivity of the echocardiographic examination is increased by thorough color Doppler flow mapping of all portions of the interventricular septum and by intravenous injection of agitated saline. All patients who are hemodynamically stable should undergo coronary angiography and ventriculography. Placement of an IABP may help to stabilize patients, particularly during diagnostic catheterization.

Postinfarction ventricular septal rupture (PIVSR) is usually a catastrophic event, with cardiogenic shock developing in 50% of the patients within 48 hours of the appearance of the ventricular septal rupture.[37-42] PIVSR usually occurs in older patients with limited coronary artery disease,[39-41] who have a paucity of collateral blood flow. In an autopsy study of patients with PIVSR, Cummings and colleagues[40] found that all infarcts in PIVSR patients were transmural, confluent, and in the distribution of one major coronary artery. Ventricular septal ruptures are equally common in association with anterior and inferior myocardial infarctions.[40] In most patients, the acute episode is the first manifestation of coronary artery disease.

Since the anterolateral papillary muscle of the mitral valve has a dual blood supply from both the left anterior descending and the circumflex coronary arteries, it rarely ruptures in patients with acute myocardial infarction. However, the posteromedial papillary muscle is supplied mainly by the right coronary artery and is thus more susceptible to rupture after inferior myocardial infarctions, which may be accompanied by right ventricular infarction.[43] Rupture of a papillary muscle trunk is associated with a fulminant course and in a few hours with death.[44] Rupture of a papillary muscle head results in severe mitral regurgitation with rapid development of acute pulmonary edema and cardiogenic shock.

Once one of these complications is detected, or in the presence of hemodynamic instability, an IABP should be inserted and the patient should be referred immediately for

TABLE 93–3. Cardiogenic Shock Due to "Extracoronary" Causes: Key Points

1. Aortic stenosis: Physical findings are not reliable. Emergency echocardiography is a must. Surgical replacement of the valve in preferred. Percutaneous balloon valvuloplasty is a viable alternative.
2. Acute aortic regurgitation: Short diastolic blow *without* the peripheral physical findings of chronic aortic regurgitation. Emergency echocardiography. Considered a surgical emergency.
3. Hypertrophic cardiomyopathy: Diagnosis is made by suspicion of aortic stenosis and confirmation with echocardiography. *Inotropes are contraindicated.* Fluid replacement and cardioversion are used if appropriate.

surgery. Although the insertion of an IABP optimizes hemodynamics and prevents development of multiple organ failure,[32, 38] most patients gradually deteriorate within a few days. The IABP should be only a temporary measure, especially in the presence of heart failure, cardiogenic shock, or any persistent or recurrent hemodynamic instability.

Although patients with PIVSR or acute mitral regurgitation secondary to rupture of a papillary muscle head may initially be stable or respond to intensive medical therapy, typically there is rapid and progressive deterioration in their hemodynamic status that is usually fatal unless emergency surgery is performed.[42, 44] Clinical and hemodynamic improvement resulting from IABP is not a reason for deferring surgery. PIVSR and acute mitral regurgitation secondary to papillary muscle rupture are surgical emergencies, and cardiogenic shock is an indication for immediate surgical repair and not for prolonged medical stabilization (see Table 93–2).

Cardiac Rupture

Sudden or rapid hemodynamic collapse occurring in a previously stable patient, especially when associated with electromechanical dissociation, should always prompt immediate suspicion of perforation of the free wall of the infarcted ventricle. Although cardiac rupture is not usually accompanied by any premonitory signs, occasionally, sudden and severe chest pain during strenuous physical activity herald it. Rarely, the ventricular perforation occurs along a tortuous, serpiginous tract, allowing for slower development of pericardial tamponade.

The clinical progression of cardiac rupture and hemopericardium consists of the rapid occurrence of severe pericardial tamponade, cardiogenic shock refractory to fluid administration, and death. Treatment should include immediate confirmation of pericardial fluid accumulation by transthoracic echocardiography followed by immediate pericardiocentesis, emergency cardiac surgery consultation and thoracotomy, administration of large amounts of fluids, and emergency cardiac repair (Table 93–3).

RIGHT VENTRICULAR INFARCTION

Thrombotic occlusion of the right coronary artery proximal to its right ventricular branches can result in ischemia or infarction of the right ventricular myocardium,[45, 46] which results in decreased right ventricular systolic function and diastolic compliance, increased right ventricular stiffness resulting in a decrease in its diastolic filling, and increased right atrial pressure, dilatation of the right ventricle, paradoxical diastolic bulging of the interventricular septum in the left ventricular cavity, and a significant decrease in the left ventricular preload (causing a decrease in cardiac output, which can lead to cardiogenic shock). Right ventricular myocardial infarction can accompany both inferior and anterior myocardial infarctions.[46] It should be suspected whenever cardiogenic shock complicates acute myocardial infarction in the presence of elevated jugular venous pressure with clear lung fields.

The diagnosis of right ventricular myocardial ischemia or infarction is made (1) by demonstrating right precordial ST-segment elevations on electrocardiography and is supported by observing right ventricular wall motion abnormalities and decreased systolic function on echocardiography[45] and (2) by meeting the hemodynamic criteria of right atrial pressure of 10 mm Hg and an 0.8 ratio of the right atrial pressure to pulmonary capillary wedge pressure.[47]

Therapy for cardiogenic shock secondary to right ventricular myocardial infarction[45, 48] should consist of an urgent attempt at restoration of brisk, antegrade, TIMI grade 3 flow in the right coronary or infarct-related artery, by either intravenous thrombolytic therapy or primary coronary angioplasty. IABP counterpulsation is indicated. Right ventricular preload should be optimized and individualized, taking into consideration the systolic function of the right ventricle and the cardiac output response to fluid administration. The failing right ventricle should be supported by positive inotropic agents. Heart rate and rhythm should be optimized to restore atrial systole, maintain the normal atrioventricular conduction sequence, and prevent excessive tachyarrhythmias or bradyarrhythmias (see Table 93–3).

AORTIC STENOSIS

The presence of shock that cannot be attributed to any specific cause and that is refractory to supportive therapy should prompt suspicion of a mechanical obstruction of the left ventricular outflow tract. Critical aortic stenosis associated with left ventricular systolic dysfunction may present as cardiogenic shock in both younger patients with bicuspid aortic valves and older patients with calcific aortic stenosis.[49–51] There may be no history of aortic stenosis, and previously some of these patients may have been summarily treated for congestive heart failure or angina pectoris.

Aortic stenosis is accompanied by left ventricular hypertrophy, increased stiffness of the left ventricle, increased myocardial oxygen consumption, prolongation of the systolic ejection period with resultant shortening of the duration of diastolic coronary blood flow, and compression of the intramyocardial blood vessels by the large mass of contracting myocardium and the high pressures generated during systole. This results in myocardial ischemia, which can be the presenting picture of these patients and which leads to further left ventricular systolic dysfunction, generating a vicious circle. In other circumstances, poorly compensated aortic stenosis may completely decompensate secondary to other causes, such as acute coronary atherosclerosis, ischemia, or infarction. Thus, other contributing causes should be sought.

In these patients auscultation can be particularly deceptive. Owing to the low cardiac output state, the accompanying tachycardia, and the multitude of extracardiac sounds in these patients, no murmurs may be heard or a faint systolic ejection murmur may be detected and either neglected or ascribed to flow (in a younger patient) or aortic sclerosis (in an older one). Echocardiography is therefore critical in the diagnosis.

Since aortic stenosis is a mechanical obstruction to the left ventricular output, it can be decreased or corrected only by a mechanical intervention. Aortic valve replacement, the modality of choice, should be undertaken as an emergency, before the development of multisystem organ failure, which is associated with high rates of surgical morbidity and mortality.[49, 52]

For these very-high-risk patients with multisystem organ failure and in those who are not judged to be surgical candidates, percutaneous balloon aortic valvuloplasty is the only available therapeutic modality that can be lifesaving, result in dramatic hemodynamic improvement, and lead to sufficient stabilization and recovery from multisystem failure, to allow them eventually to undergo aortic valve replacement (see Table 93-3).[50, 51] IABP is contraindicated, however, in patients with associated severe aortic regurgitation.

ACUTE AORTIC REGURGITATION

Cardiogenic shock can occur as a result of acute severe aortic regurgitation secondary to acute bacterial endocarditis, dehiscence of a prosthetic aortic valve, or acute dissection of the aorta. In the presence of severe acute aortic regurgitation there is marked reduction in effective forward stroke volume; marked volume overload of the left ventricle, which cannot compensate owing to the acuity of the event; significant elevation in the left ventricular end-diastolic pressure; premature closure of the mitral valve, which further diminishes cardiac output; significant elevation in pulmonary capillary wedge pressure and pulmonary venous hypertension, which results in cardiogenic shock and acute pulmonary edema.

As with critical aortic stenosis and cardiogenic shock, physical findings in patients with severe acute aortic regurgitation are deceptive. The diastolic decrescendo murmur of aortic regurgitation is abbreviated, ending well before the first heart sound, which is markedly decreased in intensity and is accompanied by an early to mid-diastolic apical murmur (the Austin Flint murmur). In addition, with acute regurgitation the classic peripheral manifestations of chronic aortic regurgitation are absent or significantly attenuated. Thus, the diagnosis of acute aortic regurgitation is frequently overlooked and its severity underestimated. Echocardiography permits rapid diagnosis and accurate assessment of the severity of acute aortic regurgitation. Severe acute aortic regurgitation is a surgical emergency. Therapy should be directed toward afterload reduction with sodium nitroprusside and myocardial positive inotropic support, in an attempt to maintain adequate systemic perfusion and a pulmonary capillary wedge pressure of about 15 to 18 mm Hg while awaiting emergency aortic valve replacement (see Table 93-3). Obviously, an IABP is contraindicated in these patients.

HYPERTROPHIC CARDIOMYOPATHY

Patients with hypertrophic cardiomyopathy have a thickened, noncompliant left ventricle and dynamic left ventricular outflow obstruction. They are thus dependent on preload and on the atrial contribution to left ventricular diastolic filling. A decrease in preload can result in hypotension, which, if not promptly and properly corrected by fluid administration or resumption of sinus rhythm, can rapidly result in cardiogenic shock. Under these conditions, failure to diagnose hypertrophic cardiomyopathy can result in administration of positive inotropic agents, which, by increasing the contractility of an already hypercontractile left ventricle and accentuating the systolic anterior motion of the mitral valve, significantly increases left ventricular outflow tract obstruction and increases the amount of mitral regurgitation, which markedly worsens the shock. This is further aggravated by the myocardial ischemia secondary to excessive myocardial oxygen demand, compression of the intramural coronary arteries, and decreased coronary perfusion pressure.[53]

Hypertrophic cardiomyopathy should be suspected in any patient with a systolic ejection murmur. A unique finding is a decrease in the arterial pulse pressure following a "post-extrasystolic" pause. Diagnosis is easily established by transthoracic echocardiography.[53]

Therapy consists of correcting fluid deficits, restoring sinus rhythm by direct current cardioversion, if necessary, in patients with paroxysmal atrial fibrillation, slowing of the ventricular rate, and decreasing left ventricular contractility with beta blockade.

MASSIVE PULMONARY EMBOLISM

(see Chapter 101)

In patients with no history of cardiopulmonary disease, acute pulmonary embolization severe enough to occlude more than 25% of the pulmonary arterial bed results in a significant acute increase in the pulmonary vascular resistance and right ventricular afterload. Acute increases in right ventricular systolic pressures result in acute right ventricular dilatation and failure, decreased left ventricular preload, paradoxical bulging of the interventricular septum in the left ventricular cavity during diastole (further interfering with filling of the left ventricle), decreased cardiac output, and cardiogenic shock. Although the finding of right ventricular systolic dysfunction is not specific to cardiogenic shock, one should suspect acute pulmonary embolization, especially when it is accompanied by echocardiographic demonstration of right ventricular mid-free wall akinesis with normal apical wall motion.[54] The echocardiographic demonstration of right ventricular dilatation in patients with acute pulmonary embolism was shown in the multicenter Management and Prognosis of Pulmonary Embolism Registry to be an independent predictor of 30-day mortality.

A review of four randomized clinical trials that compared the rate of resolution of pulmonary emboli in patients treated with rt-PA plus heparin to heparin alone revealed that treatment with rt-PA plus heparin resulted in more rapid early resolution of pulmonary embolic obstruction during the first 2 to 24 hours after treatment. Mortality rates, however, were similar, probably owing to the fact that most deaths occur from acute pulmonary embolism in undiagnosed patients or within the first hour of presentation, before therapy can be instituted.[56] Thus, in the absence of contraindications, all patients with massive pulmonary embolization complicated by shock should promptly receive intravenous thrombolytic therapy.[56] In addition, adequate right ventricular preload should be ensured and inotropic support to the failing right ventricular myocardium provided.

SUMMARY

Cardiogenic shock continues to occur in a significant portion of patients who present with acute myocardial infarction and is still associated with risk of death. It is the leading cause of death in hospitalized patients with acute myocardial infarction. Aggressive therapy should immediately be instituted and should be directed principally at reestablishing anterograde brisk TIMI grade 3 flow in the infarct-related artery, preferably by emergency primary coronary angioplasty or, if this is not readily available, by prompt intravenous administration of thrombolytic therapy. Hemodynamic support should consist of:

1. Restoration or maintenance of adequate left ventricular preload.

2. Institution of IABP counterpulsation to increase coronary arterial perfusion pressure and decrease ventricular afterload, thus reducing myocardial oxygen demand, ventricular myocardial inotropic support, administration of vasopressors to increase the mean arterial pressure, maintenance of sinus rhythm.

3. Correction of any tachyarrhythmia or bradyarrhythmia, correction of metabolic abnormalities, and maintenance of adequate oxygenation.

A high index of suspicion is necessary to determine the cause of cardiogenic shock secondary to a mechanical complication of the acute myocardial infarction or to conditions unrelated to myocardial infarction, such as critical aortic stenosis, acute severe aortic regurgitation, hypertrophic cardiomyopathy, and acute massive pulmonary embolism. Transthoracic echocardiography should be readily available, and liberally used, in these patients.

References

1. Alonso DR, Scheidt S, Post M, Killip T: Pathophysiology of cardiogenic shock: Quantification of myocardial necrosis, clinical, pathologic and electrocardiographic correlations. Circulation 1973; 48:588–596.
2. Page DL, Caulfield JB, Kastor JA, DeSanctis R, Sanders CA: Myocardial changes associated with cardiogenic shock. N Engl J Med 1971; 285:133–137.
3. Allen BS, Rosenkranz E, Buckberg GD, Davtyan H, Laks H, Tillisch J, Drinkwater DC: Studies on prolonged acute regional ischemia: VI. Myocardial infarction with left ventricular power failure. A medical/surgical emergency requiring urgent revascularization with maximal protection of remote muscle. J Thorac Cardiovasc Surg 1989; 98:691–703.
4. Beyerdoft F, Buckberg GD, Acar C: Studies on prolonged acute regional ischemia: III. Early natural history of simulated single and multivessel disease with emphasis on remote myocardium. J Thorac Cardiovasc Surg 1989; 98:368–380.
5. Beyerdord F, Acar C, Buckberg GD: Studies on prolonged acute regional ischemia: V. Metabolic support of remote myocardium during left ventricular power failure. J Thorac Cardiovasc Surg 1989; 98:567–579.
6. The GUSTO Investigators: An international randomized trial comparing four thrombolytic strategies for acute myocardial infarction. N Engl J Med 1993; 329:673–682.
7. Holmes DR Jr, Bates ER. Kleiman NS, Sadowski Z, Horgan JHS, Morris DC, Califf RM, Berger PB, Topol EJ: Contemporary reperfusion therapy for cardiogenic shock: The GUSTO-I trial experience. J Am Coll Cardiol 1995; 26:668–674.
8. Berger PB, Holmes DR, Stebbins AL, Bates ER, Califf RM, Topol EJ: Impact of an aggressive invasive catheterization and revascularization strategy on mortality in patients with cardiogenic shock in the Global Utilization of Streptokinase and Tissue Plasminogen Activator for Occluded Coronary Arteries (GUSTO-I) trial. An observational study. Circulation 1997; 96:122–127.
9. Holmes DR, Califf RM, van de Werf F, Berger PB, Bates ER, Simoons ML, White HD, Thompson TD, Topol EJ: Difference in countries' use of resources and clinical outcome for patients with cardiogenic shock myocardial infarction: Results of the GUSTO trial. Lancet 1991; 349:75–78.
10. Allen BS, Rosenkranz E, Buckberg GD, Davtyan H, Laks H, Tillisch J, Drinkwater DC: Studis on prolonged acute regional ischemia. VI. Myocardial infarction with left ventricular power failure: A medical/surgical emergency requiring urgent revascularization with maximal protection of remote muscle. J Thorac Cardiovasc Surg 1989; 98:691–703.
11. Hockman JS, Boland J, Sleeper LA, Porway M, Brinker J, Col J, Jacobs A, Slater J, Miller D, Wasserman H, Menegus MA, Talley DJ, McKinlay S, Sanborn T, LeJemtel T: Current spectrum of cardiogenic shock and effect of early revascularization of mortality: Results of an international registry. Circulation 1995; 91:873–881.
12. Eltchaninoff H, Simpfendorfer C, Franco I, Raymond RE, Caseale PN, Whitelow PL: Early and 1-year survival rates in acute myocardial infarction complicated by cardiogenic shock: A restrospective study comparing coronary angioplasty with medical treatment. Am Heart J 1995; 130:459–464.
13. Lee L, Erbel R, Brown TM, Laufer N, Meyer J, O'Neil WW: Multicenter registry of angioplasty therapy of cardiogenic shock: Initial and long-term saving. J Am Coll Cardiol 1991; 17:599–603.
14. Grassman ED, Johnson SA, Krone RJ: Predictors of success and major complications for primary percutaneous transluminal coronary angioplasty in acute myocardial infarction: An analysis of the 1990 to 1994 Society for Cardiac Angiography and Interventions registry. J Am Coll Cardiol 1997; 30:201–208.
15. O'Keefe JH, Bailey LW, Rutherford BD, Hartzler GO: Primary angioplasty for acute myocardial infarction in 1,000 consecutive patients: Results in an unselected population and high-risk subgroups. Am J Cardiol 1993; 72:107G–115G.
16. Helmcke F, Mahan EF III, Nanda NC, Jain SP, Soto B, Kirklin JK, Pacifico AD: Two dimensional echocardiography and Doppler color flow mapping in the diagnosis and prognosis of ventricular septal rupture. Circulation 1990; 81:1775–1778.
17. Karagounis L, Sorensen LG, Menlove RL, Moreno F, Anderson JI: Does thrombolysis in myocardial infarction (TIMI) perfusion grade 2 produce a most patent or a most occluded artery? Enzymatic and electrocardiographic evidence from the TEAM-2 study. J Am Coll Cardiol 1992; 19:1–190.
18. Anderson JL, Karagounis LA, Becker LC, Sorensen SG, Menlove RL: TIMI perfusion grade 3 but not grade 2 results in improved outcome after thrombolysis for myocardial infarction. Circulation 1993; 87:1829–1839.
19. Vogt A, von Essen R, Tebbe U, Feurer W, Appel K-F, Neuhaus KL: Impact of early perfusion status of the infarct-related artery on short term mortality after thrombolysis for acute myocardial infarction: Restrospective analysis of four German multicenter studies. J Am Coll Cardiol 1993; 21:1391–1395.
20. Simes RJ, Topol EJ, Holmes DR, White HD, Rutsch WR, Vahanian A, Simoons, ML, Morris D, Betriu A, Califf RM, Ross AM: Link between the angiographic substudy and mortality outcomes in a large randomized trial of myocardial reperfusion. Circulation 1995; 91:1923–1928.
21. The GUSTO Angiographic Investigators: The effects of tissue plasminogen activator, streptokinase, or both on coronary artery patency, ventricular function and survival after acute myocardial infarction. N Engl J Med 1993; 329:1615–1622.
22. Linoff AM, Topol EJ, Califf RM, Sigmon KN, Lee OK, Ohman EM, Rosenchein U, Ellis SG: Significance of a coronary artery with thrombolysis in myocardial infarction grade 2 flow "patency" (Outcome in the Thrombolysis and Angioplasty in Myocardial Infarction Trials). Am J Cardiol 1995; 75:871–876.
23. Anderson J, Karagounis L, Califf RM: Meta-analysis of five reported studies on the relation of early coronary patency grades with mortality and outcomes after acute myocardial infarction. Am J Cardiol 1996; 78:1–8.
24. Walters MI, Burn S, Houghton T, Chakraborth R, Bain R, Clark R, Kaye GC, Caplin JL, Norell MS: Cardiogenic shock: Are HEROICS justified? Circulation 1997; 96:I-31.
25. Grines CL, Browne KF, Marco J, Rothbaum D, Stone GW, O'Keefe J, Overlie P, Donohud B, Chelliah N, Timmis GC, Vliestra RE, Strzelecki M, Purchrowicz-Ochocki S, O'Neill WW: A comparison of immediate angioplasty with thrombolytic therapy for acute myocardial infarction. N Engl J Med 1993; 328:673–679.
26. Kantrowitz A, Tjonneland S, Freed PS: Initial experience with intra-aortic balloon pumping in cardiogenic shock. JAMA 1968; 203:135–140.
27. Creswell L, Rosenbloom M, Cox JL, Ferguson TD: Intraaortic balloon counterpulsation: Patterns of usage and outcomes. Ann Thorac Surg 1992; 54:11–20.
28. Anderson DR, Ohman M, Holmes DR, Col J, Stebbins AL, Bates ER, Stomel RJ, Granger CB, Topol EJ, Califf RM: Use of intraaortic balloon counterpulsation in patients with cardiogenic shock: Observations from the GUSTO-I study. J Am Coll Cardiol 1997; 30:708–715.
29. Kovack PJ, Rasak MA, Bates ER, Ohman ME, Stomel RJ: Thrombolysis plus aortic counterpulsation: Improved survival in patients who present to community hospitals with cardiogenic shock. J Am Coll Cardiol 1997; 29:1454–1458.
30. Tardiff BE, Califf RM, Morris D, Bates E, Woodlief LH, Lee KL, Green C, Ritsch W, Betriu A, Aylward PE, Topol EJ: Coronary revascularization surgery after myocardial infarction: Impact of bypass surgery on survival after thrombolysis. J Am Coll Cardiol 1997; 29:240–249.
31. Gersch BJ, Chesbro JH, Braunwald E, Lambrew C, Passamani E, Solomon RE, Ross AM, Ross R, Terrin ML, Knatterud GL: Coronary artery bypass graft surgery after thrombolytic therapy in the

Thrombolysis in Myocardial Infarction Trial, Phase II (TIMI II). J Am Coll Cardiol 1995; 25:395–402.
32. Every NR, Maynard C, Cochran RP, Martin J, Weaver DW: Characteristics, management and outcome of patients with acute myocardial infarction treated with bypass surgery. Circulation 1996; 84 (Suppl II): 81–86.
33. Kereiakes DJ, Topol EJ, George BS, Abbottsmith CW, Stack RS, Candela RJ, Oneil WW, Anderson LC, Califf RM: Favorable early and long-term prognosis following coronary bypass surgical therapy for myocardial infarction: Results of a multicenter trial. Am Heart J 1989; 118:199–206.
34. Skillington PD, Davies RH, Luff AJ, Williams JD, Dawkins KD, Conway N, Lamb RK, Shore DF, Monro JL, Ross KJ: Surgical treatment for infarct-related ventricular septal defects: Improved early results combined with analysis of late functional status. J Thoracic Cardiovasc Surg 1990; 99:798–808.
35. Hochman JS, Talley JD, Sleeper L, Col J, Miller D, Slater J, Menegus M, Forman R, White H, Aylward P, Sanborn T, Le Jemetel T: Mortality remains high when ventricular septal rupture (VSR) or acute myocardial infarction (AMI) (Abstract). J Am Coll Cardiol 1997; 30:459A.
36. Hochman JS, Talley DJ, Webb JG, Slater J, Sleeper LA, Lejemtel TH: Ventricular septal rupture (VSR) causing cardiogenic shock (CS): Clinical profile, timing and outcome (Abstract). Circulation 1997; 96:I-749.
37. Estrada-Quintero T, Uretsky BF, Murali S, Hardesty RL: Prolonged intra-aortic balloon support for septal rupture after myocardial infarction. Ann Thorac Surg 1992; 53:335–337.
38. Baillot R, Pelletier C, Trivino-Marin J, Castonguay Y: Postinfarction ventricular septal defect: Delayed closure with prolonged mechanical circulatory support. Ann Thorac Surg 1983; 35:138–142.
39. Skillington PD, Davies RH, Luff AJ, Williams JD, Dawkins KD, Conway N, Lamab RK, Shore DF, Monro JL, Ross KJ: Surgical treatment for infarct-related ventricular septal defects: Improved early results combined with analysis of late functional status. J Thorac Cardiovasc Surg 1990; 99:798–808.
40. Cummings RG, Reimer KA, Califf R, Hacke D, Boswick J, Lowe JE: Quantitative analysis of right and left ventricular infarction in the presence of postinfarction ventricular septal defect. Circulation 1988; 77:33–42.
41. Komeda M, Fremes SE, David TE: Surgical repair of postinfarction ventricular septal defect. Circulation 1990; 82 (Suppl IV): 243–247.
42. Loisance DY, Cachera JP, Poulain H, Aubry PH, Juvin AM, Galey JJ: Ventricular septal defect after acute myocardial infarction: Early repair. J Thorac Cardiovasc Surg 1980; 80:61–67.
43. Rangananthan N, Burch GE: Gross morphologic and arterial blood supply of the papillary muscles of the left ventricle. Am Heart J 1969; 77:506–516.
44. Nishiumura RA, Schaff HV, Shub C: Papillary muscle rupture complicating acute myocardial infarction: Analysis of 17 patients. Am J Cardiol 1997; 51:373–377.
45. Bates ER: Revisiting reperfusion therapy in inferior myocardial infarction. J Am Coll Cardiol 1997; 30:334–342.
46. Anderson HR, Falk E, Nielsen D: Right ventricular infarction: Frequency, size and topography in coronary heart disease: A prospective study comprising 107 consecutive autopsies from a coronary care unit. J Am Coll Cardiol 1987; 10:1223–1232.
47. Lloyd EA, Gersh BJ, Kennelly BM: Hemodynamic spectrum of "dominant" right ventricular infarction in 19 patients. Am J Cardiol 1991; 48:1016–1022.
48. Coma-Canella I, Lopez-Sendon J, Gamallo C: Low output syndrome in right ventricular infarction. Am Heart J 1979; 98:613–620.
49. Cannon RO, Rosing DR, Maron BJ: Myocardial ischemia in hypertrophic cardiomyopathy: Contribution of inadequate vasodilator reserve and elevated left ventricular filling pressures. Circulation 1985; 71:234–243.
50. Moreno PR, Jang IK, Newell JB, Block PC, Palacios IF: The role of percutaneous aortic balloon valvuloplasty in patients with cardiogenic shock and critical aortic stenosis. J Am Coll Cardiol 1994; 23:1071–1074.
51. Cribier A, Remade F, Rath P, Stix G, Letac B: Emergency balloon valvuloplasty as initial treatment of patients with aortic stenosis and cardiogenic shock. N Engl J Med 1992; 327:1452–1456.
52. Scott WC, Miller DC, Haverich A, Dawkins K, Mitchell RS, Jamieson SW, Oyer PE, Stinson EB, Baldwin JC, Shumway NE: Determinants of operative mortality for patients undergoing aortic valve replacement. J Thorac Cardiovasc Surg 1985; 89:400–413.
53. Cannon RO, Rosing DR, Maron BJK: Myocardial ischemia in hypertrophic cardiomyopathy: Contribution of inadequate vasodilator reserve and elevated left ventricular filling pressures. Circulation 1985; 71:234–243.
54. McConnell MV, Solomon SD, Rayan ME, Come PC, Goldhaver SZ, Lee RT: Regional right ventricular dysfunction detected by echocardiography in acute pulmonary embolism. Am J Cardiol 1997; 78:450–473.
55. Konstantinides S, Geibel A, Kasper W, Olschewski M, Kienast J, Iversen S, Grosser KD: Predictors of in-hospital mortality in patients with acute massive pulmonary embolism: Results of the Management and Prognosis of Pulmonary Embolism Registry (MAPPET). Circulation 1995; 94:I-572–I-593.
56. Dalen JE, Alpert JS, Hirsh J: Thrombolytic therapy for pulmonary embolism: Is it effective? Is it safe? When is it indicated? Arch Intern Med 1997; 157:2550–2556.

94

Congestive Heart Failure in Infants and Children

Bradley P. Fuhrman, MD • Lynn J. Hernan, MD

Congestive heart failure (CHF) is a clinical syndrome. It is a circulatory state in which the heart (1) is unable to meet the demands of the body for blood flow, (2) cannot meet these demands without excessive use of compensatory mechanisms, or (3) meets these demands only at the expense of excessively high ventricular filling pressures. This crudely fashioned definition is purely operational and is not concise because cardiac decompensation is not an all-or-none phenomenon. It varies from absolute exhaustion of reserve (cardiogenic shock) to reliance on minor compensatory measures such as cardiac dilatation or hypertrophy at rest, with decompensation only on exertion.

CAUSES OF CONGESTIVE HEART FAILURE

Coronary vascular occlusion is generally not the cause of CHF in infants and children, although myocardial ischemia may complicate congenital cardiac disease and may be the confounding variable on which outcome depends.[1] Some general causes of CHF are listed in Table 94–1.

In congenital cardiac malformations, CHF is often the direct result of ventricular volume overload of the heart.[2] The infant with a ventricular septal defect, for example, may have so large a left-to-right shunt across the defect that only a small fraction of left ventricular inflow (left atrial return) is ejected to the aorta. A 75% left-to-right shunt, for instance, requires that the left ventricle pump 4 units of blood for every unit that enters the aorta. In such a patient, the left ventricular volume load is massive, perhaps four times normal. The circulation, in essence, fails as a result of impaired efficiency. This requires an increase in left atrial pressure (preload) to achieve the requisite elevated left ventricular end-diastolic volume. Ultimately, the heart must enlarge (a state of hypertrophy) to pump at this greater chamber circumference,[3] making it less

TABLE 94–1. Processes Causing or Contributing to Congestive Heart Failure

Mechanism	Example
Ventricular volume overload	Ventricular septal defect
Vascular volume overload	Iatrogenic
Ventricular outflow obstruction	Aortic stenosis
Myocardial dysfunction	Myocarditis
Myocardial ischemia	Anomalous left coronary artery
Ventricular inflow restriction	Mitral stenosis
Arrhythmias	Paroxysmal atrial tachycardia
Anemia	Aplastic anemia
Hypoxia	Transposition of great vessels
Systemic hypermetabolism	Thyrotoxicosis

compliant and further increasing requisite preload. Pulmonary edema and respiratory symptoms may occur. Any exertion that requires greater aortic flow will further elevate end-diastolic volume and left atrial pressure. In fact, for every additional liter of aortic flow demanded by the body, 4 L would have to be ejected by the left ventricle. The consequent limited ability of the heart to respond to an increased demand for oxygen delivery to tissues has the appearance of "exercise intolerance."

Obstruction of a ventricle can cause CHF by exaggerating the ventricular work required to eject blood. When the metabolic cost of this work exceeds the potential of the coronary circulation to supply oxygen and substrate to the myocardium, coronary ischemia occurs.[4] Critical aortic stenosis, for instance, may cause CHF in infancy. Myocardial ischemia may lead to endocardial fibroelastosis, subendocardial infarction, and loss of myocardial function. Similarly, when the child with moderate aortic stenosis becomes an adult, calcification of the malformed valve causes progression of the obstruction and may cause ischemia, myocardial fibrosis, and CHF.[5]

Muscle dysfunction may be a primary cause of CHF in infants and children. In congenital cardiomyopathies and in myocarditis, muscle function is impaired and contractility is reduced. This limits the ability of the heart to use the Frank-Starling mechanism to augment stroke volume in response to increasing ventricular end-diastolic pressure. Excessive preload may be required to generate even a subnormal stroke volume.

Primary myocardial ischemia may cause CHF. In anomalous origin of the left coronary artery from the pulmonary artery, coronary perfusion pressure may be inadequate to perfuse the left ventricular myocardium and to support left ventricular work.[6]

Inflow restriction may contribute to symptoms by elevating the preload required to fill even the normal ventricle, as in rheumatic mitral stenosis.[7] In this situation, even minor increases in left ventricular output or small decreases in cardiac filling time (associated with tachycardia) may inordinately elevate preload and precipitate pulmonary edema.

Other causes of CHF include arrhythmias (fast or slow), anemia, hypoxia, pathologic demand for oxygen delivery (e.g., thyrotoxicosis, pyrexia), and vascular volume overload.

These mechanisms may coexist and act synergistically to produce cardiac decompensation.

Table 94–2 lists conditions that may cause CHF in infants and children. This is not an exhaustive list but serves to illustrate the diversity of conditions that may be associated with CHF in this age group.

SIGNS AND SYMPTOMS

Because of the spectrum of decompensation encompassed by the term CHF and because of the age specificity of these manifestations, presenting findings are quite variable.[1] In all age groups, CHF implies cardiac enlargement, tachycardia, and tachypnea. In the neonate, because ventricular interdependence makes left-sided and right-sided heart failure virtually inseparable, hepatomegaly is virtually always present. Exercise intolerance may appear as dyspnea on exertion or as undue fatigue in the older child, or it may interfere with feeding in the infant. Hypoxia may be a sign of pulmonary edema, in which case it is generally responsive to oxygen administration, or it may represent an associated aspect of congenital cardiac disease, such as right-to-left shunting of blood or admixture of systemic and pulmonary venous return.

Radiographic cardiomegaly may represent cardiac dilatation from ventricular volume overload in the patient with an atrial or ventricular septal defect and does not in itself establish the presence of CHF.[8] Poor contractility and reduced ejection fraction, documented by echocardiography or angiography, are often viewed as synonymous with CHF. When present, these findings clearly support a diagnosis of CHF. Their absence, however, cannot be interpreted as a guarantee that cardiac function is normal. The afterload reduction characteristic of mitral regurgitation, ventricular septal defect, or arteriovenous malformation may mask myocardial dysfunction and lend the appearance of normal contractility. Inotropic agents and sympathetic stimulation may also enhance ejection fraction and give the appearance of adequate myocardial function, although intrinsic compensatory mechanisms are no longer capable of supporting normal cardiac output.[9]

Frank cardiogenic shock is a common presentation of congenital cardiac disease. Metabolic acidosis, hypotension, poor perfusion, thready pulses, pallor, and diaphoresis are often presenting findings in ductus-dependent malformations such as coarctation, hypoplastic left-sided heart syndrome, interruption of the aortic arch, and critical aortic stenosis. This presentation is the hallmark of vein of Galen aneurysm. Cardiogenic shock is also an occasional presenting symptom in cardiomyopathy, anomalous origin of the left coronary artery, or myocarditis. In all age groups, sepsis may be accompanied by cardiogenic shock (low cardiac output, hypotension, and impaired cardiac contractility).

In infants, the age at onset of CHF is characteristic of specific lesions and provides clues to etiology. Ductus-dependent malformations generally cause CHF at the time of ductus closure (2nd to 5th day after birth.) Examples include interruption of the aortic arch and hypoplastic left heart syndrome. Large ventricular septal defects may cause CHF after pulmonary vascular resistance declines (2 to 8 weeks of age.)

TREATMENT

Treatment of CHF in infants and children is not fundamentally different from treatment in adults. (See also Chapter 89.)

TABLE 94–2. Causes of Congestive Heart Failure in Infants and Children

Congenital cardiac malformations
Congenital arteriovenous malformations
Anomalies of aortic arch
Endocardial fibroelastosis
Anomalous origin of left coronary artery
Cardiomyopathy
Myocarditis
Anemia
Congenital heart block
Tachyarrhythmias
Rheumatic fever
Kawasaki's syndrome
Endocarditis
Cardiac surgery

TABLE 94–3. Treatment of Congestive Heart Failure in Infants and Children

- Drugs that augment contractility
  - Digoxin
  - Catecholamines (dopamine, dobutamine, epinephrine, norepinephrine, isoproterenol)
  - Methylxanthines (theophylline)
  - Bipyridines (amrinone)
- Myocardial workload reduction
- Oxygen and positive end-expiratory pressure
- Diuretics
- Vascular volume expansion

There are many components to the treatment of CHF. Some are specific, such as diuresis in iatrogenic volume overload, control of hypertension in hypertensive cardiomyopathy, transfusion in severe anemia, and balloon atrial septostomy in transposition of the great arteries. The generalities of treatment are, however, readily categorized (Table 94–3).

In general, myocardial dysfunction is treated by drug therapy directed at enhancement of contractility.[10] Myocardial dysfunction occasionally responds to afterload reduction. Cautious vascular volume expansion (preload augmentation of ventricular work with the Frank-Starling mechanism) may improve cardiac output in the patient with cardiogenic shock and is a vital emergency measure. Reduction of myocardial workload is effective in all categories of CHF. This may be accomplished by bed rest, mechanical ventilation, or afterload reduction. Relief of the underlying cause of ventricular overwork should be immediately planned in the patient with surgically treatable CHF.

In certain situations, diuresis may be the mainstay of decongestive therapy. This is most commonly the case when pulmonary dysfunction contributes to symptoms and when edema, especially pulmonary edema, is itself troublesome.

Oxygen therapy is effective, insofar as it enhances arterial oxygenation, relieves dyspnea, and reduces pulmonary vascular resistance.

Volume Expansion to Enhance Cardiac Output in Cardiogenic Shock

The infant or child with cardiogenic shock may exhaust his or her Frank-Starling mechanism reserve, but this is not always the case. Severe CHF may interfere with oral fluid intake or may occur quite suddenly (as in ductus-dependent cardiac defects). This may interfere with the natural tendency of the body to retain vascular volume in the face of low cardiac output. Excessive use of diuretics may pose a similar problem. Volume expansion is, therefore, a reasonable first line of treatment in cardiogenic shock unless preload is known to be adequate.

Overzealous volume expansion can cause pulmonary edema or anasarca. It may produce myocardial edema, which can interfere with diastolic function of the heart. Pulmonary edema generally responds to positive end-expiratory pressure (PEEP). Anasarca is of little acute significance. An initial trial of volume expansion is, therefore, safe in the patient with cardiogenic shock.

Drugs That Enhance Myocardial Contractility

The general categories of inotropic agents are (1) digitalis-like agents, (2) catecholamines, and (3) amrinone-like agents. Of these, the digitalis family has the longest tradition of use for cardiac inotropy.

Digoxin

Digoxin and related compounds inhibit activity of the membrane-bound sodium potassium adenosine triphosphatase (ATPase). This raises intracellular sodium, which in turn slows the rate of exchange of intracellular calcium for extracellular sodium. The resultant rise in intracellular calcium augments contractility. This inotropic effect is not accompanied by a positive chronotropic effect. In fact, digoxin is vagomimetic and slows the heart. This may be beneficial because it lengthens diastole, allowing more time for cardiac filling. Digoxin is an effective short-term inotropic agent. Prolonged efficacy is more difficult to demonstrate. Digoxin has minimal vasomotor effects but is a modest systemic vasoconstrictor. In the critical care setting, digoxin has seen less use since the introduction of continuous catecholamine infusions because of its relatively long half-life, its predominant renal clearance, and its propensity to cause cardiac arrhythmias. This propensity of digoxin is exaggerated by hypokalemia. Diuretics, which may cause potassium depletion, add to this potential hazard of digoxin therapy.

Catecholamines

Catecholamines act through the adrenergic receptor complex. These receptors are present in myocardium and in vascular and bronchial smooth muscle. Adrenergic receptors differ in their agonist specificity (α_1 or α_2 adrenergic, β_1 or β_2 adrenergic, and D_1 or D_2 dopaminergic). They also differ in the regulatory protein used to modify activity of membrane-bound adenyl cyclase (Gs, which stimulates cyclic adenosine monophosphate [cAMP] production, and Gi, which inhibits cAMP production). Intracellular levels of cAMP determine myocardial contractility, smooth-muscle tone, and rate of spontaneous action potential formation. For instance, a β_1 receptor linked to Gs regulatory protein allows a $beta_1$ agonist to raise intracellular cAMP. Such receptors are present in myocardium and in Purkinje's cells and, consequently, when stimulated, raise heart rate and enhance contractility.

The distribution of receptors is a primary determinant of the effect of an agonist. For instance D_1 receptors, which are stimulated by dopamine, are found primarily in kidney, viscera, and coronary arteries. When stimulated, they cause renal, splanchnic, and coronary blood flow to rise and yet have no detectable effect on skin perfusion because they are not present in skin.

Another determinant of agonist effect is relative potency at each kind of receptor (Table 94–4). For instance, norepinephrine is a potent alpha agonist and a weak beta agonist. Its effect is, therefore, predominantly to constrict systemic arterioles. It is a mild inotrope. Dopamine stimulates D_1 receptors at low, intermediate, and high doses, β_1 receptors at intermediate and high doses, and α_1 receptors only at high doses.

Some general comments concerning the use of catechola-

TABLE 94–4. Adrenergic Receptors

Receptor	Action	Order of Efficacy
α_1	Vasoconstriction	Epi > NE > Dop
β_1	Inotropic, chronotropic	I, Epi, Dobut > Dop > NE
β_2	Vasodilatation and bronchodilation	I > EPi > Dobut > Dop > NE
D	Vasodilatation (renal)	Dop

Epi = epinephrine; NE = norepinephrine; Dop = dopamine; Dobut = dobutamine; I = isoproterenol.

mines to manage CHF are warranted. First, when an inotropic agent causes the heart to pump more blood at constant aortic pressure (a desired effect), cardiac workload is increased. This requires augmentation of oxygen delivery to the myocardium. For this reason, catecholamine use may be associated with myocardial ischemia, even in nonischemic cardiac disease. Second, the commonly used catecholamines—epinephrine, norepinephrine, dopamine, dobutamine, and isoproterenol—all cause tachycardia. As the heart rate rises, diastole shortens proportionally more than does systole. This can interfere with cardiac filling, thereby worsening stroke volume. Third, catecholamines are intrinsically arrhythmogenic.

Methylxanthines and Bipyridines

Methylxanthines (like theophylline) and bipyridines (like amrinone) augment contractility by elevating intracellular cAMP but by using mechanisms independent of the adrenergic receptor. Theophylline inhibits activity of all phosphodiesterases: those that "degrade" cAMP (which augments contractility) and those that "clear" intracellular cyclic guanosine monophosphate (cGMP), which is thought to decrease contractility. In the aggregate, theophylline is, nonetheless, a positive inotropic agent.

Amrinone and its congeners inhibit activity of phosphodiesterase III, which degrades cAMP only. Amrinone raises intracellular calcium, is a positive inotrope, and is a systemic vasodilator. This combination, inotropic activity and afterload reduction, may have special value in low-output states and in situations in which myocardial workload should not be excessively increased.

Treatment of Congestive Heart Failure by Reducing Cardiac Work

The burden of the heart, to meet the needs of the body for systemic oxygen and substrate delivery while supporting its own metabolic requirements, can represent a conflict of interest.[11] In cardiogenic shock, when the heart is unable to bear this burden, forcing it to perform heroics may cause myocardial ischemia, infarction, and fibrosis. Other measures that are useful in infants and children focus on reducing cardiac work to allow the myocardium to recover. This is of special importance after cardiac operations, when the heart has been injured by myocardial incision, put at risk of air embolism by opening the heart, and subjected to coronary ischemia followed by reperfusion with blood. Several of these measures are listed in Table 94-5.

Foremost among the means of reducing cardiac workload is mechanical ventilation with oxygen, coupled with sedation and, as appropriate, neuromuscular blockade.[12] Mechanical ventilation alleviates the work of breathing, which may be substantial if there is pulmonary edema or lung dysfunction. It protects the patient from risk of respiratory arrest when narcotics are used to relieve pain. Oxygen should be used to relieve arterial desaturation because desaturation wastes a fraction of the cardiac output; desaturated blood carries oxygen inefficiently. PEEP is often used to alleviate arterial desaturation in the patient with pulmonary edema. Sedation, pain relief, and neuromuscular blockade limit endogenous catecholamine secretion, reduce sympathetic vasoconstriction to pain, and prevent patient movement, which contributes to circulatory demand.

TABLE 94–5. Modalities That May Be Used to Reduce Myocardial Work

Mechanical ventilation
Sedation
Pain relief
Neuromuscular blockade
Prevent fever
Pharmacologic afterload reduction
β-blockers
Aortic balloon counterpulsation
ECMO/ECLS, LVAD, RVAD

ECMO = extracorporeal membrane oxygenation; ECLS = extracorporeal life support; LVAD = left ventricular assist device; RVAD = right ventricular assist device.

Prevention of fever reduces the metabolic demand that must be satisfied by activity of the heart. It also reduces heart rate, facilitates cardiac filling in diastole, and prevents or treats junctional ectopic tachycardia.

Pharmacologic treatment of excessive afterload may be used to reduce cardiac work to the extent that it does not impair organ perfusion, especially perfusion of the myocardium by the coronary circulation. Agents often used to reduce afterload include nitroprusside, calcium channel blockers, prostaglandin E_1, captopril, and enalapril. Myocardial work may also be limited using β-blockers, because cardiac output need not always be as great as the body appears to demand.

Devices to Support the Failing Heart

Aortic balloon counterpulsation is possible in very small children but becomes increasingly challenging as catheter size declines, heart rate rises, or myocardial function worsens. Arrhythmias interfere with this modality. Fundamentally, the underlying limitation of aortic counterpulsion is that it pumps no blood. It reduces cardiac afterload and raises diastolic myocardial perfusion pressure but only by displacing blood that has been ejected by the left ventricle.

Infants and children, like adults, can be supported using extracorporeal devices if they suffer temporary or permanent myocardial devastation. Extracorporeal membrane oxygenation (ECMO) can be useful as a means of cardiac rescue after repair of congenital cardiac malformations.[13] Some postoperative patients are unable to support their circulation despite an adequate repair, and cardiogenic shock develops. Although ECMO raises afterload in this setting by restoring adequate blood pressure (which taxes the heart), it simultaneously relieves the heart of the burden of supporting the entire circulation. At the same time, it raises coronary artery diastolic pressure. ECMO, therefore, "rests" both right and left ventricles. When ECMO is used to "rest" the heart, it must be remembered that the left ventricle may find itself unable to eject at the higher afterload afforded by the extracorporeal pump. In this setting, left atrial return (flow through the ductus arteriosus, bronchial flow, residual anterograde flow across the pulmonary valve) may pool on the left side of the heart. Pressure can, in theory, rise in the left ventricle and atrium until it equals aortic diastolic pressure. When this occurs to a clinically important degree, pulmonary edema develops. This scenario can be prevented by "venting" the left atrium to the venous return of the ECMO circuit, by administration of inotropic agents, or by atrial septectomy in selected patients. ECMO has been used with success in patients with myocarditis as well.

Other devices such as the left ventricular assist device and the right ventricular assist device can be used to move atrial return to the appropriate great cardiac vessel, completely or partially bypassing one ventricle. This does not require a membrane oxygenator and does not require systemic heparinization. In most infants and children, however, cardiogenic shock is a biventricular problem.

SUMMARY

CHF is an unstable situation. Its presence implies very limited myocardial reserve. CHF demands prompt stabilization at all ages, although treatment may be quite age or cause specific.

References

1. Talner NS: Heart failure. *In*: Moss' Heart Disease in Infants, Children and Adolescents. 3rd ed. Adams FH, Emmanouilides GC (Eds). Baltimore, Williams & Wilkins, 1989, pp 890–911.
2. Sahn DJ, Vaucher Y, Williams DC, et al: Echocardiographic detection of large left to right shunts and cardiomyopathies in infants and children. Am J Cardiol 1976; 38:73–79.
3. Gaasch WH, Levine HJ, Quinones MA, et al: Left ventricular compliance: Mechanisms and clinical implications. Am J Cardiol 1976; 38:645–653.
4. Kubler W, Katz AM: Mechanisms of early pump failure in the ischemic heart: Possible role of ATP depletion and inorganic phosphate accumulation. Am J Cardiol 1977; 40:467–471.
5. Buckberg G, Eber L, Herman M, et al: Ischemia in aortic stenosis. Am J Cardiol 1975; 35:778.
6. Takahashi M, Lurie P: Abnormalities and diseases of the coronary vessels. *In*: Moss' Heart Disease in Infants, Children and Adolescents. 3rd ed. Adams FH, Emmanouilides GC (Eds). Baltimore, Williams & Wilkins, 1989, pp 630–635.
7. Rockley CE, Edwards JE, Karp RE: Mitral valve disease. *In*: The Heart. 7th ed. Hurst JW, Schlant RL, Rockley CE, et al. (Eds). New York, McGraw-Hill, 1989.
8. Freedom RM, Benson LN: Ventricular septal defect. *In*: Neonatal Heart Disease. Freedom RM, Benson LN, Smallhorn JF (Eds). London, Springer-Verlag, 1991, p 578.
9. Sanders SP: Echocardiography. *In*: Fetal and Neonatal Cardiology. Long WA (Ed). Philadelphia, WB Saunders, 1990, p 304.
10. Notterman DA: Pharmacology of the cardiovascular system. *In*: Pediatric Critical Care. 2nd ed. Fuhrman BP, Zimmerman JJ (Eds). St. Louis, Mosby-Year Book, 1998, pp 329–346.
11. Fuhrman BP: Regional circulation. *In*: Critical Care: State of the Art. Vol 10. Fuhrman BP, Shoemaker WC (Eds). Anaheim, Calif, Society of Critical Care Medicine, 1989, pp 338–339.
12. Papo MC, Rosenkoanc ER, Hernan LJ, Fulieman EP: Critical care after surgery for congenital cardiac disease. *In*: Pediatric Critical Care. 2nd ed. Fuhrman BP, Zimmerman JJ (Eds). St. Louis, Mosby-Year Book, 1998, pp 354–370.
13. Dalton HJ, Siewers RD, Fuhrman BP, et al: Extracorporeal membrane oxygenation for cardiac rescue following surgery for congenital heart disease. Crit Care Med 1993; 21:1020–1028.

95

Conduction Disturbances and Cardiac Arrhythmias in the Critically Ill

Richard K. Shepard, MD • Andrea Hastillo, MD

Cardiac arrhythmias are common in critically ill patients. They may be triggered by a primary arrhythmogenic focus, as in atrioventricular (AV) nodal reentry tachycardia; related to a cardiac cause, as in ventricular fibrillation during an acute myocardial infarction; or in response to an illness, as in tachycardia with fever. Arrhythmias may be initially benign or life-threatening, but all must be quickly and accurately diagnosed to prevent potentially serious problems.

In every intensive care unit (ICU), monitoring of the heart rhythm is standard practice. Changes in heart rate may be harbingers of impending hemodynamic catastrophe. Thus, continuous observation of heart rate becomes an important part of the delivery of good critical care.

The major purpose of cardiac rhythm monitoring is to be able to detect abnormal rhythms as they develop. This allows treatment of either the primary arrhythmia or a change in underlying illness as soon as possible. Treatment response may be determined by constant monitoring. This may range from determining that an arrhythmia does not recur, that ectopic complexes decrease in number, or that ventricular rates in atrial fibrillation respond in a desired manner to deciding whether pacemakers are functioning properly.

ROUTINE SURVEILLANCE

Routine monitoring is accomplished with a single-lead display obtained at the bedside and displayed at the bedside and at a central monitor. A variety of leads may be used, but the one chosen should clearly display the P wave and the QRS complex. If the patient has an electronic pacemaker in place, one should select a lead that maximizes visualization of the pacemaker spike. The lead that is being used to monitor the rhythm should be recorded. Any changes in the selected lead should be noted to avoid confusion with other causes of axis shifts.

Electronic surveillance should include various warnings for high and low rates. These should always be set to supplement human surveillance in the detection of rhythm abnormalities. A good system should minimize any artifact that initiates warning systems.

Rhythms should be permanently documented on admission and at the start of each shift. A rhythm strip should be obtained and placed in the patient's chart or on the bedside flow chart, and interval measurements and diagnosis of the rhythm strip should be recorded by the nurse or monitor observer. Any changes in rhythm should be further clarified with a 12-lead electrocardiogram (ECG), because a single-lead strip may not be adequate for a full rhythm interpretation. Because rhythm strips may be lost or questions about rhythms may arise later, the ability to obtain delayed printouts, as well as real-time strips, is important.

It is important to record the initiation and termination of arrhythmias because these are where the diagnosis of the mechanism can most easily be made. For example, torsades de pointes always starts with a long-short coupling interval whereas polymorphic ventricular tachycardia does not. Mechanisms of supraventricular tachycardia (SVT) can frequently be diagnosed from both onset and termination. A ventricular fibrillation arrest may be the deterioration of primary ventricular tachycardia that may be missed if onset is not recorded.

SPECIAL TECHNIQUES

Frequently, the 12-lead ECG coupled with the monitor strip is inadequate for confirming the diagnosis of an arrhythmia. A Lewis lead or other variations of surface electrode placements can be tried to determine the rhythm. The Lewis lead is obtained by placing the patient's right arm electrode in the second right intercostal space and the left arm electrode in the fourth right intercostal space. Lead I is selected. If this is unsuccessful, one may then consider a more invasive approach: intra-atrial or esophageal electrocardiography. Each procedure requires ECG equipment that can record the surface ECG simultaneously with the intra-atrial or esophageal electrogram.

An intra-atrial lead may be placed through the jugular vein

or, less commonly, through the brachial, subclavian, or femoral vein. One can determine the location of the intravenous electrode by the configurations of the ECG, although fluoroscopy may be required.

Esophageal electrograms may be obtained if the clinician asks the patient to swallow a "pill" electrode. This may be facilitated if the patient concomitantly swallows water or gelatin. There are also catheters that may be passed in much the same way as a nasogastric tube.

LIMITATIONS OF SINGLE-CHANNEL MONITORING

There are various distinct limitations to single-channel monitoring:

1. It may not detect the full PR, QRS, or QT interval.
2. The waveforms generated may be so small that they do not consistently trigger the detection device.
3. Artifact may lead to overcounting of electrical events generated from the heart.
4. Positional changes may lead to severe axis shifts, which may be misleading if only one lead is being monitored.
5. Loose electrodes may create artifacts resembling ventricular fibrillation or asystole.
6. Other mechanical activity such as gastric suction, teeth brushing, or condensation in a delivery system may be responsible for creation of artifacts.

It is important to document artifacts on rhythm strips so that they are not confused for arrhythmias.

Whenever a question arises, and after a quick evaluation of the patient for stability, a 12-lead ECG should be obtained. One must remember that a monitor system is designed to monitor rhythms, not to measure intervals, determine axis, detect ST-T changes, or detect hypertrophy or infarction. Although a monitor lead may suggest these abnormalities, a confirmatory 12-lead ECG is usually indicated.

NORMAL CONDUCTION SYSTEM OF THE HEART

Normal electrical impulses of the heart originate in the sinoatrial (SA) node. The node lies at the anterosuperior junction of the superior vena cava and the right atrium (RA). The SA nodal cells generate spontaneous diastolic depolarizations, which result in slowly rising action potentials characteristic of calcium-dependent depolarization. The node is innervated with neural fibers from the parasympathetic system via the vagus nerve. There is also sympathetic innervation. The rate of spontaneous depolarization is modulated by both sympathetic and parasympathetic control. The intrinsic SA nodal rate is 100 to 110 beats/min in young people and declines with age, possibly because of age-related infiltration of the node with fibrous tissue. The resting heart rate is usually governed by the degree of parasympathetic tone and is less than the intrinsic heart rate.

Electrical impulses from the SA node are rapidly conducted to the rest of the atria via atrial tissue. There is no specific conduction system within the atria such as the His-Purkinje system in the ventricles. However, there is preferential conduction, with impulses propagating more rapidly along the longitudinal axis of the fibers than across the short axis.

Normally, the atria are electrically isolated from the ventricles along the AV ring. The only electrical connection between the atria and ventricles is through the AV nodal His-Purkinje conduction system. The AV node consists of a compact node located near the apex of the triangle of Koch in the atrial septum. This conducts to the His bundle, the right and left bundle branches, and the Purkinje network, which activates the ventricles. The AV junction is richly innervated by both sympathetic and parasympathetic fibers. The proximal AV node is much more sensitive to acetylcholine and atropine than the distal or compact AV node. The proximal His bundle is unresponsive to atropine. Conversely, the distal AV node and proximal His bundle are quite responsive to sympathetic stimulation.[1-4]

Adenosine affects the AV node by stimulation of a time-dependent outward potassium current. It has its primary effect on the N cells of the AV node. Verapamil has minimal effect on His-Purkinje conduction but markedly depresses AV nodal conduction by blocking slow calcium channels, which are less prominent in the distal AV node (Table 95–1).[3]

Ventricular myocardium is activated relatively synchronously via the His-Purkinje system. The activation sequence is endocardium to epicardium. The normal activation time is 80 to 100 msec, accounting for the QRS width. Widening of the QRS is usually a result of conduction block in certain portions of the His-Purkinje system or myocardial disease.

MECHANISMS OF ARRHYTHMIAS

Tachyarrhythmic abnormalities evolve from disturbances involving three mechanisms:

- *Automaticity* (impulse formation caused by spontaneous depolarization)
- *Reentry* (impulse formation caused by slowed or blocked conduction)
- *Triggered activity* (oscillations in membrane potential after an action potential results in impulse formation)

Bradyarrhythmias may be caused by abnormal automaticity or by slowed or blocked conduction. It is important to develop an understanding of the mechanism of the arrhythmia because treatment may be determined by its cause.[6]

Automaticity

Certain cells in the normal heart have an inherent ability to depolarize spontaneously and discharge repetitively. These are the *pacemaker cells* of the heart and include (1) the SA node, (2) the AV node, and (3) the His-Purkinje system.

The SA node normally discharges faster than the other sites and is the dominant pacemaker of the heart. It normally discharges at a rate of 60 to 100 beats/min. The AV nodal area's inherent rate is 40 to 60 beats/min, and the His-Purkinje system's rate is 20 to 40 beats/min. These subsidiary pacemakers are normally prematurely depolarized (relative to their inherent rate) by the faster SA node. Should the SA node fail to fire or be blocked, or should its rate slow to a level below the subsidiary pacemaker's inherent rate, the next faster subsidiary pacemaker, by default, assumes depolarization of the heart. Various disease states, drugs, and metabolic abnormalities may alter automaticity in cells possessing automaticity and may also bestow automaticity on nonpacemaker cells.

Changes in the cardiac action potential may alter automaticity and involve the following:

1. The membrane potential at the end of repolarization.
2. The rate of phase 4 depolarization.
3. The threshold potential for depolarization.

By lowering of the resting membrane potential, slowing of phase 4 depolarization, or raising of the threshold potential, automaticity is decreased. Increased parasympathetic tone,

TABLE 95–1. Antiarrhythmic Drugs: Their Doses and Uses in the Intensive Care Unit

Drug	Intravenous Loading	Intravenous Maintenance	Oral	Uses
Quinidine			Gluconate 324 to 648 mg q8–12h	AF, AFL, SVT, APD, some VT. Avoid in patients with low EF.
Procainamide	6 to 13 mg/kg at 0.2 to 0.5 mg/kg/min	2 to 6 mg/min	Procan SR 500 to 1000 mg q6h	Same as quinidine. Avoid in renal failure.
Lidocaine	1 to 3 mg/kg	1 to 4 mg/min		VT or VF. Avoid in patients with ventricular escape rhythm.
Mexilitine			150 to 300 mg q6–8h with meals	Same as lidocaine except for oral use.
Flecainide			50 to 200 mg q12h	AF, AFL, SVT. PVC suppression in patients with normal LV function. Avoid after MI.
Propafenone			150 to 300 mg q8–12h	Same as flecainide
Amiodarone	150 mg over 10 min. May repeat to total of 2 g for incessant VT or VF	1 mg/min for 6 hr, then 0.5 mg/min	800 to 1600 mg/day (dose q6–12h) for 1 to 3 wk, then 200 to 400 mg qd.	AF, AFL, SVT, VT, VF
Sotalol			80 mg q12h, titrate to maximum of 160 mg q12h	VT
Ibutilide	1 mg over 10 min. Repeat after 10 min			Acute conversion of AF or AFL to SR. Follow QT interval to avoid torsades.
Adenosine	3 to 24 mg rapid bolus			Diagnose SVT versus atrial arrhythmias. Terminate SVT.
Diltiazem	15 to 20 mg over 5 min	5 to 20 mg/hr	30 to 90 mg q6–8h	Rate control AF, AFL, AT. Treat SVT.
Esmolol	500 μg/kg over 1 min. May repeat once	50 to 200 μg/kg/min		Rate control AF, AFL, AT, inappropriate ST.

AF = atrial fibrillation; AFL = atrial flutter; APD = atrial premature depolarization; AT = atrial tachycardia; EF = ejection fraction; LV = left ventricular; MI = myocardial infarction; PVC = premature ventricular contraction; SR = sinus rhythm; ST = sinus tachycardia; SVT = supraventricular tachycardia (atrioventricular nodal or accessory pathway); VF = ventricular fibrillation; VT = ventricular tachycardia.

hyperkalemia, hypothermia, and antiarrhythmic agents decrease automaticity. Automaticity is increased (1) if the resting membrane potential is closer to the threshold membrane potential, (2) if the threshold potential is lowered, or (3) if the slope of phase 4 is increased. Clinically, increased sympathetic tone, hypokalemia, myocardial ischemia and necrosis, and cardiac stretching may increase automaticity.

Conduction

Many arrhythmias develop as a result of abnormalities of conduction. In these cases, depolarization may occur, but the impulse is not conducted normally. Conduction or propagation of the electrical impulse through the cardiac tissue depends on phase 0 and the amplitude of the action potential. If the rate of change of voltage or the height of the action potential decreases, the speed of conduction through the tissue decreases. This conduction delay may allow continued conduction but at a lower rate than normal, or conduction may be totally blocked.

Many arrhythmias result from reentry. Reentrant arrhythmias arise as a result of abnormalities of conduction. For reentry to occur, the following must take place:

1. An impulse must encounter two functionally or anatomically potential pathways exiting a common pathway, which then remerge in a more distal common pathway.
2. The impulse must fail to conduct anterogradely down one pathway (unidirectional block).
3. The impulse must conduct down the unblocked pathway but slowly enough that it finds the previously anterogradely blocked pathway now able to conduct retrogradely.

When the impulse reaches the initial site where the common pathway first split, it then conducts anterogradely as previously and keeps reestablishing itself. Alternatively, the impulse may exit the proximal common path, quickly travel down the faster pathway, and not conduct retrogradely back up the slower pathway. However, because the impulse coming down the slower pathway is not blocked, it slowly conducts anterogradely and finds the faster, earlier depolarized pathway repolarized and able to conduct retrogradely. Thus, reentrant loops are established.

Reentrant pathways may occur throughout the heart. The Wolff-Parkinson-White syndrome epitomizes reentrant arrhythmias by involving two anatomically distinct pathways: (1) the AV nodal tissue and (2) an accessory pathway.[7] Ventricular tachycardia in the setting of an old infarct scar involves reentry in the area of the scar.

Triggered Activity

Afterdepolarizations are oscillations in voltage of the membrane potential that occur after or during an action potential. These afterpotentials may be *early*, occurring before the cell has completely repolarized during phase 3 (early afterdepolarization), or *late*, occurring after complete repolarization (delayed afterdepolarization). If the afterpotential reaches threshold for depolarization, spontaneous depolarization may result. Delayed afterdepolarizations associated with digitalis and catecholamines appear to be responsible for clinical arrhythmias. There is less information about the significance of early afterdepolarizations, although they have been incriminated as a mechanism for arrhythmias seen in ventricular hypertrophy, quinidine-associated torsades de pointes, and other ventricular arrhythmias.[8-13]

SPECIFIC CARDIAC RHYTHMS

Bradyarrhythmias

Sinus Bradycardia

Sinus bradycardia is sinus rhythm with a rate lower than 60 beats/min. It is often seen in healthy individuals, especially athletes. Many cardiac drugs, including β-blockers, calcium channel blockers, digoxin, class Ia, Ic, and III antiarrhythmics, and lithium, may cause sinus bradycardia. In the older individual, the sinus node's rate of discharge may decrease, and in ischemia heightened vagal tone may precipitate sinus bradycardia. Sinus bradycardia is also seen in hypothyroidism and hypothermia. Sinus node disease or SA block may also be caused by fibrosis or inflammatory and infiltrative diseases commonly associated with sick sinus syndrome. In the ICU setting, profound sinus bradycardia may be seen with underventilation and hypoxia.

Similar to AV block, SA exit block may occur, causing pauses on the surface ECG. Because depolarization of the SA node does not cause any deflection on the surface ECG, determination of SA block is inferential. SA block is presumed to be the cause of a sudden pause if the PP interval surrounding the pause is an exact multiple of the normal sinus PP interval and no blocked premature atrial contraction (PAC) is present. SA exit block may be subdivided into two groups: *type I* (Wenckebach) SA exit block and *type II* SA exit block. Instead of measuring PR intervals, one measures PP intervals to determine that there is group beating, indicative of type I. The PP intervals should shorten, as do the RR intervals in Mobitz type I AV block, just before total block occurs. Pauses in the appearance of a P wave that do not fit into one of these types may be due to SA exit block, failure of the SA node to fire, or inability of atrial tissue to depolarize. Causes of SA exit block include medications, infiltrative diseases, fibrosis, atherosclerotic coronary disease, carotid sinus hypersensitivity, and high vagal tone.

If sinus bradycardia is responsible for an inadequate resting cardiac output or ineffective increase in cardiac output manifested by dizziness, syncope, congestive failure, or weakness, treatment should be given. In subacute situations, theophylline or propantheline may help. In acute situations, intravenous atropine is usually successful. If this fails or if a longer treatment period is necessary, intravenous isoproterenol may be used. Pacemakers are indicated for sinus node dysfunction with symptomatic sinus bradycardia. In some patients this may occur as a consequence of essential drug therapy, an example being patients receiving antiarrhythmic therapy for atrial fibrillation or SVT. If there is no AV block, temporary transvenous pacing may be employed, using the atrial rather than ventricular site to maximize stroke volume and cardiac output. Treatment of ischemia, hypoxia, and hypothyroidism and withdrawal of rate-lowering drugs must also be considered.

Sinus Arrhythmia

Sinus arrhythmia may be normal. The sinus rate is noted to vary about 10% over time, with a pattern of rhythmically increasing and decreasing rates or PP intervals. If the variation in rate is due to respirations, the atrial rate should increase with inspiration and then decrease with exhalation. Respiratory sinus arrhythmia is often a normal phenomenon readily apparent in individuals with lower sinus rates or sinus bradycardia.

Treatment is not indicated. If respirations are not causative, the sinus arrhythmia is nonrespiratory. The nonrespiratory sinus arrhythmia tends to occur in the older individual and is more likely to occur in the presence of cardiac disease. If it is related to digitalis toxicity, discontinuation of the drug is indicated.

Atrioventricular Block

First-Degree Atrioventricular Block

First-degree AV block is characterized by the presence of a prolonged PR interval greater than 0.20 second. A conducted QRS complex follows each P wave. First-degree AV block may occur in healthy individuals but may also result from ischemia, high vagal tone, and a variety of drugs, most notably certain calcium channel blockers, β-blockers, digitalis, and amiodarone. If the patient is asymptomatic, treatment is not needed. If first-degree AV block is due to drugs, dosages may need to be adjusted (see Table 95-1). In certain clinical situations, such as with endocarditis or acute myocardial infarction, the development of new first-degree AV block may alert one to potential worsening AV block. The selection of certain medications that cause AV block may be affected by preexisting first-degree AV block.[14, 15]

Second-Degree Atrioventricular Block

In second-degree AV block, some but not all P waves are conducted to the ventricles. The failure to conduct may occur at various levels, including the AV node or His-Purkinje system.

Wenckebach's Second-Degree Atrioventricular Block (Mobitz Type I)

Mobitz type I block is characterized by regular P-wave activity, single P waves not followed by a QRS, and progressive PR prolongation, with subsequent failure to conduct while the RR intervals concomitantly shorten. The conduction block most frequently occurs within the AV node. The RR interval surrounding the nonconducted P wave is less than twice the RR interval of the last conducted P wave. The degree of AV block is expressed as a ratio of P waves to QRS complexes (i.e., 4:3 indicates that every fourth P wave is not conducted). Mobitz type I AV heart block may be seen in healthy individuals. It is common in acute inferior myocardial infarction, which involves the vessel supplying the blood to the AV node.

Treatment is usually not needed, but monitoring is indicated in unstable situations that may progress, such as in acute myocardial infarction.

Mobitz Type II Second-Degree Atrioventricular Block

Mobitz type II second-degree AV block is seen less frequently than Mobitz type I and is viewed as potentially more dangerous. It may be associated with acute anterior wall myocardial infarctions and may be complicated by complete heart block with an unstable escape rhythm. Mobitz type II block demonstrates regular atrial activity with sudden failure to conduct one or more P waves. Often, the QRS complex is wider than normal, consistent with the fact that the conduction delay occurs below the bundle of His. Because of this, the PR interval of conducted beats in Mobitz type II is usually normal.

Treatment is usually necessary because the conduction abnormality lies in the distal conduction system and is often progressive. Transvenous pacing is the usual form of treatment.

In 2:1 AV block, every other P wave is conducted. This cannot be considered one of the usual two forms of second-degree AV block. On the surface ECG, sustained 2:1 AV block fulfills the criteria for neither Mobitz type I nor Mobitz type II second-degree AV block. If the 2:1 AV block is characterized by a long PR interval and a narrow QRS complex, the block is probably intra-AV nodal and a Mobitz type I. If the PR interval is normal and the QRS wide, one should suspect block distal to the bundle of His (Mobitz type II block), and backup pacing should be available even for the asymptomatic patient.

Third-Degree Atrioventricular Block

In sinus rhythm, the diagnosis of third-degree AV block is confirmed by the presence of AV dissociation with the atrial rate greater than the ventricular rate (Fig. 95-1). The atria fire independently of the ventricles, and the ventricular rate is normally controlled by an escape rhythm located below the atrium.

Common causes of complete or third-degree AV block include (1) medications, such as digitalis, selective calcium channel blockers, and β-blockers; (2) degenerative disease of the conduction system (Lev's disease and Lenegre's disease); and (3) various cardiomyopathies. It may also develop in acute myocardial infarction. If third-degree AV block is due to inferior infarction, it is usually associated with a stable junctional escape rhythm, whereas the third-degree AV block resulting from acute anterior wall myocardial infarction is likely to be associated with an unstable and unreliable ventricular escape rhythm. Endocarditis, especially of the aortic valve, may be complicated by complete heart block, as might valve replacement. Lyme disease may cause transient third-degree AV block.

Mechanisms of third-degree AV block may include increased vagal tone (inferior wall myocardial infarction), reversible slowing of conduction through the AV node (certain medications), and destruction of the conducting system (anterior wall infarction). In some instances, third-degree AV block is well tolerated at rest, although symptoms of inadequate cardiac output may occur with exercise because of the inability of the escape rhythm to accelerate properly. Other individuals may experience severe symptoms with third-degree AV block at rest.

Treatment, if indicated and depending on the urgency, may range from atropine to intravenous isoproterenol to electronic transvenous or external pacing. As noted previously, atropine does not increase the heart rate if the site of block is below the AV node.[16]

Tachyarrhythmias

Sinus Tachycardia

Sinus tachycardia is a sinus rhythm with a rate greater than 100 beats/min. The normal upper limit is about (200 − age) beats/min in most individuals. Sinus tachycardia is usually due to a problem other than increased automaticity of the SA node. Fever, pain, infection, volume depletion, heart failure, thyrotoxicosis, and certain drug toxicities should be suspected. In selecting treatment to slow the tachycardia, one should take into consideration the underlying cause and the role of the tachycardia in preserving cardiac hemodynamics. Intravenous esmolol may help to control rate. Atrial tachycardias, SVT, atrial flutter, or sinus node reentry may mimic sinus tachycardia and have different treatments. Intravenous adenosine or vagal maneuvers may aid in the differential diagnosis.

Premature Atrial Contraction

Premature atrial contractions (PACs) are common. This premature P wave often displays a configuration different from that of the normal sinus P wave. PACs usually conduct retrogradely to the SA node, causing the SA node to be depolarized prematurely. Hence, the PP interval surrounding the PAC is usually less than twice a normal sinus PP interval (noncompensatory pause). The QRS complex that follows the premature P wave is usually the same as the normal sinus-induced QRS complex. However, aberrancy may occur, and in this instance the QRS may resemble a right bundle branch block pattern.

Premature P waves may not be followed by a QRS complex (blocked PAC). These may occur in healthy hearts because of a physiologic block when a very early P-wave encounters refractoriness below the atrial tissue. Frequently, pauses in a rhythm are caused by blocked PACs, and these should be suspected. However, documentation may sometimes be difficult because the premature P wave may only minimally change the T wave on which it may superimpose. A single monitor strip may not show the blocked PAC because of the P-wave vector, and this may confuse the interpretation. A blocked PAC may be differentiated from Mobitz type II second-degree AV block because in the latter case the P wave that is blocked does not occur early.

The need for treatment of PACs is influenced by the presence of structural heart disease. If the ectopy is related to alcohol or stimulants, these should be avoided. If there is concern that the PACs are harbingers of atrial fibrillation or other potentially persistent atrial arrhythmias that might lead to hemodynamic compromise, prophylactic treatment may be considered. For example, the development of atrial fibrillation in hypertrophic cardiomyopathy or severe mitral stenosis might be followed by hemodynamic collapse. Digitalis and β-blockers can be considered to prevent a rapid ventricular response. Rarely, antiarrhythmic drugs may be used to treat symptomatic PACs.

Premature Junctional Contractions

Like the PAC, the premature junctional contraction produces a premature QRS complex that resembles the normal sinus-induced QRS and is usually associated with a noncompensatory pause. A P wave may be visible or absent altogether. If a P wave occurs, it may be found before the QRS complex, in the QRS complex, or after the QRS complex. The P-wave configuration differs from that of a normal sinus-induced P wave. It is important to recognize a P wave early before the QRS or even closely after the QRS complex to avoid a misdiagnosis of a wide QRS complex.

Atrioventricular Nodal Reentrant Tachycardia

The arrhythmias grouped together as paroxysmal supraventricular tachycardias (PSVTs), a nonhomogeneous group mechanistically, include those resulting from a concealed AV bypass tract (15% to 50%), sinus node reentry (3%), intra-atrial reentry (6%), automatic atrial tachycardia, and AV nodal reentry (50%).[17]

AV nodal reentrant tachycardia (AVNRT) requires dissocia-

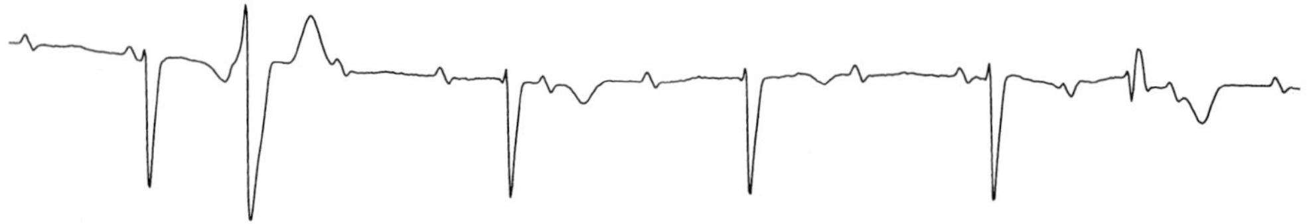

Figure 95–1. Complete heart block in a patient with a narrow complex escape rhythm and frequent ventricular ectopy. There is complete atrioventricular dissociation with "p" waves marching through. The patient received a permanent dual-chamber pacemaker.

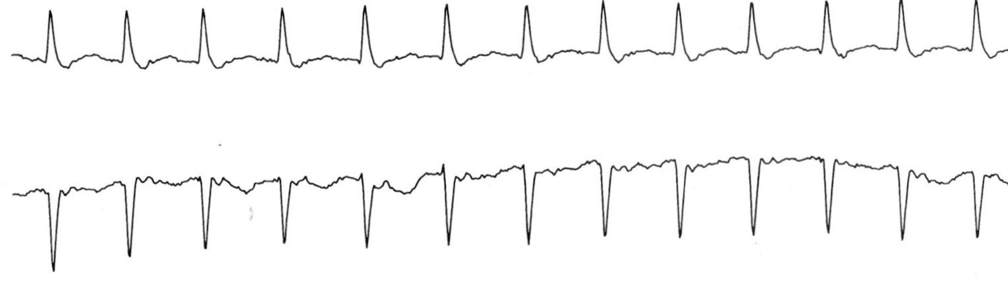

Figure 95–2. Atrioventricular node reentrant tachycardia. P waves are buried in the QRS complex. The patient was cured with a radiofrequency ablation of her slow pathway.

tion of the AV node into two functionally different pathways that form the reentrant circuit. The fast pathway has rapid conduction but has a long refractory period, whereas the slow pathway has slow conduction and a shorter refractory period. In common AV nodal reentrant tachycardia, the circuit goes down the slow pathway and back up the fast. The onset of the arrhythmia is usually abrupt and initiated by a premature complex. Termination is also usually abrupt. The QRS is regular and the complex usually narrow in the absence of a preexisting bundle branch block or intraventricular conduction delay. The rate may range from 150 to 200 beats/min, often in the higher range. P waves may be difficult to visualize and are often within the QRS complex (Fig. 95–2). P waves in the terminal QRS may manifest as a pseudo-S in leads II and III and a pseudo-R′ in lead aVR.

This arrhythmia often develops in persons with no underlying cardiac disease. The initial onset occurs by age 30 years in 50% and by age 40 years in 65% of cases. There is a 2:1 female preponderance. The rhythm is likely to be triggered in ICU patients in the setting of increased sympathetic tone and frequent PACs. The patient may sometimes describe only chest or heart "fluttering." However, at the onset of the tachycardia and before there is an adequate baroreceptor response, dizziness or even syncope may occur. Prolonged episodes may result in compromised cardiac output and heart failure symptoms. With underlying cardiac disease, hemodynamic compromise may be severe and angina precipitated.

Blocking one or both pathways in the AV node terminates the rhythm. Treatment depends on the hemodynamic status, the cause, and the recurrence rate. Severe hemodynamic compromise may require emergency cardioversion using low energy settings (20 to 50 joules [J]). Vagal maneuvers (e.g., carotid sinus massage, Valsalva's maneuver) that interrupt the reentry pathway by slowing conduction may terminate AVNRT. These may also aid in diagnosis. Sinus tachycardia may be transiently slow. Either AV nodal reentry stops, or nothing occurs. Atrial flutter may demonstrate a transient increase in AV block, and the flutter waves may be readily visualized. Atrial tachycardia with block may demonstrate further AV block. Atrial fibrillation may demonstrate a transient increase in AV block. Occasionally, ventricular tachycardia is included in the differential diagnosis of AV nodal reentry (with aberrancy); vagal maneuvers should not alter the ventricular rate.

Adenosine is a short-acting drug (seconds) that is effective in terminating AV nodal reentry tachyarrhythmias and is also used for diagnostic purposes. It causes transient complete AV block. It is administered rapidly to maximize its negative dromotropic effect (see Table 95–1).

Aminophylline is a competitive antagonist and prevents the action of adenosine. If an initial bolus of adenosine does not cause AV block, the dose should be doubled until block occurs. Atrial or ventricular pacing readily terminates the AVNRT.

Verapamil and diltiazem may also terminate the arrhythmia and may prevent reinitiation. Chronic treatment modalities may include β-blockers, Ia and Ic antiarrhythmics, amiodarone, or digitalis.[7, 18, 19] If the arrhythmia is incessant or the patient becomes stable, radiofrequency ablation (RFA) is curative (see Table 95–1).[20]

Concealed Atrioventricular Bypass Tract Tachycardia

This is the second most common cause of SVT and requires an accessory pathway (AP), somewhere along the AV ring, that bypasses the AV node and conducts only retrogradely. Normal antegrade conduction down the AV node and retrograde conduction up the bypass tract may result in a normal QRS complex with the upper rate limited by the AV node. The atria are activated ectopically at the site of the bypass tract. The onset of the tachycardia may be similar to that of AV nodal reentry tachycardia. The rate may be higher than 200 beats/min, and the P wave may be seen more than 70 msec after the QRS complex, raising the suspicion of a bypass tract. Bundle branch block ipsilateral to the site of the accessory pathway lengthens the reentrant circuit and prolongs the tachycardia cycle length by approximately 35 msec. This is diagnostic for an accessory pathway tachycardia.[17] Termination of this arrhythmia may be due to interruption of the reentrant loop at a variety of areas but most commonly at the AV node. The AV block results in a dangling retrograde P wave visible after the last QRS of the tachycardia.[7, 17, 21]

Depending on the clinical situation, treatment may require electrical cardioversion, vagal maneuvers, or drugs. Drugs used may include adenosine, verapamil, diltiazem, β-blockers, digoxin, type Ia or Ic antiarrhythmic agents, or amiodarone.[7, 22] Definitive and curative treatment is radiofrequency ablation.

Preexcitation Syndromes

Wolff-Parkinson-White syndrome (preexcitation syndrome) is characterized by early depolarization of ventricular myocardium through an accessory atrioventricular pathway (AP). These pathways are associated with reentrant tachyarrhythmias. Recognition of an accessory pathway is important for confirming the diagnosis of arrhythmias and for choosing appropriate pharmacologic or interventional therapy.[7, 23–35]

Wolff-Parkinson-White syndrome is confirmed by the surface ECG when a short PR interval, wide QRS complex, and delta wave (a slur on the initial inscription of the QRS complex) are seen (Fig. 95–3). The delta wave represents early depolarization of ventricular myocardium resulting from the use of the accessory pathway. If conduction is only through the AV node, one expects a normal PR interval, normal QRS duration, and absence of a delta wave. Conduction through the accessory pathway may vary. At times, conduction may be through the AV node alone, through the accessory pathway, or through both the AV node and the accessory pathway. Conduction through the accessory pathway may be exceedingly rapid. A reentrant loop may be formed using the AV node and the bypass tract. Antegrade conduction down the AV node and retrograde conduction back up through the bypass tract may result in orthodromic reciprocating tachycardias.

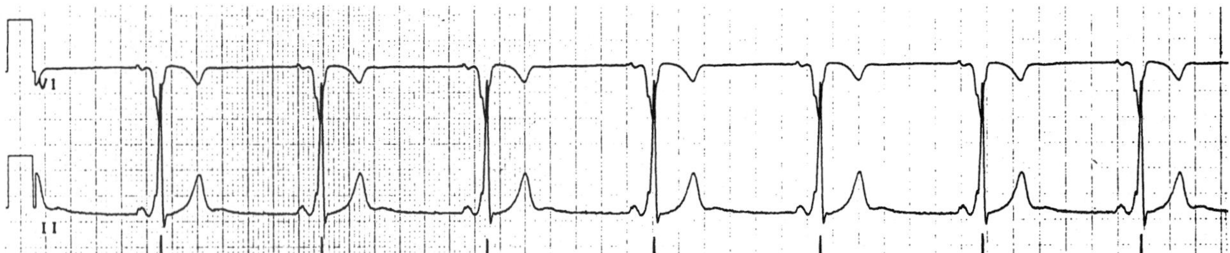

Figure 95–3. Wolff-Parkinson-White syndrome with preexcitation. The rhythm strip demonstrates a short PR interval, a slurred "delta" wave at the beginning of each QRS and a wide QRS complex.

Atrial fibrillation is frequently associated with Wolff-Parkinson-White syndrome and is usually characterized by conduction via the accessory pathway. The QRS is, therefore, widened and often quite bizarre as a result of the delta wave and the rapidity of conduction allowing a rapid ventricular response (Fig. 95–4). The mechanism for onset of the atrial fibrillation is not clearly understood. A major concern about the development of atrial fibrillation with a rapid ventricular response is its tendency to cause severe hemodynamic compromise. This is associated with a significant risk for deterioration into ventricular fibrillation. Atrial fibrillation in the hemodynamically unstable Wolff-Parkinson-White syndrome may require emergency cardioversion. Procainamide may be given intravenously in an attempt to slow anterograde conduction in the accessory pathway and terminate the atrial fibrillation as well.

AV nodal blocking drugs, including adenosine, digoxin, and verapamil, should not be given during atrial fibrillation with rapid conduction down the accessory pathway. By blocking the AV node, they may allow unopposed conduction down the accessory pathway and precipitate ventricular fibrillation. All patients with Wolff-Parkinson-White syndrome and rapidly conducting atrial fibrillation should have a curative radiofrequency ablation of their accessory pathway.

Antidromic reciprocating tachycardia involves anterograde conduction through the accessory pathway with retrograde conduction through the AV node. The QRS complex is characteristic of preexcitation. It is widened and may be confused with that in ventricular tachycardia. Multiple accessory pathways may occur in individuals with this arrhythmia. This preexcited reciprocating tachycardia may transform to atrial fibrillation followed by development of ventricular fibrillation.[24] Treatment includes cardioversion for emergency situations. Procainamide may be administered in certain situations.

Automatic Atrial Tachycardia

Automatic atrial tachycardia is due to increased automaticity and is often described in persons with cardiac or pulmonary disease, metabolic abnormalities, or digitalis toxicity. When the arrhythmia starts, it often demonstrates a warm-up as the rate of discharge gradually increases for a few beats. The P wave is usually visible and differs somewhat from the sinus-induced P wave because it is shorter in duration and more peaked. The rate of firing ranges from about 150 to 200 beats/min.

Treatment is difficult. If digitalis or another drug is incriminated as causative, it should be discontinued. Digitalis toxicity may require further treatment. Metabolic, cardiac, and pulmonary abnormalities should be treated. If the rhythm is still resistant and is not due to digitalis, β-blockers, amiodarone, or digitalis may be considered if the ventricular rate needs to be decreased.[7, 26]

Multifocal Atrial Tachycardia (Chaotic Atrial Rhythm)

Multifocal atrial tachycardia (MAT) is most commonly misinterpreted as atrial fibrillation because the RR intervals are so varied. MAT is characterized by an atrial rate greater than 100 beats/min. At least three different P waves with three different PR intervals must be present, and no single focus predomi-

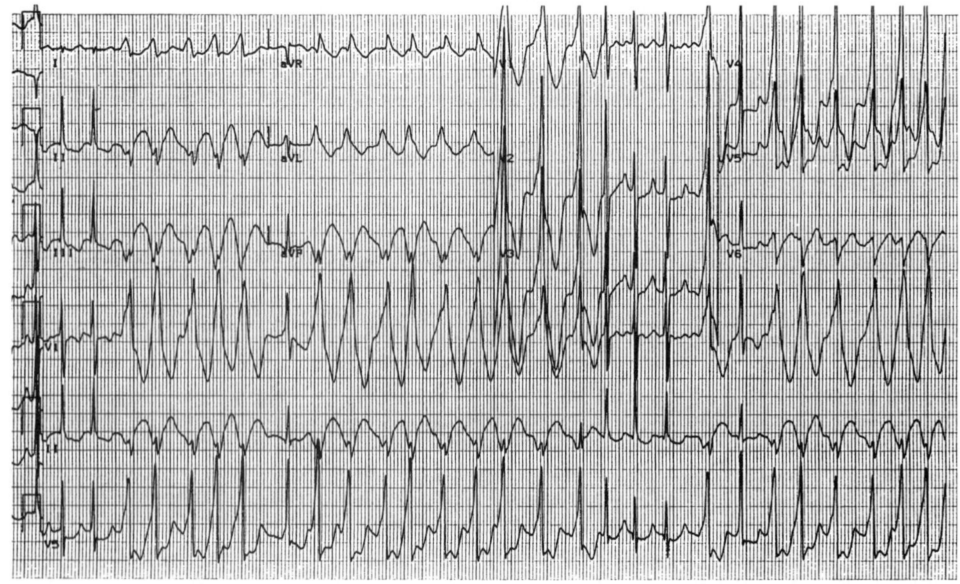

Figure 95–4. Atrial fibrillation in a patient with Wolff-Parkinson-White syndrome. Atrioventricular (AV) conduction is intermittently down the AV node and the accessory pathway (AP) leading to an irregular, bizarre, wide QRS complex. Giving an AV nodal blocking drug, such as adenosine, would lead to unopposed conduction down the AP, possibly inducing ventricular fibrillation (see text).

nates. The P waves may sometimes be misconstrued as fibrillatory waves, thus confusing the diagnosis. Increased automaticity is the underlying mechanism of MAT.

Multifocal atrial tachycardia is most commonly seen in individuals with severe decompensated lung disease. Chronic obstructive pulmonary disease and pneumonias may be complicated by this arrhythmia.

Treatment is focused on improving the underlying pulmonary process. Calcium channel blockers or amiodarone may be helpful. Digitalis may worsen the arrhythmia.[27, 28]

Atrial Fibrillation

Atrial fibrillation may occur as an intermittent, paroxysmal phenomenon or as the more typical chronic pattern. In atrial fibrillation, a variety of areas within the atrium are depolarizing in a random fashion, and reentrant loops may develop, perpetuating the arrhythmia. Conduction through the atrial tissue, entry into the AV nodal region, and conduction through the AV node are also random. Thus, depolarization of the ventricle occurs in a sporadic fashion, with the QRS complexes characteristically occurring at irregular intervals. P waves are not visible because of the disorganized atrial depolarization, although the atrial activity noted on the surface ECG may reach such magnitude that the fibrillatory waves may resemble P waves. Unless aberrancy develops or there was a preexisting bundle branch block, the QRS complex is narrow.

Aberrancy may occur, and usually the aberrant QRS complex is of a right bundle branch type. Characteristic of aberration in atrial fibrillation is *Ashman's phenomenon*; if a long RR interval is followed by a short RR interval, the QRS complex following the short RR interval may demonstrate aberrancy. This occurs because longer RR intervals (lower heart rates) are followed by longer recovery times. The subsequent shorter RR interval allows impulse conduction through the AV node but encounters a partially refractory right bundle, which allows conduction but at a lower than normal rate; hence, aberrancy results.

In some individuals, untreated atrial fibrillation may lead to hypotension, heart failure, and angina. Heart failure and hypotension may be partly due to the loss of the atrial contribution to ventricular filling, which leads to a decreased stroke volume, and to the decrease in diastolic filling time at high heart rates with a similar result. Angina may result from decreased diastolic filling time and the increased oxygen requirements caused by the increased ventricular rate.

The cause of atrial fibrillation is variable. Lone atrial fibrillation may occur without known heart disease. Systemic hypertension is the most common cause of atrial fibrillation. Other causes include atherosclerotic heart disease, valvular disease, cardiomyopathies, hyperthyroidism, and pulmonary disease. Hypoxia and a variety of drugs, including aminophylline, alcohol, and caffeine, may also precipitate atrial fibrillation. Approximately one third of patients undergoing cardiac or thoracic surgery develop atrial fibrillation postoperatively.

Treatment may require emergency cardioversion for acute decompensation, a life-threatening situation. If direct-current (DC) cardioversion is unsuccessful, intravenous (IV) amiodarone is effective at rate control and improving hemodynamics.[26] IV diltiazem or β-blockers (see Table 95–1) also control the rate. Digoxin is less effective in hyperadrenergic critically ill patients. After slowing of the ventricular response, pharmacologic attempts to convert the rhythm to sinus may be undertaken. The path taken depends on the patient's hemodynamic status, cause of the atrial fibrillation, duration of atrial fibrillation, size of the left atrium, and associated diseases such as thyrotoxicosis, atrial clot, or recent stroke.

Ibutilide is effective at normal sinus rhythm (see Table 95–1).[29] Class Ia drugs and amiodarone are also effective for both conversion to normal sinus rhythm and maintenance of normal rhythm. Because of the risk of proarrhythmias, however, class I antiarrhythmics should not be used in the long term in patients with left ventricular dysfunction.

If adequate rate control is not obtained, rate-related cardiomyopathies may develop. The patient should be referred for possible AV node ablation and permanent pacemaker implantation.[30] Patients in atrial fibrillation for more than 24 hours should receive anticoagulant therapy if there are no contraindications.

Atrial Flutter

Atrial flutter is due to macro-reentry within the atrial tissue. A frequent clinical situation involves an individual with chronic obstructive pulmonary disease (COPD), heart failure, or large atria. The flutter waves, appearing saw-toothed in the inferior leads (leads II, III, and aVF), occur at a regular frequency and with an unvarying height. This characteristic helps to differentiate flutter waves from coarse atrial fibrillatory waves. In untreated cases, the flutter waves occur about 300 times/min but vary between 220 and 350 beats/min. In the absence of AV node disease or agents that slow AV node conduction, the ventricular response is about 150 beats/min. Every other flutter wave fails to conduct through the AV node because of the AV node's inherent conduction limits.

The more classic "saw-toothed" flutter, with rates of 250 to 350 beats/min, is termed *type I* atrial flutter. *Type II* atrial flutters are frequently faster and do not inscribe the classic saw-toothed pattern. The QRS wave is usually normal in duration unless a previous bundle branch block or intraventricular conduction delay was present. Vagal maneuvers or adenosine may transiently increase block through the AV node, permitting flutter waves to be more readily visualized (Fig. 95–5).

Severe hemodynamic compromise may necessitate emergency electrical cardioversion at low energy levels of 50 to 100 J. Sometimes cardioversion of atrial flutter leads to atrial fibrillation, which may require a second shock at a higher level. Overdrive atrial pacing may terminate the atrial flutter. Atrial pacing requires placement of the electrode in the right atrium, preferably under fluoroscopic guidance. Care is needed to avoid dislodgment of the electrode into the right ventricle. Pacing starts at a rate just above the native flutter rate and is gradually increased until capture occurs, usually at a rate 20% to 30% higher than the native rate. The higher rate should be continued for several seconds and abruptly stopped to interrupt the atrial flutter. Transesophageal pacing may be used as an alternative.

One potential side effect of these modes of terminating atrial flutter is atrial fibrillation. Patients after cardiac surgery usually have temporary epicardial atrial pacing wires that can be used to diagnose and terminate atrial flutter. Drug therapy for atrial flutter includes β-blockers, verapamil, quinidine, and amiodarone.[31–33] Radiofrequency ablation of atrial flutter is curative by interruption of the reentrant circuit in the area between the tricuspid valve annulus and the eustachian ridge.[34]

Patients with atrial flutter are at risk for atrial clots, as are patients with atrial fibrillation, and may require anticoagulation. The risk of clots is increased in patients with poor left ventricular function.

Premature Ventricular Contraction

Premature ventricular contractions (PVCs) are characterized by the development of a premature QRS complex that is 0.12 second or longer in duration, different from the normally conducted QRS complex, and associated with a compensatory pause. In most instances, the PVC does not conduct retro-

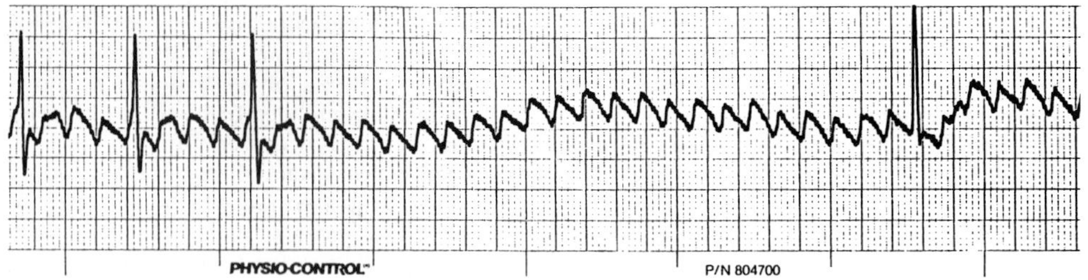

Figure 95–5. Typical atrial flutter. Flutter waves are clearly seen after 6 mg of intravenous adenosine that causes transient atrioventricular block.

gradely through the atrium to reset the SA node. Thus, the PP interval is not interrupted, and the PP interval surrounding the premature QRS complex is twice the normal sinus-induced PP interval. This is a compensatory pause. Although the P wave (which occurs on time but is not conducted because of the refractory state induced by the PVC) may occasionally be seen on the surface ECG, it is normally "hidden" in the QRS complex of the PVC.

PVCs may develop as a result of increased automaticity or reentry. They may occur in the absence of heart disease but are also commonly seen in individuals with atherosclerotic heart disease, cardiomyopathies, and nearly any form of cardiac disease. Common drugs such as caffeine, theophylline, and alcohol may induce PVCs. Infiltrative diseases must be considered and include tumors, infections, and sarcoidosis.

Treatment of isolated PVCs is controversial. During the 1990s, treatment of PVCs has clearly decreased because of the potential for severe side effects of antiarrhythmic drugs.[35] Removal of precipitating factors, correction of electrolytes (Mg^{2+} and K^+), and treatment of heart failure and ischemia are suggested. Treatment beyond this depends on the clinical situation and symptoms.

Ventricular Tachycardia

Ventricular tachycardia is the occurrence of three PVCs or more in a row. The PVCs may be of the same configuration (monomorphic) or may vary (polymorphic), and the RR intervals may be similar or diverse. In general, the diagnosis of ventricular tachycardia is made when the ventricular rate is greater than 100 beats/min (Fig. 95–6). For ventricular tachycardia in which the rate is less than 100 beats/min but greater than 50 to 60 beats/min, the term *accelerated idioventricular rhythm* is used.

Long rhythm strips may demonstrate that the atrial and ventricular rates are independent of one another. The atrial rate is usually lower than the ventricular rate. Should a P wave occur at a time when the AV node and ventricular tissue is not totally refractory, conduction from the supraventricular focus may occur, leading to a normal QRS complex or to a fusion beat. The latter QRS complex often has a configuration that merges results of supraventricular conduction and ventricular conduction.

When presented with the differential diagnosis of a SVT with aberration and ventricular tachycardia, certain characteristics on the surface ECG, as described by Wellens and colleagues, favor one diagnosis over the other.[36] AV dissociation is strongly indicative of ventricular tachycardia. Intra-atrial leads may be extremely helpful in this situation (see Fig. 95–6). A QRS duration greater than 140 msec and a superior or left superior axis also suggest ventricular tachycardia. If the QRS complex has a right bundle branch morphology, ventricular tachycardia is more likely if the QRS in lead V1 is monophasic or biphasic or if there is concordance across the precordial leads. If the QRS complex has a left bundle branch morphology, ventricular tachycardia is more likely if the QRS in lead V1 is notched in its downstroke and if it is greater than 60 msec to the nadir of the QS. It is important to differentiate SVT from ventricular tachycardia because misdiagnosis may lead to inappropriate treatment and a poor outcome.[37]

Ventricular tachycardia is associated with a number of diseases, commonly atherosclerotic heart disease and cardiomyopathy. Other abnormalities include hypoxia, hypokalemia, hypomagnesemia, digitalis toxicity, long-QT syndrome, and right ventricular dysplasia. Irritants such as right-sided heart catheters and ventricular pacemakers may also be culprits.

A variety of antiarrhythmic medications are available for treatment of ventricular tachycardia. Selection and route of

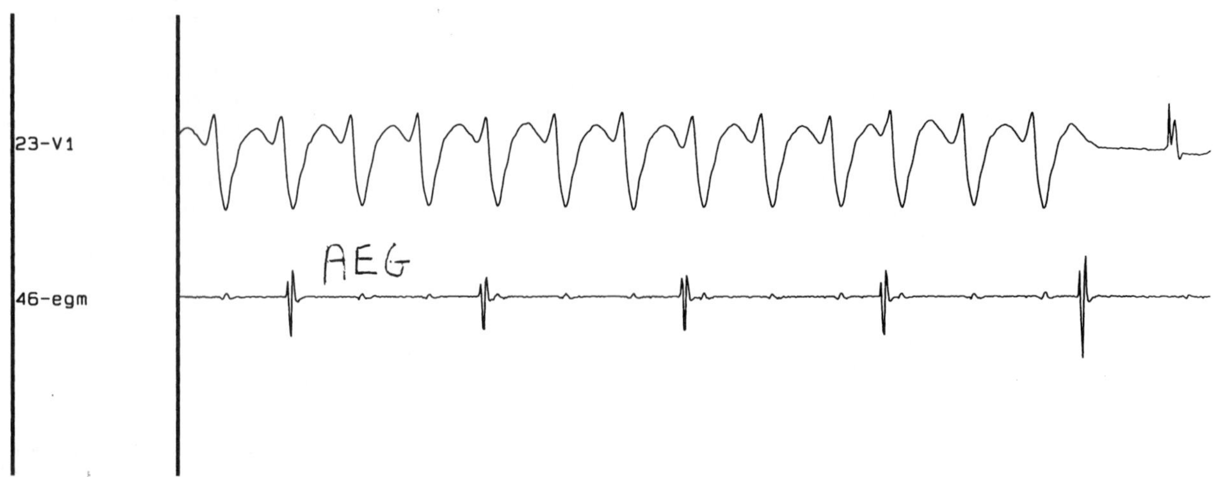

Figure 95–6. Ventricular tachycardia in a patient during an invasive electrophysiology study. An intracardiac atrial electrogram demonstrates atrial and ventricular dissociation.

administration depend on the patient's hemodynamic status and associated health problems. If the patient is hemodynamically unstable, electrical cardioversion is the first line of therapy. Symptomatic ventricular tachycardia is an indication for immediate therapy. Acute situations may require, in addition to possible cardioversion, intravenous treatment with IV procainamide, amiodarone, lidocaine, or bretylium (see Table 95–1). Intravenous β-blockade and magnesium may be helpful.

Recurrent ventricular tachycardia can be treated with transvenous pace termination. All patients with ventricular tachycardia should have electrophysiologic evaluation. Many patients benefit from an implantable cardioverter defibrillator.[38, 39] Some types of ventricular tachycardias are curable with radiofrequency ablation.

Torsades de Pointes

Torsades de pointes is a specific form of ventricular arrhythmia manifest as a rapid ventricular tachycardia with the QRS complex twisting on its axis. The ventricular rate is variable. Initiation is often by a late premature ventricular beat in a person with a long QT interval.[40] Although spontaneous termination occurs frequently, ventricular fibrillation may also develop. Torsades de pointes is often a side effect of antiarrhythmic drugs, notably type I and type III drugs in the setting of hypokalemia and hypomagnesemia. It is seen in patients with organophosphorus insecticide poisoning, liquid protein diets, and alcoholism with low potassium and magnesium levels.

Treatment requires removal of the offending agent. Either atrial or ventricular pacing may be necessary to suppress the arrhythmia. IV magnesium should be given immediately even if serum magnesium levels are normal. Potassium should be normalized. Isoproterenol infusion may be helpful by increasing the heart rate and shortening repolarization.[41–47]

Accelerated Idioventricular Rhythm

Accelerated idioventricular rhythm (AIVR) is most often observed in acute myocardial infarction. The native rhythm is usually slow, allowing this irregularity to develop. The ventricular tachycardia is usually constrained to rates of 60 to 110 beats/min. Fusion beats are common, and heart block is not present.

If necessary, treatment is aimed at carefully increasing the native rate rather than attempting to eradicate the accelerated rhythm via antiarrhythmic drugs. The latter may precipitate asystole.[48]

Ventricular Flutter

Ventricular flutter is a ventricular tachycardia with a rate of 300 beats/min or more. The QRS is usually regular but without the usual features of a QRS complex and approaching a sinusoid pattern. This rhythm abnormality is of significant hemodynamic consequence and is associated with cardiac disease. Treatment consists of direct-current cardioversion.

Ventricular Fibrillation

Ventricular fibrillation is a disorganized "rhythm." P waves are not visible. QRS complexes are not identifiable because there is no organized ventricular depolarization. Various areas of the ventricle are depolarizing, and subsequently small or even large deflections occurring at various heights and intervals are seen on the surface ECG (Fig. 95–7). If it is untreated, the deflections become smaller, and eventually all electrical activity ceases or the electrical deflection becomes so small that the tracing demonstrates a "flat" line.

Ventricular fibrillation may occur de novo in acute myocardial infarction, or it may follow an ongoing episode of ventricular tachycardia, ventricular flutter, or increased automaticity after treatment for asystole. It is also seen in patients who experience atrial fibrillation with Wolff-Parkinson-White syndrome and anterograde conduction through the accessory pathway.

Defibrillation is the first therapy. If this fails, Advanced Cardiac Life Support (ACLS) guidelines are implemented. Medications include epinephrine, followed by lidocaine, then amiodarone or bretylium. If resuscitation is successful, the underlying cause should be found and treated.

Ventricular Escape Beats

Ventricular escape beats resemble PVCs in that the QRS complex is wide and different from the QRS complex inscribed as a result of conduction from a supraventricular focus. The ventricular complex, however, is late and occurs when the ventricular focus is not depolarized before it can spontaneously repolarize. This usually occurs because the sinus node has slowed dramatically or there is AV block. Normally, the junctional escape focus, which has a higher rate of depolarization, depolarizes before the ventricular escape focus. In addition, therefore, the junctional escape focus is suppressed or slowed. The ventricular escape rate is usually less than 60 beats/min.

Ventricular escape beats or rhythms are not suppressed. They have developed not because of increased automaticity but because they have not been suppressed by normal depolarization of a faster pacemaker. The treatment that is indicated must address the causes of the sinus slowing or AV block.

NO RHYTHM (ASYSTOLE)

In asystole, there is no cardiac electrical activity. If watching a monitor strip that suddenly becomes a straight line (espe-

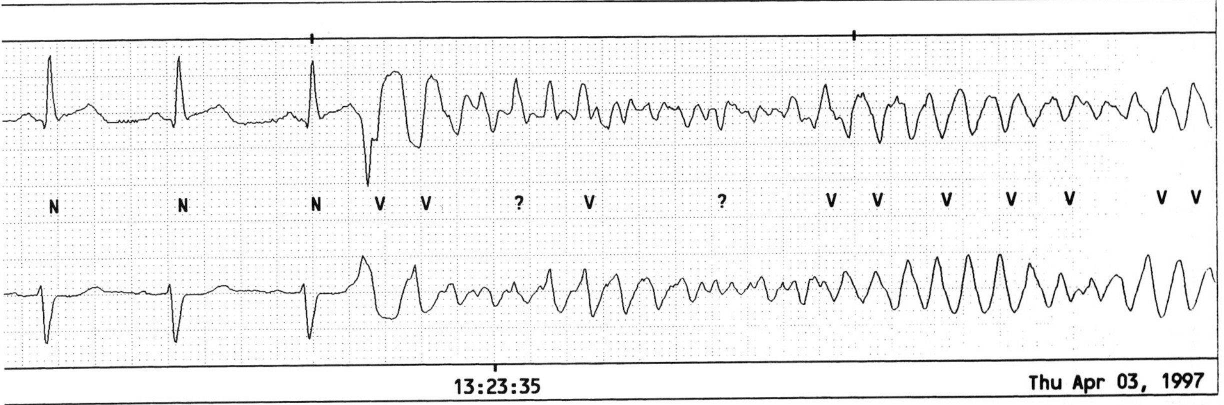

Figure 95–7. Ventricular fibrillation occurs spontaneously from sinus rhythm in this patient, who is having an acute myocardial infarction.

cially if it is quite flat), one must consider that an electrode has become dislodged. Very fine ventricular fibrillation may mimic asystole.

Treatment of asystole includes full cardiopulmonary resuscitation. Epinephrine is the first drug to be used for asystole, followed by atropine. Emergency pacing by various approaches should be considered early if the arrhythmia remains resistant to repeated medications. Attention to concomitant or precipitant drugs and metabolic abnormalities is also needed in an effort to restore a cardiac rhythm capable of sustaining the patient.

References

1. Janse MJ, van Capelle FJL, Anderson RH, et al: Electrophysiology and structure of the atrioventricular node of the isolated rabbit heart. *In:* The Conduction System of the Heart. Wellens HJJ, Lie KI, Janse MJ (Eds). Leiden, The Netherlands, Stenfert Kroese, 1976, p 296.
2. Shrier A, Adjemian RA, Munk AA: Ionic mechanisms of atrioventricular nodal cell excitability. *In:* Cardiac Electrophysiology: From Cell to Bedside. 2nd ed. Zipes DP, Jalife J (Eds). Philadelphia, WB Saunders, 1995, pp 164–172.
3. Billette J, Shrier A: Atrioventricular nodal activation and functional properties. *In:* Cardiac Electrophysiology: From Cell to Bedside. 2nd ed. Zipes DP, Jalife J (Eds). Philadelphia, WB Saunders, 1995, pp 216–225.
4. Urthaler F, Neely B, Hageman GR: Differential interaction of adrenergic and cholinergic effects on AV junctional automaticity and AV conduction. Am Heart J 1986; 112:765–770.
5. Lerman BB, Wesley RC, DiMarco JP, et al: Antiadrenergic effects of adenosine on His-Purkinje automaticity, evidence for accentuated antagonism. J Clin Invest 1988; 82:2127–2135.
6. Wit AL, Rosen MR: Pathophysiologic mechanisms of cardiac arrhythmias. Am Heart J 1983; 106:798.
7. Josephson ME, Kastor JA: Supraventricular tachycardia: Mechanisms and management. Ann Intern Med 1977; 87:346.
8. Aronson RS: Mechanisms of arrhythmias in ventricular hypertrophy. J Cardiovasc Electrophysiol 1991; 2:249.
9. Baile DS, Inoue H, Kaseda S, et al: Magnesium suppression of early depolarizations and ventricular tachyarrhythmias induced by cesium in dogs. Circulation 1988; 77:1395.
10. Rosen MR: Cellular electrophysiology of digitalis toxicity. J Am Coll Cardiol 1985; 5:22A.
11. Zipes DP: Monophasic action potentials in the diagnosis of triggered arrhythmias. Prog Cardiovasc Dis 1991; 33:385.
12. Rosen MR, Anyukhovsky EP: Arrhythmias triggered by after depolarizations. *In:* Cardiac Electrophysiology and Arrhythmias. Fisch C, Surawica B (Eds). Amsterdam, Elsevier Science, 1991, pp 67–75.
13. Davidenko JM, Cohen L, Gooddrow R, et al: Quinidine-induced action potential prolongation, early afterdepolarization and triggered activity in canine Purkinje fibers. Circulation 1989; 79:674.
14. Dreifus LS, Wanatabe Y, Haiat R, et al: Atrioventricular block. Am J Cardiol 1971; 28:371.
15. Narula OS, Scherlag BJ, Samet P, et al: Atrioventricular block: Localization and classification by His bundle recordings. Am J Med 1971; 50:146.
16. Shepard RK, Natale A, Stambler BS, Wood MA, Gilligan DM, Ellenbogen KA: Physiology of the escape rhythm after radiofrequency atrioventricular junctional ablation. Pacing Clin Electrophysiol 1998; 21:1085.
17. Josephson ME: Supraventricular tachycardias. *In:* Clinical Cardiac Electrophysiology. 2nd ed. Josephson ME (Ed). Philadelphia, Lea & Febiger, 1993, pp 181–274.
18. Waxman MB, Wald RW, Sharma A, et al: Vagal techniques for termination of paroxysmal supraventricular tachycardias. Am J Cardiol 1980; 46:655.
19. diMarco JP, Sellers TD, Lerman BB, et al: Diagnostic and therapeutic use of adenosine in patients with supraventricular tachyarrhythmias. J Am Coll Cardiol 1985; 6:417.
20. Jackman WM, Beckman KJ, McClelland JH, et al: Treatment of supraventricular tachycardia due to atrioventricular nodal reentry, by radiofrequency catheter ablation of slow-pathway conduction. N Engl J Med 1992; 327:313–318.
21. Kalbfleisch SJ, El-Atassi R, Calkins H, et al: Differentiation of paroxysmal narrow QRS complex tachycardias using the 12-lead electrocardiogram. J Am Coll Cardiol 1993; 21:85.
22. Feld GK, Nademanee K, Weiss J, et al: Electrophysiologic basis for suppression by amiodarone of orthodromic supraventricular tachycardia complicating preexcitation syndromes. J Am Coll Cardiol 1984; 3:1289.
23. Bauernfeind RA, Wyndham CR, Swiryn SP, et al: Paroxysmal atrial fibrillation in the Wolff-Parkinson-White syndrome. Am J Cardiol 1981; 47:562.
24. Bardy GH, Packer DL, German LD, et al: Preexcited reciprocating tachycardia in patients with Wolff-Parkinson-White syndrome: Incidence and mechanisms. Circulation 1984; 70:377.
25. Fujimura O, Klein GJ, Yee R, et al: Atrial fibrillation in the Wolff-Parkinson-White syndrome. *In:* Atrial Arrhythmias: Current Concepts and Management. Touboul P, Waldo AL (Eds). St. Louis, Mosby-Year Book, 1990, pp 262–269.
26. Clemo HF, Wood MA, Gilligan DM, Ellenbogen KA: Intravenous amiodarone for acute heart rate control in the critically ill patient with atrial tachyarrhythmias. Am J Cardiol 1998; 594–598.
27. Shine KI, Kastor JA, Yurchak PM: Multifocal atrial tachycardia: Clinical and electrocardiographic features. N Engl J Med 1968; 279:344.
28. Levine JH, Michael JR, Guarnieri T: Treatment of multifocal atrial tachycardia with verapamil. N Engl J Med 1985; 312:21.
29. Ellenbogen KA, Stambler BS, Wood MA, Sager PT, Wesley RC, Meissner MD, Zoble RG, Wakefield LK, Perry KT, VanderLugt CJ: Efficacy of intravenous ibutilide for rapid termination of atrial fibrillation and atrial flutter: A dose-response study. J Am Coll Cardiol 1996; 28:130–136.
30. Rodriguez LM, Smeets JL, Xie B, de Chillou C, Cheriex E, Pieters F, Metzger J, den Dulk K, Wellens HJ: Improvement in left ventricular function by ablation of atrioventricular nodal conduction in selected patients with lone atrial fibrillation. Am J Cardiol 1993; 72:1137–1141.
31. Wells JL Jr, MacLean WA, James TN, et al: Characterization of atrial flutter: Studies in man after open heart surgery using fixed atrial electrodes. Circulation 1979; 60:665.
32. Waldo AL, MacLean WA, Karp RB, et al: Entrainment and interpretation of atrial flutter with atrial pacing. Circulation 1977; 56:737.
33. Boineau JP: Atrial flutter: A synthesis of concepts. Circulation 1985; 72:249.
34. Cosio FG, Lopez GM, Goicholea A, Arribas F, Barroso JL: Radiofrequency ablation of the inferior vena cava–tricuspid valve annulus isthmus in common atrial flutter. Am J Cardiol 1993; 71:705–709.
35. Preliminary report: Effect of encainide and flecainide on mortality in a randomized trial of arrhythmia suppression after myocardial infarction. The Cardiac Arrhythmia Suppression Trial (CAST) Investigators. N Engl J Med 1989; 321:406–412.
36. Wellens HJ, Bar FW, Lie KI: The value of the electrocardiogram in the differential diagnosis of a tachycardia with a widened QRS complex. Am J Med 1978; 64:27.
37. Stewart R, Bardy GH, Green HL: Wide complex tachycardia: Misdiagnosis and outcome after emergent therapy. Ann Intern Med 1986; 104:766.
38. The Antiarrhythmics versus Implantable Defibrillators (AVID) Investigators: A comparison of antiarrhythmic drug therapy with implantable defibrillators in patients resuscitated from near fatal ventricular arrhythmias. N Engl J Med 1997; 337:1576–1583.
39. Moss AJ, Hall WJ, Cannom DS, Daubert JP, Higgins SL, Klein H, Levine JH, Saksena S, Waldo AL, Wilber D, Brown MW, Heo M: Improved survival with an implanted defibrillator in patients with coronary disease at high risk for ventricular arrhythmia. Multicenter Automatic Defibrillator Implantation Trial Investigators. N Engl J Med 1996; 335:1933–1940.
40. Kay GN, Plumb VJ, Arciniegas JG, et al: Torsades de pointes: The long-short initiating sequence and other clinical features: Observations in 32 patients. J Am Coll Cardiol 1983; 2:806.
41. Soffer J, Dreifus L, Michelson E: Polymorphous ventricular tachycardia associated with normal and long Q-T intervals. Am J Cardiol 1982; 49:2021.
42. Ludomirsky A: Q-T prolongation and polymorphous ("torsades de pointes") ventricular arrhythmias associated with organophosphorus insecticide poisoning. Am J Cardiol 1982; 49:1654.

43. Singh BN, Gaarder TD, Kanegae T, et al: Liquid protein diets and torsades de pointes. JAMA 1978; 240:115.
44. Arsenian MA: Magnesium and cardiovascular disease. Prog Cardiovasc Dis 1993; 35:271.
45. Tzivoni D, Keren A, Cohen AM, et al: Magnesium therapy for torsades de pointes. Am J Cardiol 1984; 53:528.
46. Tzivoni D, Barrai S, Schuger C: Treatment of torsades de pointes with magnesium sulfate. Circulation 1988; 77:392.
47. Smith WM, Gallagher JJ: "Les torsades de pointes": An unusual ventricular arrhythmia. Ann Intern Med 1980; 93:578.
48. Schamroth L: Ventricular extrasystoles, ventricular tachycardia, and ventricular fibrillation: Clinical-electrocardiographic considerations. Prog Cardiovasc Dis 1980; 23:13.

Additional Readings

Josephson ME: Clinical Cardiac Electrophysiology. 2nd ed. Philadelphia, Lea & Febiger, 1993.
Vlay SC: Manual of Cardiac Arrhythmias. Boston, Little, Brown & Co, 1988.
Fogoros RN: Electrophysiology Testing. Blackwell Science, 1994.

96

Cardiac Pacemakers and Implantable Defibrillators in the Intensive Care Unit Setting

Mark A. Wood, MD • Michael K. Belz, MD
Kenneth A. Ellenbogen, MD

The use of permanent pacemakers and implantable defibrillators is increasing rapidly as a result of several factors. These factors include (1) the aging of the general population, (2) expanding indications for pacemaker and defibrillator therapies, and (3) the development of entirely new devices, such as the atrial defibrillator. Most patients receiving such devices have concurrent medical illnesses. Given these factors, the admission of patients with implanted devices to the intensive care unit (ICU) must be expected as a common occurrence. It is therefore essential that intensivists who care for these patients be familiar with the basic functions of pacemakers and defibrillators. In addition, these caregivers must recognize device malfunction and situations likely to cause interactions with the implanted device.

PACEMAKERS

General Description

The function of a pacemaker is twofold: to sense intrinsic electrical cardiac events and to provide electrical stimuli to excite the myocardium in the absence of intrinsic activity. The pacemaker system consists of a battery and logic circuits, a lead for electrical continuity between the generator and the heart, and an effective lead-myocardium interface (Fig. 96–1). For both sensing and pacing functions, there are *threshold values* delineating the measured amplitude of the intracardiac electrical events for sensing and the minimum energy required to stimulate the myocardium for pacing. These values depend primarily on characteristics of the lead system and its myocardial interface, lead position, and electrical properties of the myocardium.

Because the pacemaker coordinates sensed and paced cardiac events by means of an internal clock, the time intervals between events are paramount to an understanding of pacemaker function. The *lower rate interval* is the time the pacemaker "waits" after sensed or paced events before emitting a pacing stimulus. This interval represents the slowest heart rate that the pacemaker will allow. The *upper rate interval* is the fastest that the pacemaker paces in response to sensed events (e.g., atrioventricular [AV] sequential) or to sensor input in rate-responsive pacemakers. After a sensed or paced event, sensing functions are turned off temporarily during the *refractory period* to prevent sensing far field electrical events or repolarization artifacts. The *AV delay* establishes the electronic P-R interval in dual-chamber pacing.

Each pacemaker has one or more programmable modes of operation, summarized by a standardized four-letter code. The four letters describe the chambers paced, the chambers sensed, the response to sensed events, and special functions, respectively. In this system, S represents single chamber, A represents atrium, V represents the ventricle, O represents neither chamber, I represents inhibited response, T represents triggered response, and D designates dual-chamber or dual response.

The *asynchronous mode* (SOO or VOO) paces constantly, with no sensing of intrinsic events. In most pacemakers, this mode is activated when it is exposed to an externally applied magnet. Single-chamber pacing modes are usually AAI or VVI, and they pace only when the intrinsic heart rate falls below the pacemaker's lower rate limit. Dual-chamber modes (e.g., DDD) can pace both atrium and ventricle when the intrinsic heart rate is slower than the pacemaker's programmed lower rate, but they may follow sensed atrial events with ventricular pacing at heart rates between the programmed upper and lower rates (atrial tracking). Rate-responsive pacing uses sensors incorporated into the pacemaker circuitry to modulate heart rate in patients with impaired sinus node function. These sensors may respond to body movement or vibration,

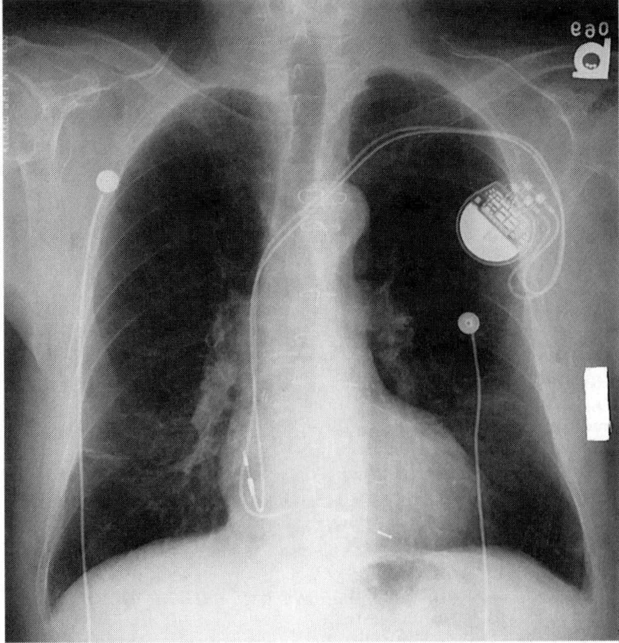

Figure 96–1. Posteroanterior chest radiograph showing a dual-chamber pacing system. The generator is implanted in the left pectoral area with an atrial lead in the right atrial appendage and a ventricular lead in the right ventricular apex.

respiratory rate, or minute ventilation. A schematic illustration of common pacemaker operation modes is shown in Figure 96–2.

Evaluation of pacemaker function requires knowledge of the pacemaker manufacturer and model as well as its programmed settings. Pacemakers may be identified as to manufacturer and model by identification cards to be carried by the patient at all times, medical records from implantation or by appearance and unique identification markings visible on chest x-ray (Fig. 96–3). Each manufacturer provides a computer-based electronic programmer to interrogate and reprogram its own pacemakers. Programming units may display intracardiac electrograms and real-time annotations of pacemaker function (marker channels), which are helpful in the diagnosis of pacemaker malfunction (Fig. 96–4).

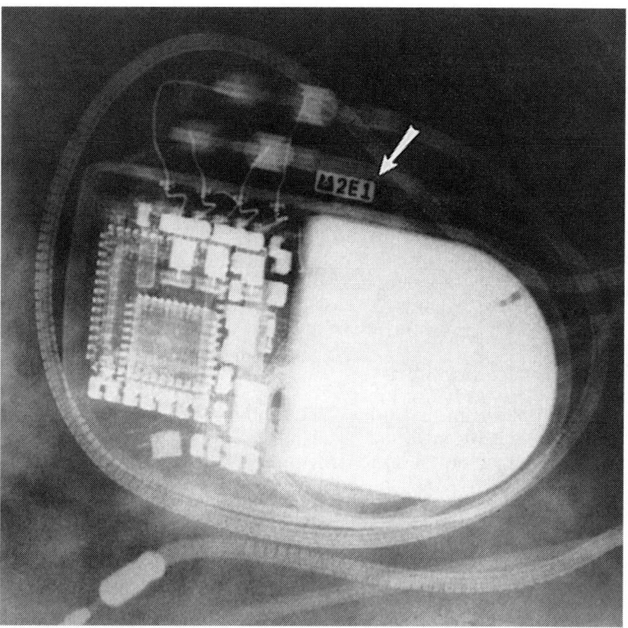

Figure 96–3. Detail of chest radiograph revealing a pacemaker identification code. The symbol and numbers 2E1 *(arrow)* identify this generator as a Medtronic Elite model No. 7084 (Minneapolis). Each manufacturer has its own unique coding that can be seen with a well-penetrated radiograph.

Pacemaker Troubleshooting

The differential diagnosis of pacemaker malfunction can be extremely difficult, especially when complex pacing modes and specialized functions are being considered. The process of troubleshooting can be greatly simplified if one recognizes that all malfunctions can be classified as either (1) failure to pace or sense or (2) inappropriate pacing or sensing.

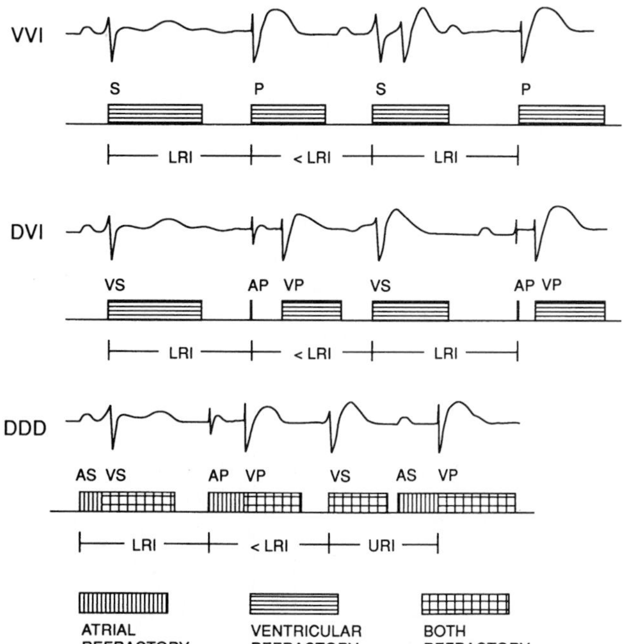

Figure 96–2. Common pacemaker modes with surface electrocardiogram lead, intracardiac events, and refractory periods illustrated. LRI = lower rate interval; URI = upper rate interval; S = sense; P = pace; A = atrium; V = ventricle.

VVI, In this mode, only ventricular signals, native or paced, are sensed by the pacemaker. If the intrinsic rate is below the programmed lower rate interval, ventricular pacing occurs at the programmed lower rate. Ventricular signals that fall within the refractory period are not sensed (fourth complex). AAI mode functions analogously with atrial sensing and pacing only.

DVI, Dual-chamber pacing with only ventricular sensing. The pacemaker is inhibited by ventricular signals only. Atrial signals neither inhibit the pacemaker nor trigger the ventricle for atrial tracking, as occurs in DDD mode.

DDD, DDD pacemakers pace both chambers and sense both atrial and ventricular events. In addition, a sensed atrial event triggers a ventricular pacing pulse if a ventricular signal is not detected within the programmed atrioventricular (AV) delay. Atrial or ventricular events that fall within their respective refractory periods are not sensed. In the last interval, the AV delay prior to ventricular pacing is prolonged beyond the programmed value to prevent ventricular pacing faster than the upper rate limit.

Failure to Capture with Pacing Stimuli Present

This problem is defined as the presence of pacemaker electrical output without capture of the myocardium (Table 96–1). A rise in pacing threshold is common during the first 4 to 6 weeks after implantation secondary to tissue reaction at the lead-myocardium interface.[1, 2] In some patients, the rise in threshold observed after implantation can exceed the maximum output of the generator. This event is described by the term "exit block." Pacemaker-dependent patients may require temporary transvenous pacing during this time. An abrupt increase in threshold or loss of capture within several days to weeks after implantation should also arouse suspicion of lead dislodgment. This finding can also be suggested by a change in the paced QRS morphology on 12-lead electrocardiogram (ECG) and may be evident on chest x-ray if one notes displacement of the lead.

Another cause of loss of capture is lead perforation of the right ventricle or right atrium. This generally presents with a high pacing threshold or complete loss of capture or abnormal sensing. Chest x-ray or echocardiography may reveal the lead outside the cardiac silhouette or may reveal pericardial effusion. Cardiac tamponade, signs of pericarditis, or diaphragmatic pacing may be present.

Other causes of increased thresholds and failure to capture include[3-7]:

- Myocardial infarction near the lead-myocardial interface
- Progressive myocardial fibrosis
- Electrolyte or metabolic derangements such as hyperkalemia, hyperglycemia, or acidemia
- Certain pharmacologic agents, including antiarrhythmic drugs (especially class Ia, Ic and III agents), mineralocorticoids, glucose with insulin, and hypertonic saline

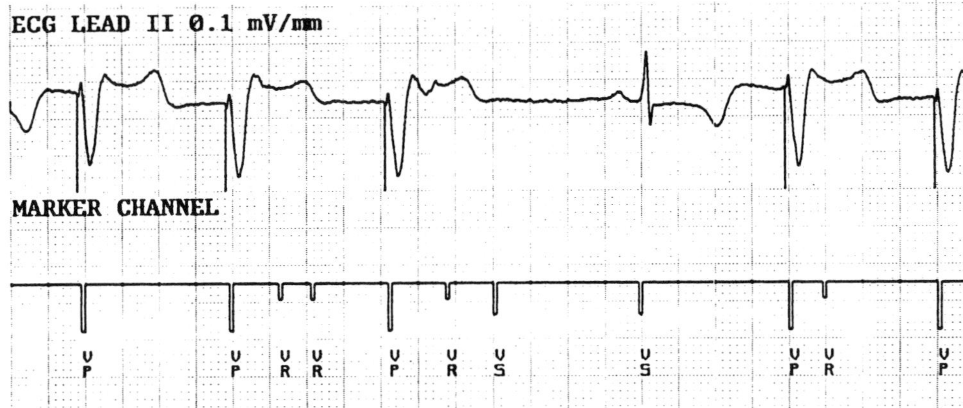

Figure 96–4. Telemetry strip from a pacemaker programmer displaying a surface electrocardiogram (ECG) lead and marker channel for a VVI pacemaker programmed to 75 beats/min. This strip demonstrates a pause in ventricular pacing after the third paced complex, resulting in a conducted sinus escape beat. This failure of ventricular pacing results from oversensing as a result of a lead insulation failure. The marker channel reveals oversensing by the device after the ventricular refractory period to produce the pause, VP = ventricle paced event; VS = ventricle sensed event; VR = ventricle event during refractory period. Events during the refractory period do not affect the function of the device.

Thresholds can also increase after direct current cardioversion.[8] Correction of metabolic derangements or discontinuation of offending agents is remedial. Elevated thresholds may be overcome by increasing the energy output of the pacemaker generator or by use of temporary pacing modalities.

Primary lead malfunction is another mechanism of loss of pacemaker capture. Leads can malfunction from either an insulation defect or a conductor fracture.[9, 10] An insulation defect effectively shunts current away from the stimulating electrode. Thus, the output must be increased in order to deliver the same amount of current to the heart. Insulation defects may be associated with pectoral muscle stimulation and low measured lead impedance on pacemaker interrogation. This problem may occur intermittently. Because insulating material is radiolucent, a chest x-ray only rarely reveals a simple insulation defect. Lead conductor fractures may be incomplete and may result in intermittent failure to pace. Palpation of the lead and generator or motion of the ipsilateral arm may reproduce the problem. Measured lead impedance may be elevated in this case, and chest x-ray findings may demonstrate lead discontinuities.

Generator battery end of life eventually results in noncapture because the battery is depleted. Battery depletion may be confirmed by pacemaker interrogation or response to magnet application.

Failure to Pace with Stimuli Absent

To categorize a pacing system malfunction as a failure to pace with stimuli absent, one must first ascertain that pacemaker output is truly absent. A 12-lead ECG is often necessary to confirm a lack of pacing stimuli, as small pacemaker spikes may be overlooked on telemetry tracings or missed completely by some digital acquisition systems. With complete lead fractures or dislodgment of the lead from the generator pacemaker, spikes may be absent as a result of complete electrical discontinuity between the generator and the body. These conditions may be apparent on the chest radiograph.

Oversensing is the sensing of signals other than true intra-

TABLE 96–1. Loss of Capture During Transvenous Cardiac Pacing

Cause	Evaluation	Solution
Catheter dislodgment or perforation	Check position on chest x-ray, paced QRS morphology, electrograms*	Reposition catheter under fluoroscopy; increase output
Poor endocardial contact	Check position on chest x-ray; check electrograms	Reposition catheter; increase output
Local myocardial necrosis or fibrosis	Check electrograms; evaluate for previous infarction	Reposition catheter; possibly increase output
Local myocardial inflammation or edema	Document adequate catheter position (chest x-ray and electrograms)	Increase output; possibly reposition
Hypoxia, acidosis, or electrolyte disturbance of drug effect (type Ia and Ic)	Check appropriate laboratory values and drug levels	Correct disturbance; reduce drug levels; increase output
Electrocautery/direct current cardioversion damaging electrodes and tissue interface	Verify recent exposure to current source	Increase output; replace or reposition catheter; possibly replace generator
Lead fracture	Check unipolar pacing thresholds	Unipolarize functional electrode or replace catheter
Generator malfunction or battery depletion	Document adequate catheter position, check battery reserve	Replace batteries or generator
Unstable electrical connections	Document adequate catheter position, check connections	Secure connections

From: Wood M, Ellenbogen K, Haines D: *In:* Ellenbogen KA (Ed): Cardiac Pacing, Boston, Blackwell Scientific Publications, 1992, p 187.
*Connect bipolar intracardiac leads to right and left arm leads of the ECG and monitor lead I.

TABLE 96–2. Oversensing During Transvenous Cardiac Pacing

Cause	Evaluation	Solution
P-wave sensing	Catheter tip near tricuspid valve on chest x-ray; check electrograms	Reposition further into right ventricular apex; reduce sensitivity
T-wave sensing	Check electrograms	Reduce generator sensitivity; possibly reposition catheter
Myopotential sensing	Check electrograms during provocative maneuvers	If electrograms unipolar, replace with bipolar system or reduce sensitivity
Electromagnetic interference	Check proper electrical grounding and isolation of patient and pacer system; possibly check electrograms	Properly ground equipment; electrically isolate patient; turn off unnecessary equipment; reduce sensitivity
Intermittent electrical contacts, unstable connections, or lead fracture	Monitor sensing during manipulation of connections and lead	Secure connections; replace lead

From Wood M, Ellenbogen K, Haines D: *In:* Ellenbogen KA (Ed): Cardiac Pacing. Boston, Blackwell Scientific Publications, 1992, p 189.

cardiac depolarizations (Table 96–2). The result is an inappropriate inhibition of pacemaker output and thus failure to pace. Pectoral muscle potentials, diaphragmatic potentials, strong electrical fields (e.g., Bovie cautery), native T waves or pacemaker stimuli in opposing chambers in dual-chamber systems are examples of signals that may be inappropriately sensed.[11-16] Temporary pacemakers placed concomitantly with permanent systems may inhibit the permanent system and vice versa. Decreasing the sensitivity of the system may eliminate oversensing, provided that intrinsic R waves continue to be sensed.

Lead problems can also result in oversensing with inhibition of output. A break in the inner insulation of an in-line coaxial bipolar lead can produce electrical signals due to contact between the inner and outer conductors. These signals are typically large, precluding a decrease in sensitivity as a management option. In the pacemaker-dependent patient, programming the system to an asynchronous or triggered mode may be the only options until the lead can be replaced.

Failure to Sense

Loss of sensing is apparent as inappropriate pacing following intrinsic electrical cardiac events or failure to track atrial activity in DDD systems. Most factors that lead to high capture thresholds and loss of capture can also result in loss of sensing. These include (Table 96–3):

- Lead dislodgment
- Lead maturation after implantation
- Perforation
- Metabolic derangements
- Antiarrhythmic drug therapy
- Myocardial infarction, insulation defects
- Conductor fractures

When battery depletion reaches critical levels, most generators revert to asynchronous pacing modes to conserve energy. Similarly, pacing generators may revert to asynchronous modes in response to high levels of electromagnetic interference from Bovie cautery, magnet application, environmental noise, or direct current cardioversion. These later noise modes can be reprogrammed to other modes while end of battery life behavior necessitates generator replacement.

True loss of sensing must be differentiated from the occurrence of intrinsic events during pacemaker refractory periods. Refractory period durations may be known by interrogation of the pacemaker.

Pacemaker-Mediated Tachycardias

Originally, the term "pacemaker-mediated tachycardia" (PMT) was used to describe the sensing of a retrograde P wave from a premature ventricular contraction (PVC) or paced ventricular event by an atrial tracking (DDD) system.[17-21] The sensed retrograde P wave triggers a ventricular pacing pulse, leading to another sensed retrograde P wave and thus an endless loop process. This form of pacemaker-mediated tachycardia can be diagnosed and terminated by reprogramming to an asynchronous mode briefly with magnet application. One can prevent recurrence by reprogramming the refractory periods so that retrograde P waves are no longer sensed.

Atrial tracking pacemakers pace the ventricle up to the maximum tracking rate in response to supraventricular tachycardias, such as atrial fibrillation, atrial flutter, sinus tachycardia, and ectopic atrial tachycardias.[22, 23] Many dual-chamber pacemakers now posses "mode switching" algorithms that automatically reset the pacemaker to a VVI mode when high atrial rates (e.g., atrial fibrillation) are detected. This function prevents inappropriate rapid ventricular pacing. When atrial arrhythmias terminate, these pacemakers automatically restore dual-chamber function. In the absence of mode switching algorithms, lowering the maximum tracking rate or reprogramming to a nonatrial tracking mode may be needed until control of the arrhythmia can be achieved with cardioversion or antiarrhythmic drugs.

Pacemaker-mediated tachycardia may also be caused by rate adaptive pacemakers in response to sensor input.[24] Two common sensors are available: vibration and minute ventilation types. These pacing systems respond to the sensor to increase paced rate in response to an increase in metabolic demand. Inappropriate responses may result from body tremors or motion stimulating increased rates with vibration sensors. Respiratory sensing pacemakers are driven to higher rates by mechanical ventilation or tachypnea. Reprogramming the pacemaker to a non-rate responsive mode is frequently necessary to eliminate inappropriate paced tachycardias and is advisable for all patients with respiratory sensing pacemakers during mechanical ventilation.

Other Problems

Damage to the generator or to the lead-myocardial interface of a pacing system can occur with external defibrillation shocks. Recently implanted leads can be dislodged by intense muscle contractions. Pacemakers may be reprogrammed to a different mode (usually VVI or VOO) by the defibrillation current. An acute rise in threshold may result from myocardial injury at the lead-myocardial interface from the defibrillation current. To minimize the risk of damage to the pulse generator, defibrillation paddles should be placed at least 10 cm from the generator and the defibrillation current path should be perpendicular to the pacemaker current path (Fig. 96–5). Use of anterior-posterior defibrillation patch positions may be useful. The pacemaker function should be monitored carefully after defibrillation or cardioversion.

Electrocautery can be sensed, and may thus inhibit or trigger pacemaker output, and can damage the generator or tissue-lead generator or lead electrodes. Electrocautery can also

TABLE 96–3. Loss of Sensing During Transvenous Cardiac Pacing

Cause	Evaluation	Solution
Lead dislodgment or perforation	Check position on chest x-ray; check unipolar or bipolar electrograms*	Reposition lead under fluoroscopy; increase sensitivity
Local tissue necrosis or fibrosis	Check unipolar or bipolar electrograms	Reposition lead; increase sensitivity
Electrodes perpendicular to depolarization wavefront, low-amplitude electrograms and/or low slew rate	Check unipolar or bipolar electrograms	Unipolarize lead or reposition; increase sensitivity
Lead fracture	Check unipolar electrograms from each electrode	Unipolarize functional electrode or replace lead
Electrocautery/direct current damaging electrode or tissue interface	Exposure to current source, check electrograms	Replace or reposition lead; increase sensitivity
Spontaneous QRS complex during refractory period of generator	Analyze appropriate ECG tracings	Do not intervene, or replace with generator having shorter refractory period
Generator malfunction	Confirm adequate electrograms and generator sensitivity settings	Replace generator or reset sensitivity
Unstable electrical connections	Confirm adequate electrograms	Secure connections

From Wood M, Ellenbogen K, Haines D: *In:* Ellenbogen KA (Ed): Cardiac Pacing, Boston, Blackwell Scientific Publications, 1992, p 188.
*Connect bipolar intracardiac leads to right and left arm leads of the ECG and monitor lead I.
ECG = electrocardiogram.

trigger failure of output in devices near end-of-battery life. Pacemaker-dependent patients may require the generators to be reprogrammed to asynchronous (or triggered) modes before surgical procedures involving electrocautery.

Central venous access lines should be placed in the contralateral subclavian vein to the pacemaker or the jugular veins to avoid trauma to the leads and infection of the device.[9] In addition, the subclavian vein containing the lead may be thrombosed, thus preventing access.

Temporary Cardiac Pacing

Indications

Temporary cardiac pacing is indicated for virtually any symptomatic or hemodynamically compromising bradyarrhythmia except in the setting of severe hypothermia, wherein refractory ventricular tachyarrhythmias may be induced. Prophylactic temporary pacing is most frequently indicated in the setting of unstable escape rhythms or during acute myocardial infarction. In acute myocardial infarction, prophylactic pacing is generally indicated for new bifascicular or trifascicular block or for alternating bundle branch block. Patients with new onset of two or more of the following—first-degree AV block, Mobitz I or II second-degree AV block, left anterior or posterior fascicular block, or right or left bundle branch block—have a 25% to 36% risk of complete heart block in the setting of an acute myocardial infarction.[25]

Modes of Pacing

The timing cycles, sensing, and pacing threshold principles described for permanent pacing also apply to temporary pacing. There are several possible modes of temporary pacing (Table 96–4):

- Esophageal
- Transcutaneous
- Transvenous
- Transthoracic

Esophageal Pacing

Esophageal pacing is generally capable of pacing only the left atrium and is thus of limited utility in emergency situations. A specialized high-output, long-pulse-width generator that delivers current through special soft bipolar leads with more than 3 cm electrode spacing is necessary.[26]

Transcutaneous Pacing

Transcutaneous pacing is a fast, simple, and generally effective initial method in brady-asystolic arrest.[27] The large pacing electrodes are placed with the *negative* electrode on the anterior chest wall over the cardiac apex or chest lead V_3 position and the *positive* patch over the posterior chest wall between the right scapula and spine. Reversal of this electrode polarity often results in failure to capture. The specialized transcutaneous pacing generator uses high current and long pulse widths and obscures unfiltered ECG monitors. Ventricular capture must be confirmed by palpation of a pulse synchro-

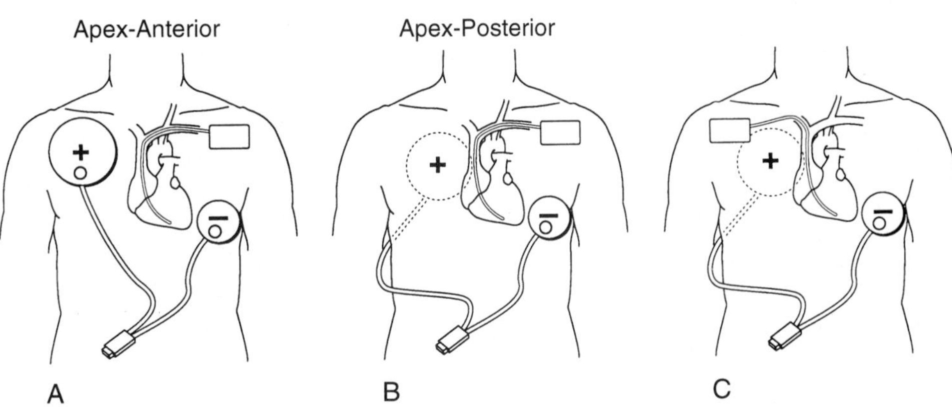

Figure 96–5. *A*, Schematic diagram of proper apical-right parasternal patch or paddle placement for external defibrillation in patients with pacemakers or pectoral defibrillators implanted in the left chest. *B* and *C*, Apical-posterior patch placement. This is the preferred configuration for patients with right-sided pacemakers, as shown in *C*.

TABLE 96–4. Comparison of Temporary Pacing Techniques

Method	Time to Initiate	Chamber Paced	Advantage	Disadvantage	Use
Transcutaneous	<1 min	Ventricle	Simple, rapid, safe	Variable capture, patient tolerance	Arrest, prophylactic
Transvenous	3–10 min	Atrium and/or ventricle	Most reliable, well tolerated long term	Invasive, time-consuming, complications	Arrest, prophylactic, maintenance
Transthoracic	10–60 sec	Ventricle	Extremely rapid, relatively simple	Complications, efficacy unproven	Arrest only
Transesophageal	Minutes	Atrium	Relatively simple, safe	Poor ventricular capture, patient tolerance	Prophylactic atrial pacing, diagnostics, termination of supraventricular tachyarrhythmia

Adapted from Wood M, Ellenbogen K, Haines D: *In:* Ellenbogen KA (Ed): Cardiac Pacing. Boston, Blackwell Scientific Publications, 1992, p 203.

nous with pacing. Maximum current is recommended initially to ensure ventricular capture in urgent situations. Pacing thresholds are generally in the range of 40 to 80 mA and are frequently uncomfortable for the patient.

Transcutaneous pacemakers pace the ventricles with hemodynamics similar to those used in endocardial VVI pacing. Transcutaneous pacing is safe and especially useful for brief prophylactic applications.

Transvenous Pacing

Transvenous pacing is the most reliable method of temporary pacing, but more operator skill and time are required compared with other methods.[27] Temporary pacing leads are best positioned in the right ventricle from a right internal jugular or left subclavian venous approach. If the patient eventually needs a permanent pacemaker, the subclavian approaches should be reserved for the permanent pacemaker implantation. The leads are directed by fluoroscopic or electrocardiographic guidance. A defibrillator should always be immediately available during lead manipulation. Ideally, atrial and ventricular capture thresholds should be less than 1 mA and atrial and ventricular sensing thresholds more than 1 mV and more than 6 mV, respectively. Temporary pacing generators capable of DVI, VVI, and DDD modes are available. Patients with ventricular systolic dysfunction or diastolic noncompliance or who have undergone recent cardiac surgery benefit hemodynamically from temporary atrioventricular sequential pacing.[28]

Lead dislodgment is the most common cause of pacing and sensing malfunction. Troubleshooting is otherwise similar to permanent pacing systems. Complications include induction of ventricular tachyarrhythmias, vascular damage, myocardial perforation, venous thrombosis, and infection.

Transthoracic Pacing

Transthoracic pacing, a rapid method of temporary ventricular pacing, is indicated only in emergent situations if other modes are not available.[27] Electrode wires are introduced percutaneously into the ventricular myocardium via a subxiphoid or parasternal approach with use of a trocar introducer. The efficacy of this method has not been established. Potential complications are numerous and include hemopericardium, pericardial tamponade, myocardial or coronary artery laceration, pneumothorax, and vascular or visceral laceration. Transthoracic wires should not be considered stable and should be replaced by transvenous pacing as soon as possible.

Temporary epicardial pacemaker wires placed at the time of cardiac surgery can be used with temporary transvenous pacing generators.[27] Atrial and ventricular wire sets permit AV sequential pacing however the thresholds typically deteriorate in the days following surgery. Reversal of lead polarity or conversion to unipolar pacing modes may be useful to maintain pacing with epicardial leads.

IMPLANTABLE CARDIOVERTER DEFIBRILLATORS

General Description

Implantable cardioverter defibrillators (ICDs) are designed to terminate malignant ventricular arrhythmias by delivering an electric shock or antitachycardia pacing to the heart.[29, 30] ICD systems are composed of defibrillation electrodes, sensing leads, and the pulse generator. Both single-chamber (ventricular) and dual-chamber (DDD) pacing defibrillator systems are available.

The sensing and pacing aspects of ICDs are similar to those as described for pacemaker systems. Shock therapy is delivered through transvenous endocardial electrode systems or, less commonly, through patch electrodes surgically positioned on the epicardial surface of the heart. Large early devices were implanted in an abdominal pocket. Current devices are small enough to permit pectoral implantation similar to that of permanent pacemakers (Fig. 96-6).

Although the detailed workings of each manufacturer's device varies, the general principles of tachycardia detection and therapy are similar. A sequence of events involves tachycardia detection, delay period, charging delay, therapy delivery, and monitoring for tachycardia termination. Heart rate is the primary parameter used by ICDs for ventricular tachycardia detection. The device continuously monitors the ventricular rate. Once the ventricular rate has exceeded a preprogrammed rate for a specified number of beats (or time duration), the ICD enters a therapy mode. There may be an initial delay of several seconds, during which time therapy may be aborted if the rhythm spontaneously terminates. After this delay, therapy is initiated according to the capabilities and programming of the device. Earlier "committed" devices charge and then deliver a shock after detection criteria are fulfilled whether or not the tachycardia terminates spontaneously (Fig. 96–7). Current "noncommitted" devices reconfirm the presence of tachycardia during charging and deliver therapy only if tachycardia persists. The time from tachycardia detection to therapy delivery may be 5 to 15 seconds.

Two modes of therapy are used by ICDs to terminate ventricular tachyarrhythmias. The first is delivery of a *depolarizing electric shock* to the heart (see Fig. 96–7). The energy required to defibrillate the heart is not an absolute value but instead follows a probability function.[29] The programmed energy delivered represents a threshold energy determined at the time of implant plus a safety factor (generally 10 joules)

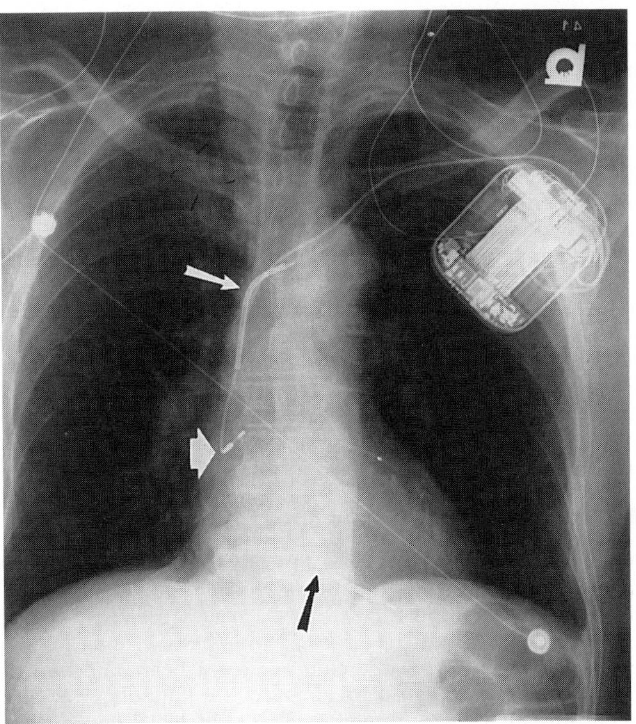

Figure 96–6. Posteroanterior chest radiograph from a patient with a transvenous pectorally implanted dual-chamber, cardioverter-defibrillator system. The ventricular lead in the right ventricular apex has two coil electrodes, one near the distal electrode and one positioned in the superior vena cava *(thin arrows)*. The atrial lead in the right atrial appendage *(broad arrow)* is used for dual-chamber (DDD) pacing and tachycardia discrimination algorithms.

to ensure a high likelihood of successful defibrillation. The defibrillation energy requirement at any particular time is influenced by characteristics of the device, impedance to current flow, presence of ischemia, drugs, and other factors. After a maximum of four to seven shocks are delivered without tachycardia termination, no further therapy is available until the device has sensed a heart rate below the tachycardia detection rate for a specified time period.

Most ICDs can also deliver *antitachycardia pacing* (ATP) as a means of terminating slower and hemodynamically tolerated ventricular tachycardias (see Fig. 96–7). This may prevent delivery of painful electric shocks, improving patient comfort and prolonging ICD battery life. If the rhythm persists or is accelerated by the pacing, shock therapy will be delivered.

For patients with ventricular arrhythmias of variable rates and hemodynamic stability, most devices deliver "tiered therapy," based on the rates of the various rhythms. For example, initial therapy for a well tolerated, relatively slow ventricular tachycardia might be antitachycardia pacing, followed by low-energy cardioversion (0.5 to 10 joules), then high-energy cardioversion (10 to 42 joules) if lower energies fail. Fast, poorly tolerated ventricular tachycardia or ventricular fibrillation should initiate shock therapy immediately. Devices capable of antitachycardia pacing are also capable of VVI or DDD pacing for bradyarrhythmias, which may follow successful tachycardia termination or for concomitant intrinsic bradyarrhythmias. Most devices have data logging capabilities to store the time, date, rate, duration, intracardiac electrograms and therapy delivered for each tachycardia detection. These data are invaluable for documenting the appropriateness of delivered therapy.

Evaluation of Recurrent Appropriate Therapy

Appropriate ICD shocks can be lifesaving, but if shocks are frequent, they are very uncomfortable for the patient and contribute to early battery depletion. Additionally, multiple episodes of ventricular tachyarrhythmias and multiple defibrillations can lead to myocardial ischemia, myocardial stunning, and worsening cardiac function.

Frequent appropriate shocks are best managed by suppression and treatment of the ventricular arrhythmia. Reversible causes of ventricular tachycardia or ventricular fibrillation should be investigated. Electrolyte abnormalities, especially hypokalemia or hypomagnesemia, should be aggressively treated. Heart failure can be associated with more frequent arrhythmias and should be optimally managed. Myocardial

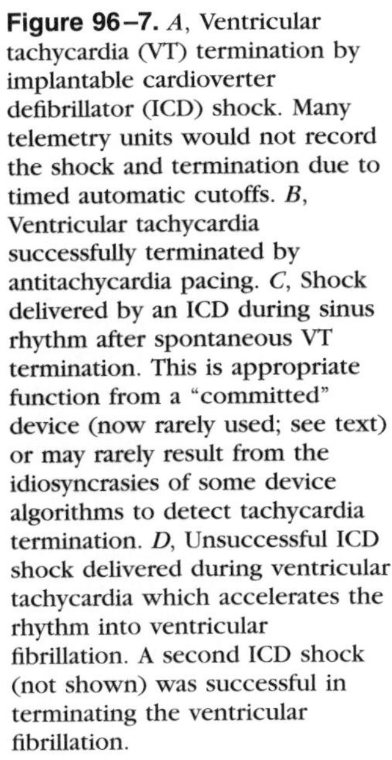

Figure 96–7. *A*, Ventricular tachycardia (VT) termination by implantable cardioverter defibrillator (ICD) shock. Many telemetry units would not record the shock and termination due to timed automatic cutoffs. *B*, Ventricular tachycardia successfully terminated by antitachycardia pacing. *C*, Shock delivered by an ICD during sinus rhythm after spontaneous VT termination. This is appropriate function from a "committed" device (now rarely used; see text) or may rarely result from the idiosyncrasies of some device algorithms to detect tachycardia termination. *D*, Unsuccessful ICD shock delivered during ventricular tachycardia which accelerates the rhythm into ventricular fibrillation. A second ICD shock (not shown) was successful in terminating the ventricular fibrillation.

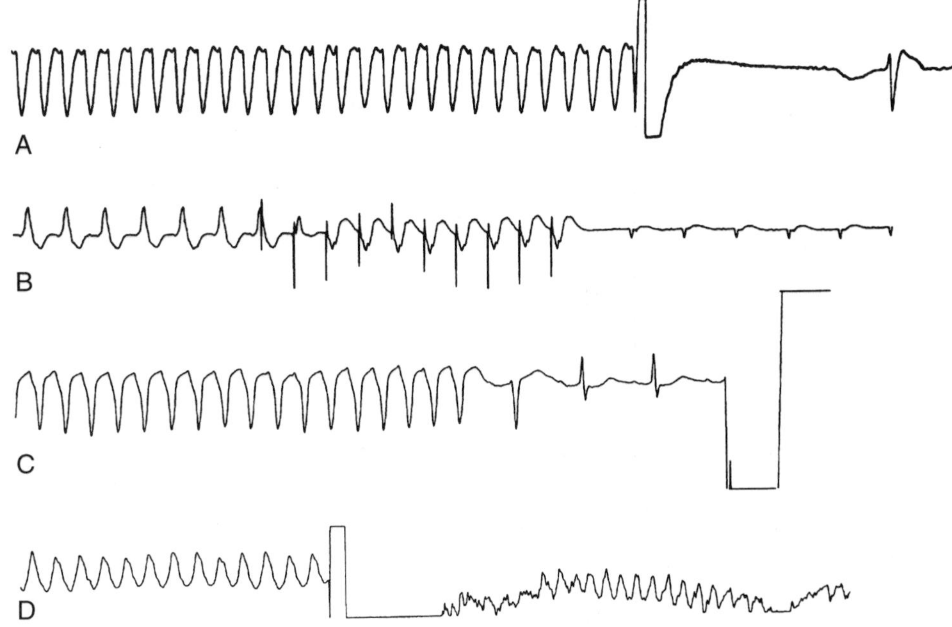

ischemia or infarction must be considered and treated. New antiarrhythmic drug therapy may be proarrhythmic, leading to multiple episodes of polymorphic ventricular tachycardia. Treatment with tricyclic antidepressant agents, phenothiazines, pentamidine, erythromycin, terfenadine, or astemizole[31-33] can lead to a prolonged QT interval in susceptible patients, precipitating torsades de pointes. Discontinuation of previously successful antiarrhythmic drug therapy may result in more frequent tachyarrhythmias.

In some patients, there is no identifiable cause of the multiple episodes of ventricular tachycardia or ventricular fibrillation. These patients require antiarrhythmic drug therapy to suppress frequent episodes. Specific antiarrhythmic drug therapy is usually empirical. Lidocaine, procainamide, bretylium, and amiodarone are rapidly acting intravenous agents effective for use in the ICU setting. Patients should be monitored during the institution of antiarrhythmic drugs for proarrhythmia (both tachyarrhythmias and bradyarrhythmias). New antiarrhythmic drugs may cause an increase in defibrillation thresholds or may slow the tachycardia rate below detection rates. Patients must therefore undergo repeated testing of the ICD after a change in antiarrhythmic drugs.

Inappropriate Therapy

Supraventricular Arrhythmias

Inappropriate therapy delivered by an ICD may be in response to supraventricular tachyarrhythmias or to electronic noise that is interpreted by the device as a ventricular tachyarrhythmia. Most ICDs use heart rate as the sole criterion to detect ventricular tachyarrhythmias. With the defibrillator, any heart rate that the device senses above its programmed cutoff rate is treated as ventricular tachycardia. Thus, supraventricular tachyarrhythmias that exceed the rate detection also initiate delivery of therapy from the device. Patients may receive inappropriate shocks for atrial fibrillation or flutter, paroxysmal supraventricular tachycardia, or even sinus tachycardia. This is not considered a device malfunction because the ICD is functioning as programmed within its limitations. Raising the cutoff rate for the detection of tachycardia may help to prevent this problem. In some patients, there is an overlap between the ventricular tachycardia rate and the rate during supraventricular tachyarrhythmias. Use of medications such as β-blockers, calcium channel blockers, or digoxin may be needed to slow the ventricular rates during these supraventricular rhythms.

Some devices incorporate special sensing algorithms to differentiate supraventricular arrhythmias from ventricular tachycardia. These features may include comparison of atrial and ventricular rates in dual-chamber ICDs, ventricular rate stability (for atrial fibrillation), and sudden onset criteria of arrhythmias. If available, these features can be activated as needed.

System Malfunctions

If a discharge is observed in a patient in sinus rhythm with no preceding tachycardia, system malfunction secondary to a lead or connector problem should be considered. Partial lead fractures or loose electrical connections between ICD generators, sensing leads, or adapters may generate electrical noise that is interpreted by the device as tachycardia. With some devices, placing a magnet over the generator elicits an audible beep with each sensed R wave. If manipulation of the device or leads brings out multiple beeps for each R wave, the device may be sensing extraneous electrical signals (e.g., noise), and generally warrants operative revision (see "double sensing" for further details).

For frequent inappropriate shocks, ICDs can be deactivated by placement of a "doughnut" (toroid) pacemaker magnet over the device. Some devices are turned off by prolonged magnet application; this is confirmed by the disappearance of beeps with each sensed R wave and replacement by a continuous tone. Other devices are deactivated only as long as the magnet is over the generator. Bradycardia pacing is generally not affected by magnet application. Device deactivation is most often necessary in the patient with rapid supraventricular arrhythmias or lead or connector malfunction to prevent multiple inappropriate shocks. The ICD should be inactivated only in a carefully monitored situation with immediately available external defibrillation capability and after consultation with physicians trained in ICD management. ICDs may also respond to external electromagnetic interference from electrocautery, diathermy, and transcutaneous electrical nerve stimulation (TENS) units. ICDs may need to be inactivated prior to surgical procedures, with provisions for intraoperative external defibrillation.

Artifacts and "Double Counting"

Another important cause of inappropriate shocks is the sensing of pacing artifacts. In patients with temporary or permanent pacemakers and ICDs, the ICD may sense the atrial or ventricular pacing artifacts as QRS complexes, leading to double counting. The ICD therefore senses a heart rate two or three times the actual heart rate. Double counting may also occur in patients with single-chamber ventricular pacemakers if the device senses both the pacing artifact and the paced QRS complex. Unipolar pacing (atrium or ventricle) is contraindicated in patients with ICDs because of the high likelihood of double counting. Bipolar pacing wires positioned in close proximity to the ICD endocardial sensing leads may also lead to double counting.

T wave sensing is another uncommon cause of this phenomenon. One can detect double counting in some devices by placing a magnet over the device and hearing two beeps for each R wave. Repositioning temporary pacing wires, deactivation of the ICD, and reliance on external cardioversion or reprogramming the sensitivity of the ICD may eliminate many causes of double counting.

Failure to Respond

The time from detection of a ventricular tachyarrhythmia to response by an ICD varies according to the device and the programmed therapy. With a long programmed detection time or delay during charging for a maximum shock, it may take 15 to 20 seconds to deliver therapy. Telemetry monitoring units may discontinue recording during this delay, leading to a misdiagnosis of "failure to respond" (see Fig. 96-7*A*). Noncommitted devices should not deliver therapy unless the ventricular tachycardia persists throughout charging and reconfirmation; thus, failure to respond to *nonsustained* ventricular tachycardia is not inappropriate.

An ICD will not respond to sustained ventricular tachycardia if the ventricular tachycardia rate is below the detection rate programmed for the device. This may be due to inappropriate programming, the emergence of a new, slower ventricular tachycardia, or ventricular tachycardias slowed by antiarrhythmic drug therapy. Reprogramming the detection rate is necessary.

Electrical signals during ventricular fibrillation may be extremely low in amplitude. These signals may be so small as to be undersensed by the pulse generator, leading to a delay or a failure to deliver therapy. In similar fashion, separate bradycardia pacemakers, temporary or permanent, may fail to sense ventricular fibrillation and will continue to pace. The pacing artifacts, as a result of their relative large size, may be sensed by the ICD as a normal, slow rhythm, thus inhibiting tachycardia therapy.

Of course, ICDs must be turned on in order to respond. As described earlier, magnets can turn off many devices in use. Patients who have come in contact with large magnets or with a magnet used in magnetic resonance imaging may have deactivated their device.

After four to seven shocks without tachycardia termination, ICDs do not deliver further therapy until termination occurs. If the physician is unaware that all therapies have failed for a given episode, failure of the device to respond may be misdiagnosed. Patients whose ventricular tachycardia or fibrillation does not convert after the maximum number of shocks or whose device fails to respond should undergo attempts at external defibrillation, coupled with cardiopulmonary resuscitative efforts, as in any patient. One should not wait for the ICD to complete delivery of therapy before beginning resuscitative measures and external defibrillation. Because epicardial patches may have an insulating effect to external shocks, different external paddle positions (e.g, anteroposterior, lateral-lateral) should be attempted if needed.

For pectorally implanted ICDs, the physician should take care to avoid external placement of paddles within 10 cm of the pulse generator.

Implantable Atrial Defibrillators

At this writing, implantable automatic atrial defibrillators are being evaluated in clinical studies in the United States.[34, 35] These devices function analogously to ventricular defibrillators in sensing and terminating sustained atrial fibrillation. The atrial defibrillator lead systems and device functions are highly variable. All systems employ a ventricular lead for shock synchronization and at least one atrial bipolar and coil electrode to sense atrial activity and deliver defibrillation shocks. Some systems also utilize a shock electrode within the coronary sinus. Combined atrial and ventricular defibrillators are also being studied in clinical trials.

Because the termination of atrial fibrillation is not urgent as with ventricular arrhythmias, these devices may have an extremely long detection time (up to hours) and may require manual activation. Escalating serial shocks, beginning with very low energies, may be tried for arrhythmia termination to enhance patient comfort. In some devices, antitachycardia atrial pacing may be available for termination of atrial flutter. In addition, some devices have complex atrial pacing algorithms in an effort to prevent atrial arrhythmia recurrences. Back-up bradycardia pacing should be available with all units.

As with pacemakers and ventricular defibrillators, care should be taken to avoid interaction between the devices and external pacemakers, external defibrillation, electrocautery and sources of electromagnetic noise.

References

1. Szabo Z, Solti F: The significance of the tissue reaction around the electrode on the late myocardial threshold. *In:* Advances in Pacemaker Technology. Schaldach M, Furman S (Eds). New York, Springer-Verlag, 1975, pp 273–285.
2. Beanlands DS, Akyurekli Y, Keon WJ: Prednisone in the management of exit block. *In:* Proceedings of the Sixth World Symposium on Cardiac Pacing. Meere C (Ed). Montreal, 1979, Chapter 18-3.
3. Lee D, Greenspan K, Edmands RE, Fisch C: The effect of electrolyte alteration on stimulus requirement of cardiac pacemakers. Circulation 1968; 38:6–124.
4. O'Reilly MV, Murnaghan DP, Williams MB: Transvenous pacemaker failure induced by hyperkalemia. JAMA 1974; 228:336.
5. Levick CE, Mizagala HF, Kerr CR: Failure to pace following high dose anti-arrhythmic therapy: Reversal with isoproterenol. PACE 1984; 7:252.
6. Dohrmann ML, Goldschlager N: Metabolic and pharmacologic effects on myocardial stimulation threshold in patients with cardiac pacemakers. *In:* Modern Cardiac Pacing, Barold SS (Ed). Mt. Kisco, NY, Futura Publishing Co, 1985, pp 161–170.
7. Hughes JC JR, Tyers GFO, Torman HA: Effects of acid-base imbalance on myocardial pacing thresholds. J Thorac Cardiovasc Surg 1975; 69:743.
8. Guarnieri T, Datorre SD, Bondke H, et al: Increased pacing thresholds after an automatic defibrillatory shock in dogs: Effects of class I and II antiarrhythmic drugs. PACE 1988; 11:1324.
9. Stokes K, Staffeson D, Lessar J, et al: A possible new complication of subclavian stick: Conductor fracture. PACE 1987; 10:748.
10. Levine PA: Clinical manifestations of lead insulation defects. J Electrophysiol 1987; 1:144.
11. Fetter J, Bobeldyk GL, Engman FJ: The clinical incidence and significance of myopotential sensing with unipolar pacemakers. PACE 1984; 7:871.
12. Gabry MD, Behrens M, Andrews C, et al: Comparison of myopotential interference in unipolar-bipolar programmable DDD pacemakers. PACE 1987; 10:1322.
13. Warnowicz-Papp MA: The pacemaker patient and the electromagnetic environment. Clin Prog Pacing Electrophysiol 1983; 1:166.
14. Sager DP: Current facts on pacemaker electromagnetic interference and their application to clinical care. Heart Lung 1987; 16:211.
15. Peter T, Harper R, Sloman G: Inhibition of demand pacemakers caused by potentials associated with inspiration. Br Heart J 1976; 38:211.
16. Barold SS, Ong LS, Falkoff MD, et al: Inhibition of bipolar demand pacemaker by diaphragmatic myopotentials. Circulation 1977; 56:679.
17. Levine PA, Selznick L: Prospective management of the patient with retrograde ventriculoatrial conduction: Prevention and Management of Pacemaker Mediated Endless Loop Tachycardias. Sylmar, Calif, Pacesetter Systems, Inc, 1990.
18. Luceri RM, Castellanos A, Zaman L, et al: The arrhythmias of dual chamber cardiac pacemakers and their management. Ann Intern Med 1983; 99:354.
19. Den Dulk K, Lindemans FW, Bar FW, et al: Pacemaker related tachycardias. PACE 1982; 5:476.
20. Rubin JW, Frank MJ, Boineau JP, et al: Current physiologic pacemakers: A serious problem with a new device. Am J Cardiol 1983; 52:88
21. Furman S, Fisher JD: Endless loop tachycardia in an AV universal (DDD) pacemaker. PACE 1982; 5:486.
22. Levine PA, Seltzer JP: AV universal (DDD) pacing and atrial fibrillation. Clin Prog Pacing Electrophysiol 1983; 1:275.
23. Greenspon AJ, Greenberg RM, Frankl WS: Tracking of atrial flutter during DDD pacing, another form of pacemaker mediated tachycardia. Pacing Clin Electrophysiol 1984; 7:955.
24. Lau C-P: Sensors and pacemaker-mediated tachycardias. *In:* Rate Adaptive Cardiac Pacing. Mt. Kisco, NY, Futura Publishing Co, 1993, pp 321–336.
25. Lamas GA, Muller JE, Turi ZG, et al: A simplified method to predict occurrence of complete heart block during acute myocardial infarction. Am J Cardiol 1986; 57:1213.
26. Deal BJ: Esophageal pacing. *In:* Clinical Cardiac Pacing. Ellenbogen KA, Kay GN, Wilkoff BL (Eds). Philadelphia, WB Saunders, 1995, pp 701–705.
27. Wood MA: Temporary cardiac pacing. *In:* Clinical Cardiac Pacing. Ellenbogen KA, Kay GN, Wilkoff BL (Eds). Philadelphia, WB Saunders, 1995, pp 687–700.
28. Hartzler GO, Malhoney JD, Curtis JJ, et al: Hemodynamic benefits of atrioventicular sequential pacing after cardiac surgery. Am J Cardiol 1977; 40:232.
29. Troup PJ: Implantable cardioverter defibrillators. Curr Probl Cardiol 1989; XIV:785.
30. Singer I (Ed): Implantable Cardioverter Defibrillators: Interventional Electrophysiology. Baltimore, Williams & Wilkins, 1977, pp 685–876.
31. Raehl CL, Patel AK, LeRoy M: Drug-induced torsade de pointes. Clin Pharm 1985; 4:675.
32. Nattel S, Ranger S, Talajic M, Lemery R, Roy D: Erythromycin-induced long QT syndrome: Concordance with quinidine and underlying cellular electrophysiologic mechanism. Am J Med 1990; 89:235.

33. Bigger JT Jr, Sahar DI: Clinical types of proarrhythmic response to antiarrhythmic drugs. Am J Cardiol 1987; 59:2E.
34. Lau CP, Tse HF, Lok NS, et al: Initial clinical experience with an implantable human atrial defibrillator. Pacing Clin Electrophysiol 1989; 20;223.
35. Ayers GM, Griffin JC: The future of defibrillators in the management of atrial fibrillation. Curr Opin Cardiol 1997; 12:12.

Bibliography

Barold SS (Ed): Modern Cardiac Pacing. Armonk, NY, Futura Publishing Co, 1985.
Ellenbogen KA (Ed): Cardiac Pacing. Boston, Blackwell Scientific Publications, 1992.
El-Sherif N, Samet P (Eds): Cardiac Pacing and Electrophysiology. 3rd ed. Philadelphia, WB Saunders, 1981.
Singer I: Implantable Cardioverter Defibrillator. Armonk, NY, Futura Publishing Co, 1994.

97

Use of Mechanical Circulatory Support Systems in Critically Ill Patients

D. Glenn Pennington, MD • Timothy E. Oaks, MD
Michael H. Hines, MD • Douglas P. Lohmann, ME

HISTORY

Mechanical devices to support the circulation have been employed over the past half century, beginning with Gibbon's[1] development of cardiopulmonary bypass in 1953. In 1957, Stuckey and colleagues[2] used cardiopulmonary bypass as a support mechanism for patients with acute myocardial infarction. Spencer and colleagues[3] used a centrifugal pump to support a patient with failing circulation after cardiac surgery. DeBakey[4] implanted the first left ventricular assist device (VAD) in 1964 in a young woman with heart failure after cardiac surgery. The introduction of the intra-aortic balloon pump (IABP) by Kantrowitz and colleagues[5] in 1968 profoundly improved the ability to maintain cardiac function in patients with cardiogenic shock. In 1969, Cooley and coworkers implanted the first total artificial heart (TAH). A bridge to transplantation as a temporary support technique was successfully accomplished with the Thoratec and the Novacor VADs in 1984 and subsequently with the Jarvik total artificial heart in 1985 and HeartMate left VAD in 1986.[7-10]

The initial goals of mechanical circulatory support were to rescue patients with cardiogenic shock and reverse myocardial injury in the acute phase. Subsequently, it became possible to support these patients for longer periods of time, thus allowing the maintenance of patients on devices until donor hearts could be available for transplantation. More recently, the concept of permanent implants has come to fruition. While intensivists have labored in intensive care units for years with patients with circulatory collapse and cardiogenic shock, the surgeon's attention was directed primarily toward weaning patients from cardiopulmonary bypass after cardiac operations. In both settings, the initial intent was to allow for recovery of native heart function by reducing the cardiac workload and thereby reducing myocardial oxygen consumption while simultaneously improving perfusion to vital organs and thus preventing vital organ injury.

This concept continues to be an important one in the treatment of surgical and nonsurgical patients who experience severe myocardial injury and subsequent pump failure. Of course, the usual measures of inotropic drug support, vasodilating drugs to unload the failing ventricle, correction of acid-base imbalance, and proper fluid volume control are critical prior to the use of mechanical circulatory support systems.

The placement of an IABP and even the institution of extracorporeal membrane oxygenation (ECMO) by portable circulatory support are now well established procedures in intensive care units and can be extremely helpful in reversing cardiogenic shock and establishing adequate perfusion. Once perfusion is established, however, the goals may differ significantly depending on the patient's circumstance.

Patients who have no realistic hope of myocardial recovery may be considered candidates for bridge to transplantation or permanent device implantation. Therefore, some of the resuscitative devices such as IABP or ECMO may actually be used as a bridge to a bridge and thus may be replaced with a more complete type of support such as a left VAD or a total artificial heart.

Patients treated with IABP and ECMO have almost always been cared for within the setting of the intensive care unit (ICU) because it is unlikely that they can be successfully managed outside the ICU environment. Conversely, VAD and TAH patients not only do well out of the ICU but may actually be discharged from the hospital. Therefore, it is appropriate to consider mechanical circulatory support systems as a whole spectrum of systems, which may be required in combination or sequentially in order to support the patient to the ultimate desired result.

The success of mechanical circulatory support can be measured in many ways, including morbidity, mortality, quality of life, and duration of support, but without the initial restoration of adequate perfusion and reversal of shock, success is beyond reach. Therefore, the critical events occurring in intensive care units often determine the ultimate outcome.

PATIENT SELECTION

Patients who are candidates for mechanical circulatory support systems vary widely but include:

1. Those in shock after cardiac operations.
2. Patients with acute myocardial infarction shock.
3. Patients with chronic heart failure and deterioration who may still be candidates for cardiac transplantation or permanent support.

Some of the difficulties in defining the clinical criteria for cardiogenic shock are related to the wide range of patients. In the initial experience with VAD applications, the patients were virtually all cardiac surgical patients in whom Norman and associates[11] described criteria for cardiogenic shock that did not respond to inotropic drugs or IABP. Modifications of these criteria have been employed in multi-institutional studies to establish the effectiveness of various devices.

The following inclusion criteria have been helpful in patients with acute cardiogenic shock:

- Cardiac index < 2 L/m^2/min
- Mean arterial pressures < 65 mm Hg
- Left or right atrial pressures > 20 mm Hg
- Urine output < 20 mL/hour
- Systemic vascular resistance > 2100 dynes · sec · cm^{-5}

These criteria describe patients in acute cardiogenic shock for whom some dramatic intervention must be made beyond drugs and the customary support, or the patients will die within 24 hours. However, other factors may apply even if the severity of the patient's condition does not actually meet these criteria. One consideration is a steady decline in the patient's condition, which suggests the prolonged need for inotropic support in an intensive care environment with a bedridden patient. Arrhythmias or impending renal failure may also justify the placement of mechanical support sooner. Of course, there must be exclusion criteria in order to ensure that valuable resources are not expended with futility. The exclusion criteria are broadly stated but can be applied in most circumstances:

- Severe renal failure (considered irreversible)
- Severe peripheral vascular disease
- Symptomatic cerebrovascular disease
- Cancer
- Severe hepatic disease
- Coagulopathy
- Severe infections resistant to therapy

More precise definitions of these inclusion and exclusion criteria are being attempted by various investigators. Similarly, there has been an attempt to define the severity of cardiogenic shock based on necessary inotropic drug regimens. In some protocols, the regimen used to indicate the need for VAD support is one of the following:

- Two or more inotropic drugs at high doses (e.g., dopamine $\geq$ 10 μg/kg/min, dobutamine $\geq$ 10 μg/kg/min, epinephrine $\geq$ 0.02 μg/kg/min)
- one inotropic drug with an IABP

Although the definitions of the specific requirements for mechanical implantation are in an evolutionary status, a moderate body of information has accumulated, making this much more effective than in the earlier years. For example, Reinhartz and colleagues[12] found that preoperative liver function was the most predictive factor of patient survival in a group of patients being bridged to transplantation with the Thoratec left VAD.

DEVICE DESCRIPTIONS

The various devices have also experienced significant evolution over the past 30 years, with improvements in technology and blood-contacting surfaces, as well as the increased implantability of the systems. Table 97-1 compares the main characteristics of the devices described next.

Intra-aortic Balloon Pump

The IABP is the most frequently used temporary left ventricular assist system. The balloon is mounted on a flexible catheter that is most commonly inserted via the femoral artery and positioned in the descending thoracic aorta. A predetermined volume of gas is pumped into the balloon during cardiac diastole and withdrawn during systole. The net result is an increase in diastolic arterial pressure and hence coronary perfusion pressure as well as a decrease in systolic arterial pressure, which decreases afterload resistance.

Extracorporeal Membrane Oxygenation or Portable Cardiorespiratory Support

The usual ECMO circuit includes venous inflow and arterial outflow tubing with a connecting bridge, a bladder, and several regulators; various infusion ports; the roller head or centrifugal pump; the oxygenator; and the heat exchanger. Unlike the circuit in cardiac surgery, the ECMO circuit has no venous reservoir in which to collect volume and from which to distribute blood if venous return temporarily drops. Instead, venous blood is collected in a small bladder, which is pressure monitored to prevent the intake and pumping of air. Collapse of the bladder indicates poor venous return, and the pump automatically stops. It will not restart until the bladder again senses adequate venous inflow. Absence of a large venous reservoir allows avoidance of high levels of anticoagulation required with full cardiopulmonary bypass, although ECMO requires moderate heparinization because of the membrane oxygenator. Thus, the ECMO circuit is a closed system in which the volume flowing in must exactly equal the volume pumped out. The ECMO system provides nonpulsatile flow. It can be used for venovenous support, which is helpful in respiratory failure, or for venoarterial support in cardiac failure. A perfusionist is required in constant attendance.

Biomedicus Centrifugal Ventricular Assist Device

The Biomedicus is one of the most commonly used centrifugal devices. Typically, centrifugal devices operate impellers or stators at high revolutions inside cone-shaped housings to produce forward blood flow. The inflow port is positioned at the top of the cone, and the outflow port exits tangentially at the bottom of the cone. The rotation imparts a centrifugal force on the blood, which drives it through the outflow port. Centrifugal pumps provide constant blood flow rather than pulsatile flow and, hence, require no valves. The cannulas originate in the right or left atria and pump the blood into the pulmonary artery or aorta, respectively. Tubing connects the cannulas to the pump and is kept as short as possible to reduce heat loss. A perfusionist usually monitors this device to adjust pump speed and prevent malfunctions because the lack of valves would allow retrograde flow. Anticoagulation is required.

Abiomed Ventricular Assist Device

The Abiomed VAD is an extracorporeal device that can be used to support the left, the right, or both ventricles simultaneously (Fig. 97-1). It uses atrial cannulas to drain the blood, which flows by gravity through tubing to the pump positioned below the level of the patient's atrium. The pump has a hard outer housing consisting of a clear polycarbonate and a flexible polyurethane blood-contacting surface. Each pump has a passive "atrial" filling chamber, an active "ventricular" chamber, and two polyurethane tri-leaflet valves. The device provides pulsatile flow through the tubing to the outflow cannula

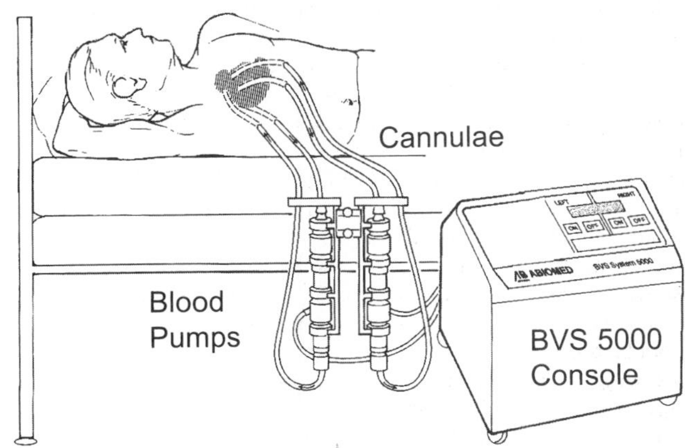

Figure 97–1. The Abiomed BVS 5000 is shown with biventricular assist devices and their connection to the control console. (Courtesy of Abiomed, Inc., Danvers, Mass.)

TABLE 97–1. Comparison of Mechanical Support Devices

Type of Device	Intra-aortic Balloon Pump	Extracorporeal Membrane Oxygenation	Biomedicus	Abiomed	Thoratec	Novacor	Heartmate	CardioWest
FDA-approved indications	Recovery or bridge	N/A	N/A	Recovery	Recovery or bridge	Bridge (investigational)	Bridge (electric-investigational)	Bridge (investigational)
Position	Intra-aortic	External	External	External	External	Internal	Internal	Internal
Ventricular support	Partial left	Complete cardiopulmonary	Left, right, or both	Left, right, or both	Left, right, or both	Left only	Left only	Left and right
Patient size	Small-Large	Small-Large	Small-Large	Small-Large	Medium-Large	Large	Large	Large
Average duration	Short	Short	Short	Intermediate	Intermediate to long	Long	Long	Long
Power source	Pneumatic	Electric	Electric	Pneumatic	Pneumatic	Electric	Electric or pneumatic	Pneumatic
Cannulation site	Peripheral arterial	Peripheral arterial and venous	Atrial	Atrial	Atrial or ventricular	Ventricular	Ventricular	N/A
Native ventricle	Remains	Remains	Remains	Remains	Remains	Remains	Remains	Removed
Anticoagulation	Not necessary	Yes	Yes	Yes	Yes	Yes	No	Yes
Patient ambulation	No	No	No	No	Yes, with assistance	Yes	Yes	Yes, with assistance
Patient discharge	No	No	No	No	No	Yes	Yes	No
Expense	$	$	$	$$	$$$	$$$$	$$$$	$$$$

FDA = Food and Drug Administration.

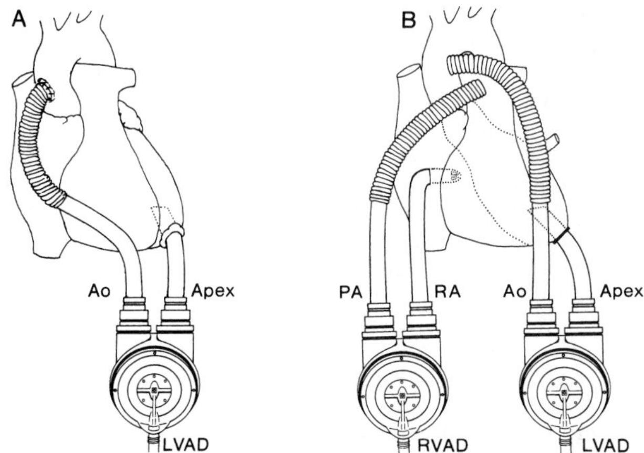

Figure 97–2. Thoratec ventricular assist device *A,* Left ventricular assist device (LVAD) with left ventricular apical (Apex) inflow and aortic (Ao) outflow. *B,* Biventricular assist devices: left VAD with the same cannulation as in *A.* Right VAD (RVAD) shows right atrial (RA) inflow and pulmonary artery (PA) outflow. (From Farrar DJ, Hill JD, Penninghm DG, et al: Preoperative and postoperative comparison of patients with univentricular and biventricular support with the Thoratec ventricular assist device as a bridge to cardiac transplantation. J Thorac Cardiovasc Surg 1997; 113: 203.)

and into the pulmonary artery or aorta. Anticoagulation is required. A console drives compressed air into the ventricular chamber to pump the blood. The console monitors and controls pump output with little intervention.

The device is preload-dependent and afterload-sensitive. The long tubing and absence of vacuum make it more dependent on preload than other devices. The device can be used in an ICU but usually does not allow the patient much mobility. It has been approved by the Food and Drug Administration (FDA) for temporary support for native cardiac recovery but not as a bridge to transplantation device.

Thoratec Ventricular Assist Device

The Thoratec VAD is a pneumatic device that is placed in a paracorporeal position. The device consists of a flexible blood sac that is actuated by alternating positive and negative air pressure. Mechanical valves are positioned in the inflow and outflow ports to ensure unidirectional blood flow. Cannulas are connected at the time of implantation to the inflow and outflow ports (Fig. 97–2). A Dacron graft is sewn to the ascending aorta and connected to the outflow port. A choice of inflow cannulas allows the option of draining blood from the left atrium or the left ventricle. Better pump flow is usually achieved with the ventricular cannula, but myocardial recovery, left ventricular geometry, left ventricular thrombus, and the surgeon's preference often influence cannula selection. The Thoratec VADs lie on the patient's abdomen, and the cannulas pierce the skin just below the 12th rib, crossing the diaphragm into the mediastinum.

The Thoratec VAD can also be used for biventricular support. The Dacron cannula can be sewn to the pulmonary artery to provide blood flow to the lungs, and blood can be withdrawn from the right atrium. Right ventricular cannulation is not usually employed because cannula obstruction has proved problematic. Generally, anticoagulation is necessary for use longer than a few days. The current system used in the United States requires a large console, which restricts patients to the hospital, but a portable system that allows for hospital discharge is being tested in Europe. Even when connected to a console, patients in the hospital can be transferred to a regular hospital floor and can be out of bed and exercise vigorously. It has been FDA-approved for temporary support for native cardiac recovery and as a bridge to transplantation.

Novacor Left Ventricular Assist Device

The Novacor Wearable Left VAD is an implanted electrical device. This device is implanted preperitoneally, posterior to the rectus abdominis muscle in the mid-upper abdomen. The cannulas cross the diaphragm to connect the heart and the device (Fig. 97–3). The inflow cannula draws blood from the left ventricle, and the outflow cannula delivers it to the aorta. Pericardial tissue valves sit just outside the inflow and outflow ports to maintain unidirectional flow. Dual pusher plates squeeze a flexible blood sac, ejecting the blood across the outflow valve.

The Novacor VAD fills passively and requires only 5 to 10 mm Hg to fill the blood sac. The device is governed by a compact controller worn on the outside of the body. A percutaneous lead connects the pump and the controller. Batteries or a monitor attaches to the controller to supply power. The monitor allows interrogation of the device. The small size of the controller and batteries allows patients to ambulate freely and to be discharged from the hospital. Anticoagulation is required. This device is approved by the FDA as a bridge to transplantation.

Heartmate Left Ventricular Assist Device

The Heartmate is available in two versions—one pneumatic and the other electric. They differ primarily in the mechanism that pumps the blood. The pneumatic version uses an external drive console that forces compressed air into the chamber until the blood sac is collapsed. In the electric version, a motor moves a pusher plate to collapse the blood sac. The electric version does not require a console; instead, a control-

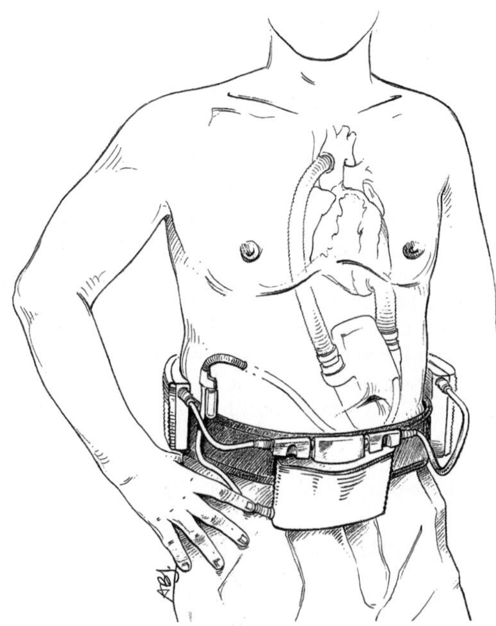

Figure 97–3. The wearable Novacor left ventricular assist device connects via a single driveline to a controller, which is worn on a belt. Primary and reserve batteries connect to the controller, also worn on a belt.

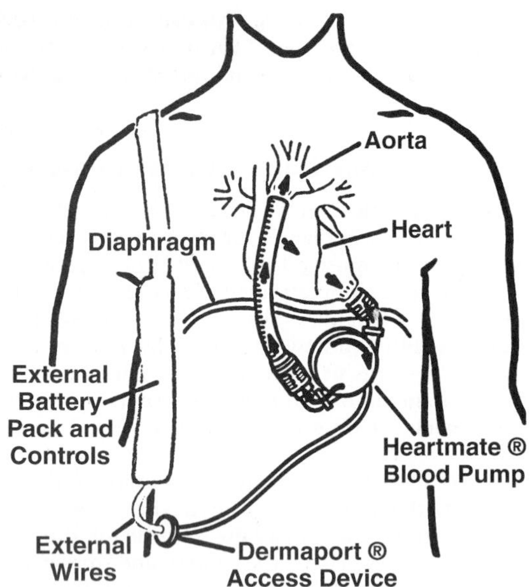

Figure 97–4. The Heartmate vented electric left ventricular assist device has a single exit site to allow connection to the external controller and batteries. (Courtesy of ThermoCardiosystems Inc., Woburn, Mass.)

ler and batteries can be worn over the shoulder, allowing greater mobility for the patient and hospital discharge (Fig. 97–4). Otherwise, the two versions are similar; each has porcine valves in the inflow and outflow conduits to ensure unidirectional flow. Each is placed preperitoneally, draining blood from the left ventricular apex and pumping it into the ascending aorta.

The unique feature of the Heartmate device is its textured blood sac and pumping chamber. These textured surfaces were designed to allow the formation of a pseudointimal lining to reduce the need for anticoagulation. Therefore, anticoagulants are not mandatory but platelet-deaggregating drugs are frequently employed. The pneumatic and electric versions are FDA-approved for bridge to transplantation.

CardioWest Total Artificial Heart

The CardioWest artificial heart is a biventricular replacement prosthesis. One pump is sewn to the patient's native right atrium and pulmonary artery, while the other connects the left atrium to the aorta. As with other pneumatic devices, compressed air is employed to squeeze the flexible blood sacs. A large console regulates the compressed air delivered to the pumps. Pneumatic tubing pierces the skin to connect the pumps and the console. The CardioWest device fits in the place of the native ventricles. Two mechanical valves in each ventricle maintain unidirectional flow. The current system requires a console, which prevents hospital discharge, but a portable system is under investigation. Anticoagulation is required. The FDA considers the CardioWest investigational as a bridge to transplantation.

RESUSCITATIVE SUPPORT

The IABP is an extremely useful device for patients in acute cardiac failure because it can be rapidly inserted percutaneously through the femoral artery in most settings, including the emergency department, cardiac catheterization laboratory, operating room, or ICU. Counterpulsation with the IABP involves the phasic displacement of blood within a fixed intravascular space. Synchronized with the cardiac cycle, it reduces blood volume in the ascending aorta during ventricular systole and augments the volume of blood in the aortic root during diastole. Abrupt reversal of cardiogenic shock may be achieved by reducing ventricular afterload and increasing diastolic coronary blood flow, thereby decreasing myocardial oxygen consumption while providing increased coronary blood flow. Positioning of the IABP above the renal arteries but below the origin of the left subclavian artery is critical.

Timing is also critical and should be adjusted to inflate the balloon on the dicrotic notch of the arterial pulse wave and deflate it just before the upstroke of the next waveform. Timing may be regulated by the R wave of the electrocardiogram (ECG), the arterial pressure trace, or a pacemaker, but extensive arrhythmias often make timing difficult. The IABP is generally considered capable of increasing cardiac output in patients with cardiogenic shock by as much as 20% to 25%, but that may not be sufficient in patients with severely depressed cardiac function. On the other hand, VADs have the capacity to capture the entire cardiac output and increase blood flow to normal levels in severe cardiogenic shock. Therefore, the IABP may provide initial resuscitation but may not be sufficient to sustain the most severely affected patients. There are also some contraindications to IABP usage, including aortic valvular regurgitation and severe aortoiliac obstruction. Complications of IABP include limb ischemia, bleeding, infection, aortic dissection or rupture, mesenteric or renal ischemia, and IABP rupture with gas embolization.

ECMO is also an effective resuscitative tool. The cardiopulmonary bypass system used to support patients in the operating room was first applied successfully in the ICU setting in 1972 for a trauma victim with respiratory failure. This system was the forerunner of the current ECMO system and is used in a variety of settings.[13] The system has been employed successfully over several days or weeks and, rarely, longer in patients with severe respiratory failure or cardiogenic shock. It has been used successfully in more than 100 United States centers, primarily for newborns with respiratory failure. The indications have now expanded to include respiratory failure in infants, children, and adults, including respiratory distress syndrome as well as circulatory support in infants and children, especially for postcardiotomy failure. Circulatory support in adults has been accomplished with ECMO as well and has been successful in postcardiotomy patients.[14]

The ECMO circuit can be applied as a venovenous system, which is appropriate for patients with pulmonary failure and adequate cardiac function, or as a venoarterial system, in which both the right and left heart are provided with some degree of bypass similar to that employed in the operating room. Because of the length of the circuit and transit time, the blood is exposed to room temperature for significant periods and patients can rapidly cool. However, heat loss can be used to induce cooling in patients with high fever, sepsis, or arrhythmias. The ECMO circuit also has the potential advantages of allowing for ultrafiltration, dialysis, plasmapheresis, drug or blood product infusion, and blood sampling, none of which are features available with VADs.

Perhaps the most important difference between the ECMO circuit and traditional cardiopulmonary bypass is that ECMO uses a true membrane oxygenator, which can be used for several days to weeks, unlike the 8-hour period that a hollow fiber oxygenator in the operating room can supply. The membrane requires a moderate level of anticoagulation and does stimulate an inflammatory response and fibrinolysis. Because of these effects, it is generally not thought to be the optimal system for postcardiotomy patients, but it can be rapidly applied as a resuscitative system in the ICU or other settings to quickly reverse cardiogenic shock. ECMO has often been used as a bridge to another more complete type of support, which does not require as vigorous an anticoagulation regimen.

POSTCARDIOTOMY SUPPORT

Most of the early experience with VADs was obtained in patients who either could not be weaned from cardiopulmonary bypass after cardiac surgery or who collapsed in the ICU and required mechanical support. The requirement for IABP after cardiac surgery is reported as high as 12%,[15] and the mortality rate in these patients ranges from 20% to 50%.[15–17] Approximately 1% of patients undergoing cardiac surgery experienced severe cardiac failure in spite of IABP and inotropic support and needed mechanical support with VADs. In our experience, which began at St. Louis University in 1978 and included Wake Forest University in 1995, 185 patients received mechanical circulatory support. Devices for postcardiotomy cardiac failure were implanted in 86 of those patients. Forty-seven received centrifugal pumps, and 39 received Thoratec pumps. In all cases, the inotropic and vasodilating drug therapy had been optimized, and in almost all cases an IABP was inserted prior to the use of the VAD. The overall survival of the postcardiotomy patients was 20%, but in the Thoratec group, 13 of 45 patients survived, for a rate of 29%. The Thoratec patients were studied under a strict protocol of the National Heart, Lung, and Blood Institute, which excluded some of the patients who were less likely to survive. The experiences of others with postcardiotomy support are similar.

From the combined registry of the ASAIO-ISHLT,*[18] 1279 patients underwent temporary circulatory support after cardiac operations and 584 patients (45.7%) were weaned from the devices, but only 323 patients (25.3%) were discharged from the hospital. In isolated center experiences, survival rates following postcardiotomy VAD support are somewhat higher than 25%, but in general the salvage should not be anticipated to exceed 50% because of the severity of the patients treated and their comorbidities. The support of postcardiotomy patients has been accomplished with a wide range of devices, including ECMO,[14] centrifugal pumps, and pulsatile VADs.[19, 20] Although there have been rare applications of the electrical, implantable devices in postcardiotomy patients, they are not currently recommended.

One important factor regarding the use of postcardiotomy devices is whether or not they can support both ventricles. Early in our experience with VADs at St. Louis University, it became apparent that right ventricular failure was often a problem in postcardiotomy patients, probably related to increased pulmonary vascular resistance, multiple transfusions, and other concomitant factors.[21] Therefore, devices that provide some support for both sides of the heart are important and include ECMO, the centrifugal VADs, the Abiomed, and the Thoratec VADs. The incidence of biventricular support in postcardiotomy patients has been high and exceeds 50% in some series. Indeed, some centers presume that postcardiotomy failure should always be supported with biventricular devices and therefore insert them in all cases. That has not been our experience, and we generally recommend implantation of a left VAD first. If adequate pump outflow can be accomplished with right-sided filling pressures below 20 mm Hg, it is often possible to support them with left devices alone. Less commonly, there have been successful applications of right VADs using IABP for left-sided support.[21, 22]

One of the primary problems with postcardiotomy support is bleeding and the need for anticoagulants. Another factor in survival following postcardiotomy support is whether or not an acute myocardial infarction has occurred. When perioperative myocardial infarction was noted, it was rare for ventricular recovery to occur and allow for survival.[23] On the other hand, patients with acute myocardial infarction shock treated with the Thoratec VAD had a moderately high rate of survival when they were also eligible for cardiac transplantation.[24]

ECMO has been successfully applied in postcardiotomy patients[14] but has a disadvantage of requiring moderate degrees of anticoagulation, which often result in bleeding. There may also be complications related to infection, or if the cannulas are inserted peripherally, problems with leg perfusion. Most investigators consider ECMO an effective support system for a limited period, such as 24 to 48 hours. Thereafter, if myocardial recovery has not occurred and the patient is a candidate for cardiac transplantation, a more complete ventricular assist system should be implanted. Therefore, ECMO has often been used as a successful bridge to a bridge.[25]

Although the overall survival rate for patients undergoing postcardiotomy support is generally low, the salvage of 25% to 30% of patients who would certainly die if not supported justifies the use of these systems. It is important that we continue to develop devices that can be applied simply and efficiently in the operating room after complex cardiac operations that will provide biventricular support when needed and do not require anticoagulation in order to prevent the bleeding complications. Furthermore, if we can identify methods of detecting which ventricles may recover, more realistic applications of these devices may be applied, particularly in patients who are not candidates for cardiac transplantation.

MECHANICAL CIRCULATORY SUPPORT PRIOR TO TRANSPLANTATION

The various types of mechanical circulatory support devices have been described earlier, and all have been successfully used in patients undergoing cardiac transplantation. The choice of device depends on many factors. For patients awaiting cardiac transplantation, the IABP is the most common choice in patients who remain hemodynamically unstable despite inotropic support. However, the IABP provides only modest support and often fails to "bridge" unstable patients to cardiac transplantation when used alone. VADs and total artificial hearts are capable of complete hemodynamic support, and their use is reserved for when inotropic and IABP support fails. Body size, body habitus, potential for myocardial recovery, presence of prosthetic valves, and need of univentricular or biventricular support all dictate which type of VAD may be used and whether a total artificial heart may be implanted. For patients with a body size smaller than 1.3 m^2, implantation of a total artificial heart may not be possible. Use of the CardioWest total artificial heart and the Novacor and Heartmate left VADs may not be possible in small patients. Fortunately, the Thoratec and the Abiomed VADs may be used in almost all adult patients.

In a few patients, some degree of myocardial recovery may be anticipated with subsequent explantation of the device. For these patients, a device that does not require ventricular cannulation may be preferable. Theoretically, damage to the apical segment of the left ventricle by ventricular cannulation impairs subsequent myocardial recovery, although that has not always been true in clinical trials. The choice of ventricular or even atrial cannulation has been a concern in patients with prosthetic aortic valves. Because ventricular cannulation theoretically captures all the cardiac output, the native ventricle may not eject blood across the aortic valve, which may lead to valve thrombosis and the potential for embolization. Atrial

*American Society for Artificial Internal Organs/International Society for Heart and Lung Transplantation.

cannulation may diminish this problem but does not ensure that the prosthetic valves will not thrombose. However, these problems may have been overestimated in the past.[26]

The most common determinant in selecting the appropriate device is the need for univentricular or biventricular support. If biventricular support is required, the total artificial heart or the appropriate VAD can be employed. However, only the Thoratec and the Abiomed devices can be used as right VADs. We prefer to use right and left Thoratec VADs in patients requiring biventricular support, although hybrid systems with a right-sided Thoratec or Abiomed VAD paired with a left-sided Novacor or HeartMate VAD have been successful.

Intra-aortic Balloon Pump as a Bridge to Cardiac Transplantation

Reemstma and colleagues[27] were the first to report the successful use of balloon counterpulsation (IABP) prior to cardiac transplantation. Since then, the IABP has been used extensively for short-term mechanical support prior to cardiac transplantation.[28-30] In a series of 43 potential transplant patients, Rosenbaum and coworkers[31] found that the IABP was an effective bridge to cardiac transplantation in patients with both ischemic and nonischemic cardiomyopathy. However, about one third of the patients continued to undergo hemodynamic deterioration while receiving IABP support, resulting in either death or the need for further circulatory support with a VAD or total artificial heart. Because the IABP is designed for temporary support (<2 weeks), it is not ideal as a bridge to cardiac transplantation. Additionally, complications associated with the use of the IABP may preclude subsequent cardiac transplantation. Complications include[32, 33]:

1. Difficulty in insertion due to peripheral vascular disease.
2. Perforation of the femoral artery, iliac artery, or aorta.
3. Thrombosis of the femoral artery with limb ischemia.
4. Embolization of thrombus or atherosclerotic plaque.
5. Aortic dissection.
6. Peripheral nerve injuries.
7. Local wound infection.
8. Sepsis.
9. Balloon rupture.

Most IABPs are inserted percutaneously via the femoral artery. Although this approach is simple and expedient, the patient must lie flat to avoid kinking of the IABP. Prolonged immobility of these already compromised patients predisposes them to pneumonia and pulmonary embolism, which may preclude transplantation. In an effort to improve patient mobility, other insertion techniques have been developed. McBride and Colleagues[34] have described IABP insertion via the axillary artery. A technique for retroperitoneal placement of an IABP that preserves patient mobility has been described by Buchanan and coworkers.[35] In their small series of four transplant candidates, the average duration of IABP support was 32 days and the longest duration of support was 86 days. Although these descriptions of alternative placement for IABP support are encouraging, most physicians believe that support with VADs or total artificial hearts is necessary when the duration of IABP exceeds 2 weeks.

Ventricular Assist Devices as a Bridge to Cardiac Transplantation

In 1978, Norman and associates[36] reported the first use of a VAD as a bridge to cardiac transplantation. Over the past 20 years, several hundred patients have been supported with various types of VADs prior to transplantation. The advantages and disadvantages of the various types of devices have been briefly mentioned. The Abiomed and Thoratec devices are versatile and can be used in most adult patients for univentricular or biventricular support. Cannulation can be accomplished through the atrium or ventricle. The Novacor and the HeartMate devices are similar, in that they can be used as left VADs only. If biventricular support were required, another type of VAD would be used to support the right ventricle. However, these devices have the advantages of being implantable and electrically driven. With the use of an electrical device with its battery pack and small console, the patient can be more mobile and even discharged from the hospital. The current cumbersome drive consoles required with pneumatic devices make hospital discharge impractical, although Thoratec is testing a portable pneumatic drive unit in Europe.

With any of these devices, there are major peri-implant complications that can influence subsequent transplantation. Bleeding complications at the time of implant may result in massive transfusion requirements and patient sensitization to the many human leukocyte antigens (HLAs) present in the blood and blood products they receive. These antibodies make subsequent donor and recipient matching problematic as well as increase the risk for acute cellular rejection once a suitable donor is found. Infectious complications as well as complications of thromboembolism may disqualify some patients for subsequent transplantation. Despite these problems, data from the Combined Registry for the Clinical Use of Mechanical Ventricular Assist Pumps and the Total Artificial Heart have shown that approximately 70% of patients supported with VADs or total artificial hearts survive to transplantation and approximately 70% of the patients who receive transplants are discharged from the hospital.[18] Similar findings have been reported by other combined series and registries.[37, 38]

The Abiomed VAD is perhaps the most simply designed of the pneumatic devices, but it is limited by being gravity-filled. This feature inhibits patient mobility to some degree. An advantage is its relatively inexpensive cost and its suitability for biventricular support. An early report of the Abiomed has demonstrated its utility by its use in six patients after transplantation, four of whom survived.[39] In Germany, Korfer and colleagues[40] reported 14 patients supported with the Abiomed device prior to cardiac transplantation, with seven long-term survivors. However, the Abiomed is not FDA-approved as a bridge to transplantation in the United States.

The Thoratec VAD has been extensively used in the United States for postcardiotomy cardiogenic shock and for bridge to cardiac transplantation. Early reports demonstrated the efficacy of this device in supporting patients prior to transplantation. In a multicenter study of 213 patients supported with the Thoratec VAD (74 left VADs, 149 biventricular VADs) as a bridge to transplantation, 141 patients underwent transplantation and 119 patients were discharged from the hospital.[41] These excellent results have been confirmed by many others.

A large experience with the pneumatic and electric HeartMate VAD has been accrued at Columbia University.[42] Over an 8-year period, 84 potential transplant recipients were supported with either the pneumatic device (52 patients) or the electric device (32 patients). The maximum duration of support was 363 days for the pneumatic device and 605 days for the electric device. In 54 patients, the device succeeded as a bridge to transplantation, whereas four patients recovered sufficient cardiac function, allowing successful explanation of the device. Four patients were still awaiting transplantation at the time of the report. Nineteen patients with the electric device were discharged to home, with a mean outpatient support of 108 days and the longest duration of support being 466 days. The majority of outpatients led reasonably normal lives. Despite these excellent results, hemorrhage, device-related infections, mechanical failures, and thromboembolism associated with infection still occurred.

Experience with the Novacor VAD parallels that of the electric Heartmate VAD. With the exception of the blood-contacting surfaces, the devices are similar in design and use. The research group at the University of Pittsburgh has accumulated 40 patients supported with the Novacor VAD as a bridge to cardiac transplantation.[43] Thirty-one patients survived to transplantation and 27 were discharged from the hospital. Other investigators have reported excellent results with the Novacor device, and most centers have an active program using the wearable console such that patients can be discharged to home to await transplantation. One such patient was supported for more than 2 years prior to explantation of the device.[44]

Total Artificial Heart as a Bridge to Cardiac Transplantation

The first attempt to bridge a patient to cardiac transplantation occurred in 1969 when Cooley and coworkers[6] used a pneumatic total artificial heart. Copeland and colleagues[9] were the first to report long-term survival with the use of the total artificial heart prior to transplantation. Since that time, different models have been used, but the largest experience has been with the CardioWest model (formerly, the Jarvik/Symbion Heart). A registry report of 171 patients demonstrated a 69% survival to transplantation[45]; however, the 1-year survival after transplantation was only 57%. Complications during implantation were common and included infection (37%), thromboembolic events (11%), renal failure (20%), severe bleeding (26%), and mechanical malfunction (4%). A similar experience was summarized by the Pittsburgh group.[46] They abandoned the use of the total artificial heart because of the complications. However, use of the CardioWest total artificial heart TAH has yielded excellent results.[47]

MECHANICAL CIRCULATORY SUPPORT AS A BRIDGE TO RECOVERY

As experience with mechanical circulatory support as a bridge to cardiac transplantation has increased, it has become apparent that a small percentage of patients recover normal or near-normal ventricular function. Isolated reports have shown that the left VAD can be removed, with subsequent preservation of ventricular function. Because donor organs are scarce, it would be beneficial to examine the potential for using mechanical circulatory support techniques to bridge patients to recovery.

Dembitsky and Coworkers[48] reported the use of successful mechanical circulatory support for noncoronary shock in patients referred for cardiac transplantation. Nine patients, eight with viral prodrome and one post partum, experienced severe heart failure and required and IABP alone (two patients), a left VAD (four patients), a biventricular VAD (two patients), or ECMO (one patient). The period of support ranged from 3 to 79 days. All patients recovered normal ventricular function, and all were in the New York Heart Association functional class I 7 months to 4.5 years after support.

Muller and colleagues[49] reported their experience from Berlin, Germany, with five patients who were successfully weaned from left VAD support. These patients were selected from a cohort of 17 patients, all of whom had idiopathic dilated cardiomyopathy, and were in the New York Heart Association functional class IV. After explantation, the patients demonstrated improvement in left ventricular ejection fraction over time as well as a decrease in the titer of antibodies directed against the β receptor. These patients were supported for 160 to 794 days, and post-explant ventricular function remained stable over the follow-up period.

An update of this experience has been presented and included 18 patients with idiopathic dilated cardiomyopathy who were weaned from left VAD support.[50] The duration of support ranged from 30 to 794 days. Although ventricular function was good in most patients, five of the 18 patients subsequently underwent transplantation because of recurrence of heart failure. Although these data representing bridge to recovery are interesting, questions regarding the mechanism of ventricular recovery, type of support necessary, and patient selection for weaning all need to be addressed.

PERMANENT IMPLANTS

Results of the bridge to transplantation experience involving pneumatic and electric VADs and total artificial hearts have demonstrated several key points. First, currently available devices are mechanically sound, with many examples of support lasting longer than 1 year. Complications of infection and stroke, although not eliminated, have been decreasing with design modification and enhanced experience. Second, most patients can be supported chronically with univentricular devices alone, meaning that chronic left ventricular support would be adequate for long-term survival. Finally, experience with the wearable VADs has demonstrated the feasibility of hospital discharge with an excellent quality of life.

Given the scarcity of donor organs, then, it is reasonable to begin long-term VAD insertion as an alternative to transplantation. In fact, the REMATCH study (Randomized Evaluation of Mechanical Assistance for the Treatment of Congestive Heart Failure) using the electric Heartmate device is now under way.[51] However, the REMATCH trial studies only patients who are not candidates for cardiac transplantation. We have speculated that a totally implantable electric VAD could compete well with the strategy of cardiac transplantation.[52] Considering the number of patients who die waiting for a transplant, the potential complications of transplantation, and the limited long-term outlook of transplant recipients as well as the anticipated immediate availability of long-term VADs, it is likely that some transplant recipients might opt for a VAD. Implantation of a VAD might not preclude later transplantation, particularly in young adults.

References

1. Gibbon GH Jr: Application of a mechanical heart and lung apparatus to cardiac surgery. Minn Med 1954; 37:171-173.
2. Stuckey JH, Newman MM, Dennis C, et al: The use of the heart-lung machine in selected cases of acute myocardial infarction. Surg Forum 1957; 8:342-344.
3. Spencer FC, Eiseman B, Trinkle JK, Rossi NP: Assisted circulation for cardiac failure following intracardiac surgery with cardiopulmonary bypass. J Thorac Cardiovasc Surg 1965; 49:56.
4. DeBakey ME: Left ventricular bypass pump for cardiac assistance: Clinical experience. Am J Cardiol 1971; 27:3-11.
5. Kantrowitz A, Tjonneland S, Freed PS, et al: Initial clinical experience with intra-aortic balloon pumping in cardiogenic shock. J Am Med Assoc 1968; 203:135-140.
6. Cooley DA, Liotta D, Hallman GL, et al: Orthotopic cardiac prosthesis for two-staged cardiac replacement. Am J Cardiol 1969; 24:723-730.
7. Hill JD, Farrar DJ, Hershon JJ, et al: Use of prosthetic ventricle as a bridge to cardiac transplantation for postinfarction cardiogenic shock. N Engl J Med 1986; 314:626-628.
8. Starnes VA, Oyer PE, Portner PM, et al: Isolated left ventricular assist as a bridge to transplantation. J Thorac Cardiovasc Surg 1988; 96:62-71.
9. Copeland JG, Levinson MM, Smith R, et al: The total artificial heart as a bridge to transplantation: A report of two cases. JAMA 1986; 256:2991-2995.

10. Frazier OH, Duncan JM, Radovancevic B, et al: Successful bridge to heart transplantation with a new left ventricular assist device. J Heart Lung Transplant 1992; 11:530–537.
11. Norman JC, Cooley DA, Igo SR, et al: Prognostic indices for survival during postcardiotomy intra-aortic balloon pumping. Methods of scoring and classification, with implications for left ventricular assist device utilization. J Thorac Cardiovasc Surg. 1977; 74:709–720.
12. Reinhartz O, Farrar DJ, Hershon JH, et al: Importance of liver function in patients supported with Thoratec ventricular assist devices as a bridge to transplantation. J Thorac Cardiovasc Surg (in press).
13. Hill D, O'Brien TG, Murray JJ, et al: Extracorporeal oxygenation for acute post-traumatic respiratory failure (shock-lung syndrome): Use of the Bramson membrane lung. N Engl J Med 1972; 286:629–634.
14. Magovern GJ: Extracorporeal life support following adult open heart surgery. *In:* ECMO: Extracorporeal Cardiopulmonary Support in Critical Care. Zwischenberger JB, Bartlett RH (Eds). Ann Arbor, Mich, Extracorporeal Life Support Organization, 1995, pp 473–488.
15. Torchiana DF, Hirsch G, Buckley MJ, et al: Intraaortic balloon pumping for cardiac support: Trends in practice and outcome, 1968 to 1995. J Thorac Cardiovasc Surg 1997; 113:758–765.
16. Naunheim KS, Swartz MT, Pennington DG: Intraaortic balloon pumping in patients requiring cardiac operations: Risk analysis and long-term follow-up. J Thorac Cardiovasc Surg 1992; 104:1654–1661.
17. Baldwin RT, Slogoff S, Noon GP, et al: A model to predict survival at time of postcardiotomy intraaortic balloon pump insertion. Ann Thorac Surg 1993; 55:908–913.
18. Mehta SM, Aufiero TX, Pae WE Jr, Miller CA, Pierce WS: Combined registry for the use of mechanical ventricular assist pumps and the total artificial heart in conjunction with transplantation: Sixth official report, 1994. J Heart Lung Transplant 1995; 14:585–593.
19. Pennington DG, McBride LR, Swartz MT, et al: Use of the Pierce-Donachy ventricular assist device in patients with cardiogenic shock after cardiac operations. Ann Thorac Surg 1989; 47:130–135.
20. Pennington DG, Bernhard WF, Golding LR, et al: Long-term follow-up of postcardiotomy patients with profound cardiogenic shock treated with ventricular assist devices. Circulation 1985; 72:II216–226.
21. Pennington DG, Merjavy JP, Swartz MT, et al: The importance of biventricular failure in patients with postoperative cardiogenic shock. Ann Thorac Surg 1985; 39:16–26.
22. Pae WE Jr, Miller CA, Matthews Y, Pierce WS: Ventricular assist devices for postcardiotomy cardiogenic shock: A combined registry experience. J Thorac Cardiovasc Surg 1992; 104:541–553.
23. Pennington DG, McBride LR, Kanter KR, et al: Effect of perioperative myocardial infarction on survival of postcardiotomy patients supported with ventricular-assist devices. Circulation 1988; 78:III110–115.
24. Hill JD, Farrar DJ, Hershon JJ, et al: Use of a prosthetic ventricle as a bridge to cardiac transplantation for postinfarction cardiogenic shock. N Engl J Med 1986; 314:626–628.
25. Muehrcke DD, McCarthy PM, Stewart RW, et al: Extracorporeal membrane oxygenation for postcardiotomy cardiogenic shock. Ann Thorac Surg 1996; 61:684–691.
26. McBride LR, Ruggiero R, Moroney DA, Powers KA, Swartz MT: Ventricular assist device support in patients with mechanical prosthetic heart valves (Abstract). J Heart Lung Transplant 1998; 17:72.
27. Reemstma K, Drusin R, Edie R, et al: Cardiac transplantation for patients requiring mechanical circulatory support. N Engl J Med 1978; 298:670–671.
28. Hardesty RL, Griffith BP, Trento A, et al: Mortally ill patients and excellent survival following cardiac transplantation. Ann Thorac Surg 1986; 41:126–129.
29. O'Connell JB, Renlund DG, Robinson JA, et al: Effect of preoperative hemodynamic support on survival after cardiac transplantation. Circulation 1988; 78:III78–82.
30. Marks JD, Karwande SV, Richenbacher WE, et al: Perioperative mechanical circulatory support for transplantation. J Heart Lung Transplant 1992; 11:117–128.
31. Rosenbaum MD, Murali S, Uretsky BF: Intra-aortic balloon counterpulsation as a 'bridge' to cardiac transplantation: Effects in nonischemic and ischemic cardiomyopathy. Chest 1994; 106:1683–1688.
32. Stavarski DH: Complications of intra-aortic balloon pumping: Preventable or not preventable? Crit Care Nurs Clin North Am 1996; 8:409–421.
33. Olsen PS, Arendrup H, Thiis JJ, et al: Intra-aortic balloon counterpulsation in Denmark 1988–1998: Early results and complications. Eur Cardiothorac Surg 1993; 7:634–636.
34. McBride LR, Miller LW, Naunheim KS, et al: Axillary artery insertion of an intraaortic balloon pump. Ann Thorac Surg 1989; 48:874–875.
35. Buchanan SC, Langenburg SC, Mauney MC, et al: Ambulatory intraaortic balloon counterpulsation. Ann Thorac Surg 1994; 58:1547–1549.
36. Norman JC, Dacso CC, Reul GJ, et al: Partial artificial heart (ALVAD) use with subsequent cardiac and renal allografting in a patient with stone heart syndrome. Artif Organs 1978; 2:413–420.
37. Piccione W: Mechanical circulatory assistance: Changing indications and options. J Heart Lung Transplant 1997; 16:S25–28.
38. Quaini E, Pavie A, Chieco S, et al: The concerted action 'Heart' European registry on clinical application of mechanical circulatory support systems: Bridge to transplant. Eur J Cardiothorac Surg 1997; 11:182–188.
39. Champsaur G, Ninet J, Vigneron M, et al: Use of the Abiomed BVS System 5000 as a bridge to cardiac transplantation. J Thorac Cardiovasc Surg 1990; 100:122–128.
40. Korfer R, El-Banayosy A, Posival H, et al: Mechanical circulatory support: The Bad Oeynhausen experience. Ann Thorac Surg 1995; 59:S56–63.
41. Farrar DJ, Hill JD, Pennington DG, et al: Preoperative and postoperative comparison of patients with univentricular and biventricular support with the Thoratec ventricular assist device as a bridge to cardiac transplantation. J Thorac Cardiovasc Surg 1997; 113:202–209.
42. DeRose JJ, Argenziano M, Sun BC, et al: Implantable left ventricular assist devices. Ann Surg 1997; 226:461–470.
43. Griffith BP, Kormos RL, Nastala CJ, et al: Results of extended bridge to transplantation: Window into the future of permanent ventricular assist devices. Ann Thorac Surg 1996; 61:396–398.
44. Loebe M, Weng Y, Muller J, et al: Successful mechanical circulatory support for more than two years with a left ventricular assist device in a patient with dilated cardiomyopathy. J Heart Lung Transplant 1997; 16:1176–1179.
45. Johnson KE, Prieto M, Joyce LD, et al: Summary of the clinical use of the Symbion total artificial heart: A registry report. J Heart Lung Transplant 1992; 11:103–116.
46. Kormos RL, Borovetz HS, Armitage JM, et al: Evolving experience with mechanical circulatory support. Ann Surg 1991; 214:471–477.
47. Arabia FA, Copeland JG, Smith RG, et al: International experience with the Cardio West total artificial heart as a bridge to heart transplantation. Eur J Cardiothorac Surg 1997; 11:S5–10.
48. Dembitsky WP, Moore CH, Holman WL, et al: Successful mechanical circulatory support for noncoronary shock. J Heart Lung Transplant 1992; 11:129–135.
49. Muller J, Wallukat G, Weng YG, et al: Weaning from mechanical cardiac support in patients with idiopathic dilated cardiomyopathy. Circulation 1997; 96:542–549.
50. Mueller J, Wallukat G, Dandel M, et al: The optimal moment for device removal in patients with a temporary cardiac assist device as a treatment of idiopathic dilated cardiomyopathy (Abstract). J Heart Lung Transplant 1998; 17:72–73.
51. Rose EA, Goldstein DJ: Wearable long-term mechanical support for patients with end-stage heart disease: A tenable goal. Ann Thorac Surg 1996; 61:399–402.
52. Pennington DG, Oaks TE, Lohmann DP: Permanent ventricular assist device support versus cardiac transplantation. Ann Thorac Surg (in press).

98

Hypertensive Crises: Emergencies and Urgencies

Janice L. Zimmerman, MD, FACP, FCCP, FCCM

Although chronic hypertension is common in the United States population, few patients present to critical care physicians with severe life-threatening elevations of blood pressure. Emphasis on early detection and treatment of hypertension has resulted in a declining incidence of hypertensive crises, but it is imperative that physicians recognize situations requiring immediate intervention and choose therapy appropriately. Many patients with hypertensive crises require the expertise of critical care physicians and the supportive care of intensive care units (ICUs).

Various terms have been used for adverse clinical conditions associated with severe hypertension. For the purpose of this chapter:

Hypertensive crises indicate the presence of severe hypertension that is potentially life-threatening. The immediacy of lowering blood pressure divides hypertensive crises into hypertensive emergencies and urgencies.

In *hypertensive emergencies*, severe hypertension is associated with new or progressive end-organ damage of the neurologic, cardiovascular, and renal systems (Table 98–1). In these situations, blood pressure should be lowered immediately to minimize organ dysfunction.

In *hypertensive urgencies,* severe hypertension is present without evidence of immediate complications (Table 98–2). Blood pressure in urgent conditions can be lowered less rapidly, usually over 24 hours.

When knowledge of prior end-organ dysfunction is not available, differentiating hypertensive emergencies from urgencies may be difficult. Accelerated hypertension is a hypertensive urgency characterized by the presence of retinal hemorrhages and exudates without papilledema.

The term *malignant hypertension* has been used in discussions of hypertensive crises to refer to pathologic, funduscopic, or clinical findings. Because of this confusion, the term malignant hypertension is not used in this chapter.

TABLE 98–1. Hypertensive Emergencies

Hypertensive encephalopathy
Acute myocardial ischemia syndromes
Unstable angina
Myocardial infarction
Acute left ventricular dysfunction
Acute aortic dissection
Acute renal insufficiency
Acute intracranial events
Hemorrhagic cerebrovascular accident
Thrombotic cerebrovascular accident
Subarachnoid hemorrhage
Excess catecholamine states
Pheochromocytoma crisis
MAOI-tyramine interaction
Antihypertensive withdrawal

MAOI = monoamine oxidase inhibitor.

TABLE 98–2. Hypertensive Urgencies

Accelerated hypertension
Perioperative hypertension
Severe hypertension associated with the following:
Congestive heart failure
Stable angina
Transient ischemic attacks
Renal failure from other causes

The physician should not rely on a specific blood pressure level to differentiate a hypertensive emergency from a less urgent situation. The rate at which blood pressure rises and the prior level of blood pressure may be more important than the absolute level.[1, 2] Although most hypertensive emergencies are associated with a diastolic blood pressure greater than 120 mm Hg, a previously normotensive patient may experience end-organ dysfunction with a diastolic blood pressure of 110 mm Hg. Conversely, patients with chronic hypertension may be asymptomatic with diastolic blood pressure greater than 120 mm Hg.

PATHOPHYSIOLOGY

Blood pressure is a function of cardiac output and systemic vascular resistance. Several factors can thus influence the development of severe hypertension. Cardiac output is determined by heart rate, filling pressure (preload), myocardial contractility, and afterload. Tachycardia does not usually result in hypertension, but acute fluid overload can produce acute hypertensive crises. Fluid overload contributes to severe hypertension in patients with renal failure, overtransfusion, or excessive use of saline infusions. Many critically ill patients have limited ability to excrete salt and water loads, so fluid balance must be carefully evaluated. Increased myocardial contractility (i.e., cocaine abuse) may result in increased cardiac output and resultant hypertension. However, autoregulation usually limits the rise in pressure by a corresponding decrease in systemic vascular resistance.

An increase in systemic vascular resistance is the common denominator in the majority of hypertensive crises. This increase is mediated by increased levels of circulating catecholamines, increased α-adrenergic activity, and activation of the renin-angiotensin-aldosterone system.[2] The rise in arterial pressure increases renal perfusion and induces a pressure natriuresis. This is important to remember, because most patients presenting with hypertensive crises tend to have relative hypovolemia. Baroreceptors are stimulated by the resultant decrease in effective arterial circulating volume and produce further increases in the α-adrenergic and β-adrenergic tone.

Although many factors can precipitate hypertensive crises (Table 98–3), an acute rise in blood pressure in patients with preexisting hypertension is most common. Other contributing factors that may affect therapeutic management must also be considered.

CLINICAL MANIFESTATIONS

The clinical findings in patients with hypertensive crises are usually nonspecific and may be related to the underlying disease or to end-organ sequelae. The clinical assessment of the patient begins with confirmation of the blood pressure measurement in both arms, using an appropriately sized cuff. This is followed by a rapid, yet detailed, evaluation of the organ systems most susceptible to damage from elevated blood pressure: the central nervous system, the cardiovascular system, and the renal system.

TABLE 98–3. Precipitating Factors for Hypertensive Crises

Preexisting hypertension	Eclampsia
Progression of disease	Collagen vascular disease
Unrecognized hypertension	Systemic lupus erythematosus
Patient's noncompliance	Progressive systemic sclerosis
Renovascular hypertension	Polyarteritis nodosa
Acute glomerulonephritis	Drugs
Parenchymal renal disease	Diet pills
Pheochromocytoma	Cocaine
Antihypertensive withdrawal	Amphetamines
Head injury	Oral contraceptives
Burns	Corticosteroids
MAOI-tyramine interactions	

MAOI = monoamine oxidase inhibitor.

Neurologic Assessment

Central nervous system involvement is suggested by complaints of headache, nausea, vomiting, visual disturbances, confusion, seizures, and focal neurologic deficits. Subtle abnormalities of mental status may be difficult to detect. A thorough examination requires inspection of the optic fundi for evidence of hypertensive retinopathy and papilledema. In the absence of other end-organ involvement, the presence of cotton-wool exudates or flame-shaped hemorrhages is compatible with a hypertensive urgency. A computed tomographic (CT) scan of the head is often necessary to rule out intracranial hemorrhage, stroke, or other lesions. Focal neurologic findings mandate an early CT scan but can be associated with hypertensive encephalopathy.

Cardiovascular Assessment

The cardiovascular consequences of severe hypertension may precipitate symptoms of anginal chest pain, dyspnea, or severe, tearing chest pain associated with acute aortic dissection. Physical findings that suggest acute left ventricular dysfunction include rales, a third heart sound, jugular venous distention, and tachycardia. Findings that may be present with aortic dissection include pulse deficits, a new murmur of aortic insufficiency, and a pericardial friction rub. An electrocardiogram is necessary for evaluating possible ischemia or infarction. A chest radiograph may indicate pulmonary edema or the nonspecific finding of a widened mediastinum, suggesting an aortic aneurysm.

Renal System Assessment

Renal involvement resulting from severe hypertension may be clinically silent with nonspecific symptoms of weakness, pedal edema, oliguria, polyuria, or hematuria. A complete assessment involves measurement of blood urea nitrogen and creatinine, as well as urinalysis with microscopic examination to detect proteinuria, hematuria, and the presence of cellular casts. The latter two findings are suggestive of glomerulonephritis as a secondary cause of hypertension. A complete blood count and electrolytes values should also be obtained. A blood smear can be examined for evidence of microangiopathic hemolytic anemia, but this is a rare finding.

GENERAL PRINCIPLES OF TREATMENT

The goal of therapy in hypertensive crises is to effect a decrease in blood pressure while maintaining organ perfusion and avoiding complications. Patients likely to experience complications of severe hypertension are also at risk for complications of lowering blood pressure. Three questions should be considered when one is deciding about the treatment of severe hypertension:

1. Should the blood pressure be lowered acutely?
2. How much should the blood pressure be lowered?
3. Which medication should be used to lower blood pressure?

The first question is the most important. Although it is important to recognize clinical situations in which blood pressure should be lowered immediately, it is also necessary to recognize when lowering the blood pressure is not indicated. A rapid but thorough clinical evaluation of the central nervous system, cardiovascular system, and renal system should provide the necessary information. In the presence of new or progressive end-organ dysfunction, a hypertensive emergency exists and blood pressure should be lowered promptly. This usually warrants ICU admission and the use of parenteral agents to lower blood pressure to safer levels in several hours. If end-organ dysfunction is not present or is unchanged from baseline, severe hypertension may represent a hypertensive urgency (see Table 98–2). In these clinical situations, oral therapy can be used to lower the blood pressure to safer levels over 24 hours. Asymptomatic patients with severe hypertension do not need immediate reductions of blood pressure.[3] These patients are best served by instituting or reinstituting an appropriate antihypertensive regimen and ensuring adequate follow-up. Physicians should not be compelled to treat an elevated blood pressure emergently in the absence of an appropriate indication.

Once the decision has been made to lower blood pressure, the second question assumes great importance. Careful consideration in determining the extent of blood pressure reduction may prevent complications. Excessive or precipitous lowering of blood pressure can result in cerebral, cardiac, or renal ischemia. Cerebral blood flow is maintained constant at 50 mL/min per 100 g of brain in normotensive patients with mean arterial pressures of 50 to 150 mm Hg by constriction and vasodilatation of cerebral arterioles. This autoregulatory mechanism adapts to higher pressures in patients with chronic hypertension because of structural changes in resistance vessels that allow toleration of elevated pressures without incurring cerebral damage (Fig. 98–1).[4] A shift to the right in the autoregulation of cerebral blood flow is also seen in elderly patients. Excessive reduction of blood pressure could easily compromise cerebral perfusion and precipitate ischemic

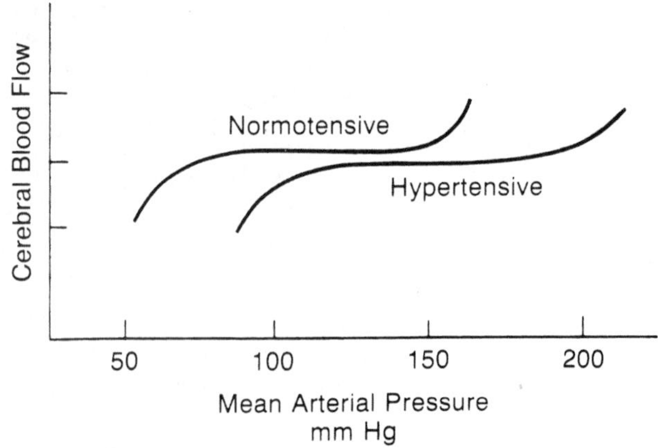

Figure 98–1. Cerebral blood flow remains constant over a wide range of pressures in normotensive individuals. This range is shifted to the right in older people and in individuals with chronic hypertension. (Courtesy of Leigh Thompson, MD, PhD.)

events in patients with altered cerebral autoregulation.[5] Similarly, coronary artery and renal blood flow can be compromised by overly aggressive blood pressure reduction.

Although various recommendations for the extent of blood pressure reduction have been proposed, each case must be treated individually. A reasonable goal for most hypertensive emergencies is to lower the mean arterial pressure by approximately 25% or to reduce the diastolic blood pressure to 100 to 110 mm Hg over a period of several minutes to hours, depending on the clinical situation. Although blood pressure should be lowered to safer levels, it is not necessary to normalize blood pressure in the first 24 to 48 hours of therapy in most situations. After the acute reduction of blood pressure with parenteral agents in hypertensive emergencies, oral medications should be instituted within 12 to 24 hours and blood pressure reduced to a normotensive level over the ensuing days to weeks.

The last question to consider is the choice of medications for lowering blood pressure. The repertoire of drugs available to clinicians today has greatly expanded. The choice of optimal intervention in hypertensive emergencies and urgencies depends on several factors. Coexisting conditions such as coronary artery disease, congestive heart failure, pulmonary disease, and renal insufficiency influence drug selection. The desired extent and rate of blood pressure reduction should be determined and appropriate drugs selected on the basis of the pharmacology of the available agents. Important considerations in choosing antihypertensive agents include the onset of action, peak effect, and duration of action. In addition, the choice of specific therapy may depend on the availability of hospital facilities and personnel to implement therapeutic regimens and safely monitor the patient. In the following text, drugs that are available for hypertensive emergencies and hypertensive urgencies are described. Specific clinical situations are addressed later.

PHARMACOTHERAPY FOR HYPERTENSIVE EMERGENCIES

Parenteral drugs available for treatment of hypertensive emergencies are summarized in Table 98-4. The ideal agent for lowering blood pressure in emergent situations should have the following characteristics:

- Rapid onset of action
- High potency
- Immediate reversibility
- Specific effect on resistance vessels without effects on other smooth muscle or cardiac muscle
- No central or autonomic nervous system effects
- Absence of tachyphylaxis
- Minimal or no adverse effects

No drug currently has all these desired characteristics. The challenge is to select the agent with the most favorable pharmacodynamic and adverse effect profile for the patient and the clinical circumstance.

Sodium Nitroprusside

Nitroprusside has been the "gold standard" for treatment of most hypertensive emergencies.[6] Although the cellular mechanism of action remains unknown, sodium nitroprusside (NTP) causes relaxation of arterial and venous smooth muscle. A controlled reduction of blood pressure is easily achieved because of the rapid onset of the hypotensive effect and the short duration of action. NTP has been used effectively for severe hypertension in encephalopathy, intracranial hemorrhage, myocardial ischemia, left ventricular failure, pheochromocytoma, dissecting aortic aneurysm, and postoperative hypertension.

The advantageous pharmacokinetic parameters of NTP can

TABLE 98–4. Parenteral Antihypertensive Agents

Drug	Class	Route	Dose	Onset of Action	Peak Effect	Duration of Effect
Sodium nitroprusside	Arteriolar and venous vasodilator	IV: infusion	0.3–10 μg/kg/min	Immediate	1–2 min	1–3 min
Labetalol	α-Adrenergic and β-adrenergic blocker	IV: bolus	20 mg, then 20–80 mg every 10 min (maximum = 300 mg)	3–5 min	10–20 min	3–6 hr
		IV: infusion	2 mg/min (maximum = 300 mg)			
Nitroglycerin	Venous >> arteriolar vasodilator	IV: infusion	5–300 μg/min	1–2 min	1–2 min	1–3 min
Nicardipine hydrochloride	Calcium channel blocker	IV: loading infusion	5–15 mg/hr	1–3 min	5–20 min (dose-dependent)	15–40 min
		IV: maintenance infusion	3–8 mg/hr			
Enalaprilat	Angiotensin-converting enzyme inhibitor	IV: bolus	0.625–1.25 mg every 6 hr	10–15 min	30 min–4 hr	6–8 hr
Diazoxide	Arteriolar vasodilator	IV: bolus	25–100 mg every 5–10 min	1–5 min	5 min	6–8 hr
		IV: infusion	7.5–30 mg/min (total dose = 300 mg)		Variable	4–12 hr
Trimethaphan camsylate	Ganglionic blocker	IV: infusion	0.5–10 mg/min	1–2 min	1–2 min	5–10 min
Phentolamine mesylate	α-Adrenergic blocker	IV: bolus	5–10 mg	1 min	3 min	10–30 min
		IV: infusion	0.2–5 mg/min			
Hydralazine	Arteriolar vasodilator	IV: bolus	5–20 mg	10–30 min	10–80 min	3–6 hr
		IV: infusion	0.5–1 mg/min			
		IM	10–40 mg			

IV = intravenous; IM = intramuscular; >> = greater than; q = every.

also result in excessive hypotension. An infusion pump must be used for administration, and the blood pressure should be closely monitored. Automated noninvasive blood pressure devices can be used, but intra-arterial blood pressure monitoring is preferred. Infusion of NTP should be initiated at a low rate (0.3 μg/kg/min) and titrated upward every few minutes.[7] If the blood pressure falls below the desired level, discontinuation of NTP results in blood pressure increases within 1 to 10 minutes.

Other potential adverse effects of NTP are related to its metabolism.[7] NTP is metabolized nonenzymatically by combining with hemoglobin to produce cyanmethemoglobin and cyanide ions. Rhodanase, a mitochondrial enzyme found predominantly in the liver, catalyzes the reaction of cyanide with thiosulfate to produce thiocyanate, which is excreted in the urine. Excess cyanide binds to cytochromes and inhibits oxidative metabolism. Renal failure can also result in thiocyanate toxicity with NTP use. Cyanide or thiocyanate toxicity usually does not pose a problem with use of NTP unless the infusion is maintained for more than 72 hours or at doses greater than 3 μg/kg/min. The maximum rate of 10 μg/kg/min should not be maintained for more than 10 minutes. Patients with renal insufficiency or hepatic disease are prone to toxicity. Cyanide levels are not generally available, but thiocyanate levels are available through referral laboratories.

In addition to close monitoring of the dose of NTP, the patient should be observed for clinical signs of cyanide toxicity such as metabolic (lactic) acidosis, confusion, or hemodynamic deterioration. Thiocyanate toxicity can manifest as abdominal pain, delirium, headache, nausea, muscle spasms, and restlessness. Some studies suggest that sodium thiosulfate infusion is effective for treating and preventing cyanide toxicity.[6] It decreases cyanide levels by acting as a sulfur donor and facilitating conversion of cyanide to thiocyanate. Hydroxycobalamin may also prevent toxicity when administered with NTP by combining with cyanide to form the nontoxic compound cyanocobalamin (vitamin B_{12}).[8] Hemodialysis is effective in eliminating thiocyanate.

Other adverse effects of NTP include rash, hypothyroidism, and, rarely, methemoglobinemia. Increased intracranial pressure has been noted with NTP in patients with mass lesions who are undergoing hypotensive surgery.

Labetalol

Labetalol is an oral and parenteral α-adrenergic and nonselective β-adrenergic blocker that reduces blood pressure by decreasing systemic vascular resistance with little or no change in cardiac output or heart rate.[9] The β-blocking effect predominates 7:1 when labetalol is administered intravenously. A controlled reduction of blood pressure is possible because of the rapid, but not abrupt, peak effect with minimum further reduction of blood pressure after an intravenous bolus or discontinuation of an infusion. Hypotension is infrequent provided the total dose remains below the recommended maximum of 300 mg. Selected cases may require prolonged infusions at reduced rates.[10]

The β-blocking properties of labetalol contraindicate its use in patients with bronchospasm, severe sinus bradycardia (heart rate $<$ 50 beats/min), greater than first-degree heart block, or decompensated congestive heart failure. Minor side effects include nausea, vomiting, paresthesias such as scalp tingling, pain at the injection site, and headache.[9] Labetalol may be particularly advantageous when intensive care facilities and intra-arterial pressure monitoring are not readily available. Labetalol has been used effectively in lowering blood pressure in hypertensive encephalopathy, myocardial ischemia, acute left ventricular dysfunction, acute neurologic syndromes, dissecting aortic aneurysm, pheochromocytoma, and eclampsia.[9, 11, 12] Labetalol is an excellent choice for control of severe hypertension associated with cocaine abuse.[13] An advantage of labetalol is the ability to convert to an oral form of the same drug.

Nitroglycerin

Nitroglycerin is a direct vasodilator, predominantly venous, that also results in coronary artery vasodilatation. Higher doses are capable of producing arterial dilatation. The intravenous form is easily titrated because of the rapid onset of action and short duration of effect, but it is much less potent than other parenteral antihypertensive agents. The favorable effects of decreasing myocardial oxygen demand by reducing preload and afterload and increasing myocardial oxygen supply by dilating coronary arteries make it particularly useful in hypertensive patients with possible myocardial ischemia. Intravenous nitroglycerin has also been used for treatment of perioperative hypertension. Side effects include headache, nausea, vomiting, bradycardia, hypotension, and rarely methemoglobinemia.

Nicardipine Hydrochloride

Nicardipine is a dihydropyridine calcium channel blocker prepared in oral or intravenous form. The intravenous form may be particularly suited for the treatment of hypertensive emergencies because of its potency, rapid onset of action, titratability, and lack of toxic metabolites. It has a direct effect on vascular smooth muscle, resulting in systemic and coronary artery vasodilatation. Nicardipine has minimal or no negative inotropic effects and usually results in increased cardiac output and left ventricular ejection fraction. Heart rate is usually not significantly increased. Nicardipine is metabolized in the liver and excreted primarily in bile and feces.

Caution should be exercised with older patients or patients with liver disease, who may have decreased hepatic metabolism. Most experience has been with loading infusions followed by maintenance infusions, but bolus administration has also been used.[14] Side effects are similar to those reported for other calcium channel blockers and include headache, flushing, lightheadedness, hypotension, tachycardia, nausea, and vomiting.[15, 16]

Most experience with intravenous nicardipine has been in the management of intraoperative and postoperative hypertension in patients with cardiac and noncardiac surgery. Nicardipine is more effective than placebo[15, 17] and as effective as nitroprusside.[18] Nicardipine effectively lowers blood pressure in severe hypertension with other causes, but reported experience in hypertensive emergencies is limited.[16, 19] Nicardipine may be an alternative to nitroprusside in many clinical situations.

Enalaprilat

Enalaprilat, an intravenously administered angiotensin-converting enzyme (ACE) inhibitor, is the active metabolite of the orally administered pro-drug enalapril. Inhibition of ACE results in vasodilation by decreasing angiotensin II vasopressor activity and decreasing aldosterone secretion. Patients with low renin hypertension may also respond to enalaprilat.[20] The response rate for enalaprilat (~60%) is lower than that for other parenteral agents and does not appear to be dose dependent.[21]

Side effects are similar to those observed with other ACE inhibitors: excessive hypotension (especially in sodium-depleted or volume-depleted patients), angioedema, impaired renal function, hyperkalemia, and cough. Although enalaprilat has been used for patients with severe hypertension and hypertensive emergencies,[20, 21] the variable response, magnitude, and duration of effect make it less attractive for use in critical situations in which reliable titration is desired.

Diazoxide

Diazoxide is a potent arterial vasodilator with little or no effect on venous capacitance. The duration of antihypertensive effect is measured in hours, but the short onset of action and short time to peak effect allow a stepwise reduction of blood pressure with repetitive bolus doses. Recommendations for minibolus administration or continuous infusion offer greater control and safety than large-bolus dosing.[22, 23]

Diazoxide evokes a reflex tachycardia and should, therefore, not be used in patients with dissecting aortic aneurysm or coronary artery disease. Precipitous drops of blood pressure may lead to myocardial and cerebral ischemia. Repetitive doses or prolonged administration may be associated with hyperglycemia, hyperuricemia, displacement of other protein-bound drugs, and salt and water retention, requiring the use of a loop diuretic. The solution is highly alkaline, so great care should be taken to avoid extravasation. The current use of diazoxide for hypertensive emergencies is limited by these serious potential adverse effects and the availability of other agents with better safety profiles.

Trimethaphan Camsylate

Trimethaphan is a titratable ganglionic blocking agent advocated for the treatment of hypertension associated with acute aortic dissection. Left ventricular ejection rate and heart rate are reduced. Adverse effects include orthostatic hypotension, urinary retention, paralytic ileus, mydriasis, and dry mouth. These effects, as well as tachyphylaxis, limit the use of trimethaphan.

Phentolamine Mesylate

Phentolamine is an α-adrenergic blocker indicated for the management of hypertensive emergencies associated with excess catecholamine levels, such as pheochromocytoma, monoamine oxidase inhibitor crises, and antihypertensive withdrawal syndrome. Side effects include hypotension, tachycardia, vomiting, and headache. Angina may also be provoked. Pheochromocytoma is rare, and the diagnosis may not be known at the time of a hypertensive emergency, but other parenteral agents (e.g., NTP and labetalol) can be used effectively.

Hydralazine

Hydralazine is a direct arteriolar vasodilator that may be administered orally, intramuscularly, or intravenously. The parenteral form is used infrequently for hypertensive emergencies because the variable response of patients and duration of action make reduction of blood pressure unpredictable. Hydralazine is contraindicated for patients with myocardial ischemia or dissecting aortic aneurysm because of reflex tachycardia, increased cardiac output, and increased myocardial oxygen consumption. Hydralazine may still have a role in blood pressure reduction in eclampsia because it improves uterine blood flow.

Esmolol

Esmolol is an ultra-short-acting α_1-adrenergic blocker. It is indicated only for the treatment of supraventricular tachycardia but may have a role in the management of perioperative hypertension.[24, 25] The decline in blood pressure results from a decrease in cardiac index, so it should not be used for patients with borderline or inadequate cardiac function. Other contraindications are the same as for labetalol. Esmolol may also be used in combination with nitroprusside to abrogate reflex tachycardia. It is unlikely that esmolol would be effective as a single agent for severe elevations of blood pressure.

Fenoldopam Mesylate

Fenoldopam is a parenteral postsynaptic dopamine-1 receptor agonist that has potential utility in hypertensive emergencies. Fenoldopam lowers blood pressure by decreasing peripheral vascular resistance through vasodilation in the renal, splanchnic, and skeletal muscle beds. A small increase in heart rate is observed and renal blood flow increases.[26, 27] Fenoldopam has a rapid onset of action (4 min) and short duration of effect ($t_{1/2}$ = 10 min), which allow administration as a continuous infusion. No toxic metabolites accumulate, and renal dysfunction has minimum impact on the pharmacokinetic parameters. Adverse effects include flushing, headache, dizziness, hypotension, tachycardia, and increased intraocular pressure.

The efficacy of fenoldopam in lowering blood pressure in patients with severe hypertension and hypertensive emergencies compares favorably with that of nitroprusside.[28] Fenoldopam may be an alternative to nitroprusside for management of hypertensive emergencies, especially in patients with renal dysfunction.

Diuretics

Diuretic agents are not indicated in the acute treatment of hypertensive emergencies unless there is clinical evidence of volume overload. As mentioned previously, most patients have sodium and volume depletion, which can be further exacerbated by diuretic use.

PHARMACOTHERAPY FOR HYPERTENSIVE URGENCIES

Drugs of potential utility for oral therapy of hypertensive urgencies are summarized in Table 98-5. Although patients with hypertensive urgencies do not usually require monitoring in an ICU, these drugs may be useful in patients hospitalized in critical care units for other reasons who require control of blood pressure elevations. A brief review of these agents is presented. More detailed information is available in other reviews.[1, 29, 30]

Nifedipine

The use of short-acting nifedipine, an oral calcium channel blocker, has decreased considerably because of concerns about excessive lowering of blood pressure. The reduction in systemic vascular resistance is associated with a mild increase in heart rate. Despite tachycardia, a simultaneous increase in coronary artery blood flow results in reduced myocardial oxygen consumption.[31] These hemodynamic effects are potentially advantageous in selected patients with myocardial ischemia or known coronary artery disease. After treatment, the mean arterial pressure decreases approximately 25%.[31, 32]

Side effects include headache, flushing, palpitations, dizziness, and hypotension.[32] A decrease in arterial oxygenation presumably related to ventilation-perfusion mismatch has been described.[33] Excessive hypotension may occur in the elderly, in patients receiving other vasodilators, and in hypovolemic patients.[31] Myocardial ischemia and cerebral ischemia have

TABLE 98–5. Oral Antihypertensive Agents

Drug	Class	Route	Dose	Onset of Action	Peak Effect	Duration of Effect
Nifedipine	Calcium channel blocker	Bite/swallow; oral	10 mg	5–15 min	15–30 min	3–5 hr
Clonidine	Central α-adrenergic agonist	Oral	0.1–0.2 mg, then 0.1 mg every 1 hr (maximum = 0.6–0.7 mg)	30–60 min	2–4 hr	3–8 hr
Captopril	Angiotensin-converting enzyme inhibitor	Oral Sublingual	6.25–25 mg	15 min 5 min	60–90 min 10–30 min	4–6 hr 2–3 hr

been reported after precipitous drops in blood pressure during treatment of severe hypertension with nifedipine.[34, 35]

Clonidine

Clonidine is a central α-adrenergic agonist that decreases sympathetic outflow and leads to a reduction in systemic vascular resistance. It has been used extensively in the treatment of hypertensive urgencies.[31, 36] It is rarely necessary to administer more than one to two doses. Precipitous drops in blood pressure are less likely with clonidine than with nifedipine. The sedative properties of clonidine may interfere with neurologic assessment of patients with encephalopathy or cerebrovascular events.[31] Other side effects include dry mouth, orthostasis, and bradycardia. A reduced dose or increase in dosing interval is necessary in the presence of renal insufficiency.

Captopril

Captopril, an oral ACE inhibitor, has been used successfully in hypertensive urgencies.[30, 37] The decrease in systemic vascular resistance is not accompanied by any significant change in heart rate or cardiac output. Hypotension may occur after the initial dose, especially in patients with sodium or volume depletion who concurrently use other antihypertensives and in those with renal vascular hypertension. Side effects with short-term use are minimal. Captopril should not be used in patients with suspected bilateral renal artery stenosis.

Other Drugs

Minoxidil and prazosin have been used for the treatment of hypertensive urgencies, but their use is not recommended because of the side effect profiles and availability of better drugs. Oral labetalol has also been used successfully in hypertensive urgencies.[9, 38]

SPECIFIC CLINICAL CONSIDERATIONS

Hypertensive Encephalopathy

Cerebral dysfunction as a result of severe hypertension mandates rapid reduction of blood pressure with a parenteral agent to prevent progression to coma and death.[39] Severe hypertension can exceed the upper limit of cerebral blood flow autoregulation and result in vasodilatation with cerebral edema. Nitroprusside is the drug of choice, with labetalol, nitroglycerin, and diazoxide as potential alternatives. The lowering of blood pressure is therapeutic as well as diagnostic, and mental status usually improves within hours. Cerebral dysfunction after the blood pressure is decreased requires consideration of other conditions such as intracranial hemorrhage, cerebral infarction, a mass lesion, trauma, or infection. Appropriate diagnostic tests (e.g., CT scanning of the head, lumbar puncture) should be performed.

Intracranial Hemorrhage, Ischemic Stroke, and Subarachnoid Hemorrhage

Treatment of severe hypertension in the setting of intracranial hemorrhage and ischemic stroke remains controversial.[39–41] The neurologic event may be the cause or consequence of elevated blood pressure. No absolute guidelines exist concerning the decision to lower blood pressure or the extent of blood pressure reduction. Severe elevations of blood pressure may cause further vascular damage, leading to increased hemorrhage, expansion of an infarct, or increased cerebral edema. However, reductions of blood pressure can lead to inadequate cerebral perfusion and ischemia, particularly in areas of altered autoregulation or areas dependent on collateral flow.[42] Careful observation of patients with mild hypertension may be all that is necessary, because blood pressure often decreases spontaneously after the acute event.[43] Moderate hypertension can be controlled with oral agents over several days. In general, severe, sustained hypertension should be treated with a parenteral drug, such as nitroprusside, nitroglycerin, labetalol, or possibly nicardipine. The effects of antihypertensive agents on cerebral blood flow, intracranial pressure, and autoregulation must be considered.[44] Careful monitoring of the neurologic status is mandatory. If the results of neurologic examination worsen as blood pressure is lowered, therapy must be discontinued or decreased and the blood pressure allowed to rise.

Preexisting hypertension is an unfavorable prognostic factor in subarachnoid hemorrhage, but treatment of hypertension after hemorrhage has not altered outcome.[45] Current therapy for subarachnoid hemorrhage includes use of the calcium channel blocker nimodipine, but the exact mechanism of the beneficial effect is unknown.[46] Guidelines recommended for the treatment of hypertension associated with subarachnoid hemorrhage are similar to those for ischemic stroke and intracranial hemorrhage. The blood pressure–lowering effects of nimodipine must be considered before instituting additional agents. Intravenous nicardipine may be an option.

Myocardial Ischemia

Sustained hypertension in patients with angina or myocardial infarction should be treated to reduce myocardial oxygen demand. Although hypertension may be initially present in one third of patients with myocardial ischemia, the blood pressure usually falls within the first 6 hours of admission without specific antihypertensive therapy.[47] The initial therapeutic maneuver should be relief of pain with sublingual nitrates, morphine sulfate, or both. If further intervention is necessary, nitroglycerin infusion addresses both hypertension and ischemia. Labetalol is another option with favorable hemodynamic effects in myocardial infarction.[12] If the hypertension is mild and a parenteral agent is not indicated, an oral β-adrenergic blocker or ACE inhibitor can be considered. Intravenous nicardipine is also a favorable antihypertensive agent for myocardial ischemia.

Nitroprusside has been used safely to lower blood pressure in myocardial ischemia, but concerns about coronary artery steal resulting in decreased collateral flow to ischemic areas make nitroglycerin and labetalol preferred agents.[48, 49] Diazoxide and hydralazine should be avoided because of reflex tachycardia.

Acute Left Ventricular Dysfunction

Acute elevations of blood pressure result in decreased compliance of the left ventricle, with resultant inadequate diastolic filling and high filling pressures leading to pulmonary edema. Alternatively, primary myocardial failure caused by systolic dysfunction with low cardiac output can be associated with hypertension resulting from catecholamine-induced peripheral vasoconstriction. An echocardiogram, if readily available, may be helpful in distinguishing systolic and diastolic dysfunction.

A significantly elevated diastolic blood pressure and the presence of hypertensive retinopathy suggest a hypertensive emergency with cardiac end-organ dysfunction. Primary myocardial failure may be suggested by a mild to moderate increase in diastolic blood pressure, absence of hypertensive retinopathy, and marked enlargement of the heart on a chest radiograph. Although differentiation of the two clinical situations may be difficult, the choice of therapy, despite the difference in pathophysiology, is similar. Nitroglycerin or nitroprusside infusions may be used in most situations. If diastolic dysfunction is suspected, overzealous reduction of filling pressures may compromise left ventricular volume. Labetalol is contraindicated in primary myocardial failure, but it has been used successfully when left ventricular dysfunction is due to the acute rise in blood pressure.

Acute Aortic Dissection

The initial treatment of a dissecting aortic aneurysm is blood pressure reduction followed by definitive surgical or medical therapy. Proximal aortic dissections or distal dissections complicated by recurrent pain, expansion, vital organ compromise, or falling hematocrit need surgical intervention. Distal aortic dissections without complications can be treated medically.

The goal of antihypertensive therapy is to lower blood pressure and reduce the shear force or rate of blood pressure rise to prevent extension of injury. Blood pressure should be reduced to the lowest level that relieves pain and allows adequate organ perfusion, usually a systolic pressure of 100 to 110 mm Hg. The most commonly used agents are a combination of nitroprusside and intravenous propranolol.[50] Alternatives include labetalol and the combination of esmolol and nitroprusside. Trimethaphan is infrequently used because of potential adverse effects, but it may be necessary for patients who are unable to tolerate α-adrenergic blockers.

Severe Preeclampsia and Eclampsia

The recommended threshold for treatment of severe hypertension in the peripartum period is a diastolic blood pressure of 110 to 105 mm Hg or lower or a mean blood pressure greater than 125 mm Hg.[51] Therapy includes delivery, if possible, and intravenous magnesium sulfate to prevent seizures. Hydralazine has been the drug of choice for blood pressure control because of the preservation of myometrial blood flow. Labetalol may be a safe and effective alternative agent.[12, 52] Oral nifedipine has been reported to be effective in a limited number of patients.[53] Because of potential adverse effects on labor and the fetus, nitroprusside, trimethaphan, and diazoxide are contraindicated.

Perioperative Hypertension

Perioperative hypertension is not classified as a hypertensive urgency, but in some circumstances emergent treatment may be required. Severe hypertension before surgery can usually be controlled with oral agents. If oral intake is precluded, parenteral agents, such as labetalol and enalaprilat, should be considered.

Intraoperative hypertension requires treatment to decrease the risk of myocardial ischemia, hemorrhage, or disruption of vascular anastomoses. Analgesic and anesthetic agents often decrease blood pressure. If blood pressure remains elevated, short-acting titratable agents, such as nitroprusside and nitroglycerin, are preferred and hypotension must be judiciously avoided. Labetalol can be used, but lower initial doses (2 to 5 mg) should be selected. Nicardipine has also been effective in treatment of intraoperative hypertension.[17]

The incidence of postoperative hypertension depends on the preoperative history of hypertension and the type of surgery performed.[54] It is usually self-limited (2 to 6 hours) but, if untreated, it can lead to complications, such as hemorrhage at the surgical site, disruption of vascular anastomoses, intracerebral hemorrhage, myocardial ischemia, and renal failure. Before antihypertensive therapy is instituted, each patient must be evaluated for the possible role of pain, anxiety, and hypothermia as a cause of elevated blood pressure.

Nitroprusside and nitroglycerin are routinely used for control of blood pressure in the postoperative period. Both drugs are amenable for use with closed-loop, computer-controlled automatic administration.[55] Nitroprusside may have disadvantages after cardiac surgery because of increases in heart rate that may increase myocardial oxygen demand and a coronary artery steal phenomenon.[48, 49] Labetalol in low doses has been used effectively for control of blood pressure after coronary artery bypass grafting.[56] Esmolol may also have a role in lowering blood pressure in the postoperative period.[24, 25] Intravenous nicardipine has compared favorably with nitroprusside for control of postoperative hypertension after cardiac and noncardiac surgery.[18]

EXCESS CATECHOLAMINE STATES

Increased levels of catecholamines leading to severe hypertension are associated with pheochromocytoma, monoamine oxidase inhibitor interactions, clonidine withdrawal, and occasionally cocaine or amphetamine abuse. Phentolamine has been the traditional treatment of choice, especially with pheochromocytoma, but other drugs, such as labetalol and nitroprusside, are also effective. Hypertensive crises resulting from interactions of monoamine oxidase inhibitors with tyramine-containing foods or sympathomimetic amines have also been treated with nifedipine.

SUMMARY

Severe hypertension mandates a rapid clinical evaluation of the central nervous system, cardiovascular system, and renal system to determine whether a hypertensive emergency or urgency exists. If rapid reduction of blood pressure is indicated, the choice of therapy and target blood pressure should be individualized on the basis of the clinical situation. Knowledge of the pharmacodynamics and adverse effects of available antihypertensive agents enables an appropriate selection for therapy. Careful monitoring is mandatory to avoid precipitous drops in blood pressure and hypoperfusion of vital organs.

References

1. Houston MC: Hypertensive urgencies and emergencies: Pathophysiology, clinical aspects and treatment. *In:* Critical Care: State of the Art. Vol 7. Chernow B, Shoemaker WC (Eds). Fullerton, Calif, Society of Critical Care Medicine, 1986, pp 151–246.
2. Houston MC: Pathophysiology, clinical aspects and treatment of hypertensive crises. Prog Cardiovasc Dis 1989; 32:99.
3. Zeller KR, Kuhnert LV, Matthews C: Rapid reduction of severe asymptomatic hypertension. Arch Intern Med 1989; 149:2186.
4. Strandgaard S: Autoregulation of cerebral circulation in hypertension. Acta Neurol Scand 1978; 57(Suppl 66):1.
5. Ledingham JGG, Rajagopalan B: Cerebral complications in the treatment of accelerated hypertension. Q J Med 1979; 48:25.
6. Cohn JN, Burke LP: Nitroprusside. N Engl J Med 1979; 91:752.
7. Physician's Desk Reference. 47th ed. Montvale, NJ: Medical Economics Data, 1993, pp 1999–2001.
8. Zerbe NF, Wagner BK: Use of vitamin B_{12} in the treatment and prevention of nitroprusside-induced cyanide toxicity. Crit Care Med 1991; 21:465.
9. MacCarthy EP, Bloomfield SS: Labetalol: A review of its pharmacology, pharmacokinetics, clinical uses and adverse effects. Pharmacotherapy 1983; 3:193.
10. Graves JW: Prolonged continuous infusion labetalol: A new alternative for parenteral antihypertensive therapy. Crit Care Med 1989; 17:759.
11. Wilson DJ, Wallin JD, Vlachakis ND, et al: Intravenous labetalol in the treatment of severe hypertension and hypertensive emergencies. Am J Med 1983; 75:95.
12. Renard M, Jacobs P, Melot C, et al: Effect of labetalol on preload in acute myocardial infarction with systemic hypertension. J Cardiovasc Pharmacol 1984; 6:90.
13. Gay GR, Loper KA: Control of cocaine-induced hypertension with labetalol. Anesth Analg 1988; 67:92.
14. Cheung DG, Gasster JL, Neutel JM, Weber MA: Acute pharmacokinetic and hemodynamic effects of intravenous bolus dosing of nicardipine. Am Heart J 1990; 119:438.
15. IV Nicardipine Study Group: Efficacy and safety of intravenous nicardipine in the control of postoperative hypertension. Chest 1991; 99:393.
16. Wallin JD, Fletcher E, Ram CVS, et al: Intravenous nicardipine for the treatment of severe hypertension. Arch Intern Med 1989; 149:2662.
17. Begon C, Dartayet B, Edouard A, et al: Intravenous nicardipine for treatment of intraoperative hypertension during abdominal surgery. J Cardiothorac Anesth 1989; 3:707.
18. Halpern NA, Goldberg M, Neely C, et al: Postoperative hypertension: A multicenter, prospective, randomized comparison between intravenous nicardipine and sodium nitroprusside. Crit Care Med 1992; 20:1637.
19. Neutel JM, Smith DHG, Wallin D, et al: A comparison of intravenous nicardipine and sodium nitroprusside in the immediate treatment of severe hypertension. Am J Hypertens 1994; 7:623.
20. Evans RR, Henzler MA, Weber EM, DiPette DJ: The effect of intravenous enalaprilat (MK-422) administration in patients with mild to moderate essential hypertension. J Clin Pharmacol 1987; 27:415.
21. Hirschl MM, Binder M, Bur A, et al: Clinical evaluation of different doses of intravenous enalaprilat in patients with hypertensive crises. Arch Intern Med 1995; 155:2217.
22. Ram CVS, Kaplan NM: Individual titration of diazoxide dosage in the treatment of severe hypertension. Am J Cardiol 1979; 43:627.
23. Garrett BN, Kaplan NM: Efficacy of slow infusion of diazoxide in the treatment of severe hypertension without organ hypoperfusion. Am Heart J 1982; 103:390.
24. Smerling A, Gersony WM: Esmolol for severe hypertension following repair of aortic coarctation. Crit Care Med 1990; 18:1288.
25. Gray RJ: Managing critically ill patients with esmolol. Chest 1988; 93:398.
26. Weber RR, McCoy CE, Ziemniak JA, et al: Pharmacokinetic and pharmacodynamic properties of intravenous fenoldopam, a dopamine$_1$-receptor agonist, in hypertensive patients. Br J Clin Pharmacol 1988; 25:17.
27. Elliott WJ, Weber RR, Nelson KS, et al: Renal and hemodynamic effects of intravenous fenoldopam versus nitroprusside in severe hypertension. Circulation 1990; 81:970.
28. Panacek EA, Bednarczyk EM, Dunbar LM, et al: Randomized, prospective trial of fenoldopam vs sodium nitroprusside in the treatment of acute severe hypertension. Acad Emerg Med 1995; 2:959.
29. DeVault GA: Hypertensive urgencies: Part 1. Sympatholytics, calcium antagonists. J Crit Illness 1991; 6:563.
30. DeVault GA: Hypertensive urgencies: Part 2. ACE inhibitors and vasodilators. J Crit Illness 1991; 6:935.
31. Houston MC: The comparative effects of clonidine hydrochloride and nifedipine in the treatment of hypertensive crises. Am Heart J 1988; 115:152.
32. Houston MC: Treatment of hypertensive urgencies and emergencies with nifedipine. Am Heart J 1986; 111:963.
33. Leeman M, Degaute J-P: Invasive hemodynamic evaluation of sublingual captopril and nifedipine in patients with arterial hypertension after abdominal surgery. Crit Care Med 1995; 23:843.
34. O'Mailia JJ, Sander GE, Giles TD: Nifedipine-associated myocardial ischemia or infarction in the treatment of hypertensive urgencies. Ann Intern Med 1987; 107:185.
35. Schwartz M, Naschitz JE, Yeshurun D, Sharf B: Oral nifedipine in the treatment of hypertensive urgency: Cerebrovascular accident following a single dose. Arch Intern Med 1990; 150:686.
36. Houston MC: Treatment of hypertensive emergencies and urgencies with oral clonidine loading and titration. Arch Intern Med 1986; 146:586.
37. Angeli P, Chiesa M, Caregaro L, et al: Comparison of sublingual captopril and nifedipine in immediate treatment of hypertensive emergencies. Arch Intern Med 1991; 151:678.
38. McDonald AJ, Yealy DM, Jacobson S: Oral labetalol versus oral nifedipine in hypertensive urgencies in the ED. Am J Emerg Med 1993; 11:460.
39. Phillips SJ, Whisnant JP: Hypertension and the brain. Arch Intern Med 1992; 152:938.
40. Spence JD, Del Maestro RF: Hypertension in acute ischemic strokes: Treat. Arch Neurol 1985; 42:1
41. Yatsu FM, Zivin J: Hypertension in acute ischemic strokes: Not to treat. Arch Neurol 1985; 42:999.
42. Meyer JS, Shimazu K, Fukuuchi Y, et al: Impaired neurogenic cerebrovascular control and dysautoregulation after stroke. Stroke 1973; 4:169.
43. Wallace JD, Levy LL: Blood pressure after stroke. JAMA 1981; 246:2177.
44. Tietjen CS, Hurn PD, Ulatowski JA, Kirsch JR: Treatment modalities for hypertensive patients with intracranial pathology: Options and risks. Crit Care Med 1996; 24:311.
45. Wijdicks EFM, Vermeulen M, Murray GD, et al: The effects of treating hypertension following aneurysmal subarachnoid hemorrhage. Clin Neurol Neurosurg 1990; 92:111.
46. Pickard JD, Murray GD, Illingworth R, et al: Effect of oral nimodipine on cerebral infarction and outcome after subarachnoid haemorrhage: British aneurysm nimodipine trial. Br Med J 1989; 298:636.
47. Gibson TC: Blood pressure levels in acute myocardial infarction. Am Heart J 1978; 96:475.
48. Flaherty JT: Comparison of intravenous nitroglycerin and sodium nitroprusside in acute myocardial infarction. Am J Med 1983; 74(Suppl 6B):53.
49. Mann T, Cohn PF, Holman BL, et al: Effect of nitroprusside on regional myocardial blood flow in coronary artery disease. Circulation 1978; 57:732.
50. Shah PK: Acute aortic dissection: Part 2. Choosing among management options. J Crit Illness 1992; 7:1075.
51. Sibai BM: Treatment of hypertension in pregnant women. N Engl J Med 1996; 335:257.
52. Silver HM: Acute hypertensive crisis in pregnancy. Med Clin North Am 1989; 73:623.
53. Scardo JA, Vermillion ST, Hogg BB, Newman RB: Hemodynamic effects of oral nifedipine in preeclamptic hypertensive emergencies. Am J Obstet Gynecol 1996; 175:336.
54. Halpern NA: Today's strategies for treating postoperative hypertension. J Crit Illness 1995; 10:478.

55. McKinley S, Cade JF, Siganporia R, et al: Clinical evaluation of closed-loop control of blood pressure in seriously ill patients. Crit Care Med 1991; 19:166.
56. Sladen RN, Klamerus KJ, Swafford MWG, et al: Labetalol for the control of elevated blood pressure following coronary artery bypass grafting. J Cardiothorac Anesth 1990; 4:210.

Hypertensive Emergencies in Infants and Children

Julie R. Ingelfinger, MD

A hypertensive emergency or crisis is determined not only by the hypertension but by the length of time blood pressure has been elevated and by the underlying clinical situation.[1] If blood pressure has increased rapidly, an immediate response to bring blood pressure under control is needed. Yet, in other situations, an underlying medical condition, such as chronic renal failure, may result in a severe accelerating increase in blood pressure that may not have been normal in the first place. Pharmacologic advances now permit effective blood pressure control in almost every instance. Nonetheless, too rapid lowering of blood pressure carries with it risks of stroke, heart failure, renal failure, and visual impairment. This chapter reviews the present understanding of hypertensive emergencies in children. An approach to management is also presented.

Table 99–1 lists blood pressure levels considered elevated and severely elevated in children.[2–4] A true hypertensive crisis or emergency necessitates that blood pressure be lowered as fast as possible (within minutes) to protect vital organ function and even life.[5, 6] Thus, the medications employed must have a rapid onset of action and must be nearly universally effective. Whenever possible, the patient should be monitored in an intensive care setting. Hypertensive urgencies, in contrast, may be approached in a more considered manner during a somewhat longer time period (e.g., 30 to 60 minutes). Although rapidly acting drugs should be used in a hypertensive urgency, intensive care unit monitoring and intra-arterial monitoring are generally not necessary. Hypertensive crisis may occur as a result of

- Accelerated or malignant hypertension with severe blood pressure elevation
- Acute change in blood pressure in a previously normotensive patient (examples would be acute glomerulonephritis, preeclampsia in a pregnant teenager, and drug-related hypertension)
- Blood pressure increase during the course of an underlying hypertension-associated medical condition

WHAT IS ACCELERATED OR MALIGNANT HYPERTENSION?

In *accelerated hypertension,* marked blood pressure increase occurs, often in association with retinopathy (grade 3 by Keith-Wagener classification, without papilledema). *Malignant hypertension* is defined by marked blood pressure elevation with severe retinopathy, often including papilledema, hemorrhages, and exudates.[7] Renal failure and heart failure will rapidly develop with untreated malignant hypertension, and the patient will succumb within days. The term *hypertensive encephalopathy* denotes central nervous system dysfunction accompanying severe hypertension.[8] Children have hypertensive encephalopathy as the most common presentation of uncontrolled or rapidly increasing blood pressure, whereas adults more often experience malignant or accelerated hypertension. Adolescents have symptoms similar to those seen in adults.

Symptoms

Severe hypertension increases the risk of end-organ damage. For example, the relative risk of intracerebral hemorrhage increases with hypertension, even in young individuals.[9] The risk of visual, cardiac, and renal damage is increased in hypertension as well.[8, 9]

Accelerating hypertension can lead to subjective visual changes with blurring and double vision, but permanent blindness can develop as a consequence of severe hypertension. Furthermore, too rapid lowering of blood pressure can also lead to irreversible visual impairment. In view of this tragic possibility, overly zealous decrease in blood pressure should be avoided.

Congestive heart failure may occur with the increased cardiac work accompanying hypertension. With effective blood pressure control, the heart failure should resolve. If blood pressure elevation remains unchecked for a long time, permanent myocardial damage may occur.

An infant or neonate with severe hypertension may have nonspecific findings. These may include irritability, poor feed-

TABLE 99–1. Severe Hypertension in Childhood*

Age	Significant Hypertension	Severe Hypertension	Hypertensive Crisis
Term neonate			
Week 1	SBP > 96 mm Hg	SBP > 106 mm Hg	?
Week 2	SBP > 104 mm Hg	SBP > 110 mm Hg	?
Infant (<2 yr)	>112/74 mm Hg	>118/82 mm Hg	145/95 mm Hg
3–5 yr	>116/76 mm Hg	>124/84 mm Hg	150/95 mm Hg
6–9 yr	>122/78 mm Hg	>130/86 mm Hg	160/100 mm Hg
10–12 yr	>126/82 mm Hg	>134/90 mm Hg	165/105 mm Hg
13–15 yr	>136/86 mm Hg	>144/92 mm Hg	175/110 mm Hg
16–18 hr	>142/92 mm Hg	>150/98 mm Hg	185/120 mm Hg

Data from the Report of the Second Task Force on Blood Pressure Control in Children, Pediatrics 1987; 79:1,[2] and Feld L: In: Gellis & Kagan's Current Pediatric Therapy, 15th ed., 1996.[3]

**Note:* These blood pressures are guidelines only, and newer data sets may revise these levels to an even lower set-point.

SBP = systolic blood pressure.

BOX 99–1
HYPERTENSIVE CRISIS

Definitions

These two definitions may overlap substantially.

Malignant Hypertension: Severe increase in blood pressure with ophthalmoscopic changes, presence of end-organ damage

Hypertensive Crisis: Severe elevation of blood pressure such that the threat of end-organ damage is imminent if it is not promptly treated

Symptoms (Variable)

- Headache
- Dizziness
- Visual changes
- Seizures
- Encephalopathy
- Accompanying signs: weight loss, thirst and polyuria, abdominal symptoms

Underlying Diagnosis (Variable)

Accelerating hypertension, malignant hypertension, hypertensive crisis—*all* can accompany almost any form of hypertension

Therapy Issues

- How fast to lower blood pressure? In first 24 hours, lower the blood pressure by one third of eventual reduction ultimately desired
- What drugs to use? Drugs that give the best control, given the circumstances
- How much investigation? As much as needed to establish the diagnosis

ing, and apparent food intolerance as well as cardiorespiratory symptoms, most typically tachypnea, cyanosis, or congestive failure. Thus, any severely ill infant must have blood pressure monitored.

An acute rise in blood pressure may cause no symptoms in older children or nonspecific findings, such as dizziness, anxiety, or headache. However, hypertensive encephalopathy may well occur before any obvious symptoms are noted. Because symptoms tend to be nonspecific, the possibility of hypertension should always be considered and either put aside or confirmed.

Pediatric patients with severe hypertension most typically present with cardiovascular and neurologic findings. The rapidity of onset and degree of blood pressure elevation will forecast whether such symptoms develop. Children who experience the gradual development of hypertension may manifest no symptoms despite remarkably high and sustained blood pressure levels. Conversely, children who have been previously normotensive may have cardiovascular or neurologic symptoms with a relatively modest blood pressure elevation when the change in blood pressure is rapid.

Pathophysiology

In accelerating hypertension, the common pathologic findings, irrespective of underlying cause, are in the vasculature, which shows fibrinoid necrosis and myointimal proliferation.[10] Thus, such marked hypertension may lead to permanent tissue damage, and the severity of the myointimal proliferation will often parallel the duration of the high blood pressure. Medial arteriolar thickening may be reversible to some extent after successful blood pressure control. However, intimal changes with marked hypertension may be irreversible and lead to irreversible narrowing of the vascular bed. Fibrinoid necrosis occurs during accelerated hypertension and may be accompanied by vascular spasm.

Failed autoregulation of the cerebral blood flow is the hallmark of hypertensive encephalopathy.[11, 12] Early symptoms include visual changes (blurring and diplopia), nausea, and severe headache. Confusion, waning degrees of consciousness, and focal neurologic changes may follow in many instances, and seizures may occur. Although children tend to have fewer retinal changes than adults do, infants are an exception and retinopathy develops quickly. Up to 20% of children have been reported to have cranial nerve palsies during hypertensive crisis. (Thus, any child with Bell's palsy should have a blood pressure assessment.)

Cerebral blood flow (CBF) is determined by the cerebral perfusion pressure (CPP) divided by the cerebral vascular resistance (CVR). CPP reflects the difference between the mean arterial pressure (MAP) and mean cerebral venous pressure (which is normally negligible unless there is intracranial hypertension). Thus:

$$CBF = MAP - CPP/CVR$$

A variety of factors affect cerebral blood flow—systemic blood pressure, blood viscosity, and sympathetic adrenergic activity. Arterial resistance is especially important and is regulated by local factors such as partial pressure of oxygen ($Pa{O_2}$), pH, and partial pressure of carbon dioxide ($Pa{CO_2}$). Decrease in pH or $Pa{O_2}$ or increase in $Pa{CO_2}$ causes vasodilatation, thus increasing cerebral blood flow. Vasoconstriction is produced by opposite changes in these variables and leads to decrease in cerebral blood flow.

Many other factors are involved in cerebral autoregulation. These include vasoactive substances such as angiotensin, endothelin, neuropeptide Y, and brain and atrial natriuretic peptides as well as adenosine and potassium ion concentration. When systemic blood pressure rises, vasoconstriction occurs because of transmitted changes in smaller cerebral arteries and arterioles. When the pressure rises above the limit of autoregulation, cerebral edema occurs because of both hypoperfusion and plasma transudation. This leads, in turn, to decreased cerebral blood flow, compression of capillaries by the edema, and symptoms of encephalopathy. Although the limit of autoregulation and pressure shifts upward in chronic hypertension, there can still be severe hypertension and symptoms. However, the phenomenon may explain why an individual with gradually increasing chronic hypertension may remain relatively asymptomatic in the face of severe hypertension. Severe hypertension also impairs the autoregulatory functions in other internal organs, including the heart, the kidney, and the eye.

Within the kidney, even a moderate increase in mean arterial pressure will change (increase) preglomerular capillary resistance while decreasing postglomerular resistance. This maintains glomerular capillary flow, but eventually glomerular hypoperfusion with azotemia and decreased urine output occurs. Accelerating hypertension can cause permanent renal impairment with necrotizing vasculitis, arteriolar spasm, and fibrin deposition in glomerular capillary walls. If blood pressure is not controlled, end-stage renal disease can result.

ETIOLOGY OF SEVERE HYPERTENSION AND HYPERTENSIVE CRISIS IN CHILDHOOD

Renal disease is the most common reason for severe hypertension in children. When Still and Cottom[13] observed patients with severe, sustained hypertension, 64% had signs of pyelonephritis. Rance and colleagues[14] found reflux nephropathy in 40% of their series. Dillon[15] reported that renal scarring from either obstructive uropathy or reflux accounted for 36% of patients with severe hypertension. Arbus and Farine[5] reported that renal disease, particularly in transplant patients, was associated with most cases of severe hypertension in their center.

However, severe hypertension can occur with *any* diagnosis that is associated with hypertension. Table 99–2 lists common causes of severe hypertension in children and is meant as a guide to those situations in which severe hypertension has most often been reported.[16] Although discussion of the pathophysiology of each entity is beyond the scope of this chapter, a few comments follow concerning several of these diagnoses.

Renal Parenchymal Disease

Hypertensive crisis may lead to renal impairment along with hematuria, proteinuria, and urinary sediment containing casts.[5] Thus, it may be difficult to distinguish antecedent renal disease in such a setting. However, the hallmarks of known renal parenchymal disease should be sought. Virtually any renal parenchymal disease can be associated with a hypertensive urgency or crisis.[5, 17, 18]

Acute glomerulonephritis[19, 20] and hemolytic-uremic syndrome[21] are relatively frequently accompanied by severe hypertension, most probably related to volume overload in the setting of decreased glomerular filtration rate and continued fluid intake or administration. Hypertensive crisis may ensue in this setting. Blood volume is usually increased, and plasma renin and aldosterone are often suppressed. In acute postinfectious nephritis, evidence of positive streptococcal serology, decreased serum complement, and a history of antecedent throat or skin infection are often, but not invariably, present. Urinary sediment frequently contains red blood cell casts, which are highly suggestive of glomerulonephritis and rarer in malignant hypertension. Many glomerular diseases can also be accompanied by severe hypertension. In hemolytic-uremic syndrome, the presence of hemolysis, thrombocytopenia, and renal dysfunction makes the diagnosis evident, particularly when there has been a prodrome of bloody diarrhea.

Although hypertension, often marked, is frequent in children with chronic glomerulonephritides,[22] hypertensive crisis is unusual. Blood pressure more commonly increases gradually, becoming progressively difficult to manage. However, particularly in the setting of fairly rapid deterioration of renal function with concomitant high salt intake, hypertensive crisis may occur. In newly detected patients, the severe hypertension may initially obscure the chronicity of the glomerular disease. However, evidence of cardiac hypertrophy or retinopathy may be present to indicate the chronicity of the situation.

Hypertensive crisis may be the first indication of chronic pyelonephritis secondary to reflux and multiple urinary tract infections.[23, 24] Scarred renal parenchyma associated with increased release of renin and other vasoactive hormones is considered a major contributing factor.

Acute, accelerating hypertension may occur in obstructive uropathy, especially in acute obstruction, and is probably due to a combination of hormonally mediated and volume-mediated factors.[25] Relieving the obstruction will make blood pressure control easier.

Marked hypertension can occur after renal trauma and may be secondary to direct vascular compromise,[26] to compression of the renal parenchyma, or to the development of an arteriovenous fistula. Thromboembolic phenomena that affect the renal arteries can also be associated with severe hypertension.[14, 18]

Cardiovascular Disease

Whereas hypertension is almost invariably associated with coarctation of the aorta, hypertensive crisis is rare in an uncorrected coarctation.[27] After repair, the phenomenon of post-coarctectomy hypertension may be associated with a hypertensive crisis.[28] This postoperative syndrome may be associated with a mesenteric arteritis, with sympathetic nervous system stimulation and consequent catecholamine release as well as renin release.

TABLE 99–2. Etiology of Severe Hypertension in Infants, Children, and Adolescents

General comment: Any condition associated with hypertension can convert to severe hypertension.

Renal

- Acute glomerulonephritides
- Chronic glomerulonephritides
- Acute and chronic pyelonephritis
- Polycystic kidney disease
- Congenital abnormalities (dysplasia, hypoplasia, cystic)
- Post-transplant hypertension
- Renal tumors (Wilms' tumor, reninoma, other)
- Obstructive uropathy
- Post-trauma, post-genitourinary surgery
- Acute tubular necrosis
- Blood transfusion in azotemic patient

Cardiovascular

- Coarctation
- Renal artery disease (stenosis, thrombosis, arteritis)
- Arteritides

Endocrine

- Pheochromocytoma
- Neuroblastoma
- Congenital adrenal hyperplasia
- Cushing's syndrome
- Hyperthyroidism
- Hyperparathyroidism
- Hyperaldosteronism

Central Nervous System

- *Any* cause of increased intracranial pressure
- Dysautonomia

Iatrogenic

- Glucocorticoid administration
- Sympathomimetic administration
- Other medications

Miscellaneous

- Immobilization (fractures, burns)
- Hypercalcemia
- Street drugs (cocaine, crack, speed)
- Other

Data from Ingelfinger JR: Pediatric Hypertension. Philadelphia, WB Saunders, 1982, pp 218–228; and Londe S: Pediatr Clin North Am 1978; 25:55.

Vasculitides are rare in children but may be accompanied by severe hypertension. This is more often severe, difficult-to-control hypertension than hypertensive crisis.[14, 15]

Renovascular disease with renal artery stenosis is usually renin mediated, and affected children may present with severe hypertension. If the renal artery disease is undiscovered or develops rapidly, hypertensive crisis may be an accompanying event.[14, 15]

Although aortic dissection is described as an unusual complication in hypertensive crisis, it would be reportable if this occurred in a child.

Centrally Mediated Hypertension

Severe hypertension may develop in the setting of centrally mediated hypertension of any cause.[29, 30] Hypertension accompanying head trauma demands great care to avoid secondary insult. It is most important in such a situation to monitor both systemic and intracranial pressure and to take every precaution to maintain cerebral blood flow.

Endocrine Hypertension

Although endocrine hypertension of all causes is relatively rare, many cases are relatively easy to diagnose; clinical findings are obvious in most instances of hyperthyroidism, Cushing's syndrome, and congenital adrenal hyperplasia. The physical findings in pheochromocytoma, although very rare, may be minimal or absent.[14, 15, 31, 32] Thus, one should always consider and rule out this diagnosis by means of determining catecholamine levels in blood and urine and by appropriate imaging studies. Pharmacologic testing with use of acute α-adrenergic blockade is not indicated because it may lower blood pressure too precipitously.

Although children with pheochromocytoma often have sustained hypertension, they may have symptoms of catecholamine overproduction, such as palpitations, sweating, weight loss, flushing, fatigue, gastrointestinal distress, and abdominal or chest pain.

Pregnancy-Induced Hypertension and Eclampsia

Teenagers who become pregnant are more likely than older women to suffer pregnancy-induced hypertension.[33] In eclampsia (blood pressure above 140/90 mm Hg with edema, proteinuria, and seizures), hydralazine may be effective, but it can lead to reflex tachycardia and increased fluid retention. Intravenous magnesium sulfate may be a safe (and long-accepted) alternative. Labetalol and β_1-selective β-receptor antagonists may also be effective and relatively safe.

To avoid angiotensin-converting enzyme (ACE) fetopathy and acute renal failure in neonates treated with ACE inhibitors, this class of medication must be avoided. Similarly, angiotensin II receptor antagonists must be avoided.

Iatrogenic and Miscellaneous Causes of Hypertensive Crisis

Hypertensive crisis has been reported after a number of surgical procedures: after orthopedic surgery to the spine or long bones, or traction[34]; after genitourinary system surgery[35]; after closure of gastroschisis[36]; and after renal transplantation.[37] Thus, blood pressure should be followed vigilantly in all such settings.

Exposure to cocaine, crack, amphetamines, and "angel dust" has been associated with hypertensive crisis.[38] In view of this, virtually any and all children presenting with acute hypertension should be screened for drug exposure or intake with a toxic screen if the cause is at all elusive.

IMMEDIATE MANAGEMENT OF HYPERTENSIVE EMERGENCIES

The optimal management of a hypertensive emergency should include close monitoring and should proceed from the emergency department to an intensive care unit.[1, 6–8] Continuous or frequent, intermittent monitoring of blood pressure permits minute-to-minute assessment of the efficacy of therapy and the need for additional steps. The child should be weighed and measured, if possible, with comparison of the present weight to a recent previous weight. The patient's fluid status must be noted, and fluid intake and output must be recorded. The initial history and physical examination should be directed at excluding drug ingestion and considering the types of hypertension that can present as hypertensive crisis. Thus, the cerebrovascular, renal, and cardiovascular status must be assessed, and target end-organ damage must be identified, if present.

Blood pressure control in the setting of hypertensive crisis is far more important than determining the precise cause of hypertension. Until blood pressure control is established, the patient should not undergo complicated or invasive tests, or be transported out of the care unit, unless it is utterly unavoidable. The astute physician should consider two things:

1. What is the most likely cause of the acute hypertension in this particular child? The answer to this question will lead to the most effective therapy.
2. Is this de novo hypertension, or is it chronic? The answer to this question dictates the rapidity with which blood pressure should be reduced.

The Neonate with Severe Hypertension

Neonatal hypertension may quickly result in end-organ damage; thus, in this age group, it is particularly important that

BOX 99–2
IMMEDIATE MANAGEMENT OF HYPERTENSIVE CRISIS

Hospitalization

- Patient should proceed from the emergency department to the intensive care unit.
- Blood pressure monitoring should be continuous.

Initial Determinations

- History and physical examination should be quickly and expeditiously performed.
- Obtain urinalysis and examine sediment.
- Check chemistry profile and complete blood count.
- Perform chest radiography and cardiography, or echocardiography.
- Obtain plasma or urine for catecholamines.
- Consider obtaining plasma renin activity before treatment.

Initial Hypotensive Therapy

- Use a short-acting drug consonant with thinking about the cause.
- Aim to lower blood pressure initially by 20% to 30% and to 30% to 40% of goal in first 1 to 2 days.

Subsequent Treatment and Evaluation

- Evaluation should proceed hand-in-hand with therapy

severe hypertension be treated before and during the diagnostic evaluation. A severely hypertensive neonate should undergo evaluation for both renovascular disease and renal parenchymal disease.[39] Ultrasonography with Doppler flow studies should demonstrate renal anatomy and assess the renal artery and vein as well as the great vessels. In general, a radionuclide renal scan will be the most expeditious study by which to examine segmental vascular flow and provide an estimate of both arterial perfusion and tissue uptake. (Although "pull-out" arteriography can identify clots on catheters and thrombi, this technique requires the administration of a contrast agent and is thus high risk. Magnetic resonance angiography is appealingly noninvasive, but it is not easily applied to the ill neonate, nor does it give the necessary definition in neonates at this time. Looking at all possibilities together, vascular studies may best be deferred).

In the neonate with a suspected coarctation, echocardiography is usually diagnostic. Cardiac catheterization is usually unnecessary, unless complex lesions are suspected. Endocrine evaluation need be performed only if there is reason to suspect endocrine disease. The most common endocrine condition associated with hypertension in the neonatal period is congenital adrenal hyperplasia, which is usually found for other reasons.

The Child or Adolescent with Severe Hypertension

Because *any* diagnosis associated with hypertension can lead to accelerated hypertension or hypertensive crisis, it is important to consider all the likely possibilities.[1] It is crucial to rule out drug exposure and to rule out pregnancy, because therapy will be altered depending on the findings around these two issues.

SPECIFIC AGENTS FOR TREATING HYPERTENSIVE EMERGENCIES AND URGENCIES

Agents with Rapid Onset

Certain medications act sufficiently rapidly to be of use in hypertensive crisis and are listed in Tables 99-3 and 99-4. Table 99-5 lists diuretics that may be helpful in avoiding fluid retention. Brief comments concerning certain of these medications follow.

Sodium Nitroprusside

Nitroprusside (Nipride, Nitropress) is particularly useful for hypertensive emergencies in children because it is virtually always effective, is easy to titrate (rapid onset and offset of action), and is generally well tolerated despite a toxic byproduct, thiocyanate.[40] Nitroprusside acts as both an arterial and a venous dilator, so it can reduce preload and afterload yet does not change cardiac output under most circumstances. Because blood pressure can drop to hypotensive levels, optimal monitoring should include infusion with a constant-speed calibrated infusion pump, measurement of intra-arterial pressure, and determination of thiocyanate levels after 24 hours. It is unusual for thiocyanate toxicity to occur unless the medication is used at a rate above 3 μg/kg/hr for more than 72 hours. (Thiocyanate levels below 10 mg/dL are usually well tolerated.)

The preparation is light-sensitive and must be infused with intravenous lines and an infusion syringe that are light-protected; it is stable for about 24 hours after reconstitution. The onset of action is within seconds, and its blood pressure effect is gone within several minutes of stopping the infusion. The initial dose should be low, 0.3 μg/kg/min, and increased with caution to a maximum of 3 μg/kg/min. Toxicity is rarely seen at the lower doses but may occur above 2 μg/kg/min. The thiocyanate toxicity has been prevented or treated with thiosulfate infusion.[40] If severe toxicity ensues, both hemodialysis and peritoneal dialysis are effective in removing the drug.

Many sources recommend thiocyanate as the drug of choice for hypertensive crisis in children.[41] Because nitroprusside does not cause sedation or somnolence, it has been recommended for hypertensive encephalopathy, despite the fact that concerns have been raised for many years[42] that it may increase cerebral vasodilatation and thus increase intracranial pressure. Fluid retention can occur, blunting the effectiveness of nitroprusside, but the concomitant administration of a loop diuretic, such as furosemide or bumetanide, prevents this.

Labetalol

Labetalol (Normodyne, Trandate) possesses both selective α-adrenergic and nonselective β-adrenergic blocking properties (ratio 1:7) and may be given intravenously for prompt but usually gradual blood pressure control. Pediatric experience with intravenous labetalol suggests that this medication is generally effective and well tolerated.[43] The medication is given as escalating boluses (initial bolus of 0.5 mg/kg during 2 minutes is doubled every 10 minutes until blood pressure control is obtained, with a maximum dose of 5 mg/kg). The onset of action is within 1 to 5 minutes, generally peaking at 5 minutes and lasting for a variable amount of time. After repeated miniboluses, reduced blood pressure can be maintained with a continuous infusion (of 0.15 to 0.30 mg/min). The precise dosage for continual infusion in children has been reached deductively and has not been approved by the Food and Drug Administration as yet.

Although labetalol has a role in treating patients with pheochromocytoma, caution should be exercised in this category of patient because exaggerated postural hypotension may occur.

Nifedipine and Other Calcium Channel Blockers

Nifedipine has been used as the pediatric hypotensive drug of choice in hypertensive urgencies and emergencies in many centers during the past several years because it is easy to administer sublingually, orally, and even rectally.[44] The medication is effective sublingually within 2 to 5 minutes, peaks in 5 to 10 minutes, and lasts for 3 to 6 hours. Headache may ensue rapidly with its use, but this is tolerable. However, there is increasing concern about the possibility of inducing cardiovascular events with this medication. More of a problem is the report that short-acting nifedipine is often associated with reflex sympathetic discharge and tachycardia. Fatal problems with tachyarrhythmias in adults with coronary insufficiency have been reported. Although there would not seem to be a risk in most children, this agent is now being used more cautiously.

Nifedipine acts to lower blood pressure primarily by peripheral vasodilatation. It is a negative inotrope, so this may be a problem. Blood pressure may drop sharply, especially in individuals who have received other blood pressure–lowering medications or who are volume depleted.

Other calcium channel blockers, such as nicardipine,[45, 46] verapamil (injectable as Isoptin),[47] nitrendipine (injectable as Cardene),[6, 7] and diltiazem (injectable as Cardizem),[6, 7] that have had their main indication for emergency use for control of cardiac arrhythmias can also be considered for emergency blood pressure control, but experience is limited in children.

Nicardipine, at a dose of 0.1 μg/kg/min, has an onset that is

TABLE 99–3. Parenteral and Sublingual Drugs for Use in Hypertensive Emergencies and Urgencies in Pediatric Patients

Medication	Route	Dosage	Onset of Action	Peak/Duration	Adverse Effects	Contraindication	Comments
Sodium nitroprusside	IV infusion	0.3–10 μg/kg/min	Immediate	1–2 min/2–3 min	Thiocyanate toxicity	Hepatic insufficiency	Photosensitive preparation; shield from light
Labetalol	IV bolus	0.5 mg/kg during 2 min; if no response, double dose and repeat every 10 min to max dose of 5 mg/kg	1–5 min	5 min/variable (generally 2–6 hr)	Postural hypotension, neurologic signs, nausea and vomiting	Bronchial asthma; congestive heart failure	
Nifedipine	SL	0.25 mg/kg every 4–6 hr	10–15 min	60–90 min/variable (usually 2–4 hr)	Vasodilation, headache, cardiac events if preceding heart failure	Cardiomyopathy; concomitant use of β-blockers; cimetidine (relative)	Cardiac concerns less relevant in children than in adults
Esmolol	IV	500 μg/kg during 30 sec, and then infusion of 25 μg/kg/min, increasing dose every 4 min to max 300 μg/kg/min	1 min	min/min	Hypotension, central nervous system effects, nausea		Good drug for hypertension intraoperatively
Enalaprilat	IV, during 5 min	0.04–0.8 mg/kg/dose (child) 0.01 mg/kg starting neonate dose	15 min	1–4 hr/variable	Hypotension, oliguria, hypokalemia	Renal failure; dehydration	If hypotension occurs, treat it with volume
Diazoxide	IV bolus	1–5 mg/kg repeated every 5–15 min until control of blood pressure	1–5 min	1–5 min/variable (usually <12 hr)	Arrhythmias, hyperglycemia, sodium and water retention	Thiazide sensitivity; diabetes; coarctation	May need diuretics to prevent fluid retention; unpredictable blood pressure drop may occur
Phentolamine	IV bolus	0.05–0.1 mg/kg	Within 30 sec	2 min/5–30 min	Tachycardia, arrhythmia, marked hypotension		Specific for pheochromocytoma

TABLE 99–4. Oral and Topical Medications Used in Hypertensive Emergencies and Urgencies

Medication Type	Drug	Route	Dosage	Adverse Effects	Contraindication	Comment
Vasodilator	Minoxidil	PO	0.2 mg/kg to start	Fluid retention, reflex tachycardia	Need to get blood pressure controlled immediately; catecholamine-mediated hypertension	May help in urgencies
	Hydralazine	PO	0.75–3.0 mg/kg/day	Vasodilation signs	Tachycardia; sensitivity to hydralazine	Unstable in suspension; consider periodic ANA testing
β-Blockers	Propranolol	PO	0.5–1.90 mg/kg/day divided every 6 hr	Bradycardia, CHF, intensification of AV block; mental depression, visual disturbances, nightmares, hallucinations; bronchospasms; gastrointestinal signs	Asthma, CHF, sinus bradycardia, liver disease, cardiogenic shock, diabetes (?), pheochromocytoma	May mask signs of hypoglycemia or hyperthyroidism; available in long-acting form
	Atenolol	PO	Once daily, 50 mg qd (adult)	Fewer side effects than nonselective β-blockers	Can consider using in patients with reactive airway disease	Relatively cardioselective
	Metoprolol	PO	1 mg/kg every 12 hr	Fewer side effects than other β-blockers	β-Blocker of choice in asthma	Relatively cardioselective
	Nadolol	PO	1 mg/kg/24 hr	Same as other β-blockers, but less severe		Longer duration of action permits once/day dosing
Angiotensin-converting enzyme (ACE) inhibitors	Captopril	PO	0.05–0.15 mg/kg/dose (low end in infants)	Hyperkalemia, proteinuria, cough, rash, marrow suppression	Use with caution in renal artery disease (bilateral), do not use in pregnancy or in anyone who has had angioneurotic edema	More rapid onset than other ACE inhibitors
	Enalapril	PO	0.05–0.15 mg/kg/day	Similar to captopril	Similar to captopril, but longer acting; not sulfur containing, so perhaps fewer side effects	
Calcium channel blockers	Nifedipine	PO	0.25 mg/kg/dose, every 4–6 hr	Vasodilatation, tachycardia, nausea, vomiting, sweating, cardiac problems	Use with caution in heart failure	Absorption not affected by food
	Verapamil	PO	4–10 mg/kg/day, given 3×/day	Similar to nifedipine		Absorption delayed by food
	Isradipine	PO	0.05–0.83 mg/kg/day	Similar to nifedipine		Can be put into suspension
α-Blockers	Prazosin	PO	1 mg to a max of 20 mg every 24 hr	Orthostatic hypotension, lethargy, sedation and fatigue	Patient receiving minoxidil	First-dose hypotension may occur
	Phenoxybenzamine	PO	0.2 mg/kg/24 hr	Orthostatic hypotension, nasal congestion		Specific for catecholamine excess
Central adrenergic stimulators	Clonidine	PO or patch	0.05 mg/kg bid to max 2.4 mg/24 hr	Lethargy, sedation, dry mouth, ? retinal degeneration		

ANA = antinuclear antibody; AV = atrioventricular; CHF = congestive heart failure.

TABLE 99–5. Diuretic Agents for Administration in Pediatric Patients

Medication	Dosage	Onset	Peak/Duration	Adverse Effects	Relative Contraindication
Furosemide (Lasix)	1–2 mg/kg (max, 6 mg/kg/24 hr)	Oral: 1–2 hr IV: 5 min (child); 1 hr (neonate)	1–2 hr/4–6 hr 30 min/2 hr (child); 1–2 hr/5–6 hr (neonate)	Hyperuricemia, hyperglycemia, hypokalemia, hyponatremia, fluid depletion, ototoxicity	Sulfonamide sensitivity, anuria, metabolic alkalosis
Ethacrynic acid (Edecrin)	1 mg/kg (max, 25 mg total/day)	Oral: ~30 min IV: 15–30 min	2 hr/6–8 hr 45 min/3 hr	Same as for furosemide; ototoxicity more	Anuria, metabolic alkalosis
Bumetanide (Bumex)					
Hydrochlorothiazide (HydroDIURIL)	2 mg/kg bid	Oral: 2 hr	4 hr/6–12 hr	Electrolyte depletion, hyperuricemia, hypoglycemia	Anuria, sulfonamide sensitivity
Spironolactone (Aldactone)	1–3.3 mg/kg every 6, 8, or 12 hr	Oral: gradual	3 days/2–3 days	Hyperkalemia, gynecomastia	Anuria, hyperkalemia, decreasing renal function
Metolazone (Zaroxolyn, Diulo, Mykrox)	1 mg/kg	Oral: gradual	Gradual	Similar to thiazide; also bloating, chest pain, chills	Anuria

immediate and a very short half-life.[45, 46] It can cause flushing, tachycardia, and headache.

Rapid injection of 5 to 10 mg of verapamil over 1 to 5 minutes in adults lowers blood pressure rapidly, peaking at 2 to 5 minutes and lasting 30 minutes to several hours. Continuous infusion rates of 3 to 25 mg/hr have also been used.[47] Although verapamil does not lead to reflex tachycardia, its use in children has not been extensive.

Diazoxide

Diazoxide, a nondiuretic benzothiadiazine, is usually given as a bolus and is nearly always effective.[48, 49] Once blood pressure has been reduced by diazoxide, it generally remains down for several hours. The initial dose is standardly 5 mg/kg all at once, as fast as possible. Because the maximum effect usually occurs within 5 minutes of injection, subsequent boluses may be given every 10 minutes or so until an effect is obtained. It is rare to see a precipitous fall in pressure. Nonetheless, it is difficult to predict the degree of blood pressure fall with this agent, particularly if diazoxide is used with other medications, such as hydralazine; marked hypotension can occur.

To avert this possibility, despite the concept that diazoxide binds to albumin and so must be given as fast as possible, some protocols with constant infusion have been successful. For example, an infusion rate of 0.25 mg/kg/min (maximum dose, 300 mg in 20 minutes) has successfully led to a smooth reduction in blood pressure.[48] Another approach has been to use smaller doses of 1 to 2 mg/kg in boluses rather than the higher dose of 5 mg/kg.[49]

The arterial vasodilatation with diazoxide often leads to sympathetic reflex tachycardia along with increased cardiac output and left ventricular contractility. The vasodilatation often causes sodium retention, so that diuretic therapy is needed as an adjunct. Hyperglycemia may occur because of inhibition of insulin release, and blood glucose level should be monitored.

Esmolol and Propranolol

Esmolol is a rapidly acting nonselective β-receptor antagonist.[50] Its action is virtually immediate, and its effect lasts up to 20 minutes or so. This agent may cause bradycardia and bronchospasm, as seen with other β-blockers. This agent has been used primarily in the operating room for control of severe hypertension. There is little direct pediatric experience with this medication.

In contrast, propranolol has an immediate effect on heart rate, yet a somewhat slower effect on blood pressure.[51] The dose is 0.01 to 0.05 mg/kg intravenously given slowly during 1 hour. The maximum dose one should use is 10 mg, and this agent should be used with cardiac monitoring. Redosing is needed every 6 to 8 hours, in general.

Intravenous Angiotensin-Converting Enzyme Inhibitors

Enalaprilat is the ACE inhibitor of choice for intravenous administration. It has had limited use in children. The dose is 0.04 to 0.08 mg/kg/dose in children and less in neonates, 0.01 mg/kg/dose.[52] The onset of action occurs within about 15 minutes, with a peak at 1 to 4 hours after infusion.

Pheochromocytoma Control

PHENTOLAMINE. Phentolamine, an α-blocker, is used at times to control hypertension from pheochromocytoma.[31] Its action is immediate, and it lasts 30 to 60 minutes. The dose is 0.1 to 0.2 mg/kg. Although this agent can also be used for diagnosing pheochromocytoma, it is *far* preferable to diagnose this tumor by use of catecholamine levels and imaging studies, avoiding the possibility that blood pressure will drop precipitously.

ADENOSINE. Adenosine, a potent and short-acting vasodilator, has been used for perioperative control of catecholamine-related hypertension at a dose of 100 μg/kg/min.[53] There is not extensive experience with this agent, but it appears to offer prompt blood pressure control in the setting of neuroblastoma or pheochromocytoma surgery.

Medications for Longer Term Preoperative Pheochromocytoma Control

PHENOXYBENZAMINE. Phenoxybenzamine is an α-blocker that is helpful in controlling blood pressure before surgery.[31] Used alone, it is moderately effective, but it is more effective used in combination with prazosin or metyrosine. Phenoxybenzamine is difficult to titrate and may take several weeks to work adequately.

METYROSINE. The catecholamine synthesis inhibitor α-methyl-*p*-tyrosine (metyrosine) has been used to control blood pressure and stabilize hemodynamic status before surgery in patients with pheochromocytoma.[54] In comparison with patients treated preoperatively with phenoxybenzamine alone, far fewer of the metyrosine-treated patients had difficulty during the operation.

Agents with Moderately Rapid Onset

Other medications that act less quickly are best used in hypertensive urgencies but less often in true hypertensive emergencies.[1, 6–8, 15] Some of these are listed in Table 99-3 and some in Table 99-4, depending on the route of delivery.

Vasodilators

HYDRALAZINE. Hydralazine may be given as an intravenous bolus or as a bolus followed by an infusion.[17] This direct arteriolar vasodilator has an onset of action in 30 minutes and lasts 4 to 12 hours, when it is effective. Reflex tachycardia, facial flushing, headache, and vomiting may occur. The bolus dose of hydralazine is 0.1 to 0.5 mg/kg intravenously (maximum, 25 mg). Alternatively, it can be given as a bolus of 0.1 mg/kg intravenously followed by an infusion of 1.5 mg/min until a response is reached (maximum, 5 mg/min). Hydralazine may lead to an unpredictable blood pressure decrease, particularly if other antihypertensive agents are "on board."

Hydralazine has been used in concert with other agents, including methyldopa, propranolol, and diuretics. Hydralazine may also be administered orally.

MINOXIDIL. Minoxidil is a potent oral vasodilator and has a fairly rapid onset of action.[17] It should not be used if pheochromocytoma is suspected. The initial dose is 0.1 to 0.2 mg/kg every 8 to 24 hours. The maximum dose for a child younger than 12 years is 50 mg/day. Although minoxidil causes headache and other symptoms of vasodilatation and may cause salt and water retention, it is occasionally helpful in urgent control of blood pressure.

Oral Angiotensin-Converting Enzyme Inhibitors

Of ACE inhibitors, captopril has a rapid onset of action and may be useful in controlling severe hypertension. It has some effect within a half-hour; given three times a day, it may help in rapid control of the hypertension seen in hypertensive urgencies.

β-Blockers

The various β-blockers listed in Table 99-4 may be helpful in blood pressure control, but these do not quickly control the hypertension. Propranolol may be given judiciously by the intravenous route but is best given orally. The other preparations are, in my view, best to administer orally. Problems are as noted in Table 99-4.

α-Blockers

Phenoxybenzamine is mentioned previously under therapy for pheochromocytoma. Prazosin (Minipress) may be helpful in patients with heart failure. The dose in children is 1 mg initially, to a maximum of 20 mg every 24 hours. The onset of action is slow, making this a drug with limited usefulness in severe hypertension.

Centrally Acting Adrenergic Stimulating Drugs

Clonidine, provided either as a tablet or as a skin patch, may be helpful in controlling severe hypertension. Somnolence and potential for rebound hypertension limit its usefulness, particularly in centrally mediated hypertensive crisis. However, this medication is helpful in drug withdrawal-related hypertension. Similarly, methyldopa (Aldomet) has limited usefulness owing to its sedating properties.

Diuretics

As listed in Table 99-5, diuretics may act as an adjunct in treating hypertensive urgencies and emergencies.

Other Agents

Fenoldopam, a selective DA_1 agonist, appears to carry promise as a parenteral agent for the treatment of hypertensive crisis.[6, 55] Fenoldopam has been reported to be as effective as sodium nitroprusside, and it is just now available in the United States. The dose in adults appears to be 0.1 to 0.6 μg/kg/min.

The α_1-blocker urapidil appears to be helpful in situations with catecholamine excess. It may have broad applicability.[6, 56] The dose is 10 to 50 mg slowly intravenously, to a maximum of 250 mg/day.

PROGNOSIS OF THE CHILD WITH HYPERTENSIVE CRISIS

Although hypertensive crisis carries the risk of mortality, the wider recognition of this problem together with the improved availability of potent antihypertensives has substantially lowered the frequency of such a dire outcome. However, hypertensive crisis still may be associated with serious and permanent sequelae, such as seizures or cortical blindness, cognitive loss, cranial nerve impairment, and hemiplegia. Furthermore, deterioration in renal or cardiac function, usually recoverable, may occur. Thus, meticulous attention to details is crucial for the best outcome.

References

1. Groshong T: Hypertensive crisis in children. Pediatr Ann 1996; 25:369.
2. Report of the Second Task Force on Blood Pressure Control in Children—1987. Task Force on Blood Pressure Control in Children. National Heart, Lung and Blood Institute. Pediatrics 1987; 79:1.
3. Feld L: Hypertension. *In:* Gellis & Kagan's Current Pediatric Therapy. Burg F, Ingelfinger JR, Wald E, Polin R (Eds). 15th ed. Philadelphia, WB Saunders, 1996, pp 158-164.
4. Update on the 1987 Task Force Report on High Blood Pressure in Children and Adolescents: A working group report from the National High Blood Pressure Education Program. Pediatrics 1996; 98:649.
5. Arbus GS, Farine M: Management of hypertensive emergencies in children. *In:* Pediatric and Adolescent Hypertension. Loggie JMH (Ed). Cambridge, UK, Blackwell Scientific Publications, 1992, pp 369-377.
6. Tepel M, Zidek W: Hypertensive crisis: Pathophysiology, treatment and handling of complications. Kidney Int 1998; 53(Suppl 64):S2.
7. Mann SJ, Atlas SA: Hypertensive emergencies. *In:* Hypertension: Pathophysiology, Diagnosis and Management. 2nd ed. Laragh JH, Brenner BM (Eds). New York, Raven Press, 1995, pp 3009-3022.
8. Jones BV, Egelhoff JC, Patterson RJ: Hypertensive encephalopathy in children. Am J Neuroradiol 1997; 18:101.
9. Hulse JA, Taylor DSI, Dillon MJ: Blindness and paraplegia in severe childhood hypertension. Lancet 1979; 2:553.
10. Adams RE, Powers WJ: Management of hypertension in acute intracerebral hemorrhage. Crit Care Clin 1997; 13:131.
11. Brewington KC 2nd, Watridge CB: Hypertensive intracranial hemorrhage. Tenn Med 1997; 90:320.
12. Strandgaard S, MacKenzie ET, Jones JV, et al: Studies on the cerebral circulation of the baboon in acutely induced hypertension. Stroke 1976; 7:287.
13. Still JL, Cottom D: Severe hypertension in childhood. Arch Dis Child 1967; 42:34.
14. Rance CP, Arbus GS, Balfe JW, et al: Persistent systemic hypertension in infants and children. Pediatr Clin North Am 1974; 21:801.
15. Dillon MJ: Modern management of hypertension. *In:* Recent Advances in Pediatrics. Meadow R (Ed). Edinburgh, Churchill Livingstone, 1984, pp 35-55.
16. Ingelfinger JR: Hypertensive emergencies and acute hypertension. *In:* Pediatric Hypertension. Philadelphia, WB Saunders, 1982, pp 218-228.
17. Ruley EJ: Hypertensive emergencies in infants and children. *In:* Textbook of Critical Care. 3rd ed. Grenvik A (Ed). Philadelphia, WB Saunders, 1992, pp 529-537.
18. Londe S: Causes of hypertension in the young. Pediatr Clin North Am 1978; 25:55.
19. Eisenberg S: Blood volume in patients with acute glomerulonephritis as determined by radioactive chromium tagged red cells. Am J Med 1959; 27:241.
20. Powell HR, Rotenberg E, Williams AL, et al: Plasma renin activity in acute poststreptococcal glomerulonephritis and the haemolytic-uraemic syndrome. Arch Dis Child 1974; 49:802.
21. Monnens L, Drayer J, De Jong M: Malignant hypertension in a child with hemolytic-uremic syndrome treated with captopril. Acta Paediatr Scand 1981; 70:583.
22. Feld LG, Lieberman E, Mendoza SA, et al: Management of hypertension in the child with chronic renal disease. J Pediatr 1996; 129:18S.
23. Holland NYH, Kotchen T, Bhathena D: Hypertension in children with chronic pyelonephritis. Kidney Int 1975; 8S:243.
24. Savage JM, Dillon MJ, Shah V, et al: Renin and blood pressure in children with renal scarring and vesicoureteric reflux. Lancet 1978; 2:441.
25. Munoz AI, Pascual JF: Arterial hypertension in infants with hydronephrosis. Am J Dis Child 1977; 131:38.
26. Grant RP, Gifford RW, Pudvan WR, et al: Renal trauma and hypertension. Am J Cardiol 1971; 27:173.
27. Bagby SP: Dissection of pathogenetic factors in coarctation hypertension. *In:* National Heart, Lung, and Blood Institute Workshop on Juvenile Hypertension. Loggie JMH, Horan MJ, Gruskin AB, Hohn AR, Dunbar JB, Havlik RJ (Eds). New York, Biomedical Information Corporation, 1984, pp 253-256.
28. Alpert BS, Bain HH, Balfe JW: Role of the renin-angiotensin-aldosterone system in hypertensive children with coarctation of the aorta. Am J Cardiol 1979; 43:828.
29. Oparil S, Chen Y-F, Berecek KH, Calhoun DA, Wyss JM: The role of the central nervous system in hypertension. *In* Hypertension: Pathophysiology, Diagnosis and Management. 2nd ed. Laragh JH, Brenner BM (Eds). New York, Raven Press, 1995, pp 713-740.
30. Brody MJ, Varner KJ, Vasquez EC, et al: Central nervous system and the pathogenesis of hypertension: Sites and mechanisms. Hypertension 1991; 18(Suppl 5):III7.
31. Turner MC, Lieberman E, DeQuattro V: The perioperative management of pheochromocytoma in children. Clin Pediatr (Phila) 1992; 31:583.
32. Stackpole RH, Melicow MM, Uson AC: Pheochromocytoma in children. J Pediatr 1963; 63:315.
33. Cunningham FG, Lindheimer MD: Hypertension in pregnancy. N Engl J Med 1992; 326:927.

34. Turner MC, Ruley EJ, Buckley KM, et al: Blood pressure elevation in children with orthopedic immobilization. J Pediatr 1979; 95:989.
35. Berens SC, Linde LM, Goodwin WE: Transitory hypertension following urologic surgery in children. Pediatrics 1966; 38:194.
36. DeLuca FG, Gilchrist BF, Paquette E, et al: External compression as initial management of giant omphaloceles. J Pediatr Surg 1996; 31:965.
37. Ingelfinger JA, Brewer ED: Pediatric post-transplant hypertension: A review of current standards of care. Child Nephrol Urol 1992; 12:139.
38. Bakir AA, Dunea G: Drugs of abuse and renal disease. Curr Opin Nephrol Hypertens 1996; 5:122.
39. Blowey DL, Warady BA, Alon U: Hypertension in the neonatal period. Child Nephrol Urol 1992; 12:113.
40. Schultz V: Clinical pharmacokinetics of nitroprusside, cyanide, thiosulphate and thiocyanate. Clin Pharmacokinet 1984; 9:239.
41. Gordillo-Paniagua G, Velascquez-Jones L, Martini R, et al: Sodium nitroprusside treatment of severe arterial hypertension in children. J Pediatr 1975; 87:799.
42. Davis RF, Douglas ME, Heenan TJ, et al: Brain tissue pressure measurement during nitroprusside infusion. Crit Care Med 1981; 9:17.
43. Bunchman TE, Lynch RE, Wood EG: Intravenously administered labetalol for treatment of hypertension in children. J Pediatr 1992; 120:140.
44. Dilmen U, Caglar MK, Senses DA: Nifedipine in hypertensive emergencies of children. Am J Dis Child 1983; 137:1162.
45. Treluyer JM, Hubert P, Jouvet P, et al: Intravenous nicardipine in hypertensive children. Eur J Pediatr 1993; 152:712.
46. Tobias JD: Nicardipine to control mean arterial pressure in a pediatric intensive care unit population. Am J Anesthesiol 1996; 23:109.
47. Tripathy N, Sahoo SK: Verapamil in hypertension. Indian Heart J 1979; 31:321.
48. Thien TA, Huysmans FTM, Gerlag PGG, et al: Diazoxide infusion in severe hypertension and hypertensive crisis. Clin Pharmacol Ther 1979; 25:795.
49. Ram CVS, Kaplan NM: Individual titration of diazoxide dosage in the treatment of severe hypertension. Am J Cardiol 1979; 43:627.
50. Wiest DB, Trippel DL, Gillette PC, et al: Pharmacokinetics of esmolol in children. Clin Pharmacol Ther 1991; 49:618.
51. Griswold WR, McNeal R, Mendoza SA: Propranolol as an antihypertensive agent for children. Arch Dis Child 1978; 53:594.
52. Wells TG, Bunchman TE, Kearns GL: Treatment of neonatal hypertension with enalaprilat. J Pediatr 1990; 117:664.
53. Sellden H, Kogner P, Sollevi A: Adenosine for per-operative blood pressure control in an infant with neuroblastoma. Acta Anaesthesiol Scand 1995; 39:715.
54. Steinsapir J, Carr AA, Prisant L, et al: Metyrosine and pheochromocytoma. Arch Intern Med 1997; 157:901.
55. Shusterman NH, Elliott WJ, White WB: Fenoldopam, but not nitroprusside, improves renal function in severely hypertensive patients with impaired renal function. Am J Med 1993; 95:161.
56. Hirschl MM, Seidler D, Zeiner A, et al: Intravenous urapidil versus sublingual nifedipine in the treatment of hypertensive urgencies. Am J Emerg Med 1993; 11:653.

100

Pericardial Tamponade

William C. Shoemaker, MD, FCCM

Cardiac tamponade is a condition produced by increased pericardial pressure from accumulation of pericardial blood or fluid that constricts the cardiac chambers and thereby limits ventricular filling, stroke volume, and cardiac output. Hemopericardium and pericardial effusions are produced by a wide variety of traumatic and medical conditions; they may progress slowly along with compensations or may develop rapidly into the acute tamponade syndrome, shock, cardiovascular collapse, cardiac arrest, and death. The lethality of tamponade depends on the volume of pericardial blood or fluid, which varies widely, and more importantly the rate of increase in this fluid.[1-9]

The major problem in acutely developing tamponade from penetrating chest and upper abdominal wounds is early recognition and correction of the hemopericardium before cardiogenic shock and cardiac arrest occur. This may entail maintenance of hemodynamic stability until the hemopericardial collection can be drained. With pericardial effusions from medical conditions, the tamponade syndrome is more likely to progress slowly; this allows more time for diagnostic procedures and trials of conservative measures.

The classic presentation of acute tamponade was described by Beck[1] as a triad: hypotension, distended neck veins, and muffled heart sounds over the precordium. Usually the diagnosis is made when only one or two features are present; the entire triad is a late event associated with cardiac arrest and high mortality.[2-5] Kussmaul's sign, another classic sign of tamponade, is jugular venous distention which paradoxically rises on inspiration; in the normal phase relationship, venous pressure falls on inspiration.

CLINICAL FEATURES

Occurrence

Table 100–1 lists the clinical conditions that produce cardiac tamponade. Although tamponade is uncommon after penetrating injuries, it may progress rapidly; if it is unrecognized or inadequately treated, it carries a high mortality. Tamponade occurs after medical conditions including lymphomas and other malignancies, tuberculosis and other bacterial effusions,

TABLE 100–1. Causes of Cardiac Tamponade

1. Penetrating trauma to the chest, back, or upper abdomen
2. Blunt trauma with fracture of left fourth, fifth, or sixth rib
3. Thrombolytic therapy
4. Lymphomas and other malignancies
5. Tuberculosis and other bacterial effusions
6. Rheumatic fever and other nonbacterial inflammatory effusions
7. Ischemic rupture of the left ventricular free wall after acute myocardial infarction
8. Postcardiac surgery
9. Perforation of the right atrium or ventricle during cardiac catheterization
10. Biopsy of the myocardial wall
11. Placement of central venous or pacemaker catheters

pericarditis with effusion, systemic lupus erythematosus, renal failure with uremia, myxedema, scleraderma, and rheumatic fever. It usually occurs insidiously and may be first recognized by chest radiologic changes.

Hemopericardium from Penetrating Injuries

Tamponade from hemopericardium after penetrating cardiac injury occurs when fluid accumulating in the pericardial sac no longer is decompressed into the pleural cavity via the pericardial rent. The incidence of tamponade is 2% of stab or gunshot wounds to the chest, back, and upper abdomen; fatal tamponade has been reported after a 1-inch stab wound in the right midaxilla.

After penetrating injury, the full clinical picture of tamponade may develop within minutes or over several days. This is because the knife or gunshot also tears the pericardial sac, which then allows the pericardial blood to decompress into the pleural cavity or mediastinum. Tamponade occurs when the egress of pericardial blood is obstructed by clots that form in the pericardial space shortly after laceration of a cardiac chamber; large clots were found in 60% of patients operated on for tamponade.[5] Although the incidence of tamponade from penetrating cardiac wounds is low, disastrous consequences occur when the diagnosis is delayed or missed in patients with rapidly expanding tamponade. The lack of specificity of vital signs, venous distention, and routine monitoring means that a high degree of suspicion should be exercised in penetrating trauma.[1-9]

Iatrogenic tamponade occurs with (1) manipulation of instruments and catheters that inadvertently perforate the auricular wall or right ventricle during cardiac catheterization or biopsy, (2) placement of pacemakers, and (3) insertion of rigid central venous catheters for nutrition or pressure recording. This form of tamponade occurs most commonly in patients with ischemic or severely diseased ventricles. In contrast to penetrating cardiac wounds, tamponade accidentally occurring after catheter manipulation may become fatal unless the tamponade is rapidly corrected by pericardiotomy and drainage. This is because there is no route for spontaneous decompression of the pericardial fluid—unlike penetrating chest wall injury that lacerates the pericardial sac and partially decompresses the pericardial blood.

Pericardial Effusion

At the other end of the temporal spectrum, effusions that occur in uremia, neoplasms, postmyocardial infarction (Dressler's syndrome), and bacterial and nonbacterial inflammatory conditions may produce tamponade slowly over weeks or months. In slowly developing patterns, the pericardial sac is able to dilate and accommodate large volumes of pericardial fluids to as much as 2 L.

Postcardiac Surgery

After cardiac surgical operations, accumulation of seromas occasionally occurs. In this case, the fluid is usually found in loculated areas either within or outside the pericardial space. When the loculations become large, whether inside or outside the confines of the pericardium, they may produce the tamponade syndrome.

CLINICAL DIAGNOSIS

The rapidly changing clinical pattern of tamponade in patients with penetrating chest or upper abdominal injuries may be described in three stages.

- *Stage 1.* The presence of tachycardia, muffled or distant heart sounds, increased area of cardiac dullness, the point of maximal impulse or P (PMI) well inside the area of cardiac dullness, and myocardial infarction central venous pressure (CVP) values of 15 mm Hg and rising suggests *early* tamponade.
- *Stage 2.* The addition of hypotension completes Beck's triad and indicates that physiologic compensations are inadequate to maintain circulatory integrity. Actually, this phase represents an *advanced* stage of the disease in which arrest is likely.
- *Stage 3.* A fall in CVP and severe hypotension suggest that circulatory deterioration is advanced and cardiac arrest is imminent. Mortality in tamponade from penetrating wounds increases from 25% without arrest to 65% after arrest.[2]

The decrease in CVP values from levels of 15 to 20 mm Hg or more together with normotension, normal heart rate, and rhythm suggests circulatory improvement without significant tamponade. Echocardiography, which is now routinely available in the emergency department, usually provides a definitive diagnosis.[10-12]

Pulsus Paradoxus

The so-called "paradoxic pulse," or pulsus paradoxus, is an exaggerated pattern of changes in arterial pressure with ventilation. By definition, pulsus paradoxus occurs when the CVP increases and the systemic arterial pressure decreases with inspiration more than 15 mm Hg; the normal variations in arterial pressures are less than 10 mm Hg and are not clearly evident by examination with stethoscope and sphygmomanometer. Pulsus paradoxus may be detectable by careful examination of the radial pulse but is more easily detected with direct recording of arterial pressures and the ventilatory cycle. It is a useful sign in slowly developing pericardial effusions but is not very useful in rapidly developing tamponade from penetrating injuries.

TABLE 100–2. Hemodynamic Values of Patients with Hemopericardium and Tamponade at the Time of the Maximum Change

Variable	Normal Values	Hemopericardium	*P* Value
Stroke index (mL/m^2)	43 ± 3	27 ± 4	<.010
Cardiac index (L/min • m^2)	3.2 ± 2	2.9 ± 0.4	NS
MAP (mm Hg)	90 ± 2	77 ± 4.5	<.025
CVP (cm H_2O)	4.4 ± 1	18.7 ± 2	<.001
Heart rate (beat/min)	90 ± 2	112 ± 4	<.001
Left ventricular stroke work (g • m/m^2)	52 ± 5	30 ± 5	<.005

MAP = mean arterial pressure; CVP = central venous pressure; NS = not significant.

Laboratory Tests

Routine chest radiographs may reveal left or right hemothorax, the most common clinical condition associated with tamponade from penetrating injuries. Hemomediastinum occasionally occurs. The "water bottle" appearance of the heart is rare in acute tamponade from penetrating cardiac injuries but may occur in slowly developing pericardial effusions from medical conditions. Pulmonary congestion is usually absent in patients with tamponade compared with the pulmonary congestion and cardiac dilatation of patients with congestive heart failure.

Computed tomography and magnetic resonance imaging of the chest accurately show small chambers of the heart and the pericardial effusion. Limited time precludes these studies in rapidly evolving tamponade after penetrating chest injuries.

Nonspecific electrocardiographic (ECG) changes include low voltage, depressed or altered ST segments, and evidence suggestive of subepicardial ischemia. The ECG patterns are rarely diagnostic of tamponade, but the test is performed routinely to rule out other cardiac conditions.

CVP values of 15 mm Hg or higher in patients with penetrating chest wounds suggest tamponade, especially if the values are rising over a short observation period.

Echocardiography provides definitive diagnostic information. Normally, sonography produces a single echo that is reflected from the posterior wall of the ventricles; two distinct echoes from this area indicate pericardial fluid, and the space between these echoes is a reflection of the volume of pericardial fluid.

Transcutaneous oxygen monitoring can warn of low flow in patients with possible tamponade.[13]

Angiocardiography with radioopaque dye outlines the right atrial lumen and the thickness of the atrial wall; wall thickness greater than 6 mm indicates increased pericardial fluid.

The diagnosis is usually made by clinical suspicion and confirmed by echocardiography. Nonclotting blood obtained by pericardiocentesis, is diagnostic, but a negative tap does not rule out the diagnosis. False-negative taps have been seen in 19% of patients with hemopericardium from penetrating chest injuries because of clotted pericardial blood.[5]

Differential Diagnosis of Elevated Central Venous Pressure

Acute tamponade must be differentiated from other conditions in which CVP is acutely elevated, such as acute right ventricular failure, chronic obstructive lung disease, constrictive pericarditis, pulmonary embolism, and acute exacerbation of chronic bronchitis. The "elevated" CVP must be differentiated from "high" CVP from excessive fluid administration, too rapid administration of fluids, abdominal distention from paralytic ileus or ascites, increased intrathoracic pressure from pneumothorax or hemothorax, airway obstruction, infusions of vasopressors, and clotted or nonfunctional CVP intravenous line.

PATHOPHYSIOLOGY

Hemodynamic Pattern of Acute Cardiac Tamponade

Preoperative hemodynamic studies of patients with acute hemopericardium and tamponade show tachycardia, hypotension, high CVP, low stroke volume, low cardiac index, and low left ventricular stroke work.[14] Compensatory responses in the early period of tamponade consist of tachycardia, increased CVP, and increased peripheral vascular resistance. The reduced cardiac output from decreased stroke volume and ventricular filling is improved by tachycardia. Increased CVP and venomotor tone returns more blood to the heart and increases ventricular filling. Blood pressure, despite falling flow, is at least partially maintained by increased peripheral vascular resistance (Fig. 100–1). Each of these compensations is part of the adrenal stress response. The hemodynamic values of patients with hemopericardium and cardiac temponade are presented in Table 100–2.

Pathologic Aspects

Penetrating cardiac injuries from knife or gunshots also tear the pericardial sac. Blood that leaks into the free pericardial

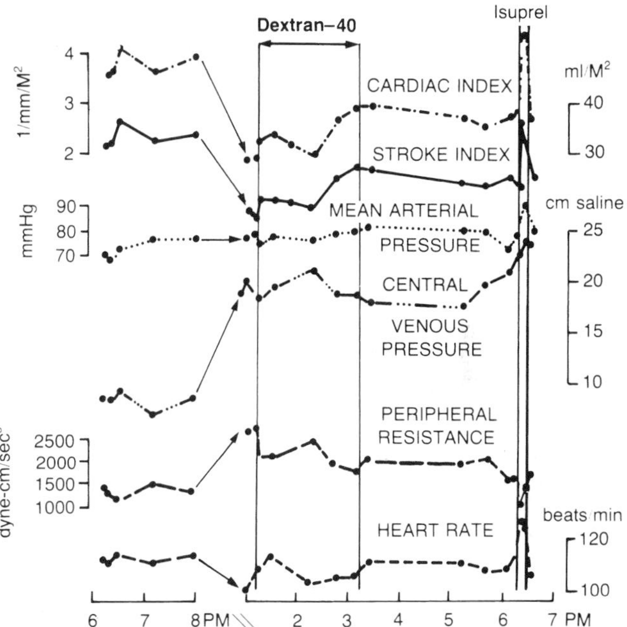

Figure 100–1. Early compensatory reactions to pericardial tamponade. A 22-year-old man was admitted to the intensive care unit 3 hours after being shot in the chest with a 22-caliber gun. The entrance wound was in the fifth intercostal space, just lateral to the midclavicular line; there was no exit wound. The findings on physical examination were otherwise normal. Radiography revealed the presence of a right hemothorax and a bullet in the posterior left side of the chest. A chest tube was placed, and 750 mL of blood was removed. After administration of 1 unit of whole blood and 750 mL of 5% plasma protein fraction, blood pressure was 100/60 mm Hg, heart rate was 110 beats per min, and the central venous pressure (CVP) was 8 cm H_2O; other hemodynamic variables were essentially normal, except for the presence of tachycardia. Initially, it was believed that the bullet had missed the heart; however, over the next few hours, the complete hemodynamic picture of cardiac tamponade developed. The stroke index fell from about 36 to 18 mL/m², cardiac output decreased from about 4 to 2 L/min · m², and CVP rose from about 10 to 22 cm H_2O. The administration of 500 mL of colloid solutions improved the stroke index and cardiac index without appreciably increasing CVP. Mean arterial pressure was maintained by the compensatory increase in peripheral resistance; the high CVP increased the effective ventricular filling pressure, and the increased heart rates tended to partially maintain blood flow. Thus, volume therapy augmented the natural compensations and almost completely restored cardiac output during the short period when the patient was being prepared for surgery. Subsequently, surgery disclosed a small hole in the pericardium, which was filled with 250 mL of unclotted liquid blood and a large, 200-mL clot. The bullet had entered the anterior left ventricle and exited posterolaterally to lie free in the pericardial sac. The ventricular perforations were sutured, and the patient recovered without complications. (From Shoemaker WC, Carey JS, Yao ST, et al: Hemodynamic alterations in acute cardiac tamponade after penetrating injuries of the heart. Surgery 1970; 67:754.)

space is quickly decompressed into the pleural space or mediastinum. Pericardial blood accumulates and produces tamponade when bleeding is sufficiently rapid that its egress from the pericardial cavity is blocked by clots that form faster than they are lysed. A rather high incidence of clots (60%) has been reported in penetrating cardiac wounds explored soon after injury.[5] Nonclotting pericardial blood, which is diagnostic of tamponade, occurs when pericardial blood has already clotted and spontaneously lysed.

The pericardial fluid, confined by the relatively unyielding pericardial sac, takes up space and exerts pressure. The intrapericardial pressure is transmitted across the cardiac wall to increase intracardiac pressures; this has proportionally greater effects on atrial and end-diastolic pressures than the ventricular systolic pressures do. The reduced filling pressure and the volume encroachment by the pericardial fluid limit ventricular filling and stroke volume. Thus, reduced stroke volume is the major circulatory defect.[8]

Physiologic Compensations and Decompensations

Secondary compensatory circulatory responses include (1) increased CVP, (2) increased heart rate, and (3) increased peripheral vascular resistance. The rise in peripheral resistance maintains blood pressure when cardiac output begins to fall, and the increased heart rate improves cardiac output when the latter is limited by stroke volume. The adrenal stress response maintains arterial blood pressure, increases peripheral resistance, further increases CVP, and augments the limited cardiac filling.

Decompensation occurs with progression of the disorder and gradually diminishing blood pressure, CVP, and peripheral vascular resistance from exhausted stress responses or overwhelming pathology (Fig. 100–2). When the adrenal stress response is exhausted, compensatory circulatory mechanisms maintaining hemodynamic stability fail. Unless promptly corrected by pericardiocentesis or surgical drainage, low cardiac output, hypotension, and acidosis further reduce the coronary and peripheral circulation and lead to further hypotension, shock, cardiac arrest, and death.[8]

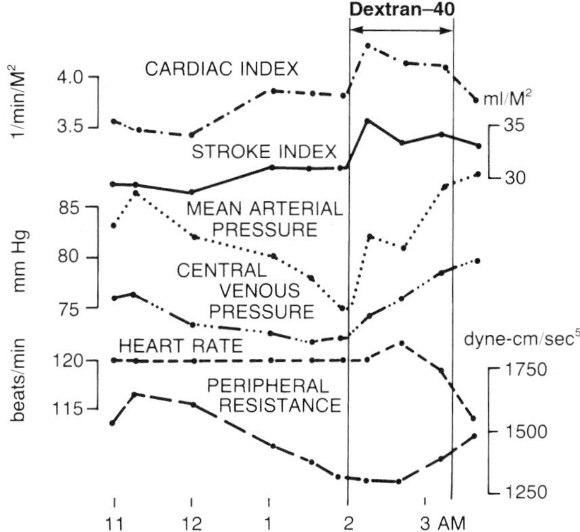

Figure 100–2. Decompensatory response to pericardial tamponade following initial improvement. A 49-year-old man was admitted to the intensive care unit 24 hours after sustaining a stab wound through the fourth intercostal space of the left anterior chest. On admission, his blood pressure was 125/70 mm Hg, heart rate was 105 beats per min, and central venous pressure (CVP) was 17 cm H_2O. Chest radiographs revealed left hemothorax; a chest tube was placed, and 700 mL of blood was removed. Pericardiocentesis yielded only 9 mL of unclotted blood. Initially, hemodynamic measurements were stable: the cardiac index was slightly above normal, the stroke index was low, mean arterial pressure was 83 to 87 mm Hg, CVP was 18 cm H_2O, and the heart rate was 120 beats per min. However, as the pH fell from 7.4 to 7.2, decompensation gradually decreased peripheral resistance, arterial pressure, and CVP. Even though CVP values were still high, volume loading with 500 mL of colloid solutions restored the mean arterial pressure and increased both the stroke index and cardiac index while the patient was being prepared for definitive surgical correction of pericardial tamponade.

Table 100–3 lists the hemodynamic effects of volume load, pericardiocentesis, and isoproterenol therapy.

THERAPEUTIC MANAGEMENT

A running account should be made at 5- to 15-minute intervals for arterial pressure, heart rate, and CVP values in suspected cases of tamponade. Hematocrit, urine output, and arterial blood gases should also be measured but at less frequent intervals.

While the patient is being prepared for surgery, a trial of volume loading usually improves the hemodynamic picture and confirms that hypovolemia and myocardial insufficiency are not the major problems. Volume loading in the face of high CVP levels is not contraindicated by high venous pressures, because tamponade is produced by inadequate ventricular filling not ventricular failure.

SURGICAL CORRECTION

Subxiphoid pericardial window may be performed through a small incision at the left lateral side of the xiphoid cartilage. The diaphragm is reflected inferiorly, the pericardium is exposed, and if blood or fluid is present, a 4 × 4 cm window of pericardium is excised and the perforation of the cardiac wall is repaired.[14, 15]

The pericardial sac may be approached through the standard left anterolateral thorocotomy at the fourth or fifth left interspace. Inspection, palpation, and ballotment of the pericardium may reveal significant amounts of pericardial fluid under pressure that, if present, may be drained by a pericardial window.

TABLE 100–3. Hemodynamic Changes Produced by Therapy

Variable	Pericardiocentesis (n = 3)	Volume Load (n = 5)	Isoproterenol (n = 3)
Stroke index (mL/m²)	+4	+8	+13
Cardiac index (L/min • m²)	+0.9	+0.7	+2.3
Mean arterial pressure (mm Hg)	+7.0	+13	+11
Central venous pressure (cm H_2O)	−2.2	+5.7	+3
Heart rate (beat/min)	+14	−1	+18
Left ventricular stroke work (g • m/m²)	+6	+16	+23

SUMMARY

Although cardiac tamponade occurs infrequently, it may be life-threatening, especially if it is recognized late after penetrating chest injury. It is usually suspected clinically, detected by echocardiography, and corrected by surgical drainage. Pericardial effusions from medical conditions usually evolve more slowly and lend themselves to conservative therapy of the underlying problem, pericardiocentesis, and surgical drainage when necessary.

References

1. Beck C: Further observations on stab wounds of the heart. Ann Surg 1942; 115:698–704.
2. Beall AC, Diethrich EB, Crawford HW: Surgical management of penetrating cardiac injuries. Am J Surg 1966; 112:686.
3. Naclerio EA: Penetrating wounds of the heart: Experience with 249 patients. Dis Chest 1964; 46:1.
4. Wilson RF, Bassett JS: Penetrating wounds of the pericardium and its contents. JAMA 1966; 195:513.
5. Yao ST, Vanecho RM, Printen KJ, et al: Penetrating wounds of the heart. Ann Surg 1968; 168:67–73.
6. Sugg WL, Rea WJ, Ecker RR, et al: Penetrating wounds of the heart: An analysis of 459 cases. J Thorac Cardiovasc Surg 1968; 56:531–545.
7. Shoemaker WC, Carey JS, Yao ST, et al: Penetrating wounds of the heart. Ann Surg 1968; 168:67–73.
8. Shoemaker WC, Carey JS, Yao ST, et al: Hemodynamic alterations in acute pericardial tamponade after penetrating injuries of the heart. Surgery 1970; 67:754–764.
9. Trinkle JK: Penetrating heart wounds. Ann Thorac Surg 1994; 38:181–182.
10. Feigenbaum H: Echocardiography. Philadelphia, Lea and Febiger, 1972.
11. Spodick DH: The pericardium: Structure, function and disease spectrum. *In:* Pericardial Diseases. Spodick DH (Ed). Philadelphia, FA Davis, 1976.
12. Aaland M, Bryan FC, Sherman R: Two dimensional echocardiogram in hemodynamically stable victims of penetrating precordial trauma. Am Surg 1994; 60:412–415.
13. Waxman K, Wong DH, O'Neal K: Early diagnosis of shock due to pericardial tamponade using transcutaneous oxygen monitoring. Crit Care Med 1987; 15:1156–1156.
14. Jimenez E, Martin M, Krukenkamp I, Barrett J: Subxiphoid pericardiotomy versus echocardiography. Surgery 1990; 108:676–680.
15. Brewster SA, Thirlby RC, Synder WH: Subziphoid window and penetrating cardiac trauma. Arch Surg 1988; 123:937–939.

101

Treatment of Massive Pulmonary Embolism

Graham F. Pineo, MD • Russell D. Hull, MBBS, MSc

Death resulting from pulmonary embolism occurs in approximately 100,000 patients per year in the United States, and pulmonary embolism contributes to the death of another 100,000 patients.[1, 2] Pulmonary embolism represents the third most common cause of cardiovascular death after acute myocardial infarction and stroke[3] and is the most common preventable cause of death in hospitalized patients.[4] Although pulmonary embolism frequently develops in hospitalized patients with one or more comorbid disorders, this condition may arise in otherwise healthy individuals after orthopedic surgery or trauma or in pregnancy.[5–8] Effective prophylaxis is available for most of these situations,[9] but venous thromboembolism can occur unexpectedly in ambulatory patients, particularly if they have been exposed to risk factors in the preceding months. When venous thromboembolism occurs, an accurate diagnosis must be established by the use of the appropriate objective tests[10] so that treatment can be instituted immediately. The first indication that venous thromboembolism has occurred may be a massive pulmonary embolus, which, unfortunately, can be fatal within a short time in up to a third of patients.[11, 12] This chapter is devoted to management of such patients with massive pulmonary embolism.

Patients with acute massive pulmonary embolism usually have a dramatic presentation, with the sudden onset of severe shortness of breath, hypoxemia, and right ventricular failure. Symptoms include central chest pain, often identical to angina; severe dyspnea; and frequently syncope, confusion, or coma. Examination reveals a patient in severe distress with tachypnea, cyanosis, and hypotension. The marked increase in pulmonary vascular resistance leads to acute right ventricular failure with the presence of large A waves in the jugular veins and a right ventricular diastolic gallop. With pulmonary hypertension, there is marked right ventricular dilatation with a shift of the intraventricular septum, decreasing cardiac output, and further decreasing coronary perfusion, and this frequently results in cardiorespiratory arrest. If these patients survive, they are acutely threatened by any further pulmonary thromboembolism.

Emergency management includes[13]:

1. Intravenous heparin.
2. Oxygen with or without mechanical ventilation, which may include positive end-expiratory pressure (PEEP).
3. Volume resuscitation.
4. Inotropic agents and vasodilators.

In addition to these supportive measures, specific treatment options include:

1. Thrombolysis.
2. Pulmonary thrombectomy with or without cardiopulmonary bypass support.
3. Transvenous catheter embolectomy or clot dissolution.
4. Insertion of an inferior vena caval filter.

THROMBOLYTIC TREATMENT

Randomized clinical trials have demonstrated that the mortality rate of patients with venous thromboembolism can be decreased by anticoagulant treatment.[11, 14, 15] A mortality rate below 5% should be achieved with intravenous heparin and oral anticoagulants, and this figure can be further reduced with the use of low-molecular-weight heparin.[16, 17] In the Prospective Investigation of Pulmonary Embolism Diagnosis (PIOPED) trial, only 10 of 399 (2.5%) patients who had angiographically confirmed pulmonary embolism died as a consequence of thromboembolism within 2 weeks of a diagnosis of angiographically proven pulmonary embolism.[18] However, patients who present with acute massive pulmonary embolism and hypotension have a mortality rate of approximately 20% even with the use of anticoagulants and other supportive measures. For such patients, the appropriate use of thrombolytic agents has a role. A high percentage of acute pulmonary emboli occur within 10 to 14 days of surgery[19–22] and, therefore, are excluded from treatment protocols utilizing thrombolytic agents. These patients may be candidates for local infusion of low-dose thrombolytic agents.[22]

Several randomized clinical trials have compared thrombolytic drugs with heparin for the treatment of pulmonary embolism.[23-28] These trials compared (1) urokinase with heparin,[23] (2) streptokinase with heparin,[24, 25] or (3) recombinant tissue-type plasminogen activator (t-PA) with heparin[26-28] in different dosage regimens that included either a bolus or chronic infusion up to 72 hours. Outcome measures for accelerated thrombolysis included quantitative measures on repeated pulmonary angiograms, quantitative scores on repeated pulmonary perfusion scans, and measures of pulmonary vascular resistance. Although all studies demonstrated superiority of thrombolysis (in particular, with t-PA) in terms of resolution of both radiographic and hemodynamic abnormalities when measured within the first 24 hours, this advantage was short-lived. Repeated perfusion scans at 5 to 7 days revealed no significant difference in the patients treated with thrombolytic agents and in those treated with heparin. Furthermore, the trials demonstrated no difference in mortality rate or in resolution of symptoms. Measurement of diffusion capacity and capillary volumes at 2 weeks and 1 year after treatment showed that patients receiving thrombolytic therapy had higher diffusion capacity and lung capillary volumes than patients receiving heparin.[29] Follow-up of 23 patients by the same group an average of 7 years after thrombolytic treatment showed that patients who had received thrombolytic therapy had lower pulmonary artery pressure and pulmonary vascular resistance than patients who had received heparin.[30] The clinical relevance of these findings, however, must await further prospective studies.

Several randomized clinical trials have compared different thrombolytic agents using different treatment protocols: (1) streptokinase versus urokinase,[31] (2) urokinase with urokinase,[32] (3) t-PA with t-PA,[33, 34] and (4) t-PA with urokinase.[35, 36] These studies again demonstrated resolution of angiographic and perfusion scan abnormalities as well as reduction of pulmonary pressure, but there was little or no difference between the regimens being compared. Again, the clinical relevance of the changes must await further study.

Three thrombolytic agents have been approved by the Food and Drug Administration (FDA) for the treatment of acute pulmonary embolism. The dosage schedules are as follows:

1. Streptokinase, 250,000 units over 30 minutes followed by 100,000 units/hr for 24 hours;
2. Urokinase, 4400 units/kg over 10 minutes followed by 4400 units/kg/hr for 12 to 24 hours;
3. Recombinant t-PA, 100 mg administered over 2 hours.

Anticoagulation with heparin or low-molecular-weight heparin is usually commenced when the activated partial thromboplastin time (aPTT) is less than twice the control value.

There does not appear to be a therapeutic advantage of any of the available thrombolytic agents, suggesting that a more modern approach to the use of streptokinase in a high-dose bolus fashion may be beneficial and less expensive. The addition of unfractionated heparin or low-molecular-weight heparin does not enhance the effect of thrombolytic agents.[27, 37]

Studies to date comparing thrombolytic therapy with heparin or studies comparing the effects of different thrombolytic agents have not shown a mortality benefit, even when results are pooled. With the appropriate use of anticoagulant therapy, the incidence of fatal pulmonary embolism is low. Therefore, mortality studies will require large numbers of patients in order to detect a mortality difference with the addition of thrombolytic therapy to anticoagulants.[38] Patients selected for clinical trials have been excluded if they are hemodynamically unstable and have significant comorbid conditions. In order to detect a mortality advantage of thrombolysis, it may be necessary to include patients who are more likely to die with acute pulmonary embolism. In order to admit such patients to studies, we must find ways to expedite the diagnostic approach to acute pulmonary embolism using alternatives to the ventilation-perfusion lung scan and pulmonary angiogram, such as two-dimensional echocardiography,[28] magnetic resonance angiography,[39] or helical computed tomographic (CT) scanning.[40, 41]

In weighing the risks and benefits of thrombolytic therapy, the main concern is related to bleeding. Data from five randomized clinical trials of thrombolytic therapy for pulmonary embolism indicated that the frequency of intracranial hemorrhage up to 14 days after thrombolytic therapy was six of 332 patients (1.9%), 95% confidence interval 0.7% to 4.1%.[42] Diastolic hypertension was identified as a risk factor for intracranial hemorrhage. The incidence of major bleeding has decreased, particularly with the use of bolus or short-term infusions and with the use of newer thrombolytic agents, but intracerebral hemorrhage continues to occur more frequently than with heparin.[19, 27, 36, 43-45]

At this time, the role of thrombolytic agents in the management of acute massive pulmonary embolism still remains controversial. Although there is a more rapid dissolution of venous thromboemboli, the risk of serious bleeding remains a concern. Until there is a clearly demonstrated benefit in both morbidity and mortality from well-controlled prospective randomized clinical trials, the question of risk and benefit will remain.[46] In the meantime, the use of thrombolytic agents has become simpler with the use of high-probability ventilation-perfusion scans or echocardiography to confirm the diagnosis, the use of short-term or bolus infusion of thrombolytic agents into peripheral veins rather than in the pulmonary artery, the elimination of monitoring by laboratory tests, and treatment in the medical ward rather than in the intensive care unit. The fact that a high number of acute massive pulmonary emboli are occurring after surgery,[8, 21, 22] even though effective prophylactic regimens against venous thromboembolism are available,[9, 47] indicates that greater efforts must be taken to ensure that these prophylactic measures are being applied in a more uniform fashion.

Death from pulmonary embolism continues to remain high in North America and in Europe, and there are differences in mortality rate by sites and ethnic background, indicating the need for further epidemiologic studies.[48]

PULMONARY EMBOLECTOMY

Pulmonary embolectomy is occasionally indicated in the management of massive pulmonary embolism. This condition is defined as the sudden occurrence of a massive embolus producing severe cardiovascular decompensation with severe hypotension, oliguria, and hypoxia refractory to aggressive treatment.[49] A somewhat more generous indication would be an obstruction of more than 50% of the pulmonary vasculature, arterial oxygen saturation less than 60 mm Hg, systolic blood pressure less than 90 mm Hg, and urine output less than 20 mL/hr.[50] Patients who have contraindications to thrombolytic therapy or who have not responded to a trial of thrombolytic therapy in some centers are considered candidates for thrombectomy. However, others suggest that a patient who survives the first 2 hours after an acute massive pulmonary embolus will probably survive with adequate medical management if no further pulmonary emboli occur. It is likely that it will be impossible to perform a randomized trial comparing thrombolytic therapy with pulmonary embolectomy, and it is difficult to compare one case series of pulmonary thrombectomy with another because the case material is often not comparable.

Early experience with the Trendelenburg procedure revealed unacceptably high mortality rates (>50%).[12, 49] With the use of cardiopulmonary bypass support, mortality rates between 16% and 57% have been reported.[50-58] In a review of

651 patients undergoing emergency pulmonary embolectomy, the survival rate was 59.3% with cardiopulmonary bypass support and 47.7% without cardiopulmonary bypass support.[49] Patients with chronic pulmonary hypertension, other medical disorders, or symptoms of more than 7 days' duration have higher mortality rates.[54, 57] Patients who have sustained a cardiac arrest before embolectomy have a higher mortality rate.[54] Greater care to avoid vasodilation at the initiation of anesthesia has decreased mortality rate.[13, 49] Pulmonary hemorrhagic infarction with reperfusion has been reported after pulmonary embolectomy.[59] Other causes of death after embolectomy include cardiogenic shock, infection, and hypoxic brain damage.[51] Pulmonary embolectomy is usually accompanied by insertion of a vena caval filter.

The role of pulmonary embolectomy remains unclear and depends in part on the ready availability of a surgical team. Patients who are not candidates for thrombolysis (e.g., those who have undergone recent surgery) or who have not responded to maximal medical therapy may be candidates for pulmonary embolectomy. However, a report of successful thrombolysis with intrapulmonary urokinase in patients treated within 10 days of surgery casts further doubt on the need for this somewhat radical procedure.[22]

PERCUTANEOUS CLOT EXTRACTION OR DISRUPTION

Pulmonary embolectomy, via a catheter suction device inserted into the jugular or femoral vein under local anesthesia, has been used in the treatment of patients with acute massive pulmonary embolism when anticoagulant therapy or thrombolysis is contraindicated.[60–64] Mortality rates of 27% and 28% were observed.[60, 63] The most common cause of death is cardiac arrest resulting from ventricular arrhythmia, right-sided heart failure, and pulmonary hemorrhage.[60, 63] Some patients in whom clot extraction was not possible have gone on to successful pulmonary embolectomy on bypass. Inferior vena caval filters are used in conjunction with catheter embolectomy.[65]

Attempts have been made to fragment pulmonary emboli with the use of conventional cardiac catheters[66] or a catheter guide wire in conjunction with pulmonary thrombolytic therapy.[67] Mechanical disruption of experimental pulmonary emboli in animals has been attempted via catheter-operated mechanical devices.[68, 69]

The practice of catheter clot extraction is currently confined to a few centers with the required expertise, and this procedure cannot be used for patients who have suffered cardiac arrest. The future role of catheter clot extraction is unclear.

INFERIOR VENA CAVAL INTERRUPTION

Early approaches to inferior vena caval interruption included ligation or plication using external clips.[70, 71] Both procedures were accompanied by an operative mortality rate of 12% to 14%, recurrent pulmonary embolism rate of 4% to 6%, and an occlusion rate of 67% to 69%.[65] Also, many patients had chronic venous insufficiency after vena caval ligation. These complications gave rise to the development of catheter-inserted intraluminal filters.

An ideal filter is one that is easily and safely placed percutaneously, is biocompatible and mechanically stable, is able to trap emboli without causing occlusion of the vena cava, does not require anticoagulation, and is not ferromagnetic (does not cause artifacts on magnetic resonance images).[72–74] Although the ideal filter does not yet exist, several of the available devices have proved useful. These include the Greenfield stainless steel filter, titanium Greenfield filter, bird's nest filter, Vena Tech filter, and Simon-Nitinol filter. In experienced hands, these devices can be quickly and safely inserted under fluoroscopic control. One novel filter can be inserted temporarily when needed, used in conjunction with thrombolytic therapy, and then removed.[75] With the available follow-up to date, the Greenfield filter has had the best performance record and any future comparative studies should use this filter as the standard.[74]

Vena caval filters are indicated mainly in the following circumstances:

1. When anticoagulant therapy is contraindicated.
2. When patients have had recurrent thromboembolism despite adequate anticoagulation.
3. As prophylactic placement in high-risk patients. This category includes patients with cor pulmonale, those with a previous history of thromboembolism who are at high risk because of such conditions as an acetabular fracture, or patients who have cancer.

For patients who have had pulmonary embolectomy either surgically or via percutaneous catheters, inferior vena caval filters should be inserted. Inferior vena caval filters are routinely inserted after surgery for chronic thromboembolic pulmonary hypertension. More controversial indications include (1) insertion during emergency surgery occurring within the first 4 weeks of initiation of anticoagulant therapy for venous thromboembolism and (2) insertion after thrombolytic therapy for acute pulmonary embolism.

In the past, the detection of a free-floating thrombus by ultrasound examination had been considered an indication for either thrombectomy or insertion of an inferior vena caval filter. A prospective study compared the clinical outcomes of patients who had either the presence or absence of a free-floating thrombus in a proximal leg vein.[76] All patients were treated with unfractionated or low-molecular-weight heparin followed by warfarin therapy. In the 3-month follow-up, there was no difference in the incidence of documented pulmonary embolism or death between the two groups. The authors conclude that anticoagulant therapy effectively prevents recurrent pulmonary embolism and that the routine insertion of inferior vena caval filters cannot be supported in patients with free-floating thrombi.[76] This finding is in keeping with an earlier observation that free-floating thrombi become attached to the vein wall rather than immobilized.[77]

In another study, patients with proximal venous thrombosis were randomized to receive an inferior caval filter or anticoagulant treatment alone; lung scanning with or without pulmonary angiography was performed on day 1 and day 10, and clinical follow-up was for 2 years.[78] All patients were given heparin, followed by oral anticoagulant therapy for 3 months. At 3-month follow-up, there was no significant difference in the incidence of pulmonary embolism, recurrent deep venous thrombosis, major bleeding, or death between the two groups. Extended follow-up at 1 and 2 years showed a higher incidence of pulmonary embolism in the control group but a higher incidence of recurrent deep venous thrombosis in the inferior vena caval filter group, with no difference in the death rates. Thus, this randomized study does not support the routine use of inferior vena caval filters in patients with proximal deep venous thrombosis.

As the filters have become safer and easier to implant, the indications have expanded somewhat. In selected patients, filters may be inserted proximal to the renal veins or in the superior vena cava. The use of filters in young individuals with a long life expectancy has been discouraged because it is not known how well the device will last in vivo. Complications of inferior vena caval filter insertion include misplacement and tilting, occasional migration and perforation, and occasional infection, but these events are rare.[65]

FUTURE PROSPECTS

More efficient anticoagulation providing optimal therapeutic levels of heparin[79] or the use of low-molecular-weight heparin[16, 17] has improved both the efficacy and safety of treatment of venous thromboembolism. Further experience with the newer thrombolytic agents using more efficient treatment protocols offers an expanded role for these agents with less serious bleeding than was seen in the past. With more efficient anticoagulation and thrombolysis, the need for pulmonary embolectomy should continue to diminish. There are new antithrombotic agents on the horizon, some of which are coming to clinical trials.[80] The more widespread use of prophylaxis for venous thromboembolism[9] should diminish the incidence of thromboembolism after surgery and in other high-risk situations. Nonetheless, the challenge confronting physicians managing patients with massive pulmonary embolism is the evidence that the mortality rate has shown little change since the 1970s despite all of these efforts.[48]

References

1. Dalen JE, Alpert JS: Natural history of pulmonary embolism. Prog Cardiovasc Dis 1975; 17:259.
2. Anderson FA, Wheeler HB, Goldberg RJ, et al: A population-based perspective of the hospital incidence and case-fatality rates of deep vein thrombosis and pulmonary embolism. The Worcester DVT Study. Arch Intern Med 1991; 151:933.
3. Bell WR, Simon TL: Current status of pulmonary thromboembolic disease: Pathophysiology, diagnosis, prevention, and treatment. Am Heart J 1982; 103:239.
4. Morrell MP, Dunhill MS: The post-mortem incidence of pulmonary embolism in a hospital population. Br J Surg 1968; 55:347.
5. Moser KM: Venous thromboembolism. Am Rev Respir Dis 1990; 141:235.
6. Coon WW, Willis PW, Keller JB: Thromboembolism and other venous disease in the Tecumseh Community Health Study. Circulation 1978; 48:839.
7. Lindblad B, Sternby NH, Bergqvist D: Incidence of venous thromboembolism verified by necropsy over 30 years. BMJ 1991; 302:709.
8. Carter CJ, Anderson FA, Wheeler HB: Epidemiology and pathophysiology of venous thromboembolism. *In:* Venous Thromboembolism: An Evidence-Based Atlas. Hull RD, Raskob GE, Pineo GF (Eds). Armonk, NY, Futura Publishers, 1996, pp 3–20.
9. Hyers TN, Hull RD, Weg JG: Antithrombotic therapy for venous thromboembolic disease. Chest 1992; 102:391S.
10. Hull RD, Secker-Walker RH, Hirsh J: Diagnosis of deep vein thrombosis. *In:* Hemostasis and Thrombosis. 2nd ed. Colman RW, Hirsh J, Marder VJ, Salzman EW (Eds). Philadelphia, JB Lippincott, 1987, p 1220.
11. Barritt DW, Jordon SC: Anticoagulant drugs in the treatment of pulmonary embolism: A controlled trial. Lancet 1960; 1:1309.
12. Donaldson GA, Williams C, Scannell JG, et al: A reappraisal of the application of the Trendelenburg operation to massive fatal embolism: Report of a successful pulmonary-artery thrombectomy using a cardiopulmonary bypass. N Engl J Med 1963; 268:171.
13. Dehring DJ, Arens JF: Pulmonary thromboembolism: Disease recognition and patient management. Anesthesiology 1990; 73:146.
14. Sevitt S, Gallagher NG: Venous thrombosis and pulmonary embolism: A clinicopathologic study in injured and burned patients. Br J Surg 1961; 48:475.
15. Hull RD, Delmore T, Genton E, et al: Warfarin sodium versus low-dose heparin in the long-term treatment of venous thrombosis. N Engl J Med 1979; 301:855.
16. Hull RD, Raskob GE, Pineo GF, et al: Subcutaneous low-molecular weight heparin compared with continuous intravenous heparin in the treatment of proximal-vein thrombosis. N Engl J Med 1992; 326:975.
17. Lensing AW, Prins MH, Davidson BL, et al: Treatment of deep venous thrombosis with low-molecular-weight heparins. Arch Intern Med 1995; 155:601.
18. PIOPED Investigators: Tissue plasminogen activator for the treatment of acute pulmonary embolism. Chest 1990; 97:528.
19. Goldhaber SZ, Morpurgo M: Diagnosis, treatment, and prevention of pulmonary embolism: Report of the WHO/International Society and Federation of Cardiology Task Force. JAMA 1992; 268:1727.
20. Goldhaber SZ: Recent advances in the diagnosis and lytic therapy of pulmonary embolism. Chest 1991; 99:173S.
21. Markel A, Manzo RA, Strandness E Jr: The potential role of thrombolytic therapy in venous thrombosis. Arch Intern Med 1992; 152:1265.
22. Molina JE, Hunter DW, Yedlicka JW, et al: Thrombolytic therapy for postoperative pulmonary embolism. Am J Surg 1992; 163:375.
23. The Urokinase Pulmonary Embolism Trial: A natural cooperative study. Circulation 1973; 47(Suppl II):II-1.
24. Tibbutt DA, Davies JA, Anderson JA, et al: Comparison by controlled clinical trial of streptokinase and heparin in treatment of life-threatening pulmonary embolism. BMJ 1974; 1:343.
25. Ly B, Arnesen H, Eie H, et al: A controlled clinical trial of streptokinase and heparin in the treatment of major pulmonary embolism. Acta Med Scand 1978; 203:465.
26. Levine M, Hirsh J, Weitz J, et al: A randomized trial of a single bolus dosage regimen of recombinant tissue plasminogen activator in patients with acute pulmonary embolism. Chest 1990; 98:1473.
27. Dalla-Volta S, Palla A, Santolicandro A, et al: PAIMS 2: Alteplase combined with heparin versus heparin in the treatment of acute pulmonary embolism: Plasminogen activator Italian multicenter study 2. J Am Coll Cardiol 1992; 20:520.
28. Goldhaber SZ, Haire WD, Feldstein ML, et al: Alteplase vs. heparin in acute pulmonary embolism: Randomised trial assessing right-ventricular function and pulmonary perfusion. Lancet 1993; 341:507.
29. Sharma GVRK, Burleson VA, Sasahara AA: Effect of thrombolytic therapy on pulmonary-capillary blood volume in patients with pulmonary embolism. N Engl J Med 1980; 303:842.
30. Sharma GVRK, Folland ED, McIntyre KM, et al: Long-term hemodynamic benefit of thrombolytic therapy in pulmonary embolic disease (Abstract). J Am Coll Cardiol 1990; 15:65A.
31. Urokinase-Streptokinase Embolism Trial: Phase 2 results. JAMA 1974; 229:1606.
32. The UKEP Study Research Group: The UKEP study: Multicentre clinical trial on two local regimens of urokinase in massive pulmonary embolism. Eur Heart J 1987; 8:2.
33. Verstraete M, Miller GAH, Bounameaux H, et al: Intravenous and intrapulmonary recombinant tissue-type plasminogen activator in the treatment of acute massive pulmonary embolism. Circulation 1988; 77:353.
34. Bolus Alteplase Pulmonary Embolism Group: Reduced dose bolus alteplase vs. conventional alteplase infusion for pulmonary embolism thrombolysis. Chest 1994; 106:718.
35. Goldhaber SZ, Kessler CM, Heit JA, et al: Recombinant tissue-type plasminogen activator versus a novel dosing regimen of urokinase in acute pulmonary embolism: A randomized controlled multicenter trial. J Am Coll Cardiol 1992; 20:24.
36. Goldhaber SZ, Kessler CM, Heit J, et al: Randomized controlled trial of recombinant tissue plasminogen activator versus urokinase in the treatment of acute pulmonary embolism. Lancet 1988; 2:293.
37. Werier J, Ducas J, Gu S, et al: Effect of low-molecular-weight heparin on recombinant tissue plasminogen activator–induced thrombolysis in canine pulmonary embolism. Chest 1991; 100:464.
38. Elliott CG: Thrombolytic therapy for acute pulmonary embolism: Can mortality be decreased? Clin Appl Thromb Hemost 1997; 3:S32.
39. Meaney JFM, Weg JH, Chenevert TL, et al: Diagnosis of pulmonary embolism with magnetic resonance angiography. N Engl J Med 1997; 336:1422.
40. Goodman LR, Curtin JJ, Mewissen MW, et al: Detection of pulmonary embolism in patients with unresolved clinical and scinti-

graphic diagnosis: Helical CT vs. angiography. AJR Am J Roentgenol 1995; 164:1369.
41. Layish DT, Tapson VF: New imaging techniques for the diagnosis of pulmonary embolism. Curr Opin Pulm Med 1997; 3:280.
42. Kanter DS, Mikkola KM, Patel SR: Thrombolytic therapy for pulmonary embolism. Chest 1997; 111:1241.
43. Levine MN, Goldhaber SZ, Califf RM, et al: Hemorrhagic complications of thrombolytic therapy in the treatment of myocardial infarction and venous thromboembolism. Chest 1992; 102:364S.
44. Anderson DR, Levine MN: Thrombolytic therapy for the treatment of acute pulmonary embolism. Can Med Assoc J 1992; 146:1317.
45. Goldhaber SZ: Evolving concepts in thrombolytic therapy for pulmonary embolism. Chest 1992; 101:183S.
46. Goldhaber SZ: Pulmonary embolism thrombolysis: A clarion call for international collaboration. J Am Coll Cardiol 1992; 19:246.
47. Collins R, Scrimgeour A, Yusuf S, et al: Reduction of fatal pulmonary embolism and venous thrombosis by perioperative administration of subcutaneous heparin. N Engl J Med 1988; 318:1162.
48. Lilienfeld DE, Chan E, Ehland J, et al: Mortality from pulmonary embolism in the United States: 1962–1984. Chest 1990; 98:1067.
49. del Campo C: Pulmonary embolectomy: A review. Can J Surg 1985; 28:111.
50. Sasahara AA, Sharma GVRK, Barsamian EM, et al: Pulmonary thromboembolism: Diagnosis and treatment. JAMA 1983; 249:2945.
51. Meyer G, Tamisier D, Sors H, et al: Pulmonary embolectomy: A 20-year experience at one centre. Ann Thorac Surg 1991; 51:232.
52. Mattox KL, Feldtman RW, Geall AC, et al: Pulmonary embolectomy for acute pulmonary embolism. Ann Surg 1982; 195:726.
53. Bauer EP, Laske A, von Segesser LK, et al: Early and late results after surgery for massive pulmonary embolism. Thorac Cardiovasc Surg 1991; 39:353.
54. Clarke DB, Abrams LD: Pulmonary embolectomy: A 25 year experience. J Thorac Cardiovasc Surg 1986; 92:442.
55. Kieny R, Charpentier A, Kieny MT: What is the place of pulmonary embolectomy today? J Cardiovasc Surg 1991; 32:549.
56. Schmid C, Zietlow S, Wagner TOF, et al: Fulminant pulmonary embolism: Symptoms, diagnostics, operative technique, and results. Ann Thorac Surg 1991; 52:1102.
57. Satter P: Pulmonary embolectomy with the aid of extracorporeal circulation. Thorac Cardiovasc Surg 1982; 30:31.
58. Gray HH, Miller GAH, Paneth M: Pulmonary embolectomy: Its place in the management of pulmonary embolism. Lancet 1988; 1:1441.
59. Brown S, Mulder D, Buckberg G: Massive pulmonary hemorrhagic infarction. Arch Surg 1974; 108:795.
60. Greenfield LJ, Langham MR: Surgical approaches to thromboembolism. Br J Surg 1984; 71:968.
61. Greenfield LJ: Vena caval interruption and pulmonary embolectomy. Clin Chest Med 1984; 5:495.
62. Greenfield LJ, Cho KJ, Proctor MC: Late results of suprarenal Greenfield vena cava filter placement. Arch Surg 1992; 127:969.
63. Timsit J-F, Reynaud P, Meyer G, et al: Pulmonary embolectomy by catheter device in massive pulmonary embolism. Chest 1991; 100:655.
64. Ponomar E, Carlson JE, Kindlund A, et al: Clot trapper device for transjugular thrombectomy from the inferior vena cava. Radiology 1991; 179:279.
65. Greenfield LJ: Evolution of venous interruption for pulmonary thromboembolism. Arch Surg 1992; 127:622.
66. Brady AJB, Crake T, Oakley CM: Percutaneous catheter fragmentation and distal dispersion of proximal pulmonary embolus. Lancet 1991; 338:1186.
67. Essop MR, Middlemost S, Skoularigis J, et al: Simultaneous mechanical clot fragmentation and pharmacologic thrombolysis in massive pulmonary embolism. Am J Cardiol 1992; 69:427.
68. Stein PD, Sabbah HN, Basha MA, et al: Mechanical disruption of pulmonary emboli in dogs with a flexible rotating-tip catheter (Kensey catheter). Chest 1990; 98:995.
69. Schmitz-Rode T, Günther RW: New device for percutaneous fragmentation of pulmonary emboli. Radiology 1991; 180:135.
70. Miles RM: Clinical evaluation of the serrated vena caval clip. Surg Gynecol Obstet 1971; 132:581.
71. Adams JT, DeWeese JA. Experimental and clinical evaluation of partial vein interruption in the prevention of pulmonary emboli. Surgery 1965; 57:82.
72. King JN, Champlin AM, Ashby RN: Vena cava filters. West J Med 1992; 156:295.
73. Becker DM, Philbrick JT, Selby JB: Inferior vena cava filters: Indications, safety, effectiveness. Arch Intern Med 1992; 152:1985.
74. Grassi CJ: Inferior vena caval filters: Analysis of five currently available devices. AJR Am J Roentgenol 1991; 156:813.
75. Thery C, Asseman P, Amrouni N, et al: Use of a new removable vena cava filter in order to prevent pulmonary embolism in patients submitted to thrombolysis. Eur Heart J 1990; 11:334.
76. Pacouret G, Alison D, Pottier JM, et al: Free-floating thrombus and embolic risk in patients with angiographically confirmed proximal deep venous thrombosis. Arch Intern Med 1997; 157:305.
77. Baldridge ED, Martin MA, Welling RE: Clinical significance of free-floating venous thrombi. J Vasc Surg 1990; 11:62–69.
78. Decousus H, Leizorovicz A, Parent F, et al: A clinical trial of vena caval filters in the prevention of pulmonary embolism in patients with proximal deep vein thrombosis. N Engl J Med 1998; 338:409.
79. Hull RD, Raskob GE, Rosenbloom D, et al: Optimal therapeutic level of heparin therapy in patients with venous thrombosis. Arch Intern Med 1992; 152:1589.
80. Salzman EW. Low molecular weight heparin and other antithrombotic drugs. N Engl J Med 1992; 326:1017.

102

Severe Heart Failure in Cardiomyopathy: Pathogenesis and Treatment

Clifford J. Kavinsky, MD, PhD • Joseph E. Parrillo, MD

The cardiomyopathies are a heterogeneous group of disorders, most often of unclear etiology, manifested as heart failure due to intrinsic disease of the cardiac muscle. The disease process is generally diffuse in character, involving all cardiac chambers. Chamber involvement is not necessarily uniform, however, and one chamber may display more extensive disease involvement than others. As a result, heart failure, the sine qua non of cardiomyopathy, may be predominantly right sided, left sided, systolic, diastolic, or a mixture thereof.[1]

Because cardiac dysfunction is considered to be a consequence of a primary myocardial disease process, heart muscle impairment occurring as a result of coronary artery disease (ischemic), hypertension, valvular heart disease, congenital disorders, or diseases of the pericardium would by definition not be grouped under the cardiomyopathy disease classification. Indeed, these disorders must effectively be ruled out when the diagnosis of cardiomyopathy is being considered. A comprehensive clinical assessment, including a detailed history, physical examination, and judicious use of currently available diagnostic modalities (electrocardiography, chest radiography, radionuclide imaging, echocardiography, and cardiac catheterization with angiography), usually allows one to identify patients with cardiomyopathies and exclude patients with other disorders. Two-dimensional and Doppler echocardiography are extremely useful in identifying patients with structural abnormalities such as congenital defects and valvular lesions. Examination of ventricular wall thickness often provides clues concerning long-standing hypertension, and findings of regional wall-motion abnormalities or aneurysm suggest antecedent ischemic heart disease. Myocardial perfusion imaging may provide evidence for myocardial ischemia or previous infarction. Finally, cardiac catheterization with coronary angiography is believed by many to be an essential diagnostic component in excluding ischemic heart disease in patients with possible cardiomyopathy.

Cardiomyopathy has been classified using a number of different methods.[1, 2] The most commonly used, that adopted by the World Health Organization (WHO), refers to cardiomyopathies as diseases solely affecting heart muscle and lacking a clearly identifiable cause.[3] Other systemic illnesses of known cause (e.g., amyloidosis, muscular dystrophy) affecting the heart would not be referred to as cardiomyopathy but, rather, as *specific heart muscle diseases* despite a clinical presentation indistinguishable from cardiomyopathy.[4] Many refer to sole cardiac muscle dysfunction of unknown cause as *idiopathic* or *primary* cardiomyopathy and that due to specific disease affecting the heart in a manner consistent with a cardiomyopathic profile as *secondary* cardiomyopathy. Such a classification scheme is both useful and appropriate because it has important pathophysiologic, prognostic, and therapeutic implications.

The WHO classification scheme describes three general categories of cardiomyopathy based on clinical, structural, functional, and hemodynamic criteria (Fig. 102–1). *Dilated cardiomyopathy*, by far the most common form, is characterized by ventricular dilatation, impairment of systolic function as evidenced by a markedly reduced left ventricular ejection fraction, and often a clinical picture of congestive heart failure (Table 102–1).

Distinguishing features of *restrictive cardiomyopathy* include normal left ventricular cavity dimensions, normal or only mildly reduced systolic function, and markedly reduced ventricular compliance, often leading to signs and symptoms of biventricular heart failure. Restrictive cardiomyopathy exhibits many similarities to pericardial constriction, and differentiating the two disorders can often be difficult.

The third category of cardiomyopathy is the *hypertrophic* form, which is due to inappropriate left ventricular hypertrophy. The hypertrophic form often involves the interventricular septum, leading to decreased compliance and impaired diastolic function. Septal hypertrophy in some cases may lead to a dynamic form of left ventricular outflow tract obstruction owing to contact between the anterior mitral valve leaflet and the hypertrophied septum, thus obstructing left ventricular outflow. This phenomenon may also be associated with systolic anterior motion of the mitral valve. Left ventricular cavity dimensions are usually normal or reduced with vigorous systolic function until late in the course of the disease. Most experts in the field believe that the cause of heart failure in hypertrophic cardiomyopathy relates more to impairment of ventricular diastolic relaxation (lusitropy) and decreased compliance rather than left ventricular dynamic outflow tract obstruction.[5]

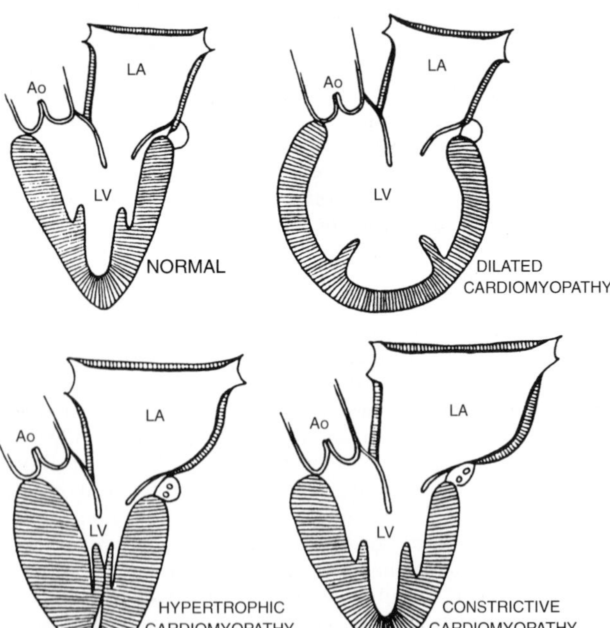

Figure 102–1. Schematic diagrams of the normal ventricle and the three types of cardiomyopathies. Table 102-1 also compares these different cardiomyopathies. (From Roberts WR, Ferrans VJ: Myocardial observations in cardiomyopathies. *In*: Myocardial Diseases. Fowler NO [Ed]. New York, Grune & Stratton, 1973.)

As can be seen in Table 102–1, the classification scheme for the cardiomyopathies is far from arbitrary and highlights structural and hemodynamic differences that must be understood in order to evaluate and treat such patients properly, particularly when the clinical presentation is one of high acuity and hemodynamic instability. Patients with cardiomyopathy are generally treated as outpatients for chronic heart failure.

Patients admitted to an intensive care unit (ICU) usually fall into two general categories. First, they may present with an acute exacerbation of heart failure, in which case it is incumbent on the critical care physician to identify both the cause of the patient's underlying chronic heart failure and the precipitating event leading to further deterioration of heart function. Such clinical information is essential for the intensivist in order to initiate effective treatment. The wrong therapeutic decision in a critically ill patient could yield disastrous results. Second, the patient may be admitted to the ICU in critical condition after a noncardiac illness has occurred. Such patients have unique management needs that must be anticipated by the critical care physician.

Whether because of increased physician awareness, improved diagnostic techniques, or a true increase in disease incidence, the number of hospitalizations and deaths attributed to cardiomyopathy is increasing.[6] The annual incidence of cardiomyopathy ranges from 0.7 to 7.5 cases per 100,000 population in developed countries.[1] In the present health care environment, in which cost-containment issues are assuming greater importance, proper recognition and treatment of cardiomyopathies and heart failure in the critical care setting are vital to optimizing outcome and efficiently using intensive care resources. This chapter reviews clinical, pathophysiologic, and diagnostic features of the cardiomyopathies. The management of patients with end-stage cardiomyopathies in an ICU is also addressed. In addition, newer therapeutic modalities, including pharmacologic and surgical interventions, are discussed, with an emphasis on improving symptoms and long-term survival.

USE OF ENDOMYOCARDIAL BIOPSY

Since Kono and Sakakibara introduced the percutaneous, transvenous technique for obtaining myocardial biopsy samples in 1962, physicians have realized that cardiac tissue samples can be obtained from patients with heart failure in a safe, nonsurgical manner.[7] The technique of transvenous endomyocardial biopsy (TEB) uses a specially designed catheter with small (1 to 2 mm in diameter), sharp-edged, cup-like forceps situated on the end and controlled by manipulation of a scissors handle at the opposite end. The biopsy catheter is introduced via a sheath situated in the femoral or internal jugular vein and, using fluoroscopic or echocardiographic guidance, is advanced to the right ventricular side of the

TABLE 102–1. Classification of the Cardiomyopathies

			Hypertrophic	
	Dilated	**Restrictive**	***Nonobstructive***	***Obstructive***
Left ventricular end-diastolic pressure	↑↑	↑↑	↑↑	↑↑
Left ventricular end-diastolic volume	↑↑	nl or ↓	nl or ↓	nl or ↓
Diastolic compliance	↑	↓↓	↓↓	↓↓
Left ventricular ejection fraction	↓↓	nl or ↑ ↓ late	nl or ↑ ↓ late	nl, ↓, ↑
Echocardiography	↑↑ LV dimension ↓↓ Ventricular systolic function AV valve regurgitation	nl or ↓ LV dimension nl Ventricular systolic function ↑ LV wall thickness and mass	nl or ↓ LV dimension nl or ↑ Ventricular systolic function Localized ↑ LV wall thickness (septum)	LV outflow tract obstruction Systolic anterior motion of mitral valve Mitral regurgitation

AV = atrioventricular; nl = normal; LV = left ventricle; ↑ = slightly increased; ↓ = slightly decreased; ↑↑ = greatly increased; ↓↓ = greatly decreased.

intraventricular septum, where multiple samples are taken (Fig. 102–2). Tissue thus obtained can then be prepared for routine histologic examination by light and electron microscopy as well as for application of immunochemical and molecular biology techniques.

In its original application, TEB was used largely to perform serial histologic evaluation of heart transplant recipients as a means of monitoring allograft rejection and the response to immunosuppressive therapy. This remains the most common and agreed-on indication for routine use of TEB. Endomyocardial biopsy is also extremely useful for monitoring the cardiotoxic effects of anthracycline chemotherapeutic agents. Endomyocardial biopsy has gained widespread use as an effective means for the diagnosis of myocarditis, particularly in patients with recent onset of symptoms of heart failure. Establishing myocarditis on biopsy specimens has been hindered in the past by interobserver variability, a lack of uniform guidelines in establishing the histologic diagnosis, and the frequently focal nature of the myocarditic process. Adoption of histologic

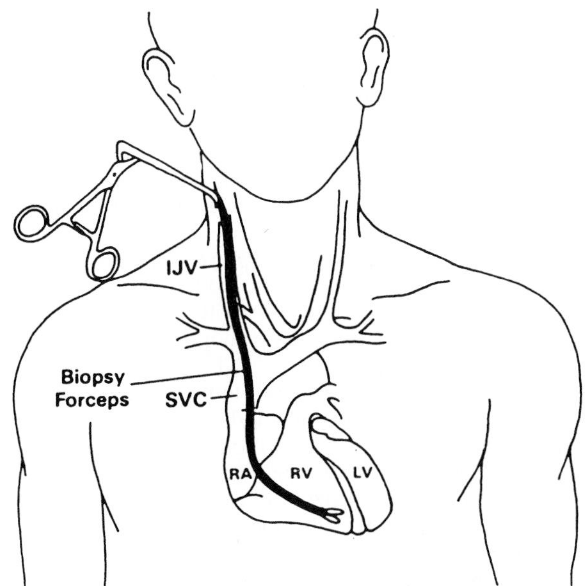

Figure 102–2. Schematic drawing of the right internal jugular vein (IJV) approach to transvenous endomyocardial biopsy of the right ventricle (RV). SVC = superior vena cava; RA = right atrium; LV = left ventricle.

grading using the Dallas criteria has helped standardize the diagnostic features of myocarditis; however, true knowledge of the value of biopsy requires prospective follow-up of a large number of patients with defined histologic myocardial inflammation.[8] The spectrum of specific diagnoses that can be established through use of TEB is summarized in Table 102–2.

The TEB can be an extremely useful diagnostic tool for evaluating and classifying patients with cardiomyopathy. Two studies examining patients with restrictive cardiomyopathy using TEB resulted in specific diagnoses, most often amyloidosis, in a substantial proportion.[9, 10] Such information also assisted in differentiating restrictive cardiomyopathy from pericardial constriction. In this manner, TEB data aided in avoiding more invasive surgical procedures, guiding future diagnostic testing, and providing important prognostic information allowing for initiation of specific therapy.

The capacity for TEB to provide useful clinical diagnostic information has been further demonstrated in 100 consecutive patients referred for TEB for heart failure of undetermined cause.[11] The biopsies were performed to establish or preclude a potential specific cause of dilated (74%) or restrictive (26%) cardiomyopathy. Figure 102–3 summarizes the diagnostic results from these 100 consecutive heart biopsies. The pathologic diagnostic information obtained was judged to be useful in clinical decision making in 54 of these 100 patients.

More recently, the widespread application of TEB to patients with cardiomyopathy and unexplained heart failure has been disputed, particularly with respect to patients with di-

TABLE 102–2. Specific Diagnoses Made by Endomyocardial Biopsy

Cardiac allograft rejection	Cardiac tumors of cardiac origin
Myocarditis	Cardiac tumors of noncardiac origin
Giant-cell myocarditis	Kearns-Sayre syndrome
Doxorubicin cardiotoxicity	Cytomegalovirus infection
Cardiac amyloidosis	Toxoplasmosis
Cardiac sarcoidosis	Henoch-Schönlein purpura
Cardiac hemochromatosis	Rheumatic carditis
Endocardial fibrosis	Chagasic cardiomyopathy
Endocardial fibroelastosis	Chloroquine cardiomyopathy
Fabry's disease of the heart	Lyme carditis
Carcinoid disease	Carnitine deficiency cardiomyopathy
Irradiation injury	Right ventricular lipomatosis
Glycogen storage disease	Hypereosinophilic syndrome

From Mason JW, O'Connell JB: Clinical merit of endomyocardial biopsy. Circulation 1989; 79:971.

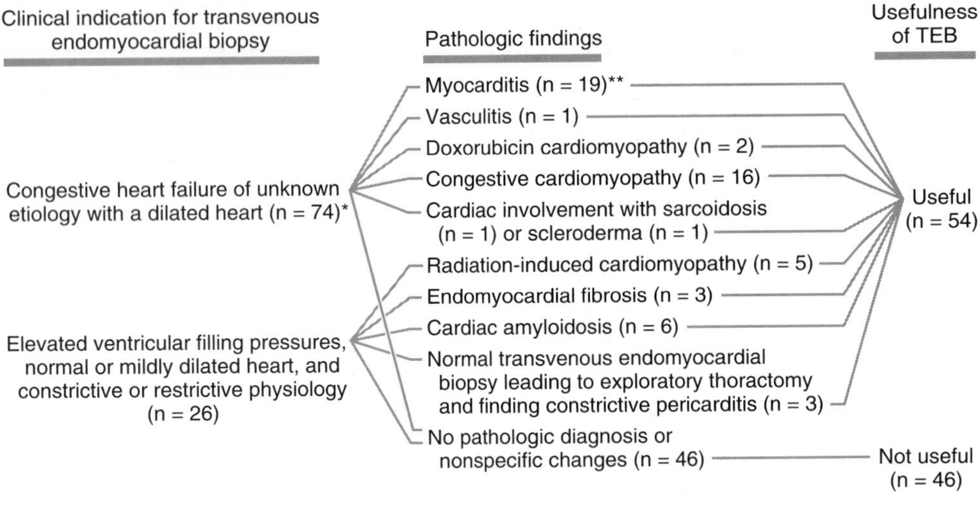

Figure 102–3. Flow diagram of the clinical indication, pathologic findings, and clinical usefulness of transvenous endomyocardial biopsy (TEB) in 100 patients. (From Parrillo JE, Aretz HT, Palacios I, et al: The results of transvenous endomyocardial biopsy can frequently be used to diagnose myocardial diseases in patients with idiopathic heart failure: Endomyocardial biopsies in 100 consecutive patients revealed a substantial incidence of myocarditis. Circulation 1984; 69:93.)

*Numbers in parentheses refer to the number of patients.

**Three patients had two diagnoses: one patient had amyloidosis and myocarditis, one patient had endomyocardial fibrosis with eosinophilic myocarditis, and one patient had vasculitis and myocarditis, so that the number of patients or indications totals 100 and the number of pathologic findings totals 103.

lated cardiomyopathy of long duration.[12] Critics of TEB argue that the yield of specific diagnostic information leading to effective therapy that improves outcome is low. It is our opinion that patients with new onset of unexplained heart failure should be considered for TEB in addition to the conventional diagnostic tests discussed previously. Numerous studies report a significant incidence of active myocarditis in patients with idiopathic dilated cardiomyopathy.[13, 14] In the previously described study of 100 patients referred for TEB for unexplained heart failure, 26% presented evidence of myocarditis (see Fig. 102–3). Certain subgroups of such patients may benefit from immunosuppressive therapy and would thus require TEB in order to identify this subset with inflammatory cardiomyopathy. In addition, cardiac biopsy also allows diagnosis of a number of other specific causes of cardiomyopathy (see Table 102–2).

TABLE 102–3. Probable and Possible Causes of Dilated Cardiomyopathy

Idiopathic Dilated Cardiomyopathy	***Metabolic/Nutritional***
Inflammatory/Myocarditis	Uremia
Infectious	Hemochromatosis
Enterovirus	Carnitine deficiency
Human immunodeficiency virus	Selenium deficiency
Toxoplasma gondii	Thiamine deficiency
Trypanosoma cruzi	Electrolyte derangements
Trichinella spiralis	***Endocrine***
Noninfectious	Thyroid disease
Transplantation rejection	Cushing's disease
Autoimmune disease	Pheochromocytoma
Pregnancy	***Hereditary***
Sarcoid	Neuromyopathic disorders
Toxic	Familial cardiomyopathy
Alcohol	***Miscellaneous***
Catecholamines	Coronary microvascular spasm
Cocaine	Decreased coronary flow reserve
Anthracycline drugs	
5-Fluorouracil	
Azidothymidine	

DILATED CARDIOMYOPATHY

Clinical and Diagnostic Findings

Dilated cardiomyopathy is myocardial disease manifested as cardiac chamber dilatation with impairment of systolic function of one or both ventricles.[15] A multitude of widely divergent inflammatory, infectious, toxic, metabolic, hereditary, and vascular disorders are associated with development of dilated cardiomyopathy (Table 102–3). However, despite the diverse causes of this disorder, many and perhaps most cases do not have a clear discernible cause and are termed *idiopathic*, although up to 25% of cases may be inherited. It is thought that dilated cardiomyopathy may represent the final common pathway, resulting as a consequence of chronic recurrent myocardial damage from a wide variety of insults (Fig. 102–4).

Most patients present with heart failure. Ventricular arrhythmias may be the sole initial presentation in a small group of patients. Another presentation of cardiomyopathy is the unexpected finding of cardiomegaly on a patient's chest radiograph that was obtained for another indication. Subsequent cardiac evaluation documents a dilated, hypocontractile ventricle. Such patients eventually have symptoms related to dilated cardiomyopathy, although it may take months or years. The overall prognosis for patients with dilated cardiomyopathy is considered later.

Patients presenting with heart failure usually complain of symptoms related to low cardiac output, such as weakness, fatigue, and decreasing exercise tolerance. Shortness of breath, dyspnea on exertion, and orthopnea appear as pulmonary vascular congestion develops. Symptoms related to right heart failure, such as increasing abdominal girth and peripheral edema, generally appear late and connote a poor prognosis. Chest pain is observed in 25% to 50% of patients with idiopathic dilated cardiomyopathy. It is believed that decreased coronary flow reserve leading to subendocardial ischemia may be partly responsible for angina-type chest pain in these patients.[16]

On physical examination, patients may demonstrate generalized wasting and pallor if the cardiomyopathy has been protracted. The systolic blood pressure may be low, with a narrow pulse pressure and pulsus alternans. Wheezing due to bronchospasm and engorgement of the bronchial vessels, as well

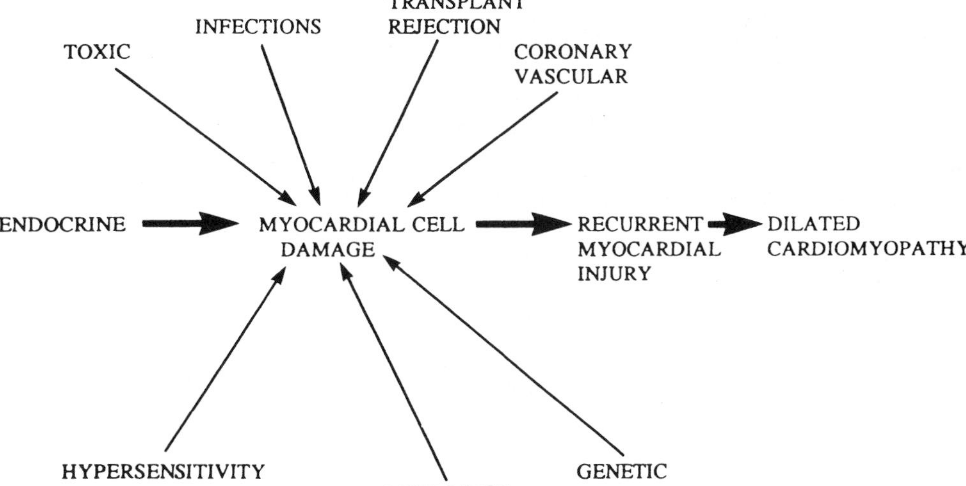

Figure 102–4. A schematic drawing summarizing the different pathways that lead to chronic myocardial injury and dilated cardiomyopathy.

as moist rales, is often noted on pulmonary examination of patients with decompensated heart failure. Pleural effusion, most often on the right side, may be detected as dullness to percussion. The apical impulse is displaced laterally. Heart sounds are often diminished, with an S_3 gallop noted at the apex. A murmur of mitral regurgitation due to left ventricular dilatation leading to nonapposition of mitral leaflets is frequently audible. With right heart dilation and failure, jugular venous distention with prominent a and v waves is present. The liver may be tender, enlarged, and pulsatile, with demonstrable hepatojugular reflux. Ascites and peripheral edema are usually found.

The heart failure of dilated cardiomyopathy is caused by a severe reduction in ventricular systolic function. Ejection fraction, a reliable measure of systolic function, is decreased (<40% to 45%) owing to impairment of contractility. Cardiac output is maintained by augmentation of heart rate and preload. Ventricular dilatation is thought to represent a compensatory response leading to increased preload and optimization of Starling forces.

A chest radiograph reveals generalized cardiomegaly and signs of pulmonary vascular hypertension. Kerley's lines, peribronchial cuffing, and interstitial and alveolar edema can also be seen. Pleural effusions are often present. The electrocardiogram may demonstrate sinus tachycardia as well as atrial or ventricular tachyarrhythmias. Conduction disturbances including atrioventricular block and bundle branch block are associated findings. Loss of anterior R-wave forces and the presence of Q waves may resemble ischemic heart disease. ST-segment and T-wave abnormalities are the rule, and P-wave changes consistent with left atrial enlargement may be noted. Twenty-four-hour Holter monitoring reveals ventricular arrhythmias, with approximately 50% of patients demonstrating nonsustained ventricular tachycardia.

Two-dimensional and Doppler echocardiography are extremely useful and gaining widespread application in the evaluation and follow-up of patients with dilated cardiomyopathy. Ventricular chamber dilatation is always present with a left ventricular end-diastolic diameter exceeding 2.7 cm/m^2. Ventricular wall thickness is normal or thin with global hypokinesis, with or without regional variation, and associated with percentage fractional shortening of less than 30%. Intracavitary thrombi may be present, usually at the apex. Doppler studies may reveal mitral or tricuspid regurgitation with pulmonary hypertension. Radionuclide ventriculography generally reveals increased end-diastolic and end-systolic volumes and diminished left ventricular ejection fraction. The right ventricle may also manifest chamber dilatation and reduced ejection fraction. Although involvement of the right ventricle is considered common in dilated cardiomyopathy, it is not always involved, and right ventricular involvement is not a reliable indicator of this disease.

Heart failure is commonly confirmed hemodynamically by the presence of elevated filling pressures, either by placement of a flow-directed pulmonary artery catheter in the ICU or during cardiac catheterization. Dilated cardiomyopathy produces a decreased stroke volume and increased left ventricular end-diastolic pressure. Mean left atrial pressure and pulmonary capillary wedge pressure (PCWP) are elevated to a degree corresponding to the extent of impairment of left ventricular systolic performance. Chronic elevation of left heart pressures may lead to moderate pulmonary vascular hypertension. Elevation of right ventricular end-diastolic and right atrial pressures signals the presence of right ventricular failure. Large v waves may be noted in the pulmonary capillary wedge tracing in patients with mitral regurgitation. In most patients with dilated cardiomyopathy, the resting cardiac output is normal or slightly decreased. Coronary angiography reveals no evidence of significant coronary artery disease. Contrast left ventriculography demonstrates global hypokinesia, sometimes with segmental wall-motion abnormalities, chamber enlargement, decreased ejection fraction, and often mitral regurgitation.

Histologic examination of myocardial tissue specimens obtained either at autopsy or by TEB generally reveals areas of interstitial and perivascular fibrosis as well as myocyte degeneration.[17] Small focal areas of mononuclear cell infiltrate are often observed along with various degrees of myocyte hypertrophy.[18]

Etiology and Natural History

When evaluating a patient with probable dilated cardiomyopathy, one should consider the specific diagnoses reviewed in Table 102–3. In most patients, however, a clear etiologic mechanism is not identifiable, and the cardiomyopathy is thus referred to as idiopathic. As previously mentioned, many investigators believe that dilated cardiomyopathy represents the end result of chronic recurrent myocardial insult due to a broad spectrum of causes (see Fig. 102–4). Dilated cardiomyopathy may result from (1) myocardial inflammation due to viral infection (coxsackievirus B, echovirus, influenza, human immunodeficiency virus [HIV]), (2) myocardial toxin (diphtheria), (3) radiation, (4) pharmacologic agents (doxorubicin [Adriamycin], azidothymidine), (5) metabolic disorders, or (6) autoimmune collagen vascular disorders.

Most bouts of myocardial inflammation due to any cause result in a self-limited illness that resolves. However, a small number of cases lead to immediate heart failure, or after a latent period, recurrent injury may lead to the late development of congestive heart failure and cardiomyopathy. Indeed, numerous studies of patients with dilated cardiomyopathy report biopsy evidence of myocarditis in a significant number of patients.[11, 13] Furthermore, enterovirus ribonucleic acid (RNA) has been detected in myocardial biopsy specimens from patients with congestive cardiomyopathy using gene amplification by polymerase chain reaction.[19] Similarly, as many as 46% of patients with acquired immunodeficiency syndrome (AIDS) are found to have histologic evidence of myocarditis at necropsy.[20]

Finally, biopsy specimens from patients with peripartum cardiomyopathy have revealed evidence of myocarditis in as many as 78%, further suggesting an acute inflammatory mechanism in this disorder.[21] Virus-induced myocardial inflammation injury may be mediated by various mechanisms, including virus-mediated cell lysis and humoral and cell-mediated autoimmunity directed against both normal myocytes (through shared epitopes) and virus-infected cardiac cells expressing structurally altered antigens or neoantigens, resulting in the development of a cardiomyopathic profile. Toxin-mediated myocardial cell injury may result in alteration of myocyte molecules, leading to formation of neoantigens to which the humoral and cell-mediated arms of the immune system respond. In addition, derangements in immune function have been reported in patients with dilated cardiomyopathy. Certain human leukocyte antigens, specifically HLA-DR4, have been shown to be significantly more common in patients with dilated cardiomyopathy. Reduced suppressor and increased helper/inducer T cell subsets have been found in these patients.[22-24] Autoantibodies directed against cardiac tissue in general and the surface β-adrenoceptor in particular have been found in the sera of patients with dilated cardiomyopathy and may be partly responsible for immune-mediated injury in this illness.[25, 26]

Besides immunologic mechanisms, other molecular mediators of impairment of cardiac performance in patients with dilated cardiomyopathy have been reported. These include structural and functional alterations in the myosin heavy and light chains as well as other myofibrillar proteins,[27] abnormalities in intracellular calcium handling, decreased density and responsiveness of myocardial β-adrenoceptors,[28, 29] and alterations in the levels of the stimulatory and inhibitory subpopulations of regulatory guanine nucleotide-binding proteins.[30, 31]

Patients with idiopathic dilated cardiomyopathy generally present with symptoms secondary to heart failure, dysrhythmias, or thromboembolic phenomena. An asymptomatic patient is occasionally identified by the finding of impaired or dilated ventricles on routine diagnostic testing. Numerous retrospective studies have served to define the natural history of this disorder as well as the prognostic factors associated with increased mortality.[32-35]

Mortality rates for idiopathic dilated cardiomyopathy are approximately 20% per year, with a 5-year mortality of 50% to 75%. In a well-defined population of 169 patients with dilated cardiomyopathy, 1- and 5-year mortality rates were 28% and 57%, respectively (Fig. 102–5).

The combination of progressive heart failure and sudden cardiac death accounts for the overwhelming majority of deaths. The 5-year point seems to define a subpopulation of patients with a more favorable long-term prognosis (see Fig. 102–5). These surviving patients, many of whom are alive

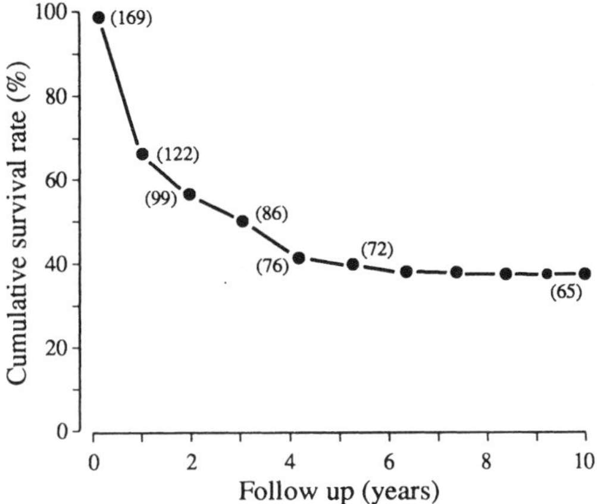

Figure 102–5. Ten-year survival curve of 169 patients with dilated cardiomyopathy. (From Diaz RA, Obasohan A, Oakley CM: Prediction of outcome in dilated cardiomyopathy. Br Heart J 1987; 58:393.)

after 10 years, generally have improvement in cardiac function to nearly normal. Thus, approximately 20% to 40% of patients with idiopathic dilated cardiomyopathy have a more favorable long-term survival, presumably because of improvement in cardiac function. Factors influencing survival in patients with idiopathic dilated cardiomyopathy (Table 102–4) generally reflect the severity of impairment in left ventricular performance and the presence of conduction abnormalities and ventricular dysrhythmias.

The presence of ventricular arrhythmias is associated with a significantly increased risk of cardiac death in general and sudden cardiac death in particular. Pooled data indicate that approximately 28% of the deaths occurring in patients with idiopathic dilated cardiomyopathy were sudden and presumably arrhythmic in character.[36] Various degrees of ventricular ectopy are noted in virtually all patients with idiopathic dilated cardiomyopathy. Nonsustained ventricular tachycardia is encountered in 35% to 83% of patients and seems to correlate with degree of left ventricular dysfunction.[37-39] Although ambulatory monitoring, electrophysiologic testing, signal-averaged electrocardiography, and monitoring of heart rate variability have aided in identifying many patients at higher risk for arrhythmic death, none of these diagnostic techniques has proved superior in detecting all patients who have dilated cardiomyopathy and who are at risk for sudden death.

Treatment

In patients with dilated cardiomyopathy, irreversible myocardial injury leading to impairment of systolic performance with

TABLE 102–4. Factors Associated with Increased Mortality in Dilated Cardiomyopathy

Increased filling pressures	Ventricular arrhythmias
Decreased ejection fraction	Intraventricular conduction delay
Mitral regurgitation	Hyponatremia
Decreased peak oxygen consumption	Presence of S_3
Increased age	Thallium 201 perfusion defects
Functional class	Requirement for permanent pacemaker
Requirement for intravenous inotropic support	Severity of myocardial biopsy findings
Elevated serum norepinephrine levels	

Data from Romeo F et al: Clin Cardiol 1989; 12:387; Saxon LA et al: Am J Cardiol 1993; 72:62; Diaz RA et al: Br Heart J 1987; 58:343; and Stevenson LW: Prog Cardiol 1989; 2:51.[32-34, 40]

resultant decrease in ejection fraction and mean arterial blood pressure sets into motion a series of compensatory mechanisms directed at maintaining cardiac output and tissue perfusion. Initially, diminished systolic function associated with enhanced ventricular compliance allows for increased end-diastolic volume with nearly normal end-diastolic pressure, resulting in optimization of preload and maintenance of stroke volume. With continued deterioration of cardiac function, optimal compliance and Starling forces are exceeded, leading to elevation in left ventricular end-diastolic and PCWP and resultant pulmonary edema. Annular dilatation leads to mitral regurgitation, further compromising forward stroke volume and exacerbating filling pressures. Reflex stimulation of the sympathetic nervous system tends to increase heart rate and systemic vascular resistance in an effort to maintain tissue perfusion. Systemic compensatory mechanisms, such as activation of the renin-angiotensin system and increased vasopressin secretion, lead to further fluid retention and vasoconstriction, which, though directed at maintaining mean arterial blood pressure, may worsen filling pressures, increase afterload, and result in increased wall stress, increased myocardial oxygen consumption, decreased stroke volume, and worsening mitral regurgitation. A cardiac index less than 2.5 L/min · m^2 and a left ventricular end-diastolic pressure greater than 27 mm Hg herald severe impairment of left ventricular function and a worse prognosis.[40]

The goals of therapy in idiopathic dilated cardiomyopathy are to improve symptoms related to heart failure and to prolong survival. In patients with decompensated heart failure in an ICU, therapy is directed at interrupting the vicious circle of progressive deterioration of cardiac function outlined earlier. The various medical and surgical therapeutic modalities currently used for patients with dilated cardiomyopathy are summarized in Table 102–5.

Diuretics and digitalis preparations together represent the most common agents used in the treatment of heart failure. Diuretics inhibit renal tubular solute reabsorption and induce salt and water excretion. The result is decreased intravascular volume, which reduces ventricular filling pressures and promotes resolution of pulmonary edema as well as signs of right-sided heart failure. Although potassium-sparing and thiazide diuretics can be effective, patients with significant decompensated heart failure usually require a loop diuretic. These drugs must be carefully titrated and given in doses sufficient to induce a brisk diuresis and reduction in filling pressures but without causing hypovolemia, prerenal azotemia, or compromise of cardiac output and mean systemic arterial pressure. In the refractory case, furosemide given as a continuous infusion can enhance urinary volume and sodium excretion with reduced toxic side-effects when compared with intermittent bolus injection.[41] Metolazone, a thiazide diuretic, may exert a synergistic diuretic effect when combined with a loop diuretic. Potassium and magnesium losses with such therapy can be substantial, and care must be taken to avoid hypokalemia and hypomagnesemia, which may contribute to digitalis toxicity and ventricular dysrhythmias. If a patient's potassium requirements remain high, a potassium-sparing diuretic, such as spironolactone, may attenuate potassium losses associated with other diuretics. Water restriction, particularly in the presence of hyponatremia, remains an important adjunct to diuretic therapy.

TABLE 102–5. Therapeutic Modalities in Dilated Cardiomyopathy

Diuretics
Digitalis glycosides
Vasodilators
Direct acting
Angiotensin-converting enzyme inhibitors
Inotropic agents
Beta-adrenergic blocking agents
Immunosuppressive agents
Anticoagulants
Antiarrhythmic therapy including implantable defibrillators
Cardiomyoplasty
Mechanical circulatory support devices
Heart transplantation
Ventricular reduction surgery

Digitalis glycosides have been used for more than 200 years for the management of congestive heart failure. Digitalis exerts both negative chronotropic and positive inotropic effects. Despite intensive debate that has spanned decades, digitalis preparations do appear to improve contractile function, augment left ventricular ejection fraction, and improve symptoms of heart failure.[42, 43] In patients with heart failure and atrial fibrillation with a rapid ventricular response, digoxin is extremely effective in slowing the heart rate, improving diastolic filling, and augmenting ventricular systolic function. Although digitalis preparations have been shown to improve systolic performance, symptoms of heart failure, and the need for hospitalization for treatment of heart failure, a survival benefit has not been demonstrated.[42] Nevertheless, digitalis remains a mainstay of therapy for patients with chronic congestive heart failure.

Vasodilators, both venous and arterial, can produce significant improvement in hemodynamics as well as in signs and symptoms of congestive heart failure by favorably decreasing preload and afterload. Such therapy decreases filling pressures and wall stress and augments ejection fraction, stroke volume, and cardiac output.[44] Critically ill patients with severe congestive heart failure refractory to conventional oral medications may be treated with intravenous nitroprusside or nitroglycerin with improvement in clinical and hemodynamic parameters but without altering survival.[45] In patients with chronic congestive heart failure, the combination of isosorbide dinitrate and hydralazine, when added to a conventional regimen of diuretics and digoxin, has been shown to improve left ventricular function and long-term survival.[46]

Angiotensin-converting enzyme (ACE) inhibitors have gained widespread use and have now become an essential part of all medical regimens for the treatment of chronic congestive heart failure. These drugs inhibit formation of angiotensin II and aldosterone and result in decreased systemic vascular resistance. Prospective randomized trials of the addition of enalapril to conventional therapy for heart failure have demonstrated improvement in signs and symptoms of heart failure as well as prolonged survival.[47, 48] The newly released angiotensin II type 1 receptor antagonists (i.e., losartan), which have been approved for use in the treatment of hypertension, are now being evaluated for the treatment of chronic heart failure either as (1) an alternative in patients intolerant of angiotensin-converting enzyme inhibitors due to cough, angioedema, renal dysfunction and hypotension or as (2) an adjunctive agent given to patients receiving ACE inhibitor therapy.[49] Preliminary clinical data suggest that these agents are well tolerated, have few adverse side effects necessitating discontinuance of therapy, and reveal a trend toward improved survival and reduced admissions to the hospital for exacerbation of heart failure.[50] At present, however, further prospective, randomized clinical trials are necessary before this class of agents can be routinely used in the treatment of chronic heart failure. Caution against the routine use of these drugs in place of conventional ACE inhibitors is warranted.

In addition to the angiotensin II receptor antagonists, clinical studies demonstrate that the dihydropyridine calcium channel blocker amlodipine may exert an additional benefit in reducing symptoms, improving exercise tolerance, and prolonging survival in patients with chronic nonischemic left ventricular dysfunction.[51] This issue remains unresolved and awaits completion of ongoing randomized trails.

Short-term administration of inotropic agents can produce sustained improvement in hemodynamic and clinical parameters in patients with dilated cardiomyopathy in severe congestive heart failure. Dobutamine, a β_1-selective sympathomimetic agent, has positive inotropic and vasodilating properties and is widely used for severely decompensated heart failure. The phosphodiesterase inhibitors amrinone and milrinone have hemodynamic effects similar to those of dobutamine.[52] In addition, chronic long-term intermittent infusion of intravenous inotropic agents may be of value in treating patients with severe congestive heart failure despite maximum medical therapy. Because both dobutamine and milrinone have been associated with excess mortality, we favor using intermittent infusions of these agents in a monitored setting.[53] Vesnarinone, another inotropic vasodilator agent, has also been shown to improve symptoms of congestive heart failure but has an adverse effect on survival.[54] Newer oral inotropic vasodilator agents such as coenzyme Q10, and pimobendan are currently being evaluated for the treatment of chronic congestive heart failure and dilated cardiomyopathy.[55, 56]

In 1975, Waagstein and colleagues reported beneficial effects of β-adrenergic blocking agents in patients with dilated cardiomyopathy, presumably by decreasing resting symptomatic tone and reversing the down-regulation of β-receptors produced by chronically elevated norepinephrine levels.[57] Widespread use of this therapy has been tempered by its potential to further suppress cardiac function owing to inherent negative inotropic effects. Even so, several large prospective clinical trials using carvedilol, a nonselective β-adrenergic receptor antagonist with α_1-blocking and antioxidant properties, have demonstrated favorable effects in diminishing the severity of symptoms, limiting progression of heart failure, and improving left ventricular function, filling pressures, and, most important, survival, when added to a conventional chronic heart failure medical regimen.[58, 59] This form of therapy needs to be initiated very slowly at low doses and titrated upward cautiously. Certain patients are intolerant of β-adrenergic blocker agents and may actually experience worsening of symptoms, necessitating discontinuation of therapy. Whether this form of therapy benefits patients hospitalized with acute onset of decompensated heart failure remains unknown and requires further study. Nonetheless, randomized trials in patients with idiopathic dilated cardiomyopathy have demonstrated that β-adrenergic blocker therapy decreases filling pressures and improves cardiac function and exercise tolerance. However, treatment with β-blockers has not yet been shown to improve survival, and their therapeutic role remains largely confined to symptomatic improvement in a subpopulation of patients with cardiomyopathy and resting tachycardia or only mild congestive heart failure.

The role of immunosuppressive agents in the treatment of idiopathic dilated cardiomyopathy is highly controversial. One prospective randomized trial of patients with idiopathic dilated cardiomyopathy and severe left ventricular dysfunction demonstrated a modest improvement in left ventricular ejection fraction in patients who had cellular infiltrates noted on myocardial biopsy and who were treated with prednisone.[60] Conversely, the myocarditis treatment trial found no benefit of immunosuppressive therapy on either left ventricular function or survival in patients with left ventricular dysfunction and biopsy-proven myocarditis.[61] Further study is required in this area, but it is likely that select patients with cardiomyopathy and a cellular infiltrate on myocardial biopsy have a myocardial inflammatory process that is responsive to immunosuppressive therapy.

Chronic anticoagulation in dilated cardiomyopathy is now widely advocated and is based on several retrospective studies suggesting an increased incidence of thromboembolic events in non-anticoagulated patients. The data are conflicting, however, and definitive resolution of this issue awaits a prospective randomized trial.[62] In the meantime, chronic warfarin administration in dilated cardiomyopathy should remain discretionary, and it is best prescribed for patients with severe atrial or ventricular dilatation, especially in the setting of atrial fibrillation.

Patients with symptomatic dilated cardiomyopathy have a 1-year mortality of 30% to 50%. Approximately half of these deaths are sudden and are believed to be secondary to malignant ventricular dysrhythmias. However, prospective identification of high-risk subsets of patients by diagnostic or clinical parameters has been disappointing. The risk of ventricular dysrhythmia and sudden death generally parallels the degree of left ventricular dysfunction. Electrolyte derangements, elevated catecholamine levels, and pharmacologic agents (such as diuretics or digoxin) can exacerbate ventricular arrhythmias in these patients.

Several published studies suggest that electrophysiologic testing may be useful in detecting patients at increased risk for sudden death.[36] In patients with documented spontaneous sustained or symptomatic monomorphic ventricular tachycardia or aborted sudden death due to ventricular tachycardia or fibrillation, amiodarone or placement of an automatic implantable cardioverter-defibrillator may reduce arrhythmic death.[63] Interestingly, amiodarone given to patients with severe heart failure improved survival independent of documented ventricular dysrhythmias.[64] However, its routine use in this setting remains controversial and necessitates further study. Conventional class Ia agents are generally contraindicated in these patients because of their significant negative inotropic and proarrhythmic effects. However, if antiarrhythmic drug therapy is used and renders a documented sustained monomorphic ventricular tachycardia noninducible on follow-up electrophysiologic testing, long-term survival is improved.[65]

For patients who have ejection fractions less than 25% and who are in severely decompensated heart failure despite maximal medical therapy, for patients with refractory ventricular dysrhythmias, and for patients dependent on intravenous inotropic agents or mechanical circulatory support devices, cardiac transplantation provides the only effective therapy for meaningful long-term survival. One- and 5-year post-transplant survival is approximately 80% and 60%, respectively. The major complications of this therapy are rejection, infection, and accelerated graft atherosclerosis. Mechanical circulatory support devices, such as ventricular assist devices and the total artificial heart, are being used in severely decompensated patients as a temporizing measure or as a bridge to transplantation. In addition, miniaturization of the power source components has allowed for the study of ventricular assist devices as permanent implants in patients who are not candidates for transplantation.

In patients who are not candidates for heart transplantation, the technique of cardiomyoplasty is being evaluated as a means of assisting cardiac function in severely impaired hearts. Several reports have demonstrated improvement in left ventricular function with a flap of synchronously contracting skeletal muscle wrapped around the failing heart.[66] Last, a new surgical technique (partial left ventriculectomy) involving resection of a wedge of myocardium, often in combination with a mitral valve replacement in an effort to reduce left ventricular chamber dimensions, has been shown in preliminary studies to increase left ventricular ejection fraction and to improve symptoms of heart failure in certain individuals as an alternative to heart transplantation.

RESTRICTIVE CARDIOMYOPATHY

Of the different forms of cardiomyopathy, restrictive cardiomyopathy is the least common. As depicted in Figure 102–1 and Table 102–1, patients with restrictive cardiomyopathy frequently present with congestive heart failure, a small or only mildly enlarged heart, and relatively preserved left ventricular systolic function. The mechanism of heart failure in restrictive cardiomyopathy is related to reduced ventricular compliance and impaired diastolic relaxation, resulting in restricted ventricular filling, high ventricular filling pressures, and reduced stroke volume despite normal systolic contractile function. The pathophysiologic mechanism leading to impaired diastolic function is related to decreased ventricular distensibility limiting diastolic filling as a result of morphologic alterations in the myocardium.

Hemodynamic measurements in restrictive cardiomyopathy reveal elevation of pulmonary and systemic venous pressures. The ventricular pressure tracing exhibits a characteristic rapid diastolic filling phase followed by an early plateau as the limits of ventricular compliance are reached (Fig. 102–6). This diastolic dip-and-plateau or square root sign is also seen in pericardial constriction, making differentiation between the two disorders difficult at times. The restriction to diastolic filling may also be noted at the atrial level, where pressures are elevated and characterized by prominent x- and y-descents. In patients with mild forms of the disease or in those whose intravascular volume is decreased secondary to diuretic therapy, the restrictive physiology described earlier may only be manifested after volume loading.

Most cases of restrictive cardiomyopathy are idiopathic. However, when evaluating a patient exhibiting restrictive physiology, one should keep in mind the secondary causes of restrictive cardiomyopathy listed in Table 102–6. Patients with restrictive cardiomyopathy generally report symptoms of dyspnea, fatigue, or chest pain.[67] Physical findings including jugular venous distention, rales, S_3 and S_4 heart sounds, ascites, and

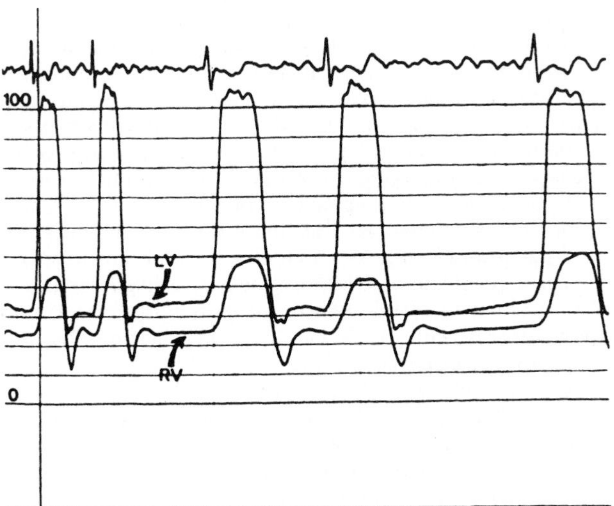

Figure 102–6. Simultaneous right and left ventricular pressure tracings from a patient with restrictive cardiomyopathy. Note the characteristic "dip-and-plateau" diastolic configuration. (From Hosenpud JD, Niles NR: Clinical, hemodynamic and endomyocardial biopsy findings in idiopathic restrictive cardiomyopathy. West J Med 1986; 144:303.)

TABLE 102–6. Classification of the Restrictive Cardiomyopathies

Primary (idiopathic)	Endomyocardial fibroelastosis
Secondary	Eosinophilic heart disease
Myocardial	Carcinoid
Amyloidosis	Radiation
Sarcoidosis	Cardiac transplant
Hemochromatosis	Anthracycline toxicity
Glycogen storage diseases	
Gaucher's disease	
Fabry's disease	
Tumor	

peripheral edema are common and due to biventricular failure. Echocardiography demonstrates small ventricular cavities with biatrial enlargement and normal or nearly normal ventricular systolic function. Atrioventricular valvular regurgitation is common. Late in the course of the disease, ventricular systolic function may deteriorate and the clinical picture may resemble that of a dilated cardiomyopathy.

In patients with suspected restrictive cardiomyopathy, pericardial constriction should be considered and effectively ruled out. Both conditions produce abnormal diastolic filling with high filling pressures and relatively spared systolic function, yet the treatment for these conditions is different. Constrictive pericarditis can be potentially cured by pericardiectomy, and restrictive cardiomyopathy can often be treated with tailored therapy directed at the underlying cause if known (e.g., amyloidosis, eosinophilic heart disease). A calcified pericardium seen on a lateral chest radiograph is suggestive of a constriction, whereas a speckled myocardium on two-dimensional echocardiography is consistent with cardiac amyloidosis. Cardiac catheterization can aid in differentiating these two disorders. Both conditions cause equalization of diastolic pressures to within 5 mm Hg of each other. The right ventricular and pulmonary artery systolic pressures are usually higher in restrictive cardiomyopathy, generally exceeding 45 mm Hg. Furthermore, the plateau of the right ventricular pressure is usually at least one third of the peak systolic pressure in pericardial constriction and less in myocardial restriction. In some cases, TEB may allow identification of a specific cause of restrictive cardiomyopathy, thereby aiding in differentiation from constrictive pericarditis. If TEB demonstrates only nonspecific changes or normal myocardium, constrictive pericarditis becomes more likely. Diagnostic evaluation by computed tomography or magnetic resonance imaging can provide accurate estimates of pericardial thickness and can aid in differentiating these diseases.[68, 69]

The prognosis for patients with restrictive cardiomyopathy is generally poor, with only approximately 10% of patients alive at 10 years. Deaths are generally due to progressive heart failure, arrhythmias, or comorbid illness. Medical therapy is often supportive, targeted at the underlying hemodynamic diastolic abnormality. Judicious use of diuretics decreases filling pressures and improves symptoms but may do so at the expense of cardiac output. Nonetheless, diuretics represent an essential component of the therapeutic regimen for restrictive cardiomyopathy, particularly in patients with congestive heart failure. Careful use of vasodilator agents or calcium channel antagonists may also provide some symptomatic benefit but may cause hypotension.

Some of the secondary forms of restrictive cardiomyopathy may be treated with more specific forms of therapy. For example, alkylating agents may be used in patients with amyloidosis, albeit with generally unsatisfactory results. Chelating agents, such as desferoxamine, can be effective in alleviating tissue iron deposition in hemochromatosis.

The *hypereosinophilic syndrome* is an uncommon cause of restrictive cardiomyopathy in which profound blood and bone marrow eosinophilia leads to multiorgan system disease, presumably due to the toxic effects produced by release of eosinophil-granule products. Although many organs are involved, almost all patient deaths are due to severe heart failure. Cardiac involvement includes myocarditis associated with intense eosinophilic infiltration, myocardial thickening, endocardial thrombus formation, and progressive endocardial fibrosis. The dense endomyocardial fibrosis and scarring lead to a hemodynamic picture of restrictive cardiomyopathy. Signs of congestive heart failure often associated with a murmur of mitral regurgitation are noted.[70]

Patients with eosinophilic heart disease often have a beneficial response to administration of corticosteroids or cytotoxic agents, particularly hydroxyurea. Such therapy may slow progression of the disease and improve symptoms as well as survival.[71] Chronic anticoagulation should be considered when ventricular thrombi are present. The course of the illness is variable. Patients with severe acute necrotizing myocarditis may rapidly drift into cardiogenic shock and death.[72] Most patients experience a more chronic, slowly progressive course of worsening heart failure.

HYPERTROPHIC CARDIOMYOPATHY

Myocardial hypertrophy occurring out of proportion to the hemodynamic load or in the absence of increased wall stress is characteristic of hypertrophic cardiomyopathy. The degree and extent of hypertrophy vary from patient to patient, with the septum and anterolateral wall involved more frequently than the posterior wall. A unique form of hypertrophic cardiomyopathy limited to the apical segments and associated with giant inverted precordial T waves is frequently encountered in patients of Japanese descent.[73] Genetic transmission of this disorder occurs in more than 50% of cases as an autosomal dominant trait with variable expression and penetrance. Myocardial hypertrophy leads to decreased ventricular cavity size and diminished lusitropic and compliance characteristics of the left ventricle, resulting in abnormal left ventricular diastolic filling. As a result, cardiac output is maintained at the expense of elevated filling pressures. Left ventricular systolic function is well preserved, and ejection fraction is often supernormal until late in the course of the disease, when approximately 10% of cases evolve to a profile more consistent with dilated cardiomyopathy.

In a minority of patients (25%), particularly those with predominant septal involvement (asymmetric septal hypertrophy), a dynamic obstruction to left ventricular outflow may exist in a way that allows a pressure gradient between the body of the left ventricle and the subaortic region during systole. The cause of the dynamic outflow obstruction is believed to be the close apposition of the hypertrophied septum and the anterior leaflet of the mitral valve. During vigorous ventricular contraction, systolic anterior motion of the mitral valve across the left ventricular outflow tract contracts the septum and impedes ventricular ejection. The obstruction to left ventricular outflow is labile and is increased by any alteration that augments ejection fraction or decreases left ventricular cavity dimension. Thus, increased contractility or decreased preload or afterload increases the outflow gradient and worsens the obstruction.

The cause of hypertrophic cardiomyopathy is unclear, but abnormal calcium regulation, genetic defects, and neurohormonal factors have been implicated.[74] Recombinant deoxyribonucleic acid (DNA) techniques have identified mutations in the long arm of chromosome 14 coding for the myosin heavy chain in several families with hypertrophic cardiomyopathy.[75, 76] Whatever the cause, the morphologic end result is myocardial hypertrophy with gross disorganization of the muscle bundles and myofibrillar disarray along with fibrosis and scar formation. Myocardial ischemia is also believed to be an important pathophysiologic mechanism and is thought to be due to abnormal narrowing of small intramural coronary arteries, impairment of coronary vascular reserve, and reduced capillary density.

Most patients with hypertrophic cardiomyopathy are asymptomatic or only mildly symptomatic. Dyspnea, chest pain, fatigue, and syncope are the most common symptoms and generally correlate with the degree of hypertrophy but not the severity of the outflow tract obstruction. Physical findings vary but may include a hyperdynamic precordium, S_4, paradoxical splitting of S_2, and a bifid carotid pulse. The systolic murmurs of hypertrophic cardiomyopathy may reflect both turbulence at the outflow tract and associated mitral regurgitation.

Echocardiography is extremely useful in evaluating patients with suspected hypertrophic cardiomyopathy. The pattern and extent of left ventricular hypertrophy, narrowing of the left ventricular outflow tract, the magnitude of the outflow tract pressure gradient, and systolic anterior motion of the mitral valve can be readily assessed. The left ventricular cavity dimensions are often decreased and associated with vigorous systolic contraction. The atria are dilated as a result of chronically elevated filling pressures and atrioventricular valvular regurgitation. The septal left ventricular wall thickness is often 1.3 to 1.5 times the thickness of the posterior wall in patients with asymmetric septal hypertrophy. Mitral regurgitation and mitral valve prolapse are common associated features. Aortic insufficiency is noted in approximately one third of patients. Cardiac catheterization reveals elevated left-sided filling pressures due to decreased left ventricular compliance. A subaortic pressure gradient may exist between the left ventricle and the aorta during systole; it can be accentuated by maneuvers that increase contractility or decrease afterload or preload. The aortic pressure tracing exhibits the classic spike-and-dome configuration in patients with outflow tract obstruction.

Therapy in hypertrophic cardiomyopathy is aimed at improving symptoms and decreasing risk of death. Pharmacologic agents that decrease filling pressure, improve left ventricular diastolic relaxation, or reduce the magnitude of the left ventricular outflow tract pressure gradient improve symptoms in this disorder. Beta-adrenergic blocking agents are the mainstay of therapy in patients with hypertrophic cardiomyopathy. Such drugs slow heart rate and lengthen the diastolic filling period, thus improving the diastolic filling abnormality associated with this condition. β-Adrenergic blocking agents also decrease myocardial oxygen consumption and improve ischemia. In patients with pulmonary congestion, careful use of diuretics may be beneficial. Calcium channel antagonists such as verapamil and to a lesser extent nifedipine and diltiazem have been postulated to improve left ventricular relaxation and ventricular diastolic filling in patients with hypertrophic cardiomyopathy with or without left ventricular outflow tract obstruction.[77] Disopyramide, presumably because of its negative inotropic effect, also improves symptoms and exercise tolerance. These agents all must be used with caution because the potential for serious side effects, such as bradycardia and hypotension, is a genuine concern.

In one study, dual-chamber pacing, carried out in patients who had hypertrophic cardiomyopathy and who did not respond to conventional medical therapy, resulted in improvement in symptoms, exercise tolerance, cardiac output, and the left ventricular outflow tract gradient.[78] Surgical therapy consisting of ventricular septal myotomy with or without myectomy has been shown to relieve the dynamic outflow tract obstruction, reduce systolic anterior motion of the mitral valve, reduce mitral regurgitation, and improve symptoms. However, because surgery carries an operative risk of 5% to 8%, such therapy is generally reserved for patients with severe symptoms despite maximum medical therapy. Mitral valve replacement usually abolishes the subaortic gradient and may be helpful in certain patients.

Patients with hypertrophic cardiomyopathy exhibit an annual mortality rate of 2% to 3%, and about half the deaths are sudden and unexpected; sudden death may be the initial presenting event. Sudden death, the most ominous complication of hypertrophic cardiomyopathy, may be due to circulatory collapse in the presence of a severe outflow tract gradient but is most often thought to be secondary to malignant ventricular arrhythmias. Factors predisposing to sudden death include age less than 30 years, a family history of hypertrophic cardiomyopathy or sudden death, syncope, and evidence of ventricular tachycardia on ambulatory monitoring. The value of electrophysiologic testing in identifying high-risk individuals is unclear and is being evaluated. Amiodarone may be of benefit in some patients with ventricular tachycardia. High-risk individuals with resuscitated cardiac arrest or documented sustained ventricular tachycardia should be considered for placement of an automatic implantable cardioverter-defibrillator.

Patients with hypertrophic cardiomyopathy are also susceptible to supraventricular tachycardia. The occurrence of atrial fibrillation may result in hemodynamic deterioration as a result of loss of the atrial contribution to left ventricular filling. Such patients benefit from aggressive treatment of their rhythm disturbance with rapid conversion to sinus rhythm.

Finally, for patients with refractory heart failure or uncontrollable dysrhythmias, cardiac transplantation remains a final consideration.

CARDIOMYOPATHIES AND THE CRITICAL CARE ENVIRONMENT

As mentioned in the introduction, certain specific problems are frequently encountered in critically ill patients with the various forms of cardiomyopathy discussed in this chapter. The pathogenetic mechanisms, diagnostic evaluations, and therapeutic modalities reviewed earlier represent a major body of information that must be well understood in order for the intensive care physician to provide optimal care to these patients.

Management of Cardiomyopathy with Invasive Hemodynamic Monitoring

Patients with severe decompensated heart failure due to cardiomyopathy are generally admitted to an ICU for diagnostic evaluation and treatment. Initially, a balloon-tipped, flow-directed pulmonary artery catheter should be placed to determine filling pressures, cardiac index, and systemic vascular resistance. Continued invasive hemodynamic monitoring aids in guiding therapy and optimizing cardiac performance.

Caring for patients with cardiomyopathy in the critical care unit requires a sophisticated understanding of fluid and pressor administration as well as the pathophysiology underlying the form of cardiomyopathy under evaluation. For example, a patient with hypertrophic cardiomyopathy with a severe dynamic outflow tract obstruction should not be treated with intravenous inotropic agents.

A first step to improving hemodynamics is to optimize preload in a way that obtains maximum cardiac index without exacerbating pulmonary edema. By using the PCWP, one can administer fluids until a PCWP of 15 to 20 mm Hg is achieved. When PCWP exceeds this level, pulmonary edema tends to occur. It should be emphasized that PCWP is a measurement of left ventricular diastolic pressure and does not necessarily reflect left ventricular volume. This is particularly true of patients with impaired diastolic relaxation or decreased compliance such as in restrictive or hypertrophic cardiomyopathy. In such patients, a small change in intravascular volume may produce a small change in ventricular volume but a large increase in ventricular filling pressure, leading to worsening pulmonary edema. These patients may best be served with treatment aimed at favorably altering lusitropic and compliance characteristics such as with β-adrenergic blockade, calcium channel antagonists, or vasodilators.

In dilated cardiomyopathy, ventricular compliance is usually increased, and one can give large amounts of fluid, increasing intraventricular diastolic volume, with a small or no change in PCWP. In these patients, one can continue to give fluid until the PCWP approaches 20 mm Hg, beyond which lung water begins to increase. Interestingly, some patients with dilated cardiomyopathy can be maintained at a higher PCWP without the development of pulmonary edema, presumably because long-standing heart failure leads to increased lymphatic drainage of extravascular pulmonary fluid. In these patients, a higher end-diastolic volume and preload can be achieved by further intravascular volume expansion to a PCWP that is high by usual standards but is well tolerated.

Patients with restrictive or hypertrophic cardiomyopathy exhibit reduced compliance and abnormal ventricular diastolic relaxation. Such patients may generally achieve a PCWP of 20 mm Hg with very little fluid supplementation. However, a subgroup of these patients may not demonstrate an increased PCWP with continued fluid administration. The response of these patients to intravascular volume expansion cannot be predicted; therefore, each patient should be given a trial of fluid administration with careful hemodynamic monitoring. In addition, echocardiography is also helpful in assessing left ventricular systolic function and valvular regurgitation and ruling out pericardial effusion and tamponade.

Perhaps more important than the absolute value for filling pressure or cardiac index are trends or changes in PCWP, cardiac output, stroke volume, or systemic vascular resistance in response to therapeutic manipulations. For example, patients with dilated cardiomyopathy may exhibit an elevated PCWP that is well matched to achieve optimal cardiac index. A small decrease in this pressure may reflect a significant decrease in left ventricular end-diastolic volume and result in decreased cardiac performance. One should monitor these changes closely and target predetermined reasonable hemodynamic goals.

Patients who have cardiomyopathy with severe impairment of heart function may present with episodes of low cardiac output characterized by severe fatigue and hemodynamic embarrassment associated with low cardiac output and evidence of end-organ hypoperfusion. Such episodes are severe and potentially life-threatening. They require admission to the ICU, invasive hemodynamic monitoring, and treatment with intravenous inotropic agents, vasopressors, diuretics, and vasodilators to prevent irreversible multiorgan system failure. Some patients improve, but others may exhibit further deterioration and become refractory to medical therapy. This latter group presents difficult ethical and practical issues regarding more aggressive means of cardiovascular support. Hemodynamic improvement can be obtained with a mechanical circulatory support device, such as intra-aortic counterpulsation balloon pumping, a ventricular assist device, or the total artificial heart. However, such therapies are temporizing measures, and endpoints for therapy need to be decided on before mechanical circulatory assist devices are applied. Such patients should

TABLE 102–7. Tailored Therapy for Heart Failure Before Transplantation

1. Measurement of baseline hemodynamics
2. Intravenous nitroprusside and diuretics tailored to hemodynamic goals:
   - Pulmonary capillary wedge pressure ≤ 15 mm Hg
   - Systemic vascular resistance ≤ 1200 dyne · s/cm^{-5} · m^2
   - Right atrial pressure ≤ 8 mm Hg
   - Systolic blood pressure ≥ 80 mm Hg
3. Definition of optimal hemodynamics by 24–48 hr
4. Titration of high-dose vasodilators as nitroprusside weaned:
   - Captopril, hydralazine, isosorbide dinitrate
5. Monitored ambulation and diuretic adjustment for 24–48 hr
6. Maintain digoxin levels 1.9–2.0 ng/dL if no contraindication
7. Detailed patient education
8. Flexible outpatient diuretic regimen including intermittent metolazone
9. Progressive walking program
10. Vigilant follow-up

From Stevenson LW: Tailored therapy before transplantation for treatment of advanced heart failure: Effective use of vasodilators and diuretics. J Heart Lung Transplant 1991; 10:468.

be urgently evaluated for heart transplantation and, if appropriate, mechanical circulatory assist devices may provide an effective bridge to transplantation therapy until a donor becomes available. An ongoing clinical trial randomizing patients with severe refractory heart failure to medical therapy, versus placement of a left ventricular assist device in individuals who are not heart transplant candidates, is designed to evaluate the feasibility and effectiveness of placing mechanical circulatory assist devices as permanent implants.

In the meantime, patients with cardiomyopathy and low-output states should be monitored with serial hemodynamic measurements and their response to fluids, vasopressors, diuretics, and inotropic agents should be closely observed in an attempt to optimize blood flow to vital organs. Determinations of mixed venous oxygen saturation and serum lactate levels provide a reliable measure of tissue perfusion. Many patients, although considered to be refractory to conventional heart failure therapy, respond to an intensive, tailored approach consisting of intravenous vasodilators and diuretics, followed by oral therapy and meticulous attention to hemodynamics and fluid balance (Table 102–7).

IMPORTANT RHYTHM DISTURBANCES

Rhythm disturbances are another special problem in patients with severe heart failure and cardiomyopathy. For example, patients with restrictive or hypertrophic cardiomyopathy may exhibit hemodynamic deterioration in the presence of atrial fibrillation owing to loss of the active atrial contribution to cardiac output. In such cases, aggressive measures to restore and maintain normal sinus rhythm should be implemented, including electrical cardioversion and use of antiarrhythmic agents.

Recurrent ventricular arrhythmias also represent a serious problem for patients with cardiomyopathy. Type 1 antiarrhythmic agents are often poorly tolerated because of their negative inotropic and proarrhythmic effects. Care should be taken to avoid electrolyte derangements, myocardial ischemia, and drug toxicity, all of which can exacerbate ventricular arrhythmias in these patients. Amiodarone can be effective for treatment of both supraventricular and ventricular arrhythmias in patients with dilated cardiomyopathy.

References

1. Abelmann WH, Lorell BH: The challenge of cardiomyopathy. J Am Coll Cardiol 1989; 3:1219.
2. Goodwin JF: Classification of nonhypertrophic cardiomyopathies. Prog Cardiol 1989; 2:3.
3. World Health Organization (WHO)/ISFC Task Force: Report of the WHO/ISFC Task Force on The Definition and Classification of Cardiomyopathies. Br Heart J 1980; 44:672.
4. World Health Organization: Cardiomyopathies: Report of a WHO Expert Committee. WHO Tech Rep Ser 1984; 697:7.
5. Stewart S, Mason DT, Braunwald E: Impaired rate of left ventricular filling in idiopathic hypertrophic subaortic stenosis and valvular aortic stenosis. Circulation 1968; 37:8.
6. Gillum RF: The epidemiology of cardiomyopathy in the United States. Prog Cardiol 1989; 2:11.
7. Kono S, Sakakibara S: Endomyocardial biopsy. Dis Chest 1963; 44:345.
8. Aretz HT, Billingham ME, Edwards WD: Myocarditis. A histopathologic definition and classification. Am J Cardiovasc Pathol 1986; 1:3.
9. French WJ, Siegel RJ, Cohen AH, et al: Yield of endomyocardial biopsy in patients with biventricular failure. Chest 1986; 90:181.
10. Schoenfeld MH, Supple EW, Dec WG, et al: Restrictive cardiomyopathy versus constrictive pericarditis: Role of endomyocardial biopsy in avoiding unnecessary thoracotomy. Circulation 1987; 75:1012.
11. Parrillo JE, Aretz HT, Palacios I, et al: The results of transvenous endomyocardial biopsy can frequently be used to diagnose myocardial diseases in patients with idiopathic heart failure: Endomyocardial biopsies in 100 consecutive patients revealed a substantial incidence of myocarditis. Circulation 1984; 69:93.
12. Mason JW, O'Connell JB: Clinical merit of endomyocardial biopsy. Circulation 1989; 79:971.
13. Dec WG, Palacios IF, Fallon JT, et al: Active myocarditis in the spectrum of acute dilated cardiomyopathies, N Engl J Med 1985; 312:885.
14. Vasiljevic JD, Kanjuh V, Seferovic P, et al: The incidence of myocarditis in endomyocardial biopsy samples from patients with congestive heart failure. Am Heart J 1990; 120:1370.
15. Manolio TA, Baughman KL, Rodcheffer R, et al: Prevalence and etiology of idiopathic dilated cardiomyopathy (summary of a national heart, lung, and blood institute workshop). Am J Cardiol 1992; 69:1458.
16. Cannon RO, Cunnion RE, Parrillo JE, et al: Dynamic limitation of coronary vasodilator reserve in patients with dilated cardiomyopathy and chest pain. J Am Coll Cardiol 1987; 10:1190.
17. Roberts WC, Siegel RJ, McManus BM: Idiopathic dilated cardiomyopathy: Analysis of 152 necropsy patients. Am J Cardiol 1987; 60:1340.
18. Ferrans VJ: Pathologic anatomy of the dilated cardiomyopathies. Am J Cardiol 1989; 64:9C.
19. Jin O, Sole MJ, Butany JW, et al: Detection of enterovirus RNA in myocardial biopsies from patients with myocarditis and cardiomyopathy using gene amplification by polymerase chain reaction. Circulation 1990; 82:8.
20. Reilly JM, Cunnion RE, Anderson DW, et al: Frequency of myocarditis, left ventricular dysfunction and ventricular tachycardia in the acquired immune deficiency syndrome. Am J Cardiol 1988; 62:789.
21. Midei MG, DeMent SH, Feldman AM, et al: Peripartum myocarditis and cardiomyopathy. Circulation 1990; 81:922.
22. Sanderson JE, Koech D, Iha D, et al: T-lymphocyte subsets in idiopathic dilated cardiomyopathy. Am J Cardiol 1985; 55:755.
23. Limas CJ, Limas C: HLA antigens in idiopathic dilated cardiomyopathy. Br Heart J 1989; 62:379.
24. Eckstein R, Mempel W, Bolte H-D: Reduced suppressor cell activity in congestive cardiomyopathy and in myocarditis. Circulation 1982; 65:1224.
25. Caforio ALP, Bonifacio E, Stewart JT, et al: Novel organ-specific circulating cardiac autoantibodies in dilated cardiomyopathy. J Am Coll Cardiol 1990; 15:1527.
26. Limas CJ, Goldenberg IF, Limas C: Autoantibodies against beta-adrenoceptors in human idiopathic dilated cardiomyopathy. Circulation Res 1989; 64:97.
27. Margossian SS, White HD, Caulfield JB, et al: Light chain 2 profile and activity of human ventricular myosin during dilated cardiomyopathy: Identification of a causal agent for impaired myocardial function. Circulation 1992; 85:1720.

28. Ungerer M, Bohm M, Elce JS, et al: Altered expression of beta-adrenergic receptor kinase and $beta_1$-adrenergic receptors in the failing human heart. Circulation 1993; 87:454.
29. Sullebarger JT, Fan T-HM, Torres F, et al: Both cell surface and internalized beta-adrenoceptors are reduced in the failing myocardium. Eur J Pharmacol 1991; 205:165.
30. Morgan HE: Cellular aspects of cardial failure. Circulation 1993; 87(Supp IV): IV-4.
31. Feldman AM, Cates AE, Veazey WB: Increase of the 40,000-mol wt pertussis toxin substrate (G-protein) in the failing human heart. J Clin Invest 1988; 82:189.
32. Romeo F, Pelliccia F, Cianfroccia C, et al: Determinants of end-stage idiopathic dilated cardiomyopathy: A multivariate analysis of 104 patients. Clin Cardiol 1989; 12:387.
33. Saxon LA, Stevenson WG, Middlekauft HR, et al: Predicting death from progressive heart failure secondary to ischemic or idiopathic dilated cardiomyopathy. Am J Cardiol 1993; 72:62.
34. Diaz RA, Obasohan A, Oakley CM: Prediction of outcome in dilated cardiomyopathy. Br Heart J 1987; 58:393.
35. Fuster V. Gersh BJ, Giuliani ER, et al: The natural history of idiopathic dilated cardiomyopathy. Am J Cardiol 1981; 47:525.
36. Tamburro P, Wilber D: Sudden death in idiopathic dilated cardiomyopathy. Am Heart J 1992; 124:1035.
37. Holmes J, Kubo SH, Cody RJ, et al: Arrhythmias in ischemic and nonischemic dilated cardiomyopathy: Prediction of mortality by ambulatory electrocardiography. Am J Cardiol 1985; 55:146.
38. Huang SK, Messer JV, Denes P: Significance of ventricular tachycardia in idiopathic dilated cardiomyopathy: Observations in 35 patients. Am J Cardiol 1983; 51:507.
39. Olshausen KV, Shafer A, Mehmel HC, et al: Ventricular arrhythmias in idiopathic dilated cardiomyopathy. Br Heart J 1984; 51:195.
40. Stevenson LW: Dilated cardiomyopathy: Principles and prognosis. Prog Cardiol 1989; 2:51.
41. Dormans TPJ, van Meyel JJM, Gerlag PGG, Tan Y, et al: Diuretic efficacy of high dose furosemide in severe heart failure: Bolus injection versus continuous infusion. J Am Coll Cardiol 1996; 28:376.
42. The Digitalis Investigation Group: The effect of digoxin on mortality and morbidity in patients with heart failure. N Engl J Med 1997; 336:525.
43. Gheorghiade M, Zarowitz BJ: Review of randomized trials of digoxin therapy in patients with chronic heart failure. Am J Cardiol 1992; 69:48G.
44. Parrillo JE: Pharmacologic Approach to the Critically Ill Patient. 2nd Ed. Baltimore, Williams & Wilkins, 1988, p 346.
45. Guiha MH, Cohn JN, Milkulic E, et al: Treatment of refractory heart failure with infusion of Nitroprusside. N Engl J Med 1974; 291:587.
46. Cohn JN, Archibald DG, Ziesche S, et al: Effect of vasodilator therapy on mortality in chronic congestive heart failure: Results of Veterans Administration Cooperative Study. N Engl J Med 1986; 314:1547.
47. The SOLVD Investigators: Effect of enalapril on survival in patients with reduced left ventricular ejection fraction and congestive heart failure. N Engl J Med 1991; 325:293.
48. The Consensus Trial Study Group: Effects of enalapril on mortality in severe congestive heart failure: Results of the cooperative North Scandinavian Enalapril Survival Study (Consensus). N Engl J Med 1987; 316:1429.
49. Azizi M, Chatellier G, Guyene TT, et al: Additive effects of combined angiotensin-converting enzyme inhibition and angiotensin II antagonism on blood pressure and renin release in sodium-depleted normotensives. Circulation 1995; 92:825.
50. Pitt B, Segal R, Martinez FA, et al: Randomised trial of losartan versus captopril in patients over 65 with heart failure: Evaluation of Losartan in the Elderly Study (ELITE). Lancet 1997; 349:747.
51. Packer M, O'Connor CM, Ghali JK, et al: Effect of amlodipine on morbidity and mortality in severe chronic heart failure. N Engl J Med 1996; 335:1107.
52. Marcus RH, Raw K, Patel J, et al: Comparison of intravenous amrinone and dobutamine in congestive heart failure due to idiopathic dilated cardiomyopathy. Am J Cardiol 1990; 66:1107.
53. Pickworth KK: Long-term dobutamine therapy for refractory congestive heart failure. Clinical Pharm 1992; 11:618.
54. Feldman AM, Bristow MR, Parmley WW, et al: Effects of vesnarinone on morbidity and mortality in patients with heart failure. N Engl J Med 1993; 329:149.
55. Beck OM, Sorensen JD, Jensen MK, et al: Effects of long-term coenzyme Q_{10} and captopril treatment on survival and functional capacity in rats with experimentally induced heart infarction. J Pharm Exp Ther 1990; 255:346.
56. Katz SD, Kubo SH, Jessup M, et al: A multicenter, randomized, double-blind, placebo-controlled trial of pimobendan, a new cardiotonic and vasodilator agent, in patients with severe congestive heart failure. Am Heart J 1992; 123:95.
57. Waagstein F, Hjalmarsou A, Varhauskus E, et al: Effect of chronic beta-adrenergic receptor blockage in congestive cardiomyopathy. Br Heart J 1975; 37:1022.
58. Packer M, Bristow MR, Cohn JN, et al: The effect of carvedilol on morbidity and mortality in patients with chronic heart failure. N Engl J Med 1996; 334:1349.
59. Colucci WS, Packer M, Bristow MR, et al: Carvedilol inhibits clinical progression in patients with mild symptoms of heart failure. Circulation 1996; 94:2800.
60. Parrillo JE, Connon RE, Epstein SE, et al: A prospective, randomized, controlled trial of prednisone for dilated cardiomyopathy. N Engl J Med 1989; 321:1061.
61. Mason JW, O'Connell JB, Herskowitz A, et al: A clinical trial of immunosuppressive therapy for myocarditis. N Engl J Med 1995; 333:269.
62. Dunkman WB, Johnson GR, Carson PE, et al: Incidence of thromboembolic events in congestive heart failure. Circulation 1993; 87(Suppl VI):VI-94.
63. Neri R, Mestroni TL, Salvi A, et al: Ventricular arrhythmias in dilated cardiomyopathy: Efficacy of amiodarone. Am Heart J 1987; 113:707.
64. Doval HC, Nul DR, Grancelli HO, et al: Randomised trial of low-dose amiodarone in severe congestive heart failure. Lancet 1994; 344:493.
65. Wilber PJ, Garan H, Finkelstein D, et al: Out-of-hospital cardiac arrest. Use of electrophysiologic testing in the prediction of long-term outcome. N Engl J Med 1982; 318:19.
66. Furnary AP, Jessup M, Moreira LFP: Multicenter trial of dynamic cardiomyoplasty for chronic heart failure. J Am Coll Cardiol 1996; 28:1175.
67. Hosenpud JD, Niles NR: Clinical, hemodynamic and endomyocardial biopsy findings in idiopathic restrictive cardiomyopathy. West J Med 1986; 144:303.
68. Isner JM, Carter BL, Bankoff MS, et al: Differentiation of constrictive pericarditis from restrictive cardiomyopathy by computed tomographic imaging. Am Heart J 1983; 105:1019.
69. Sechtem U, Higgins CB, Sommerhoff BA, et al: Magnetic resonance imaging of restrictive cardiomyopathy. Am J Cardiol 1987; 59:480.
70. Parrillo JE, Borer JS, Henry WL, et al: The cardiovascular manifestations of the hypereosinophilic syndrome. J Med 1979; 67:572.
71. Parrillo JE, Fauci AS, Wolff SM: Therapy of the hypereosinophilic syndrome. Ann Intern Med 1978; 89:167.
72. Parrillo JE: Heart disease and the eosinophil. N Engl J Med 1990; 323:1560.
73. Webb JG, Sasson Z, Rakowski H, et al: Apical hypertrophic cardiomyopathy: Clinical follow-up and diagnostic correlates. J Am Coll Cardiol 1990; 15:83.
74. Maron BJ, Borow RO, Cannon RO, et al: Hypertrophic cardiomyopathy: Interrelations of clinical manifestations, pathophysiology, and therapy (first of two parts). N Engl J Med 1987; 316:780.
75. Jarcho JA, McKenna, W, Pare P, et al: Mapping a gene for familial hypertrophic cardiomyopathy to chromosome 14q1. N Engl J Med 1989; 321:1372.
76. Geisterfer-Lowrance AA, Kass S, Tanigawa G, et al: A molecular basis for familial hypertrophic cardiomyopathy: A beta-cardiac myosin heavy chain gene missense mutation. Cell 1990; 62:999.
77. Maron BJ, Borow RO, Cannon RO, et al: Hypertrophic cardiomyopathy: Interrelations of clinical manifestations, pathophysiology, and therapy (second of two parts). N Engl J Med 1987; 316:844.
78. Fananapazir L, Epstein ND, Curiel RV, et al: Long-term results of dual-chamber (DDD) pacing in obstructive hypertrophic cardiomyopathy: Evidence for progressive symptomatic and hemodynamic improvement and reduction of left ventricular hype trophy. Circulation 1994; 90:2731.

103

Diagnosis and Therapy of Emergent Vascular Diseases

Rodney A. White, MD

The vascular patient with peripheral, cerebrovascular, or myocardial ischemia frequently has diffuse atherosclerosis that increases the risk of death postoperatively and in the long term from vascular complications.[1] These patients often have a history of excessive smoking, diabetes mellitus, or a familial predisposition to vascular diseases (e.g., an inherited tendency to hyperlipidemia). Physical findings, such as asymmetric extremities, fragile skin, hair loss, and xanthomas, are suggestive of vascular disease. Careful palpation, auscultation, Doppler segmental pressure measurement of pulses, and pulse-volume recording can indicate the severity and distribution of vascular lesions.

Contrast angiography has been the most accurate method of detecting arterial and venous disease, although Doppler and ultrasound imaging techniques, computed tomography (CT), and magnetic resonance angiography are used increasingly for less invasive and noninvasive diagnosis of vascular lesions.[2, 3] Treadmill exercise, combined with electrocardiogram (ECG) monitoring, may be used to quantitate ischemic symptoms and is particularly useful for screening patients with peripheral vascular disease for concomitant coronary artery lesions that can be corrected by surgery.[4] Newer screening methods, including isotope imaging studies, improve the assessment of ischemic coronary disease in patients who may otherwise have undetectable lesions.[5]

This chapter describes syndromes associated with acute and chronic vascular insufficiency, ischemic symptoms related to systemic inflammatory disease, complications of vascular reconstructions, and venous disorders.

ACUTE ARTERIAL INSUFFICIENCY

Patients with acute arterial occlusion resulting from trauma, embolus, or thrombosis frequently require emergency surgery to prevent irreversible tissue loss. Symptoms include pain, analgesia or anesthesia, and discoloration of the ischemic tissue.

Embolic arterial occlusion produces symptoms that vary with the origin of the embolus. Emboli originating in the heart or the ascending aorta or venous thrombi that pass from the right to left side of the heart through patent septal defects can cause central nervous system, visceral, or upper-extremity or lower-extremity symptoms, whereas emboli from the abdominal aorta and from iliofemoral or popliteal lesions affect only the lower extremities. In the *blue toe syndrome*, multiple bilateral ischemic areas in the lower leg are caused by atheromatous debris showered distally from diseased aortoiliac vessels.[6] Ischemic paralysis and hypalgesia may develop in acutely ischemic limbs as a result of neurovascular compression caused by increased fascial compartment pressure. Compartmental compression syndromes necessitate expedient decompression by fasciotomy to prevent irreversible neurovascular damage.[7] Embolic occlusion of visceral arteries may be insidious; pain, indigestion, and hematuria are often the only symptoms.

Thrombotic arterial occlusion usually occurs as a result of decreased blood flow in progressively narrowed, atherosclerotic vessels. Acute thrombosis of diseased arteries may be due to hypovolemia or a sudden decrease in cardiac output. Frequently, elderly patients with cardiac failure and an intercurrent illness may appear to have ischemic lower extremities caused by an aortic occlusion or a dissecting aneurysm. Appropriate attention to the cardiac status and fluid balance and treatment of any acute illnesses often alleviate the ischemic symptoms. Axillary arterial thrombosis occurs after intimal damage produced by repeated strain or trauma in athletes, particularly baseball pitchers, and in individuals using crutches. In rare circumstances, acute arterial thrombosis occurs in severely dehydrated children or in patients with hematologic disorders.

CHRONIC ARTERIAL INSUFFICIENCY

Although appropriate care is required to prevent complications, chronic arterial insufficiency caused by progression of atherosclerosis is infrequently a surgical emergency. Occlusion of major arteries may not cause tissue ischemia if hypertrophied collateral vessels provide adequate vascular supply. Chronic arterial occlusive disease is typically accompanied by insidious symptoms such as wasting of the extremity, hair loss, fragile skin, and pain with activity (*claudication*). Patients may complain of a burning or warm sensation in the affected extremity, which is actually cool or at normal temperature. Although nerve entrapment or inflammation also causes pain with activity, claudication caused by chronic arterial insufficiency is distinguished by consistent and reproducible symptoms.[8] Decreased exercise tolerance or prolonged recovery time suggests progression of the disease.

Because chronically ischemic limbs are easily ulcerated by local irritation, patients (especially those with diabetes) must be instructed in meticulous foot care, and any lesions should be aggressively treated. All patients with arterial insufficiency should be encouraged to stop smoking, control their diet, and immediately visit their physician if foot problems develop. Approximately 50% of patients with claudication experience decreased pain with activity if they follow these recommendations and start a supervised exercise program. The onset of rest pain heralds complications and limb loss unless surgical intervention can restore adequate oxygenation.

Figure 103–1 summarizes the steps for diagnosis and treatment of arterial ischemia.

DISEASES OF THE AORTA

Improved techniques for reconstructing the thoracic aorta and its major arterial branches have increased the importance of early, accurate diagnosis of pathologic lesions. Too often, intrathoracic aortic lesions progress and remain undiagnosed until they cause catastrophic hemodynamic problems after leakage or rupture or produce symptoms resulting from compression of adjacent structures.

In many cases, thoracic aortic aneurysms can be visualized by chest x-ray films, ultrasonography, or arteriography; however, contrast CT is the most reliable method of defining the extent of the lesions. Thoracic aneurysms may affect speech by irritating the recurrent laryngeal nerve, or they may cause dysphagia by compressing the esophagus.

Pain associated with a dissecting thoracic aneurysm may be substernal or referred to the intracapsular area. Migration of excruciating pain suggests extension of a dissection. Major arterial branches of the thoracic aorta may be occluded by extension of a subintimal dissection, causing a cerebrovascular accident or diminishing pulses in the upper extremity. Control

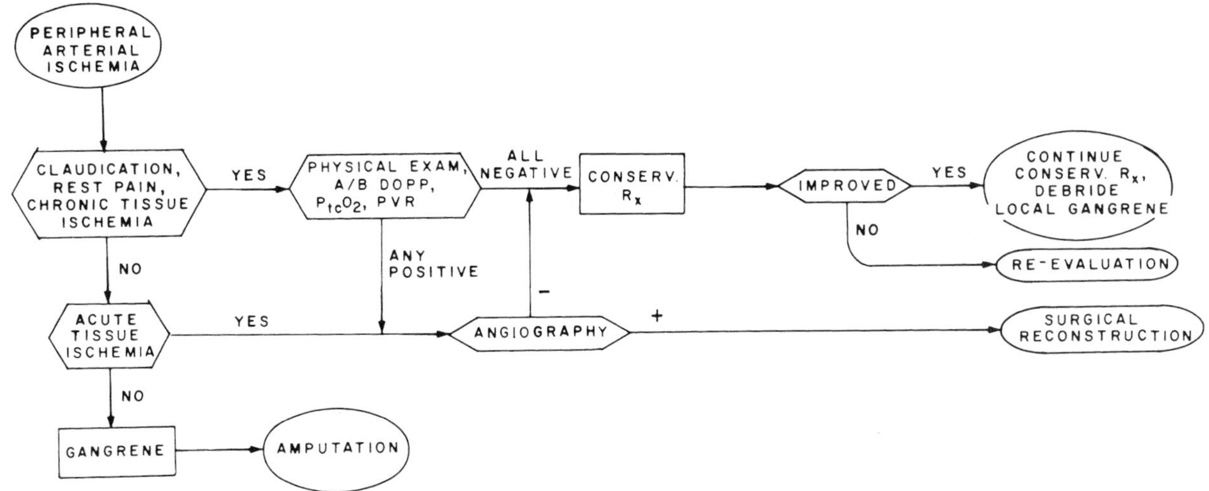

Figure 103–1. Claudication, rest pain, chronic or acute tissue ischemia, or gangrene suggests peripheral arterial ischemia. For patients with claudication, rest pain, or chronic tissue ischemia (Step 1) a physical examination, ankle/brachial artery Doppler pressure measurement (A/B Dopp), transcutaneous Po_2 ($Ptco_2$) determination, and pulse volume recording (PVR) should be performed (Step 2). Negative findings rule out arterial disease; therefore, conservative therapy plus a search for other possible etiologic factors is required. If the patient's symptoms become worse (Step 3), reevaluation is indicated. Any positive test result, (e.g., A/B Dopp < 0.6, $Ptco_2 < 70$ torr), abnormal PVR, or the presence of acute tissue ischemia (Step 4) indicates arteriography (Step 5) to determine the cause of and need for surgical reconstruction. If gangrene (Step 6) is the presenting symptom, amputation of necrotic tissue is required.

of hypertension frequently prevents further dissection. For unstable patients, immediate surgery may occasionally be the only chance for survival.

Atherosclerotic disease of the abdominal aorta and iliac arteries produces lesions that occur initially and are frequently most severe near the bifurcation of the aorta.[9] Symptomatic lesions can be reconstructed by aortoiliac or aortobifemoral bypasses using fabric prostheses that have 90% 10-year patency rates.[10] Approximately 5% of hypertensive patients can be cured by repair of renal artery obstructions. Transluminal balloon angioplasty of renal artery lesions, endarterectomy, and reconstruction are options for relief of hypertension and salvage of renal function.[11] Reduced blood flow to the hypogastric vessels has an important role in male impotence[12]; reconstructive procedures that increase flow to the pelvic vessels can restore sexual function in a significant number of patients.

Abdominal aortic aneurysms may rupture into the peritoneal cavity, a catastrophic event associated with rapid exsanguination, or they may rupture into an adjacent organ such as the vena cava, producing an aorta–vena caval fistula. Aneurysms commonly perforate posteriorly beneath the renal vessels or along the iliac artery into the retroperitoneum. Ruptured retroperitoneal aneurysms produce excruciating abdominal pain that may radiate to the groin and mimic renal colic.

Enlargement of an aneurysm to greater than 6 cm in diameter significantly increases the risk of its rupture in the near future[13]; thus, surgical correction is recommended if the patient's health is adequate. Ultrasonography provides an accurate estimate of the size of aortic aneurysms and is used to indicate the need for surgical correction. Surgery may also be indicated occasionally for postoperative patients because increased collagenase activity in the aneurysm wall of catabolic patients increases the risk of rupture.[14] Approximately 10% to 15% of abdominal aortic aneurysms extend above the renal vessels, and reimplantation of the renal arteries into the prosthesis is required.

UPPER-EXTREMITY ISCHEMIA

Upper-extremity ischemia resulting from acute arterial occlusions causes limb loss in 10% of patients with lesions in the subclavian artery, 15% with lesions in the axillary artery, and fewer than 5% with lesions in the proximal brachial artery.[15] Most acute arterial obstructions in the upper extremity are caused by trauma.

Thoracic outlet compression syndrome is caused by impingement of adjacent structures on all or part of the neurovascular supply to the upper extremity. Common causes include a cervical rib, fibrocartilaginous bands, scalene or subclavius muscle hypertrophy, upper thoracic or cervical trauma, and repeated strenuous hyperabduction of the arm. An accurate diagnosis depends on reproducing symptoms with hand exercise when the arm is abducted and externally rotated. There may be tenderness on percussion over the clavicle or brachial plexus, an audible bruit over the subclavian artery, and reduction or obliteration of pulses when the arm is in an abducted position. However, these diagnostic maneuvers are only suggestive, and many normal individuals have the same findings. Objective tests include electromyography, nerve conduction velocity tests, and arteriography.

Relief of symptoms often follows several months of a thoracic outlet exercise program.[16] In severe cases, resection of a cervical rib or the first thoracic rib or scalenectomy may relieve symptoms. Occasionally, thoracic outlet compression occurs with carpal tunnel syndrome.[17] This association should be suspected in patients with wasting of the intrinsic muscles of the hand, particularly if they have a systemic inflammatory disease.

Upper-extremity digital gangrene is infrequent but not rare. Approximately 50% of patients with digital ischemia have a correctable aneurysm, traumatic lesion, or embolic source proximal to the hand. Digital ischemia may also appear as a symptom of vasospastic or obliterative arterial disease in patients with systemic inflammatory processes. Connective tissue disorders, particularly scleroderma, are associated with progressive occlusion of medium-diameter and small-diameter arteries.

Many patients with inflammatory diseases experience Raynaud's syndrome before the onset of systemic symptoms.[18] *Raynaud's syndrome* is characterized by episodic cold-induced or stress-induced digital cyanosis, coldness, and, in severe cases, ulceration. Of patients with Raynaud's syndrome, 60% to 90% are young females with primarily vasospastic arterial disease. Older patients and males with Raynaud's syndrome typically have obstructive arterial disease. Certain occupations, particularly those involving vibratory tools or prolonged exposure to low temperatures, are associated with an increased incidence of Raynaud's syndrome.

Therapy relies on identification and treatment of the underlying inflammatory process.

CEREBROVASCULAR INSUFFICIENCY

Atherosclerosis of the extracranial carotid artery (i.e., carotid stenosis or ulceration) can cause cerebrovascular insufficiency. Transient ischemic attacks (TIAs), visual disturbances, and contralateral weakness can often be relieved by carotid endarterectomy (removal of atherosclerotic embolic and occlusive lesions at the bifurcation of the common carotid artery). Patients with less specific symptoms, such as headaches, dizziness, and unusual distribution of sensory or motor abnormalities, require extensive evaluation to document the relationship of neurologic symptoms to carotid stenosis. Patients with asymptomatic carotid lesions can be treated with antiplatelet medications instead of carotid endarterectomy; however, endarterectomy appears to reduce the incidence of subsequent stroke despite a minimally higher morbidity and mortality related to surgery in some series.[19, 20]

Flow disturbance at the carotid bifurcation is postulated as the initial stimulus for the development of carotid atheroma. Fibrous myointimal thickening is followed by hemorrhage beneath the lesion. The hematoma may significantly narrow the vessel lumen, causing an ischemic event. If the patient remains asymptomatic, the atheroma progressively thickens by a series of degenerative events, or the contents of the subintimal space may embolize, causing TIAs.[21] In the latter case, embolized atheromatous debris produces Hollenhorst's plaques on the retina, which are visible during funduscopic examination of the eye.[22] Release of the necrotic subintimal contents leaves an ulcerated plaque, which is the source of continued embolization. Arteriography may suggest an ulcerated plaque, although in some cases the ulcer endothelializes and is no longer a source of emboli. In many instances, repeated fibrosis, hemorrhage, and calcification of atheromatous lesions completely occlude the intimal carotid artery lumen.

In all cases, one should consider intracerebral and vertebral artery lesions and any other possible cause of cerebrovascular insufficiency before implicating a carotid stenosis. For example, occlusion of the first portion of the subclavian artery can cause blood to flow retrogradely from the vertebral artery to the axillary artery, precipitating cerebral ischemia during arm exercise (the *subclavian steal syndrome*).[23]

MESENTERIC ARTERIAL INSUFFICIENCY

Often the diagnosis of visceral ischemia is not made until late in the clinical course. For this reason, reported mortality rates are between 55% and 100%.[24, 25] Laboratory and noninvasive tests are not diagnostic, and the physician must always consider mesenteric insufficiency in the initial evaluation of severely ill patients with abdominal pain, particularly older patients with cardiovascular conditions. Expeditious establishment and maintenance of hemodynamic stability and arteriographic documentation of mesenteric vascular occlusion are required to reduce fatal complications.

Visceral ischemia may be acute or chronic. *Acute* insufficiency can cause nonspecific colicky pain and guaiac-positive stools, or it may produce sepsis, acidosis, and rapid hemodynamic deterioration. The symptoms of *chronic* intestinal ischemia are postprandial pain and weight loss. Approximately 40% of acute ischemic events are caused by emboli, 50% are associated with low-flow states and arterial thrombosis, and 10% or fewer are due to venous occlusion.[26]

If the vascular supply of the gut is otherwise normal, acute occlusion of the celiac or inferior mesenteric arteries is usually compensated for by extensive collateral circulation. In general, at least two of three mesenteric vessels must be significantly obstructed for occlusion of any one vessel to impair mesenteric blood flow markedly. Occasionally, acute occlusion of the inferior mesenteric artery by thrombosis or surgical ligation causes an ischemic colitis that is characterized by severe abdominal pain in the lower left quadrant, abdominal tenderness, and bloody stools.[27]

Although the superior mesenteric artery is subject to acute ischemia with either a thrombotic or embolic event, thrombosis usually results in more extensive ischemia because it occurs in severely diseased arteries and frequently involves the entire vessel. By contrast, emboli tend to lodge distal to the origin of the middle colic artery and may be found in otherwise normal intestinal vasculature. Mesenteric arterial emboli may easily require embolectomy, whereas mesenteric thrombosis often requires resection of a large segment of devitalized intestine.

Thrombosis of the superior mesenteric veins is associated with low blood flow, hypercoagulation, portal vein thrombosis resulting from portal hypertension, and splenic vein thrombosis resulting from compression or invasion by malignancy, particularly pancreatic tumors.[28] Splanchnic venous engorgement with edematous thickening of bowel loops produces a thumbprint pattern of gut folds, evident on upper gastrointestinal contrast radiography. Mesenteric venous thrombosis results in gut necrosis in 20% to 70% of patients. Mortality increases rapidly and approaches 100% if therapy is delayed longer than 12 hours after the onset of symptoms. Frequently, patients with acute mesenteric venous occlusion require thrombectomy, resection of devitalized bowel, and anticoagulation.

COMPLICATIONS OF VASCULAR SURGERY

In many instances, immediate thrombotic or hemorrhagic complications of vascular reconstructions can be corrected during the initial postoperative period. Long-term failures are related to progression of atherosclerosis, gradual thrombotic occlusion of prostheses, infection, deterioration of prosthetic grafts with false-aneurysm formation, perigraft hematoma accumulation, thrombosis caused by compression, or encroachment of a vascular reconstruction on adjacent organs. Many of these failures are insidious because occlusion of a reconstruction may not produce ischemia if hypertrophied collateral circulation can provide adequate blood supply. Unfortunately, a significant number of long-term complications result in severe ischemia, sepsis, life-threatening hemorrhage, or compromised organ function.

Most long-term failures of vascular reconstructions are related to progression of atherosclerosis or to a gradual thrombotic occlusion of a prosthetic segment. Thrombosis of arterial repairs is caused by narrowing of autogenous vein segments by arterialization of the vein wall, progressive thrombus accumulation in synthetic prostheses, infection, embolization of thrombotic deposits, and decreased flow in runoff vessels. Ankle Doppler pressure measurements every 3 months postoperatively can detect subclinical atherosclerotic or myointimal hyperplastic stenoses in lower-extremity vascular repairs. Many stenoses can be treated by surgery or transluminal balloon dilation before occlusion of the arterial reconstruction, thus restoring flow without compromising long-term patency.[29]

Graft infection frequently produces fever or sepsis and can be a life-threatening complication of vascular surgery, particularly if it occurs in synthetic or nonautogenous biologic vascular prostheses. In animals, tissue ingrowth decreases graft infection; in humans, however, vascular prostheses do not completely heal and usually only superficial wound infections that do not involve the vascular prosthesis can be treated without removing the graft.[30] Patients with cardiovascular implants undergoing invasive procedures or dental extractions should be treated prophylactically with antibiotics to avoid bacteremia.

Deterioration of vascular prosthetic materials may cause graft dilatation, false-aneurysm formation, suture line disruption, or perigraft hematoma formation. In general, any change in the configuration of a vascular reconstruction should be investigated to prevent complications.

Extra-anatomic bypasses are vascular reconstructions remote from the anatomic course of the vessel. They are usually subcutaneous or subfascial.[31] Extra-anatomic reconstructions were originally developed to revascularize the lower extremities when repair of an aortoduodenal fistula required removal of an infected aortic bifurcation graft and ligation of the aorta below the renal vessels. Blood flow to one leg is restored by placement of a prosthetic graft subcutaneously along the lateral chest wall, from the axillary artery to the ipsilateral femoral artery (i.e., axillofemoral bypass). Blood flow to the other leg is established through a second graft placed in a suprapubic subcutaneous position, from the axillofemoral reconstruction to the contralateral femoral artery (i.e., femoral-femoral bypass). Long-term function of axillobifemoral reconstructions is almost comparable to that aortobifemoral interposition prostheses.

An advantage of the extra-anatomic bypass is that the procedure can usually be performed with local or regional anesthesia in high-risk patients. A disadvantage is that subcutaneous prostheses are easily compressed while the patient is sleeping or unconscious, causing thrombosis of the graft and distal ischemia. Early recognition of thrombosis in an extra-anatomic bypass is essential because an acute thrombus can frequently be removed, restoring flow without affecting long-term patency.

Astute clinical judgment is required to detect symptoms caused by encroachment of a vascular repair on adjacent structures. Fibrous encapsulation and stiffening of a limb of an aortobifemoral prosthesis can obstruct the ureter, producing persistent flank pain resulting from hydronephrosis or renal infection.[32] Compression of the iliac vein causes unilateral lower-extremity venous hypertension, swelling, and discomfort.

Aortoduodenal fistula is a dramatic example of a vascular repair eroding into an adjacent organ.[33] Both infection and pulsation of the aortic anastomosis of an aortobifemoral reconstruction have been proposed as possible causes of the aortoduodenal communication. Aortoduodenal fistula should be suspected in patients with aortobifemoral bypasses who are experiencing massive upper gastrointestinal bleeding. These patients frequently have had a preliminary hematemesis within the previous 24 hours. Endoscopic confirmation of bleeding from the third portion of the duodenum requires immediate laparotomy to rule out this complication; aortography is usually contraindicated because it may not show the enteric communication and because immediate laparotomy is required to prevent exsanguination.

VENOUS DISEASES

Thrombophlebitis is venous thrombosis that follows inflammation of the vein wall and causes severe pain and swelling of the extremity. Venous thrombosis without inflammation of the vein wall may be asymptomatic except for mild discomfort and swelling. The incidence of venous thrombosis is increased by major injury or surgery, pregnancy, previous thrombosis, cancer, infection, varicose veins, obesity, and long periods of sitting or lying.[34] Thrombosis of the leg veins has been reported in 28% of elective surgical patients, 54% of those with hip fractures, and approximately 20% of patients treated for myocardial infarction.[35]

The three apparent causes of venous thrombosis are:

- Stasis
- Injury to the vessel wall
- Increased coagulability of the blood (Virchow's triad)

Fibrinogen radionuclide studies of hospitalized patients demonstrated that thrombi develop in areas of stasis and turbulent blood flow near venous valves.[36] Continued thrombosis occludes the vessel lumen and produces distal venous hypertension. Frequently, blood flow through the vein is restored by resorption and organization or embolization of the thrombus; however, organization of venous thrombosis destroys the valves, and recanalized veins are prone to subsequent thrombosis.

Chronic venous obstruction and valvular insufficiency are characterized by discoloration and induration of the overlying skin. If venous hypertension is greater than capillary diffusion pressure, edema develops. Tissue ischemia and venous gangrene develop if venous pressures exceed capillary perfusion pressure.

Superficial thromboses produce a bothersome lump or cord that can be treated with local care and, if necessary, excision. These thromboses are usually of no consequence unless caused by infection. By contrast, deep venous thrombosis produces severe swelling of the extremity and without treatment can lead to long-term hemodynamic problems and significant (>1 cm in diameter) pulmonary emboli.[37] The soleal veins of the lower leg are the most frequent sites of deep venous thromboses. Most soleal thromboses are asymptomatic, aside from mild calf pain; however, pain and swelling of the lower extremity increase if thrombi extend into the femoral and iliac veins. Iliofemoral venous thrombosis can produce massive swelling, pain, purpura, and a bluish discoloration of the leg called *phlegmasia cerulea dolens*. If iliofemoral thrombosis completely occludes venous outflow, venous pressure increases until venous gangrene and arterial spasm caused by local irritation result in a massively swollen and painful white leg, a condition known as *phlegmasia cerulea albicans*. This syndrome is usually associated with disseminated malignancies or sepsis. Isolated pelvic thrombi associated with pelvic inflammation or tumor invasion do not cause edema if the iliac vein remains patent.

Patients with venous thrombosis of the upper extremity require therapy if the deep veins are involved. Exertion, intravenous catheters, trauma, intravenous drug abuse, neoplastic disease, and congenital venous malformations have been described as causes of axillary-subclavian vein thromboses.[38] Intermittent subclavian vein obstruction and thrombosis can follow compression of the vein between the first rib and clavicle. Axillary-subclavian vein thromboses cause severe pain and swelling of the arm and hand, and frequently there is percussion tenderness over the clavicle and axillary vein. These thromboses can be a source of hemodynamically significant pulmonary emboli, particularly when associated with causes other than exertion.

A venous thrombus may become infected, or it may be caused by infection. Infected thromboses are usually seen in intravenous drug abusers and in debilitated patients who have had multiple intravenous catheters. Infected thromboses may be the source of systemic sepsis, endocarditis, or septic emboli. Immediate excision of the entire vein is required to prevent complications.

Venography is the most accurate method for diagnosis of significant venous thromboses, although a combination of Doppler ultrasonography and impedance plethysmography has an accuracy rate of 95% in detecting deep venous thrombosis of the leg.[39] A difference of 1.5 cm in diameter between a swollen leg and the contralateral leg offers corroborative physical evidence of venous thrombosis. Calf tenderness and Homans' sign are less reliable diagnostic signs.

Therapy for venous thrombosis ideally prevents propagation of the thrombosis, late sequelae related to destruction of venous anatomy, secondary infection, and pulmonary emboli. Destruction of the valves by the organizing thrombus increases venous pressures and ultimately leads to the *postphlebitic syndrome*, a debilitating and irreversible venous disease. There are few surgical alternatives, and therapy relies primarily on custom-fitted support stockings and meticulous skin care. Tortuous varicose veins can be removed if they are painful or unsightly, but varicosities frequently recur with persistent venous hypertension or primary venous degenerative disease. The superficial venous system should not be removed if there is deep venous occlusion, because in this instance the superficial veins are the only route for egress of blood from the extremity. Excision of varicose veins near stasis ulcers improves wound healing. In certain cases, valvuloplasty or crossover venous reconstructions can coestablish venous flow and reduce venous hypertension.[40]

FUTURE PERSPECTIVES

Vascular surgery has become a separate surgical subspecialty as direct surgical and pharmacologic approaches to therapy have developed. The pioneering vascular surgeons beginning in the 1950s discovered methods for disobliteration of occlusive atherosclerotic disease by incision of the vessel wall and surgical removal of obstructions or by use of tubular prosthetic bypasses to circumvent occluded segments. Concomitant advances in anesthetic technique, anticoagulation, and antibiotic therapy allowed reconstruction of smaller, lower-flow arteries and veins with improved instrumentation, suture materials, and operative techniques. Subsequent advances included a redefinition of the indications for surgical interventions by establishing a natural history of occlusive lesions and the outcome of surgical interventions in the peripheral and coronary circulations. The careful follow-up of patients helped to establish the data base that serves as the "gold standard" for evaluation of new therapies.

Vascular therapy continues to evolve rapidly, and the vascular surgeon can further advance the therapy of vascular diseases using new information about the biochemistry and genetics of pathologic lesions. This new information promises to enhance the understanding of the cause and development of vascular lesions and to improve the therapy for chronic ischemia and reperfusion syndromes.

Cardiovascular diagnosis and treatment are rapidly becoming more noninvasive. Ultrasonography, CT scans, magnetic resonance imaging and spectroscopy, and positron emission tomographic scans all minimize the invasive nature of the procedure and maximize the accuracy of diagnosis.[41] Special applications of these techniques provide precise anatomic, hemodynamic, and biochemical information about vascular diseases and tissue metabolism, increasing the potential for early diagnosis and treatment of lesions. Therapeutic catheter-based interventions are being evaluated to expand the treatment while potentially replacing a significant percentage of conventional surgical procedures.[42]

This rapid evolution in vascular science and surgery exemplifies the effect that technologic development has on both medicine and science. Continued, controlled experimental and clinical investigations now have the potential to improve dramatically the successful treatment of many cardiovascular disorders. This rapid advance may redefine the prevention of some diseases and the therapy of others. It is the responsibility of the scientific medical community to direct and apply our resources to maximize this evolution.

References

1. Loop FD: Combined cardiac and peripheral vascular disease. Contemp Surg 1981; 18:47.
2. Strandness DE Jr, Sumner DS, Mozersky DJ, et al: The use of ultrasonic arteriography for arterial visualization. Scand J Clin Lab Invest 1973; 31(Suppl 128):163.
3. Saloner D, Anderson C, Caputo G: Magnetic resonance imaging. *In:* Vascular Surgery: Basic Science and Clinical Correlations. White RA, Hollier L (Eds). Philadelphia, JB Lippincott, 1994, pp 477–496.
4. Stahler C, Strandness DE Jr: Ankle blood pressure response to graded treadmill exercise. Angiology 1967; 18:237.
5. deVirgilio C, Sang P, Arnell T, et al: Cardiac assessment prior to vascular surgery: Is dipyridamole-sestamibi necessary? Ann Vasc Surg 1996; 10:325.
6. Karmody AM, Powers SR, Monaco VJ, et al: "Blue toe" syndrome: An indication for limb salvage surgery. Arch Surg 1976; 111:1263.
7. Patman RD, Thompson JE: Fasciotomy in peripheral vascular surgery. Arch Surg 1970; 101:663.
8. Hines EA Jr: Some types of distress in the lower extremities simulating peripheral vascular disease. Med Clin North Am 1958; 42:991.
9. Perdue GD, Long WD, Smith RB III: Perspective concerning aortofemoral arterial reconstruction. Trans South Surg Assoc 1970; 82:330.
10. Ernst CE: Abdominal aortic aneurysm. N Engl J Med 1993; 328:1167.
11. Weibull H, Bergqvist D, Bergentz S, et al: Percutaneous transluminal renal angioplasty versus surgical reconstruction of atherosclerotic renal artery stenosis: A prospective randomized study. J Vasc Surg 1993; 16:841.
12. DePalma RC, Kedia K, Persky L: Surgical options in the correction of vasculogenic impotence. Vasc Surg 1980; 14:92.
13. Darling RC: Ruptured arteriosclerotic abdominal aortic aneurysms: Pathologic and clinical study. Am J Surg 1970; 119:397.
14. Busuttil RW, Abou-Zamzam Am, Machleder HI: Collagenase activity of the human aorta. Arch Surg 1980; 115:1373.
15. Brawley RK, Murray CR, Crisler C, et al: Management of wounds of the innominate, subclavian, and axillary blood vessels. Surg Gynecol Obstet 1970; 131:1130.
16. Peet RM, Henriksen JD, Anderson TP: Thoracic-outlet syndrome: Evaluation of a therapeutic exercise program. Proc Staff Mayo Clin 1956; 31:281.
17. Lord JW, Rosati LM: Thoracic outlet syndromes. Clin Symp 1971; 2:3.
18. Porter JM, Bardana EJ, Baur GM, et al: The clinical significance of Raynaud's syndrome. Surgery 1976; 80:756.
19. Hobson RW II, Weiss DG, Fields W, et al: Efficacy of carotid endarterectomy for asymptomatic carotid stenosis: The Veterans Affairs Cooperative Study Group. N Engl J Med 1993; 328:221.
20. Executive Committee for the Asymptomatic Carotid Atherosclerosis Study: Endarterectomy for asymptomatic carotid artery stenosis. JAMA 1995; 271:1421.
21. Imparato AM, Riles TS, Gorstein F: The carotid bifurcation plaque:

Pathologic findings associated with cerebral ischemia. Stroke 1979; 10:238.
22. Hollenhorst RW: Significance of bright plaques in the retinal arterioles. JAMA 1961; 178:23.
23. A new vascular syndrome: "The subclavian steal" (Editorial). N Engl J Med 1961; 265:912.
24. Bergan JJ, Dean RH, Conn J Jr: Revascularization in the treatment of mesenteric infarction. Ann Surg 1978; 188:721.
25. Pierce GE, Brockenbrough EC: The spectrum of mesenteric infarction. Am J Surg 1970; 119:233.
26. Ottinger LW: The surgical management of acute occlusion of the superior mesenteric artery. Ann Surg 1978; 188:721.
27. Marston A, Phiels MT, Thomas ML, et al: Ischemic colitis. Gut 1966; 7:1.
28. Warren S, Eberhard TP: Mesenteric venous thrombosis. Surg Gynecol Obstet 1935; 61:102.
29. Zarins CK, Lu C, McDonnell AE, et al: Limb salvage by percutaneous transluminal recanalization of occluded superficial femoral artery. Surgery 1980; 87:701.
30. Moore WS, Malone JS, Keown K: Prosthetic arterial graft material, influence of neointimal healing on bacteremic infectability. Arch Surg 1980; 115:1379.
31. Blaisdell FW: Symposium: Extra-anatomic vascular shunt. Contemp Surg 1979; 15:69.
32. Heard G, Hinde G: Hydronephrosis complicating aortic reconstruction. Br J Surg 1975; 62:344.
33. Kierman PD, Pairolero PC, Huber JP, et al: Aortic graft–enteric fistula. Mayo Clin Proc 1980; 55:731.
34. Coon WW, Coller FA: Some epidemiologic considerations in thromboembolism. Surg Gynecol Obstet 1959; 109:487.
35. Kakkar V: Prevention of fatal postoperative pulmonary embolism by low doses of heparin. Lancet 1975; ii:45.
36. Kakkar V: The diagnosis of deep vein thrombosis using the ^{125}I fibrinogen test. Arch Surg 1972; 104:152.
37. Barner HB, DeWeese JA: An evaluation of the sphygmomanometer cuff pain test in venous thrombosis. Surgery 1960; 48:915.
38. Harley D, White RA, Nelson RJ, et al: Pulmonary embolism secondary to upper extremity venous thrombosis. Am J Surg 1984; 147:221.
39. Sumner DS, Mattos MA: Diagnosis of deep vein thrombosis with real-time color and duplex scanning. *In:* Vascular Diagnosis. 4th ed. Bernstein EF (Ed). St. Louis, Mosby-Year Book, 1993, pp 785–800.
40. Dale WA: Crossover graft for iliofemoral venous occlusion. *In:* Venous Problems. Bergen JJ, Yao JST (Eds). Chicago, Year Book Medical Publishers, 1978, pp 411–420.
41. Cavaye DM, White RA (Eds): A Text and Atlas of Arterial Imaging. London, Chapman & Hall, 1994.
42. White RA, Fogarty TJ (Eds): Peripheral Endovascular Interventions. St. Louis, Mosby-Year Book, 1996.

104

Inotropic Therapy and the Critically Ill Patient*

Edgar R. Gonzalez, PharmD
Barbara S. Kannewurf, PharmD
Michael L. Hess, MD, FACC

Approximately 20% to 40% of patients in the intensive care unit (ICU) require inotropic support during their stay. A retrospective evaluation of the use of inotropic agents at a teaching hospital found that more than 60% of the patients received inappropriate inotropic therapy and 80% of combination inotropic regimens were deemed inappropriate. Improper use of these agents stems primarily from a poor understanding of the pharmacodynamic activities of the different agents available.

To appreciate subtle differences between inotropic agents and between vasoactive agents, it is important to understand the functions of adrenergic receptors that regulate cardiac, vascular, bronchiolar, uterine, and gastrointestinal smooth muscle tone. There are three types of adrenergic receptors:

- α-Adrenergic (α_1 and α_2)
- β-Adrenergic (β_1 and β_2)
- Dopaminergic (DA_1 and DA_2)

Sympathomimetic amines and catecholamines differ in their affinity for adrenergic receptors. Bipyridine-based agents bypass adrenergic receptors and selectively inhibit phosphodiesterase (Table 104–1).

The α_1 receptors are present in the postsynaptic region of neurons in vascular smooth muscle. Stimulation of the vascular receptor leads primarily to arteriolar vasoconstriction. The α_1 receptors in the myocardium mediate positive inotropic and negative chronotropic effects. The hierarchy of clinically available adrenergic agonists on α_1 receptors, in order of increasing potency, is phenylephrine, norepinephrine, and epinephrine.

Stimulation of β_1 receptors increases heart rate and myocardial contractility and enhances atrioventricular nodal conduction. Stimulation of β_2 receptors causes vasodilation and leads to relaxation of bronchial, uterine, and gastrointestinal smooth muscle. The β_2-receptor activity also modulates fat metabolism, promotes glycogenolysis, and drives potassium into cells. Beta$_2$-mediated hypokalemia may play an important role in the induction of arrhythmias during ischemia and may explain the beneficial effects of β-adrenergic blockade both acutely and for secondary prevention of cardiac events after myocardial infarction. Stimulation of β_2-adrenergic receptors in the kidneys releases renin from the juxtaglomerular apparatus.

Coronary arteries possess both α-adrenergic and β-adrenergic receptors. The α-adrenergic receptors predominate in the larger epicardial coronaries and β-adrenergic receptors predominate in the smaller resistance vessels of the coronary tree. Stimulation of α receptors produces coronary vasoconstriction. Postsynaptic α_2 receptors may be particularly important in mediating coronary vasospasm. Stimulation of β-adrenergic receptors generally results in coronary vasodilation. During ischemia, vasodilatory substances (e.g., adenosine

*Supported in part by a grant-in-aid from the American Heart Association to Michael L. Hess, MD.

TABLE 104–1. Adrenergic Receptor Activity of Sympathomimetic Amines*

Drug	α_1	α_2	β_1	β_2	Dopamine
Dopamine					
1–2 μg/kg/min	0	0	+	0	+ + + +
2–10 μg/kg/min	0	0	+ + + +	0	+ + + +
10–20 μg/kg/min	+ + +	0	+ + + +	0	0
Dobutamine					
2–10 μg/kg/min	+	0	+ + +	+ +	0
>10 μg/kg/min	+ +	0	+ + + +	+ + +	0
Epinephrine					
0.01–0.05 μg/kg/min	+	0	+ +	+ + +	0
>0.05 μg/kg/min	+ + +	+ + +	+ + +	+ + +	0
Norepinephrine					
0.5–3 μg/kg/min	+ + + +	+ + +	+ +	0	0
Phenylephrine					
10–50 μg/min	+ + + +	0	0	0	0
Isoproternol					
2–10 μg/min	0	0	+ + + +	+ + +	0

*β_1, contractility or inotropic activity and sinoatrial node activity (chronotropic activity); β_2, vasodilation; α_1 and α_2, vasoconstriction.

and prostacyclin) are released locally to counteract coronary vasoconstriction. Patients with coronary artery disease may have an exaggerated response to adrenergically mediated coronary vasoconstriction; therefore, α-adrenergic agonists must be used with caution, if at all, for patients with acute ischemic disease.

Stimulation of dopaminergic (DA_1) receptors produces renal, coronary, cerebral, and mesenteric vasodilation and a natriuretic response. DA_2 receptors increase norepinephrine release from sympathetic nerve endings, inhibit prolactin release, and may induce vomiting. Dopaminergic stimulation also suppresses peristalsis and may precipitate an ileus.

VASOACTIVE INOTROPES

Dopamine

Dopamine hydrochloride is a chemical precursor of norepinephrine that causes dose-dependent stimulation of dopaminergic, β_1-adrenergic, and α_1-adrenergic receptors. Dopamine also triggers the release of endogenous norepinephrine.

In low doses (1 to 2 μg/kg/min), dopamine produces vasodilation of renal, mesenteric, coronary, and cerebral arteries by direct dopaminergic stimulation. Urine output may increase, but heart rate and blood pressure are usually unchanged.

Within the dosage range 2 to 10 μg/kg/min, dopamine stimulates β_1-adrenergic receptors and increases heart rate, myocardial contractility, and cardiac output. Increases in cardiac output partially offset dopamine's α_1-adrenergic receptor–mediated arterial vasoconstriction. Dopamine at doses of 2 to 10 μg/kg/min produces minimal changes in systemic vascular resistance. In contrast, the dose-response curve of the effect of dopamine on venous capacitance is shallow.

At a dose of 2.5 μg/kg/min, dopamine produces venoconstriction and increases pulmonary arterial pressures.[1] At doses above 10 μg/kg/min, dopamine predominantly stimulates α_1-adrenergic receptors to produce widespread arterial and venous constriction. Dopamine regimens above 20 μg/kg/min produce hemodynamic effects that are similar to those of norepinephrine.[1]

Because of its hemodynamic effects, dopamine is an excellent vasopressor inotrope for patients with oliguria, hypotension, and a low cardiac output. Doses of dopamine above 2.5 μg/kg/min should be avoided for patients with elevated pulmonary pressures or elevated systemic vascular resistance and those who require inotropic support.

Dopamine is indicated for hemodynamically significant hypotension in the absence of hypovolemia. One reasonable criterion for the presence of significant hypotension is a systolic arterial pressure less than 90 mm Hg accompanied by evidence of poor tissue perfusion, oliguria, or changes in mental status. Dopamine should be used at the lowest dose that produces adequate perfusion of vital organs. The presence of increased vascular resistance, pulmonary congestion, or increased preload is a relative contraindication to the use of dopamine. In this setting, dopamine should be used in low doses (1 to 2 μg/kg/min) to enhance renal blood flow.

Experimental data for animals suggest that dopamine at a dose of 40 mg is comparable to epinephrine during closed-chest massage in its ability to increase blood pressure and improve the probability of successful resuscitation.[2] However, a later study using a prolonged model of cardiac arrest demonstrated that dopamine is less effective than epinephrine in improving hemodynamics during cardiopulmonary resuscitation (CPR).[3] During resuscitation, treatment with dopamine is usually reserved for hypotension that occurs with symptomatic bradycardia or after return of spontaneous circulation. Norepinephrine should be added if more than 20 μg/kg/min is needed to maintain blood pressure. Gonzalez and colleagues[4] studied the vasopressor response to incremental doses of intravenous epinephrine (1, 3, and 5 mg) with and without dopamine (15 μg/kg/min) in nine prehospital cardiac arrest victims. Epinephrine alone produced a significant ($P <$ .05) dose-dependent vasopressor effect on systolic and diastolic blood pressure. Concomitant administration of epinephrine and dopamine did not produce an additive vasopressor effect.[4]

In the period immediately after resuscitation, higher doses of dopamine may be required to induce the transient hypertension recommended to improve cerebral perfusion. It is important to remember that the α-adrenergic effects of dopamine, even at low infusion rates, elevate the pulmonary artery occlusive pressure and may induce or exacerbate pulmonary congestion despite a rise in cardiac output. Vasodilators (e.g., nitroglycerin or nitroprusside) can be used to reduce preload and improve cardiac output by antagonizing increases in venous and arterial resistance produced by dopamine. The combination of dopamine and nitroprusside produces hemodynamic effects similar to those of dobutamine.[5]

In shock, the initial rate of infusion for dopamine is 5 to 10 μg/kg/min. The infusion rate may be increased until blood pressure, urine output, and other parameters of organ perfusion improve. Although some patients may respond to dosages of up to 40 μg/kg/min, these high dosages of dopamine may lead to tachyarrhythmias and to depletion of endogenous norepinephrine stores with subsequent loss of vasopressor response.[4] Therefore, as with all catecholamines, the lowest infusion rate of dopamine that results in satisfactory hemodynamic performance should be used. Dopamine should be administered via a volumetric infusion pump to ensure precise flow rates. Hemodynamic monitoring is essential for proper use, and it should be instituted before or as soon as possible after initiation of treatment. Dopamine should be tapered gradually to avoid an acute hypotensive response. The risk of hypotension may be minimized if the patient is euvolemic before weaning from dopamine.

Dopamine is available for intravenous use only. The contents of one or two ampules (400 mg per ampule) should be mixed in 250 mL of 5% dextrose. This yields a concentration of 1600 or 3200 μg/mL. The initial rate of infusion is 1 to 2 μg/kg/min. A final dosage range of 5 to 30 μg/kg/min is recommended to minimize side effects. Hemodynamic monitoring is essential in patients who have ischemic heart disease or congestive heart failure and should be instituted before, or as soon as possible after, initiation of treatment with dopamine.

Dopamine increases heart rate and may induce or exacerbate supraventricular and ventricular arrhythmias. Furthermore, its venous and arterial vasoconstricting effects, even at low doses, can exacerbate pulmonary congestion and compromise cardiac output. Occasionally, these effects may warrant a dosage reduction or discontinuation of the infusion. Despite hemodynamic improvements, myocardial oxygen consumption and myocardial lactate production may increase in response to higher doses of dopamine, indicating that coronary blood supply is not sufficiently augmented to compensate for the increased cardiac work.[8] This imbalance between supply and demand would be expected to induce or exacerbate myocardial ischemia.

Nausea and vomiting are frequent side effects of dopamine, especially at high doses. Dopamine can produce cutaneous tissue necrosis and sloughing if interstitial extravasation occurs. Treatment of dopamine-induced extravasation requires discontinuation of the infusion, application of warm compresses, and intradermal administration of phentolamine.

Monoamine oxidase inhibitors, such as isocarboxazid (Marplan), pargyline hydrochloride (Eutonyl), tranylcypromine sulfate (Parnate), and phenelzine sulfate (Nardil), may potentiate the effects of dopamine.[6] Therefore, patients receiving these agents should be treated with one-tenth the usual dose of dopamine. Agents with similar hemodynamic effects (e.g., the initial effects of bretylium tosylate) may be synergistic with dopamine. Patients receiving phenytoin may experience hypotension during concomitant administration of dopamine. Dopamine may precipitate a hypertensive crisis in patients with pheochromocytoma and is contraindicated for these patients.[6] Dopamine should not be added to solutions containing sodium bicarbonate or other alkaline intravenous solutions because dopamine is slowly inactivated at alkaline pH. This reaction is slow enough that dopamine and alkaline solutions (aminophylline, phenytoin, sodium bicarbonate) that are administered over a short period can be infused through the same venous catheter.

Dobutamine

Dobutamine is a synthetic sympathomimetic amine with two active isomers. The D-isomer is a potent β-adrenergic agonist; the L-isomer is a potent α-adrenergic agonist. Experimental data suggest that dobutamine exerts its potent inotropic effect by stimulating β_1-adrenergic and α_1-adrenergic receptors in myocardium with little primary effect on peripheral vasculature.[6]

In contrast to norepinephrine and dopamine, dobutamine produces little systemic arterial or venous constriction at usual clinical doses. Dobutamine causes a reflex decrease in peripheral vascular resistance related to the increase in cardiac output. Pulmonary artery occlusive pressure is reduced.[1, 7] In addition, dobutamine increases heart rate only at higher doses. Dobutamine increases renal and mesenteric blood flow by improving cardiac output but not by dopaminergic-mediated vasodilation of the renal or mesenteric arteries. The net hemodynamic effects of dobutamine are similar to those of dopamine combined with a vasodilator such as nitroprusside.[5]

Dobutamine is an excellent agent for the treatment of left ventricular dysfunction, especially in patients with elevated pulmonary pressures and a high systemic vascular resistance. Dobutamine should not be used as a vasopressor agent to increase blood pressure in patients with hypovolemic shock or in patients with a low systemic vascular resistance.[6] The efficacy of dobutamine as a substitute for epinephrine during resuscitation has been evaluated in dogs.[2] Resuscitation was significantly more common in dogs receiving agents with potent α-adrenergic effects, such as dopamine,[5, 9] using the smallest effective dose needed to improve hemodynamics.

The hemodynamic actions of dobutamine and its lack of effect on endogenous norepinephrine release explain why it has a more favorable impact on myocardial oxygen demand than either norepinephrine or dopamine.[6] Its positive inotropic effect is balanced by increased coronary blood flow, so oxygen extraction across the heart remains unchanged.[8] However, dobutamine can produce ischemia if it increases heart rate.[9] Therefore, the dose of dobutamine should be titrated to avoid increases in heart rate greater than 10%.[10] The maximum dose is 40 μg/kg/min. Dobutamine may cause tachycardia, arrhythmias, and fluctuations in blood pressure, which can provoke myocardial ischemia, especially at higher doses. Other side effects include headache, nausea, tremor, and hypokalemia.

Isoproterenol

Isoproterenol hydrochloride is a synthetic sympathomimetic amine with pure β-adrenergic receptor agonist activity. Isoproterenol markedly increases myocardial oxygen requirements and may exacerbate or induce ischemia, especially if its potent positive chronotropic and inotropic effects are not balanced by a corresponding increase in coronary blood flow.[11] The potent positive inotropic and chronotropic effects of isoproterenol increase cardiac output, but mean arterial pressure may remain unchanged or decrease because pure β-adrenergic stimulation causes arterial vasodilation. Because isoproterenol can reduce coronary perfusion pressure despite an increase in myocardial oxygen demand, it is rarely used as an inotropic agent and is contraindicated during closed-chest massage.[12]

Newer inotropic agents (i.e., dobutamine, milrinone) that are less likely to induce ischemia and tachyarrhythmias have replaced isoproterenol as an inotrope in most clinical settings. The principal indication for isoproterenol in emergency cardiac care is for the immediate and temporary treatment of hemodynamically unstable bradycardia that is refractory to atropine in a patient with a pulse. Percutaneous or transvenous electrical pacing provides better control of the heart rate with less risk of inducing ischemia and should be initiated in preference to isoproterenol or as soon as possible after initiation of therapy with isoproterenol.

When isoproterenol is used to increase heart rate, the initial intravenous starting dose is 2 μg/min (1 mg of isoproterenol diluted in 250 mL of 5% dextrose in water [D5W]). The dose is titrated upward until the ventricular response rate is approximately 60 beats/min. In general, this takes no more than 10 μg/min. Because isoproterenol increases myocardial oxygen requirements, it should be avoided for patients with ischemic heart disease. Its potent chronotropic properties can induce serious arrhythmias, including ventricular tachycardia and fibrillation. Isoproterenol may also exacerbate tachyarrhythmias caused by digitalis toxicity and may precipitate hypokalemia.

Amrinone and Milrinone

Amrinone is a bipyridine derivative with inotropic and vasodilatory properties. Milrinone is the 2-methyl, 5-carbonitrile derivative of amrinone and differs from it in potency. Amrinone and milrinone are phosphodiesterase inhibitors that have positive inotropic, lusitropic, and vasodilator effects with little chronotropic activity.[13] Amrinone and milrinone selectively inhibit peak III cyclic adenosine monophosphate (cAMP) phosphodiesterase isoenzyme in cardiac and vascular muscle.[13, 14] The resultant increase in cAMP leads to an elevation in ionized calcium (Ca^{2+}) in the myocardium, causing positive inotropy. The dose-dependent vasodilatory effects of amrinone and milrinone are due to AMP-dependent vasodilation in vascular smooth muscle.[13] This vasodilation may further improve cardiac output by reducing systemic vascular resistance.

At higher doses, milrinone and amrinone increase myocardial filling along with the enhanced isovolumic relaxation. Furthermore, amrinone and milrinone produce a marked reduction in pulmonary arterial pressures and are the preferred inotropes for patients with left ventricular dysfunction and significant pulmonary hypertension.[13, 14] Amrinone was the first of the dipyridine derivatives developed. Its use was hampered by a long half-life and the production of thrombocytopenia. Its derivative milrinone has a much shorter half-life and is associated with a small to negligible incidence of thrombocytopenia. Milrinone has replaced amrinone as the inodilator of choice in low-cardiac-output syndromes. Arrhythmias appear to occur less frequently with milrinone than with dobutamine.

The effect of phosphodiesterase inhibitors is directly related to the amount of cAMP present in tissues. For this reason, it may be good practice to use milrinone in combination with dobutamine because dobutamine increases cAMP levels and may augment the effect of the phosphodiesterase inhibitors.[15] The phosphodiesterase inhibitors are front-line drugs for the treatment of patients with decompensated left ventricular function. They are also indicated as adjuncts to catecholamines, generally in the setting of cardiogenic shock, when tolerance to the latter is suspected, or in the setting of catecholamine intolerance.

A loading dose of milrinone (50 μg/kg) is generally required because of its relatively long half-life (2 to 3 hours), especially if no other inotrope is being administered concurrently. Patients receiving concomitant therapy with dobutamine or dopamine may be treated with amrinone or milrinone without a loading dose. Continuous infusions of milrinone are initiated at a rate of 0.25 μg/kg/min. These infusion regimens are titrated to desired hemodynamic endpoints. Milrinone infusions of up to 1 μg/kg/min may be used and produce less thrombocytopenia than amrinone.

Because the phosphodiesterase inhibitors undergo renal clearance, their elimination half-lives may be prolonged in patients with renal failure, and a reduced dosage is required for these patients. Milrinone may produce clinical improvement in patients with heart failure who become tolerant to the inotropic effects of dobutamine and is thus becoming increasingly popular as the first inotrope of choice for these patients. There is no need to taper milrinone when the drug is being discontinued.

Finally, another relative benefit of milrinone is that heart rate and myocardial oxygen consumption are not increased. This makes milrinone an excellent choice for patients with decompensated heart failure related to an ischemic cardiomyopathy.

VASOPRESSORS

Norepinephrine

Norepinephrine is a naturally occurring catecholamine that differs chemically from epinephrine only by the absence of a methyl group on the terminal amine. Epinephrine and norepinephrine are approximately equipotent in their ability to stimulate β_1-adrenergic receptors, but their effects on α_1-adrenergic and β_2-adrenergic receptors are quite different.[13, 16] Norepinephrine is a potent α-receptor agonist with no effect on β_2 receptors. Norepinephrine increases myocardial contractility because of its β_1-adrenergic effects, whereas its potent α-adrenergic effects lead to arterial and venous vasoconstriction.

Norepinephrine's positive inotropic and vasopressor effects have been used in the treatment of refractory shock. However, the increased vascular resistance induced by norepinephrine may counteract its positive inotropic effects. Because norepinephrine increases myocardial oxygen demand, it can exacerbate myocardial ischemia, especially if coronary vasoconstriction is induced by stimulation of coronary α receptors. Norepinephrine should be used with caution for patients with ischemic heart disease.

Norepinephrine is used for the treatment of hemodynamically significant hypotension. Hypotension and low systemic vascular resistance occur rarely in patients with acute myocardial infarction but are more common in patients with sepsis. Successful management requires not only support of the blood pressure but also correction of the underlying abnormalities. The combination of dobutamine and norepinephrine appears to enhance tissue perfusion more than either agent alone in patients with septic shock refractory to fluid resuscitation. Studies show that triple therapy with dobutamine (20 to 30 μg/kg/min), norepinephrine (0.5 to 1.0 μg/kg/min), and dopamine (2 to 4 μg/kg/min) improves myocardial function, enhances tissue perfusion and oxygen delivery, and maintains renal and mesenteric blood flow in patients with septic shock refractory to fluid resuscitation.[16] Patients treated in this manner tend to have improved cardiorespiratory parameters, reduced lactate production, and enhanced survival.

Norepinephrine improves blood flow and renal perfusion when used in the absence of profound acidosis in patients with septic shock refractory to fluid therapy.[16] Studies suggest that lactic acidosis may blunt the renal sparing effects of norepinephrine in patients with septic shock.[16] Therefore, norepinephrine should be used with caution in patients with lactic acidosis because norepinephrine-induced systemic vasoconstriction may adversely affect renal function in these patients.

Norepinephrine should be infused through a central venous catheter to minimize the risk of extravasation. Infusions of 2 μg/min or higher are generally used as a starting dose. The infusion rate is then titrated to achieve the desired effect, which is usually maintenance of an adequate blood pressure (a reasonable criterion is a systolic pressure of at least 90 mm Hg) at the lowest possible dose. The average adult dose is 6 to 12 μg/min. Patients with refractory shock may require norepinephrine at 3 to 5 μg/kg/min to maintain an adequate blood pressure. Norepinephrine should be administered via a volumetric infusion system that ensures a precise flow rate. The use of this drug should be viewed as a temporizing measure, and the dose should be reduced or the infusion discontinued as soon as possible. Norepinephrine should be tapered slowly to avoid abrupt and severe hypotension.

Because peripheral blood pressure measurements may be inaccurate when severe vasoconstriction is present, central intra-arterial pressure monitoring may be necessary for accurate determination of arterial pressure. If the central and peripheral pressures are the same, the use of arterial monitoring should be discontinued. When continuous invasive arterial blood pressure monitoring is not available, cuff or Doppler blood pressure should be monitored every 5 minutes during titration and then at frequent intervals depending on the patient's hemodynamic status. For patients who require vasopressor support with norepinephrine, hemodynamic monitoring should be carried out to assess changes in cardiac output, pulmonary occlusive pressure, and peripheral arterial resistance.

Norepinephrine is contraindicated when hypotension is due to hypovolemia except as a temporizing measure to maintain coronary and cerebral perfusion pressure until volume replacement can be achieved. Norepinephrine increases myocardial oxygen requirements without producing a compensatory increase in coronary blood flow. This can be deleterious in patients with myocardial ischemia or infarction. Norepinephrine may precipitate arrhythmias, especially in volume-depleted patients and those with limited myocardial reserves. Extravasation of norepinephrine produces ischemic necrosis and sloughing of superficial tissues. If extravasation occurs, phentolamine (5 to 10 mg diluted in 10 to 15 mL of saline solution) should be infiltrated into the area to antagonize the norepinephrine-induced vasoconstriction and to minimize necrosis and sloughing.

Epinephrine

Epinephrine is an endogenous catecholamine with both α-adrenergic and β-adrenergic agonist activity. In general, the following cardiovascular responses can be expected to be increased from administration of epinephrine[17]:

- Systemic vascular resistance
- Arterial blood pressure
- Electrical activity in the myocardium
- Coronary and cerebral blood flow
- Myocardial contraction
- Myocardial oxygen requirements
- Automaticity

The actions of epinephrine are dose-dependent. Low doses produce β_1-adrenergic and β_2-adrenergic stimulation. The α-adrenergic effects of epinephrine become evident at moderate doses and continue to increase in a dose-dependent manner.

Epinephrine produces favorable redistribution of blood flow during CPR. The elevation of coronary perfusion pressure after administration of epinephrine is beneficial in all forms of cardiorespiratory arrest.[17] Epinephrine is a useful vasoactive, inotropic agent for selected patients with refractory circulatory shock, for example, after cardiopulmonary bypass. The initial dose for adults is 1 μg/min titrated to desired hemodynamic response.

Epinephrine is also the drug of choice for patients with anaphylactic shock. However, epinephrine should be avoided for patients with circulatory shock caused by or exacerbated by α-adrenergic blockade because β_2-adrenergic stimulation aggravates the patient's low systemic vascular resistance. These patients require large doses of norepinephrine to counteract the underlying α-adrenergic blockade. If concurrent therapy with epinephrine is required for the treatment of anaphylactic shock in patients with α-adrenergic blockade, phenylephrine is the α-adrenergic agonists of choice because it does not stimulate β_1-adrenergic receptors.

Even at low doses of epinephrine, its positive inotropic and chronotropic effects can precipitate or exacerbate myocardial ischemia. Epinephrine and possibly other catecholamines may induce or exacerbate ventricular ectopy, especially in patients who are receiving digitalis. Autoxidation of catecholamines and related sympathomimetic compounds is dependent on pH. Contact of epinephrine with other drugs that have an alkaline pH (e.g., sodium bicarbonate) can cause autoxidation; therefore, epinephrine should not be added to infusion bags or bottles that contain alkaline solutions.

Phenylephrine

Phenylephrine is a pure α-adrenergic agonist that causes vasoconstriction with minimal cardiac activity.[18] Bradycardia has been associated with phenylephrine when used as bolus therapy to treat supraventricular tachyarrhythmia; however, this effect is thought to result from autoregulation at the baroreceptor secondary to increased blood pressure. The primary pharmacodynamic effect of phenylephrine is a dose-dependent increase in both systolic and diastolic blood pressure.[18] Phenylephrine increases afterload and may increase myocardial oxygen demand, but it does not appear to reduce coronary blood flow.[18] However, phenylephrine does reduce renal and mesenteric perfusion.

Phenylephrine is especially useful for patients who require an increase in systemic vascular resistance but who cannot tolerate increases in heart rate or contractility because of fixed coronary occlusions or tachyarrhythmias. The drug is administered intravenously as a continuous infusion at an initial rate of 0.5 μg/kg/min. The phenylephrine infusion is titrated to the desired hemodynamic response. Infusion rates of 9 μg/kg/min or higher may be required for patients with septic shock. Bolus injections of phenylephrine (2 to 5 mg) may be used to restore blood pressure acutely.

Phenylephrine should be administered into a central venous line via a volumetric infusion system that ensures a precise flow rate. Use of this drug should be viewed as a temporizing measure, and the dose should be reduced or the infusion discontinued as soon as possible. Phenylephrine should be tapered slowly to avoid abrupt and severe hypotension. Extravasation produces ischemic necrosis and sloughing of superficial tissues. If extravasation occurs, phentolamine (5 to 10 mg diluted in 10 to 15 mL of saline solution) should be infiltrated into the area to antagonize the phenylephrine-induced vasoconstriction and to minimize necrosis and sloughing.

VASODILATORS

Nitroglycerin

Nitroglycerin relaxes vascular smooth muscle by binding to specific vascular receptors and causing the formation of disulfide bonds.[19, 20] In patients with cardiogenic shock, intravenous nitroglycerin reduces left ventricular filling pressure and systemic vascular resistance.[20] The decline in ventricular volume and systolic wall tension decreases myocardial oxygen requirements and usually reduces myocardial ischemia. The net effect is an increase in cardiac output. Compared with nitroprusside, intravenous nitroglycerin produces a slightly greater reduction of preload, a smaller increase in cardiac output, and a slightly smaller reduction in afterload.[21] Nitroglycerin does not usually increase heart rate if preload is adequate.

Intravenous nitroglycerin should be administered by continuous infusion. Because nitroglycerin binds to porous polyvinyl chloride tubing, high-density polyethylene tubing has been recommended for administration of intravenous nitroglycerin preparations. In reality, because the amount of nitroglycerin administered is titrated to clinical response and not to an exact dose, there is no justification for the use of more expensive high-density tubing.

Intravenous nitroglycerin therapy is initiated at a dose of 10 to 20 μg/min. The infusion rate should be increased by 5 or 10 μg/min every 5 to 10 minutes until the desired hemodynamic or clinical response is achieved (e.g., fall in systemic vascular resistance or left ventricular filling pressure or relief of chest pain). Although a therapeutic response is usually achieved at a dose range of 80 to 200 μg/min, some patients may require a dosage of 300 to 500 μg/min.

The pharmacologic effects of nitroglycerin are dependent primarily on the patient's intravascular volume and, to a lesser extent, on the dose administered.[21] Hypovolemia blunts the beneficial effects of nitroglycerin and increases the risk of nitroglycerin-induced hypotension and paradoxical bradycardia.[21] Nitroglycerin should be administered by an infusion system that ensures a precise flow rate to minimize the risk of hypotension. When appropriate, the patient may be weaned from nitroglycerin over 4 to 6 hours as tolerated.

Headache is a common consequence of nitroglycerin therapy. Blood pressure may decrease, resulting in nausea, giddiness, faintness, or syncope. Such symptoms are often aggravated by the erect position. Hypotension in a recumbent patient often responds to elevation of the legs. Patients usually tolerate both the hypotensive effects and the headaches with chronic therapy.

Hypotension, sufficient to produce hypoperfusion, is the most serious side effect of nitroglycerin, particularly in patients in whom perfusion is impaired because of arterial obstruction. Hypotension is best treated with fluid administration and dose reduction. If bradycardia accompanies nitroglycerin-induced hypotension (i.e., vasovagal reflex arc), atropine and fluid replacement are the treatment of choice. Rapid titration of intravenous nitroglycerin in patients with cardiogenic shock requires hemodynamic monitoring to ensure efficacy and safety.[20] In rare instances, nitroglycerin may cause methemoglobinemia. Nitroglycerin-mediated reductions in pulmonary vascular resistance can lead to ventilation-perfusion mismatch and a drop in arterial oxygen pressure (Pao_2).

Sodium Nitroprusside

Sodium nitroprusside is a potent peripheral vasodilator with equal effects on arterial and venous smooth muscle.[21-23] Its effects are seen almost immediately and cease within minutes after the infusion is stopped. Nitroprusside is metabolized by red blood cells to hydrocyanic acid, which is converted to thiocyanate by the liver and excreted by the kidneys. Hepatic or renal dysfunction can affect the clearance of the drug and its potentially injurious metabolites, cyanide and thiocyanate.

Nitroprusside reduces blood pressure by lowering peripheral arterial resistance and by increasing venous capacitance and thus preload. Arterial effects are not lost even when preload is markedly diminished, although tachycardia ensues. In the absence of heart failure, cardiac output either decreases or remains unchanged.[23, 24] In patients with cardiogenic shock, nitroprusside generally increases cardiac output by diminishing vascular impedance and increasing stroke volume. The increase in stroke volume is usually sufficient to maintain the systemic blood pressure at or only slightly below the pretreatment level. In patients with left ventricular failure, nitroprusside-induced tachycardia suggests an inadequate (relative or absolute) left ventricular filling pressure. The hemodynamic improvement induced in the presence of left ventricular failure or hypertension may be of particular significance in patients with ischemic heart disease. Nitroprusside reduces myocardial work and may therefore mitigate ischemia. Unfortunately, nitroprusside may also reduce coronary perfusion to ischemic myocardium.[25, 26] This "coronary steal" phenomenon is the result of the arteriolar dilating effects of nitroprusside, which result in a lower mean difference between arteriolar pressure and left ventricular end-diastolic pressure and, therefore, reduced coronary blood flow.[25]

Numerous studies have shown improved left ventricular function, tissue perfusion, cardiac output, and clinical status in patients with low cardiac output and high systemic vascular resistance. Nitroprusside tends to reduce pulmonary occlusive pressure to a greater extent than dobutamine because of its more potent venodilating effects and its ability to enhance diastolic relaxation of the left ventricle.[22-26]

Nitroprusside is the parenteral treatment of choice for hypertensive emergencies when immediate reduction of peripheral resistance is necessary. This drug is also useful in the treatment of patients with acute left ventricular failure. Nitroprusside may be used for patients with heart failure and pulmonary congestion whose condition is acute or who are poorly controlled by diuretic therapy. In this setting, combined therapy with dopamine and nitroprusside is frequently more effective than the use of either agent alone. The net hemodynamic effects of this combination are similar to the effects of dobutamine and the combination may be less costly, although it is important to keep in mind that dobutamine is now available in a generic form.

Treatment should begin with an infusion rate of 0.1 μg/kg/min titrated to the desired endpoint. Adverse events, such as diastolic hypotension and reflex tachycardia, are generally avoided if the patient is euvolemic. Hemodynamic monitoring is essential for proper titration when treating cardiogenic shock. The average therapeutic dose of nitroprusside ranges from 0.5 to 8 μg/kg/min. Nitroprusside should be administered by an infusion system that ensures a precise flow rate.

Monitoring of central hemodynamic pressures is essential for treating cardiogenic shock for safety and for ensuring proper titration of effect. Systemic arterial pressure must be monitored frequently. Hypotension is the most common adverse reaction seen with nitroprusside. Nitroprusside-induced hypotension may precipitate myocardial ischemia, infarction, or stroke. Deterioration of the ventilation-perfusion relation and hypoxemia can occur. Elderly patients and patients with reduced intravascular volume may be more sensitive to the drug and should be treated with lower starting doses. There is controversy about the possibility that nitroprusside can reduce coronary blood flow and exacerbate ischemia despite a lower myocardial work load. In the presence of cardiogenic shock, intravenous nitroglycerin has a similar hemodynamic profile but improves ischemia, and it may be preferred over nitroprusside for patients with coronary artery disease.

Nitroprusside is metabolized to thiocyanate by the liver. Thiocyanate intoxication caused by nitroprusside is uncommon unless (1) large doses of nitroprusside are given (>3 μg/kg/min), (2) prolonged infusions (>2 to 3 days) are given, or (3) the patient has renal failure. Blood levels should be monitored when high or prolonged dosage regimens are used or renal failure is present. If thiocyanate blood concentrations remain below 10 mg/dL, continued use of the agent is usually safe. Signs of thiocyanate toxicity include tinnitus, visual blurring, changes in mental status, nausea, abdominal pain, metabolic acidosis, elevated Po_2, hyperreflexia, and seizures. Cyanide toxicity is a rare complication of nitroprusside therapy in patients with hepatic dysfunction. Prophylaxis with sodium thiosulfate and hydroxycobalamin may be beneficial in patients at high risk for cyanide toxicity (i.e., those who have liver dysfunction or renal failure or who receive nitroprusside in excess of 2 μg/kg/min continuously for more than 24 hours).[27]

SUMMARY

The correct use of inotropic therapy in the intensive care setting requires knowledge of both the pharmacology of the drug being utilized and the pathophysiology of the disease process being treated. This knowledge of the pharmacology forms the foundation for the treatment of critically ill patients.

The principal use of dopamine is for the patient with low cardiac output and oliguria or the patient with shock who requires an increase in inotropic activity and peripheral resistance to maintain perfusion, pressure, and flow. In patients with low cardiac output and oliguria, renal perfusion is improved at dopamine concentrations of 2 to 10 μg/kg/min. For patients with elevated pulmonary capillary wedge pressure and elevated systemic vascular resistance, dopamine in low doses can be combined with dobutamine at 5 to 15 μg/kg/min to improve hemodynamics. Doses of dopamine above 10 μg/kg/min produce vasoconstriction similar to that produced by norepinephrine. This makes dopamine extremely useful in the hypotensive phases of septic shock.

Dobutamine, a synthetic sympathomimetic amine, is a traditional inotrope for use in the ICU setting for patients with poor left ventricular function. At doses between 5 and 15 μg/kg/min dobutamine increases cardiac output, reduces pulmonary capillary wedge pressure, and decreases total peripheral resistance. In combination with milrinone, it can significantly reduce postcapillary pulmonary hypertension. Dobutamine can be administered peripherally, but its long-term use is limited by the development of tolerance, increased heart rate, and therefore increased myocardial oxygen consumption, which may provoke angina. Further long-term use is also limited by the development of tremor.

The use of isoproterenol, a pure beta sympathomimetic amine, is limited to emergencies requiring an increase in heart rate in patients unresponsive to atropine during preparation for pacemaker insertion. Similarly, the use of norepinephrine, a potent alpha agonist, is limited to low-output shock states for brief support until the underlying problem can be corrected. Excessive use of norepinephrine can produce intense peripheral vasoconstriction and at times has led to digital gangrene in patients.

Epinephrine produces both alpha and beta stimulation and is a drug of choice for cardiopulmonary resuscitation and the treatment of anaphylactic shock. Its use is limited by the production of myocardial ischemia and significant ventricular arrhythmias.

Milrinone is rapidly becoming the front-line drug of choice for patients with decompensated left ventricular function. It can produce biventricular afterload reduction, is a positive inotrope, does not induce tolerance, and does not increase myocardial oxygen consumption. Because of the lack of tolerance, it is now the drug of choice for patients awaiting transplantation for long periods. It is also gaining favor as an inotrope for outpatients so that patients with class III to class IV heart failure do not have to remain in the ICU.

The peripheral vasodilators nitroprusside and nitroglycerin, although not inotropic drugs, can be used in combination with inotropes or in specific emergent intensive care situations. Nitroprusside is the drug of choice in hypertensive emergencies or in combinations with dopamine for decompensated heart failure. The principal use of intravenous nitroglycerin is for the cardiac patient with ongoing ischemic pain.

Thus, knowledge of the pharmacology of these potent drugs is a must for the rational treatment of patients in critical care units. This knowledge, combined with in-depth understanding of the pathophysiology of the underlying disease process, helps to ensure increasing survival and decreased morbidity of patients in our critical care units.

References

1. Leier CV, Heban P, Huss P, Bush CA, Lewis RP: Comparative systemic and regional hemodynamic effects of dopamine and dobutamine in patients with cardiomyopathic heart failure. Circulation 1978; 58:466–475.
2. Otto CW, Yakaitas RW, Redding JS, Blitt CD: Comparison of dopamine, dobutamine, and epinephrine in CPR. Crit Care Med 1981; 9:640–643.
3. Lindner KH, Ahnefeld FW, Bowdler IM: Comparison of epinephrine and dopamine during cardiopulmonary resuscitation. Intensive Care Med 1989; 15:432–438.
4. Gonzalez ER, Ornato JP, Levine RL: Vasopressor effect of epinephrine with and without dopamine during cardiopulmonary resuscitation. Drug Intell Clin Pharm 1988; 22:868–872.
5. Keung EC, Siskind SJ, Sonnenblick EH, Ribner HS, Schwartz WJ, LeJemtel TH: Dobutamine therapy in acute myocardial infarction. JAMA 1981; 245:144–146.
6. Leier CV: Acute inotropic support. *In:* Cardiotonic Drugs. Leier CV (Ed). New York, Marcel Dekker, 1986, pp 49–84.
7. Stoner JD, Bolen JL, Harrison DC: Comparison of dobutamine and dopamine in treatment of severe heart failure. Br Heart J 1977; 39:536–539.
8. Mueller HS, Evans R, Ayers S: Effect of dopamine on hemodynamics and myocardial metabolism in man. Circulation 1978; 57:361–365.
9. Rude RE, Izquierdo C, Buja M, et al: Effects of inotropic and chronotropic stimuli on acute myocardial ischemic injury: Studies with dobutamine in the anesthetized dog. Circulation 1982: 65:1321–1328.
10. Genton R, Jaffe AS: Management of congestive heart failure in patients with acute myocardial infarction. JAMA 1986; 256:2556–2560.
11. Niemann JT, Haynes KS, Garner D, et al: Postcountershock pulseless rhythms: Response to CPR, artificial cardiac pacing, and adrenergic agonists. Ann Emerg Med 1986; 15:112–120.
12. Ditchey RV, Lindenfeld J: Potential adverse effects of volume loading on perfusion of vital organs during closed-chest resuscitation. Circulation 1984; 69:181–189.
13. Kelly R, Smith TW: Pharmacologic treatment of heart failure. *In:* Goodman and Gillman's the Pharmacological Basis of Therapeutics. 9th ed. Hardman JG, Limbird LE (Eds). New York, McGraw-Hill, 1996, pp 830–854.
14. Hilleman D: Assessing the treatment of congestive heart failure: Inotropic agents and calcium channel blockers. Pharmacotherapy 1993; 13:88S–93S.
15. Colucci WS, Wright RF, Jaski BE, et al: Milrinone and dobutamine in severe heart failure: Differing hemodynamic effects and individual patient responsiveness. Circulation 1986; 73(Suppl 3):175–183.
16. Martin C, Papazian L, Perrin G, et al: Norepinephrine or dopamine for the treatment of hyperdynamic septic shock. Chest 1993; 103:1826–1831.
17. Michael JR, Guerci AD, Koehler RC, et al: Mechanisms by which epinephrine augments cerebral and myocardial perfusion during cardiopulmonary resuscitation in dogs. Circulation 1984; 69:822–835.
18. Brown CG, Werman HA: Collective review. Adrenergic agonists during cardiopulmonary resuscitation. Resuscitation 1990; 19:1–16.
19. Awan NA, Evenson MK, Needham KE, et al: Effect of combined

nitroglycerin and dobutamine infusion in left ventricular dysfunction. Am Heart J 1983; 106:35-40.
20. Bussman WD, Schofer H, Kaltenbach M: Effect of intravenous nitroglycerin on hemodynamics and ischemic injury in patients with acute myocardial infarction. Eur J Cardiol 1978; 8:61-74.
21. Leier CV, Banbach D, Thompson MJ, et al: Central and regional hemodynamic effect of intravenous isosorbide dinitrate, nitroglycerin, and nitroprusside in patients with congestive heart failure. Am J Cardiol 1981; 48:1115-1123.
22. Parmley WW, Chatterjee K, Charuzi Y, et al: Hemodynamic effects of noninvasive systolic unloading (nitroprusside) and diastolic augmentation (external counterpulsation) in patients with acute myocardial infarction. Am J Cardiol 1974; 33:810-816.
23. Cohn JN, Franciosa JA, Francis GS, et al: Effect of short-term infusion of sodium nitroprusside on mortality rate in acute myocardial infarction complicated by left ventricular failure. N Engl J Med 1982; 306:1129-1135.
24. Durrer JD, Lie KI, Capelle FJ, et al: Effect of sodium nitroprusside on mortality in acute myocardial infarction. N Engl J Med 1982; 306:1121-1128.
25. Chiarello M, Gold HK, Leinbach RC, et al: Comparison between the effects of nitroprusside and nitroglycerin on ischemic injury during acute myocardial infarction. Circulation 1976; 54:766-773.
26. Flaherty JT: Comparison of intravenous nitroglycerin and sodium nitroprusside in acute myocardial infarction. Am J Med 1983; 74(6B):53-60.
27. Cohn JN, Burke LP: Nitroprusside. Ann Intern Med 1979; 91:752-757.

105

New Techniques in Management of the Cardiac Surgery Patient

Paul J. Corso, MD, FACS, FACC
Michael J. Hockstein, MD, FCCP

NEW APPROACHES TO ANESTHESIA

The true challenge of anesthesia in the patient undergoing cardiac surgery is to produce analgesia, amnesia, unconsciousness, and paralysis in the presence of cardiac ischemia and ventricular dysfunction. The typical medications available to the cardiac anesthesiologist include inhalational agents, narcotics, benzodiazepines, barbiturates, and paralytics. Many of the early anesthetic agents, however, caused undesired effects on the cardiovascular system. Early inhalational agents, particularly halothane, and the barbiturates cause significant myocardial depression. Halothane, in addition, sensitizes the myocardium to catecholamines, leading to arrhythmias. Morphine, the most popular narcotic available before the availability of synthetic alternatives, causes histamine release, venodilation, and hypotension when used in large doses. Thus, the earliest cardiac anesthesia, which consisted predominantly of halothane and, to a lesser degree, morphine predisposed the patient to myocardial depression and arrhythmia, particularly during times of peak catecholamine release.

Subsequent anesthetic technique consisted primarily of high-dose narcotics, benzodiazepines, and muscular paralysis. This approach reduced the myocardial depressant effects of inhalational agents (i.e., halothane) and maintained protection of the heart from sympathetic activity during laryngoscopy, intubation, and sternotomy. With the introduction of synthetic narcotics such as fentanyl and sufentanil, which are short-acting and do not cause histamine release, the untoward hemodynamic effects previously caused by high-dose morphine were eliminated. High-dose narcotics were historically followed by maintenance of anesthesia with inhalational agents, additional narcotics, muscle relaxants, and benzodiazepines. Until the early 1990s, patients were kept semiconscious for 24 hours or more postoperatively before initiation of full awakening and ventilator weaning.

However, as experience with patients undergoing cardiac surgery increased, it was found that patients could be managed with newer inhalational agents, such as isoflurane, and far less narcotic analgesia without risk to the ischemic myocardium. Isoflurane causes much less myocardial depression and does not sensitize the myocardium to catecholamines. After induction, narcotic analgesia is continued through sternotomy and inhalational agents are continued through cardiopulmonary bypass (CPB). A benefit of this new approach was faster emergence from anesthesia and far earlier extubation. Patients could be extubated as early as 2 hours after reaching the recovery room or even in the operating room (OR). Newer inhalational agents with even shorter duration of action, such as sevoflurane, may continue to shorten times of recovery from anesthesia.

Short-Acting Sedating Agents

At the end of CPB, to facilitate awakening and maintain sedation, anesthetic agents with short half-lives are used. One relatively new agent, propofol, has become popular in the operating room. This drug is a sedative-hypnotic agent provided as a lipid emulsion. It can produce a hypnotic state after a bolus of 1.5 to 2 mg/kg in as little as 40 seconds. Unconsciousness is maintained with a continuous infusion, and depth of unconscious is dependent on dose and plasma concentration. Because of its rapid metabolism (hepatic) and redistribution, patients begin to regain consciousness quickly after discontinuation of the drug, often in minutes. This pharmacodynamic profile makes it ideal as a sedating agent, especially when supplemented by narcotic analgesics. However, it is not necessary to use propofol to ensure rapid emergence from anesthesia. Any short-acting agent, alone or in combination, that can provide sedation and analgesia (such as fentanyl and midazolam) will function satisfactorily. The most important impact of the use of short-acting agents is on the ability to rapidly awaken patients in the recovery room and progress to extubation.

Regional Analgesia

For further enhancement of analgesia and facilitation of early extubation, techniques that leverage regional pain control have been used with new enthusiasm in cardiac surgery. Spinal analgesia, produced by means of a 25-gauge needle and intrathecal morphine, offers the promise of enhanced pain control with the use of less systemic narcotic. To preserve sympathetic nervous system function, no local anesthetics are used in this technique. The potential complication of this approach is extended respiratory depression if the narcotic affects the central nervous system. This technique is appropriate if CPB is used during the operation, because the risk of bleeding in the region of the dural puncture (achieved with a small-gauge needle) is minimal after heparinization for CPB. When patients are managed without CPB, another technique, epidural analgesia, can be used to produce regional pain control. In this approach, a larger-gauge needle (17-gauge) places both a narcotic (usually fentanyl) and a local anesthetic (usually bupivacaine) in the thoracic epidural space of the dermatome covering the operative site. This technique is especially useful in less invasive techniques that are performed off CPB.

MONITORING THE CARDIAC SURGERY PATIENT

Monitoring technology has certainly increased since the mid-1980s. The clinician has a wide variety of devices that can monitor physiologic systems in both an invasive or a noninvasive way. Careful selection of appropriate devices should be customized to each patient for the sake of cost effectiveness and efficacy.

Monitoring the Respiratory System

In all patients undergoing general anesthesia, oxygen saturation must be monitored noninvasively. This technology was developed for clinical use in the mid-1980s. Infrared (IR) light of two different wavelengths is used to derive the hemoglobin saturation in the arterial pulse of capillary blood.[1, 2] Calculations are based on the characteristic absorption of each wavelength for saturated and unsaturated hemoglobin. These small light-emitting diode (LED) sensors are ubiquitous and are the standard in noninvasive monitoring of oxygen saturation. The pulse oximeter will accurately report oxygen saturation, but not oxygen content, of the blood. The latter is one of the recognized shortcomings of the technology. This device, which depends on the presence of a pulse of blood coursing through peripheral tissues, can sometimes fail to "sense" the pulse, especially in cool extremities of a patient with limited cardiovascular performance. Nonetheless, this device is part of the routine monitoring that should accompany every patient. Pulse oximetry is not the only technology for measuring oxygen in the blood; there are also transcutaneous oximeters that can measure oxygen tension. However, because of the relatively long response time, the need for heated sensors, and the reliance on adequate cutaneous blood flow for operation, these devices have become more useful in measuring trends in peripheral perfusion than for measuring arterial saturation. Near infrared spectroscopy (NIRS) may soon be used as a noninvasive technology for measuring not only tissue oxygen saturation but also adequacy of oxygen delivery (via cytochrome a, a_3 concentrations, and redox potential) to muscle, myocardial, and cerebral tissue.

The complement of oxygen saturation monitoring is measurement of carbon dioxide (CO_2). The ability to measure arterial CO_2 provides objective endpoints in management of ventilation. Current noninvasive technology leverages IR absorption technology to measure exhaled CO_2.[3] The end-tidal portion of an exhaled breath contains virtually all alveolar gas (without anatomic dead space) and measurement of the carbon dioxide partial pressure ($P\text{CO}_2$) of this portion of the tidal volume most closely correlates to arterial carbon dioxide tension ($Pa\text{CO}_2$). End-tidal CO_2 monitoring is currently the standard of care in ventilation monitoring in the operating room and is of great value in the immediate postoperative period. In addition to guiding appropriate minute ventilation in the anesthetized patient, this technology facilitates weaning from the mechanical ventilator in the recovery area without the need for arterial blood. Post-CPB patients often shiver in the immediate postoperative period, generating high $Pa\text{CO}_2$. Monitoring of end-tidal CO_2 allows for titration of minute ventilation throughout this period.

There are currently numerous products on the market that integrate both pulse oximetry and end-tidal CO_2 measurement into a single portable device. There are also other devices that can measure both $Pa\text{CO}_2$ and $Pa\text{O}_2$ but through direct techniques. Currently available are small intra-arterial probes that can directly measure pH, $Pa\text{O}_2$, and $Pa\text{CO}_2$ in real time. This technology allows monitoring the effects of pharmacologic or mechanical interventions on gas exchange and acid-base balance. The probes can be easily inserted through an introducer into a radial or femoral artery and left in place while a bedside module continuously records and graphically displays changes in measurements. These devices still are expensive and lack acceptable accuracy, but future generations of devices should minimize these problems.[4]

Monitoring the Cardiovascular System

All patients have continuous three-channel electrocardiographic (ECG) monitoring. Monitoring begins in the OR and continues through the perioperative period until the patient can be managed on a nontelemetry unit. This amount of time generally totals approximately 4 days beginning with the time of operation. ECG monitoring in the immediate postoperative period is necessary for identifying high-grade atrioventricular blocks, effectiveness of external pacing, and, of course, surveillance of tachyarrhythmias. In the late postoperative period, when the risk of *new* high-grade atrioventricular block has passed, continuous ECG monitoring is necessary for identifying new-onset atrial fibrillation, a common arrhythmia in patients who undergo cardiac surgery. Monitoring equipment should include software for arrhythmia detection and retrospective analysis of rhythm disturbances.

Virtually all patients who undergo cardiovascular surgery have an arterial cannulation (or "a-line"), if technically possible, in the operating room. Arterial cannulation provides not only a real-time measurement of blood pressure but also convenient access to arterial blood for gas, hematologic, and chemical analysis. Although blood pressure can also be measured with an automated noninvasive arm cuff, this device is not an adequate substitute in either the operating room or *immediate* postoperative recovery areas. However, once the patient has demonstrated hemodynamic stability, noninvasive blood pressure monitoring provides an efficient and accurate way of monitoring blood pressure. Arterial cannulation is most commonly performed in the radial, femoral, or brachial arteries. Cannulation can also be accomplished with a small catheter through a femoral graft when no other cannulation site is available. Complications from arterial cannulation have historically been low.

Central venous access is necessary for both monitoring and drug therapy in patients undergoing cardiovascular surgery. Central venous access provides a reliable route for volume resuscitation, infusion of vasoactive medications, and infusion of other drugs, such as antiarrhythmics, insulin, and antibiotics. Because the cardiovascular system can be unpredictable, all patients should have central venous access, usually either an internal jugular vein (preferably the right) or a subclavian vein (preferably the left). The best catheter is a matter of opinion, but either a double-lumen catheter or an "introducer" (for pulmonary artery catheters) is an ideal choice.

Monitoring of cardiovascular performance—particularly central venous pressure (CVP), pulmonary artery pressure, pulmonary capillary wedge pressure (PCWP), also referred to as pulmonary artery occlusion pressure (PAOP), and cardiac output—has been a traditional component of cardiac surgery. PCWP, replacing left atrial pressure, has become the gold standard in assessment of left ventricular filling pressures. In rare instances, inflation of the catheter's balloon can lead to pulmonary artery rupture, especially in the presence of pulmonary artery hypertension, distal placement of the catheter tip, and coagulopathy. In fact, a pulmonary arterial catheter can be used effectively without PCWP data by following trends in the pulmonary artery diastolic (PAD) pressure. Because the PCWP is always less than the PAD pressure, a low PAD pressure in the presence of poor cardiovascular performance is almost certainly associated with a low PCWP.

In the absence of pulmonary artery hypertension or severe mitral regurgitation, PAD pressure correlates closely with PCWP and can be used to guide volume resuscitation when hypovolemia is suspected. However, more recent analysis of pulmonary artery catheter (PAC) use and its relationship to outcomes has called the utility of this technology into question.

The consensus on the use of the PAC by the Society of Critical Care Medicine suggests that the PAC does not reduce complications or mortality in patients at low risk in cardiovascular surgery, and its effect on the same variables in patients at high risk (clinically significant left ventricular dysfunction) is uncertain. In aortic valve surgery, the low-risk patient has uncertain reduction in complications and mortality, but the *high-risk patient does seem to reap benefit.*[5] Patients with good left ventricular function can be safely managed with a CVP monitor alone. The use of the PAC by experienced nurses and physicians can be reduced to as low as 30%. An introducer placed preoperatively provides convenient access should further definition of hemodynamic performance be needed. A PAC is placed in any patient with an ejection fraction of less than 35%, recent myocardial infarction, congestive heart failure, renal failure necessitating dialysis, or severe respiratory insufficiency as well as in any patient undergoing planned valve surgery.

Cardiac output is currently assessed by the thermodilution method with the use of the PAC. But the PAC can offer far more than cardiac output alone. Fiberoptic technology incorporated into the catheter allows for continuous measurement of mixed-venous oxyhemoglobin saturation, a valuable insight into the adequacy of oxygen delivery. Further modification of this hybrid catheter incorporates a heating filament and a rapid-response thermistor that allows for continuous measurement of cardiac output and right ventricular ejection fraction.[6] These techniques obviously require invasive access and increased cost. The later catheters have not yet attained mainstream use; nor has their use been shown to improve outcome or lessen morbidity. Although invasive monitoring is currently the standard, it may soon be replaced by a number of less invasive output devices. Current technology makes use of esophageal Doppler probes,[7] thoracic bioimpedance, and echocardiography as potential substitutes for the more invasive techniques.[8, 9]

EFFECTS OF CARDIOPULMONARY BYPASS ON THE HEMATOLOGIC SYSTEM AND BLOOD-SPARING TECHNIQUES

Effects of Cardiopulmonary Bypass on Coagulation and Platelet Function

CPB affects virtually all organ systems. The hematologic system is affected, at least in part, by the mechanical action of the pump on cellular elements, hemodilution, interaction of cellular and noncellular elements with nonbiologic surfaces, hypothermia, fibrinolysis, and anticoagulation. This causes dysfunction of platelets and of coagulation and leads to a tendency toward bleeding.[10] The degree of dysfunction and coagulopathy is related to the duration of CPB and the depth of hypothermia.[11] As CPB technology improves, untoward effects become less severe but remain present.

Physical damage to cellular elements results from pumping of blood through an extracorporeal circuit, oxygenating the blood, and recovering red blood cells (RBCs) in "cell-saving" devices. Roller pumps can cause significant hemolysis of RBCs. Newer pumping devices such as centrifugal pumps have reduced physical trauma to the RBCs. Oxygenation of blood used to occur via a bubble oxygenator. Direct contact of oxygen bubbles with blood elements causes RBC hemolysis and platelet activation.[12] This effect has been much reduced since the utilization of membrane oxygenators that prevent direct physical contact between blood and gas bubbles. Direct physical contact of blood and gas exists in "cell-saving" devices also, where a catheter drains blood from the operative field. The cell-saving device applies significant physical stresses to cellular elements during suction. Recovered cellular elements must be filtered free of debris and bubbles prior to being returned to the circulation.

Hemodilution occurs during CPB, in part due to non-blood pump primes, with approximately 2.5 L of crystalloid. Hemodilution with hematocrits between 20 and 25 allows for adequate oxygen delivery (in the presence of hypothermia) and reduces operative and postoperative transfusion needs.[13] Hemodilution, however, also causes other physiologic changes. Colloid osmotic pressure drops as much as 44%, mostly due to a 32% reduction in albumin concentrations.[14] Hemodilution also causes a significant fall (30% to 36%) in coagulation factor concentration. This dilution of clotting factors usually does not result in abnormal clotting, and factor concentration returns to normal within 48 hours.[11]

CPB subjects both cellular (i.e., RBCs, platelets) and noncellular (i.e., coagulation factors, complement) elements to nonbiologic surfaces of the pump (tubing) and oxygenator. Nonlaminar flow characteristics within the CPB system and contact with nonbiologic surfaces activate the coagulation cascade, promoting not only thrombus formation but also fibrinolysis. Activation of the fibrinolytic system likely contributes to coagulopathy seen after CPB. Most hemostatic changes due to surface contact occur within the oxygenator.[15]

Once CPB begins, the surfaces within the system become coated with an adsorbed layer of protein, 5 to 20 nm in thickness. The protein layer is composed mostly of fibrinogen. Over time, the fibrinogen is conformationally changed and replaced by cleaved high-molecular-weight kininogen. The synthetic surface does not interact with the elements of blood directly; it is the adsorbed protein layer that is responsible for interaction with formed elements, such as platelets. Platelets rapidly become activated and extend pseudopodia, adhere, aggregate, and release their granular contents (alpha, dense, and lysosomal). It is thought that severe turbulent flow can cause platelet activation as well.[16]

Upon initiation of CPB, platelet counts fall to approximately 20% of initial levels due to hemodilution, platelet adhesion to synthetic surfaces, and formation of platelet aggregates. Plasma levels of platelet factor 4 (PF4) rise, suggesting platelet activation and granule release. Platelet fibrinogen receptors decline, and platelets become less reactive to activating agents, such as adenosine diphosphate (ADP).[17] CPB causes a temporary reduction in the number of platelet glycoprotein receptors Ib, IIb, and IIa.[18] Plasmin, activated as a result of CPB, reduces the number of platelet GPIb receptors, resulting in a reduced ability of platelets to adhere.[19] After reaching a quantitative nadir shortly after the start of CPB, platelet counts begin to rise during bypass but then decline again until approximately the third postoperative day.[20] The overall effect of CPB on short-term platelet function is a *reduction* in their functionality and a *prolongation* in bleeding time.

Prior to CPB, patients are fully anticoagulated with heparin to prevent clot formation during contact with synthetic surfaces. Heparin doses are generally 400 units/kg with additional heparin to keep the activated clotting time (ACT) at least 480. At the conclusion of CPB, heparin is reversed with protamine in a dose of 1 mg/100 units of heparin. Infrequently, excessive dosage of protamine leads to enhancement rather than reversal of anticoagulation. Protamine sulfate administration can also lead to acute systemic hypotension, pulmonary hypertension, and right ventricular failure. This may be caused by too rapid an infusion or, rarely, a true immunologic reaction.

Complications related to heparinization are usually due to bleeding from inadequate reversal with protamine or to "heparin washout/rebound." In heparin washout, seen about 8 hours postoperatively, heparin sequestered in poorly perfused vascular beds is liberated in the postoperative period and causes transient anticoagulation. An alternative explanation is that active heparin is released from the heparin-protamine complex. Infrequently, heparin can cause an immunologic reaction with platelets, causing a decline in platelet count. Reexposure to heparin may then cause widespread platelet activation, leading to disastrous arterial thrombosis.[21]

Inhibition of Fibrinolysis

As a result of the costs of blood products and potential risks of transfusion-transmitted diseases, efforts must be taken to limit excessive blood loss during and after cardiac surgery. To limit the effects of CPB on the hemostatic system, physicians have devised strategies to block the activity of the fibrinolytic system and to enhance platelet activity. Three popular agents are now available to modulate the fibrinolytic system, Two are lysine analogs (ϵ-aminocaproic acid [EACA] and tranexamic acid); the other is a serine protease inhibitor. All three agents ultimately block the fibrinolytic action of plasmin. The addition of these antifibrinolytic agents can minimize CPB-induced fibrinolysis and can reduce postoperative chest tube bleeding.[22]

EACA, a synthetic monoaminocarboxylic acid the structure of which closely resembles that of lysine, acts by saturating lysine binding sites on plasminogen inhibiting conversion to the active agent, plasmin. EACA also seems to interact with fibrin, making it resistant to degradation. EACA is given as a single 5-g dose just prior to CPB.

Tranexamic acid, another inhibitor of plasminogen, is given as a 10-mg/kg dose at the time of skin incision followed by a 1-mg/kg/hr continuous dose for 12 additional hours.[23] The mechanism of action is similar to that of EACA. Prophylactic use of EACA and tranexamic acid has been shown to decrease mediastinal blood loss after cardiac surgery. However, there is no indication that use of the later agents decreases transfusion of packed red blood cells (PRBCs).[23]

Aprotinin is a serine protease inhibitor that was first isolated in 1936. It is a naturally occurring 58-amino acid polypeptide found in greatest concentrations in lung, pancreas, and parotid glands. The substance is thought to play a role in modulation of proteolytic enzymes. It inhibits plasmin by reversibly binding to the enzyme's active site, preventing degradation of fibrin or fibrinogen, ultimately retarding clot lysis. It has been utilized to successfully reduce postoperative chest tube bleeding in patients undergoing CPB.[24] Although all of these agents reduce blood *loss,* the high cost of aprotinin has limited its use except in high-risk groups, such as multiple reoperations and transplantation with previous surgery. As with other antifibrinolytics, aprotinin has not conclusively been shown to reduce blood *transfusion.* There is some concern that the use of aprotinin can reduce graft patency.[25]

LESS INVASIVE VERSUS TRADITIONAL TECHNIQUES IN CARDIAC SURGERY

Traditional cardiac surgery has evolved primarily into operations done through a median sternotomy with the use of CPB. The postoperative care protocols deal with the altered physiology that occurs due in part to the use of CPB, cross-clamping the aorta, and with the concomitant need for cardioplegia. Recently, in order to decrease complications in high-risk patients, and (even more recently) to decrease costs and recovery time, physicians have developed alternative methods to treat patients with coronary artery disease and patients with valvular pathology.

Off Bypass Surgery for Coronary Artery Disease

Because part of the risks of coronary artery bypass grafting (CABG) are related to the physiologic alterations brought on by the use of CPB, newer techniques have been developed that allow revascularization to one degree or another without the need for CPB. Long-term patency studies have not been completed, but early results are very positive. By using these methods, patients do not demonstrate the hematologic abnormalities, inflammatory response, fluid accumulation, and pulmonary dysfunction seen with traditional methods. There also does not appear to be the early myocardial dysfunction seen when the aorta is cross-clamped.

Although the number of patients who are candidates for these procedures has initially been limited, the indications are growing. Using these techniques has decreased blood utilization, strokes, and ventilator time. Time in the intensive care unit (ICU) has been decreased to hours and hospital stays vary between 48 hours and 4 days, with a commensurate decrease in cost by as much as 40%.

Alternative Methods of Cardiopulmonary Bypass and Incisions

A new system to institute CPB (Heartport) allows for peripheral cannulation and small incisions (ports) to be used to perform CABG and intracardiac repairs. These approaches eliminate or reduce the extent of median sternotomy. Although the same hematologic, inflammatory, and dilutional alterations occur with this method as seen in standard surgery, early results demonstrate a positive influence on time of recovery by use of smaller incisions. Cost savings brought on by the shorter hospital stays may not at present make up for the cost of increased OR time.

Cardiac surgery is undergoing an exciting evolution, if not revolution, because of decreasing invasions, mechanical assist devices, and alternative revascularization (transmyocardial revascularization). The care of these patients will need to evolve as well. In many situations, the use of a recovery room may well increase. At the same time, if laser revascularization and gene therapy to create neoangiogenesis pan out, greater expertise in the cardiac ICU will be needed because these therapies do not immediately fix the problem but require time to create new perfusion to the myocardium.

CARDIOVASCULAR RECOVERY ROOM

Contemporary design of the cardiovascular recovery room (CVRR) can improve the efficiency and quality of care. Although best designed specifically for the purpose of postoperative cardiovascular surgery patients, a satisfactory CVRR can be created in a variety of existing critical care areas.

Size and Location

Optimal location of the CVRR should be directly adjacent to the OR to reduce transport time to and from the OR. Patient transport is a very critical time because it occurs during a vulnerable stage in cardiovascular recovery, when blood pressure, rhythm, and pumping function of the heart can be labile. Transport back to the OR can be just as critical a time because it often occurs in the face of mediastinal bleeding, cardiac tamponade, and shock. If the CVRR is located on another floor of the hospital, an elevator of adequate size to accommodate all transport personnel (often three or more), intravenous (IV) poles and drug pumps, and balloon pumps and assist devices must be readily available. A dedicated elevator restricted from public use is best. The CVRR should also be in close proximity to blood bank, laboratory, radiologic, and respiratory services.

The size of the CVRR can vary depending upon the number of postoperative patients and their length of stay and the presence of other types of critical care patients. Typical units are designed for immediate postoperative care, with discharge the next day to a stepdown unit or other critical care setting. Other units are designed to be more comprehensive, including postoperative through extended critical care. Small units are easier to staff, can be more efficient at sharing resources, and are generally easier to manage. Large units can care for greater numbers of patients and can keep patients for more than a single day, but they are noisier and more difficult to staff and manage. The optimum size depends on the ultimate function of the unit.

Designing Functional Workspace

Dedicated CVRRs offer convenient functionality because supplemental devices (pleural drainage systems, OR equipment, intravascular catheters), medications (vasoactive agents, antiarrhythmics), and specialized monitoring (pressure monitors, continuous ECG, pulse oximetry, end-tidal CO_2) are readily available. Each bed must have suction devices and a bag-mask oxygen delivery system functional at all times that the bed is occupied. Ample room should exist between bed locations for ventilators and monitoring devices. Integrated headboards with receptacles for medical gases, electrical sockets, and suction allow for uncluttered connections of gas lines between the walls and appliances. Lighting in the CVRR must provide different levels for specific situations. Ambient light should provide satisfactory illumination so that charts and monitors can be easily read. The light should be dimmable so that a patient's sleeping can be facilitated at night. Bright lighting over the bed needs to be available for examination and procedures. Portable, directional lighting is convenient when emergency bedside exploration is required.

A complete resuscitation cart must be available, portable, and strategically located so as to be immediately available with minimal transportation. This "code cart" should contain cardiac defibrillators (with internal *and* external paddles), external pacing devices (pulse generators), resuscitation drugs, emergency surgical equipment (thoracotomy, median sternotomy, anything that would be required to open a chest and repair a problem), and intravascular catheters.

From a physician's point of view, the CVRR can never have too many supplies. Anything that is necessary for routine care and emergency operation needs to be located within open view in the CVRR. Emergency equipment should never be locked or hidden in a closet. A portable, fully stocked code cart is very useful in emergency situations (see later). All personnel should know where supplies can be found, and these resources must be checked for function, number, and expiration date on a regular basis. It is often necessary to keep duplicate supplies on the unit so they are always available. It is also convenient to have an extra ventilator and portable oxygen immediately available. From a manager's point of view, keeping ample supplies can be costly and labor intensive. It is often the shared responsibility of the nursing staff and manager to keep accurate records of supplies and their utilization.

Family visitation is necessary not only for the emotional benefit of the patient and family but also to facilitate communication between the family, physicians, and nurses. Family members should be able to visit patients soon after the patient has arrived in the CVRR. Delaying family visitation, unless absolutely necessary, can only create tension and dissatisfaction between the family and staff. It is often a good idea to provide a meeting area where staff and families can have private discussions.

Staffing

Enough cannot be said about having effective management in the CVRR. A well-functioning recovery room needs multidisciplined leadership, most often made up of a head nurse and a physician medical director. These members are responsible for daily operation, staffing, continuing education, and process improvement (quality improvement). Working under the leadership of the head nurse and medical director are clinical managers who handle routine occurrences. Nurses trained in critical and postoperative cardiovascular care should provide bedside nursing. It is far better to train and refine the skills of a consistent group of nurses than to freely assign nurses less familiar with these types of patients. This is especially true because clinical pathways such as early extubation (fast track), pain control, and chest tube and pacing wire removal need to be followed rather closely. The complement of staff in the CVRR is composed of respiratory therapists, cardiovascular and ECG technicians, secretaries, and aides. To extend the reach of a physician's care it has become common to use physician assistants or nurse practitioners. This practice has worked quite well and is a valuable adjunct to the health care team.

When a patient is initially admitted to the CVRR, it generally takes two or three nurses to get the patient settled in. A single nurse then manages the patient for the next 1 to 2 hours as long as there is hemodynamic stability. At this point, the patient is usually stable enough to be managed by a nurse caring for an additional patient. After extubation, at our institution, the nurse-patient ratio remains at 1:2. In a well-designed unit, a nurse-patient ratio of 1:3 or 1:4 can safely be achieved in 8 to 12 hours, with resultant improved efficiency and reduced cost.

Devices

A specialty unit such as a CVRR will have medical devices beyond what a typical critical care unit might have. Each bed will be equipped with a bedside monitor capable of displaying one- or two-channel ECG, three- or four-channel pressure readings, and cardiac output measurements. Additional modifications may enable the monitor to display pulse oximetry, end-tidal carbon dioxide ($ETCO_2$) and mixed venous oxygen saturation (Svo_2) and possibly to detect and record arrhythmias. Central monitoring is necessary if the nurse is out of the immediate vicinity of the patient for an extended period of time. Current monitor technology allows for alarms to be set for all measured physiologic parameters. Alarm ranges need to be set to balance sensitivity with specificity. Poorly chosen alarm ranges result in inappropriate sounding, increase noise in the unit, and likely reduce the nurse's urgency to analyze the cause of the alarm.

Unique to the cardiovascular surgery patient is the use of ventricular assist devices (VADs). These devices come in a variety of conformations, but all assist one or both ventricles. The most simplistic in application is the intra-aortic balloon pump (IABP) that can be inserted and managed at the bedside. This device occupies only a few square feet of floor space at the foot of the bed, is portable, and can be managed by the bedside nurse (with the assistance of a cardiovascular technician). This device is often placed preoperatively, such as in the catheterization laboratory and follows the patient through surgery into the CVRR. It may, however, be placed in the OR for hemodynamic instability or inability to wean from CPB. All other VADs require implantation in the OR. The "pump" can be an extracorporeal device driven by a bedside pneumatic console (such as the Abiomed). Alternatively, the "pump" can be a fully implanted device (such as the TCI HeartMate) that is driven by either a bedside pneumatic console or an external electrical source. These implanted devices are portable and take up just a few square feet of floor space at the end of the bed. Both of the latter implanted devices, however, require maintenance of a back-up console physically on the unit. All of the aforementioned devices are highly specialized and sophisticated machines. Each VAD has its own operational nuances and should only be managed by a subset of nurses familiar with its function, troubleshooting, and emergency operation.

Next to the medication pumps and pulse oximeter, the mechanical ventilator is one of the most common devices used in the CVRR. Although in most instances a ventilator does not need to provide many sophisticated modes of ventilation, occasional patients will have extraordinary gas exchange abnormalities. In these situation, it is more than just convenient to have a ventilator that can provide not only volume-controlled ventilation but also high minute ventilation, positive end-expiratory pressure (PEEP), and potentially pressure-controlled ventilation. In addition, not all patients are rapidly weaned from the ventilator and extubated. Some require a more conservative weaning schedule and perhaps the assistance of supportive modes of ventilation such as pressure support. For these reasons, the ventilators in our CVRR can provide almost any mode of ventilation necessary.

Point-of-Service Laboratories and Pharmacy

Upon admission to the CVRR, the postoperative patient has a routine battery of laboratory tests. Typical examples include a hemoglobin and hematocrit, platelet count, arterial blood gases (ABG), partial thromboplastin time (PTT), and potassium (K^+). These results are relatively useless to the patient unless they are available in a timely fashion. Correction of coagulopathy is at best empirical without prothrombin time (PT) and PTT. Transfusion can only be based on observed losses without a baseline hemoglobin and hematocrit. Oxygenation and ventilation cannot be correlated to pulse oximetry or end-tidal CO_2 without ABG. Unfortunately, a busy clinical laboratory may be unable to rapidly turn around a moderate number of admission tests in addition to its other requests. To improve turnaround time, satellite laboratories have become popular to serve specific locations. However, these satellite locations require supplemental staffing and equipment and have not been shown to be cost effective. Another alternative is to move the laboratory to the bedside, referred to as point-of-care service. Microsample technology has allowed miniaturization of laboratory equipment and accurate batteries of tests to be performed rapidly at the bedside. Although certainly convenient, the technology still requires laboratory personnel to ensure quality control. Cost savings have not clearly been demonstrated.

The CVRR must be stocked with ample supplies of pharmaceuticals. Requirements extend beyond resuscitation fluids, vasoactive agents, and antibiotics. Also required are narcotics, benzodiazepines, afterload-reducing medications, and diuretics, just to name a few. As with laboratory results, medications are not useful unless they are available in a timely fashion. Most stock medications need accurate record keeping to ensure proper availability and discourage abuse. Satellite pharmacies and even computerized dispensing equipment have facilitated access to pharmaceutical resources, but it is unclear whether this convenience will offset the cost.

TRANSPORT AND INITIAL ASSESSMENT

Materials and Personnel

Transport from the OR table to the CVRR is the first critical time period for the patient, lasting up to an hour after the chest is closed. Physiologically, the organ systems are undergoing a rewarming and reperfusion period. The body is recovering from an enzymatic assault from cytokines, prostaglandins, leukotrienes, oxygen free radicals, and complement as a result of CPB. Ventricular performance may be impaired, volume resuscitation may be incomplete, intracardiac conduction may be profoundly impaired, and bleeding may exist. Chest tubes attached to pleural collection systems will hang at the end of the bed. Large urine output, from mannitol in the CPB, diuretics, hypothermia, or the presence of intrinsic atrial natriuretic factor, may exacerbate hypovolemia. The patient may be receiving multiple inotropic agents, each delivered by a pump. VADs and electronic pulse generators may be necessary. If the patient is not already extubated, ventilation must be maintained either mechanically or by bag-mask. An endotracheal tube taped onto the face secures the airway. Oxygenation may have been difficult and positive end-expiratory pressure (PEEP) may have been necessary to maintain adequate oxygenation. Arterial and central venous catheters tether the patient, each connected by a pressure transducer. Portable electronics to monitor rhythm and pressures must accompany the patient. Moving a patient without disturbing any of the position-critical catheters requires sufficient numbers and coordination of staff.

After transport from the OR table to the bed, it generally requires three people to transport a patient safely to the CVRR. An anesthesiologist or a certified registered nurse anesthetist is generally responsible for maintaining oxygenation and ventilation, monitoring vital signs, and titrating vasoactive medications. A respiratory therapist may be available to provide hand ventilation. Portable electronic monitoring systems should provide ECG and one or two pressure-monitoring channels. In addition, an OR nurse, accompanied by a nursing assistant, assists in moving emergency drugs, VADs, and IV poles in concert with the bed. Which members of the transport team push the bed vary by institution.

Cardiopulmonary Dysfunction in the Transport Period

Two primary systems that can manifest life-threatening dysfunction during transport merit comment. The first is the pulmonary system exhibiting gas exchange abnormalities. The most common problem is desaturation on pulse oximetry. It is appropriate to restore O_2 saturation prior to transport to the CVRR if possible. This can usually be accomplished by increasing FIO_2 ensuring that endotracheal tube placement is correct, and checking that oxygen is flowing from the oxygen source. Sometimes it is beneficial to increase the PEEP to the ventilation circuit. Inadequate ventilation is infrequently noted prior to transport to the CVRR. Elevated end-tidal CO_2 suggests a true elevated $Paco_2$ and warrants increasing respiratory minute volume ($\dot{V}E$) prior to transport. This is usually achieved by increasing the respiratory rate. If the endotracheal tube

(ETT) is securely in position and pulse oximetry is above 90%, the patient is ready for transport from the point of view of the respiratory system.

The second system that can demonstrate life-threatening dysfunction is the cardiovascular system. It is best to temporarily delay transport until an acceptable cardiac performance can be achieved. The pre-transport period is not the appropriate time to *optimize* pharmacologic or mechanical support. It is best to ensure an acceptable blood pressure (systolic above 100 mm Hg), a stable rhythm, and the absence of exsanguinating mediastinal bleeding and then embark to the CVRR. The most common cause of hypotension in the early postoperative period in a patient with an otherwise well-functioning heart is bradycardia or hypovolemia. If a patient has bradycardia, pacing should commence at a rate of 80 to 100 beats/minute. In the absence of atrioventricular (AV) block, atrial pacing is preferred, but if ventricular wires are all that is present or if high-grade AV blockade is present, ventricular demand pacing at 80 to 100 beats/min should be started. If bradycardia is not present or if pacing does not improve systolic blood pressure, volume resuscitation with 250 to 500 mL of normal saline or hetastarch often improves blood pressure. If the preceding manipulations have failed to render the patient ready for transport, the addition of a vasoconstricting inotrope or further investigation will be needed prior to transport. Further details on the management of early postoperative hypotension or the care of the cardiovascular patient on inotropic support are discussed later.

One of the most challenging aspects of transporting a postoperative cardiovascular surgery patient is keeping medication pumps and assist devices functioning properly and preventing displacement. There are few words of advice other than to always have adequate personnel to push devices, keep hallways clear, use large elevators, and move slowly enough to prevent problems. A transport leader should direct movement to maximize safety.

ANTICIPATED POSTOPERATIVE COURSE

The "typical" postoperative course for a CPB patient has changed significantly over the past decade. What was once a period of observation and stabilization has become a more active period of weaning supportive therapies, removal of tubes, and mobilization out of bed. The morning after surgery the patient should be out of bed to the chair and rapidly progressing to normal activities. The dramatic change in management technique has been driven by a number of forces, including improved anesthetic technique, improved operative technique, and clinical pathways that keep the "typical" patient moving in the desired direction.

Initial Assessment and Management

Upon admission to the CVRR, the patient is transferred from the care and monitoring of the transport team to that of the CVRR staff. Mechanical ventilation is resumed and pressure, pulse oximetry, end-tidal CO_2, and ECG monitoring is transitioned to the bedside electronics. Patients are often awakening at this time, and their desires for immediate extubation and mobilization are (no fault of their own) poorly timed. To keep the patient manageable during this transitionary period, it is useful to increase sedation with an ultra short-acting agent such as propofol. Prior practices were to use longer acting narcotics, benzodiazepines, and possibly even paralysis, but this will only serve to dramatically lengthen the time until extubation. The goal is to keep the patient comfortable and manageable long enough to settle in.

Laboratory Evaluation

Initial laboratory assessment is aimed at gas exchange, oxygen-carrying capacity, serum potassium level, and coagulation. There really is no substitute for ABG determination when it comes to assessment of gas exchange. It not only provides the latter information but also identifies metabolic acidosis that may be present as well. Gradients between $PaCO_2$ and $ETCO_2$ are calculated, and $ETCO_2$ can then be used to approximate $Paco_2$. Patients usually arrive on supplemental O_2 from FIO_2 0.4 to FIO_2 1.0. If the initial O_2 saturation is above the low 90s, FIO_2 can be weaned until it is 0.4 as long as pulse oximetry remains above the low 90s. Moderate to severe abnormalities in gas exchange or acid-base balance should prompt a second ABG determination approximately 1 to 2 hours after arrival in the CVRR. In an otherwise routine postoperative CABG patient without disturbances of gas exchange, acid-base balance, or cardiac performance, additional ABG may not be necessary. Weaning and extubation can be managed exclusively with a pulse oximeter and end-tidal CO_2 monitor.

Hemoglobin should generally be kept above 8 g/dL. However, oxygen-carrying capacity needs to be assessed in view of adequacy of oxygen delivery. A well-functioning cardiovascular system can increase cardiac output enough so that oxygen delivery is adequate even if the oxygen-carrying capacity is low. If the cardiac performance cannot be increased, it may become necessary to increase oxygen-carrying capacity by way of transfusion with PRBCs to meet oxygen delivery needs. When in doubt of adequacy of oxygen delivery, check an arterial–mixed venous oxygen content difference. Values above 6 mL/dL reflect inadequate oxygen delivery.

On admission, a PTT and platelet count are obtained. These results need to be interpreted on the basis of each clinical presentation. Patients often take aspirin preoperatively, rendering the platelet function impaired but the platelet count unchanged. CPB will decrease platelet function as well and will also reduce platelet number. In the absence of active mediastinal bleeding and platelet count above approximately 50,000, platelet replacement is unnecessary. Counts below this should be reassessed in 4 to 6 hours. If there is no mediastinal output to speak of and the platelet count falls no further, it is probably safe to not transfuse platelets. Patients with an absolute platelet count below 20,000 or the presence of significant mediastinal bleeding should receive platelet transfusion. PTT can be abnormal for a number of reasons, but as with the management of platelets, it requires correction only if active mediastinal bleeding is present. Prolonged PTT can be due to the presence of heparin, inadequate reversal of heparin with protamine, factor deficiency caused by consumption or inadequate synthesis, or the presence of circulating inhibitors. It is worthwhile to check the ratio of heparin to protamine given in the OR. In the presence of mediastinal bleeding, additional protamine can be given if sufficient protamine was not initially given.

Serum potassium should be checked regularly in the postoperative period and replaced based on measured values and on expected losses in urine output. Prior to the availability of point-of-service laboratory analysis, results of serum potassium could take more than 1 or 2 hours from the time of sampling. To keep the serum potassium at a level above 4 mEq/L, potassium can be replaced based on hourly output. The scale ranges from 5 mEq K^+ for a 100-mL hourly urine output to 20 mEq K^+ for a 400-mL hourly output. The replacement (for urine output) is stopped if a 6-hour postoperative serum potassium is greater than 5.5, otherwise replacement is stopped the next morning. Now that serum potassium is rapidly available, either at the bedside or through the *stat* laboratory, potassium replacement is based on a combination of measured and expected deficits.

The Postoperative Electrocardiogram

Upon admission to the CVRR, an ECG is obtained. The cardiac rhythm is usually apparent from the bedside monitoring leads; however, the 12-lead ECG is necessary to identify new ischemic or injury currents. It is not uncommon to find small J-point elevations in many of the leads. Associated with incoving (concave) ST segments, this pattern looks similar to ECG changes seen with pericardial inflammation. Other than noting these changes, no other intervention is necessary. New, shallow, T-wave inversions are also commonly encountered, and although they could suggest ongoing ischemia, rarely progress to significant events. It is, however, our practice to empirically use IV nitroglycerin in doses of 50 to 100 μg/min as long as an acceptable mean arterial pressure (MAP) can be maintained without the necessity of adding other vasoconstrictors. Deep T-wave inversions or those associated with greater than 1 mm ST depression should be of more concern to the clinician, especially if they are new. These findings should initiate the empiric use of IV nitroglycerin, as with simple T-wave inversions, and also prompt a follow-up ECG within the next few hours. If the ECG "worsens" and the cardiac performance is less than would have been expected, further pharmacologic intervention (nitroglycerin, diltiazem) or investigation (reexploration, catheterization) may be necessary.

Prompt communication with the cardiac surgeon is needed to ensure timely, appropriate, and coordinated care. Convex ST-segment abnormalities associated with ST elevation suggest injury current. If seen in the OR, this often prompts reevaluation of grafts for patency, even if the chest already has been closed. Sometimes the injury current is occurring in a region that the surgeon thinks cannot be better revascularized, in which case little can be offered except IV nitroglycerin or balloon counterpulsation (IABP). When these changes are first noticed in the CVRR, the surgeon should be notified, even if the cardiac performance is adequate. Empiric use of IV nitroglycerin or diltiazem is often added but is of unproven benefit. Follow-up ECG in a couple of hours should be obtained to follow the course of the electrical changes. Injury current in the face of less than expected cardiac performance may represent perioperative myocardial infarction. Other common postoperative ECG findings are varieties of AV blocks and bundle branch conduction delays. Sinus bradycardia, junctional escape rhythms, and high-grade AV block are probably the most common rhythm abnormalities, but right bundle branch block (RBBB) and left bundle branch block (LBBB) are also common. These conduction abnormalities usually completely resolve by the next morning.

Chest radiographs are included in the admission assessment. It is important to confirm the position of the endotracheal tube, central and pulmonary catheters, chest tubes, and devices such as balloon pumps. Typical postoperative findings include atelectasis of the left lower lobe and degrees of interstitial edema from none to significant. Pleural effusions and mediastinal size should be noted. Sometimes a follow-up chest x-ray demonstrating enlarged cardiac shadow can be very suggestive of retained hematoma (and possibly tamponade).

Although patients are returning to the CVRR warmer than in the past (historical temperatures were 34.5°–35.5°C), some are still somewhat hypothermic (<36°C). We have found that adding warming blankets can facilitate return to euthermia. Convection (heated air systems) or conduction (warm blankets) can be used. Heated humidified cascades can be added to the ventilator circuit, but these are probably not as efficient or cost effective as the latter devices. Return to euthermia is more than just a comfort measure. All enzyme systems in the body have an optimum temperature range. Coagulation is impaired at low body temperatures.[26] We routinely actively warm our cold, bleeding patients as a part of our protocol for managing mediastinal bleeding. Active warming can be stopped when the body temperature is greater than 36.5°C.

Pain Management and Control of Sedation

Pain management and control of sedation can be extensions of anesthetic technique. The goals of early postoperative pain and sedation management are to control pain, suppress anxiety, manage agitation and movement while settling in, and allow for smooth emergence from anesthesia. In many ways this is similar to the process that occurs in standard surgical recovery rooms.

In some institutions, short-acting sedating agents (propofol, fentanyl, and midazolam) are used at the end of the case to maintain sedation until transfer to the CVRR. The use of short-acting sedating agents has greatly enhanced our ability to control consciousness in a "turn-key" fashion. Propofol, in doses of 5 to 30 μg/kg/min, can provide complete unconsciousness. Reducing the drug dose or turning the infusion off will result in rapid awakening. One key to successful CVRR management is smooth awakening from anesthesia. Once settled in, wean short-acting sedating agents gradually to allow for smooth emergence and complete consciousness *within the next 90 minutes.* Recognize that propofol and other sedating agents have no intrinsic analgesic effect. Agitation upon emergence may be due to pain, and the addition of morphine prior to awakening may smooth emergence. If patients remain agitated and unable to follow commands, it is best to maintain sedation with propofol or a narcotic for a few hours and then attempt weaning again. Long-acting benzodiazepines should be used sparingly for agitation, because they seem only to prolong the weaning process. True anxiety is best treated with benzodiazepines. Persistently agitated patients can be maintained on propofol, although adding sedating agents such as haloperidol or lorazepam can reduce the severe agitation.

Altered levels of consciousness, including agitation after 24 hours, should suggest untoward effects of CPB on the brain, cerebrovascular accident, metabolic encephalopathy, and drug withdrawal (including ethanol). Some patients take longer than expected to awaken after discontinuation of propofol. Patients may metabolize narcotics, benzodiazepines, and paralytics differently. If a patient awakens but remains weak, has a poor head lift, and has difficulty weaning from the ventilator, additional paralytic reversal agents (glycopyrrolate and neostigmine) should be given. It would be distinctly unusual for a patient to fail to awaken 12 to 18 hours after sedation and paralysis have been discontinued. Persistent agitation, focal neurologic deficits, and failure to awaken should cause a more in-depth neurologic examination and possibly a radiologic investigation.

The techniques chosen for analgesia in the CVRR must complement the techniques used in the OR. Epidural analgesia should be continued in the CVRR and not supplemented by a systemic narcotic unless the epidural is poorly functional. Breakthrough pain should be managed by increasing the dose of epidural anesthetic. Poorly functioning epidural catheters should be removed, and analgesia should be provided in an alternative way. Patients who have received spinal analgesia may present with a continuous narcotic infusion, often patient-controlled analgesia. Bolus narcotic and adjustment of basal infusion rate in this case should manage breakthrough pain.

If a patient has received neither epidural nor spinal techniques, analgesia is best accomplished with a combination of narcotic and nonsteroidal agents. Morphine is an excellent all-around choice because of its duration of action, ease of administration (IV or IM), and tolerance. Because of its ability to venodilate (reducing preload) and release histamine, morphine can potentiate hypotension in patients with marginal cardiac performance. Early use of nonsteroidal agents such as ketorolac or indomethacin can dramatically reduce postoperative pain and reduce supplemental narcotic requirement. It is our practice to give IV ketorolac or rectal indomethacin at the time of admission, prior to emergence from anesthesia. Preoperative use of nonsteroidal agents would likely enhance analgesia even further without increasing the risk of bleeding. Nonsteroidal agents can be continued into the subsequent postoperative period for pain control. When the patient is able to take medications by mouth, additional oral narcotics can be utilized to achieve analgesia.

Hypertension Assessment and Treatment

Hypertension is the most welcomed postoperative cardiac complication. In general, MAP should be kept at 70 to 80 mm Hg to protect anastomotic and cannulation sites. Blood pressure must be carefully controlled when the aorta is friable or has been repaired with pledgets. MAP is kept in the 70s for the first 4 hours and is then allowed to rise no higher than 110 mm Hg for the duration of the patient's stay in the CVRR. If a patient has known carotid disease or severe peripheral vascular disease, initial MAP may be kept in the range of 85 to 95 mm Hg to prevent end-organ ischemia.

To keep MAP in an acceptable range, a combination of IV nitroglycerin, IV nitroprusside, narcotic, or other vasodilator (hydralazine, nifedipine, enalaprilat, and captopril) is used. One must never underestimate the ability of pain to raise blood pressure. One must ensure that there is no other reason for a sudden increase in blood pressure such as hypoxemia or bolus of vasoconstrictor. All patients return from the OR with IV nitroglycerin at 50 μg/min to augment coronary blood flow. IV nitroglycerin can be used as a first-line antihypertensive in these patients by titrating the dose as high as 300 μg/min. Blood pressure response is a bit slower than using IV nitroprusside, but a rather acceptable performance as an antihypertensive agent can be achieved with a little practice. If the MAP cannot be held in the acceptable range with nitroglycerin alone, IV nitroprusside can be added or used in the place of IV nitroglycerin. Nitroprusside has a shorter half-life than IV nitroglycerin and causes a more rapid decrease and increase in blood pressure with titration. IV nitroprusside has a useful dosage range of 1 to 8 μg/kg/min. If the addition of IV nitroprusside cannot keep the MAP in a desired range, additional agents such as hydralazine or enalapril are useful. If long-term control of hypertension is required, addition of longer-acting agents such as hydralazine, β-blockers, or angiotensin-converting enzyme (ACE) inhibitors should be used to continue antihypertensive control. This longer duration therapy should begin with enough time prior to transfer from the CVRR to assure safety and effectiveness.

Management of Early Postoperative Cardiac Dysfunction

Many postoperative CABG patients require little intervention except for treatment of minor swings in blood pressure. Some, however, even when noted to have good ventricular function, require significant intervention to avoid disaster in the early postoperative period. A rapid, systematic approach reliably diagnoses and treats most problems.

"Acceptable" systolic blood pressure varies from patient to patient, depending on the presence of carotid or peripheral vascular disease, history of hypertension, or friability of the aorta. In the absence of preexisting disease, systolic blood pressure should be kept above 100 mm Hg. This value should be higher or lower in the presence of special circumstances. Similarly, an "acceptable" cardiac index depends on preexisting cardiac index, temperature of the patient, and oxygen delivery. It would be unreasonable to expect a dysfunctional ventricle preoperatively to dramatically improve unless revascularization of ischemic myocardium has awakened hibernating function.[27]

Patients who present from the OR with core temperatures below 35°C may not need a high cardiac index because of decreased metabolic rates at low body temperatures. In general, a cardiac index of 1.7 to 2.0 L/m/m^2 is acceptable during the first few hours postoperatively if the patient's core temperature is below 35.5°C. At temperatures above this, the cardiac index should exceed 2 L/m/m^2. If it is unclear whether a particular cardiac index is sufficient in a given patient at a given temperature, an arterial–mixed venous oxygen content difference can be obtained. Although the following diagnostic and therapeutic approach appears to be a serial assessment, in practice, the experienced clinician evaluates most of these points simultaneously:

- Rhythm and ventricular rate
- Adequacy of volume resuscitation
- Need for inotropic support
- Presence of mediastinal bleeding and possible tamponade
- Evidence of electrical abnormalities
- Need for mechanical support

Bradycardia, either sinus bradycardia, junctional rhythm, or high-grade atrioventricular blockade (especially after aortic valve surgery), is easily recognized on ECG and can be corrected by connecting the patient's temporary pacing wires to an electronic pulse generator. Pacing is always indicated in hypotensive patients with ventricular rates less than 60 beats/min. When the ventricular rate is 60 to 80 beats/min in a hypotensive patient, pacing (80–100 beats) can be attempted to try to reestablish acceptable blood pressure. In an emergency situation (especially when it is unclear whether atrioventricular block is present), it is best to begin *ventricular* pacing at a rate of 80 to 100 beats/min. Once a stable rhythm is established, atrial or atrioventricular sequential pacing can be initiated if these wires are available. Sometimes ventricular pacing is poorly tolerated and results in a falling blood pressure. In this situation, volume resuscitation may allow ventricular pacing to continue with better results.

Tachyarrhythmias, whether atrial or ventricular, are infrequent in the early postoperative period. Sinus tachycardia is an exception and is frequent in the early postoperative period. If present and life-threatening, they should be treated by immediate direct current (DC) cardioversion. Atrial tachyarrhythmias without hypotension can generally await definitive pharmacologic therapy. Intravenous magnesium, 2 to 4 g in patients with serum magnesium levels below 2 mEq/L, can be useful in suppressing atrial premature contractions and fibrillation.[28]

Treatment of ventricular tachyarrhythmias is somewhat more controversial. Nonsustained ventricular ectopy, such as premature ventricular contractions (PVCs), and unifocal or multifocal couplets, or triplets, do not require therapy if they do not cause hemodynamic compromise. In practice, frequently occurring couplets and triplets often beget therapy with lidocaine to reduce nurse and physician anxiety. Initially, aggressive replacement of potassium when serum level is below 4 to 4.5 mEq/L can be tried. Magnesium supplementation, as previously described, can be useful in the suppression of PVCs as well.[28]

Longer bursts of ventricular tachycardia (VT), sustained or

nonsustained, can be suppressed with lidocaine in the early postoperative period. Sustained VT with hypotension obviously requires immediate synchronized DC cardioversion. Lidocaine can be continued for 12 to 18 hours until cardiovascular stability has been demonstrated and ventricular irritability has faded. At this time, the lidocaine can be discontinued and the need for longer antiarrhythmic therapy, which is unlikely, can be assessed.

The next most common cause of early postoperative hypotension is inadequate volume resuscitation. Low CVP (<8 to 10 mm Hg), low PAD pressure (<18 mm Hg), or low PCWP (<14 to 16 mm Hg) strongly suggests this diagnosis. Rapid restoration of blood pressure by rapid infusion of 250 to 500 mL of normal saline or hetastarch is both diagnostic and therapeutic. Depending on the compliance of the heart and its inotropic state, higher filling pressures may be required to provide sufficient preload. In these situations, CVPs of 16 to 20 mm Hg, PADs of 24 to 26 mm Hg, or PCWPs of 18 to 22 mm Hg may be necessary. Rather than aiming for a particular filling pressure, it is best to try small volume challenges and remeasurement of cardiac index and blood pressure.

In general, when the PCWP is greater than 22 to 24 mm Hg, the "tank" is adequately filled and further volume resuscitation is unnecessary. In patients with right ventricular failure, CVP and pulmonary arterial pressure can be substantially elevated, even in the presence of normal left-sided filling pressures. To optimize performance in this situation, it may in fact be necessary to maintain higher right-sided pressures (CVPs 18 to 22 mm Hg). However, overdistention of the ventricle leads to increased wall tension and can worsen right ventricular ischemia. When the ventricle cannot maintain adequate performance and filling pressures are all generously elevated, the diagnosis of tamponade, especially when a ventricle described as "good" fails to perform as expected, should be considered.

If volume resuscitation is ineffective or too slow, vasoactive support should be added immediately. Although it is commonplace for phenylephrine (Neo-Synephrine) or ephedrine to be used while in the OR for temporary correction of hypotension, the choice of vasoactive medication should be based on the measurement of blood pressure, filling pressures, and cardiac index. Assuming that the patient has been adequately volume resuscitated, hypotension and low cardiac index (<2.0 to 2.2 L/m/m^2) require agents that increase inotropic state and vasomotor tone. Epinephrine or dopamine is ideal for this. Epinephrine can be started at a few micrograms per minute and titrated upward as necessary to the desired effect. Dopamine can be started at 4 μg/kg/min and titrated up to 20 to 25 μg/kg/min or until the desired effect is achieved.

When low cardiac index exists in the volume-resuscitated patient without hypotension, an agent that increases primarily inotropy and vasodilation should be used. Dobutamine or milrinone is ideal in this situation. Dobutamine can be started at 5 μg/kg/min and titrated over the next few hours up to 25 μg/kg/min until the desired effect is achieved. The rate of dose increase depends upon the urgency and degree of inotropic support needed. Milrinone can be started with a 50 μg/kg loading dose followed by a dose of 0.375 to 0.75 μg/kg/m IV continuous infusion.

When hypotension exists in the presence of a high cardiac index (>2.5 L/m/m^2) in the volume-resuscitated patient, blood pressure can be restored with a primarily vasoconstricting agent such as norepinephrine. Dosage for norepinephrine starts at 1 μg/min and should be titrated to the desired effect. The purely vasodilated patient can be managed with volume resuscitation only, but we have found that adding norepinephrine after about 2 L of resuscitation fluid simplifies management without increasing morbidity. When cardiac performance does not improve despite volume resuscitation and the addition of inotropic support, consideration for the addition of a mechanical support device, usually an IABP, needs to be made. In extreme cases, when cardiac performance is insufficient to support life, implantable VADs can be utilized.

During this resuscitation, attention should be paid to the ST morphology on the monitor or the presence of chest tube bleeding. New ST abnormalities can signify acute graft compromise and warrant reexploration. Massive chest tube output can signify surgical bleeding and deserves reexploration. As mentioned earlier, elevated filling pressures and poor cardiovascular performance may suggest cardiac tamponade. Tamponade can occur in the patient with minimal or massive mediastinal output. Some clues to tamponade include visually noticeable pulsus paradoxus seen on arterial pressure tracing (i.e., large dips in the systolic pressure) during inhalation with the ventilator, grossly distended jugular venous distention, widening cardiac silhouette on chest x-ray, and elevated CVP, PAD, and PCWP. We do not wait for "equalization of pressures." This has not been a useful pattern for diagnosis of tamponade in the postoperative cardiac patient. Uniformly elevated filling pressures in a patient with low blood pressure, low cardiac index, and a supposedly good ventricle should suggest the diagnosis. Often a history of chest tube bleeding is present, but not necessary. Subtle signs of tamponade include bleeding *through* the sternal incision and bleeding *around* the chest tube incisions. Echocardiography can be very useful to help discriminate poor left ventricular function from impaired chamber filling (as occurs in tamponade). Often a surface echocardiogram is insufficient and a transesophageal echocardiogram is necessary for accurate diagnosis.

Management of Early Postoperative Pulmonary Dysfunction

Pulmonary system dysfunction is frequent in the early postoperative period. The causes are generally ventilation-perfusion (V/Q) mismatching, intrapulmonary atelectasis, and preexisting lung disease. CPB has also been shown to increase pulmonary vascular tone and reduce pulmonary endothelial production of nitric oxide.[29] Nitric oxide used in conjunction with mechanical ventilation has been shown to reduce pulmonary hypertension and improve oxygenation, but it is unclear whether this will be a necessary and useful adjunct to therapy in the future.

The literature has also suggested that the use of vasodilators, such as IV nitroglycerin and nitroprusside, can exacerbate shunt flow through the lung by inhibiting areas of hypoxic vasoconstriction, resulting in early postoperative hypoxemia.[30] CPB also activates cytokines, prostaglandins, neutrophils, oxygen free radicals, and the coagulation-fibrinolytic system. Each of these cascades produces species that can cause direct or indirect damage to the pulmonary endothelium, leading to gas exchange abnormalities. Techniques such as leukocyte depletion (with specialized filters) and modification of oxygenators have not consistently been demonstrated to improve gas exchange or alter outcome.[31–33]

Most commonly, hypoxemia first presents as low oxygen saturation noted on pulse oximeter. Desaturation is usually corrected easily by increasing FIO_2 to the delivery system. If the patient is being manually ("bag") ventilated, the delivery device must be connected to a suitable oxygen source with *flowing* oxygen. Patients with refractory hypoxemia while on a mechanical ventilator should in general be hand-ventilated while the situation is assessed to eliminate the ventilator or its gas circuits as the problem. The patient should be auscultated for confirmation of endotracheal intubation or asymmetry of breath sounds (mucous plug, mainstem intubation, and pneumothorax). This should be followed by thorough suctioning and vigorous hand ventilation. If the patient remains hypoxemic, PEEP can be increased from 5 cm H_2O to 10 cm H_2O. Higher levels are occasionally necessary. If low oxygen saturation persists (a quick confirmation can be obtained during a check for dark red blood aspirated from arterial cannulation line), the patient is continued on 100% FIO_2 while vigorous hand ventilation is maintained. Further diagnostic evaluation should then include a chest x-ray and ABG determination. Oxygen saturation almost always increases if the preceding steps are observed. Further therapeutic maneuvers will be based on the results of diagnostic studies unless emergent intervention (such as a chest tube for suspected pneumothorax) is necessary.

Far less frequent a problem is inadequate ventilation. Elevated end-tidal CO_2 or $PaCO_2$ confirms this diagnosis. Vigorous shivering substantially increases CO_2 production and is seen in the first few hours postoperatively. This can dramatically increase $PaCO_2$ if ventilation is not increased. More likely, inadequate ventilation will be associated with a relatively low respiratory rate or low exhaled tidal volumes. Low exhaled tidal volume is usually first noted when the mechanical ventilator alarms and displays a low returned volume. First, auscultation is performed to ensure endotracheal intubation. The ventilation circuit is carefully checked to eliminate gas leakage as a problem. My clinician manually ventilates the patient with a bag device and feels for resistance to lung inflation. If resistance is present, this usually indicates a mechanical problem, such as a kinked endotracheal tube, mucus or foreign object obstruction, mainstem bronchus intubation, or tension pneumothorax or hydrothorax. If this is the case, ventilator high-pressure alarms often are triggered. Minimal resistance to lung inflation with manual ventilation may signify a leak around the endotracheal tube (ETT) cuff (listen for the leak by placing your ear over the patient's mouth) or a dislodged ETT. If no leaks are noted in the ventilatory circuit and low exhaled tidal volumes persist, check for a nasogastric tube inadvertently placed into the trachea or for large air leaks in the pleural collection system (suggesting a bronchopleural fistula). Correcting any of the preceding problems generally remedies the situation. If inadequate ventilation persists, continue the patient on 100% FIO_2 while maintaining vigorous hand ventilation. Further evaluation should then proceed and include an ABG and chest x-ray. If possible, avoid all sedating or paralyzing agents so that spontaneous ventilation, if present, can assist gas exchange.

Weaning from Mechanical Ventilation

Patients who have received "fast-track" types of anesthesia can be rapidly weaned from mechanical ventilation and extubated in the CVRR. The ideal patients for prompt extubation are awake, able to protect their airway, and without hemodynamic instability or abnormalities of gas exchange. A patient receiving low-dose vasoactive support for blood pressure or cardiac index (i.e., epinephrine or norepinephrine doses <5 μg/min or dobutamine <5 μg/kg/min) also can be included in the group for early extubation as long as cardiac performance is in fact adequate. If cardiac index has been measured, a value greater than 2 L/m/m^2 should be present. Values below this should cause the clinician to consider whether the patient's heart can provide the output necessary to support the work of breathing.

The patient should not have significant mediastinal bleeding or be considered at risk to return to the OR. A safe margin of gas exchange should also be present. PaO_2 greater than 70 mm Hg on an FIO_2 of 0.40 to 0.50 is acceptable. PEEP should be no greater than 5 cm to maintain adequate oxygenation. There should also be an absence of significant metabolic acidosis that would require the patient to have to ventilate excessively to maintain an acceptable pH. Spontaneous ventilation should be sufficient to keep $PaCO_2$ in the 40-mm Hg range or less. Safe extubation can also be accomplished with $PaCO_2$ in the low 50-mm Hg as long as the pH is above 7.30 and no significant metabolic acidosis is present.

To expedite weaning and extubation, experienced nurses and respiratory therapists specially trained in this type of clinical pathway should be on hand. Physician extenders (physician assistants and nurse practitioners) can also participate effectively in the weaning and extubation process. After the patient has settled into the CVRR, all sedating agents (such as propofol) are rapidly tapered so that the patient can be fully awake within 60 to 90 minutes from admission. If the patient remains weak by the end of this period, as assessed by a 10-second head lift and grip strength, any residual effects of paralytic agents can be reversed with neostigmine and glycopyrrolate. During this same 60- to 90-minute period, FIO_2 should be lowered from its initial value to 0.4 to 0.5 as long as the pulse oximeter demonstrates oxygen saturation in the low 90-mm Hg range or better.

As soon as the patient appears awake, weaning from ventilation can begin. Weaning requires usually only two ventilation modes, assist control (control mode ventilation [CMV], volume control [VC]) and continuous positive airway pressure (CPAP). Rarely are other modes such as pressure support necessary. Synchronized intermittent mandatory ventilation (SIMV) is almost never used in the weaning process. "Weaning parameters," that is, preextubation measurements of inspiratory forces and volumes, have not been found to be useful predictors and are not utilized.

When the patient is awake, the mode of ventilation is changed from assist/control to CPAP. The patient is observed for comfort, maintenance of effective respiratory rate (generally found to be from about 10 mm Hg into the low 20-mm Hg range), and adequate tidal volumes (generally $>$300–400 mL, depending on body size). If at any time the patient becomes agitated, drops oxygen saturation below the low 90-mm Hg range, experiences hypotension or arrhythmias, or has minute ventilation above 10 to 13 L/min or respiratory rate above 25 beats/min, the patient is returned to CMV for approximately 30 minutes. The CPAP trial can then again be attempted. If after 30 minutes on CPAP the patient does not meet any of the exclusionary criteria, the patient is suctioned and then extubated to a 4 L/min nasal cannula. If after extubation oxygen saturation cannot be maintained greater than 90%, higher flow nasal cannula or higher FIO_2 via a face mask can be utilized.

In practice, a significant proportion of patients can be extubated in the second or third hour. The preceding parameters are guidelines only; there are patients who are successfully extubated even if certain exclusionary criteria are met. The decision for extubation must be ultimately assessed on a patient-by-patient basis. Some patients take longer because of sleepiness, hemodynamic instability, gas exchange abnormalities, or just difficulty transitioning to an unassisted ventilatory mode. If after a few trials of this weaning technique the patient still cannot be extubated, an additional waiting period and possibly further investigation are warranted.

Patients who have compromised cardiac performance, even if compensated by the addition of vasoactive agents, should be considered for a more traditional, extended weaning process. The process of weaning from mechanical ventilation requires a transition of the energy source for the work of breathing from machine to the patient. The heart becomes responsible for supplying an adequate flow of energy, in the form of oxygenated blood, to the respiratory muscles. If either the demand is too great or the supply is insufficient, weaning places an unmanageable stress on the cardiopulmonary system. Any patient with ongoing shock, especially if cardiac performance is labile, or on high-dose vasoactive medications (dobutamine > 10 μg/kg/min, epinephrine or norepinephrine > 10 μg/min) should not be rapidly weaned. IABP placed preoperatively for angina or temporary pacing should not preclude early weaning and extubation.

Shivering

Shivering is a recognized syndrome that occurs in the early postoperative period. Its etiology is unclear. It can occur in patients who are hypothermic or already euthermic. Shivering may be related to the type of anesthetic technique or the depth and duration of hypothermia during CPB. Shivering causes profound increases in oxygen consumption and CO_2 production. It generally occurs within the first few hours postoperatively and is self-limited in duration from a few minutes to approximately 1 hour. It can be very uncomfortable and causes increased demands on the cardiopulmonary system. Increased oxygen demand must be met by increased oxygen supply, accomplished by increasing cardiac output. Increased CO_2 production must be met by increased minute ventilation usually accomplished by increased respiratory rate.

In the past, pharmacologic paralysis or narcotic to prevent unnecessary or harmful stress to the heart modulated shivering. However, shivering is actually far better tolerated and less deleterious than previously suspected. Increased CO_2 production can be managed by increased respiratory rate on the ventilator. If a patient has a particularly "hard" shiver, weaning and extubation can be delayed. Almost all patients tolerate mild shivering, and weaning and extubation can be accomplished concurrently. Patients with severely compromised cardiovascular performance, ongoing ischemia, or poor oxygenation should not be allowed to shiver.

Shivering can be stopped with paralyzing doses of vecuronium.[34] A narcotic should be added to enhance patient comfort. Convection blankets are also effective at reducing the incidence, duration, and severity of shivering and are used routinely in our CVRR. Cutaneous thermal input may help to modulate the shivering response and does not lead to excessive core temperature elevation.[35]

Chest Tube Drainage

Patients arriving from the OR always have at least one drainage catheter in the operative field. It may be a small Silastic catheter left in place following a minimally invasive approach, a single mediastinal tube following sternotomy without violation of the pleural spaces, or drainage tubes in the mediastinum and pleural spaces. With the addition of cell-saving techniques in the OR, "expected" chest tube output has been decreasing in recent years. The first 1 to 2 hours usually have the greatest chest tube output, typically less than 100 to 150 mL/hr. After this time, chest tube output should be less than 50 to 100 mL/hr for the next couple of hours before finally tapering off to less than 25 to 50 mL/hr or less. Infrequently, a chest tube "dump" (200 to 300 mL) of blood occurs when the patient is turned. Serial observation can determine whether significant bleeding is occurring.

The quality of the fluid must be scrutinized as well. Drainage of copious serous pleural fluid can fill up a drainage system and not represent mediastinal bleeding. Chest tubes should drain something. The absence of any output should alert clinicians to ensure that suction is correctly connected. If clot has accumulated in the tube, it should be gently stripped by hand. Infrequently, significant mediastinal bleeding decompresses into a pleural space. Inability to maintain filling pressures associated with a falling hematocrit and little chest tube output should be followed by a chest x-ray to eliminate this occult bleeding as a cause.

Each surgeon likely has a personal preference about stripping of chest tubes. Keeping the chest tubes patent is necessary to ensure prompt mediastinal evacuation. Inadequate drainage can allow blood to clot and possibly lead to tamponade. Gentle massage of the chest tube to break up clot and hand stripping of the rubber suction tube to promote drainage probably do not jeopardize the underlying grafts. If a chest tube becomes occluded and blood begins to seep up through the mediastinal wound or around the chest tube skin exit sites, clearing the tube using an embolectomy catheter is often successful at reestablishing drainage. This procedure must be done with a sterile technique. Chest tubes can drain significant amounts of air as well. There should be no leak in the tubing system up to the point of skin insertion. Large air leaks associated with inappropriately low exhaled tidal volumes may indicate a parenchymal air leak. Management of these types of problems is difficult, but one should start by aiming to keep airway pressures at a minimum and promoting spontaneous ventilation as soon as possible.

Leaving the Cardiovascular Recovery Room

An added benefit of all the techniques that speed up the weaning and extubation process is that the patient may be able to leave the CVRR after a brief observation period. Most patients have few postoperative problems that require an ICU type of intervention. To facilitate transfer to a less monitored environment, it is important to remove all tubes, catheters, and devices that are unnecessary. Chest tubes and pacing wires are often removed together if neither are being used. Temporary pacing wires can be easily removed with gentle traction (do not tug or jerk). Although occasionally the wire removal is met with resistance, clinicians should not use excessive force. Wires can be safely cut and allowed to retract below the skin surface, rather than risk ripping a heart chamber. Rarely does temporary wire removal lacerate a graft and lead to mediastinal bleeding.

Chest tubes can be removed after cumulative output is less than 150 mL in 6 hours. This allows chest tubes to be pulled in the early hours of the morning. The patient should be "dangled" at the bedside (sitting up with legs over the side of the bed) to drain any remaining mediastinal fluid. Pleural and mediastinal tubes can be removed simultaneously. The chest tube should be removed before the morning chest x-ray.

Occasionally, a pneumothorax develops after pleural tube removal. Pneumothoraces can generally be followed by serial chest x-rays. Large pneumothoraces may require replacement of the chest tube. Prior to transfer, arterial, pulmonary artery, and central venous catheters should be removed. The nasogastric tube can be removed if the patient has no nausea or vomiting. Actual transfer from the CVRR can occur as early as the next morning after surgery. Earlier transfers can also probably occur, but the admission readiness of the receiving unit is often not prepared in the late evening or early morning.

Facilitating Patient and Family Satisfaction

The patient can receive an excellent operation, expert postoperative care, and early transfer out of the CVRR. All of this effort will be unnoticed, however, and the physician's reputation can be harmed if the family is not involved the postoperative process. In fact, it is usually not a problem to allow select family members to see patients shortly after they have settled in. This gives the staff an opportunity to gather important information about the patient, including telephone numbers, and allows the family to express any concerns and ask questions. Early communication and visitation make for a more satisfied and confident family. Visitation time is also an opportunity to clearly delineate rules for visiting and telephoning. Good public relations will also provide rewards to the institution in the form of future business.

APPROACH TO PERSISTENT INADEQUATE CARDIOVASCULAR PERFORMANCE

Patients who require more than low-dose or transient vasoactive support in the postoperative period require a systematic approach to the definition and management of cardiovascular function. Only the minority of patients require persistent intervention to prevent frank shock. It is necessary to ensure that the maneuvers chosen for management do not make the existing situation worse. The approach to evaluation and management is nearly identical to that applied when patients have early, acute decompensation. In the acute period, temporary dysfunction can be managed with temporary fixes such as volume resuscitation or short-term vasoactive agents.

The management of persistent, inadequate performance generally requires a more finely balanced combination of volume resuscitation and inotropic support. An example of the latter would be the care of a postoperative aortic valve replacement patient who has persistent low filling pressures, low blood pressure, and high cardiac index. The acute management usually involves volume resuscitation, sometimes 1 to 2 L of crystalloid or colloid. The long-term management may instead add vasoconstricting agent, which will allow preservation of blood pressure without gross volume loading (or overloading). In the sections that follow, the use of inotropes, afterload reducing agents, and mechanical devices are discussed in more detail.

Assessment of Hypotension and Low Cardiac Output

Choosing Appropriate Target Performance

It is important to view cardiovascular performance as the relationship of three components: pressure, flow, and resistance. As an equation, $P = Q \times R$ oversimplifies the real-life relationship but nonetheless serves as the cornerstone to guiding therapy. It should be evident that a satisfactory value of one component of the equation, for example pressure, does not ensure that the remaining component values will be adequate. This is often the case when blood pressure in a patient is good but cardiac index is poor in the presence of high vascular resistance. Similarly, a low blood pressure and low vascular resistance may offset a seemingly good cardiac index. Clinicians often manipulate vascular resistance to augment cardiac index in favor of blood pressure.

Each patient has a minimum requirement for blood pressure and flow, and these values differ from patient to patient. Patients with greater oxygen delivery demands will require higher cardiac output, and those who have severe vascular disease may require higher blood pressure. Patients with "normal" metabolic requirements and absence of vascular disease (particularly absence of carotid disease) will tolerate cardiac index as low as 2 L/m/m^2 and MAP as low as 65 mm Hg. Patients with carotid disease should have higher MAP, probably in excess of 85 mm Hg, to prevent stroke. Patients without carotid disease, with "normally" low systolic blood pressure, may in fact tolerate systolic pressure in the 80-mm Hg range, at least in the early postoperative period. Patients with higher than usual oxygen demands, such as patients with fever or increased work of breathing, may need cardiac index in excess of 2.5 L/m/m^2. MAPs are quoted as guidelines. Target blood pressure can also aim for systolic blood pressure rather than MAP.

Appreciating Left and Right Ventricular Performance and Valvular Competence

Patients presenting for cardiovascular surgery can have global or regional wall-motion abnormalities in addition to other problems such as valvular dysfunction. Cardiomyopathy commonly causes global wall-motion abnormalities; it can also cause local pathology, such as in idiopathic hypertrophic subaortic stenosis. Hypertensive cardiomyopathy causes concentric thickening of the left ventricle, with loss of compliance. Ischemic cardiomyopathy, however, causes chamber dilation, with an increase in ventricular compliance.

Patients with infarctions in the distribution of the left anterior descending or circumflex artery (anterior or lateral myocardial infarctions) generally demonstrate left ventricular dysfunction. Infarctions in the distribution of the right coronary artery (inferior, posterior, and right ventricular wall infarctions) may demonstrate left and right ventricular dysfunction. Because of the variability of origin of the posterior descending artery and presence of collateral circulation, dysfunction of the posterior wall and apex can occur as a result of disease in either the right or the left circulation. Infarction can also cause rupture of the septum or free walls. Infarction often causes papillary muscle dysfunction or frank rupture, especially the posterior papillary muscle, leading to acute mitral regurgitation. *To logically treat the failing heart, it is necessary to identify, if possible, particular regions of the heart that are dysfunctional so that therapy can be targeted.*

Left ventricular failure is the easiest to recognize. It is usually associated with elevation in pulmonary artery occlusion pressures (or PCWP), low cardiac index, low stroke volume, and systemic hypotension. It must be distinguished from other causes of elevation in PCWP such as mitral regurgitation or low wall compliance with left ventricular hypertrophy (LVH) (see later in chapter). Severe left ventricular failure may also be associated with pulmonary edema seen on chest x-ray. Isolated right ventricular failure often shows low cardiac output and systemic blood pressure and elevated CVP and right ventricular pressure. True elevated CVP with right ventricular failure must be distinguished from severe tricuspid insufficiency. Pulmonary artery pressures are often elevated but may not be if the right ventricle, usually a much thinner structure than the left ventricle, is unable to generate such a force. PCWP may be astonishingly normal in the presence of such poor cardiac performance. In the presence of biventricular failure, cardiac output, stroke volume, and systemic pressures are low and filling pressures (CVP, PAD, and PCWP) are typically high. Tamponade should always be considered in the presence of elevations of left-sided and right-sided filling pressures.

Acute valvular incompetence can severely inhibit cardiac performance. Acute mitral valve regurgitation caused by chamber or annulus dilation, papillary muscle ischemia (especially the posterior papillary muscle), papillary muscle rupture, or ruptured chordae can result in acute failure. It can be recognized by a loud systolic murmur in the typical distribution of the mitral valve, large V waves on the PCWP tracing, pulmonary hypertension, pulmonary edema, low systemic blood pressure, and low cardiac output. It is often difficult to float the PAC into a "wedge" position. Similarly, acute tricuspid regurgitation demonstrates high CVP with V waves on tracing, low systemic blood pressure, and low cardiac output. Pulmonary artery pressure and PCWP may remain normal with isolated tricuspid regurgitation. Tricuspid regurgitation is often seen associated with right-sided endocarditis and can be exacerbated by the presence of a PAC distorting the shape and position of the valve's leaflets or by grossly elevated right ventricular pressures. Severe acute aortic valve incompetence is infrequent in the postoperative period unless its presence was unrecognized or underestimated preoperatively. In the absence of pulmonary artery hypertension, incompetence of the pulmonic valve rarely presents a clinical problem. Infrequently, acute valvular "competence," such as occurs with mitral valve repair and replacement, can result in acute ventricular decompensation. Prior to the repair of the mitral valve, the left ventricle can unload into a relatively low-pressure reservoir, the left atrium. After valve repair and replacement, the low-pressure reservoir is absent. If the left ventricle cannot accommodate the new pressure load, it will fail.

Sometimes it is impossible to specifically define which components are conspiring to limit cardiac performance, especially when there is more than one dysfunctional component. Diagnostic imaging, particularly surface echocardiography and transesophageal echocardiography, can be helpful in better defining wall function and valvular function, the presence of pericardial collections, inadequate chamber filling, and also unsuspected anomalies, such as atrial and ventricular septal defects. For these studies to be useful, a portable machine, accessible 24 hours a day with very short notice, and a person trained to read the results need to be available. A surface echocardiogram is usually performed first. It has satisfactory sensitivity and specificity to eliminate major mechanical problems such as pericardial tamponade and usually can give a satisfactory view of wall motion. If the study is technically inadequate or if doubt still exists, transesophageal echocardiography can follow.

Treatment of Inadequate Cardiac Performance

As previously discussed, the fundamentals of optimizing cardiovascular performance include the assessment and treatment of rhythm and rate, adequacy of volume resuscitation, need for inotropic support, presence of mediastinal bleeding and possible tamponade, evidence of electrical abnormalities, and need for mechanical support.

Rhythm Disturbances

Conduction and rhythm disturbances are seen regularly in the postoperative period. Their natural history is dependent on a number of factors, including the presence of preoperative conduction disturbances, effects of cardioplegia, and quality of myocardial protection. All varieties of blocks can be seen postoperatively, including AV nodal blockade and fascicular block (RBBB, LBBB, and left anterior hemiblock). If these conduction abnormalities are new postoperatively, they almost always resolve within the first 24 hours. The new presence of a new BBB (right or left) is not an ominous sign of ischemia.

Evaluation and Management of Bradycardia

Bradycardia is common postoperatively and is due to sinus bradycardia, slow dominant junctional rhythms, atrial fibrillation and flutter with slow ventricular rate, or high-grade AV block. Some bradycardias reflect preoperative conditioning or medication (especially β-blockade or digoxin). Most bradycardias are transient and resolve within 24 to 72 hours postoperatively. This is also the case with postoperative high-grade AV blockade (2° and 3°). Therapy for bradycardia depends on its impact on cardiovascular performance. Electrical pacing is almost always preferred over agents such as atropine or isoproterenol. Atropine may take too long to take effect (30 seconds to 1 minute) and the clinician has no control over any resulting tachycardia. Isoproterenol will increase the sinus rate but takes too long to mix as a drip in an emergency situation, requires a dosing pump, and is not useful for AV blockade. Fortunately, virtually all postoperative cardiovascular surgery patients have temporary epicardial pacing wires placed prior to closure of the chest. Typically, atrial leads exit the right side of the chest and ventricular leads exit the left side of the chest. One or two ground wires should be available to complete the electrical connections.

Bradycardia, in the absence of hypotension or low cardiac output, requires no intervention. For bradycardiac patients who are otherwise stable, their temporary pacing wires should be attached to a pulse generator set for demand pacing. A good initial demand rate is 60 beats/min. Patients may have quite satisfactory performance at low (<60 beats/min) heart rates, in which case the demand rate should be lowered accordingly. Atrial pacing is always preferred to ventricular pacing when AV blockade is absent because it leverages the normal sequence of chamber contraction and the conduction system. In the presence of AV block, AV sequential pacing is preferred to ventricular pacing alone, also because of the preservation of sequence of chamber contraction. Ventricular pacing should be utilized in the decompensating, bradycardiac patient without other means of pacing. When pacing wires fail and the patient remains decompensated and bradycardiac, emergency pharmacologic therapy, such as 0.5 to 1 mg atropine or 1 to 5 μg/min isoproterenol, should be utilized. If external (surface) pacing technology is available, it should be attempted.

Persistent bradycardia with shock, refractory to the preceding interventions, requires placement of an additional internal pacing device. This can be done with a traditional temporary pacing wire placed through the right internal jugular vein or by placing a specially designed pacing wire through a pace-port PAC. Pace-port catheters are extremely convenient therapeutic devices when such a situation occurs and the catheter is already in place; they are extremely difficult to place when the patient is already in shock. Pacing should be continued until bradycardia, regardless of the cause, resolves or when the intrinsic rhythm begins to compete with the pulse generator. It is appropriate to turn off the pacer every 4 to 6 hours to see whether an acceptable intrinsic rhythm has returned. When the pacer has been turned off, sometimes it takes a few minutes for the rate to pick up. (Obviously, there is no need to wait if the underlying rhythm is asystole or high-grade block with low ventricular response.) If after 72 hours bradycardia or AV block has not resolved, placement of a permanent internal pacing device should be considered.

Nonventricular Arrhythmias

Nonventricular tachycardia in the postoperative period is typically sinus or junctional. Sinus tachycardia may be due to pain, sympathetic activity, loss of preestablished β-blockade (such as preoperative β-blockade), vasoactive medications (epinephrine, dobutamine), and hypovolemia. Rates range from 100 to 150 beats per minute. Rates above this may be sinus in origin, but other diagnoses should also be entertained. Junctional tachycardia is usually slower, with a maximum rate of about 120 beats/min.

Premature atrial contractions are also common, and their abrupt onset often heralds the development of atrial fibrillation. Less frequently but more of a therapeutic problem is sustained atrial fibrillation or flutter or AV nodal reentry. Diagnosis of these rhythms is typically done by evaluation of the monitoring strip. If necessary, a 12-lead ECG should be used for confirmation. If an atrial pacing wire is available, a 12-lead ECG with V_1 attached to the atrial lead provides a powerful technique for confirming the etiology of a supraventricular tachycardia. Large P waves preceding the QRS complex in a 1:1 relationship suggest a sinus or atrial ectopic source of the rhythm. Atrial flutter shows large P waves at a rate of about 300 per minute. There is a variable relationship to the QRS complex (but typically 2:1 or 3:1, hopefully not 1:1). Atrial fibrillation shows absence of organized atrial activity and an irregular ventricular rate. If an atrial wire is unavailable, an esophageal lead, to pick up atrial activity, can be just as useful for confirming the diagnosis. When the etiology of a supraventricular rhythm is still unclear, adenosine can temporarily block the AV node to reveal flutter waves or atrial fibrillation or to terminate an AV nodal reentry rhythm.

The treatment of nonventricular tachycardia begins with recognizing hemodynamic compromise. Rapid ventricular rate reduces chamber-filling times and results in lower stroke volumes, blood pressure, and cardiac output. Tachycardia also significantly increases myocardial oxygen consumption and in the incompletely revascularized heart can precipitate ECG changes consistent with ischemia or injury. In the otherwise well-functioning early postoperative heart, it is somewhat common to see sinus rates climb into the 120 range for up to 1 or 2 hours before slowing. This rate is well tolerated and requires no intervention other than to exclude pain or hypovolemia as a cause. A 250- to 500-mL challenge with saline is usually sufficient to test for a therapeutic response. It is much less common to have sustained sinus rates in excess of 130. Again, in the presence of otherwise acceptable cardiovascular function, treatment other than analgesia or volume resuscitation is usually not needed. It is our practice not to slow otherwise stable, self-limited sinus and junctional tachycardias with agents such as calcium or β-blockers because this can change an otherwise stable situation into an unstable one.

Any rapid tachycardia originating at or above the AV node that causes hypotension requires immediate termination with synchronized DC cardioversion. This usually implies the presence of atrial fibrillation, flutter, or AV nodal reentry. Synchronized cardioversion is usually successful in restoring a sinus rhythm, but refractory non-sinus rhythms do occur. These situations are very challenging, especially in the presence of marginal cardiac performance. Definitive therapy includes control of ventricular rate and often the chemical conversion to sinus rhythm. Therapy usually involves rapid correction of electrolyte abnormalities (typically potassium and magnesium) and administration of digoxin, diltiazem, or esmolol. The latter two agents often lower blood pressure even further. AV blocking agents, such as digoxin and calcium channel blockers, should be avoided during wide complex tachyarrhythmias in the presence of known accessory conduction pathways because of the risk of potentiating the conduction down the accessory bundle. Addition of antiarrhythmic agents, typically procainamide, but more recently amiodarone, usually follows in an attempt to convert to sinus rhythm. DC cardioversion can be repeated after appropriate loading of antiarrhythmics if necessary.

The treatment of sustained, hemodynamically stable atrial fibrillation or flutter is somewhat controversial. These de novo rhythms are common and are usually self-limited, with restoration of sinus rhythm in the majority of patients by 6 weeks postoperatively. The controversy surrounds treating a well-tolerated arrhythmia with rate-controlling agents (digoxin, β-blockers, or calcium channel blockers) plus anticoagulants (warfarin to prevent atrial clot and subsequent cerebrovascular accident) versus arrhythmia control with potentially proarrhythmic drugs (procainamide). Substantial clinical data exist to support either choice. We feel that there is usually a measurable improvement in cardiac performance in sinus rhythm, often necessary in patients with impaired left ventricular function, with little increase in ventricular arrhythmia. This benefit outweighs the risks of possible cerebrovascular accident and bleeding if rate control and anticoagulation are chosen.

A reliable approach to atrial fibrillation and flutter aims to treat both ventricular response and the abnormal rhythm. Patients who have been in these arrhythmias for 48 hours or less are candidates. Patients who have chronic atrial fibrillation or flutter or de novo fibrillation or flutter for more than 48 hours should receive anticoagulation therapy with heparin and warfarin for at least 2 weeks prior to attempted cardioversion. Weight-based heparinization works well at maintaining adequate anticoagulation, while warfarin, started simultaneously, slowly raises the international normalized ratio (INR) to an acceptable level.

In patients with either atrial fibrillation or flutter, AV blockade can be achieved with IV diltiazem, titrated to a ventricular rate of 90 to 120 beats/min. Diltiazem works much more rapidly than digoxin, but both drugs, given enough time (usually a few hours for digoxin), will achieve acceptable AV blockade. Following shortly thereafter, if not simultaneously, procainamide can be loaded in the usual fashion (typically 0.75–1.25 g IV) followed by a continuous infusion of 2 mg/minute. If this fails to convert, an additional small bolus of the drug (up to 0.5 g) can be given with an increase of the continuous drip rate. If conversion still has not occurred, the dose of procainamide should be optimized based on measured serum levels of procainamide and *N*-acetylprocainamide (NAPA). A trial of DC cardioversion after optimized loading of procainamide can be done in patients with persistent atrial fibrillation. After conversion, IV procainamide can be converted to the appropriate oral form.

Quinidine preparations are avoided in our patients because there is no readily available IV form and they therefore must be given intramuscularly or orally. The oral form is notorious for causing diarrhea, an intolerable situation for a bedridden patient in an ICU. Quinidine preparations can be used in patients with renal insufficiency because procainamide in this patient population is extremely difficult to dose.

In patients with renal failure, we have recently had good experiences using amiodarone for rate control and conversion of atrial fibrillation or flutter. If after repeated trials of cardioversion, pharmacologic or electrical, the patient remains in atrial fibrillation or flutter, the therapeutic strategy changes to that of ventricular rate control and anticoagulation. As previously mentioned, weight-based heparinization works well at maintaining adequate anticoagulation while warfarin, started simultaneously, slowly raises the INR to an acceptable level.

Ventricular tachyarrhythmias are common not only in patients with coronary artery disease but also in postoperative cardiovascular surgery patients. It is far more common to see these tachyarrhythmias in patients with preexisting ventricular arrhythmias than in those without. However, the presence of myocardial ischemia or infarction can cause ventricular arrhythmias even when not present preoperatively. New myocardial ischemia due to failed revascularization, electrolyte abnormalities (particularly hypokalemia and hypomagnesemia), and the proarrhythmic effect of antiarrhythmic agents can all conspire to produce new ventricular irritability. The most common ventricular arrhythmia is the PVC. PVCs can be unifocal, multifocal, or isolated or occur in a somewhat fixed ratio of normal and abnormal beats (bigeminal or trigeminal). Ventricular arrhythmias can also occur in groups such as couplets, triplets, and nonsustained salvos of four beats or more or as a sustained VT. VT can also degenerate into ventricular fibrillation (VF). Infrequently, VF can develop spontaneously.

The urgency to treat ventricular arrhythmias depends on the severity of hemodynamic compromise. Isolated PVCs, bigeminy or trigeminy, and even infrequent couplets that do not cause a worsening in cardiovascular performance require no further treatment other than correction of hypokalemia or hypomagnesemia. Often 2 to 4 g of additional magnesium sulfate, even when the serum magnesium level is normal, can suppress these arrhythmias. If these arrhythmias need to be suppressed, such as if they result in poor cardiovascular performance or are occurring following a more sustained ventricular arrhythmia, IV lidocaine generally allows for a regular rhythm to be reestablished. Rarely, lidocaine itself is unsuccessful, in which case procainamide is an acceptable alternative. In the event of cardiovascular collapse, cardiopulmonary resuscitation (CPR) should be started immediately. DC cardioversion usually terminates the rhythm; however, VF or even asystole may follow if rapid conversion does not occur.

To say the least, performing CPR on a newly postoperative cardiac surgery patient is an unnerving experience. For adequate chest compressions, a rigid board must be placed behind the patient while standard manual compressions are administered. Volume resuscitation, inotropic support, electronic pacing, and manual ventilation must continue during attempts to restore a life-sustaining rhythm and pressure. In the presence of refractory VF or asystole, it is important to emergently reopen the chest to directly cardiovert and provide direct cardiac compressions. This is admittedly a last-ditch effort, however, to have a successful outcome (especially neurologically), restoration of adequate circulation must occur early, and reopening the chest may be the only therapeutic option. Many successful resuscitations occur this way. It is also possible to rapidly place a patient back on CPB so that stability can be restored while grafts and targets are reassessed.

Optimization of Filling Pressures

For the ventricles to perform optimally, they require an end diastolic volume that is neither too low nor too high. Underfilled ventricles lead to low stroke volume as a result of inadequate sarcomere stretch. Stroke volume continues to improve as end-diastolic volume increases up to a certain point, beyond which stroke volume does not increase and may in fact decrease. Further increases in end-diastolic volume only lead to elevated filling pressures, with subsequent congestion of right-sided or left-sided venous systems. Overdistention of the ventricles also increases the wall tension within the myocardium and can reduce diastolic blood flow, potentially increasing myocardial ischemia. The clinician's best estimation of end-diastolic volume is still the PCWP for left ventricular filling and the CVP for right-sided filling. Of course, the relationship of these pressures to the actual distending volume is a function of the ventricular compliance. As previously mentioned (see Management of Early Postoperative Cardiac Dysfunction), the optimal CVP and PCWP in the presence of normal myocardial compliance are 8 to 10 mm Hg and 14 to 16 mm Hg, respectively.

In the presence of low compliance, as in left ventricular hypertrophy, "normal" filling pressures may represent low end-diastolic filling and somewhat higher pressures may be necessary to establish adequate end-diastolic volumes. In patients with high compliance, such as a dilated cardiomyopathy, "normal" filling pressures may represent higher than normal end-diastolic filling but even higher filling pressures may be necessary to optimize stroke volume. Because of the variable nature of ventricular compliance, absolute filling pressures should not be used as guarantees of adequate ventricular filling. Rather, the trends in the filling pressures and the response of the ventricle to volume challenges should guide the clinician as to the adequacy of volume resuscitation.

Aliquots of 250 to 500 mL of saline or hetastarch given over 15 to 30 minutes are usually satisfactory volume challenges. It is a good practice to observe changes in filling pressures (especially CVP and PAD) during the volume challenge to avoid gross overload. Except in the case of right or left ventricular failure or tamponade, CVPs should not be pushed higher than 14 to 16 mm Hg and PCWP should not exceed 18 to 22 mm Hg during volume challenges.

In the case of ventricular dysfunction, filling pressures may in fact need to be pushed higher to optimize performance. After each volume challenge, the cardiac output should be reassessed. When cardiac output becomes adequate or fails to improve after volume challenge in a patient with elevated filling pressures, it is probably time to stop volume resuscitation.

The type of resuscitation fluid selected is relatively important. It is not unusual for a patient to receive 500 to 1000 mL of resuscitation fluids in the first few postoperative hours to maintain adequate cardiovascular performance. Usually, normal saline, lactated Ringer's solution, or hetastarch are the resuscitation fluids of choice. However, if a postoperative patient presents with a hematocrit in the mid or low 20s or has significant chest tube bleeding, 1500 mL of crystalloid or hetastarch resuscitation can dramatically reduce the hematocrit and therefore the oxygen-carrying capacity of the blood. It may, in fact, be necessary to provide a more balanced intravascular resuscitation that includes not only acellular fluids but also PRBCs if needed. There is no absolute hematocrit below which transfusion is necessary. This should be based on the balance between the delivery and utilization of oxygen. A patient with robust cardiac performance may tolerate a lower hematocrit than a patient with poor cardiac performance because of the former's ability to increase O_2 delivery by increasing cardiac output. In practice, a patient with a hematocrit in the low 20s, low filling pressures, and inadequate cardiovascular performance often dramatically benefits from a transfusion of 2 units of PRBCs. In addition, any resuscitation fluid short of PRBCs has a limited time that it remains in the intravascular space before leaking into the interstitium. Only 25% to 33% of saline remains in the intravascular space at the end of 1 hour. It is important to remember these characteristics of resuscitation fluids so that each can be used judiciously.

Inotropic Support

If after establishment of acceptable rhythm and adequate filling pressures cardiovascular performance is still below the desired goal, it is necessary to add inotropic support. Available agents should be selected based upon the drug's ability to affect chronotropy, inotropy, and vascular tone. These effects are mediated through direct or indirect stimulation of α, β_1 and β_2 receptors and the concentration of intracellular cyclic adenosine monophosphate (cAMP). Some of the drugs share activity with one or more receptors. Particular drug characteristics can therefore be leveraged to achieve specific cardiovascular responses.

Three *naturally occurring catecholamines* can be used pharmacologically:

- Epinephrine
- Norepinephrine
- Dopamine

These drugs must be given through a continuous IV infusion via a centrally located catheter. Extravasation of these powerful vasoconstricting agents into the skin can cause severe necrosis and sloughing of tissue. All of these agents have very short half-lives, measured in minutes.

Epinephrine is an agonist of α_1, β_1, and β_2 receptors. In clinical use, it provides a powerful chronotropic inotropic, and vasoconstricting effect. Although it is possible to see different physiologic effects as a result of dose-dependent receptor activation, it most commonly raises heart rate, blood pressure, and cardiac output as the dose is increased. Epinephrine is an excellent first-line choice to improve both blood pressure and cardiac output in the adequately volume resuscitated patient. It is also particularly useful to improve contractility in the presence of right heart failure. Because the right ventricle is frequently incompletely revascularized, right ventricular perfusion, and hence function, becomes pressor dependent. However, this drug has many side effects; it has been shown to cause hyperglycemia, tachycardia (and subsequent increased myocardial oxygen consumption), and reduced splanchnic and renal blood flow, potentiate tachyarrhythmias, and induce lactic acidosis. The lactic acidosis is due to both vasoconstriction and a change in metabolic pathways, resulting in a reduction in activity of pyruvate dehydrogenase.

Norepinephrine has many similar properties to epinephrine. It is an agonist of both α_1 and β_1 receptors. However, its hemodynamic effects are far more in favor of vasoconstriction than increased inotropy or chronotropy. It is an excellent choice when a patient with vasodilation, adequate cardiac output, and hypotension could benefit from a drug that predominately raises systemic vascular resistance (SVR). This effect, however, can cause unwanted consequences in patients with marginal cardiac output. In the latter situation, modest increases in afterload (SVR) can result in an increase in blood pressure and a simultaneous decrease in cardiac output. Norepinephrine should not be used in hypovolemic patients because of the risk of potentiating regional ischemia.

Dopamine is pharmacologically more like epinephrine in effect than norepinephrine. At very low doses, up to 2 μg/kg/min, the drug causes vasodilation of the renal and splanchnic blood vessels. This may result in increases in glomerular filtration rate and subsequent urine output. However, although controversial, low-dose dopamine does not provide either a protective or therapeutic effect in the face of acute renal failure. At higher doses, dopamine is also an excellent first-line drug to increase both blood pressure and cardiac output because of its activation of α_1 and β receptors.

Two *synthetic catecholamines* are used in clinical practice, dobutamine and isoproterenol. *Dobutamine* possesses both β_1 and β_2 properties. In a dose-dependent fashion, dobutamine causes increased heart rate, inotropy, and cardiac output and both pulmonary and systemic vasodilation. It is most commonly used in patients with low cardiac output and adequate blood pressure. It can cause systemic hypotension which can infrequently limit its use. Dobutamine is an excellent all-around inotrope in the face of poor cardiac performance.

Isoproterenol, although it is also a β_1 and β_2 agonist, is much more of a chronotrope than other catecholamines. It is useful to raise heart rate (and subsequently cardiac output) in bradycardiac patients, particularly post–heart transplant patients. It also has powerful vasodilatory properties and can be useful to lower pulmonary artery pressures. Isoproterenol can also be used as a potent inotropic agent but, because of its chronotropic and proarrhythmic effect, is used much less frequently than dobutamine.

Another class of inotropic agents functions without stimulation of *β-receptors.* Rather, these agents, phosphodiesterase inhibitors, increase intracellular cAMP, which in turn results in increased inotropic state and peripheral vasodilation. Amrinone and milrinone are the most popular of these agents. Both are given by continuous IV infusion and differ from the natural and synthetic catecholamines by having very long half-lives, measured in hours rather than minutes. The chief complications of these drugs are thrombocytopenia (greater for amrinone) and hypotension. These drugs are, however, excellent inotropic agents and can be used as first-line agents as long as the blood pressure tolerates it.

The selection of inotropic agents varies based on clinical need and clinician experience and preference. Agents that are commonly used in the OR such as phenylephrine and ephedrine have little utility in the ICU. Medications should be selected to be used alone or in combination with other vasoactive agents to achieve the desired hemodynamic effect. These medications may have been present preoperatively, may have been started in the operating room, or may need to be started new in the CVRR. Inotropic agents should be started only after appropriate control of rhythm and filling pressures have been achieved, unless life-threatening hemodynamic instability occurs or threatens. In a patient with poor ventricular function but adequate blood pressure, dobutamine is an excellent choice because of its safety profile and titratability. Phosphodiesterase inhibitors are also good choices but lack the short half-life that would allow them to be truly titratable drugs.

When hypotension and poor cardiac output are the problem, epinephrine or dopamine is an appropriate first-line choice. In patients with predominate vasodilation, hypotension, and good cardiac output, norepinephrine is an acceptable choice, although epinephrine or dopamine can be used successfully in these situations as well. Combinations of drugs can be used to provide the desired effect. Dobutamine and epinephrine or norepinephrine work well in combination. When this approach is taken, it is usually less confusing if the titration of the individual drugs is assigned to a particular hemodynamic parameter. For example, when epinephrine and dobutamine are used in combination, dobutamine should be titrated to a desired cardiac output while epinephrine is titrated for a desired blood pressure. This technique works as long as any given hemodynamic effect is not dependent on two pharmacologic agents (i.e., the cardiac output may in fact require both dobutamine and epinephrine for support).

Most patients require little more than volume resuscitation in the early postoperative period. Those who have otherwise good cardiovascular performance but are sluggish when coming off CPB may require low to moderate doses of vasoactive agents for the first 12 to 24 hours postoperatively. There are, however, those patients with poor ventricular function or in frank cardiogenic shock who require extended pharmacologic support for days or even weeks. These patients are the most challenging to manage and require careful drug titration while waiting for cardiovascular performance to improve. There are few rules to guide the tempo with which inotropic support is weaned.

A few guidelines may be helpful.

1. Pick a hemodynamic target appropriate for the patient and manipulate rate, rhythm, filling pressures, and inotropic support until that goal is reached. The greater the doses of vasoactive agents, the more likely the cardiovascular system is impaired and has reduced reserve (except with pure vasodilation, in which high doses of norepinephrine may be needed to maintain blood pressure in the presence of otherwise good cardiac performance). A more difficult path to acceptable performance should be a warning flag to delay inotrope weaning until cardiovascular function has demonstrated stability.
2. Delay weaning support until the patient is warm and any metabolic acidosis has cleared (unless the clinician feels that the acidosis is potentiated by use of epinephrine).
3. Delay weaning of mechanical ventilation in patients receiving anything greater than moderate inotropic support.

Afterload Reduction

Lowering of systemic vascular resistance (afterload reduction) is a technique that can be used in both the early and late postoperative period to augment cardiac output. It leverages the relationship between flow, pressure, and resistance but admittedly exchanges an improvement in one hemodynamic parameter for another. If the inotropic state of the heart remains constant, vasodilation can allow an increase in cardiac output and a fall in blood pressure. Usually, the gain in forward flow is more beneficial than the decrement in blood pressure. These techniques can be used in any patient with a cardiac index below the desired target as long as the patient has an MAP or a systolic blood pressure (SBP) above a value the clinician feels is a minimally acceptable pressure. Minimally acceptable pressures are MAPs in the 70s or SBPs above 95 to 100 mm Hg. These values may need to be higher in the presence of carotid or other vascular insufficiency.

In general, afterload reduction is started when the cardiac index is below 2 L/m/m^2 and the blood pressure is adequate, as previously described. Afterload reduction can (and often should) be started while the patient is on inotropic support, unless the patient requires moderate to high-dose support to maintain blood pressure.

Vasodilation is often useful when inotropes, such as epinephrine, raise blood pressure more than they raise cardiac output. The choice of vasodilating agent depends on the required duration of action and the available route for administration. An acutely ill, intubated patient on moderate (or higher) doses of inotropic support, who despite a very good blood pressure has an inadequate cardiac index, is a good candidate for afterload reduction with nitroprusside or nitroglycerin. In this instance, the IV vasodilating agent is titrated to bring the MAP into the 70s (or the SBP toward 100 mm Hg). When the target blood pressure is achieved, it is necessary to repeat the cardiac output. If the cardiac output is still below the desired target and there is no further indication for volume resuscitation or further afterload reduction, the patient requires additional inotropic support.

If the patient is extubated and is on low to moderate doses of inotropes but cannot be weaned any further because of inadequate cardiac index, oral vasodilating agents, such as captopril, are appropriate choices. Low-dose captopril (6.25 mg) is a good starting dose and usually raises cardiac index satisfactorily without unacceptable hypotension. It may take a few doses of oral vasodilating agent before the desired effect occurs. Care must be taken when using captopril in patients with increased creatinine or known renal artery stenosis. IV hydralazine can lower the blood pressure into the desired range until oral agents become effective.

Supplemental Mechanical Assist Devices

If cardiovascular performance remains unacceptable despite the optimization of rate, rhythm, filling pressures, and inotropic support, it becomes necessary to supplement the cardiovascular system with a mechanical assist device. The two major categories of assist devices are (1) balloon counterpulsation and (2) a surgically placed VAD.

Intra-aortic Balloon Counterpulsation

The intra-aortic balloon pump (IABP) is a mechanical device whose components resemble a sausage-shaped balloon secured through its long axis with a multilumen catheter. The device is inserted most commonly via a percutaneous technique into the femoral artery and advanced until the tip of the balloon lies distal to the left subclavian artery, radiographically in the aortopulmonary window. The IABP can be placed into the ascending aorta while in the OR if severe peripheral vascular disease precludes such an approach. The IABP is connected to a controlling console that monitors the intrinsic heart rate and blood pressure and uses this information to correctly time inflation and deflation of the IABP. The console uses helium (because of its low molecular weight and hence improved flow characteristics) to inflate and deflate the balloon. The console is also equipped with alarms to detect gas leakage or occlusion of the balloon.

The function of the IABP is quite simple. When timed correctly, the balloon inflates just after closure of the aortic valve, thereby increasing diastolic blood pressure and coronary blood flow. Deflation of the balloon occurs just prior to ventricular ejection and results in a fall in the aortic blood pressure, or afterload reduction, thereby facilitating the forward flow of blood. General timing is synchronized to the ECG tracing or arterial waveform from the tip of the IABP. However, manual optimization of inflation and deflation times is necessary to optimize afterload reduction and diastolic pressure augmentation. The balloon pump can fire with every, every other, or every third beat. Full support occurs when the IABP fires in a 1:1 relationship to the intrinsic rhythm. However, tachycardia (especially atrial fibrillation) can limit the ability of the IABP to remain properly synchronized. In this circumstance, it become's necessary to fire at a somewhat slower ratio of 1:2. The lower the inflation ratio the greater the chance of development of thrombus on the balloon. Systemic anticoagulation is generally not necessary when the pump fires at 1:1. If the pump is to remain at 1:3 for any extended period of time, however, heparinization should be considered to prevent distal embolization of clot.

The IABP is indicated for enhancement of cardiovascular performance refractory to the previously mentioned maneuvers, refractory angina, and optimization of afterload reduction in the presence of mitral insufficiency. Contraindications to placement include incompetence of the aortic valve, aortic dissection, and severe vascular disease at the insertion site.

Once the device has been placed, it is necessary to confirm proper placement radiographically. Balloon tips placed too high can completely or partially occlude the left subclavian or carotid artery, and balloon tips placed too low can occlude the splanchnic and renal vessels. It is also necessary to ensure that blood flow distal to the insertion point is present after completion of the procedure. This involves assessing for pulsatile arterial blood flow, either manually or by Doppler, over the popliteal, posterior tibial, and dorsalis pedis arteries. Absence of pulses associated with a cool mottled extremity requires immediate removal of the device and possible embolectomy (or other vascular repair) if acceptable perfusion does not return. Restoration of blood flow is urgent; otherwise, irreparable neurologic or muscular injury (perhaps requiring amputation) could result. The absence of an isolated dorsalis pedis or posterior tibial pulse is not necessarily reason for immediate concern if the remaining pulses are accounted for and the extremity is warm and clinically well perfused. Other complications related to the IABP include local vessel damage, bleeding with local or retroperitoneal hematoma, and clot or gas embolization.

Like other means of cardiovascular support, the IABP needs to be adjusted to perform optimally and weaned when it is no longer needed. Balloon pumps placed preoperatively for angina, "critical lesions," or catheterization misadventures can usually be weaned and removed within the first 12 to 18 hours postoperatively if the patient has adequate performance. IABPs placed for acute infarction or cardiogenic shock may need to remain in place for many days prior to attempting removal. It is a good practice to wean inotropes to moderate doses prior to removing the IABP so that in the event the cardiac performance swoons there is ample "room" available to increase dosages of vasoactive agents. Weaning of the IABP should begin with reducing the firing ratio from 1:1 to 1:2. The cardiac index can be checked shortly thereafter, and if adequate, the IABP can then be reduced again to 1:3. If the cardiac performance remains acceptable, the IABP can be removed. Some clinicians do not lower the ratio below 1:2 and will remove the IABP from this ratio if the cardiovascular performance is acceptable.

It is necessary to make sure that neither coagulopathy nor thrombocytopenia is present prior to removal. Optimally, the platelet count should be greater than 100,000, but lower counts may be tolerated if extended arterial compression is provided after removal. Balloon pumps that are placed percutaneously can usually be removed at the bedside. IABPs inserted through the thoracic aorta and those placed under direct visualization and arteriotomy need to be removed in the OR.

After removal of the IABP, the patient needs to remain supine with a compression device over the puncture site for 4 to 6 hours. Patients can be extubated while still receiving counterpulsation therapy as long as adequate cardiac reserve remains. The patient needs to remain supine, making airway management somewhat more challenging.

Ventricular Assist Device

Should hemodynamic stability fail to be achieved with the use of inotropic support and an IABP, invasive VADs can be used if appropriate therapeutic endpoints can be defined prior to placement. Cardiogenic shock may or may not be expected to improve depending on the etiology. Cardiogenic shock as a result of acute ischemia or infarct may eventually improve given enough time and support. Other causes of shock may be completely irreversible. VADs should be considered on a case-by-case basis because they can be utilized as a temporary treatment modality, as a "bridge" to eventual transplant, or in certain cases as permanent devices. Current technology in VADs is improving rapidly. Temporary devices that can support either or both ventricles (such as the Abiomed) or permanent left ventricular devices (such as the TCI HeartMate) are available; the problems of thromboembolism and infection, however, still remain.

ORGAN SYSTEM FUNCTION AFTER CARDIAC SURGERY

Neuropsychologic System

Cardiac surgery patients are at risk for neurologic complications not only in the preoperative period as a result of their cardiovascular disease but also because of the protean effects of CPB. Neurologic complications can range from subtle cognitive problems and personality changes to more significant cerebrovascular accidents. Fortunately, catastrophic, fatal intracerebral hemorrhage is infrequent, occurring in less than 0.1%; focal events such as motor or sensory deficits occur in approximately 1% to 3%; and minor clinical abnormalities occur in 5% to 10%.[36] In some patients, the neurologic deficit is manifest as severe agitation or disorientation. Focal neurologic deficits are generally easy to recognize on careful neurologic examination.

Confirmatory findings can often be found on computed tomography (CT) scan of the brain a few days after the recognition of the event. CT scans done *immediately* after the neurologic event frequently fail to demonstrate subtle areas of abnormality. This is due to insufficient passage of time to allow for changes in tissue density. Large cardiovascular accidents may be recognizable on CT even when performed early. Cognitive and personality changes are much more difficult to diagnose, especially when they are subtle, and may require sophisticated neuropsychologic testing for confirmation. Unfortunately, these tests rarely have preoperative baselines for comparison.

There are various risk factors and causes of postoperative neurologic complications. Preexisting cardiovascular disease, especially disease of the aorta and carotids, and advanced age significantly increase the risk. Surprisingly, valvular surgery does not carry a greater risk than coronary surgery.[36] The most likely etiologic mechanisms include (1) microemboli related to CPB, (2) systemic inflammation due to CPB, and (3) relative hypoperfusion. Hypoperfusion is difficult to define at the microvascular level. There are few data to define a critically low level of perfusion. Possibly, with the use of continuous EEG monitoring or near infrared spectroscopy, the clinician might be aware of possible neurologic compromise.

Microemboli have been demonstrated histologically in capillaries of brain section and can be visualized in retinal vessels on careful fundoscopic exam. Microemboli (atheroma, clot) mostly originate from the aorta, the carotid, and from the CPB device. Open cardiac procedures and the oxygenator itself present the risk of air embolization. Intracardiac debris (clot, calcium) and air can embolize if not carefully evacuated prior to restoration of aortic blood flow. Unfortunately, short of anticoagulation, little progress has been made in limiting the occurrence of microembolization.

One potentially manageable cause of neurologic injury is the systemic inflammation that accompanies CPB. CPB causes a generalized activation of leukocytes, prostaglandins, leukotrienes, coagulation factors, and cytokines. The resulting inflammatory process causes a diffuse endothelial dysfunction resulting in capillary leakage, and in the case of the brain, cerebral edema. Agents which suppress this overall inflammatory cascade, such as aprotinin, may hold promise in limiting neurologic dysfunction due to this recently recognized phenomenon.[37, 38]

Respiratory

Phrenic Nerve Dysfunction

The phrenic nerves originate from the third through fifth cervical nerves and descend toward the diaphragm, paralleling the pericardiophrenic vessels after joining them in the superior mediastinum. The phrenic nerves then proceed along the lateral surfaces of the pericardium before innervating the diaphragm. Although the diaphragm forms one continuous sheet, the two halves can operate independently. Tension developed from one half of the diaphragm may not be mechanically transmitted into tension on the contralateral side. Therefore, if one or both of the phrenic nerves are injured during cardiothoracic surgery, the injury can be manifest as profound difficulty weaning from mechanical ventilation. As long as freezing is avoided, a lower myocardial temperature enhances myocardial preservation. The optional temperature appears to be 4°C to 6°C. Topical hypothermia helps to promote uniform myocardial cooling. Topical cooling is usually achieved by chilled saline, iced saline slush, or saline ice chips. Temperatures of about 10°C are attained.

Cold-induced phrenic injuries, caused by cardiac preservation techniques, have long been implicated. Alterations in nerve function are dependent upon temperature, duration of exposure, and nerve fiber type (myelinated are more susceptible than unmyelinated). Mechanisms of injury include cold-induced inhibition of sodium-dependent adenosine triphosphatase, depressed nerve membrane electrochemical potentials, cold-induced changes in cell membrane permeability, and impaired nerve blood flow. Although functional changes can be noted immediately, pathologic changes such as demyelination and axonal degeneration occur later. Neural changes take place in the absence of serious injury to other tissues.

Other causes of phrenic nerve injury include physical trauma. The nerve may be physically transected. This risk is increased during mobilization of the internal mammary arteries (as the upper mediastinum is dissected) or when there has been prior surgery (fibrosis obscuring landmarks). Injury can also occur from hematoma formation during internal jugular vein cannulation. Stretch injury can occur from retraction of the sternum or prolonged pericardial tension. It has been suggested that vascular compromise to the phrenic nerve and diaphragm may occur with use of the internal mammary artery as a graft. The phrenic arteries arise from either the aorta or the internal mammary artery. The intercostal, internal mammary, and phrenic arteries supply the diaphragm. Dissection of the internal mammary artery can therefore adversely affect the blood supply to both the phrenic nerves and the diaphragm.

Phrenic nerve dysfunction should be considered following cardiac surgery when, in the absence of complicating factors (such as left ventricular dysfunction or preexisting lung disease), a patient cannot be weaned from mechanical ventilation or when patients develop orthopnea, exertional dyspnea, or respiratory failure requiring reintubation. If one uses radiographic findings such as left lower lobe atelectasis or an elevated hemidiaphragm to diagnose phrenic injury, the incidence has been reported as high as 73%. Unfortunately, the latter two findings are too nonspecific, and therefore the true incidence of phrenic injury is likely to be much lower. Electrophysiologic studies of the phrenic nerve, from the cervical region to the diaphragm, report incidences of approximately 10% to 12%.

Clinical assessment of the diaphragm is at best crude. Paralysis can be bilateral or unilateral (more common on the left after cardiac surgery) and often clinically silent. In bilateral diaphragmatic paralysis, inspiration is achieved by the inspiratory intercostals and accessory muscles that lower intrathoracic pressure and expand the rib cage. The flaccid diaphragm moves rostrally, pulling the abdominal contents with it. This produces the clinical finding of *paradoxical abdominal motion.* In unilateral paralysis, asymmetry of abdominal wall motion or diminution of the motion of the ipsilateral costal margin during deep inspiration may be detected. Pulmonary function studies often demonstrate reduction in vital capacity (VC) and functional residual capacity (FRC), both of which are aggravated by the supine position, and reductions in maximal inspiratory and expiratory pressures. Electrophysiology in phrenic nerve dysfunction after cardiac surgery is variable. Findings may reflect axonal loss with decreased compound action potentials on nerve conduction studies, decrease in conduction velocity, or both. Often, there is asymmetry in nerve function when comparing the right with the left phrenic nerve. Peripheral nerve conduction studies are normal.

Regardless of the diagnostic methods used to diagnose phrenic nerve dysfunction, significant morbidity, such as prolonged mechanical ventilation, develops in only a small percentage of patients with documented dysfunction. Respiratory impairment is more likely in patients with bilateral phrenic nerve dysfunction. Patients may require up to 4 or 5 months of mechanical ventilation, but the range varies from a couple of weeks to more than 2 years. Patients with unilateral phrenic nerve injury may wean faster than those with bilateral injury but in general still take a minimum of a few weeks to successfully wean from mechanical ventilation. Bilateral phrenic nerve dysfunction may also be a manifestation of a more global polyneuropathy often seen in patients with serious critical illness.

Postoperative Lung Injury

As previously noted, CPB initiates the activation of leukocytes and elaboration of cytokines, prostaglandins, leukotrienes, coagulation factors, and complement. The activity of all of these moieties can elicit a profound systemic inflammatory reaction. In the lungs, this can lead to noncardiogenic pulmonary edema. This is not always manifest in the initial 24 hours postoperatively but rather may begin well into the first or second postoperative day. The chest radiograph shows either minimal increase in interstitial markings or progressive pulmonary edema. It is sometimes difficult to distinguish this entity from fluid overload. However, PCWP (if available) is not particularly elevated. Gas exchange continues to worsen despite diuresis. The course of this entity is variable, and the patient virtually always requires high FIO_2 (0.5 to 1). In some patients, gas exchange will improve spontaneously over the next few days while supplemental O_2 and diuresis are provided. Others, however, require escalating respiratory support that may include a CPAP mask or even intubation. Patients with this severe lung injury physiologically develop acute respiratory distress syndrome (ARDS) and should be managed as such. Severe lung injury can lead to prolonged mechanical ventilation.

Extended Ventilatory Weaning and Tracheostomy

Patients who require prolonged mechanical ventilation should be started on a comprehensive weaning program as soon as cardiovascular performance (or other issues) permits safe weaning. Comprehensive weaning plans include progressive weaning trials that are evaluated regularly and extended or limited based on the patient's performance. Management of secretions, optimization of bronchodilation, treatment of infection, mobilization out of bed, and liberal encouragement are all necessary to foster weaning. Some patients, however, require mechanical ventilation for more than 2 weeks. It is our practice to continue mechanical ventilation utilizing a tracheostomy rather than an oral-endotracheal tube. The tracheostomy allows freedom of tongue and jaw, facilitating communication and swallowing. In addition, the absence of adhesive tape or other tube-securing devices is universally found to improve comfort in this patient population. We have found no significant increase in mediastinal or sternal wound infections when a tracheostomy is performed at 2 weeks, or sometimes even earlier if the situation warrants it.

Cardiovascular System

Lactic Acidosis

There is a small to moderate percentage of patients with otherwise good cardiac performance who are found to have a substantial lactic acidosis despite apparently more than adequate tissue perfusion. This severe metabolic acidemia is generally not recognizable until 1 to 2 hours after the patient arrives in the CVRR. The incidence of metabolic acidosis may range from 14% to 33% in post-CPB patients with otherwise good cardiovascular performance.[39] Previous reports of lactic acidemia occurring after cardiopulmonary bypass described inadequate delivery of oxygen (DO_2),[40–43] systemic vasodilation associated with reduced O_2 extraction (utilization defect),[44] longer and colder CPB, and hyperglycemia and altered pyruvate metabolism.[39, 45] Potential sites of lactate production include the splanchnic organs and peripheral tissues, especially in the CPB and rewarming post-CPB and early ICU period.[41–43] It has been postulated that nonpulsatile blood flow during CPB, which causes increases in angiotensin II, could exacerbate splanchnic ischemia.[46, 47] Sufficient evidence exists to identify inadequate perfusion of these sites as at least one explanation of this phenomenon.[41–43]

In our series (unpublished), acidemia occurred in patients

who had maintained sufficient cardiac performance such that global hypoperfusion would not have been expected.[39, 42, 43] Most studies have seen this phenomenon in patients who were receiving vasoactive support, particularly epinephrine. In our series, all patients who demonstrated the late acidemia had lactic acidosis (lactate level > 2.8) on admission to the CVRR. Presence of this acidemia clearly delayed timely extubation and utilized resources beyond those required by patients without acidemia. We noted no change in the mortality in these patients, as is noted elsewhere.[39]

For the most part, the lactic acidosis is a transient phenomenon, usually clearing spontaneously 6 to 12 hours postoperatively. No particular intervention is needed other than perhaps switching the epinephrine for another vasoactive agent. We have successfully utilized IV sodium bicarbonate to reduce the acidemia without negatively impacting outcome.

Gastrointestinal System

Most patients who are extubated within the first 24 hours can begin eating soon after bowel sounds return. As with any postoperative patient, the diet should begin with simple clear liquids and advance as tolerated toward solid food. However, if a patient cannot be weaned from the ventilator, attention to nutritional needs is critical. If after 24 hours the patient is not extubated and intubation is expected to continue at least another 24 hours, enteral tube feedings are begun as soon as bowel function has appeared to return. Most patients can be rapidly advanced to their nutritional goals within 24 hours. Although gastric feedings are tolerated by most patients, some patients exhibit poor gastric motility and emptying, and reaching nutritional goal is delayed because of persistently elevated gastric residual volumes. In these patients, endoscopic placement of a small-bowel feeding tube facilitates reaching nutritional goal in a timely fashion.

Complications involving the gastrointestinal (GI) system in postoperative cardiovascular surgery patients are fortunately infrequent. However, the complications that do occur can be catastrophic. The incidence of complications, including GI hemorrhage, perforated ulcer, cholecystitis, mesenteric ischemia, and hepatic failure, is 1% to 2% in post-bypass patients.[48, 49] Patients experiencing GI complications can have a mortality rate of up to 19.4%.[49] Upper GI bleeding has become less of a problem since the routine use of "ulcer prophylaxis" in the postoperative period. Sucralfate is an adequate agent and does not reduce the acidic antimicrobial environment of the stomach, as can occur with ulcer prophylaxis with H_2 blockade. Acalculous cholecystitis is another infrequent GI complication and can occur in patients with poor splanchnic circulation. Its presentation can be subtle. In the patient with right upper quadrant tenderness, fever, and leukocytosis, this diagnosis must not be overlooked. An ultrasound study of the gallbladder that demonstrates pericholecystic fluid or an abnormal HIDA scan suggestive of this diagnosis. Treatment is surgical because antimicrobial therapy in the presence of retained gangrenous tissue is rarely therapeutic.

The most devastating gastrointestinal complication is certainly bowel infarction. This process occurs mostly in patients with preexisting vascular disease who have also experienced a transient episode of poor splanchnic perfusion. The patient is usually gravely ill with a persistent acidosis and hypotension. Symptoms may be absent in the intubated, sedated patient. Physical findings and laboratory evaluation are nonspecific at best. Sometimes a lactic acidosis with modestly elevated amylase and tactate dehydrogenate associated with abdominal pain suggest the diagnosis. Flexible sigmoidoscopy or colonoscopy that demonstrates characteristic ischemic mucosa can be very suggestive as well. The only definitive way to detect and possibly treat ischemic and infarcted bowel is exploratory laparotomy. Unfortunately, even with prompt recognition and resection of dead bowel, the mortality is very high.

Renal System

In most postoperative cardiac patients, renal function is well preserved. In fact, urine output is often very high in the first few postoperative hours, necessitating volume replacement to preserve hemodynamic performance. While on CPB, patients may end up in positive fluid balance and the CPB prime often contains mannitol. There is also a fall in atrial natriuretic factor during CPB and a rapid rise to preoperative levels following CPB.[50] The combination of the latter can result in urine output of 200 to 500 mL hourly for the first few hours. The use of low-dose dopamine can also substantially enhance urine output. It may be necessary to discontinue the dopamine because of this effect on urine output. Large volumes of urine often carry significant quantities of potassium out of the body. Potassium replacement based on urine output, as described previously, can prevent potassium levels from falling too low.

Varying degrees of postoperative renal insufficiency can also occur, however. Although small, transient increases in serum creatinine are usually the extent of the renal impairment, frank acute renal failure can also occur. Certain risk factors have been identified, including age greater than 70 years, elevated preoperative serum creatinine, and low blood pressure during CPB or postoperatively.[51] As long as the patient remains nonoliguric, the patient can be effectively managed by avoidance of hypotension or hypovolemia, judicious use of IV resuscitation fluids, and careful monitoring and treatment of electrolyte abnormalities. Diuretics to keep the patient nonoliguric can enhance management of fluid balance and are usually not harmful as long as adequate intravascular volume is maintained during fluid mobilization. Diuretics should not be continued if serum creatinine continues to rise or in the presence of anuria. Some clinicians feel that unless the patient has an absolute reason to require diuretics, such as pulmonary edema, these agents are best avoided until renal function improves.

If complete renal shutdown occurs, the patient will require organ support until intrinsic function returns. Hemodialysis is well suited for this patient population only when the cardiac performance is good. In patients with hypotension requiring substantial vasoactive support, hemodialysis only further destabilizes blood pressure. There are, however, alternatives to hemodialysis in patients who are hemodynamically unstable. Continuous arteriovenous (CAVH-D) or continuous venovenous hemofiltration with dialysis (CVVH-D) are excellent alternatives and can provide not only excellent fluid removal but also some degree of dialysis. CAVH-D and CVVH-D have a much smaller effect on blood pressure than does hemodialysis and can be set up to keep the patient in positive, even, or negative fluid balance while continuously providing dialysis. These latter techniques should be considered in any hemodynamically unstable patient with appropriate vascular access that needs dialysis, ultrafiltration, or both.

Because the same risks that are associated with cardiovascular disease are also associated with renal disease, it is not surprising that a significant number of patients with chronic renal failure eventually require cardiovascular surgery. This includes the patients on hemodialysis or peritoneal dialysis. These patients can safely undergo CPB but need special attention paid to fluid balance and electrolytes in the operating room and CVRR. It is generally best to have patients well dialyzed, including the day prior to elective surgery. To simplify fluid management, patients can be ultrafiltered while on

CPB so that they enter the postoperative period in even or only slightly positive fluid balance. Patients with renal failure who are not anuric or oliguric should not receive empiric potassium replacement based on urine output in the early postoperative period. Rather, serum potassium should be checked every 6 to 8 hours for the first 24 hours and the levels should be treated as appropriate.

Infection

Postoperative infections are not uncommon in this patient population and unfortunately can contribute to increased morbidity, mortality, length of hospital stay, and cost. Despite use of operative prophylactic antibiotics, often cefazolin, vancomycin, and gentamicin, up to 21% of patients develop some nosocomial infection that may include respiratory or urinary systems, wounds, or generalized sepsis. The mortality of patients who developed nosocomial infections was significantly greater than those without (11% vs. 3%).[52] Four independent risk factors for the development of postoperative nosocomial infection are duration of mechanical ventilation, postoperative empiric antibiotic administration, duration of urinary tract catheterization, and female gender. Multiple organ system dysfunction, aortic cross-clamp time, and Acute Physiologic and Chronic Health Evaluation (APACHE II) severity of illness are the most significant independent determinants of hospital mortality.[52]

Although all postoperative infections are challenging to treat, only sternal wound infections and mediastinitis (and rarely prosthetic valve endocarditis) require prompt surgical intervention. The overall incidence of sternal wound infections in patients with median sternotomy is approximately 1%. Sternal wound infections typically present in the second or third week postoperatively but can present earlier or later. Presenting signs and symptoms may include fever, purulent drainage from the wound, instability of the sternum (including complete separation of the sternal halves), leukocytosis, and bacteremia. Patients with a recent median sternotomy and any of the preceding symptoms should have a thorough examination of the sternal wound. The examination includes palpation along the sides of the incision looking for "clicking" or gross movement or instability of the sternal halves, inspection for erythema or drainage, and a chest radiograph (looking for misalignment of the sternal wires). The combination of positive physical and laboratory findings is generally sufficient to diagnose sternal wound and mediastinal complications.

Not all sternal complications are due to infection. Sternal necrosis can occur, leading to dehiscence in the absence of true infection. It is thought that harvesting of the internal mammary artery and the presence of diabetes predispose to this occurrence. We have also seen sterile sternal dehiscence in obese patients and in patients with intractable coughing. True sternal wound infection can be of many varieties ranging from severe but superficial skin infection to deep sternal infection and mediastinitis. The responsible organisms vary by region and center, but the most typical organisms are gram-positive cocci, *Staphylococcus epidermidis* and *Staphylococcus aureus,* and a variety of gram-negative rods, including *Escherichia coli, Serratia* sp, *Pseudomonas* sp, *Enterobacter* sp, and *Klebsiella* sp. Unfortunately, the frequency of methicillin-resistant *Staphylococcus* is increasing, necessitating the use of vancomycin. Also increasing in frequency at this time is vancomycin-resistant *Enterococcus* organisms sp., for which there is no satisfactory medical therapy.

The most important aspect of therapy for sternal wound complications is open debridement of necrotic and infected tissue. Definitive closure is sometimes delayed for 24 to 48 hours and the wound is packed with sterile dressing to ensure that all necrotic or infected tissue has been removed. The type of definitive closure depends upon the presence or absence of infection and the degree of sternal destruction. Sterile sternal dehiscence with little destruction can often be managed with simple rewiring and skin closure. Wounds requiring significant sternal debridement cannot always be closed and require vascularized muscular flaps (typically *pectoralis* or *rectus*) to fill any spaces left by wound debridement.

Hematologic System

Assessment of Coagulation System in Immediate Postoperative Period

Postoperative assessment should focus on both laboratory and clinical data. Typical laboratory evaluation includes measurement of PT, PTT, and platelet count. There is probably no additional benefit in measuring both PT and PTT as opposed to PTT only. It would be unusual for a significantly elevated PT to occur in the presence of a normal PTT, especially if preoperative PT was normal and there is no factor deficiency (as could be caused by warfarin). If a PTT alone is obtained, a PT could later be obtained if necessary. As noted previously, postoperative abnormalities in PT and PTT can occur because of the dilution of factors, consumption of factors, or presence of circulating inhibitors (most often heparin). It is not necessary to obtain more sophisticated tests because significant postoperative bleeding requires prompt management and further tests will add unnecessary delay. Platelet count needs to be interpreted recognizing the acquired qualitative defect as a result of CPB. Platelet counts above 100,000 do not assure that bleeding is not due to insufficient numbers of *functioning* platelets.

Additional clinical assessment should include measurement of body temperature and measurement of the quantity and quality of chest tube output over time. Maintenance of core body temperature above 36.5°C is of key importance because enzymatic systems, especially the coagulation system, work best at euthermic temperatures. Coagulation is clearly impaired in the presence of hypothermia. Active warming with heated convection blankets is the recognized standard of practice at our institution. "Normal" chest tube output in the first few hours postoperatively varies by institution but in general should be less than 150 mL in the first hour, less than 100 mL/hr in the second and third hours, and less than 60 mL/hr in the next 2 hours. Abnormally high chest tube output can be due to coagulopathy (medical bleeding) or vascular or cardiac defect (i.e., that which can only be corrected by surgical intervention). Bleeding can also occur from "raw" surfaces such as the pericardium in a second or third CABG or valve operation. The presence of visible clot in the chest tube suggests that the patient has the ability to form clot but does not exclude coagulopathy as a cause of bleeding. Similarly, the absence of clot in the chest tube is not diagnostic of coagulopathy because brisk "surgical" bleeding may fail to show clot in the chest tubes.

Postoperative Hematologic Complications

Postoperative hematologic complications can be divided into four groups: anemia, disorders of platelets, disorders of coagulation, and postoperative bleeding.

Anemia

Postoperative hematocrit is generally in the upper 20s. The fall in hematocrit is due to hemodilution and blood loss in excess of transfusion. Rarely is the hematocrit low because of hemolysis. Optimum postoperative hematocrit depends on cardiovascular performance and oxygen consumption. Transfusion of PRBCs is based upon absolute hematocrit, insufficient delivery of oxygen that could be improved with transfusion, or empirical transfusion during active postoperative bleeding.

Transfusion based on an absolute hematocrit disregards the premise that PRBCs should be given based on measured physiologic needs (such as arteriovenous difference of oxygen content, $AVDO_2$). Young, otherwise healthy patients should tolerate a hematocrit in the low 20s if cardiac output is sufficient. However, it is our practice to transfuse PRBCs, at least in the early postoperative period, when the absolute hematocrit is less than 23 to 24. When the hematocrit is less than this number, but the patient "looks good," transfusion can be held if the $AVDO_2$ is normal (4 to 6 ml O_2/100 mL) or if there is clinical evidence of adequate oxygen delivery (absence of acidemia, good tissue perfusion and color, good urine output). When the hematocrit is more than 23 and less than 30, in the absence of active bleeding, transfusion should be based on physiologic need. If the $AVDO_2$ is greater than 6 in the presence of adequate arterial saturation, delivery of oxygen can be improved by increasing the hematocrit or increasing the cardiac output. If cardiac output is already optimized, then transfusion of PRBC is an acceptable way of increasing delivery of oxygen. In practice, the hematocrit should be raised no higher than 30 to 32. Hematocrit above this probably offers the patient no further clinical advantage.

Disorders of Platelets

As previously discussed, CPB causes a qualitative and quantitative defect to platelets. An acquired platelet functional defect is probably the most common cause of *nonsurgical* post-CPB bleeding. A few other recognized disorders deserve mention. Platelet washout is a term used to describe the situation of thrombocytopenia following massive transfusion, generally more than 10 units of PRBCs. This occurs because PRBCs are devoid of adequate numbers of functional platelets. The body has no readily mobilizable store of platelets (increased demand must be met by increased production). Massive PRBC transfusion must be supplemented by platelet transfusion, usually 4 to 6 units of random donor platelets or one single donor unit after the first 10 units of PRBCs. Further platelet transfusion should be based on measured platelet count.

Heparin-induced thrombocytopenia occurs in a mild form in 5% of all patients receiving heparin. A modest, nonprogressive drop in platelet count occurs soon after receiving heparin. The syndrome can develop with heparin in any dose, including heparin flushes, heparin in monitoring devices, or heparin bonded into medical plastics. In the absence of bleeding complications, no intervention is necessary. A more severe form occurs when platelet counts fall below 50,000 is associated with thromboembolism (venous or arterial). A heparin-dependent antiplatelet autoantibody (IgG, IgM, IgA) against specific platelet antigen (PF4) appears to be responsible. Arterial thrombosis tends to occur in smaller arteries. Therapy includes discontinuation of heparin or utilizing heparinoids (if anticoagulation must be continued). Aspirin and 6% dextran have also been used as therapies once thrombosis has occurred. In the presence of bleeding due to thrombocytopenia, platelet transfusion is appropriate.

Infrequently, post-transfusion thrombocytopenia is seen following transfusion of blood products containing platelets or platelet antigen. This most often follows PRBC transfusion. It is seen 2 to 10 days after transfusion. Platelet counts can fall to below 10,000 and stay that low for 4 weeks to 3 months. This phenomenon tends to occur in patients who have been previously exposed to platelets in blood products and is thought to be due to an immunologic host response to platelet antigen. Therapy includes corticosteroids and platelet transfusion (if there is a bleeding crisis).

Disorders of Coagulation

As previously mentioned, it is not uncommon for postoperative measurements of PT or PTT to be modestly abnormal. The abnormalities can be due to the dilution or consumption of factors or the presence of circulating inhibitors, most often heparin. Management of these abnormalities depends on the clinical manifestation of the abnormalities. Abnormal values of PT or PTT in the absence of significant chest tube bleeding usually do not require intervention. The effects of heparin are reversed with protamine after CPB, usually in the dose of 1 mg protamine for each 80 units of heparin. If less than this amount had been given, an extra 50 to 100 mg of protamine can be given. Excessive protamine, however, can potentially retard clot formation. Certainly, one of the most important interventions in the postoperative CPB patient to optimize coagulation is to ensure normal body temperature. Even if the patient returns with a temperature above 36°C, the core temperature can fall if the patient is not kept covered. When the patient's temperature is less than 36°C, active warming with heating blankets can return the patient's temperature to normal.

Postoperative Bleeding

About 3% to 5% of patients require reexploration for chest tube bleeding after open heart surgery. Bleeding occurs as a result of either inadequate mechanical hemostasis or coagulopathy. Platelet dysfunction contributes much more to bleeding than primary fibrinolysis.[10] "Expected" hourly chest tube outputs after CPB vary by institution; however, more than 200 mL in the first hour, 150 mL/hr in the second and third hours, or resumption of chest tube bleeding to more than 100 mL/hr after having been minimal requires investigation. Management of postoperative bleeding requires assessment and correction of coagulopathy, maintenance of circulating RBC mass and intravascular volume, and consideration of reexploration. These three components are carried out simultaneously and not sequentially. The risks of excessive chest tube bleeding include inadequate delivery of oxygen and pericardial tamponade.

As previously mentioned, PT, PTT, and platelet count are routinely obtained postoperatively. For these values to be of benefit, their results must be available within the first postoperative hour. It is often difficult to determine with certainty when chest tube bleeding is due to coagulopathy or to inadequate mechanical hemostasis. However, unless the rate of chest tube bleeding necessitates immediate return to the OR, patients will not return for reexploration until attempts have been made to correct coagulopathy. In the presence of significant chest tube bleeding and normal PT and PTT, it is appropriate to transfuse platelets (6 random donor units or 1 single donor unit) regardless of the platelet count (recognizing that platelets after CPB are dysfunctional). Chest tube bleeding should be treated beginning after 1 hour of excessive blood loss. It is critical not to delay intervention more than this time. Additional maneuvers such as supplemental PEEP are unproven in efficacy. If the patient's temperature is less than 36.5°C, active warming techniques should be employed.

Aspirin is now routinely used in patients with unstable angina and acute myocardial infarction. Cardiac surgical patients also frequently receive aspirin preoperatively. Aspirin irreversibly impairs platelet aggregation and thromboxane A_2 production by inhibiting cyclooxygenase activity. Thromboxane A_2 promotes vasoconstriction and platelet aggregation. The clinical effect is prolonged bleeding caused by platelet dysfunction. This effect can last for up to 7 days. Some studies have found that recent preoperative aspirin increases the need for transfusion and reoperation in CABG patients while others have not confirmed this pattern.[53] Certainly, cardiac surgery should not be delayed because of recent aspirin ingestion.[54]

Desmopressin (DDAVP), when given postoperatively to patients who received preoperative antiplatelet agents, has been shown to decrease chest tube bleeding. DDAVP can be given in doses up to 3 units/kg IV. Other studies, however, have not demonstrated this effect.[22] This reduction in chest tube bleeding has not necessarily lead to a reduction in transfusion of blood products.[55] DDAVP, an analog of vasopressin with reduced vasoconstrictor properties, is thought to work by enhancing platelet adhesion through release of von Willebrand's factor from endothelium. DDAVP can be used in conjunction with antifibrinolytic drugs or administered after CPB along with protamine. DDAVP has also been shown to reduce bleeding time in patients with hemophilia, von Willebrand's disease, uremia, cirrhosis, and congenital platelet defects.

If significant chest tube bleeding occurs in the presence of abnormal PT and PTT, it is still appropriate to transfuse platelets as a first line of therapy prior to transfusion of coagulation factors, such as fresh frozen plasma (FFP). However, in this situation, it is also prudent to give additional protamine 50 to 100 mg, especially if less than the expected dose (1 mg/80 units of heparin) was given to reverse the heparinization following CPB.

If significant chest tube bleeding continues into a second hour, it is appropriate to transfuse coagulation factors, usually 4 to 6 units of FFP, especially if initial PT and PTT were abnormal. FFP will be useful only if it can be obtained expeditiously; a delay of 90 minutes may result in return of the patient to the OR. If initial PT and PTT are normal, it may also be appropriate to transfuse FFP during the second hour of chest tube bleeding, hedging that coagulation factors are rapidly consumed in the bleeding patient.

If significant chest tube bleeding continues into a third hour, it is necessary to repeat PT, PTT, and platelet count to help guide further component replacement. "Nonsurgical" postoperative chest tube bleeding is usually due to platelet dysfunction, dilutional coagulopathy, or circulating inhibitors (e.g., heparin). Infrequently, however, primary consumptive coagulopathies such as disseminated intravascular coagulation and primary fibrinolysis are responsible for continued bleeding. These diagnoses are very difficult to make because modest abnormalities of PT, PTT, and platelet count and the presence of elevated fibrin degradation products are not unexpected post CPB. Treatment is the same regardless: transfusion of platelets and coagulation factors and usually a return to the OR to look for "surgical bleeding."

Transfusion of RBCs during chest tube bleeding is more often empiric than based on measurement of hematocrit. The reasons are as follows: bleeding is often so rapid that sampling multiple times per hour is impractical; turnaround time from moment of sampling until report of hematocrit is too slow; patients are often being resuscitated with cell-free fluids, delaying opportunity to check hematocrit; and rapid bleeding allows little time for natural homeostatic processes to restore intravascular volume so that the hematocrit may not accurately represent the RBC mass. Therefore, transfusion of RBCs is often based on blood visibly lost into the chest tubes rather than on a hematocrit.

RBCs returned to the patient are either in the form of PRBCs from the blood bank or from recovery systems such as autotransfusers. Autotransfusion devices are collection canisters placed in line with the chest tube and the water seal system. The autotransfusion canister contains a filter to remove clot and debris prior to transfusion back to the patient. Blood is collected for autotransfusion when chest tube output is brisk (approaching 200 mL/hr) and contains little clot. Chest tube output that contains too many clots often clogs the autotransfuser's filter. Blood that is collected in the autotransfuser can be returned to the patient up to 4 hours after collection began. More often, however, up to 400 mL is collected and then transfused as part of the early maintenance of circulating RBC mass. Blood collected from chest tubes is low in clotting factors and also contains fibrin degradation products. Generally, no more than 600 mL of collected blood is returned to the patient to avoid perpetuating a coagulopathy.

In the patient who is bleeding more than 200 mL/hr, empiric transfusion of two units of PRBCs should begin as soon as about 400 to 500 mL chest tube output has drained. At this point, an autotransfusion collection device should be added if not already in line. PRBCs can be transfused earlier if initial postoperative hematocrit was less than 25. It is practical to obtain follow-up hematocrits about every 2 hours, or following PRBC transfusion, so that some objective data exist to guide further transfusion. During active bleeding it is not uncommon for patients to receive cell-free fluids such as hetastarch, 5% albumin, or crystalloid to maintain hemodynamic stability. The addition of these fluids can cause an unavoidable dilutional anemia. Further transfusion should be based either on continued chest tube losses (two units of PRBC for each 400–500 mL of chest tube output) or measured hematocrit. When transfusing large quantities of cold, banked blood, it is crucial to use a high-capacity blood-warming device to avoid rapidly lowering body temperature. Rapid cooling can induce ventricular arrhythmias and inhibit coagulation. Massive PRBC transfusion also does not require empiric calcium replacement. Citrate used in the preserving banked blood remains in the plasma fraction and will not cause a clinically significant fall in blood calcium levels during massive transfusion of PRBCs. Rapid transfusion of FFP, however, does contain citrate, and there exists the potential for clinical hypocalcemia following rapid, massive administration of FFP.

Active chest tube bleeding should not be watched if refractory hypovolemic shock develops. The patient needs to return to the OR for reexploration. Patients should return to the OR if chest tube output is massive (> 500 mL in any given hour or similar volumes over short periods of time) regardless of assessment of the coagulation system. It is sometimes difficult to distinguish a "dump" of old loculated blood from active chest tube bleeding. Old sequestered blood is dark; however, venous bleeding from an atrial cannulation site can be just as dark and requires urgent intervention. Brisk bright red chest tube output can occur from a graft site or aortotomy (i.e., cannulation site). Other areas of bleeding occur from surface oozing in patients undergoing repeat cardiac surgery, from mediastinal venous bleeders, from the sternum, or infrequently from injury to the great vessels. An inadequately drained mediastinum (the pericardium is left open after CPB) can also lead to tamponade. Clot or liquid blood will prevent the heart's chambers from filling, resulting in low ejection volume, low cardiac index, and low blood pressure.

The clinician should not wait for "classic" signs of tamponade (i.e., equalization of diastolic pressures in all cardiac chambers). A keen index of suspicion in a patient with significant chest tube output, elevated CVP, elevated PAD pressure, low blood pressure and cardiac index, increased need of inotropic support, and often a pronounced pulsus paradox (best visualized on arterial line tracing) are usually all that is necessary to make the diagnosis. Surface and transesophageal echocardiography are complementary diagnostic procedures and are sometimes necessary for confirmation. Active chest tube bleeding should not be watched any longer than 2 to 3 hours after coagulopathy has been corrected. If at this point there is more than 100 mL/hr of sanguineous chest tube output, the patient should return for reexploration.

References

1. Jubran A, Tobin M: Monitoring during mechanical ventilation. Clin Chest Med 1996; 17:453–473.

2. Brown M, Vender J: Noninvasive oxygen monitoring. Clin Crit Care 1988; 4:493–510.
3. Stock MC: Noninvasive carbon dioxide monitoring. Clin Crit Care 1988; 4:511–526.
4. Venkatesh B, Hendry S-P: Continuous intra-arterial gas monitoring. Intensive Care Med 1996; 22:818–828.
5. Pulmonary Artery Catheter Consensus Conference Participants: Pulmonary Artery Catheter Consensus Conference: Consensus Statement. Crit Care Med 1997; 25:910–925.
6. Nelson L: The new pulmonary artery catheters. Crit Care Clin 1996; 12:4, 795–815.
7. Singer M: Esophageal Doppler monitoring of aortic blood flow: Beat by beat cardiac output monitoring. Int Anesthesiol Clin 1993; 31:99–125.
8. McLean AS: Needham A, Stewart D, Parkin R: Estimation of cardiac output by noninvasive echocardiographic techniques in the criticall ill subject. Anaesth Intensive Care 1997; 25:250–254.
9. Clancy T, Norman K, Reynolds R, et al: Cardiac output measurement in critical care patients: Thoracic bioimpedance versus thermodilution. J Trauma 1991; 31:1116–1121.
10. Bick RL: Physiology and pathology of hemostasis during cardiac surgery. *In:* Anticoagulation, Hemostasis, and Blood Preservation in Cardiovascular Surgery. Pifarre R (Ed). Philadelphia, Hanley & Belfus, 1993; pp. 23–46.
11. Mammen EF, Koets MH, Washington BC, et al: Hemostasis changes during cardiopulmonary bypass surgery. Semin Thromb Haemost 1985; 11:281–292.
12. Colleen C, Stenach N, Fisher CA, et al: Hollow fiber membrane oxygenator reduces platelet loss during simulated extracorporeal circulation. J Extracorporeal Technol (in press).
13. Hall TS: The pathophysiology of cardiopulmonary bypass: The risk and benefits of hemodilution. Chest 1995; 107:1125–33.
14. Webber CE, Garnett ES: The relationship between colloid osmotic pressure and plasma proteins during and after cardiopulmonary bypass. J Cardiothorac Surg 1973; 65:234–237.
15. Addonizio VP, Colman RW: Platelets and extracorporeal circulation. Biomaterials 1985; 3:9–15.
16. Addonizio VP Jr, Colman RW, Edmunds LH Jr: Effect of blood flow and surface area on platelets during extracorporeal circulation. Trans Am Soc Artif Intern Organs 1978; 24:650–655.
17. Addonizio VP Jr, Macerak EJ, Niewiarowski S, et al: Preservation of human platelets with prostaglandin E1 during in vitro cardiopulmonary bypass. Circ Res 1979; 44:350–357.
18. Musial J, Niewiarowski S, Hershock D, et al: Loss of fibrinogen receptors from the platelet surface during simulated extracorporeal circulation. J Lab Clin Med 1985; 105:514–522.
19. Adelman B, Michelson AD, Loscalzo J, et al: Plasmin effect on platelet glycoprotein Ib–von Willebrand factor interaction. Blood 1985; 65:32–40.
20. Addonizio VP: Platelet function in cardiopulmonary bypass and artificial organs. Hematol Oncol Clin North Am 1990; 4:145–155.
21. Kappa JR, Fisher CA, Cottrell ED, et al: Heparin induced platelet activation in 16 surgical patients. Diagn Manage J Vasc Surg 1987; 5:101–109.
22. Arom K, Emery R: Decreased postoperative drainage with addition of ϵ-aminocaproic acid before cardiopulmonary bypass. Ann Thoracic Surg 1994; 57:1108–1113.
23. Coffey A, Pittman J, Halbrook H, et al: The use of tranexamic acid to reduce postoperative bleeding following cardiac surgery: A double-blind randomized trial. Am Surg 1994; 61:566–568.
24. Dietrich W, Spannagl M, Jochum M, et al.: Influence of high dose aprotinin treatment on blood loss and coagulation patterns in patients undergoing myocardial revascularization. Anesthesiology 1990; 73:1119–1126.
25. Laub G, Riebman J, Chen C, et al.: The impact of aprotinin on coronary artery bypass graft patency. Chest 1994; 106:1370–1375.
26. Westaby S: Coagulation disturbance in profound hypothermia: Influence of antifibrinolytic therapy. Semin Thorac Cardiovasc Surg 1997; 9:246–256.
27. Gunning MG, Chua TP, Harrington D, et al: Hibernating myocardium: Clinical and functional response to revascularization. Eur J Cardiothoracic Surg 1997; 11:1105–1112.
28. Casthely PA, Yoganathan T, Komer C, et al: Magnesium and arrhythmias after coronary artery bypass surgery. J Cardiothorac Vasc Anesth 1994; 8:188–191.
29. Bender KA, Alexander JA, Enos JM, Skimming JW: Effects of inhaled nitric oxide in patients with hypoxemia and pulmonary hypertension after cardiac surgery. Am J Crit Care 1997; 6:127–131.
30. Wood G: Effect of antihypertensive agents on the arterial partial pressure of oxygen and venous admixture after cardiac surgery. Crit Care Med 1997; 25:1807–1812.
31. Gu YJ, de Vries AJ, Boonstra PW, Oeveren W: Leukocyte depletion results in improved lung function and reduced inflammatory response after cardiac surgery. J Thorac Cardiovasc Surg 1996;112:494–500.
32. Hurst T, Johnson D, Cujec B, Thompson D, et al: Can J Anesth 1997; 44:131–139.
33. Reeve WG, Ingram SM, Smith DC: Respiratory function after cardiopulmonary bypass: A comparison of bubble and membrane oxygenators. J Cardiothorac Vasc Anesth 1994; 8:502–508.
34. Sladen RN, Berend JZ, Fassero JS, Zehnder EB: Comparison of vecuronium and meperidine on the clinical and metabolic effects of shivering after hypothermic cardiopulmonary bypass. J Cardiothorac Vasc Anesth 1995 9:147–153.
35. Mort TC, Rintel TD, Altman F: The effects of forced air warming on post bypass central and skin temperature and shivering activity. J Clin Anesth 1996; 8:361–370.
36. Sotaniemi K: Long-term neurologic outcome after cardiac operation. Ann Thorac Surg 1995; 59:1336–1339.
37. Heyer EJ, Adams DC: neurologic assessment and cardiac surgery. J Cardiothorac Vasc Anesth 1996; 10:99–103.
38. Utley JR: Techniques for avoiding neurologic injury during adult cardiac surgery. J Cardiothorac Vasc Anesth 1996; 10:38–43.
39. Raper RF, Cameron G, Walker D, Bowey J: Type B lactic acidosis following cardiopulmonary bypass. Crit Care Med 1997; 25:46–51.
40. Harris EA, Seelye ER, Barratt-Boyes BG: Respiratory and metabolic acid-base changes during cardiopulmonary bypass in man. Br J Anaesth 1970; 42:912–921.
41. Landow L: Splanchnic lactate production in cardiac surgery patients. Crit Care Med 1993; 21:S84–S91.
42. Niinikoski J, Kutilla K: Adequacy of tissue oxygenation in cardiac surgery. Crit Care Med 1993; 21:S77–S83.
43. Takala J, Uusaro A, Parviainen I, Ruokonen E: Lactate metabolism and regional lactate exchange after cardiac surgery. New Horiz 1996; 4:483–492.
44. Raper FR, Cameron G, Walker D, Bowey J: Type B lactic acidosis following cardiopulmonary bypass. Crit Care Med 1997; 25:46–51.
45. Hampton WW, Townsend MC, Schirmer WJ, et al: Effective hepatic blood flow during cardiopulmonary bypass. Arch Surg 1989; 124:458–459.
46. Taylor KM, Bain WH, Morton JJ: The role of angiotensin II in the development of peripheral vasoconstriction during open heart surgery. Am Heart J 1980; 100:935–937.
47. Bailey RW, Bilkey GB, Hamilton ST, et al: The fundamental hemodynamic mechanism underlying gastric stress ulceration in cardiogenic shock. Ann Surg 1987; 205:597–612.
48. Yilmaz AT, Arslan M, Demirkile U, et al. Gastrointestinal complications after cardiac surgery. Eur J Cardiothorac Surg 1996; 10:763–767.
49. Perugini RA, Orr RK, Porter D, Dumas EM, Maini BS: Gastrointestinal complications following cardiac surgery: An analysis of 1477 cardiac surgery patients. Arch Surg 1997; 132:352–357.
50. Majid AA, Ch'ng AL: Atrial natriuretic peptide, diuresis and cardiopulmonary bypass. Ann Thorac Surg 1994; 57:1369–1374.
51. Leurs PB, Mulder AW, Fiers HA, Hoorntje SJ: Acute renal failure after cardiovascular surgery: Current concepts innpathophysiology, prevention and treatment. Eur Heart J 1989; 10(Suppl H):38–H42.
52. Koleff MH, Sharpless L, Vlasnik J, Pasque C, Murphy D, Fraser VJ: The impact of nosocomial infections on patient outcomes following cardiac surgery. Chest 1997; 112:666–675.
53. Bashein G, Nessly M, Rice AL, et al: Preoperative aspirin therapy and reoperation for bleeding after coronary artery bypass surgery. Arch Intern Med 1991; 151:89–93.
54. Rawitscher R, Jones J, McCoy T, Lindsley D: A prospective study of aspirin's effect on red blood cell loss in cardiac surgery. J Cardiovasc Surg 1991; 32:1–7.

55. Gratz I, Koehler J, Olsen D, Afshar M: The effect of desmopressin acetate on postoperative hemorrhage in patients receiving aspirin therapy before coronary artery bypass operations, J Thorac Cardiovasc Surg 1992; 104:1417–1422.

106

Air Embolization

Steven L. Orebaugh, MD • Ake Grenvik, MD, PhD, FCCM

Air embolization has become increasingly common and important as critical care medicine and anesthesiology have embraced invasive procedures requiring vascular access, positive-pressure ventilation (PPV), and diagnostic sampling with forceps or needles. Major operative procedures, as in cardiovascular, neurologic or transplantation surgery, also provide ready access of ambient air to the circulatory system. Entry of air or other gas into veins or arteries requires a source of gas (usually the atmosphere), a breach in the vascular wall, and a pressure gradient that favors entry of gas into the vessel. Although the clinical consequences of *venous air embolism* (VAE) and *arterial air embolism* (AAE) are quite different, *cerebral air embolism* (CAE) may result from either process, so that some overlap in presentation exists.

When air is admitted into a vessel, bubbles form in the blood, as is the case when any gas enters a liquid in volumes exceeding its solubility. Once a bubble is blood borne, its fate is relatively predictable: It may be whipped into froth, it may coalesce into larger air bubbles, or it may fracture into smaller bubbles.[1] Typically, a lining forms around gas bubbles in blood, consisting of fibrin, other plasma proteins, platelets, and phospholipids.[2] These aggregates represent foreign bodies, which may then lead to erythrocyte agglutination, microthrombi, platelet and leukocyte activation, altered blood viscosity, release of vasoactive mediators, and altered capillary permeability. The circulatory consequences of such phenomena are obstruction to blood flow, altered hemodynamics, and ischemia of any affected end organs. The specific vascular beds involved determine the clinical manifestations of VAE and AAE.

VENOUS AIR EMBOLISM

Etiology and Occurrence

As noted earlier, in order for VAE to occur, there must be a communication between the vascular lumen and the source of gas as well as a pressure gradient favoring ingress of the gas into the vessel. In the most straightforward example, air is injected through a catheter into a peripheral vein or infused inadvertently via an improperly vented intravenous set, especially when under pressure.[3] Likewise, air may enter the thoracic veins during the insertion of a central venous catheter (CVC) or use of the catheter after placement, depending on the development of subatmospheric intrathoracic venous pressure.[4-7]

Neurosurgical and head and neck procedures performed on patients in the sitting position and insufflation of air or other gases into the peritoneal cavity are other situations in which VAE frequently has been described.[7-11] Durant and colleagues[12] reported the occurrence of air embolism in the setting of maxillary sinus lavage, pneumothorax, and pneumoperitoneum. In total hip arthroplasty, VAE may produce hemodynamic disturbances, and it is difficult to distinguish from the effects of methylmethacrylate cement. Hepatic surgery, including both liver resection and transplantation, has resulted in VAE.[7] VAE is known to occur in prostate surgery and in as many as 97% of cesarean sections.[13, 14] This phenomenon may occur in any surgical procedure in which veins in the surgical field are elevated above the level of the heart. Both positive-pressure ventilation in infants with hyaline membrane disease and high peak airway pressures in adults receiving mechanical ventilation have been reported to cause VAE.[15, 16]

In the intensive care unit (ICU), VAE is most likely encountered during or after insertion of a central venous catheter. The occurrence rate of this problem varies in reports from one in 47 central venous catheter insertions to none in 355 insertions.[7, 17] However, the mortality rate of VAE is significant. By 1987, only 79 cases of central venous catheter–related VAE had been reported but 32% of these were fatal.[7]

When a central venous catheter is inserted, free communication may develop between the intrathoracic vasculature and the atmosphere. Admission of air occurs whenever intravenous pressure decreases below ambient air pressure.[18] Such negative intrathoracic venous pressure is most likely to occur with deep inspiration, dyspnea, or hypovolemia and in the upright position. During strained breathing, thoracic vein pressure may decrease to 25 mm Hg below atmospheric pressure.[7]

Numerous case reports[4-6, 17] of VAE related to catheter venous catheters exist in the medical and surgical literature. Air may enter the great veins directly after the needle is inserted if the hub is not conscientiously occluded. However, the majority of cases occur during routine use of the catheter, usually from hub fracture or disconnection.[7] Pulmonary artery catheter introducers have been reported to cause VAE as well, and it is recommended that an obturator be left in the introducer when the pulmonary catheter has been removed.[19]

Pathophysiology and Pathology

Alterations in cardiovascular and pulmonary physiology resulting from admission of air into the venous system have been well studied in animals. In 1947, Durant and coworkers[12] reported that the most important factors in determining mortality after experimental VAE in dogs were the amount of air entering the veins, the speed with which it enters, and the position of the body at the moment of embolization. However, recent canine studies utilizing invasive monitors and transesophageal echocardiography (TEE) in bolus VAE have shed doubt on the importance of position in the cardiovascular response to this phenomenon.[20]

Adornato and associates[21] distinguished the cardiovascular effects of bolus VAE from slow air infusion, as can occur with a separation of an intravenous line. With a massive bolus, these investigators noted an increase in central venous pressure (CVP), a decrease in pulmonary artery pressure (PAP), ST-segment depression, and shock. These changes were thought to be due to an "air lock" in the right ventricle, obstructing the outflow of blood. Slow, continuous infusion of air yielded an increase in both central venous pressure and pulmonary artery pressure, decreases in systemic vascular resistance and mean arterial pressure (MAP), and a surprising increase in cardiac output. Small bubbles lodge in pulmonary arterioles and create mechanical obstruction to flow, causing pulmonary arterial hypertension.[4] Pulmonary vasoconstriction results in further compromise of right heart function, as demonstrated by Berglund and coworkers[22] in a canine model subjected to slow air infusion.

Similar effects are evident in humans. Bedford and coauthors[23] evaluated 100 seated patients during neurosurgical procedures with invasive hemodynamic and precordial Doppler ultrasound monitoring. Eighty episodes of air embolism were reported. Of the 100 patients, 36 demonstrated increased pulmonary artery pressure, and only patients in this group experienced a decline in mean arterial pressure.

Air infusion rates of more than 1.8 mL/kg/min are fatal in dogs.[21] A bolus of more than 200 mL of air injected rapidly causes ventricular tachycardia and death in these animals. The volume required to cause death decreases as the rate of air entry increases. In humans, the fatal dose of air is uncertain, but estimated between 300 and 500 mL at 100 mL/sec.[4] However, much smaller amounts of air may be lethal to critically ill patients with compromised hemodynamics.

Microbubbles introduced into the pulmonary circulation result in significant ultrastructural changes and abnormalities of lung extravascular water content.[24] The bubbles themselves obstruct flow and increase pulmonary artery pressure. On the bubble's surface, a network of fibrin, platelets, red blood cells, and fat globules develops, serving to further restrict blood flow.[18] In animal models, neutrophils clump around small air bubbles in pulmonary arterioles and may attach to the endothelium of these vessels.[7, 24] This produces an increase in capillary leakage, lung lymphatic flow, and lymph protein concentration. These histopathologic and ultrastructural changes lead to significant abnormalities of pulmonary function. Lung compliance is reduced as a result of increased permeability and interstitial edema, and airway resistance is increased.[18] Abnormalities of ventilation-perfusion matching result, with increases in physiologic dead space and pulmonary shunting. These aberrations underlie the hypoxemia universally found in patients with significant VAE.

Natural History

The natural history of VAE has been well described in animal models.[7, 22] Adornato and colleagues[21] described the changes in physiology that occurred with both graded venous air infusion and bolus introduction of air. The central venous, right atrial, and pulmonary artery pressures and heart rate all increased in a dose-related fashion, with air infusion rates exceeding 0.4 mL/kg/min. At rates greater than 1.5 mL/kg/min, bradycardia supervened and cardiovascular decompensation occurred. No significant change was evident in the mean arterial pressure until a rate of 1.7 mL/kg/min had been reached, but thereafter, mean arterial pressure decreased rapidly. When canines were subjected instead to intravenous boluses of air, the central venous pressure and heart rate again increased linearly with the dose of air, whereas mean arterial pressure decreased in a dose-related manner.

Clinical Manifestations

The clinical expression of VAE varies in both severity and the organs affected (Table 106–1). In canines[21] and humans,[18] a "gasp" has been reported to follow the initial infusion of air into the pulmonary circulation, possibly a reflex response. Intrathoracic pressure is thereby decreased, facilitating greater air entry into the venous system. Patients often complain of breathlessness, lightheadedness, chest pain, or a feeling of impending doom.[4, 18]

Signs of VAE are not specific. Significant embolism results in tachypnea, tachycardia, and frequently hypotension. The only sign specific for VAE, the rare "water mill wheel" murmur, occurs late and is dependent on the presence of a large collection of air in the right ventricle.[11, 18] A harsh systolic murmur or normal heart sounds are more commonly found on examination.[7, 25] In a large proportion of patients, neurologic signs predominate. Kashuk and Penn[26] described a predominance of central nervous system manifestations in 42% of 24 instances of VAE. These manifestations included altered mental status, frank coma, and focal deficits. Whether hypoxia, hypotension, *paradoxical air embolism* (PAE), or some combination of these factors is responsible for this neurologic compromise is uncertain.

TABLE 106–1. Clinical Manifestations of Venous Arterial Embolism and Arterial Air Embolism

System	Venous Air Embolism	Arterial Air Embolism
Cardiovascular	Chest pain Coarse systolic murmur Water mill-wheel murmur Tachycardia, arrhythmias Cardiovascular	Chest pain (if coronary embolism) Arrhythmias (if coronary embolism)
Neurologic	Altered level of consciousness Acute focal deficit (paradoxical embolism)	Sudden collapse or coma Acute focal deficit Subtle cognitive abnormalities
Pulmonary	Cough, dyspnea Hypoxemia Tachypnea Rales, wheezing Gasping	Lungs not usually affected unless pulmonary injury is source
Skin	No effects	Livedo reticularis Mottling
Mucous membranes	No effects	Partial or complete tongue ischemia

In some individuals, rales or wheezing can be detected on auscultation of the lung fields minutes to hours after air embolism occurs.[11] In animal models and humans, the elevated protein content of pulmonary edema fluid together with normal pulmonary artery occlusion pressures suggests that increased vascular permeability underlies the development of extravascular lung water in VAE.[7]

Laboratory Data and Monitoring

Laboratory abnormalities vary with the severity of the embolism but lack specificity for this process. Electrocardiographic changes evident in canines include peaking of the P wave and ST-segment depression.[12] Reports of VAE in humans describe sinus tachycardia, nonspecific ST-segment and T-wave changes, and evidence of acute right ventricular strain.[27] In addition, atrial and ventricular dysrhythmias may be noted.[11] Findings on chest radiographs are usually normal initially but later may show evidence of noncardiogenic pulmonary edema. An air-fluid level in the proximal pulmonary artery or right ventricle is seen rarely (Fig. 106–1). Arterial blood gases reflect abnormalities of matching of ventilation and perfusion, usually as hypoxia, which may be profound. Hypercarbia is occasionally present.[7]

When used, invasive hemodynamic monitoring may provide further evidence of clinically important air embolism. Increases in central venous and pulmonary artery pressure are dose-dependent in animals subjected to slow air infusion.[21] However, pulmonary artery pressure may remain normal, with an increased central venous pressure, presumably due to a large air bubble trapped in the outflow tract of the right ventricle. This phenomenon occurs in animals with massive air embolism (>5 mL/kg). In one study of the occurrence of VAE in patients seated during neurosurgical procedures and

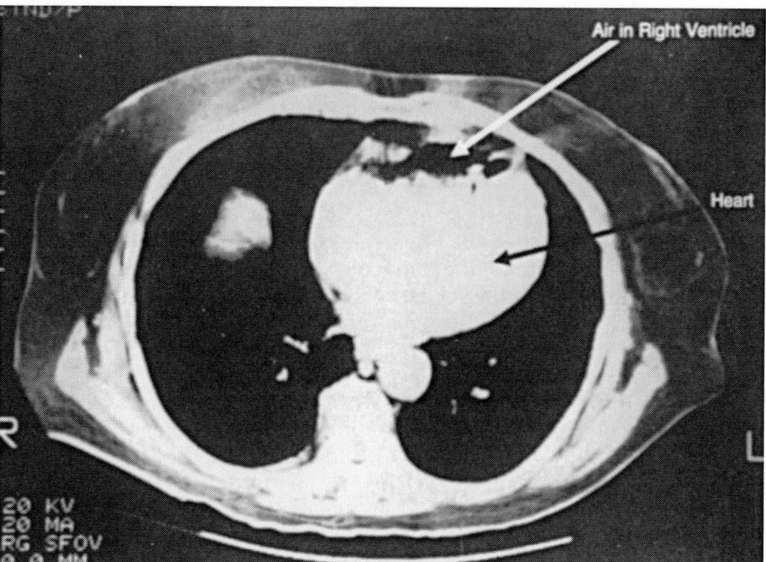

Figure 106–1. Computed tomography scan demonstrating air in the right ventricle. (From Oriscello RG, Robertello ME: Images in clinical medicine. N Engl J Med 1993; 328:855. Reprinted by permission of the New England Journal of Medicine.)

monitored with central venous catheters, 10 of 40 patients who had a VAE demonstrated an increase in central venous pressure.[25]

Bedford and coworkers[23] described the occurrence of VAE in 80 patients under similar conditions; in nearly 50%, pulmonary artery pressure became elevated. More recent data from animal investigations emphasizes the importance of elevated pulmonary artery pressure in virtually all VAE with little evidence of an "air lock," regardless of position.[28]

The utility of end-tidal carbon dioxide ($ETCO_2$) monitoring to detect significant VAE is well described, with an abrupt fall in $ETCO_2$ reflecting an increase in physiologic dead space.[11, 12] Other useful indicators of VAE include aspiration of air or foam from an indwelling central venous catheter or pulmonary artery catheter as well as ultrasonographic changes. Human and animal data have demonstrated the utility of Doppler ultrasound and precordial echocardiography. Transesophageal echocardiography, however, seems to be even more sensitive, detecting as little as 0.02 mL/kg of air in experimental scenarios,[29] and only this modality has proved useful in documenting paradoxical air embolism.[30]

Differential Diagnoses

Patients with VAE may present with a wide variety of signs and symptoms and spans a continuum of severity from insignificant to life-threatening, mandating consideration of many different entities (Table 106–2). When respiratory complaints and signs are evident, VAE must be differentiated from other causes of sudden pulmonary compromise, such as pulmonary thromboembolism, pneumothorax, acute bronchospasm, and pulmonary edema. If signs of central nervous system compromise predominate, the clinician must consider focal or global brain ischemia, hemorrhage into the parenchyma or subarachnoid spaces, hypoxia, trauma, intoxication, and hypoglycemia.

Cardiovascular compromise often dominates the clinical picture. This is usually in the form of hypotension, in which case VAE must be considered, along with other causes of obstructive shock, hypovolemia, primary cardiac dysfunction, and acute vasodilatory states, such as septic shock. VAE has also been reported to manifest as electromechanical dissociation,[31] probably a result of right ventricular outflow obstruction.

TABLE 106–2. Differential Diagnoses of Venous Air Embolism

Predominant System Affected	Differential Diagnoses
Cardiovascular	Aortic dissection
	Pericardial tamponade
	Hypovolemia
	Myocardial infarction
Neurologic	Stroke
	Intracranial bleed
	Trauma
Pulmonary	Pulmonary thromboembolism
	Tension pneumothorax
	Acute bronchospasm
	Acute pulmonary edema

Management of Venous Air Embolism

Identification of the source of air entry and immediate measures to counter this entry are the first priorities in the treatment of VAE. Subsequent management strategies are based on evidence derived from animal investigations and case reports in humans. Five areas of therapeutic intervention are discussed (Table 106–3):

- Patient positioning
- Cardiac massage
- Removal of air from the venous circulation and right atrium and right ventricle
- Reduction of bubble size
- Other measures

TABLE 106–3. Management of Venous Air Embolism

Cardiac massage: is useful in cardiac arrest due to venous air embolism.

Air retrieval: significant air retrieval is sometimes possible using a central venous catheter or direct needle puncture of the right heart in the case of cardiac arrest.

Reduced bubble size: 100% oxygen for all patients, hyperbaric oxygen may be useful in patients with severe central nervous system or cardiac manifestations.

Miscellaneous: fluorocarbon emulsions require further research to establish efficacy, cardiopulmonary bypass may be lifesaving in the moribund patient.

Durant and coauthors,[12] in their early work with air embolism in canines, demonstrated the importance of body positioning by showing that dogs had increased tolerance of air infusion when lying on their left side; however, more recent animal data appear to contradict this finding.[20] Although not validated in human clinical trials, placement of patients with suspected VAE in this position remains a cornerstone of management today.[18, 25, 32] The head-down or Trendelenburg position is recommended as well, apparently resulting in similar reduction in right ventricular outflow obstruction.[4, 20]

Closed-chest cardiac massage has been recommended as a means of forcing air from the right ventricle and into small pulmonary vessels. This measure has been documented by Ericsson and associates,[33] who used this technique to resuscitate four of five patients with severe VAE and cardiac arrest during neurosurgery. External cardiac compression has been evaluated in dogs as therapy for VAE[32] and has been found to improve survival rate as effectively as use of the left lateral decubitus position or aspiration of air from the right atrium.

More directly, air may be removed from the venous system. A comparison of intracardiac aspiration from the right ventricle versus external cardiac massage or the left lateral decubitus position in therapy of experimental VAE in dogs resulted in similar survival in all three groups but significantly more rapid resuscitation with air aspiration than with the other measures.[32] A greater proportion of injected air can be removed from the right atrium in VAE by means of a multiple orifice central venous catheter than by a pulmonary artery catheter or single-port central venous catheter, with a significantly improved survival rate.[34]

Michenfelder and colleagues[25] evaluated the utility of air retrieval in humans via right atrial catheters during 23 episodes of VAE in seated patients undergoing neurosurgical procedures. Significant air retrieval with a favorable influence on resuscitation occurred in only eight cases. Other researchers have found that air retrieval from the right atrium has had minimal impact on improving hemodynamics.[23] Nevertheless, for patients not responding to oxygen, positioning, chest compression, and Advanced Cardiac Life Support protocols, insertion of a central venous catheter or direct puncture of the chest and right atrium with a needle for air removal may be lifesaving.[20] With the patient in the supine or left lateral decubitus position, the right atrium is reached via the fifth intercostal space, 2 to 3 cm lateral to the right sternal border while a large needle is aimed in a mid-chest direction. With the patient in the Trendelenburg position, the right ventricle apex is reached from subxiphoid insertion with technique similar to pericardial puncture. If removal of gas from the heart results in return of spontaneous circulation, the possibility of creating pericardial tamponade must be considered.

To reduce the size of embolized bubbles, the physician should see that all patients with suspected VAE receive 100% oxygen; this favors nitrogen diffusion out of the bubbles. For patients under general anesthesia, nitrous oxide must be discontinued because it diffuses rapidly into all air-containing cavities in the body, including intravascular bubbles, significantly increasing their size and the obstruction they present to perfusion of vascular beds.[7, 18]

For patients not responding to these measures, hyperbaric oxygen (HBO) therapy should be considered. Although well-controlled, randomized trials comparing this therapy with other measures have not been conducted, many physicians advocate hyperbaric oxygen use on the strength of anecdotal reports of improvement in the manifestations of cerebral air embolism of venous or arterial origin after hyperbaric oxygen therapy. A review of the utility of hyperbaric oxygen is provided in Chapter 142, Section VIII.

Prophylaxis

Most clinically significant episodes of VAE are related to central venous catheters, making preventive measures particularly important when these catheters are inserted, used for infusions, or removed. Patients undergoing catheterization of the central veins should be placed in a head-down position. This position results in increased central venous pressure and reduces the likelihood of air entry through the needle or catheter.[18] After entering the vein and before inserting the guide wire with the Seldinger technique, the operator should occlude the needle hub, releasing to insert the wire only after asking the patient to perform a Valsalva maneuver or to hold the breath, timing the wire insertion to avoid the inspiratory phase of ventilation. A through-the-plunger guide wire system may reduce the risk of air embolism.

Adequate hydration should be ensured before catheter insertion to mitigate against subatmospheric venous pressure that encourages air entry during inspiration. All connections to the central venous line should be tightly sealed using Luer-Lok adapters. Placing an occlusive dressing over the catheter when in place and over the tract for 24 hours after removal also helps prevent air emboli. As with insertion, removal of the catheter in a head-down position is recommended.

In the operating room, monitoring for air embolism during high-risk procedures using precordial Doppler and capnography has become standard.[30] Avoiding surgical procedures in the seated position should reduce the incidence of VAE. Gas insufflation for diagnostic purposes should be accomplished with carbon dioxide (CO_2), not air, because this gas has a low surface tension, is absorbed quickly, and causes less obstruction to circulation if embolism occurs.[11] During cesarean section, less VAE occurs if the surgeon avoids traction or exteriorization of the uterus.[14]

Finally, if a patient experiencing air embolism can be ventilated with positive pressure, this is preferable to spontaneous breathing because it prevents unfavorable pressure gradients, permitting air entry (as during insertion of a central venous catheter). However, high peak insufflation pressure causing barotrauma may, in itself, cause VAE and must be avoided.[16]

ARTERIAL AIR EMBOLIZATION

Arterial air embolization was first reported in the medical literature by Morgagni in 1769.[37] It was not recognized as an iatrogenic complication until 1913, when AAE was observed with irrigation of empyema cavities. AAE in diving accidents was described in the 1930s but was not originally distinguished from decompression sickness.[38] Scuba diving was not yet a popular sport, and the accidents reported were related to military submarine escape training. In 30 years of Royal Navy submarine escape training, 91 cases of apparent AAE occurred in the United Kingdom.[39] More recently, an analysis of civilian scuba diving accidents occurring in Hawaii over a five year period revealed 42 cases of AAE.[40] Approximately 750 cases of AAE requiring recompression therapy occur annually in the United States, with about 100 fatalities.[41]

Etiology and Incidence

The two most common iatrogenic causes of AAE are (1) cardiopulmonary bypass (CPB) and (2) neurosurgical procedures performed with the patient in the sitting position.[37] Significant AAE related to use of cardiopulmonary bypass occurs in 0.07% to 0.11% of cases,[42] whereas asymptomatic evidence of air emboli is detected by transesophageal echocardiograms in up to 79% of cases. In neurosurgical procedures with the patient sitting upright, AAE occurs rarely and is due to paradoxical air embolism, usually in the presence of a patent foramen ovale, in contrast to the much more frequent occurrence of VAE in this setting.

Cardiopulmonary bypass presents many means by which air may gain access to the arterial circulation, most commonly related to deficiencies in the integrity of the circuit or a low level of blood in the cardiopulmonary bypass reservoir or oxygenator. In the past, the use of bubble oxygenators was an important cause of AAE, but this has become less of a problem as hollow core membrane oxygenators have become the standard. Other causes include arterial pumphead rupture, accidental disconnections, inadequate de-airing of the cardiopulmonary bypass components before operation or of the heart before resuming spontaneous circulation, air installation into the coronary arteries, and "vortexing" of air into the arterial line.[42]

Before the surge in popularity of sport diving, most AAE related to dysbaric accidents occurred in submarine escape training.[37] Improvements in technique and apparatus have reduced the dangers of this training considerably. Scuba diving now constitutes the majority of cases of noniatrogenic AAE treated in hyperbaric chambers. This is often attributed to divers with exhausted air supply who panic and ascend too rapidly without the necessary exhalation en route,[38] leading to expansion of pulmonary gas and eventual alveolar rupture with potential air admission into pulmonary veins. However, in many instances, no violation of safe diving principles is evident. Although inexperienced divers are more susceptible to AAE, this unpredictable occurrence strikes seasoned divers as well.[78]

Positive-pressure ventilation also places patients at risk for entry of air into the arterial system. Particularly in patients with inhomogeneous lung injury or chronic obstructive pulmonary disease (COPD), much of the positive-pressure inflation is directed away from the affected, poorly compliant alveoli into alveoli that are more compliant. These alveoli may rapidly overexpand, rupture, and release air into the mediastinum, predisposing to pneumothorax as well as entry of air into pulmonary capillaries or veins.[43] This may occur with ventilator insufflations, spontaneous breaths from a positive-pressure circuit, or manual bag ventilation. Stiff lungs may predispose to AAE by stenting open vascular channels disrupted by pressure, trauma, or inflammation.[43]

Other potential causes of iatrogenic AAE are surgery on the head, neck, lungs and aorta.[37, 44] AAE has also occurred in association with transthoracic lung biopsy and penetrating trauma of the chest, especially stab wounds involving the lung.[45] In addition, AAE has been described as a consequence of hepatic surgery, liver transplantation,[37] and uterine surgery.[14] Finally, radial artery catheterization for continuous blood pressure monitoring may lead to AAE, as described in a primate model by Chang and coauthors,[46] who found that more than 2 mL of air introduced during flushing of the catheter resulted in retrograde passage of air to the cerebral circulation via the ipsilateral vertebral artery.

Pathophysiology

Air may be introduced into the arterial system by three different mechanisms:

- Direct arterial air entry
- VAE with air attaining access to the arterial tree via paradoxical air embolism
- Entry of air into the pulmonary capillaries or veins by direct lung trauma

When air is present in the venous system, pulmonary air embolus can occur either by direct migration of air through the pulmonary vascular bed or by traversing an intracardiac defect, such as a patent foramen ovale or atrial septal defect.[7] The threshold of bubble size below which spillover can occur from the venous to arterial circulation through the pulmonary capillaries is reported to be 22 μm in animal studies, but larger bubbles may pass through in patients with pulmonary hypertension.

In addition to a communication between the left and right sides of the heart, a favorable pressure gradient must exist for air to enter the arterial circulation via this route. During neurosurgery with the patient in the seated position, a gradient of 5 mm Hg favoring this transseptal migration can occur. Such gradients appear to be augmented by VAE and by positive-pressure ventilation. Sudden changes in end-expiratory pressure may predispose to pulmonary air embolus because the instantaneous gradient of right-to-left atrial pressure probably determines the occurrence and direction of air movement rather than mean pressures.[47] Attempts to identify patients at risk for paradoxical air embolism preoperatively using precordial echocardiography with provocative maneuvers to demonstrate a patent foramen ovale have not been entirely successful.

As with VAE, air bubbles in the arterial circulation are typically covered by a membrane of fibrin, platelets, lipids, erythrocytes, cellular debris, and various plasma proteins.[1] The development of such a coagulum on an intravascular bubble presents a foreign body to the immune system and activates the kinin, complement, coagulation, and fibrinolytic systems, all of which may contribute to end-organ injury in AAE. In animal models, arterial injection of gas distributes rapidly to capillary beds, occluding those 30 to 60 μm in diameter.[42, 48] In the central nervous system, this leads to patchy, ischemic neuronal damage.[42] Increased capillary permeability and the loss of cerebral vascular autoregulation are prominent features of the response to experimental AAE. Some experimental models provide evidence of neuronal injury and reduced local cortical blood flow despite the absence of complete vascular obstruction, perhaps a result of activation of damaging mediators and their effect on the vasculature.[49]

Pathology

The pathologic consequences of AAE are difficult to distinguish from other ischemic events. In the brain, astrocyte and neuron swelling, vacuolation, chromatolysis, hemorrhage and necrosis identical to models of cerebral infarction are evident at necropsy.[37] Pathologists may have difficulty distinguishing evidence of cerebral air embolism (CAE) from cerebral ischemic injury accompanying profound hypotension. Both cytotoxic and vasogenic edema may result.

Natural History

The course of AAE is unpredictable. Typically, maximum end-organ dysfunction develops within seconds to minutes. The deficit may remain profound, or spontaneous improvement may occur. In animal studies, bubbles of air may disappear within minutes from capillary beds or may obstruct the capillaries for much longer periods. Smaller bubbles are quite evanescent, whereas larger ones often coalesce and persist, leading to stasis of blood flow and local tissue injury.[42] More than 50% of divers with evidence of CAE recover partially or completely before definitive therapy is instituted.[40] More profound deficits portend longer periods of recovery with less likelihood of complete resolution.[37]

Clinical Manifestations

Four clinical signs have been described as specific for significant AAE[42]:

- Skin marbling
- Reduced perfusion of all or part of the tongue
- Bloody froth emanating from a wound or needle-stick
- Air bubbles in retinal arteries

Unfortunately, these signs are not particularly sensitive.

In dysbaric diving accidents, the system most commonly affected is the central nervous system. The most frequent sign reported in submarine escape training and among scuba divers is an abrupt loss of consciousness and collapse within seconds or minutes of surfacing. This occurs in 38% to 45% of divers sustaining AAE.[40] Most episodes of loss of consciousness occurs within 10 minutes of surfacing. Other evidence of central nervous system injury includes asymmetric multiple limb weakness, sensory loss and neuropsychiatric deficits. Patients may present with cognitive abnormalities alone, and a thorough mental status examination is imperative. Severe headache is common among divers sustaining AAE.

The manifestations of AAE are diverse and may overlap considerably with the neurologic signs and symptoms of *decompression sickness*, which are often expressed as spinal cord injury with symmetric limb weakness or sensory loss. These two entities frequently coexist in divers and have been referred to as the *dysbaric syndrome*.

Cardiopulmonary bypass may cause focal, obvious neurologic deficits as a result of air bubbles or cellular debris acting as emboli, but it is much more likely to result in subtle cognitive deficits. This occurs in up to 70% of patients.[42] In patients with penetrating chest trauma, the creation of a bronchopulmonary venous fistula may be manifested by sudden cardiovascular collapse, hemoptysis, bloody foam emanating from a perforated lung or great vessel, seizures, or direct visualization of air in the coronary arteries at thoracotomy.[45] In positive-pressure ventilation, AAE may result in the dramatic onset of dysrhythmia, cerebral infarction or livedo reticularis.[43]

Laboratory Data and Monitoring

Unlike VAE, air emboli in the arterial circulation are detected largely by clinical acumen. These emboli produce few disturbances of laboratory or imaging modalities that would aid in establishing this diagnosis. However, transcranial Doppler (TCD) studies have been used successfully in monitoring for cerebral air embolism during coronary artery bypass graft procedures and carotid endarterectomy, during which AAE affecting the cerebral circulation is common but rarely clinically expressed.[50] Electroencephalographic changes occur with cerebral air embolism as well but are nonspecific and predict neurologic signs or symptoms in only half of the patients who have them.[37] Both transthoracic and transesophageal echocardiography effectively identify VAE, as does precordial Doppler monitoring, but only the transesophageal probe can detect air that crosses the interatrial septum or migrates through the pulmonary capillary bed en route to AAE. Computed tomography scanning of the brain performed within the first 24 hours after cerebral air embolism may reveal foci of air density in the brain or decreased attenuation suggestive of cerebral infarction, but findings do not correlate well with resultant clinical deficits.[51]

Differential Diagnosis

The differential diagnosis of AAE depends on the vascular beds affected and the clinical manifestations produced. The most common presentation of AAE outside the operating room is generalized neurologic compromise or focal deficit, which should lead one to consider an intracranial catastrophe, such as subarachnoid hemorrhage, intracerebral hematoma, or widespread infarction from thrombosis, atherogenic embolism, or global hypoperfusion in shock.

Management of Arterial Air Embolism

The management of AAE varies according to the setting in which it occurs. In cardiopulmonary bypass procedures, the sequence of interventions should begin immediately on detection of air embolism. The steps are as follows:

- Stopping air entry
- Compressing the carotid arteries
- Stopping the administration of nitrous oxide and substituting 100% oxygen
- Venting the aorta for air removal
- Inducing hypothermia

Anecdotal reports support the use of retrograde (venoarterial) cerebral perfusion via the cardiopulmonary bypass procedures circuit. During open-chest procedures, coronary AAE may mandate retrograde perfusion via the coronary sinus, needle puncture of the coronary arteries with direct extraction of visible air, and open-chest cardiac massage. Other interventions of potential use, but not supported by clinical trials, include administration of steroids, lidocaine, osmotic diuretics, barbiturates, and perfluorocarbons.[42]

When penetrating chest trauma is complicated by AAE via bronchovenous fistula, 100% oxygen administration should be accompanied by emergency thoracotomy and clamping of the entire hilum of the involved lung, followed by resection of the affected area, vigorous open-chest cardiac massage, and aspiration of the left ventricular apex for air or foam.[45] Air can also be aspirated form the coronary arteries if bubbles are visible within them. Emergency cardiopulmonary bypass procedures can be used in refractory cardiac arrest resulting from AAE.

Data supporting the use of hyperbaric oxygen therapy in AAE and VAE are largely anecdotal. No clinical trials have compared the efficacy of hyperbaric oxygen with supportive measures alone. Still, available clinical and experimental evidence supports use of hyperbaric oxygen in AAE once the patient has been stabilized.[42] Details of its administration appear in Chapter 142, Section VIII. Other interventions supported by animal or experimental data include the following:

- Infusion of Dextran 40 to reduce blood viscosity
- Perfluocarbons to enhance oxygen carrying capacity of the blood
- Aspirin to reduce platelet aggregation
- Lidocaine infusion to reduce neuronal injury

Prognosis

Complete resolution of neurologic deficits after AAE in divers occurs in 65% of patients treated with hyperbaric oxygen. Two thirds of these patients reach baseline neurologic status within 25 minutes[41]; relapse, however, is not uncommon.[44] Initially, these patients cannot be distinguished from those who have a lasting recovery.

Prophylaxis

Methods of preventing AAE vary with the clinical scenario. In surgical procedures utilizing cardiopulmonary bypass, the perfusionist must be observant for evidence of air in the

TABLE 106–4. Risk Factors for Venous Air Embolism and Arterial Air Embolism in an Intensive Care Unit

Positive-pressure ventilation: mechanical ventilator or continuous positive airway pressure
Central venous catheter insertion, therapy, and maintenance
Postoperative state (especially after neurosurgery and procedures requiring cardiopulmonary bypass)
Hemodialysis and other forms of extracorporeal circulation
Intra-aortic balloon pumping
Trauma victims, especially penetrating chest trauma

circuit or low blood level in the oxygenator. A low-level alarm and shutoff mechanism should be used. An air bubble detector and arterial line bubble trap are also important safety mechanisms. Vent and suction pumps should be operated at the lowest speed acceptable to avoid air transmission to the patient.[42]

Transesopheal echocardiography is frequently used to evaluate the effectiveness of de-airing procedures. Careful de-airing of the heart and pulmonary veins is essential in open-heart procedures, and an aortic vent is preferred by most surgeons. However, significant air may be sequestered in the pulmonary vessels, giving rise to detectable AAE in virtually all procedures in which the heart is opened, and half of coronary artery bypass graft procedures, despite de-airing procedures.[52] Fortunately, most of these are inconsequential.

Some patients at particular risk of paradoxical air embolus during anticipated surgery in the seated position may be identified by detection a patent foramen ovale. This is accomplished with transthoracic echocardiography while agitated saline is injected to provide contrast. A suitable maneuver is then used to increase right atrial pressure. This method, however, has not proved to be 100% sensitive in identifying individuals at risk for paradoxical air embolus.[53] Nevertheless, a positive result implies that such patients should not undergo surgery in the sitting position.[54]

In order to avert AAE related to the pulmonary dysbaric syndrome, scuba divers must be well acquainted with the physiology of hyperbaric conditions and with safe diving principles. Uncontrolled ascent must be avoided. Similarly, pulmonary overinflation with mechanical ventilation, manifested by high peak airway pressures, must be prevented. The consequences of hypoventilation and respiratory acidosis are far less injurious than the consequences of pulmonary barotrauma, which may otherwise result.[43]

Summary

Air embolism in the venous or arterial circulation may have devastating consequences. Hemodynamic disturbances predominate with VAE, whereas central nervous system compromise is the most obvious evidence of AAE. Presenting manifestations frequently are nonspecific. Identification of VAE or AAE depends on the knowledge and experience of the critical care physician, surgeon, or anesthesiologist and on awareness of those settings in which air embolism is likely (Table 106-4). Basic supportive measures, control of ventilation, 100% oxygen, and Advanced Cardiac Life Support are the cornerstones of therapy; cessation of air entry, removing air (when possible), and hyperbaric oxygen therapy are also required when indicated. Emergency cardiopulmonary bypass may also be necessary in selected cases.

References

1. Butler BD: Biophysical aspects of gas bubbles in blood. Med Instrum 1985; 19:59–63.
2. Thorsen T, Klausen H, Lie RT, et al: Bubble-induced aggregation of platelets. Undersea Hyperb Med 1993; 20:101–119.
3. Rothenberg F, Schumacher JR, Rosenthal RL: Near-fatal pulmonary air embolus from presumed inadvertent pressure placed on a partially empty plastic intravenous infusion bag. Am J Cardiol 1994; 73:1035–1036.
4. Lambert MJ: Air embolism in central venous catheterization. South Med J 2983; 75:1189–1191.
5. Peter JL, Bradford R, Gelister JK: Air embolism. Intensive Care Med 1984; 10:261–262.
6. Puri VK, Carlson RW, Bonder JJ, et al: Complications of vascular catheterization in the critically ill. Crit Care Med 1980; 8:495–499.
7. Orebaugh SL: Venous air embolism: Clinical and experimental considerations. Crit Care Med 1992; 20:1169–1177.
8. Hybels RL: Venous air embolism in head and neck surgery. Laryngoscopy 1980; 90:946–954.
9. Young ML, Smith DS, Murtagh F, et al: Comparison of surgical and anesthetic complications in neurosurgical patients experiencing venous air embolism in the sitting position. Neurosurgery 1986; 18:157–161.
10. Williamson JA, Webb RK, Rursell WJ, et al: The Australian Incidence Monitoring Study: Air embolism—an analysis of 2000 incident reports. Anaesth Intensive Care 1993; 21:638–641.
11. Lantz PE, Smith JD: Fatal carbon dioxide embolism complicating attempted laparoscopic cholecystectomy. J Forensic Sci 1994; 39:1468–1480.
12. Durant TM, Long J, Oppenheimer MJ: Pulmonary (venous) air embolism. Am Heart J 1947; 33:269–281.
13. Albin MS, Ritter RR, Reinhart R, et al: Venous air embolism during radical retropubic prostatectomy. Anesth Analg 1992; 74:151–153.
14. Weissman A, Kol S, Peretz BA: Gas embolism in obstetrics and gynecology. J Reprod Med 1996; 103–111.
15. Bower FW, Chandra R, Avery GB, et al: Pulmonary interstitial emphysema with gas embolism in hyaline membrane disease. Am J Dis Child 1973; 126:117–118.
16. Morris WP, Allen SJ, Tonnesen AS, et al: Transesophageal echocardiographic study of venous air embolism following pneumodiastinum. Intensive Care Med 1995; 21:790–796.
17. Bernard RW, Stahl WM: Subcalvian vein catheters: A prospective study. Ann Surg 1972; 173:184–190.
18. O'Quin RJ, Lakshminarayan S: Venous air embolism. Arch Intern Med 1982; 142:2173–2176.
19. Kondo D, O'Reilly LP, Chiota J: Air embolism associated with an introducer for pulmonary artery catheters. Anesth Analg 1984; 63:871–872.
20. Geissler HJ, Allen SJ, Mehlhorn U, et al: Effect of body positioning after venous air embolism. Anesthesiology 1997; 86:710–717.
21. Adornato DC, Gildenberg PL, Gerrario CM: Pathophysiology of intravenous air embolism in dogs. Anesthesiology 1978; 49:201–217.
22. Berglund E, Josephson S, Ovenfors CO: Pulmonary air embolism: Physiologic aspects. Prog Respir Res 1970; 5:259–263.
23. Bedford RF, Marshall WK, Butler A, et al: Cardiac catheters for diagnosis and treatment of venous air embolism. J Neurosurg 1981; 55:610–614.
24. Albertine KH, Winer-Kronish JP, Kioke K, et al: Quantification of damage by air emboli to lung microvessels in anesthetized sheep. J Appl Physiol 1984; 54:1360–1368.
25. Michenfelder JD, Martin JT, Allenburg BM, et al: Air embolism during neurosurgery. JAMA 1969; 208:1353–1358.
26. Kashuk JL, Penn I: Air embolism after central venous catheterization. Surg Gynecol Obstet 1984; 159:249–252.
27. Dasher WA, Weiss W, Bogen E: The electrocardiographic pattern in venous air embolism. Dis Chest 1955; 27:542–546.
28. Losasso TJ, Martino JD, Muzzi DA: Venous air embolism in the recovery room producing unexplained cardiac dysrhythmia. Anesthesiology 1990; 72:203–205.
29. Glenski JA, Cucchiara RF, Michenfelder JD: Transesophageal echocardiography and transcutaneous O_2 and CO_2 monitoring for detection of venous air embolism. Anesthesiology 1986; 74:541–545.
30. Cucchiara RF, Nugent M, Seward JB, et al: Air embolism in upright neurosurgical patients: Detection and localization by two-dimensional transesophageal echocardiography. Anesthesiology 1984; 60:353–355.

31. Gronert GA, Messick JM, Cucchiara RF, et al: Paradoxical air embolism from a patent foramen ovale. Anesthesiology 1979; 50:548-549.
32. Alvaran SB, Toung JK, Graff TE, et al: Venous air embolism: Comparative merits of external cardiac massage, intra-cardiac aspiration and left lateral decubitus position. Anesth Analg 1978; 57:166-170.
33. Ericsson JA, Gottlieb JD, Sweet RB: Closed-chest cardiac massage in the treatment of venous air embolism. N Engl J Med 1964; 270:1353-1354.
34. Colley PS, Artru AA: Bunegin-Albin catheter improves air retrieval and resuscitation from lethal venous air embolism. Anesth Analg 1987; 66:991-994.
35. Catron PW, Dutka AJ, Biondi DM, et al: Cerebral air embolism treated by pressure and hyperbaric oxygen. Neurology 1991; 41:314-315.
36. Ireland A, Pounder D, Colin-Jones DG, et al: Treatment of air embolism with hyperbaric oxygen. Br Med J 1985; 291:106-107.
37. Peirce EC: Cerebral gas embolism with special reference to iatrogenic accidents. HBO Rev 1980; 1:161-184.
38. Neuman TS, Bove AA: Combined arterial gas embolism and decompression sickness following no-stop dives. Undersea Biomed Res 1990; 17:429-435.
39. Broods GJ, Green RD: Pulmonary barotrauma in submarine escape trainees and the treatment of cerebral arterial air embolism. Aviat Space Environ Med 1986; 57:1202-1207.
40. Dizer DW: Dysbaric air embolism in Hawaii. Ann Emerg Med 1987; 16:535-541.
41. National Heart, Lung, and Blood Institute Workshop Summary: Hyperbaric oxygenation therapy. Am Rev Respir Dis 1992; 144:1414-1421.
42. Kurusz M, Butler BD, Katz J, et al: Air embolism during cardiopulmonary bypass. Perfusion 1995; 10:361-391.
43. Marini JJ, Culver BH: Systemic gas embolism complicating mechanical ventilation in the adult respiratory distress syndrome. Ann Intern Med 1989; 110:699-703.
44. Dutka AJ: A review of the pathophysiology and potential application of experimental therapies for cerebral ischemia to the treatment of cerebral arterial gas embolism. Undersea Biomed Res 1985; 12:403-421.
45. Estrera AS, Pass LJ, Platt MR: Systemic arterial air embolism in penetrating lung injury. Ann Thorac Surg 1990; 50:257-261.
46. Chang C, Dughi J, Shitabata P, et al: Air embolism and the radial arterial line. Crit Care Med 1988; 16:141-143.
47. Clayton DG, Evans P, Williams C, et al: Paradoxical air embolism during neurosurgery. Anaesthesia 1985; 40:981-989.
48. Babcock RH, Netsky MG: Respiratory and cardiovascular responses to experimental cerebral emboli. Arch Neurol 1960; 2:556-564.
49. Helps SC, Parsons DW, Reilly PL, et al: The effect of air emboli on rabbit cerebral blood flow. Stroke 1990; 21:94-99.
50. Spencer MP, Thomas HI, Nicholls SC, et al: Detection of middle cerebral artery emboli during carotid endarterectomy using transcranial Doppler ultrasonography. Stroke 1990; 21:415-423.
51. Annane D, Troche G, Delisle F, et al: Kinetics of elimination and acute consequences of cerebral air embolism. J Neuroimaging 1995; 5:183-189.
52. Tingleff J, Joyce FS, Pettersson G: Intraoperative echocardiographic study of air embolism during cardiac operations. Ann Thorac Surg 1995; 60:673-677.
53. Cucciara FR, Seward JB, Nishimura RA, et al: Identification of patent foramen ovale during sitting position craniotomy by transesophageal echocardiography with positive airway pressure. Anesthesiology 1985; 63:107-109.
54. Schwarz G, Fuchs G, Weihs W, et al: Sitting position for neurosurgery: Experience with preoperative contrast echocardiography in 301 patients. J Neurosurg Anesth 1994; 6:83-88.

PART 1

Basic Applications in Pulmonary Critical Care Medicine

107

Structural Basis of Pulmonary Function

Curtis N. Sessler, MD • Alpha A. Fowler III, MD

The human lung possesses many interacting cellular and tissue systems that act as an efficient unit, performing functions in near-automatic fashion. Low energy requirements for normal function leave the host largely unaware of the lung's ongoing metabolic activity. The transfer of oxygen from air into blood and its exchange with carbon dioxide is clearly of prime significance; however, the lung accomplishes many other tasks critical for host survival. Lung arteriolar and capillary beds autoregulate perfusion to maximize ventilation and perfusion. Lung capillaries act as "filtration devices" for systemic venous blood, preventing particulate debris from egressing to the systemic circulation. Varying cell populations in the vascular and interstitial spaces of the lung are responsible for the metabolism of vasoactive substances.

The lung's conducting airspaces (i.e., the trachea, bronchi, and bronchioles) and the vast network of alveoli are critical to the host's interaction with the environment. Respirable bacterial, viral, and parasitic organisms as well as dusts and other inorganic materials are effectively removed or neutralized in most instances by interaction with flowing mucus on ciliated epithelium or resident alveolar mononuclear phagocytes (i.e., alveolar macrophages).

Thus, the lung serves a complex array of functions to maintain homeostasis. Primary lung dysfunction or failure that results in the inability to perform these critical functions frequently leads to admission of a patient to the critical care unit. Patients initially admitted with single organ failure rapidly experience dysfunction or failure of multiple organs; this demands the rapid undertaking of therapeutic actions to support the function of multiple organs and thereby prevent long-term organ impairment or death of the host. In many instances, deterioration or failure of nonpulmonary organ function seriously affects lung physiology, resulting in compromise of lung function that ultimately leads to respiratory failure. An understanding of the basic concepts of lung function and physiology is therefore essential if a comprehensive approach to the care of the critically ill patient is to be implemented.

THE RESPIRATORY PUMP

Ventilation

Ventilation is the movement of air through the upper airways, trachea, and progressively smaller conducting airways to the gas exchange units followed by the flow of exhaled gases in the reverse direction. Inspiratory and expiratory bulk flow follows pressure gradients from high to low. Pressure gradients from the mouth to the alveoli that are necessary for inspiration are generated by the production of negative alveolar pressure relative to proximal airway pressure. At end-inspiration, elastic fibers in lung parenchyma produce a recoil pressure and generate positive-pressure gradients from the alveoli to the mouth, resulting in passive exhalation of gas. Elastic fibers and collagen within lung tissue exert forces that favor collapse of the lung. Resting tension produced by diaphragm and chest wall musculature exerts outward forces on the lung-thorax unit. At the end of passive exhalation, opposing forces governing the movement of the lungs and thoracic cavity are balanced, resulting in intrathoracic pressure equal to ambient atmospheric pressure (assuming airway patency) and thus no net gas movement. This balanced state is called *functional residual capacity*, and it usually occurs at about 50% of total lung capacity.

The Thoracic Cage and Respiratory Muscles

The energy needed for lung ventilation is supplied by the contraction of the respiratory muscles. The "respiratory pump" consists of the rib cage and its related muscles, the diaphragm, and the abdominal muscles. The rib cage consists of thoracic vertebrae, ribs, costal cartilages, and the sternum. Figure 107-1 shows the anatomic relationships and actions of the principal inspiratory and expiratory muscles.

Tidal inspiration is achieved by coordinated contraction of the diaphragm and external intercostal muscles; this generates negative alveolar pressure of -2 to -3 cm H_2O.[1] The diaphragm is the primary muscle of inspiration. It is dome-shaped, with fibers radiating from a central tendon that inserts at the xiphoid process and the upper margins of the lower six ribs.[2] Abdominal contents help maintain the diaphragm's dome shape. Diaphragmatic contraction occurs craniocaudally rather than laterally. The diaphragm is innervated by phrenic nerves arising from cervical nerve roots C-3 to C-5. Upon contraction, diaphragmatic flattening forces abdominal contents downward, increasing intrathoracic volume. In diaphragms of adults, slow fatigue-resistant type I fibers predominate[3] and permit significant repetitive work against added loads without fatiguing. Aging is associated with a reduction in diaphragm strength.[4] External intercostal muscles are innervated by the intercostal nerves arising between the first and 12th thoracic vertebrae. External intercostal muscles elevate the ribs during contraction; this increases the anteroposterior chest cavity diameter while accessory muscles of inspiration (i.e., the scalene and sternocleidomastoid muscles) splint open the upper thorax during periods of high minute ventilatory requirement.

Expiration usually occurs passively by recoil of the expanded lungs. During forced expiration, contraction of the internal intercostal and abdominal muscles produces increased intrathoracic pressure. Internal intercostal muscles are oriented at 90° to the external intercostal muscles, with contraction producing caudal rib movement. Contracting abdominal muscles produce inward movement of the abdominal wall and force the contents of the abdominal cavity and the diaphragm cranially. This results in increased pleural pressure and decreased lung volume.[5]

Over most of the range of breathing capacity, the abdominal volume change is greater than the rib cage volume change, primarily because of diaphragmatic contraction. The differ-

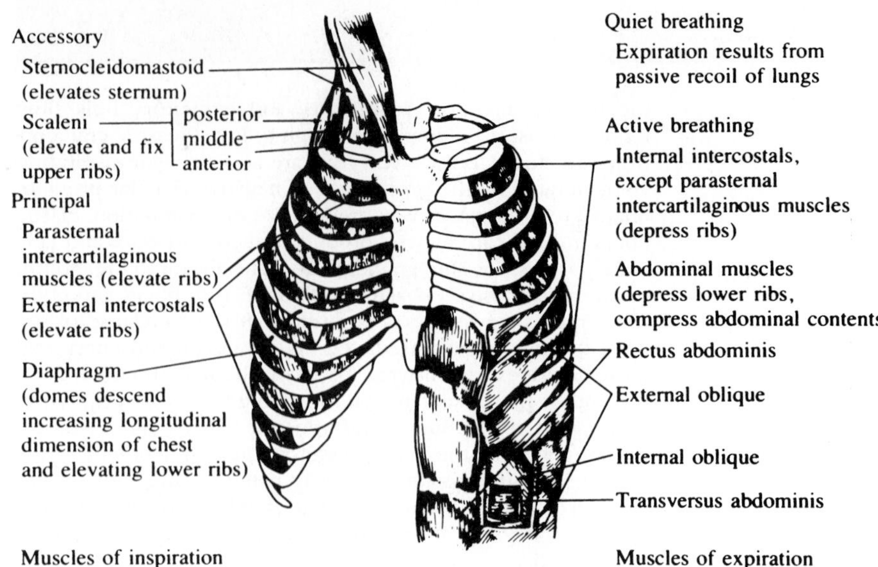

Figure 107–1. Anatomic relationship and actions of the principal inspiratory and expiratory muscles. (Adapted with permission from Garrity ER: Respiratory failure due to disorders of the chest wall and respiratory muscles. *In*: Respiratory Intensive Care. MacDonnell KF, Fahey PJ, Segal MS [Eds]. Boston, Little, Brown & Co, 1987, p 313.)

ences are more pronounced in supine rather than upright positions. At high lung volumes, however, alterations in rib cage volume predominate. With lung disease or neuromuscular dysfunction, paradoxical movement of the rib cage and abdomen occurs, and in extreme cases volume changes of other compartments must increase dramatically to compensate for the paradoxical motion and to achieve a normal tidal volume.[6] In hyperinflation caused by emphysema, the more caudal position and flattened contour of the diaphragm greatly reduce its contribution to ventilation.[7] Improvements in dyspnea and exercise ability after lung-volume reduction surgery correlate highly with a reduction in hyperinflation.[8]

Coupling of the Thorax and the Lung

The lungs and thoracic cage are coupled by a system that maintains close approximation of the structures, yet allows the smooth gliding of surfaces over one another; this minimizes frictional forces and thus the work of breathing. The pleura, a thin layer of mesothelium, lines the surface of the lung and the inner surface of the chest wall as well as the mediastinum and thoracic surface of the diaphragm. The "pleural space" between these structures contains a small amount of serous fluid and no air. The opposite resting forces of the lung (inward recoil from elastic fibers) and the chest wall (outward recoil due to tension in the muscles) create a negative pressure of -4 to -6 cm H_2O in the pleural space at functional residual capacity.[9] At end-inspiration, pressure in the pleural space may reach about -12 to -15 cm H_2O during quiet breathing and as much as -80 to -140 cm H_2O during maximum contraction of the inspiratory muscles.[10] During inspiration, negative pressure is transferred to the alveoli, creating the pressure drop required for airflow into the lungs.

AIRWAYS AND AIRFLOW

The Tracheobronchial Tree

Upon inspiration, air is filtered, warmed (37°C), and humidified by the nose, paranasal sinuses, mouth, pharynx, and larynx. Air passes through the trachea into a series of dichotomous branching bronchi and bronchioles, terminating in alveolar structures (~ 300 million). Conducting airways, which contain no gas exchange units, include 13 generations of bronchi and bronchioles that conclude with terminal bronchioles. Conducting airways combined with the upper airway account for 25% to 30% of normal tidal breaths and is referred to as "anatomic dead space." Terminal bronchioles lead to 10 subsequent generations of gas-exchanging airways, which participate both as conduits for airflow and for gas exchange. These bronchioles include transitional and respiratory bronchioles, alveolar ducts, and alveolar sacs.[11]

Airway resistance is influenced by airway geometry, flow rate, and flow characteristics. The most important variable is the *radius of the airway.* Laminar airflow is found at low flow rates through straight tubes, and resistance under these conditions is proportional to the tube length and gas viscosity and is inversely proportional to the fourth power of the radius. High flow rates or flow through irregular or branching airways produces turbulence, which causes resistance to vary with the fifth power of the airway radius. Airflow velocity is highest and most turbulent in larger airways and diminishes in smaller airways, where laminar flow patterns predominate. However, marked increases in the number of airways with each successive generation yield large increases in total cross-sectional area and, therefore, a progressive decrease in total airway resistance within distal airways. The highest airway resistances are found in large, proximal bronchi.

Airway Structure

Airway walls possess concentric layers, starting with epithelium on the luminal surface and followed by a basement membrane, lamina propria, submucosal and smooth muscle layers, and cartilage (in conducting airways only). The precise composition of airways (and thus their function) depends on the airway generation. Bronchial epithelium is primarily a pseudostratified, columnar epithelium that possesses apical cilia and goblet cells. Goblet cells, as well as mucous and serosal glands located in the submucosa, secrete a highly viscous material composed mostly of acid glycoproteins that covers the luminal surface of the conducting airways.[12] This mucus prevents desiccation of epithelium, clears inhaled particles, and performs antimicrobial function.[13] Submucosal glands are confined to the bronchi, and even though goblet cells persist into the bronchioles, they are more sparse with successive airway generations. The mucous layer is continuously propelled by the synchronized, rhythmic beating of cilia up toward the pharynx, where expectoration or swallowing occurs. Cilia diminish in number as airways diminish in caliber, becoming less dense and disappearing in the terminal or respiratory bronchioles. Clara cells account for about 15% of epithelial cells in the terminal and respiratory bronchioles of nonsmokers.[14] The many functions of Clara cells include (1) ion and liquid transport, (2) synthesis, storage, and secretion of lipids, proteins, and glycoproteins, (3) regeneration of new ciliated and new Clara cells, (4) metabolism of xenobiotic materials, and (5) secretion of bronchiolar surfactant.[15-17]

Structural support for airway patency includes cartilaginous plates in the bronchi, concentric smooth muscle, and the tethering action of radially arranged elastic fibers in the alveolar septa surrounding non–cartilage-containing bronchioles. The cartilages of the trachea and mainstem bronchi are horseshoe-shaped, whereas lobar and segmental bronchi are irregular and become smaller as the bronchial diameter diminishes. The amount and distribution of bronchial smooth muscle vary with airway caliber. In the trachea and large bronchi, muscles attach to the tips of the semicircular cartilaginous plates. In smaller bronchi, smooth muscle layers become separated from cartilage plates by loose connective tissue. In bronchioles, smooth muscle thickness diminishes as the airway caliber decreases.[18] In larger airways, muscle bundles are circular in configuration, whereas peripheral airways possess crisscrossing helical bands.

Airway smooth muscle and mucous glands are controlled by the parasympathetic nervous system and are supplied by vagus nerves.[19] Efferent nerve endings on submucosal glands include cholinergic, adrenergic, and peptidergic (e.g., vasoactive intestinal peptide) axonal profiles, with glandular secretions being stimulated more by muscarinic than by adrenergic agents.[20] Sensory receptors from the lung include large airway stretch receptors, irritant receptors, and juxtacapillary receptors, all of which are supplied by the vagus nerve. The lung also contains a component of the neuroendocrine system associated with the airways that consists of neurons and amine precursor uptake and decarboxylation (APUD) cells and cell clusters termed *neuroepithelial bodies*.[17] APUD cells contain vesicles rich in amine hormones (serotonin, dopamine, norepinephrine) and peptide hormones (vasoactive intestinal peptide, substance P, and others), but the exact function of these hormones is unknown.

Conducting airways are supplied with blood from the bronchial circulation that originates at the thoracic aorta or upper intercostal arteries near the level of the lung hila. Venous blood from the trachea and proximal bronchi enters bronchial veins, which drain into the azygos or hemiazygos vein; venous blood from more distal airways enters pulmonary venules, which ultimately drain into the left atrium and contribute to venous admixture.

At the level of the alveolus, five major cell types have been identified. The alveolar capillary membrane is 4 to 8 μm in thickness and consists of alveolar epithelium and the interstitium. Type II alveolar pneumocytes are cuboidal in shape, produce surfactant (see later), and differentiate into type I cells, which serve to cover and repopulate the alveolar surface should injury occur. Pulmonary endothelial cells lining vascular channels constitute 30% of all cells in lung parenchyma. The alveolar macrophage is a key component of lung host defense (see later) and crawls over the alveolar surfaces and distal respiratory bronchioles acting as the first-response phagocytic defense. Lung interstitium contains basement membranes, capillary endothelium, and interstitial fibroblasts critical for production of the collagen and elastin network.

SURFACTANT SYSTEM

Surfactant Structure

To prevent widespread lung collapse at resting transpulmonary pressures and avoid alterations in ventilation and perfusion, alveolar structures throughout the lung parenchyma contain a thin film of surface-active material known as *surfactant*. Surfactant is secreted by type II alveolar pneumocytes and is composed of phospholipids, neutral lipids, and surfactant-specific proteins designated SP-A, SP-B, SP-C, and SP-D. Surfactant-specific proteins exhibit a diversity of functions. Phospholipid components of surfactant are greater than 85% phosphatidylcholine.[21]

Surfactant's unique structure accounts for its surface-active function. Saturated phosphatidylcholine is the phospholipid component in the surfactant milieu, whereas SP-A is the major surfactant protein constituent.[22] SP-A, a critically important component, is primarily secreted by type II alveolar pneumocytes as a large hydrophilic, multimeric protein.[23] SP-A binds to phosphatidylcholine, promoting formation of tubular myelin-like structures from newly secreted phospholipids. Furthermore, SP-A regulates the secretion and uptake of surfactant between type II cells and alveolar structures. SP-A and SP-D are water-soluble and bind lipids. SP-A additionally is involved in organization of alveolar surfactant phospholipids.[24] SP-B and SP-C promote accelerated adsorption and spreading of surfactant phospholipids along the air-liquid interface. Recently, SP-B has been found to exhibit antibacterial and lytic properties.[24]

Surfactant Synthesis

Type II alveolar pneumocytes (type II cells) are critical to the synthesis and assembly of surfactant prior to its secretion into the alveolus. Type II cells localize to corners of alveolar structures. New evidence shows that this phenomenon occurs very rapidly as the lung undergoes maturation. By adulthood, more than 80% of type II cells have localized to alveolar corners.[25] Figure 107–2 shows that surfactant phosphatidylcholine is synthesized in the endoplasmic reticulum of type II cells and transferred to lamellar bodies intracellularly. Lamellar bodies are then secreted into alveolar spaces in tightly bound, 1-μm structures.[26]

Once they have reached the alveolus, the structures begin to "unravel" to form tubular myelin. These substances, now located in alveolar spaces, undergo a refinement process. Certain surfactant proteins initially present are likely removed, with remaining surfactant composed of dipalmitoylphosphatidylcholine, unsaturated phosphatidylcholine, and phosphatidylglycerol along with surfactant proteins. These components are necessary constituents for the promotion of adsorption of surfactant onto alveolar surfaces and for the spreading effect needed to produce a thin film across alveolar surfaces. The processes that control surfactant synthesis likely participate in

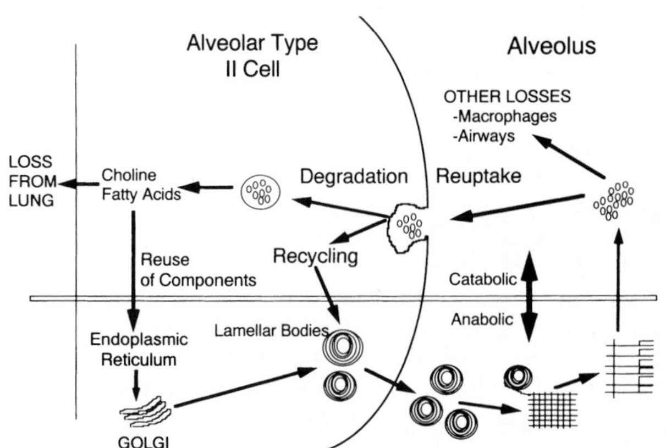

Figure 107–2. Surfactant synthesis, loss, and reuptake.

its degradation and recycling phases as well. In the lungs of adults, approximately 50% of synthesized surfactant is recycled. The processes that control turnover or degradation of surfactant remain ill defined. Excursion (inflation and deflation) of the lung during the respiratory cycle likely promotes spreading of surfactant and modulates dynamic turnover processes as well. Type II alveolar pneumocytes in this schema of metabolism remain one of the major alveolar constituents responsible for the recycling of surfactant.[27]

Surfactant Failure

The consequences of surfactant failure as observed following the onset of acute lung injury (e.g., adult respiratory distress syndrome, widespread pneumonia) are (1) widespread collapse of lung units, with resultant diffuse microatelectasis, (2) significant alterations of ventilation and perfusion with onset of arterial hypoxemia, and (3) increased work of breathing. New evidence suggests that surfactant failure results from the appearance of aqueous-soluble inhibitors of surfactant, which are likely generated within the alveolar compartment during acute inflammation. This recent research further suggests that surfactant failure cannot be accounted for on the basis of changes in phospholipid composition.[28]

Figure 107–3 shows a pressure-volume curve from normal lungs and one from lungs containing damaged surfactant. Line B shows the effects of altered compliance, with a shifting of the pressure-volume curve downward and to the right. Thus, the physiologic effect of damaged lung surfactant is the production of clinical circumstances in which significantly higher distending pressures are required to inflate the lungs to a percent that is nearly identical to predicted total lung capacity.

PULMONARY CIRCULATION

In contrast to the bronchial circulation, the pulmonary circulation is a low-pressure, high-volume system. Mean pulmonary arterial pressures average 15 mm Hg, with pulmonary vascular resistances that are one tenth of systemic vascular resistance. Whereas only 1% of systemic circulation reaches bronchial arteries, 100% of right ventricular output (5 to 6 L/min) flows through the pulmonary circulation. Pulmonary blood flow is distributed to the lungs via a dichotomous branching pulmonary arterial tree that is closely associated with the airways. In contrast, pulmonary veins are separated from airways and arteries until they reach the lung hilum. Pulmonary arterial walls are thin, reflecting the low-pressure circulation, and contain relatively little smooth muscle. Nevertheless, alteration in pulmonary vascular tone occurs with a wide variety of vasoactive substances capable of influencing pulmonary circulation. Potent pulmonary artery vasoconstrictors include histamine, serotonin, angiotensin II, and prostaglandins $F_{2\alpha}$ and E_2. Bradykinin, nitric oxide (also known as endothelial-derived relaxing factor), and prostacyclin produce vasodilatation. Accumulating evidence supports nitric oxide as the pivotal mediator of pulmonary vascular tone.[29]

Alveolar hypoxia is a common, potent stimulus for pulmonary vasoconstriction. Reduction in alveolar oxygen tension to less than 60 to 70 mm Hg promotes vasoconstriction of precapillary pulmonary arterioles, permitting redistribution of blood flow away from hypoxic areas. At very low alveolar oxygen tensions, local pulmonary blood flow is virtually absent. In contrast to alveolar hypoxia, arterial blood hypoxemia does not provoke vasoconstriction. The mechanisms underlying hypoxic pulmonary vasoconstriction are complex and appear to involve both endothelial and smooth muscle–dependent processes.[30] Putative mediators include nitric oxide, leukotrienes, prostanoids, endothelin, and components of the renin-angiotensin and natriuretic peptide systems.[29, 31] Pulmonary arteries possess distensibility properties similar to those of systemic veins and are capable of acting as a blood reservoir for redistribution to the systemic circulation in response to hydrostatic, orthostatic, and vasoactive changes.[11]

Distribution of pulmonary vascular resistance differs from that of systemic vascular resistance. Arterial and venous resistances in the lung are relatively low; this permits a proportionately larger fraction of total pulmonary vascular resistance (~ 35% to 45%) to reside in alveolar capillaries at functional residual capacity.[11] Individual microvessels (<70 μm) constrict in response to hypoxia, actions reversed by nitric oxide.[32] An important mechanism for maintaining low pulmonary vascular resistance during periods of increased pulmonary arterial or venous pressure is the recruitment and distention of underperfused capillaries.[33] Blood volume in alveolar capillaries is capable of increasing threefold above a baseline volume of 60 to 75 mL.[34] Contractile fibers and cells identified as *myofibroblasts* are present in pulmonary vasculature as far distally as the alveolar septa, where it is unclear whether they participate in the regulation of airway, vascular, or interstitial function. Alveolar pressure and lung volume may have a significant impact on pulmonary vascular resistance, with increases in resistances being observed in experimental models at low lung volumes as well as after inflation to high volumes. Compression of pulmonary capillaries with resultant increases in physiologic dead space is often present in patients subjected to high alveolar pressures. Positive-pressure ventilation with concomitant use of high levels of positive end-expiratory pressure produces this phenomenon.

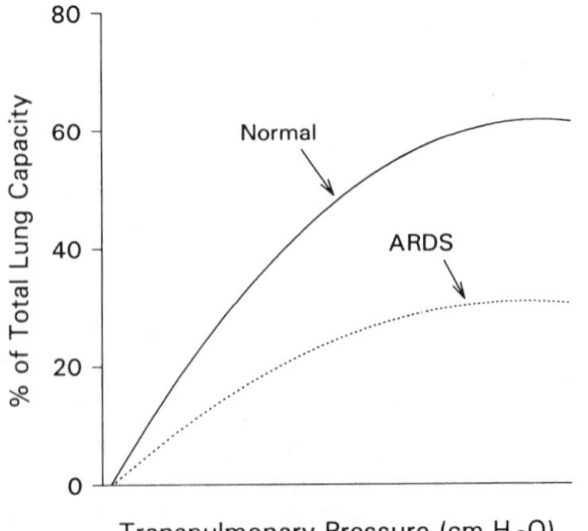

Figure 107–3. Pressure-volume curve for a person with normal lungs and for a person with lungs that contain damaged surfactant (in acute respiratory distress syndrome [ARDS]).

PULMONARY INTERSTITIUM

The airspace compartment of the lung and the vascular spaces are separated anatomically by an interstitial space. The lung's "interstitium" is a region where fluid and protein continually pass in both directions from the microvasculature into the lung tissue and from the alveolar spaces into the vascular space. Hydrostatic and oncotic pressure gradients control the magnitudes of fluid and protein passage. Intravascular water and protein must pass across the vast interstitial space from areas with lower oncotic pressures to those with higher ones to bring oncotic pressure gradients to a state of equilibrium. The interstitial space is arranged in a series of loose, binding, connective tissue fibers that contain contractile fibroblasts, immune cellular constituents, and certain neural elements.

With the structure of the interstitial space running continuously from the hilar regions of the lung to the alveolar septal structures, substantial surface area is available for fluid transport.

A large majority of protein and fluid exchange occurring in the lung's interstitial space takes place in microvascular regions. The interstitial space completely surrounds the lung microvasculature that is found in the alveolar septal spaces. Gas exchange across alveolar structures in terminal respiratory units can be greatly affected by the accumulation of interstitial fluid because of either increased left ventricular end-diastolic pressures or primary injury to the lung's microvascular surfaces. Movement of fluid and protein across lung vascular endothelial surfaces is described by the Starling equation,

$$Qf = Kf\,(Pmv - Pis) - \sigma\,(\pi mv - \pi is)$$

where Qf is the rate of filtration over time, Pis is hydrostatic pressure, Pmv is microvascular hydrostatic pressure, Pis is interstitial space hydrostatic pressure, and π is the oncotic pressure of the pulmonary microvasculature (πmv) and the interstitial space ($\pi$is). Kf is a value for fluid conductance, whereas σ is the reflection coefficient, which is thought to be equivalent to zero for small molecules such as electrolytes but equal to one for large proteins. The equation suggests that lung microvasculature is freely permeable to electrolyte-rich fluids but impermeable to large plasma proteins. Finally, the equation demonstrates that Qf, and thus an increased lung water, results from either increased hydrostatic pressure, increased permeability, or both.

Pulmonary Edema

A negative hydrostatic pressure in the interstitial space combined with tight intercellular junctions and oncotic pressure gradients promotes fluid retention within the vascular spaces of the lung. Increased hydrostatic forces caused by left ventricular failure combined with associated increases in Pmv rapidly overcome these gradients and increase interstitial water content. Entry of low-protein content, electrolyte-rich fluid is characteristic of this type of hydrostatic edema. When microvascular endothelial surfaces are injured and their integrity is thus compromised, a protein-rich fluid moves into the interstitial and alveolar spaces. This type of increased-permeability pulmonary edema characteristic of adult respiratory distress syndrome (ARDS) also is frequently associated with the movement of cellular debris into the interstitial and alveolar spaces. Edema clearance is believed to be dependent on active transport of sodium by alveolar epithelial cells.[35]

PULMONARY GAS EXCHANGE

The most important contribution of the lung is its exchange of oxygen (O_2) and carbon dioxide (CO_2) with the environment. Because human tissue possesses limited ability to store O_2 and CO_2, a continuous exchange of these gases with the environment is required to prevent tissue hypoxia and respiratory acidosis. Furthermore, gas exchange mechanisms must be able to compensate for wide variations in cellular requirements. For example, transfer of O_2 or CO_2 may increase from basal levels of from 150 to 250 mL/min to as great as 4000 mL/min during maximum exercise. To produce this range of gas exchange with minimum energy expenditure, gas and blood must be brought into apposition in volumes sufficiently great to permit rapid equilibration by means of diffusion. Diffusing capacity of the lung diminishes with advancing age, accounting for the age-dependent reduction in $Pa{O_2}$.[36]

The partial pressure of inspired O_2 ($PI{O_2}$) is determined by the pressure of all gases (the barometric pressure), water vapor pressure (47 mm Hg at 100% saturation, as present within the airways), and the fraction of inspired gases that consists of O_2:

$$PI{O_2} = 0.2093 \times (\text{barometric pressure} - 47 \text{ mm Hg})$$

Barometric pressure is 760 mm Hg at sea level and diminishes with increases in altitude. Alveolar $P{O_2}$ ($PA{O_2}$) is determined by the $PI{O_2}$ and an estimate of the amount of O_2 exchanged for arterial (a) CO_2:

$$PA{O_2} = PI{O_2} - Pa{CO_2}/R$$

R, the respiratory exchange ratio, equals the ratio of CO_2 production ($V{CO_2}$) to O_2 consumption ($\dot{V}{O_2}$) and typically ranges from 0.8 to 0.85. It is assumed that $Pa{CO_2}$, which can be measured, is equivalent to $PA{CO_2}$.

The transfer of both O_2 and CO_2 across the alveolocapillary membrane is a passive process that is accomplished by ***diffusion***. Diffusion is dependent on (1) the physical characteristics of the membrane (it is directly proportional to the area and inversely proportional to membrane thickness), (2) the characteristics of the gas (its diffusivity and solubility), and (3) the difference in the partial pressure for that gas on either side of the membrane. Adult humans possess a total gas exchange surface of approximately 70 m^2 distributed among 300 million alveoli. Alveolocapillary membrane thickness averages 1.5 μm, and its thinnest measure is only 0.2 μm. Thus, gas exchange units are ideally suited for gas exchange with a massive, virtual sheet of capillary blood in close proximity to O_2-rich alveolar air. Diffusion of O_2 is estimated at 40 mL min^{-1} mm Hg^{-1} and may increase more than threefold as increased pulmonary blood volume and pulmonary capillary recruitment improves conditions for gas diffusion.[37]

Diffusion may be impaired by (1) thickened alveolocapillary membranes, as present in pulmonary fibrosis, (2) diminished driving pressure ($PA{O_2}$), and (3) reduced equilibration time (i.e., increased cardiac output during exercise or decreased number of pulmonary capillaries). Isolated diffusion abnormalities rarely impair gas exchange unless the problem is particularly severe. Exercise reduces the time for O_2 transfer by increasing blood flow through alveolar capillaries. When combined with a thickened alveolocapillary membrane, significant hypoxemia may result. Generally, an increasing fraction of inspired oxygen ($FI{O_2}$) easily overcomes diffusion-induced hypoxemia.

The ventilation-perfusion ratio ($\dot{V}/\dot{Q}$) is a major determinant of gas exchange. $\dot{V}/\dot{Q}$ may vary from zero in lung units that are unventilated but perfused (shunt) to infinity in lung units that are ventilated but not perfused (dead space). In young individuals, the mean $\dot{V}/\dot{Q}$ is 1.0.[38] Within the lungs of normal individuals, considerable regional variability in $\dot{V}/\dot{Q}$ exists as a consequence of the effects of gravity. Both ventilation and blood flow increase in more dependent lung regions. However, blood flow increases to a greater extent such that $\dot{V}/\dot{Q}$ is less than 1.0 in these dependent regions.

At the apex of the lung in an upright individual, $\dot{V}/\dot{Q}$ exceeds 3.0 as blood flow falls more dramatically than ventilation.[39] Low $\dot{V}/\dot{Q}$ most commonly develops as a result of reduced ventilation from structural or functional abnormalities of the airways but may result from overperfusion of normally ventilated units, as is observed following pulmonary embolism.[40] High $\dot{V}/\dot{Q}$ results from underperfusion secondary to alveolar destruction or vascular obstruction. High $\dot{V}/\dot{Q}$ may be created artificially by mechanical ventilation that employs excessive positive end-expiratory pressure.

During mechanical ventilation, increased $\dot{V}/\dot{Q}$ results in hypoxemia and hypercapnia if minute ventilation is maintained without change. However, in most clinical settings in which $\dot{V}/\dot{Q}$ mismatch occurs, hypercapnia is matched by increases in expired minute ventilation ($\dot{V}E$), leading to normocapnia or even hypocapnia. The greater the degree of $\dot{V}/\dot{Q}$ inequality, the greater the $\dot{V}E$ that must be produced to maintain normal or reduced $Paco_2$. Hypoxemia resulting from $\dot{V}/\dot{Q}$ inequality responds to a varying degree to increases in FIO_2, depending on the severity of the $\dot{V}/\dot{Q}$ inequality present. When the $\dot{V}/\dot{Q}$ inequality is mild, Pao_2 increases almost linearly as FIO_2 is increased. As the degree of $\dot{V}/\dot{Q}$ inequality worsens, improving Pao_2 by O_2 administration becomes more difficult. Correction of hypercapnia requires an increase in alveolar ventilation.

The term *shunt* refers to blood entering systemic arteries without first flowing through ventilated lung units.[41] Small amounts of shunt are normally present. One per cent to 3% of venous return blood flows directly into the systemic circulation, through the bronchial and left ventricular thebesian vessels. A variety of conditions may produce considerably larger shunt fractions. Pathways for shunted blood may run through an anatomic channel, such as an atrial or ventricular septal defect, if pulmonary pressures are great enough to reverse the normal direction of blood flow. Rarely, blood may flow through pulmonary arteriovenous malformations. More commonly, however, shunts result from the passage of blood through pulmonary capillaries in contact with alveoli that are atelectatic or filled with fluid or inflammatory exudate. Increased shunt fractions result in hypoxemia, and hypercapnia rarely develops unless shunts are large and increased ventilation is prevented. Hypoxemia is relatively resistant to correction by means of the mere increase of FIO_2, especially with larger shunts. With shunt fractions of 30% and greater, administration of O_2 in concentrations as high as 100% has a minimal impact on the Pao_2.

CONTROL OF VENTILATION

Despite large variations in O_2 consumption and CO_2 production and changing environmental conditions, the respiratory system normally maintains Pao_2 and $Paco_2$ within narrow limits. These parameters are tightly regulated by the precise adjustment of ventilation that involves a complex network of feedback controls. The principal components of this network are as follows[42]:

1. *Sensors*, which gather information on blood chemistry (chemoreceptors) and mechanical actions of the lung and chest wall (mechanoreceptors).
2. A *central controller*, which processes this information and sends instructions for making short-term and long-term adjustments in accordance with metabolic needs.
3. The *controlled system*, within which respiratory muscles contract and relax in a coordinated, efficient fashion to adjust alveolar ventilation.

The major elements of respiratory control are depicted in Figure 107–4. $Paco_2$ is the single most important factor in the control of ventilation under normal conditions. In the course of daily activity, $Paco_2$ is likely maintained within 3 mm Hg, although higher levels may occur during sleep. The effects of hypoxic ventilatory drive are minimal in the day-to-day control of ventilation, although it does become critically important in patients who suffer from severe lung disease and chronic hypercapnia.

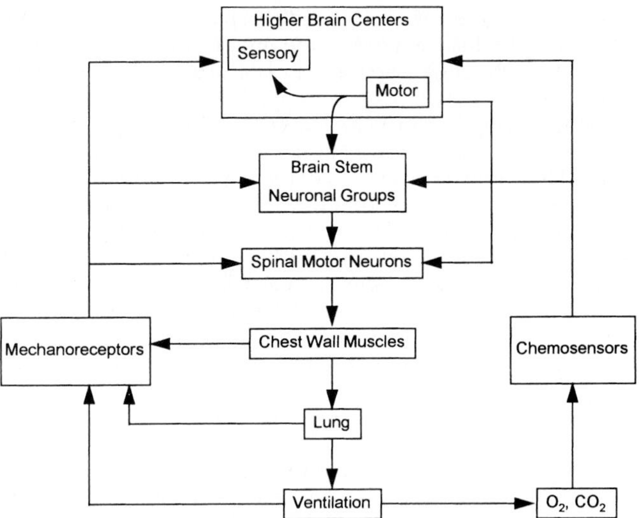

Figure 107–4. Major components of the respiratory control system. (Adapted from Strohl KP: Respiratory control. *In*: Pulmonary Critical Care Medicine. Bone RE, Dantzker DR, George RB, et al [Eds]. St. Louis, Mosby-Year Book, 1993, p 9.)

Sensors

Chemoreceptors

Central chemoreceptors are the most important receptors involved in the minute-to-minute control of ventilation. These receptors are situated near the ventral surface of the medulla and respond to changes in the hydrogen ion (H^+) concentration of the surrounding brain and extracellular fluid. In conscious humans, central chemoreceptors account for 70% to 80% of the ventilatory response to hypercapnia.[43] Extracellular fluid acid-base homeostasis is governed by the cerebrospinal fluid, local blood flow, and local cellular metabolism. Cerebrospinal fluid is separated from blood by the blood-brain barrier; this barrier is relatively impermeable to H^+ and bicarbonate ions, but CO_2 diffuses across it readily. Carbon dioxide levels in blood regulate ventilation chiefly by affecting the H^+ concentration of cerebrospinal fluid. An increase in CO_2 (and thus in extracellular fluid H^+ level) stimulates ventilation, whereas diminished levels inhibit ventilation. Increases in blood Pco_2 over a wide range cause a virtually linear increase in ventilation. Tidal volume increases first, and increases in respiratory frequency follow.

Peripheral chemoreceptors are located in carotid bodies at the bifurcation of the common carotid arteries and in aortic bodies near the aortic arch. Impulses from these chemoreceptors are carried by the ninth and 10th cranial nerves, respectively. Peripheral chemoreceptors respond primarily to hypoxemia, although carotid body receptors respond to a limited extent to hypercapnia and increased H^+ ion concentration. This response is particularly important with respect to the immediate increase in ventilation associated with metabolic acidosis.[30] Sensitivity to changes in Pao_2 begins at around 50 mm Hg; however, the maximum response occurs at a Pao_2 below 50 mm Hg.[23] Patients undergoing bilateral carotid body resection have complete loss of hypoxic ventilatory drive.

Mechanoreceptors

Three types of respiratory mechanoreceptors exist:

- Stretch receptors present in airway smooth muscles
- Irritant receptors in airway epithelium
- Juxtacapillary (J) receptors situated in the lung interstitium

Stretch receptors lie within airway smooth muscle and respond to lung distention. Impulses from stretch receptors travel along the vagus nerve via large myelinated fibers. The primary effects of activation are the inhibition of inspiration, promotion of expiration, and initiation of the Hering-Breuer reflex (a slowing of respiratory frequency due to increases in expiratory time).[31, 44] Stretch receptor activity is sustained during lung inflation. By promoting full expiration, stretch receptor activity helps to preserve inspiratory muscle function.

J receptors are believed to reside in alveolar walls near capillaries and to become activated in response to distention of pulmonary capillaries, increases in the interstitial fluid volume of alveolar walls, or exposure to chemical agents such as histamine. J-receptor impulses travel up the vagus nerve in slowly conducting, nonmyelinated fibers and result in rapid, shallow breathing. Intense stimulation may produce apnea, laryngeal closure, or both. Investigators believe that J receptors play a significant role in the sensation of dyspnea associated with pulmonary edema and interstitial lung disease.

Irritant receptors lie between airway epithelial cells and are stimulated by noxious gases (e.g., nitrogen dioxide, sulfur dioxide, and ammonia), cigarette smoke, inhaled dusts, particulate matter, cold air, and mechanical traction such as atelectasis or reduced lung compliance. Impulses travel up the vagus nerve in myelinated fibers and rapidly (within seconds) induce bronchoconstriction, coughing, and rapid, shallow breathing. The resultant pattern of breathing, in combination with cough and airway constriction, may limit penetration of noxious agents into the lung.

Intercostal muscles and the diaphragm contain muscle spindles that sense elongation of the muscle tissue and reflexly control the strength of contraction. Joint receptors and tendon receptors in the chest wall also sense movement and thus help to control ventilation. These receptors may be involved in the sensation of dyspnea that accompanies large respiratory efforts. The mechanoreceptors associated with respiratory muscles are innervated by spinal nerves and monitor changes in joint movement and in the length and tension of the muscles themselves.

The Central Controller

The central controller is located in the pons and medulla and comprises three principal neuron groups[25]:

1. The medullary respiratory center in the reticular formation of the medulla, which provides inherent rhythmicity.
2. The apneustic center in the lower pons.
3. The pneumotaxic center in the upper pons, which regulates the respiratory rate.

The interaction of cells primarily associated with inspiration and those associated with expiration produces the inherent rhythmicity of ventilation. In the event that all afferent stimuli are abolished, this rhythm continues, although somewhat irregularly.

Breathing is under voluntary control to a considerable extent, and the cortex can "override" the function of the brain stem respiratory centers within limits (i.e., with breath holding). The limbic system and hypothalamus may affect breathing patterns such as those present in highly emotional states (e.g., fear). The ventilatory response to loaded breathing is accompanied by activation of cortical and subcortical regions associated with motor control, as recently demonstrated by positron emission tomography (PET) scanning.[45]

The Controlled System

The controlled system consists of the respiratory muscles and thoracic cage (discussed earlier). Controlled ventilation is the result of highly coordinated contraction and relaxation of these muscles. Ventilation is determined by tidal volume and frequency. Tidal volume can be varied when the inspiratory time or the rate of lung inflation is changed. Each of these factors is separately controlled. Both chemical and nonchemical input affect the rate of inspiratory activity (and therefore the rate of lung inflation). In contrast, pulmonary stretch receptors and higher central nervous system structures (but not chemoreceptors) influence the duration of inspiration.[27]

This complex system of checks and balances serves to maintain smooth, efficient ventilation and gas exchange during health, yet it also responds to sudden stresses and the crisis of disease. Multiple layers of feedback compensate for disruption in one or more afferent pathways. Conflicting demands or signals (or both) coming from different receptors may in part be responsible for the production of dyspnea.

LUNG DEFENSE

Continual assault by airborne particulate matter or infectious material demands that the lung possess well-developed defense mechanisms. Primarily, respirable particles deposited on central or mainstem airways are subject to physical removal by sneeze or cough mechanisms. Secondarily, particles are subject to mucociliary clearance, which is accomplished by the continual beating of the ciliary ladder. Once impacted on ciliary structures that blanket the respiratory epithelium, particulate matter moves toward the mouth on a thin, electrolyte-rich film. The activity of mucociliary clearance is highly influenced by adequacy of bronchial circulation.[46] Clearance of particulate material and microorganisms reaching beyond these areas to the terminal airways of the lung is performed by lung phagocytes, primarily resident macrophages, and neutrophils recruited to the airspaces.

Lung Mononuclear Phagocytes

Macrophages constitute the central phagocytic defenses of the lung and represent the key resident phagocytes of the alveoli and peripheral airways that interact with various cells and molecules. Macrophages arise from circulating blood monocytes and, when mature, are capable of secreting critical substances that control multiple aspects of lung host defense (Table 107–1). Following differentiation, macrophages exhibit far greater oxidative microbicidal activity than blood monocytes.[47] The interstitial space of the lung is occupied by populations of macrophages (i.e., interstitial macrophages) with slightly dissimilar functions. Macrophages are characterized by lobulated nuclei, vacuolated cytoplasm, numerous mitochondria, and lysosomes. Alveolar macrophages are heterogeneous cell populations that exhibit varied receptor expression and kinetically different enzyme and cytokine secretion.

Macrophages can be considered mobile scavengers that are attracted to an infected focus. On arrival at the focus, macrophages ingest non-self antigens, bacteria, viruses, and fungi.

TABLE 107–1. Secretory Products of Alveolar Macrophages

Enzymes	***Platelet-Activating Factor***
Elastase	***Arachidonate Metabolites***
Plasminogen activator	Leukotrienes (LTB_4, LTC_4, LTD_4, and LTE_4)
Acid hydrolase	
Oxygen Metabolites	***C-X-C Chemokines***
Hydrogen peroxide	Interleukin-8
Superoxide anion	
Singlet oxygen	***Cytokines***
Complement Components	Interleukin-1
	Tumor necrosis factor
Enzyme Inhibitors	
Alpha$_2$-macroglobulin	

They are capable of inactivating viable, virulent encapsulated organisms. Alveolar macrophages phagocytose respirable particles from 0.5 to 3 μm in diameter. The presence of surface receptors to Fc fragments of several immunoglobulins (IgG1, IgA, IgE) and to the complement fragment C3b permits the recognition of microorganisms and is essential for phagocytosis. Through phagocytosis and the production of reactive oxygen intermediates (e.g., superoxide anion, [O_2^-]; hydrogen peroxide [H_2O_2, hydroxyl radical (•OH)]), reactive nitrogen intermediates, and proteolytic enzymes, alveolar macrophages eliminate microorganisms and particles from distal airways.[48, 49] Production of the oxygen-derived molecule hypochlorous acid (HOCl) generated through the hydrogen peroxide-myeloperoxidase system greatly enhances the killing efficiency of alveolar macrophages once phagocytosis has been accomplished.

Susceptibility of Microorganisms to Alveolar Macrophage Killing

The ability of alveolar macrophages to eliminate microbes is a function of the inoculum size and of the strain of organisms reaching the distal airways. When activated by lymphokines, alveolar macrophages are extremely active against *Pneumocystis carinii*, cytomegalovirus, *Legionella pneumophila*, and *Cryptococcus neoformans* killing through the mechanisms cited earlier.[50] Organisms such as *Mycobacterium tuberculosis* and *M. avium-intracellulare*, once phagocytosed, can survive within macrophages, able to live for long periods in the alveolar space without the presence of bactericidal antibiotics and represent the nidus of eventual infection.[51] Certain pathogens do not appear to be affected by macrophage bactericidal activity. These organisms include *Escherichia coli*, *Listeria monocytogenes*, and protein A–positive staphylococci.

Recruitment of Neutrophils to the Alveolar Space by Macrophages

Alveolar macrophages form one of the major constituents in human lung host defense. Following the onset of a high-inoculum infection, lung macrophages play a large role in orchestrating the host's response. Terashima and colleagues[52] showed that alveolar macrophages promoted the release of polymorphonuclear neutrophils (PMNs) from bone marrow when challenged by a particulate load. Similarly, macrophages recruit PMNs from the circulation to boost local host defenses within the alveolar space. Macrophages promote PMN movement into the alveolus by synthesizing and releasing lipid and peptide chemoattractant substances (Fig. 107–5). Cytokines secreted by alveolar macrophages, such as interleukin-1, interleukin-8, and tumor necrosis factor as well as the potent lipoxygenase metabolite leukotriene B_4, all serve to drive chemotaxis of PMN into a site of infection. Depletion of macrophage populations in the alveolar spaces of rats resulted in a dramatic reduction of PMN recruitment into the lungs following inoculation with gram-negative organisms (i.e., *Pseudomonas aeruginosa, Klebsiella pneumoniae*), resulting in overwhelming infection.[53, 54] During the process of migration, PMNs are activated to enhance bactericidal activity by many of these chemoattractant molecules; this provides a population of PMNs fully primed for bactericidal activity upon arrival.[55]

Bailie and colleagues[56] have underscored the critical importance of leukotrienes secreted by alveolar macrophages in a strain of mice made leukotriene (LT) deficient by gene knockout technology. LT-deficient mice exhibited severe impairments in bacterial phagocytosis and killing and significantly higher lethality following *K. pneumoniae* infection.

Role of Lymphocytes and Natural Killer Cells

Approximately 10% of nonmacrophage lung effector cells other than macrophages are lymphocytes. Five per cent of lymphocytes are plasma or B cells located in the lung parenchyma. B cells secrete IgG and IgA into the airways. These immunoglobulins play an important role in host defense. In its secretory form, IgA promotes clearance of microorganisms from the tracheobronchial tree, whereas IgG acts as an opsonic protein. Bacteria and fungi opsonized with specific IgG molecules and complement factor C3b are attacked and killed by alveolar macrophages. The factors that control the trafficking of lymphocytes to the lung are incompletely understood, and it is likely that lung macrophage populations recruit lymphocytes to the lung via the secretion of various lymphokines.

T cells are the largest population of lymphocytes in the lung. They comprise CD4 (helper) and CD8 (suppressor) cells in proportions similar to those present in the circulation. Following an infectious (bacterial, vital) or antigen challenge, T cells capable of nonspecific cytotoxicity represent a first line of defense killing in a specific fashion. If high antigen loads overwhelm these initial defenses, phagocytosis by alveolar macrophages is required. Antigen is then presented to T cells. Antigen presentation leads to the production of critical proinflammatory peptides (interleukin-1, interleukin-2, interferon-γ, tumor necrosis factor-α), which result in both the expansion of populations of specific cytotoxic lymphocytes and the recruitment of neutrophils from the circulation (Fig.

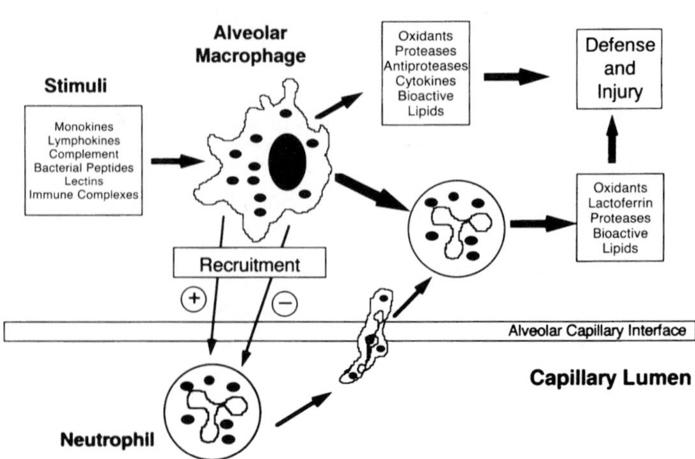

Figure 107–5. Stimulation and interaction of the alveolar macrophage and blood neutrophil in cellular recruitment and activation, which result in lung defense and lung injury.

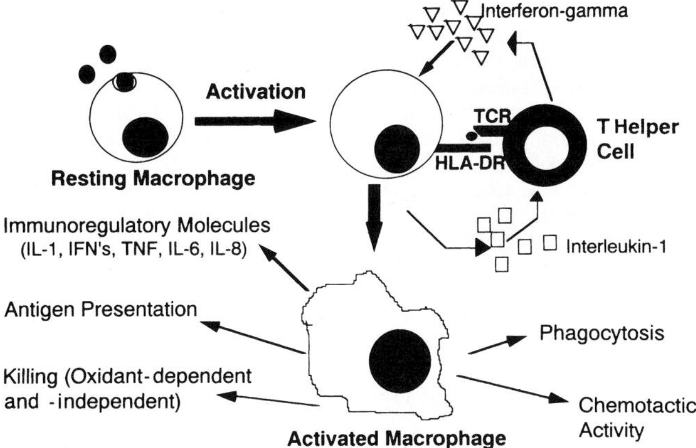

Figure 107–6. Central role of the alveolar macrophage in antigen presentation to T lymphocytes and in primary clearance of invading microorganisms. IL = interleukin; IFN = interferon; TNF = tumor necrosis factor; TCR = T cell receptor; HLA-DR = human leukocyte antigen DR.

107–6). The complex orchestration of inflammatory events described here promotes a specific response to both bacterial and viral targets.

Metabolic Functions of the Lung

It has become increasingly clear that the lung is an important site for the metabolism of circulating and locally produced substances as well as of exogenously administered agents. Lung metabolism results in alteration of exogenously administered substances modifying or enhancing their activity or, in some cases, inactivating or detoxifying metabolites. As noted earlier, the lung is exposed to the entire blood volume and has continual exposure to inhaled gases and particulate matter. Pulmonary endothelial surfaces metabolize a number of biogenic, blood-borne substances, including (1) prostaglandins of the E and F series, (2) amines, such as norepinephrine and serotonin, (3) peptides, such as angiotensin I and bradykinin, and (4) adenine nucleotides and adenosine.[57] The lungs play an important role in the regulation of circulating levels of these substances. Experimental animal and human studies have applied changes in the pulmonary uptake of these substances to address questions regarding pulmonary vascular disease and endothelial injury; the observations made in these studies may become important in clinical settings.[58, 59] Uptake and metabolism of drugs such as anesthetic agents is of clinical importance. Surfactant metabolism is also highly important in health and disease.

A variety of xenobiotic or foreign agents can produce lung damage.[39] Among the most common are (1) chemotherapeutic agents, such as bleomycin and cyclophosphamide, (2) antibiotics, such as nitrofurantoin, and (3) antiarrhythmics, such as amiodarone. The mechanisms producing injury are varied and incompletely defined but include the generation of oxygen free radicals, impairment of antioxidant systems, or the production of proinflammatory lipids, such as platelet activating factor.[60] Zitnik and colleagues[61] showed that amiodarone exerted significant effects on alveolar macrophages up-regulating production of the reactive oxygen species superoxide anion. Last, lung metabolism and the production of oxygen free radicals stand as an important intermediate step in the production of lung injury, such as that observed following ischemia-reperfusion involved in lung transplantation.[62]

References

1. Mecca RS: Pulmonary physiology. *In*: Respiratory Failure. Kirby RR, Taylor RW (Eds). Chicago, Year Book Medical Publishers, 1986, p 22.
2. Anderson WM, Zavecz JH: The chest wall, diaphragm, and mediastinum. *In*: Pulmonary and Critical Care Medicine. Bone RC, Dantzker DR, George RB, et al (Eds). St. Louis, Mosby-Year Book, 1993, pp 1-19.
3. Sieck GC: Diaphragm muscle: Structure and functional organization. Clin Chest Med 1988; 9:195.
4. Polkey MI, Harris ML, Hughes PD, Hamnegard CH, Lyons D, Green M, Moxham J: The contractile properties of the elderly human diaphragm. Am J Respir Crit Care Med 1997; 155:1560.
5. DeTroyer A, Estenne M: Functional anatomy of the respiratory muscles. Clin Chest Med 1988; 9:175.
6. Rodarte JR: Mechanics of respiration. *In*: Pulmonary and Critical Care Medicine. Bone RC, Dantzker DR, George RB, et al (Eds). St. Louis, Mosby-Year Book, 1993, pp 1-16.
7. De Troyer A: Effect of hyperinflation on the diaphragm. Eur Respir J 1997; 10:708.
8. Kuna ST, Smickley JS, Vanoye CR: Respiratory-related pharyngeal constrictor muscle activity in normal human adults. Am J Respir Crit Care Med 1997; 155:1991.
9. Agostoni E: Mechanics of the pleural space. Physiol Rev 1972; 52:57.
10. Comroe JH Jr: Physiology of Respiration. 2nd ed. Chicago, Year Book Medical Publishers, 1974.
11. Bastacky J, Hayes TL, Schmidt BV: Lung structure as revealed by microdissection. Am Rev Respir Dis 1983; 128:S7.
12. Basbaum CB, Finkbeiner WE: Mucus-producing cells of the airway. *In*: Lung Biology in Health and Disease. Vol 41. Lung Cell Biology. Massaro D (Ed). New York, Marcel Dekker, 1989, p 37.
13. Albertine KH: Structure of the respiratory system, as related to its primary function. *In*: Pulmonary and Critical Care Medicine. Bone RC, Dantzker ER, George RB, et al (Eds). St. Louis, Mosby-Year Book, 1993, pp 1-22.
14. Widdicombe JG, Pack RJ: The Clara cell. Eur J Respir Dis 1982; 63:202.
15. Massaro D: Nonciliated bronchiolar epithelial (Clara) cells. *In*: Lung Biology in Health and Disease. Lung Cell Biology. Vol 41. Massaro D (Ed). New York, Marcel Dekker, 1989, p 81.
16. Van Scott MR, Boucher RC: Current perspectives of Clara cell function. News Physiol Sci (NIPS) 1988; 3:13.
17. Walker SR, Williams MC, Benson B: Immunocytochemical localization of the major surfactant apoproteins in type II cells, Clara cells, and alveolar macrophages of rat lung. J Histochem Cytochem 1986; 34:1137.
18. Ebina M, Yaegashi H, Takahashi T, et al: Distribution of smooth muscles along the bronchial tree. Am Rev Respir Dis 1990; 141:1322.
19. Richardson JB: Recent progress in pulmonary innervation. Am Rev Respir Dis 1983; 128:S65.
20. Will JA, DiAugustine RP: Lung neuroendocrine cells and regulatory peptides: Distribution, functional studies, and implications. A symposium. Exp Lung Res 1982; 3:185.
21. Suzuki Y, Fujita Y, Kogishi K: Reconstitution of tubular myelin from synthetic lipids and proteins associated with pig pulmonary surfactant. Am Rev Respir Dis 1989; 140:75.
22. King RJ, Clements JA: Surface active materials from dog lung: Composition and physiological correlations. Am J Pathol 1972; 223:715.
23. Whitset JA, Hull W, Ross G, et al: Characteristics of human surfactant-associated proteins. Pediatr Res 1985; 19:501.
24. Johansson J, Curstedt T: Molecular structures and interactions of pulmonary surfactant components. Eur J Biochem 1997; 244:675.
25. Mensah E, Niranjan M, Kumar L, Nielsen L, Lwebuga-Muksa J: Distribution of alveolar type II cells in neonatal and adult rat lung revealed by RT-PCR in situ. Am J Physiol 1996; 271:L178.
26. Ryan US, Ryan JW, Smith DS: Alveolar type II cells: Studies on the mode of release of lamellar bodies. Tissue Cell 1975; 7:587.
27. Wright JR: Clearance and recycling of pulmonary surfactant. Am J Pathol 1990; 259:1.
28. Kennedy M, Phelps D, Ingenito E: Mechanisms of surfactant dysfunction in early acute lung injury. Exp Lung Res 1997; 23:171.

29. Singh S, Evans TW: Nitric oxide, the biological mediator of the decade: Fact or fiction? Eur Respir J 1997; 10:699–707.
30. Ward JP, Robertson TP: The role of the endothelium in hypoxic pulmonary vasoconstriction. Exp Physiol 1995; 80:793–801.
31. Cargill RI, Lipworth BJ: The role of the renin-angiotensin and natriuretic peptide systems in the pulmonary vasculature. Br J Clin Pharmacol 1995; 40:11.
32. Hillier SC, Graham JA, Hanger CC, Godbey PS, Glenny RW: Wagner WW Jr: Hypoxic vasoconstriction in pulmonary arterioles and venules. J Appl Physiol 1997; 82:1084.
33. West JB, Wagner PD: Pulmonary gas exchange in bioengineering. *In*: Bioengineering Aspects of the Lung. West JB (Ed). New York, Marcel Dekker, 1977, p 361.
34. Weibel ER: Morphometry of the Human Lung. New York, Academic Press, 1963.
35. Filippatos GS, Hughes WF, Qiao R, Sznajder JI, Uhal BD: Mechanisms of liquid flux across pulmonary alveolar epithelial cell monolayers. In Vitro Cell Dev Biol Anim 1997; 33:195–200.
36. Guenard H, Marthan R: Pulmonary gas exchange in elderly subjects. Eur Respir J 1996; 9:2573.
37. Dantzker DR: Pulmonary gas exchange. *In*: Pulmonary and Critical Care Medicine. Bone RC, Dantzker DR, George RB, et al (Eds). St. Louis, Mosby-Year Book, 1993, pp 1–13.
38. Wagner PD, Laravuso RB, Uhl RR, et al: Continuous distributions of ventilation-perfusion ratios in normal subjects breathing air and 100 per cent O_2. J Clin Invest 1974; 54:54.
39. West JB: Ventilation/Blood Flow and Gas Exchange. 3rd ed. Oxford, Blackwell Scientific Publications, 1977.
40. Dantzker DR, Brook CH, DeHart P, et al: Gas exchange in adult respiratory distress syndrome and the effects of positive end-expiratory pressure. Am Rev Respir Dis 1979; 120:1039.
41. West JB: Respiratory Physiology: The Essentials. 2nd ed. Baltimore, Williams & Wilkins, 1979.
42. Strohl KP: Respiratory control. *In*: Pulmonary and Critical Care Medicine. Bone RC, Dantzker DR, George RB, et al (Eds). St. Louis, Mosby-Year Book, 1993, p 1–16.
43. Merrill EG, Lipski J, Kubin L, et al: Origin of the expiratory inhibition of nucleus tractus solitarius inspiratory neurons. Brain Res 1983; 263:43.
44. Gautier H, Boonora M, Gaudy M, et al: Breuer-Hering inflation reflex and breathing pattern in anesthetized humans and cats. J Appl Physiol 1981; 51:1162.
45. Fink GR, Corfield DR, Murphy K, Kobayashi I, Dettmers C, Adams L, Frackowiak RS, Guz A: Human cerebral activity with increasing inspiratory force: A study using positron emission tomography. J Appl Physiol 1996; 81:1295.
46. Wagner EM, Foster WM: Importance of airway blood flow on particle clearance from the lung. J Appl Physiol 1996; 81:1878.
47. Kemmerich B, Rossing TH, Pennington JE: Comparative oxidative microbicidal activity of human blood monocytes and alveolar macrophages and activation by recombinant gamma interferon. Am Rev Respir Dis 1987; 136:266.
48. Johnson RB, Godzik CA, Cohn ZA: Increased superoxide anion production by immunologically activated and chemically elicited macrophages. J Exp Med 1978; 148:115.
49. Miles PR, Bowman L, Rengasamy A, Huffman L: Constitutive nitric oxide production by rat alveolar macrophages. Am J Physiol 1998; 274:L360.
50. Nathan CF, Murray HW, Wiebe ME, et al: Identification of interferon-gamma as the lymphokine that activates human macrophage oxidative metabolism and antimicrobial activity. J Exp Med 1983; 158:670.
51. Reynolds HY: Respiratory infections may reflect deficiencies in host defense mechanisms. Dis Mon 1985; 31:1.
52. Terashima T, Wiggs B, English D, et al: Phagocytosis of small carbon particles (PM10) by alveolar macrophages stimulates the release of polymorphonuclear leukocytes from bone marrow. Am J Respir Crit Care Med 1997; 155:1441.
53. Hashimoto S, Pittet JF, Hong K, et al: Depletion of alveolar macrophages decreases neutrophil chemotaxis to *Pseudomonas* airspace infection. Am J Physiol 1996; 270:L819.
54. Broug-Holub E, Toews GB, van Iwaarden JF, et al: Alveolar macrophages are required for protective pulmonary defenses in murine klebsiella pneumonia: Elimination of alveolar macrophages increases neutrophil recruitment but decreases bacterial clearance and survival. Infect Immun 1997; 65:1139.
55. Pennington JE, Rossing TH, Boerth LW, et al: Isolation and partial characterization of a human alveolar macrophage-derived neutrophil-activating factor. J Clin Invest 1985; 75:1230.
56. Bailie MB, Standiford TJ, Laichalk LL, et al: Leukotriene-deficient mice manifest enhanced lethality from klebsiella pneumonia in association with decreased alveolar macrophage phagocytic and bactericidal activities. J Immunol 1996; 157:5221.
57. Dawson CA, Roerig DL, Linehan JH: Evaluation of endothelial injury in the human lung. Clin Chest Med 1989; 10:13.
58. Hart CM, Block ER: Lung serotonin metabolism. Clin Chest Med 1989; 10:59.
59. Duncan CA: Lung metabolism of xenobiotic compounds. Clin Chest Med 1989; 10:49.
60. Chen J, Ziboh V, Giri SN: Up-regulation of platelet-activating factor receptors in lung and alveolar macrophages in bleomycin-hamster model of pulmonary fibrosis. J Pharmacol Exp Ther 1997; 280:1219.
61. Zitnik RJ, Cooper JAD, Rankin JA, Sussman J: Effects of in vitro amiodarone exposure on alveolar macrophage inflammatory mediator production. Am J Med Sci 1992; 304:352.
62. Jenkinson SG: Free radical effects on lung metabolism. Clin Chest Med 1989; 10:37.

108

Respiratory Muscle Function

André De Troyer, MD, PhD

The so-called respiratory muscles are those muscles that provide the motive power for the act of breathing. Although many of these muscles are involved in a variety of activities, such as speech production, cough, vomiting, and trunk motion, their primary task is therefore to displace the chest wall rhythmically to pump gas in and out of the lungs. Depending on whether their contraction expands or deflates the lungs, they may be *inspiratory* or *expiratory* muscles.

The diaphragm is the main respiratory muscle in humans, but moving the chest wall during breathing is an integrated process that involves many muscles. During spontaneous, quiet breathing in healthy individuals, the intercostal muscles of the parasternal area and the scalene muscles contract in concert with the diaphragm to expand the entire chest wall and to inflate the lungs, and relaxation of these muscles at end-inspiration allows the respiratory system to return, through its passive elastic properties, to its resting, functional residual capacity (FRC) position. During exercise, however, as the production of carbon dioxide (CO_2) by the locomotor muscles is augmented, the regulation of chest wall muscle activation becomes more complex, involving not only an increased activation of the muscles already active during resting breathing but also the recruitment of additional muscles that augment chest wall expansion (often called the "accessory muscles"). In addition, exercise hyperpnea is associated with phasic contraction of muscles that increase expiratory airflow and rhythmically bring the respiratory system below its resting volume. Although these muscles have an expiratory action on the lungs, their relaxation at end-expiration causes an increase in lung volume; in so doing, they therefore reduce the load on the inspiratory muscles and help them meet the increased ventilatory requirements.

Breathing is primarily an automatic process, and the pattern of respiratory muscle activation is, to a large extent, "hardwired" to the central respiratory controller. Therefore, essentially similar adaptations take place when the work of breathing is increased by disease. When some respiratory muscle groups are weak or paralyzed, the remaining muscles must overcome the entire resistive and elastic load; the strain imposed on them is consequently greater than normal. Similarly, when airflow resistance is abnormally elevated or when dynamic pulmonary or chest wall compliance is abnormally reduced, the inspiratory muscles must generate a greater reduction in pleural pressure to inflate the lungs. The presence of static or dynamic hyperinflation places an additional load on these muscles by making them operate at shorter than normal lengths and by reducing their ability to lower intrathoracic pressure. When breathing at rest, patients with severe obstructive or restrictive pulmonary impairment therefore use their muscles in much the same way as normal subjects do during exercise. In such patients, however, as in patients with respiratory muscle paralysis, some of the contracting muscles may have little or no beneficial effect on the act of breathing.

The respiratory muscles are structurally and functionally skeletal muscles. As with any skeletal muscle, their actions are therefore essentially determined by their anatomy and by the structures they must displace when they contract. Consequently, this chapter starts with a discussion of the basic mechanical structure of the chest wall. It next analyzes the action of each group of muscles. For the sake of clarity, the functions of the diaphragm, the intercostal muscles, the muscles of the neck, and the muscles of the abdominal wall are examined sequentially, but the most critical aspects of the interactions among these muscle groups are also emphasized. Some specific disorders are then considered, in which respiratory muscle function is altered as a result of a particular distribution of muscle weakness or chronic lung disease. The final part of the chapter discusses the issue of respiratory muscle fatigue in chronic pulmonary diseases.

CHEST WALL

The chest wall can be thought of as consisting of two compartments, the rib cage and the abdomen, separated from each other by a thin musculotendinous structure, the diaphragm[1] (Fig. 108-1). These two compartments are mechanically arranged in parallel. Expansion of the lungs, therefore, can be accommodated by expansion of the rib cage, the abdomen, or both compartments simultaneously.

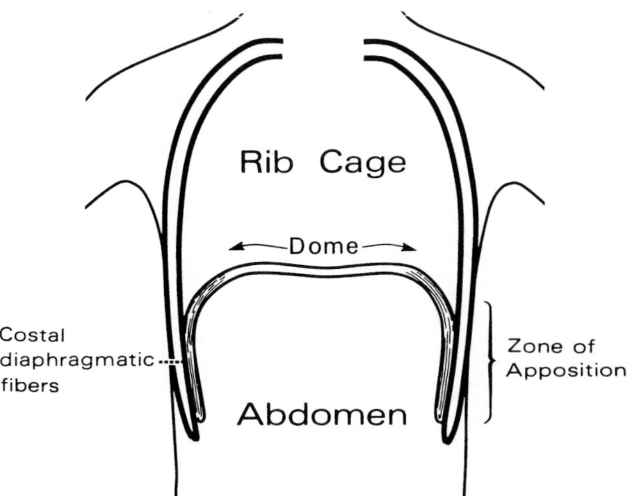

Figure 108–1. Frontal section of the chest wall at end-expiration. Note the cranial orientation of the costal diaphragmatic fibers and their apposition to the inner aspect of the lower rib cage (zone of apposition). (From De Troyer A, Loring SH: Actions of the respiratory muscles. *In:* The Thorax. 2nd ed. Vol 85. Roussos C. [Ed]. New York, Marcel Dekker, 1995, pp 535-563.)

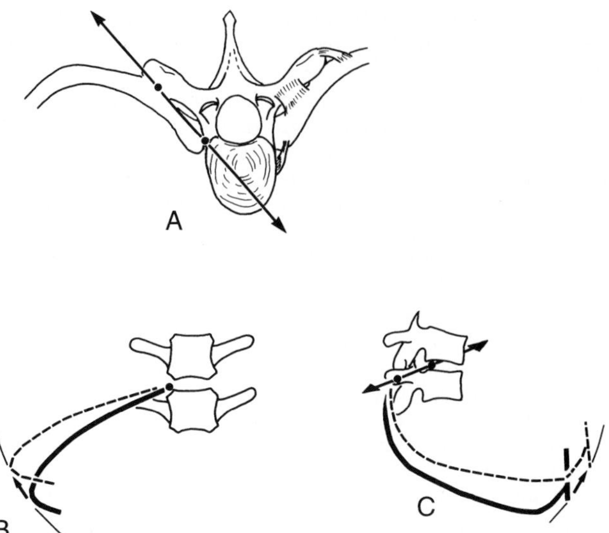

Figure 108–2. Respiratory displacements of the rib cage (*A*). Diagram of a typical thoracic vertebra and a pair of ribs (viewed from above). Each rib articulates with both the body and the transverse process of the vertebra (*closed circles*) and is bound to it by strong ligaments (*A, right*). The motion of the rib, therefore, occurs primarily through a rotation around the axis defined by these articulations (*solid line* and *double arrowhead*). From these articulations, however, the rib slopes downward and ventrally (*B* and *C*). Therefore, when the rib becomes more horizontal in inspiration (*dotted line*), it causes an increase in both the transverse (*B*) and the anteroposterior (*C*) diameter of the rib cage (*small arrows*).

Although the rib cage is a complex structure made of a series of skeletal arches, its displacements during breathing are essentially related to the motion of the ribs, and this motion is relatively straightforward. Indeed, each rib articulates by its head with the bodies of its own vertebra and the vertebra above, and by its tubercle with the transverse process of its own vertebra. The head of the rib is very closely connected to the vertebral bodies by radiate and intra-articular ligaments, such that only slight gliding movements of the articular surfaces on each other can take place. Similarly, the neck and tubercle of the rib are bound to the transverse process of the vertebra by short, strong ligaments that limit the movements of the costotransverse joint to slight cranial and caudal gliding. As a result, the costovertebral and costotransverse joints together form a hinge, and the respiratory displacements of the rib occur primarily through a rotation around the long axis of its neck,[2,3] as shown in Figure 108-2*a*. However, this axis is oriented laterally, dorsally, and caudally. In addition, the ribs are curved and slope caudally and ventrally from their costotransverse articulations, such that their ventral ends and the costal cartilages are more caudal than their dorsal part (Fig. 108-2*B* and *C*). When the ribs are displaced in the cranial direction, therefore, their ventral ends move laterally and ventrally as well as cranially, the cartilages rotate cranially around the chondrosternal junctions, and the sternum is displaced ventrally. Consequently, there is usually an increase in both the lateral diameter and the dorsoventral diameter of the rib cage (see Fig. 108-2*B* and *C*). Conversely, a displacement of the ribs in the caudal direction is usually associated with a decrease in rib cage diameters. As a corollary, the muscles that elevate the ribs as their primary action have an inspiratory effect on the rib cage, whereas the muscles that lower the ribs have an expiratory effect on the rib cage.

It is notable, however, that although every rib moves predominantly by a rotation around the long axis of its neck, the costovertebral joints of ribs 7 to 10 have less constraint on their motion than the costovertebral joints of the ribs 1 to 6. The long cartilages of ribs 8 to 10 also articulate with each other by little synovial cavities, rather than with the sternum; hence, whereas the upper ribs tend to move as a unit with the sternum, the lower ribs have some freedom to move independently.[4, 5] Both in animals and in humans, deformations of the rib cage may therefore occur under the influence of muscle contraction.

The respiratory displacements of the abdominal compartment are even more straightforward than those of the rib cage, because if one neglects the 100 to 300 mL of abdominal gas volume, its content is virtually incompressible. As a result, the abdomen behaves as a liquid-filled container, such that any local inward displacement of its boundaries results in an equal outward displacement elsewhere. Furthermore, many of these boundaries, such as the spine dorsally, the pelvis caudally, and the iliac crests laterally, are virtually fixed. Thus, the parts of the abdominal container that can be displaced are essentially limited to the ventral abdominal wall and the diaphragm. When the diaphragm contracts during inspiration (see later), therefore, its descent usually results in an outward displacement of the ventral abdominal wall; conversely, when the abdominal muscles contract, they cause, in general, an inward displacement of the belly wall, resulting in a cranial motion of the diaphragm into the thoracic cavity.

THE DIAPHRAGM

The diaphragm is anatomically unique among skeletal muscles, in that its muscle fibers radiate from a central tendinous structure (the central tendon) to insert peripherally into skeletal structures. The crural (or vertebral) portion of the diaphragmatic muscle inserts on the ventrolateral aspects of the first three lumbar vertebrae and on the aponeurotic arcuate ligaments; the costal portion inserts on the xiphoid process of the sternum and the upper margins of the lower six ribs. From their insertions, the costal fibers run cranially, so that they are directly apposed to the inner aspect of the lower rib cage (see Fig. 108–1). In standing humans at rest, this so-called zone of apposition of the diaphragm to the rib cage[6] is about 6 to 9 cm in height in the midaxillary line and occupies 25% to 30% of the total internal surface area of the rib cage. Although the older literature has suggested the possibility of an intercostal motor innervation of some portions of the diaphragm, it is now clearly established that the diaphragm's only motor supply is through the phrenic nerves, which, in humans, originate in the third, fourth, and fifth cervical segments.

Actions of the Diaphragm

As the muscle fibers of the diaphragm are activated during inspiration, they develop tension and shorten. Consequently, the axial length of the apposed diaphragm diminishes, and the dome of the diaphragm, which corresponds primarily to the central tendon, descends relative to the costal insertions of the muscle. The dome remains relatively constant in size and shape during breathing, but its descent has two effects:

1. It expands the thoracic cavity along the craniocaudal axis; hence, pleural pressure falls, and depending on whether the airways are open or closed, lung volume increases or alveolar pressure falls.

2. It produces a caudal displacement of the abdominal visceral mass and an increase in abdominal pressure, which, in turn, pushes the ventral abdominal wall outward.

In addition, because the muscle fibers of the costal diaphragm insert onto the upper margins of the lower six ribs, they also apply a force on these ribs when they contract. This force, in fact, is equal to the force exerted on the central tendon, and under normal circumstances, it is directed cranially because of the cranial orientation of the fibers (Fig. 108–3). It has, therefore, the effect of lifting the ribs and rotating them outward. The fall in pleural pressure and the increase in abdominal pressure induced by diaphragmatic contraction, however, act simultaneously on the rib cage, probably explaining why the action of the diaphragm on the rib cage has been controversial for so long.

Action of the Diaphragm on the Rib Cage

When the diaphragm in anesthetized dogs is activated selectively by electrical stimulation of the phrenic nerves, the upper ribs move caudally and the cross-sectional area of the upper portion of the rib cage decreases.[7] In contrast, the lower ribs move cranially and the cross-sectional area of the lower portion of the rib cage increases. When a bilateral pneumothorax is subsequently introduced so that the fall in pleural pressure is eliminated, isolated contraction of the diaphragm causes a greater expansion of the lower rib cage, but the dimensions of the upper rib cage now remain unchanged.[7] When contracting alone, the canine diaphragm thus has two opposing effects on the rib cage:

1. It has an expiratory action on the upper rib cage, and the fact that this action is abolished by a pneumothorax indicates that it is due to the fall in pleural pressure.

2. It has an inspiratory action on the lower rib cage. Measurements of chest wall motion (a) during phrenic nerve pacing in patients with transection of the upper cervical cord[8, 9] and (b) during resting breathing in patients who use only the diaphragm because of a traumatic transection of the lower cervical cord[10, 11] have shown that as in the dog, the diaphragm in humans has both an expiratory action on the upper rib cage and an inspiratory action on the lower rib cage.

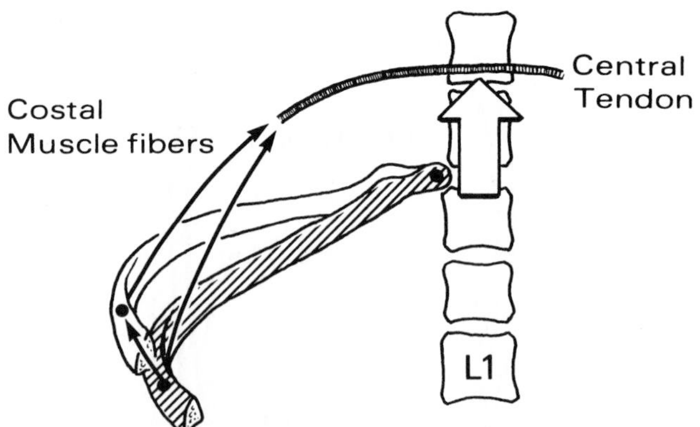

Figure 108–3. Insertional component of diaphragmatic action. During inspiration, as the fibers of the costal diaphragm contract, they exert a force on the lower ribs (*arrow*). If the abdominal visceral mass opposes effectively the descent of the diaphragmatic dome (*open arrow*), this force is oriented cranially. As a result, the lower ribs are lifted and rotate outward. (From De Troyer A: Mechanics of the chest wall muscles. *In:* Neural Control of the Respiratory Muscles. Miller AD, Bishop B, Bianchi AL [Eds]. Boca Raton, Fla, CRC Press, 1996, pp 59–73.)

Theoretical and experimental work has confirmed that the inspiratory action of the diaphragm on the lower rib cage results, in part, from the force that the muscle applies on the ribs by way of its insertions; this force is conventionally referred to as the *insertional force*.[12, 13] This inspiratory action of the diaphragm, however, is also related to its apposition to the rib cage. The zone of apposition makes the lower rib cage, in effect, part of the abdominal container, and measurements in dogs and rabbits have established that during breathing, the changes in pressure in the pleural recess between the apposed diaphragm and the rib cage are almost equal to the changes in abdominal pressure.[14] Pressure in this pleural recess rises, rather than falls, during inspiration, thus indicating that the rise in abdominal pressure is truly transmitted through the apposed diaphragm to expand the lower rib cage. This mechanism of diaphragmatic action has been called the *appositional force*.

Although the insertional and appositional forces make the normal diaphragm expand the lower rib cage, it should be appreciated that this action of the diaphragm is determined largely by the resistance provided by the abdominal contents to diaphragmatic descent (see Fig. 108-3). If this resistance is high (i.e., if abdominal compliance is low), the dome of the diaphragm descends less, so that the zone of apposition remains significant throughout inspiration and the rise in abdominal pressure is greater. Therefore, for a given diaphragmatic contraction, the appositional force is greater and the expansion of the lower rib cage is increased. Conversely, if the resistance provided by the abdominal contents is small (if the abdomen is very compliant), the dome of the diaphragm descends more easily, the zone of apposition decreases more, and the rise in abdominal pressure is smaller. Consequently, the inspiratory action of the diaphragm on the rib cage is reduced.

If the resistance provided by the abdominal contents were eliminated, not only would the zone of apposition disappear in the course of inspiration but the contracting diaphragmatic muscle fibers would also become oriented transversely inward at their insertions onto the ribs. The insertional force would then have an expiratory, rather than inspiratory, action on the lower rib cage. Indeed, when a dog is eviscerated, the diaphragm causes a decrease, rather than an increase, in lower rib cage dimensions.[7, 12, 15]

Influence of Lung Volume

The balance between pleural pressure and the insertional and appositional forces of the diaphragm is also markedly affected by changes in lung volume. As lung volume decreases from FRC to residual volume (RV), the zone of apposition enlarges, and the fraction of the rib cage exposed to pleural pressure diminishes. As a result, the appositional force increases and the effect of pleural pressure decreases, so that the inspiratory action of the diaphragm on the rib cage is enhanced. Conversely, as lung volume rises above FRC, the zone of apposition decreases, and a larger fraction of the rib cage becomes exposed to pleural pressure. The inspiratory action of the diaphragm on the rib cage is therefore diminished.[7, 12, 13]

When lung volume approaches total lung capacity (TLC), the zone of apposition all but disappears, and the diaphragmatic muscle fibers become oriented transversely inward as well as cranially. As in the eviscerated animal, the insertional force of the diaphragm is then expiratory, rather than inspiratory, in direction.

MUSCLES OF THE RIB CAGE

Intercostal Muscles

The intercostal muscles are two thin layers of muscle occupying each of the intercostal spaces; they are termed *external* and *internal* because of their surface relations, the external muscles being superficial to the internal muscles. The external intercostal muscles extend from the tubercles of the ribs dorsally to the costochondral junctions ventrally, and their fibers are oriented obliquely caudad and ventrally from the rib above to the rib below. In contrast, the internal intercostal muscles extend from the angles of the ribs dorsally to the sternum ventrally, and their fibers run obliquely caudad and dorsally from the rib above to the rib below. Thus, although the intercostal spaces in their lateral portions contain two layers of intercostal muscle running approximately at right angles to each other, the spaces contain a single muscle layer in their ventral and dorsal portions.

Ventrally, between the sternum and the chondrocostal junctions, the only fibers (also called the "parasternal intercostal muscles") are those of the internal intercostal muscles; dorsally, from the angle of the ribs to the vertebrae, the only fibers come from the external intercostal muscles. These latter fibers, however, are duplicated by a spindle-shaped muscle running in each interspace from the tip of the transverse process of the vertebra cranially to the angle of the rib caudally; this muscle is the *levator costae*. All intercostal muscles are innervated by the intercostal nerves.

Actions on the Ribs

The actions of the intercostal muscles on the ribs are conventionally regarded according to the theory proposed by Hamberger[16] in the mid-1700s. This theory is based on geometric considerations and illustrated in Figure 108-4. When an intercostal muscle contracts in one interspace, it pulls the upper rib down and the lower rib up. As the fibers of the external intercostal muscle slope obliquely caudad and ventrally from the rib above to the one below, however, their lower insertion is more distant from the center of rotation of the ribs (the vertebral articulations) than their upper insertion. When this muscle contracts, the torque acting on the lower rib is therefore greater than that acting on the upper rib, so that its net effect is to raise the ribs. The orientation of the levator costae

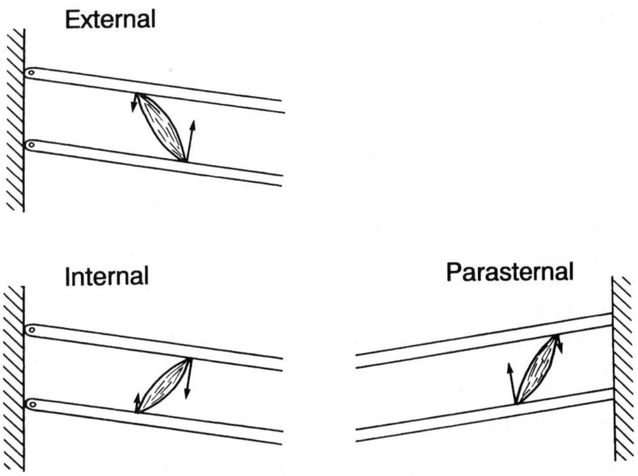

Figure 108–4. Diagram illustrating the actions of the intercostal muscles on the ribs as proposed by Hamberger (1749).[16] *Hatched area* in left panels represents the spine (*dorsal view*), and *hatched area* in the lower right panel represents the sternum (*ventral view*). The two bars oriented obliquely represent two adjacent ribs. The external and internal intercostal muscles are depicted as single bundles, and the torques acting on the ribs during contraction of these muscles are represented by arrows. (From De Troyer A: Respiratory muscle function. *In:* Respiratory Medicine. 2nd ed. Brewis RAL, Corrin B, Geddes DM, et al [Eds]. London, Bailliere Tindall, 1995, pp 125–133.)

muscle is similar to that of the external intercostal muscle, and its action is also to raise the ribs.

In contrast, the fibers of the internal intercostal muscle run obliquely caudad and dorsally from the rib above to the one below. Therefore, their lower insertion is closer to the center of rotation of the ribs than their upper insertion. As a result, when this muscle contracts, the torque acting on the lower rib is less than that acting on the upper rib, and its net effect is to lower the ribs. Hamberger[16] finally concluded that although the parasternal intercostal muscles are part of the internal intercostal layer, their action should be referred to the sternum rather than to the vertebral column; their contraction, therefore, should raise the ribs.

Several of these conclusions have received direct experimental support. When the parasternal intercostal muscles in the dog are selectively activated by electrical stimulation, they produce a cranial displacement of the ribs into which they insert and an increase in lung volume.[17] Measurements of the changes in length of the canine parasternal intercostal muscles in the different interspaces have also shown that these muscles behave like the diaphragm and invariably shorten during passive inflation; they have, therefore, a clear-cut inspiratory mechanical advantage.[18, 19] Stimulation of the levator costae muscle in a single intercostal space similarly causes a cranial displacement of the rib into which it inserts.[20]

In contrast, when either the external or the internal interosseous intercostal muscle in a single interspace is selectively stimulated in the dog, there is a mutual approximation of the adjacent ribs; however, the cranial displacement of the rib below is always greater than the caudal displacement of the rib above.[21, 22] In addition, whereas the Hamberger mechanism would predict that inflation of the relaxed respiratory system above FRC produces shortening of all the external intercostal muscles and lengthening of all the internal interosseous intercostal muscles, measurements in dogs have shown that the changes in length of these muscles are variable and largely determined by the location of the muscles along the rostrocaudal axis of the rib cage. Thus, in the rostral interspaces, these two sets of intercostal muscles tend to shorten during passive inflation, whereas in the caudal interspaces, they both tend to lengthen.[23]

The Hamberger theory is thus incomplete, and the two reasons for which it cannot entirely describe the actions of the intercostal muscles have been emphasized in two studies.[24, 25] First, this theory is based on the idea that all the ribs rotate by equal amounts around parallel axes, so that the distance between adjacent ribs remains constant. In fact, the radii of curvature of the different ribs are different, increasing from the top downward, and their rotational compliances are different as well.[19, 25] For example, in the dog, the rotational compliance of the third and fourth ribs is greater than the compliance of the more cranial and caudal ribs. As a result, both the external and internal interosseous intercostal muscles in the rostral interspaces tend to have an inspiratory mechanical advantage, and both muscle layers in the caudal interspaces tend to have an expiratory mechanical advantage.[19]

Second, the Hamberger model is planar, whereas the real ribs are curved. Consequently, the mechanical advantage of the external and internal intercostal muscles in any given interspace varies also as a function of the position of the muscle fibers along the rib. Thus, in a given rostral interspace, the inspiratory mechanical advantage of the external intercostal muscle is greatest in the dorsal region, decreases progressively as one moves around the cage, and may even be "reversed" into an expiratory mechanical advantage[25] as one approaches the sternum. The expiratory mechanical advantage of the internal intercostal muscle in a given caudal interspace is also greatest in the dorsal portion of the interspace and decreases gradually to become an inspiratory mechanical advantage in the vicinity of the sternum (parasternal intercostal muscle).

Respiratory Function

Regardless of the limitations of the Hamberger theory, a number of electromyographic (EMG) studies in dogs,[17, 26] cats,[27] and baboons[28] have clearly established that the parasternal intercostal muscles are electrically active during the inspiratory phase of the breathing cycle (Fig. 108–5). EMG recordings from intercostal muscles and nerves in these animals have also established that the external intercostal and levator costae muscles are active only during inspiration (see Fig. 108–5), whereas the internal interosseous intercostal muscles are active only during expiration.[20, 27–32]

Of interest, the inspiratory activation of the external intercostal muscles takes place predominantly in the dorsal region of the rostral interspaces,[27, 29, 32] where the muscles are thickest and have the greatest inspiratory mechanical advantage.[25] These features correspond to an inspiratory action on the rib cage, and indeed, when the diaphragm and parasternal intercostal muscles in dogs are denervated so that the external intercostal and levator costae muscles are the only muscles active during inspiration, the ribs move cranially.[20] Conversely, expiratory activation of the internal interosseous intercostal muscles is predominant in the caudal interspaces,[32] where the muscles have a greater expiratory mechanical advantage.[25] This pattern corresponds to an expiratory action on the rib cage and the lung.[33]

Although the parasternal intercostal muscles, the external intercostal muscles in the rostral interspaces, and the levator costae muscles contract together during inspiration and contribute to the inspiratory cranial displacement of the ribs, there is substantial evidence that in anesthetized animals the parasternal intercostal muscles play a larger role than the external intercostal and levator costae muscles during resting breathing. In anesthetized dogs and cats, the cranial motion of the ribs occurs together with a caudal displacement of the sternum,[4, 17, 34] and this pattern of motion results from the action of the parasternal intercostal muscles.[17] Indeed, selective stimulation of these muscles causes the sternum to move caudally, whereas both the external intercostal and levator costae muscles displace the sternum cranially.[20, 33] More important, when the canine parasternal intercostal muscles are denervated in all interspaces, the inspiratory cranial motion of the ribs is reduced by 60%, yet the inspiratory activities of the external intercostal and levator costae muscles are markedly increased.[35] Presumably, these increases in inspiratory activity reduce the decrease in cranial rib motion resulting from the denervation of the parasternal intercostal muscles. In contrast, when the canine external intercostal muscles in all interspaces are severed and the parasternal intercostal muscles are left intact, the inspiratory cranial displacement of the ribs decreases by only 10%, although the inspiratory activity of the parasternal intercostal muscles is unchanged.[35]

Normal humans breathing at rest also have inspiratory activity in the parasternal intercostal muscles and in the external intercostal muscles of the most rostral interspaces.[36, 37] Although it is difficult to compare the amounts of activity recorded in different muscles, activity in the human external intercostal muscles also appears to be less consistent and to involve fewer motor units than activity in the parasternal intercostal muscles.[36–38] This observation suggests that in humans, as in quadrupeds, the contribution of the parasternal intercostal muscles to resting breathing is greater than that of the external intercostal muscles. In contrast to the parasternal intercostal muscles, the external intercostal and levator costae muscles are abundantly supplied with muscle spindles,[31, 39]

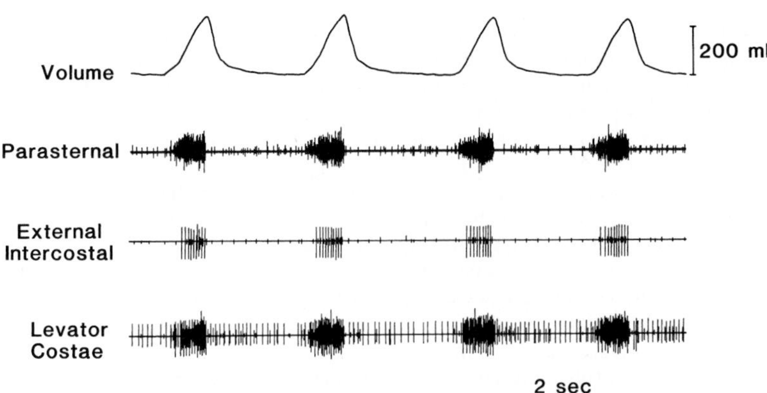

Figure 108–5. Pattern of electrical activation of the parasternal intercostal, external intercostal, and levator costae muscles in the dog during resting breathing. The trace of lung volume (increase upward) is also shown. The three muscles (recorded in the third intercostal space) are active in phase with inspiration. (From De Troyer A, Farkas GA: Inspiratory function of the levator costae and external intercostal muscles in the dog. J Appl Physiol 1989; 67:214.)

and they might therefore constitute a reserve, "load-compensating" system.[40]

Nonrespiratory Function

The insertions and orientations of the external intercostal muscles also suggest that contraction of these muscles on one side of the sternum would rotate the ribs in a transverse plane, so that the upper ribs would move forward while the lower ribs would move backward (Fig. 108-6). In contrast, contraction of the internal intercostal muscles on one side of the sternum would displace the upper ribs backward and the lower ribs forward; these muscles, therefore, would be ideally suited to twist the rib cage.

Measurements of the changes in length of these muscles during passive rotations of the thorax in anesthetized dogs have supported this idea.[23] When an animal's trunk was twisted to the left, the external intercostal muscles on the right side of the chest and the internal interosseous intercostal muscles on the left side shortened. At the same time, the external intercostal muscles on the left side and the internal intercostal muscles on the right side lengthened. The opposite pattern was seen when the animal's trunk was passively rotated to the right, with a marked shortening of the right internal and left external intercostal muscles and a lengthening of the left internals and right externals. Thus, the length of these muscles changed in the way expected if they were producing the rotations, and subsequent EMG studies in normal humans have confirmed that the external intercostal muscles on the right side of the chest are active when the trunk is rotated to the left, whereas they are silent when the trunk is rotated to the right.[41] Conversely, the internal intercostal muscles on the right side of the chest are active only when the trunk is rotated to the right. Active use of these muscles during such postural movements is also consistent with their abundant supply of muscle spindles.

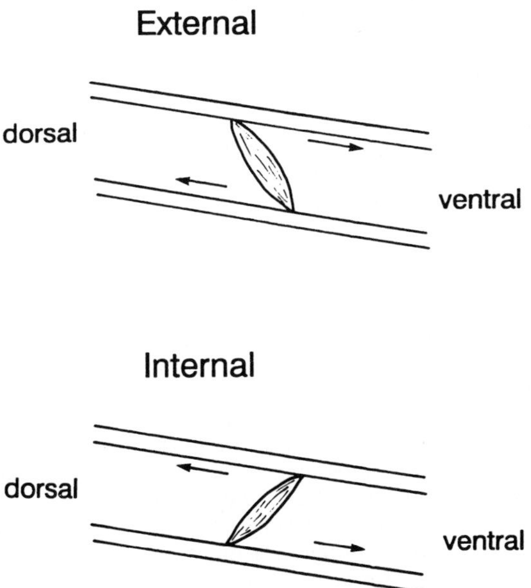

Figure 108–6. Diagram illustrating the actions of the intercostal muscles during rotations of the trunk. Lateral view of an intercostal space on the right side of the chest. The two bars oriented obliquely represent two adjacent ribs. External and internal intercostal muscles are depicted as single bundles, and *arrows* indicate the component of tension vector acting along the ribs. (From De Troyer A: Mechanics of the chest wall muscles. *In:* Neural Control of the Respiratory Muscles. Miller AD, Bishop B, Bianchi AL [Eds]. Boca Raton, Fla, CRC Press, 1996, pp 59–73.)

Triangularis Sterni

The triangularis sterni muscle, also called the transversus thoracis, is a flat muscle that lies deep to the sternum and the parasternal intercostal muscles. Its fibers originate from the dorsal aspect of the caudal half of the sternum and insert into the inner surfaces of the chondrocostal junctions of ribs 3 to 7. The muscle receives its motor supply from the intercostal nerves, and in the dog, its selective stimulation causes a caudal displacement of the ribs with a cranial motion of the sternum and a decrease in lung volume.[42]

In mammalian quadrupeds, this muscle invariably contracts during the expiratory phase of the breathing cycle, and in so doing, it pulls the ribs caudally and deflates the rib cage below its neutral (resting) position.[42] Consequently, when the muscle relaxes at the end of expiration, a passive rib cage expansion and an increase in lung volume precede the onset of inspiratory muscle contraction. In these animals, the triangularis sterni muscle thus shares the work of breathing with the inspiratory muscles and helps the inspiratory intercostal muscles, in particular the parasternal intercostal muscles, produce the rhythmic inspiratory expansion of the rib cage.[42]

Although the muscle is usually inactive in normal humans during resting breathing,[43] it also invariably contracts during voluntary or involuntary expiratory efforts such as coughing, laughing, and speech. Healthy individuals, in fact, cannot produce expiratory efforts without contracting the triangularis sterni muscle. Presumably, the muscle then acts in concert with the internal interosseous intercostal muscles to deflate the rib cage and raise pleural pressure.

Scalene Muscles

The scalene muscles in humans comprise three muscle bundles that run from the transverse processes of the lower five cervical vertebrae to the upper surfaces of the first two ribs. When these muscles are selectively activated by electrical stimulation in dogs, they produce a marked cranial displacement of the ribs and sternum and cause an increase in the rib cage anteroposterior diameter. Although the scalene muscles have traditionally been considered "accessory" muscles of inspiration, EMG studies with concentric needle electrodes have established that in normal humans, these muscles invariably contract in concert with the diaphragm and the parasternal intercostal muscles during inspiration.[38, 44, 45]

No clinical disorder causes paralysis of all the inspiratory muscles without also affecting the scalene muscles. Therefore, the isolated action of these muscles on the human rib cage cannot be precisely defined. Several observations, however, indicate that contraction of the scalene muscles is an important determinant of the motion of the sternum and the upper ribs during breathing. First, the sternum in resting humans moves cranially during inspiration. In contrast, in the dog, the scalene muscles are not active during breathing, and the sternum moves caudally rather than cranially.[17] Second, when normal subjects attempt to inspire with the diaphragm alone, there is a marked, selective decrease in scalene activity associated with either less inspiratory increase or a paradoxical decrease in anteroposterior diameter of the upper rib cage.[45] Third, the inward inspiratory displacement of the upper rib cage characteristic of quadriplegia (see later) is usually not observed when scalene muscle function is preserved after the lower cervical cord transection.[11] Because the scalene muscles are innervated from the lower five cervical segments, persistent inspiratory contraction is commonly seen in subjects with a transection at the C-7 level or below. In such subjects, the anteroposterior diameter of the upper rib cage tends to remain constant or to increase slightly during inspiration.

Sternocleidomastoid Muscles and Other Accessory Muscles of Inspiration

Many additional muscles, such as the pectoralis minor, the trapezius, the erector spinae, the serrati, and the sternocleidomastoid muscles, can elevate the ribs when they contract. These muscles, however, run between the shoulder girdle and the rib cage, between the spine and the shoulder girdle, or between the head and the rib cage. Therefore, they have primarily postural functions. In healthy individuals, these muscles contract only during greater inspiratory efforts, and, in contrast to the scalene muscles, are thus real "accessory" muscles of inspiration.

Of all these muscles, only the sternocleidomastoid muscles have been thoroughly studied. They descend from the mastoid process to the ventral surfaces of the manubrium sterni and the medial third of the clavicle, and their action in humans has been inferred from measurements of chest wall motion in patients with transection of the upper cervical cord. Indeed, the diaphragm and the intercostal, scalene, and abdominal muscles are paralyzed in such patients, but the sternocleidomastoid muscles (the motor innervation of which largely depends on the eleventh cranial nerve) are spared, and they contract forcefully during unassisted inspiration.[5, 8] In this condition, there are a marked inspiratory cranial displacement of the sternum and a large expansion of the upper rib cage, particularly in its anteroposterior diameter, but the transverse diameter of the lower rib cage decreases[5, 8] (Fig. 108–7).

ABDOMINAL MUSCLES

The four abdominal muscles that have a significant respiratory function in humans constitute the ventrolateral wall of the abdomen.

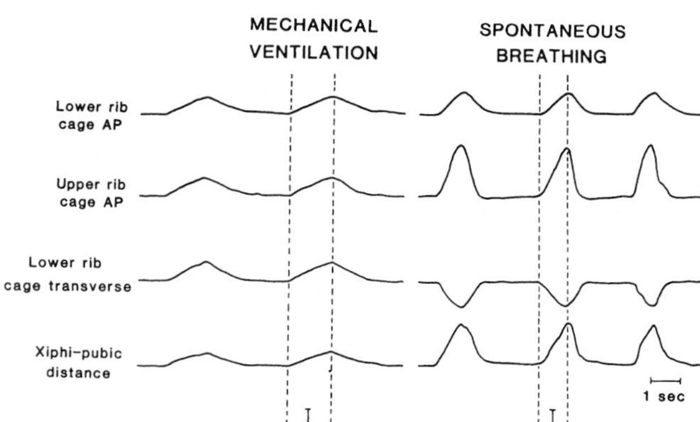

Figure 108–7. Pattern of rib cage motion during mechanical ventilation (*left*) and during spontaneous breathing (*right*) in a quadriplegic subject with a traumatic transection of the upper cervical cord (C-1). Each panel shows, from *top* to *bottom*, the respiratory changes in anteroposterior (AP) diameter of the lower rib cage, the changes in AP diameter of the upper rib cage, the changes in transverse diameter of the lower rib cage, and the changes in xiphipubic distance. Upward deflections correspond to an increase in diameter or an increase in xiphipubic distance (i.e., a cranial displacement of the sternum). I indicates duration of inspiration. During mechanical ventilation, all rib cage diameters and the xiphipubic distance increase in phase. During spontaneous inspiration, however, the xiphipubic distance and the upper rib cage AP diameter increase more than the lower rib cage AP diameter, and the lower rib cage transverse diameter decreases. (From De Troyer A: Mechanics of the chest wall muscles. *In:* Neural Control of the Respiratory Muscles. Miller AD, Bishop B, Bianchi AL [Eds]. Boca Raton, Fla, CRC Press, 1996, pp 59–73.)

The *rectus abdominis* is the most ventral of these muscles. It originates from the ventral aspect of the sternum and the fifth, sixth, and seventh costal cartilages and runs caudally along the whole length of the abdominal wall to insert into the pubis. The rectus abdominis muscle is enclosed in a sheath formed by the aponeuroses of the three muscles situated laterally.

The most superficial of these is the *external oblique*, which originates by fleshy digitations from the external surfaces of the lower eight ribs, well above the costal margin, and directly covers the lower ribs and intercostal muscles. Its fibers radiate caudally to the iliac crest and inguinal ligament and medially to the linea alba.

The *internal oblique* lies deep to the external oblique muscle. Its fibers arise from the iliac crest and inguinal ligament and then diverge to insert on the costal margin and an aponeurosis contributing to the rectus sheath down to the pubis.

The *transversus abdominis* is the deepest of the muscles of the lateral abdominal wall. It arises from the inner surface of the lower six ribs, where it interdigitates with the costal insertions of the diaphragm. From this origin and from the lumbar fascia, the iliac crest, and the inguinal ligament, its fibers run circumferentially around the abdominal visceral mass and terminate ventrally in the rectus sheath.

Actions of the Abdominal Muscles

The four muscles just described have important functions as flexors (rectus abdominis) and rotators (external oblique, internal oblique) of the trunk, but as respiratory muscles, they have two principal actions:

1. As they contract, these muscles pull the abdominal wall inward and produce an increase in abdominal pressure. The

increased pressure causes the diaphragm to move cranially into the thoracic cavity, and this motion, in turn, leads to an increase in pleural pressure and a decrease in lung volume.

2. The four muscles displace the rib cage. Their orientations and insertions on the ribs would suggest that the action of all abdominal muscles is to pull the ribs caudally and to deflate the rib cage, another expiratory action. Measurements of rib cage motion during electrical stimulation of the four abdominal muscles in dogs have shown, however, that the rise in abdominal pressure produced by these muscles also confers to them an inspiratory action on the rib cage.[46, 47] Thus, the zone of apposition of the diaphragm to the rib cage (see Fig. 108–1) allows the rise in abdominal pressure to be transmitted to the lower rib cage. In addition, by forcing the diaphragm cranially and stretching it, the rise in abdominal pressure also causes passive diaphragmatic tension. This passive tension tends to raise the lower ribs and to expand the lower rib cage in the same way as does an active diaphragmatic contraction (insertional force of the diaphragm).

The action of the abdominal muscles on the rib cage is thus determined by the balance between the insertional, expiratory force of the muscles and the inspiratory force related to the rise in abdominal pressure. Isolated contraction of the external oblique muscle in humans produces a small caudal displacement of the sternum and a large decrease in the transverse diameter of the rib cage, but the rectus abdominis, although it causes a marked caudal displacement of the sternum and a large decrease in the anteroposterior diameter of the rib cage, also produces a small increase in the transverse diameter of the rib cage.[48] The isolated actions of the internal oblique and transversus abdominis muscles on the human rib cage are not known; the anatomic arrangement of the transversus abdominis suggests, however, that among the abdominal muscles it has the smallest insertional, expiratory action on the ribs and the greatest effect on abdominal pressure. Therefore, isolated contraction of the transversus abdominis should produce little or no expiratory displacement of the rib cage.

Respiratory Function

Irrespective of their actions on the rib cage, the abdominal muscles are primarily expiratory muscles through their actions on the diaphragm and the lung, and they play important roles in activities such as coughing and speaking. When these muscles contract rhythmically in phase with expiration, however, and reduce lung volume below the neutral position of the respiratory system, their relaxation at end-expiration may promote a passive descent of the diaphragm and induce an increase in lung volume before the onset of inspiratory muscle contraction. The abdominal muscles, therefore, may also be regarded as accessory muscles of inspiration.

This inspiratory action of the abdominal muscles takes place all the time in quadrupeds, and in dogs placed in the head-up or the prone posture, the relaxation of the abdominal muscles at end-expiration accounts for up to 40% to 60% of the tidal volume.[49] Adult humans do not utilize such a breathing strategy at rest. Phasic expiratory contraction of the abdominal muscles occurs in healthy human subjects, however, whenever the demand placed on the inspiratory muscles is abnormally increased, such as during exercise or during CO_2-induced hyperpnea. It is noteworthy that in these conditions, the transversus abdominis is recruited well before activity can be recorded from either the rectus abdominis or the external oblique muscle.[50, 51] This preferential recruitment of the transversus abdominis also supports the idea that the effect of the abdominal muscles on abdominal pressure is more important to the act of breathing than their action on the rib cage.

There is a second mechanism by which the abdominal muscles can assist inspiration. Most normal human subjects, when adopting the standing posture, develop tonic abdominal muscle activity unrelated to the phases of the breathing cycle,[52] and studies in patients with transection of the upper cervical cord, in whom bilateral pacing of the phrenic nerves allows the level of diaphragmatic activation to be kept constant, have clearly illustrated the effect of this tonic abdominal contraction on inspiration.[8, 9] When the patients were supine, the unassisted paced diaphragm was able to generate an adequate tidal volume. When the patients were tilted head-up or moved to the seated posture, the weight of the abdominal viscera and the absence of abdominal muscle activity caused the belly wall to protrude. The tidal volume produced by pacing in this latter posture was markedly reduced in comparison with that in the supine posture, but the reduction was significantly smaller when a pneumatic cuff was inflated around the abdomen to mimic the tonic abdominal muscle contraction. Thus, by contracting throughout the breathing cycle in the standing posture, the abdominal muscles make the diaphragm longer at the onset of inspiration and prevent it from shortening excessively during inspiration; in accordance with the length-tension characteristics of the muscle, its ability to generate pressure is therefore increased.

RESPIRATORY MUSCLE FUNCTION IN DISEASES

Quadriplegia

As indicated earlier, the particular distribution of muscle paralysis in patients with traumatic transection of the lower cervical cord causes distinct abnormalities in the pattern of chest wall motion during breathing (Fig. 108–8). Because diaphragmatic function is preserved in these patients, the expansion of the abdomen during inspiration is associated with an expansion of the lower rib cage. In healthy subjects, however, the entire rib cage expands synchronously and uniformly, whereas the lower rib cage in quadriplegic patients expands predominantly over its lateral walls, where the area of apposed diaphragm is greater (greater appositional force).[11] In addition, the paralysis of the rib cage inspiratory muscles, in particular the scalene and parasternal intercostal muscles, is such that many quadriplegic patients at rest have an inspiratory decrease (paradoxical motion) of the anteroposterior diameter of the upper rib cage.[10, 11]

Quadriplegic patients also have complete paralysis of all the well-recognized muscles of expiration (abdominal muscles, internal intercostal muscles, triangularis sterni muscle). As a result, the expiratory reserve volume (ERV) is markedly reduced, and RV is usually greater than normal. The peak pleural pressures developed during cough are also lower than normal, and indeed, in such patients, the efficiency of cough and the clearance of bronchial secretions are severely impaired. Some studies, however, have demonstrated that most quadriplegic patients have residual expiratory muscle function as a result of the action of the clavicular portion of the pectoralis major muscle.[53] In patients with transection at the C-6 segment or below, this muscle bundle invariably contracts during voluntary expiration and during cough, and its insertions on the humerus and on the medial half of the clavicle make it displace the manubrium sterni and the upper ribs in the caudal direction when it contracts on both sides of the chest.[53] In so doing, this portion of the pectoralis major muscle produces collapse of the upper rib cage and partial emptying of the lung. In a number of patients, the clavicular portion of the pectoralis major muscle may even induce dynamic compression of the intrathoracic airways,[54] thus indicating that cough

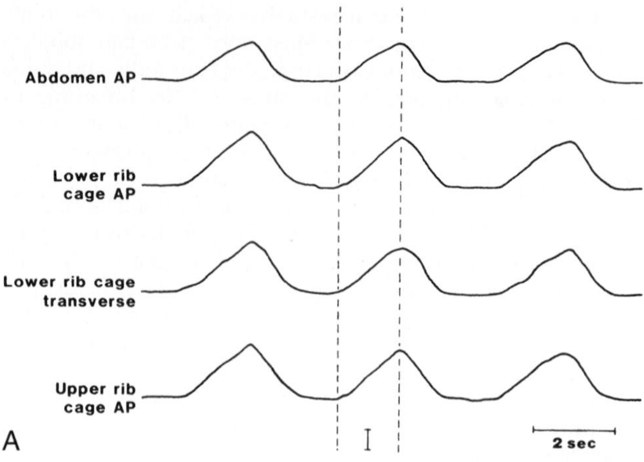

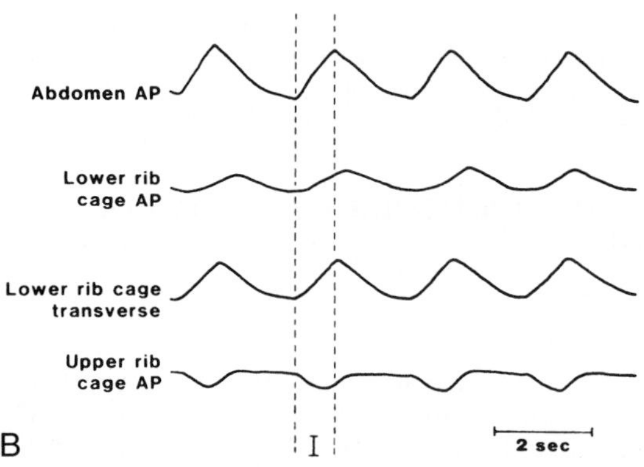

Figure 108–8. Pattern of chest wall motion in a healthy subject (*A*) and a C-5 quadriplegic patient (*B*) breathing at rest in the seated posture. The respiratory changes in anteroposterior (AP) diameter of the abdomen, lower rib cage, and upper rib cage, as well as the changes in transverse diameter of the lower rib cage, are shown. Same conventions as in Fig. 108–7. (From De Troyer A, Estenne M: The respiratory system in neuromuscular disorders. *In:* The Thorax. 2nd ed. Vol 85. Roussos C. [Ed]. New York, Marcel Dekker, 1995, pp 2177–2212.)

in this setting is not necessarily a passive phenomenon as conventionally thought.

Diaphragmatic Paralysis

Paralysis or severe weakness of both hemidiaphragms is seen usually in the context of generalized respiratory muscle weakness, but in occasional patients, the diaphragm is specifically or disproportionately affected. Selective paralysis of the diaphragm results in a compensatory increase in the activation of the inspiratory rib cage muscles, so that the inspiratory expansion of the rib cage compartment of the chest wall is accentuated.[17, 55] Also, in healthy subjects, the simultaneous contraction of the diaphragm and the rib cage inspiratory muscles causes a rise in abdominal pressure associated with a fall in pleural pressure; in the presence of diaphragmatic paralysis, however, the fall in pleural pressure is transmitted through the flaccid diaphragm such that abdominal pressure falls as well. As shown in Figure 108–9, the abdomen therefore moves paradoxically inward, opposing the inflation of the lung.[17]

Some patients also compensate for diaphragmatic paralysis by contracting the abdominal muscles during expiration, thus displacing the abdomen inward and the diaphragm cranially into the thorax. Relaxation of the abdominal muscles at the onset of inspiration may therefore result in outward abdominal motion and passive descent of the diaphragm.[56, 57] Such a contraction of the abdominal muscles during expiration seems to be particularly common in the erect patient; when present, it may remove the inspiratory inward motion of the abdomen, which is the cardinal sign of diaphragmatic paralysis on clinical examination; however, this phenomenon does not occur in the supine posture, in which the abdominal muscles usually remain relaxed during the whole respiratory cycle.

Chronic Obstructive Pulmonary Disease

Measurements of thoracoabdominal motion during breathing have shown that in patients with chronic obstructive pulmonary disease (COPD) and hyperinflation, expansion of the rib cage is relatively greater and expansion of the abdomen is smaller than in healthy subjects.[58, 59] The normal inspiratory positive swing of abdominal pressure is also attenuated,[58–60] whereas the fall in pleural pressure is larger than normal because of the greater airflow resistance and the lesser dynamic pulmonary compliance. In patients with severe disease, abdominal pressure may even become negative during inspiration, and the abdomen may move paradoxically inward, as if the diaphragm were paralyzed.[58, 59, 61] This altered pattern has

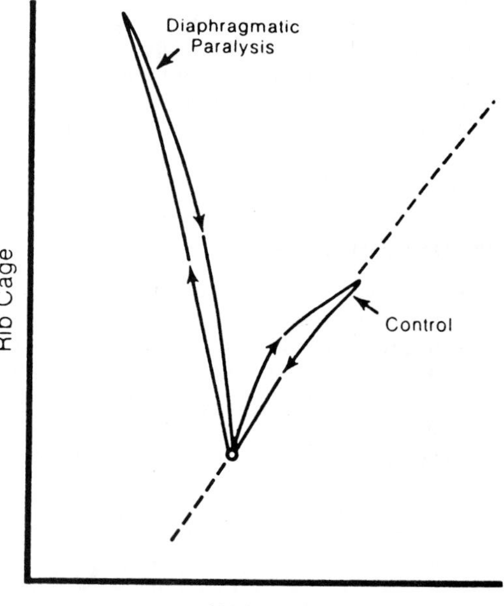

Figure 108–9. Pattern of chest wall motion during resting breathing in a supine anesthetized dog before (control) and after bilateral section of the phrenic nerves in the neck (diaphragmatic paralysis). The changes in abdominal cross section are on the abscissa (increase rightward), and the changes in rib cage cross section are on the ordinate (increase upward). The *broken line* represents the relaxation curve of the thoracoabdominal system; the *solid loops* represent tidal volume cycles; *arrows* indicate the direction of the loops; and the *open circle* corresponds to end-expiration. During breathing in the control condition, both the rib cage and the abdomen expand during inspiration and the chest wall moves on its relaxed configuration. After induction of diaphragmatic paralysis, however, the rib cage expands markedly during inspiration, but the abdomen moves paradoxically inward. (Adapted from De Troyer A, Kelly S: Chest wall mechanics in dogs with acute diaphragm paralysis. J Appl Physiol 1982; 53:373.)

led to the widespread belief that patients with severe COPD have more use of the rib cage inspiratory muscles and less use of the diaphragm than healthy subjects, possibly owing to diaphragmatic fatigue.[59, 62]

In agreement with this idea, the scalene and parasternal intercostal muscles feel tense on palpation in many patients with severe COPD. EMG studies using concentric needle electrodes have also shown that although most such patients do not contract the sternocleidomastoid or trapezius muscles when breathing at rest,[63] they demonstrate higher firing frequencies in the parasternal intercostal and scalene motor units than normal subjects.[64] The patients also have a greater number of active motor units in these two muscles. Motor units in the diaphragm, however, also demonstrate substantial increases in firing frequency during resting breathing, thus indicating that COPD is associated with an increase in neural drive not only to the rib cage inspiratory muscles but also to the diaphragm.[65] This observation suggests that the altered thoracoabdominal motion seen during inspiration in patients with COPD results from mechanical factors alone.

The diaphragm in such patients is characteristically flat and low compared with that in normal subjects, and the zone of apposition is smaller. Therefore, irrespective of the extent of neural activation, the ability of the diaphragmatic dome to descend is impaired, and hence, the rise in abdominal pressure and the outward displacement of the abdominal wall must be reduced. In some patients with severe hyperinflation, the zone of apposition has virtually disappeared, and the normal curvature of the diaphragm is even reversed, with its concavity facing upward rather than downward. The muscle fibers at their insertions on the ribs then run transversely inward rather than cranially. In this situation, contraction of the diaphragm cannot lead to any descent of the dome. Instead, the vigorous contraction of the rib cage inspiratory muscles, resulting in a greater than normal elevation of the ribs, tends to pull the diaphragm cranially and to displace the ventral abdominal wall inward. Contraction of this flat diaphragm, however, produces an inspiratory decrease in the transverse diameter of the lower rib cage (Hoover's sign).[66]

In contrast to normal subjects, many resting patients with severe COPD also have phasic expiratory contraction of the abdominal muscles, in particular the transversus abdominis muscle.[67] The neural drive to the expiratory muscles is therefore also increased, and indeed, abdominal pressure is commonly observed to increase, rather than decrease, during expiration. The expiratory contraction of the transversus abdominis muscle is thus mechanically significant, yet its benefit to the act of breathing is uncertain.

As previously described, phasic contraction of the abdominal muscles during expiration is a natural component of the response of the normal respiratory system to increased stimulation. In healthy individuals, this expiratory muscle contraction is appropriate, because it allows the work of breathing to be shared between the inspiratory and expiratory muscles. Most patients with severe COPD, however, are flow limited at rest, and so expiratory contraction of the transversus abdominis muscle is unlikely to achieve a significant increase in expiratory airflow or a significant deflation of the respiratory system below its neutral position.[67] The observation by Estenne and colleagues[68] that patients with severe restrictive ventilatory impairment due to thoracic scoliosis also have phasic expiratory contraction of the transversus abdominis muscle during quiet breathing supports the idea that the pattern of respiratory muscle activation in patients with chronic respiratory diseases is essentially an automatic response of the central respiratory controller to a greater than normal ventilatory stimulation.

RESPIRATORY MUSCLE FATIGUE

The increased neural drive to the respiratory muscles in patients with severe lung disease allows the muscles to overcome the greater than normal inspiratory load and to meet the increased pressure requirements. The ability of the muscles to lower intrathoracic pressure is reduced, however, particularly when hyperinflation makes them operate at shorter than normal lengths. As a result, the reserve available to such patients is appreciably less than that available to healthy individuals. This combination of high drive and reduced reserve for prolonged periods has generated the attractive concept, by analogy with limb muscles, that fatigue could develop in the respiratory muscles and contribute to hypercapnic ventilatory failure.[69]

Muscle Fatigue

Muscle fatigue is defined as a loss in the capacity of the muscle to develop force that is reversible by rest[70]; this latter point is important, as it distinguishes fatigue from persistent weakness. Fatigue may therefore be located peripherally in the neuromuscular apparatus (*peripheral fatigue*), or may result from an inability to maintain the necessary motor drive (*central fatigue*). The possible mechanisms of peripheral fatigue include reduced substrate supply, depletion of energy stores, and local acid-base changes; these mechanisms, in turn, depend on local blood flow. Alternatively, central fatigue may represent an important protective mechanism that avoids the adverse effects of prolonged forceful contraction on the muscle contractile machinery.

Fatigue can be induced in any limb muscle working against an increased load. It can also be observed in respiratory muscles when normal subjects are forced to breathe against increased mechanical loads, such as a very high inspiratory airflow resistance.[71] In limb muscles, evidence of fatigue is detectable with continuous contractions of approximately 15% of the maximal tension that the muscle can develop. For intermittent contractions, the fatigue threshold depends on the tension developed, the duration of each contraction, and the period of rest between successive contractions. This principle has been applied to the diaphragm by calculation of the *tension-time index* (TTdi), that is, the product of the mean transdiaphragmatic pressure (Pdi) (as a fraction of the maximal Pdi [Pdi max]) and the duty cycle (i.e., the proportion of each breathing cycle during which the diaphragm is contracting).[72] During ventilation at rest, the critical TTdi beyond which fatigue of the diaphragm is likely to develop is approximately 0.15 to 0.20. In healthy subjects, the mean Pdi during a breath is low compared with Pdi max, and so the mean Pdi can be increased about eightfold before any evidence of fatigue occurs.

Assessment

Both mechanical and EMG indices have been proposed for the recognition of muscle fatigue. The standard method for limb muscles is the measurement of muscle force during electrically induced contraction at different frequencies, which allows construction of the frequency-force relationship. As fatigue develops, muscle force declines at all stimulation frequencies; however, although the force at high-frequency stimulation recovers rapidly, the force at low-frequency stimulation recovers very slowly. This phenomenon, usually referred to as *low-frequency fatigue*, can be quantitated as a fall in the ratio of response to stimulation frequencies of 20 Hz and 50 Hz (the 20:50 ratio).

This technique has been applied successfully to the sternocleidomastoid muscle in normal subjects breathing against elevated inspiratory resistance[73] and in patients with COPD after a 12-minute walk.[74] Low-frequency fatigue was shown in both cases. The significance of this finding in COPD patients is uncertain, however, because the performance of a second 12-minute walk shortly afterward was not affected by its presence. Studies conducted during acute exacerbations of COPD also showed that the sternocleidomastoid muscle was more easily fatiguable at the time of a patient's hospital admission than during subsequent recovery, but overt fatigue was identified in only a small proportion of patients.[75]

Fatigue is also associated with a change in the frequency spectrum of the EMG during spontaneous muscle contraction. Specifically, there is an increase in amplitude of the lower-frequency components and a decrease in amplitude of the higher-frequency components. This observation has led to the suggestion that diaphragm fatigue could be quantitated by measuring the ratio of the amplitudes of signals over arbitrary ranges of higher and lower frequencies (the H/L ratio).[76] Pardy and Roussos,[77] using this index in patients with COPD, have shown that voluntary hyperventilation sufficient to reduce $Paco_2$ by 10 mm Hg was associated with a decline in the diaphragmatic H/L ratio; they therefore suggested that in such patients, a relatively small increase in ventilation could lead to the development of respiratory muscle fatigue. Unlike low-frequency fatigue, however, the H/L ratio rapidly returns to normal on recovery. Furthermore, this ratio depends on the pattern of motor unit recruitment, and its decline may therefore simply reflect an alteration in neural drive. As a result, this index has not been widely accepted as a reliable indicator of fatigue.[70]

Fatigued limb muscles also relax more slowly than normal. Fatigue of the diaphragm has therefore been quantitated from the decline in Pdi by measuring the maximum relaxation rate (MRR) or the time constant of relaxation after maximal sniffs.[78] Assuming a monoexponential decay, relaxation of the inspiratory muscles overall has also been assessed in normal subjects by measuring the rate of decline in mouth pressure after a maximal sniff.[79] However, this measurement is unreliable as a guide to changes in intrathoracic pressure in patients with abnormal pulmonary mechanics.

Respiratory Muscle Fatigue in Chronic Lung Disease

Although the force reserve available to patients with severe chronic lung diseases is less than in normal subjects, the existence of respiratory muscle fatigue during resting breathing has not been readily demonstrated. This failure may, in part, be due to the fact that the detection of chronic respiratory muscle fatigue is technically difficult.

Some investigators have reported that when patients with COPD and chronic ventilatory failure are treated with assisted ventilation, the strength of the respiratory muscles improves. This improvement has been attributed to resting of the respiratory muscles and, therefore, a reversal of chronic muscle fatigue.[80] The improved performance following assisted ventilation may well represent better patient cooperation or improved central drive, however, rather than reversal of muscle fatigue. In addition, other studies of long-term assisted ventilation in patients with hypercapnic respiratory failure have failed to demonstrate greater respiratory muscle strength, despite good evidence that the muscles were actually rested.[81]

Further investigation of chronic respiratory muscle fatigue would be best undertaken using the nonvolitional technique of *phrenic nerve stimulation* to assess diaphragmatic contractility before and after respiratory muscle rest; the technique of *cervical magnetic stimulation*[82] can be particularly useful in this regard. Measurement of the MRR of the diaphragm before and after muscle rest would also provide more direct evidence of the presence or absence of chronic diaphragmatic fatigue. It is notable, however, that although the TTdi in patients with severe COPD is higher at rest than in healthy individuals, it still lies well below the fatiguing range in most patients.[83] The TTdi at rest is also higher in hypercapnic than in eucapnic patients, but even in the severely hypercapnic, it does not exceed the fatigue threshold of 0.15.[84] Thus, even though such patients may have greater potential for the development of respiratory muscle fatigue and may actually have fatigue during acute exacerbations or during weaning trials (this question is specifically addressed in Chapter 132), the existence of chronic muscle fatigue appears unlikely. As previously emphasized, an important mechanism for avoiding the development of fatigue might be a reduction in central drive, which in turn leads to a reduction in tidal volume and to the development of hypercapnia.

References

1. Konno K, Mead J: Measurement of the separate volume changes of rib cage and abdomen during breathing. J Appl Physiol 1967; 22:407.
2. Jordanoglou J: Vector analysis of rib movement. Respir Physiol 1970; 10:109.
3. Wilson TA, Rehder K, Krayer S, et al: Geometry and respiratory displacement of human ribs. J Appl Physiol 1987; 62:1872.
4. De Troyer A, Decramer M: Mechanical coupling between the ribs and sternum in the dog. Respir Physiol 1985; 59:27.
5. De Troyer A, Estenne M, Vincken W: Rib cage motion and muscle use in high tetraplegics. Am Rev Respir Dis 1986; 133:1115.
6. Mead J: Functional significance of the area of apposition of diaphragm to rib cage. Am Rev Respir Dis 1979; 119:31.
7. D'Angelo E, Sant'Ambrogio G: Direct action of contracting diaphragm on the rib cage in rabbits and dogs. J Appl Physiol 1974; 36:715.
8. Danon J, Druz WS, Goldberg NB, et al: Function of the isolated paced diaphragm and the cervical accessory muscles in C_1 quadriplegics. Am Rev Respir Dis 1979; 119:909.
9. Strohl KP, Mead J, Banzett RB, et al: Effect of posture on upper and lower rib cage motion and tidal volume during diaphragm pacing. Am Rev Respir Dis 1984; 130:320.
10. Mortola JP, Sant'Ambrogio G: Motion of the rib cage and the abdomen in tetraplegic patients. Clin Sci Mol Med 1978; 54:25.
11. Estenne M, De Troyer A: Relationship between respiratory muscle electromyogram and rib cage motion in tetraplegia. Am Rev Respir Dis 1985; 132:53.
12. De Troyer A, Sampson M, Sigrist S, et al: Action of costal and crural parts of the diaphragm on the rib cage in dog. J Appl Physiol 1982; 53:30.
13. Loring SH, Mead J: Action of the diaphragm on the rib cage inferred from a force-balance analysis. J Appl Physiol 1982; 53:756.
14. Urmey WF, De Troyer A, Kelly SB, et al: Pleural pressure increases during inspiration in the zone of apposition of diaphragm to rib cage. J Appl Physiol 1988; 65:2207.
15. Duchenne GB: Physiologie des mouvements. Paris, Baillière, 1867.
16. Hamberger GE: De Respirationis Mechanismo et usu genuino. Jena, Germany, 1749.
17. De Troyer A, Kelly S: Chest wall mechanics in dogs with acute diaphragm paralysis. J Appl Physiol 1982; 53:373.
18. Decramer M, De Troyer A: Respiratory changes in parasternal intercostal length. J Appl Physiol 1984; 57:1254.
19. De Troyer A, Legrand A, Wilson TA: Rostrocaudal gradient of mechanical advantage in the parasternal intercostal muscles of the dog. J Physiol (Lond) 1996; 495:239.
20. De Troyer A, Farkas GA: Inspiratory function of the levator costae and external intercostal muscles in the dog. J Appl Physiol 1989; 67:2614.
21. De Troyer A, Kelly S, Zin WA: Mechanical action of the intercostal muscles on the ribs. Science 1983; 220:87.

22. Ninane V, Gorini M, Estenne M: Action of intercostal muscles on the lung in dogs. J Appl Physiol 1991; 70:2388.
23. Decramer M, Kelly S, De Troyer A: Respiratory and postural changes in intercostal muscle length in supine dogs. J Appl Physiol 1986; 60:1686.
24. Saumarez RC: An analysis of action of intercostal muscles in human upper rib cage. J Appl Physiol 1986; 60:690.
25. Wilson TA, De Troyer A: Respiratory effect of the intercostal muscles in the dog. J Appl Physiol 1993; 75:2636.
26. De Troyer A, Farkas GA: Mechanics of the parasternal intercostals in prone dogs: Statics and dynamics. J Appl Physiol 1993; 74:2757.
27. Greer JJ, Martin TP: Distribution of muscle fiber types and EMG activity in cat intercostal muscles. J Appl Physiol 1990; 69:1208.
28. De Troyer A, Farkas GA: Contribution of the rib cage inspiratory muscles to breathing in baboons. Respir Physiol 1994; 97:135.
29. Bainton CR, Kirkwood PA, Sears TA: On the transmission of the stimulating effects of carbon dioxide to the muscles of respiration. J Physiol (Lond) 1978; 280:249.
30. Sears TA: Efferent discharges in alpha and fusimotor fibres of intercostal nerves of the cat. J Physiol (Lond) 1964; 174:295.
31. Hilaire GG, Nicholls JG, Sears TA: Central and proprioceptive influences on the activity of the levator costae motoneurones in the cat. J Physiol (Lond) 1983; 342:527.
32. De Troyer A, Ninane V: Respiratory function of intercostal muscles in supine dog: An electromyographic study. J Appl Physiol 1986; 60:1692.
33. Loring SH, Woodbridge JA: Intercostal muscle action inferred from finite-element analysis. J Appl Physiol 1991; 70:2712.
34. Da Silva KMC, Sayers BMA, Sears TA, et al: The changes in configuration of the rib cage and abdomen during breathing in the anesthetized cat. J Physiol (Lond) 1977; 266:499.
35. De Troyer A: Inspiratory elevation of the ribs in the dog: Primary role of the parasternals. J Appl Physiol 1991; 70:1447.
36. Taylor A: The contribution of the intercostal muscles to the effort of respiration in man. J Physiol (Lond) 1960; 151:390.
37. Delhez L: Contribution électromyographique à l'étude de la mécanique et du contrôle nerveux des mouvements respiratoires de l'homme. Liège, Vaillant-Carmanne, Belgium, 1974.
38. Whitelaw WA, Feroah T: Patterns of intercostal muscle activity in humans. J Appl Physiol 1989; 67:2087.
39. Duron B, Jung-Caillol MC, Marlot D: Myelinated nerve fiber supply and muscle spindles in the respiratory muscles of cat: Quantitative study. Anat Embryol 1978; 152:171.
40. De Troyer A: Differential control of the inspiratory intercostal muscles during airway occlusion in the dog. J Physiol (Lond) 1991; 439:73.
41. Whitelaw WA, Ford GT, Rimmer KP, et al: Intercostal muscles are used during rotation of the thorax in humans. J Appl Physiol 1992; 72:1940.
42. De Troyer A, Ninane V: Triangularis sterni: A primary muscle of breathing in the dog. J Appl Physiol 1986; 60:14.
43. De Troyer A, Ninane V, Gilmartin JJ, et al: Triangularis sterni muscle use in supine humans. J Appl Physiol 1987; 62:919.
44. Raper AJ, Thompson WT Jr, Shapiro W, et al: Scalene and sternomastoid muscle function. J Appl Physiol 1966; 21:497.
45. De Troyer A, Estenne M: Coordination between rib cage muscles and diaphragm during quiet breathing in humans. J Appl Physiol 1984; 57:899.
46. De Troyer A, Sampson M, Sigrist S, et al: How the abdominal muscles act on the rib cage. J Appl Physiol 1983; 54:465.
47. D'Angelo E, Prandi E, Bellemare F: Mechanics of the abdominal muscles in rabbits and dogs. Respir Physiol 1994; 97:275.
48. Mier A, Brophy C, Estenne M, et al: Action of abdominal muscles on rib cage in humans. J Appl Physiol 1985; 58:1438.
49. Farkas GA, Estenne M, De Troyer A: Expiratory muscle contribution to tidal volume in head-up dogs. J Appl Physiol 1989; 67:1438.
50. De Troyer A, Estenne M, Ninane V, et al: Transversus abdominis muscle function in humans. J Appl Physiol 1990; 68:1010.
51. Abe T, Kusuhara N, Yoshimura N, et al: Differential respiratory activity of four abdominal muscles in humans. J Appl Physiol 1996; 80:1379.
52. Floyd WF, Silver PHS: Electromyographic study of patterns of activity of the anterior abdominal wall muscles in man. J Anat 1950; 84:132.
53. De Troyer A, Estenne M, Heilporn A: Mechanism of active expiration in tetraplegic patients. N Engl J Med 1986; 314:740.
54. Estenne M, Van Muylem A, Gorini M, et al: Evidence of dynamic airway compression during cough in tetraplegic subjects. Am Rev Respir Dis 1994; 150:1081.
55. Brichant JF, De Troyer A: On the intercostal muscle compensation for diaphragmatic paralysis in the dog. J Physiol (Lond) 1997; 500:245.
56. Newsom Davis J, Goldman M, Loh L, et al: Diaphragm function and alveolar hypoventilation. Q J Med 1976; 45:87.
57. Kreitzer SM, Feldman NT, Saunders NA, et al: Bilateral diaphragmatic paralysis with hypercapnic respiratory failure: A physiologic assessment. Am J Med 1978; 65:89.
58. Sharp JT, Goldberg NB, Druz WS, et al: Thoracoabdominal motion in chronic obstructive pulmonary disease. Am Rev Respir Dis 1977; 115:47.
59. Martinez FJ, Couser JI, Celli BR: Factors influencing ventilatory muscle recruitment in patients with chronic airflow obstruction. Am Rev Respir Dis 1990; 142:276.
60. Levine S, Gillen M, Weiser P, et al: Inspiratory pressure generation: Comparison of subjects with COPD and age-matched normals. J Appl Physiol 1988; 65:888.
61. Ashutosh K, Gilbert R, Auchincloss JH Jr, et al: Asynchronous breathing movements in patients with chronic obstructive pulmonary disease. Chest 1975; 67:553.
62. Cohen CA, Zagelbaum G, Gross D, et al: Clinical manifestations of inspiratory muscle fatigue. Am J Med 1982; 73:308.
63. De Troyer A, Peche R, Yernault JC, et al: Neck muscle activity in patients with severe chronic obstructive pulmonary disease. Am J Respir Crit Care Med 1994; 150:41.
64. Gandevia SC, Leeper JB, McKenzie DK, et al: Discharge frequencies of parasternal intercostal and scalene motor units during breathing in normal and COPD subjects. Am J Respir Crit Care Med 1996; 153:622.
65. De Troyer A, Leeper JB, McKenzie DK, et al: Neural drive to the diaphragm in patients with severe COPD. Am J Respir Crit Care Med 1997; 155:1335.
66. Gilmartin JJ, Gibson GJ: Mechanisms of paradoxical rib cage motion in patients with chronic obstructive pulmonary disease. Am Rev Respir Dis 1986; 134:684.
67. Ninane V, Rypens F, Yernault JC, et al: Abdominal muscle use during breathing in patients with chronic airflow obstruction. Am Rev Respir Dis 1992; 146:16.
68. Estenne M, Derom E, De Troyer A: Neck and abdominal muscle activity in patients with severe thoracic scoliosis. Am J Respir Crit Care Med 1998; 158:452.
69. Macklem PT, Roussos CS: Respiratory muscle fatigue: A cause of respiratory failure? Clin Sci 1977; 53:419.
70. Respiratory Muscle Fatigue Workshop Group: Respiratory muscle fatigue. Am Rev Respir Dis 1990; 142:474.
71. Roussos C, Macklem PT: Diaphragmatic fatigue in man. J Appl Physiol 1977; 43:189.
72. Bellemare F, Grassino A: Effect of pressure and timing of contraction on human diaphragm fatigue. J Appl Physiol 1982; 53:1190.
73. Moxham J, Wiles CM, Newham D, et al: Sternomastoid muscle function and fatigue in man. Clin Sci 1980; 59:463.
74. Wilson SH, Cooke NT, Moxham J, et al: Sternomastoid muscle function and fatigue in normal subjects and in patients with chronic obstructive pulmonary disease. Am Rev Respir Dis 1984; 129:460.
75. Efthimiou J, Fleming J, Spiro SG: Sternomastoid muscle function and fatigue in breathless patients with severe respiratory disease. Am Rev Respir Dis 1987; 136:1099.
76. Gross D, Grassino A, Ross WRD, et al: Electromyogram pattern of diaphragmatic fatigue. J Appl Physiol 1979; 46:1.
77. Pardy RL, Roussos C: Endurance of hyperventilation in chronic airflow limitation. Chest 1983; 83:744.
78. Esau SA, Bye PTB, Pardy RL: Changes in rate of relaxation of sniffs with diaphragmatic fatigue in humans. J Appl Physiol 1983; 55:731.
79. Koulouris N, Vianna LG, Mulvey DA et al: Maximal relaxation rates of oesophageal, nose and mouth pressures during a sniff reflect inspiratory muscle fatigue. Am Rev Respir Dis 1989; 139:1213.
80. Gutierrez M, Beroiza T, Contreras G, et al: Weekly cuirass ventila-

tion improves blood gases and inspiratory muscle strength in patients with chronic airflow limitation and hypercarbia. Am Rev Respir Dis 1988; 138:617.

81. Elliott MW, Mulvey DA, Moxham J, et al: Domiciliary nocturnal nasal intermittent positive pressure ventilation in COPD: Mechanisms underlying changes in arterial blood gas tensions. Eur Respir J 1991; 4:1044.
82. Similowski T, Fleury B, Launois S, et al: Cervical magnetic stimulation: A painless method for bilateral phrenic nerve stimulation in conscious humans. J Appl Physiol 1989; 67:1311.
83. Bellemare F, Grassino A: Force reserve of the diaphragm in patients with chronic obstructive pulmonary disease. J Appl Physiol 1983; 55:8.
84. Begin P, Grassino A: Inspiratory muscle dysfunction and chronic hypercapnia in chronic obstructive pulmonary disease. Am Rev Respir Dis 1991; 143:905.

109

Mechanics of the Respiratory System

John W. Kreit, MD

The primary function of the respiratory system, which consists of the lungs and chest wall, is to supply oxygen to and remove carbon dioxide from the mixed venous blood entering the lungs. For this to occur, two interrelated processes are essential: (1) *gas exchange*, the transfer of oxygen and carbon dioxide between the alveoli and the pulmonary capillary blood; and (2) *ventilation*, the repetitive movement of gas into and out of the lungs. Ventilation delivers the oxygen and removes the carbon dioxide that is exchanged across the alveolar-capillary interface.

For ventilation to occur, the respiratory system must repeatedly expand above and then return to its resting volume. This is possible only when sufficient pressure is provided to overcome three factors that oppose its movement: (1) elastic recoil, (2) viscous forces, and (3) viscoelastic forces. This chapter reviews the origins, characteristics, and measurement of each of these opposing forces as well as their interaction with the forces applied to overcome them.

OPPOSING FORCES

Elastic Recoil

Pressure-Volume Relationships

When removed from the thoracic cavity, the lungs deflate far below their resting volume in the chest, and the isolated chest wall expands outward. Any change in volume above or below these equilibrium positions requires an increasing amount of applied pressure. In essence, the lungs and chest wall behave like metal springs, each with its own resting length and *elastic recoil*.[1-4] As shown in Figure 109-1, the elastic recoil of the excised lungs increases with each volume increment and must be exactly balanced by an applied pressure (the elastic recoil pressure). Similarly, decreasing or increasing the volume of the isolated chest wall requires negative and positive pressure, respectively.

Although it is useful from a conceptual standpoint to discuss the lungs and chest wall as if they were isolated structures, they are, of course, linked together by the pressures within the pleural space. Nevertheless, the relationship between elastic recoil pressure and volume can be determined separately for the lungs and the chest wall by performing several relatively simple measurements.[1-4] A subject is instructed to exhale in a stepwise fashion after a maximal inspiration. At each point, the subject relaxes against an occluded external airway with the glottis open, and both the volume change and the pressure gradient across the lungs and chest wall are measured. These *transmural* pressures are required to balance the elastic recoil of the lungs and chest wall and are calculated by subtracting the pressure "outside" from the pressure "inside" each structure. That is, transpulmonary pressure (P_L) is the difference between alveolar (Palv) and pleural pressure (Ppl), and the gradient across the chest wall (P_W) is equal to pleural pressure minus body surface (atmospheric) pressure (Pbs):

$$P_L = Palv - Ppl \quad (1)$$

$$P_W = Ppl - Pbs \quad (2)$$

Because these measurements are performed under static conditions (i.e., there is no airflow), Palv is equal to the pressure measured at the airway opening (P_{AO}) proximal to the site of airway occlusion. Pleural pressure is approximated by measuring the pressure within the lower two thirds of the esophagus (Pes) with use of a balloon catheter. Because all pressures are referenced to it, atmospheric pressure is considered to be zero. Therefore:

$$P_L = P_{AO} - Pes \quad (3)$$

and

$$P_W = Pes \quad (4)$$

Static pressure-volume relationships obtained by use of this technique are shown in Figure 109-2.[1-4] Note that the elastic recoil pressure of the entire respiratory system (P_{RS}) at any volume is equal to the sum of the pressures generated by its two components. That is,

$$P_{RS} = P_L + P_W \quad (5)$$

Alternatively, the pressure-volume curve of the respiratory system can be determined directly during stepwise exhalation by measuring the appropriate transmural pressure at each volume. Because

$$P_{RS} = Palv - Pbs \text{ or}$$

$$P_{RS} = P_{AO} \quad (6)$$

the elastic recoil pressure of the respiratory system at any volume is simply the pressure recorded at the airway opening.[1-4]

Up to this point, pressure-volume relationships have been depicted as a single line, suggesting that a unique elastic recoil pressure exists for each volume. In fact, at any volume, elastic recoil pressure is greater during inspiration than during expiration. This property is referred to as *hysteresis*[4-7] and is illustrated in Figure 109-3. Hysteresis is exhibited by both the chest wall and the lungs, although it is much more prominent in the lungs.[7] Chest wall hysteresis is believed to result from the presence of connective tissue and muscle, which demonstrate similar properties in vitro. Lung hysteresis is due mainly to the presence of surfactant (see later), although connective tissue elements also play a role.

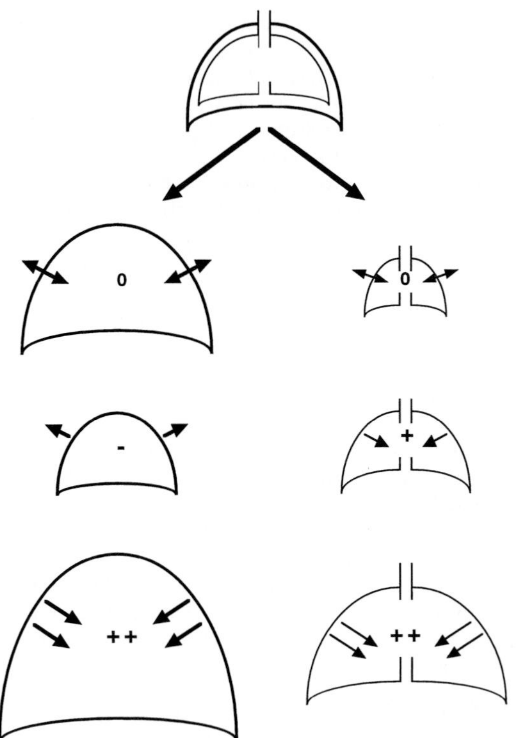

Figure 109–1. Schematic representation of the isolated lungs and chest wall. When separated from each other, the lungs deflate and the chest wall expands to reach an equilibrium volume. When volume is increased or decreased from this resting level, pressure must be supplied to overcome elastic recoil. *Arrows* illustrate the direction and magnitude of elastic recoil; 0, −, +, and + + represent the pressure required to balance it.

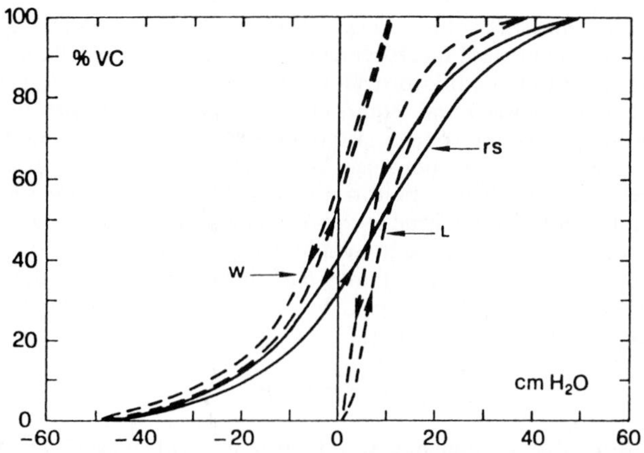

Figure 109–3. Inspiratory and expiratory static pressure-volume curves of the lungs (L), chest wall (w), and respiratory system (rs). Hysteresis is demonstrated by greater elastic recoil pressure during inspiration than during expiration. (From Agostoni E, Hyatt RE: Static behavior of the respiratory system. *In*: Handbook of Physiology: The Respiratory System. Macklem PT, Mead J [Eds]. Bethesda, Md, American Physiological Society, 1986, p 118.)

Lung Volumes

Figure 109–2 demonstrates that several commonly measured lung volumes are determined by the elastic recoil of the lungs and chest wall and by the strength of the respiratory muscles.[4]

Functional residual capacity (FRC) is the volume remaining in the lungs at the end of a passive, tidal expiration. It is the point at which the inward recoil of the lungs is exactly balanced by the outward recoil of the chest wall. Because PRS equals zero, no respiratory muscle activity is required to maintain this volume, and the FRC represents the resting or equilibrium position of the respiratory system.

Total lung capacity (TLC) is the volume present in the lungs after a maximal inspiration. It is reached when the combined elastic recoil of the lungs and chest wall is balanced by the maximum pressure that can be generated by the inspiratory muscles.

Residual volume (RV) is the volume of gas remaining in the lungs after a maximal expiration. In children and young adults, RV is determined primarily by the balance between the elastic recoil of the chest wall and maximal expiratory effort. In older adults and patients with airway and parenchymal disease, however, small airway closure, induced by increases in pleural pressure, limits the volume of gas that can be forcefully exhaled. This causes gas to be trapped within the alveoli and leads to an elevation of RV.

Vital capacity (VC) is the volume of gas that can be forcefully exhaled after a maximal inspiration. It is the difference between TLC and RV.

Compliance and Elastance

The elastic recoil of the lungs, chest wall, and respiratory system can be quantified in a number of ways. As discussed

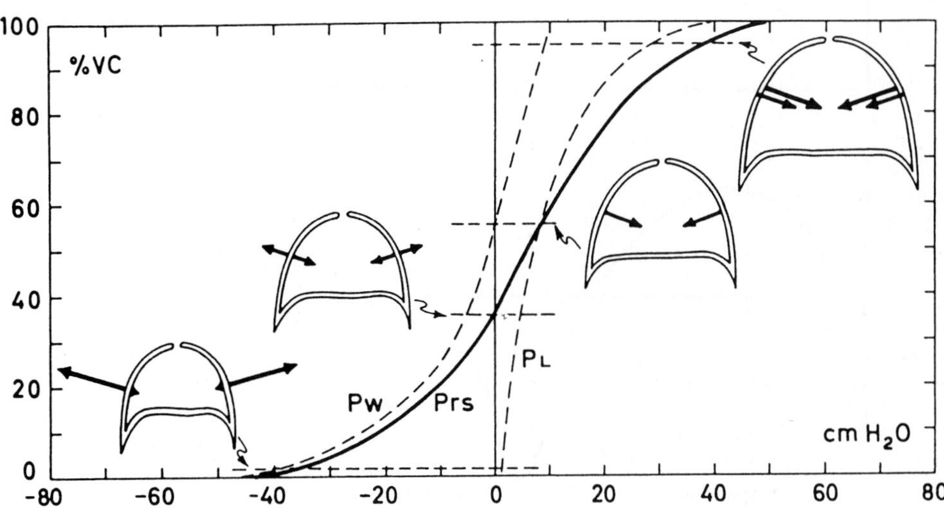

Figure 109–2. Static pressure-volume curves of the lungs (PL), chest wall (Pw), and respiratory system (Prs). From left to right, total elastic recoil pressure at residual volume, functional residual capacity, the equilibrium volume of the chest wall, and total lung capacity are shown. *Arrows* illustrate the direction and magnitude of elastic recoil. VC = vital capacity. (From Agostoni E, Hyatt RE: Static behavior of the respiratory system. *In*: Handbook of Physiology: The Respiratory System. Macklem PT, Mead J [Eds]. Bethesda, Md, American Physiological Society, 1986, p 116.)

before, pressure-volume relationships can be plotted by performing sequential measurements during stepwise exhalation. Although this method provides a great deal of information, it is time-consuming and requires both cooperation and practice on the part of the subject. Alternatively, a single measurement of pressure and volume can be made. Although it is rapid and relatively easy to perform, such a measurement provides information about elastic recoil only at a specific lung volume. A compromise between these approaches is to measure elastic recoil pressure at two volumes. The difference between these pressures (ΔP) and volumes (ΔV) can then be used to calculate the compliance (C), where

$$C = \Delta V/\Delta P \qquad (7)$$

Note that compliance varies inversely with elastic recoil. That is, when compliance is low, a given pressure increment produces only a small increase in volume (i.e., the structure is stiff), whereas a large increase occurs when compliance is high. By measuring the appropriate transmural pressures during relaxation against an occluded airway, one can determine the *static compliance* of the lungs (C_L), chest wall (C_W), and respiratory system (C_{RS}) from the following equations[1–4]:

$$C_L = \Delta V/\Delta(Pao - Pes) \qquad (8)$$

$$C_W = \Delta V/\Delta Pes \qquad (9)$$

$$C_{RS} = \Delta V/\Delta Pao \qquad (10)$$

It should be evident, in Equations 8 to 10, that static compliance is simply the slope of the pressure-volume curves shown in Figure 109–2. The static compliance of the lungs, chest wall, and respiratory system is fairly constant (i.e., there is little change in slope) over a large volume range. Near TLC and RV, however, compliance falls (i.e., the slope decreases) as the elastic elements within the lungs and chest wall reach the limits of their distensibility.

The relationship between pressure and volume may also be expressed in terms of elastance (E), where

$$E = \Delta P/\Delta V \qquad (11)$$

Because it is the reciprocal of compliance, elastance varies directly with elastic recoil. The elastance of the respiratory system and its components can be calculated simply by inverting Equations 8 to 10.

Although more commonly calculated during respiratory muscle relaxation, compliance and elastance can also be determined during active breathing.[8] As shown in Figure 109–4, because flow is zero at the end of both inspiration and expiration, we can calculate *dynamic compliance* and *elastance* by measuring both the tidal volume and the change in the appropriate transmural pressure between these two points in the respiratory cycle. Although the static and dynamic values of compliance and elastance are similar, they are not identical. The reason for this discrepancy is discussed later.

Origin of Elastic Recoil

As implied by the preceding discussion, elastic recoil is generated, in part, by elastic or distensible elements within the lung parenchyma and chest wall. On histologic examination, the alveolar septum is partitioned into three layers: the *epithelium*, which consists of type I and type II pneumocytes; the

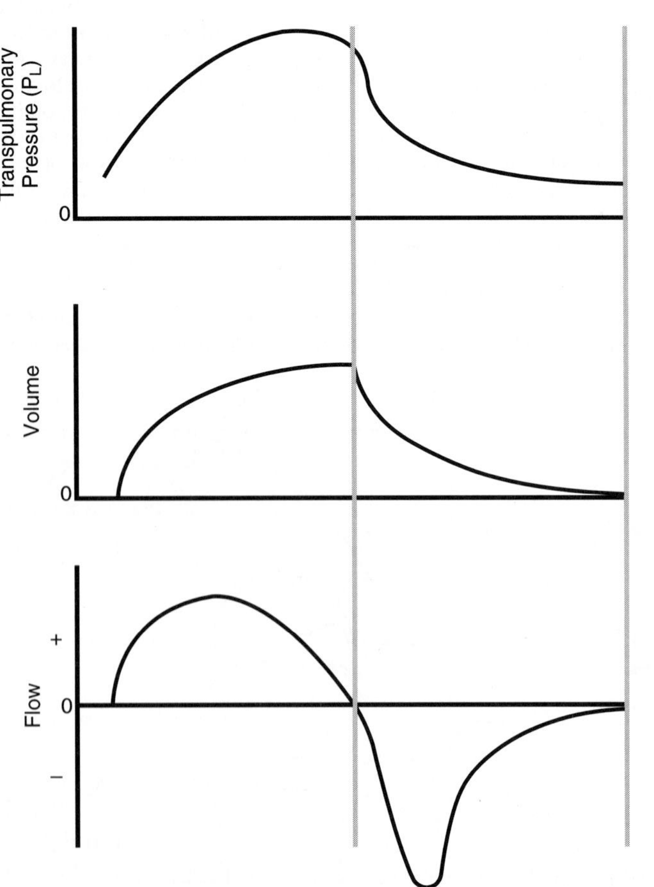

Figure 109–4. Transpulmonary pressure (P_L), volume, and flow during a spontaneous respiratory cycle. Dynamic compliance and elastance are calculated by measuring the change in volume (ΔV) and the change in pressure (ΔP) between points of zero flow.

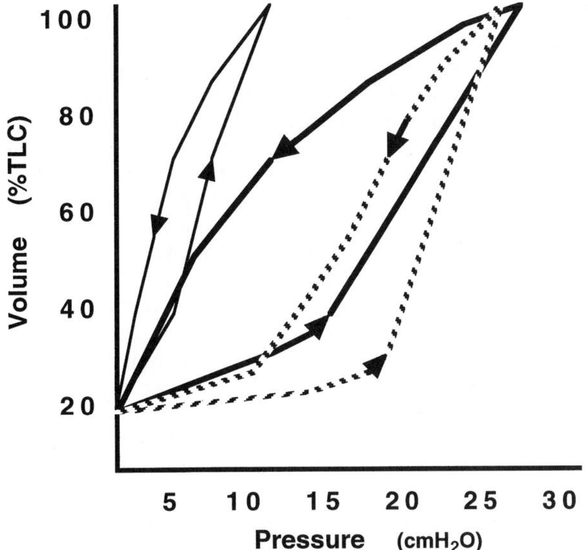

Figure 109–5. Inspiratory and expiratory pressure-volume curves in an excised normal lung *(thick line)* and in lungs rinsed with a detergent *(hatched line)* and filled with saline *(thin line)*. TLC = total lung capacity. (Adapted from Gil J, Bachofen H, Gehr P, et al: Alveolar volume-surface area relation in air- and saline-filled lungs fixed by vascular perfusion. J Appl Physiol 1979; 47:995; and Bachofen H, Gehr P, Weibel ER: Alterations of mechanical properties and morphology in excised rabbit lungs rinsed with a detergent. J Appl Physiol 1979; 47:1003.)

endothelium, which forms the walls of the alveolar capillaries; and the *interstitial space*, which separates these two layers.[9] The alveolar interstitium contains collagen and elastin fibers as well as scattered fibroblasts. Together with denser collections of collagen and elastin surrounding the airways and blood vessels, this fiber network forms the connective tissue "skeleton" of the pulmonary parenchyma. Distention of this fiber network during lung inflation requires increasing levels of applied pressure. Similarly, deformation of cartilage, muscle, and bone requires progressively increasing force as the chest wall is moved above or below its equilibrium volume. The pressures generated by distention of these connective tissue elements in the lung parenchyma and chest wall are referred to as *tissue forces*, and they are easily understood by the analogy of a metal spring.

There is, however, another important source of lung elastic recoil. Surface tension is generated by the thin layer of phospholipid, referred to as *surfactant*, that coats the alveolar epithelium.[10-12] Surface tension occurs at any gas-liquid interface. It results from the cohesive forces between molecules of the liquid and tends to reduce the gas-liquid interface to the smallest possible surface area. In the lung, these *surface forces* act to reduce alveolar size and to increase the pressure required to maintain a given lung volume. As shown in Figure 109-5, the relative importance of tissue and surface forces can be determined by examination of pressure-volume curves of saline-filled and air-filled lungs.[13, 14] In the lung filled with saline, the air-liquid interface has been eliminated and elastic recoil is produced solely by tissue forces. In the air-filled lung, both tissue and surface forces are present. It is evident from these data that surface forces are responsible for most of the elastic recoil generated by the normal lung.

Because of its air-liquid interface and spherical structure, the pressure within an alveolus should be accurately predicted by the Laplace equation:

$$P = 2T/r \qquad (12)$$

where P is the alveolar pressure, T is the surface tension of surfactant, and r is the alveolar radius. According to this equation, however, alveolar pressure due to surface forces should vary inversely with alveolar size. If this were true, elastic recoil would decrease during inspiration; and during expiration, increasing elastic recoil would lead to diffuse alveolar collapse. This, of course, does not occur.

The solution to this problem comes from two important properties of surfactant. First, unlike that of other liquids, the surface tension of surfactant is not constant but varies directly with the size of the air-liquid interface.[10-12] As alveolar volume increases, surface tension rises. This more than offsets the effect of increasing alveolar radius and allows surface forces and elastic recoil to increase with lung volume. During expiration, decreasing surface tension allows surface forces to fall, thereby decreasing elastic recoil and preventing alveolar collapse.

Second, Figure 109-5 illustrates that surfactant produces a much greater pressure-volume hysteresis than do other liquids, such as a detergent. This acts to further reduce surface forces during expiration and helps to maintain alveolar stability.[10-15] By examining the behavior of saline-filled lungs, we can see that surfactant is responsible for most of the pressure-volume hysteresis observed in the intact lung.[13, 14]

Viscous Forces

Under static conditions, maintaining the respiratory system at any point above or below its equilibrium volume requires only enough pressure to balance its elastic recoil. During the dynamic processes of inspiration and expiration, however, additional pressure must be supplied to overcome the frictional or *viscous forces* produced by the flow of gas through the airways and the movement of the lung parenchyma and chest wall.

Airway Pressure-Flow Relationships

As gas moves through the airways, pressure is required to overcome both friction at the airway surface and the cohesive forces between gas molecules. A pressure gradient must, therefore, exist between the mouth and the alveoli. This gradient may be thought of not only as the pressure needed to overcome viscous forces but also as the driving pressure required to produce flow. The magnitude of this pressure gradient depends on the flow rate, the length and caliber of the airways, and the density and viscosity of the gas. The relative importance of these factors depends on whether flow is laminar or turbulent.[16]

As illustrated in Figure 109-6, when flow is laminar, gas

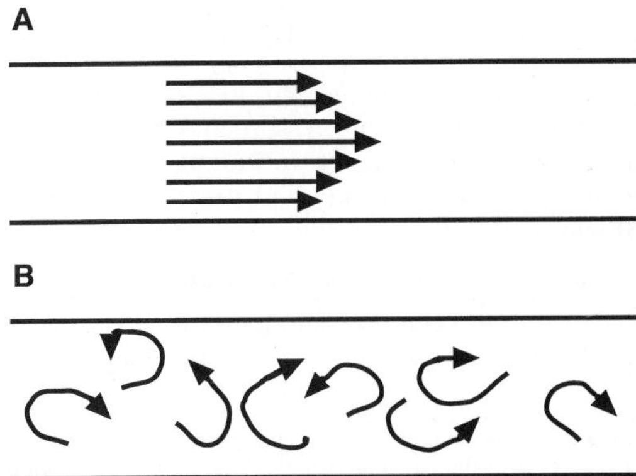

Figure 109–6. Schematic representations of laminar *(A)* and turbulent *(B)* flow.

moves in discrete cylindrical layers or laminae. Because frictional forces are greatest at the airway surface, central laminae move more rapidly than do those at the periphery, and gas flows in a conical configuration. In the presence of laminar flow, the pressure gradient (ΔP) required to produce a given flow ($\dot{V}$) is defined by Poiseuille's law:

$$\Delta P = 8\mu l\dot{V}/\pi r^4 \tag{13}$$

where μ is the viscosity of the gas and l and r are the length and radius of the airway, respectively.[16] Note that airway radius is the main determinant of driving pressure. Halving the radius will require a 16-fold increase in pressure if the same flow rate is to be maintained. Poiseuille's law states that when gas viscosity and airway length and radius are kept constant, flow is directly proportional to driving pressure. That is, the pressure-flow relationship is linear and described by the following equation:

$$\Delta P = K\dot{V} \tag{14}$$

where K is a constant that incorporates all of the other variables shown in Equation 13. Laminar flow is most likely to occur in an unbranched tube with smooth walls. Other factors that favor laminar flow are low flow rate, low gas density, and high gas viscosity.[16] *

As the airways become more branched or irregular or as gas velocity increases, the orderly characteristics of laminar flow are replaced by random, chaotic gas movement referred to as turbulent flow. When flow is turbulent, Poiseuille's law no longer applies, and the driving pressure is defined by the following equation:

$$\Delta P = fl\dot{V}^2/4\pi^2 r^5 \tag{15}$$

where f is a friction factor that incorporates gas density and viscosity.[16] Note that turbulent flow requires a much higher driving pressure than does laminar flow. This is due in part to the greater dependence of pressure on airway radius. In addition, Equation 15 indicates that driving pressure varies directly with the square of the flow rate. This means that pressure increases disproportionately with flow, and this relationship can be expressed as

$$\Delta P = K\dot{V}^2 \tag{16}$$

In the human airway, regions of fully laminar and fully turbulent flow coexist with regions that have a transitional or mixed flow pattern, and none of the equations listed accurately predicts the observed relationship between driving pressure and flow. To overcome this problem, we can combine Equations 14 and 16 to yield

$$\Delta P = K_1\dot{V} + K_2\dot{V}^2 \tag{17}$$

When flow is primarily laminar, the first term predominates, and the relationship between pressure and flow will be nearly linear. As flow becomes more turbulent, the second term assumes increasing importance, and pressure losses increase exponentially with increasing flow.

Partitioning of Viscous Pressure Losses

The relationship between flow and the viscous pressure losses produced by the components of the respiratory system is illustrated in Figure 109–7.[17, 18] Because of irregularities, protuberances, and abrupt changes in diameter, flow through the upper airway (the mouth, pharynx, and larynx) is predominantly turbulent. These structures account for approximately 35% of the pressure drop between the mouth and the alveoli at a flow rate of 1 L/sec.[17, 18] Owing to its exponential pressure-flow characteristics, this segment of the airway becomes increasingly important as flow increases (e.g., during exercise).

Viscous pressure losses in the lower airways occur predominantly in the first six generations.[19] The small airways (<2 mm in diameter) account for only about 10% of this pressure drop and for a small proportion of total airway pressure losses.[19-21] Given the marked dependence of driving pressure on airway radius (Equations 13 and 15), it may appear counterintuitive that pressure losses should decrease as the airways become smaller. The key to understanding this apparent contradiction lies in the fact that as the airways divide into smaller and smaller branches, their total number increases dramatically. Because the same volume of gas must pass through each generation of airways, flow through each individual airway must progressively slow until flow stops completely at the level of the alveolus. This reduction in gas velocity results in a progressive decrease in viscous pressure losses.

Just as viscous forces must be overcome to allow airflow between the mouth and the alveoli, pressure must also be supplied to compensate for friction produced by movement of the lung parenchyma and chest wall. Studies in dogs have indicated that the viscous pressure loss produced by lung tissue is negligible,[22, 23] and this is believed to be true in humans as well. As shown in Figure 109–7, at a flow rate of 1 L/sec, the pressure required to move the chest wall accounts for approximately 17% of the viscous pressure loss of the entire respiratory system.[17, 18] Because the pressure-flow relationship of the chest wall is linear, its contribution progressively falls with increasing flow.

Endotracheal Tubes

Like the upper airway, endotracheal tubes have nonlinear pressure-flow characteristics.[24, 25] Figure 109–8 demonstrates that the degree of nonlinearity increases dramatically as the internal diameter of the endotracheal tube decreases. This occurs because at a given flow rate, gas velocity must increase as tube diameter decreases. This leads to increasingly turbulent flow, which in turn causes disproportionate pressure

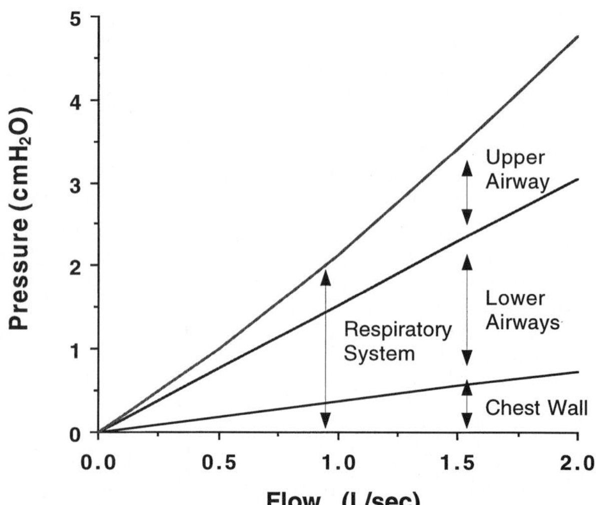

Figure 109–7. Pressure-flow relationships for the upper and lower airway and the chest wall. See text for details.

Viscosity is a measure of the resistance of a gas or liquid to movement. It is directly proportional to the strength of the cohesive forces between its molecules. *Density* is the weight per unit volume of a substance. For example, helium has a viscosity similar to that of oxygen or nitrogen but a much lower density.

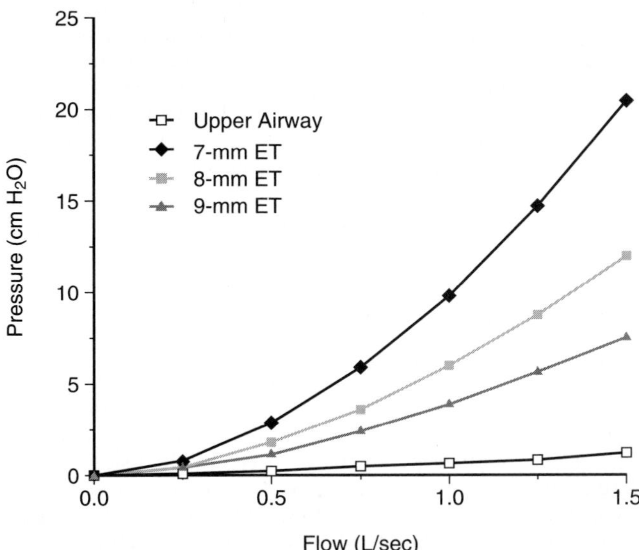

Figure 109–8. Pressure-flow relationships for endotracheal tubes (ET) with three different internal diameters compared with the normal upper airway.

losses. Although these characteristics have been well described in vitro, relatively little is known about the effect of endotracheal intubation on in vivo pressure-flow relationships. By comparing the pressure-flow characteristics of endotracheal tubes and the normal upper airway, it is evident from Figure 109–8 that endotracheal intubation should dramatically increase the pressure needed for ventilation. In fact, however, these data may actually underestimate the additional pressure required, because deformation and kinking of the endotracheal tube and partial occlusion by secretions are common in intubated patients.[26] In addition, endotracheal intubation may lead to diffuse bronchoconstriction because of stimulation of receptors in the larynx and trachea.[27]

Resistance

Just as compliance and elastance are used to quantify elastic recoil, viscous forces are conventionally expressed in terms of resistance (R), which is the ratio of driving pressure (ΔP) and flow rate:

$$R = \Delta P/\dot{V} \tag{18}$$

The resistance of the airways (R_{AW}), lung (R_L), chest wall (R_W), and respiratory system (R_{RS}) can be calculated by measuring the appropriate transmural pressure during airflow:

$$R_{AW} = (P_{AO} - P_{alv})/\dot{V} \tag{19}$$

$$R_L = (P_{AO} - P_{es})/\dot{V} \tag{20}$$

$$R_W = P_{es}/\dot{V} \tag{21}$$

$$R_{RS} = P_{AO}/\dot{V} \tag{22}$$

Since the pressure gradient across the lungs and chest wall is due in part to the elastic recoil of these structures, resistance can be calculated only when elastic recoil pressure has been subtracted from the total transmural pressure. This can be accomplished with the rapid airway occlusion technique (see later). Because of the need for respiratory muscle relaxation, however, calculating lung, chest wall, and respiratory system resistance is difficult in spontaneously breathing subjects. Airway resistance, on the other hand, can be easily measured by means of a body plethysmograph.[28]

Compliance, Elastance, and Resistance Measurements in Mechanically Ventilated Patients

Figure 109–9 illustrates the changes in pressure and flow that occur in a relaxed patient when the airway is rapidly occluded during a positive-pressure breath. During mechanical inflation, PAO, PL, and Pes increase from P0 (end-expiratory pressure) to Pmax (end-inspiratory pressure). When the airway is occluded and flow abruptly stopped, there is an immediate fall in pressure (point P1) followed by a more gradual decline that plateaus in 3 to 5 seconds (point P2). In each tracing, the difference between Pmax and P0 is the pressure required to overcome all forces opposing the movement of the total respiratory system (PAO), the airways and lung parenchyma

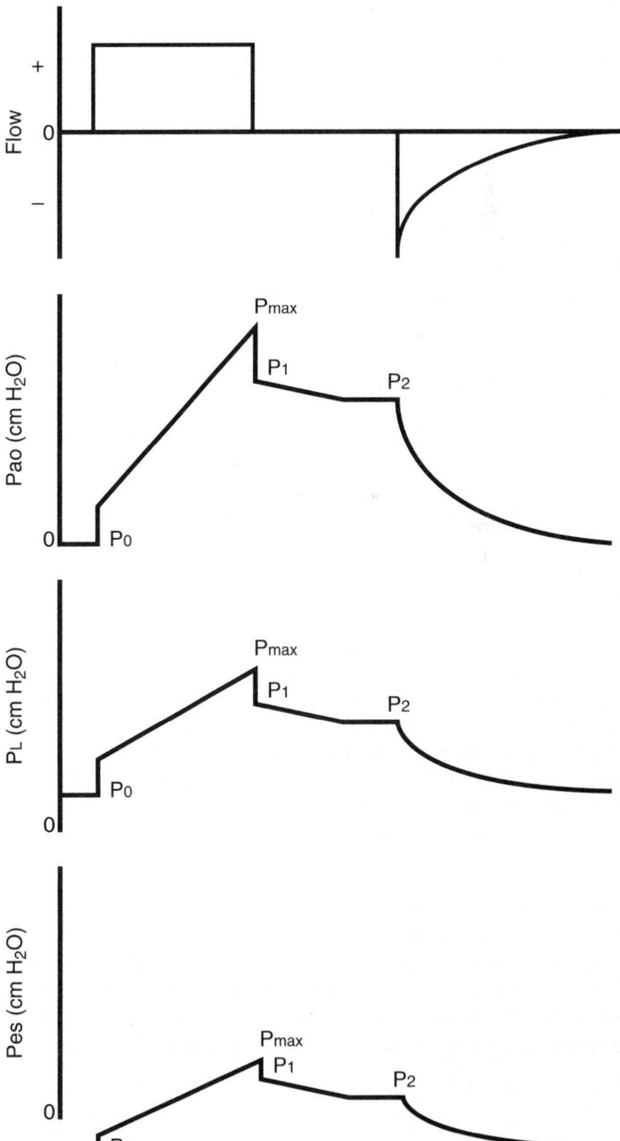

Figure 109–9. The interrupter technique. Flow and the pressure across the respiratory system (PAO), the lungs (PL), and the chest wall (Pes) are illustrated during inspiration, expiration, and end-inspiratory occlusion. See text for details.

(PL), or the chest wall (Pes), whereas the gradient between P2 and P0 is the pressure required to overcome only the elastic recoil of these structures. Because the drop from Pmax to P1 occurs immediately after the cessation of flow, this represents the pressure needed to overcome viscous forces.

With the information obtained by use of this rapid airway occlusion or "interrupter" technique, the compliance, elastance, and resistance of the respiratory system and its components can be calculated.[18, 29-33] Compliance is determined by dividing the inspired volume by the pressure gradient between P2 and P0.

$$C_{RS} = V/(P2_{ao} - P0_{ao}) \quad (23)$$

$$C_{L} = V/(P2_{L} - P0_{L}) \quad (24)$$

$$C_{W} = V/(P2_{es} - P0_{es}) \quad (25)$$

Elastance is calculated by dividing the pressure gradient by inspired volume.

By dividing the pressure drop occurring immediately after airway occlusion by the flow rate preceding it, we can determine the resistance of the respiratory system, lungs, and chest wall:

$$R_{RS} = (Pmax_{ao} - P1_{ao})/\dot{V} \quad (26)$$

$$R_{L} = (Pmax_{L} - P1_{L})/\dot{V} \quad (27)$$

$$R_{W} = (Pmax_{es} - P1_{es})/\dot{V} \quad (28)$$

Because the pressure required to overcome viscous forces of the lung parenchyma is negligible, RL is, in fact, equal to RAW.[22]

Viscoelastic Forces

In Figure 109-9, $Pmax_{ao}$ represents the total pressure required to inflate the respiratory system. If the difference between Pmax and P1 is the pressure required to overcome viscous forces, and P2 is the pressure needed to balance elastic recoil, then the gradient between P1 and P2 must be the pressure required to overcome a third factor opposing the movement of the respiratory system—the *viscoelastic forces* of the lungs and chest wall.[32-35] Viscoelasticity is a property that is common to all biologic soft tissues as well as many inorganic materials and may be understood by considering what happens when force is quickly applied to a rubber band. When the band is stretched, the pressure required to maintain its new length reaches a peak immediately after movement stops, then gradually falls to a lower level. This is referred to as stress relaxation. In the same way, movement of the respiratory system requires pressure to overcome the viscoelastic forces of the lungs and chest wall. As shown in Figure 109-9, during end-inspiratory occlusion, stress relaxation causes these forces to gradually disappear until a plateau (elastic recoil pressure) has been reached.[32-35]

The viscoelastic properties of the lung parenchyma appear to reside primarily in the network of collagen and elastin fibers that compose its connective tissue skeleton, although resting tone and contraction of interstitial fibroblasts may also play a role.[36, 37] Skeletal muscle and cartilage are responsible for the viscoelasticity of the chest wall.

Figure 109-9 also demonstrates that viscoelastic forces account for observed differences between the static and dynamic values of compliance and elastance.[31-33] When measurements are performed during active breathing (see Fig. 109-4), the pressure at end-inspiration is obtained immediately after flow reaches zero, whereas static measurements are made after a prolonged pause. This is equivalent to the difference between points P1 and P2 in Figure 109-9. Because the pressure measured during active breathing exceeds the static or plateau pressure, dynamic compliance will be less than, and dynamic elastance will be greater than, its static counterpart. During mechanical inflation, dynamic compliance (Cdyn) and elastance (Edyn) are, therefore, calculated as

$$Cdyn = \Delta V/(P1 - P0) \quad (29)$$

$$Edyn = (P1 - P0)/\Delta V \quad (30)$$

An important property of viscoelastic forces is that their magnitude varies directly with the rate of tissue expansion.[31-33, 35] This can be understood, once again, if we consider what happens when force is applied to a rubber band. If the rubber band is stretched quickly, the pressure required to achieve a given length will be higher than if it is stretched slowly, even though the plateau (or elastic recoil) pressure will be the same in both cases. If this concept is applied to the respiratory system and the pressure-time curves shown in Figure 109-9, it should be evident that P1 will be similar to P2 at low inflation rates and that P1 (and Pmax) will increase as inspiratory flow rises. This means, according to Equations 29 and 30, that dynamic compliance and elastance must also vary with the rate of inflation, a property referred to as *rate dependence* or *frequency dependence*.[31-33, 35] At low inspiratory flow rates, dynamic compliance and elastance are similar to their static values but decrease and increase, respectively, as the rate of inflation increases.

APPLIED FORCES

Inspiration

The pressure required to expand the respiratory system above its resting volume is normally provided by the respiratory muscles. When the diaphragm and accessory muscles are unable to generate sufficient force to maintain adequate ventilation, respiratory failure occurs and the pressure required for inspiration must be provided completely, or in part, by a mechanical ventilator.

Figure 109-10 illustrates the change in transpulmonary pressure,* flow, and volume during a spontaneous breath. Because PL = Pao − Pes, and Pao remains zero (atmospheric pressure) throughout the respiratory cycle, PL is simply the opposite of pleural (esophageal) pressure (i.e., PL = −Pes). Normally, PL is positive at FRC owing to the inward recoil of the lungs (see Fig. 109-2). During inspiration, PL rises further, reflecting the force provided by the respiratory muscles to overcome the elastic recoil and the viscous and viscoelastic forces of the airways and lung parenchyma. The broken line in the top panel represents the pressure required to balance lung elastic recoil, which increases with inspired volume. The difference between the solid and broken lines equals the pressure required for gas flow. These two lines converge as flow reaches zero (and viscous forces disappear) at the end of inspiration.

Figure 109-11 provides similar information during a positive-pressure mechanical breath with constant inspiratory flow.[25] Instead of transpulmonary pressure, however, the top panel shows the pressure gradient across the entire respiratory system (PRS). Because PRS = Pao − Pbs, and Pbs is equal to atmospheric pressure, PRS is equal to Pao. During mechanical inflation, viscous forces must be overcome before airflow can begin, and Pao rapidly rises before the onset of inspiratory

*Because the pressure required to expand the chest wall cannot be measured during a spontaneous breath, only transpulmonary pressure is considered.

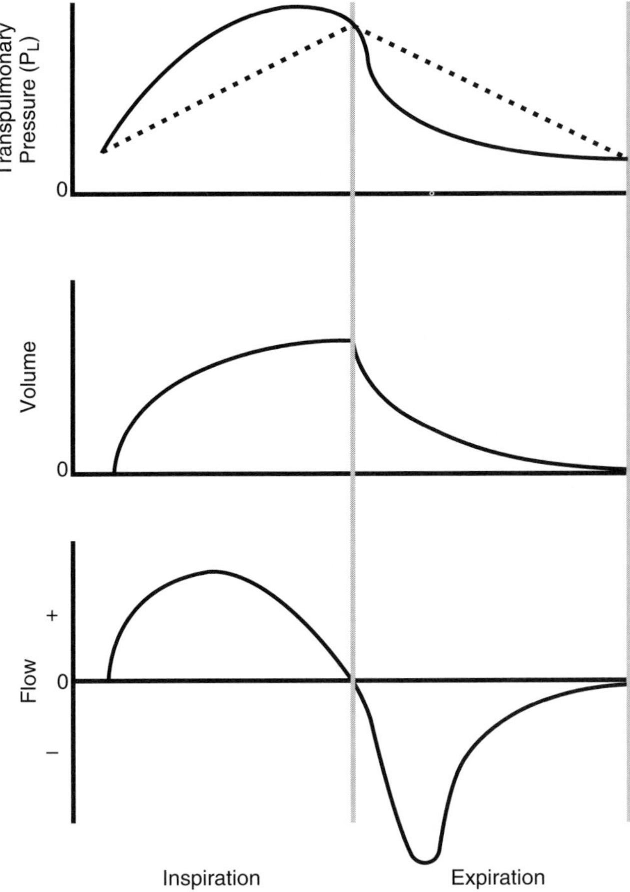

Figure 109–10. Transpulmonary pressure, volume, and flow during a spontaneous respiratory cycle. *Top panel* illustrates the total pressure required to inflate the lungs *(solid line)* as well as the pressure needed to overcome elastic recoil alone *(broken line)*.

flow. As inspiration proceeds, Pao equals the pressure required to overcome both the increasing elastic recoil of the lungs and chest wall (broken line) and the viscous forces produced by airflow and movement of the chest wall (the difference between the solid and broken lines).

Because, in this example, inspiratory flow is constant, both volume and elastic recoil increase linearly throughout inspiration, and the pressure required to overcome viscous forces is also constant.

Expiration

Passive Expiration

As gas leaves the lungs and the respiratory system returns toward its equilibrium volume, pressure must still be supplied to overcome the viscous forces produced by expiratory airflow and movement of the chest wall. When the respiratory muscles are relaxed, this pressure is provided solely by the elastic recoil of the lungs and chest wall. Figures 109-10 and 109-11 illustrate the change in pressure, flow, and volume during such a *passive* expiration. Both volume and flow decrease exponentially and elastic recoil pressure returns to zero only when expiratory flow has stopped and the respiratory system has reached its equilibrium volume. Under some circumstances, it is beneficial to terminate expiratory flow prematurely, thereby increasing end-expiratory lung volume. This can be accomplished in both spontaneously breathing and mechanically ventilated patients if sufficient pressure (positive end-expiratory pressure [PEEP]) is supplied to balance the remaining elastic recoil of the respiratory system.

Because flow is driven only by elastic recoil, the duration of a passive expiration and the shape of both the flow and volume-time curves are influenced by the compliance and resistance of the respiratory system.[38] For example, as compliance increases, driving pressure falls, thereby reducing flow and prolonging expiration. Similarly, for a given driving pressure, as resistance increases, flow falls and leads to a progressive rise in expiratory time. This dependence of expiratory flow, volume, and time on the mechanical properties of the respiratory system is conveniently expressed in terms of the product of compliance and resistance, which has the units of time (seconds) and is referred to as the time constant (τ):

$$\tau = RC \tag{31}$$

During a passive expiration, the volume remaining in the lungs (V) at any time (t), is determined by the end-inspiratory volume (Vi) and by the time constant:

$$V = Vi\, e^{-(t/\tau)} \tag{32}$$

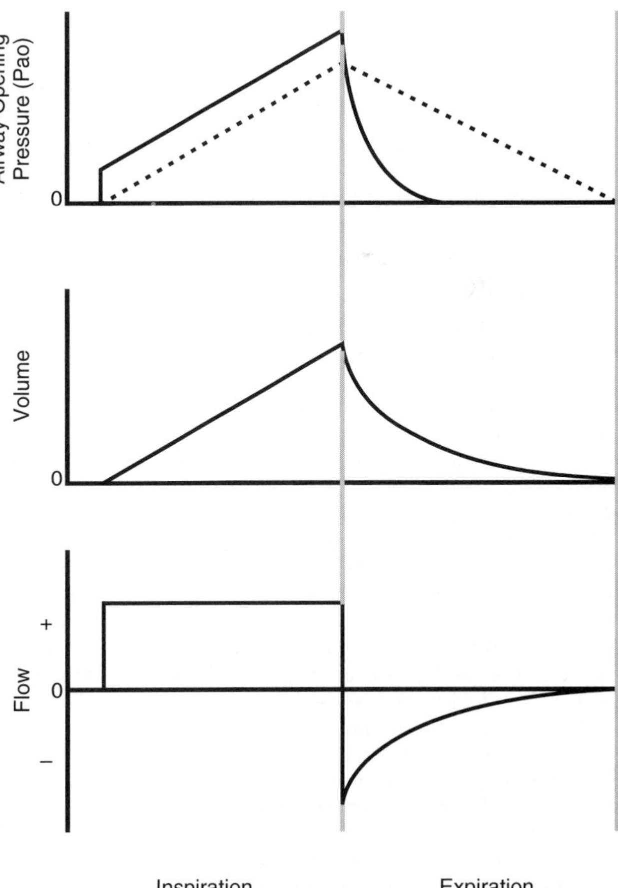

Figure 109–11. Pressure at the airway opening, volume, and flow during a mechanically ventilated breath. *Top panel* illustrates the total pressure required to inflate the lungs and chest wall *(solid line)* and the pressure required to overcome the elastic recoil of these structures *(broken line)*.

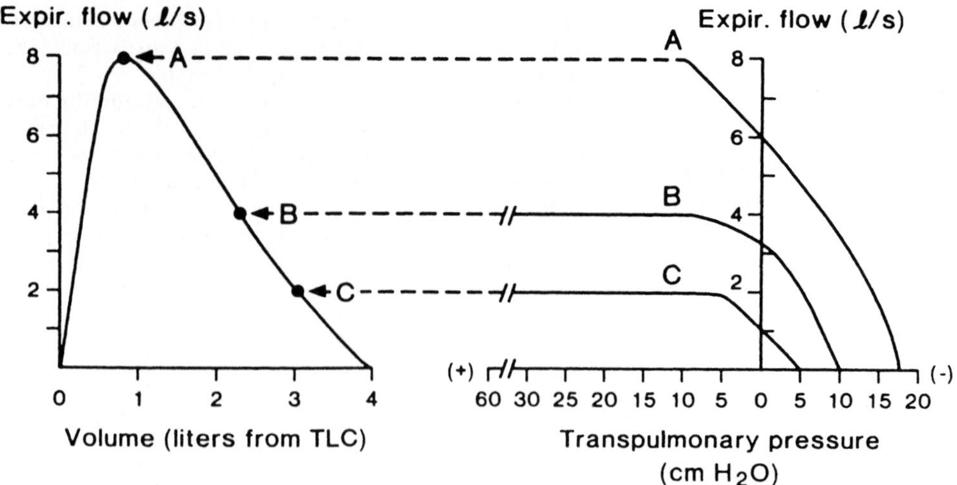

Figure 109–12. Isovolume flow-pressure curves and their relationship to the maximum expiratory flow-volume curve. TLC = total lung capacity. See text for details. (From Hyatt, RE: Forced expiration. *In*: Handbook of Physiology: The Respiratory System. Macklem PT, Mead J [Eds]. Bethesda, Md, American Physiological Society, 1986, p 296.)

where e is the base of natural logarithms, a constant equal to approximately 2.72.[38] If time is set equal to multiples of τ, Equation 32 can be simplified to:

$$V = Vi\ e^{-1}, Vi\ e^{-2}, Vi\ e^{-3}$$

or

$$V = Vi(1/e), Vi(1/e^2), Vi(1/e^3)$$

This means that during a passive expiration, 0.368 (37%), 0.135 (14%), and 0.050 (5%) of the initial volume remains in the lungs at times equal to 1, 2, and 3 time constants, respectively.[38] Because expiratory flow also decays exponentially, a similar relationship exists between initial or maximum flow and flow at any time during expiration.

$$\dot{V} = \dot{V}i\ e^{-(t/\tau)} \qquad (33)$$

Expiratory Flow Limitation

In many circumstances, of course, expiration is not passive. In the presence of high ventilation requirements or disorders affecting the mechanics of the lungs or chest wall, the expiratory muscles supply additional pressure to augment flow and shorten expiratory time. During active or *forced* expiration, however, flow does not increase indefinitely with increasing muscle effort, a property referred to as *expiratory flow limitation*.[39–42]

Figure 109–12 illustrates what happens when a subject uses more and more effort (reflected by increasing transpulmonary pressure) to exhale from several different lung volumes. At volumes greater than approximately 85% of the vital capacity, increasing effort leads to a progressive rise in expiratory flow. At lower volumes, however, a maximum flow is reached and cannot be increased regardless of how much pressure is generated by the respiratory muscles.

As suggested by Figure 109–12, if these so-called isovolume flow-pressure curves are performed at a large number of lung volumes, the relationship between maximum flow and volume can be determined over the entire vital capacity. Fortunately, we can obtain the same information simply by recording both expiratory flow and volume during a forced expiration from TLC. The usefulness of this maneuver, which is routinely performed during pulmonary function testing, is explained largely by the presence of expiratory flow limitation. Because maximum expiratory flow is fixed throughout most of the vital capacity, the downslope of this flow-volume curve and many of the measurements obtained from it are accurate and reproducible even in the absence of the patient's maximal effort. However, both the forced vital capacity (FVC) and the forced expiratory volume in 1 second (FEV_1) are influenced by the flow rates generated in the early portion of the forced expiratory maneuver and are, therefore, at least partially dependent on the patient's effort. The peak expiratory flow rate (PEFR) is, of course, largely determined by the maximum force generated during exhalation.

The Equal Pressure Point Theory

The physiologic basis of expiratory flow limitation is most easily understood in terms of the *equal pressure point concept*.[39, 40, 42] As shown in Figure 109–13, alveolar pressure is the sum of the pressure produced by lung elastic recoil and the pressure within the pleural space. This is the total pressure available to overcome the viscous forces produced during expiratory airflow. Pleural pressure surrounds both the alveoli and the intrathoracic airways and is determined by the elastic recoil of the chest wall and the activity of the expiratory muscles. During a passive expiration (panel *A*), pleural pressure remains negative, and the normal (positive) transmural pressure gradient is maintained throughout the intrathoracic airways. During a forced expiration, however, pleural pressure becomes positive (panel *B*).

Because the pressure within the airways must fall as gas moves toward the mouth (where the pressure is zero), it is evident that the pressure inside and outside the airways must eventually become equal, the so-called equal pressure point.[39, 42] It should also be evident that the airways will become narrowed at some point downstream (mouthward) from the equal pressure point if the normal transmural pressure gradient is reversed to a sufficient degree to overcome the structural forces holding them open.[40] The walls of the large airways are supported by cartilage and are relatively resistant to compression. The noncartilaginous airways, however, are easily narrowed because they have little structural rigidity and are normally supported only by the elastic recoil of the surrounding lung parenchyma.

This critical airway narrowing is responsible for expiratory flow limitation. Because resistance is high in the collapsed airway segment and much lower beyond it, expiratory flow is driven by the pressure gradient between the alveoli and this "choke point," not by the gradient between the alveoli and the mouth.[39–42] This is analogous to a waterfall, where the speed of the flowing water depends only on the slope of the riverbed, not on the height of the precipice.[40]

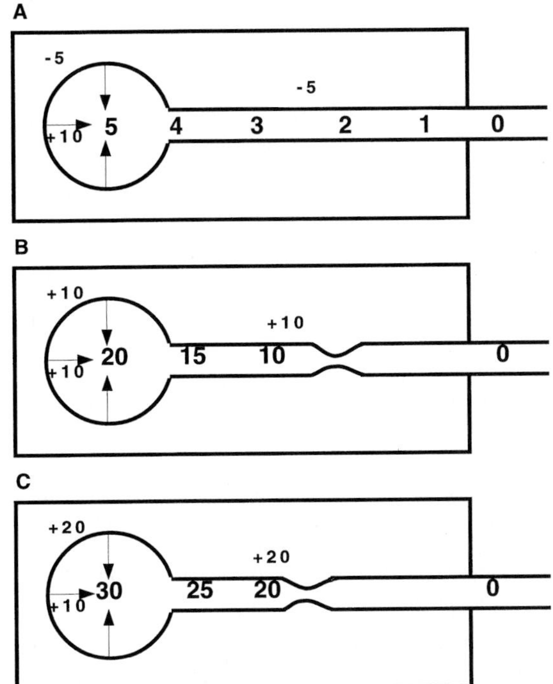

Figure 109–13. Schematic representation of the alveoli, airways, and pleural space during expiratory airflow. Each expiration is performed from the same volume with a lung elastic recoil pressure of 10 cm H_2O *(arrows)*. Panels illustrate the changes in airway pressure that occur during passive expiration *(A)* and with increasing expiratory effort (*B* and *C*).

It can be seen from panel *C* of Figure 109–13 that increasing expiratory effort (e.g., by increasing Ppl to 20 cm H_2O) serves only to move the equal pressure point and the site of airway compression closer to the alveoli. The expiratory pressure gradient and the flow rate do not change. Figure 109–13 also provides an explanation for the direct relationship between lung volume and maximum expiratory flow shown in Figure 109–12. Because intraluminal pressure at the equal pressure point is equal to Ppl, and alveolar pressure is equal to elastic recoil pressure *plus* Ppl, the expiratory pressure gradient is equal to elastic recoil pressure. This means that maximum expiratory flow is determined solely by lung elastic recoil and, therefore, varies directly with lung volume.

The Wave Speed Theory

Expiratory flow limitation may also be explained by the *wave speed theory*,[41, 42] which states that in a compliant tube, fluid or gas velocity can never exceed the speed at which pressures travel along the tube (the wave speed). In the circulation, for example, the wave speed is the rate at which the arterial pulse propagates. Wave speed varies directly with the cross-sectional area of the tube and inversely with both gas or liquid density and tube compliance. During expiration, gas moves from smaller to larger airways. This causes total cross-sectional area to decrease and leads to a progressive fall in wave speed. Because the same volume must pass through each generation of airways, however, gas velocity must increase. This is referred to as *convective acceleration* and results in a fall in airway (and transmural) pressure. During forced expiration, this decrease in pressure causes airway narrowing, which in turn causes gas velocity to increase and further decreases wave speed. Flow limitation occurs when gas velocity equals the wave speed.

RESPIRATORY MECHANICS IN PULMONARY DISEASE

Disorders of the lungs, whether affecting primarily the tracheobronchial tree or the lung parenchyma, are almost always accompanied by alterations in respiratory mechanics. It is these derangements that contribute to dyspnea and functional limitation and may, when severe, precipitate respiratory failure. On the basis of the way in which the mechanics of the respiratory system are altered, pulmonary diseases are typically divided into two broad categories—obstructive and restrictive.

Obstructive Lung Disease

Emphysema, chronic bronchitis, and asthma are by far the most common forms of obstructive lung disease. Although their pathogenesis and clinical characteristics differ, these disorders share the unifying features of airflow obstruction: airway narrowing, decreased expiratory flow, and a prolonged expiratory time. In asthma and chronic bronchitis, airway narrowing is caused by inflammation and edema of the bronchial wall and the presence of intraluminal secretions. Smooth muscle hypertrophy and bronchoconstriction are also important factors in patients with asthma. In emphysema, expiratory airway narrowing results from the destruction of alveolar septa and the subsequent loss of radial traction, which normally maintains small airway patency. Regardless of its mechanism, airway narrowing leads to an increase in viscous forces, which in turn increases airway resistance, decreases expiratory flow, and causes expiratory time to be prolonged. In emphysema, parenchymal destruction leads to loss of lung elastic recoil. This further compromises expiratory flow by reducing the driving pressure available to overcome viscous forces.

In patients with moderate-to-severe airflow obstruction, increased airway resistance and loss of lung elastic recoil predispose to extensive small airway collapse during forced expiration. This leads to elevation of RV and is referred to as *air trapping*. In addition, significant airflow obstruction is typically accompanied by an increase in the volume of gas remaining in the lungs at the end of a passive expiration. This process, known as *hyperinflation*, can result from three mechanisms.[43–45]

First, air trapping may be so severe that it limits the volume that can be exhaled during tidal breathing. Second, because the equilibrium volume of the respiratory system is determined by the opposing elastic recoil of the lungs and chest wall, loss of lung elastic recoil from emphysema leads to an increase in FRC. Finally, because of expiratory slowing, the time available for expiration may be insufficient to allow the respiratory system to return to its equilibrium volume before inspiration begins. This process is referred to as *dynamic hyperinflation*.[43–45] Because its equilibrium volume has not been reached, the elastic recoil pressure of the respiratory system remains positive. This form of PEEP is referred to as intrinsic PEEP (PEEPI)[46] or auto-PEEP[47] to distinguish it from intentionally applied extrinsic PEEP.

These alterations in the mechanics of the respiratory system account for the characteristic findings of airflow obstruction demonstrated by pulmonary function testing. The FEV_1 and the FEV_1:FVC ratio are decreased, as is expiratory flow at each lung volume. This leads to the classic "scooped out" appearance of the flow-volume curve (Fig. 109–14). Hyperinflation causes an elevation in FRC, and air trapping leads to an increase in RV, usually with a concomitant fall in VC.

Abnormal respiratory mechanics also adversely affect the function of the respiratory muscles.[43–45] Increased pressure

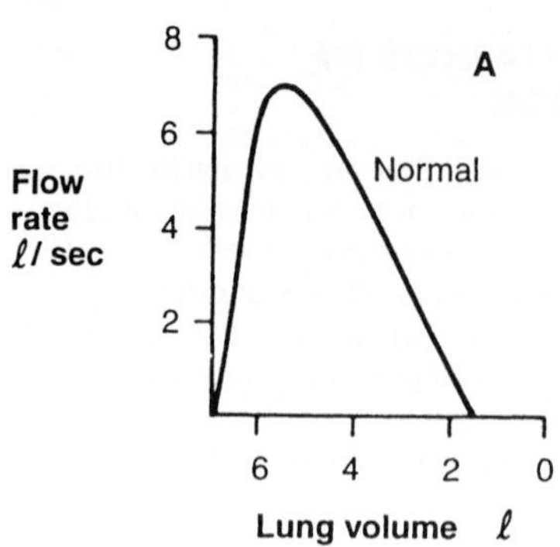

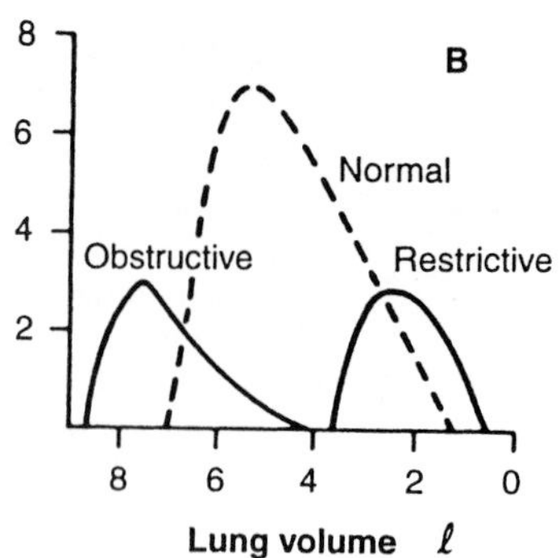

Figure 109–14. Expiratory flow-volume curves in patients with normal lungs *(A)* and in patients with obstructive and restrictive lung disease *(B)*. (From West JB: Pulmonary Pathophysiology. 5th ed. Baltimore, Williams & Wilkins, 1998, p 7.)

must be generated to overcome viscous forces, and this leads to high levels of respiratory muscle work. In addition, the ability of the diaphragm to expand the lungs and chest wall progressively falls as hyperinflation causes it to lose its normal dome-shaped configuration. Finally, PEEPI acts as a threshold load on the respiratory muscles. Because inspiration can begin only after sufficient pressure has been generated to stop expiratory flow and balance the elastic recoil of the respiratory system, the inspiratory muscles contract but do not generate airflow until this critical pressure has been reached.

Exertional dyspnea in patients with obstructive lung disease can be attributed largely to these alterations in respiratory muscle function.[48-50] As the respiratory rate rises, the work performed by the already overtaxed respiratory muscles must also increase. In addition, dynamic hyperinflation increases as the time allowed for expiration falls. This, in turn, leads to further flattening of the diaphragm and to additional increases in the threshold load placed on the respiratory muscles.

Restrictive Lung Disease

Whereas the hallmark of obstructive lung disease is an increase in viscous forces, restrictive diseases, such as interstitial fibrosis, are characterized by an increase in lung elastic recoil. Because lung volumes are determined largely by the interaction between elastic recoil and the strength of the respiratory muscles, pulmonary function testing demonstrates a decrease in FRC, RV, TLC, and VC. The fall in the VC leads to the characteristic narrowing of the flow-volume curve shown in Figure 109–14. Note that restrictive lung disease is also accompanied by a decrease in measured expiratory flow. Unlike the case with obstructive disease, however, this decrease results not from increased viscous forces or decreased elastic recoil but from a reduction in the lung volumes at which flow is being measured. Figure 109–14 illustrates that expiratory flow in restrictive disease is actually greater than normal when compared at the same lung volume. This, of course, is not surprising, because maximum expiratory flow is determined by lung elastic recoil.

Although hypoxemia and pulmonary hypertension are important factors, altered respiratory mechanics in patients with restrictive lung disease contribute significantly to dyspnea and functional limitation.[51, 52] Increased lung elastic recoil leads to a reduction in tidal volume, which must be compensated for by an increase in respiratory rate. This, combined with the increased pressure required to overcome elastic recoil, places an excessive load on the respiratory muscles. When disease is severe, these abnormalities may lead to respiratory muscle fatigue and ultimately to respiratory failure.

References

1. Rahn H, Otis AB, Chadwick LE, et al: The pressure-volume diagram of the thorax and lung. Am J Physiol 1946; 146:161.
2. Fenn WO: Mechanics of respiration. Am J Med 1951; 10:77.
3. Mead J: Mechanical properties of the lungs. Physiol Rev 1961; 41:281.
4. Agostoni E, Hyatt RE: Static behavior of the respiratory system. *In*: Handbook of Physiology. Section 3, Vol 3. Macklem PT, Mead J (Eds). Bethesda, Md, American Physiological Society, 1986, p 113.
5. Mead J, Whittenberger L, Radford EP: Surface tension as a factor in pulmonary volume-pressure hysteresis. J Appl Physiol 1957; 10:191.
6. Butler J: The adaptation of the relaxed lungs and chest wall to changes in volume. Clin Sci 1957; 16:421.
7. Sharp JT, Johnson FN, Goldberg NB, et al: Hysteresis and stress adaptation in the human respiratory system. J Appl Physiol 1967; 23:487.
8. Mead J, Whittenberger JL: Physical properties of human lungs measured during spontaneous respiration. J Appl Physiol 1953; 5:779.
9. Weibel ER: Functional morphology of lung parenchyma. *In*: Handbook of Physiology. Section 3, Vol 3. Macklem PT, Mead J (Eds). Bethesda, Md, American Physiological Society, 1986, p 89.
10. Pattle RE: Properties, function, and origin of the alveolar lining layer. Nature 1955; 175:1125.
11. Clements JA: Surface tension of lung extracts. Proc Soc Exp Biol Med 1957; 95:170.
12. Brown ES, Johnson RP, Clements JA: Pulmonary surface tension. J Appl Physiol 1959; 14:717.
13. Bachofen H, Hildebrandt J, Bachofen M: Pressure-volume curves of air- and liquid-filled excised lungs. J Appl Physiol 1970; 29:422.
14. Gil J, Bachofen H, Gehr P, et al: Alveolar volume-surface area relation in air- and saline-filled lungs fixed by vascular perfusion. J Appl Physiol 1979; 47:990.
15. Bachofen H, Gehr P, Weibel ER: Alterations of mechanical properties and morphology in excised rabbit lungs rinsed with a detergent. J Appl Physiol 1979; 47:1002.
16. Pedley TJ, Drazen JM: Aerodynamic theory. *In*: Handbook of Physiology. Section 3, Vol 3. Macklem PT, Mead J (Eds). Bethesda, Md, American Physiological Society, 1986, p 41.
17. Ferris BG, Mead J, Opie LH: Partitioning of respiratory flow resistance in man. J Appl Physiol 1964; 19:653.
18. D'Angelo E, Prandi E, Tavola M, et al: Chest wall interrupter resistance in anesthetized paralyzed humans. J Appl Physiol 1994; 77:883.
19. Pedley TJ, Schroter RC, Sudlow MF: The prediction of pressure drop and variation of resistance within the human bronchial airways. Respir Physiol 1970; 9:387.
20. Macklem PT, Mead J: Resistance of central and peripheral airways measured by a retrograde catheter. J Appl Physiol 1967; 22:395.
21. Hoppin FG, Green M, Morgan MS: Relationship of central and peripheral airway resistance to lung volume in dogs. J Appl Physiol 1978; 44:728.
22. Bates JHT, Ludwig MS, Sly PD, et al: Interrupter resistance elucidated by alveolar pressure measurement in open-chest normal dogs. J Appl Physiol 1988; 65:408.
23. Bates JHT, Abe T, Romero PV, et al: Measurement of alveolar pressure in closed chest dogs during flow interruption. J Appl Physiol 1989; 67:488.
24. Gottfried SB, Rossi A, Higgs BD, et al: Non-invasive determination of respiratory system mechanics during mechanical ventilation for acute respiratory failure. Am Rev Respir Dis 1985; 131:414.

25. Rossi A, Gottfried SB, Higgs BD, et al: Respiratory mechanics in mechanically ventilated patients with respiratory failure. J Appl Physiol 1985; 58:1849.
26. Wright PE, Marini JJ, Bernard GR: In vitro versus in vivo comparison of endotracheal tube airflow resistance. Am Rev Respir Dis 1989; 140:10.
27. Gal TJ, Suratt PM: Resistance to breathing in healthy subjects following endotracheal intubation under topical anesthesia. Anesth Analg 1980; 59:270.
28. Dubois AB, Botelho, Comroe JH: A new method for measuring airway resistance using a body plethysmograph. J Clin Invest 1956; 35:327.
29. Bates JHT, Milic-Emili J: The flow interruption technique for measuring respiratory resistance. J Crit Care 1991; 6:227.
30. Liistro G, Stanescu D, Rodenstein D, et al: Reassessment of the interruption technique for measuring flow resistance in humans. J Appl Physiol 1989; 67:933.
31. D'Angelo E, Calderini E, Torri G, et al: Respiratory mechanics in anesthetized paralyzed humans: Effects of flow, volume, and time. J Appl Physiol 1989; 67:2556.
32. D'Angelo E, Robatto FM, Calderini E, et al: Pulmonary and chest wall mechanics in anesthetized paralyzed humans. J Appl Physiol 1991; 70:2602.
33. Jonson B, Beydon L, Brauer K, et al: Mechanics of the respiratory system in healthy anesthetized humans with emphasis on viscoelastic properties. J Appl Physiol 1993; 75:132.
34. Lorino AM, Lorino H, Harf A: A synthesis of the Otis, Mead, and Mount mechanical models. Respir Physiol 1994; 97:123.
35. D'Angelo E, Prandi E, Marazzini L, Milic-Emili J: Dependence of maximal flow-volume curves on time course of preceding inspiration in patients with chronic obstructive pulmonary disease. Am J Respir Crit Care Med 1994; 150:1581.
36. Yuan H, Ingenito EP, Suki B: Dynamic properties of lung parenchyma: Mechanical contributions of fiber network and interstitial cells. J Appl Physiol 1997; 83:1420.
37. Fredberg JJ, Bunk D, Ingenito E, Shore SA: Tissue resistance and the contractile state of lung parenchyma. J Appl Physiol 1993; 74:1387.
38. Bergman NA: Properties of passive exhalations in anesthetized subjects. Anesthesiology 1969; 30:378.
39. Mead J, Turner JM, Macklem PT, et al: Significance of the relationship between lung recoil and maximum expiratory flow. J Appl Physiol 1967; 22:95.
40. Pride NB, Permutt S, Riley RL, et al: Determinants of maximal expiratory flow from the lungs. J Appl Physiol 1967; 23:646.
41. Dawson SV, Elliott EA: Wave-speed limitation on expiratory flow—a unifying concept. J Appl Physiol 1977; 43:498.
42. Hyatt RE: Expiratory flow limitation. J Appl Physiol 1983; 55:1.
43. Pinsky MR: Through the past darkly: Ventilatory management of patients with chronic obstructive pulmonary disease. Crit Care Med 1994; 22:1714.
44. Gibson GJ: Pulmonary hyperinflation: A clinical overview. Eur Respir J 1996; 9:2640.
45. Rossi A, Ganassini A, Polese G, Grassi V: Pulmonary hyperinflation and ventilator-dependent patients. Eur Respir J 1997; 10:1663.
46. Rossi A, Gottfried SB, Zocchi L, et al: Measurement of static compliance of the total respiratory system. Am Rev Respir Dis 1985; 131:672.
47. Pepe PE, Marini JJ: Occult positive end-expiratory pressure in mechanically ventilated patients with airflow obstruction. Am Rev Respir Dis 1982; 126:166.
48. DeTroyer A: Effect of hyperinflation on the diaphragm. Eur Respir J 1997; 10:708.
49. O'Donnell DE, Webb KA: Exertional breathlessness in patients with chronic airflow limitation: The role of lung hyperinflation. Am Rev Respir Dis 1993; 148:1351.
50. Eltayara L, Becklake MR, Volta CA, Milic-Emili J: Relationship between chronic dyspnea and expiratory flow limitation in patients with chronic obstructive pulmonary disease. Am J Respir Crit Care Med 1996; 154:1726.
51. Harris-Eze AO, Sridhar G, Clemens RE, et al: Role of hypoxemia and pulmonary mechanics in exercise limitation in interstitial lung disease. Am J Respir Crit Care Med 1996; 154:994.
52. Hansen JE, Wasserman K: Pathophysiology of activity limitation in patients with interstitial lung disease. Chest 1996; 109:1566.

110

Principles of Gas Exchange

Josep Roca, MD • Roberto Rodriguez-Roisin, MD

HISTORICAL BACKGROUND

The chief function of the lung is pulmonary gas exchange, which requires adequate levels of ventilation and perfusion of the alveoli. The lung must match pulmonary oxygen (O_2) uptake ($\dot{V}O_2$) and carbon dioxide (CO_2) elimination ($\dot{V}CO_2$) to the whole body metabolic O_2 consumption and CO_2 production, no matter what the O_2 and CO_2 partial pressures in the arterial blood.

During the first half of the 20th century, the heterogeneity of the alveolar ventilation-perfusion ($\dot{V}A/\dot{Q}$) ratios within the lung was identified as a factor causing hypoxemia. However, the importance of $\dot{V}A/\dot{Q}$ inequality in producing hypercapnia in patients with some forms of lung disease has only recently been described.[1,2] At the end of World War II, a crucial step toward a better understanding of the physiology of pulmonary gas exchange was the development of the three-compartment model of the lung almost simultaneously by Fenn and colleagues and Riley and Cournand. The graphic analysis of this representation of the lung provided the conceptual basis for the traditional interpretation of arterial blood gas measurements in the clinical setting (i.e., venous admixture, physiologic dead space). During the 1960s, progress in the mathematical description of the behavior of O_2 and CO_2 in the blood facilitated substantial contributions to the numerical analysis of pulmonary gas exchange. It was shown that traditional variables derived from physiologic gases (PaO_2, $PaCO_2$, alveolar-arterial PO_2 difference [$A - aPO_2$], venous admixture, and physiologic dead space) are sensitive to $\dot{V}A/\dot{Q}$ mismatch but they also vary with changes in total lung indices such as minute ventilation, cardiac output, and inspired O_2 partial pressure, as described later.[1,2] This behavior can lead to misinterpretations in the clinical setting.

The multiple inert gas elimination technique (MIGET) was developed in the early 1970s as a robust tool to obtain more information about the entire spectrum of $\dot{V}A/\dot{Q}$ distributions in the lung by measuring the exchange of six gases of different solubility in trace concentrations.[3-12] Its principle is based on the observation that the retention (or excretion) of any gas is dependent on the solubility (λ) of that gas and the $\dot{V}A/\dot{Q}$ distribution. Since the late 1980s, the use of the MIGET by several groups around the world has been key to producing a substantial amount of clinical research that has facilitated the present understanding of pulmonary gas exchange in different clinical conditions. The technique has been adequate in fostering an understanding of the basic mechanisms of PaO_2 and $PaCO_2$ abnormalities and the effects of therapeutic interventions, as described later.

The MIGET, in addition to its ability to estimate $\dot{V}A/\dot{Q}$ distributions in real lungs, provides information on other pulmonary factors causing hypoxemia (Table 110-1) and allows a numeric analysis of the influence of extrapulmonary factors on arterial PO_2, as described later. This technique provides more information concerning the role of the $\dot{V}A/\dot{Q}$ relationships on pulmonary gas exchange than previously available. It overcomes some important drawbacks of other methods, such as the topographic radioactive tracer-based techniques (venti-

TABLE 110–1. Factors Determining Arterial Hypoxemia

Intrapulmonary	Extrapulmonary
Primary Factors	
$\dot{V}A/\dot{Q}$-mismatching	Decreased ventilation
Shunt	Decreased cardiac output
Alveolar-end capillary	Decreased inspired PO_2
O_2 diffusion limitation	Increased O_2 uptake
Secondary Factors	
None	Decreased P_{50}
	Decreased Hb concentration
	Increased pH

$\dot{V}A/\dot{Q}$ = alveolar ventilation-perfusion; Hb = hemoglobin; P_{50} = PO_2 that corresponds to 50% oxyhemoglobin saturation.

lation-perfusion scans), which have limited resolution and thus underestimate the degree of $\dot{V}A/\dot{Q}$ inequality. This chapter addresses the interplay between the factors determining arterial respiratory blood gases (PaO_2 and $PaCO_2$) and the effects of different ventilatory modalities on gas exchange.

PULMONARY AND SYSTEMIC DETERMINANTS OF OXYGEN AND CARBON DIOXIDE EXCHANGE

Adequate management of patients with respiratory failure in the clinical setting requires proper assessment of pulmonary gas exchange. Partial pressures of arterial respiratory blood gases (PaO_2 and $PaCO_2$) and pH are the directly measurable variables used by most clinicians for this purpose. Although respiratory blood gases have become increasingly easy to obtain in both the intensive and the medical care setting, often the interpretation of the pathophysiologic determinants of abnormal PaO_2 or $PaCO_2$ in the clinical arena is not straightforward. This is because arterial respiratory blood gases, as indicated previously, reflect several processes. They reflect the functional conditions of the lung as a gas exchanger, thereby their intrapulmonary determinants such as ventilation-perfusion heterogeneity, intrapulmonary shunt, and alveolar end-capillary diffusion limitation for oxygen. They also reflect the conditions under which the lung operates, namely the composition of inspired gas and mixed venous blood (i.e., extrapulmonary factors).[1-6] Tables 110–1 and 110–2 show the intrapulmonary factors that may contribute individually or in combination to hypoxemia and hypercapnia as well as the extrapulmonary factors that can also influence arterial PO_2 and PCO_2. This chapter focuses essentially on the determinants of arterial PO_2 and PCO_2 in light of the results obtained with MIGET.[3, 7]

Intrapulmonary Factors

The highest efficiency of the lung as O_2 and CO_2 exchanger should be achieved when ventilation and blood flow to each individual alveolar unit are adequately balanced ($\dot{V}A/\dot{Q}$ = 1)

TABLE 110–2. Factors Determining Hypercapnia

Intrapulmonary	Extrapulmonary
$\dot{V}A/\dot{Q}$ mismatching	Decreased ventilation
	Increased carbon dioxide production
	Metabolic alkalosis

$\dot{V}A/\dot{Q}$ = alveolar ventilation-perfusion.

and, consequently, homogeneity of $\dot{V}A/\dot{Q}$ ratios among alveolar units is present. This so-called perfect lung is not seen in normal subjects because mild heterogeneity of pulmonary $\dot{V}A/\dot{Q}$ ratios is present due to gravity and a slight amount of physiologic post-pulmonary shunt (approximately 1%) due to the thebesian veins[13] draining blood flow from the coronary veins directly to the left atrium and the bronchial venous blood going to pulmonary veins.

Figure 110–1 illustrates the characteristic $\dot{V}A/\dot{Q}$ distribution in normal subjects obtained with the MIGET, which consists of narrow perfusion and ventilation distributions (second moment) centered around a $\dot{V}A/\dot{Q}$ ratio of 1.0 (first moment). Mean values for the second moment of both blood flow and ventilation distributions range from 0.35 to 0.43.[12, 13] The upper 95% confidence limit for dispersion of perfusion distribution is 0.60 and for dispersion of ventilation distribution is 0.65,[14-17] but at age 70, these are 0.70 and 0.75, respectively.[18] No (or virtually no) perfusion to $\dot{V}A/\dot{Q}$ ratios below 0.005 (shunt) is present.[12] Likewise, the amount of ventilation to $\dot{V}A/\dot{Q}$ ratios above 100 (dead space, including instrumental, anatomic, and physiologic dead space) is approximately 30%. No perfusion to lung units with $\dot{V}A/\dot{Q}$ ratios below 0.1 (low $\dot{V}A/\dot{Q}$) is observed. Similarly, ventilation to lung units with $\dot{V}A/\dot{Q}$ ratios above 10 (high $\dot{V}A/\dot{Q}$) is not present.

In most instances, $\dot{V}A/\dot{Q}$ mismatch is the predominant factor disturbing both pulmonary O_2 uptake and CO_2 output and consequently inducing hypoxemia and hypercapnia.[19, 20] Importantly, patients with $\dot{V}A/\dot{Q}$ inequality usually present with hypoxemia, not hypercapnia. This is because increased activity of central chemoreceptors provokes a rise in total ventilation (extrapulmonary factor) that returns $PaCO_2$ back to normal values but it is not as effective on PaO_2 because of the different shape of the oxygen and carbon dioxide dissociation curves.[2, 13] Particular features of uneven $\dot{V}A/\dot{Q}$ distributions in different disease states are described later. The amount of $\dot{V}A/\dot{Q}$ inequality observed in a given patient is essentially the combined end result of three distinct factors:

1. The functional consequences of pulmonary impairment caused by the underlying disease.
2. The efficiency of the ventilatory pattern (for a given minute ventilation, the combination of high tidal volume and low respiratory rate improves $\dot{V}A/\dot{Q}$ matching).
3. The magnitude of hypoxic pulmonary vasoconstriction (increased arteriolar tone in low $\dot{V}A/\dot{Q}$ areas constitutes a well-known compensatory phenomenon that reduces $\dot{V}A/\dot{Q}$ inequality).

Intrapulmonary shunt is the foremost factor causing hypoxemia in acute respiratory distress syndrome. Because shunt refers to perfusion to unventilated alveolar units ($\dot{V}A/\dot{Q}$ <0.005), it should be considered a particular condition of $\dot{V}A/\dot{Q}$ inequality. However, because of intrapulmonary shunt's pathophysiologic and therapeutic implications (hypoxemia refractory with O_2 therapy), it is considered a separate entity. Finally, alveolar-end capillary O_2 diffusion limitation is rather an uncommon cause of hypoxemia. Diffusion limitation has been demonstrated only in idiopathic pulmonary fibrosis,[21] particularly during exercise, and in the hepatopulmonary syndrome.[22]

Extrapulmonary Factors

Extrapulmonary factors of primary importance are (1) inspired O_2 fraction (FIO_2), (2) total ventilation ($\dot{V}E$), (3) cardiac output ($\dot{Q}T$), and (4) metabolic rate ($\dot{V}O_2$). The importance of FIO_2 as a key determinant of alveolar PO_2 (PAO_2), and in turn of PaO_2, is indicated by the components of the ideal alveolar gas equation:

$$P_{AO_2} = (Pb - P_{H_2O}) \cdot F_{IO_2} - Pa_{CO_2}/R + [Pa_{CO_2} \cdot F_{IO_2} \cdot (1 - R)/R]$$

where Pb is the barometric pressure, P_{H_2O} corresponds to the partial pressure of water vapor at 37°C, and R is the respiratory exchange ratio.[2, 13]

The relationships between F_{IO_2} and Pa_{O_2} are also modulated by the degree of pulmonary $\dot{V}_A/\dot{Q}$ inequality.[1, 2, 4] Total ventilation is considered an extrapulmonary factor because it is essentially set by the respiratory center (central drive). The impact of $\dot{V}_E$ on respiratory blood gases (Pa_{O_2} and Pa_{CO_2}) also varies with the degree of $\dot{V}_A/\dot{Q}$ mismatch. However, as mentioned previously, the increase in $\dot{V}_E$ is always more efficient to remove CO_2 from the blood (decrease Pa_{CO_2}) than to increase Pa_{O_2}. Because the CO_2 dissociation curve is almost linear in its working range, an increase in $\dot{V}_E$ to a lung with substantial $\dot{V}_A/\dot{Q}$ inequality continues to be effective in eliminating more CO_2. This is why arterial P_{CO_2} is so sensitive to changes in $\dot{V}_E$.[19, 20] In this regard, the equation relating P_{ACO_2} to ventilation:

$$P_{ACO_2} = K \cdot \dot{V}_{CO_2}/\dot{V}_A$$

where P_{ACO_2} is alveolar P_{O_2}, K is a constant term, $\dot{V}_{CO_2}$ is CO_2 output, and $\dot{V}_A$ is alveolar ventilation [$\dot{V}_A = \dot{V}_E \cdot (1 - V_D/V_T)$] can be meaningfully applied only to a single alveolar unit or to a homogeneous lung. This equation does not hold to describe the relationships between Pa_{CO_2} and $\dot{V}_E$ in diseased lungs because effective alveolar ventilation cannot be assessed.[19] In contrast, the nonlinear O_2 dissociation curve determines that an increase in $\dot{V}_E$ typically results in a modest gain in Pa_{O_2}. This is because the high $\dot{V}_A/\dot{Q}$ units that are operating in the "plateau" of the oxyhemoglobin dissociation curve are unable to compensate for the depressive effect on Pa_{O_2} of the low $\dot{V}_A/\dot{Q}$ units.

It is important here to emphasize the role of mixed venous P_{O_2} ($P\bar{v}_{O_2}$) and how extrapulmonary factors (other than inspired P_{O_2} and total ventilation) may contribute to reduce Pa_{O_2} through the effects on $P\bar{v}_{O_2}$. In this regard, a diminished $P\bar{v}_{O_2}$ may result from (1) a low cardiac output, (2) an increased oxygen uptake, or (3) a decreased blood oxygen content because of several alterations in the principal factors modulating the oxyhemoglobin dissociation curve. It should be noted that the impact of $P\bar{v}_{O_2}$ on arterial P_{O_2} also varies with the pattern of $\dot{V}_A/\dot{Q}$ mismatch.

In addition to the four primary extrapulmonary factors discussed previously, secondary variables such as hemoglobin concentration, hemoglobin P_{50}, body temperature, and blood acid-base status play altogether a secondary role in the clinical setting.[23] Metabolic alkalosis increases, in critically sick patients with more severe respiratory failure needing mechanical support, both intrapulmonary shunt and $\dot{V}_A/\dot{Q}$ imbalance, whereas its correction by hydrochloric acid (HCl) improves overall pulmonary gas exchange.[24] The most likely mechanism is that acidosis ameliorates the intrapulmonary determinants of hypoxemia, possibly causing an enhancement of hypoxic pulmonary areas of the lung; in contrast, shifts of the oxyhemoglobin dissociation curve related to the Bohr effect account for a marginal improvement in arterial oxygenation.[24] In a canine model of permeability pulmonary edema,[25] metabolic acidosis improved arterial oxygenation; vice versa, metabolic acidosis deteriorated it. Because cardiac output and minute ventilation remained unchanged, changes in intrapulmonary shunt and $\dot{V}_A/\dot{Q}$ mismatch, either enhancing or releasing hypoxic pulmonary vasoconstriction, respectively, mostly influenced pulmonary gas exchange.

As described by Wagner and associates,[4] it is possible to predict the arterial P_{O_2} expected from the measured $\dot{V}_A/\dot{Q}$ inequality and the particular combination of extrapulmonary factors that existed at the time of measurement. The MIGET

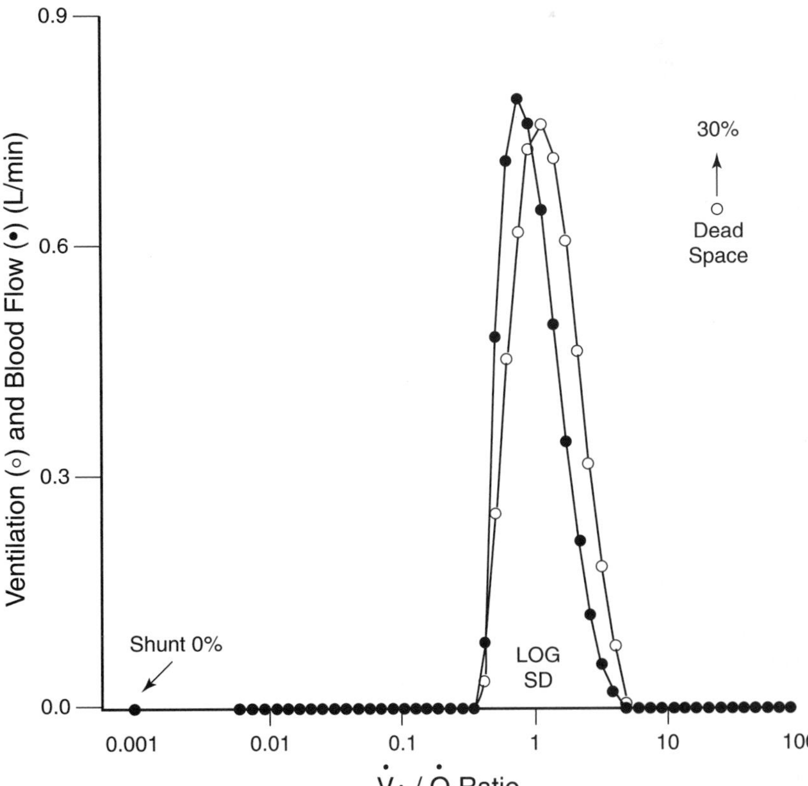

Figure 110–1. Ventilation-perfusion distributions. Ventilation *(open symbols)* and perfusion *(closed symbols)* are plotted against alveolar ventilation-perfusion ($\dot{V}_A/\dot{Q}$) ratio on a logarithmic scale in a resting young healthy subject breathing room air. LOG SD = logarithmic standard deviation.

algorithm, however, allows the observer to change any or all of the extrapulmonary factors (primary and secondary) and then to compute the expected value of arterial Po_2. Such flexibility is useful not only to understand potential expected effects of therapeutic interventions but also to separately determine the quantitative role of each extrapulmonary factor when they change between two conditions of MIGET measurement. This can be particularly useful to analyze the underlying physiologic effects of different ventilatory settings on arterial Po_2. For example, if weaning is initiated in a patient with chronic obstructive pulmonary disease (COPD), the change from mechanical ventilation to spontaneous breathing may increase cardiac output because of the increase in the preload of the right ventricle secondary to the marked increase of venous return (Fig. 110–2).[26, 27] However, possibly the $\dot{V}A/\dot{Q}$ distribution may simultaneously change for the worse because of a less efficient ventilatory pattern. The latter will be due to a fall in tidal volume together with a simultaneous increase in respiratory rate (rapid and shallow breathing) while total $\dot{V}E$ does not change.

Moreover, an eventual rise in resting O_2 uptake because of increased metabolic requirements of respiratory muscles during weaning may potentially decrease mixed venous Po_2, which in turn may have a deleterious effect on Pao_2. Arterial Po_2 will reflect the integrated effect of all these phenomena. In clinical research, one may separately analyze the effect of the increase in cardiac output. To do so is a simple matter of executing the MIGET algorithm (1) with the data during mechanical ventilation, (2) using the spontaneous breathing data with the cardiac output measured during mechanical ventilation, and (3) using all spontaneous breathing data to assess the individual influences on arterial Po_2 of each factor. By the same token, it is possible to use the $\dot{V}A/\dot{Q}$ algorithm to differentiate separately, for example, the effect of intrapulmonary shunt versus that of $\dot{V}A/\dot{Q}$ inequality on arterial Po_2.

$\dot{V}A/\dot{Q}$ INEQUALITY IN VARIOUS DISEASE CONDITIONS

Acute Lung Injury and Acute Respiratory Distress Syndrome

The pivotal mechanism of hypoxemia in acute lung injury (ALI) and acute respiratory distress syndrome (ARDS) is increased intrapulmonary shunt (20% or more of the cardiac output in ARDS). This gas exchange abnormality has been called an "all or none" phenomenon to reflect the fact that pulmonary blood flow is mainly distributed in two lung regions: those normally ventilated in proportion to local perfusion and those completely unventilated. In half of the patients there also can be a minor degree of ventilation-perfusion ($\dot{V}A/\dot{Q}$), mainly a mild to moderate amount of pulmonary perfusion distributed to areas of the lung in which ventilation is reduced (i.e., low $\dot{V}A/\dot{Q}$ areas). Dead space is increased in most of the patients with ARDS. During 100% O_2 breathing, arterial Po_2 increases modestly and there is an increase in intrapulmonary shunt, which is a finding akin to the concept of the development of reabsorption atelectasis.

The development of intrapulmonary shunt while breathing 100% O_2 concurs with the view that alveolar denitrogenation in low inspired $\dot{V}A/\dot{Q}$ ratios, called critical units, could result in a situation of absent expired ventilation, ultimately causing alveolar collapse, thereby leading to the development of reabsorption atelectasis. The small increase in arterial Po_2 on breathing 100% O_2 indicates that increased intrapulmonary shunt is the fundamental mechanism of hypoxemia in these patients. The presence of low $\dot{V}A/\dot{Q}$ ratios suggests the coexistence of alveolar units in which ventilation is reduced compared with blood flow because of increased airway resistance or the presence of alveolar spaces partially filled or both. In contrast, the increased dead space and high $\dot{V}A/\dot{Q}$ ratios, the latter of which is seen in a low percentage of patients with ARDS, may be a reflection of the use of external positive end-expiratory pressure (PEEP), ultimately leading to decreased blood flow.

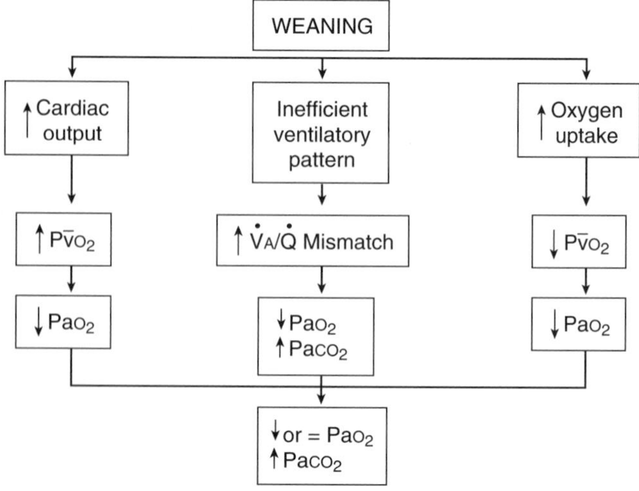

Figure 110–2. Interplay between intrapulmonary and extrapulmonary factors influencing arterial Po_2 during ventilator weaning.

Life-Threatening Pneumonia

In life-threatening pneumonia, hypoxemia is essentially determined by a considerable, although variable, amount of intrapulmonary shunt and moderate to severe $\dot{V}A/\dot{Q}$ mismatching characterized by the presence of blood flow distributed to low $\dot{V}A/\dot{Q}$ ratios. Although there is some degree of ventilation to high $\dot{V}A/\dot{Q}$ ratios in half of the patients, the amount is almost negligible; yet dead space is often increased to more than 30% of alveolar ventilation. On breathing 100% O_2, although increased intrapulmonary shunt remains unaltered, there is further $\dot{V}A/\dot{Q}$ imbalance as shown by marked deterioration of the dispersion of blood flow distribution. This suggests that the normally present hypoxic pulmonary vasoconstriction is reversed during high inspired O_2 breathing. This response also suggests that, in lungs with less diffuse lung injury than in ARDS, alveoli with low $\dot{V}A/\dot{Q}$ ratios are less prone to close during 100% oxygen breathing, probably because of the incomplete collapse of alveoli, the efficiency of collateral ventilation, or the interplay between mechanical forces within the lung. Efficacy of O_2 therapy to increase arterial Po_2 in life-threatening pneumonia depends on the relative role of low $\dot{V}A/\dot{Q}$ ratios relative to intrapulmonary shunt as factors determining arterial hypoxemia. The lower the percentage of blood flow to unventilated units (shunt), the higher the increase in arterial Po_2 with oxygen therapy. It must be taken into account that pneumonia can be both a cause of ALI and ARDS or a complication in ARDS.

Pulmonary Embolism

Patients suffering pulmonary embolism may show a wide spectrum of arterial blood gas abnormalities. Hypoxemia may range from nonexistent to severe. Gas exchange abnormalities in pulmonary embolism are essentially due to the combined effect of $\dot{V}A/\dot{Q}$ inequality and the decrease of mixed venous

PO_2. Ventilation-perfusion inequality is explained by the reduction in ventilation that ensues from the release of bronchoconstrictive agents released during embolism and by the overperfusion of some alveolar units as the result of the redistribution of pulmonary blood flow from occluded to nonoccluded regions. Furthermore, the development of areas with lung edema and atelectasis also contribute to $\dot{V}A/\dot{Q}$ inequality and, in some cases, to the presence of intrapulmonary shunt.

In cases of massive embolism causing severe pulmonary hypertension, intracardiac right to left shunt through a patent foramen may eventually occur. Hypocapnia, which is also shown in most patients, is due to hyperventilation, elicited by the presence of $\dot{V}A/\dot{Q}$ inequality or shunt. Because hypoxemia is mainly due to $\dot{V}A/\dot{Q}$ inequality, it usually can be corrected with supplemental oxygen at a reduced FIO_2 (0.24 to 0.35). The efficiency of supplemental oxygen in correcting arterial hypoxemia should be confirmed by repeating arterial blood gas measurements, because in cases where shunt is an important determinant of hypoxemia it may be necessary to increase the concentration of inspired oxygen.

Chronic Obstructive Pulmonary Disease

Acute respiratory failure during episodes of exacerbation in patients with chronic obstructive pulmonary disease (COPD) is a common complication. Whereas most episodes of acute exacerbation of COPD are of mild severity and can be treated on an outpatient basis, some patients may present with severe events, resulting in acute respiratory failure. Increased $\dot{V}A/\dot{Q}$ mismatching without a significant amount of perfusion diverted to unventilated areas (shunt) is the most prominent cause of hypoxemia in these patients.

Asthma

Gas exchange abnormalities in acute severe asthma are essentially due to increased $\dot{V}A/\dot{Q}$ inequality, which implies that hypoxemia usually can be corrected with supplemental oxygen at a reduced FIO_2.

EFFECTS OF MECHANICAL VENTILATION ON PULMONARY GAS EXCHANGE

Gravity plays a key role in adjusting alveolar ventilation and pulmonary blood flow while spontaneously breathing and during mechanical ventilation. In the awake, spontaneously breathing individual, gravity establishes a vertical gradient of pleural pressure that augments the degree of ventilation at the lung bases provided that lung volumes remain unchanged. Similarly, gravity induces hydrostatic pressure differences from the top to the bottom of the lungs so that a vertical gradient of pulmonary perfusion facilitating the lower regions is created. As a consequence, the $\dot{V}A/\dot{Q}$ ratio decreases down the lung because it is abnormally high at the top where the blood is minimal and much lower at the bottom.[2]

However, this pattern is reversed during mechanical ventilation such that regional ventilation is distributed preferentially to the nondependent regions, although the distribution of regional perfusion remains essentially unchanged. During positive-pressure ventilation, diaphragmatic movement is passive and has greater displacement in the nondependent areas, whereas the dependent zones are less compliant.[28] With mechanical ventilation, in the supine position an equal pressure is applied throughout the lung and is opposed by the hydrostatic pressure gradient of the abdomen. Yet larger mechanical breaths facilitate a more even distribution of tidal volume with a diaphragm more displaced, thus resulting in more ventilation and recruitment of the dependent regions of the lung.[28]

Inspiratory Flow Pattern

In a study by Modell and Cheney,[29] in animals with normal lungs, the accelerating and decelerating patterns had no effect on gas exchange; in contrast, the decelerating waveform contour resulted, in oleic acid-injured lungs, in a rise in PaO_2 without differences in $PaCO_2$ or hemodynamics. It has been suggested that the decelerating profile ventilated more efficiently those alveolar units with low $\dot{V}A/\dot{Q}$ ratios, hence facilitating a better intrapulmonary gas mixing. If no significant $\dot{V}A/\dot{Q}$ imbalance exists, oxygenation in all regions would be adequate without need for additional gas mixing time. When ventilatory parameters (tidal volume, inspiratory time, inspiratory-expiratory ratio, and respiratory frequency) were kept constant, in patients with respiratory insufficiency needing mechanical support, the decelerating waveform profile improved overall gas exchange as assessed by arterial blood gases and lung mechanics.[30] This amelioration of gas exchange supports the view that decelerating waveform improves both gas distribution and uptake within the lung without detrimental effect on hemodynamics. In a methacholine-induced bronchospasm porcine lung model, however, it was concluded that no inspiratory flow pattern studied offered a unique advantage for gas exchange, although peak tracheal pressure was significantly lower with decelerating flow.[31]

Positive End-Expiratory Pressure

Application of external PEEP in ARDS patients, in whom intrapulmonary shunt is the key factor disturbing pulmonary gas exchange, has been demonstrated to be an effective tool to handle refractory hypoxemia.[32-35] External PEEP increases functional residual capacity, but two different responses in terms of lung mechanics have been reported.[36] When the static volume-pressure curve at zero PEEP exhibits a concave shape with a progressive increase in slope with increasing volume, application of PEEP results in alveolar recruitment (reopening of collapsed alveoli). By contrast, in those patients exhibiting a convex volume-pressure curve at baseline (PEEP = 0), application of PEEP only enhances overdistention of the functional alveolar units but no alveolar recruitment is observed. Parallel findings of application of excessive levels of PEEP are a reduction in cardiac output, due to the increase in intrathoracic pressure, and a redistribution of extravascular lung water from alveoli to peribronchial and perivascular spaces.[37]

The effects of PEEP on $\dot{V}A/\dot{Q}$ distributions in ARDS are a reduction in shunt, broadening of the dispersion of ventilation distribution, and an increase in dead space (Fig. 110-3). The decrease in shunt can be explained by (1) reopening of collapsed alveoli with redistribution of pulmonary blood flow from severely injured (shunt) areas to poorly or normally ventilated alveolar units, (2) fall in cardiac output, and (3) the combined effect of these two mechanisms. Recruitment of alveolar units and redistribution of pulmonary blood flow within the lung are the main beneficial effects of PEEP that, in some instances, may give rise to an increase in low $\dot{V}A/\dot{Q}$ areas. All in all, with PEEP, the lung is more efficient in terms of O_2 uptake and slightly less efficient as a CO_2 exchanger. A fundamental clinical benefit of PEEP is that the changes in $\dot{V}A/\dot{Q}$ distributions allow O_2 therapy to become effective. Moreover, because PEEP decreases the amount of "critical" lung units,[32, 38, 39] high FIO_2 can be used with less likelihood of reabsorption atelectasis. However, a potential negative ef-

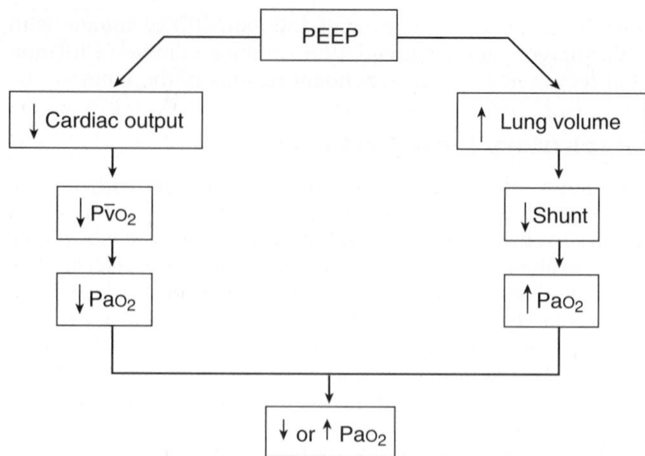

Figure 110–3. Application of external positive end-expiratory pressure (PEEP) may reduce cardiac output and increases pulmonary functional residual capacity. The impact of the intrapulmonary and systemic factors ultimately determines $Pa{O_2}$.

fect to be taken into account is that the fall in cardiac output with PEEP may facilitate a decrease in systemic O_2 delivery. It is of note that the different studies have shown some degree of individual variation in terms of the beneficial response to PEEP that cannot be predicted by the etiology of ARDS or the underlying severity of abnormal gas exchange. However, an acceptable correlation seems to exist between the characteristics of the static volume-pressure curve measured at zero PEEP and the gas exchange response to different levels of PEEP.

Application of PEEP in ARDS patients illustrates a good example of the interactions between intrapulmonary and extrapulmonary determinants of respiratory blood gases. Arterial $P{O_2}$ increases during PEEP if beneficial effects on gas exchange, essentially because of the reduction in shunt (intrapulmonary factor), are not offset by the simultaneous deleterious effect on $Pa{O_2}$ secondary to decreased cardiac output (extrapulmonary factor), which had allowed mixed venous $P{O_2}$ to decrease, other factors being equal. However, the interactions among the factors determining mixed venous $P{O_2}$ (cardiac output, tissue O_2 extraction, and arterial O_2 content) can be particularly complex in ARDS patients.

Traditionally, the use of external PEEP has been discouraged in chronic airway disease to prevent the risk of barotrauma because of excessive pulmonary hyperinflation. However, alveolar pressure in patients with acute or chronic airway disease may remain positive throughout the ventilatory cycle without any PEEP set by the ventilator, because expiratory flow limitation prevents a complete expiration within the time available to breathe out, so that both dynamic hyperinflation and intrinsic PEEP occur.[40–42] It has been shown that, in these patients, application of low values of PEEP does not increase intrathoracic pressure and lung volumes, hence preventing the risk of barotrauma, because PEEP replaces intrinsic PEEP until a critical value slightly lower than the initial intrinsic PEEP (approximately 75% to 80%) is achieved.[43–46] Under these circumstances, PEEP counterbalances intrinsic PEEP and reduces the magnitude of the inspiratory effort required either to trigger the ventilator or to resume spontaneous breathing.

The effects of two levels of PEEP, 50% and 100% of intrinsic PEEP, on $\dot{V}A/\dot{Q}$ distributions were examined by Rossi and colleagues[47] in mechanically ventilated patients with chronic airway disease during acute exacerbation. It was shown that moderate values of PEEP (50% of intrinsic PEEP) did not provoke significant changes in airway pressure, pulmonary hemodynamics, or mixed venous $P{O_2}$, whereas when PEEP equaled intrinsic PEEP (100% of intrinsic PEEP) airway pressure increased slightly but significantly. More important, application of PEEP amounting to 50% of intrinsic PEEP caused the highest improvement in overall gas exchange. A slight but significant increase in the first moment of both perfusion and ventilation distributions was observed, resulting in a mild but significant increase in $Pa{O_2}$ and in a trend to reduce $Pa{CO_2}$. Therefore, in contrast to the traditional view, these results provide further support for the use of low levels of external PEEP in mechanically ventilated patients with chronic airway disease, although caution and close adequate monitoring of the patient's condition seem to be mandatory.

Inverse I:E Ratio Ventilation

Mechanical ventilation with enlarged inspiratory time and shortened expiratory time (inverse ratio ventilation [IRV]) has been proposed as an alternative ventilatory strategy in patients with ARDS to improve gas exchange at lower than conventional lung peak distending pressure and PEEP, thereby decreasing the risk of barotrauma.[48] Three different potential mechanisms have been invoked to explain improvement of $Pa{O_2}$ with IRV: (1) higher mean airway pressure,[49] (2) intrinsic PEEP elicited by the short expiratory time,[50–53] and (3) improved distribution of inspired gas because of the low mean inspiratory flow.[54–56] However, the discrepant results obtained in clinical studies neither suggest a predominant mechanism for IRV to improve gas exchange nor provide evidence whether IRV offers any real, even short-term, benefit over conventional controlled mechanical ventilation with PEEP.[51, 53, 57–67] This is particularly true when a comparison is made at similar levels of both end-expiratory pressure and volume, while the ventilatory variables are adequately controlled.

Protective Ventilatory Strategies

It has been suggested that mechanical ventilation with (1) relatively low alveolar pressure (<25 to 30 cm H_2O), (2) low tidal volume (5 to 7 mL/kg^{-1}) compared with the values used in conventional ventilatory approaches (10 to 12 mL/kg^{-1}), and (3) application of external PEEP above the low inflection point in the static pressure-volume curve improves arterial oxygenation, protecting lung parenchyma from ventilator-induced injury. The mechanisms essentially are (1) prevention of overdistention of pulmonary units by keeping alveolar pressures at reasonably low levels and (2) relatively high levels of PEEP (above the upper inflection point) that help to recruit previously collapsed alveolar units and keep them open, avoiding mechanical stretch of pulmonary units during the ventilation cycle. Because of the low tidal volume, this ventilatory modality usually provokes well-tolerated controlled hypercapnia that, in turn, may produce a transient (24 to 48 hours) systemic vasodilator effect with increased cardiac output because of enhanced sympathomimetic activity. Interestingly, despite the increase in $Pa{CO_2}$, arterial oxygenation substantially improves. The main mechanism is a fall in intrapulmonary shunt because of recruitment of alveoli and redistribution of pulmonary blood flow from unventilated units to alveolar units with normal or low $\dot{V}A/\dot{Q}$ ratios.

A marginal, but not negligible, beneficial effect on arterial oxygenation is the increase in cardiac output. However, data on the effects of this type of ventilation on the survival rate in ARDS patients need to be compared. Further studies are also needed to assess its protective effect on pulmonary and systemic consequences of ventilator-induced injury. Finally, standardization and monitoring of this ventilatory modality in the clinical setting are still required.

Prone Position

Overall, two thirds of patients with severe ARDS can significantly improve $Pa{O_2}$ when they are turned from the supine to the prone position without major systemic and pulmonary hemodynamic changes. With computed tomography (CT), it has been shown that lung densities are mainly located in the dorsal regions and in the supine position and are redistributed characteristically to the ventral regions as soon as the patient is positioned in the prone position. The mechanism of improvement of arterial oxygenation, from supine to prone in severe ARDS, is essentially due to a decrease of intrapulmonary shunt with blood flow redistribution from nonventilated alveolar units to areas with normal $\dot{V}A/\dot{Q}$ ratios. This gas exchange improvement is accompanied by marginal hemodynamic changes.

Ventilation redistribution is the most likely factor influencing arterial oxygenation when the ARDS patient is turned to the prone position. This has been demonstrated in a canine model of the oleic acid–injured lung by measurement of regional ventilation and perfusion with isotopic techniques. Similarly, with reconstructed single photon emission computed tomography (SPECT) images of relative regional $\dot{V}A/\dot{Q}$ ratios scanned in both positions, large areas in the dorsal regions in which the relative regional $\dot{V}A/\dot{Q}$ ratios were abnormally low when supine markedly improved when the patient was moved to the prone position. With the patient turning from the supine to the prone position, the volume of lung in which the relative regional $\dot{V}A/\dot{Q}$ improved far exceeded that in which it worsened.

These findings can be interpreted in light of the changes that are supposed to occur at the pleural pressure level. The less positive pleural pressure in ventral lung regions that results in the prone position (i.e., a less gravitational pleural gradient) would cause much less lung volume below closing volume. Accordingly, the prone position would generate a transpulmonary pressure sufficient to exceed airway opening pressure in dorsal lung regions, which are precisely those where atelectasis, increased intrapulmonary shunt, and $\dot{V}A/\dot{Q}$ mismatching that are altogether more dramatically severe, without adversely affecting ventral lung regions. This would increase regional ventilation in dorsal areas, hence improving $\dot{V}A/\dot{Q}$ relationships without further deteriorating $\dot{V}A/\dot{Q}$ imbalance in the ventral regions. Other techniques for supportive therapy in ARDS, such as partial liquid ventilation, are still in an experimental phase. Extracorporeal membrane oxygenation (ECMO) and CO_2 removal ($ECCO_2R$) should be restricted to highly experienced, well-supported centers to be applied to those patients with ARDS refractory to other therapies.

PHARMACOLOGIC MANIPULATION OF $\dot{V}A/\dot{Q}$ RELATIONSHIPS

Administration of inhaled vasodilators such as nitric oxide (NO), or prostacyclin, in patients with ARDS induces a redistribution of blood flow from unventilated pulmonary units to alveoli with normal $\dot{V}A/\dot{Q}$ ratios, which results in an improvement of arterial oxygenation. The underlying mechanism is that inhaled NO does not reach areas with intrapulmonary shunt while producing vasodilation in alveolar units with normal ventilation-perfusion ratios. Moreover, because NO is rapidly inactivated by hemoglobin, no systemic vasodilator effects are observed. The majority of the potential response to inhaled NO on pulmonary gas exchange is achieved at low inspired NO concentrations (5 to 10 parts per million), whereas the response to pulmonary hypertension continues into a higher dosage range. Beneficial gas exchange response to inhaled NO can vary from patient to patient, but the response to inhaled NO seems to be essentially related with the underlying $\dot{V}A/\dot{Q}$ pattern rather than to the dosage of NO. At present, NO treatment should be considered a supportive therapy with no proven beneficial effects in the mortality rate of ARDS. Different studies show that the simultaneous administration of an intensifier of hypoxic pulmonary vasoconstriction (almitrine bysmesylate) magnifies the effectiveness of inhaled NO on gas exchange, particularly in patients with pneumonia.

NONINVASIVE POSITIVE-PRESSURE VENTILATION

The clinical interest of using noninvasive positive-pressure ventilation to prevent orotracheal intubation in patients with acute respiratory failure[68-71] as well as to manage clinically stable patients with severe restrictive ventilatory diseases has been progressively and positively accepted by both respiratory and intensive care specialists. Future applications of this ventilatory modality as a weaning strategy and its usefulness in clinically stable patients with severe obstructive ventilatory limitation are under analysis. However, the underlying mechanisms by which noninvasive ventilation reduces arterial $P{CO_2}$ and increases $Pa{O_2}$ are still controversial. Historically, three hypotheses have been suggested: (1) resting of respiratory muscles, (2) improvement in lung compliance, and (3) augmented central respiratory drive.[72]

The *rest theory* proposes that hypercapnic chronic respiratory failure is associated with chronic respiratory muscle fatigue.[73] However, the existence of the latter has never been clearly demonstrated, and no study has shown that respiratory muscle rest is necessary for improving daytime gas exchange or symptoms.[74-76] A second hypothesis postulates that noninvasive ventilation increases lung compliance, hence reopening alveolar units. Third, it also has been proposed that respiratory center sensitivity to CO_2 is blunted in these patients. Intermittent noninvasive ventilation, by preventing nocturnal hypoventilation, would allow the resetting of respiratory center sensitivity to CO_2 and daytime gas exchange improvement.[72] These last two contentions are not mutually exclusive and can contribute more or less depending upon individual clinical conditions of the patient. However, data collected in patients with COPD during an acute episode of respiratory failure[77] and in clinically stable patients with COPD or a restrictive ventilatory defect because of a chest wall abnormality[78] indicate that alternative explanations for the beneficial effect of noninvasive ventilation on respiratory blood gases should be taken into account.

These studies show that increase in total ventilation and its two components (decrease in respiratory rate and higher tidal volume) with no changes in inert gas dead space were key factors to provoke a right shift of the ventilation distribution and a reduction in its dispersion.[77, 78] Both changes may improve alveolar P_{CO_2}, hence increasing Pa_{O_2} and reducing Pa_{CO_2}. Both intrapulmonary shunt and low $\dot{V}A/\dot{Q}$ areas remained essentially unchanged during this ventilatory approach. However, there was a significant increase in the dispersion of blood flow distribution that explains the moderate increase in $A - aP_{O_2}$. Importantly, cardiac output significantly fell but its deleterious effect on mixed venous P_{O_2} was fully counterbalanced by (1) an increase in both the first moment of the perfusion and ventilation distributions (this would increase alveolar P_{O_2} and decrease alveolar P_{CO_2}, other things being equal) and (2) a trend to decrease respiratory muscle O_2 uptake.

In summary, even though the lung during noninvasive ventilation was slightly less efficient as an O_2 exchanger (both alveolar-arterial P_{O_2} difference and the dispersion of the perfusion distribution increased), arterial respiratory blood gases significantly improved by the simultaneous beneficial effect of their intrapulmonary ($\dot{V}A/\dot{Q}$ distributions) and extrapulmonary (overall ventilation, cardiac output, O_2 uptake) factors. Short-term application of noninvasive mechanical ventilation in these patients did not show evidence of alveolar recruitment. Further examination of the effects of noninvasive positive-pressure ventilation on pulmonary gas exchange needs to be done in longer serial studies in this type of COPD patient and in clinically stable subjects with a restrictive ventilatory defect, namely neuromuscular diseases, thoracic wall deformities, and hypoventilation-obesity syndrome.

ACKNOWLEDGMENTS

This work has been supported by Covant No. 96/0897 from the Fondo de Investigación Sanitaria (FIS).

References

1. West JB: Ventilation-perfusion inequality and overall gas exchange in computer models of the lung. Respir Physiol 1969; 7:88–110.
2. West JB: Ventilation-perfusion relationships. Am Rev Respir Dis 1977; 116:919–943.
3. Roca J, Wagner PD: Contribution of multiple inert gas elimination technique to pulmonary medicine: 1. Principles and information content of the multiple inert gas elimination technique. Thorax 1993; 49:815–824.
4. West JB, Wagner PD: Pulmonary gas exchange. *In:* Bioengineering Aspects of the Lung. West JB (Ed). New York, Marcel Dekker, 1977, pp 361–457.
5. Dantzker DR: The influence of cardiovascular function on gas exchange. Clin Chest Med 1983; 4:149–159.
6. Wagner PD: Ventilation-perfusion inequality in catastrophic lung disease. *In:* Applied Physiology in Clinical Respiratory Care. Prakash O (Ed). The Hague, Martinus Nijhoff, 1982, pp 363–379.
7. Light RB: Intrapulmonary oxygen consumption in experimental pneumococcal pneumonia. J Appl Physiol 1988; 64:2490–2495.
8. Wagner PD, Saltzman HA, West JB: Measurements of continuous distributions of ventilation-perfusion ratios: Theory. J Appl Physiol 1974; 36:588–599.
9. Wagner PD, Naumann PF, Laravuso RB, West JB: Simultaneous measurement of eight foreign gases in blood by gas chromatography. J Appl Physiol 1974; 36:600–605.
10. Evans JW, Wagner PD: Limits on $\dot{V}A/\dot{Q}$ distributions from analysis of experimental inert gas elimination. J Appl Physiol 1977; 36:600–605.
11. Wagner PD: Susceptibility of different gases to ventilation-perfusion inequality. J Appl Physiol 1979; 46:372–386.
12. Wagner PD, Laravuso RB, Uhl RR, West JB: Continuous distributions of ventilation-perfusion ratios in normal subjects breathing air and 100% O_2. J Clin Invest 1974; 54:54–68.
13. West JB: Ventilation/Blood Flow and Gas Exchange. 4th ed. Oxford, Blackwell Scientific Publications, 1985.
14. Gale GE, Torre-Bueno J, Moon RE, Salzman HA, Wagner PD: Ventilation-perfusion inequality in normal humans during exercise. J Appl Physiol 1985; 58:978–988.
15. Wagner PD, Gale GE, Moon RE, Torre-Bueno JE, Stolp BW, Saltzman HA: Pulmonary gas exchange in humans exercising at sea level and simulated altitude. J Appl Physiol 1986; 61:260–270.
16. Hammond MD, Gale GE, Kapitan KS, Ries A, Wagner PD: Pulmonary gas exchange in humans during normobaric hypoxic exercise. J Appl Physiol 1986; 60:1590–1598.
17. Hammond MD, Gale GE, Kapitan KS, Ries A, Wagner PD: Pulmonary gas exchange in humans during normobaric hypoxic exercise. J Appl Physiol 1985; 58:978–988.
18. Cardús J, Burgos F, Diaz O, Roca J, Barberà JA, Marrades RM, Rodriguez-Roisin R, Wagner PD: Increase in pulmonary ventilation-perfusion inequality with age in healthy individuals. Am J Respir Crit Care Med 1997; 156(2):648–653.
19. West JB: Causes of carbon dioxide retention in lung disease. N Engl J Med 1971; 284:1232–1236.
20. Weinberger SE, Schwartzstein RM, Weis JW: Hypercapnia. N Engl J Med 1989; 321:1223–1231.
21. Agustí AG, Roca J, Rodriguez-Roisin R, Gea J, Xaubet A, Wagner PD: Mechanisms of gas exchange impairment in idiopathic pulmonary fibrosis. Am Rev Respir Dis 1991; 143:219–225.
22. Rodriguez-Roisin R, Agustí AG, Roca J: The hepatopulmonary syndrome: New name, old complexities (Editorial). Thorax 1992; 47:897–902.
23. Hansen JE, Clausen JL, Levy SE, Mohler JG, Van Kessel AL: Proficiency testing materials for pH and blood gases: The California Thoracic Society Experience. Chest 1986; 89:214–217.
24. Brimouille S, Kahn RJ: Effects of metabolic acidosis on pulmonary gas exchange. Am Rev Respir Dis 1990; 141:1185–1189.
25. Brimouille S, Vachiery JL, Lejeune P, Leeman M, Melot C, Naeije R: Acid-base status affects gas exchange in canine oleic acid pulmonary edema. Am J Physiol 1991; 260:H1080–1086.
26. Torres A, Reyes A, Roca J, Wagner PD, Rodriguez-Roisin R: Ventilation-perfusion mismatching in chronic obstructive pulmonary disease during ventilator weaning. Am Rev Respir Dis 1989; 140:1246–1250.
27. Lemaire F, Teboul JL, Cinotti L, et al: Acute left ventricular dysfunction during unsuccessful weaning from mechanical ventilation. Anesthesiology 1988; 69:171–179.
28. Froese AB, Bryan AB: Effect of anesthesia and paralysis on diaphragmatic mechanics in man. Anesthesiology 1974; 41:242–245.
29. Modell HI, Cheney FW: Effects of inspiratory flow pattern on gas exchange in normal and abnormal lung. J Appl Physiol 1979; 46:1103–1107.
30. Al-Saad N, Bennet ED: Decelerating inspiratory flow waveform improves lung mechanics and gas exchange in patients on intermittent positive-pressure ventilation. Intensive Care Med 1985; 11:68–75.
31. Smith RA, Venus B: Cardiopulmonary effect of various inspiratory flow profiles during controlled mechanical ventilation in a porcine lung model. Crit Care Med 1988; 16:769–772.
32. Dantzker DR, Brook L, DeHart P, Lunch J, Weg J: Ventilation-perfusion distribution in the adult respiratory distress syndrome. Am Rev Respir Dis 1979; 120:1039–1052.
33. Matamis D, Lemaire F, Harf A, et al: Redistribution of pulmonary blood flow induced by positive end-expiratory pressure and dopamine infusion in acute respiratory failure. Am Rev Respir Dis 1984; 129:39–44.
34. Ralph DD, Robertson HT, Weaver LJ, et al: Distribution of ventilation and perfusion during positive end-expiratory pressure in the adult respiratory distress syndrome. Am Rev Respir Dis 1985; 131:54–60.
35. Coffey RL, Albert RK, Robertson HT: Mechanism of physiological dead space response to PEEP after acute oleic acid lung injury. J Appl Physiol Respir Environ Exer Physiol 1983; 55:1550–1557.
36. Ranieri MV, Giuliani R, Fiore T, Dambrosio M, Milic-Emili J: Volume-pressure curve of the respiratory system predicts effects of PEEP in ARDS: "Occlusion" versus "constant flow" technique. Am J Respir Crit Care Med 1994; 149:19–27.
37. Hopewell PC, Murray JF: Effects of continuous positive-pressure ventilation in experimental pulmonary edema. J Appl Physiol 1975; 39:672–679.
38. Dantzker DR, Wagner PD, West JB: Instability of lung units with low $\dot{V}A/\dot{Q}$ ratios during O_2 breathing. J Appl Physiol 1975; 38:886.

39. Rodriguez-Roisin R: Effect of mechanical ventilation on gas exchange. *In:* Principles and Practice of Mechanical Ventilation. Tobin MJ (Ed). New York, McGraw-Hill, 1994, pp 673–693.
40. Pepe PP, Marini JJ: Occult positive end-expiratory pressure in mechanically ventilated patients with airflow obstruction. Am Rev Respir Dis 1982; 126:166–170.
41. Rossi A, Gottfried SB, Zocchi L, Higgs BD, Lennox S, Calverley PMA, Begin P, Grassino A, Milic-Emili J: Measurement of static compliance of the total respiratory system in patients with acute respiratory failure during mechanical ventilation. Am Rev Respir Dis 1982; 131:672–677.
42. Kimball WR, Leith DE, Robins AG: Dynamic hyperinflation and ventilator dependence in chronic obstructive pulmonary disease. Am Rev Respir Dis 1982; 126:991–995.
43. Guy PC, Rodarte JR, Hubmayr RD: The effect of positive expiratory pressure on isovolume and dynamic hyperinflation in patients receiving mechanical ventilation. Am Rev Respir Dis 1987; 139:621–626.
44. Tuxen DV: Detrimental effects of positive end-expiratory pressure during controlled mechanical ventilation. Am Rev Respir Dis 1989; 140:5–9.
45. Rossi A, Brandolese R, Milic-Emili J, Gottfried SB: The role of PEEP in patients with chronic obstructive pulmonary disease during assisted ventilation. Eur Respir J 1990; 3:818–822.
46. Ranieri VM, Giuliani R, Cinnella G, Pesce C, Brienza N, Ippolito EL, Pomo V, Fiore T, Gottfried SB, Brienza A: Physiologic effects of positive end-expiratory pressure in patients with chronic obstructive pulmonary disease during acute ventilatory failure and controlled mechanical ventilation. Am Rev Respir Dis 1993; 177:5–13.
47. Rossi A, Santos C, Roca J, Torres A, Félez MA, Rodriguez-Roisin R: Effects of PEEP on $\dot{V}_A/\dot{Q}$ mismatching in ventilated patients with chronic airflow obstruction. Am J Respir Crit Care Med 1994; 149:1077–1084.
48. Marcy TW: Inverse ratio ventilation. *In:* Principles and Practice of Mechanical Ventilation. Tobin MJ (Ed). New York, McGraw-Hill, 1994, pp 319–331.
49. Gattinoni L, Marcolin R, Caspani M, Fumagali R, Mascheroni D, Pesenti A: Constant mean airway pressure with different patterns of positive pressure breathing during the adult respiratory distress syndrome. Bull Eur Physiopathol Respir 1985; 21:275–279.
50. Duncan S, Rizk N, Raffin T: Inverse ratio ventilation: PEEP in disguise? Chest 1987; 92:390–391.
51. East T, Bohm S, Wallace J, Clemmer T, Weaver L, Orme J, Morris A: A successful computerized protocol for clinical management of pressure control inverse ratio ventilation in ARDS patients. Chest 1992; 101:697–710.
52. Brandolese R, Broseghini C, Polese G, Bernasconi M, Brandi G, Milic-Emili J, Rossi A: Effects of intrinsic PEEP on pulmonary gas exchange in mechanically-ventilated patients. Eur Respir J 1992; 6:358–363.
53. Bernard G, Artigas A, Brighman K, Carlet J, Falke K, Hudson L, Lamy M, Legall J, Morris A, Spragg R: The American-European Consensus Conference on ARDS: Definitions, mechanisms, relevant outcomes, and clinical trial coordination. Am J Respir Crit Care Med 1994; 149:818–824.
54. Hubmayr R, Abel M, Rehder K: Physiologic approach to mechanical ventilation. Crit Care Med 1990; 18:103–113.
55. Manthous C, Schmidt G: Inverse ratio ventilation in ARDS: Improved oxygenation without autoPEEP. Chest 1993; 103:953–954.
56. Marini JJ: Ventilation of the acute respiratory distress syndrome: Looking for Mr. Goodmode. Anesthesiology 1994; 80:972–975.
57. Gurevitch M, Van Dyke J, Young E, Jackson K: Improved oxygenation and lower peak airway pressure in severe adult respiratory distress syndrome: treatment with inverse ratio ventilation. Chest 1986; 89:211–213.
58. Tharratt R, Allen R, Albertson T: Pressure controlled inverse ratio ventilation in severe adult respiratory failure. Chest 1988; 94:755–762.
59. Lain D, DiBenedetto R, Morris S, Van Nguyen A, Saulters R, Causey D: Pressure control inverse ratio ventilation as a method to reduce peak inspiratory pressure and provide adequate ventilation and oxygenation. Chest 1989; 95:1081–1088.
60. Abraham E, Yoshihara G: Cardiorespiratory effects of pressure controlled inverse ratio ventilation in severe respiratory failure. Chest 1989; 96:1356–1359.
61. Poelaert J, Vogelaers D, Colardyn F: Evaluation of the hemodynamic and respiratory effects of inverse ratio ventilation with a right ventricular ejection fraction catheter. Chest 1991; 99:1444–1450.
62. Chan K, Abraham E: Effects of inverse ratio ventilation on cardiorespiratory parameters in severe respiratory failure. Chest 1992; 102:1556–1561.
63. Mercat A, Graïni L, Teboul J, Lenique F, Richard C: Cardiorespiratory effects of pressure-controlled ventilation with and without inverse ratio in the adult respiratory distress syndrome. Chest 1993; 104:871–875.
64. Lessard M, Guérot E, Lorino H, Lemaire F, Brochard L: Effects of pressure-controlled with different I:E ratios versus volume-controlled ventilation on respiratory mechanics, gas exchange, and hemodynamics in patients with adult respiratory distress syndrome. Anesthesiology 1994; 80:983–991.
65. Cole A, Weller S, Sykes M: Inverse ratio ventilation compared with PEEP in adult respiratory failure. Intensive Care Med 1984; 10:227–232.
66. Zavala E, Ferrer M, Polese G, Masclans JR, Planas M, Milic-Emili J, Rodriguez-Roisin R, Roca J, Rossi A: Effects of PEEPi generated by inverse I:E ratio ventilation on pulmonary gas exchange in ARDS. Am J Respir Crit Care Med 1996; 153:A374.
67. Rossi A, Ranieri M: Positive end-expiratory pressure. *In:* Principles and Practice of Mechanical Ventilation. Tobin MJ (Ed). New York, McGraw-Hill, 1994, pp 259–303.
68. Brochard L, Isabey D, Piquet J, Amaro P, Mancebo J, Messadi AA, Brun-Buisson C, Rauss A, Lemaire F, Harf A: Reversal of acute exacerbations of chronic obstructive lung disease by inspiratory assistance with a face mask. N Engl J Med 1990; 323:1523–1530.
69. Kramer N, Meyer TJ, Meharg J, Cece RD, Hill NS: Randomized, prospective trial of noninvasive positive pressure ventilation in acute respiratory failure. Am J Respir Crit Care Med 1995; 151:1799–1806.
70. Appendini L, Patessio A, Zanaboni S, Carone M, Gukov B, Donner CF, Rossi A: Physiologic effects of positive end-expiratory pressure and mask pressure support during exacerbations of chronic obstructive pulmonary disease. Am J Respir Crit Care Med 1994; 149:1069–1076.
71. Bott J, Carroll MP, Conway JH, Keilty SEJ, Ward EM, Brown AM, Paul EA, Elliott MW, Godfrey RC, Wedzicha JA, Moxham J: Randomised controlled trial of nasal ventilation in acute ventilatory failure due to chronic obstructive airways disease. Lancet 1993; 341:1555–1557.
72. Hill NS: Noninvasive ventilation: Does it work, for whom, and how? Am Rev Respir Dis 1993; 147:1050–1055.
73. Roussos C: Function and fatigue of respiratory muscles. Chest 1985; 88:1245–1315.
74. Gay PC, Patel AM, Viggiano RW, Hubmayr RD: Nocturnal nasal ventilation for treatment of patients with hypercapneic respiratory failure. Mayo Clin Proc 1991; 66:695–703.
75. Mohr CH, Hill NS: Long-term follow-up of nocturnal ventilatory assistance in patients with respiratory failure due to Duchenne-type muscular dystrophy. Chest 1990; 97:91–96.
76. Elliot MW, Mulvey DA, Moxham J, Green M, Bronthwaite MA: Domiciliary nocturnal nasal intermittent positive pressure ventilation in COPD: Mechanisms underlying changes in arterial blood gas tensions. Eur Respir J 1991; 4:1044–1052.
77. Diaz O, Iglesia R, Ferrer M, Zavala E, Santos C, Wagner PD, Roca J, Rodriguez-Roisin R: Am J Respir Crit Care Med 1997; 156:1840–1845.
78. Ferrer M, Iglesia R, Roca J, Escarrabil J, Farrero E, Gómez FP, Farré R, Barberà JA, Rodriguez-Roisin R: Factors determining Pa_{O_2} during noninvasive ventilation in clinically stable chronic respiratory failure. Am J Respir Crit Care Med 1998; 157(3):A370.

111

Heart-Lung Interactions

Michael R. Pinsky, MD, CM, FCCP, FCCM

The heart, vasculature, and lung function as a cardiorespiratory unit delivering adequate amounts of oxygen to the tissues and removing carbon dioxide. Ventilation can profoundly alter cardiovascular function via complex processes that are reviewed in this chapter. The boundaries of the cardiovascular unit's responsiveness are defined by both cardiovascular and pulmonary factors. These include the myocardial reserve, circulating blood volume, blood flow distribution, autonomic tone, endocrinologic response, lung volume, intrathoracic pressure (ITP), and the surrounding pressures for the remainder of the circulation. That positive-pressure ventilation may influence cardiovascular function in ways not seen during spontaneous ventilation was immediately appreciated when positive-pressure ventilation was first introduced more than 50 years ago.[1]

Dramatically different hemodynamic responses to similar ventilatory maneuvers can occur between subjects when these complex influences are ignored. For example, the final response to ventilatory stress is dependent on the baseline cardiovascular state of the subject. In the most extreme of examples, maximum exercise tolerance in a young, healthy subject is limited primarily by muscle strength, endurance, and coordination rather than by minute ventilation or cardiac output. In the same subject after a disease process that compromises cardiovascular or respiratory function, such as may occur after trauma, sepsis, or acute lung injury, even simple tasks such as breathing spontaneously or sitting up in bed may be outside the realm of possibilities. Complicating this picture further, spontaneous inspiratory efforts, which can cause cardiovascular stress, may precipitate cardiopulmonary compromise in subjects in whom, before the development of respiratory dysfunction, similar ventilatory efforts had minimum hemodynamic effects. At the opposite end of this spectrum, artificial ventilation may introduce dynamic and complex changes in these interactions that neither nature nor evolution could foresee. Thus, normal adaptive autonomic reflexes may not be appropriate in the setting of artificial ventilation.

This review addresses these issues in two successive steps. First, the basic mechanisms underlying the cardiopulmonary interactions are described. Second, using these constructs, clinical trials of established and novel ventilatory therapies are examined for their observed hemodynamic effects. The goal of this development is to demonstrate that by using these constructs, reasonable predications can be made about the hemodynamic effects of ventilation in a wide variety of clinical situations. Furthermore, specific responses to ventilatory maneuvers suggest specific underlying cardiovascular conditions and accordingly may alert the physician to alter cardiovascular support.

RELATION BETWEEN AIRWAY PRESSURE, INTRATHORACIC PRESSURES, AND LUNG VOLUME

Since positive-pressure ventilation was introduced, the concept of relating hemodynamic consequences to airway pressure (Paw) has been widely accepted.[2, 3] A major source of confusion has been equating changes in Paw with changes in both pleural pressure (Ppl) and lung volume. Physicians often equate Paw with the hemodynamic effects seen because (1) Paw can be measured easily at the bedside in patients receiving mechanical ventilation, (2) mean Paw reflects mean alveolar pressure, and (3) increases in Paw qualitatively reflect increases in both lung volume and Ppl. However, the association between Paw and other variables (1) is highly variable as ventilatory patterns, airway resistance, and lung compliance change; (2) does not accurately reflect changes in pericardial pressure (Ppc), which is a primary determinant of transmural left ventricular (LV) pressure; and (3) may mislead the caregiver at the bedside into altering therapy on the basis of these wrong assumptions. Numerous studies have demonstrated that the primary determinants of the hemodynamic responses to ventilation are changes in intrathoracic pressure and lung volume,[4] not Paw. Thus, before examining heart-lung interactions, the relation between Paw, Ppl, Ppc, and lung volume needs to be addressed. To simplify the discussion, the term ITP is used to refer to a nonspecific intrathoracic surface pressure. When specific surface pressures are identified, they are referred to as either lateral chest wall, diaphragm, and juxtacardiac pleural pressures or pericardial pressure, where appropriate.

Airway Pressure, Lung Volume, and Regional Pleural Pressures

During positive-pressure inspiration, increases in lung volume tend to parallel increases in Paw. Changes in Paw are related to changes in lung volume through the interaction of airway resistance and both lung and chest compliances, as manifested by the relative increase in ITP during inspiration. Several common clinical examples serve to support this statement. If either lung or chest wall compliance changes, then Paw may change without an actual change in the size of the tidal breath. This phenomenon commonly occurs clinically with mucus plugging and "fighting" the ventilator. First, a mucous plug in a major bronchus acutely decreases the lung volume available for ventilation and induces an immediate increase in peak airway pressure during positive-pressure ventilation. Second, spontaneous ventilatory efforts out of synchrony with the mechanical ventilatory cycles (fighting the ventilator) can induce increases in Paw during mechanical breaths. Similarly, if spontaneous breaths cause ITP to decrease during positive-pressure inspiration, then both peak Paw and mean Paw decrease, whereas if bronchospasm causes airway resistance to increase, then for a constant tidal breath, both peak Paw and mean Paw increase.

As the lung expands it pushes on the surrounding structures, distorting them and causing their surface pressures to increase. Lung expansion pushes the chest wall outward, the diaphragm downward, and the cardiac fossa in upon itself. This lung expansion induces an increase in lateral wall, diaphragmatic, and juxtacardiac Ppl as well as Ppc. The degree of increase in these surface pressures in response to lung expansion is a function of the compliance and inertance of their opposing structures, which are the chest wall, diaphragm–abdominal contents, and heart, respectively.

These interactions were described by Novak and colleagues,[5] who demonstrated that the changes in Ppl induced by positive-pressure ventilation are not similar in all regions of the thorax and increase differently as inspiratory flow rate and frequency increase. Pleural pressure at the diaphragm increases least during positive-pressure inspiration, and juxtacardiac Ppl increases most (Fig. 111-1). Because the diaphragm is quite compliant, it seems reasonable that diaphrag-

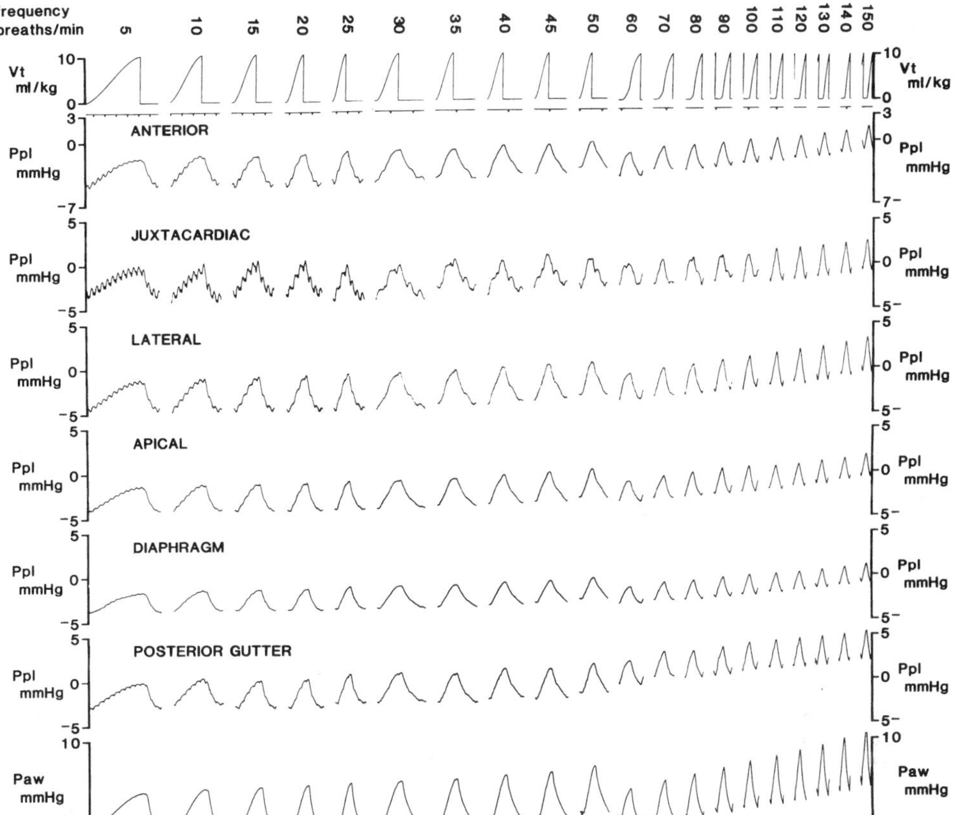

Figure 111–1. Strip-chart figure. Vt = tidal volume; Ppl = pleural pressure. (From Novak RA, Matuschak GM, Pinsky MR: Effect of ventilatory frequency on regional pleural pressure. J Appl Physiol 1995; 65:1314–1323.)

matic ITP should increase less than lateral chest wall Ppl with sudden increases in lung volume. If abdominal distention develops, as commonly occurs in the setting of sepsis, the diaphragm becomes relatively noncompliant because of the increase in abdominal pressure (Fig. 111–2). Under these conditions, Paw increases for a constant tidal breath without any change in actual lung parenchymal compliance. Thus, one may incorrectly assume that the lung is injured and becoming stiffer when, in fact, the lung compliance may be normal but chest wall compliance (here referring to the entire chest wall–diaphragm apparatus) is restricting expansion.[5] This distinction is important because increasing Paw to overcome chest wall stiffness should increase ITP more, with greater hemodynamic consequences, as described later, but should not improve gas exchange, because the alveoli are not damaged. By contrast, if lung compliance is reduced, as in acute lung injury states, similar increases in Paw should not increase ITP as much but should recruit collapsed and injured alveolar units, improving gas exchange but having less hemodynamic effects. These concepts are presently under clinical investigation.

Furthermore, a hydrostatic pressure gradient exists in the pleural space. Dependent regions have a higher baseline pressure than nondependent regions. In the supine subject, steady-state apneic Ppl values along the horizontal plane from apex to diaphragm are similar, whereas anterior Ppl is lower and posterior gutter Ppl is higher. These points are illustrated in Figure 111–3, which demonstrates regional differences in mean apneic Ppl in the intact supine dog.

It follows from this discussion that care most be taken to determine not only what types of ventilation are being compared, so as to match similar tidal volumes, but also how and where estimates of Ppl and Ppc are made. For example, if estimates of transpulmonary pressure are needed to define lung compliance and its change with recruitment maneuvers, lateral chest wall Ppl appears to reflect more accurately the pressure-volume characteristics of the intact lung.[5] Similarly, if diaphragmatic work is to be monitored, either esophageal or diaphragmatic Ppl should be used. Finally, if heart-lung interactions are being examined, juxtacardiac Ppl is the most accurate measure of Ppl, and its increases during positive-pressure inspiration would be underestimated by esophageal pressure. Because the heart is fixed within a cardiac fossa, juxtacardiac Ppl increases more than lateral chest wall or diaphragmatic Ppl.

In a related study, Pinsky and Guimond[6] demonstrated in a canine model of acute ventricular failure that the induction of heart failure was associated with a greater increase in Ppc than in juxtacardiac Ppl. Presumably, the failing heart's dilation was limited by the pericardium. With progressive increases in positive end-expiratory pressure (PEEP), juxtacardiac Ppl increased toward values similar to those in the absence of PEEP, whereas Ppc initially remained constant. When these two surface pressures became equal, further increases in PEEP increased both juxtacardiac Ppl and Ppc in parallel (Fig. 111–4). Thus, if there is a pericardial volume restraint, juxtacardiac Ppl underestimates Ppc. With sustained lung compression of the heart, however, both juxtacardiac Ppl and Ppc appear to be similar.

Regional Pleural Pressure and Lung Volume in Acute Lung Injury

The interaction of Paw, lung volume, and ITP in the setting of lung disease is complex and can be different in the same pathologic setting depending on the tidal volume, inspiratory flow rate, and ventilatory frequency. The presence of parenchymal disease and airflow obstruction and extrapulmonary

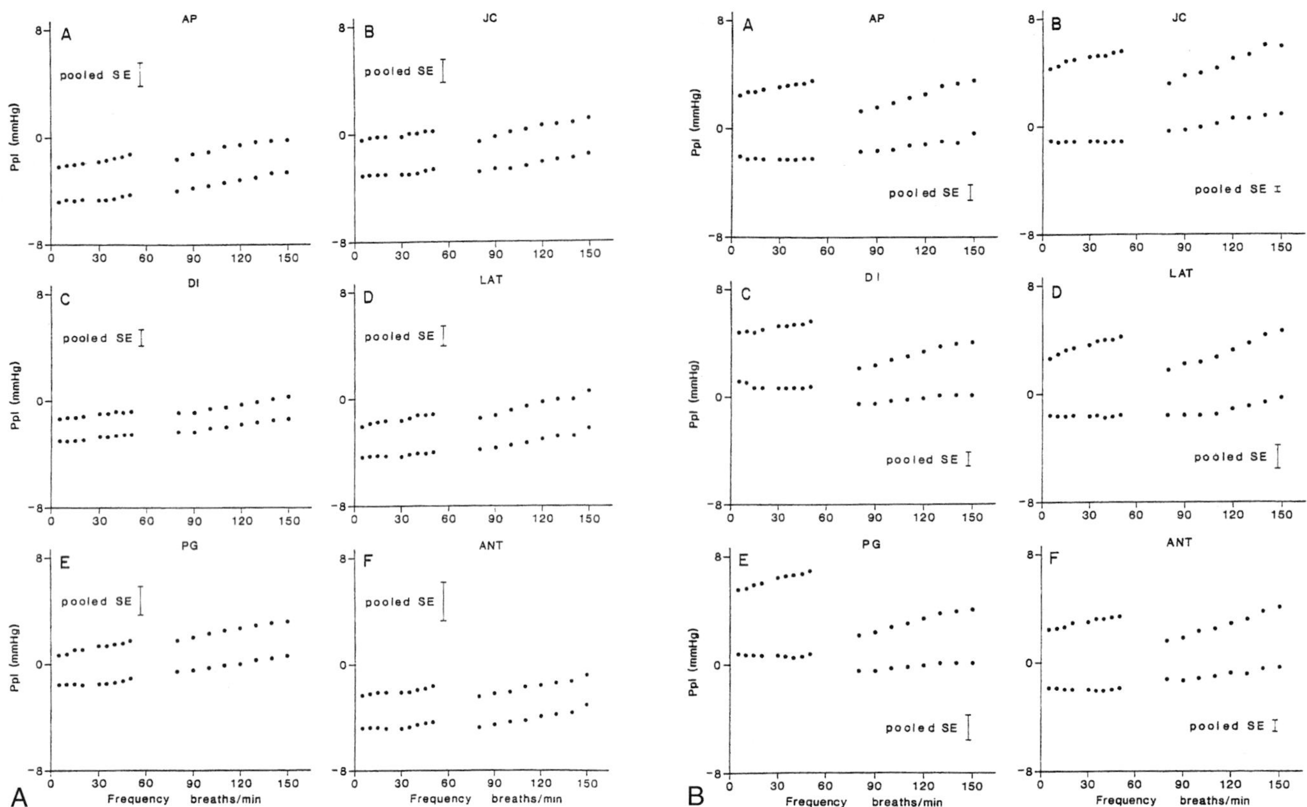

Figure 111–2. Six graphs of change in pleural pressure (Ppl) versus frequency for a constant tidal volume with the chest relaxed *(A)* and with it bound *(B)* (regions as below). (From Novak RA, Matuschak GM, Pinsky MR: Effect of ventilatory frequency on regional pleural pressures. J Appl Physiol 1995; 65:1314–1323.)

processes that directly alter chest wall–diaphragm contraction also profoundly alter these interactions. As described in Chapter 107, static lung expansion occurs as Paw increases because the transpulmonary pressure (Paw relative to ITP) increases. If lung injury induces alveolar flooding or increased pulmonary parenchymal stiffness, greater increases in Paw are required to distend the lungs to a constant end-inspiratory volume.

Romand and colleagues[7] demonstrated in an acute intact canine model that for a constant tidal volume Paw increased much more during acute lung injury than under control conditions, whereas lateral chest wall Ppl and Ppc increased similarly in both cases if tidal volume was held constant (Fig. 111–5). These data agree with the finding of O'Quinn and coworkers[8] and others that the primary determinant of the increase in Ppl and Ppc during positive-pressure ventilation is lung volume change. The data of Romand and colleagues[7] further extended this understanding by demonstrating that the increase in ITP during sustained increases in lung volume is greater than the increase in Ppc. Presumably, Ppc does not increase as much as ITP because increasing lung volume also reduces filling of the ventricles, reducing their size inside the cardiac fossa. These data also underscore the importance of measuring Ppc as the surrounding pressure for heart as lung volume changes rather than assuming that it can be approximated by juxtacardiac Ppl. To summarize, for a constant increase in lung volume, ITP increases similarly despite drastic changes in lung compliance.

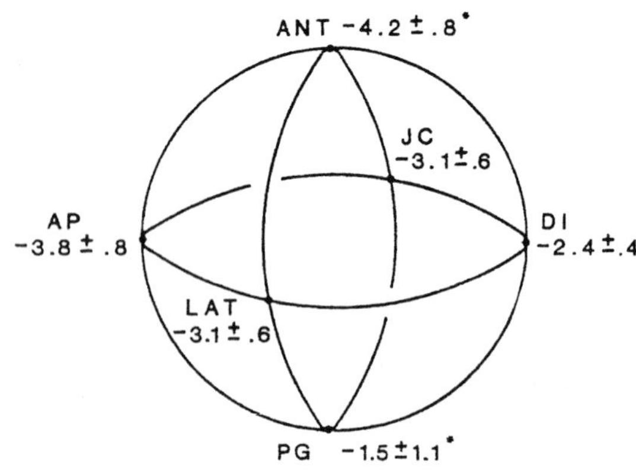

Figure 111–3. Apneic pleural pressure (Ppl) (mean ± SE) in torr for six pleural regions of the right hemothorax of an intact supine canine model. ANT = anterior; AP = apical; PG = posterior gutter; DI = diaphragmatic; JC = juxtacardiac; LAT = lateral. Ellipses represent regional measurements defining three orthogonal planes. (Modified from Novak RA, Matuschak GM, Pinsky MR: Effect of ventilatory frequency on regional pleural pressures. J Appl Physiol 1995; 65:1314–1323.)

Relation Between Airway, Pleural, and Pericardial Pressures

Because the distribution of alveolar collapse and lung compliance in acute respiratory distress syndrome is nonhomogeneous, lung distention during positive-pressure ventilation must reflect overdistention of some regions of the lung at the expense of noncompliant or poorly compliant regions. Accordingly, Paw reflects distention of lung units that were

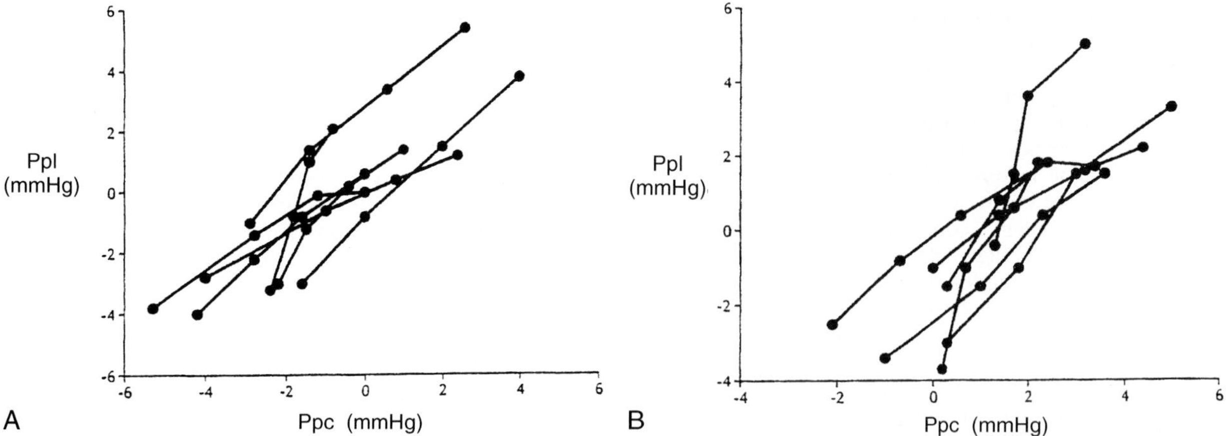

Figure 111–4. Relation between pleural pressure (Ppl), pericardial pressure (Ppc), and changes in airway pressure (Paw) for control *(A)* and acute ventricular failure *(B)* condition. (From Pinsky MR, Guimond JG: The effects of positive end-expiratory pressure on heart-lung interactions. J Crit Care 1991; 6:1–15.)

aerated before inspiration but may not reflect the degree of inflation of nonaerated lung units. As described in Chapter 116, pressure-limited ventilation assumes that this is the case and aims to limit Paw in acute lung injury states in order to prevent overdistention of aerated lung units, with the understanding that tidal volume, and thus minute ventilation, must decrease. Accordingly, pressure-limited ventilation hypoventilates the lungs, leading to "permissive" hypercapnia. From the preceding discussion, it is not surprising that in an animal model of acute lung injury, in which tidal volume was either kept constant at preinjury levels or reduced to match preinjury plateau Paw (pressure-limited ventilation), both Ppl and Ppc increased less with pressure-limited ventilation as compared with both pre–lung injury states or in acute lung injury when tidal volume remained at preinjury levels.[7]

Because acute lung injury is often nonhomogeneous, with aerated areas of the lung displaying normal specific compliance, the large increases in Paw often seen during mechanical ventilation in patients with acute lung injury should overdistend these aerated lung units.[9] Vascular structures that are

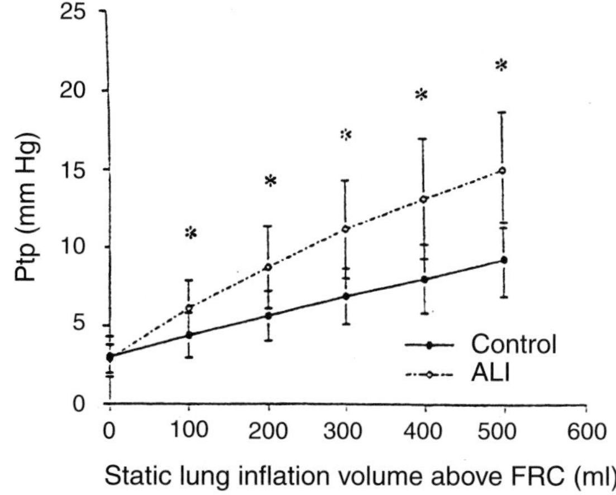

Figure 111–5. Relation between airway pressure (Paw) and tidal volume (Vt) and between pleural pressure (Ppl) and Vt in control and acute lung injury (ALI) conditions. FRC = functional residual capacity. (From Romand J, Shi W, Pinsky MR: Cardiopulmonary effects of positive pressure ventilation during acute lung injury. Chest 1995; 108:1041–1048.)

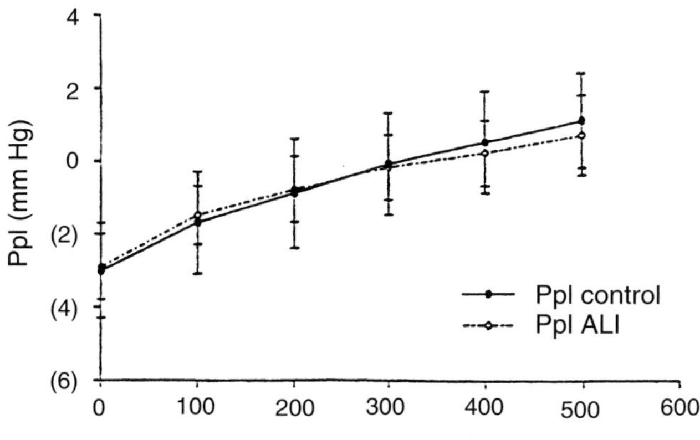

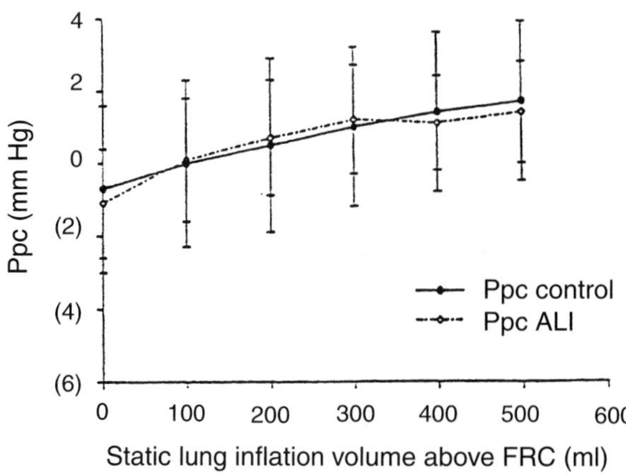

distended may have a greater increase in their surrounding pressure than collapsible structures.[10] However, Romand and colleagues[7] and Scharf and Ingram[11] have demonstrated that despite this nonhomogeneous alveolar distention, if tidal volume is kept constant, Ppl increases equally, independent of the mechanical properties of the lung. Thus, under conditions in which tidal volume is kept constant, changes in peak Paw and mean Paw reflect changes in the mechanical properties of the lungs and the patient's coordination but may not reflect changes in Ppl. Similarly, these changes in Paw may not alter global cardiovascular dynamics. Underscoring this limitation of Paw to reflect either ITP or Ppc, Pinsky and associates[12] demonstrated in postoperative patients that the percentage of Paw increase that is transmitted to the pericardial surface is not constant from one subject to the next as PEEP is increased (Fig. 111-6). Thus, one cannot predict the amount of increase in Ppc or Ppl that will occur in patients as PEEP is increased. Accordingly, assuming some constant fraction of Paw transmission to the pleural surface as a means of calculating the effect of increasing Paw on Ppl is inaccurate and potentially dangerous in management of patients.

Although it may be difficult to know the actual Ppl, it is possible to determine the change in Ppl induced by ventilation and ventilatory maneuvers. One can vary ITP by an exact amount by either inspiratory or expiratory maneuvers against an occluded airway, referred to as the Mueller and Valsalva maneuvers, respectively. Because lung volume does not change, transpulmonary pressure is constant, so the change in ITP is equal to the change in Paw.[13] Accordingly, an increase in Paw of 20 mm Hg during a Valsalva maneuver reflects an increase in ITP of 20 mm Hg, and a decrease in Paw of 20 mm Hg during a Mueller maneuver reflects a decrease in ITP of 20 mm Hg. The use of both the Mueller and Valsalva maneuvers at the bedside is a powerful diagnostic tool in assessing cardiovascular function, as described later.

Like the Mueller and Valsalva maneuvers, normal ventilatory efforts during either spontaneous or positive-pressure breathing can be used to assess the relative change in ITP in the absence of airway obstruction. Because intrathoracic vascular structures sense ITP as their surrounding pressure, dynamic and rapid swings in ITP, such as may occur during ventilation, are reflected in the intrathoracic vascular pressure swings. Both right atrial pressure and pulmonary artery diastolic pressure swings tend to follow Ppl swings closely during ventilation. Regrettably, invasive hemodynamic monitoring is necessary to obtain these data. However, as described later, these respiratory "artifacts" in the intrathoracic vascular pressure recordings can be used for diagnostic purposes. Potentially, swings in systolic arterial pressure can be used to assess swings in Ppl, assuming no LV outflow obstruction exists. Still, the use of such hemodynamic surrogates to monitor Ppl is of unproven value.

Two important limitations to the use of intrathoracic vascular and esophageal pressures to estimate Ppl or Ppc exist. First, Ppc and ITP may not be similar or increase by similar amounts with the application of positive Paw. In heart failure states, the pericardium becomes a limiting membrane.[14, 15] Operationally, this equates to Ppc exceeding juxtacardiac Ppl by the degree to which the pericardium limits biventricular dilation. Pericardial pressure is the surrounding pressure for ventricular distention such that the ventricular distending pressure equals the difference between intraluminal pressure (inside the right or left ventricle) and Ppc. Thus, estimates of Ppc made by using ITP measures may underestimate Ppc and overestimate the increase in Ppc as Paw is increased. Second, esophageal pressure is often used clinically to estimate swings in both Ppl and Ppc. Although esophageal pressure is accurate in reflecting negative swings in Ppl during spontaneous inspiration in upright-seated individuals[2] and in recumbent dogs in the left lateral position,[16] it underestimates both the positive swings in Ppl and the mean increase in Ppl seen with increases in lung volume during positive-pressure ventilation. During the Mueller and Valsalva maneuvers, however, because lung volume does not change, swings in esophageal pressure accurately reflect swings in Ppl.[2] In fact, the validity of esophageal balloon pressure recordings is often documented by demonstrating that both Paw and esophageal pressure increase by similar amounts during a Valsalva maneuver. Esophageal pressure may serve as a reasonable surrogate for Ppl or Ppc, but there are important limitations to its application in many of the disease states in which the data are needed.

In summary, Ppl is not uniform throughout the thoracic

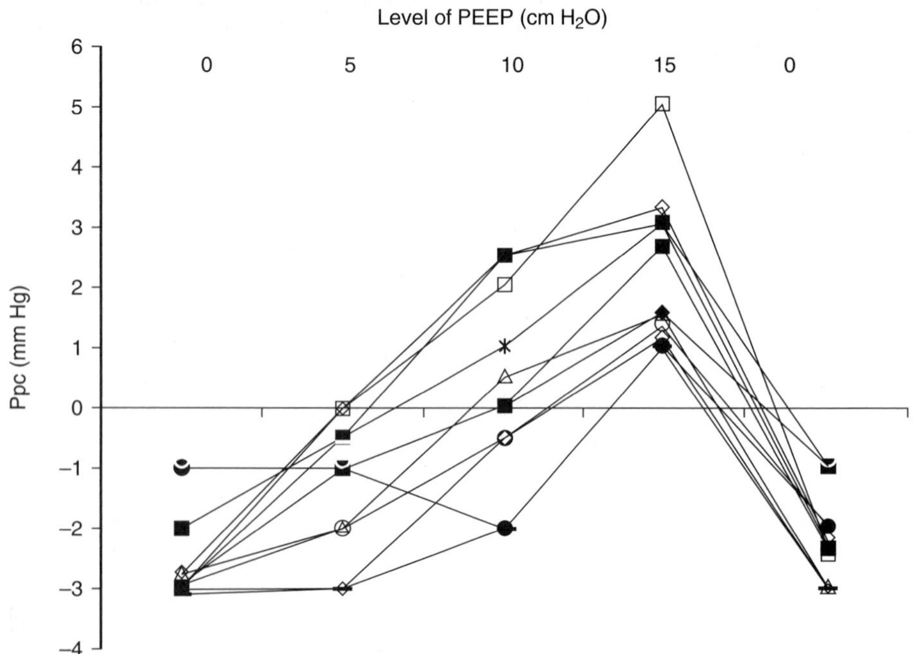

Figure 111–6. Relation between pericardial pressure (Ppc) and airway pressure in humans following cardiac surgery. Apneic levels of positive end-expiratory pressure (PEEP) were progressively increased from zero to 15 cm H_2O and then back to zero in 5 cm H_2O increments. (Created from data by Pinsky MR, et al: Estimating left ventricular filling pressure during positive end-expiratory pressure in humans. Am Rev Respir Dis 1991; 143:25-31.)

cavity and it does not vary equally with changes in lung volume from one site to another. Furthermore, Ppc and Ppl may not be similar and may not vary equally as Paw increases. Thus, much of the clinical data available is supported by animal experimental studies that can circumvent many of these limitations in deriving their measures.

During both spontaneous and conventional positive-pressure ventilation, lung volume increases in a tidal fashion, whereas ITP decreases during spontaneous ventilation and increases during positive-pressure inspiration. Thus, changes in ITP represent one of the primary determinants of the hemodynamic differences between spontaneous and positive-pressure ventilation.[17, 18] The other primary difference between spontaneous and positive-pressure ventilation involves the issue of the metabolic demand of exercising muscle, because spontaneous ventilation requires the outlay of muscular activity, referred to as the work of breathing. As a workload, spontaneous ventilation is usually associated with a minimum work of breathing. With disease, however, the work of breathing can become extremely great, compromising overall cardiovascular stability. These points are addressed in the subsequent sections of this chapter.

HEMODYNAMIC EFFECTS OF VENTILATION

Heart-lung interactions encompass a broad area. Ventilation can alter the circulation, and the circulation can have effects on ventilation. Although low pulmonary artery pressures in the setting of high alveolar pressures increase physiologic dead space, these issues are discussed in other chapters on ventilation-perfusion relations in this text and are not discussed here. We focus on the hemodynamic effects induced by ventilation and ventilatory maneuvers. These heart-lung interactions can be broadly grouped into interactions that involve three basic concepts that usually coexist to some degree in the clinical setting. To simplify the discussion of these processes, they are first discussed separately and then grouped as they relate to specific disease states and modes of ventilation.

The three basic concepts that underpin the determinants of heart-lung interactions are as follows. First, spontaneous ventilatory efforts are exercise; they require O_2, produce CO_2, and may stress the limits of adaptive circulatory mechanisms. Second, inspiration increases lung volume above end-expiratory volume; thus, some of the hemodynamic effects of ventilation may be due to changes in lung volume and chest wall expansion. Third, spontaneous inspiration decreases ITP, whereas positive-pressure ventilation increases ITP; thus, the differences between spontaneous ventilation and positive-pressure ventilation primarily reflect the differences in ITP swings and the energy necessary to produce them.

Ventilation as Exercise

Spontaneous ventilatory efforts are induced by contraction of the respiratory muscles, of which the diaphragm and intercostal muscles constitute the bulk of the tissue. With marked hyperpnea, abdominal wall muscles and muscles of the shoulder girdle also function as accessory respiratory muscles. Blood flow to these muscles is derived from several arterial circuits whose absolute flow is believed to exceed the highest metabolic demand of maximally exercising skeletal muscle under normal conditions.[19] Thus, under conditions of normal cardiovascular function, blood flow is not the limiting factor determining maximum ventilatory effort.

Although ventilation normally requires less than 5% of total O_2 delivery to meet its demand[19] and is difficult to measure at the bedside even when using calibrated metabolic measuring devices, in lung disease states in which the work of breathing is increased, such as pulmonary edema or bronchospasm, the work cost of breathing can increase metabolic demand for O_2 to 25% or 30% of total O_2 delivery.[19-22] Furthermore, if cardiac output is limited, blood flow to other organs and to the respiratory muscles may be compromised, inducing both tissue hypoperfusion and lactic acidosis.[23, 24] The institution of mechanical ventilation for ventilatory and hypoxemic respiratory failure may reduce metabolic demand on the stressed cardiovascular system, increasing venous oxygen saturation (Svo_2) for a constant cardiac output and arterial oxygen concentration (Cao_2). Intubation and mechanical ventilation, when adjusted to the metabolic demands of the patient, may dramatically decrease the work of breathing, resulting in increased O_2 delivery to other vital organs and decreased serum lactic acid levels. Under conditions in which fixed right-to-left shunts exist, the obligatory increase in Svo_2 results in an increase in the arterial partial pressure of oxygen (Pao_2) despite no change in the ratio of shunt blood flow to cardiac output. Finally, Vires and colleagues[25] demonstrated that if cardiac output is severely limited by the artificial induction of tamponade in a canine model, respiratory muscle failure develops despite high central neuronal drive, and the animals suffer respiratory death before cardiovascular standstill.

Hemodynamic Effects of Changes in Lung Volume

A change in lung volume, either inflation or deflation, alters autonomic tone and pulmonary vascular resistance. Furthermore, high lung volumes, as we shall see, interact mechanically with the heart in the cardiac fossa to limit absolute cardiac volumes, as manifest by increases in both juxtacardiac Ppl and Ppc. Each of these processes is important in determining the hemodynamic response to mechanical ventilation.

Autonomic Tone

The lungs are richly innervated with integrated somatic and autonomic fibers that originate in, traverse, and end in the thorax. These neuronal networks mediate multiple homeostatic processes through the autonomic nervous system that alter both instantaneous cardiovascular function, such as respiratory sinus arrhythmia, and steady-state cardiovascular status, such as antidiuretic hormone (ADH)–induced fluid retention. Numerous cardiovascular reflexes are centered within this network. Inflation induces immediate changes in autonomic output.

The most commonly described examples of the inflation-chronotropic responses are those that act through vagally mediated reflex arcs.[26, 27] Lung inflation to normal tidal volumes (<10 mL/kg) increases heart rate via withdrawal of parasympathetic tone. Inspiration-associated cardioacceleration is referred to as respiratory sinus arrhythmia[28] and denotes normal autonomic tone.[29] Loss of respiratory sinus arrhythmia denotes dysautonomia, and its reappearance precedes the return of peripheral autonomic control in diabetics with peripheral neuropathy.[30] However, some degree of respiration-associated heart rate change is intrinsic to the heart itself. For example, even after cardiac transplantation, when the heart demonstrates no chronotropic response to the intravenous infusion of atropine, a small degree of ventilation-associated heart rate changes persists,[31] suggesting that mechanoreceptors in the right atrium can alter sinoatrial tone. Lung inflation to larger tidal volumes (>15 mL/kg) decreases heart rate.

Pulmonary vasoconstriction may also occur through vagal reflex arcs[32] but does not appear to induce significant hemodynamic effects. Reflex arterial vasodilatation can also occur with lung hyperinflation.[26, 33–37] This inflation-vasodilatation response appears to be mediated by afferent vagal fibers because it is abolished by selective vagotomy. Interestingly, blocking sympathetic afferent fibers also blocks this reflex,[35, 38] presumably by withdrawing central sympathetic tone. This inflation-vasodilatation response is of minimum clinical significance, except during high-frequency ventilation and with hyperinflation.[26, 35]

Similarly, although humoral factors, including compounds blocked by cyclooxygenase inhibition,[39] released from pulmonary endothelial cells during lung inflation may also induce this depressor response,[40–42] these interactions do not appear to alter cardiovascular status grossly.[43] In fact, unilateral lung hyperinflation (unilateral PEEP) does not appear to influence systemic hemodynamics.[44] Interestingly, increased levels of nitric oxide were observed in the exhaled gas of rabbits ventilated at increasing tidal volumes.[32] The significance of these findings remains to be defined. Although increases in heart rate may occur with the application of PEEP and the associated decreases in cardiac output, the increases are less than those seen when cardiac output is reduced to similar degrees by hemorrhage.[32] The reasons for this difference are not known but may reflect PEEP-induced sympatholytic actions and PEEP-induced increases in arterial pressure minimizing baroreceptor stimulation.

Independent of these phasic reflex arcs, ventilation also alters control of intravascular fluid balance via hormone release. Both positive-pressure ventilation and sustained hyperinflation induced by PEEP stimulate a variety of endocrinologic responses that induce fluid retention via right atrial stretch receptors. In essence, lung distention compresses the right atrium, eliciting a sympathetic response to retaining fluid by the kidneys. Plasma norepinephrine, plasma rennin activity,[45, 46] and atrial natriuretic peptide[47] increase during positive-pressure ventilation with or without PEEP. Interestingly, when subjects with congestive heart failure were exposed to positive airway pressure in the form of nasal continuous positive airway pressure (CPAP), plasma atrial natriuretic peptide activity decreased in parallel with improvements in blood flow,[48, 49] suggesting that when hemodynamics are improved, rather than challenged by positive airway pressure ventilation, the body responds by reducing this stress response.

Determinants of Pulmonary Vascular Resistance

Tissue pressure alters vascular resistance in all vascular beds. In the lung, changes in tissue pressure reflect changes in lung volume. Thus, a major determinant of vascular resistance is directly related to changes in lung volume on a purely mechanical basis, meaning that no process extrinsic to the lungs, such as a humoral response, is required to induce the changes in pulmonary vascular resistance seen with ventilation.[17, 50–54] Lung inflation, independent of changes in ITP, primarily affects cardiac function and cardiac output by altering right ventricular (RV) afterload and both RV and LV preload.[55]

RV afterload is the maximum RV systolic wall stress during contraction,[56] which, by the law of Laplace, is equal to the radius of curvature of the right ventricle (a function of end-diastolic volume) and transmural pressure (a function of systolic RV pressure).[57] Changes in ITP that occur without changes in lung volume, as may occur with occluded respiratory efforts, do not alter the pressure gradients between the right ventricle and pulmonary artery and thus do not alter pulmonary vascular resistance. Thus, neither straining at stools (Valsalva's maneuver) nor obstructive inspiratory efforts (Mueller's maneuver) primarily affect RV afterload.

Systolic RV pressure is also transmural systolic pulmonary artery pressure (Ppa). Transmural Ppa can increase by one of two mechanisms: (1) an increase in pulmonary arterial pressure without an increase in pulmonary vasomotor tone, as may occur with either a marked increase in blood flow (exercise) or passive increases in outflow pressure (LV failure), or (2) an increase in pulmonary vascular resistance by either active changes in vasomotor tone or passive lung inflation. Commonly, any increase in transmural Ppa during positive-pressure ventilation is due to an increase in pulmonary vascular resistance, because neither instantaneous cardiac output[58] nor LV filling[13] usually increases. No matter which of these processes occurs, if transmural Ppa increases, RV ejection is impeded.[59] Furthermore, if the right ventricle does not empty as much as before, not only does stroke volume decrease[60] but its residual volume increases, limiting subsequent filling from the venous circuit.[56, 58] Such limitations to venous return usually take a few beats to become manifest. This process of decreasing RV ejection, increasing RV wall stress, and falling venous return rapidly induces acute cor pulmonale. Furthermore, if RV dilation continues, RV free wall ischemia and infarction can develop, because RV coronary perfusion cannot be sustained across such high wall stresses.[61] From this brief discussion it should be clear to the reader that acute cor pulmonale is associated with a profound decrease in cardiac output that is usually resistant to therapies that primarily increase venous return (e.g., fluid challenge). In fact, rapid fluid challenges in the setting of acute cor pulmonale can precipitate profound cardiovascular collapse related to excessive RV dilation. Accordingly, fluid resuscitation in the setting of acute RV dilation is contraindicated.

During normal end-inspiration, mild hypoxemia ($Pao_2 > 65$ mm Hg), and PEEP less than 7.5 cm H_2O, increases in transmural Ppa are less pronounced. If slight increases in transmural Ppa are sustained, however, fluid retention occurs, either by humoral mechanisms or by intravascular volume infusion,[62] resulting in an increase in RV end-diastolic volume and maintaining cardiac output constant.[57, 63]

The mechanism by which pulmonary vasomotor tone may increase is complex. If regional alveolar Po_2 (Pao_2) decreases below 60 mm Hg, local pulmonary vasomotor tone increases, reducing local blood flow.[64] This process is called hypoxic pulmonary vasoconstriction and is mediated, in part, by variations in the synthesis and release of nitric oxide by pulmonary vascular endothelial cells. These cells normally synthesize nitric oxide, a potent vasodilator, at a continual but low level to maintain a generalized pulmonary vasodilated state. This process is highly regulated and is dependent on O_2 and inhibited by acidosis. Because it is an energy-dependent process, if O_2 becomes scarce, nitric oxide is not made, and thus local pulmonary vasomotor tone increases back to the level it would have had if no nitric oxide had been around in the first place. Acidosis, alveolar hypoxia, or hypoxemia can induce inhibition of nitric oxide production in this setting.

Hypoxic pulmonary vasoconstriction is an important process in optimizing matching of ventilation to perfusion when regional impairments in ventilation exist. For example, if a lobe or entire lung is collapsed or becomes obstructed, it would be advantageous for blood flow to that region to decrease so as to minimize shunt. If alveolar hypoxia occurs throughout the lungs, however, overall pulmonary vasomotor tone increases, increasing pulmonary vascular resistance and impeding RV ejection.[56] At low lung volumes, alveoli spontaneously collapse as a result of loss of interstitial traction. This scenario is relevant to patients with acute lung injury because lung volume is reduced in acute hypoxemic respiratory failure.[65, 66] Therefore, pulmonary vascular resistance is often increased in these patients because of alveolar collapse and the resultant hypoxic pulmonary vasoconstriction.

Mechanical Ventilation–Induced Changes in Pulmonary Vascular Resistance

Mechanical ventilation can modify pulmonary vascular resistance by altering one of several mechanisms described earlier. Changes in lung volume may either reduce or increase pulmonary vascular resistance. Mechanical ventilation may reduce active pulmonary vasomotor tone by one of several related processes. Hypoxic pulmonary vasoconstrictor tone may be decreased by increasing global PaO_2 by enriching alveolar gas,[67-70] reexpanding collapsed alveolar units by increasing PaO_2 in those local alveoli,[4, 71-73] increasing alveolar ventilation and thus reversing acute respiratory acidosis[70] or merely decreasing central sympathetic output by allowing the patient in acute respiratory failure not to fight for every breath.[74, 75] Similarly, these effects need not require positive-pressure breaths as much as expansion of collapsed alveoli.[76] This expansion is usually accomplished by the addition of PEEP. Thus, if PEEP opens collapsed lung units and replenishes alveolar gas with O_2, then hypoxic pulmonary vasoconstriction is reduced, pulmonary vascular resistance decreases, and RV ejection improves. Presumably, this beneficial effect of PEEP on pulmonary vascular resistance would be greatest in the neonate, whose ability to respond to hypoxia is accentuated.

Changes in lung volume can profoundly alter pulmonary vasomotor tone by one of two mechanisms (Fig. 111-7): (1) by changing active vasomotor tone through the mechanism of hypoxic pulmonary vasoconstriction and (2) by passively compressing the alveolar vessels.[65, 72, 73] The pulmonary circulation can be separated into two groups of blood vessels depending on the pressure that surrounds them.[72] The small pulmonary arterioles, venules, and alveolar capillaries sense alveolar pressure as their surrounding pressure and are referred to as alveolar vessels. The large pulmonary arteries and veins, as well as the heart and intrathoracic great vessels of the systemic circulation, sense interstitial pressure or ITP as their surrounding pressure and can be called extra-alveolar vessels. Alveolar pressure minus ITP is the transpulmonary pressure, which, when coupled with lung compliance, defines lung distention. Increasing lung volume requires transpulmonary pressure to increase and vice versa. Thus, this extravascular pressure gradient between alveolar and extra-alveolar vessels varies with changes in lung volume. The radial interstitial forces of the lung that keep them patent[71, 77, 78] act upon the extra-alveolar vessels just as they act upon the airways. As lung volume increases, the radial interstitial forces increase, increasing the diameter of both extra-alveolar vessels and airways. As far as airways are concerned, this results in a reduction in airway resistance at higher lung volumes. Similarly, as lung volume increases, extra-alveolar vessel diameter also increases, making these vessels dilate.[79] The opposite condition with decreasing lung volume is also true. As lung volume decreases, the radial interstitial traction decreases, and the cross-sectional diameter of extra-alveolar vessels decreases, thereby increasing pulmonary vascular resistance.[68, 71] The collapse of small airways induces alveolar hypoxia. Thus, at small lung volumes, pulmonary vascular resistance is increased owing to the combined effect of hypoxic pulmonary vasoconstriction and extra-alveolar vessel collapse.

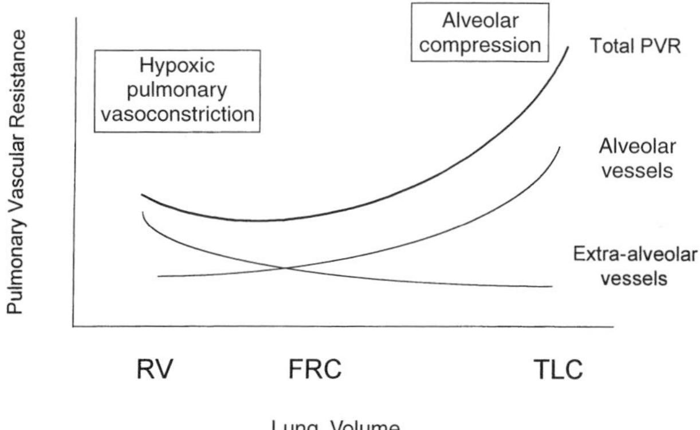

Figure 111–7. Relation between changes in lung volume and pulmonary vascular resistance (PVR), where extra-alveolar and alveolar vascular components are separated. PVR is minimum at resting lung volume or functional residual capacity (FRC). As lung volume increases toward total lung capacity (TLC) or decreases toward residual volume (RV), PVR also increases. However, the increase in resistance with hyperinflation is due to increased alveolar vascular resistance, whereas the increase in resistance with lung collapse is due to increased extra-alveolar vessel tone.

Increases in lung volume progressively increase alveolar vessel resistance, but this effect is not noticeable until lung volumes increase much above resting lung volume or functional residual capacity (FRC).[68, 80] There are two causes of the increased alveolar vessel resistance. First, the heart and extra-alveolar vessels sense ITP as their surrounding pressure, but the alveolar vessels sense alveolar pressure as their surrounding pressure. Thus, an extraluminal transpulmonary pressure gradient exists between these extra-alveolar and alveolar vessels. As lung volume increases, this pressure difference increases as well. How does all this alter pulmonary vascular resistance?

Because the intraluminal pressure in the pulmonary arteries is generated by RV ejection relative to ITP but the outside pressure of the alveolar vessels is alveolar pressure, if transpulmonary pressure increases enough to exceed intraluminal vascular pressure, the pulmonary vasculature collapses where extra-alveolar vessels pass into alveolar loci, reducing the vasculature cross-sectional area and increasing pulmonary vascular resistance. Similarly, increasing lung volume by stretching and distending the alveolar septa may also compress alveolar capillaries, although this mechanism is less well substantiated. If the cross-sectional area of the pulmonary capillaries is already reduced, the addition of abnormal hyperinflation can create significant pulmonary hypertension and may precipitate acute RV failure (acute cor pulmonale)[81] and RV ischemia.[61] Similarly, if lung volumes are reduced, increasing lung volume back to baseline levels by the use of PEEP decreases pulmonary vascular resistance.[82] Thus, PEEP may increase pulmonary vascular resistance if it induces overdistention of the lung above its normal resting volume.

Ventricular Interdependence

Changes in RV output invariably alter LV filling because the two ventricles are linked through the pulmonary vasculature. However, LV preload can also be indirectly altered by changes in RV end-diastolic volume. If RV volume increases, LV diastolic compliance decreases by the mechanism of ventricular interdependence.[83] Ventricular interdependence functions through two separate processes. First, increasing RV end-diastolic volume induces a shift of the intraventricular septum into the LV, thereby decreasing LV diastolic compliance[84] (Fig. 111-8). Thus, for the same LV filling pressure, RV dilation decreases LV end-diastolic volume and, therefore, cardiac output. This interaction is believed to be the major determinant of the phasic changes in arterial pressure and cardiac output seen in cardiac tamponade. It is referred to as *pulsus paradoxus* and can be seen in subjects with normal cardiovascular function during loaded spontaneous inspiration. However, phasic changes in arterial pressure are not commonly seen during positive-pressure ventilation.

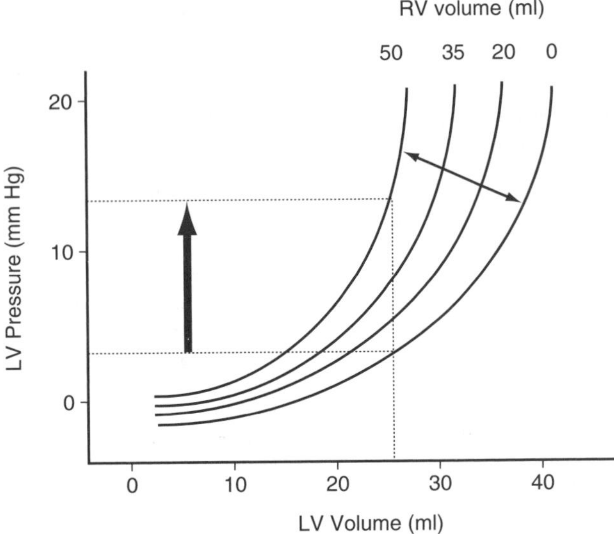

Figure 111–8. Schematic diagram representing the effect of increasing right ventricular (RV) volumes on the left ventricular (LV) diastolic pressure-volume (filling) relationship. Increases on RV volume decrease LV diastolic compliance. (From Taylor RR, Corell JW, Sonnenblick EH, Ross J Jr: Dependence of ventricular distensibility on filling the opposite ventricle. Am J Physiol 1967; 213:711–718.)

Spontaneous inspiration, by physically increasing venous return, induces an inspiration-associated RV dilation. This inspiration-associated increase in RV end-diastolic volume decreases the LV end-diastolic volume. Maintaining a relatively constant rate of venous return, by either volume resuscitation[85] or vasopressor infusion,[3] minimizes this effect. Thus, phasic changes in arterial pressure have been used as a marker of functional hypovolemia. As lung volume increases markedly, the lungs compress the heart in the cardiac fossa, limiting ventricular filling. Because most of the hemodynamic effects of hyperinflation-induced heart-lung interactions can be induced by changes in ITP alone, this aspect of heart-lung interactions is discussed in the following.

Mechanical Heart-Lung Interactions

If lung volumes increase greatly, the heart may be compressed between the two expanding lung,[86] which increases the pressure surrounding the heart. Because the chest wall and diaphragm can move away from the expanding lungs, whereas the heart, in essence, is trapped within its cardiac fossa, juxtacardiac ITP may increase more than lateral chest wall or diaphragmatic ITP.[5, 15] This compressive effect of the inflated lung can be seen with either spontaneous hyperinflation[87] or positive pressure–induced hyperinflation with PEEP.[77, 78] This decrease in "apparent" LV diastolic compliance[85] was previously misinterpreted as impaired LV contractility, because LV stroke work for a given LV end-diastolic pressure or pulmonary artery occlusion pressure is decreased.[88, 89] However, preload is more accurately defined as LV end-diastolic volume. Numerous studies have shown that when fluid resuscitation was used to return LV end-diastolic volume to its original level, both LV stroke work and cardiac output also returned to their original levels[52, 85] despite the continued application of PEEP.[90] Independent of compressive effects, expanding lungs increase the pressure surrounding the heart relative to the rest of the body. Thus, increases in ITP represent a variation in mechanical heart-lung interactions. These important processes are considered separately in the following because changing the ITP while keeping lung volumes constant can induce nearly identical responses.

Takata and colleagues[91] proposed a novel approach to understandinging mechanical heart-lung interactions. Although they use this model to describe the differences between tamponade and constrictive pericarditis on pericardial pressure using the terms "coupled" and "uncoupled" pericardial restraint, the analysis is comparable in examining the effects of hyperinflation and inspiration on cardiac fossal pressure, respectively. They proposed that pericardial stiffness (or elastance) over the right and left ventricles is different in constrictive pericarditis but similar in tamponade. Accordingly, in constrictive pericarditis changes in venous return should selectively alter RV filling, whereas in tamponade they should alter both RV and LV filling.

If we extrapolate to ventilation from the model of Takata and colleagues, it appears that tidal increases in lung volume represent "uncoupled" pericardial restraint because they selectively limit RV filling and not LV diastolic compliance. Previous workers have suggested that positive-pressure inspiration selectively decreases RV filling because the pressure gradient for systemic venous return rather than pulmonary blood flow is reduced by the increase in ITP. Although this argument is valid, as discussed in greater detail in the following section, the magnitude of the reduction in RV filling is often excessive when compared with either the increase in ITP or the decreases in the pressure gradient for systemic venous return. Using the model proposed by Takata and colleagues,[91] it can be seen that when mechanical compression of the heart occurs during inspiration, the local surface pressure over the right atrium and right ventricle may increase more than over the left atrium and left ventricle. Thus, RV filling can be selectively impaired independent of any change in the pressure gradient for systemic venous return. This would be a non–steady-state effect and would occur only during inspiration. If hyperinflation occurred, inducing a sustained increase in lung volume, then the "uncoupled" cardiac fossal restraint would become "coupled" cardiac fossal restraint.

Thus, hyperinflation, as occurs in severe asthma and with the use of excessive amounts of positive end-expiratory airway pressure, would produce a clinical picture indistinguishable from that of tamponade. Indeed, Rebuck and Read[92] made the same observation in their analysis of the hemodynamic effects of severe asthma more than 25 years ago, although they did not postulate a specific mechanism to explain this phenomenon. Presumably, the shift from uncoupled to coupled cardiac fossal restraint would occur as either absolute lung volume increased, biventricular volume increased, or both. Thus, if cardiac volumes are small and lung inflation does not overdistend the thoracic cage, as occurs under normal conditions, RV filling is primarily impeded. In congestive heart failure states and with marked lung overdistention, however, both RV filling and LV filling may be compromised by ventilation.

Hemodynamic Effects of Changes in Intrathoracic Pressure

The heart within the thorax is a pressure chamber within a pressure chamber. Therefore, changes in ITP affect the pressure gradients for both systemic venous return to the RV and systemic outflow from the LV, independent of the heart itself (Fig. 111-9). Increases in ITP, by increasing right atrial pressure and decreasing transmural LV systolic pressure, reduce these pressure gradients and thereby decrease intrathoracic blood volume. Using the same argument, decreases in ITP augment venous return and impede LV ejection, thereby increasing intrathoracic blood volume.

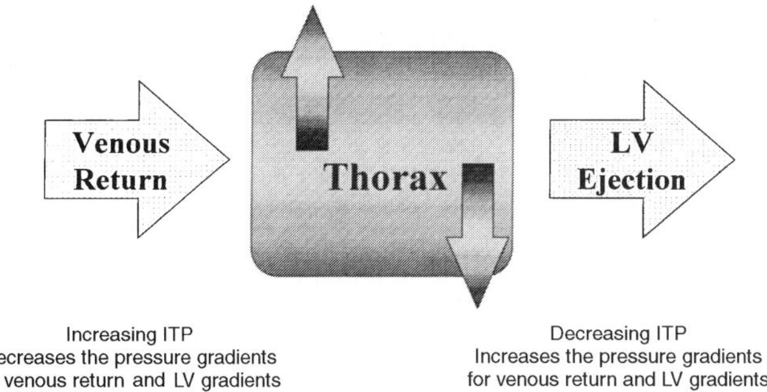

Figure 111–9. Schematic diagram of hemodynamic effects of increasing or decreasing intrathoracic pressure (ITP) on the left ventricular (LV) filling (venous return) and ejection pressure.

Systemic Venous Return

Blood flows back to the heart from the periphery through low-pressure, low-resistance venous conduits. Systemic venous flow from the venous reservoirs into the right atrium has been characterized by Guyton and coworkers.[93] As downstream right atrial pressure varies, as may occur with positive-pressure ventilation, the rate of venous return changes inversely in such a fashion as to describe a fixed upstream pressure. Pressure in the upstream venous reservoirs that can be directly measured during transient total circulatory arrest is called mean systemic pressure. Mean systemic pressure is a function of blood volume, peripheral vasomotor tone, and the distribution of blood within the vasculature.[94] Mean systemic pressure does not change rapidly during the ventilatory cycle, whereas right atrial pressure does owing to concomitant changes in ITP. Accordingly, variations in right atrial pressure represent the major factor determining the fluctuation in pressure gradient for systemic venous return during ventilation.[58, 95] With increases in ITP, as seen with positive-pressure ventilation or hyperinflation during mechanical ventilation, right atrial pressure relative to atmospheric pressure increases. As a result, the pressure gradient for systemic venous return decreases, decelerating venous blood flow,[60] decreasing RV filling, and, consequently, decreasing RV stroke volume.[58, 60, 96–103] During normal spontaneous inspiration, the converse occurs: With decreases in ITP, right atrial pressure decreases, accelerating venous blood flow and increasing RV filling and RV stroke volume[3, 18, 60, 98, 101, 104] (Fig. 111–10).

Studies of animal models have suggested that the decrease in venous return during positive-pressure ventilation may be lower than expected on the basis of the preceding scenario. Fessler and associates[105] and Takata and Robotham[106] demonstrated in an animal model that PEEP increases intra-abdominal pressure by causing the diaphragm to descend, thereby increasing the pressure surrounding the intra-abdominal vasculature. Because a large proportion of venous blood is in the abdomen, the net effect of PEEP is to increase mean systemic pressure and right atrial pressure. Accordingly, the pressure gradient for venous return may not be reduced by PEEP, especially in patients with hypervolemia.

Furthermore, Matuschak and coworkers[107] found that although PEEP decreased blood flow to the liver in proportion to the induced decrease in cardiac output in normovolemic dogs, the liver's ability to clear hepatocytic-specific compounds, such as indocyanine green, was unaltered. In fact, abdominal pressurization by diaphragmatic descent may be the major mechanism by which the decrease in venous return is minimized during positive-pressure ventilation.[108–111] Finally, when cardiac output is restored to pre-PEEP levels by fluid resuscitation[107, 112] while PEEP is maintained, liver clearance mechanisms increase above pre-PEEP levels.[113–115]

These data are consistent with a PEEP-induced alteration in intrahepatic blood flow distribution. Thus, ventilation may have less effect on venous return than originally postulated, but the effect may be more complicated than we have yet imagined. Finally, with exaggerated swings in ITP, as occur with obstructed inspiratory efforts, venous return behaves as if abdominal pressure is additive with mean systemic pressure in defining total venous blood flow.[116–119] Interest in inverse ratio ventilation has raised questions about its hemodynamic effect because its application includes a large component of hyperinflation. However, Mang and colleagues[120] demonstrated in an animal model of acute lung injury that if total PEEP (intrinsic PEEP plus extra extrinsic PEEP) was similar, there was no hemodynamic difference between conventional ventilation and inverse ratio ventilation.

Right Ventricular Filling

Under normal conditions, it is extremely difficult to document that RV filling pressure changes much as diastolic RV filling occurs. When RV filling pressure, defined as right atrial pressure minus Ppc, was directly measured in patients undergoing open-chest operations as RV volume was varied by acute volume loading, it was found to be insignificantly altered.[121] Although right atrial pressure increases with volume loading, Ppc also increases, so that RV filling pressure, defined as right atrial pressure minus Ppc, remains unchanged. Similar results were seen when RV volumes were reduced by the application

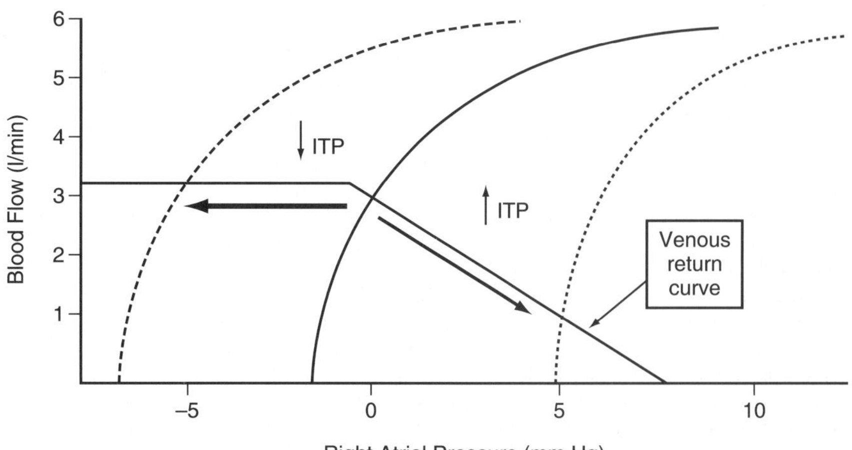

Figure 111–10. Schematic representation of the effects of increasing or decreasing intrathoracic pressure (ITP) on steady-state venous return. Changes in intrathoracic pressure alter the relation between cardiac output, venous return, and right atrial pressure. Decreases in ITP that decrease right atrial pressure to below zero relative to atmospheric pressure increase venous return by only a limited amount; increases in ITP progressively decrease venous return to a complete circulatory standstill.

of PEEP in postoperative cardiac patients.[122] These findings suggest that under normal conditions, RV diastolic compliance is high and most of the increase in right atrial pressure seen during volume loading reflects pericardial compliance and cardiac fossa stiffness more than changes in RV distending pressure. This observation implies that with RV filling, right heart sarcomere length remains constant. Presumably, conformational changes in the right ventricle more than wall stretch are responsible for RV enlargement.[14] Accordingly, changes in right atrial pressure do not follow changes in RV end-diastolic volume. When cardiac contractility is reduced and intravascular volume is expanded, RV filling pressure increases as a result of either decreased RV diastolic compliance, increased pericardial compliance, increased end-diastolic volume, or a combination of all three.

Taylor and colleagues[83] documented a curvilinear relation between RV filling pressure and volume such that as RV end-diastolic volume increased above a threshold level, RV filling pressure increased greatly. Furthermore, Pinsky and Guimond[6] demonstrated in dogs with acute ventricular failure that volume loading increased Ppc more than ITP, consistent with pericardial rather than cardiac fossal restraint. In further support of this argument, as PEEP is increased in this setting, ITP but not Ppc selectively increases until ITP equals Ppc, and then both ITP and Ppc increase equally if PEEP is increased further (see Fig. 111-4*B*). Pinsky and coworkers[12] subsequently demonstrated similar phenomena in postoperative cardiac surgery patients. PEEP, and by extension lung expansion, compresses the heart within the cardiac fossa in a fashion analogous to pericardial tamponade, but in this setting it is the expanding lungs that increase ITP, and not pericardial restraint, limiting ventricular filling.[21, 123]

Venous return, the primary determinant of cardiac output,[94] is maintained near maximum levels at rest[35, 103, 104] because RV filling occurs with minimum changes in filling pressure.[123] That is, right atrial pressure is the back pressure to venous return. Accordingly, the closer right atrial pressure is to zero relative to atmospheric pressure, the greater is the pressure gradient for systemic venous blood flow.[93, 99] For this mechanism to operate efficiently, RV output must equal venous return, otherwise sustained increases in venous blood flow would overdistend the RV, increasing right atrial pressure. Fortunately, under normal conditions of spontaneous ventilation this is not a problem because most of the increase in venous return is in phase with inspiration, decreasing again during expiration as ITP increases.[58] Similarly, the pulmonary arterial inflow circuit is highly compliant and can accept large increases in RV stroke volume without changing pressure.[60, 63] Thus, any increase in venous return is proportionally delivered to the pulmonary circuit without forcing the right ventricle to increase its force of contraction or myocardial oxygen demand.

This compensatory system rapidly becomes dysfunctional if RV diastolic compliance decreases or if right atrial pressure increases independent of changes in RV end-diastolic volume. For example, decreased RV diastolic compliance occurs with acute RV dilation or cor pulmonale (pulmonary embolism, hyperinflation, and RV infarction), which induce profound decreases in cardiac output not responsive to fluid resuscitation. Dissociation between right atrial pressure and RV end-diastolic volume occurs during either tamponade or positive-pressure ventilation. Remember that during positive-pressure inspiration, right atrial pressure is artificially increased by the increasing ITP, thus dissociating right atrial pressure from RV filling pressure. Accordingly, positive-pressure ventilation impairs normal circulatory adaptive processes that are operative during spontaneous ventilation. Furthermore, even if one restores the coupling of right atrial pressure and RV volume by using partial ventilatory support modes of ventilation, cardiac output increases only if the RV can transduce the associated increase in venous return to forward blood flow.

Thus, during weaning from mechanical ventilation, occult RV failure may be exposed and is manifest by a rapid rise in right atrial pressure and a fall in cardiac output. Because the primary effect of any form of ventilation on cardiovascular function in normal subjects is to alter RV preload by altering venous blood flow, the detrimental effect of positive-pressure ventilation on cardiac output can be minimized either by using fluid resuscitation to increase mean systemic pressure[3, 96, 116, 117] or by keeping both mean ITP and swings in lung volume as low as possible. Accordingly, prolonging expiratory time, decreasing tidal volume, and avoiding PEEP all minimize this decrease in systemic venous return to the RV.[1, 20, 58, 98-102, 124]

Because spontaneous inspiratory efforts increase lung volume by decreasing ITP, one sees an increase in venous return with spontaneous inspiration owing to the fall in right atrial pressure.[18, 50, 99-101] This augmentation of venous return is limited,[118, 119] however, because if ITP decreases below atmospheric pressure, venous return becomes flow limited as the large systemic veins collapse as they enter the thorax.[93] This flow limitation is a safety valve for the heart because ITP can decrease greatly with obstructive inspiratory efforts[36] and, if not flow limited, the right ventricle could become overdistended and fail[125] (see Fig. 111-10).

Left Ventricular Preload and Ventricular Interdependence

Changes in venous return must eventually result in directionally similar changes in LV preload, because the two ventricles function in series. For example, during a Valsalva maneuver, initially RV filling is reduced but LV filling is unaltered.[13] Then, as the strain is sustained, LV filling and cardiac output both begin to decrease.[86, 126] This phase delay in changes in output from the right ventricle to the left ventricle is exaggerated if tidal volume or respiratory rate is increased and in the setting of hypovolemia[1, 20, 53, 54, 85, 88, 89, 103, 127-131] Independent of this series interaction, direct ventricular interdependence can also occur and be clinically significant. Increasing RV volume shifts the intraventricular septum into the LV and simultaneously decreases LV diastolic compliance.

During positive-pressure ventilation, RV volumes are usually decreased, minimizing ventricular interdependence as a major factor altering hemodynamics.[83, 129-132] This effect was clearly demonstrated in humans by Jardin and coworkers,[52, 53] who showed by echocardiography that although PEEP did result in some degree of right-to-left intraventricular septal shift, the shift was small. In fact, although increases in lung volume during positive-pressure ventilation cause some septal shift, biventricular volumes usually decrease as the two ventricles are squeezed into each other.[133] Numerous investigators have shown that the decrease in cardiac output during PEEP is due to a decrease in LV end-diastolic volume and that both LV end-diastolic volume and cardiac output could be restored by fluid resuscitation[134, 135] without any measurable change in LV diastolic compliance.[85]

During spontaneous inspiration, unlike positive-pressure ventilation, RV volumes increase markedly, transiently shifting the intraventricular septum into the left ventricle[84] and decreasing LV diastolic compliance and LV end-diastolic volume.[83, 132, 136] This transient RV dilation-induced septal shift is the primary cause of inspiration-associated decreases in arterial pulse pressure, which, if greater than 10 mm Hg, is referred to as pulsus paradoxus.[18] Because spontaneous inspiratory efforts can occur during positive-pressure ventilation and especially during partial ventilatory assist, pulsus paradoxus can be seen in mechanically ventilated patients.

Left Ventricular Afterload

Left ventricular afterload is poorly defined but can be equated to systolic wall tension. Systolic wall tension, according to the Laplace equation, is proportional to the product of transmural LV pressure and the radius of curvature of the left ventricle, which itself is proportional to LV volume. As with the right ventricle, maximum LV wall tension normally occurs at the end of isometric contraction, reflecting the maximum product of LV radius of curvature (end-diastolic volume) and aortic pressure (diastolic pressure). When LV dilation exists, as in congestive heart failure, maximum LV wall stress occurs during LV ejection because the maximum product of these two variables occurs at this time. Accordingly, LV afterload varies in its definition depending on the baseline level of cardiac contractility and intravascular volume. LV ejection pressure is the transmural LV systolic pressure, which can be approximated as transmural arterial pressure. Normal baroreceptor mechanisms located in the carotid body tend to maintain arterial pressure constant with respect to atmospheric pressure, and if arterial pressure remained constant as ITP increased, then LV wall tension would decrease as well. Similarly, if transmural arterial pressure remained constant as ITP increased but LV end-diastolic volume decreased because of the associated decrease in systemic venous return usually seen with increases in ITP, LV wall tension would also decrease.[137] Thus, by either mechanism, increases in ITP decrease LV afterload. Similarly, decreases in ITP with a constant arterial pressure increase LV transmural pressure, increasing LV afterload.[13] Accordingly, unlike increases in ITP, which unload the left ventricle, decreases in ITP increase LV afterload.[138] In fact, decreasing ITP, a common occurrence during spontaneous inspiratory efforts, reflects an important cardiac stress during weaning from mechanical ventilation.[137, 139, 140] A similar argument can be given for the observed improvement in LV systolic function in patients with severe LV failure.[141, 142] Interestingly, similar "auto-EPAP" effects of expiratory grunting have been reported in infants during crying[54] and in an adult with severe LV failure.[143]

Pulsus paradoxus occurs during spontaneous inspiration under conditions of marked pericardial restraint. It may occur because of pericardial limitations, such as tamponade and constrictive pericarditis, as well as during loaded spontaneous ventilatory efforts when RV volumes swell and ITP decreases. In both cases LV stroke volume decreases.[144–148] Perhaps the most prominent mechanism creating an inspiratory decrease in both LV stroke volume and systolic arterial pressure is the increased venous return–induced transient shift of the intraventricular septum into the LV lumen owing to pericardial volume restraint, which by decreasing LV diastolic compliance transiently decreases LV end-diastolic volume. The negative swings in ITP also increase LV ejection pressure (LV pressure minus ITP), increasing the LV end-systolic volume.[13] Other influences on LV systolic function can also occur during loaded inspiratory efforts, such as with obstructive sleep apnea. These include an increase in aortic input impedance,[149] altered synchrony of contraction of the global LV myocardium,[150] and hypoxemia-induced decreased contractility.[151] Hypoxia has the added detriment of directly reducing LV diastolic compliance as well as decreasing myocardial contractile function.[152]

If ITP were to increase rapidly, as during a cough, arterial pressure would also increase by a similar amount, so that both arterial pressure relative to ITP (transmural arterial pressure or LV ejection pressure)[13] and aortic blood flow[86] would remain constant. Sustained increases in ITP, however, must eventually decrease aortic blood flow and arterial pressure because of the associated decrease in venous return.[13] Because normal baroreceptor-based homeostatic mechanisms tend to sustain a constant arterial pressure to maintain organ perfusion,[35] if ITP increased arterial pressure without changing transmural arterial pressure, the periphery would reflexively vasodilate to maintain a constant extrathoracic arterial pressure-flow relation.[128] Coronary perfusion pressure reflects the intrathoracic pressure gradient for blood flow, so it is not increased by ITP-induced increases in arterial pressure. However, compression of the coronaries by the expanding lungs may obstruct coronary blood flow. Thus, the combined decrease in coronary blood flow may induce myocardial ischemia.[153–155]

As far as LV energetics are concerned, the work performed by the contracting left ventricle increases by a similar amount with both increasing ITP above atmospheric pressure and increasing ITP from a negative value to atmospheric pressure if the absolute changes in ITP are similar. In both cases the LV ejection pressure decreases in proportion to the relative increase in ITP. However, the effect on venous return of removing large negative levels of ITP is not similar to that of adding positive ITP. Recall that once right atrial pressure becomes negative, venous return becomes flow limited. Thus, further decreases in ITP are not associated with any further increase in venous return, just a further increase in LV ejection pressure. Thus, large negative swings in ITP, as seen with vigorous inspiratory efforts in the setting of airway obstruction (asthma, upper airway obstruction, vocal cord paralysis) or stiff lungs (interstitial lung disease, pulmonary edema, and acute lung injury), selectively increase LV afterload and have been postulated to be the cause of the often observed LV failure and pulmonary edema seen in these conditions,[17, 36] especially if LV systolic function is already compromised[156, 157] (see Fig. 111-10). Similarly, removing large negative swings in ITP by either bypassing upper airway obstruction (endotracheal intubation) or instituting mechanical ventilation or PEEP-induced loss of spontaneous inspiratory efforts should selectively reduce LV afterload without significantly decreasing either venous return or cardiac output.[3, 93, 127, 141, 158, 159] Reversing this argument, weaning from mechanical ventilation, with its associated increase in both metabolic demand and LV afterload, is a form of cardiac stress testing. Although the logic of these statements is clear, neither of these observations has been documented in either animal or human experiments. Given the importance of these differential effects, with abolishing negative swings in ITP selectively reducing LV afterload in the setting of acute LV failure, this proof is clinically important.

HEMODYNAMIC EFFECTS OF VENTILATION BASED ON CARDIOPULMONARY STATUS

From the preceding discussion it should be clear that spontaneous ventilation and positive-pressure ventilation have profound hemodynamic consequences and might even have opposite effects on cardiovascular stability in different populations of patients. Furthermore, different modes of mechanical ventilatory support, by varying the degree of the patient's effort and thus changes in work of breathing and ITP as well as the level of lung volume, also alter the hemodynamic response. Schematic examples of how increasing or decreasing ITP alters the LV pressure-volume relation are depicted for conditions in which LV function is normal (Fig. 111-11) and depressed (Fig. 111-12). These figures can be used to follow the arguments developed in the subsequent text.

Still, from the preceding discussion, the following generalities hold for most modes of mechanical ventilation. In patients with markedly increased work of breathing, hypervolemia, or

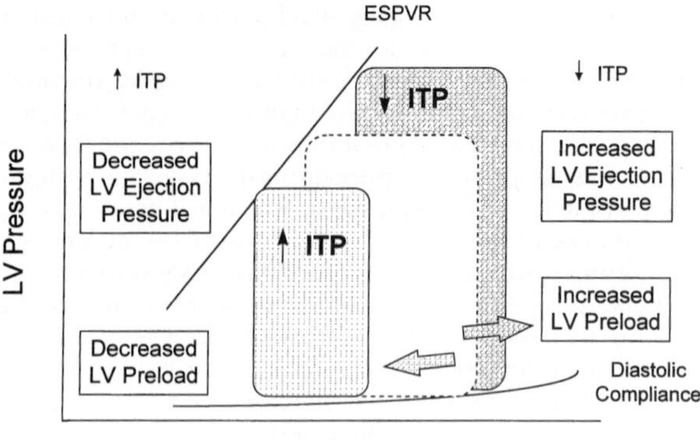

Figure 111–11. Schematic representation of the effects of changes in intrathoracic pressure (ITP) on the left ventricular (LV) pressure-volume relations when cardiac contractility is normal.

impaired LV pump function, the institution of mechanical ventilatory support can be lifesaving because of its ability to support the cardiovascular system while decreasing global O_2 demand, independent of changes in gas exchange. In patients with hypovolemia or a strong tendency to develop hyperinflation, mechanical ventilation may rapidly induce cardiovascular instability. Similarly, withdrawal of ventilatory support can be considered an exercise stress test, and if patients have limited cardiovascular reserve they may not be weaned even if their traditional weaning parameter values are acceptable.[156, 157]

The hemodynamic differences between different modes of mechanical ventilation at a constant airway pressure and PEEP can be explained by their differential effects on lung volume and ITP.[160] When two different modes of ventilation result in similar changes in ITP and ventilatory effort, their hemodynamic effects are also similar despite markedly different airway waveforms. For example, partial ventilatory support with either intermittent mandatory ventilation or pressure support ventilation resulted in similar hemodynamic responses when matched for similar tidal volumes in 20 patients after cardiac surgery.[161] Sternberg and Sahebjami[162] demonstrated that tissue oxygenation was similar in 12 stable ventilator-dependent patients when switched from assist-control to intermittent mandatory ventilation and pressure support ventilation with matched tidal volumes. Finally, high-frequency jet ventilation, when delivered at low levels, resulted in a constant cardiac output in patients with heart failure, even if the ventilation delivered was synchronous with the cardiac cycle.[163]

Acute Lung Injury

Patients with acute lung injury often require supplemental increases in airway pressure at end-expiration to maintain alveolar distention and arterial oxygenation. Clearly, positive-pressure ventilation decreases intrathoracic blood volume[99] and PEEP decreases it even more[122, 123] without altering LV contractile function.[164–166] Increases in airway pressure may not reflect increases in ITP, however, because patients with acute lung injury have varying degrees of increased lung stiffness and decreased chest wall compliance. Furthermore, it is the increase in lung volume, not airway pressure, that defines the degree of increase of ITP during positive-pressure ventilation.[7] This was shown by Singer and coworkers[164] in 18 ventilator-dependent but hemodynamically stable patients. They found that the degree of hyperinflation, not the airway pressure, determined the decrease in cardiac output. To the extent that increases in lung volume are matched with different modes of mechanical ventilation, these modes of ventilation also decrease cardiac output to a similar extent.[111, 165] However, the hemodynamic effects of hyperinflation can be counterbalanced, in part, by fluid resuscitation that restores intrathoracic blood volume to pre-PEEP levels. Similarly, when LV end-diastolic volume is returned to basal levels, as assessed by noninvasive blood pool scanning[166] or echocardiography,[167–169] cardiac output also returns to its basal level despite the continued application of PEEP. That the PEEP-induced decrease in cardiac output was due to a decreased pressure gradient for venous return was elegantly shown by Gunter and colleagues,[170] who minimized the decrease in cardiac output in ventilator-dependent septic patients by lower-body compression. If cardiac output does not increase with fluid resuscitation, then other processes, such as cor pulmonale, increased pulmonary vascular resistance, or cardiac compression, may also be inducing this cardiovascular depression.[171] The caregiver at the bedside should then focus attention on potential RV dysfunction and occult hyperinflation.

Lessard and coworkers[172] compared volume-controlled conventional ventilation with pressure-controlled and pressure-controlled inverse ratio ventilation in nine patients with acute respiratory distress syndrome (ARDS). Because ventilator settings were adjusted to keep total PEEP and tidal volume consistent between treatment arms, the changes in ITP were similar for the three therapies. Although arterial pressure was slightly lower with pressure-controlled inverse ratio ventilation than with both volume-controlled and pressure-controlled ventilation in this study, no significant hemodynamic effects were seen. Chan and Abraham[173] saw similar results in 10 patients with ARDS matched for comparable tidal volumes and total PEEP. However, when pressure control with a smaller tidal volume was compared with volume control, both Abraham and Yoshihara[174] and Poelaert and colleagues[175] found that pressure control was associated with a higher cardiac output.

Congestive Heart Failure

If cardiac output increases with the application of PEEP, then either hypoxic pulmonary vasoconstriction or LV afterload has been reduced by this maneuver. Increases in cardiac output with increases in airway pressure suggest the presence of congestive heart failure.[159, 176] Grace and Greenbaum[141] noted that adding PEEP for patients with heart failure did not decrease cardiac output and actually increased cardiac output if the pulmonary artery occlusion pressure exceeded 18 mm

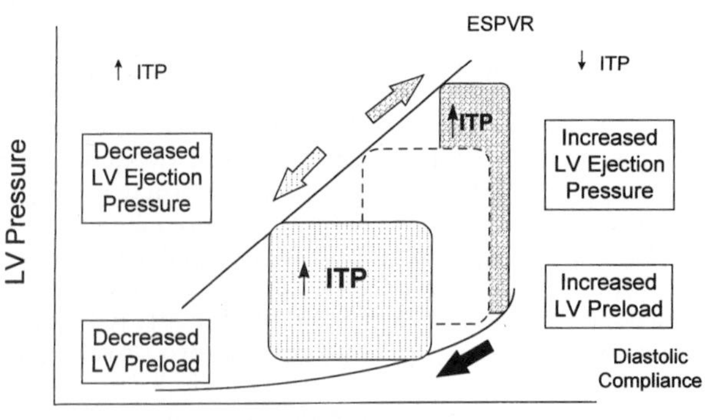

Figure 111–12. Schematic representation of the effects of changes in intrathoracic pressure (ITP) on the left ventricular (LV) pressure-volume relations when cardiac contractility is impaired and intravascular volume status is expanded. ESPVR = end-systolic pressure-volume relationship.

Hg. Similarly, Calvin and colleagues[177] noted that patients with cardiogenic pulmonary edema had no decrease in cardiac output when given PEEP. Unfortunately, PEEP may be detrimental in patients with combined heart failure and acute lung injury. PEEP can result in increased leukocyte retention in human lungs.[178] Rasanen and coworkers showed that decreasing levels of ventilatory support in patients with myocardial ischemia and acute LV failure worsened ischemia,[159, 179] and this could be minimized by preventing spontaneous inspiratory effort-induced negative swings in ITP.[158] Because weaning from mechanical ventilatory support is a form of exercise stress test, withdrawal of ventilatory support can unmask cardiac failure in otherwise stable patients with acute respiratory failure.[157, 179] Such patients may not be "weanable" from mechanical ventilator support unless supplemented with positive inotropes.[156]

The cardiovascular benefits of positive airway pressure can be seen by withdrawing negative swings in ITP, as created by using increasing levels of CPAP.[180, 181] Even CPAP levels as low as 5 cm H_2O can increase cardiac output in patients with congestive heart failure, whereas cardiac output decreases with similar levels of CPAP in both normal subjects and heart failure patients without volume overload. Nasal CPAP can accomplish the same results in patients with obstructive sleep apnea and heart failure,[182] although the benefits do not appear to be related to changes in obstructive breathing pattern.[183] Prolonged nighttime nasal CPAP can selectively improve respiratory muscle strength as well as LV contractile function in patients with heart failure.[184] These benefits are associated with reductions of serum catacholamine levels.[185]

If positive airway pressure augments LV ejection in heart failure states, then systolic arterial pressure should not decrease but actually increase compared with the value for spontaneous ventilation. This was exactly what Abel and colleagues[176] saw in 10 patients after cardiac surgery. This effect is referred to as reverse pulsus paradoxus. Perel and associates[186-188] suggested that the relation between ventilatory efforts and systolic arterial pressure may be used to determine rapidly which patients may benefit from cardiac assist by increases in ITP and which patients may not. Patients whose systolic arterial pressure increases during ventilation relative to an apneic baseline tend to have a greater degree of volume overload[187] and heart failure,[186] whereas those whose systolic arterial pressure decreases tend to be volume responsive (see Fig. 111-11).

Chronic Obstructive Pulmonary Disease

The primary hemodynamic problem seen in patients with chronic obstructive pulmonary disease (COPD) is related to hyperinflation, either that caused by loss of lung parenchyma or dynamic hyperinflation. In either case, the lungs expand, compressing the heart in the cardiac fossa, increase pulmonary vascular resistance, and impede venous return. Dynamic hyperinflation is also referred to as intrinsic PEEP. Intrinsic PEEP alters hemodynamic function in patients in a fashion similar to extrinsic PEEP. Furthermore, matching intrinsic PEEP with externally applied PEEP has no measurable detrimental hemodynamic effect,[189-191] although such matching decreases the work cost of spontaneous breathing. Furthermore, CPAP, like PEEP, has little detrimental effect in these patients when delivered below the intrinsic level of PEEP.[192] There is little hemodynamic difference between increasing airway pressure to generate a breath and decreasing extrathoracic pressure (iron lung negative-pressure ventilation). Ambrosino and coworkers[193] used negative-pressure ventilation to augment ventilation in patients with COPD and found no differences in hemodynamic response with similar levels of tidal volume.

As with patients with acute lung injury, weaning of patients with COPD taxes the cardiovascular system. Patients with severe COPD but adequate ventilatory weaning parameters may experience cardiogenic pulmonary edema during weaning.[157] The cause is probably combined volume overload and increased LV failure because LV ejection fraction decreases during such trials,[194] and after diuresis many of these patients can be subsequently weaned. The profound difficulty that bedside clinicians have in predicting weaning from mechanical ventilation, using simple measures of ventilatory reserve, airflow, and gas exchange parameters, may reflect ignorance of the patient's cardiovascular reserve and the exercise load that spontaneous breathing places on the rest of the circulation. Mohsenifar and colleagues[195] assessed the effect of weaning on gastric intramural pH (pHi) as a marker of splanchnic blood flow in 29 ventilated patients deemed ready for weaning. Patients who could not be weaned had a gastric pHi that was substantially reduced from 7.36 during intermittent positive-pressure ventilation to 7.09 during weaning. Patients who were successfully weaned showed little change in pHi (7.45 to 7.46). Thus, occult cardiovascular insufficiency may play a major role in failure to wean in critically ill patients.[196] However, this idea suggested by one clinical trial, although attractive, has not been proved conclusively.

SUMMARY

Our understanding of clinically relevant cardiopulmonary interactions has advanced far in 30 years. What was once fraught with much mystery now seems obvious. Still, complacency in the application of these principles at the bedside should be avoided. We thought we knew all there was to know about chronic obstructive lung disease 15 years ago, but the entire management schema was reversed with better understanding of dynamic hyperinflation and auto-PEEP.[191] Similarly, the exact ways in which heart-lung interactions define myocardial ejection efficiency, mechanical ejection, and myocardial O_2 requirements in both acute lung injury states and severe airflow obstruction conditions remain to be defined.

ACKNOWLEDGMENT

This work was supported in part by the Veterans Administration.

References

1. Cournaud A, Motley HL, Werko L, et al: Physiologic studies of the effect of intermittent positive pressure breathing on cardiac output in man. Am J Physiol 1948; 152:162-174.
2. Milic-Emili J, Mead J, Turner JM: Improved method for assessing the validity of the esophageal balloon technique. J Appl Physiol 1964; 19:207-211.
3. Braunwald E, Binion JT, Morgan WL, Sarnoff SJ: Alterations in central blood volume and cardiac output induced by positive pressure breathing and counteracted by metaraminol (Aramine). Circ Res 1957; 5:670-675.
4. Whittenberger JL, McGregor M, Berglund E, et al: Influence of state of inflation of the lung on pulmonary vascular resistance. J Appl Physiol 1960; 15:878-882.
5. Novak RA, Matuschak GM, Pinsky MR: Effect of ventilatory frequency on regional pleural pressure. J Appl Physiol 1988; 65:1314-1323.
6. Pinsky MR, Guimond JG: The effects of positive end-expiratory pressure on heart-lung interactions. J Crit Care 1991; 6:1-11.
7. Romand JA, Shi W, Pinsky MR: Cardiopulmonary effects of posi-

tive pressure ventilation during acute lung injury. Chest 1995; 108:1041-1048.

8. O'Quinn RJ, Marini JJ, Culver BH, et al: Transmission of airway pressure to pleural pressure during lung edema and chest wall restriction. J Appl Physiol 1985; 59:1171-1177.
9. Gattinoni, L, Mascheroni D, Torresin A, Fumagalli R, Vesconi S, Rossi GP, Rossi F, Baglioni S, Bassi F, Nastri G, Persenti A: Morphological response to positive end-expiratory pressure in acute respiratory failure. Intensive Care Med 1986; 12:137-142.
10. Globits S, Burghuber OC, Koller J, Schenk P, Frank H, Grimm M, End A, Glogar D, Imhof H, Klepetko W: Effect of lung transplantation on right and left ventricular volumes and function measured by magnetic resonance imaging. Am J Respir Crit Care Med 1994; 149:1000-1004.
11. Scharf SM, Ingram RH Jr: Effects of decreasing lung compliance with oleic acid on the cardiovascular response to PEEP. Am J Physiol 1977; 233:H635-H641.
12. Pinsky MR, Vincent JL, DeSmet JM: Estimating left ventricular filling pressure during positive end-expiratory pressure in humans. Am Rev Respir Dis 1991; 143:25-31.
13. Buda AJ, Pinsky MR, Ingels NB, et al: Effect of intrathoracic pressure on left ventricular performance. N Engl J Med 1979; 301:453-459.
14. Kingma I, Smiseth OA, Frais MA, Smith ER, Tyberg JV: Left ventricular external constraint: Relationship between pericardial, pleural and esophageal pressures during positive end-expiratory pressure and volume loading in dogs. Ann Biomed Eng 1987; 15:331-346.
15. Tsitlik JE, Halperin HR, Guerci AD, Dvorine LS, Popel AS, Siu CO, Yin FCP, Weisfeldt ML: Augmentation of pressure in a vessel indenting the surface of the lung. Ann Biomed Eng 1987; 15:259-284.
16. Marini JJ, Rodriguez RM, Lamb V: The inspiratory workload of patient-initiated mechanical ventilation. Am Rev Respir Dis 1986; 134:902-909.
17. Bromberger-Barnea B: Mechanical effects of inspiration on heart functions: A review. Fed Proc 1981; 40:2172-2177.
18. Wise RA, Robotham JL, Summer WR: Effects of spontaneous ventilation on the circulation. Lung 1981; 159:175-192.
19. Roussos C, Macklem PT: The respiratory muscles. N Engl J Med 1982; 307:786-797.
20. Grenvik A: Respiratory, circulatory and metabolic effects of respirator treatment. Acta Anaesthesiol 1966; 19(Suppl):1-122.
21. Shuey CB, Pierce AK, Johnson RL: An evaluation of exercise tests in chronic obstructive lung disease. J Appl Physiol 1969; 27:256-261.
22. Stock MC, David DW, Manning JW, Ryan ML: Lung mechanics and oxygen consumption during spontaneous ventilation and severe heart failure. Chest 1992; 102:279-283.
23. Kawagoe Y, Permutt S, Fessler HE: Hyperinflation with intrinsic PEEP and respiratory muscle blood flow. J Appl Physiol 1994; 77:2440-2448.
24. Aubier M, Vires N, Sillye G, Mozes R, Roussos C: Respiratory muscle contribution to lactic acidosis in low cardiac output. Am Rev Respir Dis 1982; 126:648-652.
25. Vires N, Sillye G, Rassidakis A, et al: Effect of mechanical ventilation on respiratory muscle blood flow during shock. Physiologist 1980; 23:1-8.
26. Glick G, Wechsler AS, Epstein DE: Reflex cardiovascular depression produced by stimulation of pulmonary stretch receptors in the dog. J Clin Invest 1969; 48:467-472.
27. Painal AS: Vagal sensory receptors and their reflex effects. Physiol Rev 1973; 53:59-88.
28. Anrep GV, Pascual W, Rossler R: Respiratory variations in the heart rate. I. The reflex mechanism of the respiratory arrhythmia. Proc R Soc Lond B Biol Sci 1936; 119:191-217.
29. Taha BH, Simon PM, Dempsey JA, Skatrud JB, Iber C: Respiratory sinus arrhythmia in humans: An obligatory role for vagal feedback from the lungs. J Appl Physiol 1995; 78:638-645.
30. Bernardi L, Calciati A, Gratarola A, Battistin I, Fratino P, Finardi G: Heart rate-respiration relationship: Computerized method for early detection of cardiac autonomic damage in diabetic patients. Acta Cardiol 1986; 41:197-206.
31. Bernardi L, Keller F, Sanders M, Reddy PS, Griffith B, Meno F, Pinsky MR: Respiratory sinus arrhythmia in the totally denervated human heart. J Appl Physiol 1989; 67:1447-1455.
32. Persson MG, Lonnqvist PA, Gustafsson LE: Positive end-expiratory pressure ventilation elicits increases in endogenously formed nitric oxide as detected in air exhaled by rabbits. Anesthesiology 1995; 82:969-974.
33. Cassidy SS, Eschenbacher WI, Johnson RL Jr.: Reflex cardiovascular depression during unilateral lung hyperinflation in the dog. J Clin Invest 1979; 64:620-626.
34. Daly MB, Hazzledine JL, Ungar A: The reflex effects of alterations in lung volume on systemic vascular resistance in the dog. J Physiol (Lond) 1967; 188:331-351.
35. Shepherd JT: The lungs as receptor sites for cardiovascular regulation. Circulation 1981; 63:1-10.
36. Stalcup SA, Mellins RB: Mechanical forces producing pulmonary edema in acute asthma. N Engl J Med 1977; 297:592-596.
37. Vatner SF, Rutherford JD: Control of the myocardial contractile state by carotid chemo- and baroreceptor and pulmonary inflation reflexes in conscious dogs. J Clin Invest 1978; 63:1593-1601.
38. Pick RA, Handler JB, Murata GH, Friedman AS: The cardiovascular effects of positive end-expiratory pressure. Chest 1982; 82:345-350.
39. Said SI, Kitamura S, Vreim C: Prostaglandins: Release from the lung during mechanical ventilation at large tidal ventilation. J Clin Invest 1972; 51:83a.
40. Bedetti C, Del Basso P, Argiolas C, Carpi A: Arachidonic acid and pulmonary function in a heart-lung preparation of guinea-pig. Modulation by P_{CO_2}. Arch Int Pharmacodyn Ther 1987; 285:98-116.
41. Berend N, Christopher KL, Voelkel NF: Effect of positive end-expiratory pressure on functional residual capacity: Role of prostaglandin production. Am Rev Respir Dis 1982; 126:641-647.
42. Pattern MY, Liebman PR, Hetchman HG: Humorally mediated decreases in cardiac output associated with positive end-expiratory pressure. Microvasc Res 1977; 13:137-144.
43. Berglund JE, Halden E, Jakobson S, Svensson J: PEEP ventilation does not cause humorally mediated cardiac output depression in pigs. Intensive Care Med 1994; 20:360-364.
44. Fuhrman BP, Everitt J, Lock JE: Cardiopulmonary effects of unilateral airway pressure changes in intact infant lambs. J Appl Physiol 1984; 56:1439-1448.
45. Payen DM, Brun-Buisson CJL, Carli PA, Huet Y, Leviel F, Cinotti L, Chiron B: Hemodynamic, gas exchange, and hormonal consequences of LBPP during PEEP ventilation. J Appl Physiol 1987; 62:61-70.
46. Frage D, de la Coussaye JE, Beloucif S, Fratacci MD, Payen DM: Interactions between hormonal modifications during PEEP-induced antidiuresis and antinatriuresis. Chest 1995; 107:1095-1100.
47. Frass M, Watschinger B, Traindl O, Popovic R, Podolsky A, Gisslinger H, Flager S, Golden M, Schuster E, Leithner C: Atrial natriuretic peptide release in response to different positive end-expiratory pressure levels. Crit Care Med 1993; 21:343-347.
48. Wilkins MA, Su XL, Palayew MD, Yamashiro Y, Bolli P, McKenzie JK, Kryger MH: The effects of posture change and continuous positive airway pressure on cardiac natriuretic peptides in congestive heart failure. Chest 1995; 107:909-915.
49. Shirakami G, Magaribuchi T, Shingu K, Suga S, Tamai S, Nakao K, Mori K: Positive end-expiratory pressure ventilation decreases plasma atrial and brain natriuretic peptide levels in humans. Anesth Analg 1993; 77:1116-1121.
50. Brecher GA, Hubay CA: Pulmonary blood flow and venous return during spontaneous respiration. Circ Res 1955; 3:40-46.
51. Goldstein JA, Vlahakes GJ, Verrier ED: The role of right ventricular systolic dysfunction and elevated intrapericardial pressures in the genesis of low output in experimental right ventricular infarction. Circulation 1982; 65:513-520.
52. Jardin F, Farcot JC, Boisante L: Influence of positive end-expiratory pressure on left ventricular performance. N Engl J Med 1981; 304:387-392.
53. Jardin FF, Farcot JC, Gueret P, Prost JF, Ozier Y, Bourdarias JP: Echocardiographic evaluation of ventricles during continuous positive pressure breathing. J Appl Physiol 1984; 56:619-627.
54. Prec KJ, Cassels DE: Oximeter studies in newborn infants during crying. Pediatrics 1952; 9:756-761.
55. Luce JM: The cardiovascular effects of mechanical ventilation and positive end-expiratory pressure. JAMA 1984; 252:807-811.

56. Maughan WL, Shoukas AA, Sagawa K, Weisfeldt ML: Instantaneous pressure-volume relationships of the canine right ventricle. Circ Res 1979; 44:309–315.
57. Sibbald WJ, Driedger AA: Right ventricular function in disease states: Pathophysiologic considerations. Crit Care Med 1983; 11:339–345.
58. Pinsky MR: Instantaneous venous return curves in an intact canine preparation. J Appl Physiol 1984; 56:765–771.
59. Piene H, Sund T: Does pulmonary impedance constitute the optimal load for the right ventricle? Am J Physiol 1982; 242:H154–H160.
60. Pinsky MR: Determinants of pulmonary arterial flow variation during respiration. J Appl Physiol 1984; 56:1237–1245.
61. Johnston WE, Vinten-Johansen J, Shugart HE, Santamore WP: Positive end-expiratory pressure potentiates the severity of canine right ventricular ischemia-reperfusion injury. Am J Physiol 1992; 262:H168–H176.
62. Sibbald WJ, Calvin JE, Holliday RL, et al: Concepts in the pharmacologic support of cardiovascular function in critically ill surgical patients. Surg Clin North Am 1983; 63:455–466.
63. Sibbald WH, Calvin J, Driedger AA: Right and left ventricular preload, and diastolic ventricular compliance: Implications of therapy in critically ill patients. *In*: Critical Care State of the Art. Vol 3. Fullerton, Calif, Society of Critical Care, 1982, pp 166–181.
64. Madden JA, Dawson CA, Harder DR: Hypoxia-induced activation in small isolated pulmonary arteries from the cat. J Appl Physiol 1985; 59:113–118.
65. Hakim TS, Michel RP, Chang HK: Effect of lung inflation on pulmonary vascular resistance by arterial and venous occlusion. J Appl Physiol 1982; 53:1110–1115.
66. Quebbeman EJ, Dawson CA: Influence of inflation and atelectasis on the hypoxic pressure response in isolated dog lung lobes. Cardiovas Res 1976; 10:672–677.
67. Brower RG, Gottlieb J, Wise RA, Permutt W, Sylvester JT: Locus of hypoxic vasoconstriction in isolated ferret lungs. J Appl Physiol 1987; 63:58–65.
68. Hakim TS, Michel RP, Minami H, Chang K: Site of pulmonary hypoxic vasoconstriction studied with arterial and venous occlusion. J Appl Physiol 1983; 54:1298–1302.
69. Marshall BE, Marshall C: A model for hypoxic constriction of the pulmonary circulation. J Appl Physiol 1988; 64:68–77.
70. Marshall BE, Marshall C: Continuity of response to hypoxic pulmonary vasoconstriction. J Appl Physiol 1980; 49:189–196.
71. Dawson CA, Grimm DJ, Linehan JH: Lung inflation and longitudinal distribution of pulmonary vascular resistance during hypoxia. J Appl Physiol 1979; 47:532–536.
72. Howell JBL, Permutt S, Proctor DF, et al: Effect of inflation of the lung on different parts of the pulmonary vascular bed. J Appl Physiol 1961; 16:71–76.
73. West JB, Dollery CT, Naimark A: Distribution of blood flow in isolated lung: Relation to vascular and alveolar pressures. J Appl Physiol 1964; 19:713–724.
74. Fuhrman BP, Everitt J, Lock JE: Cardiopulmonary effects of unilateral airway pressure changes in intact infant lambs. J Appl Physiol 1984; 56:1439–1448.
75. Fuhrman BP, Smith-Wright DL, Kulik TJ, Lock JE: Effects of static and fluctuating airway pressure on the intact, immature pulmonary circulation. J Appl Physiol 1986; 60:114–122.
76. Thorvalson J, Ilebekk A, Kiil F: Determinants of pulmonary blood volume: Effects of acute changes in airway pressure. Acta Physiol Scand 1985; 125:471–479.
77. Hoffman EA, Ritman EL: Heart-lung interaction: Effect on regional lung air content and total heart volume. Ann Biomed Eng 1987; 15:241–257.
78. Olson LE, Hoffman EA: Heart-lung interactions determined by electron beam x-ray CT in laterally recumbent rabbits. J Appl Physiol 1995; 78:417–427.
79. Grant BJB, Lieber BB: Compliance of the main pulmonary artery during the ventilatory cycle. J Appl Physiol 1992; 72:535–542.
80. Lopez-Muniz R, Stephens NL, Bromberger-Barnea B, Permutt S, Riley RL: Critical closure of pulmonary vessels analyzed in terms of Starling resistor model. J Appl Physiol 1968; 24:625–635.
81. Block AJ, Boyson PG, Wynne JW: The origins of cor pulmonale, a hypothesis. Chest 1979; 75:109–114.
82. Canada E, Benumnof JL, Tousdale FR: Pulmonary vascular resistance correlated in intact normal and abnormal canine lungs. Crit Care Med 1982; 10:719–723.
83. Taylor RR, Corell JW, Sonnenblick EH, Ross J Jr: Dependence of ventricular distensibility on filling the opposite ventricle. Am J Physiol 1967; 213:711–718.
84. Brinker JA, Weiss I, Lappe DL, et al: Leftward septal displacement during right ventricular loading in man. Circulation 1980; 61:626–633.
85. Marini JJ, Culver BN, Butler J: Mechanical effect of lung distention with positive pressure on cardiac function. Am Rev Respir Dis 1980; 124:382–386.
86. Butler J: The heart is in good hands. Circulation 1983; 67:1163–1168.
87. Cassidy SS, Wead WB, Seibert GB, Ramanathan M: Changes in left ventricular geometry during spontaneous breathing. J Appl Physiol 1987; 63:803–811.
88. Cassidy SS, Robertson CH, Pierce AK, et al: Cardiovascular effects of positive end-expiratory pressure in dogs. J Appl Physiol 1978; 4:743–749.
89. Conway CM: Hemodynamic effects of pulmonary ventilation. Br J Anaesth 1975; 47:761–766.
90. Berglund JE, Halden E, Jakobson S, Landelius J: Echocardiographic analysis of cardiac function during high PEEP ventilation. Intensive Care Med 1994; 20:174–180.
91. Takata M, Harasawa Y, Beloucif S, Robotham JL: Coupled vs. uncoupled pericardial restraint: Effects on cardiac chamber interactions. J Appl Physiol 1997; 83:1799–1813.
92. Rebuck AS, Read J: Assessment and management of severe asthma. Am J Med 1971; 51:788–792.
93. Guyton AC, Lindsey AW, Abernathy B, et al: Venous return at various right atrial pressures and the normal venous return curve. Am J Physiol 1957; 189:609–615.
94. Goldberg HS, Rabson J: Control of cardiac output by systemic vessels: Circulatory adjustments of acute and chronic respiratory failure and the effects of therapeutic interventions. Am J Cardiol 1981; 47:696–702.
95. Kilburn KH: Cardiorespiratory effects of large pneumothorax in conscious and anesthetized dogs. J Appl Physiol 1963; 18:279–283.
96. Chevalier PA, Weber KC, Engle JC, et al: Direct measurement of right and left heart outputs in Valsalva-like maneuver in dogs. Proc Soc Exp Biol Med 1972; 139:1429–1437.
97. Guntheroth WC, Gould R, Butler J, et al: Pulsatile flow in pulmonary artery, capillary and vein in the dog. Cardiovasc Res 1974; 8:330–337.
98. Guntheroth WG, Morgan BC, Mullins GL: Effect of respiration on venous return and stroke volume in cardiac tamponade: Mechanism of pulsus paradoxus. Circ Res 1967; 20:381–390.
99. Guyton AC: Effect of cardiac output by respiration, opening the chest, and cardiac tamponade. *In*: Circulatory Physiology: Cardiac Output and Its Regulation. Philadelphia, WB Saunders, 1963, pp 378–386.
100. Holt JP: The effect of positive and negative intrathoracic pressure on cardiac output and venous return in the dog. Am J Physiol 1944; 142:594–603.
101. Morgan BC, Abel FL, Mullins GL, et al: Flow patterns in cavae, pulmonary artery, pulmonary vein and aorta in intact dogs. Am J Physiol 1966; 210:903–909.
102. Morgan BC, Martin WE, Hornbein TF, et al: Hemodynamic effects of intermittent positive pressure respiration. Anesthesiology 1960; 27:584–590.
103. Scharf SM, Brown R, Saunders N, Green LH: Hemodynamic effects of positive pressure inflation. J Appl Physiol 1980; 49:124–131.
104. Scharf SM, Brown R, Saunders N, et al: Effects of normal and loaded spontaneous inspiration on cardiovascular function. J Appl Physiol 1979; 47:582–590.
105. Fessler HE, Brower RG, Wise RA, Permutt S: Effects of positive end-expiratory pressure on the canine venous return curve. Am Rev Respir Dis 1992; 146:4–10.
106. Takata M, Robotham JL: Effects of inspiratory diaphragmatic descent on inferior vena caval venous return. J Appl Physiol 1992; 72:597–607.
107. Matuschak GM, Pinsky MR, Rogers RM: Effects of positive end-

expiratory pressure on hepatic blood flow and hepatic performance. J Appl Physiol 1987; 62:1377–1383.
108. Chihara E, Hasimoto S, Kinoshita T, Hirpose M, Tanaka Y, Morimoto T: Elevated mean systemic filling pressure due to intermittent positive-pressure ventilation. Am J Physiol 1992; 262:H1116–H1121.
109. Takata M, Wise RA, Robotham JL: Effects of abdominal pressure on venous return: Abdominal vascular zone conditions. J Appl Physiol 1990; 69:1961–1972.
110. Barnes GE, Laine GA, Giam PY, Smith EE, Granger HJ: Cardiovascular responses to elevation of intra-abdominal hydrostatic pressure. Am J Physiol 1985; 248:R208–R213.
111. Lichtwarck-Aschoff M, Zeravik J, Pfeiffer UJ: Intrathoracic blood volume accurately reflects circulatory volume status in critically ill patients with mechanical ventilation. Intensive Care Med 1992; 18:142–145.
112. Brienza N, Revelly JP, Ayuse T, Robotham JL: Effect of PEEP on liver arterial and venous blood flows. Am J Respir Crit Care Med 1995; 152:504–510.
113. Sha M, Saito Y, Yokoyama K, Sawa T, Amaha K: Effects of continuous positive-pressure ventilation on hepatic blood flow and intrahepatic oxygen delivery in dogs. Crit Care Med 1987; 15:1040–1417.
114. Richard C, Berdeaux A, Delion F, et al: Effect of mechanical ventilation on hepatic drug pharmacokinetics. Chest 1986; 90:837–842.
115. Dorinsky PM, Hamlin RL, Gadek JE: Alterations in regional blood flow during positive end-expiratory pressure ventilation. Crit Care Med 1987; 15:106–115.
116. Magder S, Georgiadis G, Cheong T: Respiratory variation in right atrial pressure predict the response to fluid challenge. J Crit Care 1992; 7:76–85.
117. Terada N, Takeuchi T: Postural changes in venous pressure gradients in anesthetized monkeys. Am J Physiol 1993; 264:H21–H25.
118. Scharf S, Tow DE, Miller MJ, Brown R, McIntyre K, Dilts C: Influence of posture and abdominal pressure on the hemodynamic effects of Mueller's maneuver. J Crit Care 1989; 4:26–34.
119. Tarasiuk A, Scharf SM: Effects of periodic obstructive apneas on venous return in closed-chest dogs. Am Rev Respir Dis 1993; 148:323–329.
120. Mang H, Kacmarek RM, Ritz R, Wilson RS, Kimball WP: Cardiorespiratory effects of volume- and pressure-controlled ventilation at various I/E ratios in an acute lung injury model. Am J Respir Crit Care Med 1995; 151:731–736.
121. Tyberg JV, Taichman GC, Smith ER, Douglas NWS, Smiseth OA, Keon WJ: The relationship between pericardial pressure and right atrial pressure: An intraoperative study. Circulation 1986; 73:428–432.
122. Pinsky MR, Vincent JL, DeSmet JM: Effect of positive end-expiratory pressure on right ventricular function in man. Am Rev Respir Dis 1992; 146:681–687.
123. Jayaweera AR, Ehrlich W: Changes of phasic pleural pressure in awake dogs during exercise: Potential effects on cardiac output. Ann Biomed Eng 1987; 15:311–318.
124. Harken AH, Brennan MF, Smith N, Barsamian EM: The hemodynamic response to positive end-expiratory ventilation in hypovolemic patients. Surgery 1974; 76:786–793.
125. Lores ME, Keagy BA, Vassiliades T, Henry GW, Lucas CL, Wilcox BR: Cardiovascular effects of positive end-expiratory pressure (PEEP) after pneumonectomy in dogs. Ann Thorac Surg 1985; 40:464–473.
126. Sharpey-Schaffer EP: Effects of Valsalva maneuver on the normal and failing circulation. Br Med J 1955; 1:693–699.
127. Peters J, Kindred MK, Robotham JL: Transient analysis of cardiopulmonary interactions. II. Systolic events. J Appl Physiol 1988; 64:1518–1526.
128. Pinsky MR, Matuschak GM, Klain M: Determinants of cardiac augmentation by increases in intrathoracic pressure. J Appl Physiol 1985; 58:1189–1198.
129. Rankin JS, Olsen CO, Arentzen CE, et al: The effects of airway pressure on cardiac function in intact dogs and man. Circulation 1982; 66:108–120.
130. Robotham JL, Rabson J, Permutt S, Bromberger-Barnea B: Left ventricular hemodynamics during respiration. J Appl Physiol 1979; 47:1295–1303.
131. Ruskin J, Bache RJ, Rembert JC, Greenfield JC Jr: Pressure-flow studies in man: Effect of respiration on left ventricular stroke volume. Circulation 1973; 48:79–85.
132. Olsen CO, Tyson GS, Maier GW, et al: Dynamic ventricular interaction in the conscious dog. Circ Res 1983; 52:85–104.
133. Bell RC, Robotham JL, Badke FR, Little WC, Kindred MK: Left ventricular geometry during intermittent positive pressure ventilation in dogs. J Crit Care 1987; 2:230–244.
134. Qvist J, Pontoppidan H, Wilson RS, Lowenstein E, Laver MB: Hemodynamic responses to mechanical ventilation with PEEP: The effects of hypovolemia. Anesthesiology 1975; 42:45–53.
135. Denault AY, Gorcsan J III, Deneault LG, Pinsky MR: Effect of positive pressure ventilation on left ventricular pressure-volume relationship. Anesthesiology 1993; 79:A315.
136. Janicki JS, Weber KT: The pericardium and ventricular interaction, distensibility and function. Am J Physiol 1980; 238:H494–H503.
137. Beyar R, Goldstein Y: Model studies of the effects of the thoracic pressure on the circulation. Ann Biomed Eng 1987; 15:373–383.
138. Pinsky MR, Summer WR, Wise RA, Permutt S, Bromberger-Barnea B: Augmentation of cardiac function by elevation of intrathoracic pressure. J Appl Physiol 1983; 54:950–955.
139. Cassidy SA, Wead WB, Seibert GB, Ramanathan M: Geometric left-ventricular responses to interactions between the lung and left ventricle: Positive pressure breathing. Ann Biomed Eng 1987; 15:285–295.
140. Scharf SM, Brown R, Warner KG, Khuri S: Intrathoracic pressure and left ventricular configuration with respiratory maneuvers. J Appl Physiol 1989; 66:481–491.
141. Grace MP, Greenbaum DM: Cardiac performance in response to PEEP in patients with cardiac dysfunction. Crit Care Med 1982; 20:358–360.
142. Pinsky MR, Summer WR: Cardiac augmentation by phasic high intrathoracic support (PHIPS) in man. Chest 1983; 84:370–375.
143. Pinsky MR, Matuschak GM, Itzkoff JM: Respiratory augmentation of left ventricular function during spontaneous ventilation in severe left ventricular failure by grunting: An auto-EPAP effect. Chest 1984; 86:267–269.
144. Blaustein AS, Risser TA, Weiss JW, Parker JA, Holman L, McFadden ER: Mechanisms of pulsus paradoxus during resistive respiratory loading and asthma. J Am Coll Cardiol 1986; 8:529–536.
145. Strohl KP, Scharf SM, Brown R, Ingram RH Jr: Cardiovascular performance during bronchospasm in dogs. Respiration 1987; 51:39–48.
146. Scharf SM, Graver LM, Balaban K: Cardiovascular effects of periodic occlusions of the upper airways in dogs. Am Rev Respir Dis 1992; 146:321–329.
147. Viola AR, Puy RJM, Goldman E: Mechanisms of pulsus paradoxus in airway obstruction. J Appl Physiol 1990; 68:1927–1931.
148. Scharf SM, Graver LM, Khilnani S, Balaban K: Respiratory phasic effects of inspiratory loading on left ventricular hemodynamics in vagotomized dogs. J Appl Physiol 1992; 73:995–1003.
149. Latham RD, Sipkema P, Westerhof N, Rubal BJ: Aortic input impedance during Mueller maneuver: An evaluation of "effective strength." J Appl Physiol 1988; 65:1604–1610.
150. Virolainen J, Ventila M, Turto H, Kupari M: Effect of negative intrathoracic pressure on left ventricular pressure dynamics and relaxation. J Appl Physiol 1995; 79:455–460.
151. Garpestad E, Parker JA, Katayama H, et al: Decrease in ventricular stroke volume at apnea termination is independent of oxygen desaturation. J Appl Physiol 1994; 77:1602–1608.
152. Gomez A, Mink S: Interaction between effects of hypoxia and hypercapnia on altering left ventricular relaxation and chamber stiffness in dogs. Am Rev Respir Dis 1992; 146:313–320.
153. Abel FL, Mihailescu LS, Lader AS, Starr RG: Effects of pericardial pressure on systemic and coronary hemodynamics in dogs. Am J Physiol 1995; 268:H1593–H1605.
154. Khilnani S, Graver LM, Balaban K, Scharf SM: Effects of inspiratory loading on left ventricular myocardial blood flow and metabolism. J Appl Physiol 1992; 72:1488–1492.
155. Satoh S, Watanabe J, Keitoku M, Itoh N, Maruyama Y, Takishima T: Influences of pressure surrounding the heart and intracardiac pressure on the diastolic coronary pressure-flow relation in excised canine heart. Circ Res 1988; 63:788–797.
156. Beach T, Millen E, Grenvik A: Hemodynamic response to discontinuance of mechanical ventilation. Crit Care Med 1973; 1:85–90.

157. Lemaire F, Teboul JL, Cinoti L, Giotto G, Abrouk F, Steg G, Macquin-Mavier I, Zapol WM: Acute left ventricular dysfunction during unsuccessful weaning from mechanical ventilation. Anesthesiology 1988; 69:171-179.
158. Rasanen J, Nikki P, Heikkila J: Acute myocardial infarction complicated by respiratory failure: The effects of mechanical ventilation. Chest 1984; 85:21-28.
159. Rasanen J, Vaisanen IT, Heikkila J, et al: Acute myocardial infarction complicated by left ventricular dysfunction and respiratory failure: The effects of continuous positive airway pressure. Chest 1985; 87:156-162.
160. Pinsky MR, Matuschak GM, Bernardi L, Klain M: Hemodynamic effects of cardiac cycle-specific increases in intrathoracic pressure. J Appl Physiol 1986; 60:604-612.
161. Dries DJ, Kumar P, Mathru M, Mayer R, Zecca A, Rao TL, Freeark RJ: Hemodynamic effects of pressure support ventilation in cardiac surgery patients. Am Surg 1991; 57:122-125.
162. Sternberg R, Sahebjami H: Hemodynamic and oxygen transport characteristics of common ventilatory modes. Chest 1994; 105:1798-1803.
163. Bayly R, Sladen A, Guntapalli K, Klain M: Synchronous versus nonsynchronous high-frequency jet ventilation: Effects on cardiorespiratory variables and airway pressures in postoperative patients. Crit Care Med 1987; 15:915-923.
164. Singer M, Vermaat J, Hall G, Latter G, Patel M: Hemodynamic effects of manual hyperinflation in critically ill mechanically ventilated patients. Chest 1994; 106:1182-1187.
165. Hartmann M, Rosberg B, Jonsson K: The influence of different levels of PEEP on peripheral tissue perfusion measured by subcutaneous and transcutaneous oxygen tension. Intensive Care Med 1992; 18:474-478.
166. Dhainaut JF, Devaux JY, Monsallier JF, Brunet F, Villemant D, Huyghebaert MF: Mechanisms of decreased left ventricular preload during continuous positive pressure ventilation in ARDS. Chest 1986; 90:74-80.
167. Huemer G, Kolev N, Kurz A, Zimpfer M: Influence of positive end-expiratory pressure on right and left ventricular performance assessed by Doppler two-dimensional echocardiography. Chest 1994; 106:67-73.
168. Jardin F: PEEP and ventricular function. Intensive Care Med 1994; 20:169-170.
169. Goertz A, Heinrich H, Winter H, Deller A: Hemodynamic effects of different ventilatory patterns: A prospective clinical trial. Chest 1991; 99:1166-1171.
170. Gunter JP, deBoisblanc BP, Rust BS, Johnson WD, Summer WR: Effect of synchronized, systolic, lower body, positive pressure on hemodynamics in human septic shock: A pilot study. Am J Respir Crit Care Med 1995; 151:719-723.
171. Schuster S, Erbel R, Weilemann LS, Lu WY, Henkel B, Wellek S, Schinzel H, Meyer J: Hemodynamics during PEEP ventilation in patients with severe left ventricular failure studied by transesophageal echocardiography. Chest 1990; 97:1181-1189.
172. Lessard MR, Guerot E, Lorini H, Lemaire F, Brochard L: Effects of pressure-controlled with different I:E ratios versus volume-controlled ventilation on respiratory mechanics, gas exchange and hemodynamics in patients with adult respiratory distress syndrome. Anesthesiology 1994; 80:983-991.
173. Chan K, Abraham E: Effects of inverse ratio ventilation on cardiorespiratory parameters in severe respiratory failure. Chest 1992; 102:1556-1561.
174. Abraham E, Yoshihara G: Cardiorespiratory effects of pressure controlled ventilation in severe respiratory failure. Chest 1990; 98:1445-1449.
175. Poelaert JI, Visser CA, Everaert JA, Koolen JJ, Colardyn FA: Acute hemodynamic changes of pressure-controlled inverse ration ventilation in the adult respiratory distress syndrome: A transesophageal echocardiographic and Doppler study. Chest 1993; 104:214-219.
176. Abel JG, Salerno TA, Panos A, et al: Cardiovascular effects of positive pressure ventilation in humans. Ann Thorac Surg 1987; 43:36-43.
177. Calvin JE, Driedger AA, Sibbald WJ: Positive end-expiratory pressure (PEEP) does not depress left ventricular function in patients with pulmonary edema. Am Rev Respir Dis 1981; 124:121-128.
178. Loick HM, Wendt M, Rotker J Theissen JL: Ventilation with positive end-expiratory airway pressure causes leukocyte retention in human lung. J Appl Physiol 1993; 75:301-306.
179. Rasanen J: Respiratory failure in acute myocardial infarction. Appl Cardiopulm Pathophysiol 1988; 2:271-279.
180. DeHoyos A, Liu PP, Benard DC, Bradley TD: Haemodynamic effects of continuous positive airway pressure in humans with normal and impaired left ventricular function. Clin Sci (Colch) 1995; 88:173-178.
181. Naughton MT, Rahman MA, Hara K, Flora JS, Bradley TD: Effect of continuous positive airway pressure on intrathoracic and left ventricular transmural pressures in patients with congestive heart failure. Circulation 1995; 91:1725-1731.
182. Lin M, Yang Y-F, Chiang H-T, Chang M-S, Chiang BN, Cheitlin MD: Reappraisal of continuous positive airway pressure therapy in acute cardiogenic pulmonary edema. Chest 1995; 107:1379-1386.
183. Buckle P, Millar T, Kryger M: The effect of short-term nasal CPAP on Cheyne-Stokes respiration in congestive heart failure. Chest 1992; 102:31-35.
184. Granton JT, Naughton MT, Benard DC, Liu PP, Goldstein RS, Bradley TD: CPAP improves inspiratory muscle strength in patients with heart failure and central sleep apnea. Am J Respir Crit Care Med 1996; 153:277-282.
185. Naughton MT, Benard DC, Liu PP, Rutherford R, Rankin F, Bradley TD: Effects of nasal CPAP on sympathetic activity in patients with heart failure and central sleep apnea. Am J Respir Crit Care Med 1995; 152:473-479.
186. Baeaussier M, Coriat P, Perel A, Lebret F, Kalfon P, Chemla D, Lienhart A, Viars P: Determinants of systolic pressure variation in patients ventilated after vascular surgery. J Cardiothorac Vasc Anesth 1995; 9:547-551.
187. Coriat P, Vrillon M, Perel A, Baron JF, LeBret F, Saada M, Viars P: A comparison of systolic blood pressure variations and echocardiographic estimates of end-diastolic left ventricular size in patients after aortic surgery. Anesth Analg 1994; 78:46-53.
188. Szold A, Pizov R, Segal E, Perel A: The effect of tidal volume and intravascular volume state on systolic pressure variation in ventilated dogs. Intensive Care Med 1989; 15:368-371.
189. Ranieri VM, Giuliani R, Cinnella G, et al: Physiologic effects of positive end-expiratory pressure in patients with chronic obstructive lung disease during acute ventilatory failure and controlled mechanical ventilation. Am Rev Respir Dis 1993; 147:5-13.
190. Baigorri F, De Monte A, Blanch L, et al: Hemodynamic response to external counterbalancing of auto-positive end-expiratory pressure in mechanically ventilated patients with chronic obstructive lung disease. Crit Care Med 1994; 22:1782-1791.
191. Pinsky MR: Through the past darkly: Ventilatory management of patients with chronic obstructive pulmonary disease. Crit Care Med 1994; 22:1714-1717.
192. Ambrosino N, Nava S, Torbicki A, Riccardi G, Fracchia C, Opasich C, Rampulla C: Hemodynamic effects of pressure support and PEEP ventilation by nasal route in patients with stable chronic obstructive pulmonary disease. Thorax 1993; 48:523-528.
193. Ambrosino N, Cobelli F, Torbicki A, Opasich C, Pozzoli M, Fracchia C, Rampulla C: Hemodynamic effects of negative-pressure ventilation in patients with COPD. Chest 1990; 97:850-856.
194. Richard C, Teboul J-L, Archambaud F, Hebert J-L, Michaut P, Auzepy P: Left ventricular function during weaning of patients with chronic obstructive pulmonary disease. Intensive Care Med 1994; 20:181-186.
195. Mohsenifar Z, Hay A, Hay J, Lewis MI, Koerner SK: Gastric intramural pH as a predictor of success or failure in weaning patients from mechanical ventilation. Ann Intern Med 1993; 119:794-798.
196. Brochard L, Isabey D, Piquet J, et al: Reversal of acute exacerbations of chronic obstructive lung disease by inspiratory assistance with a face mask. N Engl J Med 1990; 323:1523-1530.

112

Assessment of Pulmonary Function in Critically Ill Patients

Charles G. Alex, MD • Martin J. Tobin, MD

The detailed assessment of pulmonary function has become essential in the evaluation of ambulatory patients with respiratory disease.[1] However, the functional assessment of critically ill patients has remained relatively rudimentary and frequently is omitted or limited to measurement of arterial blood gases. It is becoming increasingly clear that lung mechanics and respiratory muscle function are important considerations in the optimal management of ventilators and play a major role in determining the ease with which a patient can resume spontaneous respiration after a period of mechanical ventilation.[2]

The assessment of pulmonary function in the critically ill patient is of particular importance in (1) deciding whether mechanical ventilation is indicated, (2) assessing response to therapy, (3) optimizing ventilator management, and (4) deciding whether a weaning trial is indicated. In addition, management of the surgical patient is frequently enhanced by a knowledge of a patient's preoperative pulmonary function.

CLINICAL ASSESSMENT

Helpful clues regarding pulmonary performance can be derived from a detailed history and physical examination. Orthopnea may be a symptom of paralysis or severe weakness of the diaphragm and usually develops immediately when the patient assumes the supine position. This contrasts with the more gradual onset of orthopnea in patients with congestive heart failure. An impaired cough due to respiratory muscle weakness and inability to inspire deeply increases the risk of aspiration and generally precludes safe extubation.

Examination of the respiratory system is often focused on auscultatory findings; however, considerable information can be obtained from careful inspection and examination of the pattern of breathing.

An elevated respiratory rate is a sensitive indicator of respiratory dysfunction and is important in the diagnosis of impending respiratory failure.[3] Some idea of the work of breathing in relation to the patient's arterial carbon dioxide tension (Pa_{CO_2}) is helpful in making decisions regarding the institution or discontinuation of mechanical ventilation. Work of breathing (see later) is calculated as the product of changes in lung volume and transpulmonary pressure (alveolar minus pleural pressure).

Clinical estimation of tidal volume is extremely inaccurate,[4] but fortunately the extent of suprasternal and intercostal space recession provides helpful indirect evidence of increased pleural pressure swings.[5] In addition, recruitment of the accessory muscles of respiration, especially the sternomastoid muscles, indicates the patient's increased effort.

Finally, observing the pattern of rib cage and abdominal motion provides helpful information.[6] Normally, both the rib cage and abdomen expand and deflate in phase with each other during inspiration and expiration, respectively. If one compartment moves in a direction opposite to the other, this is termed *paradoxical breathing*. The degree of rib cage–abdominal paradox is a direct reflection of the level of respiratory load against which a subject is breathing.[7] In addition, the induction of marked hyperinflation in a study of healthy volunteers did not result in clinically significant abnormal rib cage–abdominal motion.[8]

Thus, noting the respiratory rate, the extent of suprasternal and intercostal recession, the presence of accessory muscle recruitment, and the degree of rib cage–abdominal paradox provides a good insight into the work of breathing being performed by the patient. More direct measurements of the work of breathing are discussed later.

RESPIRATORY NEUROMUSCULAR FUNCTION

Carbon dioxide elimination depends on adequate respiratory drive, respiratory muscle function, and coordinated chest wall movement. An abnormality of the respiratory control system should be suspected when hypercapnia exists in the following settings[9]:

1. Persistent forced expiratory volume in 1 second (FEV_1) greater than 1.3 L.
2. Normal alveolar-arterial oxygen gradient.
3. Ability to correct to normocapnia after voluntary hyperventilation.
4. Absence of respiratory muscle weakness, as indicated by the ability to generate a sufficient negative inspiratory pressure.

Respiratory Center Function

Respiratory center function is rarely measured at the bedside, although recent technologic developments have made this more feasible. One function that can be measured at the bedside is airway occlusion pressure, which is the negative pressure generated by an isometric contraction of the inspiratory muscles against an occluded airway. It bears a close relationship to the intensity of respiratory neural drive.[10, 11] The occlusion pressure is performed by transiently and surreptitiously occluding the airway during early inspiration and measuring the change in airway pressure after 0.1 second ($P_{0.1}$) before the patient reacts to the occlusion.[11] In intubated patients, this occlusion maneuver can be done at the bedside with an airway pressure transducer, a device to measure flow, and a recorder (Fig. 112–1).

Although $P_{0.1}$ values represent negative pressures, it is customary to report them in positive units, which in the normal resting subject during relaxed breathing is 0.93 ± 0.48 (SD) cm H_2O.[12] Most recently, $P_{0.1}$ has been used as a predictor of weaning outcome from mechanical ventilation. A high $P_{0.1}$ value during acute respiratory failure indicates increased respiratory drive and neuromuscular activity and, if sustained, may result in inspiratory muscle fatigue. Various investigators have demonstrated that an elevated $P_{0.1}$ value is predictive of weaning failure,[13, 14] although the threshold separating success from failure differed among the studies. Most studies found higher $P_{0.1}$ values in patients whose weaning trial failed than in patients who were successfully weaned.

Although it may appear counterintuitive that an elevated respiratory drive predisposes to ventilatory failure, in reality the high $P_{0.1}$ values reflect respiratory distress and signify the response of the respiratory center to respiratory compromise. Montgomery and coworkers[15] found that $P_{0.1}$ values were similar in patients who were successfully weaned and those whose weaning trial failed. In addition, they found that $P_{0.1}$ measurements during a hypercapnic challenge were similar in the weaning success and weaning failure groups; but hypercapnic

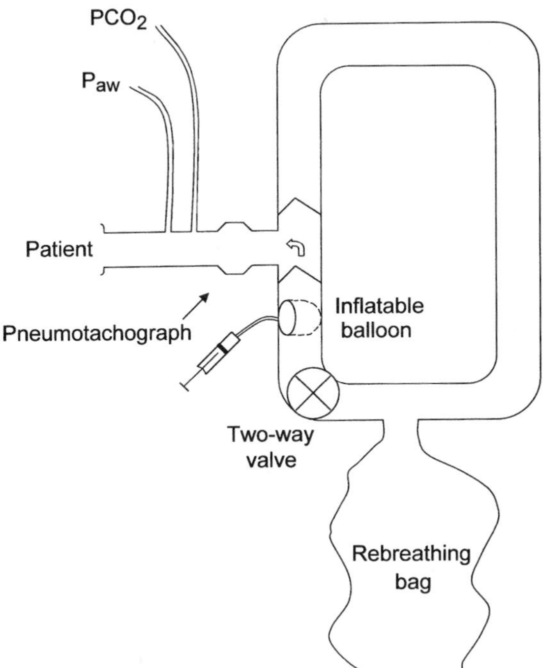

Figure 112–1. Apparatus used for measurement of airway occlusion pressure. The patient breathes through a mouthpiece attached to a one-way valve. During expiration, inflation of a balloon situated in the inspiratory circuit limb occludes this part of the circuit. Airway pressure (Paw) and end-tidal carbon dioxide P_{CO_2} are continuously recorded from ports in the airway while a pneumotachograph records airflow. A two-way valve in the circuit allows airway occlusion pressure to be measured while the patient is breathing room air or while rebreathing 7% CO_2 in O_2 from a 6- to 10-liter bag. (From Tobin MJ, Gardner WN: Monitoring of the control of breathing. *In*: Principles and Practice of Intensive Care Monitoring. Tobin MJ [Ed]. New York, McGraw-Hill, 1998, p 432.)

augmentation of $P_{0.1}$, expressed as the ratio of the carbon dioxide-stimulated $P_{0.1}$ to the baseline $P_{0.1}$, was greater in the patients who were successfully weaned. Although $P_{0.1}$ can be reliably estimated from an airway pressure tracing in mechanically ventilated patients,[16] its precise usefulness in clinical decision making in critically ill patients remains unclear.

Respiratory Muscle Function

Respiratory muscle strength is estimated by measuring respiratory pressures and is related to the number of myofibrils. Endurance is the capacity of a muscle to sustain a contractile force and is affected by muscle fiber types and blood supply. Muscle fatigue is the converse of muscle endurance and can be defined as a condition in which there is a loss in the capacity of a muscle to develop force or velocity. This results from muscle activity under load and is reversible by rest.[17]

More detailed evaluation includes measurement of maximum respiratory pressures and research techniques, such as measurements of transdiaphragmatic pressure, phrenic nerve stimulation, and tension-time index. Other simple and clinically useful methods to assess muscle performance include diaphragmatic ultrasonography and breathing pattern analysis.

Maximal Respiratory Pressures

An increased awareness of the importance of respiratory muscle function has developed during the 1990s. Respiratory muscle fatigue is now thought to be an important contributor to ventilatory failure, particularly in critically ill patients. Unfortunately, none of the laboratory techniques used to detect respiratory muscle fatigue has gained acceptance in the intensive care unit (ICU) setting; consequently, assessment of respiratory muscle function is limited to measurement of maximum respiratory pressures.[18, 19] These pressures provide a global assessment of strength of all the respiratory musculature, and the values can be subnormal in patients with neuromuscular disease at a time when spirometry remains normal.[19, 20]

Measurement

Respiratory muscle strength is assessed by measuring the maximum inspiratory and maximum expiratory pressure (PImax and PEmax, respectively) generated against an occluded airway. In the ICU setting, these measurements can be obtained readily with an inexpensive aneroid manometer.[6] The best of three efforts is commonly selected. As with other skeletal muscles, the maximum force that can be generated by the respiratory muscles is related to their degree of stretching. Inspiratory muscles generate less force as their length is decreased, such as occurs at high lung volumes in obstructive lung disease.[21] Therefore, it is important to control the lung volume at which the measurements are made. PImax is usually measured after expiration to residual volume.[22] Because of the absence of respiratory system recoil at functional residual capacity (FRC), measurements at this volume may be preferable.[21] PEmax should be measured after inspiration to total lung capacity (TLC), when the expiratory muscles are maximally stretched. In the ICU, however, the PEmax is usually not measured because it is difficult for a patient to inhale to TLC.

Published normal values of PImax and PEmax show considerable variation among reports. This variation may depend on the cohorts employed to establish the normal range and on the method used to make the measurement. Black and Hyatt[18] describe a technique using a tube connected to pressure gauges allowing a small air leak to minimize the contribution of the facial muscles to expiratory pressure. Lower values for PImax and PEmax have been found with a flanged mouthpiece versus a simple rubber tube mouthpiece.[23] With use of a flanged mouthpiece, PImax and PEmax in healthy adult men are approximately 111 ± 34 (SD) and 151 ± 68 cm H_2O, respectively.[23-25] Values are lower in women: PImax 72 ± 26 and PEmax 93 ± 30 cm H_2O. In addition, strength tends to decrease with age: PImax values are 6%, 25%, and 32% lower in men who are 31 to 35, 40 to 60, and 61 to 75 years old, respectively, compared with healthy subjects 16 to 30 years old.[26]

In ambulatory patients with neuromuscular disease but who are free of lung disease, hypercapnia is likely to develop when PImax is reduced to one third of the normal predicted value.[27] In patients with chronic obstructive pulmonary disease (COPD), hypercapnia is observed with less severe reductions in PImax (less than half normal) because of the additional problems of abnormal gas exchange and increased work of breathing.[21]

Clinical Application

PImax has been a standard measurement to predict weaning outcome in mechanically ventilated patients. Traditionally, PImax values more negative than −30 cm H_2O predicted weaning success, whereas values no lower than −20 cm H_2O predicted weaning failure.[28] However, more recent work has undermined the reliability of this measurement in ventilated patients by showing that true muscle strength is grossly underestimated.[29, 30] Moreover, most investigators have found that PImax is not reliable in discriminating between patients whose trial of weaning from mechanical ventilation fails or succeeds.[13, 31, 32]

Attention has been redirected to standardizing the method

of measuring PImax in critically ill patients. Using a valve attached to the airway to ensure that inspiration begins at a low volume and standardizing the period of occlusion to 20 seconds, Marini and colleagues[33] obtained PImax values that were approximately one third more negative than nonstandardized measurements.

Multz and coworkers[30] examined the reproducibility of this method of measuring PImax. Triplicate measurements were obtained by five experienced investigators in 14 ventilator-dependent patients. Measurements of PImax obtained at a single sitting by a single investigator showed good reproducibility: coefficient of variation, 12% ± 1%. However, there was significant variation among PImax measurements obtained by different investigators studying the same patient on the same day: coefficient of variation, 32% ± 4%. Because true inspiratory muscle strength must be equal to or greater than the highest recorded PImax, the variation in values by different investigators indicates that PImax values, even when they are obtained in a standardized manner, commonly underestimate true strength.

Respiratory Muscle Fatigue

PImax is an indicator of muscle strength rather than endurance and thus gives limited information on fatigue, which is related more to endurance. Endurance is the capacity of a muscle to sustain a contractile force and depends on muscle capillary and mitochondrial density and overall oxidative enzyme capacity.[34] The converse of endurance is fatigue, which in operational terms is the inability of a muscle to generate and sustain a required contractile force.[35]

Respiratory muscle fatigue can be central, transmission, or contractile.[35, 36] (Table 112–1). *Central fatigue* is considered present when a voluntary contraction generates less force than does electrical stimulation. In a cooperative subject, the force generated by voluntary contraction should be the same as that resulting from electrical stimulation.[35, 36] Although central fatigue has been demonstrated in some healthy subjects breathing against high respiratory loads,[37] it remains unclear whether central fatigue actually occurs in clinical situations.[36]

Transmission fatigue is thought to be due to impaired neuromuscular transmission, which is represented by a decrease in the electromyographic response to phrenic nerve stimulation. The clinical significance of transmission fatigue has yet to be resolved.

Contractile fatigue is characterized by a decrease in the contractile response to neural stimulation. This decrease in contractile response or force can occur over different frequencies of neural stimulation. Contractile fatigue is usually high-frequency or low-frequency.[36] It is likely that low-frequency fatigue is the form with greatest clinical significance because it occurs at the nerve firing frequency of normal daily activities (10 to 20 Hz). In addition, low-frequency fatigue probably results from structural damage to the respiratory muscles, and the considerable time needed for its resolution could have a negative impact on critically ill patients.[38] During brief voluntary efforts (2 to 3 seconds), nerve firing frequencies are high, with the result that force-generating ability is little affected by low-frequency fatigue.[39] Consequently, response to tests of maximum effort, such as PImax or vital capacity (VC) measurement, may not be decreased despite the presence of low-frequency fatigue.

A number of techniques, such as transdiaphragmatic pressure measurement, phrenic nerve stimulation, and determination of the tension-time index, have been used to detect the presence or development of muscle fatigue.[40]

Transdiaphragmatic Pressure

Maximum respiratory pressures do not accurately reflect performance of the diaphragm, which is the most important respiratory muscle during quiet breathing. Transdiaphragmatic pressure (Pdi), a measure of diaphragm strength, is determined from simultaneous measurements of esophageal pressure (Pes) and gastric pressure (Pga) from balloon catheters. Transdiaphragmatic pressure is calculated from the difference of Pga and Pes.

Measuring Pdi during a maximum static inspiratory effort against an occluded airway is the usual method of measuring maximum Pdi. However, many patients find it difficult to perform this maneuver, whereas most can perform a sniff. The sniff Pdi may be as effective as the maximum Pdi measurement.[41] The measurement of Pdi is especially helpful in the diagnosis of severe weakness or paralysis of the diaphragm (Fig. 112–2). In a study of eight patients with clinical features suggestive of diaphragmatic weakness, the change in Pdi during a maximum inspiration was zero in five patients and 2 to 6 cm H_2O in the remaining three patients, compared with greater than 25 cm H_2O in healthy subjects.[42]

To exclude respiratory muscle weakness as a cause of unexplained breathlessness, one should first perform other simpler tests. A decrease in VC on moving from the upright to horizontal position should suggest inspiratory muscle weakness, and PImax should be tested. A PImax greater than 80 cm H_2O in men and greater than 70 cm H_2O in women excludes clinically important muscle weakness.[43] A low PImax value could result from poor technique, and if low pressures are recorded, Pdi should then be measured with use of voluntary maneuvers or stimulation of the phrenic nerves (see following).

Phrenic Nerve Stimulation

The maximum airway pressure during voluntary maneuvers reflects the combined action of several respiratory muscle groups. The Pdi response to phrenic nerve stimulation provides the most specific assessment of diaphragmatic properties. Phrenic nerve stimulation is independent of the patient's motivation and central nervous system input and provides information on the functional integrity of the phrenic nerve *(conduction time)* and fatigue of the diaphragm. Activation is

TABLE 112–1. Diagnostic Features of Diaphragmatic Fatigue

	Voluntary Effort		Phrenic Nerve Stimulation		
Fatigue Type	***EMG Response***	***Pdi Response***	***EMG Response***	***Pdi Response***	**Direct Muscle Stimulation (Animal)**
Central	↓	↓	Normal	Normal	Normal
Transmission	↓	↓	↓	↓	Normal
Contractile	Normal	↓	Normal	↓	↓

From Tobin MJ: Respiratory monitoring during mechanical ventilation. *In*: Mechanical Ventilation. Tobin MJ (Ed). Philadelphia, WB Saunders, 1990, p 691.
EMG = electromyogram; Pdi = transdiaphragmatic pressure.

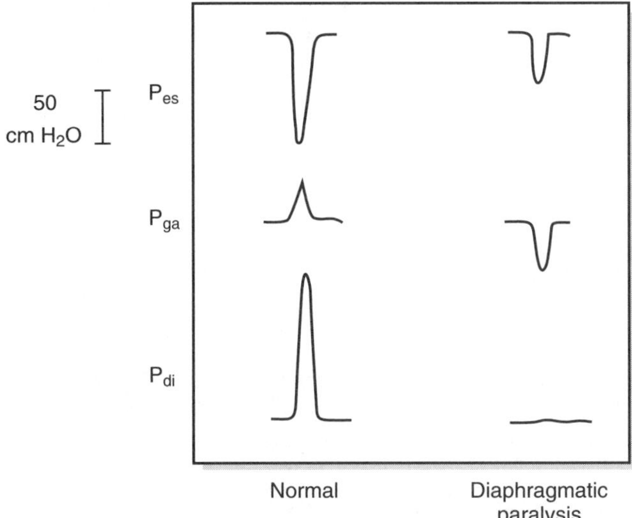

Figure 112–2. Esophageal (Pes), gastric (Pga), and transdiaphragmatic pressure (Pdi) in a normal subject and in a patient with bilateral diaphragmatic paralysis. During a maximum inspiratory effort in a patient with diaphragmatic paralysis, the loss of diaphragm function results in a lower Pes. The negative pressure generated by the other inspiratory muscles draws the flaccid diaphragm cephalad, causing a fall in Pga. (From Tobin MJ: Essentials of Critical Care Medicine. New York, Churchill Livingstone, 1989.)

more commonly achieved with an electrical stimulator, although magnetic stimulation can also be used.

Phrenic nerve conduction time is measured as the time from stimulus artifact to the onset of the diaphragmatic action potential. In healthy subjects, the mean conduction time is approximately 7 msec.[44] Prolonged or absent phrenic nerve conduction time may be observed with a mediastinal tumor, Guillain-Barré syndrome, or demyelinating diseases and after cardiac surgery and lung transplantation.

Diaphragmatic contractility can be measured by stimulation of the phrenic nerve at various frequencies. A force-frequency curve is generated by recording the Pdi at frequencies ranging from 1 to 100 Hz. A decrease in the Pdi for a given level of stimulation denotes contractile fatigue and is marked by a rightward shift of the force-frequency curve (Fig. 112–3). High-frequency fatigue is manifested by a decrease in the contractile response at high-stimulation frequencies (50 to 100 Hz), and recovery from fatigue occurs within minutes. Low-frequency fatigue occurs at low-stimulation frequencies (1 to 20 Hz), which is the operational frequency of the diaphragm. This type of fatigue is due to structural abnormalities of the muscle, and recovery may take longer than 24 hours.[38]

A less painful method of assessment of diaphragmatic fatigue is measuring the response to single supramaximal nerve stimulations at 1 Hz. The resulting pressure response of the diaphragm is commonly termed *twitch pressure*. In healthy subjects relaxing at FRC, the amplitude of twitch Pdi is about 20% to 25% of maximum tetanic stimulation.[45] In accounting for lung volume, twitch pressure responses provide a reliable means of detecting and monitoring low-frequency fatigue.[46] In a study of nine healthy subjects who had low-frequency fatigue as a result of whole-body endurance exercise, the decrease in Pdi after fatigue was similar (27% change) at stimulation frequencies of 1 and 10 Hz.[47]

Tension-Time Index

Determinants of oxygen cost of breathing and muscle fatigue are the tension developed by the respiratory muscles and the duration of respiratory muscle contraction. Bellemare and Grassino[48] have described a tension-time index (TTdi) that accounts for the contraction of the diaphragm during inspiration:

$$\text{TTdi} = \text{mean Pdi/Pdi (max)} \cdot T_I/T_{TOT}$$

where T_I/T_{TOT} is the ratio of inspiratory time to total respiratory time (duty cycle).

Normal subjects with sufficient reserve have a TTdi of 0.02 while breathing at rest. However, subjects during inspiratory resistive loading had diaphragmatic fatigue when TTdi exceeded 0.15. Similar findings were observed in a study of 31 ventilator-supported patients with COPD who underwent trials of spontaneous breathing.[49] In 17 patients who did not respond to the spontaneous breathing trial, the TTdi increased from 0.06 ± 0.01 at onset to 0.10 ± 0.01 at the end of the trial; five patients had a TTdi greater than 0.15 by the end of

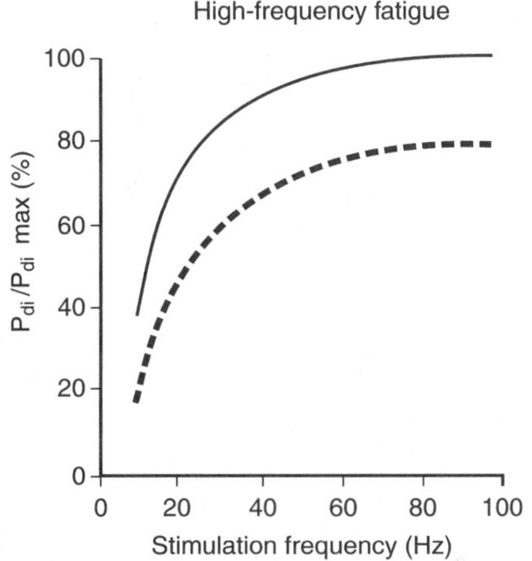

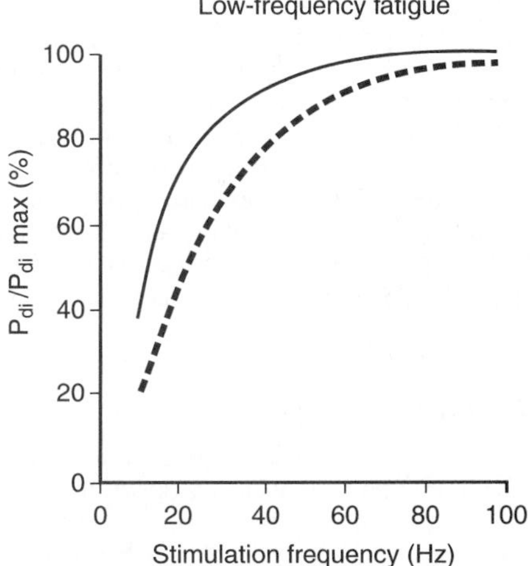

Figure 112–3. Force-frequency curves of the diaphragm. The curves are generated by stimulating the phrenic nerve at various frequencies (*x*-axis) and plotting the force output (*y*-axis) of the diaphragm measured by transdiaphragmatic pressure (Pdi). The *solid line* in both panels represents a normal force-frequency curve. *Left*, Predominantly high-frequency fatigue *(dashed line)* with a drop in force output at high frequencies. *Right*, Predominantly low-frequency fatigue *(dashed line)* with a drop in force output at low frequencies of stimulation. (From Tobin MJ [Ed]: Respiratory Monitoring. New York, Churchill Livingstone, 1991, p 145.)

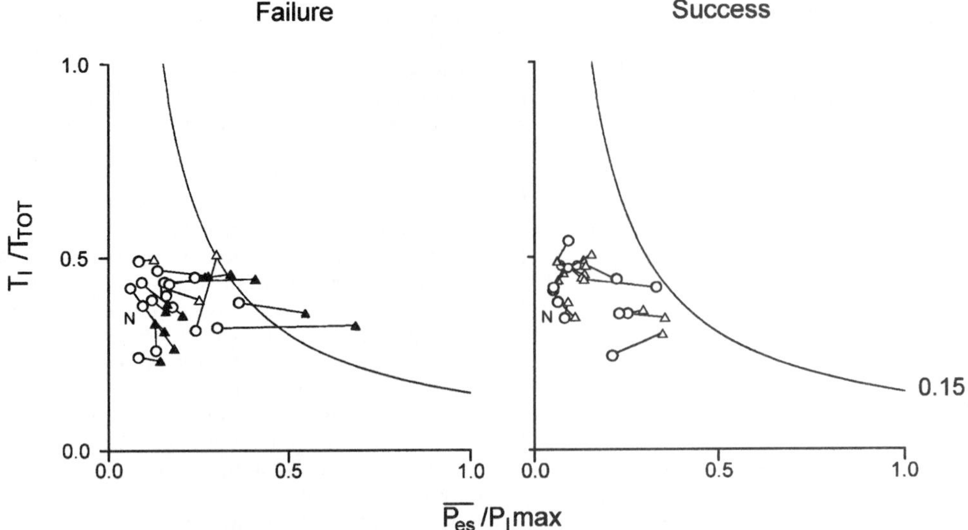

Figure 112–4. Mean esophageal pressure to maximum inspiratory pressure ratio (Pes/PImax) versus duty cycle (TI/TTOT) in 17 ventilator-supported patients with chronic obstructive pulmonary disease who did not respond to a trial of spontaneous breathing and 14 patients who tolerated the trial. The *circles* and *triangles* represent values at the start and end of the trial, respectively; *closed triangles* represent patients who showed an increase in Pa_{CO_2} during the trial. Five of the 17 patients in the treatment failure group had a tension-time index greater than 0.15 (indicated by the isopleth), suggesting respiratory muscle fatigue. N represents the value in a normal subject. (From Jubran A, Tobin MJ: Pathophysiological basis of acute respiratory distress in patients who fail a trial of weaning from mechanical ventilation. Am J Respir Crit Care Med 1997; 155:906.)

the trial. In those 14 patients who successfully tolerated the trial, there was no significant change in the TTdi (Fig. 112-4).

Diaphragmatic Ultrasonography

A relatively new and easy method to assess diaphragmatic function is diaphragmatic ultrasonography. More specifically, this technique uses ultrasonography to measure the change of diaphragm thickness during inspiration from residual volume. A close correlation between maximum Pdi and diaphragmatic thickness was observed in healthy subjects with a range of maximum Pdi from 146 to 410 cm H_2O.[50] In the ICU, the best application of diaphragmatic ultrasonography is in detecting a paralyzed diaphragm. This method has several attractive features when it is used in the ICU setting. It is portable, is noninvasive, and avoids ionizing radiation. It can be performed rapidly and provides considerable information without requiring special voluntary maneuvers.

In a study of seven patients with unilateral diaphragmatic paralysis, the paralyzed hemidiaphragm was found to be thinner than the normal hemidiaphragm (1.7 ± 0.2 and 2.7 ± 0.5 (SD) mm, respectively).[51] Likewise, five patients with bilateral diaphragmatic paralysis had thinner diaphragms than did healthy control subjects. Combining criteria of diaphragm thickness at FRC of less than 2 mm with a change in thickness during inspiration of less than 20% can be used to distinguish between a paralyzed and a functioning diaphragm[51] (Fig. 112-5).

Pattern of Breathing

Respiratory inductive plethysmography uses transducers to measure changes in inductance that are proportional to volume changes of the space over which the transducers are placed.[52] In this way, a simple analysis of respiratory timing, rib cage and abdominal motion, and changes in lung volume can be obtained.

The relationship between minute ventilation ($\dot{V}_E$) and Pa_{CO_2} provides a good indication of the demands being placed on the respiratory system. In the resting healthy adult subject, $\dot{V}_E$ is usually about 6 L/min,[53] and a value of less than 10 L/min (in the presence of normocapnia) is desirable in patients being considered for a weaning trial.[54] Because Pa_{CO_2} is determined by the relationship between alveolar ventilation and carbon dioxide production, a high $\dot{V}_E$ in the presence of hypercapnia indicates the presence of either increased carbon dioxide production or increased dead space ventilation. Conversely, hypercapnia associated with a low $\dot{V}_E$ (a less common occur-

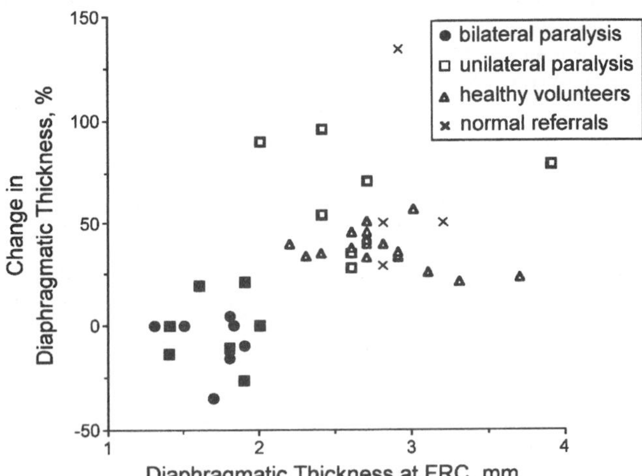

Figure 112–5. Diaphragmatic thickness (Tdi) measured at functional residual capacity (FRC) plotted against a change in Tdi during inspiration for patients with unilateral diaphragm paralysis *(open squares)*, bilateral diaphragm paralysis *(closed circles)*, functioning diaphragms in normal referrals *(crosses)*, and healthy volunteers *(open triangles)*. A paralyzed diaphragm *(solid symbols)* could be distinguished from a functioning diaphragm *(open symbols)* when the Tdi was less than 2 mm and the change in Tdi was less than 20%. (From Gottesman E, McCool FD: Ultrasound evaluation of the paralyzed diaphragm. Am J Respir Crit Care Med 1997; 155:1570.)

rence) should suggest decreased respiratory center drive, structural abnormality of the thoracic cage, or respiratory muscle dysfunction.

The measurement of $\dot{V}_E$ should be partitioned into its tidal volume (V_T) and respiratory frequency (f) components. In healthy subjects, V_T is approximately 400 mL, and higher values are observed usually under conditions of physiologic stress. The presence of a V_T that is less than 200 to 300 mL suggests that a weaning trial undertaken at that time is unlikely to have a successful outcome.[55] A low V_T is commonly combined with a high f (i.e., rapid, shallow breathing) and usually associated with hypercapnia because of increased dead space ventilation. As a way to quantify rapid, shallow breathing, an index has been devised by taking the ratio of f to V_T. In a prospective study of 100 patients,[31] it was found that a ratio lower than 100 breaths/min/L was the best predictor of successful weaning.

Accurate ventilatory measurements can be obtained with inductive plethysmography in patients requiring mechanical ventilation.[56] By recording ventilation on a breath-by-breath basis in this manner, additional information on respiratory drive and timing can be derived. Mean inspiratory flow is a measure of respiratory drive[57] and is the ratio of V_T to inspiratory time (T_I). A crude measure of airway obstruction can be obtained by calculating the ratio of T_I to the time of a single or total respiratory cycle (T_{TOT}), termed fractional inspiratory time (T_I/T_{TOT}).[58] Because the respiratory muscles are usually active only during inspiration, T_I/T_{TOT} has also been termed the duty cycle of the respiratory system, and it is an important determinant of the amount of stress being placed on the respiratory muscles.

Inductive plethysmography records the motion of the rib cage and abdomen, making it possible to detect asynchronous motion (time lag between the two compartments) and paradoxical motion (compartments moving in opposite directions).[59] Abdominal paradox, often regarded as a specific indicator of respiratory muscle fatigue, is not always associated with fatigue and is actually a better sign of increased respiratory system load.[7]

In a study of 17 ventilated patients undergoing weaning trials,[59] abdominal paradox was found to be a poor predictor of weaning outcome. Abnormal motion of the rib cage and abdomen was observed in these patients being weaned from mechanical ventilation regardless of their outcome. Patients whose weaning trials failed, however, displayed more severe asynchrony and paradox than did those who underwent successful weaning.

Finally, alterations in the end-expiratory level of an inductive plethysmography signal provide a measure of the change in FRC,[60] enabling the detection of dynamic hyperinflation or intrinsic end-expiratory pressure.[61]

RESPIRATORY MECHANICS

Vital Capacity

In the ICU, VC is the only lung volume commonly measured. VC is an effort-dependent measurement of the greatest volume of gas that a subject can exhale after maximum inspiration. The size of VC reflects the ability to inspire deeply and to cough. When performed as a forced maneuver, it is termed forced vital capacity (FVC) and is the difference between TLC (the point of maximum inspiration) and residual volume (the point of maximum expiration). Reduction in VC is observed in obstructive lung disease owing to an increase in residual volume. In patients with intrapulmonary restrictive disease, the VC is also reduced but with a decrease in TLC.

A decrease in VC is also observed with poor effort by the patient or with neuromuscular disease involving the respiratory muscles. In a study of patients with Guillain-Barré syndrome, the VC measurement was found to be a reliable predictor of respiratory failure hours before actual intubation.[62] Repeated measurements of VC did not help in predicting the need for intubation and mechanical ventilation in patients with myasthenia gravis.[63]

Timed measurements of VC, such as the FEV_1, are helpful in the diagnosis of obstructive airway disease, in which the FEV_1/FVC ratio is less than 75%. However, the FEV_1/FVC ratio is rarely measured in critically ill patients because of the patient's suboptimal effort, and the frequent presence of an endotracheal tube may contribute to erroneous results.

The normal VC is usually between 65 and 75 mL/kg, and a VC of 10 mL/kg or more has been thought to be essential for sustaining spontaneous ventilation. These values are commonly employed as outcome predictors when patients receiving mechanical ventilation are being considered for a weaning trial.[28] However, in a prospective study of 47 patients who were weaned and extubated, Tahvanainen and colleagues[29] found that a VC of 10 mL/kg was falsely positive in 18% (predicted success but actual failure) and falsely negative in 50% of the patients (predicted failure but actual success). In addition, a subsequent study has not demonstrated VC to be a useful predictor of successful weaning outcome.[64]

Compliance

For adequate ventilation to be achieved, it is necessary to overcome the elasticity of both the lungs and the chest wall. This elasticity is defined physiologically in terms of *compliance*, which is calculated as the change in volume for a given change in distending transthoracic pressure. Because this is measured at a time of zero gas flow, it is termed the *effective static compliance*. During normal spontaneous breathing, the change in thoracic volume is caused by the decrease in intrathoracic pressure consequent to respiratory muscle contraction; whereas in patients receiving mechanical ventilation, an increase in intrathoracic pressure is responsible for the volume change. In nonintubated patients, compliance is best measured with use of an esophageal balloon catheter; however, in mechanically ventilated patients, it is easily measured by ventilator transducers under passive conditions with zero gas flow.

In patients receiving mechanical ventilation and making no respiratory effort, total thoracic compliance can be estimated by dividing the volume delivered (V_T) by the distending thoracic pressure, measured as the difference between the airway opening pressure and atmospheric pressure. Measurements are performed under conditions of zero gas flow by employing an "inspiratory hold" or by occluding the expiratory port long enough to allow airway pressure to reach a constant value after 1 or 2 seconds (Fig. 112-6). This pressure, commonly termed *plateau pressure*, represents the static elastic recoil pressure of the total respiratory system at end-inflation volume. The total positive end-expiratory pressure (PEEP), the sum of applied PEEP and auto-PEEP, must be subtracted from the plateau pressure to yield the correct distending pressure.

If volume measurements are not made at the connection port of the endotracheal tube, a correction for compression volume must be made. The compression volume is a function of the internal volume of the ventilator, the in-line humidifier volume, and the volume and compliance of the circuit tubing.[65] The compression volume of commercially available circuit tubing ranges from 0.3 mL/cm H_2O (in the presence of high compliance) to 4.5 mL/cm H_2O (in the presence of low compliance) at peak airway pressure. Thus, the effective static

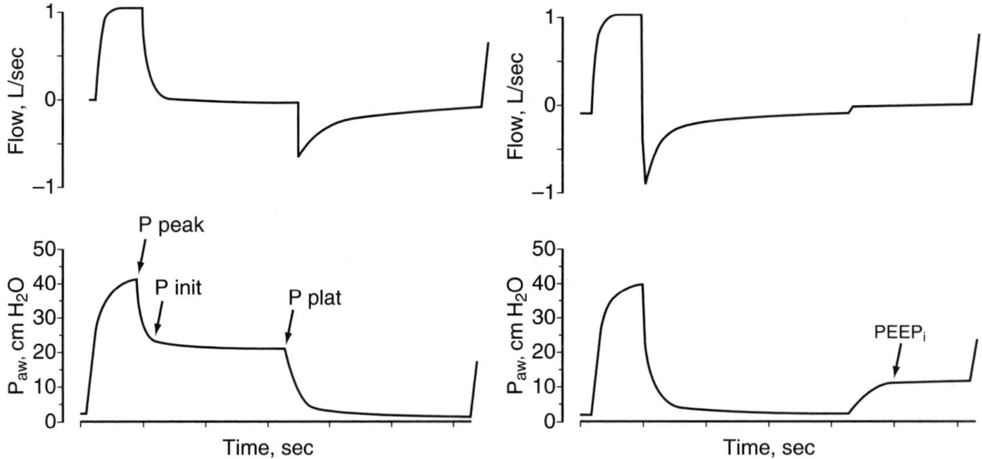

Figure 112–6. Recordings of airflow and airway pressure (Paw) showing occlusion of airway at end-inspiration *(left panel)* and end-expiration *(right panel)*. An end-inspiratory occlusion produces a rapid decline from peak pressure (P_{peak}) to a lower initial pressure (P_{init}) followed by a gradual decrease to a plateau pressure (P_{plat}). Occlusion of the airway at end-expiration produces an increase in Paw where its plateau value signifies the level of intrinsic PEEP (PEEPi). (From Dhand R, Jubran A, Tobin MJ: Efficacy of bronchodilator delivered by metered-dose inhaler in ventilator-supported patients with COPD. Am J Respir Crit Care Med 1995; 151:1827.)

compliance of the total respiratory system (CRS) is calculated as

$$\text{CRS} = \text{VT} - [(P_{plateau} - \text{PEEP}) \cdot \text{CV}]/P_{plateau} - (\text{total PEEP})$$

where $P_{plateau}$ is plateau pressure and CV is the correction factor for volume compressed in the circuit tubing. Calculations of compliance should be based on at least three breaths. The normal range of CRS in adult patients receiving mechanical ventilation is 60 to 100 mL/cm H_2O.

A decreased CRS is observed in patients having one or more of the following:

1. A reduction in the number of functioning lung units (e.g., resection, bronchial intubation, pneumothorax, pneumonia, atelectasis, or pulmonary edema).
2. Disorders of the thoracic cage (e.g., kyphoscoliosis, ankylosing spondylitis).
3. Massive pleural effusions.
4. Ascites.
5. Peritoneal dialysis.
6. Abdominal binding.

As with any measurement, care is required to avoid errors:

1. The volume-measuring device of the ventilator may be inaccurate at extremes of flow, underestimating volume at low flow rates while overestimating it at high flows.
2. Adequate tracheal cuff pressure should be ensured to avoid gas leaks.
3. Part of the volume generated by the ventilator expands the connecting tubing and is not delivered to the patient. The compliance of this tubing varies with its structure, diameter, length, and brand.[65] This factor may result in significant measurement errors in patients with stiff lungs, who typically have high airway pressures and low VT.
4. The respiratory muscles should be relaxed at the time that measurements are being made. If the patient is actively inspiring, the pressure developed by the ventilator is less than the total pressure required for thoracic inflation, and a falsely high compliance is obtained. Conversely, if the patient is "fighting" the ventilator, the total pressure developed by the ventilator is greater than that necessary to inflate the relaxed respiratory system, and a falsely low compliance is measured.
5. It is important to check for auto-PEEP (see later). Use of the plateau pressure in calculating effective static compliance is valid only if the elastic recoil pressure reaches zero at end-expiration, indicating that the elastic equilibrium point of the respiratory system has been reached. Failure to account for the level of auto-PEEP may lead to an underestimation of thoracic compliance by up to 48%.[66]

Effective dynamic compliance (Cdyn) is calculated by dividing the ventilator-delivered volume by the peak airway pressure (minus total PEEP). This index is not a measure of true thoracic compliance because the peak airway pressure also includes a resistive component, so that disorders of either the airways or the lung parenchyma (or chest wall) may cause a reduction in Cdyn. If Cdyn falls to a greater extent than CRS, an increase in airway resistance has occurred (e.g., bronchospasm, mucous plugging, saturated in-line filter, kinking of the endotracheal tube). In general, Cdyn is 50 to 80 mL/cm H_2O. In practice, alterations in the difference between peak and plateau airway pressures probably provide the best indication of change in airway resistance.

The manual measurement of thoracic compliance depends on the visualization of a single point on the ventilator pressure gauge with a considerable chance of error. Furthermore, sudden changes in the respiratory status of severely ill patients may be missed by intermittent manual measurements. Accordingly, on-line continuous monitoring of pulmonary mechanics has been advocated in the hope that such measurements might provide clues of impending respiratory failure, improve the management of ventilator performance, and aid in the critical transition between the discontinuation of ventilator support and the resumption of spontaneous breathing.

Continuous monitoring of pulmonary compliance (or resistance) requires continuous measurements of pressure and volume. Airway pressure recordings are sufficient to calculate total thoracic compliance, but calculations of pure lung compliance or resistance require a measure of pleural pressure. Esophageal pressure is usually employed as a measure of pleural pressure, and nasogastric tubes containing an attached balloon to facilitate such measurements are available.[67]

Auto–Positive End-Expiratory Pressure (Auto-PEEP)

In certain patients, the end-expiratory lung volume may exceed the predicted FRC, increasing the static recoil pressure of the respiratory system, thereby increasing alveolar pressure. This elevated alveolar pressure is termed auto-PEEP or intrinsic PEEP. Dynamic hyperinflation usually occurs in patients with airway obstruction as a result of dynamic airway collapse ("air trapping"). It also occurs in patients without dynamic airway collapse when there is insufficient time during expiration to equilibrate alveolar pressure with atmospheric pressure. This most commonly arises when minute ventilation is high with a shortened expiratory time that does not allow complete alveolar emptying. Dynamic hyperinflation may be exacerbated further by persistent inspiratory muscle activity during expiration.[68] In the absence of dynamic hyperinflation, auto-PEEP may develop solely from contraction of the expiratory muscles.[69]

In patients receiving mechanical ventilation, the presence of auto-PEEP is often referred to as "occult" PEEP because the increased alveolar pressure is not detected by the ventilator manometer since airways above the obstruction are open to atmosphere. When the expiratory port of the ventilator circuit is occluded immediately before the onset of inspiration, the alveolar pressure below the obstruction equilibrates with the entire ventilator circuit, and the level of auto-PEEP registers on the ventilator manometer (see Fig. 112-6). This technique is difficult to perform in the tachypneic patient and is most easily measured in a paralyzed patient receiving controlled ventilation. In addition, if the airway obstruction is severe, the occlusion method may not be able to overcome the obstruction and allow alveolar pressure to communicate with the manometer. This results in an underestimation of the true auto-PEEP.[70]

Another technique to assess the level of auto-PEEP in a spontaneously breathing patient uses an esophageal balloon catheter during nonoccluded breathing.[71] With this technique, auto-PEEP is determined by the drop in esophageal pressure from the start of inspiratory effort to the start of inspiratory flow. This dynamic method is based on the assumption that the change in esophageal pressure required to initiate inspiratory flow approximates the opposing end-expiratory recoil pressure (auto-PEEP). The measurements are valid only when both inspiratory and expiratory muscles are relaxed at end-expiration.

The presence of auto-PEEP has several important clinical consequences. It places the inspiratory muscles at a mechanical disadvantage so that for a given level of activity, the force output is reduced. In a hyperexpanded position, the chest wall recoils inward during inspiration, thereby opposing inflation. The maximum force output of a flattened diaphragm (shorter muscle fibers and smaller zone of apposition) is greatly reduced. Decreased muscle blood flow as a result of hyperinflation may compromise further muscle function. Auto-PEEP also poses a significant inspiratory threshold load if a patient is breathing spontaneously because a negative pressure equal to the opposing elastic recoil pressure (i.e., auto-PEEP) must be generated before inspiration can begin. Finally, pulmonary barotrauma and hemodynamic compromise are important consequences of hyperinflation.

Resistance

Airway resistance is generally measured from mechanically ventilated patients to assess bronchodilator response.[72] After rapid airway occlusion during passive constant-flow inflation, there is a fall in airway pressure from the peak pressure (P_{peak}) to a lower initial pressure ($P_{initial}$) followed by a gradual decrease to a plateau pressure ($P_{plateau}$) (see Fig. 112-6). "Minimum" airway resistance is calculated by dividing the difference between P_{peak} and $P_{initial}$ by inspiratory flow. This represents the actual resistance to airflow. "Maximum" respiratory system resistance is calculated by dividing the difference between P_{peak} and $P_{plateau}$ by inspiratory flow and includes the resistance due to viscoelastic properties of the lung.

Expiratory resistance is usually greater than inspiratory resistance in the mechanically ventilated patient because of the endotracheal tube and exhalation circuit and valve. It is more difficult to measure because of the frequent presence of airflow limitation. Significant expiratory resistance may be a determinant of dynamic hyperinflation or auto-PEEP.

Flow-Volume Curves

Expiratory flow maneuvers are difficult to perform in mechanically ventilated patients. It is more practical and useful to monitor flow-volume curves during spontaneous breathing in these patients. After passive inhalation in a relaxed patient, the elastic recoil of the total respiratory system drives exhalation. In mechanically ventilated patients, the only force opposing exhalation is respiratory system resistance, which is mainly due to the endotracheal tube. Normal subjects and patients with decreased compliance display a gradual decrease in expiratory flow throughout exhalation, whereas patients with airflow limitation display a "scooped out" pattern. These patients often have auto-PEEP that is demonstrated by an abrupt cessation of expiratory flow before the next mechanical inflation, producing a "truncated" appearance on the expiratory flow curve. Flow-volume curves have been used to follow the response to bronchodilator therapy by monitoring changes in isovolume flow.[73] In addition, a saw-toothed pattern on the inspiratory and expiratory flow-volume curves suggests the presence of airway secretions and the need for endotracheal suctioning.[74]

Work of Breathing

To achieve normal ventilation, work needs to be performed to overcome the elastic and frictional resistances of the lungs and chest wall.[75] In the physical sense, work is calculated as force multiplied by distance; in the pulmonary context, this is translated into the product of pressure and the volume of air moved in and out of the lungs. In the clinical setting, the work of breathing can be quantified in two ways: (1) estimating the mechanical work of the respiratory muscles from pressure and volume measurements and (2) estimating the metabolic cost of breathing by measuring oxygen consumption of the respiratory muscles.

We can estimate the work performed on the lungs alone during spontaneous breathing by measuring the tidal volume and the difference between pleural and airway pressure (transpulmonary pressure). Pleural pressure is best measured by an esophageal balloon catheter.[71] By use of a graphic approach with esophageal pressure-volume curves, the resistive and elastic components of inspiratory work can be determined. In the presence of increased airway resistance or decreased lung compliance, increased transpulmonary pressure is required to achieve a given tidal volume with consequent increase in the work of breathing.

During mechanical ventilation, the inability of the patient to synchronize with the ventilator adds to the work of breathing.[75] This is most likely to occur with a less sensitive trigger setting and with an inspiratory gas delivery that is insufficient to meet the patient's ventilatory demands.

During quiet breathing, the normal work of breathing is approximately 0.5 J/L or 5 J/min, where 1 J is the amount of work performed when 1 L is moved across a pressure gradient of 10 cm H_2O. Patients who are receiving mechanical ventilation should have a work/minute of less than 10 to 16 J/min and work/liter of less than 1 to 1.4 J/L before weaning is likely to be successful.[2] In a study of 10 paralyzed patients with COPD receiving mechanical ventilation, the total inspiratory work was 120% higher than in 18 normal paralyzed subjects.[76] This difference was due to increased work from hyperinflation and airway resistance apart from the endotracheal tube (Fig. 112–7).

The difference between total-body oxygen consumption during spontaneous breathing and that when the patient is relaxed and receiving mechanical ventilation estimates the respiratory workload.[77] The metabolic cost of work of breathing at rest constitutes only 1% to 3% of total oxygen consumption in healthy subjects. This may be increased considerably in patients with pulmonary disease. In a study of patients being weaned from mechanical ventilation, the average oxygen cost of breathing was 24% of the total oxygen consumption, being greater than 50% in some patients.[78] This high oxygen demand by the respiratory muscles may stress the heart and contribute to unsuccessful weaning in patients with underlying cardiac disease.

ASSESSMENT OF THE SURGICAL PATIENT

Pulmonary complications are observed commonly after surgery. Of the risk factors associated with pulmonary complications, the site of the surgical incision has long been recognized to be of major importance. Other risk factors include advanced age, pulmonary disease or symptoms, current smoking, and obesity. Therefore, preoperative assessment of pulmonary function is considered advisable in patients with these risk factors, especially if they are undergoing thoracic or upper abdominal surgery. This identifies the high-risk patient and allows careful planning of perioperative respiratory care.[79] Table 112–2 lists the important pulmonary function criteria used to identify high-risk patients undergoing either abdominal or lung resection surgery.[80]

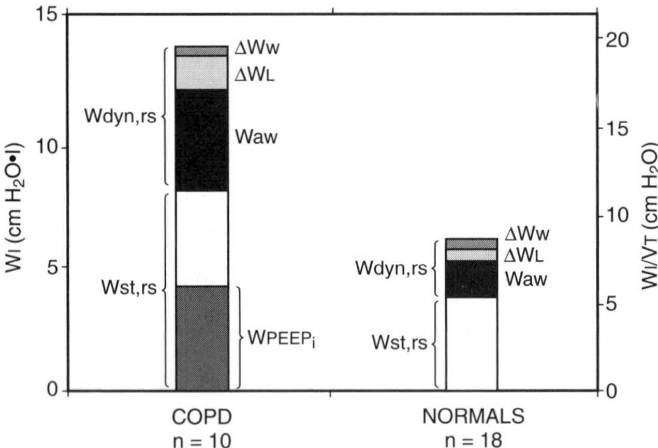

Figure 112–7. Work of breathing (WOB) during controlled mechanical ventilation. Partitioning of inspiratory work (Wi) performed by the respiratory system in 10 patients with chronic obstructive pulmonary disease (COPD) and in 18 anesthetized and paralyzed subjects. Total Wi was 120% greater in patients with COPD. Total static work of the respiratory system (Wst,rs) was greater in the COPD patients and was due mostly to static work of PEEPi (WPEEPi). Total dynamic work of the respiratory system (Wdyn,rs) was increased in the COPD patients, caused by increases in airway resistive work (Waw) and work due to viscoelastic properties of the lung (ΔWL). Viscoelastic work of the chest wall (ΔWw) was similar in the two groups. The right axis represents inspiratory work per tidal volume (Vt). (From Coussa ML, Guerin C, Eissa NT, et al: Partitioning of work of breathing in mechanically ventilated COPD patients. J Appl Physiol 1993; 75:1711.)

TABLE 112–2. Pulmonary Function Criteria Predicting High Risk in Abdominal and Thoracic Surgery

	Abdominal	Thoracic
FVC	<50% predicted	<50% predicted
FEV_1	<70% predicted	<2 L
FEV_1%	<65%	<50%
MVV	<50% predicted	<50% predicted
Pa_{CO_2}	>45 mm Hg	>45 mm Hg
$\dot{V}_{O_2}$		<15 ml/kg/min

FVC = forced vital capacity; FEV_1 = forced expiratory volume at 1 second; FEV_1%, ratio of FEV_1 to FVC; MVV = maximum voluntary ventilation; Pa_{CO_2} = arterial carbon dioxide tension; $\dot{V}_{O_2}$ = oxygen consumption.

SUMMARY

The assessment of pulmonary function in the ICU differs from that undertaken in the hospital laboratory in the nature and range of tests performed; less concentration is placed on lung volume subdivisions and flow rates and greater emphasis is given to respiratory pressures, compliance, and breathing patterns. In addition, it is becoming more evident that the continuous monitoring of pulmonary function in the critically ill patient is more useful than are intermittent measurements. Taken singly, the predictive power of many tests is somewhat low; however, combined with careful physical examination, these tests provide a better understanding of the pathophysiologic nature of the patient's pulmonary disease.

As with other diagnostic techniques in the ICU, it is difficult to demonstrate whether such measurements are cost effective or save lives. It is hoped that as greater insight is gained into the physiologic determinants of morbidity and outcome of patients, modifications of existing tests and introduction of new tests will provide greater sensitivity and specificity.

References

1. Wanner A: Interpretation of pulmonary function tests. *In*: Diagnostic Techniques in Pulmonary Disease: Part 1. Sackner MA (Ed). New York, Marcel Dekker, 1980, pp 353–426.
2. Tobin MJ, Alex CG: Discontinuation from mechanical ventilation. *In*: Principles and Practice of Mechanical Ventilation. Tobin MJ (Ed). New York, McGraw-Hill, 1994, pp 1177–1206.
3. Browning IB, D'Alonzo GE, Tobin MJ: Importance of respiratory rate as an indicator of respiratory dysfunction in patients with cystic fibrosis. Chest 1990; 97:1317.
4. Semmes BJ, Tobin MJ, Snyder JV, et al: Subjective and objective measurement of tidal volume in critically ill patients. Chest 1985; 87:577.
5. Tobin MJ, Jenouri GA, Watson H, et al: Noninvasive measurement of pleural pressure by surface inductive plethysmography. J Appl Physiol 1983; 55:267.
6. Tobin MJ: State of the art: Respiratory monitoring. Am Rev Respir Dis 1988; 138:1625.
7. Tobin MJ, Perez W, Guenther SM, et al: Does rib cage-abdominal paradox signify respiratory muscle fatigue? J Appl Physiol 1987; 63:851.
8. Jubran A, Tobin MJ: The effect of hyperinflation on rib cage-abdominal motion. Am Rev Respir Dis 1992; 146:1378.
9. Alex CG, Tobin MJ: Noninvasive respiratory monitoring. *In*: Pulmonary Disease in the Elderly Patient. Mahler DA (Ed). New York, Marcel Dekker, 1993, pp 27–60.
10. Lopata M, Lourenço R: Evaluation of respiratory control. Clin Chest Med 1980; 1:33.

11. Whitelaw WA, Derenne JP: Airway occlusion pressure. J Appl Physiol 1993; 74:1475.
12. Tobin MJ, Gardner WN: Monitoring of the control of breathing. *In*: Principles and Practice of Intensive Care Monitoring. Tobin MJ (Ed). New York, McGraw-Hill, 1998, pp 415–464.
13. Sassoon C, Mahutte CK: Airway occlusion pressure and breathing pattern as predictors of weaning outcome. Am Rev Respir Dis 1993; 148:860.
14. Capdevilla XJ, Perrigault PF, Perez PJ, et al: Occlusion pressure and its ratio to maximum inspiratory pressure are useful predictors for successful extubation following T-piece weaning trial. Chest 1995; 108:482.
15. Montgomery AB, Holle RHO, Neagley SR, et al: Prediction of successful ventilatory weaning using airway occlusion pressure and hypercapnic challenge. Chest 1987; 91:496.
16. Conti G, Cinnella G, Barboni E, et al: Estimation of occlusion pressure during assisted ventilation in patients with intrinsic PEEP. Am J Respir Crit Care Med 1996; 154:907.
17. NHLBI Workshop Summary: Respiratory muscle fatigue: Report of the respiratory muscle fatigue workshop group. Am Rev Respir Dis 1990; 142:474.
18. Black LF, Hyatt RE: Maximal respiratory pressures: Normal values and relationship to age and sex. Am Rev Respir Dis 1968; 99:696.
19. Black LF, Hyatt RE: Maximal static respiratory pressure in generalized neuromuscular disease. Am Rev Respir Dis 1971; 103:641.
20. Baydur A: Respiratory muscle strength and control of ventilation in patients with neuromuscular disease. Chest 1991; 99:330.
21. Rochester DF, Braun NMT: Determinants of maximal inspiratory pressure in chronic obstructive pulmonary disease. Am Rev Respir Dis 1985; 132:42.
22. Mortimer AJ, Sykes MK: Monitoring of ventilation. *In*: Recent Advances in Critical Care Medicine. Vol 2. Ledingham I, Hanning CD (Eds). Edinburgh, Churchill Livingstone, 1983, pp 5–28.
23. Koulouris N, Mulvey DA, Laroche CM, et al: Comparison of two different mouthpieces for the measurement of Pimax and Pemax in normal and weak subjects. Eur Respir J 1988; 1:863.
24. Vincken W, Ghezzo H, Cosio NG: Maximal static respiratory pressures in adults: Normal values and their relationship to determinants of respiratory function. Bull Eur Pathophysiol Respir 1987; 23:435.
25. Wilson SH, Cooke NT, Edwards RHT, et al: Predicted normal values for maximal respiratory pressures in Caucasian adults and children. Thorax 1984; 39:535.
26. Chen H-I, Kuo C-S: Relationship between respiratory muscle function and age, sex, and other factors. J Appl Physiol 1989; 66:943.
27. Braun NMT, Arora NS, Rochester DF: Respiratory muscle and pulmonary function in polymyositis and other proximal myopathies. Thorax 1983; 38:616.
28. Sahn SA, Lakshminarayan S: Bedside criteria for discontinuation of mechanical ventilation. Chest 1973; 63:1002.
29. Tahvanainen J, Salenpera M, Nikki P: Extubation criteria after weaning from intermittent mandatory ventilation and continuous positive airway pressure. Crit Care Med 1983; 11:702.
30. Multz AS, Aldrich TK, Prezant DJ, et al: Maximal inspiratory pressure is not a reliable test of inspiratory muscle strength in mechanically ventilated patients. Am Rev Respir Dis 1990; 142:529.
31. Yang KL, Tobin MJ: A prospective study of indexes predicting the outcome of trials of weaning from mechanical ventilation. N Engl J Med 1991; 324:1445.
32. Chatilla W, Jacob B, Guaglionone D, Manthous CA: The unassisted respiratory rate-to-tidal volume ratio accurately predicts weaning outcome. Am J Med 1996; 101:61.
33. Marini JJ, Smith TC, Lamb V: Estimation of inspiratory muscle strength in mechanically ventilated patients: The measurement of maximal inspiratory pressure. J Crit Care 1986; 1:32.
34. Faulkner JA, Maxwell LC, Ruff GL, et al: The diaphragm as muscle: Contractile properties. Am Rev Respir Dis 1979; 119(Suppl):89.
35. Aldrich TK: Respiratory muscle fatigue. *In*: The Respiratory Muscles. Tobin MJ (Ed). Philadelphia, JB Lippincott, 1990, pp 329–342.
36. Moxham J: Respiratory muscle fatigue: Mechanisms, evaluation and therapy. Br J Anesth 1990; 65:43.
37. Bellemare F, Bigland-Ritchie B: Central components of diaphragm fatigue assessed by phrenic nerve stimulation. J Appl Physiol 1987; 62:1307.
38. Laghi F, D'Alfonso N, Tobin MJ: Pattern of recovery from diaphragmatic fatigue over 24 hours. J Appl Physiol 1995; 79:539.
39. Green M, Moxham J: The respiratory muscles. Clin Sci 1985; 68:1.
40. Tobin MJ, Laghi F: Monitoring of respiratory muscle function. *In*: Principles and Practice of Intensive Care Monitoring. Tobin MJ (Ed). New York, McGraw-Hill, 1998, pp 945–966.
41. Miller J, Moxham J, Green M: The maximal sniff in the assessment of diaphragm function in man. Clin Sci 1985; 69:91.
42. Newsom-Davis J, Goldman M, Loh L, Casson M: Diaphragm function and alveolar hypoventilation. Q J Med 1976; 177:87.
43. Polkey MI, Green M, Moxham J: Measurement of respiratory muscle strength. Thorax 1995; 50:1131.
44. Mier A, Brophy C, Moxham J, Green M: Phrenic nerve stimulation in normal subjects and in patients with diaphragmatic weakness. Thorax 1987; 42:885.
45. Bellemare F, Bigland-Ritchie B: Assessment of human diaphragm strength and activation using phrenic stimulation. Respir Physiol 1984; 58:263.
46. Laghi F, Harrison M, Tobin MJ: Comparison of magnetic and electrical phrenic nerve stimulation in assessment of diaphragmatic contractility. J Appl Physiol 1996; 80:1731.
47. Babcock MA, Pegelow DF, McClaran SR, et al: Contribution of diaphragmatic power output to exercise-induced diaphragmatic fatigue. J Appl Physiol 1995; 78:1710.
48. Bellemare F, Grassino A: Effect of pressure and timing of contraction on human diaphragm fatigue. J Appl Physiol 1982; 53:1190.
49. Jubran A, Tobin MJ: Pathophysiologic basis of acute respiratory failure in patients who fail a trial of weaning from mechanical ventilation. Am J Respir Crit Care Med 1997; 155:906.
50. McCool DF, Conomos P, Benditt JO, et al: Maximal inspiratory pressures and dimensions of the diaphragm. Am J Respir Crit Care Med 1997; 155:1329.
51. Gottesman E, McCool FD: Ultrasound evaluation of the paralyzed diaphragm. Am J Respir Crit Care Med 1997; 155:1570.
52. Tobin MJ: Noninvasive monitoring of ventilaton. *In*: Principles and Practice of Intensive Care Monitoring. Tobin MJ (Ed). New York, McGraw-Hill, 1998, pp 465–495.
53. Tobin MY, Chadha TS, Jenouri G, et al: Breathing patterns: 1. Normal subjects. Chest 1983; 84:202.
54. Roussos C, Campbell EJM: Respiratory muscle energetics. *In*: Handbook of Physiology: The Respiratory System. Macklem PT, Mead J (Eds). Bethesda, Md, American Physiological Society, 1986, pp 481–509.
55. Tobin MJ, Perez W, Guenther SM, et al: The pattern of breathing during successful and unsuccessful trials of weaning from mechanical ventilation. Am Rev Respir Dis 1986; 134:1111.
56. Tobin MJ, Jenouri G, Lind B, et al: Validation of respiratory inductive plethysmography in patients with pulmonary disease. Chest 1983; 83:615.
57. Tobin MY, Mador MJ, Guenther SM, et al: Variability of resting respiratory drive and timing in healthy subjects. J Appl Physiol 1988; 65:309.
58. Tobin MJ, Chadha TS, Jenouri G, et al: Breathing patterns: 2. Diseased subjects. Chest 1983; 84:286.
59. Tobin MJ, Guenther SM, Perez W, et al: Konno-Mead analysis of ribcage-abdominal motion during successful and unsuccessful trials of weaning from mechanical ventilation. Am Rev Respir Dis 1987; 135:1320.
60. Tobin MJ, Jenouri G, Birch S, et al: Effect of positive end-expiratory pressure on breathing patterns of normal subjects and intubated patients with respiratory failure. Crit Care Med 1983; 11:859.
61. Hoffman RA, Ershowsky P, Krieger BP: Determination of auto-PEEP during spontaneous and controlled ventilation by monitoring changes in end-expiratory thoracic gas volume. Chest 1989; 96:613.
62. Chevrolet J-C, Deléamont P: Repeated vital capacity measurements as predictive parameters for mechanical ventilation need and weaning success in the Guillain-Barré syndrome. Am Rev Respir Dis 1991; 144:814.
63. Rieder P, Louis M, Jolliet P, Chevrolet JC: The repeated measurement of vital capacity is a poor predictor of the need for mechanical ventilation in myasthenia gravis. Intensive Care Med 1995; 21:663.
64. Bach JR, Saporito LR: Criteria for extubation and tracheostomy

tube removal for patients with ventilatory failure. A different approach to weaning. Chest 1996; 110:1566.
65. Hess D, McCurdy S, Simmons M: Compression volume in adult ventilator circuits: A comparison of five disposable circuits and a nondisposable circuit. Respir Care 1991; 31:1113.
66. Rossi A, Gottfried SB, Zocchi L, et al: Measurement of static lung compliance of the total respiratory system in patients with acute respiratory failure during mechanical ventilation: The effect of intrinsic positive end-expiratory pressure. Am Rev Respir Dis 1985; 131:672.
67. Tobin MJ: Monitoring respiratory mechanics in spontaneously breathing patients. *In*: Principles and Practice of Intensive Care Monitoring. Tobin MJ (Ed). New York, McGraw-Hill, 1998, pp 617–654.
68. Shee CD, Ply-song-sang Y, Milic-Emili J: Decay of inspiratory muscle pressure during expiration in conscious humans. J Appl Physiol 1985; 58:1859.
69. Ninane V, Yernault J-C, De Troyer A: Intrinsic PEEP in patients with chronic obstructive lung disease: Role of expiratory muscles. Am Rev Respir Dis 1993; 148:1037.
70. Leatherman JW, Ravenscraft SA: Low measured auto-positive end-expiratory pressure during mechanical ventilation of patients with severe asthma: Hidden auto-positive end-expiratory pressure. Crit Care Med 1996; 24:541.
71. Zin WA, Milic-Emili J: Esophageal pressure measurement. *In*: Principles and Practice of Intensive Care Monitoring. Tobin MJ (Ed). New York, McGraw-Hill, 1998, pp 542–552.
72. Dhand R, Jubran A, Tobin MJ: Efficacy of bronchodilator delivered by metered-dose inhaler in ventilator-supported patients with COPD. Am J Respir Crit Care Med 1995; 151:1827.
73. Gay PC, Rodarte JC, Tayyab M, et al: Evaluation of bronchodilator responsiveness in mechanically-ventilated patients. Am Rev Respir Dis 1987; 136:880.
74. Jubran A, Tobin MJ: Use of flow-volume curves in detecting secretions in ventilator-dependent patients. Am J Respir Crit Care Med 1994; 150:766.
75. Rossi A, Polese G, Milic-Emili J: Monitoring respiratory mechanics in ventilator-dependent patients. *In*: Principles and Practice of Intensive Care Monitoring. Tobin MJ (Ed). New York, McGraw-Hill, 1998, pp 553–596.
76. Coussa ML, Guérin C, Eissa NT, et al: Partitioning of work of breathing in mechanically ventilated COPD patients. J Appl Physiol 1993; 75:1711.
77. Hubmayr RD, Loosbrock LM, Gillespie DJ, et al: Oxygen uptake during weaning from mechanical ventilation. Chest 1988; 94:1148.
78. Field S, Kelly SM, Macklem PT: The oxygen cost of breathing in patients with cardiorespiratory distress. Am Rev Respir Dis 1982; 126:9.
79. Stein M, Cassara EL: Preoperative pulmonary evaluation and therapy for surgery patients. JAMA 1970; 211:787.
80. Gass GD, Olsen GN: Postoperative pulmonary function testing to predict postoperative morbidity and mortality. Chest 1986; 89:127.

113

Conventional Airway Access

Donna A. Castello, DO • Howard S. Smith, MD
Philip D. Lumb, MB, BS, FCCM

HISTORY

Airway patency and breathing have long been recognized to be vital for life. Vesalius[1] is credited with the earliest reports of tracheal intubation (through a tracheotomy opening) for resuscitation. The translation of his 1543 experiment is, "Life may in a matter of speaking be restored . . . an opening must be attempted in the trunk of the trachea into which a reed or cane should be put; you will then blow into this so that the lung may rise again."[2]

A similar experiment was performed by Robert Hooke[3] in 1667, in which he kept a dog alive by the "reciprocal blowing up of his lungs with bellows." He found that "upon ceasing the blast and suffering the lungs to fall and lie still, the dog would immediately fall into dying convulsing fits; but was soon revived again by renewing the fullness of his lungs with the constant blast of fresh air."[3]

John Mayow,[2, 4] a physiologist, wrote in 1674 that "on the suppression of respiration . . . the beating of the heart and, consequently, the flow of blood to the brain will necessarily be interrupted and death will ensue . . . so it appears that the air is that without which the movements of the heart cannot go on at all."

The first recognized account of tracheal intubation through the glottis was Macewen's[2, 5] work in 1880, although both nasal and oral tactile blind intubation of the trachea is probably the oldest method used and was practiced by Kite in 1785.[6, 7] Desault in the early 1800s proposed blind nasal intubation for protection of the airway in patients with laryngeal disease.[2] It was later that Kuhn described and favored nasotracheal intubation as a means of airway maintenance.[8]

Indirect laryngoscopy, developed by Manuel Garcia (a singing teacher),[6, 7] did not alleviate the difficulty of endotracheal tube (ETT) placement but did familiarize physicians with the anatomy of the pharynx and laryngeal inlet. These principles are used today with fiberoptic bundles to provide illumination of the field (fiberoptic bronchoscope [FOB] and Bullard laryngoscope).

Unlike Macewen, whose work was intended for the administration of anesthesia, Joseph O'Dwyer[9] publicized his extensive use of tracheal intubation during the diphtheria epidemics of the late 1800s. He developed ETTs that were positioned over a curved introducer, which was then removed (a forerunner of the stylet). His success prompted others, such as Maydl, Eisenmenger, Dorrance, and Van Stockum,[10] to devise ETTs with cuffs. Originally, cuffs were "milked" onto the tubes.[10] A tube with an inflatable cuff was constructed by Rowbotham[11] in 1944. Later, cuffed ETTs were used for prolonged intubation during the poliomyelitis epidemics of the 1950s and 1960s. These early cuffs led to tracheal injury, such as tracheomalacia, stenosis, and tracheoesophageal fistula. Modern ETTs may vary in their construction but most commonly are constructed of polyurethane with a low-pressure, high-volume inflatable cuff.

Direct laryngoscopy developed as the need to overcome the technical difficulty of ETT insertion was recognized in the early 1900s. Several individuals developed the laryngoscope, most notably Chevalier Jackson[12] in 1913, who streamlined the apparatus and expounded the merits of examining the larynx before intubation. As Elsberg, Janeway, Miller, MacIntosh, and a host of others practiced this technique and introduced adaptations and variations of laryngoscopes, ETTs, and nasotracheal tubes, tracheal intubation became commonplace.[6]

ANATOMY

Successful management of the airway and the potential complications related to procedures undertaken to ensure its patency requires an understanding of basic anatomic features.[13, 14]

Two external openings lead to the human airway. The nose leads to the *nasopharynx* and the mouth to the *oropharynx*. These are separated anteriorly by the palate but join posteriorly (Fig. 113–1*A*). The nasal septum divides the nasal cavity into two pyramids that contain bone, cartilage, and sinus openings and receive innervation from both the olfactory

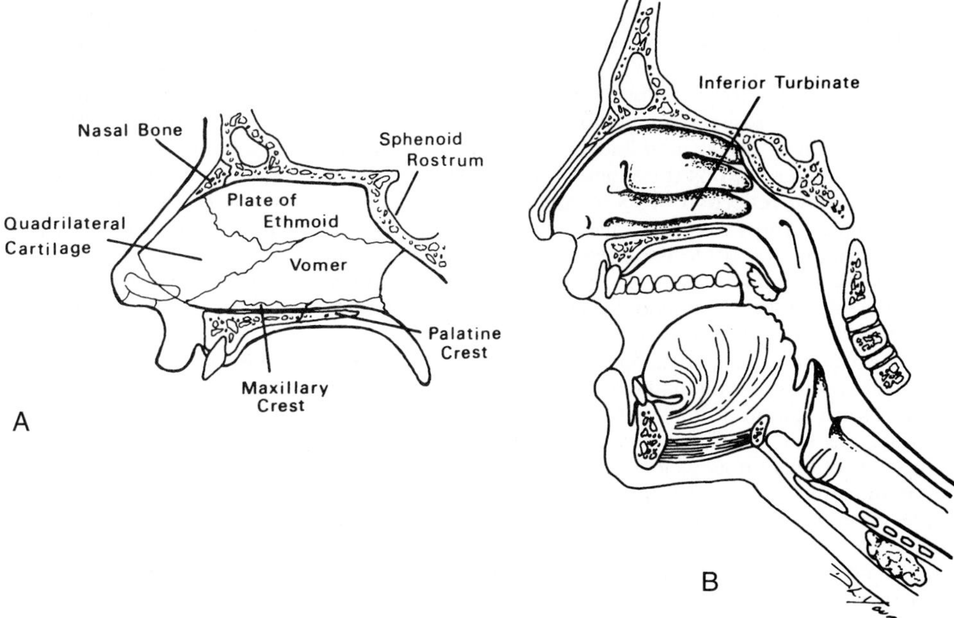

Figure 113–1. *A*, Sagittal view of the bone structure of the nose. *B*, Sagittal view of the oral and nasal airway anatomy. Note the communication of the nasopharynx and the oropharynx. (Courtesy of the Stratton Veterans Affairs Medical Center, Albany, N.Y.)

(cranial nerve I) and the trigeminal (cranial nerve V) nerves. The roof of the nose is formed by the nasal and frontal bones, the cribriform plate of the ethmoid, and the body of the sphenoid bone. The floor is formed by the maxilla and palatine bones. The medial wall is formed by septal cartilage, the vomer, and the perpendicular plate of the ethmoid (see Fig. 113–1*A*). The septum, if deviated, creates asymmetry of the nasal passages. This should be noted in planning a nasal intubation, because success will probably be greatest when attempts are made through the larger nasal passage. The lateral wall contains a portion of the ethmoid bone with three turbinate bones, superior, middle, and inferior, with the openings of the paranasal sinuses and nasolacrimal duct (see Fig. 113–1*B*). Any foreign body (nasotracheal or nasogastric tube) in proximity to these sinus openings can provoke serious infection in the intensive care unit (ICU) patient and should be removed if this occurs.

The *nasal cavity* receives its blood supply from the anterior and posterior branches of the ophthalmic artery and branches of the maxillary and facial arteries. Its venous plexus drains into sphenopalatine, facial, and ophthalmic veins. The mucous membranes that line the turbinates are extensively vascularized, and careless manipulation can lead to severe hemorrhage.

The *mouth* is bounded by the lips and cheeks externally, the gums and teeth internally, the hard and soft palate superiorly, and the mucosa inferiorly, which is connected to the tongue. The tongue, especially if large, may impede attempts at laryngeal visualization and intubation and must be swept to the left with the laryngoscope blade to afford an optimal view.

The *pharynx* is subdivided into the nasopharynx, oropharynx, and laryngopharynx. The nasopharynx follows directly from the nasal cavity above the soft palate. The oropharynx begins at the soft palate and extends to the tip of the epiglottis. It contains the pillars of the fauces (the lateral walls of the oropharynx) between which the palatine tonsils lie, an important landmark in the airway classification of Mallampati,[15] which is described later.

The *laryngopharynx* extends from the epiglottis to the cricoid cartilage. It is separated laterally from the larynx by the arytenoepiglottic folds. These lateral portions are the piriform recesses in which the inferior laryngeal nerve lies.

The laryngeal skeleton consists of several cartilages: thyroid, cricoid, epiglottic, arytenoid, corniculate, and cuneiform (the last three are paired) (Fig. 113–2).

The *thyroid cartilage* is a shield-shaped structure that does not project posteriorly and consists of right and left laminae that meet in the midline, forming the thyroid notch and thyroid prominence. The superior projections (horns) are connected to the hyoid bone, an important landmark for the performance of a superior laryngeal nerve block. Inferiorly, its attachment is the cricoid cartilage through the cricothyroid membrane.

The *cricoid cartilage* is signet ring-shaped and is connected

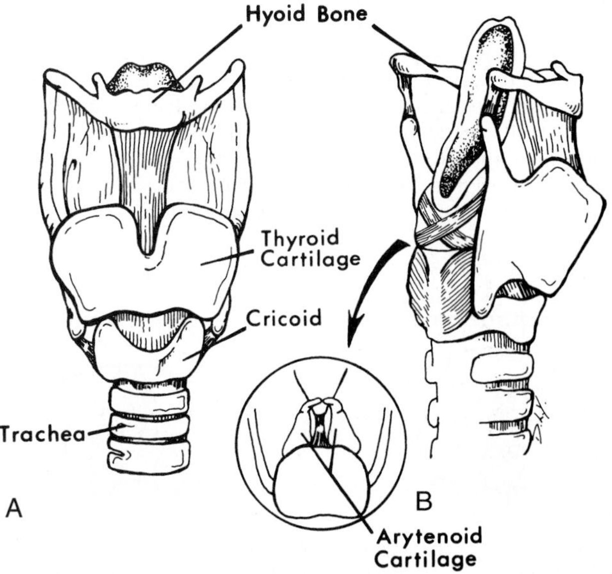

Figure 113–2. Laryngeal cartilages. *A*, Anterior view. *B*, Posterolateral view. Magnified view from the anterior aspect of the laryngeal inlet. The cuneiform and corniculate cartilages sit atop the arytenoid cartilages and are a useful landmark for identification of the glottic opening. (Courtesy of the Stratton Veterans Administration Medical Center, Albany, N.Y.)

to the first tracheal ring. Curry in 1915, and later Sellick, described posterior cricoid pressure as a useful maneuver. Curry found it useful to limit the entry of air into the esophagus during resuscitation attempts,[16] whereas Sellick noted its ability to prevent passive regurgitation of gastric contents.[17]

The *epiglottis* is leaf-shaped and covered with a membranous surface innervated by the superior laryngeal nerve (internal branch). The reflection of its membranous surface forms the depression known as the vallecula. It is here that the curved laryngoscope blade is placed to elevate the epiglottis and allow visualization of the laryngeal entrance. The aryteno-epiglottic folds join the epiglottis with the paired pyramid-shaped arytenoids. They have a synovial articular surface with the superolateral aspect of the cricoid, and each has an anterior vocal process to which attaches the vocal ligament of the cords. Disarticulation of this joint during traumatic intubation can lead to adduction of the vocal cord involved, resulting in changes in phonation as well as a decrease in the size of the airway opening.

The *corniculate cartilages* rest on the apex of each *arytenoid cartilage* along with the *cuneiform cartilage* and tubercle. The arytenoids are returned to their resting position after abduction, which is facilitated by the elastic recoil of the corniculate and cuneiform cartilages. The cuneiform and corniculate tubercles can often be seen during direct laryngoscopy and may provide a landmark to the opening of the trachea when it is impossible to bring the vocal cords into view.

The *glottis* consists of the vocal cords and space between them (rima glottidis) (Fig. 113–3). In the adult, this is the narrowest portion of the airway. The true vocal cords are covered by stratified squamous epithelium, which gives them a pearly white color when illuminated. The subglottic area begins below the vocal cords and is the narrowest area in infants and children.

The muscles of the *larynx* protect its entrance and produce changes in the quality of phonation. The extrinsic muscles elevate, depress, and constrict the pharynx. The intrinsic muscles are important for abduction, adduction, and changes in tension of the vocal cords. The only muscle that abducts the cords is the posterior cricoarytenoid muscle. Branches of the vagus (cranial nerve X) innervate the muscles of the larynx. The superior laryngeal nerve supplies only the cricothyroid muscle and provides sensory innervation to the entire mucosal surface of the larynx, piriform recess, vallecula, and base of the dorsal tongue posteriorly. Stimulation without adequate anesthesia may reflexly provoke laryngospasm. Afferent impulses transmitted to the central vagal nuclei are then carried by efferents to the intrinsic muscles of the larynx, which

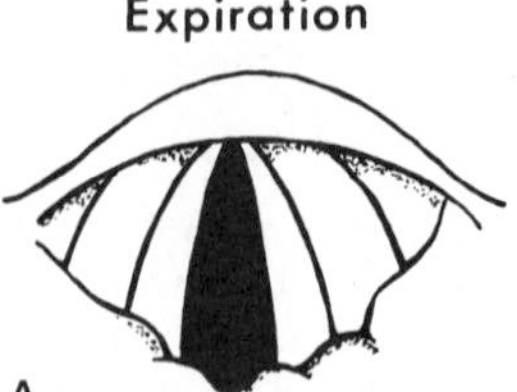

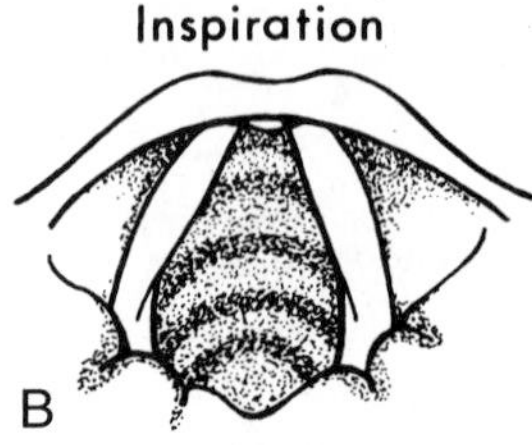

Figure 113–3. Laryngoscopic view of the glottis. *A*, Position on expiration (cadaveric position; also seen in living patients with the use of muscle relaxants or in those with bilateral cord paralysis). *B*, Position of the vocal cords during inspiration. Note the hump-like projections of the corniculate cartilages, which may provide the only landmark in identifying the laryngeal inlet in a patient with a difficult airway. (Courtesy of the Stratton Veterans Affairs Medical Center, Albany, N.Y.)

protect its entrance.[16, 18] Application of positive pressure with a mask and bag-valve device may relieve spasm in some cases. A tight mask seal is imperative for its proper application. If unsuccessful, a short-acting muscle relaxant may be administered by those skilled in its uses and complications. Because a patient may be unable to be ventilated as a result of laryngospasm followed by the use of muscle relaxants, properly trained individuals should be present to proceed quickly with alternative means of airway control whenever it is needed.

The recurrent laryngeal nerve provides motor supply to the rest of the intrinsic muscles of the larynx and sensory supply to the larynx below the vocal cords. Injury to this nerve results in paralysis of the ipsilateral vocal cord, which then lies in the cadaveric position near the midline. Bilateral paralysis of this nerve leads to vocal cord paralysis, with the cords remaining in the cadaveric position. They are seen in midline with bowing (see Fig. 113–3*A*) and not in complete opposition. This results in almost complete loss of phonation. Often, the cords become less bowed over time and voice improves, but the airway opening narrows and obstruction may ensue.

The *trachea* extends from its attachment to the cricoid cartilage to the carina where the mainstem bronchi begin. It is composed of 16 to 20 C-shaped cartilages with connective tissue between them and the tracheal muscle posteriorly, which is then in apposition to the esophagus. Obstruction of the airway may arise here from compression (mediastinal and esophageal tumors, postoperative hematoma) and foreign body ingestion.

Tracheomalacia and esophageal scarring may result from ischemic injury secondary to either trauma during intubation or overinflated cuffs. Tracheostenosis may also result from airway manipulation and postoperative changes. In the pediatric patient, lack of air leak around the ETT indicates an excessively tight fit that may lead to ischemic subglottic stenosis and tracheostenosis.

AIRWAY ASSESSMENT

A rapid assessment of the airway should be performed when management decisions involve the maintenance of airway patency and gas exchange. This should include knowledge of the patient's disease that may alter airway anatomy and its related structures (e.g., acromegaly, connective tissue disease, and other systemic diseases). A vital component of the initial assessment is consideration of the following[19]:

- Surgical and traumatic deformities of the maxillofacial bones and tissues
- Surgical scarring and fibrosis
- Laryngeal trauma and edema
- Congenital anomalies
- Airway tumors and abscesses
- Cervical spine instability, immobility, and acute injury (hematoma, paravertebral swelling)
- Tooth and jaw structure or abnormalities (temporomandibular joint syndrome, mandibular fracture, large or loose teeth, dentures)
- Diseases that may affect the airway in their pathologic destruction

In patients with obvious disease that may make ventilation or intubation difficult, it is prudent to assemble the equipment for alternative means of airway control and intubation as well as to summon those personnel with expertise in airway management.

Potential difficulties in intubation may be subtle, and unless careful initial assessment has been performed before attempts at intubation, serious complications may result, including loss of the airway, cardiac arrest, and death. In any case, the individual responsible for maintaining the airway should have an understanding of failed intubation drills (Fig. 113-4) because morbidity from the interruption of gas exchange as well as from directly mediated deleterious laryngeal reflexes (cardiovascular instability, vomiting, laryngospasm) may ensue if corrective action is not taken expediently.

Several indicators of anatomically difficult airways have been described.[15, 20-23] Of these, three are easy to perform (with certain exceptions in the ICU patient) and may together provide a reliable index for predicting difficulty in intubation.[19]

Visual grading of tongue to pharyngeal size is simple in the awake, cooperative patient. The patient should be sitting upright, with the head in the neutral position, the mouth opened as widely as possible, and the tongue protruded maximally. The airway is then classified according to the structures visible to the observer[15] (Fig. 113-5):

Class I: soft palate, fauces, uvula, anterior and posterior tonsillar pillars
Class II: soft palate, fauces, uvula
Class III: soft palate, base of uvula
Class IV: soft palate only

The ease or difficulty of laryngoscopy and subsequent intubation has been correlated with these views (Fig. 113-6). A class I airway most often provides a laryngoscopic view that includes the entire laryngeal aperture.[15, 22, 24] Patients with intermediate Mallampati airway classifications were found to have all grades of laryngoscopic view by one group of investigators.[25] The majority of those patients with class IV airways on laryngoscopy provided limited or no exposure of the laryngeal opening, with difficult intubation conditions. However, taken alone, especially in the ICU patient with the usual array of coexisting disease that may alter airway anatomy, this classification may not be clearly predictive of the degree of difficulty in intubation. The supine position, arched tongue, and phonation (patient says "Ah") may alter the view.[19]

A second bedside examination, evaluation of atlanto-occipital extension, requires a cooperative patient without cervical spine injury. Patients with unstable cervical spine injuries at C-1 and C-2 may experience neurologic damage after neck flexion or extension.[26] The patient should sit with head erect and facing forward and then extend the atlanto-occipital joint with little extension of the remainder of the cervical spine. An estimate of the angle is made by the occlusal surface of the upper teeth with the occlusal surface of the lower teeth, which should be horizontal and parallel to the ground. If no disease exists, 35° of atlanto-occipital extension is possible. Bellhouse and Doré[20] graded the reduction in joint extension and then correlated this with tongue size using a two-variable analysis to predict the difficulty in intubation.

In addition, the mandibular space can be measured as the thyromental distance (Fig. 113-7). The thyromental distance, which grades the space anterior to the larynx, is described as the number of fingerbreadths (or centimeters) between the thyroid cartilage and point of the chin and determines the acuity of the laryngopharyngeal axis. The more acute the angle, the greater the difficulty in alignment of these axes despite adequate atlanto-occipital extension.

There is a strong inverse correlation between the adequacy of the mandibular space and the pharyngeal class (Mallampati class). A low pharyngeal class coupled with a thyromental distance greater than 6 cm or horizontal mandibular length greater than 9 cm provides a low-grade direct laryngoscopic view.[21, 23, 27]

The obstetric patient deserves special mention because physiologic changes of pregnancy may make mask ventilation and intubation difficult. Of particular concern is the higher rate of failed intubation in the obstetric population undergoing cesarean section[28] compared with the general surgical patient.[29] In fact, the inability to intubate the trachea of these patients is a leading cause of maternal death.[30]

Increased extracellular fluid and plasma volume during pregnancy resulting from greater mineralocorticoid activity[31] leads to airway mucosal edema, friability, and bleeding with minimal trauma.[32] These changes are exacerbated in patients with preeclampsia and those given tocolytic agents.[33] Intubation criteria examined by one group of investigators included the pharyngeal class and tongue size, mandibular space, short neck, protruding incisors, obesity, facial edema, and swollen tongue.[34] Using multivariable analysis, these investigators found a direct correlation between the difficulty in intubation and increasing pharyngeal class, short neck, receding mandible, and protruding incisors. No correlation between facial edema and swollen tongue was found.

Parturient patients are at a greater risk for gastric aspiration as gastric acid secretion increases,[35] and in late pregnancy, gastric emptying is delayed, lower esophageal sphincter tone decreases, and intragastric pressure increases. If mask ventilation is performed, cricoid pressure should be maintained until the trachea is intubated and the tracheal tube cuff inflated.[33]

Obesity and pregnancy both contribute to a decreased functional residual capacity. In the parturient, oxygen consumption increases as well. These factors combine to lead to the rapid development of hypoxia with apnea of even short duration.

As stated previously, these criteria may be difficult to assess in some patients admitted to the ICU. Nevertheless, a rapid evaluation should be performed as equipment and personnel are assembled and plans made for alternative means of airway control and patency.

AIRWAY CONTROL

Airway maintenance remains the highest priority for those involved in acute care of patients. In those patients who are obtunded or unconscious with sudden airway obstruction, attempts to open the airway should be initiated immediately by means of the triple-airway maneuver.[36]

Head tilt with anterior displacement of the mandible (chin lift) and jaw thrust should be attempted except in the management of patients with known or suspected cervical spine instability. Although there are no outcome studies examining these maneuvers, chin lift with jaw thrust and head tilt may lead to untoward neurologic sequelae in those patients.[27] These maneuvers should be practiced until expertise is gained and repracticed at intervals to maintain the skill.

Oropharyngeal and nasopharyngeal airways (Fig. 113-8) are important adjuncts to airway control. They are designed to hold the tongue away from the posterior wall of the pharynx and should be inserted by properly trained individuals. The oral airway may be inserted either directly, with the convex side up with anterior tongue displacement, or with the convex side down and the airway then rotated 180°. Care is taken to avoid rough handling of the teeth and gums. If improperly placed, the airway increases airway obstruction by downward displacement of the tongue into the pharynx. In patients with intact upper airway reflexes, the placement of a rigid oral airway may provoke laryngospasm, vomiting, coughing, and bronchospasm.

Nasal airways are softer and better tolerated by conscious patients. Contraindications for their use are the same as those for nasotracheal intubation (Table 113-1). Insertion should be preceded by topical vasoconstrictors (i.e., phenylephrine or oxymetazoline nasal spray) and topical lidocaine. The tip should be aimed perpendicularly to the plane of the face,

Difficult Airway Algorithm

1. Assess the likelihood and clinical impact of basic management problems:

Difficult Intubation	Difficult Ventilation	Difficulty with Patient Cooperation or Consent

2. Consider the relative merits and feasibility of basic management choices:

a.	Non-surgical Technique for Initial Approach to Intubation	VS	Surgical Technique or Initial Approach to Intubation
b.	Awake Intubation	VS	Intubation Attempts After Induction of General Anesthesia
c.	Preservation of Spontaneous Ventilation	VS	Ablation of Spontaneous Ventilation

3. Develop primary and alternative strategies:

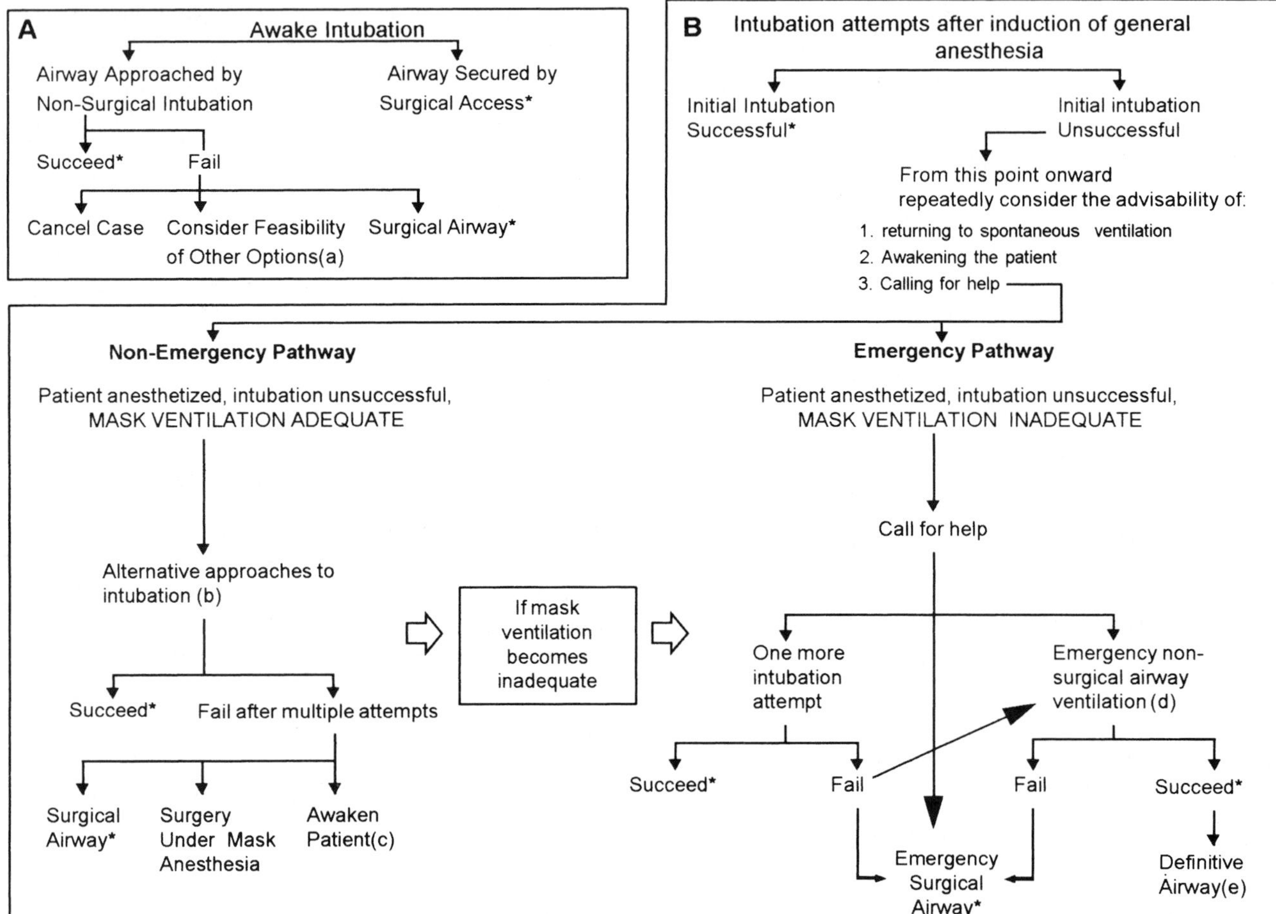

*** Confirm intubation with exhaled CO_2**

(a) Other options include (but are not limited to): surgery under mask anesthesia, surgery under local anesthesia infiltration or regional nerve blockade, or intubation attempts after induction of general anesthesia.

(b) Alternative approaches to difficult intubation include (but are not limited to): use of different laryngoscope blades, awake intubation, blind oral or nasal intubation, fiberoptic intubation, intubating stylet or tube changer, light wand, retrograde intubation, and surgical airway access.

(c) See awake intubation

(d) Options for emergency non-surgical airway ventilation include (but are not limited to): transtracheal jet ventilation, laryngeal mask ventilation, or esophageal-tracheal combitube ventilation.

(e) Options for establishing a definitive airway include (but are not limited to): returning to awake state with spontaneous ventilation, tracheotomy, or endotracheal intubation.

Figure 113–4. Algorithm for management of a difficult airway, developed by the American Society of Anesthesiologists Task Force. (From the American Society of Anesthesiologists Task Force on Management of the Difficult Airway: Practice Guidelines for Management of the Difficult Airway. Anesthesiology 1993; 78:597–602.)

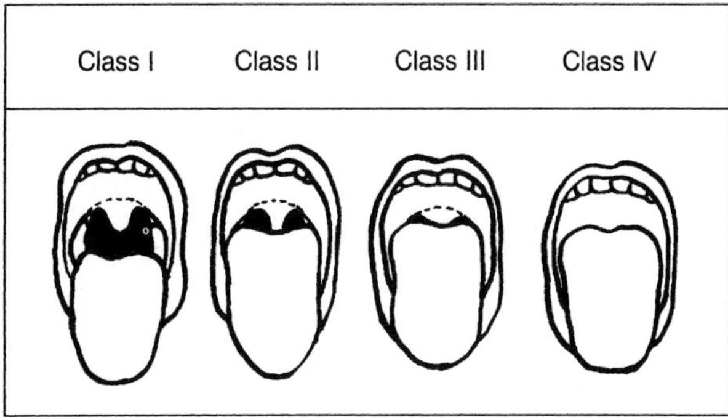

Figure 113–5. Mallampati classification of the airway. A *class I* airway affords view of the soft palate, fauces, uvula, and anterior and posterior tonsillar pillars; a *class II* airway, the soft palate, fauces, and uvula; a *class III* airway, the soft palate and base of the uvula; and a *class IV* airway, the soft palate only. (From Mallampati SR, Gatt SP, Gugino LD, et al: A clinical sign to predict difficult tracheal intubation: A prospective study. Can J Anaesth 1985; 32:429–435.)

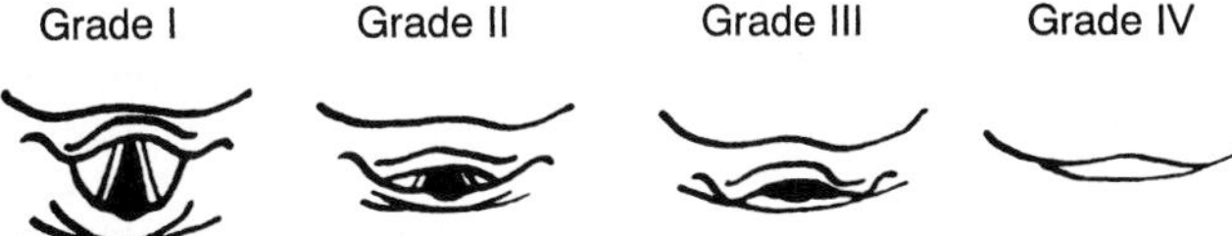

Figure 113–6. Laryngoscopic views of the laryngeal inlet. Grades I through IV show a progressive decrease in the number of structures visible. A grade I view allows inspection of the epiglottis, vocal cords, and surrounding structures. A grade IV view permits inspection of the epiglottis only. (From Cormack RS, Lehane J: Difficult tracheal intubation in obstetrics. Anaesthesia 1984; 39:1105.)

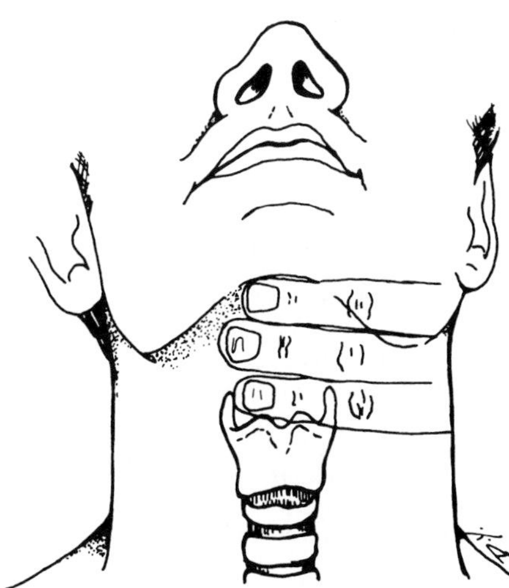

Figure 113–7. Assessment of thyromental distance. The fingers are placed such that one is touching the point of the chin and another the thyroid cartilage. The number of fingers or centimeters that span the mandibular space is the thyromental distance. (Courtesy of the Stratton Veterans Affairs Medical Center, Albany, N.Y.)

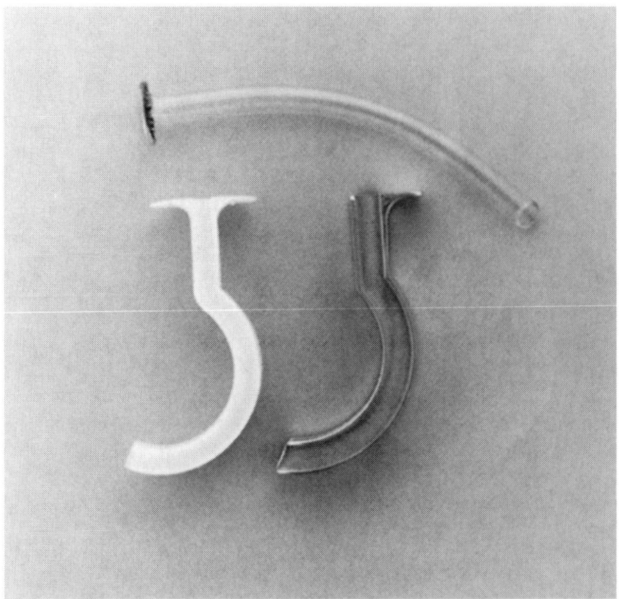

Figure 113–8. Nasopharyngeal and oral airways. *Top*, A nasopharyngeal airway. Note the angulation of the distal end. The opening should face the medial wall of the nares as the airway is inserted and advanced. *Left*, A conventional plastic oral airway. *Right*, A metal airway for use during fiberoptic bronchoscopic intubation. Note that the opening allows passage of a bronchoscope.

with the opening facing the septum and advanced with gentle downward pressure until it reaches the oropharynx. Advancement should proceed until airflow is optimal. One can test this by listening over the airway, auscultating the neck near the larynx, or feeling the flow with a hand held above the airway. Head tilt is necessary (jaw thrust may also be required) to hold the tongue away from the posterior pharyngeal wall between the airway and the laryngeal aperture[37]; therefore, these devices may not be helpful in patients with cervical spine instability.

The laryngeal mask airway (LMA) is a cuffed pharyngeal airway developed by Brain[38] in 1984 to obtain a direct connection with the patient's airway. Its use as well as that of the esophageal obturator airway (EOA) and pharyngotracheal lumen airway (PTLA) in the intensive care setting is described in another chapter.

Masks

Masks are an essential component of the airway apparatus (Fig. 113-9). Clear masks allow early visualization of regurgitation. The correct size varies from individual to individual, and a tight seal may be extremely difficult in edentulous and bearded patients. Placement of the mask over the nose and mouth while holding it in place with one hand and providing downward pressure with the thumb and first finger, at the same time raising the mandible with gentle pressure along its bony prominences (taking care not to exert pressure on the

TABLE 113–1. Contraindications to Nasal Intubation

Coagulopathy
Systemic anticoagulation
Severe intranasal disease
Basilar skull fracture
Head trauma with cerebrospinal fluid leak

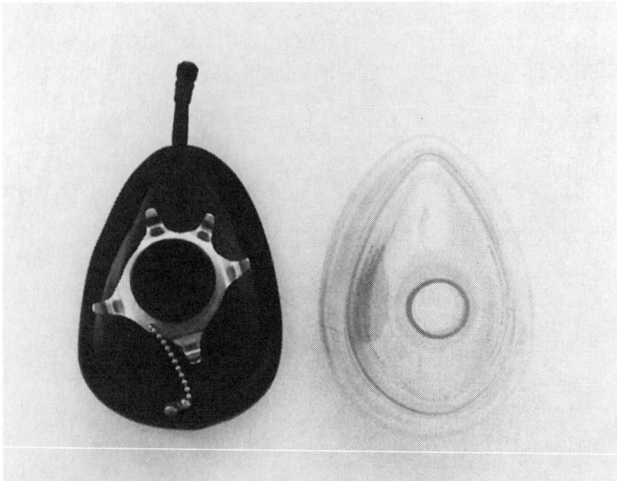

Figure 113–9. Anatomic masks. *Left*, A rubber (Saratoga) mask. Note that in this adaptation of the standard rubber mask, a chain is connected to a cover to provide for the passage of a fiberoptic scope. *Right*, A clear plastic mask that makes possible early visualization of regurgitation.

soft tissues), allows the other hand freedom for other tasks (e.g., inflation of a self-refilling bag-valve device).

Bag-Mask-Valve Units

The self-refilling bag-mask-valve unit was developed by Ruben[39] after devices by Kreiselman,[40] MacIntosh,[41] and the anesthesia bag-mask units.[42] It may be used with a mask, ETT, esophageal obturator airway, esophageal gastric tube airway (EGTA), pharyngotracheal lumen airway, combination esophagotracheal tube, tracheostomy tube, and laryngeal mask airway.

These units can deliver 100% oxygen if the reservoir is at least as large as the bag volume and the oxygen inflow rate at least equals the delivered minute volume. The bag should be squeezed and then quickly released to allow complete passive exhalation. With excessive flow rates and slow release, the valve may lock in the inspiratory position and lead to both barotrauma and decreased venous return to the heart.[37] A similar situation develops with hyperventilation and associated air trapping (auto-positive end-expiratory pressure generation), which are often seen in transport.

EQUIPMENT

Once an indication has been met for endotracheal intubation (Table 113-2), the equipment must be available immediately and checked before use to ensure proper functioning (Table 113-3). Monitoring of the patient is essential and should include a continuous visible electrocardiogram, a manual or automated blood pressure device, and continuous pulse oximetry. Peripheral intravenous access should be obtained rapidly.

As the patient is prepared for intubation (i.e., if the patient is conscious or semiconscious, a brief explanation of the plans should be conveyed to him or her), the bed is locked and positioned optimally for the laryngoscopist, topical local anesthetic and vasoconstrictor agents are applied as needed, and drugs for resuscitation are prepared. Ancillary personnel should assist in providing adequate oxygenation and necessary equipment, as previously outlined.

The equipment should be checked by the person who will assume responsibility for the initial attempt at intubation, and it should be arranged at the bedside for easy visualization and accessibility. Suction (with a Yankauer tip) should be on at 120 mm Hg negative pressure to facilitate pharyngeal suctioning as needed.

TABLE 113–2. Indications for Endotracheal Intubation*

Respiratory or ventilatory failure
Cardiac arrest
Acute respiratory distress syndrome
Pulmonary edema or embolism
Atelectasis
Neuromuscular disease or weakness (muscle relaxants, insecticides)
Pleural effusion
Near-drowning
Acute airway obstruction
Trauma
Tumor
Abscess
Infection (i.e., epiglottitis)
Coma
Tracheostenosis
Laryngeal edema
Airway protection
Trauma to upper airway
Central nervous system depressant overdose
Cerebrovascular accident
Status epilepticus
Upper airway burn or inhalation injury
Pulmonary toilet

*This list is not all-inclusive.

Laryngoscopes

A laryngoscope consists of a handle and blade. The blade contains the light source, a bulb, which should fit securely and tightly in its socket. Proper placement of the blade onto the handle results in an audible snap. The bulb should illuminate when the laryngoscope is in its position of function. Replacements should be available in case of malfunction.

TABLE 113–3. Equipment for Intubation

Mandatory Equipment
Suction Yankauer tip (large-bore tonsil tip) catheters (sized to permit passage through ETT)
Oxygen source
Bag-valve device
Masks (at least two sizes)
Oral and nasal airways
ETTs (include sizes smaller than anticipated)
Laryngoscope handle and blade (various sizes)
Syringe for cuff inflation
Stylet
Method of securing ETT (i.e., tape)
Monitors on: ECG, pulse oximetry, blood pressure cuff/device
Resuscitation drugs
Stethoscope
Highly Suggested Equipment
Tongue depressors
Local anesthetics (for topical application)
Topical vasoconstrictors
Lubricants
Intravenous access
End-tidal CO_2 monitoring

ETT = endotracheal tubes; ECG = electrocardiogram; CO_2 = carbon dioxide.

The two major classes of laryngoscope blades are curved (MacIntosh[43]) and straight (Miller[44]), respectively (Fig. 113–10). The tip of the curved blade should be placed in the vallecula and the epiglottis raised to expose the glottis. The straight blade lifts the epiglottis by lying under it. The choice of blade should depend on the experience of the laryngoscopist. Conscious patients may tolerate the MacIntosh blade better, because when it is correctly positioned in the vallecula, minimum stimulation of cranial nerves X and XII occurs. The short-handled laryngoscope[45] and the adjustable-angle laryngoscope[46] may be helpful in obese patients and in patients with large breasts and short necks. The blade lock allows adjustable positioning of the blade at various angles to the handle. This is extremely useful if the standard laryngoscope handle abuts the patient's chest on attempts to insert it.

The Bullard intubating laryngoscope (Circon ACMI, Stamford, Conn.) is a fiberoptic endoscope that uses the principles of indirect laryngoscopy to facilitate oral or nasal intubation. It has a broad, anatomically designed curved blade and introducing stylet (preshaped and easily attached to the laryngoscope), which allows easier visualization and intubation of the larynx.

The tip of the blade is placed at the base of the tongue in the vallecula or under the epiglottis, and force (minimum) is directed along the axis of the handle to obtain the desired view. The ETT can then be advanced off the intubating stylet through the glottis or, during nasotracheal intubation, advanced forward with forceps into the trachea. It is useful in patients with unstable cervical spines, because it requires no neck extension or flexion,[47] and in one author's experience it was extremely useful for intubation of patients with airway abnormalities.[48] Skills necessary for its use have to be acquired but are easily attained by those already experienced in direct laryngoscopy.[49]

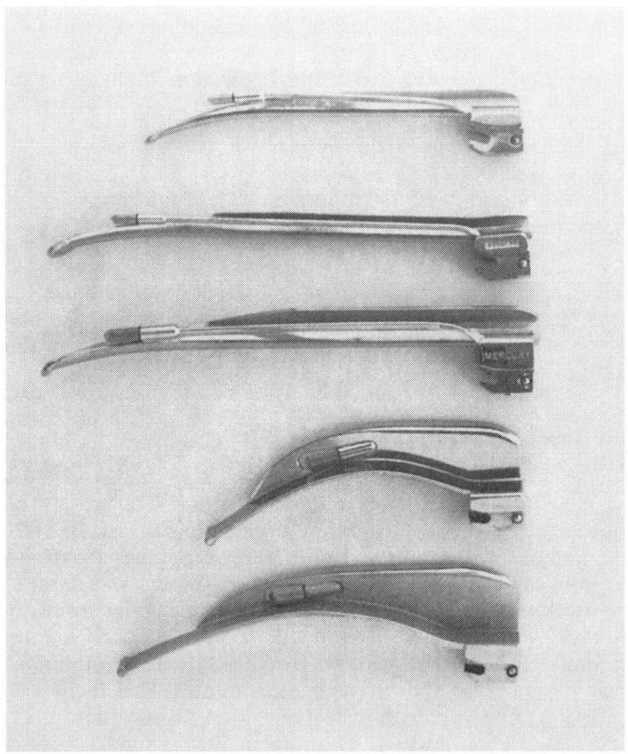

Figure 113–10. An assortment of laryngoscope blades. *From top to bottom*, Miller blades, sizes 2, 3, and 4; MacIntosh blades, sizes 3 and 4.

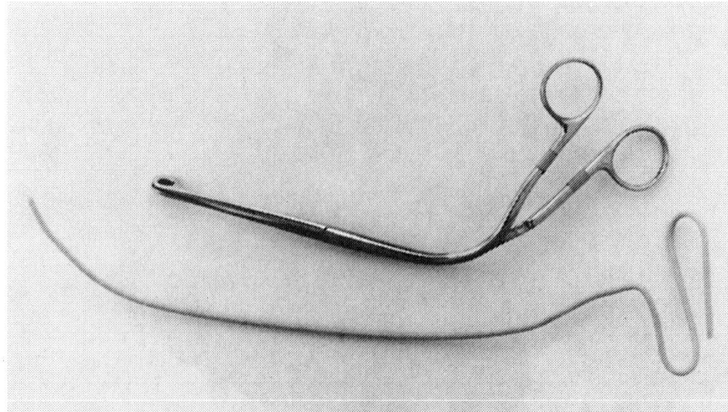

Figure 113–11. *Top*, A Magill forceps is used to advance the endotracheal tube into the trachea during orotracheal or nasotracheal intubation under direct laryngoscopy. *Bottom*, A malleable stylet should be placed inside the endotracheal tube proximal to the Murphy eye. The tube can then be manipulated into the desired position.

Stylets

Stylets have been an aid to endotracheal intubation since the curved introducers of O'Dwyer.[9] The standard stylet is composed of a malleable substance (Fig. 113–11) and is inserted into the ETT and designed to maintain its curve. Its distal end should be proximal to the Murphy's eye of the ETT and its proximal end curved over the tube to prevent inadvertent forward slippage.

Several modifications of the stylet exist. The Flex-guide (Scientific Sales International, Kalamazoo, Mich.) has a proximal thumb ring to flex its distal end, guiding it through the glottic opening.[50] The Eschmann Introducer is a gum elastic bougie introducer (Sims Surgical, Inc., Keene, N.H.) whose distal end enters the laryngeal inlet followed by ETT advancement over it.[50, 51]

The illuminating intubating stylet was introduced in 1985[52] and is a unique adjunct to intubation techniques. The Steward Tracheal Light Wand may possess advantages over its predecessors.[53] With proper position, just before entering the trachea, a glow seen in the anterior neck is diminished if the esophagus is intubated.[50] Ellis and colleagues[54] found that tracheal intubation using a lighted stylet was as fast as direct laryngoscopy and easily learned.

Endotracheal Tubes

Most ETTs (Figs. 113–12 and 113–13) are composed of sterile, nontoxic polyvinyl chloride and are marked with IT (implant tested) or Z-79 (Z-79 Committee of the American National Standards Institute) to indicate that there has been no evidence of toxicity found on testing. The internal diameter in millimeters and lengthwise centimeter markings are imprinted along the side of each tube. The selection of internal diameter should be based on the age and gender of the patients (Table 113–4) to avoid excessive pressure on the tracheal mucosa.

High-volume, low-pressure cuffs adapt to the tracheal contour as intracuff and tracheal wall pressures equilibrate, forming a leak-free seal when inflated.[55] Excessive cuff pressure causing tracheal mucosal ischemia, although less likely than with earlier cuffs (low volume), can still occur if the cuff is inflated beyond the point of no leak. Typically, 4 to 6 mL of air is sufficient to just reach the no-leak point, but tracheal cuff pressure should be obtained and the cuff volume adjusted to maintain intracuff pressure less than 25 cm H_2O.

Once the ETT is placed, the cuff inflated, and initial verifi-

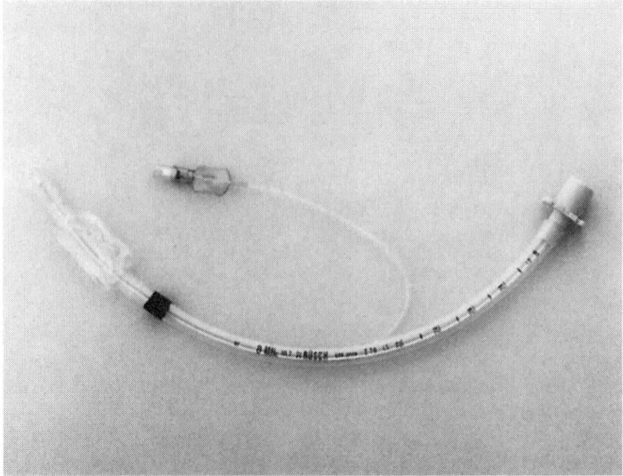

Figure 113–12. An endotracheal tube. Note the standard 14-mm adapter on the proximal end, the pilot balloon, and the cuff.

cation of placement performed (discussion follows), the tube should be secured. The lengthwise markings determine the distance from the end of the ETT to a landmark such as the lips or teeth (see Table 113–4).[56]

Esophagotracheal Double-Lumen Tube (Combitube)

With the development of the esophagotracheal double-lumen tube (Combitube), the esophageal obturator airway and the pharyngotracheal lumen airway may be obsolete. Improvement of the Combitube design has minimized previous problems with the esophageal obturator airway.[57] The Combitube is a disposable double-lumen cuffed tube with two balloons.[58, 59] Tube No. 2 (shorter clear tube) has an open distal end, and tube No. 1 (longer blue tube) has a blind distal end with pharyngeal side holes.

The Combitube is introduced blindly through the mouth, entering either the trachea or the esophagus (Fig. 113–14). It is advanced until the two proximal black rings are located between the upper and lower teeth. The pharyngeal balloon is inflated with 100 mL of air, occluding the pharynx, and the distal cuff is inflated with about 15 mL of air, occluding either the tracheal or esophageal lumen.[60] Wissler[57] recommended placing the Combitube into the esophagus under direct vision using a laryngoscope.

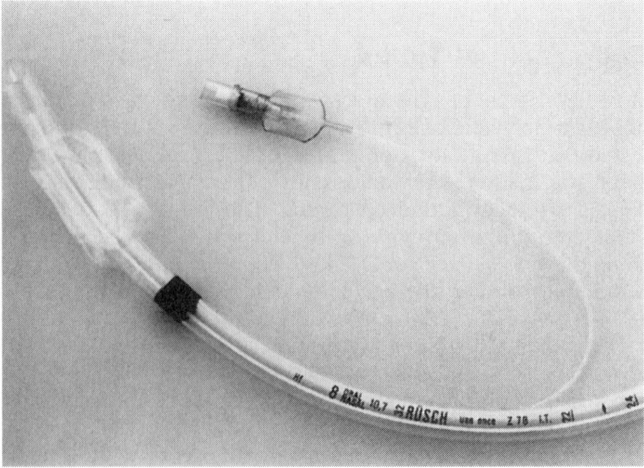

Figure 113–13. Magnification of markings on an endotracheal tube. The size (internal diameter) is marked in millimeters and expressed as a size French. The lengthwise markings indicate distance between the distal end in the midtrachea and the final secured position at the lips or teeth.

TABLE 113–4. Commonly Used Endotracheal Tube Sizes

Age	Distance from Midtrachea* to Lips/Teeth (cm)	Internal Diameter (mm)	French Gauge
Adult male	23–25	10.0	42
Adult male	23–25	9.5	40
Adult male	23–25	9.0	38
Adult male	21–25	8.5	36
Adult female	21–23	8.0, 7.5, 7.0, (6.5†, 6.0†)	34, 32, 30 (28, 26)

*Add 3 cm for nasal tubes.

†Should be available for all obstetric patients and patients with known tracheostenosis or suspected laryngeal edema.

Ventilation is initiated through tube No. 1. If the lungs inflate (bilateral chest expansion) and carbon dioxide is present by capnography and bilateral breath sounds are heard by auscultation, all without auscultation of gastric insufflation, ventilation is continued because the tube is properly placed in the esophagus (see Fig. 113–14*A*). When the Combitube is in the esophagus, tube No. 2 may be used for passage of a suction catheter into the stomach.[60]

If the lungs do not inflate (no chest expansion) and there is no evidence of carbon dioxide exhalation or breath sounds but there is auscultation of gastric insufflation, the tube is in the trachea and ventilation should immediately be switched to tube No. 2 (see Fig. 113–14*B*). Wissler[57] recommended titrating additional air to the proximal balloon (to a total of 160 mL)[61] to seal the upper pharynx and then an attempt to achieve adequate ventilation before switching to ventilation through tube No. 2.

Contraindications to use of the Combitube include the following:

1. Patients younger than 16 years of age and shorter than 5 feet.
2. Responsive patients with an intact gag reflex.
3. Patients with known esophageal disease.
4. Patients who have ingested caustic substances.

The Combitube has been used in patients with cardiac arrest[58, 59] and in cases of difficult intubation.[62–65] It may be a reasonable option in certain cases in which an ETT is unable to be placed.

AWAKE INTUBATION

Awake intubation should be considered in unfasted ("full-stomach") patients and in anticipated difficult airways. This approach is generally the safest option. In the awake state, spontaneous respiration and normal resting muscle tone protect the airway from aspiration. Under direct visualization, the awake-state airway structures clearly stand out from one another. Although safe, it may take more time and be more uncomfortable for the patient. Discomfort can be minimized with psychologic and airway preparation.[19] This includes a well-delineated explanation to the patient, topical and nerve block anesthesia, and use of an agent that minimizes orotracheal secretions.

The need for sedation should be carefully assessed individually. In preventing possible aspiration, intubation with local

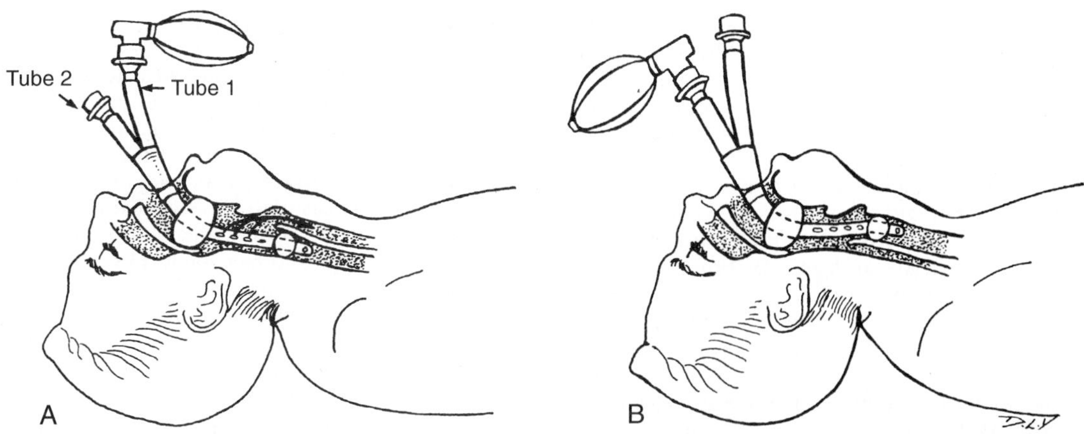

Figure 113–14. Placement of an esophageal-tracheal double-lumen tube (see text). *A*, Placement of the tube in the esophagus with the pharyngeal and distal cuffs inflated. Ventilation proceeds via the lumen of tube 1. *B*, Placement of the tube in the esophagus with the cuffs inflated. Ventilation proceeds through the lumen of tube 2. (Courtesy of the Stratton Veterans Affairs Medical Center, Albany, N.Y.)

anesthesia preparation (limited to the supraglottic region) of the airway without sedation is safer than intubation using sedation without local anesthesia.[66] If sedation is used, it should be titrated to effect. In addition, one agent should be used, and its antagonist should be immediately available (e.g., midazolam and flumazenil). One should recognize that if the use of an antagonist becomes necessary, the protective reflexes may be lost during the time required for reversal.

Various approaches of awake intubation may be used. The techniques of oral, nasal (blindly under direct laryngoscopy or with fiberoptic endoscopy), and retrograde intubation are described in the following sections.

Orotracheal Intubation

Different techniques of orotracheal intubation include:

1. Blind orotracheal intubation.
2. Orotracheal intubation under direct laryngoscopy.
3. Orotracheal intubation with fiberoptic bronchoscopy.

Orotracheal intubation should be used in patients who have absolute or relative contraindications to nasal intubation (see Table 113-1). In addition, because of the potential for nasal bleeding, the oral route is generally used in pediatric and obstetric populations. The importance of head and neck positioning cannot be overemphasized. The "sniffing position" in the supine patient is an attempt to align the axes of the mouth, pharynx, and larynx. The head is elevated about 10 cm on a pad, the base of the neck is flexed slightly, and the head is extended. Oral tubes tend to be larger than those used nasally and are advantageous in patients with excessive secretions or with a need for endotracheal toilet.

Blind Orotracheal Intubation

Blind orotracheal intubation by digital technique (without a laryngoscope) and blind orotracheal intubation with a laryngoscope (but without direct visualization of anatomic landmarks) are alternatives best reserved for experienced personnel familiar with these techniques. These techniques may be helpful in difficult intubations, especially in trauma victims (i.e., gunshot wound to face) and in cases in which all visual anatomic landmarks are obscured (e.g., by blood). If the patient is breathing spontaneously, listening to exhaled air passing from the proximal end of the ETT may aid the clinician as it can with blind nasal intubations.

Orotracheal Intubation Under Direct Laryngoscopy

The laryngoscope is generally held in the clinician's left hand, and the blade is introduced into the right side of the patient's mouth. The physician advances the blade posteriorly and toward the midline, sweeping the tongue to the left and holding it away from the visual path to the larynx. When the tonsillar fossa is reached with a curved blade, the blade is slipped into the vallecula. Traction along the axis of the laryngoscope handle will lift the base of the tongue, thereby exposing the larynx (Fig. 113-15). The upper incisors must not be used as a fulcrum. If the epiglottis is seen overhanging the larynx, the tip of the blade is advanced farther into the vallecula. If the esophagus is seen, the blade is withdrawn until the larynx comes into view.

A straight blade should be slipped under the epiglottis. If the laryngeal aperture is obscured by a large floppy epiglottis,

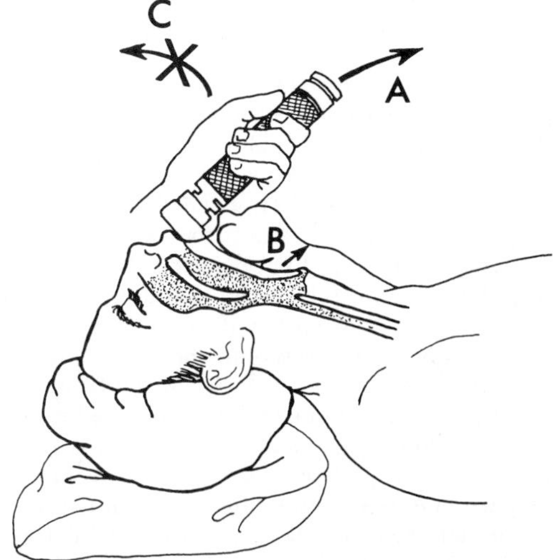

Figure 113–15. Correct alignment of the oral, pharyngeal, and laryngeal axes, with elevation of the head on a pad and head extension. The direction of force should follow the *arrows A* and *B*. If the laryngoscope force is positioned in the direction of *arrow C*, tooth damage and inadequate laryngoscopic view may result. (Adapted with permission from Roberts JT: Fundamentals of Tracheal Intubation. New York, Grune & Stratton, 1983, p 78.)

it may be helpful to pass the blade intentionally into the esophagus and then slowly withdraw it until the vocal cords are seen.

If the larynx is anterior and not well seen, applying gentle pressure dorsally on the thyroid cartilage by an assistant may help bring the vocal cords fully into view.

The glottic opening is triangular and is bounded by the true vocal cords. Often only epiglottic cartilage or the cuneiform and arytenoid projections are observed. Downward and cephalad pressure on the thyroid cartilage may bring the vocal cords into view. This position can be held by an assistant as the ETT is advanced and secured in place. In bearded patients, cloth ties ("umbilical tape") or Velcro straps may be used instead of adhesive tape.[50]

Although variation exists, the adult trachea is approximately 15 cm long.[13] The proper position of the ETT tip is roughly the middle third of the trachea with the head in a neutral position.[67] Conrady and associates[67] demonstrated that the tip of the ETT advances distally about 1.9 cm with neck flexion and is withdrawn proximally about 1.9 cm with neck extension.

Orotracheal Intubation with Fiberoptic Bronchoscopy

Although orotracheal intubation and nasotracheal intubation with fiberoptic bronchoscopy are similar, the oral route is usually more difficult. Therefore, oral fiberoptic intubation is chosen as a preferred method only when it is necessary to avoid the nasal route.

Use of the oral route permits passage of a larger ETT and is associated with less tissue trauma and bleeding,[19] although it is technically more difficult. If assisted ventilation is required, fiberoptic bronchoscopy can be continued with the use of an endoscopic mask that includes a port through which the FOB is passed[19] (see Fig. 113-9).

Careful airway preparation with anesthesia is achieved as with a nasal fiberoptic intubation (excluding the nasal passages). An airway intubator is then gently placed into the midline of the mouth (see Fig. 113-8). The ETT must be smaller than the airway intubator (e.g., an 8-mm ETT or smaller should be used with a No. 9 airway intubator). The FOB is threaded through the ETT, which sits at the external end of the FOB.[19]

The FOB and light source should be checked thoroughly and lubricated with clear lubricating fluid. An antifog agent should be applied to the lens, and the instrument should then be focused before use.[50] To enable movement of the tip, the FOB is held in an anteroposterior axis.[19] The FOB is then inserted through the airway intubator. A constant flow of oxygen maintained through the operating channel provides a higher inspired oxygen concentration and at the same time pushes mucus, blood, and secretions away from the lens.[50] A local anesthetic can be sprayed onto the vocal cords through the same channel of the FOB. The airway intubator facilitates the path to the larynx.[19] After the FOB is passed through the airway intubator, the epiglottis or vocal cords may be in view. The FOB must be maneuvered just posterior to the epiglottis and then back anteriorly until the vocal cords are in the center of the field.[50] While this view is maintained, the FOB is advanced between the vocal cords into the trachea. The ETT is passed over the FOB until it is in proper position in the trachea. The FOB is then used to confirm proper ETT position before it is removed.

Complications associated with fiberoptic bronchoscopy include hypoxemia (usually lasting between 1 and 4 hours), arrhythmias, and increased resistance to airflow.

Nasotracheal Intubation

The decision to place a nasotracheal tube in an ICU patient may be related to the presence of traumatic and surgical deformities (fractured mandible, maxillofacial surgery). Personal bias (i.e., level of comfort) of the clinician is influential, although no clear advantage in level of the patient's comfort or nursing care exists with nasotracheal intubation.[68, 69] Before this decision is made, contraindications to nasotracheal intubation should be reviewed (see Table 113-1).

Nasotracheal intubation can be performed in the awake or anesthetized patient with use of blind, direct laryngoscopic or fiberoptic (bronchoscope or Bullard laryngoscope) guidance. Awake techniques with use of nerve blocks and supplemental topical anesthesia are discussed.

After proper psychologic and sedative preparation of the conscious patient, the nasal mucosa should be anesthetized. This can be accomplished with the use of soaked cotton-tipped applicators or pledgets. If cocaine is used, a vasoconstrictor need not be applied. If not, a topical vasoconstrictor in spray form should be used after adequate absorption of the local anesthetic is ensured.

The glossopharyngeal nerve (lingual branch) and the superior laryngeal nerve (internal branch) can be blocked effectively, permitting intubation with minimal discomfort of the patient and hemodynamic alteration. These procedures are time-consuming and may have to be forgone in the emergency setting.

The superior laryngeal nerve can be blocked by either one of two techniques: internal or external. The internal block is performed by coating each piriform fossa with local anesthetic-soaked pledgets.[19] The external approach[70] involves sterile preparation of the extended neck. The hyoid bone is then palpated, displaced laterally toward the side to be blocked as a 25-gauge needle is placed on the greater cornu of this bone, walked off inferiorly, and advanced through the thyrohyoid membrane. A slight loss of resistance is felt, and 3 mL of local anesthetic is injected on either side of the membrane after negative aspiration of blood. This block should be performed bilaterally. The laryngeal epiglottis, vallecula, vestibule, arytenoepiglottic folds, and rima glottidis are anesthetized if this block is properly performed.

In addition, the lingual branch of the glossopharyngeal nerve can be blocked by injection of local anesthetic into the palatoglossal arch, where it meets the base of the tongue, with use of a 25-gauge spinal needle.[19] After negative aspiration of blood, 2 mL of 2% lidocaine should be injected in incremental doses. This should be repeated on the contralateral side. If the block is effective, the posterior third of the tongue and the pharyngeal surface of the epiglottis (vallecula) are anesthetized with all protective airway reflexes intact. If it is performed alone, care should be taken to anesthetize the larynx adequately either by spray or nebulized inhalation of local anesthetic solution, which anesthetizes the trachea as well. Care should be taken to quantify the amount of local anesthetic used to avoid systemic toxicity.

Blind nasotracheal intubation is performed through the larger naris. A tube 1 mm (internal diameter) smaller than that used for orotracheal intubation is selected and placed with the bevel facing the nasal septum. A lubricant placed on the tube will ease its passage as it is guided posteriorly and caudad into the pharynx. Slight resistance may be met as the tube passes the inferior turbinate bone of the naris. Breath sounds can be heard as the tube is advanced. As the patient reaches late inspiration, the tube should be placed through the laryngeal aperture. If the patient is breathing spontaneously and breath sounds cease during this maneuver, the tube should be withdrawn until breath sounds are again heard and then readvanced. Flexion of the neck and lateral bending toward the side of nasotracheal intubation may guide the tube into the trachea.[16]

If there are no contraindications, direct laryngoscopy or indirect laryngoscopy with the laryngeal retraction blade (Bullard laryngoscope) may facilitate nasotracheal intubation. The tube should first be guided into the pharynx, as stated previously. Then the laryngoscope is placed in the mouth with the techniques already described, a view of the laryngeal aperture is obtained, and the tube is advanced into the trachea. Magill forceps (see Fig. 113–11) may be used to grasp the distal end of the tube and guide it through the glottis. As in all endotracheal intubations, correct placement should be confirmed (see later).

Intubation of the trachea with flexible fiberoptic bronchoscopy is useful for patients with known or anticipated difficult airways or patients in whom airway and associated structure abnormalities may obscure a view of the larynx. The same preparation should precede initiation of this technique. Once preparation is completed, the lubricated FOB is inserted through the ETT, which has been placed in the oropharynx. It is then advanced into the trachea, the ETT is passed over the FOB into the trachea, the FOB is removed, and the ETT adapter is returned to its proper position. Again, confirmation of the placement should follow. This technique takes well-practiced skill and should not be performed in the emergency setting. Further descriptions of the technique are beyond the scope of this chapter.

Retrograde Intubation

The technique of retrograde intubation is suitable for the management of the difficult airway in a spontaneously breathing patient in the nonfasted state. This technique requires preparation and time to perform, and it is not ideal for emergency airway access. As always, the patient should be prepared for awake intubation (see previous discussion).

The cricothyroid membrane is punctured with an 18-gauge needle after sterile preparation of the field and skin infiltration with a local anesthetic. The bevel should be directed cephalad at an angle of approximately 45°. When the trachea is entered, as confirmed by aspiration of air, a flexible guide wire is threaded retrogradely between the vocal cords, into the pharynx, and out through the mouth. The needle is removed, and the guide wire is clamped at the skin.

The guide wire is held taut, and the ETT is advanced over the guide wire, with rotation if necessary, until it has passed between the cords into the larynx. The wire is withdrawn, and the ETT is advanced farther into the trachea.

To make the guiding system effectively stiffer and larger in diameter, one may pass the nasogastric tube anterogradely over the wire.[71]

An FOB can be used in a similar manner. The guide wire is threaded through the suction channel of the FOB, which has been passed through an ETT. The tube is positioned under direct vision, and the guide wire is removed through the proximal port of the FOB suction channel.[72]

Confirmation of Endotracheal Tube Placement

Confirmation of ETT placement is crucial. An incorrectly placed ETT is usually not a problem if it is immediately recognized.

Every tracheal intubation needs to be assessed by clinical methods. Several maneuvers and techniques make up the clinical assessment of correct ETT placement. Direct visualization of the ETT passing between the vocal cords, followed by inspection, palpation, and auscultation of the chest, is necessary. The chest wall should rise and fall with equal excursion bilaterally. Auscultation of bilateral breath sounds in the lung apices laterally is mandatory after intubation. Placement of the stethoscope bell behind the pectoralis major muscle in the axilla where chest wall mass is minimum may be preferable, especially in obese patients. Sounds may be transmitted elsewhere, yielding false-positive results. Auscultation over the epigastrium to confirm no air movement is also indicated. Visualization of water vapor with exhalation and "the feel of the bag" cannot be relied on but are part of the picture of proper tube placement, as is maintenance or improvement of preintubation oxygenation.

Clinical assessment must also be accompanied by verification of exhaled carbon dioxide. Considering the vagaries of all other methods of assessment of proper ETT placement and the simplicity and accuracy of measurement of continuous exhaled carbon dioxide, the continuous exhaled carbon dioxide technique should be employed in all patients whenever possible to confirm proper ETT placement. End-tidal carbon dioxide may be assessed with capnography (the best method), capnometry, or disposable colorimetric indicators, which change color when they are exposed to carbon dioxide. These disposable devices can be attached to the proximal end of the ETT and are used during active ventilation.

Extremely low cardiac output states may yield false-negative results because inadequate carbon dioxide is transported to the lungs to be detected in the exhaled air. Recent ingestion of carbonated fluids may yield false-positive results because carbonation may be detected as carbon dioxide; however, the signal and waveform are not maintained.

Additional techniques to confirm intubation include the use of fiberoptic bronchoscopy and the lighted stylet. An FOB passed through the ETT yields confirmation of correct placement if the tracheal rings and carina are observed. A lighted stylet advanced through the ETT to the level of the suprasternal notch transilluminates the anterior neck if the tube is in its proper position.

In 1988, Wee[73] described an esophageal detector device to help assess correct ETT placement. It is a 60-mL syringe with a catheter tip and an airtight attachment to a standard catheter mount with a 15-mm fitting. The 15-mm fitting is attached to the ETT, and aspiration with the syringe is initiated. Easy flow with minimum resistance is supportive of proper position in the trachea. Resistance to aspiration may indicate incorrect placement.[53]

Radiologic confirmation must always be performed but should not be relied on because the deleterious effects of an incorrectly placed tube will have already begun and may be irreversible before its completion. All methods to confirm ETT placement are fallible; therefore, the total picture of maintained adequate oxygenation, continuous carbon dioxide detection, and clinical assessment needs to be considered. If the clinician is uncertain of correct placement of the ETT, it should be removed and the patient ventilated by mask before any reattempts at intubation.

SPECIAL CONSIDERATIONS

Nonfasting (Full-Stomach) Patient

Considered in the nonfasting category are the following:

- Parturient patients
- The morbidly obese
- Diabetic patients with gastroparesis
- Patients who have just eaten
- Patients with known gastroesophageal reflux and hiatal hernia

- Patients with bowel obstruction, upper gastrointestinal hemorrhage, peritonitis, active nausea and vomiting, or incompetent lower esophageal sphincter
- Trauma and head-injury patients
- Patients who have diminished bowel transit time (possibly secondary to pain, narcotics, disease processes, and so on)

All of these patients are at increased risk for pulmonary aspiration of gastric contents and therefore require either a sedative-assisted, topical anesthetic "awake" intubation or a rapid-sequence induction. The extent of lung injury from aspiration is more extensive with fecal or bacterial material, particulate matter, volumes greater than 25 mL (or 0.4 mL/kg), and more acidic pH (<2.5). Pharmacologic premedication before attempts at airway management has included nonparticulate antacids (e.g., 30 mL of 0.3 mol/L sodium citrate),[74] histamine (H_2) receptor antagonists,[75] and metoclopramide (a dopamine antagonist)[76] alone or in combination.[75, 77] Metoclopramide acts as an antiemetic, accelerates gastric emptying, and increases lower esophageal sphincter pressure.

The best airway protection is afforded by a properly placed cuffed ETT. The laryngeal mask airway, esophageal obturator airway, esophageal gastric tube airway, and pharyngotracheal lumen airway do not provide adequate airway protection from regurgitation of gastric contents in the full-stomach patient.

Rapid-Sequence Induction

After checking all equipment (see earlier text and Table 113–3) and availability of a trained assistant, the clinician may proceed with preoxygenation for at least 3 minutes at high oxygen flow. If time does not permit 3 minutes of preoxygenation, four vital capacity breaths of 100% oxygen can be substituted, but this is not as effective.[78] A rapidly acting induction agent and rapidly acting muscle relaxant are administered, in sequence, and cricoid pressure is applied (Sellick's maneuver).[17] This maneuver is the application of pressure by a trained assistant with the thumb and index finger pushing on the cricoid cartilage with a dorsal and cephalad force against the sixth cervical vertebra to occlude the esophagus and prevent passive regurgitation of stomach contents. If intubation cannot be accomplished, the patient should immediately be ventilated while cricoid pressure is still held until proper ETT placement is confirmed or the patient is awake. Cricoid pressure is believed to be effective in preventing passive regurgitation of gastric contents with gastric pressures as high as 50 to 94 (mean, 74) cm H_2O.[79]

Cricoid pressure should not be released until the cuff is inflated and there is confirmation of proper ETT placement unless there is active regurgitation, at which point cricoid pressure is released and the patient is placed in Trendelenburg's position with the head turned to the side and suctioned. If intubation and ventilation cannot be accomplished (cannot intubate–cannot ventilate situation), the clinician should proceed immediately with alternative methods of securing an airway (see Fig. 113–4).[80]

Endotracheal Tube Exchange

If an ETT needs to be changed, it is prudent to use a jet stylet (especially with a difficult airway), which does not need to be removed to confirm proper ETT placement.[81] Any semirigid hollow catheter can be used as a jet stylet (e.g., tube exchanger). It is inserted through the ETT, and after the ETT is removed, the hollow catheter can be used for jet ventilation.[19] This technique can be invaluable in changing an ETT or extubating a patient with a difficult airway.[19, 82] An FOB may be used effectively as a jet stylet.[83] The FOB serves as a reintubation stylet, allowing jet ventilation, airway suctioning, and continuous oxygen administration. The FOB may also be used in a similar manner for extubation of patients in whom there is suspicion of airway injury or edema or of patients in whom access to the upper airway is limited (e.g., by halo traction).[83]

Pharmacologic Approaches to Blunt the Cardiovascular Response to Laryngoscopy and Intubation

Numerous pharmacologic agents are used to attempt attenuation of the hemodynamic responses to laryngoscopy and intubation. These include fentanyl,[84] intravenous lidocaine,[85] esmolol bolus[86] or infusion,[87] sodium nitroprusside,[88] intravenous nitroglycerin,[89] captopril,[90] labetalol,[91] alfentanil,[92] and combinations of these agents.

The Difficult Airway

Lack of gas exchange leads to morbidity and mortality, and in cases of acute airway obstruction with inability to ventilate or intubate, a plan of corrective action must progress rapidly. A difficult airway is defined as "the clinical situation in which a conventionally trained anesthesiologist experiences difficulty with mask ventilation, difficulty with tracheal intubation or both."[84]

Preparation, well-maintained airway management skills, and knowledge of the algorithm that the clinician should follow for airway maintenance are essential to the intensivist. Figure 113–4 presents the American Society of Anesthesiologists Task Force's algorithm developed to guide all clinicians who perform tracheal intubation in their medical practice. In addition, well-developed skill in other methods of airway access must be maintained.

SUMMARY

The maintenance of a patent airway and the ability to ventilate with adequate gas exchange are crucial. Airway control must be achieved rapidly to sustain a neurologically intact patient. Currently, no methods are adequate for effective rapid intravenous oxygenation. All clinicians should be familiar with the many aspects of airway management and should have a preplanned strategy when faced with emergency airway problems.

ACKNOWLEDGMENTS

We thank Ms. Jae Brady, secretary, Department of Anesthesiology, Albany Medical Center, for her excellent work with an earlier version of this chapter. We also thank Donna L. Youmans, medical illustrator, Department of Medical Media, Stratton Veterans Affairs Medical Center, Albany, N.Y., for her illustrations.

References

1. Vesalius A: De Humani Corporis Fabrica Libri Septem. Basel, Oporinus, 1543, p 658.
2. Faulconer A Jr, Keys TE: Foundations in Anesthesiology. Springfield, Ill, Charles C Thomas, 1965, pp 10–11.
3. Hooke R: On the theory of springs. Philos Trans R Soc London 1667; 2:539–540.
4. Mayow J: Tractatus Quinque Medico-Physici. Edinburgh, The Alembic Club, 1907, pp 183–210.
5. Macewen W: Clinical observations on the introduction of tracheal tubes by the mouth instead of performing tracheotomy or laryngotomy. Br Med J 1880; 2:122–124, 163–165.

6. Sykes WS: Essays on the First Hundred Years of Anaesthesia. 2nd ed. Edinburgh, Churchill Livingstone, 1982, pp 96–98.
7. Davison MH, Meredith HA: The Evolution of Anaesthesia. London, Williams & Wilkins, 1905.
8. Kuhn F: Die Pernasale Tubage. Munch Med Wochenschr 1902; 49:1456–1457.
9. O'Dwyer J: Med Rec 1887; 32:557.
10. Gillespie NA: Endotracheal Anesthesia. 2nd ed. Madison, Wisc, University of Wisconsin Press, 1948, pp 8–11, 75.
11. Rowbotham ES: An inflatable pharyngeal tube. Lancet 1944; 2:15.
12. Jackson C: The technique of insertion of intratracheal insufflation tubes. Surg Gynecol Obstet 1913; 17:507–509.
13. Ellis H, Feldman S: Anatomy for the Anaesthetist. London, Blackwell Scientific Publications, 1988.
14. Hollinshead WH: Textbook of Anatomy. 3rd ed. Hagerstown, Md, Harper & Row, 1974.
15. Mallampati SR, Gatt SP, Gugino LD, et al: A clinical sign to predict difficult tracheal intubation: A prospective study. Can J Anaesth 1985; 32:429–435.
16. Roberts JT: Fundamentals of Tracheal Intubation. New York, Grune & Stratton, 1983.
17. Sellick B: Cricoid pressure to control regurgitation of stomach contents during induction of anesthesia. Lancet 1961; 2:404–406.
18. Rex M: A review of the structural and functional basis of laryngospasm and a discussion of the nerve pathways involved in the reflex and its clinical significance in man and animals. Br J Anaesth 1970; 42:891–899.
19. Benumof JL: Management of the difficult adult airway: With special emphasis on awake tracheal intubation. Anesthesiology 1991; 75:1087–1110.
20. Bellhouse CP, Doré C: Criteria for estimating likelihood of difficulty of endotracheal intubation with Macintosh laryngoscope. Anaesth Intensive Care 1988; 16:329–337.
21. Mathew M, Hanna LS, Aldrete JA: Preoperative indices to anticipate a difficult tracheal intubation. Anesth Analg 1989; 68:51–87.
22. Samsoon GLT, Young JRB: Difficult tracheal intubation: A retrospective study. Anaesthesia 1987; 42:487–490.
23. Finucane BT, Santora AH: Evaluation of the airway prior to intubation. *In:* Principles of Airway Management. Philadelphia, FA Davis, 1988, pp 69–83.
24. Cohen SM, Zaurito CE, Segil LJ: Oral exam to predict difficult intubations: A large prospective study (Abstract). Anesthesiology 1989; 71:A937.
25. Cormack RS, Lehane J: Difficult tracheal intubation in obstetrics. Anaesthesia 1984; 39:1105–1111.
26. Hastings RH, Marks JD: Airway management for trauma patients with potential cervical spine injuries. Anesth Analg 1991; 73:471–482.
27. Patil VU, Stehling LC, Zauder HL: Techniques of endotracheal intubation. *In:* Fiberoptic Endoscopy in Anesthesia. Chicago, Year Book Medical Publishers, 1983, p 79.
28. Lyons G: Failed intubation: Six years experience in a teaching maternity unit. Anaesthesia 1985; 40:759–762.
29. King TA, Adams AP: Failed tracheal intubation. Br J Anaesth 1990; 65:400–414.
30. Morgan M: Anaesthetic contribution to maternal mortality. Br J Anaesth 1987; 59:842–855.
31. Ueland K: Maternal cardiovascular dynamics: VII. Intrapartum blood volume changes. Am J Obstet Gynecol 1976; 126:671–677.
32. Bonica JJ: Principles and Practice of Obstetric Analgesia and Anesthesia. Philadelphia, FA Davis, 1967.
33. Santos AC, Pedersen H, Finster M: Obstetric anesthesia. *In*: Clinical Anesthesia. 2nd ed. Barash PG, Cullen BF, Stoelting RK (Eds). Philadelphia, JB Lippincott, 1992, p 1278.
34. Rocke DA, Murray WB, Rout CL, et al: Relative risk analysis of factors associated with difficult intubation in obstetric anesthesia. Anesthesiology 1992; 77:67–73.
35. Murray FS, Eiskine JP, Fielding J: Gastric secretion in pregnancy. J Obstet Gynecol Br Commonw 1957; 64:373.
36. Morikawa S, Safar P, DeCarlo J: Influence of head position upon upper airway patency. Anesthesiology 1961; 22:265.
37. Safar P, Bircher-Nicholas G: Cardiopulmonary Cerebral Resuscitation. Philadelphia, WB Saunders, 1984.
38. Brain AIJ: The laryngeal mask airway: A possible new solution to airway problems in the emergency situation. Arch Emerg Med 1984; 1:229–232.
39. Ruben H: Combination resuscitator aspirator. Anesthesiology 1958; 19:408.
40. Kreiselman J: A new resuscitation apparatus. Anesthesiology 1943; 4:608.
41. MacIntosh RR: Oxford inflating bellows. Br Med J 1953; 2:202.
42. Hingson RA: Western Reserve anesthesia machine, oxygen inhalator and resuscitator. JAMA 1958; 167:1077.
43. MacIntosh R: A new laryngoscope. Lancet 1943; 1:914.
44. Miller R: A new laryngoscope. Anesthesiology 1941; 2:318.
45. Datta S, Briwa J: Modified laryngoscope for endotracheal intubation of obese patients. Anesth Analg 1981; 60:120–121.
46. Patil VU, Stehling LC, Zauder HL: An adjustable laryngoscope handle for difficult intubations (Letter). Anesthesiology 1984; 60:609.
47. Saunders PA, Geisecke AH: Clinical assessment of the adult Bullard laryngoscope. Can J Anesth 1989; 36:S118–S119.
48. Gorback MS: Management of the challenging airway with the Bullard laryngoscope. J Clin Anesth 1991; 3:473–477.
49. Borland LM, Caselbrant M: The Bullard laryngoscope: A new indirect oral laryngoscope (pediatric version). Anesth Analg 1990; 70:105–108.
50. Stehling LC: Management of the airway. *In*: Clinical Anesthesiology. 2nd ed. Barash PG, Cullen BF, Stoelting RK (Eds). Philadelphia, JB Lippincott, 1992.
51. Kidd JF, Dyson A, Latto IP: Successful difficult intubation: Use of the gum elastic bougie. Anaesthesia 1988; 43:437–438.
52. Vollmer TP, Stewart RD, Paris PH, et al: Use of a lighted stylet for guided orotracheal intubation in the prehospital setting. Ann Emerg Med 1985; 14:324–328.
53. Baskett PJF: Difficult and impossible intubation in the anaesthetic crisis. Baillieres Clin Anesthesiol 1993; 7:261–280.
54. Ellis DG, Jakvmec A, Kaplan RM, et al: Guided orotracheal intubation in the operating room using a lighted stylet: A comparison with direct laryngoscopic technique. Anesthesiology 1986; 64:823–826.
55. Dorsch JA, Dorsch SE: Understanding Anesthesia Equipment. Baltimore, Williams & Wilkins, 1984, pp 353–400.
56. Owen RL, Cheney FW: Endobronchial intubation: A preventable complication. Anesthesiology 1987; 67:255–257.
57. Wissler RN: The esophageal-tracheal Combitube. Anesth Rev 1993; 20:147–152.
58. Frass M, Frenzer R, Zdrahal F, et al: The esophageal tracheal Combitube: Preliminary results with a new airway for CPR. Ann Emerg Med 1987; 16:768–772.
59. Frass M, Frenzer R, Rauscha F, et al: Ventilation with the esophageal tracheal Combitube in cardiopulmonary resuscitation: Promptness and effectiveness. Chest 1988; 93:781–784.
60. Sheridan Catheter Corp: Package insert for the esophageal tracheal double lumen tube. Argyl, NY, Sheridan Catheter Corporation.
61. Frass M, Johnson JC, Atherton GL, et al: Esophageal tracheal Combitube (ETC) for emergency intubation: Anatomical evaluation of ETC placement by radiography. Resuscitation 1989; 18:95–102.
62. Frass M, Frenzer R, Zahler J, et al: Ventilation via the oesophageal tracheal Combitube in cases of difficult intubation. J Cardiothorac Anaesth 1987; 1:565–568.
63. Bigenzahn W, Pesau B, Frass M: Emergency ventilation using the Combitube in cases of difficult intubation. Eur Arch Otorhinolaryngol 1991; 248:129–131.
64. Eichinger S, Schreiber W, Heinz T, et al: Airway management in a case of neck impalement: Use of the oesophageal tracheal Combitube airway. Br J Anaesth 1992; 68:534–535.
65. Klauser R, Roggla G, Pidlich J, et al: Massive upper airway bleeding after thrombolytic therapy: Successful airway management with the Combitube. Ann Emerg Med 1992; 21:431–433.
66. Kopriva CJ, Eltringham RJ, Siebert PE: A comparison of the effects of intravenous Innovar and topical spray on the laryngeal closure reflex. Anesthesiology 1974; 40:596–598.
67. Conrady PA, Goodman LR, Lainge F, et al: Alteration of endotracheal tube position. Crit Care Med 1976; 4:7–12.
68. Stone DJ, Bogdonoff DL: Airway considerations in the management of patients requiring long-term endotracheal intubation. Anesth Analg 1992; 74:276–287.
69. Stauffer JL, Olson DE, Petty TL: Complications and consequence

of endotracheal intubation and tracheostomy. Am J Med 1981; 70:65–76.
70. Wedel DJ, Brown DL: Nerve blocks. *In*: Anesthesia. 3rd ed. Miller RD (Ed). New York, Churchill Livingstone, 1990, p 1429.
71. King HK, Wang LF, Khan AK, et al: Translaryngeal guided intubation for difficult intubation. Crit Care Med 1987; 15:869–871.
72. Lechman MJ, Donahoo JS, MacVaugh H: Endotracheal intubation using percutaneous retrograde guide wire insertion followed by antegrade fiberoptic bronchoscopy. Crit Care Med 1986; 14:589–590.
73. Wee MYK: The oesophageal detector device. Anaesthesia 1988; 43:27–29.
74. Gibbs CP, Spohr L, Schmidt D: The effectiveness of sodium citrate as an antacid. Anesthesiology 1982; 57:44–46.
75. Hodgkinson R, Glassenberg R, Joyce TH III, et al: Comparison of cimetidine (Tagamet) with antacid for safety and effectiveness in reducing acidity before elective cesarean section. Anesthesiology 1983; 59:86–90.
76. Murphy DF, Nally B, Gardiner J, et al: Effect of metoclopramide on gastric emptying before elective and emergency cesarean section. Br J Anaesth 1984; 56:1113–1116.
77. Manchikanti L, Marrero TC, Roush JR: Preanesthetic cimetidine and metoclopramide for acid aspiration prophylaxis in elective surgery. Anesthesiology 1984; 61:48–54.
78. Gambee AM, Hertzka RE, Fisher DM: Preoxygenation techniques: Comparison of three minutes and four breaths. Anesth Analg 1987; 66:468–470.
79. Fanning GL: The efficacy of cricoid pressure in regurgitation of gastric contents. Anesthesiology 1970; 32:553–555.
80. American Society of Anesthesiologists Task Force on Management of the Difficult Airway: Practice guidelines for management of the difficult airway. Anesthesiology 1993; 78:597–602.
81. Goskowicz R, Gaughan S, Benumof JL, et al: It is not necessary to remove a jet stylet to determine tracheal tube location. J Clin Anesth 1992; 4:42–44.
82. Bedger RC, Chang JL: A jet stylet catheter for difficult airway management. Anesthesiology 1987; 66:221–223.
83. Wheeler S, Fontenot R, Gaughan S, et al: Use of a fiberoptic bronchoscope as a jet stylet. Anesthesiol Rev 1993; 20:16–17.
84. Martin DE, Rosenberg H, Aukburg SJ, et al: Low dose fentanyl blunts circulatory responses to tracheal intubation. Anesth Analg 1982; 61:680.
85. Splinter WM, Cervenko F: Haemodynamic responses to laryngoscopy and tracheal intubation in geriatric patients: Effects of fentanyl, lidocaine and thiopentone. Can J Anaesth 1989; 36:370–376.
86. Ebert TJ, Bernstein JS, Stowe DF, et al: Attenuation of hemodynamic responses to rapid sequence induction and intubation in healthy patients with a single bolus of esmolol. J Clin Anesth 1990; 2:243–252.
87. Ebert JP, Pearson JD, Gelman S, et al: Circulating responses to laryngoscopy: The comparative effects of placebo, fentanyl and esmolol. Can J Anaesth 1989; 36:301–306.
88. Stoelting RK: Attenuation of blood pressure response to laryngoscopy and tracheal intubation with sodium nitroprusside. Anesth Analg 1979; 58:116–119.
89. Grover VK, Sharma S, Mahajan RP: Low-dose intranasal nitroglycerine attenuates pressor response (Letter). Anesthesiology 1987; 66:722.
90. McCarthy GJ, Hainsworth M, Lindsay K, et al: Pressor responses to tracheal intubation after sublingual captopril: A pilot study. Anaesthesia 1990; 45:243–245.
91. Bernstein JS, Ebert TJ, Stowe DF, et al: Partial attenuation of hemodynamic responses to rapid sequence induction and intubation with labetalol. J Clin Anesth 1989; 1:444–451.
92. Martineau RJ, Tousignant CP, Miller DR, et al: Alfentanil controls the haemodynamic response during rapid-sequence induction of anaesthesia. Can J Anaesth 1990; 37:755–761.

114

Patient-Ventilator Interactions

Neil R. MacIntyre, MD

In the acute phases of respiratory failure, near total mechanical ventilator support is required in order to provide adequate gas exchange and to unload fatigued ventilatory muscles.[1] This often requires depressing or ablating the patient's spontaneous ventilatory activity with heavy sedation or neuromuscular blockade. As gas exchange abnormalities stabilize and the neuromuscular system recovers its functional capabilities, however, ventilatory support modes that permit some degree of spontaneous ventilatory activity can be used as an alternative to controlled, total support.[2] These modes are often termed "interactive" in that patients can affect various aspects of the mechanical ventilator's functions; that is, interactive modes allow patients and ventilators to share the work of breathing.

Patient-ventilator interactions can range from simple triggering of mechanical breaths to more complex processes affecting delivered flow patterns and breath timing. Advantages to interactive modes of support versus controlled modes of support are twofold:

1. Lower ventilator pressures are generally required with interactive modes.
2. Interactive modes generally call for less sedation. This benefit, coupled with avoidance of neuromuscular blockers, may reduce long-term mental status abnormalities and muscle dysfunction.[2, 3]

Interactive modes can be either *synchronous* or *dyssynchronous* with patient efforts.[2, 3] Synchronous interactions mean that the ventilator is *sensitive* to the initiation and termination of a patient's ventilatory effort and is *responsive* to the flow characteristics of the patient's ventilatory demand.[1-3] Dyssynchronous interactions occur when ventilator gas delivery and patient efforts are not coordinated or are "out of phase." Synchronizing patient-ventilator interactions is important to avoid "imposed" muscle loading that can occur when ventilator gas delivery and patient efforts are not matched.[3, 4] Synchronous interactions prevent unnecessary ventilatory muscle oxygen consumption and often improve patient comfort, since patients are not "fighting" the ventilator.[3, 5]

The remainder of this chapter addresses patient-ventilator interactions by (1) considering the determinants of the spontaneous ventilatory drive, (2) considering ventilator sensors, and (3) reviewing the design characteristics of available interactive ventilatory support modes.

DETERMINANTS OF THE SPONTANEOUS VENTILATORY PATTERN

The ventilatory control system is located in the brain stem and receives input from several sources (Fig. 114–1).[6, 7] Among these are gas exchange sensors (i.e., pH, Pa_{O_2}), stretch receptors in the lung and thoracic cage, irritant and J receptors within the lung, cortical influences and other factors (e.g., hormonal influences, cardiac output). The output of the ventilatory control system can be characterized by the timing and

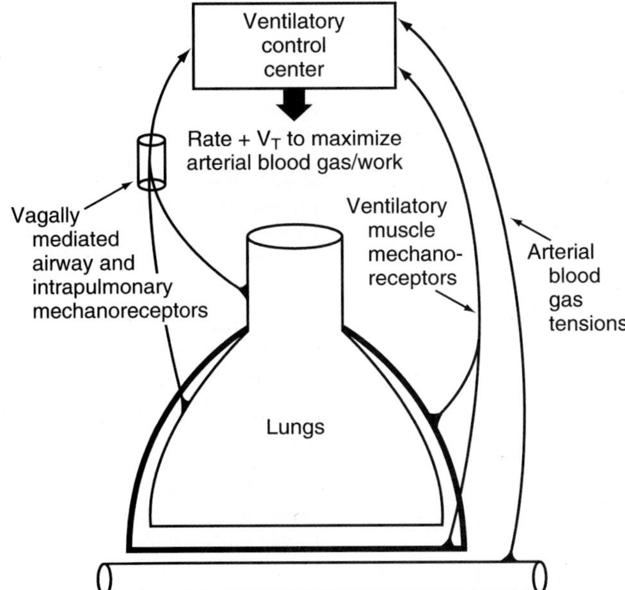

Figure 114–1. Schematic depiction of the various inputs into the ventilatory control center. Ventilatory control center output, in general, is designed to provide the best gas exchange for the least amount of work.

intensity of the phrenic nerve signal.[6-9] Timing is often described by the inspiratory time (TI) and expiratory time (TE) partitioning and the inverse of TI + TE, the respiratory frequency.[6-9] The intensity of the tidal breath signal is reflected in the electromyogram (EMG) signal, the airway occlusion pressure at 100 msec ($P_{0.1}$), the change in pressure with respect to time (dP/dt) of the inspiratory muscles, and the actual magnitude of the tidal volume.[6-9]

The overall goal of the ventilatory control system is to generate a breathing pattern that provides the best gas exchange for the least amount of ventilatory muscle energy utilization (the *minimal work concept*).[10] This simple construct, however, can be altered by the other factors already noted. Specifically, as muscles become overloaded or as irritant receptors become more active (as in dyspnea), the frequency may increase beyond the "minimal work" constraint.[7,10-14] In addition, poor cardiac function can lead to bradypnea or apnea and hyperinflation may result in a lengthening of TE in order to improve lung emptying. The ventilatory control system also responds to the effects of mechanical ventilation. For instance, as respiratory muscles become unloaded with appropriate mechanical ventilation, the abnormal mechanical input to the ventilatory control center may be lessened and an abnormal ventilatory pattern (e.g., tachypnea) may revert to a more normal one.[15] This is the physiologic basis for setting levels of mechanical ventilation according to ventilatory pattern endpoints (rate or rate/tidal volume). Similarly, the ventilatory control system may also respond to loads imposed by dyssynchronous mechanical ventilator settings. This response is often similar to the response to other causes of excess muscle loading (e.g., tachypnea, dyspnea, and abdominal paradox).

Positive end-expiratory pressure (PEEP) can also influence the ventilatory control system. Atelectasis from suboptimal applied expiratory pressure can increase inspiratory work and impair gas exchange thereby affecting patient comfort (dyspnea) and drive.[16] Conversely, excessive PEEP (either applied or intrinsic) can overdistend significant amounts of lung, putting muscles at suboptimal "resting" lengths and worsening the sense of patient discomfort.[16]

VENTILATOR TRACKING OF SPONTANEOUS EFFORT

For proper patient-ventilator synchrony, the mechanical ventilator must be able to monitor or track the patient's spontaneous ventilatory pattern.[17] This is usually done through measurements of flow or pressure at the patient's airway opening. Synchrony is then achieved by optimizing interactions with these parameters. Lung tissue elastance and airway resistance (especially the artificial airway's resistance), however, can "dampen" the magnitude of patient effort as it is transmitted to the airway sensing site. This can introduce significant lags between patient demand and gas delivery, even under the best of circumstances. Future interactive features may be improved by sensors placed in the patient's airway, the pleural space, or perhaps on the phrenic nerve itself.[18] Until such reliable sensors are developed, however, patient ventilator synchrony with current systems must rely on synchronization of the mechanical ventilator to proximal airway signals.

INTERACTIVE VENTILATOR DESIGN FEATURES

Five aspects of patient-ventilator interactions are described. The first three deal with mechanical breath parameters (Table 114–1):

- Ventilator breath triggering (trigger criteria)
- Ventilator-delivered flow pattern (target criteria)
- Ventilator flow termination (cycling criteria)
- Imposed expiratory loads
- "Back-up" ventilator breaths

Ventilator Breath Triggering

Interactive mechanical ventilation needs to sense a spontaneous effort in order to initiate gas flow (triggering).[19] This is often accomplished by detection of the drop in airway pressure that occurs with the beginning of a spontaneous effort (pressure triggering). An alternative approach is to detect the development of inspiratory flow by the patient drawing gas from the ventilator circuit (flow triggering). There is a certain inherent dyssynchrony in the triggering process, regardless of technique; this is due to several factors:

TABLE 114–1. Ventilator Breath Parameters

Common Name	Trigger	Target	Cycle
Volume control	Set ventilator timer	Set ventilator flow	Set ventilator volume
Volume assist	Patient effort	Set ventilator flow	Set ventilator volume
Pressure control	Set ventilator timer	Set ventilator pressure	Set ventilator timer
Pressure assist	Patient effort	Set ventilator pressure	Set ventilator timer
Pressure support	Patient effort	Set ventilator pressure	Flow decrease (cessation of patient effort)
Unassisted/unsupported	Patient effort	Baseline patient airway pressure	Flow decrease (cessation of patient effort)

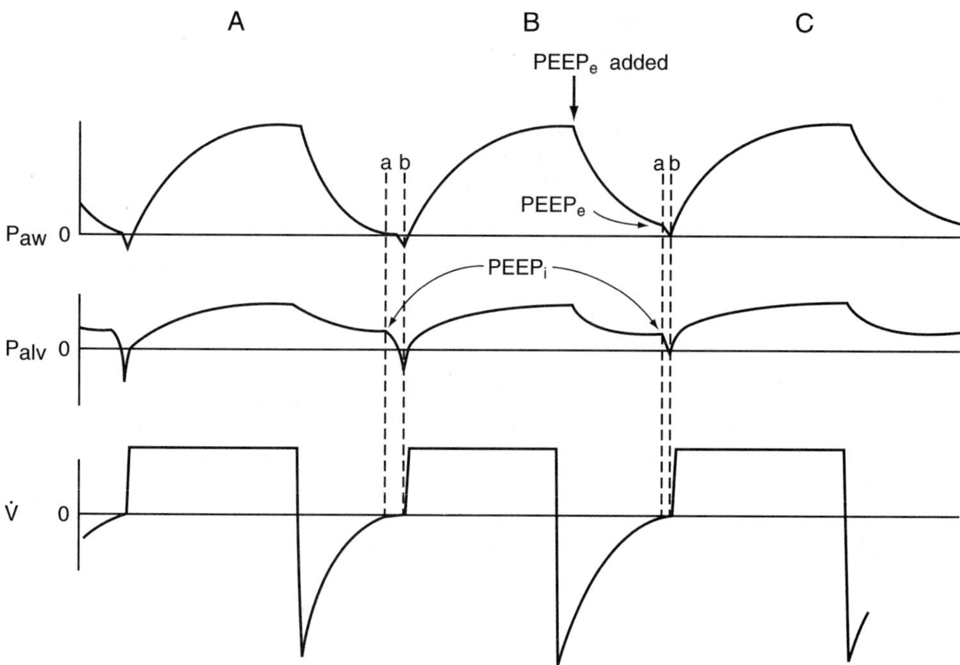

Figure 114–2. Impact of intrinsic positive end-expiratory pressure (PEEPi) on triggering. Plotted are airway pressure (Paw), alveolar pressure (Palv), and flow ($\dot{V}$) in a patient with significant PEEPi. To trigger a machine breath, alveolar pressure (Palv) must fall by the amount of PEEPi plus the set trigger sensitivity. The large drop in Palv between a and b on breaths A and B reflects this effort. The addition of extrinsic PEEP (PEEPe) downstream from dynamically compressed airways reduces the Palv − Paw gradient and attenuates the triggering effort between a and b on breath C, without a significant increase in end-inspiratory Palv.

1. A certain level of insensitivity must be put in the sensor to avoid artifacts triggering the ventilator (i.e., "auto-cycling").

2. As noted earlier, the patient's pleural pressure change is dampened as it is transmitted across lung parenchyma to the ventilator circuitry.

3. Even when the patient effort has been sensed, demand valve systems have a certain inherent delay (up to 100 msec or more) before they physically open and achieve target flow into the airway (valve responsiveness).

All of these factors can result in significant "isometric-like" pressure loads on the ventilatory muscles during the triggering process.[20] In addition, in the setting of air trapping (intrinsic PEEP), the elevated alveolar pressure at end-expiration can serve as a significant triggering threshold load on the ventilatory muscles (Fig. 114–2).[21]

Several strategies can be used to minimize the magnitude of the dyssynchrony induced during breath triggering:

1. Using ventilators with microprocessor flow controls can result in significantly better valve characteristics than those obtained on older generation ventilators.[22]

2. Continuous flow systems superimposed on the demand systems can improve demand system responsiveness in patients with high ventilatory drives, although such flows can *reduce* sensitivity in patients with very weak ventilatory drives.[20]

3. Flow-based triggers produce a more sensitive and responsive breath triggering process in mechanical lung models.[19]

4. A small amount of applied inspiratory pressure support usually increases the ventilator's initial flow delivery and can thereby improve response characteristics of the demand valve system.[19]

5. In the setting of intrinsic PEEP creating an inspiratory threshold load, applied PEEP below the intrinsic PEEP level can help to equilibrate the end-expiratory alveolar and circuit pressures and improve triggering (Fig. 114–2, right panel).[21]

6. As noted, sensors in the airways, in the pleural space, or on the phrenic nerve may improve trigger sensitivity on future systems.[18]

Ventilator-Delivered Flow Pattern

In the schema of Table 114–1, interactive breaths can be termed as follows[17]:

- Assisted (patient-triggered, ventilator-targeted, ventilator-cycled)
- Supported (patient-triggered, ventilator-targeted, patient-cycled)
- Unassisted or unsupported (patient-triggered, patient-targeted, patient-cycled)

Ventilator flow during these breath delivery strategies can be provided to meet one of three goals (Fig. 114–3):

- Full unloading of ventilatory muscles
- Partial unloading of ventilatory muscles
- No effect on ventilatory muscle loads

Synchronous flow interactions can be defined according to one of the following three goals.

Breaths Designed to Fully Unload Ventilatory Muscles

For an interactive breath to fully unload ventilator muscles, the patient should be required to only trigger the ventilator and then have the ventilator supply all of the work of the breath. It is important to remember that diaphragmatic contraction does not cease with the onset of a patient-triggered, ventilator-delivered breath.[23] The goal of synchrony during a fully unloading breath is thus to deliver adequate flow over the entire inspiratory effort to totally unload the contracting muscles. This goal can be assessed by comparing the pressure pattern of the patient-triggered breath with a machine-triggered breath (i.e., a breath occurring without patient activity). Synchronous flow delivery should produce nearly identical pressure waveforms (Fig. 114–4).

Patient-triggered breaths can be fully unloaded with either assisted or supported breaths that are either flow-targeted or pressure-targeted. The interactive flow-targeted, volume-cycled breath supplies a clinician set flow and volume in response to the patient's effort (the volume assist [VA] breath).

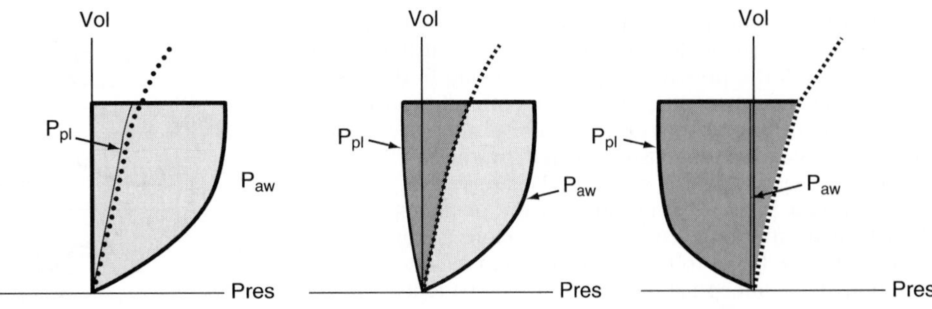

Figure 114–3. Schematic pressure-volume plots to illustrate degrees of patient muscle unloading by a ventilator-delivered positive pressure breath. In these plots, tidal volume is on the vertical axis and pressure is on the horizontal axis (pleural to left, airway to right). The *dotted line* represents the passive chest wall compliance reflected in the pleural pressure measurement. For simplicity, triggering effects on pleural and airway pressure are not depicted. The integral of pressure and volume is work and is depicted as either patient *(dark shade)* or ventilator *(light shade)* work. *Left panel,* A breath with total unloading (ventilator does all the work). *Middle panel,* A breath with partial unloading (ventilator and patients share work). *Right panel,* A breath with no unloading (patient does all the work). Partial unloading can also occur by interspersing spontaneous breaths with totally unloaded breaths (intermittent mandatory ventilation). Pres = pressure.

To fully unload ventilatory muscles, these breaths must be given with every patient effort (often with a back-up ventilator control rate). The ventilator mode is termed volume assist-control ventilation (VACV). In contrast, pressure-targeted breaths supply a clinician set airway pressure in response to the patient's effort and are either flow-cycled (pressure support [PS]) or time-cycled (pressure assist [PA]) (see cycling later). To fully unload ventilatory muscles with a pressure-targeted breath, the level of pressure must be sufficient to supply all of the work of a breath. Both PS and PA breaths can also have back-up control breaths in modes such as PS + intermittent mandatory ventilation or pressure assist-control ventilation (PACV).

Synchrony of a flow-targeted breath requires careful selection of the flow magnitude and pattern by the clinician. Arbitrary settings (e.g., constant flow of 40 to 60 L/min) are not always adequate. Indeed, in dyspneic patients receiving VACV, Marini and coworkers[23] have calculated loads of 5 to 15 joules/min (two to three times normal) from flow dyssynchrony (100% SIMV) (Fig. 114-5). Synchrony of flow-targeted breaths can be improved by careful adjustments of the set flow using both patient observations (e.g., perceived effort, tachypnea) and airway pressure/flow graphics (see Fig. 114-4). In addition, using a decelerating flow pattern may also be helpful because a patient's inspiratory effort tends to peak soon after breath initiation.

Pressure-targeted breaths may be easier to synchronize than flow-targeted breaths for two reasons.[15] First, because the

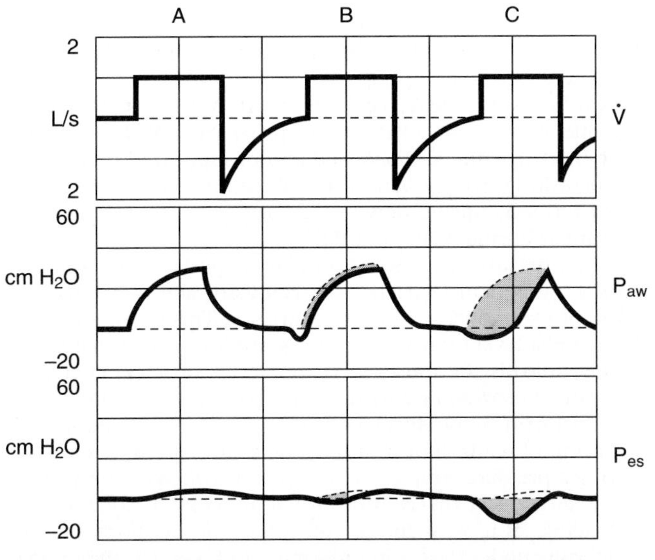

Figure 114–4. Manifestations of flow dyssynchrony of a ventilator breath. Plotted are flow *(upper panel)*, airway pressure *(middle panel)*, and pleural pressure, as reflected by esophageal pressure *(lower panel)* over a single ventilatory cycle. Breath A represents a control breath (no patient activity). Breath B represents a patient-triggered breath during which ventilator flow is adequate to fully unload the contracting ventilatory muscles. The dotted curve mimics passive breath A. As can be seen in both the airway and esophageal pressure tracings, the only appreciable difference between curve A and curve B is the triggering effort at the beginning of the breath. Breath C represents a patient-triggered breath during which ventilator flow is inadequate to fully unload the contracting ventilatory muscles. The *dotted line* again mimics the passive breath A. In contrast to the synchronous breath B, there is marked disparity in both airway and esophageal pressure tracings between breaths C and A. These differences can be quantified as a pressure time product *(shaded area)* reflecting the imposed muscle load from flow dyssynchrony.

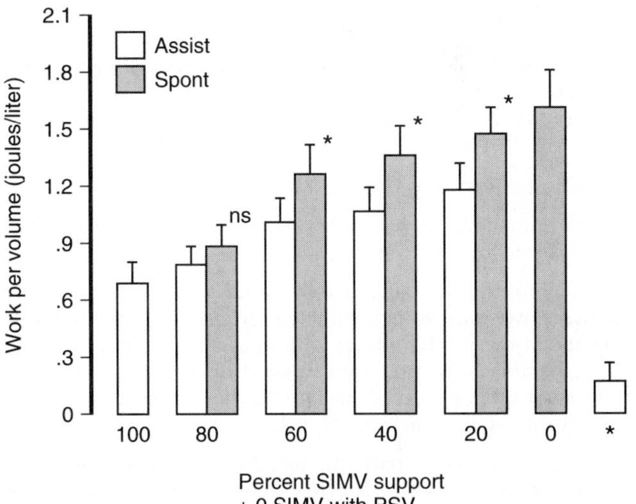

Figure 114–5. Patient work per liter of ventilation (mean inflation pressure) during the unassisted/unsupported breaths *(hatched bars)* and the ventilator-assisted breaths *(open bars)* at various levels of synchronized intermittent mandatory ventilation (SIMV) in a group of dyspneic patients. One hundred per cent SIMV support reflects volume assist control ventilation. There is significant imposed work from flow dyssynchrony during all assisted breaths in these patients, and it increases as the level of ventilator assistance (% SIMV support) is reduced. PSV = pressure support ventilation. (From Marini JJ, Smith TC, Lamb VJ: External work output and force generation during synchronized intermittent mechanical ventilation. Am Rev Respir Dis 1988; 138:1169–1179.)

ventilator has a pressure target, there is a rapid pressurization of the airway as gas is delivered with high initial flows. This tends to match the pressure changes occurring in the pleura more rapidly than that taking place with currently available set flow patterns. Second, because pressure is the independent variable, flow is continuously adjusted by the ventilator to maintain a constant airway pressure. This serves to provide a more constant pressure application to the pleural space during a patient effort and, consequently, a more continuous, or steady, pressure boost to the contracting muscles.

Although a conceptual step forward in patient-ventilator synchrony, pressure targeting has potential problems. First, ventilator-delivered initial flow (fixed by the ventilator design structure) may not be optimal in all patients.[24] Specifically, although patients with very active ventilatory drives require rapid initial flows for synchrony, patients with less active drives may demonstrate more synchronous patterns if lower initial flows are applied.[24] The capability to adjust initial flows (and thus the rate of rise to the pressure target) may be of benefit in addressing this.

Second, the pressure target for the ventilator is the proximal airway while the patient's muscle effort is actually generated in the pleural space. This separation by a series of resistive elements (i.e., endotracheal tube and airways) introduces an inherent underresponsiveness of ventilator flow to patient effort. This would be a theoretical reason for targeting ventilator pressure to the distal endotracheal tube or the pleural space instead of the ventilator circuitry. Indeed, experimental systems using carinal or pleural pressure sites for pressure targeting appear to significantly reduce imposed loading and to improve synchrony.[18, 25]

Third, because pressure targeted breaths consist only of an applied inspiratory pressure, fluctuations in patient effort and ventilatory system impedances can affect the delivered minute ventilation.

Several clinical studies have attempted to compare the synchrony effects of volume-targeted and pressure-targeted breaths.[26–28] In general, careful selection of flow and pressure settings generally can provide good patient ventilator synchrony with either breath type. In the patient with a vigorous ventilatory demand, however, many of these same studies suggest that a pressure-targeted breath may be more synchronous (Fig. 114–6).

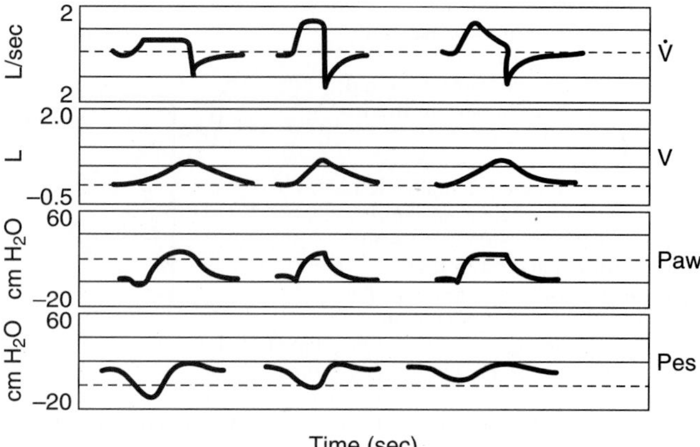

Figure 114–6. Ventilator flow ($\dot{V}_I$), tidal volume ($\dot{V}_T$), airway pressure (Paw), and esophageal pressure (Pes) tracings in a ventilated patient. *Left panels*, The patient is receiving ventilator flow set at 30 L/min to induce flow dyssynchrony. Dyssynchrony is demonstrated by a markedly negative esophageal pressure tracing during inspiration. The airway pressure tracing also appears "pulled" down. *Middle panels*, The set ventilator flow has been increased to 75 L/min, and the esophageal pressure tracing can be seen to improve. *Right panels*, A pressure-limiting feature of 22 cm H_2O above set positive end-expiratory pressure has been given. With this approach, the dyssynchronous esophageal pressure tracing can be seen to improve even further. (From MacIntyre NR, McConnell R, Cheng KG, Sane A: Patient-ventilator flow dyssynchrony: Flow limited versus pressure limited breaths. Crit Care Med 1997; 25:1671–1677.)

Breaths to Partially Unload Muscles

Partial unloading of ventilatory muscles can be provided in one of three general ways:

1. An intermittent mandatory ventilation (IMV) approach (either flow- and volume-targeted or pressure-targeted fully unloaded breaths alternating with unassisted breaths).
2. A stand-alone pressure targeted approach (partial support/assist of every breath using PS or PA breaths).
3. A mixed approach of PS + IMV.

The IMV approach partially unloads by intermittently shifting all of the work for a given effort between patient and ventilator. Synchronization of the assisted breaths during IMV has similar considerations to synchronization during VACV or PACV; however, the intermittency of breaths during IMV can add additional difficulty.[24, 29] This is because mechanical input to the ventilatory control center changes from breath to breath (i.e., unassisted breaths are alternating with assisted breaths). An "optimal" ventilatory pattern is thus impossible for the ventilatory control center to establish. This, coupled with the increased ventilatory drive intensity often associated with unassisted breaths can result in further dyssynchrony during the assisted breaths. In the patients of Marini and coauthors,[23] patient muscle work doubled during the assisted breaths as the IMV assisted breath rate was reduced to 20% of the VACV rate (see Fig. 114–5). An interesting variant of IMV, airway pressure release ventilation (APRV), holds the lung at a moderate level of inflation and provides IMV through periodic brief deflations. Unassisted and unsupported breaths can occur during both inflation and deflation phases. APRV has been termed "upside down" IMV, and synchrony issues may be similar during APRV and IMV.

The pressure-targeted approach to partial unloading requires the patient to trigger the ventilator and then share the work of every breath with the ventilator. This is accomplished by giving a level of inspiratory pressure lower than that which totally unloads the muscles. Lower levels of inspiratory pressure are thus *designed* to have the patient's ventilatory muscles perform some level of work during each assisted or supported breath. Indeed, this is how muscles are "reloaded" during a pressure-targeted weaning protocol. Synchrony under these circumstances is thus *not* a process of total muscle unloading as it was during full assist and support. Instead, synchrony under these circumstances is defined as the process of ventilator flow continuously adjusting to keep a constant pressure "bias" on the contracting ventilatory muscles.

The combined PS and IMV approach conceptually improves patient-ventilator synchrony during IMV by providing pressure support to the spontaneous efforts that alternate with pressure-targeted or volume-targeted assist/control breaths. Many of the concerns about IMV dyssynchrony noted, remain, however, and this combination mode is inherently more complex for clinicians to adjust (especially during weaning). One advantage to the PS + IMV combination is that a low IMV rate can function as a back-up if the patient's respiratory drive is unreliable.

Breaths That Do Not Affect Muscle Loads

For an interactive breath to not affect ventilatory muscle loads (i.e., the patient breathes independently), the ventilator should provide sufficient gas flow during an inspiratory effort only to maintain a constant level of airway pressure throughout the ventilatory cycle (continuous positive airway pressure [CPAP]). This interactive breath can be used during the spontaneous breaths of IMV (see earlier) or in patients not requiring ventilatory support but who need a constantly elevated airway pressure to maintain alveolar stability.

The goal of synchrony with unassisted or unsupported breaths is for the ventilator not to provide support but to ensure that adequate flow is delivered so as to minimize (or eliminate) any imposed loading. Indeed, the ideal CPAP system is one with large-bore tubing and a high continuous flow. Under these circumstances, any patient effort merely draws off the continuous flow. Because there is no sensor or valve, synchrony is less of an issue. With this type of system, however, high patient demands can exceed the continuous flow capability (inducing flow dyssynchrony) and monitoring can be difficult.

Demand valve systems, with or without a superimposed continuous flow, are a viable option for CPAP. Triggering of the valve is required, however, and the ventilator must be able to respond rapidly to the patient's effort to maintain CPAP. With any CPAP system, significant flow dyssynchrony can be detected by observing decreases in inspiratory airway pressure tracings (i.e., perfect synchrony should result in a truly constant airway pressure).

With either a continuous flow or a demand valve system, a constant airway pressure measured in the ventilator circuit during the ventilatory cycle (apparent flow synchrony) is usually *not* a constant airway pressure if it is measured at the trachea (Fig. 114-7).[18] This is because the endotracheal tube can have significant resistive properties and thus can produce an imposed load. Reducing or eliminating this load is the rationale for adding a small amount of inspiratory PS to CPAP breaths; it creates tracheal CPAP (see Fig. 114-7, the second breath). The appropriate amount of PS can be estimated from endotracheal tube size and spontaneous flow rates. A more direct approach, however, is to target the ventilator pressure to tracheal pressure (see Fig. 114-7, the third breath).[18] As noted earlier, an additional advantage to using a small amount of PS to produce tracheal CPAP is that the ventilator demand valve responsiveness is generally better when the inspiratory pressure target is above baseline values.

Ventilator Flow Termination

The process of terminating gas delivery is termed *cycling*. Synchronous cycling should be done in accordance both with patient demand and with adequacy of tidal volume. Premature termination may result in an inadequate tidal volume or in a patient continuing to demand inspiratory flow but not getting it (an inspiratory imposed load) (Fig. 114-8, left). Delayed breath termination may result in (1) excessive tidal volumes, (2) inadequate expiratory time (and consequent air trapping), (3) patients fighting the ventilator in order to "turn it off" (an expiratory imposed load), or (4) patients initiating the next inspiratory effort just as the previous machine breath has terminated (see Fig. 114-8, right).

With conventional flow-targeted, volume-cycled breaths, breath termination occurs when the set volume is reached. Synchrony is attained when an appropriate volume is set. With pressure-targeted breaths, breath termination can occur in several ways. The standard pressure support (PS) breath generally terminates at some low level of inspiratory flow (e.g., 5 L/min or 25% to 30% of peak flow). Duration and magnitude of patient effort can thus affect the TI of a PS breath. However, other factors that affect the peak flow (e.g., the pressure support level and the rate of pressure rise) can also affect TI. The response of TI to a clinician's manipulations of the PS breath can therefore be sometimes difficult to predict.[31] Usually, an adjustment in the inspiratory pressure or in the pressure rise time that results in more synchronous interactions produces a slowing of the ventilatory rate, an increase in the tidal volume, and maintenance or lengthening of the TI.[24] On the other hand, excessive inspiratory pressure levels may produce a premature termination of patient inspira-

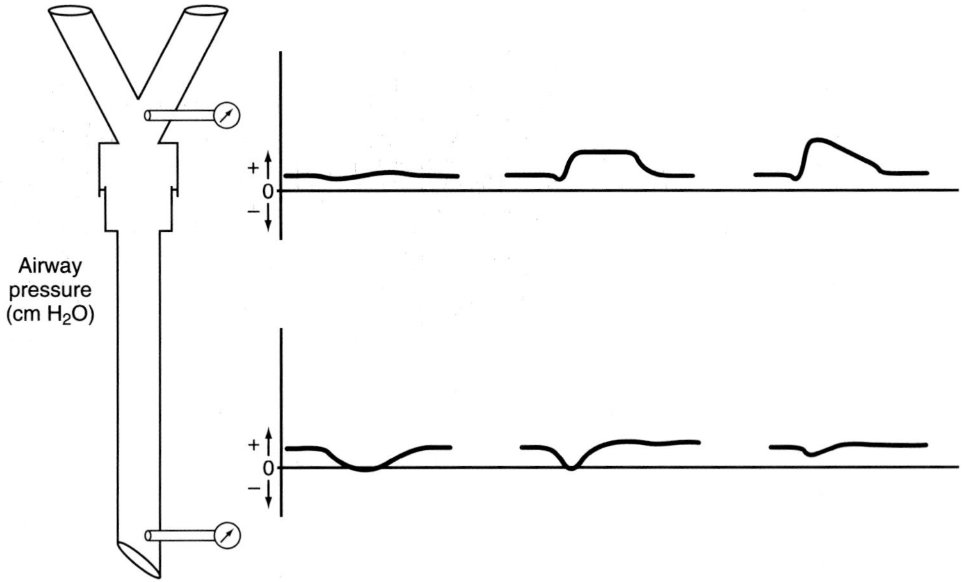

Figure 114–7. Schematic depiction of airway pressure tracings at the proximal and distal end of an endotracheal tube in which the clinical goal is to produce a continuous positive airway pressure (CPAP) of 5 cm H_2O. In the first breath, producing a CPAP of 5 cm H_2O at the proximal end of the tube results in drop in airway pressure at the distal end during patient inspiration to overcome tube resistance. Setting a pressure support (PS) level of 5 cm H_2O in the proximal airway during inspiration reduces some of the work to overcome tube resistance (second breath) and begins to produce true tracheal CPAP. Setting CPAP targeted to the distal airway, however, using a distal tube pressure sensor (third breath) actually produces a decelerating PS pattern in the proximal airway and results in true tracheal CPAP.

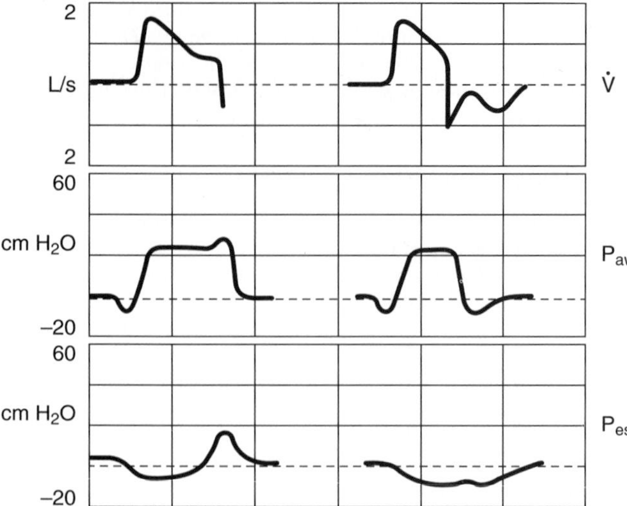

Figure 114–8. Two examples of cycling dyssynchrony. Depicted are airflow (V̇, *upper panel*), airway pressure (Paw, *middle panel*), and pleural pressure as estimated by esophageal pressure (Pes, *lower panel*). *Left panel*, Breath cycling is inappropriately delayed for patient effort. As a consequence, patient expiratory effort is evident during the latter phases of ventilator gas delivery, elevating both Paw and Pes. *Right panel*, Breath cycling is inappropriately premature for patient effort. As a consequence, Paw and Pes are lowered during the ventilator expiratory phase, resulting in reduced expiratory flow (or even additional inspiratory flow). A subsequent premature triggering of a ventilator breath may also occur ("double pumping").

tory effort or even induce an expiratory effort.[24] An excessive rate of rise and peak flow can also cause premature termination because the cycling flow (25% to 30% of peak flow) is, accordingly, too high.

Two other ways also bring about termination of an interactive pressure-targeted breath. First, one can use the pressure assist (PA) breaths (PACV with the mandatory rate set below the spontaneous rate). This allows the clinician to directly set the TI. Both total and partial muscle unloading can be provided with the PA breath. This breath may be particularly useful when a patient's partial muscle unloading with every breath is appropriate but when cycling dyssynchrony occurs using standard pressure support. Second, one can provide a back-up flow and volume guarantee during a pressure-targeted breath to ensure a minimal tidal volume.[27] This approach has been termed *volume-assured pressure support* (VAPS), or *pressure augmentation,* and may be useful in adding pressure-targeted flow features to a patient in need of full unloading with volume-guaranteed breaths. VAPS or pressure augmentation may also have utility in maintaining a minimal tidal volume in patients being weaned by pressure-targeted breaths. A similar effect can be produced through feedback control of the inspiratory pressure level to ensure a desired tidal volume (volume support or pressure-regulated volume control).

Imposed Expiratory Loads

Expiratory flow is normally generated from elastic recoil properties of the lung after termination of the inspiratory muscle activity. Expiratory muscles, however, can also contribute to expiratory alveolar pressure generation.

The only work associated with expiration should be that required to overcome airway resistance. In the ventilated patient, however, the endotracheal tube and exhalation valve assembly can produce a significant imposed load during expiration and interact with the patient's ventilatory drive accordingly.[31] Specifically, these expiratory loads can stimulate expiratory muscle contraction and affect the patient's ventilatory timing mechanism, usually prolonging TE with respect to TI and increasing dyspnea and expiratory muscle energy expenditures. Wide-bore endotracheal tubes and threshold PEEP valves (instead of flow resistive PEEP valves) are commonly used to reduce the potential dyssynchrony. Another approach involves PEEP referenced to distal endotracheal tube pressures. This approach may require the generation of a *negative* expiratory pressure in the circuit if tube resistance or expiratory flows are high.

Back-up Ventilator Breaths

The purpose of a back-up mandatory breath rate is to provide a minimal breath number guarantee during interactive modes. Several modes that call for a clinician to set the breath rate have been discussed. For instance, during volume or pressure assist control, a minimal number of mandatory breaths are guaranteed if the patient's spontaneous rate falls below the set minimum ventilator rate. IMV and APRV also provide a set number of machine breaths. "Synchronized" IMV (SIMV) allows these ventilator breaths to be patient-triggered if patient efforts are present. With SIMV, if the patient triggers the minimal number of assisted breaths, no mandatory controlled breaths are supplied.

A more sophisticated back-up rate strategy activates mandatory breaths only if a certain minute ventilation is not achieved (e.g., mandatory minute ventilation, augmented minute ventilation, apnea ventilation). These strategies provide a guaranteed certain minimum minute ventilation that can increase to near total support if patient effort deteriorates. Ventilator breath synchrony of the ventilator-delivered breaths depends on all the factors noted earlier.

FUTURE TRENDS

Future approaches to improving patient-ventilator synchrony will be aimed at making interactive ventilatory support more sensitive and responsive to patient effort. One approach to this would be to improve the ability of the ventilator to sense patient effort. Distal endotracheal tube sensors seem to be a step forward, and pleural pressure signals may be ideal.[18, 25] Clinically reliable sensors for such purposes, however, do not exist. Although such sensors are theoretically attractive, phrenic nerve output as a driving signal for the ventilator pattern is not practical now.

Improving valve sensitivity and responsiveness is also a goal. Improved valve designs with better capabilities to separate noise from patient signals coupled with low-resistance, low-compliance circuitry are goals.

Finally, an interesting alternate approach to flow-targeted or pressure-targeted breaths has been the development of a flow assist technique known as *proportional assist ventilation.*[32] This technique utilizes continuous feedback of inspiratory flow and then proportionally adjusts ventilator delivered flow according to the desired level of muscle unloading. Provided that the feedback loop is sufficiently sensitive and responsive, this approach can offer a high level of patient-ventilator synchrony. Such systems, however, are only experimental at present.

References

1. American College of Chest Physicians Consensus Group: Consensus conference on mechanical ventilation. Intensive Care Med 1994; 20:150–162.

2. MacIntyre NR: Synchronous and dys-synchronous patient ventilator interactions. *In*: Year Book of Intensive Care and Emergency Medicine. Vincent JL (Ed). Berlin, Springer-Verlag, 1992.
3. Marini JJ: Strategies to minimize breathing effort during mechanical ventilation. Crit Care Clin 1990; 6:635–661.
4. Banner MJ, Jaeger MJ, Kirby RR: Components of the work of breathing and implications for monitoring ventilator-dependent patients. Crit Care Med 1994; 22:515–523.
5. Ward ME, Corbert C, Gibbons W, Newman S, Macklen PT: Optimization of respiratory muscle relaxation during mechanical ventilation. Anesthesiology 1988; 69:29–35.
6. Berger AJ, Mitchell RA, Severinghaus JW: Regulation of respiration. (Parts I to III.) N Engl J Med 1977; 297:92–97, 138–143, 194–201.
7. Mead J: Control of respiratory frequency. J Appl Phys 1960; 15:325–336.
8. Milic-Emili J: Recent advances in clinical assessment of control of breathing. Lung 1982; 160:1–17.
9. Bellemare F, Grassino A: Effect of pressure and timing of contraction on human diaphragm failure. J Appl Physiol 1982; 53:1190–1195.
10. Luijendijk SC, Milic-Emili J: Breathing patterns in anesthetized cats and the concept of minimum respiratory effort. J Appl Physiol 1988; 64:31–41.
11. Cohen CA, Zagelbaum G, Gross D, Roussos C, Macklem PT: Clinical manifestation of inspiratory muscle fatigue. Am J Med 1982; 73:308–316.
12. Tobin MJ, Perez W, Guenther SH, et al: The pattern of breathing during successful and unsuccessful trials of weaning from mechanical ventilation. Am Rev Respir Dis 1986; 134:1111–1118.
13. Gallagher CG, Hof VI, Younes M: Effect of inspiratory muscle fatigue on breathing pattern. J Appl Phys 1986; 59:1152–1158.
14. Aubier M, Murciano D, Fournier M, Milic-Emili J, Pariente R, Derenne JP: Central respiratory drive in acute respiratory failure of patients with chronic obstructive pulmonary disease. Am Rev Respir Dis 1980;122:191–199.
15. MacIntyre NR, Leatherman NE: Ventilatory muscle loads and the frequency-tidal volume pattern during inspiratory pressure-supported ventilation. Am Rev Respir Dis 1990; 141:327–331.
16. American Association for Respiratory Care: Positive end expiratory pressure—state of the art after 20 years. Respir Care 1988; 33:417–500.
17. American Association for Respiratory Care: Consensus statement on essentials of mechanical ventilators. Respir Care 1992; 37:1000–1008.
18. Pinsky MR, Hrehocik D, Culpepper JA, Snyder JV: Flow resistance of expiratory positive pressure systems. Chest 1988; 94:788–791.
19. Sassoon CSH: Mechanical ventilator design and function: The trigger variable. Respir Care 1992; 37:1056–1069.
20. Katz J, Kraemer R, Gjerde GE: Inspiratory work and airway pressure with continuous positive airway pressure delivery systems. Chest 1985; 88:519–526.
21. Gay PG, Rodarte JR, Hubmayr RD: The effects of positive expiratory pressure on isovolumic flow and dynamic hyperinflation in patients receiving mechanical ventilation. Am Rev Respir Dis 1989; 139:621–626.
22. Hirsch C, Kacmarek RM, Stanek K: Work of breathing during CPAP and PSV imposed by the new generation mechanical ventilators: A lung model study. Respir Care 1991; 36:815–828.
23. Marini JJ, Smith TC, Lamb VJ: External work output and force generation during synchronized intermittent mechanical ventilation. Am Rev Respir Dis 1988; 138:1169–1179.
24. Ho L, MacIntyre NR: Effects of initial flow rate and breath termination criteria on pressure support ventilation: Chest 1991; 99:134–138.
25. MacIntyre NR, Nishimura M, Usada Y, et al: The Nagoya conference on system design and patient-ventilator interactions during pressure support ventilation. Chest 1990; 97:1463–1466.
26. Tokioka H, Saito S, Kosaka F: Comparison of pressure support ventilation and assist control ventilation in patients with acute respiratory failure. Intensive Care Med 1989; 15:364–367.
27. Haas CF, Branson RD, Folk LM, Campbell RS, Wise CR, Davis K, et al: Patient determined inspiratory flow during assisted mechanical ventilation. Respir Care 1995; 40:716–721.
28. MacIntyre NR, McConnell R, Cheng KG, Sane A: Patient-ventilator flow dyssynchrony: Flow-limited versus pressure-limited breaths. Crit Care Med 1997; 25:1671–1677.
29. Imsand C, Feihl F, Perret C, Fitting JW: Regulation of inspiratory neuromuscular output during synchronized intermittent mechanical ventilation. Anesthesiology 1994; 80:13–22.
30. Fiastro JF, Habib MP, Quan SF: Pressure support compensation for inspiratory work due to endotracheal tubes and demand continuous positive airway pressure. Chest 1988; 93:499–505.
31. Marini JJ, Kirk W, Culver BH: Flow resistance of the exhalation valves and PEEP devices used in mechanical ventilation. Am Rev Respir Dis 1985; 131:850–854.
32. Younes M: Proportional assist ventilation, a new approach to ventilatory support. Am Rev Respir Dis 1992; 145:114–120.

115

Controlled Mechanical Ventilation

Robert M. Kacmarek, PhD, RRT, FCCM

Conceptually, controlled mechanical ventilation or total ventilatory support implies that the patient's interaction with the ventilator is prevented or markedly minimized. That is, the majority of the work of breathing is provided by the mechanical ventilator and the patient is, essentially, passively ventilated.[1] In general, controlled ventilation is indicated in patients whose ventilatory drive is inadequate or absent, as in the postoperative setting or after an overdose, or in patients whose medical status is considered so labile that allowing the patient to interact with the ventilator results in cardiopulmonary instability, thus requiring pharmacologic depression of ventilatory drive.[2]

Removing the spontaneous ventilatory demands of the patient greatly simplifies the process of providing ventilatory support. During controlled mechanical ventilation, the ventilator is set to accomplish the goals of ventilatory support without concern for a coordinated interaction between the patient and the ventilator.[1]

PRINCIPLES OF POSITIVE-PRESSURE VENTILATION

The goals of controlled mechanical ventilation are essentially the same as those during partial ventilatory support except for the assurance of patient-ventilator synchrony, that is, the establishment of appropriate gas exchange without inducing cardiovascular compromise or ventilator-induced lung injury. Heart-lung interactions are discussed in detail in Chapter 110.

Ventilator-Induced Lung Injury

During the last decade, an abundance of experimental evidence has unequivocally demonstrated that mechanical ventilation can induce a parenchymal lung injury termed volutrauma, similar to adult respiratory distress syndrome (ARDS), as well as barotrauma.[3] Table 115-1 lists the spectrum of lung injury induced by mechanical ventilation.[4]

Parenchymal Lung Injury

Mechanical ventilation at high airway pressures has been shown in numerous species to cause parenchymal lung injury.[5-10] Webb and Tierney[5] noted gross hemorrhage edema in rats after 60 minutes of ventilation with a peak inspiratory

TABLE 115–1. The Spectrum of Lung Injury Induced by Mechanical Ventilation

Atelectasis
Alveolar hemorrhage
Alveolar neutrophil infiltration
Alveolar macrophage accumulation
Decreased compliance
Detachment of endothelial cells
Denuding of basement membranes
Emphysematous changes
Gross pulmonary edema
Hyaline membrane formation
Interstitial edema
Increased interstitial albumin levels
Interstitial lymphocyte infiltration
Intracapillary bleeding
Pneumothorax
Severe hypoxemia
Subcutaneous emphysema
Systemic gas embolism
Tension cyst formation

Modified from Kacmarek RM, Hickling KG: Permissive hypercapnia. Resp Care 1993; 38:373-387.

pressure of 45 cm H_2O (Fig. 115-1). Similar findings were reported by Hernandez and colleagues[6] in rabbits after ventilation at the same respiratory pressure. In sheep, Kolobow and associates[7] observed severe respiratory failure and pulmonary consolidation at autopsy after ventilation at 50 cm H_2O. In a series of elegant studies, Dreyfuss and coworkers[8-10] demonstrated similar injuries in rats with both negative and positive pressure (Fig. 115-2), identified transpulmonary pressure as the pressure gradient responsible for injury, and demonstrated that high airway pressure can extend preexisting lung injury.

The application of positive end-expiratory pressure (PEEP) appears to modify the injury induced by high transpulmonary pressure. Webb and Tierney[5] showed a marked reduction in the injury caused by 45 cm H_2O peak pressure when 10 cm H_2O PEEP was applied (see Fig. 115-1). Similar results (Fig. 115-3) were observed by Corbridge and associates[11] in sheep ventilated at the same peak airway pressure but different levels of PEEP (12.5 versus 2.5 cm H_2O). Muscedere and colleagues[12] in an ex vivo rat model showed that PEEP set above the lower inflection point (LIP) on the pressure-volume curve of the lung prevented injury compared with ventilation at the same peak inspiratory pressure (PIP) without PEEP or with PEEP set below the LIP. In addition, Tremblay and coworkers[13] observed lower inflammatory cytokine levels in excised normal and injured rat lungs ventilated with PEEP above the LIP compared with lungs without PEEP ventilated at high inspiratory pressures. Lungs ventilated with high airway pressures and PEEP above the LIP demonstrated intermediate levels of inflammatory cytokines.[13]

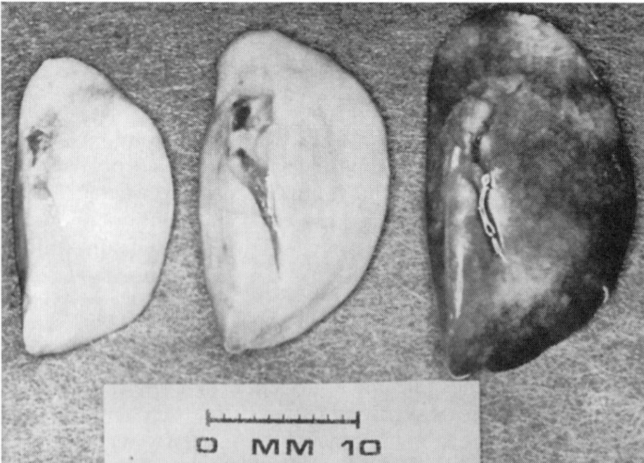

Figure 115–1. Comparison of left lungs from rats ventilated from left to right: peak inspiratory pressure, 14 cm H_20, PEEP, 0 cm H_2O; peak inspiratory pressure, 45 cm H_2O, PEEP 10 cm H_2O; peak inspiratory pressure, 45 cm H_2O, PEEP 0 cm H_2O. The perivascular groove is distended, with edema in the lung ventilated at 45/10. Gross hemorrhage edema is present in the lung ventilated with 45/0. (From Webb HH, Tierney DF; Experimental pulmonary edema due to intermittent positive pressure ventilation with high inflation end expiratory pressure. Am Rev Respir Dis 1994; 110:556-565.)

These data have led many to conclude that all patients should be ventilated with a lung-protective ventilatory strategy (LPVS),[14, 15] that is, the setting of PEEP at a sufficient level to prevent derecruitment of unstable lung units and the limiting of peak alveolar pressure to prevent overdistention of the lung. In most postoperative and overdose patients, neither of these pressure targets is an issue; however, in patients with acute lung injury and ARDS, guiding the adjustments to the ventilator on the basis of these targets may have an effect on the patient's outcome.[14, 15] Data from Nahum and coworkers[16] in dogs indicate that ventilation at low PEEP and high peak airway pressures facilitated bacterial translocation from the alveoli to the bloodstream, whereas appropriate targeting of PEEP and $P_{plateau}$ prevented translocation of bacteria. In addition, Ranieri and coworkers[17] observed that inflammatory cytokines decreased in patients with ARDS ventilated with an LPVS but increased in patients treated with conventional ventilation.

Two randomized prospective studies have been performed to evaluate conventional ventilation versus LPVS.[18, 19] In one study, Amato and colleagues[18] randomized 53 patients to conventional ventilation (volume assist-control, VT 12 mL/kg, rate set to maintain Pa_{CO_2} at 35 to 38 mm Hg, and PEEP and FIO_2 set to maintain the $Pa_{O_2} \geq 80$ mm Hg with the $FIO_2 \leq 0.6$) and an LPVS (pressure ventilation, with PEEP and peak airway pressure set by evaluation of the pressure-volume curve of the lung [see later], FIO_2 set to keep $Pa_{O_2} \geq 80$ mm Hg, and permissive hyperventilation allowed). In addition, in the LPVS group, whenever airway pressures were allowed to drop to atmospheric pressure, 35 to 40 cm H_2O continuous positive airway pressure (CPAP) was applied for 40 seconds to ensure maximal recruitment before ventilation was resumed. Twenty-eight days after enrollment, 18 patients (62%) survived in the treatment group compared with seven patients (29%) in the control group. Moreover, the incidence of barotrauma was greater in the control group (42% versus 7%, $P \leq .02$), and the weaning rate at day 28 was also higher in the treatment group (66% versus 29%, $P \leq .005$).

In a second study, Stewart and associates[19] enrolled 120 patients "at risk" for ARDS. In the control group, VT was set between 10 and 15 mL/kg with PIP limited to 50 cm H_2O; in the treatment group; VT was set at 8 mL/kg, and PIP was limited to 30 cm H_2O. In both groups, mechanical ventilation was provided with volume assist-control ventilation, and PEEP was adjusted to maintain Sa_{O_2} between 89% and 93% with FIO_2 of 0.5 or less. Respiratory mechanics were not assessed in either group. Finally, the target Pa_{CO_2} was between 35 and 45 mm Hg. No difference in survival was observed between treatment (50%) and control (53%) groups. A low incidence of barotrauma was reported in the treatment as well as in the control group (10% and 7%, respectively). A greater number of patients required dialysis (13 versus 5, $P \leq .04$) and received muscle relaxants (23 versus 13, $P \leq .05$) in the treatment than in the control group.

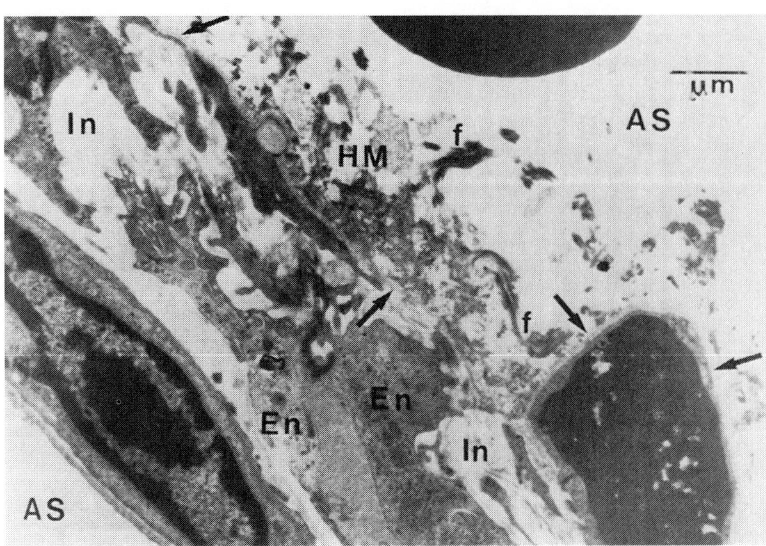

Figure 115–2. Alveolar septum (AS) with three capillaries of an adult rat after 20 minutes of ventilation at 45 cm H_2O. *Right side*, The epithelial lining is destroyed, denuding the basement membrane *(arrows)*. Hyaline membranes (HM) composed of cell debris and fibrin (f) are present. Two endothelial cells (En) of another capillary are visible inside the interstitium (In). *Lower left side*, A monocyte fills the lumen of a third capillary with a normal blood-air barrier. (From Dreyfuss D, Bassett G, Soler P, et al: Intermittent positive-pressure hyperventilation with high inflation pressure produces pulmonary microvascular injury in rats. Am Rev Respir Dis 1985; 132:880–884.)

The different results in these two studies most probably are a result of the methodology used to set PEEP and the actual $P_{plateau}$ achieved in each group.[20] In Amato's treatment group, PEEP was 16 cm H_2O or higher, and $P_{plateau}$ was 32 cm H_2O or lower. In Amato's control group and in Stewart's control and treatment groups, PEEP was less than 10 cm H_2O. In both of Stewart's groups, $P_{plateau}$ was below 30 cm H_2O; in Amato's control group, $P_{plateau}$ was above 35 cm H_2O (Fig. 115–4). Consequently, it is not surprising that Stewart and colleagues did not observe any difference in outcome between treatment and control groups. In neither group was an overinflation injury possible because of the low plateau pressure applied, and PEEP (which was not set according to the LIP) did not differ between groups. In other words, the minimal stretch aspect of an LPVS was applied to *both* groups. Mortality for both of Stewart's groups was between that of Amato's control and treatment groups. Protection from ventilator-induced lung or volutrauma injury requires PEEP set on the basis of lung mechanics and $P_{plateau}$ maximized at a level that prevents overdistention.

Barotrauma

The specific data identifying the factors that induce barotrauma are less clear than those associated with volutrauma.[21] Many agree that for barotrauma to occur, lung injury, overdistention, and high pressure are required.[22] As shown in the Amato[18] and Stewart[19] studies, as well as by data retrospectively reviewed by Weg and coworkers,[23] when $P_{plateau}$ is kept below 35 to 40 cm H_2O, the incidence of barotrauma is low. Cullen and Caldera,[24] on the other hand, reported a 44% incidence of barotrauma when peak airway pressure exceeded 70 cm H_2O, and Rouby and colleagues[25] noted during autopsy of ARDS patients that patients with barotrauma received high airway pressures (56 ± 18 cm H_2O), larger tidal volumes (12 ± 3 mL/kg), and higher FIO_2 (>0.60) for prolonged periods (8.6 ± 9.4 days). Pneumothorax is the most commonly reported acute form of barotrauma. In adult patients, the incidence varies from 0.5% to 44% of ventilated patients.[24-31]

Gas Exchange Targets

In most mechanically ventilated patients, normal gas exchange is targeted ($PaO_2 \geq 80$ mm H_2O and $PaCO_2$ 35 to 45 cm H_2O). However, in many patients with acute lung injury, ARDS, or severe asthma requiring controlled mechanical ventilation and the use of an LPVS, the maintenance of normal gas exchange targets is impossible.

PaO_2

Assuming adequate cardiac output and hemoglobin concentration, acceptable arterial oxygenation can be maintained with a PaO_2 of 60 mm Hg or higher. On occasion, PaO_2 values as low as 50 mm Hg have been considered acceptable in the most severe cases of ARDS, although adjunctive approaches to ventilatory support (prone positioning,[32] nitric oxide,[33] or

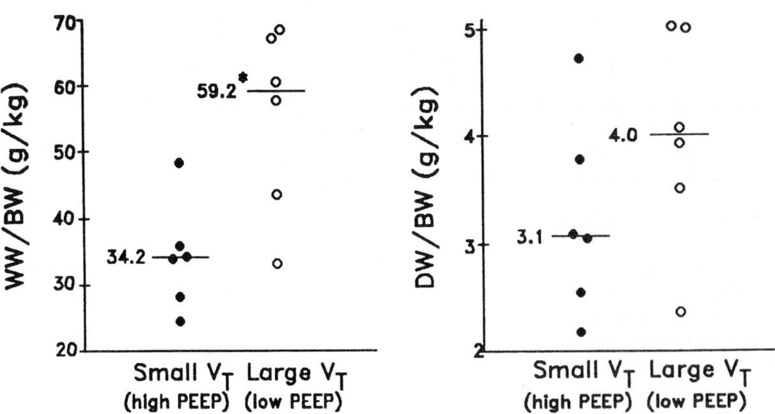

Figure 115–3. Gravimetric estimates of edema. Wet weight to body weight ratios (WW/BW) (g/kg) and dry weight to body weight ratios (DW/BW) (g/kg) with median values shown for all animals in both groups. *Asterisk* = Median WW/BW was statistically higher in the large V_T-low PEEP group by the Mann-Whitney rank sum test (P = .041). Median DW/BW ratios were not significantly different between groups. (From Corbridge TC, Wood DH, Crawford GP, et al: Adverse effects of large tidal volume and low PEEP in canine acid aspiration. Am Rev Respir Dis 1990; 142:311–315.)

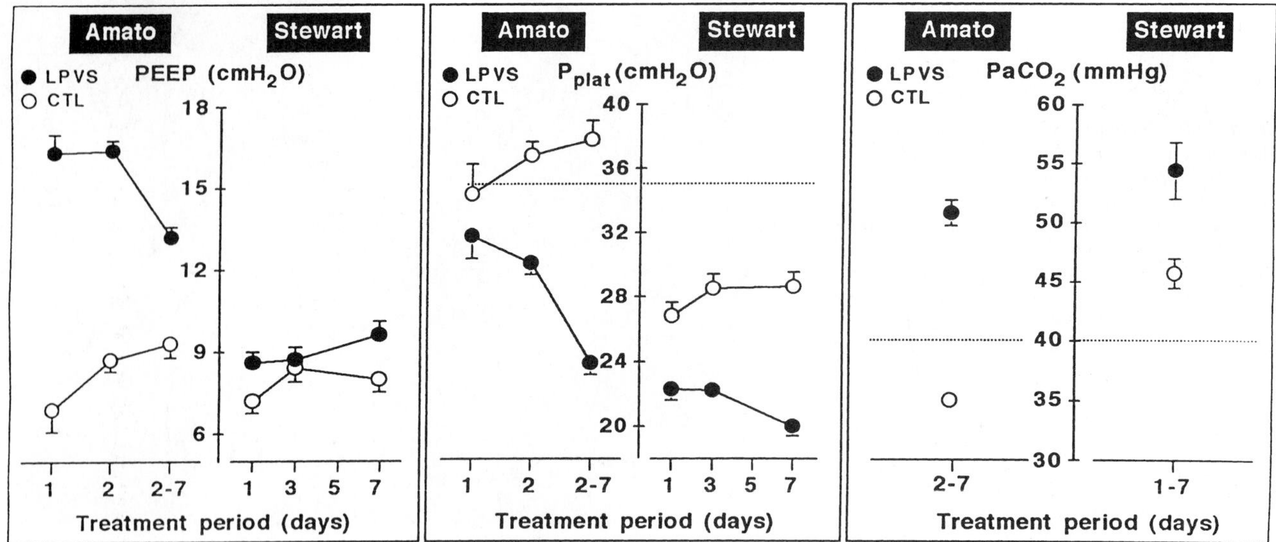

Figure 115–4. Evolution of PEEP *(left panel)*, plateau pressures *(middle panel)*, and Pa_{CO_2} *(right panel)* in studies by Amato[18] and Stewart.[19] Data (mean ± SE) are plotted for the first 7 days of each study. LPVS = lung-protective ventilatory strategy; CTL = control group. *Middle panel*, The *dashed line* represents the maximum plateau pressure recommended by the Americano-European Consensus Conference. *Right panel*, The *dashed line* represents normocapnia. There is a clear separation between the treatment and the control groups in the study by Amato and coworkers. In contrast, a lung-protective strategy was used in both groups in Stewart's study. (From Kacmarek RM, Chiche JD: Lung protective ventilatory strategies for ARDS—the data are convincing! Respir Care 1998; 43:724–727.)

high-frequency ventilation[34]) should be considered in these settings to ensure adequate tissue oxygenation.

Permissive Hypercapnia

In many ARDS and severe asthma patients, it is impossible to maintain normal carbon dioxide elimination while at the same time ventilating with a lung-protective strategy. As a result, permissive hypercapnia is a common outcome. Most would define permissive hypercapnia as a Pa_{CO_2} of 50 to 100 mm Hg as a result of limiting the level of ventilation to avoid inducing lung injury.[4] A number of case series have shown reduced barotrauma and low mortality with permissive hypercapnia,[35–39] and as discussed earlier, Amato and colleagues,[18] using an LPVS with permissive hypercapnia in a randomized controlled trial, demonstrated a lower mortality than with conventional ventilation. In a nonrandomized prospective case series of trauma patients with ARDS, patients managed with permissive hypercapnia (N = 11) had better survival (91% versus 48%, $P < .01$) but a lengthier ventilatory course (49.2 ± 15.2 versus 20.8 ± 10 days, $P < .01$) than did patients in whom Pa_{CO_2} was normalized.[39]

The potential adverse effects of an elevated Pa_{CO_2} are listed in Table 115–2. Most of the clinical problems with permissive hypercapnia occur at Pa_{CO_2} levels above 150 mm Hg.[4, 40] However, even small increases in Pa_{CO_2} cause increased cerebral blood flow; thus, permissive hypercapnia is generally contraindicated when intracranial pressure is increased.[41, 42] Elevated Pa_{CO_2} also stimulates ventilation, but patients are usually sedated and possibly paralyzed in settings in which permissive hypercapnia is considered.[39]

TABLE 115–2. Potential Adverse Physiologic Effects of Permissive Hypercapnia

Shift in the oxyhemoglobin dissociation curve to the right
Decreased alveolar P_{O_2}
Both stimulation and depression of the cardiovascular system
Central nervous system depression
Simulation of ventilation
Dilation of vascular bed
Increased intracranial pressure
Anesthesia (Pa_{CO_2} 200 mm Hg)
Decreased renal blood flow (Pa_{CO_2} 150 mm Hg)
Leakage of intracellular potassium (Pa_{CO_2} 150 mm Hg)
Alteration of the action of pharmacologic agents (a result of intracellular acidosis)

Permissive hypercapnia may adversely affect the oxygenation status of some patients. Elevated Pa_{CO_2} and low pH shifts the oxyhemoglobin dissociation curve to the right.[43] This decreases the affinity of hemoglobin for oxygen, decreasing oxygen loading in the lungs but facilitating the unloading of oxygen at the tissues.[43] As illustrated by the alveolar gas equation, an increase in the alveolar P_{CO_2} results in a decrease in alveolar P_{O_2}. For each P_{ACO_2} rise of 1 mm Hg, the P_{AO_2} decreases by about 1 mm Hg.[43]

The effect of carbon dioxide on the cardiovascular system is difficult to predict. As illustrated in Figure 115–5, carbon dioxide elicits competing responses from the cardiovascular system.[44] Carbon dioxide directly stimulates or depresses specific aspects of the cardiovascular system, but opposite effects can occur through stimulation of the autonomic nervous system.[44] It is thus difficult to predict the precise response of the cardiovascular system to permissive hypercapnia in any given patient. However, the most common response is an increase in pulmonary hypertension,[45] and potentially the most significant is myocardial depression associated with an increased cardiac output.[46] Dosages of pharmaceutical agents affecting the cardiovascular and autonomic nervous system may need to be adjusted in the presence of permissive hypercapnia, when a marked acidosis is present.[47]

The primary factor limiting permissive hypercapnia is the pH.[4, 40–42] Patients without primary cardiovascular disease or renal failure can usually tolerate a pH of 7.20 or higher, and some may tolerate an even lower pH.[36, 37, 48] The specific minimum pH acceptable needs to be determined for the individual patient. Allowing P_{CO_2} to gradually rise from the onset of ventilation permits gradual renal compensation, minimizing marked pH change. Abrupt changes in ventilatory

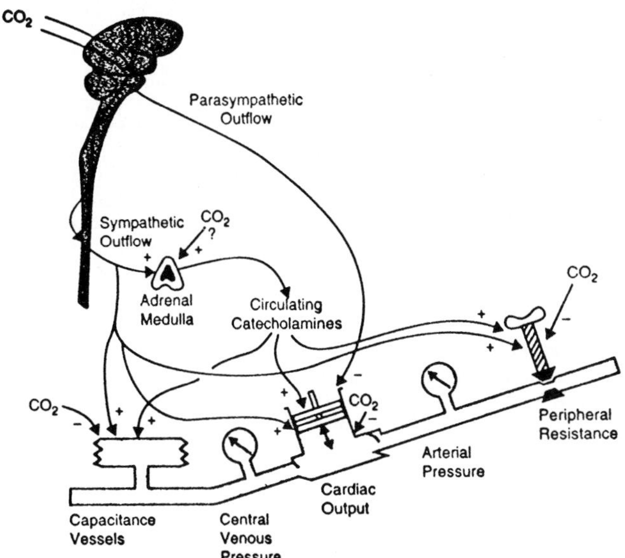

Figure 115–5. This diagram shows the complexity of the mechanisms by which carbon dioxide (CO_2) can influence the circulatory system. See text for details. (From Nunn JF [ed]: Applied Respiratory Physiology. 2nd ed. London, Butterworths & Co, 1977.)

strategies that result in rapid and marked elevation of Pa_{CO_2} are usually poorly tolerated.

MODES OF CONTROLLED VENTILATION

During controlled ventilation, as with assisted ventilation, gas can be delivered by targeting either volume or pressure.[49] Simply stated, the clinician must select either a specific volume that is delivered with each positive-pressure breath or a specific peak airway pressure that is established but not exceeded with each breath. Selection of the ventilatory target establishes the primary variable of concern when ventilatory support is applied: maintenance of ventilation with volume targeting, and avoidance of high airway pressure when pressure targeting is selected.[50]

Volume Ventilation

Modes of ventilation that are volume-targeted terminate the inspiratory phase when a preset tidal volume is delivered. This approach to cycling also defines the variables that must be set in adjusting the mechanical ventilator. The specific set of variables adjusted is dependent on the manufacturer's design; either V_T, peak flow, and flow waveform are selected, or V_T, flow waveform, and inspiratory time are adjusted.[49] With some ventilators, minute volume, inspiratory to expiratory (I:E) ratio, and flow waveform are selected. Regardless of specific ventilator design, the clinician must select parameters that define volume delivered, the time it takes to deliver the volume, and the flow waveform used during volume delivery.[51] What is not programmed by the clinician is a pressure target. When volume-targeted ventilation is selected, volume delivery and thus level of ventilation (Pa_{CO_2}) are controlled, but peak airway and peak alveolar pressure are allowed to vary on a breath-by-breath basis.[52]

Figure 115–6 illustrates the pressure, flow, and volume waveforms established during typical volume-targeted ventilation with a square wave flow pattern. Note that both pressure and volume linearly increase throughout the entire inspiratory phase. Because the flow pattern is square wave, the peak airway pressure reflects the amount of pressure necessary to overcome both compliance and resistance.[53] To identify peak alveolar pressure, an end-inspiratory hold (Fig. 115–7) must be programmed after the actual tidal volume delivery. The end-inspiratory plateau pressure is equal to peak alveolar pressure if the system gas flow rate is zero for a sufficient time to allow pressure within the lung-ventilator circuit to equilibrate (about 1 to 2 sec).[51, 54] Figure 115–8 also illustrates volume-targeted ventilation but with a decelerating flow pattern and an end-inspiratory hold. Note the difference between the pressure, volume, and flow waveforms in Figures 115–6 and 115–8 during the active gas delivery (before the end-inspiratory hold) phase. With decelerating flow, the majority of the tidal volume is delivered early in the inspiratory phase; thus, the airway pressure pattern is a square wave. For the same tidal volume, inspiratory time, ventilatory rate, and I:E ratio, a decelerating flow pattern demonstrates a lower peak airway pressure and higher mean airway pressure than does a square wave flow pattern, in spite of the fact that peak flow must be higher with decelerating flow than with square flow for the same

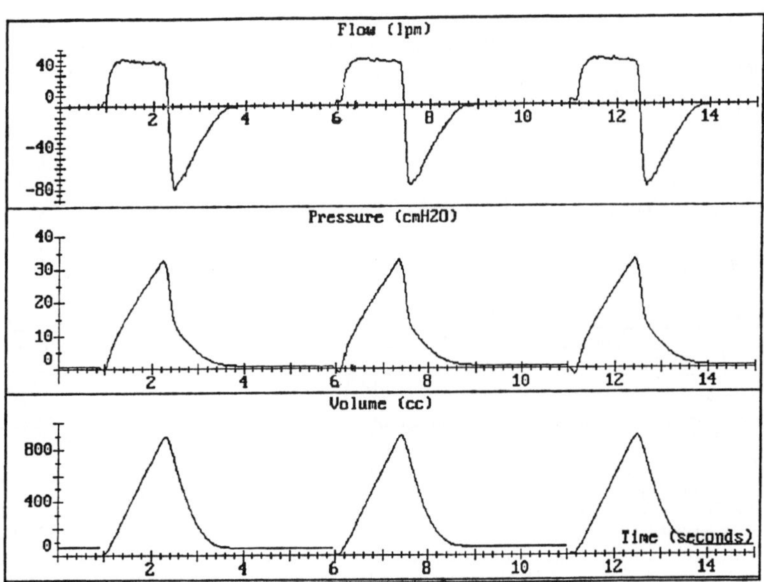

Figure 115–6. Pressure, flow, and volume versus time waveforms during volume-targeted assist-control ventilation. (From Kacmarek RM, Hess D, Stoller JD: Monitoring in Respiratory Care. St. Louis, Mosby-Year Book, 1993.)

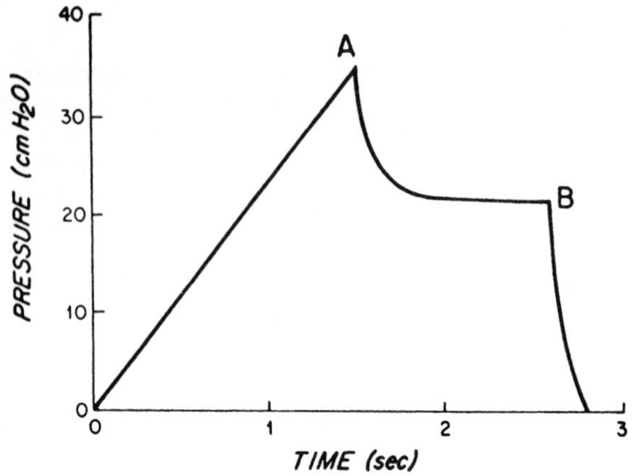

Figure 115–7. Airway pressure waveform versus time during square waveform volume-targeted ventilation with an end-inspiratory plateau. A = peak airway pressure; B = end-inspiratory plateau pressure (equivalent to peak alveolar pressure). (From Kacmarek RM, Hess D, Stoller JD: Monitoring in Respiratory Care. St. Louis, Mosby-Year Book, 1993.)

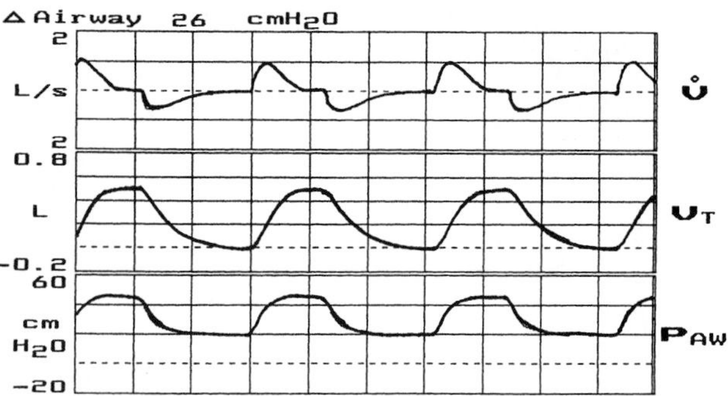

Figure 115–8. Airway (PAW), flow (V̇), and volume (VT) waveforms during volume-targeted controlled ventilation, incorporating a decelerating flow waveform and inflation hold. (From Kacmarek RM, Hess D, Stoller JD: Monitoring in Respiratory Care. St. Louis, Mosby-Year Book, 1993.)

inspiratory time.[55] However, the peak alveolar pressure will be the same if the same volume is maintained in the airway at zero flow. In Figure 115–8, peak alveolar pressure is equal to the end-inspiratory plateau pressure established just before exhalation. There is some evidence that ventilation is improved with a decelerating flow pattern compared with other flow patterns (square, sine, decelerations).[56, 57] In fact, provided appropriate inspiratory time is maintained, none of the other inspiratory flow patterns shows an advantage over the decelerating pattern.[58, 59]

Pressure Ventilation

Figure 115–9*A* and *B* depicts typical pressure-targeted, control mode ventilation. Note the similarities between Figures 115–8 and 115–9*B*. With pressure-targeted ventilation, the clinician sets the target pressure and inspiratory time or I:E ratio.[52] Because pressure is the target, tidal volume may vary from breath to breath. However, peak alveolar pressure does not exceed the targeted pressure. Pressure-targeted ventilation, although appearing similar to volume-targeted, decelerating flow ventilation, does differ from it in some fundamental aspects. With pressure control, the ventilator is designed to deliver sufficient flow at the onset of inspiration to rapidly pressurize the system to the target level,[49] after which the flow decreases, frequently exponentially, to maintain the target pressure. If inspiratory time is long enough and the impedance (resistance and compliance) of the system high enough, flow rate will reach zero before the end of the inspiratory phase (see Fig. 115–9*B*). If this occurs, the pressure target is equal to the peak alveolar pressure.[49] When pressure-targeted ventilation is selected, precise control over peak alveolar pressure is the goal; however, tidal volume and, as a result, Pa_{CO_2} may vary, depending on changes in system impedance.[56]

Tidal volume delivered in pressure-targeted ventilation is dependent on many variables. Any variable that affects the inspiratory pressure gradient or impedance of the system can alter VT (Table 115–3). As illustrated in Figure 115–9*A*, whenever inspiratory flow is greater than zero at the end of inspiration, lengthening of the inspiratory time increases tidal volume (Fig. 115–9*B*). The only setting in which tidal volume would not increase is if lengthening of the inspiratory time caused air trapping (auto-PEEP) to develop. If there is a zero flow period at the end of inspiration (Fig. 115–9*B*), lengthening of the inspiratory time will not increase VT but may result in a decrease in VT if air trapping develops.[52] Development of auto-PEEP during pressure-targeted ventilation always decreases VT because the ventilator applies the pressure-targeted level above circuit baseline pressure (atmosphere or applied PEEP).[60]

Because auto-PEEP is not recognized on a breath-to-breath basis by the ventilator, its presence results in the system's pressure immediately increasing to the auto-PEEP level once inspiration begins, essentially decreasing the applied inspira-

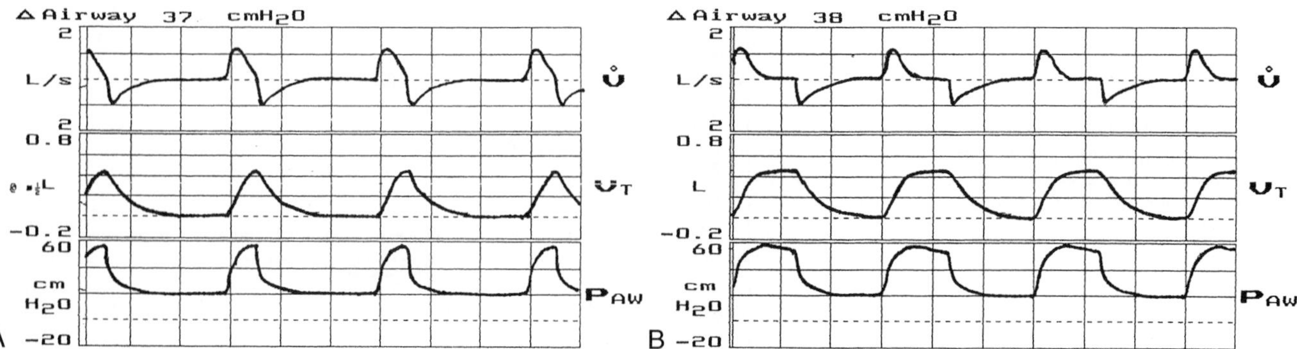

Figure 115–9. *A*, Airway pressure (PAW), flow (V̇), and volume (VT) waveforms during pressure-control ventilation. Note that inspiratory time is inadequate; flow rate has not returned to zero, nor is an inflation hold (zero flow period) observed. *B*, Results of increasing inspiratory time. Now flow returns to zero about midway through the inspiratory time period. The remaining inspiratory time illustrates an end-inspiratory hold. (From Kacmarek RM, Hess D, Stoller JD: Monitoring in Respiratory Care. St. Louis, Mosby-Year Book, 1993.)

TABLE 115–3. Factors Affecting Tidal Volume During Pressure-Targeted Ventilation

Pressure target level
Applied PEEP
Rate (auto-PEEP)
Patient–ventilator system compliance
Patient–ventilator system resistance
Inspiratory time (I:E ratio, auto-PEEP)

PEEP = positive end-expiratory pressure; I:E = inspiratory to expiratory ratio.

tory pressure gradient by a level equal to the auto-PEEP.[61] The result is always a decrease in VT. There is an optimal inspiratory time in all patients at which tidal volume delivery with pressure ventilation is maximal.[62] This inspiratory time period is dependent on the compliance and resistance of the system. The more compliant and more resistant the lung, the greater likelihood for the development of auto-PEEP, whereas the less compliant and less resistant the system, the less likely the development of auto-PEEP. In general, with obstructive lung disease, auto-PEEP can develop with much shorter inspiratory times than those seen in patients with acute restrictive lung disease.[61]

Increasing ventilatory rate with pressure ventilation may increase or decrease minute ventilation, depending on the development of air trapping and auto-PEEP. If an increase in the ventilatory rate causes auto-PEEP, VT and thus minute ventilation may decrease, increasing Pa_{CO_2}.[60]

Applied PEEP in pressure-targeted ventilation may increase or decrease VT, depending on whether it recruits lung units, improving compliance, or overdistends lung units, decreasing compliance. In general, during pressure ventilation, any factor that increases impedance (decreased compliance and increased resistance) to ventilation decreases VT, and any factor that decreases impedance increases VT.[49]

Pressure Versus Volume Ventilation

Considerable data have accumulated comparing pressure-targeted and volume-targeted ventilation.[63-70] The early data indicated that pressure-targeted ventilation was superior to volume-targeted ventilation in reference to gas exchange and pulmonary mechanics.[63, 64] However, all of these early studies were uncontrolled case series, many of which were retrospective.[63, 64] More recently, numerous well-controlled prospective animal[66] and human[65, 67-70] studies have demonstrated no difference in gas exchange or pulmonary mechanics when pressure and volume control were compared when total PEEP[65, 67-70] (applied plus auto) or mean airway pressure[66] was kept constant.

The decision to use either pressure or volume targeting depends on which of the following is of primary concern: (1) maintaining VT and Pa_{CO_2} despite airway and alveolar pressure increases, or (2) maintaining a limit on peak alveolar and airway pressure, despite allowing VT and Pa_{CO_2} to vary as system impedance varies. Table 115-4 compares volume-targeted and pressure-targeted ventilation. As illustrated in Figures 115-8 and 115-9*B*, airway pressure, flow, and volume waveforms can be set identically with pressure and volume ventilation.[71] Again, the primary difference between the two approaches is the targeting of tidal volume or system pressure. If volume control is selected, careful monitoring of peak airway pressure must occur, whereas with pressure targeting, careful monitoring of VT and minute volume is required.

With pressure targeting, it is more difficult to identify acute changes in impedance than with volume targeting. A decrease in impedance during volume ventilation normally results in high-pressure alarms being activated, and if the change in impedance is progressive, as with a tension pneumothorax, the peak airway pressure alarm continues to be activated as pressure continues to increase. With pressure targeting, an equilibrium between the peak airway pressure and the pressure inside the pneumothorax eventually occurs, limiting the change in impedance. Frequently, pneumothorax with pressure control is not identified until routine chest radiography or by concern over acutely altered blood gas values.

Volume-targeted and pressure-targeted ventilation are available on most intensive care unit (ICU) ventilators. Either is available in assist-control and control modes of ventilation, the two most common approaches to application of controlled mechanical ventilation.[72] Synchronized intermittent mandatory ventilation (SIMV) can also be applied with use of both pressure and volume targets. All three of these modes have been used to provide controlled ventilation. With assist-control ventilation and SIMV, patients not sedated to apnea can breathe at a rate higher than the set mandatory rate. With assist-control ventilation, the patient's effort triggers an additional positive-pressure breath, whereas with SIMV, the breath is unsupported.

Inverse Ratio Ventilation

Pressure control ventilation became popular in the late 1980s as a result of a number of uncontrolled case series that demonstrated improved oxygenation in ARDS patients with use of pressure control–inverse ratio (>1:1) ventilation (PCIRV).[63, 73, 74] In many of these early reports, I:E ratios as high as 3:1 were commonly employed. During the late 1980s and 1990s, a number of controlled prospective animal and human studies systematically compared PCIRV with either pressure control (PC) or volume control (VC) with normal I:E ratio.[65-70, 75, 76] None of these studies demonstrated improved oxygenation, hemodynamics, or compliance with inverse ratio ventilation (IRV); however, a number of them demonstrated a trend toward improved ventilation with IRV.[67, 69, 75, 76] Brochard's group randomly compared VC 1:2 and PC 1:2, 2:1, and 3:1 in a series of nine ARDS patients in which FIO_2, total PEEP (applied plus auto), VT, and respiratory rate were held constant between I:E ratios.[67] They noted a decrease in Pa_{O_2} ($P < .05$) with a nonsignificant decrease in mean arterial pressure and Pa_{CO_2} at inverse ratios compared with VC and PC 1:2. Mercat and associates[69] noted similar differences when PC 1:2 and VC 1:2 were randomly compared with PC 2:1 in 10 ARDS patients with FIO_2, VT, total PEEP, and respiratory rate kept constant. Pa_{O_2} was unchanged between modes; however, there was a significant ($P < .05$) decrease in cardiac index, oxygen delivery, and Pa_{CO_2} with PC 2:1 compared with both VC and PC 1:2. Most recently, in eight ARDS patients, Zavala and coworkers[75] randomly compared VC 1:2, no PEEP; VC 1:2, 8 cm H_2O PEEP; VC 2.75:1, 8 cm H_2O auto-PEEP; and PC 2.75:1,

TABLE 115–4. Pressure-Targeted Versus Volume-Targeted Ventilation

	Volume Target	Pressure Target
Peak airway pressure	Variable	Constant
Peak alveolar pressure	Variable	Constant
Tidal volume	Constant	Variable
Minimum rate	Preset	Preset
Inspiratory time	Preset	Preset
Peak flow	Constant	Variable
Flow pattern	Preset	Decelerating

8 cm H_2O auto-PEEP. They observed no difference in $Pa{O_2}$ or $Pa{CO_2}$ during VC 2.75:1 but a significant decrease ($P < .05$) in both $Pa{O_2}$ and $Pa{CO_2}$ during PC 2.75:1. In addition, using multiple inert gas analysis, they observed the highest shunt fraction and lowest dead space with PCIRV.

Much of the criticism from proponents of IRV regarding these studies has focused on the short time that inverse ratio was applied (30 to 60 min), indicating that the beneficial effects require a longer period of time. Mercat and colleagues[76] in a second study in 1997 demonstrated that there was no benefit gained over time with IRV. They randomly compared VCIRV 2:1 with VC 1:2, each applied during a 6-hour period, where V_T, respiratory rate, total PEEP, and FIO_2 were constant. Again, they observed no improvement in $Pa{O_2}$ and no difference in cardiac output but a significant improvement in $Pa{CO_2}$.

Much of the debate over the beneficial effects of IRV centers on two specific issues. First, does the lengthening of inspiratory time resulting in inverse I:E ratios improve recruitment of lung units with long opening time constants? Second, is it more beneficial to apply set PEEP on the ventilator or to establish auto-PEEP by lengthy inspiratory times? As already reviewed, none of the prospective randomized comparisons of PCIRV or VCIRV with normal I:E ratio ventilation has been able to demonstrate improved oxygenation, compliance, hemodynamics, or oxygen delivery.[65-70, 75, 76]

In most patients, when inspiratory time is increased to create an I:E ratio of 2:1 or higher, auto-PEEP develops. The question that has been debated is whether any benefit is derived by the development of auto-PEEP in preference to applied PEEP, especially when the controlled application of IRV does not appear to enhance oxygenation, compliance, or hemodynamics.

When PEEP is set on the ventilator, it is distributed equally to all lung units distal to the point of application (Fig. 115-10*A*). Auto-PEEP is not equally distributed in the lung because auto-PEEP develops as a result of local time constants (time constant = compliance × resistance) (Fig. 115-10*B*). The greater the time constant, the greater the likelihood that auto-PEEP develops, as seen in patients with chronic obstructive pulmonary disease (COPD). If this situation occurs in ARDS, the distribution of auto-PEEP is favored to lung units that are the least stiff, which results in overdistention of the most compliant lung units and underdistention of the lung units most requiring the application of PEEP.[77] This maldistribution of auto-PEEP may expose the most healthy lung units to the highest PEEP and increase the likelihood of injury. It is impos-

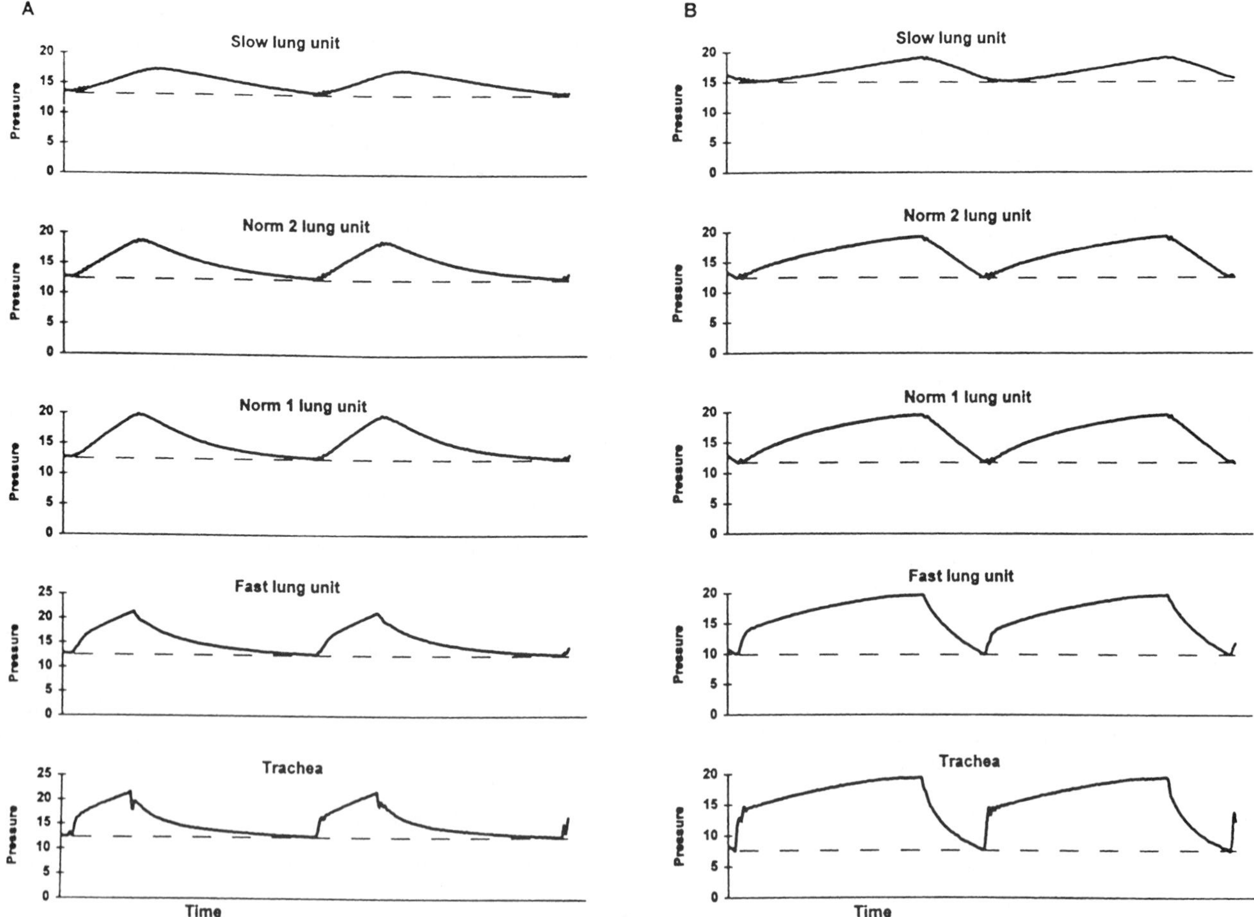

Figure 115–10. Pressure versus time tracing of the trachea and each of four lung units in a mechanical model. The slow lung unit had the longest emptying time, the fast lung unit had the quickest emptying time, and norm 1 and norm 2 had emptying times in between these. The *dotted line* represents the end-expiratory pressure (EEP) measurement. *A*, 1:3 I:E ratio ventilation: slow lung unit, EEP 13.5 cm H_2O; norm 2 lung unit, EEP 12.7 cm H_2O; norm 1 lung unit, EEP 12.6 cm H_2O; fast lung unit, EEP 12.7 cm H_2O; tracheal EEP 12.5 cm H_2O. Total system PEEP using a Braschi valve is 13.0 cm H_2O. *B*, 3:1 I:E ratio ventilation: slow lung unit, EEP 15.8 cm H_2O; norm 2 lung unit, EEP 12 cm H_2O; norm 1 lung unit, EEP 12.7 cm H_2O; fast lung unit, EEP 10.1 cm H_2O; tracheal EEP 7.5 cm H_2O. Total system PEEP using Braschi valve is 12.7 cm H_2O. (From Kacmarek RM, Kirmse M, Nishimura M, Mang M, et al: The effect of applied versus auto-PEEP on local lung unit pressure and volume in a four-unit lung model. Chest 1995; 108:1073–1079.)

sible at the bedside to evaluate the lack of uniformity of auto-PEEP distribution because its measurement, regardless of technique used, results in the measurement of the mean level of auto-PEEP in the patient's ventilator system. Figure 115-10*A* and *B* illustrates the different distributions of applied PEEP (I:E 1:3) and auto-PEEP (I:E 3:1) in a four-chamber lung model with different time constants in each chamber.[77]

AUTO-PEEP

Auto-PEEP is intrinsic PEEP or identified PEEP that develops as a result of incomplete emptying of local lung units and air trapping.[78] Two general settings increase the probability of development of auto-PEEP[79]:

- Acute or chronic pulmonary disease when dynamic airway compression is present
- A rapid respiratory rate with large VT when expiratory time is inadequate

As noted in Figure 115-11, with auto-PEEP, central airway pressure and ventilator circuit pressure do not reflect the auto-PEEP level unless an end-expiratory hold is established.[78] Thus, unless auto-PEEP is looked for, its presence is not identified. Auto-PEEP results in the same localized or global (if extensive) effects seen with applied PEEP,[78] except that it is established in lung units with high or normal compliance and normal or high airway resistance.[79] Auto-PEEP is primarily a problem in patients with intrinsic lung disease, COPD, or asthma or in patients ventilated with large minute volumes and rapid rates.

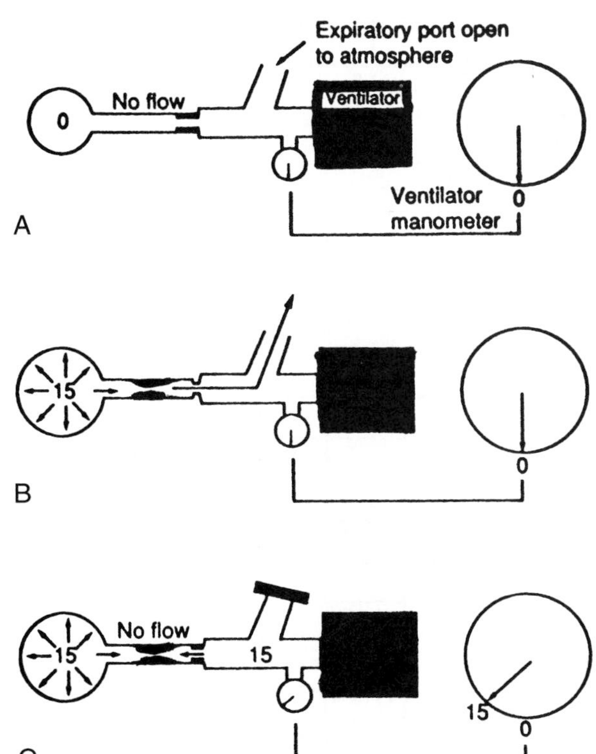

Figure 115-11. Relationship between alveolar, central airway, and ventilator circuit pressures under normal conditions and in the presence of severe dynamic airway obstruction *(A)*, with the expiratory valve open *(B)*, and with the expiratory valve occluded *(C)*. Auto-PEEP level is identified by creating an end-expiratory hold, allowing alveolar, central airway, and ventilator circuit pressure to equilibrate. During equilibration, auto-PEEP level can be read on the system manometer. (From Pepe PE, Marini JJ: Occult positive end-expiratory pressure in mechanically ventilated patients with airflow obstruction: The auto-PEEP effect. Am Rev Respir Dis 1982; 126:166-170.)

Although it is not normally an issue during controlled ventilation, patient-ventilator synchrony is adversely affected by the presence of auto-PEEP. Auto-PEEP always increases the patient's effort to trigger the ventilator[80] (Fig. 115-12). Patients must decompress the auto-PEEP present to trigger the ventilator.[81]

Identification of Auto-PEEP

Auto-PEEP can be identified from the airway pressure waveform but only after the application of an end-inspiratory hold[81] (Fig. 115-13). In general, patients must be passively ventilated to allow accurate evaluation; however, in some patients actively triggering the ventilator, an estimate of auto-PEEP is occasionally possible by use of this method.[61] The auto-PEEP reflected on the system manometer or pressure waveform is the mean auto-PEEP level because it reflects the end-expiratory equilibration pressure within the patient-ventilator system; the maximum local auto-PEEP level always exceeds that measured.[79]

Auto-PEEP measurement can occur only if no continuous system flow is present. Systems using flow triggering must be turned off or the auto-PEEP level is overestimated. During assisted or controlled ventilation, auto-PEEP can be identified but not quantified by evaluating end-expiratory flow[81] (Fig. 115-14). If end-expiratory flow has not reached zero before the next inspiration, auto-PEEP is present. However, in patients with severe dynamic airway obstruction, the end-expiratory flow may be too low to be accurately measured by the crude flow measurement technology on ventilators.

In patients with auto-PEEP, expiratory breath sounds continue until they are interrupted by inspiratory sounds, and physical examination and chest radiography show hyperinflation. In spontaneously breathing patients, the only way to accurately measure auto-PEEP is to evaluate esophageal pressure change (Fig. 115-15) during inspiration at the same time airway opening pressure or flow is evaluated.[79] With auto-PEEP, a drop in esophageal pressure occurs before flow is measured at the airway. The magnitude of the drop is equal to the auto-PEEP level. In patients activating abdominal muscles during exhalation, the estimate of auto-PEEP may be inaccurately increased.

As illustrated in Figure 115-16, the volume of gas trapped but not the auto-PEEP level can be estimated by allowing a prolonged uninterrupted expiration (30 to 60 sec).[82] This maneuver is possible only in patients who are apneic, receiving controlled ventilation. Particularly in patients with asthma whose lungs are highly compliant, adjusting the ventilator to reduce trapped volume may be more useful than attempting to measure auto-PEEP by an end-expiratory hold.[83] In some asthmatic patients, airways may completely occlude at end-expiration, and precise estimation of auto-PEEP may be impossible.[84]

In addition, because of the large intrathoracic pressure gradient that must be established to cause airflow and triggering of the ventilator in the presence of auto-PEEP, many patients are unable to trigger assisted breaths.[79] Whenever the patient's actual respiratory rate exceeds the ventilator response rate, auto-PEEP is present.

Management

Table 115-5 lists the various techniques used to minimize the level of auto-PEEP. With dynamic airway compression or secretion accumulation, aggressive bronchial hygiene and aerosolized pharmacology should be employed. In addition,

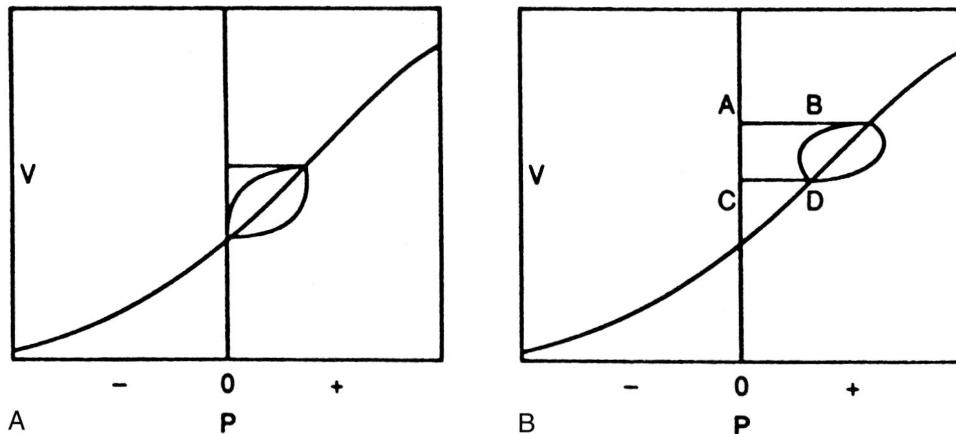

Figure 115–12. *A*, Normal spontaneously breathing esophageal pressure-volume (P-V) loop. *B*, Effect of auto-PEEP on area of P-V loop, reflecting marked increase in the effort to breathe as a result of the need to decompress the auto-PEEP prior to changing lung volume. Central airway pressure at end exhalation is depicted by C. The pressure change from C to D must occur before gas movement to the lung periphery is possible. The area of the rectangle CDBA represents the increased workload with auto-PEEP. (From Otis AB: Work of breathing. *In*: Handbook of Physiology: The Respiratory System. Vol 1. Finn WU, Rahn H [Eds]. Washington, DC, American Physiological Society, 1964.)

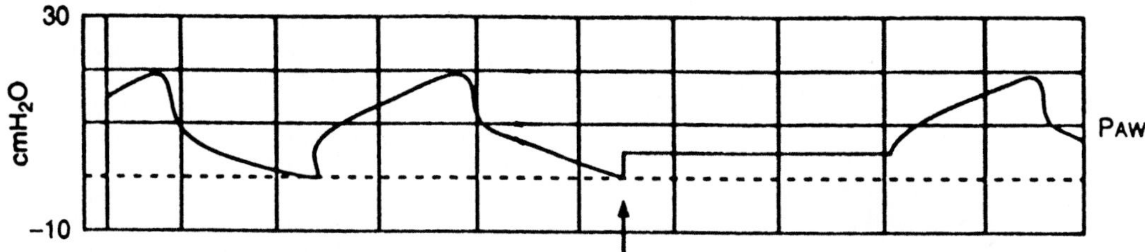

Figure 115–13. Measurement of auto-PEEP *(arrow)* using the end-expiratory hold control of an intensive care unit (ICU) ventilator. Peak airway pressure (PAW) is not affected on the inspiration following measurement because auto-PEEP is present, even though unnoticed, on every breath. (From Pierson DJ, Kacmarek RM [Eds]. Foundation of Respiratory Care. New York, Churchill Livingstone, 1992.)

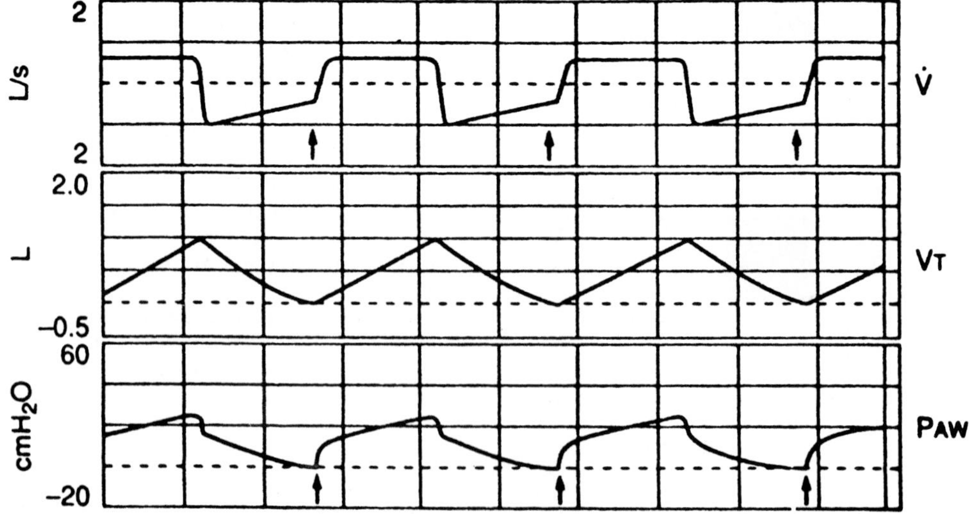

Figure 115–14. Airway pressure (PAW) and flow waveforms during volume-limited controlled ventilation in the presence of auto-PEEP. The initial airway pressure demonstrates a rapid initial increase *(arrow)*, approximating the auto-PEEP level, then gradually increasing to peak airway pressure. Expiratory gas flow does not return to zero *(arrow)* in the presence of auto-PEEP. (From Pierson DJ, Kacmarek RM [Eds]. Foundation of Respiratory Care. New York, Churchill Livingstone, 1992.)

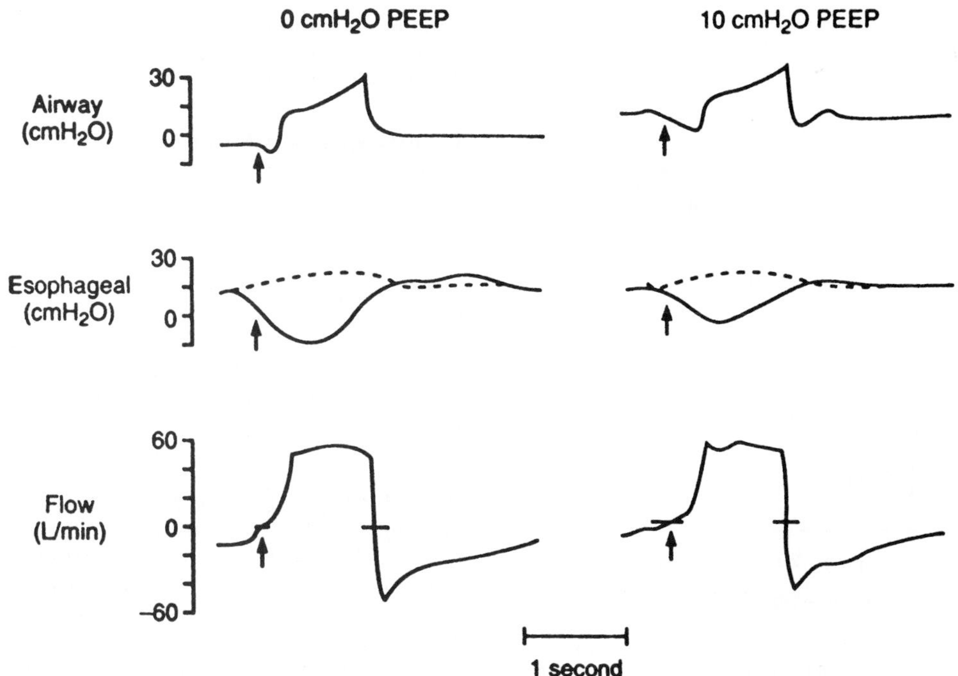

Figure 115–15. Assessment of the level of auto-PEEP in spontaneously breathing patients by evaluation of esophageal pressure change relative to either airway opening pressure or flow at airway opening. *Arrows* indicate pressure and flow change at airway opening. The change in esophageal pressure between baseline and the level that allows change in airway opening pressure or in flow is equal to the auto-PEEP level. Note the effect of 10 cm H_2O applied PEEP on the level of auto-PEEP *(left side)*. (From Smith TC, Marini JJ: Impact of PEEP on lung mechanics and work of breathing in severe airflow obstruction. J Appl Physiol 1988; 65:1488–1499.)

respiratory rate and tidal volume should be decreased to minimize minute ventilation and inspiratory time shortened to maximize expiratory time[85]; frequently, the result is permissive hypercapnia during controlled ventilation. In spontaneously breathing patients with dynamic airway closure, PEEP can be applied to balance the auto-PEEP. This allows alveolar, airway, and ventilator circuit pressure to equilibrate.[79, 86] Provided the auto-PEEP is a result of dynamic airway obstruction and applied PEEP does not exceed about 80% of the auto-PEEP, pulmonary mechanics should not be altered when PEEP is applied.[87] If peak and plateau pressures increase with volume-targeted ventilation, or if VT decreases with pressure-targeted ventilation, the applied PEEP has caused greater overdistention.

THE PRESSURE-VOLUME CURVE

A typical inspiratory pressure-volume curve of the total respiratory system in a patient with ARDS is illustrated in Figure 115-17. Two specific points on this curve have been proposed as targets for mechanical ventilation.[18, 88] The lower inflection point (LIP) or P_{flex} represents the point where compliance during inspiration improves, indicating recruitment of collapsed lung units; the upper deflection point (UDP) or P_{flex} upper indicates the point of overdistention. As discussed earlier, the LIP identifies the minimum PEEP level and the UDP the maximal peak alveolar pressure in an LPVS.

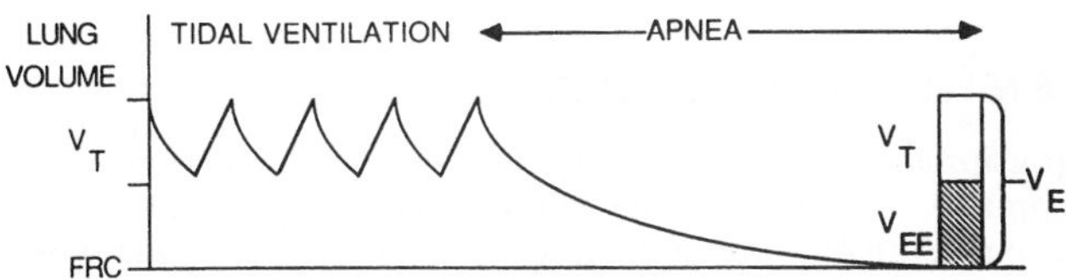

Figure 115–16. Schematic representation of the measurement of end-inspiratory volume (VEI) in a patient with acute asthma. VEE is the end-expiratory lung volume above functional residual capacity (FRC). (From Tuxon DV, Lane S: The effects of ventilatory pattern on hyperinflation, airway pressure, and circulation in mechanical ventilation of patients with severe air-flow obstruction. Am Rev Respir Dis 1987; 136:872–879.)

TABLE 115–5. Approaches Used to Modify the Level of Auto-PEEP

1. *Decrease dynamic airflow obstruction*
   - Agressive bronchodilation
   - Chest physical therapy
   - Airway suctioning
   - Large-size endotracheal tube
2. *Modify ventilatory pattern*
   - Increase expiratory time
     - Decrease rate
     - Decrease VT
   - Decrease inspiratory time
     - Increase peak inspiratory flow
     - Use low compressible volume circuit
   - Use low-rate SIMV
3. *Allow P_{CO_2} to rise above 60 mm Hg*
   - Decrease rate
   - Decrease VT
4. *Normalize pH*
   - Administer $NaHCO_3$ during metabolic acidosis
   - Avoid purposeful hyperventilation
5. *Apply PEEP/CPAP to reduce work of breathing*

CPAP = continuous positive airway pressure; PEEP = positive end-expiratory pressure; SIMV = synchronized intermittent mandatory ventilation; VT = tidal volume.

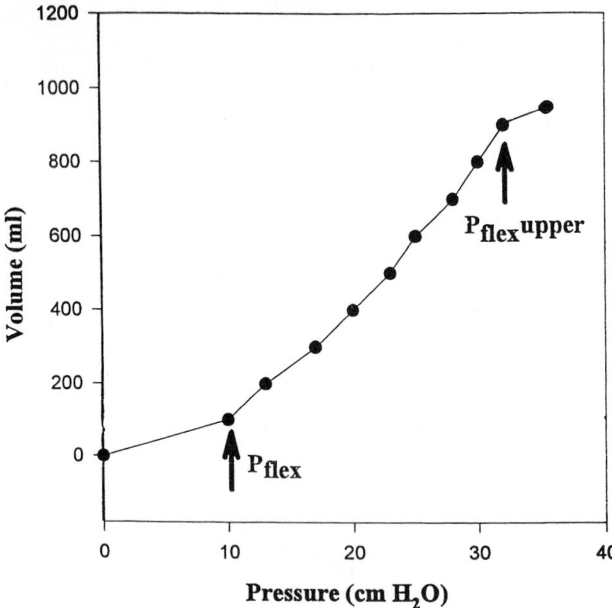

Figure 115–17. Pressure-volume curve of the total respiratory system in a patient with adult respiratory distress syndrome. P_{flex} is the lower inflection point and P_{flex}upper is the upper deflection point (UDP).

Determination of the Pressure-Volume Curve

Two approaches have been described in the literature for the determination of a pressure-volume curve in ARDS patients.[18, 88] The first is the classic *super syringe method*, and the other is the *low continuous flow method* (Fig. 115–18). During either determination, patients require heavy sedation, ideally paralysis, to ensure passive inflation. In addition, before determination, a volume history is established by repetitive breaths to the maximum volume being used during the maneuver. Small sequential (50 to 100 mL) gas volumes are then delivered, followed by a 2-second inflation hold to a maximum pressure of above 50 cm H_2O. After the data are plotted, tangents to the curve as illustrated in Figure 115–18 are drawn with the points of intersection identified as the LIP and UDP. In general, the LIP varies between about 5 and 20 cm H_2O,[18] and the UDP between 25 and 40 cm H_2O.[89] Recently, computerized programs have been developed to identify these points.[90]

In the continuous flow method, a low flow (≤15 L/min) must be delivered continuously while the airway pressure curve is recorded. Flow is continued until a peak pressure of about 50 cm H_2O is reached. A low flow is required to eliminate the effect of airways resistance. As demonstrated by Servillo and coworkers[88] using a 15 L/min flow, less than 1 cm H_2O difference exists between the LIPs and UDPs when this method is compared with a classic super syringe pressure-volume curve. The lower the flow, the less error associated with airways resistance. Amato and colleagues[18] used a continuous flow of 2 L/min to construct pressure-volume curves.

Gross estimation of both the LIP and UDP can be obtained by incremental increases in PEEP (2 cm H_2O) during either pressure control or volume control ventilation. With volume control (low constant VT setting 250 to 300 mL), end-inspiratory plateau pressures are evaluated at each PEEP level. With pressure control, VT settings at a fixed pressure control level are evaluated at each PEEP level. The key is to choose a VT or pressure control level that avoids overdistention when up to 20 cm H_2O PEEP is applied. The LIP is equal to the lowest PEEP level establishing maximum compliance, and the UDP is the highest end-inspiratory pressure before compliance begins to decrease with pressure control or volume control.

Effect of the Chest Wall

In the average patient, as illustrated in Figure 115–19, the chest wall has a minor effect on the pressure-volume curve of the total respiratory system.[89] However, in patients with large abdominal masses, in trauma patients aggressively fluid resuscitated, in patients after abdominal surgery, and in patients with thoracic deformities, chest wall compliance may be markedly reduced, leading to an underestimation of the true UDP and an overestimation of the LIP.[91, 92] That is, peak alveolar pressures higher than those predicted by the pressure-volume of the total respiratory system can be applied without causing overdistention of the lung. Although the pressure-volume relationship of the total respiratory system may also overestimate the LIP of the lung in this setting, it still identifies the minimum PEEP level needed to stabilize the lung-thoracic system. As a result, in patients in whom a decreased chest wall compliance is assumed, an esophageal balloon should be placed to allow simultaneous assessment of the chest wall and total respiratory system compliance, allowing the calculation of actual lung compliance to accurately determine the UPD.

The Expiratory Limb of the Pressure-Volume Curve

Much discussion has recently occurred regarding which limb of the pressure-volume curve of the total respiratory system is most predictive of the minimum PEEP level needed to prevent derecruitment. In an abstract, Meyer and colleagues[93] noted that to prevent derecruitment after a recruitment maneuver, PEEP higher than that predicted by the LIP on the inspiratory limb of the total respiratory system pressure-volume curve was necessary (Fig. 115–20). Harris and colleagues[90] noted that the point of maximum curvature on the expiratory curve (indicative of the pressure below which marked derecruitment occurs) was 2 to 3 cm H_2O higher than the LIP on the inflation limb.

Debate about the best value to use from the pressure-volume curve will continue until additional data are available. However, it is clear that the inspiratory pressure-volume curve of the total respiratory system identifies the minimum level of PEEP required to prevent at least partial derecruitment, although a higher level may be required in many patients. The UDP of the pressure-volume curve can be used as a gross estimate of the maximum pressure that does not cause overdistention in most patients. In those patients with clinical indications of decreased chest wall compliance, higher levels of $P_{plateau}$ can be set without increasing the probability of ventilator-induced lung injury. However, as recommended by consensus statement, a maximum $P_{plateau}$ should be targeted at about 35 to 40 cm H_2O.[94]

VENTILATOR ALARMS

Appropriate setting of alarms during controlled ventilatory support is crucial to ensure notification of potentially adverse patient-ventilator conditions. During both pressure-targeted and volume-targeted ventilation, a few specific alarms are crucial for safe management of the patient-ventilator system. Essentially, alarms should notify staff if system pressures have increased above a targeted level; if ventilatory rate, tidal volume, and minute volume have exceeded or decreased below predetermined thresholds; if a minimum system pressure is present with each breath; if PEEP is maintained; if the ventila-

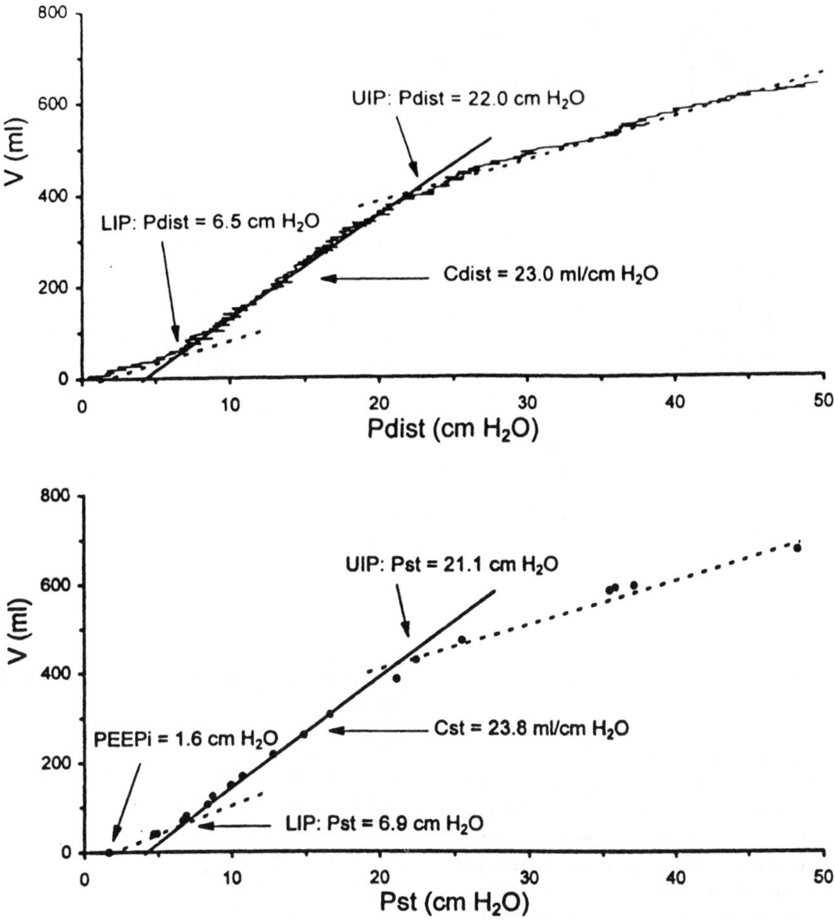

Figure 115–18. Calculation of compliance, lower inflection point (LIP) and upper deflection point (UIP) with classic super syringe method *(top panel)* and continuous flow method *(bottom panel)* in a representative patient with adult respiratory distress syndrome. A regression line of the points corresponding to the linear segment of the pressure-volume curve, defined as the range with a compliance above 80% of maximum compliance, was drawn by the computer *(solid line)*. Compliance is the slope of this line. Lines were eye-fitted through points below and above this segment *(dashed lines)*. LIP and UIP were identified as the intersections between the regression line and the latter lines. (From Servillo G, Svantesson C, Beydon L, et al: Pressure-volume curve in acute respiratory failure: automated low flow inflation versus occlusion. Am J Respir Crit Care Med 1997; 155:1629–1636.)

Figure 115–19. Static pressure-volume curves of chest wall (Ccw = *closed circles*), lung (CL = *open circles*), and total respiratory system (Crs = *squares*) obtained in one representative patient. The upper deflection point (UDP) calculated by a step-by-step regression was found at 26 cm H_2O on Crs, which corresponded to 23 cm H_2O on CL. Note the absence of UDP on the chest wall pressure-volume curve. See text for discussion. (From Roupie E, Dambrosio M, Servillo G, et al: Titration of tidal volume and induced hypercapnia in acute respiratory distress syndrome. Am J Respir Crit Care Med 1995; 152:121–128.)

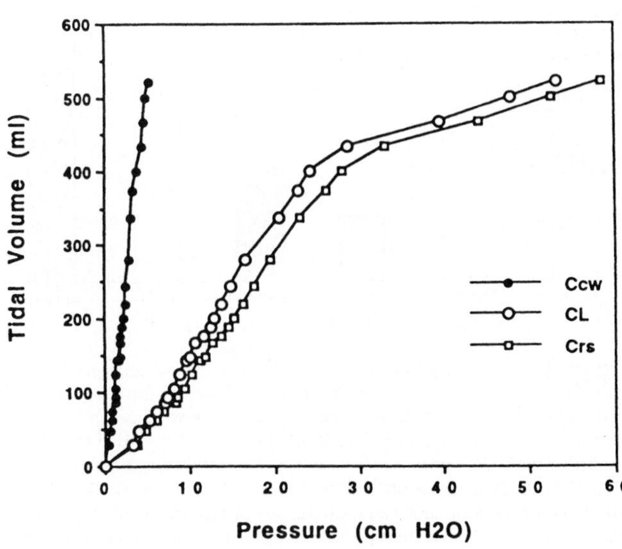

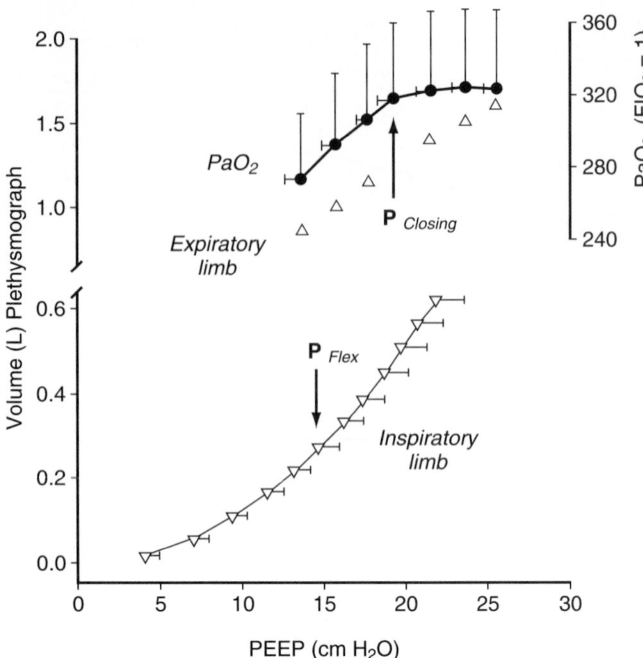

Figure 115–20. Inspiratory and expiratory limb pressure-volume curves of the total respiratory system. Inflection points on both curves are indicated. The pressure needed to prevent closure is greater than the P_{flex}. P_{flex} = inspiratory limb; P = closing expiratory limb. (From Meyer EC, Barbas CSV, Grunauer MA, et al: PEEP at P_{flex} cannot guarantee a fully open lung after a high pressure recruiting maneuver in ARDS patients (Abstract). Am J Respir Crit Care Med 1998; 157:A694).

tor is disconnected; and if the mechanical ventilator has malfunctioned.

Of concern is that the alarm algorithms currently employed on most ICU ventilators fail to differentiate the level of urgency of the alarms and make it difficult to differentiate one alarm from another or the alarms on the ventilator from those of other equipment.[95, 96] The current methodology used to activate ventilator alarms and the alarm sounds themselves can result in a low efficiency of identifying critical clinical situations, could increase the response time of personnel responding to alarms, and may actually condition ICU personnel to ignore alarms.[97]

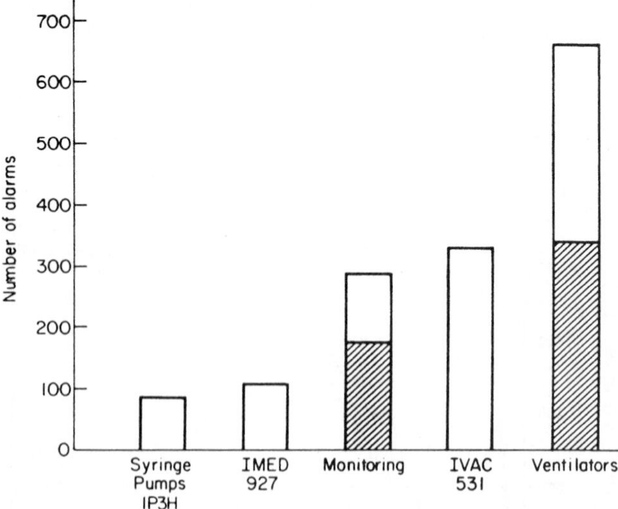

Figure 115–21. Distribution of 1455 alarms in a surgical intensive care unit occurring over a 3-week period (total/column) and the proportion simply silenced by staff (*hatched area* of column). IP3H = Vickers syringe pump model IP3H; IMED 927 = IMED infusion pump model 927; monitoring = cardiac/hemodynamic monitors; IVAC 531 = IVAC infusion pump model 531; and ventilators = Siemens Servo 900c and Cape 2000. (From O'Carroll TN: Survey of alarms in an intensive therapy unit. Anaesthesia 1986; 41:742–744.)

Alarm Overload in the Intensive Care Unit

As a result of all of the equipment used in the ICU being alarmed and each alarm having a high false-positive rate, many authors have found that more than 75% of all alarms in the ICU are false-positives.[98-102] O'Carroll[98] studied the frequency of false-positive alarms in a surgical ICU for a 3-week period. During this time, a total of 1455 alarms were recorded; however, only eight were considered potentially life-threatening. As shown in Figure 115–21, 661 of these alarms were from the mechanical ventilator.

Lawless[101] recorded the incidence of alarms in a pediatric ICU during a 7-day period. Staff were asked to record the type and number of alarms that sounded and to classify them as false, significant (resulting in a change of therapy), or induced by staff manipulation (e.g., turning, chest physiotherapy) and as a result not significant. A total of 2176 alarms were acti-

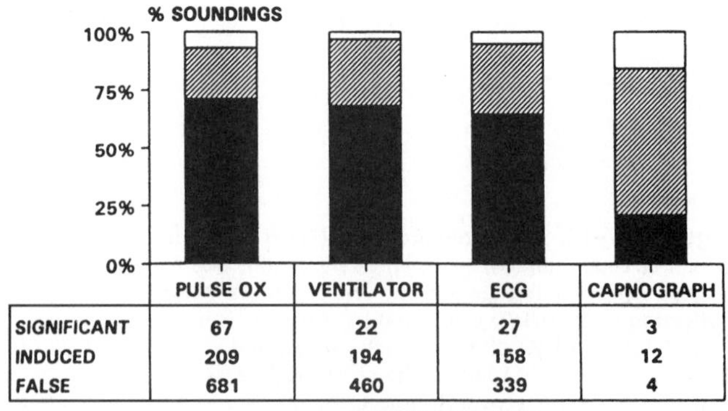

	PULSE OX	VENTILATOR	ECG	CAPNOGRAPH
SIGNIFICANT	67	22	27	3
INDUCED	209	194	158	12
FALSE	681	460	339	4

Figure 115–22. Distribution and classification of alarms tracked for 1 week in an intensive care unit. Significant alarm = need for action. *White, hatched,* and *black* portions of each bar signify significant, induced, and false alarms, respectively. Induced alarm = result of practitioner's intervention (e.g., suctioning); false alarm = false-positive alarm. (From Lawless ST: Crying wolf: False alarms in a pediatric intensive care unit. Crit Care Med 1994; 22:981–985).

TABLE 115–6. International Standards Organization (ISO) Standards for Visual Mechanical Ventilator Alarms

Alarm Category	Operator Response	Meaning	Indicator Color	Flashing Frequency	Duty Cycle
High priority	Immediate response to deal with a condition	Emergency	Red	1.4 Hz to 2.8 Hz	20% to 60% on
Medium priority	Prompt response to deal with a condition	Abnormal	Yellow	0.4 Hz to 0.8 Hz	20% to 60% on
Low priority	Awareness of condition	Change of status	Yellow	Constant (on)	100%

From International Standards Organization: Anaesthesia and Respiratory Care Alarm Signals. Part 1: Visual Alarms. ISO 9703-1, July 15, 1992.

vated; however, only 119 were considered significant (Fig. 115–22).

Tsien and Fackler[102] recorded ICU alarms during a 298-hour period, monitoring only one ICU bed at a time. Of the 2942 alarms recorded, 86% were classified as false-positive alarms; an additional 10% were classified as clinically irrelevant true-positive alarms.

A Need for More Useful Alarms

The International Standards Organization[103–105] has proposed developing ventilator alarms on the basis of three levels of urgency with both audio and visual notification when alarms are activated (Tables 115-6 and 115-7). However, the events activating each level of alarm have not been specified. MacIntyre and Day[106] have been the only ones to propose a classification system of ventilator alarms based on urgency.

Although MacIntyre and Day's classification system represents a useful first step in categorizing alarm functions into logical groupings, it is only the first step in solving the complex issue of frequent false-positive alarms. Of major concern with the current concepts associated with most alarm design and function is that they operate on a strictly on or off basis and do not allow patient-technology events to move from one level of urgency to another over time,[97, 107] that is, an event that would be classified as minor, if it lasted for a few seconds, cannot be differentiated from the same event that is occurring on a continual basis.

Smart Alarms

As is obvious from the preceding discussion or from a short exposure to the ICU, the alarms incorporated on ventilators have failed in their attempt to alert clinicians of events of true clinical significance without simultaneously identifying events that are falsely positive at a rate of nearly 10 to 1. Alarms on all ventilators need to be smarter. In addition to alarms being established on an urgency basis with a three-level visual hierarchy and having uniquely identifiable audio components, more appropriate thresholds for activation and movement from one level of urgency to another must be established. For example, a single breath violation of the high peak airway pressure alarm of the mechanical ventilator should not be identified as the highest urgency alarm, whereas a continual violation over time should activate the highest urgency alarm.

It is obvious that the one-alarm violation, one-alarm scheme used on most ventilators should end. Up-down counting algorithms, artifact filters, time delays, and movement from one level of urgency to another on the basis of frequency and length of the specific violation must be incorporated. As recommended by Sanborn,[107] alarm limit-setting can be automatically determined by specific algorithms. Built-in nomograms could provide initial boundaries subject to the practitioner's review. For ventilator rate and volume alarms, the patient's height, weight, and age could be programmed and alarms set accordingly. Once ventilation begins, statistical analysis could provide updated limits based on actual data, with currently active boundary limits being appropriately displayed.[107]

TABLE 115–7. International Standards Organization (ISO) Standards for Audio Mechanical Ventilator Alarms

Characteristic	High Priority	Medium Priority
Number of pulses in burst	5	3
Pulse spacing		
Between 1st and 2nd pulse	150–250 ms	250–500 ms
Between 2nd and 3rd pulse	150–250 ms	250–500 ms
Between 3rd and 4th pulse	150–250 ms	NA
Between 4th and 5th pulse	150–250 ms	NA
Burst spacing	2 sec	NA
Repeat time	15 sec	30 sec
Difference in amplitude between any two pulses	10 dB (A) max	10 dB (A) max

From International Standards Organization: Anaesthesia and Respiratory Care Alarm Signals. Part 2: Auditory Alarm Signals. ISO 9703-2, August 1, 1994.

References

1. Hubmayr RD: Setting the ventilator. *In*: Principles and Practice of Mechanical Ventilation. Tobin MJ (Ed). New York, McGraw-Hill, 1994, pp 191–206.
2. Hansen-Flasher JH, Braginsky S, Basile G, Lanne B: Use of sedating drugs and neuromuscular blocking agents in patients requiring mechanical ventilation for respiratory failure. JAMA 1991; 266:2870–2875.
3. Dreyfuss D, Saumon G: Ventilator-induced lung injury: Lessons from experimental studies. Am J Respir Crit Care Med 1998; 157:294–323.
4. Kacmarek R: Permissive hypercapnia. Respir Care 1993; 38:373–387.
5. Webb HH, Tierney DF: Experimental pulmonary edema due to intermittent positive pressure ventilation with high inflation pressure: Protection by positive end-expiratory pressure. Am Rev Respir Dis 1974; 110:556–565.
6. Hernandez LA, Peevy K, Moise AA, Parker JC: Chest wall restriction limits high airway pressure-induced lung injury in young rabbits. J Appl Physiol 1989; 66:2364–2368.
7. Kolobow T, Moretti MP, Fumagalli R, Mascheroni D, Prato P, Chen V, et al: Severe impairment in lung function induced by high peak airway pressure during mechanical ventilation. An experimental study. Am Rev Respir Dis 1987; 135:312–315.
8. Dreyfuss D, Soler P, Basset G, Saumon G: High inflation pressure pulmonary edema. Respective effects of high airway pressure, high tidal volume, and positive end-expiratory pressure. Am Rev Respir Dis 1988; 137:1159–1164.
9. Dreyfuss D, Basset G, Soler P, Saumon G: Intermittent positive-pressure hyperventilation with high inflation pressure produces pulmonary microvascular injury in rats. Am Rev Respir Dis 1985; 132:880–884.
10. Dreyfuss D, Soler P, Saumon G: Mechanical ventilation-induced pulmonary edema: Interaction with previous lung alterations. Am J Respir Crit Care Med 1995; 181:1568–1575.

11. Corbridge TC, Wood LD, Crawford GP, Chudoba MJ, Yanos J, Sznajder JI: Adverse effects of large tidal volume and low PEEP in canine acid aspiration. Am Rev Respir Dis 1990; 142:311–315.
12. Muscedere JG, Mullen JB, Gan K, Slutsky AS: Tidal ventilation at low airway pressures can augment lung injury. Am J Respir Crit Care Med 1994; 149:1327–1334.
13. Tremblay L, Valenza F, Ribeiro SP, Li J, Slutsky AS: Injurious ventilatory strategies increase cytokines and c-*fos* m-RNA expression in an isolated rat lung model. J Clin Invest 1997; 99:944–952.
14. Dreyfuss D, Saumon G: From ventilator-induced lung injury to multiple organ dysfunction (Editorial). Intensive Care Med 1998; 24:102–104.
15. Slutsky AS, Tremblay L: Multiple organ failure: Is mechanical ventilation a contributing factor? (Editorial) Am J Respir Crit Care Med 1998; 157:1721–1733.
16. Nahum A, Hoyt JD, Schmidt L, Moody J, Shapiro R, Marini JJ: Effect of mechanical ventilation strategy on dissemination of intratracheally instilled *Escherichia coli* in dogs. Crit Care Med 1997; 25:1733–1743.
17. Ranieri VM, Tortorella D, Detullio R, Puntillo F, Grasso S, Mascia L, et al: Limitation of mechanical stress decreases BAL cytokines in patients with ARDS (Abstract). Am J Respir Crit Care Med 1998; 157:A694.
18. Amato MB, Barbas CS, Medeiros D, Magaldi RB, Schettino GP, Lorenzi-Filho G, et al: Effect of a protective-ventilation strategy on mortality in the acute respiratory distress syndrome. N Engl J Med 1998; 338:347–354.
19. Stewart TE, Meade MO, Cook DJ, Granton JT, Hodder RV, Lapinsky SE, et al: Evaluation of a ventilation strategy to prevent barotrauma in patients at high risk for acute respiratory distress syndrome. N Engl J Med 1998; 338:355–361.
20. Kacmarek R, Chiche JD: Lung protective ventilatory strategies for ARDS—the data are convincing! Respir Care 1998; 43:724–727.
21. Pierson DJ: Complications associated with mechanical ventilation. Crit Care Clin 1990; 6:711–724.
22. Pierson DJ: Barotrauma and bronchopleural fistula. *In*: Principles and Practice of Mechanical Ventilation. Tobin MJ (Ed). New York, McGraw-Hill, 1994, pp 813–837.
23. Weg JG, Anzueto A, Balk RA, Wiedemann HP, Pattishall EN, Schorn B, et al: The relation of pneumothorax and other air leaks to mortality in the acute respiratory distress syndrome. N Engl J Med 1998; 338:341–346.
24. Cullen J, Caldera DL: The incidence of ventilator induced pulmonary barotrauma in critically ill patients. Anesthesiology 1979; 50:185–190.
25. Rouby JJ, Lherm T, Martin de Lassale E, Poete P, Bodin L, Finet JF, et al: Histologic aspects of pulmonary barotrauma in critically ill patients with acute respiratory failure. Intensive Care Med 1993; 19:383–389.
26. Petersen HP, Baier H: Incidence of pulmonary barotrauma in a medical ICU. Crit Care Med 1983; 11:67–69.
27. Rohlfing BM, Webb WR, Schlobohm RM: Ventilator-related extraalveolar air in adults. Radiology 1976; 121:25–31.
28. Pollack MM, Fields AI, Holbrook PR: Pneumothorax and pneumomediastinum during pediatric mechanical ventilation. Crit Care Med 1979; 7:536–541.
29. Hillman K: Pulmonary barotrauma. Clin Anesthesiol 1985; 3:777–782.
30. Gammon RB, Shin MS, Buchalter SE: Pulmonary barotrauma in mechanical ventilation: Patterns and risk factors. Chest 1992; 102:568–572.
31. Gammon RB, Shin MS, Grozdanovic Z, Hardin JM, Hsu CD, Buchalter SE: Clinical risk factors for pulmonary barotrauma. Am J Respir Crit Care Med 1995; 152:1235–1240.
32. Chatte G, Sab JM, Dubois JM, Sirodot M, Gaussorgues P, Robert D: Prone position in mechanically ventilated patients with severe acute respiratory failure. Am J Respir Crit Care Med 1997; 155:473–478.
33. Rossaint R, Falke KJ, Lopez F, Slama K, Pison U, Zapol WM: Inhaled nitric oxide for the adult respiratory distress syndrome. N Engl J Med 1993; 328:399–405.
34. Fort P, Farmer R, Westerman J, Johannigman JA, Beninoti W, Dolan S, et al: High frequency oscillatory ventilation for adult respiratory distress syndrome—a pilot study. Crit Care Med 1997; 25:937–947.
35. Darioli A, Perret C: Mechanical controlled hypoventilation in status asthmaticus. Am Rev Respir Dis 1984; 129:385–387.
36. Hickling KG, Henderson SJ, Jackson R: Low mortality associated with low volume pressure limited ventilation with permissive hypercapnia in severe adult respiratory distress syndrome. Intensive Care Med 1990; 16:372–377.
37. Hickling KG, Walsh J, Henderson SJ, Jackson R: Low mortality rate in adult respiratory distress syndrome using low-volume, pressure limited ventilation with permissive hypercapnia: A prospective study. Crit Care Med 1994; 22:1568–1578.
38. Hickling KG, Joyce C: Permissive hypercapnia in ARDS and its effect on tissue oxygenation. Acta Anaesthesiol Scand 1995; 39:201–208.
39. Gentilello L, Anardi D, Mock C, Arreola-Risa C, Maier RV: Permissive hypercapnia in trauma patients. J Trauma 1995; 39:846–853.
40. Bidani A, Tzouanakis AE, Cardenas VJ, Zwischenberger JB: Permissive hypercapnia in acute respiratory failure. JAMA 1994; 272:957–962.
41. Tuxen DV: Permissive hypercapnic ventilation. Am J Respir Crit Care Med 1994; 150:870–874.
42. Feihl F, Perret C: Permissive hypercapnia—how permissive should we be? Am J Respir Crit Care Med 1994; 150:1722–1734.
43. West JB: Respiratory Physiology: The Essentials. 4th ed. Baltimore, Williams & Wilkins, 1990.
44. Nunn JF: Carbon dioxide. *In*: Applied Respiratory Physiology. 2nd ed. Nunn JF (Ed). London, Butterworth & Co, 1977, pp 334–374.
45. Carpellier G, Tolh J, Walker P: Hemodynamic effects of permissive hypercapnia (Abstract). Am Rev Respir Dis 1992; 195:A527.
46. Wolley K, Lewis T, Wood L: Acute respiratory acidosis decreases left ventricular contractibility but increases cardiac output in dogs. Circ Res 1990; 100:102–106.
47. Achike F, Dai S: Cardiovascular responses to verapamil and nifedipine in hypoventilated and hyperventilated rats. Br J Pharmacol 1990; 100:102–106.
48. Hickling KG: Ventilatory management of ARDS: Can it affect the outcome? Intensive Care Med 1990; 16:219–226.
49. Kacmarek R, Hess D: Basic principles of ventilatory machinery. *In*: Principles and Practice of Mechanical Ventilation. Tobin MJ (Ed). New York, McGraw-Hill, 1994, pp 65–111.
50. Marini JJ: Pressure-controlled ventilation. *In*: Principles and Practice of Mechanical Ventilation. Tobin MJ (Ed). New York, McGraw-Hill, 1994, pp 305–317.
51. Ravenscraft SA, Burke WC, Marini JJ: Volume cycled decelerating flow: An alternate form of mechanical ventilation. Chest 1992; 101:1342–1351.
52. Kacmarek R: Management of the patient ventilator system. *In*: Foundations of Respiratory Care. Pierson DJ (Ed). New York, Churchill Livingstone, 1992, pp 973–998.
53. Truwitt JP, Marini JJ: Evaluation of thoracic mechanics in the ventilated patient. Part II: Applied mechanics. J Crit Care 1988; 3:199–213.
54. Marcy TW, Marini JJ: Inverse ratio ventilation in ARDS. Rationale and implementation. Chest 1991; 100:494–504.
55. Marcy T, Burke W, Adams A, Crooke P, Marini JC: Mean alveolar pressure is higher during ventilation with constant pressure than with constant flow or sinusoidal flow wave forms (Abstract). Am Rev Respir Dis 1990; 141:A239.
56. Abraham E, Yoshihara G: Cardiorespiratory effects of pressure controlled ventilation in severe respiratory failure. Chest 1990; 98:1445–1449.
57. Al-Saady N, Bennett ED: Decelerating flow waveform improves lung mechanics and gas exchange in patients on intermittent positive pressure ventilation. Intensive Care Med 1985; 11:68–75.
58. Baker AB, Babington PC, Colliss JE, Cowie RW: Effects of varying inspiratory flow waveform and time in intermittent positive pressure ventilation. Part 2. Br J Anaesth 1977; 49:1221–1233.
59. Baker AB, Restall R, Clark BW: Effects of varying inspiratory flow waveform and time in intermittent positive pressure ventilation: Emphysema. Br J Anaesth 1982; 54:547–554.
60. Kacmarek R: Inverse ratio ventilation (IRV) in the critically ill. Curr Opin Crit Care 1997; 3:78–83.

61. Rossi A, Ranieri VM: Positive end inspiratory pressure. *In*: Principles and Practice of Mechanical Ventilation. Tobin MJ (Ed). New York, McGraw-Hill, 1994, pp 259–304.
62. Marini JJ, Crooke PS, Truwit JD: Determinants and limits of pressure-preset ventilation: A mathematical model of pressure control. J Appl Physiol 1989; 67:1081–1092.
63. Tharratt RS, Allen R, Albertson TE: Pressure controlled inverse ratio ventilation in severe adult respiratory failure. Chest 1988; 94:755–762.
64. Gurevitch M, Van Dyke J, Young E, Jackson K: Improved oxygenation and lower peak airway pressure in severe adult respiratory distress syndrome: Treatment with inverse ratio ventilation. Chest 1986; 89:211–213.
65. Cole A, Weller S, Sykes M: Inverse ratio ventilation compared with PEEP in adult respiratory failure. Intensive Care Med 1984; 10:227–232.
66. Mang H, Kacmarek R, Ritz R, Wilson RS, Kimball W: Cardiopulmonary effects of volume and pressure controlled CPPV at various I:E ratios in an acute lung injury model. Am J Respir Crit Care Med 1995; 151:731–736.
67. Lessard MR, Guerot E, Lorino H, Lemaire F, Brochard L: Effects of pressure-controlled with different I:E ratios versus volume-controlled ventilation on respiratory mechanics, gas exchange, and hemodynamics in patients with adult respiratory distress syndrome. Anesthesiology 1994; 80:983–991.
68. Munoz J, Guerrero JE, Escalante JL, Palomino R, De La Calle B: Pressure-controlled ventilation versus controlled mechanical ventilation with decelerating inspiratory flow. Crit Care Med 1993; 21:1143–1148.
69. Mercat A, Graini L, Teboul JL, Lenique F, Richard C: Cardiorespiratory effects of pressure-controlled ventilation with and without inverse ratio in the adult respiratory distress syndrome. Chest 1993; 104:871–875.
70. Brandolese R, Broseghini C, Polese G, Bernasconi M, Brandi G, Milic-Emili J, et al: Effects of intrinsic PEEP on pulmonary gas exchange in mechanically-ventilated patients. Eur Respir J 1993; 6:358–363.
71. Kacmarek R, Hess D: Airway pressure, flow and volume waveforms and lung mechanics during mechanical ventilation. *In*: Monitoring in Respiratory Care. Kacmarek R, Hess D, Stoller JK (Eds). Chicago, Mosby-Year Book, 1993, pp 497–545.
72. Kacmarek R: Methods of providing mechanical ventilatory support. *In*: Foundations of Respiratory Care. Pierson DJ, Kacmarek R (Eds). New York, Churchill Livingstone, 1992, pp 953–971.
73. Abraham E, Yoshihara G: Cardiorespiratory effects of pressure controlled inverse ratio ventilation in severe respiratory failure. Chest 1989; 96:1356–1359.
74. Lain D, DiBenedetto R, Morris SL, Van Nguyen A, Sautlers R, Causey D: Pressure control inverse ratio ventilation as a method to reduce peak inspiratory pressure and provide adequate ventilation and oxygenation. Chest 1989; 95:1081–1088.
75. Zavala E, Ferrer M, Polese G, Masclans JR, Planas M, Milic-Emili J, et al: Effect of inverse I:E ratio ventilation on pulmonary gas exchange in acute respiratory distress syndrome. Anesthesiology 1998; 88:35–42.
76. Mercat A, Titiriga M, Anguel N, Richard C, Teboul JL: Inverse ratio ventilation (I/E = 2/1) in acute respiratory distress syndrome: A six-hour controlled study. Am J Respir Crit Care Med 1997; 155:1637–1642.
77. Kacmarek R, Kirmse M, Nishimura M, Mang H, Kimball WR: The effects of applied versus auto-PEEP on local lung unit pressure and volume in a four-unit lung model. Chest 1995; 108:1073–1079.
78. Pepe P, Marini JJ: Occult positive end-expiratory pressure in mechanically ventilated patients with airflow obstruction: The auto-PEEP effect. Am Rev Respir Dis 1982; 126:166–170.
79. Smith TC, Marini JJ: Impact of PEEP on lung mechanics and work of breathing in severe airflow obstruction. J Appl Physiol 1988; 65:1488–1499.
80. Otis AB: Work of breathing. *In*: Handbook of Physiology: The Respiratory System. Vol 1. Finn WU, Rahn H (Eds). Washington, DC, American Physiological Society, 1964, pp 868–890.
81. Kacmarek R: Positive end expiratory pressure. *In*: Foundations of Respiratory Care. Pierson DJ, Kacmarek R (Eds). New York, Churchill Livingstone, 1992, pp 891–920.
82. Tuxon D, Lane S: The effects of ventilatory pattern on hyperinflation, airway pressure, and circulation in mechanical ventilation of patients with severe airflow obstruction. Am Rev Respir Dis 1987; 136:872–879.
83. Tuxon D, William T, Scheinkestel C: Limiting dynamic hyperinflation in mechanically ventilated patients with severe asthma reduces complications. Anaesth Intensive Care 1993; 21:718–726.
84. Leatherman J, Ravenscraft SA: Low measure auto-positive end expiratory pressure during mechanical ventilation of patients with severe asthma: Hidden auto-positive end-expiratory pressure. Crit Care Med 1996; 24:541–546.
85. Auto-PEEP is common in mechanically ventilated patients: A study of incidence, severity, and detection. Respir Care 1986; 31:1069–1074.
86. Petrof BJ, Legare M, Goldberg P, Milic-Emili J, Gottfried SB: Continuous positive airway pressure reduces work of breathing and dyspnea during weaning from mechanical ventilation in severe chronic obstructive pulmonary disease. Am Rev Respir Dis 1990; 141:281–289.
87. Ranieri VM, Giuliani R, Cinnella G, Pesce C, Brienza N, Ippolito EL, et al: Physiologic effects of positive end-expiratory pressure in patients with chronic obstructive pulmonary disease during acute ventilatory failure and controlled mechanical ventilation. Am Rev Respir Dis 1993; 147:5–13.
88. Servillo G, Svantesson C, Beydon L, Roupie E, Brochard L, Lemaire F, et al: Pressure-volume curves in acute respiratory failure: Automated low flow inflation versus occlusion. Am J Respir Crit Care Med 1997; 155:1629–1636.
89. Roupie E, Dambrosio M, Servillo G, Mentec H, el Atrous S, Beydon L, et al: Titration of tidal volume and induced hypercapnia in acute respiratory distress syndrome. Am J Respir Crit Care Med 1995; 152:121–128.
90. Harris RS, Hess D, Venegas JG: Relationship of P_{flex} of the pressure-volume (PV) curve to the true inflection point of the deflation limb (Abstract). Am J Respir Crit Care Med 1998; 157:A694.
91. Ranieri VM, Brienza N, Santostasi S, Puntillo F, Mascia L, Vitale N, et al: Impairment of lung and chest wall mechanics in patients with acute respiratory distress syndrome: Role of abdominal distension. Am J Respir Crit Care Med 1997; 156:1082–1091.
92. Mergoni M, Martelli A, Volpi A, Primavera S, Zuccoli P, Rossi A: Impact of positive end-expiratory pressure on chest wall and lung pressure-volume curve in acute respiratory failure. Am J Respir Crit Care Med 1997; 156:846–854.
93. Meyer E, Barbas CS, Grunauer MA, Caramey MP, Souza R, Carvalho CRR, et al: PEEP at P_{flex} cannot guarantee a fully open lung after a high pressure recruiting maneuver in ARDS patients (Abstract). Am J Respir Crit Care Med 1998; 157:A694.
94. Slutsky AS: Mechanical ventilation: ACCP consensus conference. Chest 1993; 104:1833–1868.
95. Kerr JH: Warning devices. Br J Anaesth 1985; 57:696–708.
96. Myerson KR, Ilsey AH, Runciman WB: An evaluation of ventilator monitoring alarms. Anaesth Intensive Care 1986; 14:174–185.
97. Kacmarek R: Alarms. *In*: Cardiopulmonary Monitoring. Tobin MJ (Ed). New York, McGraw-Hill, 1998, pp 133–141.
98. O'Carroll TM: Survey of alarms in an intensive care unit. Anaesthesia 1986; 41:742–744.
99. Lockhart CH: Auditory alarms during anesthesia monitoring. Anesthesiology 1988; 69:101–109.
100. Bentt LR, Santora TA, Leverle BJ: Accuracy and utility of pulse oximetry in the surgical intensive care unit. Curr Surg 1990; 47:267–268.
101. Lawless S: Crying wolf: False alarms in a pediatric intensive care unit. Crit Care Med 1994; 22:981–985.
102. Tsien CL, Fackler JC: Poor prognosis for existing monitors in the intensive care unit. Crit Care Med 1997; 25:614–619.
103. International Standards Organization (ISO): Anaesthetic and Respiratory Care Alarm Signals. Part 1: Visual Alarms. ISO 9703-1, July 15, 1992.
104. International Standards Organization (ISO): Anaesthetic and Respiratory Care Alarm Signals. Part 2: Auditory Alarm Signals. ISO 9703-2, August 2, 1994.
105. International Standards Organization (ISO): Anaesthetic and Respiratory Equipment—Ventilator and Related Devices. ISO 9703-3, November 1, 1994.

106. MacIntyre NR, Day S: Essentials for ventilator-alarm systems. Respir Care 1992; 37:1108–1112.
107. Sanborn WG: Microprocessor-based mechanical ventilation. Respir Care 1993; 38:72–109.

116

Partial Ventilatory Assist

John J. Marini, MD

Advancing knowledge of ventilatory failure, respiratory muscle fatigue and its recovery, the pathophysiologic mechanism of severe airflow obstruction, and patient-ventilator interactions both influences the execution of partial ventilatory support and underscores the need for its expedient withdrawal. Furthermore, technologic innovations now enable the clinician to monitor patient-ventilator interactions closely and provide new options for ventilatory assistance that account better for the complex clinical physiology that characterizes the spontaneously breathing patient. This chapter reviews key management principles and alternative strategies for assisting ventilation in the intubated patient that have evolved from our improved understanding and capability. Noninvasive ventilation, a vital and expanding area of partial ventilatory support, is detailed elsewhere in this volume.

CONCEPTUAL ADVANCES IN VENTILATORY SUPPORT

Partial ventilatory support is usually required in the setting of severe airflow obstruction, neuromuscular weakness, acute lung injury, or cardiovascular compromise. The objectives of maximizing the patient's comfort, minimizing adverse patient-machine interactions, and effecting timely withdrawal of machine support ("weaning") are common to each.

Acute Airflow Obstruction

Awareness of the physiologic importance of dynamic hyperinflation in everyday clinical practice has been comparatively recent. Dynamic hyperinflation results whenever insufficient expiratory time prevents the chest from decompressing to its resting "equilibrium" volume at the end of tidal exhalation without (or despite) muscle effort. End-expiratory alveolar pressure then exceeds the pressure at the airway opening, and flow continues throughout expiration until interrupted by the next inflation cycle.[1] "Auto-PEEP," the positive difference between alveolar pressure (Pex) and the set airway pressure (PEEP) at end-exhalation that characterizes dynamic hyperinflation, is a function of the expiratory resistance to airflow, the compliance of the respiratory system, the time allowed for expiration, and the volume from which exhalation begins.[1, 2] It is referred to as auto-PEEP because it is associated with increased lung volumes at end-expiration in a manner analogous to externally applied positive end-expiratory pressure (PEEP). Although this process has been called other terms, such as occult PEEP and intrinsic PEEP, in this chapter the term auto-PEEP is used to describe this phenomenon.

The consequences of dynamic hyperinflation are linked to associated changes in lung volume and pleural pressure. During exacerbations of asthma and chronic airflow obstruction, *mean* pleural pressure is often lower than normal in patients making spontaneous breathing efforts, despite air trapping.[3] Thus, dynamic hyperinflation does not necessarily imply high mean intrathoracic (intrapleural) pressure or impaired venous return. Active expiratory muscle contraction may keep intrapleural pressure positive until the very end of exhalation, producing positive intrapleural and alveolar pressures without commensurate dynamic hyperinflation or its consequences.[4, 5] At high levels of ventilation, substantial expiratory resistance may arise in the circuitry of the machine, particularly across the endotracheal tube and exhalation valve of machines without an active expiratory valve.[6–8] Although recent technical innovations have reduced imposed resistance, ventilator circuits are still imperfect. Efforts to offset tube and valve resistance by temporarily dropping central airway pressure or controlling carinal pressure during both phases of the ventilatory cycle are methods currently under preliminary testing.[9]

Although auto-PEEP has been described in other conditions (such as acute respiratory distress syndrome [ARDS][10]) and can occur whenever minute ventilation is high enough, dynamic hyperinflation most commonly occurs during severe airflow obstruction. In this setting, expiratory resistance is often severalfold greater than inspiratory resistance, especially at end-exhalation. Expiratory resistance is often so high that expiratory flow limitation occurs during tidal exhalation.[11]

Auto-PEEP may exist *without dynamic hyperinflation* when end-expiratory airflow is driven by the expiratory muscles, and *without flow limitation* during tidal breathing, despite airways disease. Commonly, however, auto-PEEP is associated with both dynamic hyperventilation and tidal flow limitation. Dynamic hyperinflation disproportional to measurable auto-PEEP routinely occurs in patients with such severe airflow obstruction that airways serving the most compromised areas seal *completely* during the course of exhalation.[12] Undoubtedly, such "ball-valving" at least partially accounts for extreme overinflation that cannot be explained by the recorded levels of auto-PEEP during status asthma and exacerbated chronic obstructive pulmonary disease. Although often widespread, closure of this type is probably most prevalent in the dependent regions of the lung.[13] Thus, although the clinician measures only one value that averages the contributions from all open airways, auto-PEEP levels vary widely throughout the lung with "diffuse" obstructive disease.

The pathophysiologic consequences of auto-PEEP and the response to added end-expiratory pressure depend on the category of airflow obstruction.[14] Whether dynamic hyperinflation causes hemodynamically important elevations of mean intrathoracic pressure depends on the activity of the patient's ventilatory muscles.

Consequences of Auto-PEEP

Cardiovascular Sequelae

Hemodynamic consequences observed in passively inflated patients first brought the auto-PEEP phenomenon to clinical attention.[15] Indeed, auto-PEEP's adverse impact on cardiac output is greatest when spontaneous breathing efforts are minimal or absent. Alveolar overdistention increases right ventricular afterload, and when inflation occurs without vigorous muscle efforts, mean pleural pressure rises, posing a backpressure to venous return. *Transmural* pulmonary artery occlusion pressure, as a measure of left ventricular filling pressure, often declines as auto-PEEP develops under passive conditions.[15]

Alterations in the loading conditions of the heart help to explain why hypotension often develops when a spontaneously breathing patient with air trapping is sedated, intubated, and mechanically ventilated. Mean intrathoracic pressure rises as forceful ventilatory efforts end. (Hemodynamic compromise is much less likely to occur when spontaneous ventilatory efforts continue after intubation, even when these efforts are machine-assisted.) Vigorous spontaneous breathing both reduces mean intrathoracic pressure and elevates intra-abdominal pressure during the exhalation phase, thereby maintaining the pressure difference driving venous return.[16] Cardiac output is sustained at a relatively high level because of stress and the added work of breathing. Moreover, the reduced intrathoracic pressure afterloads the left ventricle and accentuates the tendency to form pulmonary edema, a factor of importance in patients already predisposed to congestive heart failure. In patients with severe airflow obstruction, spontaneous breathing increases oxygen and cardiac output demands and predisposes to pulmonary congestion. For a further discussion of these interactions, the reader is referred to Chapter 111.

Work of Breathing

Dynamic hyperinflation increases the oxygen demands on the respiratory muscles during spontaneous ventilation and boosts the ventilating pressures required during machine-assisted breathing.[17] When attempting to initiate a breath, the patient with dynamic hyperinflation encounters an inspiratory threshold load, which is an expiratory pressure that must be counterbalanced before inspiration can be initiated. During machine-assisted cycles, therefore, auto-PEEP depresses the *effective* triggering sensitivity,[18] and during spontaneous cycles, auto-PEEP adds a "residual elastic" component to the "tidal elastic" and "frictional" components of the work of breathing (Fig. 116–1).

Hyperinflation also compromises the ventilatory pump in accomplishing this increased workload. Operating from a hyperinflated position, the acutely foreshortened inspiratory muscle fibers are preloaded insufficiently to generate maximum tension. The hyperexpanded rib cage recoils inward (opposing inflation) throughout the tidal breath rather than springing outward (as it normally does) to aid in lung expansion.[19] Horizontally oriented ribs lose their normal "pump lever" and "bucket handle" actions, further compromising the effectiveness of muscle contraction. Over time, remodeling of the diaphragmatic muscle fibers helps to restore effective preload, but this process occurs slowly.[20] Moreover, the flattened diaphragm is geometrically disadvantaged. Finally, hyperinflation narrows or obliterates the "zone of apposition" with the chest wall that normally helps to expand the lower ribs during inspiration. For all of these reasons, dynamic hyperinflation can unbalance a tenuous workload–work capacity relationship.[21]

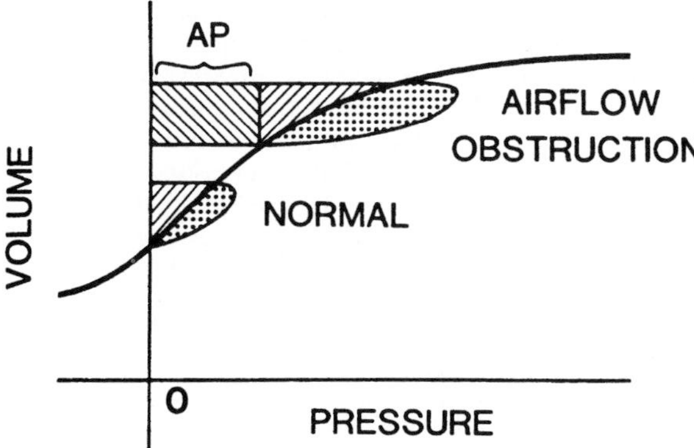

Figure 116–1. Influence of dynamic hyperinflation on the work of breathing. The *heavy solid line* is the trans-structural pressure-volume curve for the respiratory system. *Shaded areas* represent components of the work of breathing. By definition, patients with airflow obstruction expend increased frictional work *(stippled area)*. The patient with dynamic hyperinflation also experiences increased elastic work in moving a given tidal volume for two reasons: reduced compliance *(cross-hatched area)* and auto-positive end-expiratory pressure (AP). (From Marini JJ: Ventilatory management of COPD. *In:* Chronic Obstructive Pulmonary Disease. Cherniack NS [Ed]. Philadelphia, WB Saunders, 1991, p 495.)

Influence of PEEP on Dynamic Hyperinflation and Auto-PEEP

Hyperinflation may or may not worsen as PEEP is deliberately added to auto-PEEP; it depends on the mechanism for auto-PEEP generation.[14] PEEP added to a dynamically hyperinflated patient *without* expiratory muscle activity or flow limitation will cause lung volume to rise further, exacerbating the workload and compromising the pump. For some patients, however, PEEP or continuous positive airway pressure (CPAP) offers a counterspring against which the expiratory muscles may store elastic energy for release during early inspiration, allowing "work sharing" between the inspiratory and expiratory muscle groups.[22] If minute ventilation does not change, this work sharing mechanism is rendered ineffective in the presence of tidal flow limitation, because expiratory effort exacerbates the obstruction and does not assist deflation. In this setting, adding PEEP less than the original level of auto-PEEP narrows the difference between end-expiratory airway and alveolar pressures, increasing alveolar pressure little, if at all.[23] PEEP added downstream of the flow limitation site, therefore, reduces the inspiratory threshold, improves triggering sensitivity, and partially alleviates the ventilatory workload.[18] Further, it is possible that the addition of PEEP may prevent collapse of the more central airways and help reduce dyspnea in this way.[24] Because the development of auto-PEEP narrows the inspiratory pressure difference between airway and alveolar pressures, in a weak patient, PEEP that counterbalances auto-PEEP often allows a given amount of pressure support to boost tidal volume, rather than simply sparing muscle breathing workload.

As a rule, the addition of PEEP does *not* reduce chest wall dimensions or improve muscle fiber preload. However, the function of the extradiaphragmatic muscles, which are particularly important in this setting of hyperinflation, might not be as vulnerable as the diaphragm to small volume increments. Furthermore, even in the setting of expiratory flow limitation, the impact of CPAP on muscle *coordination* or on the synchrony of triggering effort with ventilator assistance may be beneficial.[25]

Weaning from Mechanical Ventilation

The need for ventilator assistance often stems either uniquely or in combination from several sources, including psychologic distress, refractory hypoxemia, and cardiovascular dysfunction.[26] The most common problem, however, is an imbalance between ventilatory demands and the ability to respond to them. An effective response requires adequate ventilatory drive and muscle endurance. Although patients are occasionally encountered in whom blunted ventilatory drive limits the pace of machine withdrawal, insufficient drive intensity is seldom the primary problem.[27] Much more often, the breathing workload overwhelms a ventilator-dependent patient who is weak, malnourished, or deconditioned. Chest wall instability, impaired muscle coordination, and hyperinflation frequently compromise ventilatory pump efficiency. Skeletal muscle strength and endurance may begin to fade within the first 3 days of total rest. Many critically ill patients experience drug-[28] or sepsis-related[29] neuromyopathy. Fortunately, most patients can be liberated quickly from controlled ventilatory support.

Prediction of Weaning Success or Failure

Power requirements necessary to move air into and out of the lungs are jointly determined by the impedance of the respiratory system, the minute ventilation requirement, and the pattern of ventilation. For a given minute ventilation, power output is minimized by increasing frequency and limiting the tidal volume. Rapid, shallow breathing, therefore, can be a fatigue-sparing adaptation to weakness or increased breathing workload. Unfortunately, as tidal volume decreases, the dead space fraction tends to rise and ventilatory efficiency falls. This obligates the tachypneic patient to either increase minute ventilation or allow hypercapnia. Whether rapid, shallow breathing proves physiologically adaptive or maladaptive depends on the extent to which inefficiency of gas exchange attenuates the benefit of reducing tidal pressure.

Ventilatory support should be withdrawn as soon as it is feasible to do so without causing physical or psychic distress. The advisability of attempting to withdraw support is a multifaceted decision based on the estimated risks and benefits of continued machine assistance. Firm guidelines have been proposed for the timing of such efforts in patients with status asthma.[30] In other, more complex situations, clear rules are often difficult to formulate. For extreme cases, it is always possible to specify some criterion that predicts weaning success or failure. The standard predictive indices (Table 116–1)—the minute ventilation requirement, the breathing pattern, and the maximum pressure developed at functional residual capacity against an occluded airway (maximum inspiratory pressure)—are usually helpful.[31]

In view of the number and interplay among the determinants of ventilator dependence, it is not surprising that isolated measures of workload or capability prove disappointing in difficult cases. A successful indicator of weanability must reflect both power demand and power reserve. Because the ventilatory pump cannot indefinitely sustain tidal pressures that exceed 40% to 50% of the true maximum isometric value (maximum inspiratory pressure),[32] well-compensated and overtaxed subjects respond differently to the same ventilatory stress. Neural outflow to the respiratory muscles may be modified in response to a potentially exhausting workload to avert energy depletion.[33] Patients in ventilatory failure may exaggerate the pattern of rapid, shallow breathing either because their response is dysfunctional or because impaired capability leaves no alternative.

Breathing pattern stabilizes soon after reloading of the respiratory system, providing the observer with near-immediate feedback. Irregularity of the breathing rhythm and disproportionate changes in respiratory rate versus tidal volume are valuable clues to distress,[34] especially when they are accompanied by tachyarrhythmia or diaphoresis, or when these signs develop or progress quickly. A brief empirical trial of spontaneous breathing under close observation (3 to 5 minutes) should be undertaken before a weaning schedule is prescribed. The frequency to tidal volume ratio quantifies rapid, shallow breathing and during the first minute of machine disconnection appears to provide a simple, yet reliable indicator of weanability.[35] This index appears to be less reliable, however, in patients with long-term machine dependence and in patients with severe airflow obstruction. Moreover, whether this frequency to tidal volume ratio criterion holds during oxygen supplementation, whether the value changes over time, and how it should be adjusted for patients different from those initially studied and described (e.g., patients with coronary disease) must be investigated further.

Preparation of the Patient

The patient's respiratory muscles must not be overtaxed, because recovery from established fatigue may require more than 24 hours.[36] Sufficient ventilatory support should be provided at night to ensure sleep quality. Whereas moderate muscle activity helps avert deconditioning and atrophy, the value of respiratory muscle training remains in doubt.

Extrapulmonary workloads, impaired cardiovascular function, anemia, fluid or electrolyte imbalance, and endocrine status must be addressed. Most modern equipment is acceptable for the moderate flows normally encountered during weaning. Yet, flow as opposed to pressure triggering may occasionally offer a slight advantage.[37, 38] Occult cardiac dysfunction is suggested when the patient cannot be weaned easily despite permissive weaning "parameters." Diuretics, antianginal medications, and inotropic support may be indicated in certain patients with underlying cardiovascular disease. Because resuming spontaneous breathing increases both the preload and afterload of the left ventricle, offsetting these changes with a well-titrated nitroprusside drip may help in selected cases as ventilatory support is withdrawn.

In patients with severe airflow obstruction, low levels of PEEP improve the workload, triggering threshold and dyspnea that accompany dynamic airway compression and auto-PEEP.[39, 40] Good arguments can be made to use at least 3 to 5 cm H_2O PEEP in all bedridden ventilated patients and to add sufficient pressure support to overcome endotracheal tube resistance during all spontaneous breathing cycles, whatever the mode. The appropriate level of pressure support to use for this purpose is a function of the tube diameter and the $\dot{V}_E$ requirement.[40] It is also good practice to briefly test the patient's reserve without either CPAP or pressure support ventilation (PSV) before extubation is attempted. To discourage atelectasis during unrelieved shallow breathing, the patient should be as upright and mobile as possible, and periodic

TABLE 116–1. Predictors of Weanability from Mechanical Ventilatory Support

	Measured Values		Clinical Observations	
Ventilation	***Strength***	***Endurance***	***Neuromuscular***	***Other***
$\dot{V}_E < 10$ L/min	MIP > -20 cm H_2O	MVV $> 2 \times \dot{V}_E$	Absence of scalene or abdominal muscle activity	$FIO_2 < 0.40$
$\dot{V}_E < 175$ mL/kg/min	$V_T > 5$ mL/kg	VC $> 2 \times V_T$		$70 <$ pulse < 120
	VC > 10 mL/kg	IEQ < 0.15		pH > 7.30
		f < 30/min	Asynchrony	MAP > 80 mm Hg
		$f/V_T < 100$	Irregular breathing	
		$P_{0.1} < 6$ cm H_2O	Rapid, shallow breathing	

$\dot{V}_E$ = minute ventilation; MIP = maximum inspiratory pressure; V_T = tidal volume; VC = vital capacity; MVV = maximum voluntary ventilation; IEQ = inspiratory effort quotient; f = ventilatory frequency; $P_{0.1}$ = inspiratory airway pressure 0.1 second after starting inspiratory efforts against an occluded airway; MAP = mean arterial pressure.

TABLE 116–2. Alternative Approaches to Weaning from Mechanical Ventilation

Primary Power Source	
Pressure Support	***Synchronized Intermittent Mandatory Ventilation***
Taper pressure support from value corresponding to VT of 7–10 mL/kg to 5 cm H_2O before extubation.	Taper number of machine breaths (7–10 mL/kg) from AMV to 2–4 breaths per minute before extubation.
Use SIMV of 1–2 breaths/min (≈10 mL/kg) to help recruit atelectatic areas.	Use pressure support of 3–8 cm H_2O for power flexibility and endotracheal tube resistance.
Use CPAP of 3–5 cm H_2O to prevent atelectasis or offset dynamic hyperinflation.	Use CPAP of 3–5 cm H_2O to prevent atelectasis or offset dynamic hyperinflation.
Ensure adequate sleep.	Ensure adequate sleep.
Challenge marginal candidates with zero pressure support and zero CPAP before extubation.	Challenge marginal candidates with zero pressure support and zero CPAP before extubation.
Consider noninvasive ventilation as a post-extubation bridge to spontaneous ventilation.	Consider noninvasive ventilation as a post-extubation bridge to spontaneous ventilation.

VT = tidal volume; AMV = assisted mechanical ventilation; SIMV = synchronized intermittent mandatory ventilation; CPAP = continuous positive airway pressure.

deep breaths (approximately 1½ to 2 times the spontaneous volume) should be encouraged or provided, for example, by synchronized intermittent mandatory ventilation (SIMV).

Weaning Technique

Despite excellent studies,[41, 42] clear superiority of any one weaning mode has not been convincingly demonstrated when each method is appropriately used in conjunction with CPAP and pressure support sufficient to offset the effects of position and endotracheal intubation (Table 116–2). Progressive *T-piece weaning* continues to be used enthusiastically, but in most centers other methods have largely supplanted this older technique. For T-piece weaning, the patient's endotracheal tube is connected to a nonvalved blow-by circuit that maintains a constant F_IO_2 but supplies no CPAP on inspiratory force to aid ventilation.

Although occasional patients express a clear preference, for most it may not matter whether pressure support or well-adjusted SIMV (with low-level pressure support to offset tube resistance) provides the machine's power as long as adequate nocturnal rest is ensured. Pressure support tends to offer the patient the flexibility to respond to changing ventilatory demands by increasing frequency, a point of clear advantage in patients with shifting $\dot{V}_E$ requirements. The machine-aided breaths of SIMV effectively overcome fluctuations in tidal impedance and auto-PEEP, but SIMV provides no reserve for changing $\dot{V}_E$ and tends to reload the patient early in the withdrawal process. In contrast, PSV tends to reload the system more evenly or even defer reloading to the later phase.[43] The flexibility to respond to changing $\dot{V}_E$ demands offered by pressure support may also be helpful at night. This reserve mechanism is less effective if there is substantial airflow obstruction or if airway pressure only builds gradually toward the targeted pressure. Moreover, if the impedance to breathing is variable (e.g., because of bronchospasm or secretion retention), the relative help offered *per breath* by a fixed level of pressure support tends to fall off.

Guidelines for the optimal pace of machine withdrawal have not been standardized. Abrupt removal of machine support works well for most patients with rapidly resolving illness and ample reserve. At least one multicenter study suggests that testing in this way, using full support between once- or twice-daily tests, may, in fact, be the most efficient weaning technique of all.[41] Yet the patient must be watched closely during these "T-piece" trials; the hours immediately after abrupt machine withdrawal can be difficult and highly dynamic.[44] Minute ventilation first rises, then falls as pump efficiency or gas exchange improves, fluids redistribute, and metabolic demands subside. Muscles gradually recondition, coordination returns, and drive adjusts to workload. The importance of making such adjustments is suggested by the reported success of biofeedback in speeding the weaning process.[45]

Graded withdrawal of support seems particularly advisable for patients who experience panic reactions, congestive heart failure, cardiac ischemia, or unusually large breathing workloads when high-level machine support is abruptly disconnected.[16, 46] It may be difficult to allow sufficient adaptation without delaying weaning progress. The frequency/tidal volume index[35] may provide guidance here, even during pressure-supported ventilation. Tolerance of a prescribed decrement in machine support can often be judged objectively at the bedside soon after the proposed change is made, allowing a suitably aggressive (but not overtaxing) schedule for the weaning protocol and minimizing the likelihood of fatigue.

Weaning management continues to be debated on many levels.[46] For example, there is no general agreement regarding the most appropriate Pa_{CO_2} to target before weaning is initiated. For a patient with ventilatory dysfunction—acute or chronic—insistence on maintaining his or her "usual" Pa_{CO_2} in the acute phase of illness forces the often weakened patient to accept the increased breathing workload, once spontaneous breathing is resumed. Newer approaches, such as mask-delivered CPAP and noninvasive intermittent ventilation (e.g., bi-level CPAP), are promising techniques to help the marginal candidate bridge the post-extubation adjustment period.[47–49]

Work of Breathing During Mechanical Ventilation

Dyspnea, breathing rhythm dyssynchrony, and high cycling pressures can result from adverse interactions between the patient and the ventilator. The total transpulmonary pressure change required per breath is a value fixed by the inspiratory flow rate, inspiratory resistance, respiratory system compliance, tidal volume, auto-PEEP (if any), and pattern of chest inflation.[50, 51] Although the machine is often capable of generating all necessary pressure, the patient and ventilator virtually always work together to accomplish the ventilatory task during patient-triggered, machine-aided cycles (Fig. 116–2).

The primary factors influencing the patient's contribution during volume-cycled mechanical ventilation are (1) ventilatory drive, (2) machine flow setting, and (3) respiratory muscle strength.[52, 53] (A debilitated patient cannot produce or sustain a large amount of ventilatory power, limiting the work he or she can do.) It follows that absolute values of work performed by the patient correlate poorly with effort relative to capability or with the relative loads of different subjects.

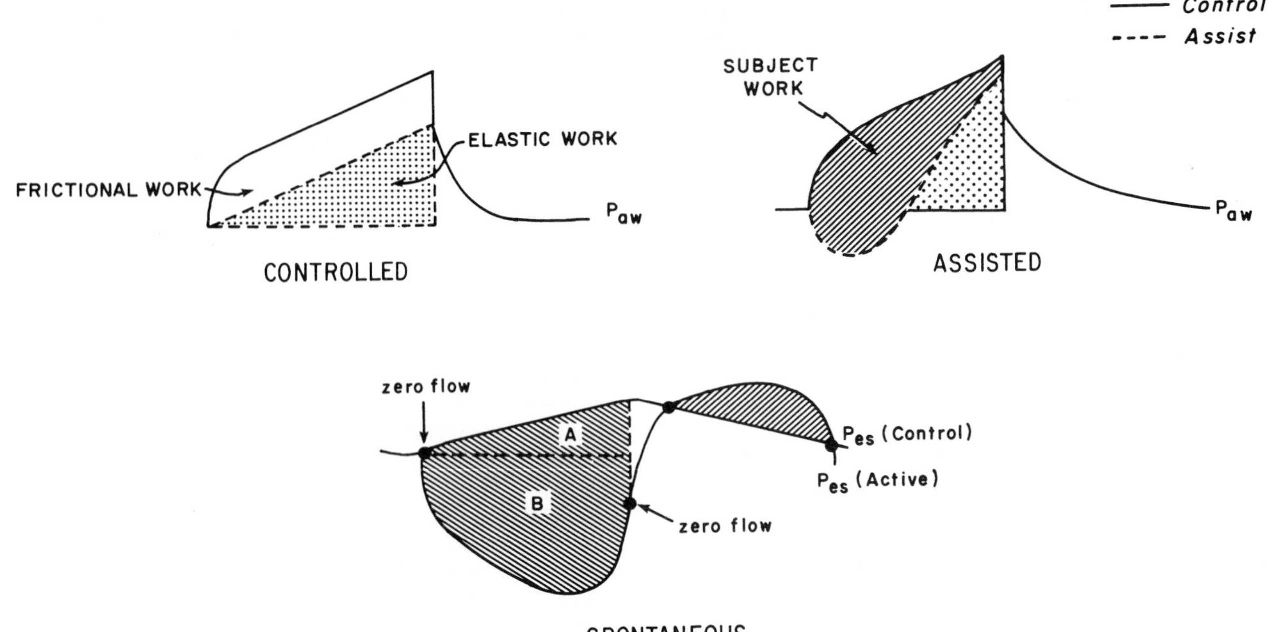

Figure 116–2. Distribution of breathing effort during the assisted and spontaneous breathing cycles of flow-controlled, volume-cycled synchronized intermittent mandatory ventilation. Under controlled conditions, the ventilator performs all frictional work against resistance and all elastic work against the recoil of the lung and chest wall. During spontaneous breathing cycles, the work to expand the chest wall (A) and all work across the lungs (B) is undertaken by the patient subject, as reflected in the difference between pleural (Pes) pressures under passive control and active conditions. During triggered machine cycles, the subject and ventilator share the workload.

Ventilatory drive is influenced by the minute ventilation requirement, the triggering sensitivity (the sum of the set pressure threshold and any imposed by auto-PEEP), and the sensation of breathlessness. In theory, if the machine delivers gas flow exactly as fast as the patient demands it, proximal airway pressure remains at the level of PEEP and the machine performs no mechanical work on the respiratory system. Conversely, if the patient relaxes immediately and completely after triggering the ventilator, almost the entire breathing workload can be accomplished by the machine (Fig. 116–3).

Because the patient's greatest demand for flow occurs in the very first part of the machine cycle, it makes sense to employ a decelerating rather than a constant flow delivery profile for the same tidal volume and inspiratory time setting. Pressure control is inherently flow decelerating; in volume control, a linearly decelerating profile can be selected as an option.[54] Although flow-regulated volume control applied with a decelerating profile may appear similar to pressure control or pressure-regulated volume control (see later) in certain patients, they are not interchangeable. If flow demands peak in midcycle, the flow-controlled decelerating waveform may not suffice, whereas a pressure-regulated waveform almost certainly would. On the other hand, patients with severe inspiratory airflow resistance may generate a flow waveform that more closely resembles a "square" profile than a decelerating one.

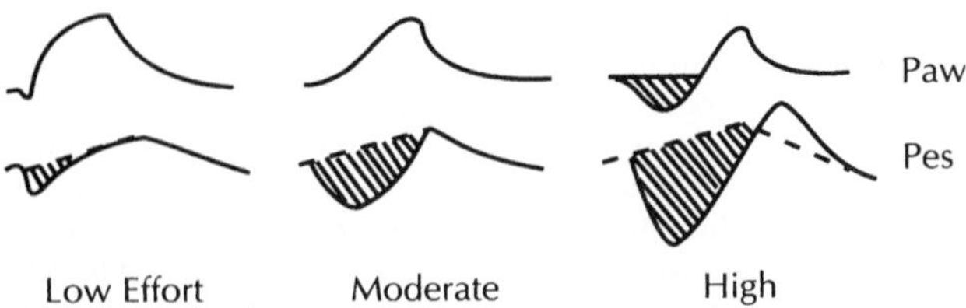

Figure 116–3. Airway (Paw) and esophageal (Pes) pressures recorded during low, moderate, and high efforts during flow-controlled, volume-cycled, assisted ventilation. The *dashed line* superimposed on the Pes tracing is the trajectory expected for passive inflation, and the *shaded region* between passive and active Pes curves reflects the patient's work of breathing. Note the reciprocal relationship between the patient's effort and airway pressure and the fact that during high effort, the patient is working against the impedance of the machine circuitry *(shaded)* during the first portion of the cycle.

A dyspneic patient helped intermittently by the ventilator (e.g., during SIMV) may exert similar effort for adjacent spontaneous and machine-aided breaths at the same overall level of machine support.[55, 56] Patients experiencing dyspnea do not adapt breathing effort quickly in response to intermittent unloading of the breathing cycle.

The work of breathing has not been extensively studied during pressure preset ventilation, but similar principles are likely to apply.[57] Pressure-supported ventilation allows the patient to control breathing cycle timing and depth. Such a *flow-cycled* mode of ventilation might be more comfortable (and result in less work by the patient) than a comparable level of flow preset, *volume-cycled* ventilation.[58, 59] Few objective data exist, however, to confirm or refute this contention. In the one study of weaning in which pressure support was compared with SIMV in the same patients, no differences in anxiety or dyspnea were detected.[60] The individual patient's preference may well vary with ventilation requirement, machine performance, and chest impedance.

Modern valving systems provide efficient gas delivery. CPAP is often associated with little additional work cost attributable to the valving or flow capacity of the system. Yet, no matter how perfectly a gas delivery system maintains the set level of end-expiratory pressure in the external circuit, the patient must contend with endotracheal tube resistance during each spontaneous breathing cycle (Fig. 116–4). Endotracheal tube resistance can be considerably higher in vivo than measured

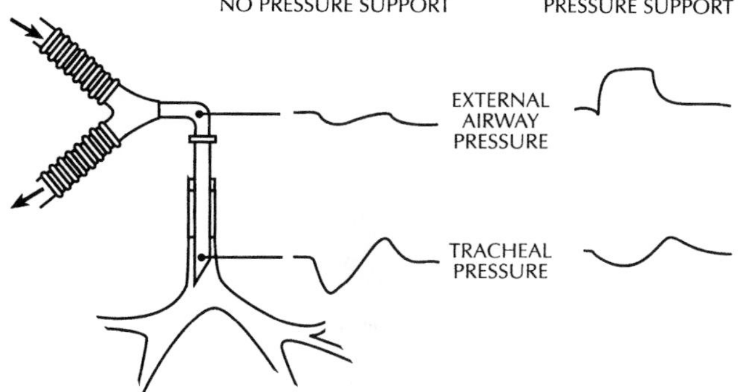

Figure 116–4. Impact of pressure support on the work presented by endotracheal tube resistance. However good the continuous positive airway pressure circuit may be, the patient must draw fresh gas through the endotracheal tube during spontaneous inspiration by generating negative intratracheal pressure *(left)*. The application of pressure support can nullify this additional breathing workload. (From Marini JJ: Work of breathing during mechanical ventilation. *In:* Update in Intensive Care and Emergency Medicine. Vol 10. New York, Springer-Verlag, 1990, pp 239–251.)

in vitro before insertion.[61] Secretions, kinks, or impingement of the endotracheal tube on the mucosal surface of the trachea can decrease the tube's effective diameter. Monitoring systems that track flow and pressure simultaneously are often instrumental in detecting such problems.[62, 63]

Inspiratory resistive work imposed by the endotracheal tube can be offset by an appropriately selected level of pressure support.[40, 64, 65] The effectiveness of a fixed level of pressure support tends to deteriorate as the ventilatory requirement increases. This occurs in part because most machines do not provide flow quickly enough at higher frequencies and because the percentage of work borne by the patient increases with the vigor of the breathing effort. A single value of airway pressure cannot provide the same *percentage* of support across a broad range of $\dot{V}E$ requirements.

However efficient pressure support may be for dealing with inspiratory tube resistance, *expiratory* resistance across the tube and exhalation valve must be overcome by elastic energy or muscle effort. Control of the tracheal pressure during both phases of the ventilatory cycle can be accomplished by sensing (or estimating) circuit pressure at the carinal end of the endotracheal tube. At least one approach to this problem (automatic tube compensation) is in the advanced stages of clinical testing.[6, 9]

MODES FOR PARTIAL VENTILATORY SUPPORT

Increased awareness of the hazards of positive-pressure ventilation, the importance of patient-ventilator interactions, and the escalating costs of inpatient care has stimulated the development of new strategies and modes for supporting machine-dependent patients. The following discussion describes the available modes of ventilatory support and gas exchange in the context of their physiologic rationale, their potential clinical indications and importance, and their shortcomings.

Established Modes of Partial Ventilatory Assistance

Four well-established modes are used in modern clinical practice:

- Assist-control (A/C)
- Synchronized intermittent mandatory ventilation (SIMV)
- Continuous positive airway pressure (CPAP)
- Pressure support ventilation (PSV)

As data are collected regarding the clinical impact of these familiar modes, it becomes clear that subtle modifications may help to achieve important therapeutic objectives.

Volume Assist/Control Ventilation

Traditionally, assist-control ventilation has been volume-cycled and delivered with a constant flow profile often provided. Linearly decelerating flow and sinusoidal flow profiles are other options. Pressure-controlled, time-cycled ventilation with its inherent exponentially decelerating flow is an analogous mode that has become popular (see later). In conventional volume assist-control, the clinician must specify tidal volume and mandatory (back-up) frequency, so that a certain level of ventilation is guaranteed—even if no spontaneous efforts are made. The clinician also sets the peak inspiratory flow target. These having been set, the inspiratory time and minimum minute ventilation are effectively set as well. (For some ventilators, back-up minute ventilation, frequency, and inspiratory time fraction are set directly, so that tidal volume and average inspiratory flow rate are the outcomes of these choices.)

When the patient controls the breathing rhythm, the back-up frequency setting is usually chosen to be 75% or 80% of the natural breathing rate. Typical initial settings for tidal volume and *average* inspiratory flow are 6 to 10 mL/kg of lean body weight and four times the maximum minute ventilation requirement. Although these guidelines are adequate for the majority, smaller tidal volumes may be appropriate if plateau pressures rise too high (see earlier). Occasional patients require other settings for maximum comfort and synchrony.

Once the breathing cycle has been triggered, the airway pressure profile that develops is a function of the flow and tidal volume settings; the impedance offered by the endotracheal tube, airways, lung, and chest wall; and the vigor of the patient's effort. The breathing work done by the patient is determined primarily by ventilatory drive and muscle strength, provided that the rate of gas delivery exceeds the patient's flow demand.[53] When the flow settings of the machine are inappropriately slow, the patient may work for part of the cycle against the flow resistance of the machine as well as against his or her own inspiratory impedance.[52] As noted before, it is prudent to consider use of the decelerating flow profile in attempting to match the patient's flow demand and limit the work of breathing. Overt dyssynchrony predictably results when the machine's attempt to deliver gas persists into the patient's expiratory cycle.

Pressure Assist-Control Ventilation ("Pressure Control")

In pressure-controlled ventilation, the ventilator provides a pressure-limited, time-cycled breath instead of a flow-limited, volume-cycled one.[2] In contrast to flow-controlled, volume-cycled ventilation, the maximum pressure experienced by any alveolus can never exceed the set airway pressure target. Tidal volume, however, varies with unchanging machine settings in response to changes in thoracic impedance and auto-PEEP. In pressure control, inspiratory flow is the variable, determined by total inflation impedance and the magnitude of difference between the pressure applied at the airway opening and the alveolar pressure.

During patient-triggered pressure control cycles, the flow response to the patient's demand is theoretically unlimited as long as the machine can maintain airway opening pressure at the targeted level. Under passive conditions, flow is inherently decelerating and opposed by any existing auto-PEEP. The decelerating flow helps to even the distribution of ventilation between lung units with differing inspiratory time constants and regional values for auto-PEEP. Moreover, the maximum pressure that can be applied to the interior of any alveolus is never higher than the set airway pressure. (Transpulmonary pressure, the difference between alveolar pressure and pleural pressure, can be higher if the patient forcefully inspires to the end of the inspiratory period.) Variations in inspiratory frequency, TI/TTOT, and lung impedance influence the tidal volume delivered, especially in patients with severe airflow obstruction. The maximum tidal volume is delivered when alveolar pressure falls to the set PEEP level at end-expiration and rises to equilibrate with set airway pressure during inspiration. The rate of rise of pressure to the targeted value influences the likelihood of end-inspiratory equilibration as well as the potential comfort of a patient who is triggering the machine.

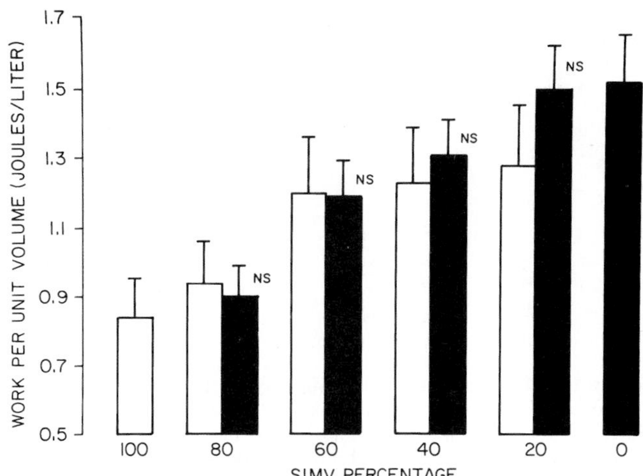

Figure 116–5. Patient's work performed per liter of ventilation during machine-aided *(open bars)* and patient-driven *(shaded bars)* cycles as the percentage of flow-controlled, volume-cycled machine breaths is withdrawn from assist-control (100%) to fully spontaneous breathing (0%). No pressure support was added to the patient-driven cycles. Note that the amount of work performed is similar for both types of cycle at any given percentage of synchronized intermittent mandatory ventilation (SIMV). (From data in Marini JJ, Smith TC, Lamb VJ: External work output and force generation during synchronized intermittent mechanical ventilation. Effect of machine assistance on breathing effort. Am Rev Respir Dis 1988; 138:1169–1179.)

Synchronized Intermittent Mandatory Ventilation

During traditional SIMV, flow-controlled, volume-cycled breaths are interspersed among unsupported spontaneous cycles at a clinician-selected rate. In many modern ventilators, pressure-controlled SIMV can also be elected. Unless the patient's underlying breathing frequency is lower than the frequency of assisted cycles, each machine cycle is initiated by the patient. SIMV can be used as a "full support" mode at high machine cycling frequencies. At lower rates, SIMV provides partial assistance in rough proportion to the relative frequency and depth of machine-aided breaths.[66] Therefore, SIMV seems a logical selection as the platform for gradually reducing machine support during the weaning process.[67]

Because spontaneous and pressurized machine-assisted cycles are intermixed, SIMV often allows adequate ventilatory support at relatively low levels of mean airway and intrapleural pressure, helping to avoid the hemodynamic compromise often encountered during controlled or assist-control ventilation.[68] Any correction of respiratory alkalosis resulting from conversion from assisted mechanical ventilation to SIMV is usually achieved at the expense of a high (occasionally overwhelming) workload for the patient.[69]

Providing a greater number of machine cycles per minute reduces the patient's total ventilatory burden.[56, 66] As already noted, however, the dyspneic patient expends a similar effort for the spontaneous and machine-aided cycles,[55, 56] as gauged by the esophageal pressure-time product, which correlates well with muscle consumption of oxygen.[70] Although pressure control or decelerating volume control may off-load better than constant flow,[57] the dyspneic patient does not appear to vary effort significantly breath-by-breath in response to the help provided by the machine (Fig. 116-5). In this sense, SIMV may not differ greatly from pressure support, a mode in which each breath is machine aided but associated with similar effort. It stands to reason, therefore, that if the peak flow setting stays unchanged as the frequency of SIMV breaths is reduced, there will be a more than proportionate increase in the patient's effort—as the patient's breathing effort and flow demand increase, less work is done by the machine per breathing cycle, and fewer breaths are assisted per minute.

Continuous Positive Airway Pressure

CPAP raises the end-expiratory lung volume from which spontaneous ventilatory efforts are initiated. To elevate pressure in an external circuit with minimum workload, the flow generator and valving mechanism must replenish the gas that flows into the patient during inspiration just fast enough to maintain steady circuit pressure, yet avoid imposing expiratory resistance. The first available CPAP devices were freestanding circuits that avoided energy-costly fluctuations of airway pressure with spring-loaded reservoirs or continuous flow systems directed through low-resistance expiratory threshold valves. Integration of demand valves into the ventilator's circuitry enabled CPAP to be applied to the spontaneous breaths of unaided breathing, SIMV, and pressure support, thereby facilitating monitoring, alarming, and ease of implementation. Poorly designed systems impose substantial resistive work during periods of high flow demand.[71] However, the latest equipment available from most manufacturers employs either sensitive valving or adequate bias flow to provide more responsive, less resistive systems[72] than those originally devised. Flow triggering may confer a marginal advantage in some systems.

CPAP should be applied to the majority of bedridden, intubated patients. In normal subjects, approximately 600 to 1200 mL of lung volume is lost in the transition from the upright to the supine position, much of it from dependent and dorsal lung units crucial to gas exchange.[73] Because atelectasis and secretion retention tend to occur at low lung volumes, modest CPAP (3 to 7 cm H_2O) can be viewed as compensatory and prophylactic. In the setting of severe airflow obstruction, CPAP may counterbalance auto-PEEP, improving the work of breathing without additional hyperinflation.[74–76] Finally, under high breathing workloads, CPAP may be used by the expiratory muscles as a counterspring against which to store elastic energy for release during inspiration (see earlier).

Pressure Support Ventilation

PSV is a pressure preset, flow-cycled mode intended to aid the spontaneous breathing cycle.[59] With most existing ventilators, the clinician chooses only the maximum level of pressure added to the airway opening after the breath is triggered. Pressure support combines with pleural pressure to constitute the transpulmonary pressure that powers inspiration. The patient retains control of the length and depth of the inspiratory cycle and, by varying the pleural pressure, influences both the percentage of the total effort provided by the machine and the flow profile of the breath. Pressurization ends when gas flow falls to some "off-switch" value (typically, 25% of the peak flow achieved earlier in the cycle or to some fixed low rate of inspiratory flow). Arbitrary pressures can be applied, and breaths of varied depth or duration can result. Previous studies have confirmed that PSV reduces the inspiratory work of breathing[58, 77, 78] and alters the shape of the work-defining pressure-volume curve.[77, 78] In patients with severe airflow obstruction, the flow profile may decelerate so slowly that the patient must actively terminate the machine's pressure by contraction of the expiratory muscles.[79]

Even if the machine could hold pressure perfectly constant in the external circuit (CPAP), generating the pressure necessary to overcome endotracheal tube resistance would remain the responsibility of the patient—unless tube resistance is offset by a phasic bias pressure (provided during inspiration by PSV). (At this time, no phasic *expiratory* assistance is yet available.) To more closely simulate the resistance of unimpeded natural breathing, PSV should be added to all spontaneous breaths during CPAP or SIMV. The pressure needed to offset endotracheal tube resistance is a function of tube caliber and flow rate. For tubes studied in vitro, this pressure ranges from 4 to 12 cm H_2O.[40] Tubes that are kinked, secretion encrusted, or poorly placed may impose greater resistance.

When used as the primary power source for weaning, PSV offers a flexibility of power response that SIMV cannot match. The ventilator's total contribution to ventilation is the product of frequency and pressure per breath. Most patients tolerate PSV and many prefer it to SIMV, but not all candidates respond well.[79-81] Each PSV-aided breath must be initiated by the patient, and the tidal volumes that result from those efforts are influenced by the changing impedance of the respiratory system. The efficacy of pressure support is sharply reduced, for example, by the development of auto-PEEP during the weaning effort.[82] Whereas a quietly breathing patient requires a gradual approach to the set pressure value to achieve comfort, the "rise time" of the pressure profile should be shortened in proportion to drive and ventilatory requirements. Although the latest generation of ventilators allow adjustment of the rise time, that setting as well as the pressure target itself should be adjusted when demands change.

As a second shortcoming, inspiratory flow tapers slowly in patients with severe airflow obstruction and those breathing through narrow endotracheal tubes. Such patients must actively decelerate flow to terminate flow delivery (trigger the "off switch") in the time dictated by their own drive center (Fig. 116–6). In other patients, the pressure profile of PSV often deviates from the optimal square configuration at high levels of ventilation or rapid breathing frequencies. In many PSV systems, delays in valve opening may cause flow delivery to lag far behind the patient's demand, severely distorting the idealized pressure waveform.[65]

Maximum flow delivery is a function of the pressure applied by PSV and the pressure developed by the patient's effort. Acting alone, the maximum flow rate achieved by the set level of pressure (P_{set}) is P_{set}/R_i, where R_i is inspiratory resistance. Flow is neither controlled nor limited by PSV—rapid flows can be generated only if P_{set} or the patient's effort is high. Largely for these reasons, the more the patient needs additional machine support, the less likely it is that the support received will be adequate.

As a final consideration, the patient may elect to take many small tidal volumes (rather than adopt a lower frequency, normal tidal volume pattern) during the weaning process to maximize the percentage of work done by the machine.[77, 78]

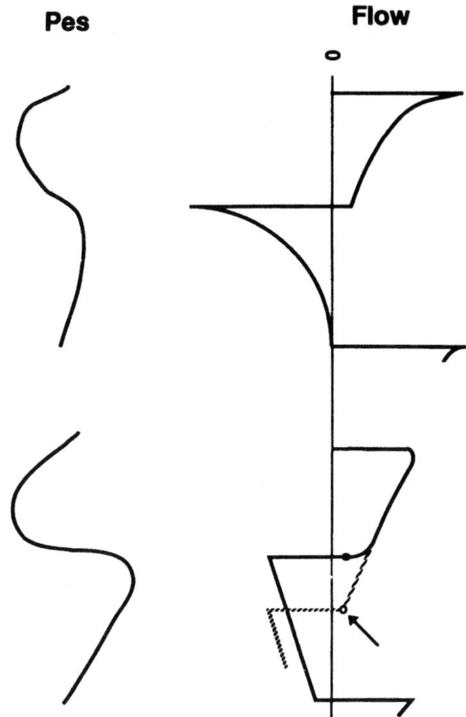

Figure 116–6. Schematic diagrams of flow and esophageal pressure (Pes) during pressure-supported ventilation. In patients with normal airway resistance and short inspiratory time constants *(left),* inspiratory flow decays rapidly. Consequently, the criterion for terminating machine pressure (here, ~ 25% of the peak value) can be met within a time frame appropriate to the patient's desired inspiratory duty cycle, without the patient's effort. Patients with long inspiratory time constants, however, such as those with chronic obstructive pulmonary disease, may require much longer to meet the pressure "off switch" criterion unless active expiratory effort is made to oppose the machine's power. The *broken line segment* is the flow profile that would have resulted in a relaxed patient. The *arrow* and *open circle* indicate the unacceptably delayed off switch that would have resulted without "fighting" the ventilator.

As a result, the reloading of the respiratory pump during weaning may simply be deferred until the latter stages of PSV withdrawal (as already noted, this contrasts sharply with SIMV).[43] Several other problems are yet to be solved. For example, the appropriate pressure target, the most desirable rate of pressure rise, and the optimal off-trigger criterion undoubtedly vary with the vigor of the patient's effort. Some of the newer modes of ventilation are geared to supplement or modify PSV to overcome these deficiencies (see later).

Innovations in Partial Ventilatory Support

Many newer modes of ventilation offer interesting options for ventilatory support, most having been designed with a distinct physiologic or clinical rationale (Fig. 116–7). With few exceptions, however, the indications, efficacy, and safety remain clinically uncertain.

Options for Ventilation

Airway Pressure-Release Ventilation and Bilevel Airway Pressure

Airway pressure-release ventilation (APRV) is a form of partial ventilatory support originally intended to offload a portion of

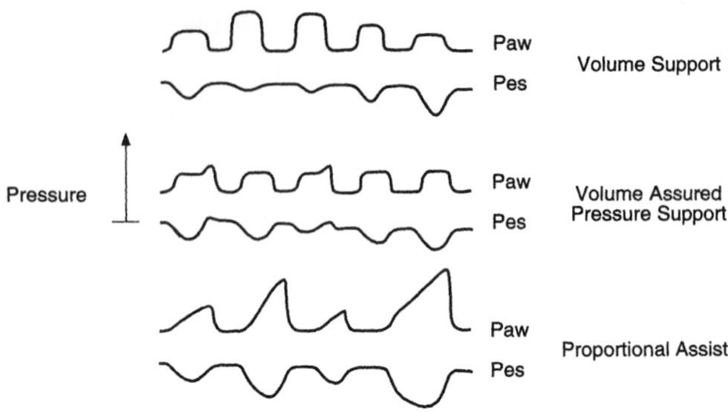

Figure 116–7. Three self-adjusting modes of partial ventilatory support (conceptual schematic). In Volume Support, pressure support is periodically increased or decreased, depending on the patient's ability to maintain tidal volume and minute ventilation targets set by the caregiver. In Volume Assured Pressure Support (also Pressure Augmentation), a fixed level of pressure support may be augmented by constant flow in the latter portion of inspiration if the patient fails to meet the preselected tidal volume target. Proportional Assist Ventilation boosts or withdraws the machine's pressure output "on-line" in direct relation to the vigor of the patient's effort as the breath evolves, thereby acting as an auxiliary set of ventilatory muscles. Paw, Pes = airway and pleural pressures. (From Marini JJ, Wheeler AW: Critical Care Medicine—The Essentials. 2nd ed. Baltimore, Williams & Wilkins, 1997, p 125.)

the work required to ventilate during a primary crisis of oxygenation.[83] APRV elevates mean airway pressure by maintaining a moderately high level of CPAP. Periodically, the airway rapidly depressurizes during a tidal deflation cycle, exhausting waste gas from the functional expiratory reserve before replacing it with fresh gas as CPAP rebuilds to the baseline level. The release pattern is repeated at a frequency selected by the clinician. Using some machines, the clinician can select the *proportion* of cycles during which release occurs, rather than the *absolute frequency* of system decompression.[84] The ventilatory support provided by APRV is a function of driving pressure (the difference between CPAP and the pressure to which airway pressure falls), the duration and frequency of release cycles, and the impedance of the thorax.[85] Synchronization of the release cycle to occur during exhalation may be important to maximize ventilatory efficiency.

This mode and its close relative, *bilevel airway pressure* (BIPAP), are analogous to SIMV in that most individual tidal breath cycles are not assisted by circuit decompression. However, these modes operate with a higher resting pressure and *reduce* rather than raise airway pressure during machine release cycles. In BIPAP, the patient breathes spontaneously for substantial periods around each of two levels of CPAP.[86] BIPAP may exhibit a time dependence—improving oxygenation gradually during hours to days.[87] BIPAP is distinct from biphasic CPAP (known commercially as Bi-PAP), a mode in which the CPAP level is varied with *each triggered cycle* between two levels. Commercial Bi-PAP can be thought of as a combination of CPAP (the lower level, termed commercially EPAP) and pressure support (the difference between the higher and lower levels). Commercial Bi-PAP is generally intended for long-term intermittent ventilatory assistance and therefore is usually implemented at relatively low pressure levels with use of a noninvasive facial or nasal appliance (see earlier).

Although the airway pressure profile generated by the machine during APRV and BIPAP closely resembles that of inverse ratio ventilation (see later), the key difference is that APRV and related techniques allow spontaneous breathing, thereby lowering the peak and mean alveolar pressures associated with a given level of ventilatory support. Allowing spontaneous breathing has an undeniable benefit in helping to promote venous return and obviating the need for deep sedation and muscle relaxants. Furthermore, spontaneous breathing is often more efficient than passive inflation in achieving alveolar ventilation and optimal ventilation-perfusion matching. The potential for overdistention and barotrauma may also be reduced, because peak *airway* pressure is limited to the CPAP applied. However, a vigorously breathing subject may intermittently be subjected to *transpulmonary* inflation pressures considerably higher than the set level of CPAP, because peak stretching pressure is the algebraic difference (absolute sum) of CPAP and intrapleural pressure. Nonetheless, if protective stretch reflexes are intact and regional "ball-valve" gas trapping can be avoided, the risk of barotrauma with this mode should remain relatively low.

Airway pressure release methods pose potential problems. To build the pressure difference needed to assist ventilation significantly, one must first raise CPAP to a moderately high level. If chest compliance is high, the respiratory muscles will be disadvantaged by the resulting hyperinflation, promoting the sensation of dyspnea that APRV is designed to relieve. (In the setting of ARDS, however, the change in *chest wall* volume may be modest.) Furthermore, as the number and duration of release cycles increase, mean airway pressure falls, a change often associated with hypoxemia. This in turn may generate the need for a compensatory increase in CPAP. Circuits must be carefully designed with valves that function properly; otherwise, an excessive breathing workload may result.

APRV has been successfully implemented in postoperative and mildly to moderately affected patients[88-90] and may eventually prove to have applications in the management of more severe forms of acute respiratory failure as well.[88] APRV was designed as a mode to partially assist patients with moderate respiratory failure. It remains open to question whether APRV will prove helpful for patients with extreme weakness, very high breathing workloads, or conditions in which release cycles are relatively ineffectual in achieving ventilation (e.g., in severe airflow obstruction).

Self-Adaptive Modes and Specialized Features

A persistent dream of the critical care specialist is to match the mechanical ventilator's output to the needs of the patient, in accordance with the physician's clinical goals. Advanced microprocessor-guided sensing and flow control technology have allowed ventilator manufacturers to respond by offering a variety of modes and features (Table 116–3) that coordinate better with the patient's flow demands and ensure the minimum tidal volumes and minute ventilations during partial ventilatory assistance that the clinician mandates. Still other approaches that are now just coming to the frontier of clinical practice and are not yet in general use (e.g., adaptive support ventilation) automate pressure regulation and flow delivery while continuously monitoring breathing pattern and ventilatory result. These modes ask the caregiver for boundary parameters (e.g., minimum minute ventilation, or maximum permitted frequency and tidal cycling pressure) but take

TABLE 116–3. Dual-Control Modes of Mechanical Ventilation

Volume-assured pressure support
Pressure augmentation
Volume support
Pressure-regulated volume control
Variable pressure support; variable pressure control
Autoflow

responsibility for optimally regulating the pressure profile or flow delivery pattern using feedback from key monitored variables to satisfy physiologically based criteria. Finally, the latest generation of machines have the potential to nullify the impedance offered by the exhalation valve and to minimize resistance through the endotracheal tube during both phases of the ventilatory cycle by actively regulating external circuit pressure, for example, automatic tube compensation (see Fig. 116-7).

Because of their longer availability and wider application, certain of the latest modes for partial ventilatory assistance deserve special consideration. "Combination" or "dual-control" modes continuously regulate the applied pressure or supplement flow as necessary to achieve a targeted minute ventilation or tidal volume.[91, 92] Dual-control modes combine pressure control and volume targeting logic to maintain the desirable features of both in the setting of changing breathing impedance or effort by the patient. These modes can provide full or partial ventilatory support and conceptually modify their operation within the confines of an individual breath (e.g., by varying the duration or flow provided) or by varying pressure output between breaths (e.g., by varying pressure support to achieve a targeted tidal volume or minute ventilation). Volume support, for example, monitors the tidal volume and ventilation rate achieved during several cycles, compares them with the targeted values, and varies the applied pressure accordingly. Failure to achieve the targeted minute ventilation or tidal volume is met by additional pressure support until the desired ventilation rate is achieved or tidal volume is met by additional pressure support until the desired ventilation rate is achieved or tidal volume exceeds 150% of the desired minimum value. Should minimum minute ventilation and minimum tidal volume be exceeded, pressure support is reduced.

Volume-assured pressure support ventilation (VAPS)[93] and augmented minute volume[94] represent another approach to accomplishing the twin objectives of allowing the patient's control of cycling rhythm while guaranteeing an appropriate tidal volume. In these modes, a flow generator operating in parallel with pressure support intervenes to complete the task of delivering the targeted tidal volume if the level of applied pressure support is insufficient to achieve it. A consequence, however, is that the ventilator determines the patient's flow pattern and may extend the inspiratory time. For many purposes, volume support and VAPS represent an advance over conventional pressure support, but they both have shortcomings that prevent them from being considered an ideal methodology for partial ventilatory support.

Insufficient clinical experience has been gathered to make a definitive assessment of the worth of these recently introduced or infrequently used innovations. Virtually all have operating characteristics that prove dysfunctional when either the patient or set-up parameters are poorly selected by the caregiver. Yet, there is a distinct need to improve the patient-machine interactions of the traditional modes, and if perfected, these newer adaptive approaches may advance comfort and safety.

Proportional Assist Ventilation

A form of ventilatory support has been developed and clinically tested that has the potential to overcome many of the coordination problems of other partial ventilatory support modes. *Proportional assist ventilation* (PAV) instructs the machine to act essentially as an "auxiliary muscle" whose vigor is controlled by the patient but whose power is adjusted by the clinician to offset flow-resistive or elastic pressure requirements.[95, 96] Pressure assistance by the machine is proportional to a variable combination of the inspired volume (the elastic assist) and the inspiratory flow rate (the resistive or frictional assist). Proportionality is accomplished by monitoring flow and volume (integrated flow), the two key components of the simplified equation of motion describing the inspiratory pressure (P) across the respiratory system[97]:

$$P = \dot{V}R + \int \dot{V}^{dt}/C$$

where $\dot{V}$ is flow and R and C are resistance and compliance of the respiratory system, respectively.

PAV is intuitively attractive, in that it yields to the patient's own neuromuscular control mechanisms and is guided by the equation of motion of the respiratory system in synchronizing the ventilator's output with the patient's continuously changing needs. Tidal volume and flow are fully controlled by the patient; the "gain factors" (volume assist percentage) and flow assist percentage that determine the elastic and flow-resistive assist proportions become the independent variables. (Although superficially similar, this control algorithm differs from other proposed approaches to amplify the patient's effort that set tidal volume and flow targets.)[98]

Thus, the machine acts to amplify the patient's own efforts; when the patient pulls harder, the machine boosts its output; as the patient relaxes, the machine cuts back in parallel. There is a continuously varying range of tidal volumes that mimics the natural breathing pattern—variation that may help to keep the lung well recruited.[99, 100] In theory, the clinician can offset any desired fraction of the frictional or elastic workload by adjusting the appropriate gain settings. It has been suggested that reflexes that normally prevent lung overdistention might also prevent barotrauma during PAV-assisted breathing. Across a wide range of gain combinations, a "runaway" condition (positive feedback) does not occur. However, runaway is possible if the gain factors are set inappropriately or if there are large, rapid changes in elastance or resistance.

No mode of partial support is without drawbacks, and PAV is no exception. Because tidal volumes and flow rates are controlled by the natural breathing rhythm, they vary continuously, and PAV requires back-up in case the patient ceases ventilatory efforts. Moreover, like pressure support, PAV does not offset auto-PEEP. As with any form of mechanical ventilation, pressure, apnea, and hypoventilation alarms must be set appropriately. Despite these reservations, PAV has the clear potential for providing appropriate ventilatory support in a variety of clinical settings ranging from acute lung injury to gradual machine withdrawal.

References

1. Kimball WR, Leith DE, Robins AG: Dynamic hyperinflation and ventilator dependence in chronic obstructive pulmonary disease. Am Rev Respir Dis 1982; 126:991-995.
2. Marini JJ, Crooke PS, Truwit JD: Determinants and limits of pressure preset ventilation: A mathematical model of pressure control. J Appl Physiol 1989; 67:1081-1092.
3. Stalcup SA, Mellins RB: Mechanical forces producing pulmonary edema in acute asthma. N Engl J Med 1977; 297:592-596.
4. Chandra A, Coggeshall JW, Ravenscraft SA, Marini JJ: Hyperpnea limits the volume recruited by positive end-expiratory pressure. Am J Respir Crit Care Med 1994; 150:911-917.
5. Ninane V, Yernault JC, de Troyer A: Intrinsic PEEP in patients with chronic obstructive pulmonary disease: Role of expiratory muscles. Am Rev Respir Dis 1993; 148(pt 1):1037-1042.
6. Banner MJ, Blanch PB, Kirby RR: Imposed work of breathing and methods of triggering a demand flow, continuous positive airway pressure system. Crit Care Med 1993; 21:183-190.
7. Gottfried SB, Rossi A, Higgs BD, et al: Noninvasive determination of respiratory system mechanics during mechanical ventilation for acute respiratory failure. Am Rev Respir Dis 1985; 131:672-677.
8. Marini JJ, Kirk W, Culver BH: Flow resistance of the exhalation

valves and PEEP devices used in mechanical ventilation. Am Rev Respir Dis 1985; 131:850-854.
9. Guttmann J, Eberhard J, Fabry B, Bertschmann W, Wolff G: Continuous calculation of intratracheal pressure in tracheally intubated patients. Anesthesiology 1993; 79:503-513.
10. Broseghini C, Brandolese R, Poggi R: Respiratory mechanics during the first day of mechanical ventilation in patients with pulmonary edema and chronic airway obstruction. Am Rev Respir Dis 1988; 138:355-361.
11. Hyatt RE: Expiratory flow limitation. J Appl Physiol 1983; 55:1-8.
12. Leatherman J, Ravenscraft S: Low measured auto-positive end-expiratory pressure during mechanical ventilation of patients with severe asthma: Hidden auto-positive end-expiratory pressure. Crit Care Med 1996; 24:541-546.
13. Shim C, Chun KJ, Williams MH Jr, Blaufox MD: Positional effects on distribution of ventilation in chronic obstructive pulmonary disease. Ann Intern Med 1986; 105:346-350.
14. Marini JJ: Should PEEP be used in airflow obstruction? Am Rev Respir Dis 1989; 140:1-3.
15. Pepe PE, Marini JJ: Occult positive end-expiratory pressure in mechanically ventilated patients with airflow obstruction. Am Rev Respir Dis 1982; 126:166-170.
16. Lemaire F, Teboul JL, Cinotti L, et al: Acute left ventricular dysfunction during unsuccessful weaning from mechanical ventilation. Anesthesiology 1988; 69:171-179.
17. Fleury BD, Murciano D, Talamo C, Aubier M, Pariente R, Milic-Emili J: Work of breathing in patients with chronic obstructive pulmonary disease in acute respiratory failure. Am Rev Respir Dis 1985; 131:822-827.
18. Smith TC, Marini JJ: Impact of PEEP on lung mechanics and work of breathing in severe airflow obstruction: The effect of PEEP on auto-PEEP. J Appl Physiol 1988; 65:1488-1499.
19. Tobin MJ: Respiratory muscles in disease. Clin Chest Med 1988; 9:264-286.
20. Similowski T, Yan S, Gauthier AP, et al: Contractile properties of the human diaphragm during chronic hyperinflation. N Engl J Med 1991; 325:917-923.
21. Macklem PT: Hyperinflation. Am Rev Respir Dis 1984; 129:1-2.
22. Martin J, Shore S, Engel LA: Effect of continuous positive airway pressure on respiratory mechanics and pattern of breathing in induced asthma. Am Rev Respir Dis 1982; 126:812-817.
23. Tobin MJ, Lodato RF: PEEP, auto-PEEP, and waterfalls. Chest 1989; 96:449-451.
24. O'Donnell DE, Sanii R, Anthonisen NR, Younes M: Effect of dynamic airway compression on breathing pattern and respiratory sensation in severe chronic obstructive pulmonary disease. Am Rev Respir Dis 1987; 135:912-918.
25. Petrof BJ, Calderini E, Legare M, Gottfried SB: Continuous positive airway pressure improves discoordinate thoracoabdominal motion during weaning in severe chronic obstructive pulmonary disease (Abstract). Am Rev Respir Dis 1989; 139:A97.
26. Marini JJ: The physiologic determinants of ventilator dependence. Respir Care 1986; 31:271-282.
27. Murciano D, Boczkowski J, Lecocguic Y, et al: Tracheal occlusion pressure: A simple index to monitor respiratory muscle fatigue during acute respiratory failure in patients with chronic obstructive pulmonary disease. Ann Intern Med 1988; 108:800-805.
28. Douglass JA, Tuxen DV, Horne M, et al: Myopathy in severe asthma. Am Rev Respir Dis 1992; 146:517-519.
29. Zochodne DW, Bolton CF, Wells GA, et al: Critical illness polyneuropathy: A complication of sepsis and multiple organ failure. Brain 1987; 110:819-841.
30. Tuxen DV, Williams TJ, Schienkestel CD, Czarny D, Bowes G: Use of a measurement of pulmonary hyperinflation to control the level of mechanical ventilation in patients with acute severe asthma. Am Rev Respir Dis 1992; 146:1136-1142.
31. Sahn SA, Lakshminarayan S: Bedside criteria for discontinuation of mechanical ventilation. Chest 1973; 63:1002-1005.
32. Bellemare F, Grassino A: Effect of pressure and timing of contraction on human diaphragm failure. J Appl Physiol 1982; 53:1190-1195.
33. Roussos C, Macklem PT: Inspiratory muscle fatigue. *In:* Handbook of Physiology. Fishman AP, Macklem PT, Mead J (Eds). Bethesda, Md, American Physiological Society, 1986, pp 511-527.
34. Tobin MJ, Perez W, Guenther SM, et al: The pattern of breathing during successful and unsuccessful trials of weaning from mechanical ventilation. Am Rev Respir Dis 1986; 134:1111-1118.
35. Yang KL, Tobin MJ: A prospective study of indexes predicting the outcome of trials of weaning from mechanical ventilation. N Engl J Med 1991; 324:1445-1450.
36. Grassino A, Macklem PT: Respiratory muscle fatigue and ventilatory failure. Annu Rev Med 1984; 35:625-647.
37. Nishimura M, Imanaka H, Yoshiya I, Kacmarek RM: Comparison of inspiratory work of breathing between flow-triggered and pressure-triggered demand flow systems in rabbits. Crit Care Med 1994; 22:1002-1009.
38. Sassoon CSH, Giron AE, Ely E, Light RW: Inspiratory work of breathing on flow-by and demand-flow continuous positive airway pressure. Crit Care Med 1989; 17:1108-1114.
39. Petrof BJ, Legare M, Goldberg P, Milic-Emili J, Gottfried SB: Continuous positive airway pressure reduces work of breathing and dyspnea during weaning from mechanical ventilation in severe chronic obstructive pulmonary disease. Am Rev Respir Dis 1990; 141:281-289.
40. Fiastro JF, Habib MP, Quan SF: Pressure support compensation for inspiratory work due to endotracheal tubes and demand continuous positive airway pressure. Chest 1988; 93:499-505.
41. Esteban A, Frutos F, Tobin MJ, et al: A comparison of four methods of weaning patients from mechanical ventilation. Spanish Lung Failure Collaborative Group. N Engl J Med 1995; 332:345-350.
42. Brochard L, Rauss A, Benito S, Conti G, Mancebo J, Rekik N, Gasparetto A, Lemaire F: Comparison of three methods of gradual withdrawal from ventilatory support during weaning from mechanical ventilation. Am J Respir Crit Care Med 1994; 150:896-903.
43. McKibben A, Chandra A, Adams AB, Marini JJ: Patterns of respiratory muscle reloading during withdrawal of pressure support ventilation (PSV) and synchronized intermittent mandatory ventilation (SIMV). Am Rev Respir Crit Care Med 1995; 151:A236.
44. Gilbert R, Auchincloss JH Jr, Peppi D, Ashutosh K: The first hours off a respirator. Chest 1974; 65:152-157.
45. Holliday JE, Hyers TM: The reduction of weaning time from mechanical ventilation using tidal volume and relaxation biofeedback. Am Rev Respir Dis 1990; 141:1214-1220.
46. Marini JJ: Weaning from mechanical ventilation. N Engl J Med 1991; 324:1496-1498.
47. Brochard L, Isabey D, Piquet J, Piedode A, Mancebo J, Messadi A, Brun-Buisson C, Rauss A, Lemaire F, Harf A: Reversal of acute exacerbations of chronic obstructive pulmonary disease by inspiratory assistance with a face mask. N Engl J Med 1990; 323:1523-1530.
48. Udwadia ZF, Santis GK, Steven MH, Simonds AK: Nasal ventilation to facilitate weaning in patients with chronic respiratory insufficiency. Thorax 1992; 47:715-718.
49. Waldhorn RE: Nocturnal nasal intermittent positive pressure ventilation with bi-level positive airway pressure (BiPAP) in respiratory failure. Chest 1992; 101:516-521.
50. Marini JJ: Work of breathing during mechanical ventilation. *In:* Update in Intensive Care and Emergency Medicine. Vol 10. Vincent JL (Ed). New York, Springer-Verlag, 1990, pp 239-251.
51. Otis AB: The work of breathing. Physiol Rev 1954; 34:449-458.
52. Marini JJ, Capps JS, Culver BH: The inspiratory work of breathing during assisted mechanical ventilation. Chest 1985; 87:612-618.
53. Marini JJ, Rodriguez RM, Lamb VJ: The inspiratory workload of patient-initiated mechanical ventilation. Am Rev Respir Dis 1986; 134:902-909.
54. Ravenscraft SA, Burke WC, Marini JJ: Volume cycled decelerating flow: An alternative form of mechanical ventilation. Chest 1992; 101:1342-1351.
55. Imsand C, Feihl F, Perret C, Fitting JW: Regulation of inspiratory neuromuscular output during synchronized intermittent mechanical ventilation. Anesthesiology 1994; 80:13-22.
56. Marini JJ, Smith TC, Lamb VJ: External work output and force generation during synchronized intermittent mechanical ventilation. Effect of machine assistance on breathing effort. Am Rev Respir Dis 1988; 138:1169-1179.
57. Cinnella G, Conti G, Lofaso F, Lorino H, Harf A, Lemaire F, Brochard L: Effects of assisted ventilation on the work of breath-

ing: Volume-controlled versus pressure-controlled ventilation. Am J Respir Crit Care Med 1996; 153:1025–1033.

58. Brochard L, Harf A, Lorino H, Lemaire F: Pressure support prevents diaphragmatic fatigue during weaning from mechanical ventilation. Am Rev Respir Dis 1989; 139:513–521.
59. MacIntyre NR: Respiratory function during pressure support ventilation. Chest 1986; 89:677–683.
60. Knebel AR, Janson-Bjerklie SL, Malley JD, Wilson AG, Marini JJ: Comparison of breathing comfort during weaning with two ventilatory modes. Am J Respir Crit Care Med 1994; 149:14–18.
61. Wright PW, Marini JJ, Bernard GR: In vitro versus in vivo comparison of endotracheal tube airflow resistance. Am Rev Respir Dis 1989; 140:10–16.
62. Jubran A, Tobin MJ: Use of flow-volume curves in detecting secretions in ventilator-dependent patients. Am J Respir Crit Care Med 1994; 150:766–769.
63. Marini JJ: Monitoring during mechanical ventilation. Clin Chest Med 1988; 9:73–100.
64. Imanaka H, Kacmarek RM, Ritz R, Hess D: Tracheal gas insufflation—pressure control versus volume control ventilation: A lung model study. Am J Respir Crit Care Med 1996; 153:1019–1024.
65. Marini JJ: Strategies to minimize breathing effort during mechanical ventilation. Crit Care Clin 1990; 6:635–661.
66. Weiss JW, Rossing TH, Ingram RH: Effect of intermittent mandatory ventilation on respiratory drive and timing. Am Rev Respir Dis 1983; 127:705–708.
67. Downs JB, Klein EF, Desautels D, Modell JH, Kirby RR: Intermittent mandatory ventilation: A new approach to weaning patients from mechanical ventilators. Chest 1973; 64:331–335.
68. Mathru M, Venus B: Ventilator-induced barotrauma in controlled mechanical ventilation versus intermittent mandatory ventilation. Crit Care Med 1983; 11:359–361.
69. Hudson LD, Hurlow RS, Craig KC, et al: Does intermittent mandatory ventilation correct respiratory alkalosis in patients receiving assisted mechanical ventilation? Am Rev Respir Dis 1985; 132:1071–1074.
70. McGregor M, Becklake M: The relationship of oxygen cost of breathing to respiratory mechanical work and respiratory force. J Clin Invest 1961; 40:971–980.
71. Gibney RTN, Wilson RS, Pontoppidan H: Comparisons of work of breathing on high gas flow and demand valve continuous positive airway pressure systems. Chest 1982; 82:692–695.
72. Samodelov LF, Falke KJ: Total inspiratory work with modern demand valve devices compared to continuous flow CPAP. Intensive Care Med 1988; 14:632–639.
73. Marini JJ, Tyler ML, Hudson LD, Davis BS, Huseby JS: Influence of head-dependent positions on lung volume and oxygen saturation in chronic airflow obstruction. Am Rev Respir Dis 1984; 129:101–105.
74. Iotti G, Braschi A: Respiratory mechanics in chronic obstructive pulmonary disease. *In:* Update in Intensive Care and Emergency Medicine. Vol 10. Vincent JL (Ed). New York, Springer-Verlag, 1990, pp 223–230.
75. Ranieri VM, Grasso S, Fiore T, Giuliani R: Auto-positive end-expiratory pressure and dynamic hyperinflation. Clin Chest Med 1996; 17:379–395.
76. Rossi A, Ganassini A, Polese G, Grassi V: Pulmonary hyperinflation and ventilator-dependent patients. Eur Respir J 1997; 10:1663–1674.
77. MacIntyre NR, Leatherman NE: Ventilatory muscle loads and the frequency-tidal volume pattern during inspiratory pressure-associated (pressure-supported) ventilation. Am Rev Respir Dis 1990; 141:327–331.
78. Tokioka S, Saito S, Kosaka F: Effect of pressure support ventilation on breathing patterns and respiratory work. Intensive Care Med 1989; 15:491–494.
79. Jubran A, Van de Graaff WB, Tobin MJ: Variability of patient-ventilator interaction with pressure support ventilation in patients with chronic obstructive pulmonary disease. Am J Respir Crit Care Med 1995; 152:129–136.
80. Specht NL, Yang SC, Killeen TS, et al: Pressure support ventilation fails to provide adequate support as a primary ventilatory mode (Abstract). Am Rev Respir Dis 1989; 139:A62.
81. Zeravik J, Borg U, Pfeiffer UJ: Efficacy of pressure support ventilation dependent on extravascular lung water. Chest 1990; 97:1412–1419.
82. Marcy TW, Marini JJ: Modes of mechanical ventilation. *In:* Current Pulmonology. Vol 13. Simmons DH, Tierney DF (Eds). Chicago, Mosby-Year Book, 1992, pp 43–90.
83. Stock MC, Downs JB, Frolichter DA: Airway pressure release ventilation. Crit Care Med 1987; 15:462–466.
84. Rouby J-J: Pressure release ventilation. *In:* Update in Intensive Care and Emergency Medicine. Vol 10. Vincent JL (Ed). New York, Springer-Verlag, 1990, pp 185–195.
85. Downs JB, Stock MC: Airway pressure release ventilation: A new concept in ventilatory support. Crit Care Med 1987; 15:459–461.
86. Baum M, Benzer H, Putensen C, et al: Biphasic positive airway pressure (BIPAP)—a new form of augmented ventilation. Anaesthetist 1989; 38:452–458.
87. Sydow M, Burchardi H, Ephraim E, Zielmann S, Crozier TA: Long term effects of two different ventilatory modes on oxygenation in acute lung injury. Comparison of airway pressure release ventilation and volume controlled inverse ratio ventilation. Am J Respir Crit Care Med 1994; 149:1550–1556.
88. Cane RD, Peruzzi WT, Shapiro BA: Airway pressure release ventilation in severe acute respiratory failure. Chest 1991; 100:460–463.
89. Garner W, Downs JB, Stock C, Rasanen J: Airway pressure release ventilation (APRV): A human trial. Chest 1988; 94:779–781.
90. Rasanen J, Cane RD, Downs JB, et al: Airway pressure release ventilation: A multicenter trial. Anesthesiology 1989; 71:A1078.
91. Al-Saady N, Bennett ED: Decelerating inspiratory flow waveform improves lung mechanics and gas exchange in patients on intermittent positive pressure-ventilation. Intensive Care Med 1985; 11:68–75.
92. Hewlett AM, Platt AS, Terry VG: Mandatory minute volume: A new concept in weaning from mechanical ventilation. Anaesthesia 1977; 32:163–169.
93. Amato MBP, Barbas CSV, Bonassa J, Saldiva PHN, Zin WA, Ribeiro de Carvalho CR: Volume-assured pressure support ventilation (VAPSV): A new approach for reducing muscle workload during acute respiratory failure. Chest 1992; 102:1225–1234.
94. MacIntyre NR, Gropper C, Westfall T: Combining pressure-limiting and volume-cycling features in a patient-interactive mechanical breath. Crit Care Med 1994; 22:353–357.
95. Younes M: Proportional assist ventilation: A new approach to ventilatory support. Am Rev Respir Dis 1991; 145:114–120.
96. Younes M: Proportional assist ventilation and pressure support ventilation: Similarities and differences. *In:* Ventilatory Failure. Marini JJ, Roussos C (Eds). New York, Springer-Verlag, 1991, pp 361–380.
97. Otis AB, Fenn WO, Rahn H: Mechanics of breathing in man. J Appl Physiol 1950; 2:592–607.
98. Lebowitz HH, Poon CS: Negative impedance ventilation (NIV): An improved inspiratory pressure support mode (Abstract). Chest 1991; 98:76S.
99. Lefevre GR, Kowalski SE, Girling LG, Thiessen DB, Mutch WA: Improved arterial oxygenation after oleic acid lung injury in the pig using a computer-controlled mechanical ventilator. Am J Respir Crit Care Med 1996; 154:1567–1592.
100. Suki B, Alencar AM, Sujeer MK, Lutchen KR, Collins JJ, Andrade JS, Ingenito EP, Zapperi S, Stanley HE: Life-support system benefits from noise. Nature 1998; 393:127–128.

117

Independent Lung Ventilation

Andrew R. Davies, MBBS, FRACP
David V. Tuxen, MD, MBBS, FRACP, DipDHM

Independent lung ventilation (ILV) is an unusual but important technique for patients with specific forms of acute, severe respiratory failure. After its first description in 1931,[1] its principal use has been for isolating one lung from the other during a thoracic surgical procedure. Since 1976, [2] it has been recognized that lungs affected differently by disease processes may benefit from different ventilatory strategies. Different tidal volumes (VT), respiratory rates (RR), and levels of positive end-expiratory pressure (PEEP) can be administered to each lung, a strategy that may enhance the management of complex pathophysiologic problems. The placement of a double-lumen tube and institution of ILV is technically complex and labor-intensive but, correctly utilized, has the potential markedly to improve gas exchange and circulation, reduce morbidity, and in some instances to be lifesaving.

The major indications for independent lung ventilation are as follows:

- Lung isolation for thoracic surgery or procedures
- Protection of one lung from the secretions of the other lung
- Separation of the ventilation of each lung owing to an asymmetric disease process

THORACIC SURGERY

Indications

Thoracic surgical procedures that require one-lung ventilation include pneumonectomy, some lobectomies, thoracic aortic surgery, thoracoscopy, and some types of esophageal surgery.[3, 4] Single-lung ventilation can be established by using either (1) a bronchial blocker or (2) a double-lumen tube. The bronchial blocker is a balloon-tipped catheter that is placed into the bronchus to be occluded—outside or within a standard cuffed endotracheal tube lumen—or passed down a specially designed second small lumen in the endobronchial tube.[5, 6] Although the bronchial-blocking technique has no independent access to the unventilated lung, it is usually preferred because it has the advantage of creating a wide-bore, low-resistance endobronchial lumen with better access to the ventilated lung for bronchoscopy and suctioning.[5] The narrow lumen in the bronchial blocker enables lung inflation, deflation, continuous positive airway pressure (CPAP), and high-frequency jet ventilation but does not allow conventional ILV.[5] One-lung or double-lung ventilation (with the blocker deflated) is possible, and the side of one-lung ventilation may be changed by switching the side of the bronchial blocker.

A double-lumen tube has the advantage of providing ILV either before or after the surgical procedure if hypoxemia is a problem, but reduced lumen diameter to the lung being ventilated is a minor disadvantage.

Pathophysiology and Positioning

Changes in body position and the presence or absence of spontaneous ventilation have important effects on the distribution of ventilation and perfusion. When a patient is transferred from the supine to the lateral decubitus position, more than 10% of perfusion shifts from the nondependent to the dependent lung, resulting in as much as two thirds of perfusion occurring through the dependent lung.[7] In the lateral decubitus position, the weight of abdominal contents displaces the dependent diaphragm upward farther than its nondependent side. During spontaneous ventilation, this confers a mechanical advantage on the dependent diaphragm, increasing ventilation to the dependent lung, although the increase is smaller than the perfusion increase, the result being increased ventilation-perfusion mismatch. A similar mismatch of ventilation and perfusion occurs when a patient is moved from the supine to the erect position.[7, 8]

When spontaneous ventilation is replaced by mechanical ventilation with the patient in the lateral decubitus position, the increased excursion of the dependent diaphragm (secondary to increased muscle contraction) is replaced by inactivity of the diaphragm, which allows the abdominal contents to retard dependent lung expansion and switches the majority (about two thirds) of ventilation to the nondependent lung.[7, 9, 10] These changes cause significant overperfusion relative to ventilation in the dependent lung (increased shunt) and overventilation relative to perfusion in the nondependent lung (increased dead space), with adverse effects on gas exchange. If the nondependent thorax is opened for surgery, the increased compliance in that lung results in a further increase in ventilation in the nondependent lung with more ventilation-perfusion mismatch.[11, 12] A right-sided thoracotomy is associated with worse oxygenation than a left-sided thoracotomy, because the left lung usually receives 10% less cardiac output than the right one.[13]

Patients with chronic airflow obstruction actually have better gas exchange in the lateral decubitus position because of the presence of dynamic hyperinflation, which resists the reduction in functional residual capacity (FRC) in the dependent lung.[13] By exclusion of the nondependent lung from ventilation during surgery, perfusion to the nondependent lung becomes a complete shunt. With hypoxic vasoconstriction, lung collapse, or surgical occlusion of blood flow to the nondependent lung, there is the potential to reduce this shunt and actually improve oxygenation. In the absence of any of these, however, gas exchange can be seriously compromised.

When the nondependent lung can be ventilated with the chest open during thoracic surgery, the effects of synchronized independent lung ventilation with equal VT to both lungs,[14] increased PEEP to the dependent lung[15-18] or to both lungs,[15, 16] or CPAP to the nondependent lung[15] can be observed. Selective application of PEEP to the dependent lung may improve dependent lung ventilation, and thus oxygenation, by improving FRC[10]; however, the increased alveolar pressure secondary to the PEEP can increase pulmonary vascular resistance in the dependent lung, leading to diversion of blood flow to the nondependent (and nonventilated) lung,[8, 19] which may offset the benefits of the PEEP for oxygenation. Thus, application of selective PEEP to the dependent lung in the lateral decubitus position needs to be considered carefully.

When a bronchial blocker and one-lung ventilation are used, PEEP can be directed to either lung. One study[15] directly compared PEEP to the dependent lung, CPAP to the nondependent lung, and a combination of both in patients positioned in the lateral decubitus position with the thorax open. PEEP to the dependent lung caused a nonsignificant oxygenation change; CPAP to the nondependent lung improved oxygenation, whereas a combination of PEEP and CPAP to each lung caused a similar improvement in oxygenation with a greater reduction in shunt fraction than nondependent CPAP. The PEEP-CPAP combination reduced cardiac output but not lower than it had been before the surgery. Variable changes in oxygenation have been demonstrated in other studies.[19–22]

When hypoxemia develops during one-lung anesthesia for thoracic surgery and the nondependent lung can be inflated, it is recommended that CPAP be applied to that lung, either alone or in combination with dependent lung PEEP at levels between 5 and 10 cm H_2O. Spontaneous or conventional mechanical ventilation is usually resumed once the surgical procedure is complete. ILV, however, has been required postoperatively by a minority of patients for persistent hypoxemia,[2, 23, 24] for bronchopleural fistulas,[25, 26] and after esophagectomy.[27]

SELECTIVE AIRWAY PROTECTION

Whole-Lung Lavage

Not long after pulmonary alveolar proteinosis was first described,[28] whole-lung lavage became established as the principal therapeutic modality.[29, 30] Lavage is now recognized to be the only effective treatment, and it is best used for patients with progressive disease.[31]

Whole-lung lavage has also been used for asthma,[32, 33] chronic obstructive pulmonary disease (COPD),[34] and cystic fibrosis.[35] Benefits were never clearly established, however, and, with improving medical treatments for these conditions, they are no longer indications for whole-lung lavage. Whole-lung lavage has also been recommended for inhalation of radioactive dust.[36] Although this is uncommon, it remains an indication.

Whole-lung lavage requires a double-lumen tube to isolate each lung. A left-sided double-lumen tube is preferred, as it is easier to place successfully. The correct position of the tube may be verified by bronchoscopic or auscultatory methods, but a nonleaking seal must be demonstrated in each lung to ensure the safety of the procedure. The patient should undergo one-lung ventilation before the procedure to ensure adequate oxygenation. Both lungs should be preoxygenated with 100% oxygen to maximize oxygenation in the ventilated lung and to minimize remaining nitrogen bubbles in the alveoli and to prevent entry of fluid into the lavaged lung.

The choice of body position is important and relates to the mechanism of hypoxemia and to the risk of fluid spillage during the procedure. Placing the patient in the lateral decubitus position with the lavaged lung dependent not only minimizes the risk of any fluid leakage during the procedure, but also maximizes blood flow to the nonventilated lung during lung emptying and hence increases hypoxemia.[37] Placing the lavaged lung in the nondependent position would minimize desaturation during the drainage phase, but the risk from fluid spillage in this position is unacceptably high.[37] As a result, the supine position is more often the best compromise between hypoxemia after fluid efflux and risk of fluid entry into the ventilated lung.

Isotonic saline (500 to 1000 mL) warmed to body temperature should then be infused through wide-bore tubing from a height of 30 cm above the midaxillary line into the lung to be lavaged.[37] Once influx of fluid is complete, one can initiate efflux by placing the drainage tube below the patient and positioning the patient to maximize gravitational forces. This step should be repeated until efflux fluid is clear, which may require 10 to 50 L of fluid.

Hypoxemia is unusual during fluid influx, because the fluid pressure in the alveoli usually exceeds the pulmonary capillary pressure, minimizing shunt through the lavaged lung.[38–40] After fluid efflux, however, restoration of blood flow to the nonventilated lung produces a large shunt and significant arterial desaturation can occur at this stage.[37, 38, 40, 41]

Should significant leakage of fluid into the ventilated lung be recognized, lavage should be ceased and drainage maximized with the patient in the lateral decubitus position with the lavaged lung dependent and the head down. Active suctioning of both lungs should be performed. If the leak is minor and oxygenation is restored, the double-lumen tube may have its airway seals reestablished and this procedure continued. If the leak is major and hypoxemia remains despite the measures described, the procedure should be abandoned. Both lungs should be ventilated and the patient returned to the supine position once fluid removal is complete. As much as 1000 mL of saline may be retained in the lavaged lung,[42] and, although this is absorbed rapidly, lung function may not improve for some hours or days.

After a successful procedure or an abandoned one, patients should be switched to double-lung ventilation via the double-lumen tube, to assess oxygenation. If oxygenation is satisfactory on a fraction of inspired oxygen (FIO_2) below 0.6, with good preoperative ventilation status, it is likely the double-lumen tube can be successfully removed. If adequate saturation requires a higher FIO_2 or if the preoperative ventilation status was marginal, the double-lumen tube may have to be replaced by a single-lumen endotracheal tube for conventional mechanical ventilation until oxygenation improves or to assess weaning. If significant desaturation remains during double-lung ventilation despite FIO_2 of 1.0 and PEEP, ILV may need to be reinstituted until oxygenation improves.

Severe hypoxemia may preclude whole-lung lavage. When severe hypoxemia is present before the procedure or if excessive desaturation occurs during one-lung ventilation, attempts at whole-lung lavage may not be safe. Under these circumstances, two alternatives exist. Extracorporeal membrane oxygenation (ECMO) may be instituted before lavage of the first lung to sustain oxygenation during the procedure.[37, 43, 44] ECMO is invasive and labor-intensive but allows whole-lung lavage to be completed in a single procedure. Bronchoscopy, with or without an inflatable cuff on the bronchoscope, is an alternative[45, 46] and can be performed with local anesthesia. Limiting lavage to a lobe or several subsegments minimizes hypoxemia during such procedures but has the disadvantage of necessitating multiple procedures.

Massive Hemoptysis

Massive hemoptysis, a medical emergency associated with high risk of mortality,[47, 48] requires prompt intervention. Bronchial carcinoma, tuberculosis, bronchiectasis, lung abscess, mycetoma, and cystic fibrosis are some common causes.[47] All are associated with tortuous, aneurysmal bronchial arteries or abnormally fragile capillary beds. There are a number of iatrogenic causes of major hemoptysis. Hemoptysis can follow procedures such as tracheostomy and transbronchial biopsy. Pulmonary artery catheters can cause massive hemoptysis by rupturing a pulmonary artery.[49] When death occurs as a result of massive hemoptysis, it is infrequently due to exsanguination and usually results from acute asphyxia. The risk of death from asphyxia is related to the rate and volume of blood loss, the severity of underlying lung disease, and the patient's capacity to cough and clear secretions.[47, 50, 51]

Management of massive hemoptysis requires urgent resuscitation, localization of the bleeding site, and measures to secure hemostasis and to isolate the bleeding lung. The patient should be administered 100% oxygen and positioned head down in the lateral decubitus position, so that the side of suspected bleeding is dependent. Simultaneous fluid resuscitation may also be necessary. Equipment for intubation should be nearby and clotting assessment urgently undertaken, with clotting factor replacement as necessary.

To localize, isolate, and control the bleeding site can be challenging. The choice of technique depends on (1) the rate of bleeding, (2) the availability of the technique, and (3) the skills of the personnel involved.

For patients with mild to moderate hemoptysis, fiberoptic bronchoscopy can allow placement of a Fogarty catheter in the appropriate lung segment.[52] Once the catheter is in position, it can be inflated to tamponade the bleeding site or merely prevent flooding of the remainder of the lung with blood. Such a patient does not necessarily require intubation. Flexible bronchoscopy also allows lavage with iced isotonic saline for identification and control of hemorrhage[47, 53] and instillation of dilute topical epinephrine when bleeding is from a proximal airway lesion.

When blood loss is moderate to massive, visibility through the flexible bronchoscope becomes extremely poor.[54] Endotracheal intubation is required. Rigid bronchoscopy is more suitable because of better suction, better visual access, and better airway control.[51, 55, 56] Like fiberoptic bronchoscopy, it allows placement of endobronchial blockers, iced saline lavage, and epinephrine instillation but also allows diathermy and placement of endobronchial tampons soaked in vasoconstrictor drugs.[51] This technique may be hampered by delays in obtaining the equipment or suitable personnel to use it and in transporting the patient to the operating room.

Selective intubation of one of the main bronchi may also be attempted. Bronchoscopic guidance is needed to localize the bleeding site, as one lung will be excluded from ventilation. Selective intubation offers reliable protection of the nonbleeding lung,[51, 54] but it has the disadvantages of permitting only one-lung ventilation and of excluding the bleeding lung from endobronchial procedures and suctioning. Bleeding must then be controlled by clot tamponade or bronchial angiography and embolization.

Intubation with a double-lumen tube has two advantages: (1) it allows isolation of the lungs as well as access and ventilation to both, and (2) it allows localization of the bleeding. Disadvantages with red rubber tubes have included (1) difficulties with insertion under adverse conditions, (2) the requirement for an experienced operator, (3) problems with suction and bronchoscopy access, and (4) high risk of tube lumen blockage with clot. Consequently, double-lumen tubes have not been recommended as an early alternative[47, 51]; however, clot occlusion of the bleeding lung is no worse than other techniques that exclude, tamponade, or obstruct the bleeding lung, and lumen-cleaning devices are available. More recently, successful use of polyvinylchloride (PVC) double-lumen tubes has been described.[50, 57]

A double-lumen tube also enables either double-lung ventilation from a single ventilator (with the ability to observe and prevent blood spreading from one circuit to the other) or ILV, which may be preferable. The latter can include administration of PEEP to the bleeding lung, which may reduce bleeding. Endobronchial therapeutic procedures can also be undertaken on the bleeding lung without compromise to the healthy lung,[50, 57] or the patient may proceed to surgery without having to risk further compromise of the nonbleeding lung during tube changes. A left-sided PVC double-lumen tube is the tube of choice.[50, 51, 57]

After isolation of the bleeding lung or segment hemostasis must be achieved. Correction of coagulopathy may be all that is required.[57] Where the bleeding lung or segment remains accessible, balloon tamponade or iced saline or epinephrine lavage may be applied via the appropriate side of the double-lumen tube. If ongoing bronchial artery hemorrhage is likely, angiographic embolization may help stanch bleeding.[58]

Surgical resection may be necessary for continued major bleeding that is not controlled by these measures. Surgical resection is associated with lower mortality rates in some series[48]; this suggests that it should not be delayed unduly when bleeding is not readily controlled. Then, ILV is almost always required during the procedure. After the bleeding lung has been resected, it is usually possible to replace the double-lumen tube with a standard endotracheal tube.

Occasionally, bleeding is so profuse that acute asphyxic arrest is imminent, a double-lumen tube is not available, and urgent endotracheal intubation is required.[47] In this circumstance, the endotracheal tube may be advanced beyond the carina (usually into the right main bronchus) and the cuff inflated so that one-lung ventilation can commence.[47] If blood does not flow out of the endotracheal tube (implying blood loss from the contralateral side), the cuff is inflated and the tube left in situ. When blood flow through the endotracheal tube continues, a Fogarty or a Foley catheter is passed to occlude the main bronchus and the tube is withdrawn as far as the trachea to ventilate the contralateral side.

Pus or Cavitating Malignancy

Markedly purulent or cavitating lung conditions (e.g., lung abscess, empyema, bronchiectasis, cavitating tuberculosis, cavitating malignant disease) are declining in frequency. When these conditions do arise, the need for thoracic surgery is also decreasing. If thoracic surgery is necessary, the patient must be positioned with the diseased lung uppermost,[1] which risks spread of infective or malignant secretions to the healthy lung. Because of this risk, double-lumen tubes have been advocated for patients who have thoracic surgery for these conditions.[1, 59] ILV may also be required during the perioperative period. Occasionally, rupture of a large abscess or cavitating lesion into an airway unrelated to thoracic surgery may threaten contralateral lung function. A double-lumen tube may confine secretions to the diseased lung and reduce unwanted effects in the contralateral one. The use of a double-lumen tube, with or without ILV, for such patients has been reported infrequently in recent years, although it clearly has a role in occasional severe cases. The limitation of a double-lumen tube in these patients is the reduced ability to drain tenacious secretions through the narrow lumen.

ASYMMETRIC LUNG DISEASE

Asymmetric lung disease can be more difficult to manage than diffuse and symmetric lung disease. When the compliance, or airway resistance, of each lung is different, normal approaches, such as changing RR, V_I, inspiratory flow rate, and PEEP, have asymmetric effects and carry the potential for adverse consequences on lung inflation, gas exchange, and hemodynamic function. Asymmetric lung disease can be categorized according to whether the primary problem is a difference in compliance or in airway resistance between the two lungs, since a different therapeutic strategy is required for each.

Asymmetric Lung Compliance

In asymmetric lung disease, when there is a major compliance difference between the two lungs, a greater proportion of V_T goes to the more compliant lung. When perfusions to each lung remain comparable, the net effect is increased shunting through the more diseased (or less compliant) lung, causing hypoxemia.

When PEEP is applied to improve oxygenation in asymmetric lung compliance, a variety of adverse effects can occur. A direct consequence of asymmetric compliance is that applied PEEP must initially expand the more compliant lung more.

PEEP at the level that would normally maximize alveolar recruitment in the less compliant lung might significantly overdistend the more compliant one and lead to increased intrathoracic pressure and mediastinal shift, and, paradoxically, cause compression of the less compliant lung. This can increase ventilation to the more normal lung and further diminish (not increase) the proportion of ventilation to the less compliant one.[60, 61]

In addition to this, PEEP-induced overdistention of the more normal lung compresses the pulmonary capillaries in that lung, diverting a greater proportion of perfusion to the collapsed, less compliant lung.[61, 62] These two effects can lead to increased dead space in the more normal lung and increased shunt in the collapsed lung and increasing arterial hypoxemia.[60]

The increased intrathoracic pressure due to hyperinflation in the more normal lung can also compress the heart and intrathoracic blood vessels, leading to reduced cardiac output and to hypotension.[63–65] The reduction in cardiac output not only leads to a further reduction in oxygen delivery but, by reducing mixed venous oxygen, also further reduces arterial oxygenation. In an animal model of asymmetric lung disease,[66] the application of PEEP to both lungs resulted in recruitment in the diseased segment, leading to improved ventilation. Concurrently, perfusion was redistributed from the "normal" lung to the diseased lung, with a net effect of no improvement in shunting or in gas exchange.

In asymmetric lung disease, all the ill effects of PEEP result from its application to the more normal lung, which compromises its potential for beneficial effects from PEEP on the more diseased lung. Application of optimal PEEP to the more diseased lung with low or no PEEP to the more normal lung has the potential to inflate and ventilate the diseased lung, thus reducing shunting without creating unwanted hyperinflation of the more normal lung and, hence, without the results of blood flow redistribution, mediastinal shift, elevation of intrathoracic pressure, and reduction in cardiac output.

Unilateral PEEP to the diseased lung in an animal model[67] (1) allows ventilation of previously nonperfused diseased lung segments while not changing blood flow distribution and (2) improves oxygenation over that afforded by bilateral PEEP.

In addition to animal model studies, numerous case reports and series now available suggest benefit from ILV for asymmetric lung compliance. The most common indication has been hypoxemia that is refractory to high oxygen concentrations and PEEP,[62] although specific PEEP-induced problems such as unilateral hyperinflation,[62, 68] barotrauma,[62, 68, 69] and deteriorating hemodynamic function[60, 62, 68] have sometimes been indications.

The causes of asymmetric compliance for which ILV has been used are pulmonary contusion,[25, 62, 68–70] aspiration,[24, 60] pneumonia,[60, 71–74] atelectasis,[23, 57, 60, 68, 74–78] asymmetric acute respiratory distress syndrome (ARDS),[79] and pulmonary embolism.[80]

Patients with pulmonary contusion have demonstrated improvements in gas exchange in response to ILV. An early study[70] reported improvement in gas exchange with spontaneous ventilation and different levels of CPAP in each limb of the circuit; however, CPAP with unassisted ventilation is now outdated because of the heavy work of breathing through the double long, narrow, tube. Others have used different levels of mechanical ventilation to each side[62, 68, 69] or unilateral high-frequency jet ventilation[25]: overall mortality was approximately 10%.

ILV has been used in patients with unilateral consolidation caused by pneumonia or aspiration injury. Although short-term oxygenation can be improved, mortality in these patients, whose disease is refractory to conventional ventilatory changes, is of the order of 70%.[24, 60, 71–74] Similarly, ILV has been reported in unilateral ARDS[79] (mortality rate of 56%) and in one patient with massive pulmonary embolism.[80]

All of the patients described above received differential PEEP, with higher levels on the affected side. The doses used were 7 to 23 cm H_2O on the affected side and 0 to 18 cm H_2O on the unaffected side.[23–25, 57, 60, 62, 68–80] In some studies V_T values in each lung were equal; in others they were smaller in the affected lung; and in only one study were greater in the affected lung.[68] In most instances the levels of PEEP were based on the clinical response of the patient. In two studies,[60, 79] the level of PEEP applied to the affected lung was determined from the compliance response of that lung to PEEP. The duration of ILV varied from 1 hour[68] to 12 days.[81]

With a slightly different approach, ILV has also been used for patients with unilateral atelectasis who failed to respond to standard mechanical ventilatory support, bronchoscopy, or both.[23, 57, 60, 68, 74–78] Often, high levels of PEEP or CPAP (up to 70 cm H_2O) have been used unilaterally for short periods. Usually, bilateral PEEP has been used,[63, 74–76] but the atelectatic lung received a larger amount, PEEP ranges being of the order of 10 to 30 cm H_2O in the affected lung and of 0 to not more than 10 cm H_2O in the less affected lung. For some patients CPAP as much as 70 cm H_2O has been applied to the atelectatic lung with spontaneous ventilation.[78] Reexpansion of the lung and improvement in oxygenation occurred without obvious lung injury. No deaths have been reported in patients with pure atelectasis, in contrast to those with other unilateral lung diseases.

Because of the infrequent use of ILV for these indications, controlled evidence is not—and is unlikely to become—available. Based on the current level of evidence, it seems appropriate to recommend the use of a double-lumen tube and ILV for asymmetric lung disease when hypoxemia is severe and refractory to, or exacerbated by, conventional mechanical ventilation maneuvers, including PEEP.

Key elements to the ILV strategy are as follows:

1. ILV can be delivered, either *synchronously* to both lungs, so that inspiration and expiration occur in each lung over the same cycle and inspiration starts simultaneously into both lungs, or *asynchronously,* so that the frequencies and timing of each breath occur in completely independent fashion in the two lungs. Asynchronous ventilation, which requires two independent ventilators, is preferred over synchronous ventilation, for which two rate-linked ventilators or a single ventilator supplying two different circuits is used, because asynchronous ventilation is simpler, more flexible, and produces no deficit in gas exchange as compared with synchronous ventilation.[24]

2. Differential PEEP with higher pressure applied to the more injured lung is the key component of this strategy. Many methods have been described for determining the PEEP required for the more injured lung, including reaching a predetermined inflection point in the lung compliance curve,[79] attaining equal lung compliance on the two sides,[60] using carbon dioxide excretion to monitor pulmonary response,[69] and simply improvement in gas exchange. Optimal PEEP based on the lower pulmonary compliance inflection point[82] may be the most appropriate objective. PEEP levels between 10 and 20 cm H_2O should be expected. Patients with refractory atelectasis may briefly require higher PEEPs to reexpand collapsed areas. Levels up to 70 cm H_2O have been reported in small numbers of patients, without adverse effects.[78] Such levels may need to be applied for only a few minutes or less and presumably carry some risk of barotrauma. Low PEEP may or may not be required for the contralateral lung, depending on its involvement in the disease process, the oxygenation

change observed after application of PEEP in the affected lung, and the effect on oxygenation and hemodynamics when PEEP is applied to this more normal lung. PEEP levels of no more than 10 cm H_2O should be used.

3. Equal VT to each lung has been the usual approach. Clinical evidence[9, 14] suggests that this is more likely to maximize gas exchange than providing either smaller or larger VT to the diseased lung; however, current ventilation strategies[82, 83] give lung injury reduction priority over optimal gas exchange. When each lung is ventilated between the optimal PEEP level and the plateau airway pressure (P_{plat}) believed to minimize overinflation (i.e., <30 to 35 cm H_2O), this may result in a lower VT in the less compliant lung.

4. Although ventilator rates to each lung need not be synchronized, similar rates are most often chosen for each lung. As with VT, lung injury reduction strategies advocate the use of lower RR[82-85] and may indicate lower RR to the more injured lung, even if the consequences of lower VT and RR in the injured lung are more hypercapnia and slightly lower arterial oxygen tension (Pa_{O_2}).

Asymmetric Lung Resistance

Airflow resistances differ principally when unilateral airway obstruction occurs. The most common causes are unilateral mechanical or chemical insult to a patient with asthma, partial occlusion of one of the major bronchi, and single-lung transplantation, all of which result in dynamic hyperinflation in the lung with airway obstruction and have the potential to raise intrathoracic pressure and compromise the nonobstructed lung, just as with asymmetric lung compliance.

Single-Lung Transplantation

Single-lung transplantation is now a popular alternative to double-lung procedures, especially for patients older than 50 years.[86-88] COPD is the most common indication for single-lung transplantation, although it is also performed for pulmonary fibrosis. Bronchiectasis, severe bilateral bullous lung disease, cystic fibrosis, and severe pulmonary vascular disease are now regarded as contraindications to single-lung transplantation.

Although lung function tests after single-lung transplantation are statistically significantly worse than those after double-lung transplantation, the difference is not large, single-lung transplantation realizes substantial improvements in quality of life,[87, 89] and there are no differences in maximum work capacity and maximum oxygen consumption.[90] Furthermore, single-lung transplantation is technically easier, has fewer complications and a better survival rate, and can benefit more recipients.[87, 89, 90]

When lung transplantation was first contemplated for COPD, single-lung transplantation was thought to be contraindicated because of the risk of dynamic hyperinflation in the native lung causing mediastinal shift[44, 87] and compromising transplant function. With or without mechanical ventilation, a nontransplant (native) lung with severe COPD undergoes dynamic hyperinflation, just as both lungs would have before transplantation,[91] but in most patients this is not a problem.

Dynamic hyperinflation in the native lung with mediastinal shift is commonly seen in the postoperative period, without lung allograft collapse, hypoxemia, or hypotension and without the need for ILV.[87, 92] This asymmetry usually decreases with time. The requirement for differential ventilation has not directly arisen in spontaneously breathing patients with a single lung transplant but can arise after reinitiation of mechanical ventilation for hypoxemia or lung transplant problems. Functional problems usually resolve when spontaneous ventilation resumes.

Problems most often arise during mechanical ventilation in the early postoperative period when there is acute injury in the allograft lung. This causes collapse and decreases compliance in the transplanted lung, which redistributes a larger portion of the ventilation to the native lung, thus hyperinflating it. As the dynamic hyperinflation increases, mediastinal shift increases, causing more collapse of the transplanted lung and more ventilation redistribution, setting up a vicious circle that can end only when the overinflation of the compliant native lung is sufficient for its alveolar pressure to match that in the injured, noncompliant allograft. Excessive hyperinflation in the native lung also increases pulmonary vascular resistance in that lung and increases intrathoracic pressure. The increased native lung pulmonary vascular resistance redistributes more cardiac output to the compromised allograft, further increasing the shunt fraction. The increased intrathoracic pressure can lead to cardiac tamponade with hypotension, tachycardia, and low cardiac output. Compromise of the lungs in this manner leads to both refractory hypoxemia and hypercapnia.

Attempts to improve the function of the transplant by increasing VT, increasing RR, reducing inspiratory flow, or adding or increasing PEEP all exacerbate dynamic hyperinflation in the native lung and thereby increase hemodynamic compromise and oxygen delivery.

Factors identified to increase the risk of dynamic hyperinflation are (1) the severity of airflow obstruction in the native lung, (2) a relatively small lung transplant for the recipient's size, and (3) perioperative injury to the donor lung. Severity of airflow obstruction directly affects the degree of hyperinflation[91]; however, in all single-lung transplantations for COPD, preoperative airway obstruction has been severe and no author has attempted to relate this fact to the requirement for ILV. When preoperative asymmetry of lung disease has been identified (e.g., by ventilation-perfusion lung scan), preferably the more severely diseased lung is replaced, although, more often such asymmetry is not obvious and the side of transplant is determined by technical preference or the side of the available donor lung.

The size of the donor lung has been identified by several authors[86, 87, 93] to be an important factor. Recipients of lungs from donors with a predicted vital capacity (VC) approximating[86] or smaller than[93] the recipient's predicted VC have needed ILV, whereas a predicted donor-recipient VC ratio of 1.4[86] or a donor lung predicted VC exceeding the recipient lung predicted VC by 2 L[87] have both been associated with no mediastinal shift after single-lung transplantation. Although most authors attribute pulmonary infiltrate in the transplanted lung to collapse secondary to contralateral dynamic hyperinflation, primary dysfunction of the allograft,[88] severe postimplantation syndrome,[93] and ARDS have been identified as major contributors to the necessity for ILV.

Early experience with single-lung transplantation confirmed these concerns.[94-97] In 20 papers reporting 118 single-lung transplantations for COPD, ILV was required by 11 (9%).[86-89, 92-107] At our hospital, a total of 73 patients have now received a single-lung transplant for COPD and 11 of them (15%) have required ILV. Need for differential ventilation after single-lung transplantation for "non-COPD" patients is rare but has been described for lymphangioleiomyomatosis[108] and for primary pulmonary hypertension, when it was used in conjunction with ECMO.[109] There are no reports, however, of patients' requiring ILV after double-lung transplantation for COPD.

In most instances when ILV has been used for single-lung transplantation, dynamic hyperinflation of the native lung and mediastinal shift have been the rule.[86, 88, 93, 99, 101, 108] The result was hypotension or collapse of the transplanted lung with

TABLE 117–1. Respiratory and Hemodynamic Variables After Single-Lung Transplantation for Chronic Obstructive Pulmonary Disease

Parameter	Initial Postoperative Values	8 hr Postoperatively	After Independent Lung Ventilation
Heart rate (beats/min)	90	120	100
Central venous pressure (mm Hg)	10	18	10
Systolic blood pressure (mm Hg)	105	85	120
Cardiac index (L/min/m^2)	2.2	1.7	3.2
FIO_2 (fraction)	0.7	1.0	0.4
PaO_2 (mm Hg)	77	55	128
PaO_2/FIO_2 ratio	110	55	320

hypoxemia, or both. One patient required ILV for a large, refractory bronchopleural fistula that arose in the native lung after single-lung transplantation and that eventually necessitated pneumonectomy in the native lung.[100] All such problems have occurred only during mechanical ventilation in the immediate or early postoperative period and have necessitated prompt, sometimes life-saving instigation of ILV. Ventilation reported under these circumstances has always involved conventional mechanical ventilation to the transplanted lung with (1) asynchronous ventilation,[86, 88, 93, 99] (2) synchronous ventilation,[101] or (3) bronchial blockade,[86] (4) PAP,[100] or (5) spontaneous ventilation[93] to the native lung. ILV has been required, sometimes for only a day,[86] but in many instances it has been used longer than a month,[88, 93, 100] with eventual resolution of the problem and a good functional result.

The typical problems can be illustrated by the case of a 57-year-old man who underwent left-sided single-lung transplantation for end-stage COPD[110] and who encountered increasing allograft compromise (due to postimplantation syndrome) during the early postoperative period while receiving mechanical ventilation with a RR of 10 breaths/min, a VT of 700 mL (8 mL/kg), 5 cm H_2O PEEP, and FIO_2 0.7. The patient experienced severe hypoxemia and cardiac tamponade (Table 117–1). Chest radiographs (Figs. 117–1 and 117–2) showed marked native lung hyperinflation, mediastinal shift, and allograft compromise. Transient addition of PEEP produced profound hypotension. Transient reduction in RR and VT improved blood pressure but produced marked arterial desaturation.

A right-sided double-lumen tube was placed to avoid the left-sided bronchial anastomosis. Independent lung ventilation was instituted. The native lung was markedly hypoventilated, with low RR and VT and no PEEP (see Fig. 117–2) to minimize dynamic hyperinflation. The transplanted lung received a higher RR, optimal PEEP, and slightly larger VT. Both physiologic parameters (see Table 117–1) and chest radiographs (see Figs. 117–1 and 117–2) improved dramatically.

The ILV strategy for dynamic hyperinflation after single-lung transplantation for severe COPD should include the following procedure:

1. *Select asynchronous ventilation as the method of choice,* principally because of the different RR and PEEP requirements of the two lungs. Introduction of these quite different ventilatory strategies to each lung and physiologic stabilization generally necessitates sedation and paralysis during the early stages. Because all single-lung transplant recipients take large doses of steroids, neuromuscular blockade must be minimized because of the risk of necrotizing myopathy.[111]

2. *Reduce dynamic hyperinflation in the native lung with preexisting severe airflow obstruction.* This is best achieved by hypoventilation. This requires low VT (<4 mL/kg), high inspiratory flow rate (e.g., 70 to 100 L/min), and a low RR (e.g., 2 to 6 breaths/min) in the native lung.[91] The degree of dynamic hyperinflation associated with this ventilatory pattern should be assessed and ventilation adjusted accordingly. This may be assessed by measuring P_{plat} during a single breath, the end-expiratory alveolar pressure (intrinsic or auto-PEEP), the

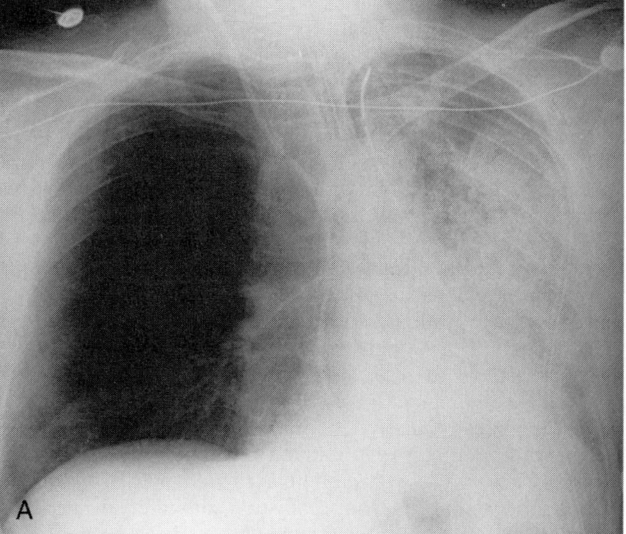

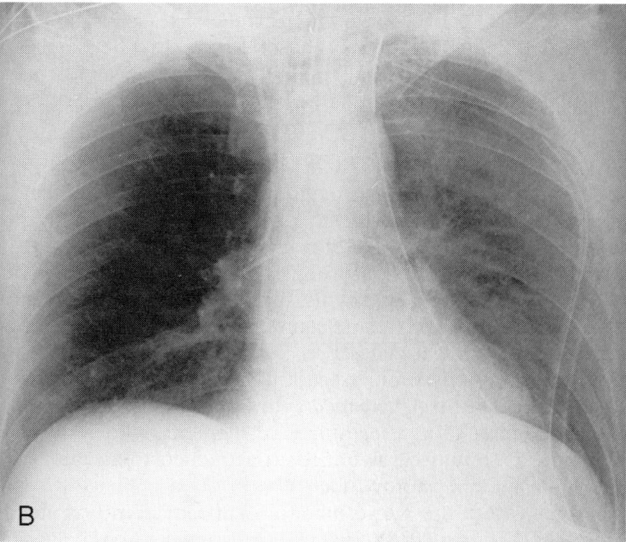

Figure 117–1. Chest x-ray study before *(A)* and after *(B)* independent lung ventilation after single lung transplantation for chronic obstructive pulmonary disease.

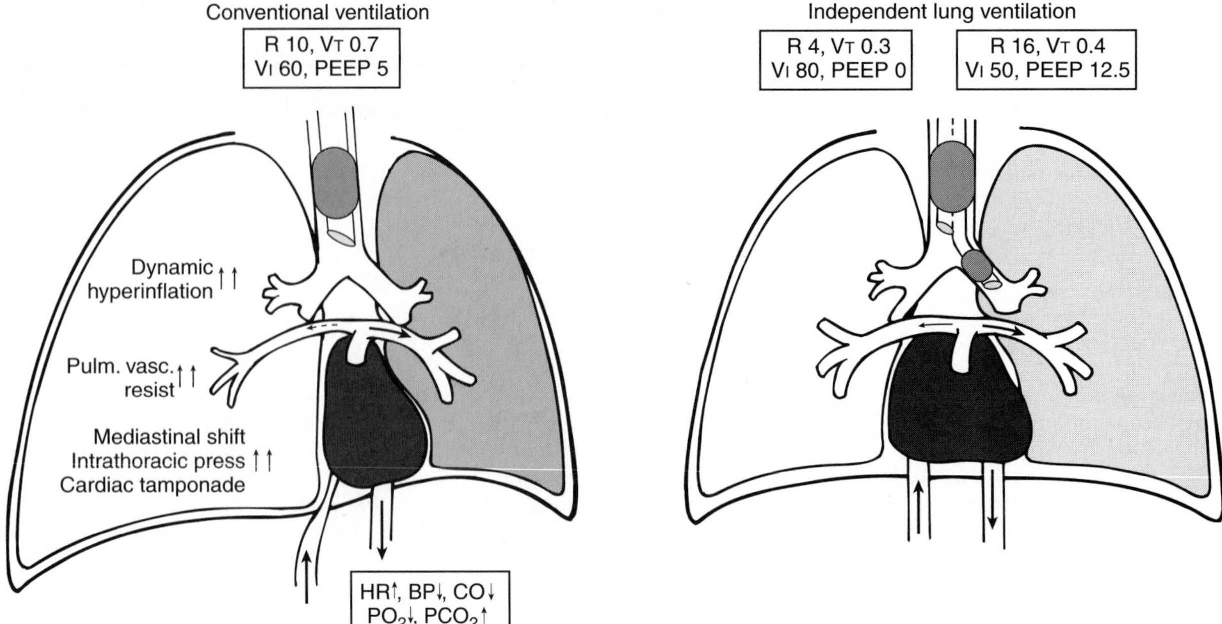

Figure 117–2. Schematic representation of major respiratory and hemodynamic effects of conventional ventilation and independent lung ventilation in the problematic patient after single lung transplantation for chronic obstructive pulmonary disease. HR = heart rate; BP = blood pressure; PEEP = positive end-expiratory pressure; CO = cardiac output.

total exhaled volume from the native lung during 30- to 60-second apnea,[91] or by observing the effects of apnea on blood pressure, central venous pressure, and heart rate. Repeating the chest film after instituting ILV also demonstrates the presence or absence of significant hyperinflation. If excessive dynamic hyperinflation is identified by any of these methods, RR should be reduced to a safe level.

3. *Expand the transplanted lung and achieve gas exchange.* This is best achieved with optimal PEEP,[82] higher RR and VT, and lower inspiratory flows, and is similar to the ventilatory approach to symmetric acute lung injury or ARDS. This requires PEEP sufficient to expand collapsed lobes and improve oxygenation, VT low enough to avoid pressure injury to the lung, and RR high enough for adequate elimination of carbon dioxide without causing flow limitation in the donor lung.

4. In contrast to other asymmetric lung diseases, when a left-sided double-lumen tube is chosen routinely, choose the tube size to cannulate the native lung in order to protect the bronchial anastomosis of the transplanted lung from injury or ischemia from the endobronchial cuff.

ILV can be withdrawn when function in the allograft lung improves and its ventilatory requirements subside. This can be assessed with a double-lumen tube in situ by ventilating both lungs with a single ventilator and a bifurcated ventilator circuit. Because spontaneous ventilation is difficult through the long narrow lumens of this tube, some patients may require reintubation with a single-lumen endotracheal tube for weaning of mechanical ventilation before extubation. Others exhibit increasing dynamic hyperinflation with double-lung ventilation and must be weaned with pressure support via the double-lumen tube already in situ. Patients who require prolonged ILV should be switched to a tracheostomy with a double-lumen tracheostomy tube.[93, 101, 112]

When data from the world literature and our own hospital are combined, they reflect a total of 214 patients who received a single-lung transplant for COPD. The mortality rate was 31%. This includes an early series[95] whose mortality rate was 100%. If this series is excluded, the mortality rate is 26%. Among patients receiving ILV, there are four known deaths (mortality rate 22%). Mortality for those patients who did not receive ILV was 34%, which suggests that such differential ventilation is not associated with worse outcomes. Thus, dynamic hyperinflation with mediastinal shift sufficient to compromise gas exchange or circulation occurs in approximately 10% of recipients of a single lung allograft for COPD. This frequency warrants routine assessment before removal of the double-lumen tube. Whenever this complication is identified, it should be treated promptly with ILV.

BRONCHOPLEURAL FISTULA

Bronchopleural fistulas are a significant complication in patients who have lung disease or need mechanical ventilation. The incidence is generally low (~2% of mechanically ventilated patients).[113] The associated mortality, however, varies from 18% to 67%,[113, 114] depending on the severity of underlying illness and the inclusion criteria for reports on this entity. There are many causes, including trauma, necrotizing pneumonia, lung abscess, tuberculosis, ARDS, COPD, thoracic surgery, mechanical ventilation, and central venous catheterization. When massive, air leakage from a bronchopleural fistula during mechanical ventilation can be a significant portion of the VT, leading to respiratory insufficiency from hypoxemia and hypercapnia. This may occur despite FIO_2 values of 1.0 and attempts to optimize ventilation. Tension pneumothorax and cardiorespiratory compromise can also result from inadequate drainage.

If the leak is small, intercostal catheterization alone is usually adequate treatment. Before ventilatory strategies are pursued, the adequacy of drainage must be carefully assessed. With larger intercostal catheters the chance of gas outflow exceeding gas inflow from the fistula, allowing successful lung inflation is much greater. In general, at least two wide-bore intercostal catheters should be in situ, both fully functioning and not compromising air drainage because of luminal clot or suboptimal placement. Wall suction should be checked to ensure it is maximizing (not retarding) gas outflow. Conventional mechanical ventilation is often manipulated to reduce mean airway pressure and thus decrease the air leakage through the fistula.[115] Measures to reduce mean airway pressure include decreasing PEEP and VT to reduce peak inspiratory pressures to below 30 cm H_2O.[116] Other management options include (1) pleurodesis, (2) thoracic surgical stapling of lung tissue, (3) positive-pleural pressure during inspiration,[117] and (4) bronchoscopic placement of occlusion catheters.[118]

High-frequency jet ventilation has reportedly been successful in a number of case reports.[114, 119] It appears to be of particular benefit for patients with a proximal fistula or normal underlying lung parenchyma,[114] although when established ARDS is present, deterioration appears more likely.[120]

ILV has been used for severe bronchopleural fistula when, despite other measures, respiratory insufficiency occurs.[26, 60, 71, 118, 121–125] Such ventilation stops VT loss from the unaffected lung, allowing it to expand and improving gas exchange. A variety of strategies can then be applied independently to the affected lung. With a double-lumen tube in position, the lung with the fistula can be ventilated with unilateral high-frequency jet ventilation[26, 114, 115] or by reducing RR, VT, or PEEP when standard ventilation is used.[24]

Because bronchopleural fistulas large enough to require ILV are rare, controlled evidence supporting such ventilation will continue to be difficult to generate. Consequently, ILV, with or without high-frequency jet ventilation, should be considered when more conservative measures have been tried.

SYMMETRIC LUNG DISEASE

It is now well recognized that apparently diffuse lung injury such as ARDS exhibits significant heterogeneity when studied by computed tomography (CT), in contrast to its apparently uniform and symmetric appearance on chest radiography.[126, 127] Collapse under its own weight of the heavy, edematous lung leads to consolidation in dependent areas and differential PEEP requirements in dependent and nondependent zones. Providing different PEEPs to dependent and nondependent zones is impossible in supine patients, but placing the patient in the lateral position creates a differential in collapse and PEEP requirements between the two lungs that can be addressed by ILV. This strategy has been used in a small number of patients placed in this position.[9, 16]

Application of greater PEEPs to the dependent lung improves perfusion matching, shunt fraction, and oxygenation without decreasing cardiac output as compared with uniform PEEP for patients positioned likewise.[9, 16] ILV has not gained any place in the treatment of symmetric lung disease, because the best physiologic results require the patient to be in the lateral decubitus position[14] and this has many practical problems with both use of two ventilators and nursing patients in the lateral decubitus position. The problem of differential collapse of dependent and nondependent lung zones in the setting of symmetric lung disease is being addressed by other measures, including optimal PEEP and an "open-lung approach,"[82] prone positioning,[128] and partial liquid ventilation.[129]

TECHNIQUE OF LUNG SEPARATION

Double-Lumen Tubes

To achieve separation of the individual lungs, it is necessary to place a double-lumen tube. In current practice, tubes are made of either red rubber or polyvinylchloride (PVC). Red rubber tubes are irritating and inflexible, require high cuff pressures to seal the airways,[130, 131] and are suitable only for short-term use. For intensive care PVC tubes are in order, which are more flexible, less irritating to the respiratory mucosa, quicker to position,[132] and seal the airway with lower cuff pressures.[131] Such tubes have better internal-external diameter ratios, a feature that enables better gas flow and easier access for suction catheters and bronchoscopy.[50]

Tubes are designed specially to be placed on either the right or the left side. The left-sided tube is appropriate for most indications, as it is easier to place properly. Because of the proximal opening of the right upper lobe bronchus, risk of occlusion of this bronchus is great.[133] When left bronchial surgery or left single-lung transplantation is performed, a right-sided tube is required.

Unlike thoracic surgical recommendations, large tube size is critical to the adequacy of long-term care, and the largest tube possible should be placed to allow adequate ventilation, bronchoscopy, and suctioning (Table 117–2). A No. 41 French tube should be the first choice for any adult.

Placement

Accurate placement of the double-lumen tube is often difficult, and some degree of expertise is required. Placement can be done blind or with a flexible bronchoscope. It is recommended that the tube be introduced with the endobronchial curvature directed anteriorly and with a rigid stylet in situ. After the tube has passed through the vocal cords, the stylet should be removed and the endobronchial curvature rotated to the appropriate side. The tube should be inserted until resistance is felt. A bronchoscope should then be passed through the tracheal lumen. Inspection then confirms that the endobronchial tube is—or is not—in the correct side and has passed for enough into the bronchus, and that the tracheal port is above the carina.[134] Correct placement can also be inferred from auscultation; however, high failure rates have been demonstrated after blind intubation.[135] Also, appropriate radiographic appearance does not ensure lung isolation.

Leak testing should be performed routinely, because correct anatomic placement does not necessarily result in lung isolation. Leaking can be tested by ventilating one lung and check-

TABLE 117–2. Choice of Size for Double-Lumen Polyvinyl Chloride Tubes

Tube Size (French)	Circumference (mm)	Lumen Diameter (mm)	Use in Thoracic Surgery	Use for Intensive Care
28	—	—	Children <40 kg	
35	38	50	Children >40 kg	
37	40	55	Small adults	
39	44	60	Medium adults (usual female size)	Small adults
41	45	65	Large adults (usual male size)	Tube of choice

Adapted from Burton NA, Watson DC, Brodsky JB, et al: Advantages of a new polyvinylchloride double-lumen tube in thoracic surgery. Ann Thorac Surg 1983; 36:78–84.

ing for gas bubbles when the other port is passed through water[136] or by checking balloon inflation when the other port has a balloon fitted to it.[137]

Complications

Most difficulties of double-lumen tubes relate to accurate positioning of the tube and failure to isolate the lung completely. Trauma to the larynx and upper airways is less common with PVC tubes than with red rubber tubes[132]; however, it occasionally occurs.[3] The fact that it is time-consuming makes placement of a double-lumen tube less useful when it is urgently needed, as with massive hemoptysis.[51] It is critical to place the right-sided tube properly. Occlusion of the right upper lobe as great as 89% has been demonstrated bronchoscopically with one type of right-sided PVC tube, and this compared with only 10% with red rubber tubes, perhaps because of the smaller right upper lobe orifice of PVC tubes.[133] This problem can be rectified by routinely using bronchoscopy for placement of right-sided tubes. Left-sided PVC tubes have also caused occasional left upper lobe occlusion.[138, 139] Extreme neck movements can alter positioning of the double-lumen tube tip as far as 7 cm, which is enough either to occlude a bronchus opening or to lose lung isolation.[140] Tracheal laceration has been reported after red rubber[34] and PVC tube[141] insertion.

High cuff pressures can be a significant problem with double-lumen tubes, as they have a low-volume, high-pressure bronchial cuff, which means that sealing the bronchial airway can lead to high pressures in the low-compliance cuff.[13] Bronchial rupture has been reported, although it appears to be more common with red rubber tubes.[142, 143] Diameters of a double-lumen tube are smaller than those of standard endotracheal tubes, so narrow-lumen suction catheters (with reduced suction efficiency) must be used. Furthermore, the length of external connections prevent the suction catheter from protruding far enough from the tip of the double-lumen tube. These problems can lead to retained secretions and lumen blockage.[72] The suction catheter should be checked against a similar-sized tube with the same external connections, to determine the extent of the suction catheter's protrusion. If this protrusion distance is inadequate, the external tubing should be shortened. Frequent bronchoscopy may be required to assist not only with sputum clearance[144] but also in determining whether if neck movements have altered the tube positioning.[140] Using two ventilators can create problems of space, gas outlet requirements, charting, and patient access. Other issues relate to increases in nursing workload.[121] Some patients also feel less comfortable with a double-lumen tube and, so, need larger doses of analgesics and sedatives. Regular patient turning for pressure care becomes more difficult and may cause loss of lung isolation.

SUMMARY

ILV now has a limited but clearly established place in the mechanical ventilation of critically ill patients, and it can be undertaken with standard mechanical ventilators. Intensivists need to be familiar with the indications and methods, so that, when the infrequent need arises, instigation of this technique, which can avoid morbidity (and sometimes mortality) is not unduly delayed.

References

1. Björk VO, Carlens E: The prevention of spread during pulmonary resection by the use of a double-lumen catheter. J Thorac Surg 1950; 20:151–157.
2. Trew F, Warren BR, Potter WA: Differential ventilation of the lungs in man. Crit Care Med 1976; 4:112.
3. Strange C: Double-lumen endotracheal tubes. Clin Chest Med 1991; 12:497–506.
4. Wilson R: Endobronchial Intubation. *In:* Thoracic Anesthesia. Caplan J (Ed). New York, Churchill Livingstone, 1983, pp 371–388.
5. Inoue H, Shohtsu A, Ogawa J, et al: New device for one-lung anesthesia: Endotracheal tube with movable blocker. J Thorac Cardiovasc Surg 1982; 83:940–941.
6. Scheller MS, Kriett JM, Smith CM, et al: Airway management during anesthesia for double-lung transplantation using a single-lumen endotracheal tube with an enclosed bronchial blocker. J Cardiothorac Vasc Anesth 1992; 6:204–207.
7. Benumof JL: Physiology of the lateral decubitus position, the open chest, and one lung ventilation. *In:* Thoracic Anesthesia. Caplan J (Ed). New York, Churchill Livingstone, 1983, pp 193–221.
8. Benumof JL: One lung ventilation: Which lung should be PEEPed? Anesthesiology 1982; 56:161–163.
9. Hedenstierna G, Baehrendtz S, Klingstedt C, et al: Ventilation and perfusion of each lung during differential ventilation with selective PEEP. Anesthesiology 1984; 61:369–376.
10. Rehder K, Wenthe FM, Sessler AD: Function of each lung during mechanical ventilation with ZEEP and with PEEP in man anesthetized with thiopental-meperidine. Anesthesiology 1973; 39:597–606.
11. Wulff KE, Aulin I: The regional lung function in the lateral decubitus position during anesthesia and operation. Acta Anaesthesiol Scand 1972; 16:195–205.
12. Nunn JF: The distribution of inspired gas during thoracic surgery. Ann R Coll Surg Engl 1961; 28:223–237.
13. Slinger P, Suissa S, Adam J, et al: Predicting arterial oxygenation during one-lung ventilation with continuous positive airway pressure to the nonventilated lung. J Cardiothorac Anesth 1990; 4:436–440.
14. Baehrendtz S, Santesson J, Bindslev L, et al: Differential ventilation in acute bilateral lung disease: Influence on gas exchange and central haemodynamics. Acta Anaesthesiol Scand 1983; 27:270–277.
15. Cohen E, Eisenkraft J, Thys DM, et al: Oxygenation and hemodynamic changes during one-lung ventilation: Effects of $CPAP_{10}$, $PEEP_{10}$, and $CPAP_{10}/PEEP_{10}$. J Cardiothorac Anesth 1988; 2:34–40.
16. Baehrendtz S, Hedenstierna G: Differential ventilation and selective positive end-expiratory pressure: Effects on patients with acute bilateral lung disease. Anesthesiology 1984; 61:511–517.
17. Baehrendtz S, Klingstedt C: Differential ventilation and selective PEEP during anaesthesia in the lateral decubital posture. Acta Anaesthesiol Scand 1984; 28:252–259.
18. Brown DR, Kafer ER, Roberson VO, et al: Improved oxygenation during thoracotomy with selective PEEP to the dependent lung. Anesth Analg 1977; 56:26–31.
19. Katz JA, Laverne RG, Fairley HB, et al: Pulmonary oxygen exchange during endobronchial anesthesia: Effect of tidal volume and PEEP. Anesthesiology 1982; 56:164–171.
20. Aalto-Setala M, Heinonen J, Salorinne Y: Cardiorespiratory function during thoracic anaesthesia: A comparison of two-lung ventilation and one-lung ventilation with and without $PEEP_5$. Acta Anaesthesiol Scand 1975; 19:287–295.
21. Capan LM, Turndorf H, Patel C, et al: Optimization of arterial oxygenation during one-lung anesthesia. Anesth Analg 1980; 59:847–851.
22. Khanam T, Branthwaite MA: Arterial oxygenation during one-lung anaesthesia. Anaesthesia 1973; 28:280–290.
23. Glass DD, Tonnesen AS, Gabel JC, et al: Therapy of unilateral pulmonary insufficiency with a double lumen endotracheal tube. Crit Care Med 1976; 4:323–326.
24. Hillman KM, Barber JD: Asynchronous independent lung ventilation (AILV). Crit Care Med 1980; 8:390–395.
25. Crimi G, Candiani A, Conti G, et al: Clinical applications of independent lung ventilation with unilateral high-frequency jet ventilation (ILV-UHFJV). Intensive Care Med 1986; 12:90–94.
26. Feeley TW, Keating D, Nishimura T: Independent lung ventilation using high-frequency ventilation in the management of a bronchopleural fistula. Anesthesiology 1988; 69:420–422.

27. Neidhardt A, Douge R, Kunegel JM, et al: Prevention of early respiratory complications in esophageal surgery by ventilation of the independent lungs. Cah Anesthesiol 1984; 32:613-616.
28. Rosen SH, Castleman B, Liebow AA: Pulmonary alveolar proteinosis. N Engl J Med 1958; 258:1123-1142.
29. Ramirez J, Kieffer RF Jr, Ball WC Jr: Bronchopulmonary lavage in man. Ann Intern Med 1965; 63:819-828.
30. Ramirez J: Pulmonary alveolar proteinosis: Treatment by massive bronchopulmonary lavage. Arch Intern Med 1967; 119:147-156.
31. Smith LJ, Katzenstein AL, Ankin MG, et al: Management of pulmonary alveolar proteinosis. Chest 1980; 78:765-770.
32. Nariman S, Bell HE: Bronchopulmonary lavage in the treatment of chronic asthma. Br J Hosp Med 1975; 14:170-172.
33. Williams NE: Bronchial lavage in asthma. Postgrad Med J 1971; 47:188-189.
34. Thompson HT, Pryor WJ, Hill J: Bronchial lavage in the treatment of obstructive lung disease. Thorax 1966; 21:557-559.
35. Rausch DC, Spick A, Kylstra JA: Lung lavage in cystic fibrosis. Am Rev Respir Dis 1970; 101:1006.
36. McClellan RO, Boyd HA, Benjamin RG, et al: Recovery of ^{239}Pu following bronchopulmonary lavage and DTPA treatment after an accidental inhalation exposure case. Health Phys 1976; 31:315-321.
37. Alfery D, Benumof J, Spragg R: Anesthesia for bronchopulmonary lavage. *In:* Thoracic Anesthesia. Caplan J (Ed). New York, Churchill Livingstone, 1983, pp 193-221.
38. Rogers RM, Szidon JP, Shelburne J, et al: Hemodynamic response of the pulmonary circulation to bronchopulmonary lavage in man. N Engl J Med 1972; 286:1230-1233.
39. Smith JD, Miller JE, Safar P, et al: Intrathoracic pressure, pulmonary vascular pressures and gas exchange during pulmonary lavage. Anesthesiology 1970; 33:401-405.
40. Alfery DD, Zamost BG, Benumof JL: Unilateral lung lavage: Blood flow manipulation by ipsilateral pulmonary artery balloon inflation in dogs. Anesthesiology 1981; 55:376-380.
41. Seidman JM, Sasahara AA: Bronchopulmonary lavage. N Engl J Med 1972; 286:1262-1263.
42. Claypool WD, Rogers RM, Matuschak GM: Update on the clinical diagnosis, management, and pathogenesis of pulmonary alveolar proteinosis (phospholipidosis). Chest 1984; 85:550-558.
43. Altose MD, Hicks RE, Edwards MW Jr: Extracorporeal membrane oxygenation during bronchopulmonary lavage. Arch Surg 1976; 111:1149-1153.
44. Cooper JD, Duffin J, Glynn MF, et al: Combination of membrane oxygenator support and pulmonary lavage for acute respiratory failure. J Thorac Cardiovasc Surg 1976; 71:304-308.
45. Brach BB, Harrell JH, Moser KM: Alveolar proteinosis: Lobar lavage by fiberoptic bronchoscopic technique. Chest 1976; 69:224-227.
46. Vast C, Demonet B, Mouveroux J: Value of selective pulmonary lavage under fibroscopic control in alveolar proteinosis. Poumon Coeur 1978; 34:305-307.
47. Strollo PJ: Hemoptysis. *In:* Critical Care. Civetta JM, Taylor RW, Kirby RR, (Ed). Philadelphia, JB Lippincott, 1988, pp 1127-1132.
48. Crocco JA, Rooney JJ, Fankushen DS, et al: Massive hemoptysis. Arch Intern Med 1968; 121:495-498.
49. Hannan AT, Brown M, Bigman O: Pulmonary artery catheter-induced hemorrhage. Chest 1984; 85:128-131.
50. Shivaram U, Finch P, Nowak P: Plastic endobronchial tubes in the management of life-threatening hemoptysis. Chest 1987; 92:1108-1110.
51. Conlan AA: Massive hemoptysis: Diagnosis and therapeutic implications. Surg Annu 1985; 17:337-354.
52. Bobrowitz ID, Ramakrishna S, Shim YS, et al: Comparison of medical v surgical treatment of major hemoptysis. Arch Intern Med 1983; 143:1343-1346.
53. Imgrund SP, Goldberg SK, Walkenstein MD, et al: Clinical diagnosis of massive hemoptysis using the fiberoptic bronchoscope. Crit Care Med 1985; 13:438-443.
54. Garzon AA, Cerruti MM, Golding ME: Exsanguinating hemoptysis. J Thorac Cardiovasc Surg 1982; 84:829-833.
55. Conlan AA, Hurwitz SS, Krige L, et al: Massive hemoptysis: Review of 123 cases. J Thorac Cardiovasc Surg 1983; 85:120-124.
56. Conlan AA, Hurwitz SS: Management of massive haemoptysis with the rigid bronchoscope and cold saline lavage. Thorax 1980; 35:901-904.
57. Miller RS, Nelson LD, Rutherford EJ, et al: Synchronised independent lung ventilation in the management of a unilateral pulmonary contusion with massive hemoptysis. J Tenn Med Assoc 1992; 85:374-375.
58. Uflacker R, Kaemmerer A, Picon PD, et al: Bronchial artery embolization in the management of hemoptysis: Technical aspects and long-term results. Radiology 1985; 157:637-644.
59. Moody JD: A method of bronchial occlusion for the prevention of transbronchial spread during lobectomy and pneumonectomy: Clinical application. J Thorac Surg 1948; 17:681-689.
60. Carlon GC, Ray C Jr, Klein R, et al: Criteria for selecting positive end-expiratory pressure and independent synchronized ventilation of each lung. Chest 1978; 74:501-507.
61. Kanarek DJ, Shannon DC: Adverse effect of positive end-expiratory pressure on pulmonary perfusion and arterial oxygenation. Am Rev Respir Dis 1975; 112:457-459.
62. Frame SB, Marshall WJ, Clifford TG: Synchronized independent lung ventilation in the management of pediatric unilateral pulmonary contusion: case report. J Trauma 1989; 29:395-397.
63. Carlon GC, Kahn R, Howland WS, et al: Acute life-threatening ventilation-perfusion inequality: An indication for independent lung ventilation. Crit Care Med 1978; 6:380-383.
64. Venus B, Pratap KS, Op'Tholt T: Treatment of unilateral pulmonary insufficiency by selective administration of continuous positive airway pressure through a double-lumen tube. Anesthesiology 1980; 53:74-77.
65. Powers SR, Mannal R, Neclerio M, et al: Physiologic consequences of positive end-expiratory pressure (PEEP) ventilation. Ann Surg 1973; 178:265-272.
66. Mink SN, Light RB, Cooligan T, et al: Effect of PEEP on gas exchange and pulmonary perfusion in canine lobar pneumonia. J Appl Physiol 1981; 50:517-523.
67. Light RB, Mink SN, Wood LDH: The effect of unilateral PEEP on gas exchange and pulmonary perfusion in canine lobar pneumonia. Anesthesiology 1981; 55:251-255.
68. Branson RD, Hurst JM, DeHaven CB: Synchronous independent lung ventilation in the treatment of unilateral pulmonary contusion: A report of two cases. Respir Care 1984; 29:361-367.
69. Zandstra DF, Stoutenbeek CP: Reflection of differential pulmonary perfusion in polytrauma patients on differential lung ventilation (DLV): A comparison of two CO_2-derived methods. Intensive Care Med 1989; 15:151-154.
70. Crimi G, Conti G, Candiani A, et al: Clinical use of differential continuous positive airway pressure in the treatment of unilateral acute lung injury. Intensive Care Med 1987; 13:416-418.
71. Parish JM, Gracey DR, Southorn PA, et al: Differential mechanical ventilation in respiratory failure due to severe unilateral lung disease. Mayo Clin Proc 1984; 59:822-828.
72. Nielsen M, Acklin L, Kelly PS: Synchronized independent lung ventilation (SILV). Progr Notes 1992; 4:6-8.
73. Powner D, Eross B, Grenvik A: Differential lung ventilation with PEEP in the treatment of unilateral pneumonia. Crit Care Med 1977; 4:170-172.
74. Lev A, Barzilay E, Geber D, et al: Differential lung ventilation: A review and 2 case reports. Resuscitation 1987; 15:77-86.
75. Bochenek KJ, Brown M, Skupin A: Use of a double-lumen endotracheal tube with independent lung ventilation for treatment of refractory atelectasis. Anesth Analg 1987; 66:1014-1017.
76. Gallagher TJ, Banner MJ, Smith RA: A simplified method of independent lung ventilation. Crit Care Med 1980; 8:396-399.
77. Miranda DR, Stoutenbeek C, Kingma L: Differential lung ventilation with HFPPV. Intensive Care Med 1981; 7:139-141.
78. Millen JE, Vandree J, Glauser FL: Fiberoptic bronchoscopic balloon occlusion and reexpansion of refractory unilateral atelectasis. Crit Care Med 1978; 6:50-55.
79. Siegel JH, Stoklosa JC, Borg U, et al: Quantification of asymmetric lung pathophysiology as a guide to the use of simultaneous independent lung ventilation in posttraumatic and septic adult respiratory distress syndrome. Ann Surg 1985; 202:425-439.
80. Zandstra DF, Stoutenbeek CP: Treatment of massive unilateral pulmonary embolism by differential lung ventilation. Intensive Care Med 1987; 13:422-424.
81. Zandstra DF, Stoutenbeek CP, van Saene HK, et al: Selective

decontamination of the digestive tract improves survival in patients receiving differential lung ventilation. Intensive Care Med 1988; 15:15–18.
82. Amato MB, Barbas CS, Medeiros DM, et al: Beneficial effects of the "open lung approach" with low distending pressures in acute respiratory distress syndrome: A prospective, randomized study on mechanical ventilation. Am J Respir Crit Care Med 1995; 152:1835–1846.
83. Tuxen DV: Permissive hypercapnic ventilation. Am J Respir Crit Care Med 1994; 150:870–874.
84. Hickling KG, Walsh J, Henderson S, et al: Low mortality rate in adult respiratory distress syndrome using low-volume, pressure-limited ventilation with permissive hypercapnia: a prospective study. Crit Care Med 1994; 22:1568–1578.
85. Bshouty Z, Younes M: Effect of breathing pattern and level of ventilation on pulmonary fluid filtration in dog lung. Am Rev Respir Dis 1992; 145:372–376.
86. Kaiser LR, Cooper JD, Trulock EP, et al: The evolution of single lung transplantation for emphysema: The Washington University Lung Transplant Group. J Thorac Cardiovasc Surg 1991; 102:333–339.
87. Patterson GA, Maurer JR, Williams TJ, et al: Comparison of outcomes of double and single lung transplantation for obstructive lung disease: The Toronto Lung Transplant Group. J Thorac Cardiovasc Surg 1991; 101:623–631.
88. Zannini P, Baisi A, Melloni G, et al: Single lung transplantation for emphysema: lessons learned on the field: The Lung Transplant Group of the Ospedale Maggiore of Milan. Int Surg 1992; 77:28–36.
89. Low DE, Trulock EP, Kaiser LR, et al: Morbidity, mortality, and early results of single versus bilateral lung transplantation for emphysema. J Thorac Cardiovasc Surg 1992; 103:1119–1126.
90. Williams TJ, Patterson GA, McClean PA, et al: Maximal exercise testing in single and double lung transplant recipients. Am Rev Respir Dis 1992; 145:101–105.
91. Tuxen DV, Lane S: The effects of ventilatory pattern on hyperinflation, airway pressures, and circulation in mechanical ventilation of patients with severe airflow obstruction. Am Rev Respir Dis 1987; 136:872–879.
92. Trulock EP, Egan TM, Kouchoukos NT, et al: Single lung transplantation for severe chronic obstructive pulmonary disease: Washington University Lung Transplant Group. Chest 1989; 96:738–742.
93. Gavazzeni V, Iapichino G, Mascheroni D, et al: Prolonged independent lung respiratory treatment after single lung transplantation in pulmonary emphysema. Chest 1993; 103:96–100.
94. Stevens PM, Johnson PC, Bell RL, et al: Regional ventilation and perfusion after lung transplantation in patients with emphysema. N Engl J Med 1970; 282:245–249.
95. Wildevuur CR, Benfield JR: A review of 23 human lung transplantations by 20 surgeons. Ann Thorac Surg 1970; 9:489–515.
96. Vanderhoeft PJ, Rocmans P, Nemry C, et al: Left lung transplantation in a patient with emphysema. Arch Surg 1971; 103:505–509.
97. Veith FJ, Koerner SK, Siegelman SS, et al: Single lung transplantation in experimental and human emphysema. Ann Surg 1973; 178:463–476.
98. Smiley RM, Navedo AT, Kirby T, et al: Postoperative independent lung ventilation in a single-lung transplant recipient. Anesthesiology 1991; 74:1144–1148.
99. Egan TM, Westerman JH, Lambert CJ, et al: Isolated lung transplantation for end-stage lung disease: A viable therapy. Ann Thorac Surg 1992; 53:590–596.
100. Novick RJ, Menkis AH, Sandler D, et al: Contralateral pneumonectomy after single-lung transplantation for emphysema. Ann Thorac Surg 1991; 52:1317–1319.
101. Harwood RJ, Graham TR, Kendall SW, et al: Use of a double-lumen tracheostomy tube after single lung transplantation. J Thorac Cardiovasc Surg 1992; 103:1224–1226.
102. Mal H, Andreassian B, Pamela F, et al: Unilateral lung transplantation in end-stage pulmonary emphysema. Am Rev Respir Dis 1989; 140:797–802.
103. Egan TM, Cooper JD: Surgical aspects of single lung transplantation. Clin Chest Med 1990; 11:195–205.
104. Thomas BJ, Siegel LC: Anesthetic and postoperative management of single-lung transplantation. J Cardiothorac Vasc Anesth 1991; 5:266–267.
105. Raffin L, Michel-Cherqui M, Sperandio M, et al: Anesthesia for bilateral lung transplantation without cardiopulmonary bypass: Initial experience and review of intraoperative problems. J Cardiothorac Vasc Anesth 1992; 6:409–417.
106. Marinelli WA, Hertz MI, Shumway SJ, et al: Single lung transplantation for severe emphysema. J Heart Lung Transplant 1992; 11:577–582.
107. Briffa NP, Dennis C, Higenbottam T, et al: Single lung transplantation for end stage emphysema. Thorax 1995; 50:562–564.
108. Popple C, Higgins TL, McCarthy P, et al: Unilateral auto-PEEP in the recipient of a single lung transplant. Chest 1993; 103:297–299.
109. Badesch DB, Zamora MR, Jones S, et al: Independent ventilation and ECMO for severe unilateral pulmonary edema after SLT for primary pulmonary hypertension. Chest 1995; 107:1766–1770.
110. Auzinger G, Tuxen DV, Davies A: Independent lung ventilation in a single lung transplant for COAD. The 22nd Australian and New Zealand Scientific Meeting on Intensive Care Medicine Handbook, October 1997; p 146.
111. Douglass JA, Tuxen DV, Horne M, et al: Myopathy in severe asthma. Am Rev Respir Dis 1992; 146:517–519.
112. Coe VL, Brodsky JB, Mark JBD: Double-lumen endobronchial tubes for patients with tracheostomies. Anesth Analg 1984; 63:882–883.
113. Pierson DJ, Horton CA, Bates PW: Persistent bronchopleural air leak during mechanical ventilation: A review of 39 cases. Chest 1986; 90:321–323.
114. Baumann MH, Sahn SA: Medical management and therapy of bronchopleural fistulas in the mechanically ventilated patient. Chest 1990; 97:721–728.
115. Powner DJ, Grenvik A: Ventilatory management of life-threatening bronchopleural fistulae: A summary. Crit Care Med 1981; 9:54–58.
116. Dennis JW, Eigen H, Ballantine TV, et al: The relationship between peak inspiratory pressure and positive end-expiratory pressure on the volume of air lost through a bronchopleural fistula. J Pediatr Surg 1980; 15:971–976.
117. Phillips YY, Lonigan RM, Joyner LR: A simple technique for managing a bronchopleural fistula while maintaining positive pressure ventilation. Crit Care Med 1979; 7:351–353.
118. Otruba Z, Oxorn D: Lobar bronchial blockade in bronchopleural fistula. Can J Anaesth 1992; 39:176–178.
119. Wippermann CF, Schranz D, Baum V, et al: Independent right lung high frequency and left lung conventional ventilation in the management of severe air leak during ARDS. Paediatr Anaesth 1995; 5:189–192.
120. Bishop MJ, Benson MS, Sato P, et al: Comparison of high-frequency jet ventilation with conventional mechanical ventilation for bronchopleural fistula. Anesth Analg 1987; 66:833–838.
121. de Bruyn GM, Prins N, Lipman J: Nursing problems encountered with asynchronous independent lung ventilation. Nurs RSA 1987; 2:16–17.
122. Dodds CP, Hillman KM: Management of massive air leak with asynchronous independent lung ventilation. Intensive Care Med 1982; 8:287–290.
123. Wendt M, Hachenberg T, Winde G, et al: Differential ventilation with low-flow CPAP and CPPV in the treatment of unilateral chest trauma. Intensive Care Med 1989; 15:209–211.
124. Benjaminsson E, Klain M: Intraoperative dual-mode independent lung ventilation of a patient with bronchopleural fistula. Anesth Analg 1981; 60:118–119.
125. Mortimer AJ, Laurie PS, Garrett H, et al: Unilateral high frequency jet ventilation: Reduction of leak in bronchopleural fistula. Intensive Care Med 1984; 10:39–41.
126. Gattinoni L, Mascheroni D, Torresin A, et al: Morphological response to positive end expiratory pressure in acute respiratory failure: Computerized tomography study. Intensive Care Med 1986; 12:137–142.
127. Gattinoni L, Presenti A, Torresin A, et al: Adult respiratory distress syndrome profiles by computed tomography. J Thorac Imaging 1986; 3:25–30.
128. Langer M, Mascheroni D, Marcolin R, et al: The prone position in ARDS patients: A clinical study. Chest 1988; 94:103–107.
129. Marini JJ: Down side up—a prone and partial liquid asset. Intensive Care Med 1995; 21:963–965.

130. Brodsky JB, Adkins MO, Gaba DM: Bronchial cuff pressures of double-lumen tubes. Anesth Analg 1989; 69:608-610.
131. Ruiz Neto PP: Bronchial cuff pressure: Comparison of carlens and polyvinylchloride (PVC) double lumen tubes. Anesthesiology 1987; 66:255-256.
132. Clapham MC, Vaughan RS: Bronchial intubation: A comparison between polyvinyl chloride and red rubber double lumen tubes. Anaesthesia 1985; 40:1111-1114.
133. McKenna MJ, Wilson RS, Botelho RJ: Right upper lobe obstruction with right-sided double-lumen endobronchial tubes; A comparison of two tube types. J Cardiothorac Anesth 1988; 2:734-740.
134. Slinger PD: Fiberoptic bronchoscopic positioning of double-lumen tubes. J Cardiothorac Anesth 1989; 3:486-496.
135. Alliaume B, Coddens J, Deloof T: Reliability of auscultation in positioning of double-lumen endobronchial tubes. Can J Anaesth 1992; 39:687-690.
136. Spragg RG, Benumof JL, Alfery DD: New methods for the performance of unilateral lung lavage. Anesthesiology 1982; 57:535-538.
137. Brodsky JB, Mark JB: Balloon method for detecting inadequate double-lumen tube cuff seal. Ann Thorac Surg 1993; 55:1584.
138. Brodsky JB, Shulman MS, Mark JB: Malposition of left-sided double-lumen endobronchial tubes. Anesthesiology 1985; 62:667-669.
139. Greene ER Jr, Gutierrez FA: Tip of polyvinyl chloride double-lumen endotracheal tube inadvertently wedged in left lower lobe bronchus. Anesthesiology 1986; 64:406.
140. Saito S, Dohi S, Naito H: Alteration of double-lumen endobronchial tube position by flexion and extension of the neck. Anesthesiology 1985; 62:696-697.
141. Wagner DL, Gammage GW, Wong ML: Tracheal rupture following the insertion of a disposable double-lumen endotracheal tube. Anesthesiology. 1985; 63:698-700.
142. Guernelli N, Bragaglia RB, Briccoli A, et al: Tracheobronchial ruptures due to cuffed Carlens tubes. Ann Thorac Surg 1979; 28:66-67.
143. Foster JM, Lau OJ, Alimo EB: Ruptured bronchus following endobronchial intubation: A case report. Br J Anaesth 1983; 55:687-688.
144. Burton NA, Watson DC, Brodsky JB, et al: Advantages of a new polyvinylchloride double-lumen tube in thoracic surgery. Ann Thorac Surg 1983; 36:78-84.

118

Continuous Gas Flow and High-Frequency Ventilation

Lorraine N. Tremblay, MD, PhD • Arthur S. Slutsky, MD

HISTORICAL PERSPECTIVE

Conventional modes of ventilatory support (e.g., volume or pressure-cycled positive-pressure mechanical ventilation) emulate human breathing patterns. In certain patients with acute lung injury, however, these techniques either cannot maintain adequate gas exchange or can do so only at precariously high pressures and volumes that injure the lung and compromise cardiovascular function. To overcome these limitations, several nonconventional techniques of ventilation have been developed, including constant (continuous) gas flow and high-frequency ventilation (i.e., ventilation at greater than physiologic frequencies).[1]

Historically, as early as 1667, Robert Hooke demonstrated that a dog could be resuscitated and kept alive by constant gas flow administered via a tracheal catheter in the absence of chest wall excursions (Fig. 118-1).[2] Multiple variations of constant gas flow ventilation were subsequently proposed, but their usefulness remained limited until the latter part of the 20th century; for although adequate oxygenation could be obtained, the animals invariably succumbed to severe respiratory acidosis within approximately 90 minutes.[3, 4] Currently, the principal application of this technique is as an adjunct to other forms of mechanical ventilation.

The history of high-frequency ventilation dates back to the observation in 1915, by Henderson and associates,[5] that panting dogs were able to maintain adequate gas exchange with tidal volumes smaller than dead space volume. It was also recognized that certain insects and hummingbirds breathed in sequence with the beat of their wings, sometimes as rapidly as 4800 breaths/min. In 1959, Emerson[6] patented a device based on his postulate that vibrating a column of gas at high frequencies would improve gas diffusion and distribution within the lungs.

The first clinical application of high-frequency ventilation was achieved in 1967 by Oberg and Sjöstrand.[7] To overcome the problem of tidal fluctuations in blood pressure with each breath, they combined use of higher than normal respiratory rates (approximately 60 breaths/min) with reduced tidal volumes, a method that later became known as ***high-frequency positive-pressure ventilation*** (HFPPV). Concurrently, Lunkenheimer and associates[8] demonstrated that ventilation could be achieved with an electromagnetic vibrator resonating at frequencies of 1380 to 2400 breaths/min (23 to 40 Hz), a technique subsequently termed ***high-frequency oscillation*** (HFO). In 1977, Klain and Smith[111] developed yet another method of ventilating at high frequencies, building on a technique previously described by Sanders,[9] which involved injecting "jets" of gases into the trachea at rates up to 600 breaths/min; this technique was termed ***high-frequency jet ventilation*** (HFJV).

As discussed later, these high-frequency ventilatory strategies, although effective, were relegated to mainly rescue therapy for patients unresponsive to conventional strategies after early clinical trials failed to demonstrate a significant advantage over conventional ventilation. There has, however, been renewed interest in HFV as a first-line option for mechanical ventilation because of (1) the promising results of several newer trials, (2) better understanding of how to optimally apply HFV, and (3) improved knowledge of the mechanisms and adverse sequelae of ventilator-induced lung injury.

THE TECHNIQUES

Both constant gas flow ventilation and high-frequency ventilation (HFV) encompass a number of different ventilatory techniques. The former comprises applications of constant gas flows in the absence of superimposed tidal volumes (e.g., apneic oxygenation or constant-flow ventilation) as well as tracheal gas insufflation used in conjunction with other ventilatory strategies; the latter consists of strategies of ventilation using greater than physiologic respiratory rates (e.g., high-frequency positive-pressure ventilation, high-frequency oscillation, high-frequency jet ventilation). Figure 118-2 depicts how the various ventilation strategies relate to another with regard to tidal volumes and respiratory rates.

Because of the use of relatively small tidal volumes in HFV and the complete absence of tidal volumes in continuous gas flow ventilation, the mechanisms of gas exchange with their use are quite different from those in conventional ventilation strategies (which use tidal volumes larger than the dead space of the lung). Movement of gases in and out of the lung occurs no longer principally by bulk flow (i.e., displacement of in-

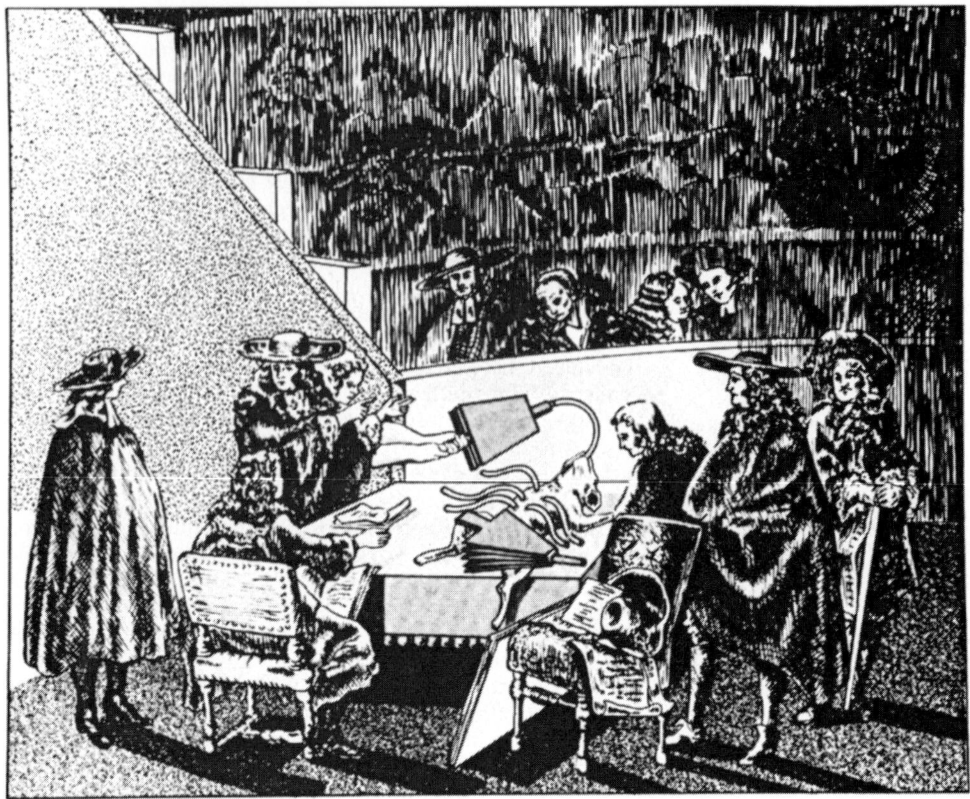

Figure 118–1. Pictorial recreation of Hooke's presentation to the Royal Society (London) in 1667. Gas was blown into the lungs at constant flow via a tracheal catheter and exited from the lungs via multiple puncture wounds in the chest wall and lungs. (From Slutsky AS: Techniques of ventilation using constant flows. Update in Intensive Care and Emergency Medicine. Vol 15: Ventilatory Failure. Marini JJ, Roussos C [Eds]. Brussels, Springer-Verlag, 1991, p 295.)

spired and expired gases) but rather via a number of other gas exchange mechanisms, including diffusion, convective streaming, pendelluft, augmented transport, and cardiogenic mixing (Fig. 118–3).[10–14] The distribution of ventilation within the lung during HFV is also different from that in conventional mechanical ventilation (CMV). At low frequencies, such as those used in CMV, the distribution of tidal ventilation is determined primarily by regional parenchymal resistance-compliance (R-C) time constants with inertance having negligible effects.[15] In contrast, at high frequencies (such as those used in HFV), the distribution of ventilation becomes less dependent on parenchymal resistance-compliance time constants and more dependent on inertance and local airway resistance.

Continuous Gas Flow

Apneic Oxygenation

As the name implies, *apneic oxygenation* is the application of 100% oxygen (O_2) at the airway opening in the absence of any tidal breaths or ventilation, following 30 to 60 minutes of ventilation with 100% O_2 to completely eliminate nitrogen (N_2) from the lungs.[16] Oxygen transport to the alveoli occurs by bulk flow because the oxygen taken up by the circulation exceeds the flux of carbon dioxide (CO_2) into the alveoli (thereby creating a subatmospheric alveolar pressure). Owing to an absence of alveolar ventilation, $Paco_2$ rises by 3 to 6 mm Hg per minute, eventually producing a severe respiratory

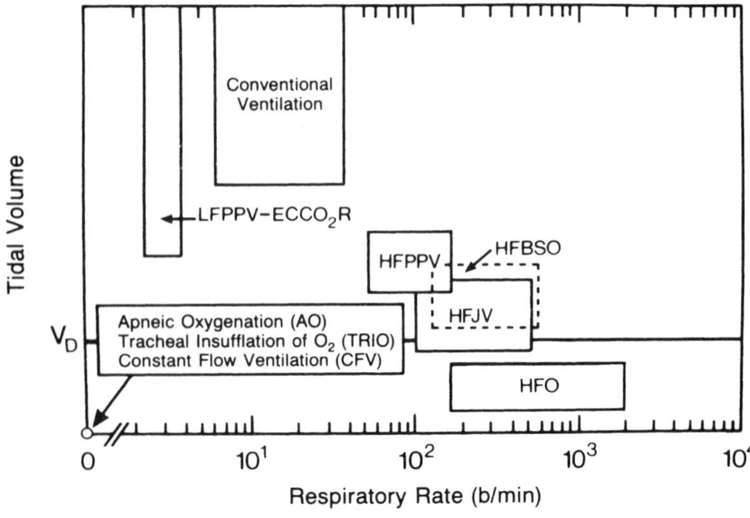

Figure 118–2. Tidal volume versus respiratory rate domain for different ventilatory strategies. Values shown are rough estimates. HFPPV = high-frequency positive-pressure ventilation; HFJV = high-frequency jet ventilation; HFBSO = high-frequency body surface oscillations; HFO = high frequency oscillations; LFPPV-ECCO$_2$R = low-frequency positive-pressure ventilation with extracorporeal carbon dioxide removal; VD = dead space volume. (From Slutsky AS: Nonconventional methods of ventilation. Am Rev Respir Dis 1988; 138:175–183.)

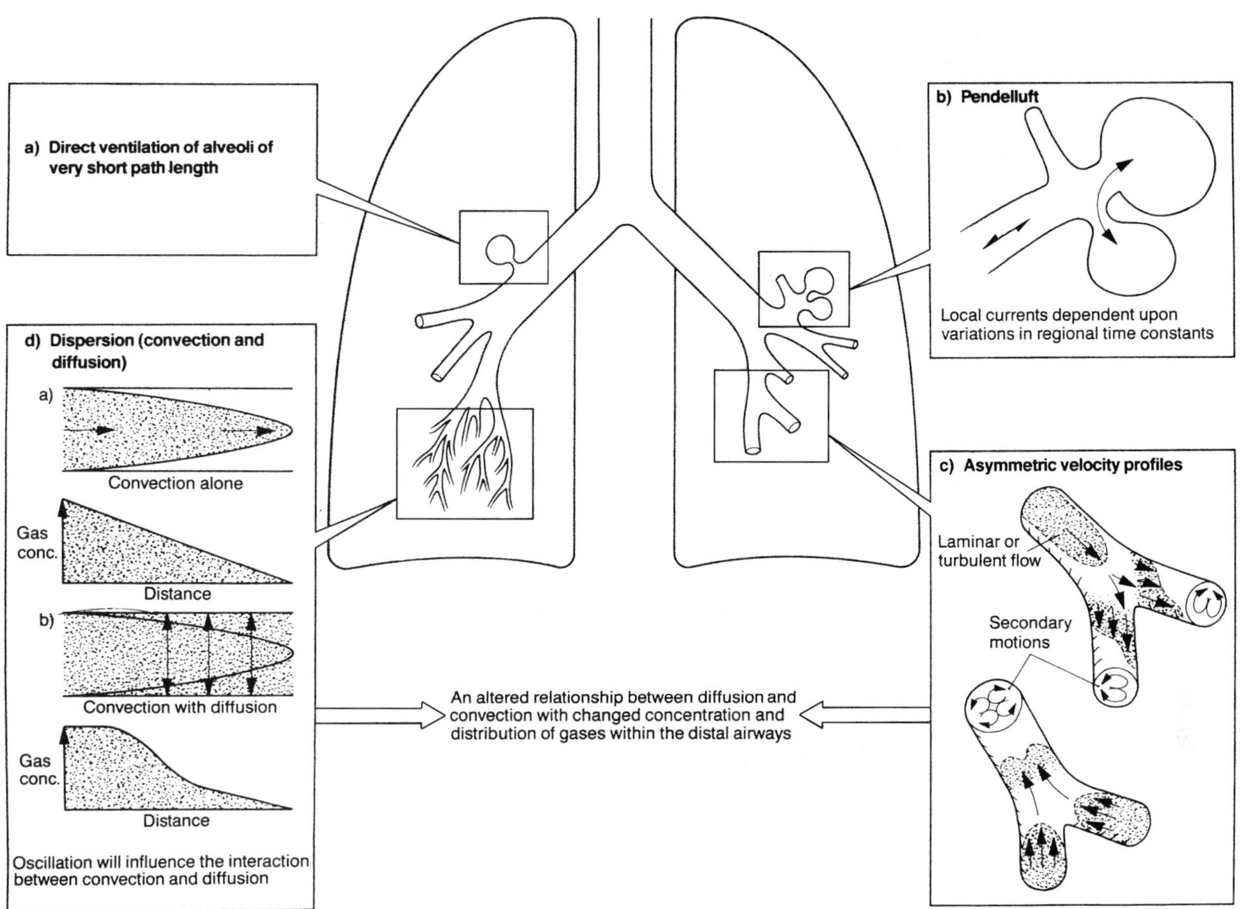

Figure 118–3. Possible mechanisms of gas dispersion in the lungs during high-frequency ventilation (HFV). (From George RJ, Geddes DM, High frequency ventilation. Br J Hosp Med 1985; 33:344–349.)

acidosis. Thus, current applications for this technique are restricted primarily to diagnosis of *brain death* (i.e., the absence of spontaneous respiration in response to hypercapnia, a potent respiratory stimulant).

Constant-Flow Ventilation

Constant-flow ventilation refers to insufflation of gases below the level of the carina at relatively high rates (1 to 3 L/min/kg).[16] In certain species, such as dogs that have a low resistance to collateral flow in the lungs, normocapnia as well as oxygenation can be achieved.[17–19] In humans, however, constant-flow ventilation is only able to provide less than 50% of the necessary alveolar ventilation.[20, 21] Hypercapnia ensues, although the rate of increase in $Pa{CO_2}$ is less than that seen with apneic oxygenation (i.e., 0.2 to 0.7 mm Hg per minute at flow rates of 0.5 to 1.6 L/min/kg).

Tracheal Gas Insufflation as an Adjunct to Mechanical Ventilation

Tracheal gas insufflation (TGI) has been found to be of use as an adjunct to either conventional or high-frequency mechanical ventilation to improve gas exchange and reduce ventilatory pressure requirements. In this technique, a catheter placed at the carina delivers a stream of gas either continuously or during a specific phase of the respiratory cycle (i.e., inspiration or expiration). Because no significant difference in CO_2 removal is found with variations in catheter position within several centimeters proximal or distal to the carina, the catheter need not be placed bronchoscopically.[22, 23] In many human studies, the catheter was introduced through a side arm adapter attached to the endotracheal tube, and its position was assessed roentgenographically. Both straight catheters and catheters with inverted tips (pointing toward the larynx) can be used. Straight catheters have proved to be more efficient at improving gas exchange, in addition to "washing out" CO_2 in the proximal airways; the turbulence generated at the catheter tip also enhances mixing of gas distally.[24, 25]

The gas flow rates used during TGI (0.1 to 0.8 L/min/kg) are lower than those used for constant-flow ventilation. CO_2 elimination can be increased by increasing TGI flows but will reach a plateau once a gas flow sufficient to completely wash out the proximal dead space during expiration is reached.[22] Monitoring of end-tidal CO_2 can be used to help guide adjustments in gas flow. If very low levels are reached (e.g., <3 mm Hg), further significant improvements in CO_2 elimination are unlikely with higher flows.

Because the gas delivered by TGI supplements the gas delivered by the ventilator, several points must be kept in mind. The first is that if the FIO_2 of the TGI differs from that of the ventilator, the FIO_2 delivered to the patient depends on both FIO_2 values and their respective contributions to the inspired tidal volume. As such, the effect on delivered FIO_2 is greatest with continuous TGI and least if phasic TGI only during expiration is used.

A second point to keep in mind is that end-expiratory lung volumes have been found to increase with TGI at higher gas flows.[24, 26] Postulated mechanisms for this finding include:

1. Back-pressure secondary to catheter flow through the endotracheal tube and expiratory circuit.

2. Decreased cross-sectional area of trachea due to the increase in expiratory resistance induced by the catheter.
3. Transfer of momentum from the jet stream of gas to the alveoli.

Studies suggest that the first two mechanisms, resulting in increased outflow resistance, are those primarily responsible for the dynamic hyperinflation seen.[24, 27] Assessment of the amount of dynamic inflation can be made using an external measure of lung volume, such as impedance plethysmography.

A third point is that catheter flow during inspiration adds to the delivered tidal volume, especially during volume-controlled modes of ventilation. An estimation of the VT due to the TGI can be made either on the basis of the duration of inspiration and the gas flow delivered or by use of inductive plethysmography.

Clinical Applications

TGI has been used as an adjunct to mechanical ventilation to reduce hypercapnia or to allow reduction of minute ventilation by the ventilator without a concomitant rise in $Paco_2$.[26, 28-30] For example, in seven patients with acute lung injury, use of TGI at rates of 6 to 8 L/min permitted decreases in VT and peak airway pressure of 25% and 20%, respectively, without changes in $Paco_2$.[28] Thus, TGI may be useful in low-pressure–low-volume lung-protective ventilatory strategies to minimize the development of hypercapnia. TGI may also be of benefit for the delivery of drugs distally into the lung, bypassing the ventilator circuit and endotracheal tube.

Complications and Limitations

Although clinical experience remains limited, a number of complications of constant-flow ventilation have been identified. One problem is bronchial mucosal injury from the stream of gas, which can be exacerbated by inadequate humidification of the gas delivered via the catheter. If the gas is not adequately humidified, prolonged TGI may also lead to inspissated secretions. Catheter tip movement ("whip") at high flows may also injure the mucosa.

Another potential problem is partial occlusion of the endotracheal tube, and interference with airway suctioning, if the catheter is passed through the endotracheal tube. If the catheter is placed adjacent to the endotracheal tube, care must be taken during placement to avoid cuff puncture. Endotracheal tubes with separate channels for TGI should obviate these difficulties.[31]

Finally, because the gas flows with TGI are relatively high, there is also a risk of barotrauma and hemodynamic compromise secondary to lung overinflation if an obstruction to gas outflow occurs.

High-Frequency Ventilation

The great interest in high-frequency ventilation in the late 1970s and 1980s was stimulated by the possibility that hemodynamic compromise and barotrauma might be minimized by the use of small tidal volumes. On the basis of a large number of animal studies, it has become clear that the best approach to use to minimize lung injury from HFO is to recruit the lung as fully as possible and then to use a mean airway pressure that ensures that the lung remains recruited.[32-38] If expressed in terms of the pressure-volume (P-V) curve of the injured lung, ventilation should occur on the descending limb of the P-V curve using pressures and volumes that avoid both overdistention and underdistention (Fig. 118–4). A number of different methods of delivering high-frequency ventilation could be used to implement this approach.

High-Frequency Positive-Pressure Ventilation

As explained earlier, HFPPV is ventilation with relatively small tidal volumes (3 to 4 mL/kg) and respiratory rates of 60 to 100 breaths/min. Optimal HFPPV is obtained through the use of a ventilator with low internal and circuit compliance and negligible compressible volume, as illustrated schematically in Figure 118–5.[39] Conventional ventilators, in most cases, cannot be used because of their high internal circuit compliances, although those equipped with external circuits using low compliance tubing have been employed on occasion.[40, 41] Breaths are given either (1) through the side arm of a pneumatic valve attached to an endotracheal tube or bronchoscope or (2) through an insufflation catheter placed in the airway. They are either pressure-controlled or volume-controlled, with inspiratory-to-expiratory (I/E) ratios usually less than 0.3. Expiration occurs passively.

Clinical Applications

HFPPV has been used during bronchoscopy and laryngoscopy and in upper airway and tracheal surgery as well as in

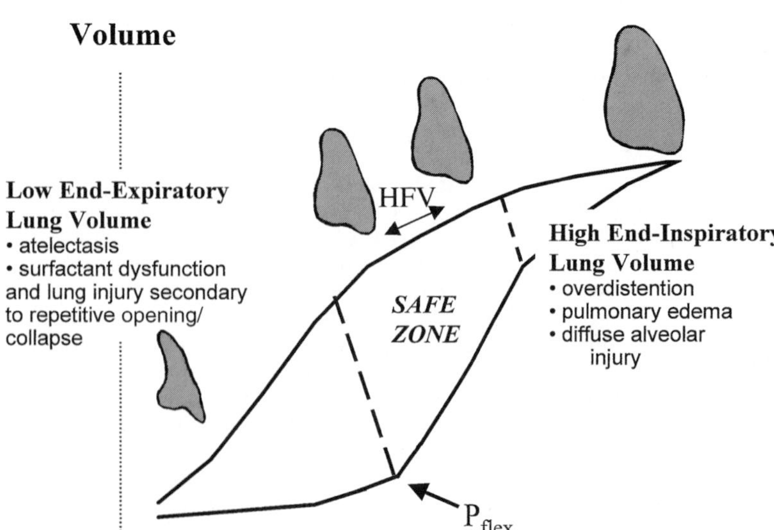

Figure 118–4. Schematic of a static P-V curve of the respiratory system. In the early phase of lung injury, an "inflection" point (depicted as P_{flex}) is sometimes seen on the inspiratory limb and is thought to represent the critical opening pressure of a large number of alveoli. Ventilation with either low end-expiratory lung volumes ($P < P_{flex}$) or high end-inspiratory lung volumes has been shown to cause lung injury. High-frequency ventilation, because of the small tidal volumes used, can be adjusted to maintain ventilation in the "safe" zone between these two extremes.

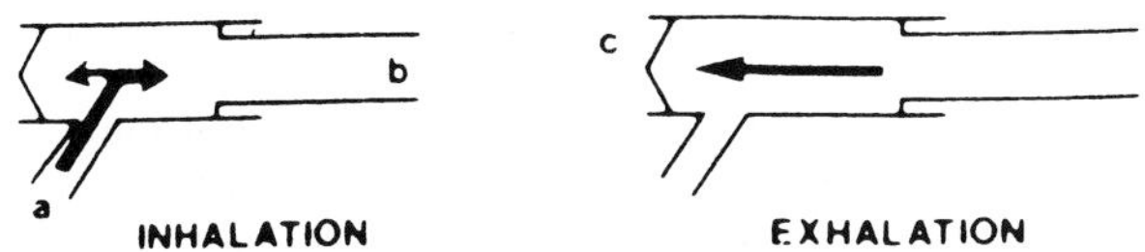

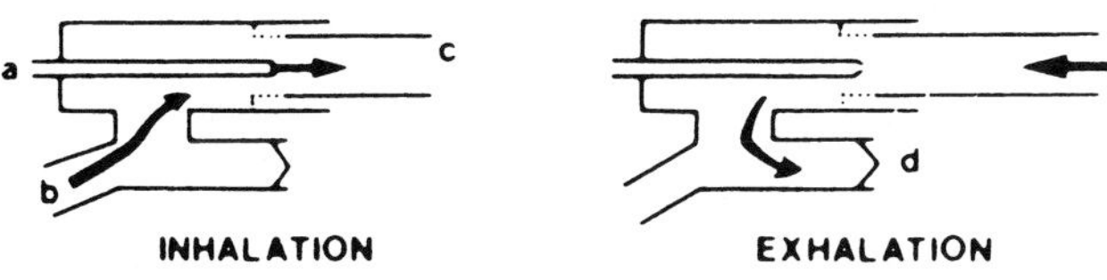

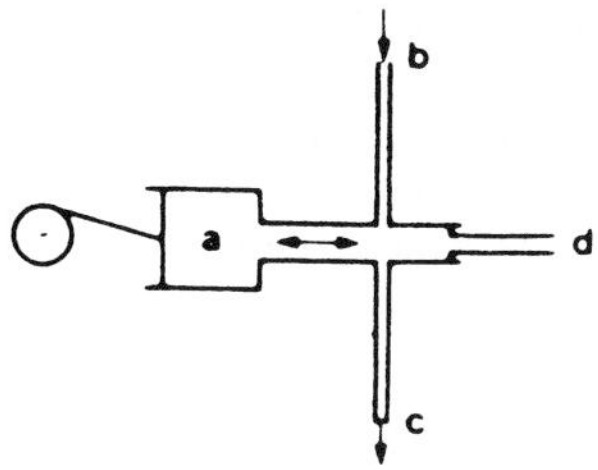

Figure 118–5. Schematic diagrams of the various modes of high-frequency ventilation. *Top,* High-frequency positive-pressure ventilation. High-pressure conditioned gas (a) is delivered during inhalation and predominantly flows through an endotracheal tube (b) to the patient with partial escape to the atmosphere. During exhalation, the gas exits through an optional one-way valve (c). *Middle,* High-frequency jet ventilator. Conditioned high-pressure gas enters from a cannula (a) at a selected level along the endotracheal tube or trachea (c). This gas entrains additional conditioned gas (b) owing to a Venturi effect. During exhalation, the gas passively exists through an optional one-way valve (d). *Bottom,* High-frequency oscillation. A piston or diaphragm (a) oscillates while fresh conditioned gas (the bias flow) enters (b) and exhaust gas exits (c) at a balanced constant rate. The bias flow ports can be positioned anywhere along the path from the external tip of the endotracheal tube to within the trachea itself (d). (From Saari AF, Rossing TH, Drazen JM: Physiological bases for new approaches to mechanical ventilation. Annu Rev Med 1984; 35:170.)

patients with respiratory failure.[42, 43] Reported advantages of HPPV over conventional pressure-controlled or volume-controlled mechanical ventilation include the following:

1. Reduced ventilator-patient asynchrony.
2. Diminished need for patient sedation.
3. Decreased cardiovascular impairment.

To date, studies demonstrating benefit in terms of minimized barotrauma or improved patient outcome are lacking.

Complications and Limitations

With HFPPV, as with any mode of mechanical ventilation, there is a risk of gas-trapping and dynamic auto-PEEP leading to hemodynamic compromise and barotrauma. Another complication that has been described, and that is dealt with in greater detail in the discussion of HFJV, is necrotizing tracheobronchitis.

High-Frequency Jet Ventilation

In HFJV, gas jets are delivered at frequencies of 100 to 600 breaths/min under high pressure (10 to 50 psi) through either a small channel incorporated within the wall of a specially designed endotracheal tube, or a 14-gauge to 16-gauge cannula passed through an endotracheal tube (or, less commonly, via a cricothyroidotomy). As illustrated in Figure 118–5, a fluidic, pneumatic, or solenoid valve regulated by a timer is used to interrupt the jet gas flow, and an ancillary circuit provides a continuous flow of humidified gas (termed "bias flow") through a side port into the endotracheal tube.

Because of the velocity of the jet stream, gas entrainment occurs. The delivered tidal volume is thus a function of both the gas volume delivered by the jet and the entrained gas volume, both of which are affected by a number of factors,[44, 45] including:

1. Position of the jet catheter.
2. The driving pressure.
3. Inspiratory time.
4. Velocity of the jet gases.
5. Velocity profile.
6. Resistance and compliance characteristics of the individual patient's lungs.

Typical tidal volumes are 2 to 5 mL/kg.

As with HFPPV, exhalation in HPJV is passive and depends on lung recoil. Auto-PEEP can occur, especially at frequencies in excess of 100 breaths/min.[46] Thus, mean airway pressure ideally should be measured at a site 5 to 10 cm distal to the jet cannula, because monitoring more proximally may result in underestimation of mean airway and alveolar pressure if dynamic hyperinflation occurs.[47] It is notable that if frequencies near that of the resonant frequency of the lung are used, alveolar pressures may become significantly greater than the pressures measured proximally.[48, 49]

The adjustments of HFJV to attain optimal ventilation differ from those used in conventional ventilation and depend on the particular ventilator used, the injector diameter, and the size of the endotracheal tube as well as patient characteristics (e.g., lung recoil, propensity to develop auto-PEEP).[50] In general, arterial oxygenation can be increased by increasing FIO_2 or lung volume. One may alter lung volume by making adjustments in PEEP (external or intrinsic) and mean airway pressures by changing driving pressures, inspiratory time, or jet frequency.[44, 51, 52]

Regulation of $Paco_2$ is a bit more complex. In general, changes in delivered tidal volume have a greater effect on CO_2 elimination than changes in frequency.[53] In fact, two studies found that increasing ventilatory frequency above 100 to 150 breaths/min often had little effect on alveolar ventilation and may actually result in a further increase in $Paco_2$ owing to a decrease in tidal volume.[53, 54] Therefore, increasing the alveolar ventilation to increase CO_2 removal is usually accomplished by a rise in tidal volume, which is determined principally by driving pressures and inspiratory time, the I/E ratio (11.1 to 0.5) having a lesser effect.[53, 54] To measure delivered tidal volume, devices such as external chest impedance or inductance bands with the appropriate frequency response characteristics are needed, because entrained gas volumes are not easily measured.

Humidification of the high-velocity jet gases poses a formidable problem but can be accomplished if a coaxial flow of saline is directed in front of the jet cannula, which results in nebulization of the saline and humidification. Entrained gases can be humidified with conventional techniques.[55]

Clinical Applications

HFJV has been found to be useful in the treatment of some, but not all, patients with bronchopleural fistulas.[56–58] It has been postulated that because at high frequencies, gas distribution is dictated preferentially by airway, rather than by parenchymal properties, HFJV leads to better alveolar ventilation compared with CMV, less gas diversion to the air leak, and, because of lower peak airway pressures, less cyclic distention of the fistula.

HFJV has also proved useful for ventilation during surgical procedures on the upper airways because it may be delivered via a small nasotracheal or orotracheal catheter, through a catheter placed percutaneously into the trachea below the level of the vocal cords, or through the side port of a rigid bronchoscope. These approaches provide adequate gas exchange while maximizing the surgical field and minimizing tidal movement without the need for a closed system.[59, 60] HFJV (and HFPPV) has also been beneficial for procedures in which lung or diaphragmatic movement must be minimized.[61, 62] In addition, percutaneous transtracheal HFJV can be used emergently in patients who cannot be intubated or who cannot be ventilated adequately by mask ventilation.[63, 64]

As a ventilatory technique for patients with acute lung injury, HFJV is the high-frequency ventilation technique being assessed in most adult clinical trials (with few pediatric applications).[65] To date, no significant advantage of HFJV over CMV has been found.[66-68] For example, Carlon and colleagues[68] prospectively assessed 309 patients randomly assigned to receive either HFJV or CMV at the onset of adult respiratory distress syndrome (ARDS). No significant difference was found between HFJV and CMV in either length of intensive care unit stay or mortality, although use of different endpoints for the two ventilatory strategies confounds interpretation of their findings. In certain patients who do not respond to conventional mechanical ventilation, HFJV has been a successful salvage technique.

Another potential indication for HFJV relates to the effects of variations in intrathoracic pressure produced by the high-frequency jet on cardiac output. Owing to smaller swings in intrathoracic pressure, HFJV has been of hemodynamic benefit in some patients.[41, 66, 69, 70] In certain patients with dilated cardiomyopathies or sepsis-related cardiac dysfunction, synchronization of the inspiratory phase of HFJV with systole may improve cardiac output.[71, 72] In such patients, the effect of higher intrathoracic pressure on reducing left ventricular wall stress along with reduced preload results in a higher left ventricular ejection fraction. There have been few trials, however, and the data from animal studies are contradictory.[72, 73] In the absence of heart failure, for example, no significant differences have been found between HFJV that is synchronous with the cardiac cycle and HFJV that is not.[74, 75] This finding has led to speculation that a brief period of HFJV that is synchronous with the cardiac cycle, in combination with continuous cardiac output assessment, may be useful to rapidly determine whether a critically ill patient is afterload-dependent or preload-dependent.[75]

Complications and Limitations

Because of the high gas flows and driving pressures used in HFJV, any obstruction of expiration can lead to a rapid increase in lung volume and intrathoracic pressure, with resultant barotrauma and cardiovascular compromise.[52, 76, 77] HFJV is therefore contraindicated in patients with airway obstruction and is not recommended for patients with increased airway resistance (e.g., chronic obstructive pulmonary disease).

Another serious complication of HFJV, seen with all modes of high-frequency ventilation, is necrotizing tracheobronchitis.[78, 79] This entity is thought to arise as a consequence of (1) injury to the mucosal lining from the "jackhammer effect" of the high-velocity gas jet and (2) inadequate humidification of the inspired gas. Improved techniques of humidification appear to have abrogated this often fatal complication.[80] Mucosal damage and air leaks can also occur as a result of injection injury if the high-pressure jet stream is directed into the mucosa.

A final limitation of HFJV relates to the unfamiliarity of personnel with the technique and the very different operating parameters and adjustments needed for its optimal use. Familiarity with the particular ventilator in use and appropriate training are needed if the benefits of HFJV are to be realized without incurring serious harm.

High-Frequency Oscillation

High-frequency oscillation differs from HFPPV and HFJV in that both the inhalation and exhalation phases are active in HFO (see Fig. 118-5). Oscillations sufficient to achieve ventilation are produced at the airway opening (standard endotracheal tubes may be used) with devices such as piston pumps,[81] high-fidelity loudspeakers,[82] or linear magnetic motors.[83, 84] Fresh gas is provided to the patient with either a bias-flow system with low impedance[81, 85] or a bias-flow system with relatively large impedance.[82, 83] Although the low-impedance system is simpler to use and allows spontaneous ventilation by the patient through the low-resistance circuit, the delivered stroke volume depends on the relative impedances of the circuit and of the patient's respiratory system. In contrast, although the high-impedance circuit is a bit more cumbersome, there is no loss of the oscillation stroke volume to the bias flow, and thus, it becomes easier to determine the delivered gas flow.[82, 83]

Ventilatory parameters that may be adjusted in HFO are:

1. Flow into and out of the ventilator circuit (which alters mean airway pressure and lung volume).
2. Pressure amplitude (e.g., 0 to 100 cm H_2O).
3. Ventilator frequency (e.g., 3 to 40 Hz).
4. Percentage duration of inspiratory time (e.g., 30% to 50%).

Typical tidal volumes generated are within the range of 0.8 to 2 mL/kg. Expiration is active because of the biphasic pressure waveform generated by the oscillator. As with HFJV, it must be kept in mind that pressures measured at the airway opening may be significantly less than those at the alveolar level.[49]

The principles of manipulating HFO to optimize gas exchange are similar in some respects to CMV. In general, oxygenation is dependent on lung volume, which is adjusted by altering mean airway pressure. CO_2 exhalation is a function of both the frequency and tidal volume used[83, 84] and is also affected by the position and flow rate of the bias flow.[86, 87] As with HFJV, factors that are not as important during conventional ventilation, such as airway compliance and lung mechanics, may also affect gas transport.[84]

Clinical Applications

A number of animal studies using different lung injury models have demonstrated significantly lower rates of lung injury, better gas exchange, and improved survival with HFO in comparison with conventional mechanical ventilation.[38, 88-91] A number of these studies also found reduced neutrophil activation and infiltration as well as lower levels of inflammatory mediators in bronchoalveolar lavage (BAL) fluid.[88-92]

Neverthless, early clinical trials of HFO,[93] especially the large HIFI Study Group trial in 1989 (a prospective randomized trial of this modality in 673 preterm neonates with infant respiratory distress syndrome),[94] failed to demonstrate any superiority of HFO over conventional mechanical ventilation. The HIFI study found no reduction in bronchopulmonary dysplasia, mortality, or level of ventilatory support required with HFO but instead an apparent increase in the incidence of pneumoperitoneum, grade 3 to 4 intracranial hemorrhage, and periventricular leukomalacia when HFO was used.

These early trials have been criticized, however, for failing to optimize lung volume prior to institution of HFO,[95, 96] a factor identified in animal studies as being important for the "beneficial" effects of HFO.[33-37] Other criticisms include prolonged periods of conventional mechanical ventilation prior to the use of HFO. In saline-lavaged (surfactant depleted) rabbits, HFO has been shown to improve gas exchange when implemented following 1 hour, but not 4 hours, of CMV.[97] Similarly, HFO has been more effective when used earlier rather than later in the course of respiratory failure in ventilated premature baboons.[98, 99]

Later, smaller trials suggest that HFO, when instituted early and optimally following lung recruitment maneuvers, may be superior to CMV.[100-103] For example, a follow-up study by the HIFI group using higher lung volumes reported significantly lower incidence of air leak syndrome and better oxygenation and ventilation with HFO than with CMV.[100] Gerstmann and colleagues[101] found that neonates randomly assigned to receive HFO had lower vasopressor requirements, needed repeat surfactant doses less frequently, needed shorter duration and lower levels of supplemental oxygenation and ventilatory support, and had lower incidences of chronic lung disease at 30 days as well as of necrotizing enterocolitis and hearing impairment.

In adults, owing to technical limitations (i.e., difficulty in developing HFO ventilators capable of generating oscillations sufficient to provide gas exchange within the much larger adult lung), few trials have compared HFO with conventional techniques. A pilot study (using a newly designed ventilator) has demonstrated that HFO was effective in improving gas exchange with no significant adverse hemodynamic effects in patients with ARDS for whom conventional ventilation failed.[104]

In summary, further studies—especially with newly developed adult HFO ventilators[104]—are needed to determine whether HFO is indeed superior to more conventional modes of ventilation. As with HFJV, there is a wealth of animal and clinical evidence that (1) HFO is as safe and effective as CMV when used properly and (2) there is a role for HFO as a rescue therapy, especially in comparison with more invasive, more labor-intensive alternatives, such as extracorporeal membrane oxygenation (ECMO).[105, 106]

Complications and Limitations

As with HFJV, the lack of familiarity with the operation of the HFO ventilator poses significant risks to the patient. The adjustments needed to optimize gas exchange differ from those for conventional ventilators, and despite active expiration, dynamic hyperinflation can occur. A meta-analysis of the nine prospective randomized controlled trials comparing HFV with CMV in neonates found no significant association between HFV and intraventricular hemorrhage; however, because of the large number of patients in the HIFI trial, a slightly higher risk of periventricular leukomalacia remained (odds ratio, 1.7).[107, 108]

FUTURE DIRECTIONS

Over the past few decades, our understanding of lung injury secondary to mechanical ventilation has grown. A consensus conference conducted in 1994 identified both lung overdistention and atelectasis as factors that predispose to further injury.[109] In a heterogeneously injured or expanded lung, such as that seen in ARDS, it becomes difficult to ensure that all regions are ventilated in the "safe" zone between these two extremes. In theory, because of the small tidal fluctuations in lung pressure and volume with high-frequency ventilation, less ventilator-associated injury and better patient outcomes should be seen. HFO also offers more flexibility than conventional ventilation for tailoring regional ventilation within the lung to meet the patient's needs while reducing the overdistention of some regions and underventilation of others.[96, 110]

Although high-frequency ventilation can, in experienced hands, be as safe and effective as conventional strategies and can, in certain cases unresponsive to CMV, be a lifesaving intervention, further clinical trials implementing the knowledge we have gained about the optimal use of HFV are needed to determine whether HFV offers any significant advantages over conventional techniques. Other avenues being explored include use of HFV or constant-flow ventilation as adjuncts with other conventional or nonconventional techniques, such as low-frequency CMV and liquid ventilation.

References

1. Slutsky AS: Nonconventional methods of ventilation. Am Rev Respir Dis 1988; 138:175–183.
2. Hooke R: Account of an experiment, made by R. Hooke, of preserving animals alive by blowing through their lungs with bellows. Philos Trans R Soc Lond 1667; 2:539–540.
3. Draper WB, Whitehead RW: Diffusion respiration in the dog anesthetized by pentothal sodium. Anesthesiology 1944; 5:262–273.
4. Frumin MJ, Epstein RM, Cohen G: Apneic oxygenation in man. Anesthesiology 1959; 20:789–798.
5. Henderson Y, Chillingsworth F, Whitney J: The respiratory dead space. Am J Physiol 1915; 38:1–19.
6. Emerson JH: Apparatus for vibrating portions of a patient's airway. U.S. Patent Office 1959, Serial No. 491,699. Patented Dec. 29.
7. Oberg PA, Sjöstrand U: Studies in blood pressure regulation: I. Common-carotid artery clamping in studies of the carotid-sinus baroreceptor control of the systemic blood pressure. Acta Physiol Scand 1969; 75:276–287.
8. Lunkenheimer PP, Rafflenbeul W, Keller H, et al: Application of transtracheal pressure oscillations as a modification of "diffusion respiration." Br J Anaesth 1972; 44:627.
9. Sanders RD: Two ventilating attachments for bronchoscopes. Del State Med J 1967; 39:170–175.
10. Slutsky AS, Drazen JM, Kamm RD: Alveolar ventilation at high frequencies using tidal volumes smaller than the anatomic dead space. *In:* Lung Biology in Health and Disease. Engel LA, Paiva M, Lenfant C (Eds). New York, Marcel Dekker, 1985, p 137.
11. Chang HK: Mechanisms of gas transport during ventilation by high-frequency oscillation. J Appl Physiol 1984; 56:553–563.
12. Pedley TJ, Corieri P, Kamm RD, et al: Gas flow and mixing in the airways. Crit Care Med 1994; 22:S24–36.
13. Fukuchi Y, Charalambos R, Macklem P, et al: Convection, diffusion and cardiogenic mixing of inspired gas in the lung: An experimental approach. Respir Physiol 1976; 26:77–90.
14. Slutsky AS, Khoo MCK, Brown R: Simulation of gas transport due to cardiogenic oscillations. J Appl Physiol 1985; 58:1331.
15. Mead J: The distribution of gas flow in the lungs. *In:* Ciba Foundation Symposium on Circulatory Mass Transport. Wolstenholme G, Knight J (Eds). London, Churchill Livingstone, 1969, p 204.
16. Slutsky AS: Techniques of ventilation using constant flows. *In:* Update in Intensive Care and Emergency Medicine. Vol 15: Ventilatory Failure. Marini JJ, Roussos C (Eds). Brussels, Springer-Verlag, 1991, p 293.
17. Lehnert BE, Oberdorster G, Slutsky AS: Constant flow ventilation of apneic dogs. J Appl Physiol 1982; 53:483–489.
18. Watson JW, Burwen DR, Kamm RD, et al: Effect of flow rate on blood gases during constant flow ventilation in dogs. Am Rev Respir Dis 1986; 133:626–629.
19. Macklem PT: Airways obstruction and collateral ventilation. Physiol Rev 1971; 51:368–436.
20. Breen PH, Sznajder JI, Morrison P, et al: Constant flow ventilation in anesthetized patients: Efficacy and safety. Anesth Analg 1986; 65:1161–1169.
21. Babinski MF, Sierra OG, Smith RB, et al: Clinical application of

continuous flow apneic ventilation. Acta Anaesthesiol Scand 1985; 29:750–752.
22. Nahum A, Ravenscraft SA, Nakos G, et al: Tracheal gas insufflation during pressure-control ventilation: Effect of catheter position, diameter, and flow rate. Am Rev Respir Dis 1992; 146:1411–1418.
23. Eckmann DM, Gavriely N: Intra-airway CO_2 distribution during airway insufflation in respiratory failure. J Appl Physiol 1995; 78:546–554.
24. Nahum A, Ravenscraft SA, Nakos G, et al: Effect of catheter flow direction on CO_2 removal during tracheal gas insufflation in dogs. J Appl Physiol 1993; 75:1238–1246.
25. Ravenscraft SA, Shapiro R, Nahum A, et al: Tracheal gas insufflation (TGI): Catheter effectiveness is determined by expiratory flush volume. Am J Respir Crit Care Med 1996; 153:1817–1824.
26. Ravenscraft SA, Burke WC, Nahum A, et al: Tracheal gas insufflation augments CO_2 clearance during mechanical ventilation. Am Rev Respir Dis 1993; 148:345–351.
27. Brampton W, Young JD: Lung volume, pressure, flow, and density relationships during constant-flow ventilation in dogs. J Appl Physiol 1993; 74:197–202.
28. Nakos G, Zakinthinos S, Kotanidou A, et al: Tracheal gas insufflation reduces the tidal volume while Pa_{CO_2} is maintained constant. Intensive Care Med 1994; 20:407–413.
29. Kuo PH, Wu HD, Yu CJ, et al: Efficacy of tracheal gas insufflation in acute respiratory distress syndrome with permissive hypercapnia. Am J Respir Crit Care Med 1996; 154:612–616.
30. Nahum A, Ravenscraft SA, Adams AB, et al: Inspiratory tidal volume sparing effects of tracheal gas insufflation in dogs with oleic acid-induced lung injury. J Crit Care 1995; 10:115–121.
31. Isabey D, Boussignac G, Harf A: Effect of air entrainment on airway pressure during endotracheal gas injection. J Appl Physiol 1989; 67:771–779.
32. Froese AB, Bryan AC: High frequency ventilation. Am Rev Respir Dis 1987; 135:1363.
33. Kolton M, Cattran CB, Kent G, et al: Oxygenation during high-frequency ventilation compared with conventional mechanical ventilation in two models of lung injury. Anesth Analg 1982; 61:323–332.
34. Froese AB, McCulloch PR, Sugiura M, et al: Optimizing alveolar expansion prolongs the effectiveness of exogenous surfactant therapy in the adult rabbit. Am Rev Respir Dis 1993; 148:569–577.
35. McCulloch PR, Forkert PG, Froese AB: Lung volume maintenance prevents lung injury during high frequency oscillation in surfactant deficient rabbits. Am Rev Respir Dis 1988; 137:1185–1192.
36. Bond DM, Froese AB: Volume recruitment maneuvers are less deleterious than persistent low lung volumes in the atelectasis-prone rabbit lung during high-frequency oscillation. Crit Care Med 1993; 21:402–412.
37. Bond DM, McAloon J, Froese AB: Sustained inflations improve respiratory compliance during high-frequency oscillatory ventilation but not during large tidal volume positive-pressure ventilation in rabbits. Crit Care Med 1994; 22:1269–1277.
38. Hamilton PP, Onayemi A, Smyth JA, et al: Comparison of conventional and high-frequency ventilation: Oxygenation and lung pathology. J Appl Physiol 1983; 55:131–138.
39. Sjöstrand U: High-frequency positive-pressure ventilation (HFPPV): A review. Crit Care Med 1980; 8:345–364.
40. Abdu-Dbai J, Flatau E, Lev A: The use of conventional ventilators for high frequency positive pressure ventilation. Crit Care Med 1983; 11:356–360.
41. Nakatsuka M, Colquhoun A, Gehr L: Right ventricular function and high-frequency positive-pressure ventilation during coronary artery bypass grafting. Ann Thorac Surg 1989; 48:263–266.
42. Borg U, Eriksson I, Sjöstrand U: High-frequency positive-pressure ventilation (HFPPV): A review based upon its use during bronchoscopy and for laryngoscopy and microlaryngeal surgery under general anesthesia. Anesth Analg 1980; 59:594–603.
43. Bjerager K, Sjöstrand U, Wattwil M: Long term treatment of two patients with respiratory insufficiency with IPPV/PEEP and HFPPV/PEEP. Acta Anaesthesiol Scand Suppl 1977; 64:55–68.
44. Guntapalli KK, Pinsky MR, Marquez J, et al: Determinants of ventilation during high frequency jet ventilation. J Crit Care 1987; 2:93–108.
45. Carlon GC, Ray C, Griffin J: Tidal volume and airway pressure on high frequency jet ventilation. Crit Care Med 1983; 11:83–89.
46. Novak RA, Matuschak GM, Pinsky MR: Effect of ventilatory frequency on regional pleural pressure. J Appl Physiol 1988; 65:1314–1323.
47. Sutton JE Jr, Glass DD: Airway pressure gradient during high-frequency ventilation. Crit Care Med 1984; 12:774–778.
48. Fredberg JJ, Keefe DH, Glass G, et al: Alveolar pressure nonhomogeneity during small-amplitude high-frequency ventilation. J Appl Physiol 1984; 57:788–800.
49. Allen JL, Fredberg JJ, Keefe DH, et al: Alveolar pressure magnitude and asynchrony during high-frequency oscillations of excised rabbit lungs. Am Rev Respir Dis 1985; 132:343–349.
50. Fredberg JJ, Glass G, Boynton B, et al: Factors influencing mechanical performance of neonatal high-frequency ventilators. J Appl Physiol 1987; 62:2485–2490.
51. Jonson B, Lachmann B: Setting and monitoring of high-frequency jet ventilation in severe respiratory distress syndrome. Crit Care Med 1989; 17:1020–1024.
52. Rouby JJ, Fusciardi J, Bourgain JL, et al: High frequency jet ventilation in post-operative respiratory failure: Determinants of oxygenation. Anesthesiology 1983; 59:281–287.
53. Rouby JJ, Simonneau G, Benhamou D, et al: Factors influencing pulmonary volumes and CO_2 elimination during high-frequency jet ventilation. Anesthesiology 1985; 63:473–482.
54. Calkins JM, Waterson CK, Hameroff SR, et al: Jet pulse characteristics for high-frequency jet ventilation in dogs. Anesth Analg 1982; 61:293–300.
55. Carlon GC, Barker RL, Benua RS: Airway humidification with high-frequency jet ventilation. Crit Care Med 1984; 12:774–778.
56. Turnbull AD, Carlon G, Howland WS, et al: High-frequency jet ventilation in major airway or pulmonary disruption. Ann Thorac Surg 1980; 32:468–474.
57. Derderian SS, Rajagopal KR, Abbrecht PH, et al: High frequency positive pressure ventilation in bilateral bronchopleural fistulae. Crit Care Med 1982; 10:119–121.
58. Bishop MJ, Benson MS, Sato T, et al: Comparison of high frequency ventilation with conventional mechanical ventilation for bronchopleural fistula. Anesth Analg 1987; 66:833.
59. Giunta F, Chiaranda M, Manani G: Clinical uses of high-frequency jet ventilation in anaesthesia. Del Med J 1967; 39:170–178.
60. el-Baz NM, Caldarelli DD, Holinger LD, et al: High frequency ventilation through a small catheter for laser surgery of laryngotracheal and bronchial disorders. Ann Otol Rhinol Laryngol 1985; 94:483–488.
61. Speiss BD, Wong CA, Tuman KJ: High frequency positive pressure ventilation for anterior thoracic spine fusion after a previous pneumonectomy. Anesth Analg 1988; 67:411–418.
62. Warner MA, Warner ME, Buck CF, et al: Clinical efficacy of high frequency jet ventilation during extracorporeal shock wave lithotripsy of renal and ureteral calculi: A comparison with conventional mechanical ventilation. J Urol 1988; 139:486–487.
63. Benumof JL, Scheller MS: The importance of transtracheal jet ventilation in the management of the difficult airway. Anesthesiology 1989; 71:769–774.
64. Nakatsuka M, MacLeod AD: Hemodynamic and respiratory effects of transtracheal high-frequency jet ventilation during difficult airway. J Clin Anesth 1992; 4:321–326.
65. Wiswell TE, Graziani LJ, Kornhauser MS, et al: High-frequency jet ventilation in the early management of respiratory distress syndrome is associated with a greater risk for adverse outcomes. Pediatrics 1996; 98:1035–1043.
66. Schuster D, Klain M, Snyder J: Comparison of high frequency jet ventilation to conventional mechanical ventilation during severe acute respiratory failure in humans. Crit Care Med 1982; 10:625–630.
67. Holzapfel L, Perrin R, Gaussorgnes P, et al: Comparison of high frequency jet ventilation to conventional ventilation in adults with respiratory distress syndrome. Intensive Care Med 1987; 13:100–105.
68. Carlon GC, Howland W, Ray C Jr, et al: High frequency jet ventilation: A prospective randomized evaluation. Chest 1983; 84:551–559.
69. Fusciardi J, Rouby JJ, Barakat T: Hemodynamic effects of high-frequency jet ventilation in patients with and without circulatory shock. Anesthesiology 1986; 65:485–491.

70. Traverse JH, Korvenranta H, Adams EM, et al: Cardiovascular effects of high-frequency oscillatory and jet ventilation. Chest 1989; 96:1400–1404.
71. Pinsky M, Marquez J, Martin D, et al: Ventricular assist by cardiac cycle-specific increases in intrathoracic pressure. Chest 1987; 91:709–715.
72. Weber A, Mathru M, Rooney M: Effect of jet ventilation on heart failure: Decreased afterload but negative response in left ventricular end-systolic pressure-volume function. Crit Care Med 1996; 24:647–657.
73. Pinsky MR, Matuschak GM, Bernardi L, et al: Hemodynamic effects of cardiac cycle-specific increases in intrathoracic pressure. J Appl Physiol 1986; 60:604–612.
74. Bayly R, Sladen A, Guntupalli K, et al: Synchronous versus nonsynchronous high-frequency jet ventilation: Effects on cardiorespiratory variables and airway pressures in postoperative patients. Crit Care Med 1987; 15:915–917.
75. Angus DC, Lidsky NM, Dotterweich LM, et al: The influence of high-frequency jet ventilation with varying cardiac-cycle specific synchronization on cardiac output in ARDS. Chest 1997; 112:1600–1606.
76. Fusciardi J, Rouby JJ, Benhamou D, et al: Hemodynamic consequences of increasing mean airway pressure during high frequency jet ventilation. Chest 1984; 86:30–34.
77. Bancalari A, Gerhardt T, Bancalari E, et al: Gas trapping with high-frequency ventilation: Jet versus oscillatory ventilation. J Pediatr 1987; 110:617–622.
78. Wiswell TE, Clark RH, Null DM, et al: Tracheal and bronchial injury in high-frequency oscillatory ventilation and high-frequency flow interruption compared with conventional positive-pressure ventilation. J Pediatr 1988; 112:249–256.
79. Boros SJ, Mammel MC, Lewallen PK, et al: Necrotizing tracheobronchitis: A complication of high-frequency ventilation. J Pediatr 1986; 109:95–100.
80. Fuchs W: Humidification techniques in high-frequency ventilation: A review. Acta Anaesthesiol Scand Suppl 1989; 90:120–123.
81. Butler WJ, Bohn DJ, Bryan AC, et al: Ventilation by high frequency oscillations in humans. Anesth Analg 1980; 59:577–584.
82. Slutsky AS, Drazen JM, Ingram RH Jr, et al: Effective pulmonary ventilation with small-volume oscillations at high frequency. Science 1980; 209:609–611.
83. Slutsky AS, Kamm RD, Rossing T, et al: Effects of frequency, tidal volume, and lung volume on CO_2 elimination in dogs by high frequency (2–30 Hz), low tidal volume ventilation. J Clin Invest 1981; 68:1475–1484.
84. Rossing T, Slutsky AS, Lehr J, et al: Tidal volume and frequency dependence of carbon dioxide elimination by high-frequency ventilation. N Engl J Med 1981; 305:1375–1379.
85. Bohn DJ, Miyasaka K, Marchak BE, et al: Ventilation by high-frequency oscillation. J Appl Physiol 1980; 48:710–716.
86. Wright K, Lyrene R, Truog W, et al: Ventilation by high frequency oscillation in rabbits with oleic acid lung disease. J Appl Physiol 1981; 50:1056–1060.
87. Rossing TH, Solway J, Saari A: Influence of the endotracheal tube on CO_2 transport during high-frequency ventilation. Am Rev Respir Dis 1984; 129:54–57.
88. Kawano T, Mori S, Cybulsky M, et al: Effect of granulocyte depletion in a ventilated surfactant-depleted lung. J Appl Physiol 1987; 62:27–33.
89. Matsuoka T, Kawano T, Miyasaka K: Role of high-frequency ventilation in surfactant-depleted lung injury as measured by granulocytes. J Appl Physiol 1994; 76:539–544.
90. Imai Y, Kawano T, Miyasaka K, et al: Inflammatory chemical mediators during conventional ventilation and during high frequency oscillatory ventilation. Am J Respir Crit Care Med 1994; 150:1550–1554.
91. Sugiura M, McCulloch PR, Wren S, et al: Ventilator pattern influences neutrophil influx and activation in atelectasis-prone rabbit lung. J Appl Physiol 1994; 77:1355–1365.
92. Takata M, Abe J, Tanaka H, et al: Intraalveolar expression of tumor necrosis factor-α gene during conventional and high-frequency ventilation. Am J Respir Crit Care Med 1997; 156:272–279.
93. Cavanagh K: High frequency ventilation of infants: An analysis of the literature. Respir Care 1990; 35:815–830.
94. HIFI Study Group: High-frequency oscillatory ventilation compared with conventional mechanical ventilation in the treatment of respiratory failure in preterm infants. N Engl J Med 1989; 320:88–91.
95. Bryan AC, Froese AB: Reflections on the HIFI trial. Pediatrics 1991; 87:565–567.
96. Froese AB: High-frequency oscillatory ventilation for adult respiratory distress syndrome: Let's get it right this time! Crit Care Med 1997; 25:906–908.
97. Suzuki H, Papazoglou K, Bryan AC: Relationship between Pa_{O_2} and lung volume during high frequency oscillatory ventilation. Acta Paediatr Jpn 1992; 34:494–500.
98. Meredith KS, deLemos RA, Coalson JJ: Role of lung injury in the pathogenesis of hyaline membrane disease in premature baboons. J Appl Physiol 1989; 66:2150–2156.
99. deLemos RA, Coalson JJ, Meredith KS, et al: A comparison of ventilation strategies for the use of high-frequency oscillatory ventilation in the treatment of hyaline membrane disease. Acta Anaesthesiol Scand Suppl 1989; 90:102–107.
100. HiFO Study Group: Randomized study of high-frequency oscillatory ventilation in infants with severe respiratory distress syndrome. J Pediatr 1993; 122:609–619.
101. Gerstmann DR, Minton SD, Stoddard RA, et al: The Provo Multicenter Early High-Frequency Oscillatory Ventilation Trial: Improved pulmonary and clinical outcome in respiratory distress syndrome. Pediatrics 1996; 98:1044–1057.
102. Clark RH, Gerstmann DR, Null DM, et al: Prospective randomized comparison of high-frequency oscillatory and conventional ventilation in respiratory distress syndrome. Pediatrics 1992; 89:5–12.
103. Arnold JH, Hanson JH, Toro-Figuero LO, et al: Prospective, randomized comparison of high-frequency oscillatory ventilation and conventional mechanical ventilation in pediatric respiratory failure. Crit Care Med 1994; 22:1530–1539.
104. Fort P, Farmer C, Westerman J, et al: High-frequency oscillatory ventilation for adult respiratory distress syndrome—a pilot study. Crit Care Med 1997; 25:937–947.
105. Clark RH, Yoder BA, Sell MS: Prospective, randomized comparison of high-frequency oscillation and conventional ventilation in candidates for extracorporeal membrane oxygenation [see "Comments"]. J Pediatr 1994; 124:447–454.
106. Varnholt V, Lasch P, Suske G, et al: High frequency oscillatory ventilation and extracorporeal membrane oxygenation in severe persistent pulmonary hypertension of the newborn. Eur J Pediatr 1992; 151:769–774.
107. Clark RH, Dykes FD, Bachman TE, et al: Intraventricular hemorrhage and high-frequency ventilation: A meta-analysis of prospective clinical trials. Pediatrics 1996; 98:1058–1061.
108. Ogawa Y, Miyasaka K, Kawano T, et al: A multicenter randomized trial of high frequency oscillatory ventilation as compared with conventional mechanical ventilation in preterm infants with respiratory failure. Early Hum Dev 1993; 32:1–10.
109. Slutsky AS: Consensus conference on mechanical ventilation: January 28-30, 1993, at Northbrook, Ill. Intensive Care Med 1994; 20:64–79.
110. Lunkenheimer PP, Salle BL, Whimster WF, et al: High-frequency ventilation: Reappraisal and progress in Europe and abroad (Editorial). Crit Care Med 1994; 22:S19–S23.
111. Klain M, Smith RB: High frequency percutaneous transtracheal jet ventilation. Crit Care Med 1977; 5:280–287.

119

Noninvasive Ventilation

Laurent J. Brochard, MD

GOALS OF TREATMENT IN ACUTE RESPIRATORY FAILURE

Noninvasive ventilation (NIV) is used in the settings of acute respiratory failure to avoid the need for endotracheal intubation and reduce the risk of complications associated with mechanical ventilation. It has been used successfully in several prospective studies in patients with various forms of respiratory failure.[1-10] Specifically, complications associated with the endotracheal intubation procedure, ventilator-associated pneumonia, and weaning difficulties with prolonged length of mechanical ventilation and of hospital stay could be substantially reduced by avoiding the need for endotracheal intubation.

Another important indication for promoting this technique is the growing number of patients who refuse endotracheal intubation[11] or in whom this intervention is not considered appropriate because of the poor underlying status and the subsequent high risk of mortality.[12] In these patients, a noninvasive technique can offer the possibility of recovering under partial ventilatory support with a low risk of complications. It may also help in postponing endotracheal intubation when the decision is difficult to take early on at admission.

PHYSIOLOGIC EFFECTS AND MECHANISMS OF ACTION

Changes in Breathing Pattern

The spontaneous breathing pattern of patients with acute ventilatory failure can be markedly abnormal and can cause respiratory acidosis. In patients with chronic obstructive pulmonary disease (COPD), rapid shallow breathing is a typical feature of acute exacerbation, resulting in alveolar hypoventilation despite preserved minute ventilation. This pattern can be modified by the use of NIV, which allows the patient to take deeper breaths with less effort. Although continuous positive airway pressure (CPAP), used to counterbalance intrinsic positive end-expiratory pressure (PEEPi), can significantly reduce the patient's effort,[13] it seems that the addition of positive inspiratory pressure, as delivered with pressure support or assist-control ventilation, is necessary to substantially alter the breathing pattern and subsequently improve carbon dioxide (CO_2) elimination. The reduction in respiratory rate and the increase in tidal volume under NIV are the best markers of the efficacy of the technique.[5, 14]

Improvement in Arterial Blood Gases

In patients with hypoxemic respiratory failure, improvement in oxygenation has often been reported,[1-4, 8, 9] but the mechanism for this improvement has not been well explored. In particular, the changes in oxygenation in many patients may be simply caused by a change in the inspired oxygen fraction. In others, improvement in functional residual capacity owing to positive end-expiratory pressure may play an important role.

In patients with hypercapnic respiratory failure, improvement of arterial blood gas disturbances can be achieved specifically through noninvasive ventilation. In patients with chronic CO_2 retention admitted for acute exacerbation, the main effect may be an improvement in oxygenation without any worsening in CO_2 retention, as usually observed in these patients with oxygen alone.[15] Improvement in oxygenation was shown in several studies, whereas improvement in P_{CO_2} and pH was much more gradual with time.[6, 16-18] In other studies, a drop in P_{CO_2} and a rise in pH toward normal values were observed within the first hour.[5, 19] The difference among studies may be explained by the severity of the patients' condition or differences in how the technique was applied. For other authors, the 2-hour response in blood gas is predictive of the further success or failure of the technique.[20]

A recent study by Diaz and coworkers[14] specifically investigated the effects of NIV on gas exchange and hemodynamics in COPD patients with acute exacerbation. During NIV, Pa_{O_2} slightly increased while Pa_{CO_2} decreased substantially, but the alveolo-arterial difference in oxygen increased slightly. This latter finding indicated that improvement in the ventilation-perfusion relationship did not play any significant role. Thus, attainment of an efficient breathing pattern rather than high inspiratory pressures should be the primary goal to improve arterial blood gases during NIV.

Reduction in Patient's Effort to Breathe

In patients with acute exacerbation of COPD, Brochard and coworkers[5] have studied the efficacy of face mask pressure-support ventilation (PSV) to reduce the patient's effort to breathe. At baseline, the transdiaphragmatic pressure swings measured in those patients were considerably higher than normal values, which suggested that these patients developed a high percentage of their maximal capacity at each breath. This situation is known to be a high risk factor for development of respiratory muscle fatigue.[21] A substantial and constant reduction in the pressure swings could be obtained under noninvasive PSV in all patients (Fig. 119–1). This finding was confirmed in further studies.[22] This physiologic effect illustrates the great potential of this technique to reverse

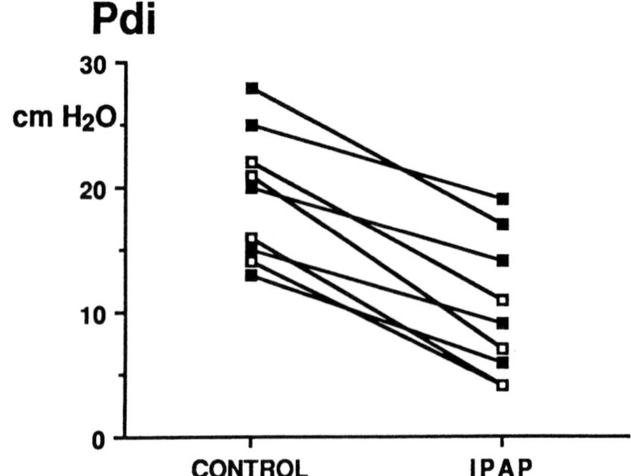

Figure 119–1. Tidal transdiaphragmatic pressure (Pdi) swings as measured in nine patients with acute exacerbation of chronic obstructive pulmonary disease, at baseline (control) and while breathing with face mask inspiratory pressure support (IPAP). (From Brochard L, Isabey D, Piquet J, et al: Reversal of acute exacerbations of chronic obstructive lung disease by inspiratory assistance with a face mask. N Engl J Med 1990; 323:1523–1530.)

acutely the deterioration of the patient's clinical status. In particular, the results of Appendini and colleagues[23] are important, showing that the combination of PSV and PEEP in patients with COPD is more efficient than each one alone in reducing diaphragmatic effort and steering the patient clear from a potential zone of fatigue.

Hemodynamic Effects

Surprisingly few data are available on the hemodynamic effects of noninvasive ventilation, which suggests that no major adverse changes are observed. In one study, PSV had no hemodynamic effect, except when positive end-expiratory pressure (PEEP) was added.[24] Thorens and colleagues[25] investigated the hemodynamic and endocrinologic effects of noninvasive ventilation, in the assist-control mode, delivered 16 to 20 hours per day in a group of 11 patients with acute worsening of chronic restrictive respiratory failure, most of whom had peripheral edema. Correction of arterial blood gas abnormalities was accompanied by a decrease in systolic and mean pulmonary arterial pressure and an increase in right ventricular ejection fraction. Cardiac index did not change. Edema subsequently decreased in all patients. Renin, aldosterone, and vasopressin remained in the normal range, whereas catecholamines and natriuretic peptides were increased. The latter decreased during NIV. Both the correction of hypercapnia and hypoxemia and the hemodynamic effects of NIV appeared to be important determinants of the subsequent loss in total body water and of the disappearance of edema.

SPECIFIC FEATURES AND LIMITATIONS

Although NIV carries many common features with the effects of assisted mechanical ventilation in the intubated trachea, it differs by some specific aspects, which require particular attention in the routine management of these patients.

The first difference is the patient-ventilator interface, which in most instances is either a full face mask covering both the nose and the mouth, or a nasal mask, which is the device predominantly used for long-term ventilation. Excellent results have been described with both type of devices.[6, 19] Nasal masks, however, can be impossible to use in patients unable to close their mouth. Leaks through the mouth make the technique inefficient,[26, 27] generate nasal congestion and increase nasal resistance,[28] or promote patient-ventilator asynchrony.[29] These masks, however, have several advantages, including more comfort than full face masks and a lower internal dead space. Several groups preferentially use full face masks because of the frequent occurrence of encephalopathy.[6, 9, 30] The peak mask pressure is an important determinant of leaks, and for this reason the use of a pressure-limited mode is sound and may explain clinical advantages reported in some studies.[30, 31] Fernandez[18] also reported that the use of PEEP in combination with PSV considerably increased leaks in a majority of patients with COPD.

Properly adapting the mask to the patient's face and smoothly starting NIV in the patient with respiratory distress are crucial features for the success of the technique. It certainly requires time and expertise, as shown by several authors.[7, 32] In addition, particular attention should be paid to avoid or minimize leaks around the mask. This may necessitate spending time at the bedside to find the patient's best fitting mask.

Finally, in most cases NIV is only an intermittent support. In almost all studies, the time spent on ventilation has ranged from 6 to 12 or 15 hours a day, particularly after the first 24 hours. Patients with a prolonged and permanent need for ventilatory support can hardly be managed with this technique, especially because it is almost never a full ventilatory support. Because it is used in awake, nonsedated patients, it requires a persistent respiratory drive to breathe.

One last specific feature is the risk of rebreathing of exhaled gas. This may be caused by some of the bilevel airway pressure devices designed for home mechanical ventilation that force the patient to exhale through holes placed on the inspiratory line. The line is usually flushed by an expiratory bias flow, the level of which is dependent on the PEEP set on the ventilator. In case of a low PEEP level or high minute ventilation, substantial rebreathing may occur. This may prevent ventilatory support from reducing $Paco_2$[33] and may cause an increase in the patient's work of breathing.[34] The use of non-rebreathing valves can reduce this problem. Because rebreathing may also be caused by the internal volume of a full face mask, special attention should be paid to this problem.

MODES OF MECHANICAL VENTILATION

Different modes of ventilation can be used. CPAP has been rigorously tested in very limited applications, although it might potentially be applied in various forms of hypoxemic respiratory failure. Cardiogenic pulmonary edema unresponsive to medical treatment is a possible application of the technique,[35] as discussed later. In patients with COPD, CPAP can potentially overcome the load imposed on the muscles by dynamic hyperinflation and auto or intrinsic PEEP.[36, 37] Experience in nonintubated COPD patients is still limited.[13, 38] PEEP combined with a mode of ventilation is commonly used for noninvasive support.[2–4, 7, 8, 39]

Several different modes of positive-pressure ventilation have been proposed, including assist-control ventilation, PSV, and assist-pressure controlled ventilation. All modes have benefits and limitations, and important clinical results have been obtained with almost all.[5, 6, 9, 19] Volume-targeted modes are more sensitive to leaks, and tidal volumes exceeding usual settings have been recommended. Because the peak mask pressure is not limited, a certain number of side effects may be favored by the use of this modality. Pressure-limited modes may help in improving tolerance. A randomized comparison between assist-control and PSV has shown that fewer side effects were observed with the latter.[30] A prospective comparative study by Girault and coworkers[31] in 15 patients with COPD and respiratory failure found again that PSV was better tolerated than assist-control ventilation, although the latter induced a greater reduction in the patient's effort. In one study,[40] the addition of PEEP to PSV did not bring any benefit.

In case of leaks during PSV, the cycling from inspiration to expiration may not be effective, because neither the flow descent nor the increase in pressure can be detected. An adjustable flow threshold may be used to solve this problem, as can the setting of an inspiratory time limit, such as the use of assist pressure-controlled ventilation.

A successful experience has also been reported using proportional assist ventilation in non-COPD patients with various forms of acute respiratory failure.[41]

The effects of all modes of ventilation may differ, however, depending on the level of ventilatory demand. Mancebo and colleagues[42] showed that in conditions of high ventilatory demand, simulated through CO_2 inhalation, ventilatory support delivered with intermittent positive-pressure breathing (IPPB) induced an extra work of breathing, which made the amount of total effort during assisted ventilation markedly superior to the situation of unassisted breathing. This suggests that the capability of the ventilatory equipment to provide flow fast enough to meet the patient's demand is critical in situations of high ventilatory demand and probably explains some failures of the technique in hypoxemic respiratory failure.

CLINICAL INDICATIONS

Patients who experience acute ventilatory failure in the absence of other organ dysfunction, without central nervous system disorders, and with no need for immediate endotracheal intubation (respiratory arrest) constitute the group of patients for whom beneficial results can be expected.

Acute on Chronic Respiratory Failure

Short-Term Efficacy

In patients with COPD, three large prospective, randomized studies demonstrated that important benefits could be obtained,[6, 7, 19] as already suggested by a number of previous studies using historical or case-control or smaller control groups.[5, 18, 30, 43] In a study by Bott and coworkers,[19] 60 patients with acute exacerbation of chronic respiratory failure were randomized to noninvasive nasal positive-pressure ventilation or to standard medical treatment. Improvement in arterial pH was significant compared with the standard group, and a reduction in breathlessness was observed in the NIV group (Fig. 119–2). A benefit in terms of mortality was also documented for the patients in the NIV group who tolerated the technique, from almost 30% to less than 5%. In a study by Kramer and associates,[7] a major reduction in the need for endotracheal intubation was observed in the treated group. This was essentially explained by the subgroup of patients with COPD. Interestingly, in this study the workload imposed on nurses and therapists was compared between the two groups and was found to be similar. Although the type and the time distribution of specific workloads differed between the two treatments, with more work needed in the first 2 hours of NIV, the total work was quite comparable.

In a study by Brochard and coworkers,[6] 85 patients were randomized with or without face mask PSV. The two groups were comparable on admission. The two groups presented with a comparable severity (based on the number of patients with frank respiratory acidosis, hypoxemia, and encephalopathy). The severity was reflected by the endotracheal intubation rate, which reached 75% of the patients in the control group.

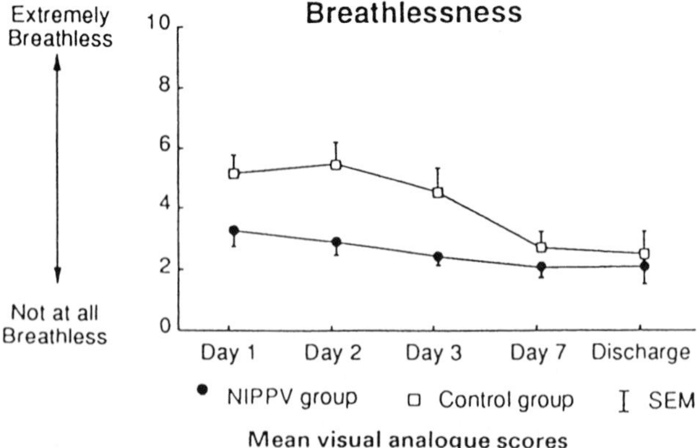

Figure 119–2. Mean score of breathlessness in two groups of patients with acute exacerbation of chronic obstructive pulmonary disease treated with noninvasive positive-pressure ventilation (NIPPV) or not treated (control group). (From Bott J, Carroll MP, Conway JH, et al: Randomised controlled trial of nasal ventilation in acute ventilatory failure due to chronic obstructive airways disease. Lancet 1993; 341:1555–1557.)

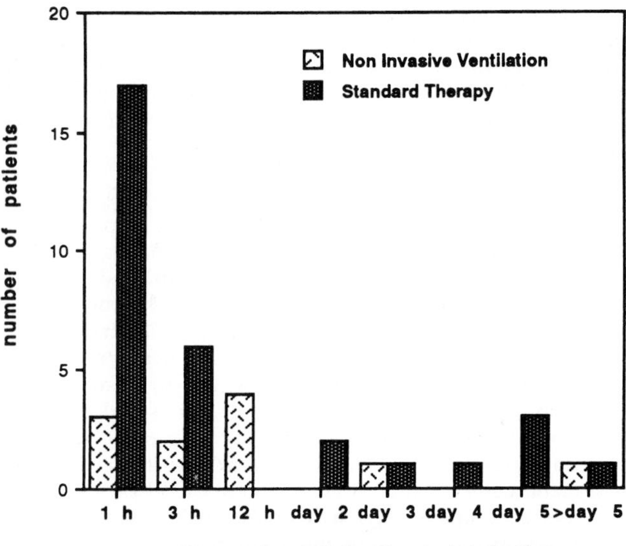

Figure 119–3. Number and time of endotracheal intubation in two groups of patients with acute exacerbation of chronic obstructive pulmonary disease, treated either with face mask inspiratory pressure support (noninvasive ventilation) or standard therapy. (From Brochard L, Mancebo J, Wysocki M, et al: Noninvasive ventilation for acute exacerbations of chronic obstructive pulmonary disease. N Engl J Med 1995; 333:817–822.)

The need for endotracheal intubation was only 25% in the new treatment group (Fig. 119–3). This reduction was associated with major differences in outcome variables. The number of patients who experienced complications during their stay in the intensive care unit (ICU), the length of hospital stay, and even the mortality rate (from 29% to 9%) all significantly decreased with the use of NIV. The study was conducted in a selected group of patients, because patients with comorbidities or requiring a specific therapy were not included.

One study by Barbé and colleagues[44] did not find any benefit of NIV in COPD patients. In contrast with the previous studies, however, the patients experienced very mild exacerbation of their disease and none among the two groups (treated or not treated with NIV) required endotracheal intubation. Therefore, this result does not contradict the previous studies but stresses that NIV is indicated when patients are at high likelihood of requiring endotracheal intubation.

Overall, major benefits were demonstrated, making this technique a first-line treatment for many of these patients.

Long-Term Effects

Confalonieri and coworkers[45] assessed the long-term outcome of 24 patients with COPD initially treated by NIV for acute exacerbation, by comparison with a historical matched control group treated initially by conventional means. Interestingly, they found that the survival rate was significantly better at 6 and 12 months in the patients treated with NIV (71% versus 50%, $P < .05$). This clearly indicated that the initial benefits of the technique were not hampered by a different rate of readmission and that the reduced duration of ventilatory assistance and of hospital stay was potentially beneficial for the patients.

Success and Failure of Treatment

It is still difficult to precisely determine which patients are unlikely to benefit from this technique and when attempts at NIV should only be brief and carefully monitored. One reason is that the efficacy of the technique certainly depends on the skill and the motivation of the staff. Several studies suggest, however, that patients who do not respond to NIV simply have the most severe condition in terms of index of acute decompensation, including hypoxemia, acidosis, and encephalopathy.[6, 46] This suggests that the technique should not be introduced too late, at a stage where either central or peripheral fatigue may be present and where total rest of the respiratory muscles is required. Several authors also suggest that the presence of pneumonia or of severe comorbidities substantially decreases the likelihood of success.[9, 27]

Cardiogenic Pulmonary Edema

Positive-pressure ventilation delivered through a face mask has been used very early in the treatment of cardiogenic pulmonary edema.[47, 48] In addition, there is a sound rationale for this technique, based on the benefits of positive-pressure mechanical ventilation in intubated patients with a failing heart, as demonstrated by Räsänen and coworkers,[49] as well as the deleterious effects of abrupt disconnection from the ventilator and the subsequent changes in intrathoracic pressure, as demonstrated by Lemaire and associates.[50] Several mechanisms are involved in this process, including reduced oxygen consumption, improvement in oxygenation through a decrease in shunt, and direct unloading of the heart resulting from the changes in intrathoracic pressure. The results of Buda and colleagues[51] suggested that large, negative intrathoracic pressure swings, such as those that can be observed during acute respiratory failure, can considerably increase left ventricle afterload. Lowering respiratory efforts and increasing intrathoracic pressure reduce the preload condition of the heart but also reduce afterload to the left ventricle. When cardiac function is essentially afterload-dependent, positive-pressure ventilation may thus result in a better cardiac performance.

The efficacy of CPAP was studied in a prospective randomized study by Bersten and coworkers.[35] In two groups of patients with asphyxic forms of cardiogenic pulmonary edema, the addition of CPAP to medical treatment significantly hastened the improvement in physiologic parameters. CPAP reduced the need for endotracheal intubation from 35% to zero. A similar benefit in such patients was again suggested later in studies using CPAP as well as other forms of positive-pressure ventilation.[2, 11, 52] Bradley and colleagues[53] were among the first to suggest that the beneficial hemodynamic effects were primarily observed in patients with elevated left filling pressures.

To better determine the mechanism of improvement, Lenique and associates[54] investigated the effects of CPAP in such patients on both the respiratory and the cardiac side. Cardiac function was slightly improved under CPAP (similar cardiac output with lower transmural filling pressures), whereas the work of breathing was markedly reduced, suggesting that the reduction of effort played a major role in the clinical benefit of CPAP.

These findings also suggested that other forms of ventilatory support, such as PSV and PEEP, may prove to be even more beneficial than CPAP.[55] This was not entirely true, however, in a prospective randomized study by Mehta and coworkers,[55] who compared CPAP and a bilevel positive-pressure ventilation. Although improvement in physiologic parameters was greater with the latter treatment, they indeed found a higher incidence of myocardial infarction in patients treated with bilevel positive-pressure ventilation. Whether this unexpected result was explained by the randomization process (with more patients admitted with ongoing myocardial infarction) or by the technique itself was unclear, however.

It is clear that CPAP, as probably other techniques able to decrease breathing workload, can be a useful adjunct to cardiac patients with acute left ventricular failure and respiratory distress caused by pulmonary edema as a means to avoid endotracheal intubation. More studies are needed to confirm and extend these findings and determine the optimal ventilatory support for severe forms of pulmonary edema.

Hypoxemic Respiratory Failure

In patients with hypoxemic respiratory failure, results are conflicting. Although a number of open studies show impressive improvement in respiratory function, few controlled data are available to assess the clinical outcome of these patients. In most of the studies, benefits seem to be preferentially observed in patients with respiratory acidosis.[41, 56] One randomized prospective trial by Wysocki and colleagues,[2] conducted in a group of patients with various causes of respiratory failure, did not find any benefit of NIV except in the subgroup with acute hypercapnia. The results of Patrick and coworkers,[41] however, using proportional assist ventilation in non-COPD patients with severe respiratory distress, suggest that searching for an optimal adjustment of the ventilatory settings may be important in these patients. Indeed, the high ventilatory demand of these patients requires a very high quality of response of the ventilator.

The largest series comes from Meduri and coworkers[9] and helps to define indications and contraindications. Patients with severe pneumonia or with the coexistence of COPD and severe left heart failure do not seem to perform as well as patients with pure COPD. Antonelli and coworkers[57] suggested that the tolerance of bronchoscopy in immunosuppressed patients could be improved by performing the procedure during NIV.

Recently, Antonelli and coworkers[58] showed that NIV delivered to hypoxemic patients at the time when they need ventilatory support could reduce complications, especially infections; length of stay; and, potentially, mortality in selected subgroups.

Weaning from Mechanical Ventilation

In patients experiencing ventilatory failure in the postextubation period or the postoperative period, interesting results have also been reported.[1–4, 8, 9, 59] Promising results have been obtained concerning shortening of the weaning period with NIV.[29] Udwadia and coworkers[60] have reported their experience in difficult to wean patients who could be separated from the ventilator using NIV. Recent results by Nava and associates[22] also show that a deliberate early extubation with a switch to face mask NIV can result in significant benefits in outcome, fewer complications, and a reduced mortality at 2 months.

SIDE EFFECTS

The side effects reported with NIV are usually of minor severity, but they may necessitate withdrawal of the technique. These include skin pressure lesions and facial pain, dry nose, eye irritation, discomfort, poor sleep, mask leakage, and gastric distention. Intolerance of the mask or poor adaptation to the patient's face may be a major limitation to the use of noninvasive ventilation. In a study by Meduri and coworkers,[8] two patients among 13 could not be adequately ventilated without major leaks and therapy was therefore withdrawn. One patient demonstrated intolerance to the mask after 2 hours of treatment. Last, two patients developed mild facial pressure necrosis at the site of the mask contact, which healed spontaneously in 2 days. Fernandez and colleagues[18] noted no significant side effects except nose pain in 14 episodes of treatment for acute respiratory failure. In a randomized study by Bott and coworkers,[19] four of the 30 patients randomized to the NIV group could not be ventilated: two because they could not cooperate, one because he was unable to breathe through his nose, and one because he requested the withdrawal of all active treatment. The study by Barbé and associates[44] found that four out of the 19 patients allocated to NIV did not tolerate it. Again, this high percentage might be put into perspective with the fact that, presumably, in this study none of the patients really needed ventilatory support. The edentulous condition has been reported as a frequent cause of treatment failure because of difficulties in proper fitting of the mask.[27] Comatose patients with inadequate protection of upper airways and patients with a frequent need to remove secretions may be difficult to treat with this technique, although these conditions do not constitute absolute contraindications in all patients.

Gastric distention seems to be uncommon with PSV when mask pressure is limited to 20 to 25 cm H_2O.[5] Therefore, routine nasogastric suctioning is not recommended. An increase in peak mask pressure augments the risk of leakage and gastric distention and necessitates tightening the mask more closely, with an increased risk of side effects.

Complications usually associated with mechanical ventilation, such as nosocomial pneumonia, thromboembolic disease, or gastrointestinal disorders, can also occur with prolonged NIV, but a much lower risk of complications is expected, as demonstrated in patients with COPD.[6]

CLINICAL BENEFITS AND CONCLUSION

In many instances, NIV can be used in patients with acute respiratory failure at high risk of requiring endotracheal intubation. This technique requires minimal equipment and can be delivered with either standard intensive care ventilators or cheaper portable turbine ventilators offering a bilevel positive airway pressure. Special attention should be paid to the specific aspects of this type of ventilation, which may be critical to the success of the technique. These include (1) avoiding leaks around the mask, (2) minimizing rebreathing, (3) ensuring optimal fitting of the mask, and (4) trying to adapt the patient to the ventilatory assistance, especially in the first couple of hours. Patients with the inability to protect the upper airway, with severe life-threatening hypoxemia, or with major associated organ dysfunction including shock are unlikely to benefit from the technique or are at high likelihood for development of complications.

In other patients, and especially in the group with acute on chronic respiratory failure, NIV has the potential to reduce several complications associated with mechanical ventilation.[6] Although there is a strong rationale[20] and several preliminary findings,[6, 61] the reduction of nosocomial pneumonia has not been fully demonstrated. It is likely, however, that the main mechanism explaining the benefits in outcome observed with NIV is the reduction of complications associated with mechanical ventilation. Subsequently, a reduction in length of hospital stay and in mortality can result from the use of NIV.

References

1. Wysocki M, Tric L, Wolff MA, Gertner J, Millet H, Herman B: Noninvasive pressure support ventilation in patients with acute respiratory failure. Chest 1995; 103:907–913.
2. Wysocki M, Tric L, Wolff MA, Millet H, Herman B: Noninvasive pressure support ventilation in patients with acute respiratory failure: A randomized comparison with conventional therapy. Chest 1995; 107:761–768.
3. Pennock BE, Kaplan PD, Carlin BW, Sabangan JS, Magovern JA: Pressure support ventilation with a simplified ventilatory support system administered with a nasal mask in patients with respiratory failure. Chest 1991; 100:1371–1376.
4. Pennock BE, Grawshaw L, Kaplan PD: Noninvasive nasal mask ventilation for acute respiratory failure: Institution of a new therapeutic technology for routine use. Chest 1994; 105:441–444.
5. Brochard L, Isabey D, Piquet J, Amaro P, Mancebo J, Messadi AA, Brun-Buisson C, Rauss A, Lemaire F, Harf A: Reversal of acute exacerbations of chronic obstructive lung disease by inspiratory assistance with a face mask. N Engl J Med 1990; 323:1523–1530.
6. Brochard L, Mancebo J, Wysocki M, Lofaso F, Conti G, Rauss A, Simonneau G, Benito S, Gasparetto A, Lemaire F, Isabey D, Harf A: Noninvasive ventilation for acute exacerbations of chronic obstructive pulmonary disease. N Engl J Med 1995; 333:817–822.
7. Kramer N, Meyer TJ, Meharg J, Cece RD, Hill NS: Randomized, prospective trial of noninvasive positive pressure ventilation in acute respiratory failure. Am J Respir Crit Care Med 1995; 151:1799–1806.
8. Meduri GU, Abou-Shala N, Fox RC, Jones CB, Leeper KV, Wunderik RG: Noninvasive face mask mechanical ventilation in patients with acute hypercapnic respiratory failure. Chest 1991; 100:445–454.
9. Meduri GU, Turner RE, Abou-Shala N, Wunderink R, Tolley E: Noninvasive positive pressure ventilation via face mask. Chest 1996; 109:179–193.
10. Padman R, Lawless ST, Kettrick RG: Noninvasive ventilation via bilevel positive airway pressure support in pediatric practice. Crit Care Med 1998; 26:169–173.
11. Meduri GU, Fox RC, Abou-Shala N, Leeper KV, Wunderink RG: Noninvasive mechanical ventilation via face mask in patients with acute respiratory failure who refused endotracheal intubation. Crit Care Med 1994; 22:1584–1590.
12. Benhamou D, Girault C, Faure C, Portier F, Muir JF: Nasal mask ventilation in acute respiratory failure: Experience in elderly patients. Chest 1992; 102:912–917.
13. Goldberg P, Reissmann H, Maltais F, Ranieri M, Gottfried SB: Efficacy of noninvasive CPAP in COPD with acute respiratory failure. Eur Respir J 1995; 8:1894–1900.
14. Diaz O, Iglesia R, Ferrer M, Zavala E, Santos C, Wagner PD, Roca J, Rodriguez-Roisin R: Effects of noninvasive ventilation on pulmonary gas exchange and hemodynamics during acute hypercapnic exacerbations of chronic obstructive pulmonary disease. Am J Respir Crit Care Med 1997; 156:1840–1845.
15. Warren PM, Flenley DC, Millar JC, Avery A: Respiratory failure revisited: Acute exacerbations of chronic bronchitis between 1961–1968 and 1970–1976. Lancet 1980; i:467–471.
16. Marino W: Intermittent volume cycled mechanical ventilation via nasal mask in patients with respiratory failure due to COPD. Chest 1991; 99:681–684.
17. Elliott MW, Steven MH, Philipps GD, Branthwaite MA: Noninvasive mechanical ventilation for acute respiratory failure. Br Med J 1990; 300:358–360.
18. Fernandez R, Blanch LP, Valles J, Baigorri F, Artigas A: Pressure support ventilation via face mask in acute respiratory failure in hypercapnic COPD patients. Intensive Care Med 1993; 19:456–461.
19. Bott J, Carroll MP, Conway JH, Klilty SEJ, Ward EM, Brown AM, Paul EA, Elliot MW, Godfrey RC, Wedzicha JA, Moxham J: Randomised controlled trial of nasal ventilation in acute ventilatory failure due to chronic obstructive airways disease. Lancet 1993; 341:1555–1557.
20. Abou-Shala N, Meduri U: Noninvasive mechanical ventilation in patients with acute respiratory failure. Crit Care Med 1996; 24:705–715.
21. Roussos C, Macklem PT: Diaphragmatic fatigue in man. J. Appl Physiol 1977; 43:198–197.
22. Nava S, Ambrosino N, Clini E, Prato M, Orlando G, Vitacca M, Brigada P, Fracchia C, Rubini F: Noninvasive mechanical ventilation in the weaning of patients with respiratory failure due to chronic obstructive pulmonary disease. A randomized, controlled trial. Ann Intern Med 1998; 128:721–728.
23. Appendini L, Patessio A, Zanaboni S, Carone M, Gukov B, Donner CF, Rossi A: Physiologic effects of positive end-expiratory pressure and mask pressure support during exacerbations of chronic ob-

structive pulmonary disease. Am J Respir Crit Care Med 1994; 149:1069–1076.

24. Ambrosino N, Rampulla C: Negative pressure ventilation in COPD patients. Eur Respir Rev 1992; 2:353–356.
25. Thorens JB, Ritz M, Reynard C, Righetti A, Vallotton M, Favre H, Kyle U, Jolliet P, Chevrolet JC: Haemodynamic and endocrinological effects of noninvasive mechanical ventilation in respiratory failure. Eur Respir J 1997; 10:2553–2559.
26. Carrey Z, Gottfried SB, Levy RD: Ventilatory muscle support in respiratory failure with nasal positive pressure ventilation. Chest 1990; 97:150–158.
27. Soo Hoo GW, Santiago S, Williams AJ: Nasal mechanical ventilation for hypercapnic respiratory failure in chronic obstructive pulmonary disease: Determinants of success and failure. Crit Care Med 1994; 22:1253–1261.
28. Richards GN, Cistulli PA, Ungar RG, Berthon-Jones M, Sullivan CE: Mouth leak with nasal continuous positive airway pressure increases nasal airway resistance. Am J Respir Crit Care Med 1996; 154:182–186.
29. Elliott M, Moxham J: Non-invasive mechanical ventilation by nasal or face mask. *In*: Principles and Practice of Mechanical Ventilation. Tobin MJ (Ed). New York, McGraw-Hill, 1994, pp 427–454.
30. Vitacca M, Rubin F, Foglio K, Scalvani S, Nava S, Ambrosino N: Noninvasive modalities of positive pressure ventilation improve the outcome of acute exacerbations in COLD patients. Intensive Care Med 1993; 19:450–455.
31. Girault C, Richard JC, Chevron V, Tamion F, Pasquis P, Leroy J, Bonmarchand G: Comparative physiologic effects of noninvasive assist-control and pressure support ventilation in acute hypercapnic respiratory failure. Chest 1997; 111:1639–1648.
32. Chevrolet JC, Jolliet P, Abajo B, Toussi A, Louis M: Nasal positive pressure ventilation in patients with acute respiratory failure: Difficult and time-consuming procedure for nurses. Chest 1991; 100:775–782.
33. Ferguson GT, Gilmartin M: CO_2 rebreathing during BiPAP ventilatory assistance. Am J Respir Crit Care Med 1995; 151:1126–1135.
34. Lofaso F, Brochard L, Hang T, Touchard D, Harf A, Isabey D: Evaluation of carbon dioxide rebreathing during pressure support with BiPAP devices. Chest 1995; 108:772–778.
35. Bersten AD, Holt AW, Vedig AE, Skowronski GA, Baggely CJ: Treatment of severe cardiogenic pulmonary edema with continuous positive airway pressure delivered by face mask. N Engl J Med 1991; 325:1825–1830.
36. Petrof BJ, Legaré M, Goldberg P, Milic-Emili J, Gottfried SB: Continuous positive airway pressure reduces work of breathing and dyspnea during weaning from mechanical ventilation in severe chronic obstructive pulmonary disease (COPD). Am Rev Respir Dis 1990; 141:281–289.
37. Smith TC, Marini JJ: Impact of PEEP on lung mechanics and work of breathing in severe airflow obstruction. J Appl Physiol 1988; 65:1488–1499.
38. Miro AM, Shivaram U, Hertig I: Continuous positive airway pressure in COPD patients in acute respiratory failure. Chest 1993; 103:266–268.
39. Meduri UG, Cook TR, Turner RE, Cohen M, Leeper KV: Noninvasive positive pressure ventilation in status asthmaticus. Chest 1996; 110:767–774.
40. Meecham Jones DJ, Paul EA, Jones PW, Wedzicha JA: Nasal pressure support ventilation plus oxygen compared with oxygen therapy alone in hypercapnic COPD. Am J Respir Crit Care Med 1995; 152:538–544.
41. Patrick W, Webster K, Ludwig L, Roberts D, Wiebe P, Younes M: Noninvasive positive-pressure ventilation in acute respiratory distress without prior chronic respiratory failure. Am J Respir Crit Care Med 1996; 153:1005–1011.
42. Mancebo J, Amaro P, Mollo JL, Lorino H, Lemaire F, Brochard L: Comparison of the effects of pressure support ventilation delivered by three different ventilators during weaning from mechanical ventilation. Intensive Care Med 1995; 21:913–919.
43. Angus RM, Ahmed AA, Fenwick LJ, Peacok AJ: Comparison of the acute effects on gas exchange of nasal ventilation and doxapram in acute exacerbations of chronic obstructive pulmonary disease. Thorax 1996; 51:1048–1050.
44. Barbé F, Togores B, Rubi M, Pons S, Maimo A, Agusti AGN: Noninvasive ventilatory support does not facilitate recovery from acute respiratory failure in chronic obstructive pulmonary disease. Eur Respir J 1996; 9:1240–1245.
45. Confalonieri M, Parigi P, Scartabellati A, Aiolfi S, Scorsetti S, Nava S, Gandola L: Noninvasive mechanical ventilation improves the immediate and long-term outcome of COPD patients with acute respiratory failure. Eur Respir J 1996; 9:422–430.
46. Ambrosino N: Noninvasive mechanical ventilation in acute respiratory failure. Eur Respir J 1996; 9:795–807.
47. Poulton EP, Oxon DM: Left-sided heart failure with pulmonary edema. Lancet 1936; 2:981–983.
48. Barach AI, Martini J, Eckman M: Positive pressure respiration and its application to the treatment of acute pulmonary edema. Ann Intern Med 1938; 12:754–795.
49. Räsänen J: Respiratory support in patients with heart failure. Bull Eur Physiopathol Respir 1987; 23:181–195.
50. Lemaire F, Teboul JL, Cinotti L, Giotto G, Abrouk F, Steg G, Macquin-Mavier I, Zapol WM: Acute left ventricular dysfunction during unsuccessful weaning from mechanical ventilation. Anesthesiology 1988; 69:171–179.
51. Buda AJ, Pinsky MR, Ingels NB, Daughters GT, Stinson EB, Alderman EL: Effect of intrathoracic pressure on left ventricular performance. N Engl J Med 1979; 301:453–459.
52. Lin M, Yang YF, Chiang HT, Chang MS, Chiang BN, Cheitlin MD: Reappraisal of continuous positive airway pressure therapy in acute cardiogenic pulmonary edema: Short-term results and long-term follow-up. Chest 1995; 107:1379–1386.
53. Bradley TD, Holloway RM, McLaughin PR, Ross BL, Walters J, Liu PL: Cardiac output response to continuous positive airway pressure in congestive heart failure. Am Rev Respir Dis 1992; 145:377–382.
54. Lenique F, Habis M, Lofaso F, Dubois-Randé JL, Harf A, Brochard L: Ventilatory and hemodynamic effects of continuous positive airway pressure in left heart failure. Am J Respir Crit Care Med 1997; 155:500–505.
55. Mehta S, Gregory DJ, Woolard RH, Hipona RA, Connolly EM, Cimini DM, Drinkwine JH, Hill NS: Randomized, prospective trial of bilevel versus continuous positive airway pressure in acute pulmonary edema. Crit Care Med 1997; 25:620–628.
56. Servera E, Perez M, Marin J, Vergara P, Castano R: Noninvasive nasal mask ventilation beyond the ICU for an exacerbation of chronic respiratory insufficiency. Chest 1995; 108:1572–1576.
57. Antonelli M, Conti G, Riccioni L, Meduri GU: Noninvasive positive-pressure ventilation via face mask during bronchoscopy with BAL in high-risk hypoxemic patients. Chest 1996; 110:724–728.
58. Antonelli M, Conti G, Rocco M, Bufi M, De Blasi RA, Vivino G, Gasparetto A, Meduri GU: A comparison of noninvasive positive-pressure ventilation and conventional mechanical ventilation in patients with acute respiratory failure. N Engl J Med 1998; 339:429–435.
59. Meduri GU, Conoscenti CC, Menashe P, Nair S: Noninvasive face mask ventilation in patients with acute respiratory failure. Chest 1989; 95:865–870.
60. Udwadia ZF, Santis GK, Steven MH, Simonds AK: Nasal ventilation to facilitate weaning in patients with chronic respiratory insufficiency. Thorax 1992; 47:715–718.
61. Guérin C, Girard R, Chemorin C, De Varax R, Fournier G: Facial mask noninvasive mechanical ventilation reduces the incidence of nosocomial pneumonia. Intensive Care Med 1997; 23:1024–1032.

120

Oxygenation Strategy

Catherine S. H. Sassoon, MD • Jeffrey P. McGovern, MD

Gas exchange in the lungs, that is, the uptake of oxygen (O_2) and the elimination of carbon dioxide (CO_2), concerns the movement and distribution of gases into the alveoli *(ventilation),* the diffusion of gases between the alveoli and blood *(diffusion),* and the volume and distribution of blood flow through the pulmonary circulation *(perfusion).* Arterial hypoxemia, therefore, may occur because of the following:

1. A decrease in inspired O_2 tension (P_{IO_2}) (at high altitude).
2. Alveolar hypoventilation resulting in a decrease in alveolar O_2 tension (P_{AO_2}).
3. Impaired diffusion at the alveoli-blood barrier.
4. Altered ventilation and perfusion distribution due to pulmonary or cardiac disease.[1]

During resting breathing, it is unusual for impaired diffusion to cause hypoxemia unless the diffusing capacity, measured with the single-breath carbon monoxide (CO) diffusion method, decreases to less than 45% of the predicted value.[2] Arterial hypoxemia may also be due to admixture of abnormally desaturated systemic venous blood, primarily in the presence of impaired gas exchange and low cardiac output.[3]

Once O_2 uptake into the pulmonary circulation is complete, O_2 is delivered into the tissues. O_2 delivery depends on multiple factors, including arterial O_2 tension (Pa_{O_2}), arterial oxygen hemoglobin saturation, hemoglobin concentration, oxyhemoglobin dissociation curve shape and position, cardiac output, and individual organ perfusion.[1] Tissue hypoxia may occur because of alterations in one or more of these factors.

Enrichment of the O_2 fraction in inspired air (FI_{O_2}) or an increase in the inspired O_2 tension (P_{IO_2}) may be of therapeutic benefit in treating diseases that manifest with hypoxemia or tissue hypoxia. O_2 therapy has been shown to have long-term benefits in the treatment of chronic hypoxemia in patients with chronic obstructive pulmonary disease (COPD).[4, 5] However, evidence of improved outcome from controlled clinical trials is not available to establish the benefit of O_2 therapy for critically ill patients. Such trials are considered unethical on the basis of the pathophysiology of hypoxemia with its consequent tissue hypoxia and grave effects on vital organ function.[6] This chapter discusses oxygenation strategies in general in relation to critically ill patients and specific clinical settings with the goal of improving hypoxemia.

INDICATIONS FOR OXYGEN THERAPY

Supplemental O_2 in acute conditions is indicated when Pa_{O_2} is less than 60 mm Hg or when the arterial oxygen hemoglobin saturation (Sa_{O_2}) is less than 90%.[1] At these values, tissue hypoxia is presumed to be present.[1] O_2 therapy is also indicated for diseases with significant tissue hypoxia despite a high Pa_{O_2}, for example, in CO poisoning (see later).[7]

GOALS OF OXYGEN THERAPY

The primary goal of O_2 therapy is to correct hypoxemia and, thereby, increase arterial O_2 content (Ca_{O_2}). In the presence of normal cardiac output (Qt), correction of hypoxemia will improve O_2 delivery (Qt $\times$ Ca_{O_2}). One measure of the ability of the lung to transfer O_2 to the capillary bed is the alveolar-to-arterial O_2 tension gradient, $P_{AO_2} - Pa_{O_2}$ or $P(A - a)O_2$. P_{AO_2} is calculated by use of the simplified alveolar gas equation, which is based on the principle of conservation of mass:

$$P_{AO_2} = FI_{O_2}(P_B - P_{H_2O}) \times Pa_{CO_2}/R$$

where P_B is barometric pressure (760 mm Hg at sea level), P_{H_2O} is water vapor pressure (47 mm Hg at 37°C), Pa_{CO_2} is arterial carbon dioxide tension, and R is a respiratory quotient estimated to be 0.8.

Both Pa_{O_2} and Pa_{CO_2} are measured from an arterial blood sample. For a healthy, young individual breathing air at sea level, the normal $P(A - a)O_2$ is 11 $\pm$ 3.1 ($\pm$SD) mm Hg, but this normal gradient increases with age[8, 9] and FI_{O_2}.[3, 8] Neither alveolar hypoventilation nor low P_{IO_2} causes an elevated $P(A - a)O_2$ gradient. On the other hand, impaired diffusion, ventilation-perfusion mismatch, shunting of blood past alveolar capillaries, and admixture of abnormally desaturated venous blood all result in an elevated $P(A - a)O_2$ gradient. Depending on the pathophysiologic mechanism of hypoxemia, O_2 therapy may or may not readily correct hypoxemia. A relatively low FI_{O_2} of less than 50% will correct hypoxemia related to all causes of hypoxemia except that due to low ventilation-perfusion mismatch and intrapulmonary or intracardiac shunt. When hypoxemia is not corrected by relatively low FI_{O_2}, the delivery of high FI_{O_2} will have to be augmented with other measures to avoid O_2 toxicity. However, some of the measures intended to avoid O_2 toxicity, for example, the application of positive end-expiratory pressure (PEEP), have been associated with barotrauma and cardiovascular compromise. Therefore, the goal of O_2 therapy is not only to correct hypoxemia but also to prevent O_2 toxicity and the complications associated with efforts to minimize the toxicity.

METHODS OF OXYGEN ADMINISTRATION

In hospitals, gas sources for both O_2 and air are available from wall lines pressurized at approximately 50 pounds per square inch (psi). Flowmeters adjusted to this pressure govern the rate of gas delivery. Standard flowmeters are calibrated to 15 L/min, but when the thumbscrew of the valve is turned wide open (flush), a much greater flow is delivered (~50 L/min). All gases exiting from these sources are dry and must be humidified to avoid desiccation of upper airway mucosa, except at low flow rates of administration.

Oxygen-enriched air may be delivered by noninvasive or invasive methods to maintain arterial hemoglobin at 88% to 90% saturation (60 mm Hg of Pa_{O_2}) (Table 120–1). Targeting Pa_{O_2} at a level greater than 60 mm Hg is unnecessary because the small increments in saturated hemoglobin do not enhance O_2 delivery to the tissues. In fact, if it is associated with a high FI_{O_2}, such a P_{AO_2} level predisposes to pulmonary O_2 toxicity and may be harmful in patients with depressed central respiratory drive or in severe COPD because of the development of acute hypercapnia (see later).[10] When hypoxemia cannot be corrected, various adjuncts to improve oxygenation may be used (see Table 120–1). These measures are discussed later (see specific clinical settings).

Noninvasive Methods of Oxygen Delivery

With all the methods of O_2 delivery listed in Table 120–1, except for the cuffed endotracheal tube, FI_{O_2} can vary, de-

TABLE 120–1. Methods of Oxygen Administration and Adjuncts to Improve Oxygenation

Noninvasive	Invasive

Nasal cannula
Face masks
  Simple face mask
  Reservoir mask
    Partial rebreather
    Non-rebreather
  Venturi mask
 	
Adjuncts to improve oxygenation
  Noninvasive positive-pressure ventilation (NPPV)
	Nasal catheter
	Transtracheal catheter
	Endotracheal tube
	Tracheostomy tube
	
	Adjuncts to improve oxygenation
	Positive-pressure ventilation
	Continuous positive airway pressure/positive end-expiratory pressure (CPAP/PEEP)
	Prone position
	Partial liquid ventilation
	Surfactant
	Nitric oxide
	Prostacyclin inhalation

TABLE 120–2. Desired and Measured Inspired Oxygen Concentration Delivered by Nasal Cannula

Flow (L/min)	Desired FIO_2	Measured FIO_2	
		*Gibson et al.**	*Schachter et al.†*
1	0.24	0.22	0.23
2	0.28	0.21–0.22	0.24
3	0.32	0.22–0.24	0.25
4	0.36		0.26
5	0.40	0.24–0.25	
10	0.52	0.30–0.46	
15	0.56	0.35–0.61	

*Data from Gibson RL, Corner PB, Beckham RW, et al: Anesthesiology 1976; 44:71–73.

†Data from Schachter EN, Littner MR, Luddy P, et al: Crit Care Med 1980; 8:405–409.

FIO_2 = inspired oxygen concentration.

pending on the patient's breathing pattern. The best choice for meeting a low-to-moderate requirement for supplemental O_2 is probably a nasal cannula (Fig. 120–1*A*). Even more important than its comfortability, the nasal cannula allows a continuous flow of O_2 while the patient is eating or expectorating as well as during routine nursing tasks, such as oropharyngeal suctioning and temperature measurement, or when one of the nostrils is occluded (e.g., resulting from use of a nasogastric tube). The continuous flow of O_2 fills the anatomic reservoir of the upper airway (i.e., the nasopharynx and oropharynx). These reservoirs empty into the lungs with each inspiration, even when the mouth is wide open. A nasal cannula, therefore, is equally effective during nose or mouth breathing.[11, 12] Flow rates of O_2 vary from 0.5 to 6 L/min. Humidification must be provided for flow rates greater than 4 L/min. At a given flow rate of O_2, the FIO_2 achieved depends on the patient's minute ventilation ($\dot{V}E$) and breathing pattern. Table 120–2 shows the desired delivered FIO_2 compared with that measured in the trachea.[13, 14] Because flow rates greater than 6 L/min are uncomfortable for most patients, a nasal cannula is unsuitable when the desired FIO_2 exceeds 0.40.

A conserving device has been added to the nasal cannula to economize O_2 delivery. A miniature reservoir is filled with O_2 during exhalation for delivery during inhalation.[15] This means of delivery is more suitable for ambulatory patients.

Face masks can be used to provide higher O_2 concentrations than the nasal cannula, because masks increase the O_2 reservoir above that of the upper airway. To achieve maximum performance from a mask, a tight seal between the mask and the patient's face is necessary, making its use somewhat uncomfortable. In practice, a snugly fitted mask is better tolerated. A face mask is also less practical than a nasal cannula, because it must be removed during the patient's and nurse's activities mentioned before, causing FIO_2 to fall during those activities.[16]

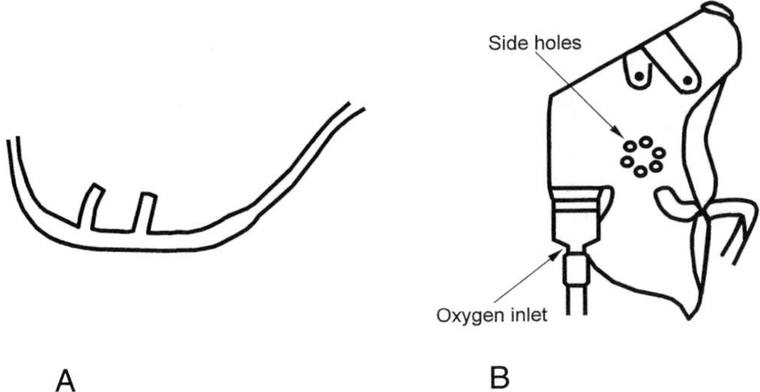

Figure 120–1. Nasal cannula *(A)* and simple face mask *(B)*. With use of the nasal cannula, the nasopharynx and oropharynx act as an oxygen reservoir. The simple face mask adds to the upper airway oxygen reservoir.

There are four common types of face masks:

- Simple face mask
- Partial rebreather mask
- Non-rebreather masks
- Venturi mask

These masks all use a moderate flow of O_2 from the wall source.

The *simple face mask* has an O_2 inlet at the base and holes at the sides for exhalation (see Fig. 120–1*B*). The FIO_2 depends on the O_2 inflow rate, the patient's tidal volume (V_T), and the inspiratory flow rate. When the peak inspiratory flow rate exceeds the O_2 inflow rate, room air is entrained around the mask and through the side holes. The FIO_2 delivered by a simple face mask varies from approximately 0.35 at 6 L/min to 0.55 at 10 L/min.[17] At an O_2 flow rate of less than 6 L/min, CO_2 can collect in the mask, effectively adding dead space (V_D).[18] In general, humidifiers are not used with simple face masks.[18]

The *partial rebreather mask* consists of a simple face mask with a collapsible reservoir bag attached to the base of the mask (Fig. 120–2*A*). O_2 flows continuously to the reservoir bag. During exhalation, about the first third of the exhaled air is returned to the reservoir bag to mix with source O_2; the remainder exits through the side holes. Thus, during inhalation, the patient rebreathes some of the exhaled air. If the O_2 inflow rate is adjusted so that the bag does not collapse during inhalation, the amount of CO_2 contaminating the reservoir bag is negligible. Although this mask allows the delivery of a higher concentration of O_2, the highest FIO_2 achievable with this device is approximately 0.60 with an O_2 inflow rate of 10 L/min.[19]

The *non-rebreather mask* is also a face mask with a reservoir bag filled with O_2 (see Fig. 120–2*B*). The difference between the partial rebreather and non-rebreather masks is the use of two sets of one-way valves. In the non-rebreather masks, one set of one-way flap valves seals the side holes during inhalation so that nearly all the inhaled gas is drawn from the reservoir bag. Another one-way valve is placed between the mask and the reservoir bag so that exhaled gas

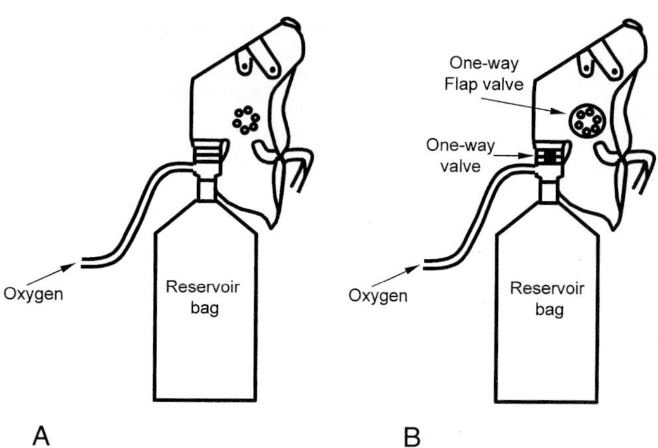

Figure 120–2. Partial rebreather *(A)* and non-rebreather *(B)* face masks. Both masks are identical, except for the use of one-way valves in the non-rebreather mask. The one-way flap valves prevent air entrainment into the mask during inhalation. The one-way valve between the mask and the reservoir bag prevents the mixing of exhaled gas and oxygen in the reservoir bag. Hence, a higher concentration of oxygen is achieved with the non-rebreather face mask than with the partial rebreather mask.

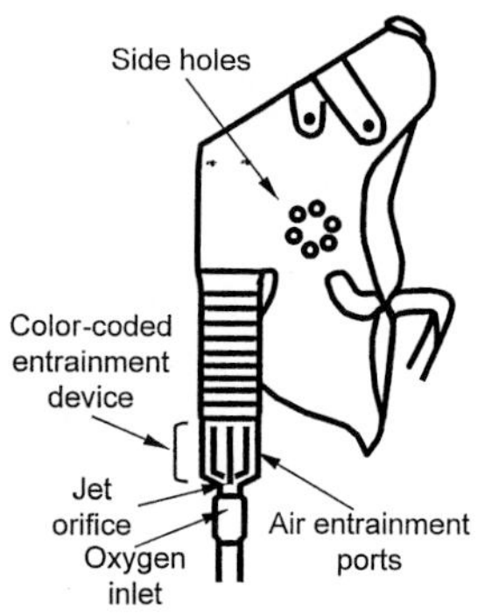

Figure 120–3. Venturi mask. This is a simple face mask with a color-coded entrainment device attachment that can deliver a set oxygen concentration at a set flow rate. The entrainment device allows delivery of fixed oxygen percentages (24%, 28%, 31%, 35%, 40%, and 50%) at set oxygen flow rates ranging from 4 to 12 L/min.

does not enter into the reservoir bag and must exit through the side holes or around the mask. Higher O_2 concentrations can generally be attained (80% to 95%) at flow rates greater than 10 L/min with the non-rebreather mask compared with the partial rebreather mask. Care needs to be taken to ensure that the reservoir bag does not collapse. Should collapse occur, the O_2 delivery rate is not sufficient to meet the $\dot{V}_E$ requirement, causing the patient to struggle against the one-way valves to entrain additional room air. Hence, a patient with a non-rebreather mask must be kept under close observation.

Non-rebreather and partial rebreather masks are used for patients with acute respiratory failure who decline endotracheal intubation, for whom a noninvasive method of O_2 delivery is the preferred choice. These masks are generally used when noninvasive positive-pressure ventilation (NPPV) has either failed or the patient does not tolerate it.

The ***Venturi mask*** is attached to a specific color-coded entrainment device that delivers a set FIO_2 at a set flow rate (Fig. 120–3). The color-coded entrainment device has various orifices of restricted sizes through which O_2 flows at high velocities or as a jet. Air is entrained at the jet site in direct proportion to the velocity with which O_2 moves through the orifice. The mixing of O_2 and air is caused by shear forces occurring at the boundary of the jet flow and not by lateral pressure at the jet orifice.[20] With the Venturi mask, the FIO_2 cannot exceed the specified value, but when the total flow of O_2 and air mixture is less than the patient's peak inspiratory flow, the FIO_2 is less than the specified value.[13] The FIO_2 delivered can range from 0.24 to 0.50. Because the FIO_2 with this method is relatively more controllable than that with other noninvasive methods of O_2 delivery, the Venturi mask is ideal for decompensated patients with COPD with CO_2 retention.

The high-flow, non-rebreather face mask system provides a constant, full-range FIO_2 from 0.21 to 1.0 (Fig. 120–4). This system requires a high-flow O_2 source. With the high-flow, non-rebreather face mask, a blending device that can generate a flow output greater than 100 L/min premixes high-pressure air and O_2 source gas. Flowmeters capable of delivering flow of 100 to 120 L/min can also be plugged directly into a standard 50-psi wall outlet to provide a high flow of O_2 and air. The O_2-enriched air is then humidified and fills a reservoir bag before it is delivered to the patient.[21] The ratio between the air and O_2 flow rates determines the FIO_2. As long as the gas flow meets the patient's $\dot{V}_E$ demand, a constant FIO_2 is provided.

One or two jet nebulizers in "tandem" can also be fitted to a non-rebreather face mask to create a high-flow system with a controlled FIO_2 from 0.28 to 1.0.[21] These jet nebulizers allow a maximum flow of 12 to 14 L/min of 100% O_2. Unfortunately, the total gas flows that are thought to result at an FIO_2

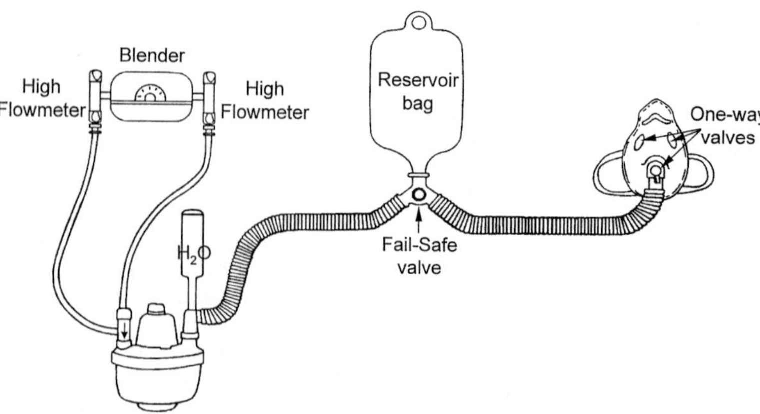

Figure 120–4. High-flow non-rebreather face mask system. This system allows premixing of air and oxygen at high source pressures and gas delivery at high flow rates exceeding the patient's peak inspiratory flow rate. A constant FIO_2 may be achieved ranging from 0.21 to 1.0, but the system requires the following equipment in addition to a face mask: a blending device, high flowmeters, a cascade humidifier, and wide-bore tubings. (Adapted from Foust GN, Potter WA, Wilson MD, et al: Shortcomings of using two jet nebulizers in tandem with aerosol face mask for optimal oxygen therapy. Chest 1991; 99:1346–1351.)

greater than 0.50 are not adequate to deliver the desired concentration of O_2. At a lower concentration of O_2, the total gas flow is high because of the high air entrainment ratios, but at a high FIO_2, the total gas flow is lower because less air is needed to achieve the high O_2 concentration. By use of a lung model, the difference between a set FIO_2 of 1.0 and the O_2 concentration analyzed at the distal airway has been estimated to range from 9% to 50%. The wide range of differences between the set and achievable FIO_2 is a function of the breathing pattern.[21]

Invasive Methods of Oxygen Delivery

Invasive methods of O_2 delivery include nasal and transtracheal catheters and endotracheal and tracheostomy tubes (see Table 120-1). A nasal catheter consists of a tube with several holes at its end, and it is placed behind the soft palate. This catheter should always be used with a humidifier. The nasal catheter is more secure than the nasal cannula but delivers similar O_2 concentrations at similar flow rates.[12] Its long-term use in the critical care setting is less popular than that of the nasal cannula because the catheter must be alternated between nostrils every 8 hours and it causes greater irritation to the nasal mucosa. Most current use is limited to short-term therapy, as might be needed in the recovery room.[19]

Transtracheal catheter O_2 delivery requires a percutaneous insertion of a small catheter into the trachea between the cricothyroid membrane and the manubrium sterni.[22] This mode of delivery is intended for long-term use in ambulatory patients with chronic hypoxemia.[22, 23] It is tolerated by most patients and has an acceptable rate of complications.[24] Its primary advantages are the conservation of O_2 achieved by reduced flow rates and decreased costs.[22, 25] In addition, the method has the benefits of improved exercise tolerance and reduced length of hospital stay for respiratory illness.[25, 26] The mechanism of improved exercise tolerance remains unclear and does not appear to be related to the correction of hypoxemia.

A cuffed endotracheal tube provides a means of O_2 administration without air entrainment. If the patient is not connected to a ventilator circuit, humidified gas is administered through either a T piece or, for a patient who has had a tracheostomy, a tracheostomy mask. When O_2 is delivered through a T piece, the FIO_2 depends on the air entrainment nebulizer system. The delivered O_2 concentration will be constant when the total flow output equals or exceeds the patient's ventilatory demand.[19] An alternative approach to maintaining a constant FIO_2 involves application of wide-bore extension tubing to the expiratory side of the T piece.[19] This creates a reservoir and avoids dilution of the inhaled gas by entrained room air. The length of the tubing depends on the source flow rate and the patient's ventilatory demand.

A tracheostomy mask is a small, open-domed hood that creates a tent-like area over the tracheostomy. The FIO_2 and humidity are variable because of room air entrainment. It is more comfortable than the T piece because it produces less traction.

MONITORING OF OXYGEN THERAPY

With the noninvasive and some of the invasive methods of O_2 delivery, FIO_2 is frequently variable and cannot be accurately determined. Furthermore, the lung gas exchange efficiency cannot be assessed unless the patient is breathing room air. Because the aim of O_2 therapy is the restoration of adequate PaO_2, direct measurement of PaO_2 or SaO_2 is necessary to assess the efficacy of the therapy. PaO_2 can be obtained from arterial blood gas analysis, which simultaneously provides information on ventilation and acid-base status. Arterial blood may be sampled intermittently as dictated by clinical conditions with blood gas analysis being performed in the laboratory.

Alternatively, arterial blood can be sampled and analyzed immediately at the bedside with on-demand extravascular fluorescent sensors placed in the arterial pressure–monitoring line.[27] For measurement of blood gas, blood is drawn into the arterial pressure line and passes the in-line sensors. After measurement, the blood is returned to the patient. The advantages of this method are that it reduces the preanalytic sampling error associated with conventional blood gas analysis, reduces blood loss because blood is flushed back into the patient, reduces the risk of infection to the patient and operator, and allows frequent blood gas analysis.[27] However, with either method, only isolated PaO_2 is obtained and used to make management decisions.

A considerable spontaneous variation in PaO_2 occurs in intensive care unit (ICU) patients who otherwise appear to be clinically stable.[28, 29] A study showed average variations in PaO_2, measured at 5-minute intervals during 1 hour, of 17.4 ± 9.0 (±SD) mm Hg[28]; a similar magnitude of variation was reported in an earlier study.[29] The degrees of spontaneous variation in PaO_2 are similar for spontaneously breathing patients and patients receiving mechanical ventilation.[28] For this reason, therapeutic decisions should probably be based not on an isolated PaO_2 value but rather on a trend value. A continuous intra-arterial blood gas analysis using intravascular sensors would allow trend monitoring of PaO_2 and could detect significant changes in oxygenation at an earlier time. Unfortunately, there are substantial technical difficulties associated with the manufacture of intravascular blood gas sensors that currently prevent the use of this technology in the ICU.[30]

Once supplemental O_2 is administered, it is customary to obtain arterial blood gas measurements after approximately 30 minutes. In a study involving 30 heterogeneous, clinically stable patients receiving mechanical ventilation, the average 90% equilibrium time ($t_{90\%}$) for PaO_2 after a 0.20 increase in FIO_2 was 6.0 ± 3.4 minutes (±SD) with a range from 1.7 to 14.3 minutes.[31] The $t_{90\%}$ is defined as the time required to reach 90% of the final equilibrated PaO_2; an exponential equation is used to describe the rise in PaO_2. For a subgroup of patients with COPD, the average $t_{90\%}$ was longer than that of patients without COPD, 7.1 minutes versus 4.4 minutes, respectively. In a mixed group of patients with and without COPD (n = 8), $t_{90\%}$ was not significantly different after 0.20 or 0.40 increase in FIO_2. The authors also examined the correlations among $t_{90\%}$ and mean blood pressure, forced expiratory volume in 1 second (FEV_1), respiratory frequency, heart rate, and initial PaO_2. Of these variables, mean arterial pressure had the highest correlation with $t_{90\%}$, followed by the inverse of FEV_1. The other variables were not significantly correlated with $t_{90\%}$. The effect of changes in FIO_2 on PaO_2 during mechanical ventilation can therefore be assessed within about 15 minutes.[31] A prolonged equilibration time might be necessary for patients with unstable hemodynamics or with severe COPD.

In contrast to the intermittent measurement of PaO_2, continuous, noninvasive measurement of SaO_2 with pulse oximetry has been widely used to monitor arterial oxygenation.[32] Pulse oximetry has become a standard part of monitoring in the ICU. The principle of operation is based on the differential absorption of red and infrared light by oxyhemoglobin and reduced hemoglobin in the pulsatile fraction of blood under the sensor probe. The percentage saturation of hemoglobin is then calculated from a nomogram derived from studies of healthy volunteers.[33] The device is self-calibrating and simple to use. In both healthy and critically ill patients with adequate arterial perfusion, pulse oximeters are generally accurate at an

TABLE 120–3. Factors Affecting the Accuracy of Pulse Oximetry Saturation

Pulse Oximetry Reading	Conditions	Reference
Falsely high (Spo_2 overestimates Sao_2)	Hypoxemia	36, 37
	Carboxyhemoglobinemia	38
	Methemoglobinemia	39
	Sickle cell crises	40
	Skin pigmentation	37
	Bright overhead fluorescent light	41
	Probe malposition*	42
Falsely low (Spo_2 underestimates Sao_2)	Intravenous dyes (methylene blue, indocyanine green, and indigo carmine)	43
	Nail polish (blue, black, or green)	44
	Chylomicron, intravenous lipids	45
No effect (Spo_2 reflects Sao_2)	Anemia	46
	Hyperbilirubinemia	47
	Cardiac arrhythmia	48
Failure to pick up signal	Low perfusion state (low cardiac output, peripheral vasoconstriction, hypothermia)	49
	Shivering	49
	Motion artifacts	50

*With probe malposition, Spo_2 overestimates Sao_2 at low Sao_2 values, but the effect may be variable, depending on the brand of the oximeter.
Sao_2 = arterial oxygen hemoglobin saturation; Spo_2 = pulse oximetry saturation.

Sao_2 of greater than 90%.[34, 35] The accuracy of pulse oximetry deteriorates when Sao_2 falls to 80% or less in spontaneously breathing healthy subjects[36] and when Sao_2 is 90% or less in mechanically ventilated patients.[37] In patients with hypoxemia, oxygen hemoglobin saturation recorded by pulse oximeter (Spo_2) systematically overestimates Sao_2. Table 120–3 lists other factors affecting the accuracy of pulse oximetry saturation reading.

Pulse oximetry is reliable for use in assessing responses to changes in FIO_2.[37] However, the commonly used target, Spo_2 of 90%, may not necessarily correlate with an adequate Pao_2 value. The optimal Spo_2 target seems to be influenced by the patient's skin pigmentation.[37] In intubated white patients, a target Spo_2 value of 92% is reliable for predicting adequate oxygenation. In black patients, a target Spo_2 of 95% is required to avoid hypoxemia. However, in some patients, this target value may also be associated with a Pao_2 of greater than 100 mm Hg, and if this Pao_2 level is associated with a high FIO_2, an Spo_2 target of 95% could result in O_2 toxicity.[37] It seems prudent to target Spo_2 at 92% or 95%, depending on the patient's skin pigmentation, at the lowest possible FIO_2.

Motion artifacts distorting the accuracy of pulse oximetry saturation readings are a frequently encountered problem in clinical practice[50] causing false alarms.[51] Currently, attempts are being made to improve the signal-to-noise ratio.[52] Another disconcerting problem in the clinical setting is a lack of knowledge among practitioners of the basic principles and interpretation of pulse oximetry readings.[53] In fact, one of the most serious problems with pulse oximetry is the false reassurance of a "normal" Spo_2 reading for a patient who is receiving supplemental O_2. Yet, the patient may have experienced deterioration in his or her clinical condition with the development of life-threatening hypercapnia and may require immediate ventilation.[54, 55]

OXYGEN THERAPY IN SPECIFIC CLINICAL SETTINGS

Acute Hypercapnic Ventilatory Failure

Patients with COPD may experience clinical deterioration characterized by hypercapnia and hypoxemia. The hypercapnia is related to the inability of the ventilatory pump to compensate for the increased load to the respiratory muscles. The hypoxemia is primarily related to ventilation-perfusion mismatch and generally responds to modest levels of supplemental O_2. The administration of excessive O_2 may result in increased $Paco_2$, particularly during acute ventilatory failure.[56, 57] This phenomenon was previously believed to be due to the O_2-induced suppression of the hypoxic drive to breathe with consequent decreased $\dot{V}E$ and increased $Paco_2$. More recent studies of patients with COPD who were clinically stable[56, 58] or during acute ventilatory failure[10, 57] demonstrated that O_2 administration led to only a small change in $\dot{V}E$ that accounted for just a small fraction of the increase in $Paco_2$. A large component of the O_2-induced hypercapnia is related to an increase in VD to VT ratio (VD/VT) or to alterations in ventilation-perfusion matching as a result of O_2-mediated airway relaxation and release of hypoxic pulmonary vasoconstriction.[57] In a computer model, the release of hypoxic pulmonary vasoconstriction and the Haldane effect have each been shown to be responsible for approximately half of the total O_2-induced increase in $Paco_2$.[59] The Haldane effect describes the increase in $Paco_2$ for a fixed CO_2 content as the Sao_2 increases. However, the Haldane effect applies to a closed system; therefore, the importance of the Haldane effect in an open system as represented by O_2-induced hypercapnia remains unclear.

During acute ventilatory failure, O_2 therapy has limited effect on hemodynamics. Patients with decompensated cor pulmonale and peripheral edema manifest depressed right ventricular contractilities with low right ventricular ejection fractions compared with those of patients without edema.[60] In these patients, the administration of O_2 did not reduce mean pulmonary artery pressure ($\overline{Ppa}$) or pulmonary vascular resistance (PVR) or improve right ventricular contractility. Similarly, in decompensated patients with COPD due to chronic bronchitis, the administration of O_2 to restore Pao_2 from an average of 36 to greater than 60 mm Hg did not change the $\overline{Ppa}$, PVR, or cardiac output.[61] O_2 delivery increased from 11.1 to 19.3 mL/kg/min. The effect of O_2 therapy seems to improve systemic O_2 delivery owing to an improvement in Sao_2 without significant changes in other hemodynamic variables.

Whereas O_2 therapy has little effect on $\overline{Ppa}$ and PVR, combined acute O_2 and nitric oxide (NO) therapy decreased $\overline{Ppa}$ and PVR and improved PaO_2 in patients with stable severe COPD.[62] Conversely, NO therapy alone has been shown to cause a significant reduction in Pao_2.[63] However, this combined therapy has not been evaluated during acute ventilatory failure.

The O_2 therapy used during acute ventilatory failure for patients with COPD is the administration of low-flow O_2 by nasal cannula or Venturi mask to achieve a Pao_2 of 60 mm Hg or an Sao_2 of 92%. Given the delicate balance between improving oxygenation and the development of hypercapnia and acidemia, the patient should not be deprived of O_2 to correct the hypoxemia. Intubation is indicated on the basis of objective undesirable effects of respiratory acidosis, that is, pH of less than 7.20, depressed mental status, or the development of cardiac arrhythmia.[64] However, on the basis of data from the comparison of NPPV and conventional treatment, NPPV significantly decreases the frequency of intubation.[65, 66]

Of the four prospective, randomized controlled studies[67-70] comparing these treatments, avoidance of endotracheal intubation was the primary outcome measure in three of them.[68-70] In two of the studies,[68, 69] in selected patients with COPD (mostly with hypercapnic respiratory failure), the number of patients requiring endotracheal intubation was significantly less with NPPV (about 30%) compared with the control group, who received conventional treatment (about 70%). The patients enrolled in the study were highly selected. In the study of Brochard and colleagues, 69% of the patients with COPD who had acute ventilatory failure were excluded from the study. In the third study, in which the investigators evaluated patients without COPD or nonhypercapnic respiratory failure, the number of patients requiring endotracheal intubation were similar between those receiving NPPV (13 of 21 patients or 62%) and conventional treatment (14 of 20 patients or 70%).[70] The high number of patients requiring intubation was related to deterioration of gas exchange, respiratory distress, and encephalopathy. NPPV seems to have less of a beneficial effect for the treatment of patients with nonhypercapnic ventilatory failure.[70] The studies suggest that in patients with COPD who present with acute hypercapnic ventilatory failure, NPPV should be in the first line of treatment along with bronchodilators, corticosteroids, and therapy for the causes of the exacerbation.

The optimal type of mask or mode of ventilation for providing NPPV is unclear. The delivery masks are either nasal or facial masks that are tightly fitted to prevent significant leakage. Both volume-cycled, assist-control (AC)[67] or pressure support ventilation (PSV) with or without PEEP have been used.[68-70] Both modes of ventilation are equally effective in decreasing the work of breathing and the patient's effort, but PSV seems to provide more comfort than AC.[71] Most ventilation modes use an inspiratory pressure of 12 to 20 cm H_2O and a PEEP of 0 to 6 cm H_2O.[65] O_2 is bled directly into the mask to achieve an Sao_2 of greater than 92%. Specific indications and contraindications, selection of patients, ventilator settings, application and discontinuation process, and adverse effects related to the use of nasal and facial masks are discussed in Chapter 119.

Inhalation of NO has beneficial effects as an adjunct of O_2 therapy in patients with adult respiratory distress syndrome (ARDS) (see later). In patients with severe COPD and secondary pulmonary artery hypertension, the inhalation of NO of 40 parts per million (ppm) decreased pulmonary artery pressure from 26 to 22 mm Hg and Pao_2 from 56 mm Hg on breathing room air to 53 mm Hg.[72] The decrease in Pao_2 resulted from worsening of ventilation-perfusion distributions. The intrapulmonary shunt on room air was small (2.7%) and was not affected on breathing NO.[72] Thus, in patients with COPD, in whom hypoxemia is caused primarily by ventilation-perfusion imbalance rather than by shunt, inhaled NO can worsen oxygenation.

Acute Asthma

During an episode of acute, severe asthma, assessment of arterial blood gases is mandatory. Pao_2 decreases with increasing airflow obstruction, but patients with severe airflow obstruction may maintain a Pao_2 of greater than 60 mm Hg.[73] In general, hypercapnia does not occur unless FEV_1 falls below 20% of its predicted value.[73] Accordingly, the development of hypercapnia in the patient with acute, severe asthma is regarded as an indicator of the severity of disease.

Unlike the case in adult asthma, Sao_2 has been a useful indicator in acute childhood asthma of poor outcome and hence of the severity of disease independent of clinical factors.[74] In 280 children with acute asthma seen in the emergency department, the Sao_2 of those who had a poor outcome was 92.7% ± 3.0% (±SD, n = 150), and the Sao_2 of those who had a good outcome was 95.4% ± 1.8% (n = 130) ($P < .01$). Poor outcome is defined as a relapse of the acute asthma or required admission. With the use of the receiver-operating characteristic (ROC), an Sao_2 of 91% was the best threshold value for predicting a worst outcome (i.e., required intravenous corticosteroid and bronchodilator treatment). The result of this study, however, was based on post hoc analysis.

The underlying mechanism of hypoxemia during acute, severe asthma is related to ventilation-perfusion mismatch with no appreciable shunt.[75, 76] In acute asthma, the administration of parenteral bronchodilators compared with the administration of inhaled beta agonist bronchodilators leads to further worsening of ventilation-perfusion matching for similar improvements in flow rates.[77] The worsened ventilation-perfusion inequality with the use of a parenterally administered bronchodilator is due to the substantial increase in cardiac output. Because of the absence of appreciable shunt, these patients readily respond to modest supplemental O_2 with correction of the hypoxemia.

O_2 therapy need not be controlled.[78] The O_2 flow rate can be as high as necessary, although as for patients with COPD it may lead to a worsening of the hypercapnia because of increased ventilation-perfusion mismatching (see earlier). In five spontaneously breathing patients with acute asthma, with a baseline FEV_1 to forced vital capacity ratio (FEV_1/FVC) of 53% and a Pao_2 of 77 mm Hg on room air, $Paco_2$ increased from an average of 37 to 40 mm Hg ($P < .05$) after 20 minutes of breathing 100% O_2.[77] Similarly, areas of low ventilation-perfusion ratio also increased significantly after high FIO_2. Yet, it seems that patients with acute asthma have little risk for development of O_2-induced hypercapnia; however, the study consisted of a small number of patients with moderate airflow obstruction. It is the hypoxemia and, to a less extent, acidosis that are detrimental.

Oxygen administration attenuates exercise-induced bronchoconstriction in patients with stable asthma. Its effects are mediated through the carotid bodies.[79] High FIO_2 may alter the airway responses to bronchoconstrictor and bronchodilator stimuli. In patients with stable asthma with a baseline Sao_2 of 96% on breathing room air, an FIO_2 of 1.0 did not potentiate the bronchodilator response of nebulized salbutamol compared with placebo.[80] The interaction between high FIO_2 and beta agonist in hypoxemic patients with acute severe asthma has not been evaluated.

Other supportive treatment modalities in acute severe asthma are primarily directed toward relief of airflow obstruction and alveolar hypoventilation and are discussed in Chapter 134.

Upper Airway Obstruction

Severe upper airway obstruction may precipitate acute ventilatory failure. The various causes include laryngeal tumors,[81-83] laryngeal edema, vocal cord dysfunction syndrome,[84] croup,[85] and post-extubation stridor.[86] Such patients manifest with respiratory distress, recruitment of accessory muscles, and inspiratory stridor. These symptoms are due to a markedly elevated airway resistance across the obstruction. The gas exchange abnormalities are characterized by acute hypercapnia with hypoxemia that is related primarily to alveolar hypoventilation. However, most of the patients from these studies had preexisting parenchymal lung disease with low ventilation-perfusion ratios resulting in concomitant increases in the $P(A - a)O_2$ gradient. Modest supplemental O_2 corrects the hypoxemia in these circumstances. The respiratory distress and alveolar hypoventilation respond rapidly to the administration of a helium-oxygen gas mixture (heliox—80% He, 20% O_2).[82, 83, 86] This is because the pressure loss due to turbulent gas flow across the obstruction is dependent on the gas density. The density of 80% He is about one third that of room air,[82, 83] and therefore heliox decreases the driving pressure across the narrowed airway. With less pressure required to move gas, airway resistance decreases.

In general, heliox comes as a premixed gas with a concentration of 80% or 70% He and 20% or 30% O_2, respectively. Because of the high diffusibility of He, heliox should be delivered through a closed system such as that with a non-rebreathing mask.[19] When a higher FIO_2 is needed, concomitant supplemental O_2 can be delivered by nasal cannula.

Heliox has been reported to be beneficial in the treatment of both diffuse airway disease associated with acute asthma[87, 88] and COPD.[89] However, these studies were uncontrolled trials. A randomized, crossover, double-blind study of 11 pediatric patients hospitalized for acute asthma (aged 5 to 18 years) reported that 15 minutes of breathing heliox (70% He, 30% O_2) did not show improvement in FEV_1, FVC, or dyspnea score.[90] Peak expiratory flow rate was significantly higher with heliox than with air (56% versus 50% of the predicted value, respectively), but the changes were small. In this group of children with acute asthma, short-term heliox treatment did not confer any benefit.

Acute Hypoxemic Respiratory Failure

An important cause of acute hypoxemic respiratory failure is ARDS. There are many associated causes of ARDS, but more recent investigation has focused on inflammatory mediators resulting in systemic inflammation.[91] "ARDS" is the term generally reserved for the severe end of the spectrum of acute lung injuries and is defined as a syndrome of inflammation and increased permeability associated with a constellation of clinical, radiologic, and physiologic abnormalities that may coexist with left atrial or pulmonary hypertension.[92]

The hypoxemia of ARDS is a result of fluid-filled alveoli and a decrease in lung volume that leads to the generation of right-to-left intrapulmonary shunts. Indeed, physiologic studies of these patients show that shunt is the predominant mechanism for the hypoxemia.[93] In these patients, decreasing the mixed venous Po_2 ($P\bar{v}o_2$) or the administration of FIO_2 of 1.0 did not influence the degree of intrapulmonary shunt.[94] Conversely, the presence of intrapulmonary shunt has two consequences[95]:

1. Pao_2 is markedly influenced by alterations in $P\bar{v}o_2$.
2. The hypoxemia is resistant to increases in FIO_2.

The clinical implications are as follows:

1. A deterioration in Pao_2 does not necessarily imply worsening of the pulmonary edema but may be related to factors that bring about an imbalance between O_2 demands and delivery. These factors include a low hemoglobin concentration, Sao_2, and cardiac output and an increase in O_2 consumption that may coexist in patients with ARDS.
2. With a large shunt, there is little increase in Pao_2 even with the administration of 100% O_2.[95] Yet, because of the shape of the oxyhemoglobin dissociation curve, for a given increase in FIO_2, Cao_2 increases are similar in the presence of a large or small shunt.[95] Because Cao_2 is an essential determinant of O_2 delivery, increasing FIO_2 with a target Sao_2 of 90% is the important initial O_2 strategy. Unfortunately, this response incurs the risk of possible O_2 toxicity because of a high FIO_2. The exact concentration of O_2 and the duration of exposure that induce lung damage in humans are unknown. However, it is prudent to limit exposure to a high FIO_2 (>60%) to as short a period as possible, and for that reason, additional methods to improve oxygenation at the lowest possible FIO_2 become necessary.

Thus, the initial O_2 strategy in patients with hypoxemic respiratory failure is to provide a high FIO_2 delivered through a non-rebreathing mask. The Pao_2/FIO_2 ratio is the best index for monitoring gas exchange abnormalities in patients with ARDS. This is because it has the least variability, particularly at FIO_2 values above 0.50 and Pao_2 values below 100 mm Hg.[96] Hypercapnia rarely occurs with the administration of high FIO_2, unless the shunt is large (>50% of cardiac output).[95] Even at these levels, the severe hypoxemia increases $\dot{V}E$, mediated partly through hypoxia-induced stimulation of peripheral chemoreceptors. The application of positive-pressure ventilation with the intent of increasing mean airway pressure and decreasing shunt is an important adjunct of O_2 therapy.[95] Mean airway pressure can be increased by increasing peak inspiratory pressure, VT, PEEP, or inspiratory time.[97]

In addition to its use in patients with hypercapnic ventilatory failure, NPPV has been applied in the treatment of patients with hypoxemic respiratory failure. In an uncontrolled study, NPPV was used for a relatively large number of patients with acute hypoxemic respiratory failure of various causes (n = 41).[98] Fourteen (34%) of the patients, including two of the three patients with ARDS, required intubation. In a prospective controlled study of patients with hypoxemic respiratory failure, the frequencies of intubation were similar for those treated with either NPPV or conventional treatment[70] (see earlier). It seems that when conventional treatment fails, invasive positive-pressure ventilation is the mainstay of O_2 therapy.

In a randomized study of 64 patients with acute hypoxemic respiratory failure treated at the outset with NPPV or conventional mechanical ventilation, NPPV was as effective as conventional mechanical ventilation in improving gas exchange in the patients who tolerated NPPV.[98a] NPPV was also associated with a lower rate of ventilator-associated pneumonia and shorter stay in the ICU. The stay was short in the ICU partly because NPPV precluded the use of sedation. However, 10 of 32 (31%) patients in the NPPV group required intubation after a mean of 15 hours.[98a] The patients who required intubation were older (mean, 62 versus 47 years) and had a higher simplified acute physiologic (SAP) score (mean, 16 versus 12) than those who tolerated NPPV. Patients with a SAP score of 16 or greater had a similar outcome irrespective of the type of ventilation.[98a]

A study advocated the use of a low VT (<6 mL/kg) and a PEEP level slightly above the lower inflection point on the static pressure-volume curve.[99] In comparison to conventional mechanical ventilation with VT of 12 mL/kg and PEEP sufficient to maintain an Spo_2 of greater than 85% (mean, 13.4; range, 6 to 20 cm H_2O), the low-VT approach improved arterial

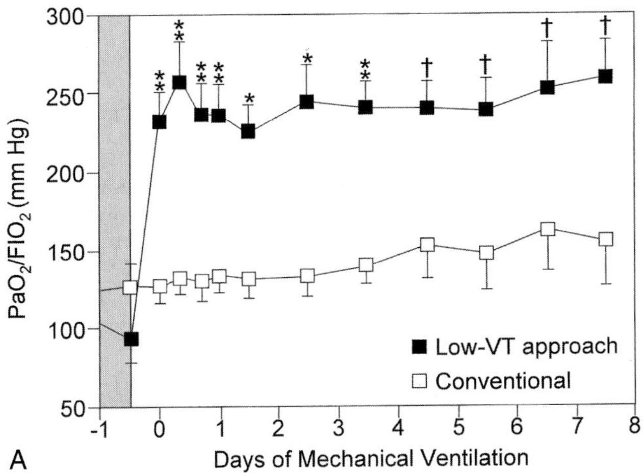

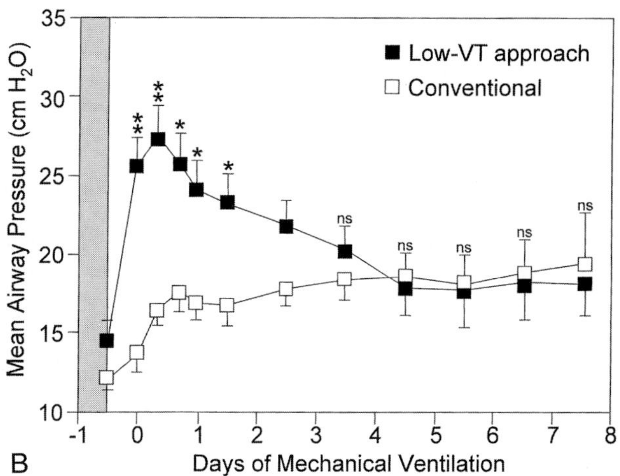

Figure 120–5. *A*, Pa_{O_2} to FIO_2 ratios during low-VT approach and conventional mechanical ventilation. The Pa_{O_2}/FIO_2 ratio increased immediately with the low-VT approach (n = 15) and remained elevated throughout the 7-day course of mechanical ventilation compared with the conventional method (n = 13). *Error bars* represent standard errors of the means. ⁑ = $P < .0004$; *, $P < .001$; †, $P < .03$ by unpaired *t*-test of values from both groups for each day. *B*, Mean airway pressures during low-VT approach and conventional mechanical ventilation. In the early course of mechanical ventilation, mean airway pressure was significantly higher with the low-VT approach compared with the conventional method. Despite similar mean airway pressures following 3 days of mechanical ventilation, Pa_{O_2}/FIO_2 remained elevated with the low-VT approach (see *A*). This suggests improvement in the underlying lung parenchymal process. *Error bars* represent standard errors of the means. ⁑ = $P < .0001$; * = $P < .02$; ns = not significant, unpaired *t*-test between both groups for each day. (From Amato MB, Barbas CS, Medeiros DM, et al: Beneficial effects of the "open lung approach" with low distending pressures in acute respiratory distress syndrome: A prospective randomized study on mechanical ventilation. Am J Respir Crit Care Med 1995; 152:1835–1846.)

oxygenation significantly.[99] In the low-VT approach, inverse ratio ventilation was applied when the FIO_2 requirement was greater than 0.50. Oxygenation, as reflected by the Pa_{O_2}/FIO_2 ratio, increased immediately with a decrease in the shunt fraction (Fig. 120–5*A*). Mean airway pressure was elevated only during the early course of mechanical ventilation, yet the improved oxygenation persisted, reflecting actual recovery of the underlying lung parenchymal process (Fig. 120–5*A* and *B*). With this approach, the average number of days for which the FIO_2 requirement was greater than 0.50 was significantly shorter, 1.1 compared with 5.1 days, than with conventional mechanical ventilation.[99] The frequencies of ventilator-induced complications, such as barotrauma or ventilator-induced pneumonia, were similar for the two modes of mechanical ventilation.

As an extension to this study, the same group of investigators have shown that the low-VT approach improved survival at 28 days (11 of 29 patients or 38% versus 17 of 24 patients or 71% in the conventional mechanical ventilation group had died) and increased the rate of weaning from mechanical ventilation.[100] In contrast to the earlier study,[99] the rate of barotrauma also decreased significantly.[100] However, factors associated with increased survival were the Acute Physiology and Chronic Health Evaluation (APACHE) II score, the mean PEEP, and the driving pressure (i.e., the difference between plateau pressure and PEEP) during the first 36 hours rather than the prevention of O_2 toxicity or the avoidance of barotrauma.

This low-VT approach allows CO_2 to rise, resulting in so-called "permissive" hypercapnia.[101] The effect of permissive hypercapnia on hemodynamics was investigated in a study of 25 patients (mean age, 32 years) with ARDS who received the low-VT approach and 23 patients who received conventional mechanical ventilation.[102] The mean increment of Pa_{CO_2} was 23 ± 11 mm Hg (±SD) from a baseline of 35 mm Hg with a maximum Pa_{CO_2} of 114 mm Hg and a minimum pH of 6.88. Permissive hypercapnia induced tachycardia, increased cardiac output and oxygen delivery, with unchanged O_2 consumption. Mean pulmonary artery pressure increased, but because of the concomitant increase in cardiac output, PVR remained unchanged. Pulmonary artery occlusion pressure also increased while systemic vascular resistance fell. In this study, the relatively high PEEP level (mean, 16.3 cm H_2O) in the low-VT group had no cardiovascular depressant effect. After approximately 36 hours, these variables were similar to those for patients receiving conventional mechanical ventilation. Hence, the effects of permissive hypercapnia on hemodynamics are short term. However, the patients were young and had no preexisting cardiovascular or neurologic disease.

As alternatives to permissive hypercapnia, several methods have been introduced to enhance CO_2 elimination. These include (1) tracheal gas insufflation,[103] (2) extrapulmonary gas exchange techniques (extracorporeal CO_2 removal [$ECCO_2R$]),[104] and (3) intra-vena caval gas exchange (IVOX).[105] Extracorporeal membrane oxygenation (ECMO) is an extrapulmonary gas exchange technique intended to oxygenate blood rather than to eliminate CO_2.[106] These methods are discussed in Chapter 123.

Other adjuncts for improving oxygenation include:

- Prone positioning[107]
- Partial liquid ventilation[108]
- Use of surfactant,[109] NO,[110] and prostacyclin[111] inhalation

Prone Positioning

In published studies[107, 112–117] with a total of 129 patients with ARDS, prone positioning improved oxygenation in 100 patients (78%) with an acceptable degree of adverse events. The criterion for improvement in Pa_{O_2} varied. Improvement gained in prone positioning was generally lost when the patient was returned to a supine position, although some responders continued to maintain better gas exchange.[107] Improvement in Pa_{O_2} was the result of a decrease in the intrapulmonary shunt fraction and better ventilation-perfusion matching.[114, 118]

The mechanism by which prone positioning improves oxygenation in ARDS relates to the decrease in the regional pleural pressure gradient from the dependent to the nondependent region. In the prone position, this gradient is lower and the dorsal (nondependent) region is exposed to a lower pleural pressure, resulting in the recruitment of previously atelectatic alveoli while perfusion is maintained.[118, 119] For that reason, it is suggested that prone positioning is most beneficial in the early stage of ARDS when lung edema and atelectasis predominate.[116]

Blanch and coworkers[116] showed that the duration of ARDS before the prone positioning was significantly shorter in responders than in nonresponders, 12 ± 16 (±SD) versus 33 ± 42 days, respectively. In an uncontrolled study, prone positioning combined with the low-V_T approach of mechanical ventilation improved survival of patients with ARDS.[117] This observation needs to be confirmed in a large, controlled study.

Partial Liquid Ventilation

Partial liquid ventilation (PLV) or perfluorocarbon-associated gas exchange (PAGE), a combined mechanical gas and liquid ventilation technique with perfluoro-octyl bromide (perflubron), holds promise as an O_2 therapy adjunct for patients with ARDS.[120] Perflubron is a liquid with high solubility for O_2 and CO_2 and has a low surface tension and nearly twice the density of water. It evaporates slowly and is distributed homogeneously. Because of the high density, airway secretions and nonadherent cellular debris tend to float on it; therefore, perflubron has a potentially cleansing action. Because of evaporation, PLV requires daily replacement of perflubron.

Perflubron improves lung mechanics by two distinct mechanisms. First, it decreases surface tension by coating the alveolar lining and maintaining alveolar stability. Second, the noncompressible fluid physically distends the alveoli and abolishes the alveolar lining–air interface, and simultaneously, blood flow is diverted to the nondependent regions. These changes result in the improvement of ventilation-perfusion mismatch and oxygenation by recruiting and maintaining recruitment of atelectatic areas and by redirecting blood flow toward the better ventilated nondependent region.[121]

A preliminary study of 10 adult patients with ARDS who were also receiving extracorporeal support found that static compliance improved and shunt fraction decreased from a median of 0.72 to 0.46 during 72 hours after initiation of PLV.[108] Complications associated with PLV were one case each of pneumothorax and mucous plug formation. The overall survival rate was 50%. Further controlled trials are needed to clarify the role of PLV in the treatment of ARDS.

Surfactant

Surfactant reduces surface tension and stabilizes alveoli. In ARDS, both the chemical composition and functional activity of the lung surfactant system are damaged.[122, 123] Surfactant therapy, therefore, is potentially beneficial for the treatment of ARDS. Two types of surfactant are available for surfactant therapy

- Natural surfactant from extract of bovine (e.g., Survanta and Alveofact) or porcine (e.g., Curosurf) lungs
- Synthetic surfactant (e.g., Exosurf)

Natural surfactant contains surfactant proteins B and C, which are important for surface and physiologic activity. Synthetic surfactant does not contain either of these proteins.

The only large controlled study of surfactant therapy has been that of Anzueto and coworkers,[109] who used aerosolized synthetic surfactant in the treatment of patients with sepsis-induced ARDS. Surfactant therapy did not offer any beneficial effects in improving oxygenation or reducing mortality compared with placebo. In an uncontrolled study of 10 patients, also with sepsis-induced ARDS, bovine surfactant (300 mg/kg of body weight) delivered through a bronchoscope increased PaO_2/FIO_2 ratios and reduced shunt fractions.[124, 125] The patients had been on mechanical ventilation for an average of 3 days (range, 1 to 7 days). In half of the patients, a repeated dose of 200 mg/kg of body weight was instilled within 18 to 24 hours because of a decline in PaO_2/FIO_2 ratio after the initial treatment. There was an 80% survival rate (8 of the 10 patients) during the course of the 14-day observation period.

In a preliminary multicenter randomized controlled study, multiple different doses of bovine surfactant were instilled through a catheter placed proximal to the carina within 48 hours of the diagnosis of ARDS.[126] The only regimen that resulted in improved oxygenation and decreased mortality compared with the control group was 100 mg/kg of body weight administered in four doses. The other two regimens studied, 50 and 100 mg/kg of body weight, each delivered in eight doses, did not show any beneficial effects. The 50 mg/kg of body weight dose induced small changes in the concentration of desaturated phosphatidylcholine. The largest dose caused the greatest changes in phospholipid levels, but the beneficial effects seemed to be offset by the large fluid volume. Natural surfactant may have a potential role as an adjunct for O_2 therapy in ARDS, but further investigations are needed to determine the optimal delivery methods, dosing amounts, and timing of administration.

Nitric Oxide

Unlike the situation for patients with COPD (see earlier), inhaled NO decreases pulmonary artery pressure and improves oxygenation in patients with ARDS.[127] NO selectively dilates pulmonary vessels without significant systemic vasodilation because NO is rapidly inactivated by avid binding to hemoglobin.[128] NO decreases pulmonary artery pressure primarily because of a decrease in capillary-venous resistance.[129]

The response to NO depends on the degree of pulmonary vasoconstriction.[130] The greater the vasoconstriction, the more pronounced is the reduction in PVR. Because of regional vasodilation, NO causes a redistribution of blood flow to the ventilated regions, thereby reducing intrapulmonary shunt and improving ventilation-perfusion mismatch and oxygenation.[110] The reduction in shunt fraction, however, is modest (<10%).[110, 131] Only a small concentration of NO (2 ppm) is required to improve PaO_2 or to decrease pulmonary artery pressure,[131] although higher concentrations of 20 to 40 ppm may be required to obtain maximum reduction in pulmonary artery pressure.[132] Long-term inhalation of NO does not induce tachyphylaxis.[132] The toxicity of NO involves elevation of the methemoglobin level and generation of nitrogen dioxide (NO_2), which is dependent on NO and O_2 concentrations.[133] A concentration of NO_2 of 2 ppm is sufficient to alter alveolar permeability, and therefore a high concentration of NO should be avoided.[131]

The effect of long-term NO inhalation on the production of NO_2 is unknown. Abrupt withdrawal of NO may cause rebound pulmonary hypertension and worsening of oxygenation.[134] NO has a promising role as an adjunct of O_2 therapy in patients with ARDS, but a large controlled clinical trial is required to determine whether NO will improve outcome.

In terms of O_2 therapy during mechanical ventilation, the delivered O_2 might be contaminated with a significant level of NO. Pinsky and coworkers[135] reported the contamination of hospital compressed air system with variable levels of NO (<1 to 6 ppm) that vary widely over time. Because mechanical ventilators use compressed air to deliver room air that is blended with pure O_2 to define variable FIO_2, this contamination is a source of occult NO inhalation. This may affect oxygenation. In fact, in postoperative patients with normal lungs, the same group of investigators showed that NO contamination in the compressed air system improved oxygenation significantly compared with values obtained when subjects breathed O_2 blended with pure N_2 for the same FIO_2.[136] Whether this level of NO and its variable level in hospital compressed air system has any physiologic or pharmacologic significance remains to be determined.

Prostacyclin

The use of aerosolized prostacyclin (PGI_2) is another technique that produces selective vasodilation and a redistribution of blood flow to well-ventilated regions.[111] In contrast to prostacyclin infusion, which dilates pulmonary vessels in both ventilated and nonventilated regions, thereby increasing intrapulmonary shunt,[110] inhaled prostacyclin decreases shunt and pulmonary artery pressure.[125] Individually titrated doses of NO (18 ppm) and prostacyclin (8 ng/kg/min) have been shown to reduce pulmonary artery pressure and intrapulmonary shunt to similar degrees.[125] More clinical experience with the application of aerosolized prostacyclin as an adjunct of O_2 therapy in patients with ARDS is necessary.

Miscellaneous Clinical Conditions

Cardiovascular Disease

Arterial hypoxemia is commonly found in the setting of acute myocardial infarction,[137] and supplemental O_2 is almost routinely ordered for such patients. Despite this practice, a controlled, double-blind study failed to show that O_2 therapy had any effects on mortality or the incidence of arrhythmia.[138] In animal experiments, supplemental O_2 (FIO_2 of 0.50) might have had, if anything, a deleterious effect rather than a beneficial one on the basis of alterations in electrolyte concentrations and water content within the ischemic myocardium.[139] However, in an animal study, 100% O_2 and reperfusion therapy reduced myocardial infarct size and improved left ventricular function compared with that of control animals breathing room air.[140] Likewise, simultaneous administration of hyperbaric O_2 and thrombolytic therapy has a synergistic effect in reducing infarct size compared with that of individual treatment alone.[141] These studies suggest that high FIO_2 (mediated by oxygen-derived free radicals) does not extend myocardial injury.

Arterial hypoxemia also developed frequently (80%) in patients with coronary artery stenosis who received premedication before coronary artery bypass surgery.[142] In this group of patients, supplemental O_2 was associated with a reduced frequency of arterial hemoglobin desaturation, but it did not reduce the frequency of myocardial ischemia.[143]

In patients with acute cardiogenic pulmonary edema, supplemental O_2 is part of the standard therapy. Furthermore, in a randomized controlled study of selective patients with acute cardiogenic pulmonary edema, the addition of continuous positive airway pressure (CPAP) of 12.5 cm H_2O to O_2 therapy improved oxygenation and cardiac function.[144] The rate of intubation also decreased significantly, from 36% of patients (18 of 50) with O_2 alone to 16% of patients (8 of 50) with O_2 therapy plus CPAP.[144] CPAP was applied for 3 hours by a face mask. All patients received pharmacologic therapy according to established guidelines. Unfortunately, hospital mortality or length of stay was not significantly different between both groups.

In another study of patients with severe congestive heart failure, the administration of 100% O_2 resulted in a decrease in cardiac output and increases in left ventricular filling pressure and systemic vascular resistance.[145] Increases in O_2 concentration (24%, 40%, and 100%) led to progressive worsening of these variables. Hyperoxia is believed to attenuate the endothelium-derived relaxing factor, leading to unfavorable hemodynamic changes.[145]

Thus, supplemental O_2 in normoxic patients with congestive heart failure may in fact be harmful. Because of the deleterious effect of hypoxemia on myocardial function,[6] we recommend O_2 therapy in patients with compromised coronary arteries or congestive heart failure with associated hypoxemia. Controlled clinical trials are needed to clarify the role of O_2 therapy with or without reperfusion in patients with acute myocardial infarction who do not experience arterial hypoxemia. Noninvasive CPAP has a potential role in the treatment of patients with congestive heart failure, but the duration of treatment and selection of patients remain to be defined.

In the treatment of patients with cardiovascular disease, we must also be attuned to the fact that hypoxemia may be worsened by the drugs used to improve myocardial function. For example, nitroglycerin may induce hypoxemia by increasing intrapulmonary shunt,[146] and dopamine and dobutamine may induce clinically significant hypoxemia by increasing both shunt and ventilation-perfusion mismatch.[147]

Liver Disease

Hepatopulmonary syndrome is a clinical condition characterized by (1) chronic liver disease (generally, but not always, cirrhosis), (2) increased $P(A - a)O_2$ gradient at rest on breathing room air, and (3) evidence of intrapulmonary vascular dilation without significant cardiopulmonary disease.[148, 149] Different mechanisms of hypoxemia are associated with different degrees of hypoxemic severity. With mild hypoxemia, ventilation-perfusion inequalities due to inadequate control of pulmonary vascular tone in response to hypoxia or hyperoxia are predominant.[150] However, as the disease progresses and hypoxemia becomes more severe, intrapulmonary shunt and O_2 diffusion limitation play an important role in the mechanism of hypoxemia.

The limitation of O_2 diffusion is termed *diffusion-perfusion defect*.[149] Because of the marked intrapulmonary vascular dilation, the diffusion distance between the alveolar gas and the center of the capillaries increases. When a person is breathing room air, the driving pressure for O_2 ($PAO_2 \cong 150$ mm Hg) is not sufficiently high to fully oxygenate the center of the capillaries, causing arterial hypoxemia. The high cardiac output characteristically seen in these patients aggravates the hypoxemia further because of the decreased time for capillary equilibration. This process is also exacerbated when the patient stands from a supine position.[151] The mechanism causing pulmonary vascular dilation is poorly understood. There is evidence from experimental studies with animals that NO may play a role.[152] One study showed a significant correlation between exhaled NO and the $P(A - a)O_2$ gradient in patients with hepatopulmonary syndrome.[153]

A modest concentration of supplemental O_2 corrects most hypoxemia, but a high concentration of O_2 is required to correct severe hypoxemia. Pharmacologic treatment (using almitrine bismesylate, somatostatin analog, indomethacin, methylene blue, or plasmapheresis) directed toward ameliorating the pulmonary vascular dilation has been disappointing.[154] Recent experience has documented the resolution of hepatopulmonary syndrome–associated hypoxemia after liver transplantation. The time to improvement of oxygenation varies postoperatively from a few days to 14 months.[155, 156] Transjugular intrahepatic portosystemic shunt may play a role but only as a palliative treatment in patients awaiting liver transplantation.[157]

Pneumothorax

In the critical care setting, pneumothorax may develop spontaneously or by way of an iatrogenic cause (e.g., subclavian catheter insertion, thoracentesis, or positive-pressure ventilation). Tube thoracostomy should be performed immediately when pneumothorax occurs during positive-pressure ventilation with associated cardiopulmonary compromise or when weaning from ventilatory support is not possible.[158] Patients with a small degree of pneumothorax (<20% of the hemithorax) who are not treated with tube thoracostomy or aspiration should receive a high concentration of O_2.[159] This is because the rate of absorption of pleural air, which is slow, 1.25% of the volume each 24 hours, is accelerated when patients are breathing a high concentration of O_2.[160–163]

In studies with animals[161] and humans,[163] supplemental O_2 increased the rate of absorption of pleural air by sixfold and fourfold, respectively. In an animal study,[164] heliox (80% He–20% O_2) increased the rate of absorption of pleural air by ninefold, a rate similar to that achieved with 100% O_2. Use of heliox could avoid the potentially serious adverse effects associated with breathing a high concentration of O_2. Clinical trials have yet to be performed to confirm these results.

Carbon Monoxide Poisoning

Carbon monoxide results from incomplete combustion of organic material. Acute CO inhalation may result from accidental (e.g., smoke inhalation) or deliberate (e.g., suicidal attempts) exposure. CO induces tissue hypoxia through the following mechanisms:

1. CO has a higher affinity for hemoglobin than O_2 does; hence, CO replaces hemoglobin and makes it unavailable for O_2 transport.
2. The O_2-hemoglobin dissociation curve shifts to the left, decreasing the unloading of O_2 at the tissue level.
3. Cytochrome in cells and myoglobin in muscle are partially inactivated.[165]

These changes result in generalized tissue hypoxia. The brain and myocardium are the most susceptible organs affected.

Whenever CO poisoning is suspected, CO-hemoglobin levels should be determined with a CO oximeter.[166] The level of CO-hemoglobin does not correlate with the clinical manifestations of CO poisoning. The CO-hemoglobin level obtained from a venous sample can be used to accurately predict the level in arterial blood,[167] and thus rapid screening of patients with suspected CO poisoning can be performed without the need for arterial puncture. In CO poisoning, Pa_{O_2}, which reflects O_2 physically dissolved in plasma, is normal unless lung complications arise. Pulse oximetry is unreliable because of a spuriously high reading of Sp_{O_2} (see Table 120–3) due to the erroneous detection of CO-hemoglobin as oxyhemoglobin.

When CO poisoning is suspected, 100% O_2 should be administered immediately through a non-rebreathing face mask without waiting for the result of the CO-hemoglobin determination. Severe poisoning may be indicated by coma, seizures, neurologic deficit, cardiovascular instability, pulmonary edema, or metabolic acidosis.[168] Although there is no consensus for grading the severity of CO poisoning, in cases of severe CO poisoning or when the CO-hemoglobin level is greater than 25%, treatment with hyperbaric O_2 is recommended.[168, 169] This recommendation is based on the shorter half-lives of CO elimination on breathing 100% O_2 (80 min) and with hyperbaric O_2 therapy at 3 atm (23 min), compared with that of breathing room air (320 min).[170] However, evidence from a study[171] did not support the superiority of hyperbaric over normobaric O_2 therapy in mild-to-moderate CO poisoning.

Conversely, in a randomized, nonblinded comparative trial of normobaric and hyperbaric O_2 therapies in patients with mild-to-moderate CO poisoning, delayed neurologic sequelae occurred in seven of the 30 (23%) patients in the normobaric group, whereas there was no evidence of delayed neurologic

TABLE 120–4. Diseases for Which Hyperbaric Oxygen Is Currently Used

Diseases for Which the Weight of Scientific Evidence Supports Hyperbaric Oxygen as Effective Therapy
Primary therapy
Arterial gas embolism
Decompression sickness
Exceptional blood-loss anemia
Severe carbon monoxide poisoning
Adjunctive therapy
Clostridial myonecrosis
Compromised skin grafts and flaps
Osteoradionecrosis prevention
Diseases for Which the Weight of Scientific Evidence Suggests Hyperbaric Oxygen May Be Helpful
Primary therapy
Less severe carbon monoxide poisoning
Adjunctive therapy
Acute traumatic ischemic injury
Osteoradionecrosis
Refractory osteomyelitis
Selective problem wounds
Radiation-induced soft-tissue injury
Diseases for Which the Weight of Scientific Evidence Does Not Support the Use of Hyperbaric Oxygen, but for Which It May Be Helpful
Adjunctive therapy
Necrotizing fasciitis
Thermal burns

From Tibbees PM, Edelsberg JS: Hyperbaric oxygen therapy. N Engl J Med 1996; 334:1642–1648.

sequelae in the hyperbaric O_2 group.[172] Delayed neurologic sequelae developed on average 6 days after poisoning and persisted for 41 days. In this study,[172] hyperbaric O_2 therapy was administered at 2.8 atm for 30 minutes followed by administration at 2.0 atm for 90 minutes.

It appears that treatment with hyperbaric O_2 reduces the frequency of delayed neurologic sequelae, but unfortunately, the study was not blinded and there was no pretreatment assessment of neuropsychological function.[173] Because hyperbaric O_2 therapy is the fastest method of reducing the potentially life-threatening effects of acute CO poisoning, patients with severe CO poisoning should receive at least one treatment with hyperbaric O_2.[168] In addition to severe CO poisoning, other therapeutic uses of hyperbaric O_2 are listed in Table 120–4.

Sickle Cell Crisis

Sickle cell anemia involves two clinical features: (1) chronic hemolysis and (2) acute, episodic vaso-occlusive crisis that may cause organ failure.

The second feature, with its associated presentation of chest pain, fever, leukocytosis, and radiographic changes consisting of pulmonary infiltrates, with or without hypoxemia, is termed the *acute chest syndrome*.[174] It is difficult to distinguish from an infectious cause. It is also an important cause of morbidity and a potentially fatal complication in adult sickle cell disease.[175] The pathophysiologic process of the acute vaso-occlusive episodes is postulated on the basis of the presence of the deoxyhemoglobin S polymer and the formation of rigid diskotic cells in the microcirculation where P_{O_2} is decreased.[176]

The initial management of sickle cell crisis consists of fluids, analgesia, and the administration of O_2 in patients with hypoxemia. Monitoring of O_2 therapy should include arterial blood gas analysis, because pulse oximetry reading provides falsely high SaO_2 during sickle cell crisis[40] (see Table 120-3). This is because of both the elevated endogenous CO-hemoglobin[166] and alterations in the O_2-hemoglobin dissociation curve.[40] The $P(A - a)O_2$ on room air has also been useful in predicting the severity of the vaso-occlusive crisis and the need for blood transfusion.[177]

The role of O_2 therapy in the absence of hypoxemia is conflicting. O_2 is a potent antisickling agent.[178] Oxygenated erythrocytes cannot sickle, and cells sickled by deoxygenation return to normal shape when they are oxygenated. An earlier study reported the benefit of O_2 therapy during sickle cell crisis,[179] but later studies did not show the beneficial effect of supplemental O_2.[180, 181] O_2 inhalation did not reduce the degree or duration of painful crisis or the requirement for analgesia. The role of O_2 therapy in the management of these patients remains to be defined.

Cluster Headache

Cluster headache is a variety of vasodilating headache characterized by one to several attacks recurring every 24 hours, during several weeks or months, with headache-free periods between each attack. Besides pharmacotherapy, treatment may include the administration of 100% O_2 through a nonrebreathing mask.

In a double-blind study comparing the breathing of O_2 with the breathing of room air, O_2 breathing relieved the subjective symptoms of headache significantly. Nine of the 16 (56%) patients who breathed O_2 experienced complete or substantial relief in 80% or more of their cluster headaches. In contrast, only one of the 14 (7%) patients who breathed room air experienced any relief. The average relief score with O_2 was also significantly higher than with room air, that is, 1.93 versus 0.77 (a higher score indicates greater relief). The benefit conferred by O_2 may be due to vasoconstriction of the involved intracranial and extracranial vessels.[182]

ADVERSE EFFECTS OF OXYGEN THERAPY

The adverse effects associated with O_2 therapy may be related to the device for O_2 administration or the high concentration of O_2. Some of the adverse effects related to the device for O_2 delivery are minor irritation of nasal mucosa (nasal cannula), conjunctivitis[183] and massive epistaxis (NPPV),[184] pneumocephalus (nasal catheter or NPPV),[185, 186] and inspissated secretions and pneumomediastinum (tracheal catheter).[22] Other complications associated with invasive mechanical ventilation, including barotrauma and volutrauma, are discussed in Chapters 114 and 115.

The administration of 100% O_2 induces hypercapnia as a result of increased ventilation-perfusion mismatch in patients with severe COPD[57] and decreases cardiac output as a result of increased systemic vascular resistance in patients with congestive heart failure[145] (see earlier). High concentration of O_2 also leads to absorption atelectasis[187] and pulmonary oxygen toxicity.[188] The development of absorption atelectasis depends on the presence of low ventilation-perfusion areas, a concomitant fall in mixed venous PO_2, a decreasing mixed venous nitrogen tension (PN_2), and a high FIO_2 greater than 0.60.[189] However, in patients with acute respiratory failure, absorption atelectasis may develop at an FIO_2 of 0.50.[190]

Hyperoxia is presumed to cause pulmonary oxygen toxicity by increasing intracellular concentration of O_2 that leads to chemical and enzymatic production of free radicals (superoxide ions $[O_2^-]$, hydroxyl ions $[OH^-]$, singlet O_2 molecules $[^1O_2]$, and hydrogen peroxide $[H_2O_2]$) at a rate that overwhelms the natural defenses of the cells (antioxidants).[188] O_2 free radicals react with and damage important biomolecules, including enzymes, membrane lipids, and nucleic acids, causing cell damage and, eventually, cell death. In baboons, the histologic changes in the early stage (40 to 66 hours of exposure to 100% O_2 at 1 atm) of O_2 toxicity consist of endothelial cell damage that progresses to increased interstitial cellularity of inflammatory cells. In the late stage (after 80 hours of exposure), extensive capillary injury, interstitial edema, bare basement membrane with fibrin deposition, type I alveolar cell destruction, and concomitant proliferation of type II cells develop.[191]

Factors contributing to the development of O_2 toxicity include

- FIO_2
- Duration of exposure
- Barometric pressure under which exposure occurs

The safe level of FIO_2 or the duration of exposure that produces O_2 toxicity in humans has not been established, but when the FIO_2 requirement exceeds 0.60, efforts should be made to improve the efficiency of pulmonary gas exchange. These include optimizing PEEP, V_T, prone positioning, and other measures mentioned before. In baboons exposed to hyperoxia, aerosolized synthetic surfactant appears to ameliorate the effect of pulmonary O_2 toxicity.[192] However, whether the administration of surfactant or exogenous antioxidants in humans would reduce hyperoxia-induced lung injury is unclear.[193]

Adverse effects of hyperbaric O_2 exposure may be related to the direct toxic effect of O_2 or the rapid pressure changes (barotrauma).[171] Pulmonary O_2 toxicity, myopia, and cataract formation may develop as a result of the direct effect of O_2. Rupture of the tympanic membrane, middle ear or sinus trauma, pneumothorax, and air embolism are adverse effects due to barotrauma.

Indiscriminate use of O_2 is dangerous; however, O_2 should never be withheld in the management of the critically ill patient because of fears of toxicity. The sequelae of hypoxemia are life-threatening, whereas O_2 toxicity takes many hours to develop.

References

1. Fulmer JD, Snider GL: American College of Chest Physicians (ACCP)–National Heart, Lung and Blood Institute (NHLBI) Conference on oxygen therapy. Chest 1984; 86:234–247.
2. Murray JF: Diffusion of gases, oxyhemoglobin equilibrium, and carbon dioxide equilibrium. *In:* The Normal Lung. 3rd ed. Murray JF (Ed). Philadelphia, WB Saunders, 1986, pp 163–182.
3. West JB, Wagner PD: Pulmonary gas exchange. *In:* Lung Biology in Health and Disease. Vol 3. Bioengineering Aspects of the Lung. West JB (Ed). New York, Marcel Dekker, 1981, pp 361–457.
4. Stuart-Harris C, Bishop JM, Clark TJH, et al: Long term domiciliary oxygen therapy in chronic hypoxic cor pulmonale complicating chronic bronchitis and emphysema. Lancet 1981; 1:681–686.
5. Nocturnal Oxygen Therapy Trials Group: Continuous or nocturnal oxygen therapy in hypoxemic chronic obstructive lung disease. Ann Intern Med 1980; 93:391–398.
6. Walley KR, Becker CJ, Hogan RA, et al: Progressive hypoxemia limits left ventricular oxygen consumption and contractility. Circ Res 1988; 63:849–859.
7. Hall J, Wood LDH: Oxygen therapy. *In:* The Lung: Scientific Foundations. Crystal RG, West JB (Eds-in-chief). New York, Raven Press, 1991, pp 2143–2153.
8. Harris EA, Kenyon AM, Nisbet HD, et al: The normal alveolar-arterial oxygen tension gradient in man. Clin Sci Mol Med 1974; 46:89–104.
9. Cerretelli P, di Prampero PE: Gas exchange. *In:* The Lung: Scientific Foundations. Crystal RG, West JB (Eds-in-chief). New York, Raven Press, 1991, pp 1565–1572.

10. Aubier M, Murciano D, Fournier M, et al: Central respiratory drive in acute respiratory failure of patients with chronic obstructive pulmonary disease. Am Rev Respir Dis 1980; 122:191-199.
11. Kory RC, Bergmann JC, Sweet RD, et al: Comparative evaluation of oxygen therapy techniques. JAMA 1962; 179:123-128.
12. Shulman M, Schmidt G, Sadove MS: Evaluation of oxygen therapy devices by arterial oxygen tension. Dis Chest 1969; 56:356-359.
13. Gibson RL, Comer PB, Beckham RW, et al: Actual tracheal oxygen concentrations with commonly used oxygen equipment. Anesthesiology 1976; 44:71-73.
14. Schachter EN, Littner MR, Luddy P, et al: Monitoring of oxygen delivery systems in clinical practice. Crit Care Med 1980; 8:405-409.
15. Tiep B: Portable oxygen therapy with oxygen conserving devices and methodologies. Monaldi Arch Chest Dis 1995; 50:51-57.
16. Nolan KM, Winyard JA, Goldhill R: Comparison of nasal cannula with face mask for oxygen administration to postoperative patients. Br J Anaesth 1993; 70:440-442.
17. Collis JM; Bethune DW: Oxygen by face mask and nasal catheter. Lancet 1967; 1:787-788.
18. Malloy R, Pierce M: Oxygen therapy. *In:* Comprehensive Respiratory Care. Dantzker DR, MacIntyre NR, Bakow ED (Eds). Philadelphia, WB Saunders, 1995, pp 499-519.
19. Scanlan CL, Thalken R: Medical gas therapy. *In:* Egan's Fundamentals of Respiratory Care. 6th ed. Scanlan CL, Spearman C, Sheldon RL (Eds). St. Louis, Mosby-Year Book, 1995, pp 702-741.
20. Scacci R: Air entrainment masks; jet mixing is how they work; the Bernoulli and Venturi principles are how they don't. Respir Care 1979; 24:928-931.
21. Foust GN, Potter WA, Wilson MD, et al: Shortcomings of using two jet nebulizers in tandem with aerosol face mask for optimal oxygen therapy. Chest 1991; 99:1346-1351.
22. Christopher KL, Spofforo BT, Petrun MD, et al: A program for transtracheal oxygen delivery. Assessment of safety and efficacy. Ann Intern Med 1987; 107:802-808.
23. Christopher KL, Spofforo BT, Brannin PK, et al: Transtracheal oxygen therapy for refractory hypoxemia. JAMA 1986; 256:494-497.
24. Hoffman LA, Johnson JT, Wesmiller SW, et al: Transtracheal delivery of oxygen: Efficacy and safety for long-term continuous therapy. Ann Otol Rhinol Laryngol 1991; 100:108-115.
25. Hoffman LA, Wesmiller SW, Sciurba FC, et al: Nasal cannula and transtracheal oxygen delivery. A comparison of patient response after 6 months of each technique. Am Rev Respir Dis 1992; 145:827-831.
26. Bloom BS, Daniel JM, Wiseman M, et al: Transtracheal oxygen delivery and patients with chronic obstructive pulmonary disease. Respir Med 1989; 83:281-288.
27. Mahutte CK, Sasse SA, Chen PA, et al: Performance of a patient-dedicated, on-demand blood gas monitor in medical ICU patients. Am J Respir Crit Care Med 1994; 150:865-869.
28. Sasse SA, Chen PA, Mahutte CK: Variability of arterial blood gas values over time in stable medical ICU patients. Chest 1994; 106:187-193.
29. Thorson SH, Marini JJ, Pierson DJ, et al: Variability of arterial blood gas values in stable patients in the ICU. Chest 1983; 84:14-18.
30. Mahutte CK: Continuous intravascular and on-demand extravascular arterial blood-gas monitoring. *In:* Principles and Practice of Critical Care Monitoring. Tobin MJ (Ed). New York, McGraw-Hill, 1998, pp 243-259.
31. Sasse SA, Jaffe MB, Chen PA, et al: Arterial oxygenation time after FIO_2 increase in mechanically ventilated patients. Am J Respir Crit Care Med 1995; 152:148-152.
32. Jubran A: Pulse oximetry. *In:* Principles and Practice of Critical Care Monitoring. Tobin MJ (Ed). New York, McGraw-Hill, 1998, pp 261-287.
33. Tremper KK, Barker SJ: Pulse oximetry. Anesthesiology 1989; 70:98-108.
34. Morris RW, Nairn M, Torda TA: A comparison of 15 pulse oximeters: Part I. A clinical comparison. Part II. A test of performance under conditions of poor perfusion. Anaesth Intensive Care 1989; 17:62-82.
35. Webb RK, Ralston AC, Runciman WB: Potential errors in pulse oximetry: II. Effects of changes in saturation and signal quality. Anaesthesia 1991; 96:207-212.
36. Hannhart B, Habere JP, Saunier C, et al: Accuracy and precision of 14 pulse oximeters. Eur Respir J 1991; 4:115-119.
37. Jubran A, Tobin MJ: Reliability of pulse oximetry in titrating supplemental oxygen therapy in ventilator-dependent patients. Chest 1990; 97:1420-1425.
38. Barker SJ, Tremper KK: The effect of carbon monoxide inhalation on pulse oximeter signal detection. Anesthesiology 1987; 67:599-603.
39. Barker SJ, Tremper KK, Hyatt J: Effects of methemoglobinemia on pulse oximetry and mixed-venous oximetry. Anesthesiology 1989; 70:112-117.
40. Craft JA, Alessandrini E, Kenney LB, et al: Comparison of oxygenation measurements in pediatric patients during sickle cell crises. J Pediatr 1994; 124:93-95.
41. Hanowell L, Eisele JH Jr, Downs D: Ambient light affects pulse oximeters. Anesthesiology 1987; 67:864-865.
42. Barker SJ, Hyatt J, Shah NK, et al: The effect of sensor malpositioning on pulse oximeter accuracy during hypoxemia. Anesthesiology 1993; 79:248-254.
43. Kessler MR, Eide T, Humayun B, et al: Spurious pulse oximeter desaturations with methylene blue injection. Anesthesiology 1986; 65:435-436.
44. Cote CJ, Goldstein EA, Fuchsman WH, et al: The effect of nail polish on pulse oximetry. Anesth Analg 1989; 67:683-686.
45. Cane RD, Harrison RA, Shapiro BA, et al: The spectrophotometric absorbance of Intralipid. Anesthesiology 1980; 53:53-55.
46. Jay GD, Hughes L, Renzi FP: Pulse oximetry is accurate in acute anemia from hemorrhage. Ann Emerg Med 1994; 24:32-35.
47. Chelluri L, Snyder JV, Bird JR: Accuracy of pulse oximetry in patients with hyperbilirubinemia. Respir Care 1991; 36:1383-1386.
48. Wong DH, Tremper KK, Davidson J, et al: Pulse oximetry is accurate in patients with dysrhythmias and a pulse deficit. Anesthesiology 1989; 70:1024-1025.
49. Clayton D, Webb RK, Ralston AC, et al: A comparison of the performance of 20 pulse oximeters under conditions of poor perfusion. Anesthesia 1991; 46:3-10.
50. Wukitsch MW, Tobler D, Pologe J, et al: Pulse oximetry: An analysis of theory, technology and practice. J Clin Monit 1988; 4:290-301.
51. Tsien CL, Fackler JC: Poor prognosis for existing monitors in the intensive care unit. Crit Care Med 1997; 25:614-619.
52. Barker SJ, Shah NK: The effects of motion on the performance of pulse oximeters in volunteers (revised publication). Anesthesiology 1997; 86:101-108.
53. Stoneham MD, Saville GM, Wilson IH: Knowledge about pulse oximetry among medical and nursing staff. Lancet 1994; 344:1339-1342.
54. Davidson JAH, Hosie HE: Limitations of pulse oximetry: Respiratory insufficiency—a failure of detection. BMJ 1993; 307:372-373.
55. Hutton P, Clutton-Brock T: The benefits and pitfalls of pulse oximetry. BMJ 1993; 307:457-458.
56. Dick CR, Liu Z, Sassoon CSH, et al: O_2-induced change in ventilation and ventilatory drive in COPD. Am J Respir Crit Care Med 1997; 155:609-614.
57. Aubier M, Murciano D, Milic-Emili J, et al: Effect of administration of O_2 on ventilation and blood gases in patients with chronic pulmonary disease during acute respiratory failure. Am Rev Respir Dis 1980; 122:747-754.
58. Sassoon CSH, Hassell KT, Mahutte CK: Hyperoxic-induced hypercapnia in stable chronic obstructive pulmonary disease. Am Rev Respir Dis 1987; 135:907-911.
59. Hanson CW III, Marshall BE, Frasch HF, et al: Causes of hypercarbia with oxygen therapy in patients with chronic obstructive pulmonary disease. Crit Care Med 1996; 24:23-28.
60. Macnee W, Wathen CG, Flenley DC, et al: The effects of controlled oxygen therapy on ventricular function in patients with stable and decompensated cor pulmonale. Am Rev Respir Dis 1988; 137:1289-1295.
61. Esteban A, Cerda E, De la Cal MA, et al: Hemodynamic effects of oxygen therapy in patients with acute exacerbations of chronic obstructive pulmonary disease. Chest 1993; 104:471-475.

62. Yoshida M, Taguchi O, Gabazza EC, et al: Combined inhalation of nitric oxide and oxygen in chronic obstructive pulmonary disease. Am J Respir Crit Care Med 1997; 155:526–529.
63. Katayama Y, Higenbottam TW, Diaz de Atauri MJ, et al: Inhaled nitric oxide and arterial oxygen tension in patients with chronic obstructive pulmonary disease and severe pulmonary hypertension. Thorax 1997; 52:120–124.
64. Feihl F, Perret C: Permissive hypercapnia. How permissive should we be? Am J Respir Crit Care Med 1994; 150:1722–1737.
65. Hillberg RE, Johnson DC: Noninvasive ventilation. N Engl J Med 1997; 337:1746–1752.
66. Jasmer RM, Luce JM, Matthay MA: Noninvasive positive pressure ventilation for acute respiratory failure. Underutilized or overrated? Chest 1997; 111:1672–1678.
67. Bott J, Carroll MP, Conway JH, et al: Randomised controlled trial of nasal ventilation in acute ventilatory failure due to chronic obstructive airways disease. Lancet 1993; 341:1555–1557.
68. Brochard L, Mancebo J, Wysocki M, et al: Noninvasive ventilation for acute exacerbations of chronic obstructive pulmonary disease. N Engl J Med 1995; 333:817–822.
69. Kramer N, Meyer TJ, Meharg J, et al: Randomized, prospective trial of noninvasive positive pressure ventilation in acute respiratory failure. Am J Respir Crit Care Med 1995; 151:1799–1806.
70. Wysocki M, Tric L, Wolff MA, et al: Noninvasive pressure support ventilation in patients with acute respiratory failure: A randomized comparison with conventional therapy. Chest 1995; 107:761–768.
71. Girault C, Richard JC, Chevron V, et al: Comparative physiologic effects of noninvasive assist-control and pressure support ventilation in acute hypercapnic respiratory failure. Chest 1997; 111:1639–1648.
72. Barbera JA, Roger N, Roca J, et al: Worsening of pulmonary gas exchange with nitric oxide inhalation in chronic obstructive pulmonary disease. Lancet 1996; 347:436–440.
73. McFadden ER, Lyons HA: Arterial blood gas tension in asthma. N Engl J Med 1968; 278:1027–1032.
74. Geelhoed GC, Landau LI, Le Souef PN: Evaluation of SaO_2 as a predictor of outcome in 280 children presenting with acute asthma. Ann Emerg Med 1994; 236:1236–1241.
75. Rodriguez-Roisin R, Ballester E, Roca J, et al: Mechanisms of hypoxemia in patients with status asthmaticus requiring mechanical ventilation. Am Rev Respir Dis 1989; 139:732–739.
76. Rodriguez-Roisin R: Gas exchange abnormalities in asthma. Lung 1990; 168(Suppl):599–605.
77. Ballester E, Reyes A, Roca J, et al: Ventilation-perfusion mismatching in acute severe asthma: Effects of salbutamol and 100% oxygen. Thorax 1989; 44:258–267.
78. Cockroft DW: Management of acute severe asthma. Ann Allergy Asthma Immun 1995; 75:83–89.
79. Schiffman PL, Ryan A, Whipp BJ, et al: Hyperoxic attenuation of exercise-induced bronchospasm in asthmatics. J Clin Invest 1979; 63:30–37.
80. Dagg KD, Thomson LJ, Ramsay SG, et al: Effect of acute hyperoxia on the bronchodilator response to salbutamol in stable asthmatic patients. Thorax 1996; 51:853–854.
81. Curtis JL, Mahlmeister M, Fink JB, et al: Helium-oxygen gas therapy. Use and availability for the emergency treatment of inoperable airway obstruction. Chest 1986; 90:455–457.
82. Lu TS, Ohmura A, Wong KC, et al: Helium-oxygen in treatment of upper airway obstruction. Anesthesiology 1976; 45:678–680.
83. Skrinskas GJ, Hyland RH, Hutcheon MA: Using helium-oxygen mixtures in the management of acute upper airway obstruction. Can Med Assoc J 1983; 128:555–559.
84. Reisner C, Borish L: Heliox therapy for acute vocal cord dysfunction (Letter). Chest 1995; 108:1477.
85. Duncan PG: Efficacy of helium-oxygen mixtures in the management of severe viral and post-intubation croup. Can Anaesth Soc J 1979; 26:206–212.
86. Rodeberg DA, Easter AJ, Washam MA, et al: Use of a helium-oxygen mixture in the treatment of postextubation stridor in pediatric patients. J Burn Care Rehabil 1995; 16:476–480.
87. Kass JE, Castriotta RJ: Heliox therapy in acute severe asthma. Chest 1995; 107:757–760.
88. Manthous CA, Hall JB, Caputo MA, et al: Heliox improves pulsus paradoxus and peak expiratory flow in nonintubated patients with severe asthma. Am J Respir Crit Care Med 1995; 151:310–314.
89. Polito A, Fessler H: Heliox in respiratory failure from obstructive lung disease. N Engl J Med 1995; 332:192–193.
90. Carter ER, Webb CR, Moffitt DR: Evaluation of heliox in children hospitalized with acute severe asthma. A randomized crossover trial. Chest 1996; 109:1256–1261.
91. Kollef MH, Schuster DP: The acute respiratory distress syndrome. N Engl J Med 1995; 332:27–37.
92. Consensus report: The American-European Consensus Conference on ARDS. Am J Respir Crit Care Med 1994; 149:818–824.
93. Dantzker DR, Brook CH, DeHart P, et al: Gas exchange in adult respiratory distress syndrome and the effects of positive end-expiratory pressure. Am Rev Respir Dis 1979; 120:1039–1052.
94. Rossaint R, Hahn SM, Pappert D, et al: Influence of mixed venous Po_2 and inspired O_2 fraction on intrapulmonary shunt in patients with severe ARDS. J Appl Physiol 1995; 78:1531–1536.
95. Dantzker DR: Gas exchange in acute lung injury. Crit Care Clin 1986; 2:527–536.
96. Gowda MS, Klocke RA: Variability of indices of hypoxemia in adult respiratory distress syndrome. Crit Care Med 1997; 25:41–45.
97. Marini JJ, Ravenscraft SA: Mean airway pressure: Physiologic determinants and clinical importance—part 1: Physiologic determinants and measurements. Crit Care Med 1992; 20:1461–1472.
98. Meduri GU, Turner RE, Abou-Shala N, et al: Noninvasive positive pressure ventilation via face mask. First-line intervention in patients with acute hypercapnic and hypoxemic respiratory failure. Chest 1996; 109:179–193.
98a. Antonelli M, Conti G, Rocco M, Bufi M, De Blasi RA, Vivino G, Gasparetto A, Meduri GU: A comparison of noninvasive positive pressure ventilation and conventional mechanical ventilation in patients with acute respiratory failure. N Engl J Med 1998; 339:429–435.
99. Amato MB, Barbas CS, Medeiros DM, et al: Beneficial effects of the "open lung approach" with low distending pressures in acute respiratory distress syndrome. A prospective randomized study on mechanical ventilation. Am J Respir Crit Care Med 1995; 152:1835–1846.
100. Amato MB, Barbas CS, Medeiros DM, et al: Effect of a protective-ventilation strategy on mortality in the acute respiratory distress syndrome. N Engl J Med 1998; 338:347–354.
101. Tuxen DV: Permissive hypercapnic ventilation. Am J Respir Crit Care Med 1994; 150:870–874.
102. Carvalho CR, Barbas CS, Medeiros DM, et al: Temporal hemodynamic effects of permissive hypercapnia associated with ideal PEEP in ARDS. Am J Respir Crit Care Med 1997; 156:1458–1466.
103. Ravenscraft SA, Burke WC, Nahum A, et al: Tracheal gas insufflation augments CO_2 clearance during mechanical ventilation. Am Rev Respir Dis 1993; 148:345–351.
104. Morris AH, Wallace CJ, Menlove RI, et al: Randomized clinical trial of pressure-controlled inverse ratio ventilation and extracorporeal CO_2 removal for adult respiratory distress syndrome. Am J Respir Crit Care Med 1994; 149:295–305.
105. Conrad SA, Eggerstedt JM, Grier LR, et al: Intravenacaval membrane oxygenation and carbon dioxide removal in severe acute respiratory failure. Chest 1995; 107:1689–1697.
106. Zapol WM, Snider MT, Hill JD, et al: Extracorporeal membrane oxygenation in severe acute respiratory failure. JAMA 1979; 242:2193–2196.
107. Chatte G, Sab JM, Dubois JM, et al: Prone positioning in mechanically ventilated patients with severe acute respiratory failure. Am J Respir Crit Care Med 1997; 155:473–478.
108. Hirschl RB, Pranikoff T, Wise C, et al: Initial experiment with partial liquid ventilation in adult patients with the acute respiratory distress syndrome. JAMA 1996; 275:383–389.
109. Anzueto A, Baughman RP, Guntupalli KK, et al: Aerosolized surfactant in adults with sepsis-induced acute respiratory distress syndrome. Exosurf Acute Respiratory Distress Syndrome Sepsis Study Group. N Engl J Med 1996; 334:1417–1421.
110. Rossaint R, Falke K, Lopez F, et al: Inhaled nitric oxide for the adult respiratory distress syndrome. N Engl J Med 1993; 328:399–405.
111. Walmrath D, Schneider W, Pitch J, et al: Aerosolized prostacycline in adult respiratory distress syndrome. Lancet 1993; 342:961–962.

112. Douglas WW, Rehder K, Beynen FJM, et al: Improved oxygenation in patients with acute respiratory failure: The prone position. Am Rev Respir Dis 1977; 115:559-566.
113. Langer M, Mascheroni D, Maecolin R, et al: The prone position in ARDS patients. A clinical study. Chest 1988; 94:103-107.
114. Pappert D, Rossaint R, Slama K, et al: Influence of positioning on ventilation-perfusion relationships in severe adult respiratory distress syndrome. Chest 1994; 106:1511-1516.
115. Fridrich P, Krafft P, Hochleutner H, et al: The effects of long term prone positioning in patients with trauma-induced adult respiratory distress syndrome. Anesth Analg 1996; 83:1206-1211.
116. Blanch I, Mancebo J, Perez M, et al: Short term effects of prone position in critically ill patients with acute respiratory distress syndrome. Intensive Care Med 1997; 23:1033-1039.
117. Stocker R, Neff T, Stein S, et al: Prone positioning and low-volume pressure-limited ventilation improve survival in patients with severe ARDS. Chest 1997; 111:1008-1017.
118. Lamm WJE, Graham MM, Albert RK: Mechanism by which the prone position improves oxygenation in acute lung injury. Am J Respir Crit Care Med 1994; 150:184-193.
119. Mutoh T, Guest RJ, Lamm WJE, et al: Prone position alters the effect of volume overload on regional pleural pressures and improves hypoxemia in pigs in vivo. Am Rev Respir Dis 1992; 146:300-306.
120. Fuhrman BP, Praczan PR, DeFrancis M: Perfluorocarbon-associated gas exchange. Crit Care Med 1991; 19:712-722.
121. Marini JJ: Evolving concepts in the ventilatory management of acute respiratory distress syndrome. Clin Chest Med 1996; 17:555-575.
122. Gregory TJ, Longmore WJ, Moxley MA, et al: Surfactant chemical composition and biophysical activity in acute respiratory distress syndrome. J Clin Invest 1991; 88:1976-1981.
123. Lewis JF, Jobe AH: Surfactant and the adult respiratory distress syndrome. Am Rev Respir Dis 1993; 147:218-233.
124. Walmrath D, Gunther A, Ghofrani HA, et al: Bronchoscopic surfactant administration in patients with severe adult respiratory distress syndrome and sepsis. Am J Respir Crit Care Med 1996; 154:57-62.
125. Walmrath D, Schneider T, Schermuly R, et al: Direct comparison of inhaled nitric oxide and aerosolized prostacycline in acute respiratory distress syndrome. Am J Respir Care Med 1996; 153:991-996.
126. Gregory TJ, Steinberg KP, Spragg R, et al: Bovine surfactant therapy for patients with acute respiratory distress syndrome. Am J Respir Crit Care Med 1997; 155:1309-1315.
127. Gerlach H, Rossaint R, Pappert D, et al: Time-course and dose-response of nitric oxide inhalation for systemic oxygenation and pulmonary hypertension in patients with adult respiratory distress syndrome. Eur J Clin Invest 1993; 23:499-502.
128. Johns RA: EDRF/nitric oxide. The endogenous nitrovasodilator and a new cellular messenger. Anesthesiology 1991; 75:927-931.
129. Rossetti M, Guenard H, Gabinski C: Effects of nitric oxide inhalation on pulmonary serial vascular resistances in ARDS. Am J Respir Crit Care Med 1996; 154:1375-1381.
130. Benzig A, Mols G, Brieschal T, et al: Hypoxic pulmonary vasoconstriction in nonventilated lung areas contributes to differences in hemodynamic and gas exchange responses to inhalation of nitric oxide. Anesthesiology 1997; 86:1254-1261.
131. Puybasset L, Rouby JJ, Mourgeon E, et al: Inhaled nitric oxide in acute respiratory failure: Dose-response curves. Intensive Care Med 1994; 20:319-327.
132. Bigatello LM, Hurford WE, Kacmarek RM, et al: Prolonged inhalation of low concentrations of nitric oxide in patients with severe adult respiratory distress syndrome. Effects on pulmonary hemodynamics and oxygenation. Anesthesiology 1994; 80:761-770.
133. Singh S, Evans TW: Nitric oxide, the biological mediator of the decade: Fact or fiction? Eur Respir J 1997; 10:699-707.
134. Lavoie A, Hall JB, Olson DM, et al: Life-threatening effects of discontinuing inhaled nitric oxide in severe respiratory failure. Am J Respir Crit Care Med 1996; 153:1985-1987.
135. Pinsky MR, Genc F, Lee KH, et al: Contamination of hospital compressed air with nitric oxide. Chest 1997; 111:1759-1763.
136. Lee KH, Tan PSK, Rico P, et al: Low levels of nitric oxide as contaminant in hospital compressed air: Physiologic significance? Crit Care Med 1997; 25:1143-1146.
137. Wilson AT, Reilly CS, Woodmansey P, et al: Oxygen therapy in myocardial infarction (Abstract). Clin Sci 1993; 84:21p.
138. Rawles JM, Kenmure ACF: Controlled trial of oxygen in uncomplicated myocardial infarction. Br Med J 1976; 1:1121-1123.
139. Weisse AB, Moore RJ, Zweil P, et al: Effects of oxygen administration and alteration in arterial P_{CO_2} on ischemic myocardial changes following experimental coronary artery ligation. Am Heart J 1982; 104:968-973.
140. Kelly RF, Hursey TL, Parrilo JE, et al: Effect of 100% oxygen administration on infarct size and left ventricular function in a canine model of myocardial infarction and reperfusion. Am Heart J 1995; 130:957-965.
141. Thomas P, Brown LA, Sponseller DR, et al: Myocardial infarct size reduction by the synergistic effect of hyperbaric oxygen and recombinant tissue plasminogen activator. Am Heart J 1990; 120:791-800.
142. Marjot R, Valentine SJ: Arterial oxygen saturation following premedication for cardiac surgery. Br J Anaesth 1990; 64:737-740.
143. Kavanagh BP, Cheng DCH, Sandler AN, et al: Supplemental oxygen does not reduce myocardial ischemia in premedicated patients with critical coronary artery disease. Anesth Analg 1993; 76:950-956.
144. Lin M, Yang YF, Chiang HT, et al: Reappraisal of continuous positive airway pressure therapy in acute cardiogenic pulmonary edema. Chest 1995; 107:1379-1386.
145. Haque WA, Boehmer J, Clemson BS, et al: Hemodynamic effects of supplemental oxygen administration in congestive heart failure. J Am Coll Cardiol 1996; 27:353-357.
146. Hales CA, Westphal D: Hypoxemia following the administration of sublingual nitroglycerin. Am J Med 1978; 65:911-918.
147. Rennotte MT, Reynaert M, Clerbaux T, et al: Effects of two inotropic drugs, dopamine and dobutamine, on pulmonary gas exchange in artificially ventilated patients. Intensive Care Med 1989; 15:160-165.
148. Lange PA, Stoller JK: The hepatopulmonary syndrome. Ann Intern Med 1995; 122:521-529.
149. Krowka MJ, Cortese DA: Hepatopulmonary syndrome. Current concepts in diagnostic and therapeutic considerations. Chest 1994; 105:1528-1537.
150. Rodriguez-Roisin R, Roca J, Agusti AGN, et al: Gas exchange and pulmonary vascular reactivity in patients with liver cirrhosis. Am Rev Respir Dis 1987; 135:1085-1092.
151. Robin ED, Laman D, Horn BR, et al: Platypnea related to orthodeoxia caused by true vascular lung shunts. N Engl J Med 1976; 294:941-943.
152. Fallon MB, Abrams GA, Luo B, et al: The role of endothelial nitric oxide synthase in the pathogenesis of a rat model of hepatopulmonary syndrome. Gastroenterology 1997; 113:606-614.
153. Rolla G, Brussino L, Colagrande P, et al: Exhaled nitric oxide and oxygenation abnormalities in hepatic cirrhosis. Hepatology 1997; 26:842-847.
154. Castro M, Krowka MJ: Hepatopulmonary syndrome. A pulmonary vascular complication of liver disease. Clin Chest Med 1996; 17:35-48.
155. Krowka MJ, Porayko MK, Plevak DJ, et al: Hepatopulmonary syndrome with progressive hypoxemia as an indication for liver transplantation: Case reports and literature review. Mayo Clin Proc 1997; 72:44-53.
156. Philit F, Wiesendanger T, Gille D, et al: Late resolution of hepatopulmonary syndrome after liver transplantation. Respiration 1997; 64:173-175.
157. Riegler JL, Lang KA, Johnson SP, et al: Transjugular intrahepatic portosystemic shunt improves oxygenation in hepatopulmonary syndrome. Gastroenterology 1995; 109:978-983.
158. Pollack MM, Fields AI, Holbrook PR: Pneumothorax and pneumomediastinum during pediatric mechanical ventilation. Crit Care Med 1979; 7:536-539.
159. Light RW: Pneumothorax. *In:* Pleural Diseases. 3rd ed. Philadelphia, Williams & Wilkins, 1995, pp 242-277.
160. Hill RC, DeCarlo DP Jr, Hill JF, et al: Resolution of experimental pneumothorax in rabbits by oxygen therapy. Ann Thorac Surg 1995; 59:825-827.
161. Chernick V, Avery ME: Spontaneous alveolar rupture at birth. Pediatrics 1963; 32:816-824.

162. Chadha TS, Cohn MA: Noninvasive treatment of pneumothorax with oxygen inhalation. Respiration 1983; 44:147-152.
163. Northfield TC: Oxygen therapy for spontaneous pneumothorax. Br Med J 1971; 4:86-88.
164. Barr J, Lushkov G, Starinsky R, et al: Heliox therapy for pneumothorax: New indication for an old remedy. Ann Emerg Med 1997; 30:159-161.
165. Coburn RF: Mechanisms of carbon monoxide toxicity. Prev Med 1979; 8:310-322.
166. Vreman HJ, Mahoney JJ, Stevenson DK: Carbon monoxide and carboxyhemoglobin. Adv Pediatr 1995; 42:303-334.
167. Touger M, Gallagher EJ, Tyrell J: Relationship between venous and arterial carboxyhemoglobin levels in patients with suspected carbon monoxide poisoning. Ann Emerg Med 1995; 25:481-483.
168. Tibbles PM, Edelsberg JS: Hyperbaric oxygen therapy. N Engl J Med 1996; 334:1642-1648.
169. Balzan MV, Agius G, Debono AG: Carbon monoxide poisoning: Easy to treat but difficult to recognize. Postgrad Med J 1996; 72:470-473.
170. Peterson JE, Stewart RD: Absorption and elimination of carbon monoxide by inactive young men. Arch Environ Health 1970; 21:165-171.
171. Tibbles PM, Perrotta PL: Treatment of carbon monoxide poisoning: A critical review of human outcome studies comparing normobaric oxygen with hyperbaric oxygen. Ann Emerg Med 1994; 24:269-276.
172. Thom SR, Taber RL, Mendiguren II, et al: Delayed neuropsychologic sequelae after carbon monoxide poisoning: Prevention by treatment with hyperbaric oxygen. Ann Emerg Med 1995; 25:474-480.
173. Olson KR, Seger D: Hyperbaric oxygen for carbon monoxide poisoning: Does it really work? (Editorial) Ann Emerg Med 1995; 25:535-537.
174. Davies SC, Luce PJ, Win AA, et al: Acute chest syndrome in sickle cell disease. Lancet 1984; 1:36-38.
175. Vichinsky EP, Styles LA, Colangelo LH, et al: Acute chest syndrome in sickle cell disease: Clinical presentation and course. Blood 1997; 89:1787-1792.
176. Ballas SK, Mohandas N: Pathophysiology of vaso-occlusion. Hematol Oncol Clin North Am 1996; 10:1221-1239.
177. Emre U, Miller ST, Rao SP, et al: Alveolar-arterial oxygen gradient in acute chest syndrome in sickle cell disease. J Pediatr 1993; 123:272-275.
178. Embury SH, Garcia JF, Mohandas N, et al: Effects of oxygen inhalation on endogenous erythropoietin kinetics, erythropoiesis, and properties of blood cells in sickle cell disease. N Engl J Med 1984; 311:291-295.
179. Reynolds JDH: Painful sickle cell crisis. Successful treatment with hyperbaric oxygen therapy. JAMA 1971; 216:1977-1978.
180. Zipursky A, Robieux AC, Brown EJ, et al: Oxygen therapy in sickle cell disease. Am J Pediatr Hematol Oncol 1992; 12:222-228.
181. Khoury H, Grimsley E: Oxygen inhalation in nonhypoxic sickle cell patients during vaso-occlusive crisis (Letter). Blood 1995; 86:3998.
182. Fogan L: Treatment of cluster headache: A double blind comparison of oxygen vs air inhalation. Arch Neurol 1985; 42:362-363.
183. Stauffer JL, Fayter NA, Mclure BJ: Conjunctivitis from nasal CPAP apparatus (Letter). Chest 1984; 84:802.
184. Strumpf DA, Harrop P, Dobbin J, Millman RP: Massive epistaxis from nasal continuous positive airway pressure therapy. Chest 1989; 95:1141.
185. Frenckner B, Ehren H, Palmer K, et al: Pneumocephalus caused by a nasopharyngeal oxygen catheter. Crit Care Med 1990; 18:1287-1288.
186. Jarjour NN, Wilson P: Pneumocephalus associated with nasal CPAP in a patient with sleep apnea. Chest 1989; 96:1425-1426.
187. Dantzker DR, Wagner PD, West JB: Proceedings: Instability of poorly ventilated lung units during oxygen breathing. J Physiol 1974; 242:72P.
188. Deneke SM, Fanburg BL: Normobaric oxygen toxicity of the lung. N Engl J Med 1980; 303:76-86.
189. Douglas ME, Downs JB, Dannemiller FJ, et al: Change in pulmonary venous admixture with varying inspired oxygen. Anesth Analg 1976; 55:688-695.
190. Register SD, Downs JB, Stock MC, et al: Is 50% oxygen harmful? Crit Care Med 1987; 15:598-601.
191. Fracica PJ, Knapp MJ, Crapo JD: Patterns of progression and markers of lung injury in rodents and subhuman primates exposed to hyperoxia. Exp Lung Res 1988; 14:869-885.
192. Huang YT, Sane AC, Simonson SG, et al: Artificial surfactant attenuates hyperoxic lung injury in primates: I. Physiology and biochemistry. J Appl Physiol 1995; 78:1816-1822.
193. Heffner JE, Repine JE: Pulmonary strategies of antioxidant defense. Am Rev Respir Dis 1989; 140:531-554.

121

Adjunctive Respiratory Therapy

Susan K. Pingleton, MD

Many primary therapies are available for critically ill patients, such as mechanical ventilation, hemodynamic support, and drugs. Other adjunctive therapies commonly used in the care of the critically ill are respiratory therapies—bronchial hygiene maneuvers designed to increase lung expansion such as incentive spirometry, orotracheal suctioning, and intermittent positive-pressure breathing (IPPB) devices (Table 121-1). Therapies to improve mucociliary clearance include chest physiotherapy and drugs such as mucolytics and bronchodilators. Newer respiratory adjunct devices include the closed-chest oscillation devices, continuous lateral rotation therapy beds, and positive expiratory pressure devices.

This chapter reviews adjunctive respiratory devices, treatments, and drugs commonly prescribed in the intensive care unit (ICU). Respiratory adjunctive therapy is useful and effective when carefully applied for clearly defined therapeutic goals.

COUGH

Cough is not only a symptom; it is also one of the lung's primary defense mechanisms. As a defense mechanism, cough has two functions: to prevent foreign material from entering the airways and to clear foreign material or excessive secretions from them. In the ICU, cough has clinical significance and consequences when it is ineffective or absent. Variables that determine the effectiveness of coughing include the thickness of the airway secretions and the velocity of air moving through the airways.[1] Once material in the airways is sufficiently thick, the effectiveness of the cough depends on

TABLE 121-1. Respiratory Adjunctive Therapies

Therapies That Increase Lung Volume
Incentive spirometry
Intermittent positive-pressure breathing
Therapies That Enhance Mucociliary Clearance
Mechanical augmentation of mucociliary clearance
Chest physiotherapy
Closed-chest oscillation technique
Positive expiratory pressure device
Suctioning
Pharmacologic augmentation of mucociliary clearance
Bronchodilators
Mucolytics

achieving a high rate of air flow and a small cross-sectional area of the airway during the expiratory phase of cough. The effectiveness of cough for a spontaneously breathing, critically ill patient or a ventilated patient about to be weaned from the ventilator is an important determinant of the course of that patient's illness. Any condition associated with decreased expiratory flow rates or reduced ability to compress airways dynamically likely will result in ineffective coughing.[2] Clinical consequences include increased probability for atelectasis, gas exchange abnormalities, and pneumonia. An ineffective cough is most likely due to respiratory muscle weakness, due either to primary neuromuscular diseases or weakness secondary to deconditioning, debilitation, or sedation. Patients with chronic obstructive pulmonary disease (COPD) also have decreased flow rates, which can impair coughing as a primary pathophysiologic aspect of the disease.

LUNG EXPANSION

When cough is ineffective, airway secretions are retained, lung volume is decreased, and atelectasis and pneumonitis can occur. In this setting, various techniques to increase lung volume are available. A lung expansion technique is one that increases lung volume or helps increase lung volume above that of usual unassisted or uncoached inspiration. Lung expansion techniques are meant to duplicate a normal sigh maneuver.[3] Although not well studied, sighs or periodic voluntary hyperinflation to near total lung capacity reverses microatelectasis.

Lung expansion techniques are indicated to prevent atelectasis and pneumonia in patients who cannot or will not perform periodic hyperinflation.[3] Such patient populations include postoperative (especially abdominal or thoracic) surgical patients and patients with respiratory disease such as COPD or neuromuscular or chest wall disorders. Adequately performed, maximum inspirations of 10 per hour while awake significantly decrease the incidence of pulmonary complications after laparotomy.[4]

Several techniques are available for lung expansion:

- Coached maximum voluntary hyperinflation
- Sustained maximal inspiration with cough
- Incentive spirometry
- Volume-oriented IPPB
- Positive end-expiratory pressure (PEEP) therapy

The incentive spirometer, a commonly used, effective, and inexpensive bronchial hygiene tool for lung expansion, provides a visual goal or incentive for patients to achieve and sustain a maximal inspiratory effort. For incentive spirometry to be effective, the patient must be awake, cooperative, motivated, and properly instructed. The goals include a vital capacity greater than 14 mL/kg.[5] Perhaps the principal reason that incentive spirometry is not effective is that it is not used frequently. Patients should be instructed and reminded by nurses to use the incentive spirometer to the assigned goal at least five times per hour by the clock.

IPPB is a form of lung expansion therapy that was widely used before it was adequately studied. IPPB therapy has fallen into disfavor, not only because of the lack of documented efficacy in a wide variety of clinical conditions but also because it is very labor-intensive and, therefore, very expensive. Also, IPPB has largely been replaced as a lung expansion technique by incentive spirometry; however, although clinical indications for the general use of IPPB are limited, it can be helpful in certain circumstances. For this therapy to be helpful, the patient's vital capacity should be less than 15 mL/kg, IPPB should increase this by at least 100%, and the therapy should have a defined endpoint.[6] The primary indication for IPPB therapy is the inability of the patient to cooperate with other lung expansion techniques. The IPPB therapy may "buy time" until the patient is able to cooperate with other therapies.

MUCOCILIARY CLEARANCE

Mucociliary clearance is another important lung defense mechanism. By action of the ciliary escalator, normal mucus is brought proximal from the distal aspects of the tracheobronchial tree, where it is either expectorated or swallowed. Ineffective mucociliary clearance leads to retention of airway secretions. Abnormalities in mucociliary clearance can result from depression of the clearance mechanisms or oversecretion in the face of normal mucus transport.

Mucus is undercleared and overproduced in smokers with or without chronic bronchitis and in asthma patients.[7,8] It is undercleared in emphysema, bronchiectasis, and cystic fibrosis, during and 4 to 6 weeks after a viral upper respiratory tract infection, during and after a period of general anesthesia due to inhalation gases and cuffed endotracheal tubes and during prolonged mechanical ventilation.[8] Prolonged mechanical ventilation alters mucociliary clearance because of the cuffed tube, high concentrations of oxygen, and injury to the tracheobronchial tree from suctioning. Initial therapies should be directed at removing the inciting cause of underclearance and overproduction of secretions. Additionally, mucociliary clearance can be enhanced by mechanical and pharmacologic therapies.

Mechanical Augmentation of Mucociliary Clearance

Chest Physiotherapy

Chest physical therapy techniques include a combination of therapeutic positioning, percussion to the chest wall over the affected area, vibration of the chest wall, and coughing. All are designed to improve and mobilize secretions, thus optimizing ventilation-perfusion ($\dot{V}/\dot{Q}$) ratios by utilizing the effects of gravity and delivering external manipulation to the thorax.

Postural drainage is a technique that utilizes different body positions to facilitate gravitational drainage of mucus from various lung segments.[5] It includes turning or rotating the body around its longitudinal axis so that the effect of gravity can enhance or minimize the movement or flow of secretions toward the central airways. External manipulation of the thorax, in the form of percussion and vibration, is used to facilitate postural drainage. Chest percussion and vibration are techniques used to loosen and mobilize secretions that are adherent to bronchial walls. The purpose of percussion is to apply kinetic energy intermittently to the chest wall and lungs. This is accomplished by rhythmically striking the thorax with cupped hands or a mechanical device placed directly over the lung segment to be drained. This generates a mechanical energy wave that is transmitted through the chest wall to the lung, where it loosens adherent mucus.[9,10] No convincing evidence demonstrates the superiority of one method over the other.

Chest physiotherapy is primarily indicated and beneficial for patients with cystic fibrosis or bronchiectasis.[11] Only patients with COPD who produce more than 30 mL of sputum per day will benefit.[12] Chest physiotherapy is also indicated for lobar atelectasis.[13] As compared to fiberoptic bronchoscopy, chest physiotherapy was more effective in resolving lobar atelectasis. It is not indicated for asthma patients.[12] Chest physiotherapy is contraindicated (1) when proper positioning cannot be performed, (2) when injuries would preclude it, or

(3) when preexisting disease processes might be exacerbated by it.[5] Specific contraindications to the Trendelenburg position include increased intracranial pressure, recent neurosurgical procedures, unclipped cerebral artery aneurysm, uncontrolled hypertension, pulmonary edema associated with congestive heart failure, increased risk for gastroesophageal reflux or aspiration, and recent eye surgery. The reverse Trendelenburg position is contraindicated in the presence of hypotension or other hemodynamic instability.

External manipulation of the thorax is contraindicated (1) in the presence of skin wounds, burns, or skin grafts; (2) thoracic or spinal injury, such as rib fractures, flail chest, pulmonary contusion, bronchopleural fistula, recent or unstable spine fractures; and (3) in the presence of severe coagulopathy or active bleeding. Complications of chest physiotherapy are infrequent but occasionally severe.[14] They include massive pulmonary hemorrhage, decreased arterial oxygen tension from positioning the "bad" lung down, rib fractures, increased intracranial pressure, decreased cardiac output, and decreased lung function, particularly with the mobilization of large amounts of secretions in a patient with an ineffective cough.

In addition to the traditional chest physical therapy techniques, alternative airway clearance methods, such as PEEP therapy, forced expiratory technique, and autogenic drainage, have shown promise in augmenting removal of large volumes of secretions from patients with cystic fibrosis, chronic bronchitis, or bronchiectasis.[15, 16] These therapies are either replacements for or adjunctive to traditional chest physiotherapy. They focus on controlled breathing and modified coughing maneuvers.

In PEEP therapy, a mask is applied tightly over the mouth and nose and a variable flow resistor adjusted to achieve a PEEP during exhalation between 10 and 20 cm H_2O.[15] This, combined with "huff" coughing, allows mobilization of peripheral secretions. Autogenic drainage is a secretion-clearing technique that combines variable tidal breathing at three distinct lung volume levels, controlled expiratory airflow, and huff coughing.[16] These techniques are most useful in spontaneously breathing patients who can cooperate with the therapy. ICU patients and those with short-term pulmonary complications are less viable candidates for alternative airway clearance methods.

High-Frequency Chest Wall Oscillation

Recently, another mechanism of augmenting mucociliary clearance has been developed. High-frequency oscillation of the chest wall produces transient increases in airflow at low lung volumes, cough-like shear forces, alterations in the physical properties of mucus, and increases in mucus mobilization.[17-20] In early studies, the device involved wrapping a modified blood pressure cuff around the lower thorax and rapidly varying the pressures in the cuff with a piston pump to produce oscillations.[17] Refinements in the technology have led to the development of an inflatable vest that fits over the patient's thorax with tubing that connects the vest to an air-pulse generator.[20] The generator produces high-frequency pressure pulses that rapidly inflate and deflate the vest, creating oscillations in the chest wall. Clinical studies of the inflatable vest have most often been conducted in patients with cystic fibrosis or chronic bronchitis, who secrete excessive mucus.[20, 21] Less information is available in mechanical ventilation patients, but data do suggest that the inflatable vest is a cost effective alternative to standard physiotherapy. Absolute contraindications include head or neck injury that has not been stabilized and active hemorrhage with hemodynamic instability.

Suctioning

Mechanical aspiration or suctioning is an important mechanism for removing bronchial secretions. Performed properly, the procedure is safe and effective; however, multiple adverse clinical consequences occur when it is performed incautiously. These include tissue trauma, laryngospasm, bronchospasm, hypoxemia, cardiac arrhythmias, respiratory arrest, cardiac arrest, atelectasis, pneumonia, misdirection of the catheter, and death.[22, 23]

Airway suction can safely be accomplished in patients with artificial airways (endotracheal or tracheostomy tubes).[5] In this situation, the patient should be ventilated with a manual resuscitation bag or six extra ventilator breaths on 100% FIO_2, "preoxygenation." This minimizes any potential hypoxemia induced by removal of the patient from an oxygen source and the application of suction to the airways. Strict aseptic technique should be observed by donning sterile gloves over freshly washed hands and using a sterile suction catheter. This catheter should be placed into the airway and advanced, without the application of a vacuum, beyond the tip of the artificial airway until it can no longer easily be advanced. The catheter should be withdrawn slightly before suction is applied. Suctioning is then accomplished by intermittent application of a vacuum and gradual withdrawal of the catheter in rotation fashion. The duration of the procedure should not exceed 20 seconds. After completion of suctioning, the patient should be manually ventilated or provided with six extra ventilator breaths with an oxygen-enriched atmosphere to ensure adequate lung reexpansion and oxygenation. Patients receiving PEEP, ideally, should not be taken off the ventilator—and thus off PEEP—during suctioning. In this instance, closed suctioning should be considered. The patient should be monitored for signs of distress, bronchospasm, hemodynamic instability, or arrhythmias throughout the entire procedure.

In closed suction catheter systems the catheter itself is shrouded in a protective sleeve that allows flexibility to advance or retract the catheter into the patient's airway without disconnecting the patient or interrupting mechanical ventilation.[24] This is operational in situations when the ventilated patient presents with an unstable hemodynamic profile and any disconnection from mechanical ventilation or intermittent discontinuation of high levels of PEEP may compromise the patient. When a similar closed-system technique is used, the patient is suctioned through the adapter that allows insertion of the suction catheter into the endotracheal tube.[25] Single-use disposable catheters without protective sheaths and multiple-use disposable catheters with protective sheaths can be used in closed tracheal suction systems.[25, 26] The latter has its own adapter and can be left in line and discarded after 24 hours. While, theoretically, the multiple-use catheter prevents cross-contamination between patients, prevents contamination of the lower respiratory tract by environmental organisms, may protect healthcare workers from contamination with infected secretions, and lowers cost, these potential advantages have yet to be verified in prospective studies.[27]

Suctioning of the tracheobronchial tree without an artificial airway in place carries several risks. Nasotracheal suctioning is rarely indicated because chest physiotherapy can be used for conscious patients and semicomatose or comatose ones with retained secretions can be intubated. Suctioning should be undertaken only in the presence of appropriate indications. The principal one is the presence of bronchial secretions that can be identified visually or with auscultation. Nasotracheal suctioning has been associated with fatal cardiac arrest and life-threatening arrhythmias, presumably due to hypoxemia, and with bacteremia.[28-31] Mucosal irritation, trauma, and bleeding can be precipitated by frequent and aggressive suctioning in the absence of bronchial secretions. Routine suction of the airway should be discouraged.

Continuous Lateral Rotation Therapy

Critically ill patients, by nature of their illness, remain in a recumbent position and immobilized for long periods. The adverse effects of prolonged immobility include atelectasis and pneumonia and are due principally to gravitational effects on blood flow and ventilation and to impairment of the normal mucociliary escalator. Continuous lateral rotational therapy delivered with a special bed has been evaluated with multiple populations of patients with diverse medical problems, including cerebrovascular disease, multiple trauma, and acute respiratory distress syndrome (ARDS).[32-37] Conflicting data exist on the effectiveness of bed rotation, in part owing to the method and the study population. While many studies demonstrate that continuous lateral rotation therapy reduces the frequency of pulmonary complications, including nosocomial pneumonia, atelectasis, and thromboembolic disease, other studies do not.[37] Moreover, the mechanisms involved are not clearly defined, and further studies are needed to determine the precise angles of turning and the frequency. However, recent clinical and pathologic data in adult baboons clearly indicate that continuous bed rotation prevents atelectasis, bronchiolitis, and bronchopneumonia, as defined pathologically, compared to control groups.[38]

Complications of continuous lateral rotation therapy include disconnection of intravascular catheters, patient intolerance, adverse effects on intracranial pressures in patients with intracranial hypertension, arrhythmias, and hemodynamic instability.[39] Absolute contraindications include unstable spinal cord injuries and traction of the arm abductors. Relative contraindications include marked agitation, severe diarrhea, a rise in intracranial pressure (ICP), a greater than 10% fall in blood pressure, and severe cardiac arrhythmias.[39]

AEROSOLS

Hypertonic saline aerosols traditionally have been used to induce expectoration of sputum for diagnostic purposes.[40] The administration of hypertonic nebulized saline can increase the mucociliary clearance of radiolabeled mucus by stimulation of productive cough, and possibly return of the administered aerosol.[41] Although effective for that purpose, there is no evidence of any therapeutic value of hypertonic saline in patients with COPD.[42] There is also little evidence that simple humidification or isotonic aerosols have an important action on mucus clearance, expect for a soothing and emollient action. In patients with asthma, administration of either hypotonic or hypertonic aerosols can induce bronchospasm.

BRONCHODILATORS

Three major classes of bronchodilators drugs are available for patients with pulmonary diseases: (1) anticholinergic drugs, (2) β_2-adrenergic agents, and (3) methylxanthines. In the ICU, as in any other clinical setting, the choice includes one or more of these drugs. Adrenegic and anticholinergic drugs are usually administered via the airway; methylxanthines must be administered systemically. In general, the airway route is favored for bronchodilators because this ensures the highest concentration of the drug in the airway and minimizes its actions elsewhere. This consideration dictates the use of an adrenergic or an anticholineric agent.

Although potency and duration of bronchodilation are often the main criteria by which bronchodilators are compared in ambulatory patients, they may be less important in mechanically ventilated patients. β-Adrenergic agents stimulate ciliary activity and promote mucociliary clearance, which is clearly important in a patient incapable of spontaneous coughing.[43] Similarly, methylxanthines may have beneficial effects not related to their bronchodilator action. They are mild respiratory stimulants and may have an inotropic effect on the respiratory muscles, both of which may contribute to the ability of a mechanically ventilated patient to be weaned from the ventilator. Pharmacologic details of each drug class are discussed elsewhere.

The majority of bronchodilator use in ICUs is for inhaled β-adrenergic agents. Two modes of delivery are available: (1) an inhalation solution given by nebulization or (2) a metered-dose inhaler (MDI).

The nebulizer consists of a disposable or reusable nebulizer and a pressurized gas (air or oxygen) source. A small volume of medication and a larger volume of diluent are placed into the nebulizer chamber. The aerosol particle size produced by a nebulizer is affected by the gas flow used to power it, the volume of solution, and the construction of the nebulizer.[44-46] Variables that affect nebulizer performance include the nebulizer brand, gas flow, and fill volume, which make it difficult to compare various results reported with such devices. Recent variations in nebulizer design that incorporate a reservoir bag to collect and suspend aerosol particles of desired therapeutic particle size, and the addition of a PEEP valve to promote better aerosol deposition have been engineered to improve nebulizer efficiency. Advocates of these design changes suggest that the result is better aerosol particle size, less systemic absorption of medication, and more medication targeted and deposited to the airways; as yet, however, no recognized clinical studies have supported this claim. In ambulatory patients, numerous studies have reported virtual equivalence between nebulizer and MDI, with or without a spacer.[44]

The MDI contains medication in suspension or solution, a metering valve, and, currently, chlorofluorocarbon propellants.[46] The drug canister is fitted to an actuator, and activation by compression of the canister into the actuator results in release of a unit dose of medication. In patients breathing spontaneously, the actuator is a mouthpiece or auxiliary spacer device, and for mechanically ventilated patients it is designed to fit into the ventilator circuit.[47] MDIs tend to spray out the medication more quickly than a spontaneously breathing patient can inhale it. As a result, much is deposited in the back of the throat or on the tongue. With appropriate use of the MDI, delivery of drug to the lower airways has been demonstrated to be approximately 10% of the total dose, an amount comparable to that delivered with the nebulizer.[44, 48] In contrast to the nebulizer, however, with which 66% of the drug is deposited in the apparatus and 2% in the mouth and stomach, MDI administration results in only 5% to 10% of drug deposition in the apparatus and 80% in the mouth and stomach.[44] Thus, local side effects and tissue toxicity occur.

Inhaler efficacy in spontaneously breathing patients is improved with spacer devices, which hold the medicine in a chamber long enough for the patient to inhale slowly and deeply once or twice. A spacer decreases the oral deposition of medicine from 80% to 8%.[49] Another cause of inefficient delivery is incoordination between actuation and inhalation. Proper inhaler technique is crucial for maximal inhaler efficacy in spontaneously breathing patients.

In terms of clinical effects, MDI and nebulizer therapy have been compared and no difference was found between peak expiratory flow rates and severity of symptoms in stable patients treated with either modality.[50] In hospitalized, spontaneously breathing patients, comparison of therapy with an MDI-spacer system and with nebulizer treatments indicated that a greater spirometric response was initially obtained with the nebulizer, but this response equalized over the period of hospitalization.[51] In mechanically ventilated patients, bronchodilator response to either an MDI placed in line or in-line nebulizer therapy was not significantly different.[52, 53] In addition to equal clinical efficacy, administrating bronchodilator therapy with MDI devices requires less "humanpower" and offers significant cost savings to the hospital.[54]

Delivery of bronchodilator drugs to patients undergoing mechanical ventilation can be effective. The use of an MDI in a ventilated patient requires that an adaptor be placed into the ventilator circuit.[47] Several commercial adaptors are available, such as chamber (reservoir, spacer) devices, in-line devices, and elbow devices. The chamber or spacer devices fit into the inspiratory limb of the circuit and act as an aerosol reservoir, and, theoretically, should allow the high initial velocity of aerosol particles to slow and the particle size to decrease. The in-line devices can be attached at any point along the inspiratory limb of the circuit. The elbow devices attach directly to the endotracheal tube and direct the aerosol into the endotracheal tube during inspiration.

MUCOLYTIC AGENTS

Tracheobronchial mucus contributes significantly to pulmonary symptoms of critically ill patients. A mucoactive drug is defined as an agent with the capability of modifying mucus production, secretion, its nature and composition, or its interactions with the mucociliary epithelium.[55] Most of the drugs used as mucolytics have been developed to reduce mucus viscosity, even though high viscosity does not significantly impair mucus clearance.[56] Other properties of mucus (particularly elasticity, deoxyribonucleic acid [DNA] content, and surface interaction of secretions with epithelium) may be more important than viscosity to effective mucus clearance. In the following discussion, the term *mucolytic* is considered synonymous with *mucoactive*. Many modalities, ranging from simple hydration to the use of bronchodilators and enzyme solutions, have been utilized to alter the characteristics of mucus, with varying results.

Although patients with COPD are encouraged to drink fluids to facilitate sputum production, few data are available to support that clinical recommendation. Whether patients were dehydrated or treated with hydration or ad lib fluid intake, hydration provided no difference in mucus volume, respiratory symptoms, or forced expiratory volume in 1 second (FEV_1).[57]

Oral expectorants (e.g., guaifenesin, bromhexine, ipecac) stimulate the gastric nerve and promote a vagally-mediated increase in airway secretions.[56] Other mechanisms of action may include a reduction in mucus velocity or enhancement of the mucociliary elevator.[56] Despite these actions, there is little evidence that oral expectorants improve lung function or subjective well-being in patients with COPD. Both bromhexine and guaifenesin improved tracheobronchial clearance but did not change lung function, the frequency of cough, emotional well-being, or the weight and content of sputum.[58]

Iodide preparations are saturated solutions of potassium iodide (SSKI), domiodol, and iodopropylidine glycerol. Iodide acts as a mucolytic by decreasing the viscosity of mucus, facilitating the breakdown of proteins by proteolytic enzymes, and increasing ciliary beat frequency.[59] SSKI may be effective, but its use is limited by side effects such as a metallic taste, rash, hyperkalemia in patients with renal insufficiency, and hypothyroidism, especially when it is used longer than 6 weeks. Domiodol is an organic iodinated mucolytic agent that improves cough intensity, sputum quantity and quality, and ease of expectoration.[60] Iodopropylidine glycerol can enhance tracheobronchial clearance and mucociliary transport in expectorating patients with chronic bronchitis. In addition, a randomized, double-blind placebo-controlled study documented improvements in cough, ease of expectoration, sense of well-being, and decreased duration of exacerbations.[61] This drug is no longer available in the United States.

True mucolytic agents are those that sever disulfide bridges, *N*-acetyl-L-cysteine (acetylcysteine), S-carboxymethyl cysteine, and 2-mercaptoethane sulfonate. They act directly on mucoproteins, thus liquefying mucus and rendering it less viscous.[56] These drugs are not approved as mucokinetic agents in the United States.

Acetylcysteine liquefies mucus and DNA. Liquefaction occurs within 1 minute after inhalation and is maximal at 5 to 10 minutes.[62] When delivered in a nebulized form it can cause bronchospasm,[63] and therefore it is usually given in combination with a β-agonist drug. This combination may obscure the determination of independent effects of acetylcysteine on mucociliary clearance.

Recombinant DNase is a new mucolytic drug recently released for use in patients with cystic fibrosis. DNA released by leukocytes is thought to contribute significantly to the viscosity of mucus in cystic fibrosis patients. Recombinant human DNase can thus be considered a mucokinetic agent that produces slight improvements in pulmonary function in patients with cystic fibrosis.[64] It can also decrease sputum adhesiveness.

No benefit of DNase has yet been demonstrated in other disorders. Studies evaluating the use of DNase in bronchiectasis unrelated to cystic fibrosis have shown no benefit on spirometry, subjective quality of life, or dyspnea.[65, 66] Studies in patients with exacerbations of COPD have shown no survival benefit.

SUMMARY

Adjunctive respiratory therapies are an important aspect of the care of critically ill patients, especially those receiving mechanical ventilation. Understanding of the role of lung defense mechanisms such as cough enables clinicians to provide therapies designed to improve lung expansion and mucociliary clearance when cough is ineffective or nonexistent. Physicians' knowledge of the indications and utilization of these drugs, devices, and therapies is important not only to prevent potential complications associated with their use but also to provide cost effective therapy. Respiratory adjunctive therapies are useful and effective when carefully applied with clearly defined therapeutic goals.

References

1. Leith DE: Cough. *In*: Respiratory Defense Mechanisms: II. Lung Biology in Health and Disease. Brain JD, Proctor DF, Redd LM (Eds). New York, Marcel Dekker, 1977, pp 545–592.
2. McCool FD, Leith DE: Pathophysiology of cough. Clin Chest Med 1987; 8:189–202.
3. Ingram RH Jr: Mechanical aids to lung expansion. Am Rev Respir Dis 1980; 122 (Suppl): 23–30.
4. Bartlett RH: Postoperative pulmonary prophylaxis: Breath deeply and read carefully. Chest 1982; 81:1–3.
5. Peruzzi WT, Smith B: Bronchial hygiene therapy. Crit Care Clin 1995; 11:79–96.
6. Shapiro BA, Kacmarek RM, Cane RD: Applying and evaluating bronchial hygiene therapy. *In*: Clinical Application of Respiratory Care. 4th ed. Shapiro BA, Kacmarek RM, Cane RD (Eds). Chicago, Mosby-Year Book, 1991, pp 85–108.
7. Sackner MA: Effect of respiratory drugs and mucociliary clearance. Chest 1978; 73(Suppl):958–961.
8. Wanner A: Clinical aspects of mucociliary transport. Am Rev Respir Dis 1977; 116:73–77.

9. Eid N, Buchheit J, Neuling M: Chest physiotherapy in review. Respir Care 1991; 36:270–282.
10. Hardy AK: A review of airway clearance: New techniques, indications, and recommendations. Respir Care 1994; 39:440–452.
11. Thomas J, Cook DJ, Brooks D: Chest physical therapy management of patients with cystic fibrosis: A meta-analysis. Am J Respir Crit Care Med 1995; 151:846–852.
12. Murray JF: The ketchup bottle method. N Engl J Med 1979; 300:1155–1157.
13. Marini JJ, Pierson DJ, Hudson LD: Acute lobar atelectasis: A prospective comparison of fiberoptic bronchoscopy and respiratory therapy. Am Rev Respir Dis 1979; 119:971–974.
14. Tyler MI: Complications of position and chest physiotherapy. Respir Care 1982; 27:458–461.
15. Mahlmeister MUJ, Fink JB, Hoffman GL: Positive-expiratory pressure mask therapy: Theoretical and practical considerations and a review of the literature. Respir Care 1991; 36:1218–1221.
16. Davidson AGF, McIlwaine PNM, Wong LTK: Comparison of positive-expiratory pressure and autogenic drainage with conventional percussion and drainage techniques. Pediatr Pulmonol 1988; 2(Suppl):132–136.
17. Gross D, Zidulka A, O'Brien C, Wight D, Fraser R, Rosenthal L, King M: Peripheral mucociliary clearance with high-frequency chest wall compression. J Appl Physiol 1985; 88:1157–1163.
18. Piquet J, Brochard L, Isabey D, De Cremoux H, Chang HK, Bignon J, Harf A: High frequency chest wall oscillation in patients with chronic air-flow obstruction. Am Rev Respir Dis 1987; 136:1355–1359.
19. King M, Phillips DM, Gross D, Vartian V, Chang HK, Zidulka A: Enhanced tracheal mucus clearance with high frequency chest wall compression. Am Rev Respir Dis 1983; 128:511–515.
20. Arens R, Gozal D, Omlin KJ, Vega J, Boyd KP, Keens TG, Woo MS: Comparison of high frequency chest compression and conventional chest physiotherapy in hospitalized patients with cystic fibrosis. Am J Respir Crit Care Med 1994; 150:1154–1157.
21. Braggion C, Cappelletti LM, Cornacchia M, Zanolla L, Mastella G: Short-term effects of three chest physiotherapy regimens in patients hospitalized for pulmonary exacerbations of cystic fibrosis: A cross-over randomized study. Pediatr Pulmonol 1995; 19:16–22.
22. Demers RR, Saklad M: Mechanical aspiration: A reappraisal of its hazards. Respir Care 1975; 20:661–663.
23. Demers RR: Complications of endotracheal suctioning procedures. Respir Care 1982; 27:453–455.
24. Mayhall CG: The Trach Care™ closed tracheal suction system: A new medical device to permit tracheal suctioning without interruption of ventilatory assistance. Infect Control Hosp Epidemiol 1988; 9:125–129.
25. Brown SE, Stansburg DW, Merrill EJ: Prevention of suctioning-related arterial oxygen desaturation. Chest 1983; 83:621–625.
26. Ritz R, Scott LR, Coyle MB: Contamination of a multiple-use suction catheter in a closed-circuit system compared to contamination of a disposable single-use suction catheter. Respir Care 1986; 31:1086–1089.
27. Taggart SA, Dovinsky NL, Sheahan JS: Airway pressures during closed system suctioning. Heart Lung 1988; 17:536–538.
28. Fineberg C, Cohn HE, Gibbon JH Jr: Cardiac arrest during nasotracheal aspiration. JAMA 1960; 174:410–414.
29. Jacquette G: To reduce hazards of tracheal suctioning. Am J Nurs 1971; 71:2362–2365.
30. Petersen GM, Pierson DJ, Hunter PM: Arterial oxygen saturation during nasotracheal suctioning. Chest 1979; 76:283–287.
31. LeFrock JL, Lainer AS, Wen-Hsien W: Transient bacteremia associated with nasotracheal suctioning. JAMA 1976; 236:1610–1615.
32. Becker DM, Gonzalez M, Gentili A: Prevention of deep venous thrombosis in patients with acute spinal cord injuries: Use of rotating treatment tables. Neurosurgery 1987; 20:675–677.
33. Demarest GB, Schmidt-Nowara WW, Vance LW: Use of kinetic treatment table to prevent the pulmonary complications of multiple trauma. West J Med 1989; 150:35–38.
34. Summer WR, Curry P, Haponk EF, Nelson S, Elson R: Continuous mechanical turning of intensive care unit patients shortens length of stay in some diagnosis related groups. J Crit Care 1989; 4:45–53.
35. Pape HC, Regel G, Borgmann RW: The effect of kinetic positioning on lung function and pulmonary hemodynamics in post traumatic ARDS. A clinical study. Injury 1994; 25:51–57.
36. Gentilello L, Thompson DA, Tonnesen AS, Hernandez D, Kapadia AS, Allen SJ: Effect of a rotating bed on the incidence of pulmonary complications in critically ill patients. Crit Care Med 1988; 16:783–786.
37. Clemmer RP, Green S, Ziegler B: Effectiveness of the kinetic treatment table for preventing and treating pulmonary complications in severely head-injured patients. Crit Care Med 1990; 18:614–617.
38. Anzueto A, Peters JI, Seidner SR, Cox WJ, Schroder W, Coalson J: Effects of continuous bed rotation and prolonged mechanical ventilation on healthy, adult baboons. Crit Care Med 1997; 25:1560–1564.
39. Sahn S: Continuous lateral rotational therapy and nosocomial pneumonia. Chest 1991; 99:1263–1267.
40. Barach AL, Bickerman HA, Beck GJ: Induced sputum as a diagnostic technique for cancer of the lungs, and for mobilization of retained secretions. Arch Intern Med 1960; 106:230–236.
41. Clarke SW, Thomson ML, Pavia D: Effect of mucolytic and expectorant drugs on tracheobronchial clearance in chronic bronchitis. Eur J Respir Dis 1980; 110(Suppl):179–183.
42. Zimet I: Pharmacologic therapy of obstructive airway disease. Clin Chest Med 1990; 11:461–467.
43. Cruz RS, Landa J, Hirsch J: Tracheal mucus velocity in normal man and patients with obstructive lung disease: Effects of terbutaline. Am Rev Respir Dis 1974; 109:458–462.
44. Kacmarek RM, Hess D: The interface between the patient and aerosol generator. Respir Care 1991; 36:952–976.
45. Kradjan WA, Lakshminarayan S: Efficiency of air compressor-driven nebulizer. Chest 1985; 87:512–516.
46. Newman SP: Aerosol generators and delivery systems. Respir Care 1991; 36:939–951.
47. Hess D: How should bronchodilators be administered to patients on ventilators? Respir Care 1991; 36:377–394.
48. Newman SP, Pavia D, Moren F: Deposition of pressurized aerosols in the human respiratory tract. Thorax 1981; 36:52–55.
49. Armitage JM, Williams SJ: Inhaler technique in the elderly. Age Ageing 1988; 17:275–278.
50. Jenkins SC, Heaton RW, Fulton TJ: Comparison for domicilary nebulized salbutamol and salbutamol from a metered-dose inhaler in stable chronic airflow limitation. Chest 1987; 91:804–807.
51. Morley TF, Marozsan E, Azppasodi SJ: Comparison of beta-adrenergic agents delivered by nebulizer vs. metered dose inhaler with Inspirease in hospitalized asthmatic patients. Chest 1989; 96:953–955.
52. Fernandez A, Lazaro A, Garcia A, Aragon C, Cerda E: Bronchodilators in patients with chronic obstructive pulmonary disease on mechanical ventilation: Utilization of metered-dose inhalers. Am Rev Respir Dis 1990; 141:164–168.
53. Gay PC, Patel HG, Nelson SB, Gilles B, Hubmayer RD: Metered dose inhaler for bronchodilator delivery in intubated, mechanically ventilated patients. Chest 1991; 99:66–71.
54. Bowton DL, Goldsmith WM, Haponik EF: Substitution of metered-dose inhalers for hand-held nebulizers: Success and cost savings in a large, acute-care hospital. Chest 1992; 101:305–308.
55. Task Group on Mucoactive Drugs: Recommendations for guidelines on clinical trials of mucoactive drugs in chronic bronchitis and chronic obstructive pulmonary impairment. Chest 1994; 106:1532–1536.
56. Richardson PS, Phipps RJ: The anatomy, physiology, pharmacology and pathology of tracheobronchial mucus secretion and the use of expectorant drugs in human disease. Pharmacol Ther (B) 1978; 3:441–447.
57. Shim C, King M, Williams MH: Lack of effect of hydration on sputum production in chronic bronchitis. Chest 1987; 92:679–683.
58. Pavia D, Thompson ML, Clarke SW: Enhanced clearance of secretions from the human lung after the administration of hypertonic saline aerosol. Am Rev Respir Dis 1978; 117:199–214.
59. Pavia D, Agnew JE, Glass JM: Effects of iodopropylidine glycerol on tracheobronchial clearance in stable, chronic bronchitic patients. Eur J Respir Dis 1985; 67:177–184.
60. Antonelli A, Carraro A, Donati C, Garrubba V: Mucolytic effects of diomidol in tracheostomized patients after total laryngectomy: Double-blind, placebo-controlled randomized pilot study with four-month follow-up. Arzneimittelforschung 1992; 42:126–135.

61. Petty TL: The National Mucolytic Study: Results of a randomized, double-blind, placebo-controlled study of iodinated glycerol in chronic bronchitis. Chest 1990; 97:75–81.
62. Swinyard EA, Pathak MA: Surface-acting drugs. *In*: The Pharmacological Basis of Therapeutics. 6th ed. Goodman, Gilman (Eds). New York, Macmillan, 1980.
63. Rao S, Wilson DW, Brooks RA: Acute effects of nebulization of *N*-acetylcysteine on pulmonary mechanics and gas exchange. Am Rev Respir Dis 1970; 102:17–22.
64. Fuchs HJ, Borowitz DS, Christiansen DH: Effect of aerosolized recombinant human DNase on exacerbations of respiratory symptoms and on pulmonary function in patients with cystic fibrosis: The Pulmozygme Study Group. N Engl J Med 1994; 331:637–641.
65. Barker A, O'Donnell A, Mallon K: Phase II trial of recombinant human DNase I in non-CF bronchiectasis. Am J Respir Crit Care Med 1995; 151:A463.
66. Wills PJ, Wodehouse T, Corkery K: Short-term recombinant human DNase in bronchiectasis. Am J Respir Crit Care Med 1996; 154:413–417.

122

Computerized Management of Mechanical Ventilation

R. Matthew Sailors, ME • Thomas D. East, PhD

This chapter reviews the current state of the art as well as future applications of computers in the management of mechanical ventilation. Four general tasks to which computers are particularly suited are as follows:

- Data acquisition and storage
- Information presentation
- Data processing and decision support
- Clinical practice improvement

We discuss the implications of these applications in the field of ventilator management, but the principles are equally applicable to all fields of medical computing.

THE CHALLENGE

Intensive care medicine has, in past decades, begun to founder in the rising flood of data available from automated monitoring equipment; microprocessor-controlled life-support equipment, such as ventilators; ever more sophisticated laboratory tests; and the plethora of minor technologic wonders that every intensive care unit (ICU) seems to collect. During morning rounds in the Shock Trauma/Intermountain Respiratory ICU at the LDS Hospital in Salt Lake City, Utah, our colleagues counted 236 different variables that could have been recorded for just one patient.[1] Dr. David Eddy summarized it best:

> *It is simply unrealistic to think that individuals can synthesize in their head scores of pieces of evidence, accurately estimate the outcomes of different options, and accurately judge the desirability of those outcomes for patients. . . . All confirm what would be expected from common sense: The complexity of modern medicine exceeds the inherent limitations of the unaided human mind.*[2]

It is no longer enough to merely display the data in a large spreadsheet or on a complex, colorful time-sequence graph. The next generation of computers for intensive care must help the clinician assimilate the myriad data and make fast and effective decisions.

HISTORY OF COMPUTERS IN MECHANICAL VENTILATION

It is ironic that the man whose name was chosen for the international unit of pressure, Blaise Pascal, was also the 17th century inventor of the first calculating machine.[3, 4] In a sense, the link between mechanical positive-pressure ventilation and computers has been there from the beginning. The introduction of the minicomputer and the microcomputer in the 1970s dramatically increased the availability of computers. It was during this era that computers first began to be routinely used in hospitals and ICUs. These initial systems typically used teletypewriters and primitive video terminals as user interfaces. The proliferation of the early personal computer (PC) and its clones in the early 1980s greatly enhanced the spread of computers in general and in the health care sector specifically. At this same time, the ratio of cost to computing power was beginning to drop. The last several years have seen this trend continue, and now anyone with $2000 can walk into a computer store and purchase a computer with hundreds of times the combined processing power of all of the computers used on the Apollo 11 spacecraft.

Why would anyone use a computer to manage mechanical ventilation? An examination of the history of computers makes it clear that they were created to (1) help the human mind deal with large amounts of information, complex mathematics, and complex data manipulation and (2) automatically perform well-defined, repetitive tasks. Few devices in medicine are as complex, as data-intensive, and as strongly associated with well-defined repetitive tasks (delivering breaths repeatedly) as a modern mechanical ventilator.

Since the late 1970s, the fundamental operation of the mechanical ventilator has been increasingly turned over to microprocessor control.[5] Besides their computing aspects, microprocessor systems provide an excellent platform upon which to build devices that can easily be modified and updated. Microprocessor-controlled systems make it easy (with software changes) to modify ventilators without changing expensive physical components. As a result, an explosion of new modes and monitoring techniques occurred during the 1980s. Automation of the routine management of mechanical ventilation has been attempted since 1953,[6] only 10 years after the first electronic digital computer was constructed. Automation of mechanical ventilation management has continued to evolve, with growing success and more areas of clinical application, over the last 40 years.[7]

OPERATION OF MECHANICAL VENTILATORS

A fundamental part of a mechanical ventilator is the section dealing with the timing and delivery of gas under positive pressure to the patient. The early mechanical ventilators used either a mechanical system or a pneumatic system to control both the timing and delivery of the gas.[5] A good example of the mechanical system was the piston pump that was driven by a motor that turned a cam shaft. The speed of the motor and the mechanical linkage between the cam and the piston determined the timing and volume of the breath. The bellows, or bag-in-box, ventilator (still in use throughout anesthesiology) is a good example of the pneumatic system, in which gas under pressure is used to compress the bellows and deliver a volume to the patient. The timing of the ventilator was controlled by pneumatic valves that switched as pressure in the circuit crossed certain thresholds.

As ventilators became more sophisticated, there was a merger of mechanical, pneumatic, and electrical systems. One of the significant advances was the use of proportional gas delivery valves, which used a high-pressure gas source to produce whatever flow or pressure profile was desired. Siemens was the first manufacturer to introduce electronic feedback control of these proportional valves (Servo 900B) to produce a variety of different flow and pressure waveforms. These servo-controlled proportional valves were really the key to the development of the variety of ventilator modes now available. Even though many of the modern ventilators introduced in the 1960s and 1970s included electronic control of the ventilator, it was not until the late 1970s that a digital computer was used to control the valves in the ventilator.

It was inevitable that digital computers would be used to operate ventilators, and it is not surprising that the first U.S. Food and Drug Administration (FDA) 510 K approval was given for a microprocessor-controlled ventilator, the Rodder Instruments ventilator (Los Altos, Calif),[7] only a few years after the initial design of a microcomputer. The Rodder ventilator was followed by the manufacture of infant ventilators with microprocessor control and then by the introduction of the Bear 5 and Puritan Bennett 7200 adult ventilators. The previous analog systems were excellent; however, they lacked the ability to be easily changed and adapted. In the electronic ventilators of the 1970s and early 1980s, adding a new mode of mechanical ventilation required the addition of all-new analog control circuits. Typically, these analog systems were not designed for such expansion. The microprocessor offered the unique ability to provide rapid and precise control of gas delivery while also running the user interface, collecting data, and monitoring ventilator performance. In addition, the computer could easily be reprogrammed to add new modes and other features. The control and operation of mechanical ventilators seemed like an ideal application for the digital microcomputer.

Figure 122-1 illustrates how microcomputers are used in a modern ventilator. The primary function of the microprocessor is to regulate the proportional valves delivering air and oxygen to the patient. Typically, these valves are closed loop-controlled. For example, to produce pressure support ventilation (PSV), the ventilator monitors airway pressure and opens or closes the valve as needed to try to maintain a desired pressure level. These fast closed loop control systems are good; however, they are not perfect, exhibiting undesired control behavior such as overshoot and ringing (Fig. 122-2). The same concept applies for volume control with a constant inspiratory flow profile. The only difference is that the proportional valve is feedback-controlled to maintain a desired flow rate. Typically, the computer in the ventilator is updating the position of the proportional valve at least every 1/100 second. In the Siemens Servo 300, the valve is adjusted every 1/1000 second.

The advantage of the closed loop controller is that the valves do not need to be linear or necessarily stable over time. What is critical is that the input to the controller, either flow or pressure, must be accurate and precise; otherwise, the entire system will be inaccurate. In addition, the control algorithm must be carefully adjusted to provide optimal performance over the operating range of the system. This adjustment is not an easy task when one considers that a ventilator (such as the Siemens Servo 300) must ventilate with tidal volumes from 2 mL up to 4 L, all with the same valve.

As can be seen from Figure 122-1, it is easy for the manufacturers to provide a variety of modes, such as pressure support, pressure control, and volume control. In several new modes of ventilation, a second feedback loop is superimposed on the existing ones for pressure support or pressure control. Figure 122-3 illustrates the new modes of volume support and pressure-regulated volume control that were introduced on the Siemens Servo 300; they include an outer feedback loop that adjusts, over several breaths, the set-point of the faster inner feedback loop. This concept has been in use since the mid-1980s in modes such as mandatory minute ventilation, in which the support level is adjusted slowly over several breaths to maintain a desired minute ventilation range. It is unclear what impact these newer ventilator modes will have on patient outcome; however, the modes represent a higher level of sophistication and complexity in control of gas delivery.

The same concepts of feedback control can be applied to the expiratory valve. The Siemens 900C ventilator uses the

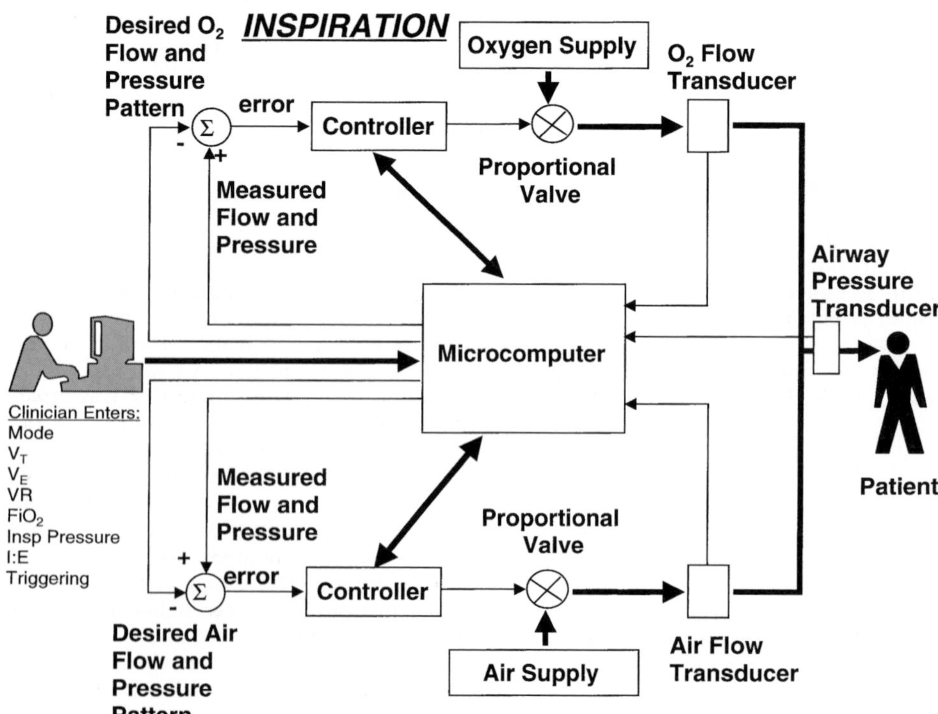

Figure 122–1. Microprocessor-controlled mechanical ventilator. The microprocessor uses data from the flow and pressure sensors as well as input from the user to determine the correct positioning of the proportional gas supply valve. There is a separate control system for air and oxygen in order to provide the desired fraction of inspired oxygen (FIO_2). V_T = tidal volume; V_E = expired minute volume; VR = respiratory volume; I:E = inspiratory to expiratory ratio.

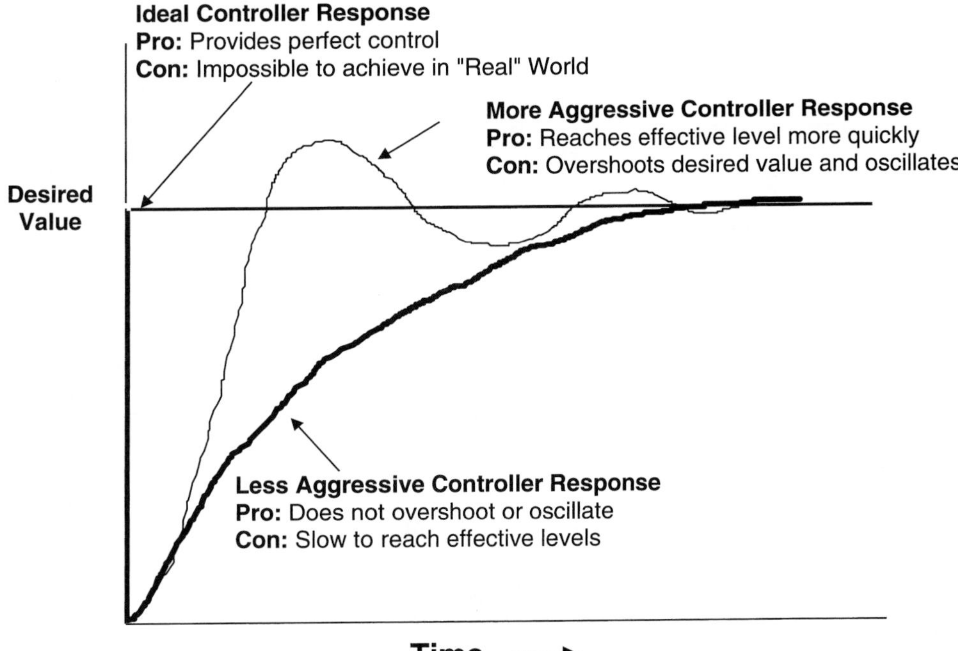

Figure 122–2. Closed loop control of the gas delivery valves is never ideal. This figure illustrates a more aggressive and a less aggressive controller in comparison to the "ideal" controller. The aggressive controller overshoots the desired value and oscillates. The less aggressive controller does not overshoot but is slow to reach the desired value.

pressure measured in the inspiratory limb of the patient circuit as feedback control to adjust the expiratory pinch valve to maintain a desired positive end-expiratory pressure (PEEP) value (Fig. 122–4). The inspiratory limb has zero flow during expiration, ensuring measurement of pressure at the patient manifold even though the pressure transducer is within the ventilator. The advantage of using a feedback-controlled valve is that a relatively simple valve and pressure sensor can be made to behave like a threshold resistor (zero resistance until pressure reaches the PEEP value; then resistance is infinite). An additional advantage is that it is easy for the microprocessor to control this expiratory valve for measurements, such as intrinsic PEEP, a measure that requires an end-expiratory hold. Not all microprocessor-based ventilators use a computer-controlled expiratory valve. For example, the Puritan Bennett 7200 uses a pneumatically controlled expiratory valve that depends only on pressures in the breathing circuit and has no computer control.

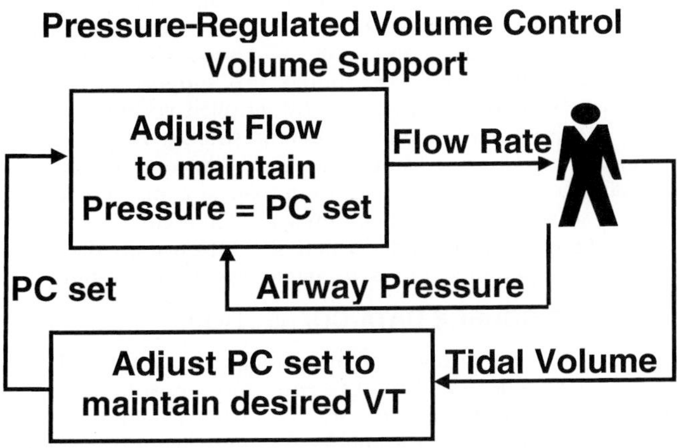

Figure 122–3. Volume support and pressure-regulated volume control are examples of double-feedback systems. The standard inner feedback loop adjusts the gas delivery valve to provide the desired pressure. An outer feedback loop adjusts the desired pressure level of the inner loop to deliver the desired tidal volume (VT).

INFORMATION SYSTEMS FOR RESPIRATORY CARE

Despite the large amount of clinical respiratory care data and the obvious difficulty in managing them in a handwritten record, respiratory care information systems have not had widespread acceptance as methods for recording information during mechanical ventilation. Much of the reason probably lies in the question of the cost justification for such systems.

Cost versus Benefit of Information Systems

The costs of information systems are typically justified on the basis of the reduction in time that hospital personnel spend charting and performing record audits, the implication being that money would be saved through reduction of staffing requirements. Andrews and colleagues[8] reported that the respiratory care charting portion of the Health Evaluation through Logical Processing (HELP) information system at LDS Hospital was associated with an 18.2% increase in personnel productivity and a 20.9% increase in work volume. Full-time equivalent staffing requirements did not change. An average of 2.6 minutes was spent on each documentation in 1984, before the respiratory care portion of the HELP system was introduced, compared with 1.37 minutes in 1992.[9] Some researchers have claimed that information systems are cost-justified on the basis of the reduction in FTE requirements that they provide; however, this claim is controversial.

Hammond and associates[10] have demonstrated that an ICU patient data management system can significantly reduce the number of errors found in paper flow charts and improve the quality, accuracy, and timely capture and retrieval of data. The same group did not, however, show a reduction in the required nursing FTE.[11] Bradshaw and coworkers[12] showed that less nursing time was spent on direct patient care (a reduction

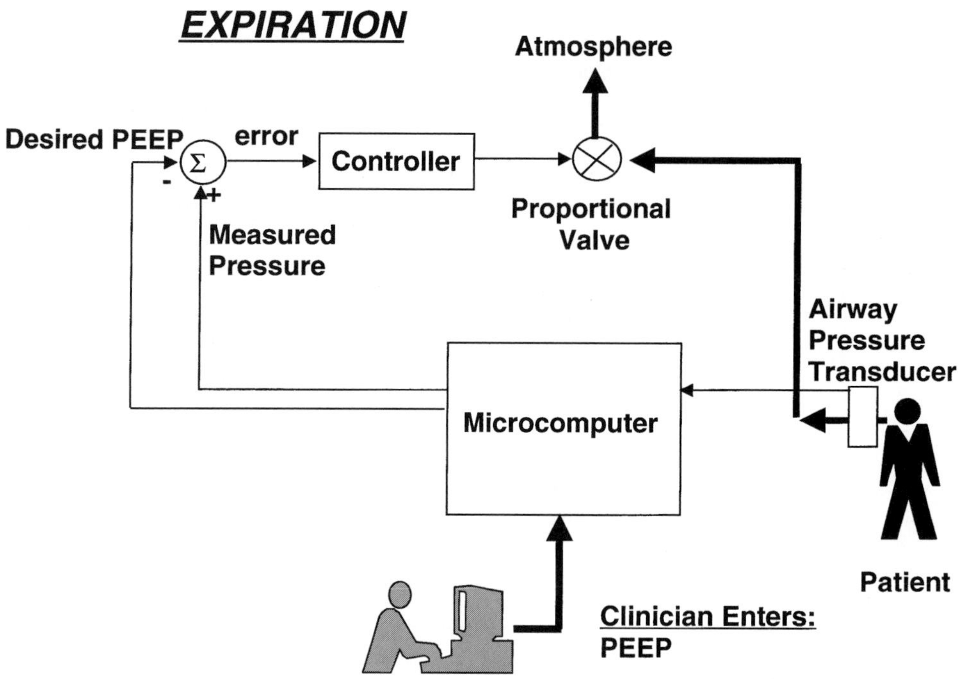

Figure 122–4. Many microprocessor-based ventilators use an active exhalation valve that is under computer control. The computer uses a feedback control system to adjust the expiratory valve to maintain the desired positive end-expiratory pressure (PEEP) level.

from 49.1% to 43.2%) and more nursing time was spent on clinical data entry (an increase from 18.2% to 24.2%).

There are many anecdotal reports of the impact of information systems on the quality of patient care, but few conclusive studies that clearly demonstrate improvement in the quality of patient care. One would assume that the improvements in the quality of the patient chart would affect the quality of patient care; however, some have estimated that it a study of at least 6000 patients would be required to statistically detect any impact on patient outcome (assuming a reduction in mortality from 16% to 14.4%).[13] It may be possible to observe an impact on the quality of patient care by looking at other intermediate indicators, such as the length of hospital stay and incidence of mistakes. It is essential that carefully designed studies be performed to evaluate the impact of information systems.

Blueprint for Success

The main problem with demonstrating efficacy of information systems for mechanical ventilation may be that the current systems that focus on automating the charting process do not really address the requirements of the clinicians in the ICU environment. What are the real needs of the clinicians (physician, nurse, and respiratory therapist) at the bedside? One need only recall the previously mentioned figure of 236 information categories counted on morning rounds for one ICU patient[1] to understand the problem. To help clinicians assimilate these data and make therapy decisions based on them, new data display concepts and expert systems must be included in new commercial products. Few computer systems for respiratory care currently provide any tools for decision support. The next generation of computer systems will have to include the following features if they are to have a significant impact on the quality of patient care:

- Data acquisition
- Data storage
- Information display
- Data processing
- Decision support

By (1) automating or streamlining repetitive or complex tasks, (2) correlating and presenting complex and potentially confusing data, and (3) tracking patient outcomes, the computer can augment clinicians' skills to improve patient care. These features and functions are examined in detail in the following discussion.

FEATURES OF A USEFUL SYSTEM

Data Acquisition and Storage

Data acquisition and storage are two of the most common roles computers play in health care delivery. Data can be acquired through manual or automatic means. In either case, the raw data that are collected must be eventually stored in some form for later use. The organization of the data base that stores the data depends greatly on how the data are to be used later. Simple display of the collected information or simple algorithmic filtering of the data (e.g., "in pulse oximeter") can be accomplished with volatile (nonpermanent) memory storage. Decision support functions generally require a more sophisticated, preferably integrated, data base. This type of complex data base should also support a common naming convention (lexicon) and controlled vocabularies, so that information from many different sources can be easily integrated to form a comprehensive view of the patient's condition. Respiratory care information systems should not merely store whatever data are presented to them; they should be designed to raise alerts when the information does not meet the requirements for reasonableness and consistency.

MULTIPLE-SOURCE DATA COLLECTION

The successful charting system must support robust multiple-source data collection. The data entry tools must (1) facilitate manual data entry, (2) support automated data acquisition, and (3) provide integrity checks for both manual and automated charting.

Manual Data Collection

Manual data entry should require no more effort than current hand charting methods and should provide benefit to the clinical users through integrity checks to improve the quality of the data. Validity of data, as discussed later, is an essential element of data collection. Data collection should take place only once and as close to the source of data generation as possible to minimize errors. Data entry mechanisms must be easy to use; this requirement implies that they be logical, rapid, and consistent. Several paradigms are being used to design manual charting systems. The two popular designs are computerized ICU flow sheet and point-in-time charting. Although the ICU flow sheet is a compact multidisciplinary chart whose paper analog is in common use, it is not necessarily the best paradigm for computerization. For comparisons of various user interfaces for data entry, see Information Display later.

Automated Data Collection

Automated acquisition of data from medical devices reduces both the time necessary to chart the information and the data entry error rate and facilitates the collection of information when care providers are not at the bedside. Several commercially available systems interface with some selected ventilators. The Puritan Bennett Clinivision interfaces directly with the manufacturer's 7200 ventilator. Manufacturers of various ICU computer systems have developed interfaces for the Puritan Bennett 7200, Siemens 900C with the 990 Servo computer module, Hamilton Amadeus, Hamilton Alveolar, Bear 5, and other ventilators with digital communication ports.[14] Because these interfaces are typically designed as custom interfaces matched specifically to the particular ventilator, they can be expensive and difficult to maintain. This means that if an existing computer system in a hospital is to be connected to the ventilators, a great deal of time and money will most likely have to be spent to accomplish the task. Thus, the vast majority of ventilators have digital communication ports that remain unused.

Several successful research systems in have interfaced ventilators with computers. Shabot and Gardner and colleagues,[15-18] at Cedar-Sinai Hospital in Los Angeles, have interfaced their Hewlett-Packard ICU computer system with the Puritan Bennett 7200 ventilator. In this system, data is sent from the ventilator only when the clinician at the bedside pushes a button or when a setting is changed. At LDS Hospital in Salt Lake City, Utah, we and our colleagues developed individual research systems that interfaced with the Siemens 900C and 900i ventilators[19-22] as well as the Hamilton Amadeus[23] and the Puritan Bennett 7200.[24] These systems are, however, the exception rather than the rule.

To facilitate automatic data acquisition from a wide variety of medical devices, a standardized Medical Information Bus (MIB) has been developed through the IEEE (Institute of Electrical and Electronics Engineers) (IEEE Standard 1073 series),[25, 26] so that all hospitals and vendors can use a common data format and easily communicate with multiple bedside devices.[16, 25-29] The MIB provides a local area network (LAN) around the patient that can interface with all bedside devices (Fig. 122–5), allowing data from each of the devices to be stored in a central data base in a common format.[30-33] The MIB differs from other standardized networks, such as Ethernet, in that it meets the unique requirements of the medical data communications environment, such as (1) association of a device with a particular patient's bedside, (2) automatic recognition of new devices placed at a bedside, and (3) automatic reconfiguration of the network.[16, 29] To this point, the greatest part of the effort of developing the MIB standard has been spent on standardizing digital communication and physical interfaces, rather than on the more clinically important standards for rejection of artifacts (see later discussion) and identification of significant events.[18]

A preliminary version of the MIB was installed at LDS Hospital and interfaced with the HELP system[18, 34, 35] and with ventilators, vital signs monitors, pulse oximeters, and intravenous (IV) infusion pumps.[17, 24, 36-38] Several studies investigating techniques for identifying artifacts and significant events have been completed.[36, 39] An IEEE 1073 Standard MIB system has been installed at McKay-Dee Hospital in Ogden, Utah, and is being used to gather data from IV pumps.[37, 38]

In one of the studies, data from the ventilator were sampled at 10-second intervals and stored in a research data base, which was then used to examine six different filters designed to eliminate artifact: moving average, moving median, two different moving exponentially weighted averages, a LOWESS (*LO*cally *WE*ighted *S*catterplot *S*moother, a robust, locally weighted regression technique[40]), and a moving LOWESS.[39] Significant events were identified as values being above a defined threshold for a specified period (both 1-minute and 3-minute thresholds were tested). The output from each of these algorithms was compared with the concurrent data in the HELP system entered by the respiratory therapist (RT) using the bedside keyboard (Fig. 122–6).[24]

There were some differences between ventilator settings charted by the respiratory therapist and the MIB. The "error" rate for manual charting of ventilator settings was 3%. Screening of these records showed that most of the difference came from "back-charting" by the RT with the wrong time stamp and the "time-delay" of the automated charting algorithms. RTs tended to enter data and stamp them with the time they "thought" was the time that the events occurred; occasionally, this time stamp was in error. The error rate for manual charting was reduced to 1% if all the errors caused by back-charting were neglected.[39]

The raw data contained a lot of *noise* (erroneous data caused by physical factors) and *artifact* (erroneous data caused by the collection method). In general, all the filtering algorithms helped to reduce artifact; however, the moving LOWESS filter performed best; the disadvantage of the moving LOWESS filter is that it requires much more computer time than a simple moving median. The moving median seemed to be the best choice, because it did not follow transient events, such as a momentary drop in reading due to probe movement or procedures (e.g., suctioning) being performed on the patient, and was relatively simple to implement.[36, 39] There were large differences in the number of events found by the filtering algorithms to be "significant" and the significant events charted manually. Two main differences were observed: (1) the respiratory therapists did not chart what occurred when they were not at the bedside and (2) when they charted, the therapists typically just recorded a "snapshot" of data for the few seconds that they were working on a ventilator, which might not have been truly representative of a patient's overall status. Table 122–1 shows an example of an automated charting algorithm, the optimized respiratory care charting algorithm developed at LDS Hospital.[18, 24, 39]

In a study[17, 18] at LDS Hospital, researchers found that instituting automated data collection reduced the ventilator setting charting errors from about 3% to near 0. For measured parameters, automated data collection found significant events that previously went undetected; however, no studies have been conducted to determine what impact these results might have on patient care. Studies conducted at LDS Hospital and McKay-Dee Hospital indicate that the use of the MIB for automated charting of IV infusion pump rate changes recorded almost twice as many rate changes per infusion in contrast to manual charting.[37, 38] When interviewed, the staff judged that the use of the MIB in this situation was "valuable" or "important" and that it "improved the timeliness, accuracy, and completeness of documentation."[37, 38] Automation of other areas of the pa-

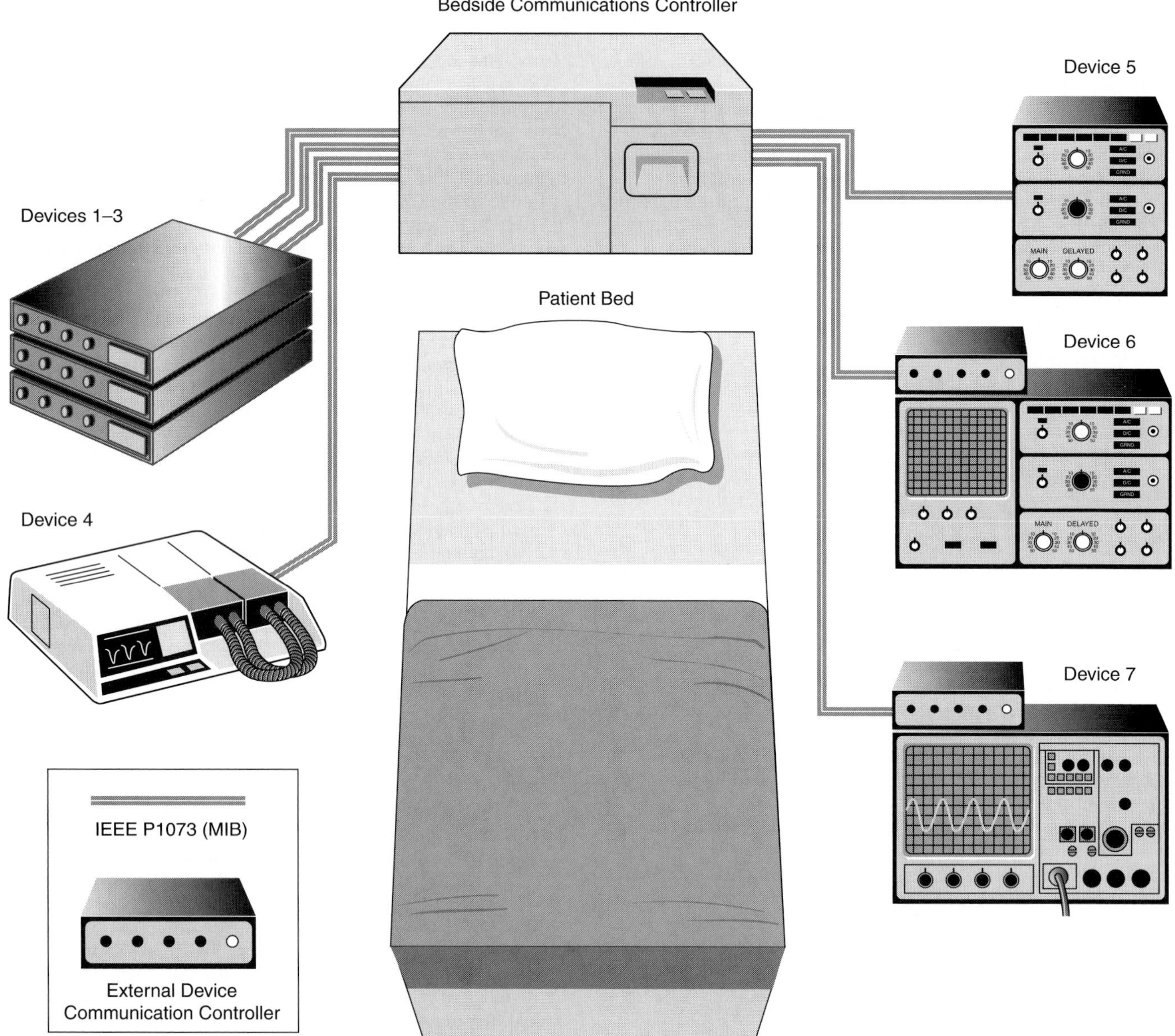

Figure 122–5. The Medical Information Bus (MIB) is a standardized (IEEE 1073) method of connecting and communicating with a variety of beside devices. The MIB allows devices to be associated with a specific location (e.g., room, bed) and provides for plug-and-play attachment of devices. The act of attaching a device to a MIB connection and turning on the device is all that is needed to alert the bedside communications controller (BCC) that a new device is attached to the network. The BCC also "knows" what type of device it is. The BCC is the interface between the beside devices and the rest of the computerized monitoring system. The BCC communicates with the attached devices through a device communications controller (DCC). The DCC may be built into the device or into an external device that translates the proprietary scheme of the device into the standard MIB scheme. The BCC itself may be connected to the rest of the computerized monitoring system with a MIB link. (From Sailors RM, East TD: The Role of the Computer in Monitoring. *In:* The Textbook of Critical Care Monitoring. Tobin MJ [Ed]. New York, McGraw-Hill, 1998.)

tient record has been shown to improve the quality of the data and reduce the amount of time spent on charting.[10]

If electronic communication with ICU equipment is to become an effective and routine part of clinical care, a standard digital communication protocol that makes it easy, both physically and electronically, to connect these devices must be adopted. More research into the elusive definitions of "artifact" and "significant events" is also needed. If the record-keeping standardization effort is to succeed, bedside clinicians must take an active part in the standardization process, because without clinical input, the process is doomed to failure. We anticipate that one day, connecting a ventilator to the computer will be as simple as plugging in a telephone and that the quality of the data will be valid and representative of the patient's true condition.

Integrity Checks

A decision is only as good as the data on which it is based. If a datum is incorrect, missing, inconsistent, or not correlated with the other pieces of data, the decision based on it is of questionable validity. Data integrity is important at all stages and in all kinds of decision making, but it is especially important when the decisions being made are about health care. Decision support systems are only as good as the data they

TABLE 122–1. Recommended Algorithm for Automated Respiratory Care Charting

1. Sample all data from ventilator every 10 seconds and hold in buffer.
2. Report any ventilator setting of more than 3 minutes' duration:
   a. Ventilation mode (MODE)
   b. Ventilator rate (V_R) or intermittent mandatory ventilation rate
   c. Tidal volume (V_T) or minute ventilation (VE)
   d. Peak inspiratory flow
   e. Inspired oxygen fraction (FIO_2)
   f. Trigger sensitivity
   g. Positive end-expiratory pressure (PEEP)
   h. Pressure support or control level
   i. Flow-by support level
   j. Flow-by sensitivity
3. Measured data:
   a. Use 3-minute moving median to filter raw data stored in buffer.
   b. Report one filtered value every hour.
   c. Report significant events:

Event	Criteria
(1) Peak pressure	Change > 10 cm H_2O *and* 3 cm H_2O < Peak Pressure < 120 cm H_2O
(2) Airway pressure	Change > 5 cm H_2O *and* 3 cm H_2O < Airway Pressure < 120 cm H_2O
(3) Plateau pressure	Change > 5 cm H_2O *and* 3 cm H_2O < Plateau Pressure < 120 cm H_2O
(4) Inspiratory/expiratory (I/E) ratio	Per cent Change > 25%
(5) Spontaneous V_T	Per cent Change > 10% *and* Change > 100 mL *and* 100 mL < Spontaneous V_T < 2500 mL
(6) Machine V_T	Per cent Change > 10% *and* Change > 50 mL *and* 100 mL < Machine V_T < 2500 mL
(7) Spontaneous V_R	Per cent change > 10% *and* Change > 5 beats/min *and* 0.5 beats/min < Spontaneous V_R < 70 beats/min
(8) Machine V_R	Per cent change > 10% *and* Change > 2 beats/min *and* 0.5 beats/min < Machine V_R < 70 beats/min

   that last for more than 3 minutes.
   d. Report all measured data values 1 minute after setting changes.

Adapted from East T, Sailors R: Clinical information systems in critical care. *In:* Clinical Information Systems. Rane M (Ed). Redmond, Wash, SpaceLabs Medical, Inc, 1997.

are given. Whether the support is based on an expert system or only on data presentation, incorrect data can lead to dangerous, even fatal, consequences.

Regardless of the method of data collection (automated or manual), checking of data integrity is the key to ensuring the quality of the data in the data base and the decisions based on that data. Data integrity should be enforced as close to the point of entry as possible. The farther from the point of entry that data integrity checks are performed, the more difficult and time-consuming the task. The concept of data integrity encompasses the following key areas[41]:

- Data completeness
- Range checking
- Referential integrity

DATA COMPLETENESS. All available data should be entered at the time they are generated; this means at the ICU bedside, in the radiology department, in the operating room, or anyplace else that patient care is performed. If values are missing, patient care can be affected. Charting by exception and default values are two methods of easing the charting burden and helping to ensure data completeness. In reviews of performance data from the use of computerized management protocols for ventilator therapy, we have found that a substantial fraction of the disagreements between decision support system and clinician were due to incomplete or missing chartings.

RANGE CHECKING. Range checking is vital to ensure correct charting of values in the computer. It is all too easy to miss the decimal point and change a pH from "7.24" to "72.4" or to transpose an oxygen saturation of "87%" to "78%." Although a clinician would recognize that the pH value of 72.4 is clearly wrong, a computer does not have the a priori knowledge necessary to make that determination. Both the correct and

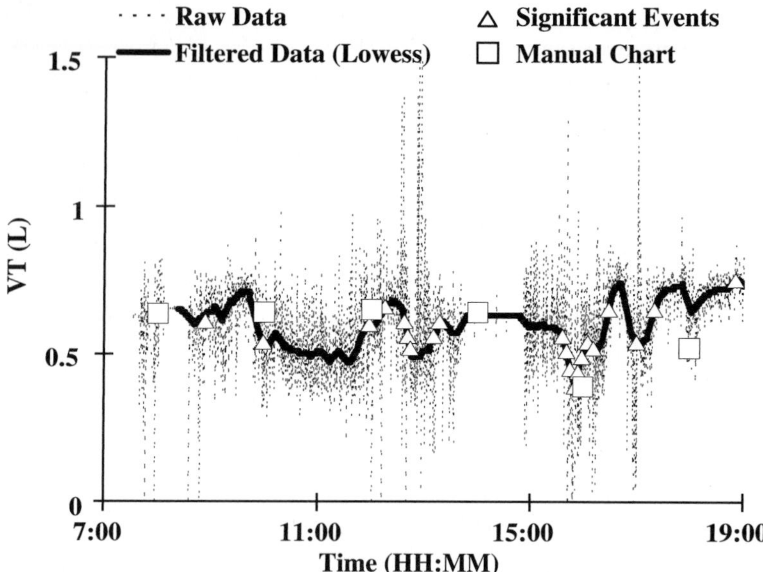

Figure 122–6. An example of tidal volume (VT) data collected at 10-second intervals from a ventilator. The effect of filtering the data with a LOWESS (*LO*cally *WE*ighted *S*catterplot *S*moother) filter is shown and only the significant events (see Table 122-1) indicated are actually stored in the patient record. The points actually recorded in the manual chart are included for comparison. (From East TD, Young WH, Gardner RM: Digital electronic communication between ventilators and computers and printers. Respir Care 1992; 37:1113–1123.)

mistyped oxygen saturations values are logically possible, but the decision based on the lower value may be vastly different from the decision based on the higher one, and in the absence of other data, neither the clinician nor the computer will be able to tell whether the numbers were transposed. Without range checking, bad data can propagate throughout the system and lead to adverse outcomes. Automated decision support aids are especially vulnerable to erroneous data.

Table 122-2 illustrates some of the range checking performed by ventilator charting screens that have been installed in LDS Hospital and other hospitals in the Intermountain Health Care, Inc., system. As the table shows, both absolute ranges and warning ranges are needed for completeness. The warning ranges may be tailored to sites and intensity of care. For example, a clinician might not be worried about an Spo_2 (oxygen saturation measured by pulse oximetry) value of 88% in an ICU patient but would be deeply concerned if a ward patient's Spo_2 value were that low; this is where the warning range applies. In neither patient, however, should a 105% Spo_2 value be charted; this error would be identified on the basis of the absolute range.

REFERENTIAL INTEGRITY. Referential integrity checking verifies that related values are consistent and rational; for example, the plateau airway pressure cannot be greater than the peak airway pressure. Table 122-3 lists some common rules for referential integrity.

We have instituted these types of integrity checks in the data collection process for our current randomized trial both at the point of entry and prior to data analysis.[41] Our data error rate (measured as the number of data that are wildly improbable or erroneous and are not found by automated checks or form-based quality assurance criteria divided by the total number of data) is currently less than 1%, compared with an estimated rate of 3% (measured as the number of data committed to our database that are wildly improbable or erroneous divided by the total number of data) in the raw data and 3% in historical controls.[39]

Multiple-View Clinical Data Repository (Integrated Data Base)

A clinical data repository contains *integrated* information from a myriad of sources: admit, discharge, and transfer

TABLE 122–2. Sample Range Checking Criteria for Siemens Servo 900c Ventilator Data Entry Screens Developed at LDS Hospital for Use in LDS Hospital and Other Intermountain Health Care, Inc., Facilities

Variable	Reasonable Low*	Reasonable High*	Absolute Low†	Absolute High†
FIO_2	0.21	1.00	0.21	1.00
Spo_2	70	100	30	100
V_E	2.0	25.0	0.5	40.0
V_R	5	80	5	120
PEEP	0	30	0	50

Adapted from East T, Sailors R: Clinical information systems in critical care. *In:* Clinical Information Systems. Rane M (Ed). Redmond, Wash, SpaceLabs Medical, Inc, 1997; and Sailors RM, East TD: The role of the computer in monitoring. *In:* The Textbook of Critical Care Monitoring. Tobin MJ (Ed). New York, McGraw-Hill, 1998.

*A warning message is generated if the entered value of the variable falls outside the Reasonable Low to Reasonable High range.

†Entering values outside the Absolute Low to Absolute High range is not allowed.

% FIO_2 = inspired oxygen fraction (percentage); Spo_2 = pulse oximetry saturation; VE = minute ventilation; VR = ventilator rate setting; PEEP = positive end expiratory pressure.

TABLE 122–3. Sample Referential Integrity Rules Used to Enforce Data Quality in Adult Respiratory Distress Syndrome (ARDS) Protocol Study Data Base*

Variable	Rule
Peak pressure	≥ Plateau Pressure
Plateau pressure	≥ PEEP and ≤ Peak Pressure
PEEP	≤ Plateau Pressure
Measured rate	≥ Set Rate
Systolic blood pressure	≥ Diastolic Blood Pressure
Diastolic blood pressure	≤ Systolic Blood Pressure
ICU admit date/time	≥ Hospital Admit Date/Time
Hospital admit date/time	≤ ICU Admit Date/Time
Date of birth	≤ Hospital Admit Date/Time

Adapted from East T, Sailors R: Clinical information systems in critical care. *In:* Clinical Information Systems. Rane M (Ed). Redmond, Wash, SpaceLabs Medical, Inc, 1997; and Sailors RM, East TD: The role of the computer in monitoring. *In:* The Textbook of Critical Care Monitoring. Tobin MJ (Ed). New York, McGraw-Hill, 1998.

*Although some rules are interrelated and may seem redundant, they are all required to handle situations in which data are not charted in the order expected or are edited at a later date.

PEEP = positive end expiratory pressure; ICU = intensive care unit.

(ADT), laboratories, radiology department, operating rooms, and outpatient clinics. Prospective reimbursement has caused a shift to performing as many tests as possible on an outpatient basis, before a patient is hospitalized, and it is essential that the data from these tests be available *and* integrated with all other data for that patient.[42, 43]

A successful clinical data repository must (1) provide data synchronization between the main data base and all source data bases and (2) guarantee accurate and timely data retrieval (less than 1-minute response time delay).[44] Data retrieval should be rapid, because most clinicians are unwilling to wait more than 3 or 4 seconds for a response from the system. The ability to present data in multiple views adds value to clinical information systems. The primary views needed for intensive care are those by patient, by provider, and by diagnosis.

By transcending the paper-based paradigm of "one patient-one record," the clinical data repository allows the information system to provide management information and outcomes measure, and to track population health among physicians, in various regions of the hospital, or by diagnosis. For example, possible sources of nosocomial infections can be easily identified by viewing microbiology results sorted according to health care provider or patient location, and the effects of a process care model can be assessed by viewing all patients with a given diagnosis. Often, with current systems, the easiest way to obtain this kind of information is to perform data analysis outside the clinical information system.[45] Other common data presentation views are of encounter-based and episode-based information. Although these views are not as important in the intensive care arena, they are necessary parts of an integrated clinical data repository, especially with the current movement toward establishing local, regional, national, and international data bases that would track all information on a patient from birth to death.[42]

Controlled Vocabulary and Clinical Lexicon

A controlled vocabulary and a clinical lexicon work symbiotically with the integrated data base to form the core of the computerized patient record. A *controlled vocabulary* eases the burden of codifying information in the data base by limiting the terms that can be used.

The *clinical lexicon* is a dictionary of concepts within the computerized patient record. Each concept is uniquely identified by a code that can be mapped into (connected with) various synonymous terms for different users. For example, the concept "arterial hemoglobin saturation, measured by pulse oximetry" could be identified by the concept code "11384," but the clinical lexicon would also know that the terms "Spo_2", "pulse ox. sat," "oximeter sat," and "HbO_2%" are synonyms for the same concept. The data base refers to concepts (e.g., "arterial hemoglobin saturation, measured by pulse oximetry") only by their concept identifiers (e.g., "11384"); thus, all data base transactions must either use this identifier or be translated by a interpreter that connects text requests with the proper concept identifier.

The clinical lexicon helps ensure against redundancy in the data base and certifies that all data base users are using a common terminology set. By limiting the terms available to the user, a controlled vocabulary makes the clinical lexicon easier to maintain and helps further reduce redundancy. The codes used in the clinical lexicon can either be publicly available codes, such as the International Classification of Diseases (ICD), or proprietary, as in the example just given and in Pointer-to-TeXT (PTXT) in the HELP system.[46] Table 122–4 lists some of the more commonly used coding schemes and their common applications.

The clinical lexicon is also well suited to multilanguage sites

TABLE 122–4. Common Coding Schemes for Medical Information

Coding Scheme	Application
ICD	Classification of inpatient diagnoses; used internationally to classify morbidity and mortality and reported to World Health Organization; used in United States for billing and reimbursement.
DRG	Classification of inpatient diagnoses; lumps similar (by cost) diagnoses into larger groups than ICD; used for billing and reimbursement in United States.
CPT	Classification of outpatient procedures for reimbursement and billing in United States.
READ	British National Health Service coding system, which covers all clinical terms and concepts
SNOMED	System from American College of Pathologists for coding clinical concepts.
UMLS	National Library of Medicine (United States) system for coding all clinical terms and concepts

Adapted from East T, Sailors R: Clinical information systems in critical care. *In:* Clinical Information Systems. Rane M (Ed). Redmond, Wash, SpaceLabs Medical, Inc, 1997; and Sailors RM, East TD: The role of the computer in monitoring. *In:* The Textbook of Critical Care Monitoring. Tobin MJ (Ed). New York, McGraw-Hill, 1998.

ICD = International Classification of Diseases; DRG = Diagnosis-Related Groups; CPT = Common Procedural Terminology; SNOMED = *S*ystematized *No*menclature of *Med*icine; UMLS = Unified Medical Language System.

and to tailoring the text output from the data base to the type of user to whom it is displayed. Thus, clinicians who speak English, Spanish, German, French, and Dutch all use the same concept identifier, even though the text each sees is in his or her own language, and although a clinician sees the concept "09023" displayed as "otitis media," the patient reading a computer-generated management plan will read the term as "ear infection."

The United States National Library of Medicine's Unified Medical Language System (UMLS) project has linked many of the current coding schemes together through a "metathesaurus," which maps concept codes from one coding system to another.[47] This is a step in the right direction, but a universal coding scheme is still necessary to eliminate the problems one faces when mapping vocabularies of different granularity (level of detail) to one another. A universal clinical lexicon and controlled vocabulary will become a 21st century version of Esperanto—a synthetic language designed to provide a common basis for communication.

Information Display

Effective and efficient data entry, data review, and use of a clinical information system require an intuitive user interface with the system. The user interface encompasses computerized interfaces for data entry and review and computer-generated reports. For the process to run efficiently, the user must be comfortable with the interface and must be able to review and enter data effectively. To this end, the user interface must be intuitive and customizable. The intuitive user interface should use common procedures and consistent visual composition and should not hinder the user with unnecessary "gimmicks." The user interface must decrease neither the efficiency of data entry nor the quality of the data.

As a start, the initial user interface configuration should give the user only the appropriate information for his or her own decision making, data charting, and review. For example, nurses should be able to both chart and review a patient's medications; ward clerks, however, do not need to chart medication delivery but should be able to review all the

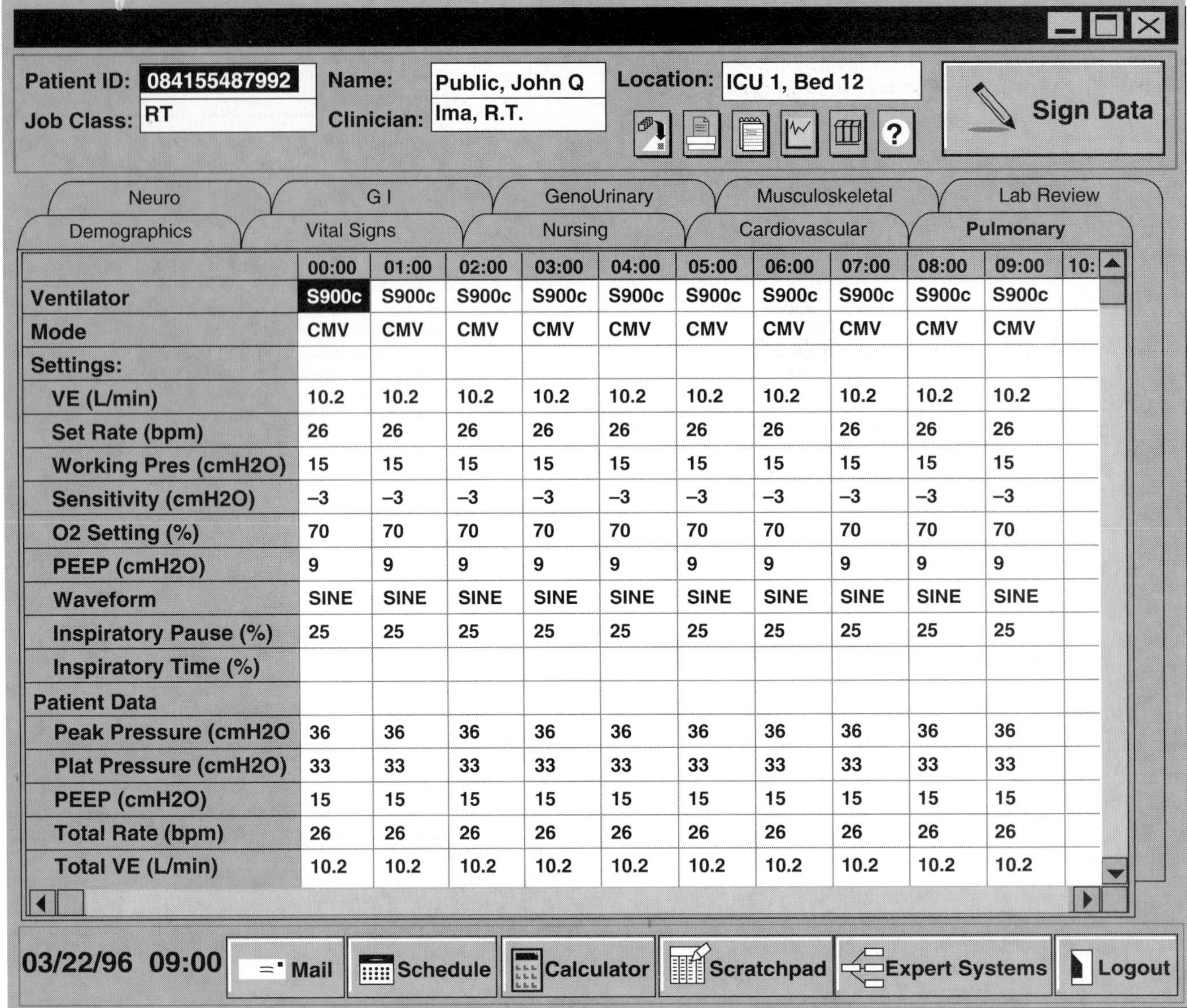

Patient ID: 084155487992 Name: Public, John Q Location: ICU 1, Bed 12

Job Class: RT Clinician: Ima, R.T.

Sign Data

Neuro | G I | GenoUrinary | Musculoskeletal | Lab Review

Demographics | Vital Signs | Nursing | Cardiovascular | **Pulmonary**

	00:00	01:00	02:00	03:00	04:00	05:00	06:00	07:00	08:00	09:00	10:
Ventilator	S900c	S900c	S900c	S900c	S900c	S900c	S900c	S900c	S900c	S900c	
Mode	CMV	CMV	CMV	CMV	CMV	CMV	CMV	CMV	CMV	CMV	
Settings:											
VE (L/min)	10.2	10.2	10.2	10.2	10.2	10.2	10.2	10.2	10.2	10.2	
Set Rate (bpm)	26	26	26	26	26	26	26	26	26	26	
Working Pres (cmH2O)	15	15	15	15	15	15	15	15	15	15	
Sensitivity (cmH2O)	–3	–3	–3	–3	–3	–3	–3	–3	–3	–3	
O2 Setting (%)	70	70	70	70	70	70	70	70	70	70	
PEEP (cmH2O)	9	9	9	9	9	9	9	9	9	9	
Waveform	SINE	SINE	SINE	SINE	SINE	SINE	SINE	SINE	SINE	SINE	
Inspiratory Pause (%)	25	25	25	25	25	25	25	25	25	25	
Inspiratory Time (%)											
Patient Data											
Peak Pressure (cmH2O	36	36	36	36	36	36	36	36	36	36	
Plat Pressure (cmH2O)	33	33	33	33	33	33	33	33	33	33	
PEEP (cmH2O)	15	15	15	15	15	15	15	15	15	15	
Total Rate (bpm)	26	26	26	26	26	26	26	26	26	26	
Total VE (L/min)	10.2	10.2	10.2	10.2	10.2	10.2	10.2	10.2	10.2	10.2	

03/22/96 09:00 Mail Schedule Calculator Scratchpad Expert Systems Logout

Figure 122–7. Characteristic flow sheet paradigm charting screen. Computerized flow sheet charting systems try to reproduce the paper intensive care unit (ICU) flowsheet with a computerized analog. (From East T, Sailors R: Clinical information in critical care. *In:* Clinical Information Systems. Rane M [Ed]. Redmond, Wash, SpaceLabs Medical, Inc, 1997.)

medications given. The user interface should also be customizable to individuals or to job categories. The customization feature should be available *only* after a user is *experienced* enough to know what does and does not work for him or her.

It has become apparent that clinicians are not adequately absorbing all of the information being offered to them by the ever more complex equipment found in a modern ICU. One of the primary functions of the information system will likely be to protect the clinician from too much information. Although data summaries and overviews play important roles in insulating the clinicians from the information overload they face every day, all data *must* be available on request through "drill-down" functions and queries.

Current State of the Art

Most clinical information systems now allow the user to view and enter data in multiple forms. The most popular forms are (1) flow sheets, (2) point-in-time displays, and (3) time-sequence graphs.

The popularity of the *flow sheet* is due to its similarity to the paper flow sheets commonly seen in ICUs; data are presented in a time-sequenced fashion (Fig. 122–7), with review and correction of previous data only a few keystrokes away. *Point-in-time* screens show a snapshot of the data from only a single point in time (Fig. 122–8). The *time-sequence* graph is used only for data display and review, not for charting (Fig. 122–9).

The majority of the commercial systems and several of the custom systems have merely reproduced the ICU flow sheet on the computer (See Fig. 122–7). Although this choice may ease the transition from pen and paper to computer, there is little evidence that it is the optimal strategy. The ICU flow sheet is a "one-stop" chart, but it is not always easy to navigate and can often contribute to the data overload faced by ICU clinicians. Merely computerizing an imperfect paper charting-and-review system does nothing to address the usability or quality of the data.

There is a disturbing trend among the systems that offer flow sheet–based charting to allow for freeform input in many fields with no quality assurance rules; the reasons cited for

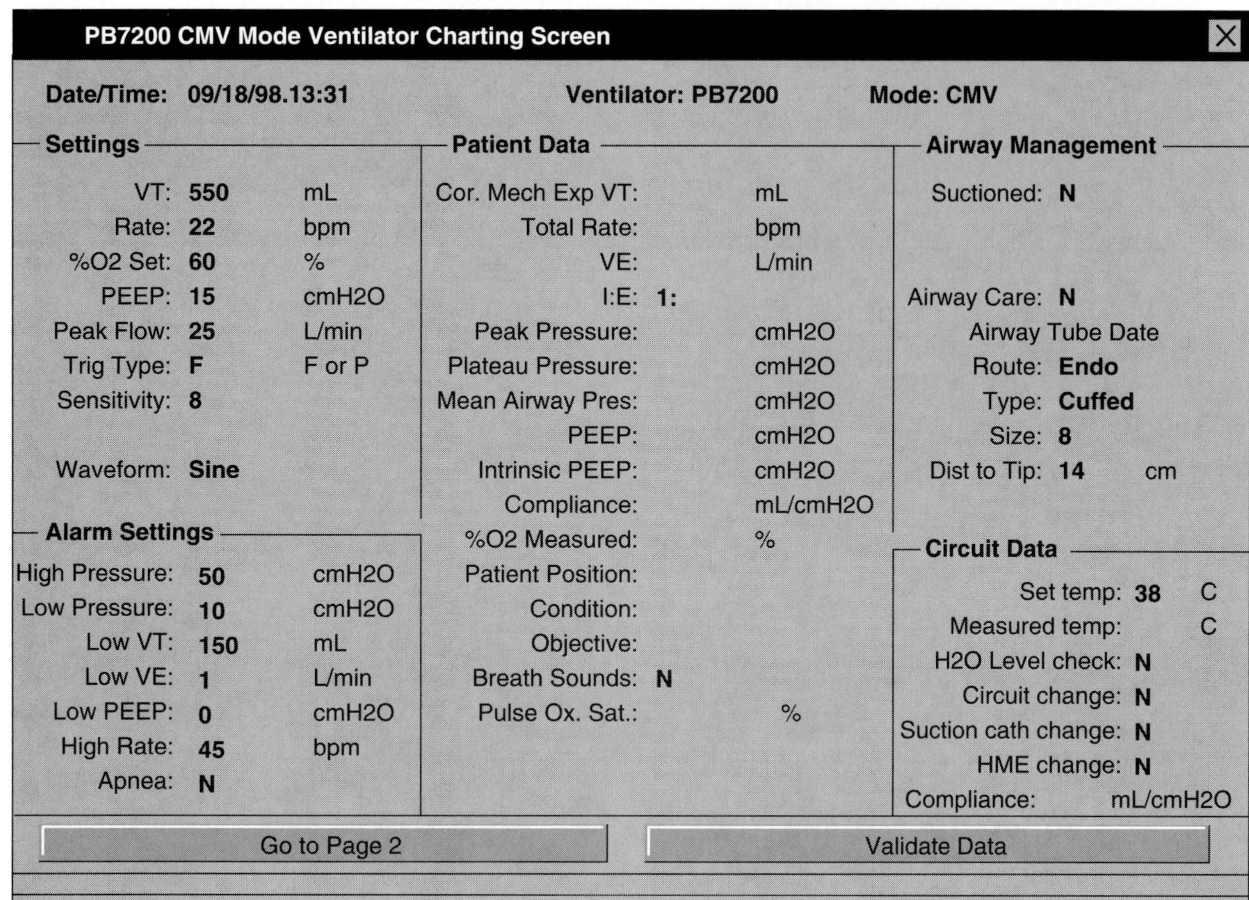

Figure 122–8. An example of a point-in-time charting screen. (From Intermountain Healthcare, Inc, 1996.)

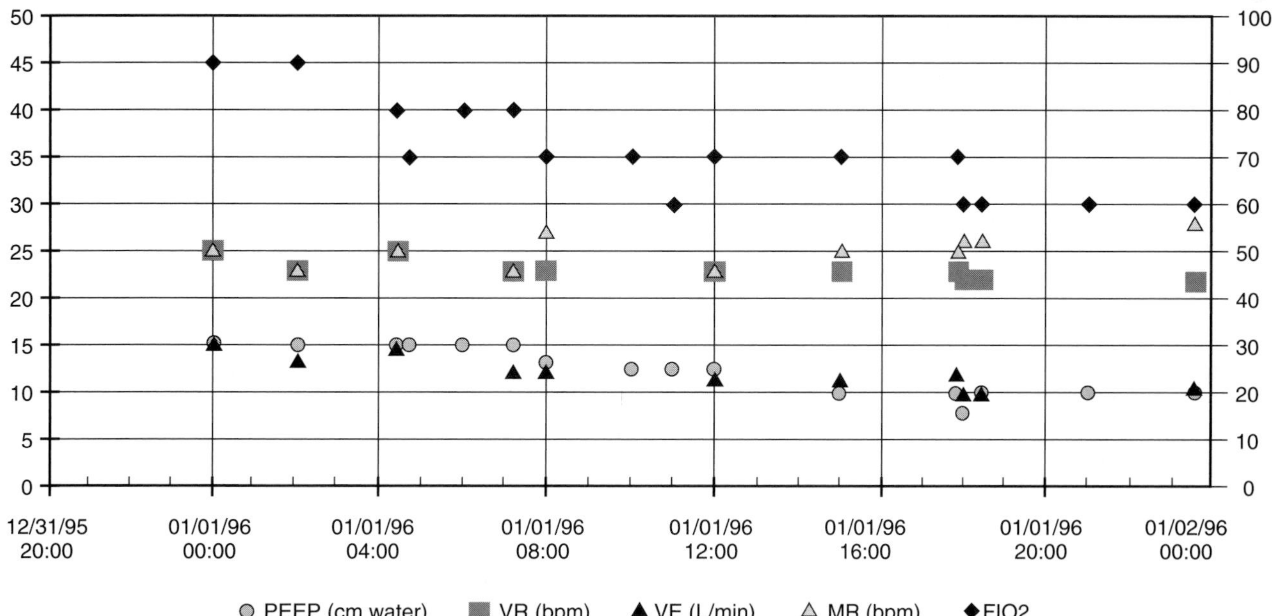

Figure 122–9. Time-sequence graph showing respiratory care data over a 24-hour period. (From East T, Sailors R: Clinical information in critical care. *In:* Clinical Information Systems. Rane M [Ed]. Redmond, Wash, SpaceLabs Medical, Inc, 1997.)

Day 1	18	19	20	21	22	23	24	01	02	03	04	05	06	07	08	09	10	11	12	13	14	15	16	17
Oxygen	70		70		70		70		70		70		70		70		70		70		70		70	
Tidal vol	0.9		0.9		0.9		0.9		0.9		0.9		0.9		0.9		0.9		0.9		0.9		0.9	
Resp rate	10.0		10.0		10.0		10.0		10.0		10.0		10.0		10.0		8.0		9.0		9.0		9.0	
Spont TV	0.0		0.0		0.0		0.0		0.0		0.0		0.0		0.0		0.0		0.0		0.0		0.0	
Spont RR	0.0		0.0		0.0		0.0		0.0		0.0		0.0		0.0		0.0		0.0		0.0		0.0	
Day 2	18	19	20	21	22	23	24	01	02	03	04	05	06	07	08	09	10	11	12	13	14	15	16	17
Oxygen	70		70		70		70		60		60		60		60		60		60		60		60	
Tidal vol	0.8		0.9		0.9		0.9		0.9		0.9		0.9		0.9		0.9		0.9		0.9		0.9	
Resp rate	9.0		9.0		9.0		9.0		9.0		9.0		9.0		9.0		9.0		9.0		9.0		9.0	
Spont TV	0.0		0.0		0.0		0.0		0.0		0.0		0.0		0.0		0.0		0.0		0.0		0.0	
Spont RR	0.0		0.0		0.0		0.0		0.0		0.0		0.0		0.0		0.0		0.0		0.0		0.0	
Day 3	18	19	20	21	22	23	24	01	02	03	04	05	06	07	08	09	10	11	12	13	14	15	16	17
Oxygen	60		60		60		70		60		60		60		60		60		50		50		50	
Tidal vol	0.8		0.9		0.9		0.9		0.9		0.9		0.9		0.9		0.9		0.9		0.9		0.9	
Resp rate	9.0		8.0		8.0		8.0		8.0		8.0		8.0		8.0		8.0		8.0		8.0		8.0	
Spont TV	0.0		0.0		0.0		0.0		0.0		0.0		0.0		0.0		0.0		0.0		0.0		0.0	
Spont RR	0.0		0.0		0.0		0.0		0.0		0.0		0.0		0.0		0.0		0.0		0.0		0.0	
Day 4	18	19	20	21	22	23	24	01	02	03	04	05	06	07	08	09	10	11	12	13	14	15	16	17
Oxygen	50		50		50		50		50		50		50		50		50		50		50		50	
Tidal vol	0.9		0.9		0.9		0.9		0.9		0.9		0.9		0.9		0.9		0.9		0.9		0.9	
Resp rate	8.0		8.0		8.0		8.0		8.0		7.0		7.0		7.0		7.0		7.0		7.0		7.0	
Spont TV	0.0		0.0		0.0		0.0		0.0		0.0		0.0		0.0		0.0		0.0		0.4		0.4	
Spont RR	0.0		0.0		0.0		0.0		0.0		0.0		0.0		0.0		0.0		0.0		1.0		1.0	
Day 5	18	19	20	21	22	23	24	01	02	03	04	05	06	07	08	09	10	11	12	13	14	15	16	17
Oxygen	50		50		50		50		50		50		50		50		50		50		50		50	
Tidal vol	0.9		0.9		0.9		0.9		0.9		0.9		0.9		0.9		0.9		0.9		0.9		0.9	
Resp rate	7.0		7.0		7.0		7.0		7.0		7.0		7.0		7.0		7.0		7.0		6.0		6.0	
Spont TV	0.4		0.4		0.4		0.4		0.4		0.4		0.4		0.4		0.4		0.4		0.4		0.4	
Spont RR	1.0		1.0		1.0		1.0		1.0		1.0		2.0		2.0		2.0		2.0		2.0		2.0	
Day 6	18	19	20	21	22	23	24	01	02	03	04	05	06	07	08	09	10	11	12	13	14	15	16	17
Oxygen	40		40		40		40		40		40		40		30		30		30		30		30	
Tidal vol	0.9		0.9		0.9		0.9		0.9		0.9		0.9		0.9		0.9		0.9		0.9		0.9	
Resp rate	6.0		6.0		6.0		6.0		6.0		6.0		6.0		6.0		6.0		6.0		6.0		6.0	
Spont TV	0.4		0.4		0.4		0.4		0.4		0.4		0.4		0.4		0.4		0.4		0.4		0.4	
Spont RR	2.0		2.0		3.0		3.0		3.0		3.0		3.0		3.0		3.0		3.0		3.0		4.0	
Day 7	18	19	20	21	22	23	24	01	02	03	04	05	06	07	08	09	10	11	12	13	14	15	16	17
Oxygen	30		30		30		30		30		30		30		30		30		30		30		30	
Tidal vol	0.9		0.9		0.9		0.9		0.9		0.9		0.9		0.9		0.9		0.9		0.9		0.9	
Resp rate	6.0		6.0		6.0		5.0		5.0		5.0		5.0		5.0		5.0		5.0		5.0		5.0	
Spont TV	0.4		0.4		0.4		0.4		0.4		0.4		0.4		0.4		0.4		0.4		0.4		0.4	
Spont RR	4.0		4.0		4.0		4.0		4.0		4.0		4.0		5.0		5.0		5.0		5.0		5.0	

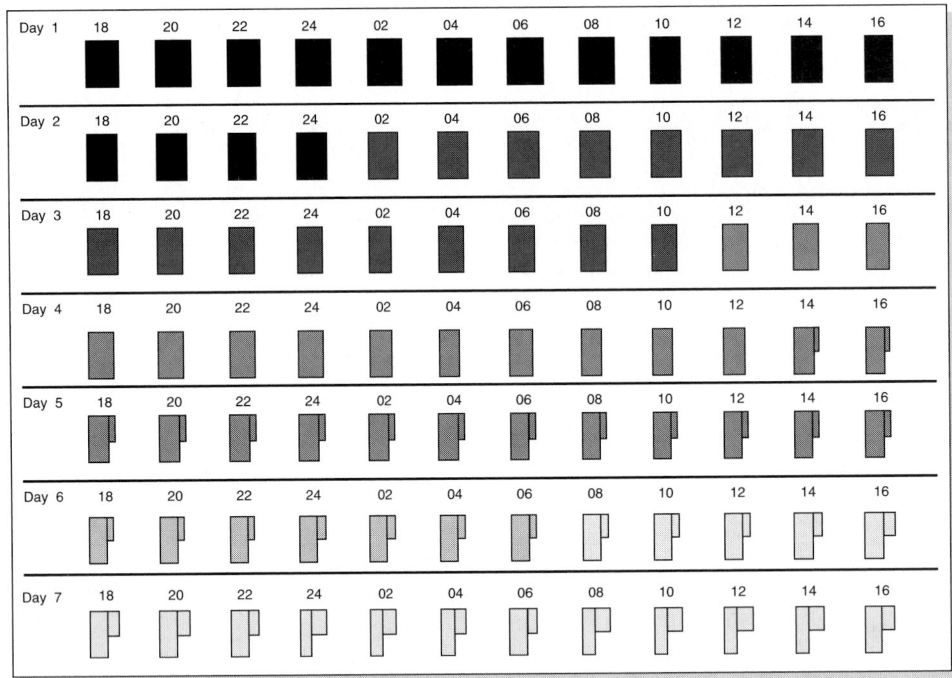

Figure 122–10. Seven days of respiratory data in both tabular and metaphor graphic form. The metaphor graphic data display uses volume rectangles to represent respiratory care data. Each charting can show up to two adjacent rectangles. The leftmost rectangle represents ventilator settings; the rightmost rectangle represents spontaneous respiration. Deeper rectangles show increased tidal volume; wider rectangles show increased rate; darker rectangles indicate higher inspired oxygen fraction. (Courtesy of William G. Cole, PhD, Information Design Seattle and Lexical Technology, Inc. Reprinted from Cole WG, Stewart JG: Human performance evaluation of a metaphor graphic display for respiratory data. Methods Inf Med 1994; 33:390–396.)

this change are to improve user acceptance and maximize customizability.[48] Freeform input results in unvalidated (no range or interfield checking) data that are often confusing to humans and useless to computerized decision support aids. For example, one nurse may mark an "X" in the box, indicating that a patient was turned; the next nurse may write "No" and a note explaining why the patient was not turned; and a third nurse may write a "0" to indicate that the patient was not turned.[49] Another common example is the charting of fractional inspired oxygen (FIO_2), which should be expressed as a decimal. Many people, however, use the terms "FIO_2" and "per cent oxygen" (which is charted as a whole number) interchangeably and chart FIO_2 as "40," for example, rather than as "0.40." Without a standard method of charting, the data are useless to a decision support tool. This problem can be rectified by using typed and coded fields (i.e., time, Boolean [true/false], integer, decimal numbers, alphabetic characters) with range and referential checking and pick lists.

"Point-in-time" displays are more appropriate for charting than for data review. A point-in-time display, as the name suggests, displays the data only as it appears at a single instant in time (see Fig. 122–8). This approach allows for less cluttered charting but displays no trend information, a lack that can make managing a patient difficult. The benefits of typed fields and pick lists described for flow sheets also apply to point-in-time displays.

"New" Display Paradigms

"Time-sequence graphs" are a staple of the health care profession. Most of the graphs used by clinicians are used primarily to call attention to trends in a patient's condition (falling Pa_{O_2} rising serum glucose, falling blood pressure). These graphs are used not as the primary charting or data review tool but to focus the clinician's attention on conditions that need to be more closely investigated. Figure 122–9 shows an example of a time-sequence graph for an ICU patient. In an advanced computerized system, the user can highlight the data points or time interval he or she wished to review and the computer would "drill down" though the data to display the data requested in the appropriate form, usually a flow sheet (see Fig. 122–7).

The time-sequence graph is often ill-suited for displaying the vast amounts of data required and generated by an ICU stay. By the time all of the laboratory results, fluid balances, respiratory therapy chartings, and vital sign data for a single patient are combined, more than 50 common pieces of data must be displayed. A different display paradigm is needed. Some researchers and clinicians are in favor of concept graphics[50, 51] or metaphor graphics (Fig. 122–10)[52–56] to represent commonly measured values such as temperature, tidal volume, and respiratory rate, whereas others suggest the use of polar graphs to quickly spot abnormalities in laboratory results (Fig. 122–11)[55, 57] and nonlinear time scales to show current and historical data on the same graph.[58, 59]

Total data abstraction is proposed by still other workers in this field. Total abstraction systems display a stylized patient form and assign various organ systems to different regions of the displayed form. Different colors or patterns indicate the status of the various organ systems (Fig. 122–12).[60] More detailed displays and charting screens can be obtained by pointing to and clicking on the appropriate regions. This approach can be extrapolated to the "virtual patient" display, in which less stylized graphics are used to show the patient's condition. The patient could be examined by selecting the appropriate part of the anatomy on the display and requesting a detailed view of the system. Figure 122–13 shows an example of this type of interface.

Information Display Summary

It is important not to confuse how well the display methodology "looks like" something from the real world with how much and how easily the information (and not just data) is conveyed.[55] No matter what type of interface a clinical information system uses, it still must fulfill the following three primary and overriding functions:

- Provide effective, correct, and efficient data entry
- Enable effective and efficient data review
- Avoid hindering the clinician with its features or problems

The best interfaces are *usually the least complex,* and are *always the easiest to use.*

Data Processing and Decision Support

Data processing is the conversion of collected data into more useful forms. Creation of reports and graphs, abstraction of information, and decision support are all data processing tasks.

Decision support is the use of the computer, at the point of care, to help the clinician make decisions about patient management. Tools for decision support must provide assistance on four levels:

1. Seamless access to information resources such as bibliographies (MEDLINE), on-line reference, and training materials.
2. Alarms and alerts.
3. Expert systems.
4. Closed loop control.

On-Line Access to Reference and Training Materials

The National Library of Medicine[61] and several research sites have been working hard on integrating reference material such as MEDLINE (accessed through tools such as GRATEFUL MED), and even full text references into the everyday work environment of the hospital. It has been suggested that eventually, context-sensitive searches would be issued automatically by information systems.[62] A clinician needing help at any point "or" would push a button and obtain both text and graphic information. This would lead to integration of the training and teaching process at the bedside with "hypermedia" tutorials and exploration of various therapies using virtual patients (Fig. 122–14).

This type of computer-based learning is not new[63, 64]; the advantages of computer-based learning as an independent learning modality were highlighted in the recommendations

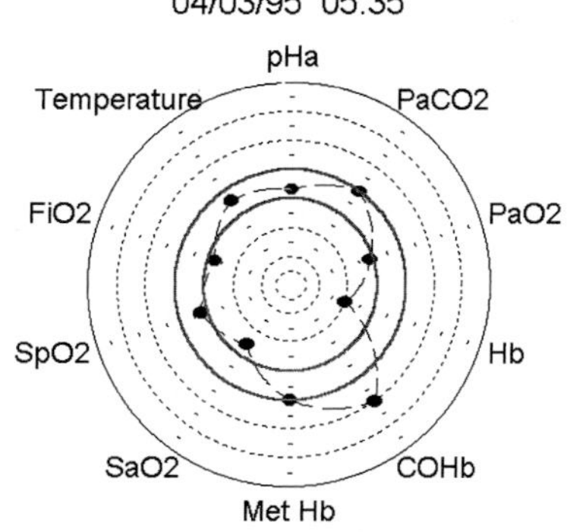

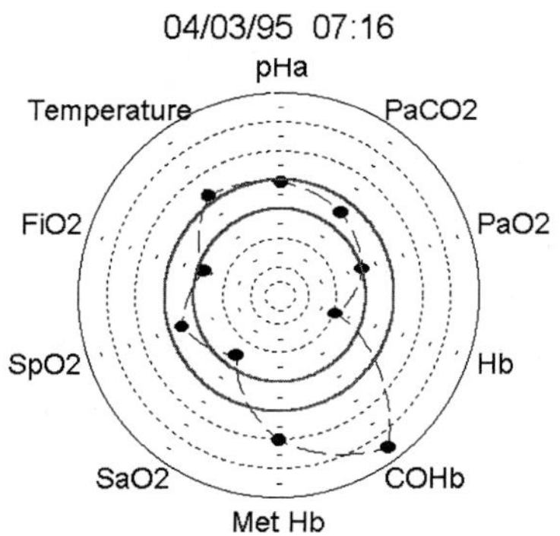

Figure 122–11. Polar graphs of arterial blood gas data. Normal ranges on each axis are represented by the solid, colored rings. The axes for each of the data are scaled independently so that the normal ranges create a pair of concentric rings. This configuration allows the clinician to determine how normal or abnormal the various laboratory measurements are by merely examining the shape of the plot of the patient's data. (After Williams BT: Some Horizons in Laboratory Computing. American Medical Informations Association Congress, 1982. Reprinted from East T, Sailors R: Clinical information systems in critical care. *In:* Clinical Information Systems. Rane M [Ed]. Redmond, Wash, SpaceLabs Medical, Inc, 1997.)

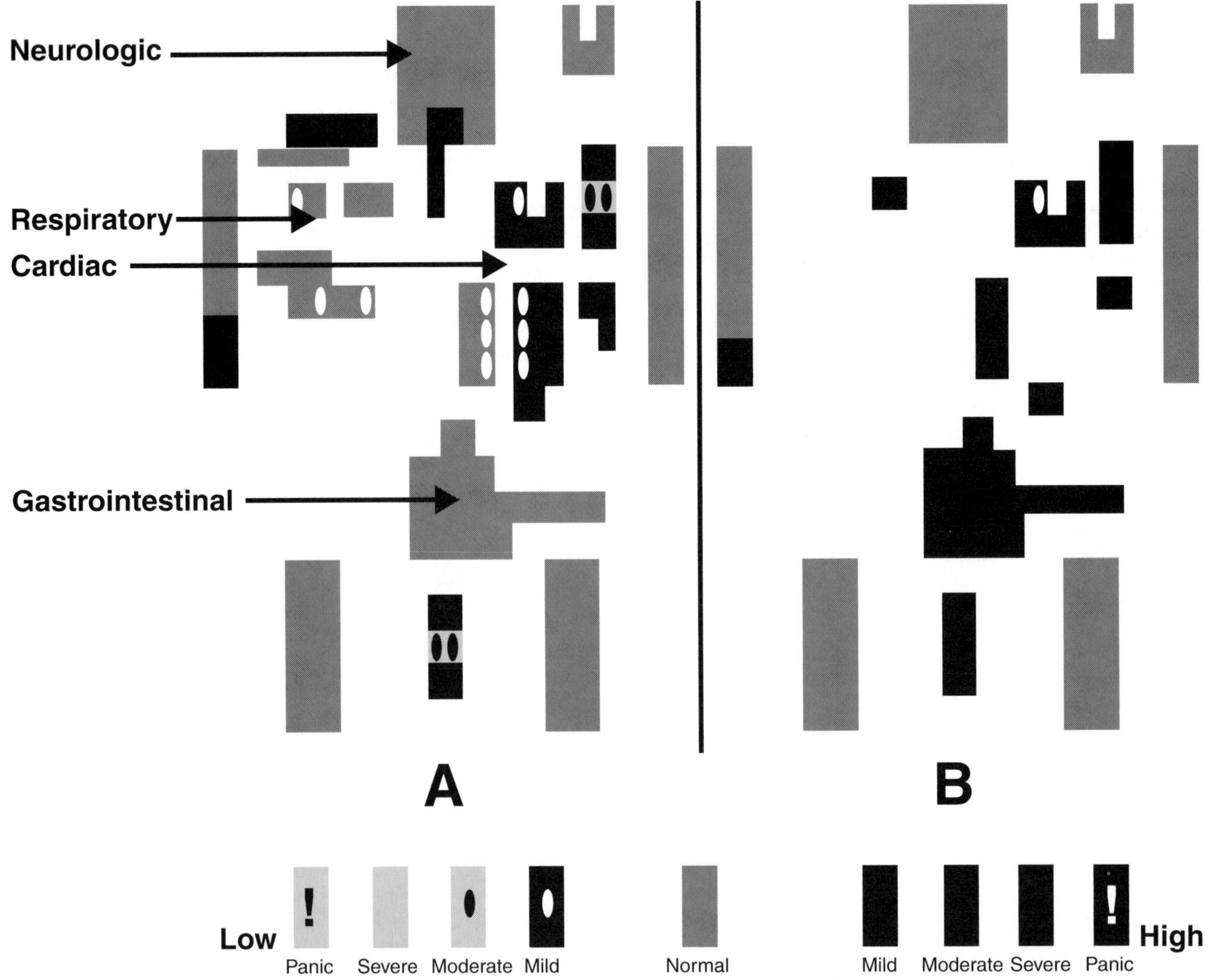

Figure 122–12. Graphical Interface for Information Cognition display of patients in an intensive care unit. The patient on the left has had a heart attack, while the patient on the right is in less critical condition. The various organ systems are represented by uniquely shaped and placed stylized shapes called Charlottes. The Knowledge Enhanced Graphic Symbols (KEGS®) indicate the status of the various organ systems. (From GIFIC Corporation, Melbourne Beach, Fla, 1996. Courtesy of Michael Lesser, MD.)

of the 1984 report of the Association of American Medical Colleges Project Panel on the General Professional Education of the Physician and College Preparation for Medicine.[65] The National Board of Medical Examiners has also begun to embrace computer-based testing as a method of evaluating fitness to practice medicine.[64, 66] Systems have already been designed for teaching pulmonary auscultation,[67] blood gas and acid/base interpretation,[68] diagnosis of chest pain,[69] diagnosis of acute respiratory failure,[70] airway management,[71] and general pulmonary system function.[72] Although the effects of these systems are inconclusive in demonstrating that computer-based learning is better than traditional training, this field is still in its infancy, and it is commonly believed that learning at the "point of care" will be far more valuable than traditional lecture and book formats.

Integrated Alarms and Alerts

Both the HELP system at LDS Hospital[12, 73-78] and the patient data management system at Cedars-Sinai Hospital in Los Angeles[76] provide alarms and alerts. Automated alarms and alerts that are generated on a wide variety of types of data can help to direct decision making. At LDS Hospital, alarms and alerts are generated for drug allergies, drug-drug interactions, drug selection and dosing,[79-83] blood ordering,[84-86] infectious disease surveillance,[75, 80, 87, 88], and organ dysfunction or critical changes in laboratory or physiologic parameters.[12, 46, 74, 75, 89] The alerts are automatically generated every time a new piece of information is entered into the system that meets the alert criteria.

To adequately perform these functions, it is essential to have an integrated data base that includes more than ICU data. For example, a respiratory care manager's alert is generated when nosocomial infections are noted in different patients served by the same respiratory therapist.[90, 91] The respiratory care department manager can then review proper policy and procedures with the therapist in the hope of reducing nosocomial infections in the future. This particular example would have required data from respiratory care charting as well as data from the microbiology laboratory. There is a high benefit-to-cost ratio for such alerting systems.[79, 84, 85]

Expert Systems

Expert systems are collections of knowledge that can be represented in the computer in a variety of different ways. The knowledge may be represented as a set of rules, such as "If A $>$ 2, then do B," or as a Bayesian probability, such as "If A $>$

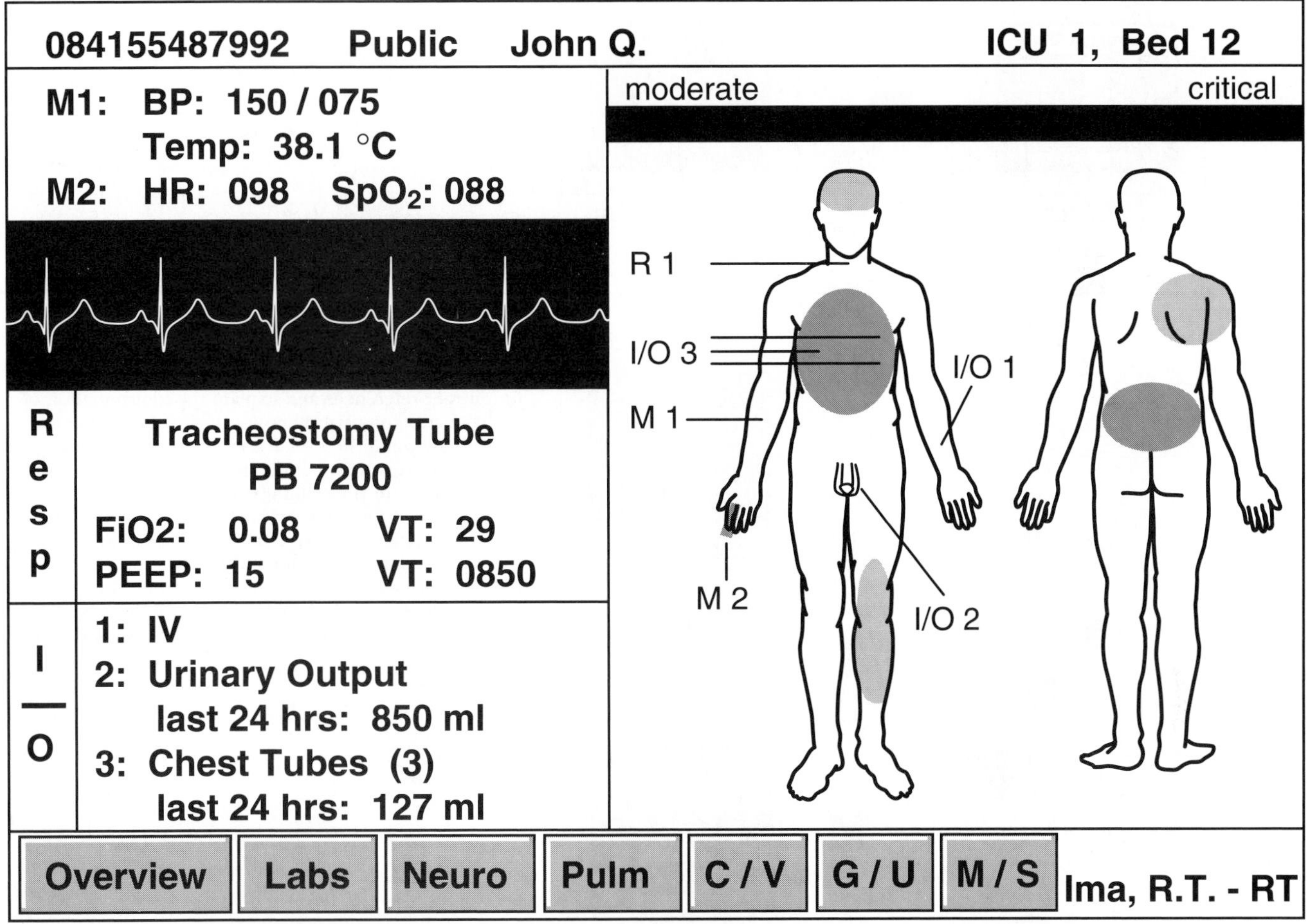

Figure 122–13. Virtual patient data charting and review screen. This screen shows an overview of the patient's status customized for a respiratory therapist. The mix of textual and graphic data can convey more information than either can individually. (From East T, Sailors R: Clinical information systems in critical care. *In:* Clinical Information Systems. Rane M [Ed]. Redmond, Wash, SpaceLabs Medical, Inc, 1997.)

2, then there is a 60% probability of B." The concept of expert systems is not new, and medical expert systems have existed for more than 20 years. Figure 122–15 illustrates the function of an expert system. The heart of the system is the *inference engine,* which applies rules from the knowledge base to data from the data base in order to generate inferences. The knowledge base contains the medical rules, heuristics, and facts, and the data base stores data and observations about the system being analyzed.

Verification and Validation

Like any other tool, expert systems must undergo verification and validation. Tests to demonstrate not only that the rules have been correctly implemented (*verification*) but also that the rules themselves are correct and complete (*validation*) should be completed and documented prior to any routine use of an expert system. Expert systems should be tested for safety against test cases and for accuracy against both test cases and the human expert's decisions.[92,93] If discrepancies are found, the knowledge base should be adjusted until the expert is satisfied with the result. Knowledge bases should not, however, be judged solely on their agreement with the expert on whom their rules are based but should also be judged on their impact on patient care or diagnostic accuracy.[94,95] In all cases, an independent evaluation of the expert system must be made.[94,96] Figure 122–16 illustrates the expert system development cycle that we and our colleagues have formalized from our experiences in this area.

Standards

In all cases, decision support aids should adhere to some sort of published standard. Whether the standard is vendor specific or from a national or international standards organization is not important, but by using a published, standard format, such as Arden Syntax,[97] the customers can develop their own expert systems without directly involving the vendor. Adherence to published standards also allows vendors to reduce development and training costs and fosters the development and dissemination of expert systems by focusing the development effort on knowledge rather than tools.

Types

In general, expert systems belong in one of two categories: *diagnostic,* those that assist or make medical diagnoses or classifications, and *therapeutic,* those that direct or carry out patient therapy.

DIAGNOSTIC EXPERT SYSTEMS. Many different diagnostic expert systems have been developed, of which QMR,[98, 99] Iliad,[100-102] and DXplain[103] are three of the most widely publicized. These are general purpose diagnostic systems to which any type of diagnostic rule can be added and that can be used for both clinical practice and medical training through various test cases and simulations.

Many special purpose diagnostic expert systems have also been developed. Systems for interpretation of blood gas data,[104-109] and for diagnosis of community-acquired pneumonia[110] and of occupational[111] and interstitial[112] lung diseases

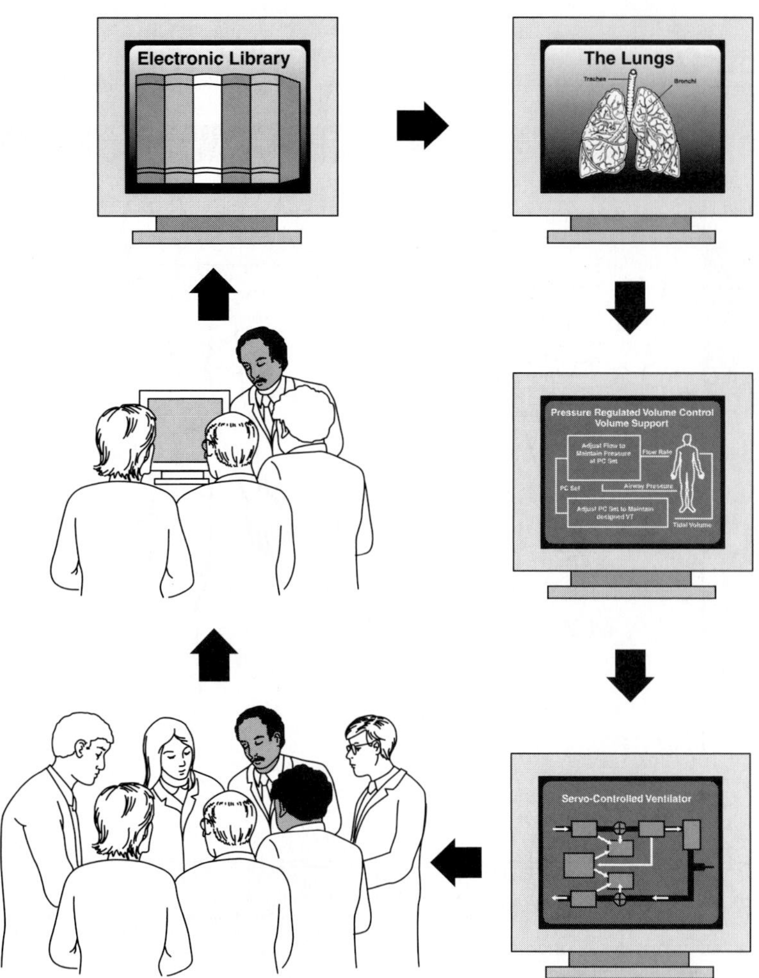

Figure 122–14. On-line reference and training example. For example, if the clinician is examining data from mechanical ventilation, the computer can issue a query for current references and explain the interpretation of the data and potential therapies. If the clinician needs help at any point, he or she can push a button and obtain both text and graphic information. There can be an integration of the training and teaching process at the bedside. If the clinician enters into a hypermedia training program, the program would describe, at the user's discretion, many different levels of pulmonary function measurements and interpretation. The hypermedia may include color images of devices and anatomy, typical auscultation sounds, graphs, and text.

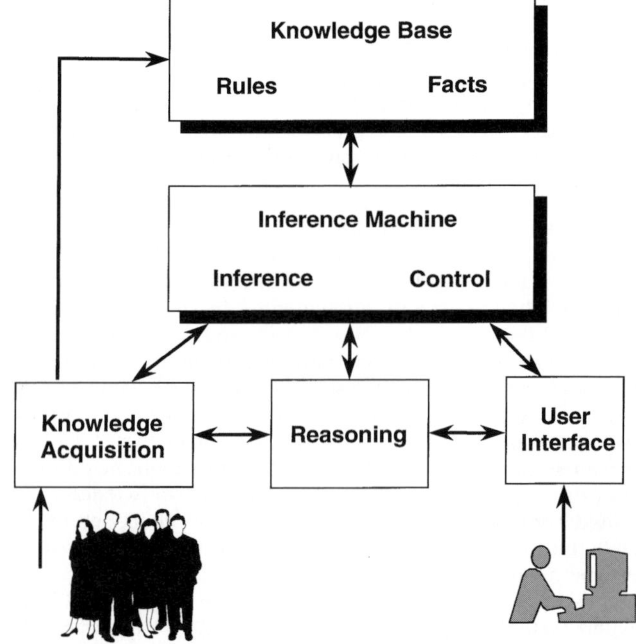

Figure 122–15. Function of an expert system. (From Klar R, Zaiss A: Medical expert systems: Design and applications in pulmonary medicine. Lung 1990; 168 [Suppl]:1201–1209.)

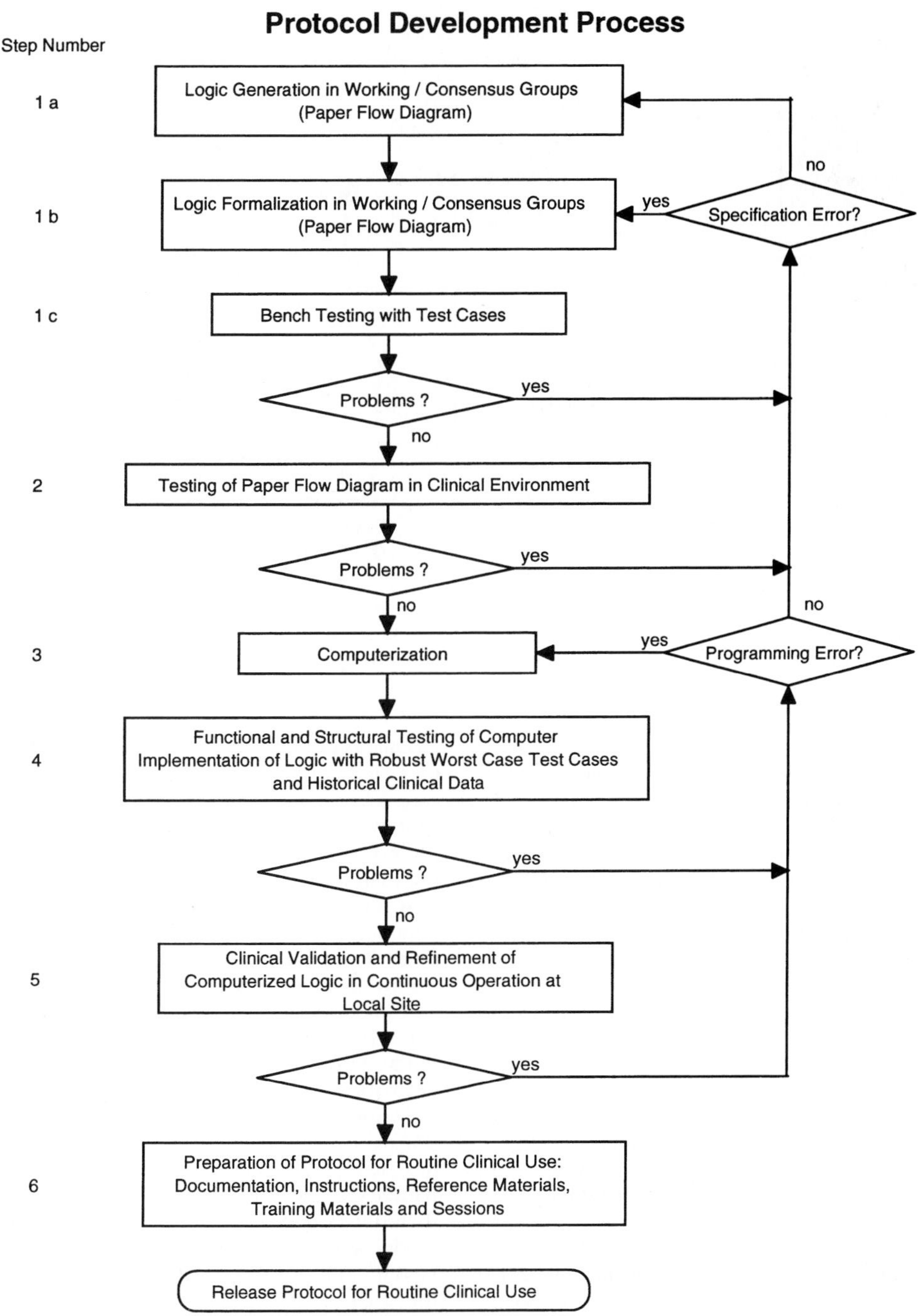

Figure 122–16. Iterative knowledge base and protocol development process. (From East T, Sailors R: Clinical information systems in critical care. *In:* Clinical Information Systems. Rane M [Ed]. Redmond, Wash, SpaceLabs Medical, Inc, 1997.)

have been described in the literature. The need for these types of systems was demonstrated by Hingston and associates,[107] who showed that although 61% of the participants at medical grand rounds believed that they knew how to interpret blood gas data, and 71% believed that an expert system was unnecessary, the physicians in attendance were able to answer only 39% of the questions regarding blood gas interpretation correctly. This type of study indicates that despite perceptions, clinicians are not capable of remembering everything in infinite detail and that bedside computerized decision support may be an important asset to patient care.

THERAPEUTIC EXPERT SYSTEMS. Many different expert systems for either directing or planning therapeutic actions have been produced and described; MYCIN,[113, 114] ONCOCIN,[115, 116] ATTENDING and its derivatives,[117-120] and ComPAS[121] are a few of the more memorably named therapeutic expert systems. Therapeutics systems have been designed to aid in planning and delivering antimicrobial therapy, chemotherapy, anesthesia, thrombolytic therapy for deep vein thrombosis, and ventilator management.[14, 117, 122-136]

The systems designed for management of mechanical ventilation have been constructed in a variety of different ways. The majority are traditional rule-based expert systems.[122, 124-126, 128, 131-133] Three good examples of these systems are the VQ-Attending, KUSIVAR, and the LDS Hospital/IHC ARDS Protocols (discussed in depth in the following case study).

VQ-Attending System. The VQ-Attending system developed by Miller[124] was designed as a critiquing system. Physicians

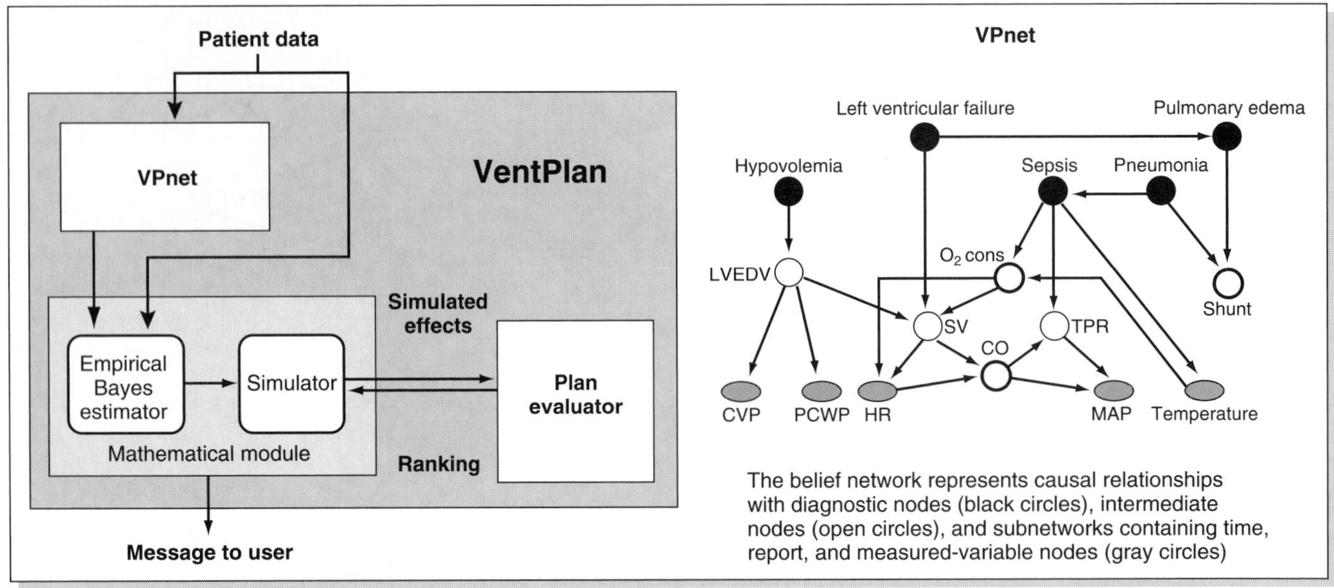

Figure 122–17. The VentPlan expert system for managing mechanical ventilation. This system was designed at Stanford University by Rutledge and coworkers.[123, 127, 137] (From Rutledge G, Thomsen G, Farr B, et al: VentPlan: A ventilator-management advisor. *In:* Clayton PD [Ed]. Symposium on Computer Applications in Medical Care. Washington, DC: IEEE Computer Society Press, 1991, pp 869–871.)

entered the current ventilator settings, blood gas data, and their suggestions for new settings. The VQ-Attending system implemented rules, frames, and semantic nets in LISP (*LIS*t *P*rocessing) programming language. It then interpreted the manually entered current data, inferred the appropriate treatment goals, and compared these findings with the physicians' suggested settings. A printed critique was provided. VQ-Attending was used as a teaching tool in anesthesiology; however, it was never put into routine clinical practice.

Kusivar System. The KUSIVAR system is an expert system designed to aid in management of adults with respiratory distress.[133] KUSIVAR was implemented in LISP language on a high-powered expert system work station (Explorer Workstation, Unisys). Knowledge was represented in the KUSIVAR system as a set of rules. A mathematical model was used to predict patient responses to a proposed therapy change. KUSIVAR has not been used in an extensive clinical trial; therefore, it is unclear what impact this system would have on patient outcome.

VentPlan System. The VentPlan system designed at Stanford University differs from most other decision support systems, in that it uses a Bayesian network and a physiologically based mathematical model to predict the impact of a recommended therapy plan[123, 127, 137, 138] (Fig. 122–17). The mathematical model, at the core of the system, consists of equations that describe a three-compartment model of the cardiopulmonary circulation. An empirical Bayesian estimator calculates the best fit for the parameters of its equations using parameter estimates and current laboratory test values. The system fit represents VentPlan's understanding of the patient's current physiologic state. A simulator then works in conjunction with the plan evaluator to determine the appropriate recommendation for the ventilator settings. The simulator uses the fitted parameters to calculate the effects of certain ventilator settings. The plan evaluator ranks the plans according to results from the simulations.

A belief network, known as VP-net, is used to calculate the prior parameter estimates for the model. Without this network, only population estimates could be used. The belief network uses hemodynamic, gas exchange, and other diagnostic information as it becomes available from the patient to update the estimates of the model parameters. This system has been evaluated with the use of data collected from 14 patients at the Palo Alto Veteran's Hospital. The results show that the concept is sound and that the estimates from the model agree well with actual data. Currently, the VentPlan system has not yet been placed in routine clinical use at the bedside.

WEANPRO System. The WEANPRO system, developed by Tong and associates,[134, 135] is a good example of an expert system designed particularly for weaning patients from mechanical ventilation (Fig. 122–18). The knowledge for the

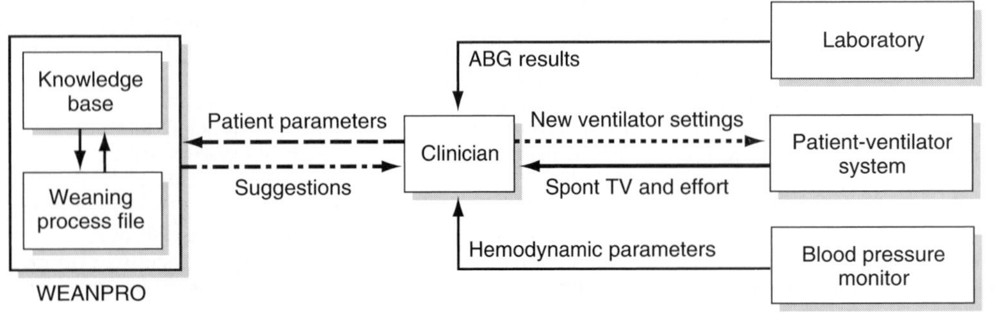

Figure 122–18. The WEANPRO system, developed by Tong,[134,135] is an expert system designed particularly for weaning patients from mechanical ventilation. (From Tong D: Weaning patients from mechanical ventilation: A knowledge based approach. *In:* Miller RA [Ed]. Proceedings Symposium on Computer Applications in Medical Care (SCAMC). Washington, DC, IEEE Computer Society Press, 1990, pp 79–85.)

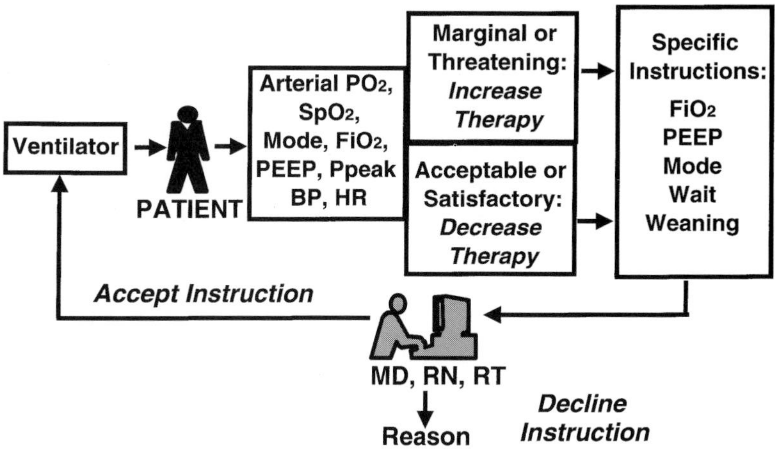

Figure 122–19. Continuous positive-pressure ventilation protocols: function of the oxygenation portion of the decision support system developed at LDS Hospital, Salt Lake City. SpO_2 = pulse oximeter saturation; FiO_2 = fraction of inspired oxygen; P_{peak} = peak pressure; BP = mean arterial blood pressure; HR = heart rate; MD = physician; RN = Registered Nurse; RT = respiratory therapist. (see East et al, 1991[128] and Morris et al, 1992.[142])

system was obtained from four domain experts (physicians who were "experts" at weaning). The knowledge base consists of 406 rules and 133 "meta facts." The system is implemented in the computer language M.1, a knowledge base development tool (Teknowledge, Inc.), and runs on any PC computer. Approximately 6 person-months of work were required to establish the system. Fifty-four patients were studied in a prospective trial. Sixteen of these patients were weaned using the WEANPRO system. Only 13 patients were successfully weaned, however; the remaining three exhibited conditions that were not adequately addressed by WEANPRO's knowledge base. WEANPRO required fewer sets of blood gas measurements (3.4 ± 0.5 versus 6.2 ± 1.9) and made more ventilator adjustments per set of blood gas measurements (1.17 ± 0.2 versus 0.8 ± 0.3) compared with the control patients. A review of the WEANPRO therapy suggestions by experts showed 96% acceptance. WEANPRO has been rewritten in MUMPS (Massachusetts General Hospital Utility Multi-Programming System), the first medically oriented programming language, and is currently in clinical use at Baptist Memorial Hospital, Memphis, Tennessee.

EXPERT SYSTEM CASE STUDY

At the LDS Hospital in Salt Lake City, Utah, the development of expert systems for management of mechanical ventilation was originally stimulated by the investigative needs of a clinical trial of extracorporeal CO_2 removal ($ECCO_2R$) for patients with adult respiratory distress syndrome (ARDS).[139-142] The intent was to develop protocols to standardize therapy[1, 22] in an attempt to increase the interpretability and credibility of our clinical trial results.[142] The protocol control goals were to ensure (1) uniformity of care, (2) equal intensity and frequency of monitoring, (3) consistent decision making logic, and (4) common therapeutic goals (e.g., Pao_2). Protocols were developed for several different ventilator modes.[14, 22, 143-145] After completion of the clinical trial in 1991, new protocols were written for ventilation and arterial pH (pH_a) control.[14, 143-145]

The protocols were developed through the use of an iterative build-test-refine cycle (similar to that shown in Fig. 122–16) that used the clinical environment as an integral part of the development process.[128, 146] We thought that this was the only way to generate a successful protocol that would handle the majority of circumstances encountered and would be acceptable to the clinical care staff. A therapy consensus committee initially consisted of 14 physicians, three nurses, one respiratory therapist, and one medical informatics expert.[22] This committee developed and refined protocol logic. All physicians agreed to forgo personal treatment style and accept the consensus recommendations that were incorporated into the protocol logic.

The operation of the protocols is demonstrated in Figure 122–19. The protocols are automatically started whenever a new pulse oximeter saturation (Spo_2) or a new Pao_2 is entered into the computer. These protocols were computerized using the HELP system at the LDS Hospital.[14, 19, 22, 128, 130, 132, 146-149] As shown in Figures 122–19 and 122–20, the computer displays instructions on the terminal at the bedside. A member of the clinical care team, typically the respiratory therapist, reads the instructions and makes the indicated ventilator setting change. This is *not* a closed-loop system; the computer never makes any adjustments of therapy directly. The clinical care team members always have the option to refuse to follow an instruction. If they refuse to follow an instruction, however, they must give a reason. The record of these reasons provides a critical feedback that permits protocol refinement.

The ability of the continuous positive-pressure ventilation (CPPV) oxygenation protocols to control care during around-the-clock application in the ICU was evaluated in a study approved by the LDS Hospital Research and Human Rights Committee. A total of 111 patients with ARDS were enrolled in the trial. ARDS was defined by the criteria listed in Table 122-5. Outcome was compared with those of two historical control groups, one from the Massachusetts General Hospital between 1978 and 1988, and one from the European Collaborative Study.[150] The CPPV oxygenation protocols were applied until patients were weaned to continuous positive airway pressure (CPAP) or died. In the first 45 patients, all instructions generated by the computerized CPPV oxygenation protocol were logged, as was the acceptance or rejection of an instruction by the clinical staff. If an instruction was not followed, the clinical staff member was asked to identify a reason from a menu.[128, 130] Figure 122–21 ummarizes these results.

Figure 122–22 summarizes the results of the CPPV oxygenation protocol used in 111 ARDS patients. The success of these CPPV oxygenation protocols clearly indicates the feasibility of using expert systems to direct management of care for critically ill patients. The

TABLE 122–5. Definition of Adult Respiratory Distress Syndrome (ARDS) Used in the Prospective Identification of Patients Included in Clinical Trials of the Computerized Decision Support System for Management of Mechanical Ventilation (Developed at LDS Hospital)

Arterial/alveolar Pao_2 ratio (a-A gradient) ≤ 0.2
or
Pao_2/FIO_2 ratio ≤ 200 mm Hg
Total static thoracic compliance (CTH) ≤ 50 mL/cm H_2O
Pulmonary artery occlusion pressure (wedge pressure) ≤ 15 mm Hg
(no evidence of heart failure or fluid overload)
Acute onset accompanied by an ARDS risk factor
Radiographic evidence of diffuse bilateral infiltrates

Adapted from East T, Sailors R: Clinical information systems in critical care. *In:* Clinical Information Systems. Redmond, Wash, SpaceLabs Medical, Inc, 1997; and Sailors RM, East TD: The role of the computer in monitoring. *In:* The Textbook of Critical Care Monitoring. Tobin MJ (Ed). New York, McGraw-Hill, 1998.

```
PUBLIC, JOHN Q.            2342123132 E907   I 03/18/86         C    47Y  M
                      A R D S   P R O T O C O L S
  Patient supported with HIGH stretch protocol.                BWP:  59.062
     Enrolled by: SMITH, JACK B                          Time:04/16 17:54

                 1. Run protocol.
                 2. Review/Acknowledge instructions
                 3. Current patient status.
                 4. Enter patient into protocol.
                 5. Remove patient from protocol.
                 6. Suspend protocol.
                 7. Resume from protocol suspension.
                 8. Barotrauma status.
```

```
PUBLIC, JOHN Q.            2342123132 E907   I 03/18/86         C    47Y  M
                      A R D S   P R O T O C O L S
  Patient supported with HIGH stretch protocol.                BWP:  59.062
                Edit options: #[A] to accept, #[R] to reject, <F7> displays past instuctions
  03/18 09:54.
        Change in tidal volume(VT) since last ABG. New ABG required to reassess patient status.
  03/18 09:54.
        Increase VT trial completed. User Cancellation.
       1. Keep ventilator rate (VR) at   29.0 bpm.......................................... A
       2. Keep tidal volume(VT) at  680.0 ml............................................... A
        Set peak flow to maintain an I:E ratio between 1:1.8 and 1:2.8.
    Acknowledged:   YOUNG, JOE Q                         Time:03/18 09:54.
  03/18 07:23.
        Change in tidal volume(VT) since last ABG. New ABG required to reassess patient status.
  03/18 05:13.
        Protocol run from ABG drawn at 04/30 05:11. PaO2= 75.1, pHa= 7.4.
        Entering a VT trial for assisting patient. This trial will attempt to reduce the rate by increasing VT.
        Continue trial if patient is stable, adequately sedated and medicated for pain. Otherwise CANCEL the trial.
       3. Keep FIO2 at   50.0 %............................................................ A
                                                                                  Page 1 of 2

    Please select 0 to 50 of the above options
```

Figure 122–20. protocol menu and instruction screen for adult respiratory distress syndrome (ARDS) from the LDS Hospital HELP system, Salt Lake City. Patient-specific instructions are provided (e.g., "Keep tidal volume (V_T) at 680.0 ml") to the bedside clinician. ABG = arterial blood gas; BWP = body weight, predicted. (From East, T, Sailors R: Clinical information systems in critical care. *In:* Clinical Information Systems. Rane M [Ed]. Redmond, Wash, SpaceLabs Medical, Inc, 1997.)

physicians, respiratory therapists, and nurses commented that the computerized protocol, which acted as "standing orders," simplified management of mechanical ventilation. The CPPV oxygenation protocols are now in routine clinical use for patients with ARDS at LDS Hospital.

As shown in Figure 122–23, the survival of patients cared for by the protocols was significantly higher than that of either of the historical control groups. This was true for all patients with ARDS as well as the two subgroups of patients with severe and less severe ARDS. Without randomized clinical trials with concurrent controls, no definitive conclusion can be drawn concerning the impact of protocol control on patient survival. Nevertheless, the outcome for patients cared for by these protocols appears at least as good as the published outcomes. This suggests that computerized protocols can be used to manage mechanical ventilation successfully and safely in critically ill patients.

Evaluation

To our knowledge, this was the first demonstration that a computerized decision support system can be used effectively in the critical care environment. Similar protocols could be used in several different arenas, as follows:

1. To control future clinical trials as part of the ongoing nationwide effort to determine efficacy of existing and new therapies.
2. To standardize the management of mechanical ventilation, an essential part of the continuous quality improvement process.
3. To provide decision support in the management of mechanical ventilation for patients with ARDS who are in a variety of settings where a clinical expert in management of ARDS is unavailable.

A randomized, controlled, prospective clinical trial is under way to objectively compare this protocol control with physician-directed care. This study will answer two questions: 1 Can a computerized decision support system be exported to other centers and used by clinicians uninvolved with its development? and Does the protocol control of mechanical ventilation have an impact on ARDS patient outcome? As part of the study, the knowledge base (protocol logic rules) was transferred from the HELP system at LDS Hospital to a PC-based ICU computer system known as ARGUS Windows. The ARGUS Windows system was installed in the surgical ICU at King Drew Medical Center in Los Angeles and used for respiratory care charting. The decision support system has been used successfully to care for five patients with ARDS in a pilot study of feasibility, but it has since been removed for hospital remodeling. A prospective randomized clinical trial to test the efficacy of computerized protocols is ongoing.

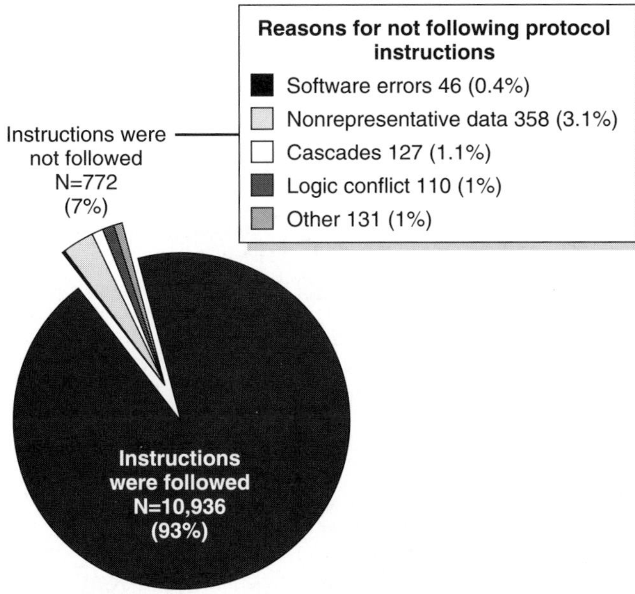

Figure 122–21. Specific reasons why the clinical staff did not follow almost 12,000 instructions in the first 45 patients with adult respiratory distress syndrome cared for within 15,520 hours using the continuous positive pressure ventilation (CPPV) oxygenation protocol. (Data from East TD, Morris AH, Wallace CJ, et al: A strategy for development of computerized critical care decision support systems. Int J Clin Monit Comput 1991; 8:263–269; and Morris AH, Wallace CJ, Clemmer TP, et al: Final Report: Computerized protocol controlled clinical trial of new therapy which includes ECCO2R for ARDS. Am Rev Respir Dis 1992; 145:A184.)

Closed Loop Control

Closed loop control is similar to an expert system, except that in the closed loop system, the computer directly adjusts the mechanical ventilator. Figure 122–24 is a typical diagram of a closed-loop controller.[151] The heart of many of the simple controllers is a proportional, integral, and differential (PID) controller. PID controllers are used frequently throughout industry for controlling many different processes.

The home thermostat and furnace are a good example of a simple closed loop control that can be used to explain PID controllers. The typical thermostat is either on, when the temperature is too cold, or off, when the temperature is too hot.

It might be possible to have a more comfortable home heated more efficiently if the furnace were hotter when the home was very cold and cooler as the home approached the desired temperature; this is the idea of *proportional control.* The disadvantage of proportional control is that it typically reaches steady state at a value that is offset from the desired set-point.

To force the system exactly to the desired set-point, one can integrate the error (the difference between the desired and actual value). Even a small error will eventually integrate into a large error over time that will force the system to the exact set-point; this is the concept of *integral control.*

Derivative control attempts to anticipate what is going to happen with the system. If the house were heating up very rapidly, it would be good for the thermostat to recognize this fact and slow down the heating process so as to not overshoot the set-point. This can be accomplished by adding some control that depends on the time rate of change of the error signal (the derivative).

Although many other closed loop controllers have been used, the PID controller remains a central element in most of them. In computerized systems, the PID controller can be represented in a recursive form that can be easily programmed.[151, 152]

An analog closed loop control system for mechanical ventilation was first introduced in 1953 by Frumin and coworkers.[6, 7] This sophisticated system included oxygen and carbon dioxide analyzers and adjusted the FIO_2 and tidal volume during anesthesia. Several other analog closed loop control systems were reported between 1953 and 1973. Coles and associates[153] introduced the first computerized closed loop controller for mechanical ventilation. This system controlled FIO_2 and tidal volume during anesthesia. Several other different systems were developed between 1975 and 1995 for closed loop control of tidal volume and ventilatory rate based on monitoring for expired CO_2.[7, 151, 154–158] Most systems were designed to maintain a desired end-tidal CO_2 value. Although all of these systems worked well, they have not had widespread clinical use because of the differences between end-tidal CO_2 and $Paco_2$ in patients who have large physiologic dead space.

Some closed loop controllers have been designed for managing oxygenation. Most of these are simple systems designed to adjust FIO_2 to produce a desired Pao_2 or Spo_2.[159–161] Morozoff and Evans[159] demonstrated in neonates that computer control was able to maintain a desired Spo_2 with more accuracy than manual control.

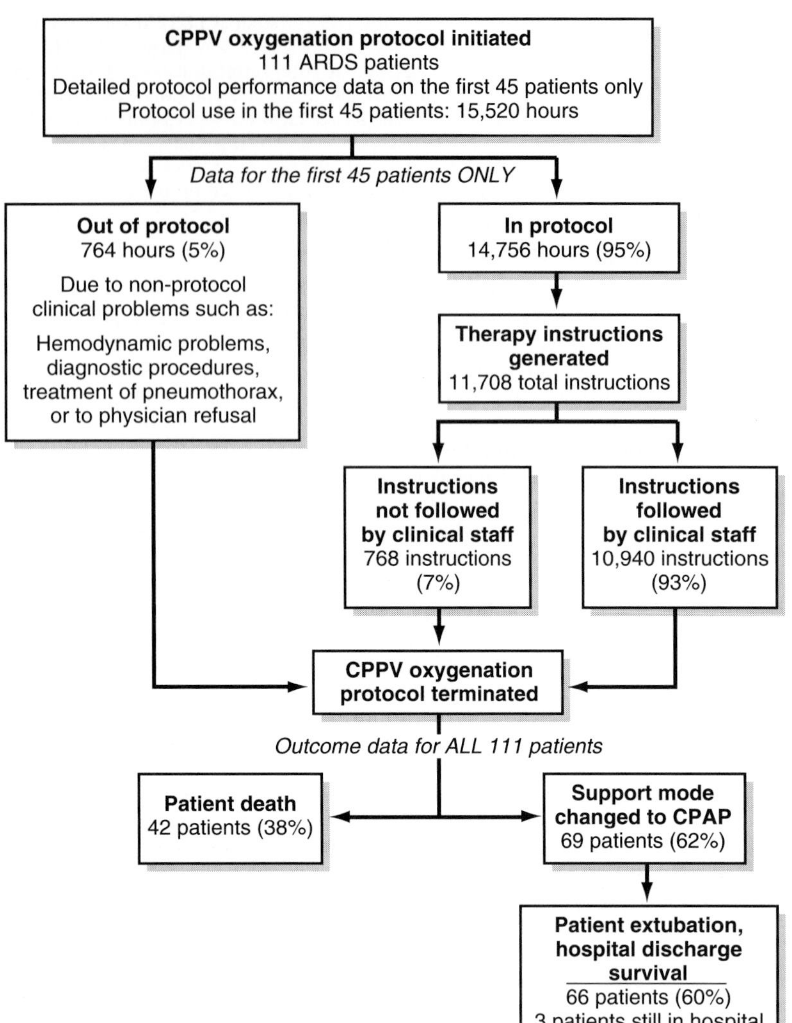

Figure 122–22. Summary of results of the continuous positive pressure ventilation (CPPV) oxygenation protocol used in 111 ARDS patients in the shock trauma intensive care unit at LDS Hospital, Salt Lake City. CPAP = continuous positive airway pressure; ARDS = adult respiratory distress syndrome. (Data from East TD, Morris AH, Wallace CJ, et al: A strategy for development of computerized critical care decision support systems. Int J Clin Monit Comput 1991; 8:263–269; and Morris AH, Wallace CJ, Clemmer TP, et al: Final Report: Computerized protocol controlled clinical trial of new therapy which includes ECCO2R for ARDS. Am Rev Respir Dis 1992; 145:A184.)

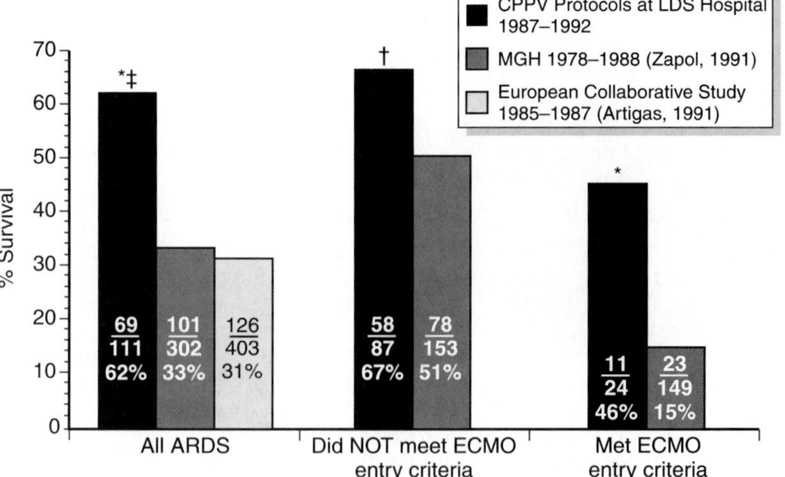

Figure 122–23. Survival results of the continuous positive pressure ventilation (CPPV) oxygenation protocol used in 111 ARDS patients in the shock trauma intensive care unit at LDS Hospital, Salt Lake City. ARDS = adult respiratory distress syndrome; ECMO = extracorporeal membrane oxygenation. (Data from East TD, et al: Int J Clin Monit Comput 1991; 8:263–269[128]; and Morris AH, et al: Am Rev Respir Dis 1992; 145:A184.[142])

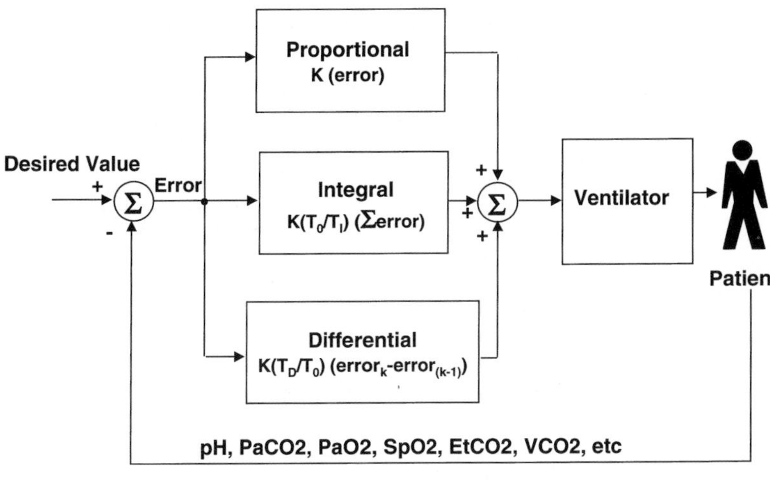

Figure 122–24. Diagram of a typical closed loop controller. The heart of many of the simple controllers is a proportional, integral, and differential (PID) controller. This controller can be easily written in a recursive form that is amenable to processing by computer. K is overall gain of the controller; T_0 is the sample interval; T_i is the integration time (essentially the integral gain constant); T_D is differential time (essentially the differential gain constant). The values of K, T_0, T_i, and T_D are adjusted to tune the controller in order to provide the best performance. When the PID equation is written in the recursive form, new gain constants q_0, q_1, and q_2 are introduced to simplify the equation. These new constants are mathematically related to the original gain constants (K,T_0,T_i, and T_D) by the equations shown.

East and associates[20] designed a system for control of PEEP based on normalizing functional residual capacity. Strickland and Hasson[136, 162] have developed a closed loop controller for weaning postoperative cardiac patients from synchronized intermittent mandatory ventilation (SIMV) with pressure support (PS). This controller decreased the SIMV rate by 2 breaths/min every 5 minutes until a rate of 2 breaths/min was reached, then decreased pressure support by 4 cm H_2O every 5 minutes, as long as the patient met the following criteria:

- Respiratory rate from 8 to 25 breaths/min
- Minute ventilation from 6 to 14 L/min
- $Spo_2 \geq 90\%$

This rule-based controller automatically adjusted a Puritan Bennett 7200 ventilator. The system was used in a 15-patient prospective randomized trial (nine patients had computer-controlled and six had manually controlled ventilators). The results showed that the computer-controlled ventilator group required significantly fewer blood gas analyses (1.4 ± 0.7 versus 7.2 ± 4.3), had shorter weaning times (18.7 ± 5.9 versus 25.6 ± 5.6 hours), and had less time spent outside acceptable VR and VT bounds (3.2 ± 2.8 versus 6.6 ± 4.1 min).[162]

This study is an interesting contrast to the previously described WEANPRO expert system developed by Tong.[134, 135] WEANPRO is far more complex, requiring hemodynamic data and a variety of other sources of data not required by the LDS Hospital protocols. The simple weaning system developed at the LDS Hospital[128] focuses on spontaneous ventilatory rate as a primary variable and Pao_2 or Spo_2 as a secondary variable. The LDS Hospital protocols have been used to successfully wean 68 patients. Despite their simplicity, the expert systems developed by Strickland and Hasson[136, 162] and at LDS Hospital appear to work as well as or better than the more sophisticated WEANPRO system. This feature reaffirms our belief in the "KIS" (Keep It Simple!) principle.

Despite the development of several very clever and sophisticated systems, none of these closed loop controllers for mechanical ventilation has had a major impact on clinical care. There are two primary reasons for the lack of general application of closed loop ventilatory control systems. First, these systems rely on input data from sensors (Pao_2, end-tidal CO_2, transcutaneous PO_2, Sao_2, etc.) that are not reliable enough to be trusted for use in a closed-loop control. Second, most of these systems were designed by engineers in the laboratory, and although they are excellent engineering exercises, they are not closely related to common clinical practice.

To address this problem, we and our colleagues[22, 131, 132] have designed a system based on well-established protocols for management of mechanical ventilation that provides continuous closed loop control of oxygenation[23] (Fig. 122–25). In this system, a Hamilton Amadeus ventilator was controlled by an Apple Macintosh SE-30 computer. A Shiley Continucath intra-arterial electrode was used to provide continuous measurement of Pao_2. Arterial oxygen saturation (Sao_2) was calculated from the Pao_2, pH, $Paco_2$, and temperature using standard equations. The size and direction of a therapy change were determined by the Pao_2 error (difference between measured and desired Pao_2. The overall gain of the controller was a function of the Sao_2. This control strategy provided an aggressive response to hypoxemia and a more conservative response to hyperoxia. The content of the therapy change was determined from a fifth dimensional quality surface that described the tradeoff between PEEP and FIO_2 changes for a specific combination of current PEEP, FIO_2, and Pao_2 values. The quality surface was generated from our extensively used protocols applied clinically in an open loop manner (see earlier discussion of expert systems).[22, 131, 132]

The controller was tested in five mongrel dogs with oleic acid lung injury. After injury, the controller was activated and the animals were monitored at 30-minute intervals for 6 hours. The controller performed as designed for all five animals, and no hazardous or failure conditions were noted. A small clinical trial of this closed loop controller has been started at the LDS Hospital to evaluate its safety and effectiveness in patients with ARDS. It is hoped that such careful management of potentially toxic therapies will improve the outcome for patients with hypoxic respiratory failure.

Because they are more rapid and accurate than the average clinician and they constantly monitor and adjust therapy, closed-loop controllers have the potential to decrease clinician workload and increase the safety and efficiency of treatment. Although the cost of these controllers remains quite high, ICU time itself is also expensive, giving closed loop controllers an economic advantage. As in other environments in which closed loop controllers have been used, humans are required

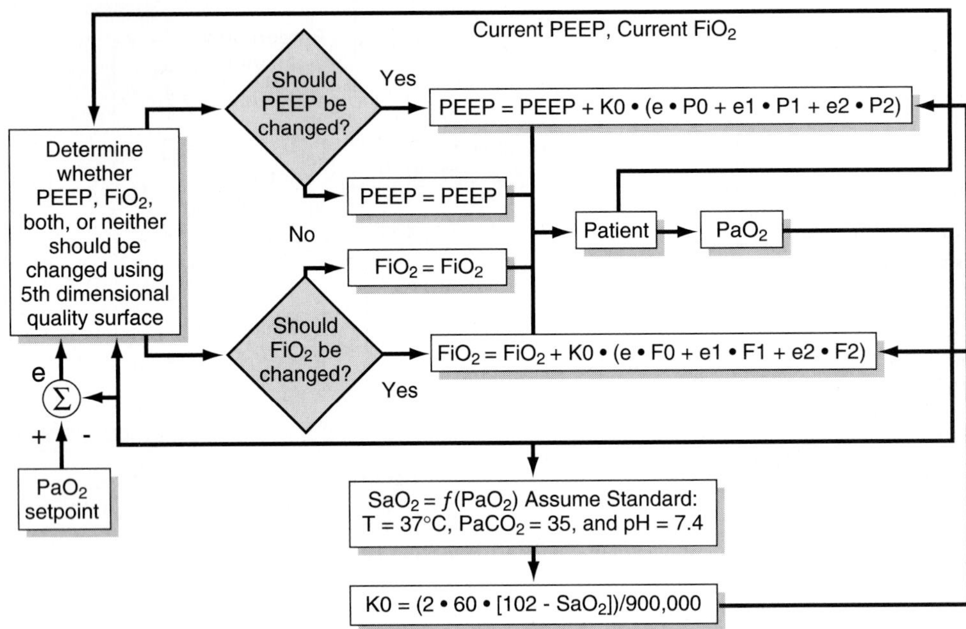

Figure 122–25. Nonlinear closed loop controller for adjusting positive end-expiratory pressure (PEEP) and fraction of inspired oxygen (FiO_2). The general concept is that the PEEP and FIO_2 are automatically adjusted to maintain Pao_2 at a desired setpoint. The size and direction of a therapy change are determined by the Pao_2 error "e" (difference between measured and desired Pao_2). A record is kept of the previous two values for the error (e1 and e2). The decision as to which variable, PEEP or FIO_2 or both, to change was determined from a fifth dimensional quality surface, which described the tradeoff between PEEP and FIO_2 changes for a specific combination of current PEEP, FIO_2, and Pao_2 values. The quality surface was generated from the clinically proven protocols. Once it has been decided which variables are to be changed, the amount of change is calculated by a proportional, integral, and differential (PID) controller. The controller uses the current (e) and previous values (e1 and e2) to calculate the actual change in PEEP or FIO_2. The PID gain constants P0, P1, P2, F0, F1, and F2 are tuned to provide the best controller performance. The overall gain of the controller (K0) was a function of the Sao_2. This provided an aggressive response to hypoxemia and a more conservative response to hyperoxia. Arterial oxygen saturation (Sao_2) was calculated from the Pao_2 (assuming pH = 7.4, $Paco_2$ = 35, and temperature = 37° C) using standard equations. (From East T: The magic bullets in the war on ARDS: Aggressive therapy for oxygenation failure. Respir Care 1993; 38:690–704.)

to oversee their safe operation. This job falls to experienced clinicians who can recognize deviations in care and respond quickly and appropriately.

Conclusion

Decision support tools are not designed to make the experienced clinician obsolete; they are designed to allow the clinician to be a more effective health care provider. With health care moving more and more toward managed or capitated care, decision support tools will become "mission-critical" components of health care delivery. Managed care is pushing clinicians to care for more patients than ever before. Decision support tools, such as expert systems, on-line references, integrated alarms and alerts, and closed loop controllers, will be necessary tools as clinicians strive to improve their delivery of health care in the managed care environment.

ACKNOWLEDGMENT

Support for research on the development of the MIB for respiratory care was initially given by Siemens Life Support Systems (Solna, Sweden) and was continued by Puritan Bennett Corporation, (Carlsbad, Calif).

Research on closed-loop control of oxygenation was supported by Hamilton Ventilators (Bonaduz, Switzerland).

Research on expert systems was supported by Intermountain Health Care, Inc., and by grants from the Deseret Foundation (LDS Hospital), the National Institutes of Health (NHLBI grant HL36787), the Agency for Health Care Policy and Research (AHCPR grant HS06594), and the Respiratory Distress Syndrome Foundation. ACT/PC Corporation (Madison, Wisconsin) and Emtek, A Motorola Corporation, are active supporters of the ongoing clinical trial of our expert systems for mechanical ventilation. The Siemens 900C ventilators, carts, and supplies were lent by Siemens Life Support Systems.

REFERENCES

1. East T: Computers in the ICU: Panacea or plague? Respir Care 1992; 37:170–180.
2. Eddy DM: Clinical decision making. JAMA 1990; 263:1265–1275.
3. Bernstein J: The Analytical Engine: Past, Present, and Future. New York, William Morrow & Co, 1981.
4. Heebink D: Computers in pulmonary medicine. Respir Care 1982; 27:793–794.
5. Sanborn W: Microprocessor-based mechanical ventilation. Respir Care 1993; 38:72–109.
6. Frumin J: Clinical use of a physiological respirator producing N2) amnesia-analgesia. Anesthesiology 1957; (18):290–299.
7. Thompson JD: Computerized control of mechanical ventilation: Closing the loop. Respir Care 1987; 32:440–446.
8. Andrews RD, Gardner RM, Metcalf SM, Simmons D: Computer charting: An evaluation of a respiratory care computer system. Respir Care 1985; 30:695–707.
9. Greenway L, Jeffs M, Turner K: Computerized management of respiratory care. Respir Care 1993; 38:42–53.
10. Hammond J, Johnson HM, Varas R, Ward CG: A qualitative comparison of paper flowsheets vs. a computer based clinical information system. Chest 1991; 99:155–157.
11. Hammond J, Johnson MH, Ward CG, et al: Clinical evaluation of a computer-based patient monitoring and data management system. Heart Lung 1991; 20:119–124.

12. Bradshaw KE, Sittig DF, Gardner RM, Pryor TA, Budd M: Computer-based data entry for nurses in the ICU. MD Comput 1989; 6:274–280.
13. Hilberman M, Kamm B, Tarter M, Osborn JJ: An evaluation of computer-based patient monitoring at Pacific Medical Center. Comput Biomed Res 1975; 8:447–460.
14. East T: Computerized management of mechanical ventilation. *In:* Textbook of Critical Care. 3rd ed. Ayres SM, Grenvik A, Holbrook PR, Shoemaker WC (Eds). Philadelphia, WB Saunders, 1994, pp 895–911.
15. Gardner RM, Sittig DF, Budd MC: The computer in the ICU: Match or mismatch? *In:* Textbook of Critical Care Medicine, 2nd ed. Shoemaker WC, Ayres S, Grenvik A, Holbrook PR, Thompson WL (Eds). Philadelphia, WB Saunders, 1989, pp 248–258.
16. Shabot MM: Standardized acquisition of bedside data: The IEEE P1073 medical information bus. Int J Clin Monit Comput 1989; 6:197–204.
17. East TD, Yang W, Tariq H, Gardner RM: The IEEE medical information bus for respiratory care. Crit Care Med 1989; 17:S80.
18. Gardner RM, Hawley WL, East TD, Oniki TA, Young HW: Real time data acquisition: Experience with the medical information bus (MIB). Proc Annu Symp Comput Appl Med Care 1991; 15:813–817.
19. East TD, Andriano KP, Pace NL: Automated measurement of functional residual capacity by sulfur hexafluoride washout. J Clin Monit 1987; 3:14–21.
20. East TD, in't Veen JCCM, Jonker TA, Pace NL, McJames S: Computer controlled positive end-expiratory pressure (PEEP) titration for effective oxygenation without frequent blood gases. Crit Care Med 1988; 16:252–257.
21. East TD, Wortelboer PJ, van Ark E, et al: Automated sulfur hexafluoride washout functional residual capacity measurement system for any mode of mechanical ventilation as well as spontaneous respiration. Crit Care Med 1990; 18:84–91.
22. East TD, Bohm SH, Wallace CJ, et al: A successful computerized protocol for clinical management of pressure control inverse ratio ventilation in ARDS patients. Chest 1992; 101:697–710.
23. East TD, Tolle CR, Farrell RM, Brunner JX: A non-linear closed-loop controller for oxygenation based on a clinically proven fifth dimensional quality surface. Crit Care Med 1991; 19:S61.
24. East TD, Young WH, Gardner RM: Digital electronic communication between ventilators and computers and printers. Respir Care 1992; 37:1113–1123.
25. Institute of Electrical and Electronic Engineers: 1073.4.1-1994 Physical Layer Interface—Cable connection IEEE Standard for Medical Device Communications. Piscataway, NJ, IEEE, 1994.
26. Institute of Electrical and Electronic Engineers: 1073.3.1-1994 Transport Profile—Connection Mode IEEE Standard for Medical Device Communications. Piscataway, NJ, IEEE, 1994.
27. Wittenber J, Shabot MM: The medical device data language for the P1073 medical information bus standard. Int J Clin Monit Comput 1990; 7:91–98.
28. Figler AA, Stead SW: The Medical Information Bus. Biomed Instrum Technol 1990; 24:101–111.
29. Nolan-Avila LS, Paganelli BE, Norden-Paul RE. The Medical Information Bus: An automated method of capturing data at the bedside. Comput Nurs 1988; 6:115–121.
30. Furst E: Cardiovascular technology. J Cardiovasc Nurs 1995; 9:24–35.
31. Gardner RM, Bradshaw KE, Hollingsworth KW: Computerizing the intensive care unit: Current status and future directions. J Cardiovasc Nurs 1989; 4:68–78.
32. McDonald CJ, Hammond WF: Standard formats for electronic transfer of clinical data (Editorial). Ann Intern Med 1989; 110:333–335.
33. Shabot MM, LoBue M, Leyerle B: An automatic PDMS interface for the Urotrack Plus 220 Urimeter. Int J Clin Monit Comput 1988; 5:125–131.
34. Gardner RM: Computerized management of intensive care patients. MD Comput 1986; 3:36–51.
35. Hawley WL, Tariq H, Gardner RM: Clinical implementation of an automated medical information bus in an intensive care unit. Proc Annu Sump Comput Appl Med Care 1988; 12:621–624.
36. Oniki T, Clemmer T, Gardner R, Johnson K: Representative charting of vital signs in an intensive care unit. Proc Annu Symp Comput Appl Med Care 1994; 18:307–311.
37. Dalto J: Automated Collection of Infusion Pump Data: Nurse Utilization and Its Effects on Clinical Data [MS thesis]. Salt Lake City, Utah, University of Utah, 1997.
38. Dalto JD, Johnson KV, Gardner RM, Spuhler VJ, Egbert L: Medical Information Bus usage for automated IV pump data acquisition: Evaluation of usage patterns. Int J Clin Monit Comput 1997; 14:151–154.
39. Young W: Automated Respiratory Care Charting: Artifact Rejection and Data Reduction [Doctoral dissertation]. Salt Lake City, Utah, University of Utah, 1993.
40. Cleveland WS, Devlin SJ: Locally weighted regression: An approach to regression analysis by local fitting. Journal of the American Statistical Association 1988; 9:596–609.
41. Carlson D, Wallace CJ, East TD, Morris AH: Verification and validation algorithms for data used in critical care decision support systems. Proc Annu Symp on Comput Appl Med Care 1995; 19:188–192
42. Stead WW: Systems for the year 2000: The case for an integrated database. MD Comput 1991; 8:103–104, 106–110.
43. Dick RS, Steen EB (Eds). The Computer-Based Patient Record: An Essential Technology for Health Care. Washington, DC, National Academy Press, 1991.
44. Stead WW, Sitting DF: Building a data foundation for tomorrow's healthcare information management systems. Int J Biomed Comput 1995; 39:127–131.
45. Shabot MM: Cedars-Sinai ICU Decision Support Tools. 1996, personal communication.
46. Kuperman GJ, Garder RM, Pryor TA: HELP: A Dynamic Hospital Information System. (Computers and Medicine. Orthner HF[Ed].) New York, Springer-Verlag, 1991.
47. Masarie FE, J., Miller RA, Bouhaddou O, Giuse NB, Warner HR: An interlingua for electronic interchange of medical information: Using frames to map between clinical vocabularies. Comput Biomed Res 1991; 24:379–400.
48. Grewal R, Arcus J, Bowen J, et al: Bedside computerization of the ICU, design issues: Benefits of computerization versus ease of paper & pen. Proc Annu Symp Comput Appl Med Care 1991; 15:793–797.
49. Higgins SB, Jiang K, Swindell BB, Bernard GR: A graphical ICU workstation. Proc Annu Symp Comput Appl Med Care 1991; 15:783–787.
50. Preiss B, Kaltenbach M, Zanazaka J, Echave V: Concept graphics: A language for medical knowledge. Proc Annu Symp Comput Appl Med Care 1992; 16:515–519.
51. Preiss B, Échavé V, Preiss SF, Kaltenbach M: UVAL-MED: A Universal Visual Associative Language for Medicine. Proc Annu Symp Comput Appl Med Care 1993; 17:262–266.
52. Cole WG: Metaphor graphics and visual analogy for medical data (workshop handout). Presented at 11th Annual Symposium on Computer Applications in Medical Care, Washington, DC, American Medical Informatics Association, 1987.
53. Cole WG: Quick and accurate monitoring via metaphor graphics. Proc Annu Symp Comput Appl Med Care 1990; 14:425–429.
54. Cole WG, Stewart JG: Metaphor graphics to support integrated decision making with respiratory data. Int J Clin Monit Comput 1993; 10:91–100.
55. Cole WG: Integrality and meaning: Essential and orthogonal dimensions of graphical data display. Proc Annu Symp Comput Appl Med Care 1993; 17:404–408.
56. Cole WG, Stewart JG: Human performance evaluation of a metaphor graphic display for respiratory data. Methods Inf Med 1994; 33:390–396.
57. Williams BT: Symposium on the role of the laboratory in clinical decision making: Part II. Perspectives on clinical decisions. Hum Pathol 1981; 12:106–111.
58. Powsner SM, Tufte ER: Graphical summary of patient status. the Lancet 1994; 344:386–389.
59. Tufte ER: Visual Explanations: Images and Quantities. Cheshire, Conn, Graphics Press, 1997.
60. Lesser MF: GIFIC: A Graphical Interface for Intensive Care. Proc Annu Symp Comput Appl Med Care 1993; 17:988.
61. Lindberg DAB, Schoolian HM: The National Library of Medicine and medical informatics. West J Med 1986; 145:786–790.
62. Cimino JJ, Johnson SB, Aguirre A, Roderer N, Clayton PD: The MEDLINE Button. Proc Annu Symp Comput Appl Med Care 1992; 16:81–85.

63. Jones A: Interactive videodisc technology: An overview for respiratory care education. Respir Care 1989; 34:890-898.
64. Clyman SG, Julian ER, Orr NA, Dillon GF, Cotton KE: Continued research on computer-based testing. Proc Annu Symp Comput Appl Med Care 1991; 15:742-746.
65. Anonymous: Physicians for the twenty-first century: Report on the Project Panel on the General Professional Education of the Physician and College Preparation for Medicine. J Med Educ 1984; 59(11, Part 2):1-208.
66. Clyman SG, Orr NA: Status report on the NBME's computer-based testing. Acad Med 1990; 65:235-241.
67. Mangione S, Nieman L, Gracely E: Comparison of computer-based learning and seminar teaching of pulmonary auscultation to first year medical students. Acad Med 1992; 67(10 Suppl):S63-S65.
68. Hess D: The hand-held computer as a teaching tool for acid-base interpretation. Respir Care 1984; 29:375-379.
69. Pincetl P, Hoffer E, Barnett O: Chest pain, an exercise in problem solving. Baltimore, Williams & Wilkins Electronic Media, 1998
70. Cyberlog: Acute Respiratory Failure. Munich, CMS-Biomedical Verlag, 1989
71. Rubens AJ: Testing airway management skills: Interactive video courseware vs ACLS instructor. Respir Care 1991; 36:849-856.
72. Dickinson C: A Computer model of human respiration. Baltimore, University Park Press, 1977.
73. Gardner RM, Cannon GH, Morris AH, Olsen KR, Price WG: Computerized blood gas interpretation and reporting system. IEEE Computer 1975; 8:39-45.
74. Bradshaw KE, Gardner RM, Pryor TA: Development of a computerized laboratory alerting system. Comput Biomed Res 1989; 22:575-587.
75. Evans RS, Gardner RM, Bush AR, et al: Development of a computerized infectious disease monitor (CIDM). Comput Biomed Res 1985; 18:103-113.
76. Shabot MM, LoBue M, Leyerle BJ, Dubin SB: Decision support alerts for clinical laboratory and blood gas data. Int J Clin Monit Comput 1990; 7:27-31.
77. Tate KE, Gardner RM, Weaver LK: A computerized laboratory alerting system. MD Comput 1990; 7:296-301.
78. Haug PJ, Gardner RM, Tate KE, et al: Decision support in medicine: Examples from the HELP system. Comput Biomed Res 1994; 27:396-418.
79. Evans RS, Pestotnik SL, Burke JP, et al: Reducing the duration of prophylactic antibiotic use through computer monitoring of surgical patients. Drug Intelligence Clin Pharmacol 1990; 24:351-354.
80. Evans RS, Burke JP, Pestotnik SL, et al: Prediction of hospital infections and selection of antibiotics using an automated hospital database. Proc Ann Symp Comput Appl Med Care 1990; 14:663-667.
81. Classen DC, Pestotnik SL. Evans RS, Burke JP: Computerized surveillance of adverse drug events in hospital patients. [see "comments"]. JAMA 1991; 266:2847-2851 [Erratum, JAMA 1992; 267:1992.]
82. Evans RS, Pestotnik SL, Classen DC, Bass SB, Burke JP: Prevention of adverse drug events through computerized surveillance. Proc Annu Symp Comput Appl Med Care 1992; 16:437-446.
83. Evans RS, Pestotnik SL, Classen DC, et al: Preventing adverse drug events in hospitalized patients. Ann Pharmacother 1994; 28:523-527.
84. Lepage ER, Gardner RM, Laud RM, Jacobson JT: Assessing the effectiveness of a computerized blood order "consultant" system. Proc Annu Symp Comput Appl Med Care 1991; 15:33-37.
85. Gardner RM, Golubjatnikov OK, Laub RM, Jacobson JT, Evans RS: Computer-critiqued blood ordering using the HELP system. Comput Biomed Res 1990; 23:514-528.
86. Gardner RM, Christiansen PD, Tate KE, Laub MB, Holmes SR: Computerized continuous quality improvement methods used to optimize blood transfusions. Proc Annu Symp Comput Appl Med Care 1993; 17:166-170.
87. Burke JP, Classen DC, Pestotnik SL, Evans RS, Stevens LE: The HELP system and its application to infection control. J Hosp Infect 1991; 18(Suppl A):424-431.
88. Evans RS, Larsen RA, Burke JP, et al: Computer surveillance of hospital-acquired infections and antibiotic use. JAMA 1986; 256:1007-1011.
89. Tate KE, Gardner RM: Computers, quality, and the clinical laboratory: A look at critical value reporting. Proc Annu Symp Comput Appl Med Care 1993; 17:193-197.
90. Morris AH: Use of monitoring information in decision making. *In:* Respiratory Monitoring. Tobin MJ (Ed). (Contemporary Management in Critical Care, vol 1. Tobin MJ, Grenvik A [Eds].) New York, Churchill Livingstone, 1991.
91. Elliot CG: Computer-assisted quality assurance: Development and performance of a respiratory care program. Qual Rev Bull J Qual Assurance 1991; 17:84-90.
92. Miller PL, Sittig DF: The evaluation of clinical decision support systems: What is necessary versus what is interesting. Med Inf (Lond) 1990; 15:185-190.
93. Hart A, Wyatt J: Evaluating black-boxes as medical decision aids: Issues arising from a study of neural networks. Med Inf (Lond) 1990; 15:229-236.
94. Hilden J, Habbema JD: Evaluation of clinical decision aids—more to think about. Med Inf (Lond) 1990; 15:275-284.
95. Wyatt J, Spiegelhalter D: Evaluating medical expert systems: What to test and how? Med Inf (Lond) 1990; 15:205-217.
96. Diamond GA, Pollock BH, Work JW: Clinician decisions and computers. *In:* Decision Support Systems in Critical Care. Shabot M, Gardner RM (Eds). (Computers in Medicine. Orthner HF [Ed].) New York, Springer-Verlag, 1994.
97. American Society for Testing and Materials: E 1460 Standard Specification for Defining And Sharing Modular Health Knowledge Bases (Arden Syntax for Medical Logic Modules). *In:* 1992 Annual Book of ASTM Standards. Vol 14.01. West Conshohocken, Pa, American Society for Testing and Materials, 1992, pp 539-587.
98. Miller RA, Pople HEJ, Myers JD: Internist-1, an experimental computer-based diagnostic consultant for general internal medicine. N Engl J Med 1982; 307:468-476.
99. Miller R, Masarie FE, Myers JD: Quick medical reference (QMR) for diagnostic assistance. MD Computing 1986; 3:34-48.
100. Warner HR J: Iliad: Moving medical decision-making into new frontiers. Methods Inf Med 1989; 28:370-372.
101. Bergeron B: Iliad: A diagnostic consultant and patient simulator [see "Comments"]. MD Computing 1991; 8:46-53. [Comment in MD Comput 1992; 9:76-78.]
102. Lau LM, Warner HR: Performance of a diagnostic system (Iliad) as a tool for quality assurance. Proc Annu Symp Comput App Med Care 1991; 15:104-108.
103. Barnett GO, Cimino JJ, Hupp JA, Hoffer EP: DXplain: An evolving diagnostic decision-support system. JAMA 1987; 258:67-74.
104. Silage DA, Maxwell C: A spirometry/interpretation program for hand-held computers. Respir Care 1983; 28:62-66.
105. Hess D, Eitel D: A portable and inexpensive computer system to interpret arterial blood gases. Respir Care 1986; 31:792-795.
106. Hess D, Silage D, Maxwell C: An arterial blood gas interpretation program for hand-held computers. Respir Care 1984; 29:756-759.
107. Hingston DM, Irwin RS, Pratter MR, Dalen JE: A computerized interpretation of arterial pH and blood gas data: Do physicians need it? Respir Care 1982; 27:809-815.
108. Gardner RM, Clemmer TP, Morris AH: Computerized medical decision-making: An evaluation in acute care. *In:* Computers in Critical Care and Pulmonary Medicine Vol 2. Prakash O (Ed). New York, Plenum Press, 1982, pp 147-150.
109. Moore MJ, Bleich HL: Consulting the computer about acid-base disorders. Respir Care 1982; 7:834-838.
110. Verdaguer A, Patak A, Sancho JJ, Sierra C, Sanz F: Validation of the medical expert system PNEUMON-IA. Comput Biomed Res 1992; 25:511-526.
111. Harber P, McCoy JM, Howard K, Greer D, Luo J: Artificial intelligence-assisted occupational lung disease diagnosis. Chest 1991; 100:340-346.
112. Asada N, Doi K, MacMahon H, et al: Potential usefulness of an artificial neural network for differential diagnosis of interstitial lung diseases: Pilot study. Radiology 1990; 177:857-860.
113. Sotos JG. MYCIN and NEOMYCIN: Two approaches to generating explanations in rule-based expert systems. Aviat Space Environ Med 1990; 61:950-954.
114. Shortliffe EH, Davis R, Axline SG, et al: Computer-based consultations in clinical therapeutics: Explanation and rule acquisition

capabilities of the MYCIN system. Comput Biomed Res 1975; 8:303–320.
115. Hickam DH, Shortliffe EH, Bischoff MB, Scott AC, Jacobs CD: The treatment advice of a computer-based cancer chemotherapy protocol advisor. Ann Intern Med 1985; 103:928–936.
116. Shortliffe EH: Update on ONCOCIN: A chemotherapy advisor for clinical oncology. Medical Inf (land) 1986; 11:19–21.
117. Miller PL: Extending computer-based critiquing to a new domain: ATTENDING, ESSENTIAL-ATTENDING, and VQ-ATTENDING. Int J Clin Monit Comput 1986; 2:135–142.
118. Miller PL: Building an expert critiquing system: ESSENTIAL-ATTENDING. Methods Inf Med 1986; 25:71–78.
119. Miller PL: Critiquing anesthetic management: The "ATTENDING" computer system. Anesthesiology 1983; 58:362–369.
120. Miller PL, Black HR: HT-ATTENDING: Critiquing the pharmacologic management of essential hypertension. J Med Syst 1984; 8:181–187.
121. Sittig DF: ComPAS: A Computerized Patient Advice System [Doctoral dissertation]. Salt Lake City, Utah, University of Utah, 1988.
122. Shahsavar N, Gill H, Wigertz O, et al: Kave: A tool for knowledge acquisition to support artificial ventilation. Comput Methods Programs Biomed 1991; 34:115–123.
123. Polaschek J, Rutledge G, Andersen S, Fagan L: Using belief networks to interpret qualitative data in the ICU. Respir Care 1993; 38:60–72.
124. Miller PL: Goal oriented critiquing by computer for ventilatory management. Comput Biomed Res 1985; 18:422–438.
125. Menn SJ, Barnett GO, Schnechel D, Owens WD, Pontoppidan H: A computer program to assist in the care of acute respiratory failure. JAMA 1973; 223:308–312.
126. Grossman R, Hew E, Aberman A: Assessment of the ability to manage patients on mechanical ventilators using a computer model. Acute Care 1984; 10:95–102.
127. Fagan L, Kunz J, Feigenbaum E, Osborn J: Representing time-dependent relations in a medical setting [Doctoral dissertation]. Stanford, Calif, Stanford University, 1980.
128. East TD, Morris AH, Wallace CJ, et al: A strategy for development of computerized critical care decision support systems. Int J Clin Monit Comput 1991; 8:263–269.
129. East TD: Role of computers in the delivery of mechanical ventilation. *In:* Principles and Practice of Mechanical Ventilation. Tobin MJ (Ed). New York, McGraw-Hill Book Co., 1993.
130. Henderson S, East TD, Morris AH, Gardner RM: Performance evaluation of computerized clinical protocols for management of mechanical ventilation in ARDS patients. Proc Annu Symp Comp Appl Med Care 1989; 13:588–592.
131. Henderson S, Crapo RO, Wallace CJ, et al: Performance of computerized protocols for the management of arterial oxygenation in an intensive care unit. Int J Clin Monit Comput 1991; 8:271–280.
132. Henderson S, Crapo RO, East TD, Morris AH, Gardner RM: Computerized clinical protocols in an intensive care unit: How well are they followed? Proc Ann Symp Comput Appl Med Care 1990; 14:284–288.
133. Rudowski R, Frostell C, Gill H: A knowledge-based support system for mechanical ventilation of the lungs: The KUSIVAR concept and prototype. Comput Methods Programs Biomed 1989; 30:59–70.
134. Tong D: Weaning patients from mechanical ventilation: A knowledge based approach. Proc Annu Symp Comput Appl Med Care 1990; 14:79–85.
135. Tong DA: Weaning patients from mechanical ventilation: A knowledge-based system approach. Comput Methods Programs Biomed 1991; 35:267–278.
136. Strickand JHJ, Hasson JH: A computer-controlled ventilator weaning system. Chest 1991; 100:1096–1099.
137. Rutledge G, Thomsen G, Farr B, et al: VentPlan: A ventilator-management advisor. Proc Annu Symp Comput Appl Med Care. 1991; 15:869–871.
138. Rutledge GW, Thomsen GE, Farr BR, et al: The design and implementation of a ventilator-management advisor. Artif Intell Med 1993; 5:67–82.
139. Morris AH, Menlove RL, Rollins RJ, Wallace CJ, Beck E: A controlled clinical trial of a new 3-step therapy that includes extracorporeal CO_2 removal for ARDS. Trans Am Soc Artif Intern Organs 1988; 11:48–53.
140. Morris AH, Wallace CJ, Clemmer TP, et al: Extracorporeal CO_2 removal therapy for adult respiratory distress syndrome patients: A computerized protocol controlled trial. Réanimat Soins Intensifs Méd Urg 1990; 6:485–490.
141. Morris AH, Wallace CJ, Clemmer TP, et al: Extracorporeal CO_2 removal therapy for adult respiratory distress syndrome patients. Respir Care 1990; 35:224–231.
142. Morris AH, Wallace CJ, Clemmer TP, et al: Final report: Computerized protocol controlled clinical trial of new therapy which includes ECCO2R for ARDS. Am Rev Respir Dis 1992; 145:A184.
143. Thomsen G, Pope D, East T, et al: Clinical performance of a rule-based decision support system for mechanical ventilation of ARDS patients. Proc Annu Symp Comput Appl Med Care. 1993; 17:339–343.
144. Morris AH: Protocol management of adult respiratory distress syndrome. New Horiz 1993; 1:593–602.
145. Morris AH: Adult respiratory distress syndrome and new modes of mechanical ventilation: Reducing the complications of high volume and high pressure. New Horiz 1994; 2:19–33.
146. Sittig DF, Pace NL, Gardner RM, Beck E, Morris AH: Implementation of a computerized patient advice system using the HELP clinical information system. Comput Biomed Res 1989; 22:474–487.
147. Sittig DF, Gardner RM, Morris AH, Wallace CJ: Clinical evaluation of computer-based respiratory care algorithms. Int J Clin Monit Comput 1990; 7:177–185.
148. Sailors RM, East TD, Wallace CJ, Morris AH: A successful protocol for the use of pulse oximetry to classify arterial oxygenation into four fuzzy categories. Proc Annu Symp Comput Appl Med Care 1995; 19:248–252.
149. East TD, Wallace CJ, Franklin MA, et al: Medical informatics academia and industry: A symbiotic relationship that may assure survival of both through health care reform. Proc Annu Symp Comput Appl Med Care. 1995; 19:243–247.
150. Artigas A, Carlet J, Le Gall JR, et al: Clinical presentation, prognostic factors, and outcome of ARDS in the European Collaborative Study (1985–1987). *In:* Adult Respiratory Distress Syndrome. Zapol WM, Lemaire F (Eds). (Lung Biology in Health and Disease: Vol 50. Lenfant C [Ed].) New York, Marcel Dekker, 1991, pp 37–63.
151. East TD: Real-time data acquisition and control. *In:* Diagnostic Methods in Critical Care: Automated Data Collection and Interpretation. Shoemaker WC, Abraham E (Eds). New York, Marcel Dekker, 1987, pp 285–310.
152. Isermann R: Digital Control Systems. Heidelberg, Germany, Springer-Verlag, 1981.
153. Coles J, Brown W, Lampard D: Computer control of respiration and anesthesia. Med Biol Eng 1973; 11:262–267.
154. Rudowski R, Skreta L, Baehrendtz S, Bokliden A, Matell G: Lung function analysis and optimization during artificial ventilation: A personal computer-based system. Comput Methods Programs Biomed 1990; 31:33–42.
155. East T, Westenskow D, Pace N, Nelson L: A microcomputer based differential lung ventilation system. IEEE Trans Biomed Eng 1982; 29:736–740.
156. Chapman F, Newell J, Roy R: A feedback controller for ventilatory therapy. Ann Biomed Eng 1985; 13:359–372.
157. Verkaaik AP, van Dijk G, Westerkamp B, Erdmann W: Gas exchange in the lung: Computer feed back controlled physiological matching of artificial ventilation. Adv Exp Med Biol 1992; 317:325–330.
158. Ohlson K, Westenskow D, Jordan W: A microprocessor based feedback controller for mechanical ventilation. Ann Biomed Eng 1982; 10:3548–3555.
159. Morozoff PE, Evans RW: Closed-loop control of SaO_2 in the neonate. Biomed Instrum Technol 1992; 26:117–123.
160. Verkaaik AP, Erdmann W, van Dijk G, Westerkamp B: On-line oxygen uptake measurement (VO_2): A computer feed-back controlled rebreathing circuit for long term oxygen uptake registration. Adv Exp Med Biol 1992; 316:195–202.
161. Tehrani FT: A microcomputer oxygen control system for ventilatory therapy. An Biomed Eng 1992; 20:547–558.
162. Strickland JJ, Hasson J: A computer-controlled ventilator weaning system: A clinical trial. Chest 1993; 103:1220–1227.

123

Extracorporeal Life Support for Respiratory Failure and Multiple Organ Failure

Harry L. Anderson III, MD • Robert H. Bartlett, MD

Extracorporeal perfusion was first used successfully as therapy for respiratory failure in 1972, when Hill and coworkers reported the recovery of a patient with the acute respiratory distress syndrome (ARDS) using prolonged extracorporeal support.[1] Since then, this type of bedside cardioperfusion technology has found use in selected neonatal, pediatric, and adult patients and is used for treatment of both respiratory and cardiac dysfunction. Extracorporeal life support (ECLS) has many other names (Table 123–1). Most designations refer to extracorporeal passage of blood through a gas exchange device, or oxygenator, and then return of blood to a major vein or artery, thus providing a unique means of assisting respiration or blood pressure (hence the term extracorporeal life support). This chapter reviews the evolution of ECLS, the current technology and management of patients, and worldwide results of ECLS for selected patient populations.

BACKGROUND

The first description of cardiopulmonary bypass dates back to 1937, when Gibbon described a system that consisted of a roller pump and a vertically mounted cylinder over which blood was pumped, allowing gas exchange of the blood with ambient gas.[2] This system was able to provide complete support of blood pressure and respiration when the pulmonary artery was occluded at the time of operation within the chest. It was with this system that cardiopulmonary bypass was born. Refinements in this technology, as applied to cardiac surgery, have led to more efficient membrane oxygenators and pumping systems and a better understanding of the interaction of blood with polymeric surfaces. Through these same avenues, ECLS was conceived, and this spin-off of cardiopulmonary bypass was modified for prolonged support of reversible heart or lung dysfunction at the bedside.

TECHNIQUE

The ECLS perfusion circuit is depicted in Figure 123–1. In a manner similar to cardiopulmonary bypass, blood is drained

TABLE 123–1. Common Acronyms for Types of Artificial Cardiac or Pulmonary Support

ECLS	Extracorporeal life support
ECMO	Extracorporeal membrane oxygenation
ECCOR or $ECCO_2R$	Extracorporeal CO_2 removal
$PECCO_2R$	Partial extracorporeal CO_2 removal
AVCOR	Arteriovenous CO_2 removal
ECLA	Extracorporeal lung assist
CPS	Cardiopulmonary support
CPB	Cardiopulmonary bypass
LVAD	Left ventricular assist device
RVAD	Right ventricular assist device
IVOX	Intravascular oxygenator

CO_2 = carbon dioxide.

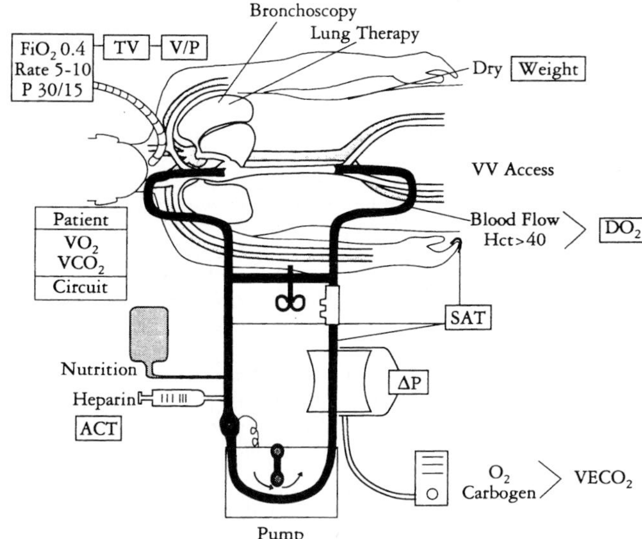

Figure 123–1. Diagram of venovenous extracorporeal life support (ECLS) perfusion circuit. Blood is drained from the right atrium by a catheter placed through the right jugular vein. Warmed and oxygenated blood is finally returned to the vena cava through a catheter placed in the right femoral vein. Parameters contained within boxes are those that are continuously monitored during ECLS. FIO_2 = inspired oxygen fraction; P = pressure; TV = tidal volume; V/P = volume/pressure, or compliance; VV = venovenous; Hct = hematocrit; Do_2 = oxygen delivery; SAT = hemoglobin saturation by oxygen; ΔP = pressure drop across membrane oxygenator; $VEco_2$ = percentage of carbon dioxide in outlet sweep gas; ACT = activated clotting time; Vo_2 = oxygen consumption; Vco_2 = carbon dioxide production. (From Anderson HL III, Steimle CM, Shapiro MB, et al: Extracorporeal life support for adult cardiorespiratory failure. Surgery 1993; 114:162.)

from the vena cava, pumped through an oxygenator device (where exchange of oxygen [O_2] and carbon dioxide [CO_2] with blood takes place), warmed by a water-jacketed heat exchanger, and then returned to a major artery (carotid, femoral, aortic arch) in the case of venoarterial bypass or to a major vein (internal jugular, femoral) in the case of venovenous bypass. Venoarterial bypass provides both cardiac (i.e., blood pressure) and respiratory support (i.e., oxygenation and ventilation), whereas venovenous bypass provides respiratory support only (cardiac function and blood pressure must be normal or nearly normal). With venovenous bypass, the venous blood is oxygenated and CO_2 is removed before reentering the venous system and mixing with venous blood from systemic circulation, raising the already low O_2 content of venous blood returning to the heart.

Cannulation

Bypass pump flow is limited by the rate at which venous blood is siphoned from a patient; therefore, the lowest-resistance configuration is selected for the drainage portion of the circuit. Large-bore, high-flow catheters are usually selected, and the internal jugular vein is usually chosen because it is the largest extrathoracic vein available by simple cutdown or by percutaneous access. Other veins that can be used for venous drainage (in order of decreasing preference) are the femoral and iliac veins (exposed by infraperitoneal dissection) as well as direct cannulation of the right atrium via thoracotomy.

Warmed, oxygenated blood is usually returned to (in decreasing order of preference) the common carotid artery, femoral artery, aortic arch, or axillary artery, in the case of venoarterial perfusion. In collateral-poor arterial beds (i.e., the leg supplied by the femoral artery, the arm supplied by the axillary artery), perfusion must also be supplied distal to the site of cannulation to prevent ischemia of the limb. With cannulation of the aortic arch through the right common carotid artery, the distal vessel is usually ligated; collateral perfusion from the external carotid, the circle of Willis, and the vertebrobasilar system prevents unilateral hemispheric cerebral ischemia. When venovenous perfusion is selected, the oxygenated blood is usually returned to the internal jugular, femoral, or iliac vein.

Vessel cannulation is usually carried out at the patient's bedside, with the assistance of an operating room team. Patients undergo systemic heparinization before catheters are inserted. Pesenti and colleagues have described venous cannulation for extracorporeal carbon dioxide removal ($ECCO_2R$) (see Respiratory Failure) by the percutaneous route,[3] and we have found this to be the preferred method of cannulation for patients with pure respiratory failure. Single-catheter venovenous systems can use a continuous-flow, double-lumen catheter or tidal flow (so-called push-pull, or to-and-fro) to propel oxygenated blood into the right atrium.[4–7] Similar techniques can be used to cannulate the femoral artery. The carotid artery is cannulated by direct exposure and distal ligation. These modifications allow cannulation using a single site and in neonates can provide total respiratory support.

ECLS Circuit Configuration

Pumping systems are of several varieties; the most common and simple is the servo-controlled roller pump. Alternatively, the centrifugal (vortex) pump has been the mainstay of many cardiac perfusion teams and can be selected for ECLS perfusion. The centrifugal pump has the advantage of a lesser requirement of regulating the pump speed by the rate of venous blood drainage from the patient, but this advantage is somewhat offset by a higher device cost, potential cavitation, and hemolysis of blood. Cavitation (creation of air bubbles) and hemolysis are of particular concern during periods of occlusion of the drainage inlet line supplying blood to the centrifugal pump head. A passively filling, servo-regulated pump has been described,[8] and a version of this pump is currently used in Europe.[6]

Oxygenators are usually of the coil membrane type (Kolobow membrane lung) or the hollow fiber type. Both types of oxygenators have undergone extensive clinical use, both short term in the operating room and for long-term perfusion. Because the need for systemic heparinization is predicated by the extensive contact of blood with foreign surfaces of the perfusion circuit, particularly in the oxygenator, significant effort is under way to perfect nonthrombogenic coating of bypass components. Heparin-bonded circuitry has enjoyed acceptance for short-term perfusion in the operating room; however, when this existing technology of heparin coating is used for long-term perfusion, leakage of plasma from the blood phase to the gas phase in the oxygenator results and limits its attractiveness.

The blood leaving the oxygenator is warmed to body temperature by a water-jacketed heat exchanger before being returned to the patient. A "bridge" connects the venous drainage limb and return limb of the ECLS circuit together, near the patient, and is occluded by a clamp during the bypass run. The bridge is opened every 15 to 20 minutes to "flash" the transiently stagnant blood within this section of tubing. This bridge has particular importance just before connecting the ECLS circuit to the patient: It allows continuous flow of blood within the circuit and avoids stagnation (and thrombus formation) of the blood prime. The bridge is also used during a "trial off" ECLS, when heart or lung recovery has occurred and extracorporeal support is temporarily removed. Blood can continue to flow within the circuit without actual disconnection of the patient and cannulas from the circuit.

Patient Management

Anticoagulation during the ECLS run is accomplished by continuous systemic heparinization and is monitored by the activated clotting time (ACT). Because ACT is a measure of the heparin effect on whole blood, it is preferred over the partial thromboplastin time (PTT) or other measures of heparin activity. Normal ACT is 90 to 120 seconds, and systemic heparinization is maintained to an ACT range of 160 to 200 seconds, usually in the range of 160 to 180 seconds. At higher ACTs, bleeding (e.g., from endobronchial, cannulation, or chest tube sites) and gross blood loss are greater; at ACT levels less than 160 seconds, the likelihood of clot formation in circuit components (especially the membrane oxygenator) increases. Perfusion of patients without systemic heparin for short periods has been described. One must plan for the eventual loss of the circuit to thrombosis and the need to replace it quickly with a new one.

Blood product administration is usually performed through the perfusion circuit, and it is usually necessary to replace the red blood cells, platelets, and clotting factors, which are normally consumed, sequestered, or lost in bulk amount (e.g., bleeding, laboratory sampling). Packed red blood cells are transfused to achieve a hematocrit of 45% to 50%, to maximize O_2 delivery from the perfusion circuit. Platelets are slowly consumed by the perfusion circuit (particularly the oxygenator) during an ECLS run, and any circulating platelets that remain are rendered dysfunctional by the extensive blood-foreign surface contact and by activation of the many inflammatory cascades within blood. A platelet level exceeding 100,000/mm^3 usually results in satisfactory hemostasis during a bypass run and a lesser likelihood of bleeding. Fresh frozen plasma or cryoprecipitate is used to replace factors consumed during extracorporeal perfusion, particularly factor II (fibrinogen), antithrombin III, and so on.

Fluids other than blood products (parenteral nutrition, intravenous fluids, intravenous medications, and others) can be similarly administered through the perfusion circuit and are concentrated as much as possible to minimize the fluid given to a patient in each 24 hours. Exquisite control of daily fluid balance can also be achieved through ultrafiltration by a minidialyzer membrane, taking advantage of the pressurized portion of the bypass circuit between the roller pump and the membrane oxygenator as the driving force for ultrafiltration through a dialyzer membrane. Slow continuous ultrafiltration (SCUF) for simple serum or fluid removal can be used, or dialysis can be added (SCUF-D),[9] a simple modification of techniques patterned after continuous hemofiltration (CAVH or CVVH).

A patient's typical course is depicted in Figure 123–2. When used for respiratory failure, ECLS allows "lung rest" from the high fraction of inspired O_2 (FIO_2) and high ventilatory pressures required to oxygenate and ventilate these patients adequately. Thus, the ventilator support is turned down to more moderate O_2 fraction, pressures, and rate. As pulmonary function improves, bypass pump flow (venoarterial or venovenous) is slowly weaned in response to increasing arterial partial pressure of oxygen (PaO_2) until support is considered to be less than 10% of the patient's metabolic needs. The ventilator is then increased to modest settings (e.g., FIO_2 of

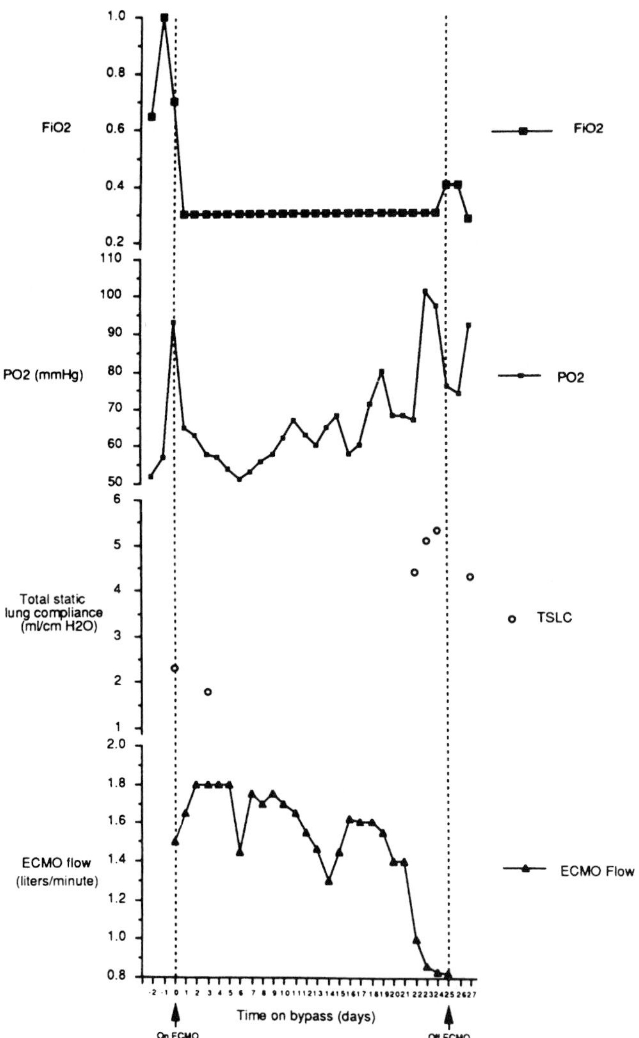

Figure 123–2. Extracorporeal life support (ECLS) course of 2-year-old infant with respiratory failure from *Varicella* pneumonia. Inspired oxygen fraction (FIO_2), arterial oxygen pressure (Po_2), total static lung compliance (TSLC), and ECLS pump flow are plotted against time. At day 25, the patient was successfully weaned from bypass and was decannulated. This patient was subsequently discharged. (From Anderson HL III, Attorri RJ, Custer JR, et al: Extracorporeal membrane oxygenation [ECMO] for pediatric cardiorespiratory failure. J Thorac Cardiovasc Surg 1990; 99:1015.)

0.5, moderate inflating pressures and minute ventilation), and the patient is "tried off" bypass if one clamps drainage and return catheters and opens the bridge, again allowing blood within the circuit to continue to circulate. If recovery of pulmonary function has been sufficient and adequate blood gases and hemodynamic parameters remain after 2 to 4 hours of a trial off, decannulation from bypass is usually considered. If not, the patient is returned to bypass support until the next trial off, usually 24 to 48 hours later. In cases of cardiac failure treated by ECLS, a trial off of venoarterial bypass is considered after cardiac function improves and blood pressure, O_2 delivery, and perfusion also improve and are sustained when pump flow is weaned. Again, a trial off of bypass is performed, after adequate cardiac preload is ensured and only minimum or moderate levels of inotropes are used.

When the decision to decannulate has been made, catheters placed percutaneously in veins are removed and the skin puncture sites closed with a simple pursestring or mattress suture. Cannulas placed operatively in vessels are removed after operative exposure of the cannulas and vessels. Veins are usually ligated after removal of surgically placed cannulas but can be repaired. Cannulated arteries supplying areas of poor collateral circulation (e.g., end-arterial beds of the femoral or axillary arteries) require primary repair (end-to-end anastomosis) or are repaired using autogenous vessel as a patch or interposition graft. Ligation of the common carotid artery is usually performed after carotid artery decannulation. Several centers have successfully performed repair of the common carotid artery in neonates after decannulation, with good results,[10, 11] although a small risk of distal embolization, pseudoaneurysm formation, or stenosis at the site of the arterial repair still remains.

Unilateral carotid artery ligation has been safely performed in thousands of neonatal, pediatric, and adult patients with virtually minimum or no morbidity, and any alternative techniques beyond simple carotid decannulation and ligation must be compared with this standard. The long-term effect of unilateral carotid ligation after treatment with ECLS is not known. The oldest surviving patient who underwent therapy with venoarterial ECLS and subsequently underwent carotid artery ligation is neurologically and developmentally normal at age 22 years. Long-term follow-up of these patients is important to discern whether (if at all) neurologic or developmental sequelae arise from unilateral carotid artery ligation.

An alternative to immediate decannulation after a trial off bypass is heparinization of the indwelling bypass cannulas after removal of the bypass circuit. A continuous infusion of a heparin-containing solution is attached to the cannulas until 12 to 24 hours have passed and the patient's condition continues to merit the removal of catheters. Should a patient's condition deteriorate before catheters are removed, with this technique a new bypass circuit can be primed and the patient can again be placed back on ECLS.

PATIENT SELECTION

Selection of Neonates

Much attention has been given to the topic of patient selection, particularly in the pediatric and adult patient population, when ECLS is considered for primary respiratory or cardiac failure. ECLS for neonates became standard therapy for neonatal respiratory failure by 1984,[12] and indications have become relatively standardized from medical center to medical center. Minimum differences exist in individual entry criteria of each center because mortality for a given level of illness in any patient varies from center to center.

Five pathophysiologic conditions (excluding congenital cardiac anomaly) of the newborn period are typically responsible for respiratory failure within the first 2 weeks of life:

- Meconium aspiration syndrome
- Respiratory distress syndrome
- Persistent pulmonary hypertension of the newborn (persistent fetal circulation)
- Pneumonia/sepsis
- Congenital diaphragmatic hernia

All of these conditions have some component of persistent fetal circulation due to elevated pulmonary vascular resistance (and pulmonary hypertension), with right-to-left shunt. Conventional therapy calls for higher FIO_2 and higher mean airway pressures by mechanical ventilation to improve oxygenation. Oxygen toxicity and barotrauma are the usual results.

Most neonatal centers select a 90% mortality threshold, as defined by physiologic and ventilatory parameters, as criteria for placement on ECLS. The oxygenation index (OI), defined as:

$$OI = \text{mean airway pressure (cm } H_2O) \times FIO_2 \times 100/Pao_2 \text{ (mm Hg)}$$

was developed as one predictor of mortality. In the authors' neonatal intensive care unit, an OI of 25 predicts a mortality of 50% and an OI of 40 predicts a mortality of 60% to 80%.

For neonates between 2.5 and 4.5 kg, without severe cardiac dysfunction, an attempt is made at placement of the double-lumen venovenous catheter, thereby sparing ligation of the carotid.

In most cases, time permits early ultrasonographic evaluation of a patient's head to rule out intracranial bleeding. Also as part of the evaluation routine, major congenital cardiac anomalies are excluded by echocardiography. Neonates with respiratory failure identified early in the disease course are usually evaluated by cranial ultrasonography and echocardiogram; in the event that urgent cannulation becomes necessary late at night, all the preparatory screening studies will have been done. Conditions that might exclude a patient from consideration for ECLS are major chromosomal aberration, major cardiac anomaly, grade II intracranial hemorrhage, and estimated gestational age less than 30 weeks or birth weight under 1 kg.

Selection of Pediatric and Adult Patients

Respiratory Failure

The pathophysiology of respiratory or cardiac failure in an older child or adult patient is much more complex when compared with the reversibility of respiratory failure in a neonate. It is clear that despite advancement in the technology of ventilators and advances in the field of respiratory care, ARDS still carries a high mortality.[13] ECLS is considered for those patients who are going to die despite the best current treatment. The challenge is to detect these patients before irreversible lung injury occurs. Indications and exclusionary criteria for older children and adult patients are listed in Table 123–2. Physiologic criteria of low static lung compliance and high transpulmonary shunt as predictors of mortality have been reverified during the years; the authors currently use Pao_2/FIO_2 consistently less than 100 despite and after optimal therapy.

Gattinoni and colleagues in Milan, Italy, have used similar entry criteria but use a different approach to ECLS (termed $ECCO_2R$), emphasizing CO_2 removal by a low-flow system (1 to 2 L/min blood flow in the circuit) and apneic oxygenation by the native lungs.[14] They have placed no limitation on the time of mechanical ventilation before institution of $ECCO_2R$, although our series suggests that the optimal time period for institution of ECLS is within 5 days of intubation.

TABLE 123–2. Indications and Contraindications for the Institution of Extracorporeal Life Support for Pediatric and Adult Patients

Indications (Despite and After Optimal Treatment)
- Total static lung compliance <0.5 $mL \cdot cm\ H_2O^{-1} \cdot kg^{-1}$
- Transpulmonary shunt >30% on inspired oxygen fraction of 0.6 or greater
- Reversible respiratory failure
- Time on mechanical ventilation <7 days

Exclusions
- Potential for severe bleeding
- Time on mechanical ventilation (>7 days is a relative contraindication for adults)
- Necrotizing pneumonia
- Poor quality of life (patients with metastatic malignancy or major central nervous system injury)
- Age (>60 years is a relative contraindication)

Once a patient has successfully been placed on ECLS, the ventilator settings can be turned down, affording true lung rest. Typical rest settings include an FIO_2 of 0.5 or less, peak pressures limited at 30 to 40 cm H_2O, positive end-expiratory pressure (PEEP) of 10 to 15 cm H_2O, and respiratory rate of 4 breaths per minute. The inspiratory period is increased, reversing the inspiratory-expiratory ratio and providing prolonged alveolar inflation.

Cardiac Failure

The use of venoarterial ECLS for support of a failing heart is an area that has only recently received renewed attention, particularly in children. Selected pathologic conditions include preoperative support of the failing heart ("bridge to transplant") or postoperative support after cardiac operation or cardiac transplantation, when cardiac index is less than 2 $L/min/m^2$. Typical reversible medical conditions treated with ECLS are myocarditis and cardiomyopathy.[9, 15, 16]

One advantage of ECLS over the use of the right ventricular assist device or the left ventricular assist device is the fact that major operation with median sternotomy is not required for cannulation, allowing rapid institution of bypass support for these patients in the intensive care unit (ICU) or emergency department. Later thoracic operation is not compromised should cardiac surgery or cardiac transplantation be necessary.

Although it appears that recent sternotomy or thoracotomy might prove to be a contraindication to institution of ECLS because of the potential for severe bleeding, the authors usually place the patient on bypass, leaving the sternum open. This method allows bedside evacuation of hematoma, minimizes the potential for cardiac tamponade, and allows easy access for correction of hemorrhage and hemothorax within the chest. For postoperative cardiac surgery patients placed on ECLS, ACT levels are maintained low (150 to 170 seconds) and platelets and fresh frozen plasma are transfused to keep platelet count greater than 100,000/mm^3 and fibrinogen level greater than 200 mg/dL.

MULTIPLE ORGAN FAILURE

In the early days of the development of the technique for respiratory failure, sepsis, septic shock, and multiple organ failure were considered to be contraindications to ECLS. Good results in neonates with systemic sepsis, however, led to trials in children and adults. Many of the patients currently treated with ECLS have combined cardiorespiratory failure complicated by shock, renal failure, coagulopathy, coma, and systemic sepsis. These patients are referred for ECLS because of respiratory failure, but the results in these patients leads us to consider ECLS for general systemic support, even before profound respiratory failure occurs. Similarly, some patients with cardiovascular collapse following prolonged hypovolemic or hemorrhage shock ("irreversible shock") have been successfully resuscitated with venoarterial perfusion while the patient recovers from myocardial stun and other organ failure.

The rationale for ECLS and multiple organ failure is similar to that for pure respiratory or cardiac failure. ECLS simply keeps the patient alive long enough to allow recovery of the failing organs, time for antibiotics and nutrition to take effect, and (in the future) direct mechanical treatment of liver failure and clearance of septic mediators.

RESULTS

To facilitate collection and exchange of information and data with regard to ECLS and extracorporeal membrane oxygen-

TABLE 123–3. Neonatal and Pediatric Extracorporeal Life Support Results Compiled by the Extracorporeal Life Support Organization (ELSO) Registry (Ann Arbor) as of July 1998

Group	Patients Reported	No. Survived	% Survival
Neonatal respiratory	13,708	10,989	80%
Pediatric respiratory	1,631	883	54%
Cardiac support	2,426	1,010	42%
Adult	606	288	48%
TOTAL	18,371	13,170	72%

ation (ECMO), an organization of health care professionals interested in ECLS was founded in 1989. The Extracorporeal Life Support Organization (ELSO) and the ELSO Registry are based at the University of Michigan and coordinate education of and multicenter studies for their member institutions. Data with respect to number of active centers, numbers of patients treated, survival, complications, and so forth are summarized each quarter for centers within the United States, in Canada, and overseas. A summary can be found in Table 123-3.

Neonatal Respiratory Failure

The largest patient experience with ECLS is for the treatment of neonatal respiratory failure, with an overall survival of 80%.[17] Survival is highest in patients with the meconium aspiration syndrome (94% survival) and lowest in neonates treated for congenital diaphragmatic hernia (58% survival). This disparity reflects the complexity of treating patients with congenital diaphragmatic hernia, whether ECLS is used as rescue therapy for deterioration in the immediate postpartum period or is used for respiratory deterioration after surgical repair of the diaphragmatic defect.

A third prospective randomized study for neonatal respiratory failure has been conducted in the United Kingdom.[18] One hundred eighty-five patients were randomized when oxygenation index reached 40. Hospital survival in patients randomized to conventional treatment was 41%, and ECMO was 70%. Patients were randomized in the primary neonatal centers; therefore, the mortality of randomization to the ECMO center included the risk of long distance transportation, treatment delay, and misdiagnosis (11 of 93 patients). The hospital survival of neonates actually treated with ECMO was 34%.

The most common physiologic complication of ECLS is bleeding, owing to the use of systemic heparinization; it occurs in as many as 20% of cases. Bleeding can be minor and easily corrected when occurring in a cannulation site or may be serious if it occurs intracranially, often mandating immediate discontinuance of ECLS. Mechanical complications with the ECLS circuit happen less frequently (e.g., failure of a membrane oxygenator or rupture of tubing) and often can be corrected with minimum disruption in the ECLS run.

Follow-up of neonates treated with ECLS has shown normal neurologic development in about 75% of patients, with the remaining 25% sustaining either minor or major neurologic handicap. Analysis of risk factors for intracranial bleeding or intraventricular hemorrhage implicated prematurity or younger gestational age.[19]

Pediatric Patients

Since 1990, the use of ECLS for the treatment of pediatric respiratory or cardiac failure has increased markedly. As more and more neonatal centers join the current list of ECLS centers, a natural transition is from neonatal ECLS to pediatric ECLS. This trend involves larger circuits with greater membrane surface area (to accommodate greater gas exchange), larger catheters, and obviously larger patients. What is not readily appreciated is the fact that the time course for non-neonatal patients on ECLS is typically 1 to 3 weeks in duration instead of only 4 to 7 days for a neonate. This longer period can involve a significant investment in hospital and medical personnel resources, with particular use of more laboratory studies and blood products and often requiring the frequent replacement of oxygenators or complete bypass circuits during these longer runs.

Typical respiratory diseases treated in pediatric patients include bacterial or viral pneumonia, aspiration, ARDS, and near-drowning. As in neonates, both venoarterial access (using the carotid artery) and venovenous access (usually with a two-catheter system) are used.

There has been no prospective randomized trial of ECLS in pediatric respiratory failure. However, Green and associates[20] conducted a double-matched pairs study using the 1991 pediatric respiratory failure data base of Timmons and colleagues.[21] Multivariate analysis of the pediatric respiratory failure data base showed that ECMO support was the only treatment variable that correlated with improved survival. On the basis of this information, Green compared 29 patients treated with ECLS with 53 other cases, matched for age, diagnosis, and severity of illness. Survival was 74% in the ECMO-treated patients and 53% with other treatment. This study is important, not only because of the implications for ECLS but also as a method for evaluating life support technology in acute lethal illness.

Cardiac diseases treated by ECLS can include heart failure before or after a cardiac operation (particularly from congenital cardiac disease or before or after cardiac transplantation), viral myocarditis, and cardiomyopathy. Approximately 25% of pediatric patients with cardiac failure are placed on ECLS in the operating room owing to the inability to be weaned from cardiopulmonary bypass.[16] Results of ECLS for the treatment of pulmonary and cardiac failure in pediatric patients are also summarized in Table 123-3.

Acute Respiratory Failure

Despite improvements in ventilator management, the overall mortality for ARDS remains approximately 40% and above 80% in severe cases. From results with neonates and children, it seems that ECLS would be ideal for these patients, but until recently, results have been discouraging. The reason is that severe ARDS in adults is often associated with necrotizing or fibrosing conditions in the pulmonary parenchyma, sepsis, multiple organ failure, and comorbid conditions associated with age.

A prospective randomized trial of venoarterial ECMO for ARDS sponsored by the National Institutes of Health from 1975 to 1977 showed only 10% survival in both groups. Now we know that the techniques used for ventilator management and ECMO in this study caused rather than prevented mortality, but the results of that study essentially stopped ECLS research for a decade. Similarly, the extracorporeal technique (low-flow ECCOR) used in the prospective study by Morris and coauthors[22, 23] is inadequate for total gas exchange support, and the survival rate (37%) is lower than the 50% to 60% reported with current techniques. However, the improved ventilator management in that study resulted in 40% survival in the ventilator management group, and this has been a major influence on changing the way that ventilators are managed in ARDS. New techniques of ECLS include percutaneous access, venovenous perfusion for primary respiratory failure, minimal bleeding, and continuous hemofiltration for management of fluids and renal failure.[24]

The concept that has evolved from all of these studies is an algorithm for general management that avoids high pressure, high oxygen ventilation, with the use of ECLS for patients who do not respond to this regimen. This approach has led to 60% to 70% survival in severe ARDS with an expected survival of 20% to 30%.[25-30] It should be emphasized that ECLS does not compete with conventional ventilation; it is an option when other modes of therapy fail. Forty per cent of patients die while on ECLS; half die because of progressive irreversible lung damage and half because of sepsis and multiple organ failure culminating in brain injury. The current research focus regarding these patients is innovative techniques, such as fluorocarbon liquid breathing to minimize lung inflammation and injury and hemodiafiltration systems to clear toxic mediators and the products of liver failure.

INNOVATIONS

As clinical application of ECLS has grown and as the indications and age groups have expanded beyond the neonate, new problems have surfaced with extracorporeal technology and support. Much attention has been directed to this question: How can we perform ECLS more safely and better? As one would expect, advances in perfusion technology for cardiac surgery cross over to many areas of ECLS, particularly with regard to the actual propulsion of blood through the bypass circuit.

Automation or servo-regulation of the ECLS system is one such advance. The ability to place a patient on ECLS and have the system wean pump flow automatically based on multiplexed physiologic information, directly input by hardwired technology that can include arterial blood gases, mixed venous oxygen saturation, and pulmonary mechanics from the ventilator, would simplify the process tremendously. Such a servo-regulated system could be attached to the patient and supervised by the one ICU nurse caring for the patient rather than having a round-the-clock ECLS specialist (the current practice) also at the bedside. Servo-regulation has been implemented successfully in the laboratory[31] and should soon find an active role for ECLS in the critical care unit.

Catheter technology, geared toward thin-wall, wire-reinforced designs (e.g., Bio-Medicus Corporation, Medtronic, Inc., Minneapolis), have simplified cannulation by percutaneous technique, as described by Pesenti and colleagues.[3, 32] These small-diameter catheters allow higher blood flow without collapse of the catheters, owing to lower intrinsic resistance and to wire reinforcing of the catheter wall. Montoya and associates described the M number, a numeric system by which catheters can be categorized according to their flow/pressure characteristics.[33] Sinard and coworkers tested perfusion catheters in use for ECLS today and determined the M number for each.[34] Knowing the required flow to support a given patient, the appropriate size, and type of catheter can be selected using the working pressure of the system and calculating the M number necessary for those constraints.

Single-site cannulation using a double-lumen catheter for venovenous bypass has been successfully used for neonatal ECLS[4, 6, 35] and in a multicenter comparison was at least as safe as venoarterial bypass.[5] Double-lumen catheters of sufficient size are not available for use in larger pediatric and adult patients. Single-site cannulation with these catheters would allow quick and easy cannulation and decannulation and would decrease bleeding from the cannulation site.[32]

Gas exchange surface technology and development of oxygenators have been primarily driven by their use in clinical cardiopulmonary bypass. Heparin coating of perfusion components has been accomplished by two manufacturing groups, Medtronic/Carmeda (Carmeda BioActive Surface, Stockholm)[36, 37] and Baxter-Bentley Laboratories (DuraFlo II, Irvine, Calif.).[38] Although heparin coating of the hollow-fiber lung has shown the greatest promise for ECLS, it is still handicapped by plasma leakage from blood to the gas phase, resulting in profuse production of soapsuds-like foam from the gas port of the oxygenator. A system that does not require full systemic heparinization would ultimately be ideal, decreasing bleeding from the patient (and reducing the need for blood transfusion).

The ideal pumping system for long-term perfusion is a continuous topic of controversy. The classic roller pump has had decades of clinical use, with advantages of relative inexpense, minimum hemolysis, and the fact that it has no spinning impeller to propel blood through the circuit. Regulation of pump speed based on venous drainage from the patient is a method of servo-regulation by which the pump is stopped when venous drainage stops (i.e., a venous return line is kinked), preventing cavitation of the stationary blood within the pump raceway. The centrifugal pump, of which the Bio-Medicus Bio-Pump is a popular model, is found in many cardiac operating rooms today. No discrete servo-control, based on venous drainage, is necessary for the centrifugal pump, obviating the need for the distensible "bladder" in the venous drainage line often used with roller pump systems. Cavitation of blood and creation of air bubbles in the blood path during inflow occlusion of the centrifugal pump pose a potential hazard. The centrifugal pump is a more expensive system owing to the magnetically coupled impeller chamber that propels the blood and must be replaced every few days. Again, neither of the pumping systems can be referred to as the perfect system.

Several European centers currently use a passively filling, roller-type pump known as the Rhone-Poulenc pump (Collin Cardio, Paris).[6] This pump system combines advantages of both the roller pump and the centrifugal pump. As venous drainage decreases or when a venous return line is occluded, the distensible pump raceway tubing collapses and no blood is moved through the pump; thus, there is no cavitation. Should a high-pressure return line become kinked or occluded, the pump raceway tubing becomes circular rather than ovoid, overcoming the occlusion of the rollers and halting propulsion of blood through the tubing. High pressures are therefore avoided, preventing tubing rupture due to high pressure within the blood return portion of the circuit. Thus, this system incorporates the benefits of the previously mentioned pumping systems without the expensive hardware that either of the two systems requires. A system incorporating these features has recently been approved by the Food and Drug Administration for use in cardiac surgery.

Pharmacologic modulation of the inflammatory and coagulation cascade has shown promise in preserving platelet number and function and in decreasing overall blood loss in patients undergoing cardiopulmonary support. Tranexamic acid, a plasmin inhibitor, has both clinically and experimentally been demonstrated to decrease blood loss and preserve platelet number and function during cardiac operation.[39, 40] Aprotinin, an inhibitor of fibrinolysis, has been shown to decrease postoperative bleeding when administered before cardiopulmonary bypass.[41] As more is learned about the coagulation and inflammatory cascades, agents that prevent their activation in blood when in contact with foreign surfaces and agents that preserve platelet number and function during bypass will make long-term ECLS perfusion safer, with less bleeding and less need for blood product transfusion.

SUMMARY

ECLS is a critical care technique that has gained popularity in recent years, particularly after its acceptance as standard therapy for neonatal respiratory failure. As the technology of ECLS has made significant advances in recent years, more complete respiratory and cardiac support and safety are now provided to patients. It is clear that in pediatric and adult patients with respiratory failure, early intervention is key to a successful outcome. ECLS technology can be expensive in terms of medical resources and personnel; however, improved results in recent years, owing to better patient selection and better understanding of pulmonary pathophysiology, make ECLS another potentially lifesaving technique in the armamentarium of critical care physicians.

References

1. Hill JD, O'Brien TG, Murray JJ, et al: Extracorporeal oxygenation for acute post-traumatic respiratory failure (shock-lung syndrome): Use of the Bramson membrane lung. N Engl J Med 1972; 286:629–634.
2. Gibbon JH Jr: Artificial maintenance circulation during experimental occlusion of the pulmonary artery. Arch Surg 1937; 34:1105.
3. Pesenti A, Gattinoni L, Kolobow T, et al: Extracorporeal circulation in adult respiratory failure. ASAIO Trans 1988; 34:43–47.
4. Anderson HL III, Otsu T, Chapman RA, et al: Veno-venous extracorporeal life support in neonates using a double lumen catheter. ASAIO Trans 1989; 35:650–653.
5. Anderson HL III, Snedecor SM, Otsu T, et al: Multicenter comparison of conventional veno-arterial access versus veno-venous double lumen catheter access in newborn infants undergoing extracorporeal membrane oxygenation. J Pediatr Surg 1993; 28:530–535.
6. Durandy Y, Chevalier JY, Lecompte Y: Single cannula veno-venous bypass for respiratory membrane lung support. J Thorac Cardiovasc Surg 1990; 99:404–409.
7. Tsuno K, Terasaki H, Tsutsumi R, et al: To-and-fro veno-venous extracorporeal lung assist for newborns with severe respiratory distress. Intensive Care Med 1989; 15:269–271.
8. Montoya JP, Merz SI, Bartlett RH: Laboratory experience with a novel, non-occlusive, pressure-regulated peristaltic pump. ASAIO J 1992; 38:M406–M411.
9. Anderson HL III, Attorri RJ, Custer JR, et al: Extracorporeal membrane oxygenation (ECMO) for pediatric cardiopulmonary failure. J Thorac Cardiovasc Surg 1990; 99:1011–1019.
10. Spector ML, Wiznitzer M, Walsh-Sukys MC, et al: Carotid reconstruction in the neonate following ECMO. J Pediatr Surg 1991; 26:357–359.
11. Taylor BJ, Seibert JJ, Glasier CM, et al: Evaluation of the reconstructed carotid artery following extracorporeal membrane oxygenation. Pediatrics 1992; 90:568–572.
12. Andrews AF, Roloff DN, Bartlett RH: Use of extracorporeal membrane oxygenation in persistent pulmonary hypertension of the newborn. Clin Perinatol 1984; 11:729–735.
13. Sloane PJ, Gee MH, Gottlieb JE, et al: A multicenter registry of patients with acute respiratory distress syndrome: Physiology and outcome. Am Rev Respir Dis 1992; 146:419–426.
14. Gattinoni L, Pesenti A, Mascheroni D, et al: Low-frequency positive-pressure ventilation with extracorporeal CO_2 removal in severe acute respiratory failure. JAMA 1986; 256:881–886.
15. Pennington GD, Swartz MT: Circulatory support in infants and children. Ann Thorac Surg 1993; 55:233–237.
16. Klein MD, Shaheen KW, Whittlesey GC, et al: Extracorporeal membrane oxygenation for the circulatory support of children after repair of congenital heart disease. J Thorac Cardiovasc Surg 1990; 100:498–505.
17. ECMO Quarterly Report (July 1998). Ann Arbor, ECMO Registry of the Extracorporeal Life Support Organization (ELSO), 1998.
18. UK Collaborative ECMO Trial Group: UK collaborative randomized trial of neonatal extracorporeal membrane oxygenation. Lancet 1996; 348:75–82.
19. Cilley RE, Zwischenberger JB, Andrews AF, et al: Intracranial hemorrhage during extracorporeal membrane oxygenation in neonates. Pediatrics 1986; 78:699–704.
20. Green TP, Timmons OD, Fackler JC, Moler FW, Thompson AE, Sweeney MF: The impact of extracorporeal membrane oxygenation on survival in pediatric patients with acute respiratory failure. Crit Care Med 1996; 24:323–329.
21. Timmons OD, Dean JM, Vernon DD: Mortality rates and prognostic variables in children with the adult respiratory distress syndrome. J Pediatr 1991; 119:896–899.
22. Suchyta MR, Clemmer TP, Orme JF, et al: Increased survival of ARDS patients: Severe hypoemia (ECMO criteria). Chest 1991; 99:951–955.
23. Morris AH, Wallace CJ, Menlove RL, et al: Randomized clinical trial of pressure controlled inverse ratio ventilation and extracorporeal CO_2 removal for adult respiratory distress syndrome. Am J Respir Crit Care Med 1994; 149:295–305.
24. Anderson HL III, Steimle CN, Shapiro MB, et al: Extracorporeal life support for adult cardiorespiratory failure. Surgery 1993; 114:161–173.
25. Manert W, Haller M, Briegel J, et al. Veno-venous extracorporeal membrane oxygenation (ECMO) with a heparin-lock bypass system: An effective addition in the treatment of acute respiratory failure. Anaesthetist 1996; 45:437–448.
26. Kolla S, Awad SA, Rich PB, Schreiner RJ, Hirschl RB, Bartlett RH: Extracorporeal life support for 100 adult patients with severe respiratory failure. Ann Surg 1997; 226:544–564.
27. Lewandowski K, Lewandowski M, Pappert D, Falke KJ: Outcome and follow-up of adults following extracorporeal life support. *In*: ECMO: Extracorporeal Cardiopulmonary Support in Critical Care. Zwischenberger J, Bartlett RH (Eds). Extracorporeal Life Support Organization, 1995.
28. Guinard N, Beloucif S, Gatecel C, et al: Interest of a therapeutic optimization strategy in severe ARDS. Chest 1997; 111:1000–1007.
29. Peek GJ, Firmin RK: Extracorporeal membrane oxygenation, a favorable outcome? Br J Anaesh 1997; 78:235–236.
30. Rich PB, Awad SS, Kolla S, et al: An approach to the treatment of severe adult respiratory failure. J Crit Care 1998; 44:26–36.
31. Merz S, Montoya PJ, Shanley CJ, et al: Implementation of a controller for extracorporeal life support (Abstract). ASAIO Trans 1993; 22:69.
32. Pesenti A, Gattinoni L, Bombino M: Long term extracorporeal respiratory support: 20 years of progress. Intensive Crit Care Dig 1993; 12:15–18.
33. Montoya JP, Merz SI, Bartlett RH: A standardized system for describing flow/pressure relationships in vascular access devices. ASAIO Trans 1991; 37:4–8.
34. Sinard JM, Merz SI, Hatcher MD, et al: Evaluation of extracorporeal perfusion catheters using a standardized measurement technique: The M-number. ASAIO Trans 1991; 37:60–64.
35. Delius RE, Anderson HL III, Schumacher RE, et al: Veno-venous compares favorably to veno-arterial access for extracorporeal membrane oxygenation in neonatal respiratory failure. J Thorac Cardiovasc Surg 1993; 106:329–338.
36. Bindslev L: Adult ECMO performed with surface-heparinized equipment. ASAIO Trans 1988; 34:1009–1013.
37. Shanley CJ, Hultquist KA, Rosenberg DM, et al: Prolonged extracorporeal circulation without heparin: Evaluation of the Medtronic Minimax oxygenator. ASAIO Trans 1992; 38:M311–M316.
38. Toomasian JM, Hsu L-C, Hirschl RB, et al: Evaluation of Duraflo II heparin coating in prolonged extracorporeal membrane oxygenation. ASAIO Trans 1988; 34:410–414.
39. Plotz FB, van Oeveren W, Aloe LS, et al: Prophylactic administration of tranexamic acid preserves platelet numbers during extracorporeal circulation in rabbits. ASAIO Trans 1987; 37:M416–M417.
40. Nakashima A, Matsuzaki K, Hisahara M, et al: Tranexamic acid decreases blood loss after cardiopulmonary bypass (Abstract). ASAIO Trans 1993; 22:64.
41. Lavee J, Raviv Z, Smolinsky A, et al: Platelet protection by low-dose aprotonin in cardiopulmonary bypass: Electron microscopic study. Ann Thorac Surg 1993; 55:114–119.

124

Fiberoptic Bronchoscopy in the Intensive Care Unit

Joseph A. Govert, MD • William J. Fulkerson, MD

Bronchoscopy was first described in 1897, when Killian removed an aspirated pork bone from a patient's right mainstem bronchus by using a rigid esophagoscope.[1] Although many practitioners improved and refined rigid bronchoscopic techniques over the ensuing 60 years, it was not until Ikeda developed the flexible fiberoptic bronchoscope in the 1960s that the use of bronchoscopy became widespread.[1] Bronchoscopy is a common procedure for patients in intensive care.[2-6] This chapter discusses the use of fiberoptic bronchoscopy in the intensive care unit (ICU), detailing its many diagnostic and therapeutic indications as well as some of its common complications.

INSTRUMENTATION

A wide variety of fiberoptic bronchoscopes and videoscopes are available commercially. Most bronchoscopes have an effective length of 600 mm. The outside diameter of the fiberoptic shaft ranges from 1.8 to 6.0 mm, with the standard adult diameter being 5.7 mm. Bronchoscopic visual fields range from 75° to 120° and can usually flex 180° and extend 130°.

Most patients undergoing bronchoscopy in the ICU are mechanically ventilated. Special endotracheal tube adapters facilitate entry of the bronchoscope into the airway without disruption of the ventilator circuit. These adapters usually consist of a unit connecting the ventilator tubing with the endotracheal tube. The adapter has a side port that is normally sealed. During bronchoscopy, a side port cap or plug opens to allow entry of the bronchoscope into the endotracheal tube without disrupting the ventilator circuit.

SEDATION AND ANALGESIA

Although many critically ill patients are heavily sedated, it is still important to ensure analgesia and sedation throughout bronchoscopy and to remember that administration of sedation and analgesia often involves different medications. Usually, topical lidocaine provides adequate analgesia, but occasionally systemic narcotics are also required. We favor short-acting benzodiazepines to obtain adequate sedation, because the effects of oversedation wear off rapidly and can be pharmacologically reversed. Although some practitioners elect not to use it, atropine (0.5 mg to 1.0 mg) is often given intramuscularly 30 minutes prior to elective bronchoscopy for prophylaxis against vasovagal reactions and to decrease airway secretions.

PHYSIOLOGIC CONSEQUENCES

Many patients in the ICU have markedly increased airway resistance owing to their underlying diseases and their intubated condition. The introduction of the bronchoscope into the airway further raises airway resistance, leading to higher airway pressures during volume ventilation. This situation may cause significant air leakage at the site of the adapter or through the bronchoscope suction channel. Very high airway pressures may surpass the pressure limits set for the ventilator, causing the ventilator pop-off valve to trigger, significantly decreasing minute ventilation. This event potentially leads to significant alveolar hypoventilation and eventually to hypoxemia.

Increased airway resistance as a result of a bronchoscope in the intubated airway also increases positive end-expiratory pressures (PEEP). In fact auto-PEEP up to 35 cm H_2O has been recorded with an adult bronchoscope in a 7.0-mm endotracheal tube.[7] However, PEEP usually remains below 20 cm H_2O in endotracheal tubes with an 8.0-mm internal diameter.[7] For this reason, Grossman and Jacobi[8] recommend using an endotracheal tube with an internal diameter of at least 8.5 mm for an adult bronchoscope with a diameter of 5.7 mm. In some circumstances, however, tubes with a diameter of 8.0 mm or even 7.5 mm may be adequate.[7, 9] When a 7.5-mm or narrower tube is in place, a pediatric bronchoscope may be used, although the suctioning of airway secretions through the pediatric bronchoscope is often quite difficult.

The presence of a bronchoscope in the airway usually leads to small increases in P_{CO_2} and decreases in P_{O_2},[7, 9] probably because a smaller tidal volume is delivered while the bronchoscope is in place.[10] Aggressive suctioning may drastically reduce the alveolar minute ventilation, leading to significant alterations in gas exchange. There are reports documenting increases in P_{CO_2} of as much as 30% and decreases in P_{O_2} of 40%.[7] Although these changes usually reverse rapidly in most patients, they may take hours to resolve in very ill patients with marked physiologic shunting.[7] For this reason, only brief periods of suctioning are generally recommended.

As a result of concerns regarding unreliable gas delivery or excessive alveolar pressure, MacIntyre and associates[11] evaluated fiberoptic bronchoscopy by means of jet ventilation. They found that the jet technique, with a 9-mm endotracheal tube, provided alveolar ventilation and airway pressures comparable to those obtained with volume-controlled ventilation prior to bronchoscopy. Fortunately, we have found that jet ventilation is rarely necessary.

Few studies have evaluated the hemodynamic consequences of fiberoptic bronchoscopy in the critically ill, but there often appears to be a significant increase in cardiac output.[7] Tachycardia is common and bradycardia occasionally occurs in the seriously ill. These changes are usually reversed within minutes after completion of the procedure.

MONITORING

The respiratory and hemodynamic consequences of fiberoptic bronchoscopy in the critically ill as well as the routine use of systemic sedation necessitate close monitoring during the procedure (Table 124-1). It is important to monitor vital signs, oxygen saturation with continuous pulse oximetry, and electrocardiographic rhythm. To help avoid difficulty with hypoxemia or hypoventilation, patients are routinely started on either volume-controlled or pressure-controlled ventilation with a fraction of inspired oxygen value (FIO_2) of 1.0 a few minutes before the procedure. In addition, some operators also increase the minute ventilation provided by the ventilator by raising the set ventilator rate and by raising the inspiratory pressure level if pressure-controlled ventilation is being used.

INDICATIONS

Airway Management

Flexible fiberoptic bronchoscopy is very useful for difficult intubations when the patient is breathing spontaneously and

TABLE 124–1. Guidelines for Fiberoptic Bronchoscopy in Mechanically Ventilated Patients

1. Use an endotracheal tube with an internal diameter of at least 8.0 mm unless a pediatric fiberoptic bronchoscope is available.
2. Increase fractional inspired oxygen (FIO_2) to 1.0 approximately 15 minutes before procedure.
3. Consider increasing tidal volume or inspiratory pressure by 20% to 30% immediately before procedure.
4. Monitor pulse, blood pressure, and respirations during procedure.
5. Monitor oxygen saturation with pulse oximeter throughout procedure.
6. Monitor electrocardiographic rhythm throughout procedure.
7. Monitor tidal volume and airway pressures throughout procedure.
8. Suction for only short periods.
9. Consider postprocedure chest radiograph if transbronchial biopsy specimens were obtained.

is stable enough to allow up to 5 minutes for the procedure. Intubation by flexible bronchoscope is contraindicated in patients with apnea or near apnea, because it is very difficult or impossible to ventilate apneic patients while one is passing the bronchoscope.[12]

Bronchoscopy may be used to assist either nasotracheal or orotracheal intubations. The nasotracheal route is generally easier, because (1) it requires less patient cooperation and (2) the angle of insertion into the larynx is less acute.[12] An 8.0-mm endotracheal tube can be inserted nasotracheally in most adults without difficulty, although some smaller patients may require a 7.0-mm tube. Technically, the procedure is easier if performed as follows:

1. The endotracheal tube is inserted transnasally into the nasopharynx initially (Fig. 124–1).
2. The bronchoscope is then passed through the endotracheal tube and beyond the vocal cords.
3. Once the bronchoscope is in place, the endotracheal tube is passed over the bronchoscope, and the bronchoscope is withdrawn.

Orotracheal intubation with a bronchoscope is more difficult; however, the advantages of the larger endotracheal tube, which can be placed orotracheally, often outweigh the disadvantages of its more difficult placement. Placement of an oral endotracheal tube often requires placement of a bite block first. There is no advantage to placement of the endotracheal tube into the oropharynx prior to insertion of the bronchoscope as in nasotracheal intubation. The endotracheal tube is loaded onto the bronchoscope prior to insertion into the oropharynx and then inserted over the bronchoscope after the bronchoscope has been passed through the oropharynx into the mid-trachea (Fig. 124–2).

Fiberoptic bronchoscopy has its greatest role in ICU airway management during the placement of a dual-lumen endotracheal tube.[12-14] The procedure is performed as follows:

1. The dual-lumen tube is inserted into the trachea under direct laryngoscopic guidance.
2. The cuff is inflated, and mechanical ventilation is initiated or resumed.
3. A pediatric bronchoscope is passed into the endobronchial lumen of the dual-lumen tube and is passed into either the right or left mainstem bronchus. Usually the left mainstem bronchus is used, because it is more difficult to obtain an adequate endobronchial cuff seal on the right owing to the short distance before the takeoff of the right upper lobe.
4. After the bronchoscope is inserted into the mainstem bronchus, the endobronchial tube is advanced into position using the bronchoscope as an obturator (Fig. 124–3).
5. The bronchoscope is withdrawn and then is passed into the tracheal lumen so that the endobronchial tube can be visualized to ensure that the endobronchial cuff is properly inflated.

Although the bronchoscope is helpful in airway management, its use is rarely necessary. In one series of bronchoscopies performed in the ICU, intubation represented only 0.5% of all indications for bronchoscopy.[5] In another series reported by Jolliet and Chevrolet,[6] ICU staff used bronchoscopy in only 12 of 17,000 consecutive intubations, of which eight were

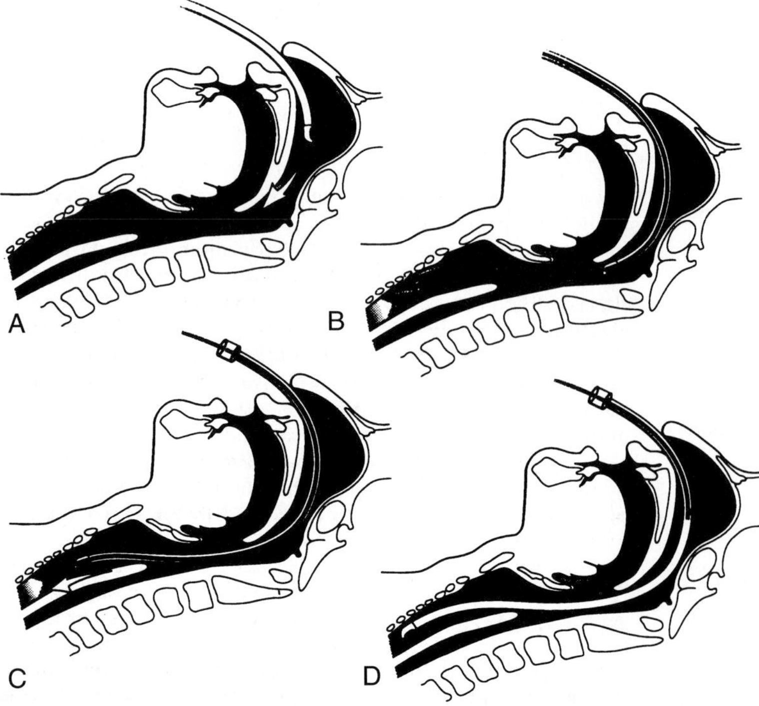

Figure 124–1. Nasotracheal intubation with the fiberoptic bronchoscope. *A,* An endotracheal tube is inserted transnasally into the posterior nasopharynx. *B,* The bronchoscope is then inserted through the endotracheal tube and passed through the vocal cords and into the midtracheal position. *C,* The endotracheal tube is then advanced, with the bronchoscope used as an obturator, into the midtracheal position. *D,* The bronchoscope is withdrawn. (Adapted from Dellinger RP: Fiberoptic bronchoscopy in adult airway management. Crit Care Med 1990; 18:883.)

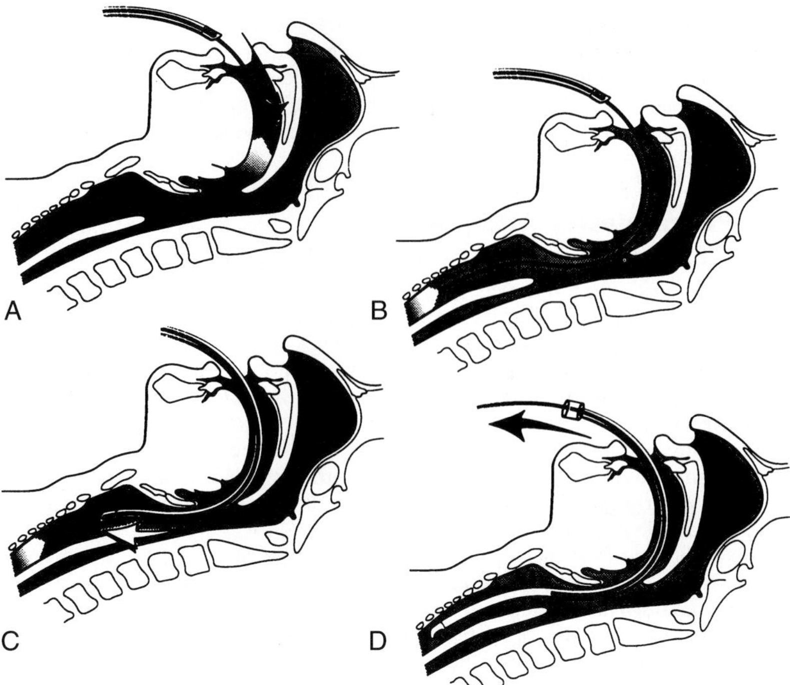

Figure 124–2. Orotracheal intubation with the fiberoptic bronchoscope. *A,* The endotracheal tube is inserted over the bronchoscope and is pushed to its proximal end. The bronchoscope is inserted orally. *B,* The bronchoscope is passed through the vocal cords into the midtracheal position. *C,* The endotracheal tube is then advanced using the bronchoscope as an obturator, into the midtracheal position. *D,* The bronchoscope is withdrawn. (Adapted from Dellinger RP: Fiberoptic bronchoscopy in adult airway management. Crit Care Med 1990; 18:883.)

performed electively and four were performed emergently. Although the elective intubations generally went smoothly, emergency intubations resulted in longer times to intubation as well as in failure to obtain an adequate airway in some instances. These researchers concluded that if a difficult intubation is anticipated, it is preferable to use the bronchoscope from the outset rather than after several unsuccessful attempts at intubation with direct laryngoscopy.

Another indication for fiberoptic bronchoscopy in airway management is for guiding the placement of percutaneous tracheostomy tubes.[15] Bronchoscopy facilitates localization of an appropriate tracheostomy site as well as verifies adequate placement of the obturators and tracheostomy tube.

Finally, patients undergoing high-frequency jet ventilation are at higher risk for necrotizing tracheitis. Repeated fiberoptic bronchoscopy may be very useful in assessment of tracheal complications in this setting; however, the extremely critical condition of many of these patients often precludes use of the procedure.[16, 17]

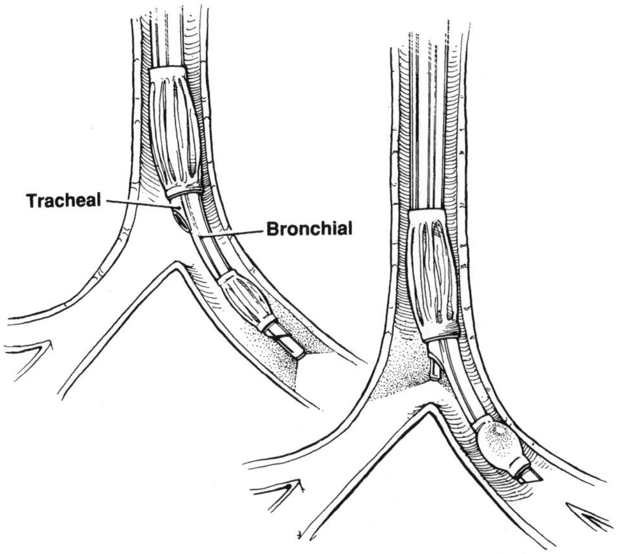

Trauma

Both blunt trauma and penetrating trauma to the chest and neck may cause injuries to the tracheobronchial tree. Except for penetrating cervical neck injuries, these injuries may be difficult to detect unless care providers maintain a high index of suspicion for them. Clinical manifestations, such as subcutaneous or mediastinal emphysema, multiple rib or clavicle injuries, and extensive chest injury with hemothorax, raise the suspicion of tracheobronchial disruption.[3] Unfortunately, symptoms such as dyspnea, cough, stridor, and hemoptysis are not always present or go unnoticed in a patient who has other, more prominent injuries or who has undergone intubation at the scene or upon arrival at the emergency department.

Fiberoptic bronchoscopy is also useful in evaluation of patients with significant risk of upper airway trauma.[18, 19] Although there is little prospective information describing the operating characteristics of bronchoscopy in traumatic upper airway injury, a retrospective series reported by Hara and Prakash[19] showed fiberoptic bronchoscopy to be of diagnostic use in 28 of 53 trauma patients. Injuries found with bronchoscopy include complete tracheal and bronchial transections and lacerations, ongoing distal hemorrhage, aspirated material, and mucous plugging. As a result of the retrospective nature

Tracheal

Bronchial

Figure 124–3. Fiberoptic-assisted insertion of a double-lumen endobronchial tube. After insertion of the double-lumen tube into the trachea via direct laryngoscopy, the bronchoscope is passed through the bronchial lumen and into the mainstem bronchus to be used as an obturator for proper placement of the endobronchial lumen (*left*). The bronchoscope is then withdrawn and passed into the tracheal lumen to assure proper positioning of the tracheal lumen and bronchial cuff (*right*). (Adapted from Dellinger RP: Fiberoptic bronchoscopy in adult airway management. Crit Care Med 1990; 18:884.)

of this series and the wide spectrum of injuries found, these researchers did not describe specific criteria for performing bronchoscopy in the evaluation of trauma patients. Rather, they suggested that the decision to perform bronchoscopy must be based on the clinical judgment of the evaluating physician.

Smoke Inhalation and Burns

In patients with burns, injury to the tracheobronchial tree initially occurs when inhaled toxins or heat contacts the upper airway mucosa.[3] Larger particles and heat generally damage the pharynx and larynx, causing edema and obstruction in the supraglottic area. Finer particles and inhaled gases often affect the more distal tracheobronchial tree or lung parenchyma, causing distal airway edema and distal obstruction or acute respiratory distress syndrome (ARDS). The upper airway inflammatory response often occurs over hours, whereas lower airway injuries progress over days, leading to delayed complications.

In patients with extensive burns or significant facial burns, emergent bronchoscopy is often necessary to evaluate for supraglottic burns and edema. In this setting, an endotracheal tube is loaded over the bronchoscope so that the tube can be inserted immediately if the fiberoptic examination reveals severe edema with significant airway obstruction. After assessing and stabilizing the upper airway, one should examine the remainder of the distal airway for signs of serious inhalation injury, such as mucosal edema, ulceration, or soot deposition in the distal airway. Although some experts advocate obtaining biopsy or brush cytology specimens from the distal airways of these patients to identify severe inhalation injury,[20, 21] others have found simple visual examination by an experienced bronchoscopist to be relatively sensitive (0.79) and highly specific (0.94) in comparison with bronchial biopsy.[22] All agree, however, that significant inhalational injury strongly predicts development of subsequent ARDS.

Hemoptysis

Patients with massive hemoptysis (variously defined as 200 to 1000 mL of expectorated blood within 24 hours) are generally considered to have an emergency. Unfortunately, few prospective trials exist to guide the management of patients with massive hemoptysis. Historically, massive hemoptysis required rigid bronchoscopy for localization and control.[23] Control of the hemoptysis was obtained by passing a Fogarty catheter through the rigid bronchoscope into the bleeding airway, then inflating it to prevent the spilling of blood into other bronchi. Once the bleeding was controlled, definitive surgical therapy with a lobectomy or pneumonectomy was performed. Occasionally, radiation therapy or laser ablation has been used to control bleeding from tumors. Some workers still strongly advocate rigid bronchoscopy for most cases of massive hemoptysis.

Unfortunately, some patients with massive hemoptysis require intubation before rigid bronchoscopy can be performed, making rigid bronchoscopy more difficult. In this setting, fiberoptic bronchoscopy may be useful in identifying the side of bleeding and can facilitate the insertion of Fogarty catheters into the bleeding lung segments to obtain emergent control of bleeding[24]; we have found, however, that this process is sometimes difficult. Once immediate control of bleeding is obtained with the fiberoptic bronchoscope, definitive treatment requires either surgery or selective bronchial artery embolization.

When it is impossible to locate the site or even the side of active bleeding, one may use the fiberoptic bronchoscope to place a dual-lumen endotracheal tube to isolate the lungs. In the case of an identified side of uncontrolled bleeding, the fiberoptic bronchoscope can guide the selective mainstem intubation of the nonbleeding lung. For stable patients with non-massive hemoptysis, fiberoptic bronchoscopy is the preferred procedure to identify the source of bleeding or at least to localize the bleeding segment so that definitive therapy can be performed.[4]

Atelectasis or Lobar Collapse

In two large series evaluating 147[5] and 198[25] ICU fiberoptic bronchoscopy procedures, the most common indication for bronchoscopy was atelectasis or lobar collapse. In one series, bronchoscopy with bronchial toilet led to full reexpansion in 20 of 28 procedures performed for atelectasis or collapse, partial reexpansion in five, and no change in three.[25] In the other series of 90 procedures, bronchoscopy removed substantial mucous plugs or nonoccluding secretions in 37 patients; only 17 of the 90 patients showed improvement in oxygenation or chest x-ray findings, however.[5]

Another small, prospective trial, published in 1979, randomly assigned 31 patients with acute lobar collapse into two groups; one received immediate bronchoscopy and standard respiratory therapy, including aggressive chest physiotherapy, and the second group received standard respiratory therapy only.[26] Although the study was underpowered, there was no statistical difference in the resolution rates of the lobar collapse between the two groups at 24 or 48 hours. Unfortunately, this study did not evaluate differences in oxygenation between the two groups.

Bronchoscopy may be more likely to relieve atelectasis in the subgroup of patients with neuromuscular disease who develop proximal atelectasis, mostly as a result of ineffective coughing. In an uncontrolled series, bronchoscopy led to improvement in atelectasis in at least 80% of the patients studied.[27] In another series, Tsao and coworkers[28] described how to insufflate air through the bronchoscope channel to reinflate a collapsed lung. With this technique, rapid and complete reexpansion occurred in 12 of their 14 patients, although these researchers did not mention whether reexpansion was maintained over the long term.

Fortunately, morbidity from bronchoscopy for atelectasis is unusual. Therefore, even though prospective data on its efficacy are lacking, we use bronchoscopy in patients with lobar collapse that has not responded to vigorous respiratory therapy and in patients with instability judged to be due to lobar or near whole lung collapse.

Foreign Body Extraction

Both flexible and rigid bronchoscopy are useful for the removal of aspirated foreign bodies. Traditionally, rigid bronchoscopy has been the preferred treatment for removing aspirated foreign objects from adults. Since the late 1970s, however, a number of reports have suggested that the flexible bronchoscope is also a valuable therapeutic option.[29–31] In the largest published series of 60 consecutive patients, 57 were managed successfully with either flexible or rigid bronchoscopy.[31] Flexible bronchoscopy succeeded in 14 of 23 patients, whereas rigid bronchoscopy succeeded in 43 of 44 patients, including six of seven patients in whom flexible bronchoscopy had failed.

Bronchopleural Fistula

Persistent bronchopleural fistula remains one of the most complex challenges for chest physicians. Most cases are characterized by a chronic air leak following a surgical procedure and result from chronic infection. The usual conservative treatment consists of management with tube thoracostomy, antimicrobial agents, and, when necessary, ventilator support emphasizing low airway pressures. If these conservative measures fail to close the fistula in 1 to 3 weeks, surgical intervention is usually required.

For patients unable to tolerate a major thoracic procedure, some experts recommend bronchoscopy to close the bronchopleural fistula endoscopically. Application of silver nitrate through the rigid bronchoscope has been successful in treating stump fistulas.[32] Flexible bronchoscopy has also been used in an attempt to isolate and close smaller, more distal fistulas.[33]

During bronchoscopy, distal bronchi are sequentially occluded with a balloon catheter passed into the airway via the flexible bronchoscope. The air leak is markedly reduced when the balloon catheter occludes the correct bronchus. After the leak is localized, endobronchial occlusion is attempted. A number of modalities, including tissue glue, fibrin glue, absorbable gelatin sponge (Gelfoam), lead plugs, and a blood patch, have all been reported to occlude bronchopleural fistulas.[32] Initial closure of the bronchopleural fistula is often possible, but in our limited experience, the fistula usually reopens within hours of the procedure.

Management of Immunocompromised Patients

Treatment of immunocompromised patients in the ICU is very challenging. This diverse population include patients who (1) have undergone transplantation, (2) are receiving immunosuppressive drugs, (3) have neutropenia, (4) have lymphopenia, or (5) have an immunodeficiency syndrome. These patients are at great risk for opportunistic infections, new or recurrent malignancies, and, in those who have received lung transplants, allograft rejection and airway complications at the site of the airway anastomosis. Flexible fiberoptic bronchoscopy is a valuable tool in the diagnosis of many of the pulmonary disorders that affect these patients.[33]

Much debate remains in the published literature regarding whether immunocompromised patients with pulmonary infiltrates should undergo bronchoscopy with bronchoalveolar lavage (BAL) alone or with additional transbronchial biopsy (TBBX). Markedly different study populations in the various published series at least partially explain the wide range of diagnostic yields for BAL and TBBX. In patients infected with human immunodeficiency virus (HIV) who have *Pneumocystis carinii* pneumonia (PCP) and who have not received PCP prophylaxis, the reported sensitivity of BAL is approximately 90%, with TBBX adding little to this value.[33] Bronchoscopy may have a lower sensitivity in patients who are receiving PCP prophylaxis, especially with inhaled pentamidine.[34] In this setting, the yield of BAL may be improved if lavage is performed in the upper lobes as well as in the middle lobe or lingula.[34, 35] In addition, TBBX may increase the sensitivity for PCP in this setting,[34] although this belief remains controversial.[36]

In series of patients with acquired immunodeficiency syndrome (AIDS), a significant proportion of whom had infections other than PCP or noninfectious conditions (such as Kaposi's sarcoma), TBBX significantly increased the yield of BAL and was recommended.[37, 38] Therefore, in HIV-infected patients who are strongly thought to have PCP and who are not receiving PCP prophylaxis, BAL alone is generally sufficient to make a firm diagnosis.[33] In patients who are receiving PCP prophylaxis or who are suspected to have a condition other than PCP, however, TBBX may increase the diagnostic yield.[34, 37, 38]

In non-HIV-infected patients who are immunocompromised, the addition of TBBX appears to have a higher sensitivity for diagnosis of infection than bronchoscopy with BAL alone.[39, 40] Special consideration must also be given, however, to the risks of transbronchial biopsy in this population. Most experts consider thrombocytopenia, with platelet counts of 50,000 cells/mm^3 or less, to be a strong contraindication to TBBX.[1, 2] Fortunately, there appears to be very little risk of bleeding from BAL even in patients with hematologic malignancy whose platelet counts are below 20,000 cells/mm^3.[41] In addition, in mechanically ventilated patients, the reported risk of pneumothorax from transbronchial biopsy is 10% to 20%.[25, 42–44]

Because the significant risks of TBBX in mechanically ventilated immunocompromised patients preclude a general recommendation for its use, the risks and benefits must be weighed in each case. One exception may be in patients undergoing high-dose chemotherapy, for whom pulmonary drug toxicity is a strong consideration. Although some reports indicate that BAL demonstrates typical cytologic changes in 40% of patients with pulmonary drug toxicity, TBBX demonstrates typical changes in alveolar cells 75% of the time and is the preferred bronchoscopic procedure.[39] Still, many patients with drug toxicity require open or thoracoscopic lung biopsy for definitive diagnosis even when bronchoscopy with TBBX is performed.

Lung transplant recipients constitute a unique subset of immunocompromised patients. In this group, allograft rejection is a common problem that causes pulmonary infiltrates and, occasionally, respiratory failure. BAL alone is insufficient to confirm diagnosis of transplant rejection. Transbronchial biopsy is approximately 80% sensitive and almost 100% specific for the diagnosis of rejection.[45] Therefore, even in mechanically ventilated transplant recipients, transbronchial biopsy is often performed to confirm the diagnosis of transplant rejection.

Fiberoptic bronchoscopy also has special utility in evaluating the airways of transplant recipients for narrowing at the allograft anastomotic site. The placement of airway stents or laser revision of these anastomotic narrowings, however, generally requires rigid bronchoscopy performed in the operating room.

Nosocomial Pneumonia

Much controversy surrounds the use of fiberoptic bronchoscopy in patients in the ICU with suspected nosocomial pneumonia (see also Chapter 145). Since its description in 1979, use of the protected specimen brush (PSB) for bronchoscopic sampling has been widely studied and is strongly advocated by many as a sensitive and specific tool for the diagnosis of nosocomial pneumonia. Similarly, BAL with quantitative cultures has also been studied extensively. Nevertheless, there is much active debate as to whether antibiotic treatment based on the results of either invasive technique is superior to empirical antibiotic therapy.[46, 47]

The published sensitivity and specificity values for PSB bronchoscopy and quantitative BAL vary widely. The sensitivity of PSB is generally reported to be in the range of 60% to 90%,[48] with some reports as high as 100%[49, 50] and some as low as 38%.[51] Quantitative BAL has a reported sensitivity of 70% to 100%.[48] For both procedures, the reported specificities vary within the same range as their sensitivities.[48] These variable results are due to many factors. In all of these studies, the invasive techniques were compared with some diagnostic "standard." Unfortunately, such standards are not consistent among studies.[48] In addition, patient populations differed markedly, with some studies including only mechanically ventilated patients, others a mixture of ventilated and nonventilated patients, and still others including only postmortem patients. Furthermore, some studies included patients who were receiving antibiotic therapy, and other studies evaluated the procedures only in patients who had stopped receiving antibiotics at least 48 to 72 hours beforehand. In studies comparing specimens obtained through PSB bronchoscopy with those from quantitative BAL, the level of agreement between results of quantitative cultures was usually only 40% to 60%.[48, 50-52] This extent of conflicts among the data makes it impossible to conclude whether either technique is superior to empirical therapy.

It is important to recognize a number of drawbacks to obtaining culture specimens through quantitative PSB or BAL. First, the most sensitive threshold for a positive result, the finding of at least 10^3 colony-forming units (CFU) per high-power field, results in some false-positive diagnoses; this fact is particularly pertinent in patients in whom the clinical suspicion of pneumonia is low.

Second, all of the invasively obtained culture specimens require at least 24 and usually 48 hours to grow. During this time, empirical antibiotic therapy is usually required, and some clinicians may be reluctant to alter antibiotic therapy 48 hours after its initiation if the patient's condition has improved.

Third, invasive techniques can lead to false-negative results if specimens are obtained (1) from an unaffected segment, (2) after a new antibiotic has been started, or (3) early in the course of pneumonia, when the bacterial burden is low. When there is a high index of suspicion for pneumonia but quantitative culture results are negative, a second bronchoscopic procedure to obtain more specimens may be necessary.[53] Finally, for bacterial pneumonia, which may have significant morbidity if left untreated, even a sensitivity of 85% reflects an unacceptably high false-negative rate.

Unfortunately, no studies have shown whether mortality, morbidity, number of ventilator-free days, or other patient outcomes are improved by the use of bronchoscopy with quantitative cultures. Therefore, at this point, it is impossible to determine the utility of bronchoscopy with quantitative BAL or PSB sampling in the diagnosis of nosocomial pneumonia. Current published recommendations range from advocating (1) widespread use of invasive quantitative procedures for culture specimen collection,[46] to (2) their use only in patients who have not received antibiotics in the preceding 48 hours,[54] to (3) no use of such procedures at all.[47]

Rigid Bronchoscopy

The few indications for using the rigid bronchoscope in the ICU include (1) management of massive hemoptysis, (2) foreign body removal, and (3) laser therapy for obstructive endobronchial tumors.[3] The main advantage of rigid bronchoscopy is establishment of an excellent airway, which permits adequate ventilation while instruments are used and suctioning is performed in the proximal airway.

Unfortunately, the rigid bronchoscope has several limitations, such as:

1. The need for general anesthesia.
2. Lack of maneuverability.
3. Inability to assess more distal airways.
4. Inability to be used in mechanically ventilated patients without removal of the endotracheal tube.

Therefore, flexible fiberoptic bronchoscopy is preferred for most indications in the ICU.

COMPLICATIONS

In addition to the physiologic alterations described previously, the following potential complications may occur in mechanically ventilated patients undergoing bronchoscopy: (1) medication reactions, (2) cardiac arrhythmia, (3) bronchospasm, (4) hypoxemia, (5) bleeding, (6) pneumothorax, (7) infection, and (8) increased intracranial pressure.

Medication Reactions

Complications due to sedative premedication or administration of topical lidocaine occur occasionally; those due to oversedation are more likely in older patients with significant underlying lung disease. In ventilated patients, complications due to sedation are rare, although hemodynamic instability is possible. Interestingly, it appears that undersedation probably carries more risk than oversedation, because patient agitation raises the risk of significant hypoxemia.[55]

Cardiac Arrhythmias

Although complications due to topical anesthetics are rare, there are reports of arrhythmia precipitated by topical anesthetic agents.[2] As a result, 300 mg of topical lidocaine is recommended as the maximum dose to the airway to avoid any significant arrhythmia.[2]

Bronchospasm

In patients who are not intubated, insertion of the bronchoscope is associated with a 0.1% to 0.4% incidence of bronchospasm or laryngospasm.[1] In the ICU, the risk of bronchospasm is undoubtedly higher, given the nature of the patient population, although no good prospective studies have demonstrated such a probability. Even for asthmatic patients, who are particularly prone to bronchospasm, a number of series show bronchoscopy to be safe.[56, 57] In acutely bronchospastic patients requiring bronchoscopy, pretreatment with a beta agonist and being prepared for emergency intubation are generally advisable.

Hypoxemia

As described earlier, some degree of hypoxemia is common in patients undergoing bronchoscopy. Published series of ICU patients undergoing bronchoscopy indicate that significant hypoxemia (defined as $Po_2 < 60$ mm Hg or O_2 saturation < 90%) develops in 5% to 20% of patients at some point during the procedure, although this hypoxemia is rarely harmful.[25, 42, 55, 58, 59]

Bleeding

Pulmonary hemorrhage occurs rarely during fiberoptic bronchoscopy. In two published series of ICU patients (99 patients and 110 patients, respectively) undergoing BAL, there were no reported cases of pulmonary hemorrhage.[58, 59] For patients undergoing TBBX, the risk is somewhat higher but still low. In the largest series published to date, only one of 83 patients undergoing transbronchial biopsy had significant bleeding (>100 mL), and only three other patients experienced between 30 mL and 100 mL of bleeding.[42] In all cases, the bleeding resolved spontaneously.

Immunocompromised patients and patients with thrombocytopenia or coagulation disorders are at higher risk for bleeding complications. For this reason, the American Thoracic Society recommends that patients have platelet counts of at least 50,000/mm³ prior to undergoing transbronchial biopsy, although it appears that BAL is safe at any platelet value.[41] If bleeding develops, intrabronchial instillation of 2-mL aliquots of epinephrine (1:10,000) may promote vasoconstriction and slow the blood flow. In addition, selective intubation and repositioning of the patient so that the bleeding lung is in the dependent position may protect the nonbleeding lung.

Pneumothorax

Pneumothorax rarely occurs in patients undergoing BAL. Even in mechanically ventilated patients undergoing BAL, the incidence of pneumothorax is reportedly less than 1%.[58, 59] When TBBX is performed, however, the incidence of pneumothorax increases to 10% to 15%.[42–44] For this reason, the risks and benefits of TBBX must be weighed carefully for every mechanically ventilated patient.

Infection

Bacteremia associated with bronchoscopy is extremely rare and does not warrant prophylactic antibiotics, even in patients with underlying valvular heart disease. Although fever higher than 101°F and parenchymal infiltrates commonly occur after bronchoscopy, these findings rarely indicate pneumonia and generally resolve without antibiotic therapy.[60, 61]

Increased Intracranial Pressure

Increased intracranial pressure occurs during bronchoscopy, even in patients who are paralyzed. In two series, however, the elevated intracranial pressure had no clinical consequences, even in patients with severe head trauma or space-occupying intracranial lesions.[62, 63] This finding apparently is related to the fact that during bronchoscopy, mean arterial blood pressure also increases, so that cerebral perfusion pressure remains relatively constant.[62]

CONTRAINDICATIONS

In an appropriate ICU setting with experienced operators, fiberoptic bronchoscopy has few if any absolute contraindications. Relative contraindications include the inability to adequately oxygenate or ventilate a patient. Although many consider recent acute myocardial infarction to be a contraindication, one series has indicated that complications are rare unless active ischemia is present.[64]

Acutely bronchospastic patients require special care. With adequate sedation, these patients have few complications during bronchoscopy; however, the bronchoscopist should always be prepared for the possibility of laryngospasm or severe bronchospasm.

Finally, severe pulmonary hypertension, coagulopathy, and thrombocytopenia (platelet count < 50,000/mm³) are relative contraindications for bronchoscopy with transbronchial biopsy. BAL appears to be safe in these patients, although there may be a higher risk of epistaxis in patients who undergo bronchoscopy by the transnasal approach.[38]

SUMMARY

Flexible fiberoptic bronchoscopy is a valuable diagnostic and therapeutic tool in the ICU. It is especially valuable in selected cases for airway management and for placement of dual-lumen endotracheal tubes. Bronchoscopy also has clear utility in evaluating hemoptysis and in confirming the diagnosis of infection or rejection in immunocompromised hosts. Although bronchoscopy is also performed commonly for nosocomial or ventilator-associated pneumonia, this use remains very controversial. It is hoped that future prospective, randomized, controlled trials will definitively demonstrate whether bronchoscopy for the collection of specimens for quantitative culture should be routinely performed in these patients. Finally, although there are few contraindications to bronchoscopy in the ICU, careful preparation and close monitoring are essential for its safe execution.

References

1. Sackner MA: Bronchofiberscopy. Am Rev Respir Dis 1975; 111:62–80.
2. Silver MR, Balk RA: Bronchoscopic procedures in the intensive care unit. Crit Care Clin 1995; 11:97–109.
3. Shennib HS, Baslaim G: Bronchoscopy in the intensive care unit. Chest Surg Clin North Am 1996; 6:349–361.
4. Dellinger RP, Bandi V: Fiberoptic bronchoscopy in the intensive care unit. Crit Care Clin 1992; 8:755–772.
5. Olopade CO, Prakash UBS: Bronchoscopy in the critical-care unit. Mayo Clin Proc 1989; 64:1255–1263.
6. Jolliet P, Chevrolet JC: Bronchoscopy in the intensive care unit. Intensive Care Med 1992; 18:160–169.
7. Lindholm C, Ollmann B, Snyder J, et al: Cardiorespiratory effects of flexible fiberoptic bronchoscopy in critically ill patients. Chest 1978; 74:362–367.
8. Grossman E, Jacobi AM: Minimal optimal endotracheal tube size for fiberoptic bronchoscopy. Anesth Analg 1974; 53:475–480.
9. Matsushima Y, Jones R, King E, et al: Alterations in pulmonary mechanics and gas exchange during routine fiberoptic bronchoscopy. Chest 1984; 86:184–188.
10. Lindholm C, Ollman B, Snyder J, et al: Flexible fiberoptic bronchoscopy in critical care medicine: Diagnosis, therapy and complications. Crit Care Med 1974; 2:250–261.
11. MacIntyre NR, Ramage JE, Follet JV: Jet ventilation in support of fiberoptic bronchoscopy. Crit Care Med 1987; 15:303–307.
12. Dellinger RP: Fiberoptic bronchoscopy in adult airway management. Crit Care Med 1990; 18:882–887.
13. Ovassapian A: Fiberoptic bronchoscope and double-lumen tracheal tubes (Letter). Anesthesiology 1983; 38:1104.
14. Hurford WE, Alfille PH: A quality improvement study of the placement and complication of double-lumen endobronchial tubes. J Cardiothorac Vasc Anesth 1993; 7:517–520.
15. Marelli D, Paul A, Manolidis S, et al: Endoscopic guided percutaneous tracheostomy: Early results of a consecutive trial. J Trauma 990; 30:433–435.
16. Kirpalani H, Higa T, Perlman M, et al: Diagnosis and therapy of necrotizing tracheobronchitis in ventilated neonates. Crit Care Med 1985; 13:792–797.
17. Tolkin J, Kirpalani H, Fitzhardinge P, et al: Necrotizing tracheobronchitis: A new complication of neonatal mechanical ventilation (Abstract). Pediatr Res 1984; 18:391.
18. Grfewal H, Rao PM, Mukerji S, et al: Management of penetrating laryngotracheal injuries. Head Neck 1995; 17:494–502.
19. Hara KS, Prakash UBS: Fiberoptic bronchoscopy in the evaluation of acute chest and upper airway trauma. Chest 1989 96:627–630.
20. Mesanes MJ, Legendre C, Lioret N: Using bronchoscopy and biopsy to diagnose early inhalation injury: Macroscopic and histologic findings. Chest 1995; 107:1365–1369.
21. Khoo AK, Lee ST, Poh WT: Tracheobronchial cytology in inhalation injury. J Trauma 1997; 42:81–85.
22. Mesanes, MJ, Legendre C, Lioret, N, et al: Fiberoptic bronchoscopy for the early diagnosis of subglottal inhalation injury: Comparative value in the assessment of prognosis. J Trauma 1994; 36:59–67.
23. Cahill BC, Ingbart DH: Massive hemoptysis: Assessment and management. Clin Chest Med 1994; 15:147–167.
24. Saw EC, Gottlieb LS, Yokoyama T, et al: Flexible fiberoptic bronchoscopy and endobronchial tamponade in the management of massive hemoptysis. Chest 1976; 70:589–591.
25. Turner JS, Willcox PA, Hayhurst FCP, et al: Fiberoptic bronchoscopy in the intensive care unit—a prospective study of 147 procedures in 107 patients. Crit Care Med 1994; 22:259–264.
26. Marini JJ, Pierson DJ, Hudson LD: Acute lobar atelectasis: A pro-

spective comparison of fiberoptic bronchoscopy and respiratory therapy. Am Rev Respir Dis 1979; 119:971-977.
27. Schmidt-Nowara WW, Altman AR: Atelectasis and neuromuscular failure. Chest 1984; 85:792-795.
28. Tsao TCY, Tsai YH, Lan RS, et al: Treatment for collapsed lung in critically ill patients: Selective intrabronchial air insufflation using the fiberoptic bronchoscope. Chest 1990; 978:435-438.
29. Zavala DC, Rhodes ML: Experimental removal of foreign bodies by fiberoptic bronchoscopy. Am Rev Respir Dis 1974; 110:357-360.
30. Lillington G, Ruhl RA, Pierce TH, et al: Removal of endobronchial foreign body by fiberoptic bronchoscopy. Am Rev Respir Dis 1976; 113:387-391.
31. Limper AH, Prakash UBS: Tracheobronchial foreign bodies in adults. Ann Intern Med 1990; 112:604-609.
32. McManigle JE, Fletcher GL, Tenholder M: Bronchoscopy in the management of bronchopleural fistula. Chest 1990; 97:135-138.
33. Kvale PA: Bronchoscopic biopsies and bronchoalveolar lavage. Chest Surg Clin N Am 1995; 6:205-221.
34. Jules-Elysee KM, Stover DE, Zaman MB, et al: Aerosolized pentamidine: Effect on diagnosis and presentation of *Pneumocystis carinii* pneumonia. Ann Intern Med 1990; 112:750-757.
35. Baughman RP, Dohn MN, Shipley R, et al: Increased *Pneumocystis carinii* recovery from the upper lobes in *Pneumocystis* pneumonia: The effect of aerosol pentamidine prophylaxis. Chest 1993; 103:426-432.
36. Baughman RP, Dohn MN, Frame PT: The continuing utility of bronchoalveolar lavage to diagnose opportunistic infection in AIDS patients. Am J Med 1994; 97:515-522.
37. Salzman SH, Smith RL, Aranda CP: Histoplasmosis in patients at risk for acquired immunodeficiency syndrome in a non-endemic setting. Chest 1988; 93:916-921.
38. Salzman SH, Schindel ML, Aranda CP, et al: The role of bronchoscopy in the diagnosis of pulmonary tuberculosis in patients at risk for HIV infection. Chest 1992; 102:143-146.
39. Stover DE, Zaman MB, Hajdu SI, et al: Bronchoalveolar lavage in the diagnosis of diffuse pulmonary infiltrates in the immunosuppressed host. Ann Intern Med 1984; 101:1-7.
40. Cazzadori A, DiPerri G, Todeschini G: Transbronchial biopsy in the diagnosis of pulmonary infiltrates in immunocompromised patients. Chest 1995; 107:101-106.
41. Weiss SM, Hert RC, Gianola FJ: Complications of fiberoptic bronchoscopy in thrombocytopenic patients. Chest 1993; 104:1025-1028.
42. O'Brien JD, Ettinger NA, Shelvin D, et al: Safety and yield of transbronchial biopsy in mechanically ventilated patients. Crit Care Med 1997; 25:440-446.
43. Pincus PS, Kallenbach JM, Hurwitz MD, et al: Transbronchial biopsy during mechanical ventilation. Crit Care Med 1987; 15:1136-1139.
44. Papin TA, Grum CM, Weg JG: Transbronchial biopsy during mechanical ventilation. Chest 1986; 89:168-170.
45. Higgenbottam T, Stewart S, Penketh A: The diagnosis of lung rejection and opportunistic infection by transbronchial lung biopsy. Transplant Proc 1987; 19:3777-3778.
46. Chastre J, Fagon JY: Invasive diagnostic testing should be routinely used to manage ventilated patients with suspected pneumonia. Am J Respir Crit Care Med 1994; 150:570-574.
47. Niedermann MS, Torres A, Sumner W: Invasive diagnostic testing is not needed routinely to manage suspected ventilator-associated pneumonia. Am J Respir Crit Care Med 1994; 150:565-569.
48. Meduri GU: Diagnosis and differential diagnosis of ventilator-associated pneumonia. Clin Chest Med 1995; 16:61-93.
49. Fagon JY, Chastre J, Hance AJ, et al: Detection of nosocomial lung infection in ventilated patients: Use of a protected specimen brush and quantitative culture techniques in 147 patients. Am Rev Respir Dis 1988; 138:110-116.
50. Chastre J, Fagon JY, Soler P, et al: Diagnosis of nosocomial bacterial pneumonia in intubated patients undergoing ventilation: Comparison of the usefulness of the bronchoalveolar lavage and the protected specimen brush. Am J Med 1988; 85:499-506.
51. Torres A, Martos A, Puig de la Bellacasa J, et al: Specificity of endotracheal aspiration, protected specimen brush and bronchoalveolar lavage in mechanically ventilated patients. Am Rev Respir Dis 1993; 147:952-957.
52. Meduri GU, Beals DH, Maijub AG, et al: Protected bronchoalveolar lavage: A new bronchoscopic technique to retrieve uncontaminated distal airway secretions. Am Rev Respir Dis 1991; 143:855-864.
53. Chastre J, Trouillet JL, Fagon JY: Diagnosis of pulmonary infections in mechanically ventilated patients. Semin Respir Infect 1996; 11:65-76.
54. Allen RM, Dunn WF, Limper AH: Diagnosing ventilator-associated pneumonia: The role of bronchoscopy. Mayo Clin Proc 1994; 69:962-968.
55. Trouillet JL, Guiguet M, Gilbert C, et al: Fiberoptic bronchoscopy in ventilated patients: Evaluation of cardiopulmonary risk under midazolam sedation. Chest 1990; 97:927-933.
56. Djukanovic R, Wilson W, Lai CK, et al: The safety aspects of fiberoptic bronchoscopy, bronchoalveolar lavage and endobronchial biopsy in asthma. Am Rev Respir Dis 1991; 143:772-777.
57. Humbert M, Robinson DS, Assoufi B, et al: Safety of fiberoptic bronchoscopy in asthmatic and control subjects and the effect on asthma control over two weeks. Thorax 1996; 51:664-669.
58. Steinberg KP, Mitchell DR, Maunder RJ, et al: Safety of bronchoalveolar lavage in patients with adult respiratory distress syndrome. Am Rev Respir Dis 1993; 148:556-561.
59. Hertz MI, Woodward ME, Gross CR, et al: Safety of bronchoalveolar lavage in the critically ill, mechanically ventilated patient. Crit Care Med 1991; 19:1526-1532.
60. Pereira W, Kovnat DM, Khan MA, et al: Fever and pneumonia after flexible fiberoptic bronchoscopy. Am Rev Respir Dis 1975; 112:59-64.
61. Standiford TJ, Kunkel SL, Streiter RM: Elevated serum levels of tumor necrosis factor after bronchoscopy and bronchoalveolar lavage. Chest 1991; 99:1529-1530.
62. Peerless JR, Snow N, Likavic MJ, et al: The effect of fiberoptic bronchoscopy on cerebral hemodynamics in patients with severe head injury. Chest 1995; 108;962-965.
63. Bajwa MK, Henein S, Kamholz SL: Fiberoptic bronchoscopy in the presence of space-occupying intracranial lesions. Chest 1993; 104:101-103.
64. Dweik RA, Mehta AC, Meeker DR, et al: Analysis of the safety of bronchoscopy after recent acute myocardial infarction. Chest 1996; 110:825-838.

PART 2

Specific Pulmonary Problems

A. ACUTE HYPOXEMIC RESPIRATORY FAILURE

125

Pathology of Acute Lung Injury

Jacqueline J. Coalson, PhD

BACKGROUND

During the late 1960s and early 1970s, the clinical syndrome of *adult respiratory distress syndrome* (ARDS) emerged. The influx of new treatment modalities had reduced the acute mortality of cardiovascular and renal failure in the intensive care setting, allowing the lung to emerge as the predominant failing organ after trauma or shock. Although Winternitz[1] had introduced the concept of diffuse alveolar damage in 1920 from studies of dogs treated with war gases, it was Liebow and colleagues,[2] especially Katzenstein and coauthors,[3] who popularized the term and noted its association with adult respiratory distress syndrome and other conditions. Before and during the years of the Vietnam War, many surgical investigators studied hemorrhagic and septic shock and described the pathologic finding of congestive atelectasis or shock lung,[4, 5] an entity that can be seen in *diffuse alveolar damage* (DAD).[6] Previous pathologists had described similar lung findings in autopsies of patients who had died of shock.[7, 8]

Following injury, repair in the lung is comparable to repair in any other organ system. It involves two distinct processes: regeneration and replacement by connective tissue. The most common regenerative response in the lung occurs when its stable epithelial cell population regenerates following mild injury and the basement membrane and underlying stroma of the lung remain intact. In this circumstance, restitution of normal structure with no trace of previous injury is expected. The most classic example of the lung's capacity to respond in this manner is lobar pneumococcal pneumonia. More commonly, however, the lung's response to injury elicits both regeneration and replacement by connective tissue.[9] A good example is DAD, a pathologic process seen in patients with *acute lung injury* (ALI) and ARDS.

DEFINITIONS

DAD is best defined as a sequential series of consistent, although nonspecific, pathologic changes in the lung that result from any of a range of injurious factors that damage endothelial cells or alveolar epithelium. Pulmonary pathologists now consider this entity to be a part of an *acute lung injury pattern* that also includes *bronchiolitis obliterans-organizing pneumonia* (BOOP) and *acute interstitial pneumonia* (AIP).[10] Each is a unique clinicopathologic condition, but they all share two microscopic features:

1. Temporal uniformity (lesions are the same age; injury and response occurred at one point in time).
2. Fibroblast proliferation.

DAD follows a *known* catastrophic event that can result in ARDS. AIP is seen in patients with an explosive onset of respiratory failure *without* a history of an initiating catastrophic event; that is, it is idiopathic and has histologic features identical to those seen in the proliferative phase of DAD (see later). The best historical example of this entity may be the original patient group described by Hamman and Rich.[11]

BOOP is an *intraluminal* reparative lesion that shows immature plugs of fibroblastic tissue within terminal and respiratory bronchioles, alveolar ducts, and alveolar airspaces. *Primary* causes of BOOP are infection, toxic inhalants, collagen vascular diseases, graft-versus-host disease, heart-lung transplantation, and an idiopathic presentation. *Secondary* BOOP occurs (1) adjacent to another pathologic process (e.g., infarct, granuloma, neoplasm, or abscess) or (2) as a component of another primary pulmonary disorder (e.g., chronic eosinophilic pneumonia or Wegener's granulomatosis).

Although the usual lung finding in patients with ARDS is diffuse alveolar damage, the lung response in some patients with ARDS may also have a BOOP component.

ETIOLOGY

One has only to read the manuscript that Weston, Liebow, and colleagues[2] published in 1972 describing DAD to appreciate the multiple etiologic factors of the disorder:

- Inhalation of chlorine, perchloroethylene, and hot mercury vapor
- Paraquat and kerosene ingestion
- Vehicular trauma and fat embolism
- Smoke and burn injury, among others

More typically in this era, the clinical syndrome of acute respiratory failure results from sepsis syndrome, pulmonary aspiration, disseminated vascular coagulation (DIC), severe pneumonia, bacteremia, long bone or pelvic fractures, and hypertransfusions (Table 125–1).

The components of the general inflammatory mechanism that lead to DAD are as follows[12]:

1. The initiating agent (e.g., endotoxin, aspiration).
2. Activation of inflammatory cascades (e.g., cytokine networks, coagulation-fibrinolysis).
3. Lung sequestration of neutrophils (up-regulation of cell surface adhesion molecules).
4. Release of neutrophilic cytotoxic products (e.g., proteases, oxygen metabolites).
5. Alveolar wall injury (e.g., endothelial and epithelial damage).

PATHOLOGY

Pathologic Phases

Three distinct phases of injury and repair in an overlapping continuum of injury are seen in patients with ARDS:

1. Acute exudative phase.
2. Proliferative phase.
3. Chronic fibrotic phase.

The sequence in which these occur in patients was documented in a number of clinicopathologic studies relating length of illness and duration of therapy to oxygen exposure,[13-18] burns,[19, 20] paraquat,[21] and others. An early report in 1974 by Nash and colleagues[19] described the sequence of pathologic findings that occurred in lungs of patients who

TABLE 125–1. Disorders Associated with Diffuse Alveolar Damage

1. Shock of any cause
2. Infections
   a. Sepsis of any type
   b. Pneumonia of any type
3. Trauma
   a. Crush, blast injury
   b. Major bone fractures
   c. Head trauma
   d. Lung contusions
   e. Fat emboli
4. Aspiration
   a. Gastric contents
   b. Hydrocarbon fluids
   c. Near-drowning (fresh and salt water)
5. Drugs
   a. Narcotic drugs
   b. Chemotherapy agents
6. Inhalational injuries
   a. Toxic chemicals (chlorine, ammonia, nitrogen dioxide)
   b. Oxygen
   c. Smoke
7. Hematotopical disorders
   a. Massive blood transfusions
   b. Disseminated intravascular coagulopathy
8. Metabolic conditions
   a. Pancreatitis
   b. Severe uremia
9. Radiation

had been treated with oxygen and ventilatory support. In 1976, Katzenstein and associates[3] popularized the term diffuse alveolar damage; 6 years later, Katzenstein and Askin[10] separated DAD histopathologically into exudative and proliferative stages.

In 1979, Pratt and associates,[18] however, reported on the pathologic findings of 59 patients with acute respiratory failure and described three patterns of lung injury that varied with the duration of respiratory failure.

1. Alveolar and septal edema and hyaline membranes were present in the first week, comparable to the *exudative* stage described by Katzenstein and Askin.[10]
2. Cell infiltration and proliferation of alveolar epithelium and fibroblasts were pathologic features evident between 7 and 10 days, comparable to the *proliferative* stage described by Katzenstein and Askin.
3. Fibrosis was seen after 2 weeks; this pattern has been called the *fibrotic* phase of DAD by Tomashefski[24] and others.[22, 23]

For completeness, a fourth phase of DAD should also be recognized—that of *resolved* DAD, but its pathologic features have not been delineated.[17, 25, 26] That the lung can undergo restitution to its normal or near-normal structure likely occurs to some degree in some patients who survive an episode of ARDS and 6 months later have normal or near-normal pulmonary function test values.[27]

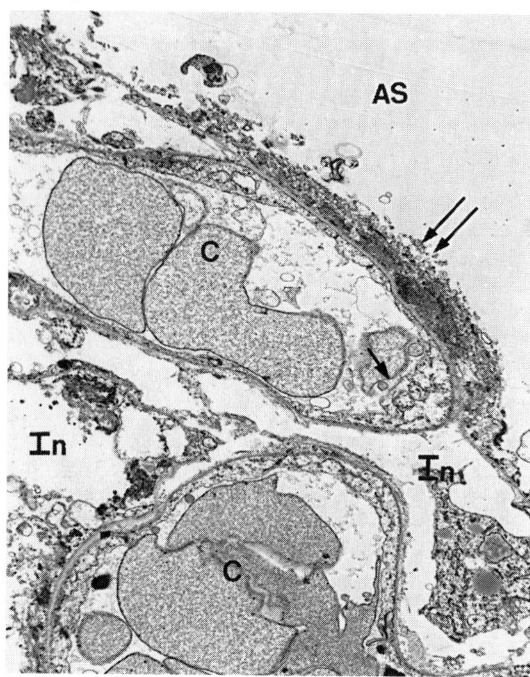

Figure 125–2. Human lung. Red blood cell ghosts and cellular remnants are in the capillary lumen (C), and the endothelium is focally edematous (*single arrow*). The degenerated type 1 epithelium is co-mingled with fibrin and proteinaceous exudate, forming a hyaline membrane (*double arrows*). The interstitium is edematous (In). AS = alveolar space. (Uranyl acetate and lead citrate, ×6800.)

Gross Pathology

Gross pathologic findings in DAD include dark, heavy, airless lungs that fill the thoracic cavities. The lungs usually weigh 2000 g or more (normal = ~800 g), and in early DAD are beefy in color, are rubbery, and ooze fluid on being cut. The lower lobes are more severely involved than the upper lobes, and the dependent portions of the lungs are more affected. Over time, the lungs become gray; they remain consolidated but show some areas of small cystic airspaces. If the lung lesions do not resolve, the cystic spaces become larger and alternate with large bands of fibrosis (adult pattern of *bronchopulmonary dysplasia* [BPD]).[28] Superimposed lesions of bronchopneumonia, abscesses, and air leak may be evident. The DAD response is believed to be a diffuse lesion throughout the lung, although considerable regional heterogeneity may be evident in some cases.[29]

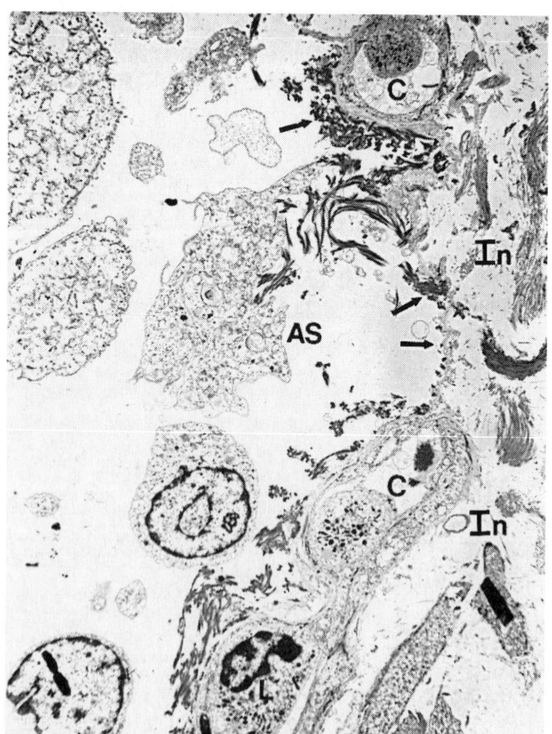

Figure 125–1. Human lung. The epithelial alveolar lining is absent; multiple fibrin strands are attached to the exposed basement membrane (arrows). The capillaries (C) contain leukocytes (L), and the endothelium is vacuolated. The interstitium (In) is widened and contains cellular fragments and connective tissue fibers. Within the alveolar space (AS), cellular fragments are present. (Uranyl acetate and lead citrate, ×3200.)

Microscopic Findings

Exudative Phase

Histopathologic findings during the 1- to 6-day exudative phase consist of vascular congestion, interstitial and alveolar edema, epithelial lifting and loss, hyaline membrane formation, and microatelectasis.

The early stage of exudative DAD involves degeneration or necrosis of alveolar lining cells, endothelium, or both[30] (Figs. 125–1 and 125–2). Considerable congestion of red blood cells (RBCs) in the capillaries results, and leukocytes and platelets are present within the capillary vessels (see Figs. 125–1 and 125–2). On examination by light microscopy, a lack of visible endothelial damage is the norm, but injured endothelium does become leaky, and a protein-rich exudate enters into the interstitial space.[30–33]

Ultrastructurally, separation of edematous endothelial cell junctions occurs.[34] Occasionally, strands of fibrin can be identified between the endothelial cells (Fig. 125–3) and in the

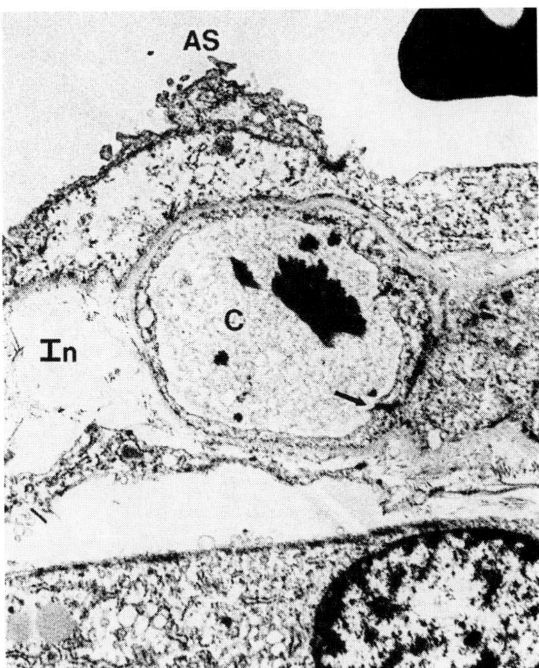

Figure 125–3. Human lung. Fibrin fragments are within the capillary lumen (C), and the endothelium is edematous focally. The intercellular junction is widened and contains fibrin (*arrow*). The interstitium is markedly edematous (In). AS = alveolar space. (Uranyl acetate and lead citrate, ×20,000.)

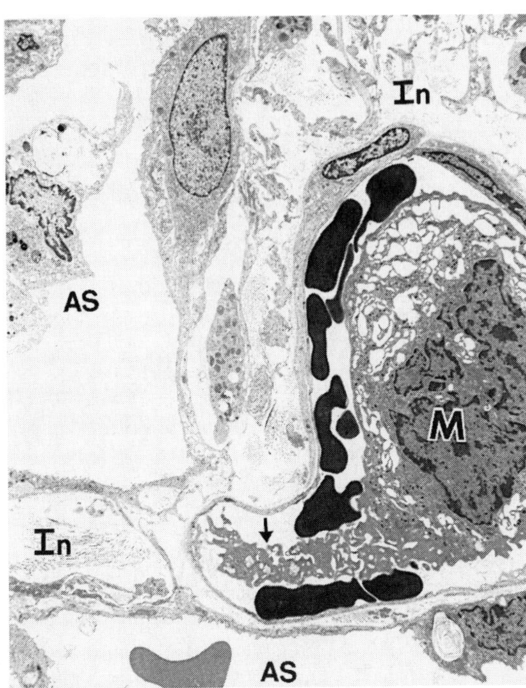

Figure 125–5. Human lung. Within the vessel, a megakaryocyte (M) with platelet formation (*arrow*) and multiple red blood cells are present. An extravasated red blood cell is in the alveolar space (AS). Increased connective tissue fibers and cells are evident within the interstitium (In). (Uranyl acetate and lead citrate, ×3000.)

subendothelial space.[35] Focal endothelial injury and death can be seen ultrastructurally, but unlike the case with the alveolar epithelium, contiguous endothelial necrosis and sloughing are rare pathologic findings[19, 33, 36] (Fig. 125–4).

In addition to degranulated platelets and neutrophils, megakaryocytes (Fig. 125–5)[37–39] and small microthrombi of platelets or fibrin can be seen within the capillaries.[40, 41] Pietra and colleagues[30] found fat emboli in capillaries during the first 5 days of the exudative phase. In larger vessels, mixed thromboemboli have been consistently seen in exudative and other phases of DAD.[42, 43]

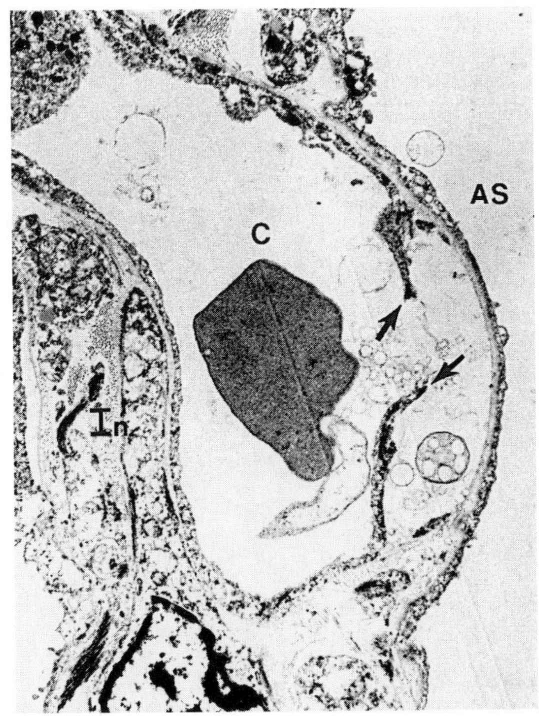

Figure 125–4. Human lung. The endothelium is disrupted (*arrows*) and lifted from the basement membrane. AS = alveolar space; In = interstitium; C = capillary. (Uranyl acetate and lead citrate, ×6200.)

Bachofen and Weibel[32] quantitated an approximate twofold increase in the interstitial volume of patients with ARDS. The edema is quite marked within the thick portion of the alveolar wall and separates the connective tissue fibers and interstitial cells.[44] Abundant fibrin strands, scattered RBCs, and a few acute inflammatory cells are invariably present in the edematous interstitium of damaged alveolar walls (see Fig. 125–2). If the proteinaceous exudate persists and is confined to the interstitium, it undergoes fibrocellular repair.

The alveolar epithelium has very tight junctions, but when it is injured sufficiently, protein-rich fluid that contains inflammatory cells, extravasated RBCs, and serum proteins, including fibrinogen, floods into the alveolar space. On light microscopy, this process is indicated by the presence of focal hemorrhages and edema fluid within the intra-alveolar space[3, 15, 31, 45] (Fig. 125–6). The protein-rich edema of DAD results from the increased permeability defect.[46]

Idell and colleagues[47] demonstrated that the bronchoalveolar lavage (BAL) fluid in patients with ARDS has an increase in total protein and procoagulant activity (attributable to the expression of tissue factor associated with factor VII; the extrinsic activation complex) and a depressed fibrinolytic activity, favoring tissue fibrin deposition and retention. Conceptually, then, during the exudative phase, the alveolar space contains material very similar to an intravascular thrombus, and many of the outcomes of an intraluminal "clot" are seen in the two processes.

If the lung injury is severe, the edematous type 1 epithelial cells undergo necrosis and desquamate, exposing the underlying basement membrane (Fig. 125–7; see Figs. 125–1 and

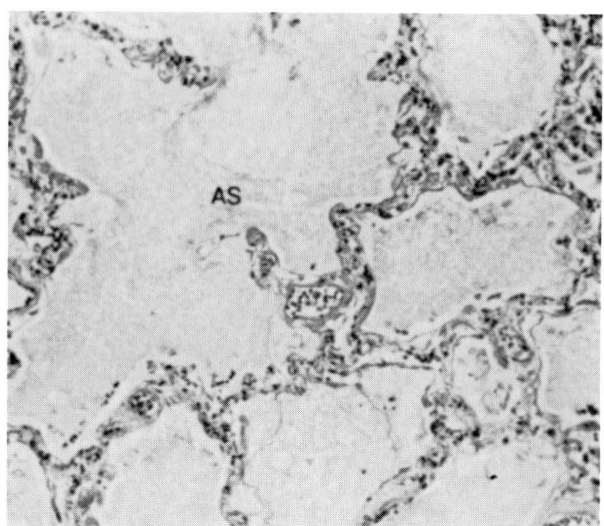

Figure 125–6. Human lung. Pulmonary edema is reflected by airspaces (AS) filled with proteinaceous material. The underlying alveolar walls are edematous, and the capillaries are congested. (Hematoxylin and eosin, ×150.)

125-2). The fibrinogen converts into fibrin and, along with necrotic cell debris and other condensed proteinaceous material, makes up the characteristic hyaline membranes, which form a "scab" over the exposed basement membranes and residual, but damaged, alveolar epithelium (Fig. 125-8). The hyaline membranes are characteristically seen at the levels of respiratory bronchiolar and alveolar ducts (Fig. 125-9)[15, 18] but can extend into the alveoli in a particularly severe lung injury. They may be seen as early as 24 hours after injury but are abundant at 4 to 7 days.[48]

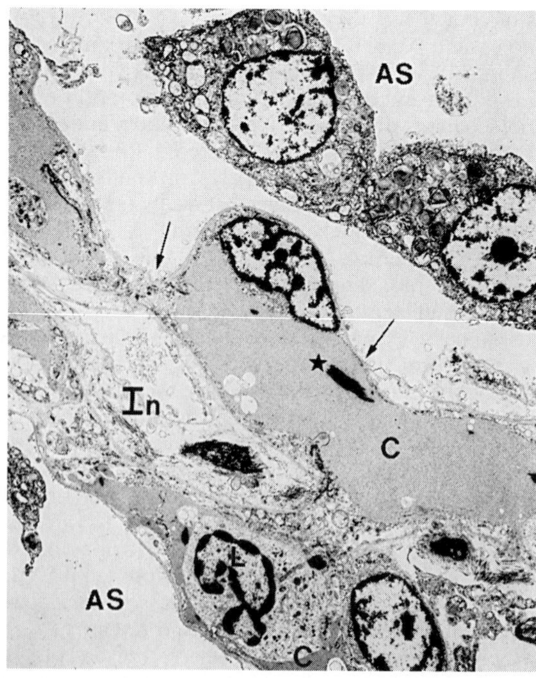

Figure 125–7. Human lung. Desquamated alveolar type 2 cells are free within the alveolar space (AS), exposing the basement membrane (*arrows*). Within the capillary (C), fibrin fragments (*star*) and leukocytes (L) are evident. The interstitium is edematous (In). (Uranyl acetate and lead citrate, ×3200.)

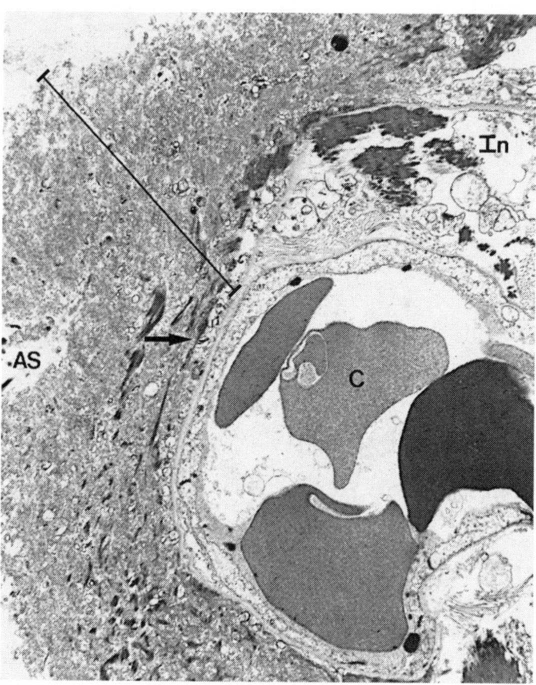

Figure 125–8. Human lung. The capillary (C) contains several red blood cells and is lined by endothelium that shows edema, prominent intercellular junctions, and surface-adherent fibrin fragments. Fibrin, degraded elastic fibers and cellular fragments are in the widened interstitium (In). The alveolar type I epithelium is disrupted and the cellular remnants, fibrin *(arrow)*, and proteinaceous exudate form a thick hyaline membrane (|——|). AS = alveolar space. (Uranyl acetate and lead citrate, ×5400.)

The high-protein permeability leak adversely affects the pulmonary surfactant system of affected lungs.[49-54] In the presence of the plasma proteins, alveolar surfactant is inactivated,[55, 56] and surfactant remnants can be identified within the proteinaceous material ultrastructurally. This surfactant abnormality or loss very likely leads to microatelectasis, which

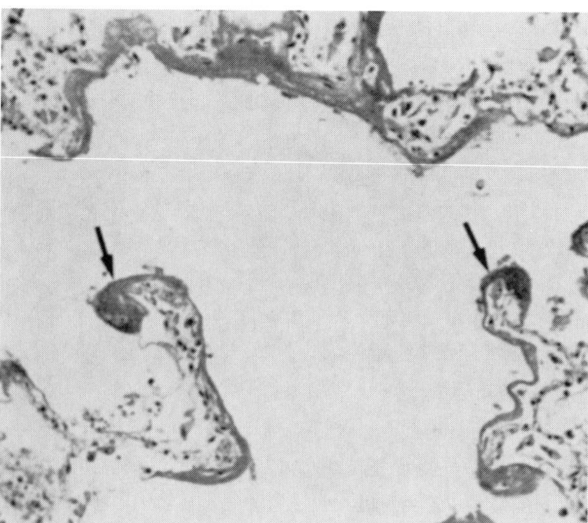

Figure 125–9. Human lung. In the alveolar duct, hyaline membranes are adhered to the ductal wall structures (*arrows*). The pulmonary parenchyma is edematous. (Hematoxylin and eosin, ×150.)

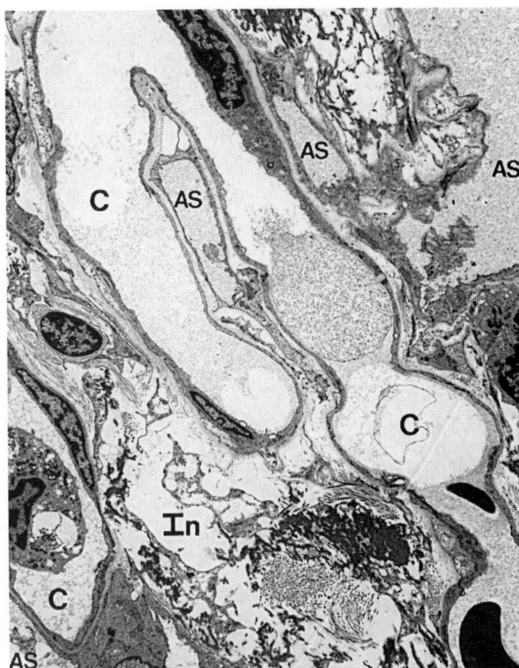

Figure 125–10. Human lung. Alveolar edema is evident in the collapsed alveolar spaces (AS). Alveolar epithelium is evident along the collapsed walls. The alveolar walls contain prominent capillaries (C). These ultrastructural changes precede the light microscopic findings of congestive atelectasis seen in Fig. 124-11. In = interstitium. (Uranyl acetate and lead citrate, ×3000.)

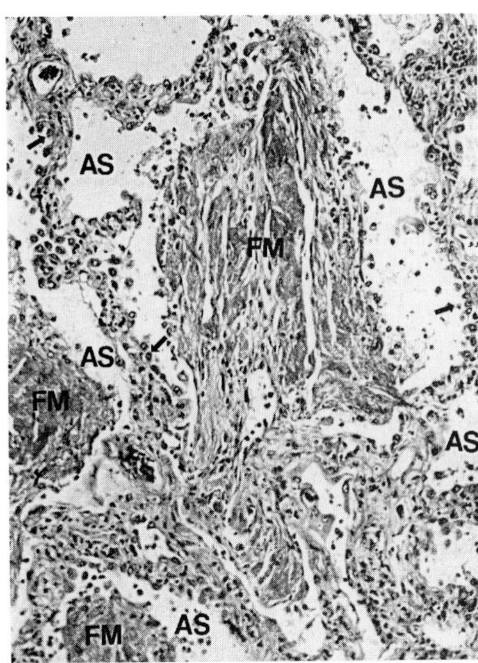

Figure 125–12. Human lung. The alveolar walls are hypercellular and contain mononuclear cells and scattered polymorphonuclear leukocytes. Within the airspace (AS), the fibrinous matrix (FM) is infiltrated with connective tissue elements. Proliferating type 2 cells line the alveolar walls (*arrows*) but not the organizing matrix within the airspace. Additional fibrinous exudates are present in other airspaces. (Hematoxylin and eosin, × 150.)

occurs in those alveoli subjacent to the alveolar ducts and respiratory bronchioles (Fig. 125-10). The process results in a light microscopic finding of ectatic alveolar ducts and respiratory bronchioles lined with prominent hyaline membranes, with adjacent alveolar walls that look quite "thickened" but are only atelectatic (Fig. 125-11).

Proliferative Phase

The proliferative phase of DAD begins within a few days after injury and becomes histologically apparent by days 5 through 7.[10] Histopathologically, it is characterized by hyperplasia of type 2 epithelial cells, an interstitial mononuclear inflammatory infiltrate and fibroproliferation, and the organization of hyaline membranes and proteinaceous exudate by mural application (Fig. 125-12). The type 2 epithelial cell is the stem cell responsible for epithelial regeneration,[57, 58] and mesenchymal cells within the interstitium participate in the reparative cellular and connective tissue fibroproliferation that occurs. Less is known about endothelial repair, but endothelial extensions are thought to repair leaks in the endothelial lining.[41]

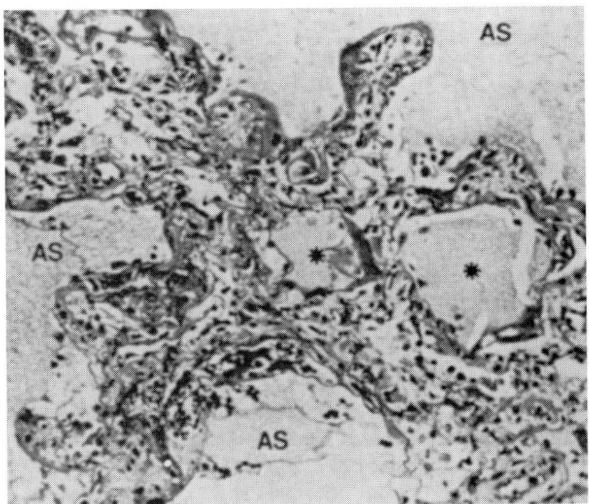

Figure 125–11. Human lung. Microatelectasis is characterized by nonuniformly sized airspaces, two of which have hyaline membranes (*asterisks*). Surrounding alveolar ducts and dilated alveoli (AS) are lined by hyaline membranes. The walls of the collapsed alveoli are thickened and hypercellular. (Hematoxylin and eosin, ×150.)

Hyperplasia and hypertrophy of type 2 epithelial cells are major components of the proliferative phase.[3, 19, 32, 59] More resistant than type 1 epithelial cells to injury, type 2 epithelial cells proliferate and cover the damaged alveolar walls and the intra-alveolar organizing exudate (Fig. 125-13). Normally, the population of type 2 cells "turns over" every 4 to 5 weeks, but after lung injury, the rate dramatically increases.[60] Type 2 epithelial cells retain microvillus processes over their cell surfaces, but they lose or have poorly developed cytoplasmic lamellar bodies during the processes of active replication, spreading, and differentiating into type 1 epithelium (see Fig. 125-10). The hyperplastic type 2 epithelial cells form a cuboidal epithelial lining layer as early as 5 days, and an alveolar lining of cuboidal type 2 cells is maximum at 14 days.[48] The vesicular nuclei in the hyperplastic type 2 cells may show lobulation and may contain large nucleoli (see Fig. 125-13), and sometimes the cells have atypical features. Occasionally, cells with squamous differentiation that contain keratin or hyaline-like material in the cytoplasm (Fig. 125-14) can line the surfaces of the damaged alveolar walls and the organizing exudate that is undergoing mural application.[24, 59]

The protein-rich edematous exudate and hyaline membranes constitute the intra-alveolar "clot" within the alveolar space that provides the provisional matrix for subsequent ingrowth of granulation tissue and intra-alveolar organization[61] (Fig. 125–15). Platelets, macrophages, and endothelial cells release a number of cytokines into the provisional matrix.[62, 63] Thus, the cytokine network not only activates the inflammatory response, usually via release of tumor necrosis factor-α (TNF-a) and interleukin-1 (IL-1), but also is critical in the establishment and maintenance of the dysregulated inflammatory and repair states of lung injury.

Cytokines, either growth factors or chemotaxins, elicit leukocyte, endothelial cell, fibroblast, and epithelial cell activation, migration, and proliferation.[61, 63, 64] Neutrophilic leukocytes emigrate into the lung and appear in the edematous interstitial spaces of alveolar walls and alveolar spaces within 24 to 36 hours after injury.[61] They are the first leukocytes to arrive, and they phagocytose debris.

The second wave of emigrating leukocytes are mononuclear cells, which persist in greater numbers as the fibroproliferative process ensues. These mononuclear cells generate a number of pro-inflammatory mediators that are important in transforming the provisional matrix into mature granulation tissue.[65, 66] Cytokines are elicited from adjacent fibroblasts and from endothelial, epithelial, and smooth muscle cells. Platelet-derived growth factor (PDGF), fibroblast growth factor (FGF), and the insulin-like growth factors (IGFs), along with some of the chemokines and interleukins, are followed by transforming growth factor-β (TGF-β) and the colony-stimulating factors (CSFs) and others as the organizing matrix undergoes chronic fibrosis.[62, 64, 67, 68] The macrophage promotes resolution of the proinflammatory activity of neutrophils by ingesting apoptotic neutrophilic leukocytes.[69]

Intramural organization of alveolar exudate is a familiar and common reparative process in the adult lung that was well defined by Spencer[70] and Liebow.[71] In this repair sequence (Figs. 125–16 to 125–18), the alveolar wall sustains an injury in which not only is type 1 epithelium lost but there is also basement membrane damage, a finding that probably precludes restitution to normal structure. The provisional matrix exudate does not undergo fibrinolysis and further resolution; rather, fibroblasts, myofibroblasts, and other cells migrate out of the damaged alveolar wall through gaps in the basement membrane into the matrix exudate and then proliferate,[59, 72] in a process comparable to the growth of granulation tissue from a vessel wall into a thrombus.

Ultimately, the organized matrix can either (1) retract into the surrounding alveolar wall and become covered by type 2 epithelial cells (accretion) or (2) occlude the alveolar space.

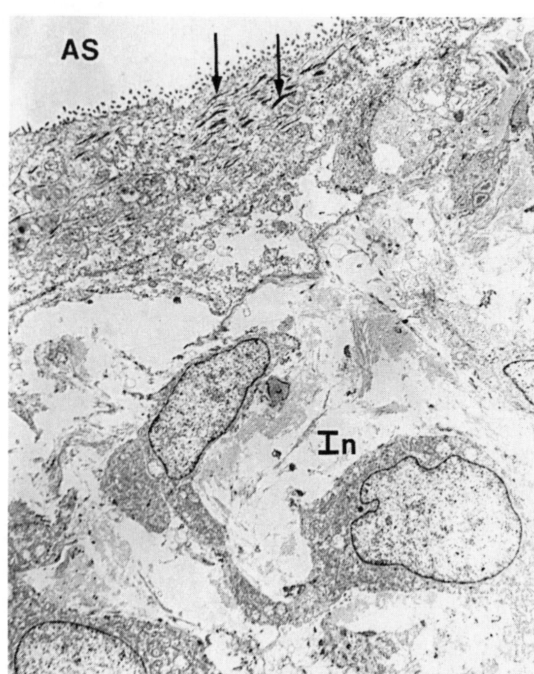

Figure 125–14. Human lung. The alveolar space (AS) is lined by a cell with microvillous projections and abundant cytoplasmic keratin or hyaline-like material indicating squamous differentiation (*arrows*). The underlying interstitium (In) is widened and contains several mononuclear cells and fibrous connective tissue. (Uranyl acetate and lead citrate, ×3200.)

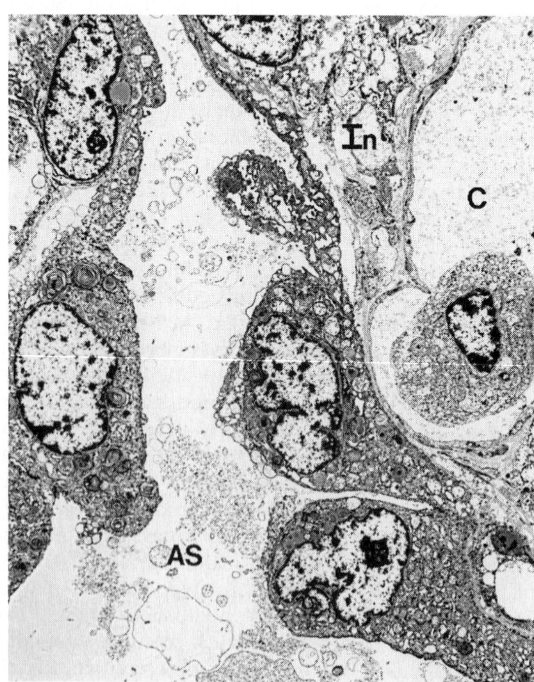

Figure 125–13. Human lung. The alveolar space (AS) is lined by hyperplastic alveolar type 2 cells. The nuclei show increased lobulation and have large vesicular nucleoli. The cytoplasmic lamellar inclusions vary in configuration and number. The interstitium (In) contains increased cells. C = capillary. (Uranyl acetate and lead citrate, ×3000.)

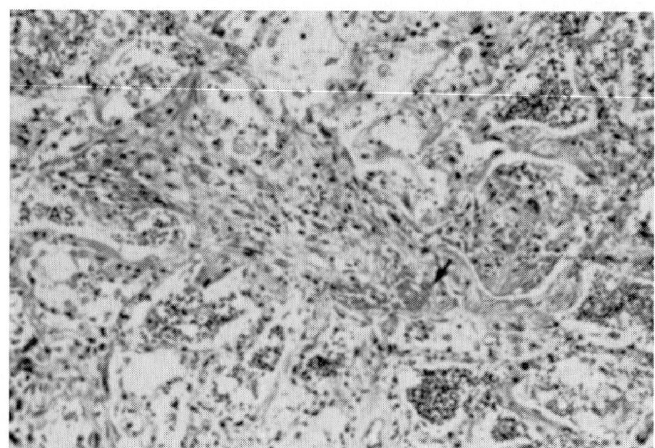

Figure 125–15. Human lung. In the proliferative phase of diffuse alveolar damage, the fibrinous matrix (*arrow*) is infiltrated with proliferating fibroblasts (F) during the process of intramural organization. Several of the alveolar spaces contain extravasated red blood cells. (Hematoxylin and eosin, ×150.)

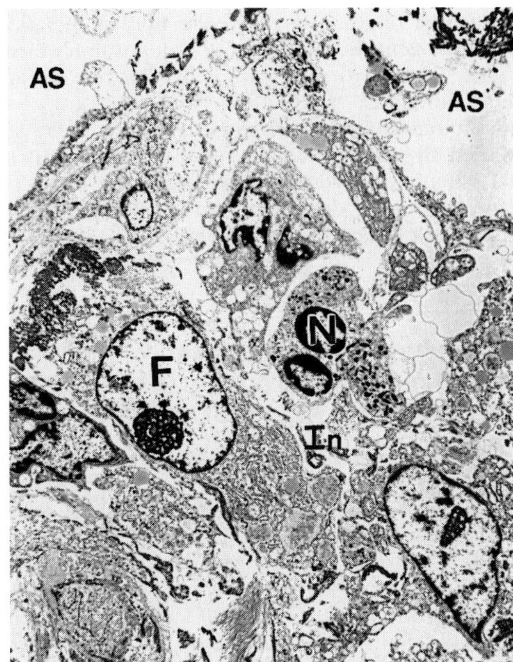

Figure 125–16. Human lung. The epithelial type 1 lining the alveolar space (AS) is destroyed focally and the underlying basement membrane is covered with fibrin fragments. The interstitium (In) shows abundant cells including neutrophils (N) and fibroblasts (F). (Uranyl acetate and lead citrate, ×3200.)

Its incorporation into the alveolar wall yields the microscopic picture of unevenly thickened alveolar walls distributed throughout the lung. The interstitial volume of the damaged alveolar wall is increased up to 10 times its normal width during this phase.[32] Although some of the collagen and extracellular matrix may be resorbed if the patient survives, it is presumed that residual scarring would remain, leaving some ARDS survivors with functional but not entirely normal lungs.

Interactions between the fibroblasts and alveolar epithelial cells occur through gaps in the basement membrane.[73, 74] Myofibroblasts that migrate through these gaps can attach to the luminal or airspace surface of the damaged basement membrane.[59, 75] As noted previously, a large number of growth factors orchestrate the coordinated interactions among varying cell types during the proliferative phase of DAD.[62, 64, 67, 68] The fibroblasts secrete a variety of extracellular matrix proteins, fibronectin, hyaluronic acid, proteoglycans, and collagens. The myofibroblasts within the intramural organizing foci are more active in the secretion of collagen than those that remain in the interstitium.[75] During the early proliferative phase of DAD, immunocytochemical staining reveals pro-collagen types 1 and 3 and fibronectin within the intra-alveolar organized foci.[75] Abnormal ratios of type 1 (normal = 60% to 70%) to type 3 (normal = 30% to 40%) collagens are seen,[76] with type 3 collagen predominating in the proliferative phase, and then type 1 as the fibrotic phase ensues. In patients who survive for more than 10 days, a twofold to threefold increase in the collagen content of the lung may be found.[77] Additional information is needed concerning the balances between the extent of cellular proliferation and the degradation activities of collagenases and other proteases within the extracellular matrix.

Studies to date have focused on the role of the myofibroblast and fibroblast in tissue repair. Angiogenesis is a prominent feature of the fibroproliferative response in other organs, but there are few substantive data concerning the angiogenic response during the proliferative and chronic fibrotic phases of DAD. It is reported that the granulation tissue within the alveolar space resembles undifferentiated mesenchyme with fibrin, a predominance of type 3 collagen, and a highly mobile and proliferative phenotype of endothelial cells that form a vascularized capillary bed.[35, 78] The vascular proliferation is needed to supply essential nutrient support for mesenchymal cell proliferation and maintenance of intra-alveolar fibrosis.[78, 79] In a series of autopsies of patients with ARDS, capillaries were evident within the intra-alveolar organizing exudate in lungs with reparative DAD (see Fig. 125–18).

For years, however, it has been thought that the organization process in the alveolar space does not show significant proliferation of capillaries. The capillary-poor response in granulation tissue within the alveolar space was noted by both Spencer[70] and Carrington[80] in their studies on *usual interstitial pneumonia* (UIP). This relative lack of capillaries was not seen in sites of the lung in which the bronchial artery was available to supply the capillary source (e.g., the remarkable capillary proliferation within the visceral pleura and interlobular septa that occurs in some interstitial pneumonias and about the airway-pulmonary artery dyads in bronchiectasis). The difference in the number of capillaries in patients with UIP versus those with proliferative DAD probably relates to the age of the organizing or organized lesion, one being days old and the other being weeks old.

Bachofen and Weibel[32] demonstrated that endothelial cells had the smallest relative volume changes in patients with ARDS and that, morphometrically, about half the lung capillaries were lost. In their study population, the most reliable index of functional impairment was the capillary-to-tissue ratio, being less than 10% of normal.

Microthrombi composed of platelets and fibrin undergo

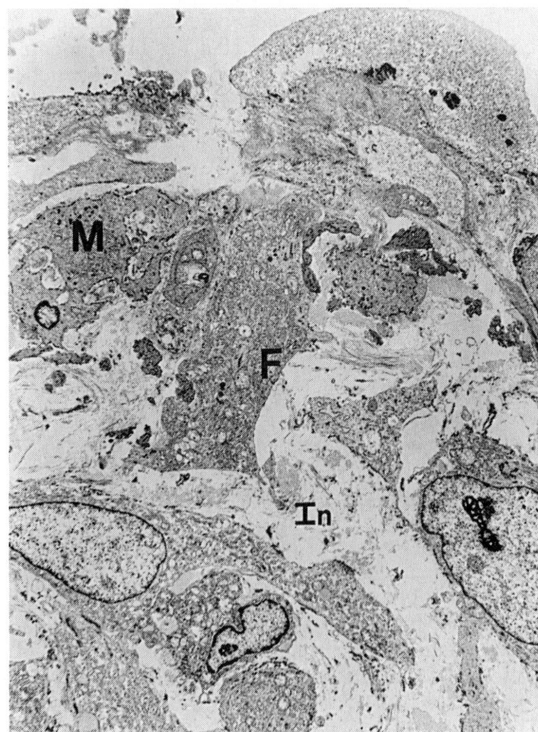

Figure 125–17. Human lung. Within the organizing matrix in the airspace, abundant fibroblasts (F), myofibroblasts (M), and extracellular matrix are evident. In = interstitium. (Uranyl acetate and lead citrate, ×3200.)

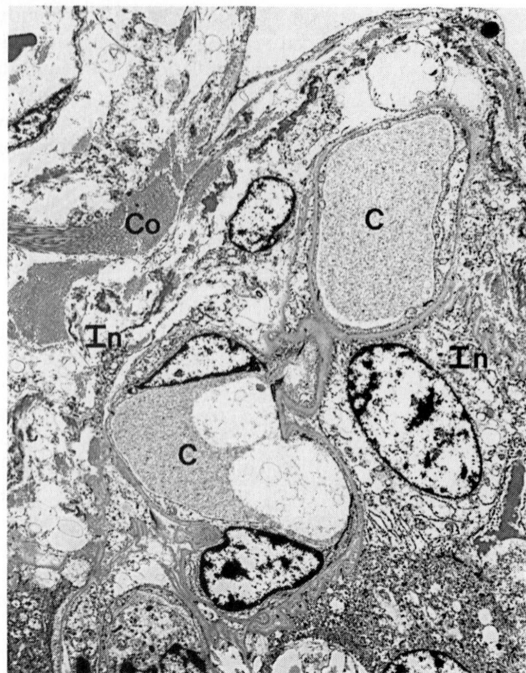

Figure 125–18. Human lung. Within the organizing matrix, several capillaries (C) are present among numerous mesenchymal cells, collagen (Co), and elastin fibers. In = interstitium. (Uranyl acetate and lead citrate, ×3000.)

organization in small arteries and intra-acinar veins.[24, 43] This process may be responsible for the reported reduction in volume and number of small arteries with external diameters of more than 1 mm.[42] Medial hypertrophy of muscular arteries occurs, and these structural changes plus the microthrombi that are usually present in the larger vessels contribute to the subsequent loss of vascular filling that has been documented on postmortem arteriograms. Clearly, the vasculogenetic-angiogenetic aspect of the lung repair process needs to be given considerable attention in the future.

An additional repair pattern seen during the reparative phase of DAD has been rediscovered and is now called *collapse* or *atelectatic induration* and *obliterative-interseptal fibrosis*.[59, 81, 82] It is implied that damaged and epithelium-denuded alveolar walls, probably through a common underlying mechanism of loss of surfactant, undergo collapse and permanent apposition (Fig. 125–19). This finding is not new; "congestive atelectasis," characterized by small areas of microatelectasis, was described in the lungs of patients and animals with hemorrhagic and septic shock many years ago.[4, 5] This repair pattern stresses the importance of the microatelectatic lesion that is always evident in DAD (see Fig. 125–19). That these sites can remain adhered and fibrose and may result in the "remodeling" of the distal airspaces is easily envisioned.

Fibrotic Phase

If the reparative phase is arrested, the lesion resolves. If the reparative phase persists, widespread fibrosis ensues in a small subset of patients. The progression of intra-alveolar fibrosis appears to be due to persistence of inflammation and a dysregulated repair response. The chronic inflammatory autoinjury of ARDS is amplified in the context of subsequent development of nosocomial pneumonia, sepsis syndrome or sepsis, multiple organ failure syndrome, and continued exposure to exogenous oxidant stress.[39, 83, 84] Any one or all of these multiple factors may contribute to the propagation of DAD by exaggerating the ongoing intra-alveolar fibroproliferation and suspected angiogenesis, along with the deposition of extracellular matrix, leading to progressive alveolar fibrosis and impaired lung function.[85, 86]

Histopathologic findings are comparable to those seen in lungs injured by other etiologic agents. Total remodeling of the distal parenchyma with cyst-like dilated airspaces, extensive connective tissue deposition, and hypertensive vascular changes are the primary features[87] (Figs. 125–20 and 125–21). There is a progressive increase in collagen with the duration of lung disease.[77]

INFLUENCE OF CHANGES IN TREATMENT MODALITIES ON DISEASE PATHOGENESIS AND EVOLUTION

As noted previously, original descriptions of ARDS emphasized that lung fibrosis constituted a major pathologic finding. Many of these reports were published when high oxygen levels and increased airway pressures were being used, and the label "oxygen toxicity" was, in retrospect, very accurate. The advent of positive end-expiratory pressure (PEEP) and continuous positive airway pressure (CPAP), lower oxygen tensions, and better ventilatory strategies in the 1970s influenced the pathology of ARDS, but the change was not documented in published pathologic studies.

A lack of severe or end-stage lung fibrosis has now been documented in the majority of patients who die of ARDS.[84, 88, 89] Until the early 1980s, it was generally believed that patients with ARDS died of hypoxemic respiratory failure with underlying proliferative fibrotic lung lesions as a consequence of the DAD process.[26] In 1986, however, a pathologic study of autopsies of 77 patients in an ARDS study population documented that more 70% of the patients had evidence of bron-

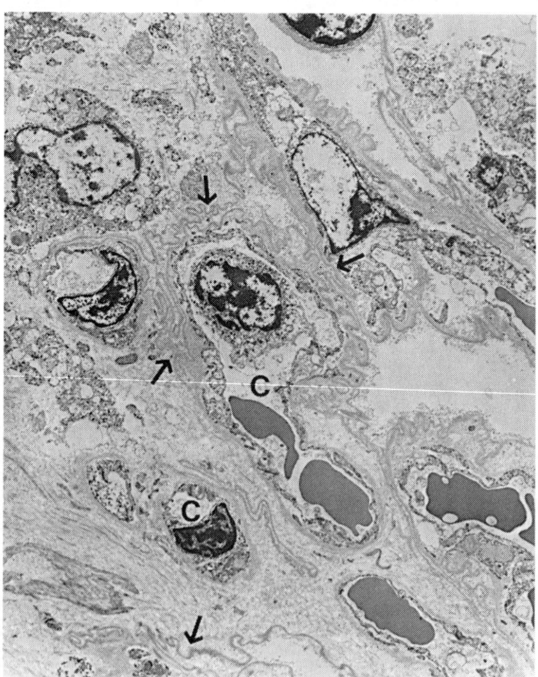

Figure 125–19. Human lung. The repair pattern of atelectatic obliteration is depicted. Collapsed alveolar walls are adhered. Note the presence of many collapsed basement membranes (*arrows*) and several capillaries (C). Alveolar lining epithelium is absent and airspaces are not evident, because they have been replaced by fibroproliferative elements. (Uranyl acetate and lead citrate, ×3000.)

chopneumonia at autopsy; in 21% of patients, bronchopneumonia was the only lung finding.[88] Only nine patients had severe pulmonary fibrosis (fibrotic phase of DAD). In this same ARDS study population, it was shown that multiple organ failure, death, and infection were highly interrelated, the most common cause of death being multiple organ failure rather than uncorrectable hypoxemia (which was the cause of death in only two of 141 patients).[83] It is now recognized that most patients with ARDS die of multiple organ failure, not respiratory failure,[83, 84, 90] and that sepsis is associated with death in 36% to 90% of patients who do not survive ARDS.[84, 89-91]

Thus, at this time, with appropriate oxygen levels and ventilatory strategies being used in intensive care units, the dual-injury pattern of hyperoxia and barotrauma-volutrauma has been diminished. This has resulted in less severe fibrosis in ARDS, but a variable fibroproliferative response does occur. Sepsis due to both gram-negative and gram-positive organisms is the leading cause of ARDS, and inflammation and the inflammatory cascade play pivotal roles in its development. The inflammatory-infection autoinjury factor is, no doubt, an important pathogenetic factor that participates in the dysregulated tissue responses seen in lungs of patients with ARDS.[12, 92, 93] Knowledge is increasing about the perturbed cellular mechanisms and signaling factors of neutrophilic-endothelial adhesive interactions that determine how cytokine-activated endothelium controls the intensity, temporal pattern, and composition of the white blood cells that are recruited into the alveolar spaces.

Recruitment and persistence of neutrophils appear to correlate with the development and severity of ARDS.[94-96] Neutrophils can initiate alveolar-capillary injury[97, 98] or amplify acute injury,[99] even if they are not required for its initiation.[93, 100, 101] At this time, much research focuses on identifying soluble mediators that might account for the lung injury in ARDS and multiple organ failure.[93, 102-104] Among those signaling factors for polymorphonuclear leukocytes, chemokines[105] are an important group; they include:

- IL-8
- Epithelial-neutrophil activating factor (ENA-78)
- Neutrophil-activating peptide (NAP-2)

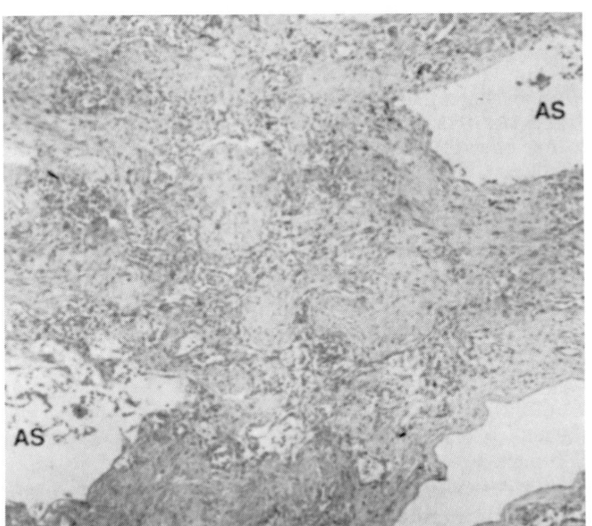

Figure 125–20. Human lung. Normal pulmonary architecture is absent in this patient specimen obtained during the fibrotic phase of diffuse alveolar damage. Only a few cystic airspaces (AS) persist; the remainder is fibrotic tissue and scattered inflammatory cells. (Hematoxylin and eosin, ×100.)

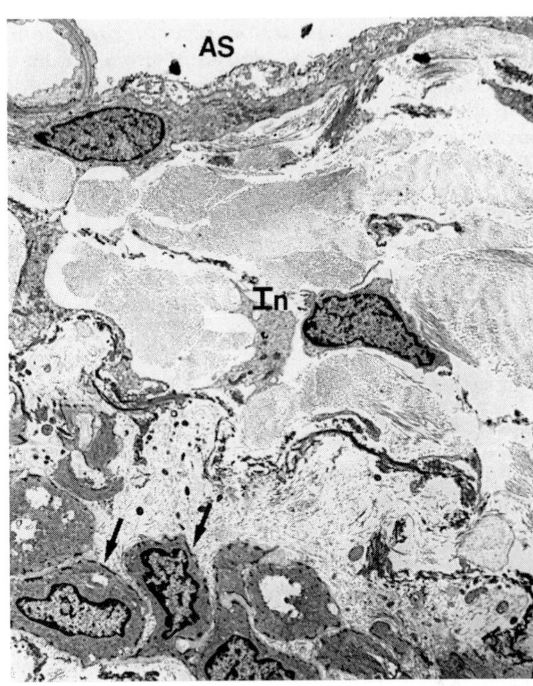

Figure 125–21. Human lung. A capillary (C) is on the surface of a severely fibrotic wall (fibrotic phase of diffuse alveolar damage). The interstitium (In) contains an abundance of collagen fibers, remnants of monocytes and myofibroblasts, and smooth muscle cells (*arrows*). AS = alveolar space. (Uranyl acetate and lead citrate, ×3300.)

- Granulocyte chemotactic protein-2 (GCP-2)
- Gro-homologs (originally described as a mitogen for melanoma cells)

ENA-78 and IL-8 may act in parallel or in sequence as signals for neutrophils in inflammatory lung injury. IL-8 is a major chemotactic factor for neutrophil recruitment, and a number of cells, including fibroblasts, epithelial cells, endothelial cells, neutrophils, and macrophages, produce it.[105] IL-8 also regulates angiogenesis in both solid tumors and chronic fibroproliferative disorders, and IL-8 levels are elevated in BAL samples from patients with ARDS.[102, 106-110] In several studies, the persistent elevation of IL-8 in the plasma or in BAL fluid of adult patients with acute lung injury predicted poor outcome,[106, 109, 111] as did elevations of IL-6.[112]

ENA-78 is present in nanograms per milliliter quantities in unconcentrated BAL fluid from patients with ARDS, and its concentration correlates with the number of neutrophils present.[103] These and other complex interactions need extensive study in humans with ARDS and sepsis and in many adult animal models of lung injury.

SUMMARY

Acute lung injury is a syndrome of pulmonary vasoconstriction, inflammation, and greater permeability of both the alveolar capillary endothelium and epithelium that results in both arterial hypoxemia resistant to oxygen therapy and the appearance of diffuse infiltrates on chest x-ray. The incidence of ARDS worldwide is 5 to 7 cases per 100,000 population. About 50% of patients with ARDS die. Although acute lung injury is caused by a variety of insults, the most common cause is sepsis. Lung injury and subsequent repair result from a complex interplay among leukocytes, soluble polypeptide mediators, and cellular and extracellular matrix networks.

DAD, the primary tissue lesion in acute lung injury, is characterized by a series of consistent though nonspecific pathologic changes that evolve through exudative, proliferative, and fibrotic phases. The progression of ARDS from the proliferative to the fibrotic phase appears to be due either to the susceptibility of the host to nosocomial infection or to the persistence of inflammation. The significance of elevated cytokine levels in lung injury needs clarification. For example, what constitutes a protective release of cytokines rather than a more massive or sustained cytokine release that may prove to be destructive to cells and tissues? The dysregulated inflammatory-reparative processes in ARDS still require intense investigation.

References

1. Winternitz M: Collected studies on the pathology of war gas Poisoning. New Haven, Yale University Press, 1920, pp 3-165.
2. Weston J, Liebow A, Dixon M, et al: Untoward effects of exogenous inhalants on the lung. J Forensic Sci 1972; 17:199-279.
3. Katzenstein A-LA, Bloor C, Liebow A: Diffuse alveolar damage: The role of oxygen, shock, and related factors. Am J Pathol 1976; 85:210-222.
4. Jenkins M, Jones R, Wilson B, et al: Congestive atelectasis: A complication of the intravenous infusion of fluids. Ann Surg 1950; 132:327-347.
5. Martin A, Soloway H, Simmons R: Pathologic anatomy of the lungs following shock and trauma. J Trauma 1968; 8:687-699.
6. Corrin B: Diffuse alveolar damage. *In*: ARDS: Acute Respiratory Distress in Adults. Evans TW, Haslett C (Eds). London, Chapman & Hall, 1996, pp 49-68.
7. Moon V: The pathology of secondary shock. Am J Pathol 1948; 24:235-273.
8. McGovern V: Shock. Pathol Annu 1971; 6:279-298.
9. Kuhn C: Patterns of lung repair. Chest 1991; 99:11S-14S.
10. Katzenstein AA, Askin FB: Diffuse alveolar damage. *In*: Surgical Pathology of Non-neoplastic Lung Disease. Philadelphia, WB Saunders, 1982, pp 9-42.
11. Hamman L, Rich A: Acute diffuse interstitial fibrosis of the lung. Bull Johns Hopkins Hosp 1944; 74:177-212.
12. Simon R, Ward P: Adult respiratory distress syndrome. *In*: Inflammation: Basic Principles and Clinical Correlates. 2nd ed. Gallin JI, Goldstein IM, Synderman R (Eds). New York, Raven Press, 1992, pp 999-1016.
13. Cederberg A, Hellsten S, Niorner G: Oxygen treatment and hyaline membranes in adults. Acta Pathol Microbiol Scand 1965; 64:450-458.
14. Pratt P: The reaction of the human lung to enriched oxygen atmosphere. Ann N Y Acad Sci 1965; 121:809-822.
15. Orell S: Lung pathology in respiratory distress following shock in the adult. Acta Pathol Microbiol Scand (A) 1971; 79:65-76.
16. Gould V, Tosco R, Wheelis R, et al: Oxygen pneumonitis in man: Ultrastructural observations on the development of alveolar lesions. Lab Invest 1972; 26:499-508.
17. Lamy M, Fallat R, Koeniger E, et al: Pathologic features and mechanisms of hypoxemia in adult respiratory distress syndrome. Am Rev Respir Dis 1976; 114:267-284.
18. Pratt P, Vollmer R, Shelburne J, et al: Pulmonary morphology in a multihospital collaborative extracorporeal membrane oxygenation project. Am J Pathol 1979; 95:191-214.
19. Nash G, Foley F, Langlinais P: Pulmonary interstitial edema and hyaline membranes in adult burn patients. Hum Pathol 1974; 5:149-160.
20. Hasleton P, McWilliam L, Haboubi N: The lung parenchyma in burns. Histopathology 1983; 7:333-347.
21. Vijeyaratnam G, Corrin B: Experimental paraquat poisoning: A histological and electron-optical study of the changes in the lung. J Pathol 1971; 103:123-129.
22. Blennerhassett J: Shock lung and diffuse alveolar damage: Pathological and pathogenetic considerations. Pathology 1985; 17:239-247.
23. Meyrick B: Pathology of the adult respiratory distress syndrome. Crit Care Clin 1986; 2:405-427.
24. Tomashefski J: Pulmonary pathology of the adult respiratory distress syndrome. Clin Chest Med 1990; 11:593-619.
25. Mittermayer C, Hassenstein J, Riede U: Is shock-induced lung fibrosis reversible? A report on recovery from "shock-lung." Pathol Res Pract 1978; 162:73-87.
26. Pratt P: Pathology of adult respiratory distress syndrome: Implications regarding therapy. Semin Respir Med 1982; 4:79-85.
27. Peters JI, Bell RC, Prihoda TJ, et al: Clinical determinants of abnormalities in pulmonary functions in survivors of the adult respiratory distress syndrome. Am Rev Respir Dis 1989; 139:1163-1168.
28. Churg A, Golden J, Fligiel S, et al: Bronchopulmonary dysplasia in the adult. Am Rev Respir Dis 1983; 127:117-120.
29. Yazdy A, Tomashefski J, Yagan R, et al: Regional alveolar damage (RAD): A localized counterpart of diffuse alveolar damage. Am J Clin Pathol 1989; 92:10-14.
30. Pietra G, Ruttner J, Wust W, et al: The lung after trauma and shock: Fine structure of the alveolar capillary barrier in 23 autopsies. J Trauma 1981; 21:454-462.
31. Teplitz C: The core pathobiology and integrated medical science of adult acute respiratory insufficiency. Surg Clin North Am 1976; 56:1091-1133.
32. Bachofen M, Weibel ER: Alterations of the gas exchange apparatus in adult respiratory insufficiency associated with septicemia. Am Rev Respir Dis 1977; 116:589-615.
33. Schnells G, Voight W, Riedl H, et al: Electron microscopic investigation of lung biopsies in patients with post-traumatic respiratory insufficiency. Acta Chir Scand Suppl 1980; 499:9-20.
34. Barrios R, Inoue S, Hogg J: Intercellular junctions in "shock lung": A freeze fracture study. Lab Invest 1977; 36:628-635.
35. Hasleton P: Adult respiratory distress syndrome—a review. Histopathology 1983; 7:307-332.
36. Bachofen M, Weibel E: Basic pattern of tissue repair in human lungs following unspecific injury. Chest (Suppl) 1974; 65:14S-19S.
37. Aabo K, Hansen K: Megakaryocytes in pulmonary blood vessels: I. Incidence at autopsy, clinicopathological relations, especially to disseminated intravascular coagulation. Acta Pathol Microbiol Scand (A) 1978; 86:285-291.
38. Corrin B: Lung pathology in septic shock. J Clin Pathol 1980; 33:891-894.
39. Hasleton P: Adult respiratory distress syndrome. *In*: Spencer's Pathology of the Lung. 5th ed. New York, McGraw-Hill, 1996, pp 375-399.
40. Bone R, Francis P, Pierce A: Intravascular coagulation associated with the adult respiratory distress syndrome. Am J Med 1976; 61:585-589.
41. Bachofen M, Weibel E: Structural alterations of lung parenchyma in the adult respiratory distress syndrome. Clin Chest Med 1982; 3:35-56.
42. Snow R, Davies P, Pontoppidian H, et al: Pulmonary vascular remodeling in adult respiratory distress syndrome. Am Rev Respir Dis 1982; 126:887-892.
43. Tomashefski J, Davies P, Boggis C, et al: The pulmonary vascular lesions of the adult respiratory distress syndrome. Am J Pathol 1983; 112:112-126.
44. Riede U, Mittermayer C, Friedburg H, et al: Morphological development of human shock lung. Pathol Res Pract 1979; 165:269-286.
45. Nash G, Blennerhassett J, Pantoppidan H: Pulmonary lesions associated with oxygen therapy and artificial ventilation. N Engl J Med 1967; 276:368-374.
46. Holter J, Weiland J, Pacht E, et al: Protein permeability in the adult respiratory distress syndrome: Loss of size selectivity of the alveolar epithelium. J Clin Invest 1986; 78:1513-1522.
47. Idell S, Gonzalez K, Bradford H, et al: Procoagulant activity in bronchoalveolar lavage in the adult respiratory distress syndrome: Contribution of tissue factor associated with factor VII. Am Rev Respir Dis 1987; 136:1466-1474.
48. Dunnill M: Pulmonary Oedema and Shock Lung. 2nd ed. New York, Churchill Livingstone, 1987, pp 23-40.
49. Petty TL, Reiss OK, Paul GW, et al: Characteristics of pulmonary surfactant in adult respiratory distress syndrome associated with trauma and shock. Am Rev Respir Dis 1977; 115:531-536.
50. Pison U, Seeger W, Buchhorn R, et al: Surfactant abnormalities

in patients with respiratory failure after multiple trauma. Am Rev Respir Dis 1989; 140:1033-1039.
51. Pison U, Overtacke U, Brand M, et al: Altered pulmonary surfactant in uncomplicated and septicemia-complicated courses of acute respiratory failure. J Trauma 1990; 30:19-26.
52. Seeger W, Pison U, Buchhorn R, et al: Surfactant abnormalities and adult respiratory failure. Lung 1990; 168(Suppl):891-902.
53. Gregory T, Longmore WJ, Moxley MA, et al: Surfactant chemical composition in acute respiratory distress syndrome. J Clin Invest 1991; 88:1976-1981.
54. Aronsen EL, Shannon JM: Epithelial injury and repair. *In*: ARDS: Acute Respiratory Distress in Adults. Evans TW, Haslett C (Eds). London, Chapman & Hall, 1996, pp 197-312.
55. Holm B, Enhorning G, Notter R: A biophysical mechanism by which plasma proteins inhibit lung surfactant activity. Chem Phys Lipids 1988; 49:49-55.
56. Holm BA, Keicher L, Liu M, et al: Inhibition of pulmonary surfactant function by phospholipases. J Appl Physiol 1991; 78:317-321.
57. Evans M, Cabral L, Stephens R, et al: Renewal of alveolar epithelium in the rat following exposure to NO_2. Am J Pathol 1973; 70:175-198.
58. Adamson I, Bowden D: The type 2 cell as progenitor of alveolar epithelial regeneration. Lab Invest 1974; 30:35-42.
59. Fukuda Y, Ishizaki M, Masuda Y, et al: The role of intra-alveolar fibrosis in the process of pulmonary structural remodeling in patients with diffuse alveolar damage. Am J Pathol 1987; 126:171-182.
60. Smith L, Brody J: Influence of methylprednisolone on mouse alveolar type 2 cell response to acute lung injury. Am Rev Respir Dis 1981; 123:459-464.
61. Clark R: The commonality of cutaneous wound repair and lung injury. Chest 1991; 99:57S-60S.
62. Snyder L, Hertz M, Harmon K, et al: Failure of lung repair following acute lung injury: Regulation of the fibroproliferative response (part 2). Chest 1990; 98:989-993.
63. Snyder L, Hwetz M, Peterson M, et al: Acute lung injury: Pathogenesis of intra-alveolar fibrosis. J Clin Invest 1991; 88:663-673.
64. Sime P, Gauldie J: Mechanisms of scarring. *In*: ARDS: Acute Respiratory Distress in Adults. Evans TW, Haslett C (Eds). London, Chapman & Hall, 1996, pp 215-231.
65. Sibille Y, Reynolds HY: Macrophages and polymorphonuclear neutrophils in lung defense and injury. Am Rev Respir Dis 1990; 141:471.
66. Henke C, Marinelli W, Jessurun J, et al: Macrophage production of basic fibroblast growth factor in the fibroproliferative disorder of alveolar fibrosis after lung injury. Am J Pathol 1993; 143:1189-1199.
67. Snyder L, Hertz M, Harmon K, et al: Failure of lung repair following acute lung injury: Regulation of the fibroproliferative response (part 1). Chest 1990; 98:733-738.
68. Bitterman P: Pathogenesis of fibrosis in acute lung injury. Am J Med 1992; 92(suppl 6A):39S-43S.
69. Haslett C: Mechanisms of resolution of lung inflammation. *In*: ARDS: Acute Respiratory Distress in Adults. Evans TW, Haslett C (Eds). London, Chapman & Hall, 1996, pp 49-68.
70. Spencer H: Chronic interstitial pneumonia. *In*: The Lung. Liebow AA, Smith DE (Eds). Baltimore, Williams & Wilkins, 1968, pp 134-150.
71. Liebow AA: Definition and classification of interstitial pneumonias in human pathology. Prog Respir Res 1975; 8:1-33.
72. Kobashi Y, Manabe T: The fibrosing process in so-called organized diffuse alveolar damage. Virchows Archiv (A) 1993; 422:47-52.
73. Brody A, Craighead J: Interstitial associations of cells lining air spaces in human pulmonary fibrosis. Virchows Arch (A) 1976; 372:39-49.
74. Adamson I, Hedgecock C, Bowden D: Epithelial cell-fibroblast interactions in lung injury and repair. Am J Pathol 1990; 137:385-392.
75. Kuhn C, Boldt J, King T, et al: An immunohistochemical study of architectural remodeling and connective tissue synthesis in pulmonary fibrosis. Am Rev Respir Dis 1989; 140:1693-1703.
76. Farjanel J, Hartmann D, Guidet B, et al: Four markers of collagen metabolism as possible indicators of disease in the adult respiratory distress syndrome. Am Rev Respir Dis 1993; 147:1091-1099.
77. Zapol W, Trelstad R, Coffey J, et al: Pulmonary fibrosis in severe acute respiratory failure. Am Rev Respir Dis 1979; 119:547-554.
78. Henke C, Fiegel V, Peterson M, et al: Identification and partial characterization of angiogenesis bioactivity in the lower respiratory tract after acute lung injury. J Clin Invest 1991; 88:1386-1395.
79. Polunovsky V, Chen B, Henke C, et al: Role of mesenchymal cell death in lung remodeling after injury. J Clin Invest 1993; 92:388-397.
80. Carrington CB: Organizing interstitial pneumonia: Definition of the lesion and attempts to devise an experimental model. Yale J Biol Med 1968; 40:352-363.
81. Katzenstein A-L: Pathogenesis of "fibrosis" in interstitial pneumonia: An electron microscopic study. Hum Pathol 1985; 16:1015-1024.
82. Burkhardt A: Alveolitis and collapse in the pathogenesis of pulmonary fibrosis. Am Rev Respir Dis 1989; 140:513-524.
83. Bell RC, Coalson JJ, Smith JD, et al: Multiple organ system failure and infection in adult respiratory distress syndrome. Ann Intern Med 1983; 99:293-298.
84. Montgomery A, Stager M, Carrico C, et al: Causes of mortality in patients with the adult respiratory distress syndrome. Am Rev Respir Dis 1985; 132:485-489.
85. Collins J, Smith J, Coalson J, et al: Variability in lung collagen amounts after prolonged support of acute respiratory failure. Chest 1984; 85:641-646.
86. Meduri G: Late adult respiratory distress syndrome. New Horiz 1993; 1:563-577.
87. Jones M, Langleben D, Reid L: Patterns of remodeling of the pulmonary circulation in acute and subacute lung injury. *In*: The Pulmonary Circulation and Acute Lung Injury. Said SI (Ed). Mount Kisco, NY, Futura Publishing, 1985, pp 137-188.
88. Coalson JJ: Pathology of sepsis, septic shock and multiple organ failure. *In*: New Horizons: Perspectives on Sepsis and Septic Shock. Sibbald WJ, Sprung CL (Eds): Fullerton, Calif, Society of Critical Care Medicine, 1986, pp 27-59.
89. Suchyta M, Clemmer T, Elliott C, et al: The adult respiratory distress syndrome: A report of survival and modifying factors. Chest 1992; 101:1074-1079.
90. Seidenfeld J, Pohl D, Bell R, et al: Incidence, site, and outcome of infections in patients with the adult respiratory distress syndrome. Am Rev Respir Dis 1986; 134:12-16.
91. Mancebo J, Artigas A: A clinical study of the adult respiratory distress syndrome. Crit Care Med 1987; 15:243-246.
92. Rinaldo J, Christman J: Mechanisms and mediators of the adult respiratory distress syndrome. Clin Chest Med 1990; 11:621-632.
93. Pittet J, Mackersie R, Martin T, et al: Biological markers of acute lung injury: Prognostic and pathogenetic significance. Am J Respir Crit Care Med 1997; 155:1187-1205.
94. Weiland J, Davis W, Holter J, et al: Lung neutrophils in the adult respiratory distress syndrome: Clinical and pathophysiologic significance. Am Rev Respir Dis 1986; 135:218-225.
95. Fowler A, Hyers T, Fisher B, et al: The adult respiratory distress syndrome: Cell populations and soluble mediators in the air spaces of patients at high risk. Am Rev Respir Dis 1987; 136:1225-1231.
96. Steinberg K, Milberg J, Martin T, et al: Evolution of bronchoalveolar cell populations in the adult respiratory distress syndrome. J Respir Crit Care Med 1994; 150:113-122.
97. Tate R, Repine J: Neutrophils and the adult respiratory distress syndrome. Am Rev Respir Dis 1983; 128:552-559.
98. Repine JE: Neutrophils, oxygen radicals, and the adult respiratory distress syndrome. *In*: The Pulmonary Circulation and Acute Lung Injury. Said S (Ed). Mount Kisco, New York, Futura Publishing, 1985, pp 249-381.
99. Rinaldo J, Borovetz H: Deterioration of oxygenation and abnormal lung microvascular permeability during resolution of leukopenia in patients with diffuse lung injury. Am Rev Respir Dis 1985; 131:579-583.
100. Boxer L, Axtell R, Suchard S: The role of the neutrophil in inflammatory diseases of the lung. Blood Cells 1990; 16:25-42.
101. Canonico A, Brigham K: Biology of acute injury. *In*: The Lung:

Scientific Foundations. 2nd ed. Crystal R, West J, Weibel E, Barne, P (Eds). Philadelphia, Lippincott-Raven, 1997, pp 2475–2498.
102. Baughman RP, Gunther KL, Rashkin MC, et al: Changes in the inflammatory response of the lung during acute respiratory distress syndrome: Prognostic indicators. Am J Respir Crit Care Med 1996; 154:76–81.
103. Goodman RB, Strieter RM, Steinberg KP, et al: Inflammatory cytokines in patients with persistence of the acute respiratory distress syndrome. Am J Respir Crit Care Med 1996; 154:602–611.
104. Schutte H, Lohmeyer J, Rosseau S, et al: Bronchoalveolar and systemic cytokine profiles in patients with ARDS, severe pneumonia and cardiogenic pulmonary oedema. Eur Respir J 1996; 9:1858–1867.
105. Kunkel S, Lukacs N, Chensue S, et al: Chemokines and the inflammatory response. *In*: Cytokines in Health and Disease. 2nd ed. Remick DG, Friedland JS (Eds). New York, Marcel Dekker, 1997, pp 121–131.
106. Miller E, Cohen A, Nagao S, et al: Elevated levels of NAP-1/interleukin-8 are present in the airspaces of patients with adult respiratory distress syndrome and are associated with increased mortality. Am Rev Respir Dis 1992; 146:427–432.
107. Chollet-Martin S, Montravers P, Gibert C, et al:. High levels of interleukin-8 in the blood and alveolar spaces of patients with pneumonia and adult respiratory distress syndrome. Infect Immun 1993; 61:4553–4559.
108. Torre D, Zeroli C, Giola M, et al: Levels of interleukin-8 in patients with adult respiratory distress syndrome. J Infect Dis 1993; 167:505–506.
109. Meduri GU, Kohler G, Headley S, et al: Inflammatory cytokines in the BAL of patients with ARDS: Persistent elevation over time predicts poor outcome. Chest 1995; 108:1303–1314.
110. Miller E, Cohen A, Matthay M: Increased interleukin-8 concentrations in the pulmonary edema fluid of patients with acute respiratory distress syndrome from sepsis. Crit Care Med 1996; 24:1448–1454.
111. Chollet-Martin S, Montravers P, Gibert A, et al: Relationship between polymorphonuclear neutrophils and cytokines in patients with adult respiratory distress syndrome. Ann N Y Acad Sci 1994; 725:354–366.
112. Roumen R, Hendriks T, van der Ven-Jongekrijg J, et al: Cytokine patterns in patients after major vascular surgery, hemorrhagic shock, and severe blunt trauma: Relation with subsequent adult respiratory distress syndrome and multiple organ failure. Ann Surg 1993; 218:769–776.

126

Pathophysiology of Acute Lung Injury

Robert W. Taylor, MD • Steven J. Trottier, MD

Acute respiratory distress syndrome (ARDS) is a broad term for catastrophic acute respiratory failure of diverse etiology and high mortality. It is commonly associated with sepsis and the multiple organ dysfunction syndrome. ARDS is generally characterized by a violent and apparently chaotic immunologic reaction leading to diffuse alveolar damage, pulmonary microvascular thrombosis, aggregation of inflammatory cells, and stagnation of blood flow through the lungs. This chain reaction gives rise to increased pulmonary capillary permeability and excessive extravascular lung water. Once started, the pathophysiologic cascade leads to intense arterial hypoxemia, pulmonary arterial hypertension, radiographic evidence of pulmonary edema, and stiff, noncompliant lungs. Implicit in the foregoing description is that ARDS is *not* a single disease but rather a pathophysiologic syndrome. Patients with increased pulmonary capillary filtration pressures causing "cardiogenic" pulmonary edema and those with chronic lung disease are characteristically excluded from this grouping for epidemiologic reasons. Experience has taught us, however, that patients with heart failure or chronic lung disease are not "protected" from ARDS; indeed, the conditions can coexist.

Ashbaugh and Petty and their colleagues[1, 2] drew attention to this syndrome and are credited with the acronym *ARDS*. Many highly accurate and interesting clinical descriptions of this syndrome, however, may be found in literature of the early 1900s.[3–6] Over the years, this form of acute respiratory failure has been referred to by many colorful and descriptive names[7] (Table 126–1). Grouping acute lung injury due to diverse causes under a single name has been questioned.[8–10] Some writers suggest that use of the term ARDS oversimplifies, creates ambiguity, and hampers research.[11] Cases fulfilling clinical criteria for ARDS might on the surface appear similar but may, in fact, have distinctly different pathophysiologic underpinnings. There is little question that use of the term is commonplace in critical care settings. We believe that the term ARDS has clinical utility because it creates a conceptual foundation on which supportive care may be based. Clinicians are advised to be mindful that the pathophysiology of this syndrome is incompletely understood and may vary according to the cause. Accepted clinical definitions of ARDS generally contain the following elements:

- Severe arterial hypoxemia
- Bilateral radiographic infiltrates consistent with pulmonary edema
- Reduced lung compliance
- Presence of a definable catastrophic event or of risk factors

Criteria for the diagnosis of ARDS used in clinical trials have varied over the years. Much of the controversy surrounding this syndrome stems from lack of precise clinical definitions. The American Thoracic Society and the European Society of Intensive Care Medicine held a consensus conference in 1994 from which uniform definitions of acute lung injury (ALI) and ARDS were developed.[12] *Acute lung injury* was defined as a syndrome of increased alveolar-capillary membrane permeabil-

TABLE 126–1. Synonyms for Acute (Adult) Respiratory Distress Syndrome

Adult hyaline membrane disease
Adult respiratory insufficiency syndrome
Congestive atelectasis
Da Nang lung
Hemorrhagic atelectasis
Hemorrhagic lung syndrome
Hypoxic hyperventilation
Postperfusion lung
Post-traumatic atelectasis
Post-traumatic pulmonary insufficiency
Progressive pulmonary consolidation
Progressive respiratory distress
Pump lung
Shock lung
Transplant lung
Traumatic wet lung
Wet lung
White lung

From Taylor RW, Duncan CA: The adult respiratory distress syndrome. Resident Med 1983; 1:17.)

ity associated with a constellation of clinical, radiologic, and physiologic findings not explained by left atrial or pulmonary capillary hypertension. Specific criteria for diagnosis of ALI are as follows:

1. Impaired arterial oxygenation with a Pa_{O_2}/FI_{O_2} ratio ≤ 300 irrespective of the level of positive end-expiratory pressure (PEEP).
2. Bilateral infiltrates on frontal chest radiograph.
3. A pulmonary artery occlusion pressure ≤ 18 mm Hg or no clinical findings suggestive of increased left atrial pressure.

The term ARDS is reserved for the more severe end of the ALI spectrum. Criteria for the diagnosis of ARDS are the same as those used for ALI, except that a Pa_{O_2}/FI_{O_2} ratio cut-off of ≤ 200 is used to confirm the diagnosis of ARDS.

The severity of ARDS is variable. A useful lung injury scoring system incorporating radiographic appearance, severity of hypoxemia, level of PEEP used, and respiratory system compliance has been described[13] (Table 126–2).

Elevations of CK-MB (the isoenzyme of creatine kinase containing muscle and brain subunits) and troponin 1 are rather sensitive and specific biochemical markers for the diagnosis of acute myocardial infarction. Likewise, marked elevations of aminotransferases suggest the presence of hepatocellular damage. Unfortunately, no such test exists to accurately diagnose or predict the outcome of ARDS. Measurement of pulmonary endothelial protein permeability has been studied but is rather cumbersome and poorly predictive of progression to ARDS.[14] Several markers of endothelial damage have been studied, including complement component C5a,[15] terminal complement complex,[16] and von Willebrand's factor antigen.[17] Although numerous cytokines circulate at increased levels in patients with ARDS, they do not predict development of this syndrome.[18–22] Various confounding problems have hindered interpretation of elevations of these markers. No simple biochemical test exists to confirm the diagnosis of ARDS convincingly or to predict outcome, but as the molecular biology of this syndrome is further unraveled, perhaps clinically useful diagnostic markers will surface.

TABLE 126–2. Components and Individual Values of the Lung Injury Score

Component		Value
Chest roentgenogram score		
No alveolar consolidation		0
Alveolar consolidation confined to 1 quadrant		1
Alveolar consolidation confined to 2 quadrants		2
Alveolar consolidation confined to 3 quadrants		3
Alveolar consolidation in all 4 quadrants		4
Hypoxemia score		
Pa_{O_2}/FI_{O_2}	>300	0
Pa_{O_2}/FI_{O_2}	225–299	1
Pa_{O_2}/FI_{O_2}	175–224	2
Pa_{O_2}/FI_{O_2}	100–174	3
Pa_{O_2}/FI_{O_2}	<100	4
PEEP score (during mechanical ventilation)		
PEEP	≤5 cm H_2O	0
PEEP	6–8 cm H_2O	1
PEEP	9–11 cm H_2O	2
PEEP	12–14 cm H_2O	3
PEEP	≥15 cm H_2O	4

The final value is obtained by dividing the aggregate sum by the number of components that were used

	Score
No lung injury	0
Mild to moderate lung injury	0.1–2.5
Severe lung injury (ARDS)	>2.5

From Murray JF, Matthay MA, Luce JM, et al: An expanded definition of the adult respiratory distress syndrome. Am Rev Respir Dis 1988;138:720.

ARDS = acute respiratory distress syndrome; Pa_{O_2}/FI_{O_2} = ratio of arterial oxygen tension to inspired oxygen concentration; PEEP = positive end-expiratory pressure.

INCIDENCE

Garber and colleagues[23] and others[24, 25] systematically reviewed the English language literature and found that the published population-based incidence of ARDS ranges from 1.5 to 5.3 per 100,000 population per year. An important part of the problem in determining exact incidence has been lack of a precise definition of ARDS prior to the American-European consensus conference.[12] The incidence appears lower when more strict criteria are applied.[26–28] On the practical side, the syndrome occurs commonly enough to consume much of a critical care practitioner's time, energy, and resources.

ETIOLOGY

Numerous, varied conditions have been causally related to ARDS (Table 126–3). Most of our therapy for ARDS remains supportive; however, in many cases, specific, targeted therapy is essential, making a thorough search for the cause critical. Risk factors for ARDS have been identified.[29, 30] Those that seem to place patients at greatest risk are sepsis (especially gram-negative septic shock), multiple emergency transfusions, near-drowning, pulmonary contusion, aspiration of gastric contents, multiple fractures, and drug overdose. Pepe and coworkers[31] reported an additive effect of risk factors; they found that ARDS developed in 25% of patients with a single risk factor, in 42% of patients with two risk factors, and in 85% of patients with three risk factors.

Important questions remain:

- Do these varied causes result in the same disease?
- Are the conditions listed in Table 126–3 directly causal, or do some of them represent epiphenomena?
- Is the pulmonary edema caused by aspiration of gastric contents the same disease as neoplastic pulmonary emboli?
- Is ARDS in the setting of gram-negative septic shock the same as ARDS associated with heroin injection?

Subsets of this syndrome with distinct molecular biologic, immunologic, and pathophysiologic features certainly exist.

Sepsis and Multiple Organ Dysfunction

The pathophysiologic processes in sepsis, septic shock, multiple organ dysfunction syndrome, and ARDS are closely linked. Many researchers believe that what we call ARDS is simply the pulmonary manifestation of a systemic inflammatory response gone askew.[32] The biology of the initiators and mediators is currently under intense investigation. ARDS develops in about 25% of patients with gram-negative sepsis and has been reported in 90% of patients with gram-negative septic shock.[33, 34]

Sepsis-induced ARDS has a higher mortality than ARDS associated with other risk factors.[35] If sepsis is the cause of ARDS, the source of infection is typically the abdomen. Sepsis is six times more likely to develop subsequently in noninfected patients with ARDS than in other patients in the intensive care unit (ICU) without ARDS. When sepsis follows ARDS, the source of infection is typically the lung.

TABLE 126–3. Conditions Associated with the Acute Respiratory Distress Syndrome

Shock	Salicylates
Septic	Chlordiazepoxide
Hemorrhagic	Colchicine
Cardiogenic	Dextran 40, 70
Anaphylactic	Ergotamine
Aspiration of Gastric Contents (Especially with a pH < 2.5)	Organophosphates
Trauma	Paraquat
Pulmonary contusion	Ritodrine
Multiple fractures	Cystosine arabinoside
Systemic inflammatory response syndrome	Bleomycin
Nonthoracic Trauma (Especially Head Trauma)	Contrast medium
Near-drowning	***Metabolic***
Burns	Renal failure
Fat embolism	Hepatic failure
Crush injury	Diabetic ketoacidosis
Infection	***Miscellaneous***
Bacterial (especially gram-negative sepsis)	Pancreatitis
Viral	Extracorporeal circulation
Fungal	Cardioversion
Mycobacterial (miliary tuberculosis)	Multiple transfusions
Parasitic	Disseminated intravascular coagulation
Inhalation of Toxic Gases and Fumes	Leukoagglutinin reaction
Oxygen (high concentration)	Eclampsia
Smoke	Chorioamnionitis
Nitrogen dioxide	Amniotic fluid emboli
Ammonia	Air emboli
Chlorine	Bowel infarction
Sulfur dioxide	Neoplastic pulmonary emboli
Cadmium	High-dose irradiation
Phosgene	Hanging
Drugs and Poisons	Airway obstruction
Cocaine	High altitude
Heroin	Autologous bone marrow transfusion
Methadone	Suction lipectomy
Barbiturates	Acute myocardial infarction
Ethchlorvynol	Volume overload
Thiazides	Baby powder inhalation
Fluorescein	Still's disease
Propoxyphene	Systemic lupus erythematosus
	Mixed essential cryoglobulinemia

Modified from Taylor RW, Duncan CA: The adult respiratory distress syndrome. Resident Med 1983; 1:17.

Trauma

Severely injured patients are at high risk for development of ARDS.[36] Both thoracic trauma and extrathoracic trauma are associated with development of ARDS. Multiple factors are operative: direct lung contusion, hemorrhagic shock, multiple transfusion, aspiration of gastric contents, head injury, infection, and long bone fractures with associated fat embolization.[37, 38] A nearly threefold incidence of ARDS occurs in the trauma patient who has sepsis.[39]

Aspiration of Gastric Contents

ARDS has been variously reported to occur in 34%[29] and in 15%[30] of patients who aspirated gastric contents. Aspiration appears to be a particularly important cause of ARDS if the pH of the inhaled material is less than 2.5;[40, 41] however, ARDS also occurs in the absence of severe acidity.[42]

Blood Transfusions

Transfusion-related acute lung injury may be caused by pulmonary microembolism with platelet-fibrin microaggregates, leukoagglutination reactions, or incorrectly crossmatched blood.[43–45] Many patients who have massive transfusion requirements may have one or more additional risk factors for ARDS, such as hemorrhagic shock, making it difficult to confidently implicate blood transfusion as the sole cause of the ARDS.

PATHOPHYSIOLOGY

The Inflammatory Response

Despite the multiple causes of ARDS, the pathophysiologic consequences are remarkably uniform. An intense inflammatory response causing acute alveolar and endothelial damage; increased vascular permeability, lung water, and protein; and deterioration in gas exchange set the stage for development of ARDS (see subsequent chapters in this section).

The initiators and mediators of the systemic inflammatory response syndrome are currently undergoing careful study.[46–49] Macrophages have an important role in recognizing initiators such as endotoxin, releasing cytokines, and modulating the inflammatory response (Table 126–4). A series of cell surface adhesion molecules (selectins, integrins, intercellular adhesion molecules) are also involved in this highly complex sequence of events. Abundant evidence suggests that the inflammatory mediators act to recruit neutrophils to the pulmonary microcirculation during the early stages of ARDS.[50–55] Indeed, the chemotactic response of neutrophils in patients with ARDS is more than twice normal.[56] Surface adhesion receptors slow and then tightly bind neutrophils to the pulmonary capillary endothelial surface. Neutrophils subsequently release many histotoxic agents in patients with ARDS.[57]

TABLE 126–4. Inflammatory Mediators in Acute Respiratory Distress Syndrome

Cytokines	Prostaglandins
Interleukins	Leukotrienes
Tumor necrosis factor	Vasoactive peptides
Interferons	Serotonin
Complement proteins	Histamine
Contact activation proteins	Platelet-activating factors
Bradykinin	
Coagulation proteins	
Thrombin	
Fibrin degradation products	

From Foner BJ, Norwood S, Taylor RW: The acute respiratory distress syndrome *In*: Critical Care. 3rd ed. Civetta JM, Taylor RW, Kirby RR (Eds). Philadelphia, Lippincott-Raven, 1997, pp 1825–1839.

Endotoxin

Lipopolysaccharide (LPS) of gram-negative bacteria is the most common and best studied initiator of the inflammatory process leading to ALI and ARDS.[58] Lipopolysaccharide-binding protein (LPB) increases in concentration more than 100-fold within 24 hours of endotoxin release into the circulation. Lipid A binds to LPB, and this complex in turn binds to CD14 receptors on macrophages, monocytes, and neutrophils. CD14 receptor binding by the LBP-LPS complex promotes transcription of genes encoding proinflammatory cytokines, such as tumor necrosis factor–α (TNF-α) and interleukins IL-1 and IL-6.

Cytokines

Secretion of cytokines into the circulation is a central feature of systemic inflammation that leads to acute lung injury.[59] TNF-α, IL-1, IL-6, and IL-8 are early-response cytokines that interact in a complex manner to initiate, sustain, and, in some cases, down-regulate the systemic inflammatory response.[60]

Selectins

Selectins are a family of molecules that promote neutrophil adhesion to the endothelial surface.[61] These single-chain glycoprotein molecules are designated E, P, and L for endothelial, platelet, and leukocyte selectin, respectively. E-selectins and P-selectins are expressed on the endothelial cell surface; L-selectin is expressed on leukocytes.[62–65]

β_2-Integrins and Intercellular Adhesion Molecule-1

The β_2-integrins are glycoproteins that are expressed on the surface of leukocytes.[66] Intercellular adhesion molecule-1 (ICAM-1) is expressed on the endothelial cell surface.

Neutrophil-Endothelium Interactions

Within minutes to hours following exposure to proinflammatory mediators, endothelial surfaces display selectins P and E. Selectin-neutrophil bonds are characteristically weak, and binding is therefore transient as shear forces within the capillary cause breakage of the bonds. The bonds are thus formed and broken repeatedly, giving rise to slowed movement and rolling of neutrophils along the endothelial surface. Simultaneous neutrophil activation promotes increased integrin expression on the cell. Because of the slowed movement, neutrophil integrins are then able to form tight bonds with ICAM-1 on the endothelial cell surface, thus promoting adhesion of the neutrophil to the endothelial cell. Once tightly adherent to the endothelial cell, neutrophils release reactive oxygen intermediates, hydrogen peroxide, and proteolytic enzymes that cause endothelial cell damage (Table 126–5).

Pulmonary Edema Formation and Microcirculatory Injury

Formation of Pulmonary Edema

Movement of water through the pulmonary capillary endothelium is determined by the balance of hydrostatic and oncotic pressures opposing one another across the membrane.[67] The Starling equation, quantitating fluid filtration across the pulmonary endothelial membrane, is written as follows:

$$Q_f = K\,(P_{CAP} - P_{INT}) - \sigma\,(\pi_{CAP} - \pi_{INT})$$

where Q_f is net transvascular fluid flow; K is filtration coefficient; P_{CAP} is pulmonary capillary hydrostatic pressure; P_{INT} is pulmonary perivascular interstitial space hydrostatic pressure; σ is the reflection coefficient (a measure of the effectiveness of the membrane in preventing flow of solute as compared to flow of water); π_{CAP} is pulmonary capillary oncotic pressure; and π_{INT} is pulmonary perivascular interstitial space oncotic pressure.

Formation of pulmonary edema in ARDS is caused by a derangement of alveolar capillary permeability.[68] Endothelial and epithelial intercellular junctions are probably the primary foci of fluid flow. Increases in both water and protein flux occur from the capillary space to the interstitial and intra-alveolar spaces at normal to low hydrostatic pressures. The exact mechanisms that lead to intercellular junctional changes are incompletely understood. Furthermore, it is not clear whether all permeability changes act through a common pathway.

Endothelial Injury

Endothelial injury has been well-studied in ALI and ARDS. Within 30 minutes of endotoxin infusion in sheep, increased interstitial edema is found.[69] Within 1 hour, electron microscopic evidence of endothelial injury can be observed.[70] Cell retraction, reduction in barrier function, and cell death occur.[71] Injured endothelial cells not only lead to a breach in barrier function but also contribute to progression of ALI by altering cell surface expression of adhesion molecules and production of prostanoids and cytokines.[72, 73]

Lung vascular reactivity is altered in acute lung injury, probably as a consequence of direct endothelial damage and recruitment of inflammatory cells. Many of the important details of the vascular smooth muscle contractile response are unknown for acute lung injury. Leukotrienes likely have an important role in the initial pulmonary hypertension seen in acute lung injury.

Epithelial Injury

Matthay[74] has described the importance of alveolar epithelial injury. Extensive morphologic damage to the epithelial barrier

TABLE 126–5. Histotoxic Neutrophil Products

Oxidants and Radicals	*Proteolytic Enzymes*
Superoxide anion	Elastase
Hydrogen peroxide	Gelatinase
Hydroxyl radical	Collagenase
Hypochlorous acid	Cathepsin
Chloramines	Lysozyme
Nitric acid	Neuraminidase
	Heparanase
Other	
Cationic proteins	

From Zimmerman G, Renzetti A, Hill R: Functional and metabolic acitivity of granulocytes from patients with adult respiratory distress syndrome. Am Rev Respir Dis 1983; 127:290.

occurs within the first 48 to 72 hours following acute lung injury. The presence of high concentrations of protein within pulmonary edema fluid in patients with ARDS confirms the presence of injury to both pulmonary endothelium and alveolar epithelium. Work from an experimental sheep model suggests that an active sodium transport mechanism is responsible for removing excess alveolar fluid.[75, 76] It appears that a sodium-potassium–adenosine triphosphatase (Na, K-ATPase) enzyme is responsible for the active removal of sodium from the basolateral surface of alveolar epithelial cells. As sodium is removed from the air spaces, chloride and water follow. β-Adrenergic therapy appears to accelerate removal of fluid from the alveolar air spaces.[77] Little information is available on pathways of fluid removal by this mechanism; it likely occurs by paracellular or transcellular routes. Alterations in pulmonary and bronchial artery blood flow do not appear to affect this mechanism.[78] The alveolar-epithelial barrier appears to be more resistant to injury than the endothelial membrane.

Ventilator-Induced Pulmonary Edema

Ventilatory strategies that apply high transalveolar stretching forces cause or extend tissue edema in experimental animals.[79-85] Failure to preserve a certain minimum end-expiratory pressure may intensify preexisting alveolar damage. The damage is thought to be secondary to shear forces associated with tidal collapse and reinflation in injured alveolar tissues.

Histologic Changes

Alveolar gas is separated from capillary hemoglobin by a very thin alveolocapillary membrane. The alveolar cells are supported by a basement membrane, as are the capillary endothelial cells. Between the basement membranes lies the interstitial space, containing interstitial fluid, connective tissue, and scattered fibroblasts. When acute lung injury occurs, the endothelium becomes increasingly permeable to fluid and protein. Interstitial fluid accumulates and soon overwhelms the lymphatic drainage system. If this pathophysiologic process progresses, interstitial edema is followed by alveolar flooding. Alveolar surface cells (type I) are sensitive to insult, and many are destroyed in the first hours to days after injury.

Within several days, the denuded alveolar basement membrane is covered with proliferating alveolar type II cells. Plasma proteins, cellular debris, fibrin, and surfactant remnants aggregate to form hyaline membranes that cover the bare basement membrane of alveoli and alveolar ducts. The normally thin alveolocapillary membrane widens, with the accumulation of more fluid, proliferating fibroblasts, plasma cells, leukocytes, and histiocytes during the course of the next week. After a week to 10 days, fibrosis of the hyaline membrane, alveolar septum, and alveolar duct may occur.[86]

These histologic changes do not occur in their entirety in all patients. In some patients, the process is arrested midstream and resolves. Why one case resolves and another progresses is not known but probably relates to the nature and severity of the original insult. Even patients with extensive fibrosis may have partial resolution of the damage.[87]

Surfactant

Surfactant is critical in maintaining normal lung function. It is secreted by alveolar type II cells and decreases surface tension as it coats the alveolar lining, serving to keep alveoli open and participating in gas exchange. Various surfactant abnormalities occur in ARDS, including an alteration in the amount of surfactant made as well as its chemical composition. Furthermore, serum proteins found in the alveolar space in ARDS inactivate surfactant. Although these surfactant abnormalities are not primary in ARDS, they promote alveolar collapse and contribute to altered gas exchange.[88, 89]

Lung Mechanics and Gas Exchange

Alveolar flooding coupled with qualitative and quantitative surfactant abnormalities leads to widespread atelectasis. Reduced functional residual capacity is a hallmark of ARDS. Fluid-filled and collapsed alveoli are difficult to expand, thus explaining the reduction in lung compliance noted in this syndrome.[90] Furthermore, increased airway resistance to gas flow has been described in some patients.[91] The severe hypoxemia that occurs in ARDS most certainly results from advanced alveolar flooding and alveolar collapse, leading to intrapulmonary shunting and areas of low ventilation-perfusion (V/Q).[92]

Extrapulmonary Organ Failure

ARDS likely represents the pulmonary expression of a systemic inflammatory process that causes dysfunction of many other organ systems[93] (Table 126–6). The mechanisms of multiple organ dysfunction are incompletely understood. Many of the mediators that lead to acute lung injury (see Table 126–4) probably are also operative in other organ dysfunctions. Leading hypotheses suggest that mediators lead to altered tissue blood flow by various mechanisms. Overperfusion of tissues with low oxygen extraction ratios may coexist with areas of relative underperfusion. Arteriovenous shunting may increase in some tissue beds, leaving affected organs underperfused. The ability to recruit capillaries at the tissue level may also be lost or diminished, further impairing the ability to adjust to local tissue needs. Direct endothelial or parenchymal injury may result in organ edema and may increase diffusion distances for oxygen and substrate delivery. Under these circumstances, the gut mucosal barrier to bacteria may be compromised, resulting in translocation of bacteria or bacterial products from the gut lumen to the systemic circulation. Thus, once initiated, the systemic inflammatory response may be perpetuated and amplified by various mechanisms.

CLINICAL FEATURES

Many of the specific clinical features of ARDS depend on the cause. Tachypnea and tachycardia usually develop in the first 12 to 24 hours after the initial insult. A clinically apparent increase in work of breathing becomes obvious. High-pitched end-expiratory crackles are heard throughout the lung fields during auscultation.

Radiographic changes become evident early in the course. An increase in interstitial markings gives way to more dense "alveolar" infiltrates as alveolar flooding occurs (Fig. 126–1). The infiltrates are typically seen diffusely; however, they may start as a focal process and then generalize.[94, 95] Several scoring systems have been developed to help quantify the increased lung water.[96, 97] Computed tomographic (CT) scanning of patients with ARDS has given us a different view of distribution patterns. Although a plain chest radiograph might suggest diffuse and uniform distribution of pulmonary edema, a CT scan suggests a more patchy distribution of infiltrates favoring the dependent portions of the lung.[98-102]

As the syndrome progresses and diffuse fibrosis ensues, the chest radiograph may have a patchy or nodular appearance. The application of positive-pressure ventilation and PEEP alters the radiographic appearance. PEEP does not decrease lung water but rather increases functional residual capacity, making the lungs appear better aerated on a chest radiograph. Careful search of the chest radiograph should be made for

TABLE 126–6. Complications Associated with Acute Respiratory Distress Syndrome

Pulmonary	***Complications Attributable to Intubation and Extubation***
Pulmonary emboli	Prolonged attempt at intubation
Pulmonary barotrauma	Intubation of a mainstem bronchus
Oxygen toxicity	Premature extubation
	Self-extubation
Gastrointestinal	***Complications Associated with Endotracheal/ Tracheostomy Tubes***
Gastrointestinal hemorrhage	Tube malfunction
Ileus	Nasal necrosis
Gastric distention	Paranasal sinus infection
Pneumoperitoneum	Tracheal stenosis
Renal	Tracheomalacia
Renal failure	Polyps
Fluid retention	Erosion
Cardiovascular	Fistulas
Invasive catheters	Airway obstruction
Arrhythmia	Hoarseness
Hypotension	***Complications Attributable to Operation of the Ventilator***
Low cardiac output	Machine failure
Infection	Alarm failure
Sepsis	Alarms silenced
Nosocomial pneumonia	Inadequate nebulization or humidification
Hematologic	***Complications Occurring During Positive Airway Pressure Therapy***
Anemia	Alveolar hypoventilation
Thrombocytopenia	Alveolar hyperventilation
Disseminated intravascular coagulation	Massive gastric distention
Other	Barotrauma
Hepatic	Atelectasis
Endocrine	Pneumonia
Neurologic	Hypotension
Psychiatric	
Malnutrition	

From Taylor RW: The adult respiratory distress syndrome. *In*: Respiratory Failure. Kirby RR, Taylor RW (Eds.). Chicago, Year Book Medical Publishers, 1986, pp 208–244.

mediastinal emphysema, subcutaneous emphysema, and pneumothorax (Figs. 126–2 and 126–3). A normal-sized cardiac silhouette sometimes helps to distinguish ARDS from "cardiogenic" pulmonary edema. Chest radiographic findings return to normal in as many as 80% of patients who survive ARDS.

TREATMENT

Complications

Numerous potential complications are associated with the treatment of patients with ARDS[103] (see Table 126–6). The staff caring for these patients must be cognizant of these complications and must respond promptly to them. Preventive measures, such as prophylaxis of deep vein thrombosis and stress ulcers, are strongly encouraged.

Experimental Therapies

Because of the intense inflammatory response in ALI and ARDS, use of anti-inflammatory therapy is theoretically attractive. Indeed, in past years, corticosteroids were commonly used for patients with these disorders. Randomized controlled trials,[104, 105] however, demonstrated that methylprednisolone was not effective in either preventing or treating ARDS in its early stages. Interest has now surfaced in the use of corticosteroids to treat the fibroproliferative stages of ARDS.[106] Randomized, controlled trials to document patient benefit are currently awaited.

Numerous other anti-inflammatory agents have been studied in patients with sepsis and ARDS (Table 126–7), but none has been associated with a reduction in mortality.[107–113]

Ketoconazole, which inhibits thromboxane A_2 synthetase, showed promise in preventing ARDS in patients at risk in a small clinical trial.[114] A large multicenter trial sponsored by the National Heart Lung and Blood Institute evaluating ketoconazole in this role is currently under way, and its results are anxiously awaited.

Surfactant is functionally abnormal in ARDS.[115] Neonates with respiratory distress syndrome clearly benefit from surfactant therapy.[116] Unfortunately, administration of surfactant to adults with ARDS has demonstrated no significant physiologic improvement or reduction in mortality.[117, 118]

The first prospective, randomized, controlled trial involving extracorporeal membrane oxygenation (ECMO) in the management of ARDS was reported in 1979.[119] Ninety patients entered the study; 48 were randomly assigned to receive conventional mechanical ventilation, and 42 to receive conventional mechanical ventilation supplemented with partial venoarterial bypass; survival rates for these groups were 8.3% and 9.5%, respectively. Enthusiasm for ECMO waned until 1986, when Gattinoni and colleagues[120] reported an impressive 49% survival rate in an uncontrolled trial using low-

TABLE 126–7. Experimental Anti-inflammatory Agents in Sepsis and Acute Respiratory Distress Syndrome*

Corticosteroids[85–87]
Prostaglandin E_1[88]
Antiendotoxin antibodies[89]
Interleukin-1 receptor antagonists[90]
Platelet-activating factor receptor antagonists[91]
Anti–tumor necrosis factor antibodies[92]
N-Acetylcysteine[93]
Ibuprofen[94]
Ketoconazole[95]

*Superscript numbers indicate chapter references.

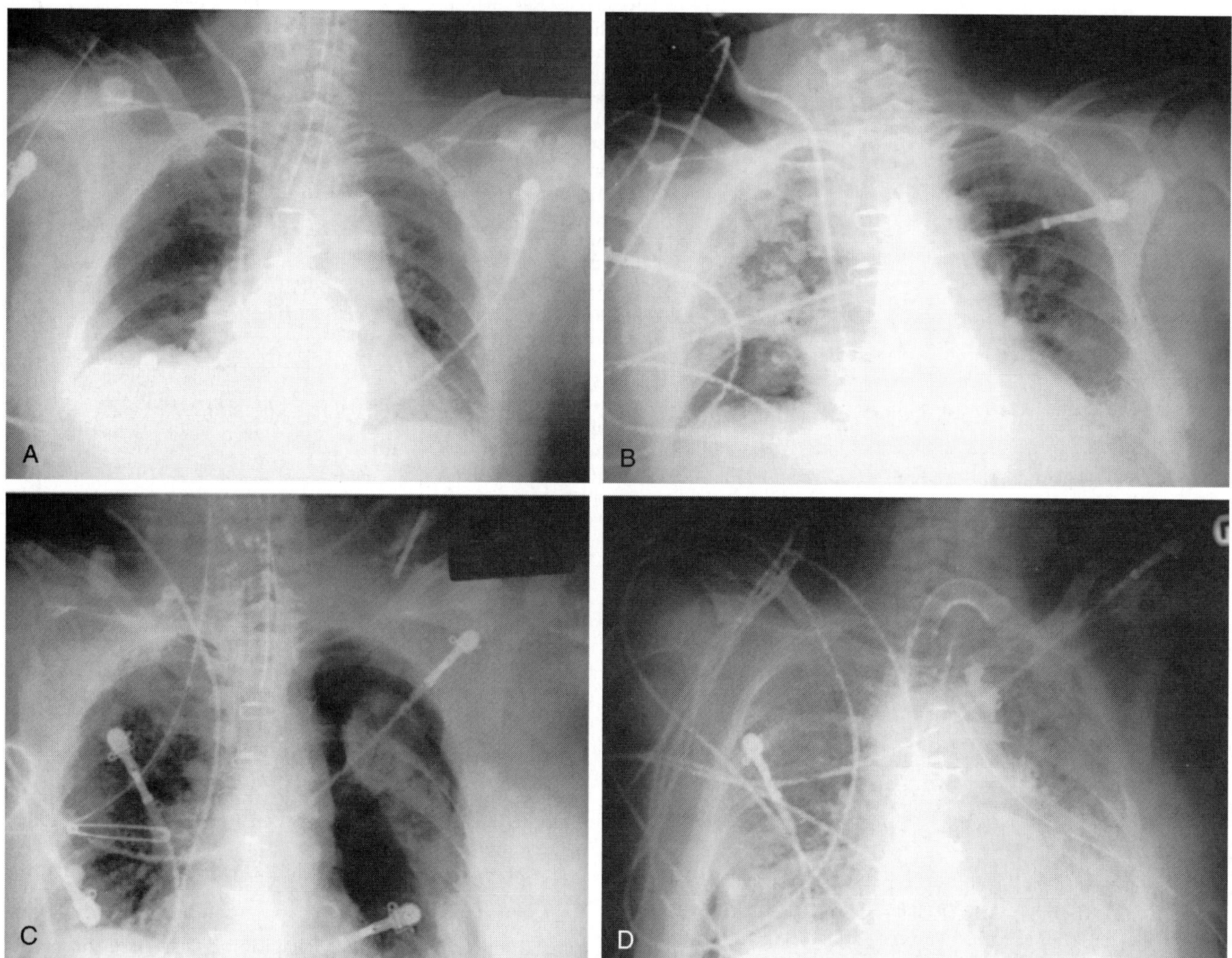

Figure 126–1. Many of the common radiographic feature of acute respiratory distress syndrome are shown in chest radiographs. All radiographs are portable (anteroposterior projection). *A*, A 62-year-old woman with a prior history of coronary artery bypass surgery underwent abdominal aortic aneurysm resection. This relatively unremarkable chest radiograph was obtained on the day of the operation immediately upon her arrival in the intensive care unit. She was extubated during the morning of the first postoperative day. *B*, Because of her increasing respiratory difficulty, this radiograph was obtained during the afternoon of the first postoperative day. Interstitial and alveolar infiltrates can be seen throughout the right lung field and in the left base. *C*, This radiograph was obtained on the 13th postoperative day. The patient remains intubated and mechanically ventilated. Diffuse infiltrates are seen throughout, and a large left pneumothorax is present. *D*, This radiograph was obtained on the 23rd postoperative day. Dense infiltrates are seen throughout all lung fields. The left lung is expanded. A left thoracostomy tube is in place. A tracheostomy tube is also in place. A small pneumothorax is present in the right costophrenic sulcus.

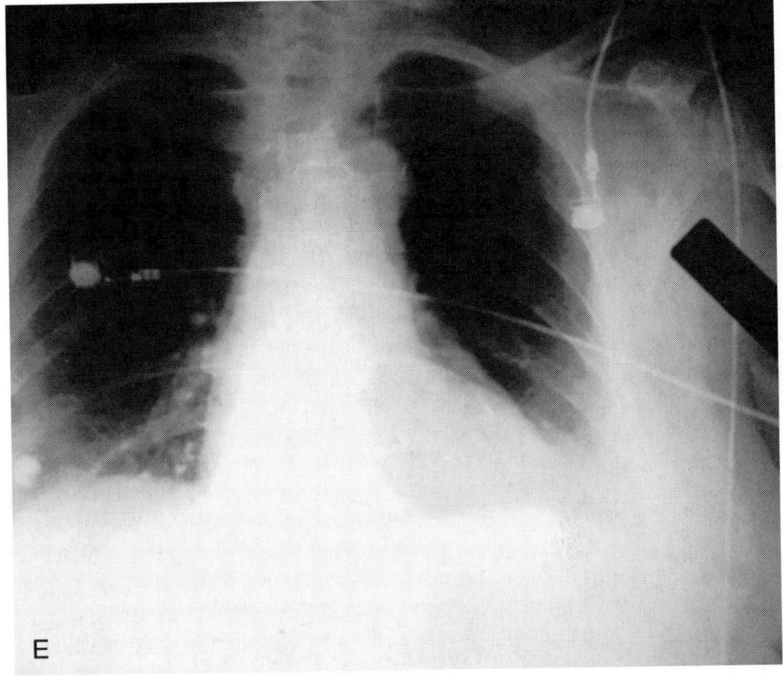

Figure 126–1 *Continued. E,* This radiograph was obtained on the 110th postoperative day. Mechanical ventilation had been discontinued, and the tracheostomy tube had been removed. The appearance of the chest radiograph returned to baseline values. One year later, this patient enjoyed an active and independent lifestyle.

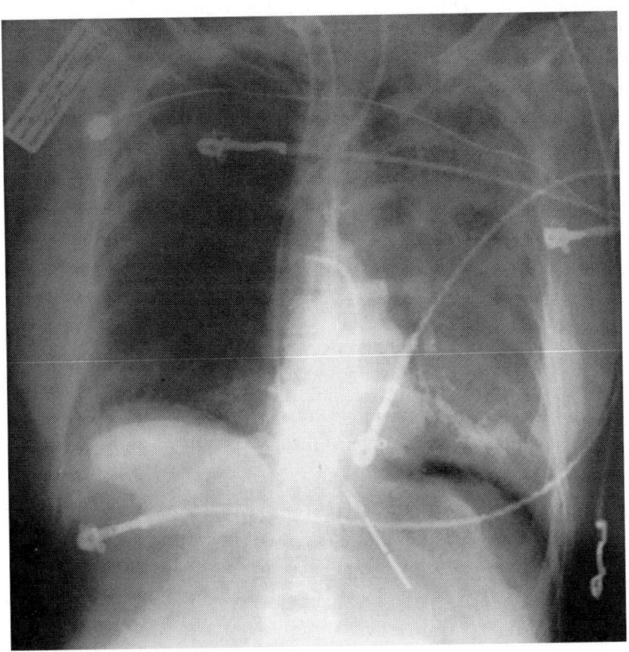

Figure 126–2. A 47-year-old woman had acute respiratory distress syndrome in association with intra-abdominal sepsis. This portable chest radiograph was taken with the patient in the supine position. Diffuse infiltrates appear more prominent on the left. Hyperlucency overlying the left uppper abdominal quadrant represents gas (pneumothorax) in the anterior costophrenic sulcus. Gas often rises to this most superior portion of the pleural space when a patient is in the supine position (deep sulcus sign).

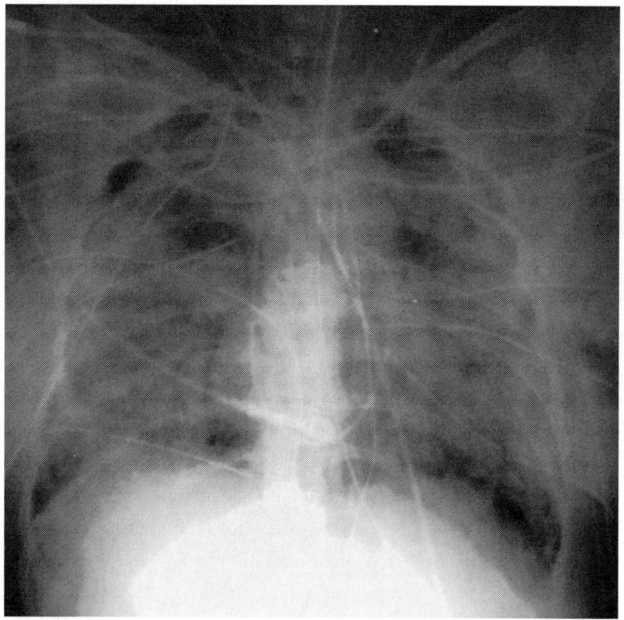

Figure 126–3. Acute respiratory distress syndrome developed in a 30-year-old woman with Crohn's disease following a small-bowel perforation and peritonitis. High peak and mean airway pressures were required. She sustained devastating barotrauma with multiple pneumothoraces. Large bronchopleural fistulas developed. A total of eight chest tubes were inserted over time in an attempt to expand her lungs. This patient died subsequent to single-organ system failure. She is one of the few patients in whom all attempts to achieve adequate oxygenation and ventilation failed.

frequency positive-pressure ventilation and extracorporeal carbon dioxide removal (venovenous LFPPV-$ECCO_2R$) with apneic oxygenation. Prospective, randomized, controlled trials comparing (1) conventional mechanical ventilation, (2) pressure-controlled inverse-ratio ventilation, and (3) LFPPV-$ECCO_2R$ with apneic oxygenation demonstrated equivalent survival rates for the three modalities.[121] Most experts recommend that extracorporeal support for ARDS should be restricted to clinical trials.[122]

Experimental therapies involving prone positioning, inhaled nitric oxide, partial liquid ventilation, and other ventilatory techniques, including pressure-controlled inverse ratio ventilation and permissive hypercapnia, are addressed elsewhere in this text.

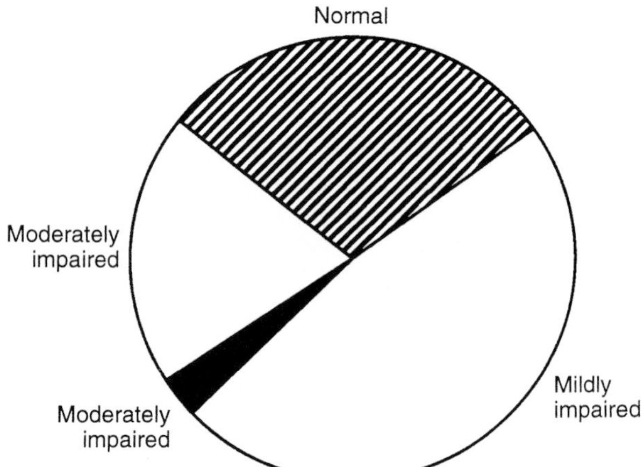

Figure 126–4. Most patients who survive acute respiratory distress syndrome have normal or mildly impaired pulmonary function when studied 1 year after development of the disorder. In this group of patients, symptoms did not correlate with pulmonary function. (Modified from Ghio AJ, Elliott CG, Crapo RO, et al: Impairment after adult respiratory distress syndrome: An evaluation based on American Thoracic Society recommendations. Am Rev Respir Dis 1989; 139:1158.)

OUTCOME

Death occurring within 3 days after the onset of ARDS is usually related to the underlying illness.[35] Later mortality in ARDS commonly results from sepsis or multiple organ failure. Irreversible respiratory failure accounts for approximately 16% of deaths in ARDS, although a rising incidence of death secondary to respiratory failure has been reported.[123] The mortality rate for ARDS is usually quoted as being in excess of 50%; later studies have suggested a rate of approximately 36%.[124, 125] A majority of patients who survive an episode of ARDS have normal or mildly impaired pulmonary function 1 year later. Symptoms are not associated with impairment of pulmonary function[126–129] (Fig. 126–4). Improvement in pulmonary function has been documented for up to 1 year after ARDS.[130]

References

1. Ashbaugh DE, Bigelow DB, Petty TL, et al: Acute respiratory distress in adults. Lancet 1967; 2:319.
2. Petty TL, Ashbaugh DG: The adult respiratory distress syndrome: Clinical features, factors influencing prognosis and principles of management. Chest 1971; 60:233.
3. Montgomery BA: Early description of ARDS. Chest 1991; 99:261.
4. Sloggett AT (Ed): Memorandum of the Treatment of Injuries in War. London, Harrison and Sons, 1915, pp 115–122.
5. Pasteur W: Massive collapse of the lung. Br J Surg 1914; 1:587.
6. Bradford JR: Massive collapse of the lung as a result of gunshot wounds with special reference to wounds of the chest. Q J Med 1919; 12:217.
7. Taylor RW, Duncan CA: The adult respiratory distress syndrome. Resident Med 1983; 1:17.
8. Fishman AP: Shock lung (a distinctive non-entity). Circulation 1973; 47:921.
9. Murray JF: The adult respiratory distress syndrome (may it rest in peace). Am Rev Respir Dis 1975; 111:716.
10. Petty TL: The adult respiratory distress syndrome: Confessions of a "lumper." Am Rev Respir Dis 1975; 111:713.
11. Rocker GM, Wiseman MS, Pearson D, et al: Diagnostic criteria for adult respiratory distress syndrome: Time for reappraisal. Lancet 1989; 1:120.
12. Bernard GR, Artigas A, Brigham KL, et al: The American-European consensus conference on ARDS definitions, mechanisms, relevant outcomes, and clinical trial coordination. Am J Respir Crit Care Med 1994; 149:818.

13. Murray JF, Matthay MA, Luce JM, et al: An expanded definition of the adult respiratory distress syndrome. Am Rev Respir Dis 1988; 138:720.
14. Jones DK: Markers for impending adult respiratory distress syndrome. Respir Med 1990; 84:89.
15. Hammerschmidt D, Weaver L, Hudson C, et al: Association of complement activation and elevated plasma-C5a with the adult respiratory distress syndrome: Pathophysiologic relevance and possible prognostic value. Lancet 1980; 1:947.
16. Langlois PF, Gawryl MS: Accentuated formation of the terminal C5b-9 complement complex in patient plasma precedes development of the adult respiratory distress syndrome. Am Rev Respir Dis 1988; 138:368.
17. Carvalho ACA, Bellman SM, Saullo VJ, et al: Altered factor VIII in acute respiratory failure. N Engl J Med 1982; 307:1113.
18. Parsons PE, Moss M, Vannice JL, et al: Circulating IL-1ra and IL-10 levels are increased but do not predict the development of acute respiratory distress syndrome in at risk patients. Am J Respir Crit Care Med 1997; 155:1469.
19. Leff JA, Parsons PE, Day CE, et al: Serum antioxidants as predictors of adult respiratory distress syndrome in patients with sepsis. Lancet 1993; 341:777.
20. Leff JA, Parsons PE, Day CE, et al: Increased serum catalase activity in septic patients with adult respiratory distress syndrome. Am Rev Respir Dis 1992; 146:985.
21. Rubin DB, Wiener-Kronish JP, Murray JF, et al: Elevated von Willebrand factor antigen is an early plasma predictor of acute lung injury in nonpulmonary sepsis. J Clin Invest 1990; 86:474.
22. Langleben D, DeMarchie M, LaPorta D, et al: Endothelin-1 in acute lung injury and the adult respiratory distress syndrome. Am Rev Respir Dis 1993; 148:1646.
23. Garber BR, Hebert PC, Yelle JD, et al: Adult respiratory distress syndrome: A systematic overview of incidence and risk factors. Crit Care Med 1996; 24:687.
24. Lung Program, National Heart and Lung Institute: Respiratory Diseases: Task Force on Problems, Research, Approaches, Needs. Bethesda, Md, U.S. Department of Health, Education and Welfare, Publication No. (NIH) 73-432. 1972, p 171.
25. Villar J, Slutsky AS: The incidence of the adult respiratory distress syndrome. Am Rev Respir Dis 1989; 140:814.
26. Webster NR, Cohen AT, Nunn JF: Adult respiratory distress syndrome: How many cases in the UK? Anesthesia 1988; 43:923.
27. Thomsen GE, Morris AH: Incidence of the adult respiratory distress syndrome in the state of Utah. Am J Respir Crit Care Med 1995; 152:965.
28. Lewandowski K, Metz J, Deutschmann C, et al: Incidence, severity and mortality of acute respiratory failure in Berlin, Germany. Am J Respir Crit Care Med 1995; 151:1121.
29. Fowler AA, Hamman RF, Good JT, et al: Adult respiratory distress syndrome: Risk with common predispositions. Ann Intern Med 1983; 98:593.
30. Hudson LD, Milberg JA, Anardi D, et al: Clinician risks for development of the acute respiratory distress syndrome. Am J Respir Crit Care Med 1995; 151:293.
31. Pepe PE, Potkin RT, Reus DH, et al: Clinical predictors of the adult respiratory distress syndrome. Am J Surg 1982; 144:124.
32. Welbourn CR, Young Y: Endotoxin, septic shock and acute lung injury: Neutrophils, macrophages and inflammatory mediators. Br J Surg 1992; 79:998.
33. Kaplan RL, Sahn SA, Petty TL: Incidence and outcome of the respiratory distress syndrome in gram-negative sepsis. Arch Intern Med 1979; 139:867.
34. Martin MA, Silverman HJ: Gram-negative sepsis and the adult respiratory distress syndrome. Clin Infect Dis 1992; 14:1213.
35. Montgomery AB, Stager MA, Carrico CJ, et al: Causes of mortality in patients with the adult respiratory distress syndrome. Am Rev Respir Dis 1985; 132:485.
36. Fulton RL, Jones CE: The cause of post-traumatic pulmonary insufficiency in man. Surg Gynecol Obstet 1975; 140:179.
37. Shoemaker WC, Appel P, Czer LSC, et al: Pathogenesis of respiratory failure (ARDS) after hemorrhage and trauma. Crit Care Med 1980; 8:504.
38. Lewis FR, Blaisdell W, Schlobohm RM: Incidence and outcome of post-traumatic respiratory failure. Arch Surg 1977; 112:436.
39. Horovitz JH, Carrico CJ, Shires GT: Pulmonary response to major injury. Arch Surg 1974; 108:349.
40. Mendelson CL: The aspiration of stomach contents into the lungs during obstetric anesthesia. Am J Obstet Gynecol 1946; 52:191.
41. Wynne JW, Modell JH: Respiratory aspiration of stomach contents. Ann Intern Med 1977; 87:466.
42. Schwartz DJ, Wynne JW, Gibbs CP, et al: Pulmonary consequences of aspiration of gastric contents at pH values greater than 2.5. Am Rev Respir Dis 1980; 121:119.
43. Popovsky MA, Chaplin HC Jr, Moore SB: Transfusion-related acute lung injury: A neglected, serious complication of hemotherapy. Transfusion 1992; 32:589.
44. Barrett J, Davidson I, Dhurandhar HN, et al: Pulmonary microembolism associated with massive transfusion: II. The basic pathophysiology of its pulmonary effects. Ann Surg 1975; 182:52.
45. Grindlinger GA, Vegas AM, Churchill WH, et al: Is respiratory failure a consequence of blood transfusion? J Trauma 1980; 20:627.
46. Chollet-Martin S, Jourdain B, Gibert C, et al: Interactions between neutrophils and cytokines in blood and alveolar spaces during ARDS. Am J Respir Crit Care Med 1996; 153:594.
47. Pugin J, Ricou B, Steinberg KP, et al: Proinflammatory activity in bronchoalveolar lavage fluids from patients with ARDS: A prominent role for interleukin-1. Am J Respir Crit Care Med 1996; 153:1850.
48. Goodman RB, Strieter RM, Martin DP, et al: Inflammatory cytokines in patients with persistence of the acute respiratory distress syndrome. Am J Respir Crit Care Med 1996; 154:602.
49. Baughman RP, Gunther KL, Rashkin MC, et al: Changes in the inflammatory response of the lung during acute respiratory distress syndrome: Prognostic indicators. Am J Respir Crit Care Med 1996; 154:76.
50. Horn JK, Lewis FR: Acute lung injury: Pathophysiology and diagnosis. *In*: Critical Care: State of the Art. Vol 12. Taylor RW, Shoemaker WC (Eds). Fullerton, Calif, Society of Critical Care Medicine, 1991, pp 1–31.
51. Sessler CN, Bloomfield GL, Fowler AA: Current concepts of sepsis and acute lung injury. Clin Chest Med 1996; 17:213.
52. Foner BJ, Norwood S, Taylor RW: The acute respiratory distress syndrome *In*: Critical Care. 3rd ed. Civetta JM, Taylor RW, Kirby RR (Eds). Philadelphia, Lippincott-Raven, 1997, pp 1825–1839.
53. Rinaldo JE, Rogers RM: Adult respiratory distress syndrome: Changing concepts of lung injury and repair. N Engl J Med 1982; 306:900.
54. Tate RM, Repive JE: Neutrophils and the adult respiratory distress syndrome. Am Rev Respir Dis 1983; 128:552.
55. Hasegawa N, Husari AW, Hart WT, et al: Role of the coagulation system in ARDS. Chest 1994; 105:268.
56. Zimmerman G, Renzetti A, Hill R: Functional and metabolic activity of granulocytes from patients with adult respiratory distress syndrome. Am Rev Respir Dis 1983; 127:290.
57. Donnelly SC, Haslett C: Cellular mechanisms of acute lung injury: Implications for future treatment in the adult respiratory distress syndrome. Thorax 1992; 47:260.
58. Schumann RR, Leong SR, Flaggs GW: Structure and function of lipopolysaccharide binding protein (LBP). Science 1990; 249:1429.
59. Darville T, Giroir B, Jacobs R: The systemic inflammatory response syndrome (SIRS): Immunology and potential immunotherapy. Infection 1993; 21:279.
60. Strieter RM, Kunkel SL, Bone RC: Role of tumor necrosis factor-α in disease states and inflammation. Crit Care Med 1993; 21:S447.
61. Bevilacqua MP, Nelson RM: Selectins. J Clin Invest 1993; 91:379.
62. Bevilacqua MP, Pober JS, Mendrick DL, et al: Identification of an inducible endothelial-leukocyte adhesion molecule. Proc Natl Acad Sci USA 1987; 84:9238.
63. Hsu-Lin SC, Berman CL, Furie BC, et al: A platelet membrane protein expressed during platelet activation and secretion. J Biol Chem 1984; 259:9121.
64. Bonfanti R, Furie BC, Furie B, et al: PADGEM (GMP-140) is a component of Weibel-Palade bodies of human endothelial cells. Blood 1989; 73:1109.
65. Anene C, Horgan MJ, Malik AB: GMP-140 (P-selectin) expression in thrombin-activated vascular endothelium in situ. FASEB J 1992; 6:14.
66. Carlos TM, Harlan JM: Membrane proteins involved in phagocyte adherence to endothelium. Immunol Rev 1990; 115:5.

67. Staub NC: Pulmonary edema. Physiol Rev 1974; 54:678.
68. Staub NC: Pulmonary edema due to increased microvascular permeability to fluid and protein. Circ Res 1978; 43:143.
69. Meyrick B, Brigham KL: Acute effects of *Escherichia coli* endotoxin on the pulmonary microcirculation of anesthetized sheep. Lab Invest 1990; 62:355.
70. Meyrick B, Ryan US, Brigham KL: Direct effects of *E. coli* endotoxin on structure and permeability of pulmonary endothelial monolayers and the endothelial layer of intimal explants. Am J Pathol 1986; 122:140.
71. Pober JC, Cotran RS: Cytokines and endothelial biology. Physiol Rev 1990; 70:427.
72. Suttorp N, Galanos C, Nuehof H: Endotoxin alters arachidonic acid metabolism in pulmonary endothelial cells. Am J Physiol 1987; 253:C384.
73. Libby P, Ordovas JM, Auger KR, et al: Endotoxin and tumor necrosis factor induce interleukin-1 gene expression in adult human vascular endothelial cells. Am J Pathol 1986; 124:179.
74. Matthay MA: Function of the alveolar epithelial barrier under pathologic conditions. Chest 1995; 105:67S.
75. Matthay MA, Landholt CC, Staub NC: Differential liquid and protein clearance from the alveoli of anesthetized sheep. J Appl Physiol 1982; 53:96.
76. Matthay MA, Berthiaume Y, Staub NC: Long term clearance of liquid and protein from the lungs of unanesthetized sheep. J Appl Physiol 1985; 59:928.
77. Berthiaume Y, Staub NC, Matthay MA: Beta-adrenergic agonists increase lung liquid clearance in anesthetized sheep. J Clin Invest 1987; 79:335.
78. Sakuma T, Pittet JF, Jayr C, et al: Alveolar liquid and protein clearance in the absence of blood flow or ventilation in sheep. J Appl Physiol 1993; 74:176.
79. Bowton DL, Kong DL: High tidal volume ventilation produces increased lung water in oleic acid injured rabbit lungs. Crit Care Med 1984; 17:908.
80. Corbridge TC, Wood LDH, Crawford GP, et al: Adverse effects of large tidal volumes and low PEEP in canine acid aspiration. Am Rev Respir Dis 1990; 142:311.
81. Dreyfuss D, Saumon G: Role of tidal volume, FRC and end-inspiratory volume in the development of pulmonary edema following mechanical ventilation. Am Rev Respir Dis 1993; 148:1194.
82. Dreyfuss D, Soler P, Basset G: High inflation pressure pulmonary edema: Respective effects of high airway pressure, high tidal volume, and positive end-expiratory pressure. Am Rev Respir Dis 1988; 137:1159.
83. Hernandez LA, Peevy KJ, Moise AA, et al: Chest wall restriction limits high airway pressure induced lung injury in young rabbits. J Appl Physiol 1989; 66:2366.
84. Kolobow T, Moretti MP, Fumigalli R, et al: Severe impairment in lung function induced by high peak airway pressure during mechanical ventilation. Am Rev Respir Dis 1987; 136:312.
85. Muscedere JG, Mullen JBM, Gan K, et al: Tidal volume at low airway pressures can augment lung injury. Am J Respir Crit Care Med 1994; 149:1327.
86. Hasleton PS: Adult respiratory distress syndrome—review. Histopathology 1983; 7:307.
87. Lakshminarayan S, Stanford RL, Petty TL: Prognosis after recovery from adult respiratory distress syndrome. Am Rev Respir Dis 1976; 113:7.
88. Pison U, Seeger W, Buckhorn R, et al: Surfactant abnormalities in patients with respiratory failure in multiple trauma. Am Rev Respir Dis 1989; 140:1033.
89. Gregory T, Longmore W, Moxley M, et al: Surfactant chemical composition and biophysical activity in acute respiratory distress syndrome. J Clin Invest 1991; 65:1976.
90. Lamy M, Fallat RJ, Koeniger E, et al: Pathologic features and mechanisms of hypoxemia in adult respiratory distress syndrome. Am Rev Respir Dis 1976; 114:267.
91. Wright PE, Bernard GR: The role of airflow resistance in patients with the adult respiratory distress syndrome. Am Rev Respir Dis 1989; 139:1169.
92. Dantzker DR, Brook CH, DeHart P, et al: Gas exchange in adult respiratory distress syndrome and the effects of positive end-expiratory pressure. Am Rev Respir Dis 1979; 120:1039.
93. Dorinsky PM, Gadek JE: Mechanisms of nonpulmonary organ failure in ARDS. Chest 1989; 96:885.
94. Johnson TH, Altman AR, McCaffree RD: Radiologic considerations in the adult respiratory distress syndrome treated with positive end-expiratory pressure (PEEP). Clin Chest Med 1982; 3:89.
95. Altman AR, Johnson TH: Roentgenographic findings: PEEP therapy, indicators of pulmonary complications. JAMA 1979; 242:727.
96. Pistolesi M, Miniati M, Milne ENC, et al: The chest roentgenogram in pulmonary edema. Clin Chest Med 1985; 6:315.
97. Halperin BD, Feeley TW, Mihm FG, et al: Evaluation of portable chest roentgenogram for quantitating extravascular lung water in critically ill adults. Chest 1985; 88:649.
98. Peruzzi W, Garner W, Bools J, et al: Portable chest roentgenography and computed tomography in critically ill patients. Chest 1988; 93:727.
99. Golding RP, Knape P, Strack Van Schijndel RJM, et al: Computed tomography as an adjunct to chest x-rays of intensive care unit patients. Crit Care Med 1988; 16:211.
100. Bombino M, Gattinoni L, Pesenti A, et al: The value of portable chest roentgenography in adult respiratory distress syndrome: Comparison with computed tomography. Chest 1991; 100:762.
101. Gattinoni L, Pesenti A, Torresin A: Adult respiratory distress syndrome profiles by computed tomography. J Thoracic Imag 1986; 1:25.
102. Maunder BJ, Shuman WP, McHugh JW, et al: Preservation of normal lung regions in the adult respiratory distress syndrome: Analysis by computed tomography. JAMA 1986; 255:2463.
103. Taylor RW: The adult respiratory distress syndrome. *In*: Respiratory Failure. Kirby RR, Taylor RW (Eds). Chicago, Year Book Medical Publishers, 1986, pp 208–244.
104. Luce JM, Montgomery AB, Marks JD, et al: Ineffectiveness of high-dose methylprednisolone in preventing parenchymal lung injury and improving mortality in patients with septic shock. Am Rev Respir Dis 1988; 138:62.
105. Bernard GR, Luce JM, Sprung CL, et al: High-dose corticosteroids in patients with the adult respiratory distress syndrome. N Engl J Med 1987; 317:1565.
106. Meduri GU, Chinn AJ, Leeper KV, et al: Corticosteroid rescue treatment of progressive fibroproliferation in late ARDS: Patterns of response and predictors of outcome. Chest 1994; 105:1516.
107. Bone RC, Slotman G, Maunder R, et al: Randomized double-blind, multicenter study of prostaglandin E_1 in patients with the adult respiratory distress syndrome. Chest 1989; 96:114.
108. Luce JM: Introduction of new technology into critical care practice: A history of HA-1A human monoclonal antibody against endotoxin. Crit Care Med 1993; 21:1233.
109. Fisher CJ, Dhainaut JF, Opal SM, et al: Recombinant human interleukin 1 receptor antagonist in the treatment of patients with sepsis syndrome: Results from a randomized double-blind, placebo-controlled trial. JAMA 1994; 271:1836.
110. Dhainaut JFA, Tenaillon A, Tulzo YL, et al: Platelet-activating factor receptor antagonist BN 52021 in the treatment of severe sepsis: A randomized, double-blind, placebo-controlled, multicenter trial. Crit Care Med 1994; 22:1720.
111. Abraham E, Wunderink R, Silverman H, et al: Efficacy and safety of monoclonal antibody to human tumor necrosis factor α in patients with sepsis syndrome: A randomized, controlled, double-blind, multicenter clinical trial. JAMA 1995; 273:934.
112. Jepsen S, Herlevsen P, Knudsen P, et al: Antioxidant treatment with *N*-acetylcysteine during adult respiratory distress syndrome: A prospective, randomized, placebo-controlled study. Crit Care Med 1992; 20:918.
113. Haupt MT, Jastremski MS, Clemmer TP, et al: Effect of ibuprofen in patients with severe sepsis: A randomized, double-blind, multicenter study. Crit Care Med 1991; 19:1339.
114. Yu M, Thomasa G: A double-blind, prospective, randomized trial of ketoconazole, a thromboxane synthetase inhibitor, in the prophylaxis of the adult respiratory distress syndrome. Crit Care Med 1993; 21:1635.
115. Veldhuizen RAW, McCaig LA, Akino T, et al: Pulmonary surfactant subfractions in patients with the acute respiratory distress syndrome. Am J Respir Crit Care Med 1995; 152:1867.
116. Horbar JD, Soll RF, Sutherland JM, et al: A multicenter random-

ized, placebo-controlled trial of surfactant therapy for respiratory distress syndrome. N Engl J Med 1989; 320:959.
117. Walmrath D, Gunther A, Ghofrani HA, et al: Bronchoscopic surfactant administration in patients with severe adult respiratory distress syndrome and sepsis. Am J Respir Crit Care Med 1996; 154:57.
118. Anzueto A, Baughman RP, Guntapalli KK, et al: Aerosolized surfactant in adults with sepsis-induced acute respiratory distress syndrome. N Engl J Med 1996; 334:1417.
119. Zapol WM, Snider MT, Hill OJ, et al: Extracorporeal membrane oxygenation in severe acute respiratory failure. JAMA 1979; 242:2193.
120. Gattinoni L, Pesenti A, Mascheroni D, et al: Low-frequency positive-pressure ventilation with extracorporeal CO_2 removal in severe acute respiratory failure. JAMA 1986; 256:881.
121. Morris AH, Wallace CJ, Menlove RL, et al: Randomized clinical trial of pressure-controlled inverse ratio ventilation and extracorporeal CO_2 removal for adult respiratory distress syndrome. Am J Respir Crit Care Med 1994; 149:295.
122. Petty TL, Bone RC, Gee MH, et al: Contemporary clinical trials in acute respiratory distress syndrome. Chest 1992; 101:550.
123. Suchyta MR, Clemmer TP, Elliot CG, et al: The adult respiratory distress syndrome: A report of survival and modifying factors. Chest 1992; 101:1074.
124. Suchyta MR, Clemmer TP, Orme JF Jr, et al: Increased survival of ARDS patients with severe hypoxemia (ECMO criteria). Chest 1991; 99:951.
125. Milberg JA, Davis DR, Steinberg KP, et al: Improved survival of patients with acute respiratory distress syndrome (ARDS): 1983–1003. JAMA 1995; 273:306.
126. Ghio AJ, Elliott CG, Crapo RO, et al: Impairment after adult respiratory distress syndrome: An evaluation based on American Thoracic Society recommendations. Am Rev Respir Dis 1989; 139:1158.
127. Elliott CG, Morris AH, Cengiz M: Pulmonary function and exercise gas exchange in survivors of adult respiratory distress syndrome. Am Rev Respir Dis 1981; 123:492.
128. Elliott CG, Rasmusson BY, Crapo RO, et al: Prediction of pulmonary function abnormalities after adult respiratory distress syndrome (ARDS). Am Rev Respir Dis 1987; 135:634.
129. Weinert CF, Cross CR, Kangas JR, et al: Health-related quality of life after acute lung injury. Am J Respir Crit Care Med 1997; 156:1120.
130. McHugh LG, Milberg JA, Whitcomb ME, et al: Recovery of function in survivors of the acute respiratory distress syndrome. Am J Respir Crit Care Med 1994; 150:90.

127

Pathophysiology and Management of Acute Respiratory Distress Syndrome After Surgery, Trauma, and Other Acute Illnesses

William C. Shoemaker, MD, FCCM

Acute respiratory distress syndrome (ARDS) after surgery, trauma, sepsis, and other acute illnesses is preventable. Moreover, it is much easier and more effective to prevent ARDS than to treat it.

This chapter summarizes the temporal relationships of blood volume, hemodynamics, oxygen transport, and cytokine patterns occurring in acutely ill postoperative and trauma patients before and after the onset of ARDS in order to elucidate the pathophysiology and to propose better therapeutic strategies. Time relationships of circulatory patterns antecedent to ARDS may have pathogenic importance, but they have not been given appropriate attention. The data reviewed here indicate that hypovolemia and inadequate or unevenly distributed blood flow results in poor tissue perfusion, tissue hypoxia, inadequate delivery of oxygen ($\dot{D}O_2$), and insufficient consumption of oxygen ($\dot{V}O_2$), which precede the appearance of ARDS and are the primary precipitating physiologic events. In essence, ARDS in previously healthy patients is the end-organ failure precipitated by tissue hypoxia from poor tissue perfusion. Therapy to prevent or rapidly treat these antecedent events can prevent postoperative and post-traumatic ARDS. Considering prior good health, the cost of care, and the increased mortality after ARDS has developed, this is a significant public health issue.

This approach is contrary to conventional thinking, which emphasizes fluid overload, pulmonary congestion, capillary leak, and a host of immunochemical mediators of systemic inflammatory response syndrome (SIRS) as the primary causes of ARDS and determinants of outcome.

CONVENTIONAL APPROACH

Clinical Description

ARDS is a frequent complication of surgery, trauma, and acute sepsis. The syndrome is defined clinically as hypoxemia (arterial oxygen tension [PaO_2] < 55 torr on room air) that is unresponsive to conservative management and that necessitates use of mechanical ventilation with increased fraction of inspired oxygen (FIO_2) for life support for more than 24 hours.[1, 2] Chest radiography may show diffuse bilateral infiltrates. The diagnosis is confirmed by a PaO_2/FIO_2 less than 200, a pulmonary venous admixture (shunt) greater than 20%, and reduced chest compliance.[3–8] ARDS most frequently occurs after surgery or trauma in patients who may have had hypotension, unstable hemodynamics, or shock during or shortly after surgery or trauma and whose fluid therapy has restored blood pressure and urine output.

The patient is usually given sufficient amounts of fluids, usually crystalloid solutions, to normalize blood pressure and urine output. Often, pulmonologists see the patients after ARDS has developed but not when the patient's lungs are normal before onset of ARDS. Diffuse infiltrates and radiographic evidence of pulmonary congestion or edema, indicating the presence of excessive fluid in the lungs, is usually interpreted as "fluid overload" from the overadministration of intravenous fluids. Fluid restriction and diuretics are usually recommended for the postoperative patient with early ARDS, almost as a knee-jerk response, because of increased interstitial and total body water. The questions rarely asked are: (1) What precisely is overloaded—intravascular or interstitial space? and (2) Which internal spaces should be kept dry?

Conventional Approach to Pathophysiology

Pulmonary edema resulting from the increased permeability of the alveolar-capillary membrane is traditionally regarded as the physiologic basis of ARDS. Increased intravascular and extracellular water with reduced protein flux produce pulmonary interstitial and alveolar edema, which in turn produces hypoxemia by interference with gas exchange.[4–12]

Evidence in support of the concept of increased endothelial permeability or capillary leak as the primary event in ARDS is usually based on three arguments. First, experimental pulmonary edema has been produced in sheep and other animals by intravenous administration of live bacteria or endotoxin.[9, 10]

Although infusions of live bacteria or endotoxin produce severe and sometimes lethal pulmonary edema, in surviving animals the edema is rapidly resolved without producing the typical ARDS radiologic or pathologic patterns.

Second, pulmonary edema is widely invoked as the principal mechanism produced in septic shock patients without cardiac problems or excessive fluid administration.[11] However, direct measurements of the presence and amount of capillary leak are not readily available under most clinical conditions. Nevertheless, capillary leak is often presumed from the clinical and radiologic appearance of pulmonary edema. Patients whose initial resuscitation and subsequent fluid therapy has been large volumes of crystalloid solutions may have immediate improvement with fluid restriction and diuretics.[13-16] It is not surprising that an overly distended interstitium occurring after resuscitation with massive crystalloid therapy may be improved after diuretic therapy if the plasma volume is not concomitantly reduced; this means, however, that diuretics may only partially correct an untoward effect of excessive crystalloid therapy rather than correct the underlying circulatory disorder. Some authors have defined *increased capillary permeability* as "pulmonary edema without cardiac failure or fluid overload."[9] Stated in its simplest form, this concept supports circular reasoning: Capillary leak may cause pulmonary edema and, therefore, pulmonary edema is due to capillary leak.

Third, evidence of capillary leak as the primary event in ARDS has been suggested by studies of biopsy and necropsy specimens. However, maldistribution of body fluids from increased pulmonary vascular permeability or capillary leak usually occurs in the late stage of ARDS. Capillary leak at this time may be inferred, but not proven, by the failure to sustain blood volume and adequate hemodynamics with fluid therapy. The crucial problems facing efforts to define capillary leaks objectively are (1) to develop methods that define and measure capillary leaks clinically and (2) to define the time between the onset of ARDS and the appearance of the leaks. Lung biopsy specimens reveal early anatomic changes immediately after the onset of respiratory failure. After hemorrhagic shock in conscious animals on the day of the ARDS diagnosis, small, patchy areas of round cell infiltration, perivascular hemorrhage, atelectasis or hyperaerated alveoli, and thickening of the alveolocapillary membrane have been observed; the lesions are confined to areas constituting as little as 5% to 10% of the lung fields.[15-17] Subsequently, on the second and third days, these areas become larger and more confluent. Not until the late stage of ARDS or at the time of autopsy does red or gray "hepatization" occur. Capillary leaks obviously do occur at this time, as evidenced by alveoli filled with pink proteinaceous fluid. In essence, capillary leak in biopsy and autopsy specimens is evidenced by pink proteinaceous fluid in the alveoli.[5, 18, 19] The problem with this argument is that late, terminal, or postmortem histologic findings reflect the results of ARDS, not its cause.

Conventional Approach to Fluid Therapy

The conventional aims of resuscitation in acute illness and ARDS are to attain normal vital signs, hematocrit, urine output, and arterial blood gas measurements while pulmonary artery (PA) occlusion pressure is maintained as low as possible. These are essentially the goals of the established Acute Cardiac Life Support (ACLS) and Acute Trauma Life Support (ATLS). After normal vital signs are achieved, the goals of therapy in ARDS consist of fluid restriction and diuretic administration, which prevent or minimize pulmonary edema by maintaining low pulmonary artery occlusion pressures. Justification for "drying the patient out" is based on:

1. Input and output records of large amounts of fluids given before the diagnosis of ARDS was made.
2. Clinical evidence of excessive fluid retention, such as peripheral edema.
3. Clinical and radiologic evidence of pulmonary congestion and edema.
4. Improvement in arterial blood gas values after administration of diuretic agents.

Critique of the Conventional Approach

The conventional approach is to maintain the patient's intravascular status on the "dry" side.[4, 8, 9, 12] However, this is more a philosophic statement of intent than an operationally useful therapeutic rule. Explicit clinical and physiologic criteria for this approach that can be used to make clinical management decisions are either lacking or have not been developed as guidelines or protocols.

Several major problems are associated with conventional concepts of fluid restriction in ARDS. The diagnosis of capillary leak is based not on direct measurements of increased capillary permeability but on clinical or radiographic evidence of pulmonary congestion. Pulmonary edema, which interferes with gas exchange, is usually considered to be compounded by excessive fluid administration where the excessive fluids have leaked into the lungs. However, Bishop and coworkers[13] and Johnson and associates[14] demonstrated that trauma patients resuscitated to supranormal $\dot{D}O_2$ and $\dot{V}O_2$ criteria, defined by values in trauma survivors prior to the development of ARDS, were given more fluids and accumulate greater fluid balances but had improved survival with fewer ARDS and other organ failures compared with the control group receiving conventional therapy. Thus, fluid restriction driven by fear of subsequent iatrogenic pulmonary edema seems an unjustified limitation in resuscitation strategies.

Pulmonary edema may be produced by many conditions, including (1) cardiac failure, (2) capillary leak, (3) hemorrhage with massive crystalloid solution replacement, (4) excessive volumes of crystalloid solutions in trauma victims, (5) low oncotic pressure from nutritional failure, (6) hypoxia of the lung tissue itself, and (7) high-altitude sickness, sepsis, decompression injury after diving, head injury, nutritional failure (e.g., kwashiorkor), and postcardiac arrest states even when no fluids are given. At autopsy, victims of combat with head injuries who died on the battlefield without having received any fluid therapy have been found to have pulmonary edema.

In postoperative, post-traumatic, and septic patients, pulmonary edema is often seen in high-risk patients who have been resuscitated with massive crystalloid infusions. Because saline solutions rapidly leave the intravascular space and equilibrate in the interstitial space, pulmonary edema is due to overexpansion of the interstitium, not to plasma volume overload that increases pulmonary capillary pressure. Peripheral and pulmonary edema reflect increased interstitial fluid volumes owing to redistribution of body water, massive crystalloid infusions, low plasma oncotic pressure, nutritional failure, increased endothelial permeability (capillary leak), lung hypoxia, or anaphylactoid reactions. In any case, fluid overload in the sense of overexpanded blood volume is infrequently the primary causative factor; in carefully measured blood volumes of a large series of ARDS patients, there were blood volume deficits of almost 1 L/m^2 in nonsurvivors and almost ¾ L/m^2 in survivors at the maximum volume.[20, 21] Hypovolemia is a major pathophysiologic factor of ARDS; pulmonary edema is an effect, not the cause of, ARDS.

The most obvious evidence against the application of fluid restriction and diuretics is the information by Bartlett and coworkers[6] that 15 years of this approach has not significantly reduced the mortality rate of patients with ARDS. Depending on associated diseases and organ failures, about 40% to 70% of ARDS patients still die. With each additional organ failure, mortality increases. Among those patients with one other organ failure, 54% died; of those with two, 72% died; of those with three, 84% died; and of those with four other organ failures, 100% died.[6] Survival rates suggest that the conventional approach to ARDS requires rethinking.

TEMPORAL PATTERNS AS AN APPROACH TO PATHOGENESIS

Time Course of Circulatory Events

The pathogenesis of ARDS should be based on objective physiologic evidence. The interacting pathologic mechanisms that contribute to lethal circulatory patterns and ARDS include: (1) hypovolemia, (2) low cardiac output, (3) anemia, (4) hypoxemia, (5) adrenomedullary and corticosteroid stress response, (6) the duration of shock or low-flow state, (7) poor tissue perfusion, (8) tissue hypoxia, (9) oxygen debt, and (10) various cascades of immunochemical mediators associated with trauma, surgery, inflammation, and sepsis.

ARDS of acute illness is produced by antecedent tissue hypoxia; this concept is supported by the demonstration of oxygen debt from circulatory deficiencies as the earliest physiologic event associated with high-risk surgical operations, major trauma, and hypovolemia. Except for ARDS caused by direct lung injury, ARDS does not materialize just as a new entity; rather, it is the end-organ failure of an antecedent hypovolemic-hypoxic event. For example, patients with postoperative or post-traumatic shock, in which blood pressure and other superficial signs of shock were corrected but the underlying tissue perfusion defect was not reversed, developed ARDS more often than their counterparts, whose tissue perfusion defect was promptly corrected. If these are indeed the precipitating events of ARDS, the present conventional approach to ARDS therapy by fluid restriction and diuretics is ill advised and possibly counterproductive.

The time course of events is a crucial factor in the determination of causality. When event "A" occurs before event "B," "A" may or may not be the cause of "B," but "B" can be excluded as the cause of the antecedent "A." However, time is often ignored in pathophysiologic evaluations and there is a dearth of information on circulatory function in the period immediately before the development of ARDS. Most clinical investigations begin to study pathogenic mechanisms after an ARDS diagnosis. More appropriate hypotheses on pathogenesis should be developed from studies of the period prior to the onset of ARDS that allow primary events to be separated from secondary, tertiary, and terminal events and by temporal description.

The following text briefly summarizes physiologic data and other evidence obtained *before* the onset of ARDS.

Blood Volume Measurements

Blood volume measurements with iodine 125–labeled albumin were reported in surgical intensive care unit (ICU) patients with ARDS.[20, 21] Figure 127–1 illustrates the blood volume deficits in 48 survivors and 47 nonsurvivors before and at the onset of ARDS. Nonsurviving ARDS patients had greater blood volume deficits at the initial observation, when maximum blood volume was observed, and at the time of onset of ARDS. Patients who died of ARDS had an average of 981 ± 52 mL blood volume deficit at its maximum; ARDS survivors had a deficit of 713 ± 56 mL; at the time that diagnostic criteria of ARDS were met, the mean blood volume deficit was 620 ± 58 mL in nonsurvivors and 401 ± 67 mL in survivors of ARDS. Those in whom ARDS did not develop had normal blood volumes ± 300 mL.

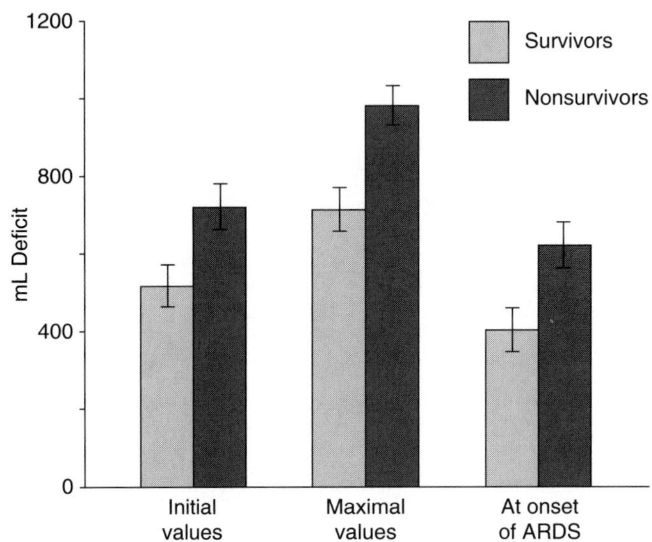

Figure 127–1. Blood volume deficits in survivors and nonsurvivors of patients with adult respiratory distress syndrome (ARDS) at time of initial values, at the time of maximal values, and at the time of onset of ARDS. *Vertical lines* on top of the bars represent SEM. (From Shoemaker WC, Appel PL, Bishop MH: Temporal patterns of blood volumes, hemodynamics, and oxygen transport in pathogenesis and therapy of postoperative adult respiratory distress syndrome. New Horiz 1993; 1:532. Copyright Williams & Wilkins, 1993.)

Although attempts were made to restore normal blood volume soon after results were known, continuing blood loss, delays in transfusion therapy, unavailability of banked blood, and the substitution of crystalloids for blood were frequent problems that delayed blood volume restoration. These data document major blood volume deficits in postoperative ARDS patients several days before criteria for diagnosis of ARDS were met. Hypovolemia was of greater intensity and lasted longer in patients who died of ARDS. Postoperative patients who did not have ARDS had relatively normal values ± 300 mL. The data clearly indicate the blood volume was not adequately restored in patients with later ARDS.

Usefulness of Pulmonary Artery Catheters in Critically Ill Patients

Although invasive PA thermodilution catheters were frequently used as the "gold standard" for monitoring critically ill ICU patients,[22] recent studies showed no advantage of the PA catheter in cardiac and other medical conditions[23–25] or in postoperative patients admitted to the ICU after organ failures had developed.[26, 27] A consensus conference[28] found insufficient evidence to fully determine whether PA catheter-guided therapy significantly alters outcome but recommended that more prospective randomized clinical trials be undertaken. Because the consensus conference did not consider time factors for therapy, they mixed early and late studies together and arrived at an ambiguous conclusion. Similarly, the European conference[71, 72] also failed to recognize the importance of time factors. In a more insightful meta-analysis, Boyd and Bennett[29]

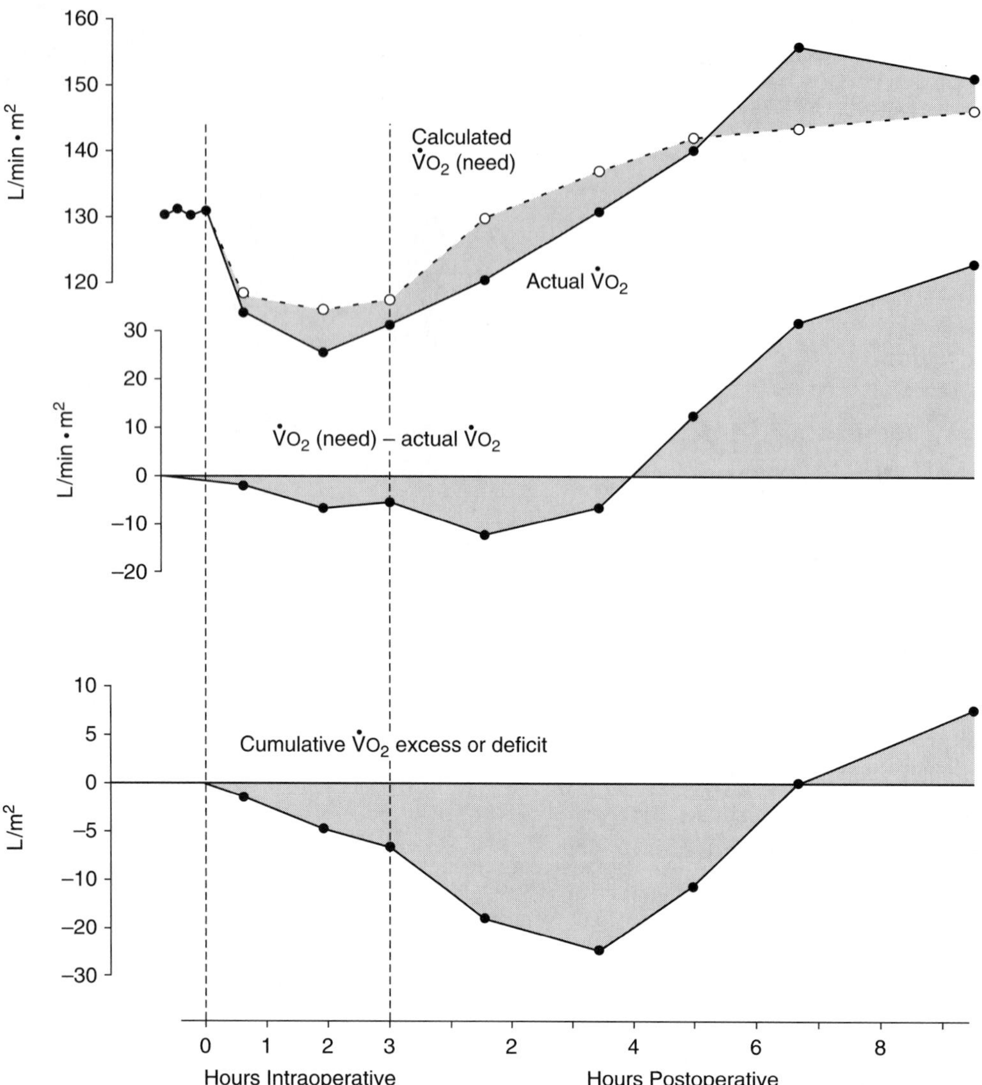

Figure 127–2. An illustrative example of the calculated oxygen consumption [$\dot{V}O_{2(need)}$] and oxygen debt. *Upper section,* Calculated $\dot{V}O_{2(need)}$ based on the patient's own $\dot{V}O_2$ corrected for temperature and anesthesia is shown by *dashed lines* and *open circles.* The actual or measured $\dot{V}O_2$ is shown by the *solid lines* and *solid dots.* The difference between them is shown by the *shaded areas. Middle section,* Rate of serially measured $\dot{V}O_2$ and the estimated need $\dot{V}O_{2(need)}$, calculated from the patient's own preoperative $\dot{V}O_2$ measurements extrapolated to the intraoperative and to the first 48-hour postoperative periods after corrections for anesthesia and temperature have been made. *Lower section,* Net cumulative oxygen deficit *(below the zero line)* or excess *(above).* (From Shoemaker WC, Appel PL, Kram HB: Role of oxygen debt in the development of organ failure, sepsis, and death. Chest 1992; 102:208–215.)

found no outcome improvement in seven prospective randomized studies of patients who entered the ICU after organ failure or sepsis had occurred, but they noted significant outcome improvement in seven other randomized studies when PA catheter–directed therapy was given early or prophylactically.[30-36]

The ineffectiveness of monitoring or optimal therapy in the late stages after appearance of organ failure is not unexpected. No amount of oxygen can restore irreversible oxygen debts, failed organs, or dead cells.

Temporal Hemodynamic and Oxygen Transport Patterns Before, During, and After High-Risk Surgery

The hemodynamic and oxygen transport patterns of 708 high-risk patients were analyzed before, during, and after surgical operations in an effort to describe the temporal responses to life-threatening trauma under conditions in which hemodynamic and oxygen variables could be measured with reasonably satisfactory reproducibility.[37] The major findings were intraoperatively reduced circulatory function, as manifested by decreased $\dot{D}O_2$, which persisted into the early postoperative period followed by improved circulatory functions, as shown by increased cardiac index (CI), $\dot{D}O_2$, and $\dot{V}O_2$ (see Chapter 8, Fig. 8–3). The postoperative increases in CI and $\dot{D}O_2$ values were greater in patients who survived hospitalization than in those who did not, particularly when these patterns were related to their own preoperative baseline values. The temporal patterns of survivors and nonsurvivors in each of the following stratifications were described in patients with and without associated cardiovascular disease:

1. Baseline CI values were normal in patients without cardiovascular disease.
2. Patients with sepsis, trauma, stress, and late cirrhosis had high preoperative baseline CI values.
3. Patients with hemorrhage, dehydration, hypovolemia, and cardiac conditions preoperatively had low CI, $\dot{D}O_2$, and $\dot{V}O_2$.

The data thus indicate that increased CI and $\dot{D}O_2$ compensate for prior circulatory deficits, tissue hypoxia, and organ dysfunction, beginning with surgical trauma.

Therapeutic goals for patients with high-risk criteria were empirically determined as the median values of CI, $\dot{D}O_2$, and $\dot{V}O_2$ at their maxima for survivors of high-risk surgery in their early postoperative course.[30, 35, 37] These values were observed to be as follows:

1. CI greater than 4.5 L/min · m^2.
2. $\dot{D}O_2$ greater than 600 mL/min · m^2.
3. $\dot{V}O_2$ greater than 170 mL/min · m^2.
4. Blood volume 500 mL greater than normal (i.e., 3.2 L/m^2 for men, 2.7 L/m^2 for women).

Target goals are higher for patients with severe trauma and for those with sepsis. To reduce the duration of tissue hypoxia, physicians should enable these goals to be reached within the first 8 to 12 hours postoperatively or after trauma.

Oxygen Debt as a Reflection of Tissue Hypoxia

Tissue hypoxia results from inadequate or unevenly distributed microcirculatory blood flow in relation to increased metabolic demands from fever, inflammatory responses, postoperative wound healing, hypovolemia, anesthesia, surgical trauma, and failure or delays in replacing blood losses. Prolonged increases in tissue hypoxia may result in multiple vital organ failure, which is the major proximate cause of death in ICU patients.

Hypoxia from inadequate tissue perfusion can be measured as an oxygen debt. Guyton and Crowell[38, 39] showed the importance of oxygen debt by measuring $\dot{V}O_2$ before and during experimental hemorrhagic shock; all dogs with an oxygen debt greater than 140 mL/kg died, whereas all those with an oxygen debt less than 100 mL/kg survived; the halfway mark between survivors and nonsurvivors was 120 mL/kg.

Oxygen Debt and Its Relationship to Mortality and Organ Failure

If tissue hypoxia from poor tissue perfusion is the major circulatory problem in acute critical illness, this hypothesis can be tested by the estimation of oxygen debt. In a consecutive series of 253 high-risk surgical patients,[40] the amount of oxygen debt was calculated from the difference between serially measured $\dot{V}O_2$ minus estimated need, $\dot{V}O_{2(need)}$, calculated from the patient's preoperative $\dot{V}O_2$ measurements, extrapolated to the intraoperative and to the first 48-hour postoperative periods after corrections for anesthesia and temperature have been made.[41] The net cumulative oxygen debt at any given time was calculated from the integrated area between the actual $\dot{V}O_2$ and the estimated $VO_{2(need)}$. Greater oxygen debts were observed in patients with organ failure than in those without organ failure, and greater oxygen debts were seen in those who died (all with organ failure) than in those who survived with or without organ failure (Figs. 127–2 and 127–3).[40]

Prospective,[37, 42–47] randomized[30–36, 48] trials demonstrated that attainment of supranormal values empirically observed in survivors significantly reduced oxygen debt, organ failure, and death in high-risk surgical patients. The data indicate that the oxygen debt of postoperative patients with organ failure (especially ARDS) was larger than that in patients without organ failure; the debt was even larger in patients who died with organ failure. Furthermore, prospective randomized trials of supranormal values of CI, $\dot{D}O_2$, and $\dot{V}O_2$ resulted in reduced oxygen debt and decreased subsequent organ failure and death.[40] The evidence indicates that oxygen debt from inadequate tissue perfusion is the primary event and that ARDS as well as other organ failures are the end-organ consequence of postoperative and traumatic shock.

Immunochemical Mediators of Adult Respiratory Distress Syndrome

The early events after hemorrhage, trauma, high-risk surgery, and other acute critical illnesses include peripheral vasoconstriction with uneven microcirculatory flow; this leaves some capillary networks with minimal flow predisposed to local hypoxia and acidosis. The endothelial surfaces of these hypoxic, acidotic, vasoconstricted capillary beds in peripheral or visceral circulations activate T-cell lymphocytes, macrophages, and other hematopoietic cells. The endothelium, activated lymphocytes, and macrophages from remote sites of injury and inflammation release various immunochemical mediators, such as tumor necrosis factor (TNF) and other cytokines, thromboxane, prostaglandins, leukotrienes, histamine and other amines, serotonin, the complement system, neuroendocrine peptides, adrenal medullary and corticoid stress hormones, platelet-activating factor, antidiuretic hormone, renin-angiotensin, endorphins, opioids, "heat shock" proteins, C-reacting proteins, and many other factors.[49]

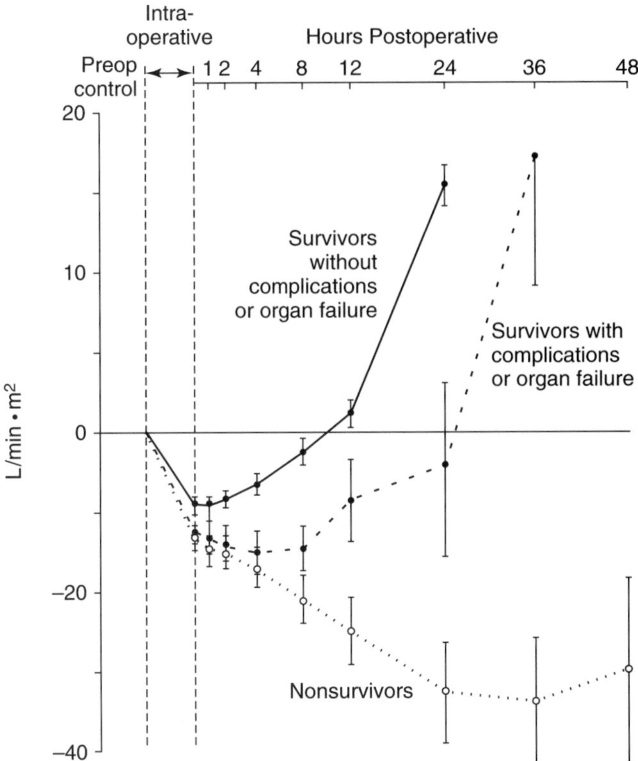

Figure 127–3. Serial measurements of cardiac index, oxygen delivery ($\dot{D}O_2$), oxygen consumption ($\dot{V}O_2$), and net cumulative oxygen debt of surviving patients with and without organ failure and nonsurviving patients with organ failure. Values were taken during preoperative *(extreme left)*, intraoperative *(second measurement to left)*, and postoperative periods. *Dots* are mean values, and the *vertical lines* are SEM. (From Shoemaker WC, Appel PL, Kram HB: Role of oxygen debt in the development of organ failure, sepsis, and death. Chest 1992; 102:208–215.)

With fluid resuscitation, these poorly perfused capillary networks are reperfused. In this process, many of these immunochemical mediators are washed out of the microcirculation and into the venous circulation, where they go directly to the lungs—the first capillary network they encounter. Here they play a major role in the development of ARDS and, subsequently, other organ failures.

It is important to distinguish the *initiators* of immunochemical response (e.g., high risk surgery, trauma, hemorrhage, hypovolemia, cardiac conditions, sepsis) from the *mediators.* The initiators may produce low flow states or uneven flow from uneven vasomotion that leaves some capillaries with little or no flow and with hypoxia and acidosis. It is obviously

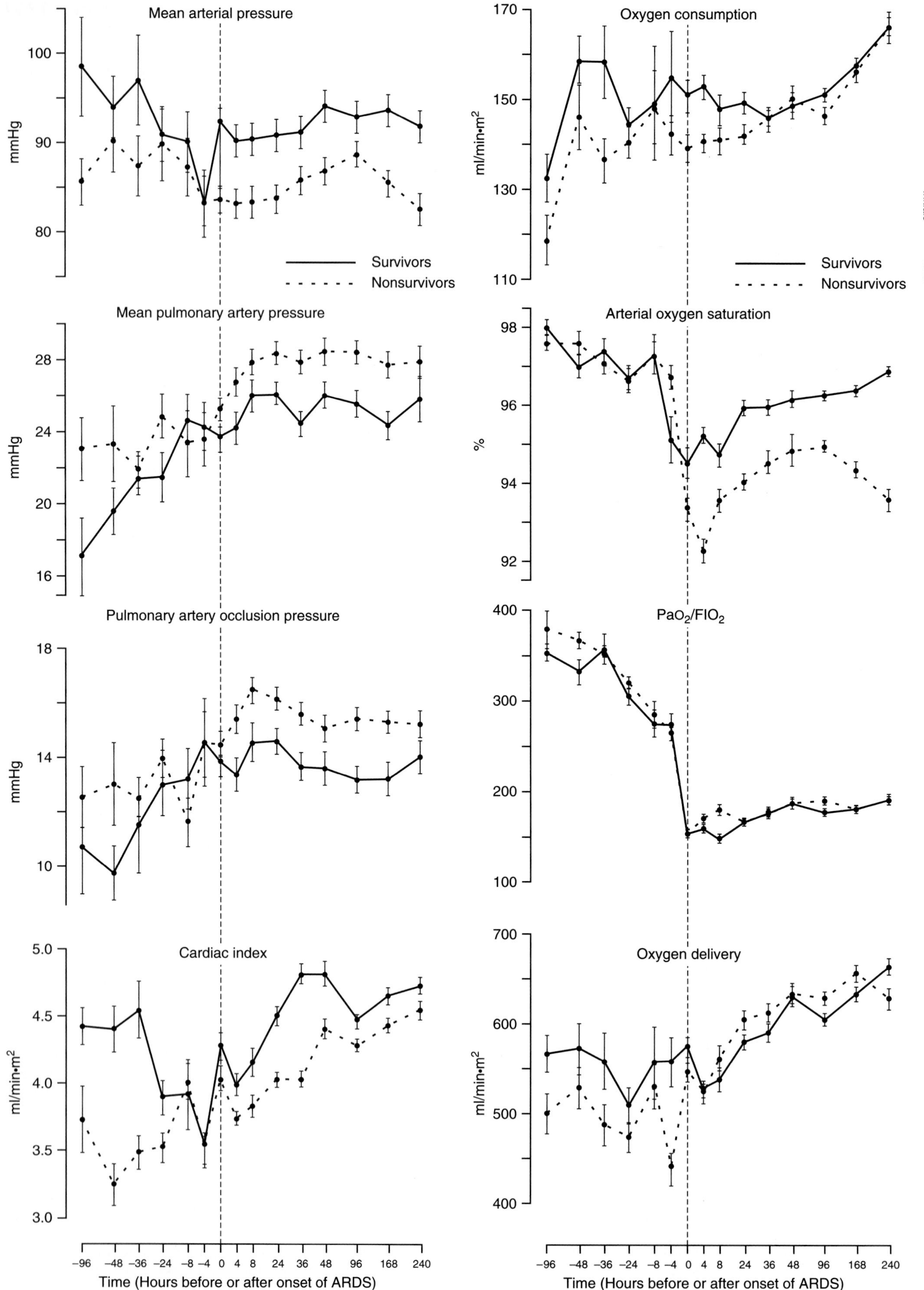

Figure 127–4. *See legend on opposite page*

easier to prevent immunochemical events from occurring in the first place than to attempt to treat their consequences, particularly organ failures that could have been prevented.

Relation of Physiologic Patterns and Tissue Hypoxia to Mediators of Organ Failure

Hypoxic, acidotic, vasoconstricted, microcirculatory endothelial surfaces trigger multiple cascades that activate T cells and produce various cytokines, including TNF and interleukins (IL-1, IL-2, IL-6, IL-8). Experimentally and clinically, the activation of IL-6, IL-8, and TNF have been demonstrated when sepsis or ARDS occurs after trauma. Increased release of these cytokines is associated with an acute-phase reaction and a hypermetabolic state.

Meade and colleagues[50] measured plasma levels of complement factors, antitoxins, and cytokines in severely traumatized patients on admission to the emergency department (ED) and at successive intervals for 48 hours; those in whom ARDS developed had initial marked reductions of CI, $\dot{D}O_2$, and $\dot{V}O_2$ in the first 4 hours after admission, but elevations of plasma IL-6 and IL-8 levels did not reach their maxima until 16 hours after the diagnostic criteria for ARDS had been met. By contrast, the trauma patients who did not develop ARDS had higher CI, $\dot{D}O_2$, and $\dot{V}O_2$ values, and lower values for pulmonary shunt and cytokines (Fig. 127–4). Thus, increased plasma cytokine levels did not *precede* occurrence of hemodynamic and oxygen transport markers or the clinical diagnostic features of ARDS.[50] However, the presence of inflammatory mediators may accelerate and augment the disorder as it occurs.

Prospective Clinical Trials to Reduce the Incidence of Adult Respiratory Distress Syndrome

The basic hypothesis that therapeutic goals should be the supranormal values empirically observed in survivors was supported in an initial trial of 252 high-risk patients. They were grouped by services, with normal values as the goals for the control service patients and with supranormal values as the therapeutic goals of a protocol service. Because it was noted that patients entering the protocol several days postoperatively had successively less and less favorable results, a randomized trial was undertaken that preoperatively allocated patients to (1) a central venous pressure (CVP) catheter group (CVP group) with normal values as goals, (2) a PA catheter group (PA control group) with normal values as goals of therapy, and (3) a PA catheter group (PA protocol group) with supranormal values as goals.[30] No significant differences in outcome were observed between the CVP group and the PA control group, both of which had normal values as their goals. This suggests that when the therapeutic intent is to maintain normal values, no real advantage is gained from the use of the PA catheter. Compared with the PA control group, the PA protocol group had fewer organ failures (one or 0.04 per patient versus 28 or 0.93 per patient, $P < .02$). There also was reduced mortality (4% versus 33%, $P < .02$), fewer hospital days (19.3 ± 2.4 versus 25.2 ± 3.4 days), fewer days in ICU (10.2 ± 1.6 versus 15.8 ± 3.1, $P < .05$) and 25% reduction in hospital costs.[30]

The hemodynamic goals were achieved with fluid therapy alone in two thirds of the protocol patients; an average of 6 to 7 L of crystalloid solutions and 3 L of starch or albumin solutions was used in the first 48 hours postoperatively. The remaining one third of patients also were given dobutamine for inotropic support, and two patients (7%) required a vasodilator because of sudden hypertensive episodes on recovery from anesthesia. The control group received about the same amount of crystalloid solutions and packed red blood cells but about one third as much colloid solutions in order to maintain normal values.[30] The concept that supranormal goals reduces the incidence of ARDS and other organ failures and thereby improves outcome has been corroborated in subsequent studies from our center and others.[29, 31, 34, 36]

Time relationships after severe trauma were studied by Bishop and coauthors,[13] who found that optimizing CI, $\dot{D}O_2$, and $\dot{V}O_2$ within 24 hours of the injury improved outcome. In prospective randomized studies, they demonstrated significantly reduced mortality from 39% to 18% ($P < .05$) and reduced incidence of organ failure from 105 in 65 control patients (1.62 ± 0.28 organ failures per patient) to 37 in 50 protocol patients (0.74 ± 0.28 organ failures per patient; $P < .01$) who achieved targeted levels of hemodynamic response early.[34]

Although a higher incidence of organ failures was observed in patients with normal values as therapeutic goals than in those with supranormal values as goals, no significant differences were seen in the incidence of other common postoperative complications.[30]

Prevention in High-Risk Surgical Patients

The incidence of postoperative organ failure and death in high-risk trauma and surgical patients was reduced by maintaining adequate tissue perfusion with optimal CI and $\dot{D}O_2$ to prevent oxygen debt.[30] Moreover, Thangathurai and associates[51] further decreased the incidence of ARDS to zero in more than 300 high-risk cancer patients per year for 3 years by maintaining tissue perfusion intraoperatively with adequate fluids (mostly colloids) and titrated doses of nitroglycerin to prevent maldistribution of microcirculatory flow, as determined by both invasive and noninvasive hemodynamic and oxygen transport monitoring. These data suggest that intraoperative oxygen debt from reduced tissue perfusion is the initiating mechanism that leads to organ failure and that monitoring can facilitate optimization of peripheral tissue oxygenation and prevent postoperative ARDS. These data underscore the concept that resuscitation in high-risk patients should occur early and not be delayed until ICU admission.

Measurement of Tissue Perfusion and Oxygenation

The transcutaneous oxygen electrode, which uses the same Clark polarographic oxygen sensor routinely used in the stan-

Figure 127–4. Data describing temporal patterns of mean arterial pressure, mean pulmonary artery (PA) pressure, PA occlusion pressure, and cardiac index (CI) *(left panel),* and oxygen consumption, $\dot{V}O_2$, arterial oxygen saturation, PaO_2/FIO_2 ratio, and oxygen delivery, $\dot{D}O_2$ *(right panel)* for 402 consecutively monitored postoperative patients with adult respiratory distress syndrome (ARDS) from 96 hours before until 10 days after diagnosis, indicated by the *vertical line.* (From Shoemaker WC, Appel PL, Bishop MH: Temporal patterns of blood volumes, hemodynamics, and oxygen transport in pathogenesis and therapy of postoperative adult respiratory distress syndrome. New Horiz 1993; 1:530. Copyright Williams & Wilkins, 1993.)

dard blood gas analyzer, accurately measures the oxygen tension of the heated skin surface. Although the oxygenation of a segment of the skin does not reflect the state of oxygenation of all tissues and organs, it has the advantage of being noninvasive and utilizing the most sensitive early warning tissue; vasoconstriction of the skin is one of the first stress responses of the shock syndromes.

Hemodynamic and Oxygen Transport Patterns Before and After Adult Respiratory Distress Syndrome

Hemodynamic patterns for 96 hours before the diagnostic criteria for ARDS were met are illustrated in Figure 127-4.[21, 51-53] Prior to the onset of ARDS, the CI in nonsurvivors was in the normal range; the CI of survivors with ARDS was significantly elevated (i.e., 4 L/min · m²) but less than the CI values of survivors without ARDS (4.5 L/min · m²). In postoperative patients with sepsis, the CI was higher; in postoperative ARDS patients without sepsis, it was 3.92 ± 0.18 L/min · m²), whereas postoperative ARDS patients with sepsis had CI values of 4.21 ± 0.15 L/min · m²) in the 96-hour period before onset of ARDS.[21]

Before ARDS onset, the mean pulmonary artery wedge pressures (PAWPs) were within acceptable limits; none of the patients had PAWPs greater than 20 mm Hg, and the mean PA pressures were well within acceptable limits for critically ill postoperative patients. In essence, according to blood volume, hematocrit, mean arterial pressure (MAP), CVP, and PA occlusion pressure, none of the patients were plasma-volume overloaded before the onset of ARDS.[21, 51-53] $\dot{D}O_2$ patterns were decreased prior to the ARDS diagnosis. $\dot{V}O_2$ was at the upper range of normal in nonsurvivors and slightly above normal but not optimal in most survivors. Pulmonary shunt increased to more than 20% at the time of ARDS diagnosis. Hypoxia to the lung per se increases pulmonary artery pressure (PAP), pulmonary vascular resistance (PVR) and pulmonary shunting by neural mechanisms; this response is similar to the well-known response of the hypoxic neonate.

After ARDS onset, hemodynamic variables tended to improve, especially CI and MAP. PAP tended to remain elevated, but the PVR index decreased as the CI increased. The PAWP remained at acceptable levels. CI, $\dot{D}O_2$, and $\dot{V}O_2$ tended to increase after mechanical ventilation, maintenance of high FIO_2 levels, and the administration of additional fluids and inotropic agents. Pulmonary shunt was usually above 30% to 40% after the onset of ARDS. In general, pulmonary shunt values were somewhat higher in nonsurvivors than in survivors.

In essence, the physiologic changes that precede the clinical diagnosis of ARDS include[21, 51-53]:

1. Hypovolemia manifested by reduced blood volume, red blood cell mass, and hematocrit.
2. Inadequate myocardial performance, as indicated by a suboptimal increase in CI response to administration of fluids and inotropic agents.
3. Inadequate tissue perfusion, as indicated by suboptimal $\dot{D}O_2$ and $\dot{V}O_2$.
4. Increased pulmonary vasoconstriction, as indicated by increased mean PAP and PVR index.

Mathematic Coupling of Oxygen Delivery and Oxygen Consumption Values

The mathematic coupling of $\dot{D}O_2$ values with $\dot{V}O_2$ values is potentially problematic because CI is a common term for the calculations of both $\dot{D}O_2$ and $\dot{V}O_2$. Obviously, if the CI is spuriously increased, the calculated $\dot{D}O_2$ and $\dot{V}O_2$ values also will be incorrectly high. Although this situation is theoretically possible, it is unlikely to be a frequent or a consistent error if careful troubleshooting and quality controls are routinely performed.

In a number of clinical conditions, changes in $\dot{D}O_2$ are not associated with similar changes in $\dot{V}O_2$, as would be the case if $\dot{D}O_2$ and $\dot{V}O_2$ were linked:

1. In the preterminal stages of nonsurvivors, fluid volume infusions and inotropes may produce appreciable $\dot{D}O_2$ changes and minimal $\dot{V}O_2$ changes, which are consistent with an oxygen debt that has become irreversible.
2. Severe cardiac conditions with limited CI responses to fluids and inotropes but reasonably good $\dot{V}O_2$ responses indicate significant oxygen debt that was at least partly reversible despite limited cardiac responsiveness.
3. In some late-stage sepsis, postoperative, and cardiac patients, small $\dot{D}O_2$ changes were associated with large $\dot{V}O_2$ responses, suggestive of large oxygen debts.
4. Early postoperative patients may have major $\dot{D}O_2$ increases with minimal $\dot{V}O_2$ changes, suggestive of good cardiac responsiveness but only small oxygen debts.
5. Infusion of packed red blood cells often stimulates major $\dot{V}O_2$ changes with minimal or insignificant CI changes.
6. Normal unstressed or preoperative patients also may have large $\dot{D}O_2$ increases with little or no $\dot{V}O_2$ response because they had little or no oxygen debt.

In essence, when $\dot{D}O_2$ and $\dot{V}O_2$ increase together, supply-dependent $\dot{V}O_2$ or an error due to coupling may be present. However, coupling cannot explain the supply-independent oxygen values; a nearly horizontal line of $\dot{D}O_2$ values plotted against their corresponding $\dot{V}O_2$ values would not be possible if $\dot{D}O_2$ and $\dot{V}O_2$ were linked (Fig. 127-5).

When carefully obtained direct Fick measurements (using measured inspired and expired oxygen concentrations together with tidal volumes) were compared with concomitant thermodilution values recorded using PA catheters with arterial and mixed venous blood gas analysis to calculate $\dot{D}O_2$ and $\dot{V}O_2$, the indirect thermodilution-calculated $\dot{V}O_2$ values closely approximated the direct Fick $\dot{V}O_2$ measurements. Confirmation of the validity of these two approaches was reported by Hankeln and associates[54] and others, who found good agreement between $\dot{V}O_2$ values, as measured with both methods.

It should be noted that the *direct Fick method,* which calculates $\dot{V}O_2$ from inspired and expired oxygen concentrations, measures a different $\dot{V}O_2$ than that calculated with the *thermodilution method*. The direct Fick method includes the metabolism of the lung itself and is particularly susceptible to error from high FIO_2 values; FIO_2 values above 0.6 use calculations based on small differences between large inspiratory and expiratory oxygen values. Furthermore, the direct Fick measurement is not reliable in rapidly changing (nonsteady) metabolic states. In such conditions, changes in the size of the oxygen pool are misinterpreted as $\dot{V}O_2$ changes. Finally, calibration of metabolic charts is time-consuming and fraught with major technical problems.

Oxygen Delivery–Oxygen Consumption Relationships in Postoperative Patients

The patterns of $\dot{D}O_2$ plotted against their corresponding $\dot{V}O_2$ values have been studied during relatively short periods of $\dot{D}O_2$ increase. A region of increasing $\dot{D}O_2$ associated with increasing $\dot{V}O_2$ values suggests *supply-dependent* $\dot{V}O_2$, whereas increasing $\dot{D}O_2$ values associated with relatively constant $\dot{V}O_2$

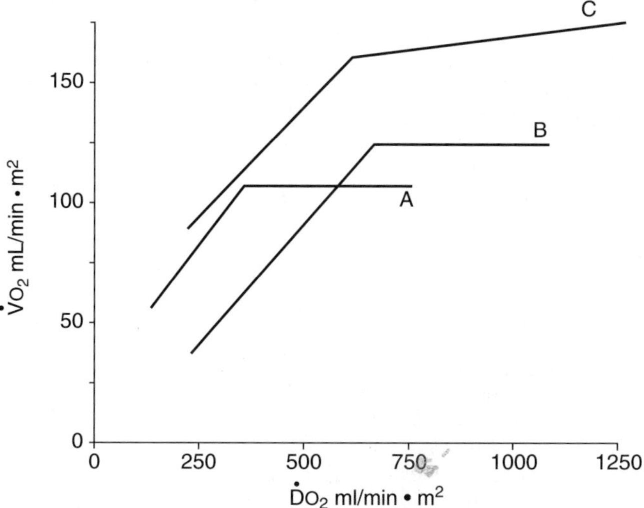

Figure 127–5. Relationship of changing oxygen delivery $\dot{D}O_2$ values to oxygen consumption $\dot{V}O_2$ values in three series of patients. *Line A*, Data of anesthetized patients coming off cardiopulmonary bypass and cardiac surgery. (Redrawn from Shibutani K, Komatsa T, Kubal K, et al: Critical level of oxygen delivery in anesthetized man. Crit Care Med 1983; 11:640.[55]) *Line B,* Data from medical septic shock patients. (Redrawn from Tuchschmidt J, Fried JC, Astiz M, et al: Elevation of cardiac output and oxygen delivery improves outcome in septic shock. Chest 1992; 102:216–220.[35]) *Line C,* Postoperative data of patients with adult respiratory distress syndrome plotted against their corresponding $\dot{V}O_2$ values during periods when both were increasing (suggesting supply dependency) and subsequently during periods when increasing $\dot{D}O_2$ values did not increase $\dot{V}O_2$ values, resulting in a plateau suggesting supply-independent $\dot{V}O_2$. (From Shoemaker WC, Appel PL, Bishop MH: Temporal patterns of blood volumes, hemodynamics, and oxygen transport in pathogenesis and therapy of postoperative adult respiratory distress syndrome. New Horiz 1993; 1:532. Copyright Williams & Wilkins, 1993.)

values suggest *supply-independent* $\dot{V}O_2$.[55-65] The capacity of tissues to maintain $\dot{V}O_2$ while $\dot{D}O_2$ is decreasing represents a compensatory peripheral circulatory response that preserves $\dot{V}O_2$ by maintaining greater oxygen extraction rates.

Several small series have found good correlations in ARDS patients but poor correlations in critically ill patients without ARDS. $\dot{V}O_2$ was found to be supply-dependent at $\dot{D}O_2$ values below 21 mL/min/kg in 10 patients with ARDS but supply-independent at $\dot{D}O_2$ values above this level.[35] This concept has been confirmed in several other series.[55-64] For example, Appel and Shoemaker[64] studied supply-dependent $\dot{V}O_2$ in a series of 127 consecutive, acute, postoperative ARDS patients. In 50 of the ARDS patients, sufficient measurements were obtained over a short time to make possible an evaluation of the presence or absence of a plateau: 29 of the 50 patients (58%) had plateaus at or near the upper end of the $\dot{D}O_2$ range, indicating supply-independent $\dot{V}O_2$ and suggesting that there had been substantial oxygen debts.

Because oxygen cannot be stored, the increased $\dot{V}O_2$ indicates greater utilization of oxygen as the body restores normal metabolism after an accumulated reversible oxygen debt. When increases in $\dot{D}O_2$ produce increases in $\dot{V}O_2$, supply-dependent $\dot{V}O_2$ suggests that either an oxygen debt was present or that nonoxidative phosphorylation processes were consuming oxygen. The relationships of $\dot{D}O_2$ to $\dot{V}O_2$ values were evaluated in a consecutive series of 238 ARDS patients before and after disease onset.[64] Supply-dependent $\dot{V}O_2$ was observed in 166 of the 238 patients (69%) who had sufficient numbers of increasing $\dot{D}O_2$ values. When $\dot{D}O_2$ was further increased with therapy, a plateau of sorts that suggested supply-independent $\dot{V}O_2$ was identified in 72% of these patients. The plateau suggested that tissue oxygen needs, which were previously rate-limited by inadequate oxygen supply, had been met and that no further increases in $\dot{V}O_2$ were needed; in essence, the patients had become $\dot{V}O_2$-supply-independent.[21, 64]

THERAPY

Most therapy for ARDS described in Section VIII (Pulmonary) is concerned with ventilatory management and is covered in subsequent chapters. The discussion here concerns fluid management of the ARDS patient.

Fluid Restriction and Diuretic Therapy

Conventional therapy in the initial resuscitation focuses on crystalloid to rapidly stabilize the cardiovascular state, but after the appearance of ARDS, the focus is on the restriction of fluids and diuretics as well as on the avoidance of colloid solution infusions. The last measure is based on the assumption that with increased endothelial permeability, the colloid solutions would leak into the lung and drag water into the lung tissue, thus worsening the ARDS. However, documentation of this occurring before or in the early period of ARDS is lacking.

Restriction of fluids and diuretic therapy have not proved effective in the overall management of ARDS. The mortality rate of 66% reported by Bartlett and coworkers[6] for a multi-institutional study was not appreciably different from the rates reported during the previous 15 years or earlier. Although patients may be more ill today than those reported in previous studies, the conventional fluid restriction approach, nevertheless, has not led to major outcome improvements. Two thirds of ARDS patients still die. Therefore, it is appropriate to reconsider the effectiveness of diuretic therapy and fluid restriction with respect to the underlying pathophysiology of ARDS based on analysis of the responses to therapy.[65-67]

Early Hemodynamic and Oxygen Transport Responses to Colloid and Crystalloid Solutions

Therapeutic goals for postoperative patients are designed to prevent tissue hypoxia and oxygen debts that lead to shock and shock lung. However, once ARDS occurs, the question of whether colloid resuscitation produces capillary leak arises. Evidence of increased capillary permeability may be observed in the physiologic responses to fluid administration at successive time periods.

In prospective, controlled, random-ordered crossover studies, the physiologic effects of the infusion of 1000 mL of crystalloid solutions were compared with those of the infusion of 100 mL of 25% albumin solution in 23 studies on 11 postoperative surgical patients in whom ARDS had developed in the previous 24 to 48 hours.[68] All patients had unmistakable evidence of respiratory distress, with shunt flow greater than 20%, alveolar-arterial difference in oxygen tension greater than 200 mm Hg, radiologic evidence of pulmonary infiltration, and mechanical ventilation as a required life-support measure for more than 48 hours. Each patient was given each fluid in random order. The 100 mL of 25% albumin solution increased plasma volume 450 mL by dragging 350 mL of interstitial water into the intravascular space. In essence, the albumin solution did not leak and the shunt fraction was unaltered.

By contrast, 1000 mL of lactated Ringer's solution given to the same patients expanded blood volume by less than 200 mL at the end of the infusion; that is, 80% of the crystalloid solution left the vascular space during the 1-hour infusion, and 40 minutes later, most of the remaining 200 mL had left the intravascular space.[68] Thus, crystalloid solutions rapidly distribute predominantly in the interstitium. When given in large quantities, crystalloid solutions can lead to both peripheral and pulmonary edema. It was concluded that in the first day or two after the ARDS diagnosis, capillary leak, if present, did not limit hemodynamic and oxygen transport responses to colloid solutions; in the middle period (48 hours to 6 days after onset), a less pronounced but significant hemodynamic and oxygen transport response occurred to colloid solutions. In the terminal stage of nonsurvivors, no significant response occurred to the infusion of colloid solutions, packed red blood cells, whole blood, or crystalloid solutions.

In any case, crystalloid solutions rapidly equilibrate into the interstitial space and provide only small transient plasma volume expansion and hemodynamic support. Moreover, they may deter tissue oxygenation by increasing the diffusion pathway through the expanded interstitium and by increasing the diffusion time of oxygen as it passes from the erythrocytes to cell mitochondria.[66, 67]

Effects of Colloid and Crystalloid Solutions on the Distribution of Body Water

If colloid solutions are deleterious and actually cause or worsen ARDS, plasmapheresis to remove plasma proteins and their replacement with the crystalloid solutions should be undertaken. However, this has already been done under rigorous experimental conditions by Guyton and Lindsey,[69] who demonstrated the importance of maintaining plasma protein levels. They depleted dogs of plasma proteins with protein-deficient diets and plasmapheresis; by increasing afterload, they found that pulmonary edema occurred at mean left atrial pressures of 13 mm Hg in depleted dogs, but pulmonary edema did not occur in control dogs until atrial pressures had reached 20 mm Hg. Clearly, there is an important contributory role in microvascular fluid shifts for maintaining near-normal plasma oncotic pressure.

Exogenously administered albumin does not act on pulmonary capillaries differently from the patient's own endogenous albumin. Rather, the infused albumin mixes in and expands the miscible albumin pool; this increases oncotic pressure and produces physiologic effects on hemodynamics, blood volume, and body water distribution. By contrast, saline infusions mix with the plasma and interstitial fluid pools. However, because capillary membranes are freely permeable to salt under normal conditions, the added saline solution rapidly equilibrates, predominately in the interstitial space. Measured with the use of radiolabeled bromide, sodium, or chloride, in the average man weighing 70 kg, the interstitial fluid volume averages 14 L, or 200 mL/kg, and the plasma volume is about 3 L, or 4 mL/kg.[70]

In major trauma, massive crystalloid infusions have been advocated in amounts up to 1 L or more per hour for the first 2 days. This inevitably leads to as much as a threefold expansion of the interstitium that may be tolerated in young, previously healthy combat casualties or street fighters. However, it is difficult to understand how this approach would benefit an older cardiac patient on a diet containing 1 g of salt per day. If massive amounts of crystalloid solutions are given to such a patient, death is likely to be attributed to the patient's trauma rather than the inappropriateness of the therapy.

When ARDS develops in patients given massive crystalloid infusions, it is likely that some improvements in arterial blood gas values occur with diuretic administration and fluid restriction, not because the ARDS was improved but because the overexpansion of the interstitium was corrected.

SUMMARY: AN ALTERNATIVE HYPOTHESIS

An alternative hypothesis has been presented for the pathogenesis and therapy of ARDS based on the temporal physiologic patterns observed before the appearance of ARDS in patients who are destined to have it after severe high-risk surgery or massive trauma. In essence, hypovolemia, low blood flow, and maldistribution of microcirculatory blood flow produce inadequate tissue perfusion and tissue hypoxia shown by inadequate $\dot{D}O_2$ and $\dot{V}O_2$ as well as significant oxygen debt. Insufficient $\dot{D}O_2$ needed to maintain body metabolism is reflected by suboptimal VO_2. Because these events take place before the clinical appearance of ARDS, they are associated with the cause, not the result, of ARDS. When tissue perfusion was maintained intraoperatively with colloids and nitroglycerin, the incidence of ARDS in high-risk cancer surgery patients was eliminated over a 3-year period.[51]

In essence, ARDS does not appear as new disease that begins with clinical manifestations of arterial hypoxemia and the need for mechanical ventilation. Rather, it is the end-organ failure of previous postoperative circulatory deficiencies: hypovolemia, microcirculatory flow maldistribution, and inadequate $\dot{D}O_2$ and $\dot{V}O_2$, which lead to postoperative shock and ARDS.

The underlying concept is that increased CI, $\dot{D}O_2$, and $\dot{V}O_2$, empirically observed in survivors, represent compensations for the basic physiologic problem of postoperative shock. Without these compensatory increases, local hypoxic areas progress to organ dysfunction and, ultimately, to organ failure. The interacting mechanisms of circulatory problems that contribute to lethal patterns include hypovolemia, a reduction in CI, anemia, hypoxemia, neural and neurohumoral components of the pituitary-adrenal stress response, various cascades of biochemical initiators and mediators, length of time in shock or low-flow states, and the amount of tissue hypoxia and oxygen debt accumulated. These data indicate that tissue oxygen debt from reduced tissue perfusion is the primary initiating physiologic response to hypovolemic shock states that subsequently lead to organ failure and death.

References

1. Ashbaugh DG, Bigelow DB, Petty TL, et al: Acute respiratory distress in adults. Lancet 1967; ii:319–323.
2. Hudson LD: Causes of ARDS: Clinical recognition. Clin Chest Med 1988; 138:720–723.
3. Murray JF, Mathay MA, Luce J, et al: An expanded definition of the adult respiratory distress syndrome. Am Rev Respir Dis 1988; 138:720–723.
4. Pepe PE: The clinical entity of adult respiratory distress syndrome: Definitions, prediction and prognosis. Crit Care Clin 1986; 2:377–403.
5. Katzenstein A-LA, Askin FB: Acute lung injury patterns. *In:* Surgical Pathology of Non-neoplastic Lung Disease. Bennington JL (Ed). Philadelphia, WB Saunders, 1990, pp 9–57.
6. Bartlett RH, Morris AH, Fairley B, et al: A prospective study of acute hypoxic respiratory failure. Chest 1986; 89:684–689.
7. Murray JF: Mechanisms of acute respiratory failure. Am Rev Respir Dis 1977; 115:1071–1078.
8. Fein AM, Lippman M, Holzman H, et al: Risk factors, incidence and prognosis of adult respiratory distress syndrome following septicemia. Chest 1978; 83:40–42.
9. Staub NC: Pulmonary edema: Physiologic approaches to management. Chest 1978; 74:559–564.
10. Brigham KL: Mechanisms of lung injury. Clin Chest Med 1982; 3:9.
11. Montgomery AB, Stager MA, Carrico CJ, et al: Causes of mortality

in patients with the adult respiratory distress syndrome. Am Rev Respir Dis 1984; 132:485–489.
12. Staub NC: Pulmonary edema: Physiologic approaches to management. Chest 1978; 74:559–564.
13. Bishop M, Shoemaker WC, Appel PL, et al: Relationship between supranormal circulatory values, time delays and outcome in severely traumatized patients. Crit Care Med 1993; 21:57.
14. Johnson KS, Bishop MH, Stephen CM, et al: Temporal patterns of radiographic infiltration in severely traumatized patients with and without adult respiratory distress syndrome. J Trauma 1994; 36:644–650.
15. Pontoppidan H, Geffin B, Lowenstein B: Acute respiratory failure in the adult. N Engl J Med 1972; 287:690–698.
16. Schuster DP: The case for and against fluid restriction and occlusion pressure reduction in adult respiratory distress syndrome. New Horiz 1993; 1:478–488.
17. Tiefenbrun J, Dikeman S, Shoemaker WC: The correlation of sequential changes in the distribution of pulmonary blood flow in hemorrhagic shock with the histopathologic anatomy. Surgery 1975; 76:618–627.
18. Katzenstein A-LA, Askin FB: Acute lung injury patterns. *In:* Surgical Pathology of Non-neoplastic Lung Disease. Bennington JL (Ed). Philadelphia, WB Saunders, 1990, pp 9–57.
19. Hogg JC, Katzenstein A-LA: Pulmonary edema and diffuse alveolar injury. *In:* Pathology of the Lung. Turlbeck WM (Ed). New York, Thieme, 1990.
20. Shippy, Appel PL, Shoemaker WC: Reliability of clinical monitoring to assess blood volume in critically ill patients. Crit Care Med 1984; 12:107–112.
21. Shoemaker WC, Appel PL, Bishop MH: Temporal patterns of blood volume, hemodynamics, and oxygen transport in pathogenesis and therapy of postoperative ARDS. New Horiz 1993; 1:522.
22. Forrester JS, Diamond GA, Swan HJC: Correlative classification of clinical and hemodynamic function after acute myocardial infarction. Am J Cardiol 1977; 39:137–145.
23. Conners AF, Jr, Speroff T, Dawson NV, Thomas C, et al: The effectiveness of right heart catheterization in the initial care of critically ill patients. JAMA 1996; 276:899–897.
24. Guyatt G, Ontario Intensive care group: A randomized control trial of right heart catheterization in critically ill patients. J Intensive Care Med 1991; 6:91–95.
25. Zion MM, Balkin J, Rosenmann D, et al: Use of pulmonary artery catheters in patients with acute myocardial infarction: Analysis of experience in 5841 patients in the SPRINT registry. Chest 1990; 98:1331–1335.
26. Hayes MA, Timmins AC, Yau EHS, et al: Elevation of systemic oxygen delivery in the treatment of critically ill patients. N Engl J Med 1994; 330:1717–1722.
27. Gattinoni L, Brazzi L, Pelosi P, et al: A trial of goal-oriented hemodynamic therapy in critically ill patients. N Engl J Med 1995; 333:1025–1032.
28. Taylor RW, and the Pulmonary Artery Catheter Consensus Conference Participants: Pulmonary Artery Catheter Consensus Conference. Crit Care Med 1997; 25:910–925.
29. Boyd O, Bennett D: Enhancement of perioperative tissue perfusion as a therapeutic strategy for major surgery. New Horiz 1996; 4:453–465.
30. Shoemaker WC, Appel P, Kram HB, et al: Prospective trial of supranormal values of survivors as therapeutic goals in high-risk surgical patients. Chest 1988; 94:1176–1186.
31. Boyd O, Grounds M, Bennett D: Preoperative increase of oxygen delivery reduces mortality in risk surgical patients. JAMA 1993; 270:2699–2704.
32. Schultz RJ, Whitfield GF, La Mura JJ, et al: The role of physiologic monitoring in patients with fractures of hip. J Trauma 1985; 25:309–316.
33. Fleming AW, Bishop MH, Shoemaker WC, et al: Prospective trial of supranormal values as goals of resuscitation in severe trauma. Arch Surg 1992; 127:1175–1181.
34. Bishop MH, Shoemaker WC, Kram HB, Ordog GJ, et al: Prospective randomized trial of survivor values of cardiac index, oxygen delivery, and oxygen consumption as resuscitation endpoints in severe trauma. J Trauma 1995; 38:780–787.
35. Tuchschmidt J, Fried JC, Astiz M, et al: Elevation of cardiac output and oxygen delivery improves outcome in septic shock. Chest 1992; 102:216–220.
36. Berlauk JF, Abrams JH, Gilmour IJ, et al: Preoperative optimization of cardiovascular hemodynamics improves outcome in peripheral vascular surgery. Ann Surg 1991; 214:289–297.
37. Shoemaker WC, Appel PL, Kram HB: Hemodynamic and oxygen transport responses in survivors and nonsurvivors of high risk surgery. Crit Care Med 1993; 21:977.
38. Guyton AC, Crowell JW: Dynamics of the heart in shock. Fed Proc 1961; 20(Suppl 9):51–56.
39. Crowell JW, Smith EE: Oxygen deficit and irreversible hemorrhagic shock. Am J Physiol 1964; 116:313–318.
40. Shoemaker WC, Appel PL, Kram HB: Role of oxygen debt in the development of organ failure, sepsis, and death. Chest 1992; 102:208–215.
41. Lowe JG, Ernst EA: The Quantitative Practice of Anesthesia: Use of the Closed Circuit. Baltimore, Williams & Wilkins, 1981, pp 146–147.
42. Hankeln KB, Senker R, Schwarten JN, et al: Evaluation of prognostic indices based on hemodynamic and oxygen transport variables in shock patients with ARDS. Crit Care Med 1987; 15:1–7.
43. Edwards JD, Brown GCS, Nightingale P, et al: Use of survivors' cardiorespiratory values as therapeutic goals in septic shock. Crit Care Med 1969; 17:1098–1103.
44. Creamer JE, Edwards JD, Nightingale P: Hemodynamic and oxygen transport variables in cardiogenic shock secondary to acute myocardial infarction. Am J Cardiol 1990; 65:1287–1291.
45. Cryer HM, Richardson JD, Longmire-Cook S, et al: Oxygen delivery in patients with adult respiratory distress syndrome who undergo surgery. Arch Surg 1989; 124:1378–1385.
46. Edwards JD: Oxygen transport in cardiogenic and septic shock. Crit Care Med 1991; 19:658–663.
47. Scalea TM, Simon HM, Duncan AO: Geriatric blunt multiple trauma: Improved survival with early invasive monitoring. J Trauma 1990; 39:129–136.
48. Yu M, Levy MM, Smith P, et al: Effect of maximizing oxygen delivery on morbidity and mortality rates in critically ill patients. Crit Care Med 1993; 21:830–838.
49. Abraham E: Physiologic stress and cellular ischemia. Crit Care Med 1991; 19:613–618.
50. Meade P, Shoemaker WC, Donnelly TJ, et al: Temporal patterns of hemodynamic oxygen transport, cytokine, and complement activity in the development of adult respiratory distress syndrome after severe injury. J Trauma 1994; 36:651–657.
51. Thangathurai D, Carbonnet C, Wo CCJ, Shoemaker WC, et al: Intraoperative maintenance of tissue perfusion prevents ARDS. New Horiz 1996; 4:466–474.
52. Shoemaker WC, Appel PL, Czer LS, et al: Pathogenesis of respiratory failure (ARDS) after hemorrhage and trauma. Crit Care Med 1980; 8:504–512.
53. Shoemaker WC, Appel PL: Pathophysiology of adult respiratory distress syndrome following sepsis and surgical operations. Crit Care Med 1985; 13:166–172.
54. Hankeln KB, Gronemeyer R, Held AM, et al: Use of continuous noninvasive measurement of oxygen consumption in patients with ARDS following shock of various etiologies. Crit Care Med 1991; 19:642–649.
55. Shibutani K, Komatsu T, Kubal K, et al: Critical level of oxygen delivery in anesthetized man. Crit Care Med 1983; 11:640–643.
56. Danek SJ, Lynch JP, Weg JD, et al: The dependence of oxygen uptake on oxygen delivery in adult respiratory distress syndrome. Am Rev Respir Dis 1980; 122:387–395.
57. Mohsenifar Z, Goldbach P, Tashkim DP, et al: Relationship between oxygen delivery and oxygen consumption in adult respiratory distress syndrome. Chest 1983; 84:267.
58. Gutierrez G, Pohil RJ: Oxygen consumption is linearly related to O_2 supply in critically ill patients. J Crit Care 1986; 1:45–53.
59. Mohsenifar Z, Amin D, Jasper AC, et al: Dependence of oxygen consumption on oxygen delivery in patients with chronic congestive heart failure. Chest 1987; 92:447–450.
60. Kariman K, Burns SR: Regulation of tissue oxygen extraction is disturbed in adult respiratory distress syndrome. Am Rev Respir Dis 1985; 132:109–114.
61. Brent BN, Matthay RA, Mohler DA, et al: Relationship between oxygen uptake and oxygen transport in stable patients with chronic obstructive pulmonary disease. Am Rev Respir Dis 1984; 129:682.

62. Dorinsky PM, Costello JL, Godek JE: Relationships of oxygen uptake and oxygen delivery in respiratory failure not due to adult respiratory distress syndrome. Chest 1988; 93:1013–1019.
63. Arnal G, Viole JP, Percival C, et al: Oxygen delivery and uptake in adult respiratory distress syndrome. Am Rev Respir Dis 1986; 133:999–1001.
64. Appel PL, Shoemaker WC: Relationship of oxygen consumption and oxygen delivery in surgical patients. Chest 1992; 102:906–911.
65. Shoemaker WC, Appel PL, Kram HB: Oxygen transport measurements to evaluate tissue perfusion and titrate therapy. Crit Care Med 1991; 19:672–681.
66. Shoemaker WC, Kram HB: Comparison of the effects of crystalloids and colloids on hemodynamic oxygen transport, mortality and morbidity. *In:* Debates in General Surgery. Simmon RS, Udeko AJ (Eds). Chicago, Year Book Medical Publishers, 1991.
67. Appel PL, Shoemaker WC: Fluid therapy in adult respiratory failure. Crit Care Med 1981; 9:862–867.
68. Hauser CJ, Shoemaker WC, Turpin I, et al: Oxygen transport responses to colloids and crystalloids in critically ill surgical patients. Surg Gynecol Obstet 1990; 150:811–818.
69. Guyton AC, Lindsey AW: Effect of elevated left atrial pressure and decreased plasma protein concentration on the development of pulmonary edema. Circ Res 1959; 7:649–655.
70. Moore FD, Olesen KH, McMurrey JD, et al: The Body Cell Mass and Its Supporting Environment: Body Composition in Health and Disease. Philadelphia, WB Saunders, 1963.
71. Artegas A, Bernard GR, Brigham RL, Carlet J, Falke K, et al: The American-European Consensus Conference on ARDS. Parts 1 and 2. Am J Respir Crit Care Med 1994; 149:818–824 and 1998; 157:1332–1347.

128

Initial Management of Acute Hypoxemia

John J. Marini, MD

The pulmonary capillaries exchange oxygen (O_2) for carbon dioxide (CO_2) across a thin gas-permeable membrane in a process fundamental to sustaining aerobic metabolism and hydrogen ion concentration (pH) homeostasis. Because different physiologic processes determine the adequacy of tissue oxygenation and CO_2 elimination, one of these functions usually takes primacy when the system begins to fail, even though dysfunctional elements of both are often present concurrently. Episodes of respiratory failure thus may logically be subclassified as oxygenation failures or ventilation failures. In this discussion I examine both primary manifestations of acute respiratory insufficiency with the aim of describing an approach to management that flows from an understanding of the underlying pathophysiology.

OXYGENATION FAILURE: DEFINITIONS

Oxygenation failure originates in one or more of the steps necessary to sustain O_2 availability for mitochondrial energy production:

1. Ventilation (the transfer of O_2 from the environment to the lungs).
2. Pulmonary O_2 exchange.
3. O_2 transport (delivery of adequate quantities of oxygenated blood to the metabolizing tissue).
4. Tissue gas exchange (utilization of O_2 and release of CO_2 by the peripheral tissues).

Tissue O_2 transport or O_2 delivery (DO_2), depends not only on lung function, as reflected in the partial pressure of arterial oxygen (PaO_2), but also on extrapulmonary factors—cardiac output (Q_T), hemoglobin (Hb) concentration, and the ability of hemoglobin to take up and release O_2:

$$DO_2 = Q_T \times CaO_2$$

In this expression, O_2 content per gram of hemoglobin (CaO_2) is determined by the following relationship (SaO_2 is the oxygen saturation of arterial blood expressed as a percentage):

$$CaO_2 = 1.36\ (Hb) \cdot SaO_2 + 0.003\ (PaO_2)$$

Cardiogenic shock, profound anemia, and carbon monoxide poisoning are clinical examples of O_2 transport failure. Laboratory abnormalities characteristic of such conditions are lactic acidosis and increased arteriovenous O_2 content gradient despite adequate arterial O_2 tension. Failure of O_2 uptake results from the inability of tissues to extract and utilize O_2. Clinical examples are septic shock, often thought to reflect a problem of microvascular distribution, and cyanide poisoning, a condition in which cytochromes vital to intracellular electron transport are inhibited. Unlike transport insufficiency, these problems of tissue uptake are distinguished by abnormally narrow arteriovenous O_2 gradients and normal or high values for mixed venous O_2 tension, saturation, and content. Like transport insufficiency, lactic acidosis is a helpful laboratory indicator of O_2 deprivation.

Despite the importance of O_2 transport and uptake, respiratory failure is generally understood to imply pulmonary dysfunction. Thus, the remainder of the present discussion focuses on the performance of the lung in oxygenating arterial blood.

MECHANISMS OF ARTERIAL HYPOXEMIA

The six mechanisms that contribute to arterial oxygen desaturation (outlined in Table 128–1) are discussed next.

Reduced Inspired Oxygen Concentration

A decrease in the partial pressure of inspired O_2 (PIO_2) occurs in response to toxic fume inhalation, in fires that consume O_2 in the combustion process, and at high altitudes.

Hypoventilation

Hypoventilation causes the partial pressure of alveolar O_2 (PAO_2) to fall when alveolar O_2 is not replenished quickly enough in the face of ongoing depletion. Although the alveolar (and arterial) partial pressures of oxygen may fall much

TABLE 128–1. Mechanisms of Arterial Hypoxemia

Low fraction of inspired oxygen (FIO_2)
Hypoventilation
Impaired diffusion
Ventilation-perfusion ($\dot{V}/\dot{Q}$) mismatch
Shunt
Desaturated mixed venous blood (in the presence of other mechanisms of hypoxemia)

faster than Pa_{CO_2} rises during the initial phase of hypoventilation or apnea, the steady-state PA_{O_2} is estimated by this simplified alveolar gas equation:

$$PA_{O_2} = PI_{O_2} - \frac{Pa_{CO_2}}{R}$$

In this equation, PI_{O_2} is the partial pressure of inspired oxygen at the tracheal level (corrected for water vapor pressure at body temperature), and R is the respiratory exchange ratio that accounts for the difference between CO_2 production and O_2 consumption at steady state (assumed to be a ratio of 0.8:1). Transiently, however, R can fall to very low values as alveolar O_2 is taken up faster than CO_2 is delivered.

Impaired Diffusion

Impaired oxygen diffusion implies incomplete equilibration of alveolar gas with pulmonary capillary blood. The clinical relevance of this potential mechanism is uncertain; however, factors that adversely affect diffusion are often encountered in practice:

- Increased distance between alveolus and erythrocyte
- Decreased O_2 gradient
- Shortened capillary transit time of red cells (e.g., high cardiac output with limited capillary reserve)

Ventilation-Perfusion Mismatch

Ventilation-perfusion ($\dot{V}/\dot{Q}$) mismatch is the most frequent contributor to clinically important O_2 desaturation. Perfused lung units that are poorly ventilated contribute to desaturation, whereas poorly perfused but well-ventilated units contribute to physiologic dead space, wasted ventilation, and a heavy workload, but not to hypoxemia. The relationship of O_2 content to Pa_{O_2}, like that of Pa_{O_2} to hemoglobin saturation, is highly curvilinear. Except under hyperbaric conditions, little additional O_2 can be loaded into blood with already well-saturated hemoglobin, no matter how high the O_2 tension in overventilated alveoli may rise. Blood streams exiting from different lung units mix gas contents (not partial pressures); consequently, overventilating some units in an attempt to compensate for others that remain underventilated cannot maintain Pa_{O_2} at a normal level unless inspired O_2 is supplemented. Thus, when equal volumes of blood from well-ventilated and poorly ventilated units mix, the blended sample will have an O_2 content halfway between the two but a Pa_{O_2} disproportionately weighted toward that of the lower $\dot{V}/\dot{Q}$ unit.

Supplemental O_2 impressively reverses hypoxemia when $\dot{V}/\dot{Q}$ mismatch, hypoventilation, or impaired diffusion is the cause. At some FI_{O_2} value, compensation is complete. In fact, after one breathes 100% O_2 for a sufficient time, only perfused units that are totally unventilated (shunt units) contribute to hypoxemia. However, when hypoxemia is caused by alveolar units with very low $\dot{V}/\dot{Q}$ ratios, relatively concentrated O_2 mixtures must be inspired before arterial oxygenation shows a noteworthy improvement.

Shunting

Shunt fraction is the percentage of the total systemic venous blood flow that effectively bypasses aerated alveoli to transfer venous blood unaltered to the arterial system. Alterations of FI_{O_2} fail to influence Pa_{O_2} significantly when shunt is the sole mechanism of hypoxemia and the *true shunt fraction* exceeds 30% (Fig. 128–1).[1, 2] In contrast, venous admixture resulting

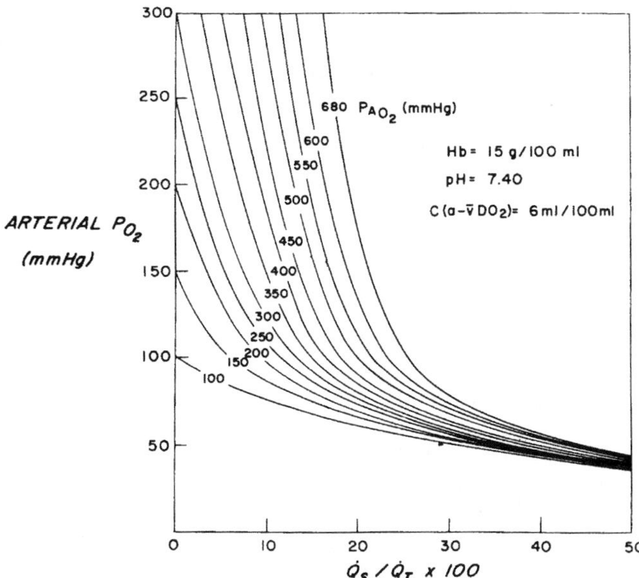

Figure 126–1. Effect of increasing shunt on arterial P_{O_2} at different fractions of inspired oxygen (FI_{O_2}). The relative effect of FI_{O_2} depends on the shunt percentage. Hb = hemoglobin. (From Dantzker DR, Sharf SM: Cardiopulmonary Critical Care. 3rd ed. Philadelphia, WB Saunders, 1998, p 45.)

from other mechanisms that cause hypoxemia of similar magnitude invariably responds to supplemental O_2. Shunting can be intracardiac, as in cyanotic right-to-left congenital heart disease, or can result from passage of blood through pulmonary arteriovenous communications. By far the most common cause of shunting, however, is airless lung.

Many indices have been devised to characterize the efficacy of O_2 exchange across the spectrum of FI_{O_2}. Although no index is ideal, the Pa_{O_2}/PA_{O_2} ratio and the alveolar-arterial oxygen tension difference (PA_{O_2}–Pa_{O_2}) are often utilized.[3] In the setting of lung disease, however, both are affected by alterations in venous O_2 content, even when the lung itself has not changed its ability to transfer O_2 to the blood.[4] Another imprecise but commonly used indicator of gas exchange is the Pa_{O_2}/FI_{O_2} ratio. In healthy adults, this ratio normally exceeds 400, whatever the FI_{O_2}. Hypoventilation and changes in the inspired O_2 concentration alter these ratios minimally in the absence of FI_{O_2}-related absorption atelectasis or cardiovascular adjustments.

Abnormal Desaturation of Systemic Venous Blood

Admixture of abnormally desaturated venous blood is an important mechanism that acts to lower Pa_{O_2} in patients with impaired pulmonary gas exchange and reduced cardiac output. Cv_{O_2}, the product of hemoglobin concentration and the oxygen saturation of venous blood (Sv_{O_2}), is influenced by cardiac output (Q), arterial oxygen saturation (Sa_{O_2}), and oxygen consumption (V_{O_2}):

$$Sv_{O_2} \sim Sa_{O_2} - [V_{O_2}/(Hb \times Q)]$$

This equation illustrates that Sv_{O_2} is directly influenced by any imbalance between V_{O_2} and O_2 delivery. Thus, anemia uncompensated by an increase in cardiac output or cardiac output insufficient for metabolic needs can cause both Sv_{O_2} and Pa_{O_2} to fall unless the lung is normal. In the normal lung,

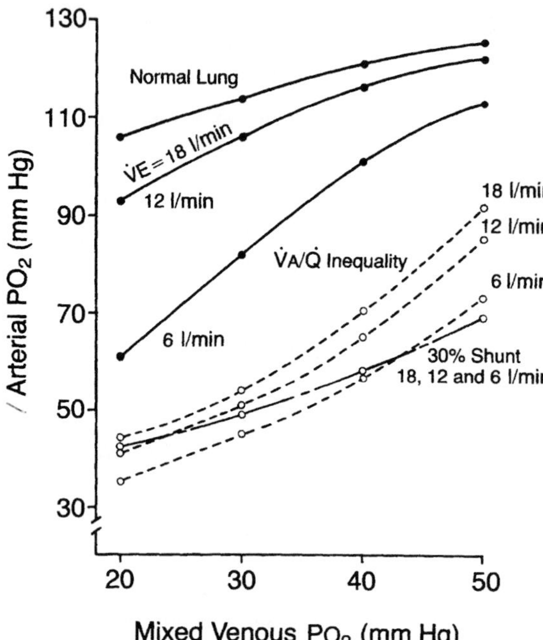

Figure 128–2. Computer simulation of the influence of changing mixed venous P_{O_2} on arterial P_{O_2} in lungs that are normal and/or impaired. Effects on arterial P_{O_2} of changes in minute ventilation and mixed venous P_{O_2} are influenced by the mechanism of transpulmonary oxygen transfer—normal, ventilation-perfusion ($\dot{V}_A/\dot{Q}$) inequality, or shunt. (From Dantzker DR, Sharf SM: Cardiopulmonary Critical Care. 3rd ed. Philadelphia, WB Saunders, 1998, p 42.)

well-ventilated alveoli have adequate oxygenation reserve to compensate for a low $S\bar{v}_{O_2}$. In healthy subjects a marked decline in $S\bar{v}_{O_2}$ without arterial hypoxemia occurs routinely during heavy exercise.

Fluctuations in $S\bar{v}_{O_2}$ tend to exert a more profound influence on Pa_{O_2} when the shunt is fixed, as in *regional* lung diseases (e.g., atelectasis), than when the shunt varies with cardiac output, as it tends to do with *diffuse* lung injury, the acute respiratory distress syndrome (ARDS).[5] Furthermore, in lungs that are normal or when hypoxemia is due to $\dot{V}/\dot{Q}$ mismatch, such variations in $S\bar{v}_{O_2}$ tend to have greater impact when minute ventilation is fixed than when it is free to increase (Fig. 128–2).[6] The severity of arterial hypoxemia tends to vary inversely with the effectiveness of hypoxic pulmonary vasoconstriction. Even when $S\bar{v}_{O_2}$ is abnormally low, Pa_{O_2} remains unaffected when all mixed venous blood gains access to well-oxygenated, well-ventilated alveoli. Abnormal $\dot{V}/\dot{Q}$ match or shunt is necessary if venous desaturation is to contribute to hypoxemia.

COMMON CLINICAL CAUSES OF HYPOXEMIA

Radiographic appearances give important clues to the appropriate management of oxygenation failure. Lung collapse (atelectasis), diffuse or patchy parenchymal infiltration, hydrostatic edema, localized or unilateral infiltration, and a clear chest radiograph are common patterns (Fig. 128–3).

Atelectasis

Classification

Morphologic type and mechanism classify atelectasis. Regional microatelectasis spontaneously develops during shallow breathing when the healthy lung is not periodically stretched beyond its usual tidal range. Plate-like atelectasis may be an exaggeration of this phenomenon secondary to regional hypodistention (e.g., pleural effusion or impaired diaphragmatic excursion). Microatelectasis and plate-like atelectasis occur most often in dependent regions.[7] Lobar collapse usually results from gas absorption in an airway plugged by retained secretions, a misplaced endotracheal tube, or a central mass. Bronchial compression and regional hypoventilation are important in some patients. Microatelectasis and plate-like atelectasis occur routinely with prolonged, uninterrupted bed rest and after operations with upper abdominal incisions.

Potential consequences of acute atelectasis are deterioration of gas exchange, pneumonitis, and increased work of breathing. Pa_{O_2} drops precipitously to its nadir within minutes to hours of a sudden bronchial occlusion, but then it improves steadily over hours to days as hypoxic vasoconstriction and altered regional forces augment pulmonary vascular resistance in the affected region. Whether an individual patient manifests hypoxemia depends much on the intensity of the hypoxic vasoconstrictive response, the abruptness of collapse, and the tissue volume involved. When small areas of atelectasis develop slowly, hypoxemia may never surface as a significant clinical problem.

Management

Mobilization is the best treatment for all types of atelectasis. Periodic sustained deep breaths (yawn equivalents) effectively reverse plate-like atelectasis and microatelectasis. Relief of chest wall pain helps to reduce splinting and enables more effective coughing. Intercostal or epidural nerve blocks with anesthetic agents, such as bupivacaine, may be effective. Epidural narcotics are also effective in certain settings. Although it seems rational, the place of positive end-expiratory pressure (PEEP) in treating established collapse has not been clarified. Retained secretions must be dislodged from the central airways. Vigorous respiratory therapy initiated soon after the onset of lobar collapse can quickly reverse most cases of atelectasis due to airway plugging.[8]

Fiberoptic bronchoscopy should be reserved for patients with symptomatic lobar collapse who lack central air bronchograms and who cannot undergo, fail to respond to, or cannot tolerate 48 hours of vigorous respiratory therapy. After reexpansion, a respiratory therapy program should be initiated to prevent recurrence.

Diffuse Pulmonary Infiltration

Severe, refractory hypoxemia may result when edema fluid or cellular infiltrates cause alveolar filling. Fluid in the interstitial spaces can cause hypoxemia as a result of compressive peribronchial edema, $\dot{V}/\dot{Q}$ mismatch, and microatelectasis; however, interstitial fluid itself does not interfere with O_2 exchange. Moreover, few clinical problems are confined exclusively to the airspaces or the interstitium. The major categories of acute disease that produce diffuse pulmonary infiltration and hypoxemia are pneumonitis (infection and aspiration), cardiogenic pulmonary edema, intravascular volume overload, and ARDS. From a radiographic viewpoint, these processes may be difficult to distinguish; however, a few features are characteristic.[9]

A prominent vascular pattern and hilar infiltrates that spare the costophrenic angles suggest volume overload or incipient cardiogenic edema. Gravitational distribution of edema is very consistent with well-established left ventricular failure or volume overload, especially when accompanied by cardiomegaly and a widened vascular pedicle. Patchy peripheral infiltrates

A Clear	B Diffuse	C Lobar	D Unilateral
Intracardiac shunt	Bronchopneumonia	Infarction	Aspiration
Pulmonary vascular shunts	BP dysplasia	Occlusion (drowned lung)	Pleural effusion
AV malformation	Hemorrhage	Lobar pneumonia	Mass and drowned lung
Cirrhosis	ARDS		Infarction
Asthma/obstructive lung disease	Hydrostatic edema		Main bronchus intubation
Pulmonary embolism	Aspiration		Mucus plug
Pneumothorax			Contusion
Head injury			Re-expansion edema
Desaturated mixed venous blood			Contralateral pneumothorax
Obesity/airway closure			Pneumonia
			Decubitus position/ hydrostatic edema

Figure 128–3. Radiographic patterns associated with hypoxemia. ARDS = acute respiratory distress syndrome.

that lack a gravitational predilection and are slow to change with position suggest permeability edema (i.e., ARDS). Septal (Kerley) lines and distinct peribronchial cuffing are common in congestive heart failure but are seldom seen in ARDS. On the other hand, prominent air bronchograms are quite unusual with hydrostatic causes but are common in ARDS and pneumonia.

Hydrostatic edema can occur in multiple settings and has different implications for prognosis and treatment. Left ventricular failure is the archetype of *hydrostatic pulmonary edema.* In this setting, signs of systemic hypoperfusion and inadequate cardiac output often accompany oxygenation failure; however, hydrostatic pulmonary edema can develop even with a normally well-compensated ventricle in patients with severe hypoalbuminemia or during transient heart dysfunction (ischemia, hypertensive crisis, arrhythmias). When the myocardium fails to relax fully during diastole (diastolic dysfunction), superimposed loading or temporary disturbances of left heart contractility (e.g., ischemia), mitral valve function, or heart rate or rhythm may cause rapid, transient alveolar flooding known as *flash pulmonary edema,* named for the impressive speed with which extensive radiographic infiltrates develop and resolve.[10]

Acute Lung Injury and Acute Respiratory Distress Syndrome

ARDS is the most severe form of acute lung injury. A general designation, it refers to all degrees of radiographically apparent, diffuse, hypoxemic lung injury. The ARDS designation is most useful when restricted to acute noncardiogenic pulmonary edema that has these characteristic features:

- Impaired compliance of the respiratory system
- Markedly reduced aerated lung volume
- Refractory hypoxemia
- Delayed resolution

Sepsis, aspiration, pneumonia, and polytrauma account for most cases of ARDS. In general, predisposing illnesses injure the alveolocapillary membrane from either the gas side (e.g., smoke inhalation, aspiration of gastric acid, pneumonia) or the blood side (e.g., sepsis, fat embolism). Typically, fewer than a third of all lung units remain aerated. Abnormally increased membrane permeability allows seepage of protein-rich fluids into the interstitial and alveolar spaces, where they directly inhibit or inactivate surfactant, contributing to widespread atelectasis as the inflammatory process degrades the lung's architecture in a three-stage process. The earliest stage of widespread edema and atelectasis (days 1 to 3) is followed by the proliferative (days 3 to 7) and resolution (after 7 days) stages.[11] Pulmonary artery occlusion pressure usually remains normal, but increased pulmonary vascular resistance and pulmonary hypertension are invariable, especially in the latter stages of severe disease. Extreme pulmonary hypertension is a very poor prognostic sign. Apart from any difference in capillary pressure, permeability edema differs from hydrostatic edema in that it resists clearance by diuretic therapy and initiates the inflammatory response, which can take weeks to recede and even longer to heal.

The response of this disease to manipulations of airway pressure (e.g., PEEP) and drugs (e.g., corticosteroids) is influenced by the stage of the process and by its cause. Still, the core pathophysiology of ARDS and the potential for further injury by misguided ventilation strategies are sufficiently similar to warrant a single treatment approach. Excessive fluids must not be given, so as to minimize lung water and improve O_2 exchange. Severe fluid restriction, on the other hand, may compromise perfusion of gut and kidneys. Appropriate nutritional support, preferably enteral, and prophylaxis for deep venous thrombosis, skin breakdown, and gastric stress ulceration should be considered for all mechanically ventilated or immobile patients.

The routine use of corticosteroids for the early phase of ARDS does not seem justified because of their adverse effects on immunity, mental status, metabolism, and protein wastage in the absence of evidence for benefit. Corticosteroids are indicated, however, for respiratory distress resulting from vasculitis, fat embolism, or allergic reactions. Corticosteroids may also be life saving in certain steroid-responsive diseases that mimic ARDS (e.g., bronchiolitis obliterans organizing pneumonia, pulmonary hemorrhage syndromes, *Pneumocystis carinii* pneumonia). Corticosteroids may help to resolve the fibroproliferative stage of ARDS, but there is still no consensus on this point.[12]

Because extravascular water accumulates readily in the setting of permeability edema, fluids should be used judiciously, in a manner consistent with adequate O_2 delivery. Liberal use of inotropes and other vasoactive drugs can be helpful in certain postoperative or post-trauma settings, but driving the cardiac output to supraphysiologic levels does *not* appear to improve the mortality rate of medical patients with ARDS.

Hypoxemia with a Clear Chest Radiograph

Patients may present with severe hypoxemia who have no major radiographic evidence of infiltration. In such cases, occult shunting and severe $\dot{V}/\dot{Q}$ mismatch are the most likely mechanisms. Intracardiac or intrapulmonary shunts, asthma and other forms of airway obstruction, low lung volume superimposed on a high closing capacity (e.g., bronchitis in a supine obese patient), pulmonary embolism, and occult microvascular communications (as in patients with cirrhosis) are potential explanations. Therapeutic vasoactive agents (nitroprusside, calcium channel blockers, dopamine) can accentuate hypoxemia from shunt or $\dot{V}/\dot{Q}$ mismatch.[13]

Unilateral Lung Disease

Marked radiographic asymmetry (see Fig. 128-3) suggests a confined set of causes, which include pneumonia, atelectasis, aspiration, and radiation injury. Most occur in characteristic clinical settings.

TECHNIQUES TO IMPROVE TISSUE OXYGENATION

Whatever the cause of hypoxemic respiratory failure, important therapeutic aims are to reverse the underlying lung disease, to improve O_2 delivery, to relieve excessive breathing workload, and to maintain electrolyte balance while preventing further damage from O_2 toxicity, barotrauma, infection, and other iatrogenic complications.

Because O_2 delivery is the product of cardiac output and the O_2 content of each milliliter of arterial blood, O_2 carrying capacity can be improved by increasing hemoglobin concentration. Increasing hemoglobin tends to elevate mixed venous O_2 saturation, as it reduces the need for any rise in cardiac output compensatory to anemia. Lower cardiac output and higher mixed venous O_2 saturation both tend to reduce venous admixture. Reversing alkalemia facilitates O_2 off-loading. As hemoglobin concentration rises, blood viscosity increases, retarding passage of erythrocytes through the capillary network. O_2 delivery can actually decline as hematocrit rises above 50%. Although the optimal hematocrit value in patients with an oxygenation crisis is not known, it is standard practice to restore it to at least 30%. More extensive supplementation increases the risk of transfusion—without proven benefit.

Oxygen Therapy

O_2 toxicity depends on both concentration and time.[14] As a rule, high concentrations of inspired O_2 can safely be used for brief periods as efforts are made to reverse the underlying process. Sustained elevations in FIO_2 (>0.6), however, result in inflammatory changes, and eventually fibrosis, in experimental animals; thus, it seems prudent to keep FIO_2 below 0.6 during the support phase of acute lung injury.

Secretion Management and Bronchodilation

Airway edema, bronchospasm, and secretion retention often contribute to hypoxemia. In intubated patients, retained secretions increase endotracheal tube resistance, risk of infection or of barotrauma, and maldistribution of ventilation. In some patients with diffuse lung injury, profound bradycardia develops during ventilator disconnections. Although hypoxemia occasionally contributes, this bradycardia is usually reflexive and responds to prophylactic (parenteral) atropine or reapplication of positive airway pressure. Circuits that do not interrupt PEEP during suctioning offer an advantage in this regard.

Reducing Oxygen Requirements

Fever, agitation, overfeeding, vigorous respiratory activity, shivering, sepsis, and anxiety can markedly increase O_2 consumption. Reducing fever may have therapeutic value, but shivering must be prevented in the cooling process. Sedatives and antipyretics make better therapeutic sense than cooling blankets.

Although muscle relaxants are a valuable adjunct to reduce O_2 consumption and improve PaO_2 in patients who remain agitated or fight the ventilator (though well sedated), lengthy paralysis must be avoided. Paralysis silences the coughing mechanism and creates a monotonous breathing pattern that encourages secretion retention in dependent regions. Protracted, unmonitored paralysis can cause weakness or devastating neuromyopathy.[15]

Repositioning

Frequent repositioning of the patient may help to preserve alveolar patency and gas exchange.[16] Prone positioning should be considered during the early phase of ARDS, as improved O_2 exchange has been confirmed in this setting. Moreover, laboratory work suggests that prone positioning may help to protect the lungs against ventilation-induced damage or barotrauma.

MECHANICAL VENTILATORY SUPPORT

Although mechanical ventilation is a cornerstone of life support, when applied inexpertly it may be associated with pulmonary and systemic infections, multisystem organ dysfunction, barotrauma, and increased mortality. In the setting of acute lung injury, high stretching forces applied repeatedly to normal or preinjured lungs ventilated without sufficient PEEP increase capillary permeability, encourage gas leaks and edema, and initiate inflammation.[17, 18] Consequently, many clinicians have revised their ventilatory priorities in attempts to prevent ventilator-induced lung injury while accomplishing adequate gas exchange.

The principal objective is to accomplish effective gas exchange at the least FIO_2 and pressure cost. The relative hazards of O_2 therapy, high-pressure ventilatory patterns, and abnormal arterial blood gases and pH, however, are controversial. Similarly, the contribution of vascular pressures and flows to iatrogenic lung injury has not yet been settled. This discussion develops a ventilatory strategy that is guided by the lessons emerging from the admittedly incomplete data base currently available (Table 128-2). Many important issues remain unresolved. The majority of information on ventilator-induced lung injury stems from experimentation with imperfect animal models of acute lung injury (ALI) and from inadequately controlled clinical reports. Although further confirmation is required, newer data from patients appear to be consistent with the mechanisms suggested by the body of laboratory evidence.

Traditional Approach to Ventilation of the Patient with Acute Respiratory Distress Syndrome

When lungs are intact and their capacity to expand remains normal (e.g., during anesthesia), tidal volumes of 10 to 15 mL/kg generate only modest alveolar pressures. In fact, large tidal volumes are often appropriate in the postoperative set-

TABLE 128–2. Ventilatory Strategies for Patients with Acute Respiratory Distress Syndrome

	Traditional	Revised
Objectives	Normal ABGs	Adequate ABGs; prevent alveolar injury; facilitate healing
Ventilation Mode Settings	Volume-cycled ventilation	Pressure-targeted ventilation
PEEP	As needed for adequate Pao_2/FIO_2	Sufficient to prevent tidal recruiting cycle and achieve adequate Pao_2/FIO_2 ratio
Tidal volume	Preset (10–15 mL/kg)	4–8 mL/kg
Peak alveolar as required for PEEP and tidal volume		No higher than a peak P_{tm} of 30–35 cm H_2O

ABGs = arterial blood gas determinations; P_{tm} = transmural alveolar pressure.

ting to prevent the microatelectasis that accompanies uninterrupted shallow breathing in the supine position.[19] Large tidal volumes are produced by healthy persons during exercise and by many spontaneously breathing patients with normal lungs, to satisfy high ventilatory demands (e.g., as of diabetic ketoacidosis). Postoperatively, the mandatory respiratory rate is usually adjusted to "normalize" pH or $Paco_2$, and sufficient PEEP is used to achieve acceptable O_2 delivery at what is assumed to be a nontoxic FIO_2, typically one less than 0.65. Reduced chest wall compliance characterizes the interval immediately after many types of thoracoabdominal surgery and, together with expansion of intravascular volume, further raises ventilation pressures.

Dating from the mid 1960s, high tidal volume, normoxic, normocapnic ventilation paradigm—generally appropriate for routine postoperative patients—developed as the standard approach to supporting most critically ill patients. Consequently, end-tidal (plateau) alveolar pressures greater than 50 cm H_2O were used then and today remain common in many intensive care units for ventilation of patients with ARDS. How best to select "optimal" PEEP remains controversial; available machine settings may not achieve all important clinical objectives.[20] Many practitioners advocate using the *least* PEEP consistent with acceptable arterial oxygenation.[21] Others rely on computations of systemic O_2 delivery or best tidal compliance to select PEEP and tidal volume. An adventuresome minority seek guidance in the contours of a static pressure-volume (P-V) curve of the respiratory system, assigning first priority to ensuring adequate lung protection.

Ventilator-Induced Lung Damage

The microscopic architecture of acute lung injury evolves continuously over its course. In the most severe cases, cellular proliferation, organization, remodeling, and fibrosis sequentially follow an initial phase of edema and atelectasis.[22] Parenchymal damage is widespread, but the nature, severity, and, perhaps, even stage of injury vary from site to site within the damaged lung. Moreover, there is compelling evidence that certain patterns of mechanical ventilation can modify the severity and nature of these pathologic findings.

Although the tough collagen framework of the previously normal lung remains relatively intact during the first days of injury, it later weakens as inflammation degrades structural proteins and, in conjunction with high airway pressure, nonuniformly remodels lung architecture. For this reason, alveolar gas tends to enter the interstitium more easily, and clinically detectable barotrauma often occurs late in the course of the disease, often well after gas exchange begins to improve.[23]

Regional Mechanics

Every form of ventilator-induced lung damage described in infants occurs in adults as well. Key clinical observations, as well as disturbing experimental data, strongly suggest that the conventional approach may place some regions of the injured lung at risk for retarded healing. Regional mechanics vary, even in the earliest phase of the process. Gravitationally dependent areas are extensively consolidated and atelectatic, whereas nondependent regions tend to aerate better, at least early in the course.[24] Regional blood flow and vascular pressures also vary. Changes of body position may alter the radiographic findings, improve gas exchange, and protect against ventilator-induced lung damage.[25–28] Perhaps 60% to 70% of patients respond to prone positioning by exhibiting significant improvement of Pao_2 during this early phase of ARDS.[28]

In severe cases of ARDS, no more than a third of all alveoli remain patent and gas-accessible. Because ventilated lung units may retain nearly normal elasticity and fragility, the apparent stiffness of the lung in the early phase of acute lung injury is better explained by fewer functioning alveoli than by a generalized increase in recoil tension.[24, 29] Tissue elastance contributes more in the later phases, when cellular infiltration is intense, edema has been reabsorbed or organized, atelectasis is less extensive, and fibrosis is under way. Large tidal volumes may subject the "baby lung" that remains to overdistention, local hyperventilation, and inhibition or depletion of surfactant.[30] Moreover, intense shearing forces can develop at the junctions of structures that are mobile (aerated lung units) with those that are immobile (owing to collapsed or consolidated alveoli, distal conducting airways). Indeed, in such a heterogeneous lung, junctional alveolar wall *tensions* may be extreme.[31] Increases in cycling frequency and duration of exposure accentuate any tendency for damage to occur.[32]

The adherent walls of collapsed small airways often require sustained high pressures to separate.[33] Once they are opened, however, somewhat lower pressures may preserve luminal patency. Differences of opening and closing pressures give rise to hysteresis of the P-V relationship (Fig. 128-4). Hysteresis is difficult to demonstrate in many patients after the first few hours to days of ventilator support.[34, 35] If the terminal airways remain closed, their unsupported walls may be subjected to forces that approach the dynamic pressures applied to more central airways, which are reinforced by cartilage. Damage to the small bronchioles occurs consistently when moderately high ventilating pressures are used (as documented in an illuminating autopsy study that detected bronchiolar dilatation, cystic changes, and/or microabscesses in the majority of patients with acute lung injury ventilated with peak airway pressures well within the range traditionally allowed).[36]

That lung damage results from overdistention has been convincingly documented.[37, 38] The severity of this *stretch injury* appears greatest when PEEP is insufficient to keep dependent lung units fully recruited. In diverse animal models, *transalveolar* cycling pressures approximating those that correspond to total lung capacity (≤30 to 35 cm H_2O) can increase permeability within a few tidal cycles and create

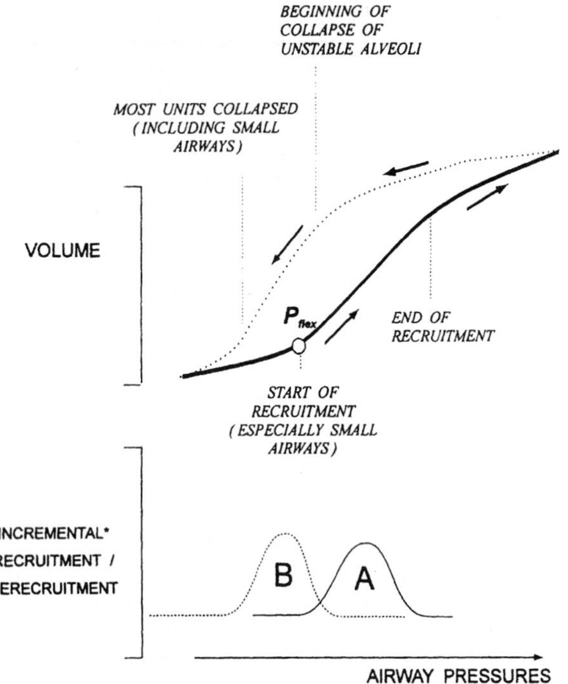

A: Frequency distribution of opening pressures (inspiration)
B: Frequency distribution of closing pressures (expiration)
(*: incremental recruitment = number of units opening at a certain pressure)

Figure 128–4. Theoretical pressure-volume loop with its expiratory *(dotted line)* and inspiratory *(solid line)* limbs. In this curve, phases 2, 3, and 4 of inspiration are merged owing to a wide distribution of opening pressures. Therefore, overdistention of elastic elements in many units that are already patent occurs at the same airway pressures at which a relatively small number of units are still being recruited. Even with the wide distributions of critical pressures across the parenchyma, the opening pressures are substantially higher than the closing pressures.

gross injury within minutes. Injurious forces can be produced by positive or negative pressure.[23, 39–41] When sustained over several days, even lower peak airway pressures (about 30 cm H_2O) damage normal lung tissues.[32]

An upper inflection point of the P-V curve of the respiratory system—suggesting regional overdistention or termination of recruitment—can be detected at peak alveolar pressures less than 28 cm H_2O in many patients with ARDS.[42] Such results are disturbing, because when acting in combination, noxious influences (e.g., alveolar pressure, inflammatory stimuli, increased FIO_2, increased vascular pressure or blood flow) may synergize. Thus, two stimuli acting in combination at low intensity can produce injury that neither could alone.[43] Moreover, preexisting lung damage (sustained before the acute episode) can predispose to ventilator-induced lung injury.[44]

Factors that affect transmural *capillary* pressure modulate microscopic injury to the endothelial membrane.[45] If this "noxious synergism" also occurs in the clinical setting, even a modest plateau pressure might be detrimental in the already damaged lung. Electron microscopic breaks in the gas-blood interface (i.e., capillary stress failure) can occur in rabbits when *transmural* capillary pressures exceed about 40 mm Hg. The transmural pressures needed to cause such damage in healthy dogs (and presumably in normal humans) appear to be considerably greater, perhaps 90 to 100 mm Hg.[46] Although *intravascular* pressures of this magnitude never occur in the clinical setting, *extramural* tensions surrounding vascular channels at the junctions of collapsed and expanding lung units could rise into this hazardous range with higher tidal volumes.[47] Furthermore, the reduced tensile strength of acutely inflamed parenchyma and microvasculature may predispose to capillary stress fracture at lower transvascular pressures. Finally, higher vascular pressures accentuate edema formation and may contribute, directly or indirectly, to hemorrhage, atelectasis, and regional shear stresses.

The Concept of Volutrauma

Peak inflation pressure is not the causative variable of ventilator-induced lung damage.[48–50] To illustrate: A lung encased in steel would not expand significantly or experience shear stress even if exposed to several atmospheres of pressure; enormous pressures (relative to atmosphere) are tolerated perfectly well in a hyperbaric chamber. Because alveolar overstretching is thought to be the key problem, *volutrauma* has been suggested as a more appropriate term than *barotrauma.*[51] In a certain sense, this newer term is more descriptive, provided that the term *volume* is understood to be ***the volume of the individual alveolus,*** whose only measurable clinical correlate is *transalveolar pressure* (PTA) (Fig. 128–5). Transalveolar pressure varies from site to site in the damaged lung, being least in dependent areas. As a practical matter, transalveolar pressure is roughly approximated by the difference between alveolar and pleural pressures. (Transmural forces, however, may be considerably greater near semirigid vascular or bronchial structures.)

In a recently injured, heterogeneous lung it may be more important to restrict the pressure *excursion* of the alveolus (the end-inspiratory–end-expiratory PTA *difference*) than the absolute PTA.[51–53] In a given patient, variations in this excursion of PTA correlate with tidal volume. It is important to understand, however, that, of themselves, large tidal volume excursions are not inherently injurious; the impact of any specific tidal volume depends not only on the tendency for end-expiratory collapse but also on the tidal pressure achieved. If tidal pressures do not approach the elastic limits of the alveolus and if PEEP is sufficient, the tidal volume (however large) may not be dangerous. In fact, failure of a "large" tidal volume to encroach upon a dangerous pressure threshold (combined with equivalent PEEP in the study and control groups) is likely

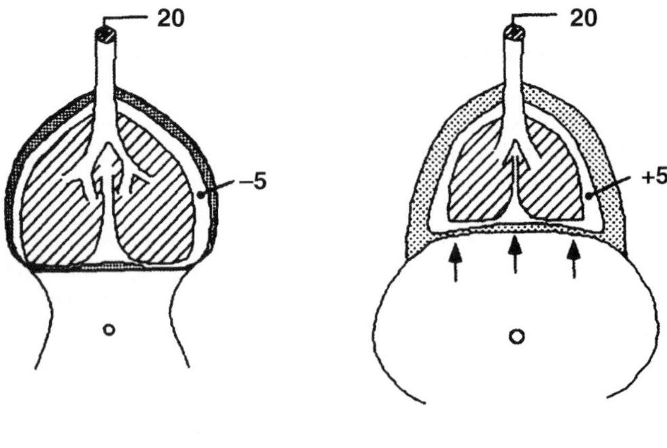

Normal **Stiff Chest Wall**

Figure 128–5. Influence of chest wall compliance on lung distention and alveolar pressure. Because alveolar distention is the major concern in avoiding ventilator-induced lung injury, alveolar pressure must be interpreted in light of the potential impact of global and regional chest wall stiffness. (From Marini JJ, Wheeler AW. Critical Care Medicine: The Essentials. 2nd ed. Baltimore, Williams and Wilkins, 1997, p 159.)

to account for the lack of difference between "low" and "high" tidal volume groups according to a recent, well-controlled clinical trial.[54]

Because the aeratable lung capacity varies greatly among patients, it may be misleading to formulate strict guidelines for tidal volume based on body weight, just as no precise rules can be formulated for narrowly fixing safe or injurious limits for plateau airway pressure. Growing scientific evidence suggests that the end-expiratory pressure and tidal volume selections are best made empirically by selecting a ventilation pattern that avoids the lower and upper inflection points of the P-V curve of the respiratory system.[51, 55, 56] When constant inspiratory flow is delivered under passive conditions, the *alveolar* P-V contour may be readily inferred under dynamic conditions, facilitating measurement of the upper inflection point.[57] Unfortunately, the contours of the static P-V curve can be influenced as much by the chest wall as by the lung. Moreover, on the lower end, regional auto-PEEP, hydraulic effects of airway liquid shift, and outward springing of the chest wall can all contribute to the lower inflection zone.

Role of End-Expiratory Volume in Lung Injury

Failure to maintain a certain *minimum* alveolar volume in the early phase of acute lung injury may accentuate lung damage.[53, 56, 58, 59] In surfactant-depleted rabbit and oleic acid–injured dog models, persisting or tidally phasic collapse causes parenchymal infiltration of the activated neutrophils believed to mediate alveolar damage.[60, 61] In animal experiments, the addition of PEEP significantly reduces alveolar hemorrhage and other histologic changes that otherwise result from high tidal pressures. This observation could help to account for the reported tolerance of certain surgical patients to the very high inspiratory pressures generated by *super PEEP* (>20 cm H_2O). Conversely, insufficient PEEP may account for the failure of "prophylactic PEEP" to avert ARDS.[62]

If the tidal range of alveolar pressures permits, collapsible units may "wink" open and closed with every tidal cycle, generating shear stresses in junctional tissues of the type already outlined. Such a "tidal recruitment" cycle is implied by data that demonstrate optimal compliance at PEEP levels, which vary inversely with tidal volume.[63] Computed tomographic densitometry data appear to confirm this possibility.[64] It must be understood, however, that PEEP responsiveness may depend greatly on the event inciting ARDS. ARDS from pulmonary causes tends to respond much less well than from extrapulmonary causes.[65]

"P_{flex}" and the Choice of PEEP

A lower inflection region on the inspiratory limb of the static P-V curve of the passive respiratory system suggests the existence of a population of alveoli at risk for excessive tidal stress. The point at which the slope of the static P-V curve stops improving rapidly with further pressure application (mathematically, when the second derivative of the least squares–fitted equation relating volume to pressure becomes zero) is known as the *P_{flex} point.* Apart from atelectasis, hydraulic factors and changing chest wall characteristics may require that higher pressures be applied along this first P-V segment. Not all patients exhibit a lower P_{flex} region, but those who do are likely to experience extensive end-expiratory atelectasis at lower PEEPs. Indeed, although alveolar recruitment occurs over an extended portion of the entire inflation span (even along the linear segment), arterial oxygenation often improves markedly as the end-expiratory pressure range just below P_{flex} is exceeded.[55]

If we acknowledge that the expiratory P-V curve may be more relevant to lung recruitment, current evidence suggests that tidal ventilation that spans the lower inflection range of pressures must be avoided. Either sufficient PEEP or the progression of disease over time obliterates the P_{flex} point and narrows the hysteresis of the P-V curve.[57, 66] It should be understood, however, that failure to identify a lower inflection zone or significant hysteresis does not imply the absence of recruitable lung. Being a composite of the behaviors of all alveoli heterogeneous lung tissue, the contours of the static P-V curve obscure very important regional differences.

Within the injured lung, opening pressures differ at different vertical levels. Alveoli in dependent regions are most susceptible to collapse, and those in nondependent regions overdistend with modest pressures. This variability of opening pressures helps account for the lower and upper inflection *zones* recorded in some (but not all) patients. In truth, however, recruitment and overdistention must occur to some extent (but in different regions) throughout the tidal cycle. The upper inflection region can as easily represent the termination of recruitment as overdistention. Whatever its magnitude, the discrepancy between opening and closing pressures is a function of the size of the tidal volume and the temporal proximity to a volume recruitment maneuver (sustained inflation to total lung capacity).

Because of marked differences in respiratory mechanics among patients with ARDS and the wide variation and rapid changeability of this syndrome, machine settings conferring optimal lung protection cannot be predetermined. Consequently, many investigators, but relatively few clinicians, inscribe the entire static P-V curve of the respiratory system, so as to determine *empirically* the tidal pressure range best positioned between collapse and overdistention. Although this is simple in concept, the pitfalls of defining the P-V relationship are many; the best technique for constructing P-V curves—and, indeed, the precise relevance of inspiratory P-V curves to tidal ventilation cycles—are not known for certain. Because volume history is important, curves inscribed by variations of tidal volume (at fixed end-expiratory pressure)[67] or of PEEP (at fixed tidal volume) do not always produce identical results. A lower inflection zone cannot always be identified[57] and when found, P_{flex} may overestimate or underestimate the least PEEP actually required to maintain alveolar stability, depending on disease, patient, and method.[61] In fact, the expiratory limb of the P-V curve may be more relevant to the PEEP values that preserve expiratory patency of the units opened or refreshed during inspiration. As a practical compromise, many practitioners rely on tidal compliance to guide PEEP and tidal volume selections. Standard calculations of tidal compliance, however, do not provide enough information.[63, 68] No method is perfectly suited in the presence of active spontaneous efforts.

Tidal Compliance and Tidal Recruitment

Tidal (or chord) compliance, the quotient of tidal volume and the difference between static pressures at the extremes of the tidal cycle, is jointly determined by PEEP and tidal volume.[69] Because the opening of collapsed units improves the calculated chord compliance, high tidal volumes in conjunction with low end-expiratory pressures can yield tidal compliance values that exceed those of a lower V-tidal volume-/higher PEEP combination. Judging from acute animal experiments, however, the former pattern may inflict more damage.[58] Under low-PEEP conditions, applying a higher tidal volume undoubtedly recruits lung units during the initial inflation cycles as the pressures needed for units reluctant to open are exceeded for the requisite time.

Although repeated opening and closing of *alveoli* is theoretically possible (when high tidal volumes are combined with low levels of PEEP), whether such events actually occur repeatedly with each tidal cycle is still controversial. Dependent alveoli are exposed to lower end-expiratory transmural forces, owing to the increased vertical gradients of pleural and interstitial pressure that characterize the edematous lung.[70] In the setting of ARDS, therefore, alveoli at the "top" of the recumbent lung tend to remain patent whatever the ventilatory pattern may be, whereas those at the "bottom" may require terminal airway pressures exceeding 30 cm H_2O to open and only modestly lower end-expiratory pressures to stabilize.[33, 71] Consequently, as transmural pressures build during inflation, alveolar recruitment may occur in the most dependent sectors. In large-animal models of ventilator-induced lung injury, histologic damage concentrates in dependent regions, where transvascular hydrostatic pressures are highest and the tendency for shear stresses, persistent collapse, and phasic tidal opening and reclosing is greatest.[72] The prone position lessens the gradient of pleural pressure and reduces the tendency for dependent atelectasis.[26, 73]

The threshold opening pressure (which may exceed 45 cm H_2O) must be applied long enough. Patency may often be preserved by pressures that are lower than those that opened the unit, depending on the type and stage of lung injury. Relatively high stretching pressures applied for 20 to 40 seconds ("recruiting maneuvers") improve lung compliance for extended periods in surfactant-depleted small animals and in human babies with the infant respiratory distress syndrome.[74] Immediately after a successful recruitment maneuver, compliance improves and the level of PEEP required to sustain an open lung becomes less. But a key question concerns the fate of these newly recruited and marginally stable units—continued patency, tidal recollapse, or eventual de-recruitment? The answer may depend in part on the level of coexisting PEEP and the period of observation.

When PEEP is insufficient, gradual deterioration of respiratory system compliance (presumably as the result of alveolar collapse) tends to occur as time passes. Although there are alternative explanations, certain alveoli recently made patent during the recruitment maneuvers may experience absorption (rather than compression) atelectasis unless the alveolar gas is continually refreshed by adequate tidal ventilation. Although used as part of an apparently successful lung-protective ventilation strategy,[75] the added value of such recruitment maneuvers in adult patients with ARDS has yet to be convincingly demonstrated. Moreover, *if* recruiting maneuvers are helpful, their optimal frequency is not known. From the limited data available, periodic recruiting maneuvers appear to be most appropriate early in the disease process, especially when relatively small tidal volumes have been used with low to moderate levels of PEEP.

Dangers of Excessive PEEP

Plateau pressures of only 25 cm H_2O often surpass the upper inflection zone of the static P-V curve of adults with ARDS.[42] Therefore, the same pressures needed to open and recruit some alveoli simultaneously overdistend others. Whether PEEP simply adds to the end-expiratory volume of units that are already open or maintains patency of unstable alveoli depends on the patient, the stage of disease, and the vertical position of the alveolus in the injured lung. Overdistention not only redirects perfusion to increase dead space; in a lung whose vascular bed is severely attenuated, alveolar distention increases pulmonary vascular resistance and mean hydrostatic pressures.

As noted earlier, high vascular pressures may accentuate edema or extend damage and thus should be avoided. It follows that when the barrier functions of the microvessels are compromised, using excessive PEEP may prove as ill advised as using insufficient PEEP in conjunction with high tidal volumes. Later on, high levels of PEEP are less effective and may encourage disruption of fragile tissues.

Pressure Limitation and Tidal Volume

Compliances for normal lung (CL), chest wall (Ccw), and total respiratory system approximate 150, 150, and 75 mL/cm H_2O, respectively, when patients lie recumbent. In ARDS, total respiratory compliance typically ranges from 15 to 30 mL/cm H_2O, values that vary with the severity of lung disease, chest wall compliance, and body size. In fixing values for maximal and minimal alveolar pressures, the pressure difference between these limits, which is the available ventilating pressure, is characteristically about 20 cm H_2O. The tidal volumes that correspond to these combinations of total respiratory compliance and ventilating pressure are, therefore, 300 to 600 mL, or for a lean 75-kg patient 4 to 8 mL/kg. Because values for lung and chest wall compliance vary through wide ranges in different patients, universal values for tidal volume and consistent pressure limits cannot be specified. When using a flow-controlled, volume-cycled mode of ventilation, therefore, tidal volume should be adjusted with guidance from plateau pressure and the response of oxygen exchange.

A recent NIH-sponsored trial of low tidal volume ventilation demonstrated a significant reduction in mortality in ARDS patients compared with those given conventional ventilation (unpublished data).

Ventilatory Alternatives

Allowing Pa_{CO_2} to rise and pH to fall during the initial stages of ARDS management may be more prudent than using high tidal cycling pressures and tidal volumes in conjunction with insufficient PEEP.[75] Whatever the controlled variable may be (flow or pressure), and whatever the cycling variable (volume or time), acceptance of upper and lower limits for alveolar pressure confines the practitioner to a maximum ventilating pressure—the difference between maximum (P_{max}) and end-expiratory airway pressures. Pressure-controlled ventilation (PCV),[76, 77] airway pressure release ventilation (BiPAP),[78, 79] and inverse ratio ventilation (IRV)[80, 81] can be considered variants of a unifying "pressure-*targeted*" strategy in which the clinician selects only four variables other than FIO_2:

- Maximum airway pressure (P_{set})
- PEEP
- Frequency (f)
- Inspiratory time fraction (duty cycle, TI/TTOT)

Permissive Hypercapnia

Retention of CO_2 may be an inevitable consequence of a *lung protective strategy* that tightly restricts applied pressure and maintains a certain minimum lung volume. Traditional guidelines for ventilator management urge the maintenance of nearly normal values for arterial blood gases, adjusting the ventilator settings for FIO_2, PEEP, and minute ventilation (VE) to achieve this objective; however, for most patients the need to maintain normocapnia has not been unequivocally demonstrated, particularly when CO_2 is retained gradually or abrupt changes in pH are avoided. It can be effectively argued that maintaining normocapnia may not be appropriate if the cost is impaired lung healing and heightened risk of extending tissue damage.[82, 83] Several reports lacking concurrent controls indicate that improved survival may be achieved by approaches that limit alveolar pressure even if normal arterial blood gases cannot be maintained.[31, 84–86] Retrospective studies suggest that "permissive hypercapnia," a strategy that allows alveolar ventilation and peak ventilatory pressures to fall and, thus, Pa_{CO_2} to rise, may reduce barotrauma and enhance survival in status asthmaticus[106] and acute lung injury.[31, 85, 86] Any basis for survival advantage has not yet been determined; however, the lung acutely damaged by stretch injury may produce inflammatory mediators transferred to the systemic circulation.[83, 87] Disruption of the lung's architecture may also promote pneumonitis or bacteremia.[88–90] One prospective study demonstrates a clear benefit for compliance and gas exchange in using a lung protective approach that allows hypercapnia.[91]

The physiologic impact of CO_2 is a function of the severity of hypercapnia and the rate of its buildup (Table 128-3).[82, 92] Although gradual elevations of Pa_{CO_2} (~5 mm Hg/hour) are usually tolerated remarkably well,[21, 82, 83] hypercapnia may not be advisable for all patients with acute lung injury. *Acute* elevations in Pa_{CO_2} increase sympathetic activity, cardiac output, and pulmonary vascular resistance; alter bronchomotor tone; impair skeletal muscle function; dilate cerebral vessels; and impair central nervous system function.[21, 92, 93] Patients with head injury, recent history of stroke, significant cardiovascular dysfunction, autonomic insufficiency, β-adrenergic blockade, or another condition that interferes with sympathetic tone and compensatory mechanisms may be rather intolerant to CO_2 retention.

Arterial pH may not closely reflect the pH of the intracellular environment. Any resulting intracellular acidosis, however, is almost certain to be less dramatic than the profound intracellular pH changes produced by ischemia. Because CO_2 affects cardiac output and vascular and bronchomotor tone, it is not certain that hypercapnia disturbs $\dot{V}/\dot{Q}$ matching or modulates the extent of lung injury and edema during the course of mechanical ventilatory support. Deep sedation or paralysis is often necessary if a patient is to tolerate permissive hypercapnia, a requirement that may be associated with impaired clearance of secretions, fluid retention, and residual muscle weakness. Moreover, permissive hypercapnia may not be advisable (or even possible to implement safely) in the setting of intercurrent *metabolic* acidosis.

Adjuncts to Ventilatory Management of Acute Respiratory Distress Syndrome

In response to the evidence that aggressive patterns of ventilation may have adverse consequences, attention has been given to techniques that accomplish effective respiratory gas exchange without further damaging the injured lung. Various methods modify the fundamental nature of ventilatory support (high-frequency ventilation, tracheal gas insufflation, partial liquid ventilation); others provide gas exchange external to the lungs (extracorporeal or intra-vena caval gas exchange), alter body position (prone positioning), or administer therapeutic agents designed to improve $\dot{V}/\dot{Q}$ matching (nitric oxide, aerosolized prostacyclin).

High-Frequency Ventilation

High-frequency ventilation (HFV) applies very small excursions of tidal alveolar pressure at extremely fast rates. Enthusiasm for HFV eventually lost momentum, as difficulty was encountered in achieving adequate ventilation and oxygenation in many patients with ARDS, and outcomes were not clearly different. As initially implemented, jet ventilation was disappointing, and, for lack of appropriate equipment, high-frequency oscillation (HFO) could not be adequately tested in adults. A prospective comparison of HFO and conventional ventilation in neonates failed to demonstrate an advantage,[94] but the methods of that trial have been seriously challenged[74] and contradicted by later studies.[17] Indeed, there has been renewed interest in HFV, as improved equipment that effectively applies higher frequencies has now become available for use in adult patients with ARDS.[95] When conducted at an appropriate lung volume and frequency, HFV seems well aligned with current principles of lung protection (maximum recruitment and minimal tidal excursions) and has a clear rationale.[96] To this point, however, superiority has been neither shown nor disproven.

TABLE 128–3. Primary Consequences of Carbon Dioxide Retention

Acute Problems
Intracellular acidosis
Nervous system dysfunction
Intracranial pressure increase
Muscle weakness
Cardiovascular dysfunction
Chronic Problems
Depressed ventilatory drive

Extrapulmonary Gas Exchange

Partial substitution for the lung's gas-exchanging function by extracorporeal membrane oxygenation (ECMO), extracorporeal CO_2 removal ($ECCO_2R$) or intra-vena caval oxygen exchange (IVOX) reduces the requirement for ventilating pressure. Although sporadically beneficial in adults with refractory hypoxemia, ECMO does not appear to be routinely helpful as a salvage technique,[97] despite its clear success in neonates.[98] In expert hands $ECCO_2R$ looked more promising,[99, 100] but in the only tightly controlled study of this approach $ECCO_2R$ currently published, routine benefit could not be demonstrated.[92] IVOX is conceptually attractive, *relatively* simple to implement, and, if perfected, may prove beneficial, especially in cases marked by hypercapnia and hypoxemia. Its first clinical trial was aborted, however, owing to unimpressive results. These exotic techniques continue to hold promise but must be further developed before they can be clinically implemented. This topic is covered further in Chapter 123.

Surfactant Administration

Following the law of Laplace, alveoli of small dimension tend to empty into communicating units of larger diameter unless surface tension can be reduced. *Surfactants,* the class of agents that stabilize alveoli otherwise vulnerable to collapse, suffer both quantitative and qualitative abnormalities in ARDS.[30, 101, 102] These alterations occur very early in the disease process and relate to both depressed synthesis and inactivation of functional surfactants by plasma proteins. Failure to prevent atelectasis further inhibits surfactant synthesis, resulting in a deleterious positive-feedback cycle. Surfactant serves numerous other biologic functions in the lung that may be instrumental in reversing the inflammatory process.[103]

Therapeutic surfactants currently available or under study vary in their composition and efficacy. To date, a controlled trial involving a synthetic surfactant lacking structural proteins revealed no change in mortality and disappointing effects on physiologic function.[104, 105] (The aerosolized method of administering the modified surfactant, however, may not have delivered a strong enough concentration to the alveolar level.) Better results might be expected were a natural surfactant given more efficiently. Exogenous surfactant may yet play a beneficial adjunctive role for carefully selected patients if it reaches recruitable alveoli in concentrations sufficient to overwhelm the inhibitory effects of exuded plasma proteins.[102, 106] It is not likely to help if the lungs are heavily consolidated or fibrotic.

Prone Positioning

The positional variation integral to normal activity in healthy patients is forgone for lengthy periods in bedridden, critically ill patients. Prone positioning is unique among the adjuncts to ventilation, as it can be implemented without cost, technical equipment, or unlicensed drugs. Although the supine posture allows direct eye contact with the caregiver and visitors, provides access to the vascular system and vital structures, and facilitates nursing care, pulmonary gas exchange of many patients with early-phase ARDS improves remarkably when they lie prone (Fig. 128–6).[28] Reduced gradients of pleural, and consequently transalveolar, pressure allow recruitment of dorsal lung units with improved $\dot{V}/\dot{Q}$ matching.[25, 27, 107] (Prone positioning may be the ultimate recruiting maneuver.) The weight of the heart, which in the supine position is borne largely by the lungs that surround it, when prone rests on the ventral rib cage and sternum, further reducing the tendency for compressive atelectasis. In some patients, modification of chest wall compliance by prone positioning redistributes transalveolar pressures and encourages ventilation of those dorsal and peridiaphragmatic regions that to open most need expansive forces. Although both the prone position and PEEP improve the distribution of ventilation during ARDS, prone positioning is less likely to redistribute blood flow to newly dependent regions. Airways serving the high-capacity dorsal regions are generally better drained in this position, as well. Although most patients respond quickly, improvement of gas exchange may take hours to develop fully.[28] Some responders to prone positioning continue to maintain better gas exchange when turned back to the supine position.

Oxygen exchange improves in about 70% of patients turned prone in the early phase of ARDS, allowing the physician to reduce both FIO_2 and PEEP. Assuming the prone position not only improves oxygenation but may protect against the dependent damage otherwise induced by the same ventilatory pattern in supine controls.[60] Based on theoretical considerations and limited personal experience, prone positioning is less likely to benefit patients with continuous pleural air leaks (especially bilateral ones). (Once the lung is surrounded by gas, the normal pleural gradient of pressure is erased or substantially altered, making the effect of prone positioning unpredictable.)

Hypotension, desaturation, and arrhythmias are unusual problems[108] that generally do not persist and can be minimized by using sedation, prior airway suctioning, and 100% O_2 during the maneuver. Continuous arterial pressure monitoring, electrocardiography, and pulse oximetry are strongly advised. Attention must also be given to preserving the position and patency of intravascular lines and endotracheal tubes during the turning process. Respiratory system compliance generally changes little in the prone conversion, but this is variable[108, 109]; tidal volume should be monitored (and adjusted if necessary) during pressure-controlled ventilation, which is influenced by any position-related changes in chest wall compliance. The optimal frequency of supine-to-prone conversions is not clear; in current practice, most experienced centers "flip" patients once or twice daily. It seems reasonable to assign the relative duration in each position in proportion to the gas exchange response (equal times when no important gas exchange difference is observed). Placing the patient prone may be less important after the first few days of treatment and probably has limited value if O_2 exchange does not improve. Occasionally, higher transpulmonary pressures applied to the inflamed dorsal regions may be responsible for lung rupture during transfer to prone positioning in late-stage ARDS.

Partial Liquid Ventilation

In clinical practice, perfluorochemicals (PFCs) are environmentally innocuous liquids at room temperature that dissolve extraordinary volumes of O_2 and CO_2.[110] Biologically inert and immiscible in both aqueous and lipid media, they cause no known tissue reaction, even during extended contact. Perfluoro-octyl bromide (Perflubron), the PFC most extensively tested, evaporates slowly, distributes homogeneously, and has both low surface tension and water-like viscosity. Perflubron is nearly twice as dense as water; airway secretions, alveolar exudate, and nonadherent cell debris tend to float on it. Its radiodensity interferes with conventional imaging.

Perflubron has the potential to keep surfactant-deficient alveoli open by two distinct mechanisms:

- Reduction of interfacial surface tension
- Physical distention by noncompressible fluid

The former property may be especially important in the infant respiratory distress syndrome, whereas the alveolar stenting effect may assume primacy in ARDS.

Partial liquid ventilation preserves the key benefits of liquid breathing while allowing gas ventilation to proceed with stan-

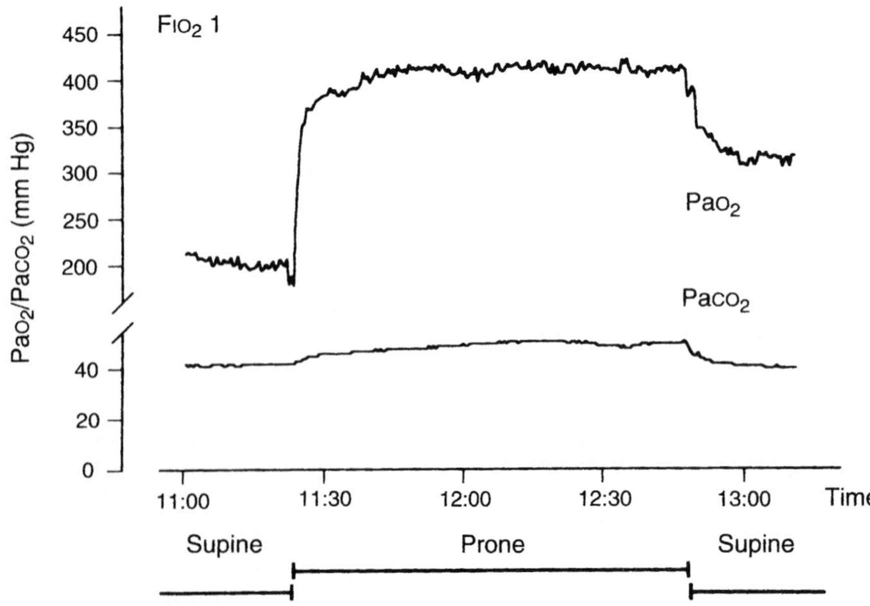

Figure 128–6. Continuous recordings of Pa_{O_2} and Pa_{CO_2} obtained in a patient with acute respiratory distress syndrome during and after position changes. Note that Pa_{O_2} increased dramatically after conversion to the prone position and that substantial improvement persisted on return to the supine position. Pa_{CO_2} increased moderately during prone positioning, possibly as a consequence of positionally reduced chest wall compliance in a patient receiving pressure targeted ventilation. (From Pappert D, Rossaint R, Slama K, et al: Influence of positioning on ventilation-perfusion relationships in severe adult respiratory syndrome. Chest 1994; 106:1511–1516.)

dard mechanical ventilators and connecting circuitry.[111-115] It is rather simple to implement. The liquid preferentially distends the dependent alveoli most in need of expansion during the initial phase of ARDS, providing the vertically graded PEEP-like effect required by the underlying disease. Simultaneously, blood flow diverts toward the better-ventilated nondependent regions. Reduced venous admixture, therefore, has at least two explanations:

- Effective oxygen exchange directly across alveolar units reopened by liquid
- Redirection of pulmonary arterial blood toward the better-ventilated nondependent regions

Partial liquid ventilation shares many characteristics with prone positioning.[116] Acting from different sides of the alveolus, both methods preferentially re-expand dorsal alveoli. Both are likely to improve regional surface tension and to redirect blood flow toward the nondependent lung. Prone positioning opens airways and improves gravitational drainage of dorsal regions; partial liquid ventilation may also help clear cellular debris, secretions, and alveolar liquids *via* the flotation mechanism. Both techniques are most effective in the early (edematous) phase of the illness. Both may protect against extension of lung damage.[113, 114, 117]

Tracheal Gas Insufflation

An alternative to allowing extreme or rapidly developing hypercapnia or to using extrapulmonary techniques for gas exchange in acute lung injury is to enhance the efficiency of CO_2 elimination at low tidal volume and cycling pressures by the tracheal insufflation of fresh gas via catheter or specialized multilumen endotracheal tube (TGI). This minimally invasive approach reduces the expiratory concentration of CO_2 in the proximal series (anatomic) dead space. During TGI-aided ventilation, fresh gas delivery occurs either throughout the respiratory cycle (continuous-flow TGI) or only during a segment of it (phasic-flow TGI).[118-124] In either mode, the crucial variable appears to be the volume of fresh gas injected per breath during expiration.[125] Low to moderate flows of fresh gas introduced near the carina dilute the proximal anatomic dead space (dead space flushing). At high catheter flow rates, turbulence generated at the catheter tip can also enhance gas mixing in regions beyond its orifice, thus contributing to CO_2 elimination.[121-123]

Modest flows of TGI can be impressively effective when the lung parenchyma is relatively normal, but the effectiveness of TGI is seriously compromised by the presence of a large alveolar dead space component (as in ARDS), because expiratory CO_2 concentration is already reduced in those settings. Despite this undeniable limitation, the efficacy of TGI-aided ventilation should be enhanced during use of a small tidal volume–permissive hypercapnia strategy, because small tidal volumes are associated with a higher percentage of series dead space and because small reductions in V_D/V_T are associated with large decreases of Pa_{CO_2} when baseline Pa_{CO_2} is much elevated.[126]

Using a similar strategy known as *intratracheal pulmonary ventilation,* Kolobow and colleagues demonstrated that adequate ventilation can be accomplished in normal sheep when seven eighths of all lung tissue has been removed, without resorting to excessive V_E and airway pressures.[127] A mouth-directed injection catheter provides all fresh gas that enters the lungs, and its innovative reverse thrust design helps to reduce alveolar pressure. These features are likely to be most important when catheter dimension and gas injection rates are high relative to airway caliber. Some encouraging preliminary clinical experience with intratracheal pulmonary ventilation has now been gathered from infants.

TGI has the clear potential to cause mucosal damage, secretion retention, and barotrauma if used improperly.[128] These effects should be mitigated by adequate humidification and injection of fresh gas via channels embedded in the walls of the endotracheal tube itself.[119] These channels can be reverse-directed or even used to provide all inspiratory gas, allowing for unidirectional (expiratory) gas flow through the main tube lumen. This may confer benefits for tube hygiene. Because of its potential to moderate the rate and extent of CO_2 retention, TGI would appear well suited as an adjunct to a pressure-targeted, lung-protective ventilatory support for ARDS.

Nitric Oxide

Inhaled nitric oxide (NO), a key biologic mediator of smooth muscle relaxation, has the therapeutic potential to dilate the pulmonary vasculature in those regions that are the best ventilated, improving the $\dot{V}/\dot{Q}$ matching in an unevenly damaged lung.[18] The recruiting effects of PEEP and prone positioning may amplify the effect of NO by opening up more of the lung to it. NO is active only locally: immediately upon exposure to hemoglobin it is quenched. Extremely low concentrations of NO achieve nearly full effect. Biologic activity is often detectable at concentrations as low as 2 parts per million (ppm), and beneficial effects are fully saturated at about 20 ppm in most patients.[129, 130]

NO's physiologic effects in ARDS are highly variable—sometimes dramatic, but often quite modest. Although the onset and offset of NO's effects (e.g., reduction of pulmonary artery pressure, improved oxygenation) are extremely rapid, gradual accommodation to its beneficial vasodilatory effects can result in rebound vasoconstriction when it is terminated abruptly. High concentrations of NO and minute quantities of its associated oxides, NO_2^{-1} and NO_3^{-2}, are histotoxic and must be avoided.

Although extremely appealing physiologically, the eventual place of NO in the management of ARDS has not yet been settled. At present, it appears most likely to benefit patients whose hypoxemia is refractory to other measures or whose pulmonary hypertension is symptomatic and accentuated by hypoxic vasoconstriction.

Inhaled Prostacyclin

Aerosolized prostacyclin is another modality designed to achieve selective vasodilation of well-ventilated areas.[114, 131] Unlike an infusion of the same drug, inhaled prostacyclin reduces (rather than increases) the pulmonary shunt fraction and pulmonary arterial pressure.[53] Aerosolized, prostacyclin appears to have relatively few side effects; however, there is very little clinical experience with this technique, and its routine clinical use thus cannot be endorsed at this time. Similarly, the value of a parentally administered enhancer of hypoxic vasoconstriction (almitrine bimesylate), used alone or combined with an inhaled agent, has been suggested but not yet confirmed.

Modes of Mechanical Ventilation for Acute Respiratory Distress Syndrome

Many choices for ventilating mode are rational as long as the practitioner follows the same guidelines for lung protection and remains alert to the potential complications of the mode in use. Pressure-targeted ventilatory modes prevent alveolar pressure from rising any higher than the selected airway pressure and in this sense are somewhat "safer" than more traditional volume-targeted modes. Because many practitioners now regard mild hypercapnia as inconsequential, pressure-preset ventilation seems especially well adapted to current priorities in ARDS management. However, volume-cycled ventilatory modes can generally be employed with identical effect, especially when delivered with a decelerating flow waveform with closely set pressure alarms and closely monitored plateau pressures.[132]

As a rule, spontaneous ventilation should be encouraged, except when oxygenation is marginal and ventilatory efforts labored. It has been argued that newer techniques, such as pressure control, pressure-regulated volume control, inverse ratio ventilation, and airway pressure release ventilation, confer advantages over more traditional approaches, but none has yet proved consistently superior to the alternatives.

A Pressure-Targeted Approach to Ventilating for Acute Lung Injury or Acute Respiratory Distress Syndrome

Although the recently published prospective Brazilian study is very encouraging,[75] additional clinical data are needed to confirm the wisdom of adopting a pressure-targeted, maximum recruitment approach. In the interim, a rational strategy for ventilating patients with acute lung injury can be formulated that is based on firm theoretical and experimental grounds (Table 128–4). Such a strategy recognizes that several mechanically distinct alveolar populations coexist in an acutely injured lung, that a poorly chosen ventilatory pattern can be damaging, and that the underlying pathophysiologic picture changes over time. This approach gives higher priority to regulating tidal transalveolar pressures (with the goal of optimizing recruitment without overdistention) than to achieving normocapnia.[29, 52, 106, 133]

Assuming that oxygen demand has been minimized and that cardiac function has been optimized, the essential strategic elements are as follows:

1. Use sufficient end-expiratory transalveolar pressure to avert tissue damage from surfactant depletion, persistent collapse, or stresses associated with repeated opening and closing of collapsible units during the tidal breathing cycle. The total PEEP applied (the sum of PEEP and auto-PEEP) should be sufficient to obliterate the *lower* inflection "point" of the P-V curve of the respiratory system, which, at tidal volumes of 7 to 8 mL/kg, generally occurs at a pressure of 12 to 20 cm H_2O in the early phase of ARDS. The appropriate PEEP value is affected by chest wall compliance and body position. In truth, there is an inflection *range* rather than a single inflection *point*, as dependent alveoli in the lower regions of the lung require greater end-expiratory alveolar pressure to maintain patency than do those above them.[24, 71] Improved arterial oxygenation tends to parallel effective recruitment, and CO_2 retention is a consequence of alveolar overdistention. Although actual construction of the P-V curve (by any of a variety of static or dynamic methods) is theoretically more appealing, for some patients it is inadvisable to eliminate spontaneous breathing efforts.

2. Because alveolar subpopulations with nearly normal elastic properties may coexist alongside flooded or infiltrated ones, avoid applying *transalveolar* pressures greater than normal lung tissue is designed to sustain at its maximum capacity (i.e., 30 to 35 cm H_2O). This pressure generally corresponds to end-inspiratory static airway pressures ("plateau pressures") of 35 to 50 cm H_2O, depending on the stiffness of the chest wall. Pressures in this range are generally sufficient to reopen closed airways. Whatever the appropriate maximal pressure setting might be for an individual patient, it seems wise to avoid the *upper* inflection range of the static P-V curve whenever possible. Incursion into this zone is signaled by deterioration of tidal compliance. This may be especially important in the later phases of ARDS, when the lung is even more fragile.

Relatively small tidal volumes often result from imposing the upper and the lower bounds on ventilatory pressure. Therefore, permissive hypercapnia should be expected, and periodic recruitment breaths (continuous positive airway pressure [CPAP] of 35 to 45 cm H_2O sustained for 15 to 40 seconds) may be needed to maintain adequate lung volume and avoid hypoxemia in some patients. Recruitment breaths must be terminated immediately if arrhythmias, hypoxemia, or hypotension develops. One interesting approach to making selections of PEEP and tidal volume is first to perform a recruiting maneuver using CPAP. Tidal ventilation is then resumed in the pressure-controlled mode with inflation pressure capped at the maximum allowed value (e.g., 40 cm H_2O). PEEP is dropped quickly to 20 to 25 cm H_2O as pressure control is raised to maintain the end-inspiratory pressure at the maximum tidal value. PEEP is then decreased gradually while maximal airway pressure is held constant (allowing V tidal volume to rise) until the point at which arterial oxygen saturation begins to fall. After a second recruiting maneuver, PEEP is then set at the next to last value. A similar attempt can then be made to reduce peak pressure and tidal volume gradually.

3. When there are contraindications, accept hypercapnia from the onset of therapy (buffered, when necessary, by judiciously infused sodium bicarbonate or another buffer) in preference to violating the guidelines of controlling alveolar pressure. Pharmacologic buffering may also be needed to allow hypercapnia when deep sedation or paralysis is not used. The strategy of permissive hypercapnia may be difficult to implement in the presence of metabolic acidosis, when other measures (e.g., dialysis) may be needed adjunctively.

4. Consider the prone position from the outset of management. When both available and necessary, adjunctive measures such as NO, tracheal gas insufflation, and partial liquid ventilation should also be contemplated.

5. After the first 3 to 5 days of treatment, begin to reduce PEEP as oxygenation allows, seeking to reduce maximum alveolar pressure and prevent alveolar rupture.

TABLE 128–4. A Lung-Protective Strategy for Ventilating Patients with Acute Respiratory Distress Syndrome

1. Tailor ventilatory strategy to the phase of the disease (generous PEEP in early stage; withdraw PEEP later).
2. Minimize oxygen demands.
3. Minimize pulmonary vascular pressures.
4. Control transalveolar pressure, not Pa_{CO_2}.
5. Maintain total end-expiratory P_{alv} (PEEP + auto-PEEP) several cm H_2O above P_{flex}. In general, this will be more than 10 cm H_2O but less than 20 cm H_2O.
6. Avoid large tidal VT and use least P_{alv} required to meet *unequivocal* therapeutic goals.
7. Hold transalveolar pressure <35 cm H_2O.
8. Consider making increases in mean P_{aw} by changing inspiratory/expiratory ratio.
9. Consider specialized adjunctive measures to improve gas exchange and oxygen delivery.*

*In addition to such standard measurements as skillful management of pulmonary vascular pressure, repositioning, and use of cardiotonic agents, specialized adjunctive measures might include (where available) such experimental methods as $ECCO_2R$ nitric oxide inhalation or intravenous or intratracheal catheter-assisted gas exchange.

P_{alv} = alveolar pressure; P_{flex} = lower inflection point of the static pressure volume relationship of the respiratory system; P_{aw} = airway pressure.

References

1. Pontoppidan H, Geffin B, Lowenstein E: Acute respiratory failure in the adult. N Engl J Med 1972; 287:690–698, 743–752, 799–806.

2. Dantzker DR, Scharf SM: Cardiopulmonary Critical Care. 3rd ed. Philadelphia, WB Saunders, 1998, pp 41–42.
3. Hess D, Maxwell C: Which is the best index of oxygenation: P (A − a) O_2, Pao_2/PAo_2, or Pao_2/FIO_2? Respir Care 1985; 30:961–968.
4. Malo J, Jameel A, Wood LDH: How does positive end-expiratory pressure reduce intrapulmonary shunt in canine pulmonary edema? J Appl Physiol 1984; 57:1002–1010.
5. Cheney FW, Colley PS: The effect of cardiac output on arterial blood oxygenation. Anesthesiology 1980; 52:496–503.
6. Dantzker DR, Scharf SM: Cardiopulmonary Critical Care. 3rd ed. Philadelphia, WB Saunders, 1998, p 45.
7. Hedenstierna G: Mechanics of the respiratory system in ARDS. Acta Anaesth Scand 1991; 95(Suppl):29–33.
8. Marini JJ, Pierson DJ, Hudson LD: Acute lobar atelectasis: A prospective comparison of fiberoptic bronchoscopy and respiratory therapy. Am Rev Respir Dis 1979; 119:971–978.
9. Milne EN, Pistolesi M, Minati M, Giuntini C: The radiologic distinction of cardiogenic and non-cardiogenic edema. Am J Roentgenol 1985; 144:879–874.
10. Grossman W: Diastolic dysfunction and congestive heart failure. Circulation 1990; 81(2 Suppl):III1–7.
11. Bernard GR, Luce JM, Sprung, CL, et al: High-dose corticosteroids in patients with the adult respiratory distress syndrome. N Engl J Med 1987; 317:1565–1570.
12. Meduri GU, Headley S, Golden E, et al: Effect of prolonged methylprednisolone therapy in unresolving acute respiratory distress syndrome. JAMA 1998; 280:159–165.
13. Colley PS, Cheney FW Jr, Hlastala MP: Ventilation-perfusion and gas exchange effects of sodium nitroprusside in dogs with normal and edematous lungs. Anesthesiology 1979; 50:489–495.
14. Klein J: Normobaric pulmonary oxygen toxicity. Anesth Analg 1990; 70:195–207.
15. Hansen-Flaschen J, Cowen J, Raps EC: Neuromuscular blockade in the intensive care unit: More than we bargained for. Am Rev Respir Dis 1993; 147:234–236.
16. Broccard AF, Marini JJ: Position and posture in acute illness. Semin Respir Criti Care Med 1997; 18:19–32.
17. Clark RH, Gerstman DR, Null DM, deLemos RA: Prospective randomized trial of high frequency oscillatory and conventional ventilation in respiratory distress syndrome. Pediatrics 1992; 89:5–12.
18. Snyder SH, Bredt DS: Biologic roles of nitric oxide. Sci Am 1992; 266:68–77.
19. Bendixen HH, Hedley-Whyte J, Laver MB: Impaired oxygenation in surgical patients during general anesthesia with controlled ventilation. N Engl J Med 1963; 269:991–997.
20. Brunet F, Jeanbourquin D, Monchi M, Mira JP, Fierobe L, et al: Should mechanical ventilation be optimized to blood gases, lung mechanics, or thoracic CT scan? Am J Respir Crit Care Med 1995; 152:524–530.
21. Carvalho CR, Barbas CS, Medeiros DM, et al: Temporal hemodynamic effects of permissive hypercapnia associated with ideal PEEP in ARDS. Am J Respir Crit Care Med 1997; 156:1458–1466.
22. Meduri GU, Belenchia JM, Estes RJ, et al: Fibroproliferation phase of ARDS: Clinical findings and effects of corticosteroids. Chest 1991; 100:943–952.
23. Gammon BR, Shin MS, Buchalter SE: Pulmonary barotrauma in mechanical ventilation: Patterns and risk factors. Chest 1992; 102:568–572.
24. Gattinoni L, Pesenti A, Bombino M: Relationships between lung computed tomographic density, gas exchange, and PEEP in acute respiratory failure. Anesthesiology 1988; 69:824–832.
25. Albert RK: One good turn. . . Intensive Care Med 1994; 20:247–248.
26. Albert RK, Leasa D, Sanderson M, et al MP: The prone position improves arterial oxygenation and reduced shunt in oleic acid-induced acute lung injury. Am Rev Respir Dis 1987; 135:628–633.
27. Gattinoni L, Pelosi P, Vitale G, et al: Body position changes redistribute lung computed tomographic density in patients with acute respiratory failure. Anesthesiology 1991; 74:15–23.
28. Pappert D, Rossaint R, Slama K, Gruning T, Falke K: Influence of positioning on ventilation-perfusion relationships in severe adult respiratory distress syndrome. Chest 1994; 106:1511–1516.
29. Marini JJ: Lung mechanics in adult respiratory distress syndrome: Recent conceptual advances and implications for management. Clin Chest Med 1990; 11:673–690.
30. Lewis JF, Jobe AH: Surfactant and the adult respiratory distress syndrome. Am Rev Respir Dis 1993; 147:218–233.
31. Lewandowski K, Slama K, Falke KJ: Approaches to improve survival in severe ARDS. *In:* Update in Intensive Care and Emergency Medicine. Vol. 16. Vincent JL (Ed). Berlin, Springer-Verlag, 1992, pp 372–383.
32. Tsuno K, Prato P, Kolobow T: Acute lung injury from mechanical ventilation at moderately high airway pressures. J Appl Physiol 1990; 69:956–961.
33. Gaver DP, Samsel RW, Solway J: Effects of surface tension and viscosity on airway opening. J Appl Physiol 1990; 69:74–85.
34. Ranieri VM, Giulani R, Fiore T, Dambrosio M, Milic-Emili, J: Volume-pressure curve of the respiratory system predicts effects of PEEP in ARDS: "Occlusion" versus "constant flow" technique. Am J Respir Crit Care Med 1994; 149:19–27.
35. Sydow M, Burchardi H, Zinserling J, Ische H, Crozier TA, Weyland W: Improved determination of static compliance by automated single volume steps in ventilated patients. Intensive Care Med 1991; 17:108–114.
36. Rouby JJ, Lherm T, Martin de Lassale E, Poète P, Bodin L, Finet JF, Callard P: Histologic aspects of pulmonary barotrauma in critically ill patients with acute respiratory failure. Intensive Care Med 1993; 19:383–389.
37. Carlton DP, Scherer RG, Cummings JS, et al: Lung overexpansion injures the pulmonary microcirculation in lambs (Abstract). Pediatr Res 1988; 23:500.
38. Egan EA: Lung inflation, lung solute permeability and alveolar edema. J Appl Physiol 1982; 53:121–125.
39. Dreyfuss D, Basset G, Soler PS, Saumon G: Intermittent positive-pressure hyperventilation with high inflation pressures produces pulmonary microvascular injury in rats. Am Rev Respir Dis 1985; 132:880–884.
40. Kolobow T, Moretti MP, Fumagalli R, Mascheroni D, Prato P, Chen V, Joris M: Severe impairment of lung function induced by high peak airway pressure during mechanical ventilation. Am Rev Respir Dis 1987; 135:312–315.
41. Mascheroni D, Kolobow T, Fumagalli R, et al: Acute respiratory failure following pharmacologically induced hyperventilation: An experimental animal study. Intensive Care Med 1988; 15:8–12.
42. Brochard L, Roudot-Thoraval F, Roupie E, Delclaux C, Chastre J, Fernandez-Mondejar E, Clementi E, Mancebo J, Factor P, Matamis D, Ranieri M, Blanch L. Rodi G, Mentec H, Dreyfuss D, Ferrer M, Brun-Buisson C, Tobin M, Lemaire F: Tidal volume reduction for prevention of ventilator-induced lung injury in acute respiratory distress syndrome. The Multicenter Trial Group on Tidal Volume Reduction in ARDS. Am J Respir Crit Care Med 1998; 158:1831–1838.
43. Hernandez LA, Coker PJ, May S, et al: Mechanical ventilation increases microvascular permeability in oleic acid injured lungs. J Appl Physiol 1990; 69:2057–2061.
44. Dreyfuss D, Soler P, Saumon G: Mechanical ventilation-induced pulmonary edema. Interaction with previous lung alterations. Am J Respir Crit Care Med 1995; 151:1568–1575.
45. Fu Z, Costello ML, Tsukimoto K, Prediletto R, Elliott AR, Mathieu-Costello O, West JB: High lung volume increases stress failure in pulmonary capillaries. J Appl Physiol 1992; 73:123–133.
46. Mathieu-Costello O, Willford CD, Fu Z, Garden RM, West JB: Pulmonary capillaries are more resistant to stress failure in dogs than in rabbits. J Appl Physiol 1995; 79:908–917.
47. Mead J, Takishima T, Leith D: Stress distribution in lungs: A model of pulmonary elasticity. J Appl Physiol 1970; 28:596–608.
48. Dreyfuss D, Soler P, Basset G, et al: High inflation pressure pulmonary edema: Respective effects of high airway pressure, high tidal volume, and positive end expiratory pressure. Am Rev Respir Dis 1988; 137:1159–1164.
49. Hernandez LA, Peevy KJ, Moise AA, et al: Chest wall restriction limits high airway pressure-induced lung injury in young rabbits. J Appl Physiol 1989; 66:2364–2368.
50. Dreyfuss D, Saumon G: Ventilator-induced lung injury: Lessons from experimental studies. Am J Respir Crit Care Med 1998; 157:294–323.
51. Dreyfuss D, Saumon G: Barotrauma is volutrauma, but which

volume is the one responsible? Intensive Care Med 1992; 18:139-141.
52. Marini JJ: Ventilating ARDS: Looking for Mr. Goodmode. Anesthesiology 1994; 80:972-975.
53. Webb HH, Tierney DF: Experimental pulmonary edema due to intermittent positive pressure ventilation with high inflation pressures: Protection by positive end-expiratory pressure. Am Rev Respir Dis 1974; 110:556-565.
54. Stewart TE, Meade, MO, Cook DJ, et al: Evaluation of a ventilation strategy to prevent barotrauma in patients at high risk for acute respiratory distress syndrome. N Engl J Med 1998; 338:355-361.
55. Matamis D, Lemire F, Harf A, Brun-Buisson C, Ansquer JC, Atlan G: Total respiratory pressure volume curves in the adult respiratory distress syndrome. Chest 1984; 86:58-66.
56. Muscedere JG, Mullen JBM, Gan K, Slutsky AS: Tidal ventilation at low airway pressures can augment lung injury. Am J Respir Crit Care Med 1994; 149:1327-1334.
57. Ranieri VM, Mascia L, Fiore T, Bruno F, Brienza A, Giuliani R: Cardiorespiratory effects of positive end expiratory pressure during progressive tidal volume reduction (permissive hypercapnia) in patients with acute respiratory distress syndrome. Anesthesiology 1995; 83:710-720.
58. Corbridge TC, Wood LDH, Crawford GP, Chudoba MJ, Yanos J, Sznajder JI: Adverse effects of large tidal volumes and low PEEP in canine acid aspiration. Am Rev Respir Dis 1990; 142:311-315.
59. McCulloch PR, Forkert PG, Froese AB: Lung volume maintenance prevents lung injury during high frequency oscillatory ventilation in surfactant-deficient rabbits. Am Rev Respir Dis 1988; 137:1185-1192.
60. Broccard AF, Hotchkiss JR, Kuwayama N, et al: Consequences of vascular flow on lung injury induced by mechanical ventilation. Am J Respir Crit Care Med 1998; 157:1935-1942.
61. Sugiura M, McCulloch PR, Wren S, Dawson RH, Froese AB: Ventilator pattern influences neutrophil influx and activation in atelectasis-prone rabbit lung. J Appl Physiol 1994; 77:1355-1365.
62. Pepe PE, Hudson LD, Carrico CJ: Early application of positive end-expiratory pressure in patients at risk for the adult respiratory distress syndrome. N Engl J Med 1984; 311:281-286.
63. Katz JA, Ozanne GM, Zinn SE, Fairley HB: Time course and mechanisms of lung-volume increase with PEEP in acute pulmonary failure. Anesthesiology 1981; 54:9-16.
64. Pelosi P, Valenza F, Crotti S, Farrario L, Cerisara M, Gattinoni L: TAC study of barotrauma (Abstract). Proceedings of the International Conference on Recent Advances in the Treatment of the Adult Respiratory Distress Syndrome. Tutzing, Germany, July 3-5, 1993.
65. Gattinoni L, Pelosi P, Suter PM, et al: Acute respiratory distress syndrome caused by pulmonary and extrapulmonary disease. Different syndromes? Am J Respir Crit Care 1998; 158:3-11.
66. Benito S, Lemaire F: Pulmonary pressure-volume relationship in acute respiratory distress syndrome in adults: Role of positive end expiratory pressure. J Crit Care 1990; 5:27-34.
67. Levy P, Similowski T, Corbeil C, Albala M, Pariente R, Milic-Emili J, Jonson B: A method for studying the static pressure-volume curves of the respiratory system during mechanical ventilation. J Crit Care 1989; 4:83-89.
68. Katz, JA, Zinn SE, Ozanne GM, Fairley HB: Pulmonary, chest wall, and lung-thorax elastances in acute respiratory failure. Chest 1981; 80:304-311.
69. Suter PM, Fairley HB, Isenberg MD: Effect of tidal volume and positive end-expiratory pressure on compliance during mechanical ventilation. Chest 1978; 73:158-162.
70. Gattinoni L, Pelosi P, Crotti S, Valenza F: Effects of positive end expiratory pressure on regional distribution of tidal volume and recruitment in adult respiratory distress syndrome. Am J Respir Crit Care Med 1995; 151:1807-1814.
71. Pelosi P, D'Andrea L, Vitale G, Pesenti A, Gattinoni L: Vertical gradient of regional lung inflation in adult respiratory distress syndrome. Am J Respir Crit Care Med 1994; 149:8-13.
72. Ravenscraft SA, Shapiro RS, Adams AB, Marini JJ: Dependent damage in ventilator induced lung injury (Abstract). Am J Respir Crit Care Med 1995; 151:A551.
73. Lamm WJE, Graham MM, Albert RK: Mechanism by which the prone position improves oxygenation in acute lung injury. Am J Respir Crit Care Med 1994; 150:184-193.
74. Bryan AC, Froese AB: Reflections on the HIFI trial. Pediatrics 1991; 87:565-567.
75. Amato MBP, Barbas CS, Medeiros DM, et al: Effect of a protective-ventilation strategy on mortality in the acute respiratory distress syndrome. N Engl J Med 1998; 338:347-354.
76. Abraham E, Yoshihara G: Cardiorespiratory effects of pressure controlled ventilation in severe respiratory failure. Chest 1990; 98:1445-1449.
77. Marini JJ, Crooke PS, Truwit JD: Determinants and limits of pressure-preset ventilation: A mathematical model of pressure control. J Appl Physiol 1989; 67:1081-1092.
78. Rouby JJ: Pressure release ventilation. *In:* Update in Intensive Care and Emergency Medicine. Vincent JL (Ed). Berlin, Springer-Verlag, 1990, pp 185-195.
79. Stock MC, Downs JB, Frolichter DA: Airway pressure release ventilation. Crit Care Med 1987; 15:462-466.
80. Cole A, Weller S, Sykes M: Inverse ratio ventilation compared with PEEP in adult respiratory failure. Intensive Care Med 1984; 10:227-232.
81. Marcy TW, Marini JJ: Inverse ratio ventilation in ARDS: Rationale and implementation. Chest 1991; 100:494-504.
82. Feihl F, Perret C: Permissive hypercapnia. How permissive should we be? Am J Respir Crit Care Med 1994; 150:1722-1737.
83. Tuxen DV: Permissive hypercapnic ventilation. Am J Respir Crit Care Med 1994; 150:870-874.
84. Darioli R, Perret C: Mechanical controlled hypoventilation in status asthmaticus. Am Rev Respir Dis 1984; 129:385-387.
85. Hickling KG, Henderson SJ, Jackson R: Low mortality associated with low volume, pressure limited ventilation with permissive hypercapnia in severe adult respiratory syndrome. Intensive Care Med 1990; 16:372-377.
86. Hickling KG, Walsh J, Henderson S, Jackson R: Low mortality rate in adult respiratory distress syndrome using low volume, pressure limited ventilation with permissive hypercapnia: A prospective study. Crit Care Med 1994; 22:1568-1578.
87. von Bethmann AN, Brasch F, Nusing R, et al: Hyperventilation induces release of cytokines from perfused mouse lung. Am J Respir Crit Care Med 1998; 157:263-272.
88. Nahum A, Hoyt J, Schmitz L, et al: Effect of mechanical ventilation strategy on dissemination of intratracheally instilled *Escherichia coli* in dogs. Crit Care Med 1997; 25:1733-1743.
89. Parker JC, Roohparvar S, Foster J, et al: High peak inspiratory pressures (PIP) affect the rate of bacterial clearance from rabbit lungs. Am Rev Respir Dis 1991; 143:a570.
90. Verbrugge SJ, Sorm V, van't Veen A, et al: Lung overinflation without positive end-expiratory pressure promotes bactermia after experimental *Klebsiella pneumoniae* inoculation. Intensive Care Med 1998; 24:172-177.
91. Amato MBP, Barbas CSV, Medeiros DM, et al: Beneficial effects of the "open lung approach" with low distending pressures in acute respiratory distress syndrome. Am J Respir Crit Care Med 1995; 152:1835-1846.
92. Kacmarek RM, Hickling KG: Permissive hypercapnia. Respir Care 1993; 38:373-387.
93. Hickling KG: Low volume ventilation with permissive hypercapnia in the adult respiratory distress syndrome. Clin Intensive Care 1992; 3:67-78.
94. HIFI Study Group: High-frequency oscillatory ventilation compared with conventional mechanical ventilation in the treatment of respiratory failure in preterm infants. N Engl J Med 1989; 370:88-93.
95. Gluck E, Heard S, Patel C, Mohr J, Calkins J: Use of ultra high frequency ventilation in patients with ARDS. A preliminary report. Chest 1993; 103:1413-1420.
96. Fort P, Farmer C, Westerman J, et al: High-frequency oscillatory ventilation for adult respiratory distress syndrome—a pilot study. Crit Care Med 1997; 25:937-947.
97. Zapol WM, Snider MT, Hill JD, et al: Extracorporeal membrane oxygenation in severe acute respiratory failure. JAMA 1979; 242:2193-2196.
98. Bartlett RH, Andrews AF, Toomasian J, et al: Extracorporeal membrane oxygenation for newborn respiratory failure: Forty five cases. Surgery 1982; 92:425-433.
99. Gattinoni L, Brazzi L, Pesenti A: Extracorporeal carbon dioxide removal in ARDS. *In:* Ventilatory Failure. Marini JJ, Roussos C (Eds). Berlin, Springer-Verlag, 1991, pp 308-317.

100. Gattinoni L, Pesenti A, Mascheroni D, et al: Low frequency positive pressure ventilation with extracorporeal CO_2 removal in severe acute respiratory failure. JAMA 1986; 256:881-886.
101. Seeger W, Pison U, Buchhorn R, et al: Surfactant abnormalities and adult respiratory failure. Lung 1990; 168(Suppl):891-902.
102. Spragg RG: Abnormalities of lung surfactant function in patients with acute lung injury: Implications for therapy. *In:* Adult Respiratory Distress Syndrome. Zapol WM, Lemaire F (Eds). New York, Marcel Dekker, 1991, pp 381-395.
103. Jobe AH, Ikegami M: Surfactant and mechanical ventilation. *In:* Physiological Basis of Ventilatory Support. Marini JJ, Slutsky AS (Eds). New York, Marcel Dekker, 1998; pp 209-229.
104. Anzueto R, Baughman K, Guntapalli K, et al: Aerosolized surfactant in adults with sepsis-induced acute respiratory distress syndrome. N Engl J Med 1996; 334:1417-1421.
105. So KL, Lachmann B: Surfactant therapy in respiratory failure. *In:* Yearbook of Intensive Care and Emergency Medicine. Vincent JL (Ed). New York, Springer-Verlag, 1995, pp 52-58.
106. Lachmann B: Open up the lung and keep the lung open. Intensive Care Med 1992; 18:319-321.
107. Langer M, Mascheroni D, Marcolin R, Gattinoni L: The prone position in ARDS patients: A clinical study. Chest 1988; 94:103-107.
108. Broccard A, Marini JJ: Effect of posture and position on the respiratory system. *In:* Yearbook of Intensive Care and Emergency Medicine. Vincent, JL (Ed). New York, Springer-Verlag, 1995, pp 165-184.
109. Pelosi P, Tubiolo D, Mascheroni D, et al: Effects of the prone position on respiratory mechanics and gas exchange during acute lung injury. Am J Respir Crit Care Med 1998; 157:387-393.
110. Faithfull NS: The role of perfluorochemicals in surgery and the ITU. Yearbook of Intensive Care and Emergency Medicine. Vincent JL, (Ed). New York, Springer-Verlag, 1994, pp 237-251.
111. Fuhrman BP, Paczan PR, DeFrancisis M: Perfluorocarbon-associated gas exchange. Crit Care Med 1991; 712-722.
112. Hirschl RB, Pranikoff T, Wise C, et al: Initial experience with partial liquid ventilation in adult patients with the acute respiratory distress syndrome. JAMA 1996; 275:383-389.
113. Hirschl RB, Tooley R, Parent AC, Johnson K, Bartlett RH: Improvement in gas exchange, pulmonary function, and lung injury with partial liquid ventilation: A study model in a setting of severe respiratory failure. Chest 1995; 108:500-508.
114. Nesti FD, Fuhrman BP, Steinhorn DM, et al: Perfluorocarbon-associated gas exchange in gastric aspiration. Crit Care Med 1994; 22:1445-1452.
115. Tutuncu AS, Akpir K, Mulder P, Erdmann W, Lachmann BK: Intratracheal perfluorocarbon administration as aid in the ventilatory management of respiratory distress syndrome. Anesthesiology 1993; 79:1083-1093.
116. Marini JJ: Down side up—a prone and partial liquid asset (Editorial). Intensive Care Med 1996; 21:963-965.
117. Broccard AF, Shapiro RS, Schmitz LL, Ravenscraft SA, Marini JJ: Influence of prone position on the extent and distribution of lung injury in a high tidal volume oleic acid model of acute respiratory distress syndrome. Crit Care Med 1997; 25:16-27.
118. Burke WC, Nahum A, Ravenscraft SA, Nakos G, Adams AB, Marcy TW, Marini JJ: Modes of tracheal gas insufflation: Comparison of continuous and phase specific gas injection in normal dogs. Am Rev Respir Dis 1993; 148:562-568.
119. Isabey D, Boussignac G, Harf A: Effect of air entrainment on airway pressure during endotracheal gas injection. J Appl Physiol 1989; 67:771-779.
120. Jonson B, Similowski T, Levy P, Vires N, Pariente R: Expiratory flushing of airways: A method to reduce dead space ventilation. Eur Respir J 1990; 3:1202-1205.
121. Nahum A, Burke WC, Ravenscraft SA, Marcy TW, Adams AB, Crooke PS, Marini JJ: Lung mechanics and gas exchange during pressure controlled ventilation in dogs: Augmentation of CO_2 elimination by an intratracheal catheter. Am Rev Respir Dis 1992; 146:965-973.
122. Nahum A, Ravenscraft SA, Nakos G, Burke WC, Adams AB, Marcy TW, Marini JJ: Tracheal gas insufflation during pressure controlled ventilation: Effect of catheter position, diameter, and flow rate. Am Rev Respir Dis 1992; 146:1411-1418.
123. Slutsky AS, Menon AS: Catheter position and blood gases during constant-flow ventilation. J Appl Physiol 1987; 62:513-519.
124. Slutsky AS, Watson J, Leith DE, Brown R: Tracheal insufflation O_2 (TRIO) at low flow rates sustains life for several hours. Anesthesiology 1985; 63:278-286.
125. Ravenscraft SA, Shapiro R, Nahum A, Burke WC, Adams AB, Nakos G, Marini JJ: Tracheal gas insufflation: Catheter effectiveness is determined by expiratory flush volume. Am J Respir Crit Care Med 1996; 153:1817-1824.
126. Nahum A, Shapiro RS, Ravenscraft SA, Adams AB, Marini JJ: Efficacy of expiratory tracheal gas insufflation in a canine model of lung injury. Am J Respir Crit Care Med 1995; 152:489-495.
127. Muller E, Kolobow T, Mandava S, Jones M, Vitale G, Aprigliano M, Yamada K: How to ventilate lungs as small as 12.5% of normal: The new technique of intratracheal pulmonary ventilation. Pediatr Res 1993; 34:606-610.
128. Shapiro RS, Ravenscraft SA, Nahum A, Adams AB, Marini JJ. Tracheal gas insufflation (TGI) cools and dries gas in the central airways. Am J Respir Crit Care Med 1995; 151:A427.
129. Pappert D, Busch T, Gerlach H, Lewandowski K, Rademacher P, Rossaint R: Aerosolized prostacyclin versus inhaled nitric oxide in children with severe acute respiratory distress syndrome. Anesthesiology 1995; 82:1507-1511.
130. Rossaint R, Falke K, Lopez F, et al: Inhaled nitric oxide for the adult respiratory distress syndrome. N Engl J Med 1993; 328:399-405.
131. Valenza F, Ribeiro SP, Slutsky AS: High volume-low pressure mechanical ventilation up-regulates IL-1-β production in an ex-vivo lung model (Abstract). Am J Respir Crit Care Med 1995; 151:A552.
132. Ravenscraft SA, Burke WC, Marini JJ: Volume-cycled decelerating flow: An alternative form of mechanical ventilation. Chest 1992; 101:1342-1351.
133. Slutsky AS: Barotrauma and alveolar recruitment (Editorial). Intensive Care Med 1993; 19:369-371.

129

Management Controversies in Acute Respiratory Distress Syndrome

Robert J. Mangialardi, MD • Gordon R. Bernard, MD

The acute respiratory distress syndrome (ARDS) was first described in 1968 as a condition associated with a wide variety of clinical events such as sepsis, multiple trauma, pneumonia, aspiration and hypovolemic shock, to name a few. Manifestations include bilateral pulmonic infiltrates, as seen on chest radiograph, and significant and poorly responsive hypoxemia. Since that time, many clinical trials have failed to demonstrate benefit versus placebo for therapies once considered promising. Some of these trials have been performed in ARDS populations, and some have been performed in patients at risk for ARDS, such as those with sepsis, burns, or multiple trauma. The failed agents have included corticosteroids (given *early* in the course of sepsis),[1-4] anti-endotoxin antibodies,[5-7] interleukin-1 (IL-1) receptor antagonists,[8] and surfactant (Table 129-1).[9]

Despite the outstanding clinical trial work that has been done, a number of controversies remain. One of the most heated of these controversies is how best to provide mechanical ventilation to these patients and whether mechanical ventilation itself causes further lung injury. This topic is under active investigation and is discussed elsewhere in this text. This chapter discusses the controversies surrounding several

TABLE 129–1. Selected Major Randomized Clinical Trials of Experimental Therapeutic Agents in Sepsis or Acute Respiratory Distress Syndrome (ARDS)

Study	Syndrome	Intervention	Comment
Bone[36]	ARDS	Intravenous PGE_1	No survival advantage to PGE_1 but may have been limited by hemodynamic effects (e.g., hypotension)
Greenman et al.[6]	Sepsis	Murine IgG monoclonal antibody to endotoxin versus placebo	No effect on mortality; antibody may have had little or no activity to neutralize endotoxin
Bernard et al.[1]	Early established ARDS	30 mg/kg methylprednisolone q6h × 4 doses versus placebo	No difference between drug and placebo in 45-day mortality or rate of ARDS reversal; small trial (only 99 patients randomized)
Fisher et al.[8]	Sepsis	Human recombinant interleukin-1 receptor antagonist versus placebo	No difference in overall mortality; molar concentration of agent may have been insufficient to block receptors consistently even with continuous infusion therapy
Anzueto et al.[9]	Early established ARDS	Aerosolized synthetic surfactant versus placebo	No difference in mortality; only 4% of aerosol reached lung
Meduri et al.[45]	Late ARDS	Methylprednisolone versus placebo	Reduced mortality in methylprednisolone (n = 16) versus placebo (n = 8) treated patients; crossover between groups allowed

PGE_1 = prostaglandin E_1; IgG = immunoglobulin G.

other important issues, namely (1) the pathophysiology of ARDS (local versus systemic disease), (2) the choice of intravenous fluid (crystalloid vs. colloid), (3) the optimal hemodynamic maintenance (wet versus dry), (4) inhaled therapies that enhance oxygenation (nitric oxide and prostaglandin E_1), and (5) *late* course therapy with corticosteroids to prevent pulmonary fibrosis.

PATHOPHYSIOLOGY: "LOCAL" VERSUS SYSTEMIC DISEASE

The definition of ARDS used in clinical trials has varied significantly over the last several years; as a result, it has frequently been difficult to compare the results of any two ARDS studies. To overcome this problem, in 1994 an expert panel of North American and European critical care specialists proposed a consensus definition of ARDS: bilateral infiltrates on chest radiograph, poor oxygenation manifest as a PaO_2/FIO_2 ratio less than 200, and no clinical evidence of heart failure.[10] The consensus conference did not require the presence of a pulmonary arterial catheter to establish the diagnosis of ARDS, but the group stipulated that the pulmonary artery occlusion pressure be less than 18 mm Hg if such a catheter is present. This new standardized definition reflects the fact that ARDS is a clinical syndrome that encompasses many diseases, some local and some systemic. This definition may apply if the patient has bilateral lung trauma with resulting contusions, diffuse lung infection, diffuse lung inflammation of any etiology, including eosinophilic pneumonia and bronchiolitis obliterans with organizing pneumonia, inhalational lung injury, aspiration, or from systemic inflammation associated with sepsis or multiple trauma.

Frequently, ARDS is referred to as a *systemic* disease, because in many series sepsis and nonpulmonary multiple trauma are the most common inciting illnesses. It should be clear, however, that patients can have a diagnosis of ARDS based on isolated lung disease. Furthermore, it is often difficult to establish whether diffuse lung infiltrates in a given patient are related to systemic illness or whether such infiltrates represent superimposed pneumonia or aspiration.

The fact that ARDS clinically encompasses both local and systemic processes is supported by epidemiologic studies. Investigators have repeatedly shown that in any particular population of ARDS patients, only a moderate fraction of these have elevated blood or bronchoalveolar lavage (BAL) cytokine levels that suggest overexuberant autoinflammation as part of the pathophysiology of lung injury.[11–16] The remainder of the patients either do not have significant inflammation as measured by proinflammatory cytokine levels, or the cytokine levels were not checked during some critical time window. Furthermore, clinicians frequently refer to ARDS as a disease of increased capillary permeability resulting in alveolar flooding. This contention is supported by animal studies in which ARDS results from increased capillary permeability when the animal receives intravenous infusions of endotoxin, tumor necrosis factor (TNF) or IL-1, agents known to be present or enumerated in human sepsis.[17]

Capillary permeability in patients with ARDS has been assessed both by radionuclide studies and by evaluation of the ratio of alveolar protein to serum protein.[18, 19] In the former method, a radiolabeled compound, such as ^{125}I-albumin, is infused peripherally and its extravasation into lung tissue is determined by placing a gamma counter over the chest wall. The rate of accumulation of counts is used as a surrogate measure of capillary permeability. In the protein method, fluid is aspirated from the endotracheal tube and its protein concentration is assessed. A high ratio of aspirate to serum protein suggests an abnormally high lung capillary permeability, whereas patients without injury have a ratio close to zero.

In both types of studies, investigators have consistently reported a wide spectrum of permeabilities in ARDS patients, ranging from near normal to greatly increased. Furthermore, these tests are rarely, if ever, used clinically to establish the presence of increased capillary permeability in patients with a diagnosis of ARDS, and such testing is not part of the consensus conference definition of ARDS.

The diverse spectrum of ARDS has important implications clinically and for clinical trials of promising new therapies. Clinicians should guard against making prognostic or therapeutic generalizations that are too broad. For instance, corticosteroids given early in the course of ARDS have not proved useful in at least three large randomized clinical trials in sepsis. However, clearly some disease processes do result in ARDS that are known to be steroid-responsive (eosinophilic pneumonia, hypersensitivity pneumonitis, idiopathic bronchiolitis obliterans with organizing pneumonia, interstitial pneumonitis associated with collagen vascular disease). Treatments aimed at blocking proinflammatory cytokines have thus far not proved useful in clinical trials, but these trials have not restricted such agents to patients with elevated serum levels of the targeted proinflammatory cytokines.[8, 20] Although antiendotoxin therapy has also failed the scrutiny of clinical trials in sepsis, some of the antibodies employed have been of marginal activity, and all of the trials have included large numbers of patients unlikely to benefit from such therapy (e.g., patients *without* positive blood cultures or with cultures positive only for gram-positive bacteria).[5-7] We must wonder if any of these studies would have had a more favorable result had the therapy been more narrowly targeted to the subgroup that the treatment was intended to address. Performing such a trial is logistically difficult, perhaps impossible, in terms of patient screening, and it would be costly in terms of recruitment time.

FLUID MANAGEMENT

There are two related controversies in ARDS management: (1) the ideal intravenous fluid, crystalloid or colloid, and (2) the ideal volume status, wet or dry.[21] Surprisingly, in a clinical syndrome whose major manifestation is pulmonary edema, a syndrome recognized for almost 30 years, no clinical trial has yet been published that directly addresses either of these two questions. On the basis of limited data available from trials in other clinical circumstances and from animal studies, cogent arguments may be made for either side of these controversies.

Most clinical trials comparing colloid to crystalloid have been performed in patients with hemorrhagic shock.[22] None of these trials demonstrated any mortality benefit of colloid over crystalloid, and there is no convincing evidence that either is superior in terms of reducing pulmonary dysfunction, ventilator duration, or length of hospital stay. The most consistent findings have been that (1) colloid resuscitation requires considerably less volume to reach the same resuscitation endpoints and (2) colloid resuscitation results in higher colloid oncotic pressure and higher serum protein and albumin levels (when the colloid used for resuscitation is albumin). We have shown that hypoproteinemia is a nearly universal finding in ARDS and have questioned whether low protein levels may contribute to the pulmonary edema through a low oncotic pressure mechanism.[23]

Although there is no published trial of colloid therapy in ARDS, there have been two published randomized trials of albumin supplementation in hospitalized patients who are hypoproteinemic. Foley and colleagues[24] randomized 40 patients with serum albumin $\leq$2.5 g/dL to receive either albumin supplementation or placebo with a goal of achieving a serum albumin level $>$ 2.5 g/dL. They found no differences in the incidence of in-hospital complications, length of stay in the intensive care unit (ICU), or length of hospital stay between the two groups.

Brown and coworkers conducted a similar randomized study in patients receiving total parenteral nutrition (TPN). Serum albumin level was $\leq$3.0 g/dL, with patients randomized to receive albumin or placebo until serum albumin exceeded 3.0 g/dL.[25] They reported a statistically significant decrease in the incidence of "pneumonia" in the treated patients. Neither of these studies specifically targeted ARDS patients, nor did they target patients who were volume-overloaded.

In both animal models of permeability pulmonary edema and in patients with ARDS, a loss of size selectivity to protein in the endothelial barrier has been demonstrated.[18] Critics of colloid therapy in ARDS argue that the protein may "leak" out of the capillary into the interstitial space and worsen edema. This argument is largely theoretical and is refuted by at least one published study. Sibbald and coauthors demonstrated that albumin administration in ARDS patients does *not* increase the flux of protein into the lung, provided that hydrostatic pressure is controlled (i.e., not increased by the albumin).[26]

What is the clinician to do in the absence of definitive data? There seems to be little compelling reason to use colloid in patients with ARDS who are not hypoproteinemic or edematous or who respond favorably to diuretics. The only clear benefit of using colloid is to reduce the fluid volume that patients receive, especially in patients when volume overload appears to be a problem. The use of colloid to increase oncotic pressure in patients with pulmonary edema is a hypothetical but unproven benefit and cannot be generally recommended.

The use of diuretic agents in patients with ARDS is also controversial. Animal models of permeability pulmonary edema reveal that the amount of lung water correlates with the hydrostatic pressure, even when the hydrostatic pressure is in the normal range; however, lung water has not consistently correlated with severity of hypoxemia.[27] Two retrospective studies in humans suggest a potential survival benefit for controlling volume.

Simmons and colleagues[28] showed that surviving patients with ARDS consistently lost weight over time during their ICU stays while nonsurvivors consistently gained weight.[28] Humphrey and associates[29] showed that ARDS patients who experienced a 25% decrease in their pulmonary artery occlusion pressures had a significantly greater survival than ARDS patients who did not experience such a reduction. Both of these studies are retrospective, and the findings may indicate that weight loss or decreasing hydrostatic pressures are simply markers for patient improvement rather than causally related to improvement. However, such a cause-and-effect relationship cannot be excluded.

Mitchell and coworkers conducted a prospective randomized trial of aggressive diuresis in pulmonary edema, a trial that included both ARDS and congestive heart failure patients.[30] The patients who were randomized to a more aggressive diuretic regimen had more rapid improvement in lung function, with fewer ventilator and ICU days, although this trend did not reach statistical significance in the subgroup with ARDS (perhaps because of insufficient sample size).

There are several theoretical arguments against the use of diuretics in ARDS patients.[31, 32] First, diuretic medications may decrease circulating volume and thus reduce cardiac output and tissue oxygen delivery. Second, lower cardiac output caused by diuresis may impair renal function, and poor renal function is a known independent predictor of poor outcome in ARDS. Third, many of these patients are in shock and require vasopressor medications or ongoing fluid challenges for hypotension, a situation that may be further compromised by diuretic use. Lung water does not correlate with oxygenation or outcome in ARDS, but additional organ system dysfunction does. To the extent that diuretics impair renal or cardiac function, they may adversely affect the outcome.

In conclusion, the proponents of any particular fluid management strategy in ARDS can point to the literature to develop cogent arguments in favor of their approach. At present, it is recognized that the definitive clinical trial to define optimal fluid management in ARDS is lacking.

INTRAVENOUS AND INHALED VASODILATORS

Role of Vasodilating Agents

Severe ARDS is associated with pulmonary hypertension, and the hypoxemia of ARDS is largely a result of venous admixture or shunting of blood through nonventilated pulmonary segments. These observations have led to the investigation of vasodilator therapies in ARDS in the hopes of reducing pulmonary hypertension and improving arterial oxygenation by decreasing venous admixture.[33] Vasodilating agents, when given intravenously, reduce pulmonary vascular resistance but also increase shunt fraction by dilating nonventilated areas of lung. If these same agents are given by the airway route, either as a gas (nitric oxide) or aerosol (prostaglandin E_1 [PGE_1]), they selectively vasodilate only ventilated lung units, thereby decreasing shunt and deadspace ventilation. Nitric oxide and PGE_1 have had additional appeal because of their potential anti-inflammatory properties. PGE_1 inhibits platelet aggregation, macrophage activation, and neutrophil chemotaxis and release of both oxygen radicals and liposomal enzymes. Nitric oxide decreases neutrophil production of hydrogen peroxide and decreases neutrophil enumeration of adhesion molecules. Nitric oxide has also been shown to decrease BAL concentrations of IL-6 and IL-8, two important proinflammatory cytokines.[34] Nitric oxide, PGE_1, and prostacyclin are all rapidly metabolized or inactivated.

Intravenous Route (Prostaglandin E_1)

Holcroft and coworkers,[35] conducting a single-center, randomized, placebo-controlled blinded trial of intravenous PGE_1 given as a continuous infusion at 30 $ng/kg^{-1} \cdot min^{-1}$, reported a statistically significant *improvement* in 30-day survival in treated patients. Bone and colleagues[36] subsequently conducted a larger multicenter randomized trial in a more diverse patient population using the same dose of PGE_1 and found a slight (but not statistically significant) *increase* in mortality in the patients treated with PGE_1. Both studies reported a transient worsening of oxygenation in treated patients, presumably because of attenuation in hypoxic vasoconstriction resulting in increased venous admixture.

Recent interest has focused on *liposomal PGE_1* which has some theoretical advantages over free PGE_1:

1. It can be given as a bolus dose rather than as a continuous infusion.
2. It can be given at a lower total dose of drug.
3. The liposomal moiety may increase the antineutrophil activity of the drug.

Abraham and coworkers conducted a small randomized trial of liposomal PGE_1 that showed statistically significant improvements in Pao_2/FIO_2 ratio at day 3, static lung compliance at day 8, and successful extubation at day 8 in the treatment group compared to the placebo group.[37]

Recent interest has also focused on *inhaled PGE_1*, which has the theoretical advantage of only dilating vessels in ventilated lung units, perhaps decreasing venous admixture and improving oxygenation. Clinical trials are pending.

Inhaled Vasodilators (Nitric Oxide, Prostacyclin)

Nitric oxide is a potent vasodilator that is rapidly inactivated by binding to hemoglobin. Several small clinical trials have demonstrated that inhaled nitric oxide in concentrations ranging from 1 to 40 parts per million (ppm) improves oxygenation by decreasing intrapulmonary shunt fraction. If this dose decreases mean pulmonary artery pressure, as well as increases right ventricular ejection fraction and cardiac output, this can result in improved oxygen delivery.[38–40]

In each of these studies, some patients responded to therapy with an increase in Pao_2 and some did not. The dose of inhaled nitric oxide that produced a favorable response varied significantly among patients. Furthermore, the response to nitric oxide varied from day to day, with some responders becoming nonresponders and vice versa.

There appears to be little risk of clinically significant toxicity through development of methemoglobinemia from nitrate combining with hemoglobin as long as the dose rate remained below 40 ppm. Surprisingly, in some responders there was no evidence of tachyphylaxis from continuous administration even when nitric oxide was given for several days. Some studies have demonstrated a rebound decrease in Pao_2, a decrease in cardiac output, and an increase in mean pulmonary artery pressure when nitric oxide is abruptly discontinued.[41] This phenomenon can be prevented by withdrawal of the agent over 15 minutes. Prostacyclin (PGI_2) has been compared to nitric oxide in clinical trials and appears to produce similar physiologic results.[42]

Future Studies

PGE_1, in either liposomal or free form, inhaled nitric oxide, and prostacyclin have not been evaluated in a large-scale randomized clinical trial that has been sufficiently powered to demonstrate a mortality benefit. So far, the demonstrated benefits of these agents are purely physiologic; they reduce intrapulmonary shunt and elevated pulmonary vascular resistance in some patients. Pending further study, routine use of these agents to treat ARDS patients cannot be recommended, but consideration of their use in difficult to oxygenate patients or patients who require a FIO_2 above 0.6 for more than 2 days seems reasonable.

STEROIDAL AND NONSTEROIDAL ANTI-INFLAMMATORY AGENTS

Several randomized, blinded, placebo-controlled clinical trials have been unable to demonstrate a survival or physiologic benefit for corticosteroids in ARDS.[1–4] This finding has been criticized because all of these trials employed corticosteroids only for brief periods (usually <48 hours) in patients with *early* ARDS. It has been long recognized that *late* ARDS is characterized by a fibroproliferative phase that may result in pulmonary fibrosis. It is believed (based on observational data) that the degree of collagen deposition in the lung interstitium is proportional to the degree and persistence of lung inflammation as measured by BAL neutrophilia and proinflammatory cytokine levels. These observations have led some to propose the use of high-dose corticosteroids in otherwise stable ARDS patients who remain ventilator-dependent after 1 week of supportive care.

There are two published retrospective observational studies of approximately 25 patients each in which high-dose corticosteroids were employed for up to 3 weeks in patients with *late* ARDS.[43, 44] Both studies reported survival rates of approximately 80% in treated patients and improvements in oxygenation and chest radiographs. Because neither study included a control group, it is unclear whether corticosteroid therapy was responsible for the good outcomes reported or whether these outcomes occurred despite the corticosteroid therapy. Some authors have suggested that abnormal gallium lung scans may be helpful in selection of patients for corticosteroid therapy, but others have shown that such abnormalities are universal in ARDS patients, thus casting doubt on the test's utility.

Corticosteroid therapy is also associated with increased risk of infection, delayed wound healing, and increased risk of gastrointestinal bleeding. These potential complications are especially worrisome in the mechanically ventilated ARDS population, already at high risk for such adverse events.

Meduri and colleagues[45] conducted a randomized, double-blind, placebo-controlled study of methylprednisolone in ARDS patients who were enrolled after 7 days of mechanical ventilation. This small study (16 treated patients, eight placebo patients) showed a dramatic reduction in mortality rate, and improvement in lung injury scores, Pa_{O_2}/FIO_2 ratio, and reduction in organ failure in the treated patients. However, several of the "placebo" patients crossed over into the treated group after 10 days, and this crossover group did not appear to receive the same benefits. In 1997, the National Institutes of Health ARDS network began a randomized, controlled trial of corticosteroids in 200 patients with ARDS who require at least 7 days of mechanical ventilation. The trial was ongoing as of 1998.

In conclusion, corticosteroids cannot be recommended in *early* ARDS based on the published clinical trials. Corticosteroids have been considered in *late* ARDS based on pathophysiologic arguments and small published series. At present, convincing clinical data are lacking to mandate their use in all ARDS patients, and corticosteroids carry some risk in this high-risk population. Until additional trials are completed, the routine use of corticosteroids in late ARDS cannot be recommended.

Nonsteroidal anti-inflammatory drugs (NSAIDs) have also received attention as possible treatment or prevention of ARDS associated with sepsis. In particular, intravenous ibuprofen (10 mg/kg every 6 hours for 48 hours) has been evaluated in patients meeting criteria for sepsis syndrome with or without ARDS.[46] Although there were reductions in fever, tachycardia, and oxygen consumption and more rapid resolution of lactic acidosis. There was no effect on development of ARDS or overall mortality.

SUMMARY

After 30 years of clinical experience with ARDS, therapy remains largely supportive. Despite this observation, the mortality rate has been declining perhaps because of improvements in supportive care and perhaps because of changing definitions of the syndrome. Numerous controversies remain unresolved, especially those relating to fluid management, vasodilator use, and late corticosteroid use in these patients. These controversies will continue to provide fertile ground for large-scale, randomized clinical trials. Until these trials are completed, the clinician needs to "resolve" the controversies individually for each ARDS patient he or she encounters.

References

1. Bernard GR, Luce JM, Sprung CL, et al: High-dose corticosteroids in patients with the adult respiratory distress syndrome. N Engl J Med 1987; 317:1565–1570.
2. Luce JM, Montgomery AB, Marks JD, Turner J, Metz CA, Murray JF: Ineffectiveness of high-dose methylprednisolone in preventing parenchymal lung injury and improving mortality in patients with septic shock. Am Rev Respir Dis 1988; 138:62–68.
3. Sprung CL, Caralis PV, Marcial EH, Pierce M, et al: The effects of high-dose corticosteroids in patients with septic shock: A prospective, controlled study. N Engl J Med 1984; 311:1137–1143.
4. Bone RC, Fisher CJJ, Clemmer TP, Slotman GJ, Metz CA, Balk RA: A controlled clinical trial of high-dose methylprednisolone in the treatment of severe sepsis and septic shock. N Engl J Med 1987; 317:653–658.
5. Chernoff AE, Granowitz EV, Shapiro L, et al: A randomized, controlled trial of IL-10 in humans: Inhibition of inflammatory cytokine production and immune responses. J Immunol 1995; 154:5492–5499.
6. Greenman RL, Schein RM, Martin MA, et al: A controlled clinical trial of E5 murine monoclonal IgM antibody to endotoxin in the treatment of gram-negative sepsis: The XOMA Sepsis Study Group. JAMA 1991; 266:1097–1102.
7. Ziegler EJ, Fisher CJJ, Sprung CL, et al: Treatment of gram-negative bacteremia and septic shock with HA-1A human monoclonal antibody against endotoxin: A randomized, double-blind, placebo-controlled trial. The HA-1A Sepsis Study Group. N Engl J Med 1991; 324:429–436.
8. Fisher CJJ, Dhainaut JF, Opal SM, et al: Recombinant human interleukin 1 receptor antagonist in the treatment of patients with sepsis syndrome: Results from a randomized, double-blind, placebo-controlled trial. Phase III rhIL-1ra Sepsis Syndrome Study Group. JAMA 1994; 271:1836–1843.
9. Anzueto A, Baughman RP, Guntupalli KK, et al: Aerosolized surfactant in adults with sepsis-induced acute respiratory distress syndrome: Exosurf Acute Respiratory Distress Syndrome Sepsis Study Group. N Engl J Med 1996; 334:1417–1421.
10. Bernard GR, Artigas A, Brigham KL, et al: The American-European Consensus Conference on ARDS: Definitions, mechanisms, relevant outcomes, and clinical trial coordination. Am J Respir Crit Care Med 1994; 149:818–824.
11. Casey LC, Balk RA, Bone RC: Plasma cytokine and endotoxin levels correlate with survival in patients with the sepsis syndrome. Ann Intern Med 1993; 119:771–778.
12. Calandra T, Gerain J, Heumann D, Baumgartner JD, Glauser MP: High circulating levels of interleukin-6 in patients with septic shock: Evolution during sepsis, prognostic value, and interplay with other cytokines. The Swiss-Dutch J5 Immunoglobulin Study Group. Am J Med 1991; 91:23–29.
13. Donnelly SC, Strieter RM, Kunkel SL, et al: Chemotactic cytokines in the established adult respiratory distress syndrome and at-risk patients. Chest 1994; 105:98S–99S.
14. Marty C, Misset B, Tamion F, Fitting C, Carlet J, Cavaillon JM: Circulating interleukin-8 concentrations in patients with multiple organ failure of septic and nonseptic origin. Crit Care Med 1994; 22:673–679.
15. Marks JD, Marks CB, Luce JM, et al: Plasma tumor necrosis factor in patients with septic shock: Mortality rate, incidence of adult respiratory distress syndrome, and effects of methylprednisolone administration. Am Rev Respir Dis 1990; 141:94–97.
16. Meduri GU, Kohler G, Headley S, Tolley E, Stentz F, Postlethwaite A: Inflammatory cytokines in the BAL of patients with ARDS: Persistent elevation over time predicts poor outcome. Chest 1995; 108:1303–1314.
17. Brigham KL: Oxidant stress and adult respiratory distress syndrome. Eur Respir J 1990; 11:482S–484S.
18. Holter JF, Weiland JE, Pacht ER, Gadek JE, Davis WB: Protein permeability in the adult respiratory distress syndrome: Loss of size selectivity of the alveolar epithelium. J Clin Invest 1986; 78:1513–1522.
19. Sibbald WJ, Driedger AA, Wells GA, Koval JJ: Clinical correlates of the spectrum of lung microvascular injury in human noncardiac edema. Crit Care Med 1983; 11:70–78.
20. Fisher CJJ, Opal SM, Dhainaut JF, et al: Influence of an anti-tumor necrosis factor monoclonal antibody on cytokine levels in patients with sepsis: The CB0006 Sepsis Syndrome Study Group. Crit Care Med 1993; 21:318–327.
21. Schuster DP: Fluid management in ARDS: "Keep them dry" or does it matter? Intensive Care Med 1995; 21:101–103.
22. Velanovich V: Crystalloid versus colloid fluid resuscitation: A meta-analysis of mortality. Surgery 1989; 105:65–71.
23. Mangialardi RJ, Wheeler AP, Bernard GR: Hypoproteinemia predicts weight gain, ventilator dependence and mortality in sepsis induced ARDS (Abstract). Am J Respir Crit Care Med 1997; 155:A504.
24. Foley EF, Borlase BC, Dzik WH, Bistrian BR, Benotti PN: Albumin supplementation in the critically ill: A prospective, randomized trial. Arch Surg 1990; 125:739–742.
25. Brown RO, Bradley JE, Bekemeyer WB, Luther RW: Effect of albumin supplementation during parenteral nutrition on hospital morbidity. Crit Care Med 1988; 16:1177–1182.
26. Sibbald WJ, Driedger AA, Wells GA, Myers ML, Lefcoe M: The short-term effects of increasing plasma colloid osmotic pressure in patients with noncardiac pulmonary edema. Surgery 1983; 93:620–633.
27. Brigham KL, Kariman K, Harris TR, Snapper JR, Bernard G, Young

SL: Correlation of oxygenation with vascular permeability-surface area but not with lung water in humans with acute respiratory failure and pulmonary edema. J Clin Invest 1983; 72:339-349.
28. Simmons RS, Berdine GG, Seidenfeld JJ, et al: Fluid balance and the adult respiratory distress syndrome. Am Rev Respir Dis 1987; 135:924-929.
29. Humphrey H, Hall J, Sznajder I, Silverstein M, Wood L: Improved survival in ARDS patients associated with a reduction in pulmonary capillary wedge pressure. Chest 1990; 97:1176-1180.
30. Mitchell JP, Schuller D, Calandrino FS, Schuster DP: Improved outcome based on fluid management in critically ill patients requiring pulmonary artery catheterization. Am Rev Respir Dis 1992; 145:990-998.
31. Marshall JC, Cook DJ, Christou NV, Bernard GR, Sprung C, Sibbald WJ: Multiple organ dysfunction score: A reliable descriptor of a complex clinical outcome. Crit Care Med 1995; 23:1638-1652.
32. Hebert PC, Drummond AJ, Singer J, Bernard GR, Russell J: A simple multiple system organ failure scoring system predicts mortality of patients who have sepsis syndrome. Chest 1993; 104:230-235.
33. Zapol WM, Rimar S, Gillis N, Marletta M, Bosken CH: Nitric oxide and the lung. Am J Respir Crit Care Med 1994; 149:1375-1380.
34. Chollet-Martin S, Gatecel C, Kermarrec N, Gougerot-Pocidalo MA, Payen DM: Alveolar neutrophil functions and cytokine levels in patients with the adult respiratory distress syndrome during nitric oxide inhalation. Am J Respir Crit Care Med 1996; 153:985-990.
35. Holcroft JW, Vassar MJ, Weber CJ: Prostaglandin E1 and survival in patients with the adult respiratory distress syndrome: A prospective trial. Ann Surg 1986; 203:371-378.
36. Bone RC, Slotman G, Maunder R, et al: Randomized double-blind, multicenter study of prostaglandin E1 in patients with the adult respiratory distress syndrome. Prostaglandin E1 Study Group. Chest 1989; 96:114-119.
37. Abraham E, Park YC, Covington P, Conrad SA, Schwartz M: Liposomal prostaglandin E1 in acute respiratory distress syndrome: A placebo-controlled, randomized, double-blind, multicenter clinical trial [see comments]. Crit Care Med 1996; 24:10-15.
38. Rossaint R, Falke KJ, Lopez F, Slama K, Pison U, Zapol WM: Inhaled nitric oxide for the adult respiratory distress syndrome. N Engl J Med 1993; 328:399-405.
39. Krafft P, Fridrich P, Fitzgerald RD, Koc D, Steltzer H: Effectiveness of nitric oxide inhalation in septic ARDS. Chest 1996; 109:486-493.
40. Rossaint R, Gerlach H, Schmidt-Ruhnke H, et al: Efficacy of inhaled nitric oxide in patients with severe ARDS. Chest 1995; 107:1107-1115.
41. Lavoie A, Hall JB, Olson DM, Wylam ME: Life-threatening effects of discontinuing inhaled nitric oxide in severe respiratory failure. Am J Respir Crit Care Med 1996; 153:1985-1987.
42. Zwissler B, Kemming G, Habler O, et al: Inhaled prostacyclin (PGI_2) versus inhaled nitric oxide in adult respiratory distress syndrome. Am J Respir Crit Care Med 1996; 154:1671-1677.
43. Meduri GU, Headley S, Tolley E, Shelby M, Stentz F, Postlethwaite A: Plasma and BAL cytokine response to corticosteroid rescue treatment in late ARDS. Chest 1995; 108:1315-1325.
44. Hooper RG, Kearl RA: Established adult respiratory distress syndrome successfully treated with corticosteroids. South Med J 1996; 89:359-364.
45. Meduri GU, Headley S, Golden E, et al: Methylprednisolone treatment (MPT) of late ARDS (Abstract). Am J Respir Crit Care Med 1997; 155:A391.
46. Bernard GR, Wheeler AP, Carmichael L, et al: Effects of ibuprofen on the physiology and survival of patients with sepsis. N Engl J Med 1997; 336:912-918.

130

Surfactant Physiology, Metabolism, Function, and Therapy

Kristine M. McCulloch, MD • Dharmapuri Vidyasagar, MD

SURFACTANT PHYSIOLOGY

Understanding the role of surfactant in pulmonary physiology and disease is important for the appropriate use of surfactant therapy in critical care medicine. The unique contributions of surfactant to the respiratory system are functions of its composition, physical behavior, and chemical properties.

Surfactant is a complex mixture of components. The chemical composition of surfactant from various mammalian species is quite similar (Table 130-1). Surfactant can be prepared from lung homogenate and from the fluid obtained by bronchoalveolar lavage (BAL). The latter represents surfactant that has been secreted into the alveoli.

Surfactant usually is isolated by differential centrifugation. It comprises approximately 90% lipid, 10% protein, and very small quantities of carbohydrate. About 50% by weight of surfactant lipid is fully saturated phosphatidylcholine, mostly dipalmitoylphosphatidylcholine (DPPC). Unsaturated phosphatidylcholines and acidic phospholipids, such as phosphatidylglycerol (PG) and phosphatidylinositol (PI), are present in smaller amounts. Approximately 10% by weight of total lipid is neutral lipid, mostly cholesterol.[1-5] Two thirds of the protein in surfactant is derived from serum.[6]

Four lung-specific nonserum proteins, SP-A, SP-B, SP-C, and SP-D, have been found in close association with surfactant phospholipids (Table 130-2).[4, 5, 7, 8]

Pulmonary gas exchange occurs at the interface between alveolar air and the extracellular fluid subphase of the alveolar lining. Surface tension is the contractile force on the alveolar surface produced by attractive forces between the molecules of the fluid subphase. The problem of alveolar stability may be understood by the LaPlace relationship for a sphere. Surface pressure (P) is directly related to twice the surface tension (T) and inversely related to the radius (R):

$$P = \frac{2T}{R}$$

The alveolar surface pressure that is generated by its surface tension is mechanically opposed by transpulmonary pressure. During expiration, transpulmonary pressure decreases and the radius and surface area of the alveolus become smaller. Unless surface tension is lowered during expiration, the pressure on the alveolar surface exceeds transpulmonary pressure and the alveolus collapses.[9, 10] Surfactant coats the alveolar surface as a monomolecular film that is capable of decreasing its molecular surface area as the alveolus contracts during expiration. The reduction of molecular surface area decreases the alveolar surface tension, thereby preventing the alveolar collapse that would be predicted from the LaPlace relationship. Surface balance measurements confirm that when a film of surfactant is compressed, surface tension decreases as surface area decreases.[2, 3, 9]

The upper limit of alveolar surface tension consistent with alveolar stability at end-expiration was calculated by King

TABLE 130–1. Biochemical Composition of Pulmonary Surfactant

Lipid	85%–90%	
Phospholipids	75%–85%	
PC	60%–70%	
DSPC	40%–45%	(DPPC >90%)
PG, PI, PE	10%–15%	
Lyso-PC, SM	5%–10%	
Neutral lipids	5%–10% (predominantly cholesterol)	
Protein	5%–10%	
Carbohydrate	5%	

PC = phosphatidylcholine; DSPC = disaturated phosphatidylcholine; PG = phosphatidylglycerol; PI = phosphatidylinositol; PE = phosphatidylethanolamine; Lyso-PC = lysophosphatidylcholine; SM = sphingomyelin; DPPC = dipalmitoyl phosphatidylcholine.

and Clements[1] using transpulmonary pressure and the rate of change of surface area with change in volume and was determined to be 10 dyne/cm. These investigators demonstrated in vitro at 37°C that surfactant lowers surface tension to less than 10 dyne/cm, shows small surface compressibility, and exhibits rapid rates of movement from a liquid subphase and of adsorption onto the air-liquid interface. These properties account for the ability of the lungs to expand from a collapsed state after just a few inflations and to maintain a residual volume at low pressures.

DPPC is the only component of surfactant with enough molecular compressibility to lower alveolar surface tension adequately and with a sufficiently slow rate of monolayer collapse to keep surface tension low and alveoli open for the duration of the respiratory cycle. The choline moiety is in the polar head group of the DPPC molecule, which is hydrophilic and thus aligns on the aqueous side of the air-liquid interface. The two fully saturated palmitic acid residues are on the opposite, nonpolar end of the DPPC molecule, which is hydrophobic and points toward the gaseous phase. The very straight, fully saturated palmitic acid chains allow close packing of the DPPC molecules. As surface area decreases, less compressible molecules may be forced out of the surface film, leaving concentrated amounts of DPPC.[2, 3, 11] Thus, DPPC is the surfactant component responsible for lowering alveolar surface tension and preventing alveolar collapse.

The ability of surfactant to form a surface film also depends on its rates of diffusion through the liquid subphase and of spread onto the air-liquid interface. By itself, DPPC diffuses and spreads slowly.[2] Thus, other surfactant components must be responsible for its rapid adsorption in vivo and in vitro. Unsaturated phosphatidylcholines, neutral lipids, and surfactant-associated proteins SP-A, SP-B, and SP-C all appear to promote adsorption of DPPC to the air-liquid interface.[2, 4, 5, 8] The poor adsorption velocity of pure DPPC may be due to the fact that it exists in the gel state at 37°C, whereas its phase transition to the liquid state occurs at 41°C. Unsaturated phosphatidylcholines and neutral lipids have phase transition

TABLE 130–2. Surfactant Proteins

Type	Monomer Size (Da)	Predominant Oligomer
SP-A	28,000–36,000	Trimer
SP-B	8,000	Dimer
SP-C	3,800	Dimer
SP-D	43,000	Trimer

temperatures of less than 37°C, and they may cause the surfactant mixture to be in the liquid phase at 37°C, thereby increasing its adsorption rate in vivo.[2, 10] SP-A also may enhance surfactant adsorption by favoring the transition of its lipids to the liquid phase at lower temperatures.[8, 10]

Surfactant is found in the type II alveolar cells in storage and secretory organelles called *lamellar bodies*. Surfactant phospholipids and surfactant-associated proteins are packed in folded layers that surround a proteinaceous core. The lamellar bodies are enclosed by a limiting membrane that participates in the exocytotic process of surfactant secretion. The limiting membrane of the lamellar body fuses with the plasma membrane of the type II cell, and surfactant is released into the extracellular fluid subphase of the alveolar lining.[2, 3, 9] After secretion, some of the lamellae are converted to tubular myelin by a calcium-dependent process of aggregation of phospholipids that is markedly enhanced by SP-A and SP-B. It is from tubular myelin that surfactant is believed to move to the air-liquid interface to form a surface film.[4, 6, 8]

The surfactant-associated proteins are found in type II alveolar cells and in the nonciliated bronchiolar cells, or *Clara cells*. These proteins are involved in various ways in surfactant physiology.

SP-A is a water-soluble protein whose structure includes a collagen-like region and a carbohydrate-binding C-terminal. SP-A does not lower surface tension. It promotes surface adsorption when added to DPPC with SP-B or SP-C or both but has no significant effect on phospholipid adsorption by itself. In the presence of calcium, SP-A enhances lipid aggregation, and thus it can promote the transformation of lamellar body contents into tubular myelin. SP-A has been shown to increase the phagocytosis of bacteria and viruses by alveolar macrophages, a function that may involve the carbohydrate-binding portion of its structure.

SP-B and *SP-C* are hydrophobic proteins. SP-B and, to a lesser extent, SP-C enhance the ability of phospholipids to reduce surface tension. SP-B or SP-C promotes surfactant adsorption and acts with SP-A to convert lamellae to tubular myelin. SP-A, SP-B, and SP-C can reduce the surfactant inactivation caused by the presence of serum proteins.

SP-D is water-soluble and is structurally similar to SP-A. Thus, it may also have a role in the binding and clearance of bacteria and viruses from the lower airways.[4, 6, 7, 8]

SURFACTANT METABOLISM

Phospholipid Synthesis

Synthesis of surfactant phospholipids occurs only in type II alveolar cells. The initial compound is glycerol-3-phosphate, which is formed from dihydroxyacetone phosphate in an adult or from glycogen in a fetus. New fatty acids may be synthesized from lactate, or circulating fatty acids can be used. Acylation of glycerol-3-phosphate by glycerol-3-phosphate acyltransferase produces palmitoyl-*sn*-glycerol-3-phosphate, which is further acylated by 1-acylglycerol-3-phosphate acyltransferase to phosphatidic acid, from which diacylglycerols are formed. When palmitoyl conconavalin A (Con A) is the principal acyl donor, disaturated phosphatidic acid predominates.

Choline is taken up efficiently by type II cells and is acted on sequentially by choline kinase and phosphocholine cytidyltransferase to form cytidine-diphosphocholine (CDP-choline). Phosphatidylcholines are formed from diacylglycerols and CDP-choline by cholinephosphotransferase. DPPC may be formed de novo by the type II cell from disaturated phosphatidic acid and CDP-choline. DPPC also can be produced by the remodeling of unsaturated phosphatidylcholines through deacylation by phospholipase A, followed either by transacylation by lysophosphatidylcholine acyltransferase or by reacylation with palmitoyl CoA.

The precursor for both PG and PI is CDP-diacylglycerol. It is formed from cytidine triphosphate and phosphatidic acid by phosphatidate cytidyltransferase. Phosphatidylglycerolphosphate, formed by CDP-diacylglycerol glycerophosphate phosphatidyltransferase, is dephosphorylated to form PG. Conversion of CDP-diacylglycerol by CDP-diacylglycerol inositol phosphatidyltransferase produces PI.[10–12]

During gestation, the relative amounts of these acidic phospholipids in pulmonary surfactant show predictable changes that have been useful in assessing fetal lung maturity. The relative quantity of PG is much lower than that of PI until about 36 weeks' gestation in a human fetus, when a sudden increase in PG synthesis causes a marked change in the ratio. This change is delayed in infants of diabetic mothers. Normally, the PG:PI ratio increases from 0.04 at 35 weeks' gestation to 1.75 at term. One reason for this change may be a decline in the amount of inositol available for synthesis of PI. Another possible explanation is that the cytidine monophosphate, formed from increased phosphatidylcholine synthesis at term, may enhance the conversion of PI to inositol and CDP-diacylglycerol, which then is available for PG synthesis. In vitro studies of human fetal lung cells have shown that glucocorticoids with prolactin or insulin increase the ratio of the rates of lamellar body synthesis of PG:PI from 0.4 to 1.6. Increased amounts of PG in pulmonary surfactant result in detectable PG in amniotic fluid, in amounts that correlate with fetal lung maturity.[11, 13]

Newly synthesized surfactant phospholipids are transferred from the endoplasmic reticulum to the Golgi apparatus. From the Golgi complex, they must be moved to the lamellar bodies. This may be accomplished by vesicular transport, in which small, dense lamellar bodies carry phospholipid from the Golgi apparatus to the large, less dense lamellar bodies.[3, 12]

Hyaline membrane disease (HMD) is primarily a result of surfactant deficiency in prematurely born infants. The developmental regulation of surfactant phospholipid synthesis is relevant to the occurrence of HMD. As in other mammals, the human fetus does not synthesize and secrete surfactant until gestation is approximately 80% complete. Although lamellar bodies are seen by 20 to 22 weeks and become numerous after 25 weeks, surfactant can be detected in amniotic fluid only after 30 to 32 weeks' gestation. Glucocorticoids increase the activities of phosphatidylcholine cytidyltransferase, cholinephosphotransferase, and possibly lysophosphatidylcholine acyltransferase and thus increase the synthesis of DPPC. Thyroid hormones, cyclic adenosine monophosphate (cAMP), prolactin, estrogen, and growth factors all have been shown to increase phospholipid synthesis by fetal lung cells. In rat, rabbit, and human fetuses, glucocorticoids and triiodothyronine (T_3) have additive or synergistic effects on phosphatidylcholine synthesis. Glucocorticoids plus cAMP analog or glucocorticoids plus theophylline (which increases cellular cAMP) are supra-additive in enhancing the rate of DPPC synthesis by fetal lung cells.

In clinical practice, the incidence of HMD in premature infants can be decreased by giving glucocorticoids to pregnant women in preterm labor. Because infants of diabetic mothers are at increased risk for HMD, studies of the effects of insulin are of interest. One study demonstrated that glucocorticoids with prolactin or insulin stimulated DPPC synthesis and surfactant secretion by human fetal lung cells better than did each hormone by itself. However, other investigators have shown that insulin antagonizes the enhancement of DPPC synthesis by glucocorticoids.[11, 13]

Protein Synthesis

Surfactant-associated proteins are synthesized in type II cells and possibly in Clara cells. Genes encoding for human SP-A, SP-B, and SP-C are located on chromosomes 10, 2, and 8, respectively. Precursor proteins are produced in the endoplasmic reticulum. Post-translational products then undergo extensive modification. The proteins are completely processed by the time they reach the lamellar bodies.[4, 12] The lipid and protein components of surfactant probably are integrated in the lamellar bodies and secreted simultaneously into the extracellular fluid subphase.[3, 10, 11]

In vitro studies of fetal lung cells demonstrate that the developmental regulation of surfactant protein synthesis is multifactorial. Low concentrations of glucocorticoids have been shown to stimulate SP-A synthesis, whereas higher concentrations are inhibitory. By contrast, glucocorticoids consistently increase SP-B and SP-C messenger ribonucleic acid (mRNA) production in a dose-dependent manner. Induction of SP-A synthesis by prostaglandin E_2 is believed to be mediated by cAMP. Analogs of cAMP and substances that increase cellular cAMP (e.g., methylxanthines, forskolin, terbutaline) increase SP-A mRNA and SP-A gene transcription. These agents have smaller, if any, effects on SP-B and SP-C synthesis. Epidermal growth factor (EGF) increases SP-A mRNA and SP-A synthesis.

The effect of insulin on SP-A synthesis is inhibitory and dose-dependent. A combination of insulin and inhibitory concentrations of glucocorticoids decreases SP-A synthesis more than does either hormone individually. In diabetic pregnancies, amniotic fluid contains significantly less SP-A than does fluid from nondiabetics. Inhibition of SP-A synthesis by insulin may contribute to the increased risk of HMD among infants of diabetic mothers. Transforming growth factor-β (TGF-B) is also an inhibitor of SP-A synthesis.[5, 14]

Secretion

The process of surfactant secretion that has been studied most extensively is the regulated release of assembled, stored surfactant from type II cells. Studies of excised lungs have shown that the phospholipid content of bronchoalveolar lavage (BAL) fluid increases when lung volume is increased. Associated decreases in lamellar body density indicate that inflation-induced increases in phospholipids result from stimulation of surfactant secretion.

Studies demonstrating that a single stretch applied to cultured type II cells results in phosphatidylcholine secretion provide further evidence that mechanical factors can stimulate surfactant secretion. Increases in cellular cAMP are known to enhance surfactant secretion, and stimulatory factors that probably act through this mechanism include β-adrenergic agents (endogenous catecholamine, isoproterenol, metaproterenol, terbutaline), methylxanthines, and adenosine compounds. Calcium ionophores, protein kinase C activators, arachidonic acid metabolites, leukotrienes, histamine, vasopressin, and intracellular alkalosis all have been shown to stimulate surfactant secretion.[14] Both baseline and stimulated surfactant secretion by type II cells are inhibited in a calcium-dependent manner by SP-A in vitro.[4, 14]

Clearance

Clearance of secreted surfactant may occur by recycling, degradation, or removal. SP-A, SP-B, SP-C, and PG stimulate the endocytotic uptake of intact, previously secreted phospholipids by type II cells. SP-A appears to be involved in the intracellular movement of these lipids to the lamellar bodies, from which they then are resecreted. Such phospholipid recycling seems to be more efficient in newborn than in adult animals. Secreted SP-A can be taken up from the fluid subphase by type II cells, but it is not clear whether it is resecreted.[4, 5, 12, 14] It appears that very little surfactant is degraded in the extracellular fluid subphase. Surfactant components can be phagocytosed by alveolar macrophages, and degradation may then occur.

Type II cells can degrade surfactant phospholipids, and radiolabeling studies have shown that these degradation products subsequently are incorporated into other lipids. Surfactant components and their degradation products have been found in very small quantities in the blood, lymph, and respiratory mucus. Radiolabeling studies have shown that some degradation products later appear in nonsurfactant lipids in the lungs or in other organs. Clearance of surfactant may be enhanced by some of the same factors that stimulate secretion, including hyperventilation and β-adrenergic agents.[14] However, SP-A enhances surfactant clearance but inhibits surfactant secretion. Thus, it has been suggested that SP-A may be an important regulator of feedback inhibition in surfactant metabolism and, as such, a prime controller of size of the surfactant pool of the extracellular fluid subphase.[4, 5, 7, 14]

Ranges of values for surfactant flux have been calculated by Wright and Clements.[3] They estimate that type II cells secrete 11% to 47% of the lamellar body surfactant pool per hour. At steady state, an equal amount of surfactant must be cleared from the alveoli. Thus, in 1 hour, 9% to 40% of the DPPC content of BAL fluid is removed from the alveoli and replaced by newly synthesized phospholipid.[3, 14]

Using radiolabeled glucose and palmitate, the half-life of DPPC initially was estimated to be 14 hours. Subsequent estimates of surfactant half-life have ranged from 17 to 90 hours and appear to vary with the phospholipid, the radiolabel, and the age and species of animal studied. Estimates of phosphatidylcholine turnover time have ranged from 3.8 to 11.1 hours and thus are more consistent with the rapid, active metabolism suggested by the surfactant flux estimates of Wright and Clements.[3, 9, 14] Pulmonary surfactant is a dynamic, continuously self-renewing system.

SURFACTANT FUNCTION

The primary function of pulmonary surfactant is to lower alveolar surface tension. As previously discussed, lowered surface tension decreases the pressure on the alveolar surface at end-expiration, when alveoli are smallest and transpulmonary pressures are lowest, and thus prevents alveolar collapse. The compliance of a lung determines the volume to which it may be expanded at a given pressure. Lowering alveolar surface tension reduces the pressure needed to inflate alveoli in accordance with the LaPlace relationship ($P = 2T/R$). Pulmonary surfactant raises compliance by lowering the pressure needed to inflate the lung to a desired volume.

The reduction of alveolar surface tension by surfactant also prevents transudation of fluid from pulmonary capillaries into the alveolar airspaces. Normally, capillary colloid oncotic pressure and intra-alveolar air pressure oppose capillary hydrostatic pressure, preventing movement of fluid into the alveoli. In the absence of surfactant, high alveolar surface tension can raise capillary hydrostatic pressure above its opposing pressures, resulting in pulmonary edema and hemorrhage. An additional function of surfactant may be a role in the defense of the lungs attributable to the ability of SP-A and possibly SP-D to bind and clear microorganisms and to stimulate alveolar macrophage activity, as already mentioned.[5, 7, 9, 11]

SURFACTANT THERAPY

Premature Infants with Hyaline Membrane Disease

In HMD, surfactant is not present in sufficient quantity to perform the functions just discussed. Surfactant deficiency results in the widespread atelectasis, poor compliance, edema, and hemorrhage that characterize the lungs of infants with HMD. The feasibility of administering surfactant to compensate for the deficiency in HMD has been of great interest to physiologists and clinicians. Initial clinical trials of exogenous artificial surfactant in human infants with HMD used aerosolized DPPC and were not successful, probably because of the poor adsorption velocity of pure DPPC that was discussed earlier. Two other exogenous artificial surfactants, a dry mixture of DPPC and PG in a 7:3 ratio and a mixture of DPPC and high-density human serum lipoprotein in a 10:1 ratio, produced inconsistent results in four clinical trials and one clinical trial, respectively, again probably as a result of adsorption rates inferior to natural surfactant.

In premature animal models of HMD, excellent therapeutic effects were demonstrated with direct tracheal instillation of natural surfactant isolated by centrifugation of BAL fluid from mature lungs. Successful clinical trials in human infants with HMD have used exogenous natural surfactant from the following sources: human amniotic fluid; bovine lung homogenates supplemented with PG or with DPPC, palmitic acid, and tripalmitoylglycerol (surfactant TA); neonatal bovine BAL fluid (calf lung surfactant extract, or CLSE, and Infasurf); and porcine lung homogenates (Curosurf). Survanta is a bovine lung-derived, reconstituted surfactant approved by the Food and Drug Administration (FDA). Efforts to develop an effective synthetic surfactant continued because of concern about possible immune sensitization of infants to foreign animal proteins present in heterologous natural surfactant. Clinical trials using a synthetic surfactant consisting of DPPC supplemented with hexadecanol and tyloxapol (Exosurf) have shown good results.[15–17] So far, only Survanta and Exosurf are approved by the FDA for clinical use in the United States (Table 130–3).

Immediate beneficial effects of surfactant therapy include improved oxygenation, lowered mean airway pressure, and improved aeration on chest radiographs. Response to treatment occurs in about 80% of infants. Causes of treatment failure include extreme prematurity, preexisting severe hypoxia, hypotension, and acidosis. Meta-analyses of the outcome differences between surfactant-treated and control infants from the reports of 35 randomized controlled trials revealed that surfactant was associated with a 30% to 40% reduction in neonatal mortality, a marked decrease in the occurrence of pneumothorax, and a decrease in the combined

TABLE 130–3. Exogenous Surfactants Currently Approved for Use in Human Infants in the United States

Surfactant	Components	Dose
Exosurf	DPPC Cetyl alcohol Tyloxapol	5 mL/kg
Survanta	Bovine lung extract DPPC Palmitic acid Tripalmitin	4 mL/kg

DPPC = dipalmitoyl phosphatidylcholine.

outcomes of bronchopulmonary dysplasia or death at 28 days. However, there were no overall decreases in the incidence of bronchopulmonary dysplasia, patent ductus arteriosus, or intracranial hemorrhage.[17, 18]

The incidence of pulmonary hemorrhage, a rare problem in premature infants, is increased by about 50% in infants who receive surfactant, and autopsy evaluations have shown extensive intra-alveolar hemorrhage to be approximately four times more common in surfactant-treated infants than in untreated control infants.[17, 19, 20] Although there had been concern that improved survival in premature infants with HMD might be associated with increased long-term morbidity, several follow-up studies have shown that surfactant treatment is associated with similar or improved late pulmonary and neurodevelopmental function in comparison with untreated controls. Serum samples from infants treated with bovine lung-derived surfactant have contained no detectable antibodies to SP-B or SP-C at 6 and 12 months of adjusted age (Table 130–4).[15–18, 21, 22]

The earliest clinical trials of exogenous surfactant involved administering it to infants in whom the diagnosis of severe HMD had already been established. Studies using this therapeutic approach have been termed *treatment* or *rescue trials*. However, animal studies showed that instillation of surfactant before the onset of ventilation resulted in better outcomes. Thus, in clinical trials, surfactant was administered in birthing areas to infants at high risk for HMD. Studies using this treatment strategy are called *prophylaxis* or *prevention trials*. In prophylaxis studies, the incidence of HMD among treated infants becomes an outcome variable. Because HMD does not actually occur in all at-risk infants, the prophylaxis approach leads to unnecessary treatment of some infants, the proportion increasing with gestational age. However, when the treatment strategy is used, HMD may be quite advanced and infants may receive significant exposure to high oxygen concentrations and ventilator trauma before surfactant is given. Because results of studies comparing prophylaxis and treatment have differed, the issue of which strategy is better remains unresolved.[17, 23–25]

The earliest studies of surfactant therapy involved single-dose treatment, but because only transient improvement often occurred, later studies usually allowed multiple doses. Trials that have compared single-dose versus multiple-dose treatments indicate lower mortality and morbidity in infants who receive multiple doses.[17, 26] However, whether retreatment should be scheduled or based on the severity of symptoms remains controversial.

Surfactant therapy for HMD usually has been administered to infants already receiving mechanical ventilation. A randomized nonblinded trial compared early initiation of nasal continuous positive airway pressure (NCPAP) alone and early NCPAP plus brief endotracheal intubation for tracheal instillation of a single dose of Curosurf in premature infants with moderate or severe HMD. Surfactant treatment was associated with a significantly higher mean ratio of arterial to alveolar oxygen tension 6 hours after randomization and lower mean incidence of subsequent mechanical ventilation.[27]

In the United States, a number of surfactant preparations were approved for open trials and thus became widely used in 1989. Exosurf was licensed for treatment of HMD in 1990, and Survanta in 1991.[15, 17] During 1990, the United States infant mortality rate decreased 6%. This was twice the annual average rate of decrease that occurred between 1980 and 1989. The large decrease in 1990 resulted from a 36% decrease in the mortality from HMD, which in turn was attributed to the widespread clinical use of surfactant therapy.[28]

A multicenter randomized trial in mechanically ventilated premature infants with HMD compared Survanta and Exosurf in 652 and 644 infants, respectively. Survanta was associated with more rapid improvement in respiratory condition. The incidence of pneumothorax was significantly higher in the group that received Exosurf. However, the combined outcomes of bronchopulmonary dysplasia (BPD) or death at 28 days of age were similar in the two treatment groups.[29]

TABLE 130–4. Clinical Outcomes of Surfactant Trials for Hyaline Membrane Disease* (Prophylaxis and Rescue; Synthetic and Natural)

Mortality	↓
Bronchopulmonary dysplasia (BPD) or death at 28 days	↓ †
Bronchopulmonary dysplasia	+/− †
Pneumothorax	↓
Patent ductus arteriosus	No effect
Intraventricular hemorrhage	No effect
SP-B, SP-C antibodies	Not found
Long-term morbidity	No effect

*Cumulative data from 35 clinical trials[17, 18] expressed in a simplified way.
†Although the combination of BPD or death at 28 days was definitely influenced by surfactant replacement, a reduction in BPD alone was not found consistently in all trials analyzed. SP = surfactant-associated protein.

Other Neonatal Respiratory Conditions

Infants with gestational ages of 34 weeks or more may be treated with extracorporeal membrane oxygenation (ECMO) for respiratory failure that is unresponsive to usual medical management. Underlying conditions that require ECMO commonly include meconium aspiration syndrome (MAS), sepsis, and persistent pulmonary hypertension of the newborn (PPHN) but, only rarely, HMD.

In one study, ECMO survivors had tracheal aspirate ratios of SP-A to total protein that increased at the same time that measurements of pulmonary compliance and aeration on chest radiographs were improving and gradual withdrawal from ECMO was being accomplished. Ratios of SP-A to total protein remained low in infants who could not be withdrawn from ECMO. The investigators speculated that ratios of tracheal aspirate SP-A to total protein reflected surfactant production in the study infants.[30]

A subsequent study demonstrated that during withdrawal from ECMO, tracheal aspirate protein concentrations decreased whereas the concentrations of SP-A, total phospholipids, and disaturated phosphatidylcholine increased. Again, it was concluded that increased surfactant production contributed to recovery from the respiratory failure that had necessitated ECMO.[31] In a blind, randomized, controlled trial of Survanta in full-term infants who had respiratory failure and were receiving ECMO, surfactant-treated infants had significantly shorter ECMO durations, better pulmonary compliance measurements, higher ratios of SP-A to total protein in tracheal aspirates, and a lower incidence of complications after ECMO.[32]

In an uncontrolled trial, multiple doses of CLSE were given to full-term newborn infants who had respiratory failure and who were not receiving ECMO. Half of the infants had underlying meconium aspiration syndrome, and half had pneumonia. Surfactant treatment was associated with improved oxygenation and lower mean airway pressures. None of the study infants died, subsequently required ECMO, developed pneumothorax, or required oxygen for longer than 2 weeks.[33]

A multicenter trial studied the effect of Survanta in 329 infants with birth weights of 2000 g or more, gestational ages ≥ 36 weeks, and respiratory failure despite mechanical ventilation with 100% oxygen as a result of MAS, sepsis, or PPHN. Within each of these three diagnostic categories, infants were randomized to receive four doses of surfactant or placebo and, if ECMO was needed, four further doses of surfactant or placebo. Infants who received surfactant were significantly less likely to require ECMO than were infants who received placebo. Mortality rates and the incidences of pulmonary, neurologic, hemorrhagic, cardiac, and infectious complications were similar in the two treatment groups.[34]

Meconium Aspiration Syndrome

Meconium aspiration syndrome occurs as a result of the aspiration of amniotic fluid that contains particulate meconium. One of the pathologic features of this syndrome is atelectasis, traditionally explained as secondary to small airway obstruction by particles of meconium. However, several experimental observations indicate that the atelectasis might instead be due to surfactant deficiency or inactivation and thus lend support to treatment of MAS with surfactant.

Classic animal experiments performed by Johnson and coworkers[35] demonstrated that when fluid was instilled and ventilated into degassed portions of the lung in vivo, later pressure-volume and surface activity studies of the excised lung showed evidence of high surface tension and low surface activity in the fluid-instilled portions. These investigators concluded that fluid in the alveoli could displace or inactivate endogenous surfactant. Later studies showed that endobronchial instillation of a filtered meconium solution caused changes in the pressure-volume relationships of excised lungs, consistent with decreased surface activity.[36]

Other investigators demonstrated increased surface tension measurements of animal lung extracts after the addition of meconium, an ether extract of meconium, or meconium free fatty acids in vitro. In vivo instillation of each of these meconium derivatives was associated with reduced oxygenation, increased mean airway pressures, and decreased pulmonary compliance measurements. Extracts from the atelectatic portions of the lungs of the experimental animals had high values when assayed for surface tension.[37]

In another study, adult rats received meconium or saline intratracheally, followed by brief mechanical ventilation, and then were allowed to breathe spontaneously for variable periods up to 72 hours. In comparison with controls that received saline, BAL fluid in the animals that received meconium showed higher alveolar cell counts and protein content at 16 hours that then progressively decreased, suggesting that meconium produced reversible exudative lung injury. BAL fluid from the meconium-instilled animals showed progressive decreases in SP-A and SP-B with a nadir at 24 hours, followed by progressive increases. These findings suggest that in addition to acute inactivation of surfactant, the lung injury produced by meconium is associated with later, reversible inhibition of surfactant protein production by type II cells.[38] An in vitro study showed that inhibition of the surface activity of CLSE by meconium solutions could be overcome by increasing CLSE concentrations.[39]

Other investigators added various meconium suspensions to Curosurf and demonstrated that meconium increased surface tension and lowered adsorption rate in a concentration-dependent manner. The degree of inhibition of surfactant function was equivalent with suspensions of meconium and its methanol-extracted, water-soluble fraction. However, similar inhibition occurred with suspensions of the chloroform-extracted meconium fraction that were 10 times more dilute, suggesting that a lipid component of meconium has the strongest inhibitory effect on surfactant function. These workers also administered filtered and nonfiltered meconium suspensions intratracheally to premature newborn rabbits and adult rats, respectively. In animals that received meconium, pulmonary compliance and blood gas pH and P_{O_2} were significantly lower, whereas blood gas P_{CO_2} and measurements of surface tension in BAL fluid were significantly higher than in control animals that did not receive meconium. Histologic examination of the lungs of animals that received meconium revealed nonuniformity of alveolar expansion with fine particles of meconium in the terminal bronchioles and alveoli of the atelectatic areas. Intratracheal administration of Curosurf (high dose or low dose) to animals that had received meconium was associated with improvements in pulmonary compliance, blood gas values, and pulmonary histology to levels similar to those in controls after high-dose Curosurf and to intermediate levels after low-dose Curosurf. After either dose of Curosurf, BAL fluid surface tension measurements in animals that had received meconium decreased to values similar to those in controls.[40–42]

Two retrospective studies of human infants with meconium aspiration syndrome found that surfactant therapy often produced immediate improvements in oxygenation.[43, 44] A prospective, randomized, controlled study of infants receiving mechanical ventilation treatment used a higher dose of Survanta (150 mg/kg) than usually is given for HMD (100 mg/kg). Treatment with Survanta or air placebo was initiated before 6 hours of age and was administered continuously over 20 minutes through a side port in the endotracheal tube adaptor. Infants could receive up to four doses of study medication. In comparison with placebo, surfactant therapy was associated with improved oxygenation that was cumulative with repeated doses, a lower incidence of air leak complications, and decreased durations of mechanical ventilation, supplemental oxygen, and hospitalization.[45]

Because the presence of meconium in the lung acts in many ways to compromise pulmonary function, the physical removal of meconium is the cornerstone of prevention and initial management of meconium aspiration syndrome. The use of pulmonary lavage with dilute surfactant solutions to accomplish both meconium removal and lowering of alveolar surface tension has shown promising results.[46, 47]

Group B Streptococcal Pneumonia

The previously discussed role of surfactant in pulmonary defense has prompted investigations of the effects of surfactant in laboratory animals with experimentally produced group B streptococcal (GBS) pneumonia. In one study, near-term newborn rabbits received either Curosurf or saline 15 minutes after intratracheal instillation of a suspension of serologic subtype Ia GBS followed by 5 hours of mechanical ventilation. GBS could be cultured from the blood of 96% of the study animals. Lungs from the surfactant-treated animals had a significantly lower number of GBS colony-forming units per gram of tissue and were significantly less likely to show inflammatory changes on histologic examination than were those from saline-treated animals.[48]

In another study, premature newborn rabbits spontaneously breathed aerosols of GBS. Animals then underwent surgical exposure of the trachea under local anesthesia and tracheal puncture for instillation of saline, one of four different surfactants, or no treatment. Four hours later, lungs from animals that had received Exosurf showed significantly fewer GBS colony-forming units than those from animals that had received no treatment, Curosurf, or human amniotic fluid–derived (HAFD) surfactant. However, 4-hour bacterial growth in Curosurf-treated or HAFD-treated animals was not significantly higher than in saline-treated or untreated controls. Comparisons between animals treated with Exosurf and those treated with Survanta, CLSE, rabbit surfactant, or saline showed no significant differences with respect to growth of GBS after 4 hours.[49]

Congenital Diaphragmatic Hernia

Studies in animal models of congenital diaphragmatic hernia (CDH) have indicated that the associated hypoplastic lungs also are compromised by surfactant deficiency. Ingestion by pregnant rats at 9 to 11.5 days' gestation of 2,4-dichlorophenyl-p-nitrophenyl (nitrofen) can produce CDH or pulmonary hypoplasia in some of the offspring. The newborn rats with CDH have significantly less total disaturated phosphatidylcholine (DSPC) in the lungs, less lung DSPC per microgram of DNA, less SP-A, and less mRNA for SP-A at 20 to 21 days' gestation in comparison with controls of the same gestational ages.[50, 51] Surgical creation of a diaphragmatic defect early in gestation in the fetal lamb results in a newborn with CDH and pulmonary hypoplasia. Pressure-volume studies of the lungs in such animals delivered at term and sacrificed before the first breath have indicated significantly lower pulmonary compliance than in litter mates without CDH. Tracheal instillation of Infasurf at delivery before the onset of breathing has been associated with significantly lower P_{CO_2} and significantly higher pH, P_{O_2}, and pulmonary compliance than in lambs with CDH that did not receive surfactant.[52]

Pulmonary Hemorrhage

A retrospective study analyzed the response of mechanically ventilated newborn infants to surfactant administered after a deterioration in respiratory condition that was associated with the appearance of blood in material obtained by tracheal suctioning. For a group of 15 such infants, surfactant therapy was followed by significant improvement in the mean oxygenation index.[53]

Early Chronic Lung Disease

A pilot study evaluated the effect of one dose of surfactant given at 9 to 30 days of age to 10 premature infants who still were receiving mechanical ventilation with 0.47 to 0.88 FIO_2 and had diffuse pulmonary haziness radiographically. Surfactant therapy was associated with significantly lower FIO_2 within 1 hour of administration and 72 hours after administration in comparison with FIO_2 at study entry.[54]

Congenital SP-B Deficiency

Inherited deficiency of SP-B can be a cause of congenital alveolar proteinosis, a rare disorder presenting with severe, progressive respiratory failure in newborn infants. Bolus therapy with SP-B–containing surfactant has not been helpful in this condition.[55, 56]

Acute Respiratory Distress Syndrome

First described in 1967, acute respiratory distress syndrome (ARDS) comprises a clinical pattern of dyspnea, tachypnea, hypoxemia despite supplemental oxygen, and poor pulmonary compliance; diffuse alveolar infiltrates on chest radiographs; and histologic findings of atelectasis, edema, hemorrhage, and hyaline membranes. ARDS was noted always to occur in association with another illness (e.g., severe trauma, pneumonia, aspiration, sepsis). Several findings in the original series of patients with ARDS were recognized as being similar to features of infants with HMD—namely, hypoxemia and acidosis before the onset of respiratory distress, low measured values for total dynamic compliance, improved oxygenation with positive end-expiratory pressure, autopsy findings of alveolar atelectasis and hyaline membranes, and high values for minimum surface tension of lung homogenates from patients. The authors of this early report speculated that ARDS was associated with loss of pulmonary surfactant.[57]

Many now believe that respiratory failure in ARDS is primarily due to pulmonary edema that is the result of increased alveolocapillary permeability. It has been proposed that complement activation leads to neutrophil aggregation. Aggregated neutrophils then generate oxygen radicals, proteases, and cytokines that cause alveolar epithelial and capillary endothelial injury.[58–60]

Studies have shown that several of the components of edema fluid are capable of inhibiting the function of pulmonary surfactant.[61, 62] It appears that protein flux across the excessively permeable alveolocapillary membrane is bidirectional because plasma concentrations of SP-B, and to a lesser extent of the larger SP-A, are elevated in patients with ARDS to values that vary directly with the severity of lung injury.[63] Comparisons of BAL fluid from patients with ARDS and controls have shown decreased quantities of PG and increased quantities of PI relative to phosphatidylcholine and decreased quantities of SP-A and SP-B relative to total protein. BAL samples from patients with ARDS demonstrate abnormally low surface activity, and measurements made on serial samples show that surface activity decreases as ARDS worsens.[59, 62]

Although the relative importance of surfactant abnormalities in the pathogenesis of ARDS still must be established, functional inactivity of surfactant probably at least contributes to the poor pulmonary compliance and atelectasis that characterize ARDS. The effect of exogenous surfactant therapy has been studied extensively in various animal models of acute lung injury. In controlled trials, exogenous surfactant has resulted in improvements in animals that have been subjected to lung lavage, bilateral cervical vagotomy, infusion of antilung serum, hyperoxia, injection of *N*-nitroso-*N*-methyl urethane, acid aspiration, viral pneumonia, or infusion of oleic acid.[59, 61] Among human patients with acute lung injury, tracheal instillation of exogenous surfactant has produced inconsistent results.

Spragg and coworkers[64] administered 4 g of Curosurf to each of six ARDS patients using a bronchoscope to instill an aliquot in each of the lobar bronchi. Treatment with Curosurf was associated with significant increases in Pa_{O_2} and in BAL phospholipid concentrations.[64] Bronchoscopic administration of natural surfactant (one to two doses of 200 to 300 mg/kg) also was used in a study of 10 patients with sepsis-induced ARDS. Surfactant therapy was associated with improvements in oxygenation and in surfactant function in samples of BAL fluid.[65]

A randomized controlled trial of Exosurf or placebo administered for 5 days by continuous aerosolization to 725 patients with sepsis-induced ARDS showed no immediate or long-term benefit of treatment with Exosurf.[66] A smaller randomized controlled trial compared a group of 16 patients with ARDS who received standard therapy only to three groups of patients with ARDS who received standard therapy plus tracheal instillation of Survanta. Eight patients received eight doses of 50 mg/kg of Survanta, 16 patients received four doses of 100 mg/kg of Survanta, and 19 patients received eight doses of 100 mg/kg of Survanta. Patients treated with four or more doses of 100 mg/kg of Survanta had significantly lower FIO_2 120 hours after beginning treatment and significantly lower mortality in comparison with control patients.[67]

ARDS has been described in pediatric patients, including full-term neonates. Approximately 1% of pediatric intensive care unit admissions are patients with ARDS, among whom the mortality rate is 50% to 60%. Reports of several small series of patients have indicated beneficial effects of surfactant therapy in pediatric ARDS, and a multicenter randomized trial is being conducted.[68–71]

SUMMARY

The understanding of surfactant physiology, function, and metabolism has been studied extensively since the 1970s. Natural surfactant derived from lungs and a synthetic surfactant have undergone extensive clinical trials in neonatal RDS. These studies have demonstrated clear effectiveness in reducing the severity of RDS, oxygen, and ventilatory requirements, and reduction of barotrauma.

Unfortunately, surfactant replacement in ARDS has not been found to be conclusively beneficial. More work needs to be done in this area. The genetic basis of surfactant deficiency and dysfunction is under extensive investigation. Surfactant protein B deficiency disease as a genetic disorder in newborn infants has been well reported as a cause of fatal RDS in several infants. Because of the phenotypic heterogeneity of the disease and multifactorial etiology, it has been difficult to pinpoint the specific gene defects in the adult RDS.

References

1. King RJ, Clements JA: Surface active materials from dog lung: II. Composition and physiological correlations. Am J Physiol 1972; 223:715.
2. King RJ: The surfactant system of the lung. Fed Proc 1974; 33:2238.
3. Wright JR, Clements JA: Metabolism and turnover of lung surfactant. Am Rev Respir Dis 1987; 135:426.
4. Weaver TE, Whitsett JA: Function and regulation of expression of pulmonary surfactant-associated proteins. Biochem J 1991; 273:249.
5. Creuwels LAJM, van Golde LMG, Haagsman HP: The pulmonary surfactant system: Biochemical and clinical aspects. Lung 1997; 175:1.
6. Hawgood S, Benson BJ, Hamilton RL Jr: Effects of a surfactant-associated protein and calcium ions on the structure and surface activity of lung surfactant lipids. Biochemistry 1985; 24:184.
7. Weaver TE: Surfactant proteins and SP-D. Am J Respir Cell Mol Biol 1991; 5:4.
8. Hawgood S, Shiffer K: Structures and properties of the surfactant-associated proteins. Annu Rev Physiol 1991; 53:375.
9. Morgan TE: Pulmonary surfactant. N Engl J Med 1971; 284:1185.
10. King RJ: Pulmonary surfactant. J Appl Physiol 1982; 53:1.
11. Harwood JL: Lung surfactant. Prog Lipid Res 1987; 26:211.
12. Haagsman HP, van Golde LMG: Synthesis and assembly of lung surfactant. Annu Rev Physiol 1991; 53:441.
13. Mendelson CR, Boggaram V: Hormonal control of the surfactant system in fetal lung. Annu Rev Physiol 1991; 53:415.
14. Wright JR, Dobbs LG: Regulation of pulmonary surfactant secretion and clearance. Annu Rev Physiol 1991; 53:395.
15. Vidyasagar D, Adeni S, Uhing MR: Surfactant replacement therapy. Perspect Crit Care 1990; 3:69.
16. Yee WFH, Scarpelli EM: Surfactant replacement therapy. Pediatr Pulmonol 1991; 11:65.
17. Jobe AH: Pulmonary surfactant therapy. N Engl J Med 1993; 328:861.
18. Soll RF, McQueen MC: Respiratory distress syndrome. *In*: Effective Care of the Newborn Infant. Sinclair JE, Bracken MB (Eds). Oxford, England, Oxford University Press, 1992, pp 327–358.
19. Raju TNK, Langenberg P: Pulmonary hemorrhage and exogenous surfactant therapy: A metaanalysis. J Pediatr 1993; 123:603.
20. Pappin A, Shenker N, Hack M, et al: Extensive intraalveolar pulmonary hemorrhage in infants dying after surfactant therapy. J Pediatr 1994; 124:621.
21. Ferrara TB, Hoekstra RE, Couser RJ, et al: Survival and follow-up of infants born at 23 to 26 weeks' of gestational age: Effects of surfactant therapy. J Pediatr 1994; 124:119.
22. Survanta Multidose Study Group: Two-year follow-up of infants treated for neonatal respiratory distress syndrome with bovine surfactant. J Pediatr 1994; 124:962.
23. Kattwinkel J, Bloom BT, Delmore P, et al: Prophylactic administration of calf lung surfactant extract is more effective than early treatment of respiratory distress syndrome in neonates of 29 through 32 weeks' gestation. Pediatrics 1993; 92:90.
24. Dunn MS: Surfactant replacement therapy: Prophylaxis or treatment? Pediatrics 1993; 92:148.
25. Egberts J, de Winter P, Sedin G, et al: Comparison of prophylaxis and rescue treatment with Curosurf in neonates less than 30 weeks' gestation: A randomized trial. Pediatrics 1993; 92:768.
26. Corbet A, Gerdes J, Long W, et al: Double-blind, randomized trial of one versus three prophylactic doses of synthetic surfactant in 826 neonates weighing 700 to 1100 grams: Effects on mortality rate. J Pediatr 1995; 126:969.
27. Verder H, Robertson B, Greison G, et al: Surfactant therapy and nasal continuous positive airway pressure for newborns with respiratory distress syndrome. N Engl J Med 1994; 331:1051.
28. Centers for Disease Control: Infant mortality: United States, 1990. MMWR Morb Mortal Wkly Rep 1993; 42:161.
29. Vermont-Oxford Neonatal Network: A multicenter, randomized trial comparing synthetic surfactant with modified bovine surfactant extract in the treatment of neonatal respiratory distress syndrome. Pediatrics 1996; 97:1.
30. Lotze A, Whitsett JA, Kammerman LA, et al: Surfactant protein A concentrations in tracheal aspirate fluid from infants requiring extracorporeal membrane oxygenation. J Pediatr 1990; 116:435.
31. Bui KC, Walther FJ, David-Cu R, et al: Phospholipid and surfactant protein A concentrations in tracheal aspirates from infants requiring extracorporeal membrane oxygenation. J Pediatr 1992; 121:271.
32. Lotze A, Knight GR, Martin GR, et al: Improved pulmonary outcome after exogenous surfactant therapy for respiratory failure in term infants requiring extracorporeal membrane oxygenation. J Pediatr 1993; 122:261.
33. Auten RL, Notter RH, Kendig JW, et al: Surfactant treatment of full-term newborns with respiratory failure. Pediatrics 1991; 87:101.
34. Lotze A, Mitchell BR, Bulas DI, et al: Multicenter trial of surfactant (beractant) use in the treatment of term infants with severe respiratory failure. J Pediatr 1998; 132:40.
35. Johnson JWC, Permutt S, Sipple JH, et al: Effect of intra-alveolar fluid on pulmonary surface tension properties. J Appl Physiol 1964; 19:769.
36. Chen CT, Toung TJK, Rogers MC: Effect of intra-alveolar meconium on pulmonary surface tension properties. Crit Care Med 1985; 13:233.
37. Clark DA, Nieman GF, Thompson JE, et al: Surfactant displacement by meconium free fatty acids: An alternative explanation for atelectasis in meconium aspiration syndrome. J Pediatr 1987; 110:765.
38. Cleary GM, Antunes MJ, Ciesielka DA, et al: Exudative lung injury is associated with decreased levels of surfactant proteins in a rat model of meconium aspiration. Pediatrics 1997; 100:998.
39. Moses D, Holm BA, Spitale P, et al: Inhibition of pulmonary surfactant function by meconium. Am J Obstet Gynecol 1991; 164:477.
40. Sun B, Curstedt T, Robertson B: Surfactant inhibition in experimental meconium aspiration. Acta Paediatr 1993; 82:182.
41. Sun B, Curstedt T, Song G-W, et al: Surfactant improves lung function and morphology in newborn rabbits with meconium aspiration. Biol Neonate 1993; 63:96.
42. Sun B, Herting E, Curstedt T, et al: Exogenous surfactant improves lung compliance and oxygenation in adult rats with meconium aspiration. J Appl Physiol 1994; 77:1961.
43. Khammash H, Perlman M, Wojtulewicz J, et al: Surfactant therapy in full-term neonates with severe respiratory failure. Pediatrics 1993; 92:135.
44. Halliday HL, Speer CP, Robertson B: Treatment of severe meconium aspiration syndrome with porcine surfactant. Eur J Pediatr 1996; 155:1047.
45. Findlay RD, Taeusch HW, Walther FJ: Surfactant replacement therapy for meconium aspiration syndrome. Pediatrics 1996; 97:48.
46. Paranka MS, Walsh WF, Stancombe BB: Surfactant lavage in a piglet model of meconium aspiration syndrome. Pediatr Res 1992; 31:625.

47. Revak SD, Cochrane CG, Merritt TA: The therapeutic effect of bronchoalveolar lavage with KL_4-surfactant in animal models of meconium aspiration syndrome (Abstract). Pediatr Res 1997; 41:265A.
48. Herting E, Jarstrand C, Rasool O, et al: Experimental neonatal group B streptococcal pneumonia: Effect of a modified porcine surfactant on bacterial proliferation in ventilated near-term rabbits. Pediatr Res 1994; 36:784.
49. Sherman MP, Campbell LA, Merritt TA, et al: Effect of different surfactants on pulmonary group B streptococcal infections in premature rabbits. J Pediatr 1994; 125:939.
50. Suen H-C, Catlin EA, Ryan DP, et al: Biochemical immaturity of lungs in congenital diaphragmatic hernia. J Pediatr Surg 1993; 28:471.
51. Mysore MR, Margraf LR, Jaramillo MA, et al: Surfactant protein A is decreased in a rat model of congenital diaphragmatic hernia. Am J Respir Crit Care Med 1998; 157:654.
52. Wilcox DI, Glick PL, Karamanoukian H, et al: Pathophysiology of congenital diaphragmatic hernia: V. Effect of exogenous surfactant therapy on gas exchange and lung mechanics in the lamb congenital diaphragmatic hernia model. J Pediatr 1994; 124:289.
53. Pandit PB, Dunn MS, Colucci EA: Surfactant therapy in neonates with respiratory deterioration due to pulmonary hemorrhage. Pediatrics 1995; 95:32.
54. Pandit PB, Dunn MS, Kelly EN, et al: Surfactant replacement in neonates with early chronic lung disease. Pediatrics 1995; 95:851.
55. Hamvas A, Nogee LM, deMello DE, et al: Pathophysiology and treatment of surfactant protein-B deficiency. Biol Neonate 1995; 67(Suppl 1):18.
56. Robertson B: New targets for surfactant replacement therapy: Experimental and clinical aspects. Arch Dis Child 1996; 75:F1.
57. Ashbaugh DG, Bigelow DB, Petty TL, et al: Acute respiratory distress in adults. Lancet 1967; 2:319.
58. Rinaldo JE, Rogers RM: Adult respiratory-distress syndrome. N Engl J Med 1982; 306:900.
59. Lewis JF, Jobe AH: Surfactant and the adult respiratory distress syndrome. Am Rev Respir Dis 1993; 147:218.
60. Fulkerson WJ, MacIntyre N, Stamler J, et al: Pathogenesis and treatment of the adult respiratory distress syndrome. Arch Intern Med 1996; 156:29.
61. Holm BA, Notter RH: Surfactant therapy in adult respiratory distress syndrome and lung injury. *In*: Surfactant Replacement Therapy. Shapiro DL, Notter RH (Eds). New York, Alan R Liss, 1989, pp 273–304.
62. Jobe AH, Ikegami M: Surfactant for acute respiratory distress syndrome. Adv Intern Med 1997; 42:203.
63. Doyle IR, Bersten AD, Nicholas T: Surfactant proteins -A and -B are elevated in plasma of patients with acute respiratory failure. Am J Respir Crit Care Med 1997; 156:1217.
64. Spragg RG, Gilliard N, Richman P, et al: Acute effects of a single dose of porcine surfactant on patients with the adult respiratory distress syndrome. Chest 1994; 105:195.
65. Walmrath D, Günther A, Ghofrani HA, et al: Bronchoscopic surfactant administration in patients with severe adult respiratory distress syndrome and sepsis. Am J Respir Crit Care Med 1996; 154:57.
66. Anzueto A, Baughman RP, Guntupalli KK: Aerosolized surfactant in adults with sepsis-induced acute respiratory distress syndrome. N Engl J Med 1996; 334:1417.
67. Gregory TJ, Steinberg KP, Spragg R, et al: Bovine surfactant therapy for patients with acute respiratory distress syndrome. Am J Respir Crit Care Med 1997; 155:1309.
68. Faix RG, Viscandi RM, DiPietro MA, et al: Adult respiratory distress syndrome in full-term newborns. Pediatrics 1989; 83:971.
69. Pfenninger J, Tschaeppeler H, Wagner BP, et al: The paradox of adult respiratory distress syndrome in neonates. Pediatr Pulmonol 1991; 10:18.
70. Paulson TE, Spear RM, Peterson BM: New concepts in the treatment of children with acute respiratory distress syndrome. J Pediatr 1995; 127:163.
71. Evans DA, Wilmott RW, Whitsett JA: Surfactant replacement therapy for adult respiratory distress syndrome in children. Pediatr Pulmonol 1996; 21:328.

131

Pulmonary Aspiration

Philip G. Boysen, MD • Jerome Modell, MD

Aspiration of gastric contents into the tracheobronchial tree, including foodstuffs and acidic fluids, can cause acute structural damage extending to the pulmonary parenchyma and producing pulmonary edema and gas exchange abnormalities. Although all obtunded patients may be at risk for aspiration, including patients who overdose on drugs or alcohol, it is a complication most often associated with the perioperative period and is especially problematic with emergency surgical procedures.[1] To ensure gastric emptying the patient undergoing an elective surgical procedure is instructed to fast (nil per os, NPO, or nothing by mouth) after midnight. In the pediatric age group, this practice has been questioned, and current recommendations allow clear fluids to be ingested until 2 hours before surgery.[2] Children are prone to aspirate many solid objects, which must be retrieved by endoscopic procedures, and to swallow various toxic substances, such as kerosene and other petroleum products.[3] Drowning and near drowning remain endemic problems, especially in children.[4]

Emergency surgical procedures must often proceed even when a patient is believed to have a "full stomach." Regional anesthetic techniques are employed whenever possible, and gastric aspiration usually can be avoided as long as the patient is conscious and mental status and upper airway function are not altered by oversedation. The approach to these patients is complicated when general anesthesia is required. In these cases, if the airway must be secured it may be necessary to perform awake intubation of the trachea or rapid-sequence induction. The recent introduction of the laryngeal mask airway is a great advance in the management of the difficult airway, but there are concerns about the incidence and magnitude of aspirations of gastric contents, and the clinical outcome when a laryngeal mask airway is used.[5,6]

The parturient is also at increased risk for gastric aspiration because of physiologic changes during pregnancy, increased volume and acidity of gastric contents, the timing and onset of labor, and the potential for difficult management of the airway.[7]

PATHOLOGY

Acidic liquid is the main cause of severe pulmonary injury after aspiration of stomach contents.[8-13] Although clear liquid aspirates with a pH greater than 2.5 can be essentially innocuous in small quantities, however, even nonacidic aspirates, particularly those containing foodstuffs, can produce severe pulmonary insufficiency.[9,14]

Most experimental work in this area has been performed with aspirates having a pH of 1.0 to 2.5. After aspiration, acid rapidly spreads throughout the lungs and produces diffuse damage that is characterized by epithelial degeneration of the bronchi, pulmonary edema, hemorrhage, isolated areas of atelectasis, necrosis of type I alveolar cells, and the presence of free laminated inclusion bodies in the pulmonary transudate.[15] Within 4 hours, acute infiltration by polymorphonuclear cells and fibrin can be seen in the alveolar space. Degeneration of type II alveolar cells and further necrosis of type I cells with detachment from the basement membrane have also been noted. Within the next 24 to 36 hours, alveolar consolidation is seen, and some of the airways show mucosal sloughing. After 48 hours, hyaline membranes appear.[15] The lung appears boggy, edematous, and hemorrhagic on gross examination. By 72 hours, resolution has begun, with regeneration of bronchial epithelium, proliferation of fibroblasts, and a decrease in acute inflammation.[16]

When clear liquids with a pH greater than 2.5 are aspirated, pulmonary edema, diapedesis of erythrocytes, separation of endothelial cells from basement membranes, and peribronchial neutrophil infiltration may occur. Compared with the aspiration of very acidic liquid, however, aspiration of nonacidic liquids causes little necrosis of alveolar cells and minimal neutrophilic infiltration. Also, the duration of injury is significantly shorter when the patient survives the acute hypoxia caused by the initial aspiration.[17]

Correlation of laboratory and clinical data after aspiration of liquids with differing pH and volume of gastric contents has been the subject of investigation.[18] Although increasing volume and decreasing pH may be problematic and associated with the degree of pulmonary damage, critical values for each variable are not easily determined. Particularly for children, methods to reduce the risk of aspiration have come into question. Having a child fast for a long time to achieve gastric emptying is not always efficacious and may itself lead to intravascular volume depletion and other problems. Similar untoward effects may occur in adult patients. For trauma patients there is usually little time to manage such problems. Thus, as an index of increased severity of parenchymal lung damage after acid aspiration it is generally agreed that the more acidic the aspirate fluid and the greater its volume, the greater the lung damage will be. This implies that morbidity and mortality after aspiration can be similarly related. Administration of a variety of agents has been suggested as a way to alter both gastric pH and gastric volume.[19]

Experimental acid aspiration of variable volumes of liquid with a pH of 1.0 has been studied in primates.[20] Aspiration of 0.4 to 0.6 mL/kg produced mild to moderate clinical and chest radiographic changes, but not death. Aspiration of volumes greater than 0.8 mL/kg produced increasingly severe pneumonitis, and 50% of the monkeys succumbed. Extrapolation of these values to adult humans approximates the critical aspirated volume of 50 mL at a pH 1.0. Although this analysis of severity in relation to the volume and acidity of gastric aspirate might considerably reduce the number of patients thought to be at risk, pH values of less than 2.5 and volumes greater than 25 mL have been promulgated by some to be indicators of severe lung damage and a protracted clinical course.[21]

Large particulate aspirates obstruct major airways. Aspiration of neutral stomach contents containing small, nonobstructing food particles can produce a prolonged inflammatory response similar to that caused by acid.[9, 22] Within 6 hours of aspiration, extensive hemorrhagic pneumonia may occur, with erythrocytes, granulocytes, and macrophages invading the alveoli and bronchi. A widespread granulomatous reaction with numerous macrophages and giant cells is present within 48 hours, and edema and infiltrating mononuclear cells thicken the alveolar walls. Obstruction of airways by small food particles does not appear to cause the reaction described above, although obstructive bronchiolitis is caused by inflammatory exudate. Within 5 days, focal areas resembling hard granulomas are present in large numbers; food particles can be identified at the center of many of these granulomas. In some cases, the smaller pulmonary vessels are occluded and have adjacent areas of hemorrhagic infarction.[7]

PHYSIOLOGY

Although any aspirated fluid can obstruct the airway and interfere with normal ventilation-perfusion patterns, the chemical burn induced by acid aspiration appears to be the most severe problem. It causes a loss of alveolocapillary integrity and exudation of fluid and protein into the interstitial spaces, the alveoli, and the bronchi.[15] The exudation causes pulmonary edema, a decrease in pulmonary compliance, an increase in lung weight, and significant intrapulmonary shunting or venous admixture.[15, 23, 24] Sufficient fluid may be lost from the circulation as pulmonary edema fluid to deplete intravascular volume and cause hypotension.[15, 23, 25]

Perhaps the most immediate and severe physiologic problem is the hypoxemia that occurs within minutes of acid aspiration.[11, 15, 16, 23, 25, 26] This hypoxemia most likely is secondary to several events:

- Reflex airway closure in response to the aspiration of fluid[24, 27, 28]
- Destruction or alteration of normal pulmonary surfactant activity[11, 28]
- Migration of fluid and protein into the damaged tissues, which causes interstitial edema and thus further pulmonary embarrassment

Even after the acute lesion has subsided, the exudate may remain in the form of hyaline membranes.

The aspiration of acid also affects the pulmonary vasculature and can cause pulmonary hypertension. Pulmonary vascular resistance (PVR) increases,[15, 29, 30] and marked constriction of pulmonary arterioles has been demonstrated arteriographically[31] and histologically after aspiration.[26] When pulmonary artery pressure is not elevated, the cause may be low intravascular volume or low cardiac output, or both.[32]

The change in PVR can be attributed to several factors. Hypoxemia, an intense stimulus to the pulmonary vascular tree, results in vasoconstriction. This is referred to as *hypoxic pulmonary vasoconstriction.* Immediately after aspiration, when gastric contents flow into the pharynx, trachea, and lung, prolonged apnea may occur. Not only does this aspiration aggravate the hypoxemia, but the resultant hypercarbia and acidosis increase the stimulus to the pulmonary vasculature and, as a result, also cause vasospasm. Accumulation of extravascular lung water results in a loss of lung volume, regardless of whether alveolar fluid accumulates. Such a lung not only is stiff and noncompliant but also exhibits lower alveolar gas volume and functional residual capacity. The end result is compression of the pulmonary microvasculature secondary to mechanical forces and hypoxic pulmonary vasoconstriction, resulting in an increase in PVR. If atelectatic, edematous areas can be reexpanded to reclaim lung volume and the PVR may return toward normal. Similarly, overexpansion of the lungs causes pressure (transmitted alveolar pressure) on the pulmonary microvasculature, which elevates PVR (see Treatment later). This indicates the strong relationship between lung volume and PVR.[20]

If PVR is elevated for any reason, hemodynamic consequences are usually immediate and severe. The right ventricle, which operates against a low impedance or pressure under normal conditions, can maintain ejection of a significant volume in order to match left ventricular output. Acute elevations in PVR overload the right ventricle, a heart chamber ill equipped to handle such changes, and may precipitate right ventricular dilatation, a decrease in right ventricular ejection fraction, and right ventricular failure (acute cor pulmonale).

If clear liquid with a pH greater than 2.5 is aspirated, the resultant lesion will not be as severe as if a highly acidic liquid had been aspirated. Reflex airway closure,[28] pulmonary edema, and changes in the surface tension characteristics of pulmonary surfactant, however, still may occur in the lungs.[33]

In summary, aspiration of significant amounts of stomach contents into the lung causes acute respiratory insufficiency, regardless of the nature of the aspirate. If the aspirate is small in volume, has a pH greater than 2.5, is free of particulate matter, and has normal tonicity, recovery may be rapid.[34] If the fluid has a pH less than 2.5, is hypertonic, or contains food particles or irritating liquid food, the inflammatory response may be prolonged. The reaction is primarily hemorrhagic, granulocytic, and narcotizing when the aspirate is acid; it is mononuclear and granulomatous when the aspirate contains food. The nature, volume, and distribution of the aspirate are all important in determining the degree of respiratory embarrassment. Although, volume for volume, acidic aspirates cause the most damage, aspiration of any material from the stomach, even of neutral pH, can be life-threatening.

DIAGNOSIS

The pathophysiology just described (i.e., hypoxemia, accumulation of perivascular, peribronchial, and alveolar lung water, loss of lung volume, and patchy or diffuse changes on the chest radiograph) is not specific for aspiration syndromes. The spectrum of changes in pulmonary function and gas exchange, commonly referred to as the *acute respiratory distress syndrome* (ARDS), can be the end result of a variety of pulmonary insults. Thus, the changes are nonspecific; the diagnosis of aspiration pneumonitis is inferred from the nature and timing of clinical events; and the clinical outcome is not necessarily obvious, making further monitoring of the patient necessary.

In a study of 172,334 consecutive patients (undergoing 215,488 anesthetics), 67 patients were identified who had bilious secretions in the tracheobronchial tree or a postoperative infiltrate not present on a preoperative chest radiograph. Fifteen of the 67 patients underwent emergency surgery, and the remaining 52 patients underwent elective procedures. In 42 of the 66 patients who survived the operation (64%), no coughing or wheezing was observed, the arterial oxygen saturation did not fall by more than 9%, and no infiltrate was seen on chest films within the first 2 hours when the question of aspiration was raised. These patients had no respiratory sequelae. Of the remaining 24 patients, 13 received mechanical ventilation for at least 6 hours; three of six patients who received ventilation longer than 24 hours died. When the index of suspicion is raised and the diagnosis is considered, intensive and careful monitoring, examination, and observation of pulmonary function for at least 2 hours are indicated.[35] Although markers to indicate aspiration of gastric contents into the lungs have not consistently been found to be useful, a recent study documented increased peptic activity in bronchoalveolar fluid within 2 hours of experimental acid aspiration syndrome.[36]

THERAPY

Prophylaxis

In many cases, aspiration of stomach contents can be avoided. The risk of aspiration in unconscious patients may be reduced by careful observation and by positioning the patient in a semiprone position with the head down. Emergency surgery perhaps carries the greatest risk. The incidence of aspiration in this setting can be reduced by the use of regional anesthesia when appropriate or by awake endotracheal intubation before induction of general anesthesia. If awake intubation is not possible, rapid-sequence induction of anesthesia with simultaneous application of cricoid pressure and intubation of the trachea with a cuffed endotracheal tube is appropriate to protect the patient's airway. Before the cuff is deflated and the endotracheal tube is removed, the patient should be awake and have normal laryngeal reflexes to protect the airway.

Cricoid pressure must be uniformly applied, to prevent regurgitation and aspiration. One study indicated that 20 newtons (N) of applied force would be adequate for an awake patient but 40 N must be applied to an unconscious patient.[37] Learning the technique and correct pressure manipulation can be enhanced with the use of teaching models. Cricoid pressure decreases lower esophageal sphincter tone, making correct application even more important.[38]

When sufficient time is available to prepare a patient for anesthesia and surgery, other therapeutic interventions may be of benefit, and concepts are changing. Although implementation of a fasting (NPO) regimen has been a long-standing practice before the administration of an anesthetic agent, it may not reduce the volume of gastric contents. Administration of clear fluids may be beneficial rather than harmful. Liberal intake of clear fluids in the 6 hours before surgery results in residual gastric volume that is similar to that after 6 hours of fasting (21 mL and 19 mL, respectively; confidence interval [CI] = −5 to +9).[39] Additionally, the pH of gastric fluid was reported to be higher in those allowed to consume fluids than in a control group of fasting subjects (2.64, as compared with 2.26; CI = −2.5 to +0.8).[39] As might be expected, patients receiving clear fluids had a lower incidence of preoperative thirst and less tendency toward dehydration. Apple juice has been used in clinical studies as the preferred clear liquid to administer to patients before surgery.[40, 41]

A variety of drugs have been studied and recommended as being efficacious in altering residual gastric volume and pH.[42–44] This includes (1) the histamine H_2 receptor antagonists (e.g., cimetidine and ranitidine), particulate and nonparticulate antacids, cholinergic receptor agonists (e.g., metoclopramide), and (2) proton pump inhibitors (e.g., omeprazole). Ranitidine is also available as an oral liquid that can be given to children.

The goal of histamine H_2 receptor therapy is to reduce gastric volume and pH. Metoclopramide facilitates gastric emptying and has a central antiemetic effect. To achieve synergism, one should give these drugs together. Their peak effect is realized between 2 and 4 hours after administration.[40] A newer histamine H_2 receptor–blocking agent, roxatidine, has a longer duration of action; a single, oral bedtime dose has an effect for 8 to 12 hours.[45] Famotidine has similarly been recommended for children.[46] When ranitidine and metoclopramide are given to adults who are given clear fluids up until 2 hours before surgery, these adults remain at low risk for aspiration.[47]

Proton pump inhibitors prevent secretion of hydrogen ions into the stomach and thus lessen gastric acidity and raise pH. For a group of pregnant women about to undergo cesarean section, a single oral dose of 80 mg of omiprazole resulted in a pH greater than 2.5 and residual gastric volume less than 50 mL in 80% of patients.[48]

The preoperative use of oral particulate antacids to reduce gastric acidity has often been recommended,[8, 49–52] although this practice has not been proven to reduce morbidity or mortality. Furthermore, if the antacid itself is aspirated, a severe persistent pulmonary lesion develops; microscopic evidence of the antacid compound can be seen in the lungs for several weeks after aspiration.[53] Orally administering either two antacid tablets (e.g., Alka-Seltzer) in 30 mL of water or a 0.3-mol/L sodium citrate solution, 30 mL, both of which are nonparticulate, also effectively buffers stomach acid without risking severe pulmonary insufficiency if the solution is aspirated.[54, 55]

Because cimetidine or ranitidine, or both, decrease the volume of gastric fluid and increase gastric pH, preoperative use of these compounds might be worthwhile for patients at risk[55, 56]; however, combination dosing of these agents has not uniformly proved superior, even though different modes of action would seem to recommend combined therapy. Intravenous ranitidine, 50 mg 30 minutes before induction, or oral doses of 150 mg twice a day, for ambulatory patients, have been suggested as monotherapy.[57, 58] Combining omeprazole with a prokinetic, such as metoclopramide,[59] or adding sodium citrate to a similar regimen[60] has been suggested for combination therapy; although a study reemphasized that, for pregnant patients, sodium citrate alone is the most efficacious therapy.[61] Therefore, a reasonable approach would be to administer oral sodium citrate to pregnant patients and combination therapy to other high-risk patients (H_2 antagonist, prokinetic agent, sodium citrate).

Finally, the nasogastric tube poses an additional risk to the patient during mechanical ventilation and tracheal intubation, presumably because the tube acts as a wicking device to move gastric contents into the oropharynx, increasing the potential for aspiration.[60] In fact, gastroesophageal reflux in patients ventilated with a nasogastric tube is common and cannot be prevented or altered by changes in body position.[62, 63]

Endotracheal Suctioning

When aspiration has occurred, the trachea should be suctioned if possible. This measure stimulates coughing, may remove some of the aspirated material, and may aid in confirming the diagnosis. Because liquid and small particulate aspirates disperse rapidly and damage the lung almost instantaneously, suctioning can remove only a portion of the aspirate and, therefore, is only the first step in therapy.

Mechanical Ventilatory Support

Severe intrapulmonary shunting causes significant venous admixture and arterial hypoxemia that must be treated immediately. Positive-pressure ventilation with positive end-expiratory pressure (PEEP) or the administration of continuous positive airway pressure (CPAP) reduces the shunt and increases the arterial oxygen tension. It also increases the rate of survival after acid aspiration. If the patient is alert and further aspiration is not a risk,[23, 31, 64–67] CPAP applied by mask may reinflate alveoli, increase functional residual capacity, and decrease the intrapulmonary shunt. If the patient is obtunded, cannot maintain a patent airway, is at risk of further aspiration, or requires mechanical breaths to remove carbon dioxide, intubation of the trachea with a high-volume, low-pressure cuffed endotracheal tube is essential. Optimal CPAP minimizes the intrapulmonary venous admixture without compromising the circulation.[68]

The concept of optimal PEEP or CPAP has been elusive because of the combined and variable effects of PEEP on pulmonary and cardiac physiology. PEEP is meant to increase lung volumes, diminish shunt, and improve oxygenation. Cardiac output must be preserved to maintain oxygen delivery. As PEEP or CPAP is increased, the resultant increase in lung volume decreases PVR as functional residual capacity returns toward normal and as oxygenation and gas exchange improve. This has the effect of decreasing impedance on the right ventricle, which improves right ventricular performance. If PEEP or CPAP results in lung hyperinflation, PVR will again increase, but by another mechanism. In this case, lung overdistention has resulted in the mechanical transmission of alveolar pressures to the pulmonary vasculature. The end result includes right ventricular dilatation, decreased right ventricular ejection fraction, and eventual impingement of left ventricular geometry due to shift of the intraventricular septum.

Further complicating therapeutic assessment is the observation that excessively high peak airway pressure may cause parenchymal lung[69, 70] damage that can persist and, thus, prolong supportive therapy.[79, 80] For this reason, mean airway pressure has been monitored as an indication of the simultaneous effect on lung inflation and alteration of hemodynamic function. Increasing inflation times to the point of reversing the normal inspiratory-expiratory ratio has been recommended as a means of increasing mean airway pressure and of avoiding high peak airway pressure while minimizing the end-expiratory pressure necessary to improve oxygenation. The patient with severe ARDS due to gastric aspiration may be included in the group recommended for low-frequency positive-pressure ventilation (with a small tidal volume) and simultaneous extracorporeal removal of carbon dioxide by venovenous bypass.[71] Under such conditions, one can maintain oxygenation by using a low level of PEEP and by performing simultaneous tracheal insufflation of oxygen. Low-frequency ventilation (24 breaths/min) with small tidal volume avoids high peak airway pressure, which is thought to be deleterious to lung healing.

To avoid hypercapnia, extracorporeal carbon dioxide removal is accomplished by venovenous bypass. Although good conceptual and theoretical data support these concepts, improved outcome has yet to be demonstrated with their use. In an experimental study of severe acid aspiration in rabbits, conventional mechanical ventilation with PEEP was compared with inverse-ratio ventilation.[72] No difference in morbidity or mortality could be demonstrated.

Bronchoscopy and Lavage

If aspiration of large particulate matter is suspected, especially if clinical and radiographic signs of localized lung volume loss are present, bronchoscopy should be performed. For a patient in severe respiratory distress after aspiration of stomach contents, bronchoscopy is a formidable and hazardous procedure. Some physicians have advocated pulmonary lavage with neutral or alkaline solutions to neutralize acid, but damage to the lung by acid is almost instantaneous and lavage is not useful unless particulate aspiration has been observed or is strongly suspected.[27] When bronchoscopy is performed, only small amounts of saline should be used to clear the airway of secretions or aspirated material. Large-volume lavage can actually compromise pulmonary function further.

Corticosteroids

Theoretically, steroid administration should decrease inflammation, stabilize liposomal membranes,[73, 74] prevent platelet and leukocyte agglutination,[75] and improve peripheral release of oxygen from erythrocytes by shifting the oxyhemoglobin dissociation curve.[76] However, no conclusive clinical or experimental data document that steroids are beneficial for patients with aspiration pneumonitis.[34] In fact, steroids administered after aspiration of food particles may interfere with normal healing.[14] For this reason, their use is not recommended.

Antibiotics

Infection in the patient who has aspirated is often difficult to document. Fever, leukocytosis, the presence of pulmonary infiltrates, and production of thick, tenacious sputum are nonspecific responses to uncomplicated chemical pneumonitis. Cultures of sputum may be misleading because samples can be contaminated by oropharyngeal flora. In general, patients with lung abscess, empyema, and pneumonia after aspiration are more likely to have organisms that reflect the oropharyngeal flora, especially anaerobic bacteria.[77, 78]

Patients with severe respiratory failure who require ventilatory support frequently harbor aerobic bacteria such as *Staph-*

ylococcus and *Pseudomonas* species.[79, 80] The effectiveness of prophylactic antibiotics is questionable: they may lead to superinfections with resistant organisms. Antibiotics should be withheld until clinical evidence of infection can be produced. Treatment can then be based on analysis of well-controlled smear and culture specimens.

Particular attention has been paid to those patients who aspirate gastric contents while in the hospital, especially to critically ill patients in intensive care units.[81] In hospitalized patients, pharyngeal colonization by gram-negative rods, which are often resistant to antibacterial therapy, develops. The bacterial flora also change during hospitalization, particularly in critically ill patients and especially in those with immune dysfunction. A gastropulmonary route of infection is thus postulated. Elevation of gastric pH during ulcer prophylaxis creates a tendency toward gastric bacterial colonization. Thus, in some patients, the stomach is a bacterial reservoir independent of changes in the oropharynx. The potential for reflux and aspiration increases the risk of parenchymal damage and the potential for superinfection.[45] In intubated intensive care patients, the risk of aspiration is increased owing to gastroduodenal reflux and regurgitation of gastric contents. Instead of gastric alkalization for prolonged periods, administration of cytoprotective anti-ulcer medication (e.g., sucralfate) may prevent infection. Acquisition of adequate culture information remains the best means of choosing appropriate antibiotic therapy when aspiration pneumonitis occurs.[77]

Intravascular Fluids Therapy

Intravascular volume lost through pulmonary edema must be restored. Furthermore, if high PEEP or CPAP is necessary, particularly combined with mechanical ventilatory breaths, venous return may decrease. This accentuates the physiologic effects of hypovolemia, and cardiac output may decrease markedly, in turn decreasing oxygen delivery. The current approach is administration of crystalloids to maintain organ perfusion as judged by clinical examination and urine output. An indwelling arterial catheter provides continuous monitoring of blood pressure and access for arterial blood specimens. Cardiac output can be monitored intermittently or continuously with pulmonary artery catheters to identify when resuscitation measures have reversed a low-flow state, if this is not evident from less invasive monitoring techniques. Similarly, mixed venous oxygen saturation can be monitored continuously, and paired with noninvasive monitoring of arterial oxygen saturation, as an index of oxygen demand versus delivery. Because pulmonary artery occlusion pressure may be artifactually elevated by the administration of PEEP, transesophageal echocardiography may be indicated to evaluate ventricular filling and contractility.

Other Therapies

Other forms of therapy have not been established as useful methods of alleviating or modifying the course of pathophysiologic changes. An experimental porcine study investigated the effect of instillation of perflubron into the airways. ARDS was induced in piglets by instilling a homogenate of gastric contents, then the piglets were randomized into a control group and a therapeutic group (perflubron instillation at 60 minutes), and given continued therapy to maintain intravascular volume. A difference in oxygenation between the two groups appeared between 2½ and 6 hours, suggesting a therapeutic window before the acute inflammatory process is manifested.[82] Although promising, the therapy remains experimental at the present time.

Chronic Aspiration Syndromes

A subset of patients not originally admitted for pulmonary aspiration syndromes, including patients undergoing mechanical ventilation, elderly patients, and patients with deglutition abnormalities, suffer from repetitive aspiration, which can lead to ongoing lung damage, infection, and sepsis. Just as in the acute syndromes, the material aspirated into the tracheobronchial tree primarily includes

- Oropharyngeal bacterial pathogens
- Inert fluids or particulate matter (e.g., foodstuffs or antacid)
- Acidic gastric contents

Patients at risk for pulmonary aspiration can be divided into those with (1) depressed sensorium, (2) neuromuscular discoordination, or (3) structural disorders of the aerodigestive system (Table 131-1)[83]. Sequelae from episodic or repetitive pulmonary aspiration thus run the gamut from acute to subacute to chronic syndromes.

Using sensitive tracer techniques with technetium 99m, Gleeson and colleagues[84] documented pulmonary aspiration of oropharyngeal contents in 10 apparently normal volunteers subjected to polysomnographic recording during a full night of sleep. The estimated quantity of the aspirate was deemed significant (0.01 to 0.2 mL) and likely to contain bacterial organisms. Although common, aspiration was not related to sleep quality or structure and had no apparent untoward consequences.

The incidence and outcome of chronic occult aspiration become more important with age. There is a direct relationship in the older age group with the high incidence of community-acquired pneumonia.[85] In the presence of documented neurologic disorders such as basal ganglia infarction the risk of pneumonia increases.[86] A separate syndrome of diffuse aspiration bronchiolitis due to chronic occult aspiration in the elderly has also been described.[87] In hospital or extended care

TABLE 131–1. Etiologic Factors in Pulmonary Aspiration Syndromes

Depressed Sensorium	Neuromuscular Discoordination	Structural Disorders of the Aerodigestive Tract
Alcoholism	Multiple sclerosis	Zenker's diverticulum
	Parkinson's disease	Achalasia
Drug overdose	Cranial neuropathy	Esophageal carcinoma
Head injury	Muscular dystrophies	Esophageal strictures
Cerebral infarction	Cerebral palsy	Gastroesophageal reflux
Cerebral hemorrhage	Cerebral infarction	Tracheoesophageal fistula
Metabolic coma	Cerebral hemorrhage	Tumors of the larynx or pharynx
Seizure disorders	Head injury	

Modified from Shifrin RY: Aspiration in patients in critical care units. Radiol Clin North Am 1996; 34:83.

facilities, nosocomial pneumonia becomes the predominant complication.[88] The necessity to care for elderly patients in such facilities often implies neurologic dysfunction, chronic organ failure, and other debilitating physical factors that preclude self-care and render them unable to mount an immune response to clear the organisms aspirated from oropharyngeal secretions.[89]

When mechanical ventilation is prolonged, the risk of pulmonary aspiration and infection increases, regardless of age. Whether the interface between the patient and the mechanical ventilator is an endotracheal or a tracheostomy tube, the risk of pulmonary aspiration is increased when normal mechanical (and immune-mediated) defense mechanisms are breached. The normal culture of oropharyngeal secretions contains mixed flora, and these organisms are not found below the larynx. Introduction of these organisms into the tracheobronchial tree does not result in infection, since the organisms are rapidly cleared and sterility is maintained. Indeed, when the laryngeal sensory deficits are observed after stroke, access to the tracheobronchial tree of any material in the oropharynx is increased, even in the absence of clinical dysphagia.[90]

Similarly, with the introduction of an endotracheal tube, a tracheostomy tube, or a feeding tube (which can wick gastric contents into the oropharynx increasing potential for aspiration into the tracheobronchial tree), the normal protection characteristic of a native airway is bypassed. Further compromising the ventilated patient, the inflated balloon at the tip of the endotracheal or tracheostomy tube results in pressure on the tracheal mucosa, interference with the function of the mucociliary escalator, and possibly alteration of the phagocytic activity of macrophages and other cellular and immune functions.[89, 91]

Over time, the ventilated patient exhibits alterations in oropharyngeal flora and becomes colonized with the gram-negative organisms common to the hospital setting, organisms that are often resistant to many antibiotics.[92] Following transcolonization of the pharynx, lower airway inoculation can occur, eventually resulting in pneumonia secondary to subclinical aspiration of the airway flora.[93]

In "tube-fed" patients, bedside diagnostic tests have been studied to document the presence of aspiration and alter therapy. Adding a dye to the enteral formula and observing tracheobronchial secretions for the color, and the use of glucose oxidase reagent strips to test the secretions for the presence of glucose, have both been questioned for efficacy, cost effectiveness, and potential harm to the patient.[89, 93-95] Finally, in addition to the pharmacologic measures mentioned above, patient position may be an effective means of prophylaxis. Elevating the head of the bed from the supine position to a 45° angle has been suggested as a simple and cost effective measure.[96]

SUMMARY

The simplest and most efficient therapy for aspiration of stomach contents is prevention. When aspiration does occur, the following steps are recommended:

1. *Suction the trachea.*
2. *Analyze arterial blood for gas tensions and pH.*
3. *Apply aggressive mechanical ventilatory support, particularly with CPAP or PEEP, and document its effectiveness by measuring blood gas parameters and shunt.*
4. *Ensure adequate fluid replacement.*
5. *Perform bronchoscopy when large particulate aspirates obstruct airways.*

We do not recommend corticosteroids, prophylactic antibiotics, or pulmonary lavage with large volumes of neutral or alkaline solutions.[55]

REFERENCES

1. Mellin-Olsen J, Fasting S, Gisvold SE: Routine preoperative gastric emptying is seldom indicated. A study of 85,594 anaesthetics with special focus on aspiration pneumonia. Acta Anaesthesiol Scand 1996; 40:1184.
2. Phillips S, Daborn AK, Hatch DJ: Preoperative fasting for paediatric anaesthesia. Br J Anaesth 1994; 73:529.
3. Lifshultz BD, Donoghue ER: Deaths due to foreign body aspiration in children: The continuing hazard of toy balloons. J Forensic Sci 1996; 41:247.
4. Noonan L, Howrey R, Ginsburg CM: Freshwater submersion injuries in children: A retrospective review of seventy-five hospitalized patients. Pediatrics 1996; 98:368.
5. Kokkinis K: The use of the laryngeal mask airway in CPR. Resuscitation 1994; 27:9.
6. Owens TM, Robertson P, Twomey C, et al: The incidence of gastroesophageal reflux with the laryngeal mask: A comparison of face mask using esophageal lumen pH electrodes. Anesth Analg 1995; 80:980.
7. Samarkandi AH, Seraj MA, el Dawlatly A, et al: The role of laryngeal mask airway in cardiopulmonary resuscitation. Resuscitation 1994; 28:103.
8. Mendelson CL: The aspiration of stomach contents into the lungs during obstetric anesthesia. Ann Obstet Gynecol 1946; 52:191.
9. Teabeaut JR II: Aspiration of gastric contents: An experimental study. Am J Pathol 1952; 28:51.
10. Taylor C, Pryse-Davies J: Evaluation of endotracheal steroid therapy in acid pulmonary aspiration syndrome (Mendelson's syndrome). Anesthesiology 1968; 29:17.
11. Awe WC, Fletcher IS, Jacob SW: The pathophysiology of aspiration pneumonitis. Surgery 1966; 60:232.
12. Bannister WK, Sattilaro AJ: Vomiting and aspiration during anesthesia. Anesthesiology 1962; 23:251.
13. Vandam LD: Aspiration of gastric contents in the operative period. N Engl J Med 1965; 273:1206.
14. Wynne JW, Reynolds IC, Hood CL, et al: Steroid therapy for pneumonitis induced in rabbits by aspiration of foodstuff. Anesthesiology 1979; 51:11.
15. Greenfield LI, Singleton RP, McCaffree DR, et al: Pulmonary effects of experimental graded aspiration of hydrochloric acid. Ann Surg 1969; 170:74.
16. Downs JB, Chapman RL Jr, Modell JH, et al: An evaluation of steroid therapy in aspiration pneumonitis. Anesthesiology 1974; 40:129.
17. Alexander IG: The ultrastructure of the pulmonary alveolar vessels in Mendelson's (acid pulmonary aspiration) syndrome. Br J Anaesth 1968; 40:408.
18. Rocke DA, Brock-Utne IC, Rout CC: At risk for aspiration: New critical values of volume and pH (Letter)? Anesth Analg 1993; 76:666.
19. Goresky CV, Finley GA, Bissonnette B, et al: Efficacy, duration, and absorption of a paediatric oral liquid preparation of ranitidine hydrochloride. Can J Anaesth 1992; 39:791.
20. Raidoo DM, Rocke DA, Brock-Utne JG, et al: Critical volume for pulmonary acid aspiration: Reappraisal in a primate model. Br J Anaesth 1990; 65:248.
21. James CF, Modell JH, Gibbs CP, et al: Pulmonary aspiration—effects of volume and pH in the rat. Anesth Analg 1984; 63:665.
22. Moran TJ: Experimental food-aspiration pneumonia. Arch Pathol 1951; 52:350.
23. Cameron JL, Caldini P, Toung JK, et al: Aspiration pneumonia: Physiologic data following experimental aspiration. Surgery 1972; 72:238.
24. Davidson JT, Rubin S, Eyal Z, et al: A comparison of the pulmonary response to the endotracheal instillation of 0.1 N hydrochloric acid and Hartman's solution in the rabbit. Br J Anaesth 1974; 46:127.
25. Lewis RT, Burgess JH, Hampson LC: Cardiorespiratory studies in critical illness: Changes in aspiration pneumonitis. Arch Surg 1971; 103:335.

26. Hamelberg W, Bosomworth PP: Aspiration pneumonitis: Experimental studies and clinical observations. Anesth Analg (Cleveland) 1964; 43:669.
27. Halmagyi DF, Colebatch HJ, Starzecki B: Inhalation of blood, saliva, and alcohol: Consequences, mechanism, and treatment. Thorax 1962; 17:244.
28. Colebatch HJ, Halmagyi DF: Reflex airway reaction to fluid aspiration. J Appl Physiol 1962; 17:787.
29. Toussaint GP, Chiu CJ, Hampson LG: Experimental aspiration pneumonia: Hemodynamics, ventilator and membrane oxygenator support. J Surg Res 1974; 16:324.
30. Fisk RL, Symes JF, Aldridge LL, et al: The pathophysiology and experimental therapy of acid pneumonitis in ex vivo lungs. Chest 1970; 57:364.
31. Booth DL, Zuidema GD, Cameron JL: Aspiration pneumonia: Pulmonary arteriography after experimental aspiration. J Surg Res 1972; 12:48.
32. Morgan BC, Abel FL, Mullins CL, et al: Flow patterns in cavae, pulmonary artery, pulmonary vein, and aorta in intact dogs. Am J Physiol 1966; 210:903.
33. Giammona ST, Modell JH: Drowning by total immersion: Effects on pulmonary surfactant of distilled water, isotonic saline and sea water. Am J Dis Child 1967; 114:612.
34. Wynne JW, Modell JH: Respiratory aspiration of stomach contents. Ann Intern Med 1977; 87:466.
35. Warner MA, Warner ME, Weber JG: Clinical significance of pulmonary aspiration during the perioperative period. Anesthesiology 1993; 78:56.
36. Badellino MM, Buckman RF Jr, Malaspina PJ, et al: Detection of pulmonary aspiration of gastric contents in an animal model by assay of peptic activity in bronchoalveolar fluid. Crit Care Med 1996; 24:1881.
37. Herman NL, Carter B, Van Decar TK: Cricoid pressure: Teaching the recommended level. Anesth Analg 1996; 83:859.
38. Chassard D, Tournadre JP, Berrada KR: Cricoid pressure decreases lower oesophageal sphincter tone in anaesthetized pigs. Can J Anaesth 1996; 43:414.
39. Phillips S, Hutchinson S, Davidson T: Preoperative drinking does not affect gastric contents. Br J Anaesth 1993; 70:6.
40. Ghignone M, Calvillo O, Quintin L: Anesthesia and hypertension: The effect of clonidine on perioperative hemodynamics and isoflurane requirements. Anesthesiology 1987; 67:3.
41. Vincent RD Jr, McNeil TJ, Spaid CL, et al: Does 360 mL of apple juice ingested before elective surgery worsen volume and acidity in patients given acid aspiration prophylaxis? J Clin Anesth 1991; 3:285.
42. Maltby JR, Sutherland AD, Sale JP, et al: Preoperative oral fluids: Is a 5-hour fast justified prior to elective surgery? Anesth Analg 1986; 65:1112.
43. Pandit SK, Kothary SP, Pandit UA, et al: Dose response study of droperidol and metoclopramide as antiemetics for outpatient anesthesia. Anesth Analg 1989; 68:798.
44. White PF: Pharmacologic and clinical aspects of preoperative medication. Anesth Analg 1986; 65:963.
45. Tryba M, Wruck G, Thole H, et al: The use of roxatidine acetate in fasting patients prior to induction of anaesthesia as prophylaxis against the acid aspiration syndrome. Drugs 1988; 35(Suppl 3):20.
46. Jahr JS, Burckart C, Smith SS, et al: Effects of famotidine on gastric pH and residual volume in pediatric surgery. Acta Anaesth Scand 1991; 35:457.
47. Strunin L: How long should patients fast before surgery? Time for new guidelines (Editorial). Br J Anaesth 1993; 70:1.
48. Moore I, Flynn RJ, Sampaio M, et al: Effect of single-dose omeprazole on intragastric acidity and volume during obstetric anaesthesia. Anaesthesia 1989; 44:559.
49. Roberts RB, Shirley MA: Reducing the risk of acid aspiration during cesarean section. Anesth Analg (Cleveland) 1974; 53:859.
50. Taylor C, Pryse-Davies J: The prophylactic use of antacids in the prevention of the acid-pulmonary-aspiration syndrome (Mendelson's syndrome). Lancet 1966; i:288.
51. Lahiri SK, Thomas TA, Hodgson RM: Single-dose antacid therapy for the prevention of Mendelson's syndrome. Br J Anaesth 1973; 45:1143.
52. Peskett WGH: Antacids before obstetric anaesthesia: A clinical evaluation of the effectiveness of mist, magnesium trisilicate BPC. Anaesthesia 1973; 28:509.
53. Gibbs CP, Schwartz DJ, Wynne JW, et al: Antacid pulmonary aspiration in the dog. Anesthesiology 1979; 51:380.
54. Gibbs CP, Spohr L, Schmidt D: The effectiveness of sodium citrate as an antacid. Anesthesiology 1982; 57:44.
55. Gibbs CP, Modell JH: Pulmonary aspiration of gastric contents: Pathophysiology, prevention, and management. *In* Anesthesia. 4th ed. Miller RD (ed). New York, Churchill Livingstone, 1994, pp 1437–1464.
56. Maliniak K, Vakil AH: Pre-anesthetic cimetidine and gastric pH. Anesth Analg (Cleveland) 1969; 58:309.
57. Rout CC, Rocke DA, Gouws E: Intravenous ranitidine reduces the risk of aspiration of gastric contents at emergency cesarean section. Anesth Analg 1993; 76:156.
58. O'Connor TA, Basak J, Parker S: The effect of three different ranitidine dosage regimens on reducing gastric acidity and volume in ambulatory surgical patients. Pharmacotherapy 1995; 15:170.
59. Orr DA, Bill KM, Gillon KR, et al: Effects of omeprazole, with and without metoclopramide, in elective obstetric anaesthesia. Anaesthesia 1993; 48:114.
60. Rocke DA, Rout CC, Gouws E: Intravenous administration of the proton pump inhibitor omeprazole reduces the risk of acid aspiration at emergency cesarean section. Anesth Analg 1994; 78:1093.
61. Stuart JC, Kan AF, Rowbottom SJ, et al: Acid aspiration prophylaxis for emergency caesarean section. Anaesthesia 1996; 51:415.
62. Russell GN, Yam PC, Tran J, et al: Gastroesophageal reflux and tracheobronchial contamination after cardiac surgery: Should a nasogastric tube be routine? Anesth Analg 1996; 83:228.
63. Orozco-Levi M, Torres A, Ferrer M, et al: Semirecumbent position protects from pulmonary aspiration but not completely from gastroesophageal reflux in mechanically ventilated patients. Am J Respir Crit Care Med 1995; 152:1387.
64. Chapman RL Jr, Downs JB, Modell JH, et al: The ineffectiveness of steroid therapy in treating aspiration of hydrochloric acid. Arch Surg 1974; 108:858.
65. Cameron JL, Sebor J, Anderson RP, et al: Aspiration pneumonia: Results of treatment by positive-pressure ventilation in dogs. J Surg Res 1968; 8:447.
66. Chapman RL Jr, Modell JH, Ruiz BC, et al: Effect of continuous positive-pressure ventilation and steroids on aspiration of hydrochloric acid (pH 1.8) in dogs. Anesth Analg (Cleveland) 1974; 53:556.
67. Pontoppidan H, Geffin B, Lowenstein E: Acute respiratory failure in the adult. N Engl J Med 1972; 287:690.
68. Downs JB, Modell JH: Patterns of respiratory support aimed at pathophysiologic conditions. *In:* ASA Refresher Courses in Anesthesiology. Vol 5. Hershey SG (Ed). Philadelphia, JB Lippincott, 1977, pp 71–85.
69. Kolobow T, Morettia MP, Fumagalli R, et al: Severe impairment in lung function induced by high peak airway pressure mechanical ventilation: An experimental study. Am Rev Respir Dis 1987; 135:312.
70. Dreyfuss D, Bassett G, Soler P, et al: Intermittent positive-pressure hyperventilation with high inflation pressures produces pulmonary microvascular injury in rats. Am Rev Respir Dis 1985; 132:880.
71. Gattinoni L, Presenti A, Marcolin R, et al: Extracorporeal support in acute respiratory failure. Intensive Med Care 1988; 5:42.
72. Sohma A, Brampton WJ, Dunnill MS, et al: Effect of ventilation with positive end-expiratory pressure on the development of lung damage in experimental acid aspiration in the rabbit. Intensive Care Med 1992; 18:112.
73. Janoff A, Weismann NG, Zweifach BW, et al: Pathogenesis of experimental shock: IV. Studies on lysosomes in normal and tolerant animals subjected to lethal trauma and endotoxemia. J Exp Med 1962; 116:451.
74. Starling JR, Rudolf LE, Ferguson W, et al: Benefits of methylprednisolone in the isolated perfused organ. Ann Surg 1973; 177:566.
75. Wilson JW: Treatment or prevention of pulmonary cellular damage with pharmacologic doses of corticosteroid. Surg Gynecol Obstet 1972; 134:675.
76. Bryan-Brown CW, Baek S, Makabali G, et al: Consumable oxygen: Availability of oxygen in relation to oxyhemoglobin dissociation. Crit Care Med 1973; 1:17.
77. Bartlett JG, Gorbach SL, Finegold SM: The bacteriology of aspiration pneumonia. Am J Med 1974; 56:202.
78. Lorber B, Swenson RM: Bacteriology of aspiration pneumonia: A

prospective study of community- and hospital-acquired cases. Ann Intern Med 1974; 81:329.
79. Arms RA, Dines DE, Tinstman TC: Aspiration pneumonia. Chest 1974; 65:136.
80. Bynum LJ, Pierce AK: Pulmonary aspiration of gastric contents. Am Rev Respir Dis 1876; 114:1129.
81. Atherton ST, White DJ: Stomach as a source of bacteria colonising respiratory tract during artificial ventilation. Lancet 1978; ii:968.
82. Nesti FD, Fuhrman BP, Steinhorn DM: Perfluorocarbon-associated gas exchange in gastric aspiration. Crit Care Med 1994; 22:1445.
83. Shifrin RY, Choplin RH: Aspiration in patients in critical care units. Radiol Clin North Am 1996; 34:83.
84. Gleeson K, Eggli DF, Maxwell SL: Quantitative aspiration during sleep in normal subjects. Chest 1997; 111:1266.
85. Kikuchi R, Watabe N, Konno T, et al: High incidence of silent aspiration in elderly patients with community-acquired pneumonia. Am J Respir Crit Care Med 1994; 150:251.
86. Nakagawa T, Sekizawa K, Arai H, et al: High incidence of pneumonia in elderly patients with basal ganglia infarction. Arch Intern Med 1997; 157:321.
87. Matsuse T, Oka T, Kida K, et al: Importance of diffuse aspiration bronchiolitis caused by chronic occult aspiration in the elderly. Chest 1996; 110:1289.
88. Pick N, McDonald A, Bennett N, et al: Pulmonary aspiration in a long-term care setting: Clinical and laboratory observations and an analysis of risk factors. J Am Geriatr Soc 1996; 44:763.
89. Matthay MA, Rosen GD: Acid aspiration induced lung injury. Am J Respir Crit Care Med 1996; 154:277.
90. Aviv JE, Sacco RL, Thomson J, et al: Silent laryngopharyngeal sensory deficits after stroke. Ann Otol Rhinol Laryngol 1997; 106:87.
91. Elpern EH, Scott MG, Petro L, et al: Pulmonary aspiration in mechanically ventilated patients with tracheostomies. Chest 1994; 105:563.
92. Estes RJ, Meduri GU: The pathogenesis of ventilator-associated pneumonia: I. Mechanisms of bacterial transcolonization and airway inoculation. Intensive Care Med 1995; 21:365.
93. Kingston GW, Phang PT, Leathley MJ: Increased incidence of nosocomial pneumonia in mechanically ventilated patients with subclinical aspiration. Am J Surg 1991; 161:589.
94. Metheny NA, Clouse RE: Bedside methods of detecting aspiration in tube-fed patients. Chest 1997; 111:724.
95. Kinsey GC, Murray MJ, Swensen SJ, et al: Glucose content of tracheal aspirates: Implications for the detection of tube feeding aspiration. Crit Care Med 1994; 22:1557.
96. Torres A, Serra-Battles J, Ros E, et al: Pulmonary aspiration of gastric contents in patients receiving mechanical ventilation: The effect of body position. Ann Intern Med 1992; 116:540.

132

Weaning from Ventilatory Support in Hypoxemic Respiratory Failure

Neil R. MacIntyre, MD

Removing a patient from mechanical ventilation has been termed *liberation, removal, discontinuation, withdrawal,* and, most commonly, *weaning.* Precision is key to discussing this process, as two distinct concepts are involved. First is the process of permanent removal from the ventilator, often with removal of the artificial airway (i.e., extubation). This is done when patients are fully capable of supporting ventilation on their own. Second is the process of gradual reduction in the level of support, often accomplished by using gradual reductions in a mode providing partial ventilatory support. This is done when patients are capable of doing some, but not all, of the necessary ventilation. "Discontinuation" refers to the first process, "weaning" to the second process.

In general, patients recovering from rapidly reversing ventilatory insufficiency or failure (e.g., recovery from anesthesia, drug overdose, asthma attack) can have the ventilator promptly discontinued. In contrast, weaning is often performed in patients with slowly resolving lung processes in the hope that having the patient perform some comfortable level of ventilatory work will accelerate muscle recovery, avoid unnecessary ventilator pressures, and require less sedation for ventilator-patient synchrony (Fig. 132–1).

WHY ARE DISCONTINUATION AND WEANING STRATEGIES IMPORTANT?

The process of ventilator discontinuation and weaning can account for 40% of the time a patient is on a ventilator.[1, 2] Proper ventilatory management during these processes is thus critical. Clearly, ventilator management should be aimed at removing the patient from ventilator support as quickly as possible. Delayed discontinuation from mechanical ventilatory support exposes patients to unnecessary risks of infection, stretch injury, sedation needs, airway trauma, and costs.[3] Weaning and discontinuation must be done with proper caution and monitoring, however, because premature withdrawal has its own problems: loss of airway protection, cardiovascular stress, suboptimal gas exchange, and muscle overload or fatigue.[3] Muscle overload and fatigue is of particular concern as it can take 24 hours or more of muscle rest (i.e., reintubation and high levels of mechanical support) for fatigued ventilatory muscles to recover.[4]

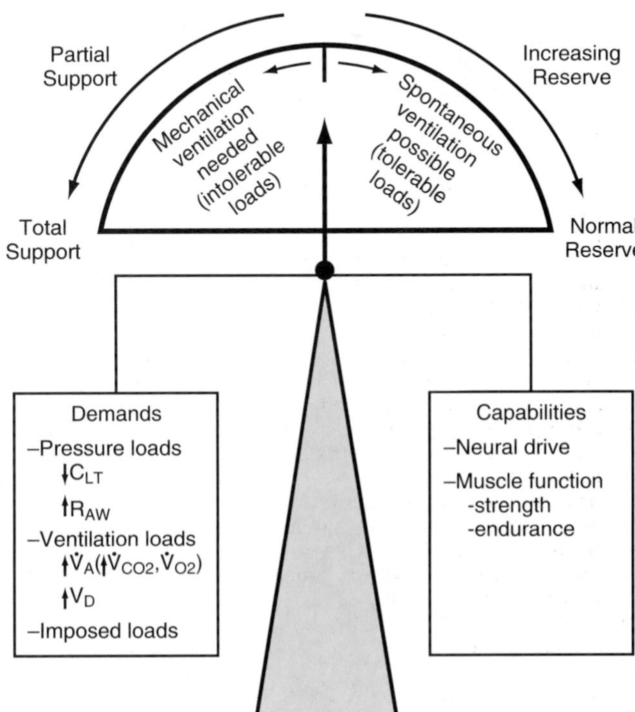

Figure 132–1. Depiction of the concept of weaning using a balance scale. When demands far exceed capabilities, total ventilator support is required; however, as loads diminish and patient capabilities improve, only partial support is required until ventilator discontinuation is possible.

TABLE 132–1. Criteria for Discontinuation of Mechanical Ventilation

Underlying disease stable or improving
$P_aO_2/FO_2 \geq 300$
Positive end-expiratory pressure ≤10 cm H_2O
Reliable respiratory drive
Stable cardiovascular status with minimal inotropes and pressors

WHEN SHOULD VENTILATOR DISCONTINUATION BE CONSIDERED?

In general, when a patient's underlying respiratory tract disease begins to stabilize and reverse, consideration for ventilator discontinuation should begin. Specific criteria are given in Table 132–1. When a patient meets these criteria, assessment for discontinuation potential is appropriate. This usually involves a number of measurements during spontaneous breathing with little or no ventilator assistance (e.g., T-piece trial or using either 1 to 5 cm H_2O continuous positive airway pressure [CPAP] or 5 to 7 cm H_2O of pressure support from the ventilator (Table 132–2).[5–8]

Some of the factors in Table 132–2 are readily obtained (e.g., vital capacity [VC], minute ventilation [MV], frequency–tidal volume ratio [f/VT], muscle force generated during 20 seconds of effort against a closed airway [maximum inspiratory force; MIF], and patient observations). Ventilator discontinuation is more likely when the MV is less than 15 L/min, the VC is more than 10 mL/kg, the f/VT is less than 105 and the MIF is less than than −25 cm H_2O.[5, 6]

Other parameters in Table 132–2 require more sophisticated measurements. For instance, an esophageal balloon to measure esophageal pressure (Pes, an estimate of pleural pressure) is necessary to assess patient muscle loads.[8] Muscle loads can be expressed as either work or pressure time products (PTPs) per breath[4, 9–12]

$$\text{work} = \int \text{Pes} \cdot V_T,$$

$$\text{PTP} = \int \text{Pes} \cdot T_I$$

TABLE 132–2. Criteria for Predicting Successful Discontinuation of Ventilation

Mechanical Factors
MV <15 L/min
MIF <−25 cm H_2O
VC> 10 mL/kg
f/VT <105
Work <5 J/min (exclusive of endotracheal tube work)
PTI <0.15
Integrated Factors
CROP index >13[7]
Weaning score based on compliance, resistance, VD/VT, $Paco_2$ and f/VT <3[8]
Weaning index (PTI × MV for $Paco_2$ of 40/VT) <4[33]
Neural network[13]
Patient Assessment
Absence of:
Dyspnea
Accessory muscle use
Abdominal paradox
Agitation, anxiety, tachycardia

MV = minute ventilation; VC = vital capacity; PTI = pressure time index; VT = tidal volume; MIF = maximal inspiratory force; f/VT = frequency: tidal volume ratio; CROP = compliance rate oxygenation pressure.

These indices of muscle load can be expressed with respect to time (i.e., work/min), to ventilation (i.e., work/L) or to maximum muscle strength (i.e., PTP/MIF). As work/min or work/L approaches normal values (5 J/min or 0.5 J/L), ventilation discontinuation becomes more likely. Multiplying the PTP/MIF by the inspiratory time fraction (TI/tot) results in the pressure time index (PTI), which can be a useful predictor of fatigue (a PTI above 0.15 predicts fatigue).[11]

Integrated factors have also been employed. The CROP index (*c*ompliance; *r*ate; *o*xygenation, *p*ressure) multiplies dynamic compliance × Pao_2/PAo_2 × MIF and divides this product by respiratory rate. A CROP index greater than 13 predicts weaning success.[7] Other integrated scores incorporate Pes load calculations[8] and may utilize neural networks.[13] Important clinical assessment criteria include subjective dyspnea, accessory muscle use, diaphoresis, tachycardia, abdominal paradox, and subjective comfort.

Analyses of receiver-operator characteristics (ROC) curves have shown none of these indices alone to be 100% sensitive and specific in predicting discontinuation success.[7] Indeed, a spontaneous breathing trial of up to 1 hour with simple observations of f/VT, dyspnea, and accessory muscle use is probably the easiest and most reliable guide for deciding the likelihood of ventilator discontinuation.[7] This procedure should probably be done daily for all patients who meet Table 132–1 criteria but who, for whatever reason, could not permanently be discontinued from the ventilator the previous day. As several studies[1, 2, 14] have shown, spontaneous breathing trials with simple clinical observations reveal that patients may be ready for successful ventilatory discontinuation, even though the complex physiologic calculation described above may not seem to support it.

The decision to perform subsequent artificial airway removal after ventilator discontinuation depends on additional considerations. First, artificial airway removal must be done only in patients who have the capability of protecting the airway. Second, the risk of potential recurrence of acute respiratory failure, and thus ventilator need, must also be assessed before the artificial airway is removed.

MANAGEMENT OF PATIENTS NOT YET READY FOR DISCONTINUATION

Causes of Inability to Discontinue Ventilation

Patients who meet Table 132–1 criteria but who cannot meet Table 132–2 discontinuation criteria pose an important management challenge. A first step would be to determine why discontinuation failed. Common causes include:

1. Respiratory drive failure involving inability of the patient to generate a reliable respiratory drive because of central nervous system (CNS) injury or drugs.[15]
2. Oxygenation failure involving rapid hemoglobin desaturation from loss of expiratory pressure or FIO_2.
3. Cardiovascular failure involving arrhythmias or hypotension from catechol release, edema formation, or coronary hypoxemia due to loss of ventilatory support.[16]
4. Muscle failure involving muscle overload from abnormal respiratory system impedances in the setting of weakened, fatigued, or metabolically disturbed muscles.[9, 17–22]

Different clinical venues may experience one form of failure more often than others. For example, the coronary care unit may see more cardiac problems, neurology units may see more respiratory drive failures. In intensive care units that deal predominantly with respiratory diseases, the most common cause of ventilator dependence is muscle loads exceeding muscle capabilities.[23]

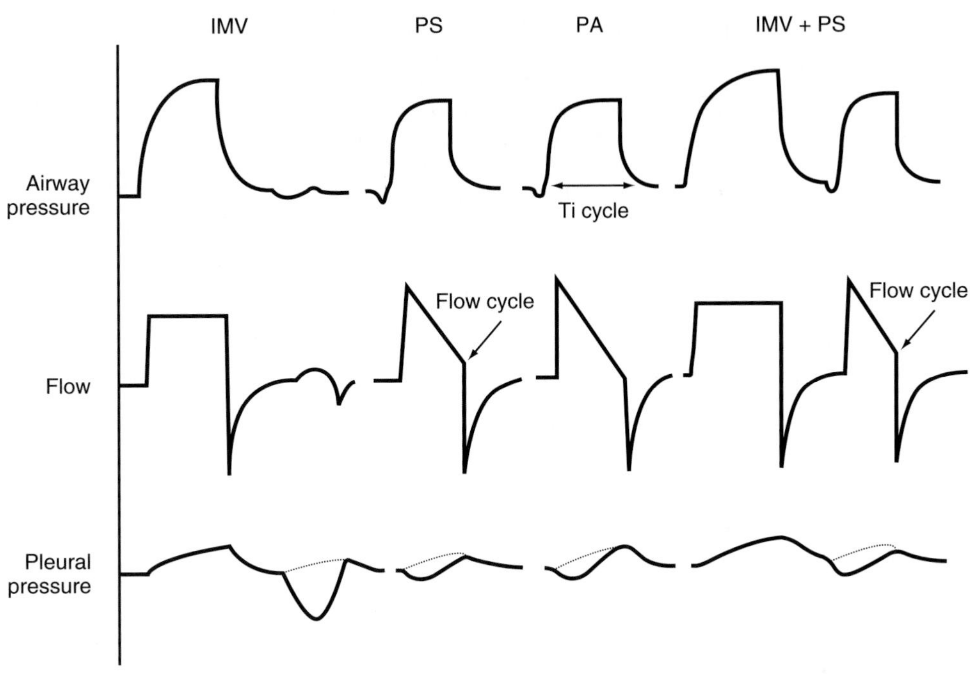

Figure 132–2. Airway pressure flow and pleural pressure patterns of commonly used modes of partial support. The shaded area reflects patient contribution to the work of breathing. *Left panel,* Intermittent mandatory ventilation (IMV) with volume assist-control breaths alternating with spontaneous unassisted breaths. *Second panel,* Pressure support (PS). A patient-triggered, pressure-targeted, flow-cycled breath provides partial support for the patient's effort. *Third panel,* Pressure assist (PA). A patient-triggered, pressure-targeted, time-cycled breath provides partial support of the patient's effort. *Last panel,* Combination of IMV and PS.

Once a cause of ventilator dependence has been determined, a management plan can be developed. This plan obviously must first focus on the cause of the ventilator dependency (e.g., improving respiratory drive, improving cardiac function, improving gas exchange). However, managing the ventilator and the patient ventilator loads can also be important in developing and maintaining optimal ventilator muscle function.

Approach to Ventilator Management

Two fundamental approaches to this exist:

- Nearly total rest with assist-control ventilation (ACV)
- Various modes of partial support

Modes of partial support generally involve either intermittent support (intermittent mandatory ventilation [IMV]) or partial support of every breath (pressure support and pressure assist [PS/PA]) (Fig. 132–2 and Table 132–3).

Near Total Rest

The conceptual advantages to near total rest with assist control are twofold. First, muscle fatigue risk is minimized with high-level support. Second, management requires no decision making other than the daily spontaneous breathing trials for discontinuation assessment. Both of these conceptual advantages require that the assist-control mode be applied in a synchronous fashion. Specifically, the trigger, the flow delivery, and the cycling criteria of the assist-control breaths must be properly synchronized to patient effort. Otherwise, high levels of imposed muscle loading can develop, which can increase the risk of fatigue. Proper ventilator settings (including consideration of pressure-targeted assist control) are thus critical, and sedation may be required to reduce imposed loads from dyssynchrony.

Partial Support

The advantages to partial support are several. First, a more gradual withdrawal may be better tolerated than periods of

TABLE 132–3. Modes of Partial Support

Mode	Description	Initial Settings	Support Weaned By:
IMV	Set number of volume or pressure-targeted assist-control breaths interspersed with spontaneous breaths (up to 10 cm H_2O PS during those breaths sometimes given to compensate for endotracheal tube resistance).	Mimic volume or pressure ACV settings with mandatory breath rate slightly below total ACV.	Reduce number of mandatory breaths.*
PS or PA	Inspiratory pressure delivered with every effort. PS terminates by flow, PA terminates on a set time.	Use pressure support mode for PS. Use pressure assist-control with rate set to 0 for PA. Mimic plateau pressure and inspiratory time of ACV.	Reduce inspiratory† pressure level.
IMV + PS	Combine IMV with >10 cm H_2O PS.	As with IMV except that PS is set between 10 cm H_2O and plateau pressure ACV.	Reduce both IMV mandatory breath rate and PS level.

*Mandatory minute ventilation (MMV) can automate this according to total minute ventilation.
†Can be automatically set by VT.
PS = pressure support; PA = pressure assit; IMV = intermittent mandatory ventilation; ACV = assist-control ventilation.

sudden total withdrawal, especially in patients who have long been on a ventilator or who may have a tenuous cardiovascular system. Second, less pressure is applied to the thorax with partial support than with total support, and there is thus potentially less lung stretch injury risk and cardiovascular compromise. Third, muscle recovery may be enhanced using partial support. This is a complex and controversial issue. Fatigued muscles need rest for recovery, but prolonged inactivity can clearly produce atrophy.[9, 24-26] An optimal balance may be to provide these types of patients with a nearly normal muscle load using a comfortable, nonfatiguing level of partial support.

In using modes of partial support to optimize muscle recovery, we must consider three issues:

- Proper balancing of aggressiveness and fatigue (Fig. 132-3)
- Patient-ventilator synchrony
- Characteristics of patient muscle loads

Aggressiveness-Fatigue Balance

When partial support modes are used, regular assessment and adjustments are mandatory for two reasons. First, weaning cannot be accomplished unless ventilatory support is reduced. This must be done carefully, however, lest too prompt a reduction precipitate fatigue. Protocols to assess patients regularly and adjust support loads accordingly are thus a vital part of any weaning strategy with partial support. Indeed, much of the variability in reported weaning studies was likely due to variability in assessment and adjustment strategies.[1, 2] Proper weaning strategy aggressiveness might be inferred by the reintubation rate (i.e., percentage of patients who are extubated but need to be reintubated within 24 to 48 hours) of a particular unit. When the reintubation rate is very low (<5%), one might wonder whether weaning practices are too cautious. In contrast, when the reintubation rate is high (>20%), one might wonder whether weaning practices are too aggressive.

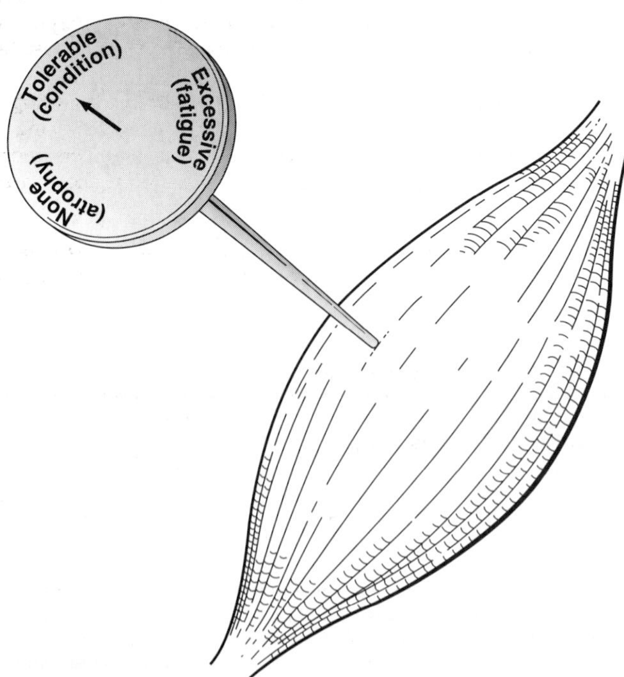

Figure 132–3. Concept of balancing aggressiveness and rest on ventilatory muscles. Excessive muscle reloading may precipitate fatigue; excessive rest may produce atrophy. Appropriate loading may enhance muscle conditioning.

Patient-Ventilator Synchrony

During partial support weaning techniques, patients must interact with the ventilator flow delivery system. Under these circumstances, these interactions must be synchronous in order to minimize unnecessary sedation, minimize unnecessary muscle work, and provide appropriate rest for sleep. Careful attention must thus be paid to proper trigger sensitivity settings and flow delivery patterns. Indeed, enhanced patient-ventilator flow synchrony is the rationale behind pressure support and pressure assist weaning strategies.[27-29]

Characteristics of Patient Loads

Muscle loads are characterized both by total load involved and by load characteristics (the pressure-volume relationship) (Fig. 132-4).[12, 27, 30, 31] Load quantity has been discussed, and the goal of weaning is to aggressively reapply tolerable, but not fatiguing, loads (see Figs. 132-1 and 132-3). Load characteristics, however, may also be important. Specifically, distortion of work characteristics to a high pressure-low volume load is clearly less efficient (i.e., work per volume of oxygen consumption falls) and probably induces fatigue more readily.[12, 23] Thus, a similar level of work performed on a lung with abnormal compliance or resistance using unassisted spontaneous breaths with high-pressure/low-volume characteristics (IMV approach) may be more fatiguing than a reconfigured patient breath using pressure-targeted breaths that "normalize" the pressure-volume relationship (PS/PA approach) (see Fig. 132-4). This is another rationale for using pressure-targeted breaths as a primary partial support technique.[27]

COMPARING THE DIFFERENT APPROACHES

Two large trials have been performed comparing T-piece/ACV, IMV, and stand-alone PS approaches to weaning (Table 132-4).[1, 2] As can be seen, one found PS to be superior and one found T piece/ACV to be superior for patients who require substantial ventilatory support for more than several days. It is obviously difficult to draw general conclusions from these studies, since the way these modes were used in each study differed greatly. For example, the study of Esteban and coworkers[1] had very aggressive T-piece weaning rules that not only produced faster weaning than the more conservative T-piece weaning rule of Brochard's group[2] but also produced an almost fourfold increase in the rate of reintubation.

There are important messages from both of these studies, however. First, weaning strategy clearly can affect outcome. Indeed, depending on strategy, weaning time could increase severalfold in these two controlled studies. Second, a weaning strategy must be aggressive. This can constitute frequent discontinuation assessments, frequent protocol-driven reduction in partial support, or both. Third, fatigue potential needs to be monitored carefully so as to minimize the risk of overaggressiveness. Finally, both studies demonstrated that substantial numbers of patients thought to be ventilator-dependent could safely be discontinued from the ventilator after successfully passing a spontaneous breathing trial. These observations, coupled with more recent reports on weaning protocols,[14, 32] reemphasize the importance of frequent (daily) assessments for discontinuation potential.

CAN WEANING BE AUTOMATED?

A number of newer ventilators supply certain feedback features that theoretically may be helpful in the weaning process

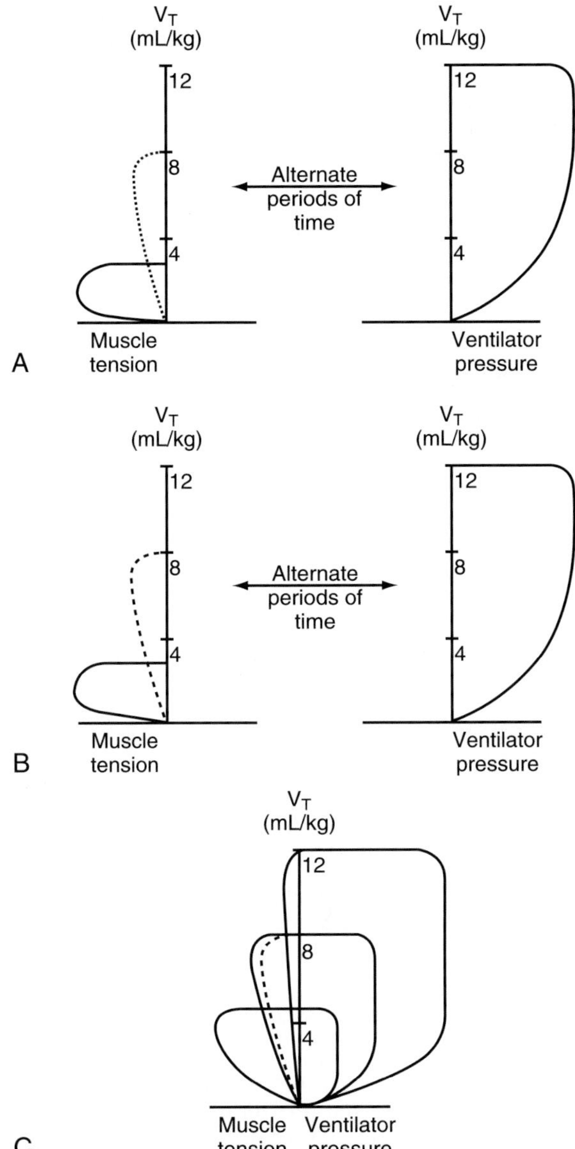

Figure 132–4. Pressure-volume diagrams illustrating the configuration of patient work during various forms of partial support. Patient effort (muscle tension) is directed leftward; ventilator-delivered pressure is directed rightward. The *dotted line* represents a normal pressure-volume work configuration. In these examples, respiratory disease has produced impedance changes that have reconfigured patient work to a high-pressure/low-volume pattern *(solid lines)*. With T-piece breathing *(A)* and intermittent mandatory ventilation *(B)*, patient work remains in this abnormal configuration during the spontaneous breaths. With pressure-targeted partial support *(C)*, ventilator assistance with every breath reconfigures patient effort to a more normal pressure-volume pattern.

(Table 132-5). An inherent problem in all of these, however, is that the input variable for machine decision making is currently only a single variable—either minute ventilation or tidal volume. As noted, many other variables (including clinical assessment) seem far more important in aggressive weaning than these two, and thus the potential utility of these current approaches seems limited. Indeed, the weaning process might actually be *delayed* if an inappropriately high minute ventilation or tidal volume is set as the target weaning variable using the available approaches in Table 132-5.

TABLE 132–4. Weaning Success Resulting from Various Ventilator Strategies

	Patients Remaining on Ventilator (%)	
	Day 5	**Day 10**
Esteban Trial[1]		
Intermittent mandatory ventilation	70	44
T piece	44	16
Pressure support	61	38
Brochard Trial[2]		
Intermittent mandatory ventilation	66	54
T piece	60	41
Pressure support	47	24

A REASONABLE APPROACH TO WEANING

Once a patient satisfies the criteria in Table 132-1, discontinuation must be considered. Although many indices can help predict, a short CPAP, low-level PS, or spontaneous breathing trial using some of the simple assessment criteria in Table 132-2 is probably the best. Patients likely to be capable of ventilator discontinuation can be identified in this fashion.

Patients who do not succeed in this trial are probably best served by a weaning protocol rather than assist-control ventilation rest. When one is designing the protocol, the approach to assessment and adjustment is probably more important than the actual partial support mode used; however, three considerations may be important in selecting mode.

1. Pressure-targeted modes do offer improved flow synchrony and more physiologic muscle loading than flow-limited volume target breaths alternating with spontaneous breaths.
2. Combining two modes of support, such as IMV and substantial pressure support, may unnecessarily complicate the weaning process; that is, two types of support must be adjusted to be aggressive.
3. If a back-up mandatory breath rate is desired, adding a breath rate to PA (i.e., pressure assist-control) or using a minimum minute ventilation back-up mode is often more comfortable than supplying irregular patterns of support with modes such as IMV.

Once the weaning process has begun, regular assessment and adjustment (e.g., every 4 hours) are mandatory to provide

TABLE 132–5. Automated Weaning Approaches

Mode	Strategy	Weaning Accomplished By
Mandatory minute ventilation	Adjusts IMV rate to ensure minimum minute ventilation	IMV rate decreased if MV maintained
Volume support	Adjusts PS level to ensure minimum V_T	PS level reduced if V_T maintained
Volume-assured pressure support/pressure augmentation	Provides a back-up flow/V_T to the PS breath	PS level reduced by clinician while machine provides "safety net" V_T

IMV = intermittent mandatory ventilation; PS = pressure support; V_T = tidal volume; MV = minute ventilation.

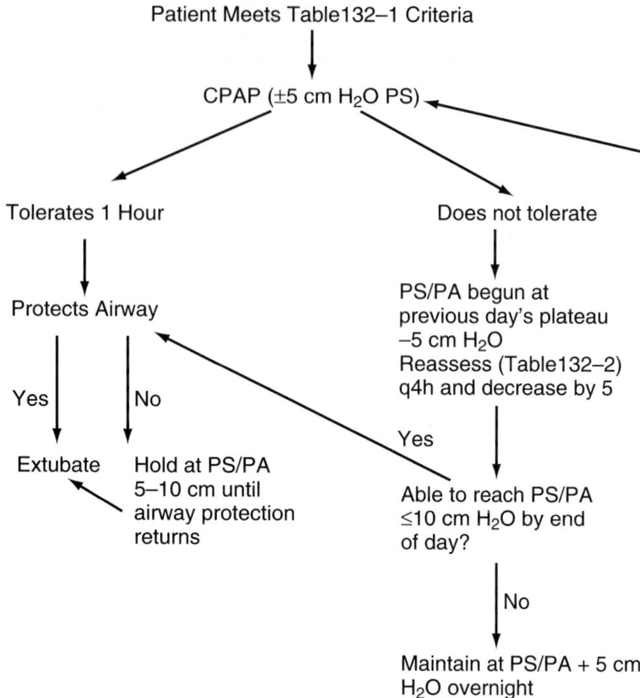

Figure 132–5. A proposed weaning strategy. PA = pressure assist; PS = pressure support.

aggressive and safe weaning. A proposed scheme is given in Figure 132-5.

SUMMARY

As shown in Table 132-4, the weaning strategy can have profound effects on ventilator length of stay. Ventilator management keys to successful weaning are (1) appropriate aggressiveness (i.e., frequent assessments and adjustments), (2) maximal patient comfort, and (3) proper muscle loading. Weaning success also depends on proper management of nutrition, psychologic needs, infection control, fluid balance, and pulmonary toilet. Although truly difficult-to-wean patients constitute only a minority of ventilated patients, their management can consume considerable intensive care unit resources.

References

1. Esteban A, Frutos F, Tobin MJ, et al: A comparison of four methods of weaning from mechanical ventilation. N Engl J Med 1995; 332:345-350.
2. Brochard L, Ramos A, Benito S, et al: Comparison of these methods of gradual withdrawal from ventilatory support during weaning from mechanical ventilation. Am J Respir Crit Care Med 1994; 150:896-903.
3. Fulkerson WJ, MacIntyre NR: Problems in Respiratory Care: Complications of Mechanical Ventilation. Philadelphia, JB Lippincott, 1991.
4. Laghi F, D'Alfonso N, Tobin MJ: Pattern of recovery from diaphragmatic fatigue over 24 hours. J Appl Physiol 1995; 79:539-546.
5. Sahn SA, Lakschminarayan MB: Bedside criteria for the discontinuation of mechanical ventilation. Chest 1973; 63:1002-1005.
6. Morganroth ML, Morganroth JL, Nett LM, et al: Criteria for weaning from prolonged mechanical ventilation. Arch Intern Med 1984; 144:1012-1016.
7. Yang K, Tobin MJ: A prospective study of indexes predicting outcome of trials of weaning from mechanical ventilation. N Engl J Med 1991; 324:1445-1450.
8. Gluck EH: Predicting eventual success of failure to wean in patients receiving long term mechanical ventilation. Chest 1996; 110:1018-1024.
9. Tobin MJ: Respiratory muscles in disease. Clin Chest Med 1988; 9:263-286.
10. Collett PW, Perry C, Engel LA: Pressure time product, flow, and oxygen cost of resistive breathing in humans. J Appl Physiol 1985; 58:1263-1272.
11. Bellemare F, Grassino A: Effect of pressure and timing or contraction on human diaphragm fatigue. J Appl Physiol 1982; 53:1190-1195.
12. MacIntyre NR, Leatherman NE: Mechanical loads on the ventilatory muscles: A theoretical analysis. Am Rev Respir Dis 1989; 139:968-973.
13. Ashutosh K, Hyukjoon L, Mohan CK, et al: Prediction criteria for successful weaning from respiratory support. Crit Care Med 1992; 20:1295-1301.
14. Ely EW, Baker AM, Dunagan DP, et al: Effect on the duration of mechanical ventilation of identifying patients capable of breathing spontaneously. N Engl J Med 1996; 335:1864-1869.
15. Argov Z, Mastaglia FL: Disorders of neuromuscular transmission caused by drugs. N Engl J Med 1979; 301:409-413.
16. Lemaire F, Teboul JL, Cinotti L, et al: Acute left ventricular dysfunction during unsuccessful weaning from mechanical ventilation. Anesthesiology 1988; 69:171-179.
17. Hussain SNA, Simkus T, Roussos C: Respiratory muscle fatigue: A cause of ventilatory failure in septic shock. J Appl Physiol 1985; 58:2033-2040.
18. Roussos CS, Macklem PT: Diaphragmatic fatigue in man. J Appl Physiol 1977; 43:189-197.
19. Agusti AGN, Torres A, Estopa R, Agustividal A: Hypophosphatemia as a cause of failed weaning: The importance of metabolic factors. Crit Care Med 1984; 12:142-143.
20. Molloy DW, Dhingra S, Solven F, et al: Hypomagnesemia and respiratory muscle power. Am Rev Respir Dis 1984; 129:497-498.
21. Bark H, Heimer D, Chaimowitz C, Mostoslowski M: Effect of chronic renal failure on respiratory muscle strength. Respiration 1988; 54:151-163.
22. Pingleton SK, Harmon GS: Nutritional management in acute respiratory failure. JAMA 1987; 257:2094-2099.
23. MacIntyre NR, Ho L: Weaning mechanical ventilatory support. Anesth Reports 1990; 3:211-215.
24. Auzueto A, Peters JI, Tobin MJ, et al: Effects of prolonged controlled mechanical ventilation on diaphragmatic function in healthy adult baboons. Crit Care Med 1997; 25:1187-1190.
25. Marini JJ: Exertion during ventilator support: How much and how important? Respir Care 1986; 31:385-387.
26. Roussos CS, Macklem PT: The respiratory muscles. N Engl J Med 1982; 307:786-797.
27. MacIntyre NR: Weaning from mechanical ventilatory support: Volume-assisting intermittent breaths versus pressure-assisting every breath. Respir Care 1988; 33:121-125.
28. Brochard L, Harf A, Lorino H, et al: Pressure support prevents diaphragmatic failure during weaning from mechanical ventilation. Am Rev Respir Dis 1989; 139:513-521.
29. MacIntyre NR, McConnell R, Cheng KC, Sane A: Pressure limited breaths improve flow dys-synchrony during assisted ventilation. Crit Care Med 1997; 25:1671-1677.
30. McGregor M, Becklake MR: The relationship of oxygen cost of breathing to respiratory mechanical work and respiratory force. J Clin Invest 1961; 40:971-980.
31. Leith DE, Bradley M: Ventilatory muscle strength and endurance training. J Appl Physiol 1976; 41:508-516.
32. Kollef MH, Shapiro SD, Silver P, et al: A randomized controlled trial of protocol directed vs physician directed weaning from mechanical ventilation. Crit Care Med 1997; 25:567-574.
33. Jabour ER, Rabil DM, Truwit JD, Rochester DF: Evaluation of a new weaning index based on ventilatory endurance and the efficiency of gas exchange. Am Rev Respir Dis 1991; 144:531-537.

133

Acute Parenchymal Disease in Childhood

Robert Katz, MD

Disorders of respiratory system structure and function with subsequent respiratory failure are a frequent cause for the admission of children to the pediatric intensive care unit. In a survey of 160 pediatric intensive care units, respiratory failure accounted for 31% of all admissions.[1] Although the management of acute parenchymal processes in infants and children is based on the same principles as that for adults, differences in physiology, etiologic agents, and technical needs exist between pediatric and adult patients; these differences are emphasized in this chapter.

ASSESSMENT OF RESPIRATORY STATUS

The manifestations of respiratory failure are not always evident, and precise assessment of a patient's ventilatory status must be based on both clinical and laboratory values. Attention should first be devoted to respiratory rate and to the pattern of breathing. The respiratory rate decreases with age and shows its greatest variability in newborn and young infants (Table 133–1). Tachypnea may be the first manifestation of respiratory distress in infants. With respect to the pattern of breathing, objective signs that indicate respiratory distress include chest wall retractions, visible use of accessory muscles, flaring of the alae nasi, and paradoxical respiratory movements. Visible contraction of the sternocleidomastoid muscles and the drawing in of the supraclavicular fossa are among the most reliable clinical signs of airway obstruction. Grunting is produced when premature glottic closure accompanies active chest wall contraction during early expiration. Infants and children grunt to increase airway pressure and, thus, functional residual capacity.

Clinical criteria also include the effects of alterations of arterial blood gas tensions and pH on other organ systems. These may include restlessness, irritability, mood changes that progress to seizures, and coma. Cardiovascular effects range from tachycardia to bradycardia, blood pressure changes, and cardiac arrest. General fatigue and excessive sweating may also be useful clinical indicators of acute respiratory failure.

Arterial blood gas measurements are almost always necessary if an accurate assessment of a child's ventilatory status is to be made. Numerous studies (mainly in adults) have shown that clinical estimation of arterial oxygen and carbon dioxide partial pressures are often unreliable. Any patient who has an unexplained sign such as confusion or cyanosis, is in an obtunded or comatose state, or has symptoms such as dyspnea, anxiety, or restlessness may have respiratory failure, and arterial blood gases should be measured.

TABLE 133–1. Normal Respiratory Rates

Age	Breaths per Minute
Newborn (after 7 days)	30
6 mo	28
1 yr	24
3 yr	22
5 yr	20
8 yr	18
12 yr	16
15 yr	14

INDICATIONS FOR INTUBATION AND MECHANICAL VENTILATION

The decision to intubate and commence mechanical ventilation should be based on assessment of clinical parameters, serial measurement of arterial blood gases, and knowledge of the natural histories of the disease process affecting a particular child.

Clinical criteria should include the status of a patient's central nervous system, hemodynamic stability, and adequacy of the work of breathing and of the overall capacity of a patient to maintain sufficient respiratory effort. Clinical signs of significant deterioration include uncontrolled restlessness, anxious expression, lack of response to physical stimuli, and limpness. Severe changes in heart rate or blood pressure, which are indicative of hemodynamic instability, are also signs that cardiopulmonary collapse may be imminent. Significant changes in the respiratory system, such as marked decrease in breath sounds, loss of the ability to cry, and apnea, are indications for securing of the airway and for providing ventilatory assessment.

Serial evaluation of arterial blood gases provides invaluable information when one must decide whether mechanical ventilation is indicated. In general, blood gas criteria for initiating mechanical ventilation in infants and children are similar to those in adults. The following are generally accepted criteria for assisting ventilation:

- Arterial carbon dioxide partial pressures that are greater than 50 to 60 mm Hg (in the absence of chronic lung disease) or that rise at a rate greater than 5 mm Hg/hr
- Partial pressure of oxygen less than 60 mm Hg
- Fraction of inspired oxygen greater than 60%

Initiating mechanical ventilation in a critically ill child may be difficult for the physician who does not treat children on a regular basis. Because uncuffed tubes are used in most infants and children, an air leak that can result in significant volume loss in the compressible spaces in the ventilator is usually present.

An approach to the initiation of mechanical ventilation in the infant and child is outlined in Figure 133–1. A fraction of inspired oxygen from 0.90 to 1.0 minimizes the risk of hypoxia. Providing positive end-expiratory pressure (PEEP) of from 3 to 5 cm H_2O tends to maintain functional residual capacity and improve oxygenation. Maintenance of an inspiratory time of at least 0.75 seconds provides even distribution of ventilation while limiting peak airway pressure. The frequency of assisted breaths depends on the age of the child:

- 20 to 25 breaths, for infants younger than 2 years of age
- 15 to 20 breaths, for children 2 to 10 years of age
- 10 to 15 breaths, for patients older than 10 years of age

Initial tidal volume is best selected on the basis of clinical judgment, which includes observation of adequate chest wall excursion and audible air entry. Usually, this will be a tidal volume of 8 to 10 mL/kg. Maintenance of adequate minute ventilation should reduce a patient's work of breathing and dyspnea. Peak pressures usually range from 20 to 35 cm H_2O, depending on the severity of the pulmonary process.

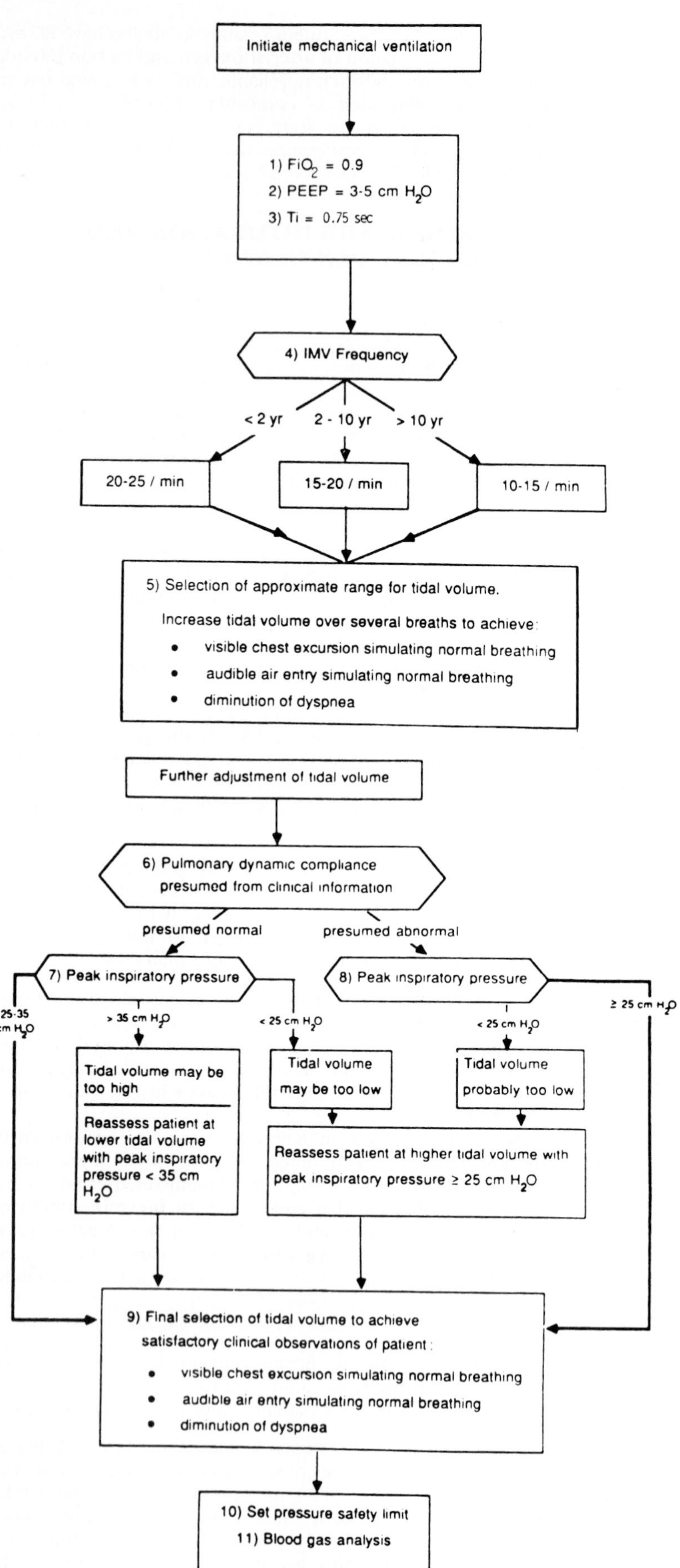

Figure 133–1. Algorithm for the initiation of mechanical ventilation in the pediatric patient. (From Kanter RK: Evaluation and stabilization of the critically ill child. Clin Chest Med 1987; 8:576–577.)

Immediately after stabilization with the ventilator has been achieved, adequacy should be assessed based on data from arterial blood gas measurement or from noninvasive modalities, such as pulse oximetry and end-tidal carbon dioxide monitoring.

PARENCHYMAL DISEASES

Viral Pneumonia

Respiratory viruses are responsible for most pediatric lower respiratory tract infections, including pneumonia. It is estimated that about 80% to 85% of cases of pediatric pneumonia are caused by viruses following direct invasion of the lower respiratory tract. Epidemiologic factors, such as the time of year and the child's age, may aid the clinician in differentiating viral from bacterial pneumonia. However, these factors do not provide much assistance in differentiating the sporadic bacterial infections that occur throughout the respiratory disease season. This becomes important when the clinician is deciding whether to initiate antibiotic therapy in a child with pneumonia.

In general, bacterial infections produce infiltrates that are well defined, involve only one lobe, and are more likely to be located in the medial or peripheral lung field. Fluid in the pleural space and abscess or pneumatocele formation are considered characteristic of bacterial infection. In contrast, infiltrates that result from viral infections are likely to be poorly defined, to involve more than one lobe, and to be located in the perihilar areas. Scattered areas of atelectasis or right upper lobe atelectasis is usually associated with viral infections.

Respiratory syncytial virus (RSV) is the most important nonbacterial pathogen to infect the respiratory tract during early life. RSV may cause bronchiolitis, pneumonia, or upper airway obstruction. Most cases of RSV infection occur in the first 3 years of life and occasionally in patients aged 5 to 7 years. At particular high risk for RSV are premature infants and infants with congenital heart disease or bronchopulmonary dysplasia. The usual illness begins with a low-grade fever and signs of upper respiratory tract infection. Coughing increases over the first 3 days of illness, and wheezing may also be present. More severe involvement develops for about 1% of infants during the first year of life and is evidenced by intercostal retractions and tachypnea.

Diagnosis of RSV infection may be made on the basis of clinical grounds in addition to knowledge of the presence of the virus in the community. Fluorescent antibody slide tests for rapid diagnosis are performed in most laboratories.

Since 1992, inhaled ribavirin (Virazole) has been available to treat infants infected with RSV who have moderate to severe disease.[2] A thorough evaluation of all the studies of ribavirin document a moderate effect at best, and many centers are no longer employing the drug except in unusual circumstances.

Bronchospasm is frequently noted in infants infected with RSV. Several studies have indicated that the status of many of these infants improves after administration of an inhaled $beta_2$ agonist, such as albuterol.[3] The usual initial dose of albuterol is 0.15 mg/kg by nebulization; administration of this dose may be repeated every 20 minutes if necessary. Nebulized racemic epinepherine may also decrease bronchial edema and improve respiratory mechanics in these infants.

Parainfluenza viruses account for about the same total morbidity as does RSV. Parainfluenza virus type 3, like RSV, may produce serious lower respiratory tract infection in infants. The clinical course and radiographic findings for patients with parainfluenza pneumonia are similar to those for RSV.

Influenza viruses are the most important causes of pneumonia that leads to hospitalization of school-age children. The morbidity rates for infants and preschool-aged children with influenza viruses are also considerable and rank just behind those for RSV and parainfluenza viruses. The clinical course of influenza virus infection is usually more abrupt and intense than the course of other respiratory viral infections. A high fever is common; older children complain of myalgia and headache. A dry, hacking cough usually precedes the development of pneumonitis. Chest radiography findings include the presence of multiple areas of atelectasis and of infiltrates that involve multiple lobes.

Influenza A virus infections can be treated with amantadine hydrochloride. Several studies have demonstrated that therapy with this drug shortens the course of uncomplicated influenza infection in otherwise healthy young adults and children if it is instituted within the first 48 hours of illness. Amantadine is not effective for the treatment of *influenza B virus* infections.

Although *adenoviruses* are an uncommon cause of pneumonia in infants and children, adenoviruses types 7, 14, and 21 are associated with severe necrotizing pneumonia and respiratory failure. Mortality rates from infections with these adenoviruses range from 10% to 17%. Most infants with severe disease are younger than 18 months of age. Clinically, the course can be very protracted, with tachypnea, cough, and wheezing persisting for weeks. Treatment is supported with mechanical ventilation, if necessary. Patients with adenovirus infections have a high incidence of residual pulmonary function abnormalities and bronchiectasis.[4]

Viral infections of the lung follow certain clinical and epidemiologic patterns; knowledge of these patterns is useful in determining proper management for the patient with pneumonia. The course of viral pneumonia is not altered by the administration of antibiotics, and bacterial superinfections are so uncommon (especially in patients with RSV infections) that the routine use of antimicrobial agents is not warranted. Most children with viral pneumonia who require intensive care are younger than 3 years of age. It is unusual for older children with viral pneumonia (except those with chronic cardiopulmonary disease) to require ventilatory assistance.

Bacterial Pneumonia

The bacterial pathogens causing pneumonia vary with the age of a patient as well as with the patient's immune status and environmental conditions. The most common of these pathogens in newborns are group B streptococci followed by gram-negative enteric bacilli and chlamydiae. In children between the ages of 1 month and 6 years, *Streptococcus pneumoniae* and *Haemophilus influenzae* B are the most common pathogens. The latter is especially likely in children between the ages of 4 months and 2 years and often is associated with bacteremia. In adolescents, *Mycoplasma pneumoniae* and *S. pneumoniae* are the most common causative agents. However, much overlap exists, and the age of the child is only one factor in elucidating the cause of the pneumonia.

It is difficult to determine the percentage of pneumonia cases that are caused by bacteria. Unless a patient is bacteremic, has pleural empyema, or has antigenuria, opportunities to establish a cause are limited. It is estimated that a causative agent is defined in less than 25% of hospitalized children with pneumonia.[5]

Although the blood culture is a specific method for establishing a cause, its results are positive only in 10% to 15% of cases and mainly in younger children with pneumonia caused by *H. influenzae, Staphylococcus aureus,* or *S. pneumoniae.* Because of the associated risks of bacteremia, cultures are warranted for any child with suspected bacterial pneumonia before antibiotic therapy is initiated. A diligent search should be made for other sites of infection (e.g., joints, pleural space, meninges), and the appropriate fluids should be collected for culture.

Staphylococcal pneumonia in infants usually develops as a primary infection of the respiratory tract or as part of a septicemic infection. Infection of the respiratory tract may rapidly produce severe distress characterized by tachypnea, grunting respirations, retractions, and cyanosis. Many infants with staphylococcal pneumonia are often gravely ill.

Diagnosis is based on a patient's history, radiography findings, and positive culture results. The radiography ray findings of staphylococcal pneumonia distinguish it from other types of pneumonia, especially in infants. Within a few hours, radiography findings can change from small infiltrative lesions to patchy consolidation, to pneumatocele and empyema formation. Pneumothorax, pyopneumothorax, and bronchopleural fistula are not uncommon. Blood culture results are positive in 9% to 25% of cases.[6] Empyema is almost universal, and cultures of pleural fluid invariably yield positive results.

Staphylococcal pneumonia is an acute medical emergency that requires early, maximum, and prolonged antibiotic therapy if tissue necrosis and the tendency for bacterial persistence, which provide a potential focus for relapse, are to be avoided. Initial treatment should be with a parenteral β-lactamase-resistant antibiotic, such as nafcillin or methicillin. Chest radiography performed daily is necessary so that possible pneumothorax, pneumatocele, empyema, or pyopneumothorax can be watched for. Pneumatoceles usually resolve spontaneously and do not necessitate needle aspiration or surgical intervention. However, if the bullae mechanically compress the trachea or mainstem bronchi, aspiration or excision may be necessary. Early closed-chest tube drainage is the preferred treatment for empyema or pyopneumothorax. This procedure is much more effective than repeated aspiration.

Despite the use of effective antimicrobial agents and the availability of intensive care, the mortality associated with staphylococcal pneumonia remains high, with most deaths occurring in infants younger than 1 year of age. For the surviving children, abnormalities revealed on radiography may persist for weeks or months; however, the prognosis for pulmonary function is excellent.

Pneumococcal pneumonia is caused by *S. pneumoniae,* the organism most frequently responsible for bacterial pneumonia. The incubation period is 1 to 3 days, and the onset of pneumonia is heralded by coughing, severe shaking, chills, and high fever. Patchy bronchopneumonia is more common than lobar consolidation, particularly during the first year of life. Pneumococcal bacteremia develops in about 25% to 33% of patients; this worsens the prognosis because it introduces extrapulmonary complications, including empyema, pericarditis, and meningitis. However, most infants with pneumococcal pneumonia do not require intensive care unless these complications develop. The treatment of choice is therapy with penicillin.

Before the introduction of the conjugated vaccine given to all infants, *H. influenzae* was an important etiologic agent of pneumonia in children between the ages of 3 months and 2 years.[6] Cases are now restricted to unvaccinated children and occasional infections with other strains of *H. influenzae.* Radiography demonstrates consolidative pneumonia in most patients. The incidence of pleural effusions, particularly empyema, appears to be high, as does the incidence of positive blood culture results. Extrapulmonary infection sites are common, and *H. influenzae* may be recovered from cerebrospinal fluid, joint fluid, or pericardial fluid in affected children. Clinically, it may be difficult to differentiate pneumonia caused by *H. influenzae* from pneumococcal or, occasionally, staphylococcal infections. About 25% of *H. influenzae* type B strains in the United States are β-lactamase producers.[7] Therefore, standard initial therapy consists of administration of one of the third-generation cephalosporins, such as cefuroxime, cefotaxime, or ceftriaxone.

Adult Respiratory Distress Syndrome

Adult respiratory distress syndrome (ARDS) is a major cause of death in children receiving intensive care for sepsis and has been associated with mortality rates of from 50% to 90%.[8-10] Septic shock, pneumonia, and near-drowning are the most common precipitating events. ARDS has been described in neonates as well.[11]

Children who are at risk for ARDS should be carefully monitored in a pediatric intensive care unit. Respiratory rates should be compared with age-related normal values (see Table 133–1). Respiratory rates consistently above normal may indicate increasing atelectasis and worsening compliance. Serial evaluation of arterial blood gases is essential if incipient pulmonary dysfunction is to be detected. The use of pulse oximeters for the continuous monitoring of saturation is extremely helpful in this setting. Indications for intubation are similar to those described previously in this chapter.

Respiratory assistance remains the keystone of supportive care for the patient with ARDS; however, despite many technologic improvements in this form of therapy, mortality rates remain high. A new generation of ventilators with microprocessor controls, continuous flow systems, and a number of different modes of ventilation are now available for the management of children with severe respiratory failure. However, it is still not clear which is the optimal approach in a child with ARDS.

The application of PEEP improves oxygenation in most patients with ARDS. The improvement in arterial oxygen partial pressure is usually due to a decrease in shunt perfusion, with occasional decreases in blood flow to areas with a low area ventilation-perfusion ratio.[15] Despite this effect of PEEP, considerable controversy exists regarding the level of PEEP to be used for ARDS patients. Although a variety of endpoints have been suggested, no data prove that one is better than another.[16] However, it is clear that the response to any PEEP increment cannot be predicted from the characteristics of the patient or of gas exchange before the application of PEEP.

It is important to apply PEEP in a controlled manner (e.g., in 3- to 5-cm H_2O increments), with arterial blood gas measurements performed 15 to 20 minutes after each increase. Ideally, 90% saturation should be achieved with a fraction of inspired oxygen of less than 0.6. With the judicious use of fluids or inotropes, cardiac function can be maintained in children subjected to high PEEP levels.[17] In fact, the highly compliant chest wall in children should lessen the transmission of positive airway pressure to the heart and great vessels.[18]

Weaning small infants and children from mechanical ventilation is complicated by the scant information available on the reliability of mechanical variables of patients in this age group. Most reports in this area have addressed weaning from mechanical ventilation after cardiovascular surgery in infants without severe parenchymal disease. Because vital capacity, peak negative pressure, and tidal volume do not usually reflect the ability to wean, intermittent mandatory ventilation is very useful in weaning these patients. Ventilator breaths should be reduced three to five at a time, and serial evaluations of respiratory rate, breathing patterns, and blood gases should be performed. A marked increase in respiratory rate, development of carbon dioxide retention, or metabolic acidosis secondary to an increase in the work of breathing is an indication that weaning should be stopped and the ventilatory rate increased. At all times, 3- to 5-cm H_2O PEEP should be used, as the absence of this physiologic level may lead to decreases in functional residual capacity and hypoxemia.

A number of new therapeutic approaches and maneuvers have been published in the management of children with respiratory failure from ARDS. Although many of these techniques show promise, their precise role in the management of the pediatric patient with severe respiratory failure has not yet been determined.

Prone Positioning

Two small studies have examined the effects of prone positioning on arterial blood gases in children with a variety of acute lung diseases. In one study of seven children with ARDS, there was a consistent improvement in oxygenation.[23] The changes in arterial $Pa{O_2}$ were seen almost immediately. The other study, which consisted of children with a variety of lung diseases, did not show results that were as consistent.[24] If turning a patient prone is done with care, complications are minimal. In patients who are severely hypoxemic, a trial of prone positioning is a reasonable step.

Pressure-Controlled Inverse Ratio Ventilation

Pressure-controlled inverse ratio ventilation (PC-IRV) has been used successfully in adults with bilateral parenchymal diseases and respiratory failure.[25] Lengthening of the inspiratory time has been used for many years in neonatal intensive care to improve oxygenation and lessen barotrauma. There have been scattered reports of the use of this technique in children with acute respiratory failure.[26, 27]

These cases have demonstrated that it is possible to ventilate children in this manner. There are not enough data to prove whether this mode of ventilation will result in decreases in mortality and/or morbidity.

High-Frequency Oscillation

High-frequency oscillation (HFO) is a mode of ventilation that uses small tidal volumes (1 to 3 mL/kg) at a very high frequency (300 to 600 breaths/min). Arnold initially demonstrated that HFO was able to be used successfully as "rescue" therapy in seven children with severe ARDS.[28] A subsequent multi-institutional randomized trial comparing HFO with conventual mechanical ventilation in children with severe respiratory failure showed reduced morbidity and mortality rates for the HFO group while adequate oxygenation was achieved without a decrease in cardiac function or increased barotrauma.[29] As a result of this study and others, HFO has become a commonly used mode of ventilation in children with severe acute respiratory failure.[30]

Nitric Oxide

Inhaled nitric oxide (NO) is a potent pulmonary vasodilator (with minimal systemic effects) and also has been shown to improve oxygenation in the setting of diffuse parenchymal disease.[31] A number of studies have examined the effects of inhaled nitric oxide in children with severe respiratory failure.[32, 33] In most studies, nitric oxide proved to be safe, although its effect on individual patients was variable and difficult to predict. Children who did respond demonstrated decreases in pulmonary artery pressure and pulmonary resistance and an improvement in oxygenation. Adverse systemic side effects were not noted in any of the studies. Although this therapy appears promising, a recent randomized controlled study in adults with ARDS—while showing an improvement in oxygenation and lack of serious side effects—did not demonstrate any effect of inhaled nitric oxide on mortality or morbidity.[34] A similar study in the pediatric population has not been performed.

Extracorporeal Membrane Oxygenation

Extracorporeal membrane oxygenation (ECMO) has been used successfully in neonates with pulmonary hypertension since the mid-1980s. As a result, there is renewed interest in applying this technique to infants and children with severe respiratory failure who are unresponsive to conventional therapy.[35] Indications for ECMO in this population are evolving but are generally thought to be alveolar-arterial gradients greater than 400 to 500 mm Hg or other measurements of severe failure of oxygenation.[36, 37] At present, there are no definitive data that the use of ECMO can alter the mortality in infants and children with severe respiratory failure.

PULMONARY CONTUSION

The types of thoracic injury that affect children depend on age and on the pediatric population studied. *Blunt chest injury* tends to be an injury of infancy and early childhood, whereas penetrating trauma is more common in adolescents. In a series of 199 patients, the incidence of blunt trauma far exceeded that of other types of trauma until the age of 13 years was reached.[20] In children older than 13 years of age, penetrating injury was more frequent and followed the adult pattern. In a series of 94 children with chest trauma reviewed by Smyth,[21] 86 had closed-chest injury and only eight sustained penetrating injuries. The most frequent cause of closed-chest injury was road traffic accidents. In 70 such cases, 68 children were pedestrians and only two were passengers in vehicles.

A *pulmonary contusion* is a blunt parenchymal injury that produces edema, hemorrhage, or desquamative alveolitis. Microscopically, the changes found in pulmonary contusion vary in degree and distribution, depending on the severity of the injury. Minimal damage produces only focal areas of interstitial edema, whereas severe injury causes a rapid intra-alveolar extravasation of blood with consolidation of the lungs.

Clinically, pulmonary contusion may lead to hypoxemia, tachypnea, reduced pulmonary compliance, and, ultimately, acute respiratory failure. Because a child's thorax is more elastic than an adult's, fractured ribs are generally less common in children than in adults even if a severe, crushing force has been exerted. Some series have documented higher mortality in patients without rib fractures; it has been postulated that fractures of the sternum or ribs expend a portion of the force applied to the chest wall and thus reduce injury to the underlying lung. Flail chest is also less common in children than in adults owing to the lower prevalence of rib fractures.

Significant thoracic injury is frequently a component of multisystemic injuries; therefore, management must address the possibility of multiple organ failure. Mortality is related to the number of organs injured. In Smyth's study,[21] 10 of the 13 deaths reported were due to nonthoracic trauma; chest trauma was the cause of death in only three children. Other studies of children have reported mortality rates from pulmonary contusion of 4% to 15%.

Initially, the clinical and radiographic appearance of the child with pulmonary contusion may be misleading. Some patients are asymptomatic and have normal chest radiographs or minimal patchy consolidation. Pulmonary contusion may be easily overlooked in the absence of rib fractures or when multiple injuries, especially those of the head or the abdomen, demand urgent attention. Concomitant pneumothorax or hemothorax may mask the underlying parenchymal damage. Auscultation of the chest may only reveal a few rales. In more severe cases, the sputum may be tinged with blood.

All children who have suffered thoracic or multiple injuries should be carefully monitored in an intensive care unit. The value of initial and serial arterial blood gas determinations cannot be overemphasized; in many instances, the severity of insult is not appreciated until blood gas analyses are performed. Although initial chest radiographs may be unremarkable, parenchymal injury, if present, is readily apparent within 24 hours. Criteria for intubation and aspects of ventilatory management are the same as those described earlier.

Secondary bacterial pneumonias are common in patients with pulmonary contusions. Infection should be suspected in patients who initially respond to treatment with an improvement in gas exchange but then deteriorate. Tracheal secretions should be obtained for Gram's staining and culturing, and appropriate antibiotics should be administered. Prophylactic antibiotic administration appears to be of little value in preventing infection following blunt or penetrating trauma.[22]

References

1. Groeger J, Guntupalli K, Strosberg M: Descriptive analysis of critical care units in the United States: Patient characteristics and intensive care unit utilization. Crit Care Med 1993; 21:279.
2. Hall CB, McBride JT, Gala CL, et al: Ribavirin treatment of respiratory syncytial viral infection in infants with underlying cardiopulmonary disease. JAMA 1985; 254:3047.
3. Schuh S, Ganny C, Reisman J: Nebulized albuterol in acute bronchiolitis. J Pediatr 1990; 117:633.
4. Becroft DM: Histopathology of fatal adenovirus infection of the respiratory tract in young children. J Clin Pathol 1967; 20:445.
5. Grossman M, Klein J, McCarthy P: Consensus: Management of presumed bacterial pneumonia in ambulatory children. Pediatr Infect Dis 1984; 3:497.
6. Yeto SD, Heller R: Acute respiratory infections. Pediatr Clin North Am 1974; 21:683.
7. Freij B: Pneumonia of known etiology. *In*: Current Therapy in Pediatric Infectious Disease. Nelson JD (Ed). New York, BC Decker, 1986, pp 25–34.
8. Lyrene R, Truog W: Adult respiratory distress syndrome in a pediatric intensive care unit: Predisposing conditions, clinical course and outcome. Pediatrics 1981; 67:790.
9. Holbrook PR, Taylor GT, Pollack MM, et al: Adult respiratory distress syndrome in children. Pediatr Clin North Am 1980; 27:677.
10. Timmons OD, Dean JM, Vernon DD: Mortality rates and prognostic variables in children with adult respiratory distress syndrome. J Pediatr 1991; 199:896–899.
11. Pfenninger J, Tschaeppeler H, Wagner BP: The paradox of adult respiratory distress syndrome in neonates. Pediatr Pulmonol 1991; 10:18.
12. Weisman JM, Rinaldo JE, Rogers RN, et al: Intermittent mandatory ventilation. Am Rev Respir Dis 1985; 127:641.
13. Christopher KL, Niff TA, Bowan JS: Demand and continuous flow intermittent mandatory ventilation systems. Chest 1985; 87:625.
14. Cox D, Niblett DJ: Studies on continuous positive airway pressure breathing systems. Br J Anaesth 1984; 56:905.
15. Ralph DD, Robertson HT, Weaver JL, et al: Distribution of ventilation and perfusion during positive and expiratory pressure in the adult respiratory distress syndrome. Am Rev Respir Dis 1985; 131:54.
16. Albert RK: Least PEEP: Primum non nocere. Chest 1985; 7:2.
17. Katz R, Pollack M, Spady D: Cardiopulmonary abnormalities in severe acute respiratory failure. J Pediatr 1984; 194:357.
18. Bryan AC, Mansell AL, Levison H: Development of the mechanical properties of the respiratory system. *In*: Development of the Lung. Hodson WA (Ed). New York, Marcel Dekker, 1977, pp 445–468.
19. Pollack MM, Fields AL, Holbrook PR: Pneumothorax and pneumomediastinum during pediatric mechanical ventilation. Crit Care Med 1979; 7:536.
20. Sinclair MC, Moore TC: Major surgery for abdominal and thoracic trauma in childhood and adolescence. J Pediatr Surg 1974; 9:155.
21. Smyth BT: Chest trauma in childhood. J Pediatr Surg 1979; 14:41.
22. Mandal AK, Montano J, Ihadepalli H: Prophylactic antibiotics and no antibiotics compared in penetrating chest trauma. J Trauma 1985; 25:639.
23. Murdock IA, Storman MO: Improved arterial oxygenation in children with adult respiratory distress syndrome: the prone position. Acta Paediatr 1994; 83:1043.
24. Numa AH, Hammer J, Newth CJL: Effect of prone and supine positions on functional residual capacity, oxygenation, and respiratory mechanics in ventilated infants and children. Am J Respir Crit Car Med 1997; 156:1185.
25. Gurevitch M, Van Dyke J, Young E, Jackson K: Improved oxygenation and lower peak airway pressure in severe adult respiratory distress syndrome: Treatment with inverse-ratio ventilation. Chest 1986; 89:211.
26. Goldstein B, Papadakos PJ: Pressure-controlled inverse-ratio ventilation in children with acute respiratory failure. Am J Crit Care 1994; 3:11.
27. Greaves TH, Cramolini GM, Walker DH, et al: Inverse-ratio ventilation in a six-year-old with severe post-traumatic adult respiratory distress syndrome. Crit Care Med 1989; 17:588.
28. Arnold JH, Truog RD, Thompson JE, et al: High frequency oscillatory ventilation in pediatric respiratory failure. Crit Care Med 1993; 21:272.
29. Arnold JH, Hanson JH, Toro-Figuero LO, et al: Prospective, randomized comparison of high-frequency oscillatory ventilation and conventional mechanical ventilation in pediatric respiratory failure. Crit Care Med 1994; 22:1530.
30. Sarnaik AP, Meert KL, Pappas MD, et al: Predicting outcome in children with severe acute respiratory failure treated with high-frequency ventilation. Crit Care Med 1996; 24:1396.
31. Nakagawa TA, Morris A, Gomez RJ, et al: Dose response to inhaled nitric oxide in pediatric patients with pulmonary hypertension and acute respiratory distress syndrome. J Pediatr 1997; 131:63.
32. Day RW, Guarin M, Lynch JM, et al: Inhaled nitric oxide in children with severe lung disease: Results of acute and prolonged therapy with two concentrations. Crit Care Med 1996; 24:215.
33. Abman SH, Griebel JL, Parker DK, et al: Acute effects of inhaled nitric oxide in children with severe hypoxemic respiratory failure. J Pediatrics 1994; 124:881.
34. Effects of inhaled nitric oxide in patients with acute respiratory distress syndrome: Results of a randomized phase II trial. Crit Care Med 1998; 96:15.
35. Moler FW, Custer JR, Bartlett RH, et al: Extracorporeal life support for severe pediatric respiratory failure: An updated experience 1991–1993. J Pediatr 1994; 124:875.
36. Green TP, Moler FW, Goodman DM: Probability of survival after prolonged extracorporeal membrane oxygenation in pediatric patients with acute respiratory failure. Crit Care Med 1995; 23:1132.
37. Moler FW, Palmisano JM, Custer JR, et al: Alveolar-arterial oxygen gradients before extracorporeal life support for severe pediatric respiratory failure: Improved outcome for extracorporeal life support-managed patients? Crit Care Med 1994; 22:620.

B. ACUTE VENTILATORY FAILURE

134

Life-Threatening Asthma

Walter J. O'Donnell, MD • Jeffrey M. Drazen, MD

The incidence of asthma and deaths due to asthma continues to increase worldwide.[1,2] Although most asthmatic patients never experience life-threatening asthma, the care of individuals with severe asthma—usually young and otherwise healthy individuals with impending or actual respiratory failure—presents a challenge to the intensivist. Appropriate treatment often, but not always, results in a salutary therapeutic outcome, whereas inappropriate treatment can lead to a complicated course or death.

DEFINITIONS

Asthma is a clinical syndrome characterized by airway inflammation and hyperresponsiveness of the airways to a variety of stimuli manifested as variable airway obstruction that resolves either spontaneously or as the result of administration of bronchodilator.[3]

Status asthmaticus is variously defined but can be summarized as evidence of persistent severe asthmatic symptoms and airways obstruction despite standard therapy for acute asthma.

Life-threatening asthma (also called "near-fatal asthma" or "potentially fatal asthma") may be referred to as asthmatic airway obstruction with ventilatory failure manifested as relative hypercapnia.

PATHOPHYSIOLOGY OF ASTHMA

Asthma as an Inflammatory Syndrome

Immunohistochemical evaluation of endobronchial biopsies performed on volunteers with mild asthma, as well as careful morphometric examination of the lungs from patients dying of status asthmaticus, has established that the airways of even mild asthmatic patients are inflamed; some data suggest that asthma severity parallels the degree of inflammation.[4,5] As shown in Table 134–1, there are three distinct components to the airway inflammation in asthma. In severe asthma the cellular characteristics of the inflammatory response are not different but they are increased in profusion. In addition, a well-established characteristic of severe asthma is the presence in the airway lumen, of highly viscous, often inspissated, secretions.

TABLE 134–1. Airway Inflammation in Asthma

Alterations in Airway Constitutive Cells
Cells, such as airway epithelial cells and mast cells, ordinarily present in the airway wall are enhanced in number and thought to adopt a proinflammatory phenotype.
Increased Numbers of Infiltrating Cells
Cells, such as eosinophils and TH_2 lymphocytes, are found in the airway wall in increased numbers.
Changes in the Noncellular Component of the Airway Wall
The airway wall is thickened beyond that which can be accounted for on the basis of the infiltrating cells alone.
There are noncellular structural alterations in the airway wall, such as changes in the basement membrane.

Alterations in Airway Constitutive Cells

It is now well established in asthma that there is both hyperplasia and hypertrophy of the cells in the airway wall, resulting in wall thickening.[6,7] Within the epithelial layer are increased numbers of surface secretory cells as well as mucous glandular hypertrophy and hyperplasia.[8,9] There is thickening of the airway smooth muscle layer.[10,11] There are increased numbers of mast cells with a proinflammatory phenotype in the airway epithelium and in the subepithelial connective tissue.[12,13] The combined effect is one that not only results in thickening of the airway wall, which promotes airway hyperresponsiveness on a simple mechanical basis,[14] but also allows for the enhanced production of *pro-phlogistic mediators* (histamine, leukotrienes [LTs], and platelet-activating factor [PAF]), and *cytokines* (interleukin-4 [IL-4], IL-5, and tumor necrosis factor-α [TNF-α]) through activation of mast cells.

Infiltration by Inflammatory Cells

The airway wall is known to be infiltrated by T lymphocytes bearing the TH_2 phenotype.[15,16] These cells have the capacity to produce IL-3, IL-4, IL-5, and granulocyte-macrophage colony-stimulating factor (GM-CSF). Although the primary signals resulting in the infiltration of the asthmatic airways by this lymphocyte subset has not been established, the net effects of these cytokines are to:

1. Promote the synthesis of immunoglobulin E (IgE).
2. Enhance the differentiation of mast cells.
3. Stimulate the differentiation and migration of eosinophils.[17,18] Indeed, infiltration by eosinophils is now recognized to be a critical component of the airway inflammation associated with asthma.[4,19]

Thickening of the Noncellular Component of the Airway Wall

The airway wall is thickened in patients with asthma. Some of the thickening can be ascribed to the cellular components already mentioned, whereas other aspects of thickening are not cellular in nature. The basement membrane is increased in thickness, with alterations in the structure of its collagen components.[7,20,21] The specific cellular events responsible for this thickening and the mechanism of collagen accumulation are not known.

Potential Schema Linking Airway Inflammation and Asthma Pathobiology

Although the anatomic alterations in the airway wall are well established, the links between the cells now known to be resident in the airway and asthma pathobiology remains speculative. A potential schema linking the known anatomic alterations with the clinical observations is shown in Figure 134–1.

As already described, an unknown stimulus results in the accumulation in the airway of lymphocytes bearing the TH_2 phenotype. The cytokines elaborated by these cells favor the synthesis of IgE and promote the recruitment of primary effector cells, most notably mast cells and eosinophils. When activated, these cells elaborate cytokines, including IL-4 and

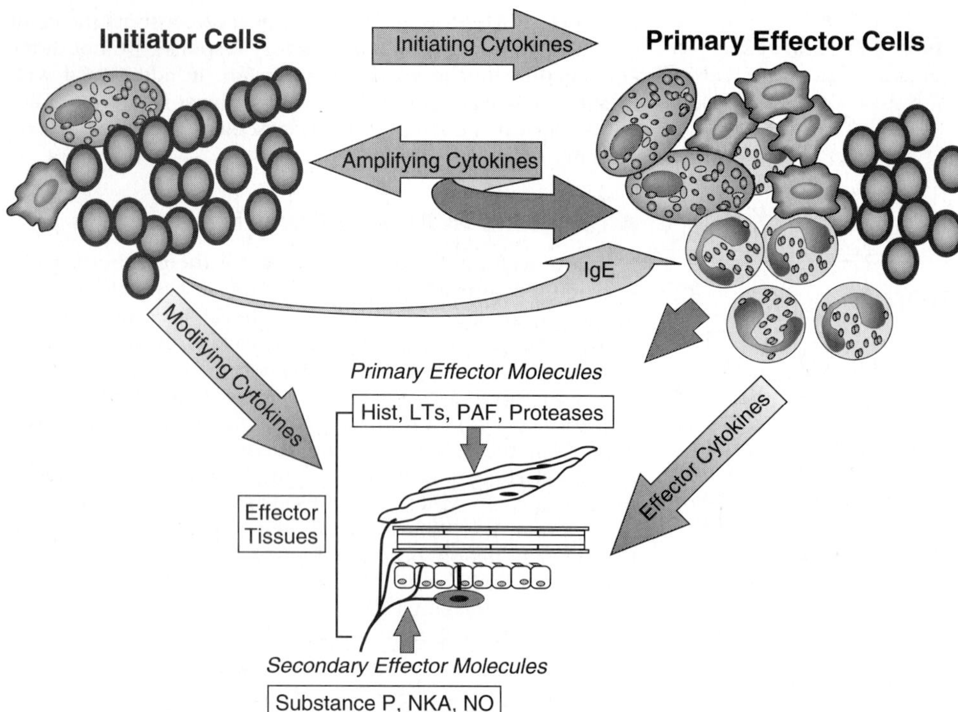

Figure 134–1. Potential schema linking airway inflammation and airway obstruction. LT = leukotriene; PAF = platelet-activating factor; IgE = immunoglobulin E.

IL-5, and mediators of inflammation, including histamine, leukotrienes, PAF, and various proteases.[22-26] The cytokines amplify the IgE and eosinophil response while the *primary effector molecules* stimulate airway smooth muscle, alter microvascular permeability and promote the release of mucins from airway glands and surface secretory cells. In addition, primary effector molecules can contribute to the inflammatory nature of the lesion; for example, PAF[25, 26] and leukotriene B_4 (LTB_4)[27, 28] are potent chemoattractants for eosinophils. As eosinophils undergo apoptosis, they release toxic proteins, further damaging airway epithelium.[29] Primary effector molecules can also stimulate sensory nerve fibers within the airway, leading to the release of *secondary effector molecules,* most notably substance P and neurokinin A. Nerve stimulation also initiates the release of both vasoactive intestinal peptide (VIP) and nitric oxide.[30-33] VIP is exclusively a *secondary inhibitory molecule;* that is, its effects are to ameliorate the actions of the pro-contractile species. Nitric oxide has a dual role both as a bronchodilator and as a proinflammatory mediator, but its precise role in status asthmaticus is not known.

In the presence of airway inflammation, as exists in status asthmaticus, not only are there more primary effector cells and, hence, more primary and secondary effector molecules; epithelial disruption also enhances antigen entry into the airway submucosa and down-regulates the cleavage of contractile neuropeptides.[30] Therefore, it is now believed that in asthma there is a primary immunologic or physical trigger that activates mast cells. This trigger leads to a series of immediate (onset, minutes to hours) and delayed (onset, hours to days) events that could account for both the rapid onset of effects as well as the slow response to treatment which characterize this disorder.

CLINICAL PRESENTATION

History

Precipitants

The most common precipitant of an acute asthmatic exacerbation is an upper respiratory tract infection, presumably viral in origin.[34] Other potential infectious etiologic factors include *Chlamydia pneumoniae* infection, which has been linked by serologic surveys to episodes of wheezing in asthmatic and nonasthmatic individuals[35] and tracheobronchitis due to *Herpes simplex*, which has been reported as a cause of refractory bronchospasm in previously nonasthmatic individuals.[36] In addition, exposure to aspirin or other nonsteroidal anti-inflammatory cyclooxygenase I inhibitors can lead to life-threatening asthma reactions in appropriately sensitive individuals.[37]

Duration

There are two common presentations of severe asthma. For most patients, before an episode of status asthmaticus, there are days to weeks of worsening asthma control and an increasing need for treatment with a beta agonist inhaler. As a result of decreased asthma control, overuse of inhaled beta agonist therapy often occurs, with many patients using medium-acting beta agonists almost continuously. The second, less common presentation occurs in a subgroup of patients with a syndrome of *sudden asphyxic asthma.* Onset of asthmatic symptoms is abrupt, and the patient presents with a "silent chest" (see later) on auscultation and progresses to severe hypercapnic respiratory failure, requiring mechanical ventilation within minutes to hours.[38, 39]

Associated Symptoms

Other symptoms of deteriorating asthma control include increasing nocturnal awakenings with breathlessness, more than a 15% decrease between peak expiratory flow determined in the evening and morning, and profound dyspnea with minimal exertion. A more atypical presentation includes a primary feature of hoarseness, cough, or nocturnal dyspnea alone.

Physical Examination

During an episode of status asthmaticus, the patient is anxious and diaphoretic and prefers to sit bolt upright; often such patients refuse to lay supine. Patients may be too breathless to furnish an adequate history. The respiratory rate is usually

25 to 30 breaths/min with a markedly prolonged expiratory phase (i.e., inspiratory/expiratory [I:E] phase ratio > 1:3). Characteristically, the accessory respiratory muscles, including the sternocleidomastoids, intercostal muscles, and abdominal muscles, are recruited during both inspiration and expiration; nasal flaring may be evident. With more severe attacks, retractions of these muscle groups and abdominal paradox (inward rather than outward movement at the onset of inspiration) may herald respiratory muscle fatigue and incipient respiratory failure.[40]

The cardiovascular examination is notable for tachycardia and pulsus paradoxus. The magnitude of pulsus paradoxus correlates with the severity of airways obstruction; inspiratory declines in systolic pressure of more than 20 mm Hg suggest severe airway obstruction.[34, 41] Auscultation of the chest reveals diffuse expiratory and inspiratory wheezes. In patients with severe bronchospasm, airflow may be so minimal as to result in an absence of wheezes; this is the so-called *silent chest sign*. More atypical auscultatory findings include rhonchi (most likely representing free mucus in the airway lumen contributing to the airflow obstruction) and focal crackles or egophony in the rare case of an coincident consolidative process, such as bacterial pneumonia.

Examination of the extremities may demonstrate eczema, consistent with the presence of an allergic diathesis in the patient. In a severe hypoxemic episode, the fingernails may be cyanotic; in simple asthma, digital clubbing should not be present. In the patient who has received chronic systemic corticosteroid therapy, cushingoid stigmata may be evident, including moon facies, centripetal fat deposition, thin extremities, and thin, easily bruised skin.

Laboratory Findings

Blood Tests

Blood eosinophilia is common.[42] Hypokalemia may occur as a result of beta agonist abuse or therapy.[43] Hypophosphatemia may also be seen, also typically in the setting of treatment; potential causes include beta agonist therapy and resolution of respiratory acidosis.[44] Hyponatremia due to inappropriate antidiuretic hormone (ADH) release has been reported.[45] Serum creatinine phosphokinase (CPK) levels, generally of the MM isozyme, may be elevated in severe asthma and have been attributed to the extreme muscular exertion required of the ventilatory muscles.[46]

Pulmonary Function Tests

In patients with inadequately controlled asthma, the peak expiratory flow rate is significantly depressed and demonstrates marked (>15% morning decrease compared with the previous evening) diurnal variation,[47] which resolves as the asthma control improves. Patients who regularly measure and record daily peak flow measurements usually document several days to weeks of depressed values and greater morning to evening differences prior to presentation. Spirometry on presentation typically evinces low flow rates, including a depressed forced expiratory volume in the first second (FEV_1), a low ratio of the FEV_1 to the forced vital capacity (FVC), and a low maximal mid-expiratory flow rate (MMEF). Plethysmographic or gas dilution measurements of lung volumes, although imperfect methods in this patient subgroup, show evidence of hyperinflation, with an increased total lung capacity, functional residual capacity (FRC) and residual volume.[48] Bronchodilator responsiveness, measured as an increase in the FEV_1 after inhalation of a beta agonist aerosol, may also be decreased or absent. With status asthmaticus, patients may be so critically ill that they cannot adequately perform the maneuvers needed to measure these indices of lung function with precision. Nevertheless, efforts should be made to record objective measures of lung function to use in assessment of the response to future treatment.

Arterial Blood Gases

Mild hypoxemia (i.e., Pa_{O_2} between 65 and 85 torr) and an increased alveolar-arterial (A − a) gradient for oxygen are common, even in mild to moderate asthma.[49] These findings have been attributed to ventilation-perfusion ($\dot{V}/Q$) mismatching caused by mucous plugging and bronchospasm. The degree of hypoxemia roughly correlates with the severity of airway obstruction and, likely as a result of the role of peripheral airways in determining overall $\dot{V}/Q$ values, shows a slower rate of resolution than does the airway obstruction.[34, 50] At the onset of therapy beta agonist therapy can aggravate, rather than ameliorate, the hypoxemia, probably by reversing hypoxic vasoconstriction and worsening $\dot{V}/Q$ mismatching.[51]

Most patients presenting with nonsevere asthma are mildly hypocapnic and therefore manifest a mild acute respiratory alkalosis. When hypercapnia occurs, it indicates severe obstruction (FEV_1 < 20% of predicted).[49] In status asthmaticus, hypercapnia (or even eucapnia) and acute respiratory acidosis on presentation or early in the course of treatment may portend an increased risk of respiratory failure. With aggressive therapy and close monitoring, however, patients in status asthmaticus presenting with normocapnia rarely progress to respiratory failure; fewer than 10% of patients presenting with hypercapnia may require mechanical ventilation, and the resolution of hypercapnia generally occurs within 8 hours in the absence of mechanical ventilation.[38]

Metabolic acidosis can occur in severe status asthmaticus; this disorder is mainly attributable to lactic acidosis from a combination of tissue hypoxia, increased work of breathing, and intracellular alkalosis, but hyperventilation-related hyperchloremic acidosis may also contribute.[52]

Sputum Examination

The sputum of an asthmatic patient in the throes of an acute attack is often laden with thick, tenacious, brownish plugs. A Gram stain of this material should be performed to exclude the possibility of a concomitant bacterial infection, particularly in the febrile patient with a productive cough. Other potential findings in the sputum include *Aspergillus* in a patient with allergic bronchopulmonary aspergillosis, Charcot-Leyden crystals (crystallized eosinophil lysophospholipase), bronchiolar casts (Curschmann's spirals) composed of cells and mucous, and Creola bodies (clusters of epithelial cells often with intact beating cilia).[53]

Thoracic Imaging

In hospitalized patients with asthma, the most common finding on the chest radiograph is hyperinflation. Clinically significant abnormalities, however, can include pneumonia, congestive heart failure, atelectasis, pneumothorax, and pneumomediastinum.[54]

Electrocardiogram

Sinus tachycardia is the most common electrocardiographic finding in patients with status asthmaticus. Other possible findings include a right axis deviation, clockwise rotation, right bundle branch, ST-segment and T-wave abnormalities, P-pulmonale, and ventricular ectopic activity.[34] This test is particularly important in the evaluation of the middle-aged or older asthmatic patient to exclude the possibility of concomitant myocardial ischemia.

MANAGEMENT

General Principles

The primary treatment of status asthmaticus includes the administration of bronchodilators to treat the airway smooth muscle spasm and systemic corticosteroids to reduce the acute local inflammatory response. Status asthmaticus is a labile condition that calls for frequent clinical and laboratory reassessment for evidence of improvement or deterioration (Table 134-2).

Primary Therapies

Beta-Adrenergic Agonists

Aerosol delivery of beta agonists by hand-held jet nebulizer, is the most common and effective method of aerosol delivery.[55] Commonly used doses of commercially available solutions (for adults) are as follows:

- Albuterol 0.5% solution (0.5 mL diluted in 2 to 2.5 mL normal saline)
- Isoetharine 1% solution (0.5 mL in 2 mL normal saline)
- Isoproterenol (0.5 mL of a 1:200 solution in 2 mL normal saline)
- Metaproterenol 5% solution (0.3 mL diluted in 2.5 mL normal saline) delivered at intervals of 20 to 30 minutes for moderately severe patients and by continuous nebulization for patients *in extremis*

Although a number of studies in small cohorts of patients have shown that mild to moderate asthma exacerbations can be treated effectively with a combination of a metered dose inhaler (MDI) and spacer device,[56] in our experience, patients with asthma severe enough to warrant hospital admission often have difficulty with the maneuvers required for proper MDI use. For the patient who is intubated and receiving mechanical ventilation, adapters are available to deliver either inhaled beta agonists by nebulizer or by MDI.

For the intubated patient with status asthmaticus who requires dangerously high ventilatory pressures, we have found that direct endotracheal administration of 1 mL of a 1 mg/mL isoproterenol solution can be used to treat refractory bronchoconstriction when all other measures have failed; this treatment should *not* be repeated. Subcutaneous injection of epinephrine or terbutaline or a continuous intravenous infusion of isoproterenol for the control of bronchospasm can precipitate adverse cardiac events in adults, such as ventricular arrhythmias and myocardial infarction, and is not recommended. Frequent or even continuous nebulization of beta agonists is preferred over systemic delivery because this approach is at least equally effective and carries less risk. In our experience, inhaled beta agonists are highly effective and we see no need for the intravenous infusion of sympathomimetic agents or magnesium sulfate.[57]

TABLE 134–2. Treatment of Life-Threatening Asthma

1. Establish diagnosis and rule out foreign body.
2. Assess severity.
   a. Auscultation for breath sounds.
   b. Pulsus paradoxus > 15 torr = severe.
   c. Electrocardiogram to rule out ischemia.
   d. Arterial blood gas.
   e. Chest x-ray.
3. Begin treatment as soon as possible.
   a. Inhaled albuterol (2 mL in nebulizer reservoir undiluted). Drive nebulizer with air-oxygen mix to obtain Sa_{O_2} of 90%.
   b. Methylprednisone (Solu-Medrol), 125 mg IV q8
4. If no response, add:
   a. Aminophylline, 5 mg/kg IV bolus, followed by 0.5 to 0.9 mg/min.
   b. Switch from albuterol to isoproterenol by medication nebulizer.
   c. Administer 80% of helium-20% oxygen if available.
5. If P_{CO_2} is greater than 50 torr or if there are physical signs consistent with respiratory muscle failure:
   a. Intubate the trachea, and institute mechanical ventilator support.
   b. Institute sedation.
   c. Consider muscular paralysis if ventilatory asynchrony exists.
   d. Aim for a P_{CO_2} between 55 and 60 torr.
   e. Titrate FI_{O_2} to achieve Sa_{O_2} of 89% to 91%.
   f. Continue preceding treatments.

Corticosteroids

Systemic corticosteroid therapy is a well-established component of the treatment regimen for status asthmaticus. Because of the high doses required and the uncertainty of oral absorption in the acute setting, these agents should be administered intravenously. Both intravenous hydrocortisone and intravenous methylprednisolone have both been demonstrated to be very effective agents in status asthmaticus. Although no comparative trials have been undertaken, there appears to be no clinical difference in the efficacy of these two agents. Methylprednisolone does have the theoretical advantage of less mineralocorticoid side effects, and can be administered by intermittent intravenous bolus rather than as a continuous intravenous drip. The optimal dose of intravenous corticosteroids to be used in status asthmaticus is undefined.[58] We prefer a regimen consisting of methylprednisolone 80 to 125 mg intravenously every 8 hours. Only when the patient is stable can a switch to oral prednisone, at a dose of 0.5 to 1 mg/kg a day, be safely initiated.

The acute adverse effects of high-dose corticosteroid therapy include gastrointestinal upset, worsening gastroesophageal reflux, hyperglycemia, and mental status changes including anxiety and psychosis. The chronic side effects are those of hypercortisolism.

Oxygen Therapy

The hypoxemia of status asthmaticus is usually mild and transient. Because supplemental oxygen promotes absorption atelectasis and has the potential to adversely effect $\dot{V}/Q$ matching,[59] the amount of oxygen administered should be titrated to yield an Sa_{O_2} *just over 90%*; higher arterial saturation levels provide no benefit and should be avoided. If severe hypercapnia and respiratory acidosis develop in the setting of oxygen therapy, the patient should be treated with mechanical ventilatory support rather than discontinuation of the oxygen therapy.

Adjunctive Therapies

Methylxanthines

The conventional rationale for the use of the methylxanthines in the treatment of acute asthma is for their bronchodilator effects; however, theophylline is at best a modest bronchodilator, with minimal additive effects to adequate inhaled beta agonist therapy. Methylxanthines have other potentially salutary properties, including the following[60, 61]:

- Inhibition of spasmogenic mediator release
- Improved diaphragmatic contractility
- Increased mucociliary transport and clearance of mucous plugs
- Decreased pulmonary arterial pressures

Because this class of drugs has a very narrow therapeutic-toxic ratio, serum concentration monitoring is required. Furthermore, to avoid the uncertainties of absorption in the critically ill patient, one should use continuous intravenous infusion delivery. The toxicity of theophylline increases significantly when the serum level exceeds 20 μg/mL, but toxic effects can occur at much lower serum concentrations:

1. *Gastrointestinal* side effects, such as nausea, vomiting, gastroesophageal reflux and diarrhea, have occurred even below a serum level of 10 μg/mL.
2. *Central nervous system* side effects include tremulousness and anxiety; seizures may occur, especially in the setting of theophylline levels over 20 μg/mL.
3. *Cardiac* side effects include supraventricular and ventricular tachyarrhythmias as well as increased atrioventricular conduction rates in patients with atrial fibrillation.

In an individual patient, there may not be a predictable progression of symptoms from gastrointestinal to central nervous system to cardiac adverse effects.

In the patient not already taking theophylline on a regular basis, an intravenous loading dose of 5 to 6 mg/kg should be administered as a bolus, followed by the immediate institution of a continuous intravenous drip at a rate of 0.5 to 0.9 mg/kg (Table 134-3). In the patient who has been receiving theophylline chronically, the loading dose should be omitted; the serum theophylline concentration should be determined prior to start of the intravenous infusion.

Because theophylline's primary locus of metabolism is the liver, other commonly used drugs can influence its rate of disappearance from the circulation. Factors known to increase theophylline clearance include the following:

1. Use of tobacco or marijuana cigarettes.
2. Treatment with rifampin, barbiturates, phenytoin, cimetidine, fluoroquinolone antibiotics, erythromycin, propranolol (although this drug should not be administered to any patient with asthma), and antiepileptic agents.
3. Concurrent asthma treatment with the 5-lipoxygenase inhibitor zileuton (Zyflo) or the *cysLT*$_1$ receptor antagonist zafirlukast (Accolate).

Disease states that impair theophylline clearance and increase the risk of toxicity include increased age, infection, congestive heart failure and hepatic disease.[61]

TABLE 134–3. Intravenous Maintenance Dose of Aminophylline

Patient Population	Age	Aminophylline Infusion Rate to Achieve Target Concentration of 10 μg/mL (mg/kg body wt · hr)
Young children	1–9 yr	1.0
Older children	9–12 yr	0.9
Adolescents (cigarette/marijuana smokers)	12–16 yr	0.9
Adolescents (nonsmokers)	12–16 yr	0.6
Adults (otherwise healthy cigarette/marijuana smokers)	16–50 yr	0.9
Adults (otherwise healthy nonsmokers)	>16 yr	0.5
Cardiac decompensation, cor pulmonale, or liver dysfunction (or a combination of these factors)	>16 yr	0.3

Adapted from Hendeles L, Weinberger M: Theophylline: A "state of the art" review. Pharmacotherapy 1983; 3:2–44.

Note: Loading doses of aminophylline average 5 to 6 mg/kg lean body weight for adult patients not currently taking methylxanthine preparations (up to 9 mg/kg lean body weight may be needed for children not currently taking methylxanthine preparations), and are administered intravenously over 20 to 30 minutes.

Anticholinergic Agents

Inhaled atropine, 0.5 to 1 mg given via a nebulizer in 2 to 3 mL of a saline solution, has been reputed to be beneficial, particularly in the patient with mucous hypersecretion or an overtly neurogenic component to the bronchoconstriction. However, some studies of inhaled atropine[62] and inhaled ipratropium bromide,[63] suggest that anticholinergic agents contribute little to the benefits of aggressive beta agonist therapy in the treatment of status asthmaticus.

Magnesium Sulfate

Several uncontrolled trials suggest that intravenously administered magnesium sulfate, even to patients with no evidence of serum magnesium deficiency, may have an additive benefit to inhaled beta agonists in the treatment of status asthmaticus. However, one randomized controlled clinical trial suggested minimal, if any, additive benefit of this treatment, and it is not recommended.[64]

Helium-Oxygen

A number of case series, of varying trial design, indicate a salutary therapeutic effect from administration of gas mixtures of 80% helium and 20% oxygen (heliox) in patients with severe asthma.[65, 66] Heliox has a beneficial effect by virtue of its lower (about one third as much) gas density compared to air or oxygen. The lower gas density decreases the pressure required to achieve a given level of gas flow in turbulent flow regimens, as may occur in the presence of airway obstruction. Therefore, even though heliox has no beneficial effect on airway obstruction per se, it allows patients to sustain their own work of breathing while treatments aimed at relieving airway obstruction are administered and thus may prevent the need for mechanical ventilatory support.

Leukotriene Pathway Modifiers

Inhibitors of the enzyme 5-lipoxygenase (zileuton) and the action of LTD_4 at its receptor (montelukast [Singulair]; pranlukast [Onon]; zafirlukast [Accolate]) are novel agents approved for the treatment of chronic persistent asthma.[67-69] Their use should be continued during a severe asthmatic attack. Even though their use has not been studied in acute severe asthma, their coadministration with other treatments at a time when oral therapies can be administered is likely to have a salutary therapeutic effect.

Other Treatments

Routine antibiotic administration in the setting of status asthmaticus, unlike exacerbations of chronic obstructive pulmonary disease (COPD), is not indicated. As mentioned, most patients usually have bronchoconstriction precipitated by a nonbacterial infection. It is conceivable that future studies may demonstrate a contributory role from *C. pneumoniae*; if so, routine administration of doxycycline or erythromycin may then be indicated. Obviously, in the rare asthma patient found to have pneumonia, antibiotic therapy directed by Gram's stain and sputum culture is indicated.

Mucolytic agents, such as *N*-acetylcysteine, can cause severe endobronchial irritation and in the setting of maximal bronchial hyperreactivity may aggravate bronchoconstriction. We favor the use of more standard therapies, such as humidification of inspired air and ensurance of adequate patient hydration, rather than the use of so-called mucolytic agents. Although the use of acute bronchoscopic lavage for removal of mucous plugs and "cleansing of the airways" has been advocated, the procedure carries a significant risk of worsened bronchospasm, barotrauma and pneumonia and is not recommended.

Antihistamines, α-adrenergic antagonists, nitroglycerin, calcium channel antagonists, cromones, and inhaled loop diuretics (e.g., furosemide) all have been found to have anti-bronchoconstrictor effects in the clinical laboratory setting. As of this writing, they have no proven clinical role in the management of status asthmaticus.

RESPIRATORY FAILURE: INTUBATION AND MECHANICAL VENTILATION

Epidemiology

Fewer than 5% of patients admitted with an acute asthmatic attack require intubation and mechanical ventilation.[70] To avoid excess morbidity and mortality, however, one must pay strictest attention to detail in the management of these patients.

General Principles of Management

Intubation and mechanical ventilation should be undertaken for a combination of clinical and laboratory data that indicate either a deterioration in the patient's status or the prolonged lack of improvement with standard therapy.

Intubation is best done in the awake patient in a nonemergent setting rather than in the setting of acute cardiopulmonary collapse. Transoral, rather than transnasal, tracheal intubation is the preferred approach in the patient with status asthmaticus; the larger endotracheal tubes permitted by this route impose less expiratory resistance to flow and should thereby have the least adverse effects on airway mechanics predisposing to auto-PEEP (positive end-expiratory pressure).[71] Since the duration of mechanical ventilatory support is usually short, the potential for airway complications caused by the larger diameter endotracheal tube should be minor.

Ventilatory support should be undertaken to provide an adequate (but not necessarily "normal") level of ventilation, enabling the drugs administered as part of a pharmacologic therapy program (described earlier) to relieve the bronchoconstriction. The severe limitation of expiratory flow in these patients, when matched with an inadequate exhalation time (either patient-generated or physician-generated) can result in dynamic hyperinflation, also known as *intrinsic PEEP* (PEEPi) or auto-PEEP. The adverse cardiopulmonary effects of this hyperinflation include depression of cardiac output, hypotension, hypercapnia, weaning failure, and, in extreme cases, cardiac arrest with electromechanical dissociation.[72, 73] To minimize the level of auto-PEEP, we favor tidal volumes of 6 to 8 mL/kg, frequencies of 10 to 12 breaths/min, and peak inspiratory flow rates of 80 to 100 L/min as initial ventilator settings; this recommendation is based on the work of Tuxen and others[74, 75] and modified by our own experience. These relatively low levels of minute ventilation permit a strategy of "permissive hypercapnia" or "controlled" hypoventilation, and are likely to result in a continued respiratory acidosis. If the systemic pH remains above 7.15, the acidosis that accompanies this ventilatory strategy need not be corrected.[76] Low levels of PEEP in amounts just adequate to match the patient's intrinsic PEEP are of value in aiding patient-ventilator synchrony during weaning.[77]

Heavy sedation is often required after institution of mechanical ventilatory support for status asthmaticus to minimize the problems of patient discomfort during controlled hypercapnia, patient-ventilator dyssynchrony, and respiratory muscle overactivity. In most cases, sedation alone is often sufficient to allow safe and effective mechanical ventilatory support. Infusion of an intravenous opiate, preferably meperidine* to avoid the potential effects of mast cell histamine release associated with morphine, decreases the sensation of air hunger in these patients and may obviate the need for neuromuscular blockade.

If ventilatory assist is difficult after administration of maximal doses of sedatives, neuromuscular blockade with a nondepolarizing muscle relaxant, such as vecuronium, may be necessary within the first 24 to 48 hours of intubation to abolish any chest wall/respiratory muscle resistance to ventilation and attain an adequate level of ventilation at the lowest possible airway pressures. Vecuronium and pancuronium are preferred over metocurine, tubocurarine, and possibly even atracurium, because vecuronium and pancuronium do not cause significant histamine release. Once the patient is paralyzed, the degree of paralysis should be titrated either by allowing the patient to partially recover movement before the next dose is administered or, preferably, by using a peripheral nerve stimulator. At least one or two twitches, rather than total paralysis with no response, should be obtained from a "train-of-four" stimulus protocol at all times.[78, 79] Prolonged neuromuscular blockade may occur in patients with renal impairment as a result of delayed clearance of these agents and their active metabolites. More important, a severe myopathy may occur even with careful monitoring.

There is reason to exercise special caution in the case of the patient with status asthmaticus; nearly all the patients affected in these reports of myopathy have also received high-dose corticosteroids in addition to more than two days of aminosteroid neuromuscular blocking agents (e.g., vecuronium, pancuronium).[80] Because barotrauma and hypotension due to hyperinflation generally occur in the first 24 hours after mechanical ventilation is begun,[73] more than 2 days of neuromuscular blockade to reduce the risk of these complications should rarely be required and should be avoided.

A number of reports[81, 82] have indicated that "noninvasive" ventilatory support with a tight-fitting mask and either varying continuous positive airway pressure (CPAP) or pressure support ventilation can prevent the need for intubation in patients with status asthmaticus. Because technical factors, such as mask application and ventilator adjustment, require substantial practical experience in order to be applied safely and effectively, this approach is recommended only in centers with extensive experience with this technique.

Hypotension

A transient drop in systolic blood pressure is common after endotracheal intubation. This hypotension can be attributed, in part, to the sedating and paralytic medications used in intubations. However, dynamic hyperinflation also renders these patients extremely sensitive to reductions in preload, as occurs at the initiation of positive-pressure ventilation. A useful maneuver for rapidly confirming the diagnosis and stabilizing such a hypotensive, hyperinflated patient is to remove the patient from ventilatory support and then administer three to four breaths/min with an FIO_2 of 1.0 using a self-inflating anesthesia bag.[83] If hemodynamic improvement occurs within

*In patients undergoing infusions or with renal impairment, accumulation of the metabolite normeperidine can lead to seizures.

1 to 2 minutes, intravenous fluid resuscitation and strategies to reduce dynamic hyperinflation should be instituted.

Other Measures

Anesthetic agents, such as isoflurane[84] and intravenous thiopental,[85] have been reported to have efficacy in refractory status asthmaticus according to several case reports. The potential mechanism of action is unclear, but most likely profound sedation and perhaps direct bronchial smooth muscle relaxation are involved. As yet, the role of anesthetic agents in the acute management of life-threatening asthma remains undefined and their use is not recommended.

Monitoring

Measurement of Respiratory System Mechanics

The peak-to-plateau pressure difference (peak inspiratory pressure minus end-inspiratory pressure, measured after a 0.2- to 0.5-second end-inspiratory pause) provides a useful, index of ongoing bronchoconstriction. The degree of dynamic hyperinflation should also be closely monitored; we can measure auto-PEEP by occluding the expiratory port of the ventilator at end expiration in a nonspontaneously breathing patient and by reading the value approximately 1 second later on the ventilator manometer,[72] or we can estimate auto-PEEP by examining real-time expiratory flow waveforms. Measurement of the total exhaled volume (which will be larger than the inspired tidal volume if there is significant auto-PEEP) is an alternative method of assessing dynamic hyperinflation. The total exhaled volume is the volume exhaled by a nonspontaneously breathing patient over 20 to 40 seconds after a tidal inspiration.[86]

Indwelling Arterial Catheter

Fluctuations and trends in blood pressure and in the degree of pulsus paradoxus, as well as repeated blood gas measurements to determine the degree of hypercapnia, often necessitate the placement of an intra-arterial cannula, preferably in the radial artery. Pulsus paradoxus is a useful indicator of airway obstruction in when large pleural pressure swings are occurring in a patient; obviously, if the patient is paralyzed or becomes so hypercarbic that respiratory drive is diminished, the utility of this index is lost.

Oximetry

Pulse oximetry allows the careful titration of supplemental oxygen to treat the common mild to moderate hypoxemia. This noninvasive method can reduce the need for frequent phlebotomy in obtaining direct arterial oxygen saturation measurements but does not provide an index of the adequacy of ventilation, as judged by the P_{CO_2}.

Capnometry

End-tidal carbon dioxide monitoring is unreliable in patients with obstructive lung disease because of increased physiologic dead space and nonuniform regional ventilation. This modality may result in a marked underestimation of the degree and, more important, the trend of hypercapnia,[87] and it cannot be recommended for routine monitoring.

Serum Chemistries

Serum electrolyte and phosphorus levels should be monitored during aggressive administration of beta agonist therapy. If intravenous theophylline is used, serum theophylline levels should be monitored to adjust the dosing.

Chest Radiography

Chest radiographs should be obtained on a frequent enough basis to ensure proper endotracheal tube position and to detect barotrauma, atelectasis, or mucous plugging and pneumonia. Emergency chest films are also important in the patient with hypotension for detecting the presence of a pneumothorax.

Pulmonary Arterial Catheterization

In the management of the typical patient with status asthmaticus and no evidence of cardiac disease, routine use of this invasive monitoring device cannot be recommended.

Course and Prognosis

Weaning

Most asthmatic patients who are intubated for status asthmaticus improve rapidly within 24 to 48 hours, with a mean duration of intubation of 3 to 5 days.[88] A trial of weaning and possible extubation should be considered when:

1. Airway pressures and auto-PEEP have fallen.
2. Secretions are minimal.
3. Bronchospasm is managed with intermittent nebulized beta agonist treatments.
4. There is no evidence of neuromuscular deficits.

Mortality

The mean mortality rate for intubation in the setting of status asthmaticus is 13.0%,[74] and at least one series has reported a rate of 22%.[88] Of note, the centers reporting no mortality for intubated patients with status asthmaticus had a large number of patients with profound hypercapnia who were managed with aggressive care short of intubation; the greatest number of complications occurred in the intubated patients.

Follow-up

Status asthmaticus severe enough to warrant admission to the intensive care unit marks the patient as being in the high-risk group for recurrent admission and possibly even death due to asthma. The groups of patients at high risk for recurrent status asthmaticus include those who use the emergency service as their primary source of asthma care[89] and individuals with low socioeconomic status.[90] Counseling and aggressive outpatient management need to be carefully arranged to avoid multiple episodes of severe asthma.

References

1. Gergen PJ, Weiss KB: The increasing problem of asthma in the United States. Am Rev Respir Dis 1992; 146:823–824.
2. Buist AS, Vollmer WM: Preventing deaths from asthma. N Engl J Med 1994; 331:1584–1585.
3. National Heart Lung and Blood Institute (NHLBI): NHLBI/WHO Workshop Report: Global Strategy for Asthma Management and Prevention. Global Initiative for Asthma. Publication No. 95-3659. Bethesda, Md, 1995.
4. Holgate ST, Roche WR, Church MK: The role of the eosinophil in asthma. Am Rev Respir Dis 1991; 143:S66–S70.
5. Pare PD, Wiggs BR, James A, Hogg JC, Bosken C: The comparative mechanics and morphology of airways in asthma and in chronic obstructive pulmonary disease. Am Rev Respir Dis 1991; 143:1189–1193.
6. Brewster CE, Howarth PH, Djukanovic R, Wilson J, Holgate ST, Roche WR: Myofibroblasts and subepithelial fibrosis in bronchial asthma. Am J Respir Cell Mol Biol 1990; 3:507–511.
7. Jeffery PK: Morphology of the airway wall in asthma and in chronic obstructive pulmonary disease. Am Rev Respir Dis 1991; 143:1152–1158 [discussion, 1161].

8. Aikawa T, Shimura S, Sasaki H, Ebina M, Takishima T: Marked goblet cell hyperplasia with mucus accumulation in the airways of patients who died of severe acute asthma attack. Chest 1992; 101:916-921.
9. Ebina MH, Yaegashi H, Chiba R, Takahashi T, Motomiya M,Tanemura M: Hyperreactive site in the airway tree of asthmatic patients revealed by thickening of bronchial muscles: A morphometric study. Am Rev Respir Dis 1990; 141:1327-1332.
10. Rodger IW: Asthma: Airway smooth muscle. Br Med Bull 1992; 48:97-107.
11. Heard BE, Jeffery PK, Kay AB: Quantitation of mast cells and eosinophils in the bronchial mucosa of symptomatic atopic asthmatics and healthy control subjects using immunohistochemistry. Am Rev Respir Dis 1991; 143:1200-1201.
12. Galli SJ: New concepts about the mast cell. N Engl J Med 1993; 328:257-265.
13. Moreno RH, Hogg JC, Pare PD: Mechanics of airway narrowing. Am Rev Respir Dis 1986; 133:1171-1180.
14. Wiggs BR, Bosken C, Pare PD, James A, Hogg JC: A model of airway narrowing in asthma and in chronic obstructive pulmonary disease [see comments]. Am Rev Respir Dis 1992; 145:1251-1258.
15. Robinson DS, Hamid Q, Ying S, Tsicopoulos A, Barkans J, Bentley AM, Corrigan C, Durham SR, Kay AB: Predominant TH2-like bronchoalveolar T-lymphocyte population in atopic asthma. N Engl J Med 1992; 326:298-304.
16. Sanderson CJ: Interleukin-5, eosinophils, and disease. Blood 1992; 79:3101-3109.
17. Renz H, Gelfand EW: T-cell receptor V elements regulate murine IgE production and airways responsiveness. Allergy 1992; 47:270-276.
18. Bousquet J, Chanez P, Lacoste JY, Barneon G, Ghavanian N, Enander I, Venge P, Ahlstedt S, Simony-Lafontaine J, Godard P: Eosinophilic inflammation in asthma. N Engl J Med 1990; 323:1033-1039.
19. Bradley BL, Azzawi M, Jacobson M, Assoufi B, Collins JV, Irani AM, Schwartz LB, Durham SR, Jeffery PK, Kay AB: Eosinophils, T-lymphocytes, mast cells, neutrophils, and macrophages in bronchial biopsy specimens from atopic subjects with asthma: Comparison with biopsy specimens from atopic subjects without asthma and normal control subjects and relationship to bronchial hyperresponsiveness. J. Allergy Clin Immunol 1991; 88:661-674.
20. Djukanovic R, Lai CK, Wilson JW, Britten KM, Wilson SJ, Roche WR, Howarth PH, Holgate ST: Bronchial mucosal manifestations of atopy: A comparison of markers of inflammation between atopic asthmatics, atopic nonasthmatics and healthy controls. Eur Respir J 1992; 5:538-544.
21. Roche WR, Beasley R, Williams JH, Holgate ST: Subepithelial fibrosis in the bronchi of asthmatics. Lancet 1989; 1:520-524.
22. Schwartz LB: Cellular inflammation in asthma: Neutral proteases of mast cells. Am Rev Respir Dis 1992; 145:S18-S21.
23. Howarth PH, Bradding P, Quint D, Redington AE, Holgate ST: Cytokines and airway inflammation. Ann N Y Acad Sci 1994; 725:69-82.
24. Leung DYM, Martin RJ, Szefler SJ, Sher ER, Ying S, Kay AB, Hamid Q: Dysregulation of interleukin 4, interleukin 5, and interferon gamma gene expression in steroid-resistant asthma. J Exp Med 1995; 181:33-40.
25. Page CP: Mechanisms of hyperresponsiveness: Platelet-activating factor. Am Rev Respir Dis 1992; 145:S31-S33.
26. Obyrne PM: Leukotrienes in the pathogenesis of asthma. Chest 1997; 111:S27-S34.
27. Wardlaw AJ, Hay H, Cromwell O, Collins JV, Kay AB: Leukotrienes, LTC_4 and LTB_4, in bronchoalveolar lavage in bronchial asthma and other respiratory diseases. J Allergy Clin Immunol 1989; 84:19-26.
28. Shindo K, Matsumoto Y, Hirai Y, Sumitomo M, Amano T, Miyakawa K, Matsumura M, Mizuno T: Measurement of leukotriene B4 in arterial blood of asthmatic patients during wheezing attacks. J Intern Med 1990; 228:91-96.
29. Persson CGA: Centennial notions of asthma as an eosinophilic, desquamative, exudative, and steroid-sensitive disease. Lancet 1997; 350:1021-1024.
30. Maggi CA, Giachetti A, Dey RD, Said SI: Neuropeptides as regulators of airway function: Vasoactive intestinal peptide and the tachykinins. Physiol Rev 1995; 75:277-322.
31. Said SI: Molecules that protect: The defense of neurons and other cells. J Clin Invest 1996; 97:2163-2164.
32. Massaro AF, Gaston B, Kita D, Fanta C, Stamler JS, Drazen JM: Expired nitric oxide levels during treatment of acute asthma. Am J Respir Crit Care Med 1995; 152:800-803.
33. Belvisi MG, Stretton CD, Yacoub M, Barnes PJ: Nitric oxide is the endogenous neurotransmitter of bronchodilator nerves in humans. Eur J Pharmacol 1992; 210:221-222.
34. Rebuck AS, Read J: Assessment and management of severe asthma. Am J Med 1971; 51:788-798.
35. Hahn DL, Dodge RW, Golubjatnikov R: Association of *Chlamydia pneumoniae* (strain TWAR) infection with wheezing, asthmatic bronchitis, and adult-onset asthma. JAMA 1991; 266:225-230.
36. Sherry MK, Klainer AS, Wolff M, Gerhard H: Herpetic tracheobronchitis. Ann Intern Med 1988; 109:229-233.
37. Szczeklik A: Aspirin-induced asthma. *In:* Asthma: Basic Mechanisms and Clinical Management. 3rd ed. Barnes PJ, Rodger IW, Thomson NC (Eds). San Diego, Academic Press, 1998, pp 607-616.
38. Wasserfallen JB, Schaller MD, Feihl F, Perret CH: Sudden asphyxic asthma: A distinct entity? Am Rev Respir Dis 1990; 142:108-111.
39. Sur S, Crotty TB, Kephart GM, Hyma BA, Colby TV, Reed CE, Hunt LW, Gleich GJ: Sudden-onset fatal asthma: A distinct entity with few eosinophils and relatively more neutrophils in the airway submucosa. Am Rev Respir Dis 1993; 148:713-719.
40. Cohen CA, Zagelbaum G, Gross D, Roussos C, Macklem PT: Clinical manifestations of inspiratory muscle fatigue. Am J Med 1982; 73:308-316.
41. Rebuck AS, Pengelly LD: Development of pulsus paradoxus in the presence of airways obstruction. N Engl J Med 1973; 288:66-69.
42. Horn BR, Robin ED, Theodore J, Van Kessel A: Total eosinophil counts in the management of bronchial asthma. N Engl J Med 1975; 292:1152-1155.
43. Gelmont DM, Balmes JR, Yee A: Hypokalemia induced by inhaled bronchodilators. Chest 1988; 94:763-766.
44. Laaban JP, Waked M, Laromiguiere M, Vuong TK, Rochemaure J: Hypophosphatemia complicating management of acute severe asthma. Ann Intern Med 1990; 112:68-69.
45. Baker JW, Yerger S, Segar WE: Elevated plasma antidiuretic hormone levels in status asthmaticus. Mayo Clin Proc 1976; 51:31-34.
46. Burki NK, Diamond L: Serum creatine phosphokinase activity in asthma. Am Rev Respir Dis 1977; 116:327-331.
47. Hetzel MR, Clark TJ, Branthwaite MA: Asthma: Analysis of sudden deaths and ventilatory arrests in hospital. Br Med J 1977; 1:808-811.
48. McFadden ER JR, Kiser R, DeGroot WJ: Acute bronchial asthma: Relations between clinical and physiologic manifestations. N Engl J Med 1973; 288:221-225.
49. McFadden ER Jr, Lyons HA: Arterial-blood gas tension in asthma. N Engl J Med 1968; 278:1027-1032.
50. Ferrer A, Roca J, Wagner PD, Lopez FA, Rodriguez-Roisin R: Airway obstruction and ventilation-perfusion relationships in acute severe asthma Am Rev Respir Dis 1993; 147:579-584. [Erratum in Am Rev Respir Dis 1993; 148(1):ff 264.]
51. Gazioglu K, Condemi JJ, Hyde RW, Kaltreider NL: Effect of isoproterenol on gas exchange during air and oxygen breathing in patients with asthma. Am J Med 1971; 50:185-190.
52. Mountain RD, Heffner JE, Brackett NC Jr, Sahn SA: Acid-base disturbances in acute asthma. Chest 1990; 98:651-655.
53. Hogg JC: Pathology of asthma. J Allergy Clin Immunol 1993; 92:1-5.
54. White CS, Cole RP, Lubetsky HW, Austin JHM: Acute asthma: Admission chest radiography in hospitalized adult patients. Chest 1991; 100:14-16.
55. Pierce RJ, Payne CR, Williams SJ, Denison DM, Clark TJ: Comparison of intravenous and inhaled terbutaline in the treatment of asthma. Chest 1981; 79:506-511.
56. Idris AH, McDermott MF, Raucci JC, Morrabel A, McGorray S, Hendeles L: Emergency department treatment of severe asthma: Metered-dose inhaler plus holding chamber is equivalent in effectiveness to nebulizer [see comments]. Chest 1993; 103:665-672.
57. Schiermeyer RP, Finklestein JA: Rapid infusion of magnesium sulfate obviates need for intubation in status asthmaticus. Am J Emerg Med 1994; 12:164-166.
58. McFadden ER: Dosages of corticosteroids in asthma. Am Rev Respir Dis 1993; 147:1306-1310.

59. Rodriguez-Roisin R, Ballester E, Roca J, Torres A, Wagner PD: Mechanisms of hypoxemia in patients with status asthmaticus requiring mechanical ventilation. Am Rev Respir Dis 1989; 139:732–739.
60. Milgrom H, Bender B: Current issues in the use of theophylline. Am Rev Respir Dis 1993; 147:S33–S39.
61. Weinberger M, Hendeles L: Theophylline in asthma. N Engl J Med 1996; 334:1380–1388.
62. Karpel JP, Appel D, Breidbart D, Fusco MJ: A comparison of atropine sulfate and metaproterenol sulfate in the emergency treatment of asthma. Am Rev Respir Dis 1986; 133:727–729.
63. Summers QA, Tarala RA: Nebulized ipratropium in the treatment of acute asthma [see comments]. Chest 1990; 97:425–429.
64. Green SM, Rothrock SG: Intravenous magnesium for acute asthma: Failure to decrease emergency treatment duration or need for hospitalization [see comments]. Ann Emerg Med 1992; 21:260–265.
65. Manthous CA, Hall JB, Caputo MA, Walter J, Klocksieben JM, Schmidt GA, Wood LD: Heliox improves pulsus paradoxus and peak expiratory flow in nonintubated patients with severe asthma. Am J Respir Crit Care Med 1995; 151:310–314.
66. Kudukis TM, Manthous CA, Schmidt GA, Hall JB, Wylam ME: Inhaled helium-oxygen revisited: Effect of inhaled helium-oxygen during the treatment of status asthmaticus in children. J Pediatr 1997; 130:217–224.
67. Busse WW: The role of leukotrienes in asthma and allergic rhinitis. Clin Exp Allergy 1996; 26:868–879.
68. Holgate ST, Bradding P, Sampson AP: Leukotriene antagonists and synthesis inhibitors: New directions in asthma therapy. J Allergy Clin Immunol 1996; 98:1–13.
69. O'Bryrne PO, Israel E, Drazen JM: Anti-leukotrienes as novel anti-asthma treatments. Ann Intern Med 1997; 127:472–480.
70. Braman SS, Kaemmerlen JT: Intensive care of status asthmaticus: A 10-year experience. JAMA 1990; 264:366–368.
71. Scott LR, Benson MS, Bishop MJ: Relationship to endotracheal tube size to auto-PEEP at high minute ventilation. Respir Care 1997; 31:1080-1082.
72. Pepe PE, Marini JJ: Occult positive end-expiratory pressure in mechanically ventilated patients with airflow obstruction: The auto-PEEP effect. Am Rev Respir Dis 1982; 126:166–170.
73. Rosengarten PL, Tuxen DV, Dziukas L, Scheinkestel C, Merrett K, Bowes G: Circulatory arrest induced by intermittent positive pressure ventilation in a patient with severe asthma [see comments]. Anaesth Intensive Care 1991; 19:118–121.
74. Williams TJ, Tuxen DV, Scheinkestel CD, Czarny D, Bowes G: Risk factors for morbidity in mechanically ventilated patients with acute severe asthma. Am Rev Respir Dis 1992; 146:607–615.
75. Tuxen DV, Williams TJ, Scheinkestel CD, Czarny D, Bowes G: Use of a measurement of pulmonary hyperinflation to control the level of mechanical ventilation in patients with acute severe asthma. Am Rev Respir Dis 1992; 146:1136–1142.
76. Feihl F, Perret C: Permissive hypercapnia. Am J Respir Crit Care Med 1994; 150:1722-1737.
77. Tan IK, Bhatt SB, Tam YH, Oh TE: Effects of PEEP on dynamic hyperinflation in patients with airflow limitation. Br J Anaesth 1993; 70:267–272.
78. Isenstein DA, Venner DS, Duggan J: Neuromuscular blockade in the intensive care unit. Chest 1992; 102:1258–1266.
79. Wheeler AP: Sedation, analgesia, and paralysis in the intensive care unit. Chest 1993; 104:566–577.
80. Hansen-Flaschen J, Cowen J, Raps EC: Neuromuscular blockade in the intensive care unit: More than we bargained for. Am Rev Respir Dis 1993; 147:234–236.
81. Patrick W, Webster K, Ludwig L, Roberts D, Wiebe P, Younes M: Noninvasive positive-pressure ventilation in acute respiratory distress without prior chronic respiratory failure. Am J Respir Crit Care Med 1996; 153:1005–1011.
82. Meduri GU, Cook TR, Turner RE, Cohen M, Leeper KV: Noninvasive positive pressure ventilation in status asthmaticus. Chest 1996; 110:767–774.
83. Hall JB, Corbridge T: Status asthmaticus in the adult: Assesment, drug therapy and mechanical ventilation. Respir Management 1991; 21:119–126.
84. Maltais F, Sovilj M, Goldberg P, Gottfried SB: Respiratory mechanics in status asthmaticus: Effects of inhalational anesthesia. Chest 1994; 106:1401-1406.
85. Grunberg G, Cohen JD, Keslin J, Gassner S: Facilitation of mechanical ventilation in status asthmaticus with continuous intravenous thiopental. Chest 1991; 99:1216–1219.
86. Tuxen DV, Lane S: The effects of ventilatory pattern on hyperinflation, airway pressures, and circulation in mechanical ventilation of patients with severe air-flow obstruction. Am Rev Respir Dis 1987; 136:872–879.
87. Morley TF, Giaimo J, Maroszan E, Bermingham J, Gordon R, Griesback R, Zappasodi SJ, Giudice JC: Use of capnography for assessment of the adequacy of alveolar ventilation during weaning from mechanical ventilation. Am Rev Respir Dis 1993; 148:339–344.
88. Mansel JK, Stogner SW, Petrini MF, Norman J: Mechanical ventilation in patients with acute severe asthma. Am J Med 1990; 89:42–48.
89. Hanania NA, David-Wang A, Kesten S, Chapman KR: Factors associated with emergency department dependence of patients with asthma. Chest 1997; 111:290–295.
90. Watson JP, Cowen P, Lewis RA: The relationship between asthma admission rates, routes of admission, and socioeconomic deprivation. Eur Respir J 1996; 9:2087–2093.
91. Hendeles L, Weinberger M: Theophylline: A "state of the art" review. Pharmacotherapy 1983; 3:2–44.

135

Acute Respiratory Failure in Patients with Chronic Obstructive Pulmonary Disease

Adelaida M. Miro, MD

Patients with chronic obstructive pulmonary disease (COPD) make up a large number of those residing in any intensive care unit (ICU), whether medical or surgical, at any given time. These patients can usually be classified into one of four groups:

1. Patients who have been admitted with an acute exacerbation of lung disease. These patients are admitted to the ICU in an attempt to maximize their medical therapy in a monitored environment and to prevent progression of respiratory failure and the subsequent need for mechanical ventilation.
2. Patients who may not have responded to inpatient medical management and now require intubation and mechanical ventilation for acute respiratory failure.
3. Patients who have chronic respiratory failure and depend on mechanical ventilation. These patients may have been admitted during an acute exacerbation but, because of their advanced lung disease and concurrent medical problems, cannot be successfully weaned from mechanical ventilation. These patients may need weeks to months for return of their ability to sustain spontaneous respiration without mechanical assistance.
4. Patients admitted to the ICU for other medical problems, such as those who have had a general surgical procedure, who, because of underlying lung disease, cannot discontinue mechanical ventilation despite recovery from their primary illness.

Patients with COPD in the ICU represent a challenge to all physicians. In the management of these complex, critically ill patients, clinical judgment often prevails over absolute, irrefutable science. Even the definition of what constitutes acute respiratory failure in these patients with chronic hypoxemia and hypercapnia is not universal. Physicians need to rely mainly on changes from the individual's previous baseline parameters to establish the diagnostic criteria for defining acute respiratory failure.

In order to manage these patients and use ICU resources optimally, we must understand the unique features of this disorder and be familiar with the underlying pathophysiologic principles that guide medical and ventilatory management.

PATHOPHYSIOLOGY

Precipitating Factors

Acute respiratory infections are the most common cause of exacerbation of COPD (Table 135–1). These respiratory infections may be confined to the upper respiratory system, such as acute tracheobronchitis, or may be more serious and debilitating pneumonias.

The clinical presentation of acute respiratory infection is often characterized by progressive worsening of symptoms, including cough, change in quantity and characteristics of sputum production, fever, and worsening dyspnea. Because these symptoms are often present in upper and lower respiratory infections, the distinction between bronchitis and pneumonia must be made by a combination of physical examination and radiographic studies. Sputum Gram staining and culture may be of only limited value, because during asymptomatic periods patients with COPD are often colonized with bacterial organisms that may eventually progress to an acute respiratory infection. More invasive diagnostic techniques, such as fiberoptic bronchoscopy with protected specimen brush and bronchoalveolar lavage with quantitative cultures, would be difficult to perform with nonintubated, dyspneic patients. Thus, these techniques should be reserved for patients already receiving mechanical ventilation and then only when the results of the procedure would lead to a potential change in therapy. Although the indications for antibiotic therapy during acute exacerbations of COPD remain controversial, most clinicians favor the use of antibiotic therapy when there is evidence of an acute upper respiratory infection. In the presence of clear-cut pneumonia, antibiotic treatment should be initiated immediately.

The choice of antibiotics should be guided by the sensitivity patterns of the microorganisms endemic to the institution that are also the most common offending organisms in this population of patients. In general, these microorganisms include *Streptococcus pneumoniae* and *Haemophilus influenzae*. Other potential organisms that should be considered include other *Streptococcus* species, enteric gram-negative bacilli, *Mycoplasma*, and *Legionella*. Although viral infections are probably quite common in this population of patients, their role in the expression of acute respiratory failure is difficult to ascertain, and most often the clinician is forced to prescribe broad-spectrum antibiotics because of the debilitated condition of the patients and the high morbidity and mortality associated with untreated infections. Issues of increasing antibiotic resistance patterns with liberal antibiotic use should be considered before antibiotics are prescribed. Diagnostic approach and antibiotic selection are addressed in the chapters on community-acquired pneumonia (see Chapter 144) and nosocomial pneumonia (see Chapter 145).

Nonpulmonary infections, such as those in the urinary tract or intra-abdominal space, should also be sought in patients with COPD who present with fever and worsening respiratory failure (see Table 135–1). Specimens of all organisms should be obtained for culture, and treatment should be based on clinical data and microbiologic culture reports.

Noninfectious causes that should be investigated as the precipitating factor are listed in Table 135–1. We must realize that the presence of cardiac arrhythmias may either precipitate acute exacerbations of respiratory failure or be a consequence of respiratory failure. For example, cardiac arrhythmias may have a variety of causes associated with abnormalities in gas exchange (hypoxemia, hypercapnia), respiratory acidosis, or electrolyte abnormalities or be drug-induced arrhythmias resulting from beta agonists or theophylline preparations. Multifocal atrial tachycardia (MAT) is seen with increased frequency in patients with acute decompensation of lung disease. This arrhythmia is characterized by a rapid, irregular rhythm with three or more distinctly different P waves and varying PR intervals in a single lead.[1] On first inspection, this rhythm may be confused with rapid atrial fibrillation, but the presence of P waves confirms the diagnosis of MAT. The etiology of this arrhythmia in acute lung disease is multifactorial, involving a combination of hypoxemia, electrolyte abnormalities, and the arrhythmogenic potential of many of the β-adrenergic bronchodilators.

Treatment is aimed at reversal of the respiratory failure and, if necessary, ventricular rate control with digitalis or calcium channel blockers, such as verapamil or diltiazem. The use of β-blockers to treat tachycardia, however, should be avoided because of their potential to exacerbate the degree of airflow obstruction.[2, 3]

The potential for corticosteroid-induced complications should always be considered with both acute and chronic steroid use. The mineralocorticoid effects of systemic corticosteroid therapy may lead to electrolyte abnormalities, especially hypokalemia and hypomagnesemia. Glucocorticoid use may also lead to hyperglycemia and difficulty in regulating blood glucose levels. Long-term steroid use can cause severe

TABLE 135–1. Precipitating Events for Acute Respiratory Failure in Patients with Chronic Obstructive Pulmonary Disease

Infections
- Pulmonary
  - Upper respiratory infections (tracheobronchitis)
  - Lower respiratory infections (pneumonia, empyema)
- Nonpulmonary
  - Urinary tract
  - Intra-abdominal (diverticulitis, abscess, perforated viscus)
  - Indwelling catheters
  - Cardiac (endocarditis)

Noninfectious Causes
- Pulmonary
  - Pneumothorax
  - Rib fractures
  - Pulmonary embolism
- Cardiovascular
  - Ischemic heart disease (angina, infarction)
  - Hypotension or shock
  - Arrhythmias
  - Cor pulmonale
  - Congestive heart failure
  - Transudative pleural effusions
- Neurologic
  - Stroke, transient ischemic attack
  - Oversedation
  - Metabolic (hypothyroid, hyponatremia)
- Gastrointestinal
  - Pancreatitis (steroid induced)
  - Perforated ulcer (steroid induced)
  - Abdominal distention (ileus, obstruction, ascites)
- Metabolic
  - Electrolyte abnormalities (hypocalcemia, hypophosphatemia, hypokalemia)
  - Endocrine (hypothyroid, hyperglycemia, hypoglycemia)

osteoporosis and a propensity for pathologic bone fractures. Steroid-induced gastric ulcers must be considered in the presence of abdominal symptoms. Furthermore, because glucocorticoids significantly reduce systemic inflammatory reactions, an intra-abdominal catastrophe (e.g., perforated ulcer or abscess) may present with few signs of systemic inflammation. Accordingly, important clinical signs of infection (such as fever, localizing signs, and rebound tenderness) may be lacking in these patients. These complications may remain unsuspected or undetected until patients have progressed to profound cardiovascular instability associated with septic shock. Maintaining a high index of suspicion for atypical presentations of serious infections is always prudent in the approach to the management of patients who receive high-dose corticosteroid therapy during acute exacerbations and also take lower doses as outpatients.

Finally, in patients with a history of systemic corticosteroid use in the past 6 months, the possibility of adrenal insufficiency should be contemplated during any acute illness. If any elective surgery is considered for patients with this history of prior corticosteroid exposure, they should receive prophylactic stress-dose corticosteroid therapy during acute interventions to prevent this complication.

Given the many pulmonary and nonpulmonary potential etiologic mechanisms of acute respiratory failure in patients with chronic airflow obstruction, it is important to maintain a broad differential diagnosis guided by history, signs, symptoms, and a thorough evaluation of all possibilities.

Respiratory Muscle Failure

The respiratory muscles may be adversely affected by COPD in many ways (Table 135–2). These factors may be seen alone or, more commonly, several may coexist. Some element of respiratory muscle fatigue is often present during acute exacerbations of COPD. Respiratory muscle fatigue, defined as inability to generate a sufficient transdiaphragmatic force during inspiration, is often due to an imbalance between respiratory supply and demand. In COPD, respiratory demand is increased by factors such as an increased work of breathing, high minute ventilation requirement (increased dead space ventilation), abnormal respiratory system mechanics (both lungs and chest wall), increased airway resistance (increased bronchomotor tone, secretions), dynamic hyperinflation (intrinsic positive end-expiratory pressure [PEEP]), and nutrition (overfeeding).[4-8] Alternatively, the ability of the respiratory system to meet these demands is decreased by such factors as decreased contractive force of mechanically disadvantaged muscles (especially the diaphragm) related to hyperinflation, abnormal gas exchange (hypoxia, hypercapnia), hemodynamic compromise, electrolyte abnormalities (hypokalemia, hypocalcemia, hypophosphatemia, hypomagnesemia), myopathy (glucocorticoids, aminoglycosides, neuromuscular blockers), and malnutrition.[9-12]

TABLE 135–2. Factors That May Adversely Affect Respiratory Muscle Function

Respiratory muscle fatigue
Glucocorticosteroids
Neuromuscular blockers
Polyneuropathy of critical illness
Muscle atrophy
Electrolyte abnormalities
Sepsis
Low cardiac output states
Malnutrition
Hypoxia and hypercapnia

Early detection of respiratory muscle fatigue is difficult to achieve at the bedside. The most sensitive methods, such as electromyography (EMG), are not usually readily available. Other clinical signs, such as tachypnea and paradoxical breathing, should raise the suspicion of impending respiratory failure. Arterial blood gas abnormalities (e.g., progressively worsening hypoxemia, hypercapnia) are insensitive and often herald an impending respiratory arrest.

Many of the medications used to treat the acute respiratory failure in patients with acute exacerbations of COPD requiring mechanical ventilation may themselves have adverse effects on neuromuscular function in general and respiratory muscle function in particular. Two frequently used medications, namely glucocorticoids and neuromuscular blocking agents, deserve special mention.

The administration of high-dose corticosteroids, as occurs frequently in patients with COPD who have acute exacerbations of disease, has also been associated with acute myopathies characterized by acute onset of (mostly) proximal limb weakness, diminished or absent deep tendon reflexes, and either normal or modestly elevated serum creatine kinase levels. Nerve conduction studies and sensory nerve action potential are normal, and EMG shows little or no abnormal spontaneous movement.[13-15] Muscle biopsy shows diffuse fiber atrophy, and electron microscopy can reveal loss of thick myosin filaments.[16-18] Chronic corticosteroid administration may also result in a chronic myopathy. Both the acute and chronic corticosteroid myopathies are slowly reversible after discontinuation of the medications.

Use of neuromuscular blocking agents is occasionally necessary during the acute management of respiratory failure to minimize peak airway pressures and reduce whole-body oxygen (O_2) consumption and carbon dioxide (CO_2) production. These agents may be given once to facilitate laryngoscopy and endotracheal intubation, or they may be given as repeated boluses or a continuous infusion to facilitate mechanical ventilation. In a study by Segredo and colleagues,[19] the administration of vecuronium for more than two consecutive days often produced severe and prolonged muscle weakness. This neuromuscular blocker is used frequently for critically ill patients because of its lack of adverse hemodynamic effects. However, it may produce severe, prolonged weakness in critically ill patients long after it is discontinued, because of high circulating levels of its active metabolite, 3-desacetylvecuronium. Renal and hepatic failures are risk factors for development of prolonged neuromuscular blockade. Therefore, the use of these drugs should be minimized whenever possible, especially in the presence of kidney and liver failure.

When repeated doses of neuromuscular agents are indicated, one may titrate the level of neuromuscular blockade by using a nerve stimulator and adjusting the doses to keep the train-of-four stimulation between one and two twitches. In one study evaluating the use of a peripheral nerve stimulator versus standard clinical dosing, use of the stimulator resulted in less neuromuscular blockers given to maintain the desired level of paralysis.[12] Furthermore, there was faster recovery of spontaneous ventilation. Others have described acute necrotizing myopathies characterized by increased serum creatine kinase levels and severe generalized weakness after the use of neuromuscular blockers and glucocorticoids.[13, 20, 21]

Drug-induced myopathies may explain the inability to wean certain patients from mechanical ventilation long after they have recovered from the primary illness. This potentially devastating and costly iatrogenic complication should also be considered in the acute and chronic care of these patients. Corticosteroids in particular, if administered during acute exacerbations of COPD, should be diligently withdrawn as clinically indicated. The use of neuromuscular blockers can be avoided by focusing attention on the adequacy of the mechanical ventilator setting[22, 23] in order to avoid patient-ventilator asynchrony and the patient "fighting" the ventilator as well as by judiciously using short-acting sedatives such as midazolam or propofol.[24, 25]

Hyperinflation

Any increase in lung volume at end-expiration above functional residual capacity (FRC), the value defined by the normal elastic properties of the lung and chest wall, is referred to as hyperinflation. Many different mechanisms can result in hyperinflation in patients with COPD. Hyperinflation can occur if the inspiratory muscles oppose lung emptying toward the end of expiration. This commonly occurs in normal subjects asked to breath at high ventilatory rates or during exercise. Similarly, during episodes of acute bronchospasm in asthmatic patients, expiratory breaking commonly occurs.[26] The reasons for this phenomenon are poorly understood, but presumably the increased lung volume minimizes the work cost of breathing because airway resistance is lower as lung volume increases. In this scenario, lung volume can return to FRC if the subject allowed it to, but no amount of increased expiratory time by itself would make hyperinflation disappear.

In healthy individuals, normal tidal breathing does not result in airway collapse or airflow limitation; however, patients with COPD exhibit dynamic airway collapse and subsequent expiratory airflow limitation during relaxed tidal breathing. This expiratory airflow limitation leads to increases in end-expiratory lung volume (EELV) above the normal FRC and produces the hyperinflation that is commonly associated with this disease.

Hyperinflation associated with expiratory airflow limitation can be caused by two separate mechanisms. First, if the airways collapse completely during exhalation, gas is trapped behind the collapsed segment. This is referred to as *air trapping*; regardless of the effort or amount of time available for exhalation, no additional gas is expired. In the second case, airways are only partially collapsed, resulting in expiratory flow limitation. Although these airway segments are flow-limited, they remain patent and can empty completely if enough expiratory time is available. Hyperinflation develops in this situation if inadequate expiratory time passes before the next breath. This is referred to as *dynamic hyperinflation*, because these lung segments continue to expel gas throughout the entire available expiratory time.[27]

With dynamic hyperinflation, because end-expiratory alveolar pressure remains positive, this process was termed "auto-PEEP" by Pepe and Marini.[7] Subsequent papers in the literature have referred to this phenomenon with other terms, including "occult PEEP," "inadvertent PEEP," and "intrinsic PEEP."[6, 7] There is no unanimity on terminology, even though all these terms describe a common phenomenon: incomplete exhalation of gas that results in an end-expiratory alveolar pressure in excess of airway pressure because of an inadequate expiratory time. Several groups, including the American Thoracic Society and the Society of Critical Care Medicine, have attempted to standardize the PEEP terminology.

When PEEP is applied at the mouth using a respiratory device, it is referred to as *extrinsic PEEP* to denote that it is extrinsic to the patient. Similarly, dynamic hyperinflation is referred to as *intrinsic PEEP* to denote that it is an intrinsic aspect of the patient and not the ventilator circuit. Although patients with expiratory flow limitation are the most susceptible to development of intrinsic PEEP, patients without any underlying lung disease are also at risk if respiratory frequency is rapid enough or the tidal volumes are large enough to prevent complete gas emptying from the lung before the next breath.[27-29]

When patients with COPD have acute decompensation of lung disease leading to acute respiratory failure, the amount of intrinsic PEEP increases with the worsening of airflow obstruction and the increase in dyspneic respiratory drive. These increases in intrinsic PEEP can lead to profound hyperinflation with all the associated adverse hemodynamic and respiratory effects (Table 135-3).

From a hemodynamic standpoint, intrinsic PEEP, by increasing lung volume, increases intrathoracic pressure. As described in the chapter on heart-lung interactions (see Chapter 111), this can adversely affect steady-state cardiac output by impeding systemic venous return to the heart in a manner identical to that of ventilator-applied extrinsic PEEP.[30, 31] Hypotension and shock may follow this decreased cardiac output. In addition, the positive alveolar pressures may be transmitted to the pulmonary vasculature, leading to a falsely elevated pulmonary artery occlusion pressure.[7] The combination of low cardiac output and elevated pulmonary artery occlusion pressure may suggest a cardiogenic cause of the hypotension, and treatment may be erroneously focused on acute heart failure.[7, 32, 33] To avoid this pitfall, it is important to recognize these potential hemodynamic effects of intrinsic PEEP and direct treatments toward improving the airflow obstruction and optimizing ventilatory strategies, as discussed subsequently.

Increases in intrinsic PEEP during acute respiratory failure may also worsen several respiratory parameters:

1. The positive alveolar pressure at end-exhalation (immediately before the subsequent inspiration) imposes an inspiratory threshold load that requires increases in the pressure generated by the inspiratory muscles. For example, if an intrinsic PEEP of 5 cm H_2O is present and the ventilator trigger sensitivity is set at -2 cm H_2O, the patient must generate a negative pressure at the mouth of -7 cm H_2O for every breath in order to open the inspiratory valves on the ventilator and receive ventilator assistance. This extra work of breathing with every breath may exceed the capability of the patient's respiratory muscle strength and reserve and, if associated with sustained respiratory muscle fatigue, ultimately impair weaning from mechanical ventilation.
2. The worsening hyperinflation with intrinsic PEEP imposes an additional mechanical disadvantage on the respiratory muscles, especially the diaphragm, which negatively affects the ability to wean the patient from mechanical ventilation. Third, hyperinflation may increase the amount of alveolar dead space and decrease CO_2 elimination efficiency.
3. One must measure the amount of intrinsic PEEP when calculating respiratory system compliance to avoid underestimation of the true value.[6]

Several methods exist for estimating the amount of intrinsic

TABLE 135–3. Adverse Effects of Auto–Positive End-Expiratory Pressure

Respiratory
Increased work of breathing
Increased dead space ventilation
Mechanical disadvantage of the respiratory muscles
Hemodynamic
False elevation of pulmonary artery occlusion pressure
Decreased venous return
Decreased cardiac output
Hypotension
Increased right ventricular afterload

PEEP in patients who are receiving mechanical ventilation (Table 135–4). One of the most commonly used is the *end-expiratory occlusion technique*. With this method, the expiratory port of the ventilator is occluded at end-expiration, immediately before the next breath would occur but during an expiratory pause.[7] If continual expiratory airflow was occurring at this moment, it would be stopped and alveolar pressure and airway opening pressure would become equal. Accordingly, any increase in the end-expiratory occlusion pressure should reflect the amount of intrinsic PEEP present. For example, if the ventilator PEEP (extrinsic PEEP) is set at 5 cm H_2O and after end-expiratory occlusion the pressure rises to 12 cm H_2O, then an intrinsic PEEP of 7 cm H_2O is present.

Several commercially available ventilators are equipped to perform an end-expiratory hold maneuver on demand in order to obtain intrinsic PEEP values more easily. If this option is not available, the end-expiratory occlusion maneuver may be performed by manually occluding the expiratory port. However, one must take care to time the expiratory port occlusion accurately. Occlusions should be made immediately before the subsequent inspiration, or air may still be leaving the lungs as part of normal expiration. Thus, if the occlusion occurs too early, this method can overestimate the amount of intrinsic PEEP present.

In ventilators with the ability to show pressures, flow, and volume graphically, intrinsic PEEP may be detected by examination of the real-time inspiratory and expiratory flows. The presence of intrinsic PEEP is confirmed if there is still ongoing expiratory flow when the subsequent inspiration begins. Disadvantages of this method are that it is qualitative and the amount of intrinsic PEEP cannot be quantified. Advantages are that it is simple to use and can provide instantaneous feedback on the effects of changes in mechanical ventilation parameters (see later) on auto-PEEP levels. Because intrinsic PEEP is the alveolar pressure at end-expiration, airway pressure must increase to this value before inspiratory flow may commence and the airway pressure when inspiratory flow starts equals the intrinsic PEEP.[6] Thus, if one simultaneously monitors airway pressure and airflow, accurate measures of intrinsic PEEP can be obtained on a breath-by-breath basis.

Another simple bedside technique for measuring intrinsic PEEP involves monitoring the peak inspiratory airway pressures as extrinsic PEEP is progressively increased. This technique is based on the physiologic premise that until the ventilator-delivered extrinsic PEEP level exceeds the intrinsic PEEP level, there is no further increase in end-expiratory lung volume and hence no increase in peak airway pressure.[34]

Other techniques have been used to quantify intrinsic PEEP, but they call for specialized equipment that may not be readily available at the bedside. One is the *inspiratory flow initiation technique*, which requires the simultaneous presence of an esophageal balloon to estimate intrathoracic pressures and a pneumotachograph to measure airflow. The amount of intrinsic PEEP is taken as the magnitude of decrease in esophageal pressure seen before inspiratory airflow is detected on the pneumotachograph.[35] The intrinsic PEEP values obtained with this technique are generally lower than those obtained with the end-expiratory occlusion technique. This discrepancy in intrinsic PEEP values is due to the fact that the occlusion technique measures an average intrinsic PEEP from all parts of the lungs, whereas the inspiratory flow method measures only the lowest value of intrinsic PEEP that must be overcome before gas begins to enter the lungs.

Finally, Hoffman and colleagues[36] used respiratory inductive plethysmography to estimate increases in end-expiratory thoracic gas volume that occurred with the addition of progressive ventilator PEEP to patients with intrinsic PEEP. They took the intrinsic PEEP value as the amount of ventilator-supplied extrinsic PEEP necessary to increase end-expiratory volume by 10% of the tidal volume. Their technique showed a good correlation ($r = .97$) with the end-expiratory occlusion technique.

TABLE 135–4. Techniques for Measuring Auto–Positive End-Expiratory Pressure

End-expiratory occlusion
Inspiratory flow initiation
Qualitative analysis of inspiratory or expiratory airflow signal
Peak airway pressure changes in response to progressive addition of ventilator PEEP
RIP end-expiratory volume change in response to progressive addition of ventilator PEEP
Measurement of exhaled volume

PEEP = positive end-expiratory pressure; RIP = respiration inductive plethysmography.

MEDICAL MANAGEMENT

There are three main goals of therapy in the acute management of respiratory failure in COPD patients:

1. Initial therapy to reverse any life-threatening complications, such as hypoxemia and cardiac arrhythmias.
2. Identification and subsequent treatment of the precipitating factors.
3. Treatment with bronchodilators and anti-inflammatory agents to reduce airflow obstruction.

Long-term therapeutic goals include successful weaning from mechanical ventilation, pulmonary rehabilitation, and optimal outpatient pharmacotherapy.

Supplemental Oxygen Administration

Patients with acute exacerbation of COPD may present with profound arterial hypoxemia. The administration of supplemental O_2 is essential to avoid life-threatening hypoxemia and cardiac arrest. However, because administration of O_2 to these patients often increases the degree of hypercapnia and respiratory acidosis, there are misconceptions and much debate regarding the goals and titration of supplemental oxygen therapy.

Administering supplemental O_2 via nasal cannula is one of the simplest techniques. For every liter per minute of O_2 flow, there is approximately an 8% increase in fractional inspired oxygen (FIO_2). For example, at 2 L/min, the FIO_2 is roughly 37% (21% from room air plus 16% from nasal cannula). The upper limit of this oxygen delivery system is approximately 6 L/min. Beyond this O_2 flow rate, there is little additional increase in the FIO_2 because of the turbulence generated within the delivery tubing and the nasopharynx. Thus, the upper limit of FIO_2 with this technique is approximately 65% to 70%.

With a conventional face mask delivery system, the volume of the mask provides an O_2 reservoir and the maximum FIO_2 delivered is approximately 70% to 80%. With both the nasal cannula and face mask, however, there is no way to monitor the precise FIO_2 because it varies with factors such as respiratory frequency, minute ventilation, entrainment of room air, and placement of delivery devices. This variability in FIO_2 makes titration of O_2 therapy to maintain adequate oxygenation while avoiding hyperoxia-induced hypercapnia difficult to achieve. Calibrated Venturi masks may offer a better alternative because they allow more precise titration of FIO_2, but these masks must be worn properly in order to achieve predictable oxygen delivery.

The mechanism of the hyperoxia-induced hypercapnia in patients with COPD has been the subject of much debate. It was generally believed that the concomitant rise in arterial oxygen pressure ($Paco_2$) with supplemental oxygen administration was due to loss of the hypoxic respiratory drive and a decrease in overall minute ventilation. However, several studies have challenged this widely held concept and have demonstrated that the increase in $Paco_2$ after administration of oxygen is due mainly to an increase in the ratio of dead space to tidal volume (VDS/VT).[37, 38]

Sassoon and colleagues[37] studied the effects of 15 minutes of hyperoxia on 17 stable, ambulatory patients with COPD. Although there was a small decrease in minute ventilation after O_2 administration, this effect was accompanied by a decrease in CO_2 production. The increase in VDS/VT accounted for 80% of the increase in $Paco_2$. The investigators also found that the severity of airway obstruction, as measured by the forced expiratory volume over 1 second (FEV_1), appeared to be a significant risk factor for the development of hyperoxia-induced hypercapnia.

Crossley and colleagues[38] studied 12 hypercapnic (mean $Paco_2$ 56 mm Hg), intubated patients with COPD and normal Pao_2 after a period of mechanical ventilation. They increased the baseline FIO_2 (0.30 to 0.40) to 0.70, which resulted in an increase in Pao_2 but no change in $Paco_2$, VDS/VT, or respiratory drive. They proposed that changes in ventilation-perfusion (V-Q) mismatching that lead to hyperoxia-induced hypercapnia are most pronounced in patients who are hypoxemic at baseline and that this response is lost after a period of mechanical ventilation with an FIO_2 that maintains Pao_2 in a normal range.

Among the general management principles for patients with acute exacerbation of COPD, it is essential to remember that correction of life-threatening hypoxemia with supplemental oxygen therapy takes precedence over the increases in $Paco_2$. Arterial oxygen saturation (Sao_2) must be corrected to minimum acceptable levels (90% oxygen saturation) regardless of the changes in $Paco_2$. The minimum acceptable Sao_2 may be higher if there is evidence of end-organ hypoxia such as coronary ischemic changes. If the respiratory acidosis continues to worsen (pH < 7.20) during O_2 administration, institution of mechanical ventilation (see later) should be strongly considered pending potential reversal of the precipitating cause. Under no circumstances should supplemental O_2 therapy be withheld or hypoxemia uncorrected simply for the sake of avoiding worsening hypercapnia. Conversely, the amount of O_2 administered should be limited to correct arterial hypoxemia without resulting in unnecessarily high O_2 tensions.

Bronchodilators

Although patients with COPD have a limited degree of reversible airflow obstruction, especially compared with those with bronchial asthma, the role of bronchodilators remains prominent in the acute and chronic management of these patients. Both β-adrenergic agonists and anticholinergic agents are effective in the management of acute exacerbation of COPD.[39, 40] Karpel and coworkers[39] showed that aerosolized ipratropium bromide and metaproterenol similarly improved FEV_1 in the same group of patients during an acute exacerbation of COPD and also when they were restudied during a clinically stable period.[40] Some studies have shown some superiority of anticholinergics over beta agonists, and the combination of both may offer some advantage over a single agent.[41]

Either method of aerosol delivery—metered dose inhaler (MDI) or nebulizer—may be used during acute exacerbations. The MDI route offers a cost advantage, but it may be difficult to administer properly to an acutely dyspneic patient. The addition of a spacer or a reservoir between the MDI device and the mouth facilitates medication delivery.[42] If a patient is still unable to use the MDI effectively, the medication can be delivered via a nebulizer attached to a mouthpiece or to a face mask.

Nebulizers can be used during the initial treatment, and the patients can then be switched over to an MDI. In intubated patients, MDI aerosols can be delivered through an adapter in the ventilator tubing and actuation of the MDI coordinated with inspiration. Because large amounts of particles are precipitated in the ventilator tubing, however, the usual dose should be increased twofold to fourfold to ensure adequate delivery of medication into the airways. Both beta agonists and ipratropium may be given as frequently as every 1 to 2 hours on the basis of response. Dosing is limited by clinical response or the development of toxicity. After stabilization, the dosage can be reduced as indicated.

The addition of theophylline during acute exacerbation of COPD adds minimal if any efficacy. One well-controlled study found no improvement in spirometry, subjective measures of dyspnea, or gas exchange when theophylline was added to aerosol bronchodilators and systemic steroids.[43] In general, initial treatment should focus on aerosolized bronchodilators, intravenous steroids, antibiotics, and O_2 administration. If patients do not improve with this regimen over 12 to 24 hours, theophylline may be added for a potential benefit. Blood theophylline levels as well as potential drug interactions with other medications must be closely monitored.

Corticosteroids

Administration of a systemic corticosteroid is usually indicated for patients with acute exacerbation of COPD that warrants hospital admission. The efficacy of systemic corticosteroids in COPD has been substantiated in several studies.

Albert and colleagues[44] studied 44 consecutive patients and showed that methylprednisolone at 0.5 mg/kg every 6 hours for 72 hours resulted in a greater improvement in FEV_1 than in patients who received placebo. Rubini and others[45] studied the acute effects of intravenous methylprednisolone (0.8 mg/kg) on respiratory mechanics in eight hypercapnic patients with acute exacerbation of COPD. Ninety minutes after the corticosteroid dose, they observed a significant reduction in inspiratory resistance and a 16% reduction in the degree of dynamic hyperinflation. They postulated that the main acute effect of systemic corticosteroids is to increase the airway caliber through a reduction in inflammatory airway secretions. Conversely, in a study by Emerman and colleagues[46] in which systemic methylprednisolone was given upon presentation to the emergency department to 96 patients with an acute exacerbation of COPD, the investigators found no benefit of steroids over placebo in FEV_1 or rate of hospitalization.

Therefore, there is still no clear consensus on the precise role of systemic corticosteroids in patients with acute exacerbation of COPD. Given the potential for rapid progression of respiratory failure and need for mechanical ventilation with its associated morbidity, however, short-term systemic corticosteroid therapy should be strongly considered for acutely ill patients who require hospitalization. This approach is especially applicable to those requiring admission to the ICU for impending or established respiratory failure.

NONINVASIVE MECHANICAL VENTILATION

Mechanical ventilatory assistance without endotracheal intubation offers the following potential advantages:

- Increased comfort of the patient
- Decreased sedation requirements

- Retention of speech and eating abilities
- Avoidance of laryngeal injury
- Preservation of upper airway defenses against aspiration and pneumonia

Several investigators have studied the use of noninvasive positive-pressure ventilation in patients with acute exacerbation of COPD.[47–54]

As previously described, one of the major precipitants of acute respiratory failure in COPD is the development of dynamic hyperinflation, which causes increased inspiratory work of breathing by imposing an added inspiratory pressure threshold. The application of continuous positive airway pressure (CPAP) at levels that approach 80% to 90%[55] of the measured intrinsic PEEP values may reduce the work of breathing without causing further hyperinflation.[55–57] The addition of positive inspiratory pressure support may further assist ventilation by increasing tidal volume, decreasing respiratory frequency, and further reducing the inspiratory work of breathing performed by the respiratory muscles.[58, 59]

Andrivet and colleagues[60] used tracheal gas insufflation (TGI) in conjunction with a minitracheotomy for 20 patients with COPD who had not responded to conventional medical management and were not considered candidates for mechanical ventilation because of advanced age, end-stage disease, or comorbid conditions. The minitracheotomy cannula was easily inserted in the majority of patients with some transient blood-tinged secretions that cleared in all patients. Patients had a statistically significant reduction in their respiratory rate from 32.2 breaths/min baseline to 29.9, 25.6, and 25.7 breaths/min at 3, 24, and 48 hours after TGI, respectively. Three hours after initiation of TGI, Pa_{CO_2} increased from 59.6 to 63.5 mm Hg, but follow-up blood gas determinations 1, 2, and 7 days later showed that Pa_{CO_2} had returned to baseline values. Although the 35% overall mortality for this series of patients is comparable to the currently predicted mortality, this new combination of techniques may be potentially beneficial to a limited subgroup of patients.

Another noninvasive ventilatory option is the external high-frequency oscillator developed by Hayek and Schonfeld.[61] In their uncontrolled study, it reduced end-tidal CO_2 and increased oxygen saturation in 20 outpatients with COPD.[62] The application of this ventilatory mode during acute exacerbations and its effect on outcome await further trials.

Although many aspects of noninvasive ventilation in acute exacerbation of COPD are still debatable, such as defining optimal candidates, cost effectiveness, labor intensiveness, and complication rates, noninvasive ventilation should be in the armamentarium of all intensivists.

CONVENTIONAL MECHANICAL VENTILATION

Initiation

The decision to initiate mechanical ventilation for patients with acute exacerbation of COPD can range from simple to complex. With patients who have life-threatening, reversible acute respiratory failure, there should not be any hesitation to institute mechanical ventilation (Table 135–5). However, often ambiguity and controversy persist about the exact timing for intubation and mechanical ventilation. Also, there is a frequent misconception that mechanical ventilation should be avoided at all costs in this population of patients because they will rapidly become "ventilator-dependent" and caretakers will "never be able to take patients off the ventilator." In addition, many controversial economic and ethical issues cloud the question of appropriateness of initiating or withholding mechanical ventilation for patients with COPD. Although the decision to initiate mechanical ventilation must be made for each patient individually, certain underlying physiologic principles should guide physicians in their ventilatory management.

TABLE 135–5. Indications for Mechanical Ventilation in Patients with Chronic Obstructive Pulmonary Disease

Progressive deterioration despite maximum medical treatment
Intractable hypoxemia or progressive hypercarbia
Reversible precipitating factors such as upper or lower respiratory tract infections
Contraindication to noninvasive mechanical ventilation
Unresponsive to noninvasive ventilation
Neurologic impairment or obtundation
Hemodynamic instability
Inability to protect airway from aspiration
Impaired secretion clearance, ineffective cough

The first consideration should be selection of the appropriate mode of mechanical ventilation. If maximum ventilatory assistance is desired to allow adequate rest and recovery of overburdened respiratory muscles by minimizing the work of breathing, assist-control or maximum pressure support ventilation should be implemented. With assist-control ventilation, every breath, whether or not it is initiated by the patient, is a ventilator-assisted breath determined by the prescribed ventilator parameters (tidal volume, inspiratory flow pattern, and rate). Tidal volumes are generally selected on the basis of the patient's weight in the range of 8 to 10 mL/kg per breath. Ventilator frequency is selected on the basis of the desired minimum level of minute ventilation. Because this parameter reflects only the minimum number of guaranteed breaths per minute, patients may exceed this rate at any time. If the goal is to minimize patient-initiated breaths, the ventilator frequency may be progressively increased until the patient's respiratory frequency is "captured" by the set ventilator rate and few, if any, breaths are patient initiated. Because a patient's respiratory drive is governed by many nonrespiratory factors, such as pain, anxiety, and agitation, however, this strategy may result in excessive levels of minute ventilation and consequently increases in hyperinflation and potentially further respiratory and hemodynamic compromise.

In patients with elevated serum bicarbonate levels (chronic metabolic alkalosis) secondary to chronic hypercapnia, acute increases in minute ventilation with a consequent rise in pH may cause a severe alkalosis that can lead to neuromuscular hyperexcitability or even tetany. Under these circumstances, anxiolytics or analgesics can be cautiously administered, remembering that these medications may cause depression of respiratory drive, obtundation, confusion, and delirium that may impede subsequent weaning from mechanical ventilation.

Providing an adequate expiratory time (Te) for the selected tidal volume should be a primary goal in the ventilatory management of patients with any type of obstructive airway disease. As can be derived from Table 135–6, Te may be increased by manipulating inspiratory flow pattern, inspiratory flow rate, tidal volume, or respiratory frequency. The inspiratory flow pattern and rate are extremely important ventilator settings that affect the work of breathing, patient-ventilator synchrony, and development of auto-PEEP or dynamic hyperinflation.

The two most commonly used flow patterns are (1) constant inspiratory flow ("square wave") and (2) decelerating flow ("ramp wave"). At similar peak flow rates, for a constant tidal volume and frequency, the inspiratory time (Ti) is always shorter and the Te is longer with the constant inspiratory flow pattern (see Table 135–6). Thus, when a longer expiration is desired, the constant flow pattern may be preferable.

TABLE 135–6. Effect of Inspiratory Flow Pattern and Rate on Peak Airway Pressure and Inspiratory-to-Expiratory Ratio

Vt (mL)	Frequency (Breaths/min)	Flow Pattern	Flow (L/min)	Paw_{pk} (cm H_2O)	I:E
800	10	Constant	50	52	1:5.0
800	20	Constant	50	52	1:2.5
800	10	Constant	100	93	1:10
800	10	Decelerating	50	40	1:2.4
800	20	Decelerating	50	40	1:0.07
400	20	Decelerating	50	22	1:2.3

I:E = inspiratory-to-expiratory ratio; Paw_{pk} = peak airway pressure; VT = tidal volume.

The peak inspiratory flow rate is usually selected by one of two methods:

1. A patient's spontaneous inspiratory peak flow is measured using software that is available with certain commonly used commercial ventilators, such as the Puritan-Bennet 7200. The ventilator peak flow should then be set to exceed the patient's measured flow by 5 to 10 L/min.
2. The patient's minute ventilation is multiplied by a factor of 4 to 5. For example, if the minute ventilation is 20 L/min, the ventilator peak flow rate is set between 80 and 100 L/min.

Correct settings of the inspiratory flow rate are important to ensure that the ventilator is providing sufficient flow to satisfy the patient's demand and promote patient-ventilator synchrony (Table 135–7). Although using lower than conventional tidal volumes and respiratory frequencies may also allow a longer Te, these ventilator manipulations are less desirable because they may negatively affect desired minute ventilation and the patient's tolerance of mechanical ventilation.

Although shortening inspiratory time with constant flow and high inspiratory flow rates increases peak airway pressure, this is not necessarily deleterious. The increase in peak airway pressure is due to the increase in inspiratory airway resistance associated with the higher inspiratory flow rates and does not necessarily reflect increasing hyperinflation. Thus, these increased peak airway pressures per se do not necessarily increase the risk of barotrauma. One study examined the effects of varying inspiratory flow rates in patients with severe obstructive disease and found that at the higher flow rates, there were a decrease in the ratio of dead space to tidal volume of 23% and an increase in Pa_{O_2} by 18%.[63]

During assist-control ventilation, although every breath is assisted by the ventilator, there may still be a considerable amount of respiratory work of breathing, mostly because of the need to open demand valves, inadequate sensitivity trigger setting, and inadequate flow rates described earlier.[64] Thus, special attention to the setting is necessary to minimize the work of breathing when patients are receiving assist-control or other forms of positive-pressure ventilation.[64–67]

The only way to ensure that no respiratory work is performed during mechanical ventilation is to administer sedatives and neuromuscular blocker agents. These interventions are not generally recommended for most cases of acute respiratory failure in patients with COPD because they are associated with several adverse effects that may further negatively affect the respiratory system. The adverse effects of this therapy may include acute myopathy, interaction with glucocorticoids in producing myopathy, prolonged neuromuscular weakness, and respiratory muscle atrophy if they are used for extended periods of time (see earlier).

TABLE 135–7. Adverse Effects Caused by Inadequate Inspiratory Flow Settings

Increased work of breathing
Subjective air hunger
Dyssynchrony or "fighting" with the ventilator
Need to administer sedatives or even neuromuscular blockers
Increased air trapping and dynamic hyperinflation caused by inadequate expiratory time
Worsening gas exchange and cardiovascular instability related to hyperinflation

Pressure support ventilation may also be used to provide maximum respiratory support and minimize the work of breathing in the management of acute respiratory failure in patients with COPD. The inspiratory assistance provided with pressure support ventilation should be titrated up until a target tidal volume of approximately 8 to 10 mL/kg per breath is achieved. With this ventilatory mode, there is no minimum back-up respiratory rate; therefore, patients must have an adequate and stable respiratory drive to avoid episodes of hypoventilation. Also, pressure support ventilation does not guarantee a constant tidal volume; instead, the delivered volume depends on the lung mechanics (resistance and compliance). Therefore, if a patient receiving pressure support ventilation has unstable lung mechanics with rapidly changing airway resistance or compliance, the set inspiratory pressure support varies the delivered tidal volumes to values that may be too large or too small for that patient.

Thus, lung mechanics, inspired tidal volumes, and minute ventilation must be closely monitored with pressure support mode. Monitoring can be achieved by having appropriate alarm settings on the ventilator to signal intrinsic changes in the patient's condition. Pressure support ventilation is usually well tolerated and subjectively comfortable for patients because of its inherent flexibility in adjusting to a patient's inspiratory efforts, inspiratory time, and intrinsic respiratory frequency.[23]

As previously discussed, there is debate about the optimal amount of supplementary oxygen to administer to patients with chronic hypercapnia because of the fear of worsening CO_2 retention and respiratory acidosis. When the degree of acute respiratory failure is severe enough to warrant endotracheal intubation and mechanical ventilation, however, a primary goal of ventilatory support must be to reverse any potential life-threatening hypoxemia, especially if there is evidence of end-organ hypoxia such as angina, arrhythmia, or obtundation. ICUs with the ability to provide continuous pulse oximetry should target keeping arterial oxygen saturation between 90% and 100%.

Previously, PEEP was not used in the ventilatory management of patients with obstructive airway disease because of the fear that increased end-expiratory airway pressures would only further distend hyperinflated lung units, promoting cardiovascular insufficiency and barotrauma. Since the 1980s, however, many studies have documented the beneficial use of PEEP in this population of patients.[6, 27, 30, 31, 34, 35] The rationale for the use of extrinsic PEEP in the management of these patients is developed in the following but can be briefly summarized as offsetting intrinsic PEEP-induced increased work of breathing.

When intrinsic PEEP is present, it increases the work of breathing by different mechanisms, two of which are:

1. The dynamic hyperinflation associated with increasing lung volume at end-expiration can cause the respiratory muscles further disadvantage by placing them in less favorable position of their length-tension relationship.[68]
2. The presence of intrinsic PEEP causes an inspiratory threshold load, such that at the onset of a spontaneous inspira-

tory effort, alveolar pressure must first be decreased by an amount equivalent to intrinsic PEEP before inspiratory flow of gas into the lungs is initiated. The work required to overcome this intrinsic PEEP inspiratory threshold is wasted, as there is no corresponding volume change. This extra respiratory workload with every breath may impair a patient's ability to be successfully weaned from mechanical ventilation.

The addition of extrinsic PEEP up to the level of intrinsic PEEP can be used for patients with acute respiratory failure and airflow limitation to offset the inspiratory pressure threshold.[30, 34, 35, 69] Under these circumstances, the amount of intrinsic PEEP present is measured as previously described. Then the ventilator-derived extrinsic PEEP can be increased to approach the measured intrinsic PEEP levels.

Ranieri and colleagues[30] studied the effects of 5, 10, and 15 cm H_2O of PEEP in patients with COPD, flow limitation, and auto-PEEP who were receiving mechanical ventilation for acute respiratory failure. In the presence of flow limitation, ventilator PEEP could be safely added at levels up to 85% of auto-PEEP values without any additional hyperinflation or deleterious effects on cardiac index or gas exchange. Similarly, Baigorri and coworkers[31] showed that no hemodynamic impairment occurs when extrinsic PEEP is increased to levels below those of intrinsic PEEP, but increasing extrinsic PEEP above these levels impairs right ventricular function and reduces cardiac output.

Guerin and colleagues[70] have described another approach to the use of extrinsic PEEP for patients with acute respiratory failure and airflow limitation caused by COPD. These authors generated inflation static volume-pressure (V-P) curves for 10 patients with 0, 5, 10, and 15 cm H_2O of PEEP. They found that the static V-P curves were S shaped and had an inflection point defining a critical pressure (Po) and volume (Vo) above which all airways were open. In their model, if end-expiratory lung volume during ZEEP (PEEP = 0) is below this Vo, some small airways are collapsed during passive exhalation, and thus there is repetitive cycling of closure and reopening of small airways with each tidal breath. Seven of their 10 patients experienced this repetitive pattern of collapse and reopening during PEEP. This cyclic collapse and reopening of airways may potentially result in ventilator-induced lung injury.[71] The repetitive collapse and reopening can be avoided by matching the end-expiratory lung volume to the critical Vo. Their study suggests that this may achieved by adjusting either ventilator-derived extrinsic PEEP to approximate intrinsic PEEP values or decreasing expiratory time so that total PEEP (ventilator PEEP plus intrinsic PEEP) equals Vo. The amount of extrinsic PEEP required to keep EELV equal to or higher than Vo varied among patients, with three patients requiring PEEP = 5 cm H_2O, three patients requiring PEEP = 10 cm H_2O, and one patient requiring 15 cm H_2O.

In contrast to the previous recommendations of Ranieri and colleagues[30] to add only 85% of the intrinsic PEEP levels, these authors recommended that ventilator-derived extrinsic PEEP should be adjusted to match Po in order to prevent lung injury. However, the static pressure-volume curves that the investigators used in this study to define Vo, Po, and EELV are somewhat cumbersome to generate, which would limit the applicability of this technique to the patient's bedside. Furthermore, no study has examined the effect of either of these ventilatory strategies on weaning from mechanical ventilation or avoidance of complications in ventilator-dependent patients with COPD.

The exact role of ventilator-derived extrinsic PEEP in patients with respiratory failure and auto-PEEP is not simple or straightforward. For example, in many studies of the effects of adding extrinsic PEEP to counteract intrinsic PEEP, patients are sedated and paralyzed with completely controlled mechanical ventilation (no spontaneous breathing). Under these circumstances, there is no benefit with respect to removing the intrinsic PEEP-induced inspiratory threshold and imposed extra work of breathing because there are no spontaneous, patient-generated breaths. In this case, one is simply substituting ventilator-derived extrinsic PEEP for intrinsic PEEP without removing the deleterious effects of hyperinflation on gas exchange and hemodynamics. Conversely, if a patient with intrinsic PEEP is breathing spontaneously, there is a rationale for adding extrinsic PEEP in order to minimize the increased work of breathing and prevent the airway collapse that often occurs in these patients.

The hemodynamic effects of adding extrinsic PEEP to patients with intrinsic PEEP are variable and somewhat unpredictable. In some circumstances, the addition of extrinsic PEEP may not necessarily induce any hemodynamic compromise. This is often the case if the level of extrinsic PEEP is less than that of intrinsic PEEP, because adding extrinsic PEEP does not affect the already increased mean intrathoracic pressures impeding systemic venous return.[7, 33]

Baigorri and colleagues[31] used a pulmonary artery catheter equipped with a rapid response thermistor that allowed measurement of right ventricular ejection fraction in 10 ventilator-dependent COPD patients. As long as the extrinsic PEEP did not exceed intrinsic PEEP levels, there were no deleterious hemodynamic effects of right ventricular function or cardiac output. When the extrinsic PEEP levels exceeded the intrinsic PEEP levels by 5 cm H_2O, however, the authors observed a reduction in right ventricular volumes and a greater than 10% reduction in cardiac output in five of the 10 patients. In the other five patients, there was no change in any variable even though the ventilator-derived extrinsic PEEP exceeded intrinsic PEEP. Thus, the hemodynamic response to the addition of PEEP for ventilator-dependent patients with COPD is variable and dependent on the baseline level of dynamic hyperinflation (intrinsic PEEP), right ventricular function, intravascular volume status, respiratory system compliance, and whether the patient is actively breathing or is fully supported by positive-pressure ventilation.

The mechanical ventilatory mode and ventilatory parameters should also be examined in attempts to maximize expiratory time and minimize the risk of dynamic hyperinflation. The size of the endotracheal tube is also an important factor in the development of intrinsic PEEP.[72] As the size of the endotracheal tube decreases below 8 mm, the resistance of the endotracheal tube progressively increases. Thus, a tube of 8 mm diameter or larger should generally be used for adults with COPD in order to minimize expiratory resistance imposed by the endotracheal tube.

Finally, priority should be always given to identification of the underlying precipitating factor and optimal medical treatment with antibiotics, bronchodilators, and systemic corticosteroids, as described earlier.

Weaning

As a patient recovers from the acute respiratory failure, the degree of mechanical ventilatory support is gradually reduced and the patient assumes a greater amount of the work of breathing. Partial respiratory support during weaning may be accomplished in several ways.

Intermittent mandatory ventilation (IMV) provides a minimum number of ventilator breaths determined by the set frequency; additional breaths beyond this minimum are unassisted. As the patient recovers and the IMV rate is decreased, the patient's respiratory workload is gradually increased until extubation is possible. The amount of pressure support assistance per breath can also be decreased to allow patients gradually to resume spontaneous work of breathing.

Finally, intermittent trials of complete spontaneous breathing, such as T-tube trials, may also allow patients slowly to resume spontaneous work of breathing. Each method has advantages and disadvantages and no study has ever definitively concluded that one technique is superior to another for weaning from mechanical ventilation.[73, 74] Therefore, which partial ventilatory support mode is used to reinstitute the patient's spontaneous respiratory workload during weaning from mechanical ventilation is largely dependent on individual and institutional practices.

OUTCOME

Mortality associated with episodes of acute respiratory failure in patients with COPD varies among studies. Overall in-hospital mortality is greater than 20%[75] in patients with COPD and acute respiratory failure who require intubation and mechanical ventilation and is greater than 50% among elderly patients.[76] Weiss and Hudson[77] found an average mortality of 43% in 11 studies of patients with an exacerbation of COPD who required mechanical ventilation. Using the Acute Physiologic and Chronic Health Evaluation (APACHE) III data base, Seneff and colleagues[78] showed that 16% of patients died while in the ICU, 32% died before hospital discharge, and more than half of patients died within 1 year. Two studies found that the mortality rate was reduced in patients with acute exacerbation of COPD who had early institution of noninvasive mask ventilation.[58, 79] Therefore, precise prediction of the outcome for individual patients is still not realistic and each case must be considered individually.

SUMMARY

The management of acute respiratory failure of patients with COPD remains challenging and complex. Successful outcomes depend on understanding of the physiologic principles that govern development and reversal of the respiratory failure. Precipitating events must be diligently sought because reversal of these events is key to reversal of the respiratory failure. An in-depth knowledge of the specific guidelines for mechanical ventilation in this specialized form of respiratory failure is needed to optimize ventilatory support while minimizing potential complications.

References

1. Wagner GS: Marriot's Practical Electrocardiography. 9th ed. Baltimore, Williams & Wilkins, 1994.
2. Greenberg YJ, Rosenfeld LE: Evaluating and managing arrhythmias in COPD. J Respir Dis 1995; 16:1099.
3. Bredikis AJ, Liebson PR: The ECG in COPD: Biventricular hypertrophy, voltage, rhythm changes. J Respir Dis 1998; 19:43.
4. Fleury B, Murciano D, Talamo C, et al: Work of breathing in patients with obstructive pulmonary disease in acute respiratory failure. Am Rev Respir Dis 1985; 131:822.
5. Broseghini C, Brandolese R, Poggi R, et al: Respiratory mechanics during the first day of mechanical ventilation in patients with pulmonary edema and chronic airway obstruction. Am Rev Respir Dis 1988; 138:355.
6. Rossi A, Gottfried SB, Zocchi L, et al: Measurement of static compliance of the total respiratory system in patients with acute respiratory failure during mechanical ventilation: The effect of intrinsic positive end-expiratory pressure. Am Rev Respir Dis 1985; 131:672.
7. Pepe PE, Marini JJ: Occult positive end-pressure in mechanically ventilated patients with airflow obstruction: The auto-PEEP effect. Am Rev Respir Dis 1982; 126:166.
8. Talpers SS, Romberger DJ, Bunce SB, et al: Nutritionally associated increased carbon dioxide production: Excess total calories vs. high proportion of carbohydrate calories. Chest 1992; 102:551.
9. Fiaccadori E, Coffrini E, Fracchia C, et al: Hypophosphatemia and phosphorus depletion in respiratory and peripheral muscles of patients with respiratory failure due to COPD. Chest 1994; 105:1392.
10. Laaban JP, Kouchakji B, Dore MF, et al: Nutritional status of patients with chronic obstructive pulmonary disease and acute respiratory failure. Chest 1993; 103:1362.
11. Juan G, Calverley P, Talamo C, et al: Effect of carbon dioxide on diaphragmatic function in human beings. N Engl J Med 1984; 310:874.
12. Rudis MI, Sikora CA, Angus A, et al: A prospective, randomized, controlled evaluation of peripheral nerve stimulation versus standard clinical dosing of neuromuscular blocking agents in critically ill patients. Crit Care Med 1997; 25:575.
13. Gooch JL, Suchyta MR, Balbierz JM, et al: Prolonged paralysis after treatment with neuromuscular junction blocking agents. Crit Care Med 1991; 19:1125.
14. Dannon MJ, Carpenter S: Myopathy with thick filament (myosin) loss following prolonged paralysis with vecuronium during steroid treatment. Muscle Nerve 1991; 14:1131.
15. al-Lozi MT, Pestronk A, Yee WC, et al: Rapidly evolving myopathy with myosin-deficient muscle fibers. Ann Neurol 1994; 35:273.
16. Chad DA, Lacomis D: Critically ill patients with newly acquired weakness: The clinicopathologic spectrum. Ann Neurol 1994; 35:257.
17. Massa R, Carpenter S, Holland P, et al: Loss and renewal of thick myofilaments in glucocorticoid-treated rat soleus after denervation and reinnervation. Muscle Nerve 1992; 15:1290.
18. Du Bois DC, Almon RR: A possible role for glucocorticoids in denervation atrophy. Muscle Nerve 1981; 4:370.
19. Segredo V, Caldwell JE, Matthay MA, et al: Persistent paralysis in critically ill patients after long-term administration of vecuronium. N Engl J Med 1992; 327:524.
20. Griffen D, Fairman N, Coursin D, et al: Acute myopathy during treatment of status asthmaticus with corticosteroids and steroidal muscle relaxants. Chest 1992; 102:510.
21. Zochodne DW, Ramsey DA, Saly V, et al: Acute necrotizing myopathy of intensive care: Electrophysiological studies. Muscle Nerve 1994; 17:285.
22. Jubran A, Van de Graaf WB, Tobin MJ: Variability of the patient-ventilator interaction with pressure support ventilation in patients with chronic obstructive pulmonary disease. Am J Respir Crit Care Med 1995; 152:129.
23. MacIntyre NR: Respiratory muscle function during pressure support ventilation. Chest 1986; 89:677.
24. Chamorro C, Latorre FJ, Montero A, et al: Comparative study of propofol versus midazolam in the sedation of critically ill patients: Results of a prospective, randomized, multicenter trial. Crit Care Med 1996; 24:932.
25. Ronan KP, Gallagher TJ, George B, et al: Comparison of propofol and midazolam for sedation in intensive care unit patients. Crit Care Med 1995; 23:286.
26. Muller N, Bryan AC, Zamel N: Tonic inspiratory muscle activity as a cause of hyperinflation in histamine induced asthma. J Appl Physiol 1981; 49:863.
27. Pinsky MR: Through the past darkly: Ventilatory management of patients with COPD (Editorial). Crit Care Med 1994; 22:1714.
28. Marini J: Should PEEP be used in airflow obstruction? Am Rev Respir Dis 1989; 140:1.
29. Bergman NA: Properties of passive exhalation in anesthetized subjects. Anesthesiology 1969; 30:378.
30. Ranieri VM, Guilano R, Cinnella G, et al: Physiologic effects of positive end-expiratory pressure in patients with chronic obstructive pulmonary disease during acute ventilatory failure and controlled mechanical ventilation. Am Rev Respir Dis 1993; 147:5.
31. Baigorri F, De Monte A, Blanch L, et al: Hemodynamic response to external counterbalancing of auto-positive end-expiratory pressure in mechanically ventilated patients with chronic obstructive pulmonary disease. Crit Care Med 1994; 22:1782.
32. Miro AM: The many disguises of PEEP. *In:* Case Studies: Tricks and Traps. Park GP, Pinsky MR (Eds). London, WB Saunders, 1997, p 59.
33. Rogers PL, Schlichtig R, Miro A, et al: Auto-PEEP during CPR: An

"occult" cause of electromechanical dissociation. Chest 1991; 99:492.

34. Smith TC, Marini JJ: Impact of PEEP on lung mechanics and work of breathing in severe airflow obstruction. J Appl Physiol 1988; 65:1488.
35. Petrof BJ, Legare P, Goldberg P, et al: Continuous positive airway pressure reduces inspiratory work of breathing and dyspnea during weaning from mechanical ventilation in severe chronic obstructive pulmonary disease. Am Rev Respir Dis 1990; 141:281.
36. Hoffman RA, Ershowsky P, Krieger BP: Determination of auto-PEEP during spontaneous and controlled ventilation by monitoring changes in end-expiratory thoracic gas volume. Chest 1989; 96:613.
37. Sassoon CS, Hassell KT, Mahutte CK: Hyperoxic-induced hypercapnia in stable chronic obstructive pulmonary disease. Am Rev Respir Dis 1987; 136:907.
38. Crossley DJ, McGuire GP, Barrow PM, et al: Influence of inspired oxygen concentration on dead space, respiratory drive, and Pa_{CO_2} in intubated patients with chronic obstructive pulmonary disease. Crit Care Med 1997; 25:1522.
39. Karpel JP, Pesin J, Greenberg D, et al: A comparison of the effects of ipratropium bromide and metaproterenol sulfate in acute exacerbations of COPD. Chest 1990; 98:835.
40. Karpel JP: Bronchodilator responses to anticholinergic and beta-adrenergic agents in acute and stable COPD. Chest 1991; 99:871.
41. Braun SR, McKenzie WN, Copeland C, et al: A comparison of the effect of ipratropium and albuterol in the treatment of chronic obstructive airway disease. Arch Intern Med 1989; 149:544.
42. Godden DJ, Crompton GK: An objective assessment of the tube spacer in patients unable to use conventional pressurized aerosol effectively. Br J Dis Chest 1981; 75:165.
43. Rice KL, Leatherman JW, Duane PG, et al: Aminophylline for acute exacerbations of chronic obstructive pulmonary disease. Ann Intern Med 1987; 107:305.
44. Albert RK, Martin TR, Lewis SW: Controlled clinical trial of methylprednisolone in patients with chronic bronchitis and acute respiratory insufficiency. Ann Intern Med 1980; 92:753.
45. Rubini F, Rampulla C, Nava S: Acute effects of corticosteroids on respiratory mechanics in mechanically ventilated patients with chronic airflow obstruction and acute respiratory failure. Am J Respir Crit Care Med 1994; 149:306.
46. Emerman CL, Connors AF, Lukens TW, et al: A randomized trial of methylprednisolone in the emergency treatment of acute exacerbations of COPD. Chest 1989; 95:563.
47. Meduri GU: Noninvasive positive pressure ventilation in chronic obstructive pulmonary disease patients with acute exacerbation (Editorial). Crit Care Med 1997; 25:1631.
48. Keenan SP, Kernerman PD, Cook DJ, et al: Effect of noninvasive positive pressure ventilation on mortality in patients admitted with acute respiratory failure: A meta-analysis. Crit Care Med 1997; 25:1685.
49. Elliot MW, Green RAM, Moxham J, et al: A comparison of different modes of noninvasive ventilatory support: Effects on ventilation and inspiratory muscle effort. Anaesthesia 1994; 49:279.
50. Kramer N, Meyer T, Meharg J, et al: Randomized, prospective trial of noninvasive positive pressure ventilation in acute respiratory failure. Am J Respir Crit Care Med 1995; 151:1799.
51. Jones DJM, Paul EA, Jones PW, et al: Nasal pressure support ventilation plus oxygen compared with oxygen therapy alone in hypercapnic COPD. Am J Respir Crit Care Med 1995; 152:538.
52. de Lucas P, Tarancon C, Puente L, et al: Nasal continuous positive airway pressure in patients with COPD in acute respiratory failure: A study of immediate effects. Chest 1993; 104:1694.
53. Servera E, Perez M, Marin J, et al: Noninvasive nasal mask ventilation beyond the ICU for an exacerbation of chronic respiratory insufficiency. Chest 1995; 108:1572.
54. Hill NS: Noninvasive ventilation: Does it work, for whom, and how? Am Rev Respir Dis 1993; 147:1050.
55. Appendini L, Patessio A, Zanaboni S, et al: Physiologic effects of positive end-expiratory pressure and mask pressure support during exacerbations of chronic obstructive pulmonary disease. Am J Respir Crit Care Med 1994; 149:1069.
56. Miro AM, Shivaram U, Hertig I: Continuous positive airway pressure in COPD patients with acute hypercapnic respiratory failure. Chest 1993; 103:266.
57. Carrey Z, Gottfried SB, Levy RD, et al: Ventilatory muscle support in respiratory failure with nasal positive pressure ventilation. Chest 1990; 97:150.
58. Brochard L, Isabey D, Piquet J, et al: Reversal of acute exacerbations of chronic obstructive lung disease by inspiratory assistance with a face mask. N Engl J Med 1990; 33:1523.
59. Brochard L, Mancebo J, Wysocki M: Noninvasive ventilation for acute exacerbations of chronic obstructive pulmonary disease. N Engl J Med 1995; 333:817.
60. Andrivet P, Richard G, Viau F, et al: Treatment of respiratory failure using minitracheotomy and intratracheal oxygenation in selected patients with chronic lung disease. Intensive Care Med 1996; 22:1323.
61. Hayek Z, Schonfeld T: External high frequency oscillation around negative baseline (EHFO-NB): Preliminary trial in humans. Proceedings of the Fifth Congress on Intensive and Critical Care Medicine. Amsterdam, Excerpta Medica, 1990, p 761.
62. Spitzer SA, Fink G, Mittleman M: External high-frequency ventilation in severe chronic obstructive pulmonary disease. Chest 1993; 104:1698.
63. Connors AF, McCaffree RD, Gray BA: Effect of inspiratory flow rate on gas exchange during mechanical ventilation. Am Rev Respir Dis 1981; 124:537.
64. Marini JJ, Capps JS, Culver BH: The inspiratory work of breathing during assisted mechanical ventilation. Chest 1985; 87:612.
65. Marini JJ, Rodriguez RM, Lamb V: The inspiratory workload of patient-initiated mechanical ventilation. Am Rev Respir Dis 1986; 134:902.
66. Marini JJ, Smith TC, Lamb VJ: External work output and force generation during synchronized intermittent mechanical ventilation: Effect of machine assistance on breathing effort. Am Rev Respir Dis 1988; 138:1169.
67. Marini JJ, Smith TC, Rodriguez RM, et al: The workload of patient-initiated mechanical ventilation. Am Rev Respir Dis 1986; 131:850.
68. Roussos C, Macklem PT: The respiratory muscles. N Engl J Med 1982; 307:78.
69. Georgopoulos D, Giannouli E, Patakas D: Effects of extrinsic positive end-expiratory pressure on mechanically ventilated patients with chronic obstructive pulmonary disease and dynamic hyperinflation. Intensive Care Med 1993; 19:197.
70. Guerin C, LeMasson S, de Varax R, et al: Small airway closure and positive end-expiratory pressure in mechanically ventilated patients with chronic obstructive pulmonary disease. Am J Respir Crit Care Med 1997; 155:1949.
71. Muscedere JG, Mullen JB, Gan K, et al: Tidal ventilation at low airway pressures can augment lung injury. Am J Respir Crit Care Med 1994; 149:1327.
72. Scott LR, Benson MS, Bishop MJ: Relationship of endotracheal tube size to auto-PEEP at high minute ventilation. Respir Care 1986; 31:1080.
73. Brochard L, Raus A, Benito S, et al: Comparison of three methods of gradual withdrawal from ventilatory support during weaning from mechanical ventilation. Am J Respir Crit Care Med 1994; 150:896.
74. Esteban A, Frutos F, Tobin MJ, et al: A comparison of four methods of weaning patients from mechanical ventilation: Spanish Lung Failure Collaborative Group. N Engl J Med 1995; 332:345.
75. Petty TL: Acute respiratory failure in COPD. *In:* Chronic Obstructive Pulmonary Disease. 2nd ed. Petty TL (Ed). New York, Marcel Dekker, 1985 p 389.
76. Swinburne AJ, Fedullo AJ, Bixby K, et al: Respiratory failure in the elderly: Analysis of outcome after treatment with mechanical ventilation. Arch Intern Med 1993; 153:1657.
77. Weiss SM, Hudson LD: Outcome from respiratory failure. Crit Care Clin 1994; 10:194.
78. Seneff MG, Wagner DP, Wagner RP, et al: Hospital and 1-year survival of patients admitted to intensive care units with acute exacerbations of chronic obstructive pulmonary disease. JAMA 1995; 274:1852.
79. Bott J, Carroll MP, Conway JH, et al: Randomised controlled trial of nasal ventilation in acute ventilatory failure due to chronic obstructive airways disease. Lancet 1993; 341:1555.

136

Weaning from Respiratory Support in Airflow Obstruction States

Kevin P. Simpson, MD • Martin Tobin, MD

More than any other technologic advance, mechanical ventilation has been identified with the development of critical care units. Although it is frequently lifesaving, mechanical ventilation poses a risk of serious complications[1, 2] and markedly increases the cost of care for ventilator-dependent patients.[3] Consequently, every effort should be made to discontinue mechanical ventilation as soon as a patient can sustain spontaneous ventilation.

In the strict literal sense, the term *weaning* refers to a gradual decrease in the level of ventilator support; in daily practice, however, the term is applied to all methods of discontinuing mechanical ventilation, including abrupt cessation.[4] Most patients tolerate the first attempt at discontinuation of ventilator support without any difficulty, and fewer than 24% experience any significant respiratory distress.[5] Nonetheless, the process of weaning constitutes a major portion of the workload in an intensive care unit (ICU) and more than 40% of the total ventilator time may be consumed by the weaning process.[6] This chapter reviews the major determinants of weaning outcome, the most commonly used predictors of weaning outcome, and methods of discontinuing mechanical ventilation.

DETERMINANTS OF WEANING OUTCOME

The pathophysiologic determinants of weaning outcome are:

- Adequacy of pulmonary gas exchange
- Performance of the respiratory muscle pump
- Psychologic factors

Adequacy of Pulmonary Gas Exchange

Attempts to restore spontaneous respiration after a period of mechanical ventilation may result in hypoxemia as a consequence of impaired pulmonary gas exchange, hypoventilation, or decreased oxygen (O_2) content of venous blood. Using the multiple inert gas technique in ventilator-supported patients, Torres and colleagues[7] found that the resumption of spontaneous breathing was associated with the development of abnormalities in the alveolar ventilation-perfusion ratio. However, a fall in PaO_2 was prevented by the associated increase in cardiac output. Unfortunately, comparable detailed investigations of gas exchange in patients in an unsuccessful weaning trial have not been conducted.

Respiratory Muscle Performance

Failure of the respiratory muscle pump is probably the most common cause of unsuccessful weaning.[8] This may result from:

- Decreased neuromuscular capacity
- Increased respiratory muscle pump load
- A combination of both factors

Decreased Neuromuscular Capacity

Respiratory Center Output

During an unsuccessful weaning trial, respiratory acidosis commonly occurs, raising the possibility that respiratory center drive may be decreased. However, indices of drive, such as airway occlusion pressure at 0.1 second ($P_{0.1}$) or mean inspiratory flow (V_T/T_I), are usually above the normal range in such patients.[9-12] Furthermore, an increase in V_T/T_I has been observed when severe alveolar hypoventilation developed during an unsuccessful weaning trial (Fig. 136–1).[9] Thus, it is doubtful that inadequate respiratory center output is primarily responsible for weaning failure in most patients.

Phrenic Nerve Function

Phrenic nerve dysfunction should be suspected in patients who have undergone coronary artery bypass surgery if weaning proves difficult in the postoperative period. Several groups of investigators have found hemidiaphragmatic paralysis in about 10% of these patients.[13] Most injuries are due to hypothermia from the topical cooling and are more common when a pericardial insulating pad is not used during surgery. Phrenic nerve dysfunction has also been reported following lung transplantation.[14] Unilateral diaphragmatic paralysis is rarely life-threatening but may make weaning difficult in the first several days after surgery. In a small number of patients, bilateral diaphragmatic paralysis may develop, resulting in prolonged ventilator dependency.

Respiratory Muscle Function

Respiratory muscle function may be impaired by various conditions commonly observed in critically ill patients.[8] These conditions are discussed in detail throughout this book, and the following text emphasizes their role during the weaning process.

Of the clinical conditions that cause a decrease in respiratory muscle strength or endurance, *hyperinflation* is one of the most important.[9] Dynamic hyperinflation often results from an altered pattern of breathing during weaning.[9] Adverse effects are numerous[8] (Fig. 136–2).

Malnutrition is particularly common in critically ill patients,[4] and up to 88% receive inadequate nutritional support. Malnutrition has a number of adverse effects on respiratory function, including decreased ventilatory response to hypoxia, a decrease in muscle mass and thickness, and a reduction in respiratory muscle strength and endurance.[4] In addition, altered host defenses predispose to nosocomial pneumonia, which can increase the load on the respiratory system.[4]

The *O_2 supply* to a muscle is decreased if cardiac output falls, the O_2 content of arterial blood decreases (hypoxemia, anemia), or O_2 extraction is impaired (sepsis).[4] Lemaire and colleagues identified hemodynamic compromise during failed weaning trials in 15 patients with chronic obstructive pulmonary disease (COPD) and cardiovascular disease.[15] After 10 minutes of spontaneous breathing, the patients showed an increase in transmural pulmonary artery occlusion pressure, cardiac index, and left and right ventricular end-diastolic volume indices; subsequently, successful weaning was achieved in nine patients after diuresis.

Several other issues can affect respiratory muscle function. Information about *hypoxic* harm to respiratory muscle function is accumulating,[4] but controversy about its precise role still exists. *Acute respiratory acidosis* may decrease contractility and endurance time of the diaphragm in healthy subjects.[16] Several *metabolic abnormalities*, including abnormalities of phosphate, potassium, calcium, and magnesium,[4] can adversely affect respiratory muscle function. *Endocrine disturbances*, such as hyperthyroidism or hypothyroidism, can also impair respiratory muscle function. Probably more relevant to the weaning situation is the use of *corticosteroid* therapy,

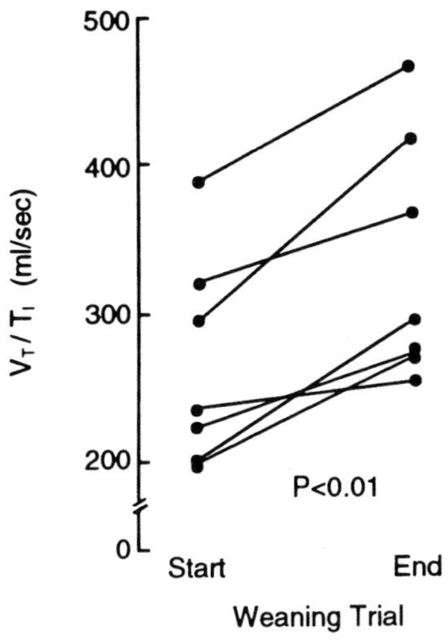

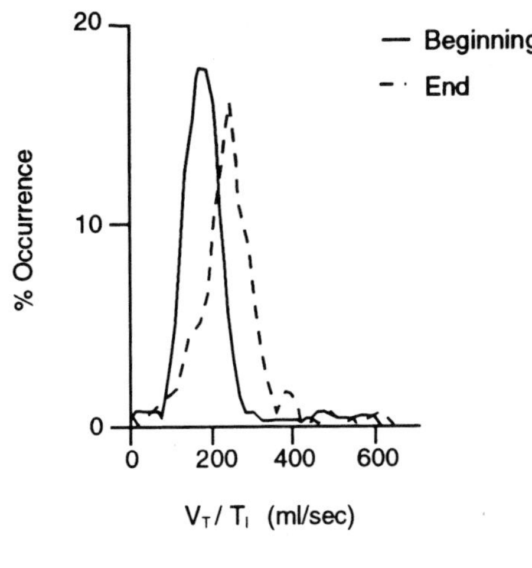

Figure 136–1. *Left panel:* Measurements of VT/TI in seven patients after a failed trial of weaning from mechanical ventilation. *Right panel:* Increase in the frequency histogram distribution of VT/TI from the onset to the end of the weaning trial in a representative patient with an unsuccessful weaning outcome ($P < .002$, Mann-Whitney U tests of medians and variability). An increase in VT/TI of this magnitude was individually observed in all but one of seven patients in the treatment failure group. (From Tobin MJ, Perez W, Guenther SM, et al: The pattern of breathing during successful and unsuccessful trials of weaning from mechanical ventilation. Am Rev Respir Dis 1986; 134:1111–1118.)

potentially leading to steroid myopathy,[17] whereas prolonged respiratory muscle weakness may occur following discontinuation of *neuromuscular blockers*.[18]

Respiratory muscle atrophy and decreased performance due to prolonged mechanical ventilation have been demonstrated in baboons,[19] but animal data may not translate well to the human condition. The respiratory muscles are not completely immobilized with mechanical ventilation, and as little as one diaphragmatic contraction daily may be enough to prevent atrophy.[20]

The development of *respiratory muscle fatigue* has long been suspected in the weaning failure patient, although unequivocal evidence is lacking. In one of the first studies to use weaning failure as a model of acute ventilatory failure, Cohen and coworkers[21] observed a shift in the power spectrum of the diaphragmatic electromyogram (EMG), which they considered to signify fatigue.[22] It is now recognized, however, that the EMG power spectrum is influenced by several factors and does not necessarily signify impaired muscle contractility.

More recently, Jubran and Tobin[23] measured tension-time index in 17 patients with COPD who did not respond to a trial of weaning from mechanical ventilation and 14 patients who tolerated such a trial and were extubated. Mean esophageal pressure (Pes) and maximum Pes were used to calculate tension-time index (TTIes). At the onset of the trial, TTIes was not different in the two groups (Fig. 136–3). However, five of the unsuccessful patients demonstrated a TTIes above 0.15 by the end of the trial, whereas no successful patient showed such a change; these data suggest that respiratory muscle fatigue may be responsible for some instances of weaning failure.

The question of whether or not weaning failure in an individual patient is due to respiratory muscle fatigue, which is associated with structural damage to the muscles, is of crucial importance for several reasons. Rest is the only means of reversing fatigue, and for the respiratory muscles this means mechanical ventilation. If respiratory muscle fatigue occurs during the course of an unsuccessful attempt to discontinue ventilator support, it is likely that the new structural injury to the muscles will impair the patient's performance and represent an additional medical complication for this patient. Trying to minimize the risk of fatigue by postponing attempts at weaning places the patient at risk for the many complications associated with mechanical ventilation. Moreover, excessive muscle rest can cause muscle atrophy,[19, 20] thus initiating a vicious circle. These issues are compounded by the lack of simple, reliable means of detecting respiratory muscle fatigue in critically ill patients. Measurement of maximum inspiratory

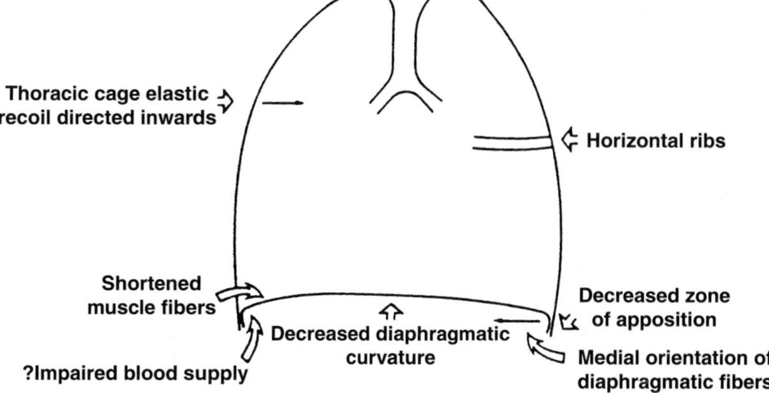

Figure 136–2. The detrimental effects of hyperinflation on respiratory muscle function. (From Tobin MJ: Respiratory muscles in disease. Clin Chest Med 1988; 9:263–286.)

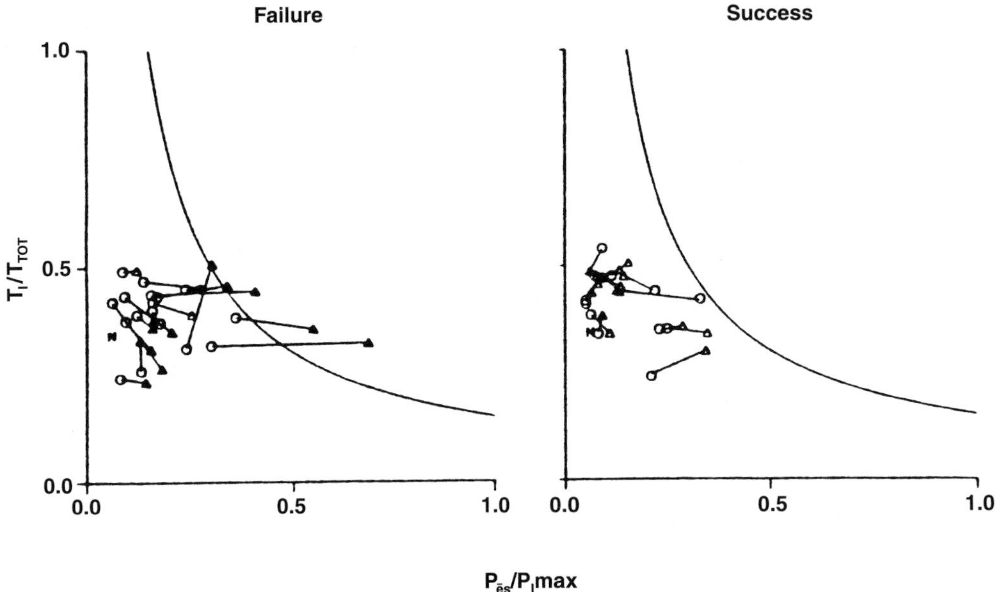

Figure 136–3. Relationship between mean esophagealpressure/maximal inspiratory pressure ratio ($P_{\bar{e}s}/P_I$max) and duty cycle (T_I/T_{TOT}) in 17 ventilator-supported patients with chronic obstructive pulmonary disease after an unsuccessful trial of spontaneous breathing and 14 patients who tolerated the trial. *Circles* and *triangles* represent values at the start and end of the trial, respectively; *closed symbols* indicate patients in whom Pa_{CO_2} increased during the trial. Five of the 17 patients in the treatment failure group had a tension time index (TTI) of >0.15 (indicated by the isopleth), suggesting respiratory muscle fatigue. N represents value in a normal subject. (From Jubran A, Tobin MJ: Pathophysiologic basis of acute respiratory distress in patients who fail a trial of weaning from mechanical ventilation. Am J Respir Crit Care Med 1997; 155:906–915.)

pressure (PImax) provides information on the strength of the respiratory muscles, but it does not quantitate a patient's susceptibility to fatigue or indicate whether or not fatigue is present. Many of the approaches employed in conducting research on fatigue in healthy volunteers, such as ability to maintain a target pressure over time, are influenced by patient motivation and cooperation and as such do not serve as satisfactory diagnostic or monitoring tools in critically ill patients. The tension-time index is elevated in both healthy volunteers at the point of diaphragmatic fatigue[24] and COPD patients who did not respond to a trial of spontaneous breathing (see earlier)[23]:

$$TTI = \text{mean } P_{br}/\text{PImax} \times T_I/T_{TOT}$$

where P_{br} reflects mean inspiratory pressure.

Interpretation of TTI, however, is confounded by a number of issues. Newer techniques, such as magnetic stimulation of the phrenic nerves,[25, 26] may answer the question of whether contractile muscle fatigue is an important mechanism of ventilator dependence and failure to be weaned.

Increased Respiratory System Load

An increase in the load on the respiratory muscle pump may result from increased ventilatory requirements or increased work of breathing. Factors causing an increase in ventilatory requirements include

- Increased CO_2 production (V_{CO_2})
- Increased dead space ventilation
- An inappropriately elevated respiratory drive

An increase in V_{CO_2} predisposes to the development of CO_2 retention, but it is never the sole cause of hypercapnia. Although inadequate respiratory drive causes hypoventilation and respiratory acidosis, an inappropriately heightened drive places excessive stress on the respiratory muscle pump and predisposes to fatigue. Several studies have shown high levels of drive in patients who could not be weaned,[9-11] but the level of drive does not appear to be inappropriate in relation to chemical stimulation.[9]

For normal ventilation to be achieved, work is performed to overcome the elastic and frictional impedances of the lungs and chest wall. In the presence of increased resistance or decreased compliance, a greater swing in pleural pressure is required to achieve a given V_T, thus resulting in increased work of breathing. In the previously mentioned study by Jubran and Tobin,[23] inspiratory resistance increased in the unsuccessful group but remained unchanged from the start of the trial in the successful group (Fig. 136–4). In addition, lung elastance was higher in the failure treatment group than in the successful group at the onset of the trial (21.2 versus 9.9 cm H_2O/L) and was more than twofold higher at the end of the trial (34.1 versus 14.0 cm H_2O/L). Furthermore, intrinsic peak end-expiratory pressure (PEEPI) was higher in the failure group than in the success group both at the onset (2.0 versus 0.7 cm H_2O) and end (4.1 versus 1.1 cm H_2O) of the trial. Clearly, the patients who were unable to initiate spontaneous breathing experienced progressive worsening of their respiratory mechanics. As a result, respiratory muscle energy expenditure, quantitated in terms of pressure-time product per minute (which was similar in the two groups at the onset of the trial), was nearly twice as high in the failure group by the end of the trial (388 versus 205 cm H_2O · sec/min).

Psychologic Factors

Psychologic factors may contribute to weaning difficulties in some patients, and feelings of insecurity, anxiety, fear, agony, and panic have been associated with dependence on mechanical ventilation.[27] Apart from a few isolated reports, little information exists on the prevalence or nature of psychologic disturbances in ventilator-dependent patients or the degree to which these disturbances contribute to ventilator dependency.

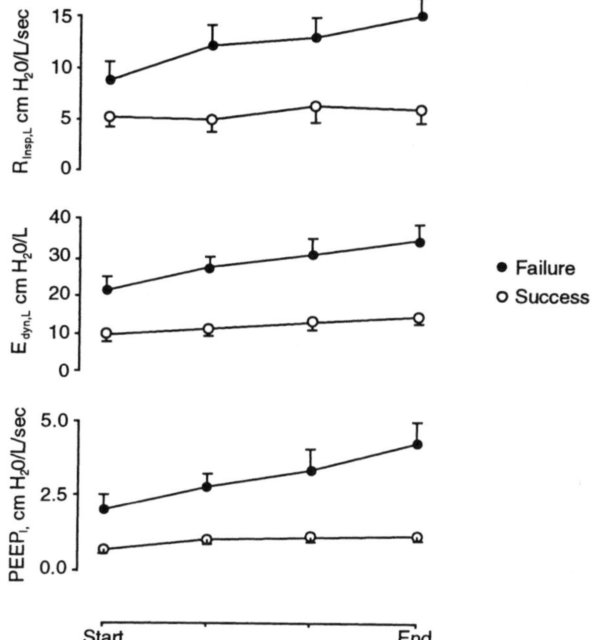

Figure 136–4. Inspiratory resistance of the lung ($Rinsp_L$), dynamic lung elastance ($Edyn_L$), and intrinsic positive end-expiratory pressure (PEEPI) during a trial of spontaneous breathing in the failure and success groups. Between the onset and the end of the trial, increases in $Rinsp_L$ ($P < .009$), $Edyn_L$ ($P < .0001$), and $PEEP_I$ ($P < .0001$) occurred in the weaning failure group, and increases in $Edyn_L$ ($P < .0006$) and $PEEP_I$ ($P < .02$) occurred in the successful group. Over the course of the trial, the unsuccessful group had higher values of $Rinsp_L$ ($P < 0.003$), $Edyn_L$ ($P < 0.0006$), and $PEEP_I$ ($P < .0009$) than in the successful group. *Bars* represent 1 standard error. (From Jubran A, Tobin MJ: Pathophysiologic basis of acute respiratory distress in patients who fail a trial of weaning from mechanical ventilation. Am J Respir Crit Care Med 1997; 155:906–915.)

PREDICTING WEANING OUTCOME

Determining the optimal time for discontinuing ventilator support can be difficult, and clinical assessment alone is not sufficient to predict weaning outcome, as shown by Stroetz and Hubmayr.[28] They studied 31 patients being weaned by gradual reductions in the level of pressure support. The physician in charge of each patient was asked to predict the patient's ability to sustain unassisted breathing without distress for 1 hour. Of 22 patients whom the physicians thought likely to fail a weaning trial, 11 were successfully weaned; of nine patients thought likely to be successfully weaned, three did not respond. Clearly, objective tests are needed to guide physicians in predicting a patient's ability to sustain spontaneous ventilation. The commonly used indices are listed in Table 136–1.

Gas Exchange

No single index of oxygenation is universally accepted to prohibit weaning, and a number of different criteria derived from arterial blood gas measurements have been proposed. The oxygenation criteria in Table 136–1 have been passed from one review article to another without systematic studies. In a study of predictors of weaning outcome, Yang and Tobin[29] found that a PaO_2:PAO_2 ratio of 0.35 provided the best separation of weaning success versus weaning failure in a preliminary "training data set" of 36 patients. However, prospective evaluation in a further 64 patients yielded a positive predictive value for this ratio of only 0.59 and a negative predictive value of only 0.53.

Maximum Inspiratory Pressure

A global assessment of respiratory muscle strength can be obtained by measuring PImax[26] at the opening of an endotracheal tube during a maximum inspiratory effort. Sahn and Lakshminarayan[30] popularized this measurement with their excellent results in 100 patients. All patients who were successfully weaned had a PImax more negative than −30 cm H_2O, and all patients who did not respond successfully had a PImax of −20 cm H_2O or less negative. Since then, however, many investigators have found PImax to be much less reliable.

Lack of patient cooperation has been cited for the poor predictive power of PImax, and thus Marini and associates[31] modified the technique. A one-way valve ensured that inspiratory efforts were made at a low lung volume while occlusion was maintained for 20 seconds. PImax gradually improved during the 20 seconds of occlusion, and values with the one-way valve were approximately one third more negative than values without it. Prospectively, however, Yang and Tobin[29] showed continued poor performance of PImax of −30 cm H_2O as a predictor of weaning outcome; its positive predictive value was only 0.58. The inability of PImax to predict weaning outcome is probably related to the fact that it is measured under static conditions, and the recorded value is probably very different than the value available to patients in a failed weaning trial. Such patients are tachypneic, have rapid flow rates, and often display dynamic hyperinflation[9]—all of which decrease the proportion of PImax that is available for force generation.[8]

Vital Capacity

Although vital capacity is commonly obtained to predict weaning, it is extremely difficult to obtain reproducible results in an intubated, critically ill patient. In addition, several investigators have reported that vital capacity does not reliably discriminate between weaning success and weaning failure patients. Accordingly, we do not recommend the measurement of vital capacity for this purpose.

Minute Ventilation and Maximum Voluntary Ventilation

In the study by Sahn and Lakshminarayan,[30] the combination of a minute ventilation of less than 10 L/min and the ability to double this value during a maximum voluntary ventilation maneuver identified all patients who could be weaned, whereas 71% of those who could not meet both criteria required continued support. However, Tahvanainen and col-

TABLE 136–1. Variables Used to Predict Weaning Success

Gas Exchange
PaO_2 of > 60 mm Hg with FIO_2 of < 0.35
Alveolar-arterial PO_2 gradient of < 350 mm Hg
PaO_2/FIO_2 ratio of > 200
Ventilatory Pump
Vital capacity of > 10–15 mL/kg body weight
Maximum negative inspiratory pressure < −30 cm H_2O
Minute ventilation < 10 L/min
Maximum voluntary ventilation more than twice resting minute ventilation

leagues[32] found a minute ventilation of 10 mL/min to be falsely positive in 11% and falsely negative in 25% of patients. The ability to double minute ventilation during a maximum voluntary ventilation maneuver was falsely positive in 5% of patients and falsely negative in 76%. Similarly, a minute ventilation of 10 L/min proved to be a misleading predictor for Yang and Tobin,[29] with positive and negative predictive values of only 0.50 and 0.40, respectively.

Airway Occlusion Pressure

The use of airway occlusion pressure as a predictor of weaning outcome has been evaluated by a number of investigations. Herrera and colleagues[10] and Sassoon and associates[11] reported that $P_{0.1}$ was elevated in all of their patients with respiratory failure and that successful weaning could be predicted by threshold values of $P_{0.1}$ less than or equal to 4.2 cm H_2O and less than 6 cm H_2O,[11] respectively. Similarly, Murciano and coworkers[12] studied 16 patients with COPD and found that the $P_{0.1}$ values for successfully weaned patients decreased substantially from the start of ventilatory support to extubation. In the patients who could not be weaned, no decrease was evident.

Rapid Shallow Breathing

Using respiratory inductive plethysmography to obtain breath-by-breath measurements, Tobin and colleagues[9] demonstrated that patients who eventually are not able to be weaned display an immediate onset of rapid shallow breathing on discontinuation of mechanical ventilation. Subsequently, Yang and Tobin[29] measured VT and respiratory frequency with a simple bedside spirometer attached to a patient's endotracheal tube while the patient spontaneously breathed room air for 1 minute. Measurements of frequency (f) and VT were combined into an index of rapid shallow breathing—the f/VT ratio. An f/VT value of 105 breaths/min per liter had positive and negative predictive values of 0.78 and 0.95, respectively, which were the highest values noted for any of the predictive indices in the study (Fig. 136-5). As a predictive index, the f/VT ratio has a number of attractive features. It is easy to measure, it is independent of a patient's effort and cooperation, it appears to be quite accurate in predicting the ability to sustain ventilation, and fortuitously, it has a "rounded off" threshold value (100) that is easy to remember. Subsequently, the ability of the f/VT to predict weaning outcome has been analyzed by a number of investigators[33-39] with varying results. Collectively, these investigations highlight the importance of strict adherence to the specifics of methodology as well as emphasize the necessity of incorporating an assessment of the pretest probability of a given outcome when any predictive index is used. The f/VT continues to be the most useful clinically applicable weaning index, although the mechanism of rapid shallow breathing in patients who cannot be weaned remains controversial.

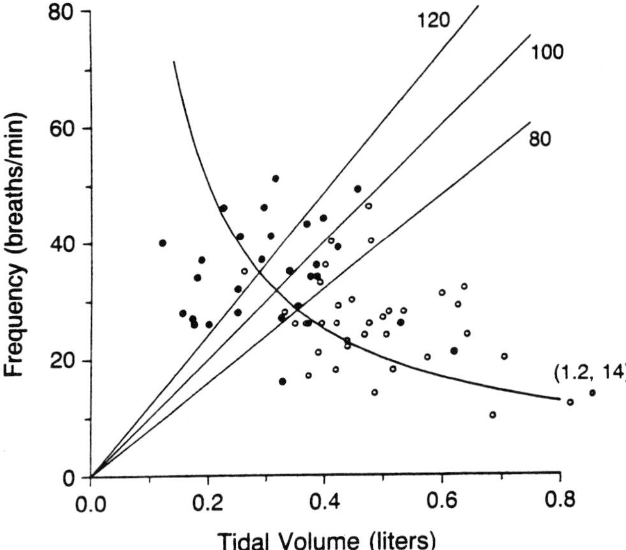

Figure 136–5. Isopleths for the ratio of frequency to tidal volume (f/VT). Different degrees of rapid shallow breathing are represented. Patients who fell to the left of the 100 breaths/min per liter isopleth had a 95% likelihood of an unsuccessful weaning trial outcome; patients who fell to the right of this isopleth had an 80% likelihood of a successful outcome. The hyperbola represents a minute ventilation of 10 L/min, a criterion commonly used to predict weaning outcome. It is apparent that this criterion was of little value in discriminating between successful patients (*open circles*) and unsuccessful patients (*solid circles*). Values for one patient (V_T = 1.2 L, f = 14 breaths/min) lay outside the graph. (From Yang K, Tobin MJ: A prospective study of indexes predicting outcome of trials of weaning from mechanical ventilation. N Engl J Med 1991; 324:1445–1450. Reproduced by permission of The New England Journal of Medicine.)

METHODS OF DISCONTINUING MECHANICAL VENTILATION

Spontaneous Breathing Trials

The ability to sustain spontaneous breathing can be tested while a patient breathes through a T-tube system[5, 40] or a continuous flow system (flow-by) available on some ventilators.[40] When a T-tube system is used, the flow of gas to the inspiratory limb should be at least twice that of the patient's spontaneous minute ventilation in order to meet the patient's peak inspiratory flow rate; an extension piece is added to the expiratory limb to prevent entrainment of room air. During a trial of spontaneous breathing, a patient's clinical status should be closely monitored by a physician, nurse, or therapist. If the signs of distress develop on physical examination, the trial is stopped and mechanical ventilation is reinstituted for at least 24 hours. The rationale behind the once-daily approach is that respiratory muscles require a prolonged period of rest in order to recover from stressful efforts.[41]

Many patients, especially those who receive ventilator support for short periods, can be extubated without prolonged weaning trials. As shown by the studies of Esteban,[5] Ely,[40] and Brochard and their coauthors,[42] most patients tolerate the first attempt at discontinuation of ventilator support without any difficulty. In each of these studies, patients were observed over a 2-hour period of spontaneous breathing and were extubated if they remained free of respiratory distress.

Intermittent Mandatory Ventilation

Patients receiving intermittent mandatory ventilation (IMV) can breathe spontaneously and receive periodic positive-pressure breaths at a preset volume and rate from the ventilator. When a patient is ready for weaning, the IMV rate is reduced in steps, usually in decrements of one to three breaths/min. If the patient does not experience distress, further decrements in the IMV rate are made until a rate close to zero is reached.

In a patient receiving IMV, it has been generally assumed that patient effort is reduced in proportion to the number of breaths delivered by the ventilator. However, some studies[4, 44, 45] have shown that a decrease in the IMV rate is accompanied by an increase in patient effort not only during the

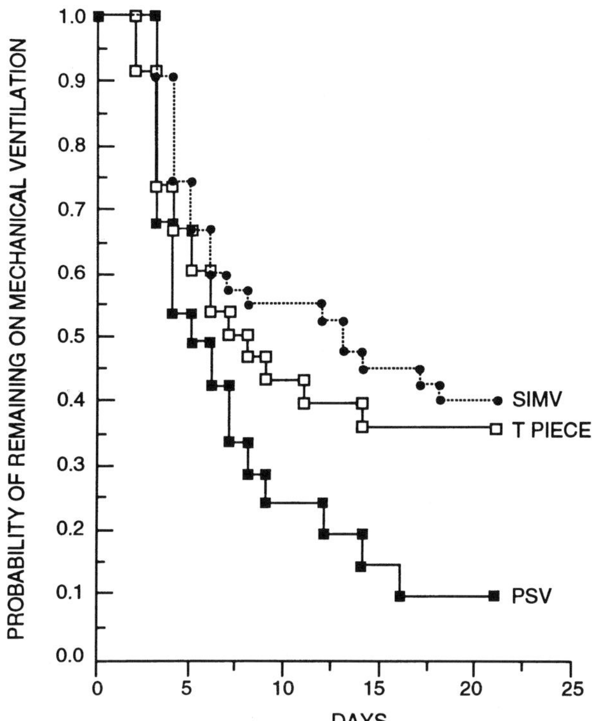

Figure 136–6. Probability of remaining on mechanical ventilation in patients with prolonged difficulties in tolerating spontaneous breathing. This probability was significantly lower for pressure support ventilation (PSV) than for either T-piece or synchronized intermittent ventilation (SIMV) (cumulative probability for 21 days; $P < .03$ with the log-rank test). (From Brochard L, Rauss A, Benito S, et al: Comparison of three methods of gradual withdrawal from ventilatory support during weaning from mechanical ventilation. Am J Respir Crit Care Med 1994; 150:896–903.)

spontaneous breaths but also during the assisted breaths. The observation that the tension-time index is commonly above the fatigue threshold for both the assisted and spontaneous breaths suggests that the common practice of using low levels of IMV may actually hinder satisfactory recovery from respiratory muscle fatigue and may therefore delay the time to successful extubation. By comparison, Leung and asociates[45] demonstrated that the pressure-time product was reduced to a greater extent during assist-control ventilation than during IMV; also, when expressed as a percentage of the maximum level of support, the latter investigators found no difference in the degree of unloading with pressure support or IMV.

Pressure Support Ventilation

Pressure support ventilation (PSV) is considered by some to be more comfortable than other ventilatory modes because patients can control the depth, length, and flow profile of each breath. PSV was once thought to be useful to "counteract" the resistive load related to the endotracheal tube during weaning trials. However, Straus and coworkers[46] demonstrated that the work of breathing during a spontaneous breathing trial and following extubation were virtually identical; accordingly, PSV should not be employed for this purpose. Weaning from PSV can be performed by gradual lowering of the level of PSV in three to six cm H_2O decrements according to patient tolerance, and extubation is commonly performed at a PSV level of 5 cm H_2O.

Comparisons of Methods of Discontinuing Mechanical Ventilation

Brochard and coauthors[42] were the first to undertake a carefully randomized controlled trial of different weaning techniques. PSV was superior to the combined results of T-tube and IMV weaning, resulting in a shorter weaning duration and a decreased ICU stay; in this study, PSV did not result in faster weaning than T-tube trials alone (Fig. 136–6).

Esteban and colleagues[5] conducted a prospective, randomized comparison of four weaning strategies involving 130 patients who had been ventilated for a mean of 7.5 days and who had not responded to an initial trial of spontaneous breathing. The time to successful extubation was less (3 days) in the groups receiving either once-daily or intermittent (multiple) daily trials of spontaneous breathing than in the groups randomized to either IMV (5 days) or PSV (4 days) weaning (Fig. 136–7). Although the conclusions differed, the studies by Brochard[42] and Esteban[5] may be viewed as complementary, in that both demonstrated that the pace of weaning depends on the manner in which a technique is employed; also, both studies agree that IMV is the least effective method of weaning.

The insight gained from these studies was extended in a randomized, controlled study by Ely and colleagues,[40] who investigated whether predictive indices combined with a trial of spontaneous breathing would hasten the pace of weaning. The patients were screened each morning for five factors: Pa_{O_2}/FI_{O_2} ratio above 200; PEEP at 5 cm H_2O or less; f/V_T at 105 breaths/min per liter; intact cough on suctioning; and absence of infusions of sedative or vasopressor agents. Patients in the intervention group (n = 149) who met all five criteria underwent a 2-hour trial of spontaneous breathing that same morning. If clinical signs of distress did not develop, according to the criteria of the studies of Brochard[42] and Esteban,[5] the trial was considered successful and the patient's physician was notified of this result. The control group (n = 151) underwent daily screening but not the spontaneous breathing trial. Although patients in the intervention group had more severe

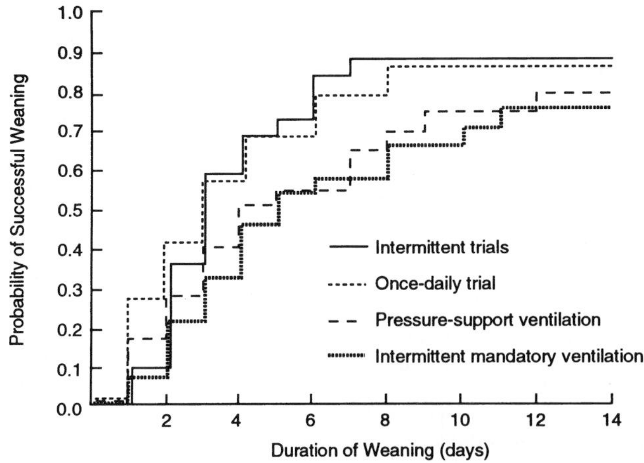

Figure 136–7. Kaplan-Meier curves of the probability of successful weaning with intermittent mandatory ventilation, pressure support ventilation, intermittent trials of spontaneous breathing, and a once-daily trial of spontaneous breathing. After adjustment for baseline characteristics in a Cox proportional-hazards model, the rate of successful weaning with a once-daily trial of spontaneous breathing was 2.83 times higher than that with intermittent mandatory ventilation ($P < .006$) and 2.05 times higher than that with pressure support ventilation ($P < .04$). (From Esteban A, Frutos F, Tobin MJ, et al: A comparison of four methods of weaning patients from mechanical ventilation. N Engl J Med 1995; 332:345–350.)

disease, with higher APACHE II and acute lung injury scores, the median duration of mechanical ventilation was 1.5 days less than in the control group (P = .003), and the rates of complications (P = .001), reintubation (P = .04), and ICU charges (P = .03) were lower.

SUMMARY

Although most patients can be easily weaned from mechanical ventilation, a substantial minority experience considerable difficulty. The major respiratory determinants of weaning outcome include respiratory muscle performance, adequacy of gas exchange, and psychologic factors. In addition, cardiac dysfunction may affect both muscle performance and gas exchange. Because weaning failure is commonly multifactorial, indices that assess a single physiologic function are frequently inaccurate in predicting weaning outcome. An index of rapid shallow breathing, the f/VT ratio, appears to be more accurate in predicting weaning outcome than traditional indices, such as maximum inspiratory pressure and minute ventilation. A variety of weaning techniques exist, and accumulating evidence indicates that measurement of predictive indices combined with a single daily trial of spontaneous breathing is the most expeditious method.

References

1. Keith RL, Pierson DJ: Complications of mechanical ventilation: A bedside approach. Clin Chest Med 1996; 17:439–451.
2. Tobin MJ: Mechanical ventilation (Review). N Engl J Med 1994; 330:1056–1061.
3. Krieger BP: Economics of ventilator care. *In:* Principles and Practice of Mechanical Ventilation. Tobin MJ (Ed). New York, McGraw-Hill, 1994, pp 1221–1232.
4. Tobin MJ, Alex CG: Discontinuation of mechanical ventilation. *In:* Principles and Practice of Mechanical Ventilation. Tobin MJ (Ed). New York, McGraw-Hill, 1994, pp 1177–1206.
5. Esteban A, Frutos F, Tobin MJ, et al: A comparison of four methods of weaning patients from mechanical ventilation. N Engl J Med 1995; 332:345–350.
6. Esteban A, Alia I, Ibanez I, et al: Modes of mechanical ventilation and weaning: A national survey of Spanish hospitals. Chest 1994; 106:1188–1193.
7. Torres A, Reyes A, Roca J, et al: Ventilation-perfusion mismatching in chronic obstructive pulmonary disease during ventilator weaning. Am Rev Respir Dis 1989; 140:1246–1250.
8. Tobin MJ: Respiratory muscles in disease. Clin Chest Med 1988; 9:263–286.
9. Tobin MJ, Perez W, Guenther SM, et al: The pattern of breathing during successful and unsuccessful trials of weaning from mechanical ventilation. Am Rev Respir Dis 1986; 134:1111–1118.
10. Herrera M, Blasco J, Venegas J, et al: Mouth occlusion pressure ($P_{0.1}$) in acute respiratory failure. Intensive Care Med 1985; 11:134–139.
11. Sassoon CSH, Te TT, Mahutte CK, et al: Airway occlusion pressure: An important indicator for successful weaning in patients with chronic obstructive pulmonary disease. Am Rev Respir Dis 1987; 135:107–113.
12. Murciano D, Boczkowski J, Lecocguic Y, et al: Tracheal occlusion pressure: A simple index to monitor respiratory muscle fatigue during acute respiratory failure in patients with chronic obstructive pulmonary disease. Ann Intern Med 1988; 108:800–805.
13. Estenne M, Yernault JC, De Smet JM, et al: Phrenic and diaphragm function after coronary artery bypass grafting. Thorax 1985; 40:293–299.
14. Sheridan PH Jr, Cheriyan A, Doud J, et al: Incidence of phrenic neuropathy after isolated lung transplantation: The Loyola University Lung Transplant Group. J Heart Lung Transplant 1995; 14:684–691.
15. Lemaire F, Teboul JL, Cinotti L, et al: Acute left ventricular dysfunction during unsuccessful weaning from mechanical ventilation. Anesthesiology 1988; 69:171–179.
16. Juan G, Calverley P, Talamo C, et al: Effect of carbon dioxide on diaphragmatic function in human beings. N Engl J Med 1984; 310:874–979.
17. Decramer M, de Bock V, Dom R: Functional and histologic picture of steroid-induced myopathy in chronic obstructive pulmonary disease. Am J Respir Crit Care Med 1996; 153:1958–1964.
18. Hansen-Flaschen J, Cowen J, Raps EC: Neuromuscular blockade in the intensive care unit: More than we bargained for. Am Rev Respir Dis 1993; 147:234–236.
19. Anzueto A, Tobin MJ, Moore G, et al: Effect of prolonged mechanical ventilation on diaphragmatic function: A preliminary study of a baboon model. Crit Care Med 1997; 25:1187–1190.
20. Muller EA: Influence of training and of inactivity on muscle strength. Arch Phys Med Rehabil 1970; 51:449–462.
21. Cohen C, Zagelbaum G, Gross D, et al: Clinical manifestations of inspiratory muscle fatigue. Am J Med 1982; 73:308–316.
22. Moxham J, Edwards RHT, Aubier M, et al: Changes in the EMG power spectrum (high-to-low) with force fatigue in humans. J Appl Physiol 1982; 53:1094–1099.
23. Jubran A, Tobin MJ: Pathophysiologic basis of acute respiratory distress in patients who fail a trial of weaning from mechanical ventilation. Am J Respir Crit Care Med 1997; 155:906–915.
24. Bellemare F, Grassino A: Effect of pressure and timing of contraction of the human diaphragm fatigue. J Appl Physiol 1982; 53:1190–1195.
25. Laghi F, Harrison MJ, Tobin MJ: Comparison of magnetic and electrical phrenic nerve stimulation in assessment of diaphragmatic contractility. J Appl Physiol 1996; 80:1731–1742.
26. Laghi F, Tobin MJ: Monitoring of respiratory muscle function. *In:* Principles and Practice of Intensive Care Monitoring. Tobin MJ (Ed). New York, McGraw-Hill, 1998, pp 497–544.
27. Bergbom-Engberg I, Haljamae H: Assessment of patients' experience of discomforts during respiratory therapy. Crit Care Med 1989; 17:1068–1072.
28. Stroetz RW, Hubmayr RD: Tidal volume maintenance during weaning with pressure support. Am J Respir Crit Care Med 1995; 152:1034–1040.
29. Yang K, Tobin MJ: A prospective study of indexes predicting outcome of trials of weaning from mechanical ventilation. N Engl J Med 1991; 324:1445–1450.
30. Sahn SA, Lakshminarayan S: Bedside criteria for discontinuation of mechanical ventilation. Chest 1973; 63:1002–1005.
31. Marini JJ, Smith TC, Lamb V: Estimation of inspiratory muscle strength in mechanically ventilated patients: The measurement of maximal inspiratory pressure. J Crit Care 1986; 1:32–38.
32. Takvanainen J, Salenpera M, Nikki P: Extubation criteria after weaning from intermittent mandatory ventilatory and continuous positive airway pressure. Crit Care Med 1983; 11:702–707.
33. Wasson JH, Sox HC, Neff RK, Goldman L: Clinical prediction rules: Applications and methodological standards. N Engl J Med 1985; 313:793–799.
34. Epstein SK: Etiology of extubation failure and the predictive value of the rapid shallow breathing index. Am J Respir Crit Care Med 1995; 152:545–549.
35. Sassoon CSH, Mahutte CK: Airway occlusion pressure and breathing pattern as predictors of weaning outcome. Am Rev Respir Dis 1993; 148:860–866.
36. Chatila W, Jacob B, Guaglionone D, Manthous CA: The unassisted respiratory rate-tidal volume ratio accurately predicts weaning outcome. Am J Med 1996; 101:61–67.
37. Jaechke RZ, Meade MO, Guyatt GH, et al: How to use diagnostic test articles in the ICU: Diagnosing wean ability using f/VT. Crit Care Med 1997; 25:1514–1521.
38. Epstein SK, Ciubotaru RL: Influence of gender and endotracheal tube size on preextubation breathing pattern. Am J Respir Crit Care Med 1996; 154:1647–1652.
39. Jacob B, Chatila W, Manthous CA: The unassisted respiratory rate/tidal volume ratio accurately predicts weaning outcome in postoperative patients. Crit Care Med 1997; 25:253–257.
40. Ely EW, Baker AM, Dunagan DP, et al: Effect on the duration of mechanical ventilation of identifying patients capable of breathing spontaneously. N Engl J Med 1996; 335:1864–1869.
41. Laghi F, D'Alfonso N, Tobin MJ: Pattern of recovery from diaphragmatic fatigue over 24 hours. J Appl Physiol 1995; 79:539–546.
42. Brochard L, Rauss A, Benito S, et al: Comparison of three methods

of gradual withdrawal from ventilatory support during weaning from mechanical ventilation. Am J Respir Crit Care Med 1994; 150:896–903.
43. Marini JJ, Smith TC, Lamb VJ: External work output and force generation during synchronized intermittent mandatory ventilation: Effect of machine assistance on breathing effort. Am Rev Respir Dis 1988; 138:1169–1179.
44. Imsand C, Feihl F, Perret C, Fitting JW: Regulation of inspiratory neuromuscular output during synchronized intermittent mechanical ventilation. Anesthesiology 1994; 80:13–22.
45. Leung P, Jubran A, Tobin MJ: Comparison of assisted ventilator modes on triggering, patient effort, and dyspnea. Am J Respir Crit Care Med 1997; 155:1940–1948.
46. Straus C, Louis B, Isabey D, et al: Contribution of the endotracheal tube and the upper airway to breathing workload. Am J Respir Crit Care Med 1998; 157:23–30.

137

Proximal Airway Disorders in the Pediatric Patient

Richard E. Weibley, MD, MPH • Luis Maldonado, MD

Airway pathology is a common problem for physicians who care for pediatric patients. The proximal airway from the nares to the carina is often involved. Although the number of different disorders that can occur in the proximal airway of pediatric patients is large, careful attention to history and physical findings coupled with an understanding of anatomy and pathophysiology should allow a clinician to localize the lesion generally and to begin treatment while investigating and defining the specific diagnosis.

ANATOMY

Developmental processes as well as absolute size differences are important to an understanding the causes of proximal airway failure and their appropriate treatment in infants, children, and adolescents. Because newborn infants have a relatively small mandible and a large tongue that crowds and fills the oropharynx, infants are primarily obligate nose breathers during quiet respiration.[1] As the midface and mandible grow, the relative difficulties of oropharyngeal breathing in infancy disappear.

The epiglottis in infancy is relatively long and stiff, U-shaped or V-shaped, and angulated approximately 45° from the anterior pharyngeal wall owing to the close proximity of the hyoid bone and thyroid cartilage.[2] As growth occurs, separation of the hyoid and the thyroid cartilage results in a more erect position of the epiglottis. By adolescence, the epiglottis assumes the flattened and flexible adult anatomy, positioned parallel to the base of the tongue.

The laryngeal structures also change with growth, moving lower in the neck with age.[1] In term infants, the laryngeal inlet is at the level of the cervical vertebral interspace C3-4; in adults, it rests at interspace C4-5. As an infant grows, the vocal cords change direction and shape with increasing length. In adults, the most narrow portion of the respiratory tract is generally the laryngeal inlet; in infants and young children, it is usually the laryngeal outlet, the inferior ring portion (arch) of the cricoid cartilage. With growth, the ring enlarges, the cricoid plate assumes a more vertical position, and this anatomic point of narrowing disappears.

Although airway diameter decreases progressively with branching of the conducting airways, total airway area steadily increases at each successive level of the tracheobronchial tree. Little decrease in individual airway diameter occurs with branching distal to the bronchiole. As the airstream moves peripherally, increases in cross-sectional area sharply reduce airflow velocity, with important physiologic implications for the distribution of airway resistance in normal and disease states.

NORMAL AND ABNORMAL PHYSIOLOGY

The proximal airway performs many functions, including filtering, warming, and humidifying air in its passage from the atmosphere to the alveoli. Perhaps the most critical physiologic characteristic of the proximal airway is its substantial contribution to total functional resistance secondary to tissue and gas movements.[3] This has implications for both acute and chronic disease states, especially in infants and young children.

Airway resistance is affected by changes in airway dimension, number, pressure, and flow. A simple formula for resistance is as follows:

$$\text{resistance} = \frac{\text{change in pressure}}{\text{flow}}$$

Thus, resistance is directly proportional to pressure changes and inversely proportional to flow changes. Poiseuille's law describes the pressure produced by laminar gas flow through a tube.[3] The radius, raised to the fourth power in the denominator of the equation, is the most important determinant of pressure and thus resistance.

Airway resistance normally changes at differing lung volumes.[3] At large volumes, the airways are distended and resistance is low. After forced expiration and near residual volume, resistance becomes infinitely high as pleural pressures close airways and flow ceases. Estimates of total lung resistance (airway and tissue) have been obtained by means of dynamic pressure-volume curves and plethysmography.[3-4] Measurements in children younger than 2 years indicate that total lung resistance is six to 20 times higher than that of adults at resting lung volumes. An infant's average nasal resistance by indirect measurements is nearly half of total respiratory resistance. Because of the rapid increase in total cross-sectional area with successive branching of conducting airways, nearly all airway resistance occurs proximal to small bronchioles. Hence, even modest reductions in the size of the most proximal airways significantly increase airway resistance, producing signs and symptoms of obstruction. This is particularly important in the smallest and youngest patients.

Normal breathing is not audible, because even during maximum inspiration and exhalation linear airflow velocity is too low to produce sound. Breathing becomes audible when narrowed air passages change the linear velocity and airflow characteristics, creating turbulence and noise. Stridor and wheezing are the hallmarks of respiratory obstruction. Understanding their pathophysiology helps a clinician to localize an obstructive lesion and direct therapy most effectively.

Abnormalities associated with proximal airway obstruction may be either acute or chronic in character. They include changes in respiratory rate, depth, inspiratory-expiratory ratio, nasal flaring, retractions, wheezing or stridor, right-sided or left-sided heart failure, and pulmonary edema. If severe obstruction is present, patients may exhibit agitation, irritability, confusion, or somnolence. Cyanosis, hypercarbia, and uncompensated respiratory or metabolic acidosis signal imminent collapse.

Supracarinal lesions commonly reveal symmetric changes throughout the respiratory cycle, whereas obstructive pathology beyond the carina creates evidence of unilateral signs and symptoms. Similarly, lesions of the extrathoracic airway are evident during the inspiratory phase of respiration, and those of an intrathoracic conducting airway are evident during exhalation. A useful general rule is that lesions causing stridor are found above the clavicle (thoracic inlet), whereas lesions associated with wheezing are located below the clavicle (intrathoracic). In rare circumstances, an inspiratory wheeze or expiratory stridor may be described. Generally, a careful physical examination coupled with a thorough history allows localization of the obstructive site.

Stridor may be loud or soft, high-pitched or low-pitched, musical or harsh. It occurs overwhelmingly in the proximal airway between the laryngeal inlet and the thoracic inlet of the trachea. In this portion of the airway, the individual forces of a relatively positive atmospheric pressure and negative intraluminal airway pressure combine to collapse the airway and obstruct airflow at the site of pathology during inspiration. The resulting airflow turbulence creates the characteristic noise of stridor.

Wheezing, most often associated with asthma and reactive airway disease, is predominantly an expiratory sound related to obstruction of the intrathoracic conducting airways. In contrast to the dynamics of the extrathoracic airway during inspiration, the intrathoracic airways are collapsed and obstructed by positive thoracic pressures and tissue elastic forces during exhalation. Wheezing is not synonymous with bronchospasm because it also arises from other obstructive airway pathologies.

Obstruction of proximal airways is associated with cardiac disease and pulmonary hypertension.[5-7] Cor pulmonale and left-sided heart failure have been documented in long-standing cases of upper airway obstructions.[6] Relief of the obstruction improves the heart failure in most cases.

Pulmonary edema has also been described in association with acute (e.g., croup, epiglottitis, strangulation, laryngospasm, laryngeal edema, and foreign bodies) and chronic upper airway obstruction.[8-11] The presence of the pulmonary edema was noted both before and after relief of the obstructive lesion. Whether it is often present (but not recognized) before the airway obstruction is relieved is of some controversy.[11] A decrease in intrathoracic and intra-alveolar pressures during obstruction causes an increased blood flow to the pulmonary vasculature, favoring the development of edema.[9]

TABLE 137–1. Common Causes of Obstruction in Pediatric Patients

Congenital
- Choanal atresia
- Craniofacial dysmorphologic features (with micrognathia and glossoptosis)
  - Pierre Robin syndrome
  - Treacher Collins syndrome
- Macroglossia
  - Beckwith's syndrome
  - Congenital hypothyroidism
  - Down's syndrome
- Laryngotracheomalacia
- Subglottic stenosis
- Vocal cord paralysis
- Laryngotracheoesophageal webs
- Vascular rings and slings
- Tracheal anomalies
- Tumors and cysts
- Metabolic: hypocalcemia
- Neurogenic: reflex laryngospasm

Acquired Obstruction
- Infectious
  - Supraglottitis
  - Laryngotracheobronchitis
  - Retropharyngeal abscess
  - Bacterial tracheitis
- Trauma
  - Foreign bodies
  - Iatrogenic
    - Postextubation
    - Postinstrumentation
    - Postoperative
  - External trauma
  - Thermal and chemical burns
- Neoplasia
  - Laryngeal papillomatosis
  - Miscellaneous tumors and nodes

DIFFERENTIAL DIAGNOSIS AND TREATMENT

Congenital Problems

Airway obstruction in pediatric patients can be easily categorized into acquired and congenital causes (Table 137–1).[12] Among the congenital lesions, three craniofacial anomalies occur most frequently: (1) Choanal atresia (2) Pierre Robin anomaly (3) Treacher Collins syndrome

Bilateral *choanal atresia,* evident in neonates with respiratory distress when the mouth is closed, is easily detected by failure of a suction catheter to pass from the nares through the nasopharynx and into the posterior pharynx. Treatment involves the placement of an oral airway followed by surgical removal of the obstructing tissue or bony plate.

Both *Pierre Robin syndrome* and *Treacher Collins syndrome* cause airway obstruction owing to mandibular hypoplasia and relative macroglossia with posterior positioning of the tongue into the nasopharynx and oropharynx. Management goals are to maintain an adequate airway until mandibular growth occurs. In the most severely affected infants, tracheostomy may be necessary to prevent the development of cor pulmonale.

Laryngotracheomalacia (LTM), also called *congenital laryngeal stridor,* is a common, transient, and generally self-limited cause of stridor due to cartilaginous immaturity and laxness in the laryngeal framework and epiglottis.[13-14] The stridor gradually resolves with growth. Endotracheal intubation or tracheostomy is rarely necessary, although symptoms may worsen dramatically with the occurrence of otherwise trivial viral upper respiratory tract infections. If a patient does not respond to conventional therapy, a new alternative is now available. The use of tracheal or bronchial stents and costocartilage or cadaveric grafts has proved helpful in severe cases.[15-18] LTM reportedly accounts for as much as 75% of congenital laryngeal pathology; however, it is probably overdiagnosed as a result of a lack of precise diagnostic criteria.[12] Patients with persistent symptoms that do not resolve with growth and maturation or with severe symptoms should be carefully evaluated for another pathologic process.

Congenital subglottic stenosis usually has its most significant point of narrowing in the area of the cricoid cartilage, 2 to 3 mm below an infant's glottis. Inflammation and swelling from secondary causes superimposed on the fixed lesion further decrease airway diameter. In infant airways, as little as 1 mm of uniform edema can reduce the airway cross-sectional area 70%, seriously limiting a child's ability to breathe.[2]

Congenital vocal cord paralysis may account for as many as 10% of congenital laryngeal disorders.[12] Bilateral or unilateral paralysis generally corresponds to central or peripheral nerve pathology. The left recurrent laryngeal nerve is more susceptible to damage associated with surgery or other congenital lesions, often cardiovascular. Bilateral vocal cord paralysis is associated with increased intracranial pressure as a result of caudal brain stem displacement and nerve root traction.[1, 12] Birth trauma may also be responsible, although in most cases the cause remains unknown. Congenital vocal cord paralysis carries a favorable prognosis for spontaneous recovery.

Aberrant aortic arch remnant vessels create vascular rings and slings with secondary compression of the esophagus or trachea.[12, 19-20] These lesions may be present as either intermittent or persistent wheezing or stridor, often in association with eating. Surgical correction is necessary for lesions causing moderate to severe obstruction associated with recurrent pneumonia, atelectasis, or failure to thrive.[3] Preoperatively, an endotracheal tube provides a secure airway.

Acquired Pathology

Infection

After the newborn period, infectious causes of upper airway obstruction are most common. Adenoidal and tonsillar hypertrophy may cause acute or chronic obstruction.[5] Potential spaces defined by fascial places serve as sites for abscess formation and airway obstruction. These occur most commonly in children older than 1 to 2 years of age and are generally bacterial, although a notable exception is the lymphoid hypertrophy associated with Epstein-Barr virus infection.[21] Acute epiglottitis (AE), laryngotracheobronchitis (LTB), and bacterial tracheitis (BT) are the most common presenting infectious causes of upper airway obstruction (Table 137-2).

Acute Epiglottitis

Also called *supraglottitis,* AE was historically most often due to *Haemophilus influenzae* type B. Currently, viral agents and group A β-hemolytic streptococci are more common etiologic agents. Widespread vaccination of infants against *H. influenzae* is dramatically lowering the incidence of life-threatening disease, including epiglottitis.[22] The clinical picture of AE is classically one of extreme respiratory distress, high fever, drooling, and dysphasia, all of abrupt onset. Unfortunately, supraglottic infections may not present with the classic picture; symptoms often mimic those of LTB or BT.

The unacceptably high mortality and morbidity associated with failure to detect AE have led to a systematized approach to diagnosis and treatment in suspected cases.[23] Patients should always be attended by someone skilled in airway management. The use of radiologic procedures such as lateral neck films should be used only for exceptional cases. At present, the accepted plan is to take the child to the operating room for visual inspection of the airway and nasotracheal intubation. specimens of the epiglottis and blood should be obtained for culture after the airway is secured and antibiotics should be instituted, ensuring coverage against β-lactamase-positive *H. influenzae*.

After intubation, patients should remain in an intensive care unit, where proper maintenance of the airway can be accomplished. An issue of some controversy concerns when to extubate patients and whether to visualize the epiglottis to aid in the decision. Although numerous studies have addressed this issue, none has provided evidence of the need for, or predictive value of, visualization.[24] Resolution of airway obstruction does not appear to correlate with resolution of fever or the size of the epiglottis.[24, 25]

Laryngotracheobronchitis

LTB is usually a mild illness not requiring critical care services. The clinical features are well recognized (see Table 137-2). For those with symptoms severe enough to warrant hospital admission, the use of a scoring system provides an objective measure of the degree of respiratory difficulty (Table 137-3).

A host of viral agents cause LTB. Parainfluenza viruses account for most cases; adenoviruses, respiratory syncytial virus, influenza virus, and measles virus are other identifiable agents. Viral LTB usually has a less rapid onset, lower fever, and less toxic appearance than AE. It also tends to occur in younger infants and children, primarily 3 months to 5 years of age.

Treatment of viral LTB is symptomatic. Mist therapy, although historically used, has never been shown to be beneficial.[26] Oxygen is indicated if hypoxemia is present. The use of adrenergic agents, primarily racemic epinephrine, is common and beneficial, although it is associated with rebound of symptoms.[27] Corticosteroid therapy has been efficacious in the treatment of LTB.[28] Helium and oxygen mixtures also have been used for LTB and other obstructive lesions.[29, 30] Of lower viscosity than nitrogen and oxygen mixtures, heliox reduces airway resistance and work of breathing.[30] At least one study

TABLE 137–2. Laryngotracheobronchitis (LTB), Acute Epiglottis (AE), and Bacterial Tracheitis (BT)

	LTB	AE	BT
History			
Age	2 mo-3 yr	3-7 yr (usually)	All ages
Onset	Gradual	Rapid	Gradual
Respiratory disease	None to moderate	Marked	Moderate-marked
Symptoms			
Dysphagia	+/−	2+	+/−
Dyspnea	+/−	2-3+	2+
Sore throat	+/−	4+	+/−
Signs			
Sound	Bark, stridor	Muffed, guttural	Bark, stridor
Secretions	Normal for age	Drooling	Normal for age
Position	Lying, sitting, standing	Sitting, leaning	Sitting
Temperature	37-38°C	38°C+	38°C+
Facies	Normal	Anxious, distressed, toxic	Anxious

TABLE 137–3. Croup Severity Scoring System

Sign	0	1	2	Individual Score
Inspiratory breath sounds	Normal	Harsh rhonchi	Delayed	______
Stridor	None	Inspiratory	Inspiratory and expiratory	______
Cough	None	Hoarse cry	Seal-like bark	______
Retractions/nasal flaring	None	Nasal flaring Suprasternal retractions	Flaring suprasternal intercostal retractions	______
Cyanosis	None	In room air	In 40% oxygen	______
			TOTAL SCORE	______

has suggested a risk of hypoxemia in small infants. Antibiotics are of no benefit in uncomplicated viral LTB.

Bacterial Tracheitis

Bacterial tracheitis, with features that overlap both LTB and AE (see Table 137–2), probably represents a bacterial superinfection complicating viral LTB.[31] Clinical symptoms begin with gradual onset of upper respiratory tract complaints, progressing to fever, toxicity, and marked distress. Laryngoscopy reveals a normal epiglottis with mucopurulent edema and copious, thick secretions requiring tracheal intubation for airway toilet and relief of obstructive symptoms. The usual pathogens are *Staphylococcus aureus, H. influenzae, Peptostreptococcus* sp. and others.[32] A few patients have been reported to develop toxic shock syndrome or acute respiratory distress syndrome (ARDS).[33] *Aspergillus* tracheobronchitis with symptomatic upper airway obstruction is also an emerging problem in human immunodeficiency virus (HIV)–infected or other immunocompromised patients.[34] Despite the concern about BT, antibiotics should not be used routinely as prophylaxis in patients with LTB.

Trauma

Trauma follows infection as the second most common cause of upper respiratory tract obstruction in the pediatric population.[35] Included are such injuries as foreign bodies, iatrogenic instrumentation injury to the laryngeal airway or recurrent laryngeal nerve, facial and laryngeal impact injuries, and chemical or thermal bums. Foreign bodies and iatrogenic, postextubation obstructive symptoms are most common.

Foreign bodies in children lodge most commonly in the major bronchi. Nuts, other food particles, and nonfood objects, such as balloons, are frequent offenders.[36–37] Toddlers are most often affected, although foreign bodies may be found from 6 months of age on into adulthood.[37] Obstruction distal to the larynx usually does not cause stridor but wheezing. Esophageal foreign bodies produce stridor or wheezing by secondary airway compression. When no aspiration history is obtained, tracheal foreign bodies often are initially misdiagnosed as viral LTB.

Foreign body removal requires close teamwork between the intensivist, pulmonologist or surgeon, and anesthesiologist. The use of inhaled bronchodilators, postural drainage, and percussion is not recommended for removal of foreign bodies because dislodgment of a distal object into the subglottic space may cause severe or total airway occlusion, a life-threatening complication.[38]

The mechanical trauma associated with intubation, instrumentation, and surgery usually causes stridor as a result of localized mucosal edema. In one study the use of dexamethasone has been shown to decrease the incidence of postextubation stridor.[39] Less commonly, ulceration, granuloma formation, webs, membranes, stenosis, necrosis, infection, or vocal cord paralysis occurs. Facial blows and neck injuries can precipitate acute respiratory difficulty through dislocation of the cricoarytenoid cartilage, hematoma or soft tissue swelling and airway compression, and laryngeal or trachea edema or disruption.[40]

Acute upper airway obstruction due to laryngeal and tracheal edema follows ingestion of acids, alkalis, and corrosive chemical substances, as well as inhalation of hot air, steam, smoke, or chemicals.[41, 42] Patients should be admitted to the hospital for observation in a setting where they can be closely monitored for signs or symptoms of airway compromise. Endoscopic examination of the airway and esophagus may be indicated in selected patients. Intravenous fluids, oxygen, and racemic epinephrine may relieve obstructive symptoms and alleviate the need for mechanical airway support. Corticosteroids, although used by some clinicians, are probably of no benefit.

Tumors

Children with tumors may present with symptoms of airway obstruction due to extrinsic compression from a mass lesion.[43] Airway support is often necessary until radiation or chemotherapy can be instituted to shrink the tumor size.

Early intubation is recommended before edema or obstruction becomes life-threatening as a result of any proximal airway lesion in childhood. It is important to realize that laryngoscopy in infants demonstrates a larynx located superiorly, a large tongue, and a hyoid bone positioned to depress the epiglottis. The epiglottis is relatively large, stiff, and U-shaped, and the airway's narrowest portion is not the glottic inlet but the subglottic space in the region of the cricoid cartilage. An endotracheal tube that passes easily between the vocal cords, but not through the cricoid ring, should be replaced with a smaller tube to avoid irritating the mucous membranes, a precipitating factor in the development of postextubation stridor and obstruction. In selected circumstances, flexible fiberoptic bronchoscopy may be the method of choice for intubation and evaluation of the airway.[44, 45]

References

1. Hengerer AS, Newburg JA: Congenital malformations of the nose and paranasal sinuses. *In:* Pediatric Otolaryngology. 2nd ed. Bluestone CD, Stool SE (Eds). Philadelphia, WB Saunders, 1990, p 727.
2. Eckenhoff JE: Some anatomic considerations of the infant larynx influencing endotracheal anesthesia. Anesthesiology 1951; 12:401.
3. Wohl MEB, Mead J: Age as a factor in respiratory disease. *In:* Kendig's Disorders of the Respiratory Tract. 5th ed. Chemick V (Ed). Philadelphia, WB Saunders, 1990, pp 175–181.
4. Bryan AC, Wohl MD: Respiratory mechanics in children. *In:* The Respiratory System: Handbook of Physiology. Section 3. Vol 3. American Physiologic Society. Fishman AP (Ed). Baltimore, Williams & Williams, 1986.
5. Sie KC, Perkins JA, Clarke WR: Acute right heart failure due to adenotonsillar hypertrophy. Int J Pediatr Otorhinolaryngol 1997; 18;41:53–58.
6. Lefaivre JF, Cohen SR, Burstein FD, et al: Down syndrome: Identification of obstructive sleep apnea. Plast Reconstr Surg 1997; 99:629–637.

7. Rosen CL: Obstructive sleep apnea syndrome (OSAS) in children: Diagnostic challenges. Sleep 1996; 19(10 Suppl):S274-S277.
8. Garyfallou GT, Costalas SK, Murphy CJ: Acute pulmonary edema in a child with spasmodic croup (Letter). Am J Emerg Med 1997; 15:211-213.
9. Guffin TN, Har-el G, Sanders A, et al: Acute postobstructive pulmonary edema. Otolaryngol Head Neck Surg 1995; 112:235-237.
10. Weiss I, Ushay HM, DeBruin W, et al: Respiratory and cardiac function in children after acute hypoxemic respiratory failure. Crit Care Med 1996; 24:148-154.
11. Kanter RK, Wachko JF: Pulmonary edema associated with upper airway obstruction. Am J Dis Child 1984; 138:356-360.
12. Maze A, Bloch E: Stridor in pediatric patients. Anesthesiology 1979; 50:132-135.
13. Thurmond M, Cote DN: Stridor in the neonate: Laryngomalacia. J La State Med Soc 1996; 148:375-378.
14. Finder JD: Primary bronchomalacia in infants and children. J Pediatr 1997; 130:59-66.
15. Filler RM, Forte V, Fraga JC, Matute J: The use of expandable metallic airway stents for tracheobronchial obstruction in children. J Pediatr Surg 1995; 30:1050-1055; discussion 1055-1056.
16. Subramanian V, Anstead M, Cottrill CM, et al: Tetralogy of Fallot with absent pulmonary valve and bronchial compression: Treatment with endobrochial stents. Pediatr Cardiol 1997; 18:237-239.
17. Kamata S, Usui N, Ishikawa, et al: Experience in tracheobronchial reconstruction with a costal cartilage graft for congenital tracheal stenosis. J Pediatr Surg 1997; 32:54-57.
18. Elliot MJ, Haw MP, Jacobs JP, et al: Tracheal reconstruction in children using cadaveric homograft trachea. Eur J Cardiothorac Surg 1996; 10:707-712.
19. Beekman RP, Beek FJ, Hazekamp MG, et al: The vale of MRI in diagnosing vascular abnormalities causing stridor. Eur J Pediatr 1997; 156:516-520.
20. Mahbouni S, Harty MP, Hubard AM, et al: Innominate artery compression of the trachea in infants (see comments). Int J Pediatr Otorhinolaryngol 1997; 38:281-284.
21. Kielmovitch IH, Keleti G, Bluestone CD, et al: Microbiology of obstructive tonsillar hypertrophy and recurrent tonsillitis. Arch Otolaryngol Head Neck Surg 1989; 115:721-728.
22. Senior BA, Radkowski D, MacArthur C, et al: Changing patterns in pediatric supraglottitis: A multi-institutional review, 1980-1992. Laryngoscope 1994; 104(11 Part 1):1314-1322.
23. Bank DE, Krug SE: New approaches to upper airway disease. Emerg Med Clin of North America 1995; 13:473-487.
24. Rothstein P, Lister C: Epiglottitis: Duration of intubation and fever. Anesth Analg 1983; 62:785-791.
25. Rowe LD: Advances and controversies in the management of supraglottitis and laryngotracheobronchitis. Am J Otholaryngol 1980; 1:235-239.
26. Bourchier D, Dawson KP, Fergusson DM: Humidification in viral croup: A controlled trial. Aust Pediatr J 1984; 20:289-293.
27. Kunkel NC, Baker MD: Use of racemic epinephrine, dexamethasone, and mist in the outpatient management of croup. Pediatr Emerg Care 1996; 12:156-159.
28. Geelhoed GC: Croup. Pediatr Pulmonol 1997; 23:370-374.
29. Tobias JD: Heliox in children with airway obstruction. Pediatr Emerg Care 1997; 13:29-32, 36.
30. Papamschou D: Theoretical validation of the respiratory benefits of helium-oxygen mixtures. Respir Physiol 1995; 99:183-190.
31. Dubin AA, Tholji A, Rambaud-Cousson A: Bacterial tracheitis among children hospitalized for severe obstructuve dyspnea. Pediatr Infect Dis J 1990; 9:293-295.
32. Brook I: Aerobic and anaerobic microbiology of bacterial tracheitis in children. Pediatr Emerg Care 1997; 13:16-18.
33. Britto J, Habibi P, Walters S, et al: Systemic complications associated with bacterial tracheitis. Arch Dis Child 1996; 74:249-250.
34. Kemper CA, Hostetler JS, Follansbee SE, et al: Ulcerative and plaque-like tracheobronchitis due to infection with *Aspergillus* in patients with AIDS. Clin Infect Dis 1993; 17:344-347.
35. Kissoon N, Dreyer J, Walia M: Pediatric trauma: Differences in pathophysiology, injury patterns and treatment compared with adult trauma. Can Med Assoc J 1990; 142:27-35.
36. Lifschultz BD, Donoghue ER: Deaths due to foreign body aspiration in children: The continuing hazard of toy balloons. J Forensic Sci 1996; 41:247-51.
37. Rimell FL, Thome A Jr, stool S, et al: Characteristics of objects that cause choking in children (see comments). JAMA 1995; 274:1763-1766.
38. Humphries CT, Wagener JS, Morgan WJ: Fatal prolonged foreign body aspiration following an asymptomatic interval. Am J Emerg Med 1988; 7:669-671.
39. Anene O, Meert KL, Uy H, et al: Dexamethasone for the prevention of postextubation airway obstruction: A prospective, randomized, double-blinded, placebo-controlled trial (see comments). Crit Care Med 1996; 24:1666-1669.
40. Fitz-Hugh GS, Powell JB: Acute traumatic injuries of the oropharynx, laryngopharynx, and cervical trachea in children. Otolaryngol Clin North Am 1970; 3:375-379.
41. Charnock EL, Meehan J: Postburn respiratory injuries in children. Pediatr Clin North Am 1980; 27:661-681.
42. Fitzpatrick JC, Cioffi WG, Cheu HW, et al: Predicting ventilation failure in children with intubation injury. J Pediatr Surg 1994; 29:1122-1126.
43. Pelton JJ, Ratner IA: A technique of airway management in children with obstructed airway due to tumor. Ann Thorac Surg 1989; 48:301-306.
44. Hinton AE, O'Connell JM, van Besouw JP, et al: Neonatal and pediatric fibre-optic laryngoscopy and bronchoscopy using the laryngeal mask airway. J Laryngol Otol 1997; 111:349-353.
45. Schellhase DE: Pediatric flexible airway endoscopy: The light in the tunnel. J Ark Med Soc 1994; 91:227-235.

138

Distal Airway Disorders in Infants and Children: Bronchiolitis and Asthma

John J. Downes, MD • Gregory J. Schears, MD

Disorders of the lower airways, the airways distal to the carina, account for much of the morbidity and mortality associated with pulmonary disease in postneonatal infants and children. Bronchiolitis and asthma rank among the leading causes of acute, reversible respiratory failure in infancy and childhood. Bronchopulmonary dysplasia (BPD), a chronic lung disease involving significant small-airway obstruction, develops as a sequela of neonatal pulmonary disorders. When experiencing a viral respiratory tract infection such as tracheobronchitis or bronchiolitis, infants with BPD often have acute respiratory failure. Together these disorders account for significant resource utilization in a busy pediatric intensive care unit (ICU).

PULMONARY DEVELOPMENT

Important maturational changes in respiratory system structure and function occur in the first 6 years of life.[1-4] In utero development of the lungs by 16 weeks' gestation normally results in formation of the permanent bronchovascular framework of the airways from the carina to the terminal bronchioles at approximately the 16th branching generation. Between 16 and 25 weeks of gestation, distal to the terminal bronchioles, the respiratory zone develops with branching respiratory bronchioles, alveolar ducts, and alveolar sacs. Blood vessels accompany these structures, including a capillary mesh that becomes adjacent to the future alveolar epithelium. By approximately 24 weeks' gestation, this process has advanced sufficiently that, when accompanied by surfactant secretion, gas exchange compatible with extrauterine survival is possible.

Rapid growth of the respiratory airways, alveolar sacs, and apposed capillaries occurs distal to the terminal bronchiole until approximately 2 years of postnatal age. Thereafter, additional branching of airways appears to be limited, although the airways increase in size as the thorax and lungs grow. Enlargement of alveolar surfaces and further alveolar septal invagination (alveolar crests) with an enclosed capillary network progressively increase the gas exchange membrane surface until age 8 to 12 years. From then until full thoracic and cardiopulmonary development in adolescence, lung growth consists primarily of enlargement of existing structures.

A fetus at term has approximately 30 million saccules, which function as immature alveoli and form a less efficient gas exchange surface than in an adult. The total lung volume and functional residual capacity are significantly smaller in relation to body mass than in a normal 8-year-old child.[3, 4] A child 8 years of age should have nearly a full adult complement of approximately 300 million alveoli.[4] Neonates and young infants, however, have oxygen consumption, carbon dioxide production, and caloric expenditure in relation to body mass that are approximately double those of an 8-year-old child or young adult. The relatively small and less efficient gas exchange surface and higher metabolic rate underlie the propensity of young infants to experience respiratory failure more often and more precipitously than older children or young adults. Available data suggest that, as the thorax expands throughout infancy and childhood, the gas exchange surface enlarges proportionately to meet the increasing demand for gas exchange associated with growth and activity.

The centrally integrated control of breathing has not fully developed in a normal newborn, even at term.[3] This immaturity of ventilatory control in term infants results in ventilatory depression or a failure to hyperventilate in the presence of hypoxia. In preterm infants, a depressed ventilatory response occurs with both hypoxia and hypercarbia. Abnormal patterns of ventilatory control, including prolonged apnea, also occur in young infants with severe acute pulmonary disorders such as bronchiolitis.[5]

In infancy and childhood, growth occurs in length and diameter of both the proximal and distal airways. Between 6 months and 5 years of age, small-airway growth surpasses proximal airway growth by as much as 30%.[3] Airway resistance in infants, when indexed to lung volume (functional residual capacity), is comparable to adult values. Pathologic processes that lead to minimal mucosal edema or excessive secretions, however, impede gas flow because of the airway's diminutive size, especially beyond the fourth order of branching. Airway smooth-muscle fibers extend from the terminal bronchiole at birth to the terminal ducts in an adult, permitting regional redistribution of gas at the intra-acinar level. Pores of Kohn and Lambert's channels, which permit gas transfer between acini, develop later in childhood; their scarcity may explain in part an infant's propensity for atelectasis.[3]

A number of factors render an infant's thoracic cage, diaphragm, and other muscles of respiration less able to meet the demands of cardiopulmonary illness than those of an adult. First, the horizontal projection of an infant's ribs from the vertebral bodies imparts a circular configuration to an infant's thorax. Unlike an adult, an infant is unable to increase thoracic volume by raising the ribs in a "bucket-handle" movement. Compared with that of an older child or adult, an infant's diaphragm is composed of less mature muscle fibers and is flatter, which limits excursions. Finally, the highly compliant cartilaginous chest wall of an infant is easily deformed during diaphragmatic contraction, especially in pathologic states. Together these structural features diminish an infant's inspiratory reserve volume in relation to metabolic rate and body mass.

Not only an infant's diaphragm but also the accessory muscles of breathing perform less effectively than in an older child under pathologic conditions that impair lung compliance or airway resistance. The composition of respiratory muscle fibers changes in the first year of life, with intercostal and diaphragmatic muscles containing 30% slow-twitch, high-oxidative (type I) fibers at term, increasing to 60% by the end of the first year. Respiratory muscle endurance has been related directly to the density of type I muscle fibers. Respiratory muscle power increases with age, as manifested by increasing maximum inspiratory and expiratory pressures.[3]

In summary, an infant faces the following physiologic compromises in comparison with an older child and an adult:

1. Higher metabolic rate and oxygen consumption but a comparable functional residual capacity, which, when combined with the normally lower blood hemoglobin concentration, results in a relatively diminished body oxygen reserve.
2. Diminished total alveolar-capillary surface for gas exchange.
3. Less mature and less powerful muscles of ventilation.
4. Very small absolute diameters of the distal airways.
5. Higher compliance of the chest wall and thus diminished chest wall stability, especially in infants younger than 6 months.

These physiologic liabilities account in great measure for the predisposition of infants with distal airway disorders to experience acute respiratory failure.

BRONCHIOLITIS

Bronchiolitis is an acute pulmonary infection, usually of viral etiology, characterized by inflammation of the bronchioles, terminal airways, and often the alveoli.[5] The disorder causes clinical signs and impaired gas exchange in children younger than 2 years of age because of the smaller lumen diameters of their distal airways. Epidemics of bronchiolitis may occur during the winter months.

The most common lower respiratory tract infection in infancy, bronchiolitis can cause acute respiratory failure in healthy full-term infants older than 3 months. Those most at risk for death or respiratory failure, however, are infants younger than 6 months postnatal age who were born prematurely and those with underlying pulmonary, cardiac, neuromuscular, or immune deficiencies.[6] The former preterm infant with BPD has proved to be especially susceptible to severe and prolonged respiratory failure during and after bronchiolitis.

Clinical Presentation

Initial findings include signs of an upper respiratory tract infection such as coryza, cough, otitis media, and fever. Partial upper airway obstruction is common with the profuse coryza. This can significantly increase the work of breathing in an infant younger than 6 months old who is an obligate nose breather. As the disease progresses, tachypnea (>40 breaths/min), retractions, wheezing, and hypoxemia develop in the severely affected infant. Apnea is a common presentation feature, particularly in patients who are young preterm infants. The mechanism of apnea remains unclear.

A typical chest roentgenogram shows hyperinflation and bronchial wall thickening but can also appear normal. The presence of perihilar infiltrates and infiltrates elsewhere makes the differentiation of atelectasis from a bacteria pneumonia difficult.

Signs of dehydration may be seen because of the effects of malaise, poor feeding, fever, and tachypnea. The disease usually runs its course in 3 to 10 days. For those more severely affected, particularly infants born before term or with the other disorders mentioned here, the course can be more prolonged, with respiratory insufficiency lasting for weeks or months.

Etiology

Estimates of the overall incidence of bronchiolitis and of the percentage of children requiring hospitalization vary greatly because uniform diagnostic criteria are lacking. Respiratory syncytial virus (RSV) is the etiologic agent in 50% to 75% of infants hospitalized with bronchiolitis in the United States.[5] A rapid enzyme-linked immunosorbent assay or immunofluorescent RSV antigen test of nasopharyngeal secretions confirms this etiology. The sensitivity of these tests compared with culture is between 80% and 90%.[6] Other organisms associated with bronchiolitis include parainfluenza virus, adenovirus, rhinovirus, mumps virus, influenza virus, and *Mycoplasma pneumoniae,* as well as coinfection with bacteria, especially *Streptococcus pneumoniae* and *Haemophilus influenzae*.[7]

RSV has an incubation period ranging from 2 to 8 days. In a normal host, viral shedding lasts 3 to 8 days.[6] Shedding can continue for weeks or months in young infants or the immunocompromised host. The virus can persist on environmental surfaces for hours and is readily transmitted between patients and hospital personnel. Nosocomial transmission is minimized by following the isolation guidelines for contact precautions of the Centers for Disease Control and Prevention (CDC).[6] Briefly, these measures includes placing infected patients in private rooms or cohorts, washing hands between patients, wearing gowns and gloves, and dedicating care equipment to individual infected patients.

Pathophysiology

The bronchospasm and mucosal edema associated with RSV bronchiolitis may be induced by a reaction to immunoglobulin E (IgE)[8] as well as to mediators released from neutrophils such as thromboxane B_2.[9] The small airways of infants who die from bronchiolitis caused by RSV infection show necrosis of respiratory epithelium. Indeed, the term "syncytium" refers to a multinucleated mass of protoplasm produced by the merging of cells, the consequence of the epithelial cell necrosis induced by this virus.[5] Extensive terminal bronchiolar and alveolar occlusion occurs because of intraluminal eosinophilic debris and peribronchiolar lymphocytic infiltration and edema. Syncytial giant cells may adhere to alveolar walls, and inclusion bodies can be found in the epithelial lining of the alveoli, bronchioles, and bronchi.[5]

Because collateral ventilation of lung units is less efficient in infants than in older children and adults, the ensuing obstruction of small airways causes atelectasis and hyperinflation, thereby profoundly decreasing dynamic compliance and mean tidal volume while mean minute volume increases because of tachypnea. The decrease in dynamic compliance that follows is augmented by uneven distribution of resistance in small peripheral airways.[10] Although elevations in both inspiratory and expiratory resistance contribute to the increased stiffness of the lung and chest wall, the increase in expiratory resistance is greater, suggesting dynamic narrowing of airways on expiration. This leads to a considerable increase in the work of breathing.[11]

The increase in arterial carbon dioxide tension ($Pa{CO_2}$) and decrease in arterial oxygen tension ($Pa{O_2}$) observed during air breathing suggest that alveolar hypoventilation contributes to the characteristic arterial hypoxemia.[12] Alveolar hypoventilation follows from an increase in the wasted ventilation (physiologic dead space) in relation to tidal volume.[12] Initially, the infant compensates by increasing both tidal volume and respiratory rate. This occurs in the presence of the increased work of breathing, and eventually the airways open or the infant fatigues and respiratory failure ensues.[12]

Differential Diagnosis

Although the diagnosis of bronchiolitis on the basis of a careful history, physical examination, and roentgenographic evaluation usually proves straightforward, the clinician should also consider other disorders that produce similar findings. The most common of these by far is asthma. A history of repeated attacks of wheezing provides the key fact indicating the likelihood of asthma and differentiating the two entities. If this is the first such episode, a brisk dilator response of the airways to a beta$_2$-agonist bronchodilator administered as an aerosol or to a single subcutaneous injection of epinephrine (0.01 mL/kg of 1:1000 dilution), combined with a familial atopic or asthmatic history, strongly suggests the diagnosis of asthma. The intense wheezing episode may have been induced, however, by a viral or bacterial respiratory infection. Other entities to be considered as causes of acute intense wheezing in infants include pertussis, foreign body aspiration, tracheal compression by a vascular ring or sling with superimposed tracheitis, cardiac failure, and inhalation of toxic fumes.

Management

Initial management of children hospitalized with bronchiolitis includes providing increased concentrations of inspired oxygen to maintain pulse oximetry ($Sp{O_2}$) levels above 90% and other monitoring. The desaturation associated with apnea can be identified with $Sp{O_2}$, and a heart rate monitor augments this surveillance. Infants often need frequent suctioning of the nares to maintain a patent airway. Feedings should be held for those with respiratory rates that exceed 60 breaths/min. Intravenous (IV) fluids (e.g., 5% dextrose in 0.45% saline at 4–5 mL/kg/hr) will meet basal and increased insensible losses to maintain adequate hydration and urine output (2 mL/kg/hr). Radial artery cannulation should be considered for children with increasing tachypnea, retractions, and $Pa{CO_2}$ levels above 50 mm Hg.

The benefit of nebulized sympathomimetic drugs in bronchiolitis has been controversial. Several studies have suggested modest relief of wheezing and tachypnea with various beta agonists,[13, 14] whereas others have noted no change.[15] Meta-analyses of the literature are in conflict on this issue.[16, 17] Clinical experience suggests that most infants do not receive a substantial benefit, but an early trial is worthwhile.

Clinical improvement with systemic corticosteroids remains even less convincing. Although there may be a reduction in hospital days for mechanically ventilated infants treated with prednisone,[18] most studies do not reflect a significant benefit of corticosteroids in bronchiolitis.[19] Similarly, anticholinergic agents do not appear to reduce wheezing in children.[20] RSV and related antiviral immune globulin (Respigam) has not been shown to be effective in the treatment of RSV bronchiolitis in children at high risk.[21] It may confer some immunologic prophylactic benefit when given by IV infusion over several months,[22] yet the monthly IV infusions become inconvenient. An RSV-specific antibody preparation, palivizumab (Synagis), given IM at monthly intervals, comparably reduces the incidence and severity of RSV bronchiolitis in infants.[22a]

Ribavirin is a nucleoside analog administered by aerosolization with in vitro activity against RSV.[6] Although an early study showed clinical efficacy,[23] a later extensive trial failed to demonstrate positive results[24] Given the cost, questionable efficacy, and safety issues involved, ribavirin is now considered appropriate only for high-risk infants hospitalized for bronchiolitis.[6]

Management of Respiratory Failure

Acute respiratory failure in infants with bronchiolitis may occur as a result of apnea or, more commonly, airway obstruction and fatigue.[12] The clinical signs of acute respiratory failure are as follows:

1. Episodes of central apnea (in infants through age 6 months).
2. Increasing respiratory rate to levels from 60 to 90 breaths/min (until exhaustion, when apnea may ensue).
3. Increasing subcostal retractions.
4. Persistent hyperinflation.
5. Diminished breath sounds.
6. Diminished alertness and reactivity.

Apneic episodes, or the other signs combined with progressive hypercapnia, call for tracheal intubation and mechanical ventilation. Large pediatric centers report an incidence of respiratory failure in infants with bronchiolitis varying from 7% to 38%.[25]

Although some clinicians have cited the benefits of continuous positive-pressure breathing applied nasally or after tracheal intubation, we recommend proceeding directly with tracheal intubation and intermittent positive-pressure mechanical ventilation. The goal is to take over most of the work of breathing and augment alveolar ventilation. Volume-preset pediatric ventilators ensure the delivery of the selected tidal volume against a high and varying airway impedance. The use of supplemental positive end-expiratory pressure appears to confer no additional benefit in bronchiolitis.[26]

Sedation of these infants with narcotics and benzodiazepines helps to provide comfort and ventilatory synchrony. Neuromuscular blockade may be necessary, especially at the onset, in an infant with extremely high airway impedance.[12] Mechanical ventilation is needed for at least 3 to 4 days and perhaps as long as several weeks. Optimizing enteral caloric intake and minimizing the duration of neuromuscular blockade facilitate postextubation recovery. Allowing a tracheal air leak around the endotracheal tube at or below 30 cm H_2O should reduce the likelihood of severe subglottic edema after extubation.

Sequelae

The mortality is approximately 2% for hospitalized children with proven RSV infection but can be much higher for immunosuppressed infants or those with congenital heart disease.[27] Although most children recover from episodes of acute bronchiolitis within 2 to 4 weeks after hospital discharge, former preterm infants with mild to moderate BPD often have more severe disease that waxes and wanes for many months. Patients who have had bronchiolitis as infants seem to be more prone to have reactive airway disease or asthma later in life.[28]

SEVERE ASTHMA AND RESPIRATORY FAILURE

Asthma, the most common chronic disease of childhood, has been defined in various ways through the centuries because of its protean and episodic manifestations. The U.S. Public Health Service National Institutes of Health Expert Panel Report (1991) on Guidelines for the Diagnosis and Management of Asthma stated:

Asthma is a lung disease with the following characteristics: (1) airway obstruction that is reversible (but not completely so in some patients) either spontaneously or with treatment; (2) airway inflammation; and (3) increased airway responsiveness to a variety of stimuli.[29]

The term *reactive airways disease* has been applied to infants with recurrent episodes of wheezing or other evidence of peripheral airway obstruction during an acute upper respiratory tract infection, as well as to older children and adolescents who experience cough and dyspnea with inhalation of cold air or the onset of vigorous exercise. Such persons are generally included in the overall spectrum of "asthma" for diagnostic and therapeutic purposes.[30]

The term *status asthmaticus* formerly denoted a severe asthmatic attack in which the intense wheezing failed to respond to routine medication as well as to two doses of subcutaneous epinephrine (0.01 mg/kg) given within a 30-minute period. Since the mid-1980s, the term has been applied less specifically or abandoned in favor of the more flexible term *acute severe asthmatic episode* (or *attack*). This term implies that intense wheezing persists despite frequent application of aerosolized beta agonists in conjunction with IV corticosteroids and sometimes systemic bronchodilators, such as subcutaneous terbutaline or IV aminophylline.

In this chapter, the term *status asthmaticus* is replaced by *severe acute asthmatic episode,* which implies a lack of response to conventional emergency therapy. The term *acute respiratory failure* refers to a severe acute asthmatic episode that leads to significant hypercapnia with a progressively rising $Pa{CO_2}$ above 45 mm Hg (the upper limit of normal for children 7 years and older). Most children who suffer an acute asthmatic episode also have hypoxemia while breathing air but have hypocapnia rather than carbon dioxide retention. Hypercapnia subsequently develops as a result of further impairment of gas flow and eventual muscular fatigue.[31]

Epidemiology

The prevalence of asthma in the total population increased 29% from 1980 to 1987 and has continued to rise in the 1990s. The most striking increment, however, occurred in the age group younger than 20 years, in whom the incidence rose 43%, from 35 to 50 per 1000 population.[29] This represents approximately 6 million to 8 million children and adolescents in the United States with asthma or reactive airways disease of some degree. Hospitalization rates for children younger than 15 years during the same period also increased 43%, from 20 to 28 per 10,000 population, and remained significantly higher than that of older asthmatic patients (16 to 18 per 10,000 population).[29]

After a decline in overall mortality resulting from asthma in the 1970s, the mortality rate for all ages increased during the 1980s but was highest for the age group 5 to 14 years.[32] Causes of these increases remain speculative. Race and socioeconomic status have a role; the prevalence, hospitalization rates, and mortality of asthma for all ages consistently prove to be many times higher among nonwhites and the urban poor.[29, 32, 33]

Nonetheless, mortality from childhood asthma is relatively low, although among severely asthmatic children it may reach 1% to 2%. In all likelihood, most of these deaths are preventable by:

1. Appropriate education of the child and family.
2. Diligent outpatient medical care.

3. Attention by all involved to the warning signs of a severe acute episode.
4. Aggressive emergency and intensive care of severe acute attacks when they develop.

Sudden Death

Sudden death caused by asthma in children and young adults appears to be increasing, although overall it remains a rare event. Case studies of these tragic events reveal certain characteristics predictive of sudden death that tend to distinguish children at higher risk from other comparably severe asthmatic patients[34, 35]:

1. A history of abrupt, unpredictable onset of intense bronchospasm, perhaps with hypoxic seizures.
2. A history of at least one progressively severe attack culminating in acute respiratory failure.
3. Self-management problems, including failure to acknowledge worsening symptoms.
4. Failure of the patient and family to adhere to the medical plan including symptom monitoring and physician notification.
5. Recent tapering or withdrawal of corticosteroids.
6. Unrecognized pneumonia.
7. Major psychologic stress or depression.

Death occurs most often but not exclusively in children who have had several emergency department visits and often one or more hospital admissions for an acute severe asthmatic episode. The time interval from onset of the attack to death may vary from minutes (sudden death) up to 2 hours (termed slow onset–late arrival death).[36, 37] The fatal hypoxic event usually occurs at home or apart from a medical facility, and emergency resuscitation proves futile. Therefore, physicians caring for survivors of asthma with respiratory failure or children with the other risk factors need to ensure that the family is properly informed of this risk of sudden death. The family must also have access to comprehensive outpatient asthma care including medication, education, and psychologic support.

Pathophysiology

The fundamental mechanisms producing a severe asthmatic episode with unresponsiveness of bronchomotor smooth muscle to catecholamines remain unclear. Any proposed theory must account for the contribution of various interacting factors,[29] including:

1. A strong familial tendency for atopy.
2. An associated immunoglobulin E response to various allergens.
3. Action of potent bronchoconstrictors released by mast cells such as histamine and the leukotrienes.
4. Levels of cyclic adenosine monophosphate (cAMP) in airway smooth-muscle cells.

These factors appear to exert their effect through cyclic nucleotides, which have a central role in regulating cell functions that modulate the asthmatic response. Decreased metabolic responses to stress and to adrenergic agents as well as bronchomotor spasm have been attributed to β-adrenergic blockade and impaired cAMP formation induced by the mediators of the allergenic response. Direct β_2-adrenergic stimulation through administration of agonist agents, which overcome the β-blockade, relaxes bronchomotor smooth muscle and improves airway conductance. This constitutes the central treatment goal in dealing with severe asthmatic episodes.

Viral respiratory infections appear to be an important inciting factor in many acute asthmatic episodes. In school-aged children with asthma, common cold viruses were associated with 80% to 85% of acute exacerbations of wheezing.[38] The predominant virus in these children is the rhinovirus. Among children younger than 2 years of age, RSV is the most common pathogen producing intense distal airway obstruction that appears as bronchiolitis.[38]

Viral infections of the airways induce local and systemic inflammatory cell responses, including enhanced release of histamine and other bronchoconstrictor mediators by pulmonary and plasma mast cells as well as basophils. In addition, infections cause an intensified late-phase response, 4 to 8 hours after the onset of wheezing, with an influx into the airways of inflammatory cells in response to the chemotactic factors released by mast cells. Viral infections also seem to enhance β-adrenergic blockade, increase cholinergic activity, and directly damage airway epithelium. Cold inspired gas, air pollutants, exercise, and emotional factors act alone or in combination to exaggerate the bronchoconstrictor responses.

Atopic phenomena, with or without infection, cause contraction of bronchial and bronchiolar smooth muscle, hypertrophy of the mucous glands and smooth muscle, and inflammatory cell infiltration and edema within the mucosa and submucosal structures. Bronchoconstriction may be direct and local or may be widespread and mediated by the vagus nerve. It involves the lung in a nonuniform fashion, causing maldistribution of gas with respect to pulmonary capillary blood flow. The small peripheral airways respond differently from the large central airways to various stimuli. In adult humans, peripheral airways dilate in response to aerosolized isoproterenol but not to atropine, whereas the central airways are dilated by atropine but respond minimally to isoproterenol. In nonsmoking adults, histamine inhalation constricts the peripheral airways, with little effect on the central airways. The airway lumen in an asthmatic patient often becomes further narrowed or occluded by viscid secretions.

In children with severe asthma, lung biopsies and autopsy specimens show that the peripheral airways are markedly obstructed by goblet cell hyperplasia, mucous plugging, eosinophilic and neutrophilic cell infiltration, and increased collagen under the mucosal basement membrane. This chronic inflammatory state sets the stage for deleterious changes in pulmonary function with onset of an acute episode. These include increased total airway resistance (mean, 370%) and residual volume (mean, 301%) and decreased 1-second forced expiratory volume (mean, 29%) and compliance (mean, 52%) (Fig. 138–1).[39] Comparable information for children with a severe asthmatic episode or respiratory failure is not available, but we can safely assume that the deviations in pulmonary function are significantly worse than in the less severe acute episodes with which this study was concerned.

Pressure from gas trapped distal to the obstructed airways combines with persistent inspiratory muscle activity during expiration and a supranormal nonchemical respiratory drive to increase residual volume and hyperinflate the chest. These changes increase both the elastic and flow-resistant components of the work of breathing. This increase, in combination with the rising minute ventilation observed early in the asthmatic episode,[40] leads to excessive inspiratory as well as expiratory efforts. The increased respiratory effort and sensation of extreme dyspnea produce fear and even terror in a child.

An infant or child in a severe acute episode of asthma incurs abnormalities in gas exchange and acid-base balance (Fig. 138–2).[40, 41] Segmental regional hyperinflation with impaired pulmonary capillary flow significantly increases physiologic dead space (wasted ventilation), as reflected in physiologic dead space/tidal volume ratios of 0.4 to 0.6 or higher.[40]

An early increase in minute ventilation, averaging two and one-half times normal resting levels, initially overcompensates for the increase in wasted ventilation and slightly reduces Pa_{CO_2}. The Pa_{O_2} while the child breathes air concomitantly falls from normal levels of 90 to 100 mm Hg to about 60 mm Hg. Hypoxemia results from maldistribution of gas with respect to blood flow within the lungs and by shunting of blood through atelectatic lung segments.

Most severe asthmatic episodes begin with moderate wheezing and various degrees of malaise. Dehydration, lack of adequate food intake, and exogenous catecholamines can result in ketonemia as well as small elevations in arterial lactate and pyruvate levels. These anions, perhaps with other organic acid anions, produce a moderate to severe nonrespiratory acidosis in 75% of children with an acute severe asthmatic attack. Acidosis and ketonemia tend to be greater in patients younger than 4 years.[40]

Unless airway resistance and wasted ventilation are decreased, the excessive work of breathing and the demand for a high minute volume, as well as hypercapnia,[31] cause respiratory muscle fatigue. The minute volume then falls toward normal resting levels, resulting in progressively severe hypercapnia (Pa_{CO_2} rising above 50 to 65 mm Hg), central nervous system irritability followed by depression, and profound respiratory failure[40, 41] (see Fig. 138-2). Progressive hypercapnia, in conjunction with a nonrespiratory acidemia and progressive arterial hypoxemia, eventually leads to severe asphyxia, with Pa_{CO_2} levels in excess of 100 mm Hg, and an arterial pH less than 7.00.[40] If alveolar ventilation is not restored, the severe acidosis and hypoxia result in cardiovascular depression, cardiac dysrhythmias, and cardiopulmonary arrest. In our experience, this sequence of events more commonly occurs, and is more likely to be lethal, in children with chronic severe asthma requiring maximum maintenance therapy. It can occur, however, in children with only moderately severe asthma who have a concurrent viral respiratory tract infection or have been exposed to a large dose of an allergen.

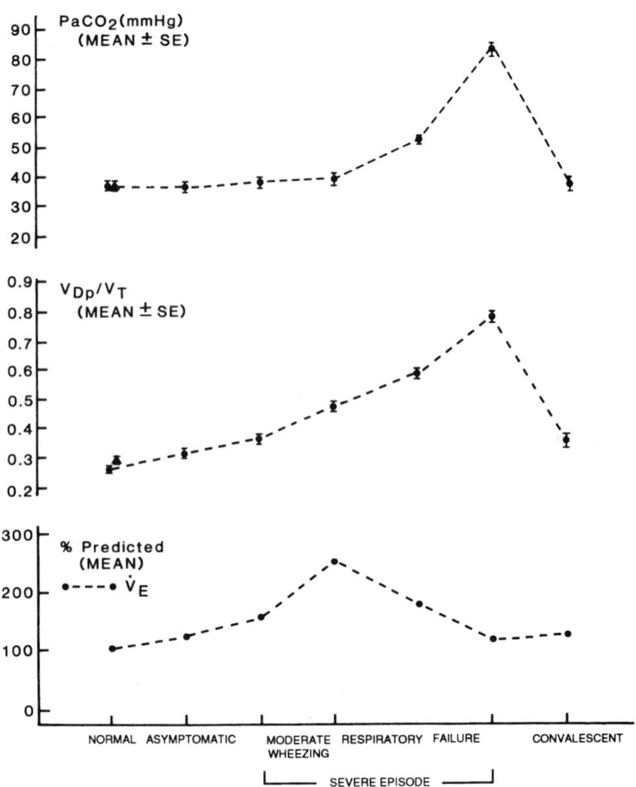

Figure 138–2. Changes in mean Pa_{CO_2}, ratio of physiologic dead space to tidal volume (V_{Dp}/V_T), and minute ventilation $\dot{V}_E$ (as a percentage of predicted) in children in various stages of an asthmatic episode compared with normal children of the same age group (7 to 14 years). The child with a severe asthmatic attack initially maintains Pa_{CO_2} at normal (compensated) levels, despite significant increases in V_{Dp}/V_T, by increasing $\dot{V}_E$ (range: 135% to 350% above predicted normal level). Acute respiratory failure (Pa_{CO_2} > 45 mm Hg) occurs when V_{Dp}/V_T approaches 0.6; respiratory muscle fatigue causes $\dot{V}_E$ to fall toward normal resting levels despite continued increases in V_{Dp}/V_T. (Data for normal mean values from Levison H, Featherby EA, Weng TR: Arterial blood gases, alveolar-arterial oxygen difference, and physiologic dead space in children and young adults. Am Rev Respir Dis 1970; 101:972; and data for asthma mean values from Downes JJ, Heiser MS: Status asthmaticus in children. *In*: Respiratory Failure in the Child. Gregory G [Ed]. New York, Churchill Livingstone, 1981, p 114.)

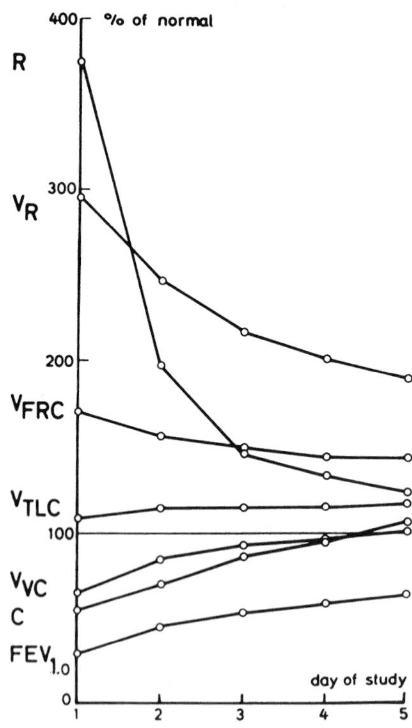

Figure 138–1. Mean values for pulmonary function tests expressed as a per cent of predicted normal values during and for 4 days following an acute asthmatic episode. R = total airways resistance; V_R = residual volume; V_{FRC} = functional residual capacity; V_{TLC} = total lung capacity; V_{VC} = vital capacity; C = total pulmonary compliance; FEV_1 = forced expiratory volume in 1 second. (From Engstrom I: Respiratory studies in children: XI. Mechanics of breathing, lung volumes, and ventilation capacity in children from attack to symptom-free status. Acta Paediatr Suppl 1964; 155:1–60.)

Diagnosis of Severe Acute Asthma and Respiratory Failure

A child with an acute, intense asthmatic episode that may lead to respiratory failure demonstrates marked dyspnea, intractable bilateral wheezing, thoracic hyperinflation, the use of accessory muscles of ventilation, and usually pulsus paradoxus (>20 mm Hg). These clinical signs are ordinarily associated with a significantly elevated clinical asthma score in any of the scoring systems used, with a score of 4 or more in our institution (Table 138–1). Children with a severe asthmatic attack should undergo a complete history evaluation and phys-

TABLE 138–1. Clinical Asthma Score

	Score*		
Clinic Signs	*0*	*1*	*2*
Oxygenation Spo_2	In air 90–97%	In air <90%	In 40% oxygen <90%
Inspiratory breath sounds	Normal	Unequal	Decreased to absent sounds
Use of accessory muscles	None	Moderate	Maximum
Expiratory wheezing	None	Moderate	Marked
Cerebral function	Normal	Depressed or agitated	Coma

Adapted from Wood DW, Downes JJ, Lecks HI: A clinical scoring system for the diagnosis of respiratory failure. Am J Dis Child 1972; 123:227. Copyright 1972, American Medical Association.

* Acute respiratory failure = score > 5, $Paco_2$ > 45 mm Hg after intermittent aerosol bronchodilator and intravenous corticosteroid therapy.

ical examination to detect preexisting infection, record the type and dosage of both immediate and long-term medications, and describe the course of events in any previous severe asthmatic episodes.[41]

A chest roentgenogram obtained at the time of hospital admission usually demonstrates considerable pulmonary hyperinflation with depression or flattening of the diaphragm as well as occasional infiltrates (atelectasis or pneumonitis) or barotrauma. A complete blood count, urinalysis, and determination of blood glucose and serum electrolyte levels aid in defining associated infection and metabolic disorders. If a patient has been receiving aminophylline, a serum theophylline level should be obtained in order to detect potentially toxic theophylline blood levels.

Acute respiratory failure usually results in the following signs: cyanosis despite administration of 40% inspired oxygen; decreased or absent inspiratory breath sounds; maximum use of the accessory respiratory muscles; intense, high-pitched expiratory wheezing; and depressed consciousness or coma. These clinical signs are ordinarily associated with a $Paco_2$ well in excess of 45 mm Hg and frequently between 65 and 100 mm Hg.

Patients with severe asthma often experience widely diverse degrees of wheezing and differ in their reactions to bronchodilators. Assessment of a child's response to therapy for a severe episode requires the following:

- Frequent observation of clinical signs (respiratory rate, heart rate, arterial pressure)
- Continuous pulse oximetry
- Repeated determinations of arterial pH and blood gas tensions

Estimates of clinical severity and the response to therapy can also be facilitated by sequential determination of the clinical asthma score (see Table 138–1). If the $Paco_2$ consistently exceeds 45 mm Hg, the child should be admitted to an ICU. Sternocleidomastoid and scalene muscle contraction and supraclavicular retraction correlate well with the severity of airway obstruction.

Continuous electrocardiogram (ECG) monitoring allows early detection of the cardiac dysrhythmias that can accompany severe hypercapnia or hypoxemia. Progressively severe distal airway obstruction usually produces pulsus paradoxus with limited right ventricular filling. Acute arterial hypotension is the common presenting sign of *tension pneumothorax*. Some of these children are moderately hypovolemic and become severely hypotensive with the initiation of positive-pressure mechanical ventilation.

Management of the Severe Asthmatic Episode

The two major treatment goals for a severe episode are as follows:

1. Increase airway conductance by relaxing airway smooth muscle, decreasing the viscosity and volume of secretions, and reducing mucosal edema.
2. Support vital functions until an effective and sustained bronchomotor response to bronchodilators returns. This requires the following measures (Table 138–2)[40, 41]:
   a. Increasing concentrations of humidified oxygen to alleviate hypoxemia.
   b. Correcting systemic dehydration with IV fluids.
   c. Restoring arterial pH to the range of 7.25 to 7.30 with IV sodium bicarbonate to prevent profound acidemia in the event of sudden hypercarbia and to elevate the threshold for cardiac dysrhythmias.
   d. Attempting to overcome the β_2-adrenergic blockade with continuous aerosolized beta agonists such as albuterol.
   e. Infusing corticosteroids intravenously to reduce inflammation and enhance responsiveness to the beta agonists.

Correction of hypoxemia with increased inspired oxygen is the most important factor in preventing cardiac arrest and major central nervous system damage in a child suffering from a severe asthmatic attack. Elevated inspired oxygen concentrations must be maintained throughout the asthmatic episode, including periods in the radiology department and during transport. Hypoxic encephalopathy continues to be a major complication and cause of death in children with a severe asthmatic episode and unrecognized respiratory failure.[36]

Bronchodilators widely used since 1985 in the initial treatment of severe asthmatic episodes in children include various aerosolized $beta_2$ agonists administered by mask inhalation, such as albuterol[42] and terbutaline.[43] In earlier years, IV amino-

TABLE 138–2. Management of Severe Acute Asthmatic Episodes: Fundamental Therapy

Oxygen (with Humidity)
Maintain Spo_2 above 90% with FIO_2 30–50% (or higher).

Intravenous Fluids
Up to twice maintenance rates until urine flow reaches 2 mL/kg/hr, then maintenance rates.

Bronchodilators
Primary: albuterol aerosolized 0.15–0.25 mg/kg per dose every 1–2 hr (0.03–0.05 mL/kg per dose in 2 mL of saline). If ineffective, use continuously (0.5 mg/kg/hr).
Secondary: ipratropium bromide 250 μg (1 mL) mixed with albuterol solution for nebulization intermittently every 20–30 min for 1 hr and then every 4 hr.

Corticosteroids
Methylprednisolone (sodium succinate) IV, 1–2 mg/kg/6 hr for 24 hr, then 1–2 mg/kg/day in three divided doses.

Buffers
If arterial pH < 7.25 and base deficit < −6 mEq/L, give intravenous $NaHCO_3$, 1–2 mEq/kg initially, followed by doses adjusted according to base deficit to maintain arterial pH > 7.30.*

Antibiotics
If bacterial infection suspected (fever, pulmonary infiltrates), intravenous broad-spectrum coverage.

* Dose $NaHCO_3$ (mEq) = base deficit × 0.3 (weight in kg).

phylline was used. The $beta_2$ agonists act in part by enhancing cAMP synthesis and thereby relaxing the airway smooth muscle; these agents also inhibit mast cell degranulation and the release of pathogenic mediators. Prior treatment with beta agonists, however, may decrease the responsiveness of an asthmatic patient to that class of drugs.[29] Nonetheless, there are no effective therapeutic options for directly relieving airway obstruction other than these agents plus corticosteroids. Aminophylline has been shown to be ineffective in acute severe asthma and is no longer recommended.[41]

The age at which bronchomotor responsiveness to beta agonists develops has not been clearly defined. Many infants younger than 6 months show little, if any, clinical response. Some infants between 6 and 20 months may respond to these agents, whereas children with reactive airways disease older than 20 months consistently respond to inhaled beta agonists with a decrease in wheezing and an improvement in airway conductance. Intermittent positive-pressure breathing by mask does not enhance this response. Aerosol droplet size ranging from 0.5 to 2 μm in diameter is necessary for effective drug deposition. The details of intermittent and continuous albuterol aerosol therapy are summarized in Tables 138–2 and 138–3. The sequence of management for progressive respiratory failure appears in Table 138–3.

Children suffering a severe asthmatic episode have limited inspiratory capacity and flow rates and may not effectively inhale drugs delivered by a conventional metered, gas-propelled aerosol (metered-dose inhaler). Furthermore, the dose per inhalation from such devices remains fixed and therefore may be inadequate for a 50-kg child but excessive for a 10-kg child. A beneficial response depends on an appropriate concentration of the drug and a sufficient peak inspiratory flow rate to permit dispersion and deposition of an effective dose in the distal airways. The duration of bronchodilation in a child with a severe asthmatic episode responding to a 5- to 10-minute aerosol treatment varies widely. Despite these drawbacks, intermittent or continuously nebulized beta agonists diluted in saline, and delivered at an appropriate gas flow rate and inspired oxygen concentration via face mask, have proved effective in most children during a severe, acute asthmatic episode (see Table 138–2).[42, 43]

Ipratropium bromide is a derivative of atropine that has twice its potency, has a 50% longer duration of bronchodilator effects, and does not cross the blood-brain barrier. It has proved beneficial in some children as an adjunctive aerosol with $beta_2$ agonists for treatment of a severe acute asthmatic episode.[44, 45]

TABLE 138–3. Management of Severe Acute Asthmatic Episodes: Respiratory Failure Management

Continuous Beta Agonist

- Continuous albuterol aerosol inhalation (0.5 mg/kg/hr)
- Continuous intravenous isoproterenol infusion (0.1 μg/kg/min to maximum of 5.0 μg/kg/min), or
- Continuous intravenous terbutaline (10 μg/kg bolus over 10 min, followed by 0.1–0.4 μg/kg/min or higher if required with increments at 10- to 20-min intervals.

Mechanical Ventilation

- Tracheal intubation (with full stomach precautions)
- Volume-preset ventilator (e.g., T-Bird, Siemens 300)
- Neuromuscular blockade (vecuronium 0.2 mg/kg bolus followed in 1 hr by 0.1 mg/kg/hr in 1 hr by infusion)
- Sedation:
  - Morphine, 0.1–0.3 mg/kg/hr or
  - Fentanyl, 2–5 μg/kg/hr and
  - Diazepam, 0.2–0.3 mg/kg/hr

Approximately 250 μg of ipratropium, together with albuterol nebulized every 20 minutes for the first hour and then every 2 to 4 hours, appears to benefit many children in an acute asthmatic episode more than albuterol alone.[41, 44–46]

As previously stated, correction of acidemia with IV sodium bicarbonate should raise the threshold for cardiac dysrhythmias, possibly enhance bronchomotor responsiveness to $beta_2$ agonists, and provide some protection against extreme acidemia in the event of sudden respiratory failure and severe hypercapnia. In our experience, the transient mild elevation of $Pa{CO_2}$ associated with a 30-minute infusion of sodium bicarbonate reverts to the preinfusion $Pa{CO_2}$ level in less than 30 minutes, but the plasma pH and bicarbonate level remain elevated. This provides, in less than an hour, the expected elevation of plasma bicarbonate level secondary to hypercapnia-induced renal bicarbonate reabsorption, which takes 12 to 24 hours to occur.

Intravenous corticosteroids have been used routinely in the treatment of severe asthmatic episodes in children for 30 years. Controlled studies support their use.[47] Corticosteroids enhance cAMP formation, and their anti-inflammatory action justifies their short-term use in every child with a severe episode. Intravenous methylprednisolone in a dose of 2 mg/kg every 6 hours appears to be more effective than other corticosteroids in ameliorating airway obstruction in asthmatic children.[48] This may be due to the drug's greater penetration into the airway epithelium and longer mean residence time in this tissue, as shown in carefully controlled animal studies.[48]

Increased potassium excretion by the kidneys is the only consistent undesirable side effect of short-term corticosteroids that we have observed. However, the hypokalemia is intensified by concurrent administration of aerosolized or IV $beta_2$ agonists, which themselves have a potent kaliuretic effect. Therefore, serum potassium levels should be determined at least every 12 hours and appropriate IV supplementation provided.

Antibiotics should be reserved for children with clinical evidence of bacterial infection such as a fever, a pulmonary infiltrate, or a history strongly suggestive of bacterial infection. When bacterial infection seems a reasonable possibility, nasopharyngeal and blood specimens should be obtained for culture and a broad-spectrum IV antibiotic initiated. A rapid respiratory viral panel analysis of nasopharyngeal secretions should be obtained to exclude RSV infection in infants with asthma.

Intravenous Isoproterenol and Other $Beta_2$ Agonists

In approximately 5% of children hospitalized for severe acute asthma, fundamental therapy, including continuous aerosolized $beta_2$-agonist inhalation, fails to relieve the intense airway obstruction and extraordinary work of breathing; respiratory failure develops with $Pa{CO_2}$ rising progressively to levels of 45 to 55 mm Hg.[40, 41] In many such patients, overcoming the apparent distal airway β-receptor blockade with high blood levels of $beta_2$ agonists has proved effective in relieving airway obstruction and reducing hypercarbia.

Three such agents used intravenously in children are albuterol, terbutaline, and isoproterenol. Intravenous albuterol has been used in Canada[49] with definite efficacy but is unavailable in injectable form in the United States. Intravenous terbutaline has not been used widely, and only a few preliminary reports of efficacy and safety have been published.[50, 51] Most of the experience in the United States with asthmatic children receiving IV beta agonists for impending respiratory failure has been with isoproterenol, despite its lack of $beta_2$ specificity and undesirable side effects in some patients.[40, 41, 52] Evidence of permanent myocardial ischemic damage with any of these beta agonists is lacking,[52] and even continuous nebulized albuterol inhalation can cause transient elevations in creatinine phosphokinase MB fraction (CPK-MB).[53]

In our practice, IV isoproterenol or terbutaline is indicated for patients with intractable airway obstruction, characterized by an asthma score of 5 or greater (see Table 138–1) and a progressively rising $Paco_2$ exceeding 45 to 55 mm Hg.[40] Both of these agents can be effective in the child with impending respiratory failure related to asthma. Their mean effective initial and maintenance dosages are comparable,[40, 50, 51] as are the mean durations of infusion required to achieve sustained improvement after discontinuing the drug. Our experience with isoproterenol indicates that 90% of nearly 200 such children treated since 1970 have experienced early and sustained clinical improvement and reduction of $Paco_2$, which enabled them to avoid mechanical ventilation. Terbutaline, with which we as well as others have limited experience, may not be as effective as isoproterenol for the child with respiratory failure and severe hypercapnia ($Paco_2 > 65$ mm Hg).

Isoproterenol has a half-life of only 2.5 to 5.0 minutes in children. It reduces distal airway resistance, $Paco_2$, and excessive ventilatory effort, usually within 2 hours. The systemic arterial hypertension that frequently accompanies the hypercapnia also declines with $Paco_2$. This gives an affected child a feeling of considerable relief.

Because of the hazards of hypoxemia, dysrhythmias, and progressive hypercapnia, IV isoproterenol should be used only in an ICU where continuous ECG monitoring, equipment and drugs for cardioversion, and personnel skilled in resuscitation are immediately available. Aminophylline infusion, if in use, should be discontinued because of its potential additive cardiac dysrhythmogenic effect in the presence of isoproterenol. Because of the need for frequent arterial blood sampling and the advantage of continuous arterial pressure monitoring, peripheral artery cannulation is advocated for these patients.

The effective peak infusion dosage of isoproterenol varies from 0.1 to 5.0 μg/kg/min and the duration from 8 hours to 5 days (mean 2 days). Because the infusion rate of a gravity drip is neither consistent nor precise, isoproterenol should be administered with a *constant infusion pump*. Although the average alveolar-arterial oxygen tension difference is not affected by the infusion of isoproterenol, transient serious decreases in Pao_2 at 30% to 40% inspired oxygen develop in about 4% of patients, requiring inspired oxygen concentrations of 60% to 85% to maintain Spo_2 at 90%.[40]

We recommend an initial dose of 0.1 μg/kg/min and determination of arterial pH and blood gas tensions at approximately 20-minute intervals. The dose is increased in increments of 0.2 to 0.4 μg/kg/min until (1) $Paco_2$ falls below 50 mm Hg or decreases at least 10% from its preinfusion levels; (2) heart rate exceeds 200 beats per minute; or (3) a clinically significant dysrhythmia develops, for example, multiple ectopic ventricular beats. An *average* dosage of 0.3 μg/kg/min produces an initial decrease in clinical score and $Paco_2$; normocapnia ($Paco_2 < 45$ mm Hg) is achieved at an *average* dosage of 0.7 μg/kg/min. Heart rate tends to stabilize or decrease after an initial rise, suggesting tachyphylaxis. Tachycardia exceeding 200 beats per minute rarely occurs, and heart rate decreases when the isoproterenol dosage is lowered.

When the $Paco_2$ has stabilized below 45 mm Hg and the clinical score is less than 4, the dosage may be decreased by 0.2 μg/kg/min at hourly intervals with determination of $Paco_2$ after each change. A dosage of 0.2 to 0.5 μg/kg/min usually needs to be maintained for 24 to 40 hours and then decreased gradually until the infusion can be discontinued. Attempts to decrease the dosage before the infusion has continued at least 12 hours are usually futile. After a dosage decrement, if the $Paco_2$ exceeds 45 mm Hg or the wheezing recurs (score increases by 1 or more), the dosage should be increased by 0.1 to 0.2 μg/kg/min.

Intravenous isoproterenol, if administered at sufficient dosage levels, reverses hypercapnia and respiratory failure in more than 90% of infants and children with a severe asthmatic episode and respiratory failure. Patients who do not achieve a sustained reduction in $Paco_2$ with isoproterenol infusion usually have a preinfusion $Paco_2$ exceeding 65 mm Hg, fever, or radiographic evidence of pulmonary infiltrates. These patients require tracheal intubation, neuromuscular blockade, and mechanical ventilation.[40]

ECG evidence suggestive of myocardial ischemia has been reported during isoproterenol infusion in asthmatic children with a severe episode and respiratory failure.[50] We have also found abnormal (>2 mm) elevation or depression of the ST segment during isoproterenol infusion in three of 24 episodes (15 patients), a 12% incidence, when monitoring with a multiple-lead ECG. The CPK-MB, determined in six of these patients, was elevated in only one of the children with an abnormal ECG. The ECG and enzyme abnormalities quickly reverted to normal in all patients when the isoproterenol was discontinued. None of these patients complained of anginal pain, and none experienced systemic arterial hypotension or cardiac dysrhythmias. Because of the concern about myocardial ischemia, we and others[52] advocate preinfusion and daily 12-lead ECGs as well as determination of serial serum CPK-MB isoenzyme levels in children receiving an isoproterenol infusion. Unless clear evidence of progressive ischemia emerges, we advocate continuing with an isoproterenol infusion in patients whose $Paco_2$ is persistently rising above 60 mm Hg despite ST segment changes. Follow-up ECG findings and CPK-MB levels quickly revert to normal when isoproterenol is stopped.

We think that the well-established risks of tracheal intubation and mechanical ventilation in asthmatic children[40] probably exceed those of possible transient myocardial ischemia associated with isoproterenol and terbutaline. For the child with impending respiratory failure (or even existing failure) caused by acute asthma, it is often possible to avoid tracheal intubation and mechanical ventilation through the appropriate use of IV beta agonists.

Mechanical Ventilation

Infants and children with severe asthma and respiratory failure who are experiencing life-threatening acute asphyxia or who are unresponsive to conventional therapy and IV isoproterenol or terbutaline require tracheal intubation and mechanical ventilation for a minimum of 12 hours and an average of 24 hours.[40] In an acutely asphyxiated asthmatic child, cyanosis, bradycardia or other dysrhythmias, or coma that fails to improve with manually assisted ventilation and oxygen calls for immediate tracheal intubation. Otherwise, tracheal intubation can be deferred until experienced personnel and optimal equipment are present.

The authors advocate a rapid IV sequence induction with ketamine and vecuronium plus cricoid pressure for laryngoscopy and orotracheal intubation. During mechanical ventilation, continued infusion of isoproterenol in an appropriate dosage partially relieves distal airway obstruction, thereby reducing the mean and peak inspiratory airway pressures required for adequate ventilation. *However, initial treatment of these patients should emphasize correction of hypoxemia and assurance of sustained, adequate delivery of oxygen to the brain and heart. Reduction of $Paco_2$ remains a secondary and subsequent goal.* Maintenance of neuromuscular blockade greatly facilitates the restoration of oxygenation and ventilation at peak inspiratory pressure (PIP) levels under 60 cm H_2O.

When arterial blood gas tensions and pH demonstrate that pulmonary gas exchange and acid-base balance have improved, a nasotracheal tube may be inserted. The nasal route provides greater security, does not hinder mouth care, and may result in less gagging and coughing after reversal of neuromuscular blockade. We have not observed sinusitis or otitis media as a consequence of short-term (<7 days) nasotracheal intubation. An adequate tracheal seal permits the development of the intratracheal pressures of 40 to 60 cm H_2O initially needed to maintain sufficient alveolar ventilation and oxygenation for survival. In patients younger than 8 years, an adequate seal can be achieved with uncuffed tubes, but the older patient usually requires a tube with a large-volume, low-pressure cuff, inflated sufficiently to prevent an audible tracheal air leak until the airway pressure exceeds 30 cm H_2O.

A volume-preset ventilator compensates more reliably than pressure-preset or time-flow cycled ventilators for changes in airway resistance and total pulmonary compliance, thus ensuring more consistent alveolar ventilation. A long inspiratory time (1.5 seconds) with a large tidal volume and low ventilatory rate minimizes the turbulence of inspiratory gas flow and tends to distribute gas more uniformly throughout the lungs. A ratio of inspiratory time to expiratory time of 1:2 to 1:3 maximizes the emptying of lung segments distal to severely obstructed airways. If the expiratory time is inadequate, progressive gas trapping in the lungs and occult positive end-expiratory pressure (auto-PEEP) increase the hazard of pneumothorax. To achieve an initial effective tidal volume of 12 to 15 mL/kg, the preset tidal volume needs to be increased by 100 to 150 mL to compensate for the volume of gas compressed within the ventilator tubing (2 to 3 mL/cm H_2O PIP).

A ventilator frequency that is approximately 50% of the predicted respiratory rate for age (~8 to 12 per minute), which allows adequate expiratory time, should produce a substantial and sustained reduction in $Paco_2$ within 6 to 12 hours.[40] Limiting PIP to 50–60 cm H_2O reduces the incidence of barotrauma but does not eliminate it. As long as arterial pH can be kept above 7.25 and $Paco_2$ below 70 mm Hg, higher PIP levels should be avoided. An inspired oxygen concentration at the minimum level (usually 40% to 70%) required to maintain Pao_2 above 75 mm Hg (Spo_2 90% to 95%) permits some nitrogen to remain in the alveoli, thus reducing the likelihood of alveolar collapse and atelectasis distal to partially obstructed airways. However, higher oxygen concentrations may be needed just to keep Pao_2 above 50 mm Hg (Spo_2 > 80%) in the rare patient.

Controlled hypoventilation, which provides appropriate oxygen delivery yet allows $Paco_2$ to remain elevated, may reduce the incidence of barotrauma.[54, 55] However, a $Paco_2$ exceeding 70 mm Hg can cause intracellular acidosis, elevate both pulmonary and systemic arterial pressures, and raise intracranial pressure. We advocate attempting to reduce the $Paco_2$ over several hours to levels below 70 mm Hg in extremely hypercapnic asthmatic children by adjusting ventilation and bronchodilator therapy with continuous nebulized albuterol or IV isoproterenol.

Neuromuscular blockade serves to coordinate patients with the ventilator so that adequate alveolar ventilation can be achieved with minimum airway pressures. Neuromuscular blockade also prevents coughing, thereby reducing the risk of barotrauma. An initial IV dose of vecuronium (0.2 mg/kg) followed by continuous IV infusion of vecuronium or pancuronium (0.1 mg/kg/hr) has proved effective for this purpose. Amnesia, sedation, and analgesia should be provided with IV narcotics (morphine, 0.1 to 0.3 mg/kg every 3 to 4 hours, or fentanyl, 1 to 2 μg/kg/hr) and sedatives (diazepam, 0.2 to 0.3 mg/kg) at 3- to 4-hour intervals. Morphine does not appear to cause symptoms associated with histamine release in these children, who have probably undergone maximum histamine release. Because of negative inotropic effects on the myocardium, ***barbiturates are not recommended.***

Chest physiotherapy, tracheobronchial toilet with saline instillation, and changes in body position facilitate the removal of tracheobronchial secretions, and may help expand previously collapsed, atelectatic lung segments, especially during the resolution phase. Gentle, slow manual ventilation with 100% oxygen before and after chest physiotherapy and tracheobronchial toilet prevents arterial hypoxemia during these procedures, which initially should be performed every 4 to 6 hours. As distal airway obstruction subsides and the bronchomotor response to catecholamines returns, mobilization of thick and voluminous secretions often requires hourly tracheobronchial toilet and chest physiotherapy. In our experience, bronchoscopy in these patients ordinarily offers no advantage over frequent tracheobronchial toilet and chest physiotherapy.

Reliable physiologic criteria for determining when to decrease and stop mechanical ventilation have yet to be established. Because attempts at assisted ventilation in asthmatic children often result in poor coordination of the patient with the ventilator, a trial of spontaneous breathing with assisted or intermittent mandatory ventilation is not recommended. Instead, the following criteria indicate that a patient can usually achieve pulmonary gas exchange without mechanical ventilation:

1. A sustained bronchomotor response to nebulized albuterol in the usual dosage or to a low dose (<0.1 μg/kg/min) of IV isoproterenol, as indicated by decreased wheezing and a reduction in PIP for more than 12 hours.
2. A chest radiograph showing reduced hyperaeration with minimal or no atelectasis.
3. A $Paco_2$ less than 45 mm Hg at a delivered minute volume less than 150% of the predicted normal.
4. A Pao_2 greater than 100 mm Hg (Spo_2 100%) at 40% inspired oxygen.

Tracheal extubation can be performed within 2 to 6 hours after spontaneous unassisted ventilation is resumed. If IV isoproterenol is being used concurrently with mechanical ventilation, it should be continued for at least 6 to 8 hours after extubation in order to ensure bronchodilatation.

Complications

Various complications may occur in children after a severe acute asthmatic episode, yet most of these are transient and, if appropriately managed, without permanent sequelae. Severe hypoxemia and acidosis, however, can lead to cardiac arrest, hypoxic encephalopathy, and death.[56]

In patients who have previously received long-term corticosteroid therapy, acute adrenocortical insufficiency can develop during the stress of a severe asthmatic episode if supplemental corticosteroids are not given. Experience demonstrates that acute respiratory failure and cardiac arrest have often been preceded by a 50% or greater decrease in maintenance corticosteroid medication within the month immediately before hospital admission.[57] As many as 70% of asthmatic children receiving IV corticosteroids and aerosolized or IV $beta_2$ agonists experience hypokalemia (<3.5 mEq/L), despite some supplementary potassium infusion.[58] Thus, in children with respiratory failure, it is necessary to monitor serum potassium closely and infuse additional potassium as indicated.

Radiographic evidence of spontaneous extrapleural air accumulation is observed in 1% of children in a severe asthmatic episode. Mechanical ventilation of children with an existing pneumothorax or pneumomediastinum can lead to massive barotrauma with cardiac tamponade and subsequent cardiac arrest. If mechanical ventilation proves necessary for these patients, the pneumothorax must first be treated with a thoracostomy tube, underwater seal, and high-volume suction. Tension pneumomediastinum requires emergent mediastinotomy with a thoracoscope by a qualified surgeon.

Tracheal intubation with mechanical ventilation in asthmatic children without previously detected barotrauma is associated with a 10% to 20% incidence of pneumothorax or pneumomediastinum, even with intentional alveolar hypoventilation and gradual reduction in Pa_{CO_2}.[58] In our experience, in the most severe episodes the PIP may need to reach a level of 70 to 80 cm H_2O in order to achieve a tidal volume sufficient to ensure an *adequate arterial oxygen content* and to gradually reduce and maintain Pa_{CO_2} at or below 70 mm Hg; this has been associated with an incidence of ventilator-related barotrauma of 10% to 15% in more than 200 patients in our pediatric ICU since 1967.[40]

Acute respiratory failure recurred in 30% of asthmatic children who experienced one severe acute episode of asthma requiring IV isoproterenol, and 16% of these patients had more than two recurrences of respiratory failure.[40] Others have observed similar rates of recurrent respiratory failure requiring mechanical ventilation in children who had severe chronic asthma with a history of corticosteroid dependence and frequent hospital admissions.

Other Therapies

Anesthetic Agents

The profound systemic arterial hypotension and cardiac dysrhythmias observed to develop with halothane in acidotic asthmatic patients have led us to conclude that inhalation anesthesia is usually unsuitable for management of severe asthma with respiratory failure. Despite numerous anecdotal case reports advocating anesthesia with halothane, isoflurane, or ketamine in acute respiratory failure related to severe asthma, the bronchodilator effects of anesthetics at safe blood levels appear to be considerably less than that of IV isoproterenol, which does not cause hypotension and rarely results in dysrhythmias.

Helium-Oxygen

A double-blind, randomized, controlled study[59] of 18 children receiving continuously nebulized albuterol for a severe acute asthmatic episode demonstrated the significant clinical efficacy of helium-oxygen (heliox, in a ratio of 80% to 20%) inhaled by mask in reducing an elevated pulses paradoxus and dyspnea index and increasing peak expiratory flows. The fundamental thesis that decreasing the density of inspired gas with helium improves flow rates in airways with turbulent flow has been known and utilized for patients with obstructive airway disorders since the 1930s.

Several problems discourage routine use of helium-oxygen in children with severe acute asthma:

1. Most of these children require supplemental inspired oxygen to correct hypoxemia, which decreases the proportional concentration of helium and its efficacy.
2. Delivery of helium, which comes in a fixed mixture, requires use of a large, bulky cylinder and additional mechanical apparatus, including a face mask.
3. Only those children with a major component of central airway obstruction are likely to benefit.

However, helium appears to be clinically effective down to concentrations of 60%,[58] and hypoxemia in most children is relieved by 40% inspired oxygen, which can be given by nasal cannula under a face mask. Also, in most severe asthmatic episodes wheezing is clearly audible, indicating that central airway obstruction with turbulent flow occurs, and reduction of gas density should be beneficial. The delivery system mechanics can be simplified by careful planning in advance with knowledgeable respiratory therapists and readily available devices.[41] Therefore, this adjunct to therapy early in the severe episode, as well as in the patient requiring tracheal intubation and mechanical ventilation,[60] deserves further clinical investigation and wider application.

Magnesium Sulfate

Magnesium sulfate ($MgSO_4$) relaxes smooth muscles, including the bronchomotor and vasomotor sites, in both children and adults. One study[61] indicated that in children with a severe asthmatic episode, $MgSO_4$, 25 mg/kg intravenously over 20 minutes, can result in improved flow rates and vital capacity without systemic hypotension. Comparisons with IV terbutaline or isoproterenol and other controlled studies need to be performed to determine the eventual role of this technique in the management of severe asthma.

SUMMARY

The proper diagnosis and management of the infant or child with acute, severe distal airway disease require a team effort involving the general pediatrician, emergency medicine and critical care physicians, the pediatric allergist, nurses, and respiratory therapists. Preplanned diagnostic and management guidelines and protocols serve to enhance effective early treatment and enable the acquisition of useful clinical experience over a period of years.[29, 40, 41] *This approach should reduce to a minimum the morbidity and mortality associated with these conditions.*

References

1. Murray JF (Ed): The Normal Lung. Philadelphia, WB Saunders, 1986, pp 1–24.
2. Weibel ER (Ed): The Pathway for Oxygen. Cambridge, Mass, Harvard University Press, 1984, p 175.
3. Scarpelli EM (Ed): Pulmonary Physiology: Fetus, Newborn, Child and Adolescent. 2nd ed. Philadelphia, Lea & Febiger, 1990, pp 215, 257.
4. Burri PH: Development and growth of the human lung. *In:* Handbook of Physiology. Sect 3. The Respiratory System. Fishman AP (Ed). Bethesda, Md, American Physiological Society, 1985.
5. Ruuskanen O, Ogra PL: Respiratory syncytial virus. Curr Probl Pediatr 1993; 23:50.
6. Peter G (Ed): Respiratory syncytial virus. *In:* 1997 Redbook, Report of the Committee on Infectious Diseases. 24th ed. Elk Village, Ill, American Academy of Pediatrics, 1997, p 443.
7. Korppi M, Leinonen N, Koskella M, et al: Bacterial co-infection in children hospitalized with respiratory syncytial virus infection. Pediatr Infect Dis 1989; 8:687.
8. Weliver RC, Sun M, Ranaldo D, et al: Predictive value of respiratory syncytial virus–specific IgE response for recurrent wheezing following bronchiolitis. J Pediatr 1986; 109:776.
9. Faden H, Kaul TN, Ogra PL: Activation of oxidative and arachidonic acid metabolism in neutrophils by respiratory syncytial virus antibody complexes: Possible role in disease. J Infect Dis 1983; 148:110.
10. Krieger I: Mechanics of respiration in bronchiolitis. Pediatrics 1964; 33:45.
11. Krieger I, Whitten CF: Work of respiration in bronchiolitis. Am J Dis Child 1964; 107:386.
12. Downes JJ, Wood DW, Striker TW, Haddad C: Acute respiratory failure in infants with bronchiolitis. Anesthesiology 1968; 29:426.

13. Klassen TP, Rowe PC, Sutcliffe T, et al: Randomized trial of salbutamol in acute bronchiolitis. J Pediatr 1991; 118:807.
14. Schuh S, Canny G, Reisman JJ, et al: Nebulized albuterol in acute bronchiolitis. J Pediatr 1990; 117:663.
15. Gadomski AM, Lichenstein R, Orton L, et al: Efficacy of albuterol in management of bronchiolitis. Pediatrics 1994; 93:907.
16. Flores G, Horwitz RI: Efficacy of $beta_2$-agonists in bronchiolitis: A reappraisal and meta-analysis. Pediatrics 1997; 100:233.
17. Kellner JD, Ohlsson A, Gadamski AM, Wang EEL: Efficacy of bronchodilator therapy and bronchiolitis. Arch Pediatr Adolesc Med 1996; 150:1166.
18. VanWoensel JBM, Wolfs TFW, vanAalderen WMC, et al: Randomized double blind placebo controlled trial of prednisone in children admitted to hospital with respiratory syncytial virus bronchiolitis. Thorax 1997; 52:634.
19. Roosevelt G, Sheehan K, Grupp-Phelan J, et al: Dexamethasone in bronchiolitis: A randomised controlled trial. Lancet 1996; 348:292.
20. Martinati LC, Boner AI: Anticholinergic antimuscarinic agents in the treatment of airways bronchoconstriction in children. Allergy 1996; 51:2.
21. Rodriguez WJ, Gruber WC, Welliver RC, et al: Respiratory syncytial virus immunoglobulin intravenous therapy for RSV lower respiratory tract infections in infants and young children at high risk for severe RSV infections. Pediatrics 1997; 99:454.
22. American Academy of Pediatrics Committee on Infectious Diseases: Respiratory syncytial virus immune globulin intravenous: Indications for use. Pediatrics 1997; 99:645.
22a. American Academy of Pediatrics Committee on Infectious Diseases: Prevention of respiratory syncytial virus infections: Indications for the use of palivizumab and update on the use of RSV-IGIV. Pediatrics 1998; 102:1211.
23. Taber LH, Knight V, Gilber BE, et al: Ribavirin aerosol treatment of bronchitis associated with respiratory syncytial virus infection in infants. Pediatrics 1983; 72:613.
24. Moler FW, Steinhart CM, Ohmit SCN, Stidham GL: Effectiveness of ribavirin in otherwise well infants with respiratory syncytial virus associated with respiratory failure. J Pediatr 1996; 128:422.
25. Lebel MH, Gauthier M, Lacroix J, et al: Respiratory failure and mechanical ventilation in severe bronchiolitis. Arch Dis Child 1989; 64:1431.
26. Smith PG, El-Khatib MF, Carlo WA: PEEP does not improve pulmonary mechanics in infants with bronchiolitis. Am Rev Respir Dis 1993; 147:1295.
27. MacDonald NE, Hall CB, Suffin SC, et al: Respiratory syncytial viral infection in infants with congenital heart disease. N Engl J Med 1982; 307:397.
28. Nobel B, Murray M, Webb MSC, et al: Respiratory status and allergy 9–10 years after acute bronchiolitis. Arch Dis Child 1997; 76:315.
29. Sheffer AL (Chair): Expert Panel Reports: Guidelines for the Diagnosis and Management of Asthma. US Dept of Health and Human Services, Public Health Service, Publication NIH 91-3042, 1991; Publication NIH 97-4051, 1997.
30. Larsen GL: Asthma in children. N Engl J Med 1992; 326:1540.
31. Yanos J, Wood LDH, Davis K, et al: The effect of respiratory and lactic acidosis on diaphragm function. Am Rev Respir Dis 1993; 147:616.
32. Weiss KB, Wagener DK: Changing patterns of asthma mortality: Identifying target populations at high risk. JAMA 1990; 264:1683.
33. McFadden ER, Gilbert IA: Asthma. N Engl J Med 1992; 327:1928.
34. Kravis L, Kolski GB: Unexpected death in childhood asthma: A review of 18 deaths in ambulatory patients. Am J Dis Child 1985; 139:558.
35. Strunk RC, Mrazek DA, Fuhrmann GSW, et al: Physiologic and psychological characteristics associated with deaths due to asthma in childhood. JAMA 1985; 254:1193.
36. Strunk RC: The fatality prone asthmatic child and adolescent. Pediatr Clin North Am 1998; 18:85.
37. Sur S, Crotty TB, Kephart GM, et al: Sudden-onset fatal asthma. Am Rev Respir Dis 1993; 148:713.
38. Heymann PW, Zambrano JC, Rakes GP: Virus-induced wheezing in children. Allergy Immunol Clin North Am 1998; 18:35.
39. Engstrom I: Respiratory studies in children: XI. Mechanics of breathing, lung volumes, and ventilator capacity in children from attack to symptom-free status. Acta Paediatr Suppl 1964; 155:1–60.
40. Downes JJ, Heiser MS: Status asthmaticus in children. *In*: Respiratory Failure in the Child. Gregory G (Ed). New York, Churchill Livingstone, 1981, pp 107–133.
41. van der Jagt EW: Contemporary issues in the emergency care of children with asthma. Allergy Immunol Clin North Am 1998; 18:211.
42. Schuh S, Parkin P, Rajan A: High versus low-dose, frequently administered, nebulized albuterol in children with severe acute asthma. Pediatrics 1989; 83:513.
43. Moler FW, Hurwitz ME, Custer JR: Improvement in clinical asthma score and Pa_{CO_2} in children with severe asthma treated with continuously nebulized terbutaline. J Allergy Clin Immunol 1988; 81:1101.
44. Reisman J, Goldes-Sebaldt M, Fazim F, et al: Frequent administration by inhalation of salbutamol and ipratropium bromide in the initial management of severe acute asthma in children. J Allergy Clin Immunol 1988; 81:16.
45. Qureshi F, Saritsky A, Lakkis H: Efficacy of nebulized ipratropium in severely asthmatic children. Ann Emerg Med 1997: 29:205.
46. Schuh S, Johnson DW, Callahan S, et al: Efficacy of frequent nebulized ipratropium bromide added to frequent high dose albuterol therapy in severe childhood asthma. J Pediatr 1995; 126:639.
47. Younger RE, Gerber PS, Herrod HG, et al: Intravenous methylprednisolone efficacy in status asthmaticus of childhood. Pediatrics 1987; 80:225.
48. Greos LS, Vichyanond P, Bloedow DC: Methylprednisolone achieves greater concentrations in the lung than prednisolone. Am Rev Respir Dis 1991; 144:586.
49. Bohn D, Kalloghlian A, Jenkins J: Intravenous salbutamol in the treatment of status asthmaticus in children. Crit Care Med 1984; 12:892.
50. Fuglsang G, Pedersen S, Borgstrom L: Dose-response relationships of intravenously administered terbutaline in children with asthma. J Pediatr 1989; 114:315.
51. Dietrich KA, Conrad SA, Romero MD; Creatinine kinase isoenzymes in pediatric status asthmaticus treated with intravenous terbutaline. Crit Care Med 1991; 19:S39.
52. Maguire JF, O'Rourke PP, Cohen SD, et al: Cardiotoxicity during treatment of severe childhood asthma. Pediatrics 1991; 88:1180.
53. Katz RW, Kelley HW, Crowley MR, et al: Safety of continuous nebulized albuterol for bronchospasm in infants and children. Pediatrics 1993; 92:666.
54. Darioli R, Perret C: Mechanical controlled hypoventilation in status asthmaticus. Am Rev Respir Dis 1984; 129:385.
55. Cox RG, Barker GA, Bohn DJ: Efficacy, results and complications of mechanical ventilation in children with status asthmaticus. Pediatr Pulmonol 1991; 11:120.
56. Newcomb RW, Akhter J: Respiratory failure from asthma: A marker for children with high morbidity and mortality. Am J Dis Child 1988; 142:1041.
57. Ruberstein S, Hindi R, Moss RB, et al: Sudden death in adolescent asthma. Ann Allergy 1984; 53:311.
58. Stein R, Canny GJ, Bohn DJ, et al: Severe acute asthma in a pediatric intensive care unit: Six years' experience. Pediatrics 1989, 83:1023.
59. Kudukis TM, Manthous CA, Schmidt GA, et al: Inhaled helium-oxygen revisited: Effect of inhaled helium-oxygen during treatment of status asthmaticus in children. J. Pediatr 1997; 130:217.
60. Gluck E, Onorato D, Castriotta R: Helium-oxygen mixtures in intubated patients with status asthmaticus and respiratory acidosis. Chest 1990; 98:693.
61. Ciarallo L, Sauer AH, Shannon MW: Intravenous magnesium therapy for moderate to severe asthma: Results of a randomized, placebo controlled trial. J Pediatr 1996; 129:809.

C. OTHER PULMONARY DISEASES

139

Pulmonary Embolism and Deep Venous Thrombosis

Peter F. Fedullo, MD

The subject of venous thromboembolism continues to engender vigorous debate despite extensive clinical and laboratory investigation into its pathogenesis, natural history, diagnosis, and treatment. The basis for this debate is clear. Venous thromboembolism represents a potentially fatal disease process with an often silent or clinically ambiguous presentation and for which a profusion of diagnostic techniques is available, most with technical and interpretive limitations. The consequence of these uncertainties is that venous thromboembolism remains a major health problem involving a wide range of medical disciplines. The best available information suggests that at least 5 million episodes of venous thrombosis occur annually in the United States, that at least 10% of these episodes lead to pulmonary embolism, and that at least 10% of those who suffer embolism—or 50,000—die each year.[1, 2] Furthermore, the incidence of venous thromboembolism and of fatal pulmonary embolism does not appear to be decreasing, a finding that probably reflects the fact that modern medicine has placed an increased population at risk for the disease and that preventive measures are not being applied to this population in an appropriate manner.

Since the late 1980s, many of the long-standing controversies surrounding the natural history, diagnosis, and treatment of venous thromboembolism have been partially or completely resolved. The persistence of a number of unresolved issues, therefore, should not be a cause for clinical cynicism. In the approach to the patient with suspected venous thromboembolism, especially one in the critical care setting, knowing what is unknown can prove invaluable to the clinical decision-making process.

PATHOGENESIS

The triad of venous stasis, alterations in coagulation, and vascular injury identified by Virchow in 1845 as risk factors for venous thromboembolism has been supported by a considerable amount of experimental evidence. The causative factors that shift the hemostatic balance toward thrombosis remained undefined in the majority of patients with venous thromboembolism. Inherited and acquired abnormalities of the coagulation and fibrinolytic systems, including isolated deficiencies of antithrombin III, protein C, protein S, and plasminogen as well as the presence of a lupus anticoagulant, had been implicated as causes of venous thrombosis.[3] However, most patients with venous thromboembolism had no identifiable coagulopathy. In a study of 227 outpatients with venous thrombosis, deficiencies of antithrombin III, protein C, and protein S were the most commonly identified disorders of the coagulation system and accounted for only 8% of the patients.[4]

In 1993, Dahlback and coworkers[5] described an inherited resistance to activated protein C. The defect responsible for this resistance, designated *factor V Leiden mutation*, was localized to a single point mutation on the factor V gene resulting in factor Va with diminished sensitivity to activated protein C. Although it was initially detected in as many as 60% of *selected* patients with venous thromboembolism, subsequent studies have detected the mutation in 10% to 20% of unselected patients.[6–8] For women suffering a thromboembolic event during pregnancy or during the postpartum period, as many as 60% are resistant to activated protein C.[9] Activated protein C resistance is also found in about one third of patients in whom venous thromboembolism develops while they are taking oral contraceptives.[9] Approximately 5% of Caucasians are carriers of the factor V Leiden mutation; the mutation appears significantly less prevalent among African and Asian populations.[10]

Hyperhomocysteinemia has also been identified as a predisposition to venous thromboembolism. Elevation of plasma homocysteine levels may be the result of genetic abnormalities, nutritional deficiencies of vitamins (B_6, B_{12}, folate), or a combination of the two. A number of studies have strongly suggested that hyperhomocysteinemia may contribute independently to the pathogenesis of venous thrombosis and that it may act synergistically with other inherited predisposing factors.[11, 12]

More recently, a sequence variation in the prothrombin gene (20210 G $\rightarrow$ A), estimated to occur in 1% to 2% of the population, appears to result in higher plasma prothrombin levels as well as in a threefold to fourfold increased risk of venous thrombosis.[13]

The identification of these inherited risk factors, with the likelihood that others exist, raises the possibility that screening for relative thromboembolic risk may be feasible in the future. However, despite these recent insights into the pathogenesis of venous thromboembolism, such an approach does not exist at present. The majority of patients at risk for venous thromboembolism do not have an identifiable inherited predisposition. Thus, in most patients, clinicians must rely on the understanding that certain clinical states resulting in venous stasis or intimal injury serve as the basis for an increased risk of venous thrombosis and pulmonary embolism. Investigators have identified these clinical states, identified in Table 139-1.[14, 15]

Because of the homogeneity of the populations studied, relative thromboembolic risk has been well defined in surgical populations. For example, it is known that approximately 50% of patients undergoing elective hip replacement and up to 70% of patients undergoing knee replacement have venous thromboembolism. In patients with multiple trauma, the incidence of venous thromboembolism approaches 50%. Relative thromboembolic risk in medical populations has been less clearly characterized. However, these risk factors are cumulative; that is, risk appears to increase in direct proportion to the number of predisposing factors present.

Data regarding the prevalence of venous thromboembolism in the intensive care setting are sparse. Hirsch and colleagues[16] reported a 33% incidence of venous thrombosis in a group of medical intensive care unit (ICU) patients despite the fact that 61% of these patients had received prophylaxis. More recently, Marik and coworkers[17] reported a 12% incidence of venous thrombosis in a cohort of 102 medical and surgical ICU patients, 92% of whom had received prophylaxis. That ICU patients are at risk for venous thromboembolism is not surprising. The diverse population of patients encountered in a critical care setting often includes those at prolonged bed rest, the elderly, patients who have experienced a traumatic injury or undergone a surgical procedure, and those with underlying cardiac disease or a malignant neoplasm.

These risk factors should be regarded as cumulative, not independent. For example, thromboembolic risk in an other-

TABLE 139–1. Thromboembolic Risk Factors

Hereditary Thrombophilias
Protein C deficiency
Protein S deficiency
Antithrombin III deficiency
Factor V Leiden mutation
Prothrombin 20210 G → A variation
Hyperhomocysteinemia
Acquired Medical Predispositions
Prior venous thromboembolism
Age >40 yr
Malignant neoplasia
Congestive heart failure
Cerebrovascular accident
Nephrotic syndrome
Estrogen therapy
Pregnancy and the postpartum period
Obesity
Prolonged immobilization
Antiphospholipid antibody syndrome
Lupus anticoagulant
Inflammatory bowel disease
Acquired Surgical Predispositions
Major thoracic or abdominal surgery requiring general anesthesia and lasting >30 min
Hip arthroplasty
Knee arthroplasty
Knee arthroscopy
Hip fracture
Major trauma
Open prostatectomy
Spinal cord injury
Neurosurgical procedures

wise healthy 45-year-old individual undergoing an elective cholecystectomy is entirely different from the risk experienced by an obese 75-year-old individual with an underlying malignant neoplasm and pelvic fracture. These considerations allow establishment of a reasonable "risk profile" in an individual patient, a profile that should influence the intensity of prophylactic initiatives.

NATURAL HISTORY AND PATHOPHYSIOLOGY

The recognition of venous thrombosis and pulmonary embolism as manifestations of a common disease entity represented a major conceptual advance in our understanding of the natural history of venous thromboembolism. Although the majority of thrombi form at the site of venous valves in the veins of the calf, the majority of pulmonary emboli arise from venous thrombi that extend into the proximal veins (popliteal and iliofemoral systems) of the lower extremities. Once a thrombus has formed, several scenarios may ensue. Thrombus behavior is a dynamic one, with extension, dissolution, and organization dependent on factors such as local blood flow and the levels of thrombogenic and fibrinolytic activity. In most patients (80%), calf thrombi resolve spontaneously, either without sequelae or with residual damage to the venous wall and valve. Approximately 20% of calf thrombi, however, extend proximally into the popliteal vein and the iliofemoral system.[18]

Available information indicates that the likelihood of embolism is strongly influenced by the location of thrombi in the veins of the lower extremity. Thrombi that remain confined to the calf appear to pose little risk of pulmonary embolism; thrombi that extend into the thigh pose a risk of embolization that approaches 50%.[19] Whatever the basis for this occurrence, many have incorrectly concluded from this information that calf-limited deep venous thrombosis represents a clinically unimportant condition. Beyond concerns related to the potential for proximal extension and embolization, preliminary data suggest that untreated calf vein thrombosis may result in a higher risk of future recurrence and in a less favorable symptomatic outcome than for those that are treated.[20, 21]

Venous thrombi capable of embolization can arise from other sites. Primary iliac or proximal femoral thrombi may develop in patients undergoing surgery involving the hip or pelvis (gynecologic or prostatic surgery). Axillosubclavian vein thrombosis may be spontaneous, resulting from congenital abnormalities of the thoracic outlet, or may be related to indwelling central venous catheters, pulmonary artery catheters, or temporary transvenous pacing wires.[22] Finally, in patients with dilated right-sided heart chambers or pulmonary arteries, thrombi can form at those sites and embolize distally into the branches of the pulmonary artery.

A series of hemodynamic and pulmonary consequences are induced once pulmonary embolism has occurred.[23, 24] The hemodynamic response to acute pulmonary embolism is a function of the degree of pulmonary vascular obstruction as well as the preexisting status of the cardiopulmonary system. Obstruction of the pulmonary vascular bed by embolism acutely increases right ventricular afterload. In patients without preexisting cardiopulmonary disease, obstruction of less than 20% of the pulmonary vascular bed results in a number of compensatory events that minimize adverse hemodynamic consequences. Recruitment and distention of pulmonary vessels occur, resulting in a normal or near-normal pulmonary artery pressure and pulmonary vascular resistance; cardiac output is maintained by increases in the right ventricular stroke volume and increases in the heart rate.

As the degree of pulmonary vascular obstruction exceeds 30% to 40%, increases in pulmonary artery pressure occur and are followed by modest increases in right atrial pressure; the Frank-Starling mechanism maintains right ventricular stroke work and cardiac output. When the degree of pulmonary artery obstruction exceeds 50% to 60%, compensatory mechanisms are overcome, cardiac output begins to fall, and right atrial pressure increases dramatically.

In patients without prior cardiopulmonary disease, a pulmonary artery mean pressure of 30 to 40 mm Hg (pulmonary artery systolic pressure of 50 to 60 mm Hg) represents severe pulmonary hypertension. With obstruction beyond 60% of the pulmonary vascular bed, the right side of the heart dilates, cardiac output falls, and hypotension develops.

The hemodynamic response to acute pulmonary embolism in patients with preexisting cardiopulmonary disease is considerably different.[23] In contrast to patients without prior cardiopulmonary disease, in whom there is a general relationship between the degree of pulmonary artery obstruction and the level of the pulmonary artery pressure, patients with prior cardiopulmonary disease demonstrate degrees of pulmonary hypertension that are disproportionate to the degree of embolic obstruction. As a result, severe pulmonary hypertension may develop in response to a relatively smaller reduction in pulmonary artery cross-sectional area. In certain patients, this may have devastating consequences; in others, the preexisting right ventricular hypertrophy may actually help prevent acute right ventricular decompensation. Thus, evidence of right ventricular hypertrophy (rather than right ventricular dilatation) associated with an estimated pulmonary artery systolic pressure in excess of 60 mm Hg in a patient with suspected embolism should suggest an element of chronic pulmonary hypertension resulting from a diverse group of etiologic possibilities (e.g., chronic thromboembolic pulmonary hypertension, valvular disease, right-to-left cardiac shunts).

The pulmonary consequences of embolism result from direct obstruction of pulmonary arterial blood flow as well as the effect of mediators released from the thrombus itself.[25] Vascular obstruction may result in increased dead space ventilation as well as in ventilation-perfusion ratio imbalance. In embolism of sufficient magnitude to lower cardiac output, a decrease in mixed venous oxygen content magnifies the effects of the normal physiologic shunt. Finally, atelectasis, perhaps related to surfactant loss, may occur. Hypoxemia due to intrapulmonary shunting may result if the pulmonary artery obstruction is incomplete or if reperfusion to the area occurs after spontaneous thrombolysis or distal migration of the thrombus.

CLINICAL PRESENTATION

The most common symptoms and physical findings of venous thrombosis include swelling, pain, erythema, and warmth. "Classic" findings, such as Homans' sign (calf pain with flexion of the knee and dorsiflexion of the ankle), Moses' sign (pain with calf compression against the tibia), and a palpable cord, occur infrequently and are nonspecific.

Multiple investigations have established that the clinical diagnosis of venous thrombosis is imprecise.[18, 26] In patients with clinical signs and symptoms suggestive of venous thrombosis, usually the diagnosis is not confirmed by venography. Although specific clinical findings can predict the presence of proximal vein thrombosis in *symptomatic* patients, most lower-extremity venous thromboses are not apparent clinically.[27]

Some investigations have also demonstrated that the diagnosis of pulmonary embolism cannot be confirmed or excluded on clinical grounds.[19, 28-31] There has been a growing awareness that the clinical presentation of pulmonary embolism may often be atypical and that embolic events can occur with minimal clinical effect. These difficulties are only accentuated in the critical care setting, in which the often subtle clinical manifestations of embolism may be obscured by elements of the patient's underlying illness.

The most comprehensive analysis of the presenting clinical findings in symptomatic patients with angiographically documented pulmonary embolism was provided by the Prospective Investigation of Pulmonary Embolism Diagnosis (PIOPED) trial.[30] In this trial, the clinical probability of embolism, based on history, physical examination, chest radiography, arterial blood gas analysis, and electrocardiographic findings, was estimated by the investigators before a ventilation-perfusion scan and pulmonary angiogram were performed. Among 90 patients in whom the clinical probability of embolism was estimated to be 80% or greater, 32% did not have angiographic evidence of pulmonary emboli. Among the 228 patients in whom the clinical probability of pulmonary embolism was considered to be 19% or less, 9% had positive angiographic findings. The majority of patients (64%) entered in the trial fell into a clinically indeterminate group in whom the incidence of angiographically confirmed embolism was 30%. Viewed from a different perspective, of the 251 patients with pulmonary embolism documented by angiography, only 24% fell into the "high clinical probability" category; and of the 635 patients with pulmonary embolism excluded by angiography, only 36% fell into the "low clinical probability" category.

These precautionary statements regarding clinical diagnosis are not meant to suggest that the presentation of clinical embolism cannot be used as a basis for clinical decision making; rather, they are meant as a reminder that the clinical presentation of pulmonary embolism, instead of being a dramatic event as commonly perceived, may often be atypical or subtle and should serve only to generate a suspicion of that diagnosis. A reliance on signs and symptoms that are considered to be classic before the decision is made to proceed to confirmatory testing will ultimately lead to underdiagnosis and unnecessary mortality.

Despite the nonspecific nature of these signs and symptoms, a review is worthwhile because clinical findings represent an essential first step in the diagnostic pathway. The presentation of pulmonary embolism can be categorized into one of three clinical syndromes[30, 32]:

1. Isolated dyspnea.
2. Pleuritic pain or hemoptysis.
3. Circulatory collapse.

In the PIOPED study, and among patients *without* preexisting cardiopulmonary disease, the syndrome of hemoptysis or pleuritic pain was the most common mode of presentation, occurring in 65% of patients; isolated dyspnea occurred in 22% and circulatory collapse in 8%.

In terms of individual symptoms, dyspnea occurred in 73% of patients, pleuritic chest pain in 66%, cough in 37%, lower-extremity edema in 28%, and hemoptysis in 13%.

In terms of individual signs, tachypnea (respiratory rate, ≥20/min) occurred in 70% of patients, rales in 51%, tachycardia in 30%, a fourth heart sound in 24%, and an increased pulmonic component of the second heart sound in 23%.

Clinically apparent venous thrombosis was present in only 11% of patients. Pulmonary embolism was rarely silent in patients without underlying cardiopulmonary disease. Dyspnea, or tachypnea, or pleuritic chest pain was present in 97% of patients; dyspnea, or tachypnea, or signs of venous thrombosis were present in 91%.

In this study, however, none of the presenting symptoms was capable of discriminating between those with positive angiograms and those with negative angiograms.[32] In terms of presenting signs, only the presence of rales, a fourth heart sound, and an increased pulmonic component of the second heart sound could differentiate between those with positive and negative angiograms. Furthermore, in patients *with* underlying cardiopulmonary disease—patients commonly encountered in an intensive care setting—the presenting symptoms and signs are frequently masked by elements of the patient's underlying illness.

Goldhaber and coworkers,[28] in a review of 1455 autopsy reports at their institution, demonstrated that none of 22 patients with pneumonia and only two of 18 patients with congestive heart failure had the diagnosis of pulmonary embolism made before death.

Therefore, in the intensive care setting, even subtle manifestations of embolism should raise clinical suspicion.[33] These include:

1. Worsening hypoxemia or *hypocapnia* in a spontaneously ventilating patient.
2. Worsening hypoxemia and *hypercapnia* in a sedated patient on controlled mechanical ventilation.
3. Worsening dyspnea, hypoxemia, and a reduction in arterial P_{CO_2} in a patient with chronic lung disease and known carbon dioxide retention.
4. Unexplained fever.
5. Sudden elevation in pulmonary artery pressure or central venous pressure in a hemodynamically monitored patient.

Owing to its nonspecific presentation, the differential diagnosis of pulmonary embolism is varied and extensive, especially in hospitalized patients with underlying cardiac or pulmonary disease. Common considerations include congestive heart failure, exacerbation of chronic lung disease, and viral pleurisy. Emboli presenting with fever, dyspnea, and chest radiographic abnormalities can easily be confused with a bacterial pneumonia. Fever is a not uncommon accompaniment of pulmonary embolism. Murray and coworkers,[34] in a review of 35 consecutive patients undergoing pulmonary angiography for suspected pulmonary embolism, found that 20 patients had fever (rectal temperature, ≥38°C) attributed solely to pulmonary embolism and that in five of these patients the peak temperature was 39°C or above.

These findings confirm that the diagnosis of pulmonary embolism based on clinical presentation is highly inaccurate and lacks specificity and that individual signs and symptoms lack sensitivity. Most physicians would have little difficulty in considering the diagnosis of pulmonary embolism in a patient presenting with the acute onset of dyspnea, pleuritic chest pain, and hemoptysis. Unfortunately, such a classic clinical presentation is rare, especially in an intensive care setting.

DIAGNOSTIC OPTIONS

Once the possibility of pulmonary embolism has been raised, confirmatory testing must be performed. Before definitive testing, a series of routine studies are usually performed. Although none has the discriminatory power to confirm the diagnosis of embolism, they do provide valuable adjunctive information, provide support for therapeutic interventions, and may confirm the presence of an alternative diagnosis.

Chest Radiography

The diverse chest radiographic findings in pulmonary embolism have been well described.[35, 36] Although the majority of patients with pulmonary embolism have abnormal chest radiographs, these abnormalities are nonspecific and therefore nondiagnostic. Among 117 patients in PIOPED without preexisting cardiac or pulmonary disease, 84% had abnormal chest radiograph results. The most common radiographic abnormalities were atelectasis and pulmonary infiltrates (68%). Although pleural effusion occurred in 48% of patients, the majority of effusions were small and involved only blunting of the costophrenic angle.[32] Findings once considered specific for embolism, such as Westermark's sign (focal areas of avascularity) and Hampton's hump (pleura-based, wedge-shaped density), have not proved to have discriminatory value.[35, 36]

A normal chest radiograph may be useful in raising the index of suspicion of pulmonary embolism in a patient with unexplained dyspnea or hypoxemia. Furthermore, the presence of cardiomegaly or prominent central pulmonary arteries on plain chest radiographs of a patient with pulmonary embolism and no prior cardiopulmonary disease suggests a higher mean pulmonary pressure and perhaps more extensive embolization than when these findings are not present.[37] The major role of chest radiography in suspected pulmonary embolism, therefore, is to exclude competing diagnoses, such as pneumothorax or rib fracture, and to evaluate the pulmonary parenchyma, essential for accurate interpretation of the ventilation-perfusion scan.

Arterial Blood Gas Analysis

Hypoxemia and a widened (A − a) Pa_{O_2} gradient are commonly considered sensitive indicators in acute pulmonary embolism. More recent reports, however, have revealed that neither has absolute diagnostic discriminant value.[38] In a subset of patients from PIOPED in whom arterial blood gas measurements were obtained while they were breathing room air, 38% of patients without prior cardiopulmonary disease, and 14% of patients with prior cardiopulmonary disease, had normal Pa_{O_2} (≥80 mm Hg), normal $P(A - a)O_2$ gradient, and normal Pa_{CO_2} (≥35 mm Hg). However, the majority of patients entered into the study had blood gas measurements obtained while they were receiving supplemental oxygen, presumably as a therapeutic intervention for hypoxemia.

Arterial blood gas analysis, therefore, has a limited role in embolism diagnosis. A normal Pa_{O_2}, although unusual, cannot absolutely exclude the diagnosis; an abnormal Pa_{O_2} is nonspecific and consistent with a variety of disease processes. Arterial blood gas analysis, of course, does have important therapeutic implications and may provide insight into the extent of thromboembolic obstruction.

Electrocardiography

Electrocardiographic abnormalities in pulmonary embolism, although they occur frequently, are diverse and nonspecific.[39, 40] The most common abnormalities are T-wave inversion and nonspecific abnormalities of the ST segment. Rhythm disturbances are uncommon and are usually confined to patients with underlying cardiac disease. Classic findings, such as $S_1Q_3T_3$, pseudoinfarction pattern, right bundle branch block, and right-axis deviation, are uncommon and usually signify massive embolism.

Echocardiography

Echocardiography may serve a valuable role in the diagnostic approach to pulmonary embolism in patients in an intensive care setting. Under appropriate clinical circumstances, the detection of right ventricular dilatation by transthoracic echocardiography, although a nonspecific finding, should suggest the possibility of embolism and lead to confirmatory testing.[41]

Of greater clinical importance, properly performed transesophageal echocardiography has demonstrated sensitivity and specificity exceeding 90% in the detection of pulmonary emboli involving the pulmonary trunk and the right and left main pulmonary arteries in patients with massive embolism.[42] Furthermore, transesophageal echocardiography has also proved valuable in the evaluation of competing diagnostic possibilities, such as right ventricular infarction, endocarditis, pericardial tamponade, and aortic dissection in patients with unexplained shock and clinical evidence of elevated central venous pressure.[43] Strong consideration, therefore, can be given to the use of transesophageal echocardiography as the initial diagnostic study in that subset of patients with suspected massive pulmonary embolism who are too ill for transportation out of the ICU, are too unstable to undergo angiography, or have an absolute or relative contraindication to the administration of a contrast agent (dye allergy, volume overload, renal insufficiency).[44] Transesophageal echocardiography is incapable of detecting emboli distal to the main pulmonary arteries. A negative study result, therefore, cannot exclude the possibility of embolism.

Hemostaseologic Assays

The development of a rapid and accurate blood test capable of confirming the diagnosis of venous thromboembolism has been the focus of considerable investigative interest. The measurement of circulating plasma cross-linked fibrin degradation products (D-dimers), alone or in combination with noninvasive lower-extremity evaluation, ventilation-perfusion scanning, or clinical probability estimates, has demonstrated the most promise.[45, 46] Unfortunately, at present, two critical deterrents limit its diagnostic use, especially in an intensive care population[47]:

1. Problems have been encountered in the development of a rapid, reproducible standardized assay.

2. A wide range of clinical conditions encountered in an intensive care setting can result in accelerated fibrinolysis and elevated D-dimer levels, severely limiting the specificity of the study.

Spiral Computed Tomography

The role of spiral computed tomography (CT) in the evaluation of pulmonary embolism remains undefined although it does demonstrate promise. Several studies have demonstrated that CT scanning is capable of visualizing central emboli (main, lobar, and segmental pulmonary arteries) with a sensitivity exceeding 85%.[48, 49] However, sensitivity appears to decline markedly when emboli are confined to the subsegmental arteries.[50] This limitation might be acceptable if emboli limited to the subsegmental arteries were rare. However, several studies have revealed that subsegmental-only emboli account for approximately 30% of all cases.[50, 51]

Given that CT scanning requires transportation of the patient and a volume of contrast agent equivalent to that administered for a pulmonary angiogram, it is my belief, based on current evidence, that CT scanning should not serve as an alternative to either ventilation-perfusion scanning or pulmonary angiography in the evaluation of the patient with suspected embolism. Of course, this recommendation may change as additional data are accumulated regarding the sensitivity and specificity of CT scanning using an angiographic "gold standard" for validation.

Lower-Extremity Evaluation

Lower-extremity venous testing can play a valuable role in the evaluation of a patient with suspected pulmonary embolism. The detection of acute, lower-extremity proximal vein thrombosis has the same therapeutic implications as does embolism per se and can be used as a basis for management. Both impedance plethysmography and duplex ultrasonography have been demonstrated to be sensitive in the detection of *symptomatic* proximal lower-extremity venous thrombosis.[52, 53] Both duplex ultrasonography and impedance plethysmography, however, lack sensitivity in the detection of calf-limited thrombi.

Impedance plethysmography, an indirect technique that measures the rate of venous outflow, is incapable of distinguishing between thrombotic and nonthrombotic causes of venous outflow obstruction. False-positive results can be caused by conditions that diminish arterial inflow (congestive heart failure, shock) or that impede venous return (right ventricular failure, obstructive lung disease, high levels of positive end-expiratory pressure)—conditions frequently encountered in an intensive care setting. Duplex ultrasonography is capable of providing anatomic visualization as well as venous flow characteristics.

A number of criteria are used for the diagnosis of acute venous thrombosis, including:

1. Noncompressibility of the vein.
2. Presence of echogenic material within the vein lumen.
3. Venous distention.
4. Loss of phasicity and augmentation of spontaneous flow.

Of these, noncompressibility appears to be the most accurate diagnostic finding, although it is incapable of differentiating acute from chronic thrombi. Recent data also suggest that most symptomatic lower-extremity venous thrombi can be detected by a simplified approach that involves compression over the common femoral and popliteal veins alone.[54, 55]

Initial enthusiasm for the study has been tempered by the recognition that duplex ultrasonography, although highly sensitive in patients with symptomatic venous thrombosis, has a considerably lower sensitivity (30% to 60%) in the detection of *asymptomatic* venous thrombosis.[56, 57] The basis for this is uncertain, although it is probably attributable to the fact that venous thrombi in asymptomatic patients tend to be smaller, less organized and hence less echogenic, and nonocclusive. However, given that both impedance plethysmography and duplex ultrasonography are simple, noninvasive studies that can be performed at the bedside, they still play a valuable role in a diagnostic strategy for embolism diagnosis.

Ideally, impedance plethysmography and duplex ultrasonography should serve complementary rather than competitive roles. Impedance plethysmography, as a low-cost, portable, accurate, and technically uncomplicated study, can serve as a rapid screening test. When positive results are encountered in a clinical situation that may cause a false-positive finding, duplex ultrasonography can be used for confirmation.

Contrast venography remains the diagnostic gold standard for venous thrombosis. The study, however, is not without shortcomings. Venous cannulation may often be difficult, especially in the presence of edema; expert interpretation is essential for accurate diagnosis; transportation of the patient is required; injection of contrast material is necessary; and venous thrombosis may be induced as a result of the study. With the exception of investigative contexts, therefore, contrast venography has played a diminished role in venous thrombosis diagnosis.[58]

Ventilation-Perfusion Scanning

Ventilation-perfusion scanning is an essential diagnostic study that continues to play a pivotal role in patients with suspected pulmonary embolism.[30] The PIOPED study provided two reassuring pieces of information:

1. A "high-probability" scan was associated with embolism in 87% of cases; coupled with a high clinical probability of embolism, the positive predictive value increased to 96%.
2. A normal scan essentially excluded the possibility of embolism.

However, the PIOPED data also provided several pieces of information that were disquieting:

1. The overwhelming majority of patients with suspected embolism did not have scan findings that fell into either a high-probability or normal category.
2. The majority of patients with embolism did *not* have a high-probability scan.
3. Most patients without embolism did *not* have a normal scan.
4. A clinically significant percentage of patients with scan findings interpreted as intermediate-probability (33%) and low-probability (16%) were subsequently demonstrated to have embolism confirmed at the time of pulmonary angiography.

An additional confounding issue is that the PIOPED and other interpretive schemes are based, at least in part, on ventilation scan findings (matched versus mismatched defects).[59] Unfortunately, unless a sophisticated exhaust venting system is available, a ventilation scan cannot be performed in an intubated, mechanically ventilated patient. In those patients who are not being mechanically ventilated, many are too dyspneic to tolerate the closed ventilation system required for the study.

These cautionary statements are not meant to imply that ventilation-perfusion scanning, or perfusion scanning alone, cannot be used in an intensive care setting.[60–62] In a study of 223 critically ill patients, 46 of whom were receiving mechanical ventilatory support, Henry and coworkers[60] determined that lung scans and clinical assessment retained their diagnostic utility and were as accurate as those obtained in noncritically ill hospitalized patients.

Further supporting a strategy of perfusion scanning alone were the results of the Prospective Investigative Study of Acute Pulmonary Embolism Diagnosis (PISA-PED), in which the interpretive criteria for embolism were based solely on the presence of wedge-shaped perfusion defects, regardless of their size, number, or association with ventilation abnormalities.[61] In this study, scans were interpreted as normal, near-normal, abnormal compatible with pulmonary embolism (PE+), and abnormal not compatible with pulmonary embolism (PE−). The sensitivity of an abnormal PE+ scan was 92%, whereas the specificity of an abnormal PE− scan was 87%. The results of this study may be limited by selection bias, however, in that patients with normal or near-normal scans did not undergo angiography, and 38% of patients with an abnormal scan did not undergo angiography for a variety of reasons.

The diagnostic approach to pulmonary embolism in patients with underlying chronic obstructive pulmonary disease (COPD), a population commonly encountered in an intensive care setting, especially remains a problem because the presentation of pulmonary embolism in this population may closely mimic an exacerbation of their underlying disease.[63] Unfortunately, the value of ventilation-perfusion scanning in these patients is even more limited than that in the general population. Lesser and coworkers,[64] in a study of 108 patients with COPD and suspected embolism, found that 60% of the ventilation-perfusion scans fell into an intermediate-probability category and that 91% fell into an intermediate-probability or low-probability category—interpretations that are considered indeterminate. However, among those few patients who had a high-probability scan or normal/near-normal scan findings, both the positive predictive value (100%) and negative predictive value (100%) were equivalent to those values in the general population.

Considerable controversy will likely continue to be generated regarding the optimal ventilation-perfusion scan interpretive scheme in patients with suspected embolism. Whatever interpretive scheme is used, ventilation-perfusion scanning can provide only three clinically useful pieces of information:

1. A normal scan essentially excludes the diagnosis of embolism.
2. A high-probability scan (multiple, mismatched segmental defects or multiple wedge-shaped defects), especially combined with a high clinical suspicion of embolism, can confirm the diagnosis under most circumstances (Fig. 139–1).
3. Scan findings interpreted to be of low or intermediate probability should be considered nondiagnostic and without sufficient power to warrant making clinical decisions.

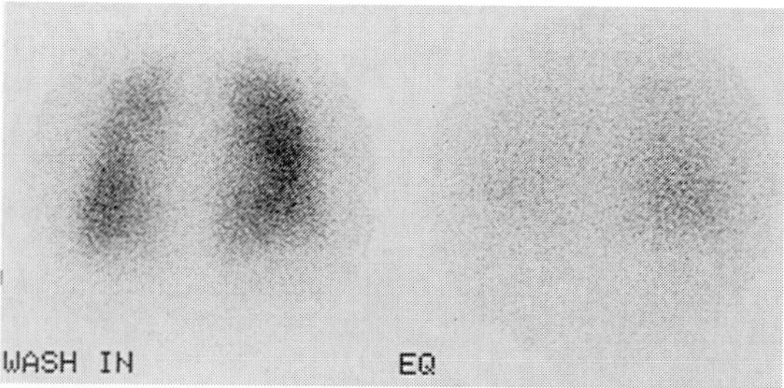

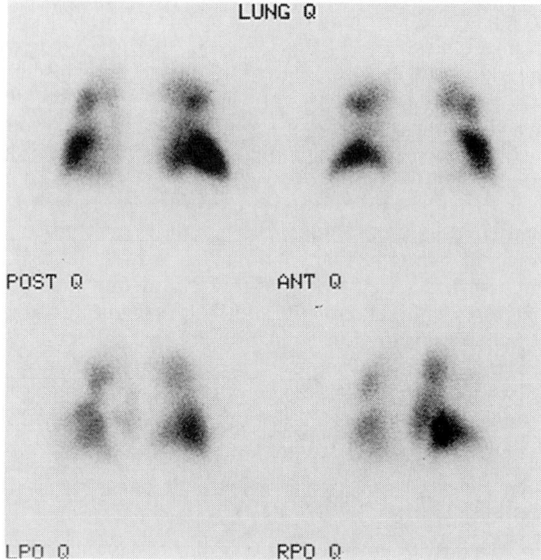

Figure 139–1. "High-probability" ventilation/perfusion scan demonstrating normal ventilation in the setting of multiple perfusion (mismatched) defects.

Pulmonary Angiography

Pulmonary angiography remains the diagnostic gold standard for pulmonary embolism (Fig. 139–2). A number of shortcomings, however, limit its use. It is expensive and invasive and entails certain risks. Furthermore, angiographic interpretation relies heavily on image quality and the observer's experience. Despite these shortcomings, current information would suggest that pulmonary angiography is substantially underused as a diagnostic tool because of the *perception* of potential risk associated with the procedure, a perception that far outweighs the actual risk.

In a review of 1111 angiographic studies performed during the PIOPED study, death occurred in five patients (0.5%); major, nonfatal complications occurred in an additional nine (0.8%).[65] Complications were not related to age, sex, the presence or absence of embolism, the level of the pulmonary artery mean pressure, or the volume of contrast material injected. The majority of patients who suffered fatal or major nonfatal complications were in critical condition with severely compromised cardiopulmonary function before the procedure.

As noted by Moser,[66] it is an odd commentary that few would advise against performance of a coronary angiogram in a patient with suspected coronary ischemia because of risk, yet the question of risk often deters pulmonary angiography in a patient with suspected embolism.

DIAGNOSTIC APPROACH

As outlined before, an almost bewildering array of diagnostic possibilities are available for patients with suspected pulmonary embolism. Diagnostic uncertainty is often accentuated in the critical care setting where the complexity of safe transportation often becomes a major determining factor in the diagnostic approach. Subsequently, management decisions are often based on incomplete clinical data and the assumed risk-benefit ratio of instituting (or withholding) anticoagulant therapy. Within the limits of clinical prudence, every attempt should be made to confirm or exclude the diagnosis of embolism. Withholding anticoagulants in a patient who has suffered an embolic event places that patient at risk for recurrent, potentially lethal events; instituting empirical anticoagulant therapy in a patient who has not suffered an embolic event

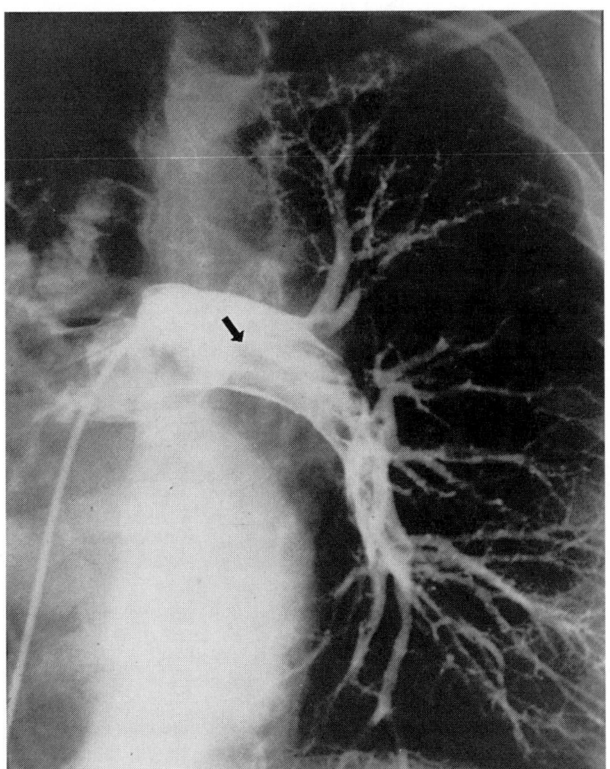

Figure 139–2. Pulmonary angiogram demonstrating extensive filling defect *(arrow)* in left main pulmonary artery and extending into upper and lower lobes.

places that patient at unnecessary risk for hemorrhagic complications.

What the clinician at the bedside must understand and accept is that a stepwise diagnostic strategy, rather than any single diagnostic technique, may be necessary to confirm or exclude the diagnosis of embolism. For certain patients in a critical care setting, attempts to confirm or exclude the diagnosis may be so fraught with risk that the only clinically feasible option, based on existing data and an informed estimate of risk-benefit, is to institute empirical therapy or to pursue a strategy of surveillance intended to prevent recurrent episodes.

Despite its limitations, ventilation-perfusion scanning, or perfusion scanning alone, should be the initial diagnostic study in patients with suspected embolism (Fig. 139–3). As noted previously, a normal perfusion scan is capable of excluding the diagnosis of embolism. A high-probability scan, in my view, can be used as a basis for therapy with the exception of three circumstances:

1. When a substantial discrepancy exists between the scan finding and the clinical impression of embolism.
2. When the institution of anticoagulant therapy in an individual patient is associated with prohibitive risk.
3. When there is a history of prior embolism and no baseline perfusion scan for comparison.

In these three groups of patients with high-probability scan findings, as well as in those with indeterminate lung scan findings (low and intermediate probability), lower-extremity venous testing should be performed. The detection of acute, lower-extremity proximal vein thrombosis, although not confirming that embolism has occurred, has the same therapeutic implications. Unfortunately, a *single*, negative lower-extremity test result is not as useful. Therefore, pulmonary angiography should be considered in any patient, especially one with preexisting cardiopulmonary compromise, with an indeterminate lung scan finding and negative lower-extremity findings. If transportation of the patient poses a significant logistical problem, transesophageal echocardiography may obviate the need for angiography by confirming the diagnosis of embolism or providing an alternative explanation for the patient's presentation.

Another potential option exists for patients with adequate cardiopulmonary reserve, indeterminate lung scan findings, and negative lower-extremity examination findings in whom pulmonary angiography cannot be safely performed. In a study of 711 patients with suspected pulmonary embolism, adequate cardiopulmonary reserve, and nondiagnostic lung scan findings, Hull and coworkers[67] demonstrated that a strategy of serial noninvasive leg studies provided a practical alternative to pulmonary angiography. In these patients, anticoagulation was withheld and noninvasive lower-extremity testing was performed at the time of presentation, on the day after presentation, and on days 3, 4, 7, 10, and 14. In those patients with nondiagnostic lung scans, 68 (9.6%) had proximal vein thrombosis at entry and were treated; in 16 additional patients (2.2%), proximal vein thrombosis was detected during serial follow-up. Of the 627 patients whose serial noninvasive study results remained negative, 12 patients returned 2 to 12 weeks later with objectively confirmed thromboembolism. Only one patient died of embolism 4 weeks later after a hemicolectomy for carcinoma.

The outcome of such a strategy in patients with underlying cardiopulmonary disease may be considerably different, and this approach may pose significant risk. This strategy does not confirm that embolism has not occurred, only that recurrence is unlikely. After their initial publication, Hull and coworkers[68] described the outcome of 77 consecutive patients with suspected embolism, low-probability lung scans, and inadequate cardiopulmonary reserve. In this cohort of patients, six patients died within days with autopsy-proven emboli; another three patients suffered nonfatal venous thromboembolic events. This study confirms the potentially lethal risk of embolism in patients with underlying cardiopulmonary disease and supports the need to repudiate a low-probability scan interpretation as one that excludes the likelihood of embolism or that is invariably associated with a favorable outcome.[69]

THERAPY

Heparin

Heparin remains the mainstay of therapy for pulmonary embolism not associated with hemodynamic compromise. With a strong suspicion of embolism based on clinical findings and laboratory tests, heparin therapy should be instituted immediately, without awaiting diagnostic confirmation, unless anticoagulation places the patient at significant risk. Although heparin can be administered by way of intermittent intravenous injection or subcutaneous injection, the optimal heparin regimen consists of a continuous intravenous administration of a dose that maintains the partial thromboplastin time between 1.5 and 2.5 times the control value.[70] This recommendation confirms earlier impressions that heparin's efficacy is related to its anticoagulant effect, as reflected by the activated partial thromboplastin time (aPTT), rather than to the absolute dose administered or to its route of administration.[71]

Some data suggest that physician practices in the administration of heparin often result in levels of anticoagulation that fall below those currently recommended in the literature. Wheeler and coworkers,[72] in a review of 65 patients with

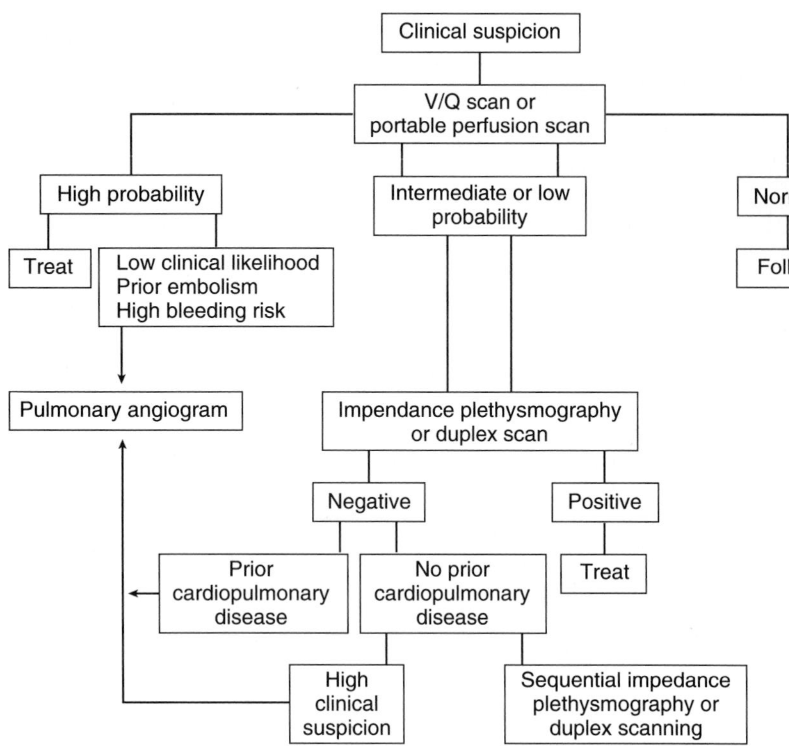

Figure 139–3. A suggested diagnostic algorithm for patients with suspected acute pulmonary embolism.

venous thromboembolism, demonstrated that only 40% of all aPTTs obtained in the first 24 hours fell within a therapeutic range and that it required 8 days before 90% of all APTTs were in a therapeutic range. Similar results were obtained by Cruickshank and coworkers.[73] These practices may be the result of concerns regarding the potential hemorrhagic complications associated with heparin use. To overcome these problems, standardized protocols for heparin administration and monitoring have been recommended. With use of these prescriptive regimens, a significant increase in the percentage of patients achieving a therapeutic aPTT within 24 hours can be realized.

Supporting the importance of achieving a therapeutic threshold as early as possible are data suggesting that a *subtherapeutic* aPTT is strongly correlated with thromboembolic recurrence whereas a *supratherapeutic* aPTT is not associated with an increased risk of clinically important bleeding complications.[70, 74] There is no direct evidence that the absolute dose of heparin or the level of the aPTT can predict the likelihood of bleeding. Rather, bleeding during heparin therapy appears to be related to the presence of concurrent illness such as renal disease, a history of heavy alcohol consumption, aspirin use, and prior surgical procedures or peptic ulcer disease. Failure to reach a therapeutic range within 24 hours appears to have long-term as well as short-term implications for thromboembolic recurrence. It has been suggested that patients who do not achieve a therapeutic threshold within 24 hours have a subsequent recurrence rate significantly higher than those who do.[75]

Many physicians, unaware of these relationships, initiate therapy with inadequate doses of heparin and then attempt to reach a therapeutic range by time-consuming, marginal increments in dose. In many instances, thrombus extension during this period of subtherapeutic anticoagulation serves to increase heparin requirements, thereby prolonging the process even further. Once a therapeutic range is reached, many "straddle" the lower therapeutic limit of aPTT in an attempt to reduce hemorrhagic risk. Fluctuations in aPTT levels can occur, and therefore a single aPTT value is not necessarily predictive of results during a 24-hour period.[76] Attempts to maintain the aPTT in a low therapeutic range on the basis of results of a single daily aPTT may result in periods of inadequate anticoagulation and an increased risk of thromboembolic recurrence. Furthermore, commercial thromboplastin reagents differ in their sensitivity to heparin so that an aPTT ratio of 1.5 obtained with a highly responsive reagent may actually not represent a therapeutic range.[77]

Given these concerns, a more prudent target for the lower limit of the aPTT ratio during heparin therapy may be 2.0 rather than 1.5, especially during the initial few days of therapy.

A number of different heparin dosing schemes have been published (Table 139–2), all of which have demonstrated the potential to reach a therapeutic threshold more rapidly than a nonstandardized approach:

1. A weight-based system that includes a bolus of 80 units/kg of heparin followed by an infusion of 18 units/kg/hr.[78]
2. A standard regimen involving a 5000-unit bolus followed by 1280 units/hr.[73]
3. A variable regimen involving a 5000-unit bolus followed by 40,000 units/day if the patient is at low risk for bleeding or 30,000 units/day if the patient is at high risk for bleeding.[74]

Each regimen includes standardized dose adjustments based on the resulting aPTT values. Whatever regimen is used, an aPTT should be obtained 6 hours after the bolus dose, 6 hours after each prescribed dose adjustment, and then on a daily basis for the duration of therapy. Because maintenance of the aPTT within a rigidly defined range does not appear to increase the efficacy or safety of the drug, frequent dosage adjustments are not necessary once the dose has been stabilized within a therapeutic range of 2.0 to 2.5 times the control value. Heparin requirements tend to decrease during the course of therapy, resulting in an increase in the level of the aPTT. For patients with heparin resistance (defined as the need for more than 40,000 units/day), monitoring heparin

TABLE 139–2. Published Standard Heparin Protocols

Dose Adjustment	Raschke et al.[78] Heparin Bolus, 80 U/kg Initial Infusion, 18 U/kg/hr		Cruickshank et al.[73] Heparin Bolus, 5000 U Initial Infusion, 1280 U/hr		Hull et al.[74] Heparin Bolus, 5000 U 40,000 U/day* Initial Infusion, 30,000 U/day†	
	aPTT (sec)	***Dose***	***aPTT (sec)***	***Dose***	***aPTT (sec)***	***Dose***
Repeat aPTT 6 hr after initiation of therapy, 6 hr after each dose change until therapeutic, then daily	<35	80 U/kg bolus; increase infusion rate by 4 U/kg/hr	<50	5000 U bolus; increase infusion rate by 120 U/hr	<45	Increase infusion rate by 120 U/hr
	35–45	40 U/kg bolus; increase infusion rate by 2 U/kg/hr	50–59	Increase infusion rate by 240 U/hr	45–54	Increase infusion rate by 120 U/hr
	46–70	No change	60–85	No change	55–85	No change
	71–90	Decrease infusion rate by 2 U/kg/hr	86–95	Decrease infusion rate by 80 U/hr	86–110	Decrease infusion rate by 120 U/hr
	>90	Hold infusion × 60 min; decrease infusion rate by 3 U/kg/hr	96–120	Hold infusion × 30 min; decrease infusion rate by 80 U/hr	>110	Decrease infusion rate by 240 U/hr
			>120	Hold infusion × 60 min; decrease infusion rate by 120 U/hr		

*Low bleeding risk.
†High bleeding risk.
aPTT = activated partial thromboplastin time.

with an antifactor Xa assay appears safe and effective and results in less escalation of the heparin dose than does monitoring with the aPTT.[79]

The complexities involved in heparin administration and aPTT monitoring may be rendered inconsequential by the introduction of low-molecular-weight heparins into clinical practice. Although it has not yet been approved for therapeutic purposes in the United States, a growing body of evidence suggests that low-molecular-weight heparin administered subcutaneously is as safe and effective as conventional heparin administered intravenously for both venous thrombosis and pulmonary embolism.[80-82] The advantage of low-molecular-weight heparins arises from their increased bioavailability and longer half-life as well as from the simplicity of their being administered subcutaneously once or twice daily without need for aPTT monitoring. Clinicians must recognize, however, that low-molecular-weight heparin preparations will not represent the panacea many envision. Standardized dosing is not possible in patients at the extremes of body weight; dose adjustments are necessary in patients with renal insufficiency because of renal clearance of the drug; the anticoagulant effect of the drug cannot be monitored easily; populations exist in which a long drug half-life is not a desirable effect (e.g., potential of high bleeding risk); the ability of protamine sulfate to reverse the anticoagulant effect remains uncertain; and drug costs are substantially higher than unfractionated heparin. Validation in ongoing clinical trials will be necessary to determine the safety, efficacy, and cost effectiveness of these agents.

Recommendations regarding the duration of heparin therapy remain undefined. Although the usual practice has been 7 to 10 days of intravenous heparin therapy, Hull and coworkers[83] demonstrated that a 5-day course of therapy in patients with proximal venous thrombosis was associated with a recurrence rate identical to that of a 10-day course. This assumes, of course, that warfarin is started early and is in a therapeutic range for two consecutive days before intravenous heparin is discontinued, an often difficult target to achieve. It is likely that a short course of intravenous heparin therapy would be similarly effective in patients with uncomplicated pulmonary embolism. However, a longer course of therapy is advisable in patients with major pulmonary embolism or massive iliofemoral venous thrombosis.

Besides bleeding, the other major complication of heparin is the development of thrombocytopenia.[84, 85] There are no predisposing factors to heparin-associated thrombocytopenia other than a history of a previous incident. The incidence of arterial thrombosis with heparin-associated thrombocytopenia appears to be low, but when it occurs, it is associated with considerable morbidity and mortality.[86]

On the basis of current data, recommendations regarding the frequency of platelet determinations during heparin therapy cannot be made. However, obtaining a baseline platelet count at 3-day intervals during heparin therapy probably represents a prudent approach. If heparin-associated thrombocytopenia develops, warfarin should be instituted and consideration given to placement of an inferior vena caval (IVC) filter. If more rapid anticoagulation than that provided by warfarin is necessary, a number of options exist that include defibrinating agents (ancrod), antithrombin drugs (hirudin and analogs), and heparinoids (danaparoid). Danaparoid has minimal cross-reactivity (5% to 10%) with unfractionated heparin and, given its ease of administration, appears to be the drug of choice in patients with heparin-associated thrombocytopenia.[87] Cross-reactivity with low-molecular-weight heparins is relatively common, and these drugs should be avoided.[88]

Thrombolytic Therapy

The use of thrombolytic agents in acute pulmonary embolism remains a subject of fervent controversy.[89-92] A number of arguments have been put forth as rationale for a wider application of thrombolytic therapy in pulmonary embolism. These include the possibility of more extensive thrombolysis than can be achieved with heparin therapy alone, an improved mortality, a decreased rate of recurrence, a decreased incidence of chronic thromboembolic pulmonary hypertension, and an improved symptomatic outcome. However, the arguments against the widespread use of thrombolytic therapy initially set forth so convincingly by Dalen[91, 92] in 1980 and again in 1997 must be considered before routine use of this class of drugs in patients with thromboembolism.

Although thrombolytic therapy (urokinase, streptokinase, or recombinant tissue plasminogen activator) can accelerate the rate of thrombolysis during the first 24 hours after treatment, there is no convincing evidence to suggest that it decreases mortality, increases the ultimate extent of resolution measured at 7 days, reduces thromboembolic recurrence rates, improves symptomatic outcome, or decreases the incidence of thromboembolic pulmonary hypertension.[92] The one issue about which there can be little controversy is that the use of thrombolytic agents is associated with a substantially increased risk of bleeding, including intracranial hemorrhage.[92, 93] Intracranial hemorrhage has occurred in 0.5% to 2.0% of patients treated with thrombolytic agents in trials evaluating the use of these agents in both pulmonary embolism and myocardial infarction.

On the basis of these data, it is my impression that the role of thrombolytic therapy in pulmonary embolism should be limited to those circumstances in which an accelerated rate of thrombolysis may be considered lifesaving (i.e., in patients with pulmonary embolism associated with hemodynamic compromise). A somewhat less absolute indication might involve a younger patient without bleeding risk who suffers an anatomically massive event. The finding of right ventricular dysfunction on echocardiography, a common accompaniment of embolism, in the absence of hemodynamic compromise should not serve as a justification for thrombolytic therapy.[94, 95] There is little basis for exposing a patient to the considerable risk of hemorrhagic complications associated with thrombolytic therapy for a disease process whose outcome is excellent with the use of heparin therapy alone. This is especially true given the recent advances that have occurred in heparin administration strategies. Some have called for more widespread use of thrombolytic therapy based on the results of nonrandomized trials.[96] However, until it has been demonstrated in a randomized trial that the use of thrombolytic therapy results in improved mortality or long-term outcome of patients, not short-term hemodynamic or angiographic improvement, compared with heparin therapy alone, such changes in the management philosophy remain unwarranted.

Inferior Vena Caval Filters

Despite their obvious hypothetical benefit, carefully controlled trials demonstrating the impact of IVC filters on pulmonary embolism recurrence rates and mortality have not been performed.[97] A large number of reports on using various filters have been published; however, they often lack clearly defined endpoints and objective criteria for pulmonary embolism recurrence and mortality. Furthermore, with rare exceptions, these studies do not allow a valid comparison among the different filter types in terms of both efficacy and complication rates. Although the data suggest that recurrent embolism and death from embolism are unusual after filter insertion, strong scientific evidence that IVC filters prevent death from pulmonary embolism is not currently available.[97]

The established indications for filter placement include the following:

1. Protection against pulmonary embolism in patients with acute venous thromboembolism in whom conventional anticoagulation is contraindicated (e.g., recent surgery, hemorrhagic cerebrovascular accident, active bleeding, heparin-associated thrombocytopenia).
2. Protection against pulmonary embolism in patients with acute venous thromboembolism in whom conventional anticoagulation has proved ineffective.
3. Protection of an already compromised pulmonary vascular bed from further thromboembolic risk (massive pulmonary embolism, chronic thromboembolic pulmonary hypertension).

With the increased ease of percutaneous filter placement, however, those indications have been expanded to include prophylaxis for patients without acute venous thrombosis but who are at high risk for its development. In several series, in fact, "prophylactic" filter placement was a more common indication than placement for "therapeutic" purposes.[98, 99] Unfortunately, this expansion in the indications for filter placement has occurred before the risks and benefits of such a strategy have been evaluated in a controlled manner. Established prophylactic options, both pharmacologic and nonpharmacologic (intermittent pneumatic compression devices), are available for most high-risk patients. Furthermore, sequential screening with duplex ultrasonography or impedance plethysmography is an option in many patients in whom the risk of venous thrombosis is thought to be especially high. Prophylactic filter placement may also induce the very problem the filter is attempting to prevent.[100]

Mortality from filter placement appears to be low regardless of what filter is used. In a review of 2557 patients undergoing filter insertion, only three deaths (0.12%) were reported.[97] Nonfatal complications of IVC filters, which occur with increased frequency and were delineated in the same review, include (1) complications relating to the insertion process, (2) venous thrombosis at the site of insertion, (3) filter migration, (4) filter erosion through the IVC wall, and (5) IVC obstruction.

The majority of clinically important complications appears to involve venous thrombosis at the insertion site and IVC obstruction. In those limited series that systematically searched for insertion site thrombosis with duplex ultrasonography, new venous thrombosis or extension of existing thrombus was detected in 22% of patients after filter insertion.[100]

Whether IVC filters should be routinely used in patients with anatomically or hemodynamically massive pulmonary embolism also remains undefined. Although the central goal of therapy in massive embolism is to relieve pulmonary vascular obstruction, the prevention of recurrence is an important secondary consideration. In this circumstance, several factors should be considered before a filter is placed:

1. There should be evidence of residual lower-extremity venous thrombosis.
2. The site of venous thrombosis must be considered. An infrarenal caval filter will not be useful if the emboli originated in the renal veins, cardiac chambers, or upper-extremity veins.
3. Finally, anticipated therapy should be considered. For example, the filter insertion site may serve as a potential site of bleeding that might hinder the anticipated use of thrombolytic therapy.

Given the reduced diameter of contemporary insertion devices and the potential risks of interrupting anticoagulant therapy in a patient with an anatomically massive embolism and residual lower-extremity thrombus, it has been my experience that anticoagulation does not have to be discontinued at the time of filter insertion.

Whether anticoagulant therapy should follow filter placement is not clear. Filter placement, although protecting the pulmonary vascular bed, does nothing to lessen the occurrence or the extension of venous thrombosis. Small thrombi can pass through patent filters or through collaterals around obstructed filters; furthermore, thrombus extension can occur through the filter itself. Data suggest that the initial benefit of IVCs for the prevention of pulmonary embolism is offset by an increased long-term risk of recurrent deep venous thrombosis, without any difference in mortality.[101] Before filter placement, the physician must be aware that this intervention is an irrevocable one. Given these considerations, anticoagulants should be used if no contraindications exist.

Pulmonary Embolectomy

The role of pulmonary embolectomy in acute, hemodynamically significant pulmonary embolism also remains controversial.[102] Although the outcome with conventional therapy is favorable for most patients with pulmonary embolism, in a subset of these patients the prognosis justifies more aggressive intervention. Patients with anatomically massive or submassive emboli who are hemodynamically compromised, who have not had a cardiac arrest, and who do not have an absolute contraindication to thrombolytic therapy should be managed initially with aggressive medical therapy (i.e., thrombolytic therapy plus heparin). Acute embolectomy might be considered in the following circumstances:

1. Patients with hemodynamically massive pulmonary embolism who have an absolute contraindication to anticoagulant or thrombolytic therapy.
2. Patients who have sustained a cardiopulmonary arrest.
3. Patients in whom aggressive medical therapy, including the use of thrombolytics, has proved ineffective.

It has been clearly demonstrated that the outcome of patients who have not sustained cardiac arrest is dramatically different from the outcome of patients who have. Gray and coworkers[103] reported a 29% mortality in 71 patients undergoing pulmonary embolectomy, 11% in those who had not sustained a cardiac arrest, and 64% in those who had.

Because the primary purpose of pulmonary embolectomy in massive embolism is to relieve the pulmonary vascular obstruction and reduce right ventricular afterload, the concept of doing so with a percutaneous device has been appealing. Several such devices designed to extract or fragment thrombi have been reported. Their role in massive pulmonary embolism remains investigative.[104, 105]

Pulmonary embolectomy for acute pulmonary embolism should not be confused with pulmonary thromboendarterectomy for chronic thromboembolic pulmonary hypertension.[106] The latter procedure is a true endarterectomy of chronic, organized, recanalized, and endothelialized thrombus in patients who have chronic pulmonary hypertension as a result of incomplete embolic resolution. Attempted pulmonary embolectomy of intraluminal thrombus in patients with chronic thromboembolic pulmonary hypertension will not reduce pulmonary vascular resistance if the distal, endothelialized obstruction is not alleviated, thereby resulting in an adverse outcome. For patients with chronic thromboembolic pulmonary hypertension, optimal evaluation, surgical intervention, and postoperative care should be provided at centers with ample experience in the care of these patients.[106]

Postembolic Prophylaxis

Early recurrence rates are sufficiently high to justify a course of long-term anticoagulation in all patients who have experienced an embolic event.[107] Two options for postembolic prophylaxis are available: warfarin sodium or adjusted-dose subcutaneous heparin.[108] On the basis of currently available information, the two options appear equally effective and safe if they are administered and monitored properly.

To be effective, the dose of subcutaneous heparin, which is administered every 12 hours, must be adjusted to maintain the aPTT at 1.5 times control value 6 hours after the administered dose. In regard to warfarin monitoring, a reliance on the absolute prothrombin time or the prothrombin time ratio may lead to either excessive or inadequate anticoagulation as a result of the considerable variability in the sensitivity of commercially available thromboplastins.

The international normalized ratio (INR), which corrects for the thromboplastin sensitivity, should be used as the means of monitoring warfarin effect.[109, 110] Therapy should be initiated with a 5-mg loading dose rather than larger doses.[111] Although a "therapeutic" INR (2.0 to 3.0) is reached sooner when larger doses are administered, this may be a consequence of a reduction in factor VII levels rather than representing a true antithrombotic effect that is thought to result from a reduction in factor II levels. Furthermore, larger doses may depress protein C activity and may result in a transient hypercoagulable state in the setting of what is considered to be a therapeutic INR range.[111]

In patients with a lupus anticoagulant, in whom the baseline INR may be elevated, the INR may not reliably reflect the level of anticoagulation. In these patients, tests that are insensitive to the lupus anticoagulant, such as the prothrombin-proconvertin time or chromogenic factor X assay, have been recommended.[112]

Substantial fluctuations can occur in vitamin K–dependent clotting factors in critically ill patients owing to factors such as erratic nutritional intake, antibiotic administration, and unpredictable gastrointestinal absorption, thereby resulting in wide swings in the INR. For this reason, use of adjusted doses of subcutaneous heparin as postembolic prophylaxis is often advisable until the patient's clinical status stabilizes.

The optimal duration of postembolic prophylaxis for patients with pulmonary embolism remains undefined. The most recent report suggests that a 6-month course of prophylactic anticoagulants after a first episode of venous thromboembolism leads to a lower recurrence rate than does treatment lasting 6 weeks. However, even beyond 6 months, recurrences occur.[106]

The difficulty in making recommendations regarding the duration of anticoagulation is the result of study design and the often diverse nature of the populations studied:

1. Patients with a well-defined predisposition for thromboembolism whose initial thromboembolic risk factor has resolved and whose ventilation-perfusion scan and noninvasive lower-extremity study findings have normalized can probably be managed with a 3-month course of anticoagulation.
2. Patients without a well-defined predisposition and those with persistent ventilation-perfusion scan defects or abnormal results on lower-extremity testing should be treated for a minimum of 6 months.
3. Patients with an ongoing predisposition should be treated until that predisposition resolves.
4. Finally, in patients with an irreversible predisposition to venous thrombosis, major ventilation-perfusion scan defects, or a history of recurrent thromboembolic events, consideration should be given to lifelong anticoagulation.[113]

Warfarin, although highly effective as postembolic prophylaxis, has no role as primary therapy in the initial management of venous thromboembolism. Unacceptable rates of thrombus extension, early recurrence, and late recurrence are associated with this intervention.[114]

Prophylaxis

There can be no better argument for the widespread use of venous thrombosis prophylaxis than that provided by the unnecessary mortality arising from pulmonary embolism and the complexity and uncertainty associated with the diagnostic and therapeutic approach to patients with suspected venous thromboembolism. If the goal is to prevent pulmonary embolism, the only effective approach is to prevent deep venous thrombosis. Despite this awareness, and despite the convincing evidence that a number of prophylactic strategies are capable of reducing the incidence not only of pulmonary embolism but of *fatal* pulmonary embolism, some surveys have demonstrated that prophylaxis is underused in patients at risk.

Anderson and coworkers,[115] in a review of 151,349 discharges from 16 acute-care hospitals, determined that 17% of the discharged patients were at risk for venous thrombosis, yet only 32% of these high-risk patients received prophylaxis. Even among patients with a prior history of pulmonary embolism, only 69% received prophylaxis during hospitalization.

Keane and coworkers,[116] in a prospective survey of the use of prophylaxis in 152 patients admitted to a medical ICU at a major teaching hospital, determined that only 33% of admitted patients received prophylaxis. Even among patients with three or more risk factors, prophylaxis was administered in only 48%.

A somewhat more encouraging perspective was provided by Ryskamp and Trottier.[117] In a retrospective review of 308 admissions to a medical-surgical ICU, 86% of patients meeting entry criteria received prophylaxis within 24 hours of admission. In those patients in whom prophylaxis was not administered, the major reason appeared to be oversight because none had an absolute contraindication to pharmacologic or mechanical prophylaxis.

Two factors appeared to contribute to this higher rate of compliance with prophylaxis: (1) the ICU was a closed unit, staffed by a limited number of critical care physicians, and (2) an educational program designed to stress the importance of prophylaxis was implemented. Supporting the need for ongoing quality assurance efforts was the finding that compliance with prophylactic measures had decreased from 97% to 86% in the absence of a structured, continuing educational program.

A number of different rationales have been proposed to explain this lack of compliance with published recommendations for prophylaxis. The overstated perception of bleeding complications associated with pharmacologic methods of prophylaxis appears to remain a deterrent. Furthermore, fatal pulmonary embolism is uncommon in any individual physician's experience, thereby diminishing the perception of risk. Finally, especially in a critical care setting, the issue of prophylaxis is often subordinated to the compelling demands of the patient's admitting diagnosis and therapy. Whatever the reason, however, increased use of prophylaxis must occur if an impact is to be made on the substantial and often unnecessary morbidity and mortality associated with venous thromboembolism.

Although a number of forms of prophylaxis have been used, four major approaches provide adequate prophylaxis in the majority of patients[15]:

- Subcutaneous heparin
- Warfarin
- Mechanical forms of prophylaxis (graduated compression stockings and intermittent pneumatic compression)
- Placement of an IVC filter

The ability of subcutaneous heparin to reduce the incidence of venous thrombosis and pulmonary embolism was defined by the International Multicentre Trial published in 1975.[118] The results of this trial confirmed that low-dose heparin prophylaxis (5000 units subcutaneously every 12 hours) was effective not only in reducing lower-extremity venous thrombosis and pulmonary embolism but also in decreasing the mortality rate from fatal pulmonary embolism in general surgical patients and was not associated with excessive bleeding risk.

Low-molecular-weight heparin preparations represent another prophylactic option. Compared with unfractionated heparin, the ability of these preparations to potentiate the inhibition of factor Xa relative to their inhibition of thrombin theoretically allows them to maintain an equivalent antithrombotic effect while minimizing their anticoagulant effect. In trials comparing the prophylactic effects of low-molecular-weight heparin with unfractionated heparin in general surgical and medical populations, low-molecular-weight heparin has not proved superior to unfractionated heparin. However, these heparin preparations appear more promising as prophylactic agents in several high-risk groups[83, 119-122]:

- Patients undergoing hip replacement
- Patients with spinal cord injury
- Patients with multiple trauma

The introduction of mechanical means of prophylaxis represented a major breakthrough in the ability to provide prophylaxis to those patients in whom pharmacologic means of prophylaxis are either contraindicated (active bleeding) or appear to pose an unacceptable hemorrhagic risk (surgery of the eye, spine, or brain). Intermittent pneumatic compression devices, in a wide range of patients, appear to be as effective as low-dose subcutaneous heparin prophylaxis in preventing lower-extremity venous thrombosis.[123] In addition to diminishing the degree of lower-extremity venous stasis, the compressive action of the pump also appears to increase fibrinolytic activity, which may contribute to their prophylactic effect.

The role of warfarin as a prophylactic agent is limited because of bleeding complications associated with its use and the need for frequent laboratory monitoring. However, warfarin has proved effective in certain high-risk patients, specifically those with hip fracture or those undergoing hip replacement. Two regimens are now widely used: small doses (1 to 2 mg) given for several days before surgery, with dose escalation to therapeutic range after surgery; and initiation after surgery.[124]

One option is available to prevent pulmonary embolism in patients at high risk who cannot be provided pharmacologic or mechanical prophylaxis. Patients with extensive trauma often fall into this category, particularly those with pelvic or lower-extremity fractures and potential internal bleeding. In such patients, prophylactic placement of an IVC filter provides protection against otherwise nonpreventable emboli.

Venous thrombosis prophylaxis, whether pharmacologic or mechanical, must be applied with several concepts in mind:

1. Prophylaxis diminishes the likelihood of venous thromboembolism but does not abolish it. Therefore, symptoms and signs suggestive of pulmonary embolism cannot be overlooked because prophylaxis has been provided.

2. Physicians who treat special populations should be familiar with the thromboembolic risk in those populations and the effective prophylactic options available.

3. The optimal application of prophylaxis involves identification of relative thromboembolic risk in an individual patient based on cumulative risk factors. A stepwise approach to prophylactic intensity would involve low-dose subcutaneous heparin or pneumatic compression devices alone in lower risk populations; higher dose subcutaneous heparin (7500 units every 12 hours), low-molecular-weight heparin, or the combination of low-dose subcutaneous heparin plus pneumatic compression devices in those at intermediate risk; and warfarin, sequential lower-extremity monitoring, or IVC filter placement in those at highest risk.

4. Finally, it has become increasingly apparent that the trend toward earlier hospital discharge has been accompanied by increased incidence of post-discharge venous thromboembolism. Thromboembolic risk does not necessarily end at the time of hospital discharge or at transfer to a lower level of care. In these patients, prophylaxis should be continued until the risk for venous thromboembolism has resolved.[125]

References

1. Dalen JE, Alpert JS: Natural history of pulmonary embolism. Prog Cardiovasc Dis 1975; 17:259–270.
2. Hansson PO, Welin L, Tibblin G, Eriksson H: Deep vein thrombosis and pulmonary embolism in the general population: The study of men born in 1913. Arch Intern Med 1997; 157:1665–1670.
3. Macik BG, Ortel TL: Clinical and laboratory evaluation of the hypercoagulable states. Clin Chest Med 1995; 16:375–389.
4. Heijboer H, Brandjes DPM, Buller HR, et al: Deficiencies of coagulation-inhibiting and fibrinolytic properties in outpatients with deep-vein thrombosis. N Engl J Med 1990; 323:1512–1516.
5. Dahlback B, Carlsson M, Svensson PJ: Familial thrombophilia due to a previously unrecognized mechanism characterized by poor anticoagulant response to activated protein C: Prediction of a cofactor to activated protein C. Proc Natl Acad Sci USA 1993; 90:1004–1008.
6. Griffin JH, Evatt B, Wideman C, Fernandez JA: Anticoagulant protein C pathway defective in majority of thrombophilic patients. Blood 1993; 82:1989–1993.
7. Koster T, Rosendaal FR, de Ronde H, et al: Venous thrombosis due to poor anticoagulant response to activated protein C: Leiden Thrombophilia Study. Lancet 1993; 342:1503–1506.
8. Ridker PM, Hennekens CH, Lindpainter K, et al: Mutation in the gene coding for coagulation factor V and the risk of myocardial infarction, stroke, and venous thrombosis in apparently healthy men. N Engl J Med 1995; 332:912–917.
9. Hellgren M, Svensson PJ, Dahlbeck B: Resistance to activated protein C as a basis for venous thromboembolism associated with pregnancy and oral contraceptives. Am J Obstet Gynecol 1995; 173:210–213.
10. Price DT, Ridker PM: Factor V Leiden mutation and the risks for thromboembolic disease: A clinical perspective. Ann Intern Med 1997; 127:895–903.
11. Heijer M, Koster T, Blom HJ, et al: Hyperhomocysteinemia as a risk factor for deep-vein thrombosis. N Engl J Med 1996; 334:759–762.
12. Mandel H, Brenner B, Berant M, et al: Coexistence of hereditary homocystinuria and factor V Leiden—effect on thrombosis. N Engl J Med 1996; 334:763–768.
13. Poort SR, Rosendaal FR, Reitsma PH, Bertina RM: A common genetic variation in the 3′-untranslated region of the prothrombin gene is associated with elevated plasma prothrombin levels and an increase in venous thrombosis. Blood 1996; 88:3698–3703.
14. Nachman RL, Silverstein R: Hypercoagulable states. Ann Intern Med 1993; 119:819–827.
15. Anderson FA, Wheeler HB: Venous thromboembolism: Risk factors and prophylaxis. Clin Chest Med 1995; 16:235–251.
16. Hirsch D, Ingenito EP, Goldhaber SZ: Prevalence of deep venous thrombosis among patients in medical intensive care. JAMA 1995; 274:335–337.
17. Marik PE, Andrews L, Maini B: The incidence of deep venous thrombosis in ICU patients. Chest 1997; 111:661–664.
18. Kakkar VV, Howe CT, Flanc C, Clark MB: Natural history of postoperative deep vein thrombosis. Lancet 1969; 2:230–232.
19. Huisman MV, Buller HR, ten Cate JW, et al: Unexpected high

prevalence of silent pulmonary embolism in patients with deep venous thrombosis. Chest 1989; 95:498-502.
20. Lagerstedt CI, Olsson CG, Fagher B, et al: Need for long-term anticoagulant treatment in symptomatic calf-vein thrombosis. Lancet 1985; 2:515-518.
21. Stradness DE, Langlois Y, Cramer M, et al: Long-term sequelae of acute venous thrombosis. JAMA 1983; 250:1289-1292.
22. Haire D: Arm vein thrombosis. Clin Chest Med 1995; 16:341-352.
23. McIntyre KM, Sasahara AA: Hemodynamic and ventricular response to pulmonary embolism. Prog Cardiovasc Dis 1974; 17:175-190.
24. McIntyre KM, Sasahara AA: The hemodynamic response to pulmonary embolism in patients without prior cardiopulmonary disease. Am J Cardiol 1971; 28:288-294.
25. Elliott CG: Pulmonary physiology during pulmonary embolism. Chest 1992; 101:163S-171S.
26. Cranley JJ, Canos AJ, Sull WJ: The diagnosis of deep venous thrombosis: Fallibility of clinical symptoms and signs. Arch Surg 1976; 111:34-36.
27. Landefeld CS, McGuire E, Cohen AM: Clinical findings associated with deep vein thrombosis: A basis for quantifying clinical judgement. Am J Med 1990; 88:382-388.
28. Goldhaber SZ, Hennekens CH, Evans DA, et al: Factors associated with the correct antemortem diagnosis of major pulmonary embolism. Am J Med 1982; 73:822-826.
29. Stein PD, Terrin ML, Hales CA, et al: Clinical, laboratory, roentgenographic, and electrocardiographic findings in patients with acute pulmonary embolism and no pre-existing cardiac or pulmonary disease. Chest 1991; 100:598-603.
30. The PIOPED Investigators: Value of the ventilation/perfusion scan in acute pulmonary embolism: Results of the prospective investigation of pulmonary embolism diagnosis (PIOPED). JAMA 1990; 263:2753-2759.
31. Monroel M, Ruiz J, Olazabal A, et al: Deep venous thrombosis and the risk of pulmonary embolism: A systematic study. Chest 1992; 102:677-681.
32. Stein PD, Terrin ML, Hales CA, et al: Clinical, laboratory, roentgenographic, and electrocardiographic findings in patients with acute pulmonary embolism and no pre-existing cardiac or pulmonary disease. Chest 1991; 100:598-603.
33. Benotti JR, Dalen JE, Alpert JS: Pulmonary embolism. *In:* Intensive Care Medicine. 2nd ed. Rippe JM, Irwin RS, Alpert JS, Fink MP (Eds). Boston, Little, Brown & Co, 1991, pp 308-314.
34. Murray HW, Ellis GC, Blumenthal DS, Sos TA: Fever and pulmonary thromboembolism. Am J Med 1979; 67:232-235.
35. Alderson PO, Martin EC: Pulmonary embolism. Diagnosis with multiple imaging modalities. Radiology 1987; 164:297-312.
36. Greenspan RH, Ravin CE, Polansky SM, et al: Accuracy of the chest radiograph in diagnosis of pulmonary embolism. Invest Radiol 1982; 17:539-543.
37. Stein PD, Athanasoulis C, Greenspan RH, Henry JW: Relation of plain chest radiographic findings to pulmonary artery pressure and arterial blood oxygen levels in patients with acute pulmonary embolism. Am J Cardiol 1992; 69:394-396.
38. Stein PD, Goldhaber SZ, Henry JW, Miller AC: Arterial blood gas analysis in the assessment of suspected acute pulmonary embolism. Chest 1996; 109:78-81.
39. Stein PD, Dalen JE, McIntyre KM, et al: The electrocardiogram in acute pulmonary embolism. Prog Cardiovasc Dis 1975; 17:247-257.
40. National Cooperative Study: The Urokinase Pulmonary Embolism Trial. Circulation 1973; 47(Suppl 2):1-100.
41. Kasper W, Geibel A, Tiede N, et al: Distinguishing between acute and subacute massive pulmonary embolism by conventional and Doppler echocardiography. Br Heart J 1993; 70:352-356.
42. Krivec B, Voga G, Zuran I, et al: Diagnosis and treatment of shock due to massive pulmonary embolism. Approach with transesophageal echocardiography and intrapulmonary thrombolysis. Chest 1997; 112:1310-1316.
43. Sohn DW, Shin GJ, Oh JK, et al: Role of transesophageal echocardiography in hemodynamically unstable patients. Mayo Clin Proc 1995; 70:925-931.
44. Gossage JR: Of emperors, emboli and echocardiography (Editorial). Chest 1997; 112:1158-1159.
45. Perrier A, Desmaris S, Goehring C, et al: D-dimer testing for suspected pulmonary embolism in outpatients. Am J Respir Crit Care Med 1997; 156:492-496.
46. Perrier A, Bounameaux H, Morabia A, et al: Diagnosis of pulmonary embolism by a decision analysis-based strategy including clinical probability, D-dimer levels, and ultrasonography. Arch Intern Med 1996; 156:531-536.
47. Moser KM: Diagnosing pulmonary embolism: D-dimer needs rigorous evaluation. BMJ 1994; 309:1525-1526.
48. Remy-Jardin M, Remy J, Deschildre F, et al: Diagnosis of pulmonary embolism with spiral CT: Comparison with pulmonary angiography and scintigraphy. Radiology 1996; 200:699-706.
49. Remy-Jardin M, Remy J, Wattinne L, et al: Central pulmonary thromboembolism: Diagnosis with spiral volumetric CT with the single breath hold technique—comparison with pulmonary angiography. Radiology 1992; 185:381-387.
50. Goodman LR, Curtin JJ, Mewissen MW, et al: Detection of pulmonary embolism in patients with unresolved clinical and scintigraphic diagnosis: Helical CT versus angiography. AJR Am J Roentgenol 1995; 164:1369-1374.
51. Oser RF, Zuckerman DA, Gutierrez FR, Brink JA: Severity of pulmonary emboli at pulmonary arteriography: Implications for spiral and ultrafast CT (Abstract). Radiology 1994; 193(P):352.
52. Heijboer H, Buller HR, Lensing AW, et al: A comparison of real-time compression ultrasonography with impedance plethysmography for the diagnosis of deep-vein thrombosis in symptomatic outpatients. N Engl J Med 1993; 329:1365-1369.
53. Huisman MV, Buller HR, ten Cate JW, Vreeken J: Serial impedance plethysmography for suspected deep venous thrombosis in outpatients. The Amsterdam General Practioner Study. N Engl J Med 1986; 314:823-828.
54. Cogo A, Lensing AWA, Prandoni P, Hirsh J: Distribution of thrombosis in patients with symptomatic deep vein thrombosis. Arch Intern Med 1993; 153:2777-2780.
55. Lensing AWA, Prandoni P, Brandjes D, et al: Detection of deep vein thrombosis by real-time B-mode ultrasonography. N Engl J Med 1989; 320:342-345.
56. Turkstra F, Kuijer PMM, van Beek EJR, et al: Diagnostic utility of ultrasonography of leg veins in patients suspected of having pulmonary embolism. Ann Intern Med 1997; 126:775-781.
57. Wells PS, Lensing AW, Davidson BL, et al: Accuracy of ultrasound for the diagnosis of deep venous thrombosis in asymptomatic patients after orthopedic surgery. A meta-analysis. Ann Intern Med 1995; 122:47-53.
58. Burke B, Sostman HD, Carroll BA, Witty LA: The diagnostic approach to deep venous thrombosis: Which technique? Clin Chest Med 1995; 16:253-268.
59. Webber MW, Gomes AS, Roe D, et al: Comparison of Biello, McNeill, and PIOPED criteria for the diagnosis of pulmonary emboli on lung scans. AJR Am J Roentgenol 1990; 154:975-981.
60. Henry JW, Stein PD, Gottschalk A, et al: Scintigraphic lung scans and clinical assessment in critically ill patients with suspected acute pulmonary embolism. Chest 1996; 109:462-466.
61. Miniati M, Pistolesi M, Marini C, et al: Value of perfusion lung scan in the diagnosis of pulmonary embolism: Results of the Prospective Investigative Study of Acute Pulmonary Embolism Diagnosis (PISA-PED). Am J Respir Crit Care Med 1996; 154:1387-1393.
62. Stein PD, Terrin ML, Gottschalk A, et al: Value of ventilation/perfusion scans versus perfusion scans alone in acute pulmonary embolism. Am J Cardiol 1992; 69:1239-1241.
63. Neuhaus A, Bentz RR, Weg JC: Pulmonary embolism in respiratory failure. Chest 1973; 73:460-465.
64. Lesser BA, Leeper KV, Stein PD, et al: The diagnosis of acute pulmonary embolism in patients with chronic obstructive lung disease. Chest 1992; 102:17-22.
65. Stein PD, Athanasoulis C, Alavi A, et al: Complications and validity of pulmonary angiography in acute pulmonary embolism. Circulation 1992; 85:462-468.
66. Moser KM: Pulmonary embolism. *In:* Textbook of Respiratory Medicine. Vol II. Murray JF, Nadel JA (Eds). Philadelphia, WB Saunders, 1988, p 1310.
67. Hull RD, Raskob GE, Ginsburg JS, et al: A noninvasive strategy for the treatment of patients with suspected pulmonary embolism. Arch Intern Med 1994; 154:289-297.

68. Hull RD, Raskob GE, Pineo GF, Brant RF: The low-probability lung scan. A need for change in nomenclature. Arch Intern Med 1995; 155:1845-1851.
69. Bone RC: The low-probability lung scan: A potentially lethal reading. Arch Intern Med 1993; 153:2621-2622.
70. Hull RD, Pineo GF: Current concepts of anticoagulation therapy. Clin Chest Med 1995; 16:269-280.
71. Hull RD, Raskob GE, Hirsh J, et al: Continuous intravenous heparin compared with intermittent subcutaneous heparin in the initial treatment of proximal vein thrombosis. N Engl J Med 1986; 315:1109-1114.
72. Wheeler RH, Jaquiss RD, Newman JH: Physician practices in the treatment of pulmonary embolism and deep venous thrombosis. Arch Intern Med 1988; 148:1321-1325.
73. Cruickshank MK, Levine MN, Hirsh J, et al: A standard nomogram for the management of heparin therapy. Arch Intern Med 1991; 151:333-337.
74. Hull RD, Raskob GE, Rosenbloom DR, et al: Optimal therapeutic level of heparin therapy in patients with venous thromboembolism. Arch Intern Med 1992; 152:1589-1595.
75. Hull RD, Raskob GE, Brant RF, et al: The importance of initial heparin treatment on long-term clinical outcomes of antithrombotic therapy. The emerging theme of delayed recurrence. Arch Intern Med 1997; 157:2317-2321.
76. Decousus HA, Croze M, Levi FA, et al: Circadian changes in anticoagulant effect of heparin infused at a constant rate. BMJ 1985; 200:341-344.
77. Baker BA, Adelman MD, Smith PA, Osborn JC: Inability of the activated partial thromboplastin time to predict heparin levels: Time to reassess guidelines for heparin assays. Arch Intern Med 1997; 157:2475-2479.
78. Raschke RA, Reilly BM, Guidry JR, et al: The weight based heparin dosing nomogram compared with a "standard care" nomogram: A randomized controlled study. Ann Intern Med 1993; 119:874-881.
79. Levine MN, Hirsh J, Gent M, et al: A randomized trial comparing activated thromboplastin time with heparin assay in patients with acute venous thromboembolism requiring large daily doses of heparin. Arch Intern Med 1994; 154:49-56.
80. The Columbus Investigators: Low-molecular-weight heparin in the treatment of patients with venous thromboembolism. N Engl J Med 1997; 337:657-662.
81. Simonneau G, Sors H, Charbonnier B, et al: A comparison of low-molecular-weight heparin with unfractionated heparin for acute pulmonary embolism. N Engl J Med 1997; 337:663-669.
82. Weitz JI: Low-molecular-weight heparins. N Engl J Med 1997; 337:688-698.
83. Hull RD, Raskob GE, Rosenbloom D, et al: Heparin for 5 days as compared with 10 days in the initial treatment of proximal venous thrombosis. N Engl J Med 1990; 322:1260-1264.
84. Landfeld CS, Beyth RJ: Anticoagulant-related bleeding: Clinical epidemiology, prediction and prevention. Am J Med 1993; 95:315-328.
85. King DJ, Kelton JG: Heparin-associated thrombocytopenia. Ann Intern Med 1984; 100:535-540.
86. Stanton PE Jr, Evans JR, Lefemine AA, et al: White clot syndrome. South Med J 1988; 81:616-620.
87. Ginsberg JS: Management of venous thromboembolism. N Engl J Med 1996; 335:1816-1828.
88. Warkentin TE, Levine MN, Hirsh J, et al: Heparin-induced thrombocytopenia in patients treated with low molecular weight heparin or unfractionated heparin. N Engl J Med 1995; 332:1330-1335.
89. Sasahara AA: The case for fibrinolytic therapy. J Cardiovasc Med 1980; 5:794-798.
90. Goldhaber SZ: Thrombolysis for pulmonary embolism. Prog Cardiovasc Dis 1991; 34:113-134.
91. Dalen JE: The case against fibrinolytic therapy. J Cardiovasc Med 1980; 5:799-814.
92. Dalen JE, Alpert JS, Hirsch J: Thrombolytic therapy for pulmonary embolism. Is it effective? Is it safe? When is it indicated? Arch Intern Med 1997; 157:2550-2556.
93. Levine MN, Goldhaber SZ, Gore JM, et al: Hemorrhagic complications of thrombolytic therapy in the treatment of myocardial infarction and venous thromboembolism. Chest 1995; 108:291S-301S.
94. Goldhaber SZ, Haire WD, Feildstein ML, et al: Alteplase versus heparin in acute pulmonary embolism: Randomized trial assessing right-ventricular function and pulmonary embolism. Lancet 1993; 341:507-511.
95. Cannon CP, Goldhaber SZ: Cardiovascular risk stratification of pulmonary embolism. Am J Cardiol 1996; 78:1149-1151.
96. Konstantinides S, Geigel A, Olschewski M, et al: Association between thrombolytic treatment and the prognosis of hemodynamically stable patients with major pulmonary embolism. Results of a multicenter registry. Circulation 1997; 96:882-888.
97. Becker DM, Philbrick JT, Selby JB: Inferior vena cava filters: Indications, safety, effectiveness. Arch Intern Med 1992; 152:1985-1994.
98. Pais SO, Tobin KD, Austin CB, Queral L: Percutaneous insertion of the Greenfield inferior vena cava filter: Experience with ninety-six patients. J Vasc Surg 1988; 8:460-464.
99. Roehm JOF, Johnsrude IS, Barth MH, et al: The bird's nest inferior vena cava filter: Initial clinical experience. Radiology 1988; 168:745-749.
100. Ferris EJ, McCowan TC, Carver DK, McFarland DR: Percutaneous inferior vena caval filters: Follow-up of seven designs in 320 patients. Radiology 1993; 188:851-856.
101. Decousus H, Leizorovicz A, Parent F, et al: A clinical trial of vena caval filters in the prevention of pulmonary embolism in patients with proximal deep-vein thrombosis. N Engl J Med 1998; 338:409-415.
102. Gray HH, Miller GAH, Paneth M: Pulmonary embolectomy: Its place in the management of pulmonary embolism. Lancet 1988; 1:1441-1445.
103. Gray HH, Morgan JM, Paneth M, Miller GAH: Pulmonary embolectomy for acute massive pulmonary embolism: An analysis of 71 cases. Br Heart J 1988; 60:196-200.
104. Greenfield LJ, Proctor MS: Role of catheter-embolectomy in treating pulmonary embolism. Semin Respir Crit Care Med 1996; 17:95-99.
105. Stein PD, Sabbah HN, Basha MA, et al: Mechanical disruption of pulmonary emboli in dogs with a flexible rotating-tip catheter (Kensey catheter). Chest 1990; 98:994-998.
106. Fedullo PF, Auger WR, Channick RN, Moser KM: Chronic thromboembolic pulmonary hypertension. Clin Chest Med 1995; 16:353-374.
107. Schulman S, Sofie-Rhedin A, Lindmarker P, et al: A comparison of six weeks with six months of oral anticoagulant therapy after a first episode of venous thromboembolism. N Engl J Med 1995; 332:1661-1665.
108. Hull R, Delmore T, Carter C, et al: Adjusted subcutaneous heparin versus warfarin sodium in the long-term treatment of venous thrombosis. N Engl J Med 1982; 306:189-194.
109. Bussey HI, Force RW, Bianco TM, et al: Reliance on prothrombin time ratios causes significant errors in anticoagulation therapy. Arch Intern Med 1992; 152:278-282.
110. Hirsh J, Poller L: The international normalized ratio. A guide to understanding and correcting its problems. Arch Intern Med 1994; 154:282-288.
111. Harrison L, Johnston M, Massicotte MP, et al: Comparison of 5-mg and 10-mg loading doses in initiation of warfarin therapy. Ann Intern Med 1997; 126:133-136.
112. Moll S, Ortel TL: Monitoring warfarin therapy in patients with lupus anticoagulants. Ann Intern Med 1997; 127:177-185.
113. Schulman S, Granqvist S, Holmstrom M, et al: The duration of oral anticoagulant therapy after a second episode of venous thromboembolism. N Engl J Med 1997; 336:393-398.
114. Brandjes DPM, Heijboer J, Buller HR, et al: Acenocoumarol and heparin compared with acenocoumarol alone in the initial treatment of proximal-vein thrombosis. N Engl J Med 1992; 327:1485-1489.
115. Anderson FA Jr, Wheeler HB, Goldberg RG, et al: Physician practices in the prevention of venous thromboembolism. Ann Intern Med 1991; 115:591-595.
116. Keane MC, Ingenito EP, Goldhaber SZ: Utilization of venous thromboembolism prophylaxis in the medical intensive care unit. Chest 1994; 106:13-22.
117. Ryskamp RS, Trottier SJ: Utilization of venous thromboembolism prophylaxis in a medical-surgical ICU. Chest 1998; 113:162-164.
118. An International Multicentre Trial: Prevention of fatal postopera-

tive pulmonary embolism by low doses of subcutaneous heparin. Lancet 1975; 2:45–51.
119. Mohr DN, Silverstein MD, Murtaugh PA, Harrison JM: Prophylactic agents for venous thrombosis in elective hip surgery. Arch Intern Med 1993; 153:2221–2228.
120. Nurmohamed MT, Rosendaal FR, Buller HR, et al: Low-molecular-weight heparin versus standard heparin in general and orthopaedic surgery: A meta-analysis. Lancet 1992; 340:152–156.
121. Green D: Prophylaxis of thromboembolism in spinal cord-injured patients. Chest 1994; 102:649S–651S.
122. Geerts WH, Jay RM, Code KI, et al: A comparison of low-dose heparin with low-molecular-weight heparin as prophylaxis against venous thromboembolism after major trauma. N Engl J Med 1996; 335:701–707.
123. Clagett GP, Anderson FA Jr, Heit J, et al: Prevention of venous thromboembolism. Chest 1995; 108:312S–334S.
124. Francis CW, Marder VJ, McCollister EC, et al: Two step warfarin therapy: Prevention of postoperative venous thrombosis without excessive bleeding. JAMA 1983; 249:374–378.
125. Planes A, Vochelle N, Darmon JY, et al: Risk of deep-venous thrombosis after hospital discharge in patients having undergone total hip replacement: Double-blind randomised comparison of enoxaparin versus placebo. Lancet 1996; 348:224–228.

140

Pulmonary Hypertension

Lewis J. Rubin, MD

The pulmonary circulation is a low-pressure circuit that accepts the entire right ventricular output at a resistance that is normally one tenth of that in the systemic circulation, even when cardiac output is increased severalfold with activity. Increases in pulmonary artery pressure lead to an increased impedance to right ventricular ejection. When afterload is increased either acutely or on a sustained basis, right-sided heart dysfunction ensues, producing symptoms that are a manifestation of the reduced cardiac output.

Cor pulmonale is best defined as pulmonary hypertension in the setting of acute or chronic respiratory disease. Right-sided heart failure occurs relatively late in the course of cor pulmonale. Indeed, patients with acute cor pulmonale may manifest few of the signs of overt right-sided heart failure with which clinicians are familiar, such as edema, ascites, or hepatomegaly.

PATHOPHYSIOLOGY

Pulmonary hypertension can be classified on the basis of the primary anatomic site in which the vascular insult originates. Left ventricular failure and left-sided valvular disease produce pulmonary artery hypertension primarily by elevating the postcapillary (venous) pressure, resulting in an increased upstream pressure to maintain flow through the lung circuit. In this setting, the gradient between the pulmonary artery diastolic and pulmonary artery occlusion or left atrial pressures is relatively small (3 to 5 mm Hg) despite the presence of pulmonary hypertension.

The total pulmonary resistance (TPR) (mean pulmonary artery pressure divided by cardiac output) is increased out of proportion to the pulmonary vascular resistance (PVR) (mean pulmonary artery pressure minus left atrial or pulmonary artery occlusion pressure divided by cardiac output), and the histopathologic changes in the arterial tree are relatively mild and potentially reversible:

$$\mathrm{TPR} = \frac{\mathrm{PAPm}}{\mathrm{CO}} \tag{1}$$

$$\mathrm{PVR} = \frac{\mathrm{PAPm} - \mathrm{PCWP}}{\mathrm{CO}} \tag{2}$$

where CO is cardiac output.

In contrast, conditions in which the pulmonary arteries and arterioles are the primary site of disease are associated with an increased pulmonary arteriovenous pressure gradient and parallel increases in TPR and PVR. The vascular abnormalities in these conditions range from mild intimal proliferation to vascular obliteration and may be highly reversible or irreversible, depending on the cause, severity, and duration.

The hemodynamic disparity in vascular resistances is helpful in differentiating the primary site and potential cause of disease in most cases, but there are two exceptions.

The first is pulmonary veno-occlusive disease, which is characterized pathologically by obliteration of the small and medium-sized pulmonary veins, yet the pulmonary artery occlusion pressure measured with a pulmonary artery flotation catheter may be normal. This occurs because the occlusion pressure reflects downstream pressure in the large pulmonary veins, which drain blood largely from those capillary-venule networks that are unaffected and that do not readily communicate with diseased capillary-venule circuits. Thus, the PVR approximates TPR in the setting of postcapillary hypertension. An occasional clue to the presence of this disease may be the measurement of disparate occlusion pressures in different regions of the lung.

Second, many patients with mitral valve disease who undergo valve replacement surgery manifest a prompt fall in pulmonary artery pressure postoperatively because of the correction of the downstream obstruction to flow. However, longstanding pulmonary venous hypertension can result in persistent precapillary hypertension, characterized pathologically by extensive arterial remodeling, despite correction of the underlying cause.

Table 140–1 shows a classification of pulmonary hypertension based on cause. Pulmonary vascular diseases resulting from disorders that primarily alter the structure or function of the lung or diseases that affect the lung circulation as part of a systemic illness are considered to be secondary forms of pulmonary hypertension. *Primary (idiopathic) pulmonary hypertension* (PPH) is a disorder in which pulmonary artery pressure is increased in the absence of a clinically demonstrable underlying cause.[1, 2]

A variety of factors contribute to the development of pulmonary hypertension in the setting of respiratory disease (Fig. 140–1). Alveolar hypoxia is a common feature of many forms of acute or chronic respiratory disease and produces selective constriction of pulmonary arteries. Hypoxic pulmonary vasoconstriction appears to be an intrinsic property of pulmonary smooth muscle cells and is dependent on both the availability of extracellular calcium and the state of the smooth-muscle cell membrane voltage-gated calcium and potassium channels.[3] Hypercapnia and acidosis, which frequently accompany chronic obstructive pulmonary disease (COPD) and may be particularly conspicuous in the setting of acute respiratory failure, potentiate the pulmonary vascular hypoxic pressor response. Although acute hypoxic pulmonary vasoconstriction is readily reversible on restoration of normal gas tensions, chronic hypoxia results in vascular remodeling, which is both slowly and incompletely responsive to correction of the derangements in ventilation and gas exchange.

Mechanical compression of the vasculature by hyperinflated

TABLE 140–1. Classification of Processes Causing Pulmonary Artery Hypertension

Diseases Affecting the Air Passages of the Lung and Alveoli
Chronic obstructive lung disease
Cystic fibrosis
Infiltrative or granulomatous diseases
Sarcoidosis
Idiopathic pulmonary fibrosis
Connective tissue diseases
Radiation
Pneumoconiosis
Upper airway obstruction
Congenital developmental defects
Adult respiratory distress syndrome
Diseases Affecting Thoracic Cage Movement
Kyphoscoliosis
Neuromuscular weakness
Sleep apnea syndrome
Idiopathic hypoventilation
Pleural fibrosis
Diseases Directly Affecting the Pulmonary Vasculature
Primary pulmonary hypertension
Granulomatous pulmonary hypertension
Toxin-induced pulmonary vascular disease
Anorectic agents
Intravenous drug use
L-Tryptophan
Cocaine
Sickle cell disease
Thromboembolic disease
Pulmonary vasculitis
Pulmonary veno-occlusive disease
Congenital heart disease
Chronic portal hypertension
Human immunodeficiency virus infection
Diseases Affecting the Pulmonary Vasculature by Extrinsic Compression
Mediastinal tumors
Aneurysms
Granuloma
Mediastinal fibrosis
Left ventricular dysfunction and left atrial hypertension

lungs may also play a role in the development of pulmonary hypertension in the setting of severe emphysema and may contribute to worsening pulmonary vascular dynamics during acute decompensations. The polycythemia that occurs in the setting of chronic hypoxemia to maximize oxygen delivery to the peripheral tissues can result in hyperviscosity, further impeding blood flow through the lung circulation. A loss of the cross-sectional surface area of the vasculature caused by widespread destruction of normal lung parenchyma may also contribute to elevations in pulmonary arterial pressure in conditions such as advanced bullous emphysema or fibrotic diseases of the lung.

Finally, thromboembolism can result in an acute decompensation in the setting of chronic cardiopulmonary disease by raising pulmonary artery pressure directly as a result of vascular obstruction by thrombus, by release of vasoactive substances at the site of thrombosis, or by worsening intrapulmonary gas exchange and potentiating hypoxic pulmonary vasoconstriction.

Elevations in pulmonary artery pressure occur frequently in patients with the acute respiratory distress syndrome (ARDS). In addition to the factors just listed, release of vasoactive mediators as a result of the underlying inflammatory process contributes to the pulmonary vascular process.[4]

A variety of connective tissue diseases can be complicated by the development of pulmonary hypertension either as part of a systemic vasculopathy or as the primary manifestation of the illness. In addition, the vasculature may be secondarily involved as a result of parenchymal lung disease, such as pulmonary fibrosis in systemic sclerosis. Pulmonary vasospasm (pulmonary Raynaud's phenomenon) has been observed during right-sided heart catheterization in some patients with connective tissue diseases, particularly among those who experience typical peripheral Raynaud's phenomenon.[5]

Pulmonary hypertension is a condition of unknown cause in which the pulmonary vasculature appears to be the exclusive target of the disease process.[1, 2] A number of conditions have been associated with this disorder:

1. Pulmonary hypertension may complicate portal hypertension possibly because of an unidentified vasotoxin that bypasses hepatic metabolism and may injure the lung circulation.[1]

2. Pulmonary hypertension has resulted from the ingestion of diet suppressants, which are chemically similar to amphetamines, suggesting the possibility that these agents either induce vasoconstriction directly or may alter the metabolism of circulating vasoactive substances, such as serotonin.[6] This potential mechanism has also been suggested to cause the pulmonary vascular disease that has occurred in patients ingesting contaminated rapeseed oil (toxic oil syndrome) and contaminated L-tryptophan.[7]

3. Extracts from the plant species *Crotalaria,* which are

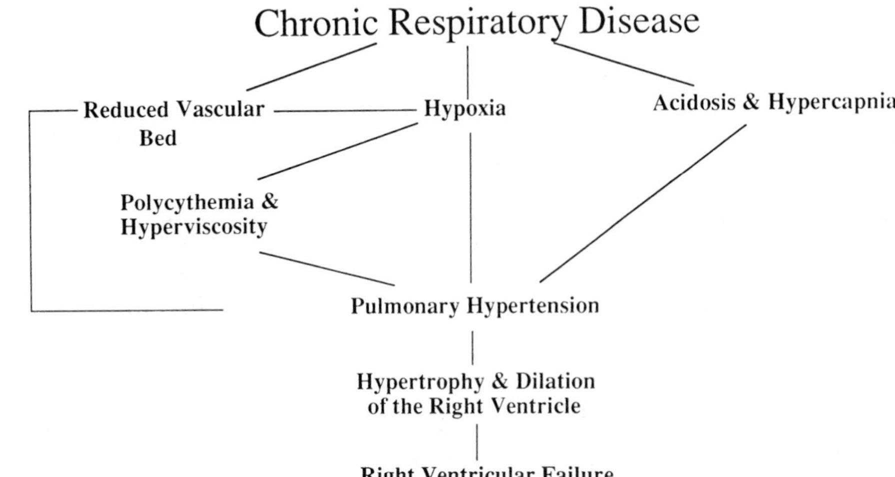

Figure 140–1. Pathogenesis of pulmonary hypertension in chronic respiratory disease (cor pulmonale).

used in parts of Africa and the Caribbean to make herbal tea, have also been implicated in the pathogenesis of PPH in several patients.[8] Furthermore, the administration of the monocrotaline derivative of this plant to laboratory animals results in a necrotizing pulmonary arteritis and the subsequent development of chronic pulmonary vascular disease.[8]

4. Cocaine, which is known to possess potent vasoconstrictor properties, has been reported to produce pulmonary hypertension that is characterized pathologically by medial hypertrophy of the muscular pulmonary arteries.[1]

5. Pulmonary vascular disease that is pathologically identical to PPH has also been observed in patients who test positive for antibodies to the human immunodeficiency virus (HIV), even in the absence of evidence of substance abuse.[1]

PPH occurs nearly twice as frequently in women as in men. Although individuals of any age may be affected, the disease is most common between ages of 20 and 50 years. Fewer than 10% of patients have a family history of PPH,[2] and it has been suggested that this disease may be transmitted genetically as an autosomal dominant trait with incomplete penetrance. The gene responsible for familial PPH has recently been localized to chromosome 2q31-32.[9]

CLINICAL MANIFESTATIONS

Patients with pulmonary hypertension typically present with nonspecific and nondiagnostic symptoms. These include exertional dyspnea, fatigue, chest pain that is often described as a substernal pressure suggestive of angina pectoris, and syncope. The last complaint is particularly noteworthy because it implies a markedly impaired cardiac output and is a poor prognostic sign. Similarly, edema or anasarca implies the presence of right-sided heart failure and portends a poor prognosis. Raynaud's phenomenon is reported to occur in up to 25% to 30% of patients with PPH,[2] although it is far more common in pulmonary hypertension secondary to connective tissue diseases. Hoarseness may result from compression of the recurrent laryngeal nerve by massively dilated proximal pulmonary arteries. A chronic, nonproductive cough may also be evident and may be due to stimulation of interstitial irritant receptors as a result of vascular enlargement.

The physical examination not only may suggest the presence of pulmonary vascular disease but also provide important clues to its cause. Examination of the jugular venous pulse may demonstrate elevation of the venous pressure, suggesting right-sided heart volume overload as well as prominent a or cv waves, indicating altered right ventricular compliance and tricuspid regurgitation, respectively. Examination of the chest may disclose abnormalities that point to an underlying specific cause of pulmonary vascular disease, such as obstructive lung disease or restriction resulting from rib cage deformities.

The findings on cardiac examination may vary, depending on the cause and severity of the process. Patients with severe, chronic pulmonary hypertension usually manifest a prominent right ventricular impulse along the parasternal region; a right-sided fourth heart sound and pulmonic component to the second heart sound (P_2) may also be palpable. In contrast, the point of maximum cardiac impulse is frequently displaced to the subxiphoid region in patients with cor pulmonale resulting from severe obstructive lung disease. Auscultation of the heart may disclose an accentuated P_2, right-sided S_4 gallop, or pulmonic ejection click. An S_3 gallop is indicative of right-sided heart failure and is a serious prognostic finding. The murmur of tricuspid insufficiency, audible along the lower right sternal border and increasing with inspiration, is a common finding in advanced pulmonary hypertension. On occasion, a murmur of pulmonic insufficiency may be heard at the left second intercostal space and the parasternal area. Fixed splitting of the second heart sound should raise suspicion of an unsuspected atrial septal defect. Short systolic bruits heard while the lungs are auscultated may be a clue to the presence of partially occlusive thrombus in the larger pulmonary arteries.[10]

Because a normal right ventricle can acutely increase systolic pressure only to a level of approximately 40 to 45 mm Hg in response to an acute vascular insult without resulting in overt right-sided heart failure and cardiogenic shock, the physical findings in acute pulmonary hypertension are usually less dramatic than the findings in established, long-standing hypertensive pulmonary vascular disease in which compensatory changes have occurred.

Peripheral cyanosis implies a markedly reduced cardiac output. Central cyanosis may indicate the presence of a right-to-left shunt, which may be due to congenital heart disease with Eisenmenger's physiology (reversal of intracardiac shunting from left-to-right to right-to-left in the setting of congenital intracardiac defect with pulmonary hypertension), pulmonary arteriovenous malformations, the opening of the foramen ovale caused by right atrial pressure and volume overload, or severe, acute lung injury. Digital clubbing does not occur in PPH, and its presence suggests that pulmonary hypertension is due to parenchymal lung disease, congenital heart disease, or hepatic cirrhosis.

DIAGNOSTIC APPROACH

A variety of laboratory tests are useful in establishing a diagnosis of pulmonary hypertension and in determining its cause.

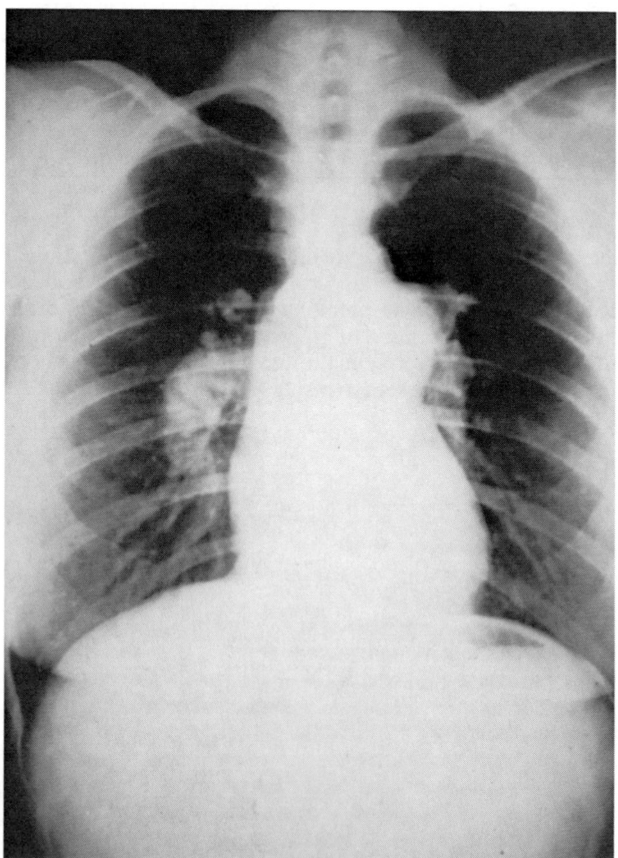

Figure 140–2. Posteroanterior chest radiograph of a patient with pulmonary hypertension. The proximal pulmonary arteries are enlarged, and the right ventricular configuration is prominent.

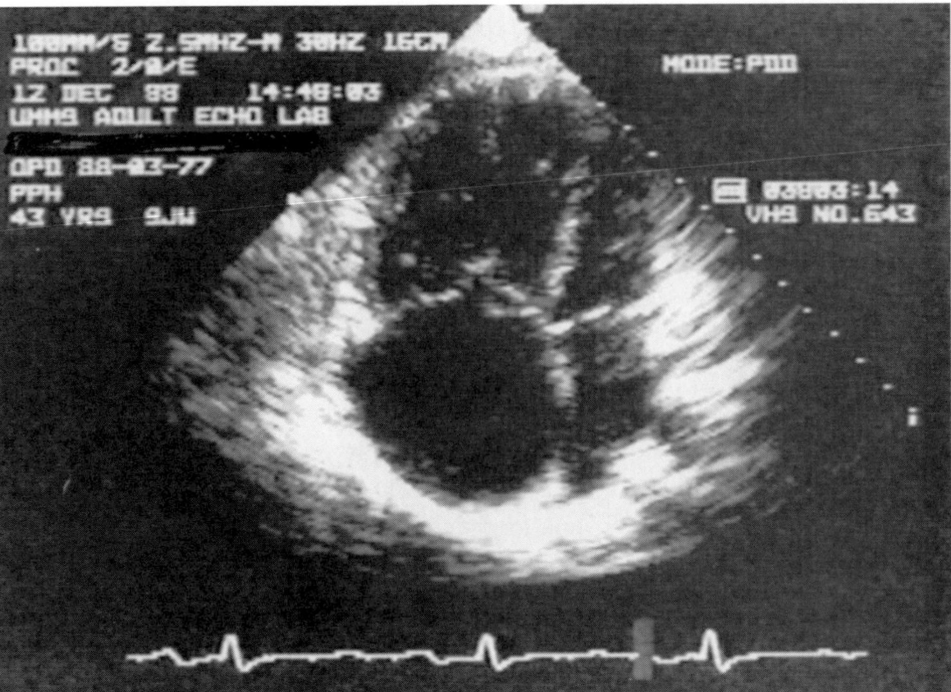

Figure 140–3. Four-chamber echocardiographic view of the heart in a patient with severe pulmonary hypertension. The right-sided heart chambers are markedly enlarged and compress the left ventricle.

Chest radiographs may disclose evidence of parenchymal lung disease or demonstrate right ventricular and pulmonary vascular prominence (Fig. 140–2). Kerley's B lines on the chest radiograph of a patient with unexplained pulmonary hypertension and a normal left side of the heart by cardiac catheterization or echocardiography suggests the presence of pulmonary veno-occlusive disease.

Electrocardiography (ECG) may show the characteristic signs of right ventricular hypertrophy, including a QRS axis greater than 110°, RSR′ complex in V_1 and V_2, and incomplete right bundle branch block. The findings are generally much less prominent in patients with underlying lung disease because of the displacement of the heart in the thorax in patients with hyperinflation and the tendency for cor pulmonale to be a milder form of pulmonary hypertension than other causes. The presence of an $S_1Q_3T_3$ pattern on the ECG strongly suggests an acute right ventricular pressure overload state, such as massive acute pulmonary thromboembolism. Prominent, peaked P waves in the inferior and right precordial leads (p pulmonale) are nonspecific findings on ECG and may appear and disappear in patients with acute, reversible airflow obstruction even in the absence of pulmonary hypertension.

Echocardiography may demonstrate right-sided chamber enlargement, flattening of the interventricular septum during systole, or the presence of coexistent left ventricular or mitral valve disease (Fig. 140–3). A pericardial effusion may also be present and is suggestive of either a connective tissue disease or right atrial pressure overload.

Doppler studies can be used to determine the presence and estimate the magnitude of tricuspid regurgitation, which may be useful in noninvasively estimating the pulmonary artery systolic pressure (Fig. 140–4).

Intravenous injection of agitated saline or hydrogen peroxide during echocardiographic study may disclose the presence and site of an intracardiac shunt (Fig. 140–5).

The severity of pulmonary hypertension correlates closely

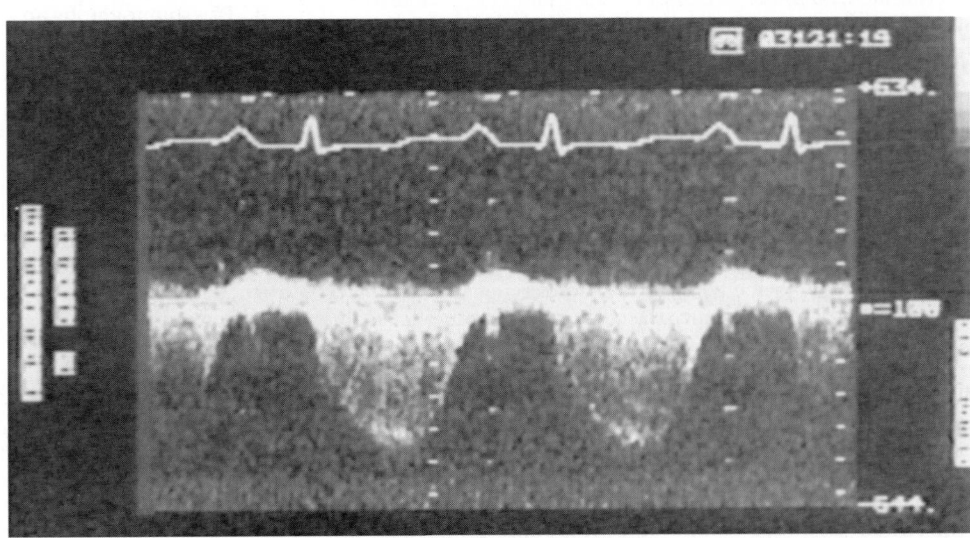

Figure 140–4. Doppler examination of the tricuspid valve showing a regurgitant jet, which can be used to estimate pulmonary artery systolic pressure.

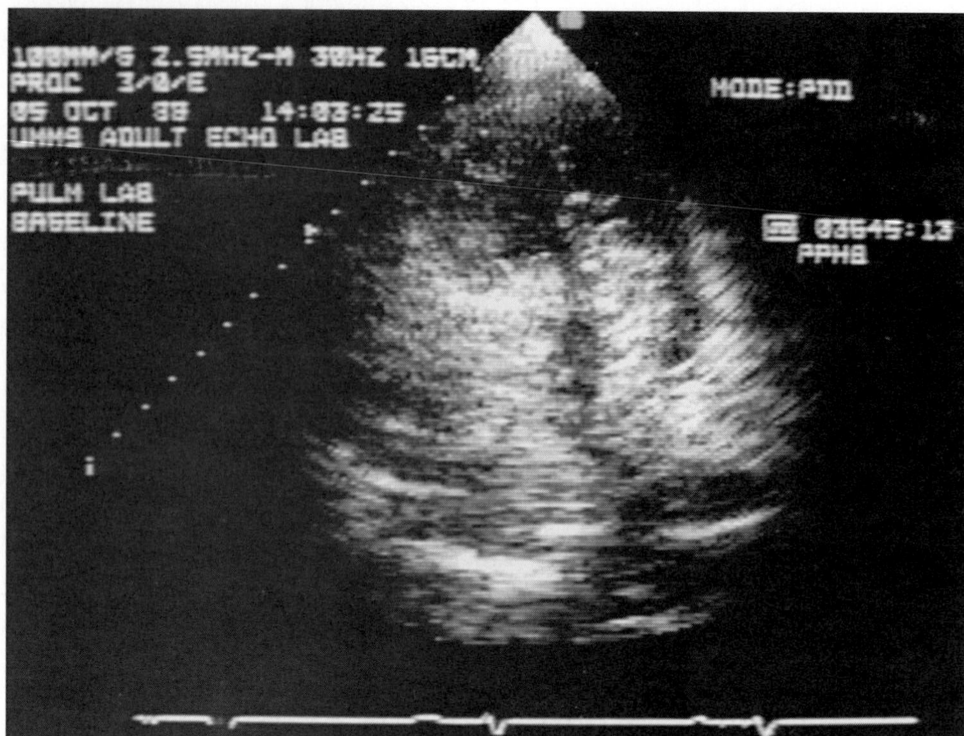

Figure 140–5. Saline contrast injection echocardiogram demonstrating the simultaneous appearance of echogenicity in both sides of the heart, indicating the presence of a right-to-left shunt.

with the degree of derangement in lung function in patients with chronic parenchymal lung disease. In general, patients with chronic airflow obstruction are likely to have concomitant pulmonary hypertension when the forced expiratory volume in 1 second falls below 1 L.[11] With chronic restrictive lung disease, pulmonary hypertension is usually present when the vital capacity or the diffusing capacity for carbon monoxide is below 50% of predicted. Patients whose partial pressure of arterial oxygen is below 55 mm Hg will generally have pulmonary hypertension, and the more severe the hypoxemia, the more severe the pulmonary hypertension is likely to be. In addition, arterial blood gas measurements taken while the patient breathes ambient air may be important not only in establishing a cause but also in guiding the initial approach to therapy. Worsening pulmonary hypertension during acute exacerbations is likely in individuals with severe, chronic parenchymal disease.

Chronic thrombotic occlusion of the pulmonary vasculature should be considered in any patient with unexplained pulmonary hypertension because it is potentially treatable by thromboendarterectomy.[10] Radioisotope lung scanning is a safe and reliable method to assess the distribution of ventilation and perfusion in the lungs, even in patients with severe pulmonary vascular disease. Patients with PPH usually manifest a homogeneous pattern of perfusion, whereas patients with chronic thromboembolism exhibit multiple perfusion defects of varying sizes. Scanning over the head or kidneys may demonstrate the presence of an unsuspected right-to-left shunt, because some of the radiolabeled tagged macroaggregated albumin bypasses the pulmonary microvasculature and gains access to the systemic circulation. Veno-occlusive disease may have a mottled appearance on perfusion scan, although this is not always the case. When a distinction between PPH and chronic thromboembolic disease cannot be made with use of noninvasive tests, the patient should undergo pulmonary arteriography. Similarly, one should consider acute pulmonary thromboembolism in a patient with chronic cor pulmonale who experiences a sudden clinical deterioration in the absence of clear signs of exacerbation of the underlying parenchymal lung disease.

Patients with pulmonary vascular disease secondary to connective tissue diseases usually have abnormal, high-titer serologic findings. Although some patients with PPH may have abnormal serologic studies as well,[2] these are usually in nonspecific patterns and at low titers. Other studies that may be useful in the diagnostic work-up of unexplained pulmonary hypertension include:

1. High-resolution computed tomographic (CT) scanning of the chest to exclude occult interstitial disease, particularly when the chest radiograph is normal but pulmonary function is substantially impaired.
2. Magnetic resonance imaging to exclude fibrosing mediastinitis.
3. Spiral CT scanning to exclude proximal thrombosis of the pulmonary vasculature.
4. Polysomnography to evaluate for the presence of sleep-disordered breathing.

Complete cardiac catheterization is recommended in patients with unexplained, severe pulmonary hypertension to exclude congenital heart disease, proximal or peripheral pulmonic stenosis, and valvular heart disease. The pulmonary artery pressure often approaches systemic levels in PPH, chronic thromboembolic disease, and connective tissue diseases and tends to be more modestly elevated in most forms of acute or chronic cor pulmonale. Hemodynamic monitoring in the critical care unit may also be useful in guiding the management of acute cor pulmonale.

In most cases, a cause for the pulmonary vascular disease can be ascertained on clinical grounds; however, for a definitive diagnosis to be made, it may be necessary to obtain a specimen of lung tissue from patients with severe pulmonary hypertension who have confusing evidence by physical examination or ancillary laboratory testing. Thoracoscopy-guided biopsy is the preferred approach. Although this method carries an increased risk of complications in patients with severe pulmonary vascular disease, it can generally be performed safely in these patients. Risk and complication rates are considerably lower compared with traditional approaches.

Transbronchial biopsy through the fiberoptic bronchoscope is not a suitable alternative to open-lung biopsy in the setting of unexplained pulmonary vascular disease because the small size of the specimens precludes establishing a pathologic diagnosis.

APPROACH TO MANAGEMENT

The management of pulmonary hypertension should initially be directed at treating the underlying cause, if one exists. Improving gas exchange and airflow in patients with cor pulmonale resulting from chronic obstructive airways disease usually ameliorates the pulmonary hypertension to some degree. Patients with interstitial lung disease and pulmonary hypertension may show marked hemodynamic improvement when lung function is improved with corticosteroid or immunosuppressive therapy.

Because hypoxia is a major contributor to both acute and chronic cor pulmonale, correcting hypoxemia is an important component of the therapeutic approach in affected patients. Although the hemodynamic effects of low-flow supplemental oxygen in patients with COPD are variable and slow in achieving their maximum,[12] survival is increased substantially when hypoxemia is corrected.[13] Patients with a stable PaO_2 of 55 mm Hg or less on breathing ambient air or a PaO_2 of 59 mm Hg or less *and* a hematocrit greater than 55%, p pulmonale on ECG, or edema should be treated chronically with supplemental oxygen using flow rates sufficient to achieve a PaO_2 greater than 60 mm Hg. Flow rates may be increased for activity or at night in patients who experience arterial desaturation with exercise or sleep, respectively. In general, PPH patients with normal resting values for PaO_2 do not manifest hemodynamic improvement with oxygen therapy.[14] However, acute deteriorations caused by further compromise of cardiac function or lower respiratory tract infections can result in hypoxemia that is poorly tolerated and should be treated aggressively. Patients with a significant right-to-left shunt do not usually experience an improvement in oxygenation to an appreciable degree with supplemental oxygen therapy.

Polycythemia, resulting from the effects of chronic hypoxia in patients with severe parenchymal lung disease or congenital heart disease, may contribute to elevations in pulmonary vascular resistance by increasing blood viscosity. Although supplemental oxygen therapy usually results in a decrease in hematocrit in these patients, this response may be incomplete.[13] Isovolemic phlebotomy to a hematocrit of 50% to 55% may reduce the degree of hyperviscosity without compromising tissue oxygen delivery.[15]

THERAPEUTIC ALTERNATIVES

Vasodilator therapy for pulmonary hypertension is based on the premise that vasoconstriction is present in some forms of pulmonary vascular disease and that these drugs may exert their vasorelaxant properties in pulmonary as well as in systemic vascular smooth muscle. Although vasodilator therapy may produce substantial hemodynamic and symptomatic improvement in some patients with chronic pulmonary hypertension, this effect is not universal, and serious adverse effects may also result. Thus, this approach to therapy should be individualized for each patient and the patient's acute and long-term responses meticulously monitored.

A variety of systemic vasodilators have been shown to reduce pulmonary artery pressure in experimentally induced pulmonary hypertension, such as:

- Hydralazine
- Calcium channel blockers (nifedipine, diltiazem, and verapamil)
- Prostaglandins E_1 and I_2 (prostacyclin)
- Adenosine
- Nitrates (nitroglycerin and nitroprusside)

These agents have also been used to treat selected patients with either primary or secondary pulmonary hypertension. A report from the National Institutes of Health–sponsored Registry on PPH suggests that approximately two thirds of patients manifest acute responses to vasodilator administration, which, if sustained, may be beneficial.[16]

The goal of vasodilator therapy is to reduce right ventricular afterload and increase cardiac output and systemic oxygen delivery. A substantial reduction in pulmonary arterial pressure concomitant with an increased stroke volume and an unchanged or minimally reduced systemic arterial pressure constitutes the optimal hemodynamic response to vasodilator administration and is frequently associated with evidence of regression of right-sided heart abnormalities by ECG, echocardiography, or catheterization[17] and improved survival.[18] This "ideal" response is seen in only 25% to 30% of patients with PPH. In the remaining 30% to 40% of "responders," cardiac output is increased in the absence of any significant change in pulmonary artery or systemic blood pressures. The decision to institute long-term vasodilator therapy in these patients should be based on individual assessment.

The major adverse effects that may result from vasodilator administration include the following[19]:

1. Systemic hypotension, which may result either from systemic vasodilation in the absence of any pulmonary vascular effect or from a reduced cardiac output caused by the negative inotropic properties of some drugs.
2. Worsening pulmonary hypertension, which is due to an increased cardiac output flowing through a vascular bed with a fixed resistance.
3. Worsening hypoxemia caused by either an increased perfusion to poorly ventilated lung units (decreased ventilation-perfusion ratio) or increased right-to-left shunting if the systemic vascular effect predominates.

Patients with right-sided heart failure appear to be at the greatest risk for adverse effects with vasodilator administration[16]; however, there are no other demographic or clinical parameters that are reliable in predicting whether a patient will respond acutely or chronically to vasodilator therapy. Because the risk of sustained adverse effects is greatest with long-acting agents, the use of potent, short-acting, titratable vasodilators to test vasoreactivity has been advocated. Prostacyclin (prostaglandin I_2), prostaglandin E_1, adenosine, acetylcholine, nitroglycerin, and nitric oxide[20] have all been used in this manner and appear to be well tolerated. The acute responses to prostacyclin and nitric oxide have been useful in predicting responsiveness to orally active drugs.[21]

Patients with severe pulmonary hypertension are at risk for fatal pulmonary thromboembolic events because of their sedentary lifestyle, venous insufficiency, and dilated right-sided heart chambers with sluggish pulmonary blood flow. Even a small vascular thrombotic occlusion can be lethal to a patient with a compromised pulmonary vascular bed that possesses the capability to neither recruit unused vessels nor dilate functional vasculature in response to an acute insult. Accordingly, prophylactic anticoagulation has been advocated for patients with severe nonthrombotic pulmonary hypertension, and survival may be improved in patients receiving anticoagulants.[18, 22] However, anticoagulant therapy is not without risk in this setting, and life-threatening side effects, including hemoptysis from spontaneously ruptured pulmonary vessels, may occur. If therapy with warfarin is contemplated, the prothrombin time should be monitored frequently and maintained at an International Normalized Ratio (INR) of approximately 1.5 to 2.5. Adjusted-dose subcutaneous heparin may be a suitable alternative to warfarin, although it is more cumbersome to administer, and its use should be reserved for patients who have a greater risk for complications with warfarin therapy. Acutely ill patients with nonthrombotic pulmonary hypertension should receive low-dose heparin subcutaneously during the acute illness.

Diuretics can be helpful in treating right-sided heart failure by reducing the degree of hepatic congestion and peripheral edema. In addition, patients with right-sided heart failure and hypoxemia resulting from a right-to-left shunt may experience improved oxygenation with diuresis owing to the reduction in the transatrial pressure gradient. However, diuretics should be used cautiously in this setting because decreasing right ventricular preload may result in a reduction in cardiac output. In addition, diuretic-induced hypokalemia and alkalosis may be poorly tolerated.

There is little role for cardiac glycosides in the acute or chronic management of pulmonary vascular disease, with the exception of supraventricular tachyarrhythmias or biventricular failure.[23] Furthermore, patients with chronic respiratory disease are at an increased risk of experiencing toxicity with these agents.[24]

Combined heart-lung transplantation had been considered the surgical treatment of choice for severe pulmonary hypertension that is refractory to medical management.[25] However, the dearth of suitable organ donors and the limited number of centers with the expertise to perform this procedure have limited its availability. Experience suggests that single or bilateral lung transplantation may result in marked hemodynamic improvement in patients with isolated pulmonary vascular disease.[26] The greater availability of donor organs for lung transplantation may enable a larger number of seriously ill patients to undergo transplantation.

Because the course of pulmonary vascular disease is variable, it is difficult to determine the ideal time to consider transplantation in an individual patient. However, patients with symptoms that substantially limit their lifestyle and that are unresponsive to medical therapy may be suitable candidates for lung transplantation. Patients with evidence of severe and irreversible right-sided heart dysfunction, significant disease affecting the left side of the heart or coronary circulation, or complex congenital cardiac defects should be considered only for combined heart-lung transplantation. Organ rejection and opportunistic infections constitute the major causes of morbidity and mortality after transplantation. It is unknown whether idiopathic diseases such as PPH will recur in transplanted lungs.

At present, the average times on a waiting list for heart-lung transplantation and for single lung transplantation are approximately 18 to 24 months and 12 to 18 months, respectively. Prostacyclin delivered by a continuous intravenous infusion with a portable infusion pump has recently been approved by the Food and Drug Administration (FDA) for use in patients with severe (New York Heart Association functional classes III and IV) PPH.[27] Chronic therapy with prostacyclin improves exercise tolerance, hemodynamics, and survival. Prostacyclin can be used as a primary mode of therapy in patients who have improvement with its use or as a bridge to transplantation in patients with limited response. The chronic effects of prostacyclin appear to be due to a beneficial effect on vascular remodeling rather than due to its vasodilator properties. Accordingly, prostacyclin should be considered in any patient with severe PPH that is refractory to medical therapy, even in the absence of acute hemodynamic responsiveness to its infusion.

Blade balloon atrial septostomy has been performed in patients with intractable right-sided heart failure. The creation of an intracardiac right-to-left shunt results in improved filling of the left side of the heart, with resultant increased systemic cardiac output. Although the shunt results in increased venous admixture and arterial desaturation, the impact of this potentially adverse phenomenon may be offset by an overall increased systemic oxygen delivery and reduction in the consequences of elevated venous pressure (i.e., ascites and anasarca).[28]

The treatment of choice for chronic thrombotic pulmonary hypertension is pulmonary thromboendarterectomy.[10] However, only organized thrombi in the proximal vessels is approachable by this technique. Preoperative evaluation should include complete pulmonary angiography to determine the site and extent of thrombosis. Marked hemodynamic improvement frequently results from successful removal of organized thrombus. Patients with acute cor pulmonale caused by massive pulmonary embolism should be evaluated for emergent embolectomy if death is imminent and if there is insufficient time for thrombolytic therapy to effect enough clot lysis to restore the integrity of the pulmonary vascular bed.

PROGNOSIS

In the settings of both chronic obstructive pulmonary disease and ARDS, the presence of cor pulmonale contributes significantly to a shortened survival.[4, 11] The 3-year survival in patients with severe airflow obstruction and a pulmonary vascular resistance three to four times normal is less than 10% to 15%.[11, 29] Survival is similarly influenced by the presence of pulmonary hypertension in chronic restrictive lung diseases and connective tissue diseases.

Mortality from PPH is, in large part, dependent on the state of the right ventricle. Patients with symptoms of severe right-sided heart dysfunction, such as syncope, and hemodynamic evidence of impaired right ventricular function, such as a reduced cardiac output or mixed venous saturation and an elevated right atrial pressure, usually succumb to the disease within 1 to 2 years.[30] Patients with milder symptoms and relatively well preserved right-sided heart function survive longer, although the course is highly variable. The impact of therapy on survival has not been addressed in large-scale, prospective studies.

References

1. Rubin LJ: Primary pulmonary hypertension. N Engl J Med 1997; 336:111–117.
2. Rich S, Dantzker DR, Ayres SM, et al: Primary pulmonary hypertension: A national prospective study. Ann Intern Med 1987; 107:216–223.
3. Yuan XJ, Goldman WF, Tod M, et al: Hypoxia reduces potassium currents in cultured rat pulmonary but not mesenteric arterial myocytes. Am J Physiol 1993; 264:L116–L123.
4. Zapol WM, Rie MA, Frikker M, et al: Pulmonary circulation during adult respiratory distress syndrome. *In:* Acute Respiratory Failure. Zapol WM, Falke KJ (Eds). New York, Marcel Dekker, 1985, pp 241–273.
5. Furst DE, Davis JA, Clements PJ, et al: Abnormalities of pulmonary vascular dynamics and inflammation in early progressive systemic sclerosis. Arthritis Rheum 1981; 24:1403–1408.
6. Abenhaim L, Moride Y, Brenot F, et al: Appetite-suppressant drugs and the risk of primary pulmonary hypertension. N Engl J Med 1996; 335:609–616.
7. Tazelaar HD, Myers JL, Drage CW, et al: Pulmonary disease associated with L-tryptophan–induced eosinophilic myalgia syndrome. Chest 1990; 97:1032–1036.

8. Dietary pulmonary hypertension. *In:* The Human Pulmonary Circulation. Harris P, Heath D (Eds). New York, Churchill Livingstone, 1977, pp 398–417.
9. Nichols WC, Kollor DL, Slovis B, et al: Localization of the gene for familial primary pulmonary hypertension to chromosome 2q31-32. Nat Genet 1997; 15:277–280.
10. Moser KM, Dailey PO, Peterson K, et al: Thromboendarterectomy for chronic, major-vessel thromboembolic pulmonary hypertension. Ann Intern Med 1987; 107:560–565.
11. Burrows B, Kettle LJ, Niden AH, et al: Patterns of cardiovascular dysfunction in chronic obstructive lung disease. N Engl J Med 1972; 286:912–918.
12. Timms RM, Khaja FU, Williams GW, et al: Hemodynamic response to oxygen therapy in chronic obstructive pulmonary disease. Ann Intern Med 1985; 102:29–36.
13. Nocturnal Oxygen Therapy Trial Group: Continuous or nocturnal oxygen therapy in hypoxemic chronic obstructive airways disease: A clinical trial. Ann Intern Med 1980; 93:391–398.
14. Morgan JM, Griffiths M, du Bois RM, et al: Hypoxic pulmonary vasoconstriction in systemic sclerosis and primary pulmonary hypertension. Chest 1991; 99:551–556.
15. Weisse AB, Moschos CB, Frank MJ, et al: Hemodynamic effects of staged hematocrit reduction in patients with stable cor pulmonale and severely elevated hematocrit levels. Am J Med 1975; 58:92–98.
16. Weir EK, Rubin LJ, Ayres SM, et al: The acute administration of vasodilators in primary pulmonary hypertension: Experience from the NIH registry on primary pulmonary hypertension. Am Rev Respir Dis 1989; 140:1623–1630.
17. Rich S, Brundage BH: High-dose calcium channel blocking therapy for primary pulmonary hypertension: Evidence for long-term reduction in pulmonary arterial pressure and regression of right ventricular hypertrophy. Circulation 1987; 76:135–141.
18. Rich S, Kaufmann E, Levy P: The effect of high doses of calcium-channel blockers on survival in primary pulmonary hypertension. N Engl J Med 1992; 327:76–81.
19. Melot C, Naeije R, Mols P, et al: Effects of nifedipine on ventilation/perfusion matching in primary pulmonary hypertension. Chest 1983; 83:203–207.
20. Rossaint R, Falke KJ, Lopez F, et al: Inhaled nitric oxide for the adult respiratory distress syndrome. N Engl J Med 1993; 328:399–405.
21. Barst RJ: Pharmacologically induced pulmonary vasodilation in children and young adults with primary pulmonary hypertension. Chest 1986; 89:497–503.
22. Fuster V, Steele PM, Edwards WD, et al: Primary pulmonary hypertension: Natural history and the importance of thrombosis. Circulation 1984; 70:580–587.
23. Mathur PN, Powles P, Pugsley SO, et al: Effect of digoxin on right ventricular function in severe chronic airflow obstruction: A controlled clinical trial. Ann Intern Med 1981; 95:283–287.
24. Green LH, Smith TW: The use of digitalis in patients with pulmonary disease. Ann Intern Med 1977; 87:459–465.
25. Reitz BA, Wallwork JL, Hunt SA, et al: Heart-lung transplantation: Successful therapy for patients with pulmonary vascular disease. N Engl J Med 1982; 306:557–564.
26. Pasque MK, Trulock EP, Kaiser LD, et al: Single lung transplantation for pulmonary hypertension: Three month hemodynamic follow-up. Circulation 1991; 84:2275–2279.
27. Barst RJ, Rubin LJ, Long WA, et al. A comparison of continuous intravenous epoprostenol (prostacyclin) with conventional therapy for primary pulmonary hypertension. N Engl J Med 1996; 334:296–301.
28. Kierstein D, Levy PS, Hsu DT, et al: Blade balloon atrial septostomy in patients with severe primary pulmonary hypertension. Circulation 1995; 91:2028–2035.
29. Traver GA, Cline MG, Burrows B: Predictors of mortality in chronic obstructive pulmonary disease. Am Rev Respir Dis 1979; 119:895–902.
30. D'Alonzo GG, Barst RJ, Ayres SM, et al: Survival in patients with primary pulmonary hypertension: Results from a national prospective registry. Ann Intern Med 1991; 115:343–349.

141

Life-Threatening Hemoptysis

David H. Ingbar, MD

Hemoptysis is an important symptom and sign of respiratory or systemic disease because it often indicates the presence of a serious or life-threatening underlying disorder. In addition, the blood in the airway or alveoli may in and of itself be life-threatening, especially in patients with other pulmonary disease. Even for experienced practitioners, hemoptysis is a concern for several reasons:

1. The clinical course of bleeding is variable and usually unpredictable.
2. There are no easy or effective treatment options at the bedside when bleeding is massive.
3. A large number of diagnoses are possible in patients presenting with hemoptysis.
4. With the decline in incidence of tuberculosis (TB) and bronchiectasis in many countries, the causes and prevalence of hemoptysis have changed. Much of the literature on hemoptysis is relatively old, and modern therapies have altered the clinical scenarios in which it is seen, especially in hospitalized patients.

Several excellent reviews of hemoptysis are available.[1-3]

In contrast to mortality from gastrointestinal bleeding, mortality from hemoptysis is rarely due to exsanguination. Rather, mortality more often arises from the accumulation of blood in functional alveoli and the lack of effective gas exchange, even after intubation and ventilation with high inspired oxygen concentrations (FIO_2). Blood can also clot within the airways and obstruct ventilation more proximally. Several factors are believed to predict higher mortality in patients with hemoptysis:

- Prior lung dysfunction
- Inability to cough out the blood
- Larger amounts or volumes of blood retained in the lung
- Rate of bleeding
- Comorbid processes
- Volume of blood lost

The term *massive hemoptysis* is commonly used to indicate that bleeding is potentially life-threatening, but there is no consensus definition of the amount of blood or rate of bleeding that should be termed "massive." This term has been used for a range of amounts from a total of 100 mL of hemoptysis to a rate of more than 300 mL expectorated over less than 6 hours. In a 1982 series from Kings County Hospital in New York City, the term *exsanguinating hemoptysis* was defined as bleeding at a rate above 150 mL/hour, or a total of greater than 600 mL.[4] The mortality rate for these patients was 75% without surgical therapy. Not surprisingly, survival was somewhat better in the surgical group; however, perioperative morbidity was high.

The overall mortality from massive hemoptysis has been examined several times since the mid-1970s. In a retrospective study of 208 patients with hemoptysis at Hadassah University Hospital from 1980 to 1995, mortality was 9% overall but ranged from 2.5% in patients with trivial amounts of hemoptysis to 38% in those with massive hemoptysis (>500 mL over

24 hours).[5] In a 7-year retrospective study in South Africa of patients with more than 200 mL of hemoptysis over a 24-hour period, the in-hospital mortality rate was 10% and did not differ between patients treated with and without surgery.[6]

In general, the mortality of patients with massive hemoptysis, defined as more than 200 mL per 24 hours, is significant and probably increases with greater rates of hemoptysis.

ANATOMIC ORIGINS OF BLEEDING

The principal sources of bleeding into the lung are as follows:

- Bronchial arteries
- Pulmonary arteries
- Pulmonary capillaries or veins
- Systemic fistulas (rarely)

Bronchial Arteries

The bronchial arteries are the source of most episodes of massive hemoptysis because, unlike in the pulmonary arteries, the blood is under systemic pressure. The bronchial arteries arise directly or indirectly from the aorta between the level of the 3rd and 8th thoracic vertebrae and exhibit considerable anatomic variation in normal individuals. In most people, two to four bronchial arteries arise either from the aorta directly or from the intercostal artery. The right bronchial artery often arises from a common right intercostal artery and commonly supplies a branch to the left bronchial artery. Of major concern, the anterior spinal artery may derive from the bronchial artery in up to 5% of patients, creating a risk for paraplegia with embolization.

The bronchial arteries supply the conducting airways, the vasa vasorum of the large pulmonary arteries, and the pleura. The bronchial veins empty into the right heart. Normally, bronchopulmonary anastomoses allow bronchial arterial blood to drain into the pulmonary veins and left heart. In chronic airway inflammation, such as bronchiectasis or cystic fibrosis, the bronchial circulation proliferates and the tortuous hypertrophic vessels are easily damaged and ruptured. The anastomoses with the pulmonary circulation increase so that the bronchial tree may supply much of the pulmonary parenchymal blood flow as well.

The bronchial arteries are the source of bleeding in most chronic parenchymal lung infections, such as lung abscess, mycetomas, and other chronic fungal infections and pulmonary TB. They also are the source in bronchogenic carcinoma, endobronchial metastases, congenital heart disease with decreased pulmonary arterial blood flow, and broncholithiasis. The bronchial veins also may account for hemoptysis, as in patients with mitral stenosis.

Pulmonary Arteries

Much less commonly, the pulmonary arteries are the source of major bleeding Arteriovenous malformations (AVMs) are supplied with blood flow from the pulmonary arteries. Hemoptysis after a pulmonary embolus or infarction also derives from the pulmonary arteries, but the amount of bleeding usually is small. The pulmonary arteries are also the source of iatrogenic hemoptysis with balloon flotation pulmonary arterial catheter–induced infarction or pulmonary artery rupture. Patients with pulmonary TB may die suddenly of rupture of a Rasmussen's aneurysm. The original pathologic studies suggested that the aneurysm occurred from dilatation of a pulmonary artery near an inflamed lung cavity that resulted in gradual expansion of the inflamed arterial wall into the free space until rupture occurred.[7] However, other authorities believe that at least some of these aneurysms of bronchial arterial origin.

In the past, it was believed that systemic arterial origin of hemoptysis was rare, but more recent arteriographic and embolization studies indicate that it accounts for up to 5% to 10% of hemoptysis in patients who have angiographic embolization.[8] Sometimes these bleeding episodes originate from congenital abnormalities or from thoracic trauma. Chronic inflammation can lead to new collateral blood supply from intrathoracic systemic arteries, including the axillary, intercostal, subclavian, and phrenic arteries. Aortic aneurysms may present with hemoptysis, but the precise anatomic pathway is not defined.

ETIOLOGY

Hemoptysis may result from a broad range of causes, and their relative frequency is shifting. In addition, sometimes bleeding from the upper gastrointestinal tract or the upper airway is easily confused with bleeding originating from the lung itself.

The broad differential diagnosis is a challenge for clinicians, especially since it is important to quickly define the cause in patients with massive hemoptysis. The frequency of the specific etiologic mechanisms varies considerably, depending on the practice setting. Apart from the Kings County Hospital series from the mid-1970s, very few large series are available to specify this range. In the South African series of 120 patients, TB accounted for 73% of patients, aspergillomas, 6%; bronchogenic carcinoma, 5%; and other lung infections, 6%. Undoubtedly, the distribution would be different at many tertiary care centers in the United States.

Infections

Infection is a common cause of hemoptysis, especially in underdeveloped countries. TB, lung abscess, and mycetomas are relatively common causes of massive hemoptysis.

Tuberculosis

TB can cause hemoptysis in several ways. Active tuberculous pneumonitis can cause hemoptysis from the bronchial circulation owing to lung parenchymal necrosis, with or without cavity formation. In patients with chronic cavitary TB, Rasmussen's aneurysms can cause sudden massive and fatal bleeding. In the era of sanitaria, sudden massive hemoptysis was a relatively common clinical mode of death. Autopsy series from the 1940s and 1950s indicate that 5% to 7% of patients with long-standing TB died of sudden, massive hemoptysis. Inactive TB can lead to hemoptysis through the residual bronchiectasis, reactivation of infection, development of a scar carcinoma, or formation of a mycetoma in an old cavity.

The course of hemoptysis from TB is usually unpredictable, and the ability to know a sentinel bleed that presages a subsequent massive bleed is possible only in retrospect. In the recent series of South African patients, approximately 50% of the TB patients had cavitary active TB while the others mainly had either noncavitary pneumonitis or bronchiectasis.

Lung Abscess

Lung abscess can also cause sudden massive hemoptysis, presumably from erosion of a bronchial vessel in the cavity wall. Fortunately, this problem has become less common. Older series report that 10% to 15% of patients with lung abscess have hemoptysis and, of these, hemoptysis is massive in 20% to 50%. This etiology has been considered an indication for early resection, although relatively few data support this recommendation.

Fungal Pulmonary Infections

Like TB, fungal pulmonary infections can lead to hemoptysis in multiple fashions. Fungal pneumonitis frequently causes hemoptysis, especially in immunocompromised hosts with poor clotting function. *Aspergillus* can do this either via direct parenchymal lung invasion or by angioinvasion with distal infarction.[8] Mucormycosis behaves similarly. Both of these fungi can have direct airway involvement with localized ulceration and bleeding. Cocciodomycosis also can lead to hemoptysis in 15% of primary infections and up to 50% of chronic cavitary infections. Blastomycosis, histoplasmosis, and cryptococcosis also may cause hemoptysis.

Mycetomas

Mycetomas are commonly accompanied by hemoptysis, with bleeding occurring at some point in up to 50% of these patients. The initial cavity may be the result of TB, sarcoidosis, an old necrotizing infection, bullous emphysema, or an old lung abscess. The chronic inflammation in the cavity wall induced by the persistent immunologic reaction leads to bronchial hypervascularity and intermittent bleeding. This can pose a major management problem, because these problems often have multifocal scarring and resection of the mycetoma may worsen lung function and lead to greater scarring and retraction, with formation of additional bullae. Aspergillomas are the most common form, but *Mucor* and rarely *Candida* also can produce fungus balls.

Bacterial and Viral Infections

Bacterial and viral infections are less common causes of significant hemoptysis, although minor amounts of bleeding can lead to blood-streaked or "rusty" sputum. Massive hemoptysis is rare in this setting unless the patient has a coagulation disorder or is taking antiplatelet or anticoagulant drugs. Primary varicella infection of the lungs can lead to moderate hemoptysis with vesicular rupture. *Serratia marcescens* may make the sputum red, resulting in pseudohemoptysis.

Parasitic Infections

Parasitic infections are the most common worldwide cause of hemoptysis, led by *Paragonimus* in Southeast Asia. Other parasites that may cause hemoptysis when they involve the lung include *Amoeba*, *Ascaris*, *Clonorchis*, *Echinococcus*, hookworm, *Strongyloides*, and *Trichinella*.

Neoplasms

Bronchogenic carcinoma leads to hemoptysis in approximately 30% to 50% of patients at some point in the course of their illness. When it is the presenting symptom, hemoptysis typically is intermittent streaking that lasts for more than 14 days, rather than massive hemoptysis. Although massive hemoptysis from bronchogenic carcinoma does not occur in a high percentage of patients (~3%), it is not a rare occurrence because bronchogenic carcinoma is relatively common.

In one series of patients from the Kansas City Veterans Administration, lung cancer patients with massive hemoptysis typically had central chest lesions with squamous cell carcinoma pathology. Massive terminal hemoptysis occurred in 3% of patients in this series.[9] Approximately 50% of these patients had evidence of cavitation on chest roentgenogram.

In rare instances, the tumor can directly invade the pulmonary vasculature or aorta, leading to rapid demise, especially if there is communication with the airway. The mechanism of hemoptysis may be erosion into airways or blood vessels, mucosal obstruction, or infection distal to obstruction.

Carcinoid Tumors

Bronchial carcinoid tumors are associated with a high frequency of bleeding because of their vascularity. Typically, they occur in younger individuals with a history of chronic cough or recurrent localized pneumonias. Most commonly, they are slowly growing polypoid tumors that are on a stalk from the wall of a large airway, but they can present as solitary peripheral pulmonary nodules. When viewed through a bronchoscope, they usually are deep red or pink owing to their rich bronchial arterial blood supply. When the tumors are visualized this way, there is controversy about the safety of endobronchial biopsy because of the risk of inducing hemorrhage.

Metastatic Cancer

Metastatic tumors involving the lung occasionally cause hemoptysis, particularly when endobronchial metastases are present. The most common primary tumors to cause significant hemoptysis are melanoma and carcinomas of the breast, colon, or kidney. Esophageal cancer rarely erodes into the lung and airways, resulting in hemoptysis and sometimes massive exsanguination. Other tumors that may be associated with hemoptysis when they metastasize to the lung are choriocarcinoma, papillary thyroid carcinoma, and osteogenic sarcoma.

Hematologic Malignancies

In patients with hematologic malignancies who undergo bone marrow transplantation, a diffuse alveolar hemorrhage syndrome commonly develops.[10] The precise cause is often unknown, but the syndrome may represent a form of lung damage related to the conditioning regimens with cytotoxic drugs or radiation, combined with subclinical infection. Sometimes alveolar hemorrhage is precipitated by a defined lung infection, particularly with fungi or viruses, but it may also occur independently. When it is an isolated problem, the patient typically improves over 2 to 4 days when treated with correction of underlying coagulopathy and high-dose of steroids. Even if these patients require mechanical ventilation, the short-term prognosis for lung recovery and extubation is very good.

Alternatively, alveolar hemorrhage in this setting may accompany the onset of the acute respiratory distress syndrome (ARDS) and the need for mechanical ventilation with very high levels of inspired oxygen. Typically, this occurs at the time of the return of neutrophils or *engraftment syndrome*. In the setting of ARDS, rapid improvement is unlikely and patients tend to be ventilator-dependent for prolonged periods and to have high mortality.

Chronic Airway Inflammation

Historically, bronchiectasis has been one of the three major causes of massive hemoptysis, and it remains significant today. In the past, it probably originated from TB, narcotizing pneumonia, or childhood viral infections, such as whooping cough. Today, with more widespread use of antibiotics and vaccines, the cause is less clear. Certainly, TB and previous lung infections remain major causes. In addition, cystic fibrosis (CF), mucociliary clearance defects, and immune deficiencies are more common causes of bronchiectasis, since people live longer with these entities.

Bronchiectasis

Bronchiectasis leads to classic symptoms of chronic cough, recurrent bronchitis, and sputum production in approximately 85% of patients, but 15% of patients have *dry bronchiectasis*, without sputum production. In this condition, the bronchial arteries are hypertrophic and ectatic with enlargement of the submucosal anastomotic plexi in the bronchial walls. Because the bleeding is from bronchial arteries, it occurs with systemic pressure. As severe bronchiectasis has become less prevalent, the classic chest roentgenogram finding of "tram tracks" now is less common. Chest computed tomography (CT) is the most sensitive diagnostic test, especially for saccular bronchiectasis. Underlying causes of bronchiectasis include (1) immunodeficiencies, including selective deficiency of IgA or some IgG subclasses, and (2) mucociliary defects, such as immotile cilia syndrome, Kartagener's syndrome, and Young's syndrome.

Cystic Fibrosis

The spectrum of clinical disease in CF has evolved markedly with more affected individuals surviving into adulthood and increased recognition of milder forms that present in the adult age range. Massive hemoptysis occurs in only 0.2% of patients with CF younger than 18 years of age but in 2.1% of those above age 18. Chronic infection and pooling of secretions rich in neutrophils lead to progressive airway damage, resulting in patchy, diffuse bronchiectasis, which in turn continues this process. Given the recurrent nature of these infections and the progressive decline in lung function with age, treatment of massive hemoptysis with bronchial artery embolization, rather than surgical resection, preserves the maximum amount of viable lung tissue.

Bronchitis

Bronchitis is a common final diagnosis in patients with small amounts of hemoptysis. In the setting of a patient with chronic obstructive pulmonary disease (COPD) with an acute infective exacerbation of bronchitis, small amounts of hemoptysis are common; however, the hemoptysis almost always is minor and disappears after several days. In patients with hemoptysis who undergo bronchoscopy, airway inflammation often is present, but it is not certain that bronchitis by itself can cause massive hemoptysis. In essence, bronchitis is a specific etiologic mechanism of exclusion as the cause of massive hemoptysis and consequently should be accepted only cautiously and after thorough evaluation.

Pulmonary Vascular Disorders

Hemoptysis commonly occurs in primary pulmonary hypertension and in long-standing secondary pulmonary hypertension, including congenital heart disease with Eisenmenger's complex. Usually, the amounts of bleeding are relatively small in the absence of anticoagulation or a coagulopathy. Presumably, the plexiform pulmonary vascular lesions can rupture when subjected to high pressure or flow. Occasionally, atherosclerotic plaques that have formed with chronic high pressure in large pulmonary vessels or small arterioles can rupture and result in massive bleeding.

Congenital pulmonary arteriovenous malformations (AVMs) are an increasingly recognized cause of hemoptysis.[11] AVMs arise gradually from abnormal capillary development late in gestation and their clinical detectability increases with age. They can occur in isolation or as part of the inherited systemic vascular disorder Osler-Weber-Rendu syndrome or hereditary hemorrhagic telangiectasia. More than 8% of patients with hereditary hemorrhagic telangiectasia have episodes of massive hemoptysis at some point in their life. Figure 141–1 demonstrates diffuse pulmonary AVMs in the right lung of a 54-year-old woman with isolated AVMs who presented with complaints of dyspnea on exertion and then had an episode of massive hemoptysis.

Pulmonary artery aneurysms can occur in the rare entities

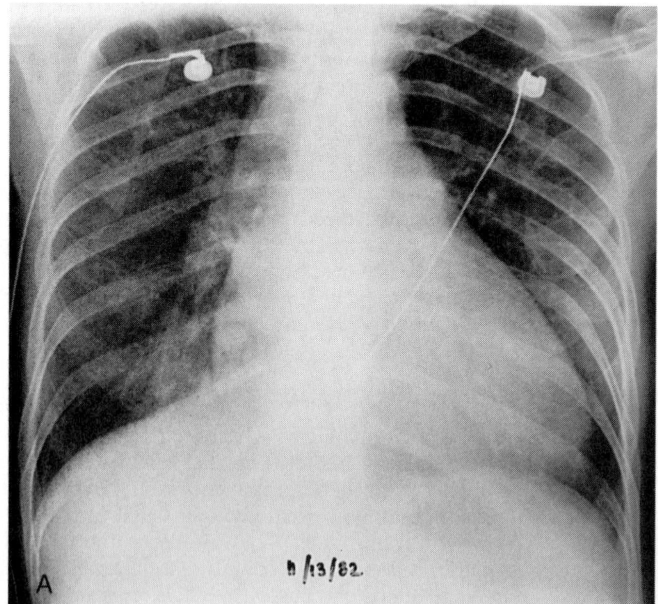

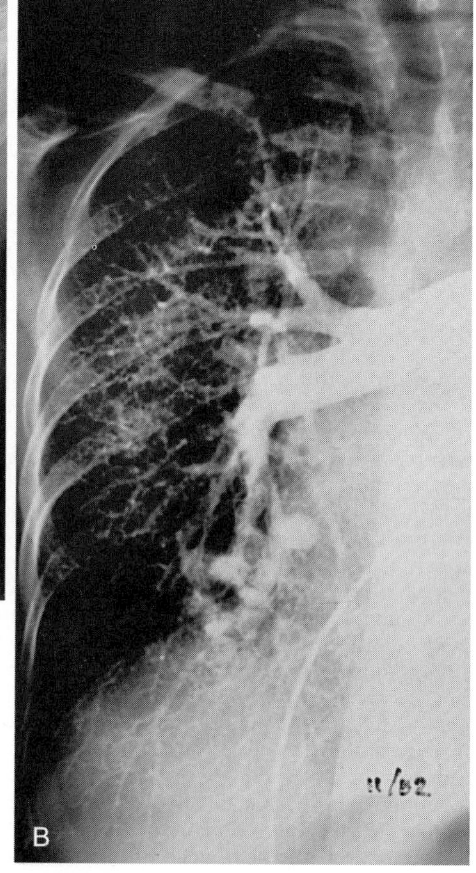

Figure 141–1. Posteroanterior chest roentgenogram *(A)* and right pulmonary arteriogram *(B)* demonstrating arteriovenous malformations (AVMs). The patient is a 54-year-old woman who presented with dyspnea on exertion and on the admitting chest roentgenogram shown. While hospitalized for evaluation, she had an episode of massive hemoptysis. A pulmonary arteriogram was taken after bronchoscopy because of the suspected nodular lesions demonstrated multiple AVMs in the right lung. She had thyrotoxicosis also, but did not have hereditary hemolytic telangiectasia.

Behçet's disease and Takayasu's arteritis. The aneurysms can rupture, resulting in massive hemoptysis.

Pulmonary emboli frequently cause scant amounts of hemoptysis, particularly as part of the pulmonary infarction syndrome. The classic presentation of this syndrome also includes pleuritic chest pain, a small bloody pleural effusion, and a small infiltrate on chest roentgenogram. Usually, hemoptysis is caused by small emboli that cause distal infarction in individuals with little underlying cardiopulmonary disease. With anticoagulation, thrombolytic therapy or an underlying coagulopathy, massive bleeding may occur.

Other Vascular and Cardiovascular Disorders

With the decline in rheumatic fever, mitral stenosis has become a rare cause of hemoptysis. The elevated left atrial pressure raises pulmonary venous and capillary pressure, eventually leading to some retrograde blood flow through bronchopulmonary anastomoses into the bronchial veins. Over time, bronchial venous calcification, which markedly elevates pulmonary capillary pressure, occurs. The dilated submucosal bronchial venous plexus easily can bleed, causing *cardiac apoplexy*, especially with infection or when vascular pressures are elevated with exertion. Bleeding typically is diffuse and can cause severe hypoxemia, which is resistant to treatment with supplemental oxygen.

Another uncommon cause of hemoptysis is a septic pulmonary embolus from right-sided infective endocarditis. Aortic aneurysms can cause small or large amounts of hemoptysis, even when they are of nontraumatic origin. The anatomic mechanism is not defined, but presumably a fistula forms between the aorta and bronchial tree.[12]

Immunologic Disorders

A variety of systemic immune disorders can lead to hemoptysis, often presenting as diffuse alveolar hemorrhage. This diagnosis can be confusing, in that patients frequently do not cough up large quantities of blood, presumably because alveolar bleeding does not activate airway irritant receptors. These entities and their specific diagnosis and management are detailed elsewhere.[13, 14]

The disorders most prominently associated with hemoptysis are systemic lupus erythematosus (SLE), Wegener's granulomatosis, and anti-basement membrane antibody (Goodpasture's) syndrome (Fig. 141-2), but hemoptysis also is associated with nonspecific systemic narcotizing vasculitis and the rare entity idiopathic pulmonary hemosiderosis. Patients with SLE may have either primarily alveolar hemorrhage or an acute lupus pneumonitis syndrome with high fever and a localized infiltrate.[15] Wegener's granulomatosis usually features nodular lesions on the chest roentgenogram, but interstitial infiltrates are the primary radiologic manifestation in 10% of patients.

Recognizing that hemoptysis is due to these disorders is important for two major reasons. First, the bleeding usually is diffuse, obviating the value of local therapies such as bronchial blockade, embolization or surgery. Second, initiation of immunosuppressive treatment may be life-saving.

The specific appropriate treatment depends on the particular diagnosis, including plasmapheresis for many patients. It has now been recognized that the histopathology accounting for hemoptysis in many of these disorders is pulmonary capillaritis. In Wegener's granulomatosis, the medium and large vessel inflammation can lead to regions of central necrosis that contribute to hemoptysis from cavitary lesions. Capillaritis and hemoptysis have been recognized to occur in other immune lung diseases, such as rheumatoid arthritis and mixed connective tissue disease.[16] The diagnostic work-up of these entities usually includes serologic studies for anti-basement membrane antibodies, antinuclear antibodies, rheumatoid factor levels, and antineutrophil cytoplasmic antibodies. Biopsy of the lung or another involved site often is essential to confirm the diagnosis and to initiate the appropriate systemic therapy.

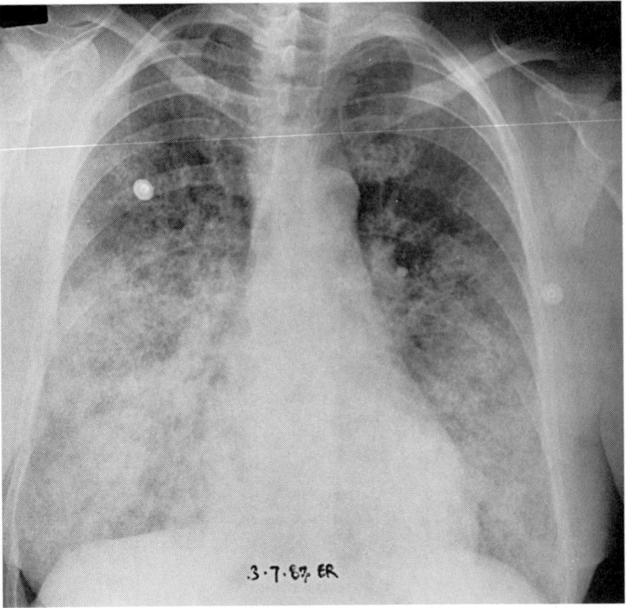

Figure 141–2. Chest roentgenogram from a patient with Goodpasture's syndrome. The patient is a 45-year-old woman who presented with shortness of breath and edema. She had acute renal and respiratory failure. She was coughing up scant amounts of blood, but the chest roentgenogram shown here was obtained. Bronchoscopy showed the presence of fresh blood in all lobar bronchi. The diagnosis was made by both anti-basement membrane antibody serology and renal biopsy immunofluorescence studies.

Miscellaneous Disorders

Patients with bullous emphysema can have the sudden onset of massive hemoptysis without any clear-cut precipitant. Presumably, infection erodes into an adjacent bronchial vessel.

Chest trauma is often accompanied by hemoptysis. In addition to the possibility of aortic aneurysm, other specific causes include ruptured bronchus, fat embolism, and blunt or penetrating chest trauma.

A variety of drugs and toxins can cause hemoptysis. Diffuse alveolar hemorrhage is reported with trimetallic anhydride exposure, anticoagulants, and penicillamine use. Exposure to solvents can precipitate Goodpasture's syndrome for unknown reasons.

Broncholithiasis or an airway foreign body may cause a highly vascular, granulomatous airway lesion that bleeds easily. When a suggestive history is present, these are important causes that should be confirmed by bronchoscopic and radiologic studies.

Other rare causes of massive hemoptysis include endometriosis, pulmonary amyloidosis, and disseminated intravascular coagulation (DIC).

Iatrogenic Hemoptysis

The three major iatrogenic causes of hemoptysis are:

- Bronchoscopy with biopsy
- Transthoracic needle biopsy
- Balloon inflation trauma from pulmonary artery catheterization

Hemoptysis from the first two causes can be reduced somewhat by careful patient selection and reversal of any bleeding tendency prior to the procedure. Pulmonary artery catheters may result in localized infarction or a pulmonary artery rupture. The diagnosis of infarction is usually suggested by a local patchy chest roentgenographic infiltrate near the tip of a catheter that is particularly distal in the lung. Patients usually have minor amounts of hemoptysis, and the lesion usually resolves gradually, with pull-back of the catheter.

In contrast, pulmonary artery rupture usually leads to massive rapid bleeding that frequently is fatal.[17] Risk factors for rupture include:

- Pulmonary hypertension
- Distal catheter tip position
- Presence of a wedge pulmonary artery waveform when the balloon is only partially inflated
- Prolonged balloon inflation

Sometimes patients can be managed conservatively with blockade therapy; at other times surgery is the only hope of saving the patient's life.

Cryptogenic Hemoptysis

Cryptogenic hemoptysis is defined as hemoptysis that does not have a specific etiology after careful diagnostic evaluation, including bronchoscopy, sputum cytology, chest roentgenogram, serologic studies, and—in the current era—a CT chest study. Even though cryptogenic hemoptysis is the final diagnosis in 5% to 10% of patients with submassive hemoptysis, it is much less common as a final diagnosis for massive hemoptysis and should be accepted only with careful scrutiny. Although most patients with submassive cryptogenic hemoptysis have an excellent prognosis, whether this applies to the much smaller population with cryptogenic massive hemoptysis is not clear.

DIAGNOSIS AND MANAGEMENT

Diagnostic Evaluation

In an ideal world, the systematic, detailed history and physical examination are the initial steps in the evaluation of hemoptysis. Based on the broad differential diagnosis, a number of specific avenues are important in the history, including:

- Travel experience
- Smoking history
- Occupation
- Recent chest trauma
- Underlying cardiopulmonary disease
- History of upper airway, sinus, or upper gastrointestinal problems
- Previous episodes of hemoptysis
- Recent infectious symptoms
- Family history of hemoptysis
- Drug usage
- Unilateral or bilateral leg swelling

It is particularly important to seek indications of upper airway or gastrointestinal sources of bleeding in the history and examination. This can be difficult, since patients with hemoptysis may describe blood welling up in the back of the throat that then is coughed out. In addition, patients with hemoptysis may swallow some of this blood, leading to positive stool guaiac tests or nasogastric aspirates. Conversely, patients with upper gastrointestinal or upper airway hemorrhage may aspirate some blood and thus blood may be present in the tracheobronchial tree. The age of the patient alters the most probable cause; younger individuals tend to have CF, congenital disorders, a foreign body, or a bronchial carcinoid; older patients are more likely to have cancer or bronchiectasis. The pattern of bleeding also is helpful in the diagnosis (see earlier). In rare instances, the history is virtually diagnostic, as when hemoptysis coincides with menses and is due to endometriosis of the airways or when there is a clear cut history of foreign body aspiration.

It is important that the clinician determine and record the rate and amount of bleeding. It is useful to obtain a historical assessment of the amount of bleeding and then to quantitate the amount of blood expectorated while the patient is in the hospital. This parameter is important, in that it guides the rate and aggressiveness of much of the diagnostic evaluation and treatment.

The physical examination generally is less helpful than the history unless telangiectasias are seen or a chest bruit suggests an AVM. The presence of crackles or wheezes over a chest region does not guarantee that this is the bleeding site, since blood may move in the bronchial tree from its origination. For example, bleeding from the right upper lobe may lead to primarily right lower lobe physical examination and chest x-ray findings due to dependent pooling. Physical findings suggestive of a deep venous thrombosis should be sought, even though the examination is not very sensitive. Nasal passages and the upper airway should be carefully examined as possible sites of bleeding or as a site of Wegener's granulomatosis.

All patients should undergo thorough laboratory tests, including a chest roentgenogram, an electrocardiogram, complete blood count, platelet count, prothrombin and partial thromboplastin times, electrolytes, blood urea nitrogen, creatinine and glucose determinations, and urinalysis.

Special diagnostic studies are often needed, such as sputum cytology, Gram stain, and specimens for culture, and examination for acid-fast bacilli and fungi. These tests should be performed early in most patients if the diagnosis is not clear. When there is a question of a primary cardiac etiology, such as congenital disease or mitral stenosis, echocardiography and sometimes right-sided or left-sided cardiac catheterization need to performed.

An echocardiogram also may be helpful in establishing the presence of significant pulmonary hypertension, demonstrating a migrating clot en passage, excluding right-sided endocarditis, and excluding intracardiac right-to-left shunts as a contributor to hypoxemia. It also may suggest the presence of an aortic aneurysm, but even transesophageal echocardiogram is not as sensitive a test as an aortogram, especially for early tears and less flagrant dissections.

Coagulation studies, including blood smears, are helpful in evaluating the possibility of hematologic malignancy, DIC, or thrombotic thrombocytopenic purpura as a cause. Sometimes bone marrow aspiration and biopsy also are necessary. Nodular pulmonary infiltrates raise a broad range of diagnostic possibilities, including infections, neoplasia or vasculitis, such as Wegener's granulomatosis. In these patients, multiple diagnostic avenues need to be pursued rapidly. For patients with diffuse x-ray changes, consistent with diffuse alveolar hemorrhage, serologic studies (including antinuclear antibody, rheumatoid factor levels, antineutrophil cytoplasmic antibody, and anti–basement membrane antibody) should be performed. Some patients require tissue biopsies with immunofluorescence studies to establish a diagnosis. Unfortunately, small bronchoscopic biopsies often do not yield enough lung tissue to confidently establish a diagnosis, especially when vasculitis is the cause. Debate remains about the need for renal or open lung biopsy in patients with pulmonary-renal syndromes. If the diagnosis can be rapidly established by serologic testing, biopsy may be obviated. If these tests cannot be rapidly available or are nondiagnostic, establishing a diagnosis and early initiation of appropriate therapy usually make the morbidity associated with biopsy worthwhile.

Approach to the Patient

Although establishing a specific diagnosis is important, with massive hemoptysis the initial focus must be to stabilize the patient. First, the following factors must be rapidly assessed as follows:

- Oxygenation
- Gas exchange
- Hemodynamic state
- Airway patency
- Ability to clear blood

In addition to vital signs, a rapid cardiopulmonary physical examination, oximetry readings, an arterial blood gas determination, and a chest roentgenogram are required immediately. If the patient is clearly in respiratory distress, intubation is performed with a large-bore (No. 8 or greater) standard endotracheal tube. If the chest roentgenogram demonstrates primarily unilateral new infiltrates, the affected side should be placed in the dependent position in order to decrease spreading of blood to the less affected side. If the patient does not need early intubation, cough suppression usually is advocated. Obviously, it is desirable to have the patient clear blood from the lungs; thus, one must walk a fine line to prevent oversedation.

Oxygen supplementation and gas humidification are usually indicated. If the patient requires intubation and is continuing to have large volumes of hemoptysis, immediate fiberoptic bronchoscopy is recommended so that the primary region of bleeding can be localized. Pulmonary and thoracic surgery consultants should be called early, and blood should be prepared for transfusion.

Evaluative blood work should be done as quickly as possible, with the clinician looking for coagulopathy and renal failure in particular. The finding of coagulopathy provides an avenue for early corrective therapy with blood products, and the presence renal failure has a major impact on the diagnostic and therapeutic approaches to be followed. Any recent use of aspirin or nonsteroidal anti-inflammatory drugs (NSAIDs) indicates the need to consider platelet transfusion. If there is any significant concern that bleeding is of upper airway or upper gastrointestinal origin, appropriate consultation should be initiated early.

If the patient continues to have major hemoptysis and the site of bleeding remains uncertain, three initial approaches are possible:

1. Placement of a double lumen endotracheal tube by an experienced individual.
2. Rigid bronchoscopy in the operating room.
3. Angiographic evaluation with embolization of abnormalities discovered.

In general, the tempo of the diagnostic work-up is secondary to the need for patient stabilization. The two goals must be judiciously interlinked, however, because specific therapy for some diagnostic entities should be initiated as early as possible.

Role of Bronchoscopy

A major question that needs to be resolved early in patients with massive hemoptysis is whether the bleeding is originating from a localized site or whther it is diffuse. Flexible fiberoptic bronchoscopy often provides the fastest answer. Usually, patients with ongoing massive hemoptysis should be intubated either before or as part of this procedure because rapid bleeding may be induced by either coughing or clot dislodgment or minor airway trauma from the bronchoscope; this may worsen oxygenation and may make bronchoscopic visualization impossible. It is important to look for lobar or segmental bronchi that have active fresh bleeding rather than for old clotting, since the latter may not represent sites of bleeding. If there is significant clotting in the airways, this may compromise oxygenation because of obstruction of major bronchi, and it may therefore be worthwhile to attempt to clear the clot because this also permits assessment of distal active bleeding. However, this step also is risky in the patient with little reserve and, therefore, must be done cautiously and selectively.

Older literature has strongly suggested rigid bronchoscopy as the procedure of choice for the patient with massive hemoptysis. The major advantage is that suctioning of large clots is much more effective, and hence visualization can be accomplished in the presence of more vigorous ongoing bleeding. It also offers some additional direct therapeutic options, such as cautery and topical application of medications. However, the practical aspects of rapid rigid bronchoscopy make it less attractive in the early management of patients with massive hemoptysis, since it usually requires a trip to the operating room, with some potential hazard, and relatively few surgeons remain skilled in this technique. When surgery is the likely definitive therapy of choice, the inconvenience of rigid bronchoscopy is less problematic since operative therapy is likely in any case. On balance, in most patients fiberoptic bronchoscopy through an endotracheal tube should be attempted first in the intensive care unit; if this step is unsuccessful in localizing bleeding, rigid bronchoscopy should be seriously considered.

In patients with massive hemoptysis that has stopped, what is the optimum timing of bronchoscopy? Few studies have carefully examined this question, but generally data indicate that early bronchoscopy has higher success in localizing the active bleeding site but may not augment or change the final diagnosis when the work-up is complete. Practically, this suggests that patients who are no longer bleeding do not always require immediate bronchoscopy, but bronchoscopy should be done within 12 to 16 hours, if not much sooner. The risk of delaying bronchoscopy is that if massive bleeding recurs in the interim, uncertainty about the bleeding side or site as well as the specific diagnosis may make management more difficult. For example, knowing the likely side of bleeding makes rational endobronchial blockade therapy a reasonable early option for many patients.

Endobronchial Blockade and Other Temporizing Therapies

If bronchoscopy localizes either the side or major bronchial site from which bleeding originates, endobronchial blockade therapy may be possible. At the time of bronchoscopy, a Fogarty catheter balloon may be placed outside the endotracheal tube (ETT) and just far enough to occlude the bronchial site of bleeding. The ETT cuff may stabilize the catheter placement; if rebleeding occurs, bronchoscopic visualization of the situation is very important. In the small series reported, the balloon was left inflated for 24 to 48 hours and the patient was observed after deflation.

Alternatively, selective intubation of either the right or left main bronchus may preserve ventilation to the nonbleeding lung while preventing spillage of blood into this side. It is easier to intubate the right main bronchus, but usually the

ETT cuff occludes the right upper lobe, thereby losing gas exchange for this lobe and the entire left lung. In contrast, if bleeding is on the right side, selective intubation of the left mainstem bronchus may be attempted using the bronchoscope as a guide. Potential complications of endobronchial blockade are ischemic mucosal injury and postobstructive pneumonia.

Other topical endobronchial therapies, such as thrombin-fibrinogen solutions, have been used in small, uncontrolled series and may help to slow bleeding temporarily. Topical epinephrine also often is used but has not been evaluated carefully. Iced saline lavage has been used but has no proven benefit and may worsen oxygenation. Endobronchial packing under direct vision during rigid bronchoscopy has not proved beneficial and presents the risks of dislodgment, obstruction, and distal infection. It is a last-ditch maneuver to be used in desperate circumstances.

Double-Lumen Endotracheal Tubes

Split lung ventilation using double-lumen endotracheal tubes is another approach to spare the nonbleeding lung and to determine which lung is the primary site of bleeding.[18] Thus, this method serves as an alternative for stabilization of the patient. The initial Carlen's double-lumen tube, which had a hook that sometimes caused carinal necrosis and laryngeal injury, has been supplanted by new versions that have either a right or left bronchial lumen and cuff and one tracheal lumen and cuff. Careful placement of the bronchial cuff is required so that it completely seals one mainstem bronchus proximally, without herniation or occlusion of other areas. If a sufficiently large double-lumen ETT can be placed so that a pediatric bronchoscope fits through each lumen, further diagnostic studies can be performed through this tube. However, use of a double-lumen ETT often poses significant practical problems:

1. These ETTs are often difficult to place safely and rapidly in the proper position, and an experienced individual must be on hand.
2. Because the ETT position can easily be dislodged, the patient must be paralyzed or sedated and must not be moved.
3. Medical and nursing staff need to know how to assess ETT and cuff placement, a complex procedure.
4. The relatively small lumen may make it difficult to remove large clots and can predispose to obstruction.

Thus, these tubes sometimes are useful as a temporizing measure, but individuals experienced in their use must be available. These tubes are most helpful for stabilizing a patient until arteriography or surgery is scheduled and, occasionally, for protection of the nonbleeding lung prior to rigid bronchoscopy, when patients are too ill for arteriography and the site of bleeding remains uncertain.

Computed Tomography of the Chest

Chest CT has been advocated as an important early diagnostic technique in patients with hemoptysis.[19, 20] This modality has the advantages of being able to detect AVMs, small bronchogenic cancer, lymphadenopathy, and other lesions frequently missed on plain chest roentgenograms and on bronchoscopy. For these reasons, chest CT is helpful in advance of bronchoscopy for submassive hemoptysis, especially in the outpatient setting. It may guide the bronchoscopist and may improve the diagnostic yield of bronchoscopy. However, chest CT may not detect smaller endobronchial lesions, including carcinomas and carcinoids. In the setting of massive hemoptysis, in which blood within the alveoli, blood clots in the airways, or blood in lung cavities are common, chest CT scans can be misleading and may result in an incorrect presumptive diagnosis. For example, a mass-like lesion in a cavity may suggest carcinoma when it is just blood within a preexisting cavity.

Thus, chest CT is helpful in selected patients with massive hemoptysis following stabilization, but it does not replace other diagnostic techniques. The one exception may be in the diagnosis of aortic aneurysms. If an aortic aneurysm is suspected, it may be worthwhile to perform a chest CT scan rather than proceed directly to aortography.

Other Radiologic Studies

Specialized tests, such as spiral chest CT angiography and newer magnetic resonance imaging scans, may identify pulmonary emboli or AVMs, but their sensitivity is not yet well established, especially for distal emboli. They may have a place in the elective work-up of the patient who has been stabilized, but they cannot yet confidently supplant other established techniques.

Arteriography and Embolization Therapy

Arteriography is gaining an increasingly important role in the management of patients with massive hemoptysis. In the hands of skilled invasive radiologists, it is able to identify sites that are the likely bleeding source and has a high success rate in stopping bleeding with embolization therapy. Because most massive bleeds originate from the bronchial arterial circulation, this usually is the first place to look for abnormal blood vessels unless either pulmonary emboli or AVMs are thought to be the cause of pulmonary arterial bleeding.

Usually, the radiologist first carefully examines the bronchial circulation. If findings are normal, the radiologist proceeds sequentially to examine the pulmonary arteries for AVMs or emboli and potential systemic collateral sources (e.g., the intercostal, internal mammary, axillary, or subclavian artery). The pulmonary arteries are the source of bleeding in 8% to 10% of patients, whereas systemic collaterals may contribute to bleeding in up to 50% of cases. A major advantage of arteriography is that this systematic approach can be applied to patients without definitive localization by bronchoscopy of either the cause or the site of bleeding. In addition, embolization is a more attractive option than surgery in patients with limited pulmonary reserve or bilateral parenchymal lung disease, such as CF, diffuse bronchiectasis, or multiple AVMs.

Bronchial arteriography is generally safe when performed by experienced radiologists. The major concern is the potential to either occlude blood flow to or embolize the anterior spinal artery, resulting in paraplegia. This risk can be minimized by carefully defining the anatomy of the spinal blood supply before embolization or distal advancement of the catheter. The rate of significant complications from bronchial arteriography is below 1%, and thus the potential benefits almost always outweigh this risk.

Occasionally, this technique cannot be safely performed because of the presence of small bronchial arteries, origin of an artery high in the thoracic aorta, or distorted mediastinal anatomy. Embolization should not be performed when the catheter tip is unstable, since systemic embolization to other organs may occur. Bronchial embolization halts bleeding in 85% to 100% of patients, even in patients with TB.[22] Embolization is relatively unsuccessful in one subgroup of patients, those with mycetomas. Hemoptysis sometimes recurs with 1 to 2 months, usually as a result of incomplete embolization of feeding nonbronchial systemic collateral vessels. Later rebleed-

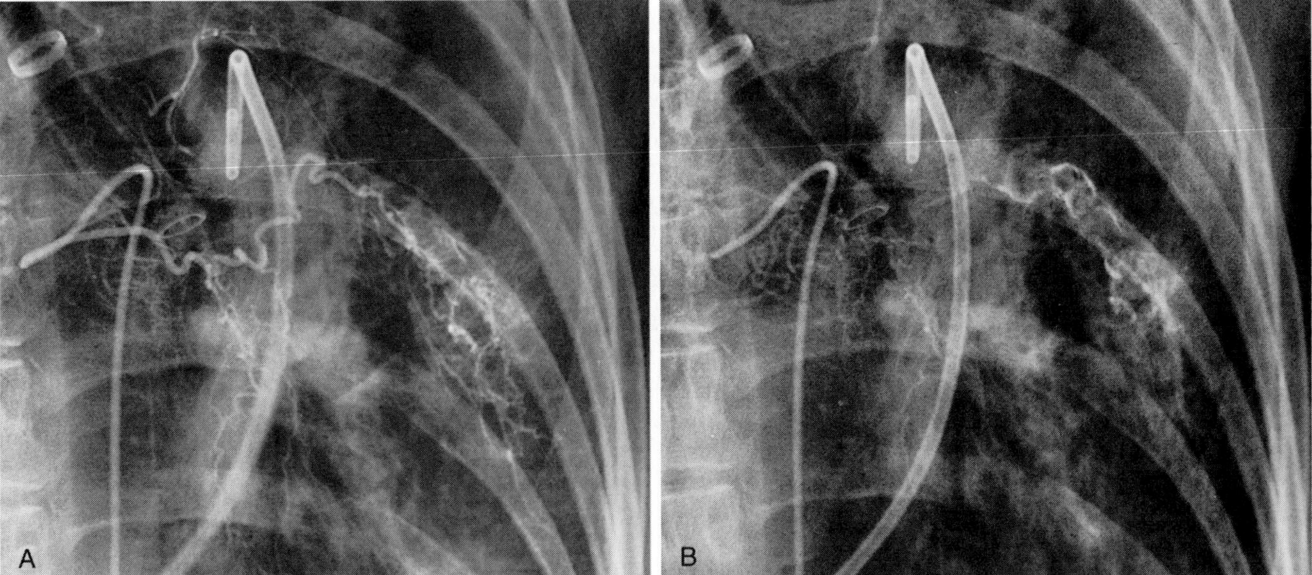

Figure 141–3. *A* and *B*, Bronchial arteriograms in a patient with bronchiectasis and massive hemoptysis. Initial injection into the bronchial artery shows a tortuous vessel and irregularity. The late view demonstrates the unusual finding of extravasation of contrast into an ectatic left upper lobe bronchus. (From Winter SM, Ingbar DH: Massive hemoptysis: Pathogenesis and management. J Intensive Care Med 1988; 3:179.)

ing, after 1 or 2 years, typically reflects new collateral recruitment into an area of chronic inflammation.

Bronchiectasis, neoplasms, CF, and other chronic inflammatory states typically have tortuous, hyperplastic bronchial arteries (Fig. 141-3). It is quite uncommon to demonstrate actual movement of radiocontrast dye from the circulation into the airways. Rather, the presence of vascular abnormalities in a region consistent with the bronchoscopically localized region of bleeding is a sufficient criterion for presumptive diagnosis and embolization. Obviously, in some diffuse lung diseases (e.g., CF), this poses a problem if bronchoscopic localization does not precede arteriography. In this situation, only if the patient is bleeding fairly briskly prior to embolization and if there is a marked decrease in bleeding after embolization of a suspected bleeding region can one be fairly confident that the actual site of bleeding has been treated.

Surgical Therapy

In the past, clinicians, especially surgeons, strongly advocated surgical therapy whenever possible for patients with massive hemoptysis. This conclusion was based on lower mortality rates (typically, 10% to 20%) compared with patients who did not undergo surgery. However, patients in the latter group usually were excluded from surgery because of their severity of illness or underlying disease. In addition, there were very high mortality (37%) and morbidity (40% to 70%) rates in patients who underwent urgent surgery. The mortality usually has been due to aspiration of blood and complications of refractory hypoxemia, whereas the major complications have been postoperative empyema and bronchopleural fistulas. More recent studies have noted generally equivalent outcomes in patients with conservative medical (including arteriography and embolization) or surgical therapy. Surgery is indicated for patients who have been unresponsive to other measures who have massive unilateral hemoptysis and adequate pulmonary reserve. As a result of the success of embolization, surgery is now being used more as an elective treatment for selected individuals rather than as emergent or urgent therapy.

Surgery is contraindicated in patients with:

- Baseline hypoxemia
- Baseline hypercapnia
- Baseline significant dyspnea
- Unresectable carcinoma
- A nonlateralized bleeding site

Diffuse lung diseases also are a relative contraindication to surgery, but it may be appropriate for some patients with bronchiectasis that is predominant in one region to undergo elective surgical wedge resection. Further long-term studies are needed to determine which patients benefit from elective surgery.

OUTCOMES

The mortality of massive hemoptysis remains quite high, with a 10% in-hospital and a 45% 6-month fatality rate in one series from South Africa.[6] A modern United States series[23] observed 46% mortality in 28 patients judged as inoperable, 50% mortality in the four patients who underwent surgical therapy, and 11% mortality in the 27 patients treated medically but who could have been surgical candidates. Clearly, mortality is highest in large-volume bleeds and in bleeding that does not respond to the medical and radiologic interventions discussed earlier. Patients at centers that do not have radiologists experienced in arteriography for hemoptysis and embolization should be transferred to regional centers if possible.

References

1. Stoller JK: Diagnosis and management of massive hemoptysis: A review. Respir Care 1992; 37:564.
2. Cahill BC, Ingbar DH: Massive hemoptysis: Assessment and management: Clin Chest Med 1994; 15:147.
3. Thompson AB, Teschler H, Rennard SI: Pathogenesis, evaluation and therapy for massive hemoptysis. Clin Chest Med 1992; 13:69.
4. Garzon AA, Cerruit MM, Golding ME: Exsanguinating hemoptysis. J Thorac Cardiovasc Surg 1982; 84:829.
5. Hirshberg B, Biran I, Glazer M, et al: Hemoptysis: Etiology, evalua-

tion and outcome in a tertiary referral hospital. Chest 1997; 112:440.
6. Knott-Craig CJ, Oostuizen JG, Rossouw G, et al: Management and prognosis of massive hemoptysis: Recent experience with 120 patients. J Thorac Cardiovasc Surg 1993; 105:394.
7. Rasmussen V: Hemoptysis, especially when fatal, in its anatomical and clinical aspects. Edinburgh Med J 1868; 14:385.
8. Albelda SM, Talbot GH, Gerson SL, et al: Pulmonary cavitation and massive hemoptysis in invasive pulmonary aspergillosis. Am Rev Respir Dis 1985; 131:115.
9. Miller RR, McGregor DH: Hemorrhage from carcinoma of the lung. Cancer 1980; 46:200.
10. Panos RJ, Barr LF, Walsh TJ, et al: Factors associated with fatal hemoptysis in cancer patients. Chest 1988; 94:1008.
11. Gossage JR, Kanj G: Pulmonary arteriovenous malformations. Am J Respir Crit Care Med 1998; 158:643.
12. Julia-Serda G, Freixinet J, Abad C, et al: Massive hemoptysis as a manifestation of fistulized thoracic aortic aneurysms into the bronchial tree. J Cardiovasc Surg 1996; 37:417.
13. Leatherman JL: Diffuse alveolar hemorrhage in immune and idiopathic disorders. *In:* Immunologically Mediated Pulmonary Diseases. Lynch JP III, DeRemee RA (Eds). Philadelphia, JB Lippincott, 1991, p 473.
14. Primack SL, Miller RR, Muller NL: Diffuse pulmonary hemorrhage: Clinical, pathologic and imaging features. AJR Am J Roentgenol 1995; 164:295.
15. Zamora MR, Warner ML, Tuder R, et al: Diffuse alveolar hemorrhage and systemic lupus erythematosus: Clinical presentation, histology, survival and outcome. Medicine 1997; 76:192.
16. Schwarz MI, Zamora MR, Hodges TH, et al: Isolated pulmonary capillaritis and diffuse alveolar hemorrhage in rheumatoid arthritis and mixed connective tissue disease. Chest 1998; 113:1609.
17. Kearney TJ, Shabot MM: Pulmonary artery rupture associated with the Swan-Ganz catheter. Chest 1995; 108:1349.
18. Strange C: Double-lumen endotracheal tubes. Clin Chest Med 1991; 12:497.
19. Naidich DP, Funt S, Ettenger NA, Arranda C: Hemoptysis: CT-bronchoscopic correlations in 58 cases. Radiology 1990; 177:357.
20. McGuiness G, Beacher JR, Harkin TJ, et al: Hemoptysis: Prospective high-resolution CT/bronchoscopic correlation. Chest 1994; 105:1155.
21. Uflacker R, Kaemmerer A, Picon PD, et al: Bronchial artery embolization in the management of hemoptysis: Technical aspects and long-term results. Radiology 1985; 157:637.
22. Ramakantan R, Bandekar VG, Gandhi MS, et al: Massive hemoptysis due to pulmonary tuberculosis: Control with bronchial artery embolization. Radiology 1997; 200:691.
23. Corey R, Hla KM: Major and massive hemoptysis: Reassessment of conservative management. Am J Med Sci 1987; 294:301.

142

Hyperbaric Oxygen in Critical Care

Richard E. Moon, MD, CM, FACP, FCCP, FRCP(C)
Guy de L. Dear, MB, FRCA • Bryant W. Stolp, MD, PhD

The value of supplemental oxygen to avert the danger of hypobaric hypoxia in high-altitude balloon flights was first recognized by Paul Bert more than 100 years ago.[1] In later years, others described the benefits of breathing supplemental oxygen at normal barometric pressure in the treatment of hypoxemia caused by lung pathology. Since the 1950s, the physiologic and pharmacologic effects of breathing oxygen at increased ambient pressure (hyperbaric oxygen [HBO] therapy) have been exploited clinically in the treatment of medical conditions other than hypoxemia.

Patients with carbon monoxide poisoning, gas embolism, decompression sickness, and necrotizing infection are often critically ill, requiring modern techniques of invasive monitoring, mechanical ventilation, and hemodynamic support during HBO therapy at pressures up to 6 atmospheres absolute (ATA) (Table 142–1). This chapter provides the background information, rationale, and practical aspects of the use of HBO treatment of these critically ill patients.

PHYSIOLOGY OF HYPEROXIA

At normal atmospheric pressure the oxygen in arterial blood is almost entirely bound to hemoglobin (Hb). At an arterial Po_2 of 90 mm Hg and Hb concentration of 12 g/dL, less than 2% of the total arterial oxygen content is in the dissolved form (0.3 mL/dL out of 16.6 mL/dL). However, during breathing of 100% O_2 at 3 ATA (arterial Po_2 > 1700 mm Hg), 24% of arterial oxygen is in the dissolved form (5.2 mL/dL out of 21.8 mL/dL [Table 142–2]).

At a constant metabolic rate and unchanged O_2 delivery to the tissue, this increase in arterial O_2 content causes a rise in tissue oxygen tension. Despite some reduction in blood flow during exposure to HBO (see later), such an increase in tissue oxygenation can be observed from direct measurements of mixed venous (see Table 142–2), transcutaneous, and tissue Po_2 and cytochrome redox state using near-infrared spectroscopy.[2]

Hyperoxia results in peripheral vasoconstriction and a reduction of tissue blood flow. During breathing of 100% O_2 at 3.04 ATA (inspired Po_2 = 2263 mm Hg), cardiac output is reduced by 13%,[3] as shown in Table 142–2. In humans breathing 100% O_2, cerebral blood flow is reduced by about 15% at 1 ATA (inspired Po_2 = 713 mm Hg) and 25% at 3.5 ATA (inspired Po_2 = 2613 mm Hg). This reduction in regional blood flow while O_2 delivery is maintained has been used therapeutically for the treatment of cerebral edema (discussed later), edema caused by crush injury,[4] and burns (discussed later). Physiologic effects of hyperbaric hyperoxia have been reviewed by Fife and Camporesi.[5]

PHARMACOLOGY OF HYPEROXIA

Antibacterial Effects

The increased oxygen tension that results from HBO therapy would be expected to be bactericidal to anaerobic bacteria, which lack antioxidant defense mechanisms. Indeed, there is ample experimental and clinical evidence that hyperbaric oxygen is useful as an adjunctive therapy in the treatment of anaerobic infection (see later).

In addition, killing of aerobic bacteria by leukocytes is related to Po_2-dependent generation of reactive oxygen species within the lysosomes. Mader and colleagues[6] have shown in vitro that phagocytic killing of *Staphylococcus aureus* by polymorphonuclear leukocytes becomes progressively impaired as ambient Po_2 is decreased from 100 to 23 mm Hg. This mechanism also appears to be important in vivo when tissue Po_2 is low, for example, in bone infections.[6] In an animal model of osteomyelitis, tobramycin had increased killing power against *Pseudomonas* when tissue oxygen tension was raised by having the animals breathe 100% O_2 at increased ambient pressure.[7] There is evidence that HBO augments the effect of penicillin in the treatment of soft-tissue streptococcal infections.[8] A review of the effects of HBO on infectious processes has been published by Park and colleagues.[9]

Cellular Effects

In addition to the physiologic effects of hyperoxia related to oxygen transport, there are some tissue effects presumably

TABLE 142–1. Range of Pressures Used in Clinical Hyperbaric Oxygen Therapy

Ambient Pressure (ATA)	Equivalent Depth: Feet of Seawater (fsw)	Equivalent Depth: Meters of Seawater (msw)	Comments
1	0	0	Sea level
2	33	10	Commonly used treatment pressure range for chronic indications
2.5	45	14	
2.8	60	18	Most commonly used initial treatment pressure for decompression illness
3.04	68	21	Duke treatment pressure for clostridial myonecrosis
6	165	50	Occasionally used for arterial gas embolism, using 21–50% O_2 for patient's breathing gas. Significant nitrogen narcosis in tenders breathing air.

ATA = atmospheres absolute.

related to cellular or subcellular mechanisms. Zamboni and colleagues[10] have described a delayed decrease in blood flow after reperfusion of myocutaneous tissue flaps. This flow reduction appears to be due to adherence of leukocytes to the endothelium of the small vessels, an effect that is significantly reduced by HBO administration. A similar flow reduction has been observed in the microcirculation of the brain after arterial gas embolism[11] and has also been attributed to leukocyte accumulation in the capillaries.[12] It has been speculated that part of the beneficial effect of HBO in arterial gas embolism might be due to prevention of such leukocyte adherence. One mechanism for this beneficial effect of HBO appears to be inhibition of leukocyte β_2-integrin function by HBO.[13]

In animal studies, HBO administration after acute carbon monoxide exposure appears to minimize the lipid peroxidation in the brain that occurs during or after removal of carbon monoxide[14] and results in more rapid repletion of brain energy store.[15]

Oxygen Toxicity

Pharmacology

Exposure of an animal to an increased partial pressure of oxygen results in higher rates of endogenous production of reactive oxygen species, including superoxide anion (O_2^-), hydroxyl radical (OH·), hydrogen peroxide (H_2O_2), and singlet oxygen, which are responsible for tissue oxygen toxicity.[16, 17] Tissue O_2 toxicity includes the following: lipid peroxidation, sulfhydryl group inactivation, oxidation of pyridine nucleotides, inactivation of Na^+-K^+ adenosine triphosphatase (ATPase), and inhibition of deoxyribonucleic acid (DNA) and protein synthesis. Toxic effects of these species depend on both dose and duration of O_2 exposure.

Organ Effects

Brain

Oxygen toxicity affects the central nervous system (CNS) to produce a wide variety of symptoms (Table 142–3). The most dramatic effect may be generalized convulsions, which most commonly occur during clinical HBO therapy when the inspired Po_2 exceeds 3 ATA. These convulsions are usually self-limited and without evidence of lasting side effects when the inspired O_2 fraction is decreased to normal levels. Factors that increase the risk of CNS oxygen toxicity include hypercapnea, exertion, and (in divers) water immersion. Although in-water convulsions in divers have been recorded at an inspired Po_2 of 1.3 ATA, convulsions during clinical HBO therapy are rare at inspired Po_2 levels less than 3 ATA. The risk of convulsions is approximately 0.02% at an inspired Po_2 of 2 ATA and about 4% at 3 ATA. At inspired Po_2 levels greater than 3 ATA, the risk of convulsions increases markedly, particularly in patients with sepsis. Mild symptoms of CNS toxicity can be managed by temporarily discontinuing the oxygen. Common symptoms such as nausea or facial paresthesias then

TABLE 142–2. Mean Blood Oxygen, Acid-Base, and Cardiovascular Responses to Hyperbaric Oxygenation*

Atmospheric Pressure (ATA)	Inspired Gas	Inspired Po_2 (mm Hg)	Alveolar Po_2 (mm Hg)	Arterial Blood: Po_2 (mm Hg)	pH	Pco_2 (mm Hg)	Cao_2 Total‡ (mL/dL)	Cao_2 Dissolved (mL/dL)	Dissolved (%)
1	Air	149	105	89	7.45	37	16.3	0.3	2
1	O_2	713	676	507	7.46	37	18.2	1.5	8
3.04	Air	474	427	402	7.45	39	17.9	1.2	7
3.04	O_2	2263	2226	1721	7.47	37	21.8	5.2	24

Venous Blood†: Po_2 (mm Hg)	pH	Pco_2 (mm Hg)	Cardiac Output (L/min)	Heart Rate (bpm)	Stroke Volume (mL)	Mean Arterial Pressure (mm Hg)	Total Peripheral Resistance (dyne · sec · cm)
41	7.42	41	6.1	75	81	89	1224
57	7.42	42	5.8	71	82	90	1280
68	7.41	44	5.7	68	85	88	1264
424	7.40	45	5.3	63	92	92	1424

*Data represent mean of 10 normal subjects from Whalen et al: Am J Cardiol 1965; 15:638–646.
†Obtained from a catheter with tip at the junction of the superior vena cava and right atrium.
‡Calculated from measured arterial Po_2, assuming hemoglobin = 12 g/dL.
ATA = atmospheres absolute; bpm = beats per minute.

TABLE 142–3. Symptoms and Signs of Central Nervous System Oxygen Toxicity

Facial pallor	Unpleasant olfactory sensations
Sweating	Unpleasant gustatory sensations
Bradycardia	Respiratory changes
Choking sensation	Panting
Sleepiness	Grunting
Depression	Hiccups
Euphoria	Inspiratory predominance
Apprehension	Diaphragmatic spasms
Changes of behavior	Severe nausea
Fidgeting	Spasmodic vomiting
Disinterest	Vertigo
Clumsiness	Fibrillation of lips
Visual symptoms	Lip twitching
Loss of acuity	Twitching of cheek and nose
Dazzle	Palpitations
Lateral movement	Epigastric tensions
Decrease of intensity	Syncope
Constriction of visual field	Convulsions
Acoustic symptoms	
Music	
Bell ringing	
Knocking	

From Clark JM: Oxygen toxicity. *In:* The Physiology and Medicine of Diving. Bennett PB, Elliott DH (Eds). Philadelphia, WB Saunders, 1993, pp 121–169.

resolve spontaneously and do not usually recur if the oxygen is restarted.

Prophylactic anticonvulsant therapy probably reduces the chance of convulsions when utilizing clinical treatment schedules with significant risk of CNS O_2 toxicity (e.g., treatment pressure > 3 ATA). In this situation, the authors' practice is to load the patient intravenously (IV) with phenobarbital as tolerated up to 12 mg/kg before HBO treatment with doses every 8 hours to maintain a serum concentration of 20 to 40 μg/mL. Phenytoin and benzodiazepines have also been used for this purpose. Anticonvulsant medication can be stopped when HBO therapy is discontinued. When using an inspired Po_2 level of 2.8 ATA or less, the risk of CNS toxicity is sufficiently low that prophylactic anticonvulsant therapy is unnecessary.

If a seizure or other manifestation of CNS O_2 toxicity occurs, the symptom is self-limited if the inspired O_2 concentration is reduced to 21%. HBO may usually be safely restarted a few minutes later, with the option of using additional prophylactic medication. During the tonic-clonic phase of a seizure, the airway may be obstructed. Therefore, it is imperative that chamber pressure not be reduced during this time in order to avoid pulmonary barotrauma and the possibility of arterial gas embolism. The occurrence of a hyperoxic seizure does not imply the development of a convulsive disorder.

HBO therapy has been associated with a significant, and sometimes severe, reduction of blood glucose in patients with diabetes. Therefore, the occurrence of an apparent hyperoxic convulsion in someone with diabetes should prompt the measurement of plasma glucose. It should be noted that when the arterial Po_2 is extremely high (e.g., during HBO therapy), bedside glucose measurement devices can be inaccurate.

Lungs

Pulmonary oxygen toxicity during HBO therapy is dose-dependent and time-dependent. It rarely occurs during routine daily or twice-daily clinical treatments of 2 hours or less with an inspired Po_2 less than 2.45 ATA. It more commonly presents during extended treatments (greater than 4 hours) of gas embolism or decompression sickness with an inspired Po_2 of 2.8 ATA. Symptoms appear initially as tracheobronchitis and progress to include burning substernal chest pain, cough, and ultimately dyspnea. Functional abnormalities include a reduction in forced vital capacity and carbon monoxide transfer factor (DLCO). Continued exposure to oxygen results in hyaline membrane formation, proliferation of type II pneumocytes, and fibrosis. Pulmonary oxygen toxicity symptoms may not be evident in patients who are sedated and mechanically ventilated. Moreover, such patients often have pulmonary infiltrates for a variety of reasons, and it may be impossible to distinguish the possible additive effects of pulmonary O_2 toxicity.

One method of qualifying pulmonary O_2 toxicity is to measure the resulting change in vital capacity. Reduction of vital capacity is related to both partial pressure of oxygen and duration of exposure in a fashion described by Lambertsen,[18] as shown in Figure 142–1. Mild symptoms of pulmonary O_2 toxicity may occur after a prolonged HBO treatment (e.g., the treatment schedule described in the U.S. Navy (USN) Diving Manual[19] (as extended USN Table 6) (see Fig. 142–6*B*), although greater exposures are necessary to cause measurable changes in pulmonary mechanics.

Reduction of the risk of pulmonary O_2 toxicity to a minimum is based on limiting the duration of exposure. Whereas the maximum safe inspired Po_2 during clinical HBO therapy is largely based on CNS O_2 toxicity limits, the duration is limited by pulmonary effects. Although the unit pulmonary toxic dose (UPTD) system (see next paragraph) may be useful as an approximate guide to the risk of pulmonary O_2 toxicity, in the awake patient the presence of burning on retrosternal chest pain is often more useful as an endpoint. Also, HBO treatment schedules that include periods of air breathing ("air breaks") interspersed between the therapeutic periods of 100% O_2 breathing dramatically reduce the rate of onset of pulmonary toxic manifestations (Fig. 142–2) and increase the overall dose of oxygen tolerated. Most symptoms of pulmonary oxygen toxicity resolve in 12 to 24 hours of air breathing.

The following equation has been used to define the UPTD:

$$UPTD = t^{m}\sqrt{\frac{0.5}{Po_2 - 0.5}} \quad \text{[Equation 1]}$$

where P is inspired Po_2 in ATA, m is an empirically derived slope constant with a value of −1.2, and t is exposure time in minutes.[20] The UPTD calculated is related to a certain reduction in vital capacity. For example, 1425 UPTD units results in approximately a 10% reduction in vital capacity and 2190 UPTD units results in about a 20% reduction. A simpler representation of the data is shown in the next equation, in which the percentage reduction in vital capacity (VC) is related to inspired Po_2 (in ATA) and minutes of exposure (t)[21]:

$$\% \Delta VC = -0.009\,(Po_2 - 0.38)\,t \quad \text{[Equation 2]}$$

The UPTD concept has proved useful in generating approximate guidelines for oxygen exposure. However, there is considerable interindividual variability in oxygen susceptibility. Moreover, other factors such as intermittent exposure, oxygen administration before HBO exposure, sepsis, tissue leukocytes, and probably a number of unknown modifiers may limit the accuracy of prediction.

Supplemental O_2 administration at 1 ATA between HBO treatments may promote the development of pulmonary O_2 toxicity. Therefore it is prudent to use the lowest safe concentration of inspired oxygen between HBO treatments. However, the effects of mild or even moderate pulmonary O_2 toxicity are usually reversible. Therefore, in life-threatening situations requiring aggressive HBO therapy, some degree of pulmonary O_2 toxicity may be acceptable (Fig. 142–3).

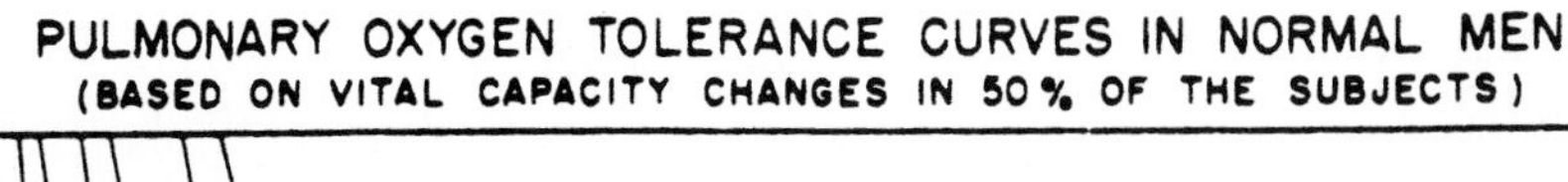

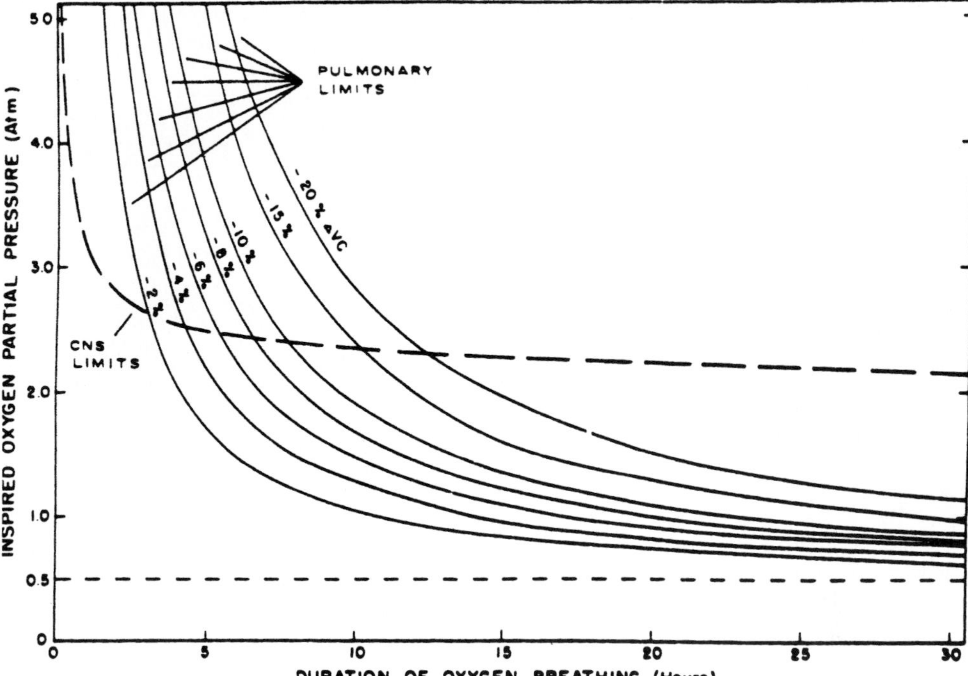

Figure 142–1. Dose-response curves for oxygen (O_2) tolerance in humans. VC = vital capacity; CNS = central nervous system. (From Clark JM: Oxygen toxicity. *In:* The Physiology and Medicine of Diving. Bennett PB, Elliott DH [Eds]. Philadelphia, WB Saunders, 1993, pp 121–169.)

There is evidence in the literature that previous exposure to some antineoplastic agents, such as bleomycin and mitomycin C, may predispose to fatal pulmonary O_2 toxicity. The risk of pulmonary O_2 toxicity caused by HBO therapy in patients with previous exposure to either of these agents is unknown, although the authors have treated several such individuals with HBO by reducing oxygen exposure during the initial treatment regimen (e.g., twice daily to daily therapy) and closely monitoring pulmonary function. Some of these individuals have an enhanced propensity to develop mild pulmonary O_2 toxicity symptoms such as retrosternal burning chest pain, but if the chemotherapy has been remote and the HBO treatment pressure is 2 ATA or less, life-threatening manifestations are rare.

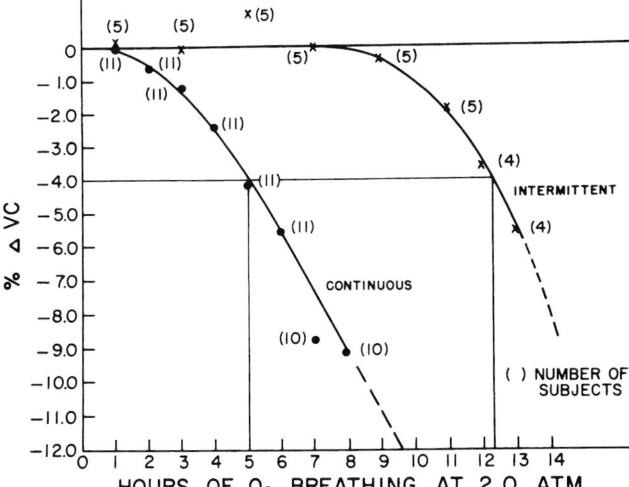

Figure 142–2. Rate of decrease of vital capacity (VC) during oxygen (O_2) exposure in normal volunteers: continuous versus intermittent exposure. Insertion of air breaks into periods of 100% O_2 breathing during hyperbaric O_2 therapy reduces the rate of development of pulmonary O_2 toxicity. (From Clark JM: Oxygen toxicity. *In:* The Physiology and Medicine of Diving. Bennett PB, Elliott DH [Eds]. Philadelphia, WB Saunders, 1993, pp 121–169.)

Eye

Repetitive HBO therapy can cause myopia, which appears to be caused by a reversible refractive change in the lens.[22] Twenty or more exposures are usually required to observe any measurable change in visual acuity, although acute deterioration can sometimes occur after only one prolonged treatment. The myopia usually resolves at a rate approximately equal to that of onset but may occasionally be only partially reversed.

Palmquist and colleagues[23] have suggested that HBO treatment may predispose to nuclear cataract formation. Although this possibility cannot be discounted, many of the patients in their study received hundreds of hours of HBO treatment, considerably more than is customary. In addition, nuclear cataracts are associated with diabetes, which is often present in patients requiring prolonged, repetitive HBO therapy.

Peripheral Nerve

After HBO exposure some patients experience paresthesias, usually in their fingers and toes. These symptoms generally occur after repetitive HBO exposures but are occasionally observed after only a single (usually prolonged) hyperbaric treatment. They normally resolve within a day or two, have no known clinical significance, and are not a reason to discontinue hyperbaric therapy.

USE OF HYPERBARIC OXYGEN FOR SPECIFIC DISEASES

Gas Embolism and Decompression Sickness

Pathophysiologic Effects of Intravascular Gas

In addition to occlusion of blood vessels, several other effects of intravascular bubbles have been observed. Histologic exami-

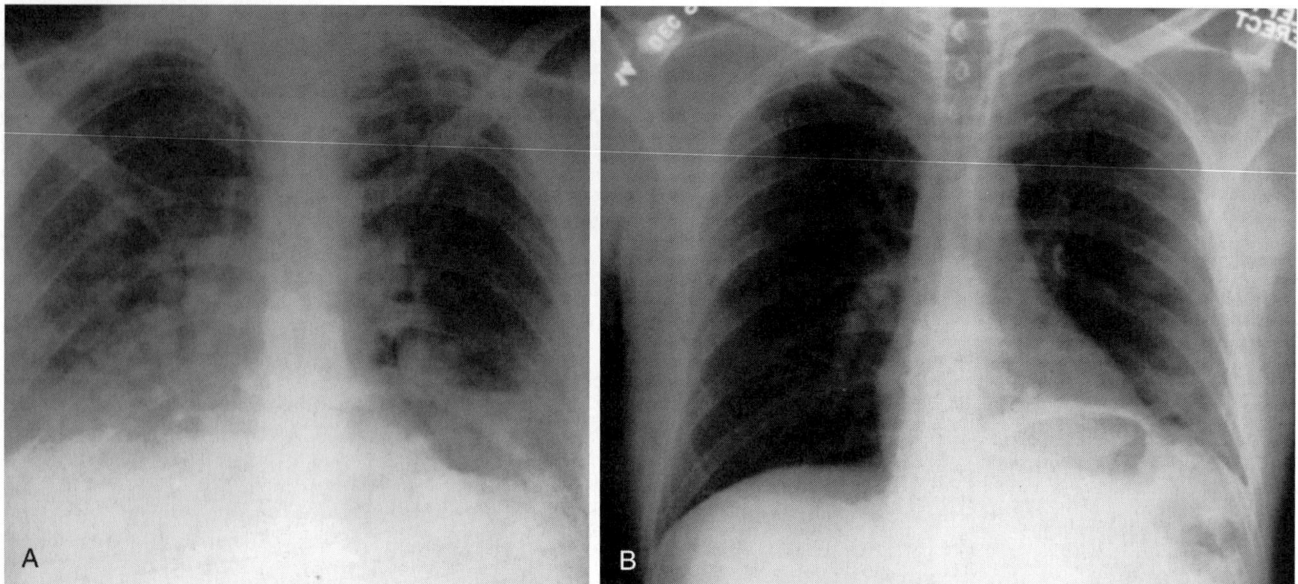

Figure 142–3. Severe pulmonary oxygen (O_2) toxicity. The patient is a 40-year-old diver who developed dense paraplegia after exceeding safe depth-time limits during a scuba dive. *A,* Bilateral pulmonary edema due to O_2 toxicity after the patient had been exposed to around 3000 units pulmonary toxic dose (UPTD), simultaneous with significant neurologic improvement. After discontinuation of supplemental O_2, symptoms resolved over the next 2 to 3 days. *B,* Radiograph of the patient in *A,* taken 2 weeks after the first one, shows an almost complete return to normal.

nation of animals subjected to decompression and autopsy studies of individuals fatally injured in dive accidents have shown that bubble-blood interactions may initiate deposition of platelets and fibrin. Even in mild decompression stress, activation and consumption of platelets may occur, as evidenced by the effect of administration of antiplatelet drugs to reduce the mild drop in platelets otherwise observed after dives.[24, 25]

Although in gas embolism platelets are rarely if ever depleted to levels that impair coagulation, histologic evidence of hemorrhage has been described with arterial gas embolism[26] and in situ formation of gas caused by supersaturation (see later) in the inner ear[27] and spinal cord.[28–30] The mechanisms have thus far not been delineated.

Helps and colleagues[31] observed in a rabbit model of arterial gas embolism that when a small volume of gas (25 μL) was injected into the cerebral circulation, the majority passed directly through the capillary network. Nevertheless, the bubbles provoked a marked dilatation of the affected pial arterioles that persisted for 90 minutes after the bubbles had disappeared and was accompanied by a delayed, progressive reduction in both cerebral blood flow and neural function. This effect is probably due to activation of leukocytes, as leukocyte-depleted animals do not demonstrate the effect.[12]

Bubble-induced endothelial injury can also cause changes in permeability. Intravenous air injection can thus produce pulmonary edema,[32, 33] which in divers is called cardiorespiratory decompression illness ("chokes," see later). Although the mechanism is not completely worked out, data for animals suggest that activation of both complement and leukocytes is involved.[34] Similarly, arterial gas embolism can cause cerebral edema.

Incubation of bubbles with serum has been demonstrated to activate complement,[35, 36] probably via the alternative pathway.[37] Evidence for complement activation in humans initiated during or after decompression from dives has been reported by several authors.[38–41] Furthermore, Ward and colleagues[42] demonstrated in rabbits a strong relationship between the degree to which the complement system could be activated in vitro by bubbles and susceptibility to decompression sickness, with decomplemented animals showing extreme resistance. Evidence that the same phenomenon may exist in humans has been published by the same investigators, who demonstrated that human divers who had high levels of complement components C3a and C5a after incubation of plasma with bubbles were also more likely to develop symptoms of decompression sickness. However, three studies have failed to confirm a correlation between intravascular bubbles and complement activation.[38, 40, 43] Moreover, in a study of rats, administration of a soluble complement receptor that neutralizes activated complement components failed to alter the susceptibility to decompression sickness after a chamber dive.[44] Whether complement activation plays a pathophysiologically significant role in gas embolism or decompression sickness remains an open question.

Regardless of the mechanisms, the most serious effect of intra-arterial gas is tissue ischemia. Thus, it is likely mechanisms of injury that have been described in thromboembolic stroke, such as the effects of oxygen free radicals,[45] excitatory neurotransmitters,[46] and activation of poly(adenosine diphosphate ribose) polymerase,[47] also apply to gas embolism.

Spectrum of Gas Embolism and Decompression Sickness

Accidental Bubble Injection

Intra-arterial injection of only small quantities of gas can occlude blood flow, producing acute stroke, myocardial infarction, or cardiac arrest. Iatrogenic arterial gas embolism is usually caused by accidental arterial injection of air during diagnostic procedures, dialysis, or cardiopulmonary bypass. Arterial gas embolism can also be caused by pulmonary overpressurization during mechanical ventilation and by penetrating lung trauma.

On the other hand, a similar volume of gas can be injected intravenously without clinical consequence because it is usually filtered by the pulmonary circulation. Careful measurement of the filtration capacity of the pulmonary capillaries has been performed in animals. Continuous infusion of gas at

0.35 mL/kg/min can result in bubbles crossing the pulmonary circulation directly[48] or traversing the interatrial septum via a patent foramen ovale. Larger amounts of intravenous gas can also totally fill the right heart and pulmonary arteries, resulting in "vapor lock." Such a situation has been most commonly described during craniotomy in the sitting position, in which air may enter the vascular system via the intraosseous sinuses. In animal studies the fatal bolus dose of gas injected IV is 4 to 5 mL/kg. Lower doses are often tolerated, although in dogs constant infusions at 0.6 mL/kg/min can cause changes in the electrocardiogram (ECG) and 2 mL/kg/min can produce severe hypotension.[49] In humans, fatalities have been recorded after IV injection of as little as 100 mL.[50, 51]

As already discussed, gas can damage the vascular endothelium and cause changes in permeability, resulting in pulmonary edema (cardiorespiratory decompression illness or chokes) or cerebral edema.

Gas Embolism in Divers

Pulmonary overpressurization is the mechanism by which arterial gas embolism occurs in scuba divers. Compressible air-containing spaces in the body decrease in size in inverse proportion to increased ambient pressure according to Boyle's law. The lung capacity during a breath-holding dive would thus be one half of the capacity at the surface at a depth equal to 2 ATA (33 feet or 10 m of seawater). During a scuba dive, gas is delivered to the diver from the scuba regulator at a pressure equal to the ambient hydrostatic pressure and supplies extra breathing gas to the lungs to restore their normal capacity at depth. During ascent from the dive, gas-containing spaces within the body must be vented of this excess gas or they tend to expand. Such spaces include bubbles within the gastrointestinal tract, paranasal sinuses, middle ear cavities, and the lungs. During ascent, gas trapped within the lung either by breath holding or by regional gas trapping (e.g., mucus plugging, bronchospasm, bullae, or blebs) therefore induces an increase in alveolar pressure. If intra-alveolar pressure exceeds tissue elastic pressure, gas may enter pulmonary capillaries. This can occur at a pressure between and 80 and 100 mm Hg.[52] Hence, a breath-holding ascent from a scuba dive as shallow as 4 to 5 feet may result in arterial gas embolism, and this has in fact been reported after a dive to a depth of 1 m.[53] Gas may also enter the pulmonary interstitium, whence it may tract into the mediastinum or the pleural space, causing pneumomediastinum or pneumothorax.

Once bubbles have entered the arterial tree, they may cause symptoms or signs related to infarction of any end-organ, including the heart. However, the most common syndromes involve the brain (see the following case history).

CASE HISTORY 1

A 21-year-old diver trainee breathed from a scuba tank in a swimming pool at a depth of 10 feet. He made a panicky ascent and when he reached the surface had a generalized convulsion. A few minutes later he regained consciousness but was hemiplegic.

This scenario illustrates a typical example of arterial gas embolism in a diver. Gas is delivered at the ambient pressure of the diver's environment (in this case approximately 1.3 ATA). Breath holding during the ascent would result in a 30% increase in lung volume. If at the start of ascent the diver had taken a full inspiration, the resulting pulmonary hyperexpansion would be sufficient to cause alveolar rupture and entry of gas into the pulmonary blood vessels.

In Situ Bubble Formation

The amount of gas that dissolves in a tissue is directly related to the gas solubility and partial pressure. When a gas is dissolved in a liquid, an acute reduction in ambient pressure may allow the gas to come out of solution and form bubbles in a fashion analogous to carbon dioxide bubbling out of a carbonated beverage when the bottle cap is removed. Symptoms related to this phenomenon were first described in the 19th century in workers who were engaged in construction of bridge abutments, tunnels, or mines. The work environment was a large inverted chamber (caisson) in an environment in which the pressure had been raised in order to prevent water from entering the open bottom. Workers breathing air under these conditions of raised barometric pressure have an increased amount of inert gas (primarily nitrogen) dissolved in their tissues. Upon decompression on leaving the work environment, many of these men developed limb pain or neurologic symptoms and some died. The condition was called the "bends," supposedly because of the similarity between the posture of afflicted caisson workers and that used during a popular 19th century dance, the "Grecian bend." This condition was subsequently described in divers and is thought to be related to bubble formation in tissues, bones, and the CNS. It can also occur in aviators who become decompressed during high-altitude flight (usually greater than 18,000 feet), although decompression illness can occur after ascent to only 8000 feet,[54] particularly if there has been scuba diving within the past 24 hours.[55]

Bubbles can form in any tissue but appear to have a predilection for the areas around joints, the spinal cord, brain, and skin. Symptoms commonly consist of joint pain, paresthesias, limb weakness, and occasionally ataxia and loss of consciousness. A list of common presenting symptoms is shown in Table 142-4. A more detailed discussion can be found in Elliott and Moon.[56]

Traditionally, in situ gas formation has been called *decompression sickness.* Decompression sickness has been classified

TABLE 142–4. Distribution of Symptoms in 1249 Cases of Decompression Illness in Recreational Divers Reported to the Divers Alert Network

Initial Symptom	%	Symptom at Any Time	%
Pain	40.7	Pain	56.7
Altered skin sensation	19.2	Altered skin sensation	52.1
Dizziness	7.8	Weakness	22.4
Extreme headache	5.7	Dizziness	18.6
Headache	5.7	Extreme fatigue	17.1
Weakness	4.8	Headache	16.1
Nausea	2.9	Nausea	13.9
Difficulty breathing	2.5	Difficulty walking	10.2
Altered level of consciousness	2.1	Difficulty breathing	8.7
Itching	1.6	Altered level of consciousness	6.9
Visual disturbance	1.5	Visual disturbance	6.4
Rash	1.1	Paralysis	6.3
Paralysis	1.0	Itching	5.0
Personality change	0.8	Restlessness	4.6
Difficulty walking	0.7	Muscle twitching	4.0
Restlessness	0.4	Rash	3.5
Muscle twitching	0.4	Urethral or anal sphincter dysfunction	3.5
Urethral or anal sphincter dysfunction	0.4	Speech disturbance	2.8
Speech disturbance	0.2	Tinnitus	1.7
Convulsions	0.2	Hearing loss	1.1
Hearing loss	0.1	Convulsions	1.0
TOTAL	100.0	Hemoptysis	0.7

From Elliott DH, Moon RE: Manifestations of the decompression disorders. *In:* The Physiology and Medicine of Diving. Bennett PB, Elliott DH (Eds). Philadelphia, WB Saunders, 1993, pp 481-505.

as *type I* (musculoskeletal, skin, lymphatic, fatigue) and *type II* (neurologic, cardiorespiratory, inner ear, shock). At one time it was believed to be important to distinguish clinically between decompression sickness and *arterial gas embolism.* This differentiation at one time had therapeutic significance because different recompression schedules were used for the two disorders. However, there has been growing recognition that the two syndromes often occur simultaneously, and generally the same treatment tables are used for both types of illness. Arterial gas embolism (in divers) and both subclasses of decompression sickness are now most commonly referred to using the umbrella term *decompression illness* (DCI).

CASE HISTORY 2

A 39-year-old man made three dives over 2 days, to depths of 104 feet, 97 feet, and 147 feet, respectively. During ascent from the third dive he noted discomfort in the area of the distal biceps tendon in one arm. The pain gradually increased in intensity, and 12 hours after surfacing he experienced paresthesias in the ipsilateral hand. Physical examination revealed no abnormality. Twenty-four hours after surfacing from his last dive, he was given HBO therapy using the schedule described in the U.S. Navy Diving Manual,[19] known as USN Table 6 (see Fig. 142-6*B*). The paresthesias resolved and the pain was reduced in intensity. The following morning, the discomfort in his arm was almost imperceptible and there were no further symptoms.

CASE HISTORY 3

A 42-year-old male diving instructor made six dives over the course of 3 days, each dive to a depth of 77 feet for about 30 minutes. During ascent (decompression) from his last dive, he noticed weakness in his legs. When he reached the surface he was disoriented and had profound weakness in his legs and his left arm. He received recompression treatment with USN Table 6A[19] (see Fig. 142-6*A*) approximately 1 hour after injury, but the abnormalities only partially resolved. After being transferred to a tertiary referral center, he was found to have cortical blindness, inability to move either leg, and profound left arm weakness. Brain computed tomography (CT) showed hypodensity at the gray-white junction of both occipital lobes and in the thalamus. He received three USN Table 6 treatments (see Fig. 142-6*B*) and then nine additional HBO treatments at 2 ATA for 2 hours each, to an endpoint of absence of stepwise improvement in neurologic function. After treatment, he was able to walk with a cane and manage his urinary sphincter dysfunction with intermittent self-catheterization.

Case 2 illustrates a typical example of mild decompression illness with two of the most common symptoms: pain and paresthesias. The absence of physical findings should not discourage the use of recompression treatment, which is usually effective even after considerable delay. Case 3 illustrates a severe case of neurologic decompression illness, with both cortical and spinal cord manifestations. If manifestations do not resolve completely after a single HBO treatment, repetitive daily or twice daily treatments are recommended, until no further incremental improvement is observed (usually no more than 5 to 10).

Treatment

Prehospital Treatment

In addition to the standard principles of resuscitation, patients should be well hydrated with either oral or intravenous fluid and administered as high a concentration of inspired oxygen as possible. Supplemental oxygen washes out blood and tissue nitrogen stores and increases tissue oxygen tension. This increases the partial pressure gradient for nitrogen to diffuse from bubbles into tissue or blood and helps in the resolution of the bubbles. Tissue hypoxia may result from vascular occlusion or pulmonary abnormalities such as aspiration, pneumothorax, or pulmonary edema caused by venous gas embolism. Supplemental O_2 therefore hastens bubble shrinkage as well as ameliorates hypoxia. In order to ensure a high inspired concentration, oxygen is best administered with a tightly fitting face mask and demand valve or, if necessary, endotracheal tube. Oxygen administered by nasal cannula or loose-fitting face mask, although undoubtedly beneficial, is probably less effective.

The head-down position was previously recommended for the treatment of arterial gas embolism on the basis that, because of buoyancy effects, residual gas in the pulmonary veins or left side of the heart might be less likely to "float to the head" and cause cerebral infarction. In addition, it was hypothesized that dilatation of the cerebral vessels secondary to hydrostatic loading would promote distal migration of bubbles and hence less cerebral ischemia. Indeed, Van Allen and coworkers[57] observed higher mortality in dogs when they were embolized in the head-up position. Furthermore, Atkinson[58] demonstrated that placement of embolized cats in a head-down position caused redistribution of bubbles in the direction of arterial flow. Anecdotal evidence that the head-down position may be beneficial in humans with arterial gas embolism has been reported by Kruse.[59] However, Butler and colleagues[60, 61] demonstrated that buoyancy has minimum importance for the distribution of either arterial or venous gas. In addition, Atkinson[58] observed a tendency for the development of cerebral edema in his cats, an observation that has been confirmed by Dutka.[62] The supine position is therefore recommended by most practitioners for conscious victims with intact airway reflexes and the lateral decubitus position for patients at increased risk for pulmonary aspiration or vomiting.

Intravenous fluid administration can reduce the severity of decompression illness in animals.[63] In severe cases of human decompression illness, hemoconcentration has been observed.[64, 65] Isotonic crystalloid or colloid solutions are recommended to reverse this process. Because hyperglycemia can increase the extent of damage in both cerebral and spinal cord injury, it is probably best to avoid glucose-containing fluids.

Physical Removal of Gas

Aspiration of gas from the superior vena cava or right atrium with an appropriately placed catheter has been lifesaving in some instances of massive venous gas embolism.[66] Removal of arterial bubbles caused by accidental injection during cardiopulmonary bypass has been performed using reversal of pump flow.[67] In most instances, however, physical removal of gas from the vascular tree is not feasible and unlikely to be complete. Furthermore, removal of bubbles would not prevent sequelae of bubble-induced endothelial damage.

Hyperbaric Treatment

An increase in the ambient pressure causes a reduction of the volume of tissue gas bubbles. For instance, recompression from 1 to 6 ATA reduces a bubble to one sixth of its original volume.

Recompression therapy remains the mainstay of treatment for tissue gas. Originally, air was used as the breathing gas during treatment. Use of air has the disadvantage that it results in additional inert gas (nitrogen) uptake, which might then promote bubble formation during the subsequent decompression.

Bert[1] demonstrated over 100 years ago that the signs of decompression illness could be resolved in experimental animals by administering supplemental O_2. Yarbrough and Behnke[68] suggested that breathing 100% O_2 during recompression therapy would lead to increased efficacy of treatment. In addition to eliminating excess inert gas uptake, oxygen breath-

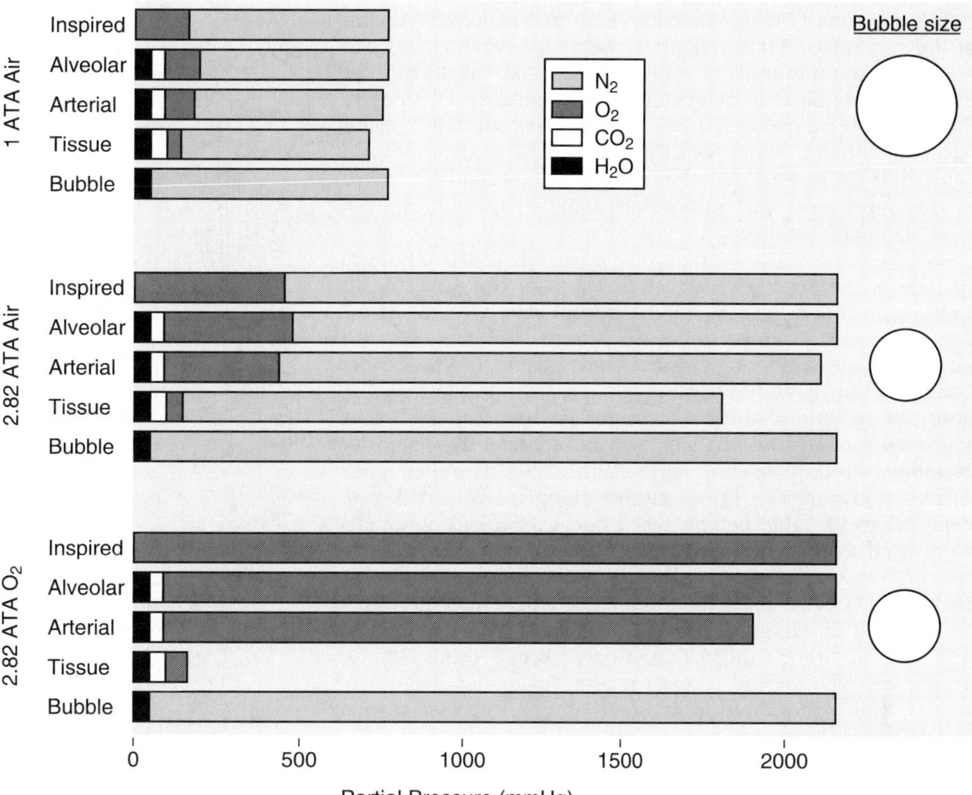

Figure 142–4. Partial pressures of gases within a bubble under various conditions. *Top panel* shows a bubble at 1 ATA while the patient breathes air. P_{N_2} in the bubble is slightly greater than that in the surrounding tissue, tending to favor resorption of the gas. Compression to 2.82 ATA increases this gradient somewhat *(middle panel)*. Breathing 100% oxygen (O_2) at 2.82 ATA *(bottom panel)* washes out nitrogen from the tissue surrounding the bubble, substantially increasing the gradient for diffusion of nitrogen and, hence, the rate of resolution of the bubble. (From Moon RE: Treatment of gas bubble disease. Probl Respir Care 1991; 4:232–252.)

ing results in a significantly greater partial pressure gradient for nitrogen to diffuse out of the bubble (Fig. 142–4). Increased arterial O_2 content could also normalize tissue oxygenation in the event of low blood flow related to bubble fibrin or platelet accumulation.

Initial recommendations for the recompression pressure are based on the empirical tradeoff between the greatest bubble size reduction and the risk of CNS oxygen toxicity. A recompression "depth" of 60 feet of seawater (fsw), equivalent to 2.82 ATA, was initially suggested as the recompression pressure for decompression illness and today remains the pressure most commonly used.

Although no controlled studies have compared the outcomes of patients treated with HBO and untreated individuals, the preponderance of evidence supports the use of recompression therapy for gas embolism and decompression sickness. Before recompression treatment was accepted as standard, large numbers of untreated cases of decompression sickness were reported by Woodward[69] and Blick.[70] Although the majority of cases of pain-only decompression illness resolved spontaneously, as did some cases of neurologic decompression illness, many others remained symptomatic or died. Keays[71] retrospectively reviewed decompression illness in treated versus untreated caisson workers. About 14% of patients who did not receive recompression therapy had residual symptoms, compared with less than 1% of patients who were treated with recompression therapy. Evidence from the Diver's Alert Network (Durham, N.C.) indicates that recreational divers with decompression illness who are treated early are less likely to have residual long-term symptoms than those treated after significant delay.[72] Similarly, a retrospective review of patients with arterial gas embolism, both iatrogenic and dive related, strongly supports the use of hyperbaric treatment.[73]

Individuals with gas embolism or decompression sickness who are treated early are more likely to have complete relief of symptoms than those treated after a delay.[72] However, delays up to several days do not preclude significant clinical improvement after recompression therapy.[74–76]

The morbidity of recompression treatment is extremely low and the efficacy high. Therefore, if appropriate recompression facilities are available, it is recommended that, unless there are extenuating circumstances, all individuals with gas embolism or decompression sickness receive hyperbaric treatment.

The decision to treat should be made only on clinical grounds. The role of supplemental diagnostic tests such as brain or spinal imaging is to exclude other pathologies such as hemorrhage if there is a high degree of suspicion that bubbles are not the cause. It has been suggested that patients with arterial gas embolism should be treated with HBO only if CT of the brain reveals air.[77] In arterial gas embolism there are HBO-responsive phenomena other than occlusion of vessels by macrobubbles. Indeed, in the authors' experience, brain imaging of patients who respond clinically to HBO shows abnormalities in a minority of cases. Unless there is a strong clinical suspicion of pathology other than arterial gas embolism that requires urgent exclusion, performing CT before treatment with HBO serves only to delay appropriate treatment.

SPECIFIC PROTOCOLS FOR GAS EMBOLISM AND DECOMPRESSION SICKNESS. The most commonly used treatment schedules ("Tables") were developed by the U.S. Navy[19] and are shown in Figures 142–5 and 142–6. Each treatment table consists of periods of 100% O_2 breathing with air breaks interspersed to minimize oxygen toxicity. The initial treatment pressure is 2.82 ATA (60 feet of seawater, fsw). After a period at that pressure, the chamber is slowly decompressed to a pressure of 1.9 ATA (30 fsw). USN Table 5 is reserved for decompression illness in which pain is the only symptom and in which symptoms are completely resolved within 10 minutes of beginning recompression.

USN Treatment Table 6 (see Fig. 142–6*B*) is a longer version of the same two-step paradigm. Additional oxygen cycles can be administered at both 60 and 30 fsw. Maximum duration at each pressure level is determined by pulmonary O_2 toxicity limits. Further details of specific treatment protocols can be found in Moon,[78] the USN Diving Manual,[19] and Moon and Gorman.[72] Consensus guidelines for evaluation and treatment of decompression illness, developed by a panel of experts, have also been published.[79]

USN Table 6A was designed for the treatment of arterial gas embolism. (see Fig. 142–6*A*). It consists of the schedule in Table 6 preceded by a 30-minute period at 6 ATA (50 msw,* 165 fsw) in an attempt to "crush" arterial bubbles. Because increasing the ambient pressure from 2.82 to 6 ATA results only in a small additional bubble diameter reduction, the utility of recompression to pressures greater than 2.82 ATA (60 fsw equivalent depth) has been questioned. The majority of animal studies do not support the use of higher pressures.[80–83] Use of 47% O_2 as the breathing gas at 6 ATA provided no measurable benefit when cortical evoked potentials were used as the endpoint in anesthetized cats.[84] In a retrospective review of cases of human decompression illness, Leitch and Green[85] concluded that clinical benefit could rarely be obtained by recompressing to a pressure higher than 2.82 ATA. On the other hand, Lee and coworkers,[86] using 40% O_2 during a 1-hour period at 6 ATA, and Thalmann[87] have presented clinical evidence in favor of using compression to 6 ATA in unresponsive or severe cases.

If a patient has serious neurologic symptoms and shows ongoing improvement during the initial period of recompression or deteriorates during decompression, *saturation* treatment can be instituted. Saturation treatment consists of an indefinite period of O_2 and air breathing at a specified treatment pressure. When the patient's clinical condition has stabilized, decompression may be commenced. All tissues in both patient and tender are assumed to be fully saturated with inert gas at the increased ambient pressure. Therefore, in order to avoid inducing decompression illness in the tender or worsening symptoms in the patient, decompression must be carried out at a significantly lower rate than in standard short recompression tables. An example of a saturation table (USN treatment Table 7) is shown in Figure 142–7.

*msw = meters sea water; fsw = feet sea water.

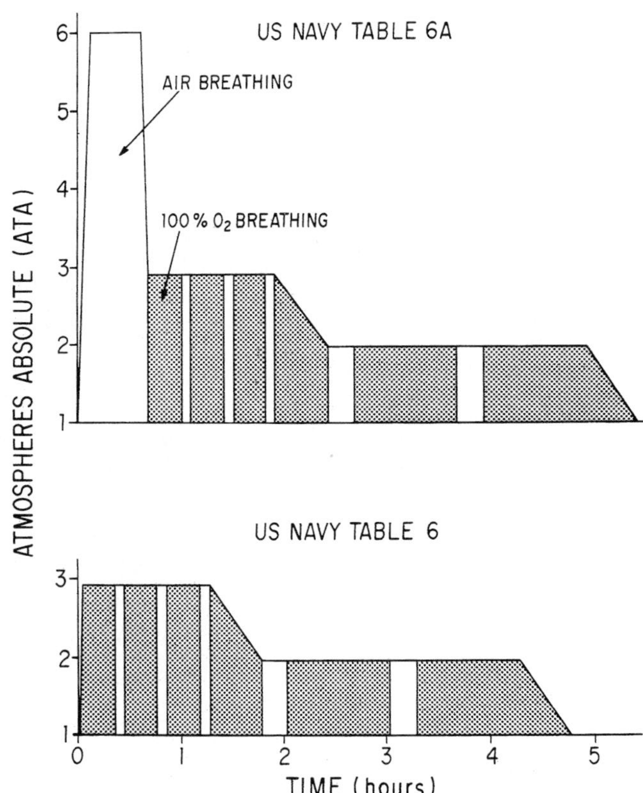

Figure 142–6. U.S. Navy treatment tables for serious decompression illness. *Top panel* shows Table 6A,[19] which was designed originally for the treatment of arterial gas embolism. Although originally designed for the patient to breathe air during the 30-minute exposure at 6 ATA, many diving physicians administer 40% to 50% oxygen (O_2) during this phase. *Bottom panel* shows U.S. Navy Table 6.[19] Additional periods of O_2 breathing can be administered at both 2.82 and 1.9 ATA ("extensions") during use of these treatment tables. The majority of recompression treatments in patients with decompression illness use U.S. Navy Table 6. If a patient does not respond completely to an initial treatment, repetitive treatments are given until no further stepwise improvement occurs. (From Moon RE: Treatment of gas bubble disease. Probl Respir Care 1991; 4:232–252.)

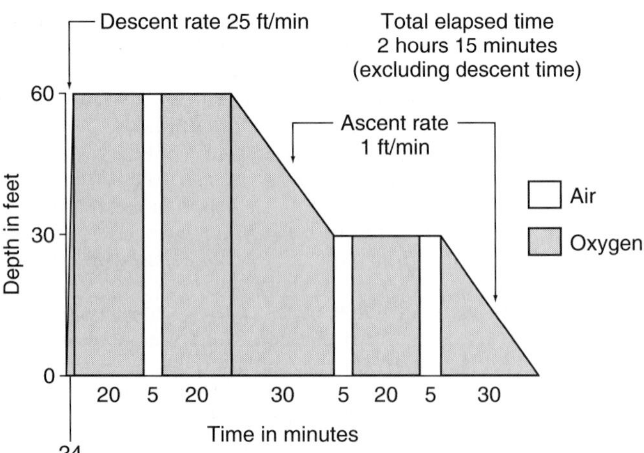

Figure 142–5. U.S. Navy Table 5.[19] This treatment table is designed for pain-only or skin bends, in which complete relief of symptoms occurs within 10 minutes of reaching the equivalent depth of 60 feet (2.82 ATA). (From Moon RE, Gorman DF: Treatment of decompression disorders. *In:* The Physiology and Medicine of Diving. Bennett PB, Elliott DH [Eds]. Philadelphia, WB Saunders, 1993, pp 121–169.)

If a single hyperbaric treatment does not resolve all symptoms, repeated treatments may produce additional improvement. The number of appropriate treatments is difficult to define and must be based on the patient's symptoms and rate of improvement during HBO therapy. Except in rare instances, the efficacy of more than five follow-up treatments is unclear and must be reassessed on an individual basis.

Adjunctive Measures

CORTICOSTEROIDS. Corticosteroids have been used both experimentally and clinically in decompression illness in various arbitrary dosages. In a retrospective review of 132 divers with arterial gas embolism,[88] use of dexamethasone was associated with a reduced relapse rate: 10.8% in treated versus 29.5% in untreated individuals. Kizer[89] reported dramatic improvement after administration of 1000 mg of IV hydrocortisone and 4 mg of dexamethasone to a diver with neurologic decompression illness whose neurologic examination results had been unchanged for 12 hours.

For a model of canine spinal decompression illness, with somatosensory evoked responses as an endpoint, Francis and Dutka[90] reported no additional benefit when methylprednisolone (20 mg/kg) was administered in addition to recompres-

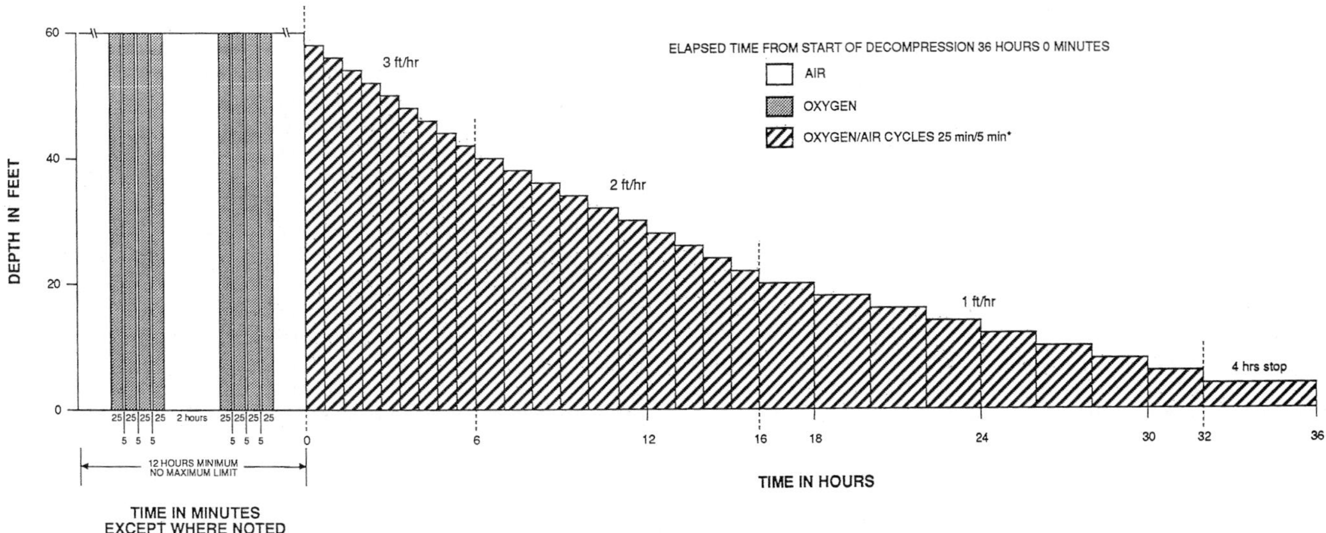

Figure 142–7. U.S. Navy Table 7 (saturation table).[19] The patient may spend an indefinite period of time at 60 feet (2.82 ATA), receiving intermittent periods of O_2 exposure. (For details on administration, see the *USN Diving Manual.*[19]) This treatment may last several days. Therefore, in order to administer this treatment, the chamber facility must have around-the-clock personnel. Two inside tenders are preferable. Control of the chamber atmosphere must be carefully maintained in order to prevent fluctuations of the levels of O_2 and carbon dioxide. (From Moon RE: Treatment of gas bubble disease. Probl Respir Care 1991; 4:232–252.)

sion treatment. In a canine study,[91] dexamethasone was administered in addition to recompression therapy after experimental embolism of anesthesized animals. There was a slight benefit of administration of dexamethasone at 1 mg/kg 3 to 4 hours before and immediately after carotid artery embolization but no effect when 2 mg/kg was administered after injection of air. Dexamethasone treatment did not prevent cerebral edema. On the other hand, the Second National Acute Spinal Cord Injury Study[92] showed that when methylprednisolone was given at a bolus dose of 30 mg/kg within 8 hours after acute spinal cord injury followed by a continuous infusion of 5.4 mg/kg/hr for 23 hours, there was significant benefit 6 months after injury. The potential value of corticosteroids administered in these high doses to patients with decompression illness is unknown.

ANTICOAGULANTS. Intravascular bubble formation induces accumulation of platelets and fibrin at the blood-bubble interface, suggesting that anticoagulant therapy may be beneficial in the treatment of decompression illness. Physicians treating injured divers have been cautions to use therapeutic anticoagulation because of the tissue hemorrhage that may accompany spinal cord and inner ear decompression illness. A variety of anticoagulants have been administered to patients with neurologic decompression illness in an attempt to minimize the secondary coagulation effects. Reeves and Workman[93] did not observe a beneficial effect of using IV heparin in experimental decompression illness in dogs. A single case report of neurologic decompression illness treated with heparin[94] indicated that there was no adverse or beneficial effect.

Nonsteroidal anti-inflammatory drugs (NSAIDs) also have antiplatelet activity and are commonly administered to patients who receive HBO therapy for pain-only decompression illness. It is not known whether this class of drugs has any benefit other than analgesia.

Despite the unknown value of anticoagulants in the treatment of decompression illness, they may have an important role in prophylaxis against deep venous thrombosis. Patients with paraplegia caused by decompression illness are at high risk for this complication,[95] and therefore low-dose subcutaneous heparin may be beneficial.

LIDOCAINE. Evans and coworkers observed both a prophylactic[96] and a therapeutic[97] effect of lidocaine on experimental arterial gas embolism in anesthetized cats. McDermott and colleagues,[98] using embolized, anesthetized cats, were unable to demonstrate a significant additive effect of lidocaine with HBO. Using a more realistic model, which included a period of transient hypertension at the time of embolization of anesthetized dogs, Dutka[62] found that when intravenous lidocaine was used in addition to recompression, recovery of cortical evoked potential amplitude was twice as great as with recompression alone.

No controlled data exist for human divers with decompression illness at the time of this writing, but reports of three individuals with decompression illness provide support for the value of lidocaine in this condition.[99, 100] Moreover, a controlled trial of lidocaine infusion after open-heart surgery supports its use for gas embolism.[101] The mechanism of action of lidocaine in gas embolism has been speculated involve reduced intracranial pressure and increased cerebral blood flow.[102]

FLUOROCARBONS. Inert gases are more soluble in fluorocarbons than in plasma. One might therefore expect IV administration of fluorocarbons to promote faster bubble resolution by providing a greater sink into which tissue and bubble nitrogen can diffuse. Indeed, Menasché and colleagues[103] found that IV infusion of the fluorocarbon FC-43 into rats allowed over three times the volume of air to be injected into the carotid artery before irreversible flattening of the electroencephalogram (EEG) occurred. Treatment of decompression illness in rats with FC-43 and 100% O_2 significantly improved survival.[104]

Conclusion

In addition to appropriate airway care and ventilatory and hemodynamic support, patients with gas embolism or decompression sickness should immediately be administered the highest available inspired O_2 concentration with sufficient isotonic intravenous fluids to restore and maintain plasma volume. Although symptoms often resolve with administration of oxygen without recompression, they frequently recur after cessation of oxygen breathing. Therefore, unless the patient's safety would be compromised (e.g., because of hemodynamic instability), recompression treatment should be administered.[79] Recompression should ideally be initiated at an ambient pressure of 2.8 ATA while administering 100% O_2. The U.S. Navy oxygen treatment tables (see Figs. 142–5 and 142–6)[19] and similar systems implemented by commercial diving companies and other navies are the most widely used treatment algorithms worldwide and, if the delay to treatment is not excessive, have a high degree of success in resolving symptoms.[87] Complete resolution is most likely to result from early hyperbaric treatment, and although complete resolution of symptoms becomes less likely with increasing delay of treatment, the available do not indicate a data maximum time after which recompression is ineffective.[79]

Poisonings

Carbon Monoxide

Carbon monoxide binds to several hemoproteins, resulting in impaired oxygen transport and utilization. Carbon monoxide binds to hemoglobin about 200 times as avidly as does O_2, resulting in decreased hemoglobin available for O_2 transport and also increased avidity of hemoglobin for O_2 (shift of the hemoglobin-oxygen dissociation curve to the left). Additional mechanisms for toxicity include binding of carbon monoxide to other intracellular proteins (e.g., myoglobin, cytochrome-*c* oxidase).[105] Piantadosi and colleagues[106] observed carbon monoxide toxicity in rats in which blood had been exchanged for fluorocarbon. During reoxygenation after exposure to carbon monoxide oxygen free radical–mediated damage may occur.[107] Carbon monoxide also binds and activates guanylate cyclase, causing enhanced synthesis of cyclic guanosine monophosphate (cGMP), which causes vascular smooth muscle to relax.[108] Vasodilatation of extracranial arteries via this mechanism is believed to be the cause of headaches commonly associated with carbon monoxide poisoning.

Acute toxicity can cause dysfunction of multiple organ systems, particularly the central nervous system. Commonly reported symptoms and signs include headache, nausea, vomiting, confusion, and loss of consciousness. A cursory neurologic examination may fail to detect cortical dysfunction caused by carbon monoxide poisoning, which can often be demonstrated by simple bedside neuropsychologic testing.[109] Late neurologic sequelae can occur, sometimes after a lucid interval of several days. Late sequelae are most likely in patients with moderate or severe poisoning. The most useful clinical information in carbon monoxide poisoning is a history of exposure and degree of functional impairment at or shortly after exposure.

The diagnosis of poisoning is based on a history of exposure to carbon monoxide from sources such as internal combustion engine exhaust, building fires, improperly adjusted gas or oil furnaces, propane or kerosene space heaters, and charcoal or gas barbecues. Inhalation of methylene chloride (paint stripper) fumes can also cause poisoning, as the compound is converted by the liver to carbon monoxide. A definitive diagnosis of carbon monoxide poisoning can be made by measuring the carboxyhemoglobin (COHb) concentration in either venous or arterial blood. Blood samples stored in an anticoagulant are stable for several days and can be transported with the patient when rescue personnel or small hospitals lack the ability to determine COHb. It should be noted that fetal hemoglobin (hemoglobin F) produces a falsely elevated reading for COHb on certain four-wavelength laboratory oximeters. In the first few weeks of life, blood from normal infants may therefore falsely appear to have 7% to 8% COHb.

Radiographic manifestations (CT and magnetic resonance imaging) of carbon monoxide poisoning include globus pallidus infarction, subcortical white matter hypodensities, cerebral cortical lesions, cerebral edema, hippocampal lesions, and loss of gray-white differentiation.[110–112] The presence of such radiographic abnormalities correlates with a poor outcome. Thus, in the clinical management of carbon monoxide poisoning, brain imaging is useful only to exclude other pathology or to provide prognostic information. Other types of imaging have been described in carbon monoxide poisoning, such as single photon emission computed tomography (SPECT). Such techniques have not yet been demonstrated to provide information that can be used for management of patients.

Pace and colleagues[113] demonstrated a relationship between the elimination half-time of COHb and the partial pressure of inspired O_2. During breathing of air at 1 ATA the half-time of COHb degradation was 214 minutes. The half-time decreased to 42 minutes during breathing of 100% O_2 at 1 ATA and to 18 minutes with 100% O_2 at 2.5 ATA, In addition to this accelerated rate of elimination of carbon monoxide from hemoglobin, removal from intracellular binding sites is enhanced by HBO treatment,[114] allowing more rapid recovery of energy metabolism.[15] During HBO the increased dissolved O_2 in the plasma can support tissue oxygenation pending elimination of carbon monoxide. This is also evidence that HBO treatment can minimize damage caused by peroxidation, which occurs after clearance of carbon monoxide.[14]

A prospective study compared normobaric O_2 with HBO in a series of carbon monoxide–poisoned patients and found no apparent benefit of HBO.[115] Unfortunately, this conclusion is not well supported by the published data, because the patients selected for this comparison were only mildly poisoned and would not have been expected a priori to have derived major benefit. Moreover, several patients were treated after a significant delay (up to 12 hours), during which time they were usually receiving supplemental O_2 which minimized a possible favorable effect of subsequent HBO.

There is now significant evidence that use of HBO in moderate to severe carbon monoxide poisoning offers significant clinical benefits. Two comparable series of patients with carbon monoxide poisoning were treated, respectively, with 100% O_2 at atmospheric pressure[116] and HBO.[117] Considering the patients who lost consciousness, in the HBO-treated group mortality was 50% lower and neurologic sequelae 80% lower than in the group treated with 100% O_2 at 1 ATA. In a prospective, randomized study of hyperbaric oxygen versus normobaric oxygen in moderately severe carbon monoxide poisoning, Thom and coworkers[118] observed a significant reduction in late neurologic sequelae in patients treated with HBO (Fig. 142–8).

Supportable indications for the use of HBO in carbon monoxide poisoning are as follows[119]:

- Peak COHb level greater than 25% at any time during the exposure. (Peak level can be estimated from the elimination half-times for carbon monoxide in air or O_2.) Although the COHb level is a useful marker of exposure, it correlates poorly with clinical outcome, and HBO should not be withheld from a symptomatic patient merely because the COHb level is low or normal.
- History of neurologic impairment, including loss of consciousness.
- Evidence of cardiac abnormalities (ischemia, arrhythmias, ventricular failure).

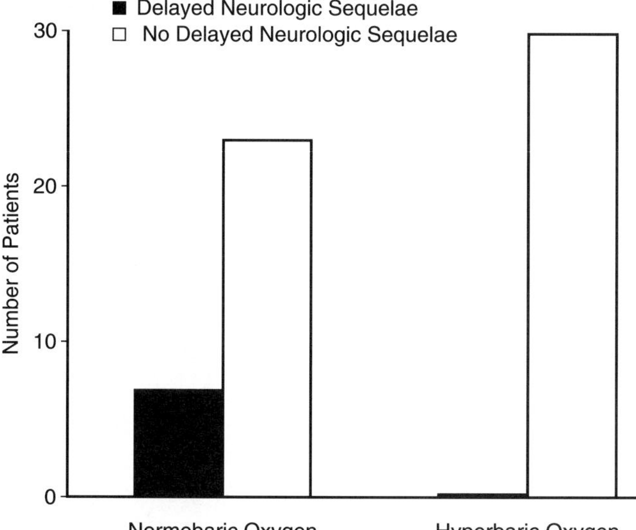

Figure 142–8. Number of patients with delayed neurologic sequelae 30 days after treatment of patients with carbon monoxide (CO) poisoning. Patients with a history of exposure to combustion products, increased blood carboxyhemoglobin (COHb) level that could not be explained by smoking, and the presence of symptoms consistent with CO poisoning were randomly assigned to receive either hyperbaric oxygen (HBO), 2.8 ATA (30 minutes) followed by 2 ATA (90 minutes), or normobaric oxygen (O_2) via nonrebreather face mask until resolution of symptoms. Patients with a history of unconsciousness were excluded. Mean COHb levels were 24.6% (HBO group) and 20.0% (normobaric group). HBO treatment began within 6 hours of removal from the source. Psychometric testing was performed on all patients immediately after either HBO or NBO treatment and after recurrence of symptoms or development of new symptoms. In asymptomatic patients, testing was performed 3 to 4 weeks after poisoning. Delayed neurologic sequelae were defined as recurrences of original symptoms or development of new symptoms in addition to deterioration in one or more subtest scores. Three of seven patients with delayed neurologic sequelae had difficulty with daily activities. Delayed neurologic sequelae were significantly more likely to occur with normobaric O_2 treatment ($P < .05$). (From Thom S, Taber R, Mendiguren J, Clark J, Hardy K, Fisher A: Delayed neuropsychologic sequelae after carbon monoxide poisoning: Prevention by treatment with hyperbaric oxygen. Ann Emerg Med 1995; 25:474–480.)

Pregnant women who fulfill these criteria or in whom there is evidence of fetal distress should also be treated. Theoretical concern about the risk of HBO in pregnancy is unfounded. Ledingham and colleagues[120] reported a 22-year-old woman with severe carbon monoxide poisoning and poor response to 100% O_2 administration at 1 ATA. She was administered 100% O_2 at 2 ATA and underwent cesarean section while in the chamber, delivering a normal child with an Apgar score of 9. Additional individual case reports,[121–123] two published series,[124, 125] and a critical review[126] provide overwhelming evidence that the major risk to the fetus is from carbon monoxide poisoning rather than HBO treatment.

Carbon monoxide–poisoned patients with unremitting nausea, vomiting, or headache despite normobaric oxygen therapy are also occasionally considered for treatment.

For treatment of carbon monoxide poisoning, HBO is customarily administered at 2 to 3 ATA for 90 to 150 minutes. Definitive studies comparing different treatment pressures and lengths of treatment have not been published. A single treatment is almost always sufficient to reduce the COHb to baseline levels. However, carbon monoxide binding to other sites cannot currently be measured, and patients with severe symptoms after a single treatment are often treated one to three more times. In addition to elimination of carbon monoxide from hemoproteins, this treatment is probably beneficial in reducing cerebral edema. HBO treatment is most likely to be effective if administered within 6 to 7 hours after exposure.

CASE HISTORY 4

A 35-year-old woman was found unconscious in her bed 48 hours after going to sleep. She was taken to the emergency department, where she was stuporous. After breathing oxygen for several minutes, she began to awaken and reported waking up several times at home with headache, nausea, and vomiting. She was unable to stand without assistance. Several small peripheral retinal hemorrhages were observed. COHb was 41% of total hemoglobin. Brain CT was normal. She was treated with oxygen at 2.5 ATA for 90 minutes with improvement. After three additional hyperbaric treatments, she was asymptomatic and neurologic examination findings were normal. The heat exchanger in her gas furnace was subsequently found to be cracked, allowing flue gas to enter the house.

This case of severe carbon monoxide poisoning is an example of accidental exposure. The retinal hemorrhages are in keeping with a prolonged exposure. A single HBO treatment probably removes all excess carbon monoxide from tissues; however, in the event of an incomplete response, most hyperbaric physicians empirically administer one to three additional treatments. A normal brain CT scan is predictive of a good recovery after HBO treatment.[111]

Cyanide

The major mode of toxicity of cyanide is interference with oxygen transport at cytochrome-*c* oxidase. Unlike carbon monoxide binding, cyanide binding with cytochrome oxidase is not dependent on Po_2. Therefore, the rationale for the use of HBO in acute cyanide poisoning is not as strong as it is for carbon monoxide poisoning, particularly given the efficacy of conventional chemical treatment with sodium nitrate and sodium thiosulfate. Hemoglobin variants caused by combination with cyanide and methemoglobin resulting from chemical treatment do not combine with oxygen. Therefore, there may be some degree of functional anemia in cyanide poisoning. If this is of sufficient magnitude to impair tissue oxygen, HBO administration could be of benefit by augmenting the quantity of O_2 dissolved in plasma. Indeed, anecdotal reports suggest efficacy of HBO in cyanide poisoning when standard chemical measures have failed.[127]

In addition to other toxic products such as carbon monoxide, cyanide is frequently produced in combustion of building materials such as plastics. Patients exposed to products of combustion frequently have significant exposure to both carbon monoxide and cyanide.

Hydrogen Sulfide

Hydrogen sulfide (H_2S) inhibits respiration at the level of the cell by reacting with cytochrome-*c* oxidase. Sulfide binding to this enzyme is not Po_2-dependent. Sulfide can also combine with hemoglobin to form sulfhemoglobin, which does not transport oxygen. Clinical manifestations of H_2S poisoning include pulmonary edema and loss of consciousness.

As with cyanide poisoning, the main rationale for use of HBO in H_2S poisoning is to overcome the reduction in O_2 transport caused by sulfhemoglobin. Anecdotal case reports suggest a beneficial effect of HBO in this toxicity.[128, 129]

Carbon Tetrachloride

Poisoning with this compound typically results in CNS and hepatic toxicity. Although experience is limited, the possible therapeutic value of HBO in this condition is exemplified by a report of a patient with circumstantial evidence of carbon monoxide poisoning who appeared to respond to treatment with HBO. There was no definitive evidence of carbon monoxide exposure, and after regaining consciousness the patient admitted to having ingested about 250 mL of carbon tetrachloride (a lethal dose) 4 hours before HBO administration.[130]

Carbon tetrachloride (CCl_4) is believed to exert its toxic effects by generation of free radicals[131] (CCl_3^- and CCl_3OO^-), which may cause lipid peroxidation. High hepatic oxygen tension has been shown to reduce the conversion of CCl_4 to its reactive metabolites, and lipid peroxidation was reduced when experimental animals poisoned with carbon tetrachloride were treated with HBO.[132]

Necrotizing Infection

Clostridial Infections

Because anaerobic bacteria lack antioxidant defenses such as superoxide dismutase, the growth of these organisms in tissue tends to be inversely related to tissue P_{O_2}. In vitro studies indicate that HBO can inhibit both clostridial growth and alpha-toxin production. An additional mechanism is a generalized increase in oxygen delivery to both infected and noninfected tissues.[133] In animal models of clostridial myonecrosis,[134–136] an independent beneficial effect of HBO, antibiotics, and surgical debridement was demonstrated. Bakker[137] found that early HBO treatment and antibiotics provided adequate time for demarcation of necrotic tissue, which could then be removed surgically. Discussing the largest published series (462 individuals) of patients with gas gangrene, with a mortality rate as low as any in the literature, Bakker and van der Kleij[138] reported that it was nearly always possible to delay definitive surgery until after one to four HBO treatments. They provided evidence that early initiation of HBO in conjunction with antibiotic therapy for patients with gas gangrene of the extremities can be limb saving and that primary amputation of the extremities is contraindicated.

Animal evidence suggesting that HBO may not be necessary has been published by Stevens and colleagues.[139] Using a mouse model of clostridial myositis, these investigators showed that HBO augmented survival when infected mice were treated with metronidazole or penicillin but not when they were treated with clindamycin, which was superior to HBO alone or either of the other antibiotics. Considering the high mortality of this rare disease and the clinical and experimental evidence supporting the use of HBO, whether this observation can be applied in the treatment of human cases of gas gangrene remains an open question.

A review of the literature comparing the outcomes of patients with clostridial infection treated with or without HBO is shown in Table 142-5. Despite the retrospective nature of the analysis, it is clear that HBO therapy is associated with lower mortality.

TABLE 142–5. Mortality in Gas Gangrene Without and With Hyperbaric Oxygen (HBO)

Author	No. of Patients	Died	Mortality (%)
Without HBO			
DeLalande et al.[174]	22	9	40.9
Freischlag et al.[175]	21	11	52.4
Gibson and Davis[176]	17	12	70.6
Hitchcock and Bubrick[177]	33	14	42.4
Kaiser and Cerra[178]	20	8	40.0
Katlic and Derkac[179]	7	5	71.4
Paillier and Labeeu[180]	20	8	40.0
Vo and Watson[181]	77	31	40.3
TOTAL	217	98	45.2
With HBO			
Bakker and van der Kleij[138]	462	54*	11.7
Caplan and Kluge[182]	34	11	32.4
Gibson and Davis[176]	29	9	31.0
Gurtner[183]	73	23	31.5
Hart and Lamb[184]	139	27	19.4
Heimbach[185]	58	3	5.2
Hirn and Niinikoski[186]	32	9	28.1
Holland et al.[136]	49	13	26.5
Nier and Kremer[187]	78	30	38.5
Rudge[188]	77	19	24.7
Shupak et al.[189]	4	1	25.0
Smolle-Juttner et al.[190]	116	17	14.7
Torda et al.[191]	9	3	33.3
Unsworth and Sharp[192]	73	15	20.5
TOTAL	1233	234	19.0

*Mortality within 4 days caused by infection. An additional 41 patients died 4 days or more after therapy from causes other than clostridial infection (e.g., pulmonary embolism, myocardial infarction, metastatic carcinoma).

HBO treatment is typically administered at 2.5 to 3 ATA, usually for 90 minutes. Two to four treatments are usually given within the first 24 hours and then two treatments daily until the patient is clinically stable and the infection is under control (usually five to 10 treatments). Many patients with coexisting small-vessel disease may benefit from additional HBO treatments in preparation for eventual skin grafting or flap coverage.

Nonclostridial Bacterial Infections

Necrotizing infection with organisms other than clostridia are often due to mixed aerobic and anaerobic bacteria. Whereas the same rationale exists for the use of HBO, many of these infections are indolent and one often cannot discern an immediate clinical improvement after a single treatment as in clostridial myonecrosis. The cornerstones of therapy in this disease are surgical debridement and antibiotic therapy. As with clostridial infections, the demarcation of viable from nonviable tissue and the beneficial effects of edema reduction may assist the surgeon during debridements.

HBO schedules are usually similar to those advocated for the treatment of clostridial infections. Empirical endpoints of treatment include resolution of the acute infection and reduction in "toxicity." In view of the subacute nature of many of these infections and lack of a well-defined endpoint, patients often receive more protracted HBO therapy, sometimes 10 to 15 treatments.

The benefit of HBO in nonclostridial necrotizing infection is suggested by a controlled trial reported by Riseman and colleagues.[140] A similar meta-analysis suggests a significant beneficial effect of HBO on clinical outcome (Table 142-6).

A point of discussion in the management of clostridial and other soft-tissue necrotizing infections is the timing of HBO versus surgery. HBO treatment provides a period during which the patient can be treated with intravenous antibiotics and appropriately fluid resuscitated before surgery, with which there is typically a significant requirement for replacement of blood and third-space fluid loss. Bakker[137] reported on a large series of patients with clostridial infections who had excellent outcomes despite delay of surgery for 24 to 48 hours.

Mucormycosis

Rhinocerebral mucormycosis is due to infection with fungi of the family Mucoraceae. These fungi grow well in an environment with a low P_{O_2}; they invade blood vessels and cause

TABLE 142–6. Mortality in Nonclostridial Fasciitis Without and With Hyperbaric Oxygen (HBO)

Author	No. of Patients	Died	Mortality (%)
Without HBO			
Brown et al.[193]	24	10	41.7
Farrell et al.[194]	11	5	45.5
Hollabaugh et al.[195]	12	5	41.7
Jarrett et al.[196]	15	8	53.3
Ledingham[197]	3	0	0.0
Mader[198]	12	6	50.0
Majeski[199]	20	10	50.0
Oh et al.[200]	28	10	35.7
Papachristodoulou et al.[201]	5	1	20.0
Pessa and Howard[202]	33	13	39.4
Pizzorno et al.[203]	11	0	0.0
Reigels-Nielsen et al.[204]	5	1	20.0
Riseman et al.[140] and Zamboni and Kindwall[205]	15	10	66.7
Rouse et al.[206]	27	20	74.1
Spimak et al.[207]	20	9	45.0
Wang and Shih[208]	18	6	33.3
Woodburn and Ramsay[209]	19	7	36.8
TOTAL	278	121	43.5
With HBO			
Aasen et al.[210]	9	1	11.1
Bakker[137]	27	5	18.5
Brown et al.[193]	30	9	30.0
Chevallier et al.[211]	13	4	30.8
Gozal et al.[212]	16	2	12.5
Hirn and Niinikoski[186]	11	1	9.1
Hollabaugh et al.[195]	13	1	7.7
Krasova et al.[213]	11	3	27.3
Langford et al.[214]	6	0	0.0
Ledingham[197]	9	8	88.9
Mader[198]	10	2	20.0
Mathieu et al.[215]	42	10	23.8
Riseman et al.[140] and Zamboni and Kindwall[205]	45	7	15.6
Torda et al.[191]	34	4	11.8
TOTAL	276	57	20.7

infarction. The impaired leukocyte function caused by hypoxia reduces killing of the organism by host defenses. This disease usually occurs in diabetic patients, is often associated with ketoacidosis, and is associated with high mortality despite ablative surgery and antifungal therapy. The rationale for HBO treatment in this disease is to increase tissue P_{O_2} and enhance leukocyte killing of the infectious agent. An exhaustive retrospective review comparing the outcomes of patients treated with or without adjunctive HBO[141] suggests a beneficial effect of HBO in this disease. Of 18 patients with bilateral disease who received amphotericin B, surgery, or both without HBO, four (22%) survived; of six who received HBO in addition to surgery and antifungal therapy, five (83%) survived (P = .007). Opinions are still divided on whether HBO should be used routinely for patients with this disease. Nevertheless, when there is clinical progression of disease despite antifungal therapy and appropriate surgery, HBO may be a useful adjunctive measure.

Head Injury

The reduction of cerebral blood flow that occurs during HBO has previously been shown to be associated with a reduction in intracranial pressure,[142] although this response to hyperoxia has been reported to be transient and does not occur when cerebral autoregulation is absent.[143]

Because of this ameliorative effect of HBO on intracranial hypertension, it has been suggested that HBO may also have a long-term beneficial effect on acute head injury. Indeed, Holbach and coworkers[144] treated 99 patients with severe head injuries using HBO. In that study, the mortality rate in the treated individuals was significantly lower than in the control subjects (33% versus 74%) and a significantly greater percentage of HBO-treated individuals made a good recovery (33% versus 6%). Rockswold and colleagues[145] studied 168 patients with head injuries who had a Glasgow Coma Scale score of 9 or less for 6 hours or more. All patients were treated with standard techniques for management of head injuries. Eighty-four patients were randomly selected to receive HBO, which was administered at 1.5 ATA for 1 hour every 8 hours for 2 weeks or until the patient was either brain dead or awake. The mortality rate of the HBO-treated patients was significantly lower (17% versus 32% of control subjects). Despite this improvement in acute mortality, the outcome at 12 months was not significantly different when the two groups of survivors were compared. Use of HBO for severe head injury is therefore investigational.

Thermal Injury

Ikeda and colleagues[146] reported on a series of patients who experienced carbon monoxide poisoning related to coal mine explosions and fire. Patients who were treated for carbon monoxide poisoning with HBO who also had burns showed more rapid healing and less infection than other burned patients who did not receive HBO. Although some studies have failed to demonstrate a beneficial effect of HBO,[147, 148] many others support its use.

Korn and colleagues[149] studied the effect of twice-daily HBO treatment at 2 ATA for 90 minutes on burn healing in guinea pigs. HBO resulted in more rapid epithelialization and return of vascularity to the burn wound. Niezgoda and colleagues[150] performed a "blinded" study of the effect of 100% O_2 versus 8.75% O_2 (normoxic sham) at 2.4 ATA on ultraviolet-irradiated blister wounds in normal volunteers. HBO resulted in significant reduction in wound size, hyperemia, and exudation. In a randomized, prospective study, Hart and colleagues[151] demonstrated that HBO treatment of patients with burns was associated with a significant reduction in healing time. Niu and colleagues[152] reported a comparative study of 266 patients with burns (affecting a mean of 34% of body surface area) treated with HBO and a control group of 609 patients who did not receive HBO (mean 36% of body surface area). Although overall mortality was not different in the groups, among patients aged 15 to 45 years with burns on 35% to 75% of the body surface area, mortality in the HBO group was significantly reduced (6.8% versus 14.8%). Cianci and associates[153] reported a controlled trial in which eight patients who received HBO treatment at 2 ATA for 90 minutes twice daily were in hospital for a mean of 20.8 days compared with 33 days for control subjects. In another report, in addition to a shorter hospital stay, HBO-treated patients had lower average hospital costs ($60,350) than control subjects ($91,960).[154]

As evidence indicating a benefit of adjunctive oxygen therapy for the treatment of burns continues to accumulate, there is growing clinical acceptance of this modality. Because many severely burned individuals require mechanical ventilation and invasive monitoring, it is important to be familiar with the techniques for management of such critically ill patients in a hyperbaric environment. Many individuals with severe burns also have carbon monoxide poisoning, which can be detected by measurement of blood COHb.

Myocardial Infarction

Increasing the blood O_2 content using HBO causes bradycardia and a reduction in cardiac output[3] (see Table 142–2) and hence cardiac work. In addition to providing additional O_2 delivery to ischemic myocardium, HBO would therefore be expected to unload the heart and reduce its O_2 requirement. Studies of awake dogs have demonstrated that even when heart rate (and hence O_2 consumption related to external cardiac work) is carefully controlled, administration of 100% O_2 at 3 ATA is associated with a 15% reduction in myocardial O_2 consumption.[155] HBO might also be expected to have salutary effects on ischemia-reperfusion phenomena that have been observed in other tissues, such as leukocyte adherence and the secondary decrease in tissue blood flow.[10] Indeed, Sterling and colleagues[156] demonstrated that after 30 minutes of left coronary occlusion in a rabbit model, HBO at 2.5 ATA reduced infarct size when administered either during or immediately after occlusion or both but not when delayed until 30 minutes after reperfusion.

Cameron and colleagues[157] demonstrated that administration of 90% O_2 at 2 ATA (arterial Po_2 508–1130 mm Hg) to 10 patients with acute myocardial infarction caused arterial pressure and systemic vascular resistance to rise (14% and 37%, respectively), cardiac output to fall (17%), and no change in cardiac work. Ashfield and Gavey[158] reported an uncontrolled series of 40 patients treated with HBO administered in continuous cycles for 4 days: 2 hours breathing 100% O_2 at 2 ATA followed by 1 hour breathing air at 1 ATA. Pain and dyspnea improved during the first HBO treatment period, worsened during the air-breathing period, and then progressively improved during successive sessions. Thurston and colleagues[159] reported a randomized, prospective trial with individuals younger than 70 years of age in which 103 patients with acute myocardial infarction (MI) were treated with HBO and compared with 105 patients treated conventionally in the same intensive care unit (ICU). HBO was administered in the same cycles of 2 hours of HBO at 2 ATA followed by 1 hour of air breathing at 1 ATA for 48 hours after entry into the study. Control patients were administered O_2 via face mask at 6 L/min. There were no complications of HBO treatment, and mortality in the HBO group was 16.5% versus 22.9% in the control subjects. Analysis of clinical subgroups revealed that differences in mortality existed only among the more severely ill patients, in whom HBO was associated with approximately a 50% lower death rate.

It was uncertain whether the apparent benefits of HBO in acute MI were due to HBO-induced enhanced oxygenation of ischemic tissue or merely to alteration of the mechanical load on the heart because of secondary effects. These trials were not followed up because of the development of pharmacologic tools for unloading the heart and use of anticoagulation, fibrinolytic agents, and interventional techniques with which to open occluded coronary arteries. Moreover, the limitations of O_2 toxicity precluded the continuous exposure to HBO that might be desired.

However, a rekindling of interest in HBO led to a new clinical trial. Shandling and colleagues[160] have published the results of a pilot study in which patients with suspected MI with symptoms of less than 6 hours' duration were treated with tissue plasminogen activator (t-PA) and randomized to receive either a single HBO treatment at 2 ATA for 1 hour or 40% O_2 via a face mask. There were no deaths in the HBO group and two (6%) in the control subjects, although the difference was not statistically significant. In the HBO group, creative phosphokinase (CPK) levels at 12 and 24 hours were 35% lower and time to pain relief was shorter (275 versus 664 minutes).

These results suggest that HBO may have a role in the treatment of acute MI. A recommendation to use HBO as routine treatment would require additional supportive data.

Other Indications

HBO has been used to support tissue oxygenation in patients with severe anemia whose blood cannot readily be cross-matched or in patients who refuse transfusion.[161] HBO has also been used to maintain arterial Po_2 during therapeutic lung lavage, during which gas exchange must be maintained in a single lung.[162] It is the routine practice of the authors to support therapeutic lung lavage under general anesthesia in a multiplace hyperbaric chamber, where hypoxemia can be quickly and safely treated by increasing the ambient pressure.

HBO is also used for a variety of nonacute conditions, listed in Table 142–7. The common theme that underlies the rationale for treatment in these conditions is insufficient tissue oxygenation. A complete review of accepted indications can be found in a biannual publication of the Undersea and Hyperbaric Medical Society.[163] Additional reference sources are listed in Greenbaum and Mathias.[164]

MECHANICS

Chambers

Hyperbaric chambers are commonly classified according to the number of individuals inside. A multiplace chamber can accommodate one or more patients along with a tender. The

TABLE 142–7. Partial List of Conditions for Which Hyperbaric Oxygen Has Been Used*

Gas-bubble disease
- Air embolism* [216, 217]
- Decompression sickness* [72]

Poisoning
- Carbon monoxide* [118, 119]
- Cyanide* [127]
- Hydrogen sulfide[129]
- Carbon tetrachloride[130]

Infections
- Clostridial myonecrosis* [138]
- Other soft-tissue necrotizing infections* [140]
- Chronic osteomyelitis* [218]
- Intracranial abcess[163]
- Mucormycosis[141]

Acute ischemia
- Crush injury* [4, 219, 220]
- Compromised skin flaps and grafts* [10]

Chronic ischemia
- Radiation necrosis* (soft tissue, radiation cystitis, and osteoradionecrosis)[221–224]
- Refractory ischemic ulcers, including diabetic ulcers* [225]

Central nervous system edema[142]

Acute hypoxia
- Support of oxygenation during therapeutic lung lavage[162, 226]
- Exceptional blood-loss anemia* (when transfusion delayed or unavailable)[161]

Thermal injury
- Burns* [150–154]

*Conditions approved by the Undersea and Hyperbaric Medical Society Hyperbaric Oxygen Therapy Committee.[163]

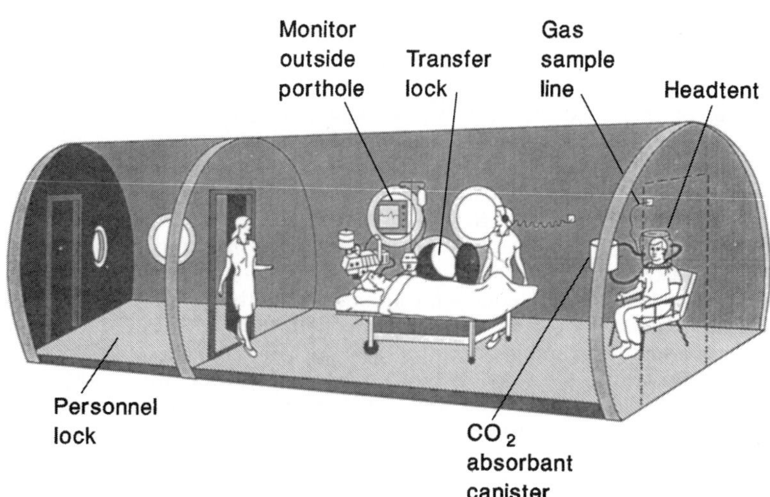

Figure 142–9. Multiplace chamber. Oxygen can be administered to the patient using a head tent (shown), endotracheal tube (shown), or a tightly fitting face mask. Many patients can be treated simultaneously. Medical personnel (tenders) accompany the patient during treatment. Additional personnel can enter the chamber using the personnel lock. Supplies can also be transferred via the transfer lock. Monitor displays are most conveniently kept outside the chamber in order to minimize electrical hazards and to prevent implosion of cathode ray tubes. Maximum pressure for multiplace chambers is usually at least 6 ATA (165 feet). Chamber atmosphere in hospital-based chambers and most other multiplace chambers is compressed air. Helium-oxygen (He-O_2) is occasionally used to compress the chamber for the treatment of divers with decompression illness sustained due to diving while breathing He-O_2. (From Moon RE, Camporesi EM: Operational use and patient monitoring in a multiplace hyperbaric chamber. Probl Respir Care 1991; 4:172–188.)

tender is typically a nurse who can provide assistance to the patient and manage intravascular monitoring catheters, obtain blood samples, manage the airway and ventilators, administer medications, and evaluate the patient. Multiplace chambers (Fig. 142–9) are usually compressed with air in order to reduce the risk of fire or explosion. Oxygen is administered to the patient with a tightly fitting face mask, head tent, or endotracheal tube. Medications, food, and blood samples can be moved into or out of the chamber using transfer locks. Prolonged treatment (up to several days) of patients with decompression illness (saturation treatment) can be accomplished using multiplace chambers. Additional personnel can also move into and out of the chamber through personnel locks. Multiplace chambers can typically be compressed to at least 6 ATA.

Monoplace chambers (Fig. 142–10), usually contructed of Plexiglas, can accommodate a single patient. They are generally compressed with 100% O_2 to a maximum operating pressure of about 3 ATA. Some practitioners have compressed these chambers with air, providing 100% O_2 to the patient via a tight-fitting mask. Connections for monitoring patients can be made via through-hull penetrators adjacent to the patient's head. Although hands-on management of patients in monoplace chambers is not possible, IV fluid administration, intravascular monitoring, mechanical ventilation, and chest tube management can all be accomplished during treatment in these units.[165] If prolonged treatments are required (e.g., USN Table 6), air breaks can be administered to the patient via a tight-fitting mask (a built-in breathing system, or "BIBS" mask) equipped with a demand valve.

Critically ill patients can be cared for more easily in multiplace chambers. Feeding and urine and stool elimination can be handled easily. On the other hand, installation of a multiplace chamber requires a specially trained staff as well as a specially designed and engineered room. Multiplace chambers are costly and require a chamber operator in addition to inside and outside tenders. Monoplace chambers, despite some practical shortcomings, are inexpensive, can be connected to standard hospital oxygen supplies, and require only one operator, who can also be a nurse.

Ventilatory Care

Important factors in the choice of a ventilator for use in a hyperbaric environment include fire hazard, simplicity, and small size. Fire hazard increases substantially when combustible materials are in contact with oxygen at high ambient pressure (see later). Therefore, it is preferable that ventilators

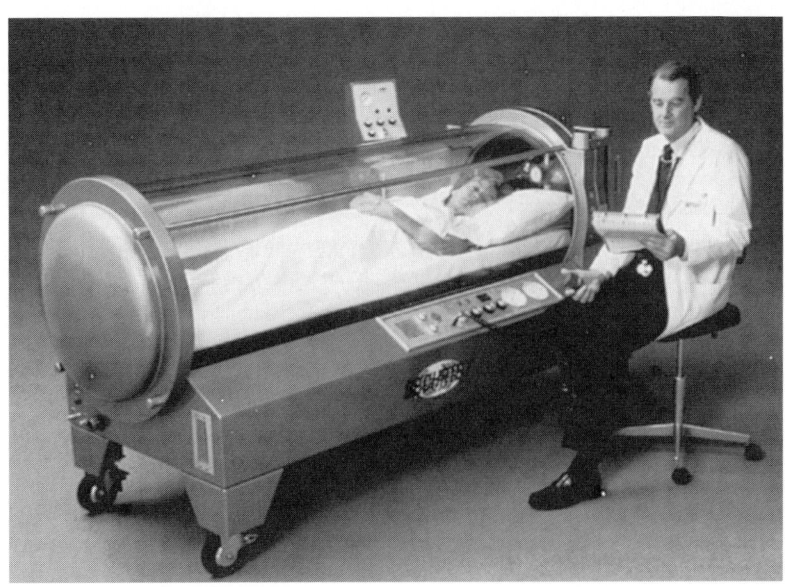

Figure 142–10. Monoplace chamber. The chamber hull is manufactured of Plexiglas, allowing direct observation of the patient. The chamber, compressed with 100% oxygen (O_2) to a maximum chamber pressure, is usually around 3 ATA. Although the patient cannot be directly accessed during treatment in the monoplace chamber, intravenous fluid administration and pressure monitoring can be accomplished with through-hole penetrators at the head of the patient.[173] Mechanical ventilation and chest tubes can also be safely managed in these chambers. (Courtesy of Sechrist Industries, Anaheim, Calif.)

be fluidically or pneumatically controlled with air rather than electrical power. Flammable lubricants should be avoided; hydrocarbons spontaneously ignite when in contact with aluminum at increased ambient Po_2. In addition, gas density increases in proportion to ambient pressure, resulting in a net rise in airway resistance. Therefore, volume-cycled ventilators are preferable. Table 142–8 summarizes a number of ventilators that have been used in hyperbaric environments.

Compression of the chamber causes a reduction in volume of any enclosed gas-containing space, including endotracheal tube cuffs. This volume reduction can be managed by continual addition of air during chamber compression. However, gas must be removed during decompression in order to avoid hyperinflation of the balloon. It is safer and easier to remove all air from the endotracheal tube cuff before compression and replace it with an appropriate volume of water.

Suction

Suction can be safely implemented using a device regulated to maintain a constant negative pressure with respect to ambient (chamber) pressure. Although endotracheal suctioning can be performed only in a multiplace chamber, nasogastric, pleural, and wound drainage suction can be applied in both types of hyperbaric chamber. When pleural suction regulators are used, unanticipated difficulties can occur because the collection compartment of such systems is a closed volume. Simonson and colleagues,[166] demonstrated that high negative pleural pressures can occur during chamber compression. Such excessive suction can be relieved by an attendant inside the chamber using the manual pressure relief valve.[166]

Intravenous Infusion Devices

Inside multiplace chambers, IV infusion of fluids contained in flexible plastic bags poses no major difficulty. The only minor adjustment is of the amount of air within the drip chamber, because the air volume tends to decrease with compression and expand with decompression. Nonvented IV fluid containers (e.g., glass bottles) can potentially be extremely dangerous, however. There is a risk of implosion during compression and of explosion during decompression. Accurate fluid administration using flow-controlled pumps is possible. IV infusion pumps or controllers that use drop counting to measure the flow rate may be inacccurate during compression and decompression because the gas within the drip chamber compresses and expands. Pumps that do not require a drip chamber for monitoring flow, for example, the Abbott Life Care 5000 Infusion Pumps (Abbott Laboratories, North Chicago, Ill.), deliver constant flow during chamber compression and decompression. Some control buttons with enclosed air spaces may malfunction at pressure, however. This can be overcome by drilling small vent holes to allow pressure equilibration. Insufflation of the cowling of electrically powered instruments inside multiplace chambers with 100% nitrogen to reduce fire risk is discussed later.

Infusion pumps supplied by line voltage are not generally used inside monoplace chambers because of the fire risk

TABLE 142–8. Ventilators Used in Hyperbaric Chambers

Ventilator	Comments	Reference
Allied Healthcare Omni-Vent Series D	Compact, time cycled, inspiratory flow variable. Has been used in monoplace chambers.	
Bennett PR-2	Controlling circuitry can be separated from the actuator and adjusted from outside the chamber.	Weaver[173]
Bird	Pressure-cycled ventilators; operating characteristics vary significantly with changes in ambient pressure.	Gallagher et al.[227]
Dräger Oxylog	Extremely compact, fluidically controlled ventilator.	
Dräger Hyperlog	Extremely compact, fluidically controlled ventilator, designed specifically for hyperbaric use.	Pelaia et al.[228]
LAMA RCH (Laboratoires de Mechanique Applique, Egly, France)	Tested to 6 ATA.	Le Masson et al.[229]
Logic-03		Degauque et al.[230]
Monaghan 225	Fluidically controlled. Satisfactory performance to 7 ATA; some slowing of rate as ambient pressure increased. Modification possible to allow compressed air actuation.	Moon et al.[231]
Ohio 550	Fluidically controlled. Preliminary testing at Duke Medical Center revealed satisfactory operation to 4 ATA.	
Penlon Nuffield 200		Lewis et al.[232]
Penlon Oxford	Successfully tested at 31 ATA.	Saywood et al.[233]
Percussionaire Corp. TXP	Time-cycled ventilator.	
PneuPAC Variant HB	Compact ventilator designed for use in monoplace chambers.	Spittal et al.[234]
Sechrist 500A	Compact fluidically controlled ventilator designed for monoplace chamber use. Some decrement in performance with changes in supply pressure, thoracic compliance, and at ambient pressure greater than 2.2 ATA.	Weaver and Strauss[165]
Siemens 900C	Sophisticated, compact, electronically controlled. Suitable only for multiplace chamber use. High oxygen levels near electrical components. Expired volume monitor may not be accurate at pressures >1 ATA.	Holcomb et al.[235]

ATA = atmospheres absolute.

associated with the 100% O_2 atmosphere. Therefore, continuous IV infusion of medications or fluids to patients inside monoplace chambers is usually performed using an infusion pump outside the chamber with tubing passed through a penetrator in the chamber hull. The controller must therefore be able to pump against the sum of the chamber transmural pressure (up to 2 ATA, or 1520 mm Hg), venous pressure, and resistance to flow within the tubing. Alternatively, an infusion bag inside the chamber can be controlled using a pneumatic cuff regulated from outside.

Arterial Blood Gas Measurement

Whereas arterial Po_2 increases along with inspired Po_2 during hyperbaric exposure, arterial pH and Pco_2 continue to be regulated by the body to about 7.4 and 40 mm Hg, respectively (see Table 142–2). Blood gas electrodes cannot be calibrated accurately at Po_2 values higher than about 700 mm Hg without pressurization of the electrodes or the entire blood gas machine. Therefore, extremely precise Po_2 measurements are best performed on a blood gas machine inside the chamber. This requires a modified blood gas instrument and analysis protocols, as well as a technician trained in this technique.

It is much more convenient to measure blood gases in samples decompressed to 1 ATA. Indeed, pH and Pco_2 can be accurately measured in such samples. However, during most routine HBO treatments, because the Po_2 is usually higher than 700 mm Hg, supersaturation of oxygen occurs during decompression and there is a tendency for bubble formation and hence for the Po_2 in the sample to decrease. Weaver and Howe[167] have shown that despite this theoretical objection, Po_2 values can be reasonably accurate if the sample is measured immediately after it has been decompressed or aspirated directly from the patient through the penetrator of a monoplace chamber. Furthermore, for clinical purposes it may not be necessary to have more than 10% to 20% accuracy under hyperbaric conditions.

Arterial Po_2 attained during hyperbaric treatment can be estimated reasonably accurately from blood gas measurements obtained at 1 ATA before treatment. Gilbert and Keighley[168] showed that the ratio of arterial to alveolar Po_2 (Pao_2/PAo_2 or a/A ratio) is reasonably constant over a range of inspired O_2 fraction from 0.21 to 1.0. In individuals with normal lungs, the a/A ratio is constant at least to an inspired Po_2 of 3 ATA. Therefore, blood gas measurement at 1 ATA can be used to predict the Po_2 under hyperbaric conditions according to the following equation:

$$Pao_2\ (\text{predicted}) = Pao_2/PAo_2 \times (760\ P_{ATA} - 47 - Paco_2) \qquad \text{[Equation 3]}$$

where Pao_2 and $Paco_2$ represent arterial O_2 and CO_2 tension and P_{ATA} is the chamber pressure in atmospheres absolute. Alveolar Po_2 is calculated from the following equation:

$$PAo_2 = (Pb - PH_2O)\,FIo_2 - PAco_2\left(FIo_2 + \frac{1 - FIo_2}{R}\right) \qquad \text{[Equation 4]}$$

where Pb is ambient pressure (usually 760 mm Hg, PH_2O is the saturated vapor pressure of water at body temperature (usually 47 mm Hg), $PAco_2$ is alveolar Pco_2 (usually assumed equal to arterial Pco_2), FIO_2 is inspired fraction of O_2, and R is the respiratory quotient (R = CO_2 elimination rate/O_2 uptake rate). R depends on diet but is usually approximately 0.8.

In the presence of lung disease, Equation 3 tends to underestimate the actual Po_2 under hyperbaric conditions. There are two reasons for this. First, Pao_2 during breathing with an inspired oxygen percentage less than 100% is affected by both ventilation-perfusion ($\dot{V}A/\dot{Q}$) mismatch and right-to-left intrapulmonary shunt (as well as, of course, intracardiac shunt), whereas during breathing of 100% O_2 $\dot{V}A/\dot{Q}$ mismatch has no influence on arterial Po_2. Second, under hyperbaric conditions, mixed venous Po_2 may be several hundred mm Hg and thus a right-to-left shunt has less tendency to produce arterial hypoxemia.

Hypercapnea results in cerebral vasodilatation, which may increase the risk of hyperoxic convulsions. It is often helpful, therefore, to measure arterial Pco_2 shortly after compression in order to ensure adequacy of ventilation. Individuals with hypercapnea under 1 ATA conditions are likely to experience an acute rise in Pco_2 when administered HBO. This is due to both a reduced respiratory drive induced by hyperoxia and relative hypoventilation because of the increased respiratory effort associated with breathing dense gas. Therefore, if hyperbaric treatment of such individuals is considered necessary, mechanical ventilation may be required.

Monitoring Patients

Monitoring of patients in a multiplace chamber should include a display that is visible to the tenders inside the chamber as well as to the outside chamber operator, nurse, or physician. Cathode-ray tubes are likely to implode at high ambient pressure. If such devices are used, it is safest to place the monitor outside the chamber facing one of the view ports. Liquid crystal display units can be used in hyperbaric chambers.

Electrical monitoring is quite easily accomplished using cables plumbed through the chamber hall. In order to isolate preamplifiers from the chamber wall, it is best to use individual shield wires for each electrode. Should a preamplifier need to be placed in the chamber, safety is enhanced if it is purged with 100% nitrogen.

Standard sphygmomanometers with stethoscopes can be used inside multiplace hyperbaric chambers. However, spillage of mercury inside a hyperbaric chamber can produce a dangerously high mercury vapor pressure. It is therefore recommended that aneroid pressure gauges be used rather than mercury-filled ones. Automatic noninvasive blood pressure monitors can be used in the hyperbaric environment provided appropriate electrical safety principles are followed.

Strain gauge pressure transducers used for invasive pressure monitoring require no modification when used under hyperbaric conditions. Whereas older diaphragm (Statham) transducers tend to be subject to baseline drift during chamber compression and decompression, the newer disposable types are acceptably stable. These transducers need to be referenced ("zeroed") to chamber pressure. A blood pressure of 120/80 mm Hg, appropriately referenced to the inside chamber pressure of 2 ATA (1520 mm Hg), would read 1640/1600 mm Hg if referenced to the outside ambient pressure. If pneumatically inflated pressure bags are used in conjunction with continuous flow pressure transducer systems, they must be further inflated on compression and deflated during decompressed in order to maintain a constant 300 mm Hg pressure. An alternative is to use a spring-loaded rather than a pneumatically pressurized device.

Blood pressure measurement can be performed inside monoplace chambers using either direct transduction of intra-arterial pressure or a variety of noninvasive methods.[165] An electronic stethoscope can be used in conjunction with a sphygmomanometer inflated from outside the chamber. Automated blood pressure devices are also available.

During compression and decompression of the chamber, pulmonary artery catheter balloon ports must be vented to the chamber atmosphere. In other words, the balloon inflation syringe must be disconnected from the inflation port. If this is not done, the balloon may be forcefully pressed against the internal port during compression, causing tearing. Failure to disconnect the syringe before decompression may lead to the balloon bursting, air embolism, and rupture of a pulmonary vessel.

Fire Hazard

The extremely high Po_2 that may be present in the chamber atmosphere or in isolated instruments (e.g., ventilators) can significantly increase the risk of fire. A systematic analysis of chamber fires indicated that before 1980 fires were frequently caused by electrical ignition. Since then, chamber fires have been caused primarily by ignition sources such as hand warmers and toys carried into the chamber by an occupant. In another instance, a preheated bed sheet caught fire when compressed to 2 ATA in a transfer lock.[169] The only survivors of chamber fires have been in chambers pressurized with air.[170]

Minimization of fire hazard may require a number of modifications of standard ICU practice. First, the inevitable increase in chamber Po_2 in multiplace facilities should be minimized. This increase in Po_2 occurs because of leakage from head tents, masks, or ventilators. Continuous monitoring of the chamber Po_2 can provide guidelines to when the chamber must be vented with air to reduce the oxygen concentration to an acceptable level (typically 23%). Sources of spark and heat should be eliminated if possible. An additional safety measure is purging of electrical instruments with 100% N_2 at a flow rate sufficient to maintain the Po_2 within the instrument at a level that does not support combustion.

The patient must be forbidden to carry sources of combustion into the chamber. These restrictions include matches, cigarette lighters, and battery-operated devices. Static electricity may possibly ignite a fire, and therefore cotton garments are safer than ones manufactured out of synthetic material. Hair grease should be removed and hydrocarbon-based salves or creams should be avoided on areas that may come into contact with increased oxygen concentrations. Petroleum-based lubricants (e.g., on stretcher wheels and other equipment) must also be replaced with fluorocarbon-based lubricants. Humidification of the breathing gas within a head tent system further reduces the fire hazard as well as making the patient more comfortable.

Sparking, which might occur when electrical instruments are plugged in or unplugged, must be avoided in the hyperbaric environment. In multiplace chambers, if the use of high-voltage (120 volts) equipment is unavoidable, sparking can be avoided or minimized if it is hard wired or at least plugged into an extension cord before compression of the chamber, with the connection securely taped to avoid accidental disconnection at pressure. An additional safety feature is the use of explosion-proof plugs, such as Arktite Series plugs (Crouse-Hinds, Division of Cooper Industries, Syracuse, N.Y.). Defibrillation is another potential source of sparking, but patients have been successfully defibrillated at pressure without causing fire. Low-resistance electrode gel or preapplied disposable defibrillator pads are likely to minimize the risk.

Electrical safety precautions must be more strict in monoplace chambers because of the considerably higher risk of ignition relates to the high oxygen environment. The voltage level in unavoidable electrical equipment, such as the communication system, is usually limited to about 5 volts. In addition, in order to prevent buildup of static charges, the patient must be grounded.

Additional safety information pertinent to both multiplace and monoplace chamber operation can be found in two volumes available from the Undersea and Hyperbaric Medical Society (Kensington, Md.).[165, 171]

Atmosphere Control

The toxic effects of trace gases depend on partial pressure. Because partial pressure increases directly with ambient pressure, trace contaminates may become toxic under hyperbaric conditions. It is important to ensure that gases that can be produced by the compressors (e.g., hydrocarbons and carbon monoxide) are at a safe level. Other trace contaminants that should be eliminated from use at pressure include alcohol from skin disinfectant solutions, mercury vapor from sphygmomanometers and glass thermometers, and other gases such as hydrogen and sulfur dioxide, which can be released from certain batteries. Many hyperbaric chamber facilities use non-alcohol-based skin disinfectant solutions. Lithium and mercury batteries are best avoided. The Gates lead acid, gelled electrolyte battery has been specifically tested to 8 ATA and verified as safe. Alkaline cells are usually considered safe.

It is also important to ensure that the gas delivered to the patient contains an appropriate concentration of O_2 and a safe concentration of CO_2. Use of a semiclosed partially recirculating gas circuit to deliver oxygen to a head tent can be associated with carbon dioxide accumulation if the recirculation rate is too low. It is the practice of many facilitates to monitor both inspired O_2 and CO_2 from the patients' head tents, particularly if semiclosed circuits are used. The inspired CO_2 pressure should be less than 3.8 mm Hg (0.5% surface-equivalent concentration); the inspired oxygen fraction should be 0.98 or higher.

Evaluation of a Patient for Hyperbaric Oxygen Therapy

Evaluation of a patient must take into consideration both the efficacy of HBO for that patient and the risk of complications or side effects.

The patient's disease must be amenable to hyperbaric therapy (see biannually published guidelines for acceptable indications available from the Undersea and Hyperbaric Medical Society[163]). It is also important that a therapeutic arterial Po_2 be attained (probably >1000 mm Hg). Conditions that may preclude attainment of a sufficiently high arterial Po_2, while employing an inspired oxygen tension (<3 ATA), include severe pulmonary disease and cyanotic heart disease.

The most common side effect of hyperbaric therapy is otic barotrauma. Patients with middle ear disease, head and neck radiation, respiratory infections, allergic rhinitis, or swallowing disorders and intubated or unconscious patients[145] may be unable to equilibrate middle ear pressure as ambient pressure is raised. This can cause pain, middle ear hemorrhage, tympanic membrane rupture, or labyrinthine (round or oval) window rupture. It is the practice of many hyperbaric physicians to perform prophylactic myringotomies on these patients. Patients likely to require more than a few treatments may benefit from tympanostomy tube placement.

The risk of pulmonary barotrauma should be assessed before instituting hyperbaric therapy. Patients with a pneumothorax may require thoracostomy. Bullous lung disease and severe airway obstruction are risk factors for pulmonary barotrauma. If possible, pulmonary function should be optimized pharmacologically before HBO treatment. With patients at increased risk for of developing pulmonary oxygen toxicity (e.g., patients who have received bleomycin or mitomycin C), the risk of acute respiratory distress syndrome (ARDS) related to HBO-induced pulmonary toxicity must be weighed against the potential benefit of hyperbaric treatment.

Commonly used treatment schedules are designed to minimize both cerebral and pulmonary oxygen toxicity. However, pulmonary O_2 toxicity can still occur, particularly if supplemental oxygen is required between treatments. There is also a risk of myopia, usually after a prolonged series of treatments (>30). This rarely influences the decision to undertake emergency HBO therapy. However, some patients who require a prolonged course of treatment may be unwilling to accept this risk if there is preexisting visual impairment.

SUMMARY

HBO therapy is the primary treatment of choice for gas embolism, decompression sickness, and severe acute carbon monoxide poisoning. It has been increasingly used as an adjunctive therapy in the treatment of patients with a variety of medical or surgical conditions in which there has been increasing evidence for improved clinical outcome. This widening use has demanded increasingly sophisticated care in this unusual environment. Although new pharmacologic therapies may obviate the need for HBO in some conditions, in the foreseeable future there will be a need to deliver oxygen at high ambient pressure to patients suffering from a selected group of conditions. Continual updating of hyperbaric technology will ensure that standards of ICU care are available in the hyperbaric environment.

References

1. Bert P: Barometric Pressure (La Pression Barométrique). Hitchcock MA, Hitchcock FA (Trans). Bethesda, Md, Undersea Medical Society, 1978.
2. Hempel FG, Jobsis FF, LaManna JL, Rosenthal MR, Saltzman HA: Oxidation of cerebral cytochrome aa_3 by oxygen plus carbon dioxide at hyperbaric pressures. J Appl Physiol 1977; 43:873-879.
3. Whalen R, Saltzman H, Holloway D, et al: Cardiovascular and blood gas responses to hyperbaric oxygenation. Am J Cardiol 1965; 15:638-646.
4. Nylander G, Lewis D, Nordstrom H, Larsson NJ: Reduction of post-ischemic edema with hyperbaric oxygen. Plast Reconstr Surg 1985; 76:596-603.
5. Fife CE, Camporesi EM: Physiologic effects of hyperbaric hyperoxia. Probl Respir Care 1991; 4:142-149.
6. Mader JT, Brown GL, Guckian JC, Wells CH, Reinarz JA: A mechanism for the amelioration by hyperbaric oxygen of experimental staphylococcal osteomyelitis in rabbits. J Infect Dis 1980; 142:915-922.
7. Mader JT, Adams KR, Sutton TE: Infectious diseases: Pathophysiology and mechanisms of hyperbaric oxygen. J Hyperb Med 1987; 2:133-140.
8. Zamboni WA, Mazolewski PJ, Erdmann D, et al: Evaluation of penicillin and hyperbaric oxygen in the treatment of streptococcal myositis. Ann Plast Surg 1997; 39:131-136.
9. Park MK, Muhvich KH, Myers RAM, Marzella L: Effects of hyperbaric oxygen in infectious diseases: Basic mechanisms. *In:* Hyperbaric Medicine Practice. Kindwall EP (Ed). Flagstaff, Ariz, Best Publishing, 1995, pp 141-172.
10. Zamboni WA, Roth AC, Russell RC, Graham B, Suchy H, Kucan JO: Morphological analysis of the microcirculation during reperfusion of ischemic skeletal muscle and the effect of hyperbaric oxygen. Plast Reconstr Surg 1993; 91:1110-1123.
11. Helps SC, Meyer-Witting M, Rilley PL, Gorman DF: Increasing doses of intracarotid air and cerebral blood flow in rabbits. Stroke 1990; 21:1340-1345.
12. Helps SC, Gorman DF: Air embolism of the brain in rabbits pretreated with mechlorethamine. Stroke 1991; 22:351-354.
13. Thom SR, Mendiguren I, Hardy K, et al: Inhibition of human neutrophil β_2-integrin-dependent adherence by hyperbaric O_2. Am J Physiol 1997; 273:C770-C777.
14. Thom S: Antagonism of carbon monoxide-mediated brain lipid peroxidation by hyperbaric oxygen. Toxicol Appl Pharmacol 1990; 105:340-344.
15. Brown SD, Piantadosi CA: Recovery of energy metabolism in rat brain after carbon monoxide hypoxia. J Clin Invest 1992; 89:666-672.
16. Gerschman R, Gilbert DL, Nye SW, Dwyer P, Fenn WO: Oxygen poisoning and x-irradiation: A mechanism in common. Science 1954; 119:623-626.
17. Freeman BA, Crapo JD: Biology of disease: Free radicals and tissue injury. Lab Invest 1982; 47:412-426.
18. Lambertsen CJ: Effects of hyperoxia on organs and their tissues. *In:* Extrapulmonary Manifestations of Respiratory Disease. Robin ED (Ed). New York, Marcel Dekker, 1978, pp 239-303.
19. Navy Department: US Navy Diving Manual. Vol 1. Revision 3: Air Diving. NAVSEA 0994-LP-001-9110. Flagstaff, Ariz, Best Publishing, 1993.
20. Clark JM: Oxygen toxicity. *In:* The Physiology and Medicine of Diving. Bennett PB, Elliott DH (Eds). Philadelphia, WB Saunders, 1993, pp 121-169.
21. Harabin AL, Homer LD, Weathersby PK, Flynn ET: An analysis of decrements in vital capacity as an index of pulmonary oxygen toxicity. J Appl Physiol 1987; 63:1130-1135.
22. Anderson B Jr, Shelton DL: Axial length in hyperoxic myopia. *In:* Underwater and Hyperbaric Physiology IX. Proceedings of the Ninth International Symposium on Underwater and Hyperbaric Physiology. Bove AA, Bachrach AJ, Greenbaum LJ Jr (Eds). Bethesda, Undersea and Hyperbaric Medical Society, 1987, pp 607-611.
23. Palmquist BM, Philipson B, Barr PO: Nuclear cataract and myopia during hyperbaric oxygen therapy. Br J Ophthalmol 1984; 68:113-117.
24. Philp RB, Inwood MJ, Ackles KN, Radomski MW: Effects of decompression on platelets and hemostasis in men and the influence of antiplatelet drugs (RA233 and VK744). Aerosp Med 1974; 45:231-240.
25. Philp RB, Bennett PB, Andersen JC, et al: Effects of aspirin and dipyridamole on platelet function, hematology, and blood chemistry of saturation divers. Undersea Biomed Res 1979; 6:127-146.
26. Waite CL, Mazzone WF, Greenwood ME, Larsen RT: Cerebral air embolism: I. Basic studies. U.S. Naval Submarine Medical Center Report 493. Panama City, Fla, U.S. Navy Submarine Research Laboratory, 1967.
27. Landolt JP, Money KE, Topliff ED, Nicholas AD, Laufer J, Johnson WH: Pathophysiology of inner ear dysfunction in the squirrel monkey in rapid decompression. J Appl Physiol 1980; 49:1070-1082.
28. Palmer AC, Blakemore WF, Payne JE, Sillence A: Decompression sickness in the goat: Nature of brain and spinal cord lesions at 48 hours. Undersea Biomed Res 1978; 5:275-286.
29. Hardman JM: Histology of decompression illness. *In:* Treatment of Decompression Illness. Moon RE, Sheffield PJ (Eds). Kensington, Md, Undersea and Hyperbaric Medical Society, 1996, pp 10-20.
30. Broome JR, Dick EJ Jr: Neurological decompression illness in swine. Aviat Space Environ Med 1996; 67:207-213.
31. Helps SC, Parsons DW, Reilly PL, Gorman DF: The effect of gas emboli on rabbit cerebral blood flow. Stroke 1990; 21:94-99.
32. Ence TJ, Gong H Jr: Adult respiratory distress syndrome after venous air embolism. Am Rev Respir Dis 1979; 119:1033-1037.
33. Ohkuda K, Nakahara K, Binder A, Staub NC: Venous air emboli in sheep: Reversible increase in lung microvascular permeability. J Appl Physiol 1981; 51:887-894.
34. Huang KL, Lin YC: Activation of complement and neutrophils increases vascular permeability during air embolism. Aviat Space Environ Med 1997; 68:300-305.
35. Ward CA, Koheil A, McCullough D, Johnson WR, Fraser WD: Activation of complement at plasma-air or serum-air interface of rabbits. J Appl Physiol 1986; 60:1651-1658.
36. Shastri KA, Logue GL, Lundgren CE: In vitro activation of human complement by nitrogen bubbles. Undersea Biomed Res 1991; 18:157-165.
37. Ward CA, McCullough D, Fraser WD: Relation between complement activation and susceptibility to decompression sickness. J Appl Physiol 1987; 62:1160-1166.

38. Zhang J, Fife CE, Currie MS, Moon RE, Piantadosi CA, Vann RD: Venous gas emboli and complement activation after deep repetitive air diving. Undersea Biomed Res 1991; 18:293-302.
39. Stevens DM, Gartner SL, Pearson RR, et al: Complement activation during saturation diving. Undersea Hyperb Med 1993; 20:279-288.
40. Hjelde A, Bergh K, Brubakk AO, Iversen OJ: Complement activation in divers after repeated air/heliox dives and its possible relevance to DCS. J Appl Physiol 1995; 78:1140-1144.
41. Pekna M, Ersson A: Complement system response to decompression. Undersea Hyperb Med 1996; 23:31-34.
42. Ward CA, McCullough D, Yee D, Stanga D, Fraser WD: Complement activation involvement in decompression sickness of rabbits. Undersea Biomed Res 1990; 17:51-66.
43. Shastri KA, Logue GL, Lundgren CE, Logue CJ, Suggs DF: Diving decompression fails to activate complement. Undersea Hyperb Med 1997; 24:51-57.
44. Broome JR, Pearson RR, Dutka AJ: Failure to prevent decompression illness in rats by pretreatment with a soluble complement receptor. Undersea Hyperb Med 1994; 21:287-295.
45. Floyd RA: Role of oxygen free radicals in carcinogenesis and brain ischemia. FASEB J 1990; 4:2587-2597.
46. Choi D: Ionic dependence of glutamate neurotoxicity. J Neurosci 1987; 7:369-379.
47. Endres M, Wang ZQ, Namura S, Waeber C, Moskowitz MA: Ischemic brain injury is mediated by the activation of poly(ADP-ribose) polymerase. J Cereb Blood Flow Metab 1997; 17:1143-1151.
48. Butler BD, Hills BA: Transpulmonary passage of venous air emboli. J Appl Physiol 1985; 59:543-547.
49. Adornato DC, Gildenberg PL, Ferrano CM, Smart J, Frost EA: The pathophysiology of intravenous air embolism in dogs. Anesthesiology 1978; 49:120-127.
50. Yeakel A: Lethal air embolism from plastic blood storage container. JAMA 1968; 204:267-268.
51. Seidelin PH, Stolarek IH, Thompson AM: Central venous catheterization and fatal air embolism. Br J Hosp Med 1987; 38:438-439.
52. Malhotra MS, Wright HC: The effects of a raised intrapulmonary pressure on the lungs of fresh unchilled cadavers. J Pathol Bacteriol 1961; 82:198-202.
53. Benton PJ, Woodfine JD, Westwook PR: Arterial gas embolism following a 1-meter ascent during helicopter escape training: A case report. Aviat Space Environ Med 1996; 67:63-64.
54. Rudge FW: A case of decompression sickness at 2,437 m (8,000 feet). Aviat Space Environ Med 1990; 61:1026-1027.
55. Vann RD, Denoble P, Emmerman MN, Corson KS: Flying after diving and decompression sickness. Aviat Space Environ Med 1993; 64:801-807.
56. Elliott DH, Moon RE: Manifestations of the decompression disorders. *In:* The Physiology and Medicine of Diving. Bennett PB, Elliott DH (Eds). Philadelphia, WB Saunders, 1993, pp 481-505.
57. Van Allen CM, Hrdina LS, Clark J: Air embolism from the pulmonary vein. Arch Surg 1929; 19:567-599.
58. Atkinson JR: Experimental air embolism. Northwest Med 1963; 62:699-703.
59. Kruse CA: Air embolism and other skin diving problems. Northwest Med 1963; 62:525-529.
60. Butler BD, Laine GA, Leiman BC, et al: Effects of Trendelenburg position on the distribution of arterial air emboli in dogs. Ann Thorac Surg 1988; 45:198-202.
61. Mehlhorn U, Burke EJ, Butler BD, et al: Body position does not affect the hemodynamic response to venous air embolism in dogs. Anesth Analg 1994; 79:734-739.
62. Dutka AJ: Therapy for dysbaric central nervous system ischemia: Adjuncts to recompression. *In:* Diving Accident Management. Bennett PB, Moon RE (Eds). Bethesda, Md, Undersea and Hyperbaric Medical Society, 1990, pp 222-234.
63. Merton DA, Fife WP, Gross DR: An evaluation of plasma volume expanders in the treatment of decompression sickness. Aviat Space Environ Med 1983; 54:218-222.
64. Brunner F, Frick P, Bühlmann A: Post-decompression shock due to extravasation of plasma. Lancet 1964; 1:1071-1073.
65. Boussuges A, Blanc P, Molenat F, Bergmann E, Sainty JM: Haemoconcentration in neurological decompression illness. Int J Sports Med 1996; 17:351-355.
66. Michenfelder JD, Martin JT, Altenburg BM, Rehder K: Air embolism during neurosurgery. An evaluation of right-atrial catheters for diagnosis and treatment. JAMA 1969; 208:1353-1358.
67. Stark J, Hough J: Air in the aorta: Treatment by reversed perfusion. Ann Thorac Surg 1986; 41:337-338.
68. Yarbrough OD, Behnke AR: The treatment of compressed air illness using oxygen. J Ind Hyg Toxicol 1939; 21:213-218.
69. Woodward CM: A History of the St. Louis Bridge. St. Louis, GI Jones, 1881.
70. Blick G: Notes on diver's paralysis. Br Med J 1909; 2:1796-1799.
71. Keays FL: Compressed air illness, with a report of 3,692 cases. Dept Med Publ Cornell Univ Med Coll 1909; 2:1-55.
72. Moon RE, Gorman DF: Treatment of the decompression disorders. *In:* The Physiology and Medicine of Diving. Bennett PB, Elliott DH (Eds). Philadelphia, WB Saunders, 1993, pp 506-541.
73. Dutka AJ: Air or gas embolism. *In:* Hyperbaric Oxygen Therapy: A Critical Review. Camporesi EM, Barker AC (Eds). Bethesda, Md, Undersea and Hyperbaric Medical Society, 1991, pp 1-10.
74. Meyers RAM, Bray P: Delayed treatment of serious decompression sickness. Ann Emerg Med 1985; 14:254-257.
75. Rudge FW, Shafer MR: The effect of delay on treatment outcome in altitude-induced decompression sickness. Aviat Space Environ Med 1991; 62:687-690.
76. Ball R: Effect of severity, time to recompression with oxygen, and retreatment on outcome in forty-nine cases of spinal cord decompression sickness. Undersea Hyperb Med 1993; 20:133-145.
77. Dexter F, Hindman BJ: Recommendations for hyperbaric oxygen therapy of cerebral air embolism based on a mathematical model of bubble absorption. Anesth Analg 1997; 84:1203-1207.
78. Moon RE: Treatment of gas bubble disease. Probl Respir Care 1991; 4:232-252.
79. Moon RE, Sheffield PJ: Guidelines for treatment of decompression illness. Aviat Space Environ Med 1997; 68:234-243.
80. Leitch DR, Greenbaum LJ Jr, Hallenbeck JM: Cerebral arterial air embolism: I. Is there benefit in beginning HBO treatment at 6 bar? Undersea Biomed Res 1984; 11:221-235.
81. Leitch DR, Greenbaum LJ Jr, Hallenbeck JM: Cerebral arterial air embolism: II. Effect of pressure and time on cortical evoked potential recovery. Undersea Biomed Res 1984; 11:237-248.
82. Leitch DR, Hallenbeck JA: Pressure in the treatment of spinal cord decompression sickness. Undersea Biomed Res 1985; 12:291-305.
83. McDermott JJ, Dutka AJ, Koller WA, Pearson RR, Flynn ET: Comparison of two recompression profiles in treating experimental cerebral air embolism. Undersea Biomed Res 1992; 19:171-185.
84. McDermott JJ, Dutka AJ, Koller WA, Flynn ET: Effects of an increased Po_2 during recompression therapy for the treatment of experimental cerebral arterial gas embolism. Undersea Biomed Res 1992; 19:403-413.
85. Leitch DR, Green RD: Additional pressurization for treating nonresponding cases of serious air decompression sickness. Aviat Space Environ Med 1985; 56:1139-1143.
86. Lee HC, Niu KC, Chen SH, et al: Therapeutic effects of different tables on type II decompression sickness. J Hyperb Med 1991; 6:11-17.
87. Thalmann ED: Principles of U.S. Navy recompression treatments for decompression sickness. *In:* Diving Accident Management. Bennett PB, Moon RE (Eds). Bethesda, Md, Undersea and Hyperbaric Medical Society, 1990, pp 194-221.
88. Pearson RR, Goad RF: Delayed cerebral edema complicating cerebral arterial gas embolism: Case histories. Undersea Biomed Res 1982; 9:283-296.
89. Kizer KW: Corticosteroids in treatment of serious decompression sickness. Ann Emerg Med 1981; 10:485-488.
90. Francis TJR, Dutka AJ: Methylprednisolone in the treatment of acute spinal cord decompression sickness. Undersea Biomed Res 1989; 16:165-174.
91. Dutka AJ, Mink RB, Pearson RR, Hallenbeck JM: Effects of treatment with dexamethasone on recovery from experimental cerebral arterial gas embolism. Undersea Biomed Res 1992; 19:131-141.
92. Bracken MB, Shepard MJ, Collins WF, et al: A randomized, controlled trial of methylprednisolone or naloxone in the treatment

of acute spinal-cord injury: Results of the Second National Acute Spinal Cord Injury Study. N Engl J Med 1990; 322:1405–1411.
93. Reeves E, Workman RD: Use of heparin for the therapeutic/prophylactic treatment of decompression sickness. Aerosp Med 1971; 42:20–23.
94. Kindwall EP, Margolis I: Management of severe decompression sickness with treatment ancillary to recompression: Case report. Aviat Space Environ Med 1975; 46:1065–1068.
95. Spadaro MV, Moon RE, Fracica PJ, et al: Life threatening pulmonary thromboembolism in neurological decompression illness. Undersea Biomed Res 1992; 19(Suppl):41–42.
96. Evans DE, Kobrine AI, LeGrys DC, Bradley ME: Protective effect of lidocaine in acute cerebral ischemia induced by air embolism. J Neurosurg 1984; 60:257–263.
97. Evans DE, Catron PW, McDermott JJ, Thomas LB, Kobrine AI, Flynn ET: Therapeutic effect of lidocaine in experimental cerebral ischemia induced by air embolism. J Neurosurg 1989; 70:97–102.
98. McDermott JJ, Dutka AJ, Evans DE, Flynn ET: Treatment of experimental cerebral air embolism with lidocaine and hyperbaric oxygen. Undersea Biomed Res 1990; 17:525–534.
99. Drewry A, Gorman DF: Lidocaine as an adjunct to hyperbaric therapy in decompression illness: A case report. Undersea Biomed Res 1992; 19:187–190.
100. Cogar WB: Intravenous lidocaine as adjunctive therapy in the treatment of decompression illness. Ann Emerg Med 1997; 29:284–286.
101. Mitchell SJ, Pellett O, Gorman DF: Cerebral protection from lidocaine during cardiac operations. Ann Thorac Surg 1999; 67:1117–1124.
102. Dutka AJ, Mink R, McDermott J, Clark JB, Hallenbeck JM: Effect of lidocaine on somatosensory evoked response and cerebral blood flow after canine cerebral air embolism. Stroke 1992; 23:1515–1520.
103. Menasché P, Pinard E, Desroches AM, et al: Fluorocarbons: A potential treatment of cerebral air embolism in open heart surgery. Ann Thorac Surg 1985; 40:494–497.
104. Spiess BD, McCarthy RJ, Tuman KJ: Treatment of decompression sickness with a perfluorocarbon emulsion (FC-43). Undersea Biomed Res 1988; 15:31–37.
105. Brown SD, Piantadosi CA: In vivo binding of carbon monoxide to cytochrome *c* oxidase in rat brain. J Appl Physiol 1990; 68:604–610.
106. Piantadosi CA, Lee PA, Sylvia AL: Direct effects of CO on cerebral energy metabolism in bloodless rats. J Appl Physiol 1988; 65:878–887.
107. Zhang J, Piantadosi CA: Mitochondrial oxidative stress after carbon monoxide hypoxia in the rat brain. J Clin Invest 1992; 90:1193–1199.
108. Marks GS, Brien JF, Nakatsu K, McLaughlin BE: Does carbon monoxide have a physiological function? Trends Pharmacol Sci 1991; 12:185–188.
109. Messier LD, Myers RA: A neuropsychological screening battery for emergency assessment of carbon monoxide poisoned patients. J Clin Psychol 1991; 47:675–684.
110. Jones JS, Lagasse J, Zimmerman G: Computed tomographic findings after acute carbon monoxide poisoning. Am J Emerg Med 1994; 12:448–451.
111. Pracyk JB, Stolp BW, Fife CE, Gray L, Piantadosi CA: Brain computerized tomography after hyperbaric oxygen therapy for carbon monoxide poisoning. Undersea Hyperb Med 1995; 22:1–7.
112. Silver DA, Cross M, Fox B, Paxton RM: Computed tomography of the brain in acute carbon monoxide poisoning. Clin Radiol 1996; 51:480–483.
113. Pace N, Strajman E, Walker E: Acceleration of carbon monoxide elimination in man by high pressure oxygen. Science 1950; 111:652–654.
114. Brown SD, Piantadosi CA: Reversal of carbon monoxide-cytochrome *c* oxidase binding by hyperbaric oxygen in vivo. Adv Exp Med Biol 1989; 248:747–754.
115. Raphael JC, Elkharrat D, Jars-Guincestre MC, et al: Trial of normobaric and hyperbaric oxygen for acute carbon monoxide intoxication. Lancet 1989; 2:414–419.
116. Krantz T, Thisted B, Strom J, Sorensen MB: Acute carbon monoxide poisoning. Acta Anaesthesiol Scand 1988; 32:278–282.
117. Norkool DM, Kirkpatrick JN: Treatment of acute carbon monoxide poisoning with hyperbaric oxygen: A review of 115 cases. Ann Emerg Med 1985; 14:1168–1171.
118. Thom S, Taber R, Mendiguren I, Clark J, Hardy K, Fisher A: Delayed neuropsychologic sequelae after carbon monoxide poisoning: Prevention by treatment with hyperbaric oxygen. Ann Emerg Med 1995; 25:474–480.
119. Piantadosi CA: The role of hyperbaric oxygen in carbon monoxide, cyanide and sulfide intoxication. Probl Respir Care 1991; 4:215–231.
120. Ledingham IM, McBride TI, Jennett WB, Adams JH, Tindal SAP: Fatal brain damage associated with cardiomyopathy of pregnancy, with notes on Caesarean section in a hyperbaric chamber. Br Med J 1968; 4:285–287.
121. Hollander DI, Nagey DA, Welch R, Pupkin M: Hyperbaric oxygen therapy for the treatment of acute carbon monoxide poisoning in pregnancy: A case report. J Reprod Med 1987; 32:615–617.
122. Van Hoesen KB, Camporesi EM, Moon RE, Hage ML, Piantadosi CA: Should hyperbaric oxygen be used to treat the pregnant patient for acute carbon monoxide poisoning? A case report and literature review. [Erratum appears in JAMA 1990; 273:2750.] JAMA 1989; 261:1039–1043.
123. Brown DB, Mueller GL, Golich FC: Hyperbaric oxygen treatment for carbon monoxide poisoning in pregnancy: A case report. Aviat Space Environ Med 1992; 63:1011–1014.
124. Elkharrat D, Raphael JC, Korach JM, et al: Acute carbon monoxide intoxication and hyperbaric oxygen in pregnancy. Intensive Care Med 1991; 17:289–292.
125. Mathieu D, Wattel F, Nevière R, Mathieu-Nolf M: Carbon monoxide poisoning: Mechanism, clinical presentation and management. *In:* Handbook on Hyperbaric Medicine. Oriani G, Marroni A, Wattel F (Eds). New York, Springer-Verlag, 1996, pp 281–296.
126. Camporesi EM: Hyperbaric oxygen therapy for CO intoxication during pregnancy. *In:* Handbook on Hyperbaric Medicine. Oriani G, Marroni A, Wattel F (Eds). New York, Springer-Verlag, 1996, pp 305–311.
127. Litovitz TL, Larkin RF, Myers RAM: Cyanide poisoning treated with hyperbaric oxygen. Am J Emerg Med 1983; 1:94–101.
128. Smilkstein MJ, Bronstein AC, Pickett HM, Rumack BH: Hyperbaric oxygen therapy for severe hydrogen sulfide poisoning. J Emerg Med 1985; 3:27–30.
129. Whitcraft DD, Bailey TD, Hart GB: Hydrogen sulfide poisoning treated with hyperbaric oxygen. J Emerg Med 1985; 3:23–25.
130. Truss CD, Killenberg PG: Treatment of carbon tetrachloride with hyperbaric oxygen. Gastroenterology 1982; 82:767–769.
131. Burkhart KK, Hall AH, Gerace R, Rumack BH: Hyperbaric oxygen treatment for carbon tetrachloride poisoning. Drug Saf 1992; 6:332–338.
132. Berk RF, Lane JM, Patel K: Relationship of oxygen and glutathione in protection against carbon tetrachloride–induced hepatic microsomal lipid peroxidation and covalent binding in the rat: Rationale for the use of hyperbaric oxygen to treat carbon tetrachloride ingestion. J Clin Invest 1984; 74:1996–2001.
133. Shoemaker W, Appel P, Kram H: Role of oxygen debt in the development of organ failure, sepsis and death in high risk surgical patients. Chest 1992; 102:208–215.
134. Hill GB, Osterhout S: Experimental effects of hyperbaric oxygen on selected clostridial species: II. In vivo studies in mice. J Infect Dis 1972; 125:26–35.
135. Demello FJ, Haglin JJ, Hitchcock CR: Comparative study of experimental *Clostridium perfringens* infection in dogs treated with antibiotics, surgery and hyperbaric oxygen. Surgery 1973; 73:936–941.
136. Holland JA, Hill CB, Wolfe WG, Osterhout S, Saltzman HA, Brown IW Jr: Experimental and clinical experience with hyperbaric oxygen in the treatment of clostridial myonecrosis. Surgery 1975; 77:75–85.
137. Bakker DJ: The Use of Hyperbaric Oxygen in the Treatment of Certain Infectious Diseases Especially Gas Gangrene and Acute Dermal Gangrene. Wageningen, Netherlands, Drukkerij Veenman BV, 1984.
138. Bakker DJ, van der Kleij AJ: Clostridial myonecrosis. *In:* Handbook on Hyperbaric Medicine. Oriani G, Marroni A, Wattel F (Eds). New York, Springer-Verlag, 1996, pp 362–385.
139. Stevens DL, Bryant AE, Adams K, Mader JT: Evaluation of therapy

with hyperbaric oxygen for experimental infection with *Clostridium perfringens.* Clin Infect Dis 1993; 17:231-237.

140. Riseman JA, Zamboni WA, Curtis A, Graham DR, Konrad HR, Ross DS: Hyperbaric oxygen therapy for necrotizing fasciitis reduces mortality and the need for debridements. Surgery 1990; 108:847-850.
141. Yohai RA, Bullock JD, Aziz AA, Markert RJ: Survival factors in rhino-orbital-cerebral mucormycosis. Surv Ophthalmol 1994; 39:3-22.
142. Sukoff MH, Ragatz RE: Hyperbaric oxygenation for the treatment of acute cerebral edema. Neurosurgery 1982; 10:29-38.
143. Ohta H, Hadeishi H, Nemoto M, Kawamura S, Hinuma Y, Suzuki E: Transient effect of hyperbaric oxygen on cerebral blood flow and intracranial pressure. J Hyperb Med 1990; 5:3-13.
144. Holbach KH, Wassmann H, Kolberg T: Verbesserte Reversibilitit des traumatischen mittelhirn syndroms bei Anwendung der hyperbaren Oxygenierung. Acta Neurochir (Wien) 1974; 30:247-256.
145. Rockswold GL, Ford SE, Anderson DC, Bergman TA, Sherman RE: Results of a prospective randomized trial for treatment of severely brain-injured patients with hyperbaric oxygen. J Neurosurg 1992; 76:929-934.
146. Ikeda K, Ajiki H, Nagao H, et al: Experimental and clinical use of hyperbaric oxygen in burns. *In:* Proceedings of the 4th International Congress on Hyperbaric Medicine. Wada J, Iwa T (Eds). Baltimore, Williams & Wilkins, 1970, pp 377-380.
147. Perrins DJD: A failed attempt to limit tissue destruction in scalds of pig skins with hyperbaric oxygen. *In:* Proceedings of the 4th International Congress on Hyperbaric Medicine. Wada J, Iwa T (Eds). Baltimore, Williams & Wilkins, 1970, pp 381-387.
148. Brannen AL, Still J, Haynes M, et al: A randomized prospective trial of hyperbaric oxygen in a referral burn center population. Am Surg 1997; 63:205-208.
149. Korn HN, Wheeler ES, Miller TA: Effect of hyperbaric oxygen on second degree burn wound healing. Arch Surg 1977; 112:732-737.
150. Niezgoda JA, Cianci P, Folden BW, Ortega RL, Slade JB, Storrow AB: The effect of hyperbaric oxygen therapy on a burn wound model in human volunteers. Plast Reconstr Surg 1997; 99:1620-1625.
151. Hart GB, O'Reilly RR, Broussard ND, Cave RH, Goodman DB, Yanda RL: Treatment of burns with hyperbaric oxygen. Surg Gynecol Obstet 1974; 139:693-696.
152. Niu AKC, Yang C, Lee HC, Chen SH, Chang LP: Burns treated with adjunctive hyperbaric oxygen therapy: A comparative study in humans. J Hyperb Med 1987; 2:75-85.
153. Cianci P, Lueders HW, Lee H, et al: Adjunctive hyperbaric oxygen therapy reduces length of hospitalization in thermal burns. J Burn Care Rehabil 1989; 10:432-435.
154. Cianci P, Williams C, Lueders HW, et al: Adjunctive hyperbaric oxygen in the treatment of thermal burns: An economic analysis. J Burn Care Rehabil 1990; 11:140-143.
155. Savitt MA, Rankin JS, Elberry JR, Owen CH, Camporesi EM: Influence of hyperbaric oxygen on left ventricular contractility, total coronary blood flow, and myocardial oxygen consumption in the conscious dog. Undersea Hyperb Med 1994; 21:169-183.
156. Sterling DL, Thornton JD, Swafford A, et al: Hyperbaric oxygen limits infarct size in ischemic rabbit myocardium in vivo. Circulation 1993; 88:1931-1936.
157. Cameron AJ, Hutton I, Kenmure AC, Murdoch WR: Haemodynamic and metabolic effects of hyperbaric oxygen in myocardial infarction. Lancet 1966; 2:833-837.
158. Ashfield R, Gavey CJ: Severe acute myocardial infarction treated with hyperbaric oxygen: Report on forty patients. Postgrad Med J 1969; 45:648-654.
159. Thurston JG, Greenwood TW, Bending MR, Connor H, Curwen MP: A controlled investigation into the effects of hyperbaric oxygen on mortality following acute myocardial infarction. Q J Med 1973; 42:751-770.
160. Shandling AH, Ellestad MH, Hart GB, et al: Hyperbaric oxygen and thrombolysis in myocardial infarction: The "HOT MI" pilot study. Am Heart J 1997; 134:544-550.
161. Hart GB, Lennon PA, Strauss MD: Hyperbaric oxygen in exceptional acute blood-loss anemia. J Hyperb Med 1987; 2:205-210.
162. Camporesi EM, Moon RE: Hyperbaric oxygen as an adjunct to therapeutic lung lavage in pulmonary alveolar proteinosis. *In:* Underwater and Hyperbaric Physiology IX. Proceedings of the Ninth International Symposium on Underwater and Hyperbaric Physiology. Bove AA, Bachrach AJ, Greenbaum LJ Jr (Eds). Bethesda, Md, Undersea and Hyperbaric Medical Society, 1987, pp 955-960.
163. Camporesi EM (Ed): Hyperbaric Oxygen Therapy: A Committee Report. Kensington, Md, Undersea and Hyperbaric Medical Society, 1996.
164. Greenbaum LJ Jr, Mathias RA: Information sources in the hyperbaric field. Probl Respir Care 1991; 4:269-272.
165. Weaver LK, Strauss MB (Eds): Monoplace Hyperbaric Chamber Safety Guidelines. Kensington, Md, Undersea and Hyperbaric Medical Society, 1997.
166. Simonson SG, Pritchard RJ, Moon RE, Stolp BW: Evaluation of two chest tube drainage systems at 2 ATA and 3 ATA. Undersea Hyperb Med 1996; 23(Suppl):124.
167. Weaver LK, Howe S: Normobaric measurement of arterial oxygen tension in subjects exposed to hyperbaric oxygen. Chest 1992; 102:1175-1181.
168. Gilbert R, Keighley JF: The arterial-alveolar oxygen tension ratio: An index of gas exchange applicable to varying inspired oxygen concentrations. Am Rev Respir Dis 1974; 109:142-145.
169. Youn BA, Gordon D, Moran C, Brown B: Fire in the multiplace hyperbaric chamber. J Hyperb Med 1989; 4:63-67.
170. Sheffield PJ, Desautels DA: Hyperbaric and hypobaric chamber fires—A 73-year analysis. Undersea Hyperb Med 1997; 24:153-164.
171. Desautels D (Ed): Guidelines for Clinical Multiplace Hyperbaric Facilities. Kensington, Md, Undersea and Hyperbaric Medical Society, 1994.
172. Moon RE, Camporesi EM: Operational use and patient monitoring in a multiplace hyperbaric chamber. Probl Respir Care 1991; 4:172-188.
173. Weaver LK: Clinical applications of hyperbaric oxygen—Monoplace chamber use. Probl Respir Care 1991; 4:189-214.
174. DeLalande JP, Perramant M, Tanguy RL: Postoperative gas gangrene: Apropos of 22 cases. Ann Anesthesiol Fr 1981; 22:351-358.
175. Freischlag JA, Ajalat G, Busuttil RW: Treatment of necrotizing soft tissue infections: The need for a new approach. Am J Surg 1985; 149:751-755.
176. Gibson A, Davis FM: Hyperbaric oxygen therapy in the management of *Clostridium perfringens* infections. N Z Med J 1986; 99:617-620.
177. Hitchcock CR, Bubrick MP: Gas gangrene infections of the small intestine, colon and rectum. Dis Colon Rectum 1976; 19:112-119.
178. Kaiser RE, Cerra FB: Progressive necrotizing surgical infections—A unified approach. J Trauma 1981; 21:349-355.
179. Katlic MR, Derkac WM: *Clostridium septicum* infection and malignancy. Ann Surg 1981; 193:361-364.
180. Pailler JL, Labeeu F: La gangrène gazeuse: Une affection militaire? Acta Chir Belg 1986; 86:63-71.
181. Vo NM, Watson S: Infections of the lower extremities due to gas forming and non-gas forming organisms. [Published erratum appears in South Med J 80: 319:1987.] South Med J 1986; 79:1493-1495.
182. Caplan ES, Kluge RM: Gas gangrene: A review of 34 cases. Arch Intern Med 1976; 136:788-791.
183. Gurtner T: Das Gasodum. Unfallchirurg 1983; 9:172-174.
184. Hart GB, Lamb RC: Gas gangrene. J Trauma 1983; 23:991-1000.
185. Heimbach RD: Gas gangrene: Review and update. HBO Rev 1980; 1:41-46.
186. Hirn M, Niinikoski J: Hyperbaric oxygen in the treatment of clostridial gas gangrene. Ann Chir Gynaecol 1988; 77:37-40.
187. Nier H, Kremer K: Der Gasbrand—Weiterhin ein diagnostiches und therapeutisches Problem. Zentralbl Chir 1984; 109:402-417.
188. Rudge FW: The role of hyperbaric oxygenation in the treatment of clostridial myonecrosis. Mil Med 1993; 158:80-83.
189. Shupak A, Halpern P, Ziser A, Melamed Y: Hyperbaric oxygen therapy for gas gangrene casualties in the Lebanon War. Isr J Med Sci 1984; 20:323-326.
190. Smolle-Jüttner FM, Pinter H, Neuhold KH, et al: Hyperbare Chirugie und Sauerstofftherapie der clostridialen Myonekrose. Wien Klin Wochenschr 1995; 107:739-741.

191. Torda AJ, Bennett MR, Torda TA: The clinical spectrum of necrotising fasciitis. Aust N Z J Med 1997; 27:440.
192. Unsworth IP, Sharp PA: An 11-year review of 73 cases managed with hyperbaric oxygen. Med J Aust 1984; 140:256-260.
193. Brown DR, Davis NL, Lepawsky M, Cunningham J, Kortbeek J: A multicenter review of the treatment of major truncal necrotizing infections with and without hyperbaric oxygen therapy. Am J Surg 1995; 167:485-489.
194. Farrell LD, Karl SR, Davis PK, Bellinger MF, Ballantine TV: Postoperative necrotizing fasciitis in children. Pediatrics 1988; 82:874-879.
195. Hollabaugh RS, Dmochowski RR, Hickerson WL, Cox CE: Fournier's gangrene: Therapeutic impact of hyperbaric oxygen. Plast Reconstr Surg 1998; 101:94-100.
196. Jarrett P, Rademaker M, Duffill M: The clinical spectrum of necrotizing fasciitis: A review of 15 cases. Aust N Z J Med 1997; 27:29-34.
197. Ledingham IM: Diagnosis, clinical course and treatment of acute dermal gangrene. Br J Surg 1975; 62:364-372.
198. Mader JT: Mixed anaerobic and aerobic soft tissue infection. *In:* Problem Wounds: The Role of Oxygen. Davis JC, Hunt TK (Eds). New York, Elsevier, 1988, pp 173-186.
199. Majeski JA: Necrotizing fasciitis. Am Fam Physician 1984; 30:221-223.
200. Oh C, Lee C, Jacobson JH: Necrotizing fasciitis of perineum. Surgery 1982; 91:49-51.
201. Papachristodoulou AJ, Zografos GN, Papastratis G, et al: Fournier's gangrene: Still highly lethal. Langenbecks Arch Surg 1997; 382:15-18.
202. Pessa ME, Howard RJ: Necrotizing fasciitis. Surg Gynecol Obstet 1985; 161:357-361.
203. Pizzorno R, Bonini F, Donelli A, Strubinski R, Medica M, Carmignani G: Hyperbaric oxygen therapy in the treatment of Fournier's disease in 11 male patients. J Urol 1997; 158:837-840.
204. Reigels-Neilsen P, Hesselfeldt-Nielsen J, Bang-Jensen E, Jacobsen E: Fournier's gangrene: 5 patients treated with hyperbaric oxygen. J Urol 1984; 132:918-920.
205. Zamboni WA, Kindwall EP: Author's reply to: Still unproved in necrotising fasciitis. BMJ 1993; 307:936.
206. Rouse TM, Malangoni MA, Schulte WJ: Necrotizing fasciitis: A preventable disaster. Surgery 1982; 92:765-770.
207. Spirnak JP, Resnick ML, Hampel N, Persky L: Fournier's gangrene: A report of 20 patients. J Urol 1984; 131:289-291.
208. Wang KC, Shih CH: Necrotizing fasciitis of the extremities. J Trauma 1992; 32:179-182.
209. Woodburn KR, Ramsay G: Retroperitoneal necrotizing fasciitis. Br J Surg 1992; 79:342-344.
210. Aasen AO, Ruud TE, Haffner J, et al: Kirurgisk behandling ved nekrotiserende fasciitis. Tidsskr Nor Laegeforen 1989; 109:2768-2772.
211. Chevallier D, Amiel J, Michetti C, Birtwisle Y, Richelme H, Toubol J: Les états gangreneux du perinée et de la sphère génitale. J Urol (Paris) 1987; 93:145-150.
212. Gozal D, Ziser A, Shupak A, Ariel A, Melamed Y: Necrotizing fasciitis. Arch Surg 1986; 121:233-235.
213. Krasova Z, Matusek A, Chmelar D: Prinos hyperbaroxie v lecbe nekrotizujici fasciitidy. Vnitr Lek 1992; 38:640-644.
214. Langford FP, Moon RE, Stolp BW, Scher RL: Treatment of cervical necrotizing fasciitis with hyperbaric oxygen therapy. Otolaryngol Head Neck Surg 1995; 112:274-278.
215. Mathieu D, Neviere R, Teillon C, Chagnon JL, Lebleu N, Wattel F: Cervical necrotizing fasciitis: Clinical manifestations and management. Clin Infect Dis 1995; 21:51-56.
216. Leitch DR, Green RD: Pulmonary barotrauma in divers and the treatment of cerebral arterial gas embolism. Aviat Space Environ Med 1986; 57:931-938.
217. Moon RE: Treatment of decompression sickness and arterial gas embolism. *In:* Diving Medicine. Bove AA (Ed). Philadelphia, WB Saunders, 1997, pp 184-204.
218. Davis JC, Heckman JD, DeLee JC, Buckwold FJ: Chronic nonhematogeneous osteomyelitis treated with adjuvant hyperbaric oxygen. J Bone Joint Surg Am 1986; 68:1210-1217.
219. Skyhar MJ, Hargens AR, Strauss MB, Gershuni DH, Hart GB, Akeson WH: Hyperbaric oxygen reduces edema and necrosis of skeletal muscle in compartment syndromes associated with hemorrhagic hypotension. J Bone Joint Surg Am 1986; 68:1218-1224.
220. Bouachour G, Cronier P, Gouello JP, Toulemonde JL, Talha A, Alquier P: Hyperbaric oxygen therapy in the management of crush injuries: A randomized double-blind placebo-controlled clinical trial. J Trauma 1996; 41:333-339.
221. Farmer JC Jr, Shelton DL, Angelillo JD, Bennett PB, Hudson WR: Treatment of radiation-induced tissue injury with hyperbaric oxygen. Ann Otol Rhinol Laryngol 1978; 87:707-715.
222. Marx RE, Johnson RP, Kline SN: Prevention of osteoradionecrosis: A randomized prospective clinical trial of hyperbaric oxygen versus penicillin. J Am Dent Assoc 1985; 111:49-54.
223. Kindwall EP: Hyperbaric oxygen's effect on radiation necrosis. Clin Plast Surg 1993; 20:473-483.
224. Bevers RF, Bakker DJ, Kurth KH: Hyperbaric oxygen treatment for haemorrhagic radiation cystitis. Lancet 1995; 346:803-805.
225. Zamboni WA, Wong HP, Stephenson LL, Pfeifer MA: Evaluation of hyperbaric oxygen for diabetic wounds—A prospective study. Undersea Hyperb Med 1997; 24:175-179.
226. Jansen HM, Zuurmond WW, Roos CM, Schreuder JJ, Bakker DJ: Whole-lung lavage under hyperbaric oxygen conditions for alveolar proteinosis with respiratory failure. Chest 1987; 91:829-832.
227. Gallagher TJ, Smith RA, Bell GC: Evaluation of mechanical ventilators in a hyperbaric environment. Aviat Space Environ Med 1978; 49:375-376.
228. Pelaia P, Volturo P, Rocco M, Mille L, Malpieri R, Spinelli V: La ventilazione meccanica in ambiente iperbarico: Valutazioni sperimentali del Draeger Hyperlog. Minerva Anestesiol 1990; 56:1371.
229. Le Masson Y, Le Pechon J-C, Barratt M, Murphy L: Ventilator for Space Station Freedom. *In:* Proceedings of the Joint Meeting on Diving and Hyperbaric Medicine. Schmutz J, Wendling J (Eds). Basle, Foundation for Hyperbaric Medicine, 1992, pp 78-82.
230. Degauque C, Lamy M, Stas M: Use of the Logic 03 for controlled ventilation in hyperbaric oxygen therapy. Acta Anaesthesiol Belg 1977; 28:251-259.
231. Moon RE, Bergquist LV, Conklin B, Miller JN: Monaghan 225 ventilator use under hyperbaric conditions. Chest 1986; 89:846-851.
232. Lewis RP, Szafranski J, Bradford RH, Smith HS, Crabbe GG: The use of the Penlon Nuffield 200 in a monoplace hyperbaric oxygen chamber: An evaluation of its use and a clinical report in two patients requiring ventilation for carbon monoxide poisoning. Anaesthesia 1991; 46:767-770.
233. Saywood AM, Howard R, Goad RF, Scott C: Function of the Oxford Ventilator at high pressure. Anaesthesia 1982; 37:740-744.
234. Spittal MJ, Hunter SJ, Jones L: The pneuPAC hyperbaric variant HB: A ventilator suitable for use within a one-man hyperbaric chamber. Br J Anaesth 1991; 67:488-491.
235. Holcomb JR, Matos-Navarro AY, Goldmann RW: Critical care in the hyperbaric chamber. *In:* Problem Wounds: The Role of Oxygen. Davis JC, Hunt TK (Eds). New York, Elsevier, 1988, pp 187-209.

143

Pleural Disease in the Intensive Care Unit

Steven A. Sahn, MD

Pleural disease is uncommonly the major reason for admission to the intensive care unit (ICU). Exceptions are a large hemothorax with hemodynamic instability and the need to monitor bleeding, secondary spontaneous pneumothorax, and large unilateral or bilateral pleural effusions that have caused acute respiratory failure.

The diagnosis may initially be missed in the critically ill patient because the disease is overshadowed by the major presenting illness that is responsible for admission to the ICU. In addition, pleural disease is frequently a subtle clinical and chest radiographic finding. A *pleural effusion* may not be detected on the supine view of the chest radiograph because diffuse alveolar infiltrates can mask the posterior layering of fluid or because bilateral effusions without parenchymal infiltrates are misinterpreted as an underexposed film or objects outside the chest. Pneumothorax may not be detected on the supine view because pleural air tends to be situated anteriorly and does not elicit the diagnostic visceral pleural line seen on an upright view. When the patient undergoing mechanical ventilation is at increased risk for barotrauma because of high peak airway pressures, the index of suspicion for pneumothorax should be heightened. If pulmonary interstitial gas (see later) or subcutaneous emphysema is detected, appropriate radiologic studies should be obtained.

RADIOLOGIC SIGNS OF PLEURAL DISEASE

Because the distribution of fluid and air in the normal pleural space tends to follow gravitational influences and because the lung has a tendency to maintain its normal shape as it becomes smaller, fluid initially accumulates between the bottom of the lung and the diaphragm, air between the top of the lung and the apex of the thorax in the upright patient. When chest radiographs are obtained in other than the erect position, free pleural fluid and air change position. In most critically ill patients, radiographs are taken in the supine or semierect positions, thereby changing the radiographic appearance of free pleural fluid and air.

Pleural Fluid

Standard Chest Radiograph

In normal humans, the anteroposterior diameter of the hemithorax is greatest at the lung base; in the supine position, therefore, the radiolucency of the lung base is equal to or greater than that in the lung apex.[1] In addition, when the patient is supine, breast and pectoral tissue fall laterally away from the lung base. Therefore, a pleural effusion should be suspected when there is increased homogeneous density over the lower lung fields in comparison to the upper lung fields. As the pleural effusion increases, the increased radiodensity involves the upper hemithorax as well. However, failure of chest wall tissue to move laterally, cardiomegaly, prominent epicardial fat pad, and lung collapse or consolidation may obscure a pleural effusion on the supine view of the radiograph. The unilateral homogeneous density can be mimicked by rotation of the patient or an off-center x-ray beam.[2] An absent pectoral muscle, prior mastectomy, unilateral hyperlucent lung, scoliosis, previous lobectomy, hypoplastic pulmonary artery, or pleural or chest wall mass may lead to a unilateral homogeneous density that mimics an effusion.

About 175 to 500 mL of pleural fluid results in blunting of the costophrenic angle on an erect view.[3] Usually, this quantity of pleural fluid can be detected on a supine view as an increased density over the lower lung zone. Inability to visualize the hemidiaphragm, absence of the costophrenic angle meniscus, and apical capping are less likely to be seen with less than 500 mL of fluid but are more likely to be recognized as the volume of fluid increases.[1]

The major radiographic finding of a pleural effusion in a supine patient is increased homogeneous density over the lower lung field that does not obliterate normal bronchovascular markings, does not show air bronchograms, and does not show hilar or mediastinal displacement until the effusion is massive (Fig. 143–1). If a pleural effusion is suspected in the supine patient, a radiograph should be obtained in the erect or lateral decubitus position for confirmation or exclusion (Fig. 143–2).

Other Radiographic Imaging

Underlying diffuse parenchymal lung disease, as is commonly found in the critically ill patient, makes the diagnosis of pleural effusion a problem and may require ultrasonography or computed tomography (CT) scanning.

Sonography

Chest sonography provides good characterization for pleural diseases and is a useful diagnostic modality for critically ill patients when they cannot be transported to the radiology department for CT. Sonographic examination is less time-consuming and less expensive than CT, can be done at the bed-

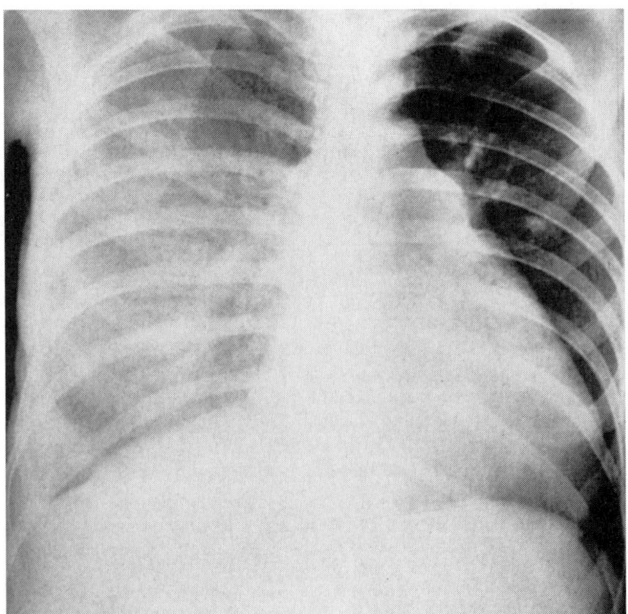

Figure 143–1. Supine chest radiograph in a patient with a large pleural effusion. An increased homogeneous density is noted over the right lung field but does not obliterate the bronchovascular markings.

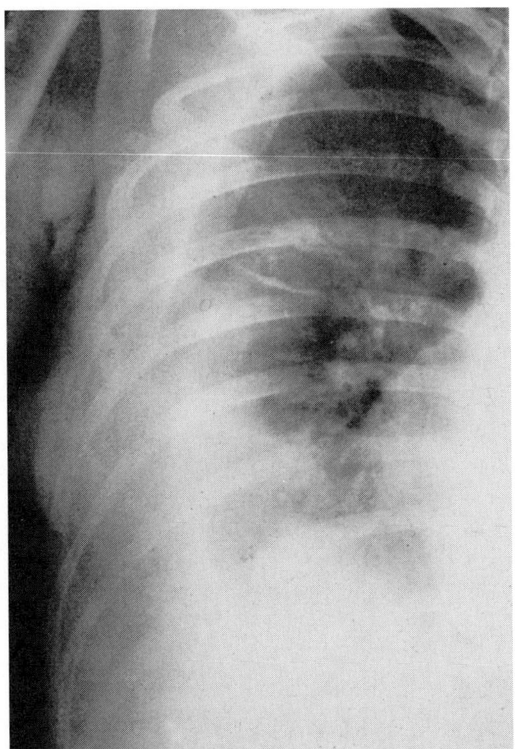

Figure 143–2. The right lateral decubitus radiograph (same patient as shown in Fig. 143-1) shows evidence of free-flowing pleural fluid and clearing of the homogeneous density.

side, and can be repeated serially. Disadvantages include (1) hindrance of the ultrasonic wave by air in either the lung or pleural space, (2) a restricted field of view, (3) inferior evaluation of the lung parenchyma compared with CT, and (4) operator dependence.[4]

Yu and colleagues found chest sonography helpful in diagnosis in 27 of 41 (66%) and in treatment in 37 of 41 (90%) critically ill patients, and it had an important influence on management in 17 of 41 (41%) patients.[5] In the same study, sonography excluded an effusion in five patients with suspected pleural fluid, confirmed the presence of effusion in eight patients, found an unsuspected effusion in three patients, and provided additional information in seven patients with effusion. Sonographic bedside thoracentesis was successful in 24 of 25 critically ill patients in the same study.

Computed Tomography

CT is recognized as providing increased resolution compared with more conventional radiographic techniques (Fig. 143-3*A* and *B*). Although moving a critically ill patient for a CT scan has potential risks, the diagnostic advantage can be justified in the stable patient when the clinical course is not compatible with the diagnosis suggested by the portable chest radiograph. In selected patients with multisystem trauma, chest CT often provides additional diagnostic information and positively affects management and outcome of the patient.[6, 7]

Pneumothorax

In the erect patient, the diagnosis of a pneumothorax is confirmed by the presence of a distinct visceral pleural line separated from the chest wall (Fig. 143-4). In the supine patient, pneumothorax gas migrates along the anterior surface of the lung, making detection on the anteroposterior projection a problem. The base, lateral chest wall, and juxtacardiac area should be carefully visualized for evidence of pneumothorax[8] (Fig. 143-5). Accumulation of air along the mediastinal parietal pleura may simulate pneumomediastinum.[9] A radiograph should be obtained with the patient in the erect or decubitus position (suspected hemithorax up) to assess for the presence of a pneumothorax.

Sonography

Ultrasonography has been found to be sensitive for the detection of pneumothorax because of its ability to detect the presence or absence of "lung sliding."[10] In individuals without

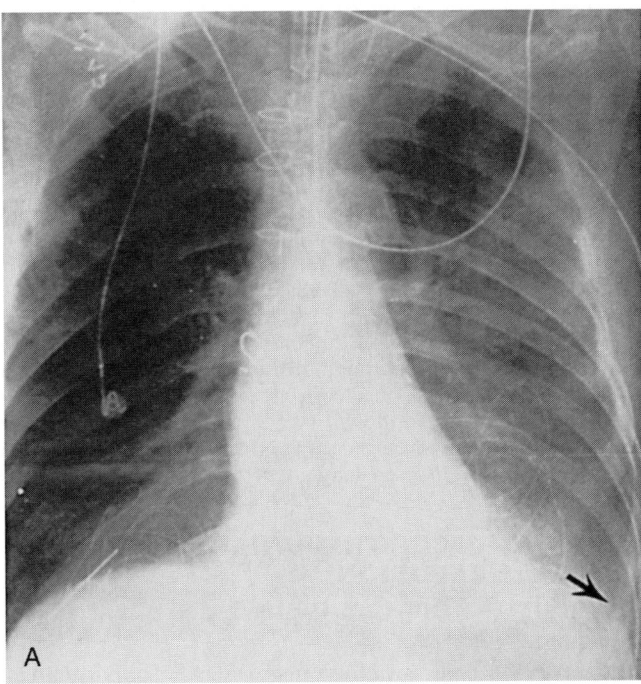

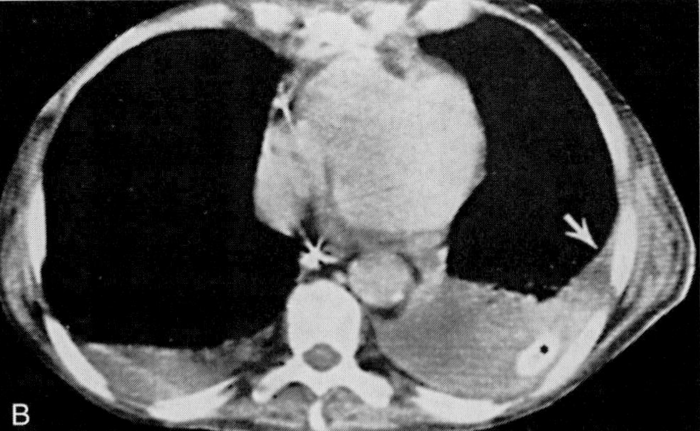

Figure 143–3. *A,* Supine patient with increased homogeneous density, left greater than right representing bilateral plerual effusions. The *arrow* denotes the meniscus sign. *B,* CT scan of the thorax at the level of the lung base several hours after the supine radiograph demonstrating a small right effusion and moderate left effusion. The *arrow* demonstrates fluid extending anteriorly into the left lateral costophrenic angle. The *asterisk* indicates a chest tube which was inserted shortly before the CT scan. (Reprinted with permission from Woodring JH: Recognition of pleural effusion on supine radiographs: How much fluid is required? AJR 1984; 142:59-64.)

pneumothorax, the "lung–chest wall interface," which represents a to-and-fro movement synchronized with respiration, can be identified. Ultrasound visualization of lung sliding is correlated with the absence of pneumothorax, and from this sign alone at least anterior pneumothorax can be excluded rapidly at the bedside of a mechanically ventilated patient. The absence of lung sliding is suggestive of but not sufficient to affirm pneumothorax.

The most common radiographic signs of tension pneumothorax are contralateral mediastinal shift, ipsilateral diaphragmatic depression, and ipsilateral chest wall expansion. Underlying lung disease may prevent total lung collapse even if tension is present. In patients undergoing mechanical ventilation, little or no midline mediastinal shift may result from the tension[11, 12]; in this case, a depressed ipsilateral diaphragm is a more reliable sign of tension than is mediastinal shift.

In patients with acute respiratory distress syndrome (ARDS), barotrauma can result in a localized tension pneumothorax with a subtle contralateral mediastinal shift, flattening of the cardiac contour, and depression of the ipsilateral hemidiaphragm.[13] Pleural adhesions and relative compressibility and mobility of surrounding structures, in addition to the supine position, probably account for these loculated tension pneumothoraces.

In 88 critically ill patients with 112 pneumothoraces, the anteromedial and subpulmonic recesses were involved in 64% of patients in the supine and semierect position.[14] Furthermore, in 30% of the pneumothoraces in this study not initially detected by the clinician or radiologist, half of the patients progressed to tension pneumothorax. Therefore, a high index of suspicion is necessary in these critically ill patients to avoid catastrophic situations.

Familiarity with atypical locations of pneumothoraces in critically ill patients (usually due to the supine or semierect position), awareness of the consequence of underlying cardiopulmonary disease, and knowledge of other risk factors contributing to misdiagnosis (e.g., mechanical ventilation, altered mental status, prolonged ICU stay, and development of pneumothorax after peak hours of physician staffing) may contribute to an improved ability to diagnose this potentially lethal problem.[15]

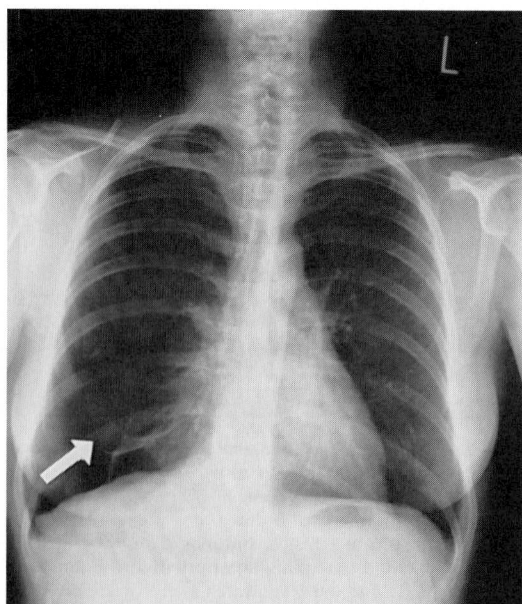

Figure 143–4. An erect posteroanterior radiograph demonstrating a right pneumothorax *(arrow)*. The slight contralateral mediastinal shift and increased distance between the ribs on the right diagnose the presence of a tension pneumothorax.

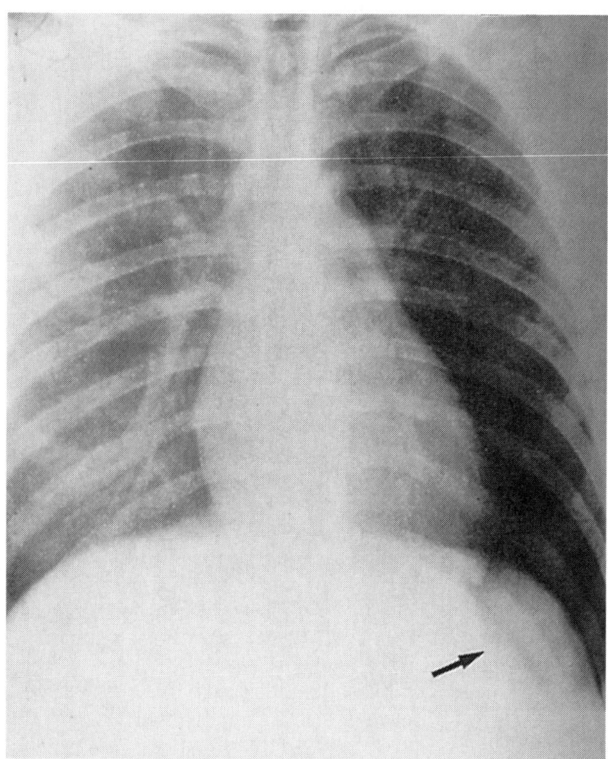

Figure 143–5. Evidence of a left pneumothorax in a supine patient. *Arrow* notes the anterior collection of air and the deep sulcus sign characteristic of pneumothorax in a supine patient. (Reprinted with permission from Rhea JL, vanSonnenberg E, McLoud T: Basilar pneumothorax in the supine adult. Radiology 1979; 133:593–595.)

Digital Radiography

Digital radiography offers some potential advantages over standard portable chest radiography in the critically ill patient. Some of the problems with portable radiographs are caused by the patient and some by technical limitations, including[16]:

1. Uncontrolled respiratory and gross body motion.
2. Limited kilovoltage and milliamperage, leading to long exposure and excessive image contrast.
3. Unavailability of phototiming, causing a reduction in image quality.
4. Difficulty in interpreting sequential images because of technical variations.

In 3500 portable digital chest radiographs in an ICU, no major problems were encountered in visualization of tubes or catheters or detection of pneumothoraces. Assessment of volume status or presence of bilateral effusions was initially a problem but improved with further experience.[16] Other studies found that radiologists detected pneumothoraces equally well on conventional radiographs and digital images printed on film but less well on electronic viewing consoles.[17, 18] In comparisons of conventional with digital images, the parameters of the systems being compared must be clearly defined because the system itself may affect the quality of the image produced.[18]

EVALUATION OF THE PATIENT WITH A PLEURAL EFFUSION

Diagnostic Thoracentesis

Indications

Patients with a pleural effusion provide the opportunity to diagnose the underlying process responsible for pleural fluid accumulation. Pleural effusions are frequently associated with disease in the chest but may also result from organ dysfunction in the gastrointestinal tract, liver, kidney, heart, or hematopoietic system.[19]

Although disease of any organ system can cause a pleural effusion in critically ill patients, the diagnoses listed in Table 143–1 represent the majority of the causes seen in ICUs. The types of pleural effusions seen in medical and surgical ICUs are similar, but some causes related to surgical (coronary artery bypass grafting, chylothorax, abdominal surgery) and nonsurgical trauma (hemothorax) represent a substantial percentage of effusions in surgical ICUs.

When a pleural effusion is suspected on physical examination and confirmed radiologically, a diagnostic thoracentesis should be performed in an attempt to establish the cause. Exceptions might be patients with a secure clinical diagnosis and only a small amount of pleural fluid, as in atelectasis, or patients with uncomplicated congestive heart failure.[19] Observation may be warranted in these situations, but thoracentesis should be performed if the clinical course is not appropriate.

When there is less than 1 cm from the pleural fluid line to the inside of the chest wall on the lateral decubitus view, the risk of thoracentesis probably outweighs the usefulness of pleural fluid analysis. If the underlying disease or pleural effusion becomes clinically important, the effusion will increase in size and allow safer thoracentesis. When fluid sampling is indicated clinically and the volume of the effusion is small, thoracentesis should be performed under ultrasound guidance in the ICU.[20] The indications for diagnostic thoracentesis are no different because the patient is in the ICU or on mechanical ventilation. Establishing the diagnosis rapidly in these critically ill patients may be more important and lifesaving than in the noncritically ill. It has been documented that even in patients on mechanical ventilation, diagnostic thoracentesis is safe if there is strict adherence to the general principles of the procedure.[21]

Pneumothorax, the most clinically important complication of thoracentesis,[22, 23] is no more likely to occur in the patient on mechanical ventilation than in the spontaneously breathing patient. If a pneumothorax does occur, the patient receiving mechanical ventilation is highly susceptible to development of a tension pneumothorax.

Contraindications

There are no absolute contraindications to diagnostic thoracentesis. If clinical judgment dictates that the information gained from pleural fluid analysis may help in diagnosis and management, thoracentesis should be performed.[24] Diagnostic thoracentesis with a small-bore needle can be performed safely in virtually any patient if meticulous technique is employed.

The major relative contraindications to thoracentesis are a patient with a bleeding diathesis or a patient receiving anticoagulation therapy. A patient with a small amount of pleural fluid and a low benefit-risk ratio also represents a relative contraindication. Thoracentesis should not be attempted through an area of active skin infection.

Complications

Complications of diagnostic thoracentesis include:

- Pain at the needle insertion site
- Bleeding (local, intrapleural, or intra-abdominal)
- Pneumothorax
- Empyema
- Spleen or liver puncture

In prospective studies, pneumothorax has been reported to occur in 4% to 30% of patients.[22, 25–27] The pneumothorax rate, however, is inversely correlated with the experience of the operator.[25] Pneumothorax caused by diagnostic thoracentesis is usually small and can often be treated expectantly or with simple aspiration. Liver or spleen puncture tends to occur when the patient is not sitting upright because movement toward recumbency causes cephalad migration of the abdominal viscera. Even if the liver or spleen is punctured with a small-bore needle, the outcome is generally favorable if the patient is not receiving anticoagulant agents and does not have a bleeding diathesis.

Therapeutic Thoracentesis

Indications and Contraindications

The primary indication for therapeutic thoracentesis is relief of dyspnea. Contraindications to therapeutic thoracentesis are similar to those for diagnostic thoracentesis. However, there appears to be an increased risk of pneumothorax,[22] which therefore makes a therapeutic thoracentesis in patients on mechanical ventilation potentially hazardous.

The technique of therapeutic thoracentesis is essentially the same as that of diagnostic thoracentesis, except that a plastic catheter, rather than a sharp tip needle, should be used. This

TABLE 143–1. Causes of Pleural Effusions in the Intensive Care Unit

Cause	Comments
Atelectasis	Small, unilateral or bilateral transudate
Congestive heart failure	Bilateral transudates, right > left
Pneumonia	Alveolar infiltrate and ipsilateral exudate
Hypoalbuminemia	Small bilateral effusions; albumin <1.5 g/dL
Pancreatitis	Small left-sided exudate
ARDS	36% incidence of pleural effusions
Pulmonary embolism	Small (<⅓ of hemithorax) ipsilateral effusion present on admission
Hepatic hydrothorax	Right-sided transudate in ESLD
Esophageal sclerotherapy	50% incidence of small effusion
Postcardiac injury syndrome	Hemorrhagic, left-sided exudate 3 weeks after surgery
EVMCV	PF/S glucose ratio >1.0 if glucose is being infused
Coronary artery bypass surgery	Left-sided hemorrhagic exudate that may persist for weeks
Spontaneous esophageal rupture	High pleural fluid salivary amylase concentration and low pH
Hemothorax	Pleural fluid/blood hematocrit ratio >0.5
Chylothorax	Surgery accounts for 25% of chylothoraces
Abdominal surgery	Effusion commonly due to atelectasis

ARDS = acute respiratory distress syndrome; ESLD = end-stage liver disease; EVMCV = extravascular migration of central venous catheter; PF/S = pleural fluid/serum.

measure reduces the risk of pneumothorax, which may occur as fluid is removed and the lung expands toward the chest wall.

The amount of fluid that can be removed safely from the pleural space at one session is controversial. Ideally, monitoring pleural pressure should dictate the amount of fluid that can be removed. As long as intrapleural pressure does not fall below -20 cm H_2O, removal of fluid can continue.[28] However, pleural liquid pressure monitoring is not done routinely. In the patient with contralateral mediastinal shift on chest radiography who tolerates thoracentesis without chest tightness, cough, or lightheadedness, several liters of pleural fluid can probably be removed safely. However, neither the patient nor the operator may be aware of a precipitous drop in pleural pressure. In patients without a contralateral mediastinal shift or with ipsilateral shift, suggesting an endobronchial obstruction or a trapped lung, the likelihood of a precipitous drop in intrapleural pressure is increased, and either pleural pressure should be monitored during thoracentesis or only a diagnostic thoracentesis should be performed (Fig. 143-6*A* and *B*).

Physiologic Effects and Complications

Improvement in lung volumes up to 24 hours after therapeutic thoracentesis does not correlate with the amount of fluid removed, despite relief of dyspnea in those patients.[29-31] Yet in some patients, maximum spirometric improvement may not occur for several days. Patients with initial negative pleural pressures and patients with marked falls in pleural pressure with thoracentesis tend to show the least improvement in pulmonary function and dyspnea after therapeutic thoracentesis because they usually have a trapped lung or major endobronchial obstruction.[28] The mechanism of dyspnea from a large pleural effusion is probably related to decreased chest wall compliance, contralateral mediastinal shift, and loss of ipsilateral lung volume in addition to neurogenic trafficking from the lung parenchyma.[30]

Complications of therapeutic thoracentesis are the same as those seen with diagnostic thoracentesis. However, three complications that are unique to therapeutic thoracentesis are hypoxemia, unilateral pulmonary edema, and hypovolemia.[24] After therapeutic thoracentesis, hypoxemia may occur despite relief of dyspnea.[32, 33] It may result from worsening ventilation-perfusion relationships in the ipsilateral lung or overt or occult unilateral pulmonary edema.

The change in $Pa{O_2}$ after therapeutic thoracentesis appears to be unpredictable[33]; some have observed a characteristic increase in $Pa{O_2}$ within minutes to hours,[29] whereas others suggest a systematic decrease in $Pa{O_2}$ that returns to prethoracentesis values by 24 hours.[32] In the largest study including 33 patients with various causes of unilateral pleural effusions, a significant increase in $Pa{O_2}$ was found 20 minutes, 2 hours, and 24 hours after therapeutic thoracentesis.[34] There was a decrease in the $P(A - a)O_2$ that was accompanied by a small but significant decrease in shunt, whereas V_D/V_T did not change. The data suggest an improved ventilation-perfusion relationship after therapeutic thoracentesis, with an increase in ventilation of parts of the lung that were previously poorly ventilated but well perfused.

The relief of dyspnea cannot be explained by improved $Pa{O_2}$. The increases have been modest, and in some cases there has been a fall in $Pa{O_2}$. Improvement in lung volumes is a constant finding after therapeutic thoracentesis but may take days or even weeks to maximize; immediate changes are usually modest and highly variable. No significant change in expiratory flow rates has been observed. Therefore, the relief of dyspnea cannot be adequately explained by changes either in lung volume or in the mechanics of breathing but may be the result of decreased stimulation of lung or chest wall receptors or of both.[30]

CAUSES OF PLEURAL EFFUSIONS

Atelectasis

Atelectasis is a common cause of small pleural effusions in comatose, immobile, pain-ridden patients in ICUs[35] and after upper abdominal surgery.[36, 37] Other causes include major bronchial obstruction from lung cancer, a mucous plug, or a foreign body. Atelectasis causes pleural fluid because of decreased pleural pressure. With alveolar collapse, the lung and chest wall separate further, creating local areas of increased negative pressure. This decrease in pleural pressure favors the movement of fluid into the pleural space, presumably from the parietal pleural surface. The fluid accumulates until the pleural-parietal pleural interstitial pressure gradient returns to normal.[19]

Pleural fluid from atelectasis is a serous transudate with a low number of mononuclear cells, a glucose concentration equivalent to that of serum, and a pH in the range of 7.45 to 7.55. When atelectasis resolves, pleural fluid dissipates during several days.

Congestive Heart Failure

Congestive heart failure (CHF) is the most common cause of all transudative pleural effusions and a common cause of pleural effusions in ICUs. Pleural effusions due to CHF are associated with increases in pulmonary venous pressure.[38]

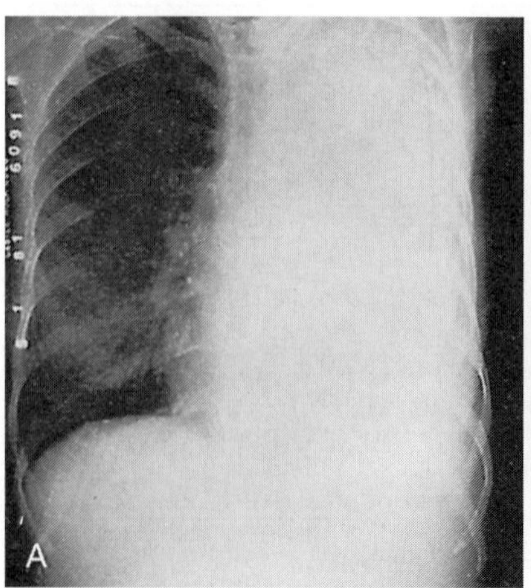

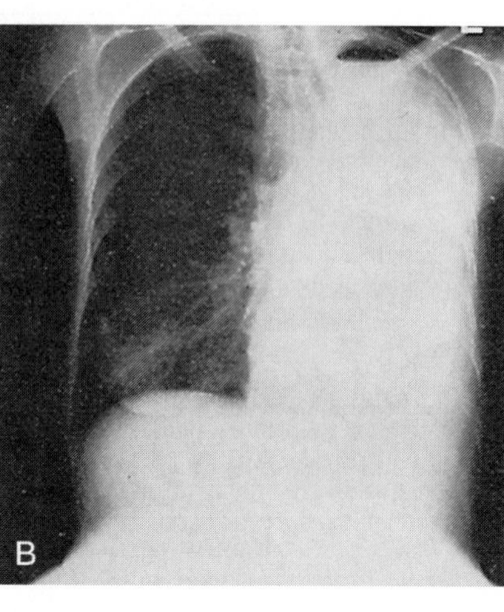

Figure 143–6. *A,* An upright radiograph in a patient with carcinoma of the left main stem bronchus. The radiograph demonstrates a homogeneous density involving the entire left hemithorax and evidence of ipsilateral mediastinal shift representing left lung collaspe and a pleural effusion. *B,* An upright radiograph immediately following therapeutic thoracentesis demonstrating further ipsilateral shift of the mediastinum due to the marked decrease in pleural pressure that occurs with substantial pleural fluid removal with an obstructed bronchus. (Reprinted with permission from Sahn SA: Pleural effusion in lung cancer. Clin Chest Med 1983; 14:189–200.)

Most patients with subacute or chronic elevation in pulmonary venous pressure (pulmonary capillary wedge pressure of at least 24 mm Hg) have evidence of pleural effusion on ultrasonography or on radiography in the lateral decubitus position. Isolated increases in systemic venous pressure, even right atrial pressures as elevated as 25 mm Hg in the chronic state, tend not to produce pleural effusions. Thus, patients with chronic obstructive pulmonary disease (COPD) and cor pulmonale rarely have pleural effusions, and the presence of pleural fluid implies another cause.

Most patients with pleural effusions secondary to CHF have the classic signs and symptoms. The chest radiograph shows cardiomegaly and bilateral small to moderate pleural effusions of similar size (right slightly greater than left). There is usually radiographic evidence of pulmonary edema, with the increasing severity of pulmonary edema increasing the likelihood of the presence and greater volume of pleural effusions.[38] The patient's records usually show intake greater than output for several days, weight gain, an increasing $P(A - a)O_2$ gradient, and, in those on mechanical ventilators, a decrease in static compliance.

The effusion is a transudate; mesothelial cells and lymphocytes account for the majority of the less than 1000 cells/μL.[19] Acute diuresis changes the transudate to an exudate in 8%[39] to 38%[40] of patients. In the afebrile patient with clinical CHF and bilateral pleural effusions of relatively equal size and an enlarged cardiac silhouette on chest radiography, the diagnosis is reasonably secure and observation is appropriate.

Thoracentesis should be performed if any of the following clinical features are present:

- Fever
- Effusions of disparate size
- A unilateral pleural effusion
- A larger effusion on the left than on the right
- Absence of cardiomegaly
- Pleuritic chest pain
- A PaO_2 inappropriate for the degree of pulmonary edema

Treatment consists of decreasing venous hypertension and improving cardiac output with diuretics, digitalis, and afterload reduction. In successfully managed heart failure, the effusions resolve during days to weeks after the pulmonary edema has cleared.

Hepatic Hydrothorax

Pleural effusions occur in approximately 6% of patients with cirrhosis of the liver and clinical ascites.[41, 42] The effusions result from movement of ascitic fluid through congenital or acquired diaphragmatic defects.[41] An effusion may occur acutely after rupture of a diaphragmatic bleb, which is formed because of defects in the muscle and collagen bundle structure at their base.

The patient usually has the classic stigmata of cirrhosis and clinically apparent ascites. With a large to massive pleural effusion, the patient may present with acute dyspnea; however, a smaller effusion may be detected only on routine chest radiography. Rarely, a massive pleural effusion may be found without clinical ascites (demonstrated only by ultrasonography), implying the presence of a large diaphragmatic defect.

The usual chest radiograph shows a normal cardiac silhouette and a right-sided pleural effusion in 70% of patients, which can vary from small to massive; effusions are less likely to be isolated to the left pleural space (15%) or are bilateral (15%).[41, 42] The pleural fluid is a serous transudate with a low nucleated cell count and a predominance of mononuclear cells, a pH greater than 7.40, a glucose level similar to that of serum, and an amylase concentration less than that of serum.[19] The fluid can be hemorrhagic because of an underlying coagulopathy or rupture of a diaphragmatic bleb.

The diagnosis is substantiated by the finding that pleural fluid and ascitic fluid have similar protein and lactate dehydrogenase (LDH) concentrations.[41] If the diagnosis is still uncertain, injection of a radionuclide into the ascitic fluid with detection on chest imaging within 1 to 2 hours supports a pleuroperitoneal communication through a diaphragmatic defect[43]; delayed demonstration of the tracer suggests that the pathogenesis of the effusion is by convection through the mesothelium.

Treatment of hepatic hydrothorax is directed at resolution of the ascites, with sodium restriction and diuresis. The effusion frequently persists unchanged until all of the ascites is mobilized. If the patient is acutely dyspneic or in respiratory failure, therapeutic thoracentesis should be done as a temporizing measure. Care should be exercised with paracentesis or thoracentesis, because hypovolemia can occur with rapid evacuation of fluid.

Chest tube insertion should be avoided; it can cause infection of the fluid, and prolonged drainage can lead to protein and lymphocyte depletion. Chemical pleurodesis is uniformly unsuccessful owing to rapid movement of ascitic fluid into the pleural space. Definitive treatment requires video-assisted thoracoscopy to patch the diaphragmatic defect followed by pleural abrasion or talc poudrage.

Hypoalbuminemia

Many patients admitted to a medical ICU have a chronic illness and associated hypoalbuminemia. When serum albumin levels are less than about 1.5 g/dL, pleural effusions are likely. Because the normal pleural space has an effective lymphatic drainage system, pleural fluid tends to be the last collection of extravascular fluid that occurs in patients with low oncotic pressure. Therefore, it is unusual to find a pleural effusion solely due to hypoalbuminemia in the absence of anasarca, which is invariably present at an albumin level less than 1.0 g/dL.[44]

Patients with hypoalbuminemic pleural effusions tend not to have pulmonary symptoms unless there is underlying lung disease because the effusions are rarely large. Chest radiography typically shows small to moderate bilateral effusions and a normal heart size. The pleural fluid is a serous transudate with a nucleated cell count of less than 1000 cells/μL, predominantly lymphocytes and mesothelial cells. The pleural fluid glucose level is similar to that of serum, and the pH is in the range of 7.45 to 7.55. The diagnosis is presumptive if other causes of transudative effusions can be excluded. The effusions resolve when hypoalbuminemia is corrected.

Iatrogenic Effusions

Extravascular migration of a central venous catheter can cause pneumothorax, hemothorax, chylothorax, or a transudative pleural effusion.[45-47] Its incidence is estimated at less than 1% but may be considerably higher. Malposition of the catheter on placement should be suspected if there is absence of blood return or questionable central venous pressure measurements.

The immediate postprocedure chest radiograph should be assessed for proper catheter placement; a catheter placed from the right side should not cross the midline. If the catheter is not in the appropriate vessel, phlebitis, perforation of a vein or the heart, or instillation of fluid into the mediastinum or pleural space can occur.

In the alert patient, acute infusion of intravenous fluid into the mediastinum usually results in new-onset chest discomfort and dyspnea. Depending on the volume and the rate with which it is introduced into the mediastinum, tachypnea, worsening respiratory status, and cardiac tamponade may ensue. The chest radiograph shows the catheter tip in an abnormal position,[48] a widened mediastinum, and evidence of unilateral or bilateral pleural effusions. The effusion can have characteristics similar to those of the infusate (milky if lipid is being given) and may be hemorrhagic and neutrophil-predominant due to trauma and inflammation. The pleural fluid to serum glucose ratio is greater than 1.0 if glucose is being infused.[46] The pleural fluid glucose concentration can fall rapidly after glucose infusion into the pleural space, probably explaining the relatively low glucose concentrations in pleural fluid compared with the infusate.[49]

Extravascular migration of a central venous catheter appears to be more common with placement in the external jugular vein, particularly on the left side. Left-sided catheters appear to put the patient at increased risk for perforation because of the horizontal orientation of the left compared with the right brachiocephalic vein. When catheters are introduced from the left side, they should be of adequate length for the tip to rest in the superior vena cava.

Free flow of fluid and proper fluctuation in central venous pressure during the respiratory cycle may not be reliable indicators of intravascular placement. This is probably because intrathoracic pressure changes are transmitted to the mediastinum and, therefore, the venous pressure catheter. Aspiration of blood or retrograde flow of blood when the catheter is lowered below the patient's heart level should confirm intravascular catheter placement. If blood cannot be aspirated and the effusate is aspirated instead, extravascular migration is ensured. The central venous catheter should be removed immediately.

If there is a small effusion, observation is warranted. If the effusion is large, causing respiratory distress, or a hemothorax is discovered, thoracentesis or tube thoracostomy should be performed.

Parapneumonic Effusions

Parapneumonic effusions often develop in patients in ICUs who have pneumonia and in patients with severe community-acquired pneumonias admitted to the ICU. The usual presentation is similar to that of the non-ICU patient with fever, chest pain, leukocytosis, purulent sputum, and a new alveolar infiltrate on chest radiography. In the elderly or debilitated patient, however, many of these findings may not be present.

The chest radiograph commonly shows a small to moderate ipsilateral pleural effusion. When the effusion is free-flowing (as demonstrated by the lateral decubitus view) and thoracentesis shows a nonpurulent, polymorphonuclear (PMN) cell–predominant exudate with a glucose level greater than 60 mg/dL, LDH concentration less than 700 IU/L, and pH of 7.30 or greater, there is a high likelihood of pleural fluid resolution during 7 to 14 days without sequelae when antibiotics alone are used (*uncomplicated effusion*).[50]

If the chest radiograph demonstrates loculation and pus is aspirated, the diagnosis of empyema is established and immediate drainage is needed. In the case of free-flowing nonpurulent fluid, if Gram's stain or culture is positive or pH is less than 7.20, with or without a glucose level less than 40 mg/dL or an LDH concentration greater than 1000 IU/L, the likelihood of a poor outcome with increased morbidity, mortality, and cost increases, and the pleural space should probably be drained.[50] Drainage can be accomplished by standard chest tube or radiographically guided catheter. With loculations, pleural space drainage should be accomplished by placement of image-guided tubes or catheters with fibrinolytic agents or empyemectomy and decortication.[51]

Today, most thoracic surgeons routinely begin with thoracoscopy. If this step is not successful, they proceed directly to a standard thoracotomy for empyemectomy and decortication.[52]

Pancreatitis

Pleuropulmonary abnormalities are commonly associated with pancreatitis, largely because of the proximity of the pancreas to the diaphragm. About 50% of patients with pancreatitis have an abnormal chest radiograph, with pleural effusions in 3% to 17%.[53] Mechanisms that may be involved in the pathogenesis of pancreatic pleural effusion include[53, 54]:

1. Direct contact of pancreatic enzymes with the diaphragm (*sympathetic effusion*).
2. Transfer of ascitic fluid through diaphragmatic defects.
3. Communication of a fistulous tract between a pseudocyst and the pleural space.
4. Retroperitoneal movement of fluid into the mediastinum with mediastinitis or rupture into the pleural space.

Ascitic amylase moves into the pleural space by these mechanisms. The pleural fluid to serum amylase ratio is greater than unity in pancreatitis because of slower lymphatic clearance from the pleural space compared with more rapid renal clearance.

The effusion associated with acute pancreatitis is usually small and left-sided (60%) but may be isolated to the right (30%) or may be bilateral (10%).[53] The patient usually presents with abdominal symptoms of acute pancreatitis.

The diagnosis is confirmed by an elevated pleural fluid amylase concentration that is greater than that in serum. A normal pleural fluid amylase concentration may be found at presentation in acute pancreatitis but increases on serial measurements. The fluid is a PMN cell–predominant exudate with glucose values approximating those of serum. Leukocyte counts are usually greater than 10,000/μL but may reach 50,000/μL. The pleural fluid pH is usually 7.30 to 7.35.[19]

No specific treatment is necessary for the pleural effusion of acute pancreatitis; the effusion resolves as the pancreatic inflammation subsides. Drainage of the pleural space does not appear to affect residual pleural damage. If the pleural effusion does not resolve in 2 to 3 weeks, pancreatic abscess or pseudocyst should be suspected.

Pulmonary Embolism

The presence of a small unilateral pleural effusion, especially in association with chest pain or dyspnea, should suggest pulmonary embolism. Pleural effusions occur in up to 50% of patients with pulmonary embolism.[55] These effusions result from several different mechanisms,[55, 56] including:

- Ischemia-induced increased pleural capillary permeability
- Imbalance in microvascular and pleural space hydrostatic pressures
- Pleuropulmonary hemorrhage

Ischemia from pulmonary vascular obstruction, in addition to release of inflammatory mediators from platelet-rich thrombi, can cause capillary leak into the lung and subsequently pleural space, explaining the usual finding of an exudative effusion. Transudates, described in approximately 20% of patients in one small series with pulmonary embolism, result from atelectasis.[56]

With pulmonary infarction, necrosis and hemorrhage into the lung and pleural space may result. More than 80% of patients with infarction have bloody pleural effusions, but more than 35% of patients with pulmonary embolism without radiographic infarction also have hemorrhagic fluid.[55] The presence of a pleural effusion does not alter the signs or symptoms in patients with pulmonary embolism. Chest pain, usually pleuritic, occurs in most patients with pleural effusions complicating pulmonary embolism and is invariably ipsilateral.[55] The chest radiograph on presentation typically shows a small, unilateral pleural effusion that occupies less than a third of the hemithorax.[55] An associated pulmonary infiltrate, representing a pulmonary infarction, is seen in approximately 50% of patients with pulmonary embolism and effusion.

Although pleural fluid analysis is variable and nondiagnostic,[56] a bloody pleural effusion suggests pulmonary embolism in the absence of chest trauma, recent cardiac injury, asbestos exposure, or malignant neoplasm.[57] The pleural fluid is hemorrhagic in two thirds of patients, but the number of red blood cells exceeds 100,000/μL in fewer than 20%.[56] The nucleated cell count ranges from less than 100 (presumably atelectatic transudates) to 50,000/μL (pulmonary infarction).[56] There is a predominance of PMNs when a thoracentesis is performed near the time of the acute symptoms and a majority of lymphocytes with later thoracentesis. The effusion due to pulmonary embolism is usually apparent (92%) on the initial chest radiograph and reaches a maximum volume during the first 72 hours.[55] Patients with pleural effusions that progress with heparin therapy after 3 days should be evaluated for a recurrent embolism, a hemothorax secondary to anticoagulation, an infected infarction, or an alternative diagnosis. When consolidation (infarction) is absent on the chest radiograph, effusions usually resolve in about 1 week; with consolidation, there is a longer resolution time, typically 2 to 3 weeks.[55]

The association of pleural effusion with pulmonary embolism does not alter therapy. Furthermore, the presence of a bloody effusion is not a contraindication to full-dose anticoagulation, because hemothorax is a rare complication of heparin therapy.[58] An enlarging pleural effusion on therapy necessitates thoracentesis to exclude hemothorax, empyema, or another cause. Active pleural space hemorrhage necessitates discontinuation of anticoagulation, tube thoracostomy, and placement of a vena caval filter.

Postcardiac Injury Syndrome

Postcardiac injury syndrome (PCIS) is characterized by the onset of fever, pleuropericarditis, and parenchymal infiltrates 3 weeks (2 to 86 days) after injury to the myocardium or pericardium.[59-61] PCIS has been described after myocardial infarction, cardiac surgery, blunt chest trauma, percutaneous left ventricular puncture, and pacemaker implantation. The incidence after myocardial infarction has been estimated at up to 4%,[59] but with more extensive myocardial and pericardial involvement, it may be higher. It occurs with greater frequency (up to 30%) after cardiac surgery.[62] The pathogenesis of PCIS remains obscure, but it probably results from autoimmune injury in patients with myocardial or pericardial damage in association with a concomitant viral illness.

The diagnosis remains one of exclusion because no specific criteria exist. It is important to confirm or exclude PCIS presumptively, for failure to make the correct diagnosis may lead to iatrogenic complications from inappropriate therapy, such as cardiac tamponade from anticoagulation for presumed pulmonary embolism and adverse effects related to antimicrobial therapy for presumed pneumonia. A single report documented higher titers of antimyocardial antibodies in pleural fluid than in serum and pleural fluid complement levels less than in serum, supporting a local immunologic pathogenesis and suggesting a diagnostic test.[63]

Pleuropulmonary manifestations are the hallmark of PCIS. The most common presenting symptoms are pleuritic chest pain (found in virtually all patients) and fever, pericardial rub, dyspnea, and rales, (found in half of all patients).[61] Hemoptysis occurs rarely, an important differential point when pulmonary embolism with infarction is in the differential diagnosis. Fifty per cent of patients have leukocytosis, and almost all have an elevated erythrocyte sedimentation rate (average, 62 mm/hr).[61]

Chest radiographic findings are abnormal in almost all patients. The most common abnormality is left-sided and bilateral pleural effusions; a unilateral right effusion is unusual.[61] Pulmonary infiltrates are present in 75% of patients and are most commonly seen in the left lower lobe.[59]

The pleural fluid is a serosanguineous or bloody exudate with a glucose level greater than 60 mg/dL and pleural fluid pH greater than 7.30. Nucleated cell counts range from 500 to 39,000/μL, with a predominance of PMNs early in the course.[61] Pericardial fluid on echocardiography is an important finding suggestive of PCIS. The pleural fluid characteristics should help differentiate PCIS from a parapneumonic effusion and CHF, but they do not exclude pulmonary embolism.

PCIS is usually self-limited. Therapy may not be required if symptoms are trivial. PCIS usually responds to aspirin or nonsteroidal anti-inflammatory agents, but some patients require corticosteroid therapy for resolution. In patients who respond, the pleural effusion resolves within 1 to 3 weeks.

Esophageal Sclerotherapy

Pleural effusions are found in 50% of patients 48 to 72 hours after esophageal sclerotherapy.[64, 65] Effusions may be unilateral or bilateral, with no predilection for side. Effusion appears more likely with larger total volumes of sclerosant injected and larger volume injected per site.[64, 65] The type of sclerosant does not appear to be a factor. The effusions tend to be small-volume, serous exudates with variable nucleated (90 to 38,000/μL) and red blood cell counts (126 to 160,000/μL) and glucose concentration similar to that of serum.[64] These effusions probably result from an intensive inflammatory reaction after extravasation of the sclerosant into the esophageal mucosa, causing mediastinal and mediastinal parietal pleural inflammation. The effusion that is not associated with fever, chest pain, or perforation is of little consequence, requires no specific therapy, and resolves in several days to weeks.[64, 65] However, late perforation may evolve in patients with apparent innocuous effusions. In patients with symptomatic effusions for 24 to 48 hours, diagnostic thoracentesis should be done and an esophagogram considered.

Acute Respiratory Distress Syndrome

The presence of pleural effusions in ARDS has not been well appreciated. In a retrospective study of 25 patients with ARDS, a 36% incidence of pleural effusions was found, a percentage similar to that found with hydrostatic pulmonary edema.[66] All patients had extensive alveolar pulmonary edema and endotracheal tube fluid that was compatible with increased permeability edema. Several experimental models of increased permeability pulmonary edema, including α-naphthylthiourea,[67] oleic acid,[68] and ethchlorvynol,[69] have been associated with pleural effusions. In both the oleic acid and ethchlorvynol models, the development of pleural effusions lagged behind interstitial and alveolar edema by several hours. In the oleic acid model, 35% of the excess lung water collected in the pleural spaces.

The pleura appears to act as a reservoir for excess lung water in both increased permeability and hydrostatic pulmonary edema. These effusions tend to be underdiagnosed clinically because the patient has bilateral alveolar infiltrates and the radiograph is taken with the patient in a supine position. Experimentally, the effusion is serous to serosanguineous, with a predominance of PMNs.[69] No specific therapy is required, and these effusions resolve as ARDS resolves.

Spontaneous Esophageal Rupture

The patient with an esophageal rupture, a potentially life-threatening event, requires immediate diagnosis and therapy. The history in spontaneous esophageal rupture is usually severe retching or vomiting or a conscious effort to resist vomiting; however, in some patients, the perforation may be silent. Early recognition of spontaneous rupture depends on correct interpretation of the chest radiograph.

Several factors influence chest radiographic findings[70]:

- The time between perforation and chest radiographic examination
- Site of perforation
- Degree of mediastinal pleural integrity

A chest radiograph taken within minutes of the acute injury is usually unremarkable. Mediastinal emphysema probably requires at least 1 to 2 hours to be demonstrated radiographically and is present in fewer than half of patients; mediastinal widening may take several hours.[71] Pneumothorax, present in 75% of patients with spontaneous rupture, indicates violation of the mediastinal pleura; 70% of pneumothoraces are on the left, 20% are on the right, and 10% are bilateral.[71] Mediastinal air is seen early if pleural integrity is maintained, whereas pleural effusion secondary to mediastinitis tends to occur later. Pleural fluid, with or without associated pneumothorax, occurs in 75% of patients. A presumptive radiographic diagnosis should be confirmed immediately. Esophagographic findings are abnormal in about 90% of patients.[72] In the upright patient, rapid passage of the contrast material may not demonstrate a small rent; therefore, the study should be done with the patient in the appropriate lateral decubitus position.[73] Chest CT may be of value in atypical cases by demonstrating mediastinal air and a small pleural effusion.

Pleural fluid findings depend on the degree of perforation and the timing of thoracentesis from injury. Early thoracentesis without mediastinal perforation shows a sterile, serous exudate with a predominance of PMNs, a pleural fluid amylase concentration less than that of serum, and pH greater than 7.30.[74] Once the mediastinal pleura tears, amylase of salivary origin appears in the fluid in high concentration.[75] As the pleural space is seeded with anaerobic organisms from the mouth, the pH falls rapidly and progressively to approach 6.00.[74, 76] Other pleural fluid findings suggestive of esophageal rupture include the presence of squamous epithelial cells and food particles.

The diagnosis of spontaneous esophageal rupture dictates immediate operative intervention. If diagnosis and treatment are accomplished appropriately within the first 24 hours with primary closure, survival is greater than 90%.[71] Delay from the time of initial symptoms to diagnosis results in a reduced survival with any form of therapy.

Hemothorax

Hemothorax (blood in the pleural space) should be differentiated from a hemorrhagic pleural effusion, because hemorrhagic pleural effusion can be the result of only a few drops of blood in serous pleural fluid. An arbitrary, but practical, definition of a hemothorax with regard to therapy is a pleural fluid to blood hematocrit ratio greater than 50%.[77] Most hemothoraces result from penetrating or blunt chest trauma.[78] Hemothorax can also result from invasive procedures (e.g., placement of central venous catheters, thoracentesis, pleural biopsy) and from pulmonary infarction, malignant neoplasm, or ruptured aortic aneurysm. Bleeding can occur from vessels of the chest wall, lung, diaphragm, or mediastinum. Blood that enters the pleural space clots, rapidly undergoes fibrinolysis, and becomes defibrinogenated; thus, it rarely causes significant pleural fibrosis.

Hemothorax should be suspected in any patient with blunt or penetrating chest trauma. If a pleural effusion is found on the admitting chest radiograph, thoracentesis should be performed immediately and the hematocrit measured on the fluid. The hemothorax may not be apparent on the initial chest radiograph because it may be small and the patient may be supine.[79] Since bleeding may be slow and may not appear for several hours,[79] it is imperative that serial radiographs be performed in these patients. The incidence of concomitant pneumothorax is high (~60%).[78, 79]

Patients with traumatic hemothorax should be treated immediately with tube thoracostomy.[78-81] Large-diameter chest tube drainage evacuates the pleural space, may tamponade the bleeding (especially if the origin is a pleural laceration), allows monitoring of the bleeding, and decreases the likelihood of subsequent fibrothorax.[81, 82] If bleeding continues without signs of slowing, thoracotomy should be performed, depending on the individual circumstances.[81] Pleural effusions occasionally occur after removal of the chest tube from traumatic hemothoraces.[83] A diagnostic thoracentesis is indicated to exclude empyema. If empyema is excluded, the pleural effusion usually resolves without specific treatment and without residual pleural fibrosis.

Hemothorax is a rare complication of anticoagulation and has been reported in patients receiving heparin and warfarin.[84] Coagulation study results are usually within the therapeutic range. The hemothorax tends to occur on the side of the pulmonary infarction. Anticoagulation therapy should be discontinued immediately, a chest tube inserted to evacuate the blood, and a vena caval filter considered.

Coronary Artery Bypass Surgery

A small left pleural effusion is virtually always present after coronary artery bypass surgery. This effusion is associated with left lower lobe atelectasis and elevation of the left hemidiaphragm on chest radiography. Left diaphragm dysfunction is secondary to intraoperative phrenic nerve injury from cold cardioplegia, stretch injury, or surgical trauma.[85-87] The larger and grossly bloody effusions tend to be associated with internal mammary artery grafting, which causes marked exudation from the bed where the internal mammary artery was harvested.[88] Furthermore, the larger and more persistent pleural effusions appear to be associated with left pleurotomy. Pleurotomy may increase pleural fluid accumulation by increasing production of fluid and decreasing lymphatic drainage from the pleural space.

The pleural fluid is a hemorrhagic exudate with a low nucleated cell count, a glucose level similar to that of serum, and a pH greater than 7.40. Rarely, a loculated hemothorax may develop with trapped lung, resulting in clinically significant restriction.[89] Some cardiovascular surgeons suggest avoiding pleurotomy, minimizing chest wall distortion during internal mammary artery harvesting, and taking special care not to injure the phrenic nerve in an attempt to decrease the volume and persistence of left pleural effusions. If a large effusion is present that qualifies as a hemothorax (see earlier), the fluid should be drained by tube thoracostomy. It is unclear whether a large hemorrhagic effusion (pleural fluid/blood hematocrit ratio $< 50\%$) needs to be drained with a needle. It is probably prudent to drain moderately large, bloody effusions to avoid the later necessity of decortication.

Abdominal Surgery

Small unilateral or bilateral pleural effusions have been known to develop within 48 to 72 hours of surgery in approximately 50% of patients who undergo abdominal surgery.[36, 37] The incidence is higher after upper abdominal surgery, in patients with postoperative atelectasis, and in patients found to have ascitic fluid at surgery.[36] Larger left-sided pleural effusions are common after splenectomy.[36] The effusion is usually exudative without a large number of nucleated cells. The pleural fluid glucose level is equivalent to that of serum, and the pH is above 7.40.[36] The effusion probably results from diaphragmatic irritation or atelectasis.

Small effusions generally do not necessitate diagnostic thoracentesis, are not of clinical significance, and resolve spontaneously. Pleural effusion from subphrenic abscess or pulmonary embolism is unlikely to occur within 2 to 3 days of surgery. The indication for diagnostic thoracentesis in this setting would be to exclude infection if the effusion is relatively large or loculated.

Chylothorax

Surgical trauma accounts for about 25% of cases of chylothorax, a rate second only to that of lymphoma.[90] The incidence of chylothorax after thoracic surgery is estimated at less than 1%,[91] but a 3% incidence has been reported after esophagectomy.[92] Virtually all intrathoracic procedures, including lobectomy and pneumonectomy and coronary artery bypass grafting, may cause chylothorax. Other iatrogenic chylothoraces can be caused by complications of prolonged central vein catheterization.[93] Nonsurgical trauma, such as penetrating and nonpenetrating neck, thoracic, and upper abdominal injuries, has also been associated with chylothorax.

When the thoracic duct is torn by stretching during surgery, chyle leaks into the mediastinum and subsequently invades the pleural space.[94] In the nonsurgical setting, penetrating injuries and fractures may directly tear the thoracic duct. Chylothorax from a central venous catheter usually involves venous thrombosis.[93]

The patient may be asymptomatic if the effusion is small and unilateral or present with dyspnea with a large unilateral effusion or bilateral effusions. The pleural fluid is usually milky, but 12% can be serous or serosanguineous,[95] with fewer than 7000 nucleated cells/μL that are virtually all lymphocytes.[19] The pleural fluid pH is alkaline (7.40 to 7.80), and triglyceride levels exceed plasma levels. Finding a pleural fluid triglyceride concentration of greater than 110 mg/dL makes the diagnosis of chylothorax highly likely.[95] If the triglyceride level is below 50 mg/dL, chylothorax is highly unlikely. Triglyceride levels of 50 to 110 mg/dL indicate the need for lipoprotein electrophoresis.[95] Demonstration of chylomicrons on electrophoresis confirms the diagnosis of chylothorax. The thoracic duct defect after trauma usually closes spontaneously within 10 to 14 days with bed rest and total parenteral nutrition to minimize chyle formation. A pleuroperitoneal shunt relieves dyspnea, recirculates chyle, and prevents malnutrition and immunocompromise.[96]

PNEUMOTHORAX

Classification

Pneumothorax literally means the presence of air *within the thorax*, but it actually refers to the presence of free air *within the confines of the chest*. However, pneumothorax is used to connote free air within the pleural space, but free air may be found in the adventitial planes of the lung (interstitial emphysema) or the mediastinum (pneumomediastinum).

Spontaneous pneumothorax occurs without an obvious cause as a consequence of the natural course of a disease process. *Primary* spontaneous pneumothorax occurs without clinical findings of lung disease. *Secondary* spontaneous pneumothorax occurs as a consequence of clinically manifest lung disease (Table 143–2). Traumatic pneumothorax results from penetrating or blunt chest injury. Iatrogenic pneumothorax occurs as an inadvertent consequence of diagnostic or therapeutic procedures.

Pathophysiology

Pressure in the pleural space is subatmospheric throughout the normal respiratory cycle, averaging −9 mm Hg during inspiration and −5 mm Hg during expiration. Because of lung elasticity, pressure in the airways is positive during expiration (+3 mm Hg) and negative during inspiration (−2 mm Hg).[97] Thus, in normal breathing, airway pressure is greater than pleural pressure throughout the respiratory cycle.

Airway pressure may be increased markedly with coughing or strenuous exercise; however, pleural pressure rises concomitantly so that the transpulmonary pressure gradient is usually not substantially changed. When there are rapid fluctuations in intrathoracic pressure, however, a large transpulmonary pressure gradient occurs transiently.

Bronchial and bronchiolar obstruction, resulting in air trapping, can substantially increase the transpulmonary pressure gradient. The alveolar walls and visceral pleura maintain the pressure gradient between the airways and pleural space. When the pressure gradient is transiently increased, alveolar rupture may occur; air enters the interstitial tissues of the lung and may enter the pleural space, resulting in a pneumothorax. If the visceral pleura remains intact, the interstitial air moves toward the hilum, resulting in pneumomediastinum.[98, 99] Because mean pressure within the mediastinum is always less than in the periphery of the lung, air would move proximally along the bronchovascular sheaths to the hilum and mediastinal soft tissues. The development of pneumomediastinum after alveolar rupture requires continual cyclic respiratory efforts, which result in slow movement of air from the ruptured alveolus along a pressure gradient to the mediastinum.[98]

TABLE 143–2. Causes of Pneumothorax Occurring in or Responsible for Admission to the Intensive Care Unit

Secondary Spontaneous Pneumothorax
Chronic obstructive pulmonary disease
Status asthmaticus
Pneumocystis carinii pneumonia
Cystic fibrosis
Pulmonary histiocytosis X
Stage IV sarcoidosis
Necrotizing pneumonia
Iatrogenic Pneumothorax
Barotrauma
Acute respiratory distress syndrome
Chronic obstructive pulmonary disease
Necrotizing pneumonia
Invasive procedures
Central venous catheters
Thoracentesis
Placement of narrow-bore enteral feeding tubes

Mediastinal air may decompress into the cervical and subcutaneous tissues or the retroperitoneum. With abrupt rise in mediastinal pressure or insufficient decompression to subcutaneous tissue, the mediastinal pleura may rupture, causing pneumothorax. Inadequate decompression of the mediastinum, rather than direct rupture of subpleural blebs into the pleural space, may be the major cause of pneumothorax.[98]

When pneumothorax occurs, the elasticity of the lung causes it to collapse. Lung collapse continues until the pleural defect seals or pleural and alveolar pressures equalize. When a ball-valve effect occurs at the site of communication between the pleural space and the alveolus, permitting only egress of air from the lung, there is a progressive accumulation of air within the pleural space, which can result in markedly increased positive pleural pressure, producing a tension pneumothorax. Tension pneumothorax compresses mediastinal structures, resulting in impaired venous return to the heart, decrease in cardiac output, and, at times, fatal cardiovascular collapse.[100, 101] Rarely, tension along the bronchovascular sheaths and in the mediastinum can cause collapse of the pulmonary arteries and veins, resulting in cardiovascular collapse.[98]

Patients with primary spontaneous pneumothorax have a decrease in vital capacity and an increase in the $P(A - a)O_2$ gradient and usually present with hypoxemia due predominantly to the development of an intrapulmonary shunt and areas of low ventilation-perfusion in the atelectatic lung.[102, 103] Hypercapnia does not occur, because there is adequate function in the uninvolved lung to maintain necessary alveolar ventilation. Patients with secondary spontaneous pneumothorax, in contrast, commonly have hypercapnia because the gas exchange abnormality caused by the pneumothorax is superimposed on lungs with preexisting abnormal pulmonary gas exchange.[104, 105]

Treatment in the Intensive Care Unit

Patients with secondary spontaneous pneumothorax may be admitted to an ICU because they have severe hypoxemic and, at times, hypercapnic respiratory failure. Patients with primary spontaneous pneumothorax rarely require ICU admission because the contralateral lung can maintain necessary alveolar ventilation and the hypoxemia can be managed with supplemental oxygen. The most common causes of pneumothoraces in ICU patients are invasive procedures and barotrauma.

Iatrogenic Pneumothorax

Central Venous Catheters

Central venous catheters are used routinely in critically ill patients for volume resuscitation, parenteral nutrition, and drug administration. Approximately 3 million central venous catheters are placed annually in the United States, and this procedure continues to be associated with clinically relevant morbidity and some mortality.[106] The morbidity and mortality associated with central venous catheter use are most commonly physician-related.[45] Pleural complications of both the acquisition of venous access and the indwelling phase of central venous catheters include pneumothorax, hydrothorax, hemothorax, and chylothorax.

In a study of mechanical complications of central venous catheters, 1.1% of 534 patients had pneumothorax.[107] This translates into approximately 36,000 pneumothoraces per year from central venous catheter insertions in critically ill patients in the United States. In the same study, none of the 405 patients had pneumothorax when the central venous catheter was replaced over a guidewire.

Both the subclavian and internal jugular routes have been associated with pneumothorax, hemothorax, chylothorax, and catheter placement into the pleural space. Cannulation of the subclavian vein is associated with a higher risk of pneumothorax ($<5\%$)[108] compared with cannulation of the internal jugular vein ($<0.2\%$)[109]; with the external jugular venous approach, pneumothorax is avoided. There is a greater risk of pneumothorax with the infraclavicular than with the supraclavicular approach to the subclavian vein. All complications of insertion, regardless of approach, can be reduced by appropriate training and experience of physicians.

Most pneumothoraces occur at the time of the procedure from direct lung puncture, but delayed pneumothoraces have been noted; therefore, it is prudent to view a chest radiograph 12 to 24 hours after the procedure. Up to half of patients with needle puncture pneumothorax may be managed expectantly without the need for tube drainage. Bilateral pneumothoraces have been reported to occur from unilateral attempts,[110] and death can occur when there is a delay in the diagnosis of pneumothorax.[111]

As stated previously, a pneumothorax may be more difficult to detect while the patient is supine. Additional views should be taken, especially if the venous cannulation does not proceed as anticipated. With any newly placed central venous catheter, a postprocedure chest radiograph should be obtained, regardless of the site cannulated, to ensure that the catheter tip is properly positioned. If a small pneumothorax is detected by chest radiography and the patient is asymptomatic and not on mechanical ventilation, the patient can be observed expectantly with repeated chest radiographs to ensure that the leak has ceased. If the patient is receiving mechanical ventilation or if the pneumothorax is large or has caused significant symptoms or gas exchange abnormalities, tube thoracostomy should be performed as soon as possible.

Barotrauma

Pulmonary barotrauma is an important clinical problem because of the widespread use of mechanical ventilation. Barotrauma occurs in about 10% of patients on mechanical ventilation and includes parenchymal interstitial gas, pneumomediastinum, subcutaneous emphysema, pneumoperitoneum, and pneumothorax.[12, 112-114] The most clinically important is pneumothorax, occurring in 1% to 15% of all patients receiving mechanical ventilation. In patients with ARDS, rates of 25% to 87% have been reported.[115, 116] The number of ventilation days, underlying disease (ARDS, COPD, necrotizing pneumonia), and use of positive end-expiratory pressure (PEEP) have an impact on the incidence of pneumothorax.[112-114, 117-120] When a pneumothorax develops in the setting of mechanical ventilation, 30% to 97% of patients have tension pneumothorax.[12, 113, 116, 117, 121]

The initial radiographic sign of barotrauma is often pulmonary interstitial gas or emphysema.[115, 121] In the early stages, however, interstitial gas may be difficult to detect radiographically. This harbinger of pneumothorax may be detected as distinct subpleural air cysts, linear air streaks emanating from the hilum, and perivascular air halos. Subpleural air cysts, most commonly seen in ARDS, tend to appear abruptly on the chest radiograph as single or multiple thin-walled, round lucencies and are most often visualized at the lung bases, medially or diaphragmatically.[122] The cysts, which may expand rapidly, are usually 3 to 5 cm in diameter. Differentiating between peripheral subpleural air cysts and a localized basilar pneumothorax may be a problem. Pleural air cysts appear to be more common in younger patients, possibly because connective tissue planes of the lung are looser in younger than in older patients.[123] The risk of tension pneumothorax is substantial in patients who have had subpleural lung cysts with continued mechanical ventilation. When mechanical ventilation is discontinued, the cyst may resolve spontaneously or become secondarily infected.

When evidence of barotrauma without pneumothorax is observed in any patient requiring continued mechanical ventilation, immediate attempts should be made to lower the plateau airway pressure. In the patient with ARDS, tidal volumes[124, 125] and inspiratory flow rates should be lowered, an attempt should be made to reduce or remove PEEP, and neuromuscular blockers and sedation should be considered.[126] In the patient with status asthmaticus, in addition to the aforementioned maneuvers, controlled hypoventilation should be accomplished.[127, 128] There is no evidence supporting the use of prophylactic chest tubes. However, the patient should be monitored closely for tension pneumothorax and provisions made for emergency bedside tube thoracostomy.

Tension Pneumothorax

Pneumothorax in the mechanically ventilated patient may present as an acute cardiopulmonary emergency, beginning with respiratory distress and, if unrecognized and untreated, progressing to cardiovascular collapse. In one report of 74 patients, the diagnosis of pneumothorax was made clinically in 45 (61%) patients on the basis of hypotension, hyperresonance, diminished breath sounds, and tachycardia.[120] The mortality rate was 7% in these patients receiving the clinical diagnosis. In the remaining 29 patients, diagnosis was delayed between 30 minutes and 8 hours, and 31% of these patients died of pneumothorax. Other series of barotrauma in the setting of mechanical ventilation have reported mortality rates of 58% to 77%.[12, 114, 118, 119]

Tension pneumothorax is lethal if diagnosis and treatment are delayed. The diagnosis should be made clinically at the bedside in the patient receiving mechanical ventilation who shows a sudden deterioration characterized by apprehension, tachypnea, cyanosis, decreased ipsilateral breath sounds, subcutaneous emphysema, tachycardia, and hypotension. The diagnosis may be a problem in the unconscious patient, the elderly patient, and the patient with bilateral tension, which may be more protective of the mediastinal structures and may lessen the impact on cardiac output.

In the unconscious or critically ill patient, hypoxemia may be one of the earlier signs of tension pneumothorax. In the patient receiving mechanical ventilation, increasing peak and mean airway pressure, decreasing compliance, and auto-PEEP should raise the possibility of tension pneumothorax. Difficulty in ventilating the patient with an Ambu bag and delivering adequate tidal volumes may be noted.

When the clinical signs and symptoms are noted in mechanically ventilated patients, treatment should not be delayed to obtain radiographic confirmation. If a chest tube is not immediately available, placement of a large-bore needle into the anterior second intercostal space is lifesaving and confirms the diagnosis, as a rush of air will be noted exiting the pleural space as the needle is inserted. An appropriately large chest tube can then be placed and connected to an adequate drainage system that can accommodate the large air leak that may develop in mechanically ventilated patients.[129]

As tension is relieved, the following effects are noted:

- Rapid improvement in oxygenation
- Increase in blood pressure
- Decrease in heart rate
- Decline in peak airway pressure

In experimental tension pneumothorax, the inability to raise cardiac output in response to hypoxemia leads to a reduction in systemic oxygen transport and a decrease in mixed venous P_{O_2}, which partially explains the cardiovascular collapse seen in these patients.[101] In mechanically ventilated patients, a decrease in cardiac output is an inevitable consequence of tension pneumothorax.

References

1. Woodring JH: Recognition of pleural effusion on supine radiographs: How much fluid is required? AJR 1984; 142:59.
2. Christensen EE, Curry TS III, Dowdey JE: An Introduction to the Physics of Diagnostic Radiology. 2nd ed. Philadelphia, Lea & Febiger, 1978, p 101.
3. Collins JD, Burwell D, Furmanski S, et al: Minimum detectable pleural effusions: A roentgen pathology model. Radiology 1975; 105:51.
4. Wiener ND, Garay SM, Leitman BS, et al: Imaging of the intensive care unit patient. Clin Chest Med 1991; 12:169.
5. Yu C-J, Yang P-C, Chang D-B, et al: Diagnostic and therapeutic use of chest sonography: Value in critically ill patients. AJR Am J Roentgenol 1992; 159:695.
6. Mirvis SE, Tobin KD, Kostrubiak I, et al: Thoracic CT in detecting occult disease in critically ill patients. AJR 1987; 148:685.
7. Peruzzi W, Garner W, Bools J, et al: Portable chest roentgenography and computed tomography in critically ill patients. Chest 1988; 93:722.
8. Greene R, McLoud TC, Stark P: Pneumothorax. Semin Roentgenol 1977; 12:313.
9. Moskowitz PS, Griscom NT: The medial pneumothorax. Radiology 1976; 120:143.
10. Lichtenstein DA, Menu Y: A bedside ultrasound sign ruling out pneumothorax in the critically ill. Lung sliding. Chest 1995; 108:1345.
11. Joffe N: The adult respiratory distress syndrome. AJR 1974; 122:719.
12. Rohlfing BM, Webb WR, Schlobohm RM: Ventilator-related extra-alveolar air in adults. Radiology 1976; 121:25.
13. Gobien RP, Reines HD, Schabel SI: Localized tension pneumothorax: Unrecognized form of barotrauma in adult respiratory distress syndrome. Radiology 1982; 142:15.
14. Tocino IM, Miller MH, Fairfax WR: Distribution of pneumothorax in the supine and semirecumbent critically ill adult. AJR 1985; 144:901.
15. Kollef MH: Risk factors for the misdiagnosis of pneumothorax in the intensive care unit. Crit Care Med 1991; 19:906.
16. Marglin SI, Rowberg AH, Godwin JD: Preliminary experience with portable digital imaging for intensive care radiology. J Thorac Imaging 1990; 5:49.
17. Elam EA, Rehm K, Hillman BJ, et al: Efficacy of digital radiography for the detection of pneumothorax: Comparison with conventional chest radiography. AJR Am J Roentgenol 1992; 158:509.
18. Humphrey LM, Fitzpatrick K, Paine SS, et al: Physician experience with viewing digital radiographs in an intensive care unit environment. J Digit Imaging 1993; 6:30.
19. Sahn SA: The pleura. Am Rev Respir Dis 1988; 138:184.
20. Lipscomb DJ, Flower CDR, Hadfield JW: Ultrasound of the pleura: An assessment of its clinical value. Clin Radiol 1981; 32:289.
21. Godwin JE, Sahn SA: Thoracentesis: A safe procedure in mechanically ventilated patients. Ann Intern Med 1990; 113:800.
22. Collins TR, Sahn SA: Thoracentesis: Clinical value, complications, technical problems, and patient experience. Chest 1987; 91:817.
23. Health and Public Policy Committee: American College of Physicians position paper: Diagnostic thoracentesis and pleural biopsy in pleural effusions. Ann Intern Med 1985; 103:799.
24. Sahn SA: Thoracentesis and pleural biopsy. *In:* Respiratory Disease in the Immunosuppressed Host. Shelhamer J, Pizzo PA, Parillo JE, Masur H (Eds). Philadelphia, JB Lippincott, 1991, p 118.
25. Bartter T, Mayo PD, Pratter MR, et al: Lower risk and higher yield for thoracentesis when performed by experienced operators. Chest 1993; 103:1873.
26. Seneff MG, Corwin W, Gold LH, et al: Complications associated with thoracocentesis. Chest 1986; 90:97.
27. Grogan DR, Irwin RS, Channick R, et al: Complications associated with thoracentesis: A prospective, randomized study comparing three different methods. Arch Intern Med 1990; 150:873.
28. Light RW, Jenkinson SG, Minh V, et al: Observations on pleural pressures as fluid is withdrawn during thoracentesis. Am Rev Respir Dis 1980; 121:799.

29. Brown NE, Zamel N, Aberman A: Changes in pulmonary mechanics in gas exchange following thoracocentesis. Chest 1978; 74:540.
30. Estenne M, Yernault J-C, Detroyer A: Mechanism of relief of dyspnea after thoracentesis in patients with large effusions. Am J Med 1983; 74:813.
31. Light RW, Stansbury DW, Brown SE: Changes in pulmonary function following therapeutic thoracentesis. Chest 1981; 80:375.
32. Brandstetter RD, Cohen RP: Hypoxemia after thoracentesis: A predictable and treatable condition. JAMA 1979; 242:1060.
33. Karetzky M, Kothari GA, Fourre JA, et al: The effect of thoracentesis on arterial oxygen tension. Respiration 1978; 36:96.
34. Perpina M, Benlloch E, Marco V, et al: The effect of thoracentesis on pulmonary gas exchange. Thorax 1983; 38:747.
35. Mattison L, Coppage L, Alderman D, Herlong J, Sahn SA: Pleural effusions in the medical intensive care unit: Prevalence, causes and clinical implications. Chest 1997; 111:1018.
36. Light RW, George RB: Incidence and significance of pleural effusion after abdominal surgery. Chest 1976; 69:621.
37. Nielsen PH, Jepsan SB, Olsen AD: Postoperative pleural effusion following upper abdominal surgery. Chest 1989; 96:1133.
38. Wiener-Kronish JP, Matthay MA, Callen PW, et al: Relationship of pleural effusions to pulmonary hemodynamics in patients with congestive heart failure. Am Rev Respir Dis 1987; 132:1253.
39. Shinto RA, Light RW: Effects of diuresis on the characteristics of pleural fluid in patients with congestive heart failure. Am J Med 1990; 88:230.
40. Chakko SC, Caldwell SH, Sforza PP: Treatment of congestive heart failure: Its effect on pleural fluid chemistry. Chest 1989; 95:798.
41. Lieberman FL, Hidemura R, Peters RL, et al: Pathogenesis and treatment of hydrothorax complicating cirrhosis with ascites. Ann Intern Med 1966; 64:341.
42. Johnson RF, Loo RB: Hepatic hydrothorax: Studies to determine the source of the fluid and report of 13 cases. Ann Intern Med 1964; 61:385.
43. Frazer IH, Lichtenstein M, Andrews JT: Pleuroperitoneal effusion without ascites. Med J Aust 1983; 2:520.
44. Adams DA: The pathophysiology of nephrotic syndrome. Arch Intern Med 1960; 106:117.
45. Scott WL: Complications associated with central venous catheters: A survey. Chest 1988; 94:1221.
46. Duntley P, Siever J, Korwes ML, et al: Vascular erosion by central venous catheters: Clinical features and outcome. Chest 1992; 101:1633.
47. Ellis LM, Vogel SB III, Copeland EM: Central venous catheter vascular erosions. Ann Surg 1989; 209:475.
48. Wechsler RJ, Byrne KJ, Steiner RM: The misplaced thoracic venous catheter: Detailed anatomical consideration. Crit Rev Diagn Imaging 1982; 21:289.
49. Ball GV, Whitfield CL: Studies on rheumatoid disease pleural fluid. Arthritis Rheum 1966; 9:846.
50. Sahn SA: Clinical commentary: Management of complicated parapneumonic effusions. Am Rev Respir Dis 1993; 148:813.
51. Ashbaugh DG: Empyema thoracis: Factors influencing morbidity and mortality. Chest 1991; 99:1162.
52. Ridley PD, Brainbridge MV: Thoracoscopic debridement and pleural irrigation in the management of empyema thoracis. Ann Thorac Surg 1991; 51:461.
53. Kaye MD: Pleuropulmonary complications of pancreatitis. Thorax 1968; 23:297.
54. Anderson WJ, Skinner DB, Zuidema GD, et al: Chronic pancreatic pleural effusions. Surg Gynecol Obstet 1973; 137:827.
55. Bynum LJ, Wilson JE III: Radiographic features of pleural effusions in pulmonary embolism. Am Rev Respir Dis 1978; 117:829.
56. Bynum LJ, Wilson JE III: Characteristics of pleural effusions associated with pulmonary embolism. Arch Intern Med 1976; 136:159.
57. Sahn SA: Pleural fluid analysis: Narrowing the differential diagnosis. Semin Respir Med 1987; 9:22.
58. Simon HB, Daggett WN, DeSanctis RW: Hemothorax as a complication of anticoagulant therapy in the presence of pulmonary infarction. JAMA 1969; 208:1830.
59. Dressler W: The post-myocardial infarction syndrome: A report of 44 cases. Arch Intern Med 1959; 103:28.
60. Engle MA, Ito T: The post-pericardiotomy syndrome. Am J Cardiol 1961; 7:73.
61. Stelzner TJ, King TE Jr, Antony VB, et al: The pleuro-pulmonary manifestations of the postcardiac injury syndrome. Chest 1983; 84:383.
62. Kaminsky ME, Rodan BA, Osborne DR, et al: Post-pericardiotomy syndrome. AJR 1982; 138:503.
63. Kim S, Sahn SA: Postcardiac injury syndrome. An immunologic pleural fluid analysis. Chest 1996; 109:570.
64. Bacon BR, Bailey-Newton RS, Connors AF Jr: Pleural effusions after endoscopic variceal sclerotherapy. Gastroenterology 1985; 88:1910.
65. Saks BJ, Kilby AE, Dietrich PA: Pleural and mediastinal changes following endoscopic injection sclerotherapy of esophageal varices. Radiology 1983; 149:639.
66. Aberle DR, Wiener-Kronish JP, Webb WR, et al: Hydrostatic versus increased permeability pulmonary edema: Diagnosis based on radiographic criteria in critically ill patients. Radiology 1988; 168:73.
67. Cunningham AL, Hurley JV: Alpha-naphthyl-thiourea-induced pulmonary oedema in the rat: A topographical and electron-microscope study. J Pathol 1971; 106:25.
68. Wiener-Kronish JP, Broaddus VC, Albertine KH, et al: Relationship of pleural effusions to increased permeability pulmonary edema in anesthetized sheep. J Clin Invest 1988; 82:1422.
69. Miller KS, Harley RA, Sahn SA: Pleural effusions associated with ethchlorvynol lung injury result from visceral pleural leak. Am Rev Respir Dis 1989; 140:764.
70. Parkin GJS: The radiology of perforated esophagus. Clin Radiol 1973; 24:324.
71. O'Connell ND: Spontaneous rupture of the esophagus. Am J Roentgenol 1967; 99:186.
72. Bladergroen MR, Lowe JE, Postlethwait RW: Diagnosis and recommended management of esophageal perforation and rupture. Ann Thorac Surg 1986; 42:235.
73. DeMeester TR: Perforation of the esophagus. Ann Thorac Surg 1986; 42:231.
74. Maulitz RM, Good JT Jr, Kaplan RL, et al: The pleuropulmonary consequences of esophageal rupture: An experimental model. Am Rev Respir Dis 1979; 120:363.
75. Sherr HP, Light RW, Merson MH, et al: Origin of pleural fluid amylase in esophageal rupture. Ann Intern Med 1972; 76:985.
76. Abbott OA, Mansour KA, Logan WD Jr, et al: Atraumatic so-called "spontaneous" rupture of the esophagus. J Thorac Cardiovasc Surg 1970; 59:67.
77. Light R: Pleural Diseases. 2nd ed. Philadelphia, Lea & Febiger, 1990, p 263.
78. Graham JM, Mattox KL, Beall AC Jr: Penetrating trauma of the lung. J Trauma 1979; 19:665.
79. Drummond DS, Craig RH: Traumatic hemothorax: Complications and management. Am Surg 1967; 33:403.
80. Beall AC Jr, Crawford HW, DeBakey ME: Considerations in the management of acute traumatic hemothorax. J Thorac Cardiovasc Surg 1966; 52:351.
81. Weil PH, Margolis IB: Systematic approach to traumatic hemothorax. Am J Surg 1981; 142:692.
82. Griffith GL, Todd EP, McMillin RD, et al: Acute traumatic hemothorax. Ann Thorac Surg 1978; 26:204.
83. Wilson JM, Boren CH, Peterson SR, et al: Traumatic hemothorax: Is decortication necessary? J Thorac Cardiovasc Surg 1979; 77:489.
84. Rostand RA, Feldman RL, Block ER: Massive hemothorax complicating heparin anticoagulation for pulmonary embolism. South Med J 1977; 70:1128.
85. Iverson L, Mittal A, Dugan D, et al: Injuries to the phrenic nerve resulting in diaphragmatic paralysis with special reference to stretch trauma. Am J Surg 1976; 132:263.
86. Marco J, Hahn J, Barner H: Topical cardiac hypothermia and phrenic nerve injury. Ann Thorac Surg 1977; 23:235.
87. Wheeler W, Rubis L, Jones C, et al: Etiology and prevention of topical cardiac hypothermia-induced phrenic nerve injury and left lower lobe atelectasis during cardiac surgery. Chest 1985; 88:680.
88. Landymore RW, Howell F: Pulmonary complications following myocardial revascularization with the internal mammary artery graft. Eur J Cardiothorac Surg 1990; 4:156.

89. Kollef MH: Trapped-lung syndrome after cardiac surgery: A potentially preventable complication of pleural injury. Heart Lung 1990; 19:671.
90. Valentine VG, Raffin TA: The management of chylothorax. Chest 1992; 102:586.
91. Ferguson MK, Little AG, Skinner DB: Current concepts in the management of postoperative chylothorax. Ann Thorac Surg 1985; 45:542.
92. Orringer MB, Bluett M, Deeb GM: Aggressive treatment of chylothorax complicating transhiatal esophagectomy without thoracotomy. Surgery 1988; 104:720.
93. Teba L, Dedhia HV, Bowen R, et al: Chylothorax review. Crit Care Med 1985; 13:49.
94. Weidner WA, Steiner RM: Roentgenographic demonstration of intrapulmonary and pleural lymphatics during lymphangiography. Radiology 1971; 100:533.
95. Staats BA, Ellefson RD, Budhan LL, et al: The lipoprotein profile of chylous and nonchylous pleural effusions. Mayo Clin Proc 1980; 55:700.
96. Little AG, Kadowaki MH, Ferguson MK, et al: Pleuroperitoneal shunting: Alternative therapy for pleural effusions. Ann Surg 1988; 208:443.
97. Killen DA, Gobbel WG Jr: Spontaneous Pneumothorax. Boston, Little, Brown & Co, 1968, p 1.
98. Macklin MT, Macklin CC: Malignant interstitial emphysema of the lungs and mediastinum as an important occult complication in many respiratory diseases and other conditions: An interpretation of the clinical literature in the light of laboratory experiments. Medicine (Baltimore) 1944; 23:281.
99. Macklin CC: Transport of air along sheaths of pulmonic blood vessels from alveoli to mediastinum: Clinical implications. Arch Intern Med 1939; 64:913.
100. Gustman P, Yerger L, Wanner A: Immediate cardiovascular effects of tension pneumothorax. Am Rev Respir Dis 1983; 127:171.
101. Hurewitz AN, Sidhu U, Bergofsky B, et al: Cardiovascular and respiratory consequence of tension pneumothorax. Bull Eur Physiopathol Respir 1986; 22:545.
102. Norris RM, Jones JG, Bishop JM: Respiratory gas exchange in patients with spontaneous pneumothorax. Thorax 1968; 23:427.
103. Moran JF, Jones RH, Wolfe WG: Regional pulmonary function during experimental unilateral pneumothorax in the awake state. J Thorac Cardiovasc Surg 1977; 74:394.
104. Dines DE, Clagett OT, Payne WS: Spontaneous pneumothorax and emphysema. Mayo Clin Proc 1970; 45:41.
105. George RB, Herbert SJ, Shames JM, et al: Pneumothorax complicating pulmonary emphysema. JAMA 1975; 234:389.
106. Food and Drug Administration Task Force: Precautions necessary with central venous catheters. FDA Drug Bull 1989; July:15.
107. Hagley MT, Martin B, Gast P, et al: Infectious and mechanical complications of central venous catheters placed by percutaneous venipuncture and over guide wires. Crit Care Med 1992; 20:1426.
108. Eerola R, Kaukinen L, Kaukinen S: Analysis of 13,800 subclavian catheterizations. Acta Anaesthesiol Scand 1985; 29:193.
109. Tyden H: Cannulation of the internal jugular vein: 500 cases. Acta Anaesthesiol Scand 1982; 26:485.
110. Weiner P, Sznajder I, Plavnick L, et al: Unusual complications of subclavian vein catheterization. Crit Care Med 1984; 12:538.
111. Adar R, Mozes M: Fatal complication of central venous catheter. Br Med J 1971; 3:746.
112. Kumar A, Pontoppidan H, Falke KJ, et al: Pulmonary barotrauma during mechanical ventilation. Crit Care Med 1973; 1:1.
113. Zimmerman JE, Dunbar BS, Klingenmaier CH: Management of subcutaneous emphysema, pneumomediastinum, and pneumothorax during respirator therapy. Crit Care Med 1975; 3:69.
114. Cullen DJ, Caldera DL: The incidence of ventilator-induced pulmonary barotrauma in critically ill patients. Anesthesiology 1979; 50:185.
115. Tocino I, Westcott JL: Barotrauma. Radiol Clin North Am 1996; 34:59.
116. Petersen GW, Baier H: Incidence of pulmonary barotrauma in the medical ICU. Crit Care Med 1983; 11:67.
117. Zwillich CW, Pierson DJ, Creagh CE, et al: Complications of assisted ventilation: A prospective study of 354 consecutive episodes. Am J Med 1974; 57:161.
118. Fleming WH, Bowen MD, Hatcher CR: Early complications of long term respiratory support. J Thorac Cardiovasc Surg 1972; 64:729.
119. de Latorre FJ, Tomasa A, Klamburg J, et al: Incidence of pneumothorax and pneumomediastinum in patients with aspiration pneumonia requiring ventilatory support. Chest 1977; 72:141.
120. Steier M, Ching N, Roberts EB, et al: Pneumothorax complicating continuous ventilatory support. J Thorac Cardiovasc Surg 1979; 67:17.
121. Johnson TH, Altman AR: Pulmonary interstitial gas: First sign of barotrauma due to PEEP therapy. Crit Care Med 1979; 7:532.
122. Albelda SM, Gefter WB, Kelley MA, et al: Ventilator-induced subpleural air cysts: Clinical, radiographic, and pathologic significance. Am Rev Respir Dis 1983; 127:360.
123. Westcott JL, Cole SR: Interstitial pulmonary emphysema in children and adults: Roentgenographic features. Radiology 1974; 111:367.
124. Snyder J, Carrol G, Schuster DP, et al: Mechanical ventilation: Physiology and application. Curr Probl Surg 1984; 21:1.
125. Suter PM, Fairley HP, Isenberg MD: Effect of tidal volume and positive end-expiratory pressure on compliance during mechanical ventilation. Chest 1978; 73:158.
126. Willetts SM: Paralysis of ventilated patients: Yes or no? Intensive Care Med 1985; 11:2.
127. Darioli E, Perret C: Mechanical controlled hypoventilation in status asthmaticus. Am Rev Respir Dis 1984; 129:385.
128. Menitove SM, Goldring RM: Combined ventilator and bicarbonate strategy in the management of status asthmaticus. Am J Med 1983; 94:898.
129. Baumann MH, Sahn SA: Tension pneumothorax: Diagnostic and therapeutic pitfalls. Crit Care Med 1993; 21:177.

144

Severe Community-Acquired Pneumonia

Jean Chastre, MD • Jean-Yves Fagon, MD, PhD
Jean-Louis Trouillet, MD

Community-acquired pneumonia (CAP) remains a potentially dreadful disease despite modern antibiotics and technology. In industrialized countries, pneumonia is the most frequent infectious cause of death among patients of all ages and the fifth or the sixth leading cause of death overall.[1-3] In-hospital mortality for pneumonia patients older than 65 years of age was 10.7 deaths per 100 discharges in 1993 in the United States.[4] In that year, more than $3.5 billion was spent on inpatient care of Medicare patients with pneumonia, according to data from the Health Care Financing Administration.[4] Although many of the patients with pneumonia who die have underlying fatal diseases, previously healthy elderly and young persons also die of pneumonia.[5,6] Therefore, more rapid identification of patients with severe pneumonia and those who are at a high risk for a complicated course and the accurate selection of appropriate antimicrobial treatment represent important clinical goals in this setting.

The aim of this chapter is to provide current information on these issues so that an updated approach to diagnosis and management can be rationally formulated. A detailed review of all diagnostic and therapeutic problems of pneumonia in the severely immunocompromised patient is beyond the scope of this report, and nosocomial infections are not included.

PROGNOSTIC FACTORS AND PREDICTION RULES FOR DETERMINING DISEASE SEVERITY

Understanding the prognosis of CAP is of particular clinical relevance, because it ranges from rapid recovery from symptoms and functional impairment to serious morbid complications and death. The ability to accurately predict medical outcomes in acute pneumonia influences patient management decisions made by physicians, including whether to hospitalize the patient (home versus hospital, versus intensive care unit [ICU]) and duration of inpatient care if the patient is hospitalized. During the past decade, the prognosis of patients with CAP has been evaluated in a large number of studies that have reported a wide range in mortality and varying predictors of mortality.[7-17] However, there is no consensus concerning the definition of *severe* pneumonia. The term has been used to characterize patients ranging from those who are in need of hospital care overall to those who require mechanical ventilation in an ICU. Therefore, it may be preferable to stratify patients into two groups: patients with severe pneumonia and those who are at high risk for severe pneumonia.

Severe pneumonia can be defined as pneumonia requiring ICU treatment. In general terms, this definition includes patients with pneumonia who require:

1. Ventilatory support, because of acute respiratory failure, inability to clear secretions, deterioration in gas exchange with hypercapnia, or persisting hypoxemia.
2. Circulatory support, because of hemodynamic instability and signs of peripheral hypoperfusion.
3. Intensive monitoring and treatment of other organ dysfunctions resulting from either a septic component of pneumonia or the underlying disease.

In 1993, the American Thoracic Society adopted a statement on the initial management of patients with CAP in which severe illness was defined by the presence of any one of the following features: an admission respiratory rate of more than 30 per minute, a PaO_2/FIO_2 ratio of less than 250 mm Hg, the need for mechanical ventilation, bilateral or multilobar infiltrates, rapidly expanding infiltrates, shock, a need for vasopressors, oliguria, or acute renal failure (Table 144-1).[18] Although this definition was based on factors known to be associated with the need for intensive care, the definition is probably too liberal. In one study, 65% of all patients admitted to the hospital were found to have at least one severe pneumonia feature.[19] To improve the specificity of the criteria, one suggestion has been to change the respiratory rate criterion to 35 breaths/min. Severe CAP probably is best defined by patients having at least two of the severe pneumonia criteria. Furthermore, in patients with coexisting medical conditions who meet the definition of severe pneumonia, transfer to the ICU should be tailored in relation to the severity and prognosis of the underlying disease.

The need for intensive care treatment is not always apparent when the patient is admitted to the hospital. This is especially true in the elderly patient, whose clinical presentation and radiographic signs are often subtle. A large number of factors have been associated with higher death rates in pneumonia. These negative predictors have in most cases been based on univariate statistical analyses, but multivariate methods have been applied in a few prospectives studies and these analyses have confirmed the independent role played by most of them.[8, 11, 14, 15] Therefore, the presence of one of these negative prognostic factors, especially on admission to the hospital, should be viewed as an indication of a high-risk patient.

Fine and colleagues[17] have systematically reviewed all the medical literature on the prognosis and outcomes of patients with CAP. The overall mortality rate for the 33,148 patients in all 127 study cohorts that were identified was 13.7%, ranging from 5.1% for the 2097 hospitalized and ambulatory patients (in six study cohorts) to 36.5% for the 788 ICU patients (in 13 cohorts). The mortality rate varied by pneumonia etiology, ranging from less than 2% to more than 30%. For the bacterial agents, the mortality rate was lower for patients with *Chlamydia psittaci* (0%), *Coxiella burnetii* (0.5%), and *Mycoplasma pneumoniae* pneumonia (1.4%) and highest for patients with *Pseudomonas aeruginosa* (61.1%), *Klebsiella* species (35.7%), *Escherichia coli* (35.3%), and *Staphylococcus aureus* pneumonia (31.8%). Mortality was 12.8% among the 11,229 patients for whom an etiologic agent was unknown. Interestingly, the wide range in mortality for most pneumonia causes was associated with the types of patients included in each cohort. For example, for patients with pneumonia attributed to *Streptococcus pneumoniae,* the mortality rate was 6.4% in the 172 hospital and ambulatory patients, 8.3% in the 2006 hospitalized patients, 18.6% in the 1145 patients identified in studies of bacteremia, and 30.7% in the 127 ICU patients.

As shown in Table 144-2, 19 factors were significantly associated with mortality based on univariate summary odds ratios: male sex, chills, pleuritic chest pain, altered mental status, dyspnea, tachypnea, hypotension, hypothermia, congestive heart failure, alcohol abuse, diabetes mellitus, immunosuppression, neoplastic disease, coronary artery disease, neurologic disease, leukopenia, bacteremia, multilobar radiographic pulmonary infiltrate, and azotemia. With the exception of two factors associated with a decreased risk of mortality, chills (odds ratio [OR], 0.4; 95% confidence interval [CI], 0.2 to 0.7) and pleuritic chest pain (OR = 0.5; 95% CI, 0.3 to 0.8), the other 17 factors were associated with a 1.3- to 5.2-fold increased risk of mortality. Increased age also had a direct association with mortality. In the 14 cohorts that evaluated the relationship between age and mortality, the mean of the differences in mean age of the deceased patients and the mean age of the survivors was 7.8 years. In contrast to information on pneumonia etiology, which often takes 48 to 72 hours to become available to clinicians, all these risk factors for mortality are readily available at initial presentation. As a result, medical practitioners could use them to help determine the initial site of care (home versus hospital, versus ICU) and the intensity of initial empirical antibiotic therapy.

Over the past decade, a variety of prognostic indices or models have been developed to predict short-term mortality in patients with CAP.[8, 9, 15, 20, 21] These models vary with respect to the patient populations studied, the statistical techniques used, and the number and type of predictors evaluated. They

TABLE 144–1. Clinical Description of Severe Pneumonia*

1. Respiratory frequency > 30 breaths/min on admission.
2. Severe respiratory failure defined by a PaO_2/FIO_2 ratio < 250 mm Hg.
3. Requirement for mechanical ventilation.
4. Chest radiograph showing bilateral involvement or involvement of multiple lobes; in addition, an increase in the size of the opacity by 50% or greater within 48 hr of admission is indicative of severe pneumonia.
5. Shock (systolic blood pressure below 90 mm Hg or diastolic blood pressure below 60 mm Hg).
6. Requirement for vasopressors for more than 4 hr.
7. Urine output lower than 20 mL/hr, or total urine output lower than 80 mL in 4 hr, unless another explanation is available, or acute renal failure requiring dialysis.

*Presence of at least one of the conditions justifies defining the pneumonia as severe.

TABLE 144–2. Prognostic Factors Associated with Mortality in 33,148 Patients with Community-Acquired Pneumonia

Type of Factor	Study Cohorts Reporting Data	Patients in Study Cohorts Reporting Data	Summary OR (95% CI)
Demographics			
Sex, male	21	17,641	1.3 (1.2–1.4)
History and Physical Examination			
Chills	4	572	0.4 (0.2–0.7)
Pleuritic chest pain	6	732	0.5 (0.3–0.8)
Cough	6	619	0.6 (0.3–1.0)
Hyperthermia, temperature ≥ 38°C	8	1,525	0.8 (0.5–1.1)
Altered mental status	8	655	2.3 (1.6–3.3)
Dyspnea	4	322	2.4 (1.0–5.6)
Tachypnea, respiratory rate ≥ 20 breaths/min	4	732	2.9 (1.7–4.9)
Hypotension, systolic blood pressure ≤ 100 mm Hg	5	1,108	4.8 (2.8–8.3)
Hypothermia, temperatures ≤ 37°C	2	602	5.0 (2.4–10.4)
Comorbid Illness			
Tobacco use	8	826	0.7 (0.4–1.1)
Prior pneumonia	3	608	0.8 (0.4–1.6)
Congestive heart failure	6	14,832	2.4 (2.1–2.6)
Pulmonary disease	6	14,911	1.0 (0.9–1.1)
Alcohol abuse	9	1,414	1.6 (1.0–2.4)
Diabetes mellitus	5	14,655	1.3 (1.1–1.5)
Immunosuppression	3	14,575	1.4 (1.0–1.9)
Neoplastic disease	12	16,168	2.8 (2.4–3.1)
Coronary artery disease	3	14,444	1.5 (1.3–1.6)
Neurologic disease	3	345	4.6 (2.3–8.9)
Laboratory and X-ray			
Leukocytosis, white blood cell count ≥ 10 × 10^9/L	8	1,214	1.3 (0.8–2.0)
Hypoxemia, Po_2 ≤ 50 mm Hg	4	346	1.2 (0.7–2.3)
Anemia, hematocrit ≤ 0.35	2	134	1.4 (0.1–23.0)
Leukopenia, white blood cell count ≤ 10 × 10^9/L	11	1,776	2.5 (1.6–3.7)
Bacteremia	30	4,984	2.8 (2.3–3.6)
X-ray infiltrate, > one lobe	6	1,227	3.1 (1.9–5.1)
Azotemia, blood urea nitrogen ≥ 7.1 mmol/L	3	394	5.2 (2.4–10.9)

Adapted from Fine MJ, Smith MA, Carson LA, et al: Prognosis and outcomes of patients with community-acquired pneumonia: A meta-analysis. JAMA 1996; 275:134–141.

CI = confidence interval; OR = odds ratio.

also differ in the goals for which they were developed. Some of the models were designed to be used by clinicians as decision-making aids, whereas others were developed as a means to adjust mortality for illness severity, for example, for assessing quality of care.

In the British Thoracic Society (BTS) study, the authors formulated a simple discriminant rule based on the three variables that were consistently associated with death.[18] The rule was considered positive when at least two of the following three factors were present:

- Respiratory rate of 30/min or more
- Diastolic blood pressure of 60 mm Hg or less
- Blood urea nitrogen of more than 7 mmol/L

A positive rule was associated with a 21-fold increase in mortality, with a specificity of 79% and a sensitivity of 88%. However, the positive predictive value was low: only 21 patients of the 108 (19%) who met the rule died.

A second rule, in which "confusion" was used instead of "blood urea nitrogen," showed even higher specificity but low sensitivity. The BTS rules have now been validated by two studies, one prospective and one retrospective.[10, 21] Unfortunately, the positive predictive values of these rules are too low to permit transfer to the ICU of all patients who meet their definition. However, these patients and those who present with one or more of the other negative prognostic factors have a higher risk for development of severe pneumonia and should be closely monitored for signs of deterioration. This monitoring should include regular checks of vital signs, mental status, fever and oxygenation, and auscultation of the lungs or chest radiography for signs of spread of the pneumonia.

While the BTS studies attempted to identify patients with a worse prognosis at the time of admission to the hospital so that they could be targeted for special attention in an ICU, the focus of other studies was just the opposite, namely, to identify those patients with pneumonia who are at lower risk of death and do not need hospital care. From the analysis of data collected on 14,199 adult inpatients with pneumonia, Fine and colleagues[23] derived a prediction rule that stratifies patients into five classes with respect to the risk of death within 30 days. This prediction rule assigns points based on age and the presence of coexisting disease, abnormal physical findings (such as respiratory rate of ≥30/min or a temperature of ≥40°C), and abnormal laboratory findings (such as a pH <7.35, a blood urea nitrogen concentration ≥30 mg/dL [11 mmol/L] or a sodium concentration <130 mmol/L) at presentation (Table 144-3). According to this point scoring system, patients 50 years of age or younger with none of the five coexisting illnesses and none of the five physical examination abnormalities listed in Table 144-3 fell into class I. Most patients in this class can safely be treated at home, provided they do not have intractable vomiting, a history of noncompliance, or other contraindications to self-care. The prediction rule defines four more treatment classes according to pre-

TABLE 144–3. Point Scoring System Permitting to Assign Patients with Community-Acquired Pneumonia to Different Risk Classes for Mortality

Characteristic	Points Assigned*
Demographic Factor	
Age	
Men	Age (yr)
Women	Age (yr) − 10
Nursing Home Resident	+10
Coexisting Illnesses	
Neoplastic disease	+30
Liver disease	+20
Congestive heart failure	+10
Cerebrovascular disease	+10
Renal disease	+10
Physical Examination Findings	
Altered mental status	+20
Respiratory rate ≥ 30/min	+20
Systolic blood pressure < 90 mm Hg	+20
Temperature < 35°C or ≥ 40°C	+15
Pulse ≥ 125/min	+10
Laboratory and Radiographic Findings	
Arterial pH < 7.35	+30
Blood urea nitrogen ≥ 30 mg/dL (11 mmol/L)	+20
Sodium < 130 mmol/L	+20
Glucose ≥ 250 mg/dL (14 mmol/L)	+10
Hematocrit < 30%	+10
Partial pressure of arterial oxygen < 60 mm Hg	+10
Pleural effusion	+10

Adapted from Fine MJ, Auble TE, Yealy DM, et al: A prediction rule to identify low-risk patients with community-acquired pneumonia. N Engl J Med 1997; 336:243–250.

*A total point score for a given patient is obtained by summing the patient's age in years (age minus 10 for women) and the points for each applicable characteristic. Mortalities for patients in risk classes I, II (≤ 70 points), III (71–90 points), IV (91–130 points), and V (>130 points) were 0.1%, 0.6%, 0.9%, 9.3%, and 27.0%, respectively.

dicted levels of mortality in a logistic regression analysis. Therefore, physicians can use the rule to estimate the probabilities of death given the presenting clinical features and to suggest where a patient should be treated.

EPIDEMIOLOGY, ETIOLOGY, AND OUTCOME OF SEVERE PNEUMONIA

Studies from Great Britain and Sweden show that 2% to 8% of patients admitted to the hospital with CAP will require ICU treatment.[3, 8, 14, 24] Slightly higher figures have been reported from the United States, Canada, and Spain.[10, 11, 25] Selected prospective studies evaluating severe CAP managed in the ICU are listed in Table 144–4.[11, 21, 25–31] Alcoholism was present in 18% to 70% of the patients, and between 36% and 75% of the patients were reported to have a preexisting chronic disease. In all studies in which the gender was reported, there was a clear predominance of males among patients, probably reflecting the high frequency of alcoholism and chronic pulmonary diseases in these populations.

Etiology

The pathogens most frequently identified among patients with severe CAP are listed in Table 144–4. These include *S. pneumoniae, Legionella,* aerobic gram-negative bacilli, *M. pneumoniae,* respiratory tract viruses, and a group of miscellaneous pathogens (*Haemophilus influenzae, Mycobacterium tuberculosis,* and endemic fungi).

Streptococcus pneumoniae

Even if its relative importance has decreased, *S. pneumoniae* remains the predominant organism in most recent studies, causing 15% to 60% of the cases of acute CAP (see Table 144–4). Studies using more aggressive laboratory methods have shown higher yields, as have studies using transtracheal aspiration to obtain uncontaminated specimens.[8, 32] In studies of bacteremic pneumococcal pneumonia, the rate of false-negative sputum results has been estimated at about 50%.[33] The BTS pneumonia research committee concluded after discriminant functional analysis of data on 148 patients with no identifiable pathogens that most of the cases were probably due to *S. pneumoniae.*[34] These data suggest that the true prevalence of *S. pneumoniae* infection is seriously underrepresented in the results of current microbiologic tests.

Advanced age, cigarette smoking, dementia, seizures, and the presence of chronic illnesses, such as chronic obstructive pulmonary disease, congestive heart failure, splenectomy, and cerebrovascular disease, have been identified as significant risk factors for the development of pneumococcal pneumonia.[35] In patients with acquired immunodeficiency syndrome (AIDS), the incidence of pneumococcal pneumonia is 5.5 to 17.5 times higher than the predicted incidence in general urban populations.[36, 37] The rate of bacteremia is higher than that for patients without human immunodeficiency virus (HIV) infection (60% versus 15% to 30%), but the mortality rate and manifestations of the disease are generally not different from those in patients without HIV infection. Overwhelming pneumococcal sepsis with disseminated intravascular coagulation has been described in asplenic patients and in patients with functional asplenia, such as those with sickle cell anemia.[38] In recent years, antibiotic-resistant *S. pneumoniae* have increasingly been identified.[39, 40] Although most of these pneumococci are only moderately resistant to penicillin, with minimal inhibitory concentrations (MICs) of 0.1 to 1 μg/mL, pneumococci highly resistant to penicillin alone and pneumococci multiresistant to various antibiotics have been found throughout the world.[39] These data underscore the need to test pneumococcal isolates on a routine basis for penicillin susceptibility.

Haemophilus influenzae

H. influenzae is now more frequently recognized as an important cause of CAP, responsible for an estimated 4% to 15% of the cases.[41] In most studies, *Haemophilus* species are ranked among the top five causes. The true incidence of this organism is, however, obscured by the difficulty encountered in isolating it from sputum and identifying it in Gram-stained sputum smears and because of the inability to distinguish true infection from colonization in earlier studies. Claims of a pathogenic relationship in individual cases are usually based on the finding of heavy or pure cultures from material obtained by transtracheal aspiration or from the Gram staining of such specimens or by identification of the organism in blood or pleural fluid cultures. The use of counterimmunoelectrophoresis to identify the antigens in sputum and blood is of uncertain efficacy because of the high incidence of colonization and the high frequency of uncategorized organisms causing disease.

In adults, *H. influenzae* infection occurs most often in compromised hosts with chronic bronchopulmonary disease, alcoholism, diabetes, or an immunoglobulin defect.[42] However, a few patients appear to be free of underlying disease. The mortality rate from bacterial *H. influenzae* pneumonia

TABLE 144–4. Prevalence (%) of Major Pathogens Associated with Severe Community Acquired Pneumonia

	Woodhead	Marrie	Feldman	Pachon	Torres	Rello	Moine	Almirall
Year	1985	1989	1989	1990	1991	1993	1994	1995
No. of patients	50	129	73	67	92	58	132	58
Unknown	18	35	22	52	48	40	28	57
Streptococcus pneumoniae	39	18	43	34	29	37	41	42
Haemophilus	—	9	—	9	—	—	13	4
Gram-negative bacilli	—	4	47	16	19	11	13	17
Staphylococcus aureus	12	13	5	3	2	—	5	—
Legionella	37	3	—	22	27	23	4	21
Mycoplasma pneumoniae	2	—	—	—	13	—	1	—
Chlamydia pneumoniae	—	—	—	3	—	—	1	4
Viruses	5	24	—	3	—	3	7	4
Others	4	28	5	12	10	25	15	8

has been estimated to be 34%, a reflection of the severity of patients' underlying illness.[42]

Treatment is complicated by the increasing incidence of ampicillin resistance, which appears to be due to the production of a β-lactamase. The degree of resistance is now estimated to be about 20% in children and 10% in adults.[43] In addition, penicillin-resistant organisms are now showing resistance to chloramphenicol, the previously recognized back-up antibiotic for ampicillin. Fortunately, the recently released second- and third-generation cephalosporins are very β-lactamase stable and most *Haemophilus* species are exquisitely sensitive.[43]

Staphylococcus aureus

S. aureus accounts for 1% to 10% of the cases of acute CAP.[3, 8, 17] The incidence of staphylococcal pneumonia has been reported to be particularly high in elderly patients institutionalized in nursing homes or during outbreaks of viral influenza.[44] In this latter situation, *S. aureus* may be responsible for up to 20% of the encountered pneumonias, even if pneumococcus remains the most frequent pathogen, accounting for about 46% of the cases in two studies.[44] A small percentage of staphylococcal pneumonia cases may result from hematogenous embolization to the lungs from primary extrapulmonary infections, usually in the setting of right-sided endocarditis or venous septic thrombophlebitis in intravenous (IV) drug abusers, in patients undergoing hemodialysis, or in patients on home IV therapy. There are no clinical or radiologic features typical of *S. aureus* pneumonia except possibly rapid cavitation of a bronchopneumonia and the development of a pleural empyema.

The diagnosis is based on identification of the organism in pleural fluid or blood or by Gram's stain. Sputum culture is unreliable because up to 40% of adults are asymptomatic carriers.

Aerobic Gram-Negative Bacilli

Aerobic gram-negative rods of Enterobacteriaceae and nonfermentative organisms are a relatively uncommon cause of CAP.[8, 17, 41] *Klebsiella pneumoniae* is most often considered, but *E. coli, P. aeruginosa, Enterobacter cloacae, Acinetobacter, Serratia* spp., *Proteus,* and many other aerobic gram-negative bacilli may also cause disease. Although these organisms can infect previously healthy patients, they are more likely to cause disease in older patients and patients with chronic underlying disease. For example, in the study by Fang and colleagues,[41] 88% of the patients with gram-negative rod pneumonia had an underlying illness, whereas only 50% of the patients with chlamydial pneumonia had a comorbid illness. Surprisingly, however, chronic obstructive pulmonary disease was the most common underlying disease in these patients with gram-negative pneumonia. For instance, pneumonia caused by *P. aeruginosa* was practically never observed except in patients with bronchiectasis or cystic fibrosis. Immunosuppression, defined as hematologic malignancy, solid tumor, neutropenia, and taking corticosteroids, was unexpectedly low (38%), but all deaths in patients with gram-negative pneumonia occurred in immunosuppressed patients. Although prior antibiotic therapy has been suggested as a predisposing factor for gram-negative pneumonia, this was corroborated for only 28% of the patients with gram-negative pneumonia, a frequency of usage that is not significantly different from that observed in other etiologies of pneumonia in one study.[41]

Legionella pneumophila

The importance of *Legionella* in causing CAP varies greatly according to the geographic area. Although incidences as high as 17% to 22% have been reported, many localities report significantly lower rates.[8, 18, 41, 45] Routine testing using selective medium for culture, direct fluorescent antibody labeling, serology (both acute and convalescent), and urinary antigen detection are crucial in uncovering the diagnosis. Community-acquired legionnaires' disease seems to be more frequent among males, people 50 years of age and older, patients requiring renal dialysis or transplantation, smokers, immunosuppressed patients, and patients with a comorbid disease, such as chronic bronchitis or diabetes mellitus.[18]

Other Etiologic Agents

Recently, *Moraxella (Branhamella) catarrhalis* has been identified as a cause of pneumonia. The overall incidence of disease caused by this bacterium is low, but it is an important pathogen in elderly patients with underlying lung disease or carcinoma.[46]

The true incidence of anaerobic etiologic mechanisms in CAP is uncertain. In some studies using invasive diagnostic methods, anaerobes have been cultured from lower respiratory tract specimens in 20% to 30% of the cases.[47] However, other reports suggest that anaerobic pneumonias account for only 3% to 4% of the cases of CAP.[8, 17, 41] Anaerobic pulmonary infections are usually recognizable by the characteristic clinical and radiographic findings. Commonly, the patient's oral hygiene is poor and he or she may have some underlying disease in which there is prior evidence of altered consciousness, a diminished gag reflex, or an abnormal swallowing mechanism (e.g., epilepsy, alcoholism, esophageal carcinoma, or drug overdose). An insidious low-grade fever is typical, and the chest radiography demonstrates segmental involvement of dependent areas of the lung, often with cavitation.

M. pneumoniae is a common cause of CAP, accounting for 10% to 20% of the infections in some studies.[8, 17] Although nearly all infections with this organism are mild, *M. pneumoniae* can also mimic bacterial pneumonia and some unusual pulmonary manifestations, such as lung abscess, lobar consolidation, or acute respiratory distress syndrome (ARDS).[48] Most laboratories do not culture *M. pneumoniae,* and the diagnosis is usually made on serologic evidence.

Chlamydia pneumoniae is a newly discovered pulmonary pathogen, which has been associated with pneumonia epidemics in teenagers, young adults, and military conscript populations.[45] In the study by Fang and colleagues,[41] this microorganism constituted 6.1% of the pneumonias and was a common etiology for pneumonia in older adults (mean age, 65 years) and patients with chronic underlying illness.

Although much more frequent in children, viral pneumonia remains a significant problem in adults. Viral pneumonia typically presents subacutely as an upper respiratory tract infection but may have an acute onset, with severe pulmonary miliary damage and ARDS. Of the viral agents associated with pneumonia in adults, influenza A and B virus and adenovirus are the most common, but respiratory syncytial virus, the predominant respiratory pathogen in infants and children, is now recognized as an etiology of pneumonia in adults. Although the number of cases is small, groups at particularly high risk appear to be the elderly and patients who are immunosuppressed.

The definitive diagnosis of viral pneumonia requires detection of the virus from sputum or nasopharyngeal swabs. Information based on serologic findings is often not clinically relevant at the time of the acute illness.

Patients with acute tuberculosis (TB) may present with a syndrome indistinguishable from acute CAP, with infiltrates involving primarily the middle and lower lung fields without apical disease.[49] On occasion, patients with TB present with a syndrome reminiscent of ARDS. Therefore, TB must be considered in patients with acute respiratory failure and fever who do not respond to the usual antibacterial therapy. This was highlighted by Bobrowitz,[50] who retrospectively identified 20 patients in whom TB was the primary cause of death but was not confirmed until autopsy.

Finally, even though a number of large series exclude HIV-infected patients, *Pneumocystis carinii* pneumonia must be considered in the differential diagnosis of severe CAP in the proper clinical setting.

In summary, recent studies have demonstrated a change in reported etiologic mechanisms for CAP. Several factors may be contributory. First, new microbial agents have been recognized and are now identifiable with readily available tests. Second, a population of patients increasingly susceptible to opportunistic infections has emerged, such as patients with AIDS or an organ transplant. Finally, in virtually every clinical series recording etiologic agents for CAP, in a sizable number of cases no specific etiology was able to be determined. This fact is probably explained for the most part by the increasing use of broad-spectrum antibiotic therapy in the community. Antibiotics given before admission decrease the ability to isolate a specific pathogen and, in particular, prevent the detection of pneumococcus.[26, 41, 45]

Outcome

The case fatality rate in severe CAP is high, ranging from 17% to more than 50% in some studies.[51] Not surprisingly, patients who were treated with mechanical ventilation had a higher mortality rate in most studies. Several prospective studies have tried to determine which clinical factors immediately after admission and during ICU stay influence outcome.[27, 28, 52] In the study by Torres and coworkers,[28] the factors found to be associated with death according to univariate analysis were the presence of a preexisting ultimately fatal disease, inadequate antibiotic treatment, requirement of mechanical ventilation, treatment with positive end-expiratory pressure or an FIO_2 above 0.6, ARDS, radiographic spread of infiltrates after admission, bacteremia, septic shock, and *P. aeruginosa* pneumonia. Of these, the multivariate evaluation selected radiographic spread, septic shock, and preexisting ultimately fatal disease, in that order, to be independently associated with death.

Interventional-related factors in the management of patients with severe CAP have a significant impact on final outcome. In particular, several studies have now reported that if the initial antibiotic regimen is inadequate or delayed in time, this was associated with higher mortality.[27, 28, 52] In a recent multicenter retrospective cohort study of 14,069 patients at least 65 years old who were hospitalized with pneumonia, Meehan and colleagues[53] demonstrated that a lower 30-day mortality was associated with antibiotic administration within 8 hours of hospital arrival (odds ratio, 0.85; 95% confidence interval 0.75 to 0.96), even in analyses that adjusted for patient risk factors and performance of other processes of care.

The value of ICU care for severe CAP has not been fully determined. In fact, it has been suggested that ICU care for severe CAP, particularly pneumococcal pneumonia with bacteremia, merely delays the time of death without altering overall mortality.[54] However, in a recent study from Cook County Hospital, the investigators demonstrated a reduction in the mortality of patients with pneumococcal bacteremia because of prompt and appropriate triage decisions that resulted in earlier admission to the ICU.[55]

CLINICAL AND RADIOGRAPHIC EVALUATION

History-taking should attempt to determine the clinical setting in which the pneumonia is occurring. Special attention should be given to pneumonia that develops in unusual settings. As previously discussed, an increased incidence of staphylococcal pneumonia has been noted during epidemics of influenza.[44] Cystic fibrosis is associated with pseudomonal and staphylococcal pulmonary infections. Recent dental work, sedative overdose, seizure, or loss of consciousness for any reason should raise the suspicion of anaerobic infection caused by aspiration of oropharyngeal bacteria.[47] Needless to say, exposure resulting from an unusual occupation or from travel must be considered (e.g., travel to a Q-fever zone or frequent handling of psittacine birds).

Patients with CAP typically present with chills, cough, sputum production, fever, and pleuritic chest pain. Mental status changes, confusion, or disorientation are also frequently observed and occur significantly more frequently in elderly patients. Although these clinical manifestations are useful in diagnosing pneumonia, individual symptoms or signs are not specific for defining the etiologic agent. Fang and colleagues[41] compared the clinical manifestations of the five most common causes (pneumococcus, *H. influenzae, Legionella, C. pneumoniae,* and gram-negative bacilli) of CAP found in their study. In contrast to previous studies, they demonstrated that abdominal pain, vomiting, relative bradycardia, neurologic changes, hyponatremia, and abnormal liver function tests did not occur significantly more frequently in pneumonia caused by *Legionella* than in those caused by other microorganisms. However, *Legionella* cases much more frequently had a temperature of at least 40°C and a slightly higher incidence of diarrhea than pneumonias of other origins. Patients with *Legionella* pneumonias were also more frequently admitted to an ICU.[41]

The atypical pneumonia syndrome includes viral, mycoplasmal, and chlamydial infections and is thought to be distinguishable from bacterial pneumonias by the presence of gradual onset, viral prodrome, absence of rigors, nonproductive cough, lower degree of fever, absence of pleurisy, absence of consolidation, low leukocyte count, and an ill-defined infiltrate on chest radiographs. Atypical pneumonia is said to be less serious and to carry a better prognosis than bacterial pneumonias. In fact, when these findings, which are considered classical for atypical pneumonias, were compared with observations made in patients with proven viral, *M. pneumoniae,* and *C. pneumoniae* infections and in patients with known bacterial pneumonia, they were essentially nonspecific.[41] Therefore, it is probably unlikely that this classification will offer sufficient specificity on which to base the selection of treatment.

The chest film may show different radiographic characteristics that can be useful in management decisions. For instance, the radiographic findings may suggest specific etiologies or conditions such as lung abscess, pneumonia caused by *P. carinii,* or TB. The radiograph can also suggest coexisting conditions such as bronchial obstruction or pleural effusions. Radiography is also useful for evaluating illness severity by identifying multilobar involvement, which is an indication of severe illness (discussed previously). However, it is unusual that the pattern of infiltrates will indicate an etiology. Although a long list of pattern-etiology associations has been developed, there are as many exceptions as there are examples of conformity to the rules. It must also be recognized that chest films are only helpful in conjunction with the clinical history and physical examination.

Studies have been done to discover whether radiographic patterns can distinguish between the various causes of pneumonia.[56, 57] A panel of six radiologists who had no prior knowledge of the clinical data were only 67% accurate in the identification of 16 bacterial pneumonias and 65% correct in nine cases of viral etiology; moreover, no consistent pattern was identified in any specific group of pneumonia.[57] In a comparative study of the radiographic features of community-acquired legionnaires' disease, pneumococcal pneumonia, mycoplasmal pneumonia, and acute psittacosis, investigators found that homogeneous opacities (airspace disease) were more frequent in legionnaires' disease and pneumococcal infection than in mycoplasmal pneumonia.[56] In both of these studies, the pattern of mycoplasmal pneumonia could be confused with airspace bacterial pneumonia in at least 50% of the cases.[56, 57]

NONINVASIVE MICROBIOLOGIC INVESTIGATION

The value of routine microbiologic tests in patients with CAP has been questioned by several experts on the basis of a number of arguments.[18] First, the bacteriology of this illness is relatively uniform (and therefore predictable), making initial empirical therapy possible. Second, initial broad-spectrum empirical therapy directed at the known spectrum of likely pathogens is associated with an improved outcome, whereas the identification of a specific etiologic pathogen has not been shown to lead to an improved outcome. Presumably, this is because the information about etiology becomes known too late in the course of the illness to reverse the effects of the initial inadequate therapy. Third, there are many controversies concerning the diagnostic value of Gram's staining and culture of expectorated sputum. Common problems are that 10% to 30% of patients have a nonproductive cough, 15% to 30% have received antibiotic treatment before hospitalization, and negative results are reported for 30% to 65% of cultures of expectorated sputum.[45] Several studies have shown that the yield of fastidious bacteria such as *S. pneumoniae* and *H. influenzae* is zero when virtually any specimen from the respiratory tract is collected after antibiotic therapy.[41, 45] Recognizing all these potential drawbacks, the American Thoracic Society in 1993 recommended that an empirical approach, not relying on extensive diagnostic testing, be used for most patients with CAP.[18]

However, the wide spectrum of possible pathogens and the fact that the cause in 20% to 80% of the patients remains unknown suggest that there is a need for a more active attitude toward the establishment of an etiologic diagnosis. The most important function of a positive diagnostic test is to allow for an optimization of the initiated empirical treatment as soon as possible after admission. In three reports, it has been stated that the use of aggressive diagnostic methods does not lower mortality.[27, 28, 58] However, none of these studies were designed to test this hypothesis. Thus, the controls consisted of patients in whom a diagnosis was not obtained despite the aggressive diagnostic methods used.

In contrast to their statement, there seemed to be definite positive effects of obtaining an etiologic diagnosis in at least two of the three studies. Sörensen and coworkers[58] obtained an etiologic diagnosis in 29 of 36 (81%) ICU-treated patients and in 19 of those within 48 to 72 hours. In 60% of patients with an early diagnosis (48 to 72 hours) and in 50% of those in which the diagnosis was obtained later, the antibiotic therapy was changed according to the results of the diagnostic tests. The case fatality rate in this series was 22%, compared with an earlier retrospective study from the same center in which, without the use of aggressive methods, an etiologic diagnosis was obtained in 50% and the case fatality rate was 47%.[24] In the study by Torres and colleagues,[28] an inadequate antibiotic treatment was clearly related to a poor prognosis. Although data are not provided for when antibiotic treatment was considered inadequate, their findings emphasize the difficulty of covering all pathogens with an empirical treatment and thus the importance of obtaining an etiologic diagnosis.

It is also of epidemiologic importance to obtain an etiologic diagnosis. Knowledge of the local epidemiology and resistance situation is necessary for correct treatment decisions. Finally, the possibility of a noninfectious cause for the pneumonia, such as pulmonary embolism, allergic alveolitis, or vasculitis, should always be considered. Of course, the latter becomes increasingly important if an etiologic diagnosis is not obtained despite the use of aggressive methods.

Sputum Examination

Despite the ongoing controversy concerning their usefulness in the initial management of patients with CAP, microscopic examination and culture of expectorated sputum are the mainstays of the laboratory evaluation of patients with CAP. These procedures are noninvasive, and whereas sputum culture requires 24 to 48 hours, Gram's staining can give valuable information in a matter of minutes that permits streamlining the initial antimicrobial treatment in many cases, provided that the specimen is carefully procured, that cytologic screening confirms the presence of lower airway secretions, and that the specimen is obtained before antibiotics are given.

In order to maximize the diagnostic yield of sputum examination, a careful methodology should be followed. First, it is imperative to obtain a proper specimen. Therefore, the patient should be carefully instructed and supervised by a physician or a respiratory therapist to obtain secretions resulting from a deep cough. Seriously ill patients and debilitated patients are often unable to follow instructions and should be assisted. One alternative for some patients unable to expectorate anything other than oropharyngeal secretions is to blindly pass a small catheter through the upper respiratory tract into the trachea to directly sample distal secretions. As a general rule, sputum specimens should be transported promptly to the laboratory for processing. Transportation delays for 2 to 5 hours at room temperature result in reduced isolation rates of pneumococci, staphylococci, and gram-negative bacilli and increased numbers of microorganisms that are indigenous to the upper respiratory tract.[43]

Only samples free of oropharyngeal contamination should be reviewed. Various criteria based on cytologic characteristics have been suggested for scoring the quality of sputum specimens.[59] In a study in which parallel cytologic and microbiologic analyses of sputa and transtracheal aspirates from patients with pneumonia were performed, Geckler and coworkers[60] found that the results of sputum culture containing more than 25 squamous epithelial cells per low-power field (magnification ×100) showed poor agreement with those of transtracheal aspiration, regardless of the number of leukocytes that were present. Such samples are therefore nondiagnostic and should be discarded. On the other hand, the presence of less than 10 epithelial cells and more than 25 leukocytes per field suggests that the specimen actually represents lower respiratory tract secretions.[59]

Gram-stained smears of acceptable specimens should then be examined under oil immersion (magnification ×1000) to determine whether bacteria of a specific or characteristic morphologic type are present. Neither the fields being examined nor any of the immediately adjacent fields should contain any squamous epithelial cells, but at least several neutrophils or alveolar macrophages should be present. The morphologic and staining characteristics of any bacteria should be recorded, and a semiquantitative estimate of their number should be made. This method has proved useful for the identification of *S. pneumoniae* in the sputum.

Rein and associates[61] have suggested that when strict criteria for Gram-stain positivity are used (predominant flora or >10 gram-positive, lancet-shaped diplococci per oil immersion field), the specificity of the technique is 85%, with a sensitivity of 62%. Whether this approach is equally useful for the identification of other bacterial causes of pneumonia remains unclear. However, Tillotson and Lerner[62] noted that gram-negative bacilli were seen in smears of all sputum specimens taken from 20 cases of *E. coli* pneumonia. Small gram-negative coccobacillary organisms are characteristic of *H. influenzae.* Staphylococci appear as gram-positive cocci in tetrads and small clusters. In contrast, the failure to detect *S. aureus* or gram-negative bacilli in the pretreatment specimen nearly completely excludes these organisms from diagnostic consideration.[45] Gram-stained smears may also support a diagnosis of atypical pneumonia or legionnaires' disease when sputum examinations repeatedly show no bacteria in a patient who has received no antimicrobial treatment prior to admission.

A variety of diagnostic techniques have been developed that provide the potential for more accurate and rapid identification of the etiologic agents of pneumonia by sputum analysis. The most frequent application of direct immunofluorescence to the examination of sputum is in the detection of *Legionella* species. Using positive cultures or antibody titers to define legionnaires' disease, Edelstein and coworkers[63] found that the sensitivity of direct immunofluorescence of respiratory tract secretions was 50%, with a specificity of 94%. Direct immunofluorescence and genetic probes may also be used to detect chlamydial species, *M. pneumoniae, M. tuberculosis,* and some viruses. Although many of these techniques are of great interest, their general applicability remains to be determined.[45]

The utility of sputum cultures as a means of establishing the agents responsible for pneumonia has been questioned. Patients with bacteremic pneumococcal pneumonia have been reported to have negative sputum cultures in 45% to 50% of the cases, even when large numbers of organisms have been noted on Gram-stained preparations.[45] Similarly, 34% to 47% of sputum cultures are negative with proven *H. influenzae* pneumonia.[43] Furthermore, cultures of expectorated sputum often yield multiple organisms, and it is difficult to tell whether these bacteria are causative or merely colonizing the upper respiratory tract. For example, contamination with gram-negative bacilli has been noted in more than 30% of sputum cultures.[45] Semiquantitative cultures, washing of sputum samples, and the use of mucolytic agents have been proposed to improve the clinical utility of sputum cultures; however, results have been variable and the practicality of these techniques for routine use is questionable. In fact, the main role of sputum cultures in clinical practice is to permit definitive identification of the organisms that are present in predominance in the Gram-stained smear and to determine their susceptibility to antibiotics. In other words, results of sputum cultures should always be used as a function of the results of the Gram staining.

Other Noninvasive Diagnostic Techniques

Approximately 20% to 30% of the patients with severe bacterial pneumonia are bacteremic, and therefore blood cultures should not be overlooked as a means of identifying the bacterial etiology of pneumonia.[45] Pleural fluid cultures, when positive, are also specific for the etiology of the underlying pneumonia.

Counterimmunoelectrophoresis and latex agglutination techniques have been used to detect *S. pneumoniae, H. influenzae,* and *Pseudomonas* antigens in sputum, urine, serum, and pleural fluid, but results have been variable and frequently disappointing. For example, detection of the pneumococcal capsular antigen by counterimmunoelectrophoresis has been reported to have a sensitivity varying from 20% to 90%, with 8% to 20% of false-positive results. Detection of *Legionella* antigens in urine seems more promising. *Legionella pneumophila* serogroup I accounts for about 70% of legionnaires' disease, and the urine antigen test has been shown to be more than 90% specific and about 90% sensitive for this pathogen.[45]

Serologic tests are used to diagnose a variety of pulmonary pathogens, including *Legionella* species, *M. pneumoniae, Chlamydia* species, and many viruses. Because these tests usually require two blood specimens drawn at a minimum of a 2-week interval, they are of help only in confirming a clinical diagnosis, not for initiating treatment.

INVASIVE DIAGNOSTIC TECHNIQUES

Of the available invasive methods for obtaining respiratory secretions, transtracheal aspiration has fallen from favor because of side effects. Bronchoscopy not only enables direct visualization of the endobronchial tree but also affords an opportunity to obtain specimens for culture and histology by various techniques directly from the site of inflammation in the lung. Initial studies concerning the reliability of specimens obtained for culture directly by suction through the inner channel have been disappointing. Bartlett and colleagues[64] demonstrated that in patients without lower respiratory tract infections, cultures of aspirates obtained during bronchoscopy were frequently contaminated, producing an average of five different bacterial species. Therefore, this type of specimen collection has the same potential drawbacks as those observed with expectorated sputum, thus stressing the importance of examining a Gram-stained preparation of bronchoscopic secretions before interpreting the results of such cultures.

The development of the protected specimen brush technique by Wimberley and associates[65] has significantly decreased, but not eliminated, this problem. This technique uses a double-catheter system with two telescoping cannulas, a distal occluding plug, and a small brush that calibrates the volume of respiratory secretions collected. Using 10^3 colony-forming units (CFU)/mL as a "breakpoint" on quantitative cultures for the determination of the clinical significance of an isolate, the protected specimen brush has been experimentally and clinically both sensitive (70% to 97%) and specific (95% to 100%) for the diagnosis of bacterial pneumonia. For example, in a study on 172 patients, Pollock and coworkers[66] found that 75 of 78 patients (96%) with a clinical diagnosis of pneumonia had a likely pulmonary pathogen in significant concentration, whereas high counts were recovered in only two of 35 control patients. As with other techniques, however, specimens obtained from patients with pneumonia who had received prior antibiotic treatment were frequently sterile, emphasizing the fact that previous treatment negates to a large extent the potential utility of this method.

Bronchoalveolar lavage, in which a segment of lung is "washed" with sterile saline, has proved to be an excellent means of confirming respiratory infections. Lavage is indeed a safe and practical method for obtaining cells and secretions from the lower respiratory tract. This technique samples a relatively large area of the lung (about 10^6 alveoli). The cells and liquid recovered can be examined microscopically immediately after the procedure and are also suitable for culture and other techniques. Bronchoalveolar lavage (BAL) is therefore now the procedure of choice for diagnosis of opportunistic pulmonary infections in immunosuppressed patients. Cytologic screening and microbiologic quantitation of BAL fluid may also enable the detection of conventional bacteria.

Thorpe and colleagues[67] performed BAL with the bronchoscope introduced either transnasally or through an endotracheal tube in a heterogeneous group of 92 hospitalized patients, 15 of whom were thought to have active bacterial pneumonia. Thirteen of the 15 patients with clinically active bacterial pneumonia had a BAL culture of more than 10^5 CFU/mL of BAL fluid, whereas none of the other patients, including those with resolving pneumonia or chronic bronchitis, had counts of more than 10^4 CFU/mL. Furthermore, Gram staining of cytocentrifuged BAL fluid was positive (one or more organisms seen per 1000 × field) only in those patients with active bacterial pneumonia.

Fiberoptic bronchoscopy is regarded as a relatively safe technique with few serious complications. Postbronchoscopy fever with increasing infiltrates may be observed. There is also a 10 to 20 mm Hg decrease in Pa_{O_2}, which could pose a problem for some patients with severe hypoxemia. Paradoxically, the risk of bronchoscopy is more important in patients not on a ventillator than in patients receiving mechanical ventilation. Therefore, in a patient already on the verge of needing assisted ventilation, the risk of worsening respiratory failure must be carefully considered. If the potential benefit of the diagnostic procedure is believed to be great, it may be preferable to perform the bronchoscopy after the patient has been safely intubated and ventilated.

Transthoracic Needle Aspiration

Percutaneous transthoracic needle aspiration enables collection of uncontaminated specimens directly from the pulmonary parenchyma for cytologic and microbiologic analyses. The use of smaller (ultrathin) gauge needles has reduced the frequency of pneumothorax as a complication.[68] Problems with the procedure include a relatively high rate of false-negative cultures and potentially serious complications in patients with severe underlying disease. This technique may be particularly attractive in children, because respiratory secretions may be difficult to obtain and transtracheal aspiration is infrequently performed.

In summary, invasive techniques are indicated only in patients with severe CAP because appropriate initial antibiotic treatment in patients with no signs of severity is associated with a good prognosis. If the patient is not receiving mechanical ventilation, the risk of performing bronchoscopy may outweigh the benefit of determining the responsible pathogens in most cases, except in deeply immunosuppressed patients. When patients are receiving mechanical ventilation, bronchoscopy using a protected specimen brush or BAL should probably be performed whenever possible, because this technique permits the clinician to safely determine the responsible organisms and therefore to select the appropriate treatment as soon as possible.

TREATMENT

To cover all pathogens that may cause severe CAP is impossible. Such treatment would have to include a broad-spectrum β-lactam antibiotic active against both *S. pneumoniae* (including resistant strains) and *P. aeruginosa,* a macrolide, trimethoprim-sulfamethoxazole, antituberculotic drugs, antifungal drugs, and antiviral drugs. Therefore, initial therapy should be based on the clues provided by clinical, epidemiologic, and radiologic evaluation and by evaluation of stained pulmonary secretions smears. In the case of a presumed bacterial pneumonia in which an etiologic agent is identified on the Gram-stained sputum smear, therapeutic decisions are greatly simplified and selection of an appropriate therapy is relatively straightforward (Table 144-5).

When the clinician is confronted with no sputum or with a

TABLE 144–5. Selection of Initial Antimicrobial Treatment in Adult Patients with Community-Acquired Pneumonia Based on Results of a Gram-Stained Sputum Smear*

Morphologic and Staining Characteristics of Predominant Bacteria	Suspected Pathogen	Presumptive Therapy
Gram-positive, oval, or lancet-shaped diplococci	*Streptococcus pneumoniae*	Penicillin G or amoxicillin
Small pleomorphic gram-negative coccobacilli	*Haemophilus influenzae*	Amoxicillin/clavulanic acid
Gram-negative, biscuit-shaped diplococci	*Moraxella catarrhalis*	Amoxicillin/clavulanic acid
Large gram-positive cocci in tetrads or clusters	*Staphylococcus aureus*	Nafcillin plus aminoglycoside
Large gram-negative encapsulated bacilli	*Klebsiella pneumoniae*	Third-generation cephalosporin plus aminoglycoside
Gram-negative rods	Enterobacteriaceae or other gram-negative bacilli	Third-generation cephalosporin† plus aminoglycoside

*Only Gram-stained smears containing ≤ 10 epithelial cells and ≥25 neutrophils under low-power magnification (×100) should be considered.
†With antipseudomonal activity in patients with bronchiectasis or cystic fibrosis.

TABLE 144–6. Recommendations for the Empirical Treatment of Severe Community Acquired Pneumonia

British Thoracic Society

Preferred regimen: erythromycin (1 g IV 4 times/day) plus a second- or third-generation cephalosporin (cefuroxime [1.5 g IV 3 times/day] or cefotaxime [2 g IV 3 times/day])

Alternative regimen: ampicillin (1 g), floxacillin (2 g), and erythromycin (1 g), all IV 4 times/day

American Thoracic Society

Regimen: (1) a macrolide (with rifampin if patient has legionellosis); (2) a third-generation cephalosporin with antipseudomonal activity or another antipseudomonal agent, such as imipenem or ciprofloxacin; and (3) an aminoglycoside

poor-quality sputum specimen or when the patient has already received prior antimicrobial treatment, the choice of antibiotics becomes more difficult. One option would be to immediately perform a fiberoptic bronchoscopy with BAL and a protected specimen brush. However, as indicated previously, these procedures are not always available on a 24-hour basis, and although they can be performed very safely in a patient who is already intubated and mechanically ventilated, they are not without risks in nonventilated patients with impending respiratory failure. In these cases, empirical therapy should be designed to treat the most likely or the most potentially lethal possibilities.

In an attempt to deal with these various issues, guidelines for the initial treatment of severe CAP were developed by the BTS[8] and the American Thoracic Society.[18] Central to these guidelines are patient-related considerations and the need to target the empirical therapy to adequately cover *S. pneumoniae,* virulent atypical pathogens such as *Legionella,* gram-negative organisms (*H. influenzae,* including β-lactamase–producing strains; *Klebsiella;* and in rare occurrences *P. aeruginosa*), and *S. aureus.* Curiously, although the two groups of experts reviewed similar data, they recommended different regimens (Table 144–6).

The BTS concluded that empirical therapy "should always cover" *S. pneumoniae.* The preferred regimen is thus a combination of erythromycin with a second-generation or third-generation cephalosporin without antipseudomonal activity. In contrast, and because of the relatively high epidemiologic risk for both *P. aeruginosa* and *Legionella* in hospitalized patients with severe CAP, combination therapy with multiple agents was deemed necessary for the American Thoracic Society. This involves a macrolide antibiotic, along with any one of a number of agents that are effective against common CAP pathogens, as well as pseudomonal species (certain third-generation cephalosporins, imipenem, ciprofloxacin), in combination with an aminoglycoside, at least during the first few days of treatment (see Table 144–6).

Fluoroquinolones (ciprofloxacin and ofloxacin) are acceptable alternatives to macrolides for legionnaires' disease and probably for *M. pneumoniae* and *C. pneumoniae* as well. Because these antimicrobial agents have excellent coverage against methicillin-sensitive *S. aureus, H. influenzae,* and gram-negative bacillary organisms, including *P. aeruginosa,* they can constitute an appropriate initial choice, especially in patients with structural lung disease (e.g., cystic fibrosis and

TABLE 144–7. Antimicrobial Agents for Community-Acquired Pneumonia Caused by Microbial Pathogens

Pathogen	Drug of Choice	Alternative Drugs	Comments
Streptococcus pneumoniae	Penicillin or amoxicillin	Cephalosporins Macrolides Doxycycline Vancomycin	For strains with intermediate levels of resistance to penicillin: high-dose penicillin, cefotaxime, or ceftriaxone For highly resistant strains: vancomycin
Haemophilus influenzae	Cephalosporin (second- or third-generation) Trimethoprim-sulfamethoxazole	Fluoroquinolone Doxycycline	β-Lactamase production with amoxicillin resistance in 20% to 30% of strains
Staphylococcus aureus	Oxacillin or nafcillin with or without gentamicin	Cefuroxime or cefazolin Vancomycin	Methicillin resistance rare in community-acquired strains
Moraxella catarrhalis	Cephalosporin (second- or third-generation) Trimethoprim-sulfamethoxazole	Macrolide Fluoroquinolone Doxycycline	β-lactamase production with ampicillin resistance in 80% to 90% of strains
Anaerobes	Clindamycin	Penicillin plus metronidazole β-lactam–β-lactamase inhibitor Penicillin or amoxicillin	Published experience limited except for penicillin and clindamycin
Gram-negative bacilli	Cephalosporin (second- or third-generation) with or without aminoglycoside	Fluoroquinolone Imipenem Antipseudomonal penicillin	In vitro sensitivity tests required
Legionella species	Erythromycin Ciprofloxacin	Clarithromycin or azithromycin	Experience extensive only with erythromycin Rifampin often added
Mycoplasma pneumoniae	Doxycycline Erythromycin	Clarithromycin or azithromycin Fluoroquinolone	
Chlamydia pneumoniae	Doxycycline Erythromycin	Clarithromycin or azithromycin Fluoroquinolone	

Adapted from Bartlett JG, Mundy LM: Community-acquired pneumonia. N Engl J Med 1995; 333:1618–1624.

bronchiectasis). However, the in vitro activity of ciprofloxacin against *S. pneumoniae* is modest, and thus this agent should never be used as a monotherapy in patients with severe CAP.

Whatever the initial antimicrobial treatment selected, if information becomes available that identifies a specific pathogen, then this one may be modified as necessary. As with any infection, once the etiologic agent is known, therapy should be given using as narrow a spectrum drug as possible to which the pathogen is susceptible (Table 144-7). Generally, considerations of drug efficacy, toxicity, cost, and compliance help in selecting the appropriate drug.

An important variable in these recommendations is the prevalence of penicillin-resistant *S. pneumoniae,* which accounts for more than 25% of pneumococcal isolates in many areas of the world[45]. Unfortunately, many of these isolates also exhibit resistance to other agents, such as macrolides and lincosamides, tetracycline, trimethoprim-sulfamethoxazole, and chloramphenicol. Most strains (~80%) have intermediate resistance ($0.1 < MIC < 2$ μg/mL) to penicillin, and uncomplicated pneumonia caused by these strains may be treated with high doses of penicillin or selected cephalosporins, such as ceftriaxone or cefotaxime. One review found that mortality due to pneumococcal pneumonia involving intermediate-resistant strains is similar to that for pneumonia involving sensitive strains, even when the treatment includes penicillins or cephalosporins.[49] However, some cases of failure may be observed, underlining the absolute necessity to precisely determine the minimal inhibitory concentration of penicillin against every *S. pneumoniae* isolate found responsible for pneumonia.

ACKNOWLEDGMENT

The authors wish to thank Agnès Failin for her invaluable help in the preparation of the manuscript.

References

1. Garibaldi RA: Epidemiology of community-acquired respiratory tract infections in adults: Incidence, etiology, and impact. Am J Med 1985; 78:32–37.
2. Woodhead MA, Macfarlane JT: Comparative clinical and laboratory features of legionella with pneumococcal and mycoplasma pneumonias. Br J Dis Chest 1987; 81:133–139.
3. Ortqvist A: Prognosis in community-acquired pneumonia requiring treatment in hospital: Importance of predisposing and complicating factors, and of diagnostic procedures. Scand J Infect Dis 1990; 65:1–62.
4. Centers for Disease Control and Prevention: Pneumonia and influenza death rates: United States, 1979–1994. MMWR Morb Mortal Wkly Rep 1995; 44:535–537.
5. Woodhead MA: Management of pneumonia. Respir Med 1992; 86:459–469.
6. Ortqvist A, Kalin M, Julander I, Mufson MA: Deaths in bacteremic pneumococcal pneumonia: A comparison of two populations: Huntington, WVa, and Stockholm, Sweden. Chest 1993; 103:710–716.
7. Fine MJ, Smith DN, Singer DE: Hospitalization decision in patients with community-acquired pneumonia: A prospective cohort study. Am J Med 1990; 89:713–721.
8. British Thoracic Society: Community-acquired pneumonia in adults in British hospitals in 1982–1983: A survey of etiology, mortality, prognostic factors and outcome. Q J Med 1987; 62:195–220.
9. Daley J, Jencks S, Draper D, Lenhart G, Thomas N, Walker J: Predicting hospital-associated mortality for Medicare patients: A method for patients with stroke, pneumonia, acute myocardial infarction, and congestive heart failure. JAMA 1988; 260:3617–3624.
10. Farr BM, Sloman AJ, Fisch MJ: Predicting death in patients hospitalized for community-acquired pneumonia. Ann Intern Med 1991; 115:428–436.
11. Marrie TJ, Durant H, Yates L: Community-acquired pneumonia requiring hospitalization: 5-year prospective study. Rev Infect Dis 1989; 11:586–599.
12. Keeler EB, Kahn KL, Draper D, et al: Changes in sickness at admission following the introduction of the prospective payment system. JAMA 1990; 264:1962–1968.
13. Kurashi NY, Al-Hamdan A, Ibrahim EM, Al-Idrissi HY, Al-Bayari TH: Community acquired acute bacterial and atypical pneumonia in Saudi Arabia. Thorax 1992; 47:115–118.
14. Ortqvist A, Hedlund J, Grillner L, et al: Aetiology, outcome and prognostic factors in community-acquired pneumonia requiring hospitalization. Eur Respir J 1990; 3:1105–1113.
15. Fine MJ, Singer DE, Hanusa BH, Lave JR, Kapoor WN: Validation of a pneumonia prognostic index using the MedisGroups Comparative Hospital Database. Am J Med 1993; 94:153–159.
16. Fine MJ, Hanusa BH, Lave JR, et al: Comparison of a disease-specific and a generic severity of illness measure for patients with community-acquired pneumonia. J Gen Intern Med 1995; 10:359–368.
17. Fine MJ, Smith MA, Carson CA, et al: Prognosis and outcomes of patients with community-acquired pneumonia: A meta-analysis. JAMA 1996; 275:134–141.
18. Niederman MS, Bass JJ, Campbell GD, et al: Guidelines for the initial management of adults with community-acquired pneumonia: Diagnosis, assessment of severity, and initial antimicrobial therapy. Am Rev Respir Dis 1993; 148:1418–1426.
19. Gordon G, Throop D, Berberian L, et al: Validation of the American Thoracic Society in hospitalized patients. Am J Respir Crit Care Med 1996; 153:A257.
20. Durocher A, Saulnier F, Beuscart R, et al: A comparison of three severity score indexes in an evaluation of serious bacterial pneumonia. Intensive Care Med 1988; 14:39–43.
21. Feldman C, Kallenbach JM, Levy H, et al: Community-acquired pneumonia of diverse aetiology: Prognostic features in patients admitted to an intensive care unit and a "severity of illness" score. Intensive Care Med 1989; 15:302–307.
22. Karalus NC, Cursons RT, Leng RA, et al: Community acquired pneumonia: Aetiology and prognostic index evaluation. Thorax 1991; 46:413–418.
23. Fine MJ, Auble TE, Yealy DM, et al: A prediction rule to identify low-risk patients with community-acquired pneumonia. N Engl J Med 1997; 336:243–250.
24. Sorensen J, Cederholm I, Carlsson C: Pneumonia: A deadly disease despite intensive care treatment. Scand J Infect Dis 1986; 18:329–335.
25. Ausina V, Coll P, Sambeat M, et al: Prospective study on the etiology of community-acquired pneumonia in children and adults in Spain. Eur J Clin Microbiol Infect Dis 1988; 7:342–347.
26. Woodhead MA, MAcFarlane JT, Rodgers FG, Laverick A, Pilkington R, Macrae AD: Aetiology and outcome of severe community-acquired pneumonia. J Infect Dis 1985; 10:204–210.
27. Pachon J, Prados MD, Capote F, Cuello JA, Garnacho J, Verano A: Severe community-acquired pneumonia: Etiology, prognosis, and treatment. Am Rev Respir Dis 1990; 142:369–373.
28. Torres A, Serra BJ, Ferrer A, et al: Severe community-acquired pneumonia: Epidemiology and prognostic factors. Am Rev Respir Dis 1991; 144:312–318.
29. Rello J, Quintana E, Ausina V, Net A, Prats G: A three-year study of severe community-acquired pneumonia with emphasis on outcome. Chest 1993; 103:232–235.
30. Moine P, Vercken JB, Chevret S, Chastang C, Gajdos P: Severe community-acquired pneumonia: Etiology, epidemiology, and prognosis factors: French Study Group for Community-Acquired Pneumonia in the Intensive Care Unit. Chest 1994; 105:1487–1495.
31. Almirall J, Mesalles E, Klamburg J, Parra O, Agudo A: Prognostic factors of pneumonia requiring admission to the intensive care unit. Chest 1995; 107:511–516.
32. Lim I, Shaw DR, Stanley DP, Lumb R, McLennan G: A prospective hospital study of the aetiology of community-acquired pneumonia. Med J Aust 1989; 151:87–91.
33. Barrett-Connor E: The nonvalue of sputum culture in the diagnosis of pneumococcal pneumonia. Am Rev Respir Dis 1970; 103:845–848.
34. Farr BM, Kaiser DL, Harrison BD, Connolly CK: Prediction of

microbial aetiology at admission to hospital for pneumonia from the presenting clinical features: British Thoracic Society Pneumonia Research Subcommittee. Thorax 1989; 44:1031-1035.
35. Lipsky BA, Boyko EJ, Inui TS, Koepsell TD: Risk factors for acquiring pneumococcal infections. Arch Intern Med 1986; 146:2179-2185.
36. Pesola GR, Charles A: Pneumococcal bacteremia with pneumonia: Mortality in acquired immunodeficiency syndrome. Chest 1992; 101:150-155.
37. Janoff EN, Breiman RF, Daley CL, Hopewell PC: Pneumococcal disease during HIV infection: Epidemiologic, clinical, and immunologic perspectives. Ann Intern Med 1992; 117:314-324.
38. Zarrabi MH, Rosner F: Serious infections in adults following splenectomy for trauma. Arch Intern Med 1984; 144:1421-1424.
39. Hofmann J, Cetron MS, Farley MM, et al: The prevalence of drug-resistant *Streptococcus pneumoniae* in Atlanta. N Engl J Med 1995; 333:481-486.
40. Pallares R, Linares J, Vadillo M, et al: Resistance to penicillin and cephalosporin and mortality from severe pneumococcal pneumonia in Barcelona, Spain. N Engl J Med 1995; 333:474-480.
41. Fang GD, Fine M, Orloff J, et al: New and emerging etiologies for community-acquired pneumonia with implications for therapy: A prospective multicenter study of 359 cases. Medicine (Baltimore) 1990; 69:307-316.
42. Trollfors B, Claesson B, Lagergard T, et al: Incidence, predisposing factors and manifestations of invasive *Haemophilus influenzae* infections in adults. Eur J Clin Microbiol 1984; 3:180-183.
43. Moxon ER: *Haemophilus influenzae In:* Principles and Practice of Infectious Diseases. 3rd ed. Mandell GL, Douglas RG Jr, Bennett JE (Eds). New York, Churchill Livingstone, 1990, pp 1722-1729.
44. Schwarzmann SW, Adler JL, Sullivan RJ, et al: Bacterial pneumonia during the Hong Kong influenza epidemic of 1968-1969: Experience in a city-county hospital. Arch Intern Med 1971; 127:1037-1041.
45. Bartlett JG, Mundy LM: Community-acquired pneumonia. N Engl J Med 1995; 333:1618-1624.
46. Slevin NJ, Aitken J, Thornleg PE: Clinical and microbiological features of *Branhamella catarrhalis* bronchopulmonary infections. Lancet 1987; 1:782-783.
47. Bartlett JG: Anaerobic bacterial infections of the lung. Chest 1987; 91:901-909.
48. Ponka A: Clinical and laboratory manifestations in patients with serological evidence of *Mycoplasma pneumoniae* infection. Scand J Infect Dis 1978; 10:271-280.
49. Khan MA, Kovnat DM, Bachus B, et al: Clinical and roentgenographic spectrum of pulmonary tuberculosis in the adults. Am J Med 1977; 62:31-38.
50. Bobrowitz ID: Active tuberculosis undiagnosed until autopsy. Am J Med 1982; 72:650-686.
51. Leeper KV: Severe community-acquired pneumonia. Semin Respir Infect 1996; 11:96-108.
52. Leroy O, Santre C, Beuscart C, et al: A five-year study of severe community-acquired pneumonia with emphasis on prognosis in patients admitted to an intensive care unit. Intensive Care Med 1995; 21:24-31.
53. Meehan TP, Fine MJ, Krumholz HM, et al: Quality of care, process, and outcomes in elderly patients with pneumonia. JAMA 1997; 278:2080-2084.
54. Hook EW, Horton CA, Schaberg DR: Failure of intensive care unit support to influence mortality from pneumococcal bacteremia. JAMA 1983; 240:1055-1058.
55. Franklin C, Hendrikson K, Weill MH: Reduced mortality of pneumococcal bacteremia after early intensive care. J Intensive Care 1994; 6:302-307.
56. MacFarlane JT, Miller AC, Smith WHR, Morris AH, Rose DH: Comparative radiographic features of community-acquired Legionnaires' disease, pneumococcal pneumonia, *Mycoplasma* pneumonia, and psittacosis. Thorax 1984; 39:28-33.
57. Tew J, Calenoff L, Berlin BS: Bacterial or nonbacterial pneumonia: Accuracy of radiographic diagnosis. Radiology 1977; 124:607-612.
58. Sörensen J, Forsberg P, Hakanson E, et al: A new diagnostic approach to the patient with severe pneumonia. Scand J Infect Dis 1989; 21:33-41.
59. Murray PR, Washington JA: Microscopic and bacteriologic analysis of expectorated sputum. Mayo Clin Proc 1975; 50:339-344.
60. Geckler RW, Gremillon DH, McAllister CK, Ellenbozen C: Microscopic and bacteriological comparison of paired sputa and transtracheal aspirates. J Clin Microbiol 1977; 6:396-399.
61. Rein MF, Gwaltney JM Jr, O'Brien WM, Jennings RH, Mandell GL: Accuracy of Gram's stain in identifying pneumococci in sputum. JAMA 1978; 239:2671-2673.
62. Tillotson JR, Lerner AM: Characteristics of pneumonia caused by *Escherichia coli.* N Engl J Med 1967; 277:115-122.
63. Edelstein PH, Meyer RD, Finegold SM: Laboratory diagnosis of Legionnaires' disease. Am Rev Respir Dis 1980; 121:317-330.
64. Bartlett JG, Alexander J, Mayhew J, et al: Should fiberoptic bronchoscopic aspirates be cultured? Am Rev Respir Dis 1976; 114:73-78.
65. Wimberley NW, Faling LJ, Bartlett JG: A fiberoptic bronchoscopic technique to obtain uncontaminated lower airway secretions for bacterial cultures. Am Rev Respir Dis 1979; 119:337-342.
66. Pollock HM, Hawkins EL Bonner IR, et al: Diagnosis of bacterial pulmonary infections with quantitative protected catheter cultures obtained during bronchoscopy. J Clin Microbiol 1983; 17:255-259.
67. Thorpe JE, Baughman RP, Frame PT, Wesseler TA, Staneck JL: Bronchoalveolar lavage for diagnosing acute bacterial pneumonia. J Infect Dis 1987; 155:855-861.
68. Torres A, Jimenez P, Puig BJ, Celis R, Gonzalez J, Gea J: Diagnostic value of nonfluoroscopic percutaneous lung needle aspiration in patients with pneumonia. Chest 1990; 98:840-844.

145

Nosocomial Pneumonia

Jean-Yves Fagon, MD, PhD • Jean Chastre, MD

Nosocomial pneumonia is thought to be the leading cause of infection acquired in the intensive care unit (ICU). Patients in the ICU have nosocomial pulmonary infection rates that are as much as five to 10 times higher than the rates in the general wards.[1-7] This nosocomial infection is associated with the highest mortality and morbidity[1-4]; about 15% of all hospital-associated deaths are directly related to hospital-acquired pneumonia.[3] However, the morbidity and mortality rates directly related to the occurrence of such infection are uncertain, ranging from 0% to more than 70% of affected patients. These variations are partly due to dramatic difference in the profile of patients admitted to and cared for in ICUs. However, most of the difference can be accounted for by the varying criteria used for diagnosis of pneumonia among studies and since the late 1970s.

Accurate diagnosis of nosocomial pneumonia is critical for both clinical research and practice, particularly the understanding of the epidemiology and pathogenesis of nosocomial pneumonia and the development of effective prophylactic and therapeutic strategies. In most hospitals, the diagnosis of pneumonia is made clinically even though it is often difficult to distinguish patients with true lung parenchymal infection from patients with only tracheobronchial airways colonization. It is highly probable that studies based only on such diagnostic criteria included some patients who did not have pneumonia. The data collected in the epidemiologic studies were further compromised by the use of sputum and tracheal secretions for microbiologic analyses, although such specimens may contain (1) organisms that normally colonize the upper respiratory tract and (2) disease-causing pathogens. During the 1980s and 1990s, bronchoscopy with bronchoalveolar lavage (BAL) and the protected specimen brush (PSB) technique have been advocated to improve the diagnosis of nosocomial pneumonia, particularly in patients receiving mechanical ventilation.[7, 8]

Definition of high-risk populations, more rapid identification of infected patients, and accurate selection of antimicrobial therapy for treatment of nosocomial pneumonia represent important clinical goals. It appears that prevention and better treatment of this infection might have a major impact on hospital-associated mortality and morbidity.

INCIDENCE

The incidence of hospital-acquired pneumonia depends on the setting in which patients are treated. The National Nosocomial Infection Study, reporting for the year 1983, recorded an annual incidence of nosocomial lower respiratory infection of approximately 0.55%.[3] The incidence was much lower in nonteaching hospitals (0.41%) and small teaching hospitals (0.46%) compared with large teaching hospitals (0.75%). The incidence of nosocomial pneumonia ranged widely among various inpatient services in the National Nosocomial Infection Study report, with highs of 0.5% to 1.0% on medical-surgical wards and lows of 0.03% to 0.3% on obstetric, gynecology, and pediatric wards. Many studies have noted an even higher incidence of nosocomial pneumonia in certain settings; for example, the incidence of nosocomial pneumonia in general ICU populations ranges from 2% to 51%.[1, 4, 5] However, most studies have reported rates between 8% and 20%.[9–21]

A large-scale, 1-day point-prevalence study of pneumonia arising in the ICU was performed on April 29, 1992, in 1417 ICUs in Europe in the context of the European Prevalence of Infection in Intensive Care (EPIC) study.[20] A total of 10,038 patients were evaluated; 2064 (20.6%) had ICU-acquired infections, including pneumonia in 967 patients (46.9%), for an overall nosocomial pneumonia prevalence rate of 9.6%. Another large-scale study conducted in 107 ICUs in Europe demonstrated a crude pneumonia incidence of 8.9%; the population studied was relatively evenly divided between medical and surgical patients, and both groups had a comparable incidence of infection.[21]

The risk of pneumonia seems to be considerably higher in the subset of ICU patients treated with mechanical ventilation. In the Study on the Efficacy of Nosocomial Infection Control (SENIC), the rate of pneumonia was 21-fold higher for patients treated with continuous ventilatory support than for patients not receiving mechanical ventilation.[3] Celis and colleagues,[13] in 120 consecutive episodes of nosocomial pneumonia and 120 controls, found that intubation independently increased the risk of nosocomial pneumonia approximately sevenfold. In the EPIC study, mechanical ventilation was identified as one of the seven risk factors for ICU-acquired infections by a logistic regression analysis.[20]

In a report from the European Cooperative Group on Nosocomial Pneumonia[21] in which all the 996 patients admitted to the 107 participating ICUs from January 17 to January 23, 1990, were observed until ICU discharge, nosocomial pneumonia developed in 89 cases for a crude incidence of 8.9%, ranging from 2% to 15% according to the participating country. In patients with no ventilatory support at ICU admission, the crude incidence of pneumonia was 4.6%; in patients who received ventilatory support at admission and in patients receiving ventilation for more than 48 hours, crude incidences were 12.6% and 21.6%, respectively, confirming that the risk of pneumonia is considerably higher in the subset of patients who are intubated and receiving mechanical ventilation.[22]

The identification of risk factors for the development of pneumonia in ICU patients was another important goal of this survey. Five baseline variables were significantly associated in multivariate analysis with acquisition of lung infection, namely:

- Presence at admission of impaired airway reflexes
- Acute Physiology and Chronic Health Evaluation (APACHE) II score higher than 16
- Mechanical ventilation
- Trauma
- Coma

The rates of nosocomial pneumonia reported in the more recent studies evaluating homogeneous groups of patients receiving mechanical ventilation are shown in Table 145–1. In their prospective investigation on pneumonia in 23 ICUs in Italy that included 724 critically ill patients who had received prolonged (>24 hours) ventilatory assistance since admission, Langer and colleagues[23] found a mean rate of 23% of nosocomial pneumonia. The incidence of nosocomial pneumonia rose from 5% in patients receiving 1 day of respiratory assistance to 68.8% in patients receiving mechanical ventilation for more than 30 days. In one study in 124 trauma patients, 67% of whom were ventilated, *early-onset* pneumonia, defined as pneumonia occurring in the first 96 hours after admission, represented 63% of the 41 pneumonias complicating the course of such trauma patients.

In the same way, in a study of a mixed population of medical, surgical, and trauma patients, all of whom were treated with mechanical ventilation, Prod'hom and coworkers[24] defined early-onset pneumonia as occurring during the first 4 days of mechanical ventilation. Overall, 53 episodes of pneumonia were observed in the 244 patients studied (22%); early-onset pneumonia represented 45% of all pneumonia episodes.[24]

TABLE 145–1. Incidence and Mortality Rate of Ventilator-Associated Pneumonia

Reference	Study Years	No. of Patients Studied	Incidence (%)	Diagnostic Criteria	Mortality Rate (%)
Salata et al.[18]	1981–1982	51	41	Clinical–autopsy	76
Craven et al.[10]	1983–1984	233	21	Clinical	55
Langer et al.[23]	1983–1984	724	23	Clinical	44
Fagon et al.[14]	1981–1985	567	9	PSB	71
Kerver et al.[30]	1986	39	67	Clinical	30
Driks et al.[17]	1986–1987	130	18	Clinical	56
Torres et al.[28]	1987–1988	322	24	Clinical–PSB	33
Baker et al.[39]	1989–1993	514	5.4	PSB–BAL	24
Kollef[32]	1992–1993	277	15.5	Clinical	37
Fagon et al.[50]	1989–1994	1118	27.5	PSB–BAL	53
Timsit et al.[51]	1990–1993	387	14.5	PSB–BAL	57

PSB = Protected specimen brush; BAL = bronchoalveolar lavage.

Using quantitative culture of specimens obtained with a PSB during fiberoptic bronchoscopy to define pneumonia in 567 ventilated patients, Fagon and associates[14] reported a nosocomial pneumonia rate of 9%. With the use of an actuarial method, the cumulative risk of pneumonia in this context was estimated to be 6.5% at 10 days and 19% at 20 days after the onset of mechanical ventilation.

In 1983, Bell and colleagues[25] evaluated the incidence of pneumonia in patients with adult respiratory distress syndrome (ARDS) as being even higher: more than 70% of the patients who had died of this syndrome had evidence of pneumonia at autopsy. In contrast, Sutherland and associates[26] suggested that pneumonia defined by quantitative bacteriology is uncommon in ARDS. In 105 ARDS patients, the majority of whom were receiving antibiotics at the time of the study, 201 bronchoscopies with the use of PSB or BAL identified pneumonia in only 16 patients (15.2%). This result is probably not of general value because the PSB technique and BAL were performed at predetermined times from day 3 to day 21 after onset of ARDS, independently of the presence of clinical signs suggestive of pneumonia.[26] Delclaux and coworkers[27] evaluated the incidence of lower respiratory tract infection in 30 patients with severe ARDS with the use of repeated quantitative cultures of a plugged telescopic catheter; they found a 60% incidence rate and estimated the incidence density to be 4.2 per 100 ventilator-days. They concluded that ventilator-associated pneumonia (VAP) is frequent and of relatively late onset (9.8 ± 5.7 days after onset of ARDS) in such patients.[27] Because of the discrepancies between studies conducted in ARDS patients, epidemiologic investigations using accurate diagnostic criteria are needed in this particular subset of mechanically ventilated patients to confirm the findings of these previous investigations.

MORTALITY

Crude mortality rates of 24% to 76% have been reported for nosocomial pneumonia at a variety of institutions (see Table 145-1). ICU ventilated patients with nosocomial pneumonia appear to have a twofold to 10-fold increased risk of mortality compared with patients without pneumonia. Stevens and colleagues[6] reported fatality rates of 50% for ICU patients with pneumonia compared with 3.5% for patients without pneumonia. Several studies have confirmed this observation in the medical ICU,[14, 28] surgical ICU,[29, 30] respiratory ICU,[31] and newborn ICU.[12]

At least four studies have evaluated mortality of VAP. Despite variations between studies that partly reflect the study populations, overall mortalities in patients with VAP were 55% compared with 25% in patients without pneumonia in the study by Craven and associates,[10] 71% and 28% in the study by Fagon and coworkers,[14] 33% and 19% in the study by Torres and colleagues,[28] and 37.5% and 8.5% in the study by Kollef,[32] corresponding to increased risks of mortality in nosocomial pneumonia patients of 2.2, 2.45, 1.7, and 4.4, respectively. In addition, nosocomial pneumonia has been identified in several studies as an important prognostic factor in different groups of critically ill patients, including cardiac surgery patients[33]; patients with acute lung injury[34] or ARDS[26]; and immunocompromised patients, such as those with acute leukemia,[35] lung transplantation,[36] or bone marrow transplantation.[37] In contrast, in patients with extremely severe medical conditions, such as those surviving cardiac arrest[38] or those with extremely severe ARDS,[27] and in trauma patients,[39-41] the occurrence of nosocomial pneumonia does not seem to significantly affect prognosis.

Although these statistics indicate that nosocomial pneumonia is a severe disease, especially in ventilator-dependent patients, previous studies have not clearly demonstrated that pneumonia actually causes increased mortality or prolongs hospitalization of these patients. Two independent factors make this important question difficult to resolve unambiguously. First, numerous studies have demonstrated that severe underlying illness predisposes intensive care patients to the development of pneumonia, and mortality rates are, consequently, high in such patients.[9, 11, 13, 19-21, 32] Therefore, it is difficult to establish whether such critically ill patients would have survived if nosocomial pneumonia had not occurred. The second factor that has hindered the accurate assessment of the excess mortality associated with nosocomial pneumonia is the difficulty in establishing a firm diagnosis (see later). Thus, the widely diverging figures reported for nosocomial pneumonia incidence and mortality rates might reflect not only differences in the populations of patients studied but also differences in the diagnostic criteria used.

In spite of these difficulties and limitations, several arguments support the presence of pneumonia as an important determinant of the poor prognosis of patients treated with mechanical ventilation. Of particular interest is the relationship between etiologic agents and mortality from nosocomial pneumonia. It is clear that the prognosis of aerobic, gram-negative bacillary pneumonia is considerably worse than that of infection with gram-positive agents.

Graybill and colleagues[15] reported 56% mortality in cases of gram-negative bacillary pneumonia and 24% in cases of gram-positive pneumonia. Death rates associated with *Pseudomonas* pneumonia are particularly high, with rates of 70% to more than 80% reported in several studies.[6, 14, 42-45] In the series reported by Fagon and associates,[14] mortality associated with *Pseudomonas* or *Acinetobacter* pneumonia was 87% compared with only 55% for pneumonias due to other organisms. The majority of patients who had pneumonia due to these multiresistant organisms had been receiving antimicrobial therapy before the onset of pneumonia. These data are confirmed by recent studies.

Kollef and associates[46] studied the effect of late-onset VAP in determining mortality in 314 patients and demonstrated that patients with VAP due to high-risk pathogens (*Pseudomonas aeruginosa*, *Acinetobacter* sp., and *Stenotrophomonas maltophilia*) had a statistically higher hospital mortality rate (65%) compared with patients with late-onset VAP due to other pathogens (31%) or compared with patients without late-onset VAP (37.4%). Describing a 7-year experience of bacteremic nosocomial pneumonia, Taylor and coworkers[47] studied 149 episodes in 145 patients and demonstrated that infections due to *P. aeruginosa* had a much higher mortality rate than those due to other pathogens (45% versus 14%; $P = .02$). Similarly, in a study comparing VAP due to methicillin-resistant *Staphylococcus aureus* with VAP due to methicillin-sensitive *S. aureus*, Rello and coworkers[48] found a mortality directly related to pneumonia of 85.7% in the case of methicillin-resistant *S. aureus* pneumonia compared with 11.9% in the case of methicillin-sensitive *S. aureus* pneumonia, with a relative risk of death equal to 20.72 in the case of methicillin-resistant *S. aureus* pneumonia. In contrast, comparison of VAP due to anaerobic bacteria with VAP due to aerobic bacteria did not show any significant difference in mortality rates (31% and 36%, respectively).[49] However, in this study by Doré and colleagues,[49] death occurred earlier when anaerobes were present (day 8 versus day 31; $P < .001$).

Other risk factors for death in ventilated patients in whom pneumonia developed have been systematically investigated only in a study by Torres and colleagues.[28] Using multiple logistic regression analysis, these authors demonstrated that worsening of the respiratory failure, presence of an ultimately or rapidly fatal underlying condition, presence of shock, inappropriate antibiotic therapy, and type of ICU in which the pneumonia developed were factors with a negative influence on the prognosis of nosocomial pneumonia.

Two methodologic solutions are theoretically available to try to elucidate the complex relationship between severity of underlying disease, occurrence of nosocomial pneumonia, and death: multivariate analysis and case-control studies.

Multivariate analysis is used to measure the independent role played by nosocomial pneumonia in inducing death. Craven and colleagues[10] found that VAP was associated with mortality on univariate analysis but was not among the seven variables identified by multivariate analysis, raising doubt as to the direct effect of lung infection on death. Similarly, Kollef,[32] performing multivariate analysis in 227 ventilated patients, failed to identify VAP as a variable independently associated with mortality. In contrast, the results of the EPIC study demonstrated that ICU-acquired pneumonia increased the risk of ICU death with an odds ratio of 1.91 (95% confidence interval [CI], 1.6 to 2.3), apart from clinical sepsis and bloodstream infections, as evidenced by a stepwise logistic regression analysis.[20]

Fagon and colleagues,[50] studying 1978 ICU patients, 1118 of whom were treated with mechanical ventilation, demonstrated that in addition to the severity of the underlying medical condition measured by the APACHE II score, the presence of organ dysfunction and the criteria of McCabe and Jackson stratifying the underlying disease as fatal, ultimately fatal, or not fatal, and nosocomial bacteremia, nosocomial pneumonia independently contributed to mortality of the ICU patient as well as to mortality of the ventilated patient. By using the Cox model as the statistical method, Timsit and coworkers[51] demonstrated that VAP, clinically diagnosed and bacteriologically confirmed, was independently associated with increased mortality (relative risk 2.1, $P < .0001$ for clinically diagnosed pneumonia; relative risk 1.7, $P = 0.01$ for bacteriologically diagnosed pneumonia).

Case-control studies are used to evaluate mortality attributable to nosocomial pneumonia, that is, the difference of the mortality rates observed between case patients (patients with pneumonia) and control subjects (patients without pneumonia). Two matched cohort studies[52, 53] of nosocomial pneumonia in which subjects were compared by demographic factors and underlying disease suggested that the relative risk of infection in inducing death, defined as the ratio of crude mortality rate of the case patients to that of the control subjects, ranged between 3.6 and 1.5, and attributable mortalities were 14.8% and 6.8%, respectively. These results, observed in patients hospitalized in general wards, were confirmed in patients treated with mechanical ventilation, except in trauma patients (Table 145–2). For example, using reliable techniques to identify patients with VAP, including PSB and BAL, Fagon and colleagues[45] undertook a cohort study in which patients who had pneumonia and control subjects were carefully matched for the severity of underlying illness and other important variables, such as age, indication for ventilatory support, and duration of exposure to risk. Their results indicated that mortality attributable to nosocomial pneumonia exceeded 25%, corresponding to a relative risk of death equal to 2.0. In cases of pneumonia due to *Pseudomonas* or *Acinetobacter* species, attributable mortality exceeded 40% and the corresponding relative risk of death was 2.50.

There are only a few reports on mortality as a result of nosocomial pneumonia in which autopsy material from patients who died during their hospital stay was analyzed. In a study of 200 consecutive hospital deaths, Gross and coworkers[54] concluded that nosocomial pneumonia contributed to 60% of the fatal infections and was the leading cause of death from hospital-acquired infection. Matching half of these patients who died in the hospital with control subjects of similar age, sex, department, primary discharge diagnosis, and severity of primary diagnosis, the same authors found that nosocomial lower respiratory tract infection occurred in 18% of the patients in the case group and in only 4% of the patients in the control group ($P < .005$). Among patients who did not have a terminal condition on admission, nosocomial infections were three times as common among those who died (46%) as among those who survived (11%); nosocomial pneumonia was present in most patients who died.[55]

Although a direct relationship between lung infection and mortality in ventilated patients has not always been formally demonstrated, a large body of evidence indicates that nosocomial pneumonia is indeed associated with mortality in excess of that due to the underlying disease alone.

MORBIDITY AND COST

It is impossible to exactly evaluate the morbidity and excess costs associated with nosocomial pneumonia. However, with respect to morbidity measures, the prolonged hospital stay as a direct consequence of pneumonia has been estimated in several studies.[45, 50–52, 56, 57] Jimenez and associates[19] demonstrated that nosocomial pneumonia extended the duration of mechanical ventilation from 10 to 32 days, and Craig and Connelly[52] found that pneumonia lengthened the ICU stay

TABLE 145–2. Mortality and Relative Risk Attributable to Nosocomial Pneumonia in Five Matched Cohort Studies

Reference	Study Years	Diagnostic Criteria	Type of Patient	Crude Mortality in Cases (%)	Crude Mortality in Controls (%)	Attributble Mortality (%)*	Risk Ratio†
Craig and Connelly[52]	1978–1979	Clinical	Non-ICU and ICU	20.4	5.6‡	14.8%	3.6
Leu et al.[53]	1982–1983	Clinical	Non-ICU	20.3	13.5§	6.8%	1.5
Fagon et al.[45]	1988–1990	PSB + BAL	Ventilated	54.2	27.1‡	27.1%	2.0
Cunnion et al.[56]	1987–1991	Clinical	Surgical ICU (95% ventilated)	55	5‡	50%	11.6
			Medical and respiratory ICU (95% ventilated)	55	7.5†	47.5%	7.3
Baker et al.[39]	1989–1993	PSB + BAL	Trauma	24	24§	0	1
Papazian et al.[58]	1989–1993	PSB	Ventilated	40	38.8§	1.2	1.3

*Defined as the crude mortality rate of controls subtracted from that of study patients.
†Defined as the ratio of crude mortality rate of study patients to that of control subjects.
‡$P < .01$ comparing cases vs. control subjects.
§Nonsignificant
BAL = bronchoalveolar lavage; PSB = protected specimen brush.

threefold. In the study by Leu and coworkers,[53] the prolonged hospital stay directly attributable to nosocomial pneumonia was 9.2 days, significantly longer than in matched control subjects. Fagon and colleagues[45] observed that the median length of stay in the ICU for the patients who had VAP was 21 days versus a median of 15 days for control subjects ($P < .02$). A mean prolongation of ICU stay of 20 days was observed for patients with pneumonia when surviving pairs were compared. Baker and coworkers[39] reported mean durations of mechanical ventilation, ICU stay, and hospital stay of 12.0, 20.5, and 43.0 days in trauma patients with pneumonia compared with 8.0, 15.0, and 34.0 days, respectively, in their matched control subjects ($P < .001$).

Analyzing the same variables, Papazian and colleagues[58] found 27.3, 32.9, and 52.5 days in case patients compared with 19.7 ($P < .05$), 24.5 ($P < .05$), and 43.2 days (NS) in patients without pneumonia. Similarly, Cunnion and associates[56] demonstrated that the mean hospital stay after admission to the ICU was greater for cases of nosocomial pneumonia in surgical ICU patients (30.0 days versus 22.3 days in control subjects) and in medical and respiratory ICU patients (40.9 days versus 23.1 days in control subjects).

These prolonged hospitalizations underscore the considerable financial burden imposed by the development of nosocomial pneumonia. Pinner and colleagues[59] estimated the average excess cost for nosocomial pneumonia to be $1255 (U.S. dollars) in 1982. In a similar study in 1985, Beyt and coworkers[60] found that the average extra cost was $2863 (U.S. dollars). For Baker and colleagues,[39] the extra hospital charges related to nosocomial pneumonia occurring in trauma patients were evaluated to be $40,000 (U.S. dollars).

ETIOLOGIC AGENTS

Etiologic agents causing nosocomial pneumonia may differ according to the population of hospital patients, the duration of hospital stay, and the specific diagnostic methods employed. *Legionella* species,[61, 62] anaerobes,[49] fungi, viruses, and even *Pneumocystis carinii* should be mentioned but are not considered to be common in the context of pneumonia acquired during mechanical ventilation. However, several of these causes may be more common and potentially underreported because of difficulties involved with the diagnostic techniques used to identify certain etiologic agents, including anaerobic bacteria[49] and viruses.[63]

In a study in which the incidence of anaerobes in 130 patients with a first episode of bacteriologically documented nosocomial pneumonia was carefully investigated with use of special precautions to preserve anaerobic conditions during PSB transport and microbiologic procedures, Doré and coworkers[49] demonstrated that this type of organism was involved in 23% of the total number of episodes. The main anaerobic strains isolated were *Prevotella melaninogenica* (36%), *Fusobacterium nucleatum* (17%), and *Veillonella parvula* (12%). The probability of recovering anaerobic bacteria was particularly high in orotracheally intubated patients and in patients in whom pneumonia occurred during the 5 days after admission to the ICU.[49]

In another study conducted during a 5-year period, Papazian and colleagues[63] identified cytomegalovirus (CMV) as a possible cause of VAP in 25 patients by using histologic examination of lung tissue obtained by autopsy or open-lung biopsy as diagnostic proof. These authors suggested that CMV should not be excluded in ICU patients as a pathogen responsible for VAP, even in patients without acquired immunodeficiency syndrome, hematologic malignant neoplasia, or immunosuppressive therapy.[63]

The importance of gram-negative bacilli as pathogens in nosocomial respiratory infections has been repeatedly documented[3-5, 14, 28, 43, 64-66] (Tables 145–3 and 145–4). Regardless of the bacteriologic method used to define the precise etiologic agent of the pneumonia, several studies have reported that more than 60% of nosocomial pneumonias are caused by aerobic, gram-negative bacilli. More recently, however, some investigators have reported that gram-positive bacteria have become increasingly important pathogens in this setting, with *S. aureus* being the predominant gram-positive isolate.

For example, *S. aureus* was the first cause of nosocomial

TABLE 145–3. Organisms Recovered from Protected Brush Specimens and Bronchoalveolar Lavage in Ventilator-Associated Pneumonia

	Fagon et al., 1984[14]	Torres et al., 1984[64]
No. of episodes of pneumonia	52	25
Gram-negative bacteria	No. (%)*	No. (%)*
Pseudomonas aeruginosa	16 (31)	7 (28)
Acinetobacter spp.	8 (15)	6 (24)
Proteus spp.	8 (15)	0
Moraxella catarrhalis	5 (10)	0
Haemophilus spp.	5 (10)	0
Escherichia coli	4 (8)	3 (12)
Klebsiella spp.	2 (4)	3 (12)
Enterobacter cloacae	1 (2)	1 (4)
Stenotrophomonas maltophilia	0	0
Legionella spp.	1 (2)	2 (8)
Miscellaneous	1 (2)	1 (4)
Gram-positive bacteria		
Staphylococcus aureus	17 (33)	5 (20)
Streptococcus pneumoniae	3 (6)	1 (4)
Other streptococci	8 (15)	4 (16)
Croynebacterium spp.	4 (8)	0
Staphylococcus epidermidis	0	1 (4)
Anaerobes	1 (2)	1 (4)
Polymicrobial flora	21 (40)	10 (40)

*Sum of percentages exceeds 100% owing to polymicrobial flora.

TABLE 145–4. Microorganisms Isolated in 129 Episodes of Ventilator-Associated Pneumonia According to Previous Antimicrobial Therapy

	Previous Antibiotics	No Previous Antibiotics
Gram-positive cocci*		
Staphylococcus aureus	6	22
Streptococcus pneumoniae	0	5
Enterococcus faecalis	0	2
Coagulase-negative staphylococci	1	1
Gram-negative bacilli		
*Haemophilus influenzae**	3	17
Pseudomonas aeruginosa†	21	3
Alcaligenes faecalis	3	4
Serratia marcescens	5	0
Proteus mirabilis	4	0
Acinetobacter calcoaceticus	3	1
Escherichia coli	0	3
Citrobacter freundii	0	1
Anaerobic flora	3	1
Fungi		
Candida species	1	1
Aspergillus species	2	0
Uncertain	13	27

Modified from Rello J, Ausina V, Ricart M, et al: Impact of previous antimicrobial therapy on the etiology and outline of ventilator-associated pneumonia. Chest 1993; 104:1230–1235.

*$P < .05$.

†$P < .01$.

pneumonia in the EPIC study, accounting for 31.7% of the 836 cases of pneumonia with identified responsible pathogens[66] (Fig. 145–1). In patients with pneumonia enrolled in the National Nosocomial Infection Study from 1985 to 1988, gram-negative bacteria accounted for six of the top seven etiologic agents identified in the survey.[67] In rank order, these organisms were *S. aureus, P. aeruginosa,* Enterobacteriaceae, *Klebsiella* spp., *Escherichia coli, Serratia marcescens,* and *Proteus* spp. As indicated in Table 145–3, the data from the study by Fagon and colleagues[14] of patients with VAP, in whom bacteriologic studies were restricted to uncontaminated specimens, confirm these results: 75% of all episodes of pneumonia included at least one gram-negative bacillus. The predominant organisms

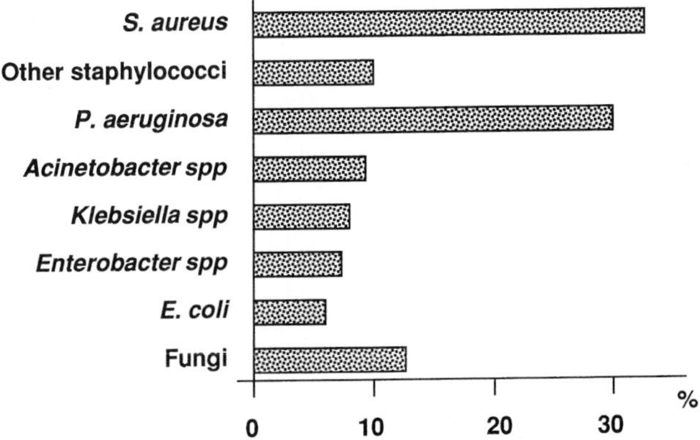

Figure 145–1. Major causative organisms for nosocomial pneumonia in the EPIC study (n = 836). (From Spencer RC: Predominant pathogens found in the European Prevalence of Infection in Intensive Care Study. Eur J Clin Microbiol Infect Dis 1996; 15:281–285.)

were *P. aeruginosa, Acinetobacter* spp., and *Proteus* spp. A relatively high rate of gram-positive pneumonias was also reported in this study, with *S. aureus* involved in 33% of cases.

Underlying diseases may predispose patients to infection with specific organisms. Patients with chronic obstructive pulmonary disease (COPD) are, for example, at increased risk for *Haemophilus influenzae* infection; cystic fibrosis increases the risk of *P. aeruginosa* and *S. aureus* infection. On the other hand, trauma and neurosurgical patients are at increased risk for *S. aureus* infection.[39, 48, 68]

In a study in which 129 episodes of nosocomial pneumonia documented by PSB specimens were prospectively included, Rello and coworkers[65] compared the distribution of infecting organisms responsible for infection according to whether or not the patients had received prior antimicrobial treatment before the onset of pneumonia. The most striking finding was that the rate of pneumonia caused by gram-positive cocci or *H. influenzae* was statistically lower in patients who had received prior antibiotics, whereas the rate of pneumonia caused by *P. aeruginosa* was statistically higher ($P < .01$) (see Table 145–4). A step-forward logistic regression analysis identified only prior antibiotic use (odds ratio = 9.2) as significantly influencing the risk of death from pneumonia. The same result was obtained when severity was included in the model. However, prior antibiotic use entirely dropped out as a significant risk factor when the etiologic agent was included in the regression equation. These observations are consistent with previous reports of nosocomial infection due to multiresistant pathogens and strongly support the fact that prior use of antibiotics is a key factor in selecting for such microorganisms.

In our experience, based on the results of a prospective study in which we documented the microorganisms responsible for infection in 135 consecutive episodes of ventilator-associated nosocomial pneumonia observed in our ICU using bronchoscopic specimens, the distribution of infecting pathogens was markedly influenced by two factors[69]:

- Duration of mechanical ventilation before the onset of pneumonia
- Previous antimicrobial therapy

Although early-onset pneumonias in patients not having received prior antimicrobial treatment were mainly caused by sensitive Enterobacteriaceae, *Haemophilus* species, methicillin-sensitive *S. aureus,* and *Streptococcus pneumoniae*, early-onset pneumonias in patients having received prior antibiotics or late-onset pneumonias in patients not having received antibiotics during the 15-day period to onset of infection were commonly caused by nonfermenting gram-negative bacilli in addition to streptococci, *Haemophilus* spp., methicillin-sensitive *S. aureus*, and Enterobacteriaceae. On the other hand, late-onset pneumonias in patients having recently received prior antimicrobial treatment were commonly caused by multiresistant pathogens, such as *P. aeruginosa, Acinetobacter baumannii,* and methicillin-resistant *S. aureus* (Table 145–5).

The high rate of polymicrobial infection in nosocomial pneumonia has been emphasized by several authors. In a study of 172 episodes of bacteremic nosocomial pneumonia reported by Bryan and Reynolds,[42] 13% of pneumonias were also caused by multiple pathogens. Similarly, using the PSB technique to establish the causative agents in 52 consecutive cases of nosocomial pneumonia in ventilated patients, Fagon and colleagues[14] found a 40% incidence of polymicrobial infection, a rate similar to that observed by Torres and coworkers[64] in a comparable population of ventilated patients.

TABLE 145–5. Bacteriology of Infection in 135 Patients with Nosocomial Pneumonia According to Duration of Mechanical Ventilation (MV) and Presence or Absence of Prior Antimicrobial (ABs) Treatment Before Infection Onset*

Microorganism	Total 254†/135‡	MV < 7 Days ABs = No 43†/24‡	MV < 7 Days ABs = Yes 21†/19‡	MV ≥ 7 Days ABs = No 32†/15‡	MV ≥ 7 Days ABs = Yes 158†/177‡
Pseudomonas spp.	15.3	0	19.0	6.2	20.9
Acinetobacter spp.	8.3	0	4.8	3.1	12.0
Enterobacteriaceae	14.1	18.5	19	21.8	10.8
Haemophilus spp.	5.9	18.6	9.5	3.1	2.5
Methicillin-resistant *Staphylococcus*	13	0	4.8	3.1	19.6
Methicillin-sensitive *S. aureus*	7.5	13.9	0	21.9	3.8
Streptococcus pneumoniae	1.6	9.3	0	0	0
Other streptococci	15	13.9	23.8	28.1	11.4
Miscellaneous	19.3	25.8	19.1	12.7	19

From Trouillet JL, Chastre J, Vuagnat A, et al: Ventilator-associated pneumonia caused by potentially drug-resistant bacteria. Am J Respir Crit Care Med 1998; 157:531–539.
*Results are expressed as percentages of the total number of microorganisms.
†Number of bacteria.
‡Number of episodes.

RISK FACTORS

Pneumonia results from microbial invasion of the normally sterile lower respiratory tract caused by either a defect in host defenses or challenge by a particular virulent microorganism or an overwhelming inoculum with complex interrelationships between host factors, treatments and procedures, and environmental factors (Fig. 145–2). A number of factors have been suspected or identified to increase the risk of pneumonia in the ICU, including those identified in the subset of mechanically ventilated patients (Table 145–6). The data indicated the following as being independently associated with nosocomial pneumonia:

1. Specific high-risk populations (patients with COPD or ARDS).
2. Patients undergoing mechanical ventilation for more than 3 days.
3. Individuals requiring intracranial pressure monitoring.
4. Patients with coma or impaired consciousness.
5. Patients with severe underlying medical conditions, as evaluated by a high APACHE II or APACHE III score or presence of organ failure.
6. Patients with specific treatment modalities or therapeutic interventions (use of H_2-blockers or antacids; previous antibiotics; use of drugs that are markers for severe underlying disease, such as dopamine, dobutamine, or barbiturate therapy; reintubation and frequent changes of ventilator circuits; bronchoscopy or nasogastric tube).

Surgery

Postsurgical patients are at increased risk for pneumonia.[9, 11, 13, 31] In a study reported in 1981 by Garibaldi and coworkers,[11] the incidence of pneumonia during the postoperative period was 17.2%. In this study, the authors stated that development of pneumonia was closely associated with preoperative markers of the severity of the underlying disease, such as low serum albumin concentration and high American Society of Anesthesiologists preanesthesia physical status classification. A history of smoking, longer preoperative stays, longer surgical procedures, and thoracic or upper abdominal operative sites were also significant risk factors for postoperative pneumonia.

In their study comparing adult critical care populations, Cunnion and associates[56] demonstrated that surgical ICU patients had consistently higher rates of nosocomial pneumonia than did medical ICU patients, with a risk ratio equal to

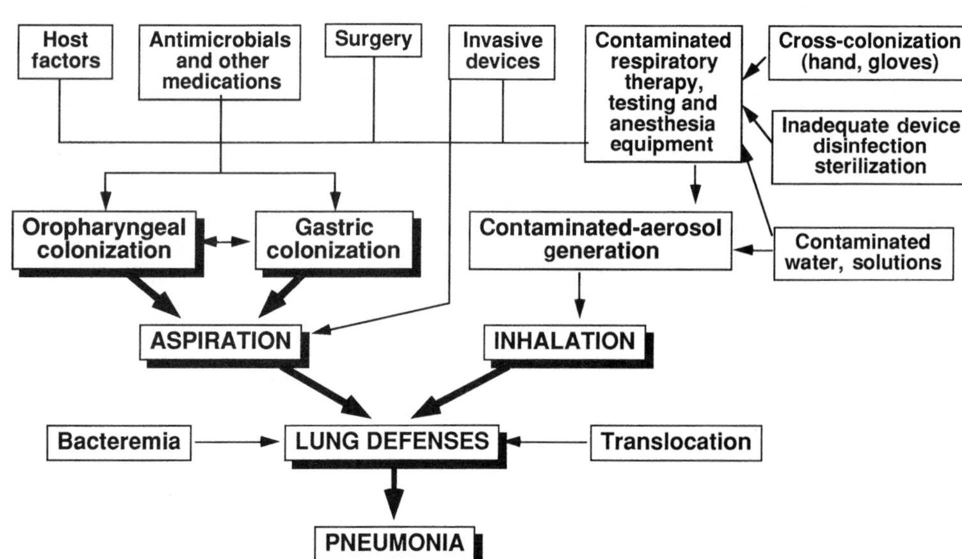

Figure 145–2. Summary of factors contributing to colonization and infection of the lower respiratory tract. (Modified from Craven DE, Driks MR: Nosocomial pneumonia in the intubated patient. Semin Respir Infect 1987; 2:20–33.)

TABLE 145–6. Independent Factor for Bacterial Nosocomial Pneumonia Identified by Multivariate Analysis in Selected Studies

Risk Factor	Reference
Ventilator-Associated Pneumonia	
• Age ≥ 60 yr	Torres et al.[28]; Kollef[32]
• COPD/PEEP/pulmonary disease	Torres et al.[28]
• Coma or impaired consciousness	Rello et al.[65]
• Intracranial pressure monitoring	Craven et al.[10]; Daschner et al.[218]
• Organ failure	Kollef[32]
• Large volume gastric aspiration	Torres et al.[28]
• Prior antibiotics	Kollef[32]
• H_2-blocker ± antacids	Craven et al.[10]
• Gastric colonization and pH	Daschner et al.[218]
• Season: fall, winter	Craven et al.[10]
• Ventilator circuit changes 24 versus 48 hr	Craven et al.[10]
• Reintubation	Torres et al.[28]
• Mechanical ventilation ≥ 2 days	Torres et al.[28]
	Daschner et al.[218]; Antonelli et al.[40]
• Tracheostomy	Daschner et al.[218]
• Supine head position	Kollef[32]
Ventilated and Nonventilated Patients	
• Age > 60 yr	Celis et al.[13]; Antonelli et al.[40]
• APACHE I > 16, APACHE II score	Chevret et al.[21]; Cunnion et al.[56]
• Trauma or head injury	Chevret et al.[21]
• Impaired airway reflexes	Chevret et al.[21]
• Coma	Chervet et al.[21]
• Bronchoscopy	Joshi et al.[9]
• Nasogastric tube	Celis[13]; Joshi et al.[9]
• Endotracheal intubation	Chevret[21]; Cunnion et al.[56]
• Upper abdominal or throacic surgery	Joshi[9]; Celis[13]; Antonelli et al.[40]
• H_2-blockers	Cook et al.[79]

COPD = chronic obstructive pulmonary disease; PEEP = positive end-expiratory pressure; APACHE = Acute Physiologic and Chronic Health Evaluation; H_2 = histamine.

2.2. Multiple logistic regression was performed to determine independent predictors for nosocomial pneumonia in the two groups; in surgical ICU patients, mechanical ventilation (>2 days) and APACHE II score were identified by the model; in medical ICU patients, only mechanical ventilation (>2 days) remained significant.[56]

Antimicrobial Agents

The use of antibiotics in the hospital setting has been associated with an increased risk of nosocomial pneumonia.[32, 44, 48, 65–71] In the study by Kollef,[32] prior antibiotic administration was identified by logistic regression analysis to be one of the four variables independently associated with VAP along with organ failure, age older than 60 years, and the patient's head positioning. In addition to this effect on the overall occurrence of VAP, prior antibiotic administration is an important factor in determining the etiology of VAP (see earlier). These so-called superinfections presumably occur as a consequence of selection for more resistant bacterial pathogens during treatment of a primary infection. In a study conducted by our group in 567 ventilated patients, patients receiving prior antimicrobial therapy were not at higher risk for development of pneumonia.[14] However, we noted that 65% of the pneumonias among patients receiving broad-spectrum antimicrobial drugs but only 19% of pneumonias among patients not having received prior antibiotics included *Pseudomonas* or *Acinetobacter* spp. as the responsible organisms.

Stress Ulcer Prophylaxis

It is widely assumed that the stomach is an important reservoir for bacteria causing nosocomial pneumonia through the gastropulmonary route of infection, especially when gastric pH is higher than bactericidal levels. In theory, patients receiving stress ulcer prophylactic agents that do not influence gastric acidity should have lower rates of gastric bacterial colonization and, consequently, a lower risk of nosocomial pneumonia. Many studies have demonstrated a direct relationship between alkaline gastric pH and gastric bacterial colonization.[72–75] For example, Hillman and coworkers[73] investigated 28 postoperative patients in the ICU. On admission to the ICU, 86% of patients showed sterile gastric juice. Two days later, the gastric juice showed colonization in 61% of patients; at this time, 43% of them had a gastric pH higher than 4. These findings were fully confirmed by Donowitz and colleagues.[75] Among the 153 ICU patients receiving antacid or cimetidine medication investigated in their study, a highly significant increase in total gastric colonization, particularly with gram-negative bacteria, was detected. Whereas the gastric juice was sterile in 65% of cases at pH below 2, at least 60% of the patients showed gastric juice colonization by gram-negative bacteria at pH above 4.[75]

However, not all studies agree that the gastropulmonary route of infection is truly operative in ICU patients.[76, 77] Bonten and associates[76] were unable to show evidence of a clear sequence of colonization from the stomach to the upper respiratory tract eventually leading to pneumonia in 14 episodes of VAP. Initial colonization with *P. aeruginosa* and *Enterobacter* species was more often demonstrated in the trachea than in the stomach, underlining that the route and mechanisms of colonization may be different according to the responsible microorganism.

Several studies have found lower rates of pneumonia for patients given a cytoprotective agent (sucralfate) rather than agents that neutralize gastric acid (antacids) or block gastric acid secretion (H_2-blockers).[17, 24, 78, 79] In a careful randomized study of 244 mechanically ventilated patients that compared stress ulcer prophylaxis with antacids, ranitidine, and sucralfate, Prod'hom and coworkers[24] confirmed the potential benefit of using sucralfate. Whereas no differences in the incidence of macroscopic gastric bleeding and early-onset (within 4 days of entry into the ICU) nosocomial pneumonia were found among the three groups, late-onset pneumonia was observed in only 5% of the patients who received sucralfate compared with 16% and 21% of the patients who received antacid or ranitidine, respectively (P = .02). Patients who received sucralfate also had a lower median gastric pH and less frequent gastric colonization compared with the other groups. Using molecular typing, 84% of the patients with late-onset gram-negative bacillary pneumonia were found to have gastric colonization with the same bacteria before pneumonia developed. In meta-analyses of the efficacy of stress bleeding prophylaxis in ICU patients, respiratory tract infection was significantly less frequent in patients treated with sucralfate compared with patients receiving H_2-blockers or antacids. Although the results have varied by the populations studied, most current data using a clinical diagnosis of VAP suggest that sucralfate provides a similar protection against stress bleeding but has a lower risk of VAP than do H_2-blockers or antacids.[78–82]

Nevertheless, the question of the potential benefit of systematic administration of a stress ulcer prophylaxis regimen to ICU patients remains unanswered. Such a therapeutic strategy is usually considered to be a standard of care; however, it probably deserves a large reevaluation in the light of recent data.[81, 83] Ben-Menachem and colleagues[83] did not find any benefit in using stress ulcer prophylactic drugs in ICU patients; the risk of hemorrhage was identical in patients with or without a prophylactic regimen. The true risk of gastrointestinal hemorrhage has been reevaluated by Cook and associates.[84] They showed that the crude risk was low, globally equal to 1.5% (95% CI, 1.0 to 2.1): 3.7% in patients with respiratory failure or coagulopathy and only 0.1% (95% CI, 0.02 to 0.5) in those with no specific risk factors.[84] These results suggest that a stress ulcer prophylaxis regimen can be administered in only a limited number of ICU patients with a documented risk of hemorrhage, and in this case, sucralfate should probably be preferred.

Endotracheal Tube and Reintubation

The presence of an endotracheal tube by itself circumvents host defenses, causes local trauma and inflammation, and increases the probability of aspiration of nosocomial pathogens from the oropharynx around the cuff. Sottile and coworkers[85] studied 25 endotracheal tubes by scanning electron microscopy and found that 96% had partial bacterial colonization and 84% were completely covered by bacteria in a biofilm or glycocalyx. The authors suggested that aggregates of bacteria in biofilm dislodged during suctioning may not be killed by antibiotics or effectively cleared by host immune defenses.[85, 86] Clearly, the type of endotracheal tube may also influence the incidence of aspiration. With low-volume, high-pressure endotracheal cuffs, an incidence of 56% was reported, which decreased to 20% with the advent of high-volume, low-pressure cuffs.[87] Leakage around the cuff allows secretions pooled above the cuff to enter the trachea.

Mahul and colleagues[88] reported a decrease in the incidence of VAP and a delay in the development of pneumonia using manual intermittent aspiration of subglottic secretions. In a later study, Valles and colleagues[89] reported that the use of continuous aspiration of subglottic secretions reduced the incidence of VAP from 39.6 episodes per 1000 ventilator-days in the control group to 19.9 episodes in the group randomized to subglottic aspiration. The effect was most dramatic during the first 2 weeks of intubation and was primarily associated with a reduction of *H. influenzae* and gram-positive cocci, such as streptococci and *S. aureus*.

In addition to the presence of endotracheal tubes, reintubation is, per se, a risk factor for nosocomial pneumonia as indicated by Torres and coworkers.[90] This result is probably related to an increased risk of aspiration of colonized oropharyngeal secretions into the lower airways in patients with glottic dysfunction or impaired consciousness after several days of intubation. Another explanation is direct aspiration of gastric contents into the lower airways, particularly when a nasogastric tube is kept in place after extubation. In their case-control study, Torres and coworkers[90] found a 47% pneumonia rate in reintubated patients compared with 4% in control subjects matched for the duration of prior mechanical ventilation ($P = .0007$).

Nasogastric Tube, Enteral Feeding, and Position of the Patient

Nearly all patients receiving mechanical ventilation have a nasogastric tube inserted to manage gastric and enteral secretions, prevent gastric distention, or provide nutritional support. The nasogastric tube is not widely considered to be a potential risk factor for pneumonia, but it may increase oropharyngeal colonization, cause stagnation of oropharyngeal secretions, and increase reflux and the risk of aspiration. Using multivariate analysis, Joshi and colleagues[9] identified the presence of a nasogastric tube as one of the three independent risk factors for nosocomial pneumonia in a series of 203 patients admitted to the ICU for 72 hours or more.

Early initiation of enteral feeding is generally regarded as beneficial in critically ill patients,[91] but it may increase the risk of gastric colonization, gastroesophageal reflux, aspiration, and pneumonia. Pingleton and associates[92] evaluated simultaneous daily gastric, tracheal, and oropharyngeal cultures in 18 ventilator-dependent patients not receiving antacids or H_2-antagonists. After enteral feeding was started, the number of gram-negative isolates increased significantly, and five patients (28%) had gram-negative rods that were first recovered in the stomach and subsequently identified in the trachea. The mechanism of transfer of gastric organisms into the trachea appears to be aspiration.

Winterbauer and coworkers[93] described a 38% incidence of aspiration in enterally fed, critically ill patients with small-bore nasogastric tubes, but all patients were fed by the bolus technique. Recent data suggest that aspiration is infrequent when small-bore feeding tubes and continuous infusion are used.[94, 95] The aspiration rate generally varies as a function of differences in the population of patients, neurologic function, type of feeding tube, location of the feeding port, and method of evaluating aspiration.[96] Clinical impression and preliminary data[97] suggest that postpyloric or jejunal feeding entails less risk of aspiration and may therefore be associated with fewer infectious complications than is gastric feeding, although this point remains controversial.[98] However, aspiration can easily occur should the feeding tube be inadvertently dislodged. A retrospective study of adult patients showed a 40% incidence of accidental dislodgment of the feeding tube.[99] This was not a population of critically ill patients, but all patients whose tube had been displaced were confused or disoriented or had altered awareness, as is frequently observed in ICU patients.

Maintaining mechanically ventilated patients with a nasogastric tube in place in the supine position is also a risk factor for aspiration of gastric contents into the lower airways. Torres and colleagues[100] injected radioactive material through a nasogastric tube directly into the stomach of 19 mechanically ventilated patients and found that mean radioactive counts in endobronchial secretions were higher in a time-dependent fashion in samples obtained while patients were in the supine position than in those obtained while patients were in the semirecumbent position. The same microorganisms were isolated from stomach, pharynx, and endobronchial samples in 32% of the specimens taken while patients were semirecumbent and in 68% of those taken while patients were in the supine position.[100] These results suggest that placing mechanically ventilated patients in the semirecumbent position is a simple and effective means to minimize aspiration of gastric contents into lower airways and hence constitutes a recommendable, no-cost prophylactic measure for those who can tolerate this position.

Such experimental results were indirectly confirmed by Kollef,[32] who demonstrated that head positioning of the supine patient during the first 24 hours of mechanical ventilation was an independent risk factor for acquiring VAP. However, a study published by the same group that demonstrated the effect of body position on aspiration of gastric contents reported disappointing results, supporting that gastroesophageal reflux in mechanically ventilated patients with a nasogastric tube occurs irrespective of body position.[101]

Respiratory Equipment

Respiratory equipment itself may act as a source of bacteria responsible for nosocomial pneumonia. In past years, the major risk of infection was associated with contaminated reservoir nebulizers, designed to deliver small-sized particles suspended in the effluent gas. These observations led to the current trends in respiratory therapy with the use of cascade humidifiers, which do not generate microaerosols. Nevertheless, respiratory equipment continues to provide a source of bacterial contamination. For example, medication nebulizers inserted into the inspiratory-phase tube of the mechanical ventilator circuit may produce bacterial aerosols after a single use.[102]

Mechanical ventilators with humidifying cascades often have high levels of tubing colonization and condensate formation that may also be risk factors for pneumonia. The rate of condensate formation in the ventilator circuit is linked to the temperature difference between the inspiratory-phase gas and the ambient temperature and may be as high as 20 to 40 mL/hour.[102]

Craven and associates[103] examined condensate colonization in 20 circuits and found a median level of 2.0×10^5 organisms/mL, and 73% of the 52 gram-negative isolates present in the patients' sputum were subsequently isolated from condensate. Because most of the tubing colonization was derived from the patients' secretions, the highest bacterial counts were present near the endotracheal tube. Simple procedures such as turning the patient or raising the bed rail may accidentally wash contaminated condensate directly into the patient's tracheobronchial tree. Inoculation of large amounts of fluid with high bacterial concentrations is an excellent way of overwhelming pulmonary defense mechanisms and producing pneumonia. Heating ventilator tubing markedly reduces the rate of condensate formation, but heated circuits are often nondisposable and are expensive. In-line devices with one-way valves to collect condensate are probably the easiest way to handle this problem. They should be correctly positioned into disposable circuits and emptied regularly. To date, no scientific evidence confirms that heated circuits reduce the incidence of VAP.

Similarly, there is not sufficient evidence to suggest that heat and moisture exchangers (HME) are superior to cascade humidifiers in terms of the risk of VAP.[104] Dreyfuss and coworkers[104] reported similar rates of pneumonia in 61 patients allocated to humidification with an HME and 70 patients with a heated humidifier (10% versus 11%, NS). When HME was used, changing the HME every 48 hours did not affect ventilator circuit colonization, and the authors suggest that the cost of mechanical ventilation may be substantially reduced without any detriment to the patient by extending the time between HME changes from 24 to 48 hours.[105] Boots and colleagues[106] confirmed that the hot-water humidifier circuit became more readily colonized by bacteria than did circuits using a bacterial-viral filtering HME, but the frequency of VAP was not affected by the humidification technique.

Interestingly, the recommendation for daily changes of ventilator circuits in patients on continuous mechanical ventilation has been abandoned in the most recent guidelines for the prevention of nosocomial pneumonia edited by the Centers for Disease Control and Prevention in 1994.[107] However, as early as 1982, Craven and associates[108] showed that the incidence of circuit contamination was not increased when the circuit was changed every 48 hours instead of every 24 hours. In recent years, several authors have reported no difference in pneumonia rates with ventilator circuit changes at 48-hour and 7-day intervals or with no change[109-112] (Table 145-7).

Sinusitis

To date, few studies have adequately compared the risk of nosocomial sinusitis in patients with various methods of intubation and the associated risk of nosocomial pneumonia.[113-116] To compare the occurrence rate of nosocomial maxillary sinusitis and pneumonia in patients who have undergone nasotracheal versus orotracheal intubation, Holzapfel and colleagues[116] randomized a total of 300 patients who required mechanical ventilation for 7 days or longer between nasal and oral endotracheal intubation. Computed tomographic evidence of sinusitis was slightly more frequently observed in the nasal group than in the oral group ($P = .08$), but this difference disappeared when only bacteriologic (quantitative culture of the aspirated material of the sinus with more than 10^3 colony-forming units [CFU]/mL) evidence of sinusitis was considered.

In a report by Rouby and coworkers,[114] the incidence of infectious maxillary sinusitis with its clinical relevance was prospectively studied in 162 consecutive critically ill patients who had been intubated and mechanically ventilated for 1 hour to 12 days before enrollment. All had a paranasal computed tomographic scan within 48 hours of admission and were divided into three groups according to the radiologic appearance of the maxillary sinuses. In patients who had no sinusitis at admission ($n = 40$), placement of endotracheal and gastric tubes to the oral route decreased the evidence of radiologic sinusitis from 95.5% to 22.5% ($P < .01$). Interestingly, an increased incidence of nosocomial pneumonia was observed in patients with infectious sinusitis with 67% of these patients who had lung infection in the days after the diagnosis of sinusitis.

This study, combined with data from other investigators, clearly identifies nasal cannulation as a major risk factor of nosocomial infection in patients requiring mechanical ventilation. Further studies are therefore required to assess whether prevention of infectious sinusitis might contribute to lowering the incidence of nosocomial pneumonia in critically ill patients.

CLINICAL OBJECTIVES OF DIAGNOSTIC STRATEGIES

More rapid identification of patients with nosocomial pneumonia and accurate selection of appropriate antimicrobial treat-

TABLE 145–7. Incidence of Ventilator-Associated Pneumonia According to the Ventilator Circuit Change Interval*

Author	Diagnostic Criteria	No. of Patients	Pneumonia Rate (%)			*P* Value
			48-Hour Change	7-Day Change	No Change	
Dreyfuss et al.[109]	PSB	63	31.4	—	28.6	.80
Hess et al.[110]	Clinical	3423	9.6	8.6	—	.51
Kollef et al.[111]	Clinical	300	24.5	28.8	—	.11
Long et al.[112]	Clinical	447	9.4	9.9	—	.90

*Incidence is expressed as number of cases of pneumonia per 1000 days.

ment represent important clinical goals in this setting. However, despite broad clinical experience with this disease and many quality papers published in the literature, the optimal management strategy for patients who have symptoms suggestive of lung infection remains controversial. Some investigators[117] advocate invasive diagnostic protocols using bronchoscopic techniques and various specialized microbiologic assays in all cases, arguing that in contrast to community-acquired pneumonia, it may be difficult to:

1. Determine whether or not pneumonia has developed in hospitalized patients.
2. Precisely identify the responsible pathogens, in the case of infection, and thereby select the optimal antimicrobial treatment.
3. Prevent resorting to broad-spectrum drug coverage in all patients suspected of having pneumonia, with the risk of favoring the emergence of multiresistant pathogens by treating patients without infection with unnecessary antibiotics.

In contrast, proponents of an empirical approach state that bronchoscopy is an invasive, time-consuming, and expensive procedure based on techniques difficult to implement in most ICUs that also results in some false-negative findings in patients with true pneumonia.[118] Furthermore, they insist that these techniques should be first validated in a prospective, randomized trial demonstrating that they improve survival or other meaningful endpoints, such as antibiotic usage, antimicrobial resistance, antibiotic complications, or costs compared with clinical diagnosis, before they can be used in clinical practice.

Halfway between these two strategies, some other investigators have proposed the use of simplified diagnostic protocols based on either quantitative cultures of endotracheal aspirates or nonbronchoscopic techniques, such as "blind" peripheral protected brushing or BAL, that would further simplify diagnostic procedures and reduce costs.[119-123]

Before these different strategies currently proposed for patients thought to have nosocomial pneumonia are examined, three points deserve further comments.

First, whereas VAP carries a significant excess morbidity and mortality,[45, 50-57] tracheobronchitis alone does not seem to be associated with a poor prognosis, and many investigators therefore agree that antimicrobial treatment of patients with tracheobronchitis alone is probably not justified. Using reliable techniques to identify patients with nosocomial pneumonia, including PSB and BAL, Fagon and colleagues[45] undertook a cohort study in which patients who had pneumonia and control subjects were carefully matched for the severity of underlying illness and other important variables, such as age, indication for ventilatory support, and duration of exposure to risk. The results clearly indicated that mortality attributable to VAP exceeded 25%, confirming other previous studies.[50-57] Interestingly, however, when the 23 pairs of patients were evaluated separately in whom the control subjects were initially suspected of having pneumonia on the basis of clinical features but for whom the diagnosis was subsequently excluded on the basis of negative PSB and BAL specimens and clinical follow-up, the authors found that the mortality rate of these control subjects with fever, pulmonary infiltrates, and purulent tracheal secretions but without pneumonia (26%) was not different from that of the entire control group (27%). Other investigators have found similar results, studying outcome of patients who were clinically suspected of having nosocomial pneumonia but in whom this diagnosis was finally excluded.[14, 18, 124] Although these patients had a lower mortality than that of patients with definite pneumonia, their mortality was identical to that observed in patients not suspected of having pneumonia.

In a study comparing patients clinically suspected of having nosocomial pneumonia with bacteriologic confirmation of *Pseudomonas* or *Acinetobacter* spp. pneumonia (PSB quantitative cultures of 10^3 CFU/mL or more) with those without bacteriologic confirmation (PSB quantitative cultures isolating less than 10^3 CFU/mL of *P. aeruginosa* or *Acinetobacter* spp.), our group found a highly significant difference in mortality rates between the two groups (73% among patients with pneumonia and 29% among patients with low bacterial burden, $P < .001$).[125] These findings support the conclusion that it is pneumonia per se that is associated with poorer survival, not the presence of fever, infiltrates, or purulent tracheal secretions.

Second, survival of patients may improve when pneumonia is correctly diagnosed and treated. Using multiple logistic regression analysis to study risk factors for death in ventilated patients in whom pneumonia developed, Torres and coworkers[28] demonstrated that inappropriate therapy was highly related to mortality with a relative odds ratio of 5.8. Similar results were also found by Celis and associates.[13] In this study, six independent risk factors for mortality were selected by logistic regression analysis: advanced age, ultimately or rapidly fatal underlying disease, high-risk microorganisms, bilateral infiltrates on the chest radiograph, presence of respiratory failure, and inappropriate antibiotic therapy, with this last factor being the most important. Because the optimal choice of antimicrobial drugs is much easier when one or several specific etiologic agents have been identified, any strategy designed to manage ventilated patients suspected of having pulmonary infection should probably be able to precisely establish the microorganisms responsible in case of infection.

Third, although appropriate antibiotics may improve survival in patients with nosocomial pneumonia, use of empirical broad-spectrum antibiotics in patients without infection is potentially harmful, facilitating colonization and superinfection with multiresistant microorganisms. Many epidemiologic investigations have clearly demonstrated a direct relationship between the use of antimicrobial agents and increased resistance found in Enterobacteriaceae and other pathogens.[126, 127]

In a study in which only episodes confirmed by positive bronchoscopic PSB specimens were prospectively included, Rello and colleagues[48] compared risk factors, clinical complications, and outcomes of mechanically ventilated patients who had nosocomial methicillin-resistant and methicillin-sensitive *S. aureus* infection in the lower respiratory tract. Methicillin-resistant *S. aureus*–infected persons were more likely to have received corticosteroids before development of infection, to have been ventilated for more than 6 days, to have been older than 25 years, or to have chronic lung disease, but the most striking finding was that all patients with methicillin-resistant *S. aureus* infection had previously received antibiotics, compared with only 21% of those with methicillin-sensitive *S. aureus* infection. These data clearly underline that the indiscriminate use of antimicrobial agents in ICU patients may have immediate but also long-term consequences, contributing to the emergence of multiresistant pathogens and increasing the risk of serious superinfections. Virtually all reports emphasize that better antibiotic control programs to limit bacterial resistance are urgently needed in ICUs and that patients without true infection should not receive antimicrobial treatment.[123, 124] Therefore, it should be made clear to physicians confronted with ICU patients clinically suspected of having nosocomial pneumonia that treating all these patients with new antimicrobial agents may lead to overtreatment in a large number of cases and, thus, to the rapid emergence of multiresistant pathogens not only in the treated patients but also in other patients hospitalized in the same unit.

In keeping with these data, most physicians would therefore

probably agree that any policy designed to evaluate patients thought to have nosocomial pneumonia should be able to achieve the following objectives:

1. To identify patients who need treatment with antibiotics for bacterial pneumonia, without delay and without missing even a few patients with infection.
2. To select the optimal antimicrobial regimen in patients with true infection, that is, to identify the causative microorganisms.
3. To withhold antimicrobial treatment in patients without pneumonia.

PATIENTS ALREADY RECEIVING ANTIMICROBIAL THERAPY

Prior antimicrobial treatment in patients clinically suspected of nosocomial pneumonia is frequently presented as a major limitation to accurate diagnosis (Fig. 145–3). In fact, as demonstrated by Johanson and colleagues[128] and other investigators,[14, 129–131] culture results of respiratory secretions are mostly not modified when pneumonia develops as a superinfection in patients who have been receiving systemic antibiotics for several days before the appearance of the new pulmonary infiltrates, the reason being that the bacteria responsible for the new infection are then resistant to the antibiotics given previously. To further evaluate the effects of antibiotic treatment received before the suspicion of pneumonia on the diagnostic yields of the PSB technique, direct examination, and culture of lavage fluid, Timsit and coworkers[131] studied two groups of ventilated patients with suspected nosocomial pneumonia; 65 patients had received antibiotics for an earlier septic episode and 96 patients had not. Bronchoscopy was always performed before any treatment for suspected pneumonia was given. As in the reports of earlier studies described before, all but two strains recovered from distal samples of patients with definite pneumonia were highly resistant to previous antibiotics. The sensitivity and specificity of each test did not differ between the two groups of patients, confirming that previous antibiotics used to treat an earlier septic episode unrelated to suspected pneumonia do not affect the diagnostic yield of the PSB and BAL techniques.

In contrast, performing microbiologic cultures of pulmonary secretions for diagnostic purposes after initiation of new antibiotic therapy in patients suspected of having nosocomial pneumonia can clearly lead to a high number of false-negative results, regardless of the way in which these secretions are obtained. In fact, all microbiologic techniques are probably of little value in patients with a recent pulmonary infiltrate who have received new antibiotics for that reason, even for less than 24 hours. In this case, a negative finding could indicate either that the patient has been successfully treated for pneumonia and the bacteria are eradicated or that the patient had no lung infection to begin with. In one study, in which follow-up cultures of protected bronchoscopic specimens were obtained in 43 cases of proven nosocomial pneumonia, 24 and 48 hours after the onset of antimicrobial treatment, nearly 40% of cultures were negative after only 24 hours of treatment and 65% after 48 hours.[132]

Similar results were obtained by Montravers and colleagues[129] in a series of 76 consecutive patients with VAP evaluated by fiberoptic bronchoscopy after 3 days of treatment. In this study, with use of follow-up PSB sample cultures to directly assess the infection site in the lung, 88% of patients had negative cultures after the onset of treatment.

These two clinical situations should be clearly distinguished before interpretation of pulmonary secretion culture results, however they were obtained (see Fig. 145–3). In the second situation, when the patient had received new antibiotics after the appearance of the signs suggesting the presence of pulmonary infection, no conclusion concerning the presence or absence of pneumonia can be drawn if culture results are negative. Pulmonary secretions therefore need to be obtained before new antibiotics are administered, as is the case for all types of microbiologic samples.

DIAGNOSTIC STRATEGY BASED ON CLINICAL EVALUATION ALONE

The classic clinical findings of pneumonia (e.g., new fever, new pulmonary infiltrate, cough, sputum production, elevated

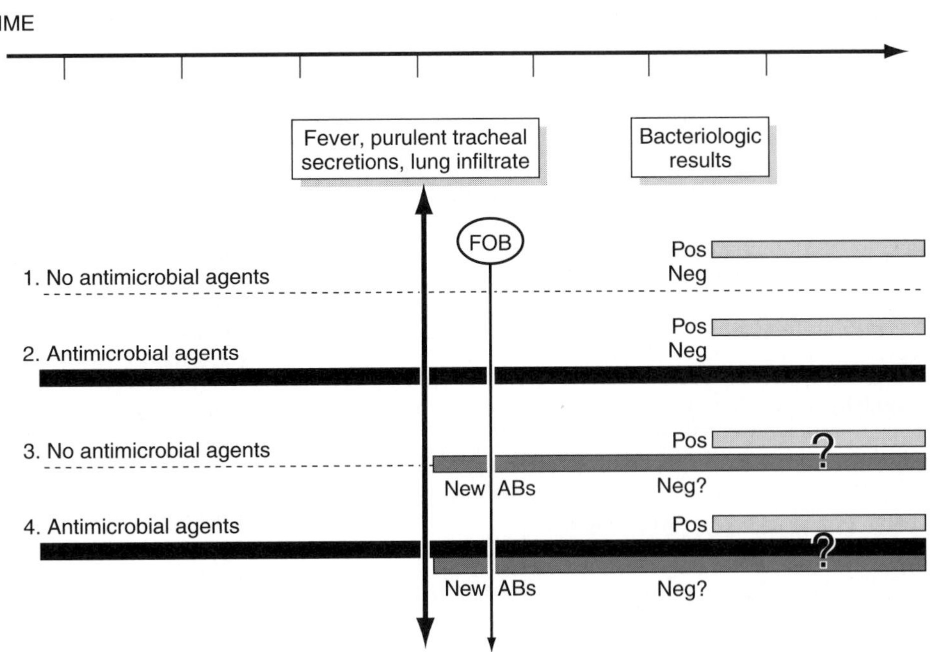

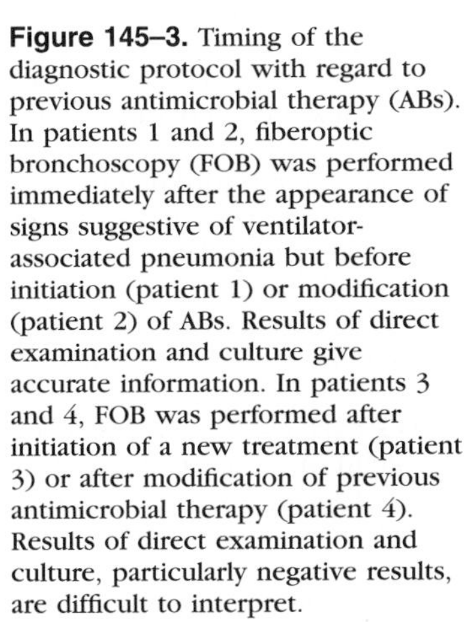
Figure 145–3. Timing of the diagnostic protocol with regard to previous antimicrobial therapy (ABs). In patients 1 and 2, fiberoptic bronchoscopy (FOB) was performed immediately after the appearance of signs suggestive of ventilator-associated pneumonia but before initiation (patient 1) or modification (patient 2) of ABs. Results of direct examination and culture give accurate information. In patients 3 and 4, FOB was performed after initiation of a new treatment (patient 3) or after modification of previous antimicrobial therapy (patient 4). Results of direct examination and culture, particularly negative results, are difficult to interpret.

leukocyte count) may not be present in the hospitalized patient with nosocomial pneumonia. Alternatively, these findings may be present but may not be caused by pneumonia. Most critically ill patients have serious underlying disease, increased oropharyngeal colonization with hospital flora, and numerous reasons for elevated body temperature and leukocytosis. Chest radiographic changes consistent with pneumonia may be caused by pulmonary edema, pulmonary infection, or atelectasis. Furthermore, microscopic evaluation and culture of tracheal secretions are frequently inconclusive because the upper respiratory tract of most ventilated patients is colonized with potential pulmonary pathogens, whether or not deep pulmonary infection is present.[71] Therefore, studies evaluating the usefulness of clinical parameters and tracheal secretions in identifying ventilated patients with nosocomial pneumonia have generally been disappointing.[133–137]

In one study conducted in 84 ventilated patients thought to have lung infection, Fagon and colleagues[135] prospectively compared the diagnostic predictions independently formulated by a team of physicians aware of all clinical, radiologic, and laboratory data, including the results of Gram-stained bronchial aspirates, with those resulting from a complete work-up including quantitative culture results of PSB specimens. The results showed that only 27 of the 84 clinically suspected patients actually had pneumonia and that the presence of pneumonia was accurately diagnosed in only 62% of the predictions. The mean value of temperature, blood leukocytes and blood lymphocytes, Pa_{O_2}/FIO_2, and radiologic score and changes in temperature, blood leukocytes, and radiologic score in the preceding 3 days were not different in patients who had pneumonia and those who did not, confirming previous data[133, 134] and the fact that no objective clinical criteria exist for differentiating patients who have pneumonia from those who do not.

Even when the clinical diagnosis of pneumonia is accurate, results of Gram's stain examination and culture of tracheal aspirates could be misleading when the appropriate antibiotics are chosen. In the study cited before, only 33% of the treatments proposed for patients subsequently diagnosed as having pneumonia proved to be effective despite the fact that the physicians who were questioned in this study usually used combination antibiotic regimens that are currently considered to be standard therapy for nosocomial pneumonia.[135] These results confirm the difficulty in selecting an initial antibiotic regimen for treatment of suspected pneumonia in hospitalized patients. Because of the emergence of multiresistant extended-spectrum β-lactamase–producing gram-negative pathogens in many institutions and the increasing role played by gram-positive bacteria, such as methicillin-resistant *S. aureus*, even a protocol combining amikacin and imipenem would not ensure adequate coverage of all cases of nosocomial pneumonia in these ICUs. In a study of 50 patients with suspected VAP who underwent a systematic diagnostic protocol designed to identify all potential causes of fever and pulmonary densities, Meduri and colleagues[137] confirmed that lung infection was present in only 42% of cases and that the frequent occurrence of multiple infectious and noninfectious processes justifies a systematic search for the source of fever in this setting.

The only two advantages of this clinical approach are its simplicity and, when all patients with a clinical suspicion of pneumonia are treated with new antibiotics, its sensitivity, alleviating the risk of not treating a patient with a true lung infection.

USE OF BRONCHOSCOPIC TECHNIQUES

Protected Specimen Brush Technique

To reduce contamination of lower airway aspirates collected by bronchoscopy, Wimberley and colleagues[138] in the late 1970s developed the PSB technique, which became commercially available in 1979. This method is in fact based on the combination of four different techniques:

1. Fiberoptic bronchoscopy to directly sample the site of inflammation in the lung.
2. A special double-catheter brush system with a distal occluding plug to reduce contamination of lower airway aspirates by the flora colonizing the proximal airways.
3. A brush to calibrate the volume of respiratory secretions obtained.
4. A quantitative culture technique to aid in distinguishing between airway colonization and serious underlying infection, with the cutoff threshold between the two set at 10^3 CFU/mL.

Because the PSB collects between 0.01 and 0.001 mL of secretions, the presence of more than 10^3 bacteria in the originally diluted sample (1 mL) represents a concentration of at least 10^5 to 10^6 CFU/mL of respiratory secretions. To obtain meaningful results with the PSB technique, however, one must follow a precise method, as summarized in an International Consensus Conference.[139]

The potential value of the PSB technique to evaluate ventilated patients suspected of having pneumonia has been extensively investigated in both human and animal studies, including five investigations in which the cultural accuracy of this technique was determined by comparison with both histologic features and quantitative cultures from the same area of the lung.[128, 130, 140–146] Many investigators have now confirmed that secretions obtained with use of this technique can ensure optimal antimicrobial treatment for most patients with pneumonia without resorting to broad-spectrum drugs in all patients clinically suspected of having pneumonia.[13, 14, 26, 45, 48, 64, 65, 119–124, 129–135, 137, 147–149] Nevertheless, some controversy persists in the literature concerning the sensitivity of this technique, especially for detecting some cases of pneumonia in patients already receiving antimicrobial treatment.[117, 118]

Four studies using a protocol based on postmortem lung biopsies have suggested that in the presence of prior antibiotic treatment, many patients with histopathologic signs of pneumonia have no or only minimal growth from lung and bronchoscopic specimen cultures.[143–146] In one study, lesions of bronchopneumonia were characterized by bacterial concentrations of more than 10^3 CFU per gram of lung tissue in only 55% of lobes, and one third of lung segments with histologic bronchopneumonia remained negative even when submitted for culture.[144]

However, several constraints specific to the evaluation of any procedure used in the diagnosis of bacterial pneumonia must be respected, even with a model in which the "gold standard" includes both histologic features and quantitative cultures of lung tissue.

First, diagnostic methods based on microbiologic techniques can only document, both qualitatively and quantitatively, the bacterial burden present in lung tissue. In no case can these techniques retrospectively identify a resolving pneumonia, at a time when antimicrobial treatment and lung antibacterial defenses might have been successful in suppressing microbial growth in lung tissue.

Second, although several studies have shown that there are at least 10^4 microorganisms per gram of tissue once bacterial infection of the lung is clinically apparent,[128, 130, 142] this assumption is valid only when patients have not received appropriate antimicrobial treatment after the onset of lung infection before lung cultures are obtained. Therefore, to evaluate the cultural accuracy of any microbiologic technique using lung cultures as the gold standard, it is absolutely imperative that no new antibiotics have been introduced during this time interval.

Third, use of histologic criteria as a reference implies that the patient did not have a lung infection before the episode to be evaluated; otherwise, it would be difficult if not impossible to distinguish a recent infection from the sequelae of the previous one and thus to correctly interpret the results of the diagnostic tools that are being evaluated.

Finally, lesions of bronchopneumonia in patients with VAP may be limited to some foci of infection in the lungs.[144] Therefore, if postmortem tissue samples are too small, the histologic diagnosis of pneumonia can be underestimated with use of this technique. On the contrary, however, because a diagnostic technique based on peripheral samplings can provide information only on the lung segment from which specimens have been taken, so-called false-negative PSB or BAL results, as defined by entire examination of the lung, can be explained by the absence of pneumonia at the very level of the sampling area.

Unfortunately, in the studies by Papazian,[146] Torres,[143] and Marquette[145] and their coworkers, many patients had pneumonia several days before their death, and lung cultures were in fact obtained during the recovery phase of the infection, at a time when antimicrobial therapy and lung antibacterial defenses might have been successful in suppressing microbial growth in lung tissue and therefore in pulmonary secretions. Even a few doses of an effective antimicrobial agent can rapidly decrease or even transiently eliminate bacterial counts in the lung and thereby invalidate all comparisons between microbiologic and histologic features of the lung.[129, 132] Interestingly, when analyses in these studies were restrained to patients with no prior antibiotics or when only lung tissue cultures were used as the gold standard, results obtained by use of bronchoscopic techniques for diagnosing nosocomial pneumonia were much better, with a sensitivity always greater than 80%.

Other studies have confirmed the accuracy of bronchoscopic techniques for diagnosing nosocomial pneumonia. In a study evaluating spontaneous lung infections occurring in baboons with permeability pulmonary edema and undergoing mechanical ventilation, Johanson and colleagues[128] found an excellent correlation between the bacterial content of lung tissue and results of quantitative culture of lavage fluid and PSB specimens. BAL recovered 74% of all species present in lung tissue, including 100% of those present at a concentration of 10^4 CFU per gram of tissue or higher. In this study, PSB specimens identified only 41% of all species recovered from lung tissue, but only microorganisms present at low concentrations in the lung were missed; 78% of species present at concentrations above 10^4 CFU per gram of tissue were correctly isolated.

Similarly, in a study of 20 ventilated patients who had not had pneumonia before the terminal phase of their disease and who had no recent changes in antimicrobial therapy, Chastre and associates[130] found that bronchoscopic PSB specimens obtained just after death were able to identify 80% of all species present in the lung, with a strong correlation between the results of quantitative cultures of both specimens. By use of a discriminative value of 10^3 CFU/mL or higher to define positive PSB cultures, this technique identified lung segments yielding 10^4 bacteria per gram of tissue or more with a sensitivity of 82% and a specificity of 89%. These findings confirm that bronchoscopic PSB samples reliably identify, both qualitatively and quantitatively, microorganisms present in lung segments with bacterial pneumonia, even when the infection develops as a superinfection in a patient already receiving antimicrobial treatment for several days.

However, three major drawbacks are still inherent in this technique:

1. Even with use of the most accurate threshold of 10^3 CFU/mL to distinguish patients with airway colonization from those with deep lung infection, a small number of false-positive results may be observed.[150]

2. Results of such cultures require 24 to 48 hours, and therefore no information is available to guide initial decisions concerning the appropriateness of antimicrobial therapy and which antibiotics should be used.

3. The PSB technique can yield negative results in patients with pneumonia in the following situations: (a) bronchoscopy performed at an early stage of infection with a bacterial burden below the concentration necessary to reach diagnostic significance, (b) specimens obtained from an unaffected segment, (c) specimens incorrectly processed, or (d) specimens obtained after initiation of a new antimicrobial therapy, as indicated before. Values within one $\log_{10}$ of the cutoff must therefore be interpreted cautiously, and fiberoptic bronchoscopy should be repeated in symptomatic patients with a negative ($<10^3$ CFU/mL) result.[124] Given the high mortality and morbidity rates of nosocomial pneumonia in ICU patients, even a low ($<15\%$) rate of false-negative results is probably unacceptable in clinical practice.

Bronchoalveolar Lavage

To overcome these drawbacks, many investigators have proposed the use of BAL to sample the suspected area in the lung. This technique is a safe and practical method for obtaining cells and secretions lining the lower respiratory tract from a large area of the lung. Many authors have now investigated the value of BAL quantitative culture in the diagnosis of pneumonia in mechanically ventilated patients.[64, 122, 128, 130, 131, 139, 148, 149, 151, 152] Although some investigators have concluded that BAL provides the best reflection of the lung's bacterial burden, both quantitatively and qualitatively, others have reported mixed results with poor specificity of BAL fluid cultures in patients with high tracheobronchial colonization. In one study from Chastre and coworkers,[130] using a protocol based on postmortem lung biopsies, the results obtained by quantitative cultures of BAL fluid proved to be as useful as those of PSB cultures.

Whatever the true usefulness of BAL quantitative cultures for a specific diagnosis of pneumonia, this technique allows harvesting of cells and secretions from a large area of the lung that can be microscopically examined immediately after the procedure to detect the presence or absence of intracellular or extracellular bacteria in the lower respiratory tract.[151] Several studies have confirmed the diagnostic value of this approach to provide rapid identification of patients with pneumonia because results are available immediately.[122, 130, 152, 153] In each study, either the Giemsa or the Gram stain was positive ($>2\%$ or 5% of BAL cells containing intracellular bacteria) in most patients with pneumonia and negative in patients without pneumonia. Furthermore, in patients with pneumonia, the morphologic appearance and Gram's staining of these bacteria were closely correlated with the result of bacterial cultures, enabling early formulation of a specific antimicrobial therapy before the results of culture were available.

We believe, therefore, that microscopic examination of BAL fluid might be easily incorporated into a protocol along with quantitative cultures of PSB samples or another reliable bronchoscopic technique to obtain uncontaminated distal secretions for cultures (Fig. 145-4). However, in a small percentage of mechanically ventilated patients, particularly in patients with severe chronic obstructive lung disease, it is virtually impossible to obtain a good return of the instilled BAL fluid. In these patients, the diagnostic value of BAL techniques is minimal and only the PSB technique can be used.

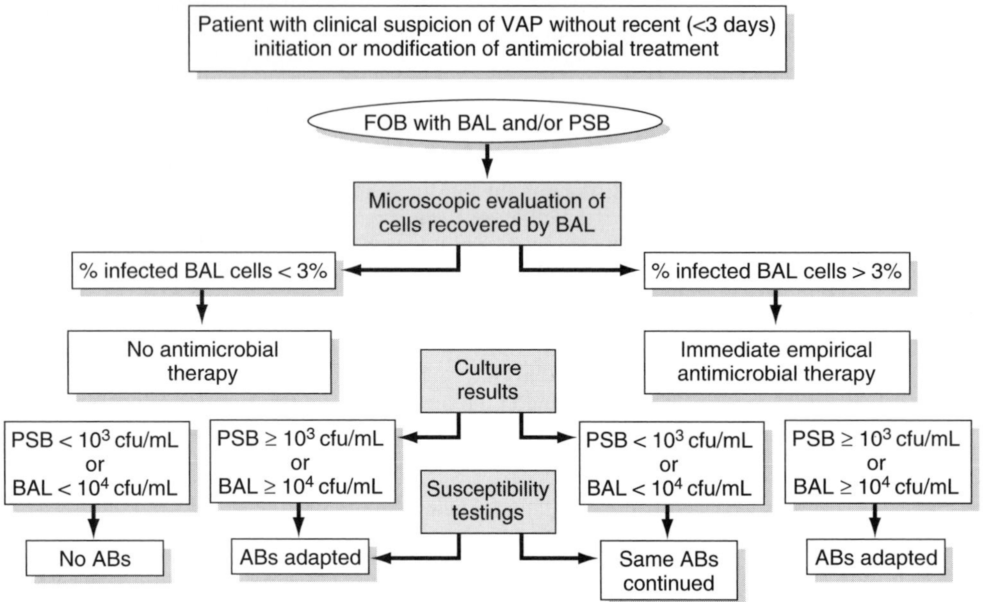

Figure 145–4. Therapeutic strategy based on results of bronchoalveolar lavage (BAL) cell examination, PSB culture, and BAL culture. VAP = ventilator-associated pneumonia; ABs = antibiotics; FOB = fiberoptic bronchoscopy.

Several potential advantages of this approach are worth emphasizing:

1. Obtaining distal pulmonary specimens from the suspected area in the lung by use of bronchoscopy with PSB and BAL is relatively simple and safe even in patients receiving mechanical ventilation for ARDS.
2. The techniques used to detect intracellular bacteria in BAL cells are easy to perform, inexpensive, and available in all hospital laboratories familiar with BAL fluid analysis.
3. Lavage may also provide useful clues for the diagnosis of other forms of respiratory failure, such as pulmonary hemorrhage or other types of infections, especially in immunocompromised patients. Clearly, the absence of detectable bacteria in BAL cells and negative quantitative PSB and BAL cultures in a patient with no recent changes in antimicrobial therapy should prompt a search for alternative explanations for respiratory dysfunction and fever.

NONBRONCHOSCOPIC TECHNIQUES

Quantitative Cultures of Endotracheal Aspirates

Although the simple qualitative culture of endotracheal aspirates is a technique with a high percentage of false-positive results because of the bacterial colonization of the proximal airways observed in most ICU patients, some studies using quantitative culture techniques suggest that culture of endotracheal aspirates may have a reasonable overall diagnostic accuracy, similar to that of several other more invasive techniques.[119, 120, 154]

In a study by Marquette and coworkers,[119] the operating characteristics of quantitative endotracheal aspirate cultures, using 10^6 CFU/mL of respiratory secretions as the interpretive cutoff point, compared favorably with those of the PSB technique, with a slightly higher sensitivity (82% versus 64%) and a lower specificity (83% versus 96%). Similarly, with use of 10^5 CFU/mL as a cutoff point for interpreting quantitative endotracheal aspirate cultures in 54 patients suspected of having pneumonia, El-Ebiary and associates[120] found that this technique represented a relatively sensitive (70%) and relatively specific (72%) method to diagnose patients with true pneumonia.

To assess the reliability of this technique, Jourdain and colleagues[154] used fiberoptic bronchoscopy with PSB and BAL to study 57 episodes of suspected lung infection in 39 ventilator-dependent patients with no recent changes in antimicrobial therapy. The operating characteristics of endotracheal aspirate cultures were calculated over a range of cutoff values (from 10^3 to 10^7 CFU/mL), and the threshold of 10^6 CFU/mL appeared to be the most accurate with a sensitivity of 68% and a specificity of 84%. However, when this threshold was applied, almost one third of the patients with pneumonia were not identified. Furthermore, only 40% of microorganisms cultured in endotracheal aspirate samples coincided with those obtained from PSB specimens. Other studies have emphasized that although quantitative endotracheal aspirate cultures can correctly identify patients with pneumonia, microbiologic results cannot be used to infer which microorganisms present in the trachea are really present in the lung.

Therefore, quantitative endotracheal aspirate cultures may be an acceptable tool for confirming the diagnosis of pneumonia when no fiberoptic techniques are available. But it must be kept in mind that this technique has several potential disadvantages:

1. Many patients may not be identified by this technique with use of the cutoff value of 10^6 CFU/mL.
2. As soon as a lower threshold is used, specificity sharply decreases and overtreatment becomes a problem.
3. Selecting antimicrobial therapy solely on the basis of endotracheal aspirate culture results can lead to either unnecessary antibiotic therapy or overtreatment with broad-spectrum antimicrobial agents. Given the potential risk of these practices in an ICU, a more rigorous diagnostic approach in such patients seems warranted whenever possible.

Quantitative Cultures of Nonbronchoscopic Distal Protected Specimens

Apparently acceptable results were recently obtained by several investigators using a nonbronchoscopic method to perform peripheral protected brushing of the lung or BAL that would further simplify the procedure and reduce costs if additional studies confirm the preliminary findings.[121-123, 155-158] For example, in a study of 78 suspected episodes of nosocomial pneumonia in 55 patients, Pham and colleagues[123] found that a protected telescoping catheter (PTC) gave results similar to those obtained with the PSB technique in 74% of cases. A major discrepancy was observed between the two techniques in only 20 episodes, including six false-negative PSB results in episodes of proven pneumonia, four possible false-positive PSB results, and 10 possible false-positive PTC results. Furthermore, blind or directed PTC samples showed a similar concordance with PSB samples taken by bronchoscopy. Similar results were obtained by Kollef and associates[158] in a study of 42 patients suspected of having VAP on the basis of clinical evidence. With use of 10^3 CFU/mL as the threshold to define a positive mini-BAL, a good diagnostic agreement was shown for quantitative cultures obtained with the PSB and mini-BAL technique (kappa statistic, 0.63; concordance, 83.3%).

Although autopsy studies indicate that pneumonia in ventilator-dependent patients has often spread into every pulmonary lobe and predominantly involves the posterior portion of the lower lobes,[143-145] two clinical studies of ventilated patients with pneumonia contradict these findings because some patients had sterile PSB specimen cultures of the noninvolved lung.[157, 159] Furthermore, in most studies that formed conclusions on the comparable sensitivities of nonbronchoscopic and bronchoscopic techniques, the overall concordance was in fact only approximately 80%, emphasizing the fact that in some patients, the diagnosis could be missed by this technique, especially in the case of pneumonia involving the upper lobes or the left lung, as demonstrated by Jorda and coworkers.[156]

Our bias is therefore to prefer bronchoscopic techniques in most patients suspected of having pneumonia to be sure not to miss the infected area in the lung and to be able to withhold antimicrobial agents with confidence in patients with negative results. However, nonbronchoscopic techniques represent a good alternative in patients with unstable conditions and in patients for whom it is not possible to delay the initiation of antimicrobial treatment while awaiting bronchoscopy.

EVALUATION OF DIAGNOSTIC STRATEGIES

The diagnosis of bacterial pneumonia in the severely ill, mechanically ventilated patient remains a difficult dilemma for the clinician. A large amount of data has evaluated the diagnostic techniques cited in the preceding discussion by use of more or less adequate methodology. However, definite response was not given by these types of studies, and considerable debate persists.

Another type of study has recently tested invasive diagnostic strategy by evaluating outcome consequences and impact on antibiotic use.[160-163] A first study by Alvarez-Lerma and the ICU-Acquired Pneumonia Study Group[160] demonstrated a high percentage (44%) of patients with clinical signs of ICU-acquired pneumonia requiring modification of initial empirical antibiotic treatment on the basis of a noninvasive diagnostic approach. Luna and colleagues[161] studied 132 patients suspected of having VAP and retrospectively compared antibiotic treatment given before BAL (performed within 24 hours of the establishment of the clinical diagnosis of VAP), immediately after BAL (without use of direct examination of liquid obtained by BAL), and after results of BAL cultures were obtained. The authors suggested that bronchoscopy can accurately define the cause of VAP but that this information becomes available too late to affect survival. Specifically, six of the 16 patients with adequate pre-BAL treatment died, versus nine of 15 patients without initiated treatment (NS) and 31 of 34 patients not adequately treated before BAL. Modifications of antimicrobial treatment made just after BAL were not, in fact, influenced by BAL results (not obtained at this time), and only comparison of treatments modified after the results of BAL cultures with those prescribed after BAL partially evaluated the "BAL impact" in this study. The pre-BAL treatment was based only on speculative knowledge. Clearly, this study does not demonstrate that BAL improves outcome and survival, but it does not demonstrate the opposite. The only documented result is that early appropriate treatment is probably better than early inappropriate treatment or delayed appropriate treatment for management of patients with true VAP.

Rello and colleagues[162] prospectively studied 113 patients with VAP and evaluated the value of bronchoscopic results in guiding antibiotic choice and influencing outcome. They demonstrated that bronchoscopic results revealed inadequate initial selection (based on clinical evaluation) of antibiotics in 24% of cases and led to a change in antibiotic treatment leading to clinical resolution in 63% of patients; in addition, bronchoscopic results permitted the reduction of the antibiotic spectrum in 6% of cases. These modifications were associated with significant reduction of related mortality (37.0% versus 15.6%, $P < .05$). In this study, the critical importance of an appropriate early antibiotic therapy was also emphasized. Bonten and associates[163] analyzed the effects of implementation of PSB and BAL bronchoscopy on antibiotic prescription. They showed that among 66 patients in whom a clinical suspicion of VAP was not confirmed by invasive procedures, only 18 (27%) were treated with antibiotics, and antibiotic therapy was withheld in 35% of the 138 patients who underwent bronchoscopy. Withholding of antibiotic therapy had no negative effect on the recurrence of clinical suspicion of VAP or on mortality rate.

To date, pending the results of randomized studies comparing the effects of these two different strategies on the outcome of ICU ventilated patients, there is no direct evidence that the use of a strategy based on the more invasive-specific samples is associated with improved outcome, reduced antibiotic usage, and decreased antibiotic resistance. However, our bias is that the use of bronchoscopic techniques to obtain PSB and BAL specimens from the affected area in the lung in patients with signs suggestive of pneumonia allows definition of a therapeutic strategy superior to that based exclusively on clinical evaluation. These bronchoscopic techniques, when they are performed before introduction of new antibiotics, enable physicians to identify most patients who need immediate treatment and help to select optimal therapy, in a manner that is safe and well tolerated by patients. On the other hand, these techniques prevent resorting to broad-spectrum drug coverage in all patients in whom development of infection is clinically suspected.

Therefore, although the true impact of this decision tree on outcome of patients has not yet been established, available data clearly suggest that being able to withhold antimicrobial treatment in some patients without infection may constitute a distinct advantage in the long term by minimizing the emergence of resistant microorganisms in the ICU. In patients with clinical evidence of severe sepsis with rapid worsening organ dysfunction, hypoperfusion, or hypotension, the initiation of antibiotic therapy should not, however, be delayed while awaiting bronchoscopy, and patients should be given immediate treatment with antibiotics. It is probably in this situation that simplified nonbronchoscopic diagnostic procedures could find their best justification, allowing distal pulmonary secretions to be obtained on a 24-hour basis, just before new antimicrobial therapy is started.

EVALUATION OF CURRENT ANTIMICROBIAL STRATEGIES

Despite many advances in antimicrobial therapy, successful treatment of patients with nosocomial pneumonia remains a difficult and complex undertaking. No consensus has been reached concerning issues as basic as the optimal antimicrobial regimen for therapy or duration of treatment. Although some investigators have recommended two-drug parenteral therapy for most cases, recent data have demonstrated the efficacy of newer β-lactam antibiotics as monotherapy for some patients. Similarly, the efficacy of endotracheal or aerosolized antibiotics as either the sole or adjunctive therapy for gram-negative pneumonia remains controversial. In fact, to date, evaluation of various antimicrobial strategies for the treatment of bacterial pneumonia in mechanically ventilated patients has been difficult for several reasons concerning clinical and bacteriologic diagnosis of VAP, as cited before.

Montravers and coworkers[129] evaluated the bacteriologic and clinical efficacy of antimicrobial therapies, selected on the basis of the etiologic microorganisms identified by cultures of PSB samples obtained during bronchoscopy, for the treatment of nosocomial bacterial pneumonia in 76 patients receiving mechanical ventilation. By use of follow-up PSB sample culture to directly assess the infection site in the lung, their results demonstrated that the administration of an antimicrobial therapy combining, in most cases, two effective agents was able to sterilize or contain the lower respiratory tract infection after only 3 days of treatment in 67 (88%) of the patients included in the study. The only two bacteriologic failures were observed in patients who did not receive adequate treatment because of errors in the selection of antimicrobial drugs. However, early superinfection due to bacteria resistant to the initial antibiotics was documented in seven patients (9%), emphasizing the need to carefully monitor the impact of treatment on the initial microbial flora for optimal management of such patients when the clinical response is suboptimal. Furthermore, results of cultures of follow-up PSB samples were well correlated with the clinical outcome noted during the 15-day observation period, making this test a good prognostic indicator in patients with nosocomial bacterial pneumonia. Although the percentage of patients with clinical improvement was 96% and 82%, in patients with sterilized or persistent low-grade infection, respectively, it was only 44% in patients with persistent high-grade infection.[129] Use of such techniques to directly sample the infection site in the lung may therefore provide, in future studies, a more rigorous evaluation of different antimicrobial strategies.

CONVENTIONAL EMPIRICAL THERAPY

Initial antimicrobial therapy often has to be selected empirically for cases of suspected pneumonia in which microscopic examination of sputum or tracheal aspirate smears does not provide a presumptive etiologic diagnosis. Because, in such cases, selected therapy must be broad enough to ensure coverage of aerobic, gram-negative bacilli, including such potentially highly resistant organisms as *P. aeruginosa, S. marcescens, Enterobacter cloacae,* and *Acinetobacter* spp., combination therapy with either an anti-*Pseudomonas* penicillin plus an aminoglycoside or an anti-*Pseudomonas* cephalosporin plus an aminoglycoside has long been the cornerstone of therapy and is currently the initial regimen recommended by many authorities in this setting.[1, 16, 164] However, treatment must not ignore the increasing role played by gram-positive bacteria, particularly in institutions in which methicillin-resistant *S. aureus* is endemic or epidemic, and vancomycin should therefore also be part of the empirical treatment in these ICUs. Additional drugs should also be considered under certain circumstances. For example, in patients with significant aspiration, adequate coverage of anaerobes should be included in the treatment regimen. Imipenem is a useful alternative for mixed aerobic-anaerobic infections. Finally, when *Legionella* species are endemic or in patients presenting with atypical pneumonia, erythromycin should be started.

FACTORS CONTRIBUTING TO BETTER SELECTION OF TREATMENT

Several important factors must be considered to better select optimal initial antibiotic therapy. These factors include the following:

- Putative causative pathogens and their patterns of antibiotic susceptibilities as observed in previous cases of nosocomial pneumonia, based on epidemiologic studies and data obtained by surveillance cultures in the same patient
- Prior duration of hospitalization or mechanical ventilation before the onset of pneumonia
- Prior usage of antimicrobial agents
- Information provided by direct microscopic examination of pulmonary secretions
- Intrinsic antibacterial activities of antimicrobial agents
- Other pharmacokinetic considerations

Etiologic Agents

As indicated before, several U.S. (National Nosocomial Infections Surveillance System) and European (EPIC study) multicenter surveys have confirmed not only the important role played by gram-negative bacteria, because such microorganisms account for six of the top 10 etiologic agents identified, but also the predominant role played by *S. aureus*, which now ranks first in most surveys.[20, 21, 66, 67] Thus, although the exact prevalence of each infecting microorganism may vary as a function of countries, hospitals, and wards concerned, a precise knowledge of the distribution of the pathogens most frequently reported to be associated with pneumonia greatly facilitates the selection of appropriate therapy as well as information about their antibiotic sensitivity patterns as previously determined.

Several epidemiologic studies of nosocomial pneumonia in patients receiving mechanical ventilation have reported an increased rate of multiresistant bacteria.[14, 19, 20, 48, 65] Many *P. aeruginosa* and *A. baumannii* strains are now class I cephalosporinase producers and are resistant to piperacillin, aztreonam, and ceftazidime. *Klebsiella pneumoniae* strains are also increasingly recognized as producers of transferable expanded-spectrum β-lactamases, which confer resistance to third-generation cephalosporins.[165] Other multiresistant aerobic gram-negative bacilli include *Stenotrophomonas maltophilia* and *Alcaligenes* spp. Unfortunately, methicillin-resistant *S. aureus* is also more and more frequently implicated as a causative pathogen in ICU patients requiring mechanical ventilation for a long time. The microbiologic trends in nosocomial pneumonia are therefore evolving toward more resistant and more difficult to treat pathogens.

Clinical Setting

As discussed before, underlying diseases may predispose patients to infection with specific organisms.

Taking into account the epidemiologic characteristics allows the definition of a more rational decision tree for selecting initial treatment in this setting. For example, the

TABLE 145–8. Definition of Severe Hospital-Acquired Pneumonia

1. Admission to intensive care unit
2. Respiratory failure, defined as the need for mechanical ventilation or the need for more than 35% oxygen to maintain an arterial oxygen saturation above 90%
3. Rapid radiographic progression, multilobar pneumonia, or cavitation of a lung infiltrate
4. Evidence of severe sepsis with hypotension and/or end-organ dysfunction:
   a. Shock (systolic blood pressure < 90 mm Hg, or diastolic blood pressure < 60 mm Hg)
   b. Requirement for vasopressors for more than 4 hr
   c. Urine output < 20 mL/hr or total urine output < 80 mL in 4 hr (unless another explanation is available)
5. Acute renal failure requiring dialysis

From American Thoracic Society: Hospital-acquired pneumonia in adults: Diagnosis, assessment of severity, initial antimicrobial therapy, and preventative strategies. Am J Respir Crit Care Med 1995; 153:1711–1725.

American Thoracic Society[164] published a Consensus Statement that provides guidelines based on assessments of disease severity, the presence of risk factors for specific organisms, and time at onset of pneumonia to guide initial antibiotic selection. Once these determinations are made, patients suspected of having nosocomial pneumonia fall into one of three groups, each with its own likely set of pathogens. These groups include the following:

1. Patients without unusual risk factors who present with mild-to-moderate pneumonia with onset at any time during hospitalization or severe pneumonia of early onset.
2. Patients with specific risk factors who present with mild-to-moderate pneumonia occurring any time during hospitalization.
3. Patients with severe pneumonia either of early onset with specific risk factors or of late onset.

Definition of severe pneumonia is given in Table 145–8; recommended therapeutic regimens in ICU patients or in patients with risk factors for pneumonia due to *P. aeruginosa* are given in Table 145–9.

On the basis of results of a prospective study in which Trouillet and coworkers[69] documented the microorganisms responsible for infection in 135 consecutive episodes of VAP using bronchoscopic specimens (see Table 145–5), a more rational decision tree for selecting initial treatment was influenced by two factors: the duration of mechanical ventilation before the onset of pneumonia and previous antimicrobial therapy; such a strategy avoids resorting to broad-spectrum drug coverage in all patients. For example, monotherapy with a second-generation cephalosporin (cefuroxime, cefamandole, cefotiam) or a combination agent in which a β-lactamase inhibitor, clavulanic acid, is added to amoxicillin would generally be an appropriate choice for most patients with early-onset pneumonia who have not received prior antimicrobial treatment (Table 145–10). In contrast, in patients who have required previous prolonged mechanical ventilation and antimicrobial treatment, a triple combination therapy with either an anti-*Pseudomonas* cephalosporin plus an aminoglycoside or imipenem plus aminoglycoside and vancomycin should be started, being aware that even such a regimen will not ensure adequate coverage of all putative pathogens (Table 145–11; see also Table 145–10).

TABLE 145–9. Patients with Severe Hospital-Acquired Pneumonia of Late Onset*

Core Organisms, Plus	Therapy
Pseudomonas aeruginosa *Acinetobacter* species	Aminoglycoside or ciprofloxacin *plus* one of the following: Antipseudomonal penicillin Combination β-lactam/β-lactamase inhibitor Ceftazidime or cefoperazone Imipenem Aztreonam†
Consider methicillin-resistant *Staphylococcus aureus*	± Vancomycin

*Excludes patients with immunosuppression.

†Aztreonam efficacy is limited to enteric gram-negative bacilli and should not be used in combination with an aminoglycoside if gram-positive or *Hemophilus influenzae* infection of concern.

From American Thoracic Society: Hospital-acquired pneumonia in adults: Diagnosis, assessment of severity, initial antimicrobial therapy, and preventative strategies. Am J Respir Crit Med 1995; 153:1711–1725.

Information Provided by Direct Examination of Pulmonary Secretions

Direct microscopic examination of pulmonary secretions is extremely important not only to identify patients with true nosocomial pneumonia but also to select appropriate treatment, especially if bronchoalveolar specimens are used to prepare cytocentrifuged Gram-stained smears. Several studies have confirmed that the morphologic characteristics and Gram staining of the bacteria disclosed by this technique are closely correlated with the results of bacterial cultures, enabling early formulation of a specific antimicrobial therapy before the results of culture are available.[122, 130, 131, 151]

Intrinsic Antibacterial Activities of Antimicrobial Agents

The interactions between bacteria and antimicrobial agents as tested in vitro by means of standard techniques are important for a therapeutic decision, although a wide variety of factors may influence the antibacterial activity of most antibiotics at the pulmonary site of infection.

The role of aminoglycosides in treating nosocomial pneumonia deserves further comment because of the existence of conflicting data. Evidence exists that aminoglycosides are more active than β-lactam antibiotics against certain resistant, gram-negative bacilli. The bactericidal mode of action, the concentration-dependent killing rate and postantibiotic effect, and the synergism with β-lactam compounds are clear advantages of these antimicrobial drugs. However, because the therapeutic ratios for aminoglycosides in serum are narrow, the

TABLE 145–10. Patients with Early-Onset Pneumonia Who Have Not Received Previous Antimicrobial Treatment

Core Organism	Monotherapy (*with one of the following*)
Streptococcus pneumoniae *Haemophilus influenzae* Sensitive enteric (non-pseudomonal) gram-negative bacilli, such as: *Escherichia coli* *Klebsiella* spp. *Proteus* spp. *Enterobacter* spp. *Serratia marcescens* Methicillin-sensitive *Staphylococcus aureus*	Penicillin/β-lactamase inhibitor combination (amoxicillin/clavulanic acid) Cephalosporin: Second generation (cefamandole, cefuroxime) Non-pseudomonal third generation (cefotaxime, ceftriaxone)

TABLE 145–11. Comparison of Patients with Early-Onset Pneumonia and Previous Antimicrobial Treatment and Patients with Late-Onset Pneumonia and No Previous Antimicrobial Treatment

Core Organisms Plus	Aminoglycoside or Ciprofloxacin (Plus one of the Following)
Pseudomonas aeruginosa	Anti-pseudomonal penicillin/β-lactamase
Stenotrophomonas maltophilia	Inhibitor combination (piperacillin/tazobactam, ticarcillin/clavulanic acid)
Multidrug-resistant enteric gram-negative bacilli such as:	Ceftazidime or cefoperazone
Enterobacter spp.	Cefepime or cefpirome
Citrobacter spp.	Imipenem
Morganella morganii	
Indole positive *Proteus* spp.	
Serratia marcescens	

penetration of circulating aminoglycosides into infected lung tissues may be insufficient to eradicate infecting organisms, and the low pH of infected airways has the potential to inactivate these agents. Consequently, these agents are now essentially used in combination with β-lactam antibiotics. To improve levels in respiratory secretions and tissues without increasing toxicity, alternative forms of application have been also investigated, such as direct instillation of aminoglycosides into the bronchial tree or single large daily dosing.[166, 167] However, further studies are necessary before the relative risks and benefits of these forms of treatment can be clearly defined.

The third-generation cephalosporins may be divided into two groups, depending on their activity on *P. aeruginosa*. For example, ceftazidime and cefoperazone exhibit excellent in vitro activity against *P. aeruginosa,* but unfortunately, these agents demonstrate a considerable loss of activity against *S. aureus* compared with other cephalosporins. Conversely, cefotaxime, ceftriaxone, cefepime, and cefpirome exhibit acceptable or good in vitro activity against *S. aureus* but relatively weak in vitro activity against *P. aeruginosa*. The third-generation cephalosporins therefore do not provide a complete solution to achieve monodrug coverage of the appropriate gram-positive and gram-negative bacterial spectrum for nosocomial pneumonia.

The in vitro spectrum of imipenem-cilastatin exceeds that of any other single agent. It provides bactericidal activity against most gram-positive cocci (except methicillin-resistant *S. aureus* and enterococci), most gram-negative bacilli including *P. aeruginosa,* and also most pathogenic anaerobes. The drawbacks for this agent, however, include reports of emergence of resistant organisms during therapy and seizures when high doses are given to patients with renal dysfunction. Furthermore, the rate of *Pseudomonas* strains resistant to imipenem is increasing. In our hospital, in 1992, 21% of 762 strains of *Pseudomonas* collected were resistant to this agent. Fortunately, 41% of these imipenem-resistant strains were sensitive to ticarcillin and ceftazidime.[168] New carbapenem agents are in development. In a multicenter randomized study, Sieger and colleagues[169] evaluated the efficacy of meropenem compared with the combination of ceftazidime with tobramycin. Satisfactory clinical responses occurred in 89% of the meropenem group and 72% of the ceftazidime-tobramycin–treated patients ($P = .04$); corresponding bacteriologic response rates were 89% and 67%, respectively ($P = .006$).

Among the currently available fluoroquinolones, ciprofloxacin is the most active against gram-negative bacteria, including *P. aeruginosa.* Methicillin-sensitive *S. aureus* is sensitive to these agents; however, resistance has readily developed in methicillin-resistant *S. aureus,* and most of these strains are now no longer sensitive to fluoroquinolones. On the other hand, anaerobic coverage is poor for currently available quinolones, and suspected anaerobic infections may therefore not respond satisfactorily. Fluoroquinolone activity against *S. pneumoniae,* enterococci, and other streptococci is also low or at best intermediate, even though these agents are concentrated intracellularly in most tissues, including bronchial mucosa, neutrophils, and alveolar macrophages, which may enhance their effectiveness against pathogens with intermediate susceptibility.

In a randomized, double-blind, multicenter study, Fink and associates[170] compared monotherapy with ciprofloxacin and imipenem for treatment of severe pneumonia in a large series of 405 patients with pneumonia. Ciprofloxacin-treated patients had a higher bacteriologic eradication rate than did imipenem-treated patients (69% versus 59%, $P = .07$) and also a significantly higher clinical response rate (69% versus 56%, $P = .02$). However, when *P. aeruginosa* was recovered from initial respiratory tract cultures, failure to achieve bacteriologic eradication and development of resistance during therapy were common in both treatment groups (67% and 33% for ciprofloxacin, and 59% and 53% for imipenem, respectively), emphasizing the fact that monotherapy, even with a potent antibiotic, can lead to a high failure rate.

Monotherapy Versus Bitherapy

Several studies have examined single-agent antibiotic therapy in nosocomial pneumonia by using a third-generation cephalosporin, or imipenem-cilastatin, or a fluoroquinolone as monodrug therapy.[169, 171–174] In general, monotherapy has proved to be a useful alternative to combination therapy, with the same success rate and without an increased rate of superinfection or colonization by multiresistant pathogens. However, most of these studies included patients with nosocomial pneumonia diagnosed on clinical grounds alone, and the efficacy of treatment was assessed with information provided by sputum or tracheal aspirate cultures and not by more specific techniques. Indeed, a more rigorous comparison of these two regimens based on follow-up PSB samples or BAL fluid cultures would be required before monotherapy could be strongly recommended for treatment of nosocomial pneumonia in patients receiving mechanical ventilation.[129] Furthermore, in patients with severe infection due to *P. aeruginosa* or other multiresistant bacteria such as *Klebsiella* species or *Acinetobacter* species, the combination of an anti-*Pseudomonas* β-lactam antibiotic with an aminoglycoside is likely to produce a much better outcome than monotherapy, as shown in several previous studies.[175, 176]

To reassess the need of combining β-lactam antibiotics with aminoglycosides for the treatment of severe infections, Cometta and associates[177] performed a prospective randomized controlled study comparing imipenem monotherapy with a combination of imipenem plus netilmicin in the empirical treatment of nosocomial pneumonia and other severe infections in non-neutropenic patients. Of the 280 patients enrolled in the study, 48% had pneumonia and required mechanical ventilation. No significant improvement in the success rate observed with imipenem monotherapy was demonstrated in patients treated with aminoglycoside. The failure rates in case of pneumonia and the number of superinfections were similar in the two treatment groups. Although the addition of netilmicin increased nephrotoxicity, it did not prevent either colonization with *P. aeruginosa* strains resistant to imipenem or clinical treatment failures due to emergence of resistant *P. aeruginosa*. Because this study included heterogeneous populations of patients with different types of infections, and given the potential inaccuracy of using only clinical criteria to diagnose lung infection, further trials will ultimately be needed to clarify all these uncertainties. In the meantime, it is probably safer to use the combination of a β-lactam antibiotic with an aminoglycoside in patients with severe nosocomial pneumonia, at least for the first days of therapy, while waiting for pulmonary secretion culture results. It may be that monodrug therapies for nosocomial pneumonia would best be reserved for infections in which *P. aeruginosa* or other multiresistant microorganisms, such as *Klebsiella*, *Enterobacter*, *Citrobacter*, *Serratia*, and *Acinetobacter* species, have been excluded as the etiologic agents.[1, 178]

Pharmacokinetic Considerations

Effective antibiotic treatment of bacterial pneumonia depends on adequate delivery of antibacterial agents to the site of infection and, therefore, scrupulous attention to optimal dosages, routes of administration, and pharmacodynamic characteristics of each agent used to treat such infection. Antibiotic levels in infected tissues are considered to be therapeutic if free drug concentrations are at least equal to the in vitro minimum inhibitory concentration for the infecting pathogen. Because of significant methodologic problems, published data concerning the penetration of most antibiotics into the lung should probably be viewed with caution, and only general trends concerning concentrations achievable at the site of the infected lung tissue can be derived from these studies.[179]

For penicillins and cephalosporins, the ratio of the drug concentration in bronchial secretions to that in serum is between 0.05 and 0.25. The fluoroquinolones have better penetration characteristics, and concentrations in bronchial secretions are between 0.80 and 2.0 times those in serum. Aminoglycosides and tetracyclines have ratios of 0.2 to 0.6. Host-related as well as drug-related factors may, however, influence the penetration of antimicrobial drugs across the blood-bronchus and alveolar-capillary barriers. In the presence of inflammation or mechanical injury, the partitioning of antimicrobial agents in tissue compartments may be altered because of increases in membrane permeability. Thus, for drugs such as β-lactams and glycopeptides, which do not cross membranes readily, penetration might increase in the presence of inflammation.[180]

Several reports published in the literature have demonstrated a relationship between serum concentrations of β-lactam or other antibiotics, the minimum inhibitory concentration of the infecting organism, and the rate of bacterial eradication from respiratory secretions in patients with lung infection, emphasizing that clinical and bacteriologic outcomes can be improved by optimizing the therapeutic regimen according to pharmacokinetic properties of the agents selected for treatment.[181, 182] In one study of 74 acutely ill patients who were treated with intravenous ciprofloxacin at dosages ranging between 200 mg every 12 hours and 400 mg every 8 hours, most of them for VAP, Forrest and colleagues[182] demonstrated, by means of multivariate analyses, that the most important independent factor for probability of cure was a pharmacodynamic variable, that is, the 24-hour area under the concentration-time curve divided by the minimum inhibitory concentration (AUIC). At an AUIC below 125, the probabilities of both clinical and microbiologic cures were 42% and 26%, respectively, whereas at an AUIC above 125, the probabilities were 80% and 82%, respectively. These findings confirm the need for targeting the dosage of antimicrobial agents used for treatment of severe pulmonary infection to the individual patient's pharmacokinetics and the susceptibilities of putative bacterial pathogens. Development of a priori dosing algorithms based on minimum inhibitory concentration, the patient's creatinine clearance and weight, and the clinician-specified AUIC target might therefore be an interesting way to improve treatment of such patients, leading to a more precise approach than current guidelines for optimal use of antimicrobial agents.

In conclusion, effective antimicrobial therapy and adequate supportive measures remain the mainstay in the treatment of nosocomial pneumonia. Persistently high mortalities for pneumonia in the critical care unit argue, however, for continued reassessment of our current modalities of therapy and definition of better protocols. More active as well as less toxic antibacterial agents are still needed, especially for some problem pathogens, such as multiresistant nonfermenting gram-negative bacilli and methicillin-resistant *S. aureus*.

However, when one or several specific etiologic agents are identified by a reliable technique such as BAL or the PSB technique, the choice of antimicrobial drugs is much easier, because the optimal treatment may be selected in the light of the susceptibility pattern of the causative pathogens without resorting to broad-spectrum drugs or risking inappropriate treatment. Great efforts should therefore be made to obtain reliable pulmonary specimens for direct microscopic examination and quantitative cultures in each patient clinically suspected of having nosocomial pneumonia before new antibiotics are administered.

PREVENTION

A number of recommendations published for the prevention of nosocomial pneumonia[183-185] are empirical rather than based on controlled observations, for several reasons, all cited before, that make evaluation of preventive measures difficult in this setting:

1. The difficulty of arriving at an accurate diagnosis of VAP (i.e., to distinguish patients with true lung infection from patients with other pathologic processes associated with tracheal colonization); only those in whom VAP subsequently develops are likely to benefit from preventive measures.
2. The difficulty of precisely determining the impact of a prophylactic measure on the overall mortality of a general population of ICU patients (i.e., to identify preventable deaths, directly attributable to nosocomial pneumonia, among all deaths occurring in a population of ICU ventilated patients).
3. The difficulty of evaluating the consequences of a preventive measure on a potentially pathogenic mechanism, for example, concerning VAP, to evaluate the exact role played by prevention or reduction of tracheal colonization in modifying the incidence of VAP.

CONVENTIONAL INFECTION CONTROL APPROACHES

Conventional infection control approaches, such as adapted unit design, staff training and motivation, barrier isolation techniques, monitoring of respiratory equipment for bacterial contamination, and active infection surveillance and reporting, effectively prevent acquisition of many pathogens and reduce infection rates in the ICU. These measures should therefore be the first steps taken in any prevention program[183-185] (Table 145-12).

TABLE 145–12. Methods of Reducing the Frequency of Nosocomial Pneumonia in Mechanically Ventilated Patients

Infection Control

1. Adapted architectural design of the ICU
2. Adequate number and quality of medical, nursing, and ancillary staffs
3. Surveillance in the ICU
4. Education and awareness programs
5. Hand washing and/or barrier precautions; removal of gloves between patient examinations
6. Check technique for suctioning patients
7. Careful suctioning of glottic secretions

General Principles

1. Treat patient's underlying disease
2. Keep patient's head elevated at 30 degrees or above
3. Reevaluate need for prophylaxis of stress, bleeding, and in case of indication, reevaluate the choice of drug
4. Assess nutritional status and need for tube feeding
5. Extubate and remove nasogastric tube as clinically indicated
6. Control use of antibiotics in the ICU
7. Use kinetic therapy, chest physiotherapy

Respiratory Care Equipment

1. At least ≥ 48-hr circuit changes (tubing and humidifier) for mechanical ventilators with humidifiers; no changes for circuits with heat-moisture exchangers
2. Careful removal and attention to tubing condensate
3. Care of in-line medication nebulizers
4. Proper disinfection of ventilator tubing bags and spirometer
5. *Caution: Never transfer equipment or devices between different patients*

Adapted from Craven DE, Steger KA, Barber TW: Preventing nosocomial pneumonia: State of the art and prospectives for the 1990s. Am J Med 1991; 91(Suppl 3B): 544–553.

ICU = intensive care unit.

SPECIFIC PROPHYLACTIC MEASURES FOR VENTILATOR-ASSOCIATED PNEUMONIA

Certain methods are proposed for preventing ventilator-associated pneumonia.

First, noninvasive ventilation is an alternative approach to the use of artificial airways to avoid infectious complications and injury of the trachea in patients with acute respiratory failure. In a study conducted in 85 patients with acute exacerbations of COPD, Brochard and coworkers[186] found that the incidence of nosocomial pneumonia was 16.6% in 42 patients treated with endotracheal intubation and mechanical ventilation compared with 4.6% in the 43 patients randomly assigned to noninvasive ventilation, suggesting that this technique can reduce the in-hospital morbidity in selected groups of patients excluding those with the most severe disease, including central nervous system disorders.

Second, placing ventilated patients in a semirecumbent position to minimize aspiration of gastric contents is a simple measure, although some practical problems can occur in unstable patients. No clinical trial has clearly shown the benefit of such a measure in reducing VAP rate; however, two indirect arguments make such a trial essential. Torres and colleagues[187] found that the supine position was associated with a major risk for aspiration of gastric contents by measuring radioactivity recovered in endobronchial secretions after technetium labeling of gastric contents. Kollef[32] showed that head positioning of the supine patient during the first 24 hours of mechanical ventilation was an independent risk factor for acquiring VAP.

Third, oscillating and rotating beds have been proposed to minimize complete immobilization that facilitates atelectasis, alters drainage secretion, and potentially predisposes to pulmonary complications including pneumonia.[188, 189] Five studies have compared continuous lateral rotational therapy with standard beds in the prevention of nosocomial pneumonia.[190–194] They included a majority of surgical or trauma patients, ventilated or not, and reported conflicting results with a significant reduction of the rate of clinically diagnosed pneumonia in two studies, principally concerning early-onset (≤5 days) pneumonia, and the duration of mechanical ventilation; however, the only study conducted in a general population of ICU patients did not show any differences in pneumonia rates but confirmed the reduction of ICU length of stay.[192] Finally, in spite of the cost of such beds, cost-benefit analyses performed in these studies suggested favorable results, mainly due to the reduction of ICU length of stay.

Fourth, continuous or intermittent aspiration of oropharyngeal secretions has been proposed as an additional care for intubated patients to avoid chronic aspiration of secretions through the tracheal cuff. In 145 ventilated patients, Mahul and coworkers[88] found that pneumonia was less frequent (12.8%) in patients whose endotracheal tube had a separate dorsal lumen for hourly suctioning of stagnant secretions above the cuff than in others (29.1%, $P < .05$) and that the development of pneumonia was delayed (16.2 days versus 8.3 days in the control group).[88] Similarly, in a 3-year prospective, randomized, controlled study, Valles and colleagues[89] documented a reduction in VAP when continuous subglottic aspiration was performed (18.4% versus 32.5% in the control group, NS; corresponding to an incidence density of 19.9 episodes per 1000 ventilator-days versus 39.6 episodes per 1000 ventilator-days, $P < .03$). However, this difference was explained exclusively by the pneumonias occurring during the first week (3 of 76 versus 21 of 77, $P < .009$), whereas the late-onset pneumonias were more frequent in the "aspiration group" (11 of 76 versus only 4 of 77 in the control group). Furthermore, detailed microbiologic analysis demonstrated that this reduction concerned only pneumonia due to *H. influenzae* and gram-positive cocci. The incidence of pneumonias due to *P. aeruginosa* or Enterobacteriaceae and mortality rates were not different between the two groups.[89]

ANTIBIOTIC PROPHYLAXIS IN THE INTENSIVE CARE UNIT

Early attempts at systemic prophylaxis of pneumonia were clearly unsuccessful.[195–198] Several authors have used prophylactic endobronchial antibiotics in an attempt to reduce the incidence of nosocomial pneumonia.[199–203] Overall, these results confirm the data obtained in 35 ventilated baboons by Johanson and coworkers,[204] who demonstrated that effective regimens of antimicrobial agents to reduce the frequency and severity of VAP required the inclusion of both intravenous and topical agents (intravenous penicillin and topical gentamicin or polymyxin B). Neither intravenous antibiotics nor topical antibiotics alone provided effective prophylaxis.

SELECTIVE DIGESTIVE TRACT DECONTAMINATION

Several groups, particularly in Europe, have used topical prophylactic antibiotics for selective decontamination of the oropharynx and gastrointestinal tract (selective digestive tract decontamination [SDD]) in patients at high risk for nosocomial pneumonia. The SDD regimen usually includes systemic antibiotic therapy, such as cefotaxime, trimethoprim, or a quinolone, and nonabsorbable local antibiotic prophylaxis consisting of a combination of an aminoglycoside, polymyxin

TABLE 145–13. Results of Meta-analysis Studies on the Effect of Selective Digestive Tract Decontamination (SDD) on the Incidence of Nosocomial Pneumonia

	Pneumonia Rate*		
Authors	*SDD* (%)	*Control* (%)	**Comment**
Vandenbroucke-Graubs[211]	7	28	OR = 0.21 (0.15–0.29), historical controls
	8	45	OR = 0.12 (0.08–0.19), concurrent controls
SDD Trialists[207]	14	29	OR = 0.37 (0.31–0.43)
Kollef[208]	7	22	Risk difference = 0.145 (0.116–0.174)
Heyland et al.[209]	—	—	RR = 0.46 (0.39–0.56)
Hurley[210]	6	28	OR = 0.18 (0.14–0.23), historical controls
	14	31	OR = 0.35 (0.30–0.42), concurrent controls

*All differences are significant.
OR = odds ratio; RR = relative risk.

B, and amphotericin.[205] Selective decontamination has been designed to prevent oropharyngeal and gastric colonization by aerobic gram-negative bacilli and *Candida* species without disturbing the anaerobic flora and has limited activity against gram-positive bacteria. The local antibiotics are applied as a paste in the oropharynx and given either orally or through the nasogastric tube. Since the original study published by Stoutenbeek and colleagues[206] in 1984, which demonstrated a decrease in overall infection rate from 81% in 59 control subjects to 16% in 63 patients receiving the SDD regimen, more than 14 historic control studies, 27 concurrent control studies including more than 5300 patients, and six meta-analyses have been published and have provided variable results, usually considered to be favorable.[207–211] However, a clear consensus of effectiveness of SDD has not been established[212, 213] owing to limitations and deficiencies of these previous studies related to (1) the use of a clinical diagnosis of pneumonia as a study endpoint, often in a nonblind study design that leads to data of uncertain value because of the possibility of subjective bias in the diagnosis of pneumonia, (2) the heterogeneity of groups of patients studied, and (3) varying oral regimens and inconstant addition of systemic administration of antibiotics (cefotaxime or ceftazidime).

Several features have arisen from SDD studies that are summarized in meta-analyses, as follows (Tables 145–13 and 145–14):

1. Decreased rates of nosocomial pneumonia in SDD groups essentially concerned pneumonia due to gram-negative bacilli; in blinded studies, the incidence of pneumonia was not always reduced, particularly when invasive methods were used to define the presence of pneumonia.

2. The potential influence of SDD on mortality rates remains inconclusive, and the majority of studies have reported an overall mortality not statistically different between treated and untreated groups of patients, although recent meta-analyses have suggested a modest reduction in mortality with the use of SDD, provided that systemic antibiotics were included in the regimen. Therefore, the usually reported epidemiologic features concerning the incidence of nosocomial pneumonia (10% to 25%), the responsibility of gram-negative bacteria in such infections (60% to 70%), and the share of the mortality rate observed in ICU patients attributable to nosocomial pneumonia (50% of 40% to 50%) suggest that the prevention of death due to gram-negative nosocomial pneumonia concerns only 1.5% to 3.5% of all ICU patients (see Incidence and Mortality, described earlier in this chapter). None of the SDD studies, including meta-analyses, included a sufficiently large population to demonstrate such a small decrease in mortality.

3. The role of SDD in the emergence of resistance and in the risk of cross-infection has been discussed[214, 215] and remains worrisome. Induced selection of resistant gram-negative organisms and increased incidence of high-level resistant enterococci or methicillin-resistant staphylococci have been observed, with an increased frequency of *Staphylococcus* spp. pneumonia.[216–218]

4. Finally, the role of SDD on the duration of mechanical ventilation, ICU stay, and hospital stay appeared limited. Increased costs were observed, resulting from the antibiotics used and from microbiologic surveillance.

At present, this approach cannot be recommended for overall populations of ICU patients, although SDD may be effective for specific populations, particularly surgical or trauma pa-

TABLE 145–14. Results of Meta-analysis Studies on the Effect of Selective Digestive Tract Decontamination (SDD) on the Mortality in the Intensive Care Unit

	Mortality Rate		
Author	*SDD* (%)	*Control* (%)	**Comments**
Vandenbroucke-Graubs[211]	25	26	OR = 0.91 (0.67–1.23), historical controls
	21	26	OR = 0.70 (0.45–1.09), concurrent controls
SDD Trialists[207]	28	30	OR = 0.90 (0.79–1.04)
Kollef[208]	24	26	Risk difference = 0.019 (−0.016–0.054)
Heyland et al.[209]	—	—	RR = 0.87 (0.79–0.97)*
Hurley[210]	24	27	OR = 0.77 (0.61–0.97,* historical controls
	26	29	OR = 0.86 (0.74–0.99),* concurrent controls

*Significant reduction of mortality rate.
OR = odds ratio; RR = relative risk.

tients rather than medical patients. More data are needed to define the patients who may benefit from this intervention.

SUMMARY

Much progress has been made in our understanding of nosocomial infections of the lower respiratory tract, but there is little evidence that significant progress has been made in either preventing these pneumonias or improving their treatment. To reduce mortality, it seems reasonable that future studies concerning ventilator-associated pneumonias should examine the determinants of infection and define "high-risk" patients in whom it will be possible to demonstrate the potential benefit of prophylactic or therapeutic measures.

ACKNOWLEDGMENT

The authors wish to thank Catherine Brun for the invaluable help in the preparation of the manuscript.

References

1. Pennington JE: Nosocomial respiratory infection. *In:* Principles and Practice of Infectious Diseases. 3rd ed. Mandell GL, Douglas RG Jr, Bennett JE (Eds). New York, Churchill Livingstone, 1990, pp 2199–2205.
2. Haley RW, Hooton TM, Culter DH, et al: Nosocomial infections in US hospitals, 1975–1976: Estimated frequency by selected characteristics of patients. Am J Med 1981; 70:947–959.
3. Horan TC, White JW, Jarvis WR, et al: Nosocomial infection surveillance. MMWR 1986; 35:175S–195S.
4. Laforce FM: Hospital-acquired gram-negative rod pneumonias: An overview. Am J Med 1981; 70:664–669.
5. Levison ME, Kaye D: Pneumonia caused by gram-negative bacilli: An overview. Rev Infect Dis 1985; 7:S656–S665.
6. Stevens RM, Teres D, Skillman JJ, et al: Pneumonia in an intensive care unit. Arch Intern Med 1974; 134:106–111.
7. Chastre J, Fagon JY: Pneumonia in the ventilator-dependent patient. *In:* Principles and Practice of Mechanical Ventilation. Tobin MJ (Ed). New York, McGraw-Hill, 1994, pp 857–890.
8. Chastre J, Trouillet JL, Fagon JY: Diagnosis of pulmonary infections in mechanically ventilated patients. Semin Respir Infect 1996; 11:65–76.
9. Joshi N, Localio AR, Hamory BH: A predictive risk index for nosocomial pneumonia in the intensive care unit. Am J Med 1992; 93:135–142.
10. Craven DE, Kunches LM, Kilinski V, Lichtenberg DA, Make BJ, McCabe WR: Risk factors for pneumonia and fatality in patients receiving continuous mechanical ventilation. Am Rev Respir Dis 1986; 133:792–796.
11. Garibaldi RA, Britt MR, Coleman ML, et al: Risk factors for postoperative pneumonia. Am J Med 1981; 70:677–680.
12. Hemming VG, Overall JC, Britt MR: Nosocomial infections in a newborn intensive care unit. N Engl J Med 1976; 294:1310–1316.
13. Celis R, Torres A, Gatell JH, Almela M, Rodriguez-Roisin R, Augusti-Vidal A: Nosocomial pneumonia: A multivariate analysis of risk and prognosis. Chest 1988; 93:318–324.
14. Fagon JY, Chastre J, Domart Y, et al: Nosocomial pneumonia in patients receiving continuous mechanical ventilation: Prospective analysis of 52 episodes with use of a protected specimen brush and quantitative culture techniques. Am Rev Respir Dis 1989; 139:877–884.
15. Graybill JR, Marshall LW, Charache P, Wallace CR, Melvin VB: Nosocomial pneumonia: A continuing major problem. Am Rev Respir Dis 1973; 108:1130–1140.
16. Craven DE, Driks MR: Nosocomial pneumonia in the intubated patient. Semin Respir Infect 1987; 2:20–33.
17. Driks MR, Craven DE, Celli BR, et al: Nosocomial pneumonia in intubated patients given sucralfate as compared with antacids or histamine type 2 blockers. N Engl J Med 1987; 317:1376–1382.
18. Salata RA, Lederman MM, Shlaes DM, et al: Diagnosis of nosocomial pneumonia in intubated intensive care unit patients. Am Rev Respir Dis 1987; 135:426–432.
19. Jimenez P, Torres A, Rodriguez-Roisin R, et al: Incidence and etiology of pneumonia acquired during mechanical ventilation. Crit Care Med 1989; 17:882–885.
20. Vincent JL, Bihari DJ, Suter PM, et al: The prevalence of nosocomial infection in intensive care units in Europe: Results of the European Prevalence of Infection in Intensive Care (EPIC) study. JAMA 1995; 274:639–644.
21. Chevret S, Hemmer M, Carlet J, Langer M, and the European Cooperative Group on Nosocomial Pneumonia: Incidence and risk factors of pneumonia acquired in intensive care units: Results from a multicenter prospective study on 996 patients. Intensive Care Med 1993; 19:256–264.
22. Cross AS, Roup B: Role of respiratory assistance devices in endemic nosocomial pneumonia. Am J Med 1981; 70:681–685.
23. Langer T, Mosconi P, Cigada M, Mandelli M, and the Intensive Care Unit Group of Infection Control: Long-term respiratory support and the risk of pneumonia in critically ill patients. Am Rev Respir Dis 1987; 140:302–305.
24. Prod'hom G, Leuenberger P, Koerfer J, et al: Nosocomial pneumonia in mechanically ventilated patients receiving antacids, ranitidine, or sucralfate as prophylaxis for stress ulcer: A randomized controlled trial. Ann Intern Med 1994; 120:653–662.
25. Bell RC, Coalson JJ, Smith JD, et al: Multiple organ system failure and infection in adult respiratory distress syndrome. Ann Intern Med 1983; 99:293–298.
26. Sutherland KR, Steinberg KP, Maunder RJ, Milberg JA, Allen DL, Hudson LD: Pulmonary infection during the acute respiratory distress syndrome. Am J Respir Crit Care Med 1995; 152:550–556.
27. Delclaux C, Roupie E, Blot F, Brochard L, Lemaire F, Brun-Buisson C: Lower respiratory tract colonization and infection during severe acute respiratory distress syndrome. Am J Respir Crit Care Med 1997; 156:1092–1098.
28. Torres A, Aznar R, Gatell JM, et al: Incidence, risk and prognosis factors of nosocomial pneumonia in mechanically ventilated patients. Am Rev Respir Dis 1990; 142:523–528.
29. Craven DE, Kuncher LM, Lichtenberg DA, et al: Nosocomial infection and fatality in medical and surgical intensive care unit patients. Arch Intern Med 1988; 148:1161–1168.
30. Kerver AJH, Rommes JH, Mevissen-Verhage EAE, Hulstaert PF, Vos A, Verhoef J: Colonization and infection in surgical intensive care patients: A prospective study. Intensive Care Med 1987; 13:347–351.
31. Costantini M, Donisi PM, Turrin MG, Diana L: Hospital acquired infections surveillance and control in intensive care services: Results of an incidence study. Eur J Epidemiol 1987; 3:347–355.
32. Kollef MH: Ventilator-associated pneumonia: A multivariate analysis. JAMA 1993; 270:1965–1970.
33. Kollef MH, Wragge T, Pasque C: Determinants of mortality and mutiorgan dysfunction in cardiac surgery patients requiring prolonged mechanical ventilation. Chest 1995; 107:1395–1401.
34. Doyle RL, Szaflanski N, Modin GW, Wiener-Kronish JP, Matthay MA: Identification of patients with acute lung injury: Predictors of mortality. Am J Respir Crit Care Med 1995; 152:1818–1824.
35. Randle CJ Jr, Frankel LR, Amylon MD: Identifying early predictors of mortality in pediatric patients with acute leukemia and pneumonia. Chest 1996; 109:457–461.
36. Egan TM, Detterbeck FC, Mill MR, et al: Improved results of lung transplantation for patients with cystic fibrosis. J Thorac Cardiovasc Surg 1995; 109:224–235.
37. Lossos IS, Breuer R, Or R, Strauss N, Elishoov H, Naparstek E, Aker M, Nagler A, Moses AE, Shapiro M, Slavin S, Engelhard D: Bacterial pneumonia recipients of bone marrow transplantation. Transplantation 1995; 60:672–678.
38. Rello J, Valles J, Jubert P, Ferrer A, Domingo C, Mariscal D, Fontanals D, Artigas A: Lower respiratory tract infections following cardiac arrest and cardiopulmonary resuscitation. Clin Infect Dis 1995; 21:310–314.
39. Baker AM, Meredith JW, Haponik EF: Pneumonia in intubated trauma patients: Microbiology and outcomes. Am J Respir Crit Care Med 1996; 153:343–349.
40. Antonelli M, Moro ML, Capelli O, De Blasi RA, D'Erico RR, Conti G, Bufi M, Gasparetto A: Risk factors for early onset pneumonia in trauma patients. Chest 1994; 105:224–228.

41. Rello J, Ausina V, Castella J, Net A, Prats G: Nosocomial respiratory tract infections in multiple trauma patients. Chest 1992; 102:525–529.
42. Bryan CS, Reynolds KL: Bacteremic nosocomial pneumonia. Am Respir Rev Dis 1984; 129:668–671.
43. Tillotson JR, Lerner AM: Characteristics of non-bacteremic *Pseudomonas* pneumonia. Ann Intern Med 1968; 118:295–307.
44. Tillotson JR, Finland M: Bacterial colonization and clinical superinfection of the respiratory tract complicating antibiotic treatment of pneumonia. J Infect Dis 1969; 119:597–624.
45. Fagon JY, Chastre J, Hance AJ, Montravers P, Novara A, Gibert C: Nosocomial pneumonia in ventilated patients: A cohort study evaluating attributable mortality and hospital stay. Am J Med 1993; 94:281–288.
46. Kollef MH, Silver P, Murphy DM, Trouillion E: The effect of late-onset ventilator-associated pneumonia in determining patient mortality. Chest 1995; 108:1655–1662.
47. Taylor GD, Buchanan-Chell M, Kirkland T, McKenzie M, Wiens R: Bacteremic nosocomial pneumonia: A 7-year experience in one institution. Chest 1995; 108:786–788.
48. Rello J, Torres A, Ricart M, et al: Ventilator-associated pneumonia by *Staphylococcus aureus:* Comparison of methicillin-resistant and methicillin-sensitive episodes. Am J Respir Crit Care Med 1994; 150:1545–1549.
49. Doré P, Robert R, Grollier G, et al: Incidence of anaerobes in ventilator-associated pneumonia with use of a protected specimen brush. Am J Respir Crit Care Med 1996; 153:1292–1298.
50. Fagon JY, Chastre J, Vuagnat A, et al: Nosocomial pneumonia and mortality among patients in intensive care units. JAMA 1996; 275:866–869.
51. Timsit JF, Chevret S, Valcke J, Misset B, Renaud B, Glodstein FW, Vaury P, Carlet J: Mortality of nosocomial pneumonia in ventilated patients: Influence of diagnostic tools. Am J Respir Crit Care Med 1996; 154:116–123.
52. Craig CP, Connelly S: Effect of intensive care unit nosocomial pneumonia on duration of stay and mortality. Am J Infect Control 1984; 12:233–238.
53. Leu HS, Kaiser DL, Mori M, Woolson RF, Wenzel RP: Hospital-acquired pneumonia. Attributable mortality and morbidity. Am J Epidemiol 1989; 129:1258–1267.
54. Gross PA, Neu HC, Aswapokee P, et al: Deaths from nosocomial infections: Experience in a university hospital and a community hospital. Am J Med 1980; 68:219–223.
55. Gross PA, Van Antwerpen C: Nosocomial infections and hospital deaths. A case control study. Am J Med 1983; 75:658–661.
56. Cunnion KM, Weber DJ, Broadhead WE, Hanson LC, Pieper CF, Rutala WA: Risk factors for nosocomial pneumonia: Comparing adult critical-care populations. Am J Respir Crit Care Med 1996; 153:157–162.
57. Freeman J, Rosner BA, McGowan JE: Adverse effects of nosocomial infection. J Infect Dis 1979; 140:732–740.
58. Papazian L, Bregeon F, Thirion X, Gregoire R, Saux P, Denis JP, Perin G, Chanel J, Dumon JF, Affray FP, Gouin F: Effect of ventilator-associated pneumonia on mortality and morbidity. Am J Respir Crit Care Med 1996; 154:91–97.
59. Pinner RW, Haley RW, Blumenstein BA, et al: High cost nosocomial infections. Infect Control 1982; 3:143–149.
60. Beyt BE, Troxler S, Cavaness J: Prospective payment and infection control. Infect Control 1985; 6:161–164.
61. Kirby BD, Snyder KM, Meyer RD, Finegold SM: Legionnaire's disease: Report of sixty-five nosocomially acquired cases and review of the literature. Medicine (Baltimore) 1980; 59:188–200.
62. Girod JC, Reichman RC, Winn WC Jr, Klaucke DN, Vogt RL, Dolin R: Pneumonic and nonpneumonic forms of legionnellosis. Arch Intern Med 1982; 142:545–547.
63. Papazian L, Fraisse A, Garbe L, et al: Cytomegalovirus. An unexpected cause of ventilator-associated pneumonia. Anesthesiology 1996; 84:280–287.
64. Torres A, de la Bellacasa JP, Xaubet A, et al: Diagnostic value of quantitative cultures of bronchoalveolar lavage and telescoping plugged catheters in mechanically ventilated patients with bacterial pneumonia. Am Rev Respir Dis 1989; 140:306–310.
65. Rello J, Ausina V, Ricart M, Castella J, Prats G: Impact of previous antimicrobial therapy on the etiology and outcome of ventilator-associated pneumonia. Chest 1993; 104:1230–1235.
66. Spencer RC: Predominant pathogens found in the European Prevalence of Infection in Intensive Care Study. Eur J Clin Microbiol Infect Dis 1996; 15:281–285.
67. Jarvis WR, Martone WJ: Predominant pathogens in hospital infections. J Antimicrob Chemother 1992; 29(A):19–24.
68. Antonelli M, Moro ML, Capelli O, et al: Risk factors for early onset pneumonia in trauma patients. Chest 1994; 105:224–229.
69. Trouillet JL, Chastre J, Vuagnat A, Joly-Guillou ML, Combaux D, Dombret MC, Gibert C: Ventilator-associated pneumonia caused by potentially drug-resistant bacteria. Am J Respir Crit Care Med 1998; 157:531–539.
70. Louria DB, Kaminski T: The effects of four antimicrobial drug regimens on sputum superinfection in hospitalized patients. Am Rev Respir Dis 1962; 85:649–665.
71. Johanson WG Jr, Pierce AK, Sanford JP, et al: Nosocomial respiratory infections with gram-negative bacilli: The significance of colonization of the respiratory tract. Ann Intern Med 1972; 77:701–706.
72. Atherton ST, White DJ: Stomach as a source of bacteria colonizing respiratory tract during artificial ventilation. Lancet 1978; 2:968–969.
73. Hillman KM, Riordan T, O'Farrell SM, Tabaqchali S: Colonization of the gastric content in critically ill patients. Crit Care Med 1982; 10:444–447.
74. du Moulin GL, Hedley-White J, Paterson DG, et al: Aspiration of gastric bacteria in antacid-treated patients: A frequent cause of postoperative colonization of the airway. Lancet 1982; 1:242–245.
75. Donowitz GL, Page ML, Mileur BL, et al: Alteration of normal gastric flora in critical care patients receiving antacid and cimetidine therapy. Infect Control 1986; 7:23–26.
76. Bonten MJ, Gaillard C, Van Tiel F, Smeets H, Van de Geest S, Stobberingh E: The stomach is not a source for colonization of the upper respiratory tract and pneumonia in ICU patients. Chest 1994; 105:878–884.
77. Torres A, El-Ebiary M, Gonzalez J, et al: Gastric and pharyngeal flora in nosocomial pneumonia acquired during mechanical ventilation. Am Rev Respir Dis 1993; 148:352–357.
78. Tryba M: Sucralfate versus antacids or H_2-antagonists for stress ulcer prophylaxis: A meta-analysis on efficacy and pneumonia rate. Crit Care Med 1991; 19:942–949.
79. Cook DJ, Laine LA, Guyatt GH, Raffin TA: Nosocomial pneumonia and the role of gastric pH: A meta-analysis. Chest 1991; 100:7–13.
80. Craven DE, Steger KA: Epidemiology of nosocomial pneumonia: New perspectives on an old disease. Chest 1995; 102:1S–16S.
81. Cook DJ, Reeves BK, Scholes LC: Histamine-2-receptor antagonists and antacids in the critically ill population: Stress ulceration versus nosocomial pneumonia. Infect Control Hosp Epidemiol 1994; 15:437–442.
82. Cook DJ, Reeve BK, Guyatt GH, et al: Stress ulcer prophylaxis in critically ill patients: Resolving discordant meta-analyses. JAMA 1996; 275:308–314.
83. Ben-Menachem T, Fagel R, Patel RV, et al: Prophylaxis for stress-related gastric hemorrhage in the medical intensive care unit: A randomized, controlled, single blind study. Ann Intern Med 1994; 121:568–575.
84. Cook DJ, Fuller HD, Gruyatt GH, et al: Risk factors for gastrointestinal bleeding in critically ill patients. N Engl J Med 1994; 330:377–381.
85. Sottile FD, Marrie TJ, Prough DS, et al: Nosocomial pulmonary infection: Possible etiologic significance of bacterial adhesion to endotracheal tubes. Crit Care Med 1986; 14:265–270.
86. Inglis TJJ, Millar MR, Jones JG, et al: Tracheal tube biofilm as a source of bacterial colonization of the lung. J Clin Microbiol 1989; 27:2014–2018.
87. Spray SB, Zuidema GD, Cameron JL: Aspiration pneumonia: Incidence of aspiration with endotracheal tubes. Am J Surg 1979; 131:701–703.
88. Mahul P, Auboyer C, Jospe R, et al: Prevention of nosocomial pneumonia in intubation patients: Respective role of mechanical subglottic secretions drainage and stress ulcer prophylaxis. Intensive Care Med 1992; 18:20–25.
89. Valles J, Artigas A, Rello J, et al: Continuous aspiration of subglottic secretions in preventing ventilator-associated pneumonia. Ann Intern Med 1995; 122:179–186.

90. Torres A, Gatell JM, Aznar E, et al: Re-intubation increases the risk of nosocomial pneumonia in patients needing mechanical ventilation. Am J Respir Crit Care Med 1995; 152:137-141.
91. Moore FA, Moore EE, Jones TN, et al: TEN versus TPN following major abdominal trauma. Reduced septic morbidity. J Trauma 1989; 29:916-923.
92. Pingleton SK, Hinthorn D, Liu C: Enteral nutrition in patients receiving mechanical ventilation. Am J Med 1986; 80:827-832.
93. Winterbauer RH, Durning RB, Barron E, et al: Aspirated nasogastric feeding solution directed by glucose strips. Ann Intern Med 1981; 95:67-68.
94. Metheny NA, Eisenberg P, Spies M: Aspiration pneumonia in patients fed through nasoenteral tubes. Heart Lung 1986; 15:256-261.
95. Treloar DM, Stechmiller J: Pulmonary aspiration in tube-fed patients with artificial airways. Heart Lung 1984; 13:667-671.
96. Pingleton SK: Enteral nutrition and infection in the intensive care unit. Semin Respir Infect 1990; 5:185-190.
97. Montecalvo MA, Steger KA, Farber HW, et al: Nutritional outcome and pneumonia in critical care patients randomized to gastric versus jejunal tube feedings. Crit Care Med 1992; 20:1377-1387.
98. Strong RM, Condom SC, Solinger MR, et al: Equal aspiration rates from postpylorus and intragastric-placed small-bore nasoenteric feeding tubes: A randomized prospective study. JPEN J Parenter Enteral Nutr 1992; 16:59-63.
99. Meer JA: Inadvertent dislodgment of nasoenteric feeding tubes: Incidence and prevention. JPEN J Parenter Enteral Nutr 1987; 11:187-189.
100. Torres A, Serra-Batlles J, Ros E, et al: Pulmonary aspiration of gastric contents in patients receiving mechanical ventilation: The effects of body position. Ann Intern Med 1992; 116:540-543.
101. Orozco-Levi M, Torres A, Ferrer M, et al: Semirecumbent position protects from pulmonary aspiration but not completely from gastroesophageal reflux in mechanically ventilated patients. Am J Respir Crit Care Med 1995; 152:1387-1390.
102. Craven DE, Lichtenberg DA, Goularte TA, et al: Contaminated medication nebulizers in mechanical ventilator circuits: A source of bacterial aerosols. Am J Med 1984; 77:834-838.
103. Craven DE, Goularte TA, Make BJ: Contaminated condensate in mechanical ventilator circuits: A risk factor for nosocomial pneumonia? Am Rev Respir Dis 1984; 129:625-628.
104. Dreyfuss D, Djedaïni K, Gros I, et al: Mechanical ventilation with heated humidifiers or heat and moisture exchangers: Effect on patient colonization and incidence of nosocomial pneumonia. Am J Respir Crit Care Med 1995; 151:986-992.
105. Djedaïni K, Billiard M, Mier L, et al: Changing heat and moisture exchangers every 48 hours rather than 24 hours does not affect their efficacy and the incidence of nosocomial pneumonia. Am J Respir Crit Care Med 1995; 152:1562-1569.
106. Boots FJ, Howe S, George N, Harris F, Faoagali J: Clinical utility of hygroscopic heat and moisture exchangers in intensive care patients. Crit Care Med 1997; 25:1707-1712.
107. Tablan OC, Anderson LJ, Arden NH, et al: Guidelines for prevention of nosocomial pneumonia. Infect Control Hosp Epidemiol 1994; 15:587-627.
108. Craven DE, Connolly MG Jr, Lichtenberg DA, et al: Contamination of mechanical ventilators with tubing changes every 24 or 48 hours. N Engl J Med 1982; 306:1505-1509.
109. Dreyfuss D, Djedaïni K, Weber P, et al: Prospective study of nosocomial pneumonia and of patient and circuit colonization during mechanical ventilation with circuit changes every 48 hours versus no change. Am Rev Respir Dis 1991; 143:738-743.
110. Hess D, Burns E, Romagnoli D, Kacmakek RM: Weekly ventilator circuit changes: A strategy to reduce costs without affecting pneumonia rates. Anesthesiology 1995; 82:903-911.
111. Kollef MH, Shapiro SD, Fraser VJ, et al: Mechanical ventilation with or without 7-day circuit changes: A randomized controlled trial. Ann Intern Med 1995; 123:168-174.
112. Long MN, Wickstrons G, Grimes A, Benton CF, Belcher B, Stamm AM: Prospective randomized study of ventilator-associated pneumonia in patients with one versus three ventilator circuit changes per week. Infect Control Hosp Epidemiol 1996; 17:14-19.
113. Heffner JE: Nosocomial sinusitis: Den of multiresistant thieves? Am J Respir Crit Care Med 1994; 150:608-609.
114. Rouby JJ, Laurent P, Gosnach M, et al: Risk factors and clinical relevance of nosocomial maxillary sinusitis in the critically ill. Am J Respir Crit Care Med 1994; 150:776-783.
115. Ahrens JF, Lejeune FE, Webre DR: Maxillary sinusitis: A complication of nasotracheal intubation. Anesthesia 1974; 40:415-416.
116. Holzapfel L, Chevret S, Madinier G, et al: Influence of long-term oro- or nasotracheal intubation on nosocomial maxillary sinusitis and pneumonia: Results of a prospective randomized clinical trial. Crit Care Med 1993; 21:1132-1138.
117. Chastre J, Fagon JY: Invasive diagnostic testing should be routinely used to manage ventilated patients with suspected pneumonia. Am J Respir Crit Care Med 1994; 150:570-574.
118. Niederman MS, Torres A, Summer W: Invasive diagnostic testing is not needed routinely to manage suspected ventilator-associated pneumonia. Am J Respir Crit Care Med 1994; 150:565-569.
119. Marquette C, Georges H, Wallet F, et al: Diagnostic efficiency of endotracheal aspirates with quantitative bacterial cultures in intubated patients with suspected pneumonia. Am Rev Respir Dis 1993; 148:138-144.
120. El-Ebiary M, Torres A, Gonzales J, et al: Quantitative cultures of endotracheal aspirates for the diagnosing of ventilator associated pneumonia. Am Rev Respir Dis 1993; 148:1552-1557.
121. Torres A, de la Bellacasa JP, Rodriguez-Roisin R, Jimenez DE, Anta MT, Agusti-Vidal A: Diagnostic value of telescoping plugged catheters in mechanically ventilated patients with bacterial pneumonia using the Metras catheter. Am Rev Respir Dis 1988; 138:117-120.
122. Pugin J, Auckenthaler R, Mili N, et al: Diagnosis of ventilator-associated pneumonia by bacteriologic analysis of bronchoscopic and nonbronchoscopic "blind" bronchoalveolar lavage fluid. Am Rev Respir Dis 1991; 143:1121-1129.
123. Pham LH, Brun Buisson C, Legrand P, et al: Diagnosis of nosocomial pneumonia in mechanically ventilated patients: Comparison of a plugged telescoping catheter with the protected specimen brush. Am Rev Respir Dis 1991; 143:1055-1061.
124. Dreyfuss D, Mier L, Le Bourdelles G, et al: Clinical significance of borderline quantitative protected brush specimen culture results. Am Rev Respir Dis 1993; 147:941-951.
125. Fagon JY, Chastre J, Domart Y, Trouillet JL, Gibert C: Mortality due to *Pseudomonas* or *Acinetobacter* species ventilator-associated pneumonia or colonization assessed by quantitative culture of protected brush specimens. Clin Infect Dis 1996; 23:538-542.
126. Neu HC: The crisis in antibiotic resistance. Science 1992; 257:1064-1073.
127. McGowan JE Jr: Antimicrobial resistance in hospital organisms and its relation to antibiotic use. Rev Infect Dis 1983; 5:1033-1048.
128. Johanson WG Jr, Seidenfeld JJ, Gomez P, De Los Santos R, Coalson JJ: Bacteriologic diagnosis of nosocomial pneumonia following prolonged mechanical ventilation. Am Rev Respir Dis 1988; 137:259-264.
129. Montravers P, Fagon JY, Chastre J, et al: Follow-up protected specimen brushes to assess treatment in nosocomial pneumonia. Am Rev Respir Dis 1993; 147:38-44.
130. Chastre J, Fagon JY, Bornet-Lecso M, et al: Evaluation of bronchoscopic techniques for the diagnosis of nosocomial pneumonia. Am J Respir Crit Care Med 1995; 152:231-240.
131. Timsit JF, Misset B, Renaud B, Goldstein FW, Carlet J: Effect of previous antimicrobial therapy on the accuracy of the main procedures used to diagnose nosocomial pneumonia in patients who are using ventilation. Chest 1995; 108:1036-1040.
132. Blavia R, Dorca J, Verdaguer R, Carratala J, Gudiol F, Manresa F: Bacteriological follow-up of nosocomial pneumonia by successive protected specimen brushes (Abstract). Eur Respir J 1991; 4:A823.
133. Andrew C, Coalson J, Smith J, Johanson WG Jr: Diagnosis of nosocomial pneumonia in acute, diffuse lung injury. Chest 1981; 80:254-258.
134. Fagon JY, Chastre J, Hance AJ, et al: Detection of nosocomial lung infection in ventilated patients: Use of a protected specimen brush and quantitative culture techniques in 147 patients. Am Rev Respir Dis 1988; 138:110-116.
135. Fagon JY, Chastre J, Hance AJ, Domart Y, Trouillet JL, Gibert C:

Evaluation of clinical judgment in the identification and treatment of nosocomial pneumonia in ventilated patients. Chest 1993; 103:547-553.

136. Wunderink RG, Woldenberg LS, Zeiss J, Day CM, Ciemins J, Lacher DA: The radiologic diagnosis of autopsy-proven ventilator-associated pneumonia. Chest 1992; 101:458-463.
137. Meduri GU, Mauldin GL, Wunderink RG, et al: Causes of fever and pulmonary densities in patients with clinical manifestations of ventilator-associated pneumonia. Chest 1994; 106:221-235.
138. Wimberley N, Faling LJ, Bartlett JG: A fiberoptic bronchoscopy technique to obtain uncontaminated lower airway secretions for bacterial culture. Am Rev Respir Dis 1979; 119:337-343.
139. Meduri GU, Chastre J: The standardization of bronchoscopic techniques for ventilator-associated pneumonia. Chest 1982; 102(Suppl 1):557S-564S.
140. Moser KM, Maurer J, Jassy L, et al: Sensitivity, specificity, and risk of diagnostic procedures in a canine model of *Streptococcus pneumoniae* pneumonia. Am Rev Respir Dis 1982; 125:436-442.
141. Higuchi JH, Coalson JJ, Johanson WG Jr: Bacteriologic diagnosis of nosocomial pneumonia in primates: Usefulness of the protected specimen brush. Am Rev Respir Dis 1982; 125:53-57.
142. Chastre J, Viau F, Brun P, et al: Prospective evaluation of the protected specimen brush for the diagnosis of pulmonary infections in ventilated patients. Am Rev Respir Dis 1984; 130:924-929.
143. Torres A, El-Ebiary M, Padro L, et al: Validation of different techniques for the diagnosis of ventilator-associated pneumonia. Am J Respir Crit Care Med 1994; 149:324-331.
144. Rouby JJ, Martin de Lassale E, Poete P, et al: Nosocomial bronchopneumonia in the critically ill: Histologic and bacteriologic aspects. Am Rev Respir Dis 1992; 148:1059-1066.
145. Marquette CH, Copin MC, Wallet F, et al: Diagnostic tests for pneumonia in ventilated patients: Prospective evaluation of diagnostic accuracy using histology as a diagnostic gold standard. Am J Respir Crit Care Med 1995; 151:1878-1188.
146. Papazian L, Thomas P, Garbe L, et al: Bronchoscopic or blind sampling techniques for the diagnosis of ventilator-associated pneumonia. Am J Respir Crit Care Med 1995; 152:1982-1991.
147. Lefcoe MS, Fox GA, Leasa DJ, Sparrow RK, McCormack DG: Accuracy of portable chest radiography in the critical care setting: Diagnosis of pneumonia based on quantitative cultures obtained from protected brush catheter. Chest 1994; 105:885-887.
148. Cook DJ, Fitzgerald JM, Guyatt GH, Walter S: Evaluation of the protected brush catheter and bronchoalveolar lavage in the diagnosis of pneumonia. J Intensive Care Med 1991; 6:196-205.
149. Middleton R, Broughton WA, Kirkpatrick MB: Comparison of four methods for assessing airway bacteriology in intubated, mechanically ventilated patients. Am J Med Sci 1992; 304:239-245.
150. Torres A, Martos J, de la Bellacasa JP, et al: Specificity of endotracheal aspiration, protected specimen brush and bronchoalveolar lavage cultures in mechanically ventilated patients without pneumonia. Am Rev Respir Dis 1993; 147:952-957.
151. Chastre J, Fagon JY, Soler P, et al: Diagnosis of nosocomial bacterial pneumonia in intubated patients undergoing ventilation: Comparison of the usefulness of bronchoalveolar lavage and the protected specimen brush. Am J Med 1988; 85:499-506.
152. Meduri GU, Beals DH, Maijub AG, Baselski V: Protected bronchoalveolar lavage. A new bronchoscopic technique to retrieve uncontaminated samples from intubated patients: A review. Crit Care Med 1994; 22:1683-1691.
153. Chastre J, Fagon JY, Soler P, et al: Quantification of BAL cells containing intracellular bacteria rapidly identifies ventilated patients with nosocomial pneumonia. Chest 1989; 95:190-192.
154. Jourdain B, Novara A, Joly-Guillou, et al: Role of quantitative cultures of endotracheal aspirates for the diagnosis of nosocomial pneumonia. Am J Respir Crit Care 1995; 152:241-246.
155. Marquette CH, Herengt F, Saulnier F, et al: Protected specimen brush in the assessment of ventilator-associated pneumonia: Selection of a certain lung segment for bronchoscopic sampling is unnecessary. Chest 1993; 103:243-247.
156. Jorda R, Parras F, Ibanez J, Reina J, Bergada J, Rawrich JM: Diagnosis of nosocomial pneumonia in mechanically ventilated patients by the blind protected telescoping catheter. Intensive Care Med 1993; 19:377-382.
157. Baughman RP, Thorpe JE, Staneck J, et al: Use of the protected specimen brush in patients with endotracheal or tracheostomy tubes. Chest 1987; 91:233-236.
158. Kollef MH, Bock KR, Richards RD, Hearns ML: The safety and accuracy of minibronchoalveolar lavage in patients with suspected ventilator-associated pneumonia. Ann Intern Med 1995; 122:743-748.
159. Belenchia JM, Wunderink RG, Meduri GU, Leeper KV: Alternative causes of fever in ARDS patients suspected of having pneumonia (Abstract). Am Rev Respir Dis 1991; 143:A683.
160. Alvarez-Lerma F, ICU-Acquired Pneumonia Group: Modification of empiric antibiotic treatment in patients with pneumonia acquired in the intensive care unit. Intensive Care Med 1996; 22:387-394.
161. Luna CM, Vujacich P, Niederman MS, Vay C, Gherardi C, Matera J, Jolly EC: Impact of BAL data on the therapy and outcome of ventilator-associated pneumonia. Chest 1997; 111:676-685.
162. Rello J, Gallego M, Mariscal D, Sondra R, Valles J: The value of routine microbial investigation in ventilator-associated pneumonia. Am J Respir Crit Care Med 1997; 156:196-200.
163. Bonten MJM, Bergmans DCJJ, Stobberingh EE, van der Geest S, De Leeuw PW, van Tiel FH, Gaillard CA: Implementation of bronchoscopic techniques in the diagnosis of ventilation-associated pneumonia to reduce antibiotic use. Am J Respir Crit Care Med 1997; 156:1820-1824.
164. American Thoracic Society: Hospital-acquired pneumonia in adults: Diagnosis, assessment of severity, initial antimicrobial therapy, and preventative strategies. Am J Respir Crit Care Med 1995; 153:1711-1725.
165. Meyer KS, Urban C, Eagan JA, Berger BJ, Rahal JJ: Nosocomial outbreak of *Klebsiella* infection resistant to late-generation cephalosporins. Ann Intern Med 1993; 119:353-358.
166. Klastersky J, Carpentier-Meunier F, Kahan-Coppens L, Thys JP: Endotracheally administered antibiotics for gram-negative bronchopneumonia. Chest 1979; 75:586-591.
167. Brown RB, Kruse JA, Counts GW, et al: Double-blind study of endotracheal tobramycin in the treatment of gram-negative bacterial pneumonia. Antimicrob Agents Chemother 1990; 34:269-270.
168. Bergogne-Berezin E: Treatment and prevention of nosocomial pneumonia. Chest 1995; 108:26S-34S.
169. Sieger B, Berman SJ, Geckler RW, Farkas SA, Meropenem Lower Respiratory Infection Group: Empiric treatment of hospital-acquired lower respiratory tract infections with meropenem or ceftazidime with tobramycin: A randomized study. Crit Care Med 1997; 25:1663-1670.
170. Fink MP, Snydman DR, Niederman MS, et al: Treatment of severe pneumonia in hospitalized patients: Results of a multicenter, randomized, double-blind trial comparing intravenous ciprofloxacin with imipenem-cilastatin. Antimicrob Agents Chemother 1994; 38:547-557.
171. Mangi RJ, Greco T, Ryan J, Thornton G, Andriolet VT: Cefoperazone versus combination antibiotic therapy of hospital-acquired infection. Am J Med 1988; 84:68-74.
172. Schentag JJ, Vari AJ, Winslade NE, et al: Treatment with aztreonam or tobramycin in critical care patients with nosocomial gram-negative rod pneumonia. Am J Med 1985; 78(Suppl 2A):34-41.
173. Rapp RP, Young B, Foster TS, Tibbs PA, O'Neal W: Ceftazidime versus tobramycin/ticarcillin in treating hospital-acquired pneumonia and bacteremia. Pharmacotherapy 1984; 4:211-215.
174. Mandell LA, Nicolle LE, Ronald AF: A multicenter prospective randomized trial comparing ceftazidime with cefazolin/tobramycin in treatment of hospitalized patients with nonpneumococcal pneumonia. J Antimicrob Chemother 1983; 12(Suppl A):S9-S20.
175. Hilf M, Yu VL, Sharp JA, Zuravleff JJ, Korvick JA, Muder RR: Antibiotic therapy for *Pseudomonas aeruginosa* bacteremia: Outcome correlations in a prospective study of 200 patients. Am J Med 1989; 87:540-546.
176. Korvick JA, Bryan CS, Farber B, et al: Prospective observational study of *Klebsiella* bacteremia in 230 patients: Outcome for antibiotic combinations versus monotherapy. Antimicrob Agents Chemother 1992; 36:2639-2644.

177. Cometta A, Baumgartner JD, Lew D, et al: Prospective randomized comparison of imipenem monotherapy with imipenem plus netilmicin for treatment of severe infections in nonneutropenic patients. Antimicrob Agents Chemother 1994; 38:1309–1313.
178. Scheld WM, Mandell GL: Nosocomial pneumonia: Pathogenesis and recent advances in diagnosis and therapy. Rev Infect Dis 1991; 13(Suppl 9):S743–S751.
179. Baldwin DR, Honeybourne D, Wise R. Pulmonary disposition of antimicrobial agents: Methodological consideration. Antimicrob Agents Chemother 1992; 36:1171–1175.
180. Lamer CH, de Beco V, Soler P, et al: Analysis of vancomycin entry into pulmonary lining fluid using bronchoalveolar lavage in critically ill patients. Antimicrob Agents Chemother 1993; 37:281–286.
181. Peloquin CA, Cumbo TJ, Nix DE, Sands MF, Schentag JJ: Evaluation of intravenous ciprofloxacin in patients with nosocomial lower respiratory tract infections. Arch Intern Med 1989; 149:2269–2273.
182. Forrest A, Nix DE, Ballow CH, Goss TF, Bermingham MC, Schentag JJ: Pharmacodynamics of intravenous ciprofloxacin in seriously ill patients. Antimicrob Agents Chemother 1993; 37:1073–1081.
183. Flaherty JP, Weinstein RA: Infection control and pneumonia prophylaxis strategies in the intensive care unit. Semin Respir Infect 1990; 5:191–203.
184. Craven DE, Steger KA, Barber TW: Preventing nosocomial pneumonia: State of the art and perspectives for the 1990s. Am J Med 1991; 91(Suppl 3B):S44–S53.
185. Faling LJ: Advances in preventing nosocomial pneumonia: Part II. Am Rev Respir Dis 1988; 137:256–258.
186. Brochard L, Mancebo J, Wysocki M, et al: Noninvasive ventilation for acute exacerbations for chronic obstructive pulmonary disease. N Engl J Med 1995; 333:817–822.
187. Torres A, Serra-Batlles J, Ros E, et al: Pulmonary aspiration of gastric contents in patients receiving mechanical ventilation: The effects of body position. Ann Intern Med 1992; 116:540–543.
188. Choi SC, Nelson LD: Kinetic therapy in critically ill patients: Combined results based on meta-analysis. J Clin Care 1992; 7:57–62.
189. O'Donohue WJ: Prevention and treatment of postoperative atelectasis. Chest 1985; 87:1–2.
190. Kelley RE, Vibuloreth, Bell L, Duncan RC: Evaluation of kinetic therapy in the prevention of complications of prolonged bed rest secondary to stroke. Stroke 1987; 18:638–642.
191. Gentilello L, Thompson DA, Tonnesen AS, et al: Effects of rotating bed on the incidence of pulmonary complications in critically ill patients. Crit Care Med 1988; 165:783–786.
192. Summer WR, Curry P, Haponik EF, Nelson S, Elston R: Continuous mechanical turning of intensive care unit patients shortens length of stay in some diagnostic-related groups. J Crit Care 1989; 4:45–53.
193. Fink MP, Helsmoortel CM, Stein KL, Lee PC, Cohn SM: The efficacy of an oscillating bed in the prevention of lower respiratory tract infection in critically ill victims of blunt trauma: A prospective study. Chest 1993; 97:132–137.
194. de Boisblanc BP, Castro M, Everret B, Grender J, Walker CD, Summer WR: Effect of air-supported, continuous postural oscillation on the risk of early ICU pneumonia in nontraumatic critical illness. Chest 1993; 103:1543–1547.
195. Lepper MH, Kofman S, Blatt N, et al: Effect of eight antibiotics used singly and in combination on the tracheal flora following tracheotomy in poliomyelitis. Antibiot Chemother 1954; 4:829–843.
196. Petersdorf RG, Merchant RK: A study of antibiotic prophylaxis in patients with acute heart failure. N Engl J Med 1959; 260:565–575.
197. Mandelli M, Mosconi P, Langer M, et al: Prevention of pneumonia in an intensive care unit: A randomized multicenter trial. Crit Care Med 1989; 17:501–503.
198. Petersdorf RG, Curtin JA, Hoeprich PD, et al: A study of antibiotic prophylaxis in unconscious patients. N Engl J Med 1957; 257:1001–1009.
199. Klick JM, du Moulin GC, Hedley-White J, et al: Prevention of gram-negative bacillary pneumonia using polymyxin aerosol as prophylaxis. J Clin Invest 1975; 55:514–519.
200. Feeley TW, du Moulin GC, Hedley-Whyte J, Bushnell LS, Gilbert JP, Feingold DS: Aerosol polymyxin and pneumonia in seriously ill patients. N Engl J Med 1975; 293:471–475.
201. Klastersky J, Huysmans E, Weerts D, Hensgens D, Daneau D: Endotracheally administered gentamicin for the prevention of infections of the respiratory tract in patients with tracheostomy: A double-blind study. Chest 1974; 65:650–654.
202. Klastersky J, Hensgens D, Noterman J, et al: Endotracheal antibiotics for the prevention of tracheobronchial infections in tracheotomized unconscious patients: A comparative study of gentamicin and aminosidine-polymyxin B combination. Chest 1975; 68:302–306.
203. Rouby JJ, Poete P, Martin de Lassale E, et al: Prevention of gram negative nosocomial bronchopneumonia by intratracheal colistin in critically ill patients: Histologic and bacteriologic study. Intensive Care Med 1994; 20:187–192.
204. Johanson WG Jr, Seidenfeld JJ, de los Santos R, Coalson JJ, Gomez P: Prevention of nosocomial pneumonia using topical and parenteral antimicrobial agents. Am Rev Respir Dis 1988; 137:265–272.
205. Van Saene HK, Stoutenbeek CP, Stoller JK: Selective decontamination of the digestive tract in the intensive care unit: Current status and future prospects. Crit Care Med 1992; 20:691–703.
206. Stoutenbeek CP, Van Saene HK, Miranda DR, Zandstra DF: The effect of selective decontamination of the digestive tract on colonization and infection rate in multiple trauma patients. Intensive Care Med 1984; 10:185–192.
207. Selective Decontamination of the Digestive Tract Trialists' Collaborative Group: Meta-analysis of randomized controlled trials of selective decontamination of the digestive tract. BMJ 1993; 307:525–532.
208. Kollef M: The role of selective digestive tract decontamination on mortality and respiratory tract infections: A meta-analysis. Chest 1994; 105:1101–1108.
209. Heyland DK, Cook DJ, Jaeschte R, Griffith L, Lee HN, Gruyatt GH: Selective decontamination of the digestive tract: An overview. Chest 1994; 105:1221–1229.
210. Hurley JC: Prophylaxis with enteral antibiotics in ventilated patients: Selective decontamination or selective cross-infection? Antimicrob Agents Chemother 1995; 39:941–947.
211. Vandenbroucke-Graubs CMJE, Vandenbroucke JP: Effect of selective decontamination of the digestive tract on respiratory tract infection and mortality in the intensive care unit. Lancet 1991; 338:859–862.
212. Brun-Buisson C: Selective decontamination in critical care: Interpreting the synthesized evidence. Chest 1994; 105:978–980.
213. Van Saene HKF, Stoutenbeek CC, Stoller JK: Selective decontamination of the digestive tract in the intensive care unit: Current status and future prospects. Crit Care Med 1992; 20:691–703.
214. Nardi G, Valentinis U, Proietti A, et al: Epidemiological impact of prolonged use of topical SDD on bacterial colonization of the tracheobronchial tree and antibiotic resistance. Intensive Care Med 1993; 19:273–278.
215. Hammond JMJ, Potgieter PD: Long-term effects of selective decontamination on antimicrobial resistance. Crit Care Med 1995; 25:637–645.
216. Gastinne H, Wolff M, Delatour F, Faurisson F, Chevret S: A controlled trial in intensive care units of selective decontamination of the digestive tract with nonabsorbable antibiotics. N Engl J Med 1992; 326:594–599.
217. Hammond JM, Potgieter PD, Saunders GL, Forder AA: A double blind study of selective decontamination in intensive care. Lancet 1992; 340:5–9.
218. Daschner F, Kappstein I, Engels I, et al: Stress ulcer prophylaxis and ventilation pneumonia: Prevention by antibacterial cytoprotective agents. Infect Control 1988; 9:59–65.

146

Partial Liquid Ventilation

Bradley P. Fuhrman, MD • Lynn J. Hernan, MD
David M. Steinhorn, MD

Ventilation-perfusion (V/Q) mismatch is the principal impediment to gas exchange in acute lung injury. Until recently, the intensivist could force air into nonreceptive lungs only and hope that this strategy would improve V/Q matching. In the past decade, new approaches that modify lung function and improve V/Q matching have been developed. Perfluorocarbon liquid ventilation is one such approach.

LIQUID BREATHING

Fish extract oxygen from the water that crosses their gills. Although oxygen is sparingly soluble in water, this method of oxygen uptake suffices. It has long been recognized that surface tension of the surfactant-deficient lung may be reduced by filling alveoli with certain fluids. These two strategies—uptake of dissolved oxygen and elimination of air-fluid interfacial surface tension—may be combined into a process known as liquid breathing. Clark and colleagues[1] have shown that mice can spontaneously breathe perfluorocarbon liquids of high oxygen solubility for periods approaching an hour before exhaustion leads to respiratory failure.

TIDAL LIQUID VENTILATION

For mammals to breathe liquid in tidal fashion for prolonged periods, two major requirements must be met: (1) a liquid must be used that possesses high solubilities for oxygen and carbon dioxide, and (2) a ventilator must be used to perform the work of breathing because of the high viscous resistance to flow of the liquid medium.

Kylstra and associates[2] have shown that dogs can be ventilated with hyperbarically oxygenated saline. Complications of this approach include pulmonary surfactant depletion and vascular volume overload. In addition to the previous requirements, to be a suitable vehicle for liquid breathing, the fluid should be nonabsorbable and a poor solvent for surfactant.

Leland Clark first identified perfluorocarbons as a class of compounds suitable for liquid breathing. Numerous impure perfluorocarbons have been studied, but only recently has a medical-grade liquid suitable for clinical applications of liquid ventilation become available (perfluorooctyl bromide, perflubron or LiquiVent, Alliance Pharmaceutical Corp., San Diego).

Devices capable of supporting liquid ventilation have been designed and tested. Such devices need not be intricate for laboratory applications and have been shown to support the very immature lung with surfactant deficiency.[3] Such a device can be used to ventilate the small lung at low alveolar pressure[4] and without impeding cardiac output.[5]

PERFLUOROCARBON-ASSOCIATED GAS EXCHANGE

A recent innovation, variously termed perfluorocarbon-associated gas exchange (PAGE) or partial liquid ventilation (PLV) has simplified the technical aspects of using perfluorocarbons in the lung. It is possible to fill the functional residual capacity (FRC) of the lungs with perfluorocarbon liquid and to "bubble oxygenate" the liquid in situ (in vivo) using a conventional gas ventilator.[6] This technique, gas ventilation of the fluid-filled lung, allows liquid to be used to recruit atelectatic lung and reduce surface tension at the alveolar lining. In expiration, the liquid FRC represents an incompressible reservoir of oxygen-occupying alveoli that would otherwise collapse and allow intrapulmonary shunting. In inspiration, tidal volumes of gas purge that reservoir of carbon dioxide and replenish the supply of dissolved oxygen after the fashion of a very efficient bubble oxygenator.

In normal piglets, PLV provides excellent gas exchange. The airway pressure excursion required to deliver a fixed tidal volume of gas to the perfluorocarbon-filled lung is no greater than that required to ventilate the dry lung.[6] It has only recently been appreciated that there is a small but consistent decline in oxygenation when the normal lung is filled with perfluorocarbon. Hernan and coworkers[7] have shown that this reduction in arterial oxygen tension is probably related in part to a diffusion barrier imposed by the perfluorocarbon liquid itself. Samples of perfluorocarbon obtained from the lung during PLV consistently have lower oxygen tension than predicted by the alveolar gas equation. It is postulated that the diffusion barrier of the perfluorocarbon generates a gradient for oxygen from the gas phase to the perfluorocarbon layer adjacent to the alveolar lining and capillary endothelium. This implies a limit to the theoretically achievable $Pa{O_2}$ during PLV. It also suggests that the alveolar lining is exposed to less oxygen when ventilated across a layer of perfluorocarbon than when ventilated "dry."

In larger animals such as sheep, oxygenation is affected by hydraulic factors as well. It has been shown that arterial oxygenation is dependent on tidal volume or peak airway pressure in the large lung.[8] This reflects the tendency of gas to gravitate to nondependent regions of fluid-filled lung when small tidal volumes and low peak airway pressures are used. In the large lung, gas exchange is often greatly enhanced by a slight increase in peak inflation pressure and tidal volume. It is now clear that FIO_2 may be adjusted during PLV without fear of alveolar nitrogen foam accumulation.[9]

It is also clear that hydraulic issues are important in the large lung but not in the small lung. In the large lung, hydraulic effects cannot be readily distinguished from consequences of lung stiffness, both of which elevate end-inspiratory airway pressure. Measurements of compliance do not reflect stiffness alone in the large lung during PLV.

In animal models, PLV is effective over prolonged treatment periods[10, 11] and recovery to gas breathing is readily accomplished. Toxicologic evidence from prolonged studies supports the suitability of perfluorooctyl bromide for PLV in patients.

MODELS OF LUNG DISEASE

Tutuncu and colleagues[12] have shown that rabbit lungs lavaged with saline to induce surfactant deficiency exchange gas more efficiently during PLV than during conventional gas ventilation. Leach and associates[13, 14] have shown this also to be the case in premature lambs with surfactant deficiency of prematurity and that PLV is compatible with exogenous surfactant therapy. Wilcox and coworkers[15] have studied lambs with surgically induced congenital left diaphragmatic hernia and have shown that this lesion (which is complicated by surfactant deficiency) is amenable to treatment by PLV. In all of these models, lung compliance is improved by the presence of perflubron within the lung. Clearly, surfactant deficiency is highly responsive to PLV.

PLV has also been applied to piglets after intratracheal instillation of meconium.[16] In this model, Thompson and associates showed that oxygenation and 6-hour survival were both substantially improved, although improvement in gas exchange was less striking and less rapid than in models of surfactant deficiency. Although meconium is thought to impair surfactant function, it is also known to obstruct distal airways. This mechanical issue contributes to the difficulty of rescuing animals after meconium instillation.

Numerous models of acute lung injury and adult respiratory distress syndrome (ARDS) have been studied. Papo and colleagues[17] showed that lung injury induced by intravenous oleic acid infusion is ameliorated by PLV. Nesti and coworkers[18] have shown that gastric aspiration-induced ARDS benefits from PLV with perflubron. Hernan and associates[8] demonstrated amelioration of acid-induced ARDS in large sheep. Improvement in histology was seen in studies by Nesti and coworkers and Papo and colleagues. Hirschl and associates[19] also documented improved histology in an oleic acid injury model treated by tidal liquid ventilation.

When the normal lung is filled with perfluorocarbon, PaO_2 falls by about 100 torr. In surfactant deficiency, oxygenation improves after instillation of perfluorocarbon and the lung then oxygenates blood as well as the normal, liquid-filled lung. This results from improved V/Q matching. In fact, PLV with perflubron makes the surfactant-deficient lung function almost as though it were normal. Surprisingly, however, several inflammatory models also behave as though the lung were made to function normally after perflubron instillation. The combination of near-normal oxygenation and near-normal histology in the study of aspiration ARDS by Nesti and colleagues and of improved histology in other recent reports of animal models of ARDS, suggests that perflubron may have anti-inflammatory effects distinct from the beneficial effects of PLV on lung function.

ANTI-INFLAMMATORY EFFECTS OF PERFLUBRON

Smith and colleagues[20] have shown that alveolar macrophages are less readily stimulated to generate free radicals and hydrogen peroxide after exposure to perflubron. Perflubron also reduces neutrophil infiltration in the acutely injured lung.[21] It reduces phagocytosis but not killing by alveolar macrophages[22] and reduces nitric oxide production by alveolar macrophages in vitro.[23] Electron micrographs of alveolar macrophages exposed to perflubron in vivo reveal vesicles (that probably represent ingested perflubron) as well as loss of villous appendages. It is possible that pinocytosis of the liquid, which might be expected to internalize (as vesicle membrane) receptor sites that are normally bound to the cell surface, reduces the surface density of receptors that trigger inflammation. It is also possible that perflubron dissolves in the macrophage's cell membrane much like a volatile anesthetic, altering membrane function. Many volatile anesthetics alter inflammation, although their predominant effect is clearly to alter neuronal surface membrane function. Effects of perflubron on the alveolar macrophage are demonstrable after in vitro exposure. Such in vitro anti-inflammatory effects of perflubron represent a discrete mechanism from "lung protective" anti-inflammatory processes (reduced volutrauma), which may also occur.

Because the clinical significance of these anti-inflammatory effects is not yet clear, there is concern that perfluorocarbons might make the lung susceptible to nosocomial infection. Steinhorn and Sajan[24] contradicted this idea, suggesting that nosocomial infection is not facilitated by the presence of perflubron. Perflubron is, in fact, a bacteriostatic environment that does not support bacterial growth.

SURFACTANT PRODUCTION

Perfluorocarbons are not miscible with aqueous solutions or gels. Surfactant is not readily soluble in perflubron. It is not likely that PLV would deplete the lung of phospholipid. Steinhorn and associates[25] have shown that, to the contrary, PLV with perflubron increases de novo synthesis of surfactant by normal lung. Similar findings apply to the immature lung studied by Leach and coworkers.[26] It has been hypothesized that lung stretch mediates these increases in surfactant synthesis.

MANAGEMENT OF SECRETIONS

Secretions are not miscible in perfluorochemicals. Early clinical experience suggested that this might be a problem during PLV. Subsequent laboratory experience has shown that secretions may be effectively debrided from the lung by saline lavage during PLV. Recovery of small volumes of saline instilled into the "dry" lung is minimal. Saline instillation may stimulate coughing and loosen proximal secretions but is not a very effective means of clearing secretions from the lung. During PLV, movement of perfluorocarbon in the airways appears to mobilize secretions toward the trachea. Tracheal instillation of saline tends to liquefy these secretions. Cessation of positive end-expiratory pressure or ventilator disconnect carries this debris forward into the trachea, where it can be removed by suctioning.

COMBINING ADVANCED RESPIRATORY THERAPIES

The clinician's use of therapies is complementary rather than exclusive. When allowable, the intensivist uses recruitment techniques to augment FRC, blood flow redistributing techniques to better match ventilation and perfusion, and lung protective strategies to prevent volutrauma. Separate approaches to pulmonary hypertension, pulmonary and extrapulmonary inflammation, and hemodynamic instability are applied as appropriate.

PLV was conceived as a recruitment strategy, a means to reduce alveolar surface tension and splint alveoli open by virtue of the liquid's weight and high density (1.95 g/mL). Its use as a means to debride the lung and to remove secretions is also a recruitment technique. Through its stimulation of surfactant synthesis, perflubron may facilitate lung expansion. PLV was intended as a means to distribute ventilation more evenly and was thus conceived as a recruitment strategy.

There is evidence that perflubron diminishes the risk of oxidative damage to the lung during experimental injury.[27] To the extent that PLV with perflubron reduces the need for oxygen and high airway pressures, it is a lung protective strategy. When lung recruitment prevents expiratory alveolar collapse, it halts the cycle of alveolar opening and closing with each breath and modulates the excessive shear forces that are believed to contribute to volutrauma. Perflubron's anti-inflammatory effects might also be viewed as lung protective.

Some of the newer modalities of respiratory support work very well together. The neonatal lamb with surgically created congenital diaphragmatic hernia is unresponsive to nitric oxide, because inhaled nitric oxide only enhances perfusion of ventilated lung. This model has too little ventilated lung to respond unless first recruited with an agent that improves alveolar ventilation. PLV makes these lungs responsive to nitric oxide.[15] High-frequency oscillatory ventilation appears to work synergistically with PLV.[28, 29] PLV also works synergistically with a combination of high-frequency oscillatory ventilation and surfactant therapy.[30]

TABLE 146–1. Physiologic Data from 13 Premature Infants Treated by Partial Liquid Ventilation (PLV) with Perflubron After Unsuccessful Surfactant Therapy

	Baseline	PLV (1 hr)	PLV (4 hr)	PLV (24 hr)
OI	41.0 ± 7.0	22.4 ± 7.1	10.4 ± 2.2	8.9 ± 2.5
$Paco_2$	66.0 ± 12	56.0 ± 5.9	45.0 ± 5.4	44.8 ± 2.1
C dyne/kg	0.22 ± 0.05	0.37 ± 0.04	0.37 ± 0.09	0.48 ± 0.19
Paw	16.6 ± 9.1	14.6 ± 0.91	12.4 ± 1.0	11.6 ± 0.89

OI = oxygenation index (mean airway pressure × 100/(Pao_2 to FIO_2 ratio); C dyne/kg = dynamic compliance (mL/cm H_2O/kg); Paw = mean airway pressure (cm H_2O).

TABLE 146–3. Outcome of 58 Adults with Acute Lung Injury or Acute Respiratory Distress Syndrome Younger Than 55 Years of Age at Enrollment*

	VFDs	Patients with >1 VFD	Mortality Rate
PLV (n = 39)	8.95 ± 1.39	61.5%	25.6%
CMV (n = 19)	4.11 ± 1.81	31.6%	36.8%

*Age < 55 yr and baseline $Pao_2/FIO_2 < 300$.
PLV = partial liquid ventilation; CMV = conventional mechanical ventilation; VFDs = ventilator-free days.

CLINICAL TRIALS OF PARTIAL LIQUID VENTILATION WITH PERFLUBRON

PLV with perflubron (LiquiVent) is an investigational technique that is now in clinical trials for regulatory approval. Results in infants with respiratory distress syndrome (RDS) attributable to surfactant deficiency have been published,[31] preliminary findings in children and adults.[33] These trials document mortality rates lower than historic controls and show physiologic improvements in gas exchange and lung compliance. However, they lack companion control populations. There have also been three small randomized, controlled neonatal trials in target populations: premature neonates with infant respiratory distress syndrome (IRDS), infants with congenital diaphragmatic hernia, and term neonates with respiratory failure. A large controlled trial has been conducted in pediatric patients with ARDS (currently under analysis). A controlled trial in adults with ARDS has been completed, and its findings have been presented.

The first corporate-sponsored study of perflubron PLV in the United States focused on the rescue of premature babies with IRDS. On average, these patients had a gestational age of 28 weeks and weighed about 1000 g. To be enrolled, a baby had to have a gestational age of 24 to 34 weeks, to have a birth weight between 600 and 2000 g, and to be less than 5 days of age. All patients were required to have been unable to respond to at least one dose of surfactant. Enrolled infants were expected to have a high risk of imminent death. The study group consisted of 13 patients who did not respond, on average, to between two and three doses of surfactant. Of these 13 patients, seven survived and did well over the long term. The physiologic response is summarized in Table 146–1.

The first pediatric Phase II trial, again, did not have a control group. On average, these patients were 4 years old and weighed about 18 kg. Most of them had pneumonia as a presenting diagnosis. At enrollment, average alveolar arterial oxygen difference was a little more than 450 torr. This difference would have predicted about a 50% risk of mortality at the time that this study was undertaken. In this group of 10 patients, eight survived. There were no serious unexpected adverse events that were deemed related to the drug.

TABLE 146–2. Demographics of 90 Adults with Adult Respiratory Distress Syndrome Randomized to Partial Liquid Ventilation (PLV) or Conventional Mechanical Ventilation (CMV)

	PLV (n = 65)	CMV (n = 25)
Age (yrs)	43 ± 2	41 ± 3
> Age 55 yr	28%	8%
Pao_2/FIO_2	178 ± 12	198 ± 22
$Pao_2/FIO_2 < 200$	62%	56%
$200 < Pao_2/FIO_2 < 300$	26%	28%

Table 146–2 shows demographics of the adult Phase II and III controlled trial. This trial compared PLV to conventional mechanical ventilation in adults with ARDS. It was intended that two patients receive PLV for every one patient randomized to conventional mechanical ventilation. The average age of this group of patients was slightly older than 40 years, but numerous patients were over 55 years of age. In the literature, it is clear that being old is disadvantageous if a person has ARDS and that mortality from ARDS is substantially higher in people older than 55 years of age than in those younger than 55 years of age. The study groups are unbalanced, in that there are more elderly patients (>55 years) in the PLV group (28%) than in the group with conventional mechanical ventilation (8%). It is also important to note that not all of these patients had ARDS. Sixty-two per cent of the patients in the PLV group and 56% in the conventional mechanical ventilation group had ARDS (a Pao_2/FIO_2 ratio <200). Some patients were not sick enough at entry to have what would be classified as acute lung injury (P/F between 200 and 300). The primary endpoints studied in this trial were ventilator-free days, the number of patients who had ventilator-free days, and the 28-day mortality rate. Mortality and ventilator-free days were different between groups in patients younger than 55 years of age who had a P/F below 300 (Table 146–3). There was a difference between the two treatments in the percentage of patients who had at least one ventilator-free day as well as a small difference in mortality.

References

1. Clark LC Jr, Gollan F: Survival of mammals breathing organic liquids equilibrated with oxygen at atmospheric pressure. Science 1966; 152:1755–1756.
2. Kylstra JA, Paganelli CV, Lanphier EH: Pulmonary gas exchange in dogs ventilated with hyperbarically oxygenated liquid. J Appl Physiol 1966; 21:177–184.
3. Shaffer TH: Gaseous exchange and acid base balance in premature lambs during liquid ventilation since birth. Pediatr Res 1976; 10:227–231.
4. Curtis SE, Fuhrman BP, Howland DF: Airway and alveolar pressures during fluorocarbon breathing in infant lambs. J Appl Physiol 1990; 68:2322–2328.
5. Curtis SE, Fuhrman BP, Howland DF, DeFrancisis M, Motoyama EK: Cardiac output during liquid (fluorocarbon) breathing in newborn piglets. Crit Care Med 1991; 19:225–230.
6. Fuhrman BP, Paczan PR, DeFrancisis M: Perfluorocarbon associated gas exchange. Crit Care Med 1991; 19:712–723.
7. Hernan LJ, Penfil S, Fuhrman BP, Dowhy MS, Rath M, Papo MC, Leach CL: Functional FiO_2 predicts alveolar Po_2 during perfluorocarbon associated gas exchange (Abstract). Crit Care Med 1996; 24(1 Suppl):A149.
8. Hernan LJ, Fuhrman BP, Kaiser R, Penfil S, Foley C, Papo MC, Leach CL: Perfluorocarbon associated gas exchange in normal and acid injured large sheep. Crit Care Med 1996; 24:475–481.
9. Hernan LJ, Fuhrman BP, Papo MC, Steinhorn DM, Leach CL, Salman N, Paczan P, Kahn B: Cardiopulmonary effects of perfluo-

rocarbon associated gas exchange at reduced oxygen concentrations. Crit Care Med 1995; 23:553-559.
10. Salman N, Fuhrman BP, Steinhorn DM, Papo MC, Hernan LJ, Leach CL, Fisher JE: Prolonged studies of perfluorocarbon associated gas exchange and of resumption of conventional mechanical ventilation. Crit Care Med 1995; 23:919-924.
11. DeLemos R, Winter D, Fields T, Doherty T, Null D Jr, Yoder B, Coalson J: Prolonged partial liquid ventilation in the treatment of hyaline membrane disease (HMD) in the premature baboon (Abstract). Pediatr Res 1994; 35:330A.
12. Tutuncu AS, Faithfull NS, Lachmann B: Comparison of ventilatory support with intratracheal perfluorocarbon administration and conventional mechanical ventilation in animals with acute respiratory failure. Am Rev Respir Dis 1993; 148:785-792.
13. Leach CL, Fuhrman BP, Morin FC III, Rath MG: Perfluorocarbon associated gas exchange (PAGE) in respiratory distress syndrome. Crit Care Med 1993; 21:1270-1278.
14. Leach CL, Holm B, Morin FC III, Fuhrman BP, Papo MC, Steinhorn DM, Hernan LJ: Partial liquid ventilation in premature lambs with respiratory distress syndrome: Efficacy and compatibility with exogenous surfactant. J Pediatr 1995; 126:412-420.
15. Wilcox DT, Glick PL, Karamanoukian HL, Morin FC, Fuhrman BP, Leach CL: Perfluorocarbon associated gas exchange improves pulmonary mechanics, oxygenation, ventilation and allows nitric oxide delivery in the hypoplastic lung congenital diaphragmatic hernia lamb model. Crit Care Med 1995; 23:1858-1863.
16. Thompson AE, Fuhrman BP, Allen J: Perfluorocarbon associated gas exchange in experimental meconium aspiration. Pediatr Res 1993; 33:239A.
17. Papo MC, Paczan P, Fuhrman BP, Steinhorn DM, Hernan LJ, Leach CL, Holm BA, Fischer JE, Khan B: Perfluorocarbon associated gas exchange improves oxygenation, lung compliance and survival in an animal model of adult respiratory distress syndrome. Crit Care Med 1996; 24:466-474.
18. Nesti FD, Fuhrman BP, Steinhorn DM, Papo MC, Hernan LJ, Duffy LC, Fischer JE, Leach CL, Paczan PR, Burak BA: Perfluorocarbon associated gas exchange (PAGE) in gastric aspiration. Crit Care Med 1994; 22:1445-1452.
19. Hirschl RB, Tooley R, Parent AC, Johnson K, Bartlett RH: Improvement of gas exchange, pulmonary function and lung injury with partial liquid ventilation: A study model in a setting of severe respiratory failure. Chest 1995; 108:500-508.
20. Smith T, Steinhorn D, Thusu K, Fuhrman B, Dandona P: A liquid perfluorocarbon decreases the in vitro production of free radicals by alveolar macrophages. Crit Care Med 1995; 23:1533-1539.
21. Colton D, Bartlett R, Gill G, Hirschl R, Johnson K: Neutrophil infiltration is reduced during partial perfluorocarbon liquid ventilation in the setting of lung injury. Surg Forum Proc 1994; XLV:668-670.
22. Steinhorn DM, Fuhrman BP, Smith T: Liquid perfluorocarbon affects phagocytosis by alveolar macrophages after in vitro exposure. Crit Care Med 1995; 23: (Suppl 1):A213.
23. Steinhorn DM, Fuhrman BP, Smith T: Perflubron decreases nitric oxide production by alveolar macrophages in vitro. Pediatr Res 1995; 27:55A.
24. Steinhorn DM, Sajan I: Partial liquid ventilation reduces colonization of the lung during experimental nosocomial pneumonia. Pediatr Res 1996; 39:54A.
25. Steinhorn DM, Fuhrman BP, Holm B, Leach C: Partial liquid ventilation enhances surfactant production. Am J Respir Crit Care Med 1996; 153:A640.
26. Leach CL, Hernan LJ, Fuhrman BP, Holm B, Morin F III, Papo MC: Partial liquid ventilation with LiquiVent increases endogenous surfactant production in premature lambs with respiratory distress syndrome. Pediatr Res 1995; 37:238A.
27. Steinhorn DM, Alijada A, Dandona P, Fuhrman B, Papo M, Thusu K: Partial liquid ventilation with perflubron decreases oxidative damage to lung during experimental injury. Crit Care Med 1996; 24: (Suppl 1):A148.
28. Smith K, Bing D, Boros S, Mammel M, Meyers P: Partial liquid ventilation using conventional and high frequency techniques. Pediatr Res 1995; 37:351A.
29. Harel Y, Toro-Figueroa LO, Vinson R, et al. HFLOV, a perfluorocarbon associated gas exchange utilizing high frequency oscillatory ventilation is feasible and may improve synergistically lung compliance in a near drowning piglet model. Pediatr Res 1995; 37:46A.
30. Leach C, Holm B, Morin F III, Papo M, Sukumar M: High frequency partial liquid ventilation and surfactant treatment in preterm lambs with respiratory distress syndrome. Pediatr Res 1996; 37:50A.
31. Leach CL, Greenspan JS, Rubenstein SD, Shaffer TH, Wolfson MR, Jackson JC, DeLemos R, Fuhrman BP: Partial liquid ventilation with perflubron in premature infants with severe respiratory distress syndrome. N Engl J Med 1996; 335:761-767.
32. Toro-Figueroa L, Curtis S, Fackler J, Fuhrman B, Hirschl R, Leach C, Meliones J, Newth C, Thompson A: Partial liquid ventilation with perflubron in premature infants with severe respiratory distress syndrome. Crit Care Med 1996; 24:A150.
33. Hirschl R, Pranikoff T, Wise C, Overbeck M, Gauger P, Schreiner R, DeMaria A, Dechert R, Bartlett R: Initial experience with partial liquid ventilation in adult patients with the acute respiratory distress syndrome. JAMA 1996; 275:383-389.

147

The Acute Abdomen

Kenneth Waxman, MD, FACS

Sir Zachary Cope, in his 1921 monograph *The Early Diagnosis of the Acute Abdomen,* eloquently outlined the importance of a carefully taken history and physical examination.[1] Despite all technologic advances, the history and physical examination remain the most important tools in the initial assessment of a patient who complains of abdominal pain. Although critically ill patients may be more difficult to evaluate, the data from their history and physical examination are, nonetheless, paramount, as this information either determines a definitive diagnosis or directs further evaluation.

During an initial assessment, the physician should obtain a thorough understanding of a patient's underlying medical problems, of the precise nature and chronicity of the abdominal pain, and of its association with related symptoms such as vomiting, diarrhea, and dysuria. In the course of a complete physical examination, the physician evaluates a patient for signs of shock, infection, cardiopulmonary disease, neurologic disorders, rectal masses or occult blood, and pelvic or genital masses or tenderness as well as for abdominal tenderness and peritoneal irritation. After this initial assessment, the following questions can be addressed:

1. Does the patient require immediate resuscitation?
2. Does the patient require invasive cardiorespiratory monitoring?
3. Are additional diagnostic tests necessary?
4. Does the patient require urgent operation?

DOES THE PATIENT REQUIRE IMMEDIATE RESUSCITATION?

Patients with acute abdominal pain often have hypovolemia because of gastrointestinal losses through vomiting or diarrhea as well as the extravascular sequestration of fluid and electrolytes in the intestinal, peritoneal, retroperitoneal, and interstitial spaces. Thus, patients with acute abdominal conditions frequently require aggressive fluid and electrolyte infusion.

Altered pulmonary function is also common in patients with acute abdominal pain. Abdominal pain and distention often limit tidal volume; this results in an increased respiratory rate and sometimes ventilatory failure. Furthermore, atelectasis and pneumonia can ensue, and this in turn can lead to hypoxia.[2] Certain acute abdominal diseases, such as pancreatitis, are particularly likely to cause hypoxia. Also, the abdominal pain itself can be caused by primary pulmonary pathology, especially lower-lobe pneumonia, pleuritis, or pulmonary infarction. Oxygenation and ventilation must therefore always be assessed and often supported in patients with abdominal pain.

Antibiotic therapy is important during the resuscitation of patients with intra-abdominal bacterial contamination or infection. Antibiotic therapy may be definitive therapy, such as in uncomplicated diverticulitis and pelvic inflammatory disease. In addition, early preoperative initiation of presumptive antibiotic therapy that is effective against suspected bacterial flora is indicated before emergency laparotomy in the setting of acute abdominal pain. One important caution, however, is that the initiation of such antibiotic therapy should generally be delayed until a definite decision to operate has been made. If the decision to operate itself is pending observation for progression of disease, antibiotic therapy is contraindicated because antibiotics may mask the signs and symptoms for which such observation is made.

Other physiologic alterations (including temperature elevation, anemia, and clotting abnormalities) also frequently require correction in the preoperative resuscitation period.

DOES THE PATIENT REQUIRE INVASIVE CARDIORESPIRATORY MONITORING?

The majority of patients with acute abdominal disease can be effectively resuscitated with the use of physical examination data, vital signs, and urine output as guidelines. For selected patients, however, early utilization of invasive monitoring may be helpful both for titrating preoperative resuscitation and for determining when the patients are best able to undergo anesthesia and operation. Patients for whom such invasive preoperative monitoring should be considered include those with severe cardiac, pulmonary, or renal disease; these patients may require precise regulation of fluid therapy and are also more likely to require afterload and contractility agents than are patients with less severe disease. Invasive preoperative monitoring is also indicated for patients with severe preoperative shock, sepsis, or blood loss because optimal titration of preoperative resuscitation may be important in determining these patients' ability to tolerate the ensuing anesthesia and operation. In each case, the time necessary to institute invasive monitoring as well as any additional time required for resuscitation must be weighed against the benefits of early operation.

The nature of preoperative monitoring depends on the particular situation. Monitoring of clinical signs and symptoms, vital signs, and urine output is sufficient to monitor resuscitation in the great majority of patients. When central venous catheterization is initiated in the emergency setting, central venous pressure is most often measured. Monitoring of central venous pressure has the advantages of simple institution and minimum equipment requirements. However, both the absolute value of central venous pressure and the response of this parameter to therapy may be misleading if used in isolation as indicators of cardiac function; thus, central venous pressure values must be interpreted with caution.[3] In selected instances, monitoring of pulmonary arterial and wedge pressures and measurement of cardiac output provide critical information and are thus justified. Again, however, in all instances care must be taken not to delay an urgent operation unduly in order to institute such monitoring. The use of noninvasive monitoring devices, which provide monitoring information rapidly with minimum risk, is extremely attractive in this setting and deserves wider application and study.[4]

ARE DIAGNOSTIC TESTS NECESSARY?

Diagnostic tests should be reserved for patients in whom indications for surgery are unclear. For patients with clear-cut signs of peritonitis requiring laparotomy, further diagnostic tests to define the precise etiology before operation are not necessary. In fact, the extra time taken to perform such diagnostic tests may delay both resuscitation and operation and thus may be harmful. Diagnostic tests should therefore be performed selectively.

Laboratory Testing

Several blood tests are frequently of importance in evaluating patients with abdominal pain. The white blood cell (WBC) count is often of diagnostic value. A mild leukocytosis (WBC count 12,000 to 20,000) is most frequently seen in patients with peritonitis; however, early in the course of disease, leukocytosis may be absent. WBC counts greater than 20,000 are seen uncommonly in peritonitis, usually only in patients with advanced intra-abdominal infection or bowel infarction.[5] Peritonitis may also be present in patients with a normal WBC count but a "left shift" (increase in the number of polymorphonuclear leukocytes), especially in elderly and debilitated patients. Finally, in patients with severe sepsis, leukopenia may supervene. Thus, although leukocytosis is characteristic of peritonitis that requires operation, a great number of exceptions exist. Although an elevated WBC count suggests a diagnosis of peritonitis, a normal count should not delay operation if history and physical examination are convincing.

Tests of the coagulation system are sometimes useful. Increased prothrombin and partial thromboplastin times and decreased platelet counts are often seen in patients with severe intra-abdominal infections.

Serum amylase determination is a useful test for patients with abdominal pain because pancreatitis, which is best treated medically, can easily be confused with other causes of peritonitis. Detection of hyperamylasemia may suggest the correct diagnosis and thus help to avoid unnecessary laparotomy; however, serum amylase values may be increased in other surgical conditions. Furthermore, serum amylase levels may not be elevated in pancreatitis, even in the presence of severe disease.[6]

Urinalysis may also be helpful in patients with abdominal pain. Pyuria may indicate the presence of a urinary tract infection, and hematuria may indicate a ureteral stone. It is also possible, however, that inflammatory processes adjacent to the kidney, ureter, or bladder are responsible for abnormal urinalysis results. Thus, abnormal urinalysis results do not rule out the need for laparotomy in patients with signs of peritonitis.

Radiologic Evaluation

If a diagnosis of peritonitis requiring operation is clear, radiologic evaluation is not necessary and may in fact delay resuscitation and operation. If the diagnosis is unclear—particularly if conditions not requiring immediate operation are in the differential diagnosis—radiologic evaluation may prove helpful. Examples of situations in which plain abdominal and chest radiographs are useful include the diagnosis of intestinal obstruction, the diagnosis of ureteral stone, and the finding of free intraperitoneal air. Gastrointestinal contrast studies may be useful in confirming a diagnosis of intestinal perforation or obstruction. Care must be taken in the emergency situation to avoid the introduction of barium into a perforated intestinal tract; water-soluble contrast agents should be utilized whenever the possibility of perforation exists. Intravenous pyelography may be indicated to differentiate ureteral obstruction as the cause of abdominal pain and to define genitourinary involvement in intra-abdominal infections.

Abdominal ultrasonography may also be useful during the evaluation of acute abdominal pain. Ultrasonography may indicate the presence of intra-abdominal fluid, blood, or abscess; help evaluate solid organs; detect abnormalities of the biliary system; and detect abdominal aortic aneurysm. Ultrasonography has the advantage of portability; that is, it may be performed at the bedside. However, with many critically ill patients, ultrasonography may be technically difficult to perform, often because of ileus. Ultrasonographic evaluation of patients with acute abdominal pain is best utilized to answer specific questions, such as:

1. Are gallstones present?
2. Are the bile ducts dilated?
3. Is there a pancreatic abscess?

Ultrasonographic examination to detect the presence of intraperitoneal blood has proved to be an efficient and effective tool in the initial assessment of trauma patients.[7]

Computed tomography (CT) is currently the most specific and sensitive test for the diagnosis of the acute abdominal conditions. CT has the ability to detect intra-abdominal fluid or blood, to determine the presence and location of intra-abdominal and retroperitoneal abscesses, and to detect abnormalities of the abdominal wall, pancreas, liver, spleen, gallbladder, genitourinary system, retroperitoneum, and, in some cases, intestine, including the appendix. A positive finding on CT is usually quite specific and allows a high degree of diagnostic certainty.[8] In addition, as the quality of CT technology continues to improve, both specificity and sensitivity of CT diagnoses are improving. CT does have disadvantages that should be considered when the decision to perform this test is being made:

1. The patient must be transported to the scanner. If the patient is critically ill and requires intensive monitoring and resuscitation, this may be difficult and risky.
2. Even the most advanced CT technique is not always sensitive in detecting abnormalities of the gastrointestinal tract; as a result, important causes of peritonitis may not be detected.
3. CT scans are expensive.

For these reasons, diagnostic CT scanning should be carefully considered and selectively performed.

Nuclear medicine imaging techniques may be useful in some instances. Iminodiacetic acid biliary scans are useful in confirming the diagnosis of acute cholecystitis in questionable cases. Ventilation-perfusion lung scans may be helpful in differentiating pulmonary embolism as the source of abdominal pain. Labeled leukocyte scans have been helpful in the evaluation of acute abdominal pain, particularly in diagnosis of appendicitis.[9]

Angiography has been indicated to evaluate for the presence of mesenteric arterial occlusion when intestinal ischemia is suspected as the cause of acute abdominal pain. Dynamic CT scanning, however, may be the better initial study.[10]

Peritoneal Lavage and Laparoscopy

Peritoneal lavage is an important diagnostic tool for patients with blunt abdominal trauma, although its usefulness for other patients with abdominal pain is less well established. For selected patients, it may be quite beneficial, particularly when an abdominal examination may be difficult to perform because of altered mental status or critical illness.[11]

Peritoneal lavage may be performed in several ways. In all cases, the bladder should be emptied by a Foley catheter and the stomach decompressed by nasogastric suction. A peritoneal dialysis catheter is then introduced. For a patient with nondistended abdomen who has not had previous abdominal surgery, a percutaneous technique may be used. After local anesthesia, an 18-gauge catheter is introduced through the midline 1 to 2 cm below the umbilicus; entry into the peritoneal cavity can be appreciated by a palpable decrease in resistance. A metal guide wire can then be passed through the catheter, over which the peritoneal dialysis catheter is introduced. Alternatively, in patients with intestinal distention or with possible intra-abdominal adhesions, it is safer to place the peritoneal catheter with a direct cut-down technique through a 2- to 4-cm incision made below the umbilicus. The linea alba is divided, and the dialysis catheter is introduced directly through an incision in the peritoneum.

After placement of the peritoneal catheter, aspiration may yield fluid for analysis. If it does not, 1000 mL of warm sterile isotonic saline solution is introduced (40 mL/kg in children). When infusion is complete, the saline bag is placed on the floor, and lavage fluid, returned by gravity, is then sent for analysis. In particular, the presence of significant numbers of red blood cells (RBCs), WBCs, or bacteria indicates the need for laparotomy.

Laparoscopy may also be useful in evaluating acute abdominal pain. Laparoscopy may be performed with either local or general anesthesia and may allow both diagnosis and treatment. The possibility of bedside diagnostic laparoscopy in the emergency department or intensive care unit (ICU) makes this procedure particularly appealing for critically ill patients.[12]

DOES THE PATIENT REQUIRE URGENT OPERATION?

Early operation is essential for a patient with acute abdominal pain who requires laparotomy. For many patients, however, a preoperative period of resuscitation is beneficial. The optimal period of time to continue this resuscitation and delay operation depends on an individual patient's physiologic response to illness and to resuscitation. Although benefit is gained by correcting preoperative deficits with resuscitation, undue operative delay may result in continued hemorrhage, obstruction, and infection and thus may contribute to a net worsening of the patient's physiologic status.

In general, acute abdominal disorders fall into three categories: (1) those that require early surgery with resuscitation performed as quickly as possible, (2) those that benefit from a definitive period of medical therapy before operation, and (3) those that are best treated nonoperatively.

Examples of conditions requiring rapid resuscitation and urgent surgery include abdominal trauma, ruptured aortic aneurysm, intestinal necrosis, ruptured ectopic pregnancy, large-intestinal obstruction, appendicitis, and perforated ulcer. Although early operation is clearly important in each of these disorders, resuscitation may need to be prolonged under certain circumstances. For example, patients with appendicitis usually require little preoperative care and are best served with early operation. A subgroup of patients with advanced appendicitis have severe generalized peritonitis, intestinal obstruction, or intra-abdominal abscess and may be critically ill on presentation. Children, older people, and patients with underlying medical diseases often fall into this category. These patients may benefit from a period of intensive preoperative resuscitation.

As another example, patients with perforated peptic ulcer may have significant peritonitis and may benefit from aggressive preoperative resuscitation. In selected patients with perforated ulcer and severe underlying illness for whom emergency operation is risky, water-soluble contrast radiography may be performed; if no intraperitoneal extravasation of contrast medium is observed, the patients can be treated nonoperatively with nasogastric suction, antibiotics, and intensive supportive care.[13]

Other conditions are best treated medically before operation. One example is gallstone pancreatitis. When pancreatitis is due to gallstones, patients should undergo cholecystectomy and, possibly, common bile duct exploration. The timing of operation remains controversial, but most investigators recommend a period of medical therapy to allow resolution of pancreatitis before operation.[14] Although such improvement occurs in most patients, a minority develop progressive pancreatitis; these patients require urgent surgery or endoscopic retrograde cholangiopancreatography (ERCP). An additional example is small-bowel obstruction. Patients with small-bowel obstruction may benefit greatly from intravenous hydration and nasogastric suction. If improvement of pain, abdominal examination, and abdominal radiography occurs within 8 to 12 hours, nonoperative management may be continued and, in some patients, operation may be avoided. If at any time signs of peritonitis, fever, or leukocytosis occur, patients must undergo prompt laparotomy. Furthermore, if progressive improvement does not occur, immediate operation is necessary.[15]

Finally, patients with abdominal pain may have conditions that cause severe illness for which intensive nonoperative care may be definitive therapy. Examples include acute pancreatitis, pelvic inflammatory disease, and severe gastroenteritis. Aggressive medical therapy and supportive intensive care are often mandatory for such patients if a successful outcome is to be achieved.[16] It is, however, important to recognize that these nonoperative conditions are easily confused with conditions for which operative therapy is necessary. It is often good medical practice to perform laparotomy under these circumstances to establish a definitive diagnosis, if this is not clear from other diagnostic studies.

INTRAOPERATIVE MANAGEMENT

Intraoperative management of patients undergoing emergency abdominal surgery requires special expertise of both anesthesiologists and surgeons.

The anesthesiologist is often at a disadvantage in having little or no time for perioperative assessment of a patient who may be seriously ill and who may also have a chronic disease that increases the risk of anesthesia. The emergency nature of the illness also increases the risk of anesthesia, for on presentation to the operating room the patient may be dehydrated and hypovolemic, may have electrolyte and acid-base disturbances, and may have acute pulmonary compromise. Of special concern is that such patients may have recently eaten or have bowel obstruction or ileus; thus, the risk of vomiting and aspiration of gastric contents may be greatly increased. This risk is even greater if the patient has been given preoperative narcotics or sedatives (which should preferably be avoided for this reason).

Of major concern during induction of anesthesia is the prevention of vomiting and aspiration. A useful technique for minimizing this risk is rapid-sequence intubation, in which the patient is quickly anesthetized, paralyzed, and intubated with a cuffed endotracheal tube. During this process, an assistant exerts cricoid pressure by pressing firmly against the anterior portion of the neck over the cricoid cartilage in order to compress the esophagus; this helps prevent aspiration of gastric contents before inflation of the endotracheal cuff.

Avoidance of cardiac decompensation and hypotension during anesthesia for emergency abdominal surgery patients may also be difficult because they may have sepsis, vasodilatation, and unrecognized hypovolemia. The appropriate choices of anesthetic agents, monitoring techniques, intraoperative fluid management, and cardiotonic or vasopressor drugs demand expert consideration by the anesthesiologist.

Sound surgical technique and judgment are also critical in the treatment of patients undergoing emergency laparotomy. Often, a number of options exist regarding the specific procedure to perform; the surgeon must choose one of these options. Optimally, these decisions are based not solely on the specific intra-abdominal pathology but also on a patient's physiologic condition. Although specific surgical approaches to the various intra-abdominal diseases cannot be discussed here, several general decisions that often affect postoperative management deserve special mention.

Bowel Anastomosis Versus Exteriorization

Although primary bowel anastomosis obviates the need for stomal care as well as for subsequent surgery for ostomy closure, the risks accompanying anastomosis must always be considered. In particular, patients with preoperative shock or sepsis, or both, may have decreased mesenteric blood flow, and thus their anastomotic blood supply may be marginal. Furthermore, patients who are severely ill and particularly those with compromised cardiorespiratory reserve would be less able to tolerate the sepsis resulting from possible anastomotic leak. Thus, when these factors are present, it is good judgment to create intestinal stomas rather than to perform intestinal anastomosis.

Wound Closure Technique

A number of factors contribute to an increased incidence of abdominal wound dehiscence and evisceration, which are often disastrous postoperative complications. These factors include shock, malnutrition, respiratory failure, recent laparotomy, steroid therapy, and intra-abdominal infection. When these factors are present, particular care should be taken in fascial wound closure, and the use of retention suture techniques should be considered.

The risks of postoperative subcutaneous wound infection should also be considered during operation. When factors such as shock, bowel obstruction, intraperitoneal contamination, and infection are present, the risk of subcutaneous wound infection is considerable. In these conditions, wound infection can be avoided by leaving the skin and subcutaneous tissues open for subsequent secondary or delayed primary closure. Again, this should be considered especially for patients who would not tolerate the sepsis of postoperative wound infection.

Intra-Abdominal Drainage

The specifics of intra-abdominal drainage remain controversial, as a number of approaches have their own advocates.[17] Several general concepts are accepted, however.

First, use of drains has negative aspects. Drains not only draw off infection from the peritoneum to the outside; they also act as conduits for bacteria to enter the peritoneal cavity. In addition, drains can erode intra-abdominal structures, causing bleeding, abscesses, or fistulas. Finally, the presence of a foreign body within the abdominal cavity may decrease the intrinsic immunologic resistance of the peritoneal cavity to infection and may impair wound healing.

Second, the entire peritoneal cavity cannot be effectively drained, as any drainage tube is relatively quickly isolated by intraperitoneal reaction. Drainage should therefore be reserved for management of localized intra-abdominal abscesses or for attempts to control fistula output through a defined outflow tract.

Third, dependent drainage is preferable. Drains should be placed in as dependent a position as possible, optimally through the flank or retroperitoneum.

Fourth, closed drainage systems may have advantages over open systems but are often prone to occlusion. The use of sump drains may help to some extent. All drainage systems, and particularly open ones, need be cared for in the postoperative period with sterile technique.

Fifth, percutaneous drains may be effective at draining selected intra-abdominal abscesses and may obviate the need for formal anesthesia and operation. When an intra-abdominal abscess is detected preoperatively, it is appropriate to consider the possibility of percutaneous drainage as an alternative to operation. When such drainage is technically feasible and when a patient does not require laparotomy to treat underlying problems, percutaneous drainage is often advantageous.

Finally, peritoneal lavage has been advocated in certain situations, such as generalized peritonitis and pancreatitis, but its application remains controversial. Although the advantages of continuously "cleansing" the peritoneal cavity seem appealing, lavage may also decrease the effectiveness of the peritoneal defense mechanisms. Net benefit of therapeutic peritoneal lavage remains to be proved.

POSTOPERATIVE CARE

It is important to recognize that many determinants of postoperative complications are already present before the postoperative period. The metabolic stress of the underlying illness, the deficits resulting from preoperative shock and sepsis, and the superimposed stress of anesthesia and operation have all occurred before the postoperative period. The patient who has undergone emergency abdominal surgery has thus already undergone such significant stress that his or her needs for survival are no longer the same as those of normal individuals. Bland and coworkers have emphasized the different physiologic needs of such patients and have described "optimal" therapeutic goals that are significantly different from "normal" physiologic states.[18] These optimal therapeutic goals reflect the requirements of postoperative emergency patients to compensate physiologically for the combined stresses of preoperative illness, shock, sepsis, anesthesia, and surgery.

Several other aspects of postoperative care deserve emphasis. Rather than wait for complications to occur, one can initiate expectant physiologic monitoring early in the postoperative period for patients at high risk for the development of complications. Early monitoring of patients at risk allows titration of postoperative therapy to achieve optimal physiologic goals. In particular, increased cardiac output, increased oxygen delivery, and increased oxygen consumption are necessary in the early postoperative period. Titration of therapy to optimize tissue oxygenation improves both cellular and organ recovery from shock and resistance to infection.[19]

Every effort must be made to prevent septic complications. Compulsive maintenance of sterile technique during insertion of indwelling catheters cannot be overemphasized. Furthermore, intravascular as well as urinary monitoring catheters should be removed as soon as possible (i.e., as soon as the information they provide is no longer essential to the patient's care).

Aggressive pulmonary care helps prevent pulmonary complications that lead to sepsis. This care should include administration of positive end-expiratory pressure and frequent suctioning with sterile technique for intubated patients and early ambulation and incentive spirometry for extubated patients.

Wound care should be meticulous. Of particular importance is avoidance of the spread of bacteria from drainage sites or wounds to other patients. Hand washing is critical in this regard.

Because surgical drains placed in the peritoneal cavity have the potential to introduce contamination as well as act as conduits for drainage, they should be removed as early as feasible. Drains placed to remove blood (e.g., splenic bed drains placed after splenectomy) may be removed after 1 day if bleeding is not evident. Drains placed to draw off secretions (e.g., drains placed after cholecystectomy) should be removed when fluid drainage ceases. Drains placed in established abscess cavities are removed by advancing them slowly as the cavity size decreases or a drainage tract becomes well established. Drains placed to control fistula output should be left in place until the fistula has closed or until a well-established tract has been formed.

Despite excellent postoperative care, an incidence of postoperative septic complications is inevitable after emergency abdominal surgery. The key to the successful management of these complications is continuing suspicion and early diagnosis. Careful daily physical examination, with particular attention devoted to the chest, abdomen, and wounds, is essential. The diagnosis of sepsis in the postoperative period can often be made before definitive culture identification on the basis of signs such as fever, hyperventilation, worsening mental status, decreased systemic vascular resistance, or deterioration of organ function.

Therapy for suspected sepsis should be instituted as early as possible, and great emphasis should be placed on signs of physiologic decompensation. Antibiotic therapy appropriate to the suspected bacteriologic flora is indicated, sometimes even before specific culture results are available. Suspected intra-abdominal sources of sepsis must be vigorously diagnosed and treated.

ACUTE ABDOMINAL COMPLICATIONS IN THE INTENSIVE CARE UNIT

The critical illness caused by acute abdominal disease has been discussed. Conversely, acute abdominal disease can also be caused by critical illness. The diagnosis and treatment of acute abdominal complications occurring in patients who are already critically ill can be difficult and deserve particular emphasis. Several such complications occur with such a frequency and have such a significant impact (particularly if unrecognized) that they deserve special mention.

Ileus

Adynamic ileus is failure of the normal peristaltic function of the intestine and is a frequent occurrence in critically ill patients. It is particularly prevalent in patients who have had shock or sepsis, possibly because of the decrease in mesenteric blood flow that results from these conditions. Patients with respiratory failure are also at risk for ileus, again perhaps because of a decrease in oxygen delivery to the gut. In addition, ileus may be an early sign of unrecognized intra-abdominal infection.[20]

Ileus in critically ill patients leads to several serious problems. First, the inability to tolerate oral or enteral feedings interferes with nutritional support. Second, the abdominal distention resulting from ileus can significantly impair pulmonary function. Third, large volumes of fluid can be sequestered in the intestinal lumen, causing hypovolemia and electrolyte disturbances. Finally, massive colonic ileus (*Ogilvie's syndrome*) can result in perforation of the colon, a disastrous complication.

The diagnosis of ileus is usually apparent when abdominal distention, nausea, and vomiting occur in postoperative patients or those with serious underlying illness. Bowel sounds are hypoactive or absent. Abdominal radiographs show distention of the small intestine and large intestine. At times, it may prove difficult to differentiate ileus from mechanical bowel obstruction; CT scanning may be most useful in this differentiation.

Early recognition and treatment of ileus are important; the more distended the intestine becomes, the less effective the peristalsis and the more prolonged the bowel dysfunction. To some extent, ileus can be prevented or minimized with optimal hemodynamic support. Correction of hypovolemia and inadequate cardiac output may restore mesenteric perfusion and improve gut motility. Electrolyte disturbances should be corrected. In particular, hypokalemia, hypophosphatemia and hypomagnesemia may intensify bowel dysfunction. An active search for intra-abdominal infection must be undertaken.

Of great importance are the early cessation of oral fluid and food intake and the initiation of nasogastric suction. Nasogastric tubes are of two types: *simple tubes* (e.g., Levine tubes), which require intermittent suction, and *sump tubes* (e.g., Salem tubes), which require constant suction. Nasogastric suction can effectively prevent intestinal distention, but tube patency must be checked frequently. Consideration should always be given to the initiation of intravenous nutritional support, because it is frequently many days before a patient is able to tolerate oral or enteral feedings.

Finally, if massive or progressive colonic distention is present, it can be effectively reversed by colonoscopic decompression and cecal perforation can be prevented.[21] If colonoscopy is not available, operative or percutaneous decompression of the cecum may be necessary.

Stress Ulcer

In the past, bleeding and perforation caused by stress ulceration of the stomach or duodenum were frequent causes of morbidity in critically ill patients. Although endoscopy continues to reveal significant mucosal injury in many ICU patients, bleeding and perforation are now uncommon because of widespread use of prophylactic antacid therapy.[22] Histamine H_2 receptor antagonists, antacids, and sucralfate are all effective in preventing complications of stress ulceration. These complications, however, do continue to occur in severely stressed and septic patients, particularly if antacid therapy is inadequate. Patients at high risk include those with head injury, multiple trauma, or burns; patients with respiratory failure receiving mechanical ventilation; and those receiving corticosteroid or nonsteroidal anti-inflammatory therapy. The most effective regimen in preventing bleeding from stress ulcers in high-risk patients is frequent titration of antacid therapy to maintain a gastric pH of 4.0 or greater.

When upper gastrointestinal bleeding does occur in the ICU, endoscopy is indicated to differentiate possible causes. If bleeding from diffuse gastric stress ulceration is identified, medical management consisting of hemodynamic resuscitation, gastric lavage, and intensive antacid therapy is usually successful. Continued bleeding may respond to intravenous administration of vasopressin. Endoscopic electrocauterization may also be helpful. If further bleeding does not respond to these measures, the prognosis is poor. Attempts at arteriographic embolization may be undertaken but are usually unsuccessful.

Operative therapy should be reserved for patients who continue to bleed despite aggressive medical management. Operation should be considered when blood loss exceeds 6 units of blood over 24 hours. Surgical options include subtotal or total gastrectomy and vagotomy and pyloroplasty or gastric resection with oversewing of gastric ulcers; such operations in the presence of bleeding in stress gastritis involve a high risk of mortality but may be lifesaving when medical management has failed.

Critically ill ICU patients with perforated gastric or duodenal ulcers also have a high risk of mortality. Perforated ulcers must be considered whenever high-risk patients experience acute abdominal pain and show peritoneal findings. Abdominal radiographs or CT scans usually demonstrate free air, but this finding may be subtle or absent in patients with extensive intra-abdominal adhesions. Early diagnosis and prompt laparotomy are essential for a successful outcome.

Acalculous Cholecystitis

Acalculous cholecystitis is due to acute biliary stasis without stone formation. It occurs most commonly in critically ill patients with prolonged illness who have had long-term intravenous hyperalimentation without oral intake and who have had shock or sepsis. Stasis of the gallbladder can be due to absent gastrointestinal stimulation, sepsis, or ischemia.

A high degree of suspicion is necessary for diagnosis of this condition because many patients are too ill to communicate their symptoms. Unexplained abdominal tenderness, ileus, and fever as well as possible abnormal liver function test results suggest the diagnosis. Bedside ultrasonography may show a distended gallbladder with a thickened wall and surrounding fluid. The gallbladder does not contract despite cholecystokinin administration. The gallbladder does not fill on iminodiacetic acid scanning, even after morphine administration.[23]

Therapy should be initiated as soon as possible after diagnosis. Options for therapy include cholecystectomy, cholecystostomy performed with local anesthesia, laparoscopic cholecystostomy, and percutaneous drainage of the gallbladder with ultrasound guidance.

Intestinal Necrosis

Ischemic intestinal necrosis may occur in critically ill patients for a variety of reasons. It may be associated with occlusive disease of the mesenteric arteries that is due to either an acute embolic event (usually associated with cardiac arrhythmias) or a low-flow state superimposed on arteriosclerotic mesenteric disease. Mesenteric ischemia is a particular risk after abdominal aortic surgery when the inferior mesenteric artery is sacrificed. Advanced pseudomembranous colitis may also progress to intestinal necrosis. Mesenteric infarction may also occur without occlusion of the arterial inflow, usually in association with severe or prolonged low-flow states and, sometimes, with mesenteric venous thrombosis.

Intestinal necrosis often presents a difficult diagnostic dilemma because patients in whom it occurs may be too ill to communicate any of their symptoms. Ileus and abdominal distention may be the only signs present. Stool may contain occult blood. Plain abdominal radiographs may show thumbprinting. Intestinal necrosis is often associated with severe systemic toxicity, fever, and significant leukocytosis. Acidosis and thrombocytopenia are also often present. When such signs occur in critically ill patients, especially in patients who have had recent arrhythmias or low-flow states, a diagnosis of intestinal necrosis should be considered. Proctosigmoidoscopy may reveal mucosal ischemia. Diagnostic peritoneal lavage is useful because it can be performed rapidly at the bedside and is quite sensitive. CT scanning is often useful in confirming the diagnosis.

Early laparotomy and bowel resection are mandatory when intestinal necrosis has occurred. If ischemic, but not necrotic, bowel is found at operation, alternatives to resection include surgical revascularization, thrombolysis and anticoagulation, and vasodilator therapy. In such cases, early planned reoperation to exclude intestinal necrosis is often necessary.

Pancreatitis

Hyperamylasemia is relatively common in critically ill patients. Serious pancreatitis, however, is unusual. When pancreatitis is severe, it is manifested by abdominal pain, ileus, hypovolemia, pulmonary failure, hypocalcemia, and multiple organ failure. Among other possible etiologic factors, inadequate blood flow may both cause and potentiate acute pancreatitis. Thus, patients with severe pancreatitis occurring in the postoperative period or superimposed on critical illness benefit from aggressive hemodynamic resuscitation to optimize cardiac output.

Fluid requirements may be enormous, hemodynamic instability is common, and respiratory failure is often severe. Intensive cardiopulmonary monitoring, optimal fluid therapy, and aggressive supportive care are essential for maximizing a patient's chances for survival. CT scanning should be performed to confirm the diagnosis of pancreatitis, to evaluate the severity of the inflammatory process, and to determine whether abscess formation amenable to drainage has occurred.

Intra-Abdominal Abscess

Intra-abdominal abscesses are a common but sometimes insidious cause of sepsis in critically ill patients. They most commonly occur after previous abdominal trauma, infection, and operation. On occasion, however, an intra-abdominal abscess, such as a hepatic or splenic abscess, may occur without prior abdominal disease, as a result of hematogenous spread from distant infection.[24]

The diagnosis of intra-abdominal abscesses in critically ill patients may be difficult, as symptoms and signs are often difficult to elicit and to interpret. A high index of suspicion is necessary for patients who are at high risk because of prior abdominal disease and operation and those who have occult sepsis. Fever, leukocytosis, and coagulopathy are additional clues. The best diagnostic test is CT, which has high sensitivity and specificity for the diagnosis of intra-abdominal abscess. Localization of abscesses with CT is also of great value in planning either percutaneous or operative drainage. If a patient is too unstable for transfer to the CT suite, bedside ultrasound imaging, if technically possible, may localize abscesses.

Treatment of intra-abdominal infection that complicates critical illness requires intensive care and judgment. Intra-abdominal infection often precipitates worsening of multiple organ function and necessitates intensification of monitoring, resuscitation, and organ support. Aggressive antibiotic therapy directed at the organisms likely to be present must be initiated. CT imaging should be performed, optimally with a plan to place percutaneous drains during the same procedure if abscesses that are amenable are identified. If intra-abdominal abscesses cannot be drained by percutaneous techniques or if a patient does not improve despite intensive support and antibiotics, exploratory laparotomy is mandatory.

References

1. Cope SZ: The Early Diagnosis of the Acute Abdomen. 14th ed. London, Oxford University Press, 1972.
2. Platell C: Atelectasis after abdominal surgery. J Am Coll Surg 1997; 185:584–592.
3. Mark JB: Central venous pressure monitoring: Clinical insights beyond the numbers. J Clin Vasc Anesth 1991; 5:163–173.
4. Shoemaker WC, Wo CC, Bishop MH, et al: Noninvasive physiologic monitoring of high risk surgical patients. Arch Surg 1996; 131:732–737.
5. Chang R, Wong GY: Prognostic significance of marked leukocytosis in hospitalized patients. J Gen Intern Med 1991; 6:199–203.
6. Winslet M, Hall C, London NJ, et al: Relation of diagnostic serum

amylase levels to aetiology and severity of acute pancreatitis. Gut 1992; 33:982–986.
7. Boulanger BR, Brenneman FD, McLellan BA, et al: A prospective study of emergent abdominal sonography after blunt trauma. J Trauma 1995; 39:325–330.
8. Taourel P, Baron MP, Pradel J, et al: Acute abdomen of unknown origin: Impact of CT on diagnosis and management. Gastrointest Radiol 1992; 17:287–291.
9. Lantto E: Investigation of suspected intra-abdominal sepsis: The contribution of nuclear medicine. Scand J Gastroenterol Suppl 1994; 203:11–14.
10. Klein HM, Lensing R, Klosterhalfen B, et al: Diagnostic imaging of mesenteric infarction. Radiology 1995; 197:79–82.
11. Mozingo DW, Cioffi WG, McManus WF, Pruitt BA: Peritoneal lavage in the diagnosis of acute surgical abdomen following thermal injury. J Trauma 1995; 38:5–7.
12. Larson GM: Laparoscopy for abdominal emergencies. Scand J Gastroenterol Suppl 1995; 208:62–66.
13. Donovan AJ, Vinson TL, Maulsby GO, et al: Selective treatment of duodenal ulcer with perforation. Ann Surg 1979; 189:627–636.
14. Patti MG, Pelligrini CA: Gallstone pancreatitis. Surg Clin North Am 1990; 70:1277–1295.
15. Bizer LS, Liebling RW, Delay HM, et al: Small bowel obstruction: The role of nonoperative treatment in simple intestinal obstruction and predictive criteria for strangulation obstruction. Surgery 1981; 89:407–413.
16. Forsmark CE, Toskes PP: Acute pancreatitis: Medical management. Crit Care Clin 1995; 11:295–309.
17. Dougherty SH, Simmons RL: The biology and practice of surgical drains. Curr Probl Surg 1992; 24:561–685.
18. Bland R, Shoemaker WC, Shabot MM: Physiologic monitoring goals for the critically ill patient. Surg Gynecol Obstet 1978; 147:833–841.
19. Sawyer RG, Pruett TL: Wound infections. Surg Clin North Am 1994; 74:519–536.
20. Dark DS, Pingleton SK: Nonhemorrhagic gastrointestinal complications in acute respiratory failure. Crit Care Med 1989; 17:755–758.
21. Jetmore AM, Timmcke AE, Gathright JB, et al: Ogilvie's syndrome: Colonoscopic decompression and analysis of predisposing factors. Dis Colon Rectum 1992; 35:1135–1142.
22. Simons RK, Hoyt DB, Winchell RJ, et al: Stress-related mucosal disease: Pathophysiology, prevention, and treatment. Crit Care Clin 1995; 11:323–345.
23. Barie PS, Fischer E: Acute acalculous cholecystitis. J Am Coll Surg 1995; 180:232–244.
24. McClean KL, Sheehan GJ, Harding GK: Intraabdominal infection: A review. Clin Infect Dis 1994; 19:100–116.

148

Severe Gastrointestinal Hemorrhage

Thomas J. Savides, MD • Dennis M. Jensen, MD

Severe gastrointestinal (GI) bleeding is defined as documented GI bleeding (i.e., hematemesis, melena, hematochezia, or positive nasogastric lavage) accompanied by either shock or orthostatic hypotension, decrease of hematocrit by 8%, or transfusion of at least 2 units of packed red blood cells. Most of these patients are admitted to intensive care units (ICUs) for resuscitation. Acute management of these patients is conducted by a team of physicians, including gastroenterologists, surgeons, and critical care specialists. Improvement in patient outcomes occurs as a result of successful medical resuscitation, precise endoscopic diagnosis, and appropriate use of therapeutic endoscopy and surgery.

INITIAL APPROACH TO THE PATIENT WITH SEVERE GASTROINTESTINAL BLEEDING

Initial Assessment

Initial patient assessment includes history, vital signs with orthostatic blood pressure determination, physical and rectal examinations, and nasogastric lavage. Patients should be asked about prior history of GI bleeding, ulcers, heartburn, liver disease, cancer, bleeding disorders, irradiation to the abdomen, aortic aneurysm repair, or other abdominal surgery. They should also be asked about use of aspirin or nonsteroidal anti-inflammatory drugs (NSAIDs), alcohol, or anticoagulants and about chest pain, syncope, weight loss, abdominal pain, vomiting, or change in bowel habits. The examiner should look for surgical scars, abdominal masses or pulsations, and signs of chronic liver disease, such as spider angiomas, palmar erythema, gynecomastia, and ascites.

One or two large-bore (14- or 16-gauge) intravenous catheters should be placed. Blood should be sent for hematocrit, platelets, prothrombin time, partial thromboplastin time, chemistry panel, and type and crossmatch for packed red blood cells. Resuscitation should be initiated simultaneously with assessment. Normal saline is infused as fast as needed to keep the systolic blood pressure above 100 mm Hg and the pulse below 100 beats/min. Patients are transfused with packed red blood cells, platelets, and fresh frozen plasma as necessary to keep the hematocrit above 24%, platelet count above 50,000/mm^3, and prothrombin time under 15 seconds. A gastroenterologist and a surgeon should be notified as soon as possible to expedite patient diagnosis and possible therapy. In hospitals with liver transplantation programs, if the patient has advanced liver disease and is a potential liver transplant candidate, the liver transplantation team should also be consulted.

Management in the Intensive Care Unit

Patients with severe GI bleeding should be admitted to an ICU or a monitored intermediate-care unit. Patients should undergo automatic blood pressure monitoring every 5 minutes if they are hemodynamically unstable and hourly if stable. Each patient should receive cardiac rhythm monitoring to observe for arrhythmias and to follow the heart rate as a sign of continued or recurrent bleeding. Laboratory-determined hematocrits (not finger-stick hematocrits, which are less reliable) should be obtained every 4 to 6 hours until the hematocrit is stable. In cases of active bleeding, an indwelling bladder catheter should be placed to help monitor fluid status. Swan-Ganz catheter monitoring is unnecessary except for patients with a history of congestive heart failure or unstable cardiac disease. Patients older than 60 years of age should also be evaluated for myocardial infarction with electrocardiograms (ECGs) and creatinine kinase measurements.

Localization of the Site of Hemorrhage

Hematemesis, coffee-grounds emesis, or a nasogastric lavage with blood or large amounts of coffee-grounds emesis indicates an upper GI source. A small amount of coffee-grounds emesis that clears easily may represent an upper GI source of bleeding or only mucosal trauma from the nasogastric tube. A clear nasogastric aspirate does not necessarily indicate a more distal GI source; 16% of patients with actively bleeding lesions have clear nasogastric aspirates.[1] The presence of bile in the nasogastric tube makes upper GI bleeding less likely but may be consistent with an upper GI source that bleeds intermittently. Guaiac tests of nasogastric aspirates are not helpful because of high rates of false-positive and false-negative test results.[2]

Use, Timing, and Complications of Endoscopy

Experienced endoscopists detect a source of upper GI bleeding in more than 90% of cases, and this facilitates simultaneous treatment via endoscopy.[1] Endoscopy should be done only when it is safe and if the information will influence patient care. Patients should be hemodynamically stable, with a heart rate of less than 100 beats/min and systolic blood pressure greater than 100 mm Hg. Respiratory insufficiency, altered mental status, or ongoing hematemesis indicates the need for endotracheal intubation before emergency endoscopy for patient stabilization and protection of the airway. Coagulopathy and thrombocytopenia should be corrected with transfusions.

Patients with active hemorrhage (i.e., bloody nasogastric lavage) should undergo urgent endoscopy after medical resuscitation. In patients with massive bleeding and shock, endoscopy can be performed in the operating room. Patients who have acute self-limited blood loss with no evidence of ongoing bleeding can undergo endoscopy within 12 hours, except those patients with cirrhosis, possible aortoenteric fistula, or evidence of rebleeding. "Middle-of-the-night" endoscopy should be avoided, if possible, because well-trained endoscopy nurses, endoscopy equipment, and surgical back-up may not be available.

Complications related to emergency endoscopy occur in up to 1% of patients.[3] The most common complications include perforation, aspiration, induced hemorrhage, medication reaction, hypotension, and hypoxia.[3] Because of the risk of aspiration, especially in encephalopathic or massively bleeding patients, prophylactic intubation for airway protection before endoscopy is often advisable.

In severe upper GI bleeding, gastric lavage with a large (No. 34 French) orogastric tube is performed to evacuate blood from the stomach to prevent aspiration and to clear the stomach of blood and clots before endoscopy. There is no value in using iced saline lavage to prevent or decrease upper GI bleeding.[4] Gastric lavage with lukewarm tap water is as safe as that with saline and significantly less expensive.[5]

In cases of suspected lower GI bleeding, patients should undergo urgent colonoscopy after rapid sulfate purge.[6] In the ICU, patients receive 4 L of polyethylene glycol (i.e., GoLYTELY) either orally or via nasogastric tube over 3 to 5 hours until the rectal effluent is clear of stool, blood, and clots. Metoclopramide, 10 mg, may be given intravenously before the purge and repeated every 3 to 4 hours to facilitate gastric emptying and reduce nausea.

Use and Timing of Angiography, Radionucleotide Studies, and Surgery

Most patients with severe GI bleeding are admitted to medical ICUs and surgical consultation. Patients who have massive hemorrhage and cannot be stabilized with ICU resuscitation should undergo urgent surgical exploration either without prior endoscopy or with emergency endoscopy in the operating room. Emergency angiography may also be used to detect and treat severe bleeding of obscure origin that was not diagnosed by upper and lower endoscopy. Radionucleotide studies are rarely needed, except in cases of intermittent bleeding of unknown origin.

UPPER GASTROINTESTINAL BLEEDING

Upper GI bleeding is a common medical emergency that accounts for more than 300,000 hospital admissions each year, or approximately 150 patients with severe upper GI bleeding per 100,000 population per year.[7] Despite advances in medical therapy, ICU care, endoscopy, and surgery, the mortality rate of 10% for severe upper GI bleeding has not changed over the past 30 years.[8, 9] The lack of decline of mortality may be explained by an increase in the proportion of elderly patients with GI bleeding who usually die of worsening of other medical problems and not of exsanguination.[8, 9]

The most common causes of severe upper GI bleeding among patients admitted to the University of California, Los Angeles (UCLA) Medical Center and the West Los Angeles Veterans Administration Medical Center are shown in Table 148–1. The frequency of causes of bleeding reflects the population served by the hospital. For example, fewer patients with bleeding ulcers and more bleeding varices and Mallory-Weiss tears are admitted to hospitals caring for greater numbers of alcoholic patients.

Bleeding is self-limited in 80% to 85% of patients with upper GI hemorrhage, even without specific therapy.[8, 10] Of the remaining 15% to 20% who continue to experience bleeding or rebleeding, the mortality rate is 30% to 40%.[1, 10] Patients at high risk for continuous bleeding or rebleeding potentially can benefit the most from acute medical, endoscopic, and surgical therapy.

PEPTIC ULCER HEMORRHAGE

Peptic ulcers are the leading cause of severe upper GI bleeding in the United States and account for 50% of bleeding episodes and approximately 100,000 hospitalizations per year.[11, 12] Poor prognostic factors in peptic ulcer bleeding are associated with increased morbidity and mortality (Table 148–2). Knowledge of these risk factors can assist physicians in identifying patients at high risk for rebleeding and in determining ICU utilization and timing of endoscopy.

Medical Therapy for Severe Peptic Ulcer Hemorrhage

No medical therapy has been found to significantly decrease transfusions, rebleeding rates, surgery rates, or mortality in

TABLE 148–1. Causes of Severe Upper Gastrointestinal Bleeding in 948 Consecutive Patients*

Diagnosis†	%
Peptic ulcer	55
Gastric or esophageal varix	14
Angioma	6
Mallory-Weiss tear	5
Tumor	4
Erosions	4
Esophagitis	4
Other	8

*All patients at the University of California, Los Angeles Medical Center, and the West Los Angeles Veterans Administration Medical Center had emergency endoscopy by the Center for Ulcer Research and Education (CURE) Hemostasis Research Group after resuscitation in an intensive care unit or monitored bed setting.

†The diagnosis was based on endoscopic findings, including stigmata of recent hemorrhage.

TABLE 148–2. Adverse Prognostic Factors in Peptic Ulcer Hemorrhage

Age greater than 60 years
Comorbid medical illness
Shock or orthostatic hypotension
Coagulopathy
Bleeding onset in hospital
Multiple transfusions required
Fresh blood in nasogastric tube
Higher lesser curve gastric ulcer (adjacent to left gastric artery)
Posterior duodenal bulb ulcer (adjacent to gastroduodenal artery)
Endoscopic finding of arterial bleeding or visible vessel

patients with severe peptic ulcer hemorrhage.[13] Although most patients with upper GI bleeding are treated with histamine$_2$ (H_2) receptor antagonists before endoscopy, randomized, placebo-controlled trials and meta-analysis indicate that H_2 blockers do not stop active bleeding or prevent acute rebleeding. One study outside the United States reported that high-dose oral omeprazole decreased the rates of rebleeding and surgery compared with placebo in patients with endoscopic nonbleeding visible vessels or adherent clots.[14] Until additional studies confirm these findings, high-dose proton pump inhibitors should not be considered standard care for patients with suspected peptic ulcer bleeding in the United States. Once the exact bleeding site is determined by endoscopy and major endoscopic stigmata are treated, the appropriate medical therapy can be instituted. Measures include stopping aspirin, NSAIDs, and anticoagulants.

Helicobacter pylori infection of the stomach is a contributing factor to the cause of peptic ulcers. Although there is a role for *H. pylori* eradication to reduce ulcer recurrence or rebleeding, there is no role for acute *H. pylori* eradication in the management of severe upper GI bleeding.

Endoscopic Therapy for Severe Peptic Ulcer Hemorrhage

The endoscopic appearance (stigmata of hemorrhage) of peptic ulcer bases and the associated risks of rebleeding are shown in Table 148–3. The patients at highest risk for rebleeding are those with active arterial bleeding, a visible vessel, or an adherent clot.[15] These are the patients who may benefit from endoscopic hemostasis. Patients with clean-based ulcers or flat spots have very low rates of rebleeding and can leave the ICU soon after endoscopy and immediately begin a regular diet.[16] Patients with oozing bleeding in the absence of a visible vessel, or with adherent clots, have an intermediate rebleeding rate of less than 20%. Treatment of these ulcers is controversial, and some endoscopists elect to treat them.

The goal of endoscopic hemostasis is to coagulate or thrombose the underlying artery. This can be done with various thermal devices, including contact probes (monopolar electrocoagulation, bipolar electrocoagulation, heater probe, argon beam coagulator) or laser devices, such as neodymium yttrium aluminum garnet (YAG) or argon. Animal studies have shown that these thermal devices are effective in coagulating arteries up to 2 mm in diameter, which is considerably larger than the arteries found in resected bleeding human peptic ulcers, which are usually less than 1 mm.[17, 18] Monopolar electrocoagulation is generally not used because of concern for excessive tissue damage. Laser is not used for acute GI bleeding because of lack of portability to the ICU and expense of the equipment. A 1989 National Institutes of Health consensus conference concluded that the two "most promising techniques" of endoscopic hemostasis for bleeding ulcers were multipolar electrocoagulation and heater probe.[19] In addition, injection therapies using epinephrine, polidocanol, or alcohol have been introduced as effective but less expensive alternatives.

Randomized controlled studies have shown that multipolar electrocoagulation probe, bipolar electrocoagulation probe, and injection therapy are all better than medical therapy alone for treating patients with peptic ulcers that have active bleeding or visible vessels in terms of reducing transfusions, length of hospital stay, and need for emergency surgery.[20–23] Table 148–4 shows the results of one such large randomized UCLA Medical Center/Center for Ulcer Research and Education (UCLA/CURE) study of multipolar electrocoagulation and heater probe compared with medical therapy alone in the treatment of peptic ulcers with active bleeding or nonbleeding visible vessels. The results of several randomized studies comparing the different thermal modalities with the injection therapy suggest that both methods have similar efficacy and safety (Table 148–5).[24, 25] The results of ongoing, randomized, controlled trials will help determine the optimal treatment techniques.

Bleeding stress ulcers that occur in either the duodenum or the stomach of severely ill inpatients in ICUs do not seem to respond as well to endoscopic therapy as do peptic ulcers that start to bleed before hospitalization.[26] The cause of these in-hospital ulcers is unknown, but the poor prognosis and high rebleeding rates are often related to impaired wound healing and multiple organ failure. Generally, patients with these lesions should be supported medically, and these ulcers heal as the patient's overall medical status improves.

TABLE 148–3. Endoscopic Appearance of Peptic Ulcer Bases After Recent Hemorrhage: Prevalence and Rate of Rebleeding*

Endoscopic Appearance (Stigmata of Hemorrhage)	Prevalence (%)	Rebleeding Rate (%)
Active arterial bleeding	10	90
Nonbleeding visible vessel	25	50
Nonbleeding adherent clot	10	25
Oozing without visible vessel	5	<20
Flat spot	15	<10
Clean ulcer base	35	<5

Data from Freeman ML: The current endoscopic diagnosis and intensive care unit management of severe ulcer and other nonvariceal upper gastrointestinal hemorrhage. Gastrointest Endosc Clin North Am 1991; 1:209–239.

*Rebleeding rates are with medical therapy alone, without endoscopic hemostasis.

TABLE 148–4. Comparison of Multipolar Electrocoagulation, Heater Probe, and Medical Therapy for Peptic Ulcers with Active Bleeding or Nonbleeding Visible Vessels

Variable	Medical Therapy (n = 41)	Electro-coagulation (n = 45)	Heater Probe (n = 41)
Initial hemostasis (%)	14	93*	95*
Rebleeding (%)	66	44	24*
Blood transfusions (units)	3.4	2.4	1.0*
Emergency surgery (%)	42	28	5*
Mortality	10	2	2

Data from Jensen DM: Heat probe for hemostasis of bleeding peptic ulcers: Techniques and results of randomized controlled trials. Gastrointest Endosc 1990; 36:S42–S49.

*$P < .05$ versus medical therapy.

TABLE 148–5. Comparison of Multipolar Electrocoagulation Versus Alcohol Injection for Peptic Ulcers with Active Bleeding or Nonbleeding Visible Vessels

Variable	Electrocoagulation (n = 31)	Injection (n = 29)	*P*
Further bleeding (%)	6.0	10.0	NS
Blood transfusions (units)	1.8	1.3	NS
Emergency surgery (%)	6.0	7.0	NS
Hospital stay (days)	5.8	7.2	NS
Mortality (%)	3.0	3.0	NS

Data from Laine L: Multipolar electrocoagulation versus injection therapy in the treatment of bleeding peptic ulcers. Gastroenterology 1990; 99:1303–1306.
NS = not significant.

Surgery for Bleeding Peptic Ulcers

Acute surgical intervention is indicated when there is an exsanguinating bleeding and the patient cannot be medically resuscitated. Patients with recurrent bleeding despite two sessions of endoscopic hemostasis should receive surgical therapy. Patients should also be referred for surgery if the endoscopist does not feel comfortable treating a very large or pulsating visible vessel (e.g., a vessel in a deep, posterior duodenal ulcer, which may represent the gastroduodenal artery). Another indication for surgery is a bleeding malignant ulcer, documented by biopsy.

VARICEAL HEMORRHAGE

Esophageal variceal bleeding related to portal hypertension is the second most common cause of severe upper GI bleeding after peptic ulcers. The acute mortality is approximately 30% with each bleed, and the long-term survival rate is less than 40% after 1 year with medical management in one large Veterans Affairs series.[27] Despite advances in medical therapy, endoscopic hemostasis, and portosystemic shunt procedures, survival rates have not improved for variceal bleeding. The exception is with liver transplantation, which can improve survival in selected patients. Survival in patients who have not received transplants is heavily influenced by the extent of underlying liver disease, with much worse survival rates for Child's class C patients than class A or B patients.

Bleeding gastric varices are a difficult therapeutic problem; unlike bleeding esophageal varices, they do not respond to most nonsurgical treatments. An exception is when isolated gastric varices are found without accompanying esophageal varices. This raises the possibility of splenic vein thrombosis, which often occurs in association with pancreatitis or pancreatic cancer. The diagnosis of splenic vein thrombosis can be made with Doppler ultrasound or angiography. Bleeding from gastric varices caused by splenic vein thrombosis is treated by splenectomy.

Medical Management of Acute Variceal Bleeding

Vasopressin can lower portal pressure by vasoconstriction of the splanchnic arteriolar bed. Although widely used for variceal bleeding, intravenous vasopressin has not been shown in clinical trials to be significantly better than placebo for hemostasis or survival.[28] Vasopressin has a high incidence of cardiac complications as a result of nonspecific vasoconstriction, which can be reduced with the simultaneous use of intravenous or sublingual nitroglycerin.

Octreotide, the long-acting analog of somatostatin, causes selective splanchnic vasoconstriction without cardiac complications. Results as to whether somatostatin is more effective than placebo in managing variceal bleeding have been mixed, but this hormone seems to be at least as effective as vasopressin and much safer.[29–31] One meta-analysis suggested that octreotide is more effective and has fewer adverse effects than vasopressin.[32] One study even showed octreotide to be as effective as sclerotherapy for initial control of variceal bleeding.[33] No studies have shown any survival benefit to patients with variceal bleeding using vasopressin or somatostatin. Given the potential ability of octreotide to control acute variceal hemorrhage and its low toxicity, octreotide appears to be the pharmacologic drug of choice for treatment of variceal hemorrhage as an adjunct to endoscopic therapy. The dose of octreotide for acute variceal hemorrhage is a 50-μg bolus followed by 50 μg/hr continuous infusion for up to 5 days.

Balloon Tamponade of Varices

Balloon tamponade of varices is seldom used today to control variceal bleeding. Because varices lie in the esophageal and gastric submucosa, they are amenable to physical tamponade. There are three types of tamponade balloons.

1. The Sengstaken-Blakemore tube has gastric and esophageal balloons, with a single aspirating port in the stomach.
2. The Minnesota tube also has gastric and esophageal balloons but has aspiration ports in the esophagus and the stomach.
3. The Linton-Nicholas tube has a single large gastric balloon and aspiration ports in the stomach and esophagus.

Most reports suggest that balloon tamponade provides initial tamponade in 85% to 98%, but variceal rebleeding recurs soon after deflating the balloon in 21% to 60% of patients.[34] The major problem with tamponade balloons is a 30% rate of serious complications such as aspiration pneumonia, esophageal rupture, and airway obstruction.[35] Patients should be intubated before placement of tamponade balloons to minimize the pulmonary complications. Clinical studies have not shown any significant difference in efficacy between vasopressin and balloon tamponade.

Endoscopic Variceal Sclerotherapy

Endoscopic variceal sclerotherapy involves injecting sclerosants into or adjacent to esophageal varices. The most commonly used sclerosants are ethanolamine oleate, sodium tetradecyl sulfate, morrhuate sodium, and ethanol. Cyanoacrylate is a glue that is very effective for both esophageal and gastric varices, but it is difficult to use and not available in the United States. Various techniques are used, with the common goal being initial hemostasis and then weekly sclerotherapy until obliteration of all varices. Esophageal varices are much more amenable to endoscopic therapy than gastric varices.

Prospective randomized trials show mixed results but suggest improved immediate hemostasis and a reduction in acute rebleeding with sclerotherapy compared with medical therapy for treatment of bleeding esophageal varices.[36–39] The complications of endoscopic variceal sclerotherapy include esophageal ulcers (which can bleed or perforate), esophageal strictures, mediastinitis, pleural effusions, aspiration pneumonia, adult respiratory distress syndrome (ARDS), chest pain, fever, and bacteremia.

Endoscopic Variceal Band Ligation

Endoscopic band ligation is a technique similar to that used in band ligation of internal hemorrhoids. A rubber band is placed over a varix, with subsequent thrombosis, sloughing, and fibrosis. Prospective, randomized, controlled trials show that endoscopic band ligation is equally effective as sclerotherapy in initial hemostasis and in reducing rebleeding rates for bleeding esophageal varices.[40, 41] Banding seems to produce fewer local complications, especially in terms of esophageal strictures. Banding may be more technically difficult to perform than endoscopic sclerotherapy during active variceal bleeding. New band ligation devices allow up to 10 bands to be placed without needing to remove the endoscope to reload the banding device.

Surgical Portosystemic Shunts

Various surgical portosystemic shunts can be performed to reduce portal venous pressure. When compared with sclerotherapy, surgical shunts significantly decrease the rebleeding rate but do not improve survival.[42–46] Some groups suggest that survival can be improved by using the combination of endoscopic sclerotherapy and surgical shunt rescue for patients who have rebleeding despite sclerotherapy.[43] Surgical shunts may be associated with increased hepatic encephalopathy and can make future liver transplantation technically more difficult. Surgical shunts do have an advantage over endoscopic techniques in terms of reducing portal hypertension to treat gastric variceal bleeding. Surgical shunts are of value in selected patients who have not had successful endoscopic therapy and who are not expected to become candidates for liver transplantation.

Radiologic Transjugular Intrahepatic Portosystemic Shunt

Transjugular intrahepatic portosystemic shunt (TIPS) is an interventional radiology procedure in which a percutaneously placed expandable metal stent is placed between the hepatic and portal veins, thereby creating an intrahepatic portosystemic shunt. TIPS seems to be effective in the short-term control of bleeding gastroesophageal varices.[47, 48] Initially envisioned to be a bridge to transplant, it is becoming used more frequently in nontransplant settings. Randomized trials comparing TIPS with endoscopic sclerotherapy mostly suggest that TIPS is more effective for long-term prevention of rebleeding.[49, 50] The main problems with TIPS are a rate of more than 50% shunt occlusion after 1 year and the development of new or worsened hepatic encephalopathy in approximately 20% of patients.[51] TIPS does not prolong survival of patients with variceal bleeding compared with endoscopic treatment. The role of TIPS for acute management of acute variceal bleeding is currently limited to patients who do not respond to endoscopic treatment.

OTHER BLEEDING UPPER GASTROINTESTINAL LESIONS

Esophagitis

In the acute setting, severe bleeding from esophagitis is treated medically with H_2 receptor antagonists followed by omeprazole when the patient is eating. There is generally no role for therapeutic endoscopy or surgery in the management of bleeding esophagitis, unless a bleeding esophageal ulcer is found.

Mallory-Weiss Tear

Mallory-Weiss tears are lacerations of the mucosa extending into the submucosa at the gastroesophageal junction, usually related to vomiting. These usually stop bleeding without therapy, but in cases of active bleeding, endoscopic therapy with bipolar electrocoagulation, heater probe, and injection therapy has been successful.[52, 53] Rebleeding is uncommon after endoscopic therapy unless patients have portal hypertension.

Dieulafoy's Lesion

Dieulafoy's lesion is an aberrant, large submucosal artery that ruptures into the upper GI tract lumen and causes massive bleeding. It usually occurs within 6 cm of the gastroesophageal junction. It is characterized by recurrent gastric hemorrhage, with no source found unless active bleeding or a visible vessel is noted. By definition, there is no surrounding ulceration. The difficulty in management of this lesion is actually identifying it during endoscopy. Once the lesion is detected, endoscopic therapy may be successful in preventing rebleeding.[54] Severe rebleeding should prompt surgical resection of the lesion.

Upper Gastrointestinal Angiodysplasia

Angiodysplasia are ectatic submucosal vessels that usually appear as cherry-red, spider-like lesions on endoscopy. The cause is unknown, but some patients have Osler-Weber-Rendu disease, chronic renal failure, or aortic stenosis. Angiodysplasia can occur in the upper and lower GI tracts and in the small intestine. Patients usually present with anemia secondary to self-limited or occult bleeding, but some may have massive bleeding. Endoscopic therapy can be used to stop bleeding and decrease transfusion rates.[55]

Upper Gastrointestinal Tumors

Upper GI tumors represent approximately 1% of severe cases of upper GI bleeding. Bleeding usually occurs from large, ulcerated, malignant esophageal or gastric tumors. Endoscopic hemostasis with heater probe, bipolar electrocoagulation, or injection can be used to control active bleeding and allow for medical stabilization of the patient before palliative surgical resection. The 1-year mortality rate was 90% for UCLA/CURE patients with severe upper GI bleeding resulting from bleeding tumors, regardless of endoscopic or surgical treatment.[56]

Aortoenteric Fistulas

Aortoenteric fistulas generally occur in patients who have undergone previous abdominal aortic artery reconstructive surgery for aneurysms. The upper portion of the aortic graft often lies in direct contact with the second portion of the duodenum and results in fistulous communication. Aortic graft infection appears to be important in the pathogenesis of the fistula. Patients usually present with an initial self-limited bleeding episode ("herald bleed") followed by an exsanguinating hemorrhage. Patients with an abdominal aortic artery graft and GI bleeding should undergo urgent upper endoscopy to attempt to identify the graft or localize the blood in the duodenum. Because the level of the fistula varies, a colonoscope or enteroscope introduced orally may be necessary to examine farther down the small bowel rather than the proximal duodenum. A computed tomographic (CT) scan with intravenous contrast, rather than an angiogram, may also help localize the fistula. Surgery is indicated in patients with documented aortoenteric fistulas. The surgeon bypasses the fistula (or removes the graft and fistula) and performs axillary femoral bypass.

SEVERE LOWER GASTROINTESTINAL BLEEDING

Severe lower GI hemorrhage occurs with an annual incidence of approximately 20 per 100,000 population, with increasing risk among the elderly.[57] Patients usually present with hematochezia and a decreased hematocrit level. Diagnosis is generally made by colonoscopy after urgent sulfate purge.[6] When internal hemorrhoids are excluded in adults, the most common causes of severe hematochezia are colonic angiomas and diverticulosis (Table 148–6). Rarely, technetium 99m red blood cell scanning or visceral angiography is necessary to detect a bleeding site.

Of ambulatory patients with acute lower GI bleeding 70% to 90% stop bleeding spontaneously. This allows for elective diagnosis and treatment in most cases. For the 10% to 30% of patients with ongoing or recurrent hematochezia, urgent diagnosis and treatment are required to control the bleeding.

In a large series of patients at UCLA Medical Center and West Los Angeles Veterans Administration Medical Center, 64% of patients with severe hematochezia required some therapeutic intervention for control of continued bleeding or rebleeding.[6] Among these patients, 39% underwent endoscopic hemostasis, 1% had angiographic embolization, and 24% underwent surgery.

Colonic Angiomas

Colonic angiomas are often found in the right colon and can be missed unless patients are resuscitated, are well prepped to clean the colon of blood and stool, and undergo a careful colonoscopic examination. As with angiomas in other parts of the GI tract, they may be associated with chronic renal failure, aortic stenosis, or Osler-Weber-Rendu disease. Individual angiomas can be coagulated endoscopically with bipolar electrocoagulation, heater probe, or YAG laser.[58] In our experience, endoscopic coagulation can control colonic angioma bleeding over the long term in 80% of patients, although 20% of these patients will have rebleeding. With repeated treatments, patients successfully treated endoscopically have a significant decrease in the frequency of bleeding episodes and the number of units of packed red blood cells transfused per year and an increase in mean hematocrit.[58] Complications of colonoscopic coagulation of angiomas occur in less than 5% of patients and include perforation, postcoagulation syndrome (pain, fever, leukocytosis), and secondary bleeding from the ulcers induced by coagulation.

TABLE 148–6. Cause of Severe Hematochezia in 80 Patients

Site of Lesion	% of Patients
Colon	74
Angiomas	30
Diverticulosis	16
Polyps or cancer	11
Colitis	9
Rectal lesions	4
Bleeding polyp stalk	3
Endometriosis	1
Upper gastrointestinal	11
Small bowel*	9
No site found	6

Data from Jensen DM, Machicado GA: Diagnosis and treatment of severe hematochezia. Gastroenterology 1988; 95:1569–1574.

*Diagnosis of small-bowel bleeding was made when upper endoscopy and colonoscopy findings were negative but fresh blood or clots were seen coming through the ileocecal valve.

Colonic Diverticular Bleeding

Colonic diverticular bleeding is usually self-limited but may be severe. When barium enema was used for diagnosis of diverticular hemorrhage in 50 patients with hematochezia requiring transfusions, 58% of patients stopped bleeding during hospitalization and had no further bleeding, 20% had recurrent bleeding in the hospital, and 22% had ongoing bleeding requiring surgery.[59] Overall, bleeding stopped with conservative management in 70% of patients. Among those patients whose bleeding stopped, 22% experienced recurrent bleeding events.

Colonoscopic treatment of bleeding diverticula has been successfully performed with heater probe, bipolar electrocoagulation, and epinephrine injection.[60] These techniques are experimental and should be reserved for experienced therapeutic endoscopists; they also need to be compared with surgical resection with long-term follow-up. However, they offer a promising new nonsurgical approach to management of diverticular bleeding in older patients who have higher morbidity or mortality from surgery.

Colon Cancer

Focal ulceration of colonic tumors can occasionally present with severe lower GI bleeding. Diagnosis and initial hemostasis can be performed with a colonoscope. Subsequent therapy may be surgical resection or palliative endoscopic laser treatment.

Ischemic Bowel Disease

Ischemic bowel disease usually is secondary to a hypotensive event, with decreased perfusion of the watershed area of the colon near the splenic flexure. However, ischemia may cause acute or chronic damage anywhere in the colon, depending on the patient's collateral circulation. Patients generally present with acute hematochezia, and urgent colonoscopy shows normal rectal mucosa with a sharp demarcation of swollen, friable tissue near the ischemic area. Ischemic lesions of the colon may resolve with medical therapy, may perforate, or may cause colonic strictures. The latter two complications necessitate surgery.

Inflammatory Bowel Disease

In rare circumstances, ulcerative colitis or Crohn's disease is accompanied by massive hematochezia. Patients with a history of ulcerative colitis that has been quiescent but suddenly becomes more active should have stool studies to exclude an infectious cause. Colonoscopy with biopsy assists in the diagnosis of inflammatory bowel disease. Acute medical therapy generally involves bowel rest, steroids, and possibly cyclosporine. Urgent colectomy is reserved for cases refractory to several days of aggressive medical management.

ACKNOWLEDGMENT

The clinical and laboratory research reported in this chapter was supported in part by National Institutes of Health (NIH) Core Grant NIDDK 41301 (Human Subjects Core) to the Center for Ulcer Research and Education, NIH RO1 Grant NIDDK 33273, and General CRC Grant M01-RR00865 (University of California, Los Angeles).

References

1. Gilbert DA, Silverstein FE, Tedesco FJ, et al: The national ASGE survey on upper gastrointestinal bleeding: III. Endoscopy in upper gastrointestinal bleeding. Gastrointest Endosc 1981; 27:94–102.

2. Layne EA, Mellow MH, Lipman TO: Insensitivity of guaiac slide tests for the detection of blood in gastric juice. Ann Intern Med 1981; 94:774–776.
3. Katon RM: Complications of upper gastrointestinal endoscopy in the gastrointestinal bleeder. Dig Dis Sci 1981; 26(Suppl):47S–54S.
4. Andrus CH, Ponsky JL: The effects of irrigant temperature on upper gastrointestinal hemorrhage: A requiem for iced saline lavage (Editorial). Am J Gastroenterol 1987; 82:1062–1063.
5. Rudolph JP: Automated gastric lavage and a comparison of 0.9% normal saline solution and tap water irrigant. Ann Emerg Med 1985; 14:1156–1159.
6. Jensen DM, Machicado GA: Diagnosis and treatment of severe hematochezia. Gastroenterology 1988; 95:1569–1574.
7. Cutler JA, Mendeloff AI: Upper gastrointestinal bleeding: Nature and magnitude of this problem in the U.S. Dig Dis Sci 1981; 26(Suppl):90S–96S.
8. Allan R, Dykes P: A study on the factors influencing mortality rates from gastrointestinal hemorrhage. Q J Med 1976; 45:533–550.
9. Silverstein FE, Gilbert DA, Tedesco FJ, et al: The national ASGE survey of upper gastrointestinal bleeding: II. Clinical prognostic factors. Gastrointest Endosc 1981; 27:80–93.
10. Fleischer D: Etiology and prevalence of severe persistent upper gastrointestinal bleeding. Gastroenterology 1983; 84:538–543.
11. Silverstein FE, Gilbert DA, Tedesco FJ, et al: The national ASGE survey on upper gastrointestinal bleeding: I. Study design and baseline data. Gastrointest Endosc 1981; 27:73–79.
12. Kurata JH, Corboy ED: Current peptic ulcer time trends: An epidemiologic profile. J Clin Gastroenterol 1988; 10:259–268.
13. Zuckerman GR, Buse PE: Current medical and surgical management of nonvariceal upper gastrointestinal bleeding. Gastrointest Endosc Clin North Am 1991; 1:263–289.
14. Khuroo MS, Yatto GN, Javid G, et. al: A comparison of omeprazole and placebo for bleeding peptic ulcers. N Engl J Med 1997; 336:1054–1058.
15. Freeman ML: The current endoscopic diagnosis and intensive care unit management of severe ulcer and other nonvariceal upper gastrointestinal hemorrhage. Gastrointest Endosc Clin North Am 1991; 1:209–239.
16. Laine L, Cohen H, Brodhead J, et al: Prospective evaluation of immediate versus delayed refeeding and prognostic value of endoscopy in patients with upper gastrointestinal hemorrhage. Gastroenterology 1992; 102:314–316.
17. Swain CP, Storey DW, Bown GS, et al: Nature of the bleeding vessel in recurrently bleeding gastric ulcers. Gastroenterology 1986; 90:595–608.
18. Johnston JH, Jensen DM, Auth D: Experimental comparison of endoscopic yttrium-aluminum-garnet laser, electrosurgery, and heater probe for canine gut arterial coagulation: Importance of compression and avoidance of erosion. Gastroenterology 1987; 92:1101–1108.
19. National Institutes of Health Consensus Development Conference: Therapeutic endoscopy and bleeding ulcers. JAMA 1989; 262:1369–1372.
20. Jensen DM: Heat probe for hemostasis of bleeding peptic ulcers: Techniques and results of randomized controlled trials. Gastrointest Endosc 1990; 36:S42–S49.
21. Laine L: Multipolar electrocoagulation in the treatment of active upper gastrointestinal hemorrhage: A prospective controlled trial. N Engl J Med 1987; 316:1613–1617.
22. Laine L: Multipolar electrocoagulation in the treatment of peptic ulcers with nonbleeding visible vessels. Ann Intern Med 1989; 110:510–514.
23. Jensen DM: Endoscopic control of non-variceal upper gastrointestinal hemorrhage. *In*: Textbook of Gastroenterology. 2nd ed. Yamada T, Alpers D, Owyang C, Powell D, Silverstein F. (Eds). Philadelphia, JB Lippincott, 1995, pp 2991–3011.
24. Laine L: Multipolar electrocoagulation versus injection therapy in the treatment of bleeding peptic ulcers. Gastroenterology 1990; 99:1303–1306.
25. Chung SC, Leung JW, Sung JY, et al: Injection or heat probe for bleeding ulcers. Gastroenterology 1991; 100:33–37.
26. Jensen DM, Machicado GA, Kovacs TOG, et al: Current treatment and outcome of patients with bleeding "stress ulcers" (Abstract). Gastroenterology 1988; 94:A208.
27. Graham DY, Smith JL: The course of patients after variceal hemorrhage. Gastroenterology 1981; 80:800–809.
28. Fogel MR, Knauer M, Andres LL, et al: Continuous intravenous vasopressin in active upper gastrointestinal bleeding: A placebo-controlled trial. Ann Intern Med 1982; 96:565–569.
29. Kravetz D, Bosch J, Teres J, et al: Comparison of intravenous somatostatin and vasopressin infusions in treatment of acute variceal hemorrhage. Hepatology 1984; 4:442–446.
30. Valenzuela JE, Schubert T, Fogel MR, et al: A multicenter, randomized, double-blind trial of somatostatin in the management of acute hemorrhage from esophageal varices. Hepatology 1989; 10:958–961.
31. Burroughs AK, McCormick PA, Hughes MD, et al: Randomized, double-blind, placebo-controlled trial of somatostatin for variceal bleeding: Emergency control and prevention of early variceal rebleeding. Gastroenterology 1990; 99:1388–1395.
32. Imperiale TF, Teran JC, McCullough AJ: A meta-analysis of somatostatin versus vasopressin in the management of acute esophageal variceal hemorrhage. Gastroenterology 1995; 109:1289–1294.
33. Sung JJ, Chung SC, Lai CW, Chan FK, Leung JW, Yung MY, Kassianides C, Li AK: Octreotide infusion or emergency sclerotherapy for variceal hemorrhage. Lancet 1993; 342:637–641.
34. Novis GH, Duys GO, Barbezat O, et al: Fibreoptic endoscopy and the use of the Sengstaken tube in acute gastrointestinal hemorrhage with portal hypertension and varices. Gut 1976; 17:258–263.
35. Conn HO, Simpson JA: Excessive mortality associated with balloon tamponade of bleeding varices: A critical reappraisal. JAMA 1967; 202:587–591.
36. Larson AW, Cohen J, Zweiban B, et al: Acute esophageal variceal sclerotherapy: Results of a prospective randomized controlled trial. JAMA 1986; 255:497–500.
37. Paquet KJ, Feussner H: Endoscopic sclerosis and esophageal balloon tamponade in acute hemorrhage from esophagogastric varices: A prospective controlled randomized trial. Hepatology 1985; 5:580–583.
38. The Copenhagen Esophageal Varices Sclerotherapy Project: Sclerotherapy after first variceal hemorrhage in cirrhosis: A randomized multicenter trial. N Engl J Med 1984; 311:1594–1596.
39. Westaby D, Hayes PC, Gimson AES, et al: Controlled clinical trial of injection sclerotherapy for active variceal bleeding. Hepatology 1989; 9:274–277.
40. Stiegmann GV, Goff JS, Michaletz-Ondey PA, et al: Endoscopic sclerotherapy as compared with endoscopic ligation for bleeding esophageal varices. N Engl J Med 1992; 326:1527–1532.
41. Laine L, El-Newihi HM, Migikovsky B, et al: Endoscopic ligation compared with sclerotherapy for the treatment of bleeding esophageal varices. Ann Intern Med 1993; 119:1–7.
42. Cello JP, Grendell JH, Crass RA, et al: Endoscopic sclerotherapy versus portacaval shunt in patients with severe cirrhosis and acute variceal hemorrhage: Long-term follow-up. N Engl J Med 1987; 316:11–15.
43. Henderson JM, Kutner MH, Millikan WJ, et al: Endoscopic variceal sclerosis compared with distal splenorenal shunt to prevent recurrent variceal bleeding in cirrhosis: A prospective, randomized trial. Ann Intern Med 1990; 112:262–269.
44. Teres J, Bordas JM, Bravo D, et al: Sclerotherapy vs. distal splenorenal shunt in the elective treatment of variceal hemorrhage: A randomized controlled trial. Hepatology 1987; 7:430–436.
45. Planas R, Boix J, Broggi M, et al: Portacaval shunt versus endoscopic sclerotherapy in the elective treatment of variceal hemorrhage. Gastroenterology 1991; 100:1078–1086.
46. Spina GP, Stantabrogio R, Opocher E, et al: Distal splenorenal shunt versus endoscopic sclerotherapy in the prevention of variceal rebleeding. Ann Surg 1990; 211:178–186.
47. Ring EJ, Lake JR, Roberts JP: Using transjugular intrahepatic portosystemic shunts to control variceal bleeding before liver transplantation. Ann Intern Med 1992; 116:304–309.
48. Rossle M, Haag K, Ochs A, et al: The transjugular intrahepatic portosystemic stent-shunt procedure for variceal bleeding. N Engl J Med 1994; 330:165–171.
49. Cello JP, Ring EJ, Olcott EW, et al: Endoscopic sclerotherapy compared with percutaneous transjugular intrahepatic portosystemic shunt after initial sclerotherapy in patients with acute variceal hemorrhage: A randomized, controlled trial. Ann Intern Med 1997; 126:858–865.
50. Rossle M, Deibert P, Haag K, et al: Randomised trial of transjugu-

lar-intrahepatic-portosystemic shunt versus endoscopy plus propranolol for prevention of variceal bleeding. Lancet 1997; 349:1043–1049.
51. Sahagun G, Benner KG, Saxon R, et al: Outcome of 100 patients after transjugular intrahepatic portosystemic shunt for variceal hemorrhage. Am J Gastroenterol 1997; 92:1444–1452.
52. Laine L: Multipolar electrocoagulation in the treatment of active upper gastrointestinal tract hemorrhage: A prospective controlled trial. N Engl J Med 1987; 316:1613–1617.
53. Kovacs TOG, Jensen DM: Endoscopic diagnosis and treatment of bleeding Mallory-Weiss tears. Gastrointest Endosc Clin North Am 1991; 1:387–400.
54. Baettig B, Haecki W, Lammer F, Jost-R: Dieulafoy's disease: Endoscopic treatment and follow up. Gut 1993; 34:1418–1421.
55. Machicado GA, Jensen DM: Upper gastrointestinal angiomata: Diagnosis and treatment. Gastrointest Endosc Clin North Am 1991; 1:241–262.
56. Savides TJ, Jensen DM, Cohen J, Randall GM, Kovacs TO, Pelayo E, Cheng S, Jensen ME, Hsieh HY: Severe upper gastrointestinal tumor bleeding: Endoscopic findings, treatment, and outcome. Endoscopy 1996; 28:244–248.
57. Longstreth GF: Epidemiology and outcome of patients hospitalized with acute lower gastrointestinal hemorrhage: A population-based study. Am J Gastroenterol 1997; 92:419–424.
58. Jensen DM, Machicado GA: Endoscopic diagnosis and treatment of bleeding colonic angiomas and radiation telangiectasia. *In*: Prospectives in Colon and Rectal Surgery. Vol 2. Schrock T (Ed). St. Louis, Quality Medical Publishing, 1989, pp 99–113.
59. McGuire HH, Haynes BW: Massive hemorrhage from diverticulosis of the colon: Guidelines for therapy based on bleeding patterns observed in fifty cases. Ann Surg 1972; 175:847–853.
60. Savides TJ, Jensen DM: Colonoscopic hemostasis for recurrent diverticular hemorrhage associated with a visible vessel: A report of three cases. Gastrointest Endosc 1994; 40:70–73.

149

Acute Hepatic Failure

Telfer B. Reynolds, MD

STAGING

Acute (fulminant) hepatic failure is defined as the rapid development (in a patient with no previous liver disease) of severe impairment of hepatic function, progressing to hepatic encephalopathy within 8 weeks of onset of the illness.[1] Invariably, bilirubin elevation and severe coagulopathy are present. Some would include in this definition patients with previously unrecognized chronic liver disease in whom a superimposed acute hepatitis develops or in whom the chronic disease abruptly changes course (as in Wilson's disease or reactivation of chronic hepatitis B). O'Grady and colleagues[2] have proposed three subdivisions of acute hepatic failure, based on different likelihoods of survival:

1. *Hyperacute*. Hepatic encephalopathy appears within 7 days of the onset of jaundice.
2. *Acute*. Encephalopathy appears between 8 and 28 days from jaundice onset.
3. *Subacute*. Encephalopathy occurs from 5 to 12 weeks after onset of jaundice.

These authors point out that, paradoxically, survival is best in the hyperacute group.

Hepatic encephalopathy is a progressive deterioration of consciousness, culminating in deep coma. For standardization in reporting, it is customary to subdivide hepatic encephalopathy into four grades (Table 149–1). In the early stages, there is mild confusion and impairment in judgment. Asterixis is prominent, and calculation deficits are easily demonstrable. In younger patients in the early stage, there is sometimes hyperactivity, dementia, or combative behavior. This manifestation may not be recognized as hepatic encephalopathy and may lead to large doses of poorly metabolized sedatives. As hepatic encephalopathy advances, there is progressive somnolence.

TABLE 149–1. Grades of Hepatic Encephalopathy

Grade	Description
I.	Slowness of thought, asterixis
II.	Drowsiness, inappropriate behavior, confusion
III.	Somnolence to semistupor, some response to stimuli
IV.	Coma, nonresponsive or minimal response to painful stimuli

ETIOLOGY

The leading causes of acute hepatic failure are (Table 149–2):

- Viral infections (hepatitis viruses A–E, herpesvirus)
- Toxic or idiosyncratic reactions to therapeutic drugs
- Metabolic disorders of obscure origin (Reye's syndrome, acute fatty liver of pregnancy)
- Toxins (*Amanita phalloides*, yellow phosphorus, *Bacillus cereus* toxin, carbon tetrachloride)
- Miscellaneous disorders, such as severe hyperthermia and prolonged hepatic ischemia

Of the known hepatitis viruses, hepatitis B is the most common cause of acute hepatic failure. Most liver research finds that hepatitis-like illness, with all known viral hepatitis serologic test markers negative, is the most common cause of acute hepatic failure.[3, 4] Whether these cases are due to an as yet undiscovered hepatitis virus is uncertain. It seems unlikely that they are due to the recently discovered hepatitis G virus, which will probably prove to be a nonpathogenic virus for humans.[5] Using polymerase chain reaction (PCR), Villamil and coworkers[6] found a positive test for hepatitis C viral-ribonucleic acid (HCV-RNA) in the serum of nine of 16 patients of this type. In Japan, two studies showed the relatively frequent presence of HCV-RNA in such patients.[7, 8] However, others have been unable to identify HCV in this setting.[3, 9]

RESULTS

Clinical Features

By definition, there are clinical signs of hepatic encephalopathy in acute hepatic failure (see Table 149–1). Jaundice is almost invariably present but is occasionally overlooked if liver disease is not suspected. Although the liver may be mildly enlarged, it is usually difficult to feel because of lack of firmness. The spleen is rarely palpable. Ascites can be present

TABLE 149–2. Etiology of Acute Hepatic Failure

Viral: Hepatitis A–E, herpesvirus

Drugs: Acetaminophen, isoniazid, halothane, phenytoin, niacin, cocaine, others

Toxins: Amanita, phosphorus, carbon tetrachloride

Miscellaneous: Hyperthermia, ischemia, Wilson's disease, microvesicular steatosis (Reye's syndrome, fatty liver of pregnancy, *Bacillus cereus,* valproate)

in patients with subacute liver failure, when jaundice has been present for several weeks before the development of hepatic encephalopathy. Such patients occasionally have vascular "spiders." With acute liver failure, the finding of any combination of vascular spiders, firm hepatomegaly, ascites, or splenomegaly suggests the presence of underlying chronic liver disease, with the superimposition of an acute process, such as acute viral hepatitis, reactivation of hepatitis B, or drug toxicity. The presence of Kayser-Fleischer rings on the iris would indicate previously unrecognized Wilson's disease.

Vital signs in acute hepatic failure are variable. There may be hypotension, a poor prognostic sign. Mild hyperventilation is common. Mild fever may be present but is not common.

Laboratory Findings

Laboratory test results invariably include marked prolongation of prothrombin time, elevation of serum bilirubin (predominantly the direct fraction), and marked to moderate elevation of serum transaminase levels. The serum lactate acid dehydrogenase (LDH) level is usually mildly to moderately elevated; if it is markedly raised, it suggests hepatic ischemia or acetaminophen toxicity as the cause of the hepatic failure.[10, 11] Renal function is usually normal early in the course of acute hepatic failure. If the serum creatinine level is elevated on presentation, acetaminophen toxicity or some other nonviral etiologic mechanism is suggested. Arterial pH with arterial blood gas measurement is useful for determining the prognosis in acetaminophen toxicity.

If the cause of the acute hepatic failure is not already known, one should request immunoglobulin M (IgM) antibody to hepatitis A, hepatitis B surface antigen, IgM antibody to hepatitis B core, antibody to HCV and HCV-RNA by PCR. If the patient has recently visited the Far East or Africa, it may be useful to request IgM antibody to hepatitis E virus. If either of the hepatitis B tests mentioned previously is positive, the possibility of acute delta hepatitis can be evaluated with IgM antibody to hepatitis D.

Prognosis

The overall prognosis of acute hepatic failure is poor, with the mortality rate approximately 80%. Mortality is age-related, with few survivors younger than 10 years of age or older than 40 years of age (Fig. 149–1). Mortality is also somewhat dependent on etiology, with above-average survival rates for acetaminophen toxicity, hepatitis A, and hepatitis B and below-average rates for idiosyncratic drug reactions, acute Wilson's disease, and acute hepatic failure of unknown cause.

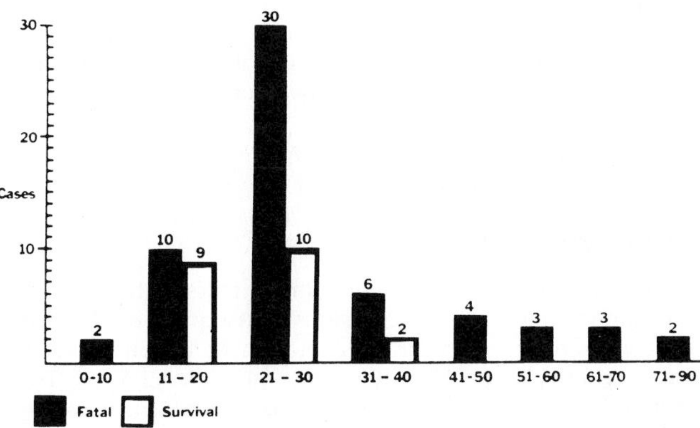

Figure 149–1. Age-specific mortality for 81 patients with fulminant hepatitis and stage IV hepatic encephalopathy, University of Southern California, Liver Unit, from 1960 to 1972. (From Redeker AG: Fulminant hepatitis. *In*: The Liver and Its Diseases. Schaffner F, Sherlock S, Leevy C [Eds]. New York, International Medical Book Corporation, 1974.)

TABLE 149–3. Factors Indicating a Poor Prognosis in Acute Hepatic Failure

1. Age <10 or >40 years
2. Etiology hepatitis non-A–E, drugs (except acetaminophen), toxins
3. Stage IV encephalopathy
4. >1 Week to development of stage III and IV encephalopathy after onset of jaundice
5. Prothrombin >3.5 (INR)
6. Creatinine >3.4 mg/dL
7. Arterial pH <7.3
8. Bilirubin >17 mg/dL
9. Factor V <20%
10. Alpha-fetoprotein <15 ng/mL

Accurate prediction of prognosis has become extremely important since the advent of hepatic transplantation for rescue therapy. Findings that suggest a poor prognosis are listed in Table 149–3. Several groups have developed prognostic indices to predict survival.[12–15] The two most widely used indexes are those from London[12] and Clichy[16] (Table 149–4). Neither are entirely satisfactory, and the prediction of need for transplantation remains somewhat problematic.

Additional factors have been suggested for predicting outcome:

1. Liver volume, as measured by computed tomography scan.[17]
2. Extent of hepatocyte necrosis on transjugular liver biopsy.[18]
3. Human hepatocyte growth factor level in serum.[19]
4. Arterial ketone body ratio.[20]
5. Hepatic galactose elimination capacity.[21]
6. Serum alpha-fetoprotein level.[22]
7. Plasma Gc protein level.[23]

None of these criteria have been applied prospectively in large groups of patients.

MANAGEMENT

Transplant Consideration

When confronted with a patient in acute hepatic failure, the physician should immediately consider the possibility that liver transplantation will be indicated. If there are no obvious contraindications to transplantation and if the procedure is not available in the institution, it may be wise to transfer the patient to a facility where transplantation is available, should the patient's condition deteriorate to the point where such surgery is indicated.

TABLE 149–4. Reasons for Withholding Transplant Surgery

1. Active sepsis
2. Adult respiratory distress syndrome
3. Prolonged increase in intracranial pressure with fixed pupils and lack of response to mannitol
4. Progressive hypotension with low cardiac index

Contraindications to transplantation include human immunodeficiency virus (HIV) infection, malignancy, and significant chronic dysfunction of the heart, lungs, or kidneys. A history of poor compliance with medical treatment or active substance abuse makes optimal follow-up after transplantation unlikely. If the patient cannot afford to pay for transplantation, is uninsured, or is ineligible for Medicaid because of residency requirements, transplantation is not feasible.

The overall survival after liver transplantation for patients with acute hepatic failure ranges from 60% to 80% in multiple reports. Data from the United Network for Organ Sharing (UNOS) show a 63% 1-year survival for 424 patients compared with 78% overall 1-year survival for patients with chronic liver disease. Clearly, a transplantation is the preferred treatment for patients likely to die with conservative treatment. However, transplantation in a patient who could survive without it is a serious mistake because the operation creates a chronic disorder in someone whose health likely would have returned to normal. In addition, because there are far fewer donor livers than transplant candidates, each inappropriate transplantation deprives a patient with chronic liver disease of the opportunity to regain health. It is very important, therefore, to identify prognostic criteria that can be relied on early in the hospital course to predict outcome.

Prediction difficulty is compounded by the fact that there is likely a 2- to 4-day waiting period after a patient with acute hepatic failure is listed before an organ becomes available. If the patient's condition improves during the waiting period, the donor liver can be passed to the next candidate on the list. If the patient's condition worsens and a complication make successful transplant outcome unlikely (see Table 149–4), the operation should be cancelled. Pending accumulation of prospective data on the reliability of some of the newer predictors of outcome (see previous topic), most centers use the predictors developed at King's College Hospital in London from a very large data base (Table 149–5). Because British-made thromboplastins are different from most American-made thromboplastins, the original criterion of prothrombin time greater than 100 seconds is not usable in America and has been replaced by an International Normalized Ratio (INR) of 6.5.

The Hepatology Group[16] at Beaujon Hospital in Clichy, France, developed a simpler set of criteria to indicate a bad prognosis and a need for transplantation in acute viral hepatitis, but it relies heavily on factor V assay, which is not available in most North American hospitals. Comparison of the London and Clichy criteria in a series of 81 patients with fulminant hepatic failure by Pauwels and colleagues[24] showed little difference in positive predictive accuracy (0.89 and 0.89) and negative predictive accuracy (0.47 and 0.36) for the London and Clichy criteria, respectively, when applied 48 hours before death. None of these patients underwent transplantation.

TABLE 149–5. Criteria for Listing for Liver Transplantation in Patients with Viral Hepatitis and Hepatic Encephalopathy

King's College Hospital (London)

1. Prothrombin: INR > 6.5

or

2. Any three of the following:
   a. Age <10 or >40 years
   b. Etiology non-A–E or any drug
   c. Bilirubin >17 mg/dL
   d. Progression from onset of jaundice to encephalopathy in >17 days
   e. Prothrombin: INR > 3.5

Beaujon Hospital (Clichy, France)

1. Low factor V
   a. <20% if age <30 years
   b. <30% if age >30 years

INR = International Normalized Ratio.

Routine Management

An intensive care unit is preferable when patients progress to grade II encephalopathy. Caloric intake should be primarily carbohydrate, either enterally or parenterally. Some physicians use branched-chain amino acid infusions to combat hepatic encephalopathy, but in my opinion their value has not been demonstrated. Fluid intake should be 1000 to 1500 mL, plus output. If lactulose is used, substantial amounts of free water can be lost rectally; this can lead to water deficit and hypernatremia if intake is not monitored closely. If the patient shows combative behavior in early hepatic encephalopathy, sedation should be minimal and limited to short-acting agents.

It is customary to give lactulose orally or by nasogastric tube to treat hepatic encephalopathy, although its value is probably limited in this setting. The dose should be titrated to produce two to three soft or liquid stools daily. Neomycin is probably best avoided because of the frequent development of renal impairment in acute hepatic failure and concern that intestinal absorption of the drug might contribute to this.

With progression to late grade II or early grade III encephalopathy, most authorities advise intubation, a nasogastric tube, a bladder catheter, arterial and central venous lines for monitoring, sedation and paralysis, and administration of a histamine$_2$ (H_2) blocker to prevent stress ulceration.

Data from King's College Hospital in London strongly support the intravenous administration of acetylcysteine, 150 mg/kg/24 hours, even in patients who do not have acetaminophen toxicity, to improve tissue oxygenation.[25] Intravenous administration is not approved by the Food and Drug Administration in the United States but is widely practiced in Europe.

Frequent monitoring of blood glucose should be routine, because hypoglycemia is common in hepatic failure. Other variables that should be monitored, in addition to hemodynamics and pulse oximetry, include prothrombin, serum electrolytes, and renal function. Replacement of phosphate and magnesium is indicated if serum levels are low. Prothrombin is one of the most valuable indices of prognosis, and a definite shortening of prothrombin time (in the absence of clotting factor administration) is a strong indication that the patient will survive. Because of the prognostic value of prothrombin time and the rarity of spontaneous bleeding in acute liver failure, I prefer to avoid routine administration of fresh frozen plasma, unless there is spontaneous bleeding or the need for an invasive procedure, such as insertion of a device for intracranial pressure measurement.

COMPLICATIONS

Hypoglycemia

Hypoglycemia occurs frequently in patients with acute hepatic failure and may have serious consequences if it goes unrecognized. It is caused by depletion of hepatic glycogen stores, together with loss of hepatic gluconeogenesis. Treatment involves continuous glucose administration, monitored by frequent finger-stick serum glucose measurements.

Infection

Prospective studies show that bacterial and fungal infections are relatively common in patients with acute hepatic failure.

With severe illness, decreased hepatic reticuloendothelial cell function, intubation, and multiple indwelling lines, this is not surprising. One study of 50 closely monitored patients by Rolando and coworkers[26] disclosed 53 bacterial infections in 40 of the patients. Respiratory and urinary tract infections were most frequent, and the predominant organisms were staphylococci, streptococci, coliforms, and fungi. Fever and leukocytosis were absent in 30% of the bacteriologically proven infections, so a high index of suspicion for infection is warranted, with frequent surveillance cultures of blood and urine. A subsequent study by Rolando and associates[27] did not show significant survival benefit from prophylactic antibiotic administration, but Salmeron and colleagues[28] found benefit from selective intestinal decontamination with antibiotics.

Renal Failure

If the etiology in acute hepatic failure is acetaminophen toxicity, renal impairment is commonly present early in the illness and presumably is due to acute renal tubular injury. Tubular injury is also frequent in acute hepatic failure caused by ischemia, hyperthermia, *A. phalloides*, yellow phosphorus, and carbon tetrachloride. With other causes, renal impairment may occur later in the course and be due to vasoconstriction of the renal microvasculature (hepatorenal syndrome). In either problem, the prognosis for recovery of renal function is excellent if the patient survives the hepatic injury. Hypovolemia and sepsis, if present, may contribute to renal impairment and should be treated vigorously.

Dialysis therapy is indicated for clinical uremia, marked hyperkalemia, or fluid overload. Arteriovenous hemodialysis is suitable for patients in satisfactory hemodynamic condition. Venovenous hemofiltration is preferable for patients with marked hypotension or evidence of cerebral edema.

Bleeding

In spite of the marked coagulopathy that is invariably present in acute hepatic failure, significant spontaneous bleeding is not very common. Gastrointestinal bleeding from mucosal stress ulcerations occurs but is rarely life-threatening. Its frequency is reduced by routine administration of an H_2 blocker or sucralfate.[29] Fortunately, intracranial hemorrhage is uncommon. Because of the great value of serial prothrombin measurements in predicting prognosis, I prefer not to administer routine prophylactic fresh frozen plasma, saving it for demonstrated bleeding or as preparation for an invasive procedure, such as placement of an intracranial pressure monitor. Thrombopenia and reduced platelet function are often present. Platelet administration may be useful when bleeding occurs.

Hypotension

Hypotension is common in hepatic failure, and refractory hypotension is an indication of a poor prognosis. As in chronic liver disease, hypotension is accompanied by peripheral vasodilatation, low systemic vascular resistance, and elevated cardiac output. Swan-Ganz catheter placement is helpful for measurement of hemodynamic indices. Pulmonary capillary wedge pressure in the range of 12 to 15 mm Hg is optimal, with administration of colloid as needed to achieve this level. Mean arterial pressure should be maintained above 50 to 60 mm Hg. If vasopressor support is required, the King's College Hospital Liver Group prefers noradrenaline, with the addition of a microcirculatory vasodilator, such as prostacyclin or acetylcysteine, to maintain tissue oxygen consumption.[30]

Cerebral Edema

Cerebral edema is the most feared complication of fulminant hepatic failure because it is difficult to treat and may result in permanent brain damage or fatal brain stem herniation. The etiologic mechanism remains problematic, although several theories for its pathogenesis exist.[31] It develops only in patients with stage IV hepatic encephalopathy. Clinical signs are not entirely reliable and include the onset of hypertension and bradycardia, increased muscle tone, dilated pupils, decerebrate rigidity, and posturing. CT can be used to exclude intracerebral hemorrhage but does not reliably detect cerebral edema.[32] Because clinical signs are not entirely reliable, many centers advocate intracranial pressure (ICP) monitoring.[33, 34] Pressure monitors can be placed in the epidural or subdural space, in direct contact with brain parenchyma, or in one of the lateral ventricles. Even with the preoperative administration of clotting factors and platelets, there is a significant risk of hemorrhage.

A questionnaire circulated by Blei and colleagues[35] reported fatal hemorrhage rates of 1%, 5%, and 4% for epidural, subdural, and parenchymal monitoring, respectively. Epidural monitoring is considered to be the least accurate of these modalities but is more widely used because it is simpler and safer. ICP levels above 30 mm Hg are of concern. A more important measurement is cerebral perfusion pressure (CPP), which is the difference between mean arterial pressure and ICP. Levels below 40 mm Hg suggest cerebral ischemia.

Modalities for the prevention and treatment of raised ICP are limited. Controlled hyperventilation has been used to lower cerebral blood flow[36] but may be counterproductive, as it may reduce cerebral oxygen supply.[37] Elevation of the head to maximize CPP is problematic; some studies favor 45° elevation, whereas others favor 20°.[38] Corticosteroid treatment has not proved useful.[39] Intravenous mannitol, 0.3 to 0.5 g/kg of body weight, given as a bolus, is effective in lowering ICP and increasing CPP in most cases, although often the effect is temporary.[40] It can be repeated as needed, although plasma osmolality should be monitored and kept below 320 mOsm/L. This may require dialysis or hemofiltration in patients with reduced renal function. If mannitol administration proves ineffective, some authorities resort to parenteral barbiturate administration in an effort to decrease cerebral oxygen demand and to prevent seizure activity.[41]

TREATMENT

Experimental Modalities

The dramatic and devastating nature of fulminant hepatic failure, and the fact that it often develops in young and otherwise healthy people, led to a number of almost desperate treatment modalities, prior to the availability of liver transplantation. The usual scenario was seemingly successful treatment in a patient or two, followed by a wave of enthusiasm, and then failure of a subsequent randomized controlled trial to confirm treatment effectiveness. From 1952 to 1987, at least 11 such treatments have been utilized (Table 149–6).

Extracorporeal Liver Assist Devices

Extracorporeal devices to assist the liver in removing accumulating toxins (charcoal hemoperfusion, polyacrylonitrile membrane dialysis, plasmapheresis, exchange transfusion) have not been beneficial in controlled trials. This suggests the need for providing some of the synthetic and biotransforming functions of the liver in any artificial liver support system.

Two bioartificial liver devices have been studied, both in animal models of acute hepatic failure and, to a limited degree,

TABLE 149–6. Historical Modalities for Treatment of Acute Hepatic Failure

1. High-dose corticosteroid (1952)
2. Exchange transfusion (1965)
3. Liver perfusion, pig (1966)
4. Cross circulation, human (1966)
5. Cross circulation, baboon (1968)
6. Total body washout (1969)
7. Large-dose hepatitis B immune globulin (1971)
8. Charcoal hemoperfusion (1973)
9. Hemodialysis with polyacrylonitrile membrane (1976)
10. Insulin and glucagon (1977)
11. Prostaglandin E (1987)

in humans.[42] Both utilize microcarrier-attached cultured hepatocytes exposed to the patient's plasma. The hepatocytes are separated from the plasma by semipermeable plastic membranes in hollow capillary tubular form, bundled together within a plastic cartridge.

The device developed by Demetriou and colleagues contains approximately 5 billion cryopreserved porcine hepatocytes attached to collagen-coated dextran microcarriers in the extratubular space of the cartilage. The patient's plasma, after being separated from the red blood cells in a mechanical separator, circulates through the hollow capillary tubes at 50 mL/min.[43] The plasma is first exposed to cellulose-coated charcoal and is oxygenated and maintained at body temperature.

A similar device developed by Sussman and coworkers[44] uses cultured human hepatocytes from an immortalized tumor cell line and locates the hepatocytes inside the capillary tubes while the patient's plasma perfuses the extratubular space. Such devices have great potential as a bridge to transplantation or, conceivably, in the absence of transplantation, to provide time for hepatic regeneration. Further improvements in design are likely, and randomized controlled trials will undoubtedly be carried out soon.

References

1. Trey C, Davidson LS: The management of fulminant hepatic failure. *In:* Progress in Liver Disease. Popper H, Schaffner F (Eds). New York, Grune & Stratton, 1970, pp 282–298.
2. O'Grady JG, Schalm SW, Willams R: Acute liver failure: Redefining the syndromes. Lancet 1993; 342:273–275.
3. Liang TJ, Jeffers L, Reddy RK, et al: Fulminant or sub-fulminant non-A, non-B viral hepatitis: The role of hepatitis C and E viruses. Gastroenterology 1993; 104:556–562.
4. Fagan EA: Acute liver failure of unknown pathogenesis: The hidden agenda. Hepatology 1994; 19:1307–1312.
5. Miyakawa Y, Mayaumi M: Hepatitis G virus: A true hepatitis virus or an accidental tourist? N Engl J Med 1997; 336:795–796.
6. Villamil FG, Hu K-Q, Yu C-H: Detection of hepatitis C virus with polymerase chain reaction in fulminant hepatic failure. Hepatology 1995; 22:1379–1386.
7. Yoshiba M, Sekiyama K, Inoue K, et al: Contribution of hepatitis C virus to non-A, non-B fulminant hepatitis in Japan. Hepatology 1994; 19:829–835.
8. Chu C, Sheen I, Liaw Y: The role of hepatitis C virus in fulminant hepatic failure in an area with endemic hepatitis A and B. Gastroenterology 1994; 107:189–195.
9. Wright TL, Hsu H, Donegan E, et al: Hepatitis C virus not found in fulminant non-A, non-B hepatitis. Ann Intern Med 1991; 115:111–112.
10. Gibson PR, Dudley FJ: Ischemic hepatitis: Clinical features, diagnosis, and prognosis. Aust N Z J Med 1984; 14:822–825.
11. Cassidy WM, Reynolds TB: Serum lactic dehydrogenase in the differential diagnosis of acute hepatocellular injury. J Clin Gastroenterol 1994; 97:439–445.
12. O'Grady JG, Alexander GJM, Hayllar KM, et al: Early indicators of prognosis in fulminant hepatic failure. Gastroenterology 1989; 97:439–445.
13. Bernuau J, Goudeau A, Poynard T, et al: Multivariate analysis of prognostic factors in fulminant hepatitis. B. Hepatology 1986; 6:648–651.
14. Christensen E, Bremmelgaard A, Bahnsen M, et al: Prediction of fatality in fulminant hepatic failure. Scand J Gastroenterol 1984; 19:90–96.
15. Takahashi Y, Kumada H, Shimizu M, et al: A multicenter study on the prognosis of fulminant viral hepatitis: Early prediction for liver transplantation. Hepatology 1994; 19:1065–1071.
16. Bernuau J, Samuel D, Durand F, et al: Criteria for emergency liver transplantation in patients with acute viral hepatitis and factor V below 50% of normal: A prospective study. Hepatology 1991; 14:49A.
17. Van Thiel DH: When should a decision to proceed with transplantation actually be made in cases of fulminant or subfulminant hepatic failure: At admission to hospital or when a donor organ is made available? J Hepatol 1993; 17:1–2.
18. Donaldson BW, Gopinath R, Wanless IR, et al: The role of transjugular liver biopsy in fulminant hepatic failure: Relation to other prognostic indicators. Hepatology 1993; 18:1370–1374.
19. Tsubouchi H, Kawakami S, Hirono S, et al: Prediction of outcome in fulminant hepatic failure by serum human hepatocyte growth factor (Letter). Lancet 1992; 340:307.
20. Saibara T, Onishi S, Sone J, et al: Arterial ketone body ratio as a possible indication for liver transplantation in fulminant hepatic failure. Transplantation 1991; 51:782–786.
21. Ranek I, Andreasen PB, Tygstrup N: Galactose elimination capacity as a prognostic index in patients with fulminant hepatic failure. Gut 1976; 17:959–964.
22. Karvountzis GG, Redekee AG: Relationship of alpha-fetoprotein in acute hepatitis to severity and prognosis. Ann Intern Med 1974; 80:156–160.
23. Lee WM, Galbraith RM, Watt GH, et al: Predicting survival in fulminant hepatic failure using serum protein Gc concentrations. Hepatology 1995; 21:103–115.
24. Pauwels A, Mostefa-Kara N, Florent C, et al: Emergency liver transplantation for acute liver failure: Evaluation of London and Clichy criteria. J Hepatol 1993; 17:124–127.
25. Harrison PM, Wendon JA, Gimson AES, et al: Improvement by acetylcysteine of hemodynamics and oxygen transport in fulminant hepatic failure. N Engl J Med 1991; 324:1852–1857.
26. Rolando N, Harvey F, Brahm J, et al: Prospective study of bacterial infection in acute liver failure: Analysis of fifty patients. Hepatology 1990; 11:49–53.
27. Rolando N, Gumson A, Wade J, et al: Prospective controlled trial of selective parenteral and enteral antimicrobial regimen in fulminant liver failure. Hepatology 1993; 17:196–201.
28. Salmeron JN, Tito L, Rimola A, et al: Selective intestinal decontamination in the prevention of bacterial infection in patients with acute liver failure. J Hepatol 1992; 14:206–285.
29. MacDougal B, Williams R: H_2 receptor antagonists in the prevention of upper gastrointestinal hemorrhage in fulminant hepatic failure. Gastroenterology 1978; 4:464–465.
30. Wendon JA, Harrison PM, Keays R, et al: Effects of vasopressor agents and eprostenol on systemic hemodynamics and oxygen transport in fulminant hepatic failure. Hepatology 1992; 15:1067–1071.
31. Blei AT: Cerebral edema and intracranial hypertension in acute liver failure: Distinct aspects of the same problem. Hepatology 1991; 13:376–379.
32. Munoz SJ, Robinson M, Northrup B, et al: Elevated intracranial pressure and computed tomography of the brain in fulminant hepatocellular failure. Hepatology 1991; 13:209–212.
33. Donovan JP, Shaw BW Jr, Lungnas AN, et al: Brain water and acute liver failure: The emerging role of intracranial pressure monitoring. Hepatology 1992; 16:265–268.
34. Lidofsky SD, Bass NM, Prager MC, et al: Intracranial pressure monitoring and liver transplantation for fulminant hepatic failure. Hepatology 1992; 16:1–7.
35. Blei AT, Olafsson S, Webster S, et al: Complications of intracranial pressure monitoring in fulminant hepatic failure. Lancet 1993; 341:157–158.

36. Ede RJ, Gimson AES, Bihari D, et al: Controlled hyperventilation in the prevention of cerebral edema in fulminant hepatic failure. J Hepatol 1986; 2:43–51.
37. Sari A, Yamashita S, Ohosita S, et al: Cerebrovascular reactivity to CO_2 in patients with hepatic or septic encephalopathy. Resuscitation 1990; 19:125–134.
38. Davenport A, Will EJ, Davison EM: Effect of posture on intracranial pressure and cerebral perfusion pressure in patients with fulminant hepatic and renal failure after acetaminophen self-poisoning. Crit Care Med 1990; 18:286–289.
39. Canalese J, Gimson AES, Davis C, et al: Controlled trial of dexamethasone and mannitol for the cerebral edema of fulminant hepatic failure. Gut 1982; 23:625–629.
40. Williams R: Classification, etiology and considerations of outcome in acute liver failure. Semin Liver Dis 1996; 16:343–348.
41. Forbes A, Alexander GJ, O'Grady JG, et al: Thiopental infusion in the treatment of intracranial hypertension complicating fulminant hepatic failure. Hepatology 1989; 10:306–310.
42. Dixit V, Gitnick G: Artificial liver support: State of the art. Scand J Gastroenterol (Suppl) 1996; 220:101–114.
43. Watanabe FD, Mullon C, Hewitt WR, et al: Clinical experience with a bioartificial liver in the treatment of severe liver failure. Ann Surg 1997; 225:484–494.
44. Sussman NL, Chong MG, Koussayer T, et al: Reversal of fulminant hepatic failure using an extracorporeal liver assist device. Hepatology 1992; 16:60–65.

150

Acute Pancreatitis

Michael L. Steer, MD

CLASSIFICATION AND PATHOLOGIC FACTORS

Pancreatitis is an inflammatory disease of the pancreas that is frequently associated with a number of other processes referred to as the causes of pancreatitis. By convention, the term *acute pancreatitis* refers to an attack involving a pancreas that was normal, both functionally and morphologically, before the onset of symptoms and that returns to normal after resolution of the attack. In contrast, the term *chronic pancreatitis* refers to a disease process in which functional or morphologic changes in the pancreas precede or follow the attack. In practice, however, the distinction between an attack of either acute or chronic pancreatitis is often difficult because, in each, the symptoms and clinical findings are frequently sudden in onset and the functional as well as the morphologic status of the gland before and after the attack is unknown. As a result, sudden-onset attacks are usually considered symptomatic of acute pancreatitis, whereas attacks characterized by long periods of waxing and waning symptoms are commonly considered symptomatic of chronic pancreatitis.

The pathologic changes of pancreatitis include interstitial edema, infiltration of inflammatory cells into the pancreas, and evidence of fat necrosis. In chronic pancreatitis, areas of fibrosis as well as atrophy of acinar tissue can also be seen. To a great extent, the morphologic changes of pancreatitis parallel the clinical severity of an attack, and, in severe cases, focal or diffuse areas of glandular necrosis are usually present. In addition, there may be thrombosis of intrapancreatic or peripancreatic vessels with intraparenchymal hemorrhage and abscess formation.

ETIOLOGY

The so-called causes[1] of acute pancreatitis are listed in Table 150–1. In any given population, roughly 80% of the cases are associated with either biliary tract stone disease or alcohol abuse and 10% to 15% of the cases have no identified cause. These latter cases are identified as "idiopathic" acute pancreatitis. In the remaining 5% to 10% of cases, patients have an attack that is associated with a variety of other processes, including periampullary tumors or other obstructing lesions, infections such as mumps or coxsackievirus, parasites such as *Clonorchis sinensis* and *Ascaris lumbricoides,* or metabolic abnormalities such as hyperlipoproteinemia or hyperparathyroidism.

Trauma to the pancreas can cause a diffuse form of acute pancreatitis as a result of pancreatic contusion or, more commonly, can lead to ductal disruption and an obstructive form of chronic pancreatitis. In such cases, the ductal disruption usually occurs near the junction between the body and tail of the pancreas, where the gland passes over the spine and can be cracked by blunt abdominal injury.

Acute pancreatitis can also follow a variety of operative procedures, including distal gastrectomy, sphincteroplasty, and common bile duct exploration. Endoscopic retrograde cholangiopancreatography is a relatively common iatrogenic cause of pancreatitis. Pancreatitis also occurs with increased frequency after either cardiac or renal transplantation and after cardiopulmonary bypass.

Acute pancreatitis can be precipitated by a variety of drugs, including the thiazide diuretics, furosemide, ethacrynic acid, azathioprine, tetracycline, estrogens, and valproic acid. Certain drugs used to treat acquired immunodeficiency syndrome (AIDS) such as pentamidine and dideoxyinosine can also cause acute pancreatitis.

PATHOGENESIS

The mechanism by which ethanol abuse leads to pancreatitis is not known. For the most part, the symptoms of pancreatitis appear only after many years of ethanol abuse and in these cases fibrosis and atrophy of the gland are already established. Evidence of exocrine or endocrine insufficiency may be present; as a result, these patients are usually given the diagnosis of chronic pancreatitis.[2] On occasion, however, an attack of pancreatitis may occur after only a brief period of ethanol abuse, and there may be no evidence of chronic morphologic or functional abnormality.

In contrast to the paucity of information concerning the events that relate ethanol abuse to pancreatitis, our knowledge concerning the pathogenesis of gallstone-related pancreatitis is much further developed. The studies of Acosta and Ledesma[3, 4] as well as those of others clearly showed that pancreatitis is triggered by stone passage into or through the terminal biliopancreatic duct.

Three theories have been advanced to explain the mechanism by which stone passage might precipitate pancreatitis. The so-called *common-channel theory* proposed by Opie[5] in 1901 suggested that a stone might occlude the biliopancreatic

TABLE 150–1. Causes of Pancreatitis

Biliary tract stones	Trauma
Ethanol abuse	Postoperative
Obstructive lesions	Drugs
Infections	Miscellaneous
Parasites	Idiopathic
Metabolic abnormalities	

duct, creating behind it a common channel through which bile might reflux into the pancreatic duct and, presumably, injure the pancreas. Objections to this theory include the observation that because pancreatic duct pressure exceeds bile duct pressure,[6] bile reflux into the pancreatic duct is unlikely. In addition, it is known that perfusion of the pancreatic duct with bile under physiologic pressures does not induce pancreatitis.[7]

The *duodenal reflux theory* suggests that stone passage through Oddi's sphincter renders that sphincter incompetent and, as a result, duodenal juices containing activated digestive enzymes can reflux through the incompetent sphincter into the pancreatic duct.[8] The currently recognized fact that the sphincter can be surgically or endoscopically divided (i.e., sphincterotomy or sphincteroplasty) without causing repeated episodes of pancreatitis certainly indicates that the duodenal reflux theory is an unlikely explanation for the development of gallstone-related pancreatitis.

The third theory and, by exclusion, the most likely explanation for the events relating stone passage to pancreatitis involves *pancreatic duct obstruction.* Presumably, either the offending stone or the edema and inflammation of the distal pancreatic duct that follow stone passage cause obstruction of the pancreatic duct. With continued secretion into the obstructed duct system, pancreatic duct hypertension would be expected. Experimental studies using various animal models of pancreatitis suggest that this could lead to intra-acinar cell activation of digestive enzyme precursors (zymogens) by the lysosomal hydrolase cathepsin-B and that this phenomenon might result in acinar cell injury and pancreatitis.[9-12]

CLINICAL PRESENTATION

History and Physical Examination

A history and physical examination[13] reveal the classic symptoms of acute pancreatitis, including abdominal pain, nausea, and vomiting. The pain typically begins abruptly and precedes the onset of nausea. It slowly increases in severity over several hours and thereafter remains constant. It is usually most severe in the epigastrium and radiates through to the midback. Frequently, the degree of discomfort is lessened by either leaning forward or assuming the knee-chest position. Patients frequently describe the pain as having a knife-like or boring character. The nausea and vomiting of an attack of pancreatitis usually persist even after the stomach has been emptied and the vomiting has become unproductive.

Patients with acute pancreatitis usually appear anxious as they constantly move about in search of a comfortable position. They may have mild, or sometimes severe, mental status alterations as a result of ethanol or drug exposure, hypotension, or hypoxemia. Jaundice is common, even in the absence of bile duct obstruction. Patients with gallstone-related pancreatitis also may have evidence of cholangitis; however, even in the absence of cholangitis, fever is often noted.

Abdominal examination usually reveals areas of tenderness as well as both voluntary and involuntary guarding. Although these changes are usually most pronounced in the epigastrium, where a mass may be felt, tenderness and guarding can also be observed elsewhere or even diffusely in the abdomen. Abdominal distention is common, and bowel sounds are frequently diminished or absent. As a result of hypovolemia and dehydration, the skin and mucous membranes may be dry, neck veins may be collapsed, and hypotension as well as tachycardia may be present. Evidence of retroperitoneal bleeding (Grey Turner's sign, Cullen's sign) is sometimes observed. Examination of the chest may reveal diminished breath sounds, especially at the bases, and evidence of pleural effusions.

Laboratory Tests

The routine laboratory tests usually show a number of nonspecific changes, including leukocytosis with a leftward shift of the differential, an elevated hematocrit, hyperglycemia, hypoalbuminemia, and an increase in the creatinine and blood urea nitrogen (BUN). Hypocalcemia, sometimes out of proportion to the degree of hypoalbuminemia, can occur. Mild elevations of the alkaline phosphatase, transaminases, and bilirubin level are common even in those without gallstone-related pancreatitis. Hypertriglyceridemia may be present in those with alcohol-related pancreatitis or pancreatitis caused by hyperlipoproteinemia.[14, 15]

Patients with acute pancreatitis usually have elevated serum and urine levels of amylase.[16, 17] Unfortunately, hyperamylasemia is not a finding that is specific to pancreatitis. Other causes of hyperamylasemia are listed in Table 150–2. Hyperamylasemia caused by perforated viscus, mesenteric infarction, bowel obstruction, or cholangitis may be particularly difficult to distinguish from hyperamylasemia caused by pancreatitis. Attempts have been made to improve the diagnostic accuracy in pancreatitis by measuring the amylase-creatinine clearance ratio, serum pancreatic amylase isoenzymes, and serum level of other pancreas-derived digestive enzymes, such as trypsinogen.[16] Unfortunately, these tests have not proved useful, and for the most part they are not widely used.

Measurement of serum lipase or urine amylase levels may be useful in identifying those patients who are first seen

TABLE 150–2. Causes of Hyperamylasemia

Pancreatic
Pancreatitis, pseudocyst, ascites
Pancreatic duct obstruction
Secretagogue stimulation
Pancreatic trauma
Endoscopic retrograde cholangiopancreatography
Pancreatic tumor
Nonpancreatic Intra-abdominal
Bowel obstruction
Perforated ulcer or viscus
Appendicitis
Bowel infarction
Salivary
Mumps
Trauma
Duct obstruction
Radiation
Pulmonary
Pneumonia
Cancer
Malignant Tumors
Lung
Prostate
Ovary
Pancreas
Breast
Genitourinary
Ovarian cyst
Ruptured ectopic pregnancy
Renal failure
Pregnancy
Prostatic disease
Miscellaneous
Burns
Diabetic ketoacidosis

several days after the onset of pancreatitis, because in those patients hyperlipasemia and hyperamylasuria may persist even after serum amylase levels have returned to normal.[16] Measurement of urine amylase levels may also aid in identifying those patients whose hyperamylasemia is caused by macroamylasemia rather than pancreatitis. In macroamylasemia, amylase is bound to an abnormal circulating protein, and as a result, urine amylase levels are very low.[18]

Routine radiographic examinations of the chest may reveal basal atelectasis and pleural effusions, which are more common on the left than on the right side. Abdominal radiographs may demonstrate pancreatic calcifications in patients with chronic pancreatitis. The gaseous pattern of a paralytic ileus is frequently noted. Routine abdominal x-ray films may also suggest displacement of various organs by an inflammatory pancreatic mass, and in patients with pancreatic abscess, retroperitoneal gas can, on occasion, be noted. In general, however, these routine radiographic studies are not of great value in the diagnosis of acute pancreatitis. Similarly, ultrasonography is of only limited value because the gaseous distention of bowel during the early stages of pancreatitis usually precludes a complete ultrasonographic examination.[19] Even in such cases, however, ultrasonographic evidence of gallbladder stones or dilated bile ducts may aid in identifying those patients whose pancreatitis is caused by gallstones.

In contrast to routine radiography and ultrasonography, computed tomography (CT) may be extremely valuable in the diagnosis and management of pancreatitis.[20] The CT scan is not limited by the presence of gas-filled loops in the upper abdomen, and it can detect the presence of relatively mild as well as severe pancreatitis. As noted later, routine CT, along with dynamic contrast-enhanced CT, may be of value in predicting the severity of an attack of pancreatitis. Finally, CT may be of value in identifying those patients mistakenly diagnosed with pancreatitis, because in such individuals the pancreas appears normal on CT.

Differential Diagnosis

Acute pancreatitis must be distinguished from the large number of other processes that can cause upper abdominal pain, nausea, and vomiting.[21] Pancreatitis frequently causes hyperamylasemia and hyperlipasemia, whereas many of the other diseases in the differential diagnosis do not cause these changes. Some diseases, such as perforated viscus, bowel obstruction, cholangitis, and mesenteric ischemia, show modest rises in circulating amylase and lipase levels, and distinguishing these processes from pancreatitis may be quite difficult.

Factors that favor the diagnosis of pancreatitis include:

1. A markedly elevated amylase level rather than the elevation of 1 to 2 times the normal value, which is seen in nonpancreatic diseases.
2. CT changes of pancreatitis.
3. Improvement after the institution of aggressive nonoperative treatment.

When doubt about the diagnosis persists, however, exploratory laparotomy for diagnostic purposes may be indicated, particularly if the patient's condition is deteriorating in spite of aggressive treatment.

Prognosis

Although only 10% to 15% of patients with pancreatitis have a severe attack, the mortality and serious morbidity among this group may exceed 50%. Identifying those individuals most likely to experience a severe attack would be helpful in allowing for comparison of various treatment strategies in prospective trials as well as in selecting those individuals who are in need of intensive care. A number of clinical, radiographic, and biochemical methods of identifying such individuals are available (Table 150–3).[22] The most widely used clinical prognostic system is that developed by Ranson and colleagues[23] (Table 150–4). Patients with fewer than three Ranson signs have a mortality rate of less than 1%; those with seven to eight prognostic signs have a mortality rate of 90%. Because of its greater flexibility, the Acute Physiologic and Chronic Health Evaluation (APACHE II) system may replace the Ranson or Imrie system for predicting the severity of an attack on clinical grounds.[24]

From a radiologic standpoint, the dynamic contrast-enhanced CT can also predict the severity of an attack. As noted by Balthazar and associates,[25] the presence of one or more pancreatic or peripancreatic fluid collections and lack of contrast enhancement of 50% of the pancreas are associated with a high probability of septic complications or death. A number of serum markers for severity have been evaluated (see Table 150–3), but the ultimate value of these tests in the management of patients with pancreatitis remains to be established. The most widely used are the C-reactive protein, polymorphonuclear elastase, and interleukin = 6 (IL-6) measurements. The ultimate value of these tests may be that low levels of these markers indicate a benign course and that, in this setting, particularly if the clinical scoring system also suggests a benign course, contrast-enhanced dynamic CT may not be needed.[22, 26]

TABLE 150–3. Prognostic Markers

Clinical
Ranson's scoring system
Imrie's scoring system
APACHE II scoring system
Radiographic
Non–contrast-enhanced computed tomography
Dynamic contrast-enhanced computed tomography
Biochemical
Polymorphonuclear elastase
C-reactive protein
Trypsinogen activation peptide
Antiprotease levels
Cytokines
Interleukin-1
Interleukin-6
Tumor necrosis factor-α

TABLE 150–4. Ranson's Criteria

On Admission
Age greater than 55 years
White blood cell count greater than 16,000/mm^3
Blood glucose level greater than 200 mg/dL
Lactate dehydrogenase level greater than 350 IU/L
Glutamic-oxaloacetic transaminase level greater than 250 SFU/dL
During Initial 48 Hours
Hematocrit decrease greater than 10%
Blood urea nitrogen rise greater than 5 mg/dL
Serum Ca^{2+} less than 8 mg/dL
PaO_2 less than 60 mm Hg
Base deficit greater than 4 mEq/L
Fluid sequestration greater than 6 L

Ca^{2+} = calcium ion; PaO_2 = partial pressure of arterial oxygen.

TREATMENT

Acute Pancreatitis

The goals of initial management in pancreatitis include establishing the diagnosis, relieving pain, and supporting fluid as well as electrolyte needs. Usually, the diagnosis can be securely established when the clinical presentation and findings are appropriate, the amylase level is markedly elevated, the CT scan is convincing, or the patient improves with appropriate treatment. On occasion, however, exploratory laparotomy may be required to establish the diagnosis when uncertainty persists, particularly if the patient does not improve with aggressive treatment.

The pain of pancreatitis may be severe, and for the most part narcotic medications are needed. In gallstone pancreatitis, meperidine (Demerol) rather than morphine should be used, because the former relaxes Oddi's sphincter whereas morphine causes contraction of the sphincter.[27]

The early stages of acute pancreatitis are frequently characterized by marked intravascular volume contraction and hypovolemia. Injury caused by the release of agents from the inflamed pancreas leads to exudation of fluid into the retroperitoneum. In addition, there is repeated vomiting and nasogastric aspiration of fluid. Overall, the lost fluid in pancreatitis usually has a plasma-like content of electrolytes and protein. Thus, although serum electrolyte concentrations may not change dramatically, a rise in hematocrit can be expected, and the magnitude of this rise may be useful in calculating fluid replacement needs. If vomiting or nasogastric fluid aspiration volumes are large, a hypochloremic alkalosis may result. On the other hand, poor tissue perfusion can favor the development of a metabolic acidosis.

Hypocalcemia or hypomagnesemia can occur either as a result of preexisting malnutrition, especially in alcoholics, or as a result of the pancreatitis itself. Usually, the hypocalcemia is merely a reflection of hypoalbuminemia, and ionized calcium levels remain normal. In severe cases of pancreatitis, however, the degree of hypocalcemia may be out of proportion to the hypoalbuminemia and may reflect a decline in ionized calcium levels. Tetany and carpopedal spasm can be seen, and, when noted, aggressive calcium and magnesium replacement should be instituted.

During the early stages of pancreatitis, the heart rate, cardiac output, and cardiac index may rise and total peripheral resistance may decline. The degree of intrapulmonary shunting may rise, and hypoxemia can develop. These changes are, most likely, caused by hypovolemia, atelectasis, and the release of vasoactive agents and cytokines from the inflamed pancreas. In severe cases, an acute respiratory distress syndrome (ARDS)–like lesion may develop and significant lung injury can occur. It has been established that close to 50% of the patients who die within the first 2 weeks after the onset of pancreatitis die as a result of pancreatitis-associated lung injury.

Treatment of the early stages of a severe attack of acute pancreatitis requires meticulous management of fluid, electrolyte, and respiratory needs. Central filling pressures and volume needs can be monitored using a Swan-Ganz catheter. The hematocrit can be used to quantitate extracellular fluid losses. An indwelling arterial catheter, used to track arterial blood gases and pH, may identify those individuals in need of endotracheal intubation and ventilatory support. Renal function can be monitored by placement of a urethral catheter. A fluid-balance flow sheet may be particularly useful in management of these complicated and seriously ill patients.

The role of peritoneal lavage in the management of patients with severe attacks of pancreatitis remains controversial. A number of uncontrolled or anecdotal reports suggested that lavage, which removes harmful agents released from the inflamed pancreas, may be beneficial. More recently, however, a randomized, multicenter study suggested that lavage does not alter the outcome of an attack.[28] The issue probably warrants further study because the randomized study used only short-term lavage, and the possibility that longer periods of lavage might be of benefit has not been adequately evaluated.[29]

The potential value of prophylactic antibiotics in the treatment of severe pancreatitis is also controversial; some studies suggested a benefit,[30] whereas others concluded that antibiotics are not beneficial. Most recent studies indicate that prophylactic antibodies are beneficial in the treatment of patients with severe pancreatitis, but it is not clear whether they improve survival or merely reduce the incidence of septic complications. Imipenem and cefuroxime are the two most commonly used agents.[30, 31] Given these uncertainties, my practice is to not administer peritoneal lavage and to confine the use of prophylactic antibiotics to patients with gallstone pancreatitis.

Many additional therapies for pancreatitis have been proposed, but the benefit of most of them remains unproven.[21, 32] These include attempts to:

1. Reduce pancreatic function using atropine, somatostatin, glucagon, or calcitonin.
2. Inhibit the activity of pancreatic digestive enzymes using aprotinin, chlorophyll-A, procainamide, or gabexate.
3. Inhibit inflammation and cytotoxicity using indomethacin or prostaglandins.

Nasogastric decompression appears to improve patient comfort but does not alter the course or severity of pancreatitis. Antacids and histamine$_2$ receptor antagonists do not appear to alter the severity of an attack, but these agents may be of value in preventing stress ulcer bleeding.

Biliary Tract Stone Disease

Most patients with gallstone pancreatitis experience only a relatively mild attack that resolves as the offending stone is either passed into the duodenum or becomes disimpacted by moving more proximally in the biliary tree. These individuals need no immediate treatment for the biliary tract stones but should eventually undergo a ductal stone clearance procedure with or without cholecystectomy to prevent repeated attacks of gallstone pancreatitis. The method of ductal stone clearance in the management of such patients can be either surgical (common duct exploration, sphincteroplasty, bilioenteric anastomosis) or endoscopic (sphincterotomy with stone extraction, lithotripsy, or stone dissolution), depending on the locally available expertise or individual preference. Most patients are now managed endoscopically. Removal of the gallbladder can usually be accomplished laparoscopically. Some evidence suggests that cholecystectomy is not mandatory, especially in high-risk patients who have only a cholangitis or pancreatitis clinical picture and who lack symptoms of acute or chronic cholecystitis.[33] Most of these individuals, if treated for ductal disease, do not require a later cholecystectomy.

Approximately 10% to 15% of patients with gallstone pancreatitis experience a severe attack. Acosta and coworkers[34] reported that the incidence of these severe attacks might be reduced by subjecting all patients with gallstone pancreatitis to early surgical duct clearance, but Kelly and Wagner[35] later reported that early surgical intervention in such patients resulted in an increased mortality rate. More recent attention has been directed to the role of early endoscopic approaches to duct clearance in such patients. Two reports[36, 37] indicated that early endoscopy with sphincterotomy and ductal clearance of stones for patients with severe gallstone pancreatitis is both safe and beneficial. It is not entirely clear whether the benefit of this approach results from the reduction in the ultimate severity of pancreatitis or, alternatively, from the relief of cholangitis.

A more recent study[38] has questioned the overall value of early endoscopic intervention in pancreatitis. On the basis of the available evidence, however, early endoscopy to clear the ductal stones seems to be the treatment of choice for individuals with severe gallstone pancreatitis, particularly in patients with jaundice or cholangitis.

Systemic Complications

The systemic complications of acute pancreatitis, for the most part, occur during the early stages of an attack. They include renal failure, respiratory failure, cardiovascular collapse, disseminated intravascular coagulopathy (DIC), and gastrointestinal bleeding. During the early stages of an attack, severe hypovolemia may result from extensive fluid losses. Vasoactive agents, proinflammatory cytokines, and activated digestive enzymes may be released into the circulation, and in a setting of hypovolemia, these agents can have profound effects on cardiac, pulmonary, and renal function.

Treatment should be directed at supporting cardiac, pulmonary, and renal function while aggressively replacing fluid losses. Close monitoring of venous filling pressure, cardiac output, urinary output, blood oxygenation, and hematocrit is critical. Endotracheal intubation or hemodialysis may be required. Theoretically, peritoneal dialysis might allow for removal of toxic agents released from the inflamed pancreas, but the value of peritoneal lavage in this setting remains controversial. Plasmapheresis may be another method of achieving the same goal. The value of these modalities is currently under investigation at several centers.

Gastrointestinal bleeding during acute pancreatitis may occur by several mechanisms, including bleeding from stress-induced gastroduodenal ulcers. In addition, there may be erosion of the peripancreatic inflammatory process into major vessels or a hollow viscus. Depletion of coagulation factors as a result of DIC can occur. Finally, portal hypertension caused by splenic or portal vein thrombosis can occur. The management of these complications of pancreatitis should be dictated by the nature of the lesion present; for the most part, however, management is similar to that used when bleeding is caused by these processes in the absence of pancreatitis.

Late Local Complications

The local complications of acute pancreatitis can be separated into two groups based on the *presence* or *absence* of infection.[39] Sterile complications include areas of pancreatic and peripancreatic necrosis, pancreatic pseudocysts, and pancreatic ascites. These lesions usually appear several days to weeks after the onset of an attack and can be identified by ultrasonography (Fig. 150–1) and CT (Fig. 150–2). CT is especially useful when dynamic contrast enhancement is used to identify areas of necrosis (Fig. 150–3). Paracentesis or thoracentesis for measurement of the amylase level in the removed fluid can identify patients with pancreatic ascites or pancreaticopleural fistulas, and endoscopic retrograde cholangiopancreatography (ERCP) in such patients can be used to localize the site of pancreatic duct disruption (Fig. 150–4).

Each of these sterile complications of pancreatitis can become secondarily infected, usually as a result of transmigration of organisms into the inflamed area from adjacent segments of the gastrointestinal tract. When infection is present, the terms *infected pancreatic/peripancreatic necrosis* and *infected pseudocyst* are usually used. The latter lesion is also frequently referred to as a *pancreatic abscess.* When the diagnosis in doubt, the presence of infection can be documented using the technique of CT-guided fine-needle aspiration.[40]

At present, the treatment of the sterile complications of pancreatitis is the subject of considerable controversy. Most surgeons prefer to avoid operation for sterile pancreatic necrosis, although some, particularly the group in Ulm, Germany, have advocated necrosectomy in such cases and claim that the procedure can lessen the overall morbidity and mortality of pancreatitis.[41] Until recently, it was generally believed that pancreatic pseudocysts greater than 6 cm in diameter and persisting longer than 6 weeks after an attack of pancreatitis should be treated by either internal or percutaneous drainage.[42] However, two reports indicated that asymptomatic pseu-

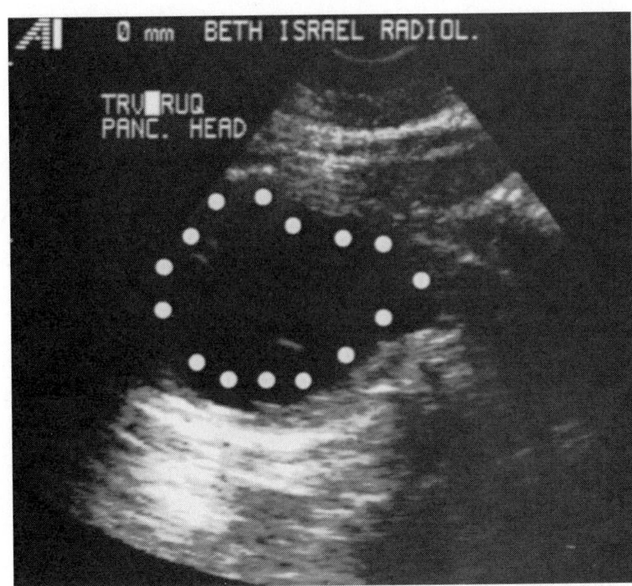

Figure 150–1. Ultrasound examination of pancreas reveals a pseudocyst (the nonechogenic area identified by *white dots*).

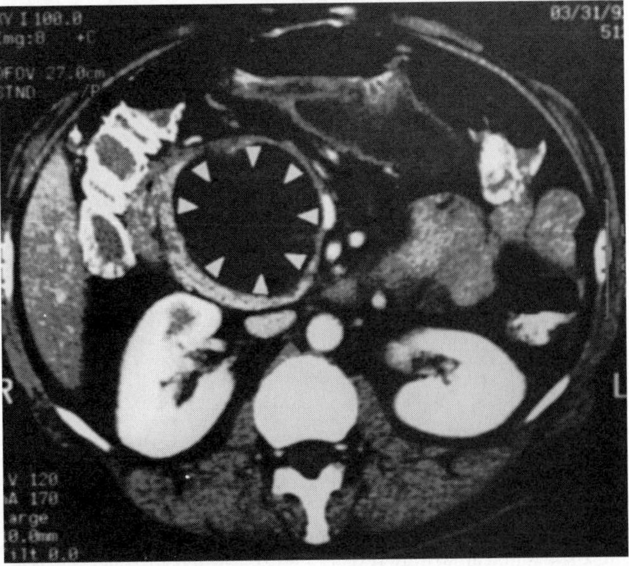

Figure 150–2. A CT image of pancreas reveals a pseudocyst (the low-density area outlined by *arrowheads*).

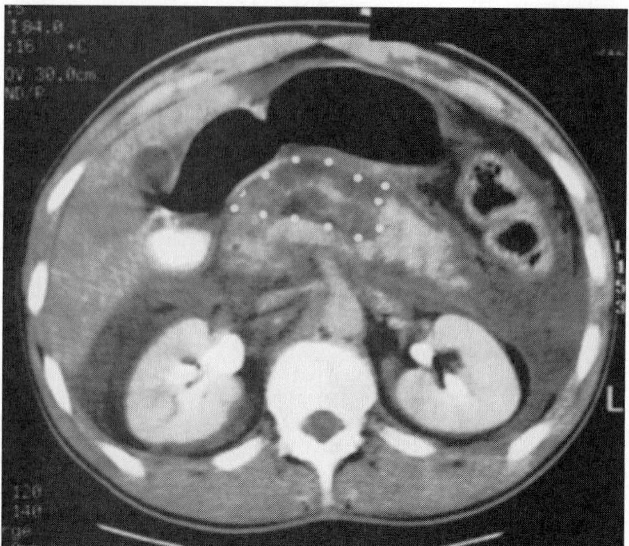

Figure 150–3. Necrosis of the pancreas. Contrast-enhanced, dynamic CT reveals an area of pancreatic underperfusion (outlined by *white dots*) around a central core of remaining perfused pancreatic tissue.

docysts, even if persistent and quite large, can be left untreated with little or no long-term morbidity.[43, 44]

In contrast to these areas of controversy, there is general agreement regarding the treatment of pancreatic ascites and pancreaticopleural fistulas. These lesions result from major pancreatic duct disruptions. In general, initial attempts to treat these lesions should include nutritional support and reduction of pancreatic secretion by the use of parenteral nutrition and administration of somatostatin.[45-47] Pancreatic duct stents, placed endoscopically across the point of duct disruption, may reduce the fluid leak.[48] If these efforts fail, treatment should include either resection of the pancreas proximal (i.e., to the left) to the ductal injury or internal drainage using a Roux-en-Y anastomosis of a jejunal limb to the site of duct disruption.

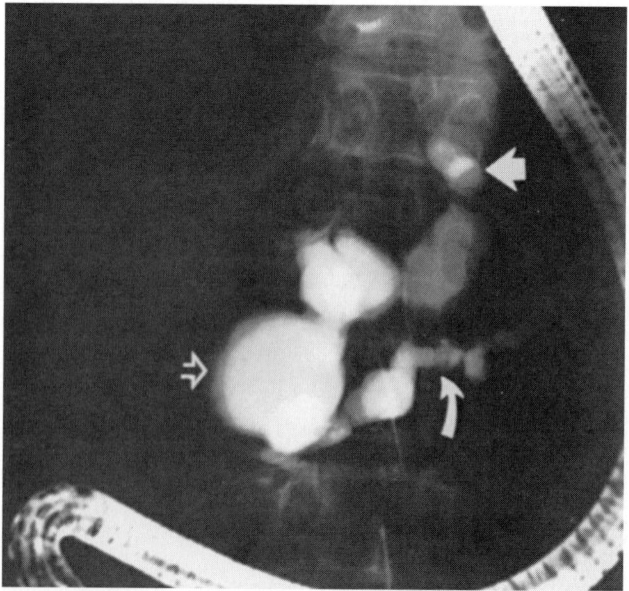

Figure 150–4. Pancreaticopleural fistula. Endoscopic retrograde cholangiopancreatography reveals a dilated pancreatic duct (*curved arrow*) filling a pseudocyst (*open arrow*) that communicates to the pleural space via a fistulous tract (*solid arrow*).

When areas of peripancreatic or pancreatic necrosis become infected, surgical intervention with debridement is almost always required.[49] The organisms recovered from such lesions include *Escherichia coli, Klebsiella, Proteus, Enterococcus, Pseudomonas,* and *Candida.*[50] Antibiotic therapy is never sufficient for treating such lesions. In addition, attempts to drain such areas nonoperatively usually fail because the infected material is putty-like and not amenable to drainage through catheters. Frequently, repeated operations for debridement are required.[49] In contrast to infected necrosis, infected pseudocysts (pancreatic abscesses) can frequently be treated by means of percutaneously placed drainage catheters because, for the most part, the infected fluid in these lesions is liquid pus, which can pass through the drainage catheters. On occasion, however, surgical intervention for debridement, drainage, or resection may be required for the treatment of pancreatic abscesses also.

References

1. Steer ML: Etiology and pathophysiology of acute pancreatitis. *In:* The Exocrine Pancreas: Biology, Pathobiology, and Diseases. 2nd ed. Go VLW, DiMagno EP, Gardner JD, et al (Eds). New York, Raven Press, 1993, pp 581–592.
2. Sarles H: Chronic pancreatitis: Etiology and pathophysiology. *In:* The Exocrine Pancreas: Biology, Pathobiology, and Diseases. Go VLW, Brooks F, DiMagno E, et al (Eds). New York, Raven Press, 1986, p 37.
3. Acosta JM, Ledesma CL: Gallstone migration as a cause of acute pancreatitis. N Engl J Med 1974; 290:484–487.
4. Acosta JL, Ross R, Ledesma CL: The usefulness of stool screening for diagnosing cholelithiasis in acute pancreatitis: A description of the technique. Am J Dig Dis 1977; 22:168.
5. Opie EL: The relationship of cholelithiasis to disease of the pancreas and fat necrosis. Am J Med Surg 1901; 12:27.
6. Menguy RB, Hallenbeck GA, Bollman JL, et al: Intraductal pressures and sphincteric resistance in canine pancreatic and biliary ducts after various stimuli. Surg Gynecol Obstet 1958; 106:306–311.
7. Robinson TM, Dunphy JE: Continuous perfusion of bile protease activators through the pancreas. JAMA 1963; 183:530–535.
8. McCutheon AD: Reflux of duodenal contents in the pathogenesis of pancreatitis. Gut 1964; 5:260–265.
9. Steer ML, Meldolesi J: The cell biology of experimental pancreatitis. N Engl J Med 1987; 316:144–150.
10. Steer ML: How and where does acute pancreatitis begin? Arch Surg 1992; 127:1350–1353.
11. Lerch MM, Saluja AK, Runzi M, et al: Pancreatic duct obstruction triggers acute necrotizing pancreatitis in the opossum. Gastroenterology 1993; 104:853–861.
12. Steer ML, Saluja AK: Experimental acute pancreatitis: Studies of the early events that lead to cell injury. *In:* The Exocrine Pancreas: Biology, Pathobiology, and Diseases. 2nd ed. Go VLW, DiMagno EP, Gardner JR, et al (Eds). New York, Raven Press, 1993, pp 489–500.
13. Silen W: Cope's Early Diagnosis of the Acute Abdomen. 15th ed. New York, Oxford University Press, 1979.
14. Fredrickson DS, Lees RS: Familial hyperlipoproteinemia. *In:* The Metabolic Basis of Inherited Disease. Stanbury JB, Wyngaarden LB, Fredrickson DS (Eds). New York, McGraw-Hill, 1966, pp 429–485.
15. Cameron JL, Crisler C, Margolis S, et al: Acute pancreatitis with hyperlipemia. Surgery 1971; 70:53–58.
16. Leavitt MD, Edkfeldt JH: Diagnosis of acute pancreatitis. *In:* The Exocrine Pancreas: Biology, Pathobiology, and Disease. Go VLW, Brooks F, DiMagno E, et al (Eds). New York, Raven Press, 1986, pp 481–502.
17. Salt WB, Schenker S: Amylase: Its clinical significance: A review of the literature. Medicine (Baltimore) 1976; 55:269–289.
18. Berk JE, Kizu H, Wilding P: A newly recognized cause for elevated serum amylase activity. J Engl J Med 1967; 277:941–945.

19. McKay AJ, Imrie CW, O'Neill J, et al: Is an early ultrasound scan of value in acute pancreatitis. Br J Surg 1982; 69:369-372.
20. Freeny PC: Incremental dynamic bolus computed tomography of acute pancreatitis. Int J Pancreatol 1993; 13:147-158.
21. Steer ML: Acute pancreatitis. *In:* Textbook of Gastroenterology. Yamada T, Alpers D, Ouyang C, et al (Eds). Philadelphia, JB Lippincott, 1991, pp 1854-1874.
22. Malfertheiner P, Dominguez-Munoz JE: Prognostic factors in acute pancreatitis. Int J Pancreatol 1993; 14:1-8.
23. Ranson JHC, Rifkind KM, Roses DF, et al: Prognostic signs and the role of operative management in acute pancreatitis. Surg Gynecol Obstet 1974; 139:69-81.
24. Larvin M, McMahon MJ: Apache-2 score for assessment and monitoring of acute pancreatitis. Lancet 1989; 2:201-205.
25. Balthazar EJ, Robinson DL, Megibow AJ, et al: Acute pancreatitis: Value of CT in establishing prognosis. Radiology 1990; 174:331-336.
26. DeBeaux AC, Goldie AS, Ross JA, Carter DC, Fearon KC: Serum concentrations of inflammatory mediators related to organ failure in patients with acute pancreatitis. Br J Surg 1996; 83:349-353.
27. Thune A, Baker RA, Saccone GT, et al: Differing effects of pethidine and morphine on human sphincter of Oddi motility. Br J Surg 1990; 77:992-995.
28. Mayer AD, McMahon MJ, Corfield AP, et al: Controlled clinical trial of peritoneal lavage for the treatment of severe acute pancreatitis. N Engl J Med 1985; 312:399-404.
29. Ranson JH, Berman RS: Long peritoneal lavage decreases pancreatic sepsis in acute pancreatitis. Ann Surg 1990; 211:708-716.
30. Pederzole P, Bassi C, Vesentini S, et al: A randomized multicenter trial of antibiotic prophylaxis of septic complications in acute necrotizing pancreatitis with imipenem. Surg Gynecol Obstet 1993; 176:480-483.
31. Saino V, Kemppainer E, Puolakkainen P, et al: Early antibiotic treatment in acute necrotizing pancreatitis. Lancet 1995; 346:663-667.
32. Steer ML: Acute pancreatitis. *In:* Gastrointestinal Emergencies. Taylor MW, Gollan J, Peppercorn MA, et al (Eds). Baltimore, Williams & Wilkins, 1992, pp 171-179.
33. Davidson BR, Neoptolemos JP, Carr-Locke DL: Endoscopic sphincterotomy for common bile duct calculi in patients with gall bladder in situ considered unfit for surgery. Gut 1988; 29:114-120.
34. Acosta JM, Rossi R, Galli OMR, et al: Early surgery for acute gallstone pancreatitis: Evaluation of a systematic approach. Surgery 1978; 83:367-370.
35. Kelly TR, Wagner DS: Gallstone pancreatitis: A prospective randomized trial of the timing of surgery. Surgery 1988; 104:600.
36. Neoptolemos JP, Carr-Locke DL, London NJ, et al: Controlled trial of urgent endoscopic retrograde cholangiopancreatography and endoscopic sphincterotomy versus conservative treatment for acute pancreatitis due to gallstones. Lancet 1988; 2:979-983.
37. Fan ST, Lai ECS, Mok FPT, et al: Early treatment of acute biliary pancreatitis by endoscopic papillotomy. N Engl J Med 1993; 328:228-232.
38. Folsch UR, Nitsche R, Ludtke R, et al: Early ERCP and papillotomy compared with conservative treatment for acute biliary pancreatitis: The German Study Group in Acute Biliary Pancreatitis. N Engl J Med 1997; 336:237-242.
39. Bradley EL: A clinically based classification system for acute pancreatitis. Arch Surg 1993; 128:586-590.
40. Gerzof SG, Banks PA, Robbins AH, et al: Early diagnosis of pancreatic infection by computed tomography-guided aspiration. Gastroenterology 1987; 93:1315-1320.
41. Beger HG, Krautzberger W, Bittner R, et al: Results of surgical treatment of necrotizing pancreatitis. World J Surg 1985; 9:972-979.
42. Bradley EL, Clements JL, Gonzales AC: The natural history of pancreatic pseudocysts: A unified coincept of management. Am J Surg 1979; 137:135-141.
43. Yeo CJ, Bastidas JA, Lynch-Nyhan A, et al: The natural history of pancreatic pseudocysts documented by computed tomography. Surg Gynecol Obstet 1990; 170:411-417.
44. Vitas GJ, Sarr MG: Selected management of pancreatic pseudocysts: Operative versus expectant management. Surgery 1992; 111:123-130.
45. Sankaren S, Walt AJ: Pancreatic ascites: Recognition and management. Arch Surg 1976; 111:430.
46. Cameron JL, Kieffer RS, Anderson WJ, et al: Internal pancreatic fistulas: Pancreatic ascites and pleural effusions. Ann Surg 1976; 184:587-593.
47. Gislason H, Growbech JE, Soreide O: Pancreatic ascites: Treatment by continuous somatostatin infusion. Am J Gastroenterol 1991; 86:519-521.
48. Kozarek RA, Ball TH, Paterson DJ, et al: Endoscopic transpapillary therapy for disrupted pancreatic duct and peripancreatic fluid collections. Gastroenterology 1991; 100:1362-1370.
49. Bradley EL: A fifteen year experience with open drainage for infected pancreatic necrosis. Surg Gynecol Obstet 1993; 177:215-222.
50. Ranson JHC: Complications of pancreatitis. *In:* Gastrointestinal Emergencies. Taylor MW, Gollan J, Peppercorn MA, et al (Eds). Baltimore, Williams & Wilkins, 1992, pp 180-192.

151

Role of the Gut in Multiple Organ Failure

Walter L. Biffl, MD • Ernest E. Moore, MD

Since the late 1980s, the gut has been recognized as central in the pathogenesis of multiple organ failure (MOF). Whereas dysfunctions of the heart, lungs, kidneys, and liver are more dramatic and easily quantifiable, gastrointestinal (GI) dysfunction is typically subtle. Formerly acknowledged for its functions of digestion and nutrient absorption and considered to be quiescent in critical illness, the gut is now known to be metabolically active, immunologically unique, and a reservoir of potentially pathogenic bacteria. In contrast to other major organ systems, the gut appears not only to be capable of provoking hyperinflammation and MOF but also to be a potential target for prevention. This chapter explores the evolution and current status of the role of the gut in the pathogenesis of MOF.

MULTIPLE ORGAN FAILURE

Systemic Hyperinflammation Model

The identification of MOF as a distinct entity dates back to 1973, when Tilney and colleagues[1] described the progressive failure of organ systems in patients after repair of ruptured abdominal aortic aneurysms. Baue[2] first suggested that there was a sequential pattern to the MOF syndrome. In 1977, Eiseman and coworkers[3] at our institution described the clinical presentation and coined the term "MOF." Once established, MOF defies our standard critical care supportive measures: mortality ranges from 40% to 100% and is related directly to the number and duration of organ failures.[4] Unfortunately, neither the incidence nor the mortality of the syndrome has improved significantly. MOF remains the leading cause of delayed mortality in the surgical intensive care unit (SICU); an epidemiologic review revealed that 61% of deaths more than 72 hours after injury in our trauma center were the result of organ failure.[5]

Early reports of MOF implicated infection as the primary etiologic factor.[6] In an influential paper, Fry and colleagues[7] in 1980 retrospectively reviewed 553 patients requiring emergent operations. Thirty-eight (7%) developed MOF; of these, 89% had sepsis, leading the investigators to conclude reasonably that MOF was a "fatal expression of uncontrolled infection." This study was pivotal in the subsequent adoption of an aggressive policy of mandatory laparotomy to search for intra-abdominal abscesses in patients with MOF. However, a provocative paper by Norton[8] in 1985 reported that drainage of intra-abdominal abscesses in critically ill patients infrequently resulted in reversal of MOF. Thus, it appeared that a localized infection could provoke MOF but an ongoing infection was not necessary to perpetuate it. At the same time, two reports from Europe emphasized that overt clinical infections were not a requisite for MOF. Faist and colleagues[9] reviewed 433 trauma patients, of whom 8% developed MOF; of these, only 59% had documented infection. Goris and colleagues[10] confirmed a focus of bacterial sepsis in only 45% of MOF patients without trauma and 33% of MOF patients with trauma.

The Two-Hit Model of Multiple Organ Failure

The systemic clinical manifestations of gram-negative bacterial infection can be mimicked by noninfectious stimuli, for example, tissue ischemia-reperfusion (I-R) or tissue disruption, that lead to a prolonged and excessive inflammatory response. To standardize communication in this area, a consensus paper by the American College of Chest Physicians and Society of Critical Care Medicine proposed definitions pertaining to the systemic inflammatory response syndrome (SIRS) and sepsis.[11] The term SIRS refers to an inflammatory response to infectious or noninfectious processes, defined as two or more of the following clinical conditions:

1. Body temperature above 38°C or below 36°C.
2. Heart rate greater than 90 beats/min.
3. Tachypnea, manifested by a respiratory rate greater than 20 breaths/min or hyperventilation indicated by an arterial carbon dioxide pressure ($Pa{CO_2}$) less than 32 mm Hg.
4. Alteration of the white blood cell (WBC) count with more than 12×10^6 cells/mm^3 or less than 4×10^6 cells/mm^3.

"Sepsis" refers to SIRS of an infectious origin.

The recognition of SIRS independent of infection stimulated several new hypotheses regarding the underlying mechanism of MOF. The focus of current thought is that MOF represents the culmination of a generalized and excessive neuroendocrine, immune, and inflammatory response—a modern "horror autotoxicus."[12] The concept that the host is destroying itself, and not being consumed by microorganisms, shifted research efforts from the detection and treatment of infections to characterization and attenuation of the inflammatory process leading to MOF.

We have proposed a "two-hit" model of MOF (Fig. 151-1). Briefly, an initial insult (first hit) "primes" the inflammatory system in such a way that a second insult (second hit) activates an unbridled systemic hyperinflammatory response. The clinical manifestation is SIRS and MOF; we believe the correlate at the cellular level is the priming and activation of polymorphonuclear leukocytes (PMNs).[13] Our Trauma Research Center has focused on the underlying pathophysiology of the first hit. A number of diverse clinical conditions have been reported to prime the inflammatory response, rendering the patient vulnerable to an activating event; in general, the priming events may be classified as inadequate tissue perfusion, extensively injured tissue, or infection. Consequently, there are several existing hypotheses regarding the genesis of SIRS, although none has been accepted wholeheartedly. One prominent theory is the "gut hypothesis," which suggests that the gut is the "motor of MOF."[14] Although the gut probably plays a key role in the pathogenesis of MOF, we believe its contribution differs in early-onset versus late-onset MOF.

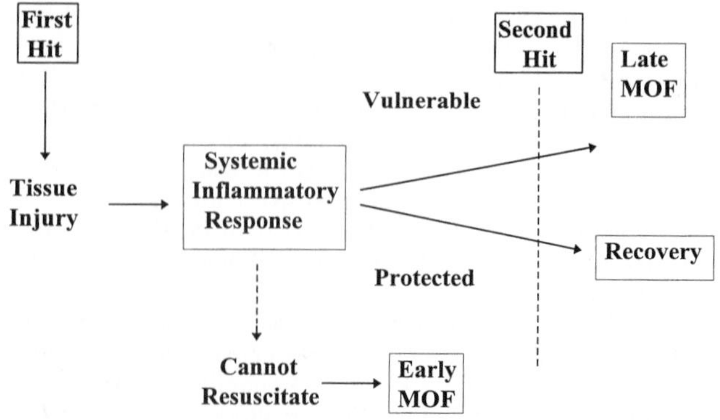

Figure 151–1. The "two-hit" model of multiple organ failure (MOF).

We have identified a bimodal pattern in the development of MOF in a large series of severely injured patients, with each group having distinct characteristics.[15] Early MOF (occurring within 72 hours of the initial insult) is rapid in onset, with indices of cellular shock identifying the patient at risk. In contrast, late-onset MOF (typically 6–8 days after injury) is insidious in onset, with infectious prominent in the pathogenesis. Consequently, we have conceptually separated the study of MOF into early onset versus late onset.

THE GUT

Gut Ischemia-Reperfusion in Early Multiple Organ Failure: The First Hit

Reactive Oxygen Metabolites

After tissue ischemia, resumption of blood flow is necessary for cellular salvage; however, reperfusion of ischemic tissues paradoxically creates more tissue injury. Reperfusion is associated with more intestinal mucosal injury than ischemia.[16] Anoxic reperfusion of ischemic tissues results in little damage.[17, 18] The formation of toxic reactive oxygen metabolites (ROMs) during reperfusion appears to be central to I-R injury. Stepwise reduction of molecular oxygen (O_2) generates different species of ROMs, including the superoxide anion radical (O_2^-), hydrogen peroxide (H_2O_2), and the hydroxyl radical (•OH), the most potent known oxidizing agent.[19] These ROMs damage membrane lipids, nucleic acids, enzymes, and receptors, resulting in impaired cellular function and eventual cell death.[20] Increases in microvascular permeability induced by I-R can be attenuated by ROM scavengers, including superoxide dismutase (SOD), catalase (an enzyme that catalyzes H_2O_2 disproportionately to H_2O and O_2), and nonenzymatic scavengers of •OH, including dimethyl sulfoxide, dimethyl thiourea, and mannitol.[19]

Xanthine oxidase (XO) is the rate-limiting enzyme in nucleic acid degradation, through which all purines are channeled for terminal oxidation. XO can generate O_2^- and H_2O_2 during the oxidation of hypoxanthine or xanthine. In healthy, nonischemic cells, XO exists predominantly as the nicotinamide-adenine dinucleotide (NAD)–dependent xanthine dehydrogenase (XD), which does not use O_2 as an electron acceptor and thus does not produce O_2^- or H_2O_2. During tissue ischemia, XD is converted to XO.[21] In comparison with other tissues, the intestinal mucosa has a tremendous capacity to oxidize hypoxanthine via XO. In humans, liver and intestine have the highest XO activity of any tissue.[22] The XO inhibitors allopurinol, oxypurinol, and pterin aldehyde all attenuate I-R–induced microvascular permeability in the gut.[19]

PMNs are a potential source of ROMs. NADPH oxidase in PMNs reduces O_2 to O_2^-. In addition, PMN-derived myeloperoxidase catalyzes the formation of hypochlorous acid (HOCl) from chloride ions and H_2O_2. HOCl is approximately 100 times as reactive as H_2O_2 as an oxidizing agent. It also reacts with primary amines to form *N*-chloro derivatives, potent oxidizing agents that are probably mediators of cellular injury.[19]

The potential role of PMNs in tissue I-R injury has been studied extensively. PMNs exist in high concentrations in intestinal mucosal tissue (10^6 PMNs per gram of tissue).[22] This population of cells is capable of producing enough O_2^- and cytotoxic enzymes (e.g., elastase, collagenase) to injure or destroy parenchymal and endothelial cells. Ischemia and, to a greater degree, reperfusion of intestine lead to a large influx of PMNs. On the basis of pretreatment with various compounds, it appears that ROMs play a role in PMN recruitment.[23, 24] Hernandez and colleagues[25] demonstrated that PMNs are the primary mediators of I-R–induced intestinal microvascular permeability. They further identified PMN adhesion to endothelium via the PMN CD11/CD18 membrane receptor as an essential component of I-R injury. Using intravital microscopy, Granger and colleagues[26] observed that I-R greatly exacerbates PMN endothelial adhesion compared with ischemia alone and demonstrated that XO-derived ROMs initiate the adherence of PMNs to endothelium.

Gut Ischemia-Reperfusion Injury Primes the Inflammatory Response

Collectively, the foregoing studies suggest that mesenteric I-R results in the generation of ROMs that attract PMNs to the intestinal microvasculature and promote their adherence to the endothelium. We have studied this phenomenon as a potential inciting event for distant organ injury.[27] In our rodent model of gut I-R, we found that 45 minutes of superior mesenteric artery (SMA) occlusion resulted in reversible liver and lung injury (as measured by microvascular albumin permeability).[28] This effect was not seen in PMN-depleted rodents, implicating PMNs in the transient injury. Our previous work had shown that depletion of XO activity by a tungsten diet decreased lung PMN accumulation after hemorrhagic shock.[29] Therefore, we investigated the role of XO in our I-R model and found that XO inactivation, like PMN depletion, abrogated the effects of I-R on distant organs.[30] In attempting to sequence the events after gut I-R, we identified XO activation as a proximal event, whose blockade attenuated accumulation of PMNs in gut, priming of circulating PMNs, and ultimately lung injury.[31]

Thus, our working hypothesis became that gut I-R initially primes the systemic inflammatory cascade and, if followed by an activating stimulus during the vulnerable primed period, results in distant organ injury. To test this hypothesis, we employed a sequential insult model: gut I-R followed by low-dose lipopolysaccharide (LPS).[32] We found that PMNs were sequestered in the lung after LPS administration, either with or without previous I-R insult. Lung injury was not seen after I-R or LPS alone but was caused by the sequential insults. Finally, there was 39% mortality in the sequential insult group, compared with 4% mortality in all other study groups. In summary, a relatively brief period of gut I-R appeared to prime the inflammatory response so that low-dose LPS exposure activated the system, resulting in distant organ injury.

Our hypothesis then became that gut I-R provokes distal organ injury via a mechanism involving priming of circulating PMNs in the reperfused splanchnic bed. PMN priming was measured as O_2^- generation and elastase release stimulated by low-dose formyl-methionylleucylphenylalanine (fMLP, 10^{-6} M) and confirmed by up-regulation of the adhesion molecule CD11b/CD18. In our I-R model, we had noted that circulating PMNs become primed at 2 hours of reperfusion.[33] To determine whether priming occurred in the splanchnic circulation, we measured priming of PMNs drawn from the splanchnic inflow (aorta) as well as the splanchnic outflow (portal vein) after 90 minutes of reperfusion. We found primed PMNs in the portal vein but not the aorta.[34]

Our next series of studies focused on the mechanism of PMN priming in the splanchnic circulation. We were interested in whether LPS was involved in PMN priming in our rodent I-R model. We measured LPS levels in the plasma of rodents after laparotomy alone and in those subjected to gut I-R, and found no difference. In addition, elimination of LPS by E5 monoclonal antibody had no effect on PMN priming after I-R.[35] We thus began our search for gut-derived inflammatory mediators capable of PMN priming. Although numerous inflammatory mediators have been implicated in SIRS and MOF, our investigations have identified two particular compounds as relevant gut-derived mediators of PMN priming: platelet-activating factor (PAF) and interleukin-6 (IL-6).

Gut-Derived Mediators

PAF is a biologically active phospholipid that is synthesized de novo continuously but may be generated to a greater degree via remodeling of membrane-bound lipids. Phospholipases catalyze the splitting of membrane phospholipids. Phospholipase A_2 (PLA_2) is designated as such because it cleaves the fatty acid (*A*cyl) group from the middle *(sn-2)* carbon of the phospholipid's glycerol backbone.[36] If the *sn*-2 acyl group is arachidonate, eicosanoid synthesis is initiated. When the remaining phospholipid has an *O*-alkyl ether in the *sn*-1 position and a phosphocholine moiety in the *sn*-3 position, lyso-PAF is formed, and PAF synthesis is subsequently initiated by a calcium-dependent acetyltransferase. PLA_2 can be activated by ROMs;[37] in addition, ROMs inhibit PAF acetylhydrolase, the enzyme that catabolizes PAF.[38] Given the high concentration of PLA_2 in intestinal mucosa, PLA_2 activation and subsequent PAF formation are a likely consequence of gut I-R.[36, 39]

PAF has many known proinflammatory effects, including PMN priming and PMN adherence to endothelium.[40–45] I-R–induced PMN adherence to endothelium can be diminished by PAF receptor antagonists.[46, 47] Few clinical studies have actually documented increases in PAF concentrations after injury, in part because of the inherent logistic difficulties in its detection and quantitation. Nevertheless, there is compelling evidence implicating PAF in postinjury hyperinflammation.[48–50] Furthermore, our finding that PAF was responsible for PMN priming in patients after both thermal and mechanical trauma[51] prompted a series of laboratory investigations. Activation of gut PLA_2 was temporally correlated with PMN priming in our rodent gut I-R model; inhibition of PLA_2 was protective against distant organ injury.[52] We subsequently confirmed PAF production in the distal small bowel after gut I-R, and a PAF receptor antagonist inhibited PMN priming in this setting.[53] Clinically, we confirmed that early postinjury PMN priming for O_2^- release occurs via a PAF mechanism.[54, 55] We also found a correlation between reduced levels of circulating PAF acetylhydrolase and the development of MOF in severely injured patients.[56]

IL-6 is considered an integral mediator of the physiologic acute-phase response to injury;[57] however, excessive and prolonged elevations of circulating IL-6 concentrations in patients after trauma, burns, and elective surgery are associated with increased morbidity and mortality.[58] An intestinal source of IL-6 after surgery and trauma has been suggested. Baigrie and colleagues[59] found significantly higher elevations of IL-6 in inferior mesenteric veins than systemic veins during and after aortic cross-clamping in patients undergoing elective aortic surgery. Similarly, Wortel and colleagues[60] detected IL-6 in higher concentrations in portal than in peripheral venous blood in patients after pancreatic and hepatic resections.

Deitch and colleagues[61] found higher IL-6 concentrations in portal than in cardiac blood after hemorrhagic shock in rats. Thus, IL-6 appears to be generated in the gut in response to systemic insults. In fact, Meyer and colleagues[62] have demonstrated IL-6 production in intestinal mucosa in vivo.

IL-6 is capable of promoting inflammation. IL-6 directly increases endothelial permeability,[63] and accumulating evidence suggests that IL-6 promotes inflammation via reprogramming of the functional repertoire of the mature PMN. We studied the effects of IL-6 on PMN cytotoxic functions in vitro and found that although IL-6 by itself does not prime PMNs for O_2^- release, it can sensitize PMNs to the priming effects of PAF.[64] Mullen and colleagues[65] have similarly demonstrated synergy between IL-6 and tumor necrosis factor-α (TNF-α) in PMN priming. IL-6 may also enhance PMN-mediated inflammation by modulating apoptosis. We have found that IL-6 delays PMN apoptosis, resulting in a larger population of nonapoptotic (surviving) PMNs with a greater collective capacity for O_2^- production than untreated PMNs.[66] The IL-6–mediated delay of PMN apoptosis could postpone the clearance of PMNs from a site of inflammation, prolong release of ROMs and proteolytic enzymes, and, consequently, aggravate PMN-mediated tissue injury, ultimately resulting in organ failure. Interestingly, IL-6 may exert its effects on the PMN via a PAF mechanism.[67, 68]

Although a direct causal link has not been made between IL-6 and MOF, an increasing body of evidence suggests that IL-6 is a pivotal component of the hyperinflammatory cascade driving SIRS. Simms and colleagues[69] studied patients with SIRS and found that PMNs had up-regulated functions during SIRS; this up-regulation persisted in patients who subsequently developed MOF. An anti–IL-6 antibody was effective in reducing PMN oxidative responses, implicating IL-6 as the primary PMN stimulant in the circulation. Gennari and colleagues[70] demonstrated that IL-6 neutralization in a murine burn model improved bacterial killing by PMNs; in addition, a correlation between IL-6 concentrations and survival time was observed. Other cytokines (e.g., TNF and IL-1) may also be generated in the gut;[71, 72] in fact, TNF has been implicated in acute lung injury after gut I-R.[73]

Although these data suggest a role for IL-1 and TNF, clinical studies have not confirmed their involvement. On the other hand, IL-6 has been consistently associated with adverse clinical outcomes. We have measured systemic IL-6, IL-8, and TNF concentrations in patients who sustained major trauma.[74, 75] The IL-6 and IL-8 concentrations were elevated immediately after injury, but the TNF concentrations were not different from those in control subjects. Similarly, Hoch and colleagues[76] found elevations of IL-6 and IL-8 in proportion to the severity of injury in trauma patients but detected no IL-1α or elevations of TNF-α. Meade and colleagues[77] also found elevated concentrations of IL-6 and IL-8 after injury but could not detect IL-1β or TNF-α at any time. In this study, both IL-6 and IL-8 concentrations remained elevated for prolonged periods in patients who developed acute respiratory distress syndrome (ARDS). In patients undergoing elective surgery, DiPadova and colleagues[78] found early increases in IL-6 after surgery but did not see increases in IL-1 or TNF. In an animal model of hindlimb I-R injury, Cipolle and colleagues[79] found IL-6 but not TNF after reperfusion.

Microbial Translocation in Late Multiple Organ Failure

In 1959, Fine and colleagues[80] advanced the observations of Walter B. Cannon, who proposed that endotoxin derived from intraluminal intestinal gram-negative bacteria was responsible for irreversible traumatic shock. Identification of the "sepsis state" associated with MOF resurrected great interest in the intestine as an occult repository of bacteria in the 1980s. This was reinforced by clinical reports of *Enterococcus, Staphylococcus*, and *Candida* bacteremias in patients who developed MOF without a focus of infection.[81–83] The concept of "gut origin septic states" was further supported by Border and colleagues[84] on the basis of observations that no septic focus could be found, either clinically or at autopsy, in more than 30% of patients who died with MOF with clinical sepsis. The mechanism by which gut-derived organisms provoke systemic sepsis was presumed to be *microbial translocation* (MT).

MT refers to the transepithelial passage of microbes or microbial products from the gut lumen to extraluminal sites. The process occurs via enterocyte uptake and transcellular passage as well as through microscopic defects in the epithelium.[85, 86] Under normal conditions, the GI tract contains 10^{12} total bacteria, including 10^9 potentially pathogenic gram-negative organisms, and enough endotoxin to kill the host many times over. The gut provides a critical barrier to exclude these pathogens via a redundant system with at least four primary components:[87]

- Resident microbial flora
- Mechanical properties
- An immune system
- The gut-liver axis

Alterations in any of these components may allow MT.

The resident microbial flora include anaerobic bacteria, which outnumber the aerobic gram-negative organisms by 100- to 1000-fold and occupy the space adjacent to the epithelial cells. The anaerobic presence prevents epithelial adherence of potential pathogens in what is termed "colonization resistance."[88] Thus, alteration of resident microbial flora by prolonged, broad-spectrum antibiotics is one potential means of promoting MT. The mucous layer provides an optimal environment for the growth of anaerobes adjacent to the epithelium. It also contains secretory immunoglobulin A (IgA), which binds bacterial cell wall antigens and prevents their adherence to intestinal epithelium. Absence of bile flow, because of biliary obstruction or administration of total parental nutrition (TPN), reduces secretory IgA in the mucous layer. Intestinal peristalsis prevents stasis and bacterial adherence to epithelium. The epithelial cells themselves provide a barrier by nature of their arrangement with desmosomes and tight junctions, but the mechanical integrity may be disrupted by intestinal ischemia.[89]

The intestinal cell-mediated immune system, referred to as gut-associated lymphoid tissue (GALT), is composed of intraepithelial and lamina propria lymphocytes, lymphoid follicles, Peyer's patches, and mesenteric lymph nodes. The immune elements serve to nullify the effects of MT by eliminating microbial organisms and their products, as well as controlling their exodus into the liver and systemic circulation. Immunosuppression that accompanies critical illness compromises this surveillance. The "gut-liver axis" primarily defends against endotoxin translocation, as bile salts bind endotoxin into detergent-like complexes intraluminally.[90] Hepatic dysfunction or bilary obstruction may allow increased levels of endotoxin into the circulation.

Extensive research employing a variety of rodent models has offered compelling evidence invoking translocation of bacteria or endotoxin in the pathogenesis of MOF after hemorrhagic shock.[91–94] Clinical investigation, however, has failed to establish a clear mechanistic role for gut MT in the pathogenesis of early-onset MOF. Indeed, considerable debate has centered around whether MT is a clinically relevant phenomenon. Human studies have documented increased intestinal permeability to low-molecular-weight, nonmetabolizable probes in sepsis,[95] burn injury,[96] major trauma,[97] hemorrhagic shock,[98] and endotoxin administration.[99] At least in the setting of major trauma and hemorrhagic shock, however, there was no demonstrable relationship to septic complications.[97] The clinical significance of MT in burned patients was further challenged by Munster and colleagues,[100] as administering polymyxin B to reduce endotoxemia did not improve sepsis scores or mortality. We performed a prospective clinical trial attempting to verify MT in patients who sustained major trauma, 30% of whom developed MOF.[74] We were unable to detect pathogenic bacteria in either portal or systemic circulation within the first 5 days after injury. In addition, we found no elevations of TNF to corroborate endotoxemia. Similar findings were reported by Peitzman and colleagues,[101] who found no evidence of MT in severely injured patients with a mortality of 16% and a major complication rate of 40%.

Selective gut decontamination (SGD) was developed on the premise that elimination of potentially pathogenic organisms from the GI tract would minimize their translocation, preventing morbidity and mortality. SGD targets aerobic gram-negative, some enteric gram-positive, and fungal organisms. Despite its theoretical benefits, SGD has not proved beneficial in reducing MOF or mortality.[102-104] Furthermore, in exchange for modest and inconsistent reductions in nosocomial pneumonia rates, it has been associated with overgrowth of resistant organisms and uniformly increased costs.[105]

In general, although there is a valid argument that MT may be underestimated, we do not believe that it is a critical event in the pathogenesis of early postinjury MOF. On the other hand, despite a paucity of clinical data, we strongly suspect that MT is a participant in late-onset MOF. Recognition of the gut as an active participant in both early and late MOF, irrespective of the specific mechanism, has led to interventions targeted specifically at the gut.

PREVENTION OF GUT-MEDIATED MULTIPLE ORGAN FAILURE

Gut-Oriented Resuscitation

The splanchnic circulation is particularly vulnerable to hypoperfusion. Several investigators have demonstrated that in low-flow states such as hemorrhagic shock, perfusion of the splanchnic bed decreases dramatically and out of proportion to the overall decrease in cardiac output.[106-108] Furthermore, the splanchnic circulation is the last to be restored after resuscitation, prompting Dantzker[109] to refer to the GI tract as the "canary of the body." The mechanism of disproportionate splanchnic vasoconstriction is probably multifactorial. Autonomic (neurally mediated α-adrenergic stimulation of postcapillary venous beds), humoral (vasopressin and angiotensin II), and local factors (prostaglandins $PGF_{2\alpha}$, PGB_2, and PGD_2, leukotrienes C_4 and D_4, thromboxane, and nitric oxide inhibition) appear to be involved.[110] In addition, motor activity and luminal distention can cause hypoperfusion of intestinal segments. The relative contribution of each factor is unclear. Although there is increased sympathetic nervous system activity in low-flow states, disproportionate splanchnic vasoconstriction is not ameliorated by α-adrenergic blockade[107] or mesenteric arterial denervation.[106] In contrast, the vasoconstriction can be abrogated by pharmacologic or surgical ablation of the renin-angiotensin axis, suggesting a primary role of the axis in mediating the effect.[111]

Prompt, aggressive resuscitation should be instituted to ensure adequate perfusion of the splanchnic circulation. Shoemaker and colleagues[112, 113] have shown that increasing oxygen delivery to supranormal levels (>600 mL/min/m²) improves the outcome of severely injured and critically ill patients. In contrast, Ivatury and colleagues[114] reported that resuscitation to supranormal levels of oxygen delivery was not as consistent in improving survival, compared with normalization of gastric intramucosal pH (pH_i) as an endpoint. In fact, there is increasing evidence that pH_i measurements have high specificity for predicting the survival of patients in the SICU.[115] Maynard and colleagues[116] found pH_i to be an earlier and more reliable predictor of outcome than cardiac index, oxygen delivery, or oxygen consumption. Low-dose dopexamine may prove a useful adjunct, as it augments splanchnic perfusion in patients with SIRS.[117] Dobutamine has also been used to improve gastric mucosal perfusion in patients treated with epinephrine for refractory shock.[118]

Nutrition as Therapy for the Gut

The gut's potential contribution to SIRS and ultimately MOF has underscored the importance of restoring the health of the gut presumptively. Thus, nutritional support via the gut, formerly a relatively low priority in the SICU, has become an early goal in SICU care. Nearly two decades ago, we began to explore the benefit of early nutritional support in injured patients. Stimulated by the 1979 report by Page and colleagues,[119] which demonstrated success with needle catheter jejunostomy (NCJ) for immediate postoperative nutritional support after elective gastrointestinal surgery, we first studied the feasibility of early NCJ feeding in patients who had sustained major abdominal trauma.[120] We found that, compared with intragastric or intraduodenal feeding, intrajejunal administration via an NCJ is a reliable way to deliver a set amount of nutrients.

To study the benefit of early nutritional support in preventing postinjury MOF, we first had to identify the patients at high risk for MOF. Our initial studies indicated that standard nutritional indices developed for elective surgical patients were not suited for this task.[121] Consequently, we devised the Abdominal Trauma Index (ATI).[122] Using the ATI to identify a homogeneous group of high-risk patients and recognizing our success with early NCJ feedings, we conducted our first prospective, randomized trial to investigate the potential benefits of early postinjury nutritional support.[123] Control patients received conventional 5% dextrose crystalloids (~100 g/day) intravenously during the first 5 postoperative days, and total parenteral nutrition (TPN) was started if they were not tolerating a regular diet at that time. The group with total enteral nutrition (TEN) had an NCJ placed just before abdominal closure, and infusion of an elemental diet was begun within 12 hours of the operation. In the enterally fed group, total lymphocyte counts were higher on day 7 and cumulative nitrogen balance was better on days 4 and 7. Most important, significantly fewer TEN patients experienced major septic complications.

Our observations that patients with major torso trauma benefit from early aggressive nutritional support are similar to those of Alexander and associates[124] in a prospective, randomized trial with major burn patients. Children with a burn size of 40% or more of the body surface area were randomized to a high-protein diet (25% of total calories as protein) or a low-protein diet (15% of total calories as protein). The total caloric load was similar in both groups, and the diets were delivered primarily by the enteral route. Patients randomized to the high-protein diet had significantly fewer bacteremic days, fewer days receiving antibiotics, and a lower mortality rate.

Enteral Versus Parenteral Nutrition

By the end of the 1980s, enteral feeding was believed to be more cost effective than TPN, but few studies were designed to test the physiologic benefits. Thus, we conducted a prospective trial[125] of patients requiring emergent laparotomy who had an ATI greater than 15 but less than 40 to receive either TEN or TPN; TPN was advanced in an isocaloric, isonitrogenous manner. Despite a slight advantage in protein-calorie intake via the parenteral route on day 5, there were no significant differences in nitrogen balance. There was, however, a significant difference in the incidence of major infections: 3% in the TEN group versus 20% in the TPN group. In addition, multiple logistic regression analysis of potential risk factors for infections identified TPN as the only independent predictor.

Kudsk and coworkers[126] confirmed these observations in an expanded prospective study. Patients with an ATI of 15 or higher were randomized to receive TEN or a similarly formulated TPN, initiated within 24 hours of injury. In contrast to the protocol in our study, TPN was advanced as tolerated (therefore more rapidly than TEN). As in our trial, patients receiving TEN experienced significantly fewer major septic complications than patients receiving TPN (14% versus 38%). Also, in this study, TPN patients experienced a significantly higher incidence of catheter-related sepsis (14% versus 2%).

Thus, two prospective, randomized clinical trials from two different investigative groups have shown the same phenomenon. Moreover, we completed a meta-analysis[127] of combined data from eight prospective, randomized clinical trials that were conducted to assess the nutritional equivalence of TEN and TPN in high-risk trauma or postoperative patients. The eight studies collectively enrolled 230 patients; 118 were randomized to TEN and 112 to TPN. Phase I meta-analysis demonstrated that (1) the data were homogenous across the study sites, (2) the combined treatment groups were comparable, and (3) significantly fewer TEN patients experienced septic complications (17% versus 44%). Phase II meta-analysis was conducted to evaluate more rigorously differences in septic complications (i.e., an intent-to-treat analysis). One or more infections developed in twice as many TPN as TEN patients (35% versus 16%).

Enteral nutrition may also prove beneficial in normalizing the immune response in critically ill patients. Although the exact mechanism of late stress-induced immunosuppression remains unclear, the current hypothesis is dysfunctional regulation of the immune response (Fig. 151-2). A traumatic insult precipitates early SIRS, but there is believed to be a concurrent effort to control systemic inflammation via a "compensatory anti-inflammatory response syndrome" (CARS).[128] For example, macrophage production of PGE_2 is increased while human leukocyte antigen HLA-DR is decreased; a shift in T-helper (Th) cells from Th1 to Th2 occurs, resulting in production of anti-inflammatory cytokines, such as IL-4 and IL-10; and PMN production of O_2^- is suppressed while elastase is augmented. This delayed immunosuppression has correlated well with the risk of secondary infections. Although various strategies for modulating this dysfunctional inflammatory response have been proposed and tested, a promising approach is the delivery via the gut of specific nutrients that exert pharmacologic immune-enhancing effects.

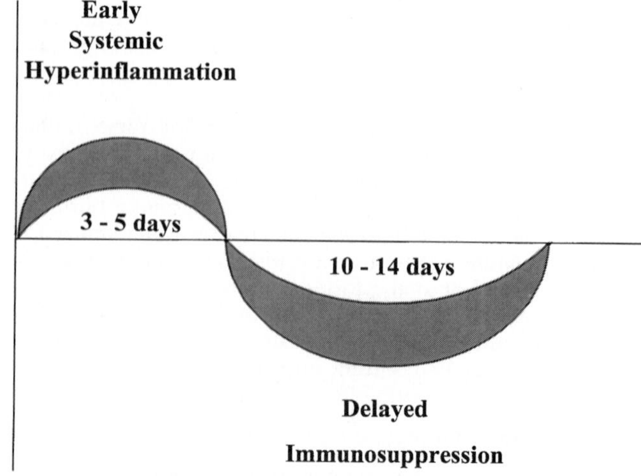

Figure 151-2. Early postinjury hyperinflammation is associated with delayed immunosuppression.

Immune-Enhancing Diets

Glutamine is the preferred fuel of the enterocyte and is thought to stimulate lymphocyte and monocyte functions.[129] It is also a substrate for the endogenous antioxidant glutathione. Arginine promotes collagen synthesis, which is required in wound healing, and increases the number of total lymphocytes as well as the proportion of Th cells. In addition, arginine has been shown to enhance delayed cutaneous hypersensitivity and lymphocyte blastogenesis.[130] Diets with low ω-6 and high ω-3 polyunsaturated fatty acid contents alter the fatty acid composition of membrane phospholipids, which in turn decrease the elaboration of arachidonate metabolites, most notably the 2-series prostaglandins (e.g., PGE_2).[131] Finally, exogenous nucleotides may be necessary in stressed states to maintain rapid cell proliferation and responsiveness.[132]

We performed a multicenter trial to determine whether additional benefits of TEN could be achieved by administering an immune-enhancing diet (IED).[133] Severely injured patients with an ATI of 18 to 40 or an Injury Severity Score (ISS) of 16 to 45 were randomized to receive an IED or control enteral diet. Both formulas were administered via NCJ within 24 hours of injury and advanced according to protocol. Both groups had similar intake volume and caloric intake on day 3 and day 7; however, because of the supplemental amino acids, the IED group received more nitrogen. The IED and control groups, however, had similar baseline and day 7 levels of serum protein, albumin, and transferrin. Thus, we believe that the extra nitrogen administered to the study group was being used for purposes other than protein synthesis. After 7 days of feeding, patients receiving the IED had significantly greater increases in T, B, and total lymphocyte counts and Th cells. Furthermore, the mean duration of ventilated days (1.9 versus 5.3), ICU days (5.3 versus 8.6), and hospital days (14.6 versus 17.2) was consistently shorter in the IED group. The key clinical finding was that the study group had significantly fewer intra-abdominal abscesses (0% versus 11%) and significantly less MOF (0% versus 11%).

There are at least seven other prospective, randomized trials in which IEDs have shown promise.[134-140] These trials have variously demonstrated improvements in immunologic functional parameters,[135, 136, 138] infectious complications,[136, 137, 139, 140] and hospital length of stay.[134, 137, 139] Collectively, these data suggest that the use of an IED for stressed surgical patients is associated with improved clinical outcome.

Pharmacologic Therapy

The best therapy for MOF is prevention. Early aggressive resuscitation, with the goal of restoring splanchnic perfusion, can minimize gut I-R injury. Nutritional support has become a pivotal issue in the care of critically ill patients, but the specific mechanisms by which early enteric feedings benefit metabolically stressed surgical patients are not clear. Prevention of acute protein malnutrition, maintenance of normal gut function, avoidance of TPN, and immunomodulation by specific nutrients may all play a role. When enteral feeding is not feasible, TPN supplementation with intravenous glutamine may enhance immunologic function as well as nitrogen balance.[141-143] In addition, growth hormone administration may serve to counter the catabolic effects of severe stress.[144, 145] Clearly, additional investigation is needed to define the pathologic as well as physiologic role of the GI tract in critical illness.

References

1. Tilney NL, Bailey GL, Morgan AP: Sequential system failure after rupture of abdominal aortic aneurysms: An unsolved problem in postoperative care. Ann Surg 1973; 178:117.
2. Baue AE: Multiple, progressive, or sequential systems failure: A syndrome of the 1970s. Arch Surg 1975; 110:779.
3. Eiseman B, Beart R, Norton L: Multiple organ failure. Surg Gynecol Obstet 1977; 144:323.
4. Knaus WA, Wagner DP: Multiple systems organ failure: Epidemiology and prognosis. Crit Care Clin North Am 1989; 5:221.
5. Sauaia A, Moore FA, Moore EE, et al: Epidemiology of trauma deaths: A reassessment. J Trauma 1995; 38:185.
6. Polk HC Jr, Shields CL: Remote organ failure: A valid sign of occult intra-abdominal infection. Surgery 1977; 81:310.
7. Fry DE, Pearlstein L, Fulton RL, et al: Multiple system organ failure: The role of uncontrolled infection. Arch Surg 1980; 115:136.
8. Norton LW: Does drainage of intraabdominal pus reverse multiple organ failure? Am J Surg 1985; 149:347.
9. Faist E, Baue AE, Dittmer H, et al: Multiple organ failure in polytrauma patients. J Trauma 1983; 23:775.
10. Goris RJA, Boekhorst TPAT, Nuytinck JKS, et al: Multiple-organ failure: Generalized autodestructive inflammation? Arch Surg 1985; 120:1109.
11. American College of Chest Physicians/Society of Critical Care Medicine Consensus Conference: Definitions for sepsis and organ failure and guidelines for the use of innovative therapies in sepsis. Crit Care Med 1992; 20:864.
12. Baue AE: The horror autotoxicus and multiple organ failure. Arch Surg 1992; 127:1451.
13. Botha AJ, Moore FA, Moore EE, et al: Postinjury neutrophil priming and activation states: Therapeutic challenges. Shock 1995; 3:157.
14. Meakins JL, Marshall JC: The gastrointestinal tract: The 'motor' of MOF. Arch Surg 1986; 121:197.
15. Moore FA, Sauaia A, Moore EE, et al: Postinjury multiple organ failure: A bimodal phenomenon. J Trauma 1996; 40:501.
16. Parks DA, Granger DN: Contributions of ischemia and reperfusion to mucosal lesion formation. Am J Physiol 1986; 250:G749.
17. Korthuis RJ, Smith JK, Carden DL: Hypoxic reperfusion attenuates postischemic microvascular injury. Am J Physiol 1989; 256:H315.
18. Perry MA, Wadhwa SS: Gradual reintroduction of oxygen reduces reperfusion injury in cat stomach. Am J Physiol 1988; 254:G366.
19. Zimmerman BJ, Granger DN: Reperfusion injury. Surg Clin North Am 1992; 72:65.
20. Southorn PA, Powis G: Free radicals in medicine. I. Chemical nature and biologic reactions. Mayo Clin Proc 1988; 63:381.
21. Batelli MG: Enzymic conversion of rat liver xanthine oxidase from dehydrogenase (D form) to oxidase (O form). FEBS Lett 1980; 113:47.
22. Granger DN: Role of xanthine oxidase and granulocytes in ischemia-reperfusion injury. Am J Physiol 1988; 255:H1269.
23. Grisham MB, Hernandez LA, Granger DN: Xanthine oxidase and neutrophil infiltration in intestinal ischemia. Am J Physiol 1986; 251:G567.
24. Suzuki M, Inauen W, Kvietys PR, et al: Superoxide mediates reperfusion-induced leukocyte–endothelial cell interactions. Am J Physiol 1989; 257:H1740.
25. Hernandez LA, Grisham MB, Twohig B, et al: Role of neutrophils in ischemia-reperfusion–induced microvascular injury. Am J Physiol 1987; 253:H699.
26. Granger DN, Benoit JN, Suzuki M, et al: Leukocyte adherence to venular endothelium during ischemia-reperfusion. Am J Physiol 1989; 257:G683.
27. Moore EE, Moore FA, Franciose RJ, et al: Postischemic gut serves as a priming bed for circulating neutrophils that provoke multiple organ failure. J Trauma 1994; 37:881.
28. Poggetti RS, Moore FA, Moore EE, et al: Liver injury is a reversible neutrophil-mediated event following gut ischemia. Arch Surg 1992; 127:175.
29. Anderson BO, Moore EE, Moore FA, et al: Hypovolemic shock promotes neutrophil sequestration in lungs by a xanthine oxidase–related mechanism. J Appl Physiol 1991; 71:1862.
30. Poggetti RS, Moore FA, Moore EE, et al: Simultaneous liver and lung injury following gut ischemia is mediated by xanthine oxidase. J Trauma 1992; 32:723.
31. Koike K, Moore FA, Moore EE, et al: Gut ischemia mediates lung injury by a xanthine oxidase–dependent neutrophil mechanism. J Surg Res 1993; 54:469.
32. Koike K, Moore FA, Moore EE, et al: Endotoxin after gut ischemia/reperfusion causes irreversible lung injury. J Surg Res 1992; 52:656.
33. Koike K, Moore EE, Moore FA, et al: Phospholipase A_2 inhibition decouples lung injury from gut ischemia-reperfusion. Surgery 1992; 112:173.
34. Franciose RJ, Moore EE, Moore FA, et al: Postischemic gut is the priming bed for PMNs. Surg Forum 1993; 44:142.
35. Koike K, Moore EE, Moore FA, et al: Gut ischemia/reperfusion produces lung injury independent of endotoxin. Crit Care Med 1994; 22:1438.
36. Anderson BO, Moore EE, Banerjee A: Phospholipase A_2 regulates critical inflammatory mediators of multiple organ failure. J Surg Res 1994; 56:199.
37. Chakraborti S, Gurtner GH, Michael JR: Oxidant-mediated activation of phospholipase A_2 in pulmonary endothelium. Am J Physiol 1989; 257:L430.
38. Ambrosio G, Oriente A, Napoli C, et al: Oxygen radicals inhibit human plasma acetylhydrolase, the enzyme that catabolizes platelet-activating factor. J Clin Invest 1994; 93:2408.
39. Otamiri T, Lindahl M, Tagesson C: Phospholipase A_2 inhibition prevents mucosal damage associated with small intestinal ischemia in rats. Gut 1988; 29:489.
40. Amould T, Michiels C, Remacle J: Increased PMN adherence on endothelial cells after hypoxia: Involvement of PAF, CD18/CD11b, and ICAM-1. Am J Physiol 1993; 264:C1102.
41. Gay JC, Beckman JK, Zaboy KA, et al: Modulation of neutrophil oxidative responses to soluble stimuli by platelet-activating factor. Blood 1986; 67:931.
42. Ingraham LM, Coates TD, Allen JM, et al: Metabolic, membrane, and functional responses of human polymorphonuclear leukocytes to platelet-activating factor. Blood 1982; 59:1259.
43. Milhoan KA, Lane TA, Bloor CM: Hypoxia induces endothelial cells to increase their adherence for neutrophils: Role of PAF. Am J Physiol 1992; 263:H956.
44. Read RA, Moore EE, Moore FA, et al: Platelet-activating factor–induced polymorphonuclear neutrophil priming independent of CD11B adhesion. Surgery 1993; 114:308.
45. Vercellotti GM, Yin HQ, Gustafson KS, et al: Platelet-activating factor primes neutrophil responses to agonists: Role in promoting neutrophil-mediated endothelial damage. Blood 1988; 71:1100.
46. Rainger GE, Fisher A, Shearman C, et al: Adhesion of flowing neutrophils to cultured endothelial cells after hypoxia and reoxygenation in vitro. Am J Physiol 1995; 269:H1398.
47. Yoshida N, Granger DN, Anderson DC, et al: Anoxia/reoxygenation-induced neutrophil adherence to cultured endothelial cells. Am J Physiol 1992; 262:H1891.
48. Mozes T, Braquet P, Filep J: Platelet-activating factor: An endogenous mediator of mesenteric ischemia-reperfusion–induced shock. Am J Physiol 1989; 257:R872.
49. Stahl GL, Bitterman H, Lefer AM: Protective effects of a specific platelet activating factor antagonist, WEB 1086, in traumatic shock. Thromb Res 1989; 53:327.
50. Stahl GL, Craft DV, Lento PH, et al: Detection of platelet-activating factor during traumatic shock. Circ Shock 1988; 26:237.
51. Pitman JM III, Thurman GW, Anderson BO, et al: Platelet-activating factor may mediate neutrophil priming following clinical burn or blunt trauma. Surg Forum 1989; 40:108.
52. Koike K, Moore EE, Moore FA, et al: Gut phospholipase A_2 mediates neutrophil priming and lung injury after mesenteric ischemia-reperfusion. Am J Physiol 1995; 268:G397.

53. Kim FJ, Moore EE, Moore FA, et al: Reperfused gut elaborates PAF that chemoattracts and primes neutrophils. J Surg Res 1995; 58:636.
54. Botha AJ, Moore FA, Moore EE, et al: Early neutrophil priming for superoxide release after injury is via a platelet activating factor mechanism. Br J Surg 1995; 82:686.
55. Botha AJ, Moore FA, Moore EE, et al: Sequential systemic platelet-activating factor and interleukin-8 primes neutrophils in patients with trauma at risk of multiple organ failure. Br J Surg 1996; 83:1407.
56. Partrick DA, Moore EE, Moore FA, et al: Reduced PAF-acetylhydrolase activity is associated with postinjury multiple organ failure. Shock 1997; 7:170.
57. Castell JV, Gomez-Lechon NJ, David M, et al: Interleukin-6 is the major regulator of acute phase protein synthesis in adult human hepatocytes. FEBS Lett 1989; 242:237.
58. Biffl WL, Moore EE, Moore FA, et al: Interleukin-6 in the injured patient: Marker of injury or mediator of inflammation? Ann Surg 1996; 224:647.
59. Baigrie RJ, Lamont PM, Whiting S, et al: Portal endotoxin and cytokine responses during abdominal aortic surgery. Am J Surg 1993; 166:248.
60. Wortel CH, van Deventer SJH, Aarden LA, et al: Interleukin-6 mediates host defense responses induced by abdominal surgery. Surgery 1993; 114:564.
61. Deitch EA, Xu D, Franko L, et al: Evidence favoring the role of the gut as a cytokine-generating organ in rats subjected to hemorrhagic shock. Shock 1994; 1:141.
62. Meyer TA, Wang J, Tiao GM, et al: Sepsis and endotoxemia stimulate intestinal interleukin-6 production. Surgery 1995; 118:336.
63. Maruo N, Morita I, Shirao M, et al: IL-6 increases endothelial permeability in vitro. Endocrinology 1992; 131:710.
64. Biffl WL, Moore EE, Moore FA, et al: Interleukin-6 potentiates neutrophil priming with platelet-activating factor. Arch Surg 1994; 129:1131.
65. Mullen PG, Windsor ACJ, Walsh CJ, et al: Tumor necrosis factor-α and interleukin-6 selectively regulate neutrophil function in vitro. J Surg Res 1995; 58:124.
66. Biffl WL, Moore EE, Moore FA, et al: Interleukin-6 delays neutrophil apoptosis. Arch Surg 1996; 113:24.
67. Biffl WL, Moore EE, Moore FA, et al: Interleukin-6 delays neutrophil apoptosis via a mechanism involving platelet-activating factor. J Trauma 1996; 40:575.
68. Biffl WL, Moore EE, Moore FA, et al: Interleukin-6 stimulates neutrophil production of platelet-activating factor. J Leukoc Biol 1996; 59:569.
69. Simms HH, D'Amico R: Polymorphonuclear leukocyte dysregulation during the systemic inflammatory response syndrome. Blood 1994; 83:1398.
70. Gennari R, Alexander JW, Pyles T, et al: Effects of antimurine interleukin-6 on bacterial translocation during gut-derived sepsis. Arch Surg 1994; 129:1191.
71. Welborn MB, Douglas WG, Abouhamze Z, et al: Visceral ischemia-reperfusion injury promotes tumor necrosis factor and interleukin-1 dependent organ injury in the mouse. Shock 1996; 6:171.
72. Altavilla D, Squadrito F, Canale P, et al: Tumor necrosis factor induces E-selectin production in splanchnic artery occlusion shock. Am J Physiol 1995; 268:H1412.
73. Caty MG, Guice KS, Oldham KT, et al: Evidence for tumor necrosis factor–induced pulmonary microvascular injury after intestinal ischemia-reperfusion injury. Ann Surg 1990; 212:694.
74. Moore FA, Moore EE, Poggetti R, et al: Gut bacterial translocation via the portal vein: A clinical perspective with major torso trauma. J Trauma 1991; 31:629.
75. Partrick DA, Moore FA, Moore EE, et al: The inflammatory profile of interleukin-6, interleukin-8, and soluble intercellular adhesion molecule-1 in postinjury multiple organ failure. Am J Surg 1996; 172:425.
76. Hoch RC, Rodriguez R, Manning T, et al: Effects of accidental trauma on cytokine and endotoxin production. Crit Care Med 1993; 21:839.
77. Meade P, Shoemaker WC, Donnelly TJ, et al: Temporal patterns of hemodynamics, oxygen transport, cytokine activity, and complement activity in the development of adult respiratory distress syndrome after severe injury. J Trauma 1994; 36:651.
78. DiPadova F, Pozzi C, Tondre MJ, et al: Selective and early increase of IL-1 inhibitors, IL-6 and cortisol after elective surgery. Clin Exp Immunol 1991; 85:137.
79. Cipolle MD, Pasquale MD, Shearer J, et al: Blunt injury augments interleukin-6 but not tumor necrosis factor in isolated, perfused rat hindlimbs. J Trauma 1994; 37:91.
80. Fine J, Frank ED, Rutenberg SH, et al: The bacterial factor in traumatic shock. N Engl J Med 1959; 260:217.
81. Garrison RN, Fry DE, Berberich S, et al: Enterococcal bacteremia: Clinical implications and determinants of death. Ann Surg 1982; 196:43.
82. Forse RA, Dixon C, Bernard K, et al: *Staphylococcus epidermidis*: An important pathogen. Surgery 1979; 86:507.
83. Solomkin JS, Flohr AB, Quie PG, et al: The role of *Candida* in intraperitoneal infections. Surgery 1980; 88:524.
84. Border JR, Hassett J, LaDuca J, et al: The gut origin septic states in blunt multiple trauma (ISS = 40) in the ICU. Ann Surg 1987; 206:427.
85. Alexander JW, Boyce ST, Babcock GF, et al: The process of microbial translocation. Ann Surg 1990; 212:496.
86. Deitch EA, Morrison J, Berg R, et al: Effect of hemorrhagic shock on bacterial translocation, intestinal morphology, and intestinal permeability in conventional and antibiotic-decontaminated rats. Crit Care Med 1990; 18:529.
87. Swank GM, Deitch EA: Role of the gut in multiple organ failure: Bacterial translocation and permeability changes. World J Surg 1996; 20:411.
88. Van der Waaij D, Berghuis-de Vries JM, Lekkerkerk-van der Wees JEC: Colonization of the digestive tract in conventional and antibiotic treated mice. J Hyg (Camb) 1971; 69:405.
89. Mardara JC: Pathobiology of the intestinal epithelial barrier. Am J Pathol 1990; 137:1273.
90. Bertok L: Physico-chemical defense of vertebrate organisms: The role of bile acids in defense against bacterial endotoxin. Perspect Biol Med 1977; 21:70.
91. Baker JW, Deitch EA, Li M, et al: Hemorrhagic shock induces bacterial translocation from the gut. J Trauma 1988; 28:896.
92. Deitch EA, Bridges RM: Effect of stress and trauma on bacterial translocation from the gut. J Surg Res 1987; 42:536.
93. Koziol JM, Rush BF Jr, Smith SM, et al: Occurrence of bacteremia during and after hemorrhagic shock. J Trauma 1988; 28:10.
94. Sori AJ, Rush BF Jr, Lysz TW, et al: The gut as source of sepsis after hemorrhagic shock. Am J Surg 1988; 155:187.
95. Ziegler TR, Smith RJ, O'Dwyer ST, et al: Increased intestinal permeability associated with infection in burn patients. Arch Surg 1988; 123:1313.
96. Deitch EA: Intestinal permeability is increased in burn patients shortly after injury. Surgery 1990; 107:411.
97. Roumen RMH, Hendriks T, Wevers RA, et al: Intestinal permeability after severe trauma and hemorrhagic shock is increased without relation to septic complications. Arch Surg 1993; 128:453.
98. Rush BF Jr, Sori AJ, Murphy TF, et al: Endotoxemia and bacteremia during hemorrhagic shock: The link between trauma and sepsis? Ann Surg 1988; 207:549.
99. O'Dwyer ST, Mitchie HR, Ziegler TR, et al: A single dose of endotoxin increased intestinal permeability in healthy humans. Arch Surg 1988; 123:1459.
100. Munster AM, Smith-Meek M, Dickerson C, et al: Translocation: Incidental phenomenon or true pathology? Ann Surg 1993; 218:321.
101. Peitzman AB, Udekwu AO, Ochoa J, et al: Bacterial translocation in trauma patients. J Trauma 1991; 31:1083.
102. Cerra FB, Maddaus MA, Dunn DL, et al: Selective gut decontamination reduces nosocomial infections and length of stay but not mortality or organ failure in surgical intensive care unit patients. Arch Surg 1992; 127:163.
103. Goris RJA, van Bebber IPT, Mollen RMH, et al: Does selective decontamination of the gastrointestinal tract prevent multiple organ failure? Arch Surg 1991; 126:561.
104. Lingnau W, Berger J, Javorsky F, et al: Selective intestinal decontamination in multiple trauma patients: Prospective, controlled trial. J Trauma 1997; 42:687.

105. Verwaest C, Verhaegen J, Ferdinande P, et al: Randomized, controlled trial of selective digestive decontamination in 600 mechanically ventilated patients in a multidisciplinary intensive care unit. Crit Care Med 1997; 25:63.
106. Adar R, Franklin A, Spark RF, et al: Effect of dehydration and cardiac tamponade on superior mesenteric artery flow: Role of vasoactive substances. Surgery 1976; 79:534.
107. McNeill JR, Srark RD, Greenway CV: Intestinal vasoconstriction after hemorrhage: Roles of vasopressin and angiotensin. Am J Physiol 1970; 219:1342.
108. Reilly PM, MacGowan S, Miyachi M, et al: Mesenteric vasoconstriction in cardiogenic shock in pigs. Gastroenterology 1992; 102:1968.
109. Dantzker DR: The gastrointestinal tract: The canary of the body? JAMA 1993; 270:1247.
110. Patel A, Kaleya RN, Sammartano RJ: Pathophysiology of mesenteric ischemia. Surg Clin North Am 1992; 72:31.
111. Bailey RW, Bulkley GB, Hamilton SR, et al: Protection of the small intestine from nonocclusive mesenteric ischemic injury due to cardiogenic shock. Am J Surg 1987; 153:108.
112. Bishop MH, Shoemaker WC, Kram HB, et al: Prospective randomized trial of survivors' values of cardiac index, oxygen delivery, and oxygen consumption as resuscitation endpoints in severe trauma. J Trauma 1996; 38:780.
113. Shoemaker WC, Appel PL, Kram HB, et al: Prospective trial of supranormal values of survivors as therapeutic goals in high risk surgical patients. Chest 1988; 94:1176.
114. Ivatury RR, Simon RJ, Havriliak D, et al: Gastric mucosal pH and oxygen delivery and oxygen consumption indices in the assessment of adequacy of resuscitation after trauma: A prospective, randomized study. J Trauma 1995; 39:128.
115. Doglio GR, Pusajo JF, Egurrola MA, et al: Gastric mucosal pH as a prognostic index of mortality in critically ill patients. Crit Care Med 1991; 19:1037.
116. Maynard N, Bihari D, Beale R, et al: Assessment of splanchnic oxygenation by gastric tonometry in patients with acute circulatory failure. JAMA 1993; 270:1203.
117. Maynard ND, Bihari DJ, Dalton RN, et al: Increasing splanchnic blood flow in the critically ill. Chest 1995; 108:1648.
118. Levy B, Bollaert P-E, Lucchelli J-P, et al: Dobutamine improves the adequacy of gastric mucosal perfusion in epinephrine-treated septic shock. Crit Care Med 1997; 25:1649.
119. Page CP, Carlton PK, Andrassy RJ, et al: Safe, cost-effective postoperative nutrition: Refined formula diet via needle catheter jejunostomy (NCJ). Am J Surg 1979; 133:939.
120. Moore EE, Dunn EL, Jones TN: Immediate jejunostomy feeding: Its use after major abdominal trauma. Arch Surg 1981; 116:681.
121. Moore EE, Jones TN: Nutritional assessment and preliminary report on early support of the trauma patient. J Am Coll Nutr 1983; 2:45.
122. Moore EE, Dunn EL, Jones TN, et al: Penetrating abdominal trauma index. J Trauma 1982; 21:439.
123. Moore EE, Jones TN: Benefits of immediate jejunal feeding after major abdominal trauma: A prospective randomized study. J Trauma 1986; 26:874.
124. Alexander JW, Macmillan BG, Stinnett JD, et al: Beneficial effects of aggressive protein feeding in severely burned children. Ann Surg 1980; 192:505.
125. Moore FA, Moore EE, Jones TN, et al: TEN versus TPN following major abdominal trauma: Reduced septic morbidity. J Trauma 1989; 29:916.
126. Kudsk KA, Croce MA, Fabian TC, et al: Enteral versus parenteral feeding: Effects on septic morbidity following blunt and penetrating abdominal trauma. Ann Surg 1992; 215:503.
127. Moore FA, Feliciano DV, Andrassey RJ, et al: Early enteral feeding, compared with parenteral, reduces postoperative septic complications: The results of a meta-analysis. Ann Surg 1992; 216:1992.
128. Bone RC: Sir Isaac Newton, sepsis, SIRS, and CARS. Crit Care Med 1996; 24:1125.
129. Souba WW, Klinberg VS, Plumley DA, et al: The role of glutamine in maintaining a healthy gut and supporting the metabolic response to injury and infection. J Surg Res 1990; 48:383.
130. Barbul A, Lazarou SA, Efron DT, et al: Arginine enhances wound healing and lymphocyte immune responses in humans. Surgery 1990; 108:331.
131. Alexander JW, Saito H, Ogle CK, et al: The importance of lipid type in diet after burn injury. Ann Surg 1986; 204:1.
132. Van Buren CT, Kulkarni A, Fanslow WC, et al: Dietary nucleotides, a requirement for helper/inducer T lymphocytes. Transplantation 1985; 40:694.
133. Moore FA, Moore EE, Kudsk KA, et al: Clinical benefits of an immune-enhancing diet for early postinjury enteral feeding. J Trauma 1994; 37:607.
134. Bower RH, Cerra FB, Bershadsky B, et al: Early enteral administration of a formula supplemented with arginine, nucleotides, and fish oil in intensive care unit patients: Results of a multicenter, prospective, randomized clinical trial. Crit Care Med 1995; 23:436.
135. Cerra FB, Lehman S, Konstantinides N, et al: Improvement in immune function in ICU patients by enteral nutrition supplemented with arginine, RNA and menhaden oil independent of nitrogen balance. Nutrition 1991; 7:193.
136. Daly JM, Liberman MD, Goldfine J, et al: Enteral nutrition with supplemental arginine, RNA and omega-3 fatty acids in patients with operation: Immunologic, metabolic and clinical outcome. Surgery 1992; 56:112.
137. Gottschlich MM, Jenkins M, Warden GD, et al: Differential effects of three enteral dietary regimens on selected outcome variables in burn patients. JPEN J Parenter Enteral Nutr 1990; 14:225.
138. Kemen M, Senkal M, Homann H-H, et al: Early postoperative enteral nutrition with arginine-ω-3 fatty acids and ribonucleic acid–supplemented diet versus placebo in cancer patients: An immunologic evaluation of Impact. Crit Care Med 1995; 23:652.
139. Kudsk KA, Minard G, Croce MA, et al: A randomized trial of isonitrogenous enteral diets after severe trauma: An immune-enhancing diet reduces septic complications. Ann Surg 1996; 224:531.
140. Senkal M, Mumme A, Eickhoff U, et al: Early postoperative enteral immunonutrition: Clinical outcome and cost-comparison analysis in surgical patients. Crit Care Med 1997; 25:1489.
141. Burke DJ, Alverdy JC, Aoys E, et al: Glutamine-supplemented total parenteral nutrition improves gut immune function. Arch Surg 1989; 124:1396.
142. Hammarqvist F, Wernerman J, Ali R, et al: Addition of glutamine to total parenteral nutrition after elective abdominal surgery spares free glutamine in muscle, counteracts the fall in muscle protein synthesis, and improves nitrogen balance. Ann Surg 1989; 209:455.
143. O'Riordain MG, Fearon KCH, Ross JA, et al: Glutamine-supplemented total parenteral nutrition enhances T-lymphocyte response in surgical patients undergoing colorectal resection. Ann Surg 1994; 220:212.
144. Byrne TA, Morrissey TB, Gatzen C, et al: Anabolic therapy with growth hormone accelerates protein gain in surgical patients requiring nutritional rehabilitation. Ann Surg 1993; 218:400.
145. Wolf RF, Pearlstone DB, Newman E, et al: Growth hormone and insulin reverse net whole body and skeletal muscle protein catabolism in cancer patients. Ann Surg 1992; 216:280.

152

Clinical Assessment of Renal Function

Anton C. Schoolwerth, MD, MSHA • Todd W. B. Gehr, MD

Abnormalities in renal function constitute a major problem in critical care units. It is estimated that 5% to 15% of patients in intensive care units (ICUs) experience acute deterioration in renal function.[1, 2] Conversely, renal dysfunction adds substantially to the morbidity and mortality of these patients. Moreover, changes in renal function directly affect drug disposition. Thus, a means to assess renal function is essential for optimal management. The glomerular filtration rate (GFR) is the standard measure of renal function. It reflects overall renal functional capacity and, in renal failure, correlates with structural damage to the kidney. This chapter reviews selected aspects of renal physiology with an emphasis on measurement of renal function, consequences of altered function, and approaches to improving renal function. The focus is on measurement and optimization of GFR and renal blood flow (RBF).

RENAL BLOOD FLOW

Under physiologic conditions, blood flow to the kidneys is 20% of cardiac output. This is a high rate of blood flow (~1 to 1.2 L/min), a particularly remarkable value in that the kidneys make up only 0.5% of total body weight. The high blood flow rate is due, at least in part, to the unique anatomic arrangement of the renal vasculature, with the interlobar and arcuate vessels offering little resistance to flow. This, in turn, is due to the fact that the interlobular arteries originate from the arcuates in a parallel arrangement and that the afferent arterioles also arise in a parallel arrangement from the interlobular vessels. It is this parallel arrangement that accounts for the low resistance because the total resistance of n equal parallel paths, each with a resistance R, is R/n^3. Major resistance vessels in the kidney are the afferent and efferent arterioles that bound the glomerular capillary network. Although total resistance is a function of resistance across each of these vessels, it is a unique feature of the kidney that variations in the individual resistances across the afferent and efferent arterioles, respectively, may lead to alterations in glomerular capillary pressure and, hence, in GFR.

Despite a wide range of perfusion pressures, RBF and GFR are maintained relatively constant, a process described as autoregulation. The term *autoregulation* generally refers to the relative constancy of GFR over a range of perfusion pressures but also refers to the regulation of RBF. Emphasis has been placed on the preglomerular vasculature, mainly the afferent arterioles, as the major site at which renal perfusion is regulated. However, studies also suggest that the larger vessels, such as the interlobular vessels, may respond to a variety of vasoactive stimuli and participate in an autoregulatory phenomenon. A variety of hypotheses have been generated to explain the autoregulatory response of the kidney with respect to RBF. There is evidence to suggest mediation by neural, humoral, or intrarenal factors that regulate the renal circulation.[4] The list of neurohumoral factors that may potentially regulate renal hemodynamics is growing rapidly; emphasis has been placed on several known mediators of this process.

The renin-angiotensin pathway has a significant effect on renal hemodynamics. Renin, elaborated in the juxtaglomerular cells, may be released in response to a decrease in renal perfusion pressure and to altered sodium chloride delivery to the ascending limb and macula densa cells. Increased renin secretion in turn leads to augmented angiotensin II (AII) formation at the local nephron level. AII in turn affects renal vascular resistance by an effect on both the afferent and efferent arterioles, with the effect predominating on the latter vessels.

Renal eicosanoids also affect renal hemodynamics. Eicosanoids are biologically active fatty acid products of arachidonic acid and are synthesized in the kidney in response to a variety of stimuli, with local release and effect on the renal vasculature. Stimulation of the cyclooxygenase pathway and prostaglandin synthetases leads to the formation of endoperoxides (PGG_2, PGH_2), prostaglandins (PGD_2, PGE_2, $PGF_{2\alpha}$, PGI_2), and thromboxane A_2 (TXA_2). Leukotrienes are synthesized by another major pathway involving the enzyme lipoxygenase. In the kidney, the major products of arachidonic acid metabolism are PGE_2 and PGI_2 and, to a lesser extent, $PGI_{2\alpha}$. These compounds have a predominant effect to relax renal vascular smooth muscle and lead to vasodilatation, whereas TXA_2 is a vasoconstrictor prostanoid. It is believed that in disease states endogenous vasodilator prostaglandins serve a protective function to maintain renal perfusion and GFR in response to vasoconstrictor stimuli, including AII and enhanced sympathetic nervous system activity. In contrast, release is inhibited by nonsteroidal anti-inflammatory drugs.

Other vasoactive compounds that affect the renal circulation include the plasma and glandular kallikreins and kinins and endothelium-derived vasoactive factors, such as nitric oxide and endothelin.[4] Among the catecholamines, α- and β-adrenergic agonists are known to affect renal vascular tone by causing vasoconstriction and vasodilatation, respectively. In addition, dopamine in low doses leads to renal vasodilatation. Emphasis has more recently been placed on atrial natriuretic peptide and purinergic agents, such as adenosine. The effect is likely to be influenced by changes in salt intake and extracellular fluid volume as well as by hydration status. For example, the influence of AII on renal hemodynamics is greater in sodium depletion, which also activates the sympathetic nervous system. In response to mild nonhypotensive hemorrhage, renal hemodynamics are relatively well maintained. However, with further reductions in volume associated with a more severe hemorrhage, renal ischemia, mediated by activation of the renin-angiotensin system, renal efferent adrenergic nerves, and circulating catecholamines, may occur.[4]

Finally, modification of dietary protein and amino acid intake may affect renal hemodynamics. Dietary protein intake in excess of 1 g/kg/day has been associated with renal vasodilatation, as have infusions of casein hydrolysates and amino acids.[5, 6] Conversely, chronic consumption of a low-protein diet may be associated with renal vasoconstriction.

Measurement of Renal Blood Flow

RBF is measured conventionally by the clearance of infused para-aminohippurate (PAH), which is cleared almost totally from the arterial plasma by both filtration and secretion. Thus, its clearance approximates the rate of renal plasma flow (RPF):

$$RPF = U_{PAH} \cdot V/P_{PAH}$$

where U_{PAH} and P_{PAH} refer to urine and plasma PAH concentration, respectively, and V is urine flow rate in milliliters per minute.

RBF can be estimated by correction for the hematocrit (Hct):

$$RBF = RPF/[1 - Hct]$$

Although available, this test is rarely utilized in clinical practice. In fact, direct quantitation of RPF and RBF is rarely indicated outside of research studies; however, sometimes it is necessary to document that the kidneys are being perfused. In this case, one of three additional methods[3] may be utilized:

- Selective arteriography
- Doppler ultrasonography
- External radionuclide scanning

Because the latter two methods are noninvasive, they are preferred. With respect to the nuclide study, until recently, scanning was usually performed utilizing ^{131}I-iodohippurate sodium; however, the poor radiocharacteristics of ^{131}I limit its use in renal imaging.[7] More recently, other agents, such as ^{127}I-orthoiodohippurate and technetium (^{99m}Tc)-L,L-ethylenedicysteine may prove to be superior.[7, 8]

Clinical Correlates

Although a significant body of data has been obtained to indicate a complex relationship between neurocirculatory factors and renal hemodynamics, several points can be made from a clinical perspective. Optimization of cardiac output and extracellular fluid (ECF) volume, including the intravascular space, is essential for the maintenance of renal perfusion. Particularly because the effects of vasoactive compounds such as AII and catecholamines are accentuated in the face of renal hypoperfusion and volume contraction, attention should be directed to an assessment of ECF volume, with correction of any deficits, and to optimizing cardiac function. Frequently, pharmacologic agents have been employed to maintain renal perfusion in situations in which this may be compromised. Specifically, there has been widespread use of so-called low-dose or renal dose dopamine infusions. This is based on the observation that in low doses ($<$3 μg/kg/min) dopamine leads to renal vasodilatation.[10] At higher doses, renal vasoconstriction may occur.

The beneficial effects of dopamine infusion have not been documented in patients who are depleted of sodium chloride and volume, and the use of dopamine has not been shown to be effective beyond a short period of infusion.[9–11] That is, infusions of renal dose dopamine for 24 to 36 hours may be beneficial in the appropriate circumstance, but there is no evidence supporting the long-term use of this agent. Thus, justification for prolongation of its use beyond several days is not supported by available data. Furthermore, reports suggest that adverse outcomes may be associated with the use of dopamine.[11] Beyond anecdotal evidence, there are no compelling data to support the use of other potential vasodilator substances such as prostaglandins. Although high-protein feeding and amino acid infusions may increase renal hemodynamics by an undefined mechanism, there is no justification for utilizing these therapies solely from a hemodynamic point of view.[5, 6]

GLOMERULAR FILTRATION RATE

Of the 500 to 700 mL of plasma delivered per minute to the kidneys (corresponding to a renal blood flow of 1–1.2 L/min), approximately 20% to 25% is filtered. Glomerular filtration is a major function of the kidney and averages approximately 130 mL/min/1.73 m^2 in normal males and 120 mL/min/1.73 m^2 in females. Estimation or direct assessment of GFR remains one of the most important measurements of renal function and is widely utilized in clinical practice.

Measurement of Glomerular Filtration Rate

GFR is classically measured as the clearance of inulin (C_{in}), a fructose polymer with a mean molecular weight of approximately 5 kD. Because this substance is not present endogenously, it must be given by constant infusion following a loading dose. Inulin is available commercially but is expensive, often difficult to obtain, and cumbersome to utilize. As a result, inulin clearances are rarely used in clinical practice except for research protocols. Although inulin is generally measured chemically, ^{3}H-labeled and ^{14}C-labeled inulin are also available but are expensive.

More recently, other radiolabeled nuclides have been found to be satisfactory substitutes for inulin and have advantages in the measurement of GFR.[7, 8, 12, 13] Particularly ^{99m}Tc-labeled diethylenetriamine pentaacetic acid (DTPA) and ^{125}I- or ^{131}I-labeled iothalamate clearances closely approximate the inulin clearance.[14, 15] ^{99m}Tc-DTPA has been utilized and found to give measurements that correlate closely with C_{in} in ICU patients.[16, 17] In addition, the clearance of gentamicin has been utilized in a limited fashion to measure GFR.[18, 19] At the present time, it is not common for GFR to be measured directly. Rather, GFR is estimated by the endogenous creatinine clearance or serum creatinine determination (see later).

The normal values for GFR given previously apply for individuals from the teenage years through approximately 35 years of age. Thereafter, GFR declines in most individuals. Whereas this decline was formerly thought to occur at a relatively constant rate of approximately 10 mL/min per decade,[20–22] more recent data, obtained in a longitudinal fashion, indicate that this reduction is not so predictable.[23] In addition, a circadian rhythm for GFR has been described.[24, 25] GFR is maximal in the daytime, whereas a minimum value during the night has been found in normal individuals. Whether this circadian pattern of GFR occurs in critically ill hospitalized patients is not known.

CREATININE CLEARANCE AND SERUM CREATININE

Creatinine Clearance

The endogenous creatinine clearance (C_{cr}) enjoys widespread use as a reasonable gauge of GFR when great precision is not demanded; it rarely is in clinical practice. The use of creatinine as a marker of GFR has the advantage that creatinine is endogenously produced and is easily measured by inexpensive methods. Creatinine, like inulin, is freely filtered and absorbed not at all or to a minimum extent. However, creatinine is secreted, and the contribution of secretion to total excretion is greater as the GFR decreases and serum creatinine rises. At GFRs below 40 mL/min, C_{cr} exceeds C_{in} by 50% to 100%.[14, 26] When GFR is significantly depressed and it is deemed important to get a more precise measurement of GFR, one of the previously mentioned methods to estimate GFR directly might be utilized. Additionally, because C_{cr} overestimates GFR and the clearance of urea underestimates GFR, the mean value of simultaneously obtained creatinine and urea clearances has been shown to provide a close estimation of C_{in} when the latter is below 20 mL/min.[27]

Because cimetidine competes with creatinine for tubular

secretion (see later), administration of cimetidine may increase the accuracy both of creatinine clearance in 24-hour collections (when given for several days beforehand) and of 4-hour, water-loaded clearances.[28-30] This effect has been used to obtain a more accurate estimate of GFR. Specifically, C_{cr} obtained in the presence of cimetidine (400 mg as a priming dose followed by 200 mg every 3 hours) yielded values that closely approximated C_{in}.[28, 29] Volume expansion in humans causes a small rise in GFR, whereas volume depletion, severe heart failure, hypotension, anesthesia, surgery, trauma, sepsis, and even mild intestinal bleeding without frank hypotension may depress GFR substantially.

Various methods are available to measure creatinine. Creatinine is frequently measured using the Jaffé alkaline picric acid reaction. Although this method is widely utilized, this reaction also measures other chromogens, which may lead to a false elevation in the estimated serum creatinine (S_{cr}) measurement. Substances such as acetoacetate (in ketoacidosis), pyruvate, ascorbate, 5-flucytosine, certain (but not all) cephalosporin antibiotics, and very high urate artifactually raise S_{cr} in normal subjects by 0.5 to 2 mg/dL.[31-37] These substances are excreted into the urine but contribute trivially compared with overall urine creatinine (U_{cr}). Thus, noncreatinine chromogens affect the S_{cr} but have little effect on the U_{cr}.

In individuals with normal renal function, the contribution of serum noncreatinine chromogens to raising the S_{cr} is approximately equal to the contribution of secretion to creatinine excretion such that the C_{cr} closely approximates GFR. As GFR decreases, the contribution of noncreatinine chromogens to the total measured S_{cr} becomes less than the secreted moiety and the C_{cr} overestimates GFR to a greater extent. Direct enzymatic creatinine measurements are not affected by noncreatinine chromogens. Very high levels of serum glucose (>1000 mg/dL) and 5-flucytosine may interfere with the enzymatic reaction, whereas high levels of bilirubin (>5 mg/dL) affect the autoanalyzer method[35] and lead to falsely low S_{cr} values. It is therefore important to know the method by which a given laboratory measures S_{cr}. Competing for the same proximal tubular organic base secretory site as creatinine, certain pharmacologic agents may suppress this process and lead to a rise in S_{cr}. Trimethoprim, probenecid, and cimetidine, but not ranitidine, are organic bases that inhibit creatinine secretion competitively and can result in a mild elevation in S_{cr}, usually 0.5 mg/dL or less.[38-41]

As with all clearance methods, the C_{cr} is subject to errors that may amount to as much as 10% to 15% or more. In addition to potential problems in estimating S_{cr} and urine creatine, errors in timing of urine collection, incomplete collection, and inaccurate measurement of urine volume are other factors that contribute to errors.[42] Although 24-hour urine creatine clearances have been widely utilized, no specified time period is required for the clearance to be obtained. In fact, shorter collection periods of several hours may be more accurate in patients passing adequate amounts of urine (not oliguric), particularly if the patient is not in a steady state (see later). To reduce errors in volume measurement, one can induce a water diuresis in stable subjects prior to beginning the test,[43] although this is rarely practical in the ICU setting. Nevertheless, because many ICU patients have indwelling Foley catheters, it should be possible for accurately timed urine collections to be obtained and for C_{cr} to be measured with reasonable accuracy.

Serum Creatinine

Because of the practical and technical problems in obtaining estimates of GFR by clearance methods, renal function is most commonly estimated by following the S_{cr} in hospitalized patients. Creatinine is formed nonenzymatically from creatine and phosphocreatine in muscle cells and is normally present in the serum at a concentration of 0.8 to 1.4 mg/dL in adults and 0.3 to 0.6 mg/dL in children and pregnant subjects. The actually measured S_{cr} depends on the method of measurement, as discussed previously, GFR, rate of creatinine production, volume of distribution (e.g., S_{cr} is lower in anasarca), and extent of its tubular secretion and intestinal degradation.[3] Because creatinine production is closely related to muscle mass, S_{cr} is generally less in females than in males and decreases as muscle mass is lost with aging or with debilitating illnesses.

The relationship between S_{cr} and C_{cr} (and hence GFR) can be described by a rectangular hyperbola[42]; however, this relationship applies in the steady state and assumes a constant rate of creatinine production (Fig. 152–1). Thus, a doubling of the S_{cr} reflects a 50% decrease in C_{cr}, a fourfold increase in S_{cr}, a 75% drop in GFR, and so on. As creatinine production may not remain constant, S_{cr} may underestimate the decrease in GFR in critically ill patients who have a decrease in muscle mass secondary to an ongoing catabolic state. Moreover, it should be appreciated that S_{cr} is an insensitive marker of change early in the course of renal disease. Thus, a 33% fall in GFR may raise the S_{cr} from 0.8 to 1.2 mg/dL, a value that is still within the normal range. If the prior value is not known, this fall in GFR may go unrecognized.

S_{cr} provides a close estimate of GFR only in the steady state. With an abrupt decrease in GFR, as may occur in acute renal failure, creatinine production would be expected to continue unchanged, but because of the decrease in GFR, creatinine excretion will be impaired. As a result, the S_{cr} increases until a new steady state is obtained, at which time the amount of creatinine produced equals the amount filtered (GFR · S_{cr}) and excreted (U_{cr}·V). Depending on the extent of damage and decrease in GFR, it may take several days for a new steady state to be achieved (Fig. 152–2). Therefore, following an

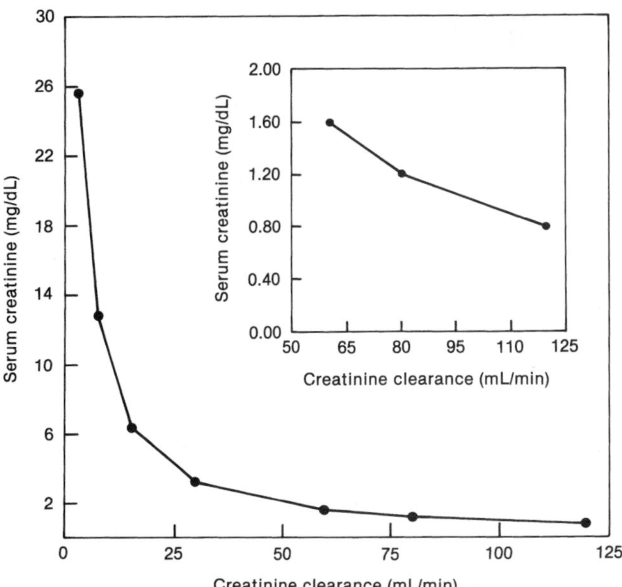

Figure 152–1. Relationship between creatinine clearance and serum creatinine. In the steady state, the serum creatinine should increase twofold for each 50% reduction in creatinine clearance. Inset represents an enlarged view of the changes in serum creatinine as creatinine clearance decreases from 120 to 60 mL/min. If serum creatinine is 0.8 mg/dL when the creatinine clearance is 120 mL/min, creatinine clearance can decrease by 33% such that the increased serum creatinine is still within the normal range.

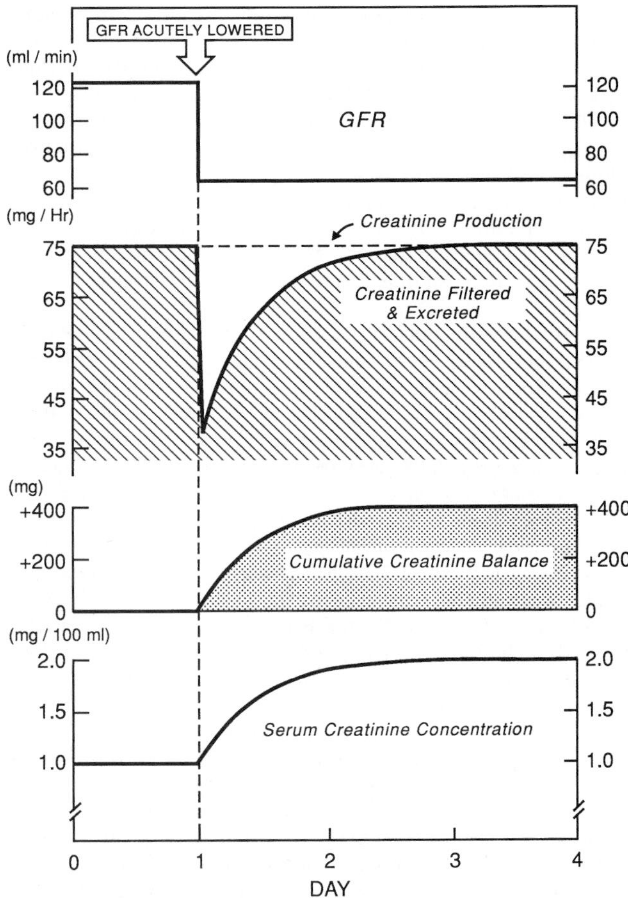

Figure 152–2. Expected changes in serum creatinine resulting from an acute fall in the glomerular filtration rate (GFR) and attainment of a new steady state. Between days 0 and 1, the patient is excreting all the creatinine that is produced and serum creatinine is stable at 1 mg/dL. A 50% reduction in GFR on day 1 results in an abrupt fall in filtered (and, therefore, excreted) creatinine. Release of creatinine from muscle remains constant; as a result, creatinine is retained and its serum concentration is increased. As the creatinine concentration rises progressively, filtered (and excreted) creatinine also increases until the excreted creatinine returns to control levels and matches creatinine production. This new steady state (days 3 to 4) is achieved by doubling of serum creatinine concentration, which maintains the filtered creatinine load at control levels in the face of halving of the GFR. A larger decrease in GFR would lead to a greater increase in the steady state (e.g., a 90% reduction in GFR would lead to a 10-fold rise in serum creatinine) and would take a longer time to achieve. (From Kassirer JP: Clinical evaluation of kidney function–glomerular function. N Engl J Med 1971; 285:385. Reprinted with permission from *The New England Journal of Medicine*.)

insult leading to an abrupt decrease in GFR, the S_{cr} rises progressively over the next several days. This should not be interpreted as a new insult each day but, rather, that a steady state has not yet been obtained. While the S_{cr} is changing, its absolute value cannot be used as an accurate measure of the decrease in GFR. If an accurate measurement of GFR is needed during this time, a short C_{cr} can be obtained.

A variety of equations have been developed to estimate C_{cr} based on the S_{cr} without collection of urine. These equations generally take into consideration muscle mass (estimated as body weight), sex (males having a higher GFR than females), and age. Aging, hepatic diseases, excessive muscle wasting, severe muscular atrophy or dystrophy, hyperthyroidism, paralysis, and chronic glucocorticoid therapy have been associated with reduced creatinine generation.[17] In addition, particularly at low levels of GFR, correction for nonrenal creatinine metabolism is also recommended.[44, 45] One of the most commonly utilized equations is that developed by Cockcroft and Gault.[46]

$$C_{cr} = \frac{(140 - \text{age}) \cdot \text{lean wt in kg}}{72 \cdot S_{cr}}$$

where age is expressed in years. The preceding expression is used for men. The formula for women is the preceding formula multiplied by 0.85.

The reliability of this equation as a measure of GFR has been assessed in patients with diabetes,[52] pregnant women with renal disease,[47] obese individuals,[48] elderly individuals,[49, 50] and black Americans with hypertensive renal disease.[51] It has also been assessed in critically ill patients.[52] These studies have indicated that the accuracy of GFR estimates using the Cockcroft-Gault equation is similar to, or greater than, 24-hour C_{cr} and the precision is better. This equation seems to be most accurate for estimating GFR when the latter is in the range of 10 to 100 mL/min.[43, 48, 51, 52] An accurate prediction of GFR was derived by Walser and colleagues[53] in patients with advanced renal disease ($S_{cr} > 2$ mg/dL) as follows:

For males,

$$\text{GFR} = 7.57\ [\text{Cr}]^{-1} - 0.103\ \text{age} + 0.096\ \text{weight} - 6.66$$

For females,

$$\text{GFR} = 6.05\ [\text{Cr}]^{-1} - 0.08\ \text{age} + 0.08\ \text{weight} - 4.81$$

where creatinine (Cr) is expressed in millimoles, age in years, and weight in kilograms. More precision was obtained by including a value for 24-hour urinary urea nitrogen, as a measure of protein intake.[53]

Serum Urea Nitrogen

Less accurate as a marker of GFR than the S_{cr}, serum urea nitrogen (SUN) (or blood urea nitrogen) is still used extensively in clinical practice to estimate renal function. Although this was the earliest available indicator of renal function, several other factors should be appreciated regarding the use of this substance. Urea, like creatinine, is freely filtered and is retained in the blood as GFR falls. However, in contrast to creatinine, urea may be reabsorbed to a significant extent, its excretion tending to be increased with increasing urine flow rates, whereas its excretion is reduced when tubular fluid reabsorption is enhanced. Of greater importance, urea production is more variable than creatinine. Produced in the liver, urea increases with high protein intake, amino acid infusions, and hypercatabolic states. In addition, endogenous sources of protein such as absorbed hemoglobin from gastrointestinal bleeding may contribute to increased urea synthesis. Even at a constant GFR, SUN may rise in subjects on high protein intake and fall with protein restriction or on refeeding of previously starved, nonhypercatabolic subjects.

Several pharmacologic agents also may affect urea nitrogen formation. Tetracyclines may lead to an increase in SUN by an antianabolic effect without any detectable change in GFR, whereas glucocorticoids and severe illnesses or trauma do the same by inducing endogenous protein hypercatabolism. Because of the widespread use of hyperalimentation in ICU patients, an impairment in renal function is often associated with a marked disproportion in the elevation of SUN compared with S_{cr}. For this reason, the issue is raised as to whether SUN elevation itself poses an important threat to the patient if the GFR is in a range that should not lead to enhanced morbidity by itself. In those circumstances, it is useful to measure the rate of urea appearance (or generation) in order to estimate whether other factors, such as gastrointestinal bleeding, excessive amino acid infusions, and protein administration, are contributing to the increase in SUN above that expected by the decrease in GFR.[44, 45] Urea nitrogen (UN) appearance can be determined from urine urea nitrogen (UUN), SUN, and body weight as follows:

$$\text{UN} = \text{UUN} \cdot \text{V} + \Delta \text{ body pool UN}$$

where UUN · V is 24-hour UN excretion, and

$$\Delta \text{ body pool UN} = 0.6 \cdot \text{nonedematous weight (kg)} \cdot \Delta\text{SUN/day}$$

If the weight is changing,

$$\Delta \text{ body pool UN} = (0.6 \cdot \text{nonedematous weight} \cdot \Delta\text{SUN}) + (\Delta \text{ weight} \cdot \text{final SUN})$$ [44, 45]

Nitrogen balance (BN) is equal to

$$\text{BN} = \text{IN} - \text{UN} - \text{NUN}$$

where IN is urea nitrogen intake and NUN is nonurea nitrogen excretion.[45]

NUN, which includes fecal nitrogen, urinary creatinine, uric acid, and unmeasured nitrogen, averages 0.031 g nitrogen/kg/day.[45] The data obtained from the above measurements may be quite useful in evaluating the cause of disproportionate elevations in SUN. If the patient is in a steady state (with a stable weight and SUN), BN = 0, and IN can be estimated from UN + NUN.[45] Because catabolism, except for *severe* trauma and burns, is usually 2 to 4 g nitrogen/day, additional conclusions can be drawn if the patient is not in the steady state. For example, if it is known that IN is less than UN + NUN, gastrointestinal bleeding with or without excess catabolism would be suggested. Similarly, one can evaluate if the increase in [SUN] is a reflection of excessive exogenous protein and amino acid administration (usually > 1.5 g/kg/day; g UN 0.16 = g protein or amino acids). If IN is above UN, such as in severe liver disease, the clinician might more carefully evaluate changes in weight and SUN as well as clearances, because the latter may be more severely depressed than initially suspected.

SODIUM BALANCE AND EXTRACELLULAR FLUID VOLUME

Sodium is the primary cation of the ECF, present in a concentration of 140 to 142 mmol/L. The volume of the ECF is approximately 20% of total body weight and represents a third of total body water. Regulation of ECF volume is governed by factors regulating sodium balance and sodium excretion. The reader is referred to several excellent reviews on this topic.[54, 55] For the purposes of this discussion, several factors are emphasized. Under physiologic conditions and in the steady state, sodium balance pertains, and the amount of sodium excreted equals that which enters the body by oral and intravenous routes. Sodium excretion and the fraction of filtered sodium that is excreted (FE_{Na}) can be readily determined. Absolute sodium excretion is measured as the product of the urine sodium concentration and the urine volume,

$$\text{Na}^+ \text{ excretion} = (U_{Na} \cdot V)$$

FE_{Na} can be determined as follows:

$$FE_{Na} = U_{Na} \cdot V/GFR \cdot S_{Na}$$

For practical reasons, the C_{cr} (= $U_{cr} \cdot V/S_{cr}$) is used to estimate GFR, such that

$$FE_{Na} = U_{Na} \cdot V/U_{cr} \cdot V/S_{cr} \cdot S_{Na}$$

Because the V term in the numerator and denominator cancels out,

$$FE_{Na} = U_{Na}/S_{Na} \cdot S_{cr}/U_{cr}$$

Thus, FE_{Na} can be calculated from the sodium and creatinine determined in a random urine sample and serum (or plasma) simultaneously. The resulting calculation is expressed as a percentage by multiplying by 100. This test is of value in the setting of acute renal failure to aid in distinguishing a prerenal from renal parenchymal etiology.[56] It is not usually helpful in aiding in the diagnosis of urinary tract obstruction or in the presence of underlying chronic renal insufficiency. The reason for the difficulty in interpretation in chronic renal insufficiency can be illustrated by the following considerations. At a GFR of 130 mL/min and a dietary sodium intake of 3 g of sodium (130 mmol), an individual in sodium balance will excrete 0.5% of the filtered load (FE_{Na} = 0.5%). For sodium balance to be maintained at lower levels of GFR with the same sodium intake, FE_{Na} must be increased progressively. Successive decreases in GFR by 2 from 130 would result in an FE_{Na} of 1%, 2%, 4%, and 8%, respectively. Thus, interpretation of the FE_{Na} in a patient with acute renal failure superimposed on chronic renal insufficiency is problematic unless the prior steady-state FE_{Na} is known; this is rarely the case.

The fractional excretion of chloride (FE_{Cl}) has been suggested to be more accurate than that of sodium in aiding in distinguishing prerenal from parenchymal causes of acute renal failure.[57] This is particularly so in the situation in which acute renal failure occurs with simultaneous metabolic alkalosis. If the urine contains substantial amounts of bicarbonate urinary pH (U_{pH} > 7), sodium excretion increases to maintain electroneutrality. Under these circumstances, the FE_{Na} may give misleading information but the FE_{Cl} can be used to obtain the same information.

Although urinary sodium excretion can be used to help make determinations with respect to ECF volume under certain circumstances, this may be fraught with potential errors. No laboratory test is available to provide this information. Rather, the astute clinician must rely on bedside evaluation complemented, where appropriate, with measurements of central venous pressure and pulmonary capillary wedge pressure to assist in making determinations with respect to ECF volume status. For example, a low FE_{Na} (<1%) in the setting of acute renal failure usually indicates a decrease in renal perfusion but does not provide information on the status of the patient's ECF volume. Because a low FE_{Na} can be seen with either ECF volume contraction or severe congestive heart failure, these conditions must be distinguished at the bedside. Moreover, sometimes (see Chapter 153 on acute renal failure) a low FE_{Na} exists even in the presence of parenchymal renal disease, such as acute glomerulonephritis, severe burn, and radiocontrast nephropathy. Finally, administration of potent diuretic agents can alter the FE_{Na} and may result in misleading interpretations. For this reason, urine samples should be obtained before diuretics are administered.

A few additional points are worthy of note with respect to diuretic use. There is now ample evidence that in a patient in positive sodium balance, diuretic therapy should not be utilized without simultaneously restricting sodium intake, including intravenous saline, if negative sodium balance and reduction in edema fluid are desired.[58] In general, this requires restriction of dietary sodium intake, usually to less than 2 g of sodium per day (0.88 mmol) if the patient is in edema-forming state. Although a diuresis can be affected even with liberal sodium intake, this requires higher doses of diuretics and more frequent administration of these agents. The coexistence of hyponatremia should not deter clinicians from restricting sodium intake but, rather, should cause them to address solute-free water intake as well. Of course, under certain circumstances, obligatory intakes make it difficult to achieve optimal restriction to assist diuresis. That is, with various pharmacologic drips, blood products, and feeding regimens necessary in acutely ill patients in the ICU, this may become a difficult problem. Under those circumstances, increasing doses of diuretics, including continuous infusions of loop diuretics, may be required.

References

1. Jochimsen F, Schafer JH, Maurer A, et al: Impairment of renal function in medical intensive care: Predictability of acute renal failure. Crit Care Med 1990; 18:480.
2. Menashe PI, Ross SA, Tottlieb JE: Acquired renal insufficiency in critically ill patients. Crit Care Med 1988; 16:1106.
3. Oken DE, Schoolwerth AC: The kidneys. *In:* Laboratory Medicine: The Selection and Interpretation of Clinical Laboratory Studies. Noe DA, Rock RC (Eds). Baltimore, Williams & Wilkins. 1994, pp 401–461.
4. Arendshorst WJ, Navar LG: Renal circulation and glomerular hemodynamics. *In:* Diseases of the Kidney. 6th ed. Vol 1. Schrier RW, Gottschalk CW (Eds). Boston, Little, Brown & Co, 1997, pp 59–106.
5. Bergstrom J, Ahlberg M, Alvestrand A: Influence of protein intake on renal hemodynamics and plasma hormone concentrations in normal subjects. Acta Med Scand 1985; 217:189.
6. Bosch JP, Saccaggi A, Lauer A, et al: Renal functional reserve in humans. Am J Med 1983; 75:943.
7. Dondi M, Fanti S: Determination of individual renal function through noninvasive methodologies. Curr Opin Nephrol Hypertens 1995; 4:520.
8. Bubeck B: Radionuclide techniques for the evaluation of renal function: Advantages over conventional methodology. Curr Opin Nephrol Hypertens 1995; 4:514.
9. Szerlip HM: Renal-dose dopamine: Fact and fiction. Ann Intern Med 1991; 115:153.
10. Denton MD, Chertow GM, Brady HR: Renal-dose dopamine for the treatment of acute renal failure: Scientific rationale, experimental studies and chemical trials. Kidney Int 1996; 49:4.
11. Chertow GM, Sayegh MH, Allgren RL, Lazarus JM: Is the administration of dopamine associated with adverse outcomes in acute renal failure? Am J Med 1996; 101:49.
12. Blaufox MD: Measurement of renal function. Curr Opin Nephrol Hypertens 1995; 4:503.
13. Blaufox MD, Aurell M, Bubeck B, Fommei E, Piepsz A, Russell C, Taylor A, Thomsen HS, Volterrani D: Report of the Radionuclides in Nephrourology Committee on Renal Clearance. J Nucl Med 1996; 37:1883.
14. Shemesh O, Golbetz H, Riss JP, et al: Limitations of creatinine as a filtration marker in glomerulopathic patients. Kidney Int 1985; 28:830.
15. Blaufox MD: Radionuclide techniques for the diagnosis of urinary tract disease. *In:* Contemporary Issues in Nephrology. Vol 25. Diagnostic Techniques in Renal Disease. Narins RG, Stein JH (Eds). New York, Churchill Livingstone, 1992, pp 305–329.
16. Wharton WW, Sondeen JL, McBiles M, et al: Measurement of glomerular filtration rate in ICU patients using ^{99m}Tc-DTPA and inulin. Kidney Int 1992; 42:174.
17. Robert S, Zarowitz BJ: Is there a reliable index of glomerular filtration rate in critically ill patients? Drug Intell Clin Pharmacol 1991; 25:169.
18. Salazar DE, Corcoran GB: Predicting creatinine clearance and renal drug clearance in obese patients from estimated fat-free body mass. Am J Med 1988; 84:1053.
19. Zarowitz BJ, Robert S, Peterson EL: Prediction of glomerular filtration rate using aminoglycoside clearance in critically ill medical patients. Ann Pharmacother 1992; 26:1205.
20. Davies DF, Shock NW: Age changes in glomerular filtration rate, effective renal plasma flow and tubular excretory capacity in adult males. J Clin Invest 1950; 29:496.
21. Rowe JW, Andres R, Tobin JD, et al: The effect of age on creatinine clearance in men: A cross-sectional and longitudinal study. J Gerontol 1976; 31:155.
22. Kafetz K: Renal impairment in the elderly: A review. J R Soc Med 1983; 76:398.
23. Epstein M: Aging and the kidney. J Am Soc Nephrol 1996; 7:1106.
24. Koopman MG, Koomen GCM, Krediet RT, et al: Circadian rhythm of glomerular filtration rate in normal individuals. Clin Sci (Colch) 1989; 77:105.
25. Van Acker BAC, Koomen GCM, Koopman MG, et al: Discrepancy between circadian rhythms of inulin and creatinine clearance. J Lab Clin Med 1992; 120:400.
26. Bauer JH, Brooks CS, Burch RN: Clinical appraisal of creatinine clearance as a measurement of glomerular filtration rate. Am J Kidney Dis 1982; 2:337.
27. Lubowitz H, Slatopolsky E, Shankel S, et al: Glomerular filtration rate: Determination in patients with chronic renal disease. JAMA 1967; 199:252.
28. Hilbrands LB, Artz MA, Wetzels JFM, et al: Cimetidine improves the reliability of creatinine as a marker of glomerular filtration. Kidney Int 1991; 40:1171.
29. Rocci ML Jr, Vlasses PH, Ferguson RK: Creatinine serum concentrations and H_2-receptor antagonists. Clin Nephrol 1984; 22:214.
30. Marcen R, Serrano P, Teruel JL, Rivera ME, Mitjavila M: Oral cimetidine improved the accuracy of creatinine clearance in transplant patients on cyclosporine (Abstract). Transplant Proc 1994; 26:2624.
31. Gerard SK, Khayam-Bashi H: Characterization of creatinine error in ketotic patients: A prospective comparison of alkaline picrate methods with an enzymatic method. Am J Clin Pathol 1985; 84:659.
32. Molitch ME, Rodman E, Hirsch CA, et al: Spurious serum creatinine elevations in ketoacidosis. Ann Intern Med 1980; 93:280.
33. Cruickshank AM, Shenkin A: A comparison of the effect of acetoacetate concentration on the measurement of serum creatinine using Technicon SMAC II, Beckman Astra and enzymatic techniques. Ann Clin Biochem 1987; 24:317.
34. Mascioli SR, Bantle JP, Freier EF, et al: Artifactual elevation of serum creatinine level due to fasting. Arch Intern Med 1984; 144:1575.
35. Levey AS, Perrone RD, Madias NE: Serum creatinine and renal function. Annu Rev Med 1988; 39:465.
36. Kroll MH, Elin RJ: Mechanism of cefoxitin and cephalothin interference with the Jaffe method for creatinine. Clin Chem 1983; 29:2044.
37. Kroll MH, Koch TR, Drusano GL, et al: Lack of interference with creatinine assays by four cephalosporin-like antibiotics. Am J Clin Pathol 1984; 82:214.
38. Berglund F, Killander J, Pompeius R: Effect of trimethoprim-sulfamethoxazole on the renal excretion of creatinine in man. J Urol 1975; 114:802.
39. Odlind B, Hällgren R, Sohtell M, et al: Is ^{125}I iothalamate an ideal marker for glomerular filtration? Kidney Int 1985; 27:9.
40. Dubb JW, Stote RM, Familiar R, et al: Effect of cimetidine on renal function in normal man. Clin Pharmacol Ther 1978; 24:76.
41. Van Acker BAC, Koomen GCM, Koopman MG, et al: Creatinine clearance during cimetidine administration for measurement of glomerular filtration rate. Lancet 1992; 340:1326.
42. Kassirer JP: Clinical evaluation of kidney function–glomerular function. N Engl J Med 1971; 285:385.
43. Lemann J, Bidani AK, Bain RP, Lewis EJ, Rohde RD: Use of the

serum creatinine to estimate glomerular filtration rate in health and early diabetic nephropathy. Am J Kidney Dis 1990; 16:236.
44. Maroni BJ, Steinman TI, Mitch WE: A method for estimating nitrogen intake of patients with chronic renal failure. Kidney Int 1985; 27:58.
45. Mitch WE: Restricted diets and slowing the progression of chronic renal insufficiency. *In:* Nutrition and the Kidney. 2nd ed. Mitch WE, Klahr S (Eds). Boston, Little, Brown & Co, 1993, pp 243–262.
46. Cockcroft DW, Gault MH: Prediction of creatinine clearance from serum creatinine. Nephron 1976; 16:31.
47. Quadri KHM, Bernardini J, Greenberg A, Laifer S, Syed A, Holley JL: Assessment of renal function during pregnancy using a random urine protein to creatinine ratio and Cockcroft-Gault formula. Am J Kidney Dis 1994; 24:416.
48. Cochran M, St. John A: A comparison between estimates of GFR using [^{99m}Tc] DTPA clearance and the approximation of Cockcroft and Gault. Aust N Z J Med 1993; 23:494.
49. O'Connell MB, Dwinell AM, Bannick-Mohrland SD: Predictive performance of equations to estimate creatinine clearance in hospitalized elderly patients. Ann Pharmacother 1992; 26:627.
50. Sokoll LJ, Russell RM, Sadowski JA: Establishment of creatinine clearance reference values for older women. Clin Chem 1994; 40:2276.
51. Toto R, Kirk K, Coresh J, Jones C, Appel L, Campese V, Olutade B, Agodoa L: Evaluation of serum creatinine for estimating glomerular filtration rate in African Americans with hypertensive nephrosclerosis: Results from the African-American Study of Kidney Disease and Hypertension (AASK) Pilot Study. J Am Soc Nephrol 1997; 8:279.
52. Robert S, Zarowitz BJ, Peterson EL, Dumler F: Predictability of creatinine clearance estimates in critically ill patients. Crit Care Med 1993; 21:1487.
53. Walser M, Drew HH, Guldan JL: Prediction of glomerular filtration rate from serum creatinine concentration in advanced chronic renal failure. Kidney Int 1993; 44:1145.
54. Miller JA, Tobe SW, Skorecki KL: Control of extracellular fluid volume and pathophysiology of edema formation. *In:* The Kidney. 5th ed. Vol 1. Brenner BM, Rector FC Jr (Eds). Philadelphia, WB Saunders, 1996, pp 817–872.
55. Reeves WB, Andreoli TE: Tubular sodium transport. *In:* Diseases of the Kidney. 6th ed. Vol 1. Schrier RW, Gottschalk CW (Eds). Boston, Little, Brown & Co, 1997, pp 127–162.
56. Espinel CH: The FE test: Use in the differential diagnosis of acute renal failure. JAMA 1976; 236:579.
57. Anderson RJ, Gross PA, Gabow P: Urinary chloride concentration in acute renal failure. Miner Electrolyte Metab 1984; 10:92.
58. Wilcox CS, Mitch WE, Kelly RA, et al: Response of the kidney to furosemide: I. Effects of salt intake and renal compensation. J Lab Clin Med 1983; 102:450.

153

Prevention of Acute Renal Failure

Rinaldo Bellomo, MB BS (HONS), MD, FRACP
Claudio Ronco, MD

Acute renal failure (ARF) is a common complication of critical illness.[1] Although its incidence varies according to its definition, approximately 10% to 20% of patients in intensive care units (ICUs) appear to develop a clinically important degree of renal dysfunction, with an overall population incidence of approximately 1 per 1000 per year.[2] On the other hand, if one focuses on severe renal failure alone (renal failure severe enough to require some form of acute renal replacement therapy), its incidence is approximately 4% to 6% of all ICU admissions with an overall incidence of 1 per 10,000 people per year (Australian and New Zealand Intensive Care Society Acute Renal Failure Survey: Unpublished data, 1997).

Clearly, no matter how one classifies this disorder or what epidemiologic figures one considers, ARF is a major and common condition in critically ill patients that requires important adjustments in drug dosage and overall management strategy, as well as the introduction of complex and costly extracorporeal techniques of organ support.

Because of these considerations and because the treatment of established ARF is essentially supportive, the major thrust of ARF management should be directed toward its prevention. In addition, because in most critically ill patients ARF is due to prerenal factors, prevention of prerenal ARF is the most common therapeutic goal of critical care physicians. Such prevention is the focus of this chapter (other causes of ARF, including nephrotoxins, are discussed elsewhere in this section).

PATHOGENESIS OF ACUTE RENAL FAILURE

A large body of evidence[3-5] supports the following concepts: (1) prerenal ARF initially occurs through the final common pathway of medullary ischemia,[6] (2) such ischemia is initially functional in nature,[6] and (3) its occurrence is, in part, sustained by the activation of the tubuloglomerular feedback response.[7]

In order to understand the primacy of medullary ischemia in the pathogenesis of ARF, one must understand why the outer medulla is uniquely sensitive to ischemia. The outer medulla is the site where most countercurrent solute transport takes place and creates the tissue solute gradients necessary to achieve urine concentration. The outer medulla is also the site of significant energy-dependent solute transport (thick ascending portion of the loop of Henle). Because countercurrent solute transport involves oxygen as well as cations and anions, there is a progressive and severe desaturation of arterial blood as the renal circulation follows the loop of Henle through the vasa recta down into the outer medulla. Thus, the tension of oxygen in the tissues and blood surrounding the thick ascending loop of Henle is in the range 10 to 15 mm Hg; that is, this segment of the kidney lives in an ischemic penumbra[8] (Fig. 153–1).

This level of near-hypoxia is at a site of relatively high oxygen consumption (because of the energy cost of solute movement across the tubule cells of the loop of Henle). The combination of relatively high oxygen consumption and low oxygen delivery makes the outer medulla highly sensitive to any event that would reduce oxygen delivery to the kidney (hypotension, low cardiac output, sepsis, hemorrhage, systemic hypoxia, and the like). The kidney, therefore, despite receiving a large part of the cardiac output, becomes exquisitely sensitive to changes in perfusion.

This paradox can be explained by the fact that most renal blood flow is directed at the kidney's blood purification function (glomerulus) and is effectively shunted away from the tubules themselves, which are the site of organ oxygen consumption. This unique arrangement can be seen either as the price the kidney pays for being able to concentrate urine or, teleologically, as a means by which the kidney ceases to function during high-stress situations, thus immediately interrupting any further loss of fluid at a time when circulating volume is to be maintained at all costs (flight-or-fight reaction). In either case, the kidney is set up to "fail" under stressful conditions, or, as some have argued, acute renal failure should be more correctly named "acute renal success,"[9] as the kidney acts in accordance with what it has evolved to achieve.

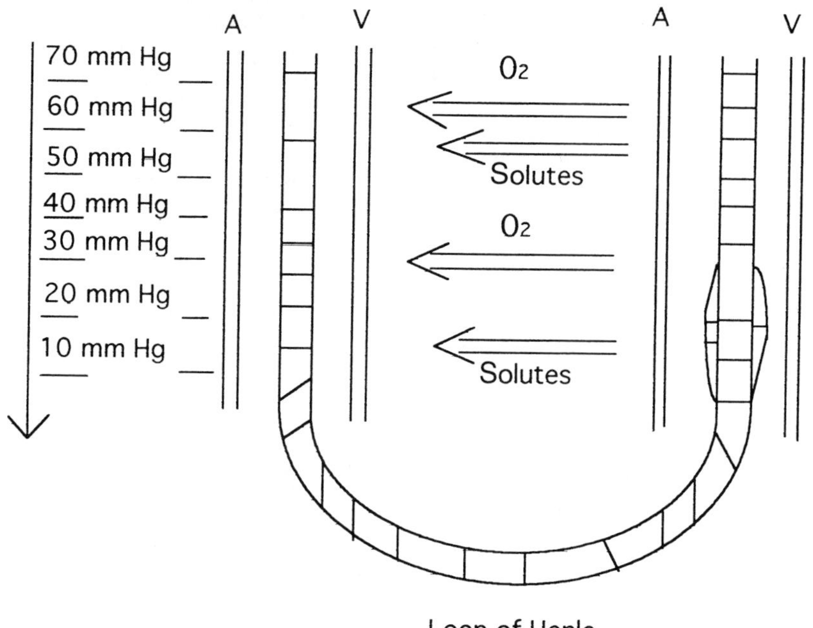

Figure 153–1. Diagram illustrating the changes in tissue oxygen tension in the outer medulla. As arterial blood runs along the arterial vasa recta (A), solute and oxygen move by countercurrent transfer to their venous (V) counterparts. This leads to a rapid fall in arterial oxygen tension, down to a partial pressure of 10 to 20 mm Hg at the level of the thick ascending portion of the loop.

TUBULOGLOMERULAR FEEDBACK

Much evidence supports the concept[7, 10] that the initial steps that lead to a decrease in glomerular filtration rate (GFR) and the onset of oliguria are due to a stereotyped response to decreased oxygen delivery to the medulla. This response is called tubuloglomerular feedback (TGF) (Fig. 153-2). TGF is a physiologic mechanism that links GFR (the major determinant of solute delivery to the outer medulla) to the energy state of the tubules in the medulla.

When there is an imbalance between oxygen delivery and oxygen consumption in the ascending loop of Henle, tubular adenosine triphosphate (ATP) stores are depleted and adenosine is released. Adenosine is a powerful afferent arteriolar

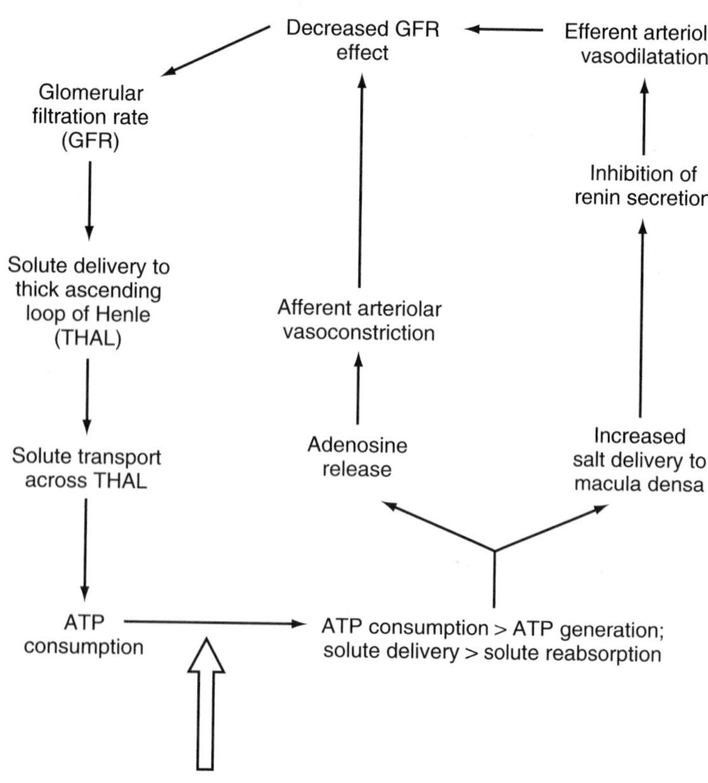

Figure 153–2. The tubuloglomerular feedback (TGF) loop. Glomerular filtration rate (GFR) regulates solute delivery to the thick ascending loop of Henle (THAL). Most of THAL's adenosine triphosphate (ATP) consumption is related to solute transport. When ischemia occurs, ATP stores are depleted and solute absorption cannot meet solute delivery. Adenosine is released, and as solute is not absorbed, more of it is delivered to the macula densa, which is adjacent to THAL. Adenosine induces afferent arteriolar vasoconstriction and increased salt delivery to the macula densa inhibits renin production and induces efferent arteriolar vasodilatation. These vascular tone changes induce a decrease in GFR, which in turn decreases solute delivery to THAL with a decrease in its oxygen consumption. The loop is thus closed.

vasoconstrictor and its biologic effect is to decrease intraglomerular pressure, thus decreasing GFR. The decrease in GFR, in turn, decreases solute delivery to the medulla, resulting in decreased medullary work and a trend toward restoring the balance between oxygen delivery and consumption.[10] Tubular oxygen consumption and oxygen delivery are therefore linked in an attempt to prevent severe tubular hypoxia and cell death while homeostasis is being restored.

Unfortunately, if the ischemia persists, even this compensatory mechanism is overcome, structural cell injury develops, and the decrease in GFR is maintained and amplified. In this regard, severe sepsis is a particular pathophysiologic state in which medullary ischemia is also sustained by intense renal vasoconstriction. This intense renal vasoconstriction is mediated by both endotoxin directly and a multitude of soluble mediators released systemically and locally in response to infection.[11] In the setting of sepsis, therefore, renal injury results from hypotension and intense vasoconstriction and compensatory mechanisms are insufficient to maintain medullary oxygenation. When compensatory mechanisms fail, the patient moves from a functional decrease in GFR to established irreversible renal failure (so-called acute tubular necrosis) with cell death, tubular swelling, tubular obstruction, and interstitial and tubular edema.

PRINCIPLES OF RENAL PROTECTION

From the preceding discussion, one can see that prompt and complete restoration of adequate medullary oxygenation should be the rational basis for renal protection during so-called prerenal ARF. Such restoration of medullary oxygenation must initially rest upon restoration of global renal perfusion, because we do not yet know of any mechanisms that selectively and predictably redirect blood flow to the medulla. In order to return blood flow to normal or simply increase it, one must understand the three major determinants of renal blood flow: (1) cardiac output, (2) intravascular volume, and (3) renal perfusion pressure.

Cardiac Output

In the normal human, increasing cardiac output increases renal blood flow and decreasing cardiac output decreases renal blood flow. When these oscillations are within the normal cardiac output range, autoregulatory mechanisms come into play that minimize such fluctuations in renal perfusion. When the cardiac output falls below normal levels, however, the kidney is unable to compensate, renal blood flow decreases, and renal dysfunction occurs. In critically ill patients with prerenal acute renal dysfunction, it is therefore important to maintain a normal cardiac output. This support of the cardiac output may simply require intravenous fluid administration in some cases or, in others, it may require the full gamut of cardiovascular support including continuous infusion of inotropic drugs, insertion of an intra-aortic balloon counterpulsation device, or application of a ventricular assist device.

Despite these physiologic considerations, there has never been any randomized controlled study comparing a given level of cardiac output support to another (i.e., normal vs. supranormal) in critically ill patients with pre-renal renal dysfunction.

Intravascular Fluid Expansion

A large body of experimental data,[12] as well as some controlled data for humans,[13] supports the concept that intravascular fluid expansion with sodium-containing solutions protects the kidney at risk for prerenal renal failure. It is likely that the mechanisms of protection under these circumstances involve the maintenance of or an increase in renal blood flow. Because of the importance of adequate intravascular fluid resuscitation, it is therefore mandatory to monitor the state of intravascular fluid repletion with great care in patients with prerenal renal dysfunction. In many critically ill patients, this involves invasive monitoring of the right atrial pressure and, in a large proportion, even more aggressive forms of invasive monitoring such as measurement of the pulmonary arterial occlusion pressure with a standard right heart catheter and measurement of the right ventricular end-diastolic volume by means of a fast-response thermistor right heart catheter.

At this time, the effect of fluid resuscitation in the prevention of renal injury before an ischemic insult is sustained by controlled evidence. No data, however, are available to indicate that a certain degree of intravascular filling (right atrial pressure $>$ 15 mm Hg, for instance) is more protective to the kidney with early prerenal dysfunction than a lesser degree of intravascular filling (right atrial pressure $>$ 10 mm Hg and $<$ 12 mm Hg). Clinical judgment, therefore, continues to play a major part in the management of fluid therapy in patients with prerenal ARF.

Renal Perfusion Pressure

Although, in general, there is strong awareness among clinicians of the need to provide adequate fluid resuscitation and maintain a normal or increased cardiac output in patients with signs of early prerenal renal dysfunction, the impact of hypotension on renal blood flow is less commonly emphasized.[14] This lack of emphasis is unfortunate because maintenance of an adequate renal perfusion pressure (RPP) is paramount in maintaining renal blood flow, as in the following equation:

$$\text{RPP} = \text{mean arterial blood pressure} - \text{interstitial renal pressure}$$

The kidney, like other end-organs, autoregulates its own blood flow within set boundaries despite changes in arterial blood pressure. For instance, if the blood pressure decreases somewhat, as would happen on standing from a lying position, a number of compensatory mechanisms are set into motion to maintain renal blood flow and GFR. Equally, if the blood pressure rises, reflexes are induced that trigger changes in blood vessel tone. Such changes, in turn, decrease GFR and renal blood flow toward normal. In this range of blood pressures, the kidney is said to be operating within its "autoregulation plateau"[15] (Fig. 153–3). When the fall in blood pressure exceeds this compensatory mechanism, however, there is a rapid decrease in GFR and renal blood flow (see Fig. 153–3). It is not widely appreciated that, in the normal mammalian kidney, such loss of autoregulation of renal blood flow generally occurs at a mean blood pressure of 75 to 80 mm Hg and that the loss of GFR autoregulation occurs at a mean arterial blood pressure of approximately 80 to 85 mm Hg.[16, 17] In states of long-standing hypertension or intense vasoconstriction (such as sepsis), autoregulation may fail at even higher mean arterial blood pressures. Once acute renal failure has developed, autoregulation may even be lost altogether.[18] In addition, if the backup pressure to renal perfusion is increased[19] (organ edema or, more important, states of increased intra-abdominal pressure), major decreases in renal blood flow are likely to occur even with a mean arterial pressure above 85 to 90 mm Hg.

In light of this knowledge, once cardiac output has been restored and intravascular filling has been optimized, the blood pressure must be attended to and maintained within the

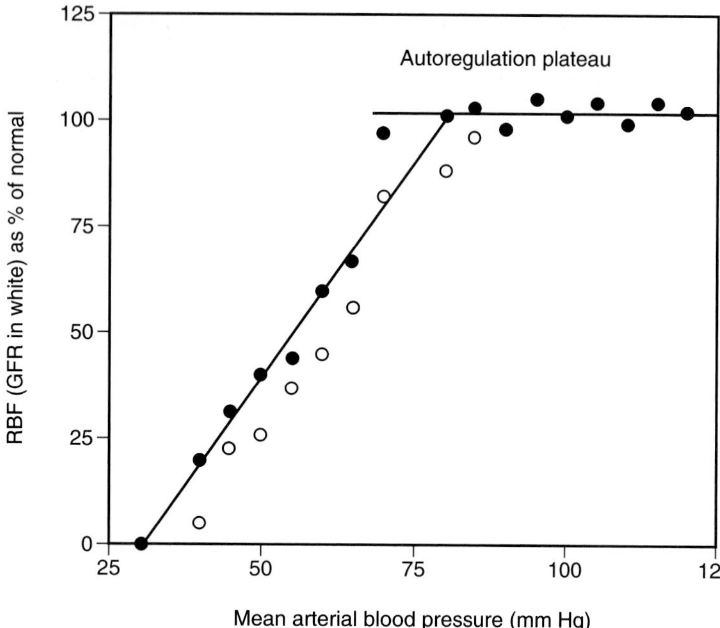

Figure 153–3. Diagram summarizing the pressure/flow relationship for the mammalian kidney. Once the mean arterial blood pressure falls below 75 to 80 mm Hg, renal blood flow rapidly decreases, so that even at a mean blood pressure of approximately 60 mm Hg, renal blood flow is a little more than 50% of its normal value.

autoregulation range if one is to avoid hypotension-induced medullary hypoxia. In the first instance, the correction of hypotension is often achieved with the administration of intravenous fluids. In many critically ill patients, however, particularly those with hyperdynamic septic shock, once optimal intravascular filling has been achieved, the mean arterial blood pressure may still remain low despite the presence of a high cardiac output. In most of these patients with hyperdynamic septic shock, there is evidence of persistent prerenal renal dysfunction. Such renal dysfunction is likely to be, in part, sustained by inadequate renal perfusion pressure. Correction of this hypotensive state with vasopressor agents such as norepinephrine has been shown to improve renal function and protect the kidney from further injury.[20, 21] There are no controlled studies to tell us whether a strategy aimed at maintaining a given mean arterial blood pressure (85 to 90 mm Hg) in hyperdynamic septic shock would protect the kidney more effectively than one that accepted a lower mean systemic pressure (70 to 75 mm Hg).

Because an imbalance between medullary oxygen supply and demand is likely to be the initial mechanism of prerenal ARF, there is a biologic rationale not only for increasing renal blood flow but also for administering drugs that decrease medullary oxygen consumption. Loop diuretics, by blocking solute resorption in the loop of Henle, significantly decrease medullary oxygen consumption and should protect the kidney from further injury. Ex vivo experiments and animal studies[22, 23] clearly support the concept that loop diuretics protect kidneys exposed to ischemic injury. Human studies of sufficient statistical power, however, have not been conducted to show whether these benefits translate into clinically important advantages.[24-26] Thus, the role of loop diuretics in the prevention of renal injury remains uncertain.

DRUGS USED FOR RENAL PROTECTION

Over the years, several drugs have been proposed as having a beneficial effect on the kidney suffering from prerenal injury (Table 153–1). The most common approach with these drugs is probably the continuous infusion of so-called low-dose dopamine (2 μg/kg/min). At this dose, dopamine has been shown to increase renal blood flow in the normal mammalian kidney.[12] Its action on renal blood flow is believed to be secondary to selective stimulation of dopaminergic receptors in the kidney, resulting in renal vasodilatation. In addition, dopamine has been demonstrated to be a proximal tubular diuretic. Thus, its administration can be expected to increase urine output independent of any effect on renal perfusion. Despite many years of clinical use of dopamine, it remains highly controversial[27] whether it does indeed induce a degree of renal protection in patients at risk for or experiencing a prerenal insult. Randomized controlled studies of selected populations[28-30] have so far failed to show any benefit. Such trials, however, have been hindered by lack of statistical power. A small crossover study[31] has even suggested that low-dose dobutamine improves creatinine clearance in critically ill patients whereas low-dose dopamine does not. A large study with sufficient power is necessary to gain a better understanding of the role of this drug in critically ill patients.

Mannitol has also been used for the purpose of renal protection, particularly in surgical patients about to experience a prerenal renal insult. The biologic rationale for its administration is related to its ability to induce diuresis, decrease cell swelling, scavenge free radicals, and induce intrarenal prostaglandin production and vasodilatation.[12] There are currently no controlled animal or human studies to support its use, however, and a randomized controlled study of patients receiving a radiocontrast agent demonstrated an increase in renal injury with its administration.[13] Mannitol cannot be currently recommended for renal protection in humans.

Calcium antagonists have been shown to protect the kidney from ischemic injury ex vivo and in animal experiments.[32] Their protective action is thought to be secondary to blockage of calcium influx during or after ischemic injury. Because calcium influx is one of the major mechanisms of cell damage during postischemic reperfusion, prevention of such influx can be expected to decrease tubular damage. Ex vivo studies and animal studies support a protective role for these agents during prerenal insults. Their effectiveness in humans has been shown in the context of renal transplantation, in which calcium antagonists appear to decrease the incidence and severity of post-transplantation acute tubular necrosis.[33, 34] For critically ill patients with multiple organ failure and severe

TABLE 153–1. Type and Level of Evidence Supporting the Use of Various Drugs for Renal Protection

Drug	Biologic Rationale	Ex Vivo Studies	Animal Studies	Uncontrolled Human Data	Positive Random Controlled Trial in Humans	Level of Evidence
Dopamine	Yes	No	Yes	Yes	No	II-III
Dobutamine	Yes	No	No	Yes	No	III
Norepinephrine	Yes	No	No	Yes	No	II-III
Furosemide	Yes	Yes	Yes	Yes	No	III
Mannitol	Yes	Yes	Yes	Yes	No	III
Prostaglandins	Yes	Yes	Yes	Yes	No	III
Atrial natriuretic peptide analogs	Yes	Yes	Yes	Yes	No	III
Theophylline	Yes	No	Yes	Yes	No	III
Sodium loading	Yes	No	Yes	Yes	No	III

sepsis or septic shock, the administration of these agents, which induce significant hypotension, cannot be recommended because the risks (refractory hypotension) are likely to be greater than the benefits.

Adenosine antagonists may have a role in protecting the kidney from ischemia. Their mechanism of action would be based on counteracting the exaggerated tubuloglomerular feedback response triggered by medullary ischemia. Such a TGF response, although initially beneficial and protective, may sustain oliguria or anuria unnecessarily once adequate hemodynamic resuscitation has been accomplished. Theophylline (a competitive adenosine receptor antagonist) administered at low doses by continuous infusion has, in fact, been shown to be protective in animal models of renal ischemia.[35, 36] Controlled human studies have yet to be performed to determine whether this drug is effective in the clinical arena.

Prostaglandins are major regulators of intrarenal blood flow distribution and participate in the autoregulation of renal blood flow. Their inhibition with nonsteroidal anti-inflammatory drugs in patients with precarious renal perfusion can result in the development of ARF. Several animal experiments support the concept that prostaglandin E_2 (PGE_2) administration plays a protective role during renal ischemia.[37] Unfortunately, no randomized controlled studies have been performed in humans to determine whether there is a clinically significant beneficial effect.

Atrial natriuretic peptide (ANP) potentially has clinically important beneficial effects on the human kidney. It may increase renal blood flow, and it clearly increases glomerular ultrafiltration and induces afferent arteriolar vasodilatation. Ex vivo and animal studies indeed suggest that ANP or ANP analogs are protective during experimental ARF.[38] These protective effects, however, have to be weighed against the systemic hypotensive effects of ANP. It may, therefore, be necessary to administer this agent with concomitant vasopressor support.

A multicenter, placebo-controlled randomized trial with sufficient power of anaritide, an ANP analog, in patients with acute tubular necrosis has shown no overall benefit in the prevention of dialysis-requiring renal failure.[39] Subgroup analysis, however, suggested a benefit in patients with oliguria (urine output < 400 mL/day) at the time of administration. Further studies are needed and may demonstrate a role for this agent in the prevention of ARF.

Experimental work has also shown the presence of an intrarenal ANP analog. This substance, called urodilatin, has been shown to induce renal vasodilatation and to be protective in animal models of renal ischemia.[40] Pilot human studies are under way to define the role of this agent in the protection of the ischemic kidney.

Stimulation of renal α receptors can be demonstrated to occur in stress states and to induce a decrease in GFR. Prevention of such vasoconstriction in patients known to be at risk of renal injury may be protective to the kidney. Clonidine, a central α-receptor antagonist, may attenuate such vasoconstriction and has been administered before surgery to patients undergoing cardiopulmonary bypass.[41] Preliminary results suggest that clonidine may have a beneficial role in this setting. In this preliminary trial, however, patients receiving placebo had a longer time on bypass, so it is not yet clear what the role of clonidine is in this setting.

The peptide endothelin is released during endotoxemia, hypoxia, or exposure to nephrotoxins and appears to lead to strong renal vasoconstriction. It is likely to have an important role in the pathogenesis of ARF. Initial experimental studies using antiendothelin antibodies and endothelin receptor antagonists have already demonstrated that blocking the action of endothelin has a beneficial effect on the ischemic kidney.[42, 43] It is likely that human studies using endothelin antagonists will be performed in the near future.

SUMMARY

Prevention of ARF caused by prerenal factors is one of the major therapeutic goals the critical care physician faces in his or her everyday practice. Such prevention rests upon the principle that outer medullary ischemia should be avoided or attenuated. This goal can be rationally achieved by rapidly and aggressively correcting hemodynamic imbalances and promptly restoring cardiac output, intravascular filling, and arterial blood pressure to adequate levels. Such restoration may require invasive hemodynamic monitoring and the use of inotropic or vasopressor drugs. Once such measures have been undertaken, a number of pharmaceutical agents have been proposed for the purpose of protecting the kidney. None of these agents can be recommended on the basis of the available scientific evidence (see Table 153-1). Several new agents, however, show promise in the area of renal protection, and evidence from randomized controlled trials of sufficient statistical power is being gathered to support or counter their use in critically ill patients.

References

1. Lins RL, Chew SL, Daelemans R: Epidemiology of acute renal failure. *In*: Acute Renal Failure in the Critically Ill. Bellomo R, Ronco C (Eds). Berlin, Springer-Verlag, 1995, pp 147–159.
2. Feest TG, Round A: Incidence of severe acute renal failure in adults: Results of a community based study. BMJ 1993; 306:481–483.
3. Brezis M, Epstein FH: Pathophysiology of acute renal failure. *In*: Toxicology of the Kidney. 2nd ed. Hook JB, Goldstein RS (Eds). New York, Raven, 1993, pp 129–152.
4. Brezis M, Rosen S, Spokes K, et al: Substrates induce hypoxic

injury to medullary thick limbs of isolated rat kidneys. Am J Physiol 1986; 251:F710–F717.
5. Brezis M, Rosen S, Silva P, et al: Selective vulnerability of the medullary thick ascending limb to anoxia in isolated perfused rat kidney. J Clin Invest 1984; 73:182–190.
6. Heyman SH, Fuchs S, Brezis M: The role of medullary ischemia in acute renal failure. New Horiz 1995; 3:597–607.
7. Osswald H, Muhlbauer B, Schenk F: Adenosine mediates tubuloglomerular feedback response: An element of metabolic control of kidney function. Kidney Int 1991; 39:S128–S131.
8. Epstein FH: Oxygen and renal metabolism. Kidney Int 1997; 51:381–385.
9. Thurau K, Boylan JW: Acute renal success: The unexpected logic of oliguria in renal failure. Am J Med 1976; 61:308–315.
10. Schurek H-J, Johns O: Is tubuloglomerular feedback a tool to prevent nephron oxygen deficiency? Kidney Int 1997; 51:386–392.
11. Badr KF, Kelley VE, Rennke HG, et al: Roles of thromboxane A_2 and leukotrienes in endotoxin-induced acute renal failure. Kidney Int 1986; 30:474–480.
12. Bersten AD, Holt AW: Prevention of acute renal failure in the critically ill patient. *In*: Acute Renal Failure in the Critically Ill. Bellomo R, Ronco C (Eds). Berlin, Springer-Verlag, 1995, pp 122–146.
13. Solomon R, Werner C, Mann D, D'Elia J, Silva P: Effects of saline, mannitol, and furosemide on acute decreases in renal function induced by radiocontrast agents. N Engl J Med 1994; 331:1416–1420.
14. Bersten AD, Holt AW: Vasoactive drugs and the importance of renal perfusion pressure. New Horiz 1995; 3:650–661.
15. Knox FG, Spielman WS: Renal circulation. *In*: Handbook of Physiology. Sect 2. The Cardiovascular System. Vol III. Sheppard JT, Abboud FM (Eds). Bethesda, Md, American Physiological Society, 1983, pp 183–217.
16. Shipley RE, Study RS: Changes in renal blood flow, extraction of inulin, glomerular filtration rate, tissue pressure, and urine flow with acute alterations in renal artery pressure. Am J Physiol 1951; 167:676–688.
17. Schmid HE, Garrett RC, Spencer MP: Intrinsic hemodynamic adjustments to reduced renal pressure gradients. Circ Res 1964; 14(Suppl I):170–177.
18. Kelleher SP, Robinette JB, Conger JD: Sympathetic nervous system in the loss of autoregulation in acute renal failure. Am J Physiol 1984; 246:F379–F386.
19. Kron IL, Harman PK, Nolan SP: The measurement of intra-abdominal blood pressure as a criterion for abdominal re-exploration. Ann Surg 1984; 199:28–30.
20. Martin C, Papazian L, Perrin G, et al: Norepinephrine or dopamine for the treatment of septic shock. Chest 1993; 103:1826–1831.
21. Redl-Wenzel EM, Armbruster C, Edelmann G, et al: The effects of norepinephrine on hemodynamics and renal function in severe septic shock states. Intensive Care Med 1993; 19:151–154.
22. Brezis M, Rosen S, Silva P, Epstein FH: Transport activity modifies thick ascending limb damage in the isolated perfused kidney. Kidney Int 1984; 25:65–72.
23. Hanley MJ, Davidson K: Prior mannitol and furosemide infusion in a model of ischemic acute renal failure. Am J Physiol 1981; 241:F556–F564.
24. Kleinknecht D, Ganeval D, Gozalez-Duque LA, et al: Furosemide in acute renal failure: A controlled trial. Nephron 1976; 17:51–58.
25. Brown CB, Ogg CS, Cameron JS: High dose furosemide in acute renal failure: A controlled trial. Clin Nephrol 1981; 15:90–96.
26. Lucas CE, Zito JG, Carter KM, et al: Questionable value of furosemide in preventing renal failure. Surgery 1977; 82:314–320.
27. Thompson BT, Cockrill BA: Renal-dose dopamine: A siren song? Lancet 1994; 344:7–8.
28. Baldwin L, Henderson A, Hickman P: Effect of postoperative low-dose dopamine on renal function after elective major vascular surgery. Ann Intern Med 1994; 120:744–747.
29. Swygert TH, Roberts LC, Valek TR, et al: Effect of intraoperative low-dose dopamine on renal function in liver transplant patients. Anesthesiology 1991; 75:571–576.
30. Myles PS, Buckland MR, Schenk NJ, et al: Effect of renal dose dopamine on renal function following cardiac surgery. Anaesth Intensive Care 1993; 21:56–61.
31. Duke GJ, Briedis JH, Weaver RA: Renal support in critically ill: Low-dose dopamine or low-dose dobutamine? Crit Care Med 1994; 22:1919–1925.
32. Schrier RW, Arnold PE, Van Putten VJ, et al: Cellular calcium in ischemic acute renal failure: Role of calcium entry blockers. Kidney Int 1987; 32:313–321.
33. Duggan KA, Macdonald GJ, Charlesworth JA, et al: Verapamil prevents post transplant oliguric renal failure. Clin Nephrol 1985; 24:289–291.
34. Wagner K, Albrecht S, Neumayer HH: Prevention of post transplant acute tubular necrosis by the calcium antagonist diltiazem: A prospective randomized study. Am J Nephrol 1987; 7:287–291.
35. Gouyon G-B, Guignard J-P: Theophylline prevents the hypoxemia-induced renal hemodynamic changes in rabbits. Kidney Int 1988; 33:1078–1083.
36. Oken DE, Reilly KM: Total prevention of glycerol-induced acute renal failure with adenosine-receptor blockade. Kidney Int 1989; 35:415–419.
37. Paller MS, Manivel JC: Prostaglandins protect kidneys against ischemic and toxic injury by a cellular effect. Kidney Int 1992; 42:1345–1354.
38. Weinmann M: Natriuretic peptides and acute renal failure. New Horiz 1995; 3:624–633.
39. Allgren RL, Marbury TC, Rahman SN, et al: Anaritide in acute tubular necrosis. N Engl J Med 1997; 336:828–834.
40. Endlich K, Forssmann W-G, Steinhausen M: Effects of urodilatin in the rat kidney: Comparison with ANF and interaction with vasoactive substances. Kidney Int 1995; 47:1558–1568.
41. Kulka PJ, Tryba M, Zenz M: Preoperative $alpha_2$-adrenergic receptor agonists prevent the deterioration of renal function after cardiac surgery: Results of a randomized controlled trial. Crit Care Med 1996; 24:947–952.
42. Kon V, Badr KF: Biological actions and pathophysiologic significance of endothelin in the kidney. Kidney Int 1991; 40:1–12.
43. Mino N, Kobayashi M, Nakajima, et al: Protective effect of a selective endothelin receptor antagonist, BQ-123, in ischemic acute renal failure in rats. Eur J Pharmacol 1992; 221:77–83.

154

Adult Acute and Chronic Renal Failure

Todd W. B. Gehr, MD • Anton C. Schoolwerth, MD, MSHA

Acute renal failure (ARF) describes any abrupt and almost complete cessation of renal function. Chronic renal insufficiency (CRI) describes the irreversible reduction in renal function that is usually progressive in nature and ultimately leads to chronic renal failure (CRF). End-stage renal disease (ESRD) is applied to the patient with CRF who also requires some type of renal replacement therapy (e.g., dialysis or renal transplantation). Although ARF is more relevant to critical care, patients with CRI, dialysis patients, and renal transplant patients all present with unique critical care requirements.

Renal hypoperfusion resulting in functional or prerenal renal failure, urinary tract obstruction, and acute renal parenchymal damage produce characteristic responses that form the basis of diagnostic and therapeutic approaches. It is customary to refer to acute renal parenchymal failure in mechanistic terms (acute tubular necrosis, vasomotor nephropathy), although these terms are not entirely accurate.[1] Some of the confusion in terminology is due to the fact that ARF has a variety of causes, the most common of which are listed in Table 154–1. ARF and CRF are discussed in general terms;

TABLE 154–1. Causes of Renal Failure

1. *Glomerulopathy* (especially necrotizing, proliferative, membranoproliferative, rapidly progressive)
   - Streptococcal or other bacterial infection
   - Viral infection
   - Lupus erythematosus
   - Goodpasture's syndrome
   - Eclampsia
   - Mixed cryoglobulinemia
2. *Vascular and thrombotic disease*
   - Malignant hypertension
   - Wegener's granulomatosis
   - Hypersensitivity angiitis
   - Periarteritis nodosa
   - Thrombotic thrombocytopenic purpura
   - Hemolytic-uremic syndrome (cyclosporine, tacrolimus, mitomycin, cocaine, quinine, conjugated estrogen)
   - Postpartum acute renal failure
   - Disseminated intravascular coagulation (cortical necrosis)
   - Scleroderma
   - Acute allograft rejection
   - Fat or cholesterol embolism
   - Renal venous-vena caval thrombosis
   - Post-traumatic renal arterial thrombosis or avulsion
   - Aortic coarctation, dissection, or thrombosis
   - Renal artery dysplasia
3. *Interstitial disease*
   - Allergic (penicillins, cephalosporins, sulfonamides, rifampin, NSAIDs, thiazides, furosemide, cimetidine, phenytoin, allopurinol, ciprofloxacin), postinfectious, or idiosyncratic interstitial nephritis
   - Fulminating pyelonephritis (infants)
   - Papillary necrosis
4. *Functional (pre)renal failure*
   - Severe volume depletion
   - Shock
   - Sepsis
   - Trauma
   - Heart failure
   - Alteration in renal hemodynamics (NSAIDs, angiotensin-converting enzyme inhibitors, cyclosporine, tacrolimus, interleukin-2, amphotericin B, radiocontrast agents)
5. *Acute renal parenchymal failure* (acute tubular necrosis, vasomotor nephropathy)
   - All causes of functional renal failure (e.g., nephrotic syndrome, sepsis, hemorrhage, vomiting, diarrhea, hypotension) if not adequately treated
   - Blunt trauma, burns, surgery, fractures
   - Intravascular hemolysis
   - Heat stroke
   - Malaria
   - Snake bite
   - Electric shock
   - Dissecting aneurysm (e.g., Marfan's, homocystinuria)
   - Septicemia
   - Rhabdomyolysis
   - Antibiotics (aminoglycosides, amphotericin B, pentamidine)
   - Mercury, bismuth, phosphorus, lead, carbon tetrachloride, ethylene gycol, methanol, mushrooms, Lysol
   - Methoxyflurane, cyclosporine, tacrolimus, intravenous immune globulin
   - Chemotherapeutic agents (cisplatin, methotrexate, foscarnet)
   - Uric acid
6. *Hepatorenal syndrome*
7. *Urinary obstruction*
   - Ureter, bladder, or urethra (due to inflammation, stone, blood clot, urate crystallization, tumor, retroperitoneal mass, hemorrhage or fibrosis)
   - Intratubular obstruction (acyclovir, sulfonamides, oxalate and uric acid crystals)
8. *Bladder rupture*

NSAIDs = nonsteroidal anti-inflammatory drugs.

urinary tract obstruction and five specific ARF causes that are particularly germane to critical care are discussed in detail. These include ARF associated with cardiac failure and sepsis, interstitial nephritis, hepatorenal syndrome, myoglobinuric ARF (rhabdomyolysis), and pulmonary-renal syndromes.

ACUTE RENAL FAILURE

Clinical Presentation

ARF is commonly induced by shock, sepsis, or trauma and is characterized by an abrupt decrease in the glomerular filtration rate (GFR). Oliguria (defined as a urine output below 400 mL/day) is typical,[2] although nonoliguric ARF is increasingly common.[3] Whether oliguria is present or not, the urine volume is constant from day to day and, once renal failure is fully developed, usually does not increase significantly even when large dose of diuretics are administered. However, the urine output may decrease in parallel with blood pressure and cardiac output if the patient is intermittently hypotensive.

The GFR remains fixed at a low level up to the time of recovery. As a result, the serum creatinine concentration rises steadily by 1 to 4 mg/dL per day. It would be atypical for the serum creatinine concentration to rise 2 mg/dL on the first day, fall slightly on the next, and then rise 0.5 mg/dL during the next day. Such behavior is, however, common in ARF secondary to functional (prerenal) renal failure and in urinary outflow obstruction.

Although renal failure may last 3 or 4 weeks in a few patients, renal function usually begins to improve after 10 to 12 days.[2] In general, nonoliguric renal failure is of significantly shorter duration than oliguric renal failure, often lasting only 5 to 6 days.[3] In both, recovery is heralded by an initially small increase in urine volume that rises on successive days to reach 1 to 2 L/day or more. Massive diuresis of 3 to 5 L/day during the recovery period is no longer common, probably because aggressive dialysis now prevents the severe fluid overload and high blood urea nitrogen (BUN) concentration that were commonplace in the predialysis era.

Total anuria is so atypical of uncomplicated ARF that its presence for more than 2 or 3 days in a hemodynamically stable patient should prompt consideration of urinary outflow obstruction, compromise of the major renal vessels, renal cortical necrosis, glomerular or small-vessel disease, or ruptured bladder as a possible cause.

Symptoms associated with urinary outflow obstruction may be insidious and often depend on the acuteness of the obstruction. When ARF occurs, pain localized to the flank and costovertebral angle that may be referred to the groin or genital area is common. Pain is an exception when the obstruction is chronic, however. Associated symptoms may include hypertension, sepsis, and gastrointestinal symptoms. Both symptoms and ARF are rapidly alleviated when the obstruction is corrected. If the obstruction is of a chronic nature, recovery of renal function will depend on the extent of permanent renal parenchymal damage. In either case, a postobstructive diuresis may ensue owing to an inability of the kidney to concentrate the urine (nephrogenic diabetes insipidus).

Etiology

ARF occurs most commonly in a setting of surgery, trauma, sepsis, hypotension, hemolytic reaction, or poisoning. Unfortunately, a number of these predisposing factors may be present concomitantly in critically ill patients.

Once common, obstetric complications (such as intrapartum and postpartum hemorrhage, placenta previa, and abruptio placentae) still produce ARF in a small but significant number of patients. Septic abortion, especially when it is attended by clostridial endometritis, is the leading cause of ARF in areas of the world where contraception and medically supervised abortion are not readily available.[4] Transfusion accidents, formerly a major contribution to the syndrome, likewise have become uncommon as blood banking techniques for the detection of ABO and Rh mismatch have improved. Hemolytic crises due to glucose 6-phosphate dehydrogenase deficiency[5] and paroxysmal nocturnal hemoglobinuria[6] are rare potential causes of the syndrome. Other uncommon causes associated with hemolysis include intra-amniotic infusions of hypertonic saline,[7] intracervical instillation of various solutions for self-induced abortions,[8] intravenous glycerol therapy for cerebral edema,[9] snakebite,[10] malarial blackwater fever,[11] and acute arsine poisoning.[12]

A variety of industrial and household chemicals may produce both severe acute illness and ARF. Carbon tetrachloride, ethylene glycol (antifreeze), methanol, trichloroethylene (dope solvent), toluene, paraquat, and chlordane have been among the most commonly incriminated culprits in the past but appear to have become less common offenders since their dangers have become widely known. Industrial exposure to these compounds and certain heavy metals (especially mercury and lead) is still a problem. Some poisons exert a direct nephrotoxic effect; others, such as *Amanita* mushroom and carbon tetrachloride poisoning, cause ARF as the result of severe volume depletion and cardiovascular collapse.[13, 14]

Antibiotics, particularly the aminoglycoside antibiotics, continue to be a frequent cause of ARF. With the exception of streptomycin, aminoglycoside antibiotics are universally nephrotoxic when they are given in sufficiently high doses for an extended time. These agents are excreted almost exclusively by the kidney, predominantly through glomerular filtration, and have a relatively low therapeutic index. Their dosage must be carefully adjusted in the setting of renal insufficiency. The half-life of gentamicin in serum of normal human subjects is approximately 2 hours, whereas that in renal tissue of the same individuals is about 4 days.[15] The concentration of the drug in renal tissue thus increases inexorably with each injection. With careful dosing, the tissue concentration usually does not reach a frankly toxic level during a typical 5- to 7-day course of treatment, although small changes in renal function may be seen even when the peak and trough concentrations of these antibiotics have been consistently in the acceptable range.[16] The potential for nephrotoxicity seems to be about the same with gentamicin and amikacin, but it may be less with tobramicin, which has a distinctly lower rate of tissue accumulation.[17] Nevertheless, tobramicin is still a potent nephrotoxin and must be used with the same dosing precautions as for gentamicin and amikacin.

The degree of renal functional impairment produced by the aminoglycoside antibiotics ranges from mild renal insufficiency, with a maximum serum creatinine concentration of perhaps 1.5 to 3 mg/dL, to frank renal failure that is indistinguishable from typical ARF. Even if it is not certain that mild renal insufficiency in hemodynamically unstable patients is caused by aminoglycoside toxicity, further use of these agents before the full return of renal function should be avoided if possible. On the other hand, dialysis is far preferable to fatal sepsis. In general, the incidence or severity of aminoglycoside nephrotoxicity can be minimized by carefully limiting the duration of antibiotic therapy, adjusting the dose according to the patient's renal function, and maintaining adequate volume throughout the treatment period. In most cases, alternative antibiotics can be safely employed.

Another commonly used antibiotic, amphotericin, also inevitably causes renal damage. As with aminoglycosides, the occurrence of renal dysfunction is dose dependent, with cumulative doses of 2 to 3 g being necessary before important toxicity occurs.[18] Hypokalemia, hypomagnesemia, and renal acidification and concentrating defects commonly precede reductions in GFR.[19]

ARF that follows the intravenous administration of radiographic contrast agents ranges from mild nonoliguric reductions in GFR to irreversible renal failure. In normal subjects, the incidence is probably less than 2%.[20] Particularly in the intensive care unit (ICU) setting, predisposing risk factors lead to a much higher incidence. Preexisting renal insufficiency is probably the most important of these risk factors, but diabetes mellitus, multiple myeloma, intravascular volume depletion, the amount of contrast material used, age, and congestive heart failure are additional important risk factors.[21] The use of nonioidinated contrast materials may reduce the incidence of this serious complication, although studies to date do not suggest this.[22]

Finally, ARF is increasingly encountered in patients with hematologic malignant neoplasms and acquired immunodeficiency syndrome. The underlying illness may cause ARF either directly or indirectly; but more commonly, medications that are employed during therapy, such as cyclophosphamide, methotrexate, cisplatin, foscarnet, pentamidine, antibiotics, and immune globulin, lead to ARF.[23, 24]

Pathogenesis

The pathogenic mechanisms responsible for ARF have been the subject of debate ever since the syndrome first became widely recognized some 50 years ago. A number of mechanisms have been proposed to explain the cessation of glomerular filtration characteristic of this syndrome; these are based on a variety of animal models of ARF,[25] four of which are intratubular obstruction, tubular backleak of filtrate, filtration failure related to disturbed renal hemodynamics, and reduction in glomerular permeability.

Although these mechanisms explain the reduction in filtration, the predisposing cellular abnormalities have not been well characterized. Depletion of cellular adenosine triphosphate (ATP), the release of reactive oxygen species, the role of complement activation, neutrophil infiltration, and the role of renal growth factors are currently being actively investigated.[26]

It is likely that no one mechanism explains this syndrome because measures aimed at preventing this syndrome (diuresis, vasodilators) invariably fail. In addition, the type of renal injury may be an important determinant of a particular mechanism. Combinations of mechanisms are probably necessary to explain the pathogenesis of this complex syndrome, although the renal tubule epithelial cell's susceptibility to ischemic injury may be central to our understanding.[27]

Differential Diagnosis

The diagnostic approach to a patient with reduced renal function is outlined in Figure 154–1. The approach should be used for all patients to avoid missing a potential reversible diagnosis. As shown, it is useful to determine the time course of the reduction in renal function, acute versus chronic, and then to categorize the cause of the renal failure as functional (prerenal), renal parenchymal, or urinary tract obstruction.

Acute Versus Chronic Renal Failure

On admission to the hospital, severely ill patients often have an elevated serum creatinine concentration, which may be recent (ARF) or long-standing (CRI). In the latter case, the patient may have been unaware of a kidney problem, because chronic renal disease usually does not produce obvious symptoms except when it is associated with renal colic, dysuria, gross hematuria, or anuria. Instead, renal disease may be discovered when the patient seeks medical care either for unrelated reasons or because of the dramatic and life-threatening complications that develop during ESRD.

Because ARF usually causes the serum creatinine concentration to increase about 1 to 3 mg/dL per day, a patient admitted for an acute illness of 1 or 2 days' duration who has a serum creatinine level of 10 to 12 mg/dL or more either has had ARF considerably longer than the history would suggest or has chronic renal disease that may have gone unrecognized. A *careful history* may be helpful in distinguishing between these possibilities. Most forms of ARF are associated with a sudden and marked reduction in urine volume that patients may not report unless they are specifically asked. By contrast, nocturia is an almost universal hallmark of chronic renal disease, and its absence or recent development strongly favors a relatively acute process. A long history of difficulties with

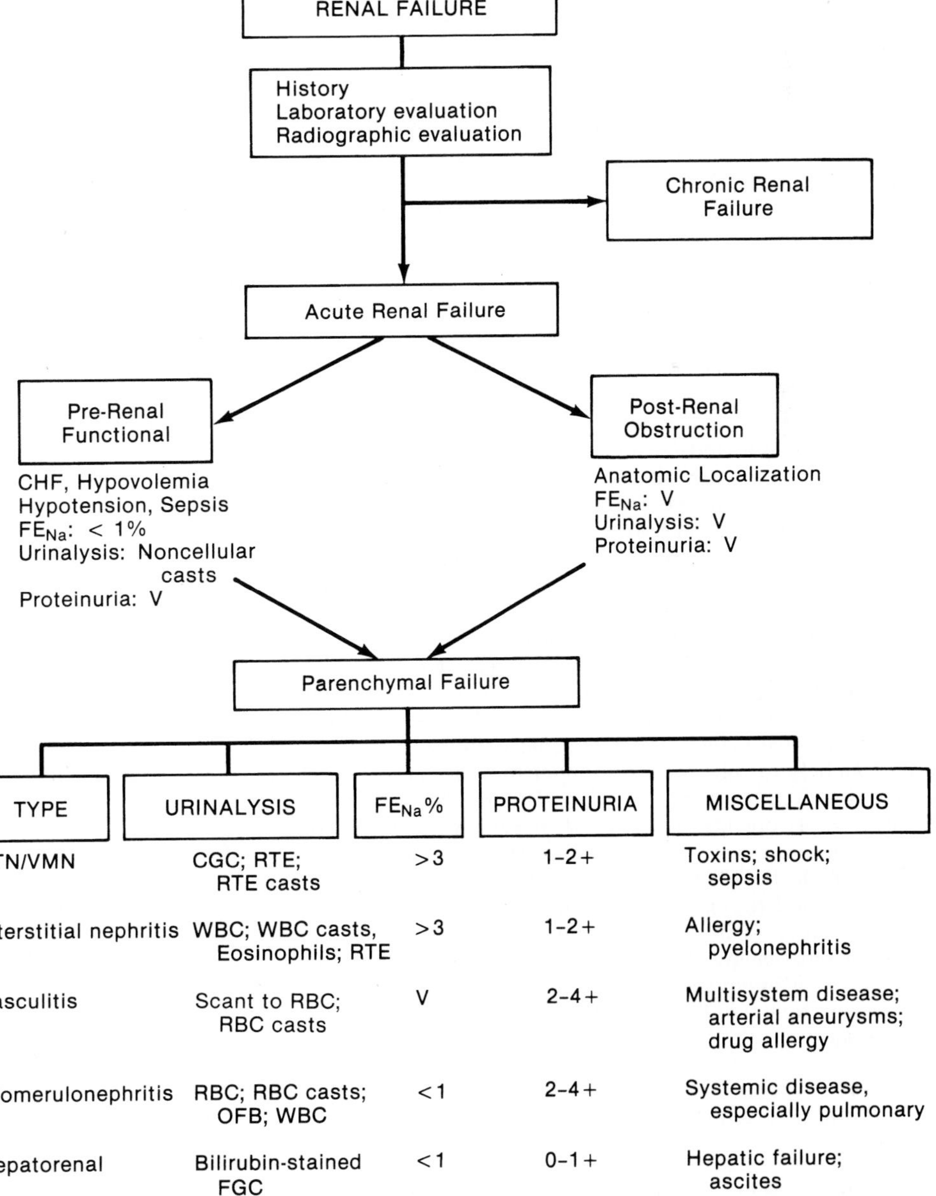

TYPE	URINALYSIS	FE_{Na}%	PROTEINURIA	MISCELLANEOUS
ATN/VMN	CGC; RTE; RTE casts	>3	1-2+	Toxins; shock; sepsis
Interstitial nephritis	WBC; WBC casts, Eosinophils; RTE	>3	1-2+	Allergy; pyelonephritis
Vasculitis	Scant to RBC; RBC casts	V	2-4+	Multisystem disease; arterial aneurysms; drug allergy
Glomerulonephritis	RBC; RBC casts; OFB; WBC	<1	2-4+	Systemic disease, especially pulmonary
Hepatorenal	Bilirubin-stained FGC	<1	0-1+	Hepatic failure; ascites

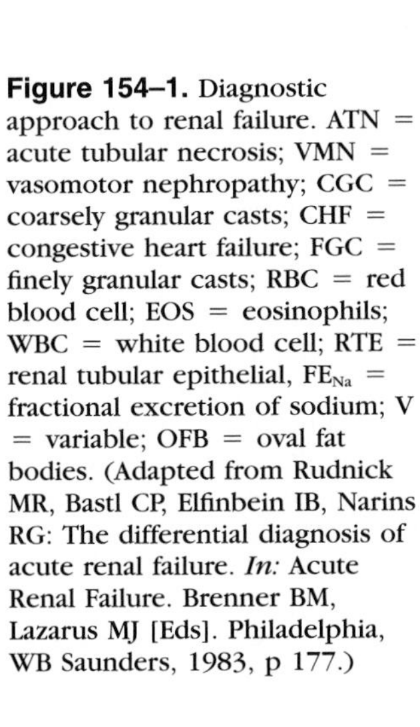

Figure 154–1. Diagnostic approach to renal failure. ATN = acute tubular necrosis; VMN = vasomotor nephropathy; CGC = coarsely granular casts; CHF = congestive heart failure; FGC = finely granular casts; RBC = red blood cell; EOS = eosinophils; WBC = white blood cell; RTE = renal tubular epithelial, FE_{Na} = fractional excretion of sodium; V = variable; OFB = oval fat bodies. (Adapted from Rudnick MR, Bastl CP, Elfinbein IB, Narins RG: The differential diagnosis of acute renal failure. *In:* Acute Renal Failure. Brenner BM, Lazarus MJ [Eds]. Philadelphia, WB Saunders, 1983, p 177.)

micturition (e.g., hesitancy, urgency, dribbling, or incontinence in particular) suggests chronic bladder outflow obstruction as the cause of renal dysfunction. Suggestive of chronic renal involvement are a history of any form of renal disease, proteinuria, or abnormal urinary sediment; repeated bouts of dysuria and other symptoms of pyelonephritis; long-standing and severe hypertension; prior abdominal or pelvic irradiation for the treatment of malignant disease; diabetes of many years' duration or other systemic diseases that commonly cause CRF; repeated passage of renal stones; chronic analgesic ingestion; and family history of polycystic kidney disease, Alport's syndrome, or other hereditary renal disease.

On physical examination, patients with CRF frequently display a highly characteristic, yellow-tan, sallow coloration of the skin that is not found in the acutely uremic patient. Although pruritus is often an extremely bothersome symptom in ARF as well as in CRF, the association of both old and new pruritic excoriations of the skin is an unmistakable sign of chronicity. Symptomatic renal osteodystrophy with pain and difficulty in walking are hallmarks of chronic, but not of acute, renal failure. Nerve deafness or keratoconus may indicate CRF due to Alport's syndrome, and large cystic kidneys found on abdominal palpation provide almost prima facie evidence of polycystic kidney disease. A lax rectal sphincter and perianal anesthesia are hallmarks of a neurogenic bladder; a palpable bladder or an impaired ability to initiate or sustain urination suggests bladder outflow problems. Marked prostatic enlargement in men, cervical or pelvic malignant neoplasms in women, or a rectal mass in a patient of either sex may be clues to the existence and cause of chronic obstructive uropathy.

Few laboratory determinations are helpful in distinguishing ARF from CRF, although normocytic, normochromic anemia, when the serum creatinine concentration has not yet reached 6 mg/dL, favors a chronic process. The serum electrolyte profile can be equally abnormal in the two conditions. ARF frequently causes a rapid depression of calcium concentration and an increase in phosphorus concentration comparable to that found in CRF, and acidosis may be severe in acutely ill, hypercatabolic patients early in the course of ARF. Urinary sodium, potassium, and creatinine concentrations are usually indistinguishable in the two conditions; urine concentrating capacity is equally affected and the fraction of filtered sodium excreted (FE_{Na}) is high in both.

An abdominal radiograph or ultrasound examination can be helpful. First, the kidney typically is notably enlarged 2 days or more after the onset of ARF and usually has normal echogenicity, whereas most forms of CRF result in small, abnormally echogenic kidneys. Both maneuvers can detect nephrocalcinosis and staghorn calculi found in some forms of CRF as well as ureteral stones that might be the cause of acute obstructive renal failure. The ultrasonic examination is now used routinely to rule out acute upper urinary tract obstruction.[28] However, the typical hydronephrotic dilatation of the renal pelvis is not invariably found in patients with proven acute upper tract obstruction.[29] Therefore, the ultrasound procedure should be followed by direct urologic assessment by cystoscopy and retrograde pyelography when obstruction is strongly suspected in a patient with no obvious alternative cause for renal failure. X-ray studies of the outer clavicle and hands can document the presence of osteomalacia and other changes of long-standing hyperparathyroidism that are not seen in ARF.

ARF Due to Renal Parenchymal Failure Versus Functional (Prerenal) Renal Failure

Severe volume depletion reduces both GFR and renal blood flow. The assessment of volume status is the first step in differentiating the cause of ARF. This important subject is covered in detail in Chapter 153.

The accurate assessment of urine volume is of obvious importance in the evaluation of ARF. Anuria refers to the most severe reduction of urine volume and includes volumes of 100 mL/day or less. Oliguria describes a reduction of urine volume to 100 to 400 mL/day. In the past, polyuria described urine volumes of greater than 400 mL/day in the setting of ARF, but the term nonoliguria is often applied instead to the ARF patient with urine volumes between 400 mL and 2 L/day. Polyuria is now applied to the patient with greater than 3 L/day.

Anuria may result from complete urinary tract obstruction, bilateral cortical necrosis, acute glomerulonephritis or vasculitis, or bilateral renal arterial or venous occlusion. The presence of alternating anuria and polyuria is strongly suggestive of intermittent urinary tract obstruction. Although most cases of ARF result in oliguria, anuria is more common than was once thought. Whereas transient episodes of reversible anuria lasting up to 6 hours can occur with hypotension and dehydration, sustained anuria argues against the presence of functional renal failure.

Oliguria may occur with any type of ARF. When oliguria accompanies functional renal failure, the urine is concentrated and has a low sodium content. With usual solute loads of 500 to 600 mOsm/day and normal urinary concentrating ability of 1200 mOsm/L, a urine volume of 400 to 500 mL is necessary to maintain solute balance. Therefore, a urine volume of less than 400 to 500 mL/day will result in the accumulation of excess solute (BUN, creatinine). In critically ill patients, the usual solute load may be increased dramatically owing to increased catabolism and parenterally administered nutrition. This large solute load may increase the obligatory urine volume to above 1 L/day, so even with nonoliguric or polyuric volumes, accumulation of excess solute may occur.

Otherwise normal subjects with purely functional renal failure excrete a concentrated urine that has a vanishingly low urine sodium concentration, a urine to plasma (U/P) creatinine ratio far higher than 20, a high urine osmolality, and a benign urinary sediment. The fractional excretion of sodium (FE_{Na}), defined in Chapter 152, is probably the best single indicator of renal function and is usually below 1%. There is no difficulty in separating such individuals from those with ARF on this basis alone (see Fig. 154–1). However, the situation often becomes blurred in volume-depleted patients with preexisting renal disease as well as in the elderly, whose capacity to maximally conserve sodium and to concentrate the urine appropriately may be severely blunted by benign nephrosclerosis.[30] In these patients, urine sodium concentration and the U/P creatinine and osmolality ratios may approach those expected in ARF, despite marked volume depletion, significant hypotension, or cardiac failure. Prompt return of renal function after correction of volume abnormalities, or a salutary response to diuretics, often proves the functional origin of renal failure that otherwise might be mistaken for atypical ARF.

Assessment of the urine's composition may be complicated if the patient has received potent diuretics in the preceding 12 hours or is undergoing an osmotic diuresis maintained by glycosuria or mannitol infusions; even in the presence of serious volume depletion, the urine sodium concentration is likely to be much higher than it would otherwise be, whereas the osmolality and U/P creatinine ratio may be reduced. Recently administered infusions of radiologic contrast medium exert the same osmotic effect, and irrigation of the bladder with either a glucose or saline solution grossly distorts the composition of urine obtained soon thereafter. Thus, these considerations must be kept in mind in interpreting the pathophysiologic connotations of the urine's composition. Furthermore, urine sodium, osmolality, and U/P creatinine values that typify functional renal failure may be encountered with any parenchymal renal disease that greatly reduces renal perfusion while largely sparing tubular function, such as hepatorenal syndrome, vasculitis, or glomerulonephritis, despite evidence of euvolemia or even plasma volume expansion.

Chemical and microscopic examination of the urine offers valuable diagnostic clues in the evaluation of ARF. A positive reaction for blood with orthotoluidine-impregnated dipsticks indicates the presence of heme pigment, in the form of myoglobin seen in rhabdomyolysis, free hemoglobin seen in transfusion reaction and hemolytic anemia, or red blood cells (RBCs). A positive result and the absence of RBCs on microscopic examination support the first two diagnoses, which can be confirmed by more specific laboratory methods. The quantity and quality of protein are also helpful. Minimum proteinuria characterizes functional renal failure and urinary tract obstruction. Glomerular disease leads to selective albuminuria, whereas ARF and acute interstitial nephritis lead to nonselective proteinuria.[31] Light-chain proteinuria, as seen in multiple myeloma, causes ARF and can be determined by urinary immunoelectrophoresis.

The urinary sediment in functional renal failure and urinary tract obstruction tends to be unimpressive and often consists of increased numbers of hyaline and finely granular casts. Large numbers of tubular epithelial cells, free and in casts, and many coarsely granular casts characterize the urinary sediment in ARF due to parenchymal failure. Inflammatory diseases of the kidney—glomerulonephritis, vasculitis, or interstitial nephritis—result in RBCs and white blood cells free or in casts in the urine. The importance of identifying these cellular elements in the urine cannot be overstated.

Important Causes of Acute Renal Failure in the Critical Care Setting

ARF Associated with Cardiac Failure, Hypoxia, or Sepsis

Hemodynamic instability due to cardiac failure, hypoxia, or sepsis occurs commonly in the intensive care setting, all the more so with the advent of sophisticated life-support systems. Indeed, sepsis has been identified as an important predisposing factor in up to one third of patients who have ARF.[32] The normal kidney responds to heart failure in much the same way as it does to uncomplicated volume depletion: the GFR and renal blood flow fall modestly, urinary sodium excretion is reduced, and the urine osmolality is high. The urinary sediment should be relatively benign in the absence of chronic renal disease, but in contrast to the volume-depleted state, the elevated central venous pressure and decreased renal perfusion in heart failure may cause a significant degree of proteinuria.

Despite normal or hyperdynamic cardiac function, sepsis is often associated with reductions in renal function. As with the kidney in heart failure, the urinary characteristics suggest functional or prerenal renal failure. The etiology of this renal vasoconstriction remains unknown but may be related to the stimulation of a number of recently discovered vasoconstrictor substances, such as endothelin and arachidonic acid derivatives.[33]

As blood pressure is reduced, glomerular filtration is maintained through autoregulatory mechanisms. Autoregulation is apparently blunted in many elderly patients and those with underlying renal disease, especially after severe surgical trauma or during sepsis. In this population, systemic hypotension or compromised cardiac output may cause large reductions in renal perfusion and glomerular filtration that suggest the development of ARF. The true etiology becomes apparent if the patient retains the capacity to conserve sodium appropriately and concentrate the urine, exhibits either spontaneous fluctuations in urine volume or an increased urine output in response to diuretic agents or an improved blood pressure, and rapidly recovers renal function after hemodynamic instability is reversed. As in volume depletion, patients with preexisting renal disease may not show the expected urinary characteristics, making the differentiation from ARF more difficult. This sequence of events is common after cardiovascular surgery, especially in patients who require vasopressor and inotropic agents for several days postoperatively.

Unlike simple volume depletion, for which the underlying basis of renal dysfunction can usually be corrected easily, heart failure, sepsis, and hypoxia often do not immediately respond to treatment. Additional synergistic factors, such as the use of aminoglycoside antibiotics, may also be important.[34] It is not unusual for these patients to present a baffling clinical picture that suggests ARF and may last for many days. However, the rate of rise in serum creatinine concentration may be inconstant; there may be a clear improvement in urine volume or a smaller rise in serum creatinine on days when the hemodynamic status is ameliorated; there may be some modest response to diuretics, and the urine volume may fluctuate significantly from day to day. All of these features are highly atypical of acute renal parenchymal failure. Nevertheless, dialytic therapy may be required for treatment of progressive volume overload, hyperkalemia, acidosis, or worsening azotemia. The true basis of renal failure in such patients may be confirmed only retrospectively as hemodynamic abnormalities are finally corrected.

Acute Interstitial Nephritis

Patients in an ICU receive a variety of medications, often for an extended period. Some of these, the penicillin-related β-lactam antibiotics in particular, cause ARF that differs both clinically and mechanistically from that associated with ischemia or aminoglycoside antibiotics.[35, 36] Methicillin, ampicillin, nafcillin, oxacillin, amoxicillin, carbenicillin, cefotaxime, cephradine, and cephalexin are not nephrotoxic and produce renal failure only in certain susceptible individuals, usually after at least 10 days of treatment. There is usually no prior history of penicillin allergy.

ARF caused by acute interstitial nephritis has a distinct clinical presentation that is typified by patients exposed to methicillin.[37] Fever is almost invariably present but, unfortunately, is often shrugged off as part of the infectious process for which the antibiotic was originally prescribed. Microscopic hematuria is also characteristic; only about one third of all cases have gross hematuria. Morbilliform or maculopapular rash, with or without arthralgias, can suggest a possible immune basis for renal failure, but rashes are found in no more than half of all cases. A blood smear reveals peripheral eosinophilia in perhaps three quarters of the patients, but it often does not persist beyond 1 to 3 days and so may be missed. However, sterile pyuria, frequently profuse, and eosinophiluria are evident as long as there is mononuclear and eosinophilic cell infiltration in the renal interstitium. Proteinuria is often present but usually not massive, and erythrocyte casts are more suggestive of an allergic vasculitis or other causes of renal failure. Bilateral flank pain is a common complaint; when it is coupled with fever and pyuria, it not infrequently can lead to an erroneous initial diagnosis of acute pyelonephritis. However, acute pyelonephritis almost never causes ARF unless it is complicated by urinary obstruction, septic shock, severe volume depletion, or acute papillary necrosis.

Although hematuria, fever, rash, eosinophilia, and eosinophiluria are hallmarks of allergic interstitial nephritis due to any of the β-lactam antibiotics, the variability of these findings in individual patients makes the recognition of the entity somewhat difficult unless it is routinely considered in the differential diagnosis of ARF. The patient's past and present drug intake would be carefully scrutinized, each of the classic presenting features looked for, and further work-up initiated if necessary. Skin biopsy can often definitively identify the origin of even relatively innocent-looking rashes, and a Wright's or Hansel's stain of the urinary sediment can establish the presence of eosinophiluria. Most commonly, 30% or more of the leukocytes in urine will be eosinophils,[35] but any degree of eosinophiluria in a patient with unexplained renal failure is worthy of note. An intensely positive gallium scan can be helpful to separate this entity from ARF,[35] but renal biopsy may still be required for a definitive diagnosis.

A host of other agents also cause an acute interstitial nephritis but without all of the characteristic clinical manifestations of the penicillin-related drugs. Cimetidine, rifampin, virtually any of the nonsteroidal anti-inflammatory agents, allopurinol, trimethoprim-sulfamethoxazole, furosemide, thiazide diuretics, phenytoin, and barbiturates are but a few of the many medications that have been incriminated. Although rash, fever, pyuria, or flank pain may signal a reaction to these agents, peripheral eosinophilia and eosinophiluria are generally absent when interstitial nephritis is caused by these drugs.

Once the diagnosis of interstitial nephritis is made, the patient's entire medication list should be carefully scrutinized. No penicillin-related drug should be continued or prescribed, especially because their use is rarely essential and there is no easy way to identify which drug is the actual culprit. The same is true of the thiazide and loop diuretics. Of course, decisions must be individualized in patients receiving essential anticonvulsive and antiarrhythmic medications. There is no consensus on the necessity of corticosteroid therapy; however, because treatment usually lasts only a few days, many nephrologists prescribe steroids.

Hepatorenal Syndrome

Although the pathogenesis of the hepatorenal syndrome remains unknown, the combination of systemic vasodilatation and renal vasoconstriction results in a dramatic reduction in renal function that often portends a grave prognosis.[38] The term was originally applied to patients in whom ARF developed after hepatobiliary surgery, but hepatorenal syndrome is now reserved for those patients who have ARF associated with hepatic failure from any cause and portal hypertension.[39] If patients have chronic liver failure, they will often have the physical signs of their disease: ascites, spider angiomas, palmar erythema, splenomegaly, hypothermia, and cachexia. Jaundice is usually present, although the severity bears no relationship to the degree of renal insufficiency.[40] Hypotension is a late development in most instances. Oliguria is a characteristic feature. Cardiac dysfunction may be an important concomitant disorder that is usually secondary to alcohol-induced cardiomyopathy. The fact that many cases occur in hospitalized patients points to iatrogenic initiators of the syndrome. These include volume depletion induced by diuretics, paracentesis, or gastrointestinal bleeding; drugs, the most important of which are nonsteroidal anti-inflammatory drugs; and infection of any kind.

Laboratory studies confirm the presence of advanced liver dysfunction with elevations of prothrombin time, reduction of the serum albumin and cholesterol concentrations, and increased bilirubin concentration.[41] Concentrations of serum urea nitrogen (BUN) and creatinine are sometimes difficult to interpret in the patient with liver failure. BUN levels tend to be low in cirrhotic patients because of both reduced protein intake and hepatic urea synthesis. Creatinine is also low owing to reduced muscle mass characteristic of this population of patients. Falsely low serum creatinine values may result from assay interference by high bilirubin concentrations. Normal or high-normal concentrations of BUN or creatinine may in fact indicate a significant reduction in renal function.

Urinary electrolyte values are suggestive of functional renal failure (urinary sodium, <10 mEq/L; U/P creatinine, >20; FE_{Na}, $<1\%$, urinary osmolarity, >450 mOsm/L). Even in patients who have typical ARF, urinary electrolyte values continue to indicate a prerenal state. Microscopic examination of the urine reveals many bilirubin-stained hyaline and granular casts; the sediment is typically acellular.

Exclusion of reversible causes of ARF is essential when the physician is faced with the patient with liver and renal failure. Once obstruction is ruled out, differentiating hepatorenal syndrome from functional renal failure is difficult. Central hemodynamic monitoring may be useful, but the parameters are often difficult to interpret because of tense ascites. A low pulmonary capillary wedge pressure and cardiac output should prompt efforts at volume repletion. An empirical trial of colloid infusion is often indicated to exclude functional renal failure, although these infusions are not without their risks.[42]

Therapy for hepatorenal syndrome has, for the most part, been unsuccessful.[43] Systemic vasoconstrictors have been employed to counter the systemic vasodilatation that is characteristic of this syndrome, but they are only of transient or negligible benefit.[44] On the other hand, renal vasodilator agents have also been used to counter the intense renal vasoconstriction seen in hepatorenal syndrome. Dopamine, prostaglandins, saralasin, phentolamine, isoproterenol, acetylcholine, and thromboxane synthetase inhibitors are but a few of these that have been used unsuccessfully to restore renal function.[45–47] Ornipressin, a unique compound possessing renal vasodilatory and systemic vasoconstrictive properties, has been used successfully to restore renal function in decompensated cirrhosis.[48]

A number of other therapies have also been tried, but all have little or transient benefit (paracentesis with or without colloid infusion, portosystemic shunt[49]) or exchange "renal death" for another form of complication, such as hemorrhage or sepsis. Dialysis has been employed in these patients[50] but should be reserved for those patients who are expected to demonstrate recovery of their liver failure, have other causes of ARF, or are awaiting liver transplantation. Cadaveric liver transplantation offers the best chance of curing both the hepatorenal syndrome and the liver failure.[51]

Because the therapy for hepatorenal syndrome is usually ineffective, prevention is the key in caring for patients with decompensated liver disease. Measures that should be employed include avoiding vigorous diuresis (0.5 kg/day in those patients without peripheral edema); treating hemorrhage early and aggressively; removing ascitic fluid cautiously with hemodynamic monitoring (large-volume paracentesis with albumin replacement is often more effective than high doses of diuretics[52]); using lactulose wisely to avoid heavy diarrhea; and finally, avoiding the use of nephrotoxic drugs, such as aminoglycosides (even neomycin) and nonsteroidal anti-inflammatory agents.

Myoglobin-Induced Acute Renal Failure (Rhabdomyolysis)

Myoglobinuric ARF remains an important cause of ARF in the critical care setting.[53] Although its course is typical of other forms of ARF, several distinctive clinical features and therapeutic interventions make this cause of ARF unique. The causes of myoglobinuric ARF are summarized in Table 154–2 and are

TABLE 154–2. Causes of Myoglobinuric Acute Renal Failure

Traumatic	Nontraumatic
"Crush injury"	Myopathy
Seizures	Phosphorylase deficiency
Strenuous exercise	Phosphofructokinase deficiency
Ischemia	Myxedema
Status asthmaticus	Dermatomyositis/polymyositis
Delirium tremens	Drug
Air embolism	Alcohol, narcotics, cocaine
Electric shock	Sedatives, amphetamines, lysergic acid diethylamide (LSD)
	Salicylate, clofibrate
	Lovastatin
	Metabolic
	Hyperpyrexia
	Hyperosmolarity
	Hypokalemia, hypophosphatemia
	Carbon monoxide poisoning
	Idiopathic paroxysmal hemoglobinuria
	Diabetic ketoacidosis
	Water intoxication
	Toxins
	Tetanus
	Typhoid
	Staphylococcal
	Snake/insect

divided into traumatic and nontraumatic. "Crush" injury and ischemia make up the majority of these important causes, which include sustained strenuous exercise, drug overdose, carbon monoxide poisoning, inherited glycogen storage diseases, and electrolyte abnormalities.[54] Ethanol intoxication is, in fact, a frequent forerunner of rhabdomyolysis and myoglobinuric ARF even in the absence of overt muscle injury[55]; the attendant hypomagnesemia, hypokalemia, and hypophosphatemia found so commonly in chronic alcoholic patients are likely to be contributing factors.

The characteristic clinical presentation results from the large quantity of muscle necrosis with its attendant delivery of intracellular contents into the extracellular space. Hyperkalemia, hyperuricemia, and hyperphosphatemia are much more pronounced than with typical ARF.[56, 57] Hypocalcemia is also common and is most likely related to deposition of calcium salts within necrotic muscle,[58] although skeletal resistance to parathyroid hormone[59] and altered vitamin D metabolism[60] have also been implicated. Creatinine is often elevated out of proportion to the BUN concentration and may rise more than the usual 1 mg/dL per day.[57] A BUN/creatinine ratio lower than the usual 10 may suggest the presence of rhabdomyolysis. Examination of the urine reveals darkly pigmented, coarsely granular casts and tubular cell casts. As mentioned previously, a positive dipstick reaction for blood in the face of negative findings on microscopic examination for blood is good evidence of myoglobin in the urine. Evidence of muscle necrosis is invariably present with elevation of creatine kinase and aldolase, lactate dehydrogenase, and alkaline phosphatase activities. Concomitant volume depletion and hypotension are important factors contributing to the development of the ARF.

Therapy is first directed toward prevention. Aggressive, early fluid replacement is essential to prevent intratubular cast formation. Mannitol and furosemide have been employed in this regard, although evidence for their effectiveness is scant. Alkalinization of the urine with volume repletion is probably the most useful maneuver,[61] although no prospective clinical trials have been performed. Care must be exercised if oliguric ARF develops because mannitol or sodium bicarbonate therapy can precipitate pulmonary edema. Dialysis is often necessary for the treatment of hyperkalemia well before there are other indications for dialysis. As renal recovery occurs, hypercalcemia may become a problem as calcium is mobilized from muscle.

Pulmonary-Renal Syndrome

A diverse number of systemic immunologic diseases may present with both ARF and acute pulmonary disease. Although Goodpasture's syndrome is the best known of these, systemic lupus erythematosus (SLE), Wegener's granulomatosis, polyarteritis nodosa (both classical and microvascular), sarcoidosis, and right-sided endocarditis may present with similar characteristics.[62–65] Although a detailed description of each of these diseases is beyond the scope of this chapter, recognition of this group of diseases is important for directing therapy that is often lifesaving.

The presentation of these patients may be dominated by either the pulmonary disease or the renal disease. The pulmonary disease may vary from mild, patchy infiltrates to life-threatening, diffuse hemorrhage. ARF is frequently accompanied by hypertension and evidence of volume expansion. Examination of the urine often reveals albuminuria, RBCs, and RBC casts. Because the renal tubules are often unaffected early in the course of the disease, the urine will be concentrated and urine sodium low. FE_{Na} is often less than 1%. Later in the course of the disease, renal ischemia results in tubular dysfunction and the customary urinary indices.

Serologic evaluation may be helpful in establishing a diagnosis. Anti–glomerular basement membrane antibody in Goodpasture's syndrome,[66] anti–neutrophil cytoplasmic antibodies (C(PR3)-ANCA or P(MPO)-ANCA) in Wegener's granulomatosis and polyarteritis,[67] and antinuclear antibodies for SLE[68] are sensitive and specific markers for these diseases. Less specific but still helpful in diagnosis are hepatitis B antigen status,[69] complement activity,[70] and cryoglobulins.[71] These serologic markers may also be helpful in observing patients once treatment has begun. Although serologic evaluation is often helpful, there may be some delay in obtaining results because specialized laboratories are often used. Therefore, pathologic diagnosis is imperative owing to the diversity of diseases that can present in this dramatic manner. Percutaneous renal biopsy may be too hazardous, and open biopsy of the kidney is often necessary. Angiography is helpful in establishing the diagnosis of polyarteritis nodosa, therefore precluding the need for renal biopsy.

Therapy, if initiated before oliguria develops or dialysis is necessary, is often effective in reversing the renal and pulmonary disease. "Pulse" intravenous methylprednisolone, cytotoxic drugs such as cyclophosphamide or azathioprine, and plasma exchange are the treatments of choice for Goodpasture's syndrome,[72] whereas steroids and cyclophosphamide are the preferred therapies for Wegener's granulomatosis, polyarteritis nodosa, and SLE.[64] Pulse steroids may be particularly effective in controlling the diffuse pulmonary hemorrhage in all of these diseases. Because of the potential for reversibility, rapid diagnosis and treatment are imperative.

Prognosis for Recovery and Survival

The major determinant of survival in the patient with ARF is the number and severity of concomitant illnesses.[73] Intensive supportive care in the ICU make death directly due to the complications of renal failure a rarity; death occurs primarily from infectious, cardiovascular, or respiratory complications.[73] Mortality rates, unfortunately, remain high in patients with ARF, ranging from approximately 20% in obstetric patients to 50% to 60% in postoperative and trauma patients.

Although there may be some improvement in survival in postsurgical and traumatic ARF, it is generally acknowledged that survival has reached a plateau.[74] This lack of improvement is most likely related to both an increase in the age of the population and the occurrence of multiorgan failure.[75] When ARF is a part of multiorgan failure, mortality approaches 100%.[73] Urine volume in patients with ARF also has an impact on survival. Patients with nonoliguric ARF have a significantly lower mortality rate than do those patients with either oliguric or anuric ARF.[76, 77] This difference is related to a reduction in the number of complications in the nonoliguric patients.[78]

Prevention and Treatment

Because ARF is usually not immediately reversible, prevention remains the most effective tool. When the patient is at risk for development of ARF because of disordered hemodynamics rather than nephrotoxins, prompt and full restoration of blood volume and adequate cardiovascular support are the key prophylactic tools. The dramatic reduction in post-traumatic ARF occurring during the Vietnam War in comparison to the Korean War is mainly attributed to rapid volume resuscitation delivered in the field.[79] Reliance on mannitol, loop diuretics, or vasopressor agents without considering the underlying abnormality is not wise. Careful monitoring of both the serum creatinine and the serum antibiotic concentrations and maintaining optimal renal function whenever aminoglycoside agents are given may limit the incidence and severity of renal toxicity.

The use of diuretics, particularly furosemide, to prevent, ameliorate, or speed recovery in ARF continues to be a controversial subject. Although there are few controlled studies on the effects of furosemide on human ARF, these studies show that furosemide increases urine volume,[80] occasionally reduces the need for dialysis,[81] but has no effect on clinical outcome.[80] The detrimental effects of furosemide or ethacrynic acid, such as permanent deafness and volume depletion, should be weighed against the small and inconsistent benefit of their use.

Mannitol, dopamine, calcium channel blockers, angiotensin-converting enzyme inhibitors, atrial natriuretic peptide, ATP, magnesium chloride, prostaglandins, heparin, and thyroxine have also been employed in human ARF, but their benefit continues to be speculative.

Once ARF becomes established, therapy should be directed toward the prevention of complications (Table 154–3). Complications may arise rapidly in the hypercatabolic patient or more subtly in the nonoliguric patient with significant residual renal function. Meticulous attention to fluid and electrolyte balance, drug use, and nutritional support will prevent many of these complications. Unfortunately, even with meticulous attention, patients with sepsis, multiorgan failure, or trauma often have life-threatening complications, such as hyperkalemia, acidosis, or volume overload.

Without aggressive nutritional support, loss of body mass can be extreme in these catabolic patients. Few controlled studies are available concerning the role of parenteral nutrition in ARF. The ones performed have generally shown a beneficial effect of amino acid infusions on ARF recovery but have not shown a significant benefit in terms of overall survival of patients.[82, 83] Although enteral nutrition is the preferred route of administration, parenteral nutrition is often necessary because of a poorly functioning gastrointestinal tract in many critically ill patients. The prescription for calories and protein is dependent on the severity of the illness as well as on whether dialysis is required. In the situation in which oliguria is expected to be brief (1 to 3 days), the goal should be to minimize tissue breakdown through supplying the minimum nutritional requirements. Restriction of fluid and protein may in these cases avoid the need for dialysis.

In the situation of prolonged oliguric ARF, the administration of calories and protein can be more generous because dialysis is invariably required. Even with dialysis, though, the overzealous administration of amino acids, fluid, and glucose may overwhelm the capacity of routine hemodialysis and lead to fluid overload or uremia.

Because recovery from ARF may be delayed, dialysis therapy is often necessary to both prevent and treat complications as they arise. Indications for dialysis are listed in Table 154–4, but dialysis is often initiated well before the development of these complications. Clearly, dialysis therapy has made a significant impact on improving survival in some patients with ARF.[84] Although there is some debate on the appropriate "intensity" of dialysis, most studies support the use of early aggressive dialysis.[85] However, a study showed little benefit of intensive dialysis on survival of patients.[86]

Dialysis therapy should be modified to fit the particular needs of the patient. There are currently four modalities that may be used, each offering certain advantages to the particular patient. Intermittent hemodialysis is the most widely used form of dialysis but may be difficult to perform in the hemodynamically unstable ICU patient. Continuous renal replacement therapies, such as peritoneal dialysis, continuous arteriovenous hemo(dia)filtration, continuous venovenous hemo(dia)filtration, and slow continuous ultrafiltration, all offer unique advantages to these unstable patients.[87] Specific advantages and disadvantages are summarized in Table 154–5. Technologic advances in dialysis equipment have made dialysis safer, although meticulous attention is necessary to avoid dialysis complications. Dialysis-induced hypotension, a complication that may prolong the course of ARF,[88] excessive or inappropriate systemic anticoagulation, and dialysis-induced electrolyte disturbances, such as hypokalemia or alkalosis, can worsen the ICU patient's condition.

TABLE 154–3. Complications of Acute Renal Failure

1. *Metabolic:* hyperkalemia, acidosis, hypocalcemia, hyperphosphatemia, hyperuricemia, hypermagnesemia, insulin resistance, malnutrition
2. *Cardiovascular:* pulmonary edema, arrhythmias, hypertension, pericarditis
3. *Neurologic:* asterixis, myoclonus, confusion, somnolence, coma, seizures, nonspecific electroencephalographic changes
4. *Gastrointestinal:* nausea, vomiting, gastritis/duodenitis, anorexia, ileus
5. *Hematologic:* platelet dysfunction, factor VII dysfunction, anemia
6. *Infectious:* pneumonia, septicemia, urinary tract infection, indwelling catheter-related infection

TABLE 154–4. Indications for Dialysis

Uremia*
Fluid overload
Pericarditis
Hyperkalemia
Hyponatremia†
Hypercalcemia/hyperphosphatemia
Platelet dysfunction
Metabolic acidosis or alkalosis
Neurologic symptoms (confusion, seizures)

*Blood urea nitrogen concentration greater than 100 mg/dL and serum creatinine concentration greater than 10 mg/dL serve as rough guidelines.

†The rapid correction of serum sodium concentrations may be harmful owing to osmolality shifts.

TABLE 154–5. Advantages and Disadvantages of Renal Replacement Therapy in Patients with Acute Renal Failure

Modality	Advantages	Disadvantages
Hemodialysis	Efficient, rapid Preferred for hyperkalemic and catabolic patients Citrate/NaCl flush No anticoagulation	Hemodynamically stressful Technically complicated Special personnel required
Peritoneal dialysis	Simple No vascular access No anticoagulation Preferred for hemodynamically unstable patients	Inefficient, slow Glucose load Not for patients with previous abdominal surgery
CAVH(D)	Simple No specialized personnel Preferred for hypotensive patients Large fluid intake possible	Arterial access Anticoagulation Blood pressure-dependent
CVVH(D)	No arterial access Preferred for hypotensive patients Large fluid intake possible More dependable blood flow	Anticoagulation Specialized equipment Specialized ICU nurse training
SCUF	Fluid removal only Preferred for hypotensive patients	Poor clearance Anticoagulation

CAVH(D) = continuous arteriovenous hemo(dia)filtration; CVVH(D) = continuous venovenous hemo(dia)filtration; SCUF = slow continuous ultrafiltration; ICU = intensive care unit.

SPECIAL CONSIDERATIONS IN PATIENTS WITH CHRONIC RENAL INSUFFICIENCY OR FAILURE

The ICU patient with chronic, stable renal insufficiency presents special clinical problems. Not only are these patients more susceptible to the development of acute deterioration in their renal function, but all aspects of their care—nutritional and fluid support, drug therapy, and diagnostic testing—are affected by the presence of renal dysfunction.

The first consideration in these patients is preservation of renal function. To this end, maintenance of extracellular volume status is of primary importance to ensure adequate renal perfusion. But because of the kidney's reduced ability to excrete salt and water, care should be exercised in administering fluid to these patients. Central pressure monitoring may be helpful if not necessary to direct this fluid administration. In patients who are volume depleted, the indiscriminate use of vasopressor drugs may also depress renal perfusion and worsen renal function.

Hypertension is a common feature in CRI, and the incidence increases as renal function worsens. Stage 4 hypertension (blood pressure above 210/120) may cause rapid deterioration of renal function, particularly when CRI exists, and should be treated aggressively. Because drugs administered orally are often not practical in the ICU, parenteral antihypertensive medications are often necessary. Sodium nitroprusside is the most potent of these and has the advantage of rapid onset of action and short half-life. Unfortunately, metabolic by-products, cyanide and thiocyanate, have long half-lives and accumulate in renal insufficiency. Toxicity may occur within 48 hours and includes metabolic acidosis, confusion, hyperreflexia, and seizures. Other parenteral antihypertensive medications can be used as alternatives and include methyldopa, labetalol, esmolol, hydralazine, and enalaprilat. The hypotensive effects of these drugs may be extreme and must be avoided, particularly in CRI patients.

Finally, the prevention of renal deterioration in the ICU setting depends on the judicious use of drugs and diagnostic tests. Drug toxicity is often enhanced in CRI patients owing to altered drug disposition as well as to increased susceptibility. Some drugs, such as aminoglycoside antibiotics, amphotericin, and cyclosporin A, may cause predictable decreases in renal function that should be monitored carefully. Avoiding these drugs may not be possible, so the determination of blood concentrations is essential to prevent toxicity. Radiocontrast agents should be avoided, if possible, because preexisting renal insufficiency is a predisposing factor for the development of ARF.

Many of the drugs used in the ICU are excreted in the urine as intact drug or metabolite; with diminished function, these drugs or metabolites often accumulate. Vigilance is therefore necessary to avoid serious toxicity. Most ICUs rely on hospital pharmacy services to help in this vigilance, although the daily review and educated use of medications by the physicians caring for the patient are essential to good ICU care.

References

1. Oken DE: Nosologic considerations in the nomenclature of acute renal failure. Nephron 1971; 8:505.
2. Swan RC, Merrill JP: The clinical course of acute renal failure. Medicine (Baltimore) 1953; 32:215.
3. Anderson RJ, Linas SL, Berns AS, et al: Nonoliguric acute renal failure. N Engl J Med 1977; 296:1134.
4. Chugh KS, Singhal PC, Sharma BK, et al: Acute renal failure of obstetric origin. Obstet Gynecol 1976; 48:642.
5. Guluti PD, Rizva SNA: Acute reversible renal failure in G-6-PD deficient siblings. Postgrad Med J 1976; 52:83.
6. Hartmann RC, Auditore JV: Paroxysmal nocturnal hemoglobinuria 1: Clinical studies. Am J Med 1959; 27:389.
7. Eisner GM, Piver JS: Acute renal failure after therapeutic abortion by intra-amniotic saline administration. N Engl J Med 1968; 279:360.
8. Thomas TA, Galizia EJ, Wensley RT: Termination of pregnancy with Utus paste: Report of a fatal case. Br Med J 1975; 1:375.
9. Hagvenik K, Gordon E, Lins LE, et al: Gycerol-induced haemolysis with haemoglobinuria and acute renal failure: Report of three cases. Lancet 1974; 1:78.
10. Warrell DA, Ormerod LD, Davidson NM: Bites by puff-adder *(Bitis arietans)* in Nigeria, and value of antivenom. Br Med J 1975; 4:697.
11. Rosen S, Hano JE, Inman MM, et al: The kidney in blackwater fever: Light and electron microscopic studies. Am J Clin Pathol 1968; 49:358.
12. Muehrcke RC, Pirani CL: Arsine-induced anuria: A correlative

clinicopathological study with electron microscopic observations. Ann Intern Med 1968; 68:853.
13. Grossman CM, Malbin B: Mushroom poisoning: A review of the literature and report of two cases caused by a previously undescribed species. Ann Intern Med 1954; 40:249.
14. Sinicrope RA, Gordon JA, Little JR, et al: Carbon tetrachloride nephrotoxicity: A reassessment of pathophysiology based upon urinary diagnostic indices. Am J Kidney Dis 1984; 3:362.
15. Schentag JJ, Cumbo TJ, Jusko WJ, et al: Gentamicin tissue accumulation and nephrotoxic reactions. JAMA 1978; 240:2067.
16. Plaut ME, Schentag JJ, Jusko WJ: Aminoglycoside nephrotoxicity: Comparative assessment in critically ill patients. J Med 1979; 10:257.
17. de Rosa F, Buoncristiani U, Capitanucci P, et al: Tobramycin: Toxicological and pharmacological studies in animals and pharmacokinetic research in patients with varying degrees of renal impairment. J Int Med Res 1974; 2:100.
18. Butler WT, Bennett JE, Alling DW, et al: Nephrotoxicity of amphotericin B: Early and late effects in 81 patients. Ann Intern Med 1964; 61:175.
19. Cooper K, Bennett WM: Nephrotoxicity of common drugs used in clinical practice. Arch Intern Med 1987; 147:1213.
20. Byrd L, Sherman RL: Radiocontrast-induced acute renal failure: A clinical and pathophysiologic review. Medicine (Baltimore) 1979; 58:270.
21. Weisberg LS, Kurnik PB, Kurnik BRC: Risk of radiocontrast nephropathy in patients with and without diabetes mellitus. Kidney Int 1994; 45:259.
22. Schwab SJ, Hlatky MA, Pieper KS, et al: Contrast nephrotoxicity: A randomized controlled trial of a nonionic and an ionic radiographic contrast agent. N Engl J Med 1989; 320:149.
23. Harris KP, Hattersley JM, Feehally J, Walls J: Acute renal failure associated with haematological malignancies: A review of 10 years experience. Eur J Haematol 1991; 47:119.
24. Rao TK, Friedman EA: Outcome of severe acute renal failure in patients with acquired immunodeficiency syndrome. Am J Kidney Dis 1995; 25:390.
25. Bonventre JV: Mechanisms of ischemic acute renal failure. Kidney Int 1993; 43:1160.
26. Thadhani R, Pascual M, Bonventre JV: Acute renal failure. N Engl J Med 1997; 334:1448.
27. Brezis M, Rosen S, Epstein FH: Acute renal failure. *In:* The Kidney. 4th ed. Brenner BM, Rector FC Jr (Eds). Philadelphia, WB Saunders, 1991, pp 1011–1015.
28. Ellenbogen PH, Scheible FW, Talner LB, et al: Sensitivity of gray scale ultrasound in detecting urinary tract obstruction. Am J Roentgenol 1978; 130:731.
29. Rascoff JH, Golden RA, Spinowitz BS, et al: Non-dilated obstructive uropathy. Arch Intern Med 1983; 143:696.
30. Sporn IN, Lancestremere RG, Papper S: Differential diagnosis of oliguria in aged patients. N Engl J Med 1962; 267:130.
31. MacLean PR, Robson JS: Unselective proteinuria in acute ischaemic renal failure. Clin Sci 1966; 30:91.
32. Werb R, Linton AL: Aetiology, diagnosis, treatment and prognosis of acute renal failure in an intensive care unit. Resuscitation 1979; 29:95.
33. Badr KF: Sepsis-associated renal vasoconstriction: Potential targets for future therapy. Am J Kidney Dis 1992; 20:207.
34. Zager RA: Endotoxemia, renal hypoperfusion, and fever: Interactive risk factors for aminoglycoside and sepsis-associated acute renal failure. Am J Kidney Dis 1992; 20:223.
35. Murray KM, Deane WR: Review of drug-induced acute interstitial nephritis. Pharmacotherapy 1992; 12:462.
36. Paller MS: Drug-induced nephropathies. Med Clin North Am 1990; 74:909.
37. Baldwin DW, Levine BB, McCluskey RT, et al: Renal failure and interstitial nephritis due to penicillin and methicillin. N Engl J Med 1968; 29:1245.
38. Levy M: Hepatorenal syndrome. Kidney Int 1993; 43:737.
39. Arroyo V, Gines P, Gerbes AL, et al: Definition and diagnostic criteria of refractory ascites and hepatorenal syndrome in cirrhosis. International Ascites Club. Hepatology 1996; 23:164.
40. Baldus WP, Feichter RN, Summerskill WHJ, et al: The kidney in cirrhosis. II: Disorders of renal function. Ann Intern Med 1964; 60:366.
41. Baldus WP, Feichter RN, Summerskill WHJ, et al: The kidney in cirrhosis. I: Clinical and biochemical features of azotemia in hepatic failure. Ann Intern Med 1964; 60:353.
42. Reynolds TB, Lieberman FL, Redeker AF: Functional renal failure with cirrhosis. Medicine (Baltimore) 1967; 46:191.
43. Epstein M: Hepatorenal syndrome: Emerging perspectives of pathophysiology and therapy (Editorial). J Am Soc Nephrol 1994; 4:1735.
44. Sugarman HJ, Berkowitz HD, Miller KD: Metaraminol in "hepatorenal syndrome." N Engl J Med 1971; 285:180.
45. Barnardo DE, Baldus WP, Maher FT: Effects of dopamine on renal function in patients with cirrhosis. Gastroenterology 1970; 58:524.
46. Zusman RM, Axelrod L, Tolkoff-Rubin N: The treatment of the hepatorenal syndrome (HRS) with intrarenal administration of prostaglandin E. Prostaglandins 1977; 13:814.
47. Zipser RD, Kronborg I, Rector W, et al: Therapeutic trial of thromboxane synthesis inhibition in the hepatorenal syndrome. Gastroenterology 1984; 87:1228.
48. Lenz K, Hortnag LH, Drum LW: Beneficial effect of 8-ornithin vasopressin in renal dysfunction in decompensated cirrhosis. Gut 1989; 30:90.
49. Moskovits M: The peritoneovenous shunt: Expectations and reality. Am J Gastroenterol 1990; 85:917.
50. Keller F, Heinze H, Jochimsen F, et al: Risk factors and outcome of 107 patients with decompensated liver disease and acute renal failure (including 26 patients with hepatorenal syndrome): Role of hemodialysis. Ren Fail 1995; 17:135.
51. Iwatsuki S, Popovtzer MM, Corman JL, et al: Recovery from "hepatorenal syndrome" after orthotopic liver transplantation. N Engl J Med 1973; 289:1155.
52. Gines P, Arroyo V, Quintero E, et al: Comparison of paracentesis and diuretics in the treatment of cirrhotics with tense ascites. Gastroenterology 1987; 93:234.
53. Zager RA: Rhabdomyolysis and myohemoglobinuric acute renal failure. Kidney Int 1996; 49:314.
54. Gabow PA, Kaehny WD, Kelleher SP: The spectrum of rhabdomyolysis. Medicine (Baltimore) 1982; 61:141.
55. Rubin E, Kantz AM, Lieber CS, et al: Muscle damage produced by chronic alcohol consumption. Am J Pathol 1976; 291:807.
56. Grossman RA, Hamilton RW, Morse BM, et al: Nontraumatic rhabdomyolysis and acute renal failure. N Engl J Med 1974; 291:807.
57. Chugh KS, Nath IV, Ubroi HS, et al: Acute renal failure due to non-traumatic rhabdomyolysis. Postgrad Med J 1979; 55:386.
58. Akmal M, Goldstein DA, Telfer N, et al: Resolution of muscle calcification in rhabdomyolysis and acute renal failure. Ann Intern Med 1978; 89:928.
59. Massry SG, Arieff AI, Coburn JW, et al: Divalent ion metabolism in patients with acute renal failure. Studies on the mechanism of hypocalcemia. Kidney Int 1974; 5:437.
60. Pietrek J, Kokot F, Jadwiga K: Serum 25-hydroxyvitamin D and parathyroid hormone in patients with acute renal failure. Kidney Int 1978; 13:178.
61. Ron D, Taitelman MD, Michaelson MD, et al: Prevention of acute renal failure in traumatic rhabdomyolysis. Arch Intern Med 1984; 144:277.
62. Duncan DA, Drummond KN, Michael AF, Wernier RL: Pulmonary hemorrhage and glomerulonephritis. Ann Intern Med 1964; 62:920.
63. Eagen JW, Memoli VA, Roberts JL, et al: Pulmonary hemorrhage in systemic lupus erythematosus. Medicine (Baltimore) 1978; 57:545.
64. Jennette JC, Falk RJ: Small-vessel vasculitis. N Engl J Med 1997; 337:1512.
65. Allegri L, Olivetti G, David S, et al: Sarcoid granulomatous nephritis with isolated and reversible renal failure. Nephron 1980; 25:207.
66. Wilson CB, Dixon FJ: Anti–glomerular basement membrane antibody induced glomerulonephritis. Kidney Int 1973; 3:74.
67. Falk RJ, Jennette JC: ANCA small-vessel vasculitis. J Am Soc Nephrol 1997; 8:314.
68. Emlen W, Pisetsky D, Taylor R: Antibodies to DNA: A perspective. Arthritis Rheum 1986; 29:1417.
69. Ronco P, Verroust P, Mignon F, et al: Immunopathological studies of polyarteritis nodosa and Wegener's granulomatosis: A report of 43 patients with 51 renal biopsies. Q J Med 1983; 52:212.

70. Lloyd W, Schur PH: Immune complexes, complement and anti-DNA in exacerbations of systemic lupus erythematosus (SLE). Medicine (Baltimore) 1981; 60:208.
71. Gamble CN, Ruggles SW: The immunopathogenesis of glomerulonephritis associated with mixed cryoglobulinemia. N Engl J Med 1978; 299:81.
72. Lockwood C, Boulton-Jones J, Lowenthal R, et al: Recovery from Goodpasture's syndrome after immunosuppressive treatment and plasmapheresis. Br Med J 1975; 2:252.
73. Bullock ML, Umen AJ, Finkelstein M, Keane WF: The assessment of risk factors in 462 patients with acute renal failure. Am J Kidney Dis 1985; 5:97.
74. DuBose TD Jr, Warnock DG, Mehta RL, et al: Acute renal failure in the 21st century: Recommendations for management and outcomes assessment. Am J Kidney Dis 1997; 29:793.
75. Eisman B, Beart R, Norton L: Multiple organ failure. Surg Gynecol Obstet 1977; 144:323.
76. Baek SM, Makabali GG, Shoemaker WC: Clinical determinants of survival from postoperative renal failure. Surgery 1975; 140:685.
77. Rasmussen H, Ibels LS: Acute renal failure: Multivariate analysis of causes and risk factors. Am J Med 1982; 73:211.
78. Anderson RJ, Linas SL, Berns AS, et al: Nonoliguric acute renal failure. N Engl J Med 1977; 296:1134.
79. Whelton A, Donadio JV: Post-traumatic acute renal failure in Vietnam. Johns Hopkins Med J 1969; 124:95.
80. Minuth AN, Terrell JB, Suki WN: Acute renal failure: A study of the course and prognosis of 104 patients and of the role of furosemide. Am J Med Sci 1976; 271:317.
81. Fries D, Pozet N, Dubois N, Traeger J: The use of large doses of furosemide in acute renal failure. Postgrad Med J 1971; 47:18.
82. Abel RM, Beck CH Jr, Abbott WM, et al: Improved survival from acute renal failure after treatment with intravenous essential L-amino acids and glucose. Results of a prospective double-blind study. N Engl J Med 1973; 288:695.
83. Baek SM, Makabali GG, Bryan-Brown CW, et al: The influence of parenteral nutrition on the course of acute renal failure. Surg Gynecol Obstet 1975; 141:405.
84. Kleinknecht D, Jungers P, Chanard J, et al: Uremic and non-uremic complications in acute renal failure: Evaluation of early and frequent dialysis on prognosis. Kidney Int 1972; 1:190.
85. Conger JD: A controlled evaluation of prophylactic dialysis in post-traumatic acute renal failure. J Trauma 1975; 15:1056.
86. Gillum DM, Dixon BS, Yanover MJ, et al: The role of intensive dialysis in acute renal failure. Clin Nephrol 1986; 25:249.
87. Forni LG, Hilton PJ: Continuous hemofiltration in the treatment of acute renal failure. N Engl J Med 1997; 336:1303.
88. Kelleher SP, Robinette JB, Miller F, Conger JD: Effect of hemorrhagic reduction in blood pressure on recovery from acute renal failure. Kidney Int 1987; 31:725.

155

Renal Replacement Therapy in the Intensive Care Unit

William Silvester, MD • Glenn Chertow, MD
Claudio Ronco, MD
Rinaldo Bellomo, MB BS (HONS), MD, FRACP

THE NEED FOR RENAL REPLACEMENT THERAPY

In patients with severe acute renal failure (ARF), the blood purification function of the kidneys is lost. Because of this functional loss, several components of homeostasis are affected. Loss of excretion of toxic metabolites and of nitrogen waste products causes azotemia, uremic encephalopathy, gastrointestinal symptoms and bleeding, neuropathy, myopathy, bone marrow suppression, severe platelet dysfunction, pericarditis, and cutaneous manifestations of uremic toxemia. Loss of adequate excretory function of sodium and water causes fluid retention, peripheral edema, and pulmonary edema. Loss of the ability to excrete potassium and control acid-base balance leads to progressive hyperkalemia and marked metabolic acidosis. Inability to excrete phosphate results in hyperphosphatemia and hypocalcemia with possible tetany. Catabolism is enhanced in severe renal failure, and the administration of nitrogen for the purpose of nutritional support further accelerates the rate of development of uremia. If no artificial kidney treatment is provided, slowly but inexorably, the patient loses consciousness and frequent myoclonic jerks develop. Later on, recurrent seizures develop and, finally, physiologic deterioration progresses until death occurs.

If survival is to be achieved in the setting of severe ARF, a procedure that replaces excretory renal function and restores homeostasis becomes necessary. Over the last 50 years, various techniques have been developed to achieve these goals; they include (1) intermittent hemodialysis (IHD), (2) peritoneal dialysis (PD), and (3) more recently, continuous hemofiltration (CHF) techniques, also known as continuous renal replacement therapy (CRRT). All of the techniques rely on the principle of achieving solute and water removal through a semipermeable membrane that is either artificial (hemodialysis and hemofiltration) or natural (peritoneum). During such removal, unwanted solutes and water are discarded, and any undesirable solute or water loss is replaced with a fluid of appropriate composition.

This chapter reviews the various forms of renal replacement therapy (RRT) as they are applied to the care of critically ill patients in a modern intensive care unit (ICU) and describes the principles, biologic rationales, and evidence concerning their use in the field of critical care medicine.

PRINCIPLES OF RENAL REPLACEMENT THERAPY

In order to administer or understand the prescription and practical execution of RRT in the ICU, one needs to understand the fundamental principles regulating the movement of water (the solvent), metabolites, electrolytes, toxins, drugs, and other water-soluble components of plasma (the solutes) across semipermeable membranes (Fig. 155–1). The principal mechanisms of fluid and solute transport across semipermeable membranes are diffusion, convection, and ultrafiltration.

During *diffusion,* the movement of solute depends on its statistical tendency to reach the same concentration in the available distribution space on each side of the membrane. The practical result is the passage of solutes from the compartment with the higher concentration to the compartment with the lower concentration[1] (Fig. 155–1). Solute transport under these circumstances can be described by the following formula:

$$Jd = DTA\ (dc/dx) \qquad \text{[Equation 1]}$$

where Jd is the diffusive solute flux, D is the diffusion coefficient, T is the temperature of the solution, A is the surface area of the membrane, dc is the concentration gradient between the two compartments, and dx is the thickness of the membrane.

If the permeability of the membrane is limited by its porosity to molecules less than 500 daltons in molecular weight, diffusive clearance applies only to solutes with a molecular weight less than 500 daltons.

During *convection,* however, the movement of solute across a semipermeable membrane takes place in conjunction with

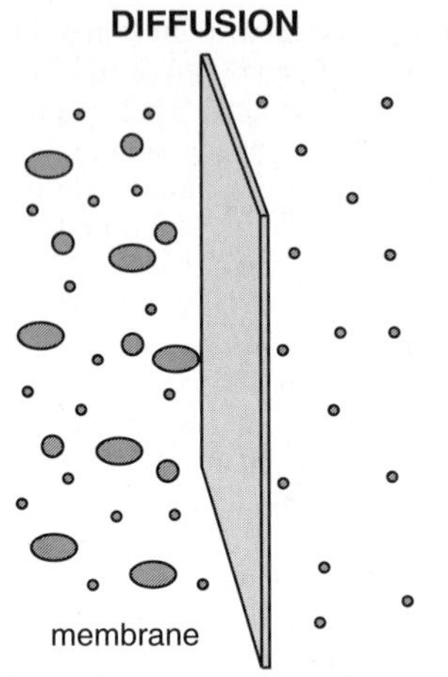

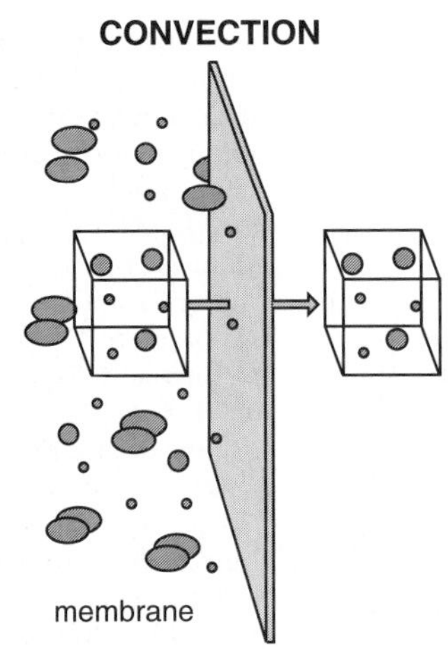

Figure 155–1. Mechanisms of solute removal. The two mechanisms of solute movement across a semipermeable membrane are shown. Diffusion operates through a concentration gradient, while convection moves solutes by means of pressure and solvent drag. Convection removes larger molecules more effectively.

significant amounts of ultrafiltration and water transfer across the membrane (see Fig. 155–1). To state this definition another way: During convection, solute is "carried" by solvent, as the solvent (water) is pushed across the membrane (a process called ultrafiltration; see later) in response to a transmembrane pressure gradient according to the following formula.

$$Qf = Km \times TMP = Km\,(Pb - Puf - p) \qquad \text{[Equation 2]}$$

where Qf is the ultrafiltration rate, Km is the coefficient of permeability of the membrane, TMP is the transmembrane pressure, Pb is the hydrostatic pressure of blood, Puf is the hydrostatic pressure in the ultrafiltrate compartment, and p is the oncotic pressure of blood.

Once ultrafiltration occurs, each solute is carried to the other side of the membrane at a particular rate according to its membrane rejection coefficient (σ). In standard semipermeable membranes used for renal replacement therapy, σ is essentially 1 for albumin (complete rejection and no movement across the membrane) and close to 0 for small solutes such as urea (easy transfer across the membrane).

Assuming a relation of $S = 1 - \sigma$, we can derive the so-called sieving coefficient for a solute (S), which is inversely correlated to the membrane rejection coefficient. In clinical practice, the sieving coefficient is measured as the ratio between the concentrations of solute in the ultrafiltrate and in plasma water. In convective treatments, therefore, the transport (Jc) of solute X is described by the following formula:

$$Jc = UF\,[X]_{UF} \qquad \text{[Equation 3]}$$

where UF is the volume of ultrafiltrate and $[X]_{UF}$ is the concentration in the ultrafiltrate of solute X.

From this equation, we can derive the formula that describes clearance during convective treatment:

$$Kc = Qf\,[X]_{UF}/[X]P_w \qquad \text{[Equation 4]}$$

where Qf is the ultrafiltration rate and $[X]_{UF}/[X]P_W$ is the ratio of the solute concentration in the ultrafiltrate and plasma water, or the sieving coefficient (S).

From Equation 4, we can easily see that when S is 1, clearance is equal to the ultrafiltration rate.

Despite the preceding distinctions, diffusion and convection often act simultaneously, and it is almost impossible to physically divide these transport mechanisms. All one can say is that under certain operative circumstances, convective transport is the dominant mechanism of solute movement and under other operative circumstances, diffusive transport dominates instead. In some situations, the two modes of solute transport occur simultaneously and in near equal proportions (hemodiafiltration).[3]

Ultrafiltration is a process by which plasma water and crystalloids are separated from whole blood across a semipermeable membrane in response to a transmembrane pressure gradient. The process is governed by the following formula:

$$Qf = Km \times TMP \qquad \text{[Equation 5]}$$

where Qf is the ultrafiltration rate (mL/min); Km is the membrane ultrafiltration coefficient, derived from the ratio Qf/TMP and expressed in (mL/hr) $\times$ (m²/mm Hg), and TMP is the transmembrane pressure gradient generated by the pressures on both sides of the membrane, as described by the following equation:

$$TMP = Pb - Puf - p \qquad \text{[Equation 6]}$$

where Pb is the hydrostatic pressure in the blood compartment, Puf is the hydraulic pressure in the ultrafiltrate/dialysate compartment, and p is the oncotic pressure generated by proteins.

The hydrostatic pressure in the blood compartment depends, of course, on blood flow. The greater the blood flow, the greater the transmembrane pressure. In a spontaneous ultrafiltration system based on convective clearance, therefore, measures that maximize blood flow maximize ultrafiltrate production and solute clearance. Equally, measures that raise the negative pressure on the ultrafiltrate compartment of the membrane also increase ultrafiltration, as do measures that decrease oncotic pressure (*predilution,* or the administration of replacement fluid before the filter). As ultrafiltration proceeds and plasma water is ultrafiltered, hydrostatic pressure is lost and oncotic pressure is gained. Thus, if the filter is long enough, a condition of filtration-pressure equilibrium is achieved, whereby the oncotic pressure is equal to or greater than transmembrane pressure, and ultrafiltration ceases. In modern filters, however, this is rarely, if ever, the case. The relationship between transmembrane pressure and oncotic pressure determines the *filtration fraction* (i.e., the fraction of plasma water that is removed from blood during hemofiltration). The optimal filtration fraction for patients with a hematocrit value of approximately 30% is in the range of 20%

to 25%. This level of filtration prevents excessive hemoconcentration at the filter outlet, which otherwise would promote filter clotting.

If ultrafiltration is obtained by applying a negative pressure generated by a pump (volumetric or peristaltic) to the ultrafiltration side of the filtering membrane, attention must be paid to the maintenance of both a safe filtration fraction and a transmembrane pressure in the range specified by the manufacturer of the pump. If this is not done, filter clotting becomes likely, and the membrane may rupture.

MEMBRANES

Different membranes are employed during RRT: They can be *cellulose-based* or *synthetic.*[4]

Cellulose-Based Membranes

Cellulose-based membranes (cuprophane, hemophan, cellulose acetate) are generally considered "low-flux" membranes, that is, membranes with a permeability coefficient to water (Km) of less than 10 mL/hr × mm Hg/m^2. These membranes are very thin (5 to 15 μm of wall thickness) and have a symmetric structure with uniform porosity. They are strongly hydrophilic.

Synthetic Membranes

Synthetic membranes (polysulphone, polyamide, polyacrylonitrile) are high-flux membranes with a Km > 30 mL/hr × mm Hg/ m^2. Wall thickness ranges between 40 and 100 μm with an asymmetric structure composed of an inner skin layer and a surrounding sponge layer. Synthetic membranes have large pores (10 to 30,000 daltons) and are hydrophobic.

Because they have high sieving coefficients for solutes in a wide range of molecular weights, synthetic membranes are much more suitable for convective treatments. Filtration rates are always high when synthetic membranes are used. An associated significant amount of convection results from such rates of filtration (Fig. 155–2). Thus, when synthetic membranes are used, extracorporeal RRT is not adequately defined by the use of the term "hemodialysis"; such treatment should be more suitably named *hemodiafiltration* (if replacement solution is needed) or *high-flux dialysis* (if a filtration-backfiltration mechanism is present and no replacement is required).[5] Specific terms should be applied to different treatments according to their characteristics and mechanisms of operation.

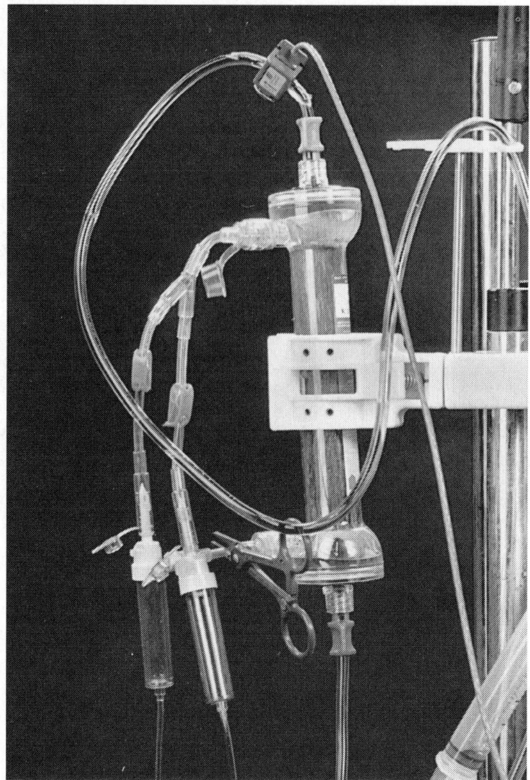

Figure 155–2. A standard hemofilter, used for continuous venovenous hemofiltration with controlled ultrafiltrate. The membrane is synthetic (polyacrylonitrile). Ultrafiltrate is pumped off, the dialysate port is clamped (with scissor clamp), and a Doppler flow probe is placed at the filter outlet to monitor blood flow. IV = intravenous.

BLOOD ACCESS AND EXTRACORPOREAL CIRCUIT DESIGN

Extracorporeal blood treatments require vascular access and a specific extracorporeal circuit design. Two different approaches are in use for extracorporeal treatments, arteriovenous and venovenous modes.

Arteriovenous Mode

In arteriovenous (AV) circulation, the arteriovenous pressure gradient of the patient is the driving force moving blood through the circuit. An artery and a vein are cannulated with large-bore catheters (size 10 to 14 French), and no blood pumps are used.[6–9] Maximum care is taken to avoid unnecessary resistances along the length of the circuit. Therefore, large and short catheters, short blood lines, and short filters are used. Three-way stopcocks, narrow connections, and kinking are carefully avoided. In arteriovenous mode, the determinants of ultrafiltration are different from those generally considered in pumped circulations. Hematocrit, plasma protein concentration (oncotic pressure), and the distance between the filter and the ultrafiltrate collection system become critical factors. In this system, blood flow generally ranges between 50 and 150 mL/min. In some patients, vascular access may require the surgical construction of a Scribner shunt. Under these circumstances, blood flows tend to be between 60 and 80 mL/min.

Venovenous Mode

Venovenous (VV) circulation requires a roller pump in the prefilter line segment as well as a drip chamber in the line returning the blood from the filter (Figs. 155–3 and 155–4). Either two central veins are cannulated or a single central vein is cannulated with a double-lumen catheter. Double-lumen catheters are now available on the market, are of size 11.5 to 13.5 French, can be easily inserted percutaneously by the Seldinger technique, and come in different designs (Fig. 155–5).

Site of Placement for Vascular Access Catheters

In a critically ill patient, the site of choice for the insertion of a double-lumen catheter is usually determined by the patient's underlying disease. For example, the patient with coagulopathy is more safely managed with a femoral catheter, that

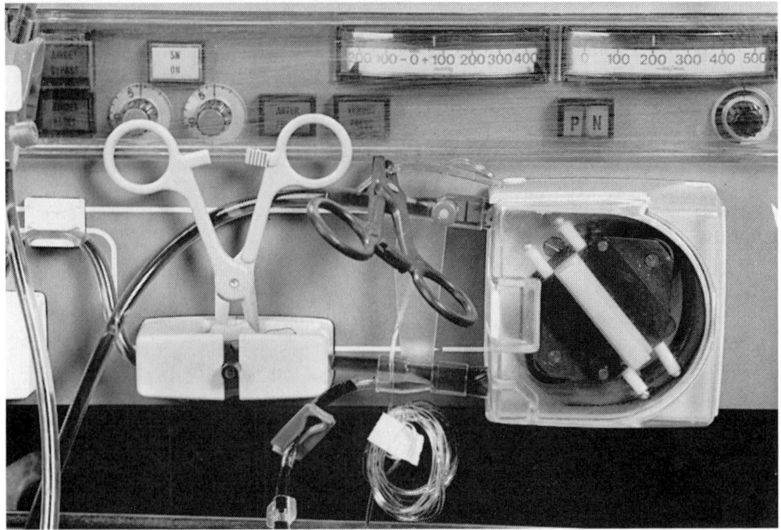

Figure 155–3. Peristaltic pump for continuous venovenous renal replacement therapy in operation. Blood flow is set at 200 mL/m, the venous pressure gauge is recording a pressure of about 75 mm Hg, and the arterial alarm pillow (marked by white scissor clamp) is used to detect catheter outflow problems.

site being more amenable to compression in the event of inadvertent arterial puncture. Similarly, access in the patient who has severe pulmonary disease or who requires positive-pressure ventilation for some other reason may be more safely established at the femoral site, to avoid the risk of pneumothorax associated with internal jugular or subclavian catheter placement of the catheter. A femoral catheter, however, may be more prone to infection than a upper extremity line, and it also limits the patient's mobility, because sitting up in bed or ambulating increases the risk of catheter malfunction and local bleeding. The immobility with femoral placement of a catheter may also impair wound healing and delay overall physical and nutritional rehabilitation.

There is increasing evidence that prolonged cannulation of the subclavian vein with dialysis catheters can promote venous stenosis at that site. This concern has tempered enthusiasm for the subclavian approach, particularly because subclavian stenosis could impede the creation of a permanent arteriovenous fistula or graft in the corresponding arm, an important outcome in the event that the patient's renal function does not recover.

If the anticipated duration of dialysis exceeds 2 to 3 weeks, a surgically placed internal jugular catheter may be preferred to a percutaneous catheter, because the tunneled position and Dacron cuff used in such a catheter may reduce the risk of infection (and may be associated with more reliable blood flows). Some practitioners would delay placement of an internal jugular catheter in intubated patients because of the fear of bacterial colonization and infection related to orotracheal secretions.

Careful local management is critical to catheter performance. The site should be kept sterile at all times and should be used only for hemodialysis. Heparin at 7500 units is rou-

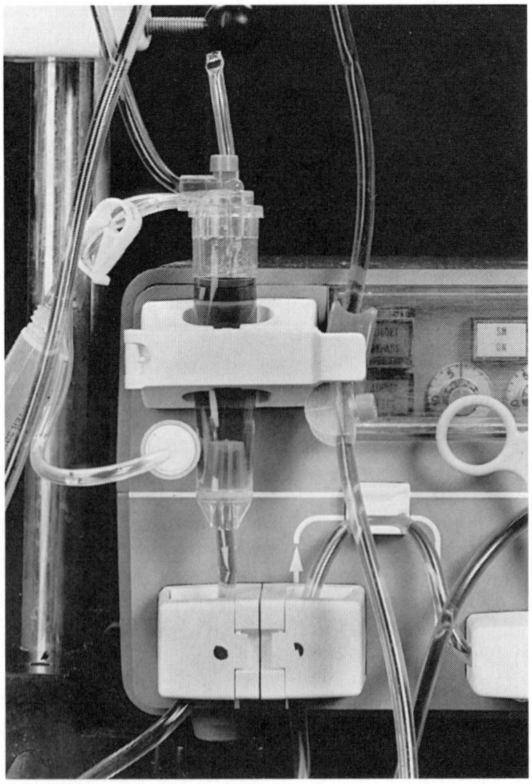

Figure 155–4. Drip chamber to prevent air embolism. The way in which the venous pressure transducer transmits pressure from the top of the chamber (post filter) is shown. A post filter clamp is triggered by air in the chamber.

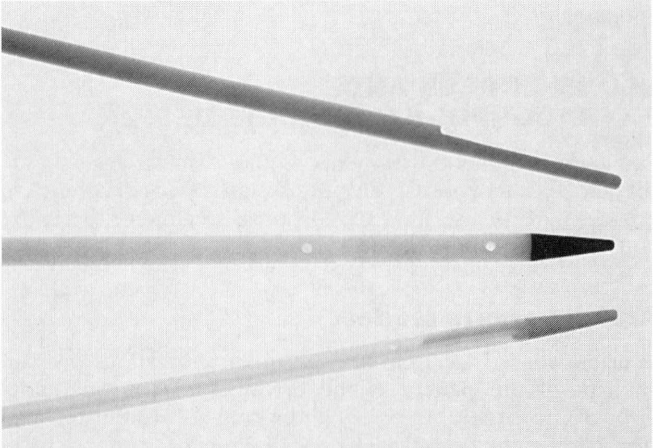

Figure 155–5. Catheter tips with three different designs for double-lumen temporary vascular access hemodialysis catheters. Note the difference in the profile of the tips and in the "arterial" outflow lumen for the delivery of blood to the peristaltic pump.

tinely instilled into each catheter lumen after the completion of the dialysis session. If, in spite of the heparin, the catheter becomes occluded with thrombus or fibrin, urokinase at 5000 units may be instilled for 20 to 30 minutes, to achieve thrombolysis with negligible systemic absorption.

The common feature of all double-lumen catheters is the presence of one lumen that functions as the "arterial" or outflow limb of the circuit and a second lumen that functions as the "venous" or inflow limb of the circuit. Blood lines can be longer than in arteriovenous circuits, and pressure measurements are required before the pump and after the filter to ensure safe use of the blood pump and avoid any damage to the cannulated vein. In this system, blood flow can usually be kept between 150 and 200 mL/min.

In patients receiving long-term hemodialysis who have acute complications, the cannulas of a plastic catheter can be used when a preexisting vascular access such as arteriovenous fistula or Scribner shunt is present; this, however, is an unusual situation. Finally, in peritoneal dialysis, access for treatment is obtained by the surgical (preferably) or percutaneous insertion of an intra-abdominal Tenckhoff catheter.

DIALYSATE AND FLUID REPLACEMENT DELIVERY SYSTEMS

In continuous hemodialysis and hemodiafiltration, a dialysate flow rate between 10 and 30 mL/min is generally considered sufficient.[10] Dialysate can be delivered by gravity, by means of a single or coupled infusion pumps, or by a roller pump (Fig. 155-6). The same system can be applied to the dialysate and ultrafiltrate outlet line in order to achieve fluid control. In continuous high-flux dialysis, a pair of pumps is required to maintain the ultrafiltration control effective. Sterile dialysate can be recirculated or run in a single pass.

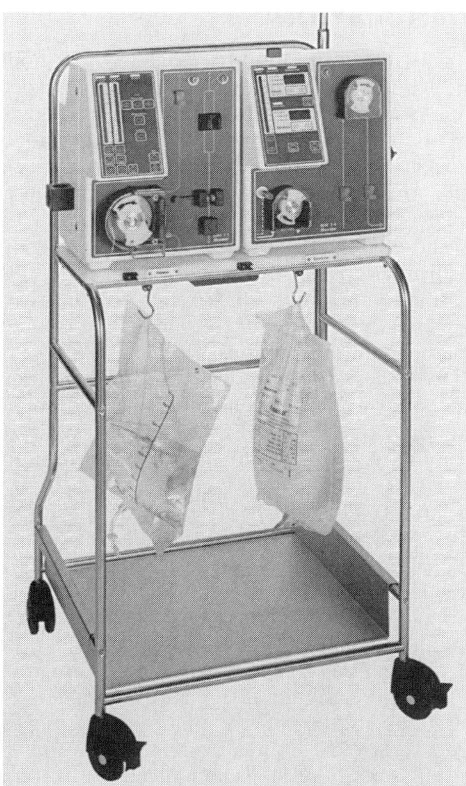

Figure 155–6. Standard machine for continuous renal replacement therapy and the delivery of dialysate or replacement fluid. Note the 5-liter replacement fluid and discarded fluid bags, which are weighed electronically with high precision in order to achieve the desired fluid balance.

When replacement solution is needed to maintain the patient's fluid balance (continuous arteriovenous or venovenous hemofiltration or hemodiafiltration), substitution fluid can be infused in either postdilutional or predilutional mode or both. Postdilution is preferred in arteriovenous-driven circulation and it can be achieved by gravity, even though infusion pumps or other balancing devices are often utilized.[11, 12] Predilution is preferred in pump-driven circulations and whenever a reduction of the blood viscosity may help to achieve a longer filter survival and less heparin infusion. The use of pumps to control fluid replacement and removal is growing, because it offers the advantage of decreasing nursing workload.[13] It is otherwise possible to operate in a spontaneous system of filtration with replacement being based on frequent (at least hourly) measurements of ultrafiltrate production. Sterile replacement and dialysate fluids for hemofiltration are now commercially available.

TECHNIQUE AND NOMENCLATURE

It is important for the critical care physician to understand and appreciate the differences among renal replacement therapies and the reasons for the relatively complex nomenclature that surrounds them. The following definitions reflect the principles and technical requirements of the various types of RRTs as agreed on during a 1996 consensus conference.[14]

Hemodialysis. This term refers to a prevalently diffusive treatment in which blood and dialysate are circulated in countercurrent mode and a low-permeability, cellulose-based membrane is employed. The ultrafiltration rate is approximately equal to the scheduled weight loss. This treatment can be performed intermittently (intermittent hemodialysis [IHD], for example, for 4 hours three times per week), daily (2 to 4 hours)[15] or continuously, in either arteriovenous mode (continuous arteriovenous hemodialysis [CAVHD]) or venovenous mode (continuous venovenous hemodialysis [CVVHD]).[16]

Peritoneal Dialysis. This term refers to a predominantly diffusive treatment in which blood circulating along the capillaries of the peritoneal membrane is exposed to dialysate. Access is obtained by the insertion of a peritoneal catheter, which allows the abdominal instillation of dialysate. Movement of solute and water is achieved by means of variable gradients of concentration and tonicity generated by the dialysate. This treatment can be performed intermittently or continuously.[18]

Hemofiltration (HF). This is an essentially convective treatment, with highly permeable membranes. The ultrafiltrate produced is replaced completely or in part by a sterile solution of water and electrolytes, thus achieving both blood purification and fluid control. Any net fluid loss results from the difference between ultrafiltration and reinfusion rates (no dialysate is used). This treatment can be performed intermittently (30 L per session three times per week), daily (10 to 30 L exchange) or continuously in either arteriovenous mode (CAVH) or venovenous mode (CVVH) (12 to 30 L of plasma water exchange per day).[19]

Hemodiafiltration. In this treatment, diffusion and convection are combined with the use of a highly permeable membrane. Blood and dialysate are circulated as in hemodialysis, but typically, an ultrafiltration rate in excess of the scheduled weight loss is produced (Fig. 155-7). To achieve fluid balance, a sterile solution of water and electrolytes is reinfused at an adequate rate. This treatment can be performed intermittently (3 to 4 hours and 9 to 15 L exchange per session three times per week), daily (3 hours and 9 L exchange), or continuously

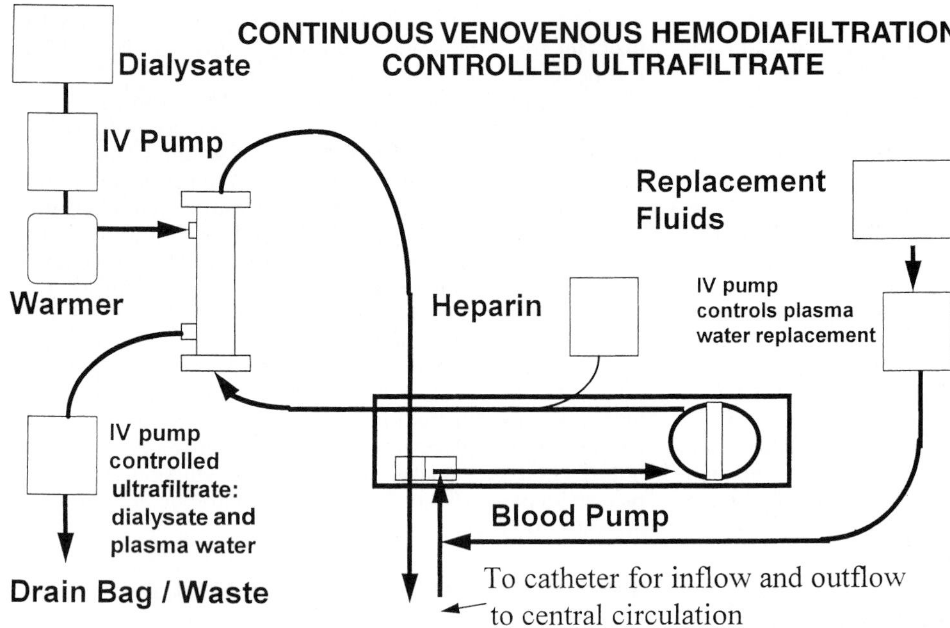

Figure 155–7. Diagram of a continuous venovenous hemodiafiltration system with pump-off control of effluent.

in either arteriovenous mode (CAVHDF) or venovenous mode (CVVHDF).[20-24]

High-Flux Dialysis. This treatment utilizes highly permeable membranes in conjunction with an ultrafiltration control system. Blood and dialysate are circulated as in hemodialysis. With the high permeability coefficient of the membrane, however, ultrafiltration would exceed the required patient weight loss. Therefore, a positive pressure is applied to the dialysate compartment to reduce the amount of ultrafiltration (UF) and to avoid the need for replacement solution. Owing to the peculiar structure of hollow-fiber dialyzers, filtration takes place in the proximal part of the filter, and backfiltration occurs in the distal part of the filter. Diffusion and convection, therefore, are still combined, because the high filtration rate occurring in the proximal part of the dialyzer is masked by a backfiltration occurring in the distal part. Replacement is avoided because it takes place inside the filter through the mechanism of backfiltration. Such backfiltration implies that, during HFD, dialysate must be sterile and pyrogen free.[5]

Ultrafiltration. In this treatment, fluid removal is the main target of therapy. Highly permeable filters are used, and fluid is removed from the body without being replaced by any solution. Ultrafiltration can be performed intermittently or daily, and a maximum of 3 L per session is generally removed in a period of 4 to 6 hours. In clinical practice, UF has been used in sequence with hemodialysis to improve cardiovascular tolerance. In critically ill patients, UF can be performed continuously at very low filtration rates (1 to 2 mL/min) with or without the addition of dialysate—slow, continuous ultrafiltration (SCUF) or slow, continuous ultrafiltration without dialysate (SCUF-D)—to remove edema fluid. Both arteriovenous and venovenous modes can be used.[25]

Plasmapheresis (PF). This treatment uses special plasma filters. The molecular weight cutoff of the membrane in such filters is much higher than that of hemofilters. Plasma as a whole is filtered, and blood is reconstituted by the infusion of plasma products such as fresh frozen plasma, or albumin. This treatment is performed in an attempt to remove proteins or protein-bound solutes that cannot be removed by simple hemofiltration.[26, 27]

Hemoperfusion. In this treatment, blood is circulated on a bed of coated charcoal powder to remove solutes by adsorption. The technique is specifically indicated in cases of poisoning or intoxication with agents that can be effectively removed by charcoal, such as theophylline. This treatment commonly causes platelet and protein fraction depletion and therefore is utilized only in specific cases under intensive and continuous monitoring.[28]

ANTICOAGULATION

All forms of RRT expose blood to contact with a nonbiologic surface and, therefore, activate the clotting cascade. At the same time, it is imperative for the function of any extracorporeal circuit, such as those needed for RRT, that blood not clot within it for a period sufficient to perform the procedure in question. For these reasons, anticoagulation for the extracorporeal circuit is desirable and, at times, necessary to perform RRT safely and effectively.

Several approaches to anticoagulation during RRT have been described, and most of them rely on the use of heparin.[29, 30] Heparin can be given to achieve systemic anticoagulation if no contraindications exist. In many critically ill patients, however, systemic anticoagulation is undesirable. In these patients, low-dose heparin (5 to 10 IU/kg/hour) can be administered into the circuit in a prefilter or predialyzer position. Such therapy is often sufficient to perform intermittent hemodialysis or to achieve an adequate circuit life (approximately 24 hours) during CRRT and has the advantage of inducing very little change in the patient's risk of bleeding.

In some patients, more aggressive anticoagulation of the dialyzing or filtering membrane may be necessary, along with the need to avoid systemic anticoagulation. In these patients, "regional" anticoagulation is often effective. Such "regional" anticoagulation can be achieved by the premembrane administration of heparin at full anticoagulation doses and the postmembrane administration of protamine to reverse its effects prior to the return of blood to the patient. Typically, this process results in a heparin-protamine ratio of 100 IU to 1 mg, both given by continuous infusion.[29]

Another form of "regional" anticoagulation is based on the use of citrate to achieved chelation of calcium and the postmembrane administration of a calcium infusion to reestablish blood coagulability.[31] This approach is very effective but it requires specially made dialysate and the addition of calcium, and is associated with the development of alkalosis. Its use offers a major advantage in patients thought to have serious heparin-induced thrombocytopenia. In very-high-risk patients, such as those with severe liver coagulopathy, it is possible to perform RRT without any coagulation at all and still achieve adequate circuit performance and patient survival.[29] Low-molecular-weight heparin can also be used to maintain circuit function, but limited controlled data are available on its usefulness in comparison with standard heparin.

INITIATING AND MAINTAINING RENAL REPLACEMENT THERAPY

Many intensive care specialists believe that RRT is best initiated early in the course of the patient's ilness. This view holds that it is physiologically unsound and clinically dangerous to wait for any of the complications of uremia to develop before dialytic therapy is undertaken. Now that CRRT is available and hemodynamic instability can, therefore, be avoided, little morbidity is associated with initiating RRT early, even in the sickest of patients. There are no scientific studies, however, to help the physician decide when to start RRT. Time-honored criteria are usually descriptors of uremic complications. Such criteria deserve some detailed discussion if a conservative approach to management is preferred.

Fluid Overload

Acute renal failure may result in extravascular volume expansion (e.g., peripheral edema, ascites, pleural effusions) as well as intravascular volume expansion (e.g., hypertension, pulmonary congestion), largely because of the reduced capacity of the injured kidney to excrete sodium, which is often compounded by the administration of 2 L/day or more of various drugs and other therapies (e.g., blood products, parenteral alimentation) in the ICU. Although the extravascular manifestations of volume overload can occasionally be dramatic, they are uncommonly of sufficient morbidity to warrant urgent dialytic intervention. Exceptions to this rule are patients with anasarca (usually >10 kg in excess of dry weight), in whom UF may be required to allow for adequate wound healing, extubation, or enteral feeding. More often than not, however, extracellular volume overload is accompanied by intravascular overload, which is indicated by an elevated central venous pressure or pulmonary capillary wedge pressure, mandating dialysis or UF to optimize cardiopulmonary function.

Acute renal failure with oliguria has traditionally been defined as a daily urine output of less than 400 mL/day. Even among patients with nonoliguric ARF, however, there may be significant volume retention, particularly in patients with preexisting states of sodium avidity, such as congestive heart failure, hepatic cirrhosis, and sepsis syndrome. Volume overload is often iatrogenic and may be exacerbated following the recognition of ARF. In the absence of intravascular monitoring, parenteral fluid challenges are often attempted in patients with ARF to correct suspected hypovolemia or other reductions in renal perfusion. These fluid challenges may ultimately result in pulmonary congestion, especially in patients with concurrent cardiac or pulmonary insufficiency. The sodium salts contained in various medications (e.g., semisynthetic penicillins), alkali administration (e.g., sodium bicarbonate), and parenteral or enteral alimentation can also contribute to volume overload.

Patients with prolonged hospitalization, particularly in the setting of infectious or inflammatory disease with catabolism, can undergo significant changes in body composition that indirectly lead to hypervolemia if the shift in body water from the intracellular to the extracellular compartment is unrecognized. For example, a patient with necrotizing pancreatitis may be hypercatabolic, and his or her nutritional needs may not be met by standard enteral or parenteral nutritional formulations. Such a patient can be expected to lose up to 0.5 to 1.0 kg of lean body mass per day. The proportional reduction in body cell mass (visceral and somatic protein plus intracellular water) may be even more dramatic.[32] Thus, stable body weight in a critically ill ICU patient with ARF may be indicative of substantial extracellular volume overload.

A diuretic challenge can be undertaken in all patients with hypervolemia before ultrafiltration or dialysis is initiated. A loop diuretic, such as furosemide (200 to 400 mg) or bumetanide (5 to 10 mg) can be administered intravenously in combination with a thiazide agent, such as chlorthiazide (250 to 500 mg) or oral metolazone (5 to 10 mg), if initial attempts at inducing diuresis with loop agents alone are unsuccessful. Aminophylline (125 to 250 mg) or low-dose dopamine (1 to 2 mg/kg/min)[33] may be added to the diuretic regimen, in an attempt to augment renal perfusion and increase natriuresis.

The efficacy of a loop diuretic may be enhanced over time by continuous low-dose intravenous infusion (e.g., furosemide, 10 to 40 mg/hour)[34] or by its administration in combination with salt-poor albumin.[35] Even in the absence of an adequate diuretic effect, the vasodilatory effect of parenteral furosemide may ameliorate the symptoms of pulmonary congestion by increasing venous capacitance.[36] Additionally, the use of topical or intravenous nitrates and parenteral narcotic analgesic agents (e.g., morphine sulfate) should be considered to control dyspnea while dialysis is being arranged.

Ultrafiltration can be accomplished by intermittent hemodialysis, continuous hemofiltration or hemodiafiltration, or peritoneal dialysis. Patients with massive volume overload (>20 kg in excess of dry weight) may be optimally managed with continuous renal replacement therapy, especially in the presence of systemic hypotension requiring pressor agents.[37] More modest degrees of volume overload, however, can usually be effectively managed with either isolated UF or UF with IHD, depending on the need for solute clearance. These "conventional" dialytic methods are more widely available in most settings and do not require around-the-clock monitoring by ICU nursing staff. Improvements in IHD techniques (e.g., bicarbonate dialysate, sodium modeling, sequential ultrafiltration-hemodialysis, and UF profiling) have made IHD efficient and safe for the management of symptomatic hypervolemia with ARF in the majority of cases in the ICU.

Hyperkalemia

Hyperkalemia sufficient to cause disturbances of cardiac conduction may complicate ARF in the critically ill. Typically, individuals with primary disorders associated with hypercatabolism and tissue breakdown are at highest risk; they include patients with concurrent rhabdomyolysis, hemolytic anemia, disseminated intravascular hemolysis, gastrointestinal hemorrhage, and tumor lysis syndrome. Hyperkalemia can be aggravated by drugs such as nonsteroidal anti-inflammatory (NSAIDs), angiotensin-converting enzyme (ACE) inhibitors, angiotensin receptor antagonists, nonselective β-blockers (e.g., propranolol, nadolol), trimethoprim-sulfamethoxazole, and potassium-penicillin preparations. Efforts to direct extracellular potassium excess into the intracellular compartment with insulin and glucose, nebulized or subcutaneous $beta_2$ agonists,[38] and sodium bicarbonate are effective management strategies for the short term, but they do not reduce the total body potassium burden. Although loop or thiazide diuretic therapy can promote kaliuresis in normal individuals, this response may be blunted or absent in patients with ARF. An enterally administered cation exchange resin is an efficient potassium binder (sodium polystyrene sulfonate, 50 to 60 g every 1 to 2 hr PO or PR),[39] but its use may be limited in postoperative patients or in patients with ileus or gastrointestinal hemorrhage.

The rapid removal of potassium is one of several advantages of intermittent hemodialysis, compared with peritoneal dialysis or the other continuous renal replacement therapies. The maximum rate of potassium removal by peritoneal dialysis is approximately 12 mEq/hr,[40] whereas intermittent hemodialysis with maximum blood and dialysate flows is three to four times as efficient. Although the time-averaged small solute clearance achieved with hemodiafiltration can meet or exceed that achieved with intermittent hemodialysis, the capacity of HDF to remove a large quantity of potassium rapidly is limited.

When hyperkalemia is accompanied by electrocardiographic abnormalities (e.g., peaked T waves, prolonged QRS complex, absence of P waves), it is advisable to initially utilize a potassium dialysate concentration of 2 to 3 mEq/L and subsequently to lower it in order not to expose the patient to a dialysate that is potassium-free in an effort to limit the risk of ventricular ectopy.[41]

Uremia

Unlike pulmonary edema or hyperkalemia, which can be readily identified, the clinical consequences of uremia may be difficult to detect in the intensive care unit. For example, encephalopathy, a clinical hallmark of uremia, is common among critically ill ICU patients and may be due to advanced hepatic failure, medication-related effects, sleep disturbance, or "ICU psychosis." Likewise, asterixis, neuromuscular irritability, impaired cognition, somnolence, stupor, and coma can be observed in critically ill patients from multiple causes (e.g., side effects of narcotic analgesics). Pericarditis, another complication of uremia, may be seen after cardiac surgery or myocardial infarction or as a complication of infectious (e.g., pneumonia), neoplastic (e.g., carcinoma of the breast or lung), or autoimmune (e.g., systemic lupus erythematosus) disease.[42] Pulmonary infiltrates associated with uremia can mimic the adult respiratory distress syndrome, independent of the effects of volume overload. Uremia can also lead to a bleeding diathesis due to platelet malfunction, although underlying coagulopathy (e.g., disseminated intravascular coagulation [DIC] associated with multiple organ failure), stress gastritis, or anticoagulant and antiplatelet drugs are equally if not more likely culprits.

Although non-nephrology consultants might hope to place the blame for a variety of the preceding complications on ARF, it is extremely important to recognize that the blood urea nitrogen (BUN) value is a relatively poor surrogate for uremia. Increased levels of BUN ("azotemia") can result from catabolism (endogenous due to infection or other stress, or augmented by drugs, such as glucocorticoids or tetracyclines), gastrointestinal bleeding, or protein overfeeding, without a dramatic reduction in glomerular filtration rate. Isolated azotemia is not a cause of encephalopathy, bleeding diathesis, or other major uremic complications; rather, it can be a marker of the severity of illness. Albeit imperfect, the serum creatinine concentration (or urinary creatinine clearance) is a much better indicator of renal function in the critically ill patient.

Central nervous system complications of uremia generally improve most rapidly with dialysis,[43] often with one or two treatments; others usually improve over several days, regardless of the dialytic modality.

Acidemia

Metabolic acidosis almost invariably accompanies ARF, as endogenously generated organic acids are retained and the kidney suffers from a diminished ability to retain bicarbonate and to maximally acidify the urine. Among critically ill patients, acidosis may be exacerbated by hypoventilation, diarrhea, and an errant (chloride-rich) composition of intravenous fluids and alimentation.

Metabolic acidosis is usually well tolerated until the systemic pH declines below 7.20. Less severe acidemia may have untoward metabolic effects[44] but can usually be corrected conservatively. The administration of alkali (e.g., sodium bicarbonate) is usually sufficient to match endogenous acid production in the nonhypercatabolic patient. More severe acidemia (pH less than 7.20) may be associated with cardiovascular dysfunction.

Alkali therapy for patients with lactic acidosis due to low cardiac output or hypoxemic states may be contraindicated, because the administration of sodium bicarbonate in this subgroup of critically ill patients can paradoxically worsen intracellular acidosis.[45] Dichloroacetate and other agents touted as potential medical treatments for severe lactic acidosis have yielded disappointing results.[46] RRT is usually indicated if severe acidemia is not readily reversed. Hemodynamic instability should be anticipated in these patients, and either efforts aimed at reducing hemodialysis-associated hypotension should be considered (see later) or CRRT should be used.

Bicarbonate has replaced acetate as the dialysate base in virtually all uses of intermittent hemodialysis. This is in contrast to PD and CRRT, in which lactate is the most commonly used base. Although modifications of the CRRT prescription can be made to provide either a citrate-based replacement solution or a "customized" bicarbonate-based dialysate to patients with ARF and lactic acidosis, some practitioners may opt for IHD in this subpopulation.

Relative Indications

Disorders of calcium, magnesium, and uric acid only rarely require dialytic management. Modest levels of hypocalcemia often accompany ARF and can usually be treated effectively with intravenous or oral calcium supplementation if hyperphosphatemia (and the risk of metastatic calcification) is not present. Hypercalcemia is usually managed with volume expansion and loop diuretics; if hypercalcemia is refractory to such measures, treatment with biphosphanates, corticosteroids, or other agents may be required, depending on the etiology of the disorder. It is noteworthy that hypercalcemia can itself exacerbate renal dysfunction by its direct vasoconstrictive effect. If hypercalcemia is severe and unresponsive to conservative therapy, a modified dialysate calcium concentration should be formulated (0 to 1.5 mEq/L) and IHD should be initiated. IHD offers the most rapid and efficient correction of calcium excess among the available dialytic modalities. CRRT, however, is also effective in smoothly lowering serum calcium concentrations.

When magnesium toxicity results in respiratory depression, as with massive ingestion of magnesium-containing antacid preparations, IHD can be performed with a magnesium-free dialysate. Similarly, uric acid can be effectively removed by dialysis or CRRT in the setting of tumor lysis with ARF. Usually, allopurinol, volume expansion, and alkalinization allow for the conservative management of this syndrome.

A different and more aggressive approach to the above problems, however, has been advocated for use in the ICU patient, in whom maintenance of homeostasis is an important therapeutic goal.[47] According to such an approach, prevention is superior to treatment, early intervention is desirable, and CRRT offers the ideal form of RRT. More "intensivist-minded" and less nephrologically oriented views of RRT in the ICU hold that different criteria for initiating RRT in the ICU should now be considered (Table 155–1).

Once RRT has been instituted, there is no scientifically established biochemical or clinical measure of so-called dialytic adequacy. Most clinicians using CRRT, however, seek to maintain a urea concentration of less than 30 mmol/L and, preferably, less than 25 mmol/L. Normalization of electrolyte, phosphate, and calcium levels is also pursued. The ideal therapy should be able to achieve these goals with a minimum of morbidity and at reasonable cost. The ideal dialysis dose in critically ill patients, however, remains unclear, and we still have little information on the relationship between the "dose" of dialysis and outcomes in ARF. Moreover, the gap between dialysis prescribed and dialysis delivered, which may be in excess of 20% or more in end-stage renal disease (ESRD),[48] may be even more pronounced with ARF, owing to hemodynamic instability, reduced blood flow (Qb) shortened dialysis time because of scheduled procedures or diagnostic tests, and suboptimal vascular access, usually a temporary catheter prone to recirculation.

Conger[49] performed a prospective study of "prophylactic" dialysis in ARF aboard a naval hospital ship stationed near Viet Nam in 1970. Patients were prospectively matched for type and severity of trauma and then assigned to receive one of two dialysis regimens: an "intensive" treatment, in which patients were dialyzed to maintain the BUN and creatinine concentrations below 70 and 5 mg/dL, respectively, or a "conservative" treatment, in which dialysis was not provided unless the BUN value was in excess of 150 mg/dL, as long as other complications (e.g., hyperkalemia) could be adequately controlled with conservative measures. Five of eight patients in the intensive treatment group survived, compared with two of 10 patients in the conservative treatment group, a beneficial trend that did not reach statistical significance. Hemorrhage, gram-negative septicemia, and peritonitis were less commonly seen in the intensive therapy group. Despite its small sample size, this study is most notable for being the first assessment of differing dialysis strategies using nonhistorical control subjects.

Gillum and associates[50] conducted a study in which patients with ARF were randomly assigned in pairs matched by ARF etiology to receive either intensive treatment (dialysis to maintain predialysis blood urea nitrogen and serum creatinine concentrations below 60 mg/dL and 5 mg/dL, respectively) or a "nonintensive" treatment (dialysis to maintain the corresponding values 100 mg/dL and 9 mg/dL, respectively). The timing of dialysis was roughly controlled for by requiring that a patient have a serum creatinine concentration of at least 8 mg/dL before being randomly assigned for treatment. Assignments to treatment were not blinded for either physicians or patients. By design, the causes of ARF were similar in the two groups, as were patient age, the proportions of males and females, presence of oliguria, nutritional parameters, and other clinical factors reported. Seven of 17 (41%) patients in the intensive treatment group survived their hospitalization for ARF, compared with nine of 17 (53%) in the nonintensive treatment group. Hemorrhage and septicemia were less commonly seen in the intensive treatment group. None of these differences reached statistical significance; however, this study had very limited statistical power.

Preliminary reports from a study being conducted by Paganini and colleagues[51] are worth noting. In the first report, these researchers examined the influence of dialytic modality (IHD versus CRRT; not randomly allocated) in 856 critically ill patients with ARF. Among the 280 patients treated with IHD, there was no significant association between prescribed dialysis dose and the odds of death. Mortality was strongly associated with severity of illness and comorbidity. In a later report, patients were categorized into risk quartiles on the basis of an institution-specific severity of illness and comorbidity score.[52] Dialysis dose was not associated with mortality at either extreme (very low or very high) of risk. Mortality was reduced, however, in intermediate-risk patients treated with more intensive dialysis, defined as a urea reduction ratio in excess of 58% in patients in IHD, and a time-averaged urea concentration below 45 mg/dL in patients treated with CRRT. Renal recovery and other outcomes were not reported.

Schiffl and coworkers[53] have reported on preliminary results of a randomized clinical trial in which 72 patients with ARF were randomly assigned to receive either daily or alternate-day IHD. Mortality was significantly reduced in the daily IHD group (21% versus 47%). When patients at the extremes of dose were compared, mortality was 57% in patients with time-clearance product (Kt/V) of less than 3, compared with 16% in patients with Kt/V greater than 6. These data are provocative but require confirmation elsewhere.

On the basis of data derived from patients with ESRD, and on limited data in ARF, it can be concluded that more dialysis is better. The prescription should be individualized. Patients who are hypercatabolic or who experience large obligate fluid intake will likely need daily IHD for control of azotemia and hypervolemia. Until a more refined tool is available, it is reasonable to use the urea reduction ratio (pre-BUN minus post-BUN, divided by pre-BUN × 100), aiming for at least 65% to 70% per session, corresponding to a time-clearance product (Kt/V) of roughly 1.2 per treatment, or 4.2 per week assuming alternate-day therapy. This goal should be higher in hypercatabolic patients. The dangers of using moderate or low BUN or creatinine levels (potentially the result of low dietary protein intake and diminished somatic protein mass, respectively) as measures of treatment adequacy cannot be overemphasized.

TABLE 155–1. Modern Indications for Initiating Renal Replacement Therapy (RRT) in Critically Ill Adult Patients*

1. Oliguria (urine output < 200 mL/12 hr)
2. Anuria or extreme oliguria (urine output < 50 mL/12 hr)
3. Hyperkalemia ($[K^+]$ > 6.5 mmol/L and rising)
4. Severe acidemia (pH < 7.1)
5. Azotemia ([urea] > 30 mmol/L or [creat] > 300 μcmol/L)
6. Pulmonary edema
7. Uremic encephalopathy
8. Uremic pericarditis
9. Uremic neuropathy or myopathy
10. Severe dysnatremia ($[Na^+]$ > 160 or <115 mmol/L)
11. Hyperthermia
12. Drug overdose with filterable toxin (e.g., lithium, vancomycin, procainamide)
13. Anasarca
14. Diuretic-resistant cardiac failure
15. Imminent or ongoing massive blood product administration

**Note:* The presence of one of these criteria is sufficient to initiate RRT. The simultaneous presence of two of these criteria makes the prompt initiation of RRT highly desirable. The presence of three criteria makes the prompt initiation of RRT mandatory. In all of these cases, continuous RRT is the preferred approach.

SPECIFIC ISSUES RELATED TO INTERMITTENT HEMODIALYSIS

Which Dialyzer?

The chemical composition and porosity of hollow-fiber dialyzers are of growing interest to nephrologists as more is learned about accumulated products in uremia and the immunologic consequences of the blood-dialyzer contact. These effects may be particularly important for patients with ARF, in whom the kidneys, which are often ischemic owing to surgery, shock, or sepsis or are otherwise affected by cytokines or nephrotoxins, may be especially vulnerable to immunologic or other secondary injuries.

Commonly used dialyzers are composed of a variety of materials, including regenerated cellulose, modified cellulose (e.g., cuprophane, hemophan, cellulose acetate), and newer synthetic materials, such as polymethylmethacrylate, polyamide, polysulfone, and polyacrilonitrile. These materials vary widely in capacity for solute transport (i.e., flux) and UF and extent of interaction with cellular and soluble components of the blood (i.e., biocompatibility) as well as cost (synthetic membranes are more expensive).

It is noteworthy that IHD has been associated with several potentially adverse biophysical and inflammatory changes in the human, including enhanced cell surface expression of leukocyte adhesion molecules (LAMs) such as MAC-1 and LAM-1,[54] stimulation of synthesis of reactive oxygen species such as superoxide,[55] systemic release of thromboxane,[56] and augmented monocyte elaboration of interleukin-1, interleukin-6, and tumor necrosis factor.[57, 58] Many of these molecules are abundant in multiple organ failure, although the effect of their modulation by hemodialysis remains unknown. Cuprophane hemodialyzers appear to initiate these processes more than synthetic dialyzers.[59]

Two 1994 prospective trials have explored the role of the dialysis membrane in critically ill patients with ARF, comparing cuprophane with polymethylmethacrylate or polyacrylonitrile.[60, 61] In terms of patient survival, neither study reached conventional levels of statistical significance, although the sample sizes were relatively small, and the trends toward better patient survival with noncellulose membranes were impressive (57% versus 37% in one study[60]). Furthermore, the proportion of patients who recovered renal function was significantly higher, and the time to renal recovery significantly shorter, in patients dialyzed with noncellulose membranes.

Nearly all hollow-fiber dialyzers used in IHD share the capacity to efficiently remove small solutes such as potassium and urea. Dialyzers are considered either "low flux" or "high flux" according to their hydraulic permeability and their ability to transport compounds of molecular weights exceeding 10,000 daltons, so-called *middle molecules.* Perhaps the most widely studied of these molecules is β_2-microglobulin, a protein implicated in the development of dialysis-related amyloidosis (but of unknown relevance in ARF). High-flux dialyzers are capable of removing or binding the anaphylatoxins C3a and C5a[62] as well as inflammatory cytokines such as tumor necrosis factor-α (TNF-α), and interleukin-1,[63] so that greater membrane porosity may affect common mediators of critical illness. Nevertheless, it is difficult to separate the specific effects of membrane flux from the concordant effects of biocompatibility. One potential disadvantage of high-flux dialyzers is that the larger pore configuration may permit the backfiltration of bacterial cell wall products (e.g., lipopolysaccharide) from unsterile dialysate. Whether "protective" mediators are lost in larger quantity is unknown. At present, therefore, there is limited evidence to support or refute the use of high-flux membranes in ARF.

Which Dialysate?

One of the major advantages of IHD is the ability to individualize therapy for the patient with ARF with regard to duration, drugs, dialyzer, delivery system, and dialysate. This capacity has made IHD more effective and safer for critically ill patients. In the following discussion, we review separately each of the dialysate components and its relevance in the management of ARF.

In general, dialysate is infused within the dialyzer (surrounding the hollow fibers) countercurrent to blood flow (Qb) to maximize solute clearance. Dialysate flow rates (Qd) of 500 mL/min are typically used, in excess of the 15 to 30 mL/min rate used in most CRRT regimens. In IHD, solute clearance can be augmented by dialysate flow rates of up to 500 mL/min in the presence of blood flow rates (generated via a pump-driven system) of 250 to 350 mL/min. Given the biophysical limitations of a double-lumen temporary dialysis catheter, Qb rates in excess of 400 mL/min are generally not achieved; investigations in patients with ESRD have suggested that increases in Qd above 500 mL/min yield little if any benefit in solute clearance without Qb of 400 mL/min or more.[64]

Sodium

Sodium is the main determinant of dialysate osmolality. Dialysate sodium concentration typically ranges from 135 to 145 mEq/L. Lower dialysate sodium concentrations can attenuate hypertension and thirst but can also contribute to the development of cerebral edema, an especially undesirable effect in critically ill patients. Patients with ARF associated with systemic hypotension may benefit from dialysate sodium concentrations in the range of 140 to 148 mEq/L, which may lessen the hypotensive effect of diffusive dialysis.[65]

During IHD, osmotically active solutes (e.g., urea nitrogen) are removed, resulting in a relative reduction in extracellular osmolality. This phenomenon leads to further loss of extracellular fluid into the intracellular space, with the potential for hemodynamic instability. Maintaining dialysate sodium concentration at or above the serum sodium concentration (usually ~140 mEq/L) attenuates this hemodynamic effect in most patients. Although a higher dialysate sodium concentration can lead to thirst and polydipsia, resulting in layer interdialytic weight gain in patients with ESRD, these potential complications are of less concern in the acute setting.

Newer dialysate delivery systems permit on-line adjustment of dialysate sodium concentration, a capacity that may stabilize hemodynamics in critically ill patients. "Sodium modeling" is accomplished through the use of variable dilution proportioning systems, rather than a fixed dialysate solute-water ratio. Typically, the initial sodium concentration is 145 to 150 mEq/L, to allow for more vigorous ultrafiltration with less systemic hypotension; a step, linear, or exponential reduction is made toward 138 to 140 mEq/L near the end of the session. Although a reduction in dialysate sodium concentration from 145 to 150 mEq/L down to 130 to 135 mEq/L in as little as 2 to 3 hours has been modeled, little is known about the potential central nervous system consequences of such a practice, and randomized trials of this technique in ARF are lacking. Sodium concentration modeling reduces the frequency of hypotension during ultrafiltration without a decrease in time committed to diffusive clearance (see sequential ultrafiltration hemodialysis); however, it is unclear whether the technique is safer or more effective than treatment with a fixed dialysate concentration of 140 to 145 mEq/L.

Potassium

The capacity for rapid removal of potassium is one of the major advantages of IHD over PD and CRRT. Still, the extent of potassium removal is unpredictable and widely variable among individuals. The major reason for the variability is that only a small fraction of the total body potassium is present in the extracellular space, and the flux of potassium from the intracellular to the extracellular space, the source of the majority of potassium removed,[66] depends on patient-specific and dialysate-specific factors.[67] As a result of this flux from intracellular to extracellular compartment after dialysis, a potassium rebound occurs, leading to a higher serum potassium concentration at 1 to 2 hours after the completion of treatment. It is consequently unwise to monitor the immediately postdialysis potassium concentration as a measure of the adequacy of potassium removal, and supplements should not be administered until sufficient time has elapsed for the rebound to occur.

Another practical implication of the double-pool distribution of potassium is that optimal potassium removal is achieved with daily IHD treatments rather than protracted treatments given every other day, particularly in patients with excess potassium delivery (e.g., because of transfusion) and in patients with excess potassium or generation; (e.g., due to tissue catabolism). The integrity of the vascular access is another important patient-specific component of potassium removal. Poorly functional catheters tend to recirculate blood (i.e., a small fraction of the blood volume is cleansed repeatedly, whereas the majority of the blood volume is ineffectively dialyzed).

In addition to these patient-specific variables, the composition of other dialysate elements (e.g., glucose, alkali) alters the extent of potassium removal. It is probably inadvisable to deliver glucose-free dialysate to critically ill patients, given the potential risks of hypoglycemia, particularly in individuals with hepatic dysfunction. Nevertheless, the use of glucose-free dialysate can augment potassium clearance by up to 30%, by minimizing insulin release and transcellular potassium uptake. Rapid increases in systemic pH, as may occur in acidemic patients started on bicarbonate-buffered dialysis, augment transcellular potassium uptake, resulting in diminished potassium dialysance. Effects of the potassium gradient on base transfer have also been observed. With a 1-mEq increase in the blood:dialysate potassium gradient, the uptake of bicarbonate is reduced by 50 mEq (roughly equivalent to 50 mL of an 8.4% sodium bicarbonate solution). Therefore, the correction of acidemia in a critically ill patient with ARF is diminished if severe hyperkalemia necessitates the use of a 0 to 1 mEq/L dialysate potassium concentration.

Since many factors contribute to the efficiency of potassium removal with IHD, the initial dialysate potassium concentration is usually chosen empirically. For patients with severe hyperkalemia (i.e., potassium concentration higher than 7 to 8 mEq/L), a final dialysate potassium concentration of 0 to 1 mEq/L is often required to maintain intradialytic potassium concentrations below 5 to 6 mEq/L. The patient should be started on a dialysate potassium concentration of 2 to 3 mEq/L for 30 minutes to 1 hour to attenuate the rate of reduction of extracellular potassium concentration, which may be the most important determinant of the risk of arrhythmia. Patients without hyperkalemia are best served with dialysate potassium concentrations in the range of 3- to 4 mEq/L, especially if urine output is sustained. Finally, one should consider gastrointestinal losses of potassium (e.g., through diarrhea, nasogastric suction) when planning the IHD prescription.

Alkali

Bicarbonate is the principal base used in IHD. In past years, acetate rather than bicarbonate was routinely employed. However, acetate acts as a direct peripheral vasodilator and myocardial depressant, characteristics that make it particularly undesirable in the critically ill patient. Furthermore, patients with hepatic failure or underperfused skeletal muscle may have diminished capacity for acetate (as well as citrate and lactate) metabolism, potentially leading to hypotension, nausea, vomiting, and transient worsening of metabolic acidosis.[68] This complication appears to be more common in women, in elderly patients, and in malnourished patients.[69]

There are two important disadvantages to the use of bicarbonate-buffered dialysate, although both can be readily managed. First, bicarbonate forms insoluble salts with calcium and magnesium after prolonged exposure in solution. Second, bicarbonate-based solutions support the growth of certain hydrophylic gram-negative bacteria, including *Pseudomonas, Xanthomonas, Acinetobacter,* and *Flavobacterium* species.[70] Therefore, a bicarbonate solution is usually mixed daily from a powdered source, obviating the need for storage, and is safely added to other dialysate components by a computerized delivery system.

The concentration of bicarbonate in dialysate is usually around 35 mEq/L. This concentration allows for correction of acidemia in most patients. In patients with preexisting alkalosis (e.g., secondary to nasogastric suction), either the concentration of bicarbonate should be reduced or, if optimal solute clearance is not paramount, the intensity of dialysis should be diminished, so that excessive alkalemia (with accompanying hypoventilation and hypoxemia) does not occur. Finally, intravenous fluids and alimentation should be adjusted accordingly (e.g., more or less chloride or acetate) after the initiation of IHD.

Glucose

Historically, the dialysate glucose concentration was decreased to help control hyperglycemia in patients with diabetes mellitus or increased to enhance the ultrafiltration. Today, most patients with ARF receive a dialysate glucose concentration of 200 mg/dL, a safe "middle ground."

Glucose-free dialysate should be avoided in patients with ARF. Aside from the loss of calories, ARF may predispose a patient to hypoglycemia because of impaired renal gluconeogenesis along with diminished clearance of endogenous (or exogenous) insulin. Patients with concomitant hepatic failure and those receiving sulfonylureas (e.g., glyburide, glipizide) are at increased risk for this complication.

Calcium

Hypocalcemia is a common complication of acute and chronic renal failure. As with chronic renal failure, hypocalcemia associated with ARF may be due to phosphate retention, impaired formation of 1,25-OH cholecalciferol, and skeletal resistance to the calcemic effects of parathyroid hormone. Hypocalcemia may be particularly severe in patients with ARF associated with rhabdomyolysis and tumor lysis syndrome, because of calcium-phosphate binding and deposition, or in patients with pancreatitis, owing to calcium–fatty acid "soap" formation. Patients with alkalemia (pH 7.45 or more) are at higher risk of hypocalemic complications, including seizures and cardiac arrhythmias, because of a relative reduction in ionized calcium concentration.

The dialysate calcium concentration should be individualized in all cases. In practice, a value of 2.5 mEq/L is often selected. Dialysate calcium concentrations of 3 to 3.5 mEq/L are usually needed to correct hypocalcemia and to maintain vascular tone during the IHD procedure. Indeed, it has been determined that to achieve positive calcium balance during hemodialysis, the dialysate calcium concentration must be at least 3.5 mEq/L.[71]

For the rare patient with multiple myeloma or milk-alkali syndrome complicated by ARF, the dialysate calcium concentration may need to be reduced to 1 to 2 mEq/L.

Magnesium

Formerly largely ignored, magnesium has now been given closer attention as a potentially important determinant in critical illness. Hypomagnesemia has been implicated in the pathogenesis of atrial[72] and ventricular[73] arrhythmias and as a regulator of bronchial smooth muscle tone in asthma and chronic obstructive pulmonary disease.[74] Renewed interest in this cation has led to more frequent monitoring of blood levels and more liberal parenteral and enteral supplementation, despite the fact that serum levels are known to be poorly predictive of total body stores.

Because the kidneys are the predominant site of magnesium excretion, mild to moderate hypermagnesemia is commonly observed in association with ARF. A dialysate magnesium concentration of 1.0 mEq/L is usually employed. Magnesium-free dialysate is manufactured and might be preferred in rare patients with severe hypermagnesemia and respiratory failure. Nephrotoxic ARF due to amphotericin B, cisplatin, ifosfamide, or aminoglycosides can be associated with hypomagnesemia. In these cases, most practitioners would carefully give supplements of oral or intravenous magnesium rather than increasing the magnesium concentration of the dialysate.

Complications

Major complications of IHD in the setting of ARF are listed in Table 155–2. The most common complication is systemic hypotension, which results from the removal of extracellular fluid with UF and from the vasodilation due to diffusive solute clearance and blood membrane interactions (see earlier). Iatrogenic hypotension can be promoted by the injudicious use of antihypertensive agents or vasodilators either during or immediately before or after the dialysis session. Many popular antihypertensive agents have been formulated as long-acting preparations or have prolonged elimination with renal dysfunction and are commonly prescribed for ICU patients with cardiovascular disease. Avoiding the administration of these medications during the 4 or more hours before dialysis (depending on drug half-life) may attenuate hypotension, particularly in preload-dependent patients who require UF. Patients should be carefully evaluated for occult blood loss (e.g., retroperitoneal hemorrhage after femoral line placement), new cardiovascular complications, and pericardial disease, since uremic pericarditis can predispose to cardiac tamponade.

More often, hypotension results from the underlying disease process (e.g., sepsis, cardiogenic shock) and can be exacerbated by the IHD procedure. The IHD regimen can be modified in several ways to attenuate procedure-related hypotension. The UF rate can be reduced to allow for more gradual recruitment of interstitial fluid into the vascular space, although the total dialysis time may need to be longer to accommodate overall UF requirements. The dialysate sodium concentration should be maintained at or above 140 mEq/L, and, if tolerated, the dialysate can be cooled to 35°C to 36°C to promote peripheral vasoconstriction.[75]

Sequential ultrafiltration-hemodialysis is a practical and effective modification of IHD in patients with ARF. This technique is based on the observed improvement in vascular and cardiac hemodynamics during the temporal and physical segregation of UF and solute clearance.[76] When UF is performed in concert with diffusive dialysis, the compensatory increase in peripheral vascular resistance appears to diminish, perhaps in relation to the diffusive loss of osmotically active substances and to transcellular fluid and electrolyte shifts. In contrast, when UF is performed alone, it is usually accompanied by an increase in peripheral vascular resistance, such that up to 2 L/hour or more can be removed without systemic hypotension.[77] Although some convective clearance is provided during the UF phase of sequential ultrafiltration-hemodialysis (in practice usually 60 to 90 minutes), it is important to maintain a diffusive phase long enough to achieve the desired level of solute clearance.

TABLE 155–2. Major Complications of Intermittent Hemodialysis

Systemic hypotension
Arrhythmia
Hypoxemia
Hemorrhage
Infection
Line-related complications (e.g., pneumothorax)
Seizure/dialysis dysequilibrium
Pyrogen reaction or hemolysis
(?) Delay in recovery of renal function

Nutritional Support

Acute renal failure, particularly when associated with sepsis, trauma, or multiple organ failure, can be marked by increased energy expenditure and protein catabolism. The optimal means of providing nutrients to such patients, given concerns about urea generation, uremia, and extracellular volume overload, have been elusive. Indeed, the widespread use of parenteral nutrition in the course of ARF has led to the increasingly frequent need to initiate dialysis because of obligate nutrition-related fluid administration.

When possible, enteral nutrition is preferred, as it allows for reduced fluid administration compared with total parenteral nutrition (TPN), and eliminates the need for a dedicated central venous catheter. Low-electrolyte formulas are available, some designed specifically for patients with renal disease. More important, the potential risks of central venous catheter–associated bacteremia and fungemia are reduced. Likewise, enteral feeding may preserve intestinal mucosal integrity and limit the translocation of gram-negative bacteria and endotoxin.[78, 79]

In spite of considerable experience in providing nutritional support to patients with ARF for more than two decades, the optimal parenteral nutrition formulation for patients with ARF is unknown. An early, oft-cited study compared hypertonic glucose alone with a solution containing essential amino acids and demonstrated better survival and higher rates of return of renal function with the latter solution.[80] However, no significant differences in survival, renal recovery, or laboratory evidence of nitrogen balance were seen in several subsequent studies that examined modifications of the type (essential versus nonessential or mixed) and quantity of amino acid supplement provided.[81–83]

At present, we recommend the administration of at least 1.2 g protein and 25 to 35 kcal/kg/day for patients with ARF who require dialysis; substantially more protein and calories may be needed in patients with sepsis or multiple organ failure. Efforts to quantify protein needs, by calculation of urea appearance or protein catabolic rate, may help to guide administration of protein or amino acid therapy. Although amino acids are lost during IHD, parenteral nutrition should not be withheld before or during IHD; approximately 90% of infused amino acids are retained even during treatment.[84]

CONTROVERSIES IN THE CHOICE OF RENAL REPLACEMENT THERAPY IN THE INTENSIVE CARE UNIT

No randomized controlled trial has been published to guide the clinician in choosing the best form of RRT for a given critically ill patient. Not surprisingly, in the absence of such a trial, there is much controversy and disagreement concerning the choice of RRT in the ICU. In the adult population, however, it is fair to say that peritoneal dialysis is now only uncommonly used in developed countries. This lack of application is due to several factors, including (1) insufficient solute clearance,[85] (2) limited control of hyperkalemia, (3) a high incidence of peritonitis, (4) poor fluid removal, (5) unpredictable fluctuations in glycemia, (6) abdominal leaks, and (7) respiratory dysfunction. Because of these factors, the major controversy pertains to the preferential use of CRRT versus IHD. This controversy has generally divided practitioners according to national or regional lines, with Australian and European intensivists increasingly adopting CRRT and American nephrologists choosing to remain with IHD. Although this controversy is likely to remain unresolved, some observations may assist the intensivist in appreciating the pros and cons of the options available.

First, hemodialysis is often (15% to 20% of the time) associated with hypotension in critically ill patients, and such hypotension is most severe in patients whose cardiovascular status is most unstable.[60, 86, 87] The physiologic cost of such hypotension is clinically significant because IHD may precipitate ischemia in specific organs, such as the recovering kidneys, which have temporarily lost pressure-flow autoregulation. Such ischemia can be seen histologically as fresh ischemic lesions occurring with each session of IHD.[88, 89] These lesions delay renal recovery. The other major concern regarding episodic fluid removal with IHD is the intermittent fluid overload that occurs between treatments. In the extreme case, this can be unacceptable, as is the case for oliguric patients with ARDS, who do not easily tolerate excess extravascular water. CRRT is the obvious choice in such patients; indeed, CRRT may also improve the respiratory function in patients with multiple organ failure and acute lung injury.

An important practical benefit of CRRT is its ability to continuously remove as much fluid as desired; this feature particularly affects patient nutrition, which can be delivered without restriction.[90, 91] The importance of feeding the critically ill patient adequately has been borne out by studies demonstrating a correlation between mortality and a progressive calorie deficit[92] as well as an association between patient morbidity and cumulative protein intake. The advantages of the CRRT techniques are that they (1) can clear urea adequately, even in septic patients,[91] and (2) provide sufficient nutritional support, even in those who are hypercatabolic. Compared with IHD, both CAVHD and CVVHD are superior in delivering the required daily nutrients. As an aside, it should be noted that using bio-incompatible membranes may increase protein catabolism.[93] The daily loss of free amino acids and nitrogen during CRRT is similar to that seen during a 4-hour hemodialysis session (~1 to 2 g) or 10% of the usual daily intake[94] (Fig. 155-8). Last, CRRT also reduces energy expenditure by cooling the febrile patient and no hormonal or trace element losses of significance take place. Vitamin losses are also minimal, except for vitamin C, which is lost in the amount roughly equivalent to its recommended daily allowance (Fig. 155-9).

There are now several reports on the utility of hemofiltration for heart failure that is resistant to diuretics. Such cases often respond well to continuous UF with a rise in cardiac index while avoiding a fall in arterial pressure. These hemodynamic improvements are due to a change in preload, which optimizes myocardial contractility on the Starling curve. Many patients with congestive cardiac failure that does not respond to conventional therapy are now successfully treated in this way.[95]

The rationale for using CRRT is to achieve a physiologic, progressive removal of fluid and solute. The cumulative clearance of urea and creatinine by a continuous method is superior (clinically and statistically) to that achieved by IHD applied up to four times per week, even in septic patients Indeed, IHD six times per week would be necessary to achieve the same uremic control seen with standard CRRT.[96] The net result is that, in practice, uremic control is clearly superior during CRRT.[97] As argued previously, several lines of evidence suggest that better uremic control may translate into clinically important benefits.

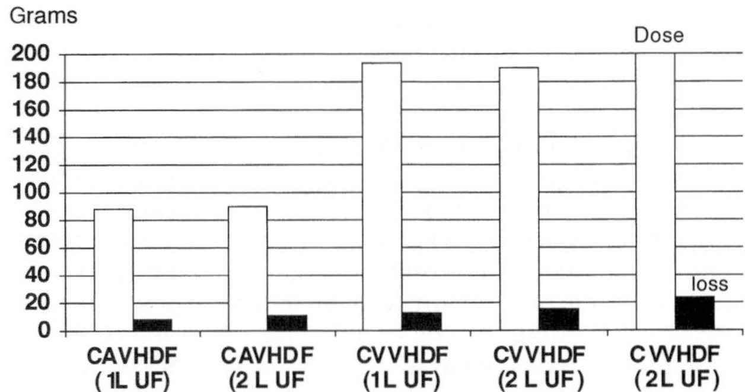

Figure 155–8. Histogram illustrating daily amino acid losses in relation to administered amount during various techniques of continuous renal replacement therapy. As can be seen, amino acid losses represent a small fraction of the administered amount. UF = ultrafiltrate; CAVHDF = continuous arteriovenous hemodiafiltration; CVVHDF = continuous venovenous hemodiafiltration.

The disadvantage of the faster, diffusive clearance of solute with IHD is that it causes solute dysequilibrium, because solute is extracted from the intravascular space by the dialyzer at a rate substantially faster than the movement of solute from the intracellular and interstitial compartments. A well-recognized phenomenon in dialysis for chronic renal failure, such dysequilibrium is responsible for brain edema[98] and has even more pronounced ill effects in critically ill patients, particularly those with increased intracranial pressure.[99] In high-risk patients, rapid solute movements may cause herniation and death. CRRT, however, does not induce such surges in intracranial pressure and maintains cerebral perfusion pressure.[99] CRRT is, therefore, the treatment of choice in all patients with or at risk for cerebral edema.

Other practical considerations regarding differences between CRRT and IHD include thermal loss, anticoagulation, and patient mobilization. The ability to cool febrile patients may be beneficial, as it is often accompanied by amelioration

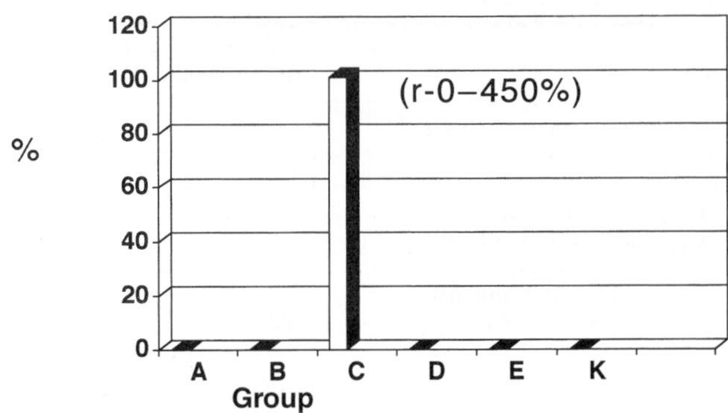

Figure 155–9. Diagram illustrating daily vitamin losses during continuous venovenous hemofiltration. As can be seen, there are no significant losses of vitamins except for vitamin C, which is lost in amounts close to the recommended daily allowance (RDA).

of tachycardia and vasodilation.[100] Because this effect conceals some clinical signs of infection, however, the clinician should have a lower threshold for suspicion of ongoing sepsis in patients so treated.

Anticoagulation of the hemofiltration circuit with heparin is safe and adequate in the vast majority of patients. In those at risk of bleeding, various alternative approaches are used, including low-dose heparin, regional heparinization, low-molecular-weight heparin, prostacyclin, citrate, and no anticoagulation. It is not uncommon to find that persisting difficulties with circuit clotting are due to problems with vascular access. These problems can occur irrespective of whether continuous or intermittent treatment is being employed. Overall, the need for anticoagulation does not pose a sufficient obstacle to the use of CRRT instead of IHD.

Once a patient starts to improve, the focus of patient management begins to swing toward physical rehabilitation, including mobilization both within the bed and out of the bed. To achieve mobilization in patients who still depend on RRT, it may be appropriate to change to IHD, given that hemodynamic stability will have returned and that only biocompatible filters will be used. Dialysis may then be potentially more in tune with the overall management than CRRT.

Despite the demonstrable benefits of using CRRT in critically ill patients, there are some who believe that, in the absence of a proven effect on mortality, IHD should be regarded as the standard approach. The difficulty, however, is that to demonstrate such a difference would require a multicenter study evaluating more than a thousand randomly grouped patients with standardization of other aspects of clinical management. Two attempts have been made to conduct such studies. Both have had difficulty with methodology, randomization, and recruitment of patients; neither has yet been published in full, and neither has achieved conclusive results so far. Unless it is shown that hemofiltration can influence the outcome of sepsis, patients will still survive, or die of, the underlying disease. Furthermore, as more ICUs change to using CRRT, such a trial will be increasingly difficult to undertake.

Of all the patients in intensive care, those who are receiving RRT and have multiple organ failure have the poorest prognosis and yet cost the most. It is, therefore, important to consider the costs of treatments used in these patients, including renal replacement. Although the principles of cost estimation apply generally, they must be calculated for individual institutions and ICUs to account for local factors, such as salaries, costs of replacement of dialysate fluids, methods of anticoagulation, and rates of depreciation on equipment purchased. As an example, Table 155–3 sets out the estimated costs of providing CVVHD or IHD as the RRT for an ICU patient for 1 week. The calculations shown, for the ICU of Guy's Hospital, London, in 1994, were based on the following assumptions:

- The CVVH hemofilters and circuits survive 28 hours (probably an underestimation, overvaluing the cost of CRRT).
- Critically ill patients would receive IHD at least four times per week (this may be an underestimation, thereby undervaluing the cost of IHD).
- Heparin is used for anticoagulation with both methods.
- The costs are estimated for one patient for 1 week. The renal unit dialysis machine would be in the ICU for only half of its possible daytime use; hence, only half of its depreciation and maintenance costs are taken into account.
- Critically ill patients would undergo dialysis with a biocompatible synthetic filter rather than a cellulose-based filter.
- The ICU nurse would set up, prime, and run the CVVHD for his or her own patient or would receive assistance from nurses within the ICU (a standard in all units using CRRT).

The costs of the two methods are very close, with IHD being only 6% cheaper. CAVHD would be cheaper overall because a blood pump would not be required, however, CAVHD may not be as efficient as IHD and is not as suitable for patients with coagulopathy or peripheral vascular disease, and the weekly cost of CAVHD is only marginally lower than that of IHD, from the initial capital outlay for the blood pump.

Such costs have also been considered by van Bommel and associates[101] amd Moreno and colleagues[102] who concluded that CAVHD was more expensive than IHD; these authors recognized, however, that significant limitations made their comparisons inaccurate. They noted that "the actual difference is reduced somewhat as the costs of dialysis machines and water treatment systems were not considered. Moreover, to achieve azotemic control similar to that achieved with CAVHD, the frequency of IHD would have to be increased, thus increasing costs. The apparent prolongation of ARF with IHD represents a further increase in total costs." Furthermore, cheaper cellulose-based filters were used with IHD. In a proper assessment of the cost effectiveness of different treat-

TABLE 155–3. Comparative Costs (in Pounds Sterling)* of Renal Replacement Therapy (RRT) at Guy's Hospital Intensive Care Unit (ICU)

Item	Continuous Venovenous Hemodialysis	Intermittent Hemodialysis
Filter life/frequency of change	28 hours	4 times/wk
Vascular access	Quinton catheter	Quinton catheter
Machine	Hospal BSM22	Gambro AK10/100; only 50% usage in ICU
Purchase cost	£3,500	£14,000
Depreciation over 8 years (per annum)	£438	£1750
Maintenance (per annum)	£300	£1050
Total (per week)	***£14***	***£27***
Consumables		
Circuit/filter (per week)	Hospal AN69 @ £40; 6 filters = ***£240***	Hospal AN69 @ £40; 4 filters = ***£160***
Dialysis/replacement (per week)	Fluid @ £7/5 litres; 50 litres/day = ***£490***	Electrolyte/bicarbonate concentrate × 4 @ £12.50 = ***£50***
Staffing	Nothing extra	Renal unit nurse @ £115/session × 4 = ***£460*** per week
Total (per week)	***£744***	***£697***

*The approximate conversion rate from pound sterling to U.S. dollars is $1.40 per £1.

ments, it is imperative to quantify real costs in monetary terms, and to determine the benefits or effectiveness of each treatment on the basis of clinical outcome. Finally, structural issues (nursing ratios in ICU, availability of commercially made replacement fluid, and so on) are likely to determine costs in a given intitution. Data from a randomized controlled trial do indeed show that complete renal recovery is significantly more common with CRRT than with IHD, suggesting hidden costs associated with an IHD-based approach.[103]

Finally, many patients with ARF have severe sepsis. In these patients, the demostrated ability of CRRT to remove putative mediators of organ dysfunction may represent yet another reason for its preferential application.[104, 105] Investigations in animals and humans suggest that if hemofiltration is to have an additional role in the management of sepsis, the rate of plasma water exchange will have to be increased.[106, 107] It is possible that the effect of CRRT in sepsis may improve survival in patients with sepsis-associated ARF.[108]

SUMMARY

The physician caring for critically ill patients with severe ARF now needs to be aware of myriad issues and to understand the implications of changes in the area of renal replacement technology.[109] *It is likely that the application of CRRT will continue to grow in intensive care units around the world and that the intensivist will be called upon to play a more important role in its prescription and execution. Furthermore, as the knowledge base in this area of medicine expands, it is increasingly desirable for such physicians involved in what can be now called "critical care nephrology"*[110] *to develop a unique level of expertise in order to improve patient outcomes. Because artificial renal support remains a large component of the practice of critical care and may expand to become the adjunctive management of septic shock, the critical care physician can no longer partly neglect it or completely delegate its prescription and execution to others. To move forward, we need to focus attention on this component of the care of critically ill patients, and cooperation between nephrologists and intensivists must be strongly promoted; only then will we see mortality rates in the population decline significantly.*

References

1. Kolff WJ. The artificial kidney—past and future. Circulation 1957; 15:285–291.
2. Henderson LW, Besarab A, Michaels A, Bluemle LW Jr: Blood purification by ultrafiltration and fluid replacement (diafiltration). Trans Am Soc Artif Intern Organs 1967; 17:216–224.
3. Henderson LW, Lilley JJ, Ford CA, Stone RA: Hemodiafiltration. J Dial 1977; 1:211–217.
4. Konstantin P: Newer membranes: Cuprophan versus polysulfone versus polyacrylonitrile. Contemp Issues Nephrol 1993; 27:63–78.
5. Ronco C, Bellomo R: Continuous high-flux dialysis: An efficient renal replacement. *In:* 1996 Yearbook of Intensive Care and Emergency Medicine. Vincent JL (Ed). Berlin, Springer-Verlag, 1996, pp 690–698.
6. Kramer P, Wigger W, Rieger J, Matthaei D, Scheler F: Arteriovenous hemofiltration: A new and simple method for treatment of overhydrated patients resistant to diuretics. Klin Wochenschr 1977; 55:1121–1125.
7. Lauer A, Saccaggi A, Ronco C, Belledonne M, Glabman S, Bosch JP: Continuous arteriovenous hemofiltration in the critically ill patient. Ann Intern Med 1983; 99:455–460.
8. Ronco C, Brendolan A, Bragantini L, Feriani M, Chiaramonte S, Fabris A, La Greca G: Continuous arteriovenous hemofiltration. Contrib Nephrol 1985; 48:70–78.
9. Bartlett R, Bosch JP, Paganini EP, Geronemus R, Ronco C: Continuous arteriovenous hemofiltration. Trans Am Soc Artif Intern Organs 1987; 38:345–350.
10. Bosch JP, Ronco C: Continuous arteriovenous hemofiltration. *In:* Replacement of Renal Function by Dialysis. Maher JF (Ed). Dordrecht, Kluwer Academic Publishers, 1989, pp 347–361.
11. Golper TA, Ronco C, Kaplan AA: Continuous arteriovenous hemofiltration: Improvements, modifications and future directions. Semin Dial 1988; 1:50–54.
12. Kaplan AA: Predilution versus postdilution for continuous arteriovenous hemofiltration. Trans Am Soc Artif Intern Organs 1985; 31:28–31.
13. Bellomo R, Ronco C: Circulation of the continuous artificial kidney: Bloodflow, pressures, clearances, and the search for the best. *In:* Circulation in Native and Artificial Kidneys. Ronco C, Artigas A, Bellomo R (Eds). Basel, S. Karger, 1997, pp 354–365.
14. Bellomo R, Ronco C, Mehta R: Nomenclature for continuous renal replacement therapies. Am J Kidney Dis 1996; 28:S2–S7.
15. Buoncristiani U, Quitaliani G, Cozzari M: Daily dialysis: Long term clinical-metabolic results. Kidney Int Suppl 1988; 24:S137–S140.
16. Geronemus R, Schneider M: Continuous arteriovenous hemodialysis: A new modality for treatment of acute renal failure. Trans Am Soc Artif Intern Organs 1984; 30:610–614.
17. Sigler MH, Teehan BP, Valkenburgh DV: Solute transport in continuous hemodialysis. A new treatment for acute renal failure. Kidney Int 1987; 32:562–570.
18. Nolph KD: Peritoneal dialysis. *In:* The Kidney. Brenner BM, Rector FC (Eds). Philadelphia, WB Saunders, 1986, pp 1791–1845.
19. Bellomo R: Choosing a therapeutic modality: Hemofiltration vs. hemodialysis vs. hemodiafiltration. Semin Dialysis 1996; 9:88–92.
20. Ronco C, Fecondini L, Gavioli L, Conz P, Milan M, Dell'Aquila R, Bragantini L, Brendolan A, Chiaramonte S, Crepaldi C, Feriani M, La Greca G: A new blood module for continuous renal replacement therapies. Int J Artif Organs 1983; 17:14–18.
21. Ronco C: Arteriovenous hemodiafiltration (A-VHDF): A possible way to increase urea removal during CAVH. Int J Artif Organs 1985; 8:61–62.
22. Ronco C: Continuous renal replacement therapies for the treatment of acute renal failure in intensive care patients. Clin Nephrol 1993; 40:187–198.
23. Bellomo R, Boyce N: Acute continuous hemodiafiltration: A prospective study of 110 patients and a review of the literature. Am J Kidney Dis 1993; 21:508–518.
24. Bellomo R, Parkin G, Boyce N: Acute renal failure in the critically ill: Management by continuous veno-venous hemodiafiltration. J Crit Care 1993; 8:140–144.
25. Fauchaid P, Kolbjorn F, Amlie J: An evaluation of ultrafiltration as treatment of therapy resistant cardiac edema. Acta Med Scand 1988; 219:47–52.
26. Barzilay E, Kessler D, Berlot G, et al: Use of extracorporeal supportive techniques as additional treatment for septic induced multiple organ failure patients. Crit Care Med 1989; 17:634–637.
27. Stegmayr BG: Plasmapheresis in severe sepsis or septic shock. Blood Purif 1996; 14:94–101.
28. Winchester JF: Hemoperfusion. *In:* Replacement of Renal Function by Dialysis. Maher JF (Ed). Dordrecht, Kluwer Academic Publishers, 1989, pp 439–459.
29. Bellomo R, Teede H, Boyce N: Anticoagulant regimens in acute continuous hemodiafiltration. Intensive Care Med 1993; 19:329–332.
30. Ward DM, Mehta R: Extracorporeal management of acute renal failure patients at high risk of bleeding. Kidney Int 1993; 4:S237–S244.
31. Mehta RL, McDonald BR, Aguilar MM, et al: Regional citrate anticoagulation for continuous arteriovenous hemodialysis in critically ill patients. Kidney Int 1990; 38:976–981.
32. Ziegler T, Young L, Manson J, Wilmore D: Metabolic effects of recombinant human growth hormone in patients receiving parenteral nutrition. Ann Surg 1988; 208:6–16.
33. Denton MD, Chertow GM, Brady HR: Renal-dose dopamine for the treatment of acute renal failure: A review of the rationale and results of experimental and human studies. Kidney Int 1996; 49:4–14.
34. Rudy DW, Voelker JR, Greene PK, Esparza FA, Brater DO: Loop

diuretics for chronic renal failure: A continuous infusion is more efficacious than bolus therapy. Ann Intern Med 1991; 115:360–366.
35. Inoue M, Okajima K, Itoh K, Ando Y, Watanabe N, Yasaka T, Nagase S, Morino Y: Mechanism of furosemide resistance in analbuminemic rats and hypoalbuminemic patients. Kidney Int 1987; 32:198–203.
36. Anderson C, Shahvari M, Zimmerman J: The treatment of pulmonary edema in the absence of renal function—a role for sorbitol and furosemide. JAMA 1979; 241:1008–1110.
37. Mehta R: Therapeutic alternatives to renal replacement for critically ill patients in acute renal failure. Semin Nephrol 1994; 14:64–82.
38. Hohnloser S, Verrier R, Lown B: Influence of beta$_2$-adrenoceptor stimulation and blockade on cardiac electrophysiologic properties and serum potassium concentration in the anesthetized dog. Am Heart J 1987; 113:1066–1070.
39. Flinn R, Merrill J, Wlezant W: Treatment of the oliguric patient with a new sodium exchange resin and sorbitol. N Engl J Med 1961; 264:111–114.
40. Brown T, Ahern D, Nolph K: Potassium removal with peritoneal dialysis. Kidney Int 1973; 4:67–69.
41. Hou S, McElroy P, Nootens J, Beach M: Safety and efficacy of low-potassium dialysate. Am J Kidney Dis 1989; 13:137–143.
42. Marini PV, Hull AR: Uremic pericarditis: A review of incidence and management. Kidney Int Suppl 1975; 2:S163–S166.
43. Locke S, Merrill J, Tyler H: Neurologic complications of acute uremia. Arch Intern Med 1961; 108:75–83.
44. Mitch WE, May RC, Maroni BJ, Druml W: Protein and amino acid metabolism in uremia: Influence of metabolic acidosis. Kidney Int 1989; 36:S205–S207.
45. Androgue H, Rashad M, Gorin A, Yacoub J, Madias N: Assessing acid-base status in circulatory failure: Differences between arterial and central venous blood. N Engl J Med 1989; 320:1312–1315.
46. Stacpoole PW, Wright EC, Baumgartner TG, Bersin RM, Buchalter S, Curry SH, Duncan CA, Harman EM, Henderson GN, Jenkinson S: A contolled clinical trial of dichloroacetate for treatment of lactic acidosis in adults: The Dichloroacetate-Lactic Acidosis Study. N Engl J Med 1992; 327:1564–1569.
47. Bellomo R, Ronco C: Acute renal failure in the intensive care unit: Adequacy of dialysis and the case for continuous therapies. Nephrol Dial Transplant 1996; 11:424–428.
48. Parker TF: Trends and concepts in the prescription and delivery of dialysis in the U.S. Semin Nephrol 1992; 12:267–275.
49. Conger JD: A controlled evaluation of prophylactic dialysis in post-traumatic acute renal failure. J Trauma 1975; 15:1056–1063.
50. Gillum DM, Dixon BS, Yanover MJ, Kelleher SP, Shapiro MD, Benedetti RA, Dillingham MI, Paller MS, Goldberg JP, Tomford R, Gordon JA, Conger JD: The role of intensive dialysis in acute renal failure. Clin Nephrol 1986; 25:249–255.
51. Paganini EP, Tapolyai M, Goormastic M, Sakai K, Heyka R, Moreno L, Lee JC, Koslowski L: Patient outcome in ICU acute renal failure requiring dialytic support is related to both comorbidity and delivered dialysis dose. *In:* Acute Renal Failure in the 21st Century. Bethesda, Md, National Institute of Diabetes and Digestive and Kidney Diseases, 1996.
52. Paganini EP, Halstenberg WK, Goormastic M: Risk modeling in acute renal failure requiring dialysis: The introduction of a new model. Clin Nephrol 1996; 46:206–211.
53. Schiffl H, Lang SM, Konig A, Held E: Dose of intermittent hemodialysis and outcome of acute renal failure: A prospective randomized study (Abstract). J Am Soc Nephrol 1997; 8:290A.
54. Himmelfarb J, Zaoui P, Hakim R: Modulation of granulocyte LAM-1 and MAC-1 during dialysis: A prospective randomized controlled trial. Kidney Int 1992; 41:388–395.
55. Himmelfarb J, Lazarus J, Hakim R: Reactive oxygen species production to monocytes and polymorphonuclear leukocytes during dialysis. Am J Kidney Dis 1991; 17:271–276.
56. Cheung A, Baranowski R, Wayman A: The role of thromboxane in cuprophan-induced pulmonary hypertension. Kidney Int 1987; 31:1072–1079.
57. Shaldon S, Lonnemann G, Koch K: Cytokine relevance in biocompatibility. Contrib Nephrol 1989; 79:227–236.
58. Schindler R, Lonnemann G, Shaldon S, Koch K, Dinarello C: Transcription, not synthesis, of interleukin-1 and tumor necrosis factor by complement. Kidney Int 1990; 37:85–93.
59. Canivet E, Lavaud S, Wong T, Guenounou M, Willemin J, Potron G: Cuprophane but not synthetic membrane induces increases in serum tumor necrosis factor-alpha levels during hemodialysis. Am J Kidney Dis 1994; 23:41–46.
60. Hakim RM, Wingard RL, Parker RA: Effect of the dialysis membrane in the treatment of patients with acute renal failure. N Engl J Med 1994; 331:1338–1342.
61. Schiffl H, Lang SM, Konig A, Strasser T, Haider MC, Held E: Biocompatible membranes in acute renal failure: Prospective case-controlled study. Lancet 1994; 344:570–572.
62. Jorstad S: Generation and removal of anaphylatoxins during hemofiltration with 5 different membranes. Blood Purif 1988; 6:325–335.
63. Bellomo R, Tipping P, Boyce N: Continuous venovenous hemofiltration with dialysis removes cytokines from the circulation of septic patients. Crit Care Med 1993; 21:522–526.
64. Leypoldt JK, Cheung AK, Agadoa LY, Daugerdae JT, Greene T, Keshaviah PR: Hemodialyzer mass transfer-area coefficients for urea increase at high dialysate flow rates: The Hemodialysis (HEMO) Study. Kidney Int 1997; 51:2013–2017.
65. VanStone JC, Bauer J, Carey J: The effect of dialysate sodium concentration on body fluid distribution during hemodialysis. Trans Am Soc Artif Intern Organs 1980; 26:383–386.
66. Ward R, Wathen R, Williams T, Harding G: Hemodialysate composition and intradialytic metabolic, acid-base, and potassium changes. Kidney Int 1987; 32:129–135.
67. Sherman R, Hwang E, Bernhole A, Eisinger R: Variability in potassium removal by hemodialysis. Am J Nephrol 1986; 6:284–288.
68. Henrich W: Hemodynamic instability during hemodialysis. Kidney Int 1986; 30:605–612.
69. Vinay P, Prud'homme M, Vinet B, Cournoyer G, Degoulet P, Leville M, Gougoux A, St-Louis-G, Lapierre L, Piettre Y: Acetate metabolism and bicarbonate generation during hemodialysis: 10 years of observation. Kidney Int 1987; 31:1194–1204.
70. Ebben J, Hirsh D, Luchmann D, Collins A, Keshaviah P: Microbiologic contamination of liquid bicarbonate concentrate for hemodialysis. Trans Am Soc Artif Intern Organs 1987; 33:269–273.
71. Raman A, Chong Y, Sreenevasan G: Effects of varying dialysate calcium concentrations on the plasma calcium fractions in patients on dialysis. Nephron 1976; 16:181–187.
72. Vliskin S, Belhassen B, Sheps D, Laniado S: Clinical and electrophysiologic effects of magnesium sulfate on paroxysmal supraventricular tachycardia and comparison to adenosine triphosphate. Am J Cardiol 1992; 70:870–885.
73. Roden D: Magnesium treatment of ventricular arrhythmias. Am J Cardiol 1989; 63:43G–46G.
74. Skobeloff E, Spivey W, McNamara R, Greenspon L: Intravenous magnesium sulfate in the treatment of acute asthma in the emergency department. JAMA 1989; 262:1210–1213.
75. Sherman R, Faustino E, Bernholc A, Eisinger R: Effect of variations in dialysate temperature on blood pressure during hemodialysis. Am J Kidney Dis 1984; 4:66–68.
76. Shinaberger J, Brautbar N, Miller J, Gardner P: Successful application of sequential hemofiltration followed by diffusion dialysis with standard dialysis equipment. Trans Am Soc Artif Intern Organ 1978; 24:677–681.
77. Asaba H, Bergstrom J, Furst P, et al: Sequential ultrafiltration and diffusion as alternatives to conventional hemodialysis. Proc Clin Dial Transplant Forum 1976; 6:129–135.
78. Langkamp-Henken B, Glezer J, Kuosk K: Immunologic structure and function of the gastrointestinal tract. Nutr Clin Pract 1992; 7:100–108.
79. Haglund U: Systemic mediators released from the gut in critical illness. Crit Care Med 1993; 21:S15–S18.
80. Abel RM, Beck CH, Abbott WM, Ryan JA, Barnett GO, Fischer JE: Improved survival from acute renal failure after treatment with intravenous essential l-amino acids and glucose. N Engl J Med 1973; 288:695–699.
81. Blumenkrantz M, Kopple J, Koffler A, Kamdar A, Healy M, Feinstein-E, Massry S: Total parenteral nutrition in the management of acute renal failure. Am J Clin Nutr 1978; 31:1831–1840.
82. Feinstein El, Blumenkrantz MJ, Healy M, Koffler A, Silberman

H, Massry SG, Kopple JD: Clinical and metabolic responses to parenteral nutrition in acute renal failure. Medicine 1981; 60:124-137.
83. Mirtallo J, Schneider P, Mavko K, Ruberg R, Fabri P: A comparison of essential and general amino acid infusions in the nutritional support of patients with compromised renal function. JPEN J Parenter Enter Nutr 1982; 6:109-113.
84. Wolfson M, Jones MR, Kopple JD: Amino acid losses during hemodialysis with infusion of amino acids and glucose. Kidney Int 1982; 21:500-506.
85. Howdieshell TR, Blalock WE, Bowen PA, Hawkins ML, Hess C: Mangement of post-traumatic acute renal failure with peritoneal dialysis. Am Surg 1992; 6:378-382.
86. Zucchelli P, Santoro A: Dialysis-induced hypotension: A fresh look at pathophysiology. Blood Purif 1993; 11:85-98.
87. Manns M, Sigler MH, Teehan BP: Intradialytic renal hemodynamics: Potential consequences for the management of the patient with acute renal failure. Nephrol Dial Transplant 1997; 12:870-873.
88. Kelleher SP, Robinette JB, Conger JD: Effect of hemorrhagic reduction in blood pressure on recovery from acute renal failure. Am J Physiol 1984; 246:F379-F386.
89. Conger JD: Does hemodialysis delay recovery from acute renal failure? Semin Dial 1990; 3:146-148.
90. Bellomo R, Ronco C: Nutrition au cours de l'insuffisance rénale aigue. Nutr Clin Metabol 1997; 11:499-509.
91. Bellomo R, Seacombe J, Daskalakis M, et al: A prospective comparative study of moderate versus high protein intake for critically ill patients with acute renal failure. Rl Fail 1997; 19:11-20.
92. Mault JR, Kresowik J, Deckerk RE, Arnoldi DK, Swartz RD, Bartlett RH: Continuous arteriovenous haemofiltration: The answer to starvation in acute renal failure. Trans Am Soc Artif Intern Organs 1984; 30:203-208.
93. Alverstrand A, Gutierrez A, Wahren J, Begstrom J: Protein catabolism in sham hemodialysis: The effect of different membranes. Blood Purif 1987; 5:269-275.
94. Kierdorf H, Kindler J, Sieberth RH: Nitrogen balance in patients with acute renal failure treated by continuous hemofiltration. Nephrol Dial Transplant 1986; 1:72-77.
95. Coraim FI, Wolner E: Continuous hemofiltration for the failing heart. New Horiz 1995; 3:725-731.
96. Clark WR, Macias WL: Azotemia control by extracorporeal therapy in patients with acute renal failure. New Horiz 1995; 3:688-698.
97. Bellomo R, Ronco C: Acute renal failure in the intensive care unit: Adequacy of dialysis and the case for continuous therapies. Nephrol Dial Transplant 1996; 11:424-428.
98. La Greca G, Biasioli S, Chiaramonte S, et al: Studies on brain density in hemodialysis and peritoneal dialysis. Nephron 1982; 31:146-150.
99. Davenport A: The management of renal failure in patients at risk of cerebral edema/hypoxia. New Horiz 1995; 3:717-724.
100. Manns M, Maurer E, Evering HG: Thermal energy balance during continuous venovenous hemofiltration. Blood Purif 1998; 16:101.
101. van Bommel EFH, Leunissen K, Weimer W: Continuous renal replacement therapy for critically ill patients: An update. J Intensive Care Med 1994; 9:265-280.
102. Moreno L, Heyka RJ, Paganini EP: Continuous renal replacement therapy: Cost considerations and reimbursement. Semin Dial 1996; 9:209-214.
103. Hoyt DB: CRRT in the area of cost containment: Is it justified? Am J Kidney Dis 1997; 30:S102-S104.
104. Bellomo R, Tipping P, Boyce N: Tumor necrosing factor clearances during veno-venous hemodiafiltration in the critically ill. Trans Am Soc Artif Intern Organs 1991; 37:322-323.
105. Bellomo R: Continuous hemofiltration as blood purification in sepsis. New Horizons 1995; 3:732-738.
106. Grootendorst AF, van Bommel EFH, van der Hoven B, et al: High-volume hemofiltration improves hemodynamics in endotoxin-induced shock in the pig. J Crit Care 1992; 7:67-75.
107. Cole L, Bellomo R, Baldwin I: A randomized cross-over study of the hemodynamic effects of high volume hemofiltration in patients with septic shock. Blood Purif 1998; 16:113-114.
108. Bellomo R, Farmer M, Wright C, Parkin G, Boyce N: Treatment of sepsis-associated severe acute renal failure with continuous hemodiafiltration: Clinical experience and comparison with conventional dialysis. Blood Purif 1995; 13:246-254.
109. Bellomo R, Mehta R: Acute renal replacement in the intensive care unit: Now and tomorrow. New Horiz 1995; 3:760-767.
110. Ronco C, Bellomo R: Critical care nephrology: The time has come. Nephrol Dial Transplant 1998; 13:264-267.

156

Drug-Kidney Interactions

George J. Kaloyanides, MD, FACP

The subject of drug-kidney interactions is important to the critical care specialist from several perspectives. In the first place, it is well established that patients admitted to the hospital in general[1, 2] and to the intensive care unit (ICU) in particular are at risk for development of acute renal failure (ARF).[3] Among the causes of ARF, drugs have been implicated as a major contributory factor.[1-3] Thus, it behooves the intensivist to be informed about current concepts concerning the pathogenesis and prevention of drug-induced ARF. Second, adverse drug reactions rank high on the list of complications sustained by hospitalized patients and frequently cause serious morbidity and even mortality.[4] Adverse drug reactions are common in patients with acute or chronic renal failure. It is widely recognized that the dosing of renally excreted drugs must be adjusted in patients with impaired kidney function, but in practice, such adjustments, if undertaken at all, are frequently suboptimal.[5] Less well appreciated is the fact that renal failure is also associated with alterations in drug binding to protein and with changes in drug metabolism by the liver. Both effects, either singly or in concert, can lead to adverse drug reactions. Moreover, patients with renal failure commonly suffer from comorbidities for which multiple drugs are prescribed, thereby further elevating the risk of adverse drug reactions and interactions in this population of patients. An additional level of complexity is superimposed if the patient's renal failure requires support with one of the various renal replacement therapies, which may necessitate further adjustments in drug dosing, depending on the extent to which a drug is removed during dialysis.

All of these factors make safe and effective pharmacotherapy in the population of patients with renal failure a challenging task for the most astute and seasoned intensivist. In the first part of this chapter, current concepts concerning the pathogenesis and prevention of drug-induced ARF are reviewed. In the second part of this chapter, principles of drug prescribing in patients with renal disease are discussed, and general guidelines for drug adjustments in patients with renal failure are provided with emphasis on those drugs commonly used in the ICU.

DRUG-INDUCED ACUTE RENAL FAILURE

Major Mechanisms of Drug-Induced Acute Renal Failure

Table 156-1 summarizes the four major mechanisms by which drugs may cause ARF.[6] Among these, the most common cause is renal hypoperfusion secondary to low or suboptimal sys-

TABLE 156–1. Major Mechanisms of Drug-Induced Acute Renal Failure

Mechanism	Examples
Renal hypoperfusion	
Low systemic blood pressure	Diuretics, vasodilating agents, ACE inhibitors
Direct renal vasoconstriction	NSAID, amphotericin B, radiocontrast agents
Acute tubular necrosis	Aminoglycosides, β-lactams, amphotericin B
Intratubular obstruction	Sulfadiazine, acyclovir
Allergic interstitial nephritis	β-Lactam antibiotics, NSAID

From Kaloyanides GJ: Drug-induced acute renal failure. *In:* Acute Renal Failure in the Critically Ill. Update in Intensive Care and Emergency Medicine. Vol 20. Bellomo R, Ronco C (Eds). Berlin, Springer-Verlag, 1995, p 178.

ACE = angiotensin-converting enzyme; NSAID = nonsteroidal anti-inflammatory drug.

temic blood pressure occurring in a clinical setting of excessive diuretic or vasodilator therapy, especially in elderly patients with unrecognized occlusive renovascular disease. In the early stage, these agents give rise to the syndrome of prerenal ARF, the diagnosis of which is supported by a urine sodium concentration of less than 20 mmol/L, a fractional sodium excretion (FE_{Na}) below 1.0%, a urine/plasma (U/P) creatinine ratio greater than 40, and a U/P osmolality higher than 1.4. This syndrome can also be induced by drugs that stimulate renal vasoconstriction.

A second major mechanism of drug-induced ARF is acute tubular necrosis (ATN). The diagnosis of ATN is supported by a urine sodium concentration greater than 40 mmol/L, an FE_{Na} above 1.5%, a U/P creatinine of less than 20, a U/P osmolality below 1.2, and findings of muddy brown casts and tubular epithelial cells in the urinary sediment.

A third major mechanism of drug-induced ARF is intratubular obstruction caused by the precipitation of drug. This diagnosis is supported by the findings of drug crystals in the urine usually accompanied by red blood cells.

A fourth major mechanism of drug-induced ARF is allergic interstitial nephritis (AIN). This diagnosis is suggested by findings of hematuria and pyuria with eosinophiluria and confirmed by renal biopsy.

Risk Factors for Drug-Induced Acute Renal Failure

Drug-induced ARF in an ICU setting typically occurs in a patient with multiple predisposing factors.[6] Table 156–2 lists those factors, acting singly or often in combination, that magnify the risk of ARF in patients exposed to a nephrotoxic drug.

Paramount among these predisposing factors is renal hypoperfusion irrespective of cause because it impairs the renal excretion of drugs, and this may result in prolonged exposure of the kidney to toxic quantities of drug or metabolite. Prolonged renal hypoperfusion carries the additional risk of causing ischemic injury to tubular cells, and even subclinical degrees of ischemic injury magnify the nephrotoxic potential of drugs.

The risk associated with advanced age is related in part to the fact that the elderly patient is more likely to experience hemodynamic instability with renal hypoperfusion and ischemia. In addition, failure to appreciate the age-related decline of kidney function that is often not reflected by the prevailing blood urea nitrogen (BUN) and serum creatinine concentrations may lead to inappropriate dosing of potentially nephrotoxic drugs. The age-related loss of renal reserve and reduced capacity for renal tubular cell regeneration also contribute to the heightened risk that accompanies advanced age. Similar mechanisms contribute to the increased risk associated with chronic renal insufficiency.

Finally, exposure to two or more potentially nephrotoxic agents, which is not uncommon in the ICU, may lead to a synergistic interaction. Details concerning specific drug interactions and related risk factors are discussed in the following pages.

ACUTE RENAL FAILURE CAUSED BY SPECIFIC DRUGS

Antibacterial Agents

Aminoglycoside Antibiotics

Aminoglycoside antibiotics are polycations with a net charge ranging between +4.47 for neomycin and +2.39 for amikacin.[7] Consequently, these drugs are highly hydrophilic and poorly absorbed across the intestinal mucosa. After parenteral administration, they are distributed in an apparent volume slightly greater than extracellular fluid and eliminated without metabolic transformation through the kidneys by glomerular filtration.[7]

The nephrotoxicity of these drugs relates to the fact that a small fraction of filtered drug is transported into proximal tubular cells by receptor-mediated endocytosis and subsequently accumulates within the lysosomal compartment, where it resides with a half-life measured in days and impairs lysosomal function.[7] When the concentration of drug within renal proximal tubular cells reaches a critical threshold, clinical signs of nephrotoxicity become evident.[6, 8] These include increased urinary excretion of low-molecular-weight proteins, lysosomal and brush border enzymes, tubular epithelial cells, white blood cells, and casts. It usually takes 7 days or more of drug therapy before nonoliguric ARF appears in pure aminoglycoside nephrotoxicity. An earlier onset of ARF may occur in the presence of complicating factors, such as renal hypoperfusion or sepsis.

The incidence of aminoglycoside nephrotoxicity as defined by strict criteria has varied between 7% and 36%, with the higher incidence observed in critically ill patients.[6, 8] Established risk factors for aminoglycoside toxicity, in addition to those listed in Table 156–2, include the following[6, 8]:

- Daily dose
- Interval and duration of aminoglycoside therapy

TABLE 156–2. Risk Factors for Drug-Induced Acute Renal Failure

Renal hypoperfusion
Volume depletion
Low cardiac output states
Systemic vasodilatation
Sepsis
Advanced age
Chronic disease
Renal insufficiency
Cardiac disease
Liver disease
Hypertension
Peripheral vascular disease
Diabetes mellitus
Exposure to multiple potentially nephrotoxic agents

- The specific aminoglycoside administered
- Hypokalemia
- Hypomagnesemia
- Metabolic acidosis
- Concurrent exposure to amphotericin B, vancomycin, cisplatin, furosemide, and radiocontrast agents

Many of these risk factors are potentially modifiable by the clinician, and appropriate steps should be undertaken to do so whenever possible. Total daily drug dose is an obvious risk factor, as is the duration of therapy. Because these drugs are eliminated virtually exclusively by the kidneys, the dose must be reduced in proportion to the decline of kidney function. Animal studies have shown that administration of the total daily dose of drug as a single dose is less nephrotoxic than is administration of the same amount of drug in equally divided doses.[9] Studies in humans have established that a single daily dose of drug is as efficacious as or more therapeutically efficacious than equally divided daily dosing.[10–14] Importantly, the incidence of nephrotoxicity is no greater with single daily dosing, and several studies suggest that it may be less.[12, 13] (Thus, Table 156-5 [see later] provides guidelines for single daily dosing.)

Frequent monitoring of plasma concentrations is recommended to ensure that therapeutic concentrations are achieved and toxic levels are avoided. Comparative studies in humans suggest that the rank order for clinical nephrotoxicity is gentamicin > tobramycin > amikacin > netilmicin.[6, 8] This knowledge should be taken into consideration in prescribing an aminoglycoside for a patient at increased risk for nephrotoxicity.

β-Lactam Antibiotics

The penicillins, cephalosporins, and carbapenems are the β-lactam antibiotics. This class of drugs may cause ARF secondary to acute proximal tubular cell necrosis or AIN.[6, 15, 16] The rank order of nephrotoxicity potential as defined in animal studies is cephaloglycin > cephaloridine >> cefaclor > cefazolin > cephalothin >>> cephalexin, ceftazidime, and penicillins that are not nephrotoxic.

The nephrotoxic potential of these drugs is determined by the extent to which they undergo concentrative uptake by the organic transport system of proximal tubular cells and their intrinsic reactivity with mitochondrial targets that cause inhibition of mitochondrial respiration. The overall incidence of severe nephrotoxic ARF is low, especially with the third-generation cephalosporins. As with other antibiotics, high doses and prolonged therapy elevate the risk of nephrotoxicity, as do renal ischemia and endotoxemia. Several studies suggested that aminoglycoside antibiotics potentiated the nephrotoxicity of first-generation cephalosporins; no such effect has been observed with third-generation cephalosporins.[15, 16] Because these drugs are excreted primarily by the kidneys, most require some dose modification in patients with severe renal impairment (see Table 156-5).

Vancomycin

The rise in the incidence of methicillin-resistant staphylococcal infections has stimulated increased clinical use of this glycopeptide. Because vancomycin is poorly absorbed from the gastrointestinal tract, it must be administered intravenously for the treatment of systemic infections. More than 95% of the drug is eliminated unchanged in the urine.[6, 17] Therefore, the dose must be modified in patients with renal failure.

Animal studies have demonstrated that vancomycin causes ototoxicity and nephrotoxicity.[6, 18] In humans, the incidence of nephrotoxic ARF associated with vancomycin administered as sole therapy ranges between 5% and 15%.[6, 19] The risk of nephrotoxic ARF is augmented when vancomycin is administered in combination with aminoglycoside antibiotics.[20] In high-risk patients, monitoring of blood levels is recommended to ensure that therapeutic concentrations are achieved and toxic concentrations are avoided.[21]

Antifungal Agents

Amphotericin B

Amphotericin B, a polyene antibiotic, remains the drug of choice for the treatment of many systemic fungal infections. Its clinical use is associated with a number of toxic side effects, including ARF.[6] The toxicity of this drug has been attributed to its ability to increase membrane permeability to small cations by forming membrane pores estimated to be composed of eight molecules of drug alternating with eight molecules of cholesterol.[22] Amphotericin binds preferentially to ergosterol, the major sterol of fungi, and increased membrane permeability through pore formation is thought to be the mechanism responsible for the selective toxicity of this and similar drugs for fungi.[23]

Because it is poorly absorbed across the gastrointestinal tract, amphotericin B is given by intravenous infusion. The drug's volume of distribution in pharmacokinetic studies[24, 25] is about 4 L/kg. Up to 95% of the drug in serum is bound to protein, primarily beta-lipoprotein. The liver, where up to 41% of administered drug can be recovered, is the major depot site for amphotericin B. Only 6% is found in the lungs and 2% in the kidneys. No metabolites have been identified. The elimination of amphotericin B from serum is described by a triexponential curve with a half-life of 24 hours, 48 hours, and 15 days, respectively. Less than 10% of an administered dose is recovered in the urine. Nevertheless, for reasons still unclear, the kidney is the major site of toxicity.

The incidence of amphotericin B nephrotoxicity increases as a function of the following[26, 27]:

- Daily drug dose
- Duration of therapy
- Number of potentiating risk factors, prominent among which are chronic renal insufficiency; sodium depletion; renal hypoperfusion; and concomitant exposure to aminoglycoside antibiotics, diuretics, cyclosporine, or radiocontrast agents

The clinical expression of amphotericin B nephrotoxicity is dominated by the appearance of azotemia and creatininemia, which may occur early in the course of drug administration and initially reflects a reversible depression of renal blood flow (RBF) and glomerular filtration rate (GFR) secondary to an increase in renal vascular resistance.[6, 26] Depolarization of vascular smooth muscle secondary to pore formation has been postulated as the basic mechanism responsible for the increase in renal vascular resistance.[28] With prolonged therapy, depression of renal function may persist owing to the development of frank tubular cell injury and possibly vascular injury. Abnormalities of tubular cell function may appear, including distal renal tubular acidosis, hypokalemia and hypomagnesemia secondary to renal tubular wasting of these cations, and loss of urine concentrating capacity. The urine sediment commonly contains many red blood cells, white blood cells, tubular epithelial cells, and casts. Although most of these abnormalities are potentially reversible after the drug is discontinued, full recovery may be delayed for a number of months or some degree of renal insufficiency may persist, especially with prolonged therapy.

The clinician should minimize those factors known to potentiate the risk of nephrotoxicity. For example, the risk of nephrotoxicity was observed to increase by 1.8-fold for each increment of 0.1 mg/kg in the daily dose of amphotericin B, by 15-fold if renal insufficiency was present before the initiation of therapy, and by 12.5-fold if diuretics were given during the course of therapy.[27] Vigorous sodium loading reduces the risk of nephrotoxicity. In the presence of chronic renal insufficiency, a reduction in the daily dose or changing the dosing to every other day is recommended. Deoxycholate, the vehicle in which amphotericin B is suspended, contributes to the cytotoxicity.[29] When amphotericin B is administered in a lipid-containing formulation, the incidence and severity of nephrotoxicity are reduced.[30]

Antiprotozoal Agents

Pentamidine

In the era before the acquired immunodeficiency syndrome (AIDS), pentamidine therapy was complicated by ARF in about 25% of cases. Individuals with AIDS treated with pentamidine for *Pneumocystis carinii* pneumonia (PCP) have a higher incidence of ARF[6, 31] as well as of other adverse drug reactions.[32] The mechanism of ARF is not known. Although less than 5% of the daily dose is excreted in the urine each day, the drug has been shown to be concentrated in the kidneys.[6]

Pentamidine nephrotoxicity presents as nonoliguric ARF 7 to 10 days after the initiation of therapy.[6, 33] Urinalysis reveals mild proteinuria, microscopic hematuria, pyuria, and cylindruria. In most cases, the ARF is of mild to moderate severity. On occasion, it is severe and necessitates dialysis support. Hyperchloremic metabolic acidosis and hyperkalemia may develop out of proportion to the level of azotemia. Hypomagnesemia secondary to renal tubular wasting has been observed.[34, 35] Recovery of renal function usually begins within a week after discontinuation of therapy with return to baseline within several weeks. Chronic renal failure, volume depletion, and concomitant therapy with nephrotoxic drugs increase the risk for nephrotoxicity.[6, 33] Some authors recommend increasing the dosing interval in patients with renal failure to minimize the risk of nephrotoxicity.[36]

Sulfadiazine

Sulfadiazine is a first-generation sulfonamide that continues to be used today in combination with pyrimethamine for the treatment of *Toxoplasma* encephalitis.[6, 33, 37] Because of limited solubility in acid urine, this drug along with its major metabolite has a propensity to cause obstruction secondary to the intratubular precipitation of crystals. Renal insufficiency associated with renal colic, hematuria, and crystalluria complicate therapy in 5% of cases. This complication can be reversed and prevented by forced diuresis and alkalinization of the urine.

Co-trimoxazole

The combination of trimethoprim and sulfamethoxazole (TMP-SMZ) is used as an alternative to pentamidine for the treatment of PCP. An increase in the serum creatinine concentration is commonly observed with this agent because of inhibition of tubular secretion of creatinine by trimethoprim.[38] The magnitude of this effect is most pronounced in individuals with an elevated baseline serum creatinine concentration due to chronic renal insufficiency. Failure of the BUN to rise in proportion to the rise in serum creatinine should alert one to the correct diagnosis.

Although sulfamethoxazole is far more soluble than the first-generation sulfonamides, the intravenous administration of co-trimoxazole in high doses for the therapy of PCP carries a finite risk of ARF secondary to crystal deposition of the parent drug or a metabolite.[39] In addition, sulfonamides as a group are known to cause hypersensitivity vasculitis and AIN.[6]

Antiviral Agents

Acyclovir

This agent is eliminated primarily through the kidneys by glomerular filtration and tubular secretion. Because of the low solubility of acyclovir, rapid intravenous therapy may cause ARF secondary to the intratubular precipitation of acyclovir crystals.[6, 33] The clinical expression of nephrotoxicity ranges from asymptomatic azotemia to severe renal failure with renal colic. High drug dose, rapid infusion, and low urine volume predispose to the development of this complication.

Foscarnet

This agent is excreted unchanged in the urine by glomerular filtration and tubular secretion. ARF, often accompanied by hypomagnesemia, hypocalcemia, hypophosphatemia, and hypokalemia, is the major complication of therapy with this drug.[6, 33] The cause of toxicity has not been established. Saline loading reduces the incidence and the severity of ARF.[40]

Indinavir

Nephrolithiasis secondary to crystal deposition has been reported as a complication of therapy with this new protease inhibitor, which has limited solubility.[41] Hydration to augment urine output is recommended.

Cidofovir

Nephrotoxicity is a common complication of intravenous therapy with this nucleotide analog of cytosine. Concomitant probenecid administration and saline loading mitigate this risk.[42]

Radiocontrast Agents

The radiocontrast agents in clinical use are water-soluble compounds that are excreted by glomerular filtration. The expanded use of these agents in diagnostic and therapeutic procedures has been accompanied by an increase in radiocontrast-induced nephropathy (RCIN).[6] The incidence of RCIN, defined as a rise in the serum creatinine concentration of more than 50% above baseline levels or more than 1 mg/dL, is negligible in patients with normal renal function; in the presence of one or more risk factors (chronic renal insufficiency, diabetes mellitus, congestive heart failure, renal hypoperfusion, high volume of radiocontrast, repeated exposure to radiocontrast, exposure to other nephrotoxic agents), the incidence may exceed 50%.[43] The single most important risk factor is chronic renal insufficiency (serum creatinine concentration, >1.5 mg/dL), and the more severe the renal insufficiency, the greater the risk. The risk is potentiated by the combination of diabetes mellitus and renal insufficiency.

The clinical expression of RCIN typically begins with a rise in the serum creatinine concentration evident by 24 to 48 hours after the injection of dye.[6, 44] In most cases, the rise in serum creatinine reaches a peak within 5 days and returns to baseline level within 10 days. In more severe cases, the serum creatinine concentration may not peak until 7 to 10 days and may not return to baseline level until 21 days after the procedure. Some patients may require dialysis support.

The pathogenesis of RCIN has not been unequivocally established. Renal vasoconstriction mediated by endothelin, by adenosine, and by the high osmolality of the radiocontrast agent has been implicated in the process and is potentiated by inhibition of release of endogenous renal vasodilators (nitric oxide and prostaglandins).[6, 44] A direct toxic effect of these agents on tubular epithelial cells possibly mediated by oxygen free radicals may also play a role.

The prevention of RCIN begins with an assessment of the risk-benefit ratio. In patients with advanced renal failure (serum creatinine concentration, >4 mg/dL), the risk of precipitating a decline of kidney function that requires the initiation of dialysis therapy must be weighed against the value of the information to be gained from the radiographic procedure. In high-risk patients, alternative imaging techniques should be considered. Medications should be systematically reviewed to eliminate, if possible, drugs known to potentiate RCIN. Extracellular volume deficits should be repaired and renal function optimized before the procedure. Careful consideration should be given to limiting the volume of dye and to spacing multiple procedures whenever possible. Nonionic radiocontrast agents have been shown to be less nephrotoxic than high osmolar agents when they are administered to azotemic patients with or without diabetes mellitus[45] and, therefore, should be included in the strategy for preventing this complication.

Finally, it is standard practice to "hydrate" patients at risk for RCIN before the procedure. Various protocols using saline infusion with and without mannitol and with and without a diuretic have been recommended,[44] but only recently was a prospective and randomized trial conducted to compare the efficacy of three protocols in preventing RCIN.[46] Patients with stable chronic renal insufficiency (mean serum creatinine concentration, 2.1 mg/dL) scheduled to undergo coronary angiography were randomized to one of three treatment protocols. All patients received 0.45% NaCl infused at 1 mL/kg per hour for 12 hours before and continuing for 12 hours after the procedure. In addition, one group of patients was infused with 25 g of mannitol in 0.45% NaCl during the 1-hour period before the procedure, and a second group was infused with 80 mg of furosemide in 0.45% NaCl during the 30 minutes before the procedure. The third group received only 0.45% NaCl. The incidence of RCIN (defined as an increase in serum creatinine of 0.5 mg/dL or more) was 11% in the saline-only group, 28% in the saline-mannitol group, and 40% in the saline-furosemide group. Calcium channel blockers, adenosine receptor antagonists, and vasodilators have also been recommended as prophylactic measures against RCIN.[44]

Nonsteroidal Anti-inflammatory Drugs

The therapeutic efficacy of nonsteroidal anti-inflammatory drugs (NSAIDs) is linked to their potency as inhibitors of cyclooxygenase activity, the first enzymatic step in the synthesis of prostaglandins from arachidonic acid. A number of adverse effects on kidney function may occur as a direct result of the pharmacologic action of these drugs.[6, 47–49] These include ARF secondary to reversible renal vasoconstriction, which may progress to ischemic ATN; and fluid and electrolyte abnormalities, that is, sodium and water retention, hyponatremia, and hyporenin-hypoaldosteronism with hyperkalemia and metabolic acidosis. In addition, these drugs are a major cause of AIN, which is frequently accompanied by the nephrotic syndrome.[6, 47] Long-term use of these drugs has been linked to the development of chronic interstitial nephritis secondary to papillary necrosis.[6, 47]

Renal prostaglandins modulate kidney function at several levels.[49] Prostaglandin I_2 (PGI_2) and prostaglandin E_2 (PGE_2) are vasodilators that modulate the vasoconstricting actions of angiotensin II, norepinephrine, endothelin, and arginine vasopressin on the afferent and efferent arterioles. PGI_2 modulates renin secretion by the juxtaglomerular cells. PGE_2 inhibits sodium transport along the thick ascending limb of Henle's loop and antagonizes vasopressin's action on water transport along the collecting duct. Prostaglandins also play an important role in the adaptive hyperfiltration of residual nephrons that accompany all forms of chronic renal failure. In healthy individuals, inhibition of prostaglandin synthesis has little discernible impact on kidney function or electrolyte balance. On the other hand, individuals who suffer from an absolute or relative decline of effective circulating volume as a consequence of diuretic therapy, gastrointestinal losses, congestive heart failure, liver disease with ascites, or hypoalbuminemic states in which there is heightened stimulation of the renin-angiotensin system, the sympathetic nervous system, and other vasoconstrictor mechanisms to support systemic hemodynamics are at increased risk for complications from NSAID therapy. Under these clinical circumstances, the vasodilator prostaglandins play a critical role in antagonizing renal vasoconstricting stimuli and maintaining RBF and GFR. Inhibition of prostaglandin synthesis in these clinical settings may provoke a sharp decline of RBF and GFR and sodium and water excretion.

The typical clinical picture is that of prerenal azotemia manifested by a variable elevation of the BUN/creatinine ratio and a low FE_{Na}.[6, 47–49] However, in high-risk individuals (i.e., those of advanced age with underlying heart, liver, or kidney disease), a severe decline of kidney function may occur and signify the development of ischemic ATN secondary to intense renal vasoconstriction. In patients with chronic renal failure, NSAIDs may precipitate end-stage renal disease. In most cases, however, discontinuation of the drug leads to reversal of ARF. In some patients, the clinical picture is dominated by sodium retention, edema formation, and escape from control of antihypertensive medication. Because these drugs inhibit renin secretion, hyperkalemia may be a prominent finding, especially in patients with chronic renal failure, in patients with diabetes mellitus, and in patients taking potassium-sparing diuretics.

All NSAIDs have the potential to cause these complications. Of particular relevance to the ICU setting is ketorolac, an NSAID commonly used for pain control to avoid the complications of opiates. This agent has the same potential to cause renal dysfunction as do the other NSAIDs.[50, 51] ICU patients, because of the severity of their illness that often involves multiorgan dysfunction, are especially likely to have complications from ketorolac. This drug, like most NSAIDs, is metabolized in the liver to an inactive metabolite. In the case of ketorolac, however, the metabolite is an unstable acylglucuronide conjugate that is excreted primarily by the kidneys.[48] In the setting of renal insufficiency, the metabolite accumulates in plasma and undergoes hydrolysis to reform the active drug, thereby magnifying the risk of renal complications. Close monitoring of renal function in these patients is essential.

ARF in patients receiving NSAIDs may also result from AIN.[6, 47, 52] This complication is usually observed after more than several months of therapy, although it has been observed in rare cases after only 1 week of therapy. The clinical expression of AIN secondary to NSAIDs is typically devoid of signs of hypersensitivity, such as fever, rash, eosinophilia, and eosinophiluria. Renal insufficiency accompanied by nephrotic-range proteinuria with or without nephrotic syndrome is highly suggestive of AIN. Kidney biopsy is required to establish the diagnosis. Discontinuation of the drug is followed by recovery or improvement of function during several weeks to several months. The effectiveness of steroid therapy in promoting recovery has not been established.

Angiotensin-Converting Enzyme Inhibitors

Angiotensin-converting enzyme (ACE) inhibitors are widely used in the treatment of hypertension, congestive heart failure, and glomerular diseases of the kidney. Soon after the release of this class of drugs, a syndrome of functional ARF was described occurring most commonly in patients with bilateral renal artery stenosis or with renal artery stenosis of a solitary kidney.[47, 53] Subsequently, this syndrome was recognized in patients treated with these drugs for heart failure.[47, 53]

The pathogenesis of functional ARF relates to the important physiologic role angiotensin II plays in regulating efferent arteriolar tone and maintaining constant glomerular capillary hydraulic pressure to support glomerular filtration. Inhibition of angiotensin II formation leads to dilatation of the efferent arteriole. In the normal kidney, the afferent arteriole reflexly dilates to maintain constant glomerular capillary pressure and filtration rate. However, in the clinical setting of renal artery stenosis, which constitutes a fixed preglomerular resistance, the afferent arteriole is unable to compensate for the fall in efferent arteriolar resistance. Consequently, glomerular capillary pressure falls, resulting in a fall in GFR. If systemic blood pressure declines in response to the ACE inhibitor, the renal microcirculatory changes are accentuated. Similar hemodynamic alterations occur in patients treated with these drugs for heart failure who frequently have diffuse atherosclerotic disease involving the kidneys, which becomes functionally significant when low systemic arterial pressure is pursued for afterload reduction. Those patients with renal insufficiency before initiation of therapy with ACE inhibitors are at increased risk for functional ARF.[53] Discontinuation of the drug usually leads to recovery of renal function to baseline.

Another potential complication of therapy with ACE inhibitors is hyperkalemia. This usually occurs in combination with some other predisposing factor, such as chronic renal insufficiency, diabetes mellitus, or concomitant therapy with potassium-sparing diuretics, potassium supplements, or NSAIDs.[53]

Because the half-life of these drugs is prolonged in renal failure, the starting dose of these drugs should be reduced in patients with impaired kidney function (see Table 156-5). In high-risk patients, a short-acting drug is recommended. Angiotensin II receptor antagonists have the same potential to disturb kidney function as do ACE inhibitors.

DRUG THERAPY IN KIDNEY FAILURE

General Pharmacokinetic Concepts

The pharmacologic effect of a drug depends on the concentration and duration of drug or active metabolite delivered to specific cell receptors. Pharmacokinetics is the science of ascertaining the concentration profile of a drug in a biologic fluid, most commonly plasma, over time. The concentration/time profile of a drug in plasma is commonly referred to as the area under the curve (AUC) and is determined by the amount and route of drug administered, the extent and rate of drug absorption (bioavailability), the volume of distribution of the drug, the amount of drug bound to plasma proteins, the rate of drug metabolism or biotransformation, and the rate of drug excretion.[54]

Bioavailability

Bioavailability is defined as the fraction of orally administered drug that reaches the systemic circulation. It is dependent on the amount of drug absorbed across the gastrointestinal tract and the amount of drug that undergoes first-pass elimination by the liver or less commonly by the gut mucosa.

Bioavailability can be determined by comparing the AUC after oral administration with the AUC after intravenous administration of a drug. A number of factors may influence gastrointestinal absorption of drug. These include the chemical and physical formulation of the drug, gastric pH, the functional and structural integrity of the intestinal tract, and the presence of food or other drugs in the gastrointestinal tract. Renal failure may depress the absorption of drugs as a consequence of increased gastric pH caused by buffering by ammonia generated from urea, uremia-associated vomiting, or uremia-associated enteropathy. Edema of the intestinal wall due to hypoalbuminemia or volume overload may also impede drug absorption. Calcium salts or aluminum-containing agents administered for the purpose of binding dietary phosphate may form complexes with drugs (e.g., ciprofloxacin) and, thereby, inhibit absorption.

Volume of Distribution

The volume of distribution (V_d) of a drug represents the apparent volume of plasma in which the drug would have to be distributed to achieve the observed plasma concentration. V_d is commonly expressed in units of liters per kilogram of lean body weight. Drugs that are tightly bound to plasma proteins have a V_d that approximates the volume of extracellular fluid. In the case of drugs that are lipid soluble or bind avidly to tissue proteins, the V_d may exceed total body water.

Knowledge of V_d is useful in estimating the loading dose of a drug required to achieve a desired plasma concentration (C_p) after intravenous bolus administration. In renal failure, the V_d for a given drug may be altered as a consequence of expansion or contraction of body fluid compartments, malnutrition with depletion of protein and lipids, or retention of products that interfere with drug binding to plasma or tissue proteins. For example, in advanced renal failure, the V_d of digoxin is reduced by 30% to 40%, so that the loading dose should be reduced accordingly.[55]

Intercompartmental Transfer Coefficient

Some drugs behave pharmacokinetically as if they were distributed in a single homogeneous compartment, the volume of which commonly exceeds that of extracellular fluid. Other drugs behave pharmacokinetically as if they were distributed in two and occasionally three compartments.

In the more common two-compartment open model, drugs enter and are eliminated from a central compartment that consists of the intravascular volume along with a component of the interstitial volume derived from highly perfused organs such as the lungs, the kidneys, and the heart. Drug distributes between the central compartment and the larger peripheral compartment at a rate defined by the intercompartmental transfer coefficient. Both the size of the peripheral compartment and the rate at which drug is transferred to the central compartment influence the quantity of drug eliminated from the body during hemodialysis.

Plasma Protein Binding

The extent to which a drug is tightly bound to plasma proteins is a major determinant of V_d. It also determines the pharmacologic efficacy of a given dose of drug because drug bound to plasma proteins is pharmacologically inactive. Acidic drugs bind primarily to albumin. Basic drugs bind primarily to α_1-acid glycoprotein.

In renal failure, the binding of many acidic drugs to albumin is reduced,[56] possibly because of competitive inhibition by retained organic acids or metabolites. The net effect is an increase in the fraction of pharmacologically active drug. This may lead to misinterpretation of the total serum concentration of a drug like phenytoin, which because of reduced plasma protein binding in patients with renal failure is typically prescribed at a dose to maintain a lower total plasma concentration, whereas the unbound fraction remains unchanged. If a laboratory measures only total drug concentration, the result may mislead a clinician to increase the dose of phenytoin, and this could result in the development of toxicity. Basic drugs bind mainly to α_1-acid glycoprotein, which is often elevated in renal failure[57] and may result in increased binding of these agents.

Drug Metabolism

Most drugs undergo metabolic transformation, which alters their pharmacologic activity before elimination from the body. Multiple enzymes participate in this process, and these have been classified under two broad categories. *Phase I reactions* include oxidations, hydroxylations, reductions, and hydrolyses. For example, cytochrome P_{450} microsomal enzymes compose a family of heme proteins that participate in the oxidation and hydroxylation of xenobiotics. Phase I reactions may generate highly reactive and potentially toxic metabolites because of their ability to induce oxidative stress or to bind to macromolecules. Phase I reactions are usually coupled to *phase II reactions,* such as glucuronidation, sulfation, acylation, methylation, and glutathionation. Phase II reactions usually generate highly polar, water-soluble, and biologically inactive products that are excreted in the urine or in the bile. Whereas the largest capacity for the biotransformation of drugs resides in the liver, other organs including the kidneys contribute to this process.

Renal failure alters the hepatic clearance of certain drugs.[58, 59] In some cases, hepatic clearance is augmented; in other cases, hepatic clearance is depressed (Table 156–3). Increased hepatic clearance may result from decreased binding of drug to plasma protein, which results in a greater fraction of active drug available for transport and metabolism by the liver. Induction of specific cytochrome P_{450} enzymes, possibly by metabolites that accumulate in uremia, has been postulated as the mechanism underlying the increased hepatic clearance of certain drugs (e.g., phenytoin and nifedipine). Depression of hepatic clearance of drugs in renal failure may result from multiple mechanisms. The accumulation of inactive drug metabolites may depress the hepatic clearance of the parent drug by competitive inhibition of drug uptake or of enzymatic biotransformation. Retention of uremic toxins or depletion of critical cofactors may lead to depressed activity of drug-metabolizing enzymes.

The possibility that renal failure may depress the synthesis or accelerate the degradation of certain drug-metabolizing enzymes warrants investigation. An apparent reduction in hepatic clearance may result from increased enterohepatic recirculation of parent drug (e.g., oxazepam[60]), regenerated by the hydrolysis within the intestine of glucuronide conjugates normally excreted in the urine. Increased regeneration of parent drug may also occur in extracellular fluid as a consequence of the reversal of labile conjugated derivatives (e.g., ketorolac[48]) or by a shift in the equilibrium of oxidation-reduction reactions (e.g., ketanserin[61]).

TABLE 156–3. Altered Hepatic Metabolism of Drugs in Kidney Failure

Metabolism Increased	Metabolism Decreased
Antipyrine	Bufuralol
Cefpiramide	Erythromycin
Fosinopril	Metoclopramide
Nifedipine	Nicardipine
Phenytoin	Nimodipine
Sulfadimidine	Nitrendipine
	Oxprenolol
	Propranolol
	Verapamil

Modified from Elston AC, Bayliss MK, Park GR: Effect of renal failure on drug metabolism by the liver. Br J Anaesth 1993; 71:282.

Plasma Drug Clearance

Plasma drug clearance (Cl) is defined as the volume of plasma cleared of a drug per unit time. The principal organs responsible for clearing a drug from plasma are the liver and the kidneys. The liver plays the major role in the biotransformation of drugs, after which the metabolites are eliminated either in bile or in urine. In some cases, drug is excreted in bile or urine without any metabolic transformation. Total plasma clearance (Cl_T) is defined by Equation 1:

$$Cl_T = Cl_H + Cl_R + Cl_x \quad (1)$$

where Cl_H equals hepatic clearance, Cl_R equals renal clearance, and Cl_x equals the contribution of the remaining organs and tissues to the clearance of a drug. In most cases, Cl_x is negligible and can be ignored.

Hepatic clearance is defined by Equation 2:

$$Cl_H = Q_H \cdot E_H \quad (2)$$

where Q_H equals hepatic blood flow and E_H equals hepatic extraction ratio, which is the fraction of drug removed from the blood during its passage through the liver. E_H is defined by Equation 3:

$$E_H = (C_a - C_v) / C_a \quad (3)$$

where C_a equals the drug concentration in hepatic arterial blood and C_v equals the drug concentration in hepatic venous blood. The hepatic extraction ratio also includes the removal of drug from portal venous as well as arterial blood. Some orally administered drugs undergo a high first-pass inactivation/elimination rate because of a high rate of drug extraction from portal venous blood. Drugs with a high hepatic extraction ratio, such as propranolol, exhibit clearance rates that are sensitive to changes in hepatic blood flow. The extent of protein binding and the intrinsic hepatic transport and metabolic rates are important determinants of hepatic drug clearance.

Renal clearance is defined by Equation 4:

$$Cl_R = Q_R \cdot E_R \quad (4)$$

where Q_R equals renal blood flow and E_R equals the renal extraction ratio. The renal extraction ratio of a drug or metabolite is determined by the net effect of several mechanisms: the extent to which the drug or metabolite is filtered across the glomerular capillaries, the extent to which the drug or metabolite undergoes active or passive tubular secretion, the extent to which filtered or secreted drug or metabolite undergoes active or passive absorption as it courses through the tubules, and the extent to which the drug is metabolized by tubular epithelial cells. Renal clearance can also be determined by measuring the rate of excretion of drug in urine according to Equation 5:

$$Cl_R = (C_U \cdot V_U) / C_P \quad (5)$$

where C_U and C_P define the concentration of drug in urine and plasma, respectively, and V_U defines urine volume per unit time.

By far the most important effect of renal failure is to decrease the drug elimination rate, especially of those agents excreted exclusively or principally by the kidneys without prior metabolic transformation. The renal clearance of such drugs is usually reduced in direct proportion to the reduction in GFR. Aminoglycoside antibiotics and digoxin serve as examples of drugs that in the absence of appropriate dose reductions accumulate to toxic concentrations in renal failure. Drugs eliminated by renal tubular secretion may exhibit a greater reduction in renal clearance than that predicted by the depression in GFR owing to the accumulation in renal failure of organic acids that compete with weakly acidic drugs for access to transport proteins. For those drugs eliminated partially by the liver as well as by the kidneys, renal failure may cause little or no change in the rate of drug elimination because the liver may be able to augment its rate of drug clearance, as is the case for fosinopril[62] and for cefpiramide.[63] On the other hand, in the presence of impaired hepatic function, even minor depression of kidney function may result in major reductions in total drug clearance.

In addition to playing a major role in elimination of unmodified drug, the kidneys are the principal route for the excretion of many drug metabolites. Predictably, renal failure leads to the accumulation in extracellular fluid of these metabolites, some of which are pharmacologically active and may produce undesirable side effects. Examples of active metabolites that accumulate in renal failure are listed in Table 156–4. The kidneys have the capacity to metabolize certain drugs by phase I and phase II reactions. Loss of this metabolic function in parallel with the loss of renal excretory function may contribute to the derangements in pharmacokinetics.

Plasma Drug Half-life

The rate of decline in plasma drug concentration (C_p) as a function of time (t) can be determined by Equation 6:

$$-\,dC_p/dt = k_e \cdot C_p \qquad (6)$$

where d is the rate of change, and k_e is the first-order elimination rate constant with the dimension of reciprocal time (e.g., min^{-1}, hr^{-1}). It denotes the constant fraction of residual drug eliminated per unit of time. Knowing the value of k_e permits calculation of the concentration of drug remaining in plasma at a specific time, according to Equation 7:

$$C_p = C_0 \cdot e^{-kt} \qquad (7)$$

where C_0 is the concentration of drug in plasma at time zero. The half-life ($t_{1/2}$) of a drug is defined as the time it takes for the plasma drug concentration to decline by 50% and can be determined by Equation 8:

$$t_{1/2} = \ln (C_0 / 0.5C_0) / k_e = \ln 2 / k_e = 0.693 / k_e \qquad (8)$$

The $t_{1/2}$ is a dependent pharmacokinetic variable, the value of which is determined by V_d and by Cl_T according to Equation 9:

$$t_{1/2} = 0.693\,(V_d \cdot IBW / Cl_T) \qquad (9)$$

where IBW stands for ideal body weight. A change in the half-life of a drug may result from a change in the volume of distribution or most commonly from a change in drug clearance by the liver or the kidneys. Knowledge of the $t_{1/2}$ is useful in estimating the time it will take to achieve a steady-state concentration of drug (five half-lives) in the absence of a loading dose and in determining the appropriate drug dosing interval, which usually is once every half-life. For drugs with pharmacokinetics conforming to a two-compartment open model, the relevant parameter is the $t_{1/2\beta}$, which is derived from the elimination phase as opposed to the distribution phase of a drug. For drugs that are excreted principally by the kidneys, the $t_{1/2}$ will be prolonged to a degree inversely proportional to the depression of kidney function. Knowledge of the magnitude of change in the $t_{1/2}$ of a drug together with knowledge of the V_d of the drug provides the basis for making decisions about drug dose adjustments in kidney failure.

General Guidelines

Application of these general guidelines to individual patients with kidney failure should be undertaken only after due consideration of a number of factors known to influence pharmacokinetics and pharmacodynamics. These factors include the patient's age, volume status, nutritional status, metabolic status, physiologic status of critical organ systems, and concurrent medications. A clearly defined rationale that includes a systematic evaluation of the risk-benefit ratio should be undertaken before therapy is instituted with any drug. Although this principle is applicable to all patients, it is especially important in the patient with acute or chronic renal failure because these patients are at increased risk for adverse drug reactions and nephrotoxic injury.[3] Knowledge of the cause or causes of the renal failure is of critical importance to the risk-benefit analysis. If a patient's renal failure is thought

TABLE 156–4. Active or Toxic Metabolites That Accumulate in Kidney Failure

Drug	Metabolite	Effect
Narcotics/Analgesics		
Morphine	Morphine 3- and 6-glucuronide	Prolonged sedation
Pethidine	Norpethidine	Seizures, prolonged sedation
Propoxyphene	Norpropoxyphene	Depressed cardiac conduction
Cardiovascular Drugs		
Acebutolol	Diacetolol	β-Receptor blockade
Methyldopa	Methyldopa-*O*-sulfate	Hypotension
Procainamide	*N*-Acetylprocainamide	Cardiac toxicity
Sodium nitroprusside	Thiocyanate	Neurotoxicity
Miscellaneous Drugs		
Allopurinol	Oxypurinol	Hypersensitivity reactions
Diazepam	Desmethyldiazepam	Prolonged sedation
Pancuronium	3-Hydroxypancuronium	Prolonged paralysis, myopathy
Vecuronium	3-Hydroxyvecuronium	Prolonged paralysis, myopathy

Modified from Bellomo R: Drug-kidney interactions. *In:* Textbook of Critical Care. 3rd ed. Shoemaker WC (Ed). Philadelphia, WB Saunders, 1995, p 1056.

to be related to exposure to a specific agent, it would be prudent to avoid other agents from the same drug class.

A clinically sound and practical approach to drug prescription in renal failure requires knowledge of:

- The degree of renal dysfunction
- The effect of renal dysfunction on the pharmacokinetics of the drug
- The required change in drug dose or interval to achieve an efficacious and nontoxic plasma drug concentration
- The effect of renal replacement therapies on drug elimination

Estimating Glomerular Filtration Rate

GFR is the single best estimate of kidney function. In the clinical situation, GFR can be estimated from the creatinine clearance, the determination of which can be performed by measuring the amount of creatinine excreted in the urine during a precise time interval, typically 12 or 24 hours, and dividing this value by the simultaneously measured serum creatinine concentration according to Equation 6. Because of time constraints, this method is often cumbersome and inconvenient. An alternative approach suitable for patients with a documented stable serum creatinine concentration[64] is to estimate the creatinine clearance according to Equation 10:

$$Cl_{CR} = (140 - \text{age}) \cdot (\text{IBW}) / 72 \cdot \text{serum creatinine} \qquad (10)$$

where age is expressed in years, ideal body weight in kilograms, and serum creatinine in milligrams per deciliter. To estimate the creatinine clearance in women, the value calculated by this equation is multiplied by 0.85. Ideal body weight for men is calculated as 50 kg plus 2.3 kg for each 2.5 cm (1 inch) of body height over 152 cm (5 feet). For women, ideal body weight is calculated as 45.5 kg plus 2.3 kg per 2.5 cm over 152 cm. In the case of a patient whose serum creatinine is unstable, it would be prudent to directly measure the creatinine clearance. If the serum creatinine is rising more than 0.5 mg/dL per day, it signifies severe depression of GFR, typically below 10 mL/min.

Estimating Loading Dose

The loading dose is the amount of drug administered as the first dose to rapidly achieve the desired therapeutic concentration of drug. It requires knowledge of the volume of distribution (V_d) of the drug and the desired plasma concentration (C_p) of the drug and is calculated by use of Equation 11:

$$\text{Loading dose} = C_p \cdot V_d \cdot \text{IBW} \qquad (11)$$

As a general rule, the volume of distribution of drugs is not greatly altered by renal failure. However, if renal failure is accompanied by generalized edema or ascites, then for drugs that are distributed primarily in extracellular fluid, an increase in the loading dose may be warranted. In the absence of a loading dose, peak drug concentrations will be achieved by the fifth maintenance dose administered at an interval equal to the plasma half-life of the drug. Patients with kidney failure should receive a normal loading dose of a drug followed by a maintenance dose adjusted for the severity of the kidney failure.

Estimating Maintenance Dose

The maintenance dose is equal to the amount of drug eliminated from the body during the time interval between drug doses. It can be calculated as the product of the fraction of drug excreted and the loading dose of drug according to Equation 12:

$$\begin{aligned}&\text{Maintenance dose} = \\ &[C_p - (C_p \cdot e^{-kt})] \cdot V_d \cdot \text{IBW} = \\ &(1 - e^{-kt}) \cdot (C_p \cdot V_d \cdot \text{IBW})\end{aligned} \qquad (12)$$

For drugs administered at an interval equal to the $t_{1/2}$, the maintenance dose is equal to half the loading dose. If renal failure decreases the elimination rate, the clinician has the option of administering the same maintenance dose and prolonging the interval between drug doses or of reducing the maintenance dose and keeping the interval between doses constant, or a combination of the two. For example, if a drug is normally administered every 8 hours and renal failure prolongs the $t_{1/2}$ by a factor of 2, the clinician could choose to give the same maintenance dose every 16 hours or give half the standard maintenance dose every 8 hours. The choice may be influenced by such factors as the importance of achieving a specific peak concentration of drug in plasma to obtain the desired therapeutic benefit, the importance of avoiding high trough levels to obviate potential toxicity, or the convenience of the dosing interval. By reducing the maintenance dose and keeping the dosing interval constant, the peak concentration of drug in plasma will be lower and the trough concentration will be higher than those achieved by maintaining the drug dose constant and prolonging the interval.

For drugs administered by constant infusion, the rate can be calculated as the product of the desired steady-state plasma concentration of drug (C_{ss}) and the total clearance rate (Cl_T), or the product of C_{ss}, the elimination rate constant (k_e), and the volume of distribution (V_d) as shown in Equation 13:

$$\begin{aligned}\text{Infusion rate} &= C_{ss} \cdot C_T \\ &= C_{ss} \cdot (k_e \cdot V_d \cdot \text{IBW})\end{aligned} \qquad (13)$$

Thus, a 50% reduction in total clearance would dictate a 50% reduction in the infusion rate to maintain the same steady-state plasma concentration of drug.

Drug Therapy in Patients Receiving Renal Replacement Therapy

Patients with end-stage renal disease may receive one of three renal replacement therapies:

- Conventional intermittent hemodialysis with or without hemofiltration
- Continuous hemofiltration with or without hemodialysis
- Continuous or intermittent peritoneal dialysis

Each of these therapies may promote the removal of drugs from the body, although the rate of drug removal varies significantly among these techniques. Effective drug therapy requires that maintenance dosimetry take into consideration the amount of drug eliminated from the body during the interval in which a patient is receiving a specific renal replacement therapy.

Conventional Hemodialysis

Drug removal during hemodialysis is accomplished primarily by diffusion, the rate of which is determined by the permeability of the dialysis membrane to the drug, the surface area of the membrane, and the concentration gradient of unbound drug between blood and dialysis fluid.[65] Drugs that have a molecular weight (MW) less than 500, are less than 90% protein bound, and have a low volume of distribution are most likely to undergo significant elimination during hemodialysis. The rate of elimination is augmented by increasing the blood flow rate, the dialysate flow rate, and the membrane surface area. If hemofiltration is performed during hemodialysis, an additional moiety of drug is removed by convection. The rate of drug removal during hemodialysis can be expressed as the dialyzer clearance (Cl_{HD}) and quantitated by Equation 14:

$$\begin{aligned} Cl_{HD} &= (Q_{Bi} \cdot C_{Bi}) - (Q_{Bo} \cdot C_{Bo}) / C_{Bi} \\ &= (Q_{Do} \cdot C_{Do}) / C_{Bi} \end{aligned} \tag{14}$$

where Q_{Bi} equals the rate of blood flow entering the dialyzer, Q_{Bo} equals blood flow rate leaving the dialyzer, C_{Bi} equals the concentration of drug in blood entering the dialyzer, C_{Bo} equals the concentration of drug in blood leaving the dialyzer, Q_{Do} equals the dialysate flow rate leaving the dialyzer, and C_{Do} equals the concentration of drug in the dialysate leaving the dialyzer.

Equation 14 is valid for single-pass dialysate flow where the concentration of drug in the dialysate (C_{Di}) entering the dialyzer equals zero. The equation is valid also if hemofiltration is performed during hemodialysis. The ultrafiltration rate (Q_{UF}) equals the difference between Q_{Bi} and Q_{Bo} or the difference between Q_{Do} and Q_{Di}. In the case of drugs whose hemodialysis clearance is not known, it can be estimated by use of the clearance of urea (Cl_{urea}) in Equation 15[65]:

$$Cl_{HD} = Cl_{urea} \cdot (60 / MW_{drug}) \tag{15}$$

Continuous Renal Replacement Therapies

Continuous renal replacement therapies include continuous arteriovenous hemofiltration (CAVHF) or venovenous hemofiltration (CVVHF), which use highly porous membranes that permit the convective transport of solutes with molecular weights up to 20,000. Consequently, significant quantities of large-molecular-weight drugs may be eliminated by these techniques.[66, 67] The clearance of a drug during hemofiltration (Cl_{HF}) is determined by the product of the sieving coefficient (SC) of the membrane with respect to the drug and the ultrafiltration rate (Q_{UF}) as defined by Equation 16:

$$Cl_{HF} = SC \cdot Q_{UF} \tag{16}$$

The sieving coefficient defines the ability of the drug to permeate the membrane and can be estimated by Equation 17:

$$SC = 2C_{UF} / (C_{Bi} + C_{Bo}) \tag{17}$$

where C_{UF} is the concentration of drug in the ultrafiltrate, C_{Bi} is the concentration of solute in blood entering the hemofilter, and C_{Bo} is the concentration of solute in blood leaving the hemofilter. The major factor determining the sieving coefficient of a drug is the extent of its binding to plasma proteins. However, under conditions of high ultrafiltration rates, the amount of drug removed may be less than that predicted by the sieving coefficient because of the constraint on transport imposed by the formation of a concentrated layer of plasma proteins adjacent to the membrane. The impact of hemofiltration on drug elimination will be greatest for those drugs that have a low volume of distribution, low plasma protein binding, and low nonrenal clearance. In contrast to hemodialysis, molecular weight is not a major determinant of drug elimination by hemofiltration because the molecular weight of most drugs in use clinically is significantly below the molecular weight cutoff of the hemofilter membrane.

Continuous arteriovenous hemodiafiltration (CAVHDF) or continuous venovenous hemodiafiltration (CVVHDF) combines the convective transport of hemofiltration and the diffusive transport of slow hemodialysis with dialysate flow rates typically between 1 and 3 L/hr. The contribution of slow hemodialysis to total drug elimination during CAVHDF and CVVHDF has been examined by a number of investigators.[66–69] From such studies, it is clear that the results are influenced by a number of variables, including the dialysate flow rate, ultrafiltration rate, extent of protein binding of drug, and membrane permeability and surface area. In the absence of specific information about these variables, it is not possible to provide specific recommendations about drug adjustments for patients undergoing CAVHDF or CVVHDF. The general guideline given in Table 156-5 for these patients is based on the equivalent creatinine clearance that is estimated as the sum of the ultrafiltration rate and 0.5 × the dialysate flow rate (Q_D) for flow rates up to 3 L/hr (50 mL/min). Sieving coefficients may be estimated as $1 - f_b$, where f_b equals the fraction of drug bound to plasma proteins (see Table 156-5).

Peritoneal Dialysis

The number of patients with end-stage renal disease treated by continuous ambulatory peritoneal dialysis (CAPD) or continuous cycling peritoneal dialysis (CCPD) has grown substantially in recent years. Thus, it can be anticipated that an increasing number of these patients will be encountered in the ICU. Drug removal during peritoneal dialysis is less efficient than that achieved by hemodialysis owing in part to the low permeability of the peritoneal membrane and low dialysate flow rates, which for a standard regimen of 10 L of dialysate per 24 hours is equivalent to a dialysate flow rate of 7 mL/min. Assuming urea in plasma fully equilibrates with the dialysate, this will generate a urea clearance of only 7 mL/min. This number may be augmented by increasing the number of exchanges and by promoting net ultrafiltration of fluid. However, from a practical perspective, urea clearances are unlikely to exceed 15 mL/min. Drug clearance by peritoneal dialysis (Cl_{PD}) can be estimated by the relationship expressed by Equation 18[70]:

$$Cl_{PD} = Cl_{urea} \cdot (60 / MW_{drug})^{1/2} \tag{18}$$

In addition to molecular weight, the amount of drug removed by peritoneal dialysis is critically dependent on its volume of distribution and the extent of its binding to plasma proteins. Thus, drug dose adjustments for patients receiving CAPD or CCPD are approximately the same as for patients with a creatinine clearance of 10 mL/min or less (see Table 156-5).

Table 156-5 contains guidelines for drug dose adjustments in adult patients with kidney failure ranging from mild to end-stage renal disease requiring renal replacement therapy. These guidelines reflect the author's synthesis of recommendations by drug manufacturers and published pharmacokinetic studies. Space constraints do not permit citation of the large number of original papers that provide the foundation for these guidelines; however, these can be found among references 36, 65 to 69, and 71 to 89. In applying these guidelines, the clinician needs to take into consideration a number of patient-specific factors (enumerated earlier) besides the degree of kidney function impairment that may dictate further modification of drug dosimetry. Moreover, it behooves the clinician to monitor plasma drug levels to fine-tune drug dose adjustments. From inspection of Table 156-5, it is evident that antimicrobial agents compose the largest drug class that requires dose modification. Those antibiotics that do not require dose modification in renal failure are listed in Table 156-6 along with common agents from other major drug groups.

TABLE 156–5. Pharmacokinetic Data and Guidelines for Adjusting Drug Dosage in Adults with Renal Failure

Drug	MW	Protein Binding (%)	V_d (L/kg)	$t_{1/2}$ (hr) Normal/ESRD	Renal Excretion (%) (intact drug and active metabolite)	Usual Dose in Normal Renal Function	Method	Maintenance Dose Adjustments for Kidney Failure* — Estimated Creatinine Clearance (mL/min) >50	>10 <50	<10	HD	CAPD/CCPD	CRRT	Comments
Antibacterial Antibiotics														
AMINOGLYCOSIDES														
Amikacin	585.6	<5	0.25	2–3/80	95	15 mg/kg q 24 h	D and I	7.5–12 mg/kg q 24 h	1.5–6 mg/kg q 24 h	1.5–3 mg/kg q 48 h	5–7 mg/kg AD	150–200 mg IV/IP qd	Dose for Cl_{CR} = UFR + 0.5 Q_D†	Nephro/ototoxic; monitor levels
Gentamicin	496.6	<5	0.25	2–3/60	95	4.5 mg/kg q 24 h	D and I	2.4–3.6 mg/kg q 24 h	0.5–2.3 mg/kg q 24 h	0.5–1 mg/kg q 48 h	1–1.5 mg/kg AD	30–40 mg IV/IP qd	Dose for Cl_{CR} = UFR + 0.5 Q_D	Nephro/ototoxic; monitor levels
Netilmicin	475.6	<5	0.22	2–3/72	95	6 mg/kg q 24 h	D and I	3.1–4.8 mg/kg q 24 h	0.6–3.0 mg/kg q 24 h	0.6–1.2 mg/kg q 48 h	1.2–1.8 mg/kg AD	30–40 mg IV/IP qd	Dose for Cl_{CR} = UFR + 0.5 Q_D	Nephro/ototoxic; monitor levels
Streptomycin	581.6	30	0.26	2–3/110	70	15 mg/kg q 24 h + AD	D and I	7.5 mg/kg q 24 h	7.5 mg/kg q 24–72 h	7.5 mg/kg q 72–96 h	5–7 mg/kg AD	150–200 mg IV/IP qd	Dose for Cl_{CR} = UFR + 0.5 Q_D	Ototoxic
Tobramycin	467.5	<5	0.25	2–3/60	95	4.5 mg/kg q 24 h	D and I	2.4–3.6 mg/kg q 24 h	0.5–2.3 mg/kg q 24 h	0.5–1 mg/kg q 48 h	1–1.5 mg/kg AD	30–40 mg IV/IP qd	Dose for Cl_{CR} = UFR + 0.5 Q_D	Nephro/ototoxic; monitor levels
CARBAPENEM														
Imipenem/cilastatin	317.4	20	0.38	1/4	70	0.5 g q 6 h	D and I	250–500 mg q 6–8 h	250–500 mg q 8–12 h	125–250 mg q 12 h	125–250 mg q 12 h + AD	125–250 mg q 12 h	Dose for Cl_{CR} = UFR + 0.5 Q_D	↑ Risk of seizures in ESRD
CEPHALOSPORINS														
Cefazolin	454.5	80	0.20	1.9/70	80	1–2 g q 8 h	D and I	1–2 g q 8 h	1–2 g q 12–24 h	0.5–1 g q 24 h	0.5–1 g q 24 h + AD	0.5 g q 12 h	Dose for Cl_{CR} = UFR + 0.5 Q_D	
Cefepime	534.5	16	0.30	2.2/14	85	1–2 g q 12 h	D and I	1–2 g q 12 h	1–2 g q 24 h	0.5–1 g q 24 h	0.5–1 g q 24 h + AD	0.5–1 g q 24 h	Dose for Cl_{CR} = UFR + 0.5 Q_D	
Cefotaxime	455.5	37	0.25	1.7/11	60	1–2 g q 8 h	D and I	1–2 g q 8–12 h	1–2 g q 12–24 h	1 g q 24 h	1 g q 24 h + AD	1 g q 24 h	Dose for Cl_{CR} = UFR + 0.5 Q_D	
Cefoxitin	427.5	70	0.20	1/23	85	1–2 g q 8 h	D and I	1–2 g q 8–12 h	1–2 g q 12–24 h	1–2 g q 24–48 h	0.5–1 g q 24 h + AD	1 g q 24 h	Dose for Cl_{CR} = UFR + 0.5 Q_D	
Ceftazidime	546.6	15	0.25	1.7/25	85	1–2 g q 8 h	D and I	1–2 g q 8–12 h	1–2 g q 12–24 h	1–2 g q 24–48 h	0.5–1 g q 24 h + AD	0.5–1 g q 24 h	Dose for Cl_{CR} = UFR + 0.5 Q_D	
Cefuroxime	242.0	33	0.30	1.3/22	95	0.75–1.5 g q 8 h	I	0.75–1.5 g q 8 h	0.75–1.5 g q 8–12 h	0.75–1.5 g q 24 h	0.75–1.5 g q 24 h + AD	0.75–1.5 g q 24 h	Dose for Cl_{CR} = UFR + 0.5 Q_D	
PENICILLINS														
Ampicillin	349.4	15–25	0.30	1.3/20	70	0.5–2 g q 6 h	I	0.5–2 g q 6–8 h	0.5–2 g q 8–12 h	0.5–2 g q 12–24 h	0.5–1 g q 24 h + AD	0.5–1 g q 24 h	Dose for Cl_{CR} = UFR + 0.5 Q_D	
Methicillin	380.4	30–50	0.30	0.5–1/4–6	80	1–2 g q 4 h	I	1–2 g q 4–6 h	1–2 g q 6–8 h	1–2 g q 8–12 h	1–2 g q 12 h	1–2 g q 12 h	Dose for Cl_{CR} = UFR + 0.5 Q_D	
Mezlocillin	539.6	16–42	0.20	1.2/6	60–70	1.5–4 g q 4–6 h	I	1.5–4 g q 4–6 h	1.5–4 g q 6–8 h	1.5–4 g q 8–12 h	1.5–4 g q 12 h	1.5–4 g q 12 h	Dose for Cl_{CR} = UFR + 0.5 Q_D	Decrease dose for liver disease
Penicillin G	334.4	45–68	0.35	0.6/6–12	85	0.5–4 × 10^6 U q 4 h	I	0.5–4 × 10^6 U q 4–6 h	0.5–4 × 10^6 U q 6–12 h	0.5–4 × 10^6 U q 12–24 h	0.5–4 × 10^6 U q 12–24 h + AD	Dose for Cl_{CR} <10	Dose for Cl_{CR} = UFR + 0.5 Q_D	
Piperacillin	517.6	16–22	0.25	0.6–1.3/5	80–90	3–4 g q 4–6 h	I	3–4 g q 4–6 h	3–4 g q 6–8 h	3–4 g q 8–12 h	3–4 g q 12 h + AD	3–4 g q 12 h	Dose for Cl_{CR} = UFR + 0.5 Q_D	
Ticarcillin-clavulanate	384.4	45–65	0.21	0.9–1.3/16	80–90	3.1 g q 4 h	D and I	3.1 g q 4–6 h	2 g q 6–8 h	2 g q 12 h	2 g q 12 h +3.1 g AD	2 g q 12 h	Dose for Cl_{CR} = UFR + 0.5 Q_D	
QUINOLONES														
Ciprofloxacin	331.4	20–40	2.5	3–5/6–12	50–70	400 mg IV q 12 h	D and I	400 mg IV q 12 h	200–300 mg IV q 12 h	200 mg IV q 12 h	400 mg IV q 24 h	200 mg IV q 12 h	Dose for Cl_{CR} = UFR + 0.5 Q_D	
Ofloxacin	361.4	25	2.5	4–8/25–48	>90	200–400 mg IV q 12 h	D and I	200–400 mg IV q 12 h	100–200 mg IV q 12 h	100 mg IV q 12 h	200 mg IV q 24 h	100 mg IV q 12 h	Dose for Cl_{CR} = UFR + 0.5 Q_D	
MISCELLANEOUS														
Aztreonam	435.4	56	0.15	1.3–2.2/8	58–74	1–2 g q 8 h	D and I	1–2 g q 8 h	1–1.5 g q 8–12 h	0.5–1 g q 12 h	0.5–1 g q 12 h + AD	0.5–1 g q 12 h	Dose for Cl_{CR} = UFR + 0.5 Q_D	
Clarithromycin	748.0	70	3.0	6/22	15	0.5–1 g q 12 h	D	0.5–1.0 g q 12 h	0.25–0.75 g q 12 h	0.25–0.5 g q 12 h	0.25–0.5 g q 12 h	0.25–0.5 g q 12 h	Dose for Cl_{CR} = UFR + 0.5 Q_D	
Erythromycin	733.9	70–85	0.8	2/5	15	250–500 mg q 6–12 h	D	250–500 mg q 6–12 h	250–500 mg q 6–12 h	125–250 mg q 6–12 h	125–250 mg q 6–12 h	125–250 mg q 6–12 h	Dose for Cl_{CR} = UFR + 0.5 Q_D	Ototoxic with high dose in ESRD

Table continued on following page

TABLE 156–5. Pharmacokinetic Data and Guidelines for Adjusting Drug Dosage in Adults with Renal Failure

Drug	MW	Protein Binding (%)	V_d (L/kg)	$t_{1/2}$ (hr) Normal/ESRD	Renal Excretion (%) (intact drug and active metabolite)	Usual Dose in Normal Renal Function	Method	Maintenance Dose Adjustments for Kidney Failure*						Comments
								Estimated Creatinine Clearance (mL/min)						
								>50	>10 <50	<10	HD	CAPD/CCPD	CRRT	
Metronidazole	171.2	<20	0.75	6–8/12–20	<20	7.5 mg/kg q 6 h	I	7.5 mg/kg q 6 h	7.5 mg/kg q 6–8 h	7.5 mg/kg q 12 h	7.5 mg/kg q 12 h + AD	7.5 mg/kg q 12 h	Dose for Cl_{CR} = UFR + 0.5 Q_D	Metabolites ↑ in ESRD
Teicoplanin	934.0	90	0.76	20–70/240–380	>50	6 mg/kg q 24 h	I	6 mg/kg q 24 h	6 mg/kg q 48 h	6 mg/kg q 72 h	6 mg/kg q 72 h	6 mg/kg q 72 h	Dose for Cl_{CR} = UFR + 0.5 Q_D	Ototoxic
Tetracycline	444.4	25–65	1.5	6–12/57–120	48–60	250–500 mg q 6 h	I	250–500 mg q 8–12 h	250–500 mg q 12–24 h	Avoid	Avoid	Avoid	Avoid	
Trimethoprim / Sulfamethoxazole	290.3 / 253.3	40–70 / 65	1.6 / 0.25	8–11/>26 / 10–13/>50	50–60 / 10–25	2.5–5 mg/kg / 12.5–25 mg/kg IV q 6–12 h	I / I	2.5–5 mg/kg / 12.5–25 mg/kg IV q 6–12 h	2.5–5 mg/kg / 12.5–25 mg/kg IV q 12–24 h	2.5–5 mg/kg / 12.5–25 mg/kg IV q 24 h	2.5–5 mg/kg / 12.5–25 mg/kg IV q 24 h	2.5–5 mg/kg / 12.5–25 mg/kg IV q 24 h	Dose for Cl_{CR} = UFR + 0.5 Q_D / Dose for Cl_{CR} = UFR + 0.5 Q_D	
Vancomycin	1449.2	30	0.65	4–8/>150	>95	1 g q 12 h	I	1 g q 12–24 h	1 g q 24–96 h	1 g q 4–7 d	1 g q 4–7 d	1 g q 4–7 d	Dose for Cl_{CR} = UFR + 0.5 Q_D	Nephrotoxic; monitor levels
Antifungal Antibiotics														
Amphotericin	924.1	95	4	24/24	<10	0.3–0.8 mg/kg q 24 h	I	0.3–0.8 mg/kg q 24 h	0.3–0.8 mg/kg q 24–36 h	0.3–0.8 mg/kg q 48 h	Dose for Cl_{CR} <10	Dose for Cl_{CR} <10	Dose for Cl_{CR} <10	Nephrotoxic
Fluconazole	303.6	12	0.85	22–30/100	80	200–400 mg q 24 h	D	200–400 mg q 24 h	100–200 mg q 24 h	100 mg q 24 h	200 mg AD	100 mg q 24 h	Dose for Cl_{CR} = UFR + 0.5 Q_D	
Flucytosine	129.1	<10	0.6	3–6/75–250	80–90	37.5 mg/kg q 6 h	D and I	37.5 mg/kg q 8–12 h	37.5 mg/kg q 12–24 h	20 mg/kg q 24 h	20 mg/kg q 24 h	20 mg/kg q 24 h	Dose for Cl_{CR} = UFR + 0.5 Q_D	Monitor levels
Antiparasitic Antibiotics														
Pentamidine	340.4	69	3	29/118	<5	4 mg/kg q 24 h	I	4 mg/kg q 24 h	4 mg/kg q 36–48 h	4 mg/kg q 48 h	4 mg/kg q 48 h	4 mg/kg q 48 h	4 mg/kg q 48 h	Nephrotoxic
Sulfadiazine	250.3	20–55	0.3	5–7/32	40–60	0.5–2 g q 6 h	I	0.5–2 g q 6 h	Avoid	Avoid	Avoid	Avoid	Avoid	ARF from crystal deposition
Antituberculous Antibiotics														
Cycloserine	102.1	<5	0.19	10/>25	60–70	250 mg q 12 h	I	250 mg q 12 h	250 mg q 18–24 h	250 mg q 24–36 h	ND	ND	ND	CNS toxicity; monitor levels
Ethambutol	204.3	8–22	2.3	3.3/7–15	80	15 mg/kg q 24 h	I	15 mg/kg q 24 h	15 mg/kg q 24–36 h	15 mg/kg q 48 h	15 mg/kg AD	15 mg/kg q 48 h	Dose for Cl_{CR} = UFR + 0.5 Q_D	Optic neuritis
Antiviral Agents														
Acyclovir	225.2	9–33	0.8	2–3/20	75–85	5–10 mg/kg IV q 8 h	D and I	5–10 mg/kg q 8–12 h	5–10 mg/kg q 12–24 h	2.5–5 mg/kg q 24 h	2.5–5 mg/kg q 24 h	2.5–5 mg/kg q 24 h	Dose for Cl_{CR} = UFR + 0.5 Q_D	ARF from crystal deposition
Amantadine	151.3	67	5–7	12–24/200	>90	200 mg q 24 h	D and I	100–200 mg q 24–36 h	100 mg q 36–72 h	100 mg q 7 days	100 mg q 7 days	100 mg q 7 days	100 mg q 7 days	
Didanosine	236.0	<5	54	1.5/4.5	20–55	200 mg q 12 h	D and I	200 mg q 12 h	200 mg q 24 h	100 mg q 24 h	100 mg q 24 h + AD	100 mg q 24 h	Dose for Cl_{CR} = UFR + 0.5 Q_D	
Ganciclovir	204.2	<5	0.55	3.1/30	>90	5 mg/kg q 12 h	D and I	2.5–5 mg/kg q 12 h	1.25–2.5 mg/kg q 24 h	1.25 mg/kg q 48–72h	1.25 mg/kg AD	1.25 mg/kg q 48–72h	Dose for Cl_{CR} = UFR + 0.5 Q_D	Monitor levels
Lamivudine	229.3	36	1.3	6/15–35	70	150 mg q 12 h	D and I	150 mg q 12 h	100–150 mg q 24 h	25–50 mg q 24 h	ND	ND	ND	
Zalcitabine	211.2	<4	0.55	1.6/>8	60–80	0.75 mg q 8 h	I	0.75 mg q 8 h	0.75 mg q 12–18 h	0.75 mg q 24 h	ND	ND	ND	
Zidovudine	267.3	36	1.5	1.1/1.4–3	15–25	200 mg q 8 h	I	200 mg q 8 h	200 mg q 8 h	100 mg q 8 h	100 mg q 8 h + AD	100 mg q 8 h	Dose for Cl_{CR} = UFR + 0.5 Q_D	

Cardiovascular Agents

ACE INHIBITORS													
Benazepril	424.0	95	1.5	20/30	85	10–40 mg q 24 h	D	10–40 mg q 24 h	10–30 mg q 24 h	5–20 mg q 24 h	5–20 mg q 24 h	5–20 mg q 24 h	Dose for Cl_{CR} = UFR + 0.5 Q_D	
Captopril	217.3	30	0.7	1–3/40	80	12.5–25 mg q 8 h	D and I	12.5–25 mg q 8–12 h	12.5–25 mg q 12–24 h	12.5–25 mg q 24 h	12.5–25 mg q 24 h	12.5–25 mg q 24 h	Dose for Cl_{CR} = UFR + 0.5 Q_D	
Enalapril	368.4	55	—	11–24/34–60	80	10–40 mg q 24 h	D	10–40 mg q 24 h	5–20 mg q 24 h	2.5–10 mg q 24 h	2.5–10 mg q 24 h	2.5–10 mg q 24 h	Dose for Cl_{CR} = UFR + 0.5 Q_D	
Lisinopril	405.5	<5	1.4	12.6/40–50	90	10–40 mg q 24 h	D	10–40 mg q 24 h	5–20 mg q 24 h	2.5–10 mg q 24 h	2.5–10 mg q 24 h	2.5–10 mg q 24 h	Dose for Cl_{CR} = UFR + 0.5 Q_D	
Quinapril	475.0	97	—	1–2/6–15	60	10–40 mg q 24 h	D	10–40 mg q 24 h	10–30 mg q 24 h	5–20 mg q 24 h	2.5–10 mg q 24 h	2.5–10 mg q 24 h	Dose for Cl_{CR} = UFR + 0.5 Q_D	
Ramipril	416.5	55–70	—	6–10/15–30	35	2.5–20 mg q 24 h	D	2.5–20 mg q 24 h	2.5–10 mg q 24 h	2.5–5 mg q 24 h	2.5–5 mg q 24 h	2.5–5 mg q 24 h	Dose for Cl_{CR} = UFR + 0.5 Q_D	
ANTIARRHYTHMIA AGENTS													
Bretylium	414.4	<10	1.3	5–10/>30	>90	LD: 5–30 mg/kg MD: 5–10 mg/kg q 6 h	D	MD: 5–10 mg/kg q 6 h	2.5–5 mg/kg q 6 h	1.25–2.5 mg/kg q 6 h	1.25–2.5 mg/kg q 6 h	1.25–2.5 mg/kg q 6 h	Dose for Cl_{CR} = UFR + 0.5 Q_D	LD unchanged; adjust MD
Disopyramide	339.5	50–65	0.9	4–9/17–43	42–62	150 mg q 6 h	D and I	100 mg q 6 h	100 mg q 8–12 h	100 mg q 24 h	100 mg q 24 h	100 mg q 24 h	Dose for Cl_{CR} = UFR + 0.5 Q_D	Active metabolite ↑ in ESRD
Procainamide (NAPA)	235.3	15 (10)	2.2 (1.6)	3–5/6–10 (6–8/>40)	50–60 (15–35)	12.5 mg/kg q 6 h	D and I	12.5 mg/kg q 6–8 h	6–9 mg/kg q 8–12 h	3–6 mg/kg q 12–24 h	3–6 mg/kg q 12–24 h + AD	3–6 mg/kg q 12–24 h	Dose for Cl_{CR} = UFR + 0.5 Q_D	Monitor NAPA and procainamide levels
Tocainide	192.3	10–20	2.2	13/>20	30–50	400–600 mg q 8 h	D and I	400–600 mg q 8–12 h	400–600 mg q 12–24 h	200–300 mg q 24 h	200–300 mg q 24 h	200–300 mg q 24 h	Dose for Cl_{CR} = UFR + 0.5 Q_D	
β-BLOCKING AGENTS													
Acebutolol (active metabolite: diacetolol)	236.4	11–25	1.2	3–4/6–12 (7–11/17–54)	10–17 (65)	200–400 mg q 12–24 h	D and I	200–400 mg q 12–24 h	100–200 mg q 12–24 h	100–200 mg q 24–48 h	100–200 mg q 24–48 h	100–200 mg q 24–48 h	Dose for Cl_{CR} = UFR + 0.5 Q_D	Active metabolite ↑ in ESRD
Atenolol	266.3	<5	0.7	6/>27	>90	50–100 mg q 12–24 h	D and I	50–100 mg q 12–24 h	25–50 mg q 12–24 h	25–50 mg q 24–48 h	25–50 mg q 24–48 h	25–50 mg q 24–48 h	Dose for Cl_{CR} = UFR + 0.5 Q_D	
Nadolol	309.4	20–30	1.9	14–24/45	70	80–160 mg q 24 h	D	80–160 mg q 24 h	40–80 mg q 24 h	20–40 mg q 24 h	20–40 mg q 24 h	20–40 mg q 24 h	Dose for Cl_{CR} = UFR + 0.5 Q_D	
Sotalol	272.4	0	2.0	7.5–15/>30	>90	80–160 mg q 12 h	D and I	80–160 mg q 12 h	40–80 mg q 12–24 h	20–40 mg q 24–48 h	20–40 mg q 24–48 h	20–40 mg q 24–48 h	Dose for Cl_{CR} = UFR + 0.5 Q_D	
CARDIAC GLYCOSIDES													
Digoxin	780.9	20–30	5–8	34–44/>100	70	LD: 10–15 μg/kg MD: 2.5–5.25 μg/kg/day	D and I	MD: 2–4 μg/kg q 24 h	0.6–2.6 μg/kg q 24–48 h	0.6–1.3 μg/kg q 48–72 h	Dose for Cl_{CR} <10	Dose for Cl_{CR} <10	Dose for Cl_{CR} = UFR + 0.5 Q_D	↓ LD in RF; monitor levels
H_2-BLOCKING AGENTS													
Cimetidine	252.3	15–20	1.0	1.5–2/5	50–75	300 mg IV q 6–8 h	D	300 mg IV q 6–8 h	300 mg IV q 8–12 h	300 mg IV q 12 h	300 mg IV q 12 h	300 mg IV q 12 h	Dose for Cl_{CR} = UFR + 0.5 Q_D	Inhibits liver microsomal enzymes
Famotidine	337.4	15–20	1.3	2.5–4/12–24	65–80	20 mg IV q 12 h	D and I	20 mg IV q 12 h	20 mg IV q 24 h	10 mg IV q 24 h	10 mg IV q 24 h	10 mg IV q 24 h	Dose for Cl_{CR} = UFR + 0.5 Q_D	
Ranitidine	314.4	10–20	1.6	2–3/7–14	40–70	50 mg IV q 6–8 h	I	50 mg IV q 6–8 h	50 mg IV q 12–16 h	50 mg IV q 24 h	50 mg IV q 24 h	50 mg IV q 24 h	Dose for Cl_{CR} = UFR + 0.5 Q_D	
MISCELLANEOUS DRUGS													
Allopurinol (active metabolite: oxypurinol)	136.1	<5	0.5	1–3/1–3 (18–30/125)	10 (50–60)	300 mg q 24 h	D	200–300 mg q 24 h	100–200 mg q 24 h	100 mg q 48 h	100 mg AD	100 mg q 48 h	Dose for Cl_{CR} = UFR + 0.5 Q_D	
Phenobarbital	232.2	20–45	0.85	48–144/160	20–25	100–300 mg q 24 h	D	100–300 mg q 24 h	75–200 mg q 24 h	50–150 mg q 24 h	50–150 mg q 24 h + AD	50–150 mg q 24 h	Dose for Cl_{CR} = UFR + 0.5 Q_D	Monitor levels

*The recommended maintenance dose adjustments assume that the patient receives a standard loading dose.

†This formula is valid only for dialysate flow rates of 3 L/hr or less.

MW = molecular weight; V_d = volume of distribution; $t_{1/2}$ = half-life of drug in plasma; ESRD = end-stage renal disease; D = dose reduction method; I = interval prolongation method; HD = conventional hemodialysis; CAPD = continuous ambulatory peritoneal dialysis; CCPD = continuous cycling peritoneal dialysis; CRRT = continuous renal replacement therapies (see text); Cl_{CR} = creatinine clearance; UFR = ultrafiltration rate; Q_D = dialysate flow rate; LD = loading dose; MD = maintenance dose; ACE = angiotensin-converting enzyme; ARF = acute renal failure; CNS = central nervous system; RF = renal failure; AD = after hemodialysis; ND = no data; IP = intraperitoneal.

TABLE 156–6. Drugs That Usually Do Not Require Dosage Adjustments for Kidney Failure

Drug Class	Drug Name
Antibiotics	
Antibacterial	Azithromycin, cefoperazone, ceftriaxone, chloramphenicol, clindamycin, dicloxacillin, doxycycline, minocycline, nafcillin, rifampin
Antifungal	Griseofulvin, itraconazole, ketoconazole, miconazole
Antiparasitic	Pyrimethamine
Anticonvulsants	Carbamazepine, ethosuximide, phenytoin, valproic acid
Cardiovascular Agents	
ACE inhibitors	Fosinopril
Adrenoceptor blockers	Clonidine, doxazosin, guanabenz, prazosin, terazosin
Antiarrhythmics	Adenosine, amiodarone, lidocaine, lorcainide, moricizine, propafenone
β-Blockers	Esmolol, labetalol, metoprolol, penbutolol, pindolol, propranolol, timolol
CCBs	Amlodipine, diltiazem, felodipine, isradipine, nicardipine, nifedipine, nimodipine, nisoldipine, nitrendipine, verapamil
Glycosides	Digitoxin
Vasodilators	Diazoxide, minoxidil
CNS Agents	
Barbiturates	Hexobarbital, pentobarbital, secobarbital
Benzodiazepines	Alprazolam, clonazepam, diazepam, flurazepam, temazepam, triazolam
Miscellaneous	Chlorpromazine, haloperidol, tricyclic antidepressants

ACE = angiotensin-converting enzyme; CCBs = calcium channel blockers; CNS = central nervous system.

References

1. Hou SH, Bushinsky DA, Wish JB, et al: Hospital acquired renal insufficiency: A prospective study. Am J Med 1983; 74:243.
2. Shusterman N, Strom BL, Murray TG, et al: Risk factors and outcome of hospital-acquired acute renal failure. Am J Med 1987; 83:65.
3. Menashe PI, Ross SA, Gottlieb JE: Acquired renal insufficiency in critically ill patients. Crit Care Med 1988; 16:1106.
4. Brennan TA, Leape LL, Laird NM, et al: Incidence of adverse events and negligence in hospitalized patients. N Engl J Med 1991; 324:370.
5. Cantu TG, Ellerbeck EF, Yun SD, et al: Drug prescribing for patients with changing renal function. Am J Hosp Pharm 1992; 49:2944.
6. Kaloyanides GJ: Drug-induced acute renal failure. *In:* Acute Renal Failure in the Critically Ill. Update in Intensive Care and Emergency Medicine. Vol 20. Bellomo R, Ronco C (Eds). Berlin, Springer-Verlag, 1995; p 178.
7. Kaloyanides GJ: Renal pharmacology of aminoglycoside antibiotics. *In:* Kidney, Small Proteins, and Drugs. Contributions to Nephrology. Vol 42. Bianchi C, Bertelli A, Duarte CG (Eds). Basel, Karger, 1984; p 148.
8. Kaloyanides GJ, Bosmans J-L, De Broe ME: Antibiotic- and immunosuppression-related renal failure. *In:* Diseases of the Kidney. 6th ed. Schrier RW, Gottschalk CW (Eds). Boston, Little, Brown & Co, 1997, p 1115.
9. Gilbert DN: Once daily aminoglycoside therapy. Antimicrob Agents Chemother 1991; 35:399.
10. Blaser J, Konig C: Once daily dosing of aminoglycosides. Eur J Clin Microbiol Infect Dis 1995; 14:1029.
11. Munckhof WJ, Grayson ML, Turnidge JD: A meta-analysis of studies of the safety and efficacy of aminoglycosides given either once daily or as divided doses. J Antimicrob Chemother 1996; 37:645.
12. Barza M, Ioannidis JPA, Cappelari JC, et al: Single or multiple daily doses of aminoglycosides: A meta-analysis. BMJ 1996; 312:338.
13. Nicolau DP, Wu AHB, Finocchiaro S, et al: Once-daily aminoglycoside dosing: Impact on requests and costs for therapeutic drug monitoring. Ther Drug Monit 1996; 18:263.
14. Bailey TC, Little JR, Littenberg B, et al: A meta-analysis of extended-interval dosing versus multiple daily dosing of aminoglycosides. Clin Infect Dis 1997; 24:786.
15. Tune BM: Renal tubular transport and nephrotoxicity of beta lactam antibiotics: Structure-activity relationships. Miner Electrolyte Metab 1994; 20:221.
16. Tune BM: The nephrotoxicity of beta-lactam antibiotics. *In:* Toxicology of the Kidney. 2nd ed. Hook JB, Goldstein RS (Eds). New York, Raven Press, 1993; p 257.
17. Moellering RC, Krogstad DJ, Greenblatt DJ: Pharmacokinetics of vancomycin in normal subjects and in patients with reduced renal function. Rev Infect Dis 1981; 3(Suppl):S230.
18. Wold JS, Turnipseed SA: Toxicology of vancomycin in laboratory animals. Rev Infect Dis 1981; 3(Suppl):S224.
19. Appel GB, Given DB, Levine LR, et al: Vancomycin and the kidney. Am J Kidney Dis 1986; 8:75.
20. Rybak MJ, Albrecht LM, Burke SC, et al: Nephrotoxicity of vancomycin, alone and with an aminoglycoside. J Antimicrob Chemother 1990; 26:679.
21. Degatta MDF, Calvo MV, Hernandez JM, et al: Cost-effectiveness analysis of serum vancomycin concentration monitoring in patients with hematologic malignancies. Clin Pharmacol Ther 1996; 60:332.
22. Bolard J: How do the polyene macrolide antibiotics affect cellular membrane properties? Biochim Biophys Acta 1986; 864:257.
23. Brajtburg J, Powderly WG, Kobayashi GS, et al: Amphotericin B: Current understanding of mechanisms of action. Antimicrob Agents Chemother 1990; 34:183.
24. Atkinson AJ Jr, Bennett JE: Amphotericin B pharmacokinetics in humans. Antimicrob Agents Chemother 1978; 13:271.
25. Christiansen KJ, Bernard EM, Gold JWM: Distribution and activity of amphotericin B in humans. J Infect Dis 1985; 152:1037.
26. Branch RA: Prevention of amphotericin B–induced renal impairment: A review of the use of sodium supplementation. Arch Intern Med 1988; 148:2389.
27. Fisher MA, Talbot GH, Maislin G, et al: Risk factors for amphotericin B–associated nephrotoxicity. Am J Med 1989; 87:547.
28. Sawaya BP, Weihprecht H, Campbell WR, et al: Direct vasoconstriction as a possible cause for amphotericin B–induced nephrotoxicity in rats. J Clin Invest 1991; 87:2097.
29. Zager RA, Bredl CR, Schimpf BA: Direct amphotericin B–mediated tubular toxicity: Assessment of selected cytoprotective agents. Kidney Int 1992; 41:337.
30. Kauffman CA, Carver PL: Antifungal agents in the 1990s: Current status and future developments. Drugs 1997; 53:539.
31. Lachaal M, Venuto R: Nephrotoxicity and hyperkalemia in patients with AIDS treated with pentamidine. Am J Med 1989; 87:260.
32. O'Brien JG, Dong BJ, Coleman RL, et al: A 5-year retrospective review of adverse drug reactions and their risk factors in human immunodeficiency virus–infected patients who were receiving intravenous pentamidine therapy for *Pneumocystis carinii* pneumonia. Clin Infect Dis 1997; 24:854.
33. Berns JS, Cohen RM, Stumacher RJ, et al: Renal aspects of therapy for human immunodeficiency virus and associated opportunistic infections. J Am Soc Nephrol 1991; 1:1061.
34. Shah GM, Alvaredo P, Kirschenbaum MA: Symptomatic hypocalcemia and hypomagnesemia with renal magnesium wasting associated with pentamidine therapy in a patient with AIDS. Am J Med 1990; 89:380.
35. Gradon JD, Fricchione L, Sepkowitz D: Severe hypomagnesemia associated with pentamidine therapy. Rev Infect Dis 1991; 13:511.
36. Bennett WM, Aronoff GR, Golper TA, et al: Drug Prescribing in Renal Failure—Dosing Guidelines for Adults. 3rd ed. Philadelphia, American College of Physicians, 1993, p 33.
37. Molina J-M, Belenfant X, Doco-Lecompte T, et al: Sulfadiazine-induced crystalluria in AIDS patients with toxoplasma encephalitis. AIDS 1991; 5:587.
38. Kainer G, Rosenberg AR: Effect of co-trimoxazole on the glomerular filtration of healthy adults. Chemotherapy 1981; 27:229.

39. Buchanan N: Sulfamethoxazole, hypoalbuminemia, crystalluria and renal failure. Br Med J 1978; 21:172.
40. Deray G, Martinez K, Katlama C, et al: Foscarnet nephrotoxicity: Mechanism, incidence, and prevention. Am J Nephrol 1989; 9:316.
41. Daudon M, Estepa L, Viard JP, et al: Urinary stones in HIV-1 positive patients treated with indinavir. Lancet 1997; 349:1294.
42. Lea AP, Bryson HM: Cidofovir. Drugs 1996; 52:225.
43. Lautin EM, Freeman NJ, Schoenfeld AH, et al: Radiocontrast-associated renal dysfunction; Incidence and risk factors. AJR Am J Roentgenol 1991; 157:49.
44. Rudnick MR, Berns JS, Cohen RM, et al: Contrast media-associated nephrotoxicity. Semin Nephrol 1997; 17:15.
45. Rudnick MR, Goldfarb S, Wexler L, et al: Nephrotoxicity of ionic and nonionic contrast media in 1196 patients: A randomized trial. Kidney Int 1995; 47:254.
46. Solomon R, Werner C, Mann D, et al: Effects of saline and furosemide on acute decreases in renal function induced by radiocontrast agents. N Engl J Med 1994; 331:1416.
47. Palmer BF, Henrich WL: Nephrotoxicity of nonsteroidal anti-inflammatory agents, analgesics, and angiotensin converting enzyme inhibitors. *In:* Diseases of the Kidney. 6th ed. Schrier RW, Gottschalk CW (Eds). Boston, Little, Brown & Co, 1997, p 1167.
48. Murray MD, Brater DC: Renal toxicity of nonsteroidal anti-inflammatory drugs. Annu Rev Pharmacol Toxicol 1993; 323:435.
49. Schlondorff DD: Renal complications of nonsteroidal anti-inflammatory drugs. Kidney Int 1993; 44:463.
50. Haragsim L, Dalal R, Bagga H, et al: Ketorolac-induced acute renal failure: Report of three cases. Am J Kidney Dis 1994; 24:578.
51. Feldman HI, Kinman JL, Berlin JA, et al: Parenteral ketorolac: The risk for acute renal failure. Ann Intern Med 1997; 126:193.
52. Porile JL, Bakris GL, Garella S: Acute interstitial nephritis with glomerulopathy due to nonsteroidal anti-inflammatory agents: A review of its clinical spectrum and effects of steroid therapy. J Clin Pharmacol 1990; 30:468.
53. Textor SC: Renal failure related to angiotensin-converting enzyme inhibitors. Semin Nephrol 1997; 17:67.
54. Godin DV: Pharmacokinetics: Disposition and metabolism of drugs. *In:* Principles of Pharmacology and Clinical Application. Munson PL, Mueller RA, Bruse GA (Eds). New York, Chapman Hall, 1995, p 39.
55. Koup JR, Jusko WJ, Elwood CM, et al: Digoxin pharmacokinetics: Role of renal failure in dosage regimen design. Clin Pharmacol Ther 1975; 18:9.
56. Reidenberg MM, Drayer DE: Alteration of drug-protein binding in renal disease. Clin Pharmacokinet 1984; 9(Suppl):18.
57. Docci D, Bilancioni R, Pistocchi E, et al: Serum α_1-acid glycoprotein in chronic renal failure. Nephron 1985; 39:160.
58. Elston AC, Bayliss MK, Park GR: Effect of renal failure on drug metabolism by the liver. Br J Anaesth 1993; 71:282.
59. Park GR: Molecular mechanisms of drug metabolism in the critically ill. Br J Anaesth 1996; 77:32.
60. Odar-Cederlof I, Vessman J, Alran G: Oxazepam disposition in uremic subjects. Acta Pharmacol Toxicol 1977; 20(Suppl I):52.
61. Barendregt JN, Van Peer A, Van Der Hoeven JG, et al: Ketanserin pharmacokinetics in patients with renal failure. Br J Clin Pharmacol 1990; 29:715.
62. Hui KK, Duchin KL, Kripalani KL: Pharmacokinetics of fosinopril in patients with various degrees of renal function. Clin Pharmacol Ther 1991; 49:457.
63. Conte JE: Pharmacokinetics of cefpiramide in volunteers with normal or impaired renal function. Antimicrob Agents Chemother 1987; 31:1575.
64. Cockcroft DW, Gault MH: Prediction of creatinine clearance from serum creatinine. Nephron 1976; 15:31.
65. Maher JF: Pharmacokinetics in patients with renal failure. Clin Nephrol 1984; 21:39.
66. Bressolle F, Kinowski J-M, de la Coussaye JE, et al: Clinical pharmacokinetics during continuous hemofiltration. Clin Pharmacokinet 1994; 26:457.
67. Reetze-Bonorden P, Bohler J, Keller F: Drug dosage in patients during continuous renal replacement therapy: Pharmacokinetic and therapeutic considerations. Clin Pharmacokinet 1993; 24:362.
68. Vincent HH, Vos MC, Akcahuseyin E, et al: Drug clearance by continuous haemofiltration. Blood Purif 1993; 11:99.
69. Keller E: Pharmacokinetics during continuous renal replacement therapy. Int J Artif Organs 1996; 19:113.
70. Lasrich M, Maher JM, Hirszel P, et al: Correlation of peritoneal transport rates with molecular weight: A method for predicting clearances. J Am Soc Artif Intern Organs 1979; 2:107.
71. Seyffart G: Drug Dosages in Renal Insufficiency. Dordrecht, The Netherlands, Kluwer Academic Publishers, 1991.
72. Golper TA, Vincent HH, Gleason JR, et al: Drug removal during high-efficiency and high-flux hemodialysis. *In:* Hemodialysis: High Efficiency Treatments. Contemporary Issues in Nephrology. Vol 27. Bosch JP, Stein JH (Eds). New York, Churchill Livingstone, 1993, p 175.
73. Golper TA, Vincent HH, Kroh UF: Drug use in critically ill patients with acute renal failure. *In:* Acute Renal Failure in the Critically Ill. Update in Intensive Care and Emergency Medicine. Vol 20. Bellomo R, Ronco C (Eds). Berlin, Springer-Verlag, 1995, p 407.
74. Shuler C, Golper TA, Bennett WM: Prescribing drugs in renal disease. *In:* The Kidney. 5th ed. Brenner BM, Rector FC Jr (Eds). Philadelphia, WB Saunders, 1996, p 2653.
75. Swan S, Bennett WM: Use of drugs in patients with renal failure. *In:* Diseases of the Kidney. 6th ed. Schrier RW, Gottschalk CW (Eds). Boston, Little, Brown & Co, 1997, p 2962.
76. Paton TW, Cornish WR, Manuel MA, et al: Drug therapy in patients undergoing peritoneal dialysis. Clin Pharmacokinet 1985; 10:404.
77. Maher JF: Influence of continuous ambulatory peritoneal dialysis on elimination of drugs. Perit Dial Bull 1987; 7:159.
78. Keller E, Reetze P, Schollmeyer P: Drug therapy in patients undergoing continuous peritoneal dialysis: Clinical pharmacokinetic considerations. Clin Pharmacokinet 1990; 18:104.
79. Taylor CA, Abdelrahman E, Zimmerman SW, et al: Clinical pharmacokinetics during continuous ambulatory peritoneal dialysis. Clin Pharmacokinet 1996; 31:293.
80. Cotterill S: Antimicrobial prescribing in patients on haemofiltration. J Antimicrob Chemother 1995; 36:773.
81. Eckhardt A, Borner K, Keller F, et al: Dosage adjustment of antiinfective therapy in patients with renal impairment. Int J Clin Pharmacol Ther 1997; 35:99.
82. Vos MC, Vincent HH, Yzerman EPF, et al: Drug clearance by continuous haemodiafiltration: Results with the AN-69 capillary haemofilter and recommended dose adjustments for 7 antibiotics. Drug Invest 1994; 7:315.
83. Kihara M, Ikeda Y, Shibata K, et al: Pharmacokinetic profiles of intravenous imipenem/cilastin during slow hemodialysis in critically ill patients. Clin Nephrol 1994; 42:193.
84. Keller E, Bohler J, Bussegrawitz A, et al: Single dose kinetics of piperacillin during continuous arteriovenous hemodialysis in intensive care patients. Clin Nephrol 1995; 43(Suppl 1):S20.
85. Berl T, Wilner KD, Gardner M, et al: Pharmacokinetics of fluconazole in renal failure. J Am Soc Nephrol 1995; 6:242.
86. Boulieu R, Bastien O, Bleyzac N: Pharmacokinetics of ganciclovir in heart transplant patients undergoing continuous venovenous hemodialysis. Ther Drug Monit 1993; 15:105.
87. Burger DM, Meenhorst PL, Beijnen JH: Concise overview of the clinical pharmacokinetics of dideoxynucleoside antiviral agents. Pharm World Sci 1995; 17:25.
88. Knupp CA, Hak LJ, Coakley DF, et al: Disposition of didanosine in HIV-seropositive patients with normal renal function or chronic renal failure: Influence of hemodialysis and continuous ambulatory peritoneal dialysis. Clin Pharmacol Ther 1996; 60:535.
89. Gladziwa U, Klotz U: Pharmacokinetics and pharmacodynamics of H-2 receptor antagonists in patients with renal insufficiency. Clin Pharmacokinet 1993; 24:319.

157

Acute Renal Failure in Infants and Children

Claudio Ronco, MD • Massimo Ronconi, MD
Rinaldo Bellomo, MB BS (HONS), MD, FRACP

Acute renal failure (ARF) in infants and children may result from a variety of pathophysiologic events and is characterized by a sudden impairment of renal function with consequent decrease in urine output (<1 mL/kg/hr in the newborn) and a parallel increase in blood levels of urea nitrogen, creatinine, and other waste products.[1-3]

The main cause of ARF in infancy is renal hypoperfusion due to acute volume depletion, perinatal asphyxia, severe hypotension, and septic shock. In children, other causes become more common; they include volume depletion secondary to gastroenteritis, parenchymal renal disease, obstruction of renal outflow, and renal or systemic infection. Fluid and electrolyte imbalances are commonly present, and metabolic-acidosis is often associated with other alterations of intermediary metabolism. Another common cause of ARF in children is acute tubular necrosis (ATN) secondary to abdominal or cardiac surgery. All of these pathologic conditions are aggravated in children by the small size of the patient and the low tolerance to homeostatic imbalances. For these reasons, ARF often represents a remarkable management challenge when it occurs in children and may become even more complex to treat when it occurs in premature or term neonates.

DEFINITION

Acute renal failure is defined as an acute and transient decrease in glomerular filtration rate (GFR). Depending on the site of the primary disorder (circulation, renal parenchyma, or urinary outflow tract), the etiology of ARF can be classified as prerenal, intrinsic, or postrenal, respectively (Tables 157-1 and 157-2).

Prerenal failure, or so-called vasomotor nephropathy, accounts for more than one third of the pediatric cases of ARF.[4] Although ARF due to parenchymal disease may require dialytic treatment, and postrenal failure may require surgical removal of the obstruction, prerenal failure is usually reversible if treated early. Ideally, situations leading to prerenal failure can be anticipated and the precipitating factors corrected before the development of intense renal vasoconstriction and cell damage.

PATHOPHYSIOLOGY

Prerenal Acute Renal Failure

The kidney is normally able to withstand relatively large changes in perfusion pressure without a change in renal blood flow or GFR. This self-protecting process is known as *autoregulation*. Prerenal ARF occurs when autoregulation fails to maintain a normal GFR in response to diminished renal perfusion.[5]

Prolonged hypoperfusion leads to the development of ischemic parenchymal damage and a transition from functional to established renal failure with permanent impairment of GFR.

TABLE 157–1. Causes of Acute Renal Failure

Prerenal (Hypovolemia, Hypotension, Hypoperfusion)
- Severe dehydration or hemorrhage
- Burns, septic shock
- Pancreatitis, peritonitis, ascites
- Cardiac surgery, major trauma
- Osmotic diuresis associated with diabetes mellitus
- Respiratory distress syndrome
- Diabetes insipidus
- Hepatorenal syndrome

Renal (Intrinsic)

PRIMARY GLOMERULAR DISEASES
- Acute poststreptococcal nephritis
- Membranoproliferative glomerulonephritis
- Rapidly progressive glomerulonephritis of unknown cause

SYSTEMIC DISEASE WITH RENAL INVOLVEMENT
- Systemic lupus erythematosus, hemolytic-uremic syndrome
- Bacterial endocarditis
- Vasculitides, Henoch-Schönlein purpura

METABOLIC, DRUGS, TOXINS
- Hypersensitivity reactions
- Antibiotics (aminoglycosides, methicillin, amphotericin)
- Metal or chelating agents (lead, gold, platinum, ethylenediaminetetraacetic acid)
- Organic solvents (carbon tetrachloride, ethylene glycol, methanol, toluene)
- Oxalic acid, uric acid
- Massive hemolysis (hemoglobinuria)
- Rhabdomyolysis (myoglobinuria)
- Radiocontrast dyes
- Antihypertensive medications (captopril)

INFILTRATING DISEASES
- Tumor
- Pyelonephritis

VASCULAR
- Renal artery thrombosis or embolus
- Renal vein thrombosis

Postrenal (Either Bilateral Ureteral, or Bladder Outlet Obstruction)
- Obstruction from stones, blood clots, tumor
- Congenital obstructive uropathy

The response to decreased perfusion also involves a marked increase in the reabsorption of solutes and water throughout the nephron. Relative preservation of GFR in the presence of diminished renal blood flow results in an increased filtration fraction, defined as GFR divided by renal plasma flow.[6] The associated enhancement of the peritubular oncotic pressure results in increased proximal tubular reabsorption of sodium and fluid.[7] Renin secretion is stimulated, thereby increasing aldosterone production and ultimately increasing sodium reabsorption along the cortical and medullary collecting tubule.[8] Greater renal sympathetic nerve activity may also play a part by decreasing both renal blood flow and GFR, directly enhancing renal tubular sodium and water reabsorption and increasing renin release.[9] The release of antidiuretic hormone (ADH) in response to an ineffective circulatory volume also increases water reabsorption in the collecting tubule.[10]

The net result of the preceding responses to volume depletion is a decreased rate of urine formation (oliguria), a decreased urinary sodium concentration, and an increased urine osmolality, all of which characterize prerenal ARF. Occasionally, a patient with prerenal ARF can have normal urine flow rates and isosthenuria if the urine-concentrating ability is impaired because of decreased ADH release or decreased renal response to ADH[11, 12] (so-called polyuric ARF). For polyuric as

TABLE 157–2. Causes of Acute Renal Failure in Neonates

Prerenal—Hypovolemia or Renal Hypoperfusion

- Asphyxia
- Respiratory distress syndrome
- Dehydration
- Hemorrhage (maternal antepartum, twin-to-twin transfusion, intraventricular bleeding, hemolytic disease)
- Sepsis
- Cardiac disease (patent ductus arteriosus, aortic coarctation)
- Polycythemia (hyperviscosity)
- Administration of converting enzyme inhibitor to mother
- Indomethacin

Renal

ACUTE TUBULAR NECROSIS

- Persistent prerenal disturbances
- Nephrotoxins
  - Nephrotoxic antibiotics, e.g., aminoglycosides, contrast agents
- Myoglobinuria, hemoglobinuria, hyperuricemia

VASCULAR DISORDERS

- Renal vein thrombosis
- Renal artery thrombosis
- Aortic thrombosis
- Disseminated intravascular coagulation

CONGENITAL RENAL ANOMALY

- Dysplasia
- Hypoplasia
- Polycystic kidney
- Agenesis

Postrenal

CONGENITAL ANOMALY

- Ureteral or urethral obstruction
- Neurogenic bladder
- Megacystis-megaureter

well as oliguric ARF, rapid resolution of azotemia occurs when the underlying cause for renal hypoperfusion is corrected.

Intrinsic Renal Failure

Abrupt decreases in GFR and tubular cell dysfunction (azotemia, isosthenuria, excessive urinary sodium excretion) are the characteristic features of intrinsic renal failure. Acute renal parenchymal disorders (glomerular or renovascular disease, vasculitis, interstitial nephritis, and intrarenal crystal deposition) and renal failure resulting from ischemic or nephrotoxic insult are both part of this form of ARF. The severity of hypoxic-ischemic insult determines the spectrum of renal damage, which ranges from mild tubular dysfunction and acute tubular necrosis to renal infarction with corticomedullary necrosis.[13] Any cause of prerenal failure or obstructive renal failure, if sustained, can eventually develop into intrinsic ARF.

Malformations of the kidney or of the genitourinary tract are occasional causes of intrinsic ARF in the newborn. The lesions must either be bilateral or involve a solitary kidney to cause ARF. Renal agenesis, renal dysplasia, and polycystic kidney disease are the most common malformations. Congenital infections, including syphilis and toxoplasmosis, have been associated with renal failure. Severe acute pyelonephritis may also progress to ARF. Nosocomial infection due to *Candida* species is becoming more common in neonatal intensive care units. *Candida* pyelonephritis has been reported to cause anuria and ARF in newborns.[14]

Vascular disorders, such as aortic and renal artery thrombosis, renal venous thrombosis, and disseminated intravascular coagulation (DIC), may lead to ARF. Aortic and renal artery thrombosis, in particular, are possible complications of umbilical artery catheterization.[15, 16] Renal venous thrombosis occasionally occurs with severe prerenal failure but is most commonly seen in infants of diabetic mothers.[17] DIC or intrarenal coagulation is another important vascular cause of intrinsic ARF.[18]

Several nephrotoxins can induce ARF. Clinical studies have shown that aminoglycosides are nephrotoxic to neonates and children.[19, 20] Such nephrotoxicity was demonstrated by a delay in the postnatal fall in serum creatinine, a delay in postnatal maturation of GFR, or a decrease in creatinine clearance in aminoglycoside-treated infants. Nephrotoxicity can also occur with the administration of indomethacin, a drug used to promote the closure of a patent ductus arteriosus. The decrease in renal prostaglandin production due to indomethacin leads to decreases in renal blood flow and GRF.[21, 22] Transient oliguria or ARF can ensue.[23, 24] Decreased renal prostaglandin production also potentiates the effect of vasopressin, leading to fluid retention, oliguria, and hyponatremia.[25] Amphotericin B affects the kidneys by reducing renal blood flow and GFR. It also has a direct effect on tubular cells, leading to hypokalemia and renal tubular acidosis.[26] Radiocontrast agents have also been reported to cause renal failure in neonates and children.[27]

Renal failure in the fetus and newborn can be caused by drugs prescribed during pregnancy. An alarming number of cases of severe disturbance of fetal and neonatal renal function (oligohydramnios, pulmonary hypoplasia, long-lasting neonatal anuria) have been revealed by reviews of the use of angiotensin-converting enzyme (ACE) inhibitors for the treatment of hypertension in pregnancy.[28, 29] Maternal use of nonsteroidal anti-inflammatory drugs has been associated with fetal renal failure.[30]

Intrinsic ARF may occur through intrarenal obstruction. Uric acid nephropathy involves precipitation of uric acid or monosodium urate crystals in renal tubules.[31] Uric acid nephropathy is associated with hypoxia and perinatal asphyxia.[32] Intrarenal obstruction and ARF are also associated with severe myoglobinemia and myoglobinuria, resulting from rhabdomyolysis due to severe perinatal asphyxia[33] and to massive hemoglobinuria from severe intravascular hemolysis.[34]

Obstructive (Postrenal) Renal Failure

Although some obstructive malformations are considered to be reversible causes of renal failure, a large percentage of infants with obstructive lesions also have renal dysplasia.[35] Extrinsic compression on the urinary collecting system from a large mass, such as a sacrococcygeal teratoma or hematocolpos may cause obstructive renal failure.[36] Intrinsic obstruction within the urinary collecting system can occur with urinary calculi or fungus balls.[37, 38] Neurogenic bladder can also lead to obstructive renal failure.

CLINICAL MANIFESTATIONS AND BIOCHEMICAL ABNORMALITIES

The presenting signs and symptoms of ARF may be obscured or modified by the disease responsible for its development. Clinical findings related to renal failure include pallor (anemia), diminished urine output, edema (salt and water overload), hypertension, vomiting, and lethargy (uremic encephalopathy).

A careful history may help define the cause of ARF. Vomiting, diarrhea, and fever suggest dehydration and prerenal azotemia, but these symptoms may also precede the development of the hemolytic-uremic syndrome or renal vein thrombosis. Antecedent skin or throat infection suggests post-streptococcal glomerulonephritis. A rash may be found in systemic lupus erythematosus (SLE) or anaphylactoid purpura. A history of exposure to chemicals and medications should be sought. Flank masses suggest renal vein thrombosis, tumors, cystic disease, or obstruction.

Laboratory abnormalities include:

1. Elevated serum concentrations of blood urea nitrogen (BUN) and creatinine.
2. Anemia. With the rare exception of blood loss, the anemia is usually dilutional or hemolytic, as seen in SLE, renal vein thrombosis, and the hemolytic-uremic syndrome.
3. Leukopenia (lupus).
4. Thrombocytopenia (lupus, renal vein thrombosis, hemolytic-uremic syndrome, cardiopulmonary bypass, and DIC).
5. Hyponatremia. Hypervolemia in oliguric ARF may dilute serum sodium, hemoglobin, and protein concentrations. Conversely, diuresis during the recovery phase of oliguric renal failure may produce abnormally high serum concentrations if water losses are not adequately replaced.
6. Hyperkalemia (common in oliguric ARF and potentially severe). The adverse effects of hyperkalemia are potentiated by concomitant hyponatremia, hypocalcemia, hypomagnesemia, and digitalis use. Hyperkalemia in a patient with ARF should be monitored with serial electrocardiography: severe hyperkalemia causes peaking of the T waves, with shortening of the QT interval, followed by prolongation of the QRS complex, atrioventricular block, flattening and then disappearance of the P wave, the appearance of a sine wave, and finally, ventricular fibrillation or asystole. Spurious hyperkalemia corresponds to a serum potassium value that is more than 0.5 mEq/L or greater than the plasma value, and may occur in patients with thrombocytosis. Hyperkalemia is uncommon in nonoliguric ARF.
7. Metabolic acidosis. This finding may appear early in ARF and can be particularly intractable in children with reduced perfusion or with a hypermetabolic state. In the critically ill child, such acidosis may be complicated by respiratory acidosis due to concomitant pulmonary injury, infection, or edema.
8. Hypocalcemia: Although hypocalcemia may develop early after the onset of ARF, tetany is uncommon.
9. Hyperphosphatemia: This finding is common, but phosphate levels rarely exceed 2 mmol/L.
10. Hypermagnesemia: Also common in ARF, but it is usually moderate and asymptomatic.
11. Depressed serum protein C *level*: This finding is seen in post-streptococcal glomerulonephritis, lupus, and membranoproliferative glomerulonephritis.
12. Antibodies: Antibodies may be detected in the serum to streptococcal (poststreptococcal glomerulonephritis), nuclear (lupus), or basement membrane (Goodpasture's disease) antigens.

DIAGNOSIS

The diagnosis of ARF is based on the presence of azotemia. The nitrogenous compounds most commonly measured in clinical practice are BUN and serum creatinine. However, because the BUN is affected by factors other than nitrogen excretion by the kidney, it is an unreliable single indicator of renal function. Serum creatinine is relatively unaffected by extrarenal factors and therefore is a better indicator of glomerular function. Extrarenal factors that affect blood urea nitrogen and creatinine concentrations are shown in Table 157-3.

Analysis of urine composition can be used to assess renal tubule cell function and distinguish prerenal from intrinsic renal failure. Radiologic tests are used to detect urinary tract obstruction and renovascular occlusion.

Plasma Creatinine

Normal values for plasma creatinine vary with age and gender, reflecting dependence on muscle mass and maturation of renal function.[39, 40] Unfortunately, a variety of noncreatinine chromogens (ketones, cephalosporins) can artificially elevate plasma creatinine values by interfering with standard photometric assays.[41, 42] Plasma creatinine concentrations vary inversely with GFR, because creatinine excretion by glomerular filtration typically equals creatinine production by skeletal muscle. Children with chronic malnutrition or muscle wasting may have a lower plasma creatinine value than predicted for height or age as a result of reduced muscle mass. An isolated plasma creatinine value reflects GFR only during steady-state conditions and cannot be used to quantify abrupt changes in glomerular filtration. In general, a progressive rise in plasma creatinine of at least 0.5 mg/dL/day indicates an acute reduction of GFR.

Blood Urea Nitrogen

Urea and BUN are two other plasma solutes that can be used to estimate glomerular filtration. Plasma concentrations of urea tend to vary inversely with GFR, because urea is excreted primarily via glomerular filtration. Changes in urea production or excretion, however, can alter BUN levels in the absence of any change in glomerular filtration, making it unreliable, under many circumstances, for estimation of GFR. High protein intake, gastrointestinal tract bleeding, and hypercatabolic states are common conditions in which the BUN level is elevated out of proportion to any change in GFR (see Table 157-3).

Urea excretion is governed by both glomerular filtration and tubular reabsorption. Normally, approximately 40% of

TABLE 157–3. Extrarenal Factors Affecting Blood Urea Nitrogen and Creatinine Concentrations

	Increased By	Decreased By
Blood urea nitrogen	High-protein diet Starvation Gastrointestinal hemorrhage Dehydration Corticosteroid administration Hypercatabolic states (fever, sepsis)	Low-protein diet High-calorie diet Liver disease Hypometabolism Hyperlipidemia
Creatinine	Rhabdomyolysis Dehydration	Loss of muscle mass (amputations, dystrophy, atrophy) Burns Hyperlipemia, hyperbilirubinemia

TABLE 157–4. Urinary Indices Suggestive of Prerenal or Intrinsic Renal Failure

	Child		Neonate	
Index	***Prerenal***	***Intrinsic***	***Prerenal***	***Intrinsic***
Urine flow rate	Variable	Variable	Variable	Variable
Urine osmolality (mOsm/kg H_2O)	>500	<350	>400	<400
Urine/plasma osmolar ratio	>1.3	<1.1	>1.3	≤1.0
Urine/plasma creatinine ratio	>40	<20	>30	<10
Fractional excretion of sodium (%)	<1	>2	<2.5	>2.5

filtered urea is reclaimed by passive diffusion. Conditions resulting in decreased intravascular volume or renal hypoperfusion increase tubular water reabsorption and lead to urea retention in the absence of a significant alteration in glomerular filtration (prerenal azotemia). When the BUN:creatinine ratio exceeds 20, an increase in either production or tubular reabsorption of urea should be suspected.

Urine Volume

Although oliguria has been traditionally considered a major sign of ARF, it is now clear that urine flow rate is not a reliable reflection of renal function. Up to 80% of adults and 50% of infants with ARF do not have oliguria, and any of the three major types of renal failure (prerenal, intrinsic, postrenal) can occur in an oliguric or nonoliguric form.[43–45] Although urine volume has limited diagnostic value in acute azotemia, it is an important prognostic factor. The severity and duration of ARF as well as morbidity and mortality are usually diminished in nonoliguric renal failure.[43, 44]

Urine Composition

Urine composition is a valuable diagnostic tool (Table 157–4). It is essential to obtain a urine sample as soon as renal disease is suspected, prior to diagnostic or therapeutic maneuvers. Routine dipstick evaluation and microscopic urinalysis are mandatory. Decreased concentrating ability is probably the most consistent defect in intrinsic ARF and provides an early sign of impending acute renal insufficiency.[46]

Most children with intrinsic ARF have isosthenuria, reflecting inability to either concentrate or dilute urine because of tubular cell damage. Urine osmolality is a more reliable measure of concentrating ability than specific gravity, because the former is unaffected by extraneous solutes. The use of urine-plasma osmolar ratios excludes the possibility that changes in plasma osmolality are responsible for altering urine osmolality without reflecting the true tubular concentrating ability. Because of the effect of low protein intake and urea excretion on urine osmolality, such evaluations are of questionable value in newborn infants and malnourished children.[47] In these situations, other measures of renal tubule reabsorptive capacity, such as urine-plasma creatinine ratios, can be used.

Fluid Challenge

The administration of a fluid challenge is probably one of the most practical and useful diagnostic tests for differentiating prerenal from intrinsic renal failure.[48, 49] The fluid challenge should employ enough isotonic (preferably also iso-oncotic) solution to expand intravascular volume or return it to normal status. In certain critically ill children, invasive monitoring may be necessary to assess the adequacy of such a fluid challenge. In addition, a colloid solution is more likely to lead to a rapid return of the intravascular volume to the desired levels.

The initial amount of fluid may consist of 15 to 20 mL/kg of isotonic solution or approximately 5 to 7 mL/kg of colloid solution. If oliguria continues, intravenous furosemide, 2 to 3 mg per kg, should be given, usually over 1 hour, to be followed by an infusion of 0.1 to 0.3 mg/kg/hr for 3 to 4 hours.

If there is no diuresis or urine output is low (<1 mL/kg/hr in the newborn) within 4 to 6 hours and the patient is clinically euvolemic, intrinsic renal failure should be suspected. If fluid challenge and furosemide are unsuccessful in reversing oliguric renal failure or if there is nonoliguric renal failure, a blood specimen should be obtained so that the following laboratory tests can be performed: BUN, creatinine (Cr), uric acid, serum sodium (Na), potassium, chloride, bicarbonate, glucose, calcium, phosphorus, and platelet count. If urine can be obtained, a urinalysis, urine culture, and spot urine sample for measurements of sodium, creatinine, and osmolarity should be performed. Once the results are available, a clearer diagnostic picture can be obtained.

Urinary Indices

A variety of urinary indices are available to help differentiate prerenal from intrinsic renal failure (Table 157–5), but none has the therapeutic advantage or practical diagnostic reliability of the fluid and diuretic challenge. The most useful urinary indices are the fractional excretion of filtered sodium (Fe_{NA}) and the renal failure index (RFI). Each is calculated from a spot urine and serum specimen as follows:

$$Fe_{NA} = \frac{\text{urine Na/serum Na}}{\text{urine Cr/serum Cr}} \times 100$$

$$RFI = \frac{\text{urine Na}}{\text{urine Cr/serum Cr}}$$

Fe_{NA} describes two functions of intact renal tubules: reabsorption of water and sodium from glomerular filtrate.[50, 51] The major value of this measurement lies in its ability to accurately distinguish rapidly reversible azotemia caused by renal hypoperfusion (prerenal ARF) from intrinsic renal failure.

The interpretation of Fe_{NA} in neonatal renal failure is complicated by maturational changes in renal sodium handling. Although urinary indices are highly sensitive for intrinsic renal

TABLE 157–5. Urinary Indices of Acute Renal Failure in the Term Infant

	Prerenal	**Intrinsic**
Urine osmolality (U_{osm}) (mOsm/L)	>400	<400
Fractional excretion of sodium (Fe_{NA}) (%)	<3	>3
Renal failure index (RFI)	<3	>3
Response to fluid challenge and furosemide	Increased urine output	No effect

failure, they may have poor specificity because some neonates, especially very-low-birth-weight infants with prerenal failure may have values overlapping those attributed to intrinsic renal failure.[52] There are other problems with urinary indices in the newborn. Premature infants of less than 32 weeks' gestation may normally have Fe_{NA} values greater than 5%,[53] and there are no definite values for Fe_{NA} in premature infants with intrinsic renal failure.[54]

Renal Imaging

Occasionally, radiodiagnostic studies are needed to clarify the cause of acute azotemia. These procedures are most helpful if either urinary tract obstruction or occlusion of major renal blood vessels is suspected.

The widespread availability of ultrasonography and radionuclide scanning has eliminated the need to use intravenous pyelography in ARF, thus avoiding the risks of radiation exposure, radiocontrast-induced anaphylaxis, and nephrotoxicity. Ultrasonography should be the initial imaging procedure in infants when either intrinsic or obstructive ARF is suspected.[55] Ultrasonography can accurately describe the presence or absence of kidneys as well as their size and shape, hydronephrosis, renal calculi, and bladder distention and thickness. When renal failure due to urinary outlet obstruction is likely, voiding cystourethrography is recommended to detect posterior urethral valves and other causes of lower urinary tract obstruction and vesicoureteral reflux.

Radionuclide Scanning

Radionuclide renal scans are an excellent means of assessing renal perfusion and function and thus complement the anatomic information obtained from ultrasonography.[56, 57] Advantages of radionuclide scanning include the absence of known systemic effects, a relatively low radiation dose, and the ability to visualize the kidneys despite low GFR.

Technetium 99m diethylenetriaminepentaacetic acid (^{99m}Tc-DTPA) can provide most of the information required for pediatric renal studies. Initial transit of the radionuclide through the kidneys reflects renal perfusion, whereas activity between 1 and 3 minutes after injection is a measure of functioning renal mass. Clearance of ^{99m}Tc-DTPA is by glomerular filtration, with no significant tubular excretion or renal parenchymal retention. Thus, its rate of clearance provides an accurate measure of GFR. Its high concentration in the urine allows excellent visualization of the urinary collecting system. Because of its low retention in the renal cortex, this agent may fail to delineate small cortical lesions.

Technetium 99m glucoheptonate may be used when better visualization of the renal cortex is desired. Because approximately 10% of the injected dose is retained in renal tubule cells, delayed imaging provides excellent visualization of renal cortex anatomy.

Similarly, technetium 99m dimercaptosuccinic acid (^{99m}Tc-DMSA) may be used to delineate renal structure because 60% to 70% of this agent remains within the renal cortex.

Ultrasonography

Improvements in ultrasound technology have introduced a new technique to study renal blood flow without the invasiveness and exposure to radioisotopes required for radionuclide scans. Duplex ultrasonography combines B-mode ultrasound imaging with pulsed Doppler ultrasound. Such technology has been used to assess renal blood flow velocity patterns at the bedside for the critically ill patient.[58] The absence of diastolic flow may have prognostic significance. In one study of older infants and children with ARF due to hemolytic-uremic syndrome, diuresis was reported to have occurred within 24 to 48 hours after diastolic Doppler ultrasound shifts returned to normal.[59] Further clinical investigation is needed to determine the place of renal duplex Doppler ultrasound in the evaluation of the infant with ARF.

PREVENTION AND CONSERVATIVE MANAGEMENT

Correct diagnosis and the identification and early removal of the causes responsible for ARF are the first steps in the prevention or, at least, reduction of the renal tissue damage. Prompt restoration of circulating plasma volume is most important in preventing the evolution of prerenal azotemia into a frank acute tubular necrosis. It is also important to avoid or remove possible nephrotoxins. At the same time, the correct and early diagnosis of any underlying renal disease may further help trigger the necessary therapeutic interventions.

Once ARF has become established, maintenance of homeostasis is a vital therapeutic goal. Homeostasis is achieved by preventing or correcting all biochemical, metabolic, and clinical abnormalities associated with ARF. Fluid and electrolyte balance should be achieved by appropriate intravenous fluid replacement and accurate control of the fluid losses; calcium, phosphate, and acid-base derangements must be promptly corrected, as should anemia, hypotension, and severe catabolism.

Fluid and Electrolyte Balance

The maintenance of fluid and electrolyte balance must be individualized. Body weight should be checked carefully, and accurate charting of fluid intake and output should be performed. Fluid and electrolyte losses may come from urine output, gastrointestinal losses, cavity drainage, or insensible losses. In patients receiving mechanical ventilation, fluid management may need to be altered.

Considerable controversy exists regarding the use of so-called nephroprotective medications in patients with prerenal ARF.[60, 61] Intravenous mannitol has been suggested to reduce the incidence of ARF in patients with impending oliguria. The suggested benefits are based on the action of mannitol as a pharmacologically inert osmotic agent to maintain a high urine flow together with reduced endothelial cell swelling and renin secretion. Unfortunately, there are no controlled animal or human studies to support the use of mannitol in this setting. Improved urine flow can be achieved with the use of high doses of intravenous furosemide. Possible ototoxicity and combined toxicity with other agents must, however, be taken into account. Dopamine, at doses of 2 to 3 µg/kg/min (so-called low-dose dopamine) may be infused alone or in combination with furosemide to increase urine flow and possibly to improve renal blood flow. Such treatment is not, however, supported by controlled studies.

Hyperkalemia

Cell damage may lead to significant increases of extracellular potassium levels. Hyperkalemia, however, may also occur because of oliguria, catabolism, and fever or because of functional alterations in potassium intracellular-extracellular concentration induced by acidosis.

Hyperkalemia is a potentially fatal complication of ARF, and patients should be closely monitored when the serum potassium exceeds 5 mEq/L. Hyperkalemia may be treated (1) by reducing potassium intake, (2) by shifting the ion into the intracellular compartment, or (3) by removing potassium from the body via natural or artificial pathways. Intravenous 2.5% calcium gluconate (2 mL/kg) reduces membrane excitability and the dangerous effects of hyperkalemia on cardiac rhythm. This intervention does not reduce the potassium concentration and must therefore be followed by other measures intended to decrease serum potassium levels, such as the administration of dextrose with insulin, inhaled salbutamol, a combination of salbutamol and insulin with dextrose, sodium bicarbonate infusion in the presence of acidosis, or cation exchange resin administration (1 g/kg). For the last measure, sorbitol can be given as a cathartic agent to prevent constipation or retention of resin. Resins exchange sodium for potassium, and they may produce significant sodium and water retention. This complication must be watched for in the case of repeated administrations.

When hyperkalemia becomes intractable and potentially life-threatening (serum potassium > 6.5 to 7 mmol/L), hemodialysis or peritoneal dialysis becomes necessary. Continuous renal replacement therapies are also indicated because they provide correction of acidosis and at the same time tend to normalize the intracellular-extracellular concentration gradients for potassium.

Hyperphosphatemia

Phosphate binders are often administered orally to control hyperphosphatemia. Calcium carbonate in powder can also be used as a chelating agent. During all of these interventions, continuous monitoring of the calcium × phosphate product must be carried out to avoid soft-tissue calcifications.

Acidosis

Intravenous sodium bicarbonate or the use of other buffers is helpful in the treatment of moderate to severe acidotic states. The neonate may be unable to adequately metabolize lactate or other buffers; therefore, lactate levels should be monitored when lactate solutions are used as buffers for peritoneal dialysis.

Anemia

When severe anemia is present, blood transfusion may be required. It should be performed with great care in order to avoid hypertension or pulmonary congestion.

Hypertension

Hypertension may occur during ARF and should be promptly treated with appropriate antihypertensive drugs or by reducing volume overload through induced diuresis or extracorporeal fluid and sodium removal.

Nutrition

Any conservative therapy is not complete if adequate nutritional support is not provided. Enteral or parenteral nutrition should include sufficient caloric intake and administration of protein with high biologic value. This practice not only reduces catabolism but also decreases the level of immunosuppression and anergy. To maintain a zero or positive nitrogen balance, 1.5 to 2 g of protein per kg of body weight should be administered daily. In case of enteral nutrition, osmotic diarrhea must be avoided. If parenteral nutrition is provided, remarkable plasma osmotic changes may occur; they should be prevented by careful monitoring of electrolyte concentrations. Concentrated solutions should be administered only via a central venous catheter. For a patient receiving peritoneal dialysis, the caloric intake provided by glucose reabsorption via the peritoneal route should be taken into account.

SUBSTITUTIVE THERAPY

When conservative measures are insufficient to maintain a child or infant in an acceptable condition of homeostasis, the substitution of renal function by dialytic techniques becomes mandatory. Unique problems may arise owing to the small size of the patient.

Although pediatric hemodialysis is generally performed in only a few specialized pediatric centers, peritoneal dialysis and continuous renal replacement therapies are more widely used with success. For this reason, more detailed descriptions of these two latter techniques are presented in this chapter.

Peritoneal Dialysis

Peritoneal dialysis has represented the treatment of choice for pediatric ARF for many years. It is relatively safe and easy to perform, and it yields acceptable clinical results. Peritoneal dialysis overcomes the typical problems related to extracorporeal hemodialysis, such as the need for a specialized center and staff, the need for a vascular access, and the possible complications of hemodialysis (e.g., dialysis dysequilibrium syndrome).

Kinetics of Peritoneal Transport

The overall peritoneal surface area in the child or infant is almost two times that in the adult (383 cm^2/kg in the neonate versus 177 cm^2/kg in the adult). For this reason, peritoneal transport has been suggested to be more efficient in children than in adults. However, very few studies have been performed to analyze in detail the characteristics of solute and water transport across the peritoneal membrane in children and neonates. Popovich and colleagues have compared the peritoneal transport characteristics in children and adults, reaching some interesting conclusions. The use of hypertonic peritoneal dialysis solutions generates different amounts of ultrafiltration but does not increase solute transport. Furthermore, although different amounts of ultrafiltration can be obtained using 1.5% or 4.25% glucose solutions, the average response to hypertonic peritoneal dialysis is lower in children than in adults.

The explanation for the preceding phenomena may be (1) the lower effective surface area available for peritoneal exchange in children, in whom the bladder occupies a greater space in the abdominal cavity; (2) the lower effective capillary blood flow per unit of surface area; and (3) the higher permeability of the membrane with a consequent rapid dissipation of the osmotic gradient secondary to a fast glucose reabsorption. The last hypothesis is supported by the frequent observation of hyperglycemia in patients undergoing peritoneal dialysis.

The mass transfer area coefficients for urea and creatinine in the child are similar to or even greater than those observed in the adult, leading to a remarkable efficiency of small solutes clearance during peritoneal dialysis in the child. In the case of marked hyperpermeability of the peritoneal membrane, rapid exchanges instead of long dwell times should be performed to reduce glucose and fluid reabsorption.

The tension of the abdominal wall and intraperitoneal pressure should be monitored in some cases to avoid interferences with the processes of ultrafiltration and of lymphatic reabsorption, the latter representing an important route of fluid reabsorption from the peritoneal cavity.

Practical Aspects

To perform peritoneal dialysis in children with ARF, the institution of an intraperitoneal access is necessary. It can be achieved by percutaneous puncture or by surgical insertion of a peritoneal catheter. In both cases, flexible polytetrafluoroethylene (Teflon) cannulas are used to permit instillation of the peritoneal dialysis solution into the abdominal cavity and its subsequent drainage. Infusion and drainage peritoneal fluid can be performed manually with volumetric or gravimetric control systems or can be performed with the help of cyclers or special automated peritoneal dialysis machines.

In all cases, flows and dwell times should be chosen after a peritoneal equilibration test is performed. The solution must be warmed to avoid thermal hypothermia. In the case of average permeability, both long dwell time and rapid exchanges can be adequate. In the case of a hyperpermeable peritoneal membrane, short rapid exchanges should be performed. For the peritoneal membrane with low permeability, volume dwell times can be slightly increased. The infusion volumes may vary from 20 to 50 mL/kg per exchange, on the basis of the compliance of the peritoneal cavity and the rate of ultrafiltration.

Several measures aimed at maintaining homeostasis are often necessary. They include frequent monitoring of blood pressure and central venous pressure to adjust the infusion of fluids and to choose the most appropriate solution for the dialytic exchanges.

Clinical Aspects and Indications

Peritoneal dialysis can be effectively used to achieve blood purification in anuric patients. Urea and creatinine are efficiently removed together with larger molecules, such as phosphates and drugs. Under normal conditions, 1 to 2 L of solution per day represents an adequate amount to achieve efficient blood purification in the neonate. If the child is larger or older, or if rapid exchanges are performed, 3 to 6 L/day should be employed.

Peritoneal dialysis can remove significant amounts of potassium if potassium-free solutions are used. Severe hypernatremia may occur from excessive dehydration induced by hypertonic glucose; the patient should be monitored for this complication so as to prevent it.

Metabolic acidosis can be corrected by the infusion of sodium bicarbonate (1 to 2 mEq/kg) or by the use of peritoneal dialysis with lactate-containing solutions. Bicarbonate-based solutions have become commercially available and may be used in patients with lactate intolerance.

During peritoneal dialysis, an overall intake of at least 100 to 150 cal/kg/day is advisable to reduce catabolism; 1 to 2 g/kg/day of proteins with high biologic value should be provided.

Complications

The complications of peritoneal dialysis can be technical or clinical. Technical complications can be related to peritoneal access function, fluid balance errors, reduction of treatment efficiency, clogging of the catheter, and one-way obstruction of the catheter.

Clinical complications are related to possible bowel perforation, fluid balance errors, lactate intolerance, respiratory problems related to abdominal distention, protein losses, hyperglycemic and hyperosmolar syndromes, and, above all, peritonitis.

All of these complications can usually be prevented or successfully managed and do not represent absolute contraindications to the continuation of peritoneal dialysis treatment.

Hemodialysis

As previously noted, hemodialysis, hemofiltration, and hemodiafiltration should be available in specialized pediatric centers. These techniques require the presence of a dialysis nurse, specialized medical staff, and appropriate equipment. Once these requirements are met, the hemodialysis treatment in the child is not significantly different from that in the adult, especially if the child is older than 3 years of age. For younger children, most centers have today moved to the use of continuous renal replacement therapies because of their higher level of safety, easy institution, and simple monitoring requirements.

Continuous Renal Replacement Therapies

Advances in technology have made intermittent hemodialysis possible even in small patients. This technique, however, is difficult and is not routinely applied.[62] Peritoneal dialysis has been used for blood purification in infants and has produced satisfactory clinical results.[63] Neonatal ARF, however, is commonly associated with severe cardiovascular instability, respiratory problems, and other medical complications that preclude hemodialysis because of the induction of severe hemodynamic instability.[64] Equally, peritoneal dialysis may become technically impossible or undesirable in patients with recent abdominal surgery or skin infection. Moreover, severe fluid overload cannot always be effectively treated by peritoneal dialysis because of the low ultrafiltration efficiency seen with this therapy.[65] In all of these conditions, an alternative treatment is needed.

Continuous arteriovenous hemofiltration (CAVH) is a simple method of blood purification and body fluid control that was originally described by Kramer and associates[66] in 1977. In this technique, a small hemofilter is connected to an artery and a vein, and the simple arteriovenous hydrostatic gradient generated by the heart moves the blood through the circuit, producing slow continuous ultrafiltration. Blood purification is achieved mainly by convection. Replacement of ultrafiltrate by substitution solutions contributes to lower solute levels in the blood. No pumps are used in the classic method, and the system operates with low blood flows and low transmembrane pressures.[67-72] CAVH has been widely used in adults as an alternative treatment for critically ill patients.[73-75]

Simplicity, rapid application, and good clinical tolerance are the main advantages of the technique. CAVH is also a reliable treatment for infants and children.[76-78] In these smaller patients, the technique has special advantages in terms of the low priming volume of the extracorporeal circuit, low rate of heparinization,[79] low blood flow, and slow continuous removal of isotonic fluid. The use of CAVH in adults has been almost abandoned in favor of continuous venovenous hemofiltration (CVVH). Although CVVH is a more efficient technique, the use of a blood pump and the more complex layout of the extracorporeal circuit make CVVH somewhat less suitable for infants and neonates. Thus, according to many experts, either CAVH or continuous arteriovenous hemodiafiltration (CAVHDF), if countercurrent dialysate delivery is used to increase solute clearance, is still the treatment of choice.

Vascular Access

Vascular access in CAVH is the source of blood for the extracorporeal circuit and generates the hydrostatic gradient that moves the blood through the filter.[80]

Shortness and large diameter of the cannulas are critical for achieving a good blood flow while avoiding unnecessary pressure loss. Flexibility without reduction of the inner lumen of the cannula and good clinical tolerance are other important features of an ideal vascular access.

Umbilical vessels can be used in the neonate with appropriate catheters. This type of access cannot be used for a long time, however, and cannot be used at all in patients older

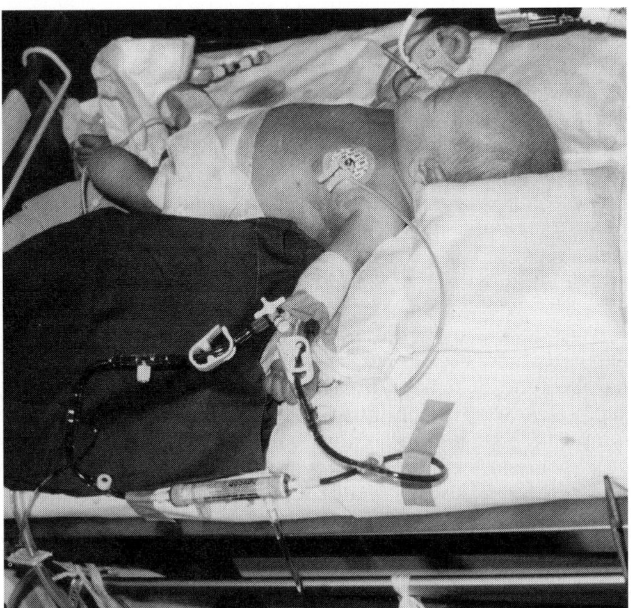

Figure 157–1. Typical example of extracorporeal circuit for continuous arteriovenous hemofiltration. Resistance of the circuit is reduced by short blood lines in order to avoid unnecessary pressure loss and blood flow reduction.

than 4 to 5 days.[81, 82] Brachial or femoral artery cannulation may be used (Fig. 157–1). Surgical isolation of the artery is preferred in order to avoid hematomas or hemorrhagic complications. Generally, 18-gauge to 20-gauge, flexible Teflon cannulas 20 to 25 mm long are employed. The cannulas should be fixed to the skin to avoid accidental disconnection or unwanted folding with reduction of blood flow. In larger children, percutaneous cannulation of the brachial or femoral artery can be performed with the standard Seldinger technique.

In the newborn, the mean arterial pressure (usually ranging from 35 to 50 mm Hg) generally yields a blood flow of 15 to 50 mL/min during CAVH.[83]

Cannulation of the brachial or femoral artery in infants may lead to distal hypoperfusion or even occlusion of the vessels. Although long-term complications are seldom observed, acute occlusion may on occasion lead to proximal propagation of clot and severe limb ischemia. For this reason, limb perfusion must be rigorously monitored.

The jugular or subclavian vein is the most common route for venous return. Standard connections for fluid infusion (e.g., those for parenteral nutrition and central venous pressure measurement), however, are extremely thin and too long for CAVH. Short lines with large inner diameters (18-gauge) are useful to reduce resistance.[80–83]

In some cases, two veins, or a double-lumen catheter, can be used with a blood pump to perform venovenous hemofiltration. This approach reduces the risk of arterial bleeding and may guarantee a stable blood flow rate with a constant performance of the treatment. In this case, however, the priming volume of the extracorporeal circuit is larger, and it is advisable to start the procedure with a prefilled circuit containing anticoagulated blood.

Extracorporeal Circuit

Standard pediatric hemodialysis lines (inner diameter, 0.3 cm) can be modified in order to obtain arterial and venous lines for CAVH. However, commercially available blood tubings have been especially created for CAVH in infants. The arterial line should be as short as possible to avoid unnecessary pressure drops along the length of the circuit. Because CAVH operates at low pressures, a loss of 5 to 10 mm Hg may seriously affect ultrafiltration rate and, consequently, treatment efficiency. For the same reason, a hemofilter with very low end-to-end pressure drop is required and short connections with adequate diameter should be employed between the venous line and the jugular cannula. The arterial line should have one port for continuous heparin infusion and another port for arterial blood sampling. The sampling port can also be used for pressure measurements or for the use of the filter in a predilutional mode.[83–87]

The venous line must have a port for the infusion of replacement solutions and a port for venous blood sampling, which can also be used for pressure measurements. At the inlet and outlet of the circuit, wide-bore three-way taps should be placed in order to exclude the patient's circulation during rinsing of the filter with heparinized saline solution. Folding of the arterial and venous lines should be carefully avoided during treatment.[88, 89]

When a blood pump is used in CVVH, two veins are cannulated and a constant blood flow is provided by the pump. At blood flows between 20 and 80 mL/min, pressure-sensitive blood modules are strongly recommended to avoid any damage to the vessels. A blood module specifically designed for CVVH in neonates has been made available (HP150, Medica-Medolla, Mo., Italy).[90] Even though specifically designed blood pumps are now appearing on the market, the technique of CVVH in very small babies is still cumbersome and should be undertaken only by skilled personnel and trained teams.

ARF is observed in approximately 10% to 20% of neonates treated with extracorporeal membrane oxygenation (ECMO) or extracorporeal carbon dioxide (CO_2) removal ($ECCO_2R$). A hemofilter can be incorporated into these circuits, thus permitting adequate fluid balance during treatment.[91] The hemofilter can also be used as a hemoconcentration device after open heart surgery.

Filters

The availability of adequate filters is the key point in performing CAVH in infants. New, commercially available filters (minifilters) are designed to operate with minimal end-to-end pressure drop during CAVH in infants. Their low resistance is their main feature, since high flows are obtained even at very low perfusion pressures. The blood path appears adequate to operate in conditions of arteriovenous driven circulation. In such conditions, ultrafiltration ranges between 0.5 and 2 mL/min. The minifilters may in fact reach ultrafiltration rates between 0.5 and 1.5 mL/min for transmembrane pressure (TMP) values between 20 and 70 mm Hg and a blood flow of 20 mL/min with a plateau value at 2.0 to 2.5 mL/min. At similar pressures, the minifilters display ultrafiltration rates significantly higher (3 to 4 mL/min) when the blood flow exceeds 50 mL/min.

In such filters, filtration pressure equilibrium (hydrostatic = oncotic) does not occur and low filtration fractions are obtained. This permits an extended filter life span and lower heparin requirement compared with those observed in hemofilters for adults.[92, 93]

The new minifilters have two ports in the ultrafiltrate compartment, permiting the use of a countercurrent flow of dialysate. In this case, the treatment is called CAVHDF, because both diffusive and convective transports are present. In this treatment, dialysate flows of up to 10 mL/min can be usefully employed.[94, 95] These new minifilters are now manufactured by Minntech Corporation in the United States. Other hemofilters for children have also been developed (Gambro FH22, Gambro, Sweden; Hospal, Lyon, France), widening the choice available to the physician.[96]

Solute Removal and Membrane Characteristics

Asymmetric synthetic polysulfone, polyamide, or AN 69S membranes are commonly employed in CAVH-CVVH filters. The process of convective transport is quite similar to the physiologic function of the human glomeruli. In CAVH, this property results in an ultrafiltrate with the same characteristics as plasma water.[97, 98]

In our experience with CAVH, no reduction in membrane permeability has been noted after as much as 86 hours of treatment.[21] Periodic lavages of the filter with small quantities of heparinized saline may help prevent the negative effect of protein "concentration polarization."[80, 82, 83, 93]

CAVH and CVVH take their maximum advantage from convective removal of solutes, that is, from high filtration rates and high sieving coefficients. When dialysis fluid is circulated in the filters (CAVHDF or CVVHDF), a mixed diffusive-convective transport takes place, with a consequent enhancement of small solute clearance.[95-97]

Because a remarkable amount of thermal energy can be lost through the hemofilter, it is advisable to warm the dialysis solution when a countercurrent configuration is chosen. In CAVHDF, in fact, the hemofilter acts as a heat exchanger, and hypothermia may represent a possible complication.

Anticoagulation in CAVH

Preparation of the filter for CAVH treatment is extremely important to its function and duration during therapy.[79] The filter and circuit should be rinsed with 1000 mL of heparinized saline solution (5000 IU of heparin/L). During the washing procedure, the venous line and the ultrafiltration line should be clamped periodically in order to remove all air bubbles from the system.

Because the population treated with CAVH is often at risk of bleeding, the main goal of anticoagulation is to achieve an adequate local effect without any systemic consequence. Whole-blood activated clotting time and partial thromboplastin time must be carefully monitored.[79, 81, 83] If the pretreatment coagulation value is within normal limits, a bolus of heparin (100 IU per kg of body weight) can be administered. The neonate usually metabolizes heparin rapidly, and coagulation parameters return to normal after less than 1 hour. This practice, therefore, ensures a maximal anticoagulant effect during the first minutes of contact between blood and membrane, a feature that may be critical for subsequent filter function. A continuous heparin infusion of 5 to 10 IU per kg of body weight per hour is then generally adequate to maintain effective extracorporeal anticoagulation with minimal systemic effects.[81] This amount must be adjusted case by case, however, because the rate of heparin metabolism may vary significantly in the newborn. At infusion rates between 5 and 8 IU/per kg of body weight per hour maximal anticoagulation is achieved in the filter with minimal effects in the systemic circulation. This anticoagulation level achieves good filter life.

Periodic flushing of the circuit with saline helps to assess the condition of the filter and to ensure the complete absence of clots. To avoid acute fluid overload during this procedure, the patient circulation must be excluded from the circuit using the three-way taps.

Substitution Fluids

The removal of large amounts of ultrafiltrate from the patient (1 to 2 L/day) requires the administration of substitution fluids. Depending on the patient's requirements, ultrafiltrate can be replaced in part, in whole, or even in excess. The replacement solution can be administered by manual, semiautomatic, or completely automatic systems, with the rate of replacement regulated on the basis of the ultrafiltration rate during the antecedent 15-minute period. Particular care has to be placed in obtaining the scheduled fluid balance because of the high sensitivity of the neonate to even small variations in body fluid balance and composition. In our experience, a simple gravimetric control system (EQUALINE, Medica–Medolla, Mo., Italy) is safe and reliable for precise fluid balance during CAVH over a prolonged period.[98]

The composition of the replacement fluid must be adapted to the metabolic requirements of and the electrolyte imbalances recorded for the patient. In our experience, lactate-containing replacement solutions used for chronic hemofiltration are adequate in the majority of patients. Because of enzyme deficiency and consequent lactate intolerance in immature babies, bicarbonate-containing replacement solutions may become necessary. If bicarbonate solutions are needed, calcium and magnesium must be administered separately. The composition of these solutions can be manually modified as far as potassium content is concerned. Finally, such fluids can be safely used also as dialysate for hemodiafiltration treatments.

Indications for and Clinical Management of CAVH

CAVH is not a substitute for any of the dialytic therapies already in use, but it complements them as a further modality of renal replacement therapy. The simplicity of the technique allows rapid application and easy monitoring, even when hemodialysis or peritoneal dialysis cannot be used because of technical or logistic problems.

The clinical tolerance to and the peculiar operational characteristics of CAVH, however, permit its use when other types of treatment might be dangerous or contraindicated (severe cardiovascular instability, multiple organ failure, abdominal surgery, septic shock.)[99, 100] In these cases, we consider CAVH the treatment of first choice. When "surgical" ARF develops after abdominal or cardiac surgery, peritoneal dialysis is contraindicated because of the risk of leakage and infections. In patients with severe cardiovascular instability, hemodialysis is contraindicated. Among the medical causes of ARF, renal hypoperfusion due to hemorrhage, volume depletion, and sepsis are the most common. The unstable hemodynamics of the patient with such a disorder often preclude any intermittent treatment. Under such circumstances, continuous therapies are generally well tolerated, and monitoring is easily carried out. Duration of treatment may vary from a few hours to several days or weeks. The rate of complications related to the treatment is generally low. In some cases, CAVHDF must be utilized in conjunction with CAVH to improve treatment efficacy.

Fluid Overload

Fluid overload with pulmonary edema in the newborn may be due to ARF or cardiac failure or may be iatrogenic (excessive fluid intake in the case of oliguria). Under these conditions, CAVH may effectively reduce fluid overload if a constantly negative fluid balance is maintained. The slow and continuous removal of isotonic fluid is generally well tolerated and produces a reduction in preload and a negative sodium balance. This process may be responsible for the observed decrease in peripheral vascular resistance and the increase in cardiac index with consequent stability of arterial blood pressure.[101-106] Finally, maintenance of cardiovascular stability and intravascular blood volume may help restore renal perfusion.[81-101]

Electrolyte and Acid-Base Derangements

The manipulation of extracellular fluid achievable with CAVH permits the treatment of several electrolyte derangements. Hyponatremia, hypernatremia, hypercalcemia, and hyperkalemia can be managed by changing the composition of the replacement solution. The speed of correction depends on the ultrafiltration rate and on the amount and composition of substitution fluid. During a single day, CAVH may produce 1 to 2 L of ultrafiltrate (five to ten times the circulating volume in a neonate weighing 3 kg). Furthermore, if we assume a body water pool of about 2000 mL, an average ultrafiltration of 2000 mL in 24 hours achieves a daily purification index (liters of clearance/liters of body water) above 1.

This relatively high turnover of fluid can be used to vary not only the concentration but also the absolute body content of some electrolytes. For instance, hyperkalemia can be corrected with CAVH. Potassium removal is directly related to ultrafiltrate production. CAVH is also a reliable treatment for hypercalcemia or in acute renal failure associated with alkalosis, in which hemodialysis or peritoneal dialysis might worsen the clinical condition of the patient. In CAVHDF, efficiency depends on the dialysate composition and the flow. The kinetics of solute transport is similar to that of hemodialysis, and a final solute balance is sometimes difficult.[101-104]

Hypocalcemia may occur in the newborn from immaturity of the parathyroid glands, especially during an exchange transfusion. Seizures may than appear, requiring the urgent administration of calcium. Calcium solutions may induce thrombophlebitis. During CAVH, however, calcium supplements can be diluted in the replacement solution, which is then rapidly distributed in the venous circulation. In the absence of seizures, calcium gluconate supplementation can be scheduled as an addition to the replacement solution, and a continuous infusion can be provided at the rate of 5 mg/kg/hr. Calcium solutions are incompatible with sodium bicarbonate solutions, and separate bags must be used.

Hypomagnesemia may occur if phenytoin is given to the mother for the treatment of toxemia in pregnancy. Treatment with 1% magnesium sulfate should not exceed 5 to 10 mL at the rate of 0.5 to 1 mL/min. Ultrafiltrate losses should be considered.

In acid-base derangements, different situations should be considered. Bicarbonate loss during CAVH can easily be measured directly in the ultrafiltrate or by using the following formula:

$$HCO_{3(f)} = UF \times HCO_{3(s)} \times 1.124$$

where $HCO_{3(f)}$ is the bicarbonate concentration in the ultrafiltrate; $HCO_{3(s)}$ is the bicarbonate concentration in the serum; UF is the total amount of ultrafiltrate; and 1.124 is the average sieving coefficient for bicarbonate.

When CAVH is applied without substitution fluid in order to reduce the patient's fluid overload, bicarbonate losses are compensated by the reduction of the body volume distribution for the buffer, and the serum concentration does not change significantly. When replacement solutions are infused to maintain body fluid balance, however, the amount lost in the ultrafiltrate must be replaced. Finally, when CAVH is used to correct metabolic acidosis, the amount of bicarbonate in the replacement solution must exceed the amount lost in the ultrafiltrate.

Conclusion

When correction of water, electrolyte, or acid-base derangements is required, the following factors must be considered for all the solutes in order to achieve the desired physiologic targets:

- Rate of ultrafiltration and replacement
- Initial plasma concentrations and rate of production
- Amount lost in the ultrafiltrate
- Other losses (insensible loss in incubator, fever-induced losses, and the like)
- Contents of the replacement solution

Removal of Urea and Metabolic Balance

Despite the remarkable amount of ultrafiltration, treatment may sometimes fail to achieve metabolic balance. The identical compositions of ultrafiltrate and plasma water and the purely convective nature of the treatment limit the efficiency of CAVH in removal of small molecules. The limited efficiency of CAVH is most evident in severely catabolic patients. Several strategies can then be used when urea nitrogen generation rates exceed 1.2 to 1.8 g/day. First, ultrafiltration rate should be maximized. Second, protein catabolic rate and urea generation should be reduced. To achieve a positive nitrogen balance and control of BUN level, early parenteral or enteral nutrition should be instituted.

Nutritional supplementation in the newborn must be carried out with special attention to the patient's fluid and electrolyte requirements. Glucose solutions and mixed essential and nonessential amino acid solutions should be provided in order to obtain an energy intake of about 100 to 150 cal/kg/day and adequate dietary protein. In some cases, even these steps are inadequate.

The new filters can increase daily ultrafiltration to up to 4 L with the use of a blood pump. Furthermore, they have a second port in the ultrafiltrate compartment. Dialysate fluid can thus be administered at countercurrent flow into the ultrafiltration compartment performing continuous arteriovenous or venovenous hemodiafiltration. This procedure improves efficiency of the treatment by adding diffusive transport to convection. If the dialysate circulates at flows of 2 to 3 mL/min, it is still possible to have a concentration of solutes in the dialysate close to that of plasma (equilibrium dialysis). Under these conditions, clearance equals dialysate flow, and treatment efficiency treatment can be doubled.[101-104]

Monitoring and Complications of CAVH

Although CAVH is a safe and simple method, technical or clinical complications may occur during the treatment.

Clinical Complications

There has been concern about the occurrence of depletion syndromes (e.g., nonspecific loss of vitamins, amino acids, hormones) as well as hypophosphatemia with CAVH. None of our patients has experienced any of these complications, possibly because we provided specific parenteral nutrition support during treatment. Electrolyte and acid-base imbalances can occur if inappropriate replacement solutions are prescribed. Bleeding episodes can be observed if excessive doses of heparin are given. Hypervolemia or hypovolemia may also occur with errors in fluid balance. We suggest the use of micromethods for blood chemistry determinations in order to avoid iatrogenic anemia. When necessary, blood transfusions can be provided via the replacement solution infusion port. Finally, drug dosage should be varied according to target plasma concentrations, protein binding, and molecular size of the drug; all of these parameters affect the pharmacodynamics of the molecule during CAVH.

Technical Complications

Blood loss can occur if a hollow fiber develops a leak. This potential problem is negligible in CAVH because of the low pressures operating in the system. Should it occur, however, the high visibility of the red blood cells in the filtrate renders the problem rapidly detectable, and a rapid filter exchange can be scheduled. When ultrafiltration rates drop below 0.5 mL/min, a general inspection of the filter, blood access, blood lines, and patient arterial pressure should be carried out. If clotting in the fibers is suspected, flushing can be performed using 50 to 100 mL of heparinized solution, via the three-way taps to exclude the patient's circulation. If this measure is unsuccessful, the filter should be replaced. Finally, air embolism is impossible in this system, which operates under conditions of positive pressure. Special care must be taken, however, when umbilical vessels are used for blood access or when a blood module is utilized for CVVH. In our experience, the use of a pressure-sensitive blood module permitted the detection of increases in the end-to-end pressure drop in the filter due to fibers' clotting, so that the unit could be replaced before significant reductions of efficiency had occurred.

Conclusion

Continuous arteriovenous hemofiltration can be used as an alternative treatment in infants and children as well as in adults.[100-104] The small size of the patients may present special problems. Clinical experience so far suggests that such technical problems can be overcome. CAVH is simple, safe, and effective for conditions in which hemodialysis or peritoneal dialysis is contraindicated. These features make it a new dialytic therapy in the neonate. The development of devices especially designed for CAVH in infants will certainly increase its future use. Deeper knowledge of the mechanisms involved in acute renal failure, septic shock, and multiple organ failure will further encourage the use of continuous therapies in the critically ill patient, not only for blood purification purposes but also for the removal of possible mediators of tissue and organ injury.[105, 106]

SUMMARY

Acute renal failure is a severe clinical condition that is further complicated in small children by several peculiar problems typical of a pediatric population. Early diagnosis, prevention, conservative measures, and renal replacement therapies are all part of a common approach that must be promptly implemented in these high-risk patients.

The outcome may vary significantly according to the underlying disease, the severity of illness, and the time of intervention. New technologic advances can help the clinician to improve the quality of treatment and the speed of diagnosis. A multidisciplinary approach is also desirable in the care of these patients in order to achieve the best possible outcomes and to practice at the highest levels of competence in each single branch of intensive care medicine and nephrology.

References

1. Donkerwolcke RA, Chantler C, Brojer MJC: Paediatric dialysis. *In:* Replacement of Renal Function by Dialysis. Drukker W, Parsons FM, Maher JF (Eds). Boston, Martinus Nijhoff, 1983, pp 514-535.
2. Knochel J. Biochemical, electrolyte and acid-base disturbances in acute renal failure. *In:* Acute Renal Failure. Brenner BM and Lazarus JM (Eds). Philadelphia, WB Saunders, 1983, pp 568-585.
3. Stokke T, Kettler D: Komplikationen der kontinuierlichen arteriovenosen Hemofiltration. Anaesthesist 1985; 34:528-533.
4. Loirat C, Guesnu M: Insuffisanse rénale aiguë. *In:* Néphrologie Pédiatrique. Royer P, Habib R, Mathieu H, et al (Eds). Paris, Flammarion Médecine Science, 1983, pp 415-424.
5. Kon V, Ichikawa I: Research seminar: Physiology of acute renal failure. J Pediatr 1984; 105:351-355.
6. Navar LG: Renal autoregulation: perspectives from whole kidney and single nephron studies. Am J Physiol 1978; 234:F357-363.
7. Skorecki KL, Brenner MB: Body fluid homeostasis in man. Am J Med 1981; 70:77-81.
8. Davis JO, Freeman RH: Mechanisms regulating renin release. Physiol Rev 1976; 56:1-9.
9. Kon V, Yared A, Ichikawa I: Role of renal sympathetic nerves in mediating hypoperfusion of renal cortical microcirculation in experimental heart failure and acute extracellular fluid volume depletion. J Clin Invest 1989; 76:1913-1917.
10. Schrier RW, Berl T, Anderson RJ: Osmotic and nonosmotic control of vasopressin release. Am J Physiol 1979; 236:F321.
11. Anderson RJ, Schrier RW: Clinical spectrum of oliguric and nonoliguric acute renal failure. *In:* Contemporary Issues in Nephrology, Vol 6. Acute Renal Failure. Brenner BM, Stein JM (Eds). New York, Churchill Livingstone, 1980, pp 1-22.
12. Dixon BS, Anderson RJ: Nonoliguric acute renal failure. Am J Kidney Dis 1989; 6:71-77.
13. Dauber IM, Krauss AN, Symchych PS, et al: Renal failure following perinatal anoxia. J Pediatr 1976; 88:851-855.
14. Khan MY: Anuria from *Candida* pyelonephritis and obstructing fungal balls. Urology 1983; 21:421-423.
15. Adelman RD: The hypertensive neonate. Clin Perinatol 1988; 15:567-585.
16. Bauer SB, Feldman SM, Gellis SS, et al: Neonatal hypertension: A complication of umbilical artery catheterization. N Engl J Med 1975; 293:1032-1033.
17. Avery ME, Oppenheimer EH, Gordon HH: Renal-vein thrombosis in newborn infants of diabetic mothers. N Engl J Med 1957; 256:1134-1138.
18. Assadi F, Delivoria-Papadopulos M, Pereira G, et al: Fibrinogen degradation products in acute renal failure of the newborn. Clin Nephrol 1983; 19:74-81.
19. Adelman RD, Wirth F, Rubio T: A controlled study of the nephrotoxicity of mezlocillin and amikacin in the neonate. Am J Dis Child 1987; 141:1175-1178.
20. Adelman RD, Wirth F, Rubio T: A controlled study of the nephrotoxicity of mezlocillin and gentamicin plus ampicillin in the neonate. J Pediatr 1987; 111:888-893.
21. Van Bel F, Guit GL, Schipper J, et al: Indomethacin-induced changes in renal blood flow velocity waveform in premature infants investigated with color Doppler imaging. J Pediatr 1991; 118:621-626.
22. Cifuentes RF, Olley PM, Balfe JW, et al: Indomethacin and renal function in premature infants with patent ductus arteriosus. J Pediatr 1979; 95:583-587.
23. Rennie JM, Cooke RWI: Prolonged low dose indomethacin for persistent ductus arteriosus of prematurity. Arch Dis Child 1991; 65:55-58.
24. Vert P, Bianchetti G, Marchal F, et al: Effectiveness and pharmacokinetics of indomethacin in premature newborns with patent ductus arteriosus. Eur J Clin Pharmacol 1980; 18:83-88.
25. Gordillo-Paniagua G, Velasquez-Jones L: Acute renal failure. Pediatr Clin North Am 1976; 23:817-821.
26. Roberts RJ: Drug Therapy in Infants: Pharmacologic Principles and Clinical Experience. Philadelphia, WB Saunders, 1984, p 82.
27. Gilbert EF, Khoury GH, Hogan GR, et al: Hemorrhagic renal necrosis in infancy: Relationship to radio-opaque compounds. J Pediatr 1970; 76:49-53.
28. Hanssens M, Keirse MJNC, Vankelecom F, et al: Fetal and neonatal effects of treatment with angiotensin-converting enzyme inhibitors in pregnancy. Obstet Gynecol 1991; 78:128-135.
29. Rosa FW, Bosco LA, Graham CF, et al: Neonatal anuria with maternal angiotensin-converting enzyme inhibitors. Obstet Gynecol 1989; 74:371-374.
30. Bavoux F: Non-steroidal anti-inflammatory drugs and fetal toxicity. Presse Med 1992; 21:1909-1912.
31. Ravio KO: Neonatal hyperuricemia. J Pediatr 1976; 88:625-630.
32. Stapleton FB, Jones DP, Green RS: Acute renal failure in neonates: Incidence, etiology, and outcome. Pediatr Nephrol 1987; 1:314-320.
33. Roberts DS, Haycock GB, Dalton RN, et al: Prediction of acute renal failure after birth asphyxia. Arch Dis Child 1990; 65:1021-1028.
34. Merlob P, Litwin A, Lazar L, et al: Neonatal ABO incompatibility complicated by hemoglobinuria and acute renal failure. Clin Pediatr 1990; 29:219-222.
35. Bernstein J: The morphogenesis of renal parenchymal maldevelopment (renal dysplasia). Pediatr Clin North Am 1971; 18:395-407.
36. Nakayama DK, Killian A, Hill LM, et al: The newborn with

hydrops and sacrococcygeal teratoma. J Pediatr Surg 1991; 26:1435–1438.
37. Noe HN, Bryant JF, Roy S III, et al: Urolithiasis in preterm neonates associated with furosemide therapy. J Urol 1984; 132:93–94.
38. Eckstein CW, Kass EJ: Anuria in a newborn secondary to bilateral uteropelvic fungus balls. J Urol 1982; 127:109–110.
39. Arant BS: Renal disorders of the newborn infant. *In:* Contemporary Issues in Nephrology, Vol 12. Pediatric Nephrology. Tune B, Mendoza S (Eds). New York, Churchill Livingstone, 1980, pp 111–115.
40. Schwartz GJ, Haycock GB, Chir B, Spitzer A: Plasma creatinine and urea concentrations in children: Normal values for age and sex. J Pediatr 1976; 88:828–833.
41. Assadi FK, John EG, Fornell L, Rosenthal IM: Falsely elevated serum creatinine concentration in ketoacidosis. J Pediatr 1985; 107:562–570.
42. Saah AJ, Koch TR, Drusano GL: Cefoxitin falsely elevates creatinine levels. JAMA 1982; 247:205–210.
43. Dixon BS, Anderson RJ: Nonoliguric acute renal failure. AM J Kidney Dis 1985; 6:71.
44. Chevalier RL, Campbell F, Brendridge AN: Prognostic factors in neonatal acute renal failure. Pediatrics 1984; 74:265–272.
45. Grylock L, Medani C, Holtzen C, et al: Nonoliguric acute renal failure in the newborn. Am J Dis Child 1982; 136:518–523.
46. Brezis M, Rosen S, Silva P, Epstein FH: Renal ischemia: A new perspective. Kidney Int 1984; 26:375–381.
47. Kuttnig M, Zobel G, Ring E: Nitrogen and amino acid balance during total parenteral nutrition and continuous arteriovenous hemofiltration in critically ill anuric children. Child Nephrol Urol 1991; 11:74–80.
48. Anand SK: Acute renal failure. *In:* Diseases of the Newborn. Taeusch HW, Ballard RA, Avery ME (Eds). Philadelphia, WB Saunders, 1991, pp 894–906.
49. Shaffer SE, Norman ME: Renal function and renal failure in the newborn. Clin Perinatol 1989; 16:199–218.
50. Steiner RW. Interpreting the fractional excretion of sodium. Am J Med 1984; 77:699–704.
51. Earley LE, Friedler RM: Renal tubular effects of ethacrynic acid. J Clin Invest 1964; 43:1495–1502.
52. Ellis EN, Arnold WC: Use of urinary indexes in renal failure in the newborn. Am J Dis Child 1982; 136:615–617.
53. Siegel SR, Oh W: Renal function as a marker of human fetal maturation. Acta Pediatr 1976; 65:481–485.
54. Anderson RJ, Berl T, McDonald KM, et al: Evidence for an in vivo antagonism between vasopressin and prostaglandin in the mammalian kidney. J Clin Invest 1975; 56:420–426.
55. Boineau FG, Rothman J, Lewy JE: Nephrosonography in the evaluation of renal failure and masses in infants. J Pediatr 1975; 87:195–201.
56. Ash JM, Antico VF, Gilday DL, Houle S: Special considerations in the pediatric use of radionuclides for kidney studies. Semin Nucl Med 1982; 12:345–350.
57. Sherman RA, Byun KJ: Nuclear medicine in acute and chronic renal failure. Semin Nucl Med 1982; 12:265–270.
58. Wong SN, Lo RNS, Yu ECL: Renal blood flow pattern by noninvasive Doppler ultrasound in normal children and acute renal failure patients. J Ultrasound Med 1989; 8:135–141.
59. Patriquin HB, O'Regan S, Robitaille P, et al: Hemolytic-uremic syndrome: Intrarenal arterial Doppler patterns as a useful guide to therapy. Radiology 1989; 172:625–628.
60. Morris CR, Alexander EA, Bruns SJ: Restoration and maintenance of glomerular filtration by mannitol during hypoperfusion of the kidney. J Clin Invest 1972; 51:1555–1559.
61. Prandota J: High doses of furosemide in children with acute renal failure: A preliminary retrospective study. Int J Urol Nephrol 1991; 23:383–388.
62. Trachtman H, Hackney P, Tejani A: Pediatric hemodialysis: A decade's (1974–1984) perspective. Kidney Int Suppl 1986; 30:S15–S22.
63. Potter DE, San Luis E, Wippler JE, Portale AA: Comparison of continuous ambulatory peritoneal dialysis and hemodialysis in children. Kidney Int Suppl 1986; 30:S11–S14.
64. Myers BD, Moran SM: Hemodynamically mediated acute renal failure. N Engl J Med 1986; 314:97–103.
65. Balfe JW: Peritoneal dialysis. *In:* Pediatric Nephrology. 2nd ed. Holliday MA, Barratt IM, Vernier RC (Eds). Baltimore, Williams & Wilkins, 1987, pp 814–822.
66. Kramer P, Wigger W, Rieger J, Matthaei D, Scheler F: Arteriovenous hemofiltration: A new and simple method for treatment of overhydrated patients resistant to diuretics. Klin Wschr 1977; 55:1121–1125.
67. Lauer A, Saccggi A, Ronco C, et al: Continuous artriovenous hemofiltration in the critically ill patient. Ann Intern Med 1983; 99:455–461.
68. Olbricht CJ, Schurek HJ, Stolte H, Koch KM: The influence of vascular access modes on the efficiency of CAVH. *In:* Continuous Arteriovenous Hemofiltration. Sieberth HG, Mann H (Eds). Basel, Karger, 1985, pp 14–24.
69. Jenkins RD, Harrison HL, Jackson EC, Fink JE: Continuous renal replacement in infants and toddlers. Contrib Nephrol 1991; 93:245–249.
70. La Greca G, Fabris A, Ronco C: Continuous Arteriovenous Hemofiltration. *In:* Proceedings of the International Symposium on Continuous Arteriovenous Hemofiltration, Vicenza. La Greca G, Fabris A, Ronco C (Eds). Milano, Wichtig Ed, 1986.
71. Ronco C, Brendolan A, Bragantini L, La Greca G: Self limited dehydration during CAVH. Blood Purif 1984; 2:88–93.
72. Ronco C, Brendolan A, Bragantini L, La Greca G: Studies on blood flow dynamics and ultrafiltration kinetics during continuous arteriovenous hemofiltration. Blood Purif 1986; 4:220–226.
73. Ronco C, Brendolan A, Bragantini L, La Greca G: Continuous arterio-venous hemofiltration. Contrib Nephrol 1985; 48:70–78.
74. Bartlett R, Bosch JP, Paganini EA, Geronemus R, Ronco C: Continuous arterio-venous hemofiltration. Trans Am Soc Artif Intern Organs 1987; 38:345–352.
75. Paganini EP: Acute Continuous Renal Replacement Therapy. Boston, Martinus Nijhoff, 1986.
76. Ronco C, Brendolan A, Bragantini L, La Greca G: Treatment of acute renal failure in newborns by continuous arteriovenous hemofiltration. Trans Am Soc Artif Intern Organs 1985; 41:634–638.
77. Lieberman KV, Nardi L, Bosch JP: Treatment of acute renal failure in an infant using continuous arterio-venous hemofiltration. 1985; 106:646–649.
78. Ronco C, Brendolan A, Bragantini L, La Greca G: Treatment of acute renal failure in the newborn by continuous arteriovenous hemofiltration. Kidney Int 1986; 29:908–915.
79. Zobel G, Trop M, Muntean W, Ring E, Gleispach H: Anticoagulation for continuous arteriovenous hemofiltration in children. Blood Purif 1988; 6:90–95.
80. Olbricht CJ, Schurek HJ, Tytul S, Muller C, Stolte H: Comparison between Scribner shunt and femoral catheters as vascular access for continuous arteriovenous hemofiltration. *In:* Arteriovenous Hemofiltration. Kramer P (Ed). Berlin, Springer-Verlag, 1985; pp 57–66.
81. Ronco C, Bosch JP, Lew S: Technical and clinical evaluation of a new hemofilter for CAVH: Theoretical concepts and practical applications of a different blood flow geometry. *In:* Proceedings of the International Symposium on Continuous Arteriovenous Hemofiltration, Vicenza, 1986. La Greca G, Fabris A, Ronco C (Eds). Milano, Wichtig Ed, 1986, pp 55–61.
82. Golper TA, Ronco C, Kaplan AA: Continuous arterio-venous hemofiltration: Improvements, modifications and future directions. Semin Dial 1988; 1:50–54.
83. Pallone TL, Peterson J: Continuous arteriovenous hemofiltration, an in vivo simulation. Trans Am Soc Artif Intern Organs 1987; 33:304–308.
84. Ronco C, Brendolan A, Borin D, et al: Continuous arterio-venous hemofiltration in newborns. *In:* Proceedings of the International Conference on Continuous Arteriovenous Hemofiltration, Aachen. Sieberth H, Mann H (Eds). Basel, Karger, pp 76–79.
85. Kramer P: Limitations and pitfalls of continuous arteriovenous hemofiltration. *In:* Arteriovenous Hemofiltration. Kramer P (Ed). Heidelberg, Springer-Verlag, 1985, pp 206–211.
86. Ronco C, Fecondini L, Gavioli L, et al: A new blood module for continuous renal replacement therapies. Int J Artif Organs 1994; 17:29–33.
87. Stolar CJ, Snedecor SM, Bartlett RH: Extracorporeal membrane oxygenation and neonatal respiratory failure: Experience from

the extracorporeal life support organization. J Pediatr Surg 1991; 26:563–571.

88. Bosch JP, Ronco C: Continuous arteriovenous hemofiltration. *In:* Replacement of Renal function by Dialysis. 3rd ed. JF Maher (Ed): Dordrecht, The Netherlands, Kluwer Academic, 1989, pp 347–361.
89. Pappenheimer AM Jr: Passage of molecules through capillary walls. Physiol Rev 1953; 33:387–423.
90. Geronemus R, Schnaider N: Continuous arteriovenous hemodialysis. *In:* Proceedings of the Third International Symposium on Acute Continuous Renal Replacement Therapy. Paganini E, Geronemus R (Eds). Fort Lauderdale, Fla, March 15–17, 1987, pp 77–85.
91. Ronco C: Arterio-venous hemodiafiltration (AVHDF): A possible way to increase urea removal during CAVH. Int J Artif Organs 1985; 8:61–62.
92. Ronco C: Continuous renal replacement therapies and the polyamide membrane. Contrib Nephrol 1992; 96:111–123.
93. Ronco C, Brendolan A, Bragantini L, La Greca G: Solute and water transport during continuous arterio-venous hemofiltration. Int J Artif Organs 1987; 10:179–184.
94. Brendolan A, Ronco C, Crepaldi C, Feriani M, Milan M, Fecondini L, La Greca G: Clinical use of a new fluid balancing system: A useful complement to continuous replacement therapies. J Nephrol 1993; 6:149–152.
95. Ronco C, Burchardi H: Management of acute renal failure in the patient critically ill. *In:* Pathophysiologic Foundations of Critical Care. Dhainaut JF, Pinsky M (Eds). Baltimore, Williams & Wilkins, 1993, pp 630–676.
96. Ronco C: Continuous arterio-venous hemofiltration: Optimization of technical procedures and new directions. *In:* New Perspectives in Hemodialysis, Peritoneal Dialysis, Arteriovenous Hemofiltration and Plasmapheresis. Horl WH, Schollmeyer P (Eds). New York, Plenum Press, 1987, pp 167–181.
97. Zobel G, Ring E, Kuttnig M, Grubbauer HM: Continuous arterio-venous Hemofiltration versus continuous veno-venous hemofiltration in critically ill pediatric patients. Contrib Nephrol 1991; 93:257–260.
98. Zobel G, Ring E, Kuttnig M, Grubbauer HM: Five years experience with continuous extracorporeal renal support in pediatric intensive care. Intensive Care Med 1991; 17:315–319.
99. Ronco C, Brendolan A, Bragantini L, La Greca G: Arteriovenous hemodiafiltration associated with continuous arteriovenous hemofiltration: A combined therapy in the hypercatabolic patient. *In:* Proceedings of the International Symposium on Continuous Arteriovenous Hemofiltration, Vicenza. La Greca G, Fabris A, Ronco C (Eds). Milano, Wichtig Ed, 1986, pp 171–183.
100. Geronemus R, Schneider N: Continuous arterio-venous hemodialysis: A new modality for treatment of acute renal failure. Trans Am Soc Artif Intern Organs 1984; 30:610–613.
101. Sigler M, Teehan BP: Solute transport in slow continuous arterio-venous hemodialysis: An improved method for treating acute renal failure. *In:* Proceedings of the Third International Symposium on Acute Continuous Renal Replacement Therapy, Fort Lauderdale, Fla, March 15–17, 1987, pp 78–85.
102. Zobel G, Stein JI, Kuttnig M, Beitzke A, Metzler H, Riegler B et al: Continuous extracorporeal fluid removal in children with low cardiac output after cardiac operations. J Thorac Cardiovasc Surg 1991; 101:593–597.
103. Ronco C: Acute renal failure in the neonate: Treatment by continuous renal replacement therapies. *In:* Acute Renal Failure in the Critically Ill. Bellomo R, Ronco C (Eds). Heidelberg, Springer-Verlag, 1995, pp 246–265.
104. Ronco C, Parenzan L: Acute renal failure in infancy: Treatment by continuous renal replacement therapy. Intensive Care Med, 1995; 21:490–499.
105. Bellomo R, Tipping P, Boyce N: Tumor necrosing factor clearances during veno-venous hemodiafiltration in the critically ill. Trans Am Soc Artif Intern Organs 1991; 37:322–323.
106. deVries I, van Deventer SJH, Debetes J: Endotoxin induced cytokines in human septicemia. Adv Exp Med Biol 1990; 256:635–640.

158

Bone Marrow Transplantation

Edward D. Ball, MD • Elana J. Bloom, MD
Albert D. Donnenberg, PhD
Steven M. Pincus, MD, PhD • Witold B. Rybka, MD
Margarida de Magalhaes-Silverman, MD

Bone marrow transplantation (BMT) is increasingly used in the treatment of certain malignant as well as nonmalignant disorders (Table 158–1). The basic strategy is to give very high doses of drugs or radiation or both to ablate malignant cells or the host's lymphohematopoietic system, followed by infusion of normal stem cells. The source of these cells can be a human leukocyte antigen (HLA)–identical sibling or a partially or fully HLA-identical related donor or matched unrelated donor (MUD); with these sources, the process is *allogeneic* BMT. A twin donor is sometimes used (*syngeneic* transplant). In *autologous* BMT, the recipient's bone marrow or blood-derived stem cells are used. The choice between an autologous or allogeneic BMT depends on many issues, including the disease state, the availability of a suitable donor, and the risk-benefit analysis for each patient.

The age of BMT recipients has been increasing. Allogeneic BMT is now performed in patients as old as 65 years. Autologous BMT can be performed in patients as old as 70 years.

This chapter reviews the major indications and problems associated with BMT and attempts to address the main issues in treatment of patients undergoing BMT.

INDICATIONS

The indications for BMT are steadily growing. This modality was first applied to the leukemias and immune deficiency disorders (including aplastic anemia), but the indications have expanded to include lymphoma, solid tumors, and genetic diseases. As BMT becomes safer, the indications and the numbers of patients treated will most likely continue to increase. Some of the current indications for BMT are shown in Table 158–1.

Acute Leukemia

Complete remission (CR) rates of 70% to 80% are achieved in patients with acute myelogenous leukemia (AML). Cure of AML can be obtained only with additional therapy. Direct comparisons of the different modalities of treatment for patients with AML in first CR have been difficult to assess. Autologous or allogeneic transplantation from an HLA-identical sibling yields better leukemia-free survival results than those with standard chemotherapy in patients with AML in first CR. Patients experiencing a relapse from chemotherapy, however, can undergo transplantation or other salvage regimens, resulting in similar levels of overall survival.[1, 2] It is increasingly suggested that prognostic information such as the karyotypes of the AML cells be taken into account.

Patients who suffer a relapse can often achieve a second CR with further induction chemotherapy, but they are rarely cured. Patients undergoing transplantation in second or subsequent CR or early relapse have a 30% to 50% disease-free survival (DFS) rate after allogeneic or autologous BMT.[3]

For adults with acute lymphoblastic leukemia (ALL), CR rates of 75% to 95% can be obtained using intensive regimens. The use of allogeneic BMT in first CR in adults with ALL is also controversial.[4] An analysis in the International Bone Marrow Transplant Registry showed 5-year leukemia-free survival probabilities of 38% with chemotherapy alone and 44% with allogeneic BMT. Some groups, however, recommend allogeneic BMT for adults who have certain high-risk factors and ALL in first CR. As with AML, patients with ALL who suffer relapse or those who have resistant disease have a poor prognosis. About 30% of these patients may be salvaged by allogeneic BMT. Autologous BMT for ALL yields fewer long-term periods of DFS. The National Marrow Donor Program reported on the use of MUD transplants in acute leukemia (AML and ALL). The probability of DFS at 1.5 years was 45% in 58 patients in first and second CR and 19% in 98 patients with more advanced disease.

TABLE 158–1. Disorders Treated with Bone Marrow Transplantation

Malignant Disorders	*Nonmalignant Disorders*
Acute leukemia	Aplastic anemia
Chronic myelogenous leukemia	Immunologic disorders
Myelodysplastic syndrome	Hemoglobinopathies
Lymphomas	Metabolic disorders
Solid tumors	
Multiple myeloma	

Lymphomas

Most data on BMT in lymphoma are from autologous BMT; relatively few HLA-identical transplants are reported.[5] Patients who have aggressive non-Hodgkin's lymphoma and are not cured with the initial chemotherapy regimen have a poor outcome. During the past few years, high-dose chemotherapy with autologous or allogeneic BMT has been increasingly used.[5–8] Patients whose tumor fails to respond initially to chemotherapy have an extremely poor prognosis even when high-dose chemotherapy is used.[7, 8] Patients who achieve an initial complete response and then suffer relapse are those in whom the results of high-dose chemotherapy are most encouraging. An important trial of the use of high-dose therapy versus standard-dose therapy as salvage treatment for patients with relapsed but chemotherapy-sensitive diffuse aggressive lymphoma has been reported.[6] The event-free survival (12% versus 46%) and overall survival (32% versus 53%) favored transplant.

In advanced Hodgkin's disease, high-dose chemotherapy with bone marrow rescue has been used.[9] Results from retrospective studies have shown efficacy of this strategy in disease refractory to front-line therapy, in early relapse, and even in second or subsequent CR.

Chronic Myelogenous Leukemia

BMT using marrow from related donors or MUD is the only known curative therapy for chronic myelogenous leukemia (CML).[10] When bone marrow from HLA-identical siblings are used, 50% to 65% of patients with CML in the chronic phase can be cured. When patients undergo transplantation in the accelerated phase of CML, however, only 15% to 30% are expected to be cured. If BMT is performed in patients whose disease is in blast crisis, approximately 10% of the patients are expected to have long-term DFS. Best results with allogeneic BMT in CML are obtained in persons who are younger than 20 years and who receive a transplant while their disease is in the chronic phase within the first year of diagnosis. For patients who do not have an HLA-identical sibling, BMT with an HLA-identical MUD is an option.[11] The data on 102 consecutive patients who had CML and who received an allogeneic BMT from an MUD have been published. A 29% DFS at 2½ years was observed. Interest has been expressed in the possibility that patients with CML may be cured by high-dose chemotherapy followed by autologous rescue with bone marrow or blood-derived stem cells.[12] Data from numerous sources suggest that benign Philadelphia chromosome-negative hematopoietic stem cells exist with their malignant counterparts in a vast majority of patients with CML.

Aplastic Anemia

Among nonmalignant disorders, the largest number of allogeneic BMTs have been carried out for the treatment of severe aplastic anemia. With supportive treatment alone, only 20% to 30% of patients with severe aplastic anemia are alive 2 years after diagnosis.[13] If an allogeneic BMT from an HLA-identical donor is performed soon after the diagnosis in a nontransfused patient, the long-term survival exceeds 80%. Transfused patients have a probability of survival of about 60% to 70%. BMT from HLA-identical MUD has also been performed in patients with severe aplastic anemia. A report from five centers on 40 unrelated BMTs for severe aplastic anemia reported a 28% survival rate.

Myelodysplastic Syndrome

Patients with myelodysplastic syndrome (MDS) represent a treatment challenge. No specific effective therapy currently exists for this syndrome. Allogeneic BMT has been used in patients who have myelodysplastic syndrome, are younger than 50 years, and have a histocompatible donor.[14] DFS at 3 years is estimated at 45%. Autologous BMT has been tested in a few patients whose MDS has transformed into acute leukemia, but early results are not encouraging.

Multiple Myeloma

The concept of high-dose chemotherapy with or without stem cell support was introduced in the early 1980s to treat patients with multiple myeloma.[15]

Several uncontrolled studies of high-dose treatment with autologous stem cell transplantation and two controlled randomized trials comparing transplantations with standard chemotherapy have been reported.[16, 17] In most studies, the median survival has been superior to that seen with conventional chemotherapy, and small numbers of patients are alive with no disease almost 8 years after transplant.

Even so, most patients with myeloma are not cured, and new strategies such as repeated autografting and post-transplant immunotherapy (interferon alpha) seem to have additional benefit with respect to survival and freedom from progression of disease.

Allogeneic transplantation has also been used. Although some patients are cured, the mortality of the procedure approaches 50%.

Germ Cell Tumors

In approximately 30% of patients with germ cell tumors, the disease relapses or is unresponsive to first-line chemotherapy. For patients who do not experience a complete response to initial induction therapy or for whom standard-dose salvage chemotherapy fails, dose-intensive therapy with autologous BMT is an option. A review of the published literature shows that this approach results in a durable, complete response (3 to 42 months) in about 10% to 20% of heavily pretreated patients and represents a curative option in patients who otherwise would die of their disease.

Breast Cancer

Metastatic breast cancer is essentially incurable. The overall median survival of afflicted women is about 2 years. High-dose chemotherapy followed by autologous BMT or peripheral stem cell rescue has been used in patients with metastatic, hormone-unresponsive breast cancer. When such a strategy is used in heavily pretreated patients with refractory metastatic disease, the results are dismal and the responses obtained are not durable. The latest generation of clinical studies of high-dose chemotherapy has consisted of a standard-dose induction regimen implemented to the point of maximum response, followed by the administration of high-dose chemotherapy as consolidation.[18, 19] The complete response rate achieved with this strategy is about 50%, and 20% to 30% of women are in continuous complete response with a follow-up interval of 18 to 40 months from the time of BMT.

On the basis of the high complete response rates and durable remissions in patients with metastatic disease, trials of primary or adjuvant intensive therapy and autologous BMT were initiated in patients with locally advanced breast cancer (inflammatory or stage III or stage II disease with more than 10 positive nodes). These women have 85% probability of relapse within 10 years. Randomized trials assessing the efficacy of dose-intensive therapy and autologous BMT in stage II (with 10 or more positive nodes), stage III, and Stage IV breast cancer are under way. One relatively small randomized trial has shown a survival benefit for patients with metastatic disease treated with high-dose therapy and stem cell rescue compared with standard dose chemotherapy.[20]

Other Solid Tumors

Intensive therapy with autologous BMT has been tried for patients with other solid tumors. Trials of dose-intensive therapy for sarcomas, gliomas, and malignant melanomas have not shown any significant benefit. Early results for high-dose chemotherapy with BMT or peripheral stem cell rescue in patients with ovarian cancer or neuroblastoma are encouraging, however.

MANIPULATION OF THE GRAFT

Tumor Cell Purging

Because autologous BMT may contain occult tumor cells that could contribute to relapse, various methods to deplete tumor cells from autografts have been developed. Purging of bone marrow is commonly used in autologous BMT for leukemia, lymphoma, neuroblastoma, and breast cancer. The most commonly used methods use chemical agents or monoclonal antibodies (mAbs).

Cyclophosphamide congeners, including mafosfamide and 4-hydroperoxycyclophosphamide (4-HC), have been extensively used for bone marrow purging in the leukemias,[21] lymphoma, and breast cancer.[22] These compounds are cytotoxic to both lymphoid and myeloid leukemia cells, including normal colony-forming cells (hematopoietic progenitors). Long-term bone marrow cultures indicate that earlier progenitor cells are spared, and clinical BMT has shown that bone marrow repopulation after myeloablative therapy does occur. Purging with 4-HC has been applied to autologous BMT in AML, ALL, breast cancer, and lymphoma.

A large number of murine mAbs reactive with antigens present on hematopoietic and solid tumors are available for purging of malignant cells from BM.[23] Complement-mediated (C′) lysis has been the most commonly used method of achieving tumor cell lysis with mAbs. Repeated treatment with mAbs and C′ is capable of removing four to six logs of tumor cells.[24] It is important that the mAb not react with and destroy large numbers of normal bone marrow hematopoietic progenitor cells.

Monoclonal antibody purging has been used for the treatment of AML, ALL, lymphoma, breast cancer, and neuroblastoma. Patients who have AML and undergo transplantation with autologous bone marrow purged with two mAbs (PM-81 and AML-2-23) in second and third CR experienced a 3-year DFS of 50%.[3, 25] Similarly, patients with malignant lymphoma undergoing autologous BMT with bone marrow that had been purged with B1 and B4 mAbs and C′ had a 50% probability of remaining disease free 37.8 months after BMT. Purging was monitored by polymerase chain reaction, focusing on the bcl2 transcript.[26] If the polymerase chain reaction was not rendered negative after purging, the relapse rate was much higher.

An alternative method of purging involves the use of magnetic microspheres, or magnetic colloids. The method consists of reacting the target cells with mAb followed by incubation with antimouse immunoglobulin–coated immunomagnetic beads. Alternatively, the mAb may be conjugated or absorbed onto the immunomagnetic beads directly. The magnetized cellular particles are then passed over a magnet, which removes the magnetized particles and allows the unbound cells to pass through into a collection system. This method has also been applied to the removal of lymphoma cells, small-cell carcinoma of the lung cells, neuroblastoma cells, and breast carcinoma cells.[26, 27]

Another alternative to BM purging is to enrich for hematopoietic stem cells. This may be accomplished using mAb to the CD34 antigen, which is expressed on hematopoietic progenitor cells and probably the true stem cell.[28] Immunoabsorption column–based approaches using the CD34 mAb 12.8 to enrich for hematopoietic progenitors for autologous BMT have been developed. Enriched $CD34^+$ cells have been successfully used to reconstitute bone marrow after myeloablative chemotherapy in patients with metastatic breast cancer and neuroblastoma.[29, 30]

The evaluation of bone marrow purging is problematic because relapse can occur from failure to eradicate cells both in vivo and in vitro. Evaluation of purging in lymphoma is aided by the common existence of the translocation t(14;18) with rearrangement of the bcl-2 proto-oncogene. Relapse was found to be more common in cases of malignant lymphoma in which residual disease was still present, as shown by polymerase chain reaction amplification of the t(14;18) breakpoint after bone marrow purging with mAb and C′.[26] Genetically tagged bone marrow cells from patients with AML were present in leukemia cells at relapse, suggesting that occult leukemia cells in the bone marrow are capable of contributing to relapse.[31]

T Cell Depletion

Elimination of mature T lymphocytes from the bone marrow allografts by various methods has markedly reduced the incidence and severity of acute and chronic graft-versus-host disease (GVHD). The incidence of acute GVHD has been reduced to 10% to 11% in recipients of T cell–depleted HLA-matched bone marrow grafts. Significant reductions have also been noted in partially matched familial and MUD transplant recipients. To date, elimination of this life-threatening complication through allograft T cell depletion has not lived up to its potential for improving the overall success of allogeneic BMT. Higher incidence of graft failure and increased leukemic relapse in some diseases, most notably CML, have offset the advantages of GVHD ablation to the extent that in the aggregate, DFSs in T cell–depleted and T cell–replete allogeneic BMT are similar. This observation suggests that T cell depletion, as currently practiced, may not be equally indicated in all instances of allogeneic BMT. Factors such as the source of the graft (partially matched familial or MUD) or a patient's age can affect GVHD incidence, severity, or consequent morbidity and mortality. Thus, T cell depletion may be of significant benefit for particular diseases or risk groups.

Various methods have been proposed for T cell depletion. Among the most widely used are mAb-based negative selection techniques, separation based on lectin-mediated agglutination, and physical separation by size and density. Remarkably, similar success in elimination of acute GVHD has been reported for all of these processes, providing that they achieved a T cell reduction on the order of 2 logs. Interpretation of reported differences in the incidence of T cell depletion–related complications are hampered by differences in patient selection and the small sample size of diagnosis-specific groups in individual studies.

Monoclonal Antibody–Based Methods

Monoclonal antibodies represent an important tool for graft processing. Monoclonal antibodies directed against determinants expressed on T cells and T cell subsets as well as non-T lymphocytes have been used alone and in combination in clinical trials. They include OKT3 (anti-CD3); Campath-1 (CDw52); anti-CD2, anti-CD3, anti-CD4, anti-CD5, anti-CD6, and anti-CD8 plus Tp44; CT2 (anti-CD2); anti-CD6 plus anti-CD8[32]; anti-CD2, anti-CD5 plus anti-CD7; anti-CD5 alone; and anti-CD8 alone.[33] Several different mAb-based techniques are available for T cell depletion; they include incubation with complement, antiglobulin-conjugated magnetic beads, conjugation to immunotoxins, and conjugation to solid-phase substrates. Positive selection of $CD34^+$ progenitor cells has also been used in the allogeneic BMT setting for T cell depletion.[34] Most of these methods, when optimally applied, yield a depletion of two to three orders of magnitude[35] and thus are sufficient to prevent GVHD in the majority of HLA-matched BMTs.

Soybean Agglutinin and E-Rosette Depletion

Agglutination using a lectin derived from soybeans (SBA) formed the basis for the first clinically successful implementation of BMT with lymphocyte-depleted bone marrow. Preclinical experiments using human bone marrow revealed that the majority of clonogenic myeloid cells are SBA-negative and that SBA could be used to agglutinate and deplete a wide variety of lineage-committed cells, including lymphocytes. Addition of a second round of depletion using treated sheep red blood cells, which bind to T cells via the T cell-specific surface determinant CD2, permitted up to 3 logs of T cell depletion. The SBA-positive fraction is irradiated and infused with the SBA-negative/E-rosette–negative fraction (about 5×10^7 cells/kg).

Elutriation

Counterflow centrifugal elutriation (CCE) separates cells on the basis of size and density. It takes advantage of the observation that the majority of myeloid clonogenic cells can be isolated in a "large-cell" fraction that is depleted of lymphocytes. The method is rapid and reproducible and does not destroy the lymphocyte-rich fractions. Protocols initiated at the Johns Hopkins Oncology Center and the Pittsburgh Cancer Institute have standardized the level of lymphocyte depletion by adding back a specified number of lymphocytes determined on the basis of a recipient's ideal body weight. The rationale is to recover some of the beneficial effects of graft lymphocytes (promotion of engraftment, antileukemic effect) while preventing GVHD. At a dose of 0.5×10^6 lymphocytes per kilogram,[36] no patients receiving bone marrow from a matched sibling died of or developed organ GVHD (grade II) or chronic GVHD. The incidence of grade 1 GVHD was 15%. Stable engraftment occurred in 95% of patients. Overall actuarial 2-year survival for 60 high-risk patients receiving CCE-engineered bone marrow was 50%. In data combined from two published trials of CCE-lymphocyte depletion,[36, 37] DFS depended on the original diagnosis: 60% (at 24 months) in acute leukemias but only 21% in CML.[37] Use of elutriation in the MUD setting required greater peritransplant immunosuppression to prevent graft rejection.[38]

GRAFT-VERSUS-HOST DISEASE

GVHD is a complication of transplantation unique to allogeneic BMT. It occurs if the following requirements are met[22]:

1. Immunologically competent donor T lymphocytes are present in the graft.
2. These cells recognize host alloantigens as incompatible.
3. The host lacks immunocompetence to mount an effective immunologic reaction (i.e., rejection) against these attacking cells.

This process may occur even if a donor is an HLA-identical sibling and in vitro testing by mixed lymphocytic culture is nonreactive. GVHD increases in frequency and severity with the use of a MUD, however, presumably because of histocompatibility differences undetected by current HLA testing. GVHD in syngeneic (identical twin) and autologous BMT may also occur. It is thought to be due to autoreactivity (i.e., failure to develop mechanisms of self-tolerance).

Effector Cells and Target Antigens

Unmanipulated bone marrow allografts typically contain 2 to 5 billion mature T cells. Peripheral stem cell grafts can contain up to 10 times this number. Animal data and clinical experience indicate that the effector cells that mediate acute GVHD make up a potent but small subpopulation of these mature T cells. In animal models of major histocompatibility complex (MHC)–mismatched allogeneic BMT, $CD8^+$ T cells are responsible for GVHD directed against MHC class I differences, and $CD4^+$ T cells account for MHC class II–specific disease.

In humans, the majority of allogeneic BMTs performed to date have relied on the availability of fully MHC-matched sibling donors. Despite this fact, more than half of the recipients of grafts obtained from these matched sibling donors develop clinically significant GVHD. The target antigens of such responses are presumed to be minor histocompatibility determinants. Although animal models provide support for the GVHD directed against minor histocompatibility antigens, the absence or presence of GVHD cannot be predicted solely on the basis of such genetic disparities. Among patients who underwent second allogeneic BMT with bone marrow from the same matched sibling donor, GVHD outcomes in the first and second transplants were often discordant.[39]

Incidence and Risk

Despite modern serologic and molecular HLA typing techniques to confirm compatibility of donor and recipient, GVHD continues to be a major cause of morbidity and mortality associated with BMT. Clinically significant GVHD incidence is 45% (25%–70%) in patients receiving HLA-identical sibling bone marrow and occurs in virtually all recipients of incompatible or MUD bone marrow. Risk factors for development of GVHD include HLA disparity, female-to-male (donor-recipient) transplant, older patient age, and prophylaxis regimens or T cell depletion used for prevention of GVHD. In addition, the type of leukemia, viral infections, cytomegalovirus (CMV) status, HLA type, donor alloimmunity (through pregnancy or transfusion), splenectomy, and T cell dose have been reported to affect the risk of GVHD.[40]

The spectrum of GVHD encompasses two forms: acute GVHD and chronic GVHD. They are distinctive with respect to rate of progression, time of onset, and response to treatment. Because acute GVHD may be the greatest risk factor for developing chronic GVHD, however, prevention of both forms is logical.

Prophylaxis of GVHD consists of immunosuppressive agents such as corticosteroids, methotrexate, cyclosporine, and tacrolimus. Methotrexate and cyclosporine are effective in preventing GVHD, and a combination of the two drugs is better than either drug alone, resulting in improved survival. The addition of corticosteroids to methotrexate, cyclosporine, or antithymocyte globulin is more effective than any single-drug therapy.

Administration of intravenous immunoglobulin and elimination of T lymphocytes from the donor bone marrow before transplantation (T cell depletion) have been associated with a reduction in the incidence of GVHD. Total elimination of GVHD in patients with leukemia may cause loss of graft-versus-leukemia effect, resulting in higher relapse rates and adverse effects on long-term survival. Current research efforts are also directed toward elimination of GVHD without compromising the graft-versus-leukemia effect.

Acute Graft-Versus-Host Disease

Clinical Manifestations

Acute GVHD, which generally occurs within the first 100 days after allogeneic transplant, may affect the skin, gastrointestinal (GI) tract, and liver. The first manifestation is often an erythematous maculopapular rash involving face, neck, palms, and soles, associated with pain or tingling of the extremities. This may be accompanied by fever and flu-like symptoms. The rash may be localized or may involve the entire body, with formation of bullae and desquamation. Insensible fluid loss and superinfection are critical care issues in the presence of epidermolysis in GVHD. The characteristic progression of rash (distal to proximal), pruritus, and onset coinciding with early engraftment help a clinician differentiate acute GVHD from drug eruptions, chemotherapy effect, and infectious skin diseases. Nevertheless, biopsy is mandatory to confirm the diagnosis.

Immunopathology

Cutaneous acute GVHD is signified histologically by epidermal necrosis and dyskeratosis as well as perivascular mononuclear cell infiltration of the dermis and lower epidermis. Although immunohistochemical studies have identified the preponderance of these mononuclear cells as T lymphocytes,[41] natural killer (NK) cells have also been observed. Attempts to characterize the T cell–target cell interactions underlying GVHD have led to identification of intercellular adhesion molecules

TABLE 158–2. Clinical Staging of Acute Graft-Versus-Host Disease

	Organ Site		
Stage	***Skin***	***Liver***	***Gut***
I	<25% of body surface area	Bilirubin 2–3 mg/dL	Diarrhea 500–1000 mL/day
II	25%–50% of body surface area	Bilirubin 3–6 mg/dL	Diarrhea 1000–1500 mL/day
III	Generalized	Bilirubin 6–15 mg/dL	Diarrhea >1500 mL/day
IV	Desquamation	Bilirubin >15 mg/dL	Ileus

and HLA-DR expression on keratinocytes as well as the detection of T cells bearing a determinant associated with skin localization. The hypothesis that epidermal destruction is mediated directly by cytotoxic T cells is supported by the observation that a high proportion of CD8$^+$ T cells detected in cutaneous GVHD lesions are serine protease–positive (i.e., putative cytotoxic effector cells). Despite this evidence, a controlled prospective study failed to reveal differences in the distribution of lymphocytes in skin biopsy samples from recipients of bone marrow autografts and recipients of allografts (with and without acute GVHD).

Intestinal GVHD manifests as secretory, often bloody diarrhea with cramping abdominal pain, nausea, and vomiting. Even when oral intake is stopped, high stool volumes (several liters per day) persist. (This diarrhea may overlap temporally with that caused by chemotherapy-induced damage to mucosa.) Stool studies reveal no pathogens and few, if any, leukocytes. Superimposed viral or fungal infection is not rare and must also be ruled out. Radiologic studies (generally not required for diagnosis) reveal a thickened bowel wall, loss of haustral markings, and rapid transit time. Computed tomography scans show thickened bowel. Histologic confirmation of GVHD is necessary and may be achieved through sigmoidoscopy. The upper GI tract may, however, also be involved (with or without symptoms of anorexia, dyspepsia, or food intolerance); therefore, upper and lower endoscopic biopsies are recommended.[42, 43]

Liver involvement may occur simultaneously or may follow the onset of rash by several days, with elevated bilirubin and alkaline phosphatase levels and subsequent elevation of transaminases. Differential diagnosis includes veno-occlusive disease (VOD) of the liver, gallstones, and cholestasis caused by total parenteral support or drugs (including cyclosporin). If coagulation and platelet support are adequate, histologic confirmation by liver biopsy should be made in equivocal cases such as those without diagnostic skin or gut histology.

Clinical staging of each organ site (Table 158–2) and grading (Table 158–3) of overall GVHD status use relatively gross measurements yet have significant prognostic value, with grades III and IV being associated with significant mortality.

Treatment

Although literature on and trials of GVHD prophylaxis abound, fewer studies have been conducted for treatment of GVHD, and results are less than satisfactory. Once established, GVHD is difficult to cure. Corticosteroids (methylprednisolone, 2–5 mg/kg/day IV in divided doses) and intravenous cyclosporine together are first-line treatments, but overall response rates are less than 50% for grades III and IV GVHD.[44] Complete response rates of 20% are found with conventional prophylaxis therapy for acute GVHD in MUD transplant recipients.[45] Infections, fluid retention, and hyperglycemia during high-dose steroid therapy may further compromise these patients. If therapy is unsuccessful, initial treatment of GVHD second-line therapies may include tacrolimus (formerly called FK-506), antithymocyte globulin, anti-T cell mAb (OKT3), mycophenolate mofetil, and clofazimine.[46] Results have varied, but skin and gut GVHD may be responsive to second-line therapy; however, only skin GVHD shows appreciable rates of CR (up to 40% to 50%). Octreotide acetate (Sandostatin), a synthetic somatostatin analog useful in some secretory diarrheal diseases, has been beneficial as an adjunct therapy for acute GVHD of the intestine.[47] Critical care management of patients with GVHD includes total parenteral nutrition support (to avoid a catabolic state) and slow reintroduction of low-fat, lactose-free diets; a formal "GVHD diet" has been proposed for this purpose.

The effect of acute GVHD on immune reconstitution has been difficult to assess. The disorder typically occurs at a time when T cell responses are markedly reduced, and it is treated by prompt initiation of immunosuppressive therapy. These agents exert variable effects on the adoptive transfer of donor immunity. Experimental immunization of bone marrow donors and recipients was undertaken to determine the effects of two immunoprophylactic regimens independent of GVHD. These studies indicated that the combination of cyclosporine and methylprednisolone did not prevent transfer of donor responses to recall antigens but virtually eliminated transfer of primary immunity to novel antigens. In contrast, cyclophosphamide plus methylprednisolone spared responses to a novel antigen (sheep erythrocytes) but blunted the transfer of tetanus toxoid–specific memory cells. It is not clear whether (1) GVHD-induced immunopathology results in greater susceptibility to infection or (2) the presence of viral infections in the early post-BMT period predisposes to acute GVHD.

With these caveats in mind, we should note that the pace of T cell and B cell reconstitution is retarded in patients with GVHD. The retardation may be explained in part by alloimmune alteration of lymph node architecture.[48] Chronic GVHD is clearly immunosuppressive and is often accompanied by systemic effects on the immune system, such as dysregulation of immunoglobulin synthesis, lymphopenia, and functional asplenism. Because patients with significant chronic GVHD are at greatest risk of significant bacterial infections, immunization with pneumococcal, meningococcal, and *Haemophilus influenzae* type B vaccines is desirable. Although no information on the efficacy of immunization in this group is available, it would predictably be considerably lower than the efficacy in patients without chronic GVHD. Successful immunization with tetanus and diphtheria toxoids has been reported in a proportion of patients with chronic GVHD.[49]

TABLE 158–3. Clinical Grade of Graft-Versus-Host Disease

Grade	Features
I	Skin + to + +; no gut or liver involvement
II	Skin + to + + +; gut + *or* liver + (or both)
III	Skin + + to + + +; gut + + to + + + *or* liver + + to + + + (*or* both)
IV	Any organ + + + +

Autologous Graft-Versus-Host Disease

Anecdotal reports of GVHD-like skin rashes in autologous BMT have been confirmed by the later observation that a syndrome indistinguishable from cutaneous GVHD can be reproducibly elicited by administration of cyclosporine in the post-BMT period. Ongoing clinical trials are designed to determine whether this GVHD-like syndrome is associated with an antileukemic effect as it appears to be in allogeneic BMT.[50]

Chronic Graft-Versus-Host Disease

Clinical Manifestations

Chronic GVHD (Table 158–4), a late complication of allogeneic BMT, occurs in 60% of patients surviving more than 100 days after BMT. The incidence of chronic GVHD may be higher in patients undergoing transplantation with allogeneic peripheral blood stem cells.[51] This syndrome resembles an autoimmune disorder involving lacrimal and salivary glands, with dry eyes and mouth (Sjögren-like syndrome), and skin fibrosis, with damage to adnexal structures (sweat glands, hair follicles, subcutaneous nerves) and hyperpigmentation or hypopigmentation of the skin. The GI tract may be involved, leading to lichenoid oral mucosal changes, esophageal constriction with web formation, malabsorption, weight loss, and liver function abnormalities of cholestasis. Muscles and joints may be involved, resulting in myositis, polyserositis, and joint contractures. These manifestations may be chronically debilitating, but pulmonary involvement with bronchiolitis obliterans is most life-threatening.[52]

The bone marrow graft and immune system are often affected by GVHD. Thrombocytopenia is correlated with poor outcome of chronic GVHD,[53] and immunoglobulin replacement may be helpful in preventing recurrent infections.

Treatment

Treatment of chronic GVHD has relied largely on steroids. A regimen of alternating-day steroids and cyclosporine has been proposed for refractory disease. More potent or additional immunosuppression, however, is often needed for this chronic, debilitating disorder. Tacrolimus has been used successfully at the University of Pittsburgh in patients with severe chronic GVHD, including severe liver GVHD and bronchiolitis obliterans.[54] Other agents and modalities are thalidomide, ursodeoxycholic acid, photopheresis, and psoralin ultraviolet A.[55]

New Approaches

Prediction of Graft-Versus-Host Disease

The ability to predict the outcome of GVHD would offer obvious advantages in donor selection and in choice of prophylactic strategy. The use of an assay involving cocultivation of primed donor lymphocytes with a patient's skin[56] has permitted prospective identification of patients with a sixfold higher relative risk of acute GVHD of stage II or greater. A positive or inconclusive result in this skin explant assay has been used as an inclusion criterion for a clinical trial of T cell depletion.[56] Another approach has been to assess the ability of bone marrow donors to mount mixed lymphocyte reactions against histocompatibility antigens expressed on "third-party" transformed B cell lines. This entirely nonspecific evaluation of donor alloreactivity identified patients with a 4.5-fold relative risk of development of GVHD of stages II to IV. Other potential predictors of GVHD are tumor necrosis factor-α (TNF-α) levels during the conditioning regimen[57] and helper T cell response to recipient keratinocytes.[58]

Once BMT has been performed, careful monitoring of the clinical parameters used to stage acute GVHD can provide information about the likelihood of disease progression. Peak values for extent of rash, bilirubin level, and daily stool output were usually reached earlier than 40 days after BMT. In 69 patients with biopsy-proven acute GVHD, the magnitude of these peak values was predictive of disease progression.

Graft Engineering

In graft engineering, bone marrow grafts with defined hematopoietic and immunologic characteristics are formulated. Current examples of graft engineering are efforts to control the T cell dose, to augment the stem cell content of T cell–depleted allografts, and to eliminate specific T cell subsets. In the last category are exclusion of $CD5^+$ T cells (and consequent inclusion of $CD5^-$ mature T cells and NK cells), exclusion of $CD8^+$ T cells (and inclusion of $CD4^+$ T cells and $CD8^-$ NK cells),[33] and exclusion of $CD4^+$ T cells (and inclusion of NK cells and $CD8^+$ T cells). As the diversity of approaches demonstrates, these attempts are only first approximations of the ultimate goal, which is to formulate a preparation that reliably and rapidly engrafts, has enhanced antitumor and antimicrobial activity, and is tolerant of the host. Although benefit may be derived from further manipulating bone marrow ablative or postgrafting immunosuppressive regimens, it is likely that the next significant increment in clinical benefit will require refinements in graft engineering and post-transplant immunotherapy. Grafts may be rigorously T cell–depleted and subsequently repleted with specific T cell subsets from freshly isolated donor cells or may be selected after in vitro stimulation. Additionally, immunotherepeutic T cells may be administered to mediate graft versus leukemia and antimicrobial effects after the patient has recovered from cytotoxic therapy.

TABLE 158–4. Classification of Chronic Graft-Versus-Host Disease

Limited

- Localized skin involvement
- Hepatic dysfunction

Extensive

- Generalized skin involvement
- Local skin and/or hepatic dysfunction plus:
  - Liver with histology of cirrhosis or chronic aggressive hepatitis
  - Eye involvement
  - Oral mucosa or salivary gland
  - Other target organ involvement

INFECTIOUS COMPLICATIONS OF BONE MARROW TRANSPLANTATION

Despite advances in the management of infectious complications of BMT, infections remain the most common cause of morbidity and mortality after BMT.[59] The infections most commonly developing after BMT occur during specific periods that are related to the immunocompetence of the patient and are termed the *early, middle,* and *late* periods of infectious risk (Table 158–5).

The *early period* after BMT is marked by severe neutropenia, lymphopenia, mucositis, and gastroenteritis due to the toxicity of the chemotherapy and radiation therapy. Further immunosuppression due to the prophylactic measures used to prevent acute GVHD also increase the infectious risk in allogeneic BMT. Common pathogens during the first month after BMT are *Staphylococcus, Streptococcus,* gram-negative enterics, herpes simplex virus (HSV), and *Candida.* After mucositis and neutropenia have resolved, the risk of bacterial

TABLE 158–5. Peak Incidence of Infections After Bone Marrow Transplantation

Early (<30 Days)	Middle (30–100 Days)	Late (>100 Days)
Staphylococcus	*Aspergillus*	Pneumococcus
Streptococcus	*Pneumocystic carinii*	*Haemophilus influenzae*
Gram-negative enterics	*Toxoplasma gondii*	Varicella-zoster virus
Candida albicans	Cytomegalovirus	
Herpes simplex virus	Adenovirus	
	JK virus	

infection decreases. Humoral and cellular immunodeficiencies persist for long periods after BMT, however, and are especially severe in patients being treated for acute or chronic GVHD. The *middle period,* from engraftment until 100 days after BMT, is characterized by infections due to CMV, *Pneumocystis carinii,* and *Aspergillus* species. During the *late period* after BMT, herpes zoster and encapsulated bacterial infections are prominent. In the absence of chronic GVHD, cellular and humoral immunity return to normal over 1 to 2 years.

Major reductions in infectious complications after BMT have been achieved by using the strategies of prophylactic and empirical antibiotic therapy.[60] Reverse isolation and strict hand washing are other approaches that are generally accepted as standard practice to decrease nosocomial transmission of infection. The use of chlorhexidine and nystatin mouthwashes also reduces the infectious risk posed by mucositis due to the suppression of oral flora.

Bacterial Infections

Gram-positive bacteria remain common causes of morbidity in BMT and occasional causes of mortality. The use of multilumen central venous catheters has resulted in lower incidence of staphylococcal bacteremia. Furthermore, the widespread use of prophylactic antibiotics for gram-negative bacteria has led to a relative increase in the frequency of bacteremia due to gram-positive isolates. The prophylactic use of vancomycin has been very effective in reducing documented gram-positive infections.[61] Streptococcal bacteremia also occurs commonly in neutropenic patients who are not receiving prophylactic antibiotic coverage for gram-positive organisms.[62] Sepsis and death due to *Streptococcus mitis* have been reported in neutropenic patients after BMT. Risk factors are severe mucositis, young age, and lack of prophylaxis for gram-positive organisms. Therefore, initiation of gram-positive coverage at first neutropenic fever is highly recommended if prophylaxis is not used. Sinopulmonary pneumococcal infections commonly occur in the late period after BMT, owing to the impairment in opsonization and functional asplenia. Prophylaxis with trimethoprim-sulfamethoxazole given several days a week prevents this complication.

Neutropenic patients are especially prone to infections due to gram-negative bacteria. The mucositis and gastroenteritis present during neutropenia allow easy access of enteric organisms into the bloodstream. Historically, the first neutropenic fever was caused by *Escherichia coli, Klebsiella, Pseudomonas,* or other facultative anaerobes. Neutropenic patients with BMT must be given broad-spectrum gram-negative antibiotic coverage at the first sign of fever. Traditionally, a semisynthetic penicillin or an antipseudomonal cephalosporin has been combined with an aminoglycoside. The nephrotoxicity of the aminoglycoside can be avoided by the use of either imipenem-cilastatin or double-β-lactam regimens. The two approaches have been demonstrated to be of equal effectiveness to aminoglycoside-containing regimens for empirical initial therapy in febrile neutropenic patients.[63, 64]

Because of the frequency and severity of gram-negative infections in neutropenic hosts, much effort has been devoted to developing effective prophylaxis against then. The agents with the greatest success in achieving gram-negative prophylaxis are the fluoroquinolones. The effectiveness of oral ciprofloxacin prophylaxis after BMT compared with placebo was demonstrated in a small randomized trial.[65] In a large randomized trial that contained significant numbers of neutropenic BMT recipients with hematologic malignancies, ciprofloxacin was found to be superior to norfloxacin in decreasing the incidence of documented gram-negative bacteremia. The patients receiving ciprofloxacin also had a lower incidence of neutropenic fevers. The prophylactic antibiotic can be discontinued at the time of first neutropenic fever when broad-spectrum gram-negative coverage is initiated, or, if a patient remains afebrile, when neutropenia resolves.

Fungal Infections

Recipients of BMT are at high risk for mucositis or invasive fungal infections due to neutropenia. They are often receiving therapy with corticosteroids and have an indwelling central venous catheter. The most common pathogens are *Candida* species, especially *Candida albicans,* and *Aspergillus* species. Less commonly encountered are fusaridiosis and mucormycosis.

Antifungal therapy continues to rely on amphotericin B; however, the response of documented aspergillosis to amphotericin B in a neutropenic host is rather poor. Survival and response rates are improved when amphotericin B is begun empirically in patients with febrile neutropenia that does not respond to broad-spectrum antibacterial antibiotics.[65] Because of the toxicity of standard amphotericin B, numerous efforts have been made to find alternatives. Liposomal formulations of amphotericin B have significantly less toxicity yet appear to retain activity. Liposomal amphotericin B used prophylactically in recipients of BMT has been studied in randomized trials and found to be well tolerated, to decrease fungal colonization, and to reduce the incidence of systemic fungal infections.[66]

Fluconazole has been efficacious as antifungal prophylaxis for *Candida* when started at the beginning of neutropenia.[53] The overall frequency of *Candida* colonization and infection was markedly reduced compared with retrospective controls. Interestingly, higher incidence of *Candida krusei* infections resistant to fluconazole has been reported.[67, 68] An alternative to fluconazole may be itraconazole, which has activity against *Aspergillus* in vitro, but whether it will be as effective clinically as amphotericin is not yet known.

Viral Infections

The herpesviruses are the most common causes of viral infection in BMT recipients. Members of the herpesvirus family are CMV, HSV, varicella-zoster virus (VZV), human herpesvirus 6, and Epstein-Barr virus; these infections are usually caused by reactivation of dormant virus. Other viruses that may cause infection after BMT are the BK and JC viruses, adenovirus, and respiratory syncytial virus. Post-BMT viral hepatitis is much less common than in the past, owing to the screening of blood products for hepatitis C.

The most common infectious cause of death after allogeneic BMT is CMV infection. The most life-threatening presentation is CMV pneumonia, which has been fatal in as many as 85% of affected patients. CMV can also cause gastroenteritis, bone marrow suppression, hepatitis, and, less commonly, retinitis and encephalitis. CMV infection may be manifested only by fever and viremia. Most CMV infections occur during the middle period of infectious risk. CMV infections develop in more than half of CMV-seropositive patients if no prophylaxis is used. Other risk factors for CMV infection are severe GVHD and the use of total-body irradiation in the preparative regimen for BMT. The risk of CMV infection in seronegative patients can be eliminated by the use of a seronegative bone marrow donor and of seronegative blood products for transfusion.[69] Another major warning sign of CMV pneumonia is the development of CMV viremia in surveillance blood cultures.[70]

The definitive diagnosis of CMV pneumonia can be difficult to obtain because a lung biopsy is usually required. The presence of viral inclusion bodies in cytology specimens obtained by bronchoalveolar lavage (BAL) or the culture of CMV from BAL fluid is sufficient for a presumptive diagnosis of CMV pneumonia in patients with interstitial pneumonitis.

Treatment of CMV pneumonia has been more satisfying since the demonstration that the combination of ganciclovir and intravenous immune globulin can reduce the mortality of this infection.[71] Patients in whom therapy is initiated early are most likely to benefit. Research efforts have attempted to identify patients with early CMV infections and to target them for treatment. One approach was to perform BAL on all asymptomatic patients on day 35 after BMT. In this study, asymptomatic CMV infection of the lungs was identified as a major risk factor for CMV pneumonia.[72] Patients who were randomly assigned to receive prophylactic ganciclovir did not experience CMV pneumonia. Another study[72a] used CMV excretion at any site as a basis for random assignment to receive placebo or ganciclovir therapy. The researchers of this study concluded that early treatment with ganciclovir reduced CMV disease and improved survival.

Two trials of ganciclovir prophylaxis for all patients seropositive for CMV have been reported. In both studies, patients were randomly assigned to receive ganciclovir or placebo at the time of engraftment.[73, 74] In one study, ganciclovir was also given for 1 week before BMT.[73] Both studies demonstrated a decrease in the incidence and severity of CMV infection in the patients receiving ganciclovir.[73, 74] Also in both studies, neutropenia was identified as the major toxicity associated with ganciclovir therapy. Despite the reduction in incidence of significant CMV disease, survival was not improved by the prophylactic use of ganciclovir. Therefore, the best approach to treating BMT recipients who are seropositive for CMV has yet to be determined. The use of hematopoietic growth factors in combination with ganciclovir may abrogate the neutropenia caused by this drug. An alternative to ganciclovir may be foscarnet. This agent lacks bone marrow toxicity and has been demonstrated to be effective for CMV retinitis in patients with acquired immunodeficiency syndrome. Foscarnet is currently undergoing clinical trials in recipients of BMT.

HSV infection had previously been a common complication in BMT recipients for several weeks after engraftment. With the common use of prophylactic acyclovir, HSV infections are usually not encountered until prophylaxis has ended. Both oral and genital HSV infections occur. Reinstitution of acyclovir is generally effective therapy. In a case report, an acyclovir-resistant HSV infection in a BMT recipient was successfully treated with foscarnet. Human herpesvirus 6 infection has also been identified as a possible pathogen in pediatric and adult patients.[75] Isolation of the virus is associated with fever, skin rash, and bone marrow suppression.

Shingles develops in approximately one third of BMT recipients who are seropositive for VZV, generally during the late period after BMT. The frequency of VZV infection appears to be similar in allogeneic and autologous BMT recipients.[76] Disseminated disease and involvement of multiple dermatomes are more common presentations in BMT recipients compared with the general population. Acyclovir is effective therapy and should be given intravenously in complicated cases. If oral acyclovir is used, the patient must be monitored closely for any progression of lesions.

BK virus and JC virus are occasional causes of cystitis after BMT during the middle period of infectious risk. BK viruria is much more common and is associated with hemorrhagic cystitis.[77] Adenovirus is associated with interstitial pneumonia with the same time-course as CMV. No effective therapy for adenovirus pneumonia has been found, and this infection is usually fatal. Respiratory syncytial virus can cause an upper respiratory tract infection and pneumonia and did cause an outbreak in a BMT center. Ribavirin has generally been used to treat this infection, although it is not clear whether the drug is effective in this setting.

Protozoal Infections

P. carinii is a common pathogen in immunocompromised hosts and can cause lethal pneumonia in BMT recipients. *P. carinii* pneumonia (PCP) usually occurs during the middle period after BMT.[78] Patients at highest risk are those who have not received prophylaxis for PCP or in whom prophylaxis was discontinued.

Affected patients present with a cough, fever, and dyspnea, and an interstitial process is detected on chest radiograph. In order to confirm the diagnosis, it is necessary to obtain BAL fluid or a lung biopsy sample. Trimethoprim-sulfamethoxazole remains the treatment of choice for PCP. The use of adjunctive corticosteroids has improved survival in patients with acquired immunodeficiency syndrome (AIDS) and PCP and should be considered in BMT recipients with moderate or severe pneumonia. Survival remains poor, with only one third of patients surviving PCP.[78] Survival is improved in patients in whom therapy is initiated promptly, in those who develop PCP more than 6 months after BMT, and in those in whom *P. carinii* is the only pathogen identified.

Toxoplasmosis is an occasional cause of death after BMT, with 31 cases reported in the literature as of 1992.[79] A high index of suspicion should be maintained when patients present with central nervous system (CNS) symptoms such as hemiplegia, meningitis, and confusion. Unfortunately, some present with nonspecific signs, such as fever alone, and the diagnosis is not made until autopsy. Almost all cases occur in patients who are seropositive for *Toxoplasma gondii* before BMT or for whom serologic status was not determined. Because most donors were seronegative in the reported cases, reactivation of latent infection appears to be the principal cause of disease. Most infections develop during the second or third month after BMT.

The diagnosis is confirmed by parasitemia, brain biopsy, or autopsy in most cases. Isolation of *T. gondii* from cerebrospinal fluid or BAL fluid has also been reported. Therapy with pyrimethamine-sulfadiazine can be successful, but patients who respond to this therapy are at risk for relapse.

NONINFECTIOUS COMPLICATIONS

A significant proportion of the complications of BMT arise from the toxicity of the chemotherapy and irradiation used in BMT induction regimens. In fact, it is the intent of most such regimens to approach but not to exceed lethal dose, limiting toxicity for organ systems other than the BM. In addition, the toxicity of supportive treatments compounds the complexity of the situation. The success of BMT, then, depends on successfully maintaining patients through such critical complications. Intensive care facilities are used aggressively to achieve these ends.

Specific end-organ toxicities may be the primary source of dysfunction or may complicate dysfunction due to other toxicities. Each major toxicity must be judged individually in terms of reversibility when one is developing a therapeutic plan. The combination of all toxicities and their inter-relationships define the practical issues of the success of acute supportive therapy.

Neurologic Complications

Neurologic complications are common after BMT, affecting as many as 70% of both adults and children.[80] The majority of these patients experience reversible metabolic encephalopathy. Autopsy studies have established the importance of cerebrovascular lesions, including hematoma, hemorrhagic necrosis, and infarction. Nonbacterial thrombotic endocarditis is the most common cause of embolization.

Acute CNS toxicity can be encountered with the initial cytoreductive regimen. Mechlorethamine is particularly toxic; its acute manifestations are confusion, disorientation, headache, hallucinations, lethargy, tremor, paraplegia, seizure, and vertigo. Later manifestations include personality change, confusion, seizure, diplopia, and dementia. Radiologic studies reveal ventricular enlargement and cerebral atrophy, and electroencephalograms show diffuse slowing. Carmustine can also be associated with direct CNS toxicity. Busulfan induces seizures, and two thirds of patients show epileptiform activity on electroencephalography despite prophylaxis.

Irradiation can produce a reversible syndrome of somnolence associated with lethargy, irritability, headache, low-grade fever, GI disturbance, and depression. *Lhermitte's sign* (pain in the lower extremities upon flexion of the neck) has been observed after irradiation and BMT. A particularly devastating complication of irradiation and intrathecal methotrexate is multifocal leukoencephalopathy, an extensive irreversible demyelination of the cerebral white matter associated with cerebral atrophy.[81] Late cognitive dysfunction resulting from irradiation has been reported in both children and adults.[82]

Cyclosporine is associated with several CNS toxicities. Seizures occur in association with the hypomagnesemia produced by cyclosporine. Reversible abnormalities include mental confusion, a motor spinal cord syndrome, a cerebellar ataxia–like syndrome,[83] and optic disk edema. Concurrent use of cyclosporine and corticosteroids is associated with a syndrome of hypertension, severe visual disturbances, including blindness, seizures, and occipital lobe density, as well as changes on computed tomography scanning or nuclear magnetic resonance imaging of the brain.[83] A common association is noted between cyclosporine therapy and the presence of microangiopathic hemolytic anemia. These abnormalities usually clear after cessation of cyclosporine; however, this agent has been resumed subsequently at reduced dose without recurrence of these abnormalities.

Acute demyelinating polyneuropathy can occur de novo or can be exacerbated after BMT.[84] In addition, autonomic neuropathy has also been observed.

Mucosal and Gastrointestinal Complications

Oral and GI mucositis is a common, severe complication of intensive cytotoxic therapy.[85] Nausea and diarrhea accompany administration of both high-dose chemotherapy and irradiation but diminish rapidly after delivery of the agent is completed. Extensive mucosal ulceration develops during the 10 to 14 days after treatment, however, leading to recurrence of both symptoms.

Pain in the oropharynx can be debilitating, requiring massive narcotic analgesia. In both adolescents and adults, use of patient-controlled analgesia improves palliation of pain and decreases analgesic requirements.[86] Topical antibiotic treatment leads to suppression of bacterial and fungal mouth flora but does not alter the course of mucositis.[87] The airway can be compromised by secretions and local edema. In severe cases, tracheal intubation can be very difficult.

Involvement of the GI tract leads to diarrhea, abdominal pain, and intestinal bleeding.[88] Ulceration of the GI tract produces cholera-like fluid losses. The severe intestinal ulceration is commonly associated with sepsis, and necrotizing enterocolitis accompanies the most severe cases. The severe thrombocytopenia present throughout this phase complicates GI bleeding. Despite its severity, this complication is usually self-limited, resolving promptly with restoration of adequate neutrophil and platelet levels.

Pulmonary Complications

Although infections are the predominant cause of severe pulmonary toxicity after BMT, similar dysfunction has been attributed directly to chemotherapy and irradiation.[89] Drug-induced interstitial pneumonia can occur with cyclophosphamide, carmustine, and busulfan. Idiopathic interstitial pneumonia, which complicates the use of total-body irradiation, depends on total dose. Lung shielding to attenuate the total dose to the lung has been effective in decreasing the rate of this complication.[90] High irradiation dosages may increase the incidence of idiopathic interstitial pneumonia, although the overall incidence of interstitial pneumonia is not affected. Prior radiotherapy to the chest associated with the use of total-body irradiation increases the risk of interstitial pneumonia.

Treatment of interstitial pneumonia is generally ineffective. Patients requiring ventilatory support show reversibility of disease only if rapid extubation, within 4 days, is possible. Progressive interstitial pneumonia is uniformly fatal. Pulmonary function testing before BMT can identify patients at increased risk,[91] and post-BMT monitoring of diffusing capacity[92] or the detection of increased lung density on computed tomography may allow early diagnosis in affected patients.

Diffuse alveolar hemorrhage produces a syndrome of progressive dyspnea, hypoxia, cough, and diffuse consolidation on chest radiograph. It is differentiated from interstitial pneumonia by a very early onset in the post-BMT course and by the finding of hemorrhage on BAL. This complication is generally fatal, although it has been reversed with high-dose corticosteroids.[93]

Cardiac Complications

The major cardiac complications of BMT are also related to the dose-limiting toxicity of cytotoxic therapy. Cyclophosphamide, at 200 mg/kg, is dose limiting for the heart. Higher doses can cause myocardial edema, fibrosis, and cellular hypertrophy[94] as well as fibrinous pericarditis. Patients with more rapid in vivo activation of cyclophosphamide are more prone to toxicity.[82] A similar complication is seen with ifosfamide at doses of 10 to 18 g/m^2.[95] Severely affected individuals develop intractable congestive failure, usually in the first 2 weeks after BMT. In others, the changes are subclinical, consisting of an increase in left ventricular mass and impaired systolic and diastolic left ventricular function. These changes return to normal 1 year after BMT.

Many patients will have had extensive therapy with anthracyclines before undergoing BMT. The myocardial fibrosis can lead to a baseline deficit that is subsequently exacerbated by fluid overload or compromised pulmonary function. Congestive heart failure can be a component of interstitial pneumonia or hepatic VOD. In this setting, strict attention must be given to the risk of fluid overload.

Nonbacterial thrombotic endocarditis following BMT occurs at a higher frequency in autopsy series than in clinical reports, being found in approximately 8% of patients.

Hepatic Complications

Hepatic VOD is a severe liver injury characterized by progressive fibrous obliteration of the lumina of small intrahepatic venules associated with centrilobular hepatocyte degeneration and sinusoidal fibrosis, resulting in portal hypertension and liver failure. An injury to the endothelium is followed by activation of coagulation. Risk factors include preexisting liver disease and elevated serum levels of glutamate-oxalate transaminase before BMT as well as the use of methotrexate,[96] busulfan,[97] carmustine, and mitomycin C.

The diagnosis of hepatic VOD, when made on clinical grounds, is accurate in approximately 20% of patients.[98] The exact definition of the clinical criteria for hepatic VOD is important, because slight alterations in definition can lead to observed differences of 8% to 32% in the same group of patients.[99] Patients in whom early mortality rates are high are identified by the occurrence of hyperbilirubinemia greater than 34 mmol/L before day 21 after BMT, together with two of the following three features: hepatomegaly, weight gain greater than 5% of baseline, and ascites.[86] The diagnosis is confirmed by biopsy, but this procedure is often precluded by the unstable condition of the patient, including the presence of increased platelet consumption attributed to this disorder.[100] Endovenous biopsy offers an alternative. Sonograms of the liver and portal circulation showing abnormalities of flow may help in establishing the diagnosis.

Prophylactic therapy has been attempted with heparin, prostaglandin E_1, and ursodiol, a hydrophilic bile salt, with initially promising results, although a larger trial of heparin has not confirmed benefit. Thrombolytic therapy with recombinant human tissue plasminogen activator can reverse established severe VOD.[101]

Nodular regenerative hyperplasia, which can be confused with hepatic VOD, is a more common disorder after BMT. Although severe hepatic VOD is associated with high mortality, nodular regenerative hyperplasia usually has a benign course.

Renal Complications

Acute renal failure commonly occurs after allogeneic BMT.[102] Simple doubling of the serum creatinine level occurs in 53% of patients, and as many as 24% require dialysis. The potential for drug interactions is great. Cyclosporine nephrotoxicity is noted more commonly after BMT than after heart transplantation,[103] possibly indicating an interaction of cyclosporine with the cytoreductive regimens used in BMT. The use of amphotericin B in addition to cyclosporine markedly increases the risk of renal failure. In autologous BMT, acute renal failure can occur with infusion of large amounts of hemolysate in the cryopreserved bone marrow.[104] Late renal failure has been attributed to radiation nephritis. The onset of renal insufficiency, anemia, and hypertension occurs at a median of 9 months after BMT.

A common complication of high-dose cyclophosphamide, hemorrhagic cystitis affects not only the bladder but also the renal pelvis and ureters.[105] The use of either sodium-2-mercaptoethane sulfonate (Mesna) or forced saline diuresis during cyclophosphamide administration decreases the incidence and severity of this complication.[106, 107] Bladder irrigation via an indwelling catheter has been ineffective.

Hematologic Complications

Hemolytic-uremic syndrome, characterized by intravascular hemolysis, thrombocytopenia, and renal failure, can arise in association with both cyclosporine and tacrolimus. In addition, this syndrome has been noted after autologous BMT.[108] The outcome in severe cases is usually fatal. Treatment with vincristine and plasma exchange has generally provided transient benefit.

Allogeneic platelet sensitization requires strategies for platelet matching to allow adequate support. In an acute care setting, this issue can frequently be a difficult problem, because the usual adequate hemostatic levels of 50,000 or 100,000 platelets per microliter are difficult to achieve and maintain. This situation complicates respiratory management, causing pulmonary and CNS hemorrhage. Coagulopathy complicating thrombocytopenia can be attributed to vitamin K deficiency secondary to the use of broad-spectrum antibiotics or liver failure.

Endocrine and Metabolic Complications

Endocrine dysfunction following BMT has been studied primarily in children. Compensated hypothyroidism occurs in approximately 25% of children at a median time of 1 year after BMT. Growth hormone deficiency can be the cause of growth retardation. Sterility occurs with irradiation regimens in postpubertal individuals, and delay of secondary sexual characteristics is observed in children receiving a transplant before puberty. The extensive use of corticosteroids in the immediate post-BMT period and the multiplicity of organ systems showing abnormal signs make acute adrenal insufficiency hard to assess. Acutely ill patients should be assessed for adequacy of corticosteroid replacement.

The immediate post-BMT period is also associated with severe metabolic stress secondary to anorexia, mucositis, enteritis, and infection. Prophylactic total parenteral mutrition has been useful to manage this complication. A combination of partial parenteral nutrition and enteral nutrition has also been used successfully.[108] The total energy requirements for such support are uncertain. Although the normal practice is to exceed basal energy expenditure, replacement at basal levels is sufficient to maintain body weight and serum albumin with less derangement of sodium and potassium balance. Increasing the nitrogen dose without increasing calories can improve maintenance of body weight. Glutamine supplementation of parenteral nutrition can attenuate the fluid retention and expansion of the extracellular fluid compartment commonly encountered with standard parenteral formulations. In addition, nitrogen balance is improved and the incidence of infection is decreased with glutamine supplementation.[109]

INTENSIVE CARE CONSIDERATIONS

BMT units are generally organized as acute care settings dedicated to the management of the complications of high-dose chemoradiotherapy as well as the consequences of prolonged myelosuppression. The onset of severe renal, cardiac, or pulmonary failure usually necessitates an escalation of intervention, often leading to intubation and mechanical ventilation. The extent and duration of intensive care support must be chosen on the basis of the reversibility of each process affecting a patient. Seemingly severe complications involving bone marrow failure before expected engraftment, such as acute renal failure and acute sepsis, can in fact be reversed with adequate supportive care.

Invasive monitoring by intra-arterial catheterization and pulmonary artery catheterization can be maintained in the setting of neutropenia and thrombocytopenia, provided that strict sterile precautions are observed and adequate hemostasis is achieved. If possible, coagulopathy should be reversed, and a platelet count of 50,000/mL should be maintained. Because these levels cannot always be achieved, however, care should be taken to optimize these parameters as much as possible and to achieve effective local hemostatic control.

Reverse isolation and full neutropenic precautions are often compromised in an acute care setting. An attempt should be made to maintain them while patients remain neutropenic. However, once neutropenia is resolved, continued isolation techniques should focus on preventing nosocomial infections in an immunocompromised host, such as *P. carinii* and CMV infections, rather than continued precautions aimed at neutropenia alone. Segregation of BMT recipients from other infected patients in an intensive care unit is important.

The occurrence of multiple irreversible organ failure should be considered differently, because acute support has little success in this setting. Failure of more than three organ systems, septic shock, and mechanical ventilation are associated with a high mortality.[110] In patients with respiratory failure, prolonged ventilatory support for more than 4 to 7 days is generally associated with a fatal outcome.[111, 112]

SUMMARY

BMT is increasingly used successfully to treat various malignant as well as nonmalignant diseases. The toxicity of BMT has been reduced by the use of antibiotics, better transfusion support, more informed use of cytoreductive agents, prophylaxis of GVHD, the use of cytokines and peripheral blood stem cells, and earlier selection of patients for BMT. Limitations continue to be the difficulty in controlling GVHD and relapse of malignant diseases. Current research on the use of cytokines, immunomodulatory agents, new preparative regimens, and identification of histocompatibility antigens offer the hope of continued improvement in outcomes. Moreover, BMT is likely to become a means of correcting certain genetic diseases by gene transfer approaches.[113]

References

1. Zittoun RA, Mandelli F, Willemze R, et al: Autologous or allogeneic bone marrow transplantation compared with intensive chemotherapy in acute myelogenous leukemia. N Engl J Med 1995; 322:217.
2. Harousseau JL, Cahn JV, Pignon B, et al: Comparison of autologous bone marrow transplantation and intensive chemotherapy as postremission therapy in adult acute myeloid leukemia. Blood 1997; 90:2978.
3. Selvaggi KJ, Wilson J, Mills LE, et al: Improved outcome for high-risk acute myeloid leukemia patients using autologous bone marrow transplantation and monoclonal antibody purged bone marrow. Blood 1994; 83:1698.
4. Zhang M-J, Hoelzer D, Horowitz M, et al: Long-term follow-up of adults with acute lymphoblastic leukemia in first remission treated with chemotherapy or bone marrow transplantation: The Acute Lymphoblastic Leukemia Working Committee. Ann Intern Med 1995; 123:428.
5. Sheperd JD, Barnett MJ, Connors JM, et al: Allogeneic bone marrow transplantation for poor prognosis non-Hodgkin's lymphoma. Br Med J 1993; 12:591.
6. Philip T, Guguelmi C, Hagenbeek A, et al: Autologous bone marrow transplantation as compared with salvage chemotherapy in relapses of chemotherapy-sensitive non-Hodgkin's lymphoma. N Engl J Med 1995; 333:1540.
7. Martelli M, Vignetti M, Zinzani P, et al: High-dose chemotherapy followed by autologous bone marrow transplantation versus dexamethasone, cisplatin, and cytarabine in aggressive non-Hodgkin's lymphoma with partial response to front-line chemotherapy: A prospective randomized multicenter study. J Clin Oncol 1996; 14:534.
8. Verdenck LF, van Putten WLJ, Hapenbeek K, et al: Comparison of CHOP chemotherapy with autologous bone marrow transplantation for slowly responding patients with aggressive non-Hodgkin's lymphoma. N Engl J Med 1995; 332:1045.
9. Bierman PJ, Vose JM, Armitage JD: Autologous transplantation for Hodgkin's disease: Coming of age? Blood 1994; 83:1161.
10. Thomas ED, Clift R: Indications for marrow transplantation in chronic myelogenous leukemia. Blood 1989; 73:861.
11. McGlave P, Bartsh G, Anasetti C, et al: Unrelated donor marrow transplantation therapy for chronic myelogenous leukemia: Initial experience of the National Marrow Donor Program. Blood 1993; 81:453.
12. McGlave PB, DeFabritiis P, Deisseroth A, et al: Autologous transplants for chronic myelogenous leukemia: Results from eight transplant groups. Lancet 1994; 342:1486.
13. Doney K, Leisenring W, Storb R, Appelbaum FR: Primary treatment of acquired aplastic anemia: Outcomes with bone marrow transplantation and immunosuppressive therapy. Ann Intern Med 1997; 126:107.
14. Schultz AB, Geller RB, Hillyer CD: The role of bone marrow transplantation in the treatment of myelodysplastic syndromes. J Hematother 1995; 4:323.
15. Barlogie B, Alexamau R, Dicke KA, et al: High-dose chemoradiotherapy and autologous bone marrow transplantation for resistant multiple myeloma. Blood 1987; 70:869.
16. Attal M, Harousseau JL, Stoppa AM, et al: A prospective, randomized trial of autologous bone marrow transplantation and chemotherapy in multiple myeloma. Intergraph Français du myelome. N Engl J Med 1996; 335:97.
17. Bensinger WI, Rowley SD, Demirer T, et al: High-dose therapy followed by autologous hematopoietic stem-cell infusion for patients with multiple myeloma. J Clin Oncol 1996; 14:1447.
18. Antman K, Ayash L, Elias A, et al: A phase II study of high-dose cyclophosphamide, thiotepa, and carboplatin with autologous marrow support in women with measurable advanced breast cancer responding to standard-dose therapy. J Clin Oncol 1992; 10:102.
19. Peters WP, Ross M, Vredenburgh JJ, et al: High-dose chemotherapy and autologous bone marrow support as consolidation after standard-dose adjuvant therapy for high-risk primary breast cancer. J Clin Oncol 1993; 1:1132.
20. Bezwoda WR, Seymour L, Dansey RD: High-dose chemotherapy with hematopoietic rescue as primary treatment for metastatic breast cancer: A randomized trial. J Clin Oncol 1995; 13:2483.
21. Yeager A, Kaizer H, Santos G, et al: Autologous bone marrow transplantation in patients with acute nonlymphocytic leukemia using ex-vivo marrow treatment with 4-hydroperoxycyclophosphamide. N Engl J Med 1986; 315:141.
22. Shpall E, Bast RJ, Joines W, et al: Immunomagnetic purging of breast cancer from bone marrow for autologous transplantation. Bone Marrow Transplant 1991; 7:145.
23. Ball E: Immunophenotyping of acute myeloid leukemia cells. Clin Lab Med 1990; 10:721.
24. Howell A, Fogg-Leach M, Davis B, et al: Continuous infusion of complement by an automated cell processor enhances cytotoxicity of monoclonal antibody sensitized leukemia cells. Bone Marrow Transplant 1989; 4:317.
25. Ball ED, Rybka WB: Autologous bone marrow transplantation for adult acute leukemia. Hematol Oncol Clin North Am 1993; 7:201.
26. Gribben J, Freedman A, Neuberg D, et al: Immunologic purging of marrow assessed by PCR before autologous bone marrow transplantation for B-cell lymphoma. N Engl J Med 1991; 325:1525.
27. Vredenburgh J, Simpson W, Memoli V, et al: Reactivity of anti-CD15 monoclonal antibody PM-81 with breast cancer and elimination of breast cancer cells from human bone marrow by PM-81 and immunomagnetic beads. Cancer Res 1991; 51:2451.

28. Civin C, Strauss L, Brovall C, et al: Antigenic analysis of hematopoiesis: III. A hematopoietic progenitor cell surface antigen defined by a monoclonal antibody raised against KG-1a cells. J Immunol 1984; 133:157.
29. Berenson RJ, Bensinger WI, Hill RS, et al: Engraftment after infusion of CD34+ marrow cells in patients with breast cancer or neuroblastoma. Blood 1991; 77:1717.
30. Shpall EJ, LeMaistre CF, Holland K, Ball E, Jones RB, Saral R, Jacobs C, Heimfeld S, Berenson R, Champlin R: A prospective randomized trial of buffy coat versus CD34-selected autologous bone marrow support in high-risk breast cancer patients receiving high dose chemotherapy. Blood 1997; 90:4313.
31. Brenner MK, Rill DR, Moen RC, et al: Gene-marking to trace origin of relapse after autologous bone-marrow transplantation. Lancet 1993; 341:85.
32. Patterson J, Prentice HG, Brenner MK, et al: Graft rejection following HLA matched T-lymphocyte depleted bone marrow transplantation. Br J Haematol 1986; 63:221.
33. Champlin R, Ho W, Gajewski J, et al: Selective depletion of CD8+ T lymphocytes for prevention of graft-versus-host disease after allogeneic bone marrow transplantation. Blood 1990; 76:418.
34. Stockschlader M, Hassan HT, Zeller W, Kruger W, Clausen J, Loliger C, Dieck AT, Kroger N, Link H, Kabisch H, Hossfeld DK, Zander A: Allogeneic transplantation with CD34+-selected cells. Leuk Lymphoma. 1997; 25:145.
35. Poynton C: T cell depletion in bone marrow transplantation. Bone Marrow Transplant 1988; 3:265.
36. Wagner JE, Santos GW, Noga SJ, et al: Bone marrow graft engineering by counterflow centrifugal elutriation: Results of a phase I–II clinical trial. Blood 1990; 75:1370.
37. Noga SJ, Wagner JE, Santos GW, et al: Allograft lymphocyte-dose modification with counterflow centrifugal elutriation (CCE): Effects on chronic GVHD and survival in a case/control study. Blood 1991; 78:227.
38. Neudorf SML, Rybka W, Ball E, Blatt J, Bloom E, Corey S, deMagalhaes-Silverman M, Koehler M, Lister J, Mierski J, Mirro J, Pincus S, Wilson J, Wollman M, Donnenberg AD: The use of counterflow centrifugal elutriation for the depletion of T cells from unrelated donor bone marrow. J Hematother 1997; 6:351.
39. Gale RP, Horowitz MM, Butturini A, et al: What determines who develops graft-versus-host disease: The graft or the host (or both)? Bone Marrow Transplant 1992; 10:99.
40. Weisdorf D, Hakke R, Blazar B, et al: Risk factors for acute graft-versus-host disease in histocompatible donor bone marrow transplantation. Transplantation 1991; 51:1197.
41. Sloane JP, Thomas JA, Imrie SF, et al: Morphological and immunohistological changes in the skin in allogeneic bone marrow recipients. J Clin Pathol 1984; 37:919.
42. Roy J, Snover D, Weisdorf S, et al: Simultaneous upper and lower endoscopic biopsy in the diagnosis of intestinal graft-versus-host disease. Transplantation 1991; 51:642.
43. Weisdorf DJ, Snover DC, Haake R, et al: Acute upper gastrointestinal graft-versus-host disease: Clinical significance and response to immunosuppressive therapy. Blood 1990; 76:624.
44. Martin PJ, Schoch G, Fisher L, et al: A retrospective analysis of therapy for acute graft-versus-host disease: Initial treatment. Blood 1990; 76:1464.
45. Roy J, McGlave PB, Filipovich AH, et al: Acute graft-versus-host disease following unrelated bone marrow transplantation: Failure of conventional therapy. Bone Marrow Transplant 1992; 10:77.
46. Hiraoka A, Masaoka T, Asano S, et al: Phase II study of FK506 for allogeneic bone marrow transplantation. Bone Marrow Transplant 1992; 10:707.
47. Ely P, Dunitz J, Rogosheske J, et al: Use of a somatostatin analogue, octreotide acetate, in the management of acute gastrointestinal graft-versus-host disease. Am J Med 1991; 90:707.
48. Sale GE, Anderson P, Browne M, et al: Abnormal CD4:CD8 ratios and delayed germinal center reconstitution in lymph nodes of human graft recipients with graft-versus-host disease (GVHD): An immunohistological study. Exp Hematol 1992; 20:1017.
49. Ljungman P, Wilkund-Hammarsten M, Duraj V, et al: Response to tetanus toxoid immunization after allogeneic bone marrow transplantation. J Infect Dis 1990; 162:496.
50. Hess AD, Thoburn CJ: Immunobiology and immunotherapeutic implications of syngeneic/autologous graft-versus-host disease. Immunol Rev 1997; 157:111.
51. Storek J, Gooley R, Siadak M, Bensinger WI, Maloney DG, Chauncey TR, Flowers M, Sullivan KM, Witherspoon RP, Rowley SD, Hansen JA, Storb R, Appelbaum FR: Allogeneic peripheral blood stem cell transplantation may be associated with a high risk of chronic graft-versus-host disease. Blood 1997; 90:4705.
52. Holland HK, Wingard JR, Beschorner WE, et al: Bronchiolitis obliterans in bone marrow transplantation and its relationship to chronic graft-v-host disease and low serum IgG. Blood 1988; 72:621.
53. Sullivan KM, Witherspoon RP, Storb R, et al: Prednisone and azathioprine compared with prednisone and placebo for treatment of chronic graft-v-host disease: Prognostic influence of prolonged thrombocytopenia after allogeneic marrow transplantation. Blood 1988; 72:546.
54. Tzakis AG, Abu-Elmagd A, Fung JJ, et al: FK 506 rescue in chronic graft-versus-host disease after bone marrow transplantation. Transplant Proc 1991; 23:3225.
55. Vogelsang G, Farmer ER, Hess AD, et al: Thalidomide for the treatment of chronic graft-versus-host disease. N Engl J Med 1992; 326:1055.
56. Darmstadt GL, Donnenberg AD, Vogelsang GB, et al: Clinical, laboratory, and histopathologic indicators of the development of progressive acute graft-versus-host disease. J Invest Dermatol 1992; 99:397.
57. Remberger M, Ringden O, Markling L: TNF-alpha levels are increased during bone marrow transplantation conditioning in patients who develop acute GVHD. Bone Marrow Transplant 1995; 15:99.
58. van Dijk AM, Otten HG, Kessler FL, de Boer M, de Gast GC: Detection of keratinocyte-specific helper T-lymphocyte precursor cells for prediction of acute graft-versus-host-disease. Transplant Proc 1997; 29:720.
59. Karp J, Merz W, Dick J, et al: Strategies to prevent or control infections after bone marrow transplants. Bone Marrow Transplant 1991; 8:1.
60. Attal M, Schlaifer D, Rubie H, et al: Prevention of gram-positive infections after bone marrow transplantation by systemic vancomycin: A prospective, randomized trial. J Clin Oncol 1991; 9:865.
61. Valteau D, Hartmann O, Brugieres L, et al: Streptococcal septicaemia following autologous bone marrow transplantation in children treated with high-dose chemotherapy. Bone Marrow Transplant 1991; 7:415.
62. Rolston KV, Berkey P, Bodey GP, et al: A comparison of imipenem to ceftazidime with or without amikacin as empiric therapy in febrile neutropenic patients. Arch Intern Med 1992; 152:283.
63. Winston D, Ho W, Bruckner D, et al: Beta-lactam antibiotic therapy in febrile granulocytopenic patients: A randomized trial comparing cefoperazone plus piperacillin, ceftazidime plus piperacillin, and imipenem alone. Ann Intern Med 1991; 115:849.
64. Lew MA, Kehoe K, Ritz J, et al: Prophylaxis of bacterial infections with ciprofloxacin in patients undergoing bone marrow transplantation. Transplantation 1991; 51:630.
65. Karp JE, Merz WG, Charache P: Response to empiric amphotericin B during antileukemic therapy–induced granulocytopenia. Rev Infect Dis 1991; 13:592.
66. Tollemar J, Ringden O, Andersson S, et al: Prophylactic use of liposomal amphotericin B (AmBisome) against fungal infections: A randomized trial in bone marrow transplant recipients. Transplant Proc 1993; 25:1495.
67. Goodman JL, Winston DJ, Greenfield RA, et al: A controlled trial of fluconazole to prevent fungal infections in patients undergoing bone marrow transplantation. N Engl J Med 1992; 326:845.
68. Wingard J, Merz W, Rinaldi M, et al: Increase in *Candida krusei* infection among patients with bone marrow transplantation and neutropenia treated prophylactically with fluconazole. N Engl J Med 1991; 325:1274.
69. Bowden RA, Slichter SJ, Sayers MH, et al: Use of leukocyte-depleted platelets and cytomegalovirus-seronegative red blood cells for prevention of primary cytomegalovirus infection after marrow transplant. Blood 1991; 78:246.
70. Ljungman P, Aschan J, Azinge JN, et al: Cytomegalovirus viraemia and specific T-helper cell responses as predictors of disease after allogeneic marrow transplantation. Br J Haematol 1993; 83:118.
71. Emanuel D, Cunningham I, Jules-Elysee K, et al: Cytomegalovirus

pneumonia after bone marrow transplantation successfully treated with the combination of ganciclovir and high-dose intravenous immune globulin. Ann Intern Med 1988; 109:777.
72. Schmidt GM, Horak DA, Niland JC, et al: A randomized, controlled trial of prophylactic ganciclovir for cytomegalovirus pulmonary infection in recipients of allogeneic bone marrow transplants. N Engl J Med 1991; 324:1005.
72a. Goodrich JM, Mori M, Gleaves CA, Du Mond C, Cays M, Ebeling DF, Buhles WC, DeArmond B, Meyers JD: Early treatment with ganciclovir to prevent cytomegalovirus disease after allogeneic bone marrow transplantation. N Engl J Med 1991; 325:1601.
73. Winston DJ, Ho WG, Bartoni K, et al: Ganciclovir prophylaxis of cytomegalovirus infection and disease in allogeneic bone marrow transplant recipients. Ann Intern Med 1993; 118:179.
74. Goodrich JM, Bowden RA, Fisher L, et al: Ganciclovir prophylaxis to prevent cytomegalovirus disease after allogeneic marrow transplant. Ann Intern Med 1993; 118:173.
75. Drobyski WR, Dunne WM, Burd EM, et al: Human herpesvirus-6 (HHV-6) infection in allogeneic bone marrow transplant recipients: Evidence of a marrow-suppressive role for HHV-6 in vivo. J Infect Dis 1993; 167:735.
76. Schuchter LM, Wingard JR, Piantadosi S, et al: Herpes zoster infection after autologous bone marrow transplantation. Blood 1989; 74:1424.
77. Arthur RR, Shah KV, Charache P, et al: BK and JC virus infections in bone marrow transplants. J Infect Dis 1988; 158:563.
78. Tuan IZ, Dennison D, Weisdorf DJ: *Pneumocystis carinii* pneumonitis following bone marrow transplantation. Bone Marrow Transplant 1992; 10:267.
79. Derouin F, Devergie A, Auber P, et al: Toxoplasmosis in bone marrow–transplant recipients: Report of seven cases and review. Clin Infect Dis 1992; 15:267.
80. Patchell RA, White CL III, Clark AW, et al: Neurologic complications of bone marrow transplantation. Neurology 1985; 35:300.
81. Thompson CB, Sanders JE, Flournoy N, et al: The risks of central nervous system relapse and leukoencephalopathy in patients receiving marrow transplants for acute leukemia. Blood 1986; 67:195.
82. Andrykowski MA, Altmaier EM, Barnett RL, et al: Cognitive dysfunction in adult survivors of allogeneic marrow transplantation: Relationship to dose to total body radiation. Bone Marrow Transplant 1990; 6:269.
83. Reece DE, Frei-Lahr DA, Shepherd JD, et al: Neurologic complications in allogeneic bone marrow transplant patients receiving cyclosporin. Bone Marrow Transplant 1991; 8:393.
84. Eliashiv S, Brenner T, Abramsky O, et al: Acute inflammatory demyelination polyneuropathy following bone marrow transplantation. Bone Marrow Transplant 1991; 8:315.
85. Carl W, Higby DJ: Oral manifestations of bone marrow transplantation. Am J Clin Oncol 1985; 8:81.
86. Hill HF, Mackie AM, Coda BA, et al: Patient-controlled analgesic administration: A comparison of steady-state morphine infusions with bolus doses. Cancer 1991; 67:873.
87. Epstein JB, Vickars L, Spinelli J, et al: Efficacy of chlorhexidine and nystatin rinses in prevention of oral complications in leukemia and bone marrow transplantation. Oral Surg Oral Med Oral Pathol 1992; 73:682.
88. Wolford JL, McDonald GB: A problem-oriented approach to intestinal and liver disease after marrow transplantation. J Clin Gastroenterol 1988; 10:419.
89. Masaoka T, Ramsay NK, Rimm AA, et al: Risk factors for interstitial pneumonia following bone marrow transplantation for severe aplastic anemia. Br J Haematol 1989; 71:535.
90. Labar B, Bogdanic V, Nemet D, et al: Total body irradiation with or without lung shielding for allogeneic bone marrow transplantation. Bone Marrow Transplant 1992; 9:343.
91. Ghalie R, Szidon JP, Thompson L, et al: Evaluation of pulmonary complications after bone marrow transplantation: The role of pretransplant pulmonary function tests. Bone Marrow Transplant 1992; 10:359.
92. Milburn HJ, Prentice HG, duBois RM: Can lung function measurements be used to predict which patients will be at risk of developing interstitial pneumonitis after bone marrow transplantation? Thorax 1992; 47:421.
93. Chao NJ, Duncan SR, Long GD, et al: Corticosteroid therapy for diffuse alveolar hemorrhage in autologous bone marrow transplant recipients. Ann Intern Med 1991; 114:145.
94. Kupari M, Volin L, Suokas A, et al: Cardiac involvement in bone marrow transplantation: Electrocardiographic changes, arrhythmias, heart failure and autopsy findings. Bone Marrow Transplant 1990; 5:91.
95. Ayash LJ, Wright JE, Tretyakov O, et al: Cyclophosphamide pharmacokinetics: Correlation with cardiac toxicity and tumor response. J Clin Oncol 1992; 10:995.
96. Quezado ZM, Wilson WH, Cunnion RE, et al: High-dose ifosfamide is associated with severe, reversible cardiac dysfunction. Ann Intern Med 1993; 118:31.
97. Essell JH, Thompson JM, Harman GS, et al: Marked increase in veno-occlusive disease of the liver associated with methotrexate use for graft-versus-host disease prophylaxis in patients receiving busulfan/cyclophosphamide. Blood 1992; 79:2784.
98. Meresse V, Hartmann O, Vassal G, et al: Risk factors for hepatic veno-occlusive disease after a high-dose busulfan-containing regimen followed by autologous bone marrow transplantation: A study in 136 children. Bone Marrow Transplant 1992; 10:135.
99. Blostein MD, Paltiel OB, Thibault A, et al: A comparison of clinical criteria for the diagnosis of veno-occlusive disease of the liver after bone marrow transplantation. Bone Marrow Transplant 1992; 10:439.
100. Rio B, Andreu G, Nicod A, et al: Thrombocytopenia in veno-occlusive disease after bone marrow transplantation. Blood 1986; 67:1773.
101. Bearman SI, Lee JL, Baron AE, McDonald GB: Treatment of hepatic venocclusive disease with recombinant human tissue plasminogen activator and heparin in 42 marrow transplant patients. Blood 1997; 89:1501.
102. Zager RA, O'Quigley J, Zager BK, et al: Acute renal failure following bone marrow transplantation: A retrospective study of 272 patients. Am J Kidney Dis 1989; 13:210.
103. Nizze H, Mihatsch MJ, Zollinger HU, et al: Cyclosporine-associated nephropathy in patients with heart and bone marrow transplants. Clin Nephrol 1988; 30:248.
104. Smith DM, Weisenburger DD, Bierman P, et al: Acute renal failure associated with autologous bone marrow transplantation. Bone Marrow Transplant 1987; 2:195.
105. Efros M, Ahmed T, Choudhury M: Cyclophosphamide-induced hemorrhagic pyelitis and ureteritis associated with cystitis in marrow transplantation. J Urol 1990; 144:1231.
106. Hows JM, Mehta A, Ward L, et al: Comparison of mesna with forced diuresis to prevent cyclophosphamide induced haemorrhagic cystitis in marrow transplantation: A prospective randomised study. Br J Cancer 1984; 50:753.
107. Shepherd JD, Pringle LE, Barnett MJ, et al: Mesna versus hyperhydration for the prevention of cyclophosphamide-induced hemorrhagic cystitis in bone marrow transplantation. J Clin Oncol 1991; 9:2016.
108. Rabinowe SN, Soiffer RJ, Tarbell NJ, et al: Hemolytic-uremic syndrome following bone marrow transplantation in adults for hematologic malignancies. Blood 1991; 77:1837.
109. Mulder PO, Bouman JG, Gietema JA, et al: Hyperalimentation in autologous bone marrow transplantation for solid tumors: Comparison of total parenteral versus partial parenteral plus enteral nutrition. Cancer 1989; 64:2045.
110. Ziegler TR, Young LS, Benfell K, et al: Clinical and metabolic efficacy of glutamine-supplemented parenteral nutrition after bone marrow transplantation: A randomized, double-blind, controlled study. Ann Intern Med 1992; 116:821.
111. Torrecilla C, Cortes JL, Chamorro C, et al: Prognostic assessment of the acute complications of bone marrow transplantation requiring intensive therapy. Intensive Care Med 1988; 14:393.
112. Afessa B, Tefferi A, Hoagland HC, et al: Outcome of recipients of bone marrow transplants who require intensive-care unit support. Mayo Clin Proc 1992; 67:117.
113. Blau HM, Springer ML: Gene therapy—a novel form of drug delivery. N Engl J Med 1995; 333:1204.

159

Diagnosis and Management of Bleeding Disorders

Nils U. Bang, MD, PhD

Approximately 80,000 patients in the United States die every year as a result of uncontrollable generalized bleeding arising from congenital or acquired coagulation defects. In contrast, thrombotic disorders remain the leading causes of death in the United States and most of the Western world. Most commonly, death is caused by thrombi formed at sites of atheromatous lesions that result in heart attacks and strokes; venous thromboembolism also contributes a sizeable number of fatalities. Considered together, generalized bleeding problems and thrombotic disorders occur in all specialties of medicine and surgery. Rapid establishment of an accurate diagnosis and institution of correct therapy represent the major challenges facing critical care physicians today.

The information gained from a careful history and physical examination almost never suffices to establish a correct diagnosis of an unknown bleeding disorder or a suspected case of venous thromboembolism. The final diagnosis of coagulopathies is made in the laboratory. To choose and to order the proper laboratory tests and then to interpret the results correctly, a critical care physician must have substantial knowledge of the principal physiologic features of normal hemostasis as well as the pathophysiology of bleeding disorders and thrombotic events.

NORMAL HEMOSTASIS

In simplistic terms, the cessation of bleeding from a severed blood vessel occurs in two well-defined phases. At the site of vascular injury, blood platelets come in contact with subendothelial connective tissue, most notably microfibrils[1] and collagen.[2] Although platelets do not adhere to normal endothelial cells, they have a strong affinity for subendothelial connective tissue, particularly collagen, and they stick to collagen exposed when a vessel is severed. Contact with collagen activates platelets, setting in motion a series of complex events: the generation of the prostaglandin thromboxane A_2[3] and activation of the cyclic adenosine monophosphate (cAMP) and the inositol triphosphate–diacylglycerol messenger systems.[4–6] The net result is the secretion from the platelet of most substances normally stored in the so-called alpha granules and dense bodies readily visible in the platelet by electron microscopy. Released substances include adenine nucleotides, particularly adenosine diphosphate, catecholamines, serotonin, and thromboxane A_2, all substances that cause platelets to aggregate (i.e., cause more platelets to stick to the platelets already adhering to the collagen of the vessel wall).[7] A platelet plug is eventually formed, constituting a temporary seal of the injured vessel.

For this seal to become permanent, stabilized fibrin must form in and around the platelet plug. The activated platelet undergoes dramatic membrane changes, making possible the assembly of clotting factors on the platelet surface that cooperatively generate large quantities of thrombin,[8] the enzyme ultimately responsible for clotting of fibrinogen. Thrombin also is a potent activator of platelets, which attracts more platelets to the aggregate and further consolidates the seal.

Thrombin and activators of platelets also activate a key platelet membrane glycoprotein (GP) complex, GP IIb-IIIa, on platelet surfaces. GP IIb-IIIa molecules interact with sticky plasma protein molecules, most notably fibrinogen (see later). One fibrinogen molecule connecting two activated GP IIb-IIIa complexes will stick adjacent platelets together; this action represents the essential final event of the platelet aggregation process.

It is easy to comprehend, then, that patients can bleed for three different reasons, as follows:

1. The platelets may be too scarce; therefore, insufficient platelets are available to form the initial hemostatic plug.
2. Platelets may be present in normal numbers but function abnormally. These platelets either adhere poorly to subendothelial connective tissue or activate sluggishly, thereby slowing or abolishing the formation of an aggregate.
3. If a patient's fibrin-forming mechanism is abnormal, the initial hemostatic plug forms normally; however, if no fibrin is available to reinforce the primary plug, platelets deaggregate, the plug washes away, and rebleeding is likely to occur.

If a patient is admitted with a history or physical findings of spontaneous hemorrhages into the skin (petechiae and ecchymoses), mucous membrane bleeding, including nosebleeds, or bleeding from the gastrointestinal tract, thrombocytopenia or a platelet function disorder should be considered. If, on the other hand, a patient appears with a history of physical findings of bleeding into the muscles, bones, or joints, a defect in the fibrin-forming mechanism may be primarily suspected. These guidelines are not without exception, and the precise diagnosis requires a laboratory examination.

PLATELET DISORDERS

Quantitative Platelet Disorders

If a platelet count of less than 50,000 to 100,000 cells/mm^3 is detected and found to be decreased on evaluation of the peripheral blood smear, a bone marrow examination should be conducted early in any patient with atypical features or in patients older than 60 years or if splenectomy is being considered. This bone marrow examination serves to estimate the bone marrow megakaryocytes to aid in the diagnosis of megakaryocytic versus amegakaryocytic thrombocytopenia.

The major causes of decreased bone marrow megakaryocytes (Table 159–1) include:

1. Bone marrow infiltration by metastatic tumors, leukemic cells, and sometimes infectious granulomas.
2. Bone marrow dysplasia.
3. Bone marrow aplasia secondary to exposure to chemicals or drugs, with thiazide diuretics and ethanol heading the list, in addition to ionizing radiation.

Megakaryocytic thrombocytopenia can, on rare occasions, be congenital or hereditary. Conditions producing thrombocytopenia at birth include constitutional aplastic anemia (Fanconi's syndrome)[9] and certain types of thrombocytopenia with congenital malformations as well as sex-linked thrombocytopenia (Wiskott-Aldrich syndrome).[10] Megaloblastic anemia secondary to folic acid or vitamin B_{12} deficiency produces ineffective megakaryocytopoiesis and, in severe cases, a sharply reduced number of megakaryocytes in the bone marrow.[11] Likewise, severe iron deficiency anemia, which is commonly accompanied by thrombocytopenia, can occasionally result in ineffective megakararyocytopoiesis and decreased numbers of megakaryocytes in the bone marrow.

TABLE 159–1. Amegakaryocytic Thrombocytopenias

Bone Marrow Infiltration with:
- Tumor cells
- Leukemic cells
- Infectious granulomas (rare)

Bone Marrow Dysplasia

Myeloproliferative Disorders
- (Myelofibrosis)

Bone Marrow Aplasia
- Primary
- Secondary to chemicals or drugs (e.g., thiazide diuretics, ethanol), ionizing radiation

Hereditary Disorders
- Fanconi's syndrome
- Thrombocytopenia with congenital malformations
- X-linked thrombocytopenia (Wiskott-Aldrich syndrome)

Ineffective Megakaryocytopoiesis
- Vitamin B_{12} deficiency
- Folate deficiency
- Iron deficiency (rare)

Infections

Many bacterial, viral, and rickettsial infections are complicated by thrombocytopenia. Several mechanisms have been implicated, including suppression of platelet production and increased platelet destruction. The demonstration of thrombocytopenia in the infected patient must always prompt an evaluation for disseminated intravascular coagulation (see later). Thrombocytopenia is common in patients with acquired immunodeficiency syndrome (AIDS) and is seen in patients with only serologic evidence of human immunodeficiency virus (HIV).[12]

If a bone marrow examination demonstrates a normal or increased number of megakaryocytes, several differential diagnostic possibilities are considered (Table 159–2). Thrombocytopenia can occur because of altered distribution of platelets. Normally, 20% of platelets reside in the spleen and 80% circulate in the blood. When the spleen is substantially enlarged for various reasons, the splenic pool increases (i.e., the number of platelets sequestered in the spleen rises).[13] Depending on the severity of splenomegaly, the normal blood-to-spleen platelet distribution of 80% to 20% can be reduced or, in severe cases, reversed. The enlarged spleen may cause a reduction in the platelet count because of simple redistribution between peripheral and splenic pools. Patients with splenomegaly, as encountered in portal hypertension, also show evidence of enhanced platelet destruction by the spleen, or *hypersplenism.* Both platelets and red blood cells can be mechanically destroyed during cardiopulmonary bypass procedures.[14] Finally, platelets can be destroyed in the circulation through immune mechanisms (Table 159–3).

TABLE 159–2. Megakaryocytic Thrombocytopenias

1. Altered distribution of platelets (splenomegaly)
2. Enhanced destruction of platelets in the circulation
   a. Disseminated intravascular coagulation
   b. Thrombotic thrombocytopenic purpura
   c. Hypersplenism
   d. Prosthetic heart valves
   e. Immune thrombocytopenias

TABLE 159–3. Immune Thrombocytopenias

Secondary to
- Multiple transfusions (isoantibodies)
- Drugs
- Post-transfusion (in PL1-negative individuals, alloantibodies)
- Lymphomas
- Chronic lymphocytic leukemia
- Collagen vascular disease
- Viral infections (acute "ITP")

Idiopathic Thrombocytopenic Purpura

Thrombotic Thrombocytopenic Purpura and Hemolytic-Uremic Syndrome

Thrombotic thrombocytopenic purpura (TTP) and its close relative the hemolytic-uremic syndrome (HUS) are rare disorders in which platelets are consumed through deposition in the microcirculation. HUS is a clinical syndrome consisting of the triad of hemolytic anemia, thrombocytopenia, and acute renal failure. Substantial evidence exists for a common association between HUS and certain cytotoxin-producing bacterial agents, particularly *Escherichia coli* serotype O157:H7.[15, 16] An episode of gastroenteritis that is frequently hemorrhagic precedes the onset of HUS in about 90% of cases. Upper respiratory infections have also been noted.[16] The infectious phase is followed several weeks later by signs of acute renal failure, thrombocytopenia, and microangiopathic hemolytic anemia.

The diagnosis of TTP is suspected if a patient is admitted with a constellation of renal impairment, central nervous system manifestations, fever, hemolytic anemia, and thrombocytopenia. At presentation, 80% of patients may be expected to have a triad consisting of hemolytic anemia, thrombocytopenia, and neurologic dysfunction that can start as a sudden change in personality or mental status. One third of patients present with a picture that includes renal dysfunction and fever. Elevated lactate dehydrogenase (LDH) correlates well with TTP-HUS and is higher than for other hemolytic anemias. Prodromal bloody diarrhea, although not nearly as common as in HUS, is occasionally seen in TTP. Although a common etiologic denominator for these two syndromes has not been established, it is strongly suspected that TTP and HUS are closely related variants of the same disease entity. There appears to be higher incidence of TTP and HUS among patients with a diagnosis of HIV. Most of the patients respond well to plasma exchange. If this standard regimen is unsuccessful, salvage splenectomy produces complete response in most cases.

Idiopathic Autoimmune Thrombocytopenic Purpura

The diagnosis of idiopathetic autoimmune thrombocytopenic purpura (ITP)[17] is primarily one of exclusion.[17] Before the diagnosis is made, collagen vascular disease, especially systemic lupus erythematosus (SLE), leukemia, and lymphomas must be rigidly excluded. About 90% of cases of acute ITP occur in children and are characterized by an abrupt onset of severe thrombocytopenia with a benign course, resolving in more than 80% of cases within 6 weeks to 6 months. A viral illness commonly precedes it. Ten per cent of acute cases occur in adults, and these patients also recover irrespective of treatment.

Treatment of Acute ITP

What constitutes the optimal treatment regimen in acute ITP, the criteria for initiating treatment, and the predictors for response to treatment are questions under active discussion. Guidelines for diagnosis and treatment for acute ITP in an adult or children include the following measures: Severe hemorrhage with thrombocytopenia in an adult or pediatric patient warrants intervention, the administration of immunoglobulin G (IgG), 1 g/kg intravenously (IV) for one dose, or parenteral glucocorticoids (e.g., methylprednisolone, 30 mg/kg/day) for up to 3 days in adults and children. Some but not all researchers recommend platelet transfusions. Adults with platelet counts at certain levels more commonly have hemorrhagic complications than children with similar platelet numbers. Hospitalization is also recommended for adults and children without major bleeding when the platelet count is less than 20,000 cells/mm^3. When mucous membrane bleeding that may require intervention is present, follow-up must be adequate and appropriate. There is strong disagreement regarding splenectomy, even in children with severe bleeding at presentation.

Children with acute ITP and with platelet counts greater than 20,000 cells/mm^3 who are asymptomatic may be observed initially. In contrast, observation as initial treatment of an adult is recommended only if the platelet count is greater than 50,000 mm^3 and the patient is asymptomatic or displays only minor purpura and ecchymoses and is without a risk factor, such as hypertension, peptic ulcer disease, age older than 60 years, or vigorous life style. No consensus has been reached allowing recommendation for one method of treatment in adults whose platelet counts lie between 20,000 and 50,000 cells/mm^3 even if they are asymptomatic.

Treatment of Chronic ITP

Whereas ITP in childhood is usually acute and transient, the condition in adults is usually chronic. Antibodies are usually directed against circulating platelets, but megakaryocyte damage may also occur in some patients. The first-line treatment in adult ITP is corticosteroid therapy followed by splenectomy, but fewer than 10% of patients are cured by short-term corticosteroid therapy alone. Platelet count increases to 50,000 to 100,000 cells/mm^3 usually within 7 to 14 days, although up to 6 weeks may be required. In most of these patients, however, thrombocytopenia recurs during tapering of the steroid dosage.

The next step is splenectomy. Approximately 70% of patients achieve a normal platelet count after splenectomy, and 10% to 20% of splenectomized patients are found to have less severe thrombocytopenia after splenectomy than before. The operative mortality from splenectomy is less than 1%. An important part of an early splenectomy failure or later relapse of disease is the presence of an auxiliary spleen, which can usually be detected by radionuclide scanning using iridium-labeled platelets. Patients with immune thrombocytopenia commonly have underlying diseases, such as SLE and rheumatoid arthritis. Of some concern in splenectomized patients are the long-term complications of overwhelming bacterial septicemia, particularly pneumococcal septicemia; however, in patients who have undergone splenectomy for ITP, this risk may be relatively low. Perioperative bleeding complications are relatively uncommon even for severely thrombocytopenic patients. Thus, platelet transfusions are usually not given. In patients who have previously received corticosteroid therapy, therapy is usually reinstituted during surgery to prevent adrenal insufficiency.

Among patients who remain severely thrombocytopenic after splenectomy (10% to 20% in the adult population), many treatments have been suggested, but most are only partly successful or are unsuccessful. Most researchers today recommend azathioprine, vincristine, or cyclophosphamide. Azathioprine therapy has resulted in complete or partial remissions in 40% to 50% of patients in whom splenectomy failed to ameliorate ITP.

Drug-Induced Immune Thrombocytopenia[18]

Most hematology textbooks provide lists of hundreds of drugs implicated in drug-induced immune thrombocytopenia, the most important offenders being quinidine and quinine. Sulfonamides are also common offenders. The thrombocytopenia is often accompanied by bleeding. Treatment of drug-induced immune thrombocytopenia consists of immediate discontinuation of the drug and, in patients with severe thrombocytopenia or bleeding, addition of IV IgG. Platelet transfusions can be given, but the benefit of corticosteroids is uncertain.

Heparin-Induced Thrombocytopenia

Heparin-induced thrombocytopenia (HIT) has been reported at widely different frequencies in different populations,[19, 20] but it is probably the most common drug-induced thrombocytopenia. According to most authorities, it occurs in approximately 5% of patients receiving heparin derived from porcine intestinal mucosa and slightly more commonly in patients receiving heparin derived from bovine lung. Thrombocytopenia occurs with unfractionated heparin and low-molecular-weight heparin[21] and also with synthetic antithrombotic glycosaminoglycans, such as pentosan polysulfate.

The clinical picture of HIT differs from that of other drug-induced thrombocytopenia. When heparin is the cause of thrombocytopenia, bleeding is relatively uncommon, but venous or arterial thromboses are common features. In all carefully examined cases of HIT the antigen may be a complex between the highly positively charged protein platelet factor 4 (PF_4) and heparin. PF_4 is secreted from activated platelet and is also found on cell membranes combined with heparan or heparin sulfate molecules. When these heparin-PF_4 complexes interact with specific antibodies, platelets and endothelial cells are destroyed, resulting in intravascular thrombosis. Platelet-rich white clots that adhere to the vessel wall are characteristic of HIT.

Two tests are available in the diagnosis of the syndrome: (1) an immunoassay specific for heparin-PF_4 antibodies and (2) a test that quantifies the ability of heparin to release radioactive carbon–labeled serotonin from platelets. The immunoassay for antibodies to heparin-PF_4 has improved the diagnosis of HIT and may have predictive value in monitoring heparin therapy.

For treating the syndrome, there is no universal agreement other than discontinuing heparin. Low-molecular-weight heparin is not recommended if unfractionated heparin appears to be the culprit because cross-reactivity occurs in vitro and more often in vivo. The compound danaparoid sodium, a non-heparin mixture of sulfated glycosaminoglycans, is preferred by most experienced clinicians. The specific antithrombin hirudin (recombinant) has been claimed to be useful and effective in isolated instances, but its availability in the United States is limited.

Post-transfusion Purpura[22]

Although ITP accounts for most of the immune-mediated cases of thrombocytopenia seen in adults, an acquired, potentially life-threatening cause of thrombocytopenia is post-transfusion purpura (PTP). This disorder represents an immune response to certain platelet surface antigens resulting in platelet destruction. PTP generally occurs as an anamnestic response in an individual previously exposed to blood products through transfusion or pregnancy; however, PTP occurs on rare occasions in naive individuals as a primary immune response.

The basic clinical presentation is usually sudden bleeding with the onset of thrombocytopenia within 1 to 14 days after transfusion in a recipient whose acute serum specimen contains antibodies to platelets of normal donors or who has the platelet antigen PLA-I (HPA-I A). If a platelet product used in a transfusion happens to contain antibodies against the recipient's platelet antigen, PTP can result.

Qualitative Platelet Disorders

Three major types of functional platelet syndromes are recognized:

- Defective or absent protein complex
- Defective or absent GPIG-V-IX
- von Willebrand disease

Integrins are glycoprotein receptor-like surface protein complexes that typically stick individual cells together to make organs or tissues. A major integrin concerned with platelet function is GPIIb-IIIa.[23] Genetic molecular abnormalities can cause the absence of GPIIb-IIIa, giving rise to Glanzmann's thrombasthenia. The lack of functional GPIIb-IIIa molecules in this disorder prevents the platelets from binding fibrinogen molecules, an event necessary for normal platelet aggregation.

The second integrin defect, dysfunction or absence of GPIG-V-IX, results in the Bernard-Soulier syndrome. GPIG-V-IX uses von Willebrand factor (see later) to bridge platelets to vascular connective tissue.

The third type of disorder, von Willebrand's disease, represents not a primary platelet disorder but, rather, a defect of a cofactor protein, the von Willebrand factor. As mentioned previously, von Willebrand factor promotes platelet adhesion by interacting with the GPIG-V-IX integrin on the platelet surface,[24] bridging this structure to vascular connective tissue.

The exact diagnosis of a platelet function disorder, and especially the many subtypes of von Willebrand's disease, requires a specialized coagulation laboratory and a hematology consultation. In the acute setting, having established the diagnosis, the physician can use platelet transfusions. In most instances, a concentrate of von Willebrand factor found in cryoprecipitate from normal plasma is helpful. One should keep in mind that cryoprecipitate is contraindicated in certain subtypes of von Willebrand's disease. An alternative that has become available is recombinant von Willebrand factor protein.

Drug-Induced Platelet Dysfunction

Of far greater clinical significance than congenital platelet disorders are the drug-induced platelet functional disorders. Platelet dysfunction can be caused by many classes of commonly used drugs, including the nonsteroidal anti-inflammatory agents (with aspirin heading the list), β-blockers, slow calcium channel blockers, local anesthetic-type antiarrhythmic drugs, and a number of commonly used β-lactam antibiotics.

DISORDERS OF THE COAGULATION SYSTEM

Normal Blood Coagulation

Figure 159-1 represents the classic concepts of the coagulation system.[25, 26] According to international agreement, individual coagulation proteins are assigned Roman numerals, and their activated counterparts have Roman numerals plus the letter *a*. Blood coagulation is best viewed as a chain reaction involving serine proteases and cofactors.

The clotting factor serine proteases normally circulate as inactive proenzymes. When the first enzyme of the coagulation cascade is activated, the activated serine protease makes a clip and splits certain peptide bonds in the next proenzyme link in the chain, thereby activating it; from this sequence of conversions of the inactive zymogen precursors to active serine protease through limited proteolysis, the enzyme thrombin finally emerges. Thrombin makes four clips in the fibrinogen molecule, the soluble plasma protein precursor of fibrin, converting fibrinogen into fibrin monomer. Fibrin monomer in turn spontaneously lines up with other fibrin molecules in a polymerization reaction, producing the network gel fibrin.

Classically, two pathways of coagulation are recognized, an intrinsic pathway and an extrinsic pathway. The intrinsic pathway is so named because it operates strictly with components contained in the blood. The extrinsic pathway is so named because it requires, in addition to blood components, a tissue factor available in many cells, including monocytes and endothelial cells. For certain steps in the chain reaction—that is, conversion of factor IX into factor IXa by factor XIa or VIIa; conversion of factor X to factor Xa by Factor IXa or factor VIIa; and conversion of prothrombin (factor II) to thrombin (factor IIa)—phospholipid bilayer membranes and ionized calcium (Ca^{2+}) are required. Intrinsic as well as extrinsic blood coagulation does not occur without Ca^{2+}.

Key steps in the coagulation reaction occur on cell surfaces. These interphase phenomena can take place on platelets, monocytes, polymorphonuclear leukocytes, and even endothelial cells. The system operates very poorly in solution unless phospholipid liposomes, substituting for the cell bilayer membrane, are added. Table 159-4 depicts the biochemical classification of proteins involved in blood coagulation. The final substrate in the reaction is fibrinogen, which is converted into fibrin by thrombin.

The enzymes involved in coagulation are serine proteases, close relatives of trypsin, chymotrypsin, and plasmin, with the exception of factor XIII, or fibrin-stabilizing factor, which is a transpeptidase, an enzyme capable of forming new peptide

TABLE 159-4. Blood Coagulation Proteins

	Enzymes		
Final Substrate	***Transpeptidase***	***Serine Proteases***	***Cofactors***
Fibrinogen	Factor XIII	Factor XII	High-molecular-weight kininogen
		Prekallikrein	
		Factor XI	
		Factor IX	Factor VII
		Factor X	Factor V
		Factor VII	Tissue factor
		Factor II	

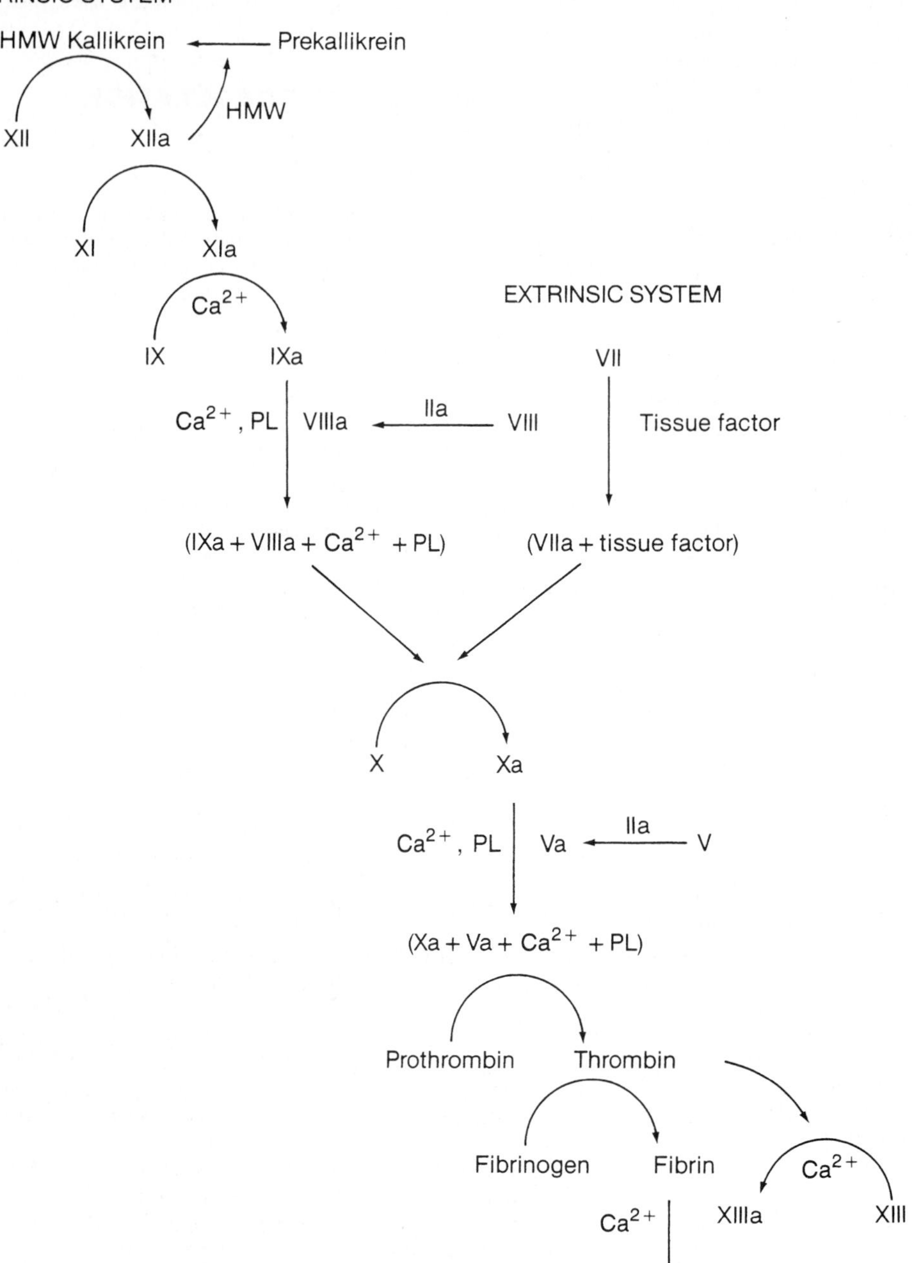

Figure 159–1. Diagram of the coagulation system (see text).

bonds. This enzyme introduces new peptide bonds into fibrin, making the fibrin clot mechanically stronger as well as more resistant to degradation by proteolytic enzymes. The serine proteases of the system are factor XII, or Hageman factor, prekallikrein, factors XI, IX, X, and VII, and factor II, or prothrombin.

In addition, the system makes use of cofactor proteins that in themselves posses no enzymatic activity but that are of critical importance in the activation of the individual clotting factors of the cascade. Cofactors exist in the circulation as relatively inactive precursors that are activated by serine proteases, usually thrombin. The activated serine proteases, the activated cofactor, and the zymogen to be activated must align in a spatially correct fashion in the presence of Ca^{2+} on the cell surface to produce optimal enzyme kinetics for the interactions. Membrane surfaces or phospholipid micelles and calcium ions, through conversion of cofactor V to Va and cofactor VIII to VIIIa, enhance thrombin generation approximately 500,000-fold. A major role of thrombin is to produce more thrombin through this highly effective self-generating system.

These classic theories of blood coagulation, the cascade or waterfall hypotheses, have not stood the test of time. It has become apparent that the sharp distinction between the intrinsic and extrinsic pathways in blood coagulation cannot be maintained.[27] It was first observed that factor VIIa of the extrinsic pathway activates not only factor X but also factor IX of the intrinsic pathway; factor IXa then activates factor X to Xa. This is an important discovery because it is difficult to explain the major bleeding problems arising in hemophilia A (factor VIII deficiency) or hemophilia B (factor IX deficiency) with the classic theory. The extrinsic pathway, according to the old theory, enters at the level of factor X, producing clotting in the absence of either factor VIII or factor IX.

Figure 159-2 depicts the more recent concept, which places heavy emphasis on the extrinsic pathway. In this scheme, tissue factor in consort with factor VIIa activates factors IX and X. Factor VIIa combined with tissue factor also activates factor VII. A major new inhibitor in the system (tissue factor pathway inhibitor [TFPI]) has been identified, cloned, and expressed and its complete primary structure has been determined. The activity of TFPI, like the activity of antithrombin III, is substantially increased by heparin. It should also be noted from Figure 159-2 that thrombin, the final enzyme in the coagulation cascade, can generate more thrombin by activating factor XI to factor XIa and also, as mentioned, through activation of the cofactors VIII and V. It is through these mechanisms that thrombin initially can generate 500,000-fold more thrombin through positive feedback loops.

According to the new scheme of coagulation, in the early phases of the intrinsic pathway, also known as the contact phase, the activation of factor XII to XIIa and of factor XI to XIa are assigned only a secondary role in blood coagulation. However, Hageman factor (factor XII) appears to play a significant role in the activation of other systems, such as the prekallikrein-kinin system, which is important in acute and chronic inflammation; the fibrinolytic enzyme system, which results in the dissolution of fibrin clots; and, perhaps, the complement system.

Clinical Considerations

In the practical diagnosis of an unknown defect of hemostasis, as previously mentioned, petechiae, ecchymoses, and mucous membrane bleeding with or without bleeding elsewhere point to a quantitative or qualitative platelet disorder. If a patient is admitted with inappropriate bleeding into muscles, bones, or joints, however, the physician should primarily suspect a defect in the fibrin-forming mechanism. If there is a positive family history, the disorder may be one of the inherited hemophilias; if the history suggests otherwise, the cause may be one of the acquired coagulation disorders.

It is essential to obtain a detailed history for a constitutional bleeding disorder, for several reasons. Most inherited bleeding disorders, certainly hemophilias A and B (factor VIII and factor IX deficiency, respectively) exist in all degrees of severity. The textbook descriptions of these disorders largely refer to severe hemophilia, in which frequent spontaneous hemorrhages into joints and tissues lead to crippling joint deformities.

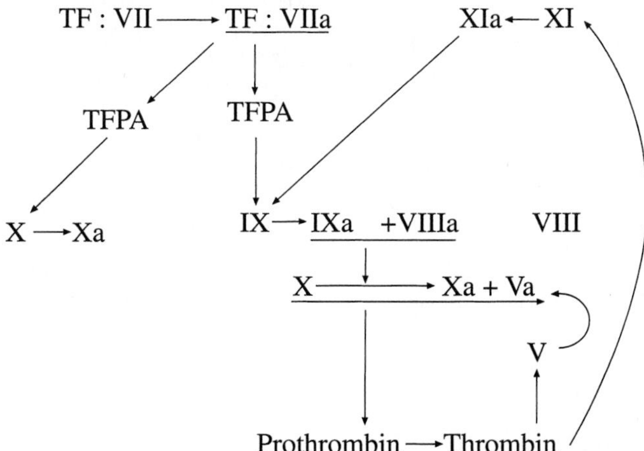

Figure 159–2. Relevant steps in blood coagulation, current concepts. Tissue factor (TF) can convert factor VII to VIIa. Factor VIIa converts factor X to Xa and factor IX to IXa, leading to increased thrombin generation. Note also positive feedback loops in thrombin generation via conversion of factor VIII to VIIIa, factor V to Va and factor XI to XIa. Tissue factor pathway inhibitor (TFPI), an important inhibitor in this system, is capable of inhibiting factors VIIa and Xa. The inhibitory effect of TFPI is augmented by heparin.

The clinical course of the mild to moderate cases of hemophilia is much less appreciated; the diagnosis of these cases commonly is not made until serious or even life-threatening hemorrhage appears as a result of surgery or a major injury, to the surprise of the patient as well the physician. In evaluating a bleeding history, it is therefore important to ask detailed, specific questions about surgery and trauma. It has been shown that many normal healthy people consider their bleeding or bruising excessive. It is also established that patients with mild or moderate abnormalities, as seen, for instance, in von Willebrand's disease and platelet function disorders such as storage pool disease, may not be recognized as having excessive bleeding symptoms. Von Willebrand's disease is the most common hereditary bleeding disorder, and studies have shown that one third to one half of people known to have either von Willebrand's disease or platelet function defects do not identify themselves as having a bleeding disorder.

When interviewing patients with recurrent bleeding problems, the physician should suspect hemophilia or other constitutional bleeding disorders in a patient whose bleeding lasts more than 24 hours after surgery. When obtaining a history for the neonatal period, it is important to remember that even severe hemophiliacs often endure the major trauma of delivery without bleeding complications. This protection of the newborn is not caused by transplacental transfer of maternal clotting factors, because clotting factors in severe hemophiliacs were demonstrated to be totally absent in cord blood. This protection lasts for the first week or two of the child's life, and circumcision performed in a hemophiliac during the first few days of life may not cause excessive bleeding. The first symptom is tendency to bruising occurring within the first 3 to 6 months of life; toward the end of the first year, an affected child becomes more susceptible to injuries, and this is the time when serious bleeding abnormalities begin to occur in severely afflicted individuals.

Several points about the family history also need to be emphasized. The two major types of hemophilia, A and B, are transmitted by the sex-linked recessive mode of inheritance. When a male carries the abnormal gene located in the X chromosome, he is affected by the disease, when a female carries the abnormal gene, she is a carrier. Therefore, all daughters of an affected man are carriers because they inherit his abnormal X chromosome. None of his sons is affected, however, because they derive the single X chromosome from their mother.

The offspring of a female carrier have a 50% chance of inheriting the abnormal X chromosome, which causes disease in the male and a carrier state in the female. Hemophilia A and hemophilia B are the only two congenital bleeding disorders transmitted in this manner. Deficiencies in all other clotting factors as well as platelet function disorders are inherited by other mechanisms. Thus, all congenital bleeding disorders with the exception of hemophilia A and B affect males and females equally. However, 25% to 30% of cases of hemophilia A and about 20% of cases of hemophilia B appear de novo, that is, with a *negative* family history. These de novo cases are almost always severe and must represent gene mutations in recent generations.

Thus, the diagnosis of a constitutional clotting factor deficiency can never be made on the basis of history or physical examination alone; a series of simple laboratory tests is required for the diagnosis to be unequivocally established.

Figure 159-3 is a simplified scheme that divides the clotting reactions into three boxes. Clotting factors in *Box No. 1,* factors XII, XI, IX, and VIII (in addition to prekallikrein and high-molecular-weight kininogen), are the four factors strictly involved in the intrinsic mechanism. *Box No. 2* contains only one clotting factor, factor VII, the only factor needed in the extrinsic but not the intrinsic pathway. *Box No. 3* contains four factors (X, V, II, and I). These factors are required in the final activation steps that are common for both pathways, extrinsic and intrinsic. This box system, although not in agreement with today's concepts, which emphasize the extrinsic pathway, is convenient because it explains how to use two simple routine clotting tests—the prothrombin time (PT) test and the activated partial thromboplastin time (aPTT) test—to help in establishing the diagnosis of an unknown constitutional bleeding disorder.

To determine the PT, it is necessary to mix the patient's plasma, a source of the tissue factor necessary to activate the extrinsic mechanism, and calcium ions (Fig. 159-4). Prolongation of PT denotes that the extrinsic pathway is no longer intact. The affected factor may be one of five:

- Proconvertin, or factor VII
- Stuart factor, or factor X
- AC (accelerator) globulin, or factor V
- Prothrombin, or factor II
- Fibrinogen, or factor I.

The PT does not measure factors that are concerned strictly with the intrinsic mechanism:

- Hageman's factor, or factor XII
- PTA (plasma thromboplastic antecedent), or factor XI
- Christmas factor, or factor IX
- Antihemophilic globulin, or factor VIII

Factors VIII and IX, which are deficient in the more common forms of hemophilia, are not registered by an abnormal PT.

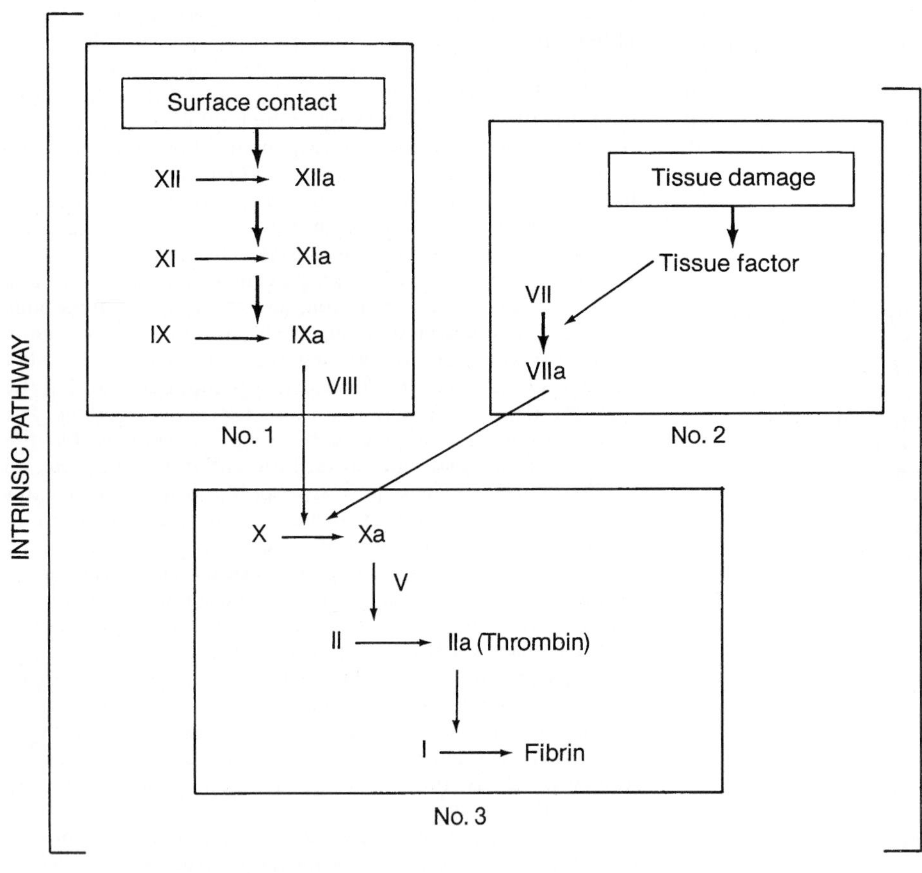

Figure 159–3. A simplified scheme of the clotting mechanism (see text).

CLOTTING FACTORS MEASURED IN THE PTT	CLOTTING FACTORS MEASURED IN THE PRO-TIME
Hageman (XII)	Proconvertin (VII)
PTA (XI)	Stuart factor (X)
PTC (IX)	Ac globulin (V)
AHG (VIII)	Prothrombin (II)
Stuart (X)	Fibrinogen (I)
Ac globulin (V)	
Prothrombin (II)	
Fibrinogen (I)	

	POSSIBLE COAGULATION DEFECT
Patient 1. Pro-time normal, PTT prolonged	XII, XI, IX, VIII
Patient 2. Pro-time prolonged, PTT normal	VII
Patient 3. Pro-time prolonged, PTT prolonged	X, V, II, I

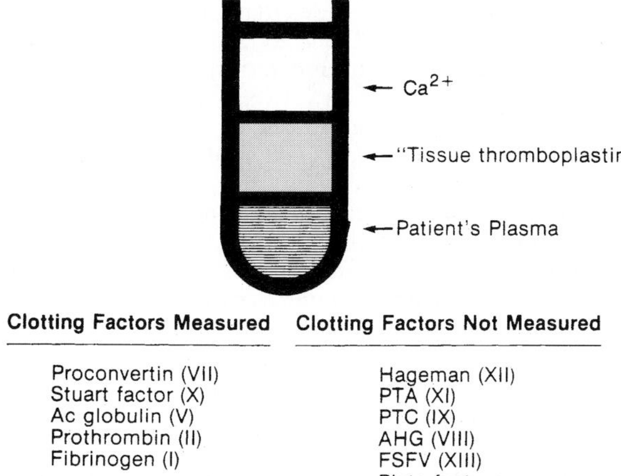

Figure 159–4. Principles of the prothrombin time test.

Thus, the PT is perfectly normal in patients suffering from either hemophilia A or hemophilia B.

For the aPTT test, one must mix the patient's plasma and phospholipid liposomes, mimicking the cell membrane phospholipid bilayer, and calcium ions, without which intrinsic and extrinsic clotting is impossible (Fig. 159-5). Negatively charged substances, such as kaolin, celite, and ellagic acid, are also added to maximally activate Hageman's factor, thereby ensuring maximum activation of the intrinsic coagulation mechanism. Prolongation of the partial thromboplastin time (PTT) means a deficiency somewhere along the intrinsic pathway; one link in the chain is weak or missing. For instance, deficiencies of both factor VIII and factor IX in hemophilia A and hemophilia B result in prolongation of the aPTT. The test becomes particularly valuable if combined with the PT.

The simplified coagulation scheme depicted in Figure 159-3 shows the three possible permutations that may be encountered in evaluating a patient with an unknown constitutional bleeding disorder. If, for instance, a patient has a normal PT and a prolonged aPTT, factor deficiencies in Boxes 2 and 3 are excluded. The defect must be among factors XII, XI, IX, and VIII, in Box 1, all of which are strictly concerned with the intrinsic clotting mechanism. If the patient has a prolonged PT and a normal aPTT, abnormalities along the intrinsic pathway are excluded; that is, clotting factors contained in Boxes 1 and 3. The only clotting factor abnormality producing this permutation is a deficiency in factor VII. If both the PT and the aPTT are prolonged, the defect must lie somewhere in that part of the activation sequence that is common to both pathways; that is, the clotting factors contained in Box 3, clotting factors X, V, II, and I.

To identify the defect further, we make use of the so-called substituted aPTT (Fig. 159-6). If the PT is normal and the aPTT is grossly abnormal, a physician would suspect abnormal activities of one of four clotting factors strictly operative along the intrinsic pathway contained in Box 1, factors VIII, IX, XI, and XII. Illustrated in Figure 159-6 is the approach to differentiating among deficiencies of factor VIII and factor IX, hemophilia A and hemophilia B. The patient's plasma, previously shown to produce a prolonged aPTT, is admixed with plasmas known to be severely deficient in factor VIII and factor IX. In the specialized laboratory, appropriate reagents from patients with known clotting factor deficiencies or plasma specimens from which a specific clotting factor has been removed through immunoabsorption are stored away in the freezer. High-quality reagents for these diagnostic tests are readily available through commercial sources.

To differentiate between deficiencies of factor VIII and factor IX, one must add to the unknown plasma, in turn, plasma deficient in factor VIII or factor IX. If the prolonged aPTT is corrected with hemophilia A plasma, the patient must suffer from hemophilia B. If, however, the prolonged aPTT is corrected with hemophilia B plasma but not with hemophilia A plasma, the patient must have hemophilia A. If no correction occurs with either hemophilia A or hemophilia B plasma, the patient likely has deficiencies of either factor XI or XII; this can be checked in the same fashion, by performing aPTT tests on mixtures of aliquots of the patient's plasma and plasma grossly deficient in factor XI or XII.

If the PT as well as aPTT is abnormal, one should return to the clotting factors in Box 3, the clotting factors common to both the extrinsic and intrinsic pathways. Using the same substitution strategy, the physician tests the patient's plasma for aPTT in a system mixed with plasma deficient in factors V, X, and II.

Congenital or acquired deficiency in fibrinogen is readily quantified in the test system in which excess thrombin is added to the patient's plasma; fibrinogen can then be measured by a calibration curve and a standard plasma sample of predetermined fibrinogen content. In mild hemophilia, the aPTT is occasionally at the upper limit of normal or marginally prolonged. In these cases, specific factor assays must be used. Clotting factor assays are variants of the aPTT that essentially measure the extent to which a patient's plasma corrects the defect of a plasma known to contain zero or near-zero levels of the clotting factor to be determined.

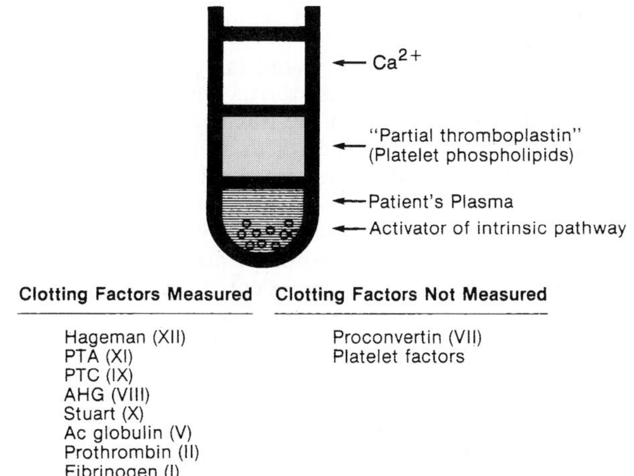

Figure 159–5. Principles of the activated partial thromboplastin time test.

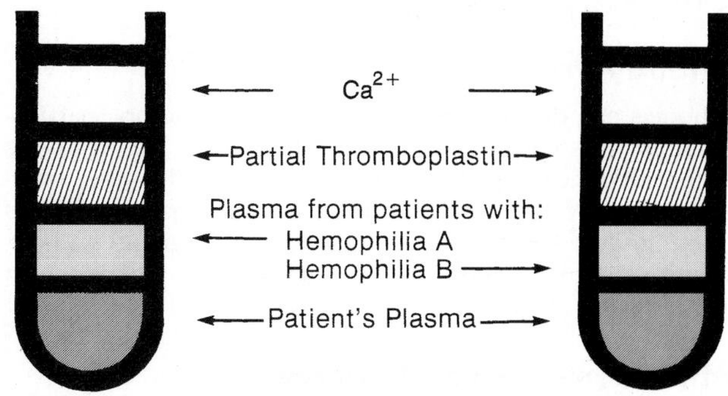

Figure 159–6. Differential diagnosis between hemophilia A and hemophilia B (see text).

Unfortunately, factor assays are not universally available in small hospital laboratories. Factor assays are not difficult to set up and standardize; without the availability of such tests, an emergency physician may occasionally face a serious dilemma when instituting correct therapy in if the diagnosis of mild hemophilia has not been confirmed and if the patient bleeds uncontrollably after trauma or during surgery. Such patients usually have mild hemophilia A or B that may not be symptomatic until the patient suffers major trauma or undergoes major surgery. The treatment of patients with hemophilia is difficult and is usually performed in special hemophilia centers with special laboratory facilities and special equipment for the handling of these often complex cases.

Treatment of the Hemophilias[28]

For the emergency department physician whose institution does not have a hemophilia center, a few ground rules may be useful. The hemostatically effective plasma levels of each coagulation factor are different, depending on volume of distribution and biologic half-life of the protein. The dose of any replacement factor is calculated in units, one unit being the activity of a given coagulation factor in 1.0 mL of pooled fresh frozen human plasma.

The biologic half-life (t½) of factor VIII in plasma is between 8 and 12 hours, including the initial decline in levels due to equilibration with extravascular pools. For hemostasis to be achieved in mild hemorrhage, the level of Factor VIII should be 0.3 units/mL plasma. For major hemorrhagic complications, 0.5 units/mL is needed. For life-threatening bleeding or surgery, levels of 0.8 to 1 unit per mL should be achieved.

A simple, reliable means of dose calculation is to estimate that each unit of factor VIII per kilogram of body weight yields a 2% rise in plasma factor VIII levels. This general rule applies to all factor VIII preparations, the crude as well as the more highly purified or recombinant preparations. Similar guidelines apply to factor IX preparations. Although the t½ is approximately 24 hours and the minimum hemostatic level (0.1 to 0.25 units/mL) is significantly lower than estimated values for factor VIII, approximately 25% to 50% of the administered doses are lost during the equilibration phase. A simple dose calculation can be made: Each unit of factor IX infused per kilogram of body weight yields a 1% rise in plasma factor IX (0.01 units/mL).

Factor IX preparations can be crude, comprising in addition to factor IX the other vitamin K clotting factors (II, VII, and X), and these crude preparations can be used in treatment not only for hemophilia B but also for rare hemophilias caused by factor II, VII, and X deficiencies. Such preparations are also useful in patients who have received an overdose of oral anticoagulants or who have severe liver disease. These situations can lead to dangerously low levels of factors II, VII, IX and X. A highly purified recombinant factor IX preparation (Benefix) has also become available.

Antibody Problems

Antibodies can develop to all known clotting factors, particularly in patients with severe hemophilia A or B. The diagnosis and the identification of such antibodies as well as the treatment are frustrating and complicated problems that should not be undertaken in the emergency department without access to a hematologist who has substantial experience in handling these problems.

Antiphospholipid Antibodies

Antiphospholipid antibodies[29] are most generally known as lupus anticoagulants, probably a misnomer because antibodies to phospholipid-protein complexes that interfere with clotting tests are not restricted to SLE. They are commonly encountered during and after viral, bacterial, or fungal infections, and they can be associated with drugs (e.g., phenothiazines and synthetic penicillins). They are observed in certain malignancies, such as hairy cell leukemia and lymphoproliferative disorders.

The antigens against which antibodies occur are complexes between proteins and negatively charged phospholipids; the best studied are beta$_2$ glycoprotein 1 and prothrombin-phospholipid complexes. These complexes can generate antibodies of the IgG, IgA, and IgM classes, which in turn can prolong both the PT and aPTT. These changes almost never result in clinical bleeding, in contrast to clotting factor deficiencies, but do cause prolongation of the common clotting tests. The lupus anticoagulant is important to recognize not only because it produces spurious warning signals for bleeding but also because antiphospholipid antibodies carry a relative high risk for venous as well as arterial thrombosis and other problems, such as recurrent miscarriage.

To distinguish between a lupus anticoagulant and factor deficiencies, we usually make up mixtures of equal parts patient plasma and normal plasma. If a prolonged PT or aPTT in the patient plasma is corrected by mixture, a lupus anticoagulant can usually be ruled out. Other tests, such as the diluted Russel's viper venom test, can be helpful in establishing the diagnosis.

The Routine (Presurgical) Screen

It is common in most surgical departments to require standard coagulation tests prior to surgery to guard against undetected hemostatic problems. Most surgeons engaging in significant surgical procedures would insist on a PT, an aPTT, and a platelet count; sometimes bleeding time measurements are also requested. Most laboratories today use the so-called International Normalized Ratio (INR) rather than the PT. The INR is a ratio between the patient's PT and the PT from a normal plasma pool, usually with a correction factor that reflects the strength of the tissue thromboplastin used in the test. With newer reagents introduced, both the PT and the aPTT can vary significantly from laboratory to laboratory, and close collaboration between the pathologist and the emergency physician is necessary to correctly interpret tests results. The bleeding time is commonly requested but has limited predictive value; it is labor-intensive, is not easily standardized, and therefore is not encouraged in this institution.

LIVER DISEASE

The coagulation defects encountered in severe chronic liver disease are complex and multifactorial. The liver synthesizes all procoagulant proteins, with the possible exception of factor VIII, and decreased synthesis of these proteins may itself result in serious coagulation defects and bleeding problems. The synthesis of the vitamin K-dependent procoagulants is usually affected the earliest, followed by that of factors V, XI, and XII. Cholestasis and malabsorption may further suppress the biosynthesis of vitamin K-dependent clotting factors. Most clinicians recommend a single test dose of 5 to 10 mg of vitamin K to establish whether the clotting defect is, in part, correctable. Fibrinogen biosynthesis is maintained at normal levels until the very end, so a low level of fibrinogen in a patient without symptoms or signs of disseminated intravascular coagulation (DIC) is of grave prognostic significance. Clotting factor VIII levels always remain normal or elevated, even in end-stage liver disease, and low levels of factor VIII in liver disease strongly suggest the complication of DIC.

A perplexing coagulation defect in liver disease is acquired dysfibrinogenemia, which was first demonstrated in patients with hepatoma but is also demonstrated in a sizable number of patients with cirrhosis of the liver.[30] The abnormal fibrinogen in liver disease is more heavily glycosylated than normal fibrinogen, with a sharp increase in total hexose, hexosamine, and sialic acid levels. This abnormal protein converts normally to fibrin monomer, but polymerization of fibrin monomer is slow and inefficient. Because all clotting tests depend on the rate of appearance of a fibrin clot, an abnormal fibrinogen level can produce spuriously low values in clotting tests such as PT and aPTT. The diagnosis of dysfibrinogenemia is made in the special laboratory through the use of the so-called thrombin clotting time and the measurement of fibrinogen through chronometric assays and immunoassays.

DISSEMINATED INTRAVASCULAR COAGULATION[31]

Once considered a complication encountered occasionally in obstetric practice, DIC is now a more commonly noted hematologic complication that occurs in association with disease states treated by the entire spectrum of medical and surgical specialties. Today, with improved laboratory techniques, it has become apparent that DIC exists in varying degrees of severity, ranging from life-threatening, acute, and severe to mild or more chronic.

In *acute* DIC, deposition of fibrin in the microcirculation and consumption of clotting factors and platelets occur more quickly than they can be synthesized by the liver and bone marrow. Consequently, the levels of circulating, consumable clotting factors (fibrinogen and factors V, VIII, XIII, and II) and circulating platelets sharply decrease. Compensatory fibrinolytic mechanisms are almost always operative; as a consequence, high levels of fibrinogen-fibrin split products are readily demonstrable in the serum of patients with acute DIC.

In *chronic* DIC, fibrin deposition and consumption of clotting factors are thought to proceed more slowly, to permit hepatic synthesis of clotting factors and even bone marrow production of platelets to keep pace. The body possesses an impressive capability for the compensatory production of platelets and clotting factors to maintain adequate hemostasis. Thus, the bone marrow can generate 10 times the usual number of platelets, and the liver can synthesize at least five times the amount of fibrinogen it produces under normal baseline conditions. The rate of synthesis may occasionally exceed the consumption rate, net results are the higher than normal levels of fibrinogen and factors V, VIII, and XIII and normal or only mildly depressed platelet counts.

In chronic DIC states, compensatory fibrinolytic mechanisms are also active, producing high levels of fibrinogen-fibrin split products in the circulation. Unless suitable measurements for fibrinogen-fibrin split products are performed, the diagnosis of chronic DIC cannot be made in a significant number of cases.

Table 159-5 summarizes the many clinical situations in which DIC can be encountered as a complication, underscoring the magnitude of the problem.

TABLE 159–5. Disease States Associated with Disseminated Intravascular Coagulation

Category	Clinical Situation
Obstetric complications	Abruptio placentae Amniotic fluid embolism Dead fetus syndrome Eclampsia (preeclampsia?) Placenta previa Placenta accreta Abortion (hypertonic saline solution) Hydatid mole Extrauterine pregnancy Forceps delivery Normal delivery
Tissue trauma	Major surgery Major trauma and burns Fat embolism Rejection of transplants Heat stroke
Hemolytic processes	Transfusion of mismatched blood Drowning Acute hemolysis secondary to infection Immune mechanisms Acid ingestion
Malignant neoplasms	Solid tumors Leukemias, lymphomas
Snakebites	Acute myocardial infarction (usually associated with cardiogenic shock)
Cardiovascular system	Circulatory collapse from any cause Severe progressive strokes Aortic aneurysms and Kasabach-Merritt syndrome (local intravascular coagulation)
Chronic liver disease	
Infections	
Bacterial	Gram-negative meningococcal and pneumococcal septicemia
Rickettsial	Rocky Mountain spotted fever
Viral	Hemorrhagic smallpox, hemorrhagic fevers (Thai, Korean, and others)
Mycotic	Acute histoplasmosis
Parasitic	Malaria (particularly falciparum)
Miscellaneous	Acute and chronic renal disease (?) Collagen vascular disorders Thrombotic thrombocytopenic purpura (?) Hemolytic-uremic syndrome (?) Purpura fulminans Acute pancreatitis Allergic vasculitis Amyloidosis Polycythemia vera Thrombocythemia Ulcerative colitis

From Bang NU: Disseminated intravascular coagulation. *In:* Laboratory Evaluation of Coagulation. Triplett DA (Ed). Chicago, American Society of Clinical Pathologists Press, 1982, pp 210–249.

Pathogenesis

Whenever substantial and traumatic tissue damage or large areas of tissue necrosis occur, the possibility of complicating DIC must always be kept in mind. Tissue factor may not enter blood vessels from surrounding damaged tissues, but it can arise when cells in direct contact with circulating blood (i.e., monocytes and endothelial cells) are triggered to synthesize and express tissue factor on their cell membranes. This is most likely the mechanism responsible for the common occurrence of DIC in endotoxemia, and it may also be implicated in numerous other inflammatory states in which cytokines, such as interleukin-1 (IL-1) and tumor necrosis factor (TNF), are synthesized and secreted.

Other mechanisms implicated in DIC are the release of thromboplastin-like substances from red blood cells during acute hemolysis, particularly after transfusion of mismatched blood, and the secretion of certain proteases from leukemic or solid tumor cells capable of bypassing the normal coagulation mechanisms through direct activation of factor X. Such proteases have been demonstrated particularly in acute promyelocytic leukemia, which carries an almost 100% risk for DIC.

A very high incidence of DIC is also found in mucinous adenocarcinomas. In patients with solid tumors, DIC is usually chronic, and the hemorrhagic tendency is usually mild, but major vessel thrombosis is a common complication.

Disseminated Intravascular Coagulation Versus Primary Fibrinolysis

It has previously been reported that blood obtained from some patients clotted in the test tube but soon liquefied again. Subsequently, the connection was established between enhanced levels of fibrinolytic activity and bleeding under these conditions. In these clinical situations, the designation of pathologic or primary fibrinolytic states became popular. It has become increasingly obvious from critical reviews of previously published cases that the diagnosis of a primary fibrinolytic state is untenable in most cases; many investigators seriously question whether the bleeding resulting from primary fibrinolysis is a bona fide clinical entity. Most cases previously reported as primary fibrinolysis were later interpreted as being fibrinolysis secondary to DIC.

Today, most workers in the field tend to regard DIC as the primary event and fibrinolysis as the compensatory physiologic repair mechanism. Depending on the magnitude of the fibrinolytic response (i.e., whether it is feeble or whether it grossly overshoots), we may encounter a clinical picture in which either DIC or fibrinolysis predominates; however, an element of each process—clotting and lysis—is almost always present.

Disseminated Intravascular Coagulation in Liver Disease

Coagulation problems in acute and chronic parenchymal liver disease are numerous and difficult to sort out. Several mechanisms are responsible, for example (1) suppression of synthesis of procoagulant proteins, (2) thrombocytopenia secondary to hypersplenism, (3) acute ethanol intoxication and folate deficiency, and (4) the inability of the severely injured liver to clear activated clotting factors and fibrinolytic enzymes from the circulation.

Although some have questioned the existence of DIC syndrome associated with severe acute and chronic liver disease, most clinicians today are convinced that DIC occurs with some frequency in liver disease, often representing a serious complication. Arguments in favor of the occurrence of the DIC syndrome in acute and chronic parenchymal liver disease are increased levels of fibrinogen-fibrin degradation products and shortened fibrinogen survival that is improved by heparin.

Diagnosis

In the acute forms of DIC, the diagnosis is strongly suspected from the findings of a combination of low-level fibrinogen, a prolonged prothrombin time, and an APTT reflecting both low levels of consumable clotting factors V, VIII, and II and thrombocytopenia. To substantiate the diagnosis, a test for fibrinogen-fibrin split products in serum by immunoassay (e.g., Thrombo-Wellco test) is necessary. A more specific test, the D-dimer test, is replacing the Thrombo-Wellco test. The D-dimer test quantifies a fragment of fully polymerized, cross-linked fibrin fragment arising from active fibrinolysis. This fragment is claimed to be pathognomonic for DIC and major vessel thrombosis.

In confirming the diagnosis of the chronic forms of DIC, one cannot rely on low levels of fibrinogen, prolonged PT and aPTT, and a low platelet count. All of these variables may be normal or nearly normal, and the diagnosis can be made only through the demonstration of high levels of fibrinogen and fibrin split products in serum. Additional tests have been suggested to reflect the presence of soluble fibrin complexes in plasma, which are soluble intermediates between fibrinogen and fibrin.

High levels of fibrinogen-fibrin split products are not specific for DIC. In large aortic aneurysms, fibrin is being deposited and dissolved with rapid turnover, thereby producing high circulating levels of fibrinogen-fibrin split products. Similarly, in the giant hemangioma of the Kasabach-Merritt syndrome, fibrin turnover is rapid enough to sharply elevate the levels of fibrin degradation products.

Fibrinogen-fibrin degradation products are elevated commonly in various acute and chronic glomerular disorders, most likely reflecting localized intravascular coagulation in renal glomeruli. Elevations of fibrinogen-fibrin split products should not be considered evidence of DIC in the setting of acute or chronic renal disease. The one important exception to this rule is acute renal failure associated with shock from gram-negative septicemia or other causes in which renal glomeruli represent only one of many target organs for microcirculatory thrombosis. Of special importance is the recognition that DIC occurs as a complication of gram-negative septicemia due to septic abortion, because pregnant women are at very high risk for development of bilateral renal cortical necrosis in conjunction with DIC.

Clinical Features

In acute DIC, bleeding combined with multiple organ failure is usual. Frequent bleeding problems are severe gastrointestinal bleeding, hematuria, oozing from venipuncture sites, and large areas of ecchymosis. These bleeding problems are often accompanied by acute renal failure. Chronic DIC, as observed in certain malignancies, usually produces mild bleeding problems (with the exception of metastatic cancer of the prostate, which usually produces the more acute picture of DIC). Chronic DIC is often complicated by major vessel thrombosis, commonly deep vein thrombosis or pulmonary embolism, which characteristically responds poorly to heparin or oral anticoagulant therapy and tends to be recurrent. In some instances, thrombosis of medium-sized arteries can occur, leading to gangrene of the lower extremities. Chronic DIC is occasionally accompanied by heavy fibrin deposition in renal glomeruli and the development of renal failure.

Treatment[32]

The most controversial issue in DIC is therapy, and the controversies remain so deep that it is impossible to make specific recommendations at this time. Through the late 1950s, the recommended treatment was replacement with whole fresh blood, platelets, clotting factors such as fibrinogen, and fresh frozen plasma that contained, in addition to fibrinogen, clotting factors V and VIII. In the 1950s, attention was focused mainly on the fibrinolytic component of DIC states; for that reason, the fibrinolytic enzyme system inhibitor ε-aminocaproic acid (EACA) (Amicar) was introduced as the specific treatment of choice for patients with hypofibrinogenemic hemorrhage.

Although initial case reports of the use of EACA were encouraging, subsequent experience has taught us differently.

TABLE 159–6. Retrospective Analysis of Results of Heparin Treatment in Disseminated Intravascular Coagulation

	After Heparin Therapy		
Type	***Total No. of Patients***	***No. Improved***	***No. Unchanged, Deteriorated, Died***
Acute			
Meningococcal septicemia, Waterhouse-Friderichsen syndrome	3	2	1
All other causes (mainly cirrhosis and/or gram-negative septicemia)	41	6	35
Chronic			
Major vessel thrombosis (mainly solid tumors)	12	7	5

Modified from Bang NU: Disseminated intravascular coagulation. *In:* Laboratory Evaluation of Coagulation. Triplet DA (Ed). Chicago, American Society of Clinical Pathologists Press, 1982, pp 210–249.

Between 1959 and 1968, I personally treated 51 patients with DIC with EACA, with an 80% failure rate. Serious complications were occasionally encountered in the form of major vessel thrombosis, particularly thrombotic strokes; on two occasions, patients with cirrhosis of the liver and hypofibrinogenemic hemorrhage lapsed into hepatic coma during treatment with EACA. It is likely that this complication occurs because EACA effectively competes with essential amino acids for transmembrane transport. Today there is almost universal agreement that EACA has little, if any, role in the treatment of DIC states.

In the early 1960s, treatment with heparin was instituted on the basis of reasoning that heparin would block the fundamental problem of enhanced clotting activity. Heparin, given in doses ranging from 150 to 600 $U \cdot kg^{-1} \cdot day^{-1}$ and usually in combination with suitable replacement measures, was the mainstay of treatment of DIC syndromes during the next 10 to 15 years. Widespread use of heparin was based almost entirely on anecdotal material, isolated case reports, and small uncontrolled clinical trials. A prospective controlled clinical trial has never been performed, and even retrospective analyses are rare.

Table 159-6 is a retrospective analysis of the outcome of heparin treatment in DIC from the author's laboratory, based on records from Indiana University Hospitals from 1966 to 1974.[32] This series of cases has been divided into three categories: two categories of patients with severe acute DIC and one category of patients with chronic DIC. Patients in all three groups received heparin in full dosages comparable to those given to patients with acute pulmonary embolism. One group of patients with acute DIC included those with meningococcal septicemia and the Waterhouse-Friderichsen syndrome, a specialized form of DIC producing bilateral adrenal cortical necrosis. This group contained only three patients, but in view of the grave prognosis in these cases, it was encouraging to note two survivors; similar encouraging results have been reported by others. A second, larger group was composed of patients with acute severe DIC due to various causes. Most of these patients had cirrhosis of the liver or gram-negative septicemia.

The series encompassed only six obstetric and surgical cases; for the whole group, the failure rate in heparin-treated patients was 90%. Twelve patients with chronic DIC were given treatment with heparin. Most had solid tumors, often presenting with deep vein thrombosis and mild bleeding diathesis with laboratory evidence of chronic DIC. These 12 patients with chronic DIC fared somewhat better. Among the 12 patients, definitive improvement was observed in 7 after treatment with heparin. On the basis of these studies, heparin as treatment in acute DIC has been largely abandoned at Indiana University Hospitals; currently, heparin is used only in patients with chronic DIC who have concurrent major vessel thrombosis.

Culled from past failures and newer information, Table 159-7 summarizes the different modalities of treatment of DIC. The one most important principle in the treatment of DIC agreed on by all workers in the field is to treat the underlying cause. Effective treatment of an obstetric emergency or gram-negative septicemia is by far the most effective treatment of DIC; in most instances, specific forms of treatment for DIC itself, such as heparin, need not be considered. One additional issue that has been resolved with reasonable certainty is that EACA, the fibrinolytic enzyme inhibitor, has little if any role in the treatment of DIC.

In acute DIC, with the possible exception of the special case of meningococcal septicemia, the author concluded from previously mentioned data that the therapeutic approach used

TABLE 159–7. Therapy for Disseminated Intravascular Coagulation (DIC)

When Indicated	Treatment	Degree of Certainty
Always	Treat underlying disease when possible	Established
Almost never	ε-Aminocaproic acid (Amicar)	Established
Chronic DIC, with major vessel thrombosis	Heparin, full dose	Reasonable
Acute DIC	Substitution therapy and full-dose heparin	Most uncertain
	Antithrombin III preactivated with small doses of heparin in sufficient quantity to correct calculated antithrombin III deficiency	Speculative
	Platelet function inhibitors to prevent release of platelet factor 4	Speculative
	Cold-insoluble globulin to improve reticuloendothelial function	Speculative

earlier—full-dosage heparin combined with various replacement measures—is an unsatisfactory solution. The theoretic alternative of replacement of antithrombin III–heparin cofactor, which is often sharply reduced in DIC, in combination with low-dose heparin remains largely speculative. It is believed, however that the approach of treating DIC with purified antithrombin and low-dose heparin should be tested in controlled clinical trials in an attempt to improve what has been a truly dismal record.

References

1. Fauvel F, Grant ME, Legrand YJ, et al: Interaction of blood platelets with microfibrillar extract from adult bovine aorta: Requirement for von Willebrand factor. Proc Natl Acad Sci U S A 1983; 80:551.
2. Barnes MJ, Bailey AJ, Gordon JL, MacIntyre ED: Platelet aggregation by basement membrane–associated collagens. Thromb Res 1980; 18:375.
3. Hammarstrom S, Falaradeau P: Resolution of prostaglandin endoperoxide synthase and thromboxane synthase of human platelets. Proc Natl Acad Sci USA 1977; 74:3691.
4. Haslam RJ: Roles of cyclic nucleotides in platelet function. Ciba Found Symp 1975; 35:121.
5. Brass LF, Joseph SK: A role for inositol triphosphate in intracellular Ca^{2+} mobilization and granule secretion in platelets. J Biol Chem 1985; 260:15172.
6. O'Rourke FA, Halenda SP, Zavoico GB: Inositol 1,4,5-triphosphate-induced releases Ca^{2+} from a Ca^{2+}-transporting membrane vesicle fraction derived from human platelets. J Biol Chem 1985; 260:956.
7. Holmsen H, Weiss HJ: Secretable storage pools in platelets. Annu Rev Med 1979; 30:119.
8. Tracy PB, Eide LL, Mann KG: Human prothrombinase complex assembly and function on isolated peripheral blood cell populations. J Biol Chem 1985; 260:2119.
9. McIntosh S, Breg WR, Lubiniecki AS; Fanconi's anemia: The preanemic phase. Am J Pediatr Hematol Oncol 1979; 1:107.
10. Perry GS, Spector BD, Schuman LM, et al: The Wiskott-Aldrich syndrome in the United States and Canada (1892–1979). J Pediatr 1980; 97:72.
11. Dameshek W, Valentine EH: The sternal marrow in pernicious anemia. Arch Pathol 1937; 23:159.
12. Walsh C, Krigel R, Lennette E, Karpatkin S: Thrombocytopenia in homosexual patients. Ann Intern Med 1985; 103:542.
13. Karpatkin S: The spleen and thrombocytopenia. Clin Haematol 1983; 12:591.
14. George JN, Pickett EB, Saucerman S, et al: Platelet surface glycoproteins: Studies of resting and activated platelets and platelet membrane microparticles in normal subjects, and observations in patients during acute respiratory distress syndrome and cardiac surgery. J Clin Invest 1986; 78:340.
15. Ashenazi S: Role of bacterial cytotoxins in hemolytic uremic syndrome and thrombotic thrombocytopenic purpura. Annu Rev Med 1993; 44:11.
16. Thompson CE, Damon L, Ries CA, Linker CA: Thrombotic microangiopathies in the 1980's: Clinical features, response to treatment, and the impact of the human immunodeficiency virus epidemic. Blood 1992; 80:1890.
17. George JN, Woolf SH, Raskob GE, et al: Idiopathic thrombocytopenic purpura: A practice guideline developed by explicit methods for the American Society of Hematology. Blood 1996; 88:3.
18. Murphy WG, Kelton JG: Idiosyncratic drug-induced thrombocytopenia. Curr Stud Hematol Blood Transf 1988; 54:71.
19. Greinacher A: Antigen generation in heparin-associated thrombocytopenia: The nonimmunologic type and the immunologic type are closely linked in their pathogenesis. Semin Thromb Hemost 1995; 21:106–116.
20. Arnout J: The pathogenesis of the antiphospholipid syndrome: A hypothesis based on parallelism with heparin-induced thrombocytopenia. © F.K. Schattuer Verlagsgesellshaft mbh (Stuttgart) 1996; 75:536.
21. Siegbahn A, Y-Hassan S, Boberg J, et al: Subcutaneous treatment of deep venous thrombosis with low molecular weight heparin. A dose finding study with low-molecular-weight heparin-Novo. Thromb Res 1989; 55:767.
22. Mueller-Eckhardt C: Post transfusion purpura. Br J Haematol 1986; 64:419.
23. Coller BS, Seligsohn U, Zivelin A, et al: Immunologic and biochemical characterization of homozygous and heterozygous Glanzmann thrombasthenia in the Iraqui-Jewish and Arab populations of Israel: Comparison of techniques for carrier detection. Br J Haematol 1986; 62:723.
24. Du X, Beautler L, Ruan C, et al: Glycoprotein Ib and glycoprotein IX are fully complexed in the intact platelet membrane. Blood 1987; 69:1524.
25. Macfarlane RG: An enzyme cascade in the blood clotting mechanism and its function as a biological amplifier. Nature 1964; 202:498.
26. Davie EW, Ratnoff OD: Waterfall sequence for intrinsic blood clotting. Science 1964; 145:1310.
27. Osterud B, Bajaj MS, Bajaj P: Sites of tissue factor pathway inhibitor (TFPI) and tissue factor expression under physiologic and pathologic conditions. Thromb Haemost 1995; 73:873.
28. Gill JC, Montgomery RR: Principles of therapy for coagulation factor deficiencies. *In:* Hematology of Infancy and Childhood. 4th ed. Nathan DG, Oski FA (Eds). Philadelphia, WB Saunders, 1993, pp 1796–1818.
29. Shapiro SS: The lupus anticoagulant/antiphospholipid syndrome. Annu Rev Med 1996; 47:533.
30. Bang NU: Hepatoma with Dysfibrinogenemia: Check sample. American Society of Clinical Pathology Check Sample Series, Thromb Haemost 1980. pp 80–82.
31. Bick RL: Disseminated intravascular coagulation: Objective clinical and laboratory diagnosis, treatment, and assessment of therapeutic response. Semin Thromb Haemost 1996; 22:69.
32. Bang NU: Disseminated intravascular coagulation. *In:* Laboratory Evaluation of Coagulation. Triplett DA (Ed). Chicago, American Society of Clinical Pathologists Press, 1982, pp 210–249.

160

Bleeding Disorders of Childhood

David H. Ebb, MD • Gordon L. Bray, MD

Prompt restoration of adequate hemostasis in a bleeding child requires both an understanding of the basic elements of normal coagulation and a familiarity with the array of pathologic states that are common in children. This chapter provides a logical framework for the assessment and management of abnormal bleeding in children, with special emphasis on aspects of the hemostatic mechanism that are unique to children.

Although a carefully obtained history and physical examination may define an acquired cause of acute hemorrhage (e.g., infection, liver disease, or inadvertent ingestion of anticoagulant medications), no antecedent event may have occurred that suggests a bleeding tendency in the young patient with an inherited disorder of hemostasis. An otherwise healthy infant or child may never have encountered a hemostatic challenge sufficient to unmask an underlying bleeding disorder. Even the most exhaustive patient and family history may not identify a hemostatic disorder inherited in an autosomal recessive manner or one that is the result of a germline mutation in one or both parents. In addition, postnatal development of the hemostatic system over the first 3 to 4 years of life is associated with levels of coagulation factors that are different from adult standards. Failure to account for the physiologic differences in hemostasis between children and adults may lead to misdiagnosis and improper management of children who have excessive bleeding.

MAJOR COMPONENTS OF NORMAL HEMOSTASIS

The normal response to vascular injury includes reflex vasoconstriction, formation of a platelet plug that adheres to exposed subendothelial connective tissues (*primary hemostasis*), and consolidation of the platelet plug within a meshwork of polymerized fibrin (*coagulation mechanism*). Most causes of excessive bleeding can be classified according to whether either or both of these hemostatic components are abnormal. Defects in primary hemostasis result from either abnormal platelet function or decreased platelet number. Abnormal coagulation reflects accelerated degradation of fibrin, resulting in inadequate clot stabilization, or it reflects decreased availability or function of one or more coagulation proteins. The distinction between primary hemostasis and coagulation is useful for a theoretical understanding of the hemostatic mechanism. In vivo, both occur simultaneously and are interdependent (Fig. 160–1).

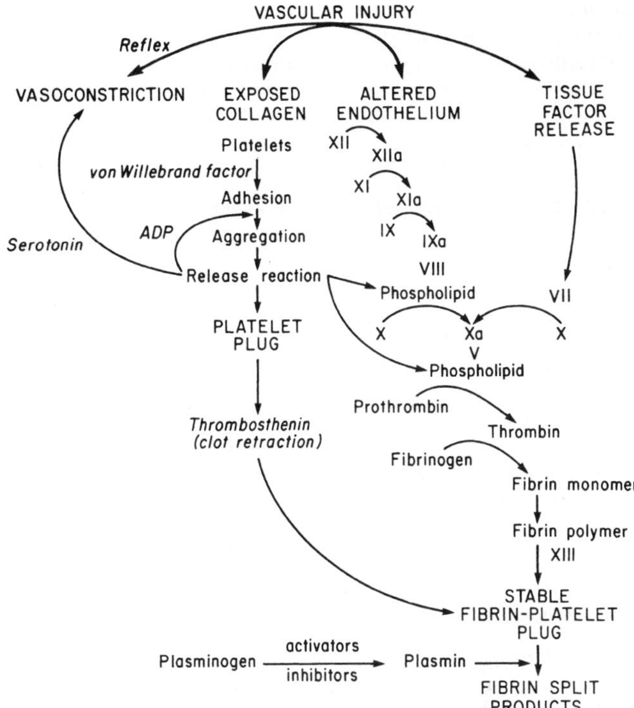

Figure 160–1. Diagrammatic representation of the hemostatic mechanism. (From Lusher JM: Diseases of coagulation: The fluid phase. *In:* Hematology of Infancy and Childhood. 3rd ed. Nathan DG, Oski FA [Eds]. Philadelphia, WB Saunders, 1987, p 1294.)

INHERITED DISORDERS OF PRIMARY HEMOSTASIS

Thrombocytopenias

Normal platelet number is the same in infants, young children, and adults. Platelet production begins at the end of the first trimester, with normal adult levels (150,000 to 450,000/mm^3) established by 30 weeks' gestation.[1] Under normal circumstances, platelets are released into the plasma as anuclear cell fragments derived from polyploid megakaryocytes in the bone marrow. The circulating platelet has an average life span of 10 days.[2] Quantitative defects are caused by:

- Decreased production (e.g., bone marrow failure syndromes)
- Increased consumption (e.g., hemorrhage, disseminated intravascular coagulation [DIC])
- Peripheral destruction (e.g., immune-mediated processes)
- Splenic pooling

Constitutional disorders of platelet production are relatively rare. Thrombocytopenia may present in early infancy as an isolated hematologic finding (e.g., amegakaryocytic thrombocytopenia) or as part of a syndrome marked by other phenotypic abnormalities (e.g., Wiskott-Aldrich syndrome or thrombocytopenia with absent radii syndrome). Aregenerative thrombocytopenia may also arise later in childhood as the initial hematologic manifestation of bone marrow failure. Syndromes causing such failure include Fanconi's aplastic anemia and dyskeratosis congenita.[3]

Wiskott-Aldrich syndrome is an X-linked disorder characterized by thrombocytopenia, eczema, progressive immunodeficiency involving both cellular and humoral immunity, and increased predisposition to lymphoid malignancies.[4] Platelets from patients with Wiskott-Aldrich syndrome are small, have decreased numbers of dense granules, and exhibit shortened survival. Hemorrhage and overwhelming infection are the commonest causes of early mortality in patients with Wiskott-Aldrich syndrome. Allogeneic bone marrow transplantation is curative of both the platelet and immunologic defects for patients who have a human leukocyte antigen-matched donor.[5] Splenectomy brings about a long-term increase in platelet number and size at the cost of an increased risk of bacterial sepsis.[6] Patients who are unable have a sustained response to splenectomy may respond to a combination of intravenous gamma G immunoglobulin (IgG), high-dose steroids, and vinca alkaloids, administered on an intermittent basis (Bray, 1987, unpublished data).

The thrombocytopenia with absent radii syndrome is characterized by forearm abnormalities, including absence or hypoplasia of the radii or ulnae, cardiac malformations in nearly one third of cases, transient leukemoid reactions, and thrombocytopenia that presents within the first 4 months of life.[7] Examination of bone marrow aspirates from affected infants reveals a marked decrease or absence of megakaryocytes, often in the presence of myeloid hyperplasia. Hemorrhagic complications tend to occur during the first year of life, with a bleeding-related mortality rate of 35%.

Platelet transfusions are the only intervention available for managing bleeding in these children. To avoid allosensitization and refractoriness to platelet concentrates, one should reserve platelet transfusions for use in the acutely bleeding patient. Neither splenectomy nor pharmacologic intervention (steroids, intravenous IgG) is useful in this syndrome.[7] Interestingly, the platelet count begins to rise spontaneously after the first year of life, and thrombocytopenia partially or completely resolves. Affected children do not show an increased risk of bone marrow aplasia or malignancy.

Fanconi's aplastic anemia resembles thrombocytopenia with absent radii in its initial presentation, which includes thrombocytopenia and skeletal abnormalities involving the upper extremities. In contrast to patients with thrombocytopenia with absent radii, those with Fanconi's anemia typically present with thrombocytopenia at a mean age of 8 years and invariably progress to complete bone marrow failure over a period of months to years. In addition, patients have an increased predisposition to the development of malignancies (particularly myeloid leukemias) and often demonstrate radial anomalies that include the absence of thumbs.[3]

In addition to hematologic and skeletal abnormalities, one third of patients with Fanconi's anemia have renal anomalies. Cytogenetic studies reveal markedly increased spontaneous and mutagenic agent-induced chromosomal breaks, which is the single most reliable diagnostic finding. Because bone marrow transplantation is the treatment of choice, administration of blood products should be reserved for emergent situations in transplant candidates. Platelets should be administered only for acute bleeding.

Disorders of Platelet Function

Children with normal platelet counts who present with hemorrhage may have a qualitative defect in platelet function. Functional abnormalities may arise as a result of the following:

1. Defects in platelet membrane glycoproteins (e.g., glycoprotein Ib, glycoprotein IIb/IIIa) that mediate platelet-vessel wall and platelet-platelet interactions.
2. Deficient or qualitatively abnormal plasma protein ligands (e.g., von Willebrand's factor [vWF], fibrinogen) required for effective platelet adhesion and aggregation.
3. Platelet granule deficiencies.
4. Abnormalities in the generation of thromboxane A_2, the most potent physiologic agonist of platelet aggregation.

von Willebrand's Disease

vWF is a large, multimeric molecule that circulates in a noncovalent complex with factor VIII. The gene for vWF has been localized to the short arm of chromosome 12.[8] Binding of vWF to platelet membrane glycoprotein Ib is essential for effective platelet adhesion to exposed subendothelial collagen in damaged vessel walls.[9] Because vWF is the carrier protein for factor VIII, decreased levels of vWF can result in correspondingly low levels of factor VIII and in prolongation of the activated partial thromboplastin time (aPTT). vWF is synthesized in endothelial cells and megakaryocytes, where it is packaged in platelet alpha granules. Release of vWF from endothelial cell storage pools (e.g., Weibel-Palade bodies) can be induced by thrombin, epinephrine, and vasopressin analogs (e.g., desmopressin acetate [DDAVP]).[9]

von Willebrand's disease (vWD) is a group of disorders in which quantitative or qualitative abnormalities of vWF cause impaired adhesion of platelets to exposed subendothelial surfaces at sites of vascular injury. This defect in primary hemostasis underlies the bleeding diathesis observed in patients with vWD. Although patients with vWD have variable bleeding severity, affected patients typically present with easy bruisability, recurrent epistaxis, and other mucous membrane bleeding. Menorrhagia in postpubescent girls may lead to chronic blood loss and iron deficiency anemia. Excessive hemorrhage may follow surgery, dental procedures, or trauma, and even mild head injury carries a risk of intracranial hemorrhage.

vWD is usually inherited in an autosomal dominant fashion, and males and females are affected in equal numbers. A small subset of patients with a severe form of the disease exhibit an autosomal recessive pattern of inheritance. Hemarthrosis and muscle hematomas characteristic of the hemophilias (see later) are features of this severe (type III) variant of the disease.[9]

Diagnosis and Classification

Evaluation of the patient with suspected vWD should include (1) a platelet count; (2) assays of factor VIII activity, vWF antigen, ristocetin cofactor activity, and ristocetin-induced platelet aggregation; and (3) analysis of vWF multimeric composition by sodium dodecyl sulfate (SDS) agarose gel electrophoresis (Table 160–1). Use of the template bleeding time has fallen out of favor because of its lack of sensitivity, difficulties in obtaining consistently reproducible results, and the risk of permanent scarring. Differentiating vWD subtypes is essential because the choice of therapy for bleeding depends on the specific subtype present.

Type I

Approximately 80% of vWD patients have type I disease, which is characterized by decreased amounts of structurally and functionally normal vWF.[10] Type I vWD is the subtlest form of the disease, in which the bleeding time may be prolonged in only 50% of cases.[10] Plasma levels of factor VIII, vWF antigen, and ristocetin cofactor activity are decreased proportionately in type I vWD, and SDS agarose gels demonstrate normal vWF multimeric structure.[11]

Type II

According to the revised classification scheme for vWD, all patients with type II variants suffer from a qualitative defect

TABLE 160–1. Results of Laboratory Studies in Patients with von Willebrand's Disease

	von Willebrand's Disease			
Laboratory Test	***Type I***	***Type IIa***	***Type IIb***	***Type III***
Bleeding time	Normal or prolonged	Usually prolonged	Usually prolonged	Always prolonged
Factor VIII:C	Normal or mildly decreased	Normal or mildly decreased	Usually normal	Always markedly decreased*
vWF antigen (Laurell assay)	Normal or mildly decreased	Normal or mildly decreased	Usually normal	Usually absent
Ristocetin-induced platelet aggregation	Usually normal	Usually decreased	Increased†	Markedly decreased to absent
Ristocetin cofactor activity	Normal or mildly to moderately decreased‡	Moderately to markedly decreased	Usually mildly to moderately decreased	Markedly decreased to absent
vWF multimeric analysis in SDS agarose gels	All MW multimers present and decreased proportionately	Absent of high and intermediate MW multimers; normal or increased low MW multimers	Absence of high MW multimers; normal or increased low and intermediate MW multimers	Lack of *all* MW multimers (high, intermediate, and low)

From Bray GL: Inherited and acquired disorders of hemostasis. *In:* Textbook of Pediatric Critical Care. Holbrook PR (Ed). Philadelphia, WB Saunders, 1993, pp 783–801.

*Levels of factor VIII:C in most patients with type III vWD are comparable with those exhibited by patients with moderate-to-severe factor VIII deficiency.

†A diagnostic feature of type IIb vWD is the ability of low concentrations of ristocetin (0.2–0.3 mg/mL) to cause aggregation in platelet-rich plasma.

‡Patients with type I vWD usually have proportionate decreases in plasma levels of VIII:C, vWF antigen, and ristocetin cofactor activity.

MW = molecular weight; SDS = sodium dodecyl sulfate; vWD = von Willebrand's disease; vWF = von Willebrand's factor.

in vWF.[12] Patients with subtype IIa have decreased or absent high-molecular-weight vWF multimers. These patients almost always exhibit prolonged bleeding times and have markedly diminished ristocetin cofactor activity, although levels of factor VIII activity and vWF antigen are usually normal. Patients with subtype IIb have mildly decreased ristocetin cofactor activity, and they demonstrate a distinctive *increase* in platelet aggregation when platelet-rich plasma is incubated in the presence of low-dose ristocetin.[9, 11] Aggregation of autologous, platelet-rich plasma in response to low-dose ristocetin administration reflects the increased affinity of abnormal, type IIb vWF for platelet membranes and distinguishes type IIb vWD from types I and IIa.

Type III

Type III vWD is the most severe form of the disease, affecting 1% to 3% of patients. Hemorrhagic complications are similar to those observed in patients with moderate hemophilia.[13] This variant is characterized by the complete absence of vWF antigen and ristocetin cofactor activity.

Treatment and Prevention of Bleeding

Management of bleeding complications in patients with vWD requires prompt increase of vWF activity in plasma either by infusion of exogenous vWF or by stimulation of release of endogenous stores. DDAVP is the treatment of choice for bleeding in most patients with type I and in some patients with type IIa vWD.[14] DDAVP stimulates the release of vWF from Weibel-Palade bodies in endothelial cells. Because it is not a blood product, its use does not incur a risk of blood-borne viral infection. When administered intravenously (0.3 μg/kg over 15 to 30 minutes in 30 to 50 mL of normal saline) or subcutaneously, DDAVP stimulates a rapid, threefold to fivefold increase in factor VIII, vWF antigen, and ristocetin cofactor activity. Repetitive use of DDAVP over short intervals leads to the development of tachyphylaxis due to depletion of endogenous vWF stores, thereby limiting its subsequent effectiveness. Frequent dosing can also lead to water retention and hyponatremia. For these reasons, DDAVP should be given no more frequently than once daily and serum electrolyte levels should be carefully monitored. Patients with type III vWD do not respond to DDAVP because they have no endogenous stores of vWF to mobilize. DDAVP is relatively contraindicated in patients with type IIb because it stimulates the secretion of functionally abnormal vWF that promotes intravascular platelet aggregation and thrombocytopenia.[14]

Until fairly recently, cryoprecipitate was the most commonly administered form of plasma-derived replacement therapy for those patients with vWD for whom DDAVP was ineffective or contraindicated. The use of cryoprecipitate, however, has fallen into disfavor because of concerns regarding the risk of exposure to human immunodeficiency virus (HIV) or hepatitis from infusions of untreated plasma products. Most hematologists now employ one of several virally attenuated factor VIII concentrates (e.g., Humate-P, Alphanate), which contain hemostatic levels of structurally normal vWF.[15] Therapeutic monitoring and dosing guidelines remain controversial for these vWF-containing concentrates. Because vWF content is not specified on the factor VIII concentrate labels, we generally administer concentrate at a starting dose of 50 units/kg of factor VIII concentrate.[16]

Defects in Platelet Membrane Glycoprotein Receptors

Bernard-Soulier Syndrome

Patients with Bernard-Soulier syndrome lack platelet membrane glycoprotein Ib, which mediates adhesion of platelets to subendothelium through the binding of vWF. This syndrome is characterized by moderate-to-severe mucocutaneous bleeding that presents early in life. Laboratory findings include mild-to-moderate thrombocytopenia, unusually large platelets noted on peripheral blood film, and prolonged bleeding time. In vitro assays of platelet aggregation reveal a normal response to adenosine diphosphate, epinephrine, and collagen as well as a decreased response to thrombin. Platelets from individuals with Bernard-Soulier syndrome fail to aggregate in the presence of ristocetin.[17]

Therapy for the bleeding patient with Bernard-Soulier syndrome is limited to platelet transfusions. However, because transfused platelets possess glycoprotein Ib, platelet concentrate use frequently results in the development of alloantibodies to glycoprotein Ib and subsequent refractoriness to platelet transfusions.[18]

Glanzmann's Thrombasthenia

Glanzmann's thrombasthenia is an autosomal recessive disorder characterized by prolonged bleeding time and early-onset mucocutaneous bleeding, despite a normal platelet count. Platelets from individuals with Glanzmann's thrombasthenia lack the membrane glycoprotein IIb-IIIa complex required for fibrinogen-mediated platelet-platelet interaction. Platelets in patients with this disorder adhere normally to injured vessel walls but are unable to extend the primary platelet plug by aggregating with each other. These platelets do not aggregate in vitro in the presence of physiologic agonists (adenosine diphosphate, epinephrine, thrombin, collagen) but do respond to the antibiotic ristocetin.[17] The same pattern of bleeding prolongation and impaired platelet aggregation is observed in patients with congenital afibrinogenemia, although this disorder is easily distinguished from Glanzmann's thrombasthenia by measurement of fibrinogen levels.

Hemorrhagic complications in patients with Glanzmann's thrombasthenia are treated with platelet transfusions. The risk of antiglycoprotein IIb-IIIa alloantibody formation in these patients mandates a cautious approach to the use of platelet concentrates.[18] Menorrhagia in postpubescent females often responds to treatment with oral contraceptives.

Platelet Granule Deficiencies

Absence or deficiency of platelet granules can produce a mild-to-moderate bleeding diathesis. Normal platelets contain three types of storage organelles: alpha granules, dense granules, and lysosomes. The constituents of alpha granules include platelet factor 4, β-thromboglobulin, platelet-derived growth factor, fibrinogen, factor V, vWF, and high-molecular-weight kininogen. Dense granules are rich in adenosine diphosphate and adenosine triphosphate and contain serotonin, phospholipase, and calcium.[19]

Gray Platelet Syndrome

Individuals with gray platelet syndrome are severely deficient or completely lacking in alpha granules. Elevations of platelet factor 4 and β-thromboglobulin in plasma suggest that this syndrome is the result of a packaging defect rather than an intrinsic inability to synthesize alpha-granule constituents. The clinical features of gray platelet syndrome include mild thrombocytopenia, prolonged bleeding time, and abnormal, thrombin-induced platelet aggregation and secretion.[19]

Dense-Granule Deficiency

Patients with dense-granule deficiency often have a history of easy bruising, epistaxis, gingival or gastrointestinal bleeding, menorrhagia, and excessive bleeding after surgical procedures. Platelets from some individuals with dense-granule defects have a concomitant deficiency of alpha granules. Characteristic laboratory findings include prolongation of bleeding time and failure to have a second wave of aggregation when platelets are stimulated by adenosine diphosphate or epinephrine.[7, 19]

Treatment of hemorrhagic complications requires the infusion of platelet concentrates.

ACQUIRED DISORDERS OF PRIMARY HEMOSTASIS

Acquired disorders of primary hemostasis include both quantitative and functional platelet defects. Acquired thrombocytopenias are a consequence of impaired production, peripheral sequestration, or accelerated platelet destruction by immune or nonimmune mechanisms. Immune-mediated platelet destruction is caused by the binding of IgG, or less commonly by IgM and complement, resulting in the subsequent clearance of sensitized platelets by the reticuloendothelial system.

Neonatal Thrombocytopenia

Most often, thrombocytopenia in premature and full-term neonates is a consequence of accelerated platelet destruction due to infection or immune-mediated mechanisms. Severe thrombocytopenia can occur in infants who are infected by any of the TORCH (*to*xoplasmosis, *r*ubella, *c*ytomegalovirus, or *h*erpes simplex) viruses or HIV-1. Bacterial sepsis can trigger DIC and platelet consumption by acceleration of platelet adhesion to damaged blood vessels. Consumptive thrombocytopenia also occurs in the setting of birth asphyxia, preeclampsia, hyperbilirubinemia treated with phototherapy, meconium aspiration, neonatal respiratory distress syndrome, persistent pulmonary hypertension, necrotizing enterocolitis, or cyanotic congenital heart disease.[20]

For all of these conditions, acute bleeding is treated or prevented with platelet transfusions while the underlying disorder is being investigated and corrected. *Platelet concentrates must be irradiated to minimize the risk of graft-versus-host disease.*

Neonatal Immune Thrombocytopenia

Isolated thrombocytopenia in an otherwise healthy newborn should raise suspicion of an immune-mediated mechanism. Discrimination between alloimmune and isoimmune thrombocytopenia is essential for the selection of a suitable platelet donor for the neonate.

Alloimmune thrombocytopenia is the result of transplacental passage of maternal antiplatelet autoantibody. In such situations, the mother's platelet count is usually decreased but may be normal. The duration of thrombocytopenia in the infant is a function of the persistence of maternal antibody in the neonate's circulation. Because IgG has a half-life of 21 days, the infant's thrombocytopenia generally resolves within several days to weeks after parturition.[20]

Most infants born to mothers with immune thrombocytopenic purpura (ITP) are not severely thrombocytopenic and require no intervention other than close observation. In the event of life-threatening hemorrhage, platelet transfusions may promote hemostasis, although a sustained increment in platelet count may not occur because of the rapid clearance of sensitized donor platelets. For the severely thrombocytopenic newborn at risk for life-threatening hemorrhage, infusion of IgG (1 g/kg/day for 2–3 days), either alone or in conjunction with corticosteroid administration (prednisolone, 2 mg/kg), may be the most effective therapy.[1]

Isoimmune thrombocytopenia occurs in infants whose mothers have normal platelet counts and no bleeding history. Hemorrhagic complications, such as gastrointestinal bleeding, hematuria, and hemoptysis, frequently occur in conjunction with a platelet count of less than $20 \times 10^9/L$. The occurrence of intracranial hemorrhage in approximately 15% of severely thrombocytopenic newborns represents the greatest source of morbidity in affected infants.[20]

Isoimmune thrombocytopenia is the result of maternal exposure to paternally derived antigens on fetal platelets that are not present in the same allelic form on maternal platelets. Maternal sensitization to foreign-platelet antigens results in the formation of antibodies directed against fetal platelets. Transplacental passage of antibodies results in fetal and neonatal thrombocytopenia. Human platelet antigen-1 (HPA-1, formerly designated PL^{A1}) is the most commonly implicated platelet antigen, causing 75% of cases of isoimmune thrombocytopenia. This antigen is found on the surface of platelets in 98% of the general population but is missing from the platelets of mothers with affected newborns.[21] First-born infants are affected in nearly 50% the cases. Maternal sensitization along with an attendant risk of antenatal intracranial hemorrhage can occur at any time during pregnancy.[22]

Infants born with platelet counts of less than $30 \times 10^9/L$ should be treated with platelet transfusions from a donor of HPA-1a antigen-negative status. The best source of HPA-1a–negative platelets is usually the patient's mother.[1] Isoimmune thrombocytopenia usually resolves within the first month of life.

Immune Thrombocytopenic Purpura

ITP affects about 20,000 children in the United States annually and has a peak incidence between 2 and 5 years of age. Patients commonly present with acute onset of petechiae and purpura, often 1 to 3 weeks after a nonspecific viral illness. Approximately 25% to 30% of affected children present with epistaxis, 5% of cases are complicated by gastrointestinal bleeding, and central nervous system (CNS) hemorrhage complicates 0.5% to 1% of cases.[23] Petechiae and purpura are the commonest findings on physical examination, and splenomegaly has been reported in 10% to 20% of patients. In contrast to adult-onset ITP, in which women are more commonly affected, no gender predilection exists in the pediatric form of the disease.

Laboratory Findings

Of all patients with ITP, 80% have with platelet counts below $40 \times 10^9/L$.[7] Review of the peripheral blood film reveals decreased numbers of abnormally large platelets. Results of coagulation studies (prothrombin time [PT], aPTT, fibrinogen, fibrin degradation products) are always normal. Examination of bone marrow aspirates typically reveals normal to increased numbers of megakaryocytes, consistent with increased platelet turnover. Although debate continues about the role of bone marrow aspiration in the diagnosis of acute ITP, many pediatric hematologists continue to perform this study as part of their evaluation of ITP.[24] While bone marrow aspiration appears to be unnecessary for the diagnosis and treatment of children with typical features of ITP,[25] this investigation is strongly recommended for children with atypical features, including a history of bone pain, palpable organomegaly, or neutropenia with or without anemia.[26] Bone marrow aspiration is also recommended in children with thrombocytopenia of greater than 6 months in duration, in children who fail to respond to intravenous (IV) IgG, and prior to initiating therapy with corticosteroids. In cases of life-threatening bleeding, IV IgG and IV high-dose corticosteroids (Solu-Medrol, 30 mg/kg) may be given concurrently.

Natural History

More than 80% of children with ITP experience remission within several months of presentation of the disease. Chronic ITP is defined as a platelet count below 100×10^9/L for longer than 6 months.[18] The pathogenesis of the acute and chronic forms of childhood ITP differs, with chronic ITP more closely resembling the adult form of the disease. Increased levels of platelet-associated IgG are found in approximately 90% of children with ITP; most of the immunoglobulin in patients with acute ITP is not platelet-specific autoantibody.[23] Some studies suggest that high levels of platelet-associated IgG may reflect the rapid turnover of platelets and the mobilization of IgG from alpha granules to the platelet membrane. Hence, elevated platelet-associated IgG levels are primarily a consequence, not a cause, of increased thrombolysis.[27] The temporal association of viral illness with the onset of acute ITP suggests that the latter may be triggered by antigen-antibody complexes adsorbed to the platelet membrane, prompting platelet clearance by reticuloendothelial system macrophages.[18, 28]

The onset of chronic ITP may be more insidious than that of the acute form, often presenting without a history of a viral prodrome. Ten per cent to 20% of children with new-onset ITP ultimately have chronic disease, with the greatest risk occurring in children older than 10 years of age.[18] The pathogenesis of chronic ITP involves the formation of platelet-specific autoantibodies that bind to antigenic determinants on the platelet surface.[18]

Treatment

The debate among pediatric hematologists regarding the need for treatment of acute ITP in childhood reflects the generally benign nature of the disease and the high incidence of spontaneous recovery. This course is in contrast to that of adult ITP, in which 60% to 80% of patients ultimately require splenectomy.[23] The most commonly employed treatment options include oral prednisone, intravenous IgG administration, and more recently, anti-D.[29, 30] For the acutely bleeding child, IgG (1 g/kg/day IV for 1 to 3 days) is the treatment of choice because of its rapid onset of action. Most children treated with IV IgG respond with an increase in platelet count within 1 week of initiation of therapy.

The mechanisms of action of intravenous IgG and corticosteroids remain incompletely understood. The effect of intravenous IgG may be mediated through the blockade of Fc receptors on macrophages, which prevents recognition and phagocytosis of opsonized platelets, or through idiotype–anti-idiotype interactions.[23] The mechanism of action of corticosteroids is even less well understood, although it appears to be multifactorial. Independent of their effect on platelet number, steroids may reduce bleeding risk in the thrombocytopenic patient by increasing microvascular stability.[2] Steroid-mediated increased platelet survival and subsequent resolution of thrombocytopenia have been attributed to suppression of antibody production by B lymphocytes and inhibition of phagocytosis of antibody-sensitized platelets.[7]

Platelet transfusions are indicated only in patients with life-threatening (e.g., CNS) hemorrhage. Donor platelets offer minimal benefit because of their rapid sensitization and subsequent clearance by the host reticuloendothelial system. In addition, donor platelets may stimulate alloantibody formation. If CNS bleeding requires neurosurgical evacuation, the patient should be prepared for emergency splenectomy and should be treated with IV IgG and bolus methylprednisolone administration.[18] Intraoperative infusion of platelet concentrates after interruption of the splenic blood supply maximizes the recovery and life span of donor platelets before craniotomy is performed. Because patients with ITP produce platelets at two to three times the rate of normal individuals, many patients exhibit a rapid increase in platelet count after ligation of the splenic pedicle.

Management guidelines for the thrombocytopenic child without active bleeding are less clear. We recommend that children with platelet counts of less than 20 to 30×10^9/L be treated with prednisone at an initial dose of 2 mg/kg/day for 1 to 3 weeks, followed by a gradual weaning of the dosage over 1 to 3 weeks. Because prolonged therapy with steroids can lead to fluid retention, osteoporosis, growth retardation, cushingoid features, and acne, children who either do not improve or cannot sustain improvement when steroids are weaned should be treated with intermittent doses of IV IgG or anti-D (50 μg/kg IV—*only effective in Rh+ individuals*) to maintain a platelet count of at least 30 to 40×10^9/L.[29] Splenectomy may be considered for the child with chronic ITP (see later). Because of the high risk of postsplenectomy sepsis, splenectomy should be deferred, if possible, until affected children are 6 years of age. All patients should receive the polyvalent pneumococcal vaccine before splenectomy and penicillin prophylaxis after splenectomy.

Splenectomy leads to partial or complete remission of thrombocytopenia in approximately 75% of patients with chronic ITP.[31] Recurrence of thrombocytopenia after splenectomy is performed should prompt a search for an accessory spleen or spleens. Treatment options for splenectomy nonresponders include periodic infusions of IgG, alternate-day administration of steroids, or administration of vinca alkaloids (vincristine or vinblastine), cyclophosphamide, cyclosporine, IgG anti-D, or interferon-α.[31]

Human Immunodeficiency Virus–Related Thrombocytopenia

Thrombocytopenia is a relatively common manifestation of HIV-1 infection. Although multiple etiologies exist for thrombocytopenia in patients with acquired immunodeficiency syndrome (e.g., infections, drugs), asymptomatic HIV-1–infected patients frequently experience a syndrome that is analogous to ITP. Although platelet-associated IgG levels are uniformly elevated in HIV-1–related ITP, the pathophysiology of platelet destruction is complex and multifaceted. Accelerated platelet destruction in homosexual men has been attributed to the adsorption of circulating immune complexes to platelet membranes, prompting their clearance by reticuloendothelial system macrophages. ITP in HIV-1–infected intravenous drug users results from a combination of platelet-bound immune complexes and platelet-specific autoantibody formation. In HIV-1–infected people with hemophilia, ITP is predominantly a consequence of autoantibodies directed against platelet membrane glycoproteins.[23] Most patients exhibit normal to increased numbers of megakaryocytes on examination of bone marrow aspirates. Some thrombocytopenic patients exhibit decreased numbers of megakaryocytes in bone marrow, or ineffective thrombopoiesis, or both, which may be a consequence of HIV-1 infection of megakaryocytes or deposition of immune complexes on their surfaces.[32]

Therapeutic options for patients with HIV-related thrombocytopenia are similar to those previously outlined for ITP. For bleeding patients, IV IgG administration is frequently effective, although increases in platelet count are transient, generally lasting 7 to 10 days. Corticosteroids are effective in a significant number of patients, although the effect is often not sustained. Steroid therapy may be complicated by the development of oropharyngeal candidiasis, reactivation of latent herpesvirus infection, and accelerated $CD4^+$ lymphocyte depletion. Zidovudine may be the most effective medical therapy for patients with thrombocytopenia. The rapid rise in platelet count observed after the initiation of zidovudine has been attributed to its antiviral effect.[33] Splenectomy is reserved for patients who do not respond to any of the aforementioned medical approaches.

Miscellaneous Causes of Acquired Thrombocytopenia

Infection

Thrombocytopenia is a common complication of systemic viral and bacterial infections, affecting 20% to 30% of patients with bacterial septicemia. Typically, the mechanism for development of thrombocytopenia is accelerated platelet clearance. Elevated levels of platelet-associated IgG and decreased platelet survival in both bacterial and viral (particularly Epstein-Barr virus) infections suggest an immune complex–mediated cause for the thrombocytopenia. Increased adhesion of platelets to exposed subendothelial surfaces of damaged blood vessels may contribute to thrombocytopenia in patients with bacterial sepsis.[7] Many patients with sepsis-associated thrombocytopenia do not experience concomitant consumptive coagulopathy.

Bone Marrow Infiltration

Thrombocytopenia secondary to decreased platelet production can result from the replacement of normal bone marrow by neoplastic or other infiltrative processes, such as the leukemias, neuroblastoma, and myeloproliferative, storage, and granulomatous disorders. Decreased production and increased consumption of platelets are associated with the virus-associated hemophagocytic syndrome, which is most frequently a consequence of acute cytomegalovirus or Epstein-Barr virus infection. Virus-associated hemophagocytic syndrome is characterized by histiocytic hyperplasia, sequestration of circulating platelets in the spleen and liver, and phagocytosis of hematopoietic precursors by medullary histiocytes.[34]

Pharmacologic Agents

Thrombocytopenia can be caused by decreased production or increased consumption of circulating platelets. The marrow-suppressive effects of chemotherapeutic agents used to treat cancer are well characterized and predictable. Thrombocytopenia secondary to myelosuppressive medications is treated with infusions of platelet concentrates in patients with active bleeding or in those with platelet counts of less than 10×10^9/L. A higher threshold for platelet transfusion (20×10^9/L) is recommended for patients with brain tumors.[35]

Drug-mediated platelet consumption is usually idiosyncratic and typically results from an immune-mediated mechanism. Thrombocytopenia usually occurs days to weeks after the introduction of the offending drug. Reexposure to the causative medication after resolution of the thrombocytopenia leads to a prompt decrease in platelet count. Specific mechanisms underlying the development of drug-induced thrombocytopenia[7] include:

1. Binding of drug-antidrug antibody complexes to platelets.
2. Binding of the drug directly to the platelet surface, prompting antibody attachment to the drug-platelet complex.
3. Formation of platelet membrane neoantigens caused by binding of the drug to the platelet surface.
4. Formation of drug-induced platelet autoantibodies (e.g., those caused by methyldopa, quinidine, interferon).

Although many drugs have been implicated in the development of drug-induced thrombocytopenia, this complication occurs most commonly in patients taking heparin. Quinidine, the penicillins, digoxin, valproic acid, and cimetidine have also been implicated in the development of idiosyncratic thrombocytopenia.[7, 36] Heparin is unique because of its ability to cause life-threatening arterial thrombosis with thrombocytopenia and because of the tendency for the thrombocytopenia to improve in some instances, despite continuation of heparin therapy. Heparin-induced thrombocytopenia occurs a mean of 10 days after its initiation; more commonly, it appears in patients taking higher doses and in those treated with bovine preparations. If arterial thrombosis develops, heparin therapy should be immediately discontinued. A combination of low-molecular-weight heparin and antifibrinolytic therapy may be an effective alternative therapy in patients with arterial thrombosis until oral anticoagulants reach effective plasma levels.[36] In children with mild thrombocytopenia, heparin therapy may be continued; however, careful attention should be paid to the platelet count, and transition to oral anticoagulant therapy should be initiated as soon as possible.

Therapy for drug-induced thrombocytopenias consists of stopping the offending drug as soon as possible.[7]

Miscellaneous Causes of Platelet Dysfunction

Uremia

Hemorrhagic complications in uremic patients arise from impaired platelet–vessel wall interactions. Qualitative defects in plasma vWF and decreased levels of platelet vWF are believed to be the primary causes of uremic bleeding.[37] Additional factors contributing to the increased bleeding include platelet granule defects and impairment of platelet aggregation resulting from high concentrations of uremic retention products. Alterations in vessel wall endothelium lead to increased production of the platelet antagonist prostacyclin (prostaglandin I_2).[38] Patients characteristically exhibit petechiae, purpura, mucous membrane bleeding, prolonged bleeding times, and abnormal platelet aggregation.

Anemia has also been identified as a contributor to the hemostatic impairment occurring in uremic patients. Elevations in hematocrit value, achieved either through red blood cell transfusions or through the use of recombinant human erythropoietin, can lead to shortened bleeding time and decreased bleeding tendency. Increasing the hematocrit value to 30% may lead to displacement of circulating platelets toward the vessel wall, thereby facilitating their contact with the endothelium and improving hemostasis.[38]

Uremic bleeding diathesis is most effectively managed with a combination of dialysis and maintenance of an adequate hematocrit value.[38] In patients with persistent bleeding after dialysis or in those who are at high risk for hemorrhagic complications from elective surgery, bleeding risk can be further reduced with infusions of cryoprecipitate or DDAVP. Both measures increase plasma vWF levels, transiently decrease bleeding time, and probably reduce bleeding tendency.[14]

Extracorporeal Oxygenation

Children supported by cardiopulmonary bypass or extracorporeal membrane oxygenation (ECMO) are at risk for hemostatic derangements that can lead to excessive intraoperative and postoperative bleeding. Potential defects include impaired platelet function, mild (dilutional) thrombocytopenia, increased fibrinolysis, and inadequate neutralization of the anticoagulant heparin. Hypothermia can exacerbate thrombocytopenia as a result of splenic and hepatic platelet pooling, which is reversed when body temperature is normalized.[39]

Platelet dysfunction appears to be the primary cause of postoperative bleeding complications. As platelets pass through the oxygenator apparatus, they may undergo partial activation and may secrete their granular contents, causing partial depletion of alpha granules.[39] Platelet function is further impaired by plasma membrane–receptor defects that compromise the binding of plasma protein ligands, such as fibrinogen and vWF. The severity of platelet dysfunction appears to vary in proportion to the duration of bypass. Postoperative platelet transfusions are usually sufficient to control hemorrhage for all patients except those (~3%) who require surgical reexploration.[40] Controlled, randomized studies using preoperative infusions of the serine protease inhibitor aprotonin or intraoperative infusions of DDAVP in adults have demonstrated shortened bleeding times and decreased blood loss after cardiopulmonary bypass.[40, 41] Although these therapeutic adjuncts appear promising, their role in children remains to be established.

Pharmacologic Agents

Drug-induced platelet dysfunction rarely causes spontaneous hemorrhage unless it is superimposed on an underlying hemostatic disorder, such as thrombocytopenia or hemophilia. The most noteworthy drug effects on platelet function (e.g., those resulting from aspirin or nonsteroidal anti-inflammatory drug administration) are mediated through inhibition of platelet cyclooxygenase activity. Inactivation of cyclooxygenase inhibits the production of thromboxane A_2, a potent platelet agonist. The semisynthetic penicillins and cephalosporins can produce variable defects of in vitro platelet aggregation that are dose and duration dependent.[18]

The clinical significance of these observations is unclear. Although inhibition of platelet function may be therapeutically desirable in specific contexts (e.g., prevention of recurrent myocardial infarction or stroke), unwanted platelet dysfunction is treated by withdrawal of the causative agent. Drugs that interfere with platelet function should be avoided, if possible, in patients with underlying congenital or acquired hemostatic deficits (Table 160–2).

TABLE 160–2. Commonly Used Drugs That Prolong Bleeding Time or Decrease In Vitro Platelet Aggregation

Antiplatelet Agents
Aspirin
Dipyridamole
Sulfinpyrazone
Ticlopidine
Antibiotics
Semisynthetic penicillins
Cephalosporins
Nonsteroidal Anti-inflammatory Agents
Ibuprofen
Naproxen
Indomethacin
Phenylbutazone
Miscellaneous
Heparin
Dextran sulfate
Glyceryl guaiacolate
Ethyl alcohol
Valproic acid
ω_3-J Polyunsaturated fatty acids
Phenothiazines

From Bray GL: Inherited and acquired disorders of hemostasis. *In:* Textbook of Pediatric Clinical Care. Holbrook PR (Ed). Philadelphia, WB Saunders, 1993, pp 783–801.

INHERITED COAGULOPATHIES

Development of the Coagulation Mechanism

Clotting and fibrinolytic proteins are detectable in fetal plasma as early as 10 to 11 weeks of gestation, with the levels of most coagulation proteins rising in proportion to gestational age.[42] Although most coagulation plasma proteins approach adult levels by the time an individual is 6 months of age, as a group they exhibit discordant developmental patterns.[43] For example, the mean levels of factor VIII, vWF, and fibrinogen approximate the normal adult range by 30 weeks' gestation. In contrast, the levels of vitamin K–dependent coagulation proteins (factors II, IX, and X and protein C) are significantly lower, ranging from 40% to 66% of adult mean levels in full-term infants.[44] Significant differences exist also in neonatal, early childhood, and adult levels of the contact activation clotting factors (newborns have 30% to 50% of adult mean levels at term), the major coagulation protease inhibitors (protein C, protein S, antithrombin III, and heparin cofactor II), and the activators and inhibitors of fibrinolysis.[44, 45] Some investigators have suggested that the lower risk for thrombosis in early childhood may be the result of the nearly twofold higher levels of the minor coagulation protease inhibitor, alpha$_2$-macroglobulin.[45] The relative infrequency of thrombosis in children may also result from lower levels of prothrombin, which alter the kinetics of clot formation in a protective manner.

Not surprisingly, in view of the physiologic differences in individual factor levels at different stages of development, results of coagulation screening tests must be interpreted in the context of age-specific norms. During the first 6 months of life, the acceptable upper limit of the aPTT is greater than in adults. This discrepancy is the result of the aforementioned age-dependent difference in concentration of the contact activation factors (factor XII, factor XI, high-molecular-weight kininogen, and prekallikrein). In contrast, upper-limit norms for PT are stable from shortly after birth through adulthood, reflecting the attainment of adult levels of factor VII within the first week of life.[43] Recently established age-adjusted norms for factor levels and coagulation screening tests should improve diagnostic accuracy and enhance the appropriateness of interventions based on these assays. Table 160–3 lists the age-adjusted normal values for various components of the coagulation mechanism.

Hemophilias

Patients with hemophilia characteristically exhibit bleeding into joints and muscles after either minimal or no trauma. In all individuals with hemophilia, bleeding is the result of delayed thrombin generation, which in turn results in deficient clot formation.

Hemophilia A (factor VIII deficiency) and hemophilia B (factor IX deficiency) account for most inherited coagulopathies. Factor VIII deficiency is the cause of 80% to 85% of all cases of hemophilia, occurring in 1 in 5000 male births. Ten per cent to 15% of hemophilia results from factor IX deficiency, which occurs in 1 in 25,000 males. Nearly one third of newly diagnosed patients with hemophilia have no family history of coagulopathy, reflecting the common occurrence of spontaneous mutation in the genes for factors VIII and IX.[46–48] Because the clinical manifestations of hemophilias A and B are indistinguishable, the correct diagnosis depends on the results of specific assays for factors VIII and IX.

The frequency and severity of bleeding episodes in people with hemophilia are largely a function of the baseline coagulation factor level. Activity levels measure endogenous factor availability relative to a reference standard that is 100% of

TABLE 160–3. Reference Values for Coagulation Tests in the Healthy Full-Term Infant During the First 6 Months of Life

Coagulation Test*	Day 1 (mean/range)	Day 5 (mean/range)	Day 30 (mean/range)	Day 90 (mean/range)	Day 180 (mean/range)	Adult (mean/range)
PT	13.0/10.1–15.9†	12.4/10.0–15.3†	11.8/10.0–14.3†	11.9/10.0–14.2†	12.3/10.7–13.9†	12.4/10.8–13.9
INR	1.00/0.53–1.62	0.89/0.53–1.48	0.79/0.53–1.26	0.81/0.53–1.26	0.88/0.61–1.17	0.89/0.64–1.17
aPTT	42.9/31.3–54.5	42.6/25.4–59.8	40.4/32.0–55.2	37.1/29.0–50.1†	35.5/28.1–42.9†	33.5/26.6–40.3
TCT	23.5/19.0–28.3†	23.1/18.0–29.2	24.3/19.4–29.2†	25.1/20.5–29.7†	25.5/19.8–31.2†	25.0/19.7–30.3
Fibrinogen (g/L)	2.83/1.67–3.99†	3.12/1.62–4.62†	2.70/1.62–3.78†	2.43/1.50–3.79†	2.51/1.50–3.87†	2.78/1.56–4.00
Procoagulation factors						
II (U/mL)	0.48/0.26–0.70	0.63/0.33–0.93	0.68/0.34–1.02	0.75/0.45–1.05	0.88/0.60–1.16	1.08/0.70–1.46
V (U/mL)	0.72/0.34–1.08	0.96/0.45–1.45	0.98/0.62–1.34	0.90/0.48–1.32	0.91/0.55–1.27	1.06/0.62–1.50
VII (U/mL)	0.66/0.28–1.04	0.89/0.35–1.43	0.90/0.42–1.38	0.91/0.39–1.43	0.87/0.47–1.27	1.05/0.67–1.43
VIII (U/mL)	1.00/0.50–1.78†	0.88/0.50–1.54†	0.91/0.50–1.57†	0.79/0.50–1.25†	0.73/0.50–1.09	0.99/0.50–1.49
IX (U/mL)	0.53/0.15–0.91	0.53/0.15–0.91	0.51/0.21–0.81	0.67/0.21–1.13	0.86/0.36–1.36	1.09/0.55–1.63
X (U/mL)	0.40/0.12–0.68	0.49/0.19–0.79	0.59/0.31–0.87	0.71/0.35–1.07	0.78/0.38–1.18	1.06/0.70–1.52
XI (U/mL)	0.38/0.10–0.66	0.55/0.23–0.87	0.53/0.27–0.79	0.69/0.41–0.97	0.86/0.49–1.34	0.97/0.67–1.27
XII (U/mL)	0.53/0.13–0.93	0.47/0.11–0.83	0.49/0.17–0.81	0.67/0.25–1.09	0.77/0.39–1.15	1.08/0.52–1.64
XIIIa (U/mL)	0.79/0.27–1.31	0.94/0.44–1.44†	0.93/0.39–1.47†	1.04/0.36–1.72†	1.04/0.46–1.62†	1.05/0.55–1.55
XIIIb (U/mL)	0.76/0.30–1.22	1.06/0.32–1.90	1.11/0.39–1.73†	1.16/0.48–1.84†	1.10/0.50–1.70†	0.97/0.57–1.37
vWF (U/mL)	1.53/0.50–2.87	1.40/0.50–2.54	1.28/0.50–2.46†	1.18/0.50–2.06	1.07/0.50–1.97	0.92/0.50–1.58
PK (U/mL)	0.37/0.18–0.69	0.48/0.20–0.76	0.57/0.23–0.91	0.73/0.41–1.05	0.86/0.56–1.16	1.12/0.62–1.62
HMWK (U/mL)	0.54/0.06–1.02	0.74/0.16–1.32	0.77/0.33–1.21	0.82/0.30–1.46†	0.82/0.36–1.28†	0.92/0.50–1.36

Modified from Andrew M, Paes B, Milner R, et al: Development of the human coagulation system in the full-term infant. Blood 1987; 70:165–172.

*All factors except fibrinogen are expressed as U/mL, where pooled plasma contains 1.0 U/mL. All reference values are expressed as mean and range, which encompass 95% of the population. Between 40 and 77 samples were assayed for each value for the newborn. Some measurements were skewed because of a disproportionate number of high values. The lower limit, which excludes the lower 2.5% of the population, has been given.

†Values that are indistinguishable from those of the adult.

aPTT = activated partial thromboplastin time; HMWK = high-molecular-weight kininogen; INR = international normalized ratio; PK = prekallikrein; PT = prothrombin time; TCT = thrombin-clotting time; vWF = von Willebrand's factor.

normal (100 IU/dL). Patients with factor levels greater than 5% of normal are mildly affected and bleed only in response to significant trauma or surgery. Severely affected patients with less than 1% of normal activity are prone to frequent, spontaneous episodes of bleeding.[46] Because mean factor VIII levels in normal newborns are within the normal adult range, the diagnosis of factor VIII deficiency, regardless of severity, is generally easy in early infancy.[43] In contrast, factor IX levels consistent with mild deficiency overlap with those observed in normal newborns, potentially complicating the diagnosis of mild hemophilia B shortly after birth.[43]

Bleeding Manifestations

Many children with hemophilia, particularly those who are mildly or moderately affected, do not experience abnormal bleeding during the first year of life. The onset of abnormal bleeding often coincides with the attainment of motor development milestones, such as crawling or walking.[46] Some hemophilic infants initially present with significant bleeding after a forceps-assisted delivery or circumcision. The absence of abnormal bleeding after circumcision does not rule out the diagnosis of hemophilia, since only 30% of infants bleed excessively after this procedure.[13] As the child becomes increasingly mobile during the second year of life, the incidence of musculoskeletal bleeding generally increases. Typical presentations include excessive cutaneous bruising, bleeding from the nose and mouth, muscle hematomas in the extremities, and hemarthroses, most often involving the knees, elbows, and ankles.

Potentially life-threatening complications of hemophilia include CNS, retropharyngeal, or retroperitoneal hemorrhage and bleeding associated with episodes of multiple trauma or with surgery undertaken without adequate factor replacement. The incidence of CNS hemorrhage in patients with hemophilia varies from 2.6% to 13.8%, with a case fatality rate ranging from 20% to 50%. Chronic neurologic deficits (seizure disorder, cognitive or motor deficits) occur in up to 50% of patients who survive CNS bleeding.[49]

Intracranial bleeding in infants and children usually follows head trauma. In a large, retrospective study of infants with hemophilia, nearly 2% experienced CNS hemorrhage related to birth trauma either during or shortly after delivery, and an additional 1.9% exhibited intracranial hemorrhage within the first 4 weeks of life.[50] Because CNS bleeding is a relatively common problem in newborns, particularly in premature infants, the possibility of an inherited factor deficiency may be overlooked. Thus, levels of factors VIII and IX should be assayed in any male infant with intracranial bleeding, regardless of whether a history of trauma or birth asphyxia is elicited.

Bleeding into the retropharyngeal space can lead to asphyxia as a result of extrinsic compression of the upper airway. This complication may occur rapidly in infants because of their small upper-airway diameter. Older children may present with complaints of sore throat, dysphagia, or hoarse speech. Presenting manifestations in infants and toddlers may include nasal flaring, labored respirations, and inspiratory stridor suggestive of upper-airway obstruction. Diagnostic findings include abnormal widening of the retropharyngeal soft tissue shadow on lateral neck x-ray studies and increased lucency of the retropharyngeal soft tissues on computed tomography (CT).[51]

Retroperitoneal hemorrhage occurring after blunt trauma to the abdomen or flank can lead to cardiovascular collapse as a result of extensive bleeding into the retroperitoneal space. Clinical manifestations include diffuse tenderness over the abdomen and back, accompanied by signs and symptoms of intravascular volume loss. Blood in the retroperitoneal cavity can be identified by either ultrasound or abdominal CT scan.[46, 52]

Limb-threatening bleeding complications of hemophilia include compartment syndromes caused by hematomas that compress neurovascular bundles. Bleeding into the iliopsoas muscle may be difficult to diagnose because of the localization of pain to the groin or lower abdomen, mimicking either hemarthrosis of the hip or acute appendicitis. Patients typically present with flexion and external rotation of the hip on the involved side. Compression of the femoral nerve can result in paresthesias along the anterior aspect of the thigh, quadriceps muscle paresis, and diminished patellar reflexes. Plain x-ray studies of the abdomen often reveal loss of the psoas muscle shadow.

The presence of a hematoma can be confirmed with retroperitoneal ultrasound.[13, 46] Compartment syndrome can also arise in the forearm. Expanding intramuscular hematomas can compress the median and ulnar nerves, resulting in significant functional deficits in the hand.[46]

Treatment

Guidelines

Therapy for hemophilia-related bleeding depends on several factors:

1. Severity of the factor deficiency.
2. Location, severity, and duration of the hemorrhagic event.
3. Half-life of the coagulation product infused.
4. Issues that may alter the pharmacokinetics of factor replacement, such as the presence of an inhibitor.

Products available for the treatment of bleeding in patients with hemophilia A include lyophilized factor VIII concentrates (either plasma-derived or recombinant) and DDAVP.

Factor VIII concentrates are available in either intermediate or high purity. *Intermediate-purity* products have relatively low specific activity (<15 IU/mg of protein) and often contain variable quantities of fibrinogen, fibronectin, and vWF. *High-purity* factor VIII, either recombinant or plasma-derived, is prepared by monoclonal antibody–affinity chromatography and contains only factor VIII and pasteurized human albumin, which is added as a stabilizer. Plasma from several thousand donors who are screened for HIV-1 and hepatitis B and C virus infection are required for each lot of factor VIII concentrate manufactured.

Factor VIII concentrates are either pasteurized or treated with a solvent-detergent suspension to inactivate lipid-enveloped viruses that may have eluded detection in the screening process. The combination of screening, purification, and viral inactivation measures has nearly eliminated the risk of viral transmission from the use of factor concentrates. Risk of infection by human blood-borne viruses is nonexistent when recombinant factor VIII is employed.[53–56] In light of these advances in purity and safety, replacement therapy for hemophilia A–related bleeding has moved away from the use of single-donor cryoprecipitate and toward the *exclusive* use of virally inactivated, plasma-derived, or recombinant factor VIII preparations.[57]

The in vivo recovery, biologic half-life, and hemostatic effectiveness of high-purity products are comparable to those of intermediate-purity preparations. Infusion of 1 U/kg of factor VIII usually results in a 2% increment in plasma factor VIII level 30 minutes after infusion, and the factor has a biologic half-life ranging from 12 to 15 hours.[46] Less than the expected recovery or half-life suggests the presence of an inhibitor to factor VIII.

As noted earlier, DDAVP carries no risk of blood-borne viral infection because it is not derived from human plasma. Infusion of DDAVP (0.3 μg/kg) generally increases factor VIII levels to three to five times baseline levels. Patients with moderate to severe factor VIII deficiency do not exhibit an adequate therapeutic response to DDAVP for most bleeding events.[14] Potential candidates for treatment (i.e., patients with baseline factor VIII levels ≥ 10% to 15% of normal) should receive DDAVP infusion to assess the extent of their response. Once the magnitude of response has been documented, the indication for DDAVP is determined by the severity of the bleeding episode and the desired plasma factor VIII level. DDAVP is not recommended for the treatment of life-threatening hemorrhage.[14, 58]

Therapeutic options for patients with factor IX deficiency include infusion of fresh frozen plasma (FFP) and factor IX concentrates of intermediate or high purity. FFP provides 1 U/mL of factor IX activity. In view of its low specific activity and the fluid limitations frequently imposed on critically ill children, FFP is often impractical as a means of factor IX replacement therapy. In general, FFP use is limited to the treatment or prophylaxis of minor bleeding complications that require no more than a 10% to 15% increment in factor IX activity over baseline levels.[58]

Until recently, prothrombin complex concentrates (PCCs) were the only alternative to FFP for factor IX replacement therapy. In addition to factor IX, PCCs contain significant amounts of other vitamin K–dependent clotting proteins (factors II and X) and small quantities of activated clotting proteins. Factors II and X have in vivo half-lives that exceed that of factor IX, leading to accumulation of these procoagulants when repeated doses of PCCs are used. Frequent infusions of PCCs carry a risk of thromboembolic complications and DIC that may be caused by the accumulation of activated clotting proteins and supraphysiologic levels of factors II and X in plasma.[59] The risk of thrombosis is greatest in patients receiving large amounts of PCCs over a short period of time and in those with other risk factors for hypercoagulability, such as polycythemia, prolonged immobility, or advanced liver disease. The risk of thromboembolic complications may be decreased by the addition of heparin, given as 5 IU/mL of reconstituted factor concentrate or 100 IU of heparin per 500 IU of factor IX.[60, 61] In view of the risk for thrombosis with PCCs, their use should be avoided in newborns.

Currently, two licensed high-purity factor IX preparations provide highly specific activity for factor IX and decreased concentrations of non–factor IX proteins. These preparations are recommended for use in patients who require surgery, who have chronic liver disease, or who have sustained substantial crush injuries requiring prolonged factor replacement and immobilization.[59, 62] Available options for factor IX replacement have recently increased with the licensure of Benefix, a recombinant factor IX preparation. Although the absence of infectious risk makes this recombinant product an appealing option, clinicians should be aware that pharmacokinetic studies have demonstrated in vivo factor IX recovery that is only 70% of the level achieved with a comparable dose of high-purity, plasma-derived factor IX concentrate.[63] Thus, 20% to 30% more recombinant factor IX must be infused to achieve desired plasma levels.

The recovery and half-life of factor IX differ from those of factor VIII. Thirty minutes after infusion of 1 IU/kg of factor IX, plasma levels rise by only 1%. The biologic half-life of factor IX is 18 to 24 hours.[46, 60]

Major Bleeding Events and Preparation for Surgery

Patients with life-threatening or limb-threatening hemorrhage require prompt correction of factor activity to 80% to 100% of normal, and maintenance of factor levels in the range of 50% to 100% is usually indicated for several days to weeks thereafter. Patients with CNS bleeding should receive 2 weeks of uninterrupted factor replacement therapy. These individuals are at risk for rebleeding into the CNS for up to 6 months after the initial event.[58]

For patients with hemophilia A, 100% correction is achieved with a loading dose of 50 IU/kg of factor VIII, followed by repeated infusions of 25 IU/kg every 12 to 15 hours. Alternately, a continuous infusion of factor VIII at a dose of 2 to 3

U/kg/hr may be delivered after the initial loading dose.[58] Response to factor replacement should be carefully monitored both by clinical assessment and by regular assays of plasma factor VIII levels. The management of major bleeding events in patients with hemophilia B is analogous to that of hemophilia A, requiring 80% to 100% correction of factor IX activity. This goal is usually achieved with a loading dose of 80 to 100 IU/kg of factor IX, followed by 40 to 50 U/kg every 18 to 24 hours.[13] When PCCs are used, patients should be closely monitored for evidence of DIC and thrombosis because of the significant levels of activated factors VII, X, and prothrombin contained in these preparations. In light of the improved safety profile of the high-purity factor IX concentrates, these preparations are preferred to PCCs when available.[64]

Preparation for surgical procedures follows similar guidelines for factor replacement as outlined for life-threatening hemorrhages. All surgical candidates should be screened preoperatively for the presence of inhibitors to prevent potentially life-threatening bleeding due to suboptimal intraoperative factor recovery and half-life (discussed later). For major surgery, postoperative factor replacement should allow for maintenance of factor levels that are 50% of normal for 5 to 7 days, followed by levels of at least 30% for an additional week.[13]

Non–Life-Threatening Hemorrhage and Minor Invasive Procedures

Less aggressive measures are required for the treatment of routine hemarthrosis and hematomas or for the preparation for minor surgical procedures, such as tooth extractions. For children undergoing dental extractions or presenting with gingival bleeding, adjunctive therapy with an antifibrinolytic agent (ε-aminocaproic acid or tranexamic acid) is often sufficient to maintain hemostasis after an initial infusion of factor concentrate. Antifibrinolytic therapy has not proved useful for the treatment of hemarthrosis. Use of these adjunctive measures is contraindicated in the setting of hematuria. Because of the increased risk of thrombosis, use of antifibrinolytic therapy in patients receiving PCCs should be deferred or avoided.[58] Specific dosing recommendations for both routine and major hemorrhagic events or surgical procedures are summarized in Table 160–4.

Complications

INHIBITORS. Approximately 22% to 33% of patients with hemophilia A and 2% to 3% of those with hemophilia B develop alloantibodies against factors VIII and IX, respectively.[65–67] Alloantibodies neutralize the functional activity of infused clotting proteins, resulting in the partial or complete failure of factor replacement therapy. Inhibitors occur principally in patients with moderate-to-severe factor deficiency (i.e., <5% factor activity), and most of these patients are initially identified in childhood or adolescence. Inhibitors are quantitated in a Bethesda assay, in which 1 U of inhibitory activity is the amount capable of neutralizing 50% of the factor activity present in a 1:1 mixture of patient and normal plasma that is incubated at 37°C for 2 hours.[68, 69]

Strategies for the treatment or prevention of bleeding in patients with inhibitors depend on:

- Inhibitor titer at the time of the bleeding event
- Presence or absence of an anamnestic response when the patient is challenged with the deficient clotting factor
- Type and severity of hemorrhage

TABLE 160–4. Treatment of Specific Hemorrhages in Hemophilia

Type of Bleeding	Hemophilia A	Hemophilia B
Hemarthrosis*	20 U/kg FVIII concentrate†, 15 U/kg if treated early. Repeat dose the following day if bleed is severe.	30 U/kg FIX concentrate‡; 20 U/kg if treated early.
Muscle or significant subcutaneous hematoma	20 U/kg FVIII concentrate; may need treatment every other day until bleed is well controlled.	30 U/kg FIX concentrate; may need treatment every 2 or 3 days until bleeding is well controlled.†
Mouth, deciduous tooth, or tooth extraction	20 U/kg FVIII concentrate; antifibrinolytic therapy; remove loose deciduous tooth.	30 U/kg concentrate; antifibrinolytic therapy§; remove loose deciduous tooth.
Epistaxis	Pressure for 15–20 min; pack with petroleum jelly gauze; antifibrinolytic therapy; 20 U/kg FVIII concentrate if aforementioned therapy fails.	Pressure for 15–20 min; pack with petroleum jelly gauze; antifibrinolytic therapy; 30 U/kg FIX concentrate if aforementioned therapy fails (4 h after antifibrinolytic dose).
Major surgery, life-threatening hemorrhage (e.g., CNS, GI, airway)	50 U/kg FVIII concentrate, then 25 U/kg q 12 h or continuous infusion to maintain FVIII >50 U/dL for 5–7 d, then >30 U/dL for 5–7 d.	80 U/kg FIX concentrate, then 20–40 U/kg every 12–24 h to maintain FIX >40 U/dL for 5–7 days, then >30 U/dL for 5–7 days.‡
Iliopsoas hemorrhage	50 U/kg FVIII concentrate, then 25 U/kg every 12 h until patient is asymptomatic, then 50 U/kg every other day for a total of 10–14 d.‖	80 U/kg FIX concentrate, then 20–40 U/kg every 12–24 h to maintain FIX > 40 U/dL until patient is asymptomatic, then 30 U/kg every other day for a total of 10–14 days.‡‖
Hematuria	Bed rest; 1½ × maintenance fluids; if bleeding is not controlled in 1 or 2 days, 20 U/kg FVIII concentrate; if bleeding is not controlled, prednisone if patient's status is HIV-negative.	Bed rest; 1½ × maintenance fluids; if bleeding is not controlled in 1 or 2 days, 30 U/kg FIX concentrate; if bleeding is not controlled, prednisone if patient's status is HIV-negative.

Modified from Gill JC, Montgomery RR: Principles of therapy for hemostasis factor deficiencies. *In:* Hematology of Infancy and Childhood. 4th ed. Nathan DG, Oski FA (Eds). Philadelphia, WB Saunders, 1993, p 1799.

*For hip hemarthrosis, orthopedic evaluation for possible aspiration is advisable.

†For mild or moderate hemophilia, DDAVP, 0.3 μg/kg, should be used instead of FVIII concentrate if patient is known to respond with a hemostatic level of FVIII; if repeated doses are given, monitor FVIII levels for tachyphylaxis.

‡If repeated doses of prothrombin complex concentrate are used to replace FIX, add heparin, 100 units per 500 units of FIX, and monitor antithrombin III and DIC parameters. When highly purified FIX concentrates are available, they are preferred. When Benefix (recombinant FIX) is used, recommended doses should be increased by 120% to 150%.

§Do not give antifibrinolytic therapy until 4–6 hours after a dose of FIX concentrate.

‖Repeat radiologic assessment before discontinuation of therapy.

CNS = central nervous system; DDAVP = desmopressin acetate; DIC = disseminated intravascular coagulation; F = factor; GI = gastrointestinal; HIV = human immunodeficiency virus; FVIII = factor VIII; FIX = factor 9.

Patients who demonstrate a brisk anamnestic response after repeated exposure to infused factor are described as "high responders." In contrast, patients with inhibitors that are low in titer (<10 Bethesda units) and that do not rise significantly after repeated exposure to the deficient factor are referred to as "low responders." Low responders can spontaneously lose antibody or can evolve into high responders, and high responders can revert to low-responder status.[58]

Life-threatening hemorrhage in low responders can usually be managed by infusion of higher than normal doses of the deficient factor (e.g., bolus with 100 U/kg of factor VIII, followed by continuous infusion of 10 to 20 U/kg/hr) as a means of overwhelming the effects of the inhibitor. Factor levels should be monitored at 1 and 4 hours after the bolus infusion and then at least once daily to determine the efficacy of the dosing schedule.[58] Patients who respond well to this regimen initially may later not benefit, necessitating a switch to a different therapeutic approach.

Few universally accepted guidelines exist for the management of bleeding in high responders. Although several potential treatment modalities exist for these patients, none predictably and consistently arrests (or prevents) bleeding.[62, 67] Management of bleeding complications in patients with high-responder inhibitors should always be carried out in consultation with a hematologist (preferably in a hemophilia treatment center) who is familiar with available treatment modalities.[68-76]

TRANSFUSION-TRANSMITTED INFECTIONS. Since the first reported cases of acquired immunodeficiency syndrome (AIDS) in people with hemophilia, infection by human blood-borne viruses (principally HIV-1 and hepatitis C virus) has emerged as the greatest cause of mortality in patients with hemophilia.[77, 78] In a 1989 review, approximately 80% of patients with severe factor VIII deficiency and 40% to 50% of patients with severe factor IX deficiency have HIV-1 infection.[77] A more recent review of treatment-related infectious complications in hemophiliacs reported a 53% rate of HIV seropositivity.[79, 80] More than 80% of patients with severe hemophilia are seropositive for hepatitis C virus; most of these patients have chronic hepatitis C virus infection and thus are at significant risk for development of chronic active hepatitis, cirrhosis, and hepatocellular carcinoma over the course of years to decades.[74, 81, 82]

Other Inherited Coagulation Factor Deficiencies

Deficiencies of the contact activation factor XII, prekallikrein, or high-molecular-weight kininogen are rare conditions that cause a prolonged aPTT but do not predispose to abnormal bleeding. No specific measures are indicated in the critical care management of patients with a deficiency of one of these proteins. Deficiency of factor XI is inherited in an autosomal fashion and occurs most frequently in individuals of Ashkenazi Jewish descent. Levels of factor XI of less than 30% are associated with postoperative or post-traumatic bleeding complications. Because neither the degree of aPTT prolongation nor the baseline level of factor XI correlates well with the risk of bleeding, factor XI replacement is recommended for patients with levels of factor XI that are less than 30% of normal who require surgery.[13]

Deficiencies of prothrombin, fibrinogen, or factors V, VII, X, and XIII are inherited in an autosomal fashion. All are associated with abnormal bleeding, with the severity and risk of hemorrhage reflecting the extent of deficiency. Deficiency of factor V, factor X, fibrinogen, or prothrombin is associated with prolongation of both the PT and the aPTT. Isolated prolongation of PT is characteristic of factor VII deficiency. Abnormal bleeding occurs in patients with prothrombin levels of less than 30% and factor VII levels of less than 15% to 20%. Bleeding secondary to prothrombin deficiency usually responds to infusions of FFP or PCCs.[13] Likewise, factor VII-deficient patients can be treated with either FFP or lyophilized concentrates that contain high levels of factor VII.[13, 14]

Clinically significant hypofibrinogenemia (<75 mg/dL) may become apparent in the neonatal period, with gastrointestinal bleeding or extensive hematoma formation related to birth trauma, or later in life, with excessive postsurgical bleeding or wound dehiscence. Both FFP and cryoprecipitate can be used for fibrinogen replacement, although cryoprecipitate is a more concentrated source of this protein.[13] Severe deficiency of factor XIII (<1% of normal) is associated with impaired clot stability. Clinical manifestations include prolonged oozing after separation of the umbilical stump, easy bruisability, mucous membrane bleeding, and poor wound healing. Patients with factor XIII deficiency have normal PT, aPTT, and thrombin time. Diagnosis depends on the demonstration of abnormally rapid clot lysis in the presence of 5 mol/L urea or 1% monochloroacetic acid.[13]

ACQUIRED COAGULOPATHIES

Vitamin K Deficiency

Vitamin K is a cofactor that is required for the normal post translational γ-carboxylation of prothrombin, factor VII, factor IX, factor X, protein C, and protein S. In vitamin K–deficiency states, these coagulation proteins do not bind calcium normally, a prerequisite for their normal activation and function.[12] Factors contributing to vitamin K deficiency in the newborn include low placental transfer of vitamin K, low concentrations of vitamin K in breast milk, and lack of vitamin K_2 synthesis by intestinal flora at birth.[45] Symptomatic vitamin K deficiency generally presents within the first days to weeks of life in the form of hemorrhagic disease of the newborn. Early hemorrhagic disease of the newborn presents at or shortly after birth with the occurrence of cephalhematomas and intracranial, intrathoracic, or intra-abdominal hemorrhage. It is usually a consequence of maternal ingestion of vitamin K antagonists (e.g., warfarin, anticonvulsants, antituberculous medications) before delivery.[57]

Classic hemorrhagic disease of the newborn arises within the first week of life, often with cutaneous bruising, gastrointestinal bleeding, or excessive hemorrhage after circumcision in breast-fed infants who do not receive vitamin K at birth.[57] The lower frequency of this disorder in formula-fed infants reflects the higher concentration of vitamin K in proprietary formulas compared with breast milk.[45] The routine administration of vitamin K at birth (0.5 to 1 mg IM) has significantly reduced the incidence of classic hemorrhagic disease of the newborn. Delayed hemorrhagic disease of the newborn may occur as late as 3 months of age, regardless of whether vitamin K is given at birth. It typically occurs in infants who are exclusively breast-fed and have a prolonged diarrheal illness or who are receiving broad-spectrum antimicrobial therapy. These infants commonly present with ecchymoses, mucous membrane bleeding, or excessive oozing after venipuncture.[45]

Hemorrhagic complications caused by vitamin K deficiency can occur in older infants and in children as a result of fat malabsorption states (e.g., cystic fibrosis, celiac disease) or in children who are supported by total parenteral nutrition that lacks vitamin K supplementation.[57] Vitamin K deficiency may also present after the accidental or deliberate ingestion of warfarin-containing compounds (e.g., Coumadin, rodenticides) and carries an attendant risk of bleeding that can last for days to months.[21, 60]

Patients with vitamin K deficiency should be treated with

parenteral vitamin K_1 (e.g., phytonadione [AquaMEPHYTON]), given subcutaneously or by slow intravenous infusion at a dose of 1 to 5 mg. Resolution of bleeding symptoms is generally rapid (within 4 to 6 hours) and usually precedes improvement in the results of coagulation screening studies. Any infant or child with life-threatening hemorrhage caused by vitamin K deficiency should also receive FFP to rapidly increase vitamin K–dependent clotting factor levels.[57]

Liver Disease

The coagulopathy that accompanies advanced liver disease reflects the liver's role in the production and regulation of most proteins required for normal coagulation. In addition to decreased biosynthesis of essential coagulation proteins, other contributors to impaired hemostasis in patients with advanced liver disease include[83]:

- Low-grade DIC due to diminished clearance of activated clotting factors
- Thrombocytopenia due to hypersplenism
- Increased fibrinolysis
- Platelet dysfunction secondary to increased concentrations of fibrin degradation products.

Improved hemostasis in patients with liver failure can be achieved by infusions of FFP and cryoprecipitate. Correction of the PT and aPTT to 1.5 times their control values or less is usually sufficient to allow for minor diagnostic procedures, such as liver biopsy. Coagulation factor replacement with FFP and cryoprecipitate is only a temporizing measure in the treatment or prevention of excessive hemorrhage secondary to liver disease. Supplemental vitamin K administration is rarely successful unless a significant biliary obstructive component is present that leads to decreased absorption of dietary vitamin K.[60]

DISORDERS OF HEMOSTASIS INVOLVING PLATELETS AND CLOTTING FACTORS

Disseminated Intravascular Coagulation

DIC is the term given to describe the pathologic activation of the coagulation and fibrinolytic pathways that results in the systemic depletion of procoagulant, anticoagulant, and fibrinolytic proteins. The disorder carries an attendant risk of hemorrhage, thrombosis, or both. Common conditions that lead to DIC in children are summarized in Table 160-5.

Pathophysiology

DIC is triggered by two major mechanisms[84]:

1. Vascular endothelial cell injury.
2. Parenchymal tissue damage leading to the exposure of tissue factor.

Injury to vascular endothelium results in the release of tissue plasminogen activator and the exposure of subendothelial adhesive proteins to circulating platelets and clotting factors. Plasma contact with negatively charged, subendothelial matrix leads to activation of factor XII and initiation of the intrinsic coagulation pathway. Activated factor XII (XIIa) mediates the activation of kallikrein from prekallikrein and hydrolyzes plasminogen to plasmin. Kallikrein catalyzes the cleavage of bradykinin from high-molecular-weight kininogen. Bradykinin is a powerful vasodilator that plays an integral role in the development of the hypotension that is often associated with DIC.[84]

TABLE 160–5. Conditions That Commonly Trigger Acute Disseminated Intravascular Coagulation in Children

Neonatal Disorder
Intrauterine infections
Maternal toxemia
Abruptio placentae
Hyaline membrane disease, meconium aspiration
Necrotizing enterocolitis
Infections
Bacterial sepsis (either gram-positive or gram-negative)
Falciparum malaria
Rickettsial infections (e.g., Rocky Mountain spotted fever)
Disseminated fungal infections
Systemic viral infections (e.g., herpesvirus infections)
Other Illnesses
Hypovolemic shock
Acute (hypergranular) promyelocytic leukemia
Intravascular hemolytic transfusion reactions
Extensive burns or trauma
Intracranial injuries (e.g., gunshot wounds)
Hyperthermia or hypothermia
Proteolytic snake venoms (e.g., *Echis carinatus*)
Localized Consumptive Coagulopathy
Kasabach-Merritt syndrome (giant hemangioma, disseminated intravascular coagulation)
Hyperacute renal allograft rejection
Dead fetus syndrome

From Bray GL: Inherited and acquired disorders of hemostasis. *In:* Textbook of Pediatric Critical Care. Holbrook PR (Ed). Philadelphia, WB Saunders, 1993, pp 783–801.

Parenchymal tissue injury and necrosis result in the release of membrane-bound tissue factor that binds and activates factor VII; factor VIIa–tissue factor complex in turn activates factors X and IX. Both mechanisms lead to the generation of circulating thrombin, which cleaves fibrinogen to soluble fibrin and activates platelet factors V, VIII, and XIII. This combination of events results in hypofibrinogenemia, thrombocytopenia, depletion of plasma procoagulant levels, and activation of fibrinolysis. As a result, patients with DIC exhibit increased risk of hemorrhage, formation of microthrombi, or both, resulting in ischemic tissue damage.[84]

Clinical Manifestations

Petechiae and purpura are the most consistent clinical manifestations of DIC, followed by mucosal bleeding from the nasopharynx the gastrointestinal tract and the genitourinary tract. Hemorrhage into the CNS or pulmonary parenchyma may complicate cases of DIC that are especially severe and fulminant. Ischemia resulting from thrombus formation in distal extremities can lead to the gangrene and tissue sloughing that is characteristic of purpura fulminans. Ischemic thrombosis of the renal vasculature results in acute cortical necrosis and chronic renal failure. Bleeding complications of DIC are usually treated more successfully than are thrombotic complications, which frequently result in long-term functional disability, organ failure, or both.[85]

Diagnosis

Acute DIC is accompanied by varying degrees of thrombocytopenia, hypofibrinogenemia, and increased concentrations of fibrin degradation products in plasma. These conditions typically lead to prolongation of PT and aPTT.[85] Levels of prothrombin, factor V, and factor VIII are most frequently reduced in DIC. Levels of factor VIII are useful in discriminating between DIC and the coagulopathy associated with liver failure:

factor VIII levels are typically normal or elevated in most patients with liver failure.[12] Examination of the peripheral blood smear may reveal erythrocyte injury and fragmentation secondary to microangiopathic hemolysis.[85]

Treatment

The cornerstone of therapy for DIC is correction of its underlying cause. Life-threatening hemorrhagic complications can be averted with platelet transfusions in patients with severe thrombocytopenia (platelet count <20,000/mm³). Infusions of FFP and cryoprecipitate are indicated for severe hypofibrinogenemia. Anticoagulation with heparin may be beneficial in patients with DIC in whom thrombosis predominates (e.g., those with purpura fulminans).[86] Anecdotal evidence suggests that heparin may ameliorate or prevent DIC in patients with acute promyelocytic leukemia if therapy is initiated before the start of chemotherapy.[87] Intracranial hemorrhage should be regarded as an absolute contraindication to the use of heparin.

The licensure of antithrombin III concentrates has generated interest in their potential usefulness in the treatment of DIC. In a randomized trial comparing antithrombin III with heparin, antithrombin III significantly shortened the duration of DIC and improved survival in cases of advanced shock.[88] Although the role of antithrombin III concentrates in DIC has not been clearly defined, they appear to be most effective when endogenous antithrombin III levels are <70% of normal.[88-90]

DIAGNOSTIC APPROACH TO THE BLEEDING CHILD

In addition to the history and physical examination, several principles are useful in guiding the diagnostic evaluation in a child with abnormal bleeding. The presence of petechiae and purpura or mucosal bleeding suggests disorders of primary hemostasis (i.e., deficits in platelet number or function). Hemorrhages involving muscles and joints with swelling and impaired range of motion suggest the presence of coagulation factor deficiencies (Table 160–6).[91] Hemorrhagic complications that initially present in infancy or early childhood in an otherwise healthy child suggest an inherited rather than acquired cause.[91] Initial laboratory evaluation of a suspected bleeding disorder should include screening studies, such as a platelet count and determinations of PT, aPTT, and bleeding time. Examination of the peripheral blood smear may reveal the presence of platelet aggregates, a common finding in patients with spurious or anticoagulant-induced thrombocytopenia. Review of the peripheral smear may also reveal platelets that are abnormally large (e.g., ITP, Bernard-Soulier syndrome) or abnormally small (e.g., Wiskott-Aldrich syndrome).

Despite its shortcomings, the bleeding time test remains the best available test of platelet function in vivo. Results should be interpreted cautiously because they may be influenced by medications that interfere with platelet function. A normal bleeding time does not preclude a defect in primary hemostasis in a child with a strong personal or family history

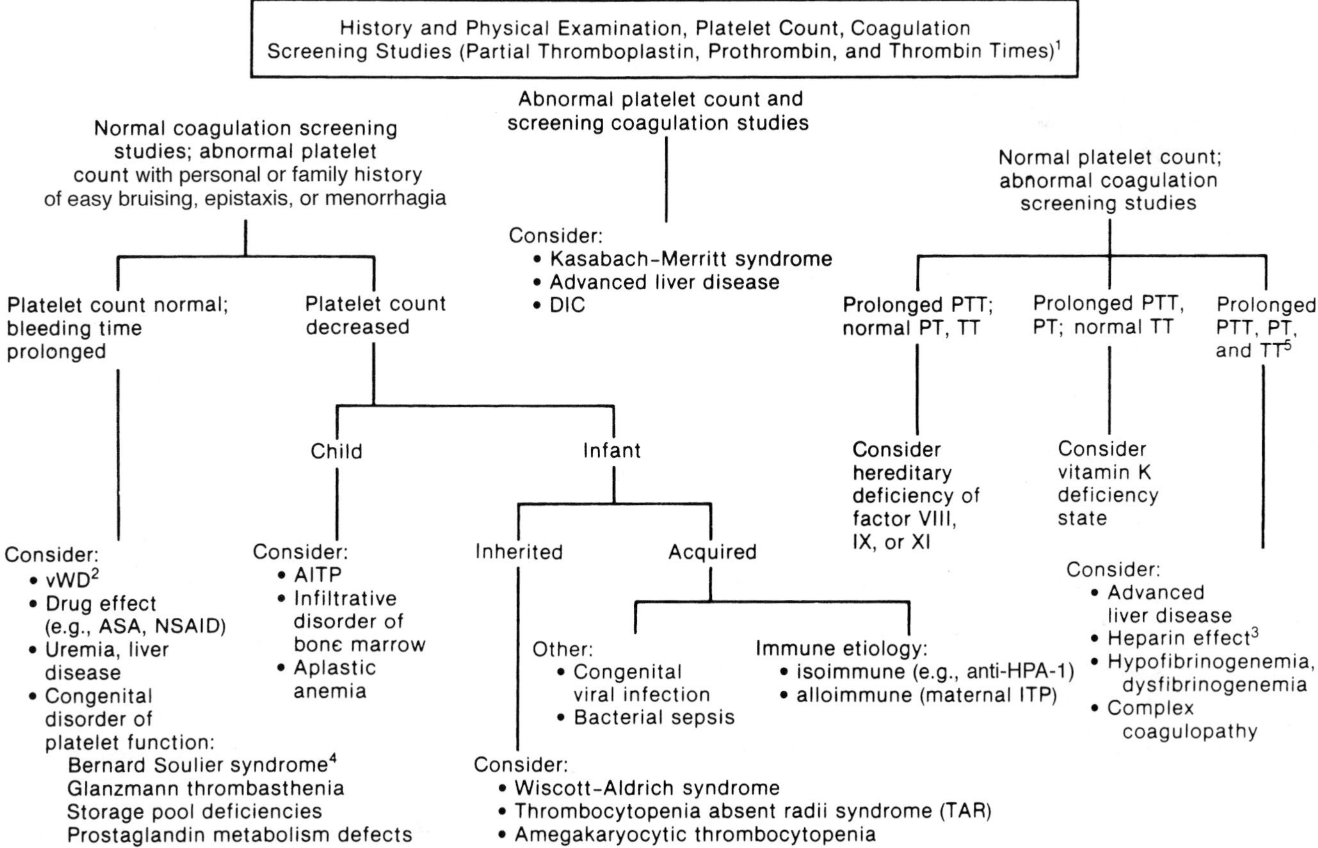

Figure 160–2. Algorithmic approach to the infant or child with a suspected bleeding disorder. (From Bray GL: Inherited and acquired disorders of hemostasis. *In:* Textbook of Pediatric Critical Care. Holbrook PR [Ed]. Philadelphia, WB Saunders, 1993, p 799.)

TABLE 160–6. Clinical Features of the Two Main Groups of Hemostatic Disease

Clinical Findings	Platelet or Vascular Defects	Plasma Coagulation Defects
Common hemorrhagic symptoms	Epistaxis; petechiae; purpura; ecchymoses; gastrointestinal hemorrhage; menorrhagia	Deep tissue hemorrhages, especially hemarthroses and intramuscular bleeds
Bleeding from superficial cuts and abrasions	Often profuse and prolonged	Usually mild
Bleeding from deep cuts, lacerations, dental extractions	Onset immediate; often permanently arrested with local pressure; seldom rebleeds	Onset often delayed; not permanently controlled by local pressure; rebleeding likely to occur several hours after removal of local pressure
Spontaneous bleeding	Usually superficial; small and multiple loci of involvement	Usually a single locus; large and deep-seated hematomas or hemarthroses

From Stuart M, Kelton J: The platelet: Quantitative and qualitative abnormalities. *In:* Hematology of Infancy and Childhood. 3rd ed. Nathan DG, Oski FA (Eds). Philadelphia, WB Saunders, 1987, p 1347.

of a bleeding disorder. Screening tests for the assessment of coagulation include PT, aPTT, and thrombin time. Heparin-contaminated samples drawn from indwelling catheters can significantly alter the results of these studies. For this reason, plasma for coagulation studies should be obtained by peripheral venipuncture whenever possible to ensure plasma sampling uncontaminated by heparin.

Figure 160–2 provides an algorithmic approach to the evaluation of bleeding disorders in children.

References

1. Andrew M: Neonatal hematology. *In:* Hematology of Infancy and Childhood. 4th ed. Nathan DG, Oski FA (Eds). Philadelphia, WB Saunders, 1993, pp 115–153.
2. Hawiger J, Handin R: Structure and function of platelets. *In:* Hematology of Infancy and Childhood. 4th ed. Nathan DG, Oski FA (Eds). Philadelphia, WB Saunders, 1993, 1512–1533.
3. Alter BP, Young NS: The bone marrow failure syndromes. *In:* Hematology of Infancy and Childhood. 4th ed. Nathan DG, Oski FA (Eds). Philadelphia, WB Saunders, 1993, pp 216–316.
4. Perry GS IV, Spector BD, Schumann LM, et al: The Wiskott-Aldrich syndrome in the United States and Canada (1892–1979). J Pediatr 1980; 97:72.
5. Corash L, Shafer L, Blaese RM: Platelet-associated immunoglobulin, platelet size, and the effect of splenectomy in the Wiskott-Aldrich syndrome. Blood 1985; 65:1439.
6. Lum LG, Tubergen DG, Corash L, et al: Splenectomy in the management of the thrombocytopenia of the Wiskott-Aldrich syndrome. N Engl J Med 1980; 302:892.
7. Stuart MJ, Kelton JG: The platelet: Quantitative and qualitative abnormalities. *In:* Hematology of Infancy and Childhood. 3rd ed. Nathan DG, Oski FA (Eds). Philadelphia, WB Saunders, 1987, pp 1343–1478.
8. Ginsburg D, Bowie EJW: Molecular genetics of von Willebrand disease. Blood 1992; 79:2507.
9. Nichols WC, Ginsburg D: von Willebrand disease. Medicine 1997; 76:1.
10. Werner EJ: Von Willebrand disease in children and adolescents. Pediatr Clin North Am 1996; 43:683.
11. Montgomery RR, Coller BS: von Willebrand disease. *In:* Hemostasis and Thrombosis. Colman RW, Hirsh J, Marder VJ, et al (Eds). Philadelphia, JB Lippincott, 1994, pp 1134–1147.
12. Sadler JE: A revised classification of von Willebrand disease. Thromb Haemost 1994; 71:520.
13. Montgomery RR, Scott JP: Hemostasis: Diseases of the fluid phase. *In:* Hematology of Infancy and Childhood. 4th ed. Nathan DG, Oski FA (Eds). Philadelphia, WB Saunders, 1993, pp 1605–1650.
14. Manucci PM: Desmopressin (DDAVP) in the treatment of bleeding disorders: The first 20 years. Blood 1997; 90:2515.
15. Manucci PM, Tenconi PM, Castaman G, et al: Comparison of four virus-inactivated plasma concentrates for treatment of severe von Willebrand disease: A cross-over randomized trial. Blood 1992; 79:3130.
16. Menarche D, Aronson DL: New treatments of von Willebrand disease: Plasma derived von Willebrand factor concentrates. Thromb Haemost 1997; 78:566.
17. McEver RP: The clinical significance of platelet membrane glycoproteins. Hematol Oncol Clin North Am 1990; 4:87.
18. Beardsley DS: Platelet abnormalities in infancy and childhood. *In:* Hematology of Infancy and Childhood. 4th ed. Nathan DG, Oski FA (Eds). Philadelphia, WB Saunders, 1993, pp 1561–1604.
19. Rao AK: Congenital disorders of platelet function. Hematol Oncol Clin North Am 1990; 4:65.
20. Homans A: Thrombocytopenia in the neonate. Pediatr Clin North Am 1996; 43:737.
21. Buchanan GR: Hemorrhagic diseases. *In:* Hematology of Infancy and Childhood. 3rd ed. Nathan DG, Oski FA (Eds). Philadelphia, WB Saunders, 1987, pp 104–127.
22. Goldman M, Filion M, Proulx C, et al: Neonatal alloimmune thrombocytopenia. Transfus Med Rev 1994; 8:123.
23. Bussel JB: Autoimmune thrombocytopenic purpura. Hematol Oncol Clin North Am 1990; 4:179.
24. Dubansky AS, Oski FA: Controversies in the management of acute idiopathic thrombocytopenic purpura: A survey of specialists. Pediatrics 1986; 77:49.
25. Halperin DS, Doyle JJ: Is bone marrow examination justified in idiopathic thrombocytopenic purpura? Am J Dis Child 1988; 142:505.
26. George JN, Woolf SH, Raskob GE, et al: Idiopathic thrombocytopenic purpura: A practice guideline developed by explicit methods for the American Society of Hematology. Blood 1996; 88:3.
27. George JN: Platelet IgG: Its significance for the evaluation of thrombocytopenia and for understanding the origin of alpha-granule proteins. Blood 1990; 76:859.
28. Karpatkin S: HIV-1–related thrombocytopenia. Hematol Oncol Clin North Am 1990; 4:193.
29. Scaradavou A, Woo B, Woloski BMR, et al: Intravenous anti-D treatment of immune thrombocytopenic purpura: Experience in 272 patients. Blood 1997; 89:2689.
30. Blanchette V, Imbach P, Andrew M, et al: Randomised trial of immunoglobulin G, intravenous anti-D, and oral prednisone in childhood acute immune thrombocytopenic purpura. Lancet 1994; 344:703.
31. Medeiros D, Buchanan GR: Current controversies in the management of idiopathic thrombocytopenic purpura. Pediatr Clin North Am 1996; 43:757.
32. Northfelt DW, Mitsuyasu RT: Hematologic complications of HIV infection. *In:* Pediatric AIDS: The Challenge of HIV Infection in Infants, Children and Adolescents. Pizzo PA, Wilfert CM (Eds). Baltimore, Williams & Wilkins, 1991, pp 337–345.
33. Coyle TE: Hematologic complications of human immunodeficiency virus infection and the acquired immunodeficiency syndrome. Med Clin North Am 1997; 81:449.
34. McClain K, Gehrz R, Grierson H, et al: Virus-associated histiocytic proliferations in children. Am J Pediatr Hematol Oncol 1988; 10:196.
35. Beutler E: Platelet transfusions: The 20,000/mL trigger. Blood 1993; 81:1411.
36. Warkentin TE, Levine MN, Hirsh J, et al: Heparin-induced thrombocytopenian patients treated with low molecular weight heparin or unfractionated heparin. N Engl J Med 1995; 332:1330.

37. Gralnick HR, McKeown LP, Williams SB, et al: Plasma and platelet von Willebrand factor defects in uremia. Am J Med 1988; 85:806.
38. Carvalho AC: Acquired platelet dysfunction in patients with uremia. Hematol Oncol Clin North Am 1990; 4:129.
39. Haskes LA: Bleeding after cardiopulmonary bypass. N Engl J Med 1986; 314:1446.
40. Salzman EW, Weinstein MJ, Weintraub MD, et al: Treatment with desmopressin acetate to reduce blood loss after cardiac surgery. N Engl J Med 1986; 314:1402.
41. Bidstrup BP, Royston D, Sapsford TN, et al: Reduction in blood use after cardiopulmonary bypass with high dose aprotinin (Trasylol). J Thorac Cardiovasc Surg 1989; 97:364.
42. Andrew M, Castle V, Sagal S, et al: Clinical impact of neonatal thrombocytopenia. J Pediatr 1987; 110:457.
43. Andrew M, Paes B, Milner R, et al: Development of the human coagulation system in the full-term infant. Blood 1987; 70:165.
44. Andrew M, Paes B, Johnston M: Development of the hemostatic system in the neonate and young infant. Am J Pediatr Hematol Oncol 1990; 12:95.
45. Andrew M, Vegh P, Johnston M, et al: Maturation of the hemostatic system during childhood. Blood 1992; 80:1998.
46. Brettler DB, Levine PH: Clinical Manifestations and Therapy of Inherited Coagulation Factor Deficiencies. *In:* Hemostasis and Thrombosis. 3rd ed. Colman RW, Hirsh J, Marder VJ, Salzman EW (Eds). Philadelphia, JB Lippincott, 1994, pp 167–183.
47. Hoyer LW: Hemophilia A. N Engl J Med 1994; 330:38.
48. Furie B, Limentani SA, Rosenfeld CG: A practical guide to the evaluation and treatment of hemophilia. Blood 1994; 84:3.
49. Bray GL, Luban NLC: Hemophilia presenting with intracranial hemorrhage. Am J Dis Child 1987; 141:1215.
50. Goldsmith JC, Kletzel M: Risk of birth-related intracranial hemorrhage in hemophilic newborns: Results of a North American survey (Abstract). Blood 1990; 76(suppl):167a.
51. Bray GL, Nugent D: Hemorrhage involving the upper airway in hemophilia. Clin Pediatr (Phila) 1986; 25:436.
52. Forbes CD, Madhok R: Genetic disorders of blood coagulation: Clinical presentation and management. *In:* Disorders of Hemostasis. 2nd ed. Ratnoff OD, Forbes CD (Eds). Philadelphia, WB Saunders, 1991, pp 141–202.
53. Lusher JM: Viral safety and inhibitor development associated with monoclonal antibody–purified F VIII C. Ann Hematol 1991; 63:138.
54. Lusher JM, Arkin S, Abildgaard CF, et al: Recombinant factor VIII for the treatment of previously untreated patients with hemophilia A. N Engl J Med 1993; 328:453.
55. Bray GL: Recent developments in the biotechnology of plasma-derived and recombinant coagulation factor VIII. J Pediatr 1990; 117:503.
56. Bray GL, Gomperts ED, Courter S, et al: A multicenter study of recombinant factor VIII (Recombinate): Safety, efficacy, and inhibitor risk in previously untreated patients with hemophilia A. Blood 1994; 83:2428.
57. Bray GL: Normal and disordered coagulation in the neonate. Transfus Sci 1991; 12:231.
58. Gill JC, Montgomery RR: Principles of therapy for coagulation factor deficiencies. *In:* Hematology of Infancy and Childhood. 4th ed. Nathan DG, Oski FA (Eds). Philadelphia, WB Saunders, 1993, pp 1796–1818.
59. Kim HC, McMillan CW, White GC, et al: Purified factor IX using monoclonal immunoaffinity technique: Clinical trials in hemophilia B and comparison to prothrombin complex concentrates. Blood 1992; 79:568.
60. Lusher JM: Diseases of coagulation: The fluid phase. *In:* Hematology of Infancy and Childhood. 3rd ed. Nathan DG, Oski FA (Eds). Philadelphia, WB Saunders, 1987, pp 1293–1342.
61. Winter M: The practical management of hemophilia. Blood Rev 1992; 6:174.
62. Maunucci PM, Bauer KA, Gringeri A, et al: No activation of the common pathway of the coagulation cascade after a highly purified factor IX concentrate. Br J Haematol 1991; 79:766.
63. White GC, Beebe A, Nielsen B: Recombinant factor IX. Thromb Haemos 1997; 78:261.
64. DiMichele D: Hemophilia 1996: New approach to an old disease. Pediatr Clin North Am 1996; 43:709.
65. Ehrenforth S, Kreuz W, Scharrer I, et al: Incidence of development of factor VIII and factor IX inhibitors in haemophiliacs. Lancet 1992; 339:594.
66. Gilles JG, Jacquemin MG, Saint-Remy JMR: Factor VIII inhibitors. Thromb Haemost 1997; 78:641.
67. Kasper CK: Treatment of factor VIII inhibitors. *In:* Progress in Hemostasis and Thrombosis. Coller BS (Ed). Philadelphia, WB Saunders, 1989, pp 57–86.
68. Kasper CK, Aledort LM, Counts RB, et al: A more uniform measurement of factor VIII inhibitors. Thromb Diath Haemorrh 1975; 34:869.
69. Kessler CM: An introduction to factor VIII inhibitors: Their detection and quantitation. Am J Med 1991; 91(suppl 5A):15.
70. Hay CRM, Lozier JN, Lee CA, et al: Safety profile of porcine factor VIII and its use as hospital and home-therapy for patients with hemophilia A and inhibitors: The results of an international survey. Thromb Haemost 1996; 75:25.
71. Sjamsoedin LJ, Heijnen L, Mauser-Bunschoten EP, et al: The effect of activated prothrombin-complex concentrate (FEIBA) on joint and muscle bleeding in patients with hemophilia A and antibodies to factor VIII. N Engl J Med 1981; 305:717.
72. Hedner U, Glazer S: Management of hemophilia patients with inhibitors. Hematol Oncol Clin North Am 1992; 6:1035.
73. Schmidt ML, Gamerman S, Smith HE, et al: Recombinant activated factor VII (rFVIIa) therapy for intracranial hemorrhage in hemophilia A patients with inhibitors. Am J Hematol 1994; 47:36.
74. Bloom AL: Progress in the management of hemophilia. Thromb Haemost 1991; 66:166.
75. Nilsson IM: The management of hemophilia in patients with inhibitors. Transfus Med Rev 1992; 6:285.
76. Kessler CM, Ludlam CA: The treatment of acquired factor VIII inhibitors: Worldwide experience with porcine factor VIII concentrate. Semin Hematol 1993; 30(Suppl 1):22.
77. Pierce GF, Lusher JM, Brownstein AP, et al: The use of purified clotting factor concentrates in hemophilia. JAMA 1989; 261:3434.
78. Roberts HR: The treatment of hemophilia: Past tragedy and future promise. N Engl J Med 1989; 321:1188.
79. Troisi CL, Hollinger B, Hoots WK, et al: A multicenter study of viral hepatitis in a United States hemophilic population. Blood 1993; 81:412.
80. Schreiber GB, Busch MP, Kleinman SH, et al: The risk of transfusion-transmitted viral infections. N Engl J Med 1996; 334:1685.
81. Cuthbert JA: Southwestern Internal Medicine Conference: Hepatitis C. Am J Med Sci 1990; 299:346.
82. Alter HJ, Purcell RH, Shih JW, et al: Detection of antibody to hepatitis C virus in prospectively followed transfusion recipients with acute and chronic non-A, non-B hepatitis. N Engl J Med 1989; 321:1494.
83. Mannucci PM, Forman SP: Hemostasis and liver disease. *In:* Hemostasis and Thrombosis. Colman RW, Hirsh J, Marder VJ, et al (Eds). Philadelphia, JB Lippincott, 1982, pp 595–601.
84. Marder VJ, Feinstein DI, Francis CW: Consumptive thrombohemorrhagic disorders. *In:* Hemostasis and Thrombosis. 3rd ed. Colman RW, Hirsh J, Marder VJ, et al (Eds). Philadelphia, JB Lippincott, 1994, pp 1023–1063.
85. Bick RL: Disseminated intravascular coagulation and related syndromes: A clinical review. Semin Thromb Hemost 1988; 14:299.
86. Feinstein DI: Treatment of disseminated intravascular coagulation. Semin Thromb Hemost 1988; 14:351.
87. Lisiewicz J: DIC in acute leukemia. Semin Thromb Hemost 1988; 14:343.
88. Vinazzer H: Therapeutic use of antithrombin III in shock and disseminated intravascular coagulation. Semin Thromb Hemost 1989; 15:347.
89. Fourrier F, Chopin C, Huart J-J, et al: Double-blind, placebo-controlled trial of antithrombin III concentrates in septic shock with disseminated intravascular coagulation. Chest 1993; 104:882.
90. Fourrier F, Jourdain M, Tournois A, et al: Coagulation inhibitor substitution during sepsis. Intensive Care Med 1995; 21(Suppl):264.
91. White GC II, Marder VJ, Colman RW, et al: Approach to the bleeding patient. *In:* Hemostasis and Thrombosis. 3rd ed. Colman RW, Hirsh J, Marder VJ, et al (Eds). Philadelphia, JB Lippincott, 1994, pp 1134–1147.

161

Diagnosis and Treatment of Venous Thromboembolism

Russell D. Hull, MBBS, MSc • Graham F. Pineo, MD
Gary E. Raskob, MSc, PhD

Venous thromboembolism (venous thrombosis, pulmonary embolism, or both) usually complicates the course of sick, hospitalized patients but may also affect ambulant and otherwise apparently healthy individuals.[1-3] Pulmonary embolism remains the most common preventable cause of hospital death and is responsible for approximately 150,000 to 200,000 deaths per year in the United States. Most patients who die of pulmonary embolism succumb suddenly or within 2 hours of the acute event, before therapy can be initiated or can take effect.[4] Effective prophylaxis against venous thromboembolism is now available for most high-risk patients.[5-7] Prophylaxis of the disease is more effective in preventing death and morbidity from venous thromboembolism than treatment.

PATHOPHYSIOLOGY

Venous thrombi are composed predominantly of fibrin and red blood cells and have a variable platelet and leukocyte component. The formation, growth, and dissolution of venous thromboemboli represent a balance between thrombogenic stimuli and protective mechanisms. The factors that predispose to the development of venous thromboemboli are:

1. Venous stasis.
2. Activation of blood coagulation.
3. Vascular damage.

The protective mechanisms that counteract these thrombogenic stimuli include:

1. The inactivation of activated coagulation factors by circulating inhibitors (e.g., antithrombin III, a_2-macroglobulin, $alpha_1$ antitrypsin, and activated protein C).
2. Clearance of activated coagulation factors and soluble fibrin polymer complexes by the reticuloendothelial system and by the liver.
3. dissolution of fibrin by fibrinolytic enzymes derived from plasma and endothelial cells and digestion of fibrin by leukocytes.

Various risk factors predispose to the development of venous thromboembolism (Table 161-1).

Pulmonary embolism originates from thrombi in the deep veins of the leg in 90% or more of patients.[8-12] Other less common sources include the deep pelvic veins, the renal veins, the inferior vena cava, the right ventricle, and the axillary veins. Most clinically important pulmonary emboli arise from thrombi in the popliteal or more proximal deep veins of the leg. Pulmonary embolism occurs in 50% of patients with objectively documented proximal vein thrombosis; many of these emboli are asymptomatic.[8] Usually, only part of the thrombus embolizes, and 50% to 70% of patients with angiographically documented pulmonary embolism have detectable deep venous thrombosis of the legs at the time of presentation.[9]

CLINICAL FEATURES

The clinical features of venous thrombosis include leg pain, tenderness and swelling, a palpable cord, discoloration, venous distention, prominence of the superficial veins, and cyanosis. The clinical diagnosis of venous thrombosis is highly nonspecific, because none of the symptoms or signs is unique and each may be a result of nonthrombotic disorders. Patients with relatively minor symptoms and signs may have extensive deep venous thrombi, whereas those with florid leg pain and swelling, suggesting extensive deep venous thrombosis, may have negative results on objective testing. Thus, objective testing is mandatory to confirm or exclude a diagnosis of venous thrombosis.[10-13]

The clinical presentation of pulmonary embolism depends on the size, location, and number of emboli, and on the patient's underlying cardiorespiratory reserve. The clinical manifestations of acute pulmonary embolism generally can be divided into several syndromes that overlap considerably:

1. Transient dyspnea and tachypnea in the absence of other associated clinical manifestations.
2. Pulmonary infarction or congestive atelectasis (also known as ischemic pneumonitis or incomplete infarction), which includes pleuritic chest pain, cough, hemoptysis, pleural effusion, and pulmonary infiltrates on the chest x-ray.
3. Right ventricular failure associated with severe dyspnea and tachypnea.
4. Cardiovascular collapse with hypotension, syncope, and coma (usually associated with massive pulmonary embolism).
5. Less common and highly nonspecific clinical features, including confusion and coma, pyrexia, wheezing, resistant cardiac failure, and unexplained arrhythmia.

It is now widely accepted that the clinical diagnosis of pulmonary embolism is highly nonspecific. Multiple studies indicate that in more than 50% of all patients with clinically suspected pulmonary embolism the diagnosis is not confirmed by objective testing.[9, 14-16] Therefore, objective testing is mandatory to confirm or exclude the presence of pulmonary embolism.[14-16]

TABLE 161–1. Factors Predisposing to the Development of Venous Thromboembolism

Clinical Risk Factors
Surgical and nonsurgical trauma
Previous venous thromboembolism
Immobilization
Malignant disease
Heart disease
Leg paralysis
Age (>40 yrs)
Obesity
Estrogens
Parturition
Inherited or Acquired Abnormalities
Factor V Leiden
Protein C deficiency
Protein S deficiency
Antithrombin III deficiency
Hyperhomocysteinemia
Prothrombin 20210A
Dysfibrinogenemia
Heparin-induced thrombocytopenia

DIAGNOSIS

Objective Tests for the Diagnosis of Venous Thrombosis

Various ancillary tests (e.g., chest x-ray, arterial blood gas determination, electrocardiography) and laboratory tests (e.g., serum lactate dehydrogenase levels) have a role in the diagnosis of venous thromboembolism, but they all lack sensitivity and specificity for pulmonary embolism. The main role of these tests is to rule out other conditions that may mimic pulmonary embolism, such as acute myocardial infarction, or pneumothorax.

Objective tests used in the diagnosis of *venous thrombosis* include impedance plethysmography (IPG), B-mode ultrasonography, duplex ultrasonography, color-flow ultrasonography, and ascending venography. Objective tests used in the diagnosis of *pulmonary embolism* include ventilation-perfusion lung scanning and pulmonary angiography.

Venography

Venography is the standard objective method for the diagnosis of venous thrombosis. Venography is a difficult technique to perform well, and considerable experience is required to execute adequately and to interpret accurately. Certain venographic abnormalities have been used as criteria for the diagnosis of acute deep venous thrombosis.[13] The most reliable of these is the presence of an intraluminal filling defect that is constant in all x-ray films and is seen in numerous projections. Other venographic abnormalities, such as nonfilling of a segment of the deep venous system or nonfilling of the entire deep venous system above the knee, may be caused by technical artifacts, particularly if the dye is injected too far proximally into the dorsal foot vein. These artifacts may then be interpreted either as caused by thrombus (because the vein is not filled) or as normal (because a filling defect is not seen). The common femoral, external iliac, and common iliac veins may not be adequately filled by ascending venography, which can lead to an incorrect diagnosis based on inadequate venography. In the case of nonfilling of an entire segment of the deep venous system, the diagnosis of acute or recurrent venous thrombosis must depend on the use of other tests, such as IPG and ultrasonography.[17]

Numerous problems are related to venography. Even in the best of circumstances, it may be impossible to cannulate a vein on the dorsum of the foot, making ascending venography impossible on one or both legs. If filling of the common femoral or iliac systems is inadequate, femoral venography may be necessary.

Venography is associated with some clinically troublesome side effects. Pain may occur in the foot while dye is being injected, or delayed pain may occur in the calf 1 or 2 days after injection. The procedure may be complicated by superficial phlebitis and even deep venous thrombosis in a small percentage of patients with normal results on venography (1% to 2%).[12, 17] Other less common complications of venography include (1) hypersensitivity to the radiopaque dye and local skin and (2) tissue necrosis due to extravasation of dye at the injection site. Both non-ionic and high ionic contrast media may cause or aggravate renal insufficiency in patients at risk for these complications, such as those with established renal disease, hypertension, heart failure, diabetes, or multiple myeloma.[19, 20] The risks of venography must be carefully weighed in such circumstances and reviewed with the patient before venography is performed.

Impedance Plethysmography

IPG is sensitive and specific for proximal vein thrombosis in symptomatic patients, but it is insensitive to calf vein thrombosis.[21-23] In patients with clinically suspected venous thrombosis, positive IPG results can be used to make therapeutic decisions in the absence of clinical conditions known to produce false-positive results. A normal result excludes the diagnosis of proximal vein thrombosis but does not exclude calf vein thrombosis. This potential limitation can be overcome by serial IPG evaluations. The use of serial IPG is based on the concept now confirmed by clinical observation that calf vein thrombi are clinically important only when extension into the proximal veins occurs, at which point detection with IPG is possible.

The effectiveness and safety of IPG have been evaluated by prospective clinical trials in patients with clinically suspected venous thrombosis. According to the data provided by these studies, the following recommendations can be made[10, 21, 23]:

1. A positive result on IPG is highly predictive of acute proximal vein thrombosis (positive predictive value >90%).
2. Withholding anticoagulant therapy is safe in symptomatic patients who have negative results by serial IPG for 10 to 14 days.

Although IPG has a high sensitivity and specificity for the detection of symptomatic venous thrombosis, it lacks sensitivity for the detection of asymptomatic venous thrombosis in patients who have had surgery, such as total hip replacement, or in trauma patients. In such circumstances, the only reliable method for the detection of deep venous thrombosis is bilateral ascending venography.

IPG has certain limitations. False-positive results may occur in patients with disorders that interfere with arterial inflow or venous outflow. These disorders include severe congestive cardiac failure, constrictive pericarditis, severe arterial insufficiency, hypotension, and external compression of veins. Most of these disorders are readily recognized clinically. False-positive results may also occur if the test is performed incorrectly or if the patient is not relaxed. The test cannot be performed on some patients, such as those who are in plaster casts or who cannot be adequately positioned because of immobilization or pain.

Ultrasonography

Venous imaging using real-time, B-mode ultrasound with or without Doppler assessment is an established technique for the evaluation of patients with clinically suspected deep venous thrombosis.[24-29] Prospective studies have shown that the single criterion of vein compressibility is highly sensitive and specific for the detection of proximal vein thrombosis (sensitivity and specificity, both >95%).[24-29] Other criteria, such as echogenicity and change in venous diameter during a Valsalva maneuver, are less useful for this purpose. The visualization of an echogenic band is highly sensitive but is nonspecific (specificity, 50%).[25] The percentage of change in venous diameter during a Valsalva maneuver is both insensitive and nonspecific.[25]

Real-time, B-mode venous ultrasonography is insensitive for the detection of isolated calf vein thrombosis, and, like IPG, serial testing using this method is required to detect proximal extension. B-Mode venous ultrasound may fail to detect isolated iliac vein thrombi. This is a practical clinical limitation in patients in whom isolated vein thrombosis is common, such as pregnant patients with clinically suspected venous thrombosis.

Ultrasound imaging and IPG are both highly sensitive and specific in the diagnosis of proximal vein thrombosis in symptomatic patients. Ultrasonography is more reliable than IPG for detecting proximal vein thrombosis in patients with increased central venous pressure or arterial insufficiency. Ultrasonography can be used in patients whose leg is in a plaster cast or external fixation, who are in traction, or who have had leg amputation.

Both IPG and Doppler ultrasonography have high sensitivity and specificity for the diagnosis of proximal vein thrombosis in symptomatic patients, but both lack sensitivity and specificity for the detection of asymptomatic venous thrombosis in patients who have undergone surgery.[30, 31] Ultrasonography is more readily available, and, as the cost outlay for the equipment decreases, it has supplanted IPG as the most widely used noninvasive test for the detection of venous thrombosis.

Objective Tests for the Diagnosis of Pulmonary Embolism

Perfusion Lung Scanning

Perfusion lung scanning is the key diagnostic test for patients with suspected pulmonary embolism. A normal perfusion scan result excludes clinically important pulmonary embolism.[32-34] An abnormal perfusion scan result, however, is nonspecific and may occur in conditions that produce either increased radiographic density (e.g., pneumonia, atelectasis, and pleural effusion) or regional reduction in ventilation (e.g., chronic obstructive lung disease, acute asthma, bronchial mucus plugs, and bronchitis, all of which are frequently associated with normal radiographic results).

Ventilation imaging was introduced to improve the specificity of an abnormal perfusion scan result by differentiating embolic occlusion of the pulmonary vasculature from perfusion defects occurring secondary to a primary disorder of ventilation.[35-37] This basic premise (i.e., that perfusion defects that ventilate normally [ventilation-perfusion mismatch]) is due to pulmonary embolism, whereas matching ventilation-perfusion abnormalities are due to other conditions has been shown to be incorrect by prospective clinical trials.[34, 38]

Ventilation lung scanning is helpful only if the perfusion defect is segmental or greater and is associated with ventilation mismatch; such patients have a high probability (86%) of pulmonary embolism confirmed by pulmonary angiography.[9, 34-38] Other abnormal findings on lung scans, such as matching ventilation-perfusion defects (either segmental or subsegmental, or "low-probability"), subsegmental defects with ventilation mismatch, or perfusion defects that correspond to an area of increased density on chest radiography (indeterminate perfusion scan), are associated with a 20% to 40% frequency of pulmonary embolism.[9, 34, 38] These scan patterns are nondiagnostic. Further investigations, including pulmonary angiography and objective tests for venous thrombosis, are therefore required in patients who have nondiagnostic ventilation-perfusion scan findings.[9, 16, 34, 38, 39]

Pulmonary angiography, or venography, or both, should be used when other approaches are unavailable or inconclusive. The morbidity associated with these tests is substantially less than that arising from unnecessary anticoagulant therapy and inappropriate hospitalization.

Pulmonary Angiography

Pulmonary angiography is the accepted diagnostic reference standard for pulmonary embolism.[40-42] The diagnosis is established if an intraluminal filling defect is constant on multiple films or if abrupt termination (cutoff) of a vessel greater than 2 to 5 mm in diameter occurs and is constant on multiple films.[40, 41] Other abnormalities, such as oligemia, vessel pruning, and loss of filling of small vessels, are nonspecific and occur in many conditions, including pneumonia, atelectasis, bronchiectasis, emphysema, and pulmonary carcinoma.[40, 41]

In recent years, the diagnostic resolution of pulmonary angiography has been markedly improved, and the risk to the patient decreased, by the use of selective catheterization and repeated injections of small volumes of dye. This technique is safe in the absence of severe chronic pulmonary hypertension or severe cardiac or respiratory decompensation.[43] Clinically significant complications, including tachyarrhythmias, endocardial or myocardial injury, cardiac perforation, cardiac arrest, and hypersensitivity reactions to contrast medium, occur in up to 3% to 4% of patients.[40, 43]

Spiral Computed Tomography and Magnetic Resonance Imaging

Spiral computed tomography (CT) scanning and magnetic resonance imaging (MRI) are potentially promising techniques for the diagnosis of pulmonary embolism. To date, however, these tests have been evaluated only in relatively small series of selected patients. The initial results are promising, but further large prospective studies incorporating consecutive patients with suspected pulmonary embolism are required to validly determine the sensitivity and specificity of these tests for pulmonary embolism. Before clinical recommendations are made, the safety of withholding anticoagulant treatment in patients with suspected pulmonary embolism who have negative findings by either spiral CT or MRI should be demonstrated by a prospective study incorporating long-term follow-up.

Diagnosis and Management of Pulmonary Embolism Based on Objective Testing for Proximal Deep Venous Thrombosis

At least 80% of patients with pulmonary embolism have thrombi originating in the lower leg veins.[8, 9, 11] Because of the diagnostic inaccuracy of noninvasive tests for pulmonary embolism, particularly in patients with nondiagnostic lung scan results, the concept of using objective tests for the detection of proximal venous thrombosis in the legs was developed for suspected pulmonary embolism.[14-16, 44] This combined strategy for the diagnosis and treatment of pulmonary embolus or venous thrombosis (e.g., venous thromboembolism) has been applied in prospective clinical trials.

Noninvasive tests, such as IPG and B-mode venous ultrasonography, have advantages because they are free of morbidity and are readily repeatable. Proximal vein thrombosis is revealed by IPG in 10% to 25% of patients with nondiagnostic results on ventilation-perfusion scans. This diagnostic ability has important implications for management: untreated or inadequately treated proximal vein thrombosis is associated with a high risk (20% to 50%) of recurrent venous thromboembolism.

A positive result on venography or noninvasive testing is an indication for therapy; however, the venographic result is negative in approximately 30% of patients with angiographically documented pulmonary embolism.[9] Two possible explanations exist for this finding. First, pulmonary embolism may have originated from a source other than the deep veins of the legs. Alternatively, the emboli may have originated from the deep veins of the legs but all or most of the thrombus embolized, leaving no residual thrombosis detectable at the time of presentation.

Patients with abnormal but nondiagnostic lung scan results and negative objective test results for venous thrombosis require pulmonary angiography to confirm or exclude pulmonary embolism. This diagnostic modality may, however, be impractical or unavailable. In patients who do not have severely limited cardiac or respiratory reserve, serial objective testing for proximal vein thrombosis is an alternative approach, based on the concept that clinically important recurrent pulmonary embolism is unlikely (<1%) in the absence of proximal vein thrombosis. This concept is supported by the findings of studies of the natural history of venous thrombosis and by clinical trials of noninvasive testing in patients with symptoms or signs suggesting deep venous thrombosis.[10, 21, 23] Prospective studies indicate that the use of serial objective testing for proximal vein thrombosis is an effective and practical alternative to pulmonary angiography in patients with nondiagnostic lung scan results who have adequate cardiorespiratory reserve.[44-46]

Measurement of D-Dimer in Plasma

The measurement of the fibrin breakdown product D-dimer is a promising approach that has the potential to make an important impact on the diagnosis of venous thromboembolism. Since the test is highly nonspecific and is positive in many disorders associated with fibrin deposition, the value of this test lies in the ability of a negative result to exclude the presence of clinically important venous thromboembolism.

Results from research laboratories using an enzyme-linked immunosorbent assay (ELISA) show that this test is highly sensitive for the presence of acute venous thrombosis or pulmonary embolism. A negative result by the D-dimer ELISA has high negative predictive value. The practical application of D-dimer in clinical practice requires a simplified test that will be widely available and will provide results in a sufficiently short period of time to be useful to the clinician. Promising initial results have been obtained using a latex assay or the simplified test known as SimpliRed, which suggests these tests may have high sensitivity for acute venous thromboembolism and may be useful as an exclusionary test. However, lower sensitivities have also been reported.

Finally, further studies are required to document the safety of withholding anticoagulant treatment in patients with suspected venous thromboembolism and negative D-dimer results. If the clinician has access to measurement of D-dimer from a laboratory that has documented a high sensitivity (>95%), this test may be a useful addition in the diagnostic work-up. For most centers, however, further studies are needed to determine the ultimate place of the D-dimer in clinical management.

TREATMENT: ANTICOAGULANT THERAPY

Anticoagulant drugs (heparin, warfarin, or both) are the mainstay of the management of venous thromboembolism. This chapter emphasizes the role of heparin and warfarin in the treatment of thromboembolism and does not discuss the role of thrombolysis, thrombectomy, or vena caval filters (see Chapter 101).

The objectives of treatment in patients with venous thromboembolism are to prevent (1) death from pulmonary embolism, (2) recurrent venous thromboembolism, and (3) the *postphlebitic syndrome.*

Heparin

Unfractionated heparin from either porcine or bovine sources has been available for clinical use for several decades. Although heparin has been studied extensively, much remains uncertain about its mode of action, particularly the non-anticoagulant properties, and some of the complications have only recently been better understood.[47] Because of the problems and complications related to heparin therapy, there has been great interest in the use of the low-molecular-weight heparins in a variety of clinical settings.

The anticoagulant activity of unfractionated heparin depends on a unique pentasaccharide that binds to antithrombin III (AT III) and potentiates the inhibition of thrombin and activated factor X (Xa) by AT III.[48-50] About one third of all heparin molecules contain the unique pentasaccharide sequence regardless of whether they are low or high in molecular weight fractions. It is the pentasaccharide sequence that confers the molecular high affinity for AT III.[49, 51] The remaining two thirds of heparin have minimal anticoagulant activity at the therapeutic concentrations that are used clinically.

To inhibit thrombin, heparin must form a bridge between thrombin and AT III but for the inhibition of factor Xa this bridging is not necessary.[50, 51] Molecules of heparin with fewer than 18 saccharide units are unable to bind thrombin and AT III simultaneously and as a result cannot catalyze thrombin inhibition.[52] Heparin fragments with smaller numbers of saccharide units are capable of catalyzing the inhibition of factor Xa by AT III, provided that the high-affinity pentasaccharide sequence is present. Unfractionated heparin cannot inhibit thrombin bound to fibrin, whereas the specific antithrombin agents do so.[53] Heparin does not inhibit factor Xa bound to platelets.[54]

Heparin also catalyzes the inactivation of thrombin by another plasma cofactor (cofactor II), which acts independently of AT III.[55] Heparin has a number of other effects. Those related to the anticoagulant effects of heparin include:

- Release of tissue factor pathway inhibitor[56]
- Binding to numerous plasma and platelet proteins
- Endothelial cells and leucocytes[48, 57]
- Suppression of platelet function[54]
- Increased vascular permeability[58]

Monitoring of Heparin Therapy: Therapeutic Range

Clinical trials have established the need for initial heparin treatment in patients with proximal vein thrombosis.[59, 60] Randomized clinical trials have shown that an adequate intensity of heparin treatment is required to prevent recurrent venous thromboembolism.[59, 60] This finding establishes both the need to monitor the anticoagulant response to heparin and the need to titrate the heparin dose in the individual patient because the anticoagulant response to a standard dose of heparin varies widely among patients.[61-65]

It has become common clinical practice to adjust the heparin dose to maintain the result of the activated partial thromboplastin time (aPTT) within a defined therapeutic range. Over the years, this therapeutic range has evolved based on clinical custom to the use of an upper and lower limit, which is an aPTT of 1.5 to 2.5 times the control value. This compares to a heparin blood level of 0.2 to 0.4 units/mL by protamine sulfate titration and to .035 to 0.70 by the more commonly used anti-factor Xa assay.[65] The use of an aPTT ratio of 1.5 as the lower limit of the therapeutic range is supported by data from clinical trials. In contrast, until recently, no firm evidence was reported from clinical trials to provide clear guidelines on the upper limit of the therapeutic range. The use of an upper limit and the clinical practice of reducing the heparin dose when the aPTT exceeds this limit have been based on clinical custom and the intuitive belief that this practice will minimize the risk of bleeding. Indeed, the dose of heparin given has been cited as one of the risk factors for bleeding during heparin therapy, but this observation was based on retrospective studies.

Data from rigorously designed clinical trials have become available that enable firm recommendations to be made about the appropriate therapeutic range for the aPTT.[61] The findings

TABLE 161–2. Heparin Protocol

1. *Administer initial intravenous heparin bolus:* 5000 U.
2. *Administer continuous intravenous heparin infusion:* commence at 42 mL/hr of 20,000 U (1680 U/hr) in 500 mL of two thirds dextrose and one third saline (a 24 hr heparin dose of 40,320 U), except in the following patients (commence infusion at a rate of 31 mL/hr [1240 U/hr, a 24-hr dose of 29,760 U]):
   a. Patients who have undergone surgery within the previous 2 weeks.
   b. Patients with a previous history of peptic ulcer disease or gastrointestinal or genitourinary bleeding.
   c. Patients with recent stroke (i.e., thrombotic stroke within 2 weeks previously).
   d. Patients with a platelet count <150 × 10^9/L.
   e. Patients with miscellaneous reasons for a high risk of bleeding (e.g., hepatic failure, renal failure, or vitamin K deficiency).
3. *Adjust heparin dose by use of the aPTT:* The aPTT test is performed in all patients as follows:
   a. 4-6 hours after initiation of heparin; the heparin dose is then adjusted according to the nomogram shown in Table 161–3.
   b. 4-6 hours after the first dosage adjustment.
   c. Then, as indicated by the nomogram for the first 24 hours of therapy.
   d. Thereafter, once daily, unless the patient has a subtherapeutic aPTT,* in which case the aPTT test is repeated 4-6 hr after the heparin dose is increased.

*Subtherapeutic = aPTT <1.5 times the mean normal control value for the thromboplastin reagent being used.

aPTT = activated partial thromboplastin time; IV = intravenous; U = units; L = liter.

indicate that failure to exceed the lower limit (aPTT ratio, 1.5) is associated with an unacceptably high risk of recurrent venous thromboembolism; however, no association exists between supratherapeutic aPTT responses and the risk of bleeding.[61] The use of a prescriptive approach or protocol for administering intravenous heparin therapy has been evaluated in three studies in patients with venous thromboembolism.[61, 63, 64]

In one clinical trial for the treatment of proximal venous thrombosis, patients were given either intravenous heparin alone followed by warfarin sodium, or intravenous heparin and simultaneous warfarin.[61] The heparin nomogram is summarized in Tables 161–2 and 161–3. Only 1% and 2% of the patients were subtherapeutic with respect to aPTT for more than 24 hours in the heparin group and in the heparin and warfarin group, respectively. Recurrent venous thromboembolism (objectively documented) occurred infrequently in both groups (7%), rates similar to those previously reported. These findings demonstrated that subtherapy was avoided in most patients and that the heparin protocol resulted in effective delivery of heparin therapy in both groups.[61]

In the other clinical trial, a weight-based heparin dosing nomogram was compared with a standard-care nomogram[64] (Table 161–4.) Patients on the weight-adjusted heparin nomogram received a starting dose of 80 U/kg as a bolus and 18 U/kg/hour as an infusion. Patients on the standard-care nomogram received a bolus of 5000 U followed by 1000 U/hour by infusion. The heparin dose was adjusted to maintain an aPTT of 1.5 to 2.3 times control. In the weight-adjusted group, 89% of patients achieved the therapeutic range within 24 hours compared with 75% in the standard-care group. The risk of recurrent thromboembolism was more frequent in the standard-care group, supporting the previous observation that subtherapeutic heparin during the initial 24 hours is associated with a higher incidence of recurrences. This study included patients with unstable angina and arterial thromboembolism in addition to venous thromboembolism, suggesting that the principles applied to a heparin nomogram for the treatment of venous thromboembolism may be generalizable to other clinical conditions.[64]

These findings are strongly supported by a randomized trial that compared intravenously administered heparin with orally administered anticoagulants alone for the initial treatment of patients with proximal vein thrombosis.[60] The latter treatment group, by the nature of the treatment, have an inadequate aPTT for at least the first 48 hours because the onset of the anticoagulant effect of oral anticoagulants is delayed. Recurrent venous thromboembolism occurred in 11 of 55 patients (20%) treated with oral anticoagulants alone, compared with three of 50 patients (6%) who received initial intravenous heparin that was adjusted to maintain the aPTT above 1.5 times the control value (P = .032).

New information about the upper limit of the therapeutic range for the aPTT has also become available.[61] Clinical outcomes were evaluated in patients with proximal vein thrombosis who were randomly assigned to receive initial treatment with either intravenous heparin alone or intravenous heparin with simultaneous warfarin sodium. Both regimens proved adequate in almost all patients, but the combined heparin and warfarin group received more intensive anticoagulation and most of these patients exceeded the predefined upper limit (aPTT ratio, 2.5) for sustained periods of time. Thus, 69 of 99 patients (69%) in the group who received combined therapy had a supratherapeutic value (ratio > 2.5) that persisted for 24 hours or more compared with 24 of 100 patients (24%) who received heparin alone ($P < .001$).

Despite this more intense therapy in the combined group, bleeding complications occurred with similar frequency in the

TABLE 161–3. Intravenous Heparin Dose: Titration Nomogram for Activated Partial Thromboplastin Time (aPTT)

	IV Infusion		
aPTT	***Rate Change (mL/hr)***	***Dose Change (U/24 hr)****	***Additional Action***
<45	+6	+5760	Repeated aPTT test† in 4-6 hr
46-54	+3	+2880	Repeated aPTT test in 4-6 hr
55-85	+0	0	None‡
86-110	−3	−2880	Stop heparin sodium treatment for 1 hr; repeated aPTT test 4-6 hr after heparin treatment is restarted
>110	−6	−5760	Stop heparin treatment for 1 hr; repeated aPTT test 4-6 hr after heparin treatment is restarted

From Hull RD, Raskob GE, Rosenbloom D, et al: Optimal therapeutic level of heparin therapy in patients with venous thrombosis. Arch Intern Med 1992; 152:1589.
*Heparin sodium concentration, 20,000 U in 500 mL = 40 U/mL.
†With the use of Actin-FS thromboplastin reagent (Dade, Mississauga, Ontario).
‡During the first 24 hours, repeated aPTT test in 4-6 hours. Thereafter, the aPTT is determined once daily unless subtherapeutic.

TABLE 161–4. Weight-Based Nomogram for Initial Heparin Therapy

Initial Dose	80 U/kg bolus, then 18 U/kg/hr
aPTT <35 sec (<1.2 × control)*	80 U/kg bolus, then 4 U/kg/hr
aPTT, 35–45 sec (1.2–1.5 × control)	40 U/kg bolus, then 2 U/kg/hr
aPTT, 46–70 sec (1.5–2.3 × control)	No change
aPTT, 71–90 sec (2.3–3.0 × control)	Decrease infusion rate by 2 U/kg/hr
PTT >90 sec (>3.0 × control)	Hold infusion 1 hr, then decrease infusion rate by 3 U/kg/hr

Reproduced with permission from Raschke RA, Reilly BM, Guidry JR, et al: The weight-based heparin dosing nomogram compared with a "standard care" nomogram. Ann Intern Med 1993; 119:874–881.
*Figures in parentheses show comparisons with control.
aPTT = activated partial thromboplastin time; PTT = partial thromboplastine time; U = unit; kg = kilogram; hr = hour.

two groups: nine of 99 patients in the group given combined therapy (9.1%), compared with 12 of 100 patients (12.0%) in the group given heparin alone. Importantly, bleeding complications occurred in eight of 93 patients (8.6%) who had supratherapeutic findings. Major bleeding occurred in three of 93 patients (3.2%) who had supratherapeutic aPTT findings (relative risk, 0.3; $P = .09$). Major bleeding occurred in 11% of patients considered to be at high risk but in only 1% of those considered to be at low risk ($P = .007$). These findings demonstrate a lack of association between a supratherapeutic aPTT (ratio > 2.5) and the risk of clinically important bleeding complications.

Subcutaneous Heparin Compared with Continuous Intravenous Heparin

In the past, numerous randomized trials compared the effectiveness and safety of heparin given by the subcutaneous and continuous intravenous routes.[66, 67] Investigators have concluded that subcutaneously administered heparin is as effective and as safe as intravenously administered heparin.[67] However, this meta-analysis has been criticized because of the selection of studies for review and because of the lack of data on aPTT values in patients receiving subcutaneous heparin.[68] In view of the well-established need to achieve a lower limit of the aPTT therapeutic range, heparin given by the subcutaneous route is not recommended in the initial treatment of proximal vein thrombosis.

Subcutaneous Adjusted-Dose Heparin for Long-Term Treatment

Adjusted-dose subcutaneous heparin is the long-term anticoagulant regimen of choice in pregnant patients, in certain patients at high risk of bleeding, and in patients who return to geographically remote areas in which long-term anticoagulant monitoring is unavailable or impractical (in whom the heparin dose is adjusted during the first few days of long-term therapy and then fixed).[69] The starting dose of long-term subcutaneous heparin is determined from the patient's initial intravenous heparin dose requirement.

A starting subcutaneous dose equivalent to one third of the patient's 24-hour intravenous heparin dose is administered every 12 hours. The subcutaneous dose is adjusted during the first few days of long-term therapy to maintain the mid-interval aPTT (determined 6 hours after injection) at 1.5 times the control value. This level of anticoagulant response is usually achieved with a dose of 8000 to 12,000 U every 12 hours (mean dose, 10,000 U every 12 hours). In pregnant patients, larger doses may be required, and continued monitoring is desirable because of changes in heparin requirements throughout the course of pregnancy.

Complications of Heparin Therapy

The main side effects of heparin therapy include (1) bleeding, (2) thrombocytopenia, and (3) osteoporosis. Patients at particular risk are those who have had recent surgery or trauma or who have other clinical factors which predispose to bleeding on heparin, such as peptic ulcer, occult malignancy, liver disease, hemostatic defects, age greater than 65 years, and female gender.[70]

Bleeding

The management of bleeding in patients taking heparin depends on the location and severity of bleeding, the risk of recurrent venous thromboembolism, and the level of aPTT. Heparin should be discontinued temporarily or permanently. Patients with recent venous thromboembolism may be candidates for insertion of an inferior vena caval filter. If urgent reversal of heparin effect is required, protamine sulfate can be administered.

Thrombocytopenia

Heparin-induced thrombocytopenia is a well-recognized complication of heparin therapy, usually occurring within 5 to 10 days after heparin treatment has started.[71–73] Approximately 1% to 2% of patients receiving unfractionated heparin experience a fall in platelet count to less than the normal range or a 50% fall in the platelet count within the normal range. In most cases, this mild to moderate thrombocytopenia appears to be a direct effect of heparin on platelets and is of no consequence. However, approximately 0.1% to 0.2% of patients receiving heparin experience an immune thrombocytopenia mediated by immunoglobulin G (IgG) antibody directed against a complex of platelet factor 4 and heparin.[74] The development of thrombocytopenia may be accompanied by arterial or venous thrombosis, which may lead to serious consequences, such as death or limb amputation. The diagnosis of heparin-induced thrombocytopenia, with or without thrombosis, must be made on clinical grounds because the assays with the highest sensitivity and specificity are not readily available and have a slow turnaround time.[74–78]

When the diagnosis of heparin-induced thrombocytopenia is made, heparin in all forms must be stopped immediately.[73] For patients requiring ongoing anticoagulation, several alternatives exist: warfarin therapy, insertion of an inferior vena caval filter, the use (where available) of the defibrinogenating extract of snake venom, ancrod (Arvin),[79] the heparinoid danaparoid,[80] and, more recently, a specific antithrombin, hirudin[81] or argatroban.[82] Most of the reports in case series have included the use of Arvin[79] or danaparoid,[80] but clinical trials are under way to assess the efficacy and safety of the specific antithrombin agents. Danaparoid may cross-react in patients with heparin-induced thrombocytopenia.

Osteoporosis

Osteoporosis has been reported in patients receiving unfractionated heparin in doses of 20,000 U/day (or more) for more than 6 months.[47] Demineralization can progress to the fracture of vertebral bodies or long bones, and the defect may not be entirely reversible. Hypersensitivity to heparin is uncommon and may take the form of a skin rash or, less commonly, anaphylaxis. Alopecia has been reported as a rare complication of heparin therapy. Serum transaminase levels may be moderately raised. Heparin-induced hypoaldosteronism is recognized but rare. Rarely, a bluish discoloration of the toes, associated with a burning sensation, has been reported.[47]

Neutralization of Heparin Anticoagulant Effect

The anticoagulant effect of heparin can be immediately neutralized by intravenous injection of protamine sulfate. The appropriate neutralizing dose depends on the dose of heparin, its route of administration, and the time it is given. If protamine sulfate is used within minutes of an intravenous heparin injection, a full neutralizing dose (1 mg protamine sulfate per 100 U of heparin) should be given.[47] Because the plasma half-life of intravenously administered heparin is approximately 60 minutes, an injection of protamine sulfate in a bolus of more than 50 mg is seldom required. An occasional hypotensive response to protamine sulfate has been reported; therefore, it should be injected slowly over a 10- to 30-minute period.

Treatment with protamine sulfate may need to be repeated because protamine is cleared more quickly than heparin from the blood. After subcutaneous injection of heparin is administered, repeated small doses of protamine may be required because of prolonged heparin absorption from the subcutaneous depot.

Low-Molecular-Weight Heparin and Heparinoids

Since the early 1980s, a number of low-molecular-weight heparin fractions of unfractionated heparin have become available for clinical use.[83] The low-molecular-weight heparins are manufactured from unfractionated heparin (usually of porcine origin) by controlled depolymerization using either chemical (nitrous oxide, alkaline hydrolysis, or peroxidative cleavage) or enzymatic (heparinase) techniques.[84] The low-molecular-weight fractions have a molecular weight between 4000 and 6000, with 60% of the polysaccharide chains having a molecular weight between 2000 and 8000. The various low-molecular-weight heparins differ in terms of mean molecular weight, glycosoaminoglycans content, and anticoagulant activity in terms of anti-X_a and anti-II_a activity.[84-91] The various fractions have different pharmacologic profiles in terms of bioavailability, plasma clearance, and release of tissue factor pathway inhibitor. In experimental models, they have different antithrombotic and hemorraghic properties.[84-91] The low-molecular-weight heparins currently available for commercial use are shown in Table 161-5 along with the method of production, molecular weights, and anti-X_a to anti-II_a ratio.

Because the low-molecular-weight heparins are different compounds with distinct pharmacologic properties[84-89] and because different regimens have been used in clinical trials, it is considered inappropriate to use meta-analyses for comparing the effects of low-molecular-weight heparin with placebo, unfractionated heparin, dextran, or warfarin. Despite the various differences between the low-molecular-weight heparins, the clinical outcomes in clinical trials have been similar particularly in prophylactic studies using lower doses. With the higher doses used in treatment of thrombotic disorders, it is possible that differences in outcomes may become apparent.

It is hoped that the low-molecular-weight heparins will result in fewer serious complications, such as bleeding,[91-94] osteoporosis,[95-98] and heparin-induced thrombocytopenia[99] compared with unfractionated heparin. Evidence is accumulating that these complications are, indeed, less serious and less frequent with the use of low-molecular-weight heparin.

Low-molecular-weight heparin has not been approved for the prevention or treatment of venous thromboembolism in pregnancy. These drugs do not cross the placenta,[100, 101] and small case series suggest they may be both effective and safe.[101-105] At present, however, the standard treatment for venous thromboembolism in pregnancy is twice-daily, adjusted-dose subcutaneous unfractionated heparin.[106] The low-molecular-weight heparins all cross-react with unfractionated heparin and can therefore not be used as alternative therapy in patients with heparin-induced thrombocytopenia. The heparinoid danaparoid possesses a 10% to 20% cross-reactivity with heparin, and it can be safely used in patients who have no cross-reactivity.[80]

The low-molecular-weight heparins differ from unfractionated heparin in numerous ways. Of particular importance are the following:

1. Increased bioavailability[87, 88] (>90% after subcutaneous injection).
2. Prolonged half life[84, 87] and predictable clearance enabling once-daily or twice-daily injection.[107]
3. Predictable antithrombotic response based on body weight permitting treatment without laboratory monitoring.[97]

Other possible advantages are (1) their ability to inactivate platelet bound factor X_a,[108] (2) resistance to inhibition by platelet factor 4,[54, 57] and their decreased effect on platelet function[54] and vascular permeability[58] (possibly accounting for fewer hemorraghic effects at comparable antithrombotic doses).[91-93]

Low-Molecular-Weight Heparin in the Treatment of Proximal Venous Thrombosis

In the treatment of established venous thromboembolism, low-molecular-weight heparin given by subcutaneous injection has a number of advantages over continuous intravenous unfractionated heparin; doses can be given by once-daily or twice-daily subcutaneous injection, and the antithrombotic response to low-molecular-weight heparin is highly correlated with body weight, permitting administration of a fixed dose without laboratory monitoring.

In a number of early clinical trials (some of which were

TABLE 161–5. Properties of Commercial Low-Molecular-Weight Heparins

Trade Name	International Nonproprietary Name (INN)	Method of Production	Mean Molecular Weight
Innohep	Tinzaparin	HD	5866
Fragmin	Dalteparin	NAP	5819
Lovenox	Enoxaparin	AH	4371
Fraxiparine	Nadroparin	NAP	4855
Reviparin	Clivarin	NAP	4653
Normiflo	Ardeparin	PC	6000

HD = heparinase digestion; NAP = nitrous acid depolymerization; AH = alkaline hydrolysis; PC = peroxidative cleavage.

dose-finding), low-molecular-weight heparin given by subcutaneous or intravenous injection was compared with continuous intravenous unfractionated heparin, with repeated venography at days 7 to 10 being the primary endpoint.[109-114] These studies demonstrated that low-molecular-weight heparin was at least as effective as unfractionated heparin in preventing extension or increasing resolution of thrombi on repeated venography.[109-114]

More recently, the more relevant clinical outcomes of recurrent venous thromboembolism or death during follow-up have been used as endpoints.[115-119]. These studies are not all comparable, because (1) different regimens of low-molecular-weight heparins were used, (2) not all studies ensured that adequate intravenous heparin therapy was given or properly monitored, and (3) some studies entered patients with distal as well as proximal deep vein thrombosis. Only one study was double-blinded. Low-molecular-weight heparin was given for 6 to 10 days, with warfarin therapy starting either on day 2[115] or on days 7 to 10.[116-119] Warfarin was continued for 3 months, with the target International Normalized Ratio (INR) range 2.0 to 3.0. The INR is the PT ratio obtained by testing a given sample using the WHO reference thromboplastin. For practical clinical purposes, the INR for a given plasma sample is equivalent to the PT ratio obtained using a standardized human brain thromboplastin known as the Manchester Comparative Reagent, which has been widely used in the United Kingdom. The outcomes in terms of recurrent venous thromboembolism, major bleeding, and mortality for five clinical trials using clinical endpoints are summarized in Table 161-6.

The clinical trial by Hull and coworkers[115] was a double-blinded randomized study of 432 patients. Each received either once-daily subcutaneous low-molecular-weight heparin (tinzaparin) or unfractionated heparin by continuous intravenous infusion using a validated heparin nomogram to ensure adequate heparinization. Warfarin was started on day 2 and continued for 3 months with a targeted INR of 2 to 3. Patients receiving low-molecular-weight heparin experienced fewer recurrent events, and the rates of major bleeding and death were significantly lower than in the patients receiving the unfractionated heparin. None of the other clinical trials demonstrated a statistically significant decrease in any of these clinical events. When the results of this trial and that of Prandoni and associates[116] were pooled, there was a striking decrease in mortality in the patients receiving low-molecular-weight heparin, particularly in patients with cancer.[120]

A cost effectiveness analysis indicated that low-molecular-weight heparin was cost effective when compared with continuous intravenous heparin under the study protocol conditions because monitoring was not necessary and there were fewer complications requiring rehospitalization and treatment.[121] These findings were verified by a sensitivity analysis. It was estimated that 37% of patients receiving low-molecular-weight heparin could have been discharged on day 2, which would have further increased the cost effectiveness of the low-molecular-weight heparin.[121]

Two studies indicate that in selected patients low-molecular-weight heparin treatment can be administered safely out of the hospital.[122, 123] Patients who met the entry criteria were randomized to receive twice-daily, low-molecular-weight heparin either entirely out of the hospital or with early discharge or continuous intravenous heparin in the hospital. Warfarin therapy was started on day 1 or 2 and continued for 3 months. Both studies showed equivalence with respect to the incidence of recurrent venous thromboembolism, major bleeding, and mortality rates.[122, 123] In these studies, 31% and 33% of patients with proximal venous thrombosis were eligible for entry. Whether out-of-hospital treatment can be more widely applied in the treatment of proximal venous thrombosis awaits further study.

It appears that low-molecular-weight heparin can be used safely for the treatment of acute non–massive pulmonary embolism as well.[124, 125] Studies are under way to assess the effectiveness and safety of treatment with low-molecular-weight heparin for 3 months compared with standard heparin and warfarin therapy, and for the treatment of proximal venous thrombosis in pregnancy comparing once-daily, low-molecular-weight heparin with twice-daily, adjusted-dose subcutaneous unfractionated heparin.

Oral Anticoagulant Therapy

There are two distinct chemical groups of oral anticoagulants:[126]

- 4-Hydroxy coumarin derivatives (e.g., warfarin sodium)
- Indane-1, 3-dione derivatives (e.g., phenindione).

The coumarin derivatives are the oral anticoagulants of choice because they are associated with fewer nonhemorrhagic side effects than the indanedione derivatives.

The anticoagulant effect of warfarin is mediated by the inhibition of the vitamin K–dependent gamma-carboxylation of coagulation factors II, VII, IX, and X.[126, 127] This results in the synthesis of immunologically detectable but biologically inactive forms of these coagulation proteins. Warfarin also inhibits the vitamin K–dependent gamma-carboxylation of proteins C and S.[128] Protein C circulates as a proenzyme that is activated on endothelial cells by the thrombin-thrombomodulin complex to form activated protein C. Activated protein

TABLE 161–6. Randomized Trials of Low-Molecular-Weight Heparin versus Unfractionated Heparin for In-hospital Treatment of Proximal Deep Vein Thrombosis: Long-Term Follow-up

Reference	Treatment	Recurrent Venous Thromboembolism No. (%)	Major Bleeding No. (%)	Mortality No. (%)
Hull et al.[70]	Tinzaparin	6/213 (2.8)	1/213 (0.5)*	10/213 (4.7)*
	Heparin	15/219 (6.8)	11/219 (5.0)	21/219 (9.6)
Prandoni et al.[71]	Fraxiparine	6/85 (7.1)	1/85 (1.2)	6/85 (7.1)
	Heparin	12/85 (14.1)	3/85 (3.8)	12/85 (14.1)
Lopaciuk et al.[72]	Fraxiparine	0/74 (0)	0/74	0/74
	Heparin	3/72 (4.2)	1/72 (1.4)	1/72 (1.4)
Simonneau et al.[73]	Enoxaparin	0/67	0/67	3/67 (4.5)
	Heparin	0/67	0/67	2/67 (3.0)
Lindmarker et al.[74]	Dalteparin	5/101 (5.0)	1/101	2/101 (2.0)
	Heparin	3/103 (2.9)	0/103	3/103 (2.9)

*$P < .05$ versus heparin.

C in the presence of protein S inhibits activated factor VIII and activated factor V activity.[128] Therefore, vitamin K antagonists, such as warfarin, create a biochemical paradox by producing an anticoagulant effect due to the inhibition of procoagulants (factors II, VII, IX, and X) and a potentially thrombogenic effect by impairing the synthesis of naturally occurring inhibitors of coagulation (proteins C and S).[128] Heparin and warfarin treatment should overlap by 4 to 5 days when warfarin treatment is initiated in patients with thrombotic disease.

The anticoagulant effect of warfarin is delayed until the normal clotting factors are cleared from the circulation, and the peak effect does not occur until 36 to 72 hours after drug administration.[129] During the first few days of warfarin therapy, the prothrombin time (PT) reflects mainly the depression of factor VII ($t^{1/2}$, 5 to 7 hours). Equilibrium levels of factors II, IX, and X are not reached until about 1 week after the initiation of therapy.

The use of small initial daily doses (e.g., 5 to 10 mg) is the preferred approach for initiating warfarin treatment. The dose-response relationship to warfarin therapy varies widely between individuals, and therefore the dose must be carefully monitored to prevent overdosing or underdosing.

A number of drugs interact with warfarin. Critical appraisal of the literature reporting such interactions indicates that the evidence substantiating many of the claims is limited.[130] Nonetheless, patients must be warned against taking any new drugs without the knowledge of their attending physician.

Laboratory Monitoring and Therapeutic Range

The laboratory test most commonly used to measure the effects of warfarin is the one-stage PT test. The PT is sensitive to reduced activity of factors II, VII, and X but is insensitive to reduced activity of factor IX. Confusion about the appropriate therapeutic range has occurred because the different tissue thromboplastins used for measuring the PT vary considerably in sensitivity to the vitamin K–dependent clotting factors and in response to warfarin.[131] Rabbit brain thromboplastin, which is widely used in North America, is less sensitive than standardized human brain thromboplastin, which has been widely used in the United Kingdom and other parts of Europe. A PT ratio of 1.5 to 2.0 using rabbit brain thromboplastin (i.e., the traditional therapeutic range in North America) is equivalent to a ratio of 4.0 to 6.0 using human brain thromboplastin.[131] Conversely, a twofold to threefold increase in the PT using standardized human brain thromboplastin is equivalent to a 1.25- to 1.5-fold increase in the PT using a rabbit brain thromboplastin, such as Simplastin or Dade-C.[131]

In order to promote standardization of the PT for monitoring oral anticoagulant therapy, the World Health Organization (WHO) developed an international reference thromboplastin from human brain tissue and recommended that the PT ratio be expressed as the INR.[127]

Warfarin is administered in an initial dose of 5.0 to 10 mg per day for the first 2 days, and the daily dose is then adjusted according to the INR. Heparin or low-molecular-weight heparin therapy is discontinued on the 4th or 5th day following initiation of warfarin therapy, provided that the INR is prolonged into the recommended therapeutic range (INR, 2.0 to 3.0) for at least 2 consecutive days.[127] Because some individuals may metabolize the drug quickly or slowly, selection of the correct dosage of warfarin must be individualized. Therefore, frequent INR determinations are required initially to establish therapeutic anticoagulation.

Once the anticoagulant effect and patient's warfarin dose requirements are stable, the INR should be monitored every 1 to 2 weeks throughout the course of warfarin therapy for venous thromboembolism. If there are factors that may produce an unpredictable response to warfarin (e.g., concomitant drug therapy),[130] however, the INR should be monitored more frequently to minimize the risk of complications due to poor anticoagulant control.

Long-Term Treatment

Patients with established venous thrombosis or pulmonary embolism require long-term anticoagulant therapy to prevent recurrent disease. Warfarin therapy is highly effective and is preferred in most patients.[131] Adjusted-dose, subcutaneous heparin is the treatment of choice when long-term oral anticoagulants are contraindicated, such as in pregnancy. Adjusted-dose, subcutaneous heparin, or unmonitored low-molecular-weight heparin therapy has been used for the long-term treatment of patients in whom oral anticoagulant therapy proves to be very difficult to control.[69] In patients with proximal vein thrombosis, long-term therapy with warfarin reduces the frequency of objectively documented recurrent venous thromboembolism from 47% to 2%.[131]

The use of a less intensive warfarin regimen (INR 2.0 to 3.0) markedly reduces the risk of bleeding from 20% to 4% without loss of effectiveness in comparison with a more intensive warfarin regimen.[131] With the improved safety of oral anticoagulant therapy using a less intensive warfarin regimen, there has been renewed interest in evaluating the long-term treatment of thrombotic disorders.

In clinical trials in patients with atrial fibrillation, oral anticoagulant treatment has been given safely with a low risk of major bleeding complications (1% to 2% per year).[132] In trials such as these, the safety of oral anticoagulant treatment depends heavily on the maintenance of a narrow therapeutic INR range. When the INR falls below the therapeutic range, the incidence of thrombotic stroke increases; when the INR exceeds a level of 3.5 to 5.0, the incidence of major hemorrhage markedly increases. These and other studies have emphasized the importance of maintaining careful control of oral anticoagulant therapy, particularly with the use of anticoagulant management clinics if oral anticoagulants are to be used for extended periods.

Data from clinical trials have documented an unacceptably high incidence of recurrent venous thromboembolism, including fatal pulmonary embolism, during the long-term clinical course of patients with proximal deep vein thrombosis who are treated according to the current practice with intravenous heparin for several days, followed by oral anticoagulant treatment for 3 to 6 months. This has created renewed interest in longer-term treatment of venous thromboembolism.[18, 133-137]

Three groups of patients who have a particularly poor prognosis have been identified[138, 139]:

1. Patients with idiopathic, recurrent venous thromboembolism.
2. Patients who are carriers of genetic mutations which predispose to venous thromboembolism, such as the factor V Leiden mutation.
3. Patients with cancer.

Duration of Treatment After a First Episode of Deep Vein Thrombosis

It has been recommended that all patients with a first episode of venous thromboembolism receive warfarin therapy for 12 weeks. Attempts to decrease the treatment to 4 weeks[140, 141] or 6 weeks[136] resulted in higher rates of recurrent thromboembolism in contrast to either 12 or 26 weeks of treatment (11% to 18% recurrent thromboembolism in the following 1 to 2 years). Most of the recurrent thromboembolic events occurred in the 6 to 8 weeks immediately after anticoagulant treatment was stopped, and the incidence was higher in patients with continuing risk factors, such as cancer and immobilization.[136, 141] Treatment with oral anticoagulants for 6 months reduced the incidence of recurrent thromboembolic events, but there was a cumulative incidence of recurrent events at two years (11%) and an ongoing risk of recurrent thromboembolism of approximately 5% to 6% per year.[136]

In patients with a first episode of idiopathic venous thromboembolism treated with intravenous heparin followed by warfarin for 3 months, continuation of warfarin for 24 months led to a significant reduction in the incidence of recurrent venous thromboembolism compared with placebo.[142] This continued risk of recurrent thromboembolism, even with 6 months of treatment after a first episode of deep vein thrombosis, has encouraged the development of clinical trials evaluating the effectiveness of long-term anticoagulant treatment beyond 6 months.

Duration of Treatment in Patients with Recurrent Deep Vein Thrombosis

In a multicenter clinical trial, Schulman and coauthors randomized patients with a first recurrent episode of venous thromboembolism to receive either 6 months of or a continued course of oral anticoagulants indefinitely, with a targeted INR of 2.0 to 2.85.[137] The analysis was reported at 4 years. In the patients receiving anticoagulants for 6 months, recurrent thromboembolism occurred in 20.7%, compared with 2.6% of patients on the indefinite treatment ($P < .001$). However, the rates of major bleeding were 2.7% in the 6-month group but 8.6% in the indefinite-course group. In the indefinite group, two of the major hemorrhages were fatal; in the 6-month group, there were no fatal hemorrhages. This study showed that extending the duration of oral anticoagulants for approximately 4 years resulted in a significant decrease in the incidence of recurrent venous thromboembolism but with a higher incidence of major bleeding. Without a mortality difference, the risk of hemorrhage versus the benefit of decreased recurrent thromboembolism with the use of extended warfarin treatment remains uncertain and will require further clinical trials.

For patients experiencing a first episode of venous thromboembolism, long-term anticoagulant therapy should be continued for at least 3 months using oral anticoagulants to achieve an INR of 2.0 to 3.0.[143]

For patients with recurrent venous thromboembolism or a continuing risk factor, such as immobilization, heart failure, and cancer, anticoagulants should be continued for a longer time and possibly indefinitely, particularly for patients with more than one recurrent episode of thrombosis.[143]

For patients with genetic mutations predisposing to venous thromboembolism, such as the factor IV Leiden mutation, AT III, protein C, or protein S deficiency, or the presence of a lupus anticoagulant, anticoagulant treatment may be required for more than 3 months. Until further information from randomized clinical trials is available, firm recommendations cannot be made.[143]

Adverse Effects

Bleeding

The major side effect of oral anticoagulant therapy is bleeding.[144] Bleeding during well-controlled oral anticoagulant therapy is usually due to surgery or other forms of trauma, or to local lesions, such as peptic ulcer or carcinoma.[144] Spontaneous bleeding may occur if warfarin sodium is given in an excessive dose, resulting in marked prolongation of the INR; this bleeding may be severe and even life-threatening. The risk of bleeding can be substantially reduced by adjustment of the warfarin dose to achieve a less intense anticoagulant effect than has traditionally been used in North America (INR, 2.0 to 3.0; PT, 1.25 to 1.5 times control value obtained using a rabbit brain thromboplastin).[131]

Nonhemorrhagic Effects

Nonhemorrhagic side effects of oral anticoagulant therapy differ according to whether coumarin derivatives (e.g., warfarin sodium) or indanediones are administered. Such side effects are uncommon with coumarin anticoagulants, and the coumarins are therefore the oral anticoagulants of choice.

Coumarin-induced skin necrosis is a rare but serious complication that calls for immediate cessation of oral anticoagulant therapy.[145, 146] This condition usually occurs between 3 and 10 days after therapy has commenced; it is more common in women and most often involves areas of abundant subcutaneous tissues, such as the abdomen, buttocks, thighs, and breast. The mechanism of coumarin-induced skin necrosis, which is associated with microvascular thrombosis, is uncertain but appears to be related, at least in some patients, to depression of protein C level. Patients with congenital deficiencies of protein C may be particularly susceptible.

Fetal Defects

Oral anticoagulants cross the placenta and may cause fetal malformations when used during pregnancy.[147-149] Two specific fetopathic syndromes are associated with oral anticoagulant administration during pregnancy.

Treatment with oral anticoagulants during the 6th to 12th weeks of gestation may induce the syndrome of *warfarin embryopathy* in the fetus. This syndrome consists of skeletal abnormalities ranging from stippled epiphyses to frank skeletal hypoplasia. Although most of the reported cases have occurred in infants of mothers receiving warfarin, this syndrome has also been reported to result from phenindanedione or acenocoumarin administration. Oral anticoagulant administration during the second or third trimester may result in central nervous system abnormalities in the fetus, including *abnormalities of the ventricular system* (Dandy-Walker malformation), dorsal midline dysplasia, and optic atrophy. Therefore, the use of oral anticoagulants is contraindicated at any time during pregnancy, and the drugs should not be used in women planning a pregnancy.

Adjusted-dose heparin can safely be given throughout pregnancy in patients with venous thromboembolism, and from this observation, indications have been extrapolated to include patients requiring anticoagulation to prevent systemic embolism from prosthetic heart valves.[148]

Factors That Interact with the Effects of Oral Anticoagulant Therapy

A large number of drugs interact with oral anticoagulants and may produce either a prolongation or a reduction in the anticoagulant effect.[130] Special care should be taken to adjust the dose of oral anticoagulants during the time that other drugs are being taken, to minimize the risk of inadequate anticoagulant control.

Increased sensitivity to oral anticoagulants occurs in patients with vitamin K deficiency or impaired liver function, and in those with thyrotoxicosis due to the more rapid metabolism of the vitamin K-dependent clotting factors.[127]

Management of Surgical Patients Receiving Long-Term Oral Anticoagulant Therapy

Physicians are commonly confronted with the problem of managing oral anticoagulants in individuals who require temporary interruption of treatment for surgery or other invasive procedures.[150-155] In the absence of data from randomized clinical trials, recommendations can be made based only on cohort studies, retrospective reviews, and expert opinions. The most common conditions requiring long-term anticoagulant therapy are atrial fibrillation, mechanical or prosthetic heart valve replacement, and venous thromboembolism.[156] For each of these conditions, the risk of arterial or venous thromboembolism, when anticoagulants have been discontinued, must be weighed against the risk of bleeding if intravenous heparin is applied before or after the surgical procedure or if oral anticoagulant therapy is continued at the therapeutic level.

The possible choices based on the risk-benefit assessment in the individual patient include[157]:

1. Discontinuing warfarin for 3 to 5 days before the procedure to allow the INR to return to normal and then restarting therapy shortly after surgery.
2. Reducing the warfarin dose to maintain an INR in the lower or subtherapeutic range during the surgical procedure.
3. Discontinuing warfarin and treating the patient in the hospital with intravenous heparin before and after the surgical procedure until warfarin therapy can be reinstituted.

Low-molecular-weight heparin is now being used in some of the circumstances.

In a review[156] that attempted to estimate the risks and benefits of temporary discontinuation of oral anticoagulants and the temporary use of heparin in patients with different conditions requiring oral anticoagulation, further revised recommendations were made. Until further randomized clinical trials are carried out in these patients, no firm recommendations can be made, but these guidelines have proved useful in clinical practice.

Antidotes

The antidote to a vitamin K antagonist is vitamin K. If an excessive increase of the INR occurs, the treatment depends on the degree of the increase and whether or not bleeding has occurred:

1. If the increase is *mild* and the patient is not bleeding, no specific treatment is necessary other than reduction in the warfarin dose. The INR can be expected to decrease during the next 24 hours with this approach.
2. With more *marked* increase of the INR in patients who are not bleeding, treatment with small doses of vitamin K, given either orally or by subcutaneous injection (2.5 to 5.0 mg), may be considered.
3. With *very marked* increase of the INR, particularly in a patient who is either actively bleeding or at risk for bleeding, the coagulation defect should be corrected.

Reported side effects of vitamin K include flushing, dizziness, tachycardia, hypotension, dyspnea, and sweating.[127] Intravenous administration of vitamin K should be performed with caution to avoid inducing an anaphylactoid reaction. The risk of anaphylactoid reaction can be reduced by slow administration of intravenous vitamin K, at a rate no faster than 1 mg/min. In most patients, intravenous administration of vitamin K produces a demonstrable effect on the INR within 6 to 8 hours and corrects the increased INR within 12 to 24 hours. Because the half-life of vitamin K is less than that of warfarin sodium, a repeated course of vitamin K may be necessary. If bleeding is severe or life-threatening, vitamin K therapy can be supplemented with fresh frozen plasma.

References

1. Dismuke SE, Wagner EH: Pulmonary embolism as a cause of death: The changing mortality in hospitalized patient. JAMA 1986; 255:2039.
2. Dalen JE, Alpert JS: Natural history of pulmonary embolism. Prog Cardiovasc Dis 1975; 17:259.
3. Anderson FA, Wheeler HB, Goldberg RJ, et al: A population-based perspective of the hospital incidence and case-fatality rates of deep vein thrombosis and pulmonary embolism. Arch Intern Med 1991; 151:933.
4. Donaldson GA, Williams C, Scanell J, et al: A reappraisal of the application of the Trendelenburg operation to massive fatal embolism. N Engl J Med 1963; 268:171.
5. Consensus Conference: Prevention of venous thrombosis and pulmonary embolism. JAMA 1986; 256:744.
6. International Multicentre Trial: Prevention of fatal postoperative pulmonary embolism by low doses of heparin. Lancet 1975; ii:45.
7. Hyers TN, Hull RD, Weg JG: Antithrombotic therapy for venous thromboembolic disease. Chest 1992; 102:391S.
8. Moser KM, LeMoine JR: Is embolic risk conditioned by location of deep venous thrombosis? Ann Intern Med 1981; 94:439.
9. Hull RD, Hirsh J, Carter CJ, et al: Pulmonary angiography, ventilation lung scanning, and venography for clinically suspected pulmonary embolism with abnormal perfusion lung scan. Ann Intern Med 1983; 98:891.
10. Huisman MV, Buller HR, ten Cate JW, et al: Serial impedance plethysmography for suspected deep-vein thrombosis in outpatients: The Amsterdam general practitioner study. N Engl J Med 1986; 314:823.
11. Nicolaides AN, Kakkar VV, Field ES, et al: The origin of deep vein thrombosis: A venographic study. Br J Radiol 1971; 44:653.
12. Hull RD, Hirsh J, Sackett DL, et al: Clinical validity of a negative venogram in patients with clinically suspected venous thrombosis. Circulation 1981; 64:622.
13. Rabinov K, Paulin S: Roentgen diagnosis of venous thrombosis in the leg. Arch Surg 1972; 104:134.
14. Bone RC: Ventialtion/perfusion scan in pulmonary embolism: "The emperor is incompletely attired." J Am Med Assoc 1990; 263:2794.
15. Secker-Walker RH: On purple emperors, pulmonary embolism, and venous thrombosis. Ann Intern Med 1983; 98:1006.
16. Kelley MA, Carson JL, Palevsky HI, et al: Diagnosing pulmonary embolism: New facts and strategies. Ann Intern Med 1991; 114:300.
17. Hull RD, Secker-Walker RH, Hirsh J: Diagnosis of deep vein thrombosis. *In:* Thrombosis and Hemostasis: Basic Principles and Clinical Practice. 2nd Ed. Colman RW, Hirsh J, Marder VJ, et al (Eds). Philadelphia, JB Lippincott, 1987, p 1220.
18. Hull RD, Carter CJ, Jay RM, et al: The diagnosis of acute, recurrent deep-vein thrombosis: A diagnostic challenge. Circulation 1983; 67:901.
19. Parfrey PS, Griffiths SM, Barrett BJ, et al: Contrast material-induced renal failure in patients with diabetes mellitus, renal insufficiency or both. N Engl J Med 1989; 320:143.
20. Schwab SJ, Hlarky MA, Pieper KS, et al: Contrast nephrotoxicity: A randomized controlled trial of a nonionic and an ionic radiographic contrast agent. N Engl J Med 1989; 320:149.
21. Hull RD, Hirsh J, Carter CJ, et al: A randomized trial for noninvasive diagnostic testing for clinically suspected deep-vein thrombosis: The diagnostic efficacy of impedance plethysmography. Ann Intern Med 1985; 102:21.
22. Hull RD, Taylor DW, Hirsh J, et al: Impedance plethysmography: The relationship between venous filling and sensitivity and specificity for proximal-vein thrombosis. Circulation 1978; 58:898.
23. Huisman MV, Buller HR, ten Cate JW, et al: Management of clinically suspected acute venous thrombosis in outpatients with serial impedance plethysmography in a community hospital setting. Arch Intern Med 1989; 149:511.
24. Cronan JJ, Dorfman GS, Scola FH, et al: Deep venous thrombosis: US assessment using vein compressibility. Radiology 1987; 162:191.
25. Lensing AWA, Prandoni P, Brandjes D, et al: Detection of deep vein thrombosis by real-time B-mode ultrasonography. N Engl J Med 1989; 320:342.
26. Pedersen OM, Aslaksen A, Vik-Mo H, et al: Compression ultrasonography in hospitalized patients with suspected deep venous thrombosis. Arch Intern Med 1991; 151:2217.
27. Vaccaro JP, Cronan JJ, Dorfman GS: Outcome analysis of patients

with normal compression US examinations. Radiology 1990; 175:645.
28. Heijboer H, Brandjes D, Lensing AWA, et al: Efficacy of realtime B-mode ultrasonography versus impedance plethysmography in the diagnosis of deep vein thrombosis in symptomatic outpatients. Arch Intern Med 1992; 152:1901.
29. Rose SC, Zwiebel WJ, Nelson BD, et al: Symptomatic lower extremity deep venous thrombosis: Accuracy, limitations, and role of color duplex flow imaging in diagnosis. Radiology 1990; 173:639.
30. Ginsberg JS, Caco CC, Brill-Edwards P, et al: Venous thrombosis in patients who have undergone major hip or knee surgery: Detection with compression US and impedance plethysmography. Radiology 1991; 181:651.
31. Davidson B, Elliott GC, Lensing AWA: Low accuracy of color Doppler ultrasound to detect proximal leg vein thrombosis during screening of asymptomatic high-risk patients. Ann Intern Med 1992; 117:735.
32. Kipper MS, Moser KM, Kortman KE, et al: Long-term follow-up of patients with suspected pulmonary embolism and a normal lung scan. Chest 1985; 82:411.
33. Hull RD, Raskob GE, Coates G, et al: Clinical validity of a normal perfusion lung scan inpatients with suspected pulmonary embolism. Chest 1990; 97:23.
34. PIOPED Investigators: Value of the ventilation/perfusion scan in acute pulmonary embolism: Results of the Prospective Investigation of Pulmonary Embolism Diagnosis (PIOPED). JAMA 1990; 263:2753.
35. Alderson PO, Rujanavech N, Secker-Walker RH, et al: The role of ^{133}Xe ventilation studies in the scintigraph detection of pulmonary embolism. Radiology 1976; 120:633.
36. McNeil BJ: Ventilation-perfusion studies and the diagnosis of pulmonary embolism: Concise communication. J Nucl Med 1980; 21:319.
37. Biello DR, Mattar AG, McKnight RC, et al: Ventilation-perfusion studies in suspected pulmonary embolism. Am J Radiol 1979; 133:1033.
38. Hull RD, Hirsh J, Carter CJ, et al: Diagnostic value for ventilation-perfusion lung scanning in patients with suspected pulmonary embolism. Chest 1985; 88:819.
39. Sasahara AA, Sharma GVRK, Parisi AF: New development in the detection and prevention of venous thromboembolism. Am J Cardiol 1979; 43:1214.
40. Dalen JE, Brooks HL, Johnson LW, et al: Pulmonary angiography in acute pulmonary embolism, indications, techniques, and results in 367 patients. Am Heart J 1979; 81:175.
41. Bookstein JJ, Silver TM: The angiographic differential diagnosis of acute pulmonary embolism. Radiology 1974; 110:25.
42. Novelline RA, Oksana HB, Athanasoulis CA, et al: The clinical course of patients with suspected pulmonary embolism and a negative pulmonary arteriogram. Radiology 1978; 126:561.
43. Mills SR, Jackson DC, Older RA, et al: The incidence, etiologies and avoidance of complications of pulmonary angiography in a large series. Radiology 1980; 136:295.
44. Stein PD, Hull RD, Saltzman HA, et al: Strategy for diagnosis of patients with suspected acute pulmonary embolism. Chest 1993; 103:1553.
45. Hull RD, Raskob GE, Coates G, et al: A new non-invasive management strategy for patients with suspected acute pulmonary embolism. Arch Intern Med 1989; 149:2549.
46. Hull RD, Raskob GE, Ginsberg JS, et al: A definitive noninvasive strategy for the management of patients with suspected pulmonary embolism. Arch Intern Med 1993; 154:289.
47. Hirsh J, Raschke R, Warkentin TE, et al: Heparin: Mechanism of action, pharmacokinetics, dosing considerations, monitoring, efficacy, and safety. Chest 1995; 108:258S.
48. Lane DA: Heparin binding and neutralizing protein. *In:* Heparin, Chemical and Biological Properties, Clinical Applications. Lane DA, Lindahl U (Eds). London, Edward Arnold, 1989, pp 363-391.
49. Lindahl U, Backstrom G, Hook M, et al: Structure of the antithrombin-binding site of heparin. Proc Natl Acad Sci USA 1979; 76:3198.
50. Lindahl U, Thunberg L, Backstrom G, et al: Extension and structural variability of the antithrombin-binding sequence in heparin. J Biol Chem 1984; 259:12368.
51. Rosenberg RD, Lam L: Correlation between structure and function of heparin. Proc Natl Acad Sci USA 1979; 76:1218.
52. Casu B, Oreste P, Torri G, et al: The structure of heparin oligosaccharide fragments with high anti-(factor X_a) activity containing the minimal antithrombin III-binding sequence. Biochem J 1981; 197:599.
53. Weitz JI, Hudoba M, Massel D, et al: Clot-bound thrombin is protected from inhibition by heparin–antithrombin III but is susceptible to inactivation by antithrombin III–independent inhibitors. J Clin Invest 1990; 86:385.
54. Salzman EW, Rosenberg RD, Smith MH, et al: Effect of heparin and heparin fractions on platelet aggregation. J Clin Invest 1980; 65:64.
55. Tollefsen DM, Majerus DW, Blank MK: Heparin cofactor II: Purification and properties of a heparin-dependent inhibitor of thrombin in human plasma. J Biol Chem 1982; 257:2162.
56. Hoppensteadt D, Walenga JM, Fasanella A, et al: TFPI antigen levels in normal human volunteers after intravenous and subcutaneous administration of unfactionated heparin and low molecular weight heparin. Thromb Res 1995; 77:175.
57. Barzu T, Molho P, Tobelem G, et al: Binding of heparin and low molecular weight heparin fragments to human vascular endothelial cells in culture. Nouv Rev Fr Haematol 1984; 26:243.
58. Blajchman MA, Young E, Ofosu FA: Effects of unfractionated heparin, dermatan sulfate and low molecular weight heparin on vessel wall permeability in rabbits. Ann N Y Acad Sci 1989; 556:245.
59. Hull RD, Raskob GE, Hirsh J, et al: Continuous intravenous heparin compared with intermittent subcutaneous heparin in the initial treatment of proximal-vein thrombosis. N Engl J Med 1986; 315:1109.
60. Brandjes DPM, Buller HR, Heijboer H, et al: Comparative trial of heparin and oral anticoagulants in the initial treatment of proximal deep vein thrombosis. N Engl J Med 1992; 327:1485.
61. Hull RD, Raskob GE, Rosenbloom D, et al: Optimal therapeutic level of heparin therapy in patients with venous thrombosis. Arch Intern Med 1992; 152:1589.
62. Wheeler AP, Jaquiss RD, Newman JH: Physician practices in the treatment of pulmonary embolism and deep-venous thrombosis. Arch Intern Med 1988; 148:1321.
63. Cruickshank MK, Levine MN, Hirsh J, et al: A standard heparin nomogram for the management of heparin therapy. Arch Intern Med 1991; 151:333.
64. Raschke RA, Reilly BM, Guidry JR, et al: The weight-based heparin dosing nomogram compared with a "standard care" nomogram. Ann Intern Med 1993; 119:874.
65. Brill-Edwards P, Ginsberg S, Johnston M, et al: Establishing a therapeutic range for heparin therapy. Ann Intern Med 1993; 119:104.
66. Pini M, Pattachini C, Quintavalla R, et al: Subcutaneous vs intravenous heparin in the treatment of deep venous thrombosis—a randomized clinical trial. Thromb Haemost 1990; 64:222.
67. Hommes DW, Bura A, Mazzolai L, et al: Subcutaneous heparin compared with continuous intravenous heparin administration in the initial treatment of deep vein thrombosis. Ann Intern Med 1992; 116:279.
68. Moser KM, Fedullo PF: Subcutaneous compared with intravenous heparin for deep vein thrombosis. Ann Intern Med 1992; 117:265.
69. Hull R, Delmore T, Carter C, et al: Adjusted subcutaneous heparin versus warfarin sodium in the long-term treatment of venous thrombosis. N Engl J Med 1982; 306:189.
70. Campbell N, Hull RD, Brant R, et al: Aging and heparin-related bleeding. Arch Intern Med 1996; 156:857.
71. Kelton JG: Heparin-induced thrombocytopenia. Haemostasis 1986; 16:173.
72. Warkentin TE, Kelton JG: Heparin-induced thrombocytopenia. Prog Hemost Thromb 1991; 10:1.
73. Boshkov LK, Warkentin TE, Hayward CPM, Andrew M, Kelton JG: Heparin-induced thrombocytopenia and thrombosis: Clinical and laboratory studies. Br J Haematol 1993; 84:322.
74. Arepally G, Reynolds C, Tomaski A, et al: Comparison of PF4/heparin ELISA assay with the ^{14}C-serotonin release assay in the diagnosis of heparin-induced thrombocytopenia. Am J Clin Pathol 1995; 104:648.

75. Kelton JG, Sheridan D, Brian H, et al: Clinical usefulness of testing for a heparin-dependent platelet aggregation factor in patients with suspected heparin-associated thrombocytopenia. J Lab Clin Med 1984; 103:606.
76. Greinacher A, Michels I, Kiefel V, Mueller-Eckhardt C: A rapid and sensitive test for diagnosing heparin-associated thrombocytopenia. Thromb Haemost 1991; 66:734.
77. Chong BH, Burgess J, Ismail F: The clinical usefulness of the platelet aggregation test for the diagnosis of heparin-induced thrombocytopenia. Thromb Haemost 1993; 69:344.
78. Kelton JG: The laboratory diagnosis of heparin-induced thrombocytopenia: Still a journey, not yet a destination (Editorial). Am J Clin Pathol 1995; 104:611.
79. Demers C, Ginsberg JS, Brill-Edwards P, et al: Rapid anticoagulation using ancrod for heparin-induced thrombocytopenia. Blood 1991; 78:2194.
80. Magnani HN: Heparin-induced thrombocytopenia (HIT): An overview of 230 patients treated with Orgaran (Org 10172). Thromb Haemost 1993; 70:554.
81. Nand S: Hirudin therapy for heparin-associated thrombocytopenia and deep vein thrombosis. Am J Hematol 43:310, 1993.
82. Matsuo T, Kario K, Chikahira Y, et al: Treatment of heparin-induced thrombocytopenia by use of argatroban, a synthetic thrombin inhibitor. Br J Haematol 1992; 82:627.
83. Hirsh J, Levine MN: Low molecular weight heparin. Blood 1992; 79:1.
84. Fareed J, Walenga JM, Hoppensteadt D, et al: Comparative study on the in vitro and in vivo activities of seven low-molecular weight heparins. Haemostasis 1988; 18 (Suppl 3):3.
85. Bara L, Samama MM: Pharmacokinetics of low molecular weight heparins. Acta Chir Scand 1988; 543:65.
86. Briant L, Caranobe C, Saivin S, et al: Unfractionated heparin and CY216. Pharmacokinetics and bioavailabilities of the anti-factor X_a and II_a: Effects of intravenous and subcutaneous injection in rabbits. Thromb Haemost 1989; 61:348.
87. Anderson L-O, Barrowcliffe TW, Holmer E, et al: Molecular weight dependency of the heparin potentiated inhibition of thrombin and activated factor X: Effect of heparin neutralization in plasma. Thromb Res 1979; 115:531.
88. Fareed J, Walenga JM, Racanelli A, et al: Validity of the newly established low molecular weight heparin standard in cross referencing low molecular weight heparins. Haemostasis 1988; 3(Suppl):33.
89. Barrowcliffe TW, Curtis AD, Johnson EA, et al: An international standard for low molecular weight heparin. Thromb Haemost 1988; 60:1.
90. Holmer E, Soderberg K, Bergqvist D, et al: Heparin and its low molecular weight derivatives: Anticoagulant and antithrombotic properties. Haemostasis 1986; 16(Suppl 2):1–7.
91. Carter CJ, Kelton JG, Hirsh J, et al: The relationship between the hemorrhagic and antithrombotic properties of low molecular weight heparins and heparin. Blood 1982; 59:1239.
92. Cade JF, Buchanan Mr, Boneu B, et al: A comparison of the antithrombotic and haemorrahagic effects of low molecular weight heparin fractions: The influence of the method of preparation. Thromb Res 1984; 35:613.
93. Andriuoli G, Mastacchi R, Barnti M, et al: Comparison of the antithrombotic and hemorrhagic effects of heparin and a new low molecular weight heparin in the rat. Haemostasis 1985; 15:324.
94. Lensing AW, Prins MH, Davidson BL, et al: Treatment of deep venous thrombosis with low-molecular-weight heparins. Arch Intern Med 1995; 155:601.
95. Monreal M, Lafoz E, Salvador R, et al: Adverse effects of three different forms of heparin therapy: Thrombocytopenia, increased transaminases, and hyperkalaemia. Eur J Clin Pharmacol 1989; 37:415.
96. Monreal M, Vinas L, Monreal L, et al: Heparin-related osteoporosis in rats: A comparative study between unfractionated heparin and a low molecular weight heparin. Haemostasis 1990; 20:204.
97. Matzsch T, Bergqvist D, Hedner U, et al: Effects of low molecular weight heparin and unfragmented heparin on induction of osteoporosis in rates. Thromb Haemost 1990; 63:505.
98. Shaughnessy SG, Young E, Deschamps P, Hirsh J: The effects of low molecular weight and standard heparin on calcium loss from fetal rat calvaria. Blood 1995; 86:1368.
99. Warkentin TE, Levine MN, Hirsh J, et al: Heparin-induced thrombocytopenia in patients treated with low-molecular-weight heparin or unfractionated heparin. N Engl J Med 1995; 332:1330.
100. Forestier F, Daffos F, Capella-Pavlovsky M: Low molecular weight heparin (PH 10169) does not cross the placenta during the second trimester of pregnancy: Study by direct foetal blood sampling under ultrasound. Thromb Res 1984; 34:557.
101. Andrew M, Cade J, Buchanan MR, et al: Low-molecular weight heparin does not cross the placenta (Abstract). Thromb Haemost 1983; 50:225.
102. Omri A, Delaloye FJ, Andersen H, et al: Low-molecular-weight heparin Novo (LHN-1) does not cross the placenta during the second trimester of pregnancy. Thromb Haemost 1989; 61:55.
103. Melissari E, Parker CJ, Wilson NV, et al: Use of low molecular weight heparin in pregnancy. Thromb Haemost 1992; 68:652.
104. Sturridge F, de Swiet M, Letsky E. The use of low molecular weight heparin for thromboprophylaxis in pregnancy. Br J Obstet Gynaecol 1994; 101:69.
105. Wahlberg, TB, Kher A: Low molecular weight heparin as thromboprophylaxis in pregnancy: A retrospective analysis from 14 European clinics. Haemostasis 1994; 24:55–56.
106. Ginsberg JS, Hirsh J: Use of antithrombotic agents during pregnancy. Chest 1995; 108:305S.
107. Boneu, B, Caranobe C, Cadroy Y, et al: Pharmacokinetic studies of standard unfractionated heparin, and low molecular weight heparins in the rabbit. Semin Thromb Hemost 1988; 14:18.
108. Boneu B, Buchanan MR, Cade JF, et al: Effects of heparin, its low molecular weight fractions and other glycosaminoglycans on thrombus growth in vivo. Thromb Res 1985; 40:81.
109. Bratt G, Tornebohm E, Granqvist S, Aberg W, Lockner D: A comparison between low molecular weight heparin (KABI 2165) and standard heparin in the intravenous treatment of deep venous thrombosis. Thromb Haemost 1985; 54:813.
110. Holm HA, Ly B, Handeland GF, Abildgaard U, et al: Subcutaneous heparin treatment of deep venous thrombosis: A comparison of unfractionated and low molecular weight heparin. Haemostasis 1986; 16:30.
111. Albada J, Nieuwenhuis HK, Sixma JJ: Treatment of acute venous thromboembolism with low molecular weight heparin (Fragmin): Results of a double-blind randomized study. Circulation 1989; 80:935–40.
112. Bratt G, Aberg W, Johansson M, Tornebohm E, et al: Two daily subcutaneous injections of Fragmin as compared with intravenous standard heparin in the treatment of deep venous thrombosis (VDT). Thromb Haemost 1990; 64:506.
113. Harenberg J, Huck K, Bratsch H, Stehle G, et al: Therapeutic application of subcutaneous low-molecular-weight heparin in acute venous thrombosis. Haemostasis 1990; 20(Suppl 1):205.
114. Siegbahan A, Y-Hassan S, Boberg J, Bylund A, et al: Subcutaneous treatment of deep venous thrombosis with low molecular weight heparin: A dose finding study with LMWH-Novo. Thromb Res 1989; 55:267.
115. Hull RD, Raskob GE, Pineo GF, et al: Subcutaneous low-molecular-weight heparin compared with continuous intravenous heparin in the treatment of proximal-vein thrombosis. N Engl J Med 1992; 326:975.
116. Prandoni P, Lensing AW, Buller HR, et al: Comparison of subcutaneous low-molecular-weight heparin with intravenous standard heparin in proximal deep-vein thrombosis. Lancet 1992; 339:441.
117. Lopaciuk S, Meissner AJ, Filipecki S, et al: Subcutaneous low-molecular-weight-heparin versus subcutaneous unfractionated heparin in the treatment of deep vein thrombosis: A Polish multicentre trial. Thromb Haemost 1992; 68:14.
118. Simonneau G, Charbonnier B, Decousus H, et al: Subcutaneous low-molecular-weight heparin compared with continuous intravenous unfractionated heparin in the treatment of proximal deep vein thrombosis. Arch Intern Med 1993; 153:1541.
119. Lindmarker P, Holmstrom M, Granqvist S, Johnsson H, Locner D: Comparison of once-daily subcutaneous Fragmin with continuous intravenous unfractionated heparin in the treatment of deep venous thrombosis. Thromb Haemost 1994; 72:186.
120. Green D, Hull RD, Brant R, Pineo GF: Lower mortality in cancer patients treated with low-molecular-weight versus standard heparin. Lancet 1992; 339:1476.

121. Hull RD, Raskob GE, Rosenbloom D, et al: Treatment of proximal vein thrombosis with subcutaneous low-molecular-weight heparin vs. intravenous heparin. An economic perspective. Arch Intern Med 1997; 157:289.
122. Levine M, Gent M, Hirsh J, et al: A comparison of low-molecular-weight heparin administered primarily at home with unfractionated heparin administered in the hospital for proximal deep vein thrombosis. N Engl J Med 1996; 334:677.
123. Koopman MMW, Prandoni P, Piovella F, Ockelford PA, et al: Treatment of venous thrombosis with intravenous unfractionated heparin administered in the hospital as compared with subcutaneous low-molecular-weight heparin administered at home. N Engl J Med 1996; 334:682.
124. Meyer G, Brenot F, Pacouret G, et al: Subcutaneous low-molecular-weight heparin Fragmin versus intravenous unfractionated heparin in the treatment of acute non massive pulmonary embolism: An open randomized pilot study. Thromb Haemost 1995; 74:1432.
125. Simonneau G, Sors H, Charbonnier B, et al: Once daily low molecular weight heparin tinzaparin vs. unfractionated heparin in the treatment of acute pulmonary embolism. Thromb Haemost 1997; 3080:753.
126. Freedman MD: Oral anticoagulants: Pharmacodynamics, clinical indications and adverse effects. J Clin Pharmacol 1992; 32:196.
127. Hirsh J, Dalen JE, Deykin D, Poller L, Bussey HI: Oral anticoagulants: mechanism of action, clinical effectiveness, and optimal therapeutic range. Chest 1995; 108:231S.
128. Clouse LH, Comp PC: The regulation of haemostasis: The protein C system. N Engl J Med 1986; 314:1298.
129. O'Reilly RA, Aggeler PM: Studies on coumarin anticoagulant drugs: Initiation of warfarin therapy without a loading dose. Circulation 1968; 38:169.
130. Wells PS, Holbrook AM, Crowther R, Hirsh J: Warfarin and its drug/food interactions: A critical appraisal of the literature. Ann Intern Med 1994; 121:676.
131. Hull R, Hirsh J, Jay R, et al: Different intensities of oral anticoagulant therapy in the treatment of proximal-vein thrombosis. N Engl J Med 1982; 307:1676.
132. Laupacis A, Albers G, Dalen J, et al: Antithrombotic therapy in atrial fibrillation. Chest 1995; 108:352S.
133. Prandoni P, Lensing AWA, Cogo A, et al: The long-term clinical course of acute deep venous thrombosis. Ann Intern Med 1996; 125:1.
134. Beyth RJ, Cohen AM, Landefeld CS: Long-term outcomes of deep vein thrombosis. Arch Intern Med 1995; 155:1031.
135. Franzeck UK, Schaich I, Jager KA, et al: Prospective 12 year follow-up study of clinical and hemodynamic sequelae after deep vein thrombosis in low-risk patients (Zurich study). Circulation 1996; 93:74.
136. Schulman S, Rhedin AS, Lindmarker P, et al: A comparison of six weeks with six months of oral anticoagulation therapy after a first episode of venous thromboembolism: Duration of Anticoagulation Trial Study Group. N Engl J Med 1995; 332:1661.
137. Schulman S, Granqvist S, Holmstrom M, et al: The duration of oral anticoagulant therapy after a second episode of venous thromboembolism. N Engl M Med 1997; 336:393.
138. Prandoni P, Lensing A, Buller H, et al: Deep vein thrombosis and the incidence of subsequent symptomatic cancer. N Engl J Med 1992; 327:1128.
139. Simioni P, Prandoni P, Lensing AWA, et al: The risk of recurrent venous thromboembolism in patients with an Arg[506] — Glu mutation in the gene for factor V (factor V Leiden). N Engl J Med 1997; 336:339.
140. Research Committee of the British Thoracic Society. Optimum duration of anticoagulation for deep vein thrombosis and pulmonary embolism. Lancet 1992; 340:873.
141. Levine MN, Hirsh J, Gent M, et al: Optimal duration of oral anticoagulant therapy: A randomized trial comparing four weeks with three months of warfarin in patients with proximal deep vein thrombosis. Thromb Haemost 1995; 74:606.
142. Kearon C, for the LAFIT Investigators: Two years of warfarin vs. placebo following three months of anticoagulation for a first episode of idiopathic venous thromboembolism (VTE), (Abstract). Thromb Haemost 1997; 69:767.
143. Hyers T, Hull R, Weg J: Antithrombotic therapy for venous thromboembolic disease. Chest 1995; 108:335S.
144. Levine MN, Raskob GE, Hirsh J: Hemorrhagic complications of long term anticoagulant therapy. Chest 1989; 95(Suppl 2):26S.
145. Grimaudo V, Gueissaz F, Hauert J, et al: Necrosis of skin induced by coumarin in a patient deficient in protein S. Br Med J 1989; 298:233.
146. Becker CG: Oral anticoagulant therapy and skin necrosis: Speculation on pathogenesis. Adv Exp Med Biol 1987; 214:217
147. Hall JG, Pauli RM, Wilson KM: Maternal and fetal sequelae of anticoagulation during pregnancy. Am J Med 1980; 68:122
148. Ginsberg JS, Hirsh J: Use of antithrombotic agents during pregnancy. Chest 1995; 100:305S.
149. Iturbe-Alessio I, del Carmen Fonseca M, Mutchinik O, et al: Risks of anticoagulant therapy in pregnant women with artificial heart valves. N Engl J Med 1986; 315:1390.
150. Rustad H, Myhre E: Surgery during anticoagulant treatment. Acta Med Scand 1963; 173:115.
151. McIntyre H: Management during dental surgery of patients on anticoagulants. Lancet 1966; 2:99.
152. Tinker JH, Tarhan S: Discontinuing anticoagulant therapy in surgical patients with cardiac valve prostheses. JAMA 1978; 239:738.
153. Katholi RE, Nolan SP, McGuire LB: The management of anticoagulation during noncardiac operations in patients with prosthetic heart valves. Am Heart J 1978; 96:163.
154. Bodnar AG, Hutter AM: Anticoagulation in valvular heart disease preoperatively and postoperatively. Cardiovasc Clin 1984; 14:247.
155. Eckman MH, Beshansky JR, Duranad-Zaleski I, et al: Anticoagulation for noncardiac procedures in patients with prosthetic heart valves. JAMA 1990; 263:1513.
156. Kearon C, Hirsh J: Management of anticoagulation before and after elective surgery. N Engl J Med 1997; 336:1506.
157. Stein PD, Alpert JS, Copeland JG, et al: Antithrombotic therapy in patients with mechanical and biological prosthetic heart valves. Chest 1995; 108:371S.

162

Intensive Care of the Cancer Patient

Graziano C. Carlon, MD

A quick review of information on the Internet regarding official statistics on the prevalence and outcome of malignancies (http://www.cancer.org) provides a bewildering volume of data. It is possible, however, to derive a few generic conclusions:

1. The incidence of cancer in the population is increasing.
2. The prevalence of cancer as a cause of death is increasing.[1]
3. The long-term survival of individuals with cancer is increasing at a significant rate.[2]
4. The probabilities of long-term survival have significantly increased even for types of malignancies most likely to require major surgical procedures (lung, esophagus, pancreas) or treatments that affect the immune system (leukemia, lymphoma).

These findings are not contradictory, because an aging population, in whom many other causes of death have been prevented, is more susceptible to cancer. The findings do hold, however, important implications for most physicians, including those practicing in intensive care units (ICUs).

First, most medical practitioners will be involved in the treatment of patients with malignancies. For critical care specialists, the justification for applying extraordinary therapeutic and life-support interventions increases with a higher expectation of worthwhile palliation, prolonged survival, and even complete cure for malignancies and stages of disease once considered rapidly and inexorably lethal. Life-threatening complications can be associated with the malignancy itself or can appear as side effects of treatment. An acute event may be the first manifestation of the disease or may occur while the patient is being actively treated. Finally, illnesses common to the general population may also affect cancer patients at any time, and a relationship to the underlying malignancy should not be automatically assumed.

This chapter describes complications of cancer and its treatment that may result in urgent consultation for admission to an ICU. Both the major categories of malignancies and the most important therapeutic modalities are reviewed.

LIFE-THREATENING COMPLICATIONS OF CANCER

Hematologic Malignancies

Hematologic malignancies rarely present as acute events requiring immediate intensive care. Usually, patients are admitted to the ICU for supportive treatment of complications that have developed during therapy. Aggressive management of complications is justified by continuous improvement in the results of treatment. For instance, 5-year survival in childhood leukemia was 4% in 1970 and in 1998 exceeded 70%, because of advances in chemotherapy and bone marrow transplantation. The more benign forms of Hodgkin's disease show comparable cure rates, and the rate of permanent remission exceeds 50% for non-Hodgkin's lymphoma. These results have been largely achieved through aggressive treatment modalities that carry their own risks of significant complications that may require intensive care.

Leukemias

Bleeding, sepsis, and neurologic dysfunction are occasional initial manifestations of acute leukemia that may require advanced life support. Principal means of treatment include replacement of blood volume; administration of coagulation factors, including platelets; and antibiotics. Resistance to infections is extremely limited, and antibiotics should be administered without delay at the first suspicion of bacterial contamination.[3]

The recommended therapeutic regimen remains controversial. Some authors still recommend a broad-spectrum coverage with three or more antibiotics, including aminoglycosides, penicillins active against gram-negative bacteria, agents that provide adequate coverage of staphylococcal species, third-generation and fourth-generation cephalosporins, and quinolones. Others suggest that, in many cases, single-agent treatment should be attempted first to minimize both end-organ damage and the development of resistant bacterial strains.[4-6] The actual selection of specific agents should depend on patterns of sensitivity and antibiotic susceptibility in each hospital.[7]

Fungal infections can also be devastating in these patients. Antifungal therapy with intravenous amphotericin B, possibly supplemented by imidazoles (fluconazole, ketoconazole, itraconazole),[8-10] should be instituted early in patients who do not improve rapidly with antimicrobial therapy, but the mortality rate is very high when fungal dissemination to vital organs has occurred (Figs. 162-1 and 162-2).[11-13] Infestation by opportunistic and parasitic organisms as well as by viral infections may also be suspected. Coverage with antiviral agents, trimethoprim or pentamidine,[14] and antitubercular drugs, for typical and atypical mycobacteria,[15, 16] should be entertained in patients who continue to deteriorate.[17, 18] The addition of granulocyte colony-stimulating factor (G-CSF) is also recommended to reduce the frequency and severity of infection.[19]

Central venous, pulmonary artery, and systemic arterial access should be obtained only when clinically necessary, by use of the strictest aseptic precautions.[20] The risks of infection associated with indwelling catheters are well known. The lowest infection rates occur with implantable devices, especially those that are completely submerged under the skin, although they cannot be used for monitoring.[21] Once in place, catheters should not be manipulated. Clinical studies have indicated that routine catheter substitution does not prevent infections and may even increase the risk of bacterial contami-

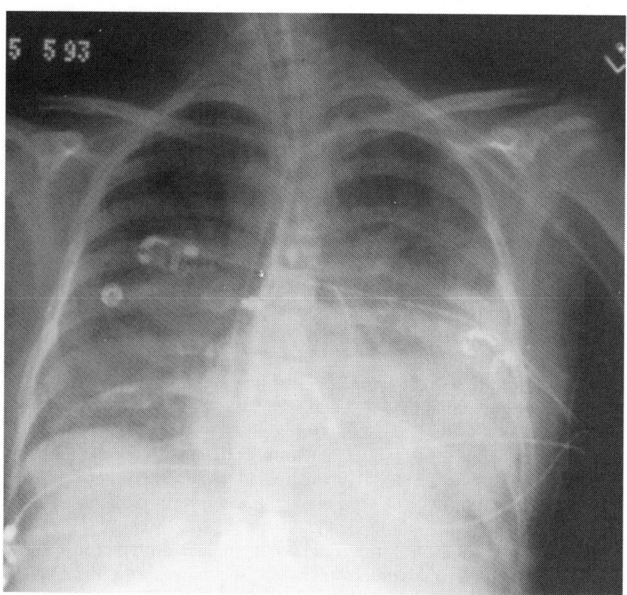

Figure 162–1. Chest radiograph of a patient with severe, disseminated fungal infection. The radiographic picture suggests the presence of pulmonary infiltrates.

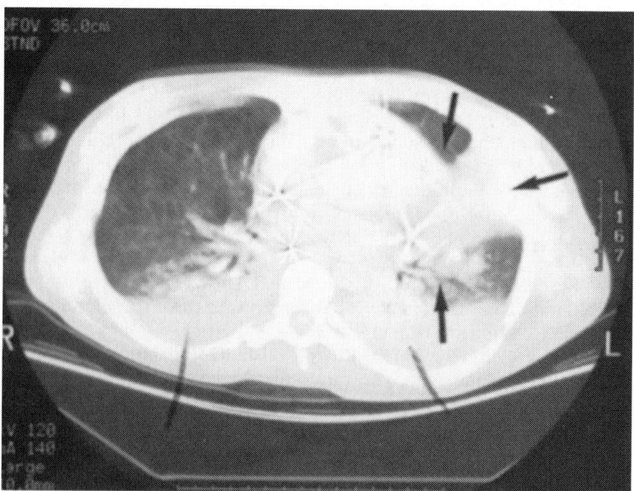

Figure 162–2. CT scan of the chest from the patient in Figure 162-1. The fungal mass is penetrating the pericardium and invading the myocardium.

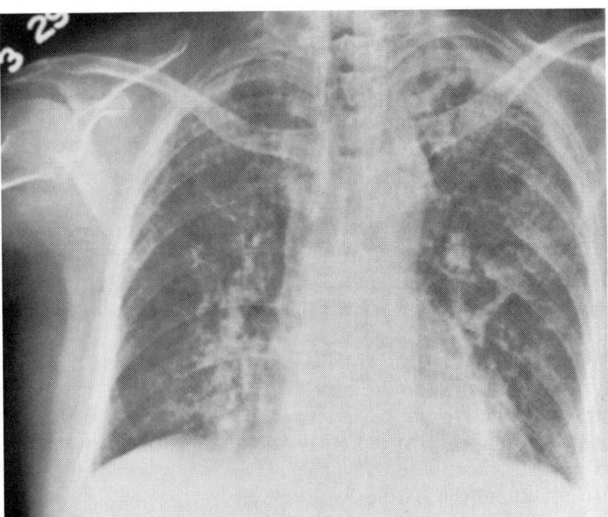

Figure 162–3. Chest radiograph of a patient with diffuse bilateral modular infiltrates. The radiographic findings cleared within a few days, subsequent to combination chemotherapy for the underlying acute myeloblastic leukemia.

nation; accordingly, this practice should no longer be recommended.[22] If a catheter must be replaced, insertion at a new site causes fewer infectious but higher mechanical complications compared with guide wire substitution at the same site. Depletion of accessible insertion sites also must be considered.[23, 24] It is not possible to make generic recommendations, and the needs of each patient should be considered individually.[25, 26]

Respiratory failure with hypoxemia and increased pulmonary venous admixture requiring mechanical ventilation and positive end-expiratory pressure (PEEP) is a particularly serious event in leukemic patients.[27] Occasionally, respiratory failure may be the first manifestation of the disease and may improve after chemotherapy (Fig. 162–3).[28] Radiographic evidence may be scanty because dense infiltrates do not usually develop in the absence of white blood cells. The diagnosis is based on the absence of positive culture specimens, the identification of leukemic cells in bronchoalveolar lavage fluid (BAL), and the rapid improvement seen on chest x-ray evaluation and in respiratory function after chemotherapy. More commonly, lung infiltrates are expressions of local or systemic sepsis, drug toxicity, hypersensitivity, or fluid overload. Acute respiratory distress requiring mechanical ventilation for more than 72 to 96 hours is associated with a mortality rate of 60% to 70% in these patients,[29] a figure that does not differ from those reported for the general population.[30]

Pulmonary parenchymal bleeding is a severe complication of the thrombocytopenia and other coagulation abnormalities frequently seen with systemic malignancies. Treatment includes replacement of clotting factors and early institution of mechanical ventilation.[31]

Acute promyelocytic leukemia is often associated with disseminated intravascular coagulation (DIC). Most authors recommend continuous intravenous infusion of low-dose heparin (7 to 10 U/kg/hr) and cautious replacement of coagulation factors. The dangers of the disease and its therapy justify admitting patients to an ICU for close monitoring during the early phases of management. Because these patients are severely thrombocytopenic, sensitivity to heparin may be disproportionately increased, and frequent determination of partial thromboplastin time is required to regulate dosage. Often, DIC subsides after the first course of chemotherapy.[32]

Renal infiltrates, although common in patients with acute leukemia, rarely cause serious deterioration of renal function. Because many patients with systemic malignancies have reduced total body muscle mass, indices of renal function (e.g., serum creatinine) should be interpreted with caution. Nephrotoxic chemotherapy or antibiotics contribute to renal dysfunction, and dosages must be adjusted according to measured creatinine clearance and serum levels. A method that has proved effective is daily determination of creatinine clearance on the basis of 3-hour urine collections.[33]

Hyperviscosity syndromes, as seen in plasma cell myeloma, occasionally cause renal failure. Plasmapheresis rapidly reverses the associated symptomatology, but chemotherapy is needed to control the progression of the disease.

Lymphomas

Malignant lymphoma in the mediastinum can compress the superior vena cava, causing signs and symptoms of frightening gravity. Although usually slowly progressive, with ample time for the development of adequate collateral circulation, acute superior vena caval occlusion is a medical emergency that requires immediate intervention with radiation therapy, chemotherapy, or both.[34] Dramatic resolution may be seen in as little as 12 to 24 hours. Depending on the severity of the symptoms, a biopsy may not be possible before treatment begins. Whenever possible, however, specimens should be obtained first to confirm the histologic diagnosis and to guide subsequent treatment.

Infiltration of lung parenchyma by lymphoma is common and can be confused with chronic pulmonary infiltrates. Although the infiltration rarely causes respiratory failure severe enough to require mechanical ventilation, massive hemorrhage secondary to vascular invasion has been observed.

Expansion of the tumor into, and infiltration of, other organs such as the stomach has also been described in patients with lymphomas. Massive bleeding is difficult to control both because surgical removal may be impossible and because effective therapy may result in rapid necrosis of the malignant infiltrate, precipitating hemorrhage or perforation.

Myelomas

The kidneys are often severely affected by multiple myeloma, particularly of the light-chain variety; renal failure, once established, is usually not reversible.[35]

Hypercalcemia, a complication of myeloma and of tumors that metastasize to bones, may cause obtundation, coma, and—in extreme cases—respiratory or cardiac arrest. Treatment includes intravenously administered balanced saline solutions to facilitate calcium elimination by increasing glomerular filtration and intravenous furosemide (5 to 20 mg), which selectively inhibits calcium reabsorption.[36] Salmon calcitonin (80 to 150 U/kg given at 8- to 12-hour intervals) can rapidly lower serum calcium levels, but its usefulness is limited by early tachyphylaxis.[37] Corticosteroids (100 to 300 mg/day of hydrocortisone) are also useful in the treatment of hypercalcemia secondary to osteolytic processes. The antineoplastic antibiotic mithramycin effectively lowers calcium level through inhibition of osteoclast activity, but its action does not begin until 18 to 24 hours after administration, it has the potential of severe hypocalcemia, and it is often accompanied by a precipitous fall in platelet count.[38]

More recently, biphosphonates have been successful in lowering serum calcium levels.[39–41] Many patients with myeloma are severely malnourished and have low serum albumin levels; therefore, the ionized fraction of serum calcium represents a higher percentage of the total value. Estimation of ionized calcium concentration from the McLean-Hastings nomograms

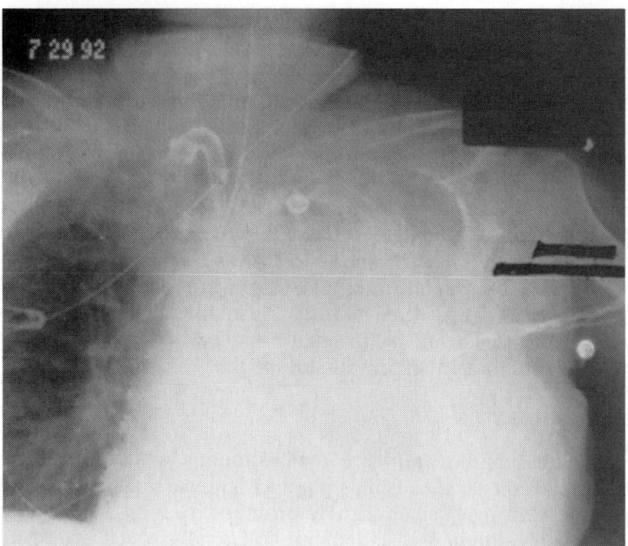

Figure 162–4. Chest radiograph of a patient with obstruction of the left mainstem bronchus secondary to adenocarcinoma of the lung. A brief period of support on mechanical ventilation allowed palliative laser vaporization of the obstruction and several months of survival for the patient.

is far less accurate than direct determination with an ion-selective electrode.

Solid Tumors

Serious emergencies related to solid tumors or their treatment may arise at any time during the course of the disease. They commonly represent a terminal event, and decisions on the degree of support that should be given must include considerations of the likelihood of worthwhile palliation.

Central nervous system (CNS) metastases are sometimes associated with coma and respiratory depression. Rapid resolution of symptoms is achieved with pharmacologic doses of steroids, preferably dexamethasone (24 to 100 mg/day given in four divided doses), followed by surgical excision, if appropriate, and whole-brain radiation therapy. The 2-year survival rate of patients with solitary brain metastasis from lung adenocarcinoma is as high as 40%.[42] Because at least temporary palliation can be obtained, ICU admission is justified in the absence of widespread disease.

Malignant invasion of the major bronchi or the trachea can usually be palliated by interstitial brachytherapy, external beam radiation, or vaporization with the neodymium:yttrium aluminum garnet laser.[43] Intubation through the tumor or into the contralateral uninvolved bronchus may be required for support until the occlusion is at least partially relieved (Fig. 162–4).

Malignant mediastinal adenopathy can cause superior vena caval occlusion. Radiotherapy or chemotherapy is associated with considerable improvement in patients with lymphomas, but it is of short-term benefit in most solid tumors. Invasion of the heart chambers by metastatic lesions is rare but almost invariably fatal (Figs. 162–5 and 162–6).

Severe hepatic dysfunction rarely occurs with primary or metastatic disease, because 80% of the parenchyma can be replaced without appreciable change in laboratory values. Liver failure is invariably an irreversible terminal event.[44]

Renal failure from parenchymal invasion occurs rarely in solid tumor patients. Bilateral ureteral obstruction from malignant disease in the pelvis is more common and leads to hydronephrosis and renal failure. Percutaneous or direct surgical relief of obstruction is often followed by massive postobstructive diuresis, which requires careful fluid and electrolyte replacement to avoid further renal damage.

CHEMOTHERAPY

During the past two decades, impressive advances have been made in the development of chemotherapeutic agents, increasing both the efficacy of the drugs and the spectrum of disease covered. Few neoplasms are completely unresponsive to drug therapy. Chemotherapy alone may provide long-term or complete control of disease in acute childhood leukemias, choriocarcinoma, Hodgkin's disease, and testicular carcinoma. Many other cancers have shown improved survival and dis-

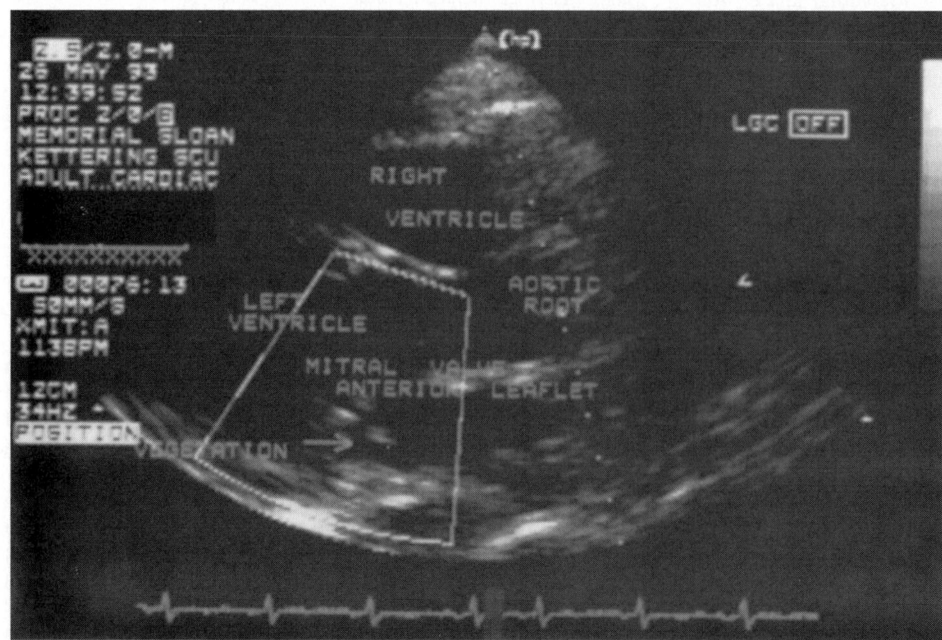

Figure 162–5. Echocardiograph of a patient with a cardiac lesion that was initially interpreted as a bacterial vegetation; at autopsy, the lesion was revealed to be a metastatic lesion from a rhabdomyosarcoma.

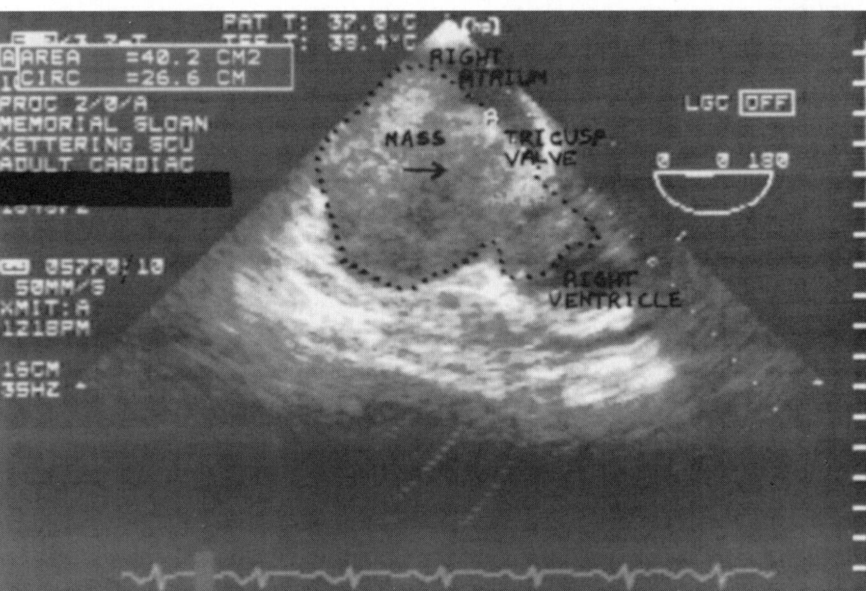

Figure 162–6. Rare, pedunculated metastatic lesion from a peripheral rhabdomyosarcoma, invading the right atrium and the posterior leaflet of the tricuspid valve. An attempt to remove the mass under bypass was unsuccessful. The patient received a palliative anastomosis between the right innominate vein and the pulmonary artery to relieve blood flow obstruction.

ease-free intervals as a result of chemotherapy used alone or in conjunction with surgery and radiotherapy.

Conceptually, chemotherapeutic agents should selectively destroy neoplastic cells by interfering with pathways of metabolism not shared by their normal counterparts. Unfortunately, such specificity is difficult to achieve, and healthy cells are also damaged during therapy. Drugs used in combination can have additive side effects that may be potentiated by other factors, such as malnutrition, prior radiation therapy, and surgery. Accordingly, critical care physicians should be familiar with the complications of commonly used chemotherapeutic agents.

Alkylating Agents

Alkylating agents form covalent bonds with preformed nucleic acids, and this interferes with their action.

Mechlorethamine

The prototype of this class of drug is mechlorethamine (nitrogen mustard), which is used primarily to treat disseminated Hodgkin's disease. Mechlorethamine causes nausea, vomiting, and bone marrow suppression.

Busulfan

Busulfan is used in the treatment of chronic myeloid leukemia. It is associated with an irreversible interstitial lung fibrosis that develops after months or even years of therapy. When busulfan is administered with nitrosoureas, however, its toxicity can be accelerated and lung fibrosis may develop within a few weeks.[45]

Cyclophosphamide

Cyclophosphamide, one of the most versatile chemotherapeutic agents, is useful in the treatment of hematologic malignancies as well as solid tumors, neuroblastomas, and carcinomas of the breast, testis, lung, ovary, endometrium, and prostate. Although usually safe, it can cause diffuse interstitial lung fibrosis after a few months to several years of therapy.[46] Respiratory failure associated with lung fibrosis is characterized by an inability to increase lung volume or to recruit collapsed alveoli despite increasing airway pressure. The high airway pressures caused by inelastic and fibrotic lung parenchyma frequently result in barotrauma. High-frequency jet ventilation has been useful in some patients, enabling the maintenance of satisfactory gas exchange, but the ultimate prognosis of these patients remains dismal.[47]

Cyclophosphamide is associated with myocardial toxicity when cumulative doses exceed 1800 to 2000 mg/mm^2.[48] Active metabolites of cyclophosphamide are excreted in the urine, where they reach concentrations that are damaging to the bladder mucosa, causing severe hemorrhagic cystitis. Because cyclophosphamide increases water reabsorption by distal renal tubules and collecting ducts, hydration alone may not maintain a sufficient diuresis without the use of mannitol or other diuretics. Cyclophosphamide and other alkylating agents deplete plasma cholinesterase, probably by interfering with hepatic synthesis, thereby prolonging the duration of action of local anesthetics and depolarizing neuromuscular blocking drugs. Resolution of muscle paralysis after anesthesia may be prolonged unless this effect is considered.

Chlorambucil, Melphalan

Chlorambucil and melphalan are oral agents that cause myelosuppression and minimal nausea or vomiting. Melphalan is used to treat multiple myeloma and breast and ovarian carcinomas, and chlorambucil is used to treat the nodular forms of non-Hodgkin's lymphoma, chronic lymphatic leukemia, and ovarian carcinoma.[49]

Antimetabolites

Antimetabolites interfere with nucleic acid synthesis of new nucleic acids in actively dividing cells, such as those of the hematopoietic system. Most, if not all, antimetabolites cause severe myelosuppression and present the risk of life-threatening sepsis or hemorrhage.

Methotrexate

Methotrexate competitively inhibits the action of folic acid, preventing nucleic acid formation and cellular replication. It is used to treat choriocarcinomas, acute lymphatic leukemia, sarcomas, and breast and lung carcinomas. Methotrexate is highly toxic to the liver, and serial liver biopsies have been recommended for early identification of liver damage during prolonged therapy. Renal failure has also been reported and is usually reversible. Mucositis and exfoliative dermatitis are common, and fluid loss or sepsis may follow loss of large areas of skin. Pulmonary toxicity, usually of modest severity, characterized by mild nondesquamative alveolitis and noncaseating granulomas, has been observed.[50] More severe respiratory complications, however, have also been reported, leading to acute respiratory failure.[51] Intrathecal administration to control central nervous system involvement in childhood leukemia also has the potential for tissue damage. Folinic acid (citrovorum rescue factor) is given to minimize these toxic effects.

5-Fluorouracil

5-Fluorouracil, a pyrimidine antimetabolite, is the chemotherapeutic agent of choice for neoplasms of the gastrointestinal tract and is used in combination with other drugs in breast cancer. It is primarily complicated by myelosuppression. An analog, 5-fluorodeoxyuridine, sometimes causes severe diarrhea that necessitates fluid and electrolyte support.

Vinca Alkaloids

Vincristine, Vinblastine

Vincristine and vinblastine, alkaloids derived from plants of the periwinkle family, impair the synthesis of cellular microtubules. They are an effective treatment for Hodgkin's and non-Hodgkin's lymphomas, acute lymphoblastic leukemia, and some solid tumors, including Wilms' tumor and sarcomas. They are administered intravenously and are highly toxic to both the peripheral and the central nervous systems. Both the sensory and the motor neurons are affected, as are nonmyelinated sympathetic fibers. Orthostatic hypotension related to the loss of sympathetic tone is a common complication of vincristine administration. Prolonged ileus can develop after vincristine or vinblastine therapy and is usually a self-limiting complication that responds to conservative measures, although cecal dilatation may require emergency cecostomy or colonoscopic decompression to avoid perforation.

At high doses, vinca alkaloids are powerful antidiuretics and can cause an inappropriate antidiuretic hormone syndrome, leading to severe hyponatremia. Severe skin necrosis develops with subcutaneous extravasation.[52]

Vinorelbine

Vinorelbine is a new vinca alkaloid, used alone or more often in combination, for the treatment of pulmonary malignancies.[53] The most severe complication is bone marrow suppression, which usually is rapidly reversible after cessation of treatment or administration of G-CSF. There have been reports, however, of acute pulmonary toxicity[54] following high-dose administration of the drug, alone or in association with mitomycin C.

Antineoplastic Antibiotics

Doxorubicin

Doxorubicin is an effective treatment for tumors of the ovary, colon, breast, testicles, stomach, thyroid, and bladder. It is also effective against lymphomas, sarcomas, multiple myeloma, and acute myeloblastic leukemia. Its liposome-encapsulated form has been effectively used in the treatment of liver metastases from colorectal cancer.[55] Toxicities associated with doxorubicin include myelosuppression, stomatitis, alopecia, and severe skin necrosis if extravasation occurs (Fig. 162–7).

The most serious complication of this drug is the irreversible cardiomyopathy that often develops when doses exceed 550 mg/m^2.[56] Patients who have also received chest irradiation may be more sensitive to the drug.[57] With lower amounts, swelling of myofibril cytoplasm may cause temporary deterioration of cardiac function. Continued therapy causes further myocardial injury, leading to vacuolization, cellular necrosis, and eventually, fibrosis. Patients should be followed up with serial echocardiograms, electrocardiography-gated radionuclide scans, or endomyocardial biopsy. Information obtained from electrocardiographic (ECG) tracings is usually nonspecific and identifies the presence of irreversible lesions only. Myelosuppression can be profound, consisting of absolute granulocyte counts below 250 mm^3 and platelet counts below 20,000 mm^3 for 14 to 21 days after doses of 90 to 120 mg/m^2 are administered; occasionally, pancytopenia may last as long as 5 weeks.

Treatment of cardiac failure, once established, is difficult. Digitalis toxicity can develop rapidly because the number of cardiac receptors available to bind the drug is decreased by necrosis of myocardial cells. Other oral inotropes, such as amrinone, cause unacceptable side effects and are no longer used clinically.[58] Some benefits have been reported with the oral inotrope vasodilator flosequinan, but complications are also being observed with long-term administration of this agent.[59, 60]

Treatment of patients with heart failure secondary to anthracycline administration is best handled by afterload reduction;

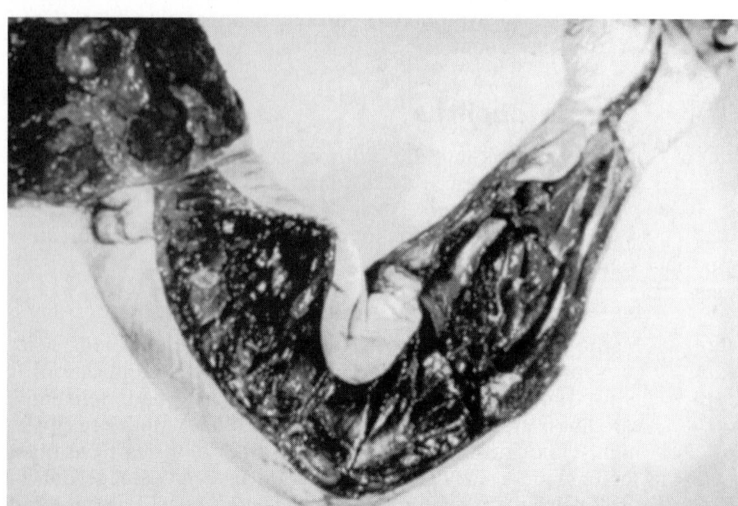

Figure 162–7. Fascial necrosis involving an entire arm following local extravasation of doxorubicin.

oral and intravenous angiotensin-converting enzyme II (ACE II) inhibitors can be helpful if blood pressure and renal function can be satisfactorily maintained.[61] Satisfactory results in preventing cardiac damage from athrocydines have been obtained with the simultaneous administration of dexrazoxane.[62] However, the beneficial effects of that drug have been often used to increase the dosage of doxorubicin, thus increasing its antineoplastic effects but maintaining comparable levels of cardiac toxicity.

Epirubicin

Epirubicin is a parent compound to doxorubicin. As with other anthracyclines, such as daunorubicin, idarubicin, and mitoxantrone, the hope of lower cardiac toxicity has not been supported by clinical evidence.[63]

Actinomycin D

Actinomycin D is an effective treatment for Wilms' tumors, choriocarcinoma, neuroblastoma, and rhabdomyosarcoma; it is also effective in the combination chemotherapy of Ewing's sarcoma. Actinomycin D is defined as a "radiomimetic agent" because its modality of action is similar to that of ionizing radiation. When administered after radiation therapy, actinomycin D may reactivate or aggravate radiation-induced side effects, such as skin erythema, vascular necrosis, and radiation pneumonitis. A similar recall effect has also been described after therapy with other antineoplastic agents.[64] Severe nausea and vomiting, cardiac toxicity, and bone marrow suppression also occur. Veno-occlusive disease of the liver has also been reported. Supportive therapy is required to prevent lethal respiratory or renal failure.[65]

Streptozotocin

Streptozotocin is used in the treatment of malignant pancreatic islet cell tumors. It has a beneficial effect on hypoglycemia and, experimentally, in colonic adenocarcinoma. Its most serious toxicity is renal failure, which can be irreversible.[66]

Mithramycin

Mithramycin is used to treat patients with metastatic testicular tumors other than seminoma. Toxic side effects include hemorrhage, hepatic toxicity, renal damage, hypocalcemia, stomatitis, and fever.

Mitomycin C

Mitomycin C has proved to be moderately effective against gastric and colon carcinomas. Major toxicities include nausea, diarrhea, and delayed bone marrow suppression. The drug is also commonly used as an adjuvant treatment, before surgery, in patients with adenocarcinoma of the lung. In some cases, however, severe respiratory failure has developed postoperatively, with diffuse alveolar infiltrates, extreme hypoxemia, and an often rapidly lethal progress despite aggressive life support.[67, 68] Endothelial injury leading to hemolytic uremic syndrome has also been reported.[69]

Bleomycin

Bleomycin is effective against solid tumors of the head and neck, lymphomas, and epidermoid tumors of the esophagus. It is exceptionally beneficial for the treatment of dysgerminomas when it is infused in high doses and in combination with other chemotherapeutic agents. The most common complication of bleomycin therapy is acute interstitial pneumonitis, which is usually associated with cumulative doses greater than 350 mg/m^2;[70] however, severe respiratory failure has been reported after doses as low as 100 mg/m^2.

The histopathology is characterized by alveolar and interstitial infiltrates, which are more prominent at the bases.[71] Fibrotic nodules have also been reported.[72] Diffusion abnormalities and restrictive lung disease persist 4 to 9 months after cessation of treatment. Although pulmonary function test results usually return to normal within 12 months of therapy, the lungs remain abnormally susceptible to nonspecific noxious agents, such as high levels of inspired oxygen and fluid overload.[73, 74] No increase in toxicity has been observed by simultaneous administration of G-CSF.[75]

In patients with hypersensitivity to bleomycin, a single dose may cause severe exfoliative dermatitis, which occasionally results in sloughing of large areas of skin. In immunosuppressed patients, the consequences of this complication are obvious, and treatment follows all the dictates for management of massive second-degree and third-degree body burns.

Taxanes

Considerable enthusiasm has greeted the introduction of a new class of antineoplastic agent, the taxanes. These substances are the most promising representatives of antimicrotubular chemotherapy, an approach that directly interferes with mitosis during cell division.[76] Paclitaxel (Taxol), the first taxane used in humans, was initially applied to the treatment of ovarian cancer; more recently, it has been used for metastatic breast cancer, non–small cell lung cancer, and dysgerminomas. Phase I trials are being proposed for other neoplasms as well. Taxanes may represent the major new drug category of the 1990s, as platinum compounds were in the 1980s and anthracyclines in the 1970s.

Initially, the use of paclitaxel was limited because the substance could be obtained only from the bark of the partially endangered California yew tree.[77] For several years now, however, a paclitaxel derivative, docetaxel (Taxotere), with a nearly identical antitumoral activity, has been obtained from the renewable needles of the American and European yew trees,[78] thus rapidly increasing the number of patients who can be treated with taxanes.

Taxane administration has not been associated with specific organ injury, even though patients have complained of many problems, such as neurologic deficits and typhlitis.[79] The main complication associated with taxanes has been severe bone marrow suppression, which is usually the dose-limiting problem but can be controlled by simultaneous administration of G-CSF.[80–83] Some authors have reported severe postoperative bronchopulmonary complications in patients who have received paclitaxel or docetaxel for lung cancer, alone or in combination with other drugs or radiation therapy, as adjuvant preoperative treatment. Although the evidence is still anecdotal, the evolution of respiratory failure in affected patients is dramatic and often rapidly lethal, resembling the injury observed after mitomycin or bleomycin (Figs. 162–8 to 162–10).[84] Some complications may also be related to the solvent medium, ricinic acid; early phase I trials were occasionally suspended until treatment for hypersensitivity to ricinic acid was added.[85]

Tamoxifen

Tamoxifen has been used for many years in the treatment of metastatic breast cancer. Renewed interest has developed because of a large, prospective study that is attempting to determine its efficacy in the prophylaxis of breast cancer in high-risk individuals. Even though no life-threatening complications have been reported after tamoxifen administration, its proposed administration to healthy individuals requires especially close monitoring for unexpected complications.[86]

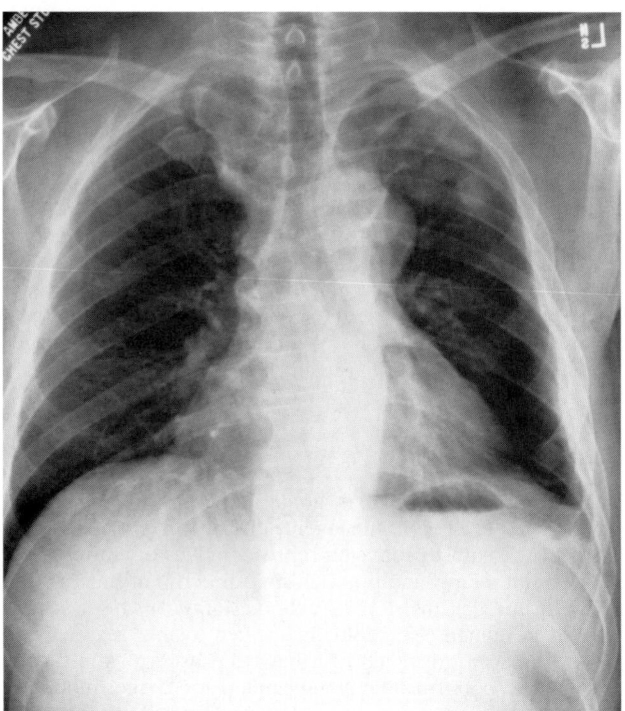

Figure 162–8. Chest radiogram of a patient who had received docetaxel (Taxotere) and mitomycin C in preparation for a pneumonectomy for mesothelioma. There are no obvious parenchymal abnormalities, and the preoperative pulmonary function tests were within normal limits.

Miscellaneous Agents

Nitrosoureas

The nitrosoureas carmustine, lomustine (chloroethyl-cyclohexyl-nitrosourea [CCNU]), and methyl-CCNU probably act as alkylating agents. They are among the few substances that have activity against brain tumors because they are lipid soluble and can cross the blood-brain barrier. CCNU is effective in the treatment of lymphomas, and carmustine is effective in lymphomas, multiple myeloma, and oat cell carcinoma. Methyl-CCNU is being investigated as a treatment for gastrointestinal carcinomas. Nitrosoureas induce severe myelotoxicity, which is the dose-limiting factor. Myelosuppression is prolonged (4 to 5 weeks) and is potentiated by repeated doses. Hepatotoxicity and pulmonary hypersensitivity have been reported.

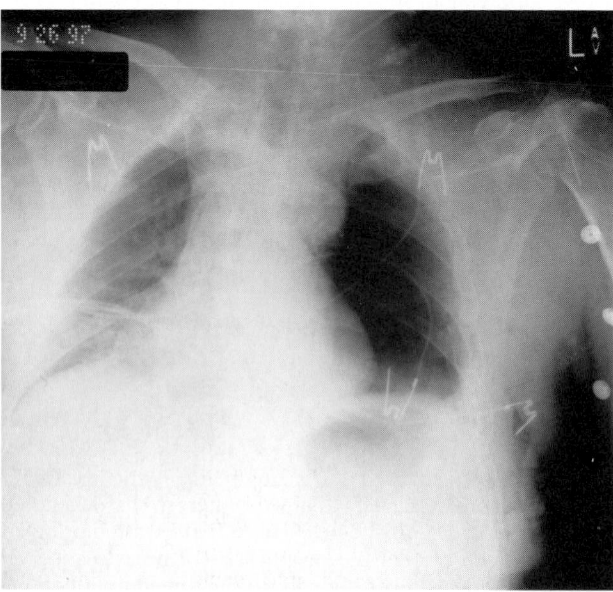

Figure 162–9. Chest radiogram of the same patient 24 hours after surgery. Alveolar infiltrates are noted at the right base. Arterial blood gas determinations showed moderately severe hypoxemia.

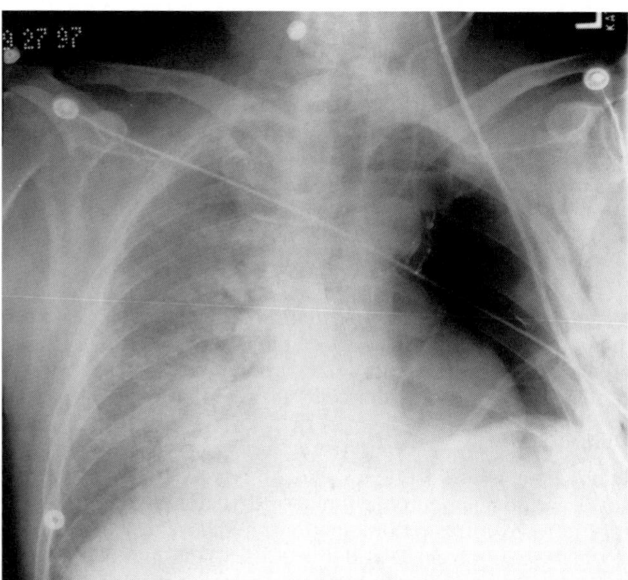

Figure 162–10. Chest radiogram of the same patient 48 hours after surgery. Extensive alveolar infiltrates occupy the entire right lung. Arterial blood gas measurements showed severe hypoxemia despite aggressive diuresis and tracheobronchial toilette. The patient required intubation and mechanical ventilation and died after 20 days of support.

Cisplatin

Another agent, *cis*-diamminedichloroplatinum (formerly, *cis*-platinum) is an effective treatment for testicular, ovarian, bladder, and head and neck cancers and for soft-tissue sarcomas and lymphomas.[87] Synergy between cisplatin and other agents, particularly doxorubicin (Adriamycin), has been shown experimentally. This drug is nephrotoxic and invariably causes some deterioration of renal function. Failure to maintain high urinary flow (>2 mL/kg/hr) for 24 to 48 hours after administration of cisplatin results in a high incidence of acute tubular necrosis that is often irreversible. Isolated reports have been published of cardiac failure and seizures following cisplatin administration.[88] New platinum compounds, such as carboplatinum, have been associated with fewer renal and neurologic side effects.

Procarbazine

Procarbazine, an oral agent, is used to treat lymphomas, brain tumors, melanoma, and oat cell carcinoma. Toxicities include nausea, vomiting, bone marrow suppression, and skin rash.

L-Asparaginase

L-Asparaginase is useful only in the treatment of acute lymphoblastic leukemia. It can cause severe but reversible depression of albumin synthesis,[89] central nervous system abnormalities, anorexia, nausea, vomiting, and pancreatitis. Anaphylactic reactions, sometimes extremely severe, occur in 5% to 20% of patients.

DTIC

Dimethyl triazeno imidazole carboxamide is used intravenously in the treatment of malignant melanoma, but antineoplastic activity has also been observed in lymphomas, sarcomas, and oat cell carcinoma. Its side effects include nausea, vomiting, delayed myelosuppression, and a flu-like syndrome.

Interferon

Human lymphocytic interferon, which has been synthesized by human cells for protection from viral infections, has become the subject of intensive clinical studies in the past few years. Previously available only in minute quantities, interferon can now be obtained from the microorganism *Escherichia coli* by recombinant deoxyribonucleic acid (DNA) techniques.[90] Interest in interferon is based on the theory that some malignancies may be induced by virally mediated changes in cellular nucleic acids. Patients treated with interferon may require ICU admission because of complications of their underlying disease. Serious side effects of interferon administration include hypotension, weakness, bone marrow suppression, and hyperthermia.[91] Supportive therapy and discontinuation of treatment are often required to reverse the symptoms.

Gemcitabine

Gemcitabine (2′,2′-difluorodeoxycitidine), alone or in combination with other agents, has been found effective against a variety of solid tumors, especially non–small cell lung cancers.[92, 93] There have been reports, however, of severe lung toxicity, similar to that observed after administration of mitomycin C. Treatment is supportive, with fluid restriction, increased FIO_2, and mechanical ventilation when necessary.[94] Steroids have been empirically used, with no convincing clinical evidence that they improve the course of the lung injury.

ATRA

all-*trans*-retinoic acid (ATRA) is used in the treatment of acute promyelocytic leukemia.[95] It causes severe bone marrow suppression and has been associated with other severe end-organ damage, including renal, hepatic, cardiac, and respiratory failure. Indeed, the complications of ATRA administration can be summarized in the *retinoic acid syndrome,* which consist of fever, dyspnea, weight gain, and pulmonary, pleural, and cardiac effusions. Other findings occasionally described are lower extremity edema.[96, 97] Steroids and, more recently, α-tocopherol have been used to limit toxicity.[98]

Antiangiogenic Agents

The observation that angiogenesis plays an important role in the progression of many metastatic lesions has led to the development of substances that specifically inhibit the growth of new capillaries. Treatment with angiogenic agents is still experimental and has been used in the management of neuroblastoma. No specific adverse effects have been reported thus far.[99]

Amifostine

Amifostine is a substance with the generic ability to act as a scavenger of free radicals. It has been proposed as an antidote to cell damage caused by a variety of antineoplastic drugs, including alkylating agents, platinum compounds, and vinca alkaloids.[100, 101] Its clinical use has been associated with reduced complications, but its potential to interfere with the efficacy of chemotherapy requires further investigation.

Cytokines

Because cancer represents uncontrolled cellular development, some research has focused on the utilization of substances that interfere with cellular growth and multiplication. Furthermore, destruction of cancerous and other abnormal cells is a task usually accomplished by T lymphocytes. Therapeutic opportunities may exist through the improvement of the ability of lymphocytes to attack cancer cells.

Tumor necrosis factor (TNF) is probably generated by activated macrophages[102] and can now be produced in large quantities by recombinant DNA methodology. In human applications, TNF has caused serious febrile reactions[103] and severe metabolic acidosis, at times lethal. Despite these adverse effects, TNF has shown some antineoplastic activity in various solid tumors, thus opening a new avenue in antineoplastic research therapy. Patients receiving TNF may require admission to the ICU for treatment of consequent hypotension and renal failure.

Adoptive Immunotherapy

Interleukin and *lymphokine-activated killer cells* are used alone or, more often, in combination in the treatment of aggressive malignancies, including hepatomas and melanomas. Severe sequelae, ranging from renal failure to cardiovascular collapse and respiratory failure, have been reported and may precipitate admission to the ICU.[104–106]

Recent research has demonstrated the involvement of *cytokines* in the pathogenesis of septic shock; these findings may explain the similarity of symptoms observed after exogenous administration of these drugs for antitumoral purposes with the classic manifestation of septic shock.[107] This modality of cancer treatment is promising because it is based on the enhancement of natural defenses against cancer; however, caution is needed until all potential side effects have been identified.

Clinical Drug Trials

The most common chemotherapeutic agents, their indications, and the major complications associated with their administration have been described. New agents are continuously being developed, and their introduction into clinical use follows a precise methodology that is designed to acquire extensive clinical information while minimizing potential complications. Three phases can be identified in the development process.

Phase I Drugs

Experimental chemotherapeutic agents that have proved effective in animal models are introduced through a phase I trial. A drug is administered at predetermined doses to patients who have not responded to all other forms of therapy, regardless of the underlying disease. The dangers of taking these agents are substantial:

1. Organ damage in human beings may be more severe than in experimental animals.
2. Systems and organs not affected in animals may be injured in humans.
3. Unpredictable reactions may develop at any time.

In most institutions, patients who receive phase I drugs are not considered candidates for admission to the ICU. A delicate ethical problem develops when a patient whose disease had been considered irreversible exhibits a positive response to a phase I drug and subsequently develops life-threatening complications as a consequence of the therapy administered. Refusing advanced life support may result in iatrogenic death while the underlying disease is improving. The balance between allocation of scarce ICU resources, patient rights, and potential benefits originating from better understanding of the therapy should be assessed on an individual basis. Inflexible restrictive rules should be avoided.

Phase II Drugs

Phase II drugs are agents that have proved effective in phase I studies. During phase II trials, drugs are tested in specific types of malignancy, and their efficacy is quantitatively determined.

A major risk for patients receiving a phase II drug is toxicity that occurs as doses are carefully escalated. Unexpected complications can arise during phase II trials, as evidenced by events that followed trials of two agents that have since been withdrawn because of unacceptable side effects. Succinylated *Acinetobacter* glutaminase asparaginase, a metabolic inhibitor similar to L-asparaginase, had demonstrated antineoplastic activity in acute leukemia. In humans, however, treatment with high doses resulted in severe metabolic acidosis secondary to lactate accumulation. Coma, possibly caused by inhibition of glutamic acid synthesis or generation of false neurotransmitters, also developed. Although both conditions were reversible with appropriate therapy (respiratory support, hydration, and bicarbonate administration), the benefits did not justify the risks of side effects, and the use of the drug was abandoned.

2,3′-Deoxycoformycin was also introduced for the treatment of acute leukemias. Unexpected toxic effects included severe renal and respiratory failure that required hemodialysis and mechanical ventilation. The pulmonary complications suggested hypersensitivity pneumonitis and resolved within 48 hours with high-dose steroid therapy.[108] None of the complications observed with high doses of these two agents had been anticipated from the results of animal experiments and phase I trials.

Treatment with phase II drugs presents the same ethical problems as treatment with phase I drugs. Allocation of an ICU bed must be evaluated in each individual case.

Phase III Drugs

Substances that have successfully completed a phase II trial are compared with standard therapy for efficacy. Unexpected complications are uncommon at this stage, and patients enrolled in phase III trials should be considered for admission to ICUs.

Combination Chemotherapy

Whereas single-agent chemotherapy was the common treatment modality during the early phases of drug management of neoplasms, current protocols are based on the use of multiple agents in combination, each with a different mechanism of action and toxicity. Neoplasms in which combination chemotherapy has proved successful include Hodgkin's disease, diffuse non-Hodgkin's lymphomas, acute leukemias, and disseminated testicular and breast tumors.

When such protocols are designed, the following criteria apply:

1. Each drug should have some antitumoral activity when used alone.
2. Each drug should have a different mechanism of action.
3. Toxic effects should not be additive, so that each drug may be used at full dose.

Despite these precautions, however, more serious complications may still develop when multiple drugs are administered simultaneously. Patients receiving aggressive combination therapy are therefore more likely to require admission to an ICU than patients receiving single agents. In some centers, oncology wards include intermediate care units, where intensive nursing care can be provided.

Adjuvant Chemotherapy

Solid tumors that have been successfully resected are the subject of prospective trials to determine whether chemotherapy agents, used alone or in combination, are effective in preventing local or systemic recurrence. This concept is known as *adjuvant therapy,* but results to date are not as encouraging as it had been hoped. Toxicity is related to the dosage schedule and the agents used.

RADIATION THERAPY

Radiation therapy alone can be curative for stage I Hodgkin's disease or early breast cancer. More commonly, it is used in association with surgery, chemotherapy, or both to achieve local or regional control. Radiation therapy is also useful for the symptomatic relief of metastatic bone diseases, multiple brain metastases, and spinal cord compression.

Factors such as bulk, site, growth rate, and vascularity determine the responsiveness of a tumor to ionizing radiation. The sensitivity of adjacent tissues to high-energy particles is often the limiting factor in treatment. In recent years, the availability of computerized techniques to define the field of radiation and of more accurate methods to deliver the ionizing particles has increased the effective dose that can be safely administered and has greatly reduced the incidence of complications.

The diseases in which radiation therapy can offer definitive cure, prolongation of life, or worthwhile palliation are many, but potentially dangerous side effects must always be considered because all tissues, particularly those with higher cell turnover rates, are subject to injury. Radiation damage is characterized histologically by diffuse microvascular thrombosis with necrosis of surrounding tissues, thereby explaining such diverse complications of radiation therapy as myocardial infarction, renal failure, skin necrosis, and injury to major vessels, such as the thoracic and abdominal aorta.[109]

Critical care physicians should be familiar with the extraordinary range of morbid changes associated with radiation therapy because complications may develop into life-threatening circumstances that require ICU admission. *Radiation pneumonitis* is probably the most common adverse effect of ionizing radiation that may require ICU support. Developing 3 to 6 months after treatment, it may lead to acute respiratory failure or to permanent functional limitation from interstitial fibrosis.

Injuries to other organs may also occur, precipitating frustrating problems of management that fortunately are rarely life-threatening. The gastrointestinal tract is highly susceptible to radiation injury. Severe malabsorption and diarrhea, with marked derangement of fluid and electrolyte balance, may follow a course of radiation therapy. Although the process is usually self-limiting and reversible, it may progress for weeks and months after termination of therapy. In a few extreme cases, patients otherwise cured become permanently unable to tolerate enteral feedings and must be supplemented by total parenteral nutrition. The most catastrophic complications pertain to obstruction, bleeding, enteric fistulas, or perforation, which often require emergency surgery.

Some antineoplastic agents (cyclophosphamide, methotrexate, doxorubicin, actinomycin D, bleomycin, carmustine) may cause a *recall phenomenon* when given to a patient who has been exposed to radiation; injury, sometimes severe, develops in organs irradiated months and even years earlier.[110, 111] Damage during the initial course of therapy is often not apparent at the time of treatment.

The CNS and the peripheral nervous system are not immune from radiation damage. These tissues have a rich capillary network and are extremely susceptible to oxygen deprivation.

Brain necrosis, transverse necrotizing myelitis, paraplegia, and tetraplegia have been associated with radiation therapy.

Steroid administration can limit most adverse side effects of radiation therapy. Although radiation pneumonitis can be entirely eliminated by simultaneously administered steroid treatment,[112] a recall phenomenon almost invariably occurs once steroids are withdrawn. The pneumonic process is then as severe or more severe than if steroids had never been given. Resumption of steroids is the only option and often must be continued for life. At present, a consensus advises against the prophylactic use of steroids.[113]

HYPERTHERMIA

There is experimental and, to a lesser degree, clinical evidence that elevated body temperature is more damaging to cancerous than normal tissues. This susceptibility has been identified for the cells of many solid tumors and systemic malignancies. Therapeutic exploitation of this selective sensitivity has been the subject of recent laboratory investigations and some cautiously enthusiastic clinical trial results. After the insertion of an arteriovenous shunt, blood is circulated through an extracorporeal heat exchanger, and body temperature is raised to 41.5° to 42°C for 2 to 4 hours. Life-threatening complications may develop quite rapidly at these temperatures, and close observation is mandatory. Admission to an ICU or another comparable location may be advisable prior to treatment.

The response of major organ systems to controlled hyperthermia has been carefully investigated. Pulmonary artery catheterization and thermodilution cardiac output measurements have indicated that cardiac compromise is uncommon, even in patients with a history of heart disease.[114] Minor arrhythmias have been reported and are attributed to the significant electrolyte imbalance that may occur with hyperthermia. Hypokalemia can be severe and is sustained by the hyperventilation and respiratory alkalosis that are induced by elevated temperature and increased potassium loss through the urine.

Hemolysis has not been detected, but coagulation abnormalities, including increased prothrombin time, partial thromboplastin time, and decreased platelet count, are commonly reported. Measurement of fibrin degradation products indicates a modest but continuous process of DIC. Patients with extensive metastatic liver disease are reported to have a high incidence of serious complications from hyperthermia. Acute myelopathy and irreversible demyelinization have developed, resulting in limb paralysis.[115] Cellular phagocytosis is decreased when temperature exceeds 41.5°C, and patients become more susceptible to bacterial infections.

For most patients under the care of experienced clinicians and with very close monitoring, hyperthermia is a safe, although experimental, form of therapy. Despite several years of applications, however, indications for hyperthermia have not been expanded. The role of this form of therapy may remain limited,[116, 117] even though clinical investigations are continuing.[118, 119]

References

1. Kimmick GG, Fleming R, Muss HB, Balducci L: Cancer chemotherapy in older adults: A tolerability perspective. Drugs Aging 1997; 10:34.
2. Davies HA, Wales JK: The effects of chemotherapy on the long-term survivors of malignancy. Br J Hosp Med 1997; 57:215.
3. Dekker AW, Rozenberg-Arska M, Sixma JJ, et al: Prevention of infection by trimethoprim-sulfamethoxazole plus amphotericin B in patients with acute nonlymphocytic leukemia. Ann Intern Med 1981; 95:555.
4. Aparicio J, Oltra A, Llorca C, Montalar J, Herranz C, Gomez-Codina J, Pastor M, Munarriz B: Randomized comparison of ceftazidime and imipenem as initial monotherapy for febrile episodes in neutropenic cancer patients. Eur J Cancer 1996; 32A:1739.
5. Wacker P, Halperin DS, Wyss M, Humbert J: Early hospital discharge of children with fever and neutropenia: A prospective study. J Pediatr Hematol Oncol 1997; 19:208.
6. Gilbert C, Meisenberg B, Vredenburgh J, Ross M, Hussein A, Perfect J, Peters WP: Sequential prophylactic oral and empiric once-daily parenteral antibiotics for neutropenia and fever after high-dose chemotherapy and autologous bone marrow support. J Clin Oncol 1994; 12:1005.
7. Hidalgo M, Hornedo J, Lumbreras C, Trigo JM, Gomez C, Perea S, Ruiz A, Hitt R, Cortes-Fumes H: Lack of ability of ciprofloxacin-rifampin prophylaxis to decrease infection-related morbidity in neutropenic patients given cytoxic therapy and peripheral blood stem cell transplants. Antimicrob Agents Chemother 1997; 41:1175.
8. Ehninger G, Schuler HK, Sarnow E: Fluconazole in the prophylaxis of fungal infection after bone marrow transplantation. Mycoses 1996; 39:259.
9. Minguez Minguez F, Lima JE, Garcia MT, Prieto J: Effects of antifungal pretreatment on the susceptibility of *Candida albicans* to human leukocytes. Chemotherapy 1997; 43:346.
10. Maschmeyer G, Hiddermann W, Link H, Cornely OA, Buchheidt D, Glass B, Adam D: Management of infections during intensive treatment of hematologic malignancies. Ann Hematol 1997; 75:9.
11. Bohme A, Hoelzer D: Liposomal amphotericin B as early empiric antimycotic therapy of pneumonia in granulocytopenic patients. Mycoses 1996; 39:419.
12. Tollemar J, Ringden O, Andersson S, et al: Prophylactic use of liposomal, amphotericin B (AmBisome) against fungal infections: A randomized trial in bone marrow transplant recipients. Transplant Proc 1993; 25:1495.
13. Nolte FS, Parkinson T, Falconer DJ, Dix S, Williams J, Gilmore C, Geller R, Wingard JR: Isolation and characterization of fluconazole- and amphotericin B–resistant *Candida albicans* from blood of two patients with leukemia. Antimicrob Agents Chemother 1997; 41:196.
14. Warren E, George S, You J, Kazanjian P: Advances in the treatment and prophylaxis of *Pneumocystis carinii* pneumonia. Pharmacotherapy 1997; 17:900.
15. Engervall P, Kalin M, Bjorkholm M: Disseminated tuberculosis treated with amikacin in a patient with acute myelocytic leukemia. Acta Oncol 1997; 36:444.
16. Brettle RP: *Mycobacterium avium intracellulare* infection in patients with HIV or AIDS. J Antimicrob Chemother 1997; 40:156.
17. Emmanoulides C, Glaspy J: Opportunistic infections in oncologic patients. Hematol Oncol Clin North Am 1996; 10:841.
18. de Lalla F: Antibiotic treatment of febrile episodes in neutropenic cancer patients: Clinical and economic considerations. Drugs 1997; 53:789.
19. Aviles A, Guzman R, Garcia EL, Talavera A, Diaz-Maqueo JC: Results of a randomized trial of granulocyte colony-stimulating factor in patients with infection and severe granulocytopenia. Anticancer Drugs 1996; 7:392.
20. Vost J, Longstaff V: Infection control and related issues in intravascular therapy. Br J Nurs 1997; 6:846.
21. LaQuaglia MP, Lucas A, Thaler HT, et al: A prospective analysis of vascular access device-related infections in children. J Pediatr Surg 1992; 27:840.
22. Groeger JS, Lucas AB, Coit D, et al: A prospective randomized evaluation of the effect of silver impregnated subcutaneous cuffs for preventing tunneled chronic venous access catheter infections in cancer patients. Ann Surg 1993; 218:206.
23. Cook D, Randolph A, Kernerman P, Cupido C, King D, Soukup C, Brun-Buisson C: Central venous catheter replacement strategies: A systematic review of the literature. Crit Care Med 1997; 25:1417.
24. Taber SW, Bergamini TM: Long-term venous access: Indications and choice of site and catheter. Semin Vasc Surg 1997; 10:130.
25. Hoch Jr: Management of the complications of long-term venous access. Semin Vasc Surg 1997; 10:135.

26. Raad II, Fraschini G: Intravascular device–related infections in cancer patients. Cancer Treat Res 1995; 79:211.
27. Bodey GP: Pulmonary infiltrates in acute leukemias. Chest 1979; 75:298.
28. Prakash UB, Divertie MB, Banks PM: Aggressive therapy in acute respiratory failure from pulmonary infiltrates. Chest 1979; 73:345.
29. Carlon GC, Howland WS, Ray C, et al: High frequency jet ventilation: A prospective randomized evaluation. Chest 1983; 84:551.
30. Cunningham AJ: Acute respiratory distress syndrome: Two decades later. Yale J Biol Med 1991; 64:387.
31. Snow RM, Miller WC, Rice DL, et al: Respiratory failure in cancer patients. JAMA 1979; 241:2039.
32. Rosenthal RL: Acute promyelocytic leukemia associated with hypofibrinogenemia. Blood 1963; 21:495.
33. Carlon GC, Scheiner E, Colaco FM, et al: Nephrotoxic antibiotics in patients with renal failure: Guidelines for debilitated patients. Crit Care Med 1979; 7:1.
34. Perez CA, Present CA, Van Amburg AL III, et al: Management of superior vena cava syndrome. Semin Oncol 1978; 5:123.
35. Martinez-Maldonado M, Yium DM, Suki WM, et al: Renal complications of multiple myeloma: Pathophysiology and some aspects of clinical management. J Chronic Dis 1971; 24:221.
36. Suki WM, Yium JJ, Von Minden M, et al: Acute treatment of hypercalcemia with furosemide. N Engl J Med 1970; 282:839.
37. Vaughn CB, Vaitkevicius VK: The effects of calcitonin in hypercalcemia in patients with malignancy. Cancer 1974; 34:1268.
38. Godfrey TE: Mithramycin for hypercalcemia of malignant disease. Calif Med 1971; 115:1.
39. Burckhardt P, Thiebaud D, Perey L, et al: Treatment of tumor-induced osteolysis by APD: Recent results. Cancer Res 1989; 116:54.
40. Theiault RL: Management of hypercalcemia in breast cancer. Oncology 1990; 4:43.
41. Clemens MR, Fessele K, Heim ME: Multiple myeloma: Effect of daily dichloromethylene biphosphate on skeletal complications. Ann Hematol 1993; 66:141.
42. Posner JB: Neurologic complications of systemic cancer. Med Clin North Am 1971; 55:265.
43. Joyner LR, Maran PG, Sarama R, et al: Neodymium-YAG laser treatment of intrabronchial lesions. Chest 1985; 87:418.
44. Fortner JC, McLean B, Kim DK, et al: The seventies evolution in liver surgery for cancer. Cancer 1981; 47:2162.
45. Hankins DG, Sander S, MacDonald FM, et al: Pulmonary toxicity recurring after a six week course of busulfan therapy and after subsequent therapy with uracil mustard. Chest 1978; 73:415.
46. Friedman MA, Carter JB: Serious toxicities associated with chemotherapy. Semin Oncol 1978; 5:193.
47. Carlon GC, Kahn RC, Howland WS, et al: Clinical experience with high frequency jet ventilation. Crit Care Med 1981; 9:1.
48. Pierri MK: Heart disease and cancer. *In:* Critical Care of the Cancer Patient. Howland WS, Carlon GC (Eds). Chicago, Year Book Medical Publishers, 1985, pp 61–85.
49. Chabner BA, Myers CE, Olivero VT: Clinical pharmacology of anticancer drugs. Semin Oncol 1978; 4:165.
50. Rosenow EC III: The spectrum of drug-induced pulmonary disease. Ann Intern Med 1972; 77:977.
51. Salaffi F, Manganelli P, Carotti M, Subiaco S, Lamanna G, Cervini C: Methotrexate-induced pneumonitis in patients with rheumatoid arthritis and psoriatic arthritis: Report of five cases and review of the literature. Clin Rheumatol 1997; 16:296.
52. Gottlieb RJ, Cottner J: Vincristine induced bladder atony. Cancer 1971; 28:674.
53. Mencoboni M, Lerza R, Castello G, Arboscello E, Barsotti BP, Cerruti A, Ballarino P, Botta M, Bogliolo G, Pannacciulli I: Feasibility and toxicity of combination chemotherapy with ifosfamide, vinorelbine, cisplat versus ifosfamide, vinorelbine in patients with advanced non small cell lung cancer. Anticancer Res 1997; 17:2795.
54. Raderer M, Kornek G, Hejna M, Vorbeck F, Weinlaender G, Scheithauer W: Acute pulmonary toxicity with high-dose vinorelbine and mitomycin C. Ann Oncol 1996; 7:973.
55. Cay O, Kruskal JB, Nasser I, Thomas P, Clouse ME: Liver metastases from colorectal cancer: Drug delivery with liposome-encapsulated doxorubicin. Radiology 1997; 205:95.
56. Bristow MR, Mason JW, Billingham ME, et al: Doxorubicin cardiomyopathy evaluation by phonocardiography, endomyocardial biopsy and cardiac catheterization. Ann Intern Med 1978; 88:168.
57. Pihkala J, Saarinen UM, Lundstrom U, Virtanen K, Virkola K, Siimes MA, Pesonen E: Myocardial function in children and adolescents after therapy with anthracyclines and chest irradiation. Eur J Cancer 1996; 32A:97.
58. Leier CV: Current status of non-digitalis positive inotropic drugs. Am J Cardiol 1992; 69:120G.
59. Barnett DB: Flosequinan. Lancet 1993; 341:733.
60. Noble J, Farrer M, McComb JM: Flosequinan and arrhythmogenesis. Lancet 1993; 341:1100.
61. Swedberg K: Reduction in mortality by pharmacological therapy in congestive heart failure. Circulation 1993; 87:IV126.
62. Hellmann K: Cardioprotection by dexrazoxane (Cardioxane; ICRF 187): Progress in supportive care. Support Care Cancer 1996; 4:305.
63. Luck HJ, Du Bois A, Thomssen C, Lisboa B, Untch M, Kohler G, Hecker D: Paclitaxel and epirubicin as first-line therapy for patients with metastatic breast cancer. Oncology (Huntingt) 1997; 11 (4 Suppl 3):34.
64. Einhorn L, Krause M, Horseback N, et al: Enhanced pulmonary toxicity with bleomycin and radiotherapy in oat cell lung cancer. Cancer 1976; 37:2414.
65. Kullendorff CM, Bekassy AN: Hepatic veno-occlusive disease in Wilms' tumor. Eur J Pediatr Surg 1996; 6:338.
66. Moertel CG, Reitmier RJ, Schutt AJ, et al: Phase II study of streptozotocin (NSC-85998) in the treatment of advanced gastrointestinal cancer. Chemotherapy Rep 1971; 55:303.
67. Okuno SH, Frytak S: Mitomycin lung toxicity: Acute and chronic phases. Am J Clin Oncol 1997; 20:282.
68. Castro M, Veeder MH, Malliard JA, Tazelaar HD, Jett JR: A prospective study of pulmonary function in patients receiving mitomycin. Chest 1996; 109:939.
69. Groff JA, Kozak M, Boehmer JP, Demko TM, Diamond JR: Endotheliopathy: A continuum of hemolytic uremic syndrome due to mitomycin therapy. Am J Kidney Dis 1997; 29:280.
70. Luna MA, Bedrossian CWM, Lichtiger B, et al: Interstitial pneumonitis associated with bleomycin therapy. Am J Clin Pathol 1972; 58:501.
71. Bernet JM, Reich JD: Bleomycin. Ann Intern Med 1979; 90:945.
72. Ben Arush MW, Roguin A, Zamir E, el-Hassid R, Pries D, Gaitini D, Dale A, Postovsky S: Bleomycin and cyclophosphamide toxicity simulating metastatic nodules to the lungs in childhood cancer. Pediatr Hematol Oncol 1997; 14:381.
73. Goldiner PL, Carlon GC, Cvitkovic E, et al: Factors influencing morbidity and mortality in patients treated with bleomycin. Br Med J 1978; 1:1664.
74. Gilson AJ, Sahn SA: Reactivation of bleomycin lung toxicity following oxygen administration. Chest 1985; 88:304.
75. Saxman SB, Nichols CR, Einhorn LH: Pulmonary toxicity in patients with advanced-stage germ cell tumors receiving bleomycin with and without granulocyte colony stimulating factor. Chest 1997; 111:657.
76. Rowinsky EK, Onetto N, Canetta RM, et al: Taxol: The first of the taxanes, an important new class of antitumor agents. Semin Oncol 1992; 19:646.
77. Runowicz CD, Wiernik PH, Einzig AI, et al: Taxol in ovarian cancer. Cancer 1993; 71:1591.
78. Bissett D, Setanoians A, Cassidy J, et al: Phase 1 and pharmacokinetic study of taxotere (RP 56976) administered as a 24-hour infusion. Cancer Res 1993; 53:523.
79. Pestalozzi BC, Sotos GA, Choyke PL, et al: Typhlitis resulting from treatment with taxol and doxurubicin in patients with metastatic breast cancer. Cancer 1993; 71:1797.
80. Rosenthal DI, Okani O, Corak J, Kavanaugh D, Kamen B, Vuitch FM, Gazdar AF, Greiner J, Frenkel EF, Carbone DP: Seven-week continuous-infusion paclitaxel plus concurrent radiation therapy for locally advanced non–small cell lung cancer: A phase I study. Semin Oncol 1997; 24(Suppl):S12-96.
81. Mattson K, Saarimen A, Jekunen A: Combination treatment with docetaxel (Taxotere) and platinum compounds for non–small cell lung cancer. Semin Oncol 1997; 24(Suppl):S14-5.
82. Shapiro JD, Millward MJ, Rischin D, Davison JD, Michael M, Francis PA, Ganju V, Toner GC: Activity and toxicity of docetaxel

(Taxotere) in women with previously treated metastatic breast cancer. Aust N Z J Med 1997; 27:40.
83. Georgoulias V, Kourousis C, Androulakis N, Kakolyris S, Papadakis E, Bouros D, Apostolopoulou F, Georgopoulou T, Agelidou M, Souglakos J, Halkiadakis G, Hatzidaki D: Docetaxel (Taxotere) and vinorelbine in the treatment of non–small cell lung cancer. Semin Oncol 1997; 24(Suppl):S14-9.
84. Bonomi P, Faber LP, Warren W, Lincoln S, LaFollette S, Sharma M, Recine D: Postoperative bronchopulmonary complications in stage III lung cancer patients treated with preoperative paclitaxel-containing chemotherapy and concurrent radiation. Semin Oncol 1997; 24(4 Suppl 12):S12-123.
85. Chang AY, Kim K, Glick J, et al: Phase II study of Taxol, merbarone and piroxantrone in stage IV non–small-cell lung cancer: The Eastern Cooperative Oncology Group. J Natl Cancer Inst 1993; 85:388.
86. Rubens RD: Metastatic breast cancer and its complications. Curr Opin Oncol 1992; 4:1050.
87. Einhorn LH, William SD: The role of *cis*-platinum in solid tumor therapy. N Engl J Med 1979; 330:284.
88. Rosenzweig M, Von Hoff DD, Slavik M, et al: *Cis*-diamminedichloroplatinum. Ann Intern Med 1977; 86:803.
89. Haskell CM, Canellos GI, Loventhal BD, et al: L-Asparaginase toxicity. Cancer Res 1968; 24:74.
90. Sherwin SA, Mayer D, Ochs JJ, et al: Recombinant leukocyte A interferon in advanced breast cancer. Ann Intern Med 1983; 98:598.
91. Scott G, Secher DS, Flowers D, et al: Toxicity of interferon. Br Med J 1981; 282:1345.
92. van Moorsel CJ, Veerman G, Bergman AM, Guechev A, Vermorken JB, Postmus PE, Peters GJ: Combination chemotherapy studies with gemcitabine. Semin Oncol 1997; 24(2 Suppl 7):S7-17.
93. Cortes-Funes H, Martin C, Abratt R, Lund B: Safety profile of gemcitabine, a novel anticancer agent in non–small cell lung cancer. Anticancer Drugs 1997; 8:582.
94. Pavlakis N, Bell DR, Millward MJ, Levi JA: Fatal pulmonary toxicity resulting from treatment with gemcitabine. Cancer 1997; 80:286.
95. Mandelli F: New strategies for the treatment of acute promyelocytic leukemia. J Intern Med Suppl 1997; 740:23.
96. Cull GM, Eikelboom JW, Cannell PK: Exacerbation of coagulopathy with concurrent bone marrow necrosis, hepatic and renal dysfunction secondary to all-*trans* retinoic acid therapy for acute promyelocytic leukemia. Hematol Oncol 1997; 15:13.
97. Larrea L, de la Rubia J, Jimenez C, Martin G, Sanz MA: Cardiac tamponade and cardiogenic shock as a manifestation of all-*trans* retinoic acid syndrome: An association not previously reported. Haematologica 1997; 82:463.
98. Dimery IW, Hong WK, Lee JJ, Guillory-Perez C, Pham F, Fritsche HA Jr, Lippman SM: Phase I trial of alpha-tocopherol effects on 13-*cis*-retinoic acid toxicity. Ann Oncol 1997; 8:85.
99. Nagabuchi E, VanderKolk WE, Une Y, Ziegler NM: TNP-470 antiangiogenic therapy for advanced murine neuroblastoma. J Pediatr Surg 1997; 32:287.
100. Foster-Nora JA, Siden R: Amifostine for protection from antineoplastic drug toxicity. Am J Health Syst Pharm 1997; 54:787.
101. Tannehill SP, Mehta MP, Larson M, Storer B, Pellet J, Kinsella TJ, Schiller JH: Effect of amifostine on toxicities associated with sequential chemotherapy and radiation therapy for unresectable non–small-cell lung cancer: Results of a phase II trial. J Clin Oncol 1997; 15:2850.
102. Zacharchuck CM, Drysdale BE, Mayer MM, et al: Macrophage-mediated cytotoxicity: Role of a soluble macrophage cytotoxic factor similar to lymphotoxin and tumor necrosis factor. Proc Natl Acad Sci USA 1983; 80:6341.
103. Khan A: Preclinical and phase I clinical trials with lymphotoxin. *In* Human Lymphokines. New York, Academic Press, 1982, pp 621-630.
104. Redman BG, Flaherty L, Martino S, et al: Effect of calcium replacement on the hemodynamic changes associated with high dose interleukin-2 therapy. Am J Clin Oncol 1992; 15:340.
105. Feinfeld DA, D'Agati V, Dutcher JP, et al: Interstitial nephritis in a patient receiving adoptive immunotherapy with recombinant interleukin-2 and lymphokine-activated killer cells. Am J Nephrol 1991; 11:489.
106. Farrell MM: The challenge of adult respiratory distress syndrome during interleukin-2 immunotherapy. Oncol Nurs Forum 1992; 19:475.
107. Giroir BP: Mediation of septic shock: New approaches for interrupting the endogenous inflammatory cascade. Crit Care Med 1993; 21:780.
108. Kahn RC, Carlon GC, Miller D, et al: Acute respiratory failure due to 2,3′-deoxycoformycin. Intensive Care Med 1982; 8:101.
109. Moreynolds RA, Gold GL, Roberts WC: Coronary heart disease after mediastinal irradiation for Hodgkin's disease. Am J Med 1976; 60:39.
110. Schreml W, Bargon G, Anger B, et al: Progrediente Lungfibrose unter Kombinationstherapie mit BCNU. Blut 1978; 36:353.
111. Lamoureux KB: Increased clinically symptomatic pulmonary radiation reactions with adjuvant chemotherapy. Cancer Chemother Res 1974; 58:705.
112. Casciari RJ, Berman JJ, Glauser FL: Acute febrile illness associated with bilateral pulmonary infiltrates after irradiation in a patient with Hodgkin's disease. South Med J 1977; 70:345.
113. Wara WM, Phillips TL, Margolis LW, et al: Radiation pneumonitis: A new approach to the derivation of time-dose factors. Cancer 1973; 32:547.
114. Bull JM, Lees D, Schuette W, et al: Whole body hyperthermia: A phase I trial of a potential adjuvant to chemotherapy. Ann Intern Med 1979; 90:317.
115. Douglas MA, Parks LC, Bebin J: Sudden myelopathy secondary to therapeutic total-body hyperthermia after spinal cord irradiation. Med Intell 1977; 304:583.
116. Yoshikawa T, Kokura S, Tainaka K, et al: The role of active oxygen species and lipid peroxidation in the antitumor effect of hyperthermia. Cancer Res 1993; 53:2326.
117. Ben-Yosef R, Kapp DS: Persistent and/or late complications of combined radiation therapy and hyperthermia. Int J Hyperthermia 1992; 8:733.
118. Feyerabend T, Steeves R, Wiedemann GJ, Richter E, Robins HI: Rationale and clinical status of local hyperthermia, radiation, and chemotherapy in locally advanced malignancies. Anticancer Res 1997; 17:2895.
119. Feyerabend T, Steeves R, Wiedemann GJ, Weiss C, Wagner T, Richter JL, Robins HI: Local hyperthermia, radiation, and chemotherapy in locally advanced malignancies. Oncology 1996; 53:214.

163

Surgical Problems in the Critically Ill Oncologic Patient

Robert J. Downey, MD
Joseph Espat, MD • F. Ida Hsu, BA

Surgical problems affecting patients with cancer are similar to those seen in the general population but also include conditions arising as a consequence of the neoplasm or anti-neoplastic therapies. Patients with malignancies who have received, or are receiving, cytotoxic agents exhibit increased susceptibility to complications, as well as decreased healing capability. As such, there should be as short a delay as possible between the (often minimal) presenting symptoms, evaluation, and subsequent interventions.

This chapter covers aspects of the surgical care of the patient with malignancy, including (1) thoracic conditions, such as pericardial tamponade, superior vena caval obstruction, airway obstruction, and hemoptysis; (2) abdominal conditions, such as abdominal pain in the neutropenic patient, and bowel obstruction, perforation, and hemorrhage in the patient with malignancy; (3) anesthetic implications of the cardiopulmonary effects of antineoplastic agents; and (4) management of possibly infected central venous catheters.

THORACIC EMERGENCIES

Superior Vena Caval Obstruction

Obstruction of the superior vena cava (SVC) may be the first presentation of lung carcinoma, metastatic disease to the chest, or mediastinal disease (e.g., lymphoma or thymoma). It may also occur in patients with previously diagnosed malignant disease or with benign disease such as sclerosing mediastinitis (often due to histoplasmosis) or caval thrombi associated with indwelling central venous access devices. Patients with caval obstruction usually exhibit swelling, cyanosis of the head, neck, upper chest, and one or both upper extremities. Edema of the conjunctiva, jugular venous distention, and visible distention of subcutaneous venous collaterals may be noted above the level of the obstruction. Depending on the location of the tumor mass, one may see an associated Horner's syndrome, recurrent nerve palsy, or airway obstruction.

Careful questioning of the patient may elicit nonspecific symptoms, such as pain, headache, cough, dysphagia, nausea, vomiting, drowsiness, and vertigo.[1] These symptoms may be more severe in the supine position and patients will often have begun sleeping on several pillows or even in a chair prior to being seen by a physician.

The clinical presentation is dramatic, and physicians often conclude that SVC obstruction is an oncologic emergency; however, it is usually not a life-threatening event unless there is coexisting airway compromise and respiratory failure[2] or unless it occurs in the neutropenic patient with a head and neck or upper extremity infection.

Once the diagnosis of SVC obstruction is suspected, confirmation can be obtained by radiologic, ultrasound, or nuclide techniques. Chest radiographs often suggest a superior or anterior mediastinal mass in patients with clinical SVC compression. SVC venography has been replaced by the thoracic computed tomogram (CT) with intravenous contrast administered from one or both arms. In addition to demonstrating diminished flow through the SVC and the presence of chest wall and mediastinal collaterals, CT often delineates mediastinal and hilar disease and may help in differentiating neoplasm from inflammatory conditions such as mediastinal fibrosis.

Duplex imaging of the upper extremities may demonstrate diminished flow; however, because it does not often suggest the etiology, it is not preferred to CT images. In the critically ill patient who cannot be transported, the diagnosis of caval obstruction may be confirmed if a short-lived isotope, such as technetium 99 phosphate, is injected into a peripheral vein prior to scanning of the thorax with a portable nuclear camera, or with bedside duplex imaging.

Therapeutic steps aimed at relieving symptoms include establishing venous access from a vein below the diaphragm, usually a saphenous or femoral vein line, for the administration of both fluids and medications. The patient's head and affected upper extremities should be elevated above 45° to favor hydrostatic drainage of venous blood. A diuresis should be effected in order to diminish venous pressures. Systemic heparinization is often instituted in order to prevent progression of obstruction or to diminish the risk of pulmonary emboli, but the degree to which these ends are achieved is not clear. Indwelling central venous lines at the site of occlusion are usually removed, as this seems to both speed the rate of resolution of the thrombus and to decrease the likelihood of recurrence. In some malignancies, high-dose corticosteroids may decrease edema and inflammation of the tumor and, similarly, may be of benefit during radiation therapy.

Therapeutic steps undertaken to relieve the extrinsic compression of the cava are based on knowledge of the malignant tissue type and relative sensitivity to radiation or chemotherapy. A careful search for evidence of extrathoracic disease should be undertaken with intent of biopsy, as this can probably done more safely than a procedure performed in the presence of engorged vessels of the mediastinum. If no extrathoracic disease can be found, tissue is obtained from the thorax, usually by fine-needle aspiration, bronchoscopy, supraclavicular node biopsy, Chamberlain procedure, or mediastinoscopy.

The mainstay of treatment for extrinsic malignant disease has been radiation therapy; more recently, angiographically placed intracaval stents have proved effective, although, in our experience, rarely necessary. Collateral flow usually appears to relieve the symptoms of obstruction after a while during which the measures just mentioned can be implemented to offer symptomatic relief.

Oropharyngeal and Tracheal Obstruction

Upper airway obstruction may result from:

1. Extrinsic invasion of the trachea, as seen with thyroid carcinoma.
2. Intrinsic lesions, such as bulky supraglottic, glottic, or oropharyngeal tumors.
3. External compression of the trachea, as by lymphoma.

Sudden upper airway obstruction is uncommon with cancer of the head and neck. Tumors of the larynx, pharynx, thyroid, and base of the tongue are usually slowly growing, and obvious symptoms of airway compromise are evident before an emergency situation develops. During a thorough head and neck examination, care should be taken to minimize trauma to large friable tumors because bleeding may lead to complete airway obstruction. Examination may reveal tachycardia, tachypnea, and, occasionally, a significant pulsus paradox. Obstruction due to a bulky oropharyngeal or thyroid carcinoma may be best managed by elective tracheostomy. If the obstruction is due to an external compression of the trachea by lymphoma or other tissue highly sensitive to radiation or chemotherapy, nasal or orotracheal intubation alone may be used to maintain airway patency in anticipation of a rapid reduction in tumor mass.[3]

Life-threatening intrathoracic airway obstruction occurs often with primary or secondary lung malignancies or with mediastinal tumors, such as Hodgkin's and non-Hodgkin's lymphoma. Intrathoracic airway obstruction should be suspected when a patient complains of dyspnea, wheezing, or chest discomfort. Chest examination may reveal a prolonged expiratory time and wheezing. Respiratory symptoms may occasionally be unilateral, and chest radiographs reveal asymmetric lung fields, particularly if end-inspiratory films are compared with end-expiratory images. For stable patients, a flow-volume loop should be performed, the characteristic finding being flattening of the expiratory loop. If bronchoscopy is necessary either as a diagnostic or a therapeutic step, we favor flexible bronchoscopy with the patient awake performed in the operating room; rigid bronchoscopy should be available, and an anesthesiologist should be present. Once the location and severity of the obstruction are clear, further steps, such as intubation above or beyond the obstruction, can be undertaken. If mechanical ventilation is employed, hemodynamic compromise due to asymmetric ventilation and air trapping may lead to significant increases in airway pressure distal to the obstruction, with secondary mediastinal shift with altered venous return to the heart, or to barotrauma-associated pneumothorax.

Therapy for intrathoracic airway obstruction is guided by the specific malignancy. *Lymphoma* may present with bulky mediastinal and hilar adenopathy, causing airway compression. As this tumor is extremely sensitive to radiation and chemotherapy and may regress rapidly regardless of initial size, every attempt to maintain ventilation in these patients is warranted. *Metastatic* and *primary tumors* of the lung may also present with intrathoracic obstruction.

Small-cell carcinoma of the lung often is associated with extensive mediastinal nodal disease. As such, the airway compression is due to extrinsic compression and even erosion into the tracheobronchial tree. Because small cell cancer responds well to radiation treatment, further steps are not usually undertaken.

For *non-small-cell carcinoma* of the lung and *metastatic disease* to the lung from a extrathoracic site, some combination of radiation (either external beam or endobronchial), chemotherapy, surgical resection, flexible or rigid bronchoscopy with mechanical debridement, laser ablation, or stent placement may be required. During the procedure, it is reasonable to obtain cultures of secretions distal to an obstruction to guide antibiotic therapy should a pneumonia become apparent later.

Prior to an attempt at surgical correction, a detailed discussion with the patient and family is mandatory. The talk should outline (1) the possibilities of an inability to extubate if intubation is required for the procedure; (2) intraoperative bleeding, which may lead to inability to ventilate in the operating room; (3) or development of pneumonia several days later. All decisions must be made with the knowledge that, for many malignancies leading to intrathoracic airway obstruction, the prognosis for long-term survival is poor.

Hemoptysis

Bleeding into the airway is an imminent threat to life, first, because of the risk of drowning, and second, because of the risk of subsequent pulmonary infection. A significant number of cases (probably a majority) are due to benign causes,[4] but the discussion here will focus on the management of the patient with malignant disease causing hemoptysis. Because patients with malignant disease are often malnourished, relatively inactive, often sedated, and possibly with previously compromised pulmonary reserve, their ability to tolerate significant pulmonary insults is decreased, and management needs to be both expeditious and effective to prevent the sequelae of respiratory insufficiency.

Massive hemoptysis is usually held to be more than 200 to 600 mL over 24 hours, although in practice this volume is difficult to quantitate. Appropriate questions to ask a patient with hemoptysis are the character (blood streaking of sputum or clots), the frequency per day, and the number of days that it has been present. The ability of the patient to maintain a clear airway should be evaluated, focusing on the level of consciousness and the effectiveness of the cough. Possible predisposing factors, such as the use of aspirin, Coumadin, or underlying coagulopathies, should be considered.

Malignant disease in the thorax may lead to airway bleeding in one of several ways:

1. The necrotic tissues of a primary lung carcinoma may themselves bleed.
2. The tissues may erode into the pulmonary vasculature.
3. The tumor may extrude into the central tracheobronchial tree, where the raw surface may ooze.
4. Involvement of mediastinal lymph nodes may erode into the trachea or main stem bronchi, with bleeding from the exposed surfaces.

Metastatic disease involving the lung is visible endobronchially by bronchoscopy in 2% to 3% of cases; these exposed surfaces with abnormal vasculature are prone to bleeding.

The management of the patient with known malignant disease and hemoptysis must be individually tailored. The patient with massive hemoptysis that threatens the ability to adequately perform gas exchange should be placed with the side suspected as the source down and taken to the operating room for emergency rigid bronchoscopy. Although it may be difficult to verify the side that is the source of the bleeding, patients themselves are often remarkably aware and can identify the problem. Patients with lesser amounts of bleeding may be managed more deliberately. Flexible bronchoscopy[5] localizes the bleeding site in more than 90% of patients and further guides therapy.

We favor an initial evaluation in the awake patient with the flexible bronchoscope, thus ensuring that the entire trachea to the level of the vocal cords is examined. The rigid bronchoscope, the yttrium:aluminum:garnet (YAG) laser, a No. 4 French venous Fogarty balloon, epinephrine solution, and a double-lumen tube should all be available. Once the site of bleeding is localized, it may be managed by irrigation with the epinephrine solution (or even direct injection through either a Wang needle or a brachytherapy seed implantation needle) or application of a laser. Bleeding that does not respond to these measures may be controlled with placement of a Fogarty catheter proximal to the bleeding to allow isolation of the bleeding site from the remainder of the lung.[6–8] At all times, one must keep in mind that the major concern in the patient with hemoptysis is the "good lung"; it is very easy to become distracted by the bleeding site, only to ignore the clots occluding the contralateral lung

The alternative to endobronchial treatment is angiographic treatment, which, because of a high rate of recurrent bleeding, is usually reserved, in our institution, for the patient unable to undergo general anesthesia. Initial success rates have been reported as being as high as 80%; the major risk, other than ongoing bleeding during the procedure, is occlusion of the anterior spinal artery[9]

Again, all therapeutic decisions must be made with the patient's overall prognosis in mind. For example, the decision to intubate a patient must be made with a clear understanding as to whether the patient is likely to be extubated, and this must be communicated to the patient and the family. Similarly, some bleeding episodes (usually secondary to malignancies metastatic to the lung) are best controlled with lung resection; such an undertaking involving a thoracotomy must be begun with the patient's overall outlook and desires in mind.

Pericardial Tamponade

The possible presence of a hemodynamically significant pericardial effusion should be considered in any patient with a previously diagnosed malignancy and new hemodynamic instability or respiratory difficulty. Malignancy is present in the pericardium in 15% to 20% of cancer patients in postmortem examination.[10] Pericardial disease can develop in cancer patients for a number of reasons, including infectious processes, and as a complication of treatments such as radiation or chemotherapy. Most pericardial effusions in cancer patients are malignant in origin. Metastasis to the pericardium is possible with most malignancies and is common in patients with lung or breast carcinomas, leukemias, and Hodgkin's and non-Hodgkin's lymphomas. Malignancy is also the most common cause of cardiac tamponade in patients without previously suspected cancer.[11] Unfortunately, the prognosis on diagnosis of a malignant pericardial effusion is fairly dismal, since involvement of the pericardium generally indicates advanced disease.[12]

Normal pericardial fluid is an ultrafiltrate of plasma with similar electrolyte composition but a lower protein content, although the albumin ratio is higher due to its lower molecular weight and ease of transmembrane transport. Pathologic pericardial effusions are usually exudates resulting from inflammatory processes or are remnants of normal transudate that is not reabsorbed back into the venous circulation if lymphatics are blocked. Both types of fluid have a higher protein content compared with normal pericardial fluid; while the former is simply similar in composition to plasma, the latter is filled with the higher-molecular-weight proteins that are not easily reabsorbed into the venous capillaries and that normally need to find their way back via the lymphatic system.[13-15] Both inflammation and blockage of lymphatics occur with the presence of malignant cells in the pericardium. Thus, malignant (and infectious) effusions usually contain large amounts of fibrin and protein content, whereas noninflammatory transudate, as may occur in congestive heart failure, has much less protein and no fibrin or blood. Hemorrhagic exudates are also more likely with severe infections and malignancies.

Currently, the most sensitive and least invasive method for detecting pericardial effusions is echocardiography. This modality can detect effusions as small as 15 mL, can characterize the volume of an effusion, and can demonstrate the presence of fibrin bands and pericardial masses, loculations, thickened pericardial membranes, chamber compression, and dilatation of the inferior vena cava.[11, 16] It has not been clearly established whether such information can be used to identify a pericardial effusion as likely to be malignant or benign. The ability to define the disease processes at the root of an effusion is critical, because both overall prognosis and the treatment choice may be altered.[5] In a number of studies, prognosis was found to be more dependent on the cause of the effusion and the extent of the underlying disease than on subsequent treatment.[12, 17, 18] For a debilitated, hemodynamically unstable patient prone to complication and facing a limited outlook even with the best of available therapies, extensively invasive intervention may often be deemed inappropriate.

To correlate various echocardiographic signs with the presence of either benign or malignant pericardial effusion in order to determine whether echocardiographic findings may reliably characterize an effusion as one or the other and to examine the sensitivity and specificity of pericardial fluid cytology or pericardial tissue histology in establishing the diagnosis of malignancy, we reviewed the records of 25 patients with pericardial fluid or tissue submitted for analysis from January 1, 1993, to December 30, 1994, at Memorial Sloan-Kettering Cancer Center (MSKCC).[19] Patients were divided into two groups: those with malignant, and those with benign effusions. The diagnosis of malignant pericardial effusion was made when cytologic examination of pericardial fluid or pathologic examination of pericardial tissue demonstrated the presence of malignant cells. The effusion was confirmed as malignant in 13 of the 25 patients (52%), while both fluid cytologic findings and pericardial tissue were benign in 12. Of the patients with intrapericardial malignancy, eight demonstrated positive cytology but negative pathology; two negative cytology but positive pathology; and three positive cytology and positive pathology. Specimens were obtained from pericardial fluid in eight patients (five patients with malignant effusion, three with benign effusion). None of the specimens were positive for bacterial or fungal infection; specimens from the remaining patients were not submitted for culture.

Nine of the malignant effusions (69%) were classified as large, as were six of the benign effusions (50%). Cardiac tamponade, as evidenced by moderate to severe collapse of one or more chambers, was more common in patients with malignant effusions than with benign effusions. The presence or absence of fibrin bands, loculations, pericardial masses, or inferior vena cava dilatation, however, could not be correlated convincingly with the eventual characterization of an effusion as malignant or benign.

A pericardial effusion may result from a number of processes, the most common being malignant involvement of the pericardial cavity. Effusion may also be a benign sequela of inflammatory processes, chemotherapy, or radiation.[20] Other less frequent causes are autoimmune processes, renal failure, trauma, and hypothyroid conditions.[13] In the presence of a known malignancy, accurate determination of the disease processes at the root of an effusion is important for a number of reasons.

First, prognosis is dramatically altered with a diagnosis of malignant cells in the pericardium. In one series, only 17% of 29 patients with a diagnosis of malignant pericardial effusion or tamponade survived for 1 year compared with 95% of 21 patients with benign effusions.[21] In another series, the 5-year survival rate was 60% among patients with nonmalignant effusions who were treated with a left anterior thoracotomy and pericardial window. Only 20% of similarly treated patients with malignant effusions were alive after 2 years.[22] In no study that we reviewed did a patient with a malignant pericardial effusion survive for longer than 4 years, no matter what the form of treatment. The long-term survival among the patients in this study was limited due to the extent of their underlying disease; the patients with benign effusions, however, did have a median survival of 2.75 times longer than those with malignant effusions after pericardial window placement.

Second, the initial presentation of an extracardiac malignancy may be pericardial effusion or tamponade. Certainly, in these patients it is important to learn the etiologic mechanism of the effusion both quickly and accurately in order to determine an appropriate course of treatment for the primary disease.[23, 24]

Third, the treatment of an effusion may differ according to etiology. Initial relief of the symptoms of pericardial effusion is most often, most quickly, and most safely achieved with percutaneous pericardiocentesis with echocardiographic guidance.[25] In many cases, complete drainage can be achieved over several days with an indwelling catheter, although without additional therapy, malignant effusions often recur.[12, 25] The use of an indwelling catheter allows one to wait for diagnostic results before subjecting a patient to a thoracotomy; it also provides a route for administration of agents into the pericardial cavity, if needed.[26]

Pericardiocentesis also provides fluid material for cytologic analysis, with a reported sensitivity of 84% to 87%.[23, 24, 27] False-positive results are rare.[20, 27] In our study, 11 of 13 malignant cases of were confirmed by positive cytology; 13% to 16% (two of 13 in our study) of malignant pericardial effusions, however, would currently remain undetected without the use of a more invasive method of diagnosis, such as pericardial biopsy or pathologic examination of the specimen. The concurrent use of carcinoembryonic antigen (CEA) measurements with cytologic examination has been reported to elevate the diagnostic rate of pericardiocentesis to 100% and may obviate the need to obtain tissue, but this method has not been widely adopted.[28]

The procedures for obtaining pericardial tissue range from a percutaneous subxiphoid pericardiotomy[29] to a thoracotomy with the creation of a pleuropericardial window or complete pericardiectomy.[22, 30] While these procedures simultaneously (principally) serve as long-term treatment for recurring pericardial effusion, they can be accompanied by significant morbidity and mortality, especially when general anesthesia and positive-pressure ventilation are used. A procedure performed through a thoracotomy, for example, may be accompanied by an approximate 8% risk of immediate mortality.[13, 23, 12] To understand the risks of the procedures, we must understand the underlying pathophysiology. The body compensates for obstruction to venous return by increasing venous volume. Instituting positive-pressure ventilation increases the obstruction to venous return, and a marginally compensated patient can suffer hemodynamic collapse during induction. For this reason, it is our practice to have the attending surgeon present, and often scrubbed, with the patient prepared and draped during induction of anesthesia. It is not often commented on that, given the large increases in venous volume that occur as compensation for cardiac compression, rapid drainage of pericardial fluid by either catheter or open procedures is unwise because it may precipitate either acute pulmonary edema or right ventricular failure once the venous volume can freely return to the heart and lungs. We prefer to perform catheter drainage rather than surgically create a pericardial window, since the catheter allows for better control over rate of removal.[31, 32] Removal is usually performed at a rate of 50 to 100 mL/hour. After surgical creation of a pericardial window, a diuretic agent should be administered, preferably initiated in the operating room. It is not uncommon for patients to eliminate 2 to 4 L of urine over the 12 to 24 hours after relief of a severe hemodynamically significant pericardial effusion.

Because of the limited life expectancy of patients with metastatic involvement of the pericardium, pericardiocentesis is useful for symptomatic relief even if it is associated with a higher long-term recurrence rate. If the tumor is known to be chemosensitive or radiosensitive, malignant effusion can often be treated with the appropriate systemic chemotherapy, local introduction of chemotherapeutic agents into the pericardial sac, or thoracic radiotherapy if the patient has not already received previous thoracic irradiation.[10, 13, 25, 27, 33, 34, 35]

In 1973, Lokich reported that 50% of such patients were "successfully" treated with thoracic irradiation.[33] Sclerotherapy with the intrapericardial instillation of cytostatic agents, such as tetracycline or radioactive chromic phosphate, through an indwelling catheter can also be effective for recurrent pericardial effusion and less invasive than creation of a pericardial window.[18, 36, 37] This treatment, however, is advised only in cases of malignant pericardial effusion due to the unestablished risks of long-term constrictive pericarditis. While the technique is painful and may cause a febrile reaction and cardiac arrhythmias, it may also impede tumor cell dissemination as a result of its cytotoxic effects.[36, 37]

Biran and colleagues[34] advise pericardiectomy for malignant effusions only if fluid reaccumulates more rapidly than drainage by indwelling catheter or repeated pericardiocentesis can control, since the general condition of these patients is usually poor. As Hancock has phrased it, because patients have endured "multiple surgical procedures and other protracted and difficult therapeutic programs, it is desirable as a general rule to limit the number of surgical procedures [these patients] are asked to undergo."[20, 34] Avoiding the additional risk of anesthesia in these hemodynamically unstable patients may confer survival benefits because the mean survival of patients treated conservatively (11.7 months) seems to be longer than the mean survival of those treated with a pericardial window (6.4 months).[35] In contrast, constrictive pericarditis, as seen with radiation-induced pericarditis, is regularly treated with corticosteroids or primary pericardiectomy.[33, 34]

INDWELLING CATHETER–RELATED SEPSIS IN THE NEUTROPENIC PATIENT

Indwelling central venous catheters have become a standard of cancer care and have given rise to potential life-threatening, catheter-related sepsis in the immune-compromised patient. The incidence of device-related infection is as much as 2.7% to 60% for all devices, depending on the type of device, the criteria used for the diagnosis of the device-related infection, and the underlying disease.[38-40] At our center, the number of infections per 1000 device days is 2.77 for tunneled catheters but only 0.21 for implanted ports.[40]

Although a great deal has been written about the care and management of temporary central venous access catheters in the general medical population, only limited data are available relevant to the management of permanent catheters in neutropenic patients, with neutropenia an independent risk factor for the development of catheter-related sepsis.[39, 40] Various strategies to reduce insertion site or catheter infections have been proposed, most notably related to aseptic insertion and the maintenance of a sterile field during subsequent use.

The evaluation of a febrile patient must include careful examination of the catheter insertion site, in addition to a thorough physical examination, in order to identify the source of infection. Erythema, representing cellulitis, or suppurative drainage is a clear indication of infection, but subcutaneously tunneled catheters my result in no external sign of infection.

In the febrile patient, we advocate transcatheter blood cultures along with simultaneous peripheral blood cultures to evaluate the catheter as a nidus of infection. Microbiologic isolates from devices in patients with a device-related bacteremia at our center tend to be gram-negative bacilli with tunneled catheters, while gram-positive cocci predominate in patients with implanted port devices.[40] Attempts to sterilize permanent or indwelling catheters with a 10- to 14-day organism-specific course of antibiotics has previously been advocated; however, we favor the removal of any culture-positive temporary central line as well as any indwelling catheter or port when the patient is hemodynamically unstable, when there is evidence of a catheter tunnel or port pocket infection, for septic emboli, or when associated with fungal or *Staphylococcus aureus* septicemia.[40]

When devices in close proximity to or within an abscess cavity are removed, the cavity or tunnel is left open to drain and is treated with wet-to-dry loose packing and dressing changes every 6 to 8 hours. Specimens of the cavity and catheter tip should be obtained for culture to confirm or redirect the antibiotic therapy. Temporary venous access should be obtained while the patient is being treated for the infection. Absolute requirements before placement of another permanent catheter should include negative blood cultures in an afebrile patient who has completed antibiotic therapy.

TREATMENT-RELATED END ORGAN TOXICITY: PERIOPERATIVE IMPLICATIONS

During the preoperative evaluation of the patient with malignancy, specific attention should be paid to the possible side-effects of previously administered chemoradiotherapy, with particular attention to the cardiac and pulmonary effects. The total dose and field of radiation should be quantified, as should the dose and schedule of previously administered cytotoxic agents, such as doxorubicin (Adriamycin) or bleomycin. Knowledge of the timing of the last chemotherapy cycle will enable accurate planning in order to avoid a neutropenic nadir.

Adriamycin is a cytotoxic anthracycline antibiotic that binds to nucleic acids and can be considered a representative agent for a discussion of cardiac chemotherapy toxicity. Cardiac toxicity occurs with increasing frequency in patients who have received a cumulative Adriamycin dose of 450 mg/m^2.[43] Clinically, the patient may describe worsening exercise tolerance, orthopnea, or lower-extremity edema that suggest the diagnosis of congestive heart failure of cardiomyopathy. Physical findings may include an S_3 gallop, jugular venous distention, hepatomegaly, or lower-extremity pitting edema. Chest radiographs may demonstrate cardiomegaly, pleural effusions, or pulmonary edema. Further cardiac evaluation, including echocardiography, is warranted in patients who have received Adriamycin in order to assess and possibly optimize cardiac performance.[44-46]

Bleomycin, a mixture of cytotoxic glycopeptides, inhibits deoxyribonucleic acid, ribonucleic acid, and protein synthesis and has been demonstrated to cause interstitial pulmonary fibrosis, particularly in patients with preexisting lung disease and prior thoracic irradiation.[47-49] Pathologic evaluation of lung tissue from patients with bleomycin toxicity reveals septal thickening with fibrosis, atypical type II pneumocytes, and pulmonary endothelial injury.[50] A history of nonproductive cough and physical findings of bibasilar rales may be present. If cough and rales are found, evaluation should include a chest radiograph (although physical findings often precede radiographic evidence of damage) and pulmonary function tests (PFTs), including arterial blood gas measurements, spirometry, and diffusing capacity of carbon monoxide (DLCO). PFTs may demonstrate restrictive airway disease, an increased (A − a) gradient, and decreased DLCO in these patients (one of the earliest markers alerting to the potential of bleomycin-induced pulmonary toxicity).[47-51] Reversal of acute bleomycin toxicity with high-dose corticosteroids has been reported, and their role as routine perioperative treatment remains under evaluation.[52] Other chemotherapy agents have been found to cause bone marrow suppression, gastrointestinal disturbances, metabolic derangement, or neurologic sequelae and are discussed in Chapters 162 and 164.

Radiation therapy is being used more frequently as a primary or adjuvant modality for the treatment of thoracic malignancies. Independently or synergistically with chemotherapeutic agents, radiotherapy has been demonstrated to result in pulmonary fibrosis.[50] Symptoms can be either acute or chronic, manifesting either during therapy or many months after completion. Patients who demonstrate findings consistent with pulmonary toxicity following chemotherapy or radiation should be managed with the lowest possible fraction of inspired oxygen in order to minimize synergistic oxygen toxicity. Specifically, the fraction of inspired oxygen therapy has been recommended not to exceed 0.3 (30%).[53]

ABDOMINAL PAIN IN THE NEUTROPENIC PATIENT

Abdominal pain in neutropenic patients is a common symptom leading to surgical evaluation. Differentiating abdominal pain requiring surgical intervention from pain of a self-limited nature can be difficult. Classic clinical and laboratory parameters useful in the evaluation of the general population may be of more limited value in the cancer patient who has recently undergone cytotoxic therapy. Fever, nausea, vomiting, or abdominal pain may arise as a consequence of antineoplastic therapy and as such is a less reliable symptom in the cancer patient. Leukocytosis normally seen during an inflammatory or infectious processes may be absent in the neutropenic patient. Knowledge of the differential diagnosis and judicious use of radiographic imaging studies facilitate accurate diagnosis and corrective interventions. Abdominal pain in the neutropenic patient may be the result of present or previous therapy or the malignant process itself. The causes of abdominal pain can be broadly grouped as due to inflammation, obstruction, or perforation.[54]

Neutropenic enterocolitis (NE), also termed typhlitis, ileocecal syndrome, or enteropathy of neutropenia, is a cause of abdominal pain essentially unique to the patient receiving cytotoxic chemotherapy.[54, 55] The common presenting symptoms include diffuse abdominal pain that may localize to the right lower quadrant with or without rebound tenderness, fever, nausea, vomiting, and diarrhea (occasionally bloody) and can be as extreme as florid sepsis. The differential diagnosis includes acute appendicitis, neutropenic enterocolitis, pseudomembranous colitis, and ischemic colitis.[54]

The typical patient with NE is leukemic, approaching or at neutropenic nadir 7 to 14 days after initiation of the therapy.[55, 56] Cytosine arabinoside (Ara-c) therapy alone or in combination with other agents has been the regimen most frequently associated with this syndrome.[55-58] NE is reported to occur in 2.6% of adults[59] with leukemia undergoing treatment and is found in 12% of autopsy specimens.[60] Abdominal pain in the neutropenic leukemia patient has been reported to occur 35% to 62% of the time, with significant morbidity and mortality when urgent abdominal surgery is required.[61, 62] While NE has been most frequently reported in leukemia patients, it has also been described in patients with aplastic anemia, cyclic neutropenia, and recently in patients undergoing bone marrow transplantation.[62-65]

Etiologic mechanisms have been suggested from the demonstrated susceptibility of the right colon to injury from Ara-c.[66, 67] Although NE may affect the entire colon, the reason for the common finding of injury to the right colon alone is unknown.[68] Violation of mucosal integrity with subsequent focal ulceration is thought to be secondary to underlying ischemia, leading to both abdominal pain and the entry of bacteria into the systemic circulation with the development of sepsis.

Surgical evaluation with subsequent radiographic evaluation helps to guide the appropriate therapy. Plain radiographs are nonspecific in most patients; however, the findings of intestinal pneumatosis or free intraperitoneal air warrant surgical exploration. Oral contrast imaging studies are of limited value and should be avoided, as they may complicate the management of intra-abdominal spillage in the presence of bowel perforation. Abdominal CT scan may demonstrate specific findings of ileocecal wall thickening, mural edema, pneumatosis, abscess, or pericolonic fluid.[69]

The clinical course of neutropenic enterocolitis may be self-limited with pain, fever, and gastrointestinal discomfort responsive to supportive management.[54, 70] Conservative management of the patient at this juncture should consist of broad-spectrum antibiotic coverage, including an anaerobic agent (metronidazole), intravenous hydration, bowel rest with parenteral nutrition, and nasogastric decompression. Patients who either do not improve or whose condition worsens over 24 to 48 hours or who have clinical or radiographic appearance of obstruction should be considered for laparotomy.[71] CT scan evidence of a localized abscess is usually best managed by percutaneous drainage rather than laparotomy, but this decision must be individualized. The patient with findings strongly suggestive of perforation should undergo laparotomy. Appreciation for the potential severity of this disease process can be demonstrated from the reported mortality in these patients. Surgical management of neutropenic enterocolitis has a reported mortality of 21%, while medical management alone has resulted in a 48% mortality rate in a reported series, suggesting a clear role for surgical intervention.[72]

The surgical treatment for NE is determined by findings at the time of laparotomy. Usually, intraoperative abdominal examination reveals a predominant right colon distribution of affected bowel; nonperforated, edematous bowel does not require resection and should be managed expectantly.[73-75] Abscess noted during laparotomy should be drained and the peritoneal cavity generously irrigated. Careful examination of the bowel, with a search for obvious or microperforation, is important to identify the source of abdominal contamination. Perforation has been managed both by resection and diversion[72-74] or resection and primary anastomosis.[76] Although no data are presently available, proximal diversion and distal mucous fistula can be supported as a safe approach for the management of perforation in the complicated immunologically challenged patient.

Pathologic examination of surgical specimens has revealed normal-appearing serosa with mural edema and varying degrees of mucosal ulceration.[77] Organisms obtained for culture at the time of surgery from the affected bowel or abscess are usually gram-negative enteric flora and have been correlated with blood culture isolates in 40% of these patients,[78-80] a finding that may explain the recurrent episodes of sepsis in these patients. Postoperatively, the patient will require total parenteral nutrition.

The role of recombinant hematopoietic stimulation therapies in the neutropenic patient, such as granulocyte colony-stimulating factor (G-CSF) and granulocyte macrophage colony-stimulating factor (GM-CSF) are under investigation; the literature suggests a benefit for these patients.[63]

Gastrointestinal (GI) obstruction may have a functional or a mechanical origin. What at initial presentation may appear to be a functional obstruction may in fact represent an early or progressing mechanical problem. Ileus following surgery is a common occurrence and usually resolves spontaneously with conservative care alone, including nasogastric decompression, and after correction of underlying metabolic abnormalities. Narcotic medications are almost universally used in the care of cancer patients and can lead to an adynamic bowel. Serial abdominal examination and radiographs may warn of the development of bowel distention and may lead to interventions that prevent the development of dramatic complications, such as aspiration or perforation.

Following previous laparotomy, radiation enteritis[81] and adhesions[82] are common benign causes of mechanical intestinal obstruction in up to one third of obstructions occurring in the cancer patient population. Without clear evidence of a malignant cause of obstruction, no limitations on surgical treatment should be placed on these patients because of a presumed poor outcome. Malignant obstructions from recurrence or new malignancy represent as many as 60% of abdominal obstructions and almost invariably require surgical intervention.[83-86] Only about one third of these patients with malignant obstructions derive long-term relief from laparotomy and bypass.[85, 86] In patients with known intra-abdominal carcinomatosis who present with obstruction, operation is generally futile and carries a perioperative mortality approaching 50%.[85, 86] Palliation by percutaneous endoscopic gastrostomy (PEG) to drain GI secretions is recommended for these patients, but individualized management is emphasized.[87]

Perforation of the GI tract may occur as the result of benign conditions (peptic ulcer, diverticulitis), from primary or metastatic tumor, or as the consequence of antineoplastic treatment. Tumor-associated GI perforations have been reported as 66% of all perforations in one cancer patient series.[88] Bowel perforations have been reported in patients with metastasis to the gut, including such varied malignancies as melanoma, lung carcinoma, or breast carcinoma. Patients undergoing cytotoxic chemotherapy in whom neutropenic enterocolitis develops have also been reported to have GI perforations.[89]

Non-Hodgkin's lymphoma of the GI tract represents a disease whose treatment is in evolution. Previously, surgery was necessary for the diagnosis, staging, and treatment of this disease; however, endoscopic examination and biopsy have been demonstrated to reliably establish the diagnosis. As such, the initial treatment of gastric lymphoma has become chemotherapy and adjuvant radiation with resection, with curative intent reserved for selected patients.[91, 92]

Historically, there has been concern for the potential of fatal hemorrhage and perforation following the nonsurgical management of a rapidly responding transmural malignancy. While this concern may have been overstated in this specific disease, the potential for hemorrhage and perforation in the cancer patient should not go unrecognized.[92-95]

New abdominal pain or discomfort in a patient who is undergoing or has recently begun chemotherapy for a GI malignancy, such as gastric lymphoma, should be thoroughly evaluated for perforation. Although abdominal pain (ranging from acute discomfort to steadily increasing pain) is the main initial symptom, the patient may complain of thirst and demonstrate a low urine output and tachycardia from hypovolemia of third-space fluid, which worsens with progressive peritonitis. Physical findings demonstrate a distended abdomen varying with the degree of intra-abdominal free air and abdominal discomfort and that ranges from localized tenderness to extreme guarding with rebound that progresses as the peritonitis worsens.

Standard abdominal radiographs, with the addition of a left lateral decubitus film, may demonstrate free intraperitoneal air, the hallmark of a perforated hollow viscus. Isolated gastric perforation usually leads to laparotomy, and the intraoperative findings (size of the perforation, peritoneal soiling, and extent of organ viability) determine extent of the procedure performed. Limited areas of perforation may be amenable to primary repair or omental patch closure; however, a larger area of organ damage may require partial or total gastrectomy.[96]

Peptic ulcer disease and gastritis are the most frequent causes of intestinal bleeding in the cancer patient. Hemorrhage arising directly from necrotic tumor is rare. More often, hemorrhage occurs as a consequence of thrombocytopenia or coagulopathies or following an invasive procedure. Primary GI lymphomas and metastatic disease to the GI tract are most commonly associated with hemorrhage.[97]

The initial approach to these patients should be the same as for patients with presumed benign disease. While the patient is undergoing resuscitation, including specific therapies to correct underlying hematologic or coagulation deficits, identification of the site of hemorrhage should be attempted. Hematemesis occurs with bleeding proximal to the ligament of Treitz, and confirmation of the bleeding site should be attempted by upper endoscopy. Identification of lower GI bleeding can be evaluated by rigid proctoscopy or flexible colonoscopy. Tagged red blood cell scan and angiography are useful in the localization of colonic sites of hemorrhage. CT scan can best evaluate extraluminal sites, and the most frequent location is the retroperitoneum. Attempts to control bleeding should be guided by the patient's overall condition, prognostic outlook, and the specific cause of bleeding. These efforts can range from correction of underlying coagulopathy and endoscopic coagulation alone to selective angiographic embolization or surgical intervention.[97-99]

While uncommon, the inclusion of perforation and hemorrhage in the differential, during the evaluation of abdominal pain or unexplained rapid deterioration in the cancer patient, may be lifesaving.

References

1. Simpson JR, Perez CA, Presant BJ, et al: Superior vena cava syndrome. *In:* Oncologic Emergencies. Yabro JW, Bornstein RS (Eds). New York, Grune & Stratton, 1981, pp 43–72.
2. Ahman F: A reassessment of the clinical implications of the superior vena caval syndrome. J Clin Oncol 1984; 2:8.
3. Strong EW: Head and neck emergencies: Life threatening emergencies in the cancer patient. Part II. Curr Probl Cancer 1979; 4:36.

4. Conlan AA, Hurwitz SS, Krige L, Nicolaou N, Pool R: Massive hemoptysis: A review of 123 cases. J Thorac Cardiovasc Surg 1983; 85:120.
5. Slecky PA: Evaluation of hemoptysis through the bronchoscope. Chest 1978; 73:741.
6. Saw EC, Gottlieb LS, Yokoyama T, et al: Flexible fiberoptic bronchoscopy and endobronchial tamponade in the management of massive hemoptysis. Chest 1976; 70:589.
7. Gottlieb LS, Hillberg R: Endobronchial tamponade therapy for intractable hemoptysis. Chest 1975; 67:482.
8. Freitag L: Development of a new balloon catheter for management of hemoptysis with bronchofiberscopes. Chest 1993; 103:593.
9. Uflacker I, Kaemmerer A, Neves C, et al: Management of massive hemoptysis by bronchial artery embolization. Radiology 1983; 146:627.
10. Hawkins JW, Vacek JL: What constitutes definitive therapy of malignant pericardial effusion? "Medical" versus surgical treatment. Am Heart J 1989; 118:428.
11. Groeger JS, Keefe D: Cardiac tamponade. *In:* Critical Care of the Cancer Patient. 2nd ed. Groeger JS (Ed). St. Louis: Mosby-Year Book, 1991; pp 250–260.
12. Markiewicz W, Borovik R, Ecker S: Cardiac tamponade in medical patients: Treatment and prognosis in the echocardiographic era. Am Heart J 1986; 111:1138.
13. Press OW, Livingston R: Management of malignant pericardial effusion and tamponade. JAMA 1987; 257:1088.
14. Spodick DH: Diseases of the pericardium. *In:* Cardiology: An Illustrated Text/Reference. Chatterjee K, Cheitlin MD, Karliner J, et al (Eds). New York, Gower Medical Publishing, 1991; pp 10.38–10.64.
15. Memon A, Zawadski ZA: Malignant effusions: Diagnostic evaluation and therapeutic strategy. Curr Probl Cancer 1981; 5:3.
16. Horowitz MS, Schultz CS, Stinson EB, Harrison DC, Popp RL: Sensitivity and specificity of echocardiographic diagnosis of pericardial effusion. Circulation 1974; 50:239.
17. Wilkes JD, Fidias P, Vaickus L, Perez RP: Malignancy-related pericardial effusion. Cancer 1995; 76:1377.
18. Martini N, Freiman AH, Watson RC, Hilaris BS: Intrapericardial instillation of radioactive chromic phosphate in malignant pericardial effusion. Am J Roentgenol 1977; 128:639.
19. Hsu FI, Keefe D, Desiderio D, Downey RJ: Echocardiographic and surgical correlation of pericardial effusions in patients with malignant disease. J Thorac Cardiovasc Surg 1998; 115:1215.
20. Hancock EW: Neoplastic pericardial disease. Cardiol Clin 1990; 8:673.
21. Levine MJ, Lorell BH, Diver DJ, Come PC: Implications of echocardiographically assisted diagnosis of pericardial tamponade in contemporary medical patients: Detection before hemodynamic embarrassment. J Am Coll Cardiol 1991; 17:59.
22. Olsen PS, Sorensen C, Anderson HO: Surgical treatment of large pericardial effusions: Etiology and long-term survival. Eur J Cardiothorac Surg 1991; 5:430.
23. Muir KW, Rodger JC: Cardiac tamponade as the initial presentation of malignancy: Is it as rare as previously supposed? Postgrad Med J 1994; 70:703.
24. Fraser RS, Viloria JB, Wang N-S: Cardiac tamponade as a presentation of extracardiac malignancy. Cancer 1980; 45:1697.
25. Vaitkus PT, Herrmann HC, LeWinter MM: Treatment of malignant pericardial effusion. JAMA 1994; 272:59.
26. Wei JY, Taylor GJ, Achuff SC: Recurrent cardiac tamponade and large pericardial effusions: Management with an indwelling pericardial catheter. Am J Cardiol 1978; 42:281.
27. Zipf RE, Johnston WW: The role of cytology in the evaluation of pericardial effusions. Chest 1972; 62:593.
28. Tatsuta M, Yamamura H, Yamamoto R, Ichii M, Iishi H, Noguchi S: Carcinoembryonic antigens in the pericardial fluid of patients with malignant pericarditis. Oncology 1984; 41:328.
29. Santos GH, Frater RWM: The subxiphoid approach in the treatment of pericardial effusion. Ann Thorac Surg 1977; 23:467.
30. Miller JI, Mansour KA, Hatcher CR: Pericardiectomy: Current indications, concepts, and results in a university center. Ann Thorac Surg 1982; 34:40.
31. Shenoy MM, Dhar S, Gittin R, Sinha AK, Sabado M: Pulmonary edema following pericardiectomy for cardiac tamponade. Chest 1984; 86:647.
32. Downey RJ, Bessler M, Weissman C: Acute pulmonary edema following pericardiocentesis for chronic cardiac tamponade secondary to trauma. Crit Care Med 1991; 19:1323.
33. Lokich JJ: The management of malignant pericardial effusions. JAMA 1973; 224:1401.
34. Biran S, Brufman G, Klein E, Hochman A: The management of pericardial effusion in cancer patients. Chest 1977; 71:182.
35. Smith FE, Lane M, Hudgins PT: Conservative management of malignant pericardial effusion. Cancer 1974; 33:47.
36. Davis S, Rambotti P, Grignani F: Intrapericardial tetracycline sclerosis in the treatment of malignant pericardial effusion: An analysis of 33 cases. J Clin Oncol 1984; 2:631.
37. Shepherd FA, Morgan C, Evans WK, Ginsberg JF, Watt D, Murphy K: Medical management of malignant pericardial effusion by tetracycline sclerosis. Am J Cardiol 1987; 60:1161.
38. Tacconelli E, Tumbarello M, Pittiruti M, Leone F, Lucia MB, Cauda R, Ortona L: Central venous catheter–related sepsis in a cohort of 366 hospitalized patients. Eur J Clin Microbiol Infect Dis 1997; 16:203.
39. Howell PB, Walters PE, Donowitz GR, Farr BM: Risk factors for infection of adult patients with cancer who have tunneled central venous catheters. Cancer 1995; 75:1367.
40. Groeger JS, Lucas AB, Thaler HT, et al: Infectious morbidity associated with long term venous access devices in patients with cancer. Ann Intern Med 1993; 119:1168.
41. Ginsberg SJ, Comis RL: The pulmonary toxicity of antineoplastic agents. Semin Oncol 1982; 9:34.
42. Von Hoff DD, Rozencweig M, Piccart M: The cardiotoxicity of anticancer agents. Semin Oncol 1982; 9:23.
43. Chan KK, Chleboski RT, Myron-Tonn HS, et al: Clinical pharmacokinetics of adriamycin in hepatoma patients with cirrhosis. Cancer Res 1980; 40:1263.
44. Billingham ME, Mason JW, Bristow MR, Daniels JR: Anthracycline cardiomyopathy monitored by morphologic changes. Cancer Treat Rep 1978; 62:865.
45. Lipshultz SE, Dolan SD, Gelber RD, Perez-Atayde AR, Sallan SE, Sanders SP: Late cardiac effects of doxorubicin therapy for acute lymphoblastic leukemia in childhood. Engl J Med 1991; 324:808.
46. Minow RA, Benjamin RS, Lee ET, Gottlieb JA: Adriamycin cardiomyopathy risk factors. Cancer 1977; 39:1397.
47. Parvinen LM, Kilkku P, Maekinen E, et al: Factors affecting the pulmonary toxicity of bleomycin. Acta Radiol 1983; 22:417.
48. Klein DS, Wilds PR: Pulmonary toxicity of antineoplastic agents: Anaesthetic and postoperative implications. Can Anaesthesiol Soc J 1983; 30:399.
49. Waid-Jones MI, Coursin DB: Perioperative considerations for patients treated with bleomycin. Chest 1991; 99:993.
50. Todd NW, Peters WP, Ost AH, Roggli VL, Piantadosi CA: Pulmonary drug toxicity in patients with primary breast cancer treated with high-dose combination chemotherapy and autologous bone marrow transplantation. Am Rev Respir Dis 1993; 147:1264.
51. Sorensen PG, Rossing N, Rorth M: Carbon monoxide diffusing capacity: A reliable indicator of bleomycin-induced pulmonary toxicity. Eur J Respir Dis 1985; 66:333.
52. Maher J, Daly PA: Severe bleomycin lung toxicity: Reversal with high dose corticosteroids. Thorax 1993; 48:92.
53. Goldiner PL, Carlon GC, Cvitokovik E, et al: Factors influencing post-operative morbidity and mortality in patients treated with bleomycin. Br Med J 1978; 1:664.
54. Scott-Conner DEH, Fabrega AJ: Gastrointestinal problems in the immunocompromised host: A review for surgeons. Surg Endosc 1996; 10:959.
55. Starnes H, Moore G, Mentzer S, et al: Abdominal pain in neutropenic cancer patients. Cancer 1986; 57:616.
56. Keidan R, Ganning J, Gatenby R, et al: Recurrent typhlitis: A disease resulting from aggressive chemotherapy. Dis Colon Rectum 1989; 32:206.
57. Vlasveld L, Zwaan F, Fibbe R, et al: Neutropenic enterocolitis following treatment with cytosine arabinoside-containing regimens for hematological malignancies: A potentiating role for amsacrine. Ann Hematol 1991; 62:129.
58. Wade D, Douglass H, Nava H, et al: Abdominal pain in neutropenic patients. Arch Surg 1990; 125:1119.
59. Mower W, Hawkins J, Nelson E: Neutropenic enterocolitis in adults with acute leukemia. Arch Surg 1986; 121:571.

60. Steinberg D, Gold J, Brodin A: Necrotizing enterocolitis in leukemia. Arch Intern Med 1973; 131:538.
61. Glenn J, Funkhouser W, Schneider P: Acute illnesses necessitating urgent abdominal surgery in neutropenic cancer patients: Description of 14 cases and review of the literature. Surgery 1989; 105:778.
62. Martell R, Jacobs P: Surgery for the acute abdomen in adults with leukemia. Postgrad Med J 1986; 62:915.
63. Weinberger M, Hollingsworth H, Feuerstein I, et al: Successful surgical management of neutropenic enterocolitis in two patients with severe aplastic anemia. Arch Intern Med 1993; 153:107.
64. Mehta J, Nagler A, Or R, et al: Neutropenic enterocolitis and intestinal perforation associated with carboplatin-containing conditioning regimen for autologous bone marrow transplantation. Acta Oncol 1992; 31:591.
65. Or R, Mehta O, Nagler A, et al: Neutropenic enterocolitis associated with autologous bone marrow transplantation. Bone Marrow Transplant 1992; 9:383.
66. Plunkett W, Liliemark JO, Estey E, et al: Saturation of ara-CTP accumulation during high-dose ara-C therapy: Pharmacologic rationale for intermediate-dose ara-C. Semin Oncol 1989; 14(Suppl 1):159.
67. Chabner BA: Cytosine arabinoside. *In:* Pharmacologic Principles of Cancer Treatment. Chabner BA (Eds). Philadelphia, WB Saunders, 1982; pp 387–401.
68. Skibber J, Matter G, Pizzo P, et al: Right lower quadrant pain in young patients with leukemia. Ann Surg 1987; 206:711.
69. Grick M, Maiale C, Crass J, et al: Computed tomography of neutropenic colitis. Am J Radiol 1984; 143:763.
70. Villar H, Warneke J, Peck M, et al: Role of surgical treatment in the management of complications of the gastrointestinal tract in patients with leukemia. Surg Gynecol Obstet 1987; 165:217.
71. Moir C, Scudamore C, Benny W: Typhlitis: Selective surgical management. Am J Surg 1986; 141:563.
72. Ettinhausen S: Collagenous colitis, eosinophilic colitis and neutropenic colitis. Surg Clin North Am 1993; 73:993.
73. Dosik G, Luna M, Valdivieso M, et al: Necrotizing colitis in patients with cancer. Am J Med 1979; 67:646.
74. Kingry R, Hobson R, Muir R: Cecal necrosis and perforation with systemic chemotherapy. Am Surg 1973; 39:129.
75. Geelhoed G, Kane M, Dale D, et al: Colon ulceration and perforation in cyclic neutropenia. J Pediatr Surg 1973; 3:379.
76. Anderson P: Neutropenic enterocolitis treated by primary resection with anastomosis in a leukemic patient receiving chemotherapy. Aust N Z J Surg 1993; 63:74.
77. Newbold K: Neutropenic enterocolitis: Clinical and pathological review. Dig Dis 1989; 7:281.
78. Coleman N, Speirs G, Khan J, et al: Neutropenic enterocolitis associated with *Clostridium tertium.* J Clin Pathol 1983; 46:180.
79. Pouwels MJ, Donnelly JP, Raemaekers JM, Verweij PE, de Pauw BE: *Clostridium septicum* sepsis and neutropenic enterocolitis in a patient treated with intensive chemotherapy for acute myeloid leukemia. Ann Hematol 1997; 74:143.
80. Sadullah S, Nages K, Johnston D, McCullough JB, Murray F, Cachia PG: Recurrent septicemia in a neutropenic patient with typhlitis. Clin Lab Haematol 1996; 18:215.
81. Tsioulias GJ, De Cosse JJ: Radiation enteritis: Diagnosis and treatment. *In:* Cancer Surgery. Mckenna RJ, Murphy GP (Eds): Philadelphia, JB Lippincott, 1994, pp 201.
82. Ellis CN, Boggs HW Jr, Slagle GW, Cole PA: Small bowel obstruction after colon resection for benign and malignant diseases. Dis Colon Rectum 1991; 34:367.
83. Osteen RT, Guyton S, Steele G Jr, Wilson RE: Malignant intestinal obstruction. Surgery 1980; 87:611.
84. Gallick HL, Weaver DW, Sacha RJ, et al: Intestinal obstruction in cancer patients: An assessment of risk factors and outcome. Am Surg 1986; 8:434.
85. Annest LS, Jolly PC: The results of surgical treatment of bowel obstruction caused by peritoneal carcinomatosis. Am Surg 1979; 45:718.
86. Lau PWK, Lorentz TG: Results of surgery for malignant bowel obstruction in advanced, unresectable, recurrent colorectal cancer. Dis Colon Rectum 1993; 36:61.
87. Stellato TA, Shenk RR: Gastrointestinal emergencies in the oncology patient. Semin Oncol 1989; 16:521.
88. Ferrara JJ, Martin EW, Care LC: Morbidity of emergency operations in patients with metastatic cancer receiving chemotherapy. Surgery 1982; 92:605.
89. Alt B, Glass RR, Sollinger H: Neutropenic enterocolitis in adults: Review of the literature and assessment of surgical intervention. Am J Surg 1985; 149:405.
90. Kemeny M, Brennan M: The surgical complications of chemotherapy in cancer patients. Curr Probl Surg 1987; 24:609.
91. Rabbi C, Aden E, Cavazzini G, Cantor M, Gorghieri ME, Pari F, Zamagni D, Mambrini A, Amadori M, Smerieri F: Stomach preservation in low-and high-grade primary gastric lymphomas: Preliminary results. Haematologica 1996; 81:15.
92. Cooper DL, Doria R, Salloum E: Primary gastrointestinal lymphomas. Gastroenterologist 1996; 4:54.
93. Talamonti M, Dawes C, Joehol R, et al: Gastrointestinal lymphoma. Arch Surg 1990; 125:972.
94. Weingard D, Decosse J, Sherlock P, et al: Gastrointestinal Lymphoma: A 30-year review. Cancer 1982; 49:1258.
95. List A, Greer J, Cousar J, et al: Non-Hodgkin's lymphoma of the gastrointestinal tract: An analysis of clinical and pathologic features affecting outcome. J Clin Oncol 1988; 6:1125.
96. Ono K, Matsumura S, Sakamoto K, Kobayashi S, Kamano T, Iwasaki R: A case of gastric malignant lymphoma with perforation during chemotherapy. Gan To Kagaku Ryoho 1997; 24:105–108.
97. Lightdale DJ, Kurtz RC, Boyle CC, et al: Cancer and upper gastrointestinal tract hemorrhage: Benign causes of bleeding demonstrated by endoscopy. JAMA 1973; 226:139.
98. Haim N, Leviov M, Ben-Arieh Y, Epelbaum R, Frieidin N, Reshef R, Ben-Shahar M: Intermediate and high-grade gastric non-Hodgkin's lymphoma: A prospective study of non-surgical treatment with primary chemotherapy, with or without radiotherapy. Leuk Lymphoma 1995; 17:321.
99. Randall J, Obeid M, Blackledge G: Hemorrhage and perforation of gastrointestinal neoplasms during chemotherapy. Ann R Coll Surg Engl 1986; 68:286.

164

Medical Complications in the Patient with Cancer

Rafael Barrera, MD • Jeffrey S. Groeger, MD

Continually developing chemotherapeutic agents, novel approaches to radiation therapy, more aggressive bone marrow transplantation protocols, and immunologic therapies have changed the course of cancer care. Once thought to be a fatal disease, cancer may now be curable or at least controlled to extend life by years. Life extension in a patient with malignancy may come at great expense, with therapy-related morbidity or with quality of life deteriorating as the disease progresses.

Predictors of intensive care unit (ICU) mortality are few for the cancer population. Cohorts of patients with respiratory failure who receive mechanical ventilation, who have disease progression, who undergo allogeneic bone marrow transplantation, or who have poor performance status tend to do poorly. Yet these variables, as in all outcome models, work well for a population and poorly for an individual.[1] As with an acute life-threatening event, indications for ICU support should be based on (1) the probability of surviving the acute illness and (2) the anticipated duration and quality of life after discharge from the hospital as well as (3) the patient's wishes.

In this chapter, we focus on the clinical conditions, complications, and treatment of patients with cancer that might require ICU admission.

HYPERCALCEMIA AND ELECTROLYTE ABNORMALITIES

Malignancy accounts for approximately 45% of all cases of hypercalcemia and develops in up to 20% of all cancer patients. Patients with a serum calcium level exceeding 13 mg/dL or a clinical picture consistent with hypercalcemia warrant urgent intervention and evaluation and may need a monitored environment.[2]

Malignancies and primary hyperparathyroidism may coexist in the critically ill cancer patient. Combined, they account for approximately 90% of all cases of hypercalcemia. Distinguishing between hypercalcemia secondary to malignancy and primary hyperparathyroidism is usually confirmed by measuring the serum parathyroid hormone (PTH) level. Most patients with primary hyperparathyroidism have elevated serum concentrations of PTH, yet approximately one fourth of cancer patients with hypercalcemia also have elevations of PTH.[3] Incorporating the measurement of PTH with that of total or ionized serum calcium identifies primary hyperparathyroidism in a majority of cases.[4, 5] Breast and lung carcinomas account for 80% of cases of malignancy-associated hypercalcemia; hematologic malignancies, such as multiple myeloma and lymphoma, account for most of the remaining 20%.[2, 6, 7] About 30% of patients with multiple myeloma experience hypercalcemia during the course of their disease as a result of increased bone resorption and renal insufficiency.[8, 9] Hospitalized patients in whom hypercalcemia develops usually have malignancies.

A complete differential diagnosis of hypercalcemia includes abnormal renal function, sarcoidosis, thyrotoxicosis, vitamin D or A intoxication, long-term incapacitation, milk-alkali syndrome, adrenal insufficiency, and some medications (tamoxifen, thiazides).

Although various tumors associated with hypercalcemia of malignancy have been described, it is interesting to note that there is no single unifying mechanism for this syndrome.[6, 10] Local bone-resorbing factors may be responsible in the hematologic malignancies; in solid tumors with advanced bone metastasis, however, there is extensive local bone destruction. Secretion of PTH-like proteins (PLPs) by the tumor is the mechanism of increased bone resorption in some other solid tumors.[5, 11–18]

Osteoclast-activating factor, interleukins, interferon gamma, and tumor necrosis factor may act independently or synergistically in the pathophysiology of hypercalcemia.[19] Any renal insufficiency associated with a major change in calcium homeostasis can lead to hypercalcemia in a patient with increased bone resorption because of decrease in the filtered calcium load.

Diagnosis

There are no signs and symptoms pathognomonic of hypercalcemia. The clinical manifestation of the hypercalcemic syndrome is commonly related to the rapidity of the rise in calcium rather than to the absolute serum concentration. Patients with hypercalcemic crisis present with such neurologic signs as somnolence, lethargy, and general weakness. Psychotic behavior, ocular abnormalities, stupor, and coma, and, occasionally, localizing signs found at neurologic examination may also be present. Patients may have nausea and vomiting and, rarely, hypertension.[2] All of these signs may disappear with therapy that lowers the patient's serum calcium level.[20]

The clinical syndrome of hypercalcemia can easily be confused with the terminal features of the underlying malignancy or with the side effects of treatment. Some patients may be asymptomatic or may have nonspecific complaints. Other times patients have abdominal pain, lethargy, dehydration, and renal failure.

In rare cases, peptic ulcer disease or pancreatitis has been described as the presenting clinical picture. A rapid rise in the serum calcium levels impairs the kidney's ability to concentrate urine. Nephrogenic diabetes insipidus secondary to hypercalcemia leads to dehydration and electrolyte abnormalities with associated polydipsia. Contraction alkalosis leading to dehydration and further renal damage can cause patients to deteriorate rapidly. In the patient with multiple myeloma, the renal failure can be devastating. Hypercalcemia of malignancy is rarely associated with nephrocalcinosis and nephrolithiasis.

Critical elevations of the serum calcium concentration are not usually associated with significant hemodynamic alterations other than dehydration.[6] Electrocardiographic (ECG) changes associated with hypercalcemia can be shortening of the QT interval, bradycardia, and nonspecific T-wave abnormalities. Hypokalemia-associated cardiac arrhythmias are usually seen when the calcium level is greater than 14 mg/dL.[21] Massive diuresis may exacerbate this problem.

Either abnormal binding proteins or the presence of hypoalbuminemia may lead to inaccurate estimates of the ionized fraction of calcium. In the patient with cancer or another critical illness who has hypoalbuminemia, ionized calcium becomes a larger fraction of the total serum calcium, and therefore, total calcium measurements may understate the severity of hypercalcemia. Measurement of ionized calcium correlates best with the signs and symptoms of hypercalcemia. Although ionized calcium levels increase with acidosis and decrease with alkalosis, these changes are usually minimal and have no clinical significance.[22]

Treatment

The only effective way of helping patients with hypercalcemia of malignancy is treatment of the tumor. The measures to decrease the calcium level (specifically, therapy to inhibit osteoclast-mediated bone resorption) as well as treatment to increase urinary calcium excretion should be started in patients who present with severe symptoms.[12, 23, 24]

Rehydration to replenish intravascular volume in these patients usually increases urinary calcium secretion by 100 to 300 mg/day.[24, 25] A urine output of more than 1.5 mL/kg/hr is ideal. Calciuresis is enhanced by a provoked natriuresis. Rehydration with calciuresis may offer transient reduction in ionized calcium, and therapy must be instituted to correct the underlying process of excessive bone resorption. The contribution of furosemide to the urinary excretion of calcium remains unclear, as does the optimal dose. Careful attention is given to volume and to electrolyte repletion, especially potassium, sodium, and phosphorus. The rate of administration of intravenous fluid should be determined by the severity of the clinical picture. Obviously, all agents capable of precipitating hypercalcemic crisis should be discontinued.

Pharmacologic agents used in the management of hypercalcemia are as follows:

- Plicamycin, an inhibitor of ribonucleic acid (RNA) synthesis in osteoclasts[25–29]
- Calcitonin, a peptide hormone that inhibits bone resorption and also increases renal excretion of calcium[30, 31]
- Gallium nitrate, which inhibits bone resoption[32, 33]
- Biphosphonates (etidronate sodium and pamidronate sodium), which inhibit bone resorption[19, 34–36]

Calcitonin, a synthetic polypeptide of 32 amino acids, decreases plasma calcium levels by inhibiting bone resorption.[37] Up to 8 IU/kg given IV, SC, or IM every 12 hours usually produces a partial and mild lowering of the calcium level and helps promote urinary calcium excretion. This agent is nontoxic, well tolerated, and useful in patients with congestive heart failure or renal failure, who cannot tolerate large amounts of intravenous fluids and forced diuresis. The effect is rapid but, unfortunately, transient. Tachyphylaxis may occur with its continued use.

Administered in doses of 25 μg/kg IV over 4 to 12 hours, *plicamycin* lowers serum calcium levels in about 48 hours, and the effect usually lasts 4 to 6 days.[37] This agent's mechanism of action appears to be direct action on osteoclasts with retardation of bone resorption rather than promotion of calciuresis. Reduction of bone resorption occurs without affecting the rate of bone accretion. Most patients achieve normocalcemic status after a single injection. Thrombocytopenia, mild reversible hepatic dysfunction, hemorrhagic diathesis, and nephrotoxicity may all follow the administration of plicamycin, although usually with higher doses and repeated administration.[38] Plicamycin should be used with calcitonin for life-threatening hypercalcemia, because calcitonin, though less effective, has a significantly more rapid onset of action.

Intravenous phosphates lower calcium levels in a dose-dependent manner. They are extremely toxic and are associated with extraskeletal calcification of the lung, kidney, or both.[2, 24] Deaths have been associated with phosphate therapy, which should be used to lower serum calcium levels only when all other therapies either have failed or are contraindicated.

Gallium nitrate inhibits bone resorption and increases the calcium content of bone.[39, 40] Administered at a daily dose of 200 mg/m^2 for 5 days, gallium nitrate lowers serum calcium to normal levels in approximately 85% of cancer patients. This agent is well tolerated and is associated with a decrease in serum concentration of phosphorus. Serum calcium levels decrease dramatically, but symptoms of hypocalcemia usually do not occur. Caution is warranted in patients with preexisting renal disease, because gallium nitrate is a heavy metal. The concomitant use of nephrotoxic agents should be avoided.

Etidronate disodium and *pamidronate disodium,* structural analogs of pyrophosphate, are inhibitors of osteoclastic bone resorption. The principal action of diphosphonates in the treatment of hypercalcemia associated with malignant neoplasms is the reduction of abnormal bone resorption with no direct antineoplastic activity. Etidronate is administered as an infusion of 7.5 mg/kg slowly over 4 to 6 hours for 3 consecutive days. With this regimen, more than 50% of patients obtain normalization of serum calcium levels. Pamidronate, a highly effective second-generation biphosphonate derivative, is administered as a single 60-mg dose over 4 to 6 hours.[41–43] When the corrected serum calcium value exceeds 13.5 mg/dL, the pamidronate dose is increased to 90 mg. A minimum of 7 days should elapse to fully evaluate the effect of pamidronate before retreatment is considered. Most patients given diphosphonates achieve normal corrected serum calcium levels. Special attention must be paid to phosphate levels when biphosphonates are used, because pamidronate is often associated with hypophosphatemia, whereas etidronate usually produces hyperphosphatemia. Biphosphonate treatment is safe and well tolerated as a palliative treatment of osteolytic bone metastases.[44]

Glucocorticoids, although unpredictable, may be of some benefit for the treatment of hypercalcemia in steroid-responsive tumors, such as multiple myeloma and non-Hodgkin's lymphoma. Their mechanism of action is thought to be inhibition of the growth of neoplastic lymphoid tissue. Usually, patients with nonhematologic cancers do not respond to glucocorticoids. Responses to glucocorticoids may take 7 to 14 days, and, therefore, one cannot count on their being useful in acute situations.[10, 24, 45]

No single therapy for acute hypercalcemia can be used in all clinical settings. Treatment has to be tailored for specific patients' needs, with the various causes of hypercalcemia and the urgency of the situation taken into consideration.[46–55]

ACUTE TUMOR LYSIS SYNDROME

Etiology

Renal and metabolic complications may result from the rapid destruction of bulky neoplasms that are highly sensitive to chemotherapy or radiation. Patients at risk for tumor lysis syndrome should be admitted to the ICU for close monitoring and prompt correction of electrolyte abnormalities, such as hyperkalemia, hyperuricemia, hyperphosphatemia, and hypocalcemia, either associated with or without acute renal failure.[56–60] The gravity of complications is related to baseline renal function, the bulk of the tumor, and the rapidity of cell lysis. This syndrome is seen with Burkitt's lymphoma and other lymphomas, in acute and chronic leukemia, and in lung and breast cancer.[58–60] Acute renal failure (ARF) is a consequence of the precipitation of uric acid or calcium phosphate crystals in the renal tubules.[56, 57] If the release of uric acid occurs more slowly, uric acid stones forming in the renal pelvis may lead to ureteral obstruction.

Patients with bulky abdominal disease, markedly elevated plasma lactate dehydrogenase levels, evidence of renal dysfunction, or metabolic alterations require careful monitoring and renal protection during the induction of antineoplastic therapy. Dialysis should be initiated early when metabolic abnormalities or ARF is present.

Release of potassium or phosphates from the destroyed tumor cells can lead to hyperkalemia and hyperphosphatemia. These metabolic disturbances may cause life-threatening arrhythmias and sudden death. Rapid release of intracellular phosphorus results in reciprocal depression of serum calcium and, possibly, metastatic precipitates of calcium phosphate. Hypocalcemia may cause tetany, a prolonged QT interval, and ventricular arrhythmias.

Treatment

Hyperkalemia is treated in standard fashion with glucose, insulin, and exchange resins. When necessary, bicarbonate infusion is given, but alkalosis may further lower ionized calcium levels. The solubility of uric acid in this state increases, as well as the risk for calcium phosphate precipitation.[61–63] Calcium should not be administered unless there is a positive Chvostek or Trousseau sign. Administration of calcium in the presence of an elevated calcium-phosphorus product may produce metastatic calcifications. Hyperphosphatemia usually occurs, and phosphate-binding antacids should be started prior to therapy. Hyperuricemia appears secondary to increased metabolism of purines. Patients might be dehydrated as a result of anorexia, poor oral intake, gastrointestinal symptoms, and insensible losses secondary to fever, further raising the uric acid levels. Uric acid deposition as crystals associated with profound hyperphosphatemia and hypocalcemia, causing intratubular obstruction, is a major pathogenic factor in the renal lesion of tumor lysis.

When tumor lysis is anticipated, predicted potassium, phosphorus, calcium, uric acid, magnesium, arterial pH, creatinine, and blood urea nitrogen (BUN) levels should be measured at least every 6 to 8 hours for the first 72 hours after cancer therapy is started and then twice daily. It remains difficult to predict which patients need close monitoring for possible development of this syndrome, because its occurrence is not confined to one subtype of non-Hodgkin's lymphoma. Only patients with high serum LDH levels were found to be at higher risk in some series.[62, 63]

The clinician's role is to protect the patient against ARF with vigorous hydration and maintenance of a urine output of at least 2 mL/kg/hr. If saline hydration alone does not achieve this goal, an infusion of dopamine, 1.5 μg/kg/min, is useful in initiating and maintaining urine flow.[64] If this is unsuccessful, patients may be given either an intravenous bolus or a continuous infusion of furosemide. Mannitol, at 12.5 g of a 25% solution, can also be used. Mannitol is preferred when intravascular volume is decreased, whereas furosemide is used in patients with normal or elevated intravascular volume. Diuresis can be maintained by continuous infusion of furosemide, 3 to 5 mg/kg/day, or mannitol, 5 g/hr. Urine losses in excess of total volume infused hourly are replaced with dextrose 2.5% with 0.45% saline, allowing for insensible fluid losses. Careful attention to fluid retention, as evidenced by progressive weight gain and accumulation of edema, is mandatory. As with the management of any severe fluid and electrolyte disorder, the clinician may consider the insertion of a flow-directed pulmonary artery catheter to help direct fluid management to maintain the diuresis.[64, 65]

Allopurinol, 10 mg/kg/day PO or IV, is given to control hyperuricemia by decreasing uric acid production. While the patient remains hyperuricemic, the urine pH can be maintained at or greater than 7 with IV sodium bicarbonate to provide maximal solubility of urate. Alkalinization of the urine has its problems, because an alkaline pH, although increasing the solubility of uric acid, also raises the risk for calcium phosphate precipitation.[61-63] Bicarbonate administration can be discontinued when serum uric acid is normalized or when the arterial pH is greater than 7.5. Acetazolamide, 250 mg to 500 mg IV, alkalinizes the urine without administration of bicarbonate.

Hydration remains important in preventing xanthine crystallization and stone formation; xanthine excretion is increased with use of allopurinol.[57] Hypertonic glucose and insulin, administered intravenously, or the initiation of total parenteral nutrition may help control hyperphosphatemia and hyperkalemia. Dialysis should be initiated if oliguria develops or there is significant hyperkalemia or other electrolyte imbalance. Extreme hyperkalemia has been reported in the critically ill patient with this syndrome because of the rapid and unpredictable rate of tumor lysis. Electrolyte abnormalities, especially hyperkalemia, should be aggressively treated with measures aimed at removing potassium from the body, not at shifting it into cells to lower the serum level[66-71] (Table 164-1).

TABLE 164–1. Prevention and Management of the Metabolic Complications of Acute Tumor Lysis

Control of Hyperuricemia
Begin allopurinol
Urine Alkalinization
Maintain urine pH ≥ 7
$NaHCO_3$
Acetazolamide
Discontinue urinary alkalinization once hyperuricemia is corrected or arterial pH > 7.5
Forced Diuresis
Maintain urine flow at 2 ml/kg/hr
Initiate low-dose dopamine and diuretics
Fluid Balance
Avoid fluid overload
Strict records of intake and output
Obtain daily weights
Administer furosemide
Monitoring Blood Components
Serum electrolytes, blood urea nitrogen, creatinine, uric acid, calcium, phosphorus
Magnesium q 6–8 hr during the first 72 hr following chemotherapy
Acute Hyperkalemia
Glucose and insulin infusion
Kayexalate and furosemide when indicated
Hyperphosphatemia
Oral aluminum-containing antacids

OBSTRUCTIVE SYNDROMES: SUPERIOR VENA CAVA OBSTRUCTION

Superior vena cava (SVC) obstruction may be the first presentation of lung carcinoma or lymphoma or may develop in the patient with previously documented neoplastic disease. This clinical presentation is often dramatic and suggests that SVC obstruction is an oncologic emergency; however, this is not a life-threatening event unless there is coexisting airway compromise and respiratory failure.[72-92]

A more complete description of obstructive syndromes is presented in Chapter 163.

NEUROLOGIC SYNDROMES: SPINAL CORD COMPRESSION

Spinal cord compression is a nonfatal yet devastating complication of malignant disease.[93-95] Fifty percent of the cases of metastatic epidural compression in adults arise from breast, lung, or prostate cancer; the other cancers are lymphoma, melanoma, renal cancer, sarcoma, and multiple myeloma.[95-97] Most cases of cord compression are due to epidural metastasis.[98-103] Thoracic compression occurs in 70%, lumbar in 20%, and cervical in 10% of cases.[101] Approximately 10% of cases are caused by direct extension into the intravertebral space of lymphomatous lymph nodes arising within the retroperitoneal space. Intramedullary metastases account for less than 4% of all cases.[103] Vertebral subluxation or spinal subdural hematomas are other causes of cord compression in the cancer patient.[101] The vertebral column, the most common site of skeletal metastasis, is the involved site in 40% of patients who die of cancer.[104, 105]

Pressure on the spinal cord decreases blood supply to the area of compression with resulting edema of the cord, occlusion and stasis of the epidural venous plexus, and ischemia of the neural tissue, leading to neurologic deterioration. Animal models of metastatic epidural compression demonstrated that compression of the vertebral venous plexus causes vasogenic cord edema, venous hemorrhage, loss of myelin, and ischemia.[106, 107]

Diagnosis

Pain, either motor or sensory neurologic symptoms, and bowel or bladder dysfunction may all be associated with epidural spinal cord compression. Symptoms may be present from hours to days to even longer periods before the diagnosis is confirmed by imaging studies.[99] If untreated, this syndrome inexorably progresses to paralysis, sensory loss, and sphincter incontinence. The most important factors determining prognosis are the level of the lesion and the speed of diagnosis and initiation of treatment.

Pain is almost always present. Complaints of localized pain can occasionally be misleading if there is cancerous involvement of other vertebral bodies that produces pain without cord compression. Pain is usually persistent and can worsen with movement, straining, or even coughing. The discomfort is also worse with lying down. Pain is usually in the involved vertebral body. Neck flexion and straight leg raising often reproduce symptoms in the area affected. Bilateral involvement is very common with thoracic disease. The mechanism of the pain may involve stretching or compression of pain-conducting nerve fibers situated in the anterior and posterior spinal ligaments, in the annulus of the intervertebral disk, and in the dura and the apophyseal joints.[99-100] The pain in this syndrome appears first and is usually followed by neurologic deficits. Once a neurologic deficit appears, it can evolve to paraplegia over a time.[95]

Most patients complain of weakness or numbness. On physical examination, more than 80% of patients have demonstrable motor loss, bowel or bladder sphincter deficits, and sensory deficits. Herpes zoster, clinically apparent at the site of extradural compression, has also been described.[99]

The onset of new back pain, even with a normal neurologic examination in any patient with cancer, warrants a radiographic investigation by computed tomography (CT), magnetic resonance imaging (MRI), or myelogram.[103, 105] Radiologic studies of the vertebral bodies demonstrate abnormalities in two thirds of patients with new pain. If the neurologic exam and the radiographs are normal, the clinician may choose careful observation.[101] MRI is the diagnostic imaging of choice because it affords excellent delineation of bone, soft tissue, cord, and tumor. The resolution of tissues by MRI is important in defining radiation port therapy and is especially useful when surgery is planned.

Treatment

A diagnosis of epidural cord compression mandates immediate therapy, particularly in the patient with rapidly evolving neurologic signs. For most patients, corticosteroids and radiation therapy are the mainstays of treatment, but interest is developing again in a surgical solution because of excellent results with anterior decompression. The dosage of dexamethasone, the most common corticosteroid used, remains controversial. Some recommend doses as low as 4 mg four times a day, although laboratory data have shown a dose-related benefit with high-dose dexamethasone. Other workers suggest dexamethasone, 100 mg IV, followed by 24 mg IV every 6 hours for 72 hours, and then tapered over 2 weeks; this regimen offers substantial amelioration of pain for the majority of patients, often within hours.[99, 101, 108] The larger doses are used in patients with profound or rapidly progressive neurologic injury, the lower doses in patients with mild or equivocal signs.[108]

Consultation for external beam radiation therapy to the involved area should be obtained immediately. There appears to be no difference in outcome between radiation therapy alone and combined surgery-radiotherapy. The concept that radiation alone might be the initial treatment for most patients with metastatic cord compression is being accepted.[109-115] Surgery should not be considered in the patient who presents with paraplegia because the outlook for neurologic recovery is dismal. Laminectomy has been associated with an increased morbidity, including spinal instability.[116] When diagnosis is in doubt, the nature of the tumor is unknown, or a bone protrusion is causing the block, surgery is indicated. Relapse after radiation therapy, when no further radiation can be administered, and progression of symptoms despite ongoing irradiation also are indications for surgery, preferably by an anterior approach.[102-116]

Some controversies remain in the treatment of these patients with cancer and spinal cord compression, but neurologic function can be preserved in most patients if the diagnosis is made when the earliest clinical manifestations appear or abnormalities in diagnostic imaging are seen, and especially if treatment is initiated early, before neurologic injury occurs.[108]

PERICARDIAL DISEASES

Malignancy is the most common cause of cardiac tamponade in cancer patients. Cardiac tamponade may also follow constrictive pericarditis induced by inflammatory process or irradiation. Hemopericardium can be seen in patients with thrombocytopenia.

Primary neoplasms of the myocardium and pericardium are uncommon, but metastatic disease to the pericardial space is very common in patients with lung or breast carcinomas, leukemias, and Hodgkin's or non-Hodgkin's lymphoma.[117-121] Malignancy is the cause of approximately 50% of all cases of cardiac tamponade in medical patients. Idiopathic pericarditis, radiation-related pericarditis or subacute effusive constrictive pericarditis, hemorrhagic or purulent pericarditis, and restrictive myopathies must all be considered in the differential diagnosis.[122, 123] Clinical syndromes observed include dysrhythmias, especially supraventricular, pericarditis, and diastolic cardiac failure.

Pericardial effusions may become quite large and may remain relatively hemodynamically asymptomatic; however, the enlarged pericardial sac will eventually compress surrounding structures such as the airway, leading to symptoms such as a cough and dypsnea in most patients. Other symptoms that appear are chest pain, fever, edema, and nonspecific complaints.[124-127] Symptoms of incipient hemodynamic compromise include a sense of fullness in the head and neck, and vague gastrointestinal distress as a result of visceral engorgement. Eventually, signs of more significant hemodynamic impairment ensue, such as tachycardia, narrow pulse pressure, pulsus paradoxicus, and, eventually, systolic hypotension.

Chest radiographs are helpful if an enlarged cardiac silhouette without pulmonary congestion is seen. Because small amounts of pericardial fluid can be hemodynamically very significant, a normal chest radiograph does not rule out the presence of a significant effusion. ECG changes are nonspecific; sinus tachycardia, ST-segment elevation, or electrical alternans may be seen. Echocardiography, which has become the imaging technique of choice, can document pericardial effusions as small as 20 mL. Tamponade is suggested by the findings of right ventricular and atrial compression as well as plethora of the inferior vena cava without fluctuation in size during the respiratory cycle. CT of the chest can detect an effusion as small as 50 mL in the pericardial sac but does not provide hemodynamic information.[128]

Right heart catheterization may reveal elevation and equalization of central pressures. Diagnostically, the most significant echocardiographic findings are right ventricular (RV) diastolic collapse or right atrial (RA) collapse persisting in late systole. Marked increase in respiratory variation of the mitral flow may be detected by Doppler echocardiography. Right-sided heart catheterization shows equalization of RA, RV, and pulmonary artery diastolic pressures at 10 mm Hg or higher. The right atrium tracing shows a prominent x descent (systolic) and decreased y descent (diastolic). The use of esophageal echocardiography may prove with time to assist with diagnosis and treatment.

For management of critical tamponade, a substernal paraxyphoid approach for pericardiocentesis is the procedure of choice.[129-131] Some researchers recommend attaching an ECG lead to the needle to observe a current of injury if the ventricle wall is entered. There are multiple possible ways to effectively drain the pericardial fluid,[124-133] including creation of a window either through a subxiphoid incision, a limited left anterior thoracotomy, or thoracoscopically; catheter drainage under echocardiographic guidance; and, less commonly, percutaneous balloon pericardiostomy, and placement of a pericardial-peritoneal shunt or window.[134-141]

Many workers in this field recommend the creation of a pericardial window either by thoracotomy or by thoracoscopy.[142] Video-assisted thoracoscopy might offer an alternative to anterior thoracotomy for patients whose initial subxiphoid procedure failed, but many questions remain unanswered regarding the best procedure.[142-145] There are now various reports documenting the effectiveness of pericardial window formation by percutaneous balloon pericardiostomy.[146-157] In severely thrombocytopenic patients, pericardiostomy performed in the operating room should be considered.[157, 158]

PULMONARY PROBLEMS

Pulmonary Complications of Chemotherapy

Acute toxicities of anticancer therapies require rapid recognition and treatment and support in an ICU. The management of affected patients has become complex, secondary to the nature of the complications. The use of different support medications, such as granulocyte colony-stimulating factor (G-CSF), have altered the toxicities associated with these agents and allowed the development of different therapeutic approaches for patients with cancer. It is often difficult to ascribe toxicity to a single agent because chemotherapy is usually administered in complex regimens. Many agents have cumulative dosage levels, but idiosyncratic reactions can also occur. The diagnosis of pulmonary drug toxicity is usually a diagnosis of exclusion.[159]

Pulmonary toxicity, both acute and chronic, is seen increasingly with numerous antineoplastic agents.[160] Respiratory failure may manifest as an acute hypersensitivity reaction, as chronic insidious pulmonary fibrosis, and, rarely, as noncardiogenic pulmonary edema.[161] Symptoms can appear immediately or months after termination of therapy, as seen with acute radiation-induced pneumonitis. Synergistic toxicity also occurs (e.g., radiation with bleomycin, 5-fluorouracil with mitomycin, and bleomycin with G-CSF).

Bleomycin

The parenchymal pulmonary damage caused by bleomycin is probably secondary to oxidant-mediated damage to the alveolar and capillary endothelium. Bleomycin causes a spectrum of syndromes, from pneumonitis to chest pain to fibrosis. Patients with a history of bleomycin therapy and respiratory failure should ideally be managed with as low an FIO_2 value as clinically possible, because oxygen is synergistic with bleomycin, worsening toxicity. Mortality from bleomycin pulmonary toxicity ranges from 1% to 7%, patients with pneumonitis or fibrosis having a worse outcome.[162-166]

Mitomycin

Mitomycin in combination with vinca alkaloids has come into wide use in the treatment of ovarian, breast, and small-cell lung cancer. Acute dyspnea associated with hypoxemia and bronchospasm has been reported 1 to 2 hours after administration of the vinca alkaloids. Bilateral rales and wheezing are common. Pulmonary toxicity occurs in up to 12% of patients given this treatment. Additional radiation or combination therapy with other agents can increase the rate of toxicity to around 35%.[164, 167]

An acute dyspnea syndrome can occur in up to 4% of patients; it is characterized by acute dyspnea without cough, chest pain, hemoptysis, and sputum production. Physical examination reveals tachypnea, rales, rhonchi, or wheezing. The chest roentgenogram demonstrates bilateral interstitial infiltrates, and arterial blood gas analysis usually reveals hypoxemia. Symptoms usually resolve within 12 to 24 hours and are treated with supplemental oxygen, bronchodilators, and, occasionally, steroids. If the patients are challenged with this chemotherapeutic agent and the syndrome recurs, both mitomycin and vinblastine therapy must be stopped. About 20% of patients require intubation secondary to severe symptomatology and hypoxemia. The etiology of this acute dyspnea syndrome is unknown.[168]

Pulmonary mitomycin toxicity in rare cases can produce unusual pulmonary reactions that mimic the microangiopathic hemolytic anemia syndrome, hemolytic-uremic syndrome, noncardiogenic pulmonary edema, and pulmonary hemorrhage. The outcome in affected patients is poor, in that over 90% have a fatal outcome.[169, 170]

All-*trans*-Retinoic Acid

All-*trans*-retinoic acid (ATRA) has dramatically changed the therapy of acute promyelocytic leukemia (APL). ATRA is of great interest to intensivists because of the "retinoic acid syndrome." Approximately 25% of patients treated with ATRA have experienced a syndrome characterized by fever, respiratory distress, radiographic pulmonary infiltrates, pleural effusions, and weight gain. The onset of reaction has appeared as early as the second day of treatment and as late as the third week. Clinically, this syndrome resembles a "capillary leak syndrome."

Several patients have experienced progressive hypoxemia, requiring mechanical ventilation with high positive end-expiratory pressure (PEEP) support. Most of the patients have expired with multiple organ failure despite obvious hematologic improvement. The few patients who survived needed prolonged mechanical ventilation, usually 2 to 3 weeks. All patients required invasive hemodynamic monitoring. Autopsy has revealed extensive infiltration of myeloid cells into lungs, skin, kidney, liver, and lymph nodes. Although leukocytosis is commonly observed with this syndrome, the reaction may occur with a normal leukocyte count in up to one third of cases.

The cause of this syndrome is unknown, although several mechanisms have been proposed, including release of vasoactive cytokines, increased expression of adhesion molecules on myeloid cell surfaces, and acquisition of migratory properties by leukemic cells as they undergo differentiation. Early recognition of this syndrome, especially of unexplained dyspnea, weight gain, and fever, is critical; the appearance of these signs should prompt immediate steroid therapy (dexamethasone, 10 mg IV every 12 hours for 3 days). Leukapheresis effectively reduces the peripheral leukocyte count but has not been shown to ameliorate the syndrome.[171-173]

Pulmonary Infections

A chapter on infections in the immunocompromised host is found elsewhere in this book (see Chapter 61); it is worth mentioning here some critical elements of pulmonary infections in patients with cancer. Infections must always be included in the differential diagnosis of respiratory compromise in any patient with cancer.

In neutropenic patients with leukemia who have not received chemotherapy, *Staphylococcus aureus* and *Streptococcus pneumoniae* are the most common cause of pneumonia. Later in the course of chemotherapy, gram-negative bacilli and mixed infections are more common. The longer the patient is neutropenic, the greater the risk of invasive fungal pneumonia, particularly by *Aspergillus*.[173-177]

Cytomegalovirus (CMV) pneumonia is common within patients with T cell defects, especially recipients of bone marrow transplantation. Risk is highest in patients who are CMV-seropositive, who receive CMV seropositive blood products, or who have graft-versus-host disease. CMV pneumonia is usually a reactivation.[178-180]

Pneumocystis carinii pneumonia is a cause of morbidity and death in patients who have malignancy and are immunosupressed.[181, 182]

Pulmonary Hemorrhage

Pulmonary hemorrhage usually manifests as dyspnea, and cough with or without hemoptysis. Thrombocytopenic patients with cancer are especially at risk. Concomitant infection may be present in some cases and may trigger the bleeding. Chest films usually show a fine granular pattern but may also show infiltrates if the patient is severely tachypneic, hypoxemic, and actively coughing and bleeding. The detection of hemosiderin-laden macrophages in the sputum or bronchoalveolar lavage (BAL) specimens indicates that blood has been present in the alveolar spaces long enough for it to have been broken down by alveolar macrophages. Many patients with pulmonary hemorrhage require intubation with mechanical ventilation. Although the disease may be self-limiting in many of the immune-mediated disorders, the syndrome is often fatal in patients with bone marrow transplants and those with hematologic malignancies. Correction of coagulation abnormalities and platelet transfusions are the mainstays of therapy.[183]

Pulmonary Leukostasis

Pulmonary leukostasis occurs because of accumulation of leukemic cells in small arterioles of the lung. This accumulation occurs if white blood cell counts are greater than 100,000 cells/mm^3 in myeloid leukemias, especially chronic myelogenous leukemia (CML) (rarely in lymphoid leukemias). Chest x-ray findings usually show diffuse infiltrates but may be normal. Leukostasis may occur in brain vessels and may cause lethargy, change of mental status, and coma. Arterial blood gas measurements are inaccurate in this condition, because oxygen is metabolized rapidly by the high numbers of leukocytes in the test tube. Pulse oximetry is more accurate and reliable for monitoring oxygen saturation in this situation. Cytoreduction is achieved by either chemotherapy, particularly with hydroxyurea, or a single leukapheresis, which may reduce the white blood cell count by 20% to 60%.[184]

Bronchiolitis Obliterans and Organizing Pneumonia

Bronchiolitis obliterans and organizing pneumonia is a well-described syndrome affecting some patients with cancer. This syndrome is defined in histologic terms as an intraluminal fibrosing lung lesion affecting the distal airways, alveolar ducts, and peribronchial alveolar spaces. This entity has been reported in collagen vascular disorders, after ingestions of toxins, after infection, and specially after bone marrow transplantation.

Patients can present with cough, fever, and dypsnea. Abnormal breath sounds are heard in a majority of patients. Hypoxemia is common in post-transplant patients, because they present with a rapid progressive airflow obstruction. The chest x-ray reveals diffuse peribronchial and interstitial infiltrates with pleural thickening. An open lung biopsy is necessary to make a prompt diagnosis. Corticosteroids and bronchodilators have been used with various degrees of success.[185-188]

CARDIAC TOXICITY

Anthracyclines

Cardiac toxicity is seen with anthracycline antibiotics such as adriamycin. Acute adriamycin toxicity occurs during or after infusion. Long-term administration may be associated with subclinical ventricular dysfunction or overt congestive heart failure (CHF). Acute toxicities of anthracyclines are uncommon but can manifest as ECG abnormalities in up to 40% of the patients and is higher in patients with abnormal pretreatment tracings. Sudden death occurs in 1% of the patients within a few days of administration of this agent. The most common abnormalities appear to be nonspecific ST-T changes, sinus tachycardia, premature atrial and ventricular contractions, and a low-voltage QRS complex. Arrhythmias are usually benign, and ECG changes are self-limited and transient, not requiring discontinuation of the drug.

Myocarditis-pericarditis is another aspect of the toxicity. It seems to occur in younger patients and appears within 3 to 4 days. The clinical course varies from complete recovery to rapid demise. Transient deterioration of left ventricular function usually occurs in older patients after a low cumulative dose and appears within 10 days. The decision to continue treatment should be made on a individual basis.[189, 190] In general, patients who have clinical evidence of cardiac deterioration should not be candidates for further chemotherapy.

Patients with anthracycline-induced cardiomyopathy present clinically as having classic congestive heart failure. Chronic toxicity, presenting as cardiomyopathy, is dose-related myocardial injury and is the most prominent toxic effect. This syndrome has been described in up to 20% of patients receiving around 600 mg/m^2 of doxorubicin.[191] The treatment of these patients is essentially the same as in any cardiomyopathy, that is, manipulation of preload, afterload, and contractility.[192-195]

Bleomycin

Chest pain mimicking myocardial infarction or pulmonary emboli is reported, though rarely, with infusions of bleomycin.[196, 197] Bleomycin has been associated with Raynaud's phenomenon and with coronary atherosclerosis in several young men treated for testicular carcinoma.[198, 199]

5-Fluorouracil

Chest pain with coronary spasm and ischemic changes on ECG progressing to myocardial infarction are seen with continuous infusion of 5-fluorouracil.[198] The myocardial ischemic syndrome has a spectrum of clinical presentation ranging from silent ST-segment changes on ECG to angina and myocardial infarction and even sudden death syndrome. Segmental and global hypokinesia as well as arrhythmias have been observed. Most of the reactions are acute, occurring during infusion or shortly afterward, and are transient.[200, 201] Nitrates and calcium channel blockers have been used as antischemic prophylaxis. Patients rarely experience adverse cardiac effects after the third treatment cycle, suggesting that there is no cumulative effect of this drug.[202-204]

Cyclophosphamide

Cyclophosphamide is ordinarily lethal at doses above 50 to 100 mg/kg, although this amount is routinely administered as preparation for bone marrow transplantation. A potential side effect is a severe hemorrhagic myocarditis.[203] The ventricular dysfunction is significantly worse in patients who have received prior anthracyclines or mediastinal radiation. Adverse reactions range from transient ECG changes with asymptomatic elevations in cardiac enzymes to cases of CHF, pericardial effusion, coronary artery vasculitis, and fatal hemorrhagic myocardial necrosis.[204] Invasive monitoring to optimize hemodynamic function maybe required. Early recognition is paramount in the treatment of this syndrome. Doxorubicin given concomitantly with cyclophosphamide can potentiate the cardiotoxicity of the former.

Interleukin-2

Interleukin-2 (IL-2) is an immunoregulator that initiates proliferation of activated T cells, among other properties. Most of the initial studies reported a significant incidence of cardiovascular complications, such as systemic hypotension and tachycardia. IL-2 has been associated with capillary leak syndrome secondary to increased vascular permeability, which can lead to extravasation and loss of vascular tone. IL-2 can cause hypotension by reducing the systemic vascular resistance. It is also at times associated with cardiac arrhythmias, myocardial depression, pulmonary edema, and pericardial effusion.[205, 206] Medical management of capillary leak syndrome consists of careful hemodynamic monitoring and then use of vasopressors to maintain organ perfusion. Hemodynamic stability returns 48 hours after discontinuation of the drug.

Paclitaxel

Paclitaxel is another chemotherapy agent that has cardiotoxic effects such as hypotension in 25% of subjects and transient bradycardia in up to 12% of patients. Rare cardiac events associated with this agent are myocardial infarction, CHF, atrial fibrillation, and diminished left ventricular ejection fraction.[207, 208] Most of the cardiotoxic reactions to paclitaxel seem to occur within hours of infusion, resolving shortly after the drug is discontinued but recurring if the treatment is reinstituted. The cardiac toxicity does not appear to be cumulative.[209-211]

CENTRAL VENOUS ACCESS INFECTIONS

Long-term use of tunneled Hickman-type cuffed catheters and fully implanted port devices are used for long-term central venous accesses. Infection is common in patients with venous access devices and can be divided into exit site infection, tunnel tract or port pocket infection, and device-related bacteremia or fungemia.

Catheter-related infection occurs five times more often than port infections, with a 12-fold difference when assessed according to incidence of morbidity per device-day. Differences for bacteremia or fungemia are even more dramatic, with a 21-fold difference between catheters and ports on a risk per day basis.[212]

Initial antibiotic therapy for device-related bacteremia or fungemia should be based on knowledge of the patient's host defenses, the presence or absence of neutropenia, and the type of device. The experience at our center is that the majority of cases of catheter-related bacteremia or fungemia can be sterilized with antibiotics without the need to remove the device. Specific predictors of treatment success are not available. Development of one device-related bacteremia cannot predict a second infection, nor does the organism of the first infection help predict the second organism when a second infection occurs. Antibiotic sterilization of ports after diagnosis of device-related bacteremia or fungemia is usually also successful without device removal.

Ports are most often placed in patients with solid tumors, and gram-positive cocci are the predominant pathogens in port pocket infections at our institution. Clinicians should always consider the removal of any device in which there is evidence of septic emboli, refractory hypotension, persistent culture positivity without eradication of infection as evidenced by decreasing serial colony forming units, and when the device is no longer required for therapy. Controversy exists when septicemia is due to *S. aureus* or a fungal infection.

The mechanism of catheter tunnel infection remains uncertain, because it can arise on a catheter segment on either side of the Dacron cuff and need not be associated with septicemia or with exit site infection. The incidence of tunnel infection is low, accounting for less than 2% of all catheter-related infections; however, it can be associated with catastrophic local morbidity or mortality and invariably requires device removal. Port pocket infections, usually caused by gram-positive cocci, suggest direct inoculation or migration of organisms along the accessing needle as the primary mechanism. Regardless of the underlying disease, virtually all port pocket infections have been caused by *S. aureus* and require device removal.[213, 214]

Site infection can range from a small infection easily managed with local care and topical antibiotics to a more aggressive infection with progression to cellulitis, tunnel or pocket infection, and septicemia. Findings of erythema and exudate may be subtle in the neutropenic, immunosuppressed patient. If possible, in patients with port site infections, the Huber point needle should be removed and an intravenous access remote from the site should be established for delivery of antibiotics until all signs of site infection have resolved.

INVASIVE PROCEDURE: IN THE IMMUNOCOMPROMISED AND THROMBOCYTOPENIC PATIENT

A platelet count of 100,000 cells/mm^3 or higher is preferred for the performance of surgical or major invasive procedures. Central venous cannulation and pulmonary artery catheter placement can be performed safely with platelet counts as low as 50,000 cells/mm^3 without platelet transfusion. The nature and the magnitude of complications associated with central venous catheterization are related to the invasiveness of the procedure, the operator's experience, and the patient's clinical condition. Thrombocytopenic patients with cancer present a dilemma for central venous access. Some investigators consider the safest site, with the least potential for bleeding complications, to be a percutaneous approach into the external jugular vein or the anterior cubital fossa, or even the femoral approach. The incidence of contamination is high.

Thrombocytopenia is not an absolute contraindication for any procedure. The complication rate in a study of patients with platelet counts less than 20,000 cells/mm^3 was similar to those in patients with normal platelet counts. In experienced hands, these procedures can be performed with platelet counts less than 20,000 cells/mm^3 with platelet transfusion coverage. Judicious selection of the procedure site and rigid attention to the technical details of the procedure minimize the potential for complications.[215, 216]

References

1. Groeger J, Lemeshow S, Price K, et al: Multi-center outcome study of cancer patients admitted to the the intensive care unit: A probability of mortality model. J Clin Oncol 1998; 16:761-770.
2. Myers WPL: Differential diagnosis of hypercalcemia and cancer. CA 1977; 27:258-272.
3. Nussbaum SR, Zahradnik RJ, Lavigne JR, et al: Highly sensitive two-site immunoradiometric assay of parathyroid, and its clinical utility in evaluating patients with hypercalcemia. Clin Chem 1987; 33:1364-1367.

4. Boyd JC, Ladenson JH: Value of laboratory tests in the differential diagnosis of hypercalcemia. Am J Med 1984; 77:863-872.
5. Broadus A, Mangin M, Ikeda K, et al: Humoral hypercalcemia of cancer: Identification of a novel parathyroid hormone-like peptide. N Engl J Med 1988; 319:556-562.
6. Cogan MG, Covey GM, Arieff AL, et al: Central nervous system manifestations of hyperparathyroidism. Am J Med 1978; 65:963-970.
7. Fisken RA, Health DA, Somers S, et al: Hypercalcemia in hospital patients: Clinical and diagnostic aspects. Lancet 1981; 1:202-207.
8. Kanis JA, Yates AJP, Russell RGG: Hypercalcemia and skeletal complications of myeloma, *In:* Multiple Myeloma and Other Paraproteinaemias. Delamora IW (Ed). Edinburgh, Churchill Livinstone, 1986; pp 307-322.
9. Side L, Fahie-Wilson MN, Mills MJ: Hypercalcemia due to calcium binding IgM paraprotein in Waldenström's macroglobulinaemia. J Clin Pathol 1995; 48:961-962.
10. Steward AF, Horst R, Deftos L, et al: Biochemical evaluation of patients with malignancy-associated hypercalcemia: Evidence for humoral and non humoral groups. N Engl J Med 1980; 330:1377-1386.
11. McDonnell GD, Dunstan CR, Evans RA, et al: Quantitative bone histology in the hypercalcemia of malignant disease. J Clin Endocrinol Metab 1982; 55:1066-1072.
12. Mundy GR: Hypercalcemia of malignancy revisited. J Clin Invest 1988; 82:1-6.
13. Orloff JJ, Wu TL, Stewart AF: Parathyroid hormone-like proteins: Biochemical responses and receptor interactions. Endocr Rev 1989; 10:476-494.
14. Yarbro JW, Bornstein RS (Eds): Oncologic Emergencies. New York, Grune & Stratton, 1981.
15. Attie MF: Treatment of hypercalcemia. Endocrinol Metab Clin North Am 1989; 18:807-828.
16. Leung SC, Rosenblatt M, Nissensoon RA: Parathyroid hormone-like protein from human renal carcinoma cell: Structural and functional homology with parathyroid hormone. J Clin Invest 1987; 80:1803-1807.
17. Mosely JM, Kubota M, Diefenbach-Jagger H, et al: Parathyroid hormone-related protein purified from a human lung cancer cell line. Proc Natl Acad Sci USA 1987; 84:5048-5050.
18. Stewart AF, We T, Goumas D, et al: *N*-Terminal amino acid sequence of two novel tumor-derived adenylate cyclase-stimulating proteins: Identification of parathyroid hormone-like and parathyroid hormone-unlike domains. Biochem Biophys Res Commun 1987; 146:672-678.
19. Mundy GR, Ibbotson KJ, D'Souza SM: Tumor products and the hypercalcemia of malignancy. J Clin Invest 1985; 76:391-394.
20. Nainby-Luxmoore JC, Langford HG, Nelson NC, et al: A case-comparison study of hypertension and hyperparathyroidism. J Clin Endocrinol Metab 1982; 55:303-306.
21. Bilezikian JP: Management of acute hypercalcemia. N Engl J Med 1992; 326:1196-1202.
22. Hoff HE, Smith PK, Winkler W: Electrocardiographic changes and concentrations of calcium in serum following intravenous injection of calcium chloride. Am J Physiol 1938; 125:162-165.
23. Warrell RP Jr, Bockman RS: Metabolic emergencies. *In:* Cancer: Principles and Practice of Oncology. DeVita VTY, Hellman S, Rosenberg SA (Eds). Philadelphia, JB Lippincott, 1989, pp 1986-2003.
24. Gaskin JH: Hypercalcemia in cancer patients (Letter). N Engl J Med 1976; 294(9):500.
25. Kiang DT, Loken MK, Kennedy BJ: Mechanism of the hypocalcemic effect of mithramycin. J Clin Endocrinol Metab 1979; 48:341-344.
26. Stewart AF: Therapy of malignancy-associated hypercalcemia. Am J Med 1983; 74:475-480.
27. Perlia CP, Gubisch NJ, Wolter J, Edelberg D, Dederick MM, Taylor SG: Mithramycin treatment of hypercalcemia. Cancer 1970; 25:389-394.
28. Minkin C: Inhibition of parathyroid hormone stimulated bone resorptionin vitro by the antibiotic mithramycin. Calcif Tissue Res 1973; 25:249-257.
29. Kiang DT, Loken MK, Kennedy BJ: Mechanism of the hypocalcemic effect of mithramycin 1979; 48:341-344.
30. Silva OI, Becker KL: Salmon calcitonin in the treatment of hypercalcemia. Arch Intern Med 1973; 132:337-339.
31. Hoskins DJ, Gilson D: Comparison of the renal and skeletal actions of calcitonin in the treatment of severe hypercalcemia of malignancy. Q J Med 1984; 53:359-368.
32. Warrell RP, Bockman RS, Coonley CJ, Isaacs M, Staszewski H: Gallium nitrate inhibits calcium resorption from bone and is effective treatment for cancer-related hypercalcemia. J Clin Invest 1984; 73:1487-1490.
33. Bockman RS, Boskey AL, Blumenthal NC, Alcock NW, Warrell RP: Gallium increases bone calcium and crystalline perfection of hydroxyapatite. Calcif Tissue Int 1986; 39:376-381.
34. Fitton A, McTavish D: Pamidronate: A review of its pharmacological and therapeutic efficacy in resorptive bone disease. Drugs 1991; 41:289-318.
35. Ritch PS: Treatment of cancer related hypercalcemia. Semin Oncol 1990; 17(Suppl 5):26-33.
36. Jacobs TP, Gordon AC, Silberberg SJ, et al: Neoplastic hypercalcemia: Physiologic response to intravenous etidronate disodium. Am J Med 1987; 82(S2A):42-50.
37. Silva OL, Becker KL: Salmon calcitonin in the treatment of hypercalcemia. Arch Intern Med 1973; 132:337-339.
38. Green L, Donehower RC: Hepatic toxicity of low doses mithramycin in hypercalcemia. Cancer Treat Rep 1984; 68:1379-1381.
39. Warrell RP, Skelos A, Alcock N, et al: Gallium nitrate for acute treatment of cancer related hypercalcemia: Clinicopharmacological and dose response analysis. Cancer Res 1986; 46:4208-4212.
40. Warrell RP, Israel R, Fisone ME, et al: Gallium nitrate for acute treatment of cancer related hypercalcemia: A randomized double-blind comparison to calcitonin. Ann Intern Med 1988; 108:669-674.
41. Glover D, Lipton A, Keller A, et al: Intravenous pamidronate disodium treatment of bone metastases in patients with breast cancer: A dose-seeking remedy. Cancer 1994; 74:2949-2955.
42. Hortobagyi GN, Theriault RL, Porter L, et al: Efficacy of pamidronate in reducing skeletal complications in patients with breast cancer and lytic bone metastases. N Engl J Med 1996; 335:1785-1791.
43. Hasling C, Charles P, Mosekilde L: Etidronate disodium in the management of malignant related hypercalcemia. Am J Med 1987; 82(Suppl 2A):51-54.
44. Kanis JA, Urwin GH, Gray RES, et al: Effects of intravenous etidronate disodium on skeletal and calcium metabolism. Am J Med 1987; 82(Suppl 2A):55-70.
45. Wood AJJ: Management of acute hypercalcemia. N Engl J Med 1992; 326:1156-1203.
46. Mundy GR, Martin TJ: The hypercalcemia of malignancy: Pathogenesis and management. Metabolism 1982; 31:1247-1277.
47. Foster J, Querusio L, Burchard KW, Gann DS: Hypercalcaemia in critically ill patients. Ann Surg 1985; 202:512-518.
48. Lind L, Ljunghall S: Critical care hypercalcaemia a hyperparathyroid state. Expl Clin Endocrinol 1992; 100:148-511.
49. Lord RCC: Critical care hypercalcaemia. Ann Clin Biochem 1997; 34:111-113.
50. Nussbaum S, Zahradnik R, LaVigne J, et al: Highly sensitive two-site immunoradiometric assay of parathyroid hormone and its clinical utility in evaluating patients with hypercalcemia. Clin Chem 1987; 33:1364-1367.
51. Palmer FJ, Nelson JC, Bacchus H: The chloride-phosphate ratio in hypercalcemia. Ann Intern Med 1974; 80:200-204.
52. Rude RK, Sharp CF, Fredericks RS, et al: Urinary and nephrogenous adenosine 3′,5′-monophosphate in the hypercalcemia of malignancy. J Clin Endocrinol Metab 1981; 52:765-771.
53. Aldinger KA, Samaan NA: Hypokalemia with hypercalcemia: Prevalence with significance in treatment. Ann Intern Med 1977; 87:571-573.
54. Di Contanzo F, Gori S, Tonato M, et al: Vindesine and mitomycin C in chemotherapy: Refractory advanced breast cancer. Cancer 1986; 57:904-907.
55. Ralston SH, Patel U, Fraser WD, et al: Comparison of three intravenous biphosphonates in cancer-associated hypercalcemia. Lancet 1989; 2:1180-1182.
56. Flombaum CD: Electrolyte and renal abnormalities. *In:* Critical Care of the Cancer Patient. Groeger JS (Ed). St. Louis, Mosby-Year Book, 1991, p 140.

57. Simpson DP, Wen SF, Chesney RW: Fluid and electrolyte abnormalities due to tumors, their products or metabolites. *In:* Cancer and the Kidney. Rieselbach RE, Garnick MB (Eds). Philadelphia, Lea & Febiger, 1982; pp 534–590.
58. Band PR, Silverberg DS, Henderson JF: Xanthine nephropathy in patients with lymphosarcoma treated with allopurinol. N Engl J Med 1970; 283:354–357.
59. Arseneau JC, Bagley CM, Anderson T, et al: Hyperkalemia, a sequel to chemotherapy of Burkitt's lymphoma. Lancet 1973; 1:10–14.
60. Zusman J, Brown DM, Nesbit ME: Hyperphosphatemia, hyperphosphaturia, and hypocalcemia in acute lymphoblastic leukemia. N Engl J Med 1973; 289:1333–1340.
61. Masera G, Jankovic M: The tumor lysis syndrome: Case report and review of the literature. Ann Oncol 1997; 8:97–100.
62. Hande K, Garrow G: Acute tumor lysis syndrome in patients with high-grade non-Hodgkin lymphoma. Am J Med 1993; 94:133–140.
63. Hoffman V: Tumor lysis syndrome: Implications for nursing. Home Health Nurse 1996; 14:595–600.
64. Parker S, Carlon GC, Isaacs M, et al: Dopamine administration in oliguria and oliguric renal failure. Crit Care Med 1981; 9:630–632.
65. Arrambide K, Toto R: Tumor lysis syndrome. Semin Nephrol 1993; 13:273–279.
66. Lynch RE, Kjellstrand CM, Coccia PF: Renal and metabolic complications of childhood non-Hodgkin's lymphoma. Semin Oncol 1978; 4:325–334.
67. Jones DP, Mahmoud H, Chesney RW: Tumor lysis syndrome: Pathogenesis and management. Pediatr Nephrol 1995; 9:206–212.
68. Razis E, Arlin ZA, Ahmed T, et al: Incidence and treatment of tumor lysis syndrome in patients with acute leukemia. Acta Haematol 1994; 91:171–174.
69. Chasty RC, Liu-Yin JA: Acute tumor lysis syndrome. BJ Hosp Med 1993; 49:488–492.
70. Bilgrami SF, Fallon BG: Tumor lysis syndrome after combination chemotherapy for ovarian cancer. Med Pediatr Oncol 1993; 21:521–524.
71. Haller C, Dhadly M: The tumor lysis syndrome. Ann Intern Med 1991; 114:808–809.
72. Ahman F: A reassessment of the clinical implications of the superior vena caval syndrome. J Clin Oncol 1984; 2:8–12.
73. Yellin A, Rosen A, Reichter N, Liebman Y: Superior vena cava syndrome: The myth—the facts. Am Rev Respir Dis 1990; 141:1114–1118.
74. Abner A: Approach to the patient who presents with superior vena cava obstruction. Chest 1993; 103:394S–397S.
75. Woodyard TC, Mellinger JD, Vann KG, Nisebaum J: Acute superior vena cava syndrome after central venous catheter placement. Cancer 1993; 71:2621–2623.
76. Nishino M, Tanouchi I, Ito T, et al: Echographoic detection of latent severe thrombotic stenosis of the superior vena cava and innominate vein in patients with a pacemaker: Integrated diagnosis using sonography, pulse Doppler and color flow. Pacing Clin Electrphysiol 1997; 20:946–9452.
77. Ito T, Tanouchi J, Kawabata M, et al: Superior vena cava syndrome due to a permanent transvenous pacing lead. Jpn Circ J 1996; 60:707–709.
78. Kim HJ, Kim HS, Chung SH: CT diagnosis of superior vena cava syndrome: Importance of collateral vessels. AJR Am J Roentgenol 1993; 161:539–542.
79. Martionoli C, Cittadini G, Gandolfo N, Crespi G, De Caro G, Derchi LE: Superior vena cava stents: Doppler US of the internal mammary veins to detect collateral flow-preliminary observations. Radiology 1997; 20:865–870.
80. Kishio K, Sonomura T, Mitsuzane K, et al: Self-expandable metallic stent therapy for superior vena cava syndrome: Clinical observations. Radiology 1993; 189:531–535.
81. Shepherd FA: Intrathoracic complications of malignancy and its treatment. Curr Opin Oncol 1995; 7:150–157.
82. Ostler PJ, Clarke DP, Watkinson AF, Gaze MN: Superior vena cava obstruction: A modern management strategy: Clin Oncol 1997; 9:83–89.
83. Ez CA, Presant BJ, et al: Superior vena cava syndrome. *In:* Oncologic Emergencies. Yabro JW, Bornstein RS (Eds). New York, Grune & Stratton, 1981, pp 43–72.
84. Strong EW: Head and neck emergencies. Life threatening emergencies in the cancer patient. Part II. Curr Probl Cancer 1979; 4:36–41.
85. Turner MO, Patel A, Ginsburg S, FitzGerald JM: Bronchodilator delivery in acute airflow obstruction: A meta-analysis. Arch Intern Med 1997; 157:1734–1744.
86. Adolph MD, Oliver AM, Dejak T: Death following adult respiratory distress syndrome and multiorgan failure following acute upper airway obstruction. Ear Nose Throat J 1994; 73:324–327.
87. Hosai SA, Fisher JA, Freeman JL: Mediastinal obstruction of the trachea. J Otolaryngol 1995; 24:139–142.
88. DeVane GG: Acute postoperative pulmonary edema. CRNA 1995; 6:110–113.
89. Guffin TN, Har-el G, Sanders A, Lucente FE, Nash M: Acute postobstructive pulmonary edema. Otolaryngology 1995; 122:235–237.
90. Ninane V: Endoscopic management of acute respiratory failure related to tracheobronchial malignancies. Support Care Cancer 1995; 3:418–421.
91. Courey MS: Airway obstruction. The problem and its causes. Otolaryngol Clin North Am 1995; 28:673–684.
92. Hosal SA, Fisher JA, Freeman JL: Mediastinal obstruction of the trachea. J Otolaryngol 1995; 24:139–142.
93. Lewis DW, Packer RJ, Raney B, Rak IW, Belasco J, Lange B: Incidence, presentation and outcome of spinal cord disease in children with systemic cancer. Pediatrics 1986; 78:438–443.
94. Kim RY, Spencer SA, Meredith RF, et al: Extradural spinal cord compression: Analysis of factors determining functional prognosis-prospective study. Radiology 1990; 176:279–282.
95. Gilbert RW, Kim JH, Posner JB: Epidural spinal cord compression from metastatic tumor: Diagnosis and treatment. Ann Neurol 1978; 3:40–51.
96. Constans JP, de Divitilis E, Donzelli R, Spaziate R, Mader JF, Haye C: Spinal metastases with neurological manifestations: Review of 600 cases. J Neurosurg 1983; 59:111–118.
97. Stark RJ, Henson RA, Evans S: Spinal metastases: A retrospective from a general hospital. Brain 1982; 105:189–213.
98. Barr LR, Nealon N: Neurologic complications. *In:* Critical Care of the Cancer Patient. Groeger JS (Ed). St. Louis, Mosby-Year Book 1991, pp 226–235.
99. Gilbert RW, Kim JH, Posner JB: Epidural spinal cord compression from metastatic tumor: Diagnosis and treatment. Ann Neurol 1978; 3:40.
100. Greenberg HS, Kin JH, Posner JB: Epidural spinal cord compression from metastatic tumor: Results with a new treatment protocol. Ann Neurol 1980; 8:361.
101. Rodichok L, Harper GR, Ruckdeschell JC, et al: Early diagnosis of spinal epidural metastasis. Am J Med 1981; 70(6):1181–1188.
102. Siegel T, Siegal T, Robin G, et al: Anterior decompression of the spine for metastatic epidural compression: A promising avenue of therapy? Ann Neurol 1982; 11:28.
103. Edelson RN, Chernik NL, Posner JB: Spinal subdural hematomas complicating lumbar puncture. Arch Neurol 1974; 31:134.
104. Ruff RL, Lanaka DJ: Epidural metastases in prospectively evaluated veterans with cancer and back pain. Cancer 1989; 63:2234–2241.
105. O'Rourke, George CB, Redmond J, et al: Spinal computed tomography and computed tomographic matrizamide myelography in the early diagnoses of metastatic disease. J Clin Oncol 1986; 4:576–583.
106. Manabe S, Tanaka H, Higo Y, Park P, Ohno T, Tateishi A: Experimental analysis of the spinal cord compressed by spinal metastases. Spine 1989; 14:1308–1315.
107. Kato A, Ushio Y, Hayakawa T, Yamada K, Ikeda H, Mogami H: Circulation disturbances of the spinal cord with epidural neoplasm in rats. J Neurosurg 1985; 63:260–265.
108. Byrne T: Spinal cord compression from epidural metastases. N Engl J Med 1992; 614–619.
109. Maranzano E, Latini P, Perrucci E, Beneventi S, Lupattelli M, Corga E: Short course radiotherapy (8Gy ×2) in metastatic spinal cord compression: An effective and feasible treatment. Int J Radiat Oncol Biol Phys 1997; 38:1037–1044.
110. Maranzano E, Latini P: Effectiveness of radiation therapy without

surgery in metastatic spinal cord compression: Final results from a prospective trial. Int J Radiat Oncol Biol Phys 1995; 32:959-967.
111. Siegel T, Siegal T: Current considerations in the management of neoplastic spinal cord compression. Spine 1989; 14:223-228.
112. Bates T: A review of local radiotherapy in the treatment of bone metastases and cord compression. Int J Radiat Oncol Biol Phys 1992; 23:217-221.
113. Hill M, Richards M, Gregory W, Smith P, Rubens R: Spinal cord compression in breast cancer: A review of 70 cases. Br J Cancer 1993; 68:969-973.
114. Koehler P: Use of corticosteroids in neuro-oncology. Anticancer Drugs 1995; 1:19-33.
115. Sorensen S, Helweg-Larsen S, Mouridsen H, Hansen H: Effect of high dose dexamethasone in carcinomatous metastatic spinal cord compression treated with radiotherapy: A randomized trial. Eur J Cancer 1994; 30:22-27.
116. Gokaslan Z: Spine surgery for cancer. Current Opi Oncol 1996; 8:178-181.
117. Pierri MK: Heart disease. *In:* Critical Care of the Cancer Patient. Groeger JS (Ed). St. Louis, Mosby-Year Book, 1991, pp 64-85.
118. Griffiths GC: A review of primary tumors of the heart. Prog Cardiovasc Dis 1965; 7:465-469.
119. Berge T, Sievers J: Myocardial metastases: A pathological and electrocardiographic study. Br Heart J 1986; 30:383-390.
120. Goodwin JF: Symposium on cardiac tumors: Introduction: The spectrum of cardiac tumors. Am J Cardiol 1968; 21:307-313.
121. Theologides A: Neoplastic cardiac tamponade. Semin Oncol 1958; 5:181-192.
122. Hancock EW: Subacute effusive-constrictive pericarditis. Circulation 1971; 43:183-192.
123. Brosius FC, Waller BF, Roberts WC: Radiation heart disease: Analysis of 16 young (aged 15-32 years) necropsy patients who received over 3,500 rads to the heart. Am J Med 1981; 70:519-530.
124. Vaitkus PT, Howard C, Herrman HC, Martin M, Le Winter MM: Treatment of malignant pericardial effusion. JAMA 1994; 272:59-64.
125. Laham RJ, Cohen DJ, Simons M: Pericardial effusion in patients with cancer. J Am Coll Cardiol 1994; 21:275A.
126. Fincher RE: Malignant pericardial effusion as the initial manifestation of malignancy. Am J Med Sci 1993; 305:106-110.
127. Okamoto H, Shinkai J, Yamakido M, Saijo N: Cardiac tamponade caused by primary lung cancer and the management of pericardial effusion. Cancer 1993; 71:93-98.
128. Chong HH, Plotnick GD: Pericardial effusion and tamponade: Evaluation, imaging, modalities and management. Compr Ther 1995; 21:378-385.
129. Vora AM, Lokhandwala YY, Kale PA: Echocardiography guided creation of ballon pericardial window. Catheter Diagn 1992; 25:164-165.
130. Mack MJ, Aronoff RJ, Acuff TE, Douthit MB, Bowman RT, Ryan WH: Present role of thoracoscopy in the diagnosis and treatment of disease of the chest. Ann Thorac Surg 1992; 54:403-409.
131. Sastic JW, Stalter KD, Goddard RL: Laparoscopic pericardial window. J Laparoendosc Surg 1992; 2:263-266.
132. Naunheim KS, Kesler KA, Fiore AC, et al: Pericardial drainage. Eur J Cardiothorac Surg 1991; 5:99-104.
133. Park JS, Restschler R, Wilbur D: Surgical management of pericardial effusion in patients with malignancies. Cancer 1991; 67:76-80.
134. Moores DW, Allen KB, Faber LP, et al: Subxiphoid pericardial drainage for pericardial tamponade. J Thorac Cardiovasc Surg 1995; 109:546-551.
135. Liu HP, Chang CH, Lin PJ, Hsieh HC, Chang JP, Hsieh MJ: Thorascopic management of effusive pericardial disease: Indications and technique. Ann Thorac Surg 1994; 58:1695-1697.
136. Hingorani AD, Bloomberg TJ: Ultrasound-guided pigtail catheter drainage of malignant pericardial effusions. Clin Radiol 1995; 50:15-19.
137. DiSegni E, Lavee J, Kaplinsky E, Vered Z: Percutaneous balloon pericardiostomy for treatment of cardiac tamponade. Eur Heart J 1995; 16:184-187.
138. Ziskind AA, Pearce AC, Lemmon CC, et al: Percutaneous balloon pericardiotomy for the treatment of cardiac tamponade and large pericardial effusions: Description of technique and report of the first 50 cases. J Am Coll Cardiol 1993; 21:1-5.
139. Rabinovic R, Szewczyk D, Ovadia P, Greenspan JR, Sivalingam JJ: Candida pericarditis: Clinical profile and treatment. Ann Thorac Surg 1997; 63:1200-1204.
140. Wang N, Feikes JR, Mogansen T, Vyhmeister EE, Bailey LL: Pericardioperitoneal shunt: Alternative treatment for malignant pericardial effusion. Ann Thorac Surg 1994; 57:289-292.
141. Olson JE, Ryan MB, Blumenstock DA: Eleven years' experience with pericardial-peritoneal window in the management of malignant and benign pericardial effusions. Ann Surg Oncol 1995; 2:165-169.
142. Moores DWO, Dziuban SW: Pericardial drainage procedures. Chest Surg Clin North Am 1995; 5:359-373.
143. Kasana M, Fiocco M: Thorascopic pericardiectomy. Surg Laparosc Endosc 1995; 5:202-204.
144. Frank MW, Prystowsky J, Soper W: Laparoscopic pericardiotomy, biopsy, and external drainage. J Laparoendosc Surg 1995; 5:113-117.
145. Yim A, Ho J: Video-assisted subxyphoid pericardiectomy. J Laparosc Surg 1995; 5:193-198.
146. Vassilopoulos PP, Nikolaidis K, Filopoulos E, Griniatosos J, Efremidou A: Subxyphoidal pericardial window in the management of malignant pericardial effusion. Eur J Surg Oncol 1995; 21:545-547.
147. Law DA, Haque R, Jain A: Percutaneous balloon pericardiotomy: Non-surgical treatment for patients with cardiac tamponade. W V Med J 1997; 93:310-312.
148. Kouvaras G, Polydorou A, Hatziantoniou G: Percutaneous balloon pericardiotomy for management of cardiac tamponade in a patient with lung cancer and large pericardial effusion. Acta Cardiol 1994; 49:549-553.
149. Di Segni E, Lavee J, Kaplinsky E, Vered Z: Percutaneous balloon pericardiostomy for treatment of cardiac tamponade. Eur Heart J 1995; 16:184-187.
150. Galli M, Politi A, Pedretti F, Castiglioni E, Zerboni S: Percutaneous balloon pericardiotomy for malignant pericardial tamponade. Chest 1995; 108:1499-1501.
151. Maher EA, Shepherd FA, Todd TJR: Pericardial sclerosis as the primary management of malignant pericardial effusion and cardiac tamponade. J Thorac Cardiovasc Surg 1996; 112:673-643.
152. Liu G, Crump M, Goss P, Dancey J, Shepherd F: A prospective comparison of the sclerosing agents doxycycline and bleomycin for the primary management of malignant pericardial effusion and cardiac tamponade. J Clin Oncol 1996; 14:3141-3147.
153. Lin MT, Yang PC, Luh KT: Constrictive pericarditis after sclerosing therapy with mitomycin for malignant pericardial effusion: Report of a case. J Formos Med Assoc 1994; 93:250-252.
154. Downey RJ, Bessler M, Weissman C: Acute pulmonary edema following pericardiocentesis for chronic cardiac tamponade secondary to trauma. Crit Care Med 1991; 19:1323-1325.
155. Downey RJ, Keefe D, Groeger J, JS, Desiderio D: Correlation of echocardiographic, cytologic, and histologic findings of pericardial effusions in patients with malignancy. Chest 1995; 108:150S.
156. Cooper JP, Oliver RM, Currie P, Walker JM, Swanton RH: How do the clinical findings in patients with pericardial effusions influence the success of aspiration? Br Heart J 1995; 73:351-354.
157. Shepherd F: Malignant pericardial effusion. Curr Op Oncol 1997; 9:170-174.
158. Ball JB, Morrison WL: Cardiac tamponade. Postgrad Med J 1997; 73:141-145.
159. Zitnik R: Drug-induced lung disease: Cancer chemotherapy agents. J Respir Dis 1995; 16:855-865.
160. White DA, Orenstein M, Godwin TA, et al: Chemotherapy-associated pulmonary toxic reactions during treatment of breast cancer. Arch Intern Med 1984; 144:953-956.
161. Cooper JA Jr, White DA, Matthay RA: Drug-induced pulmonary disease: State of art. Am Rev Respir Dis 1986; 133:321-340.
162. Goldiner PL, Carlon GC, Cvitkovic E, et al: Factors influencing post-operative morbidity and mortality in patients treated with bleomycin. Br Med J 1978; 1:1664-1667.
163. Jules-Elysee K, White DA: Bleomycin-induced pulmonary toxicity. Clin Chest Med 1990; 11:1-20.
164. Kriesman H, Wolkove N: Pulmonary toxicity of antineoplastic therapy. Semin Oncol 1992; 19:508-520.

165. Van Barnevel PWC, Sleijfer DT, van der Mark TW, et al: Natural course of bleomycin-induced pneumonitis. Am Rev Respir Dis 1987; 135:48–51.
166. Lei KIK, Leung WT, Johnsen PJ: Serious complications in patients receiving recombinant G-CSF factor during BACOP chemotherapy for aggressive non-Hodgkin's lymphoma. Br J Cancer 1994; 70:1009–1013.
167. Twohig KJ, Matthay RA: Pulmonary effects of cytotoxic agents other than bleomycin. Clin Chest Med 1990; 11:31–54.
168. Pisters K, Rivera P, Kris M: Acute toxicities of cancer therapy. *In:* Critical Care of the Cancer Patient. Groeger JS (Ed). St. Louis, Mosby-Year Book, 1991.
169. Torra R, Poch E, Torras A, et al: Pulmonary hemorrhage as a clinical manifestation of hemolytic-uremic syndrome associated with mitomycin C therapy. Chemotherapy 1993; 39:453–456.
170. Rivera MP, Kris MG, Gralla RJ, et al: Syndrome of acute dyspnea related to combined mitomycin plus vinca alkaloid chemotherapy. Am J Oncol 1995; 18:245–250.
171. Frankel SR, Eardley A, Lauwers G, Weiss M, Warrell R: The retinoic acid syndrome in acute promyelocytic leukemia. Ann Intern Med 1992; 117:292–296.
172. Warrell RP, Frankel SR, Miller WH, et al: Differentiation therapy of acute promyelocytic leukemia with tretinoin (all-*trans* retinoic acid). N Engl J Med 1991; 324:1385–1393.
173. Wiley IS, Firkin FC. Reduction of pulmonary toxicity by prednisolone prophylaxis during all-*trans* retinoic acid treatment of acute promyelocytic leukemia. Leukemia 1996; 9:774–778.
174. Benezra D, Kiehn TE, Gold J, et al: Prospective study of infections in indwelling central venous catheters using quantative blood cultures. Am J Med 1988; 85:495–498.
175. Hughes WT, Armstrong O, Bodey OP, et al: Guidelines for the use of use of antimicrobial agents in neutropenic patients with unexplained fever. J Infect Dis 1990; 161:381–396.
176. Pizzo PA: Management of fever in patients with cancer and treatment induced neutropenia. N Engl J Med 1993; 328:1323–1332.
177. Sugar AL: Empiric treatment of fungal infection in the neutropenic host. Arch Intern Med 1990; 150:2258–2264.
178. Chan CK, Hyland RH, Hutcheon MA: Pulmonary complications following bone marrow transplantation. Clin Chest Med 1990; 11:323–332.
179. Emanuel D, Cunningham L, Jules-Elysee K, et al: CMV pneumonia after BMT successfully treated with the combination of ganciclovir and high dose intravenous immune globulin. Ann Intern Med 1988; 109:777–782.
180. Sing Ming C, Chan C, Kasupski G, Chamberlain D, Fyles G, Messner H: Long term sequelae after recovery from CMV pneumonia in allogenic BMT recipients. Chest 1992; 101:1000–1004.
181. Stover D, Greeno R, Gagliardi A: The use of a simple exercise test for the diagnosis of PCP in patients with AIDS. Am Rev Respir Dis 1989; 139:1343–1346.
182. Stover DE, White DA, Romano PA, Gellen RA, Robeson WA: Spectrum of pulmonary disease associated with the acquired immune deficiency syndrome. Am J Med 1985; 78:429–37.
183. Dalen JE, Haffajee CI, Alpert JS, Howe JP, Ockene IS, Paraskos JA: Pulmonary embolism, pulmonary hemorrhage and pulmonary infarction. N Engl J Med 1977; 296:1431–1435.
184. de Fiter, Schuur J, Potter BJ, Kingman WP, Schweitzer MJ: Acute cardiorespiratory failure as presenting symptom of chronic lymphocytic leukemia. N J Med 1996; 49:33–37.
185. Izumi T, Kitaichi M, Nishimura K, Nagai S: Bronchiolitis obliterans and organizing pneumonia. Chest 1992; 102:715–719.
186. King T: Bronchiolitis obliterans: Keys to diagnosis and management. Immunol Allergy Pract 1989; 472:17–23.
187. Epler G, Colby T, McLoud T, Carrington C, Gaensler E: Bronchiolitis obliterans organizing pneumonia. N Engl J Med 1985; 312:152–8.
188. Colby TV: Pathologic aspects of bronchiolitis obliterans organizing pneumonia. Chest 1992; 102:38S–43S.
189. Lipshultz SE, Lipsitz SR, Mone SM, et al: Female sex and higher drug dose as a risk factors for late cardiotoxicity effects of doxorubicin therapy for childhood cancer. N Engl J Med 1995; 332:1738–1743.
190. Young RC, Ozols RF, Myers CE: The anthracycline antineoplastic drugs. N Engl J Med 1981; 305:159–163.
191. Praga C, Beretta G, Vigo PI, et al: Adriamycin cardiotoxicity: A survey of 1273 patients. Cancer Treat Rep 1979; 63:827–834.
192. Moreg JS, Oylon DJ: Outcome of clinical congestive heart failure induced by anthracycline chemotherapy. Cancer 1992; 70:637–641.
193. Von Hoff DD, Layard MW, Basa P, et al: Risk factors for doxorubicin induced congestive heart failure. Ann Intern Med 1979; 91:710–717.
194. Basser RL, Green MD: Complications of treatment: Strategies for prevention of anthracycline cardiotoxicity. Cancer Treat Rev 1993; 19:57–77.
195. Lipshultz SE, Colan SD, Gelberg RD, et al: Late cardiac effect of doxorubicin therapy for acute lymphoblastic leukemia in childhood. N Engl J Med 1991; 82:1109–1115.
196. LaBianca R, Beretta G, Clerici M, et al: Cardiac toxicity of 5-FU: A study on 1083 patients. Tumori 1982; 68:505–510.
197. White DA, Schwartzberg LS, Kris MG, et al: Acute chest pain syndrome during bleomycin infusions. Cancer 1987; 59:1582–1585.
198. Gottdiener JS, Mathisen DJ, Borer JS, et al: Doxorubicin cardiotoxicity: Assessment of late left ventricular dysfunction by radionuclide cineangiography. Ann Intern Med 1981; 94:430–435.
199. Malcom D: Bleomycin induced injury to the hands. J Med Soc N J 1978; 75:314–316.
200. Edwards GS: Long-term treatment with *cis*-dichlorodiamine-platinum-vinblastine-bleomycin: Possible association with severe coronary artery disease. Cancer Treat Rep 1979; 63:551–552.
201. Akhtar SS, Salim KP, Bano ZA: Symptomatic cardiotoxicity with high dose 5-fluorouracil infusion: A prospective study. Oncology 1993; 50:441–444.
202. Keefe DL, Roistacher N, Pierri MK: Clinical cardiotoxicity of 5-fluorouracil. J Clin Pharmacol 1993; 33:1060–1070.
203. Mills BA, Roberts RW: Cyclophosphamide-induced cardiomyopathy. Cancer 1979; 43:2223–2226.
204. Braveman AC, Antin JH, Plappert MT, et al: Cyclophosphamide: New dosing regimens. J Clin Oncol 1991; 9:1215–1223.
205. Du Bois JS, Udelson JE, Atkins MB: Severe reversible global and regionalventricular dysfunction associated with high-dose interleukin-2 immunotherapy. J Immunol 1995; 18:119–123.
206. Rosenberg SA, Lotze MT, Muul LM, et al: Observations on the systemic administration of autologous lymphokine-activated killer cells and recombinant interleukin-2 to patients with metastatic cancer. N Engl J Med 1985; 313:1485–1492.
207. Kenyon J (Ed): Paclitaxel: A promising addition to the antineoplastic armamentarium. Drugs Ther Perspect Rational Drug Sel Use 1995; 5:1–5.
208. Eisenhauer EA, ten Bokkel Huinink WW, Swenerton KD, et al: European-Canadian randomized trial of paclitaxel in relapsed ovarian cancer: High dose vs low-dose and long vs short infusion. J Clin Oncol 1994; 12:2654–666.
209. Gottdiener JS, Aplebaum FR, Ferrans J, et al: Radiation-induced cardiac disease. Am Heart J 1995; 129:1193–1196.
210. Applefeld MM, Slawson RG, Hall-Craigs M, et al: Delayed pericardial disease after radiotherapy. Am J Cardiol 1981; 47:210–213.
211. Gottdiener JS, Katin MJ, Borer JS, Bacharach SL, Green MV: Late cardiac effects of therapeutic mediastinal irradiation: Assessment by echocardiography and radionucleotide angiography. New Engl J Med 1983; 308:569–572.
212. Groeger J, Lucas A, Thaler H: Infectious morbidity associated with long-term use of venous access devices in patients with cancer. Ann Intern Med 1993; 119:1168–1174.
213. Coit DG, Turnbull AD: A safe technique for placement of implantable access devices in patients with thrombocytopenia. Surg Gynecol Obstet 1988; 167:420–431.
214. Hagely MT, Martin B, Traeger S: Infectious and mechanical complications of central venous catheters placed by percutaneous venipuncture and over a guide wire. Crit Care Med 1992; 20:1426–1430.
215. Barrera R, Mina B, Huang Y, Groeger J: Acute complications of central line placement in profoundly thrombocytopenic cancer patients. Cancer 1996; 78:2025–2030.
216. Foster PF, Moore LR, Sankary HN, Ashman MK, Williams JW: Central venous catheterization in patients with coagulopathy. Arch Surg 1992; 127:273–275.

165

Neuropathophysiology

W. Andrew Kofke, MD, FCCM

Neural function is essential to human existence. Thus, loss of any neural element in the course of a critical illness represents a major loss. Neurons or supporting elements may be lost in a small, virtually unnoticeable manner, or there may be widespread selective neuronal loss or tissue infarction. Based on the notion that neural function is the essence of acceptable survival from critical illness, it is crucial for critical care management to include consideration of neural viability and of the impact on the nervous system and interactions of the primary diseases and therapeutics.

There are numerous clinical scenarios wherein a critically ill patient may present with a primary neurologic illness. In a general sense, these scenarios often involve ischemia, trauma, or neuroexcitation. In the potential progression to brain death, each of these may include a period of decreased cerebral perfusion pressure (CPP), usually due to elevated intracranial pressure (ICP), eventually compromising cerebral blood flow (CBF) sufficiently to produce permanent neuronal loss and whole brain death. In the process, a variety of biochemical pathways play major roles. There are several such distinct yet interrelated pathways that ultimately produce neuronal death. In this chapter, I review these concepts, moving from adverse biochemical or genetic processes, physiologic factors, and ICP considerations to clinical scenarios.

BIOCHEMICAL PATHWAYS: INFARCT VERSUS SELECTIVE CELL LOSS WITH ISCHEMIA

Generally, the progression to brain death includes a period of cerebral ischemia. Indeed, cerebral ischemia is a major contributor to permanent neuronal loss, regardless of the original presenting problem. Ischemia produces many pathophysiologic responses (Fig. 165-1), which lead to combinations of:

1. *Cell and tissue edema.* Edema arises from increases in intracellular osmoles (including sodium and other factors) producing water shifts into the cell.[1] This cell edema presumably compromises regional perfusion, worsening the ischemia. Moreover, edema can occur in the interstitium (vasogenic edema) with breakdown of the blood-brain barrier, and the vasculature promotes movement of fluid from the vasculature into the tissue,[1] further compromising regional perfusion.

2. *Activation of acute autolytic processes.* Although the biochemical response to decreased energy supply is described later in more detail, in summary the increase in inappropriate second messengers, most notably calcium, produces a response to activate biochemical processes that lead to cell death. A major factor in this process is decreased pH,[2,3] which is associated with relatively rapid *tissue necrosis,* including many neural cell elements. In addition, release of excitatory amino acids[4] contributes to both tissue necrosis and selective cell loss in the brain after ischemic insults.

3. *Apoptosis.* Apoptosis is a genetically programmed function to ensure the appropriate numbers of cells in the brain and is an important process in normal development.[5] However, in addition to acute destructive processes due to other mechanisms, apoptosis clearly plays a role in the pathologic response to brain injury. Even with apparently satisfactory return of blood flow and energy supply, without immediate structural damage, cell death can occur several days later. Apoptosis is thought to contribute to this delayed lesional maturation through linkage to adverse genetic processes related to activation of "suicide" genes in cells. This is generally associated with *selective cell loss.*[6] Free radicals and other mediators are thought to be important contributors to this process.[7]

4. *Inflammation.* Hematogenous inflammatory cells are constantly present in the blood, perfusing all tissues. Such cells may cross the blood-brain barrier and may be activated to induce an inflammatory response in the central nervous system (CNS). This response includes proinflammatory cytokines with up-regulation of endothelial adhesion molecules and production locally of cytokines, which may further exacerbate the process by locally increasing the number of inflammatory cells and their mediators.[8]

Data from animal models of ischemia have provided some insight into the pathogenesis of neuronal death due to cerebral ischemia. The primary event is energy failure. With total cessation of brain blood flow, normal subjects lose consciousness within 7 seconds, and electroencephalographic (EEG) activity ceases by 10 seconds.[9] In canine models, brain adenosine triphosphate (ATP) is depleted to less than 20% of baseline amount at 5 minutes of no blood flow.[10]

Recirculation after ischemic periods as long as 60 minutes in animal models is associated with return of brain high-energy phosphates to greater than 90% of baseline values; however, this restoration of energy metabolism does not correlate with functional recovery.[11] Such observations led to a search for other causes of neurologic deficit after cerebral ischemia.

Pathologic studies have indicated a heterogeneous susceptibility among neurons to ischemia-mediated death. Selectively vulnerable neurons have been identified, and in rodents a hierarchy of vulnerability among neuron types has been reported. Furthermore, the observation that neurons die hours to days after the ischemic insult, has inspired the concept of delayed maturation of a lesion, possibly with postischemic continuation of potentially reversible pathophysiologic processes.[12,13] Subsequent reports have indicated that ischemia-susceptible neurons are innervated by dopaminergic or glutamatergic (excitatory) fibers.[14,15] Such observations clearly suggest a relationship between glutamate-mediated synaptic transmission and postischemic neuronal death.

Ischemia is associated with a massive increase in extracellular levels of excitatory neurotransmitters (Fig. 165-2).[4] The most injurious are thought to be dicarboxylic amino acids such as glutamate; however, other neurotransmitters may also play a role.[14,15] Neurotransmitter release stimulates metabotropic G protein–coupled receptors[16] and agonist-gated ionotropic receptors (Fig. 165-3).[17] Metabotropic receptors activate phospholipase C, which results in production of phospholipid-derived second messengers, inositol 1,4,5-triphosphate (IP_3) and diacylglycerol (DAG).[18] DAG stimulates protein kinase C (PKC)[19] and IP_3,[20] leading to a further increase in intracellular calcium from intracellular stores (ryanodine receptors on endoplasmic reticulum play a role here).[21]

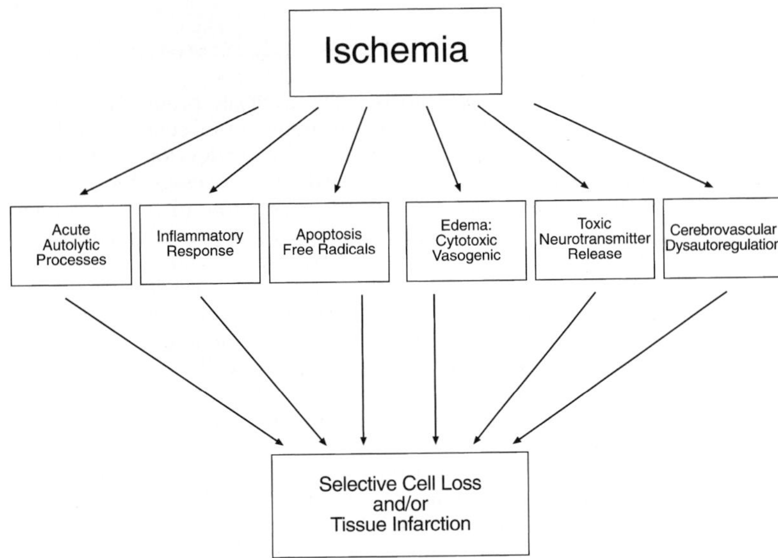

Figure 165–1. Multiple events occur consequent to an ischemic insult. The specific events occurring and the final outcome will vary according to the duration and depth of ischemia. Many processes continue after ischemia has been resolved.

"Ionotropic" receptors[17] permit sodium and calcium influx, which can promote cell swelling. Thus, massive increases in intracellular calcium occur that are due to both exogenous and endogenous entry (e.g., from endoplasmic reticulum). This allows activation of calcium-dependent protein kinase[22] and a variety of other enzyme systems that cause a cellular response, including alterations in gene expression.[23] This gene expression can take hours to arise and likely accounts for the delay in observable injury in particularly vulnerable neurons.[12, 13, 24] If the severity of the ischemia is substantial enough in terms of duration or decrement in blood flow, however, the cells will simply die acutely, with maturation becoming irrelevant.

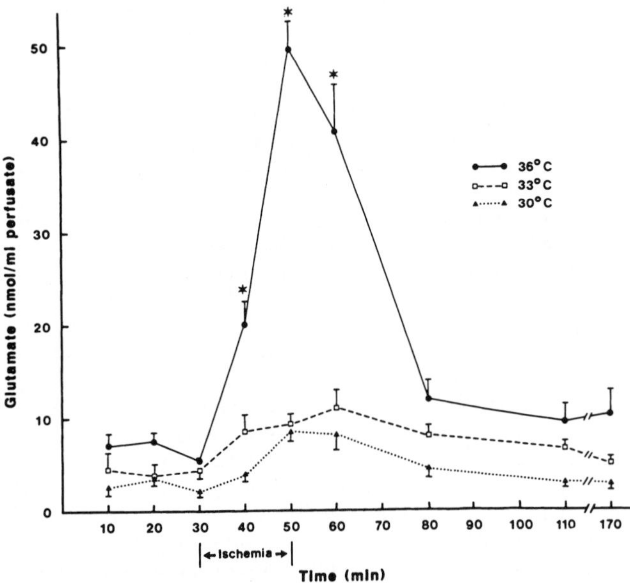

Figure 165–2. Extracellular glutamate concentration rises significantly during and after cerebral ischemia. Glutamate is thought to promote adverse intracellular processes, leading to exacerbation of the ischemic deficit. Mild hypothermia attenuates the increased glutamate concentration. (From Busto R, Globus MY, Dietrich WD, et al: Effect of mild hypothermia on ischemia-induced release of neurotransmitters and free fatty acids in rat brain. Stroke 1989; 20:904–910.)

A host of intranuclear events also occur consequent to cerebral ischemia. They include elaboration of immediate early genes[25] and heat shock proteins.[26] There are undoubtedly many other genetic responses that have yet to be determined (Fig. 165–4).

Increased intracellular osmolarity arises with cerebral ischemia.[27] In addition, vascular and cell membranes may become disrupted or disintegrate. The combination of these factors sets the stage for brain edema.[1] With perfusion of the border zones around the ischemic zone, peri-infarct edema forms.[28] This may further compromise perfusion of this already marginally perfused zone. Indeed, in this low-flow area perfusion may be insufficient to fully support aerobic metabolism yet may be sufficient to supply substrates for edema formation, such as sodium and glucose.[29] There may also be an accumulation of neutrophils in an inflammatory response to this edema.[8]

A variety of other factors also contribute to the neurochemical pathogenesis of cerebral infarction. They include agents that increase vascular permeability such as interleukin 1, bradykinin, serotonin, histamine, arachidonic acid, and free radicals. Many of these mediators may be released locally by neutrophils.[8]

PHYSIOLOGIC PATHWAYS AND EXACERBATING FACTORS

Elevated Intracranial Pressure

Physiology

The brain, spinal cord, cerebrospinal fluid (CSF), and blood are encased in the protective but noncompliant skull and vertebral canal, constituting a nearly incompressible system (Fig. 165–5). In a totally incompressible system, pressure would rise linearly with increased volume; however, there is capacitance in the system, which is thought to be provided by the intervertebral spaces. Once this capacitance is exhausted, the ICP increases dramatically with increased intracranial volume.

Based on the relation CBF = (MAP − ICP)/CVR, the concern is raised mathematically that increasing ICP is associated with decrements in CBF. However, the effect of increasing ICP on CBF is not straightforward, as mean arterial pressure (MAP) may increase with ICP elevations[30] and cerebral vascular resistance (CVR) adjusts with decreasing cerebral perfusion pres-

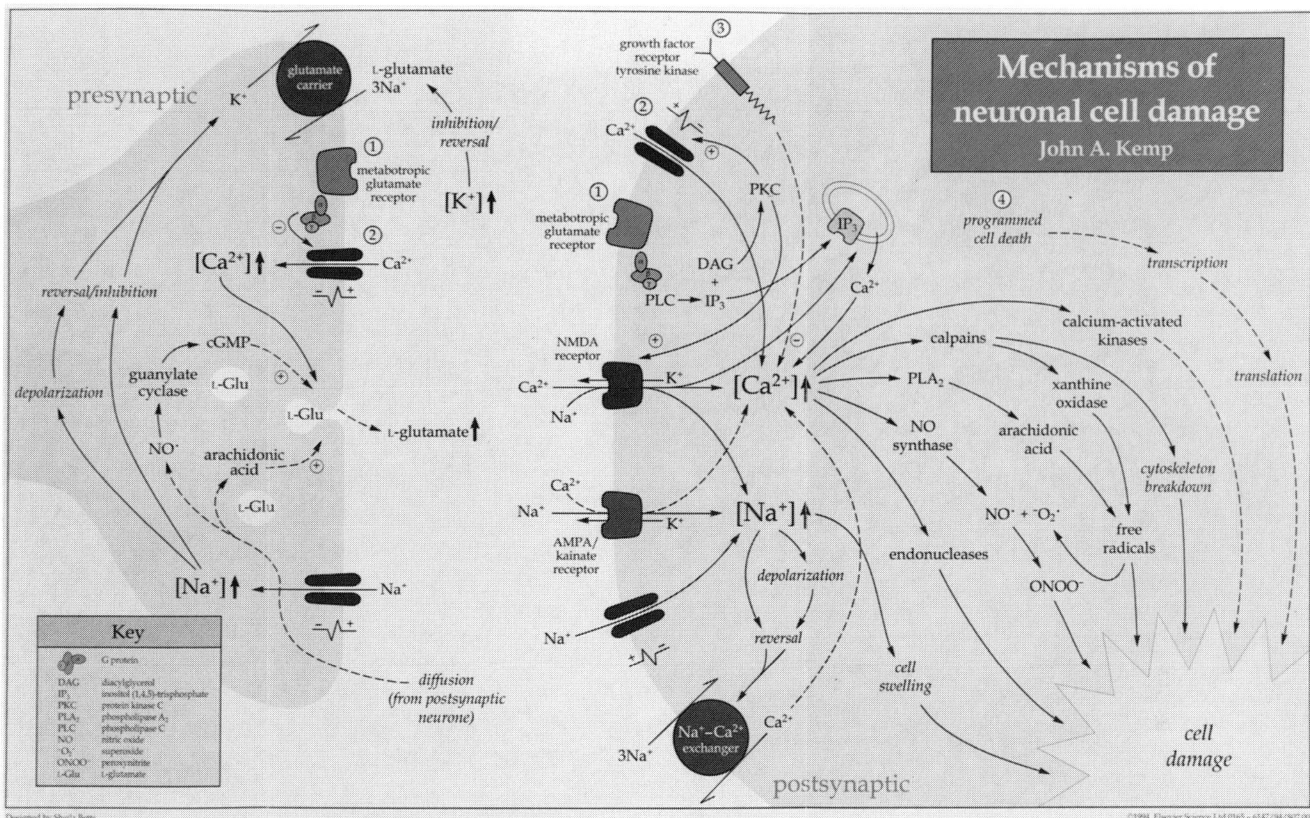

Figure 165–3. Excitatory amino acid receptors. *1,* Metabotropic glutamate receptors mGlu1 and mGlu5 couple to phospholipase C (PLC), whereas mGlu2, mGlu3, mGlu4, and mGlu7 are candidates for presynaptic inhibitory effects. All subtypes may have both presynaptic and postsynaptic effects. *2,* Different subtypes of calcium channels (e.g., N, P, and O but not L) may regulate glutamate release within different, and even the same, pathways. The subtypes may also be differentially located on the dendrites and soma of postsynaptic neurons. *3,* It is not clear how growth factors exert their protective effects, but it has been suggested that they "stabilize" intracellular calcium concentrations. *4,* Apoptosis may play a role in some forms of neuronal degeneration that occur following certain types of insults. (From Kemp JA: Mechanisms of neuronal cell damage. Trends Pharmacol Sci 1994; vol 15. With permission from Elsevier Science.)

sure (CPP) (increasing cerebral blood volume [CBV]) to maintain CBF until vasodilatation is maximal.[31, 32] This is thought to occur at CPP below 50 mm Hg, although considerable individual heterogeneity in this value is observed. Thus, increasing ICP initially is often associated with vasodilatation or increasing MAP to maintain CBF without a nutritive decrement.

Normal ICP is less than 10 mm Hg. ICP in excess of 20 mm Hg is generally treated with ICP-reducing agents[33]; however this is an epidemiologically derived action. Head trauma studies have indicated that patients with ICP above 20 mm Hg generally do poorly,[33] although simply elevating ICP above 20 mm Hg (in experimental animals) is not necessarily associated with decrements in CBF or with permanent sequelae, provided the above noted compensatory mechanisms are operative.[34]

Nonetheless, increasing ICP due to mass lesions or obstruction of CSF outflow can exhaust compensatory mechanisms and compromise CBF. Initially, distal runoff of the cerebral circulation decreases. As the process progresses, the normally continuous (through systole and diastole) cerebral perfusion becomes discontinuous (i.e., systolic perfusion only) (Fig. 165–6).[35] Further compromise of CPP results in anaerobic metabolism, exacerbation of edema, and ultimately intracranial circulatory arrest.[35] Thus, when ICP increases, early recognition is important to determine whether a lethal sequence of events is starting.

Contributors to Intracranial Hypertension

Brain

The brain normally occupies about 80% of the space within the skull, but its volume can be increased by edema. The two types of edema, *cytotoxic* and *vasogenic,* refer to swelling produced by cellular and vascular processes, respectively.[1] Any edema can increase ICP; such edema can be heterogeneously distributed so that pressure gradients occur, resulting in a variety of herniation syndromes.

Cerebrospinal Fluid

CSF is generated in the choroid plexus and absorbed in the arachnoid villi. Normally, an equilibrium exists between production and absorption. Disruption of this equilibrium can lead to increased ICP with hydrocephalus, the condition of an excess of fluid in all or part of the CSF system in the brain.

Hydrocephalus is generally categorized as *communicating* or *noncommunicating.* In communicating hydrocephalus, the CSF circulation between the site of CSF production and absorption is intact; however, abnormally decreased absorption or increased production results in accumulation of CSF. In noncommunicating hydrocephalus the pathways are blocked so that CSF cannot circulate to the convexity of the brain to be absorbed. This results in accumulation of CSF in the ventricles, producing distention.[36]

Blood

CBV is an important contributor to variations in ICP, in part owing to the wide variations in CBV that can occur with

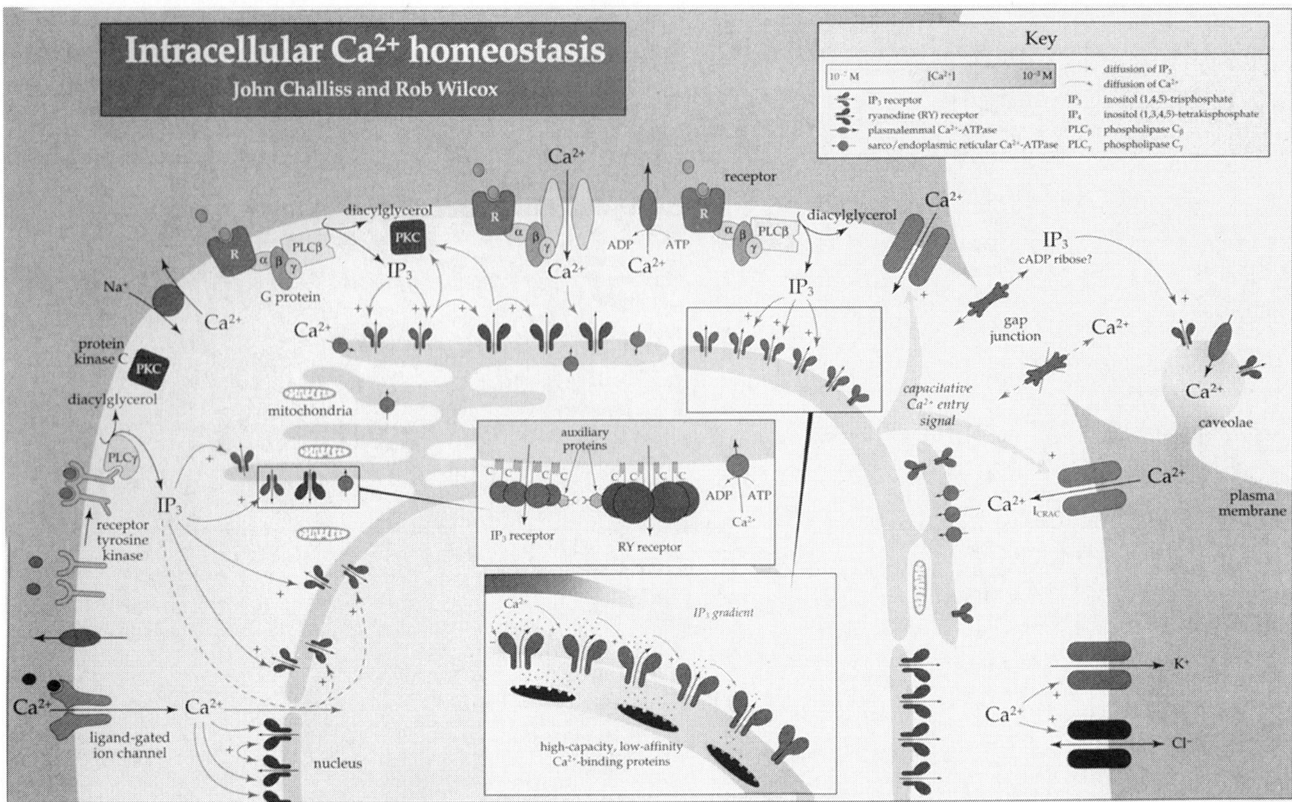

Figure 165–4. Intracellular calcium homeostasis. Most cells maintain a low cytoplasmic free Ca^{2+} concentration compared with that of the extracellular environment. The cell also contains organelles that possess a releasable Ca^{2+} store. Ca^{2+} gradients are maintained principally by Ca^{2+}-ATPases, located in the plasma membrane or in the endoplasmic reticular membrane. A variety of extracellular cues alter cellular activity by increasing $[Ca^{2+}]i$. The strict control of $[Ca^{2+}]i$ and the highly ordered structure of the cytoplasm (owing to Ca^{2+} binding proteins limiting diffusion of Ca^{2+}) make this signaling mechanism attractive with respect to the sophistication of the information transmitted (e.g., spatiotemporal encoding).

The source of Ca^{2+} utilized to increase $[Ca^{2+}]i$ varies considerably among cell types. It is generally accepted that extracellular Ca^{2+} is quantitatively the most important source for Ca^{2+} signaling in neurons (although mobilization of Ca^{2+} from stored Ca^{2+} by influx-induced activation of ryanodine receptors is also important). By contrast, in some cell types, mobilization of Ca^{2+} stored by IP_3 appears to be the principal mechanism. In the latter case, attention has focused on the mechanisms by which Ca^{2+} store depletion can activate a plasma membrane Ca^{2+} conductance pathway, which facilitates Ca^{2+} store repletion. A number of mediators have been proposed for the regulation of the Ca^{2+} release-activated Ca^{2+} current, including IP_3, IP_4, cyclic nucleotides, GTPases, and Ca^{2+} influx factor.

The maintenance and exploitation of the Ca^{2+} gradient exact a considerable energetic cost. Thus, even brief cellular energy deficits can have catastrophic consequences. Although a number of mechanisms appear to have evolved to deal temporarily with Ca^{2+} overload (e.g., mitochondrial uptake), all cells can be irreversibly damaged by persistently elevated $[Ca^{2+}]i$. (From Challis J, Wilcox R: Intracellular Ca^{2+} homeostasis. Trends Pharmacol Sci 1996; 17:80.)

normal physiologic homeostasis and with the effects of drugs and disordered physiology. When CBV increases secondary to increased CBF, this can produce a dramatic increase in ICP if intracranial compliance is abnormal; however, unlike ICP elevation due to increased CSF volume, edema, or a tumor, in which decreased CBF is expected, this variety of ICP increase is often produced by increased CBF, making the significance of the ICP elevation unclear.

Another mechanism of increased CBV is obstruction of venous outflow. This results in brain engorgement and CBV-mediated increased ICP but without increased CBF.[37]

Masses

The fourth cause of increased ICP is a mass lesion. These masses can be in the form of hematoma or neoplastic tumors. In both cases, the faster the onset of the mass effect, the more acute the rise in ICP. Evidently compensatory mechanisms in intracranial compliance can allow large, slow-growing masses to arise in the brain without elevating ICP. On the other hand, similar-sized masses, arising acutely, are associated with symptomatic increases in ICP.

Two Types of Intracranial Hypertension

There are two types of intracranial hypertension, categorized according to CBF: *hyperemic* and *oligemic* (Fig. 165–7). In the normal state, increases in CBF are not associated with increased ICP, as capacitive mechanisms compensate for the CBV-mediated increased intracranial volume. In the situation of disordered intracranial compliance, however, small increases in intracranial volume produce significant increases in ICP.[31, 32]

This finding, however, suggests an important issue. Elevated ICP has traditionally been a concern because it indicates that cerebral perfusion might be jeopardized. It is unclear whether it is appropriate to be concerned about high ICP–induced intracranial oligemia when the cause of the high ICP is intracranial hyperemia with associated increased CBV. There have been no detailed examinations of this question, although some studies allow reasonable inferences to be made about the significance of hyperemic intracranial hypertension.

Hyperemia

For many years, it has been known that abrupt noxious stimuli briefly increase ICP in the setting of decreased intra-

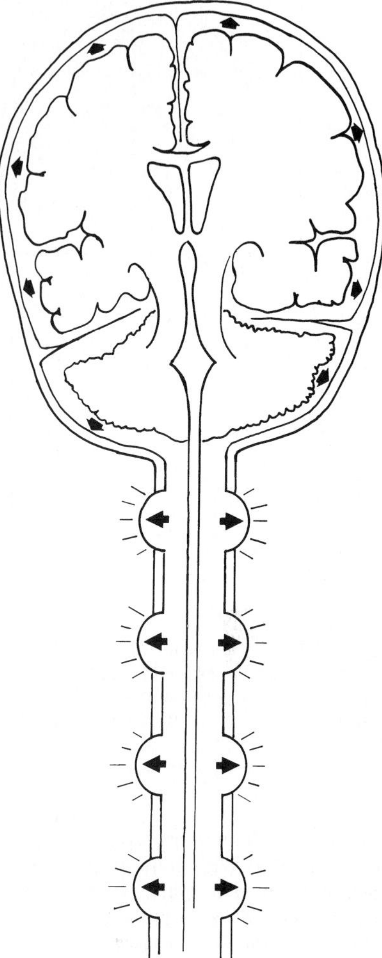

Figure 165–5. The brain, spinal cord, and blood are encased in the skull and vertebral canal, thus constituting a nearly incompressible system. System capacitance is thought to be provided via intervertebral spaces. (From Kofke W, Yonas H, Wechsler L: Neurologic intensive care. *In:* Textbook of Neuroanesthesia. Albin M [Ed]. New York, McGraw-Hill, 1997.)

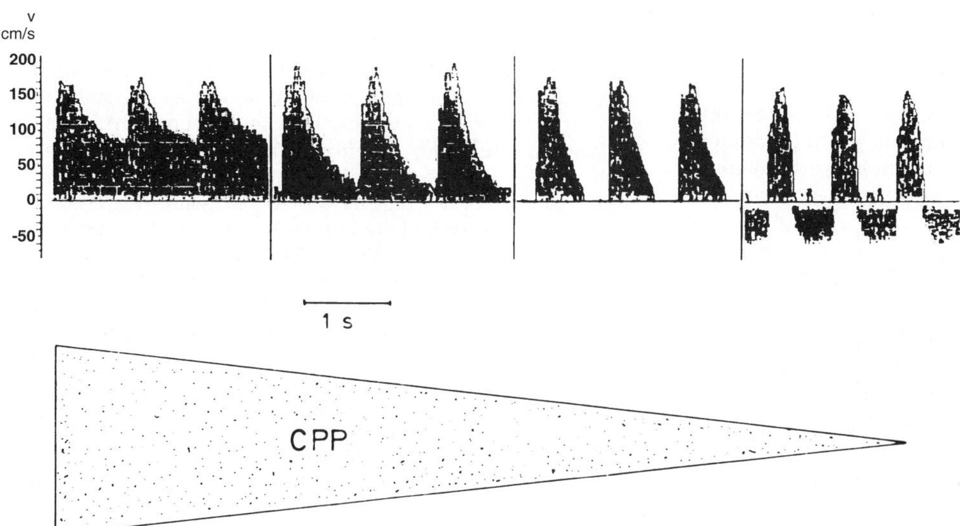

Figure 165–6. Progression of transcranial Doppler (TCD) waveforms with decreasing cerebral perfusion pressure after head injury. Progression is apparent from a normal-appearing TCD waveform to intracranial hypertension sufficient to induce intracerebral circulatory arrest. (From Hassler W, Steinmetz H, Gawlowski J: Transcranial Doppler ultrasonography in raised intracranial pressure and intracranial circulatory arrest. J Neurosurg 1988; 68:745.)

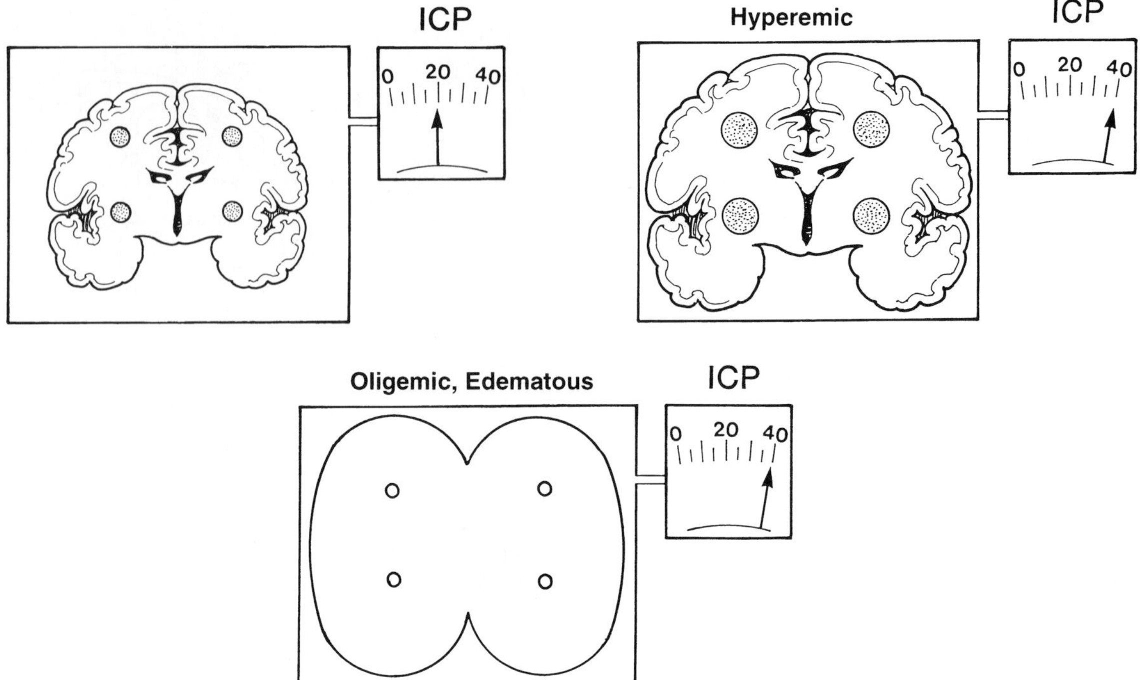

Figure 165–7. Two types of intracranial hypertension. From a baseline condition, intracranial pressure (ICP) can increase in two ways. One is via an increase in cerebral blood volume associated with reflex vasodilation due to moderate blood pressure decreases. The second mechanism of intracranial hypertension is via malignant brain edema or other expanding masses encroaching on the vascular bed to produce intracranial ischemia. (From Kofke W, Yonas H, Wechsler L: Neurologic intensive care. *In:* Textbook of Neuroanesthesia. Albin M [Ed]. New York, McGraw-Hill, 1997, pp 1247–1347.)

cranial compliance. Studies have revealed that such situations are associated with hyperemia, strongly suggesting that brief hyperemic intracranial hypertension is not a dangerous situation[38]; however, it is reasonable to be concerned about such hyperemia, for three reasons:

1. Elevated ICP due to hyperemia in one portion of the brain may increase ICP to compromise CBF in other areas of the brain where CBF is marginal.
2. Increased pressure in one area of the brain may produce gradients that might lead to a herniation syndrome.
3. There is theoretical concern that inappropriate hyperemia might predispose the brain to worse edema or hemorrhage, as with hyperperfusion syndromes.

Thus, hyperemic intracranial hypertension has the theoretical potential to be deleterious, but this has yet to be demonstrated. For brief periods, as during intubation or other limited noxious stimuli, it has been suggested (but not proven) that it may not be problematic.[39]

Oligemia

In contrast, oligemic intracranial hypertension is associated with compromised cerebral perfusion and is clearly deleterious.[35] This finding is supported by the high mortality rate observed in head trauma patients whose ICP rises due to brain edema with decrements in CBF.[33, 40] Transcranial Doppler and CBF studies of these patients have demonstrated that CBF is low and perfusion is discontinuous during the cardiac cycle (see Fig. 165–6).[33, 40] Moreover, jugular venous bulb data indicate that oxygen extraction is markedly increased, suggesting loss of reserve with anaerobic metabolism.[40] In this setting, noxious stimuli can further increase ICP, producing the situation of hyperemic intracranial hypertension added to oligemic, intracranial hypertension. Presumably, in this setting the hyperemic rise in ICP acts to further reduce regional cerebral blood flow (rCBF) in compromised areas of brain edema and may contribute to vasogenic edema (see Fig. 165–7).

Blood Pressure Effects on Intracranial Pressure: Plateau Waves

Lundberg, in a pioneering 1960 study,[41] monitored ICP in hundreds of patients, identifying characteristic pressure waves. One category of these waves has been identified as *plateau waves,* known to be associated with increased CBV (Fig. 165–8).[31] Such waves occur when the ICP abruptly increases to systemic blood pressure levels for about 15 to 30 minutes, occasionally accompanied by neurologic deterioration.

Rosner and Becker[32] synthesized the data and convincingly suggested that intracranial blood volume dysautoregulation is responsible for plateau waves. They induced mild head trauma in cats and intensively monitored the animals after the insult. With normal fluctuations in blood pressure within the normal range, they observed that mild blood pressure decrements to a mean of approximately 70 to 80 mm Hg preceded the development of plateau waves (Fig. 165–9).

CBV in normally autoregulating brain tissue increases as blood pressure decreases; however the increase in CBV is nonlinear. There is an exponential increase in CBV as perfusion pressure decreases to about 80 mm Hg and below (Fig. 165–10).[32] A small decrease in blood pressure, although in the normotensive range, produces exponential increases in CBV in a setting of abnormal intracranial compliance with the ICP at the elbow of the ICP–intracranial volume curve. Thus, a small decrease in blood pressure introduces an exponential CBV change upon an exponential ICP relation, so that ICP increases abruptly and significantly. Plateau waves spontaneously resolve with a hypertensive response or with hyperventilation, which acts to oppose the increase in CBV. Clearly, to develop a plateau wave there must be a portion of the brain

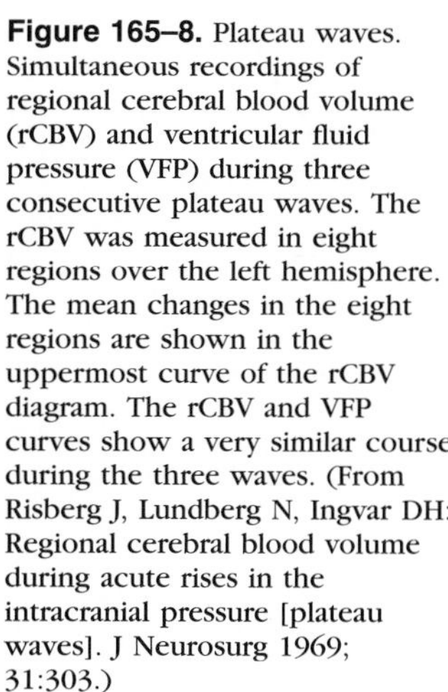

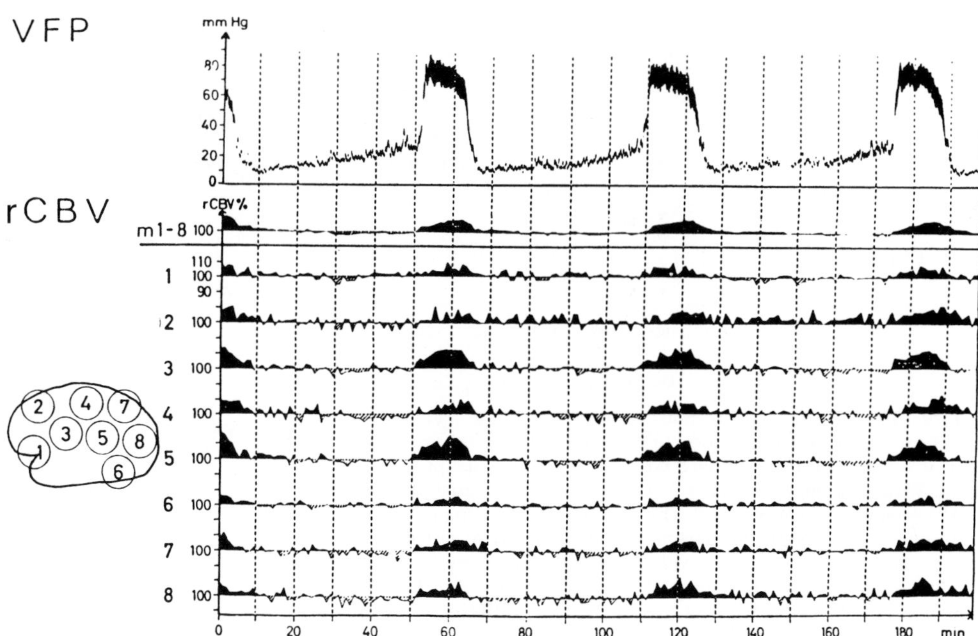

Figure 165–8. Plateau waves. Simultaneous recordings of regional cerebral blood volume (rCBV) and ventricular fluid pressure (VFP) during three consecutive plateau waves. The rCBV was measured in eight regions over the left hemisphere. The mean changes in the eight regions are shown in the uppermost curve of the rCBV diagram. The rCBV and VFP curves show a very similar course during the three waves. (From Risberg J, Lundberg N, Ingvar DH: Regional cerebral blood volume during acute rises in the intracranial pressure [plateau waves]. J Neurosurg 1969; 31:303.)

with normally reactive vasculature in the presence of other brain areas with a mass effect and elevated ICP, a situation of heterogeneous autoregulation. In addition to preventing and treating plateau waves, the physician must maintain MAP in the range of 80 to 100 mm Hg in patients with high ICP.

Conversely, hypertension can also increase ICP. Typically, within the normal autoregulatory range changes in blood pressure have no effect on ICP; however, with brain injury and associated vasoparalysis, blood pressure increases mechanically produce cerebral vasodilatation, increasing ICP (Fig. 165–11).[42] It appears that either increasing or decreasing blood pressure can increase ICP, suggesting the presence of an optimal CPP value for ICP, probably 80 to 100 mm Hg, although this has not been definitively determined experimentally (Figs. 165–12 and 165–13).

Positive End-Expiratory Pressure and Intracranial Hypertension

Positive end-expiratory pressure (PEEP) ventilation can increase ICP in two ways. The first is through impedance of

Figure 165–9. In an animal head trauma model, a trivial-appearing and transient decrease in systemic arterial blood pressure in the setting of borderline cerebral perfusion pressure (CPP) precipitates sufficient cerebral vasodilatation to markedly increase intracranial pressure (ICP). Restoration of CPP is associated with abolition of the plateau wave. (From Rosner MJ, Becker DP: Origin and evolution of plateau waves: Experimental observations and a theoretical model. J Neurosurg 1984; 60:312.)

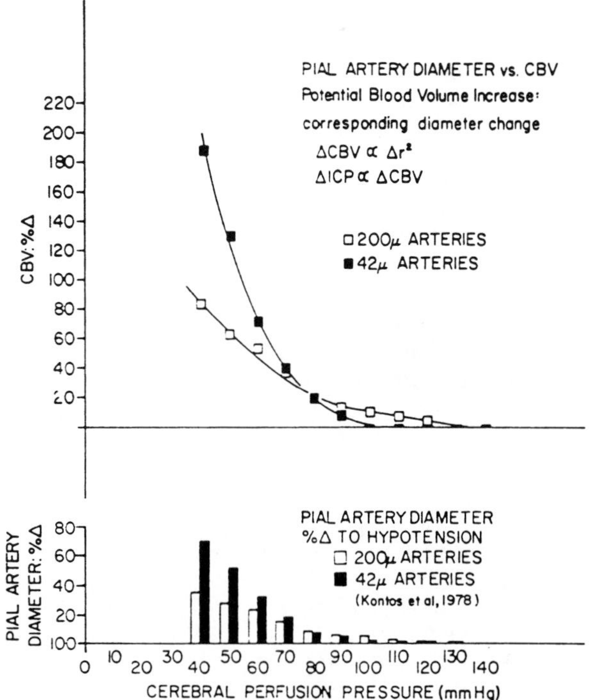

Figure 165–10. Cerebral vasodilatation occurs exponentially as cerebral perfusion pressure is reduced. CBV = cerebral blood volume; ICP = intracranial pressure. (From Rosner MJ, Becker DP: The etiology of plateau waves: A theoretical model and experimental observations. *In:* Intracranial Pressure V. Ishii S, Nagai H, Brock M [Eds]. New York, Springer-Verlag, 1983, p 301.)

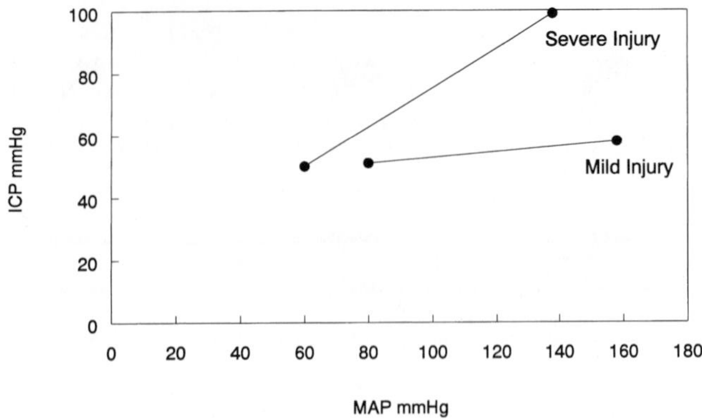

Figure 165–11. Intracranial response to hypertension in patients with head injury. Normally, blood pressure changes within the normal autoregulatory range have no effect on intracranial pressure (ICP). With brain injury, however, increases in mean arterial pressure (MAP) produce increases in ICP with this effect more pronounced with more severe injury. Presumably, this effect is due to distention of vasoparalyzed blood vessels, with a consequent increase in cerebral blood volume. (Data from Matakas F, Von Waechter R, Knupling R, Potolicchio SJ Jr: Increase in cerebral perfusion pressure by arterial hypertension in brain swelling: A mathematical model of the volume-pressure relationship. J Neurosurg 1975; 42:282. Reproduced from Kofke W, Yonas H, Wechsler L: Neurologic intensive care. *In:* Textbook of Neuroanesthesia. Albin M [Ed]. New York, McGraw-Hill, 1997, pp 1247–1347.)

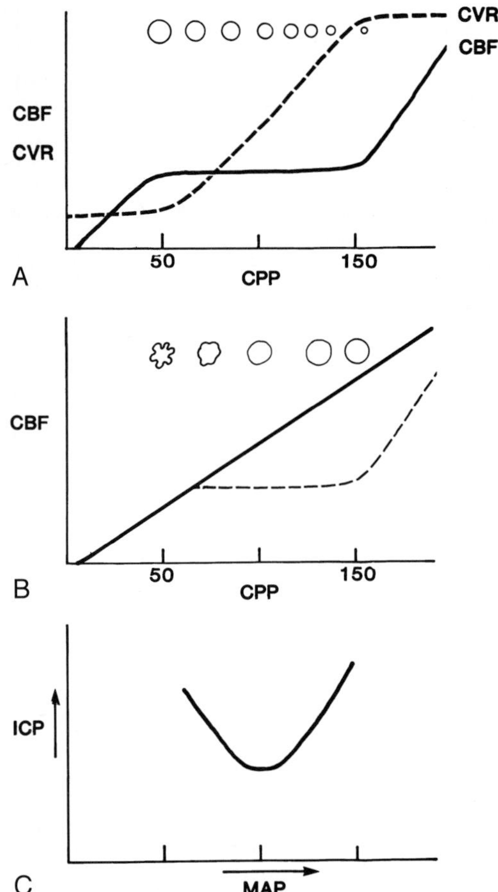

Figure 165–12. Cerebral perfusion pressure (CPP) versus cerebral blood flow (CBF) and cerebrovascular resistance (CVR). *A,* Blood flow is normally maintained constant through changes in CVR, depicted as changes in vascular diameter (and thus cerebral blood volume [CBC]) in the figure. CBV varies inversely with CPP. *B,* With vasoparalysis due to injury, CVR does not change with CPP variations, such that CBF and CBV vary directly with CPP. *C,* In the situation of decreased intracranial compliance, both of these factors in *A* and *B* may interact to increase intracranial pressure (ICP). Normally, autoregulating tissue as in *(A)* predisposes to CBV-mediated ICP elevation with decreasing blood pressure, whereas vasoparalyzed tissue *(B)* predisposes to CBV-mediated ICP elevations with increasing blood pressure, leading to the notion of an ICP optima (~80 to 100 mm Hg) with varying CPP. (From Kofke W, et al: Neurologic intensive care. *In:* Textbook of Neuroanesthesia. Albin M [Ed]. New York, McGraw-Hill, 1997, pp 1247–1347.)

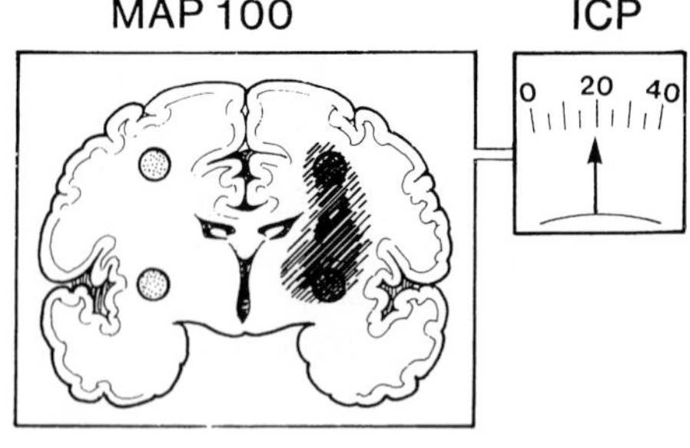

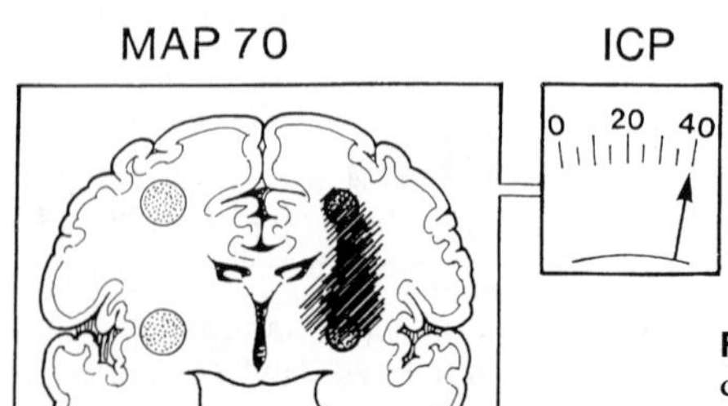

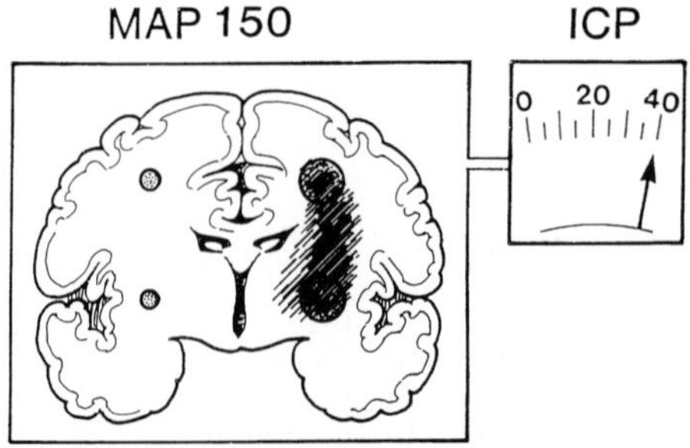

Figure 165–13. In the setting of heterogeneous autoregulation in the brain, conditions may predispose to cerebral blood volume–mediated increases in intracranial pressure (ICP) with both increases or decreases in blood pressure. MAP = mean arterial pressure.

Low PEEP → ↓CO → ↓BP → ↑CBV → ↑ICP

High PEEP → ↑CVP → ↑P_{SS} > ICP → ↑ICP

Figure 165–14. Two mechanisms of positive end-expiratory pressure (PEEP)-mediated increases in intracranial pressure (ICP). Addition of PEEP decreases cardiac output (CO) and blood pressure (BP) leading to a reflex increase in cerebral blood volume (CBV). If cerebral perfusion pressure is marginal with heterogeneous autoregulation, this can lead to further increases in ICP. Conversely, to increase sagittal sinus pressure to an extent sufficient to further increase ICP, which is already elevated, one must apply PEEP levels at or greater than the ICP. P_{ss} = sagittal sinus pressure.

venous return, increasing cerebral venous pressure and ICP. The second is through decreased blood pressure and reflex increase of CBV increasing ICP (Fig. 165–14). The latter is likely the most common mechanism, as Huseby and colleagues[43] suggest that cerebral venous effects only occur with very high PEEP.

Shapiro and colleagues[44] demonstrated increases in ICP in head-injured humans during intracranial hypertension with application of PEEP (Fig. 165–15). Examination of their data suggests that the most profound decreases in CPP occurred in patients with PEEP-induced decrements in MAP. This is consistent with the notion put forth by Rosner and Becker[32] that decreases in blood pressure increase CBV and ICP.

Aidinis and coworkers[45] in studies of cats confirmed these observations in a more controlled setting. In addition, they assessed the role of pulmonary compliance, finding that decreased pulmonary compliance induced by oleic acid injections reduces the effect of PEEP in increasing ICP. When PEEP is likely to be needed, with decrements in pulmonary compliance, such observations indicate that any adverse effects on ICP are less likely to be manifested. This may be related to observations that hemodynamic effects of PEEP are less apparent with noncompliant lungs,[45, 46] so that hypotension-mediated increases in CBV do not occur.

The intuitive notion that PEEP increases cerebral venous pressure to increase ICP is not as straightforward as it initially may seem. For PEEP to increase cerebral venous pressure to levels that increase ICP, the cerebral venous pressure must at least equal the ICP. Thus, the higher the ICP, the higher PEEP must be to have such a direct hydraulic effect on ICP. This concept was nicely proven by Huseby's group[43] in dog studies, when PEEP was increased progressively with different starting levels of ICP (Fig. 165–16). It is important to note that they

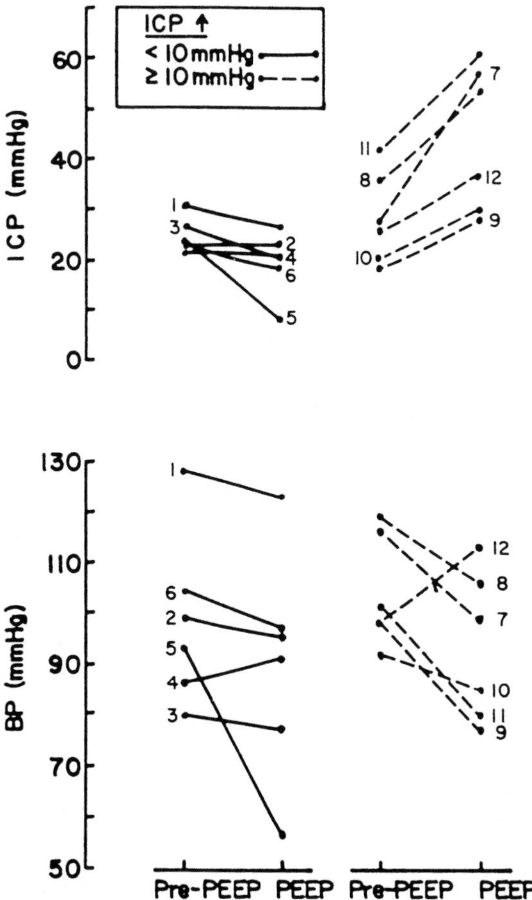

Figure 165–15. Intracranial pressure (ICP) and arterial blood pressure (BP) before and with the application of PEEP (4 to 8 cm H_2O) in severely head-injured patients. The patients are divided arbitrarily into two groups: those with an ICP increase equal to or above 10 mm Hg, and those with ICP gains below 10 mm Hg. PEEP-induced blood pressure decreases appear to be more marked in patients sustaining larger ICP increases. (From Shapiro HM, Marshall LF: Intracranial pressure responses to PEEP in head-injured patients. J Trauma 1978; 18:254.)

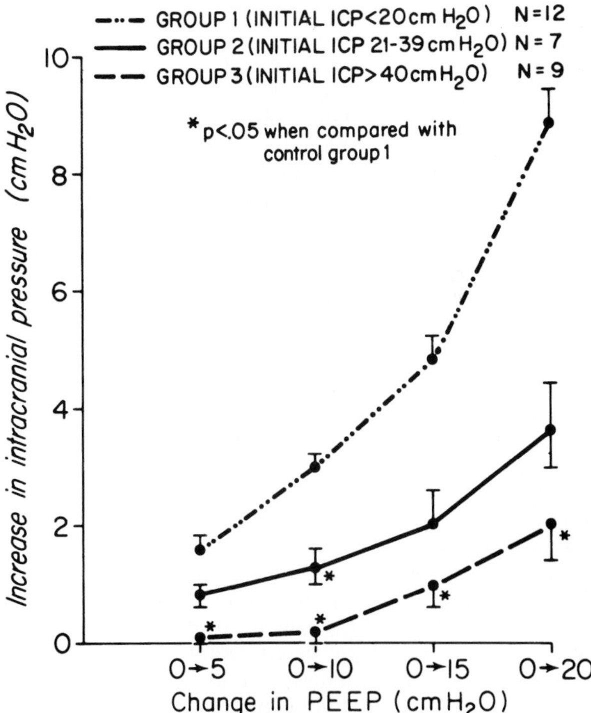

Figure 165–16. Increases in intracranial pressure (ICP) with positive end-expiratory pressure (PEEP) in dogs. Values are mean ± standard error of the mean. Group 1 included 12 animals with an initial intracranial pressure (ICP) less than 20 cm H_2O, Group 2 included seven animals with an initial ICP of 21 to 39 cm H_2O, and Group 3 included nine animals with an initial ICP above 40 cm H_2O. Blood pressure was maintained constant in all animals. With blood pressure maintained constant, the most significant increases in ICP occurred in the animals with the lowest starting ICP level. (From Huseby JS, Luce JM, Cary JM, et al: Effects of positive end-expiratory pressure on intracranial pressure in dogs with intracranial hypertension. J Neurosurg 1981; 55:704.)

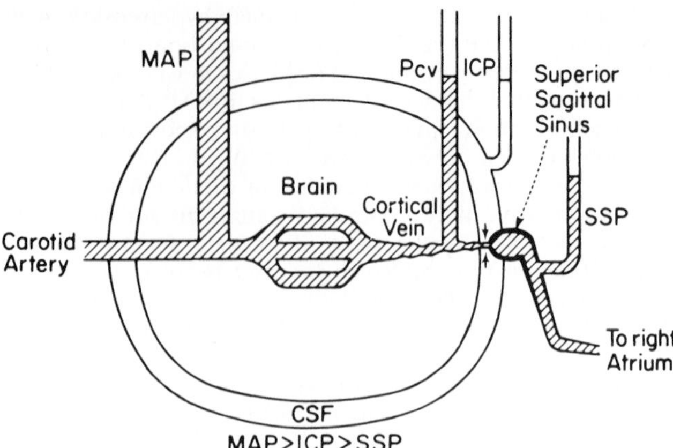

Figure 165–17. Schematic illustration of the intracranial space during raised intracranial pressure (ICP). *Arrows* indicate the position of the hypothesized Starling resistor. Here, the mean arterial pressure (MAP) is greater than ICP, which is greater than sagittal sinus pressure (SSP). Cortical vein pressure (Pcv) cannot fall below ICP, and thus flow is dependent on MAP-ICP and independent of small changes in SSP. (From Huseby JS, Luce JM, Cary JM, et al: Effects of positive end-expiratory pressure on intracranial pressure in dogs with intracranial hypertension. J Neurosurg 1981; 55:704.)

prevented PEEP-induced decrements in blood pressure, thus avoiding any reflex increases in CBV. They suggested a hydraulic model to better conceptualize this (Fig. 165–17). For example, if all of a 10-cm H_2O PEEP application was transmitted to the cerebral vasculature, which is unlikely given the decreased pulmonary compliance associated with the need for such PEEP, ICP is affected only if it is below 10 cm H_2O (7.7 mm Hg), increasing to a level no higher than the applied PEEP. This presupposes no PEEP-induced arterial pressure decrement.

Effects of Antihypertensive Therapy on Intracranial Pressure

ICP can be influenced by antihypertensive drugs. In general, vasodilator drugs such as nitroprusside,[47–49] nitroglycerin,[50] and nifedipine[51] can be expected to increase ICP. Conversely nonvasodilator antihypertensive drugs, generally sympatholytic drugs (e.g., trimethophan), or beta-adrenergic–blocking drugs (e.g., esmolol, labetalol)[52] can be expected to have little or no effect on ICP. These observations suggest that the rise in ICP due to vasodilators is caused by increased CBF with an attendant increase in CBV. The increase in ICP thus does not threaten ischemia, although herniation and hyperperfusion syndromes may occur and might be problematic. There has been a report of neurologic deterioration with nitroprusside use despite no change in blood pressure.[49] Another consideration in the use of vasodilators is their propensity to increase plasma catecholamines reflexly.[53] Such increases in plasma catecholamines may be deleterious to marginally perfused injured brain tissue.[54–56]

Hyperemia

Hyperperfusion Syndromes

In a variety of clinical situations, CBF may be inappropriately increased for a given blood pressure. In extreme cases, vasoparalysis is present and CBF becomes a more or less linear function of blood pressure. Such hyperperfusion syndromes may occur (1) early in severe hepatic encephalopathy,[57] (2) 2 to 3 days after severe head injury,[40] (3) after resection of large arteriovenous malformations (AVMs),[58] (4) after carotid endarterectomy of severely stenotic lesions with poor collaterals, (probably after cerebral arterial thrombolysis),[101, 102] and (5) possibly during administration of cerebral vasodilators at high systemic blood pressure.

Fulminant hepatic failure produces widespread physiologic changes, including altered cerebral physiology.[57] Aggarwal and coworkers[57] have systematically examined cerebral hemodynamics and metabolism in severe hepatic encephalopathy and during recovery after hepatic transplantation. They have identified phases that are traversed in the course of going from normal cerebral physiology to brain death. Patients initially demonstrate elevated CBF with normotension. This is usually followed by hyperemic (high CBF or CBV) intracranial hypertension, then by edema with oligemic intracranial hypertension, and finally by intracranial circulatory arrest and brain death. The data clearly suggest that the hyperemia may be deleterious, possibly contributing to subsequent development of cerebral edema. This is supported by observations that the cerebral edema seems to be prevented by use of barbiturates and hyperventilation during the hyperemic phase.

Several investigators, examining cerebrovascular physiology after severe head trauma have observed that patients with severe head injury initially have normal or low CBF. This finding is followed a few days later by increased CBF, which is associated with intracranial hypertension.[40] This hyperemia may contribute to subsequent oligemic intracranial hypertension.

The concept of normal perfusion pressure breakthrough indicates hyperperfusion at normal blood pressure (e.g., after resection of a large AVM), when the remaining blood vessels lack the ability to clamp down normally and regulate blood flow, resulting in abnormally high regional CBF. The pathogenesis is thought to be related to chronic arterial hypotension proximal to the AVM. The larger the AVM, the lower the MAP the patient is used to, with the cerebral vasculature locally down-regulating the CBF-MAP autoregulatory relation. Removing the AVM abruptly exposes the cerebral arterial vessels and arterioles to pressure never before experienced.[59]

Thus, even though blood pressure is within normal limits, the pressure-naive vasculature is unable to autoregulate and the physiology of malignant hypertension may ensue to cause cerebral edema or hemorrhage. This is an attractive hypothesis that makes physiologic sense; however, observations of Young and coworkers[60] report that autoregulation of the vascular bed after AVM resection is generally intact, indicating that vasoparalysis due to chronic hypotension may not be the most important contributor to normal perfusion pressure breakthrough.

One cause of neurologic deterioration after carotid endarterectomy is cerebral edema or hemorrhage. This situation is rather unusual, but the presence postoperatively of a unilateral throbbing headache suggests that it may be present. Blood flow studies reveal such patients to have cerebral hyperemia associated with removal of a large proximal obstruction. While normotension is usually tolerated well, hypertension probably increases the risk of hemorrhage, especially when there was a preoperative cerebral infarction. Similar to the AVM situation, vasculature that has acclimated to low proximal pressure now is presented with arterial pressure that is much higher, although within the epidemiologic norm.[61]

After thrombolysis of a cerebral artery, one important source of morbidity is edema or hemorrhage of the reperfused territory. With reperfusion of the ischemic tissue, hyperemia occurs for a time. When it is sustained, irreversible endothelial damage has probably occurred and the patient is at risk for secondary edema or hemorrhage, particularly if the depth of ischemia is sufficient to produce early changes on computed tomography (CT).[62]

Vasodilators such as nitroprusside are frequently used for severe arterial hypertension. When CBF is measured, nitroprusside has minimal CBF effect with induced hypotension[63]; however, no data are available on its CBF-CBV effects with treatment of hypertension. Such vasodilators are known to cause an increase in ICP,[64] suggesting an element of cerebral hyperemia. This finding is supported by reports of cerebral dysautoregulation induced by nitroprusside.[65] The extent of this ICP elevation and hyperemia[63, 66] appear to decrease as blood pressure decreases. This notion is supported by observations during neurosurgery of cerebral swelling when nitroprusside is administered.[67] When it is used for induced hypotension during neurosurgery, the brain is noted to be flaccid with no evident hyperemia. Thus, cerebral vasodilators can produce a cerebral *dysautoregulation-hyperperfusion syndrome,* the extent of which is likely dependent on blood pressure. Their use has not yet been reported to be associated with exacerbation of cerebral edema or hemorrhage.

All of these syndromes describe a clinical course in humans consisting of inappropriate hyperemia for a given blood pressure followed by cerebral edema or hemorrhage. This suggests that the failure of autoregulation at normal pressure results in exposure of arterioles and capillaries to unacceptably high pressure. This then disrupts the blood-brain barrier with consequent transudation of fluid or frank bleeding.

Hyperthermia

Temperature management can be critical to neurointensive care. In animal models, hyperthermia has been shown to have deleterious effects on outcome after cerebral ischemia,[68] head trauma,[68] and seizure.[69] Conversely, mild hypothermia has been shown to be protective.[70] It is of interest that the extent of hypothermia required to produce protection is modest—in the 32° to 36°C range. The extent of protection is not adequately explained by reduction in cerebral metabolic rate,[71] suggesting that hypothermia has additional beneficial effects such as decreased free radical production or reduction in neurotransmitter neurotoxicity[72] (see Fig. 165–2).

In a multicenter trial with head trauma patients, moderate hypothermia, in preliminary reports, conferred cerebral protection when applied within 6 hours of the insult and maintained for 24 to 48 hours.[70] There have been no clinical trials to assess hypothermia in humans with cerebral ischemia or seizure, although a survey of neuroanesthesiologists in North America indicated that it is now used routinely in many medical centers during neurosurgery.[73]

Gas Exchange

Cerebrovascular reserve is compromised in many intracranial pathologic processes. Normally, the brain compensates for decrements in supplies of oxygen and substrates by vasodilating to maintain or increase flow.[74] Animal experiments indicate that it is possible to produce a condition of compromised cerebrovascular reserve and increased risk of cerebral infarction. For example, occlusion of one carotid artery or inducing moderate hypoxemia does not produce symptoms, because cerebral vasodilatation occurs to compensate. Indeed, some contend that arterial hypoxemia, occurring with normal cerebral vascular compensatory mechanisms, does not cause brain damage. Of course, one contributing factor to this notion is that hypoxic myocardial dysfunction produces circulatory collapse and death such that isolated posthypoxic (without ischemia) neuronal injury cannot occur. With hypoxemia added to carotid occlusion, or vice versa, however, a stroke may occur because compensatory mechanisms are already fully mobilized and cannot accommodate the further decrease in oxygen supply.[75] Clinical examples of variants of this situation abound.[76] Such examples of attenuated cerebrovascular reserve include cerebral edema, hypoxemia, carotid artery stenosis, peri-infarct penumbra, and anemia. In each of these situations, although not easy to quantitate, it is clear that added situations of compromised oxygen supply to the brain risk neuronal injury.

Arterial carbon dioxide partial pressure ($Paco_2$) changes have a profound impact on CBF. Normally, CBF varies linearly with $Paco_2$ between 20 and 60 mm Hg.[77] $Paco_2$-mediated changes in CBF occur with corresponding changes in CBV. Thus, in situations of abnormal intracranial compliance, where small changes in intracranial volume have large ICP effects, decreased $Paco_2$ decreases ICP, and increased $Paco_2$ increases ICP.

The primary concern with elevated ICP is that it may be associated with cerebral oligemia. Thus, these effects of $Paco_2$ on ICP are paradoxical; that is, decreased $Paco_2$ decreases ICP but at the expense of decreasing CBF (Fig. 165–18), the very entity that is desired to be maintained.[78]

Minhas and coworkers[79] reported that mild hyperventilation in brain-injured patients produced dangerous perilesional CBF decrements. However, Gupta's group,[80] using tissue measures of oxygen perfusion in brain-injured humans, reported sequential increases in tissue oxygen tension ($Ptio_2$) with decreasing $Paco_2$ with an optimum at 26 to 30 mm Hg. Nonetheless, data from head trauma studies indicate that routine use of hyperventilation can worsen outcome.[81] Conversely, allowing hypercapnia to occur, although it leads to increased ICP, is associated with increased CBF. These observations pertain to normally autoregulating tissue. The CBF effects in injured brain tissue can be unpredictable. For example, allowing $Paco_2$ to increase CBF in autoregulating brain areas, by increasing ICP, may compromise flow in other injured and already fully vasodilated areas.

Finally, despite observations that hyperglycemia exacerbates ischemic brain damage, there is evidence that mild acidosis can be protective in the brain.[4, 82] This is thought to be due to antagonism of the *N*-methyl-D-aspartate (NMDA) glutamate receptor. If these initial studies in vitro are relevant to clinical care, hyperventilation, in addition to decreasing CBF, may have adverse biochemical effects.

Hyperglycemia

Hyperglycemia has been associated with exacerbation of brain damage with both head trauma and cerebral ischemia,[83–85] but it is not a straightforward issue. Clearly, neuronal damage after global cerebral ischemia is exacerbated by hyperglycemia.[86] Some studies have suggested that a blood glucose level over 120 mg/dL is deleterious in stroke patients[83]; however, subsequent studies suggested a threshold of around 180 mg/dL for subhuman primates subjected to global ischemia.[86] Clearly, blood glucose concentration greater than 400 mg/dL causes striking worsening of neurologic outcome with global ischemia.[84, 87]

With focal cerebral ischemia, the situation is less clear. Animal and human studies have shown variously, that brain damage is worsened, not affected, or lessened with hyperglycemia.[88–92] One report by Prado and colleagues[92] in rats suggested that the deciding factor in worsening brain damage

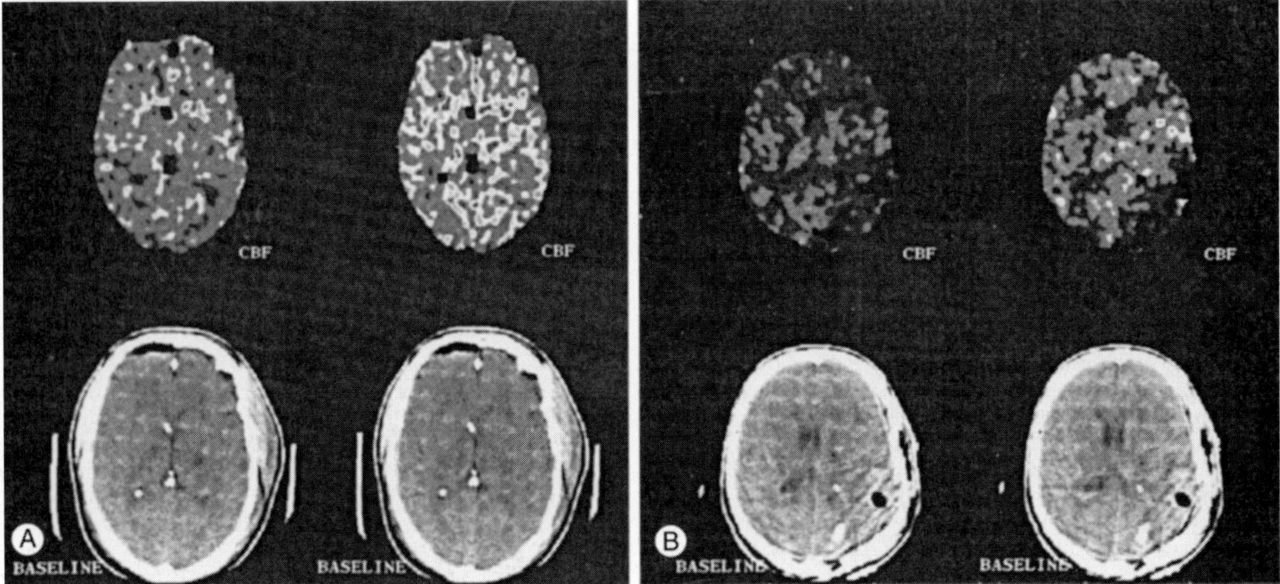

Figure 165–18. Effects of hyperventilation on cerebral blood flow (CBF) and two examples of disparate effects of hyperventilation on CBF. Both figures are stable xenon CBFs in head trauma patients with and without hyperventilation. Brighter shading indicates higher CBF. CT images are indicated in the lower figures, and CBF maps are in the upper figures. *A*, P_{CO_2} was decreased from 39 to 29 mm Hg. The baseline scan *(right)* shows hyperemia, and the hyperventilated scan *(left)* shows CBFs of approximately 30 mL/100 g/min, probably acceptable flows. *B*, P_{CO_2} was decreased from 46 to 30 mm Hg. The baseline CBF *(right)* has only marginally acceptable CBF. The effect of hyperventilation *(left)* was to produce widespread areas of CBF less than 20 mL/100 g/min, probably unacceptable flows. (From Kofke W, Yonas H, Wechsler L: Neurologic intensive care. *In:* Textbook of Neuroanesthesia. Albin M [Ed]. New York, McGraw-Hill, 1997, pp 1247–1347.)

with hyperglycemia is whether there is collateral flow. Areas of the brain with minimal or no collaterals were not affected or were improved with hyperglycemia. Brain areas with a continued trickle of flow sustained worse damage. Presumably, the continued substrate supply in oligemic (not ischemic) areas allowed greater accumulation of organic acids in the cells, leading to greater brain damage.[2, 88] Unfortunately, these observations are difficult to apply clinically to individual patients with focal ischemia.

In two animal models of status epilepticus, hyperglycemia had neither deleterious nor protective effects.[93, 94] The model used by Swan and coworkers[94] produced limbic system damage, whereas Kofke and colleagues[93] used a model that produced substantia nigra damage. Seizure-induced nigral damage in rats is associated with hypermetabolic lactic acidosis,[95] which was not exacerbated with hyperglycemia. The fact that nigral damage was not exacerbated with hyperglycemia suggests that metabolic acidosis may not be the sole factor in the development of brain damage after seizure.

Sepsis

In animal models, sepsis is known to decrease CBF while increasing cerebral metabolic rate and disrupting the blood-brain barrier.[96] In addition, it can decrease blood pressure in a manner that may not be tolerated well by the brain with abnormal cerebrovascular reserve. Sepsis-induced decreases in blood pressure can turn an area of cerebral oligemia into one of ischemic cerebral infarction.

Sodium

Hypernatremia

Hypernatremia can occur in neurointensive care patients from nonketotic diabetic coma, dehydration from lack of fluids or from diuretics, inappropriate hypertonic fluid administration, diabetes insipidus, or panhypopituitarism.[97] It can be associated with thirst, irritability, seizures, intracranial hemorrhage, or coma, although the rate of increase in sodium concentration is thought to be an important determinant of the clinical presentation. For example, a sodium level of 170 mEq/L can be associated with few neurologic symptoms if the rise occurs over a prolonged period.

Diabetes insipidus can occur when disease processes affect the pituitary or its vascular supply. It should be expected when urine output is inappropriately increased. Typically, urine output can increase abruptly to greater than 1 Liter/hour and may be associated with severe hypernatremia and hypovolemic hypotension. Diagnosis of diabetes insipidus is based on continued output of dilute urine in the context of hypertonic serum. Specific gravity of urine will be close to 1.001 with osmolarity less than 200 mOsm/L despite serum osmolarity that may be greater than 320 mOsm/L.[98]

Hyponatremia

Hyponatremia can be due to the syndrome of inappropriate secretion of antidiuretic hormone (SIADH), so-called cerebral salt wasting, or excessive free water administration. SIADH is generally associated with hypervolemia, and cerebral salt wasting is associated with hypovolemia. Both syndromes may be associated with elevated urine sodium concentrations, making differentiation between the two syndromes difficult in routine clinical practice.[99] Rapidly increasing the sodium concentration can produce permanent neurologic damage from central pontine myelinolysis.[100]

Catecholamines

Subarachnoid hemorrhage (SAH) is an entity particularly notable for catecholamine effects, some of which will be described; however, catecholamine effects also occur with increased ICP, stroke, head trauma, or any compromise of midbrain or hindbrain oxygen delivery.

Serum catecholamine levels increase dramatically after SAH, notably peaking at the same time as the peak incidence of post-SAH vasospasm, with symptom development corresponding to serum catecholamine levels.[101-104] This leads to the notion that hypothalamic injury with excessive catecholamine release may be an important factor in the genesis of post-SAH spasm and stroke.[102] Several lines of evidence further support this hypothesis:

1. The cerebral vasculature is invested somewhat with adrenergic nerves. With SAH the adrenergic receptors in the cerebral vessels decrease in number.[105, 106] This suggests that denervation hypersensitivity may be occurring such that the increase in humoral catecholamines with SAH produces spasm in hyper-reacting vessels.
2. Catecholamine release after SAH is sufficient to produce electrocardiographic (ECG) changes[101, 107] with ventricular wall motion abnormalities[108, 109] and myocardial injury.[110, 111]
3. Treatment of humans with SAH with β- and α-adrenergic antagonists is associated with an improvement in neurologic outcome (Fig. 165-19)[55] and ECG abnormalities.[108]
4. In animal models, selective destruction of hindbrain adrenergic nuclei with cephalad projections prevents the development of vasospasm.[111] Moreover, laboratory studies indicate an important role for vasopressin in vasospasm, because vasospasm cannot be produced in vasopressin-deficient rats.[112]
5. Animal data with cerebral ischemia models provide strong support for the notion that catecholamines can exacerbate cerebral ischemia. Compared to hemorrhage-induced hypotension, ischemic damage was decreased with hypotension induced through the use of ganglionic blockade with hexamethonium,[54] central adrenergic blockade with α_2 agonists,[56] and angiotension-converting enzyme (ACE) inhibition.[113] Rats treated with hemorrhage alone sustained increased exogenous catecholamine concentrations. To test the hypothesis that these catecholamines contributed to brain damage, some of the animals treated with hexamethonium also received intravenous (IV) catecholamine infusions. Reversal of the hexamethonium brain protective effect was observed in these animals (Fig. 165-20).[54]
6. Brain protection (Fig. 165-21) has been observed in laboratory studies with preischemic[114] and preseizure[115] treatment using reserpine, a drug that depletes presynaptic catecholamine stores.

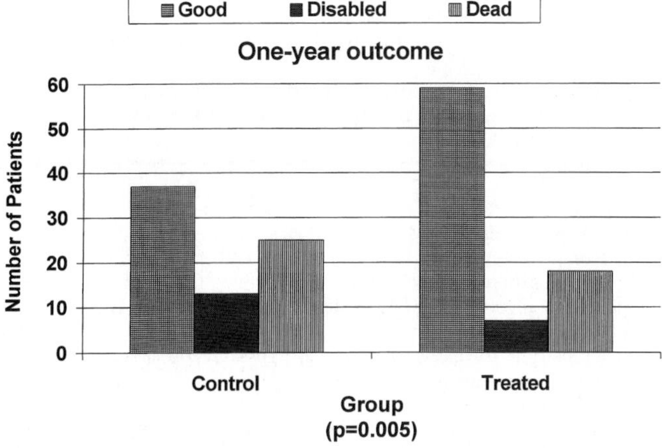

Figure 165–19. Beta blockade in patients with subarachnoid hemorrhage. Patients were randomly treated with propranolol or placebo. Neurologic outcome was better in patients undergoing beta blockade. (Based on data from Neil-Dwyer G, Walter P, Cruickshank JM: Beta-blockade benefits patients following a subarachnoid hemorrhage. Eur J Clin Pharmacol 1985; 28[Suppl]:25.)

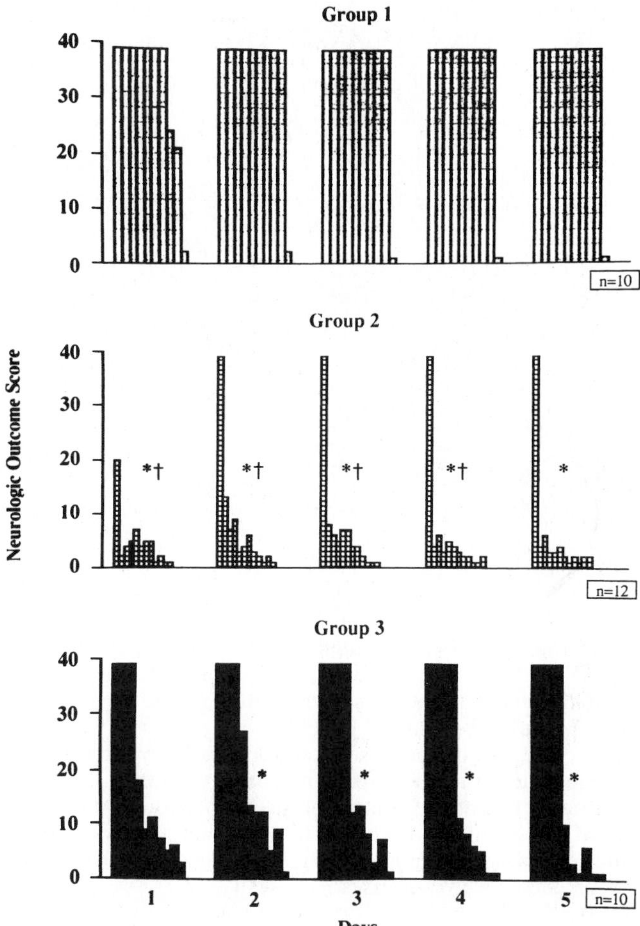

Figure 165–20. Neurologic deficit scores after incomplete focal cerebral ischemia in rats over a 5-day examination period. Each bar represents the neurologic score for each rat (*$P < .05$ versus group 1; †$P < .05$ versus group 3). The rats are ranked according to total outcome score in descending order (0 = normal). Cerebral ischemia was induced with occlusion of one carotid artery with hemorrhagic hypotension. Group 1 rats received no vasoactive drugs, group 2 rats received preischemic hexamethonium, and group 3 rats received hexamethonium plus intravenous epinephrine and norepinephrine. Protection was conferred by hexamethonium in a catecholamine-reversible manner. (From Werner C, Hoffman WE, Thomas C, et al: Ganglionic blockade improves neurologic outcome from incomplete ischemia in rats: Partial reversal by exogenous catecholamines. Anesthesiology 1990; 73:923.)

7. Application of catecholamines directly to nonischemic cortical tissue has also been observed to have neurotoxic potential.[116]

CLINICAL PATHWAYS

Stroke

Subarachnoid Hemorrhage

Incidence

Autopsy studies indicate that as many as 5% of people may harbor aneurysms.[117] Data from a cooperative aneurysm study suggest that about 80% of SAHs arise from aneurysmal rupture.[118] Estimates of the incidence of SAH vary from 3.9 to 19.4 per 100,000 per year,[117, 118] accounting for 6% of all strokes.[119] Mortality from SAH differs considerably among reports—from 3% to 5% in patients in good clinical condition

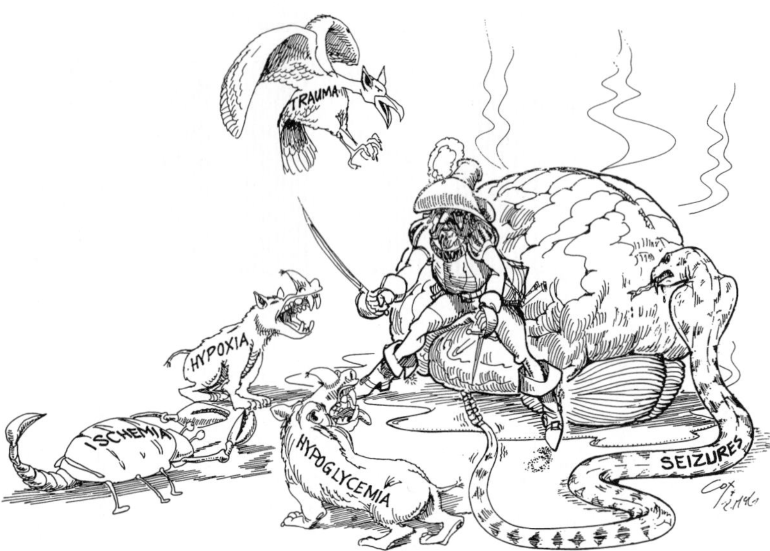

Figure 165–21. Brain protection.

to as high as 68%, overall mortality being approximately 23%.[117, 119, 120] Of the survivors, more than half sustain major disability and 64% of those who return home never regain their premorbid quality of life.[121]

Several types of aneurysms can rupture. They are classified as saccular, atherosclerotic, mycotic, traumatic, and dissecting.[117] The risk of rupture seems to increase as the diameter of the aneurysm exceeds 10 mm. Giant aneurysms (>25 mm) constitute 5% of all aneurysms.[122] Finally, multiple aneurysms occur in 13% of cases.[123]

Ictus

The initial bleeding episode is associated with a transient increase in ICP to systemic levels. This has two predominant effects. The first is a decrement in the level of consciousness, with coma occurring in 45%. Usually, the loss of consciousness is brief, but in 10% of cases it can last days.[124] The second effect of high ICP, presumably, is cessation of the egress of blood from the arterial rupture to promote clot formation.

Subsequent to the bleed, a complex series of events can occur. These include rebleeding, hydrocephalus, catecholamine release, and vasospasm (which can produce a delayed neurologic deficit). Extracranial complications can also contribute to postbleed morbidity and contribute to neurologic problems.

Rebleeding

The probability of rebleeding is about 4% the first day after the initial bleed and about 1.5% per day thereafter. Overall, the incidence of rebleeding is reportedly 19% during the first 2 weeks, 64% by the end of the first month, and 78% 8 weeks after the initial bleed.[125, 126] Several predisposing factors for rebleeding have been identified[126]:

- Female gender
- Admission within the first day after SAH (implying that survival outside the hospital for longer periods selects more stable patients)
- Poor neurologic grade
- Poor general medical condition
- Systolic blood pressure greater than 170 mm Hg

Other factors have also been identified based on theoretical considerations or observations (Table 165–1). Rebleeding is associated with a mortality rate of 48% to 78%.[125, 127]

Hydrocephalus

Based on temporal considerations, hydrocephalus can be divided into three categories: acute, subacute, and delayed (Table 165–2).[128, 129] The ventricular dilatation arises secondary to the effects of fresh blood in the CSF, which can fill the ventricles, block the aqueduct of Sylvius, fill and obstruct the fourth ventricle, fill the subarachnoid cisterns, or block the arachnoid villi. This results in obstruction of CSF circulation or reabsorption leading to hydrocephalus, increased ICP, and depressed level of consciousness.

Intraventricular hemorrhage in association with SAH is associated with worse outcome when hydrocephalus occurs.[130] The cause of this is obstruction of egress of CSF from the ventricles and obstruction of absorption in the arachnoid villi. The likelihood of hydrocephalus correlates with the amount of blood evident on CT.[129] The overall mortality when hydrocephalus occurs is reportedly 64%.[130] Even with ventricular drainage, mortality can remain quite high.[130] Most such patients are admitted with a poorer neurologic grade. The morbidity is related to herniation and to decrements in CBF, which may already be compromised. Hydrocephalus can occur at any time after SAH. It occurs acutely in 20% of patients[129] and

TABLE 165–1. Risk Factors for Rebleeding from a Ruptured Aneurysm During the First 14 Days After Subarachnoid Hemorrhage (SAH)

Risk Factors
Female gender
Advanced age (>70 yr)
Short interval after SAH (days 0–1)
Poor Hunt/Hess grade
Poor systemic medical condition
Moderate to severe systolic hypertension (170–240 mm Hg)
Lumbar puncture
Ventriculostomy to relieve intracranial hypertension associated with systemic hypertension
Infusion of mannitol
Abrupt interruption of antifibrinolytic therapy (inducing rebound in plasma fibrinolytic activity)
Intubation without adequate anesthesia, neuromuscular blockade, or sedation

Adapted from Espinosa F, Weir B, Noseworthy T: Nonoperative treatment of subarachnoid hemorrhage. *In* Neurological Surgery, 3rd ed. Yeomans JR (Ed). Philadelphia, WB Saunders, 1990, pp 1661–1689.

TABLE 165–2. Acute Hydrocephalus After Subarachnoid Hemorrhage

Category	Time to Onset	Presentation
Acute	Hours	Abrupt coma
Subacute	Few days	Gradual decline in mental status
Delayed	Weeks to years	Dementia, gait apraxia, bladder incontinence

subacutely or chronically in 15% to 20%.[125] Permanent CSF diversion is required in 5% to 10% of patients after SAH.[125]

Catecholamines and Glutamate

It is clear that both dicarboxylic amino acid (e.g., glutamate) and catecholamine neurotransmitters have neurotoxic potential.[4, 116, 131, 132] Perhaps equally important are reports of a positive interaction between glutamate and catecholamines.[133] Corticostriatal glutamatergic neurons[134–136] stimulate striatal release of dopamine.[133, 135] Moreover, kainic acid (an excitatory amino acid) administration elevates extracellular dopamine levels.[137] Presynaptic regulation of dopaminergic terminals involves glutamate receptors.[138, 139] This interaction is further supported by observed protective effects of hexamethonium[54] and reserpine[140] against ischemic brain damage. Such observations, examined in the context of SAH and other hyperadrenergic neurologic states, logically suggest that increased brain interstitial catecholamine concentration is associated with increased glutamate release, which may contribute to exacerbation of brain damage.

Vasospasm

The genesis of vasospasm is extremely complex and appears to be multifactorial. Some 3 to 21 days after SAH, more often after 4 to 14 days, comes the period of post-SAH vasospasm. The peak incidence is between days 6 and 8 after SAH.[141, 142] The actual incidence of post-SAH vasospasm varies in the literature between 15% and 76%. The true incidence is probably in the 30% to 40% range.[117, 119, 125] Delayed cerebral ischemia due to delayed vascular narrowing remains one of the most frightening and devastating causes of stroke in a patient who otherwise is recovering well from SAH and surgery. Of patients who develop vasospasm about 30% sustain an ischemic deficit[143, 144] and about 7% to 17% go on to have permanent neurologic deficit or death.[121, 141]

The pathogenesis of vasospasm has been correlated clinically with the amount of blood in the basal cisterns adhering to basal cerebral arteries.[129, 141, 142, 145] In further support of this are observations that in vivo and in vitro application of blood to cerebral arteries produces contraction of the vessels.[146, 147] Several studies have examined the many components of blood for their potential to produce vasospasm.[146] Most of these components do cause spasm, although no single spasmogen has been identified to be the sole cause. Similarly, numerous studies have examined many of the chemicals in the blood, determining that they can cause spasm of cerebral arteries in the experimental situation.[146] Other potential contributors to vasospasm include mechanical wall disruption, inflammation, and free radicals.[146]

The cerebral vasculature maintains appropriate tone through the interplay of many factors. Important in this homeostasis is the balance between endothelin and nitric oxide. Endothelin is a potent vasoconstrictor,[148] and nitric oxide is a short-lived potent vasodilator.[149] Oxyhemoglobin is known to bind nitric oxide.[150] Thus, with degradation of the erythrocytes in the CSF, the basal cerebral arteries are exposed to oxyhemoglobin, which may bind nitric oxide, resulting in spasm.[146, 151] Further support for this cause comes from studies of nitric oxide infused into the vasospastic arteries of monkeys, relieving the spasm.[152]

Serum catecholamine levels increase dramatically after SAH, peaking at the same time as the peak incidence of vasospasm after SAH with symptoms corresponding to serum catecholamine levels.[101–104] Hypothalamic injury with excess catecholamine release may be an important factor in the genesis of post-SAH spasm.[102, 153]

SAH is associated with a decrease in rCBF and cerebral metabolic rate of oxygen ($CMRO_2$), even with a good clinical grade and without vasospasm.[146, 154] Nonetheless, many studies have shown a relationship between decreased rCBF and the presence of vasospasm, particularly when vasospasm is severe or there are focal deficits.[154, 155] The decrease in rCBF is accompanied by an increase in CBV,[154] suggesting that the large proximal vessel constriction is accompanied by small distal vessel dilatation.

Data indicate that the vasospasm-mediated decreased rCBF and accompanying decrease in cerebral metabolic rate (CMR) are uncoupled.[155] The extent of the uncoupling of vascular control from metabolic needs is so severe that decrements in rCBF sufficient to cause ischemic stroke can occur.[125, 156] In nonsurvivors of SAH, as many as 45% developed a stroke after the SAH.[157, 158] Thus, vasospasm represents an extreme form of cerebral dysautoregulation, one severe enough to persist in spite of persistent and severe anaerobic metabolism.

Seizures

During the acute phase after SAH, up to 26% of patients have seizures.[159] Moreover, some 13% to 15% go on to have epilepsy as a chronic complication of the SAH, the incidence increasing to 30% when the SAH arises from a middle cerebral artery (MCA) aneurysm, presumably because of proximity to the temporal lobe. In addition, the incidence increases from 5% in those without neurologic deficit to 41% in those with such deficits.[160]

Extracranial Complications

A variety of extracranial complications arise as direct consequences of the SAH. These include abnormalities in cardiovascular, pulmonary, endocrine, and electrolyte homeostasis. Many of these abnormalities can be traced to the post-SAH hyperadrenergic state or hypothalamic dysfunction.

Systemic hypertension is common after SAH[161] and is most likely related to elevated catecholamines and renin secondary to hypothalamic disturbance.[107, 162] Other causes include intracranial hypertension, preexisting essential hypertension, seizures, vomiting, pain, bladder distention, agitation, or vasospasm. Hypertension, in addition to rebleeding, is associated with a higher incidence of vasospasm and death.[163]

Cardiac arrhythmias are observed in almost all patients after SAH,[107, 108, 164] and ECG changes suggestive of myocardial ischemia occur in 50% to 80% of patients after SAH.[101, 107, 164] The arrhythmias can be severe or life-threatening in 20%.[164] A rather diverse array of ECG changes can occur (Table 165–3), many of them indicative of myocardial ischemia. It is likely that these changes are more than simple artifacts. Ventricular wall motion abnormalities consistent with myocardial ischemia have been observed after SAH, particularly with poorer neurologic grades.[109] In addition, creatine phosphokinase (CPK) isoenzyme elevations indicative of myocardial infarction have been reported,[110] and at postmortem examination myocardial necrosis has been documented in association with SAH.[165]

Neurogenic pulmonary edema is a rare complication of SAH, having been ascribed to the brief period of severe intracranial hypertension associated with the initial bleeding or the postbleeding surge in catecholamine levels.[166–168] After

TABLE 165–3. Electrocardiographic Abnormalities After Subarachnoid Hemorrhage

Prominent P waves
Prolonged or shortened PR interval
Broad, inverted, or flattened T waves
Q-T prolongation or shortening
ST-segment elevation or depression
Prominent or inverted U waves
Pathological Q waves
S in V_1 and R in V_5 combined > 35 mm
Rhythm disturbances

Adapted from Adams HP, Love BB: Medical management of aneurysmal subarachnoid hemorrhage. *In:* Stroke: Pathophysiology, Diagnosis, and Management. 2nd ed. Barnett HJM, Mohr JP, Stein BM, Yatsu FM (Eds). New York, Churchill Livingstone, 1992, pp 1029–1054.

SAH, increases in blood-borne vasogenic substances may occur. These substances promote permeability of the pulmonary vasculature so that pulmonary edema occurs at lower than normal hydrostatic pressures.[166, 168]

After SAH, abnormalities in fluid and sodium homeostasis occur in about 33% of patients.[169] Both hypovolemia and hyponatremia are commonly observed. The clinical presentation may appear consistent with SIADH. In the past, such patients typically were treated with fluid restriction,[170] which in retrospect would be expected to aggravate hypovolemia and increase blood viscosity, both undesirable after SAH. More recent studies indicate that both fluid and sodium are lost after SAH,[99, 171, 172] indicating that the hyponatremia is not a straightforward issue of dilution due to excessive water retention. Declines in blood volume have been observed using tracer techniques.[171] In addition, the kidneys cannot retain sodium,[172] consistent with observed increases in atrial natriuretic factor,[172, 173] constituting the so-called cerebral salt wasting syndrome.[99, 161, 172] Atrial natriuretic factor levels in plasma peak 3 days after SAH and then fall by 7 days after the SAH.[172, 173] Hypokalemia occurs frequently after SAH and is most likely due to vomiting, elevated circulating catecholamines, corticosteroids, renin, or diuretic use.

Fever is a common concomitant of SAH.[174, 175] The etiologic mechanism is unclear. Nonetheless, fever can be one indicator of developing vasospasm.[175] Unfortunately, patients with SAH commonly have undergone instrumentation of the vasculature, bladder, brain, or trachea, all of which can independently cause infection with accompanying fever. In addition, these patients may have other potential causes of fever, including deep vein thrombosis, biliary stasis, and multiple drug therapy. The presence of fever in this patient group is made more serious by the fact that fever dramatically exacerbates the consequences of cerebral ischemia,[67] as can occur with vasospasm.

Intracerebral Hemorrhage

Multiple epidemiologic studies performed after the advent of CT indicate that the incidence of intracerebral hemorrhage (ICH) is 12 to 15 per 100,000 per year and accounts for 8% to 13% of all strokes.[176, 177] Before the age of 45 years, the incidence is less than 2 per 100,000. With each 10 years above that, the incidence progressively increases to 350 per 100,000 for persons 80 years or older.[177] In the Rochester 32-year study, ICH increased with age, male gender, and hypertension. The primary risk factor for ICH is hypertension.[177, 178] It has been reported as a preexisting condition in 72% to 81% of ICHs.[179] This is further supported by observations of left ventricular hypertrophy[180] and significantly higher admission blood pressures with ICH than in other types of stroke.[181] However, other conditions can also predispose to ICH. These include blood dyscrasias, vascular malformations, and tumors, accounting for about 25% of ICHs.[182] Others have suggested that hypertension accounts for only 50% of ICHs,[183] not 75%, as was earlier reported.[179] With time and better control of hypertension the incidence of ICH has decreased, indicating that hypertension is a controllable risk factor for ICH.[176, 184] The use of anticoagulants increases the risk of ICH sixfold.[185] Amyloid angiopathy accounts for most lobar hemorrhages.[186]

With the onset of blood leak from an intracranial vessel, blood accumulates locally under arteriolar pressure, injuring adjacent vessels, which then leak, destroying parenchyma locally, displacing intact neural structures, and dissecting away from the initial bleeding site. High arterial pressure and brain atrophy promote enlargement of the hematoma; however, local tissue pressure increase combined with elevated ICP tends to limit the size of the enlarging hematoma.[187] The bleeding focus has been described pathologically as *fibrin globes* or *bleeding globes.*[178, 188] The bleeding is thought generally to be an abrupt monophasic event that usually lasts only minutes.[178, 181, 189] Symptoms and signs are then due to increased ICP, disruption of local neural function, and brain edema[187]; however, recent anecdotes and reports of clinical series indicate that secondary enlargement of the hemorrhage can occur.[178, 190]

Specific vascular abnormalities that may contribute to or cause intracerebral hematomas have been identified, although the presence of other factors is still a possibility. Fibrinoid necrosis, lipohyalinosis, and microaneurysms of brain blood vessels have been implicated. Fibrinoid necrosis refers to observations of fibrin-platelet masses observed primarily at the interface between hematoma and surrounding brain tissue. Such fibrin globes seem to cover areas of disruptions in small arteries.[191] Lipohyalinization is a degenerative process of subintimal accumulation of lipid and proteinaceous material in the walls of small arteries associated with focal necrosis and inflammation.[191–193] Charcot-Bouchard miliary microaneurysms are also seen in patients with ICH and are associated with lacunar infarcts.[189, 193]

ICHs have been categorized pathologically based on size as *petechial, small, large,* and *massive.* An ICH is considered massive when it is greater than 3 cm in the cerebrum, greater than 2 cm in the cerebellum, and greater than 1 cm in the brain stem.

The anatomic site of ICH has been described in a number of reports.[178, 191] The approximate frequencies are shown in Table 165–4. The anatomic location is also thought to provide some etiologic information.

Ischemic Stroke

The pathophysiologic biochemical processes underlying cerebral ischemia were reviewed earlier in this chapter. Patients

TABLE 165–4. Anatomic Site, Frequency, and Etiology of Intracerebral Hematomas

Location	Frequency (%)	Usual Causes
Caudate/putamen	35–50	Hypertension
Subcortical white matter	30	AVM, saccular aneurysm, neoplasm, blood dyscrasia, drug abuse, amyloid angiopathy, hypertension
Cerebellum	16	Hypertension, AVM, blood dyscrasia
Thalamus	10–15	Hypertension
Pons	5–12	Hypertension, AVM

AVM = arteriovenous malformation.

with ischemic stroke, particularly those with thrombotic stroke, often present with a history that includes risk factors for stroke, including hypertension, smoking, heart disease, and diabetes. In addition, a history of transient ischemic attacks (TIAs) is common, particularly with thrombotic stroke. Patients present with focal signs that usually come on abruptly and may have progressed from the time of onset.

Ischemic infarcts in the brain are due to one of three mechanisms of vascular insufficiency:

- Cerebral arterial hypotension (hemodynamic infarct)
- Embolism
- Thrombosis

However, 30% to 40% of patients cannot be readily categorized and are considered to have infarction of unknown origin.[196, 197]

Cerebral arterial hypotension occurs with systemic hypotension resulting in CPP below 60 mm Hg; however, it can also occur with focal intracranial vascular stenosis, so that a patient who is systemically normotensive may exhibit symptomatic intracranial hypotension. This situation also occurs when hypertensive patients taking antihypertensive therapy develop ischemic signs as blood pressure is reduced.

Cerebral embolism arises from clots originating in the left chamber of the heart, aorta, or carotid artery, or from venous thromboembolism with right-to-left passage through the heart. Several categories of patients are particularly prone to embolic stroke; these conditions include:

- Atrial fibrillation
- Ventricular wall motion abnormalities (e.g., recent myocardial infarction, ventricular aneurysm, cardiomyopathy)
- Valvular diseases
- Septal defects
- Carotid or aortic disease
- Proximal thrombosis throwing emboli distally
- Hypercoagulation states

Embolism is suggested when there are multiple brain infarcts in different arterial territories. Most of these infarcts involve cortical structures and tend to involve MCA territory. Cardioembolic strokes are thought to account for about one third of ischemic strokes.[194]

Thrombotic stroke occurs when a thrombosis arises in a patent artery. Atherothrombotic strokes occur secondary to arteriosclerotic narrowing of a cerebral vessel with superimposed development of a thrombus, which may propagate distally. Atherothrombotic strokes are thought to account for two thirds of ischemic strokes.[194] Typically, the vessel was previously stenotic from atherosclerosis and the low-flow state, with perhaps nonlaminar flow predisposing to thrombotic occlusion of the artery with ischemia to distal tissues.[195] Cerebral venous sinus thrombosis can also cause ischemic infarction. Lacunar strokes, a subcategory of atherothrombotic strokes, are small infarcts due to occlusion of small penetrating arteries of the brain that tend to branch at 90 degrees from the parent artery and supply the deep white and gray matter of the cerebral hemispheres.

Ischemic stroke has a variety of presentations, which vary according to the vascular territory being disrupted (Table 165–5).[196] The brain's vascular supply can be divided into the *anterior circulation,* arising from the carotid arteries, and the *posterior circulation,* arising from the vertebrobasilar arteries. Strokes secondary to internal carotid artery occlusion can be due to low flow or distal embolus and can present with a spectrum of symptoms from infarction of the entire anterior cerebral artery (ACA) and MCA territories to silent occlusion.

MCA symptoms vary according to which MCA division has been occluded:

Superior division MCA stroke usually presents with hemiparesis (face and arm more than leg), hemisensory loss, mutism or motor aphasia, and dysarthria.

Inferior division MCA stroke may present with Wernicke's aphasia (left hemisphere) without hemiparesis, homonymous hemianopia, neglect, dressing apraxia, and constructional apraxia (right hemisphere).

MCA stem occlusion produces contralateral hemiplegia, hemisensory loss, global aphasia, homonymous hemianopia, and gaze preference.

Anterior cerebral artery occlusion produces contralateral weakness and sensory loss in the foot and leg more than arm, grasp reflex, incontinence, and transcortical motor aphasia.

Posterior cerebral artery occlusion causes contralateral homonymous hemianopia, sensory loss, hemiparesis (usually transient), and memory loss. In dominant-hemisphere posterior cerebral artery (PCA) infarcts, a syndrome of alexia (inability to read) without agraphia (inability to write) may occur.

Basilar artery occlusion produces brain stem signs such as cranial nerve palsies, gaze palsies, internuclear ophthal-

TABLE 165–5. Ischemic Stroke Signs and Symptoms by Site*

Site	Signs and Symptoms
Internal carotid artery	With adequate collaterals, none Wide range of contralateral deficits, depending on collaterals and mechanism: monoparesis, hemiparesis, sensory deficit, language difficulty; ipsilateral transient monocular blindness
Middle cerebral artery	M1 occlusion: contralateral hemiplegia, hemisensory deficit, homonymous hemianopsia; gaze preference and aphasia (dominant stroke); and nondominant parietal syndrome (nondominant stroke). With intact surface collaterals only motor deficit may be seen, or none. Distal occlusions produce partial syndromes.
Anterior cerebral artery	Contralateral leg weakness and sensory deficit. Sometimes involvement of proximal muscles of contralateral arm. Cognitive impairment. Grasp responses
Vertebral artery	Lateral medullary infarct (also from occlusion of PICA): vertigo, nausea, vomiting, dysphagia, ipsilateral cerebellar ataxia, ipsilateral Horner's syndrome, decreased pain and temperature sensation on ipsilateral face and contralateral legs, arms, and trunk.
Basilar artery	Deficits of variable severity: none, transient ischemic attacks, brain stem infarction. Dizziness, vertigo, nystagmus, "locked in," coma, cranial nerve palsies.
Posterior cerebral artery	Contralateral homonymous visual field deficit. Alexia without agraphia (dominant hemisphere). Thalamic-sensory loss with proximal lesion; sometimes transient hemiplegia.

Data from Barnett HJM et al (Eds): Stroke. Pathophysiology, Diagnosis, and Management 2nd ed., New York, Churchill-Livingstone, 1992, and Adams RD, Victor M: Cerebrovascular diseases. In: Principles of Neurology. 5th ed. Adams RD, Victor M (Eds). New York, McGraw-Hill, 1993.

*Onset of signs and symptoms is usually abrupt but not always. The deficits can either progress or remit in the first 24 hours.

PICA = posterior inferior cerebral artery.

moplegia (paresis for eye adduction), bilateral long tract signs (motor or sensory), coma, and cerebellar ataxia. Lower and midbasilar arterial occlusions are usually due to thrombosis. In the upper basilar artery, embolus is more common.

Coma in association with stroke is an important stroke subset in the intensive care unit. Coma tends to occur when there is loss of function of both cerebral hemispheres or the reticular activating system in the midbrain and upper pons. Thus, strokes producing decrements in flow to these areas depress consciousness. Bilateral cerebral ischemia is uncommon upon presentation with focal ischemia of only one hemisphere unless there is hypotension, previous infarction of the other hemisphere, or emboli to both hemispheres. Such patients tend to present "responsive"; however, when the stroke is large enough and significant post-stroke swelling occurs, elevations in ICP can compromise perfusion to the brain stem or the other hemisphere, leading to a comatose state. Conversely, patients with significant basilar ischemia involving the reticular activating system may present initially comatose and remain so unless there is early recanalization of the obstructed artery. Patients who present with cerebellar hemorrhage or infarction may be responsive; however, the cerebellum may swell. There is little room for edema formation in the posterior fossa, and obstructive hydrocephalus can arise secondary to occlusion of the fourth ventricle. Thus, a limited amount of swelling can lead precipitously to a comatose state after cerebellar infarction or hemorrhage.

Coma can also be produced by nonischemic events with stroke, one of the most significant being seizures. Such an occurrence can appear to be occult if the patient is having nonconvulsive seizure activity or if the seizure was not witnessed and the patient is exhibiting a postictal depression of consciousness. Other causes of coma that may be associated with stroke are sepsis, electrolyte disturbances, hyperosmolar states, hypoglycemia, Wernicke's encephalopathy, hepatic encephalopathy, and toxic states.[197]

It is estimated that 4% to 10% of stroke patients develop secondary seizure.[198] Age, gender, or side of the stroke appear to have no effect on occurrence of these seizures. Some 50% to 60% of seizures occur in the first 24 hours after the onset of the stroke; 7% to 8% by the end of the first month; and the remainder, later. About 50% of the seizures are grand mal (i.e., tonic-clonic), convulsions. Simple partial seizures occur in 37% to 47% and status epilepticus in 6% to 8%.[198] Hemorrhage tends to increase the risk of seizure. In general, infarct-associated seizure occurs when the infarct involves the cortex of the parietal lobe or motor cortex. When seizure follows stroke it is associated with increased risk of mortality, from 21% to 31%.[198]

About 20% of ischemic stroke patients exhibit worsening of the initial deficit within 4 days of onset of symptoms.[199] It is likely that such stroke progression is secondary to enlargement of the intravascular clot that causes the stroke, providing a logical rationale for the use of heparin. However, other factors, such as increasing peri-infarct edema or superimposed oxygenation and metabolic disturbances, can also contribute to secondary worsening, as can hemorrhagic conversion of the infarct. Elevated ICP can be a cause of delayed deterioration after stroke. Indeed, a patient may be admitted fully conscious with a large deficit related to hemispheric ischemia yet be dead within days because of swelling and herniation of the infarcted brain and surrounding tissue. In general, the more extensive the stroke the greater is the chance of intracranial hypertension.

Like intracranial hemorrhage and SAH,[110, 200] ischemic stroke is associated with a significantly increased incidence of cardiac arrhythmias, ventricular ectopy being most common.[201, 202] These ECG changes portend a poorer prognosis.[203] In addition, 11% of patients with ECG changes show elevations in cardiac isoenzymes,[204] an observation associated with doubling of mortality.[205] These consequences are probably related to stroke-induced elevations of blood catecholamines.[108, 200, 206] It is apparent that ECG changes in stroke patients are not mere artifacts.

Laboratory studies have provided evidence that an ischemic stroke produces a central ischemic core surrounded by a penumbra where blood flow is reduced and pressure-dependent (via collateral vessels). This dependence of blood flow on perfusion pressure is supported by clinical observations in stroke patients.[207] Such data suggest that it may not be safe to decrease blood pressure in a stroke patient in the absence of compelling indications.

Seizures*

Status epilepticus is defined as (1) more than 30 minutes of continuous seizure activity or (2) two or more sequential seizures without full recovery of consciousness between convulsions.[208, 209] An urgent approach to seizure control is supported by observations of seizure-associated brain damage in humans[210] and by animal studies showing uncontrolled status epilepticus for 20 minutes or longer to be associated with neuronal damage.[211, 212] Thus, generalized convulsive status epilepticus is considered a neurologic emergency.

Epilepsy is a rather heterogeneous disease with a diverse array of pathogenetic mechanisms. Seizures can arise as a result of abnormalities in (1) regulation of neural circuits, (2) the balance between excitation and inhibition, (3) extracellular potassium homeostasis, and (4) genes. These will be briefly reviewed. Several excellent recent reviews provide more detailed summaries.[213-215] Many of the mechanisms suggested for the genesis of seizures are only hypotheses, but they have been proposed in the context of ample experimental support to make them credible.

The CNS exists in a delicate equilibrium between depression and excitation. Pathologic processes that disrupt it can lead to seizure. This is the overriding concept that seems to be common to all theories of the pathogenesis of epilepsy.

Anatomic Circuit Mechanisms

Seizure activity is generated and propagated by specific neural macrocircuits. Such circuits often exist in a state of interactive modulation of their respective functions. An excitatory pathway, in addition to sending afferents to a given structure, may also be modulated by another structure that modulates the originating excitatory source. One example of this in rat models is the substantia nigra. Available evidence indicates that it acts as a gating mechanism to modulate, via GABA-ergic efferents, excitation in other brain structures.[216]

Uncontrolled seizure activity produces selective neuronal loss, which, one theory suggests, leads to disruption of the inhibitory-excitatory balance subsequently to favor recurrent seizures. Hippocampal sclerosis has long been associated with epilepsy. Resection of this injured area of the hippocampus substantially decreases seizure tendency. This suggests that an initial seizure damages the hippocampus, which leads to further seizures and worse hippocampal damage, further predisposing to seizure. Thus, a single inciting clinical event, such as a febrile seizure, may lead to this positive feedback cycle and epilepsy.[217]

*Adapted from Kofke WA, Dasheff RM, Tempelhoff R: J Neurosurg Anesth 1997; 9:349-372.

Two theories have been suggested to account for this phenomenon of seizures begetting epilepsy. The first is the "dormant basket cell hypothesis."[218] Temporal lobe seizure leads to selective loss of excitatory cells in the hippocampus. These cells excite GABA-ergic interneurons to modulate the effects of the exciting afferent cell and other excitatory cells in the hippocampus. Thus, a paradoxical effect may arise wherein loss of excitatory cells results in more excitation owing to synaptic dysinhibition. The second hypothesis, the "mossy fiber–sprouting hypothesis," holds that increased dentate granule cell excitability is due to pathologic rearrangement of neuronal circuitry consequent to seizure-induced damage.[219] With the loss of the mossy cell, the granule cell, rather than forming synapses with the mossy cell, "synapses on itself," so that the granule cell is more likely to overrespond to excitatory input.[213] The anatomic basis for this observation has been reported in animal models[219, 220] and in specimens from humans with epilepsy.[219-221]

Local Imbalance Between Excitation and Inhibition

Excitation-inhibition imbalance is basically the mechanism of epileptogenesis with neuronal microcircuit abnormalities. Several mechanisms are important at the level of neurotransmitters and receptors that can contribute to this imbalance. Enhanced function of the NMDA receptor has been identified in some animal models,[222] and it is thought to be related to a novel NMDA receptor type.[222] Consistent with these observations in animals are reports of enhanced excitatory amino acid receptor function in tissue from epileptic humans.[223] Conversely, there is experimental evidence that indicates that the efficacy of GABA stimulation to increase chloride conductance (an important inhibitory membrane effect) decreases in kindled epileptic rats.[224] Congruent observations, decreased GABA-A and benzodiazepine receptor binding, and reduced benzodiazepine receptors, have also been made in humans with epilepsy.[225] Microdialysis studies indicate increased release of excitatory amino acids in animal models[226] and in humans with epilepsy[227]; however, it is not clear whether these observations are causative or a secondary effect of seizures.

Extracellular Potassium

The role of potassium in epilepsy has been very nicely reviewed and synthesized by McNamara.[213] Elevated extracellular potassium has been observed in vivo in seizure models in animals.[228] Whether such increases in extracellular potassium are causing seizures or are an epiphenomenon has been questioned.[229] Studies in vitro have suggested that elevated extracellular potassium may be an important contributor to initiation and propagation of seizures.[230] The evidence is most supportive of the notion that high extracellular potassium levels are an important contributor to propagation of seizures, for example after an interictal spike. The theory proposed suggests that a variety of epileptogenic events are consequent to elevated extracellular potassium[230]:

- Partial depolarization, shifting the membrane potential closer to the spike threshold
- Attenuating post-burst hyperpolarizing afterpotential, which normally limits repetitive firing
- Reduction of the GABA-B component of the inhibitory postsynaptic potential (IPSP), which is mediated by potassium efflux[231] while reducing the GABA-A component of the IPSP[232]
- Swelling of cells via reduced potassium efflux,[233] further increasing extracellular potassium concentration through decreased size of the extracellular space and further increasing neuronal synchronization[213]
- Depolarization induced by extracellular potassium-promoting NMDA receptor activation[234]

Genes

Inherited forms of epilepsy account for at least 20% of all cases.[235] Several animal models of genetic epilepsy have been described that identify a variety of gene mutations that can cause epilepsy. Indeed, some reports localize certain human epileptic conditions to a specific chromosome.[236] Studies of twins with epilepsy with a 65% concordance for penetrance of an epilepsy phenotype provide further support for the notion of a strong genetic influence on its development.[215] These studies clearly indicate that the genesis of epilepsy can be multifactorial and that several genetic abnormalities most certainly underlie the predisposition to develop epilepsy.

Trauma

Pathophysiology

Brain trauma can be produced by several mechanisms. There are many categories of brain trauma: penetrating injury, hematoma effects, contusion, and white matter shear. The specific effects of such disruption depend to a great extent on the anatomic site. Isolated cortical or white matter lesions tend to produce focal deficits. Injuries to the midbrain and hindbrain or diffusely and bilaterally to the cerebral hemispheres tend to have global effects on the level of consciousness. Penetrating injury produces irreversible structural abnormalities. Contusion and hematoma produce abnormalities that may resolve. White matter shear occurs as a result of inertia between brain structures that disrupts neural circuitry.[237] Such lesions *may* be suggested by the presence of petechial lesions on CT; however, when the lesions are not demonstrated by CT the diagnosis depends on the extent of clinical improvement, which is less than would be expected from the initial imaging studies.

Brain trauma results in widespread abnormalities in brain anatomy, perfusion, metabolism, and function. With closed head trauma, to which this discussion will be limited, the initial impact results in mechanical disruption of the integrity of cellular and supporting tissue membranes.[238, 239] Subsequently, numerous secondary phenomena result that can cause the patient's condition to deteriorate.[240, 241] Blood and edema fluid accumulate as normal compartmentation is disrupted. Secondary ischemia then assumes principal pathophysiologic importance.

As ischemia develops, a variety of adverse biochemical processes occur. Many are due to the mechanical disruption and secondarily are exacerbated by ischemia. These biochemical events include release of free radicals[242] with lipid peroxidation, excitatory amino acids,[243] inflammatory mediators,[244] production of metabolic acidosis,[245] and other effects that compromise the neurologic outcome. As time passes microcirculatory disturbances related to edema and blood-brain barrier disruption occur with abnormalities in substances that regulate blood flow. In addition, it is thought that areas of vasospasm may occur, perhaps related to the presence of free blood in the CSF or locally around parenchymal blood vessels.[246]

Initially, CBF is depressed, subsequently resulting in hyperemia. After that, CBF returns to normal with resolution of membrane abnormalities or progresses to zero with infarction, because hyperemia may act to exacerbate the edema.[49, 247]

With edema and hemorrhage, the intracranial volume of blood and brain tissue can increase. This results in increased ICP.[33, 247, 248] Regional or global ICP increases progressively with edema, resulting in lower CBF, an oligemic form of intracranial hypertension that can lead to permanent brain damage. With head injury, cerebral dysautoregulation with altered intracranial compliance results in hyperemia that is manifested as high ICP (i.e., hyperemic ICH), which is exacerbated by increased blood pressure (and distention of injured vessels), fever, cerebral stimulants, cerebral vasodilators, and noxious or painful stimuli. With respect to whole brain function hyperemic intracranial hypertension probably does not have the same dire significance as the oligemic type; however, the intracranial hypertension may produce regional exacerbation of the brain damage ultimately sustained in injured brain areas where perfusion is tenuous (see Physiologic Pathways and Exacerbating Factors earlier).

SUMMARY

Brain damage can arise from a variety of seemingly disparate neurologic disease states—ischemia, seizures, and trauma, among others. At the biochemical level there appears to be significant commonality among these conditions. Observations in humans and in animal models indicate involvement of acidosis, excitatory amino acids, apoptosis, autolytic processes, and brain edema. Moreover, elevated ICP typically occurs as these conditions progress. With episodes of elevated ICP, it is important to distinguish hyperemic causes (i.e., high CBV) from oligemic ones. Any brain injury is significantly affected by the extracranial environment. Such extracranial factors include temperature, gas exchange, glucose, sepsis, sodium, and catecholamines.

The notion of delayed maturation of a neural lesion suggests that post-insult therapies and external factors may affect the ultimate outcome. Significant advances have been made in understanding the pathogenesis of neural death after ischemia, trauma, and seizures; however, few specific therapies are available that can reliably and safely prevent biochemical progression of a neurologic lesion. Nonetheless, there is a nascent clinical effort that uses this information about neuropathophysiology to develop brain-protective therapies for humans.

References

1. Klatzo I: Evolution of brain edema concepts. Acta Neurochir 1994; 60(Suppl):3-6.
2. Sapolsky RM, Trafton J, Tombaugh GC: Excitotoxic neuron death, acidotic endangerment, and the paradox of acidotic protection. Adv Neurol 1996; 71:237-244; discussion, 244-245.
3. Tombaugh GC, Sapolsky RM: Evolving concepts about the role of acidosis in ischemic neuropathology. J Neurochem 1993; 61:793-803.
4. Benveniste H: The excitotoxin hypothesis in relation to cerebral ischemia. Cerebrovasc Brain Metab Rev 1991; 3:213-245.
5. Weller M, Schulz JB, Wullner U, Loschmann PA, Klockgether T, Dichgans J: Developmental and genetic regulation of programmed neuronal death. J Neural Transm 1997; 50(Suppl):115-123.
6. Choi DW: Ischemia-induced neuronal apoptosis. Curr Opin Neurobiol 1996; 6:667-672.
7. Citron BA, Zhang SX, Smirnova IV, Festoff BW: Apoptotic, injury-induced cell death in cultured mouse murine motor neurons. Neurosci Lett 1997; 230:25-28.
8. Lassman H: Basic mechanisms of brain inflammation. J Neural Transm 1997; 50(Suppl):183-190.
9. Rossen R, Kabat H, Anderson JP: Acute arrest of cerebral circulation in man. Arch Neurol Psychiatr 1943; 50:510-528.
10. Michenfelder JD, Theye RA: The effects of anesthesia and hypothermia on canine cerebral ATP and lactate during anoxia produced by decapitation. Anesthesiology 1970; 33:430-439.
11. Ljunggren B, Ratcheson RA, Siesjo BK: Cerebral metabolic state following complete compression ischemia. Brain Res 1974; 73:291-307.
12. Pulsinelli WA, Brierley JB, Plum F: Temporal profile of neuronal damage in a model of transient forebrain ischemia. Ann Neurol 1982; 11:491-498.
13. Kofke WA, Garman RH, Stiller R, Rose M, Janosky M: Striatal extracellular dopamine levels are not increased by hyperglycemic exacerbation of ischemic brain damage in rats. Brain Res 1994; 633:171-177.
14. Ingvar M: Seizure-induced damage in the substantia nigra pars reticulata: Lesions in the frontal cortex prior to the seizure period mitigate the damage. Exp Brain Res 1989; 75:369-374.
15. Buisson A, Callebert J, Mathieu E, Plotkine M, Boulu RG: Striatal projection induced by lesioning the substantia nigra of rats subjected to focal ischemia. J Neurochem 1992; 59:1153-1157.
16. Gilman AG: G proteins: Transducers of receptor-generated signals. Ann Rev Biochem 1987; 56:615-649.
17. Alexander SPH, Peters JA: 1997 receptor and ion channel nomenclature. Trends Pharmacol Sci Suppl 1997; 1-84.
18. Nishizuka Y: The role of protein kinase C in cell surface signal transduction and tumour promotion. Nature 1984; 308:693-698.
19. Bell RM: Protein kinase C activation by diacylglycerol second messengers. Cell 1986; 45:631-632.
20. Berridge MJ, Irvine RF: Inositol phosphates and cell signalling. Nature 1989; 341:197-205.
21. Marks AR: Intracellular calcium-release channels: Regulators of cell life and death. Am J Physiol 1997; 272:H597-H605.
22. Schulman H, Lou LL: Multifunctional Ca^{+2}/calmodulin-dependent protein kinase: Domain structure and regulation. Trends Pharm Sci 1989; 14:62-66.
23. Sheng M, McFadden G, Greenberg M: Membrane depolarization and calcium induce c-fos transcription via phosphorylation of transcription factor CREB. Neuron 1990; 4:571-582.
24. Coyle JT, Bird SJ, Evans RH, et al: Excitatory amino acid neurotoxins: Selectivity, specificity, and mechanisms of action. Neruro-sci Res Prog Bull 1981; 19:331-427.
25. Akins PT, Liu PK, Hsu CY: Immediate early gene expression in response to cerebral ischemia. Friend or foe? Stroke 1996; 27:1682-1687.
26. Gaspary H, Graham SH, Sagar SM, Sharp FR: HSP70 heat shock protein induction following global ischemia in the rat. Brain Res Mol Brain Res 1995; 34:327-332.
27. Matsuoka Y, Hossmann KA: Brain tissue osmolality after middle cerebral artery occlusion in cats. Exp Neurol 1982; 77:599-611.
28. Gotoh O, Asano T, Koide T, et al: Ischemic brain edema following occlusion of the middle cerebral artery in the rat. I. The time course of the brain water, sodium, and potassium contents and blood-brain barrier permeability to ^{125}I-albumin. Stroke 1985; 16:101-109.
29. Kato H, Kogure K, Sakamoto N, Watanabe T: Greater disturbance of water and ion homeostasis in the periphery of experimental focal cerebral ischemia. Exp Neurol 1987; 96:118-126.
30. Cushing H: Concerning a definite regulatory mechanism of the vaso-motor centre which controls blood pressure during cerebral compression. Johns Hopkins Hosp Bull 1901; 290-292.
31. Risberg J, Lundberg N, Ingvar DH: Regional cerebral blood volume during acute rises in the intracranial pressure (plateau waves). J Neurosurg 1969; 31:303-310.
32. Rosner MJ, Becker DP: Origin and evolution of plateau waves: Experimental observations and a theoretical model. J Neurosurg 1984; 50:312-324.
33. Miller JD, Becker DP, Ward JD, Sullivan HG, Asams WE, Rosner MJ: Significance of intracranial hypertension in severe head injury. J Neurosurg 1977; 47:503-516.
34. Giulioni M, Ursino M, Alvisi C: Correlations among intracranial pulsatility, intracranial hemodynamics, and transcranial Doppler wave form: Literature review and hypothesis for future studies. Neurosurgery 1988; 22:807-812.
35. Hassler W, Steinmetz H, Gawlowski J: Transcranial Doppler ultrasonography in raised intracranial pressure and in intracranial circulatory arrest. J Neurosurg 1988; 68:745-751.
36. von Haken MS, Aschoff AA: Acute obstructive hydrocephalus.

In: NeuroCritical Care. Hacke W, Hanley DF, Einhaupt KM, et al (Eds). New York, Springer-Verlag, 1994, p 869.

37. Bederson JB, Wiestler OD, Brustle O, Roth P, Frick R, Yasargil MG: Intracranial venous hypertension and the effects of venous outflow obstruction in a rat model of arteriovenous fistula. Neurosurgery 1991; 29:341-350.
38. Kofke WA, Dong ML, Bloom M, Policare R, Janosky J, Sekhar L: Transcranial Doppler ultrasonography with induction of anesthesia for neurosurgery. J Neurosurg Anesthesiol 1994; 6:89-97.
39. Michenfelder JD: The 27th Rovenstine Lecture: Neuroanesthesia and the achievement of professional respect. Anesthesiology 1989; 70:695-701.
40. Jaggi JL, Obrist WD, Gennarelli TA, Langfitt TW: Relationship of early CBF and metabolism to outcome in acute head injury. J Neurosurg 1990; 72:176-182.
41. Lundberg N: Continuous recording and control of ventricular fluid pressure in neurosurgical practice. Acta Psychiatr Neurol Scand 1960; 36(Suppl 149):1.
42. Matakas F, Von Waechter R, Knupling R, Potolicchio SJ Jr: Increase in cerebral perfusion pressure by arterial hypertension in brain swelling: A mathematical model of the volume-pressure relationship. J Neurosurg 1975; 42:282-289.
43. Huseby JS, Luce JM, Cary JM, Pavlin EG, Butler J: Effects of positive end-expiratory pressure on intracranial pressure in dogs with intracranial hypertension. J Neurosurg 1981; 55:704-705.
44. Shapiro HM, Marshall LF: Intracranial pressure responses to PEEP in head-injured patients. J Trauma 1978; 18:254-256.
45. Aidinis SJ, Lafferty J, Shapiro HM: Intracranial responses to PEEP. Anesthesiology 1976; 45:275-286.
46. Harken AH, Brennan MF, Smith B, et al: The hemodynamic response to positive end-expiratory ventilation in hypovolemic patients. Surgery 1974; 76:786-793.
47. Griswold WR, Roznik V, Mendoza SA: Nitroprusside induced intracranial hypertension. JAMA 1981; 246:2679-2680.
48. Overgaard J, Skinhoj E: A paradoxical cerebral hemodynamic effect of hydralazine. Stroke 1975; 6:402-410.
49. Marsh ML, Shapiro HM, Smith RW, et al: Changes in neurologic status and intracranial pressure associated with sodium nitroprusside administration. Anesthesiology 1979; 51:336-338.
50. Dohi S, Matsumoto M, Takahashi K: The effects of nitroglycerin on cerebrospinal fluid pressure in awake and anesthetized humans. Anesthesiology 1981; 54:511-514.
51. Hayashi M, et al: Treatment of systemic hypertension and intracranial hypertension and intracranial hypertension in cases of brain hemorrhage. Stroke 1988; 19:314-321.
52. Van Aken H, Puchstein C, Schweppe M-L, et al: Effect of labetalol on intracranial pressure in dogs with and without intracranial hypertension. Acta Anaesth Scand 1982; 26:615-619.
53. Stanek B, Zimpfer M, Fitzal S, Raberger G: Plasma catecholamines, plasma renin activity and haemodynamics during sodium nitroprusside-induced hypotension and additional beta-blockage with bunitrolol. Eur J Clin Pharmacol 1981; 19:317-322.
54. Werner C, Hoffman WE, Thomas C, Miletich DJ, Albrecht RF: Ganglionic blockade improves neurologic outcome from incomplete ischemia in rats: Partial reversal by exogenous catecholamines. Anesthesiology 1990; 73:923-929.
55. Neil-Dwyer G, Walter P, Cruickshank JM: Beta-blockade benefits patients following a subarachnoid hemorrhage. Eur J Clin Pharmacol 1985; 28(Suppl):25-29.
56. Hoffman WE, Kochs E, Werner C, Thomas C, Albrecht RF: Dexmedetomidine improves neurologic outcome from incomplete ischemia in the rat. Reversal by the alpha 2-adrenergic antagonist atipamezole. Anesthesiology 1991; 75:328-332.
57. Aggarwal S, Kramer D, Yonas H, Obrist W, Kang Y, Martin M, Policare R: Cerebral hemodynamic and metabolic changes in fulminant hepatic failure: A retrospective study. Hepatology 1994; 19:80-87.
58. Batjer HH, Devous MD Sr, Meyer YJ, Purdy PD, Samson DS: Cerebrovascular hemodynamics in arteriovenous malformation complicated by normal perfusion pressure breakthrough. Neurosurgery 1988; 22:503-509.
59. Young WL, Solomon RA, Prohovnik I, Ornstein E, Weinstein J, Stein BM: ^{133}Xe blood flow monitoring during arteriovenous malformation resection: A case of intraoperative hyperperfusion with subsequent brain swelling. Neurosurgery 1988; 22:765-769.
60. Young WL, Kader A, Prohovnik I, Ornstein E, Fleischer LH, Ostapkovich N, Jackson LD, Stein BM: Pressure autoregulation is intact after arteriovenous malformation resection. Neurosurgery 1993; 32:491-496.
61. Reigel MM, Hollier LH, Sundt TM Jr, Peipgras DG, Sharbrough FW, Cherry KJ: Cerebral hyperperfusion syndrome: A cause of neurologic dysfunction after carotid endarterectomy. J Vasc Surg 1987; 5:628-634.
62. del Zoppo GJ: Thrombolysis in acute stroke. Neurologia 1995; 10(Suppl 2):37-47.
63. Henriks C, Harmsen A, Christensen P, Sorensen MB, Lester J, Paulson OB: Controlled hypotension with sodium nitroprusside: Effects on cerebral blood flow and cerebral venous blood gases in patients operated for cerebral aneurysms. Acta Anaesth Scand 1983; 27:62-67.
64. Cottrell JE, Patel KP, Ransahoff JR, et al: Intracranial pressure changes induced by sodium nitroprusside in patients with intracranial mass lesions. J Neurosurg 1978; 48:329-331.
65. Weiss MH, Spence J, Apuzzo ML, Heiden JS, McComb JG, Kurze T: Influence of nitroprusside on cerebral pressure autoregulation. Neurosurgery 1979; 4:56-59.
66. Candia GJ, Heros RC, Lavyne MH, Zervas NT, Nelson CN: Effect of intravenous sodium nitroprusside on cerebral blood flow and intracranial pressure. Neurosurgery 1978; 3:50-53.
67. Theard MA, Cheng MA, Crowder CM, Tempelhoff R: Control of blood pressure during intracranial procedures: Comparison between nicardipine and nitroprusside (Abstract). J Neurosurg Anesth 1997; 9:388.
68. Dietrich WD: The importance of brain temperature in cerebral injury. J Neurotrauma 1992; 9(Suppl 2):S475-S485.
69. Blennow G, Brierley JB, Meldrum BS, Siesjo BK: Epileptic brain damage: The role of systemic factors that modify cerebral energy metabolism. Brain 1978; 101:687-700.
70. Marion DW, Penrod LE, Kelsey SF, Obrist WD, Kochanek PM, Palmer AM, Wisniewski SR, DeKosky ST: Treatment of traumatic brain injury with moderate hypothermia. N Engl J Med 1997; 336:540-546.
71. Nemoto EM, Klementavicius R, Melick JA, Yonas H: Effect of mild hypothermia on active and basal cerebral oxygen metabolism and blood flow. Adv Exp Med Biol 1994; 361:469-473.
72. Busto R, Globus MY, Dietrich WD, Martinez E, Valdes I, Ginsberg MD: Effect of mild hypothermia on ischemia-induced release of neurotransmitters and free fatty acids in rat brain. Stroke 1989; 20:904-910.
73. Craen RA, Gelb AW, Eliasziw M, Lok P: Current anesthetic practices and use of brain protective therapies for cerebral aneurysm surgery at 41 North American centers (Abstract). J Neurosurg Anesthesiol 1994; 6:303.
74. Kogure K, Scheinberg P, Reinmuth OM, Fujishima M, Bustro R: Mechanisms of cerebral vasodilation in hypoxia. J Appl Physiol 1970; 29:223-229.
75. Levine S: Anoxic-ischemic encephalopathy in rats. Am J Pathol 1960; 36:1.
76. Hojer-Pedersen E: Effect of acetazolamide on CBF in subacute and chronic cerebrovascular disease. Stroke 1987; 18:887-891.
77. Tominaga S, Strandgaard S, Uemura K, Ito K, Kutsuzawa T: Cerebrovascular CO_2 reactivity in normotensive and hypertensive man. Stroke 1976; 7:507-510.
78. Stringer WA, Hasso AN, Thompson JR, Hinshaw DB, Jordan KG: Hyperventilation-induced cerebral ischemia in patients with acute brain lesions: Demonstration by xenon-enhanced CT. Am J Neuroradiol 1993; 14:475-484.
79. Minhas PS, Menon DK, Herrod NJ, et al: Cerebral ischemia associated with hyperventilation: A PET study (Abstract). J Neurosurg Anesth 1997; 9:380.
80. Gupta AK, Gupta S, Swart M, Al-Rawi P, Hutchinson P, Kirkpatrick P: Comparison of brain tissue oxygen with jugular venous oxygen saturation during hyperventilation in head-injured patients (Abstract). J Neurosurg Anesth 1997; 9:399.
81. Muizelaar JP, Marmarou A, Ward JD, et al: Adverse effects of prolonged hyperventilation in patients with severe head injury: A randomized clinical trial. J Neurosurg 1991; 75:731-739.
82. Leahy JC, Chen Q, Vallano ML: Chronic mild acidosis specifically reduces functional expression of *N*-methyl-D-aspartate receptors and increases long-term survival in primary cultures of cerebellar granule cells. Neuroscience 1994; 63:457-470.

83. Pulsinelli WA, Levy DE, Sigsbee B, Scherer P, Plum F: Increased damage after ischemic stroke in patients with hyperglycemia with or without established diabetes mellitus. Am J Med 1983; 74:540–544.
84. Siemkowicz E: Hyperglycemia in the reperfusion period hampers recovery from cerebral ischemia. Acta Neurol Scand 1981; 64:207–216.
85. De Salles AA, Muizelaar JP, Young HF: Hyperglycemia, cerebrospinal fluid lactic acidosis, and CBF in severely head-injured patients. Neurosurgery 1987; 21:45–50.
86. Lanier WL, Stangland KJ, Scheithauer BW, Milde JH, Michenfelder JD: The effects of dextrose infusion and head position on neurologic outcome after complete cerebral ischemia in primates: Examination of a model. Anesthesiology 1987; 66:39–48.
87. Siemkowicz E, Gjedde A: Post-ischemic coma in rat: Effect of different pre-ischemic blood glucose levels on cerebral metabolic recovery after ischemia. Acta Physiol Scand 1980; 110:225–232.
88. Sieber FE, Traystman RJ: Special issues: Glucose and the brain (Review). Crit Care Med 1992; 20:104–114.
89. Zasslow MA, Pearl RG, Shuer LM, Steinberg GK, Lieberson RE, Larson CP Jr: Hyperglycemia decreases acute neuronal ischemic changes after middle cerebral artery occlusion in cats. Stroke 1989; 20:519–523.
90. de Courten-Myers G, Myers RE, Schoolfield L: Hyperglycemia enlarges infarct size in cerebrovascular occlusion in cats. Stroke 1988; 19:623–630.
91. Nedergaard M: Mechanisms of brain damage in focal cerebral ischemia (Review). Acta Neurol Scand 1988; 77:81–101.
92. Prado R, Ginsberg MD, Dietrich WD, Watson BD, Busto R: Hyperglycemia increases infarct size in collaterally perfused but not end-arterial vascular territories. J Cereb Blood Flow Metab 1988; 8:186–192.
93. Kofke WA, Ahdab-Barmada M, Rose M, Clyde C, Nemoto E: Substantia nigra damage after flurothyl-induced seizures in rats worsens after post seizure recovery: No exacerbation with hyperglycemia. Neurol Res 1993; 15:333–338.
94. Swan JH, Meldrum BS, Simon RP: Hyperglycemia does not augment neuronal damage in experimental status epilepticus. Neurology 1986; 36:1351–1354.
95. Ingvar M, Folbegrova J, Siesjo BK: Metabolic alterations underlying the development of hypermetabolic necrosis in the substantia nigra in status epilepticus. J Cereb Blood Flow Metab 1987; 7:103–108.
96. Ekstrom-Jodal B, Haggendal E, Larsson LE: CBF and oxygen uptake in endotoxic shock: An experimental study in dogs. Acta Anaesth Scand 1982; 26:163–170.
97. Oh MS, Carroll HJ: Disorders of sodium metabolism: Hypernatremia and hyponatremia (Review). Crit Care Med 1992; 20:94–103.
98. Buonocore CM, Robinson AG: The diagnosis and management of diabetes insipidus during medical emergencies. Endocrin Metab Clin North Am 1993; 22:411–423.
99. Maroon JC, Nelson PB: Hypovolemia in patients with subarachnoid hemorrhage: Therapeutic implications. Neurosurgery 1979; 4:223–226.
100. Laureno R, Kapp BI: Pontine and extrapontine myelinolysis following rapid correction of hyponatremia. Lancet 1988; 1:1439–1441.
101. Cruickshank JM, Neil-Dwyer G, Stott AW: Possible role of catecholamines, corticosteroids, and potassium in production of electrocardiographic abnormalities associated with subarachnoid hemorrhage. Br Heart J 1974; 36:697–706.
102. Loach AB, Benedict CR: Plasma catecholamine concentration associated with cerebral vasospasm. J Neurol Sci 1980; 45:261–271.
103. Cruickshank JM, Neil-Dwyer G, Brice J: Electrocardiographic changes and their prognostic significance in subarachnoid hemorrhage. J Neurol Neurosurg Psychiatry 1974; 37:755.
104. Neil-Dwyer G, Cruickshank J, Stott A, Brice J: The urinary catecholamine and plasma cortisol levels in patients with subarachnoid haemorrhage. J Neurol Sci 1974; 22:375–382.
105. Fraser RAR, Stein BM, Barrett RE, Pool JL: Noradrenergic mediation of experimental cerebrovascular spasm. Stroke 1970; 1:356–362.
106. Peerless SJ, Kendall MJ: The innervation of the cerebral blood vessels. *In:* Subarachnoid Hemorrhage and Cerebrovascular Spasm. Smith RR, Robertson JT (Eds). Springfield, Ill, Charles C Thomas, 1975, pp 38–54.
107. Marion DW, Segal R, Thompson ME: Subarachnoid hemorrhage and the heart. Neurosurgery 1986; 18:101–106.
108. Cruickshank JM, Neil-Dwyer G, Lane J: The effect of oral propranolol upon the ECG changes occurring in subarachnoid hemorrhage. Cardiovasc Res 1975; 9:236–245.
109. Kono T, Morita H, Kuroiwa T, Onaka H, Takatsuka H, Fujiwara A: Left ventricular wall motion abnormalities in patients with subarachnoid hemorrhage: Neurogenic stunned myocardium. J Am Coll Cardiol 1994; 24:636–640.
110. Kolin A, Norris JW: Myocardial damage from acute cerebral lesions. Stroke 1984; 15:990–943.
111. Svengaard NA, Brismar, Delgado TJ, Rosengren E: Subarachnoid haemorrhage in the rat: Effect on the development of vasospasm of selective lesions of the catecholamine systems in the lower brain stem. Stroke 1985; 16:602–608.
112. Svendgaard NA, Delgado TJ, Arbab MAR: Catecholaminergic and peptidergic systems underlying cerebral vasospasm: CBF and CMRgl changes following an experimental subarachnoid hemorrhage in the rat. *In:* Cerebral Vasospasm: Proceedings of the Charlottesville Conference, April 29–May 1, 1987. Wilkins RH (Ed). New York, Raven Press, 1988, p 175.
113. Werner C, Hoffman WE, Kochs E, Rabito SF, Miletich DJ: Captopril improves neurologic outcome from incomplete cerebral ischemia in rats. Stroke 1991; 22:910–914.
114. Busto R, Harik SI, Yoshida S, Scheinberg P, Ginsberg MD: Cerebral norepinephrine depletion enhances recovery after brain ischemia. Ann Neurol 1985; 18:329–336.
115. Kofke WA, Garman RH, Garman R, Rose M: Opioid neurotoxicity: Role of neurotransmitter systems (Abstract). J Neurosurg Anesthesiol 1995; 7:321.
116. Stein SC, Cracco RG: Cortical injury without ischemia produced by topical monoamines. Stroke 1982; 13:74–83.
117. Mohr JP, Kistler JP, Fink ME: Intracranial aneurysms. *In:* Stroke: Pathophysiology, Diagnosis, and Management. 2nd ed. Barnett HJM, Mohr JP, Stein BM, Yatsu FM (Eds). New York, Churchill Livingstone, 1992, pp 617–644.
118. Sahs AL: Preface. *In:* Aneurysmal Subarachnoid Hemorrhage. Report of the Cooperative Study. Sahs AL, Nibbelink DW et al (Eds). Baltimore, Urban and Schwarzenberg, 1981, p xvii.
119. Mohr JP, Kase CS: Cerebral vasospasm. Rev Neurol 1983; 139:99–113.
120. Popovic EA, Siu K: Ruptured intracranial aneurysms: A 12-month prospective study. Med J Aust 1989; 150:496–497, 500–501.
121. Ropper AH, Zervas NT: Outcome one year after subarachnoid hemorrhage from cerebral aneurysm. J Neurosurg 1984; 60:909–915.
122. Morley TP, Barr HWK: Giant intracranial aneurysms: Diagnosis, course, and management. Clin Neurosurg 1968; 16:73–94.
123. Fairburn B: "Twin" intracranial aneurysms causing subarachnoid hemorrhage in identical twins. Br Med J 1973; 1:210–211.
124. Findlay JM, Weir BK, Kanamaru K, Espinosa F: Arterial wall changes in cerebral vasospasm. Neurosurgery 1989; 25:736–745.
125. Espinosa F, Weir B, Noseworthy T: Nonoperative treatment of subarachnoid hemorrhage. *In:* Neurological Surgery. 3rd ed. Youmans JR (Ed). Philadelphia, WB Saunders, 1990.
126. Torner JC, Kassell NF, Wallace RB, Adams HP: Preoperative prognostic factors for rebleeding and survival in aneurysm patients receiving antifibrinolytic therapy: Report of the cooperative aneurysm study. Neurosurgery 1981; 9:506–513.
127. Nishioka H, Torner JC, Goettler LC: Cooperative study of intracranial aneurysms and subarachnoid hemorrhage: A long-term prognostic study: II. Ruptured intracranial aneurysms managed conservatively. Arch Neurol 1984; 41:1142–1146.
128. Heros RC: Acute hydrocephalus after subarachnoid hemorrhage. Stroke 1989; 20:715–717.
129. Black P McL: Hydrocephalus and vasospasm after subarachnoid hemorrhage from ruptured intracranial aneurysms. Neurosurgery 1986; 18:12–16.
130. Mohr G, Ferguson G, Khan M, Malloy D, Watts R, Benoit B, Weir B: Intraventricular hemorrhage from ruptured aneurysm: Retrospective analysis of 91 cases. J Neurosurg 1983; 58:482–487.

131. Globus MY, Busto R, Dietrich WD, et al: Intra-ischemic extracellular release of dopamine and glutamate is associated with striatal vulnerability to ischemia. Neurosci Lett 1988; 91:36–40.
132. Nevander G, Ingvar M, Lindvall O: Mechanisms of epileptic brain damage: Evidence for a protective role of the noradrenergic locus coeruleus system in the rat. Exp Brain Res 1986; 63:439–442.
133. Romo R, Cheramy A, Godeheu G, Glowinski J: In vivo presynaptic control of dopamine release in the cat caudate nucleus: III. Further evidence for the implication of corticostriatal glutamatergic neurons. Neuroscience 1986; 19:1091–1099.
134. Rothe F, Wolf G: Changes in glutamate-related enzyme activities in the striatum of the rat following lesion of corticostriatal fibres. Exp Brain Res 1990; 79:400–404.
135. Garcia-Munoz M, Young SJ, Groves PM: Terminal excitability of the corticostriatal pathway: I. Regulation by dopamine receptor stimulation. Brain Res 1991; 551:195–206.
136. Garcia-Munoz M, Young SJ, Groves PM: Terminal excitability of the corticostriatal pathway: II. Regulation by glutamate receptor stimulation. Brain Res 1991; 551:207–215.
137. Arvin B, Chapman AG, Meldrum BS: Monoaminergic activity and excitotoxicity: An approach using microdialysis. *In:* Excitatory Amino Acids. Meldrum BS, Moroni F, Simon RP, Woods JH (Eds). New York, Raven Press, 1991.
138. Barbeito L, Cheramy A, Godeheu G, Desce JM, Glowinski J: Glutamate receptors of the quisqualate-kainate subtype are involved in the presynaptic regulation of dopamine release in the cat caudate nucleus in vivo. Eur J Neurosci 1990; 2:304.
139. Roberts PJ, Anderson SD: Stimulatory effect of L-glutamate and related amino acids on 3H-dopamine release from rat striatum: An in vitro model for glutamate actions. J Neurochem 1979; 32:1539–1545.
140. Busto R, Harik SI, Yoshida S, Scheinberg P, Ginsberg MD: Cerebral norepinephrine depletion enhances recovery after brain ischemia. Ann Neurol 1985; 18:329–336.
141. Kassell NF: The natural history and treatment outcome of SAH: Comments derived from the national cooperative aneurysm study. *In:* Calcium Antagonists: Possible Therapeutic Use in Neurosurgery. Battye R (Ed). New York, Raven Press, 1983, p 24.
142. Weir BK: Pathophysiology of vasospasm. Int Anesthesiol Clin 1982; 20:39–43.
143. Mohr JP, Kase CS: Cerebral vasospasm. Rev Neurol 1983; 139:99–113.
144. Sundt TM Jr: Management of ischemic complications after subarachnoid hemorrhage. J Neurosurg 1974; 43:418–425.
145. Kistler JP, Crowell RM, Davis KR, Heros R, Ojemann RG, Zervas NT, Fisher CM: The relation of cerebral vasospasm to the extent and location of subarachnoid blood visualized by CT scan: A prospective study. Neurology 1983; 33:424–436.
146. Wilkins RH: Cerebral vasospasm. Crit Rev Neurobiol 1990; 6:51–77.
147. Echlin FA: Spasm of basilar and vertebral arteries caused by experimental subarachnoid hemorrhage. J Neurosurg 1965; 23:1–11.
148. Adner M, Jansen I, Edvinsson L: Endothelin-A receptors mediate contraction in human cerebral, meningeal, and temporal arteries. J Autonom Nerv Syst 1994; 49(Suppl):S117–S121.
149. Aldasoro M, Martinez C, Vila JM, Medina P, Lluch S: Influence of endothelial nitric oxide on adrenergic contractile responses of human cerebral arteries. J Cereb Blood Flow Metab 1996; 16:623–628.
150. Kim HW, Greenburg AG: Ferrous hemoglobin scavenging of endothelium derived nitric oxide is a principal mechanism for hemoglobin mediated vasoactivities in isolated rat thoracic aorta. Artif Cells, Blood Substit Immobil Biotechnol 1997; 25:121–133.
151. Kanamaru K, Waga S, Kojima T, Fujimoto K, Niwa S: Inhibition of endothelium dependent relaxation by hemoglobin and cerebrospinal fluid from patients with aneurysm subarachnoid hemorrhage: A possible mechanism and relation to cerebral vasospasm. *In:* Cerebral Vasospasm: Proceedings of the Charlottesville Conference, April 29–May 1, 1987. Wilkins RH (Ed). New York, Raven Press, 1988, pp 163–168.
152. Afshar JK, Pluta RM, Boock RJ, Thompson BG, Oldfield EH: Effect of intracarotid nitric oxide on primate cerebral vasospasm after subarachnoid hemorrhage. J Neurosurg 1995; 83:118–122.
153. Crompton MR: Hypothalamic lesions following the rupture of cerebral berry aneurysms. Brain 1963; 86:301–304.
154. Grubb RL Jr, Raichle ME, Eichling JO, Gado MH: Effects of subarachnoid hemorrhage on cerebral blood volume, blood flow, and oxygen utilization in humans. J Neurosurg 1977; 46:446–453.
155. Powers WJ, Grubb RL Jr, Baker RP, Mintun MA, Raichle ME: Regional CBF and metabolism in reversible ischemia due to vasospasm: Determination by positron emission tomography. J Neurosurg 1985; 62:539–546.
156. Robertson EG: Cerebral lesions due to intracranial aneurysms. Brain 1949; 72:150–185.
157. Crompton MR: The pathogenesis of cerebral infarction following the rupture of cerebral berry aneurysms. Brain 1964; 87:491–510.
158. Birse SH, Tom ML: Incidence of cerebral infarction associated with ruptured intracranial aneurysms: A study of 8 unoperated cases of anterior cerebral aneurysm. Neurology 1960; 10:101–106.
159. Germano I: Seizures and epilepsy after subarachnoid hemorrhage. *In* Subarachnoid Hemorrhage: Pathophysiology and Management. Bederson JB (Ed). American Association of Neurological Surgeons, Park Ridge, Ill, 1997, pp 117–126.
160. Keranen T, Tapaninaho A, Hernesniemi J, Vapalahti M: Late epilepsy after aneurysm operations. Neurosurgery 1985; 17:897–900.
161. Adams HP, Love BB: Medical management of aneurysmal subarachnoid hemorrhage. *In:* Stroke: Pathophysiology, Diagnosis, and Management. 2nd ed. Barnett HJM, Mohr JP, Stein BM, Yatsu FM (Eds). New York, Churchill Livingstone, 1992, pp 1029–1054.
162. Neil-Dwyer G, Walter P, Shaw HJH, et al: Plasma renin activity in patients after a subarachnoid hemorrhage: A possible predictor of outcome. Neurosurgery 1980; 7:578–582.
163. Disney L, Weir B, Grace M, Roberts P: Trends in blood pressure, osmolality, and electrolytes after subarachnoid hemorrhage from aneurysms. Can J Neurol Sci 1989; 16:299–304.
164. Estanol Vidal B, Badui Dergal E, Cesarman E, et al: Cardiac arrhythmias associated with subarachnoid hemorrhage: Prospective study. Neurosurgery 1979; 5:675–680.
165. Koskelo P, Punsar S, Sipila W: Subendocardial hemorrhage and ECG changes in intracranial bleeding. Br Med J 1964; 1:1479–1480.
166. Touho H, Karasawa J, Shishido H, et al: Neurogenic pulmonary edema in the acute stage of hemorrhagic cerebrovascular disease. Neurosurgery 1989; 25:762–768.
167. Weisman SJ: Edema and congestion of the lungs resulting from intracranial hemorrhage. Surgery 1939; 6:722.
168. Theodore J, Robin ED: Pathogenesis of neurogenic pulmonary oedema. Lancet 1975; 2:749–751.
169. Wijdicks EFM, Vermeulen M, Hijdra A, van Gijn J: Hyponatremia and cerebral infarction in patients with ruptured intracranial aneurysms: Is fluid restriction harmful? Ann Neurol 1985; 17:137–140.
170. Crowell RM, Zervas NT: Management of intracranial aneurysm. Med Clin North Am 1979; 63:695–713.
171. Widjicks EFM, et al: Volume depletion and natriuresis in patients with a ruptured intracranial aneurysm. Ann Neurol 1985; 18:211–216.
172. Diringer M, Ladesnon PW, Stern BJ, et al: Plasma atrial natriuretic factor and subarachnoid hemorrhage. Stroke 1988; 19:1119–1124.
173. Rosenfeld JV, Barnett GH, Sila CA, et al: The effect of subarachnoid hemorrhage on blood and CSF atrial natriuretic factor. J Neurosurg 1989; 71:32–37.
174. Simpson RK Jr, Fischer DK, Ehni BL: Neurogenic hyperthermia in subarachnoid hemorrhage. South Med J 1989; 82:1577–1578.
175. Rousseaux P, Scherpereel B, Bernard MH, Graftieaux JP, Guyot JF: Fever and cerebral vasospasm in ruptured intracranial aneurysms. Surg Neurol 1980; 14:459–465.
176. Frankowski RF: Epidemiology of stroke and intracerebral hemorrhage. *In:* Intracerebral Hematomas. Kaufman HH (Ed). New York, Raven Press, 1992, pp 1–11.
177. Brott T, Thalinger K, Hertzberg V: Hypertension as a risk factor for spontaneous intracerebral hemorrhage. Stroke 1986; 17:1078–1083.

178. Kase CS, Mohr JP, Caplan LR: Intracerebral hemorrhage. *In:* Stroke: Pathophysiology, Diagnosis, and Management. 2nd ed. Barnett HJM, Mohr JP, Stein BM, Yatsu FM (Eds). New York, Churchill Livingstone, 1992, pp 561-616.
179. Mohr JP, Caplan LR, Melski JW, et al: The Harvard Cooperative Stroke Registry: A prospective registry. Neurology (NY) 1978; 28:754-762.
180. Brewer DB, Fawcett FJ, Horsfield GI: A necropsy series of non-traumatic cerebral hemorrhages and softenings, with particular reference to heart weight. J Pathol Bacteriol 1968; 96:311.
181. Ojemann RG, Mohr JP: Hypertensive brain hemorrhage. Clin Neurosurg 1976; 23:220-244.
182. McCormick WF, Rosenfield DB: Massive brain hemorrhage: A review of 144 cases and an examination of their causes. Stroke 1973; 4:946.
183. Brott T, Thalinger K, Hertzberg V: Hypertension as a risk factor for spontaneous intracerebral hemorrhage. Stroke 1986; 17:1078-1083.
184. Broderick JP, Phillips SJ, Whisnant JP, O'Fallon WM, Bergstralh EJ: Incidence rates of stroke in the eighties: The end of the decline in stroke? Stroke 1989; 20:577-582.
185. Furlan AJ, Whisnant JP, Elveback LR: The decreasing incidence of primary intracerebral hemorrhage: A population study. Ann Neurol 1979; 5:367-373.
186. Gilles S, Brucher JM, Khoubesserian P, Vanderhaeghn JJ: Cerebral amyloid angiopathy as a cause of multiple intracerebral hemorrhages. Neurology 1984; 4:730.
187. Caplan LR: Clinical features of spontaneous intracerebral hemorrhage. *In:* Intracerebral Hematomas. Kaufman HH (Ed). New York, Raven Press, 1992, pp 31-48.
188. Fisher CM: Pathological observations in hypertensive cerebral hemorrhage. J Neuropathol Exp Neurol 1971; 30:536-550.
189. Herbstein DJ, Schaumburg HH: Hypertensive intracerebral hematoma: An investigation of the initial hemorrhage and rebleeding using chromium 51-labeled erythrocytes. Arch Neurol 1974; 30:412-414.
190. Broderick JP, Brott TG, Tomsick T, et al: Ultraearly evaluation of intracerebral hemorrhage. J Neurosurg 1990; 72:195-199.
191. Kaufman HH, Schochet SS: Pathology, physiology, and modeling. *In:* Intracerebral Hematomas. Kaufman HH (Ed). New York, Raven Press, 1992.
192. Feigin I, Prose P: Hypertensive fibrinoid arteritis of the brain and gross cerebral hemorrhage. Arch Neurol 1959; 1:98-110.
193. Rosenblum WI: Miliary aneurysms and "fibrinoid" degeneration of cerebral blood vessels. Hum Pathol 1977; 8:133-139.
194. Grotta JC: Acute stroke management: Diagnosis (Part I). *In:* Grotta JC et al (Eds). Stroke: Clinical Updates 3:17, 1993, National Stroke Association, Englewood, Colo.
195. Garcia JH, Ho K-L, Caccamo DV: Pathology of stroke. *In:* Stroke: Pathophysiology, Diagnosis, and Management. 2nd ed. Barnett HJM, Mohr JP, Stein BM, Yatsu FM (Eds). New York, Churchill Livingstone, 1992, pp 125-146.
196. Adams RD, Victor M: Cerebrovascular diseases. *In:* Principles of Neurology. 5th ed. Adams RD, Victor M (Eds). New York, McGraw-Hill, 1993, p 669.
197. Frank JI, Biller J: Coma in focal cerebrovascular disease: An overview. *In:* Grott JC et al (Eds). Stroke: Clinical Updates. 3:9, 1992, National Stroke Association, Englewood, Colo.
198. Bladin CF, Willmore J: Seizures after stroke. *In:* Grotta JC, et al (Eds). Stroke: Clinical Updates 5:5, 1994, National Stroke Association, Englewood, Colo.
199. Rothrock JF, Hart RG: Antithrombotic therapy in cerebrovascular disease. Ann Intern Med 1991; 11:885-895.
200. Dimant J, Grob D: Electrocardiographic changes and myocardial damage in patients with acute cerebrovascular accidents. Stroke 1977; 8:448-455.
201. Myers MG, Norris JW, Hachinski VC, et al: Cardiac sequelae of acute stroke. Stroke 1982; 13:838-842.
202. Norris JW, Froggart GM, Hachinski VC: Cardiac arrhythmias in acute stroke. Stroke 1978; 9:392-396.
203. Lavy S, Yaar I, Melamed E, Stern S: The effect of acute stroke on cardiac functions as observed in an intensive care unit. Stroke 1974; 5:775-780.
204. Norris JW, Hachinski VC, Myers MG, et al: Serum cardiac enzymes in stroke. 1979; 10:548-553.
205. Adams HP, Brott TG, Crowell RM, et al: Guidelines for the management of patients with acute ischemic stroke. A statement for health care professionals form a special writing group of the stroke council, American Heart Association. Stroke 1994; 25:1901-1914.
206. Myers MG, Norris JW, Hachinski VC, et al: Plasma norepinephrine in stroke. Stroke 1981; 12:200-204.
207. Meyer JS, Shimazu K, Fukuuchi Y, et al: Impaired neurogenic cerebrovascular control and dysautoregulation after stroke. Stroke 1973; 4:169-186.
208. Delgado-Escueta AV, Wasterlain C, Treiman DM, et al: Current concepts in neurology: Management of status epilepticus. N Engl J Med 1982; 306:1337-1340.
209. Treatment of convulsive status epilepticus: Recommendations of the Epilepsy Foundation of America's Working Group on Status Epilepticus. JAMA 1993; 270:854-859.
210. Corsellis JA, Bruton CJ: Neuropathology of status epilepticus in humans. Adv Neurol 1983; 34:129-139.
211. O'Connell BK, Towfighi J, Kofke WA, et al: Neuronal lesions in mercaptopropionic acid-induced status epilepticus. Acta Neuropathol 1988; 77:47-54.
212. Towfighi J, Kofke WA, O'Connell BK: Substantia nigra lesions in mercaptopropionic acid-induced status epilepticus: A light and electron microscopic study. Acta Neuropathol 1989; 77:612-620.
213. McNamara JO: Cellular and molecular basis of epilepsy. J Neurosci 1994; 14:3413-3425.
214. Kofke WA, Tempelhoff R, Dasheiff RM: Anesthetic implications of epilepsy: I. Epilepsy, status epilepticus and epilepsy surgery. J Neurosurg Anesth 1997; 9:349-372.
215. Loscher W: Basic aspects of epilepsy. Curr Opin Neurol Neurosurg 1993; 6:223-232.
216. Garant DS, Gale K: Substantia nigra-mediated anticovulsant actions: Role of nigral output pathways. Exp Neurol 1987; 97:143-159.
217. Sagar HJ, Oxbury JM: Hippocampal neuron loss in temporal lobe epilepsy: Correlation with early childhood convulsions. Ann Neurol 1987; 22:334-340.
218. Sloviter RS: Feedforward and feedback inhibition of hippocampal principal cell activity evoked by perforant path stimulation: GABA-mediated mechanisms that regulate excitability in vivo. Hippocampus 1991; 1:31-40.
219. Tauck DL, Nadler JV: Evidence of functional mossy fiber sprouting in hippocampal formation of kainic acid-treated rats. J Neurosci 1985; 5:1016.
220. Cavazos JE, Golarai G, Sutula TP: Mossy fiber synaptic reorganization induced by kindling: Time course development, progression, and permanence. J Neurosci 1991; 11:2795.
221. Sutula T, Cascino G, Cavazos J, et al: Mossy fiber synaptic reorganization in the epileptic human temporal lobe. Ann Neurol 1989; 26:321-330.
222. Martin D, McNamara JO, Nadler JV: Kindling enhances sensitivity of CA3 hippocampal pyramidal cells to NMDA. J Neurosci 1992; 12:1928-1935.
223. Avoli M: Excitatory amino acid receptors in the human epileptogenic neocortex. Epilepsy Res 1991; 10:33-40.
224. Tietz EI, Chiu TH: Regional GABA-stimulated chloride uptake in amygdala kindled rats. Neurosci Lett 1991; 123:269-272.
225. McDonald JW, Garofalo EA, Hood T, et al: Altered excitatory and inhibitory amino acid receptor binding in hippocampus of patients with temporal lobe epilepsy. Ann Neurol 1991; 29:529-541.
226. Minamato Y, Itano T, Tokuda M, et al: In vivo microdialysis of amino acid neurotransmitters in the hippocampus in amygdaloid kindled rats. Brain Res 1992; 573:345.
227. Ronneengstrom E, Hillered L, Flink R, et al: Intracerebral microdialysis of extracellular amino acids in the human epileptic focus. J Cereb Blood Flow Metab 1992; 12:873-876.
228. Fisher RS, Pedley TA, Moody WJ, et al: The role of extracellular potassium in hippocampal epilepsy. Arch Neurol 1976; 33:76-83.
229. Lux HD, Heinemann U, Dietzel I: Ionic changes and alterations in the size of the extracellular space during epileptic activity. Adv Neurol 1986; 44:619-639.
230. Traynelis SF, Dingledine R: Potassium-induced spontaneous elec-

trographic seizures in the rat hippocampal slice. J Neurophysiol 1988; 59:259-276.
231. Solis JM, Nicoll RA: Pharmacological characterization of GABA-B-mediated responses in the CA1 region of the rat hippocampal slice. J Neurosci 1992; 12:3466.
232. Chamberlin NL, Dingledine R: GABAergic inhibition and the induction of spontaneous epileptiform activity by low chloride and high potassium in the hippocampal slice. Brain Res 1988; 445:12-18.
233. Dietzel I, Heineman U, Hofmeier G, et al: Transient changes in the size of the extracellular space in the sensorimotor cortex of cats in relation to stimulus-induced changes in potassium concentrations. Exp Brain Res 1980; 40:432-439.
234. Dingledine R, McBain CB, McNamara JO: Excitatory amino acids in epilepsy. Trends Pharmacol Sci 1990; 11:334.
235. McNamara JO: The neurobiological basis of epilepsy. Trends Neurosci 1992; 15:357-359.
236. Dumer M, Sander T, Greenberg DA, et al: Localization of idiopathic generalized epilepsy on chromosome 6p in families of juvenile myoclonic epilepsy patients. Neurology 1991; 41:1651-1655.
237. Maxwell WL, Watt C, Graham DI, Gennarelli TA: Ultrastructural evidence of axonal shearing as a result of lateral acceleration of the head in non-human primates. Acta Neuropathol 1993; 86:136.
238. Nevin C: Neuropathologic changes in the white matter following head injury. J Neuropathol Exp Neurol 1967; 26:77.
239. Nilsson B, Ponten U, Voigt G: Experimental head injury in the rat: Part 1. Mechanics, pathophysiology, and morphology in an impact acceleration trauma model. J Neurosurg 1977; 47:241-251.
240. Wald SL, Shackford SR, Fenwick J: The effect of secondary insults on mortality and long-term disability after severe head injury in a rural region without a trauma system. J Trauma 1993; 34:377-381.
241. Graham DI, Adams JH, Doyle D, Ford I, Gennarelli TA, Lawrence AE, Maxwell WL, McLellan DR: Quantification of primary and secondary lesions in severe head injury. Acta Neurochir 1993; 57(Suppl):41-48.
242. Braughler JM, Hall ED: Involvement of lipid peroxidation in CNS injury. J Neurotrauma 1992; 9(Suppl)1:S1-S7.
243. Palmer AM, Marion DW, Botscheller ML, Swedlow PE, Styren SD, DeKosky ST: Traumatic brain injury-induced excitotoxicity assessed in a controlled cortical impact model. J Neurochem 1993; 61:2015-2024.
244. Kochanek PM: Ischemic and traumatic brain injury: Pathobiology and cellular mechanisms. Crit Care Med 1993; 21(9 Suppl):S333-S335.
245. Marmarou A: Intracellular acidosis in human and experimental brain injury. J Neurotrauma 1992; 9(Suppl 2):S551-S562.
246. Martin NA, Doberstein C, Zane C, Caron MJ, Thomas K, Becker DP: Posttraumatic cerebral arterial spasm: Transcranial Doppler ultrasound, CBF, and angiographic findings. J Neurosurg 1992; 77:575-583.
247. Obrist WD, Langfitt TW, Jaggi JL, et al: CBF and metabolism in comatose patients with acute head injury: Relationship to intracranial hypertension. J Neurosurg 1984; 61:241-253.
248. Unterberg A, Kiening K, Schmiedek P, Lanksch W: Long-term observations of intracranial pressure after severe head injury: The phenomenon of secondary rise of intracranial pressure. Neurosurgery 1993; 32:17-23.

166

Brain Function Monitoring

Donald J. Deyo, DVM • Verna Yancy, MD
Donald S. Prough, MD

Despite the frequency in intensive care units (ICUs) of patients with acute traumatic and ischemic brain diseases, clinical neurologic monitoring remains rudimentary. Often, only systemic hemodynamics and gas exchange are monitored, an approach that is adequate only in patients in whom cerebral vascular resistance (CVR), mean arterial pressure (MAP), and arterial oxygen content (Cao_2) are within physiologic ranges. In many ICUs, the only brain-specific monitor is intracranial pressure (ICP). Although clinical experience suggests that morbidity and mortality might be altered by measurement and therapeutic alteration of cerebral blood flow (CBF) and cerebral metabolism in some neurologically injured patients, no data confirm the general clinical utility of neurologic monitoring.

This chapter reviews the techniques currently available for cerebral function monitoring and summarizes information about the use of those techniques in common neurologic and neurosurgical diseases. The following three basic questions form the background for any consideration of brain monitoring:

1. In what diseases is the proportion of patients in whom avoidable injury will develop sufficiently large to justify extensive (and potentially expensive) application of neurologic monitoring devices?
2. Under what circumstances do blood pressure, $Paco_2$, Pao_2, and body temperature provide insufficient information about the adequacy of cerebral oxygen delivery (CDo_2 = [CBF] • Cao_2)?
3. Under what circumstances does more precise information about the adequacy of cerebral oxygen delivery permit therapeutic interventions that improve outcome?

GOALS OF BRAIN MONITORING

Monitoring devices potentially contribute to reductions in morbidity and mortality by providing physiologic data that can be integrated into a more effective therapeutic plan. Neurologic monitoring can be divided into two distinct categories (Table 166-1): The first category, which comprises electroencephalography (EEG) and evoked potential (EP) monitoring, defines a neurologic ischemic threshold based on electrophysiologic dysfunction. The second category, which comprises monitors of ICP, CBF, and cerebral metabolism, provides quantitative or semiquantitative physiologic information that can potentially define a threshold for changing treatment. Nevertheless, few data quantify the relationship between monitored variables and the risk of preventable neurologic injury. Changes in electrophysiologic variables that correlate with various levels of CBF and neurologic outcome are summarized in Table 166-2.

CEREBRAL ISCHEMIA

Virtually all neurologic monitors detect actual or possible *cerebral ischemia,* defined as CDo_2 insufficient to meet meta-

TABLE 166–1. **Brain Function Monitors**

Cerebral Perfusion*	Cerebral Oxygen Extraction*	Cerebral Function†
Cerebral blood flow	Jugular bulb saturation	Electroencephalogram Processed Raw
Cerebral blood flow velocity Intracranial pressure	Near-infrared spectroscopy	Evoked potentials

*Variable relationship between monitored data and cerebral ischemia.
†Electrophysiologic dysfunction present at ischemic threshold.

bolic needs. Cerebral ischemia is traditionally characterized as *global* or *focal* and *complete* or *incomplete.* Most global cerebral insults, such as hypotension, hypoxemia, and cardiac arrest, are readily detected by systemic monitors. Therefore, brain-specific monitors can provide additional information primarily in situations, such as stroke, subarachnoid hemorrhage (SAH) with vasospasm, and traumatic brain injury (TBI), in which focal cerebral oxygenation may be impaired despite adequate systemic oxygenation and perfusion.

The severity of ischemic brain damage is proportional to the magnitude and duration of CDo_2 reductions. In monkeys, potentially reversible paralysis develops if regional CBF declines below about 23 mL · 100 g^{-1} · min^{-1}.[1] Infarction of brain tissue, however, requires that CBF remain below 18 mL · 100 g^{-1} · min^{-1}.[1] The tolerable duration of more profound ischemia is inversely proportional to the severity of reduction in CBF.

TECHNIQUES OF NEUROLOGIC MONITORING

Brain monitors directly or indirectly assess cerebral perfusion, cerebral oxygen extraction, or cerebral function (see Table 166–1). Brain monitors can be classified in terms of the validity of the measurements performed and in terms of the ease with which monitored information can be incorporated into the clinical reasoning process (Table 166–3). The design and utilization of monitoring devices necessitate tradeoffs among various performance characteristics. For instance, a monitor with high positive predictive value (i.e., that falls outside threshold values only when cerebral ischemia is unequivocally present) is unlikely to be sufficiently sensitive to detect less profound ischemia. A monitor that is highly sensitive to changes in cerebral oxygenation frequently warns of small changes that are unlikely to produce brain injury.

If a cerebral monitor detects ischemia, all that is known is that cerebral oxygenation in the region of brain that is assessed by that monitor has fallen below a critical threshold. Because more severe ischemia produces neurologic injury in less time, it is impossible to predict with certainty whether changes in function will be followed by cerebral infarction. In addition, if regional ischemia involves structures that do not participate in the monitored function, infarction could develop without warning.

Systemic Monitoring

Blood pressure monitoring, pulse oximetry, and body temperature provide important data about the adequacy of global brain oxygenation and the vulnerability of the brain to ischemic injury. The initial step in ensuring adequate CDo_2 is the maintenance of adequate Cao_2, which in turn depends on hemoglobin (Hb) concentration and arterial oxygen saturation (Sao_2); therefore, both hypoxemia and anemia can reduce CDo_2. The second step is the maintenance of adequate CBF. Increases in CBF to some extent can compensate for decreases in Cao_2.

In normal persons, CBF is controlled by metabolic demand, pressure autoregulation, $Paco_2$, and Cao_2. In the normal "coupled" relationship, CBF depends on the cerebral metabolic rate for oxygen ($CMRo_2$), which varies directly with body temperature and with the level of brain activation. Because of the phenomenon of pressure autoregulation, changes in cerebral perfusion pressure (CPP) in the normal cerebral vasculature do not alter CBF over a range of pressures of 50 to 130 mm Hg.[2] After experimental brain injury, the ability of the cerebral vasculature to increase CBF in response to decreasing CPP is impaired.[3] If $Paco_2$ is halved, CBF is acutely halved; if $Paco_2$ doubles, CBF doubles. In response to decreasing Cao_2, CBF increases, whether the reduction is secondary to a decrease in Hb or in Sao_2.[4, 5] As Sao_2 decreases as a result of a decrease in Pao_2, jugular venous bulb oxygen saturation ($Sjvo_2$) also decreases (Fig. 166–1*A*).[6] The correlation is most evident below a Pao_2 of approximately 60 mm Hg, the Pao_2 value at which Sao_2 is 90% and below which saturation rapidly decreases. In contrast, as Hb concentration is reduced by normovolemic hemodilution, $Sjvo_2$ remains constant (Fig. 166–1*B*).[6]

Recognition of the importance of temperature regulation in patients with neurologic injury has been growing. Experimental and clinical data now suggest that relatively small changes in body temperature may change outcome in patients with

TABLE 166–2. **Clinical, Pathophysiologic, and Monitoring Thresholds in Cerebral Ischemia**

CBF (mL · 100 g^{-1} · min^{-1})	Clinical Threshold	Pathophysiologic Changes	Monitored Changes
50	Normal		
23	Reversible paralysis		EEG slowing, EP change
20		Na^+/K^+ pump dysfunction	
18	Infarction		EEG flat
15			EP absent
10		K^+ efflux, Ca^{2+} influx	

Ca^{2+} = calcium ion; CBF = cerebral blood flow; EEG = electroencephalogram; EP = evoked potential; K^+ = potassium ion; Na^+ = sodium ion.

TABLE 166–3. Brain Monitor Characteristics: Glossary

Term	Definition
Bias	Average difference (positive or negative) between monitored values and "gold standard" values.
Precision	Standard deviation of the differences (bias) between the measurements.
True-positive fraction	Probability that the monitor will identify patients at risk for preventable secondary injury.
False-positive fraction	Probability that the monitor will demonstrate the possibility of preventable second injury in patients not at risk.
True-negative fraction	Probability that the monitor will not demonstrate the possibility of preventable secondary injury in patients not at risk.
False-negative fraction	Probability that the monitor will not demonstrate the possibility of preventable secondary injury in patients at risk.
Interventional threshold	The value used to separate acceptable (i.e., no ischemia present) from unacceptable (i.e., ischemia present).
Speed	The time elapsed from the onset of risk of preventable secondary injury until the monitor recognizes the possibility.

stroke or TBI. Mild hypothermia (34°C) decreases the basal component of $CMRO_2$ more than the active component by reducing membrane permeability to sodium ion (Na^+) and potassium ion (K^+).[7] Brain protection by hypothermia was once considered a dose-dependent function of body temperature, with substantial benefit obtained only from reduction to temperatures of 26 to 28°C, such as have been commonly used during cardiopulmonary bypass. In rats subjected to global ischemic[8] or traumatic[9] insults, however, mild hypothermia (30 to 33°C) provided substantial protection, whereas increases of a few degrees above normal worsened outcome. In experimental global ischemia, brain hypothermia attenuated histopathologic damage, inhibited release of the excitotoxin glutamate during ischemia, and reduced hydroxyl radical generation during reperfusion.[10] In head-injured patients, a randomized clinical trial demonstrated that reduction of temperature to 33 to 34°C within 10 hours of TBI and continuing for 24 hours significantly improved outcome in patients with Glasgow Coma Scale (GCS) scores of 5 to 7 on admission to the hospital.[11]

Neurologic Examination

Neurologic examination quantifies changes in consciousness and focal brain dysfunction. The GCS has become popular as a brief, reproducible estimate of level of consciousness in critically ill patients. The score should be supplemented by recording pupillary size and reactivity and the status of focal neurologic findings. Although a finding of impaired consciousness is nonspecific, recognition of changing consciousness may warn of a variety of treatable conditions, including progression of intracranial hypertension, developing vasospasm in patients after SAH, delayed post-traumatic intracranial hematomas, and systemic complications of intracranial pathology such as hyponatremia, hypoxemia, and hypercarbia.

Neuroimaging

Cerebral computed tomographic (CT) scans, magnetic resonance imaging (MRI) scans, and radionuclide scans do not function as monitors per se. Rather, they are indicated as responses to the suspicion of a new or progressive anatomic lesion, such as a subdural or intracerebral hematoma, that will require an alteration in treatment. Both CT and MRI scanning provide static, discontinuous data and require moving a critically ill patient out of the ICU. CT scans obtained at the time of admission to the hospital, however, can provide valuable prognostic information. Marshall and colleagues[12] predicted outcome of head-injured patients in relation to four grades of increasingly severe diffuse brain injury and the presence of evacuated or nonevacuated intracranial mass lesions. Normal CT scans at admission in patients with GCS scores of less than 8 are associated with a 10% to 15% incidence of ICP elevation[13-15]; however, the risk of ICP elevation increases in patients older than 40 years, patients with unilateral or bilateral motor posturing, and patients with systolic blood pressure less than 90 mm Hg.[13]

Although MRI scans often provide better resolution than CT

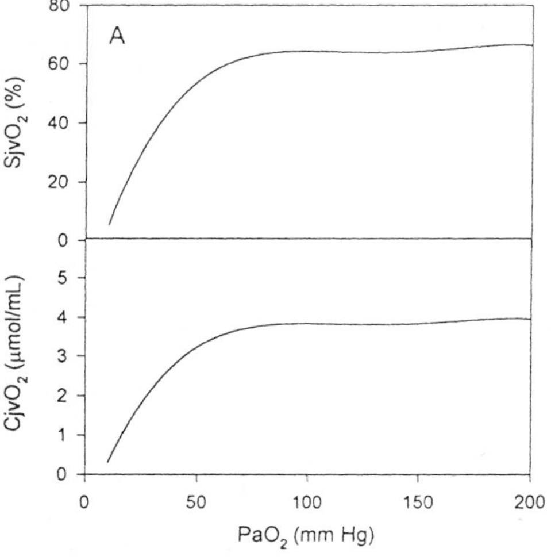

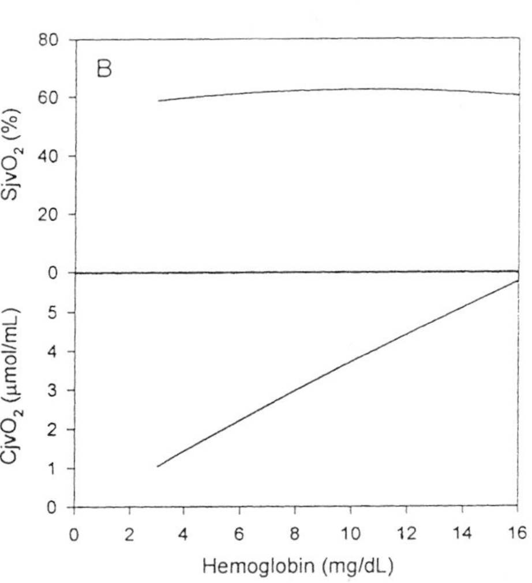

Figure 166–1. Changes in jugular venous bulb oxygen saturation ($SjvO_2$) and jugular venous bulb oxygen content ($CjvO_2$) in normal subjects as PaO_2 is reduced (*A*) or as normovolemic anemia is induced (*B*). The influence of decreasing PaO_2 below 60 mm Hg is a consequence of the steep slope of the oxyhemoglobin dissociation curve below a PaO_2 of 60 mm Hg and an SaO_2 of 90%. (From Feldman Z, Robertson CS: Monitoring of cerebral hemodynamics with jugular bulb catheters. Crit Care Clin 1997; 13:51–77.)

scans, the powerful magnets are incompatible with ferrous metals, a ubiquitous component of life-support equipment. Advances in MRI technology, such as diffusion-weighted imaging (DWI), may provide some information about brain function.[16, 17] Because of the incompatibility of MRI with ferrous metals, MRI-compatible ventilators and monitors have been developed.[18] Techniques have been described for improving the ventilation of critically ill patients undergoing MRI scanning.[19] In patients with clinical evidence of brain death, CBF studies (the initial component of radionuclide brain scans) can document cessation of CBF and have generally replaced repeated EEG for confirmation of brain death.[20]

Cerebral Blood Flow Monitoring

The first quantitative clinical method of measurement of CBF, the Kety-Schmidt technique,[21] calculated global CBF from the difference between the arterial and jugular bulb saturation curves of an inhaled, inert gas. Later techniques used extracranial gamma detectors to measure regional cortical CBF from washout curves after intracarotid injection of a radioisotope such as xenon 133 (^{133}Xe).[22] Carotid puncture was avoided by techniques that measured cortical CBF after inhaled[23] or intravenous administration of ^{133}Xe, using gamma counting of exhaled gas to correct clearance curves for recirculation of ^{133}Xe. Among the obstacles to wider use of ^{133}Xe clearance are technical complexity, cumbersome regulations governing radionuclides, and the sustained stable conditions (5 to 15 minutes) required to perform a single measurement.

Because xenon is radiodense, saturation of brain tissue increases radiographic density in proportion to CBF. Imaging of the brain after equilibration with stable xenon provides a regional estimate of CBF that includes deep brain structures.[24] Clinical studies using stable xenon CT have provided data that prompted a radical revision of the conventional understanding of CBF after TBI, by demonstrating that one third of patients had evidence of cerebral ischemia within 8 hours of trauma.[25] However, the requirement for an extended motionless interval in the CT scanner has inhibited wider use of this technique in head-injured patients.

In most patients, arterial flow velocity can be readily measured in intracranial vessels, especially the middle cerebral artery (MCA), using transcranial Doppler (TCD) ultrasonography. Doppler flow velocity ultrasonography uses the frequency shift, proportional to velocity, observed when sound waves are reflected by moving red blood cells. Blood moving toward the transducer shifts the transmitted frequency to higher frequencies; blood moving away, to lower frequencies. Velocity is a function of both blood flow rate and vessel diameter. If diameter remains constant, changes in velocity are proportional to changes in CBF; however, intersubject differences in flow velocity correlate poorly with intersubject differences in CBF.[26] Entirely noninvasive, TCD measurements can be repeated at short intervals or even applied continuously. Further clinical research is necessary, however, to define those situations in which the excellent capacity for rapid trend monitoring can be exploited.

Intracranial Pressure Monitoring

Intracranial pressure functions as the outflow pressure for the cerebral circulation, according to the following equation:

$$CPP = MAP - ICP$$

when ICP exceeds jugular venous pressure. Because the skull is not distensible, the brain, cerebrospinal fluid (CSF), and cerebral blood volume have little room to expand without increasing ICP. Although CBF cannot be directly inferred from knowledge of MAP and ICP, severe increases in ICP reduce both CPP and CBF.

The symptoms and signs of intracranial hypertension are neither sensitive nor specific. Usually, the physical findings associated with increasing ICP become apparent only when intracranial hypertension has become sufficiently severe to injure the brain. Because ICP cannot otherwise be adequately assessed, direct measurement and monitoring of ICP has become a common intervention. Currently, one of three sites—one of the lateral ventricles, the subdural space, or the brain parenchyma—is usually used. Because pressure gradients may exist among various sites, it may be advantageous to monitor in or adjacent to the more severely damaged hemisphere. The problems associated with ICP monitoring can be divided generally into three categories: (1) risks to patients (i.e., intracranial hemorrhage, cortical damage, and infection), (2) inaccurate data, and (3) inappropriate use or misinterpretation of data.

Ventricular catheterization, performed under strict aseptic technique, is the method of choice for ICP monitoring and CSF drainage in patients with acute intracranial hypertension and excess CSF. Intraventricular catheters may be difficult to place, however, if cerebral edema or brain swelling has compressed the ventricular system. Intraventricular monitoring can be performed with hollow catheters that are fluid-coupled to external pressure transducers or with catheters that are transducer tipped (Camino Laboratories, San Diego, Calif.). Fiberoptic catheters are less susceptible to short-term malfunction than conventional, fluid-filled catheters.[27] All fluid-coupled systems that passively connect to external transducers must be "zeroed" at the level of the external auditory meatus.

Intracranial pressure monitoring from the subdural space is usually carried out with fluid-coupled bolts, fluid-coupled subdural catheters, or fiberoptic transducer-tipped catheters. Because subdural bolts are open tubes facing end-on against the brain surface, brain tissue may herniate into the system, obstructing the system and potentially damaging the brain cortex. The fiberoptic system, when inserted subdurally, cannot be calibrated after insertion but demonstrates acceptably low drift.[27] In a series of 46 patients monitored with fiberoptic catheters in the intraparenchymal (43 patients) or intraventricular (3 patients) position, 12% of catheters developed broken components, 8.6% required repositioning for erroneous readings, and 3.4% were complicated by epidural hematomas.[28]

In addition to revealing frankly increased ICP, monitoring can also demonstrate pathologic waveforms and reduced intracranial compliance. B waves, cycling at a rate of 2 to 4 per second with an amplitude of approximately 10 mm Hg, warn of possible decompensation of reserve. Plateau waves, or A waves, which have long been recognized as a sign of impending intracranial catastrophe, consist of cyclic increases in ICP, often 50 mm Hg or higher and lasting as long as 15 to 30 minutes.[29]

Cerebral Oxygenation

Several measurements of cerebral oxygenation have been evaluated clinically. The most extensively used is $Sjvo_2$, which reflects the adequacy of CBF much as systemic "mixed venous" oxygenation reflects the adequacy of cardiac output. In contrast to monitoring of ICP and CPP, which provide minimal information concerning the ability of CDo_2 to support $CMRo_2$,[30] $Sjvo_2$ directly reflects the balance between these variables. Cerebral blood flow, $CMRo_2$, Cao_2, and jugular venous oxygen content ($CjvO_2$) are related according to the following equation:

$$CMRO_2 = CBF\ (CaO_2 - CjvO_2)$$

This equation suggests the likely changes in other variables as any variable is altered. As CBF decreases, both $SjvO_2$ and $CjvO_2$ decrease (Fig. 166–2*A*).[6] As $CMRO_2$ decreases, $SjvO_2$ and $CjvO_2$ remain constant, because CBF decreases in parallel with $CMRO_2$ (Fig. 166–2*B*).

Mixed cerebral venous blood, like mixed systemic venous blood, is a global average and may not reflect marked regional hypoperfusion. Therefore, abnormally low $SjvO_2$ (i.e., <50%, compared with a normal value of 65%) suggests the possibility of cerebral ischemia, but normal or elevated $SjvO_2$ does not prove adequate cerebral perfusion. Clinically, intermittent jugular venous bulb blood analysis or continuous oximetric monitoring has detected unexpected cerebral desaturation that otherwise would have gone unnoticed.

To insert a jugular venous bulb catheter, one can locate the internal jugular vein through the use of external anatomic landmarks and a "seeker" needle, as for antegrade passage of central venous catheters or pulmonary artery catheters; however, the catheter is directed toward the mastoid process, below which lies the jugular venous bulb. A skull radiograph can confirm the position just superior to the base of the skull. The jugular bulb catheter should be placed in the dominant jugular vein; that is, the jugular vein that when compressed produces the greater increase in ICP or the vein on the side of the larger jugular foramen as detected by CT.[31]

Oxygen saturation can be monitored continuously in the jugular bulb using a fiberoptic catheter. Because oxyhemoglobin and deoxyhemoglobin absorb light differently, $SjvO_2$ can be determined from differential absorbance. The highest rate of desaturation episodes occurs in patients with intracerebral hematomas, closely followed by those with SAH. In patients with TBI, the number of jugular desaturations is strongly associated with poor neurologic outcome; even a single desaturation episode is associated with a doubling of the mortality rate (Table 166–4).[32]

Several more complex applications of jugular venous oxygen monitoring have been proposed. *Cerebral extraction of oxygen* (CEO_2), which Cruz and colleagues[33] defined as the difference between SaO_2 and $SjvO_2$, provides a more meaningful calculation than the cerebral arteriovenous oxygen content difference ($A - VDO_2$) in the presence of acute anemia. Another concept, termed *cerebral hemodynamic reserve* (CHR), is defined as the ratio of percentage change in global CEO_2 (reflecting the balance of $CMRO_2$ and CBF) to percentage change in CPP.[34] This latter equation attempts to integrate cerebral hemodynamics and metabolism with intracranial compliance. Cruz[34] found that CHR decreased as intracranial compliance decreased, even as a consequence of minor elevations in ICP. Theoretically, this variable may allow more precise management of cerebral hemodynamics in patients with reduced intracranial compliance.

TABLE 166–4. Relationship Between the Frequency of Jugular Venous Desaturations and Neurologic Outcome in Patients with Traumatic Brain Injury

No. Desaturations*	No. Patients†	Mortality (%)	% Dead/PVS/SD‡
0	70	17	55
1	27	41	74
>1	19	68	90

Modified with permission from Gopinath SP, Robertson CS, Contant CF, et al: Jugular venous desaturation and outcome after head injury. J Neurol Neurosurg Psychiatry 1994; 54:717–723.

*The number of desaturation episodes occurring in individual patients.

†The number of patients with each number (0, 1, or >1) of desaturations.

‡PVS = in persistent vegetative state; SD = left with severe disability.

Another promising technique for monitoring the adequacy of CDO_2 is direct assessment of brain tissue oxygenation. One important weakness of $SjvO_2$ monitoring is that the global measurement provides no information about regional tissue oxygenation. Only relatively profound ischemia causes $SjvO_2$ to decrease to less than the accepted critical threshold of 50%. Even severe regional ischemia may not result in desaturation if venous effluence from other regions is normally saturated, in part because blood flow returning from ischemic regions is by definition less per volume of tissue than flow from well-perfused regions. One potential means of obtaining data that reflect regional oxygenation is the use of intracranial probes that monitor regional (r) PO_2, PCO_2, and pH.[35] Modified from probes designed to be inserted through arterial catheters to continuously monitor arterial blood gases, the intracranial probes can be placed through multiple-lumen ICP monitoring bolts. Although these probes provide no information about remote regions, they nevertheless provide continuous information about the region that is contiguous to the probe.

Perhaps the best monitor of brain oxygenation would be a noninvasive device that functions for the brain like a pulse

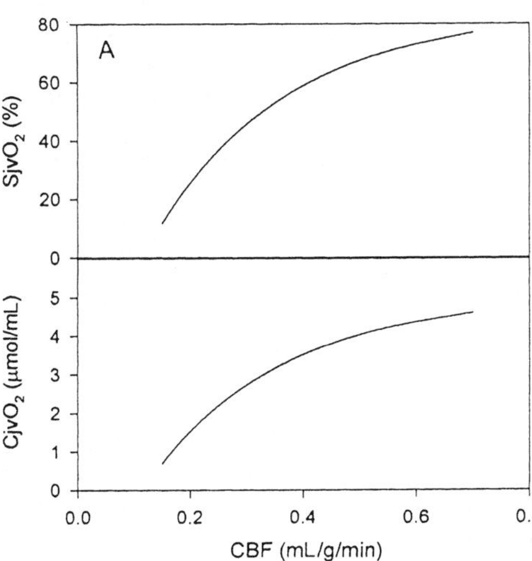

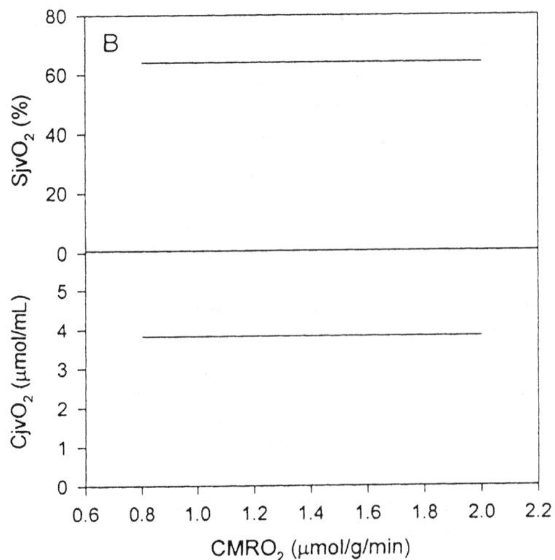

Figure 166–2. Changes in jugular venous bulb oxygen saturation ($SjvO_2$) and jugular venous bulb oxygen content ($CjvO_2$) in normal subjects as cerebral blood flow (CBF) is reduced (*A*) or as the cerebral metabolic rate for oxygen ($CMRO_2$) decreases (*B*). (From Feldman Z, Robertson CS: Monitoring of cerebral hemodynamics with jugular bulb catheters. Crit Care Clin 1997; 13:51–77.)

oximeter functions for systemic oxygenation. Near-infrared spectroscopy (NIRS) may eventually offer the opportunity to assess the adequacy of brain oxygenation continuously and noninvasively. In this technique, near-infrared light penetrates the skull and, during transmission through or reflection from brain tissue, undergoes changes in wavelength that are proportional to the relative concentrations of oxygenated and deoxygenated Hb in the tissue beneath the field.[36] The absorption (A) of light by a chromophore (i.e., hemoglobin) is defined by Beer's law, as follows:

$$A = abc$$

where a = the absorption constant; b = path length of the light; and c = concentration of the chromophore.

Extensive preclinical and clinical data demonstrate that NIRS detects qualitative changes in brain oxygenation[37–39] (Fig. 166–3). Despite promise, however, many problems remain with the technology.[40, 41] Brain saturation measured using NIRS correlated poorly with continuous $Sjvo_2$ in patients with severe closed head injury,[42] although the technique seemed promising for detecting desaturation during carotid endarterectomy[43] and cardiopulmonary bypass.[44] Technical challenges to quantification of the signal include (1) difficulty in determining the path lengths of reflected lights of different wavelengths and (2) estimating the relative proportions of arterial, venous, and capillary blood in the field. Therefore, validation studies suggest that NIRS may be more useful for monitoring trends than for actual quantification of brain tissue oxygenation[45, 46] (Fig. 166–4).

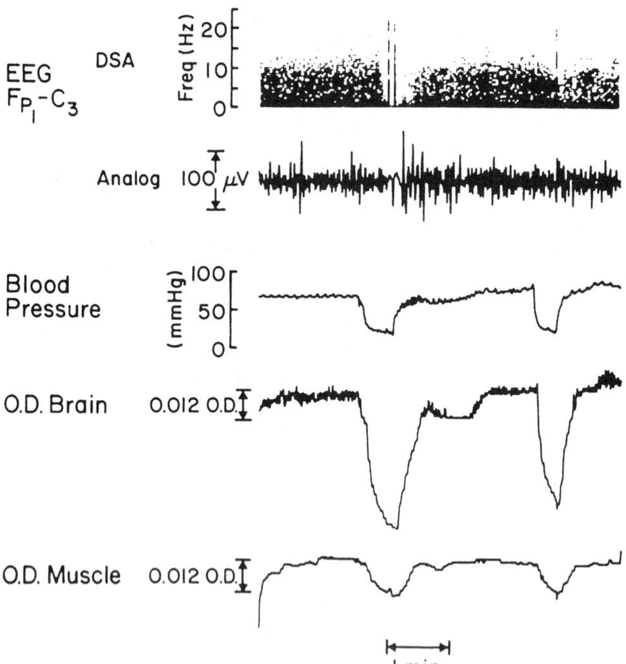

Figure 166–3. Electroencephalographic (EEG; density spectral array [DSA] display), analog EEG, blood pressure, and near-infrared spectroscopic estimation (O.D. [optical density]) of hemoglobin saturation in brain and muscle during an episode of ventricular fibrillation in a patient undergoing implantation of an automatic implantable defibrillator. With abrupt cessation of cerebral circulation, O.D. in brain and muscle declined abruptly. After an interval of absent circulation, defibrillation restored perfusion. The post-defibrillation increase in O.D. in brain may represent transient postischemic hyperemia. (From Smith DS, Levy W, Maris M, et al: Reperfusion hyperoxia in brain after circulatory arrest in humans. Anesthesiology 1990; 73:12–19.)

Electrophysiologic Monitoring

The cortical EEG, altered by mild cerebral ischemia and abolished by profound cerebral ischemia, can be used to indicate potentially damaging hypoperfusion. Although the EEG has not been used extensively in critically ill patients, it may be useful (1) in patients thought to have isolated seizures or status epilepticus, (2) in defining the depth or the type of coma, and (3) in documenting focal or lateral intracranial abnormalities.

In the ICU, electrical noise from equipment such as monitors and nearby computers may interfere with technically adequate tracings. Continuous EEG recording is cumbersome owing to the sheer volume of data (300 pages per hour of hard copy on as many as 16 channels). Therefore, various software programs have been designed to compress the data. If the complex waveform, consisting of four frequency ranges, delta (<4 Hz), theta (4 to 8 Hz), alpha (8 to 13 Hz), and beta (>13 Hz), is filtered and digitized, rapid Fourier analysis of the digitized data can determine the relative amplitude present in each frequency band. Data can then be displayed in formats such as the compressed spectral array (CSA) or density spectral array (DSA).[47, 48]

Sensory EPs, which include somatosensory evoked potentials (SSEPs), brain stem auditory evoked potentials (BAEPs), and visual evoked potentials (VEPs), can be used as qualitative threshold monitors to detect severe neural ischemia. Whereas the EEG records the continuous, spontaneous activity of the brain, EPs evaluate the responses of the brain to specific stimuli.

To record SSEPs, the clinician applies a stimulus to a peripheral nerve, usually the median nerve at the wrist, by a low-amplitude current of approximately 20 msec in duration. The resultant sensory (afferent) nerve stimulation is sufficient to provoke a slight thumb twitch. Repeated identical stimuli are applied, and signal averaging is used to visualize the reproducible evoked responses while removing the highly variable background EEG. Evoked potentials are described in terms of (1) the amplitude of individual peaks and (2) the delay (*latency*) from stimulus administration to the appearance of specific portions of the waveform. Because peripheral nerve stimulation can be uncomfortable, SSEPs are usually obtained in comatose patients. SSEPs are unaffected by neuromuscular blocking agents.

The sensitivity of EP monitoring is similar to that of EEG monitoring. Evoked potentials, especially BAEPs, are relatively robust, although they are modified by sedatives, narcotics, and anesthetics, as well as by trauma, hypoxia, or ischemia. Because obliteration of EPs occurs only under conditions of profound cerebral ischemia or mechanical trauma, EP monitoring is one of the most specific ways in which to assess neurologic integrity. However, neurologic deficits occur that have not been predicted by changes in EPs,[49] and severe changes in EPs may not be followed by neurologic deficits. The former finding probably represents damage to tissue that has not been part of the conducting pathway for the monitored response; the latter finding presumably reflects ischemia of either insufficient duration or insufficient magnitude to produce cell death.

Extensive use of electrophysiologic techniques in the ICU has been limited by three factors:

- Expensive equipment
- The requirement for highly trained technicians
- The need for clinical sophistication in the art of pattern recognition

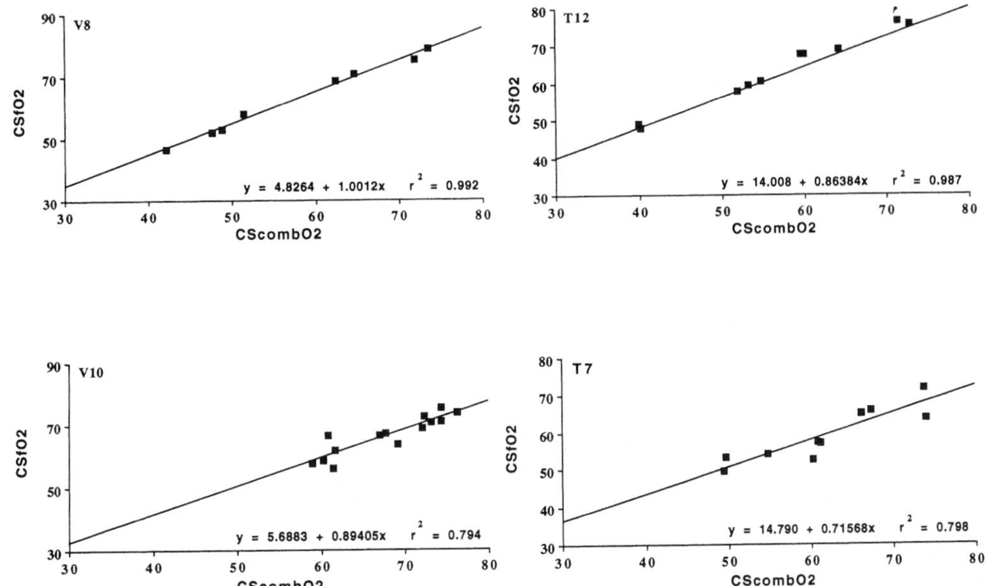

Figure 166–4. Cerebral oximeter signal (CS_fO_2) and calculated brain oxygen saturation ($CS_{comb}O_2$ = 0.25 × SaO_2 + 0.75 × $SjvO_2$) are closely correlated (r^2 = 0.798 to 0.987) in individual subjects for the training group (subjects T12 and T7) and validation group (r^2 = 0.798 to 0.992) (subjects V8 and V10). However, the agreement between the measured and calculated values is imprecise. The number in the *upper left* corner represents the individual subject identities. T = training set; V = validation set. The best and worst examples are represented. (From Pollard V, Prough DS, DeMelo AE, et al: Validation in volunteers of a near-infrared spectroscope for monitoring brain oxygenation in vivo. Anesth Analg 1996; 82:269–277.)

Nevertheless, some research centers have used electrophysiologic monitoring as an integral part of a battery of monitors in patients with severe intracranial hypertension.[50]

Neurochemical Monitoring

Neurochemical monitoring via microdialysis allows assessment of the chemical milieu of cerebral extracellular fluid and provides valuable information about neurochemical processes in various neuropathologic states. In addition, microdialysate reflects the metabolic response to treatment modalities such as hypothermia, CSF drainage, and barbiturate administration. Both cerebral ischemia and trauma are associated with substantial increases in energy-related metabolites, such as lactate, adenosine, inosine, and hypoxanthine, as well as neurotransmitters such as glutamate, aspartate, dopamine, and gamma-aminobutyric acid (GABA).[51] The magnitude of release of these substances correlates with the extent of ischemic damage.[52] The lactate-pyruvate ratio in dialysate correlates with the glutamate concentration[53]; at lactate-pyruvate ratios less than 20 to 25 (close to the normal range of 15 to 20), glutamate concentrations were low, whereas at moderately elevated lactate-pyruvate ratios of 40 or more, glutamate levels increased. This finding suggests that (1) there is a threshold relationship between cerebral energy failure and glutamate levels in cerebral extracellular fluid and (2) the lactate-pyruvate ratio could be used as an indicator of disturbances in brain energy metabolism.

SPECIFIC NEUROLOGIC AND NEUROSURGICAL DISEASES

A variety of powerful techniques, all of which can be performed at the bedside of the critically ill patient, are available for assessing the cerebral circulation. The next step in the evolution of neurologic monitoring necessitates the development of physiologically and pharmacologically sound protocols for goal-directed therapy. These protocols must then be carefully tested to determine whether they can reduce morbidity and mortality in patients with critical neurologic illnesses. To a limited extent, progress toward these goals has been made in TBI and ischemic neurologic disease.

Traumatic Brain Injury

The conventional view of the cerebral circulation after TBI is that some head-injured patients demonstrate depressed levels of both $CMRO_2$ and CBF (i.e., flow and metabolism are *coupled*), whereas other patients, especially those who are young, demonstrate *uncoupling,* with CBF substantially in excess of $CMRO_2$ (also termed *luxury perfusion*).[54] In one study, nearly 90% of patients 18 years or younger demonstrated cerebral hyperemia at some point during intensive monitoring.[55]

The Cerebral Circulation

The traditional understanding of the post-traumatic cerebral circulation has undergone substantial revision, however, on the basis of data suggesting that cerebral ischemia may be particularly common within the first few hours after injury. Bouma and associates[56] reported that CBF, as measured with ^{133}Xe, was less than a critical value of 18 mL · 100 g^{-1} · min^{-1} in one third of measurements made within 6 hours of injury in 106 head-injured patients. Within the first few hours after injury, CEO_2 also was high, but it returned toward normal within 24 hours. Follow-up studies using stable xenon CT confirmed cerebral ischemia in one third of patients within 8 hours of TBI.[25] Cerebral vascular resistance, which is substantially greater than normal in many patients in the first few hours after injury,[25, 56] may produce profound cerebral hypoperfusion if hypotension also develops. Lower CBF correlates with poorer outcome, after adjustment is made for confounding variables, in head-injured patients.[57]

The regional distribution of CBF is more variable in head-injured patients than in healthy individuals.[58] Nonsurviving patients and patients who will survive in a persistent vegetative state commonly demonstrate regional CBF values less than 20 mL · 100 g^{-1} · min^{-1}, especially in the frontal and parietal lobes.[59] Low flow in arterial boundary regions in the frontoparietal cortex, often secondary to high ICP, predicts poor neurologic outcome.[60] CBF may be less than 20 mL · 100 g^{-1} · min^{-1} in some brain regions, however, even in some patients who progress to good recovery.

In many patients studied more than 24 hours after TBI, reduced CBF appeared not to represent cerebral ischemia but rather to represent appropriate coupling between low $CMRO_2$ and low CBF.[54] Such patients may be vulnerable to excessive vasoconstriction during acute hyperventilation. In nearly 20% of patients, a wide A − VDO_2 developed during hyperventilation, suggesting that hyperventilation therapy should be accompanied by an estimate of the adequacy of cerebral perfusion. Data from a controlled clinical trial suggested that routine hyperventilation was not beneficial and might have been harmful,[61] perhaps because of regional ischemia.

Experimental and clinical data suggest that CBF after head trauma may be pressure-dependent at levels of CPP normally associated with unchanged CBF. In experimental animals, CBF measured after TBI using radiolabeled microspheres was found to be poorly maintained in response to hemorrhagic hypotension.[62] In one third of patients after TBI in another series, CBF passively changed as CPP changed.[63] In these patients, CBF may not increase to normal even at high levels of CPP. Even mild TBI (GCS scores of 13 to 15) was associated in another series with impaired autoregulation in eight of 29 patients.[64] In children, either abnormally high or abnormally low CBF was found to be associated with impaired autoregulation.[65] Lam and associates[66] correlated outcome with impairment of autoregulation (assessed using laser Doppler flowmetry) in severely head-injured patients; five patients with intact autoregulation had good outcomes, in contrast to good outcome in only four of 10 patients with transient impairment and nine deaths and two severe disabilities in 11 patients with persistent loss of autoregulation.

TCD ultrasonography has been used to identify moderate and severe cerebral vasospasm after head injury[67, 68]; in one series, all patients with severe vasospasm (five of eight patients with vasospasm in a total group of 30 head-injured patients) had traumatic SAH.[67] Increased flow velocity is common after head injury and may be due to vasospasm (decreased vascular diameter) or hyperemia (increased CBF). $SjvO_2$ can also be used to distinguish between these two entities, because decreased CBF is associated with low $SjvO_2$, and increased CBF is associated with increased $SjvO_2$.[50]

If CBF measurements are unavailable, calculation of the CEO_2 or lactate extraction may provide clinically useful information regarding the adequacy of cerebral perfusion.[69] Excessive regional vasoconstriction represents a possible mechanism for the reported worsening of outcome[61] in patients hyperventilated after head trauma in comparison with those maintained at a higher level of $PaCO_2$.

Conceptually, much of the management of patients with acute head injuries is intended to maintain adequate CBF. However, CBF is not routinely measured. Most cerebral circulatory information is inferred from knowledge of MAP and $PaCO_2$ and from measurement of ICP. Intracranial pressure monitoring is usually considered to be a fundamental part of the care of patients with severe closed head injury (i.e., those with GCS scores ≤ 8).[70] Severe intracranial hypertension is the primary cause of death in more than 10% of severely injured patients, and ICP above 20 mm Hg increases morbidity in those who survive.[71] Although many neurosurgeons believe that aggressive monitoring and control of ICP improves outcome in severe head injury,[72] other data suggest the possibility that concurrent changes in management, rather than ICP monitoring, explain the improvement.[73, 74]

Guidelines

In head-injured patients, clinicians have applied systematic, though institutionally specific, protocols for avoidance of intracranial hypertension and for reduction of increased ICP when a threshold of 15 or 20 mm Hg is exceeded. In particular, decisions about diuretics, hyperventilation, position changes, and additional diagnostic procedures may be determined by ICP information. The information is considered necessary in patients in whom neuromuscular blocking agents are administered as part of treatment to reduce ICP, because of the inability to perform a comprehensive neurologic examination. If intracranial hypertension is refractory to conventional therapy, ICP monitoring is one of the alternative techniques used to control barbiturate coma.[75]

A consensus committee formed by the Brain Trauma Foundation and the American Association of Neurological Surgeons has published standards, guidelines, and options for the use of ICP monitoring in TBI.[76] Although the committee found insufficient data to support a treatment standard, they did develop several guidelines, as follows:

1. Intracranial pressure monitoring is appropriate in patients with an abnormal admission CT scan and severe head injury (GCS score 3 to 8) after cardiopulmonary resuscitation for cardiac arrest.
2. Intracranial pressure monitoring is appropriate in patients with severe head injury and a normal CT scan if two or more of the following features are noted at admission: age above 40 years, unilateral or bilateral motor posturing, and systolic blood pressure below 90 mm Hg.
3. ICP monitoring is not indicated in patients with mild or moderate head injury.

The consensus committee also provided a guideline for treatment of ICP at a threshold of 20 to 25 mm Hg and suggested as an option that treatment of ICP should be corroborated by frequent clinical examination and CPP data.

After analysis of available ICP monitoring technology, the committee ranked devices, on the basis of their accuracy, stability, and ability to drain CSF, in the following order[76]:

1. Intraventricular devices, including fluid-coupled catheters and catheter-tip pressure transducers.
2. Parenchymal catheter-tip transducers.
3. Subdural devices, including catheter-tip transducers and fluid-coupled catheters.
4. Subarachnoid fluid-coupled devices.
5. Epidural devices.

Robertson and coworkers[69] reported extensive experience in head-injured patients with monitoring of the A − VDO_2. In a series of 100 patients, measurements of the cerebral arteriovenous differences of lactate and oxygen content could be used to predict CBF and to differentiate patients with patterns consistent with ischemia or infarction, normal CBF, cerebral hyperemia, and compensated hypoperfusion[69] (Fig. 166–5).

Regional Oxygenation Probes

Zauner and colleagues[35] have reported their experience with a probe that measures rPO_2, $rPCO_2$, and rpH. The probe uses optical fibers to measure pH and PCO_2 and a miniaturized Clark electrode to measure PO_2. Through a triple-lumen subarachnoid bolt, these researchers inserted (1) an intracranial pressure monitor; (2) a probe to monitor rPO_2, $rPCO_2$, and rpH

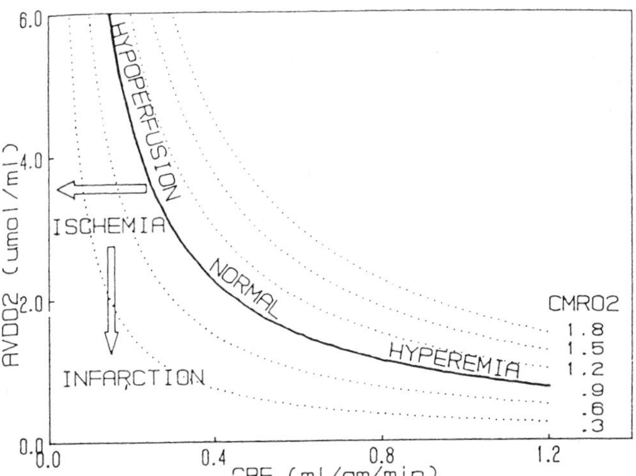

Figure 166–5. Conceptual model of the relationship between cerebral blood flow (CBF) and cerebral metabolism in comatose, head-injured patients. In nonischemic brain, the cerebral arteriovenous oxygen content difference ($A-VDo_2$) and CBF vary reciprocally as illustrated by the solid curve, representing a cerebral metabolic rate of oxygen ($CMRo_2$) averaging 1.5 μmol/g/min. In the presence of cerebral ischemia/infarction *(open arrows),* $A - VDo_2$ and CBF have an unpredictable relationship. (From Robertson CS, Narayan RK, Gokaslan ZL, et al: Cerebral arteriovenous oxygen difference as an estimate of cerebral blood flow in comatose patients. J Neurosurg 1989; 70:222–230.)

(Paratrend 7; Diametrics Medical Inc., Roseville, Minn.); and (3) a microdialysis probe (CMA Microdialysis, Acton, Mass.) to monitor regional concentrations of glucose and lactate. In 24 severely head-injured patients, rPo_2 values less than 20 mm Hg correlated strongly with poor outcome (Fig. 166–6). In individual cases, trends in regional blood gas tensions and glucose and lactate levels appeared to reflect improving or deteriorating tissue metabolic status (Fig. 166–7).

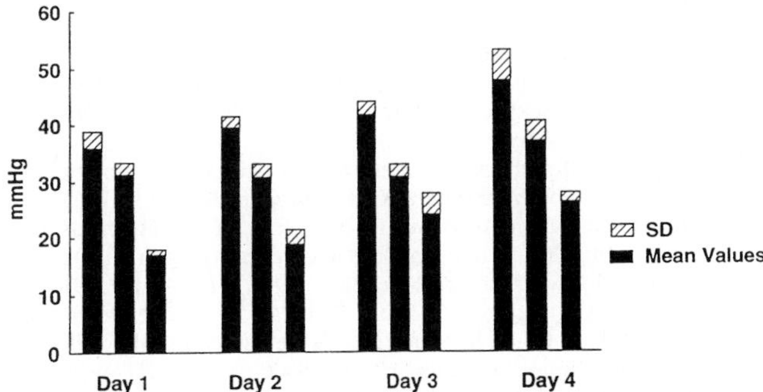

Figure 166–6. Bar graph of the time course of mean regional brain oxygen tension levels (± SD, in mm Hg). Patients were divided into three groups according to outcome. Group I (first column for each day) represents patients in the Good Recovery category of the Glasgow Outcome Scale; Group II (second column for each day) represents patients in the categories of Moderate Disability or Severe Disability; Group III (third column for each day) represents patients in the categories of Persistent Vegetative State or Death. (From Zauner A, Doppenberg EMR, Woodward JJ, et al: Continuous monitoring of cerebral substrate delivery and clearance: Initial experience in 24 patients with severe acute brain injuries. Neurosurgery 1997; 41:1082–1093.)

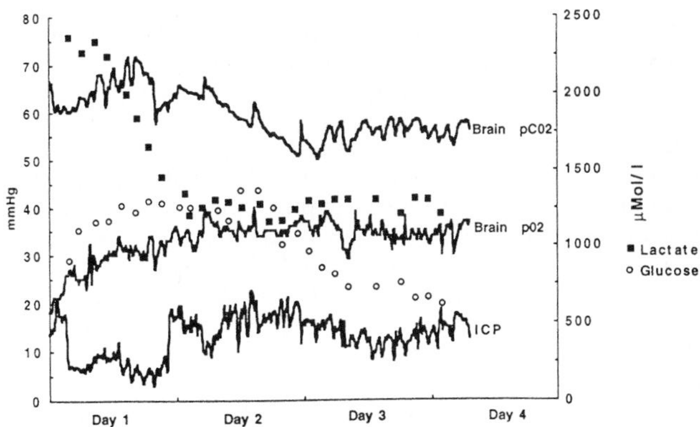

Figure 166–7. Line graph of changes in regional brain Po_2 and Pco_2 measured using a regional intracranial probe (Paratrend 7; Diametrics Medical, Inc., Roseville, Minn.); and regional concentrations of glucose and lactate measured using a microdialysis probe (CMA Microdialysis, Acton, Mass.). In this 24-year-old man with an admission Glasgow Coma Scale score of 7, brain lactate and Pco_2 rapidly decreased over the first day of intensive care and Po_2 increased. ICP = intracranial pressure. (From Zauner A, Doppenberg EMR, Woodward JJ, et al: Continuous monitoring of cerebral substrate delivery and clearance: Initial experience in 24 patients with severe acute brain injuries. Neurosurgery 1997; 41:1082–1093.)

Near-Infrared Spectroscopy

In general, NIRS has no established role in the management of head-injured patients; however, it has been used to localize post-traumatic intracranial hematomas.[77]

Electroencephalography and Evoked Potential Monitoring

Sloan[48] has concisely reviewed the application of EEG and EP monitoring in TBI. In head-injured patients, EP monitoring has been used as a diagnostic and prognostic aid. BAEPs correlate less well with clinical outcome than cortical SSEPs, the disappearance of which is a particularly ominous prognostic sign.[78] Multimodality EPs improve the prognostic accuracy of the clinical examination and measurement of ICP.[50, 79]

Microdialysis Techniques

Using microdialysis, both experimental and clinical investigations of TBI have documented the release of lactate and of the excitatory amino acids (EAAs) glutamate and aspartate. In a series of 15 head-injured patients, those having peak lactate concentrations below 1.0 mM had good recoveries, whereas all of those with poor outcome (severe disability, persistent vegetative state, or death) had peak lactate levels exceeding 1.0 mM.[80] In general, glutamate and aspartate release fluctuates proportionately. In one study of 17 head-injured patients, EAA concentrations increased six to 50 times the normal level in those with focal contusions and 20 to 50 times normal in those with secondary ischemic events.[81] Excitatory amino acid release and ICP were also correlated, especially if ICP exceeded 40 mm Hg for sustained intervals in conjunction with CPP of less than 40 mm Hg.[82] Brief ($<$5 minutes) increases in ICP or decreases in CPP, however, did not influence release of EAAs.

Ischemic Neurologic Disease

Neurologic monitoring in patients with nontraumatic, ischemic neurologic and neurosurgical conditions has been less extensive than in patients with traumatic coma. If CBF cannot increase, adequate oxygenation is maintained by increasing oxygen extraction until that compensatory mechanism is exhausted. At the point at which further increases in extraction are no longer possible, lactate production increases and $CMRO_2$ decreases (see Fig. 166-5). After cardiac arrest, some patients have postischemic hypoperfusion but $CMRO_2$ tends to be proportionately reduced.[83] Because the cerebral vasodilator nimodipine increased CBF and improved neurologic outcome in animals after complete cerebral ischemia, immediate post-resuscitation administration of nimodipine was investigated in patients; however, neurologic outcome was not improved.[84] In some patients, CBF, measured using ^{133}Xe, actually increases markedly within 24 to 48 hours after cardiac arrest, and the increase is associated with poor prognosis.[85]

Neurologic deterioration after SAH often represents cerebral vasospasm. Although CBF decreases, vasospasm reduces blood vessel diameter, thereby increasing flow velocity in the MCA.[86] As vasospasm resolves (and CBF increases), velocity decreases. In patients randomly assigned to receive nicardipine (a calcium entry blocker) or placebo after SAH, the incidence of vasospasm, as reflected in mean MCA flow velocities exceeding 120 cm/sec, was 23% in the nicardipine group versus 49% in the placebo group.[87] Elevated MCA velocity has also been used to determine the success of angioplasty in treating intracranial vasospasm.[88] Nevertheless, some investigators find TCD ultrasonography to be of questionable value, in that it fails to predict delayed ischemic deficits[89] even if more sophisticated pulsatility indices are used.[90]

Intracranial Pressure Monitoring

ICP monitoring has been applied in diverse acute ischemic and nonischemic neurologic conditions, including SAH and anoxic cerebral insult.[91] In nontraumatic brain disease, data defining the impact of ICP monitoring on outcome are more fragmentary and less convincing than those available for traumatized patients.

Electroencephalographic Monitoring

Because of the sensitivity of the EEG to drug effects, either unprocessed or processed EEG monitoring can be used to assess sedation in critically ill patients. It can also provide early evidence of seizure activity or cerebral ischemia. Quantitative EEG monitoring has been used to identify delayed ischemic deficits after SAH, occasionally before clinical deterioration.[92] Serial EEGs have been employed to improve prognostication in children with nontraumatic coma; the worst prognostic finding was low-amplitude activity or electrocerebral silence.[93]

Alpha-coma, unconsciousness associated with an EEG pattern resembling normal wakefulness occurring after brain stem stroke or hypoxic or anoxic cerebral injury, suggests a poor prognosis. Using a CSA display of EEG data, Cant and Shaw[94] monitored 51 patients and reported that persistence or return of a peak of activity in the theta or alpha frequency bands within 10 days of the onset of coma was associated with a favorable recovery. In contrast, patients in whom such a peak was lost were likely to die or to experience residual neurologic damage. In patients comatose from a mixture of traumatic and ischemic injuries, an alternating pattern of CSA activity was associated with a more favorable outcome.[95]

Evoked Potential Monitoring

When EPs are used for brain and spinal cord monitoring, they are intended to detect deterioration in neurologic function at a time when corrective action may still reverse changes. To a limited extent, EPs have been used to facilitate diagnosis and prognostication in ischemic and hypoxic brain injury. Central conduction time is prolonged in humans who have ischemic complications of SAH.[96] With impending brain death, cortical SSEPs disappear first; BAEPs disappear only when brain death is imminent.[97] Persistence of the medullary components of the SSEP, at a time when the cortical components are no longer present, confirms brain death. In children, absence of the cortical components of SSEPs with preserved brain stem function suggests the likelihood of a persistent vegetative state.[98]

SSEPs persist, though in altered form, during barbiturate administration; BAEPs are resistant to the effects of barbiturates.[99] *Central conduction time,* a measure of the time required to transmit the response to a stimulus from the periphery to the cortex, appears to be unaffected even by high levels of barbiturates.[100] Therefore, EPs assist in assessing neurologic status even in patients who are in barbiturate coma.

SUMMARY

During the 1990s, brain monitoring has substantially advanced. Widespread use of transcranial Doppler studies has contributed to evaluation of vasospasm in SAH and, to a lesser extent, in TBI. Equipment for monitoring ICP has improved, and guidelines have been developed for the use of ICP monitoring in TBI. Great progress has been made in assessment of cerebral oxygenation; jugular venous bulb catheterization and regional oxygen saturation measurements promise to provide continuous useful information about the adequacy of CBF. Meanwhile, continued advances in NIRS suggest that a clinically useful monitor will ultimately be developed. Microdialysis techniques have provided fascinating insights into brain metabolism and the role of neurotransmitters in brain injury. Continued progress may well result in protocols that can be tested and will improve neurologic outcome in patients with critical neurologic illness.

References

1. Jones TH, Morawetz RB, Crowell RM, et al: Thresholds of focal cerebral ischemia in awake monkeys. J Neurosurg 1981; 54:773-782.
2. Strandgaard S, Paulson OB: Cerebral autoregulation. Stroke 1984; 15:413-416.
3. DeWitt DS, Prough DS, Taylor CL, et al: Reduced cerebral blood flow, oxygen delivery, and electroencephalographic activity after traumatic brain injury and mild hemorrhage in cats. J Neurosurg 1992; 76:812-821.
4. Phillis JW, Preston G, DeLong RE: Effects of anoxia on cerebral blood flow in the rat brain: Evidence for a role of adenosine in autoregulation. J Cereb Blood Flow Metab 1984; 4:586-592.
5. Tommasino C, Moore S, Todd MM: Cerebral effects of isovolemic hemodilution with crystalloid or colloid solutions. Crit Care Med 1988; 16:862-868.
6. Feldman Z, Robertson CS: Monitoring of cerebral hemodynamics with jugular bulb catheters. Crit Care Clin 1997; 13:51-77.
7. Nemoto E, Klementavicius R, Melick J, et al: Effect of mild hypothermia on active and basal cerebral oxygen metabolism and blood flow. Adv Exp Med Biol 1994; 361:469-473.
8. Dietrich WD, Busto R, Alonso O, et al: Intraischemic but not postischemic brain hypothermia protects chronically following global forebrain ischemia in rats. J Cereb Blood Flow Metab 1993; 13:541-549.
9. Clifton GL, Jiang JY, Lyeth BG, et al: Marked protection by moderate hypothermia after experimental traumatic brain injury. J Cereb Blood Flow Metab 1991; 11:114-121.
10. Globus M, Alonso O, Dietrich W, et al: Glutamate release and free radical production following brain injury: Effects of posttraumatic hypothermia. J Neurochem 1995; 65:1704-1711.
11. Marion DW, Penrod LE, Kelsey SF, et al: Treatment of traumatic brain injury with moderate hypothermia. N Engl J Med 1997; 336:540-546.
12. Marshall LF, Marshall SB, Klauber MR, et al: A new classification of head injury based on computerized tomography. J Neurosurg 1991; 75:S14-S20.

13. Narayan RK, Kishore PRS, Becker DP, et al: Intracranial pressure: To monitor or not to monitor? A review of our experience with severe head injury. J Neurosurg 1982; 56:650-659.
14. Lobato RD, Sarabia R, Cordobes F, et al: Posttraumatic cerebral hemispheric swelling. Analysis of 55 cases studied with computerized tomography. J Neurosurg 1988; 68:417-423.
15. Eisenberg HM, Gary HE, Jr, Aldrich EF, et al: Initial CT findings in 753 patients with severe head injury: A report from the NIH Traumatic Coma Data Bank. J Neurosurg 1990; 73:688-698.
16. Le Bihan D, Turner R: Diffusion and perfusion. *In:* Magnetic Resonance Imaging. Stark D, Bradley W (Eds). Chicago, Mosby-Year Book, 1991, pp 335-371.
17. Prichard JW, Rosen BR: Functional study of the brain by NMR. J Cereb Blood Flow Metab 1994; 14:365-372.
18. Smith MC, Summers P, Padayachee TS: A variable pitch oxygen saturation indicator designed for use in the magnetic resonance environment. Physiol Meas 1994; 15:401-406.
19. Rotello LC, Radin EJ, Jastremski MS, et al: MRI protocol for critically ill patients. Am J Crit Care 1994; 3:187-190.
20. Korein J, Braunstein P, Kricheff I, et al: Radioisotopic bolus technique as a test to detect circulatory deficit associated with cerebral death: 142 studies on 80 patients demonstrating the bedside use of an innocuous IV procedure as an adjunct in the diagnosis of cerebral death. Circulation 1975; 51:924-939.
21. Kety SS, Schmidt CF: The nitrous oxide method for the quantitative determination of cerebral blood flow in man: Theory, procedure and normal values. J Clin Invest 1948; 27:476-483.
22. Olesen J, Paulson OB, Lassen NA: Regional cerebral blood flow in man determined by the initial slope of the clearance of intra-arterially injected ^{133}Xe: Theory of the method, normal values, error of measurement, correction for remaining radioactivity, relation to other flow parameters and response to $PaCO_2$ changes. Stroke 1971; 2:519-540.
23. Obrist WD, Thompson HK, Jr, Wang HS, et al: Regional cerebral blood flow estimated by ^{133}xenon inhalation. Stroke 1975; 6:245-256.
24. Tachibana H, Meyer JS, Okayasu H, et al: Changing topographic patterns of human cerebral blood flow with age measured by xenon CT. Am J Roentgenol 1984; 142:1027-1034.
25. Bouma GJ, Muizelaar JP, Stringer WA, et al: Ultra-early evaluation of regional cerebral blood flow in severely head-injured patients using xenon-enhanced computerized tomography. J Neurosurg 1992; 77:360-368.
26. Bishop CCR, Powell S, Rutt D, et al: Transcranial Doppler measurement of middle cerebral artery blood flow velocity: A validation study. Stroke 1986; 17:913-915.
27. Crutchfield JS, Narayan RK, Robertson CS, et al: Evaluation of a fiberoptic intracranial pressure monitor. J Neurosurg 1990; 72:482-487.
28. Yablon JS, Lantner HJ, McCormack TM, et al: Clinical experience with a fiberoptic intracranial pressure monitor. J Clin Monit 1993; 9:171-175.
29. Lundberg N, Troupp H, Lorin H: Continuous recording of the ventricular fluid pressure in patients with severe acute traumatic brain injury. J Neurosurg 1965; 22:581-590.
30. Cruz J, Raps EC, Hoffstad OJ, et al: Cerebral oxygenation monitoring. Crit Care Med 1993; 21:1242-1246.
31. Goodman JC, Gopinath SP, Valadka AB, et al: Lactic acid and amino acid fluctuations measured using microdialysis reflect physiological derangements in head injury. Acta Neurochir 1996; 67:37-39.
32. Gopinath SP, Robertson CS, Contant CF, et al: Jugular venous desaturation and outcome after head injury. J Neurol Neurosurg Psychiatry 1994; 57:717-723.
33. Cruz J, Jaggi JL, Hoffstad OJ: Cerebral blood flow and oxygen consumption in acute brain injury with acute anemia: An alternative for the cerebral metabolic rate of oxygen consumption? Crit Care Med 1993; 21:1218-1224.
34. Cruz J: Cerebral oxygenation—monitoring and management. Acta Neurochir 1993; 59:86-90.
35. Zauner A, Doppenberg EMR, Woodward JJ, et al: Continuous monitoring of cerebral substrate delivery and clearance: Initial experience in 24 patients with severe acute brain injuries. Neurosurgery 1997; 41:1082-1093.
36. Pollard V, Prough DS: Cerebral oxygenation: Near-infrared spectroscopy. *In:* Principles and Practice of Intensive Care Monitoring. Tobin MJ (Ed). New York, McGraw-Hill, 1998, pp 1019-1033.
37. Smith DS, Levy W, Maris M, et al: Reperfusion hyperoxia in brain after circulatory arrest in humans. Anesthesiology 1990; 73:12-19.
38. Delpy DT, Arridge SR, Cope M, et al: Quantitation of pathlength in optical spectroscopy. Adv Exp Med Biol 1989; 248:41-46.
39. Delpy DT, Cope M, van der Zee P, et al: Estimation of optical path length through tissue from direct time of flight measurement. Phys Med Biol 1988; 33:1433-1442.
40. Hirtz DG: Report of the National Institute of Neurological Disorders and Stroke workshop on near infrared spectroscopy. Pediatrics 1993; 91:414-417.
41. Villringer A, Planck J, Hock C, et al: Near infrared spectroscopy (NIRS): A new tool to study hemodynamic changes during activation of brain function in human adults. Neurosci Lett 1993; 154:101-104.
42. Unterberg A, Rosenthal A, Schneider GH, et al: Validation of monitoring of cerebral oxygenation by near-infrared spectroscopy in comatose patients. *In:* Neurochemical Monitoring in the Intensive Care Unit. Tasubokawa T, Marmarou A, Robertson C, et al (Eds). New York, Springer-Verlag, 1995, pp 204-210.
43. Williams IM, Picton A, Farrell A, et al: Light-reflective cerebral oximetry and jugular bulb venous oxygen saturation during carotid endarterectomy. Br J Surg 1994; 81:1291-1295.
44. Konishi A, Kikuchi K: Cerebral oxygen saturation (rSO_2) during open heart surgery and postoperative brain dysfunction. Masui 1995; 44:1322-1326.
45. Pollard V, Prough DS, DeMelo AE, et al: Validation in volunteers of a near-infrared spectroscope for monitoring brain oxygenation in vivo. Anesth Analg 1996; 82:269-277.
46. Pollard V, Prough DS, DeMelo AE, et al: The influence of carbon dioxide and body position on near-infrared spectroscopic assessment of cerebral hemoglobin oxygen saturation. Anesth Analg 1996; 82:278-287.
47. Levy WJ, Shapiro HM, Maruchak G, et al: Automated EEG processing for intraoperative monitoring: A comparison of techniques. Anesthesiology 1980; 53:223-236.
48. Sloan TB: Electrophysiologic monitoring in head injury. New Horiz 1995; 3:431-438.
49. Lesser RP, Raudzens P, Luders H: Postoperative neurological deficits may occur despite unchanged intraoperative somatosensory evoked potentials. Ann Neurol 1986; 19:22-25.
50. Chan KH, Dearden NM, Miller JD, et al: Multimodality monitoring as a guide to treatment of intracranial hypertension after severe brain injury. Neurosurgery 1993; 32:547-553.
51. Hillered L, Persson L, Ponten U: Neurometabolic monitoring of the ischaemic human brain using microdialysis. Acta Neurochir 1990; 102:91-97.
52. Hillered L, Persson L, Carlson H, et al: Excitatory amino acids: Basic pharmacology to clinical evaluation. Clin Neuropharmacol 1992; 15:695-696.
53. Hillered L, Persson L: Microdialysis for neurochemical monitoring in human brain injury. *In:* Neurochemical Monitoring in the Intensive Care Unit. Tsubokawa T, Marmarou A, Robertson C, et al (Eds). New York, Springer-Verlag, 1995, pp 59-63.
54. Obrist WD, Langfitt TW, Jaggi JL, et al: Cerebral blood flow and metabolism in comatose patients with acute head injury. Relationship to intracranial hypertension. J Neurosurg 1984; 61:241-253.
55. Muizelaar JP, Marmarou A, DeSalles AAF, et al: Cerebral blood flow and metabolism in severely head-injured children: Part 1. Relationship with GCS score, outcome, ICP, and PVI. J Neurosurg 1989; 71:63-71.
56. Bouma GJ, Muizelaar JP, Choi SC, et al: Cerebral circulation and metabolism after severe traumatic brain injury: The elusive role of ischemia. J Neurosurg 1991; 75:685-693.
57. Robertson CS, Contant CF, Gokaslan ZL, et al: Cerebral blood flow, arteriovenous oxygen difference, and outcome in head injured patients. J Neurol Neurosurg Psychiatry 1992; 55:594-603.
58. Cold GE: Cerebral blood flow in the acute phase after head injury: Part 2. Correlation to intraventricular pressure (IVP), cerebral perfusion pressure (CPP), $PaCO_2$, ventricular fluid lac-

tate, lactate/pyruvate ratio and pH. Acta Anaesthesiol Scand 1981; 25:332-335.
59. Overgaard J, Mosdal C, Tweed WA: Cerebral circulation after head injury: Part 3. Does reduced regional cerebral blood flow determine recovery of brain function after blunt head injury? J Neurosurg 1981; 55:63-74.
60. Overgaard J, Tweed WA: Cerebral circulation after head injury: Part 4. Functional anatomy and boundary-zone flow deprivation in the first week of traumatic coma. J Neurosurg 1983; 59:439-446.
61. Muizelaar JP, Marmarou A, Ward JD, et al: Adverse effects of prolonged hyperventilation in patients with severe head injury: A randomized clinical trial. J Neurosurg 1991; 75:731-739.
62. DeWitt DS, Prough DS, Taylor CL, et al: Regional cerebrovascular responses to progressive hypotension after traumatic brain injury in cats. Am J Physiol 1992; 32:H1276-H1284.
63. Bouma GJ, Muizelaar JP, Bandoh K, et al: Blood pressure and intracranial pressure-volume dynamics in severe head injury: Relationship with cerebral blood flow. J Neurosurg 1992; 77:15-19.
64. Jünger EC, Newell DW, Grant GA, et al: Cerebral autoregulation following minor head injury. J Neurosurg 1997; 86:425-432.
65. Muizelaar JP, Ward JD, Marmarou A, et al: Cerebral blood flow and metabolism in severely head-injured children: Part 2. Autoregulation. J Neurosurg 1989; 71:72-76.
66. Lam JMK, Hsiang JNK, Poon WS: Monitoring of autoregulation using laser Doppler flowmetry in patients with head injury. J Neurosurg 1997; 86:438-445.
67. Martin NA, Doberstein C, Zane C, et al: Posttraumatic cerebral arterial spasm: Transcranial Doppler ultrasound, cerebral blood flow, and angiographic findings. J Neurosurg 1992; 77:575-583.
68. Steiger HJ, Aaslid R, Stooss R, et al: Transcranial Doppler monitoring in head injury: Relations between type of injury, flow velocities, vasoreactivity, and outcome. Neurosurgery 1994; 34:79-86.
69. Robertson CS, Narayan RK, Gokaslan ZL, et al: Cerebral arteriovenous oxygen difference as an estimate of cerebral blood flow in comatose patients. J Neurosurg 1989; 70:222-230.
70. Ward JD: Intracranial pressure monitoring. *In:* Critical Care: State of the Art. Fuhrman BP, Shoemaker WC (Eds). Fullerton, Calif, The Society of Critical Care Medicine, 1989, pp 173-185.
71. Miller JD, Becker DP, Ward JD, et al: Significance of intracranial hypertension in severe head injury. J Neurosurg 1977; 47:503-516.
72. Saul TG, Ducker TB: Effect of intracranial pressure monitoring and aggressive treatment on mortality in severe head injury. J Neurosurg 1982; 56:498-503.
73. Colohan AR, Alves WM, Gross CR, et al: Head injury mortality in two centers with different emergency medical services and intensive care. J Neurosurg 1989; 71:202-207.
74. Stuart GG, Merry GS, Smith JA, et al: Severe head injury managed without intracranial pressure monitoring. J Neurosurg 1983; 59:601-605.
75. Eisenberg HM, Frankowski RF, Contant CF, et al: High-dose barbiturate control of elevated intracranial pressure in patients with severe head injury. J Neurosurg 1988; 69:15-23.
76. Brain Trauma Foundation, American Association of Neurological Surgeons, Joint Section on Neurotrauma and Critical Care: Guidelines for the management of severe head injury. J Neurotrauma 1996; 13:641-734.
77. Gopinath SP, Robertson CS, Grossman RG, et al: Near-infrared spectroscopic localization of intracranial hematomas. J Neurosurg 1993; 79:43-47.
78. Ganes T, Lundar T: EEG and evoked potentials in comatose patients with severe brain damage. Electroencephalogr Clin Neurophys 1988; 69:6-13.
79. Anderson DC, Bundlie S, Rockswold GL: Multimodality evoked potentials in closed head trauma. Arch Neurol 1984; 41:369-374.
80. Goodman JC, Robertson DP, Gopinath SP, et al: Measurement of lactic acid and amino acids in the cerebral cortex of head-injured patients using microdialysis. *In:* Neurochemical Monitoring in the Intensive Care Unit. Tsubokawa T, Marmarou A, Robertson C, et al (Eds). New York, Springer-Verlag, 1995, pp 78-83.
81. Bullock R, Zauner A, Tsuji O, et al: Patterns of excitatory amino acid release and ionic flux after severe human head trauma. *In:* Neurochemical Monitoring in the Intensive Care Unit. Tsubokawa T, Marmarou A, Robertson C, et al (Eds). New York, Springer-Verlag, 1995, pp 64-71.
82. Bullock R, Zauner A, Myseros J, et al: Evidence for prolonged release of excitatory amino acids in severe human head trauma: Relationship to clinical events. Ann N Y Acad Sci 1995; 765:290-297.
83. Beckstead JE, Tweed WA, Lee J, et al: Cerebral blood flow and metabolism in man following cardiac arrest. Stroke 1978; 9:569-573.
84. Roine RO, Kaste M, Kinnunen A, et al: Nimodipine after resuscitation from out-of-hospital ventricular fibrillation: A placebo-controlled, double-blind, randomized trial. JAMA 1990; 264:3171-3177.
85. Cohan SL, Mun SK, Petite J, et al: Cerebral blood flow in humans following resuscitation from cardiac arrest. Stroke 1989; 20:761-765.
86. Aaslid R, Huber P, Nornes H: Evaluation of cerebrovascular spasm with transcranial Doppler ultrasound. J Neurosurg 1984; 60:37-41.
87. Haley EC, Kassell NF, Torner JC: A randomized trial of nicardipine in subarachnoid hemorrhage: Angiographic and transcranial Doppler ultrasound results: A report of the Cooperative Aneurysm Study. J Neurosurg 1991; 78:537-547.
88. Hurst RW, Schnee C, Raps EC, et al: Role of transcranial Doppler in neuroradiological treatment of intracranial vasospasm. Stroke 1993; 24:299-303.
89. Laumer R, Steinmeier R, Gönner F, et al: Cerebral hemodynamics in subarachnoid hemorrhage evaluated by transcranial Doppler sonography: Part 1. Reliability of flow velocities in clinical management. Neurosurgery 1993; 33:1-9.
90. Steinmeier R, Laumer R, Bondár I, et al: Cerebral hemodynamics in subarachnoid hemorrhage evaluated by transcranial Doppler sonography: Part 2. Pulsatility indices: Normal reference values and characteristics in subarachnoid hemorrhage. Neurosurgery 1993; 33:10-19.
91. Tasker RC, Matthew DJ, Helms P, et al: Monitoring in non-traumatic coma: Part I. Invasive intracranial measurements. Arch Dis Child 1988; 63:888-894.
92. Labar DR, Fisch BJ, Pedley TA, et al: Quantitative EEG monitoring for patients with subarachnoid hemorrhage. Electroencephalogr Clin Neurophys 1991; 78:325-332.
93. Tasker RC, Boyd S, Harden A: Monitoring in non-traumatic coma: II. Electroencephalography. Arch Dis Child 1988; 63:895-899.
94. Cant BR, Shaw NA: Monitoring by compressed spectral array in prolonged coma. Neurology 1984; 34:35-39.
95. Karnaze DS, Marshall LF, Bickford RG: EEG monitoring of clinical coma: The compressed spectral array. Neurology 1982; 32:289-292.
96. Symon L, Hargadine J, Zawirski M: Central conduction time as an index of ischaemia in subarachnoid hemorrhage. J Neurol Sci 1979; 44:95-103.
97. Garcia-Larrea L, Bertrand O, Artru F, et al: Brain-stem monitoring: II. Preterminal BAEP changes observed until brain death in deeply comatose patients. Electroencephalogr Clin Neurophys 1987; 68:446-457.
98. Frank LM, Furgiuele TL, Etheridge JE, Jr: Prediction of chronic vegetative state in children using evoked potentials. Neurology 1985; 35:931-934.
99. de Weerd AW, Groeneveld C: The use of evoked potentials in the management of patients with severe cerebral trauma. Acta Neurol Scand 1985; 72:489-494.
100. Hume AL, Cant BR, Shaw NA: Central somatosensory conduction time in comatose patients. Ann Neurol 1979; 5:379-384.

167

Postoperative Confusion

Jill D. Kaplan, MD • Allan H. Ropper, MD

Confusion in the hours and days after surgery is a common condition that is often overlooked or is attributed to an underlying dementia or to the ill-defined "intensive care unit (ICU) psychosis." Perhaps the most common complication following surgery in older persons, confusion is associated with higher mortality and complication rates, longer lengths of hospital stay, greater need for long-term care, and higher cost.[1-3] The incidence of this syndrome is likely to increase as the population that requires routine surgery ages and as improved techniques allow older and sicker patients to undergo these procedures.

The list of conditions associated with postoperative confusion is extensive because it occurs in association with numerous circumstances. This is especially true in the elderly, in whom confusion is more common as a sign of illness than is fever, pain, or tachycardia.[1] The relatively stereotypic mental status changes of the acute confusional state reflect a response to any number of pathogenic changes that affect the cerebral cortex.[4, 5] This ambiguity is reflected in the frustration of pursuing the evaluation for confusion, an exercise that often fails to establish a definite single cause. It should be stated at the outset that postoperative confusion is uncommonly caused by a primary neurologic illness; rather, a combination of toxic or metabolic abnormalities is more often responsible, overt examples being drug effects or withdrawal, electrolyte imbalance, hypoxia, acid-base disorders, hepatic and renal failure, hyperglycemia or hypoglycemia, and cardiac or pulmonary insufficiency.[5-7] An acute confusional state may also represent the initial or the only sign of a serious medical illness, such as acute myocardial infarction, pulmonary embolism, pneumonia, or sepsis. Furthermore, the agitated patient may remove sutures, intravenous lines, or nasogastric tubes, impairing care and nutrition or leading to a fall and a complicating fracture or a subdural hematoma.

In this chapter, we review the terminology of postoperative confusion, discuss the factors associated with the condition, and describe how to evaluate a confused postoperative patient. The interested reader is also directed to a recent text that treats this subject in detail.[7a]

DEFINITION

Postoperative confusion is a bewildering topic, in part because of the nearly 30 different terms used to describe the syndrome. *Encephalopathy, organic brain or mental syndrome, acute brain failure, beclouded state* or *beclouded dementia, delirium,* and *acute confusional state* (ACS) all describe similar constellations of mental status changes, at the root of which is confused thinking and behavior. Even the most widely used terms—*ACS* and *delirium*—are not universally employed, with neurologists favoring the former, and psychiatrists and gerontologists the latter.

We use *confusion* to denote a state characterized principally by a disturbance of global attention and inability to maintain a coherent stream of thought. Disorientation, distractibility, inability to register events and to recall them later, and an unreasonable behavior are the salient features. Rapid fluctuations may occur from one hour to the next, and symptoms usually worsen nocturnally, a phenomenon that has been colorfully termed *sundowning.* Although diminished alertness and reduced motor activity are common, the opposite, irritability and restlessness may also occur. In advanced stages, confusion is accompanied by decreased alertness or drowsiness, then progressing to stupor and, finally, coma if the underlying problem worsens. *Stupor* is a state from which a patient can be aroused only by vigorous and repeated stimuli. In *coma,* the patient appears asleep and is unarousable.

We prefer to preserve the term *delirium* for a state of confusion with excessive motor and autonomic nervous system activity, but in deference to current common usage, it may be used interchangeably with ACS. In delirium, perceptual disturbances are prominent, as in the prototype delirium tremens; vivid hallucinations and delusions, insomnia, and motor agitation give the state a distinctive appearance. Tremulousness and jerky movements may be present, but are not always seen, along with dilated pupils, flushed face, tachycardia, and diaphoresis.

INCIDENCE AND ASSOCIATED FACTORS

The incidence and risk factors for postoperative confusion are not well established despite a sizable literature on the subject. Discrepancies between studies have been accounted for by differences in diagnostic criteria, patient selection, study design, and types of surgery. For example, mental status changes have reportedly followed coronary artery bypass in 3%[8] to 79%[9] of patients; following orthopedic surgery in 28%[10] to 61%[2]; and following lung transplantation in up to 73%.[11] Most reports have found no greater likelihood of cognitive impairment after surgery involving the cardiac chambers than after coronary bypass,[12-15] but others have disagreed.[16] Two specific problems in interpreting the literature arise because (1) some studies have sought delicate changes in cognitive functioning by utilizing sophisticated neuropsychologic tests and (2) many studies lack preoperative mental and neurologic evaluations and therefore overestimate the extent of change in elderly patients. Nonetheless, certain features of the postoperative state emerge consistently and form the basis for a clinical approach. A number of conditions and medications seem relatively common offenders, but at best, they are associated with ACS and not always clearly causal.

Cardiac Surgery

Studies of cardiac procedures, the surgery most commonly assessed for neurologic complications, have reported widely varying results. Prospective series cite a rate of postoperative confusion between 11% and 34% of patients,[12-17] whereas retrospective studies almost certainly give falsely low figures below 3%.[8, 18, 19] Many studies have used a battery of neuropsychologic tests to measure cognitive impairment,[9, 12, 13, 18, 20] but they do not specifically address the presence of clinically evident confusion or delirium. Although 79% of patients undergoing coronary bypass were found to have postoperative cognitive deterioration by formal testing in one large study, more than half of the patients denied mental difficulty and were clinically asymptomatic.[9]

Age, Dementia, and Alcohol Consumption

More useful have been several large prospective studies that found older age and previous excessive alcohol consumption to be associated with cognitive impairment after cardiac[21] and noncardiac[22] surgery. In one of these studies, postoperative delirium occurred in 9% of 1341 patients after orthopedic, general or gynecologic surgery; the condition was associated with (1) age older than 70 years, (2) self-reported alcohol abuse, (3) poor prior cognitive or functional state, and (4) markedly abnormal preoperative serum sodium, potassium, or glucose concentration. Noncardiac thoracic surgery and aortic aneurysm surgery were overrepresented. These associations are not surprising, because advanced age, alcohol abuse, poor cognitive and physical functioning, and abnormal laboratory values were found to be similarly associated with cognitive impairment in numerous studies of hospitalized patients, both surgical[23] and nonsurgical.[3, 24] These latter studies found that the elderly were particularly susceptible to confusion in the presence of fever, infection, or psychoactive drug therapy, and these notions have found their way into general medical thinking.

Psychoactive and Anticholinergic Drugs

Psychoactive medicines in particular, which are known to increase the risk of falls and hip fractures,[25, 26] have also been implicated as causing confusion.[2, 3, 10, 13, 27-30] The administration of narcotics has been associated with ACS in two of the largest prospective studies of patients primarily with medical illnesses.[3, 23] Of this group of drugs, meperidine has been most consistently associated with delirium in postoperative patients,[30] putatively because it has much more potent anticholinergic activity than other narcotics.[31] Noteworthy in this same study was the finding that anticholinergic drugs (antihistamines, tricyclic antidepressants, antiemetics, and certain neuroleptics) were not associated with confusion, although their low rates of use limited the certainty of the conclusions. Benzodiazepines, particularly the long-acting agents (chlordiazepoxide, diazepam, and flurazepam) were associated by the same authors with delirium; this association was less evident with the shorter-acting agents (oxazepam, lorazepam, triazolam, midazolam, and temazepam).

In other studies, however, drugs with anticholinergic effects have indeed been associated with confusion.[2, 3, 10, 17, 27-29] In a study of postcardiotomy delirium, most of the 34% of patients in whom delirium developed had high serum levels of anticholinergic drugs, whereas those who remained cognitively normal had low levels. As anticholinergic drug levels increased, progressive impairment of cognitive function occurred on the "Mini-Mental State" examination.[17] Anticholinergic eye drops were thought to have contributed to the 16% incidence of delirium after cataract surgery.[32]

Operative and Postoperative Technical Factors

The importance of intraoperative technical factors during cardiac surgery in the genesis of ACS has been controversial. Cardiopulmonary bypass time[12, 14, 15, 20] prolonged aortic cross-clamp time,[11, 13] low mean arterial pressure of 40 to 60 mm Hg,[12, 14, 15, 18, 20, 33] and hematocrit value[14] have not been related to postoperative mental status changes in most studies, but others have reported a correlation with perfusion time longer than 2 hours,[13, 18] operation lasting more than 7 hours,[13] minimum hemoglobin level,[20] or major unanticipated intraoperative events, such as massive bleeding.[18]

Conflicting evidence has also been reported regarding postoperative events associated with confusion after cardiac surgery. Hypotension[20] and the postoperative use of pressors[14] have been associated with cognitive impairment in some series, but the use of an intra-aortic balloon pump (a marker for hypotensive and severely ill patients) has not been a factor,[8, 20] except in one study.[14]

The ACS that followed cardiac transplantation was most often due to systemic infection in a study in which neurologic complications developed in 54% of patients.[34] Alternatively, high cyclosporine levels and cardiopulmonary bypass were predictive of confusion after lung transplantation in a small retrospective study in which delirium developed in most patients.[11]

Other Associations

Some researchers have correlated a history of depression[2, 29] with the development of confusion after orthopedic surgery; however, this has been disputed. In one study of 124 patients undergoing coronary artery bypass graft, depressed mood showed no correlation with prior cognitive decline.[35] Previous stroke was shown to be a risk factor for confusion in a study of 71 patients with old stroke who underwent coronary artery bypass surgery.[36] Old stroke deficits reappeared in nearly 27% of patients and worsened in nearly 9% of study subjects, although no new lesions were found by computed tomography scanning. Most of the patients had made a nearly complete recovery before discharge or within 6 months.[36]

As discussed later, Young and associates,[40] have expanded the concept of sepsis as causing a specific encephalopathy. Few studies of postoperative cases address this connection in any depth.

The state characterized by cortical seizures with inevident convulsions ("spike-wave stupor") has received considerable attention and has been associated at high frequency to drowsiness and stupor in medical ICU patients, but its importance in postoperative patients is not known. Also, certain drugs, such as imipenem and lidocaine, may produce the same state in susceptible patients.

Conclusion

To summarize, there is little cohesion regarding the causes of the postoperative confusional, state but certain features, highlighted in the next section, seem consistent enough among various studies to allow for an intelligent approach. In many cases, two or more factors conspire to disorder mentation in an individual patient (e.g., older age *and* medications, or prior stroke *and* alcoholism). The incidence and associated factors depend on the diagnostic criteria used to define the mental status abnormalities, but also on the patient population, the type of surgery, and the study design. Only prospective investigations will help to clarify risk factors and prevalence, and even then, a panoply of causes will need to be addressed systematically.

A CLINICAL APPROACH

Accurate mental status and neurologic examination ideally begin *before* the patient becomes confused; that is, preoperatively. A history from the patient and the family is invaluable, specifically through answers to questions about alcohol consumption, prior strokes, or cognitive abilities (whether the patient can balance a checkbook, shops alone, and drives). The presence of overtly "lateralizing" findings, such as hemiparesis, that suggest a prior stroke are harbingers of postoperative confusion. This information is valuable later, when the physician tries to decipher which physical findings are new. The same information can be gleaned from interviewing the family once ACS has supervened, but this approach is often awkward, because the physician (surgeon) asking the questions is simultaneously explaining the confusional state to the family in an attempt to allay their fears about brain damage and permanent mental illness. The clinical approach to the evaluation of postoperative confusion is outlined in Table 167–1.

General Examination

In the postoperative period, the examination begins by observing the patient casually for asymmetries of movement, gaze preference, or neglect of visual space. If no "focal" or lateralizing motor or sensory signs are present, a stroke or a primary neurologic process is unlikely, with a few exceptions.

Vital signs can provide an important clue to diagnosis. Fever should not be attributed to atelectasis without a thorough search for an infection. The neck should be examined for meningismus. Alcohol or barbiturate intoxication, extracellular fluid depletion, and myxedema may cause hypothermia. Decreased respiratory rate may point to barbiturate or morphine toxicity or, rarely, to hypothyroidism, whereas tachypnea suggests pneumonia, pulmonary edema, or diabetic or uremic acidosis. Although hyperventilation can result from brain stem lesions, it is most commonly a compensation for primary pulmonary dysfunction. *Cheyne-Stokes breathing,* a regular crescendo-decrescendo cycle between apneic periods, occurs commonly in patients with deep bilateral cerebral lesions or with a massive supratentorial lesion, but it is also common in metabolic disturbances and congestive heart failure. Hypotension is common in depressed alertness, particularly in patients with sepsis, internal hemorrhage, diabetes, myocardial infarction, or alcohol or barbiturate intoxication. Hypertensive encephalopathy is an infrequent cause of postoperative confusion. When increased blood pressure is combined with bradycardia, known as the *Cushing response,* increased intracranial pressure from a cerebral hemorrhage is likely. The stigmata of chronic alcoholism, such as spider telangiectasias, palmar erythema, hepatosplenomegaly, and caput medusae, may be evident; these make hepatic encephalopathy or a withdrawal state suspect as the cause of ACS.

TABLE 167–1. Examination of the Confused Patient

History (from Family and Patient)

- Baseline mental status (balances checkbook, shops independently, and drives) and known diagnosis of dementia
- Previous medical illnesses (diabetes mellitus, heart disease, or liver disease)
- Previous stroke
- Previous psychiatric history
- Substance abuse (alcohol, sedative-hypnotics)

General Physical Examination

- Vital signs (respiratory pattern, e.g., Cheyne-Stokes, hyperventilation)
- Evidence of acute or chronic systemic illness
- Nuchal rigidity
- Evidence of head trauma

Neurologic Examination

MENTAL STATUS EXAMINATION

- Level of consciousness (e.g., is hyperalert, alert, lethargic, stuporous, or comatose)
- Attention (repeats number strings and can give months or days in reverse order)
- Language (comprehends yes/no questions and conveys meaning without errors)
- Memory (remembers details of hospitalization or a short story)
- Visuospatial (draws a clock or shows spatial neglect)

CRANIAL NERVES

- Pupillary reaction and size
- Extraocular movements (gaze preference)
- Facial symmetry

MOTOR SYSTEM

- Pronator "drift" of outstretched supinated arms
- Fine finger movements (touch thumb to each finger rapidly)
- Gait (walks on steady base with good step length)
- Spontaneous adventitious movements (e.g., tremor, myoclonus, clonic movements)
- Asterixis

Mental Status Examination

The examination of cognition can be directed by initial global observations of behavior and can be abbreviated if language or attention deficits are obvious. Further assessment should be systematic and should include a narrative description of the level of consciousness, of attention, language, memory, and visuospatial skills if the patient's sustained attention can be captured. The following details may be helpful in establishing the severity of the deficit and following its progress.

Level of Consciousness and Affect

The physician should begin by noting the patient's ability to attend to commands and to the environment, because abnormalities in these areas limit the interpretation of cognitive tests that follow. It is extremely useful to test attention in a formal manner (number string repetition is typically used), as described later, rather than by casual observation. Speech and writing may appear incoherent or comprehension may appear impaired in the inattentive patient, leading to the mistaken diagnosis of aphasia, amnesia, or inability to calculate. The affect should also be considered; a lack of concern about a deficit may be a sign of right parietal lobe stroke, frontal lobe disease, or underlying depression.

Attention

Asking the patient either to repeat spoken number strings or to recite the months of the year in reverse order, or the days of the week, easily tests attention. The normally functioning person should be able to repeat a sequence of at least six digits forward and four digits backward, after hearing them recited at the rate of 1 per second.[37] Serial subtraction of 7 from 100 is a less consistent measure of attention but is expected of a fully awake and attentive patient.

Language

Formal language testing is not necessary if the patient can understand the examiner and can convey meaning through fluent speech without malformed or inappropriate words, the latter termed *paraphasias.* If the patient is aphasic, testing of spontaneous speech output, comprehension, repetition, naming, reading, and writing should be performed. Comprehension is best tested with questions requiring "Yes" or "No" responses, such as "Do monkeys fly?" or "Does April come before March?" Naming difficulty in isolation (anomia) is not helpful for localization, because it occurs with metabolic derangements as well as with aphasia.

Memory

The patient's memory can be examined informally through questions about current events or the hospitalization. If this information is accurate, no further probing is needed. The patient is given three words or a short story to recall and then should be asked to repeat the information until able do so without prompting. Memory (the retention of learned information) cannot be tested unless the information is first registered, so it is futile to assess memory if attention is not normal. *Wernicke's disease,* seen mostly in alcoholics, is characterized by nystagmus, gaze palsies, gait ataxia, and mental confusion. Although Wernicke's disease and Korsakoff's psychosis are associated with thiamine deficiency, the latter may also appear in patients with lesions of the diencephalon or temporal lobes. A korsakoffian type of impairment of retentive memory may also be a late feature of anoxic encephalopathy.

Visuospatial Ability

Visuospatial skills, which reflect right parietal lobe function, can be tested by asking the patient to copy a picture of a solid cube onto a piece of paper or to write numbers inside a large circle (of at least a 5-inch diameter, to detect a spatial neglect) that represents a clock.[37] As with memory, defective attention profoundly disorders these more complex abilities, and overinterpretation of testing abnormalities is common.

The Somatic Neurologic Examination

The neurologic examination can be directed toward three key areas: the eyes, the face, and motor function. Asymmetries in these areas may point to a focal brain lesion. The pupils and their reaction to light, ocular movements, visual fields, optic disks, and symmetry of facial movements should be assessed. Normal pupils indicate that the midbrain is intact, which is usually the case in patients with drug intoxication and metabolic disorders. Exceptions include opiate intoxication, which, as is well known to all clinicians, causes pinpoint pupils that barely react to light, and atropinic drug excess, which causes dilated and fixed pupils. Visual fields can be assessed by noting whether the patient blinks to threat from either side.

The integrity of the motor system (more specifically the corticospinal tracts) can be determined by having the patient hold the arms outstretched, with the palms upward, and then observing for pronation (drift). Slowness of fine finger movements, such as tapping on the thumb with the index finger, are more refined indications of corticospinal tract abnormality. If the patient can arise from a chair unassisted and walk on heels and toes, important leg weakness is unlikely.

Tremor, myoclonus, and asterixis are significant clues to a toxic or metabolic state, and each occurs in 15% to 25% of patients who are encephalopathic from sepsis.[38] *Tremor* refers to a regular, rhythmic oscillation of a part of the body around a fixed point, usually in one plane. The tremor of metabolic encephalopathy is coarse and less regular, occurring at a rate of 8 to 10 per second, and is usually absent at rest.[39] Sudden, nonrhythmic, asymmetric twitching of parts or groups of muscles signifies *myoclonus,* which is particularly common in the postanoxic and uremic states or with the use of haloperidol. Widespread lightning-like contractions, or *myoclonus multiplex,* can be triggered by sensory stimuli, such as loud noises, or by an abrupt touch to the body, and usually indicates a severe metabolic disturbance or cortical damage from hypoxia.

Arrhythmic lapses of sustained posture, or *asterixis,* are elicited by asking the patient to hold the arms outstretched with the hands dorsiflexed at the wrists. Asterixis occurs not only in its originally described form with hepatic encephalopathy but also with hypercapnia, uremia, and other metabolic and toxic encephalopathies, and is exaggerated after phenytoin administration. In all these cases, the sign is bilateral. Unilateral asterixis is most often an indication of a subtle hemiparesis on the side without the flapping movement, but thalamic lesions are also an uncommon cause (in which case the asterixis is on the side opposite the lesion).

Finally, as mentioned earlier, increasing attention has been given to inevident seizures as the cause of diminished alertness. Subtle indications of this condition include eyelid twitching, ocular jerking to one side, head turning, and subtle and intermittent convulsive movements in the limbs and an electroencephalogram is required for confirmation.

Laboratory Analysis and Imaging

Three neurologic studies are useful, in different circumstances, for the evaluation of the confused patient: (1) cranial computed tomography or magnetic resonance imaging, (2) lumbar puncture, and (3) electroencephalography (EEG).

Computed tomography (or magnetic resonance imaging) provides important information if asymmetries are present on the somatic neurologic examination or if a focal process is suspected, such as a subdural hematoma following a fall. Computed tomography is advisable before the lumbar puncture in such cases, or if intracranial bleeding is suspected on the basis of sudden unresponsiveness, hemiparesis, or the Cushing response.

Lumbar puncture is, of course, imperative if bacterial meningitis is a consideration. This issue arises most often after neurosurgical procedures but should not be neglected in any febrile and confused patient. It is often stated that meningitis may occur in the absence of a stiff neck if the patient is unresponsive, but deep coma is generally required to obliterate this defensive reaction. The physician should record the opening cerebrospinal pressure (a common omission in modern practice) before sending the fluid specimens for cell count analysis in the first and fourth specimen tubes and the other tubes for glucose, protein, and bacteriologic analyses.

The EEG is a useful and underutilized diagnostic tool in patients with postoperative confusion. Several conditions that cause confusion have differing effects on the EEG, even though slowing of the background rhythm is common in almost all patients with alterations of consciousness. Barbiturates and other sedatives may induce a high frequency (beta rhythm) in the EEG, whereas delirium tremens and Wernicke-Korsakoff syndrome cause surprisingly little or no change. Bilaterally synchronous, large, sharp "triphasic waves" are characteristic of hepatic encephalopathy but may also appear in patients with renal or pulmonary failure. Sharp waves, or "spikes" (fast waves of high amplitude), may be detected if seizures underlie the confusion, a condition thought by some to be quite common in the ICU but actually infrequent in our experience. A normal EEG in a patient whose responses are slow and who is inattentive supports the diagnosis of depression or catatonia, whereas mild but diffuse slow-wave abnormalities may occur with profound dementia. Major asymmetries of EEG background rhythms indicate an underlying structural lesion such as ischemic stroke, cerebral hemorrhage, or subdural hematoma.

Laboratory tests should generally include determinations of serum electrolytes, glucose, and calcium levels; white blood cell count; hematocrit value; and both urine and serum toxin screenings. Additional laboratory tests that may be useful in selected circumstances are determinations of arterial blood gases and ammonia and phosphate levels; liver and thyroid function tests; coagulation screenings; blood and urine cultures; urinalysis; electrocardiography; and chest x-ray. Occasionally, a blood culture reveals bacteremia in a patient with no other indications of sepsis.

DIFFERENTIAL DIAGNOSIS

The array of conditions associated with postoperative confusion is extensive, as previously emphasized; a list of such considerations appears in Table 167–2.

TABLE 167–2. Differential Diagnosis of Brain Dysfunction in Critical Care Patients (Ludwig's Differential Diagnosis of the Confusion-Delirium-Dementia-Coma Complex)

General Cause	Specific Causes
Vascular	Hypertensive encephalopathy; cerebral arteriosclerosis; intracranial hemorrhage or thromboses; circulatory collapse (shock); systemic lupus erythematosus; polyarteritis nodosa; thrombotic thrombocytopenic purpura
Infectious	Encephalitits; meningitis; general paresis; human immunodeficiency virus
Neoplastic	Space-occupying lesions such as gliomas, meningiomas, abscesses
Degenerative	Senile and presenile dementias such as Alzheimer's or Pick's dementia, Huntington's chorea, Wilson's disease
Intoxication	Chronic intoxication or withdrawal effect of sedative-hypnotic drugs such as bromides, opiates, tranquilizers, anticholinergics, dissociative anesthetics, anticonvulsants
Congenital	Epilepsy; postictal states; aneurysm
Traumatic	Subdural and epidural hematomas; contusion; laceration; postoperative trauma; heat stroke
Intraventricular	Normal-pressure hydrocephalus
Vitamin deficiency	Deficiencies of thiamine (Wernicke-Korsakoff), niacin (pellagra), vitamin B_{12} (pernicious anemia)
Endocrine-metabolic	Diabetic coma and shock; uremia; myxedema; hyperthyroidism, parathyroid dysfunction; hypoglycemia; hepatic failure; porphyria; severe electrolyte or acid-base disturbances; remote side effect of carcinoma; Cushing's syndrome; Wilson's disease
Metals	Heavy metals (lead, manganese, mercury); carbon monoxide; toxins
Anoxia	Hypoxia and anoxia secondary to pulmonary or cardiac failure, anesthesia, anemia
Depression, other	Depressive pseudodementia; hysteria; catatonia

From Ludwig AM: Principles of Clinical Psychiatry. New York, Free Press, 1980, p 234.

As a first approximation, the absence of focal findings suggests that the primary source of the ACS is not a structural brain lesion. In such cases, tremor, asterixis, or myoclonus indicate a toxic or metabolic etiology. Postoperative hypoxia, infection, hyperglycemia, metabolic acidosis or alkalosis, renal or hepatic failure, hyponatremia, and drug intoxication or withdrawal are conditions without lateralizing signs that are commonly associated with ACS. Thiamine deficiency, which is responsible for the symptoms of the Wernicke-Korsakoff syndrome, may produce confusion in the undernourished patient, especially after the administration of glucose.

Infections usually do not cause focal neurologic findings unless there has been a previous underlying stroke. The most common diagnostic error in this regard made by physicians in one retrospective cardiac transplantation study was to ascribe unrecognized central nervous system infection to metabolic disturbances or to "intensive care unit psychosis."[34] Neurologic disorders occurred in more than 50% of the transplant recipients, and infection was the most common cause.

The term *septic encephalopathy* has been introduced by Young and colleagues[40] to denote the mental status changes that accompany systemic infection in the absence of other organ failure. This concept has achieved great credibility as further studies have been conducted. Clinical or EEG evidence of diffuse cerebral dysfunction has been found in more than 70% of patients with positive blood cultures.[40] Often, a polyneuropathy also becomes evident as the confusional state abates ("critical illness polyneuropathy"), and affected patients may have unexplained difficulty in weaning from mechanical ventilation.[40]

Medications are, of course, the most commonly cited causes of postoperative confusion. Drug toxicity is especially common in the patient with a compensated dementia, impaired renal or hepatic function, or a known higher sensitivity to medications. Anticholinergic drugs, such as atropine, antihistamines, and antiparkinsonian agents, are most often implicated,[2, 3, 17, 27, 28] as discussed earlier. Cimetidine may produce confusional states,[41, 42] but this agent also inhibits the cytochrome P_{450} enzyme system and thus increases the toxicity of drugs metabolized by the liver, such as bendzodiazepines, barbiturates, lidocaine, and narcotic analgesics.[43] Mental status abnormalities have occurred in 5% of patients given 40 mg/day of prednisone and in up to 20% of patients given 80 mg/day.[43] Corticosteroids are particularly likely to produce a psychosis or delirium with the confusional state. Drugs commonly associated with postoperative confusion are listed in Table 167-3.

Patients with structural neurologic causes of postoperative confusion usually have focal signs, except those with meningitis, encephalitis, with widespread emboli from endocarditis, and with a few syndromes resulting from numerous small strokes, as discussed later. It should be pointed out that toxic or metabolic derangements, especially hypoglycemia or hyperglycemia, may also on occasion cause focal signs. Focal findings result from a subdural hematoma, suspected if there has been a fall, or with anticoagulants or a blood dyscrasia.

Two particular stroke syndromes, right middle cerebral artery infarction and left posterior cerebral artery infarction, may manifest as confusion, with other associated features of the stroke often being difficult to detect in the inattentive patient.[44–47] Visual field loss, hemisensory deficit, inability to read (but ability to write), and anomia that is most severe for colors are seen after bilateral or dominant-hemisphere posterior cerebral artery strokes.[44] Signs of right middle cerebral artery strokes are visual field defects, neglect of visual stimuli on the left side of space, and, slight drift of the outstretched left arm, or mild left face and hand weakness.[45, 46]

MECHANISMS AND PATHOPHYSIOLOGY

Such a wide diversity of conditions is associated with postoperative confusion that a common pathophysiology is unlikely.

TABLE 167–3. Drugs Commonly Used Postoperatively That May Be Associated with a Confusional State

Anticholinergic agents	Methyldopa
Anticonvulsants	Metoclopramide
Antihistamines	Metronidazole
Benzodiazepines	Narcotic agents
Captopril	Nitroprusside sodium
Cephalosporins	Nonsteroidal anti-inflammatory agents
Cimetidine	Penicillin†
Ciprofloxacin	Procainamide
Clonidine	Propranolol
Corticosteroids*	Quinidine sulfate
Digitalis	Ranitidine
Imipenem-cilastin†	Theophylline†
Ketoconazole	Trimethoprim-sulfamethoxazole
Lidocaine†	

*Prone to cause psychotic or manic features.
†Prone to cause seizures.

Cerebral metabolism is reduced in all metabolic disorders that produce decreased consciousness. A subsequent reduction in synthesis of neurotransmitters and especially of acetylcholine has been theorized.[48] Interference with cholinergic transmission also occurs as a result of exposure to toxins and drugs that produce confusional states, such as antihistamines, antidepressants, neuroleptics, and antiparkinsonian drugs. Raised serum levels of anticholinergic drugs were found in most of the 34% of patients in one study in whom postcardiotomy delirium developed, whereas those who remained cognitively normal had low levels.[20] Drugs such as alcohol, barbiturates, phenytoin, and phenothiazines exert direct effects on neuronal membranes in the cerebrum and diencephalon,[6] where impairment of the reticular activation system may reduce arousal.

The mental status changes associated with infection may be due to bacterial products or to cytokines (messengers released from macrophages and lymphoctes during sepsis).[38, 49] Cytokines may directly affect brain function, increase procoagulant activity, cause capillary leakage with tissue edema, and alter the blood-brain barrier.[38] None of these disorders has been substantiated, however.

Focal brain lesions of the inferior posterior parietal, temporal, or inferior frontostriatal region of the right middle cerebral artery[45–47] or of the posterior hippocampus, parahippocampal, or occipitotemporal gyri of the left posterior cerebral artery territory[44] also cause ACS, as alluded to earlier. Strokes in these areas usually result from emboli, most often of a cardiac source.[46] It has been speculated that the attention deficit resulting from these strokes is caused by the disconnection of limbic structures from cortical input.[44–46]

TREATMENT

Therapy of postoperative confusion is generally aimed at reversible medical disorders, but symptomatic treatment may also be needed to protect the agitated patient from injury. Fluid and electrolyte balance, blood volume, perfusion pressure, oxygenation, and infection all require close attention postoperatively. "Polypharmacy" should be avoided, and all nonessential drugs, especially those with psychoactive properties, should be withdrawn. Around-the-clock acetaminophen or nonsteroidal anti-inflammatory drug therapy may significantly reduce narcotic requirements. Sedative-hypnotic drugs should generally be avoided unless alcohol or benzodiazepine withdrawal is being treated.

Agitation is best controlled by nonpharmacologic means whenever possible, with the following measures:

- Encourage the presence of a family member
- Explain all procedures in detail
- Arrange nursing procedures to maximize uninterrupted sleep
- Keep the patient's room dimly lit at night and well lit in the daytime
- Replace the patient's eyeglasses or hearing aid to avoid loss of sensory cues.

Haloperidol and olanzapine are useful for rapid control of agitation when nonpharmacologic measures fail. Because these two antipsychotic medications have minimal effects on respiration and blood pressure, they are ideal for severely ill patients with cardiovascular or respiratory diseases.

The initial intravenous dose of haloperidol varies with the degree of delirium: 0.5 to 2 mg for mild agitation; 2 to 5 mg for moderate agitation; and 10 to 20 mg, given slowly, for severe agitation.[43] If given intravenously, heparin infusions should be stopped because heparin sodium forms a precipitate when it is combined with haloperidol lactate; intravenous lines or heparin locks should be flushed with 0.9% saline before and after haloperidol infusion. Because the onset of action is delayed 10 to 30 minutes, repeated doses should be given at intervals of no less than 20 to 30 minutes. The dose may be repeated if the desired effect is not achieved 30 to 60 minutes after the initial dose. If the agitated delirium is still uncontrolled 30 minutes after the second dose, the initial dose should be doubled and can be given every 30 minutes until the patient is calm. Alternatively, if the patient is severly agitated, each successive dose may be doubled and given every 30 minutes until the patient is calm.[43]

Haloperidol administered intravenously rarely causes extrapyramidal symptoms, such as occur after its oral administration.[43] Dystonic reactions, usually involving face and neck respond to anticholinergic therapy (e.g., diphenydramine or benztropine).

The newer drug olanzapine offers some advantage, in that its selective dopamine blockade avoids some of the extrapyramidal side effects of haloperidol and phenothiazines. We have found it particularly useful for "sundowning," but its use in the postoperative state has not been extensively studied. Also, in its usual oral dose of 5 to 10 mg it is not rapidly acting and more suited to subacute and chronic confusional states.

Neuroleptics (phenothiazines, haloperidol) are not the ideal treatment for anticholinergic delirium, hepatic encephalopathy, or alcohol or benzodiazepine withdrawal. They are also contraindicated in coma. Anticholinergic drugs should be discontinued and supportive care provided in patients with anticholinergic delirium; parenteral physostigmine may be useful in life-threatening cases but can cause side effects, such as cardiac arrhythmias and respiratory depression. In hepatic encephalopathy, a short-acting benzodiazepine that requires little liver degradation (e.g., oxazepam) is recommended. Benzodiazepines are still the drugs of choice in the treatment of alcohol or benzodiazepine withdrawal.

PROGNOSIS

Several factors are often simultaneously responsible for postoperative confusion, but because they are reversible with time, the patient is usually left without residual damage. Cognitive shortcomings not previously noted by the family, however, may suddenly become apparent. In elderly patients, usually a considerable delay (days to months) occurs between the resolution of the underlying metabolic derangement or drug effect and the recovery of mental function. Furthermore, elderly patients[5] and patients with anoxic brain damage may not regain a normal mental state or return to their original level of functioning.

References

1. Lipowski ZJ: Delirium in the elderly patient. N Engl J Med 1989; 320:57.
2. Gustafson Y, Berggren D, Brannstrom B, et al: Acute confusional states in elderly patients treated for femoral neck fracture. J Am Geriatr Soc 1988; 36:525.
3. Francis J, Martin D, Kapoor WN: A prospective study of delirium in hospitalized elderly. JAMA 1990; 263:1097.
4. Chedru C, Geschwind N: Disorders of higher cortical functions in acute confusional states. Cortex 1972; 8:395.
5. Mesulam MM: Disordered mental states in the postoperative period. Urol Clin North Am 1976; 3:199.
6. Adams RD, Victor M, Ropper AH: Principles of Neurology. 6th ed. New York, McGraw-Hill, 1997.
7. Heilman KM, Valenstein E, Watson RT: Behavioral aspects of neurological disease: Attentional, intentional, and emotional disorders. *In:* Clinical Neurology. Joynt RJ (Ed). Philadelphia, JB Lippincott, 1990, pp 1–35.

7a. Young GB, Ropper AH, Bolton CF (Eds). Coma and Impaired Consciousness. New York, McGraw-Hill, 1998.
8. Coffey CE, Massey EW, Roberts KB, et al: Natural history of cerebral complications of coronary artery bypass graft surgery. Neurology 1983; 33:1416.
9. Shaw PJ, Bates D, Cartlidge NEF, et al: Early intellectual dysfunction following coronary bypass surgery. Q J Med 1986; 58:59.
10. Rogers MP, Liang MH, Daltroy LH, et al: Delirium after elective orthopedic surgery: Risk factors and natural history. Int J Psychiatry Med 1989; 19:109.
11. Craven JL: Postoperative organic mental syndromes in lung transplant recipients. J Heart Lung Transplant 1990; 9:129.
12. Townes BD, Bashein G, Hornbein TF, et al: Neurobehavioral outcomes in cardiac operations. J Thorac Cardiovasc Surg 1989; 98:774.
13. Savagneau JA, Stanton BA, Jenkins CD, et al: Neuropsychological dysfunction following elective cardiac operation. J Thorac Cardiovasc Surg 1982; 84:585.
14. Breuer AC, Furlan AJ, Hanson MR, et al: Central nervous system complications of coronary artery bypass graft surgery: Prospective analysis of 41 patients. Stroke 1983; 14:682.
15. Kornfeld DS, Heller SS, Frank KA, et al: Delirium after coronary artery bypass surgery. J Thorac Cardiovasc Surg 1978; 76:93.
16. Slogoff S, Girgis KZ, Keats AS: Etiologic factors in neuropsychiatric complications associated with cardiopulmonary bypass. Anesth Analg 1982; 61:903.
17. Tune LE, Damlouji N, Holland A, et al: Association of postoperative delirium with raised serum levels of anticholinergic drugs. Lancet 1981; ii:651.
18. Sotaniemi KA, Juolasmaa A, Hokkanen ET: Neuropsychological outcome after open-heart surgery. Arch Neurol 1981; 38:2.
19. Coupal P, Morin P, Paiement B: Delirium after surgery with extracorporeal circulation. Can J Anaesth 1981; 28:350.
20. Shaw PJ, Bates D, Cartlidge NEF, et al: An analysis of factors predisposing to neurological injury in patients undergoing coronary bypass operations. Q J Med 1989; 72:633.
21. Roach GW, Kanchuger M, Mangano CM, et al: Adverse cerebral outcomes after coronary bypass surgery. N Engl J Med 1996; 335:1857.
22. Marcantonio ER, Goldman L, Mangione CM, et al: A clinical prediction rule for delirium after elective noncardiac surgery. JAMA 1994; 271:134.
23. Schor JD, Levokoff SE, Lipsitz LA, et al: Risk factors for delirium in hospitalized elderly. JAMA 1992; 267:827.
24. Inouye SK, Viscoli CM, Horwitz RI, et al: A predictive model for delirium in hospitalized elderly medical patients based on admission characteristics. Ann Intern Med 1993; 119:474.
25. Ray WA, Griffin MR, Schaffner W, et al: Psychotropic drug use and the risk of hip fracture. N Engl J Med 1987; 316:363.
26. Tinetti ME, Speechley M, Ginter SF: Risk factors for falls among elderly persons living in the community. N Engl J Med 1988; 319:1701.
27. Golinger RC, Peet T, Tune LE: Association of elevated plasma anticholinergic activity with delirium in surgical patients. Am J Psychiatry 1987; 144:1218.
28. Greenblatt DJ, Shader RI: Anticholinergics. N Engl J Med 1973; 288:1215.
29. Berggren D, Gustafson Y, Eriksson B, et al: Postoperative confusion after anesthesia in elderly patients with femoral neck fractures. Anesth Analg 1987; 66:497.
30. Marcantonio ER, Juarez G, Goldman L, et al: The relationship of postoperative delirium with psychoactive medications. JAMA 1994; 272:1518.
31. Eisendrath SJ, Goldman B, Douglas J, et al: Meperidine-induced delirium. Am J Psychiatry 1987; 144:1062.
32. Chung F, Lavelle PA, McDonald S, et al: Cognitive impairment after neuroleptanalgesia in cataract surgery. Anesth Analg 1989; 68:614.
33. Gold JP, Charlson ME, Williams-Russo P, et al: Improvement of outcomes after coronary artery bypass. J Thorac Cardiovasc Surg 1995; 110:1302.
34. Hotson JR, Pedley TA: The neurological complications of cardiac transplantation. Brain 1976; 99:673.
35. McKhann GM, Borowicz LM, Goldsborough MA, et al: Depression and cognitive decline after coronary artery bypass. Lancet 1997; 349:1282.
36. Redmond JM, Greene PS, Goldsborough MA, et al: Neurologic injury in cardiac surgical patients with a history of stroke. Ann Thorac Surg 1996; 61:42.
37. Mesulam MM: Principles of Behavioral Neurology. Philadelphia, FA Davis, 1988.
38. Young CB, Bolton CF: The neurology of sepsis. Neurol Chron 1992; 2:1.
39. Plum F, Posner JB: The diagnosis of stupor and coma. Philadelphia, FA Davis, 1982.
40. Young GB, Bolton CF, Austin TW, et al: The encephalopathy associated with septic illness. Clin Invest Med 1990; 13:297.
41. Adler LE, Sudju L, Wilets G: Cimetidine toxicity manifested as paranoia and hallucinations. Am J Psychiatry 1980; 137:1112.
42. Schentag JJ, Cerra FB, Calleri G: Pharmacokinetic and clinical studies in patients with cimetidine-induced mental confusion. Lancet 1979; i:177.
43. Fish DN: Treatment of delirium in the critically ill patient. Clin Pharmacokinet 1991; 10:456.
44. Devinsky O, Bear D, Volpe BT: Confusional states following posterior cerebral artery infarction. Arch Neurol 1988; 45:160.
45. Mesulam MM, Waxman SG, Geschwind N, et al: Acute confusional states with right middle cerebral artery infarctions. J Neurol Neurosurg Psychiatry 1976; 39:84.
46. Caplan LR, Kelley M, Kase CS, et al: Infarcts of the inferior division of the right middle cerebral artery: Mirror image of Wernicke's aphasia. Neurology 1986; 36:1015.
47. Mori E, Yamadori A: Acute confusional state and acute agitated delirium. Arch Neurol 1987; 44:1139.
48. Engel GL, Romano J: Delirium, a syndrome of cerebral insufficiency. J Chronic Dis 1959; 9:260.
49. Dinarello CA: Interleukin-1 and the pathogenesis of the acute-phase response. N Engl J Med 1984; 311:1413.

168

Evaluation of Coma

Joerg-Patrick Stübgen, MD, FRCPC • Fred Plum, MD

Altered states of consciousness are a common reason for visits to the emergency room and admission to intensive care units. Few problems are more difficult to manage than the unconscious patient, because the potential causes of an altered mental status are considerable and the time for diagnosis and effective intervention is short. *Consciousness* may be defined as the state of awareness of the self and the environment. The phenomenon of consciousness depends on two intact and interdependent physiologic and anatomic components: (1) arousal (or wakefulness) and its underlying neural substrate, the *ascending reticular activating system* (ARAS) and diencephalon, and (2) awareness, which requires the functioning cerebral cortex of both hemispheres. Most disorders that acutely disturb consciousness are, in fact, impairments of arousal that create circumstances under which the brain's capacity for consciousness cannot be accurately assessed; in other words, failure of arousal makes it impossible to test awareness.

Alterations of arousal may be transient, lasting only several seconds or minutes (following seizures, syncope, and cardiac dysrhythmia), or sustained, lasting several hours or longer. Four terms are used to describe disturbed arousal of a patient.

Alert refers to a normal state of arousal.

Stupor describes a state of spontaneous unarousability in which strong external stimuli can transiently restore wakefulness. Stupor implies evidence that at least a limited degree of appropriate cognitive activity accompanies the arousal, even if transient.

Coma is characterized by an uninterruptable loss of the capacity for arousal. The eyes are closed, sleep-wake cycles disappear, and even vigorous stimulation produces no evidence of appropriate psychologic reaction. At best, only reflex responses can be elicited.

Lethargy describes a range of behavior between arousal and stupor.

Only the terms *alert* and *coma* have enough precision to be used without further qualification; possibly, coma has gradations in depth, but this cannot be accurately assessed once the patient is no longer responsive to external stimuli. Stupor and coma reflect an acute or subacute brain insult. The cerebral reserve capacity is large; therefore, altered consciousness reflects diffuse and bilateral cerebral dysfunction, failure of the brain stem–thalamic ARAS, or both. All alterations in arousal should be regarded as acute and potentially life-threatening emergencies.

The evaluation of a comatose patient demands a systematic approach with appropriate, directed diagnostic and therapeutic endeavors; time should not be wasted on irrelevant considerations. Urgent steps are required to prevent or minimize permanent brain damage from reversible causes. Patient evaluation and treatment must necessarily occur simultaneously. Such a systematic approach demands an understanding of the pathophysiology of consciousness and the ways in which it may be deranged.

ANATOMY, PATHOLOGY, AND PATHOPHYSIOLOGY

Consciousness depends on an intact ARAS in the brain stem and adjacent thalamus, which acts as the alerting or awakening element of consciousness, together with a functioning cerebral cortex of both hemispheres, which determines the content of that consciousness.[1] The ARAS lies within a more or less isodendritic core that extends from the medulla through the tegmentum of the pons to the midbrain and primitive, paramedian thalamus. The system is continuous caudally with the reticular intermediate gray matter of the spinal cord and rostrally with the subthalamus, the hypothalamus, the anterior thalamus, and the basal forebrain.[2]

The ARAS itself arises within the rostral pontine tegmentum and extends across the mesencephalic tegmentum and its adjacent intrathalamic nuclei. ARAS functions and interconnections are considerable and likely contribute more than only a cortical arousal system. The specific role of the various links from the reticular formation to the thalamus has yet to be fully identified.[3] Furthermore, the cortex feeds back on the thalamic nuclei to contribute an important self-cycling loop that amplifies arousal mechanisms.[4, 5]

The ascending arousal system contains cholinergic, monoaminergic, and gamma-aminobutyric acid (GABA) systems, none of which has been identified as the singular arousal neurotransmitter.[6, 7] It follows that acute structural damage to or metabolic-chemical derangements of either the ascending brain stem–thalamic activating system or the thalamocortico-thalamic loop are capable of altering the aroused, attentive state. Consciousness depends on the continuous interaction between the mechanisms that provide arousal and awareness. The brain stem and thalamus provide the activating mechanism, and the cerebrum provides full cognition and self-excitation. Content of consciousness can best be regarded as the amalgam and integration of all cognitive function that resides in the thalamocortical circuits of both hemispheres. Altered awareness arises from disruption of this cortical activity by diffuse pathology. Focal lesions of the cerebrum can produce profound deficits, such as aphasia, alexia, amnesia, and hemianopsia, but only diffuse bilateral damage, sparing the ARAS and diencephalon, can lead to wakeful unawareness. Thus, there are two kinds of altered consciousness:

- Altered arousal due to dysfunction of the ARAS-diencephalon
- Altered awareness due to bilateral diffuse cerebral hemisphere dysfunction

Four major pathologic groupings can cause such severe, global, acute reductions of consciousness[1, 8]:

1. In the presence of diffuse or extensive multifocal bilateral dysfunction of the cerebral cortex, the cortical gray matter is diffusely and acutely depressed or destroyed. Concurrently, cortical-subcortical physiologic feedback excitatory loops are impaired, with the result that brain stem autonomic mechanisms become temporarily, profoundly inhibited, producing the equivalent of acute "reticular shock" below the level of the lesion.
2. Direct damage to a paramedian upper brain stem and posterior-inferior diencephalic ascending arousal system blocks normal cortical activation. Anatomically, the affected structures lie predominantly in the paramedian gray matter, extending roughly from the level of the nucleus parabrachialis of the pontine tegmentum forward as far as the ventral posterior hypothalamus and the adjacent pretectal area.
3. Widespread disconnection between the cortex and subcortical activating mechanisms acts pathophysiologically to produce effects similar to both preceding conditions.
4. Diffuse disorders, usually metabolic in origin, concurrently affect both the cortical and subcortical arousal mechanisms, although to a different extent according to the cause.

Structural Lesions Causing Coma

Intracranial mass lesions that produce coma may be located in the supratentorial or infratentorial compartments. From either location, impaired arousal or coma can be produced by compression of the brain stem–hypothalamic activating mechanisms secondary to swelling and displacement of deep-lying intracranial contents; the ultimate event may occur either from halting of axoplasmic flow or from production of sustained neuronal depolarization because of ischemia or hemorrhage.

Factors that contribute to the degree of loss of arousal include the rate of development, the location, and the ultimate size of the lesion. Cerebral mass lesions distort the intracranial anatomy, thereby altering the cerebrospinal fluid circulation and brain blood supply. These changes result in a larger bulk of injured tissue and a reduction in intracranial compliance. Intercompartmental pressure gradients result in herniation syndromes that are not necessarily associated with large increases in intracranial pressure (ICP). Recently sustained or evolving mass lesions may disturb cerebral vascular autoregulation, resulting in abrupt, brief vasodilation; this, in turn, causes recurrent increases in ICP (pressure waves), thereby further compromising cerebral blood supply to injured regions.

Supratentorial Lesions

Two herniation syndromes demonstrate the mechanism by which supratentorial lesions produce coma, central herniation and uncal herniation. The rate of evolution of a mass dictates whether the anatomic distortion precedes (in slowly evolving lesions) or parallels the deterioration in the patient's wakefulness. Downward transtentorial herniation can be central or predominantly unilateral.

Central herniation results from (1) caudally displaced deep midline supratentorial masses, (2) large space-occupying hemisphere lesions, or (3) large unilateral or bilateral compressive extra-axial lesions and leads to compression of the ARAS. The progressive rostral-caudal pathologic and clinical stages of the herniation syndromes are outlined by Plum and Posner.[1]

Pathologically, bilateral symmetric displacement of the supratentorial contents occurs through the tentorial notch into the posterior fossa. Alertness is impaired early, pupils become small (to 3 mm) and reactive, and bilateral upper motor neuron signs develop. Cheyne-Stokes breathing, grasp reflexes, roving eye movements, and depressed escape of oculocephalic reflexes are the clinical manifestations.

In the absence of effective therapy at this diencephalic stage, herniation progresses caudally to compress the midbrain, leading to a deep coma and fixed, midposition (3 to 5 mm) pupils, signifying both sympathetic and parasympathetic interruption. Spontaneous eye movements cease, and oculovestibular and oculocephalic reflexes become difficult to elicit. Spontaneous extensor posturing may occur. Once this stage is reached, full recovery becomes unlikely. As the caudal compression-ischemia process advances, pontine and medullary function are destroyed, resulting in bizarre breathing patterns and the absence of reflex eye movements. *Finally, autonomic cardiovascular and respiratory functions cease as medullary centers fail.*

Uncus herniation results from laterally placed hemisphere lesions, particularly of the temporal lobes, that cause side-to-side cerebral displacement as well as transtentorial herniation. Focal hemisphere dysfunction (hemiparesis, aphasia, seizures) precedes unilateral (usually ipsilateral) compression paralysis of the third cranial nerve. An early sign of uncus herniation is an ipsilateral or, less often, contralateral enlarged pupil that responds sluggishly to light, followed by a fixed, dilated pupil and an oculomotor palsy characterized by an eye turned downward and outward.[1] The ipsilateral posterior cerebral artery may become compressed as it crosses the tentorium, resulting in ipsilateral occipital lobe ischemia. If the herniation progresses, the temporal lobe compresses the midbrain, with loss of consciousness and bilateral or contralateral extensor posturing. Ipsilateral to the intracranial lesion, a hemiparesis may develop if the opposite cerebral peduncle becomes compressed against the contralateral tentorial edge (Kernohan's notch). Abnormal brain stem signs become symmetric, and herniation proceeds in the same pattern seen with central herniation, as rostrocaudal brain stem displacement progresses.

Infratentorial Lesions

Infratentorial lesions cause coma by displacement, compression, or direct destruction of the pontomesencephalic tegmental activating system. Displacement of the medulla downward sufficient to push the brain stem and cerebellar tonsils into the foramen magnum *causes cardiorespiratory collapse.* Acute intrinsic lesions of the brain stem, usually hemorrhagic or ischemic, cause abrupt onset of coma and are associated with abnormal neuro-ophthalmologic findings. Pupils may be either pinpoint, as a result of disruption of pontine sympathetic pathways, or dilated, as a result of destruction of the third cranial nerve nuclei or intra-axial exiting fibers. Dysconjugate eye movements and nystagmus occur, and vertical eye movements are relatively spared. Ocular bobbing signifies pontine damage. Upper motor neuron signs develop and patients may become quadriplegic; flaccidity in the upper extremities and flexor withdrawal responses in the lower extremities often accompany midbrain-pontine damage.

Pathologically, *basilar artery occlusion* leads to asymmetric ischemia of the brain stem, with involvement of the ARAS and the neighboring densely packed neuropil as well as the descending and ascending motor and sensory tracts. Thrombosis of the rostral basilar artery leads to infarction of the midline thalamic nuclei and brief coma without other obvious brain stem signs. Hemorrhage into the ventral pons sometimes spares consciousness but produces neuro-ophthalmologic signs and motor dysfunction. Extension of the hemorrhage into the rostral pontine tegmentum results in stupor, coma, or death.

Basilar artery migraine may produce altered consciousness by interfering with arterial blood flow in basilar artery tributaries. Rapidly developing, extensive central pontine myelinolysis may cause coma by extension into the pontine tegmentum. Other intrinsic brain stem lesions (e.g., tumor, abscess, granuloma, demyelination) tend to progress slowly and usually spare arousal mechanisms; however, they may reduce attention and other cognitive functions, leading to severe psychomotor retardation.

Extra-axial posterior fossa lesions cause coma by direct compression of the ARAS in the brain stem and in the diencephalon by upward transtentorial herniation. Compression of the pons may be difficult to distinguish from intrinsic lesions but is often accompanied by headache, vomiting, and hypertension due to a Cushing reflex. Upward herniation at the midbrain level is initially characterized by coma, reactive miotic pupils, asymmetry or absence of caloric eye responses, and decerebrate posturing; caudal-rostral brain stem dysfunction then occurs, with midbrain failure and midposition, fixed pupils.[9] Causes of brain stem compression include cerebellar hemorrhage, infarction and abscess, primary rostral brain stem hemorrhages, rapidly expanding cerebellar or fourth ventricular tumors, and less commonly, infratentorial epidural or subdural hematomas. Drainage of the lateral ventricles aimed at relieving obstructive hydrocephalus associated with posterior fossa masses may potentially precipitate acute upward transtentorial herniation.[10, 11]

As mentioned previously, downward herniation of the cerebellar tonsils through the foramen magnum causes acute medullary dysfunction and *abrupt respiratory and circulatory collapse.* Less severe impaction of the tonsils in the foramen magnum may lead to obstructive hydrocephalus and consequent bihemispheric dysfunction with an altered arousal. Accompanying manifestations are headache, nausea, vomiting, lower cranial nerve signs, vertical nystagmus, ataxia, and irregular breathing. Lumbar puncture in this setting carries a risk of catastrophic consequences.[10]

Nonstructural Disorders Causing Coma

Nonstructural disorders, such as metabolic and toxic disturbances, produce coma by diffusely depressing the function of the brain stem and cerebral arousal mechanisms. The onset of coma can be abrupt, as with toxic drug ingestion, surgical-level anesthesia, or cardiac arrest, or it may evolve slowly after a period of confusion and inattention.

The chief manifestations of metabolic encephalopathy are disturbances in arousal and cognitive function. Other findings are abnormalities of the sleep-wake cycle, autonomic disturbances, and abnormal respiratory variations depending on the cause of the encephalopathy. The most helpful distinguishing clinical feature of a diffuse encephalopathy is the preservation of the pupillary light response, the only exceptions being an overdose of anticholinergic agents, near-fatal anoxia, and self-initiated malingering. Except for the last, lack of pupillary reactivity requires a search for an underlying structural lesion. The neurologic examination shows a decreased level of arousal and a widespread cognitive decline. Deeply comatose patients without brain stem or hemisphere function and no known cause for coma must be assumed to have suffered accidental or intentional self-poisoning. Metabolic disturbances of arousal and thinking particularly affect elderly patients who suffer serious systemic illnesses or who have undergone complicated surgery.

Metabolic encephalopathy is clinically characterized by multilevel central nervous system dysfunction. At onset, abnormalities in cognition are at least as severe as the disturbance of arousal. Misperception, disorientation, multimodality hallucinations, concentration and memory deficits, and, occasionally, hypervigilance may progress to profound stupor and coma. The patient's level of arousal and consciousness often fluctuates between examinations. Motor abnormalities, if present, usually are symmetric and bilateral. Patients often experience tremor, asterixis, and multifocal myoclonus. Spontaneous motor activity ranges from hypoactivity (in cases of sedating drug or endogenous metabolic disturbances) to hyperactivity (after drug withdrawal or overdose of stimulating agents, such as cocaine and phencyclidine). Seizures occasionally occur, particularly after alcohol or drug withdrawal, and particularly in patients with established cortical pathology. Focal seizures may occur even without structural disease in patients with hypoglycemia, hepatic encephalopathy, uremia, abnormal calcium levels, or toxin ingestion. Autonomic disregulation, including hypothermia, occurs with hypoglycemia, myxedema, and sedative drug overdose. Hyperthermia occurs in withdrawal states, particularly delirium tremens, anticholinergic drug overdose, infection, neuroleptic malignant syndrome, and malignant hyperthermia.

COMA-LIKE BEHAVIORAL STATES

Several different behavioral states appear similar to, and can be confused with, coma. Differentiation of such states from true coma has important diagnostic, therapeutic, and prognostic implications. Moreover, coma is not a permanent state; patients who survive initial coma may evolve through and into these altered behavioral states. All patients who survive beyond the stage of acute, systemic complications reawaken and either proceed to recovery (with no or varying degrees of disability) or survive in a vegetative state.

Vegetative State

The *vegetative state* can be defined as wakefulness without awareness and is the consequence of various diffuse brain insults.[1, 12] It may be a transient phase through which patients in coma pass as the cerebral cortex recovers more slowly than the brain stem. Clinically, patients in a vegetative state appear to be awake and to have cyclic sleep patterns; however, they do not show evidence of cognitive function or learned behavioral responses to external stimuli. Such patients may demonstrate spontaneous eye opening and eye movements and stereotypical facial and limb movements; however, they are unable to demonstrate speech or comprehension, and they lack purposeful activity. Patients in the vegetative state generate normal body temperature; usually have normally functioning cardiovascular, respiratory, and digestive systems; but are doubly incontinent.

The vegetative state should be termed "persistent" at 1 month after injury and "permanent" at 3 months after nontraumatic injury or 12 months after a traumatic injury.[13, 14] Extended observation of the patient is required to assess behavioral responses to external stimulation and to demonstrate cognitive unawareness. The electroencephalogram (EEG) is never isoelectric but shows various patterns of rhythm and amplitude, inconsistent from one patient to the next. Normal EEG sleep-wake patterns are absent.

Locked-In Syndrome

In the *locked-in syndrome,* patients retain or regain arousability and self-awareness but, because of extensive bilateral paralysis (in other words, deefferentation), can no longer communicate except in severely limited ways. Such patients suffer bilateral ventral pontine lesions with quadriplegia, horizontal gaze palsies, and lower cranial nerve palsies; voluntarily, they are capable only of vertical eye movements or blinking.[1] Sleep may be abnormal, with marked reduction in non–rapid eye movement (REM) and REM sleep phases.

The most common etiology of the locked-in syndrome is pontine infarction due to basilar artery thrombosis, but pontine hemorrhage, central pontine myelinolysis, and brain stem mass lesions also occur. Neuromuscular causes include severe, acute inflammatory demyelinating polyradiculoneuropathies; myasthenia gravis; botulism; and neuromuscular blocking agents. In these peripheral disorders, upward gaze is not selectively spared.

Akinetic Mutism

Akinetic mutism describes a rare subacute or chronic state of altered behavior in which an alert-appearing patient is both silent and immobile but not paralyzed.[15] External evidence of mental activity is unobtainable. The patient usually lies with the eyes open and retains cycles of self-sustained arousal, giving the appearance of vigilance. Skeletal muscle tone can be normal or hypertonic but is usually not spastic. Movements are rudimentary even in response to unpleasant stimuli. Affected patients are usually doubly incontinent.

Lesions that result in akinetic mutism may vary widely. One pattern consists of bilateral damage to frontal lobe or limbic-cortical integration with relative sparing of motor pathways. Vulnerable areas involve both basal medial frontal areas. Somewhat similar behavior also can follow incomplete lesions of the deep gray matter (paramedian reticular formation of the posterior diencephalon and adjacent midbrain), but patients with such lesions usually suffer double hemiplegia and act slowly yet are not completely akinetic or noncommunicative.

Catatonia

Catatonia is a symptom complex associated most often with psychiatric disease. This behavioral disturbance is characterized by stupor or excitement and variable mutism, posturing, rigidity, grimacing, and catalepsy. Catatonia can be caused by a variety of illnesses, both psychiatric (affective more than psychotic) disorders and structural or metabolic diseases (toxic and drug-induced psychosis, encephalitis, and alcoholic degeneration). Psychiatric catatonia may be difficult to distinguish from organic disease because affected patients often appear lethargic or stuporous rather than totally unresponsive. Such patients also may have a variety of endocrine or autonomic abnormalities.

Patients in catatonic stupor do not move spontaneously, and they appear unresponsive to the environment despite what seems to be a normal level of arousal and consciousness. This impression is supported by a normal neurologic examination and a subsequent recall of most events that took place during the unresponsive period. Patients in catatonic stupor usually lie with the eyes open and may not blink in response to visual threat, but the physician can usually elicit optokinetic responses. The pupils are semidilated and reactive to light, oculocephalic reflexes are absent, and vestibulo-ocular testing evokes normal nystagmus. Patients may hypersalivate and may be doubly incontinent. Passive movement of the limbs meets with waxy flexibility, and catalepsy is seen in 30% of patients. Choreiform jerks of the extremities and facial grimaces are common. The EEG, in both catatonic excitement and stupor, most often shows a reactive, low-voltage, fast normal record rather than the slow record seen in a comatose patient.

APPROACH TO COMA

The initial approach to stupor and coma is based on the principle that all alterations in arousal are acute, life-threatening emergencies. The patient must be evaluated and treated simultaneously, because urgent steps are required to prevent or minimize permanent brain damage from reversible causes. Serial examinations are needed, with accurate documentation to determine any change in the patient's state. Appropriate management decisions (therapeutic and diagnostic) must be made rapidly.

The clinical approach to an unconscious patient logically entails the following steps:

1. Emergency treatment.
2. History (from relatives, friends, and emergency medical personnel).
3. General physical examination.
4. Neurologic profile, the key to categorizing the nature of coma.
5. Specific management.
6. Prediction of outcome.

Emergency Management

The initial assessment of a patient in coma or deep stupor must focus on the vital signs to determine the appropriate resuscitation measures; the diagnostic process begins later. Urgent, and sometimes empirical, therapy must be given to avoid additional brain insult.

Oxygenation

Oxygenation must be assured by the establishment of an airway and ventilation of the lungs. The threshold for intubation should be low in the comatose patient, even if respiratory function is sufficient for proper ventilation and oxygenation: The level of consciousness may deteriorate and breathing may decompensate suddenly and unexpectedly. An open airway must be ensured and must be protected from aspiration of vomitus and blood. During preparation for intubation, maximal oxygenation can be ensured by suction of the upper airway, gentle extension of the neck, elevation of the jaw, and manual ventilation with oxygen using a mask and bag. Maximal oxygenation ("bagging") and 1 mg atropine help to prevent cardiac dysrhythmias. If severe neck injury is a possibility or has not been excluded, intubation should be performed by the most skilled practitioner present without extension of the patient's neck. A brief neurologic examination is mandatory prior to the administration of sedation required for intubation.

The key points of the "rapid neurologic exam" are as follows[16]:

- Hand drop from over the head (to assess for malingering or hysterical loss of consciousness)
- Pupillary size and response to light
- Abnormal eye movements (active dysconjugate, unilaterally paralytic, passively induced, or none at all)
- Grimacing, withdrawal from noxious stimulation
- Abnormal plantar response (unilateral or bilateral Babinski's sign)

Mask-and-bag assisted ventilation should be continued during the neurologic examination if necessary. Neuromuscular blockade required for patient management and care should be deferred until the neurologic examination is completed (3 to 5 minutes). Signs of arousal or inadequate sedation are dilated, reactive pupils, copious tears, diaphoresis, tachycardia, systemic hypertension, and elevated pulmonary artery pressure. For neurologic monitoring, head computed tomography (CT) may need to be performed more than once.

Respiration

Respiratory excursions should be evaluated; arterial blood gas measurement is the only certain method to determine adequate ventilation and oxygenation. Pulse oximetry is useful, however, because it provides immediate, continuous information regarding arterial oxygen saturation. The comatose patient ideally should maintain a $Pa{O_2}$ greater than 100 mm Hg and a $Pa{CO_2}$ between 34 and 37 mm Hg. The patient should *not* be hyperventilated to a $Pa{CO_2}$ of less than 35 mm Hg, because this process constricts brain arteries. Positive end-expiratory pressure should be avoided if increased ICP is suspected. A nasogastric tube should be placed to facilitate gastric lavage and prevent regurgitation.

Circulation

Circulation should be maintained to ensure adequate cerebral perfusion. Appropriate resuscitation fluid is lactated Ringer's solution; normal saline is also used when high ICP is suspected. A mean arterial pressure of about 100 mm Hg is adequate and safe for most patients. While venous access is being obtained, blood samples should be collected for anticipated tests (Table 168–1). Hypotension should be treated by replacement of any blood volume loss and use of vasoactive agents (preferably dopamine). Elevated blood pressure should be judiciously managed with hypotensive agents that do not substantially raise ICP through their vasodilating effect. (Labetalol, hydralazine, and titrated nitroprusside infusion are the favored agents for managing uncontrollable hypertension.) For most situations, systolic blood pressure should be maintained at 150 to 160 mm Hg and diastolic blood pressure at 90 to 100 mm Hg. Urine output should be at least 0.5 mL/kg per hour; accurate measurement requires bladder catheterization.

Glucose and Thiamine

Hypoglycemia is a common cause of altered consciousness; glucose (25 g as a 50% solution) should be given intravenously immediately after blood specimens have been collected for baseline evaluation. Empirical glucose treatment will prevent hypoglycemic brain damage and outweighs the theoretical risks of additional harm to the brain in hyperglycemic, hyperosmolar or anoxic coma. Thiamine (100 mg) must be given with the glucose infusion to prevent precipitation of Wernicke's encephalopathy in malnourished, thiamine-depleted patients. Rarely, an established thiamine deficiency can cause coma.

Seizures

Repeated generalized seizures damage the brain and must be stopped. Initial treatment should include intravenous benzodiazepines, such as lorazepam (2 to 4 mg) or diazepam (5 to 10 mg). Seizure control can be maintained with intravenous phenytoin (18 mg/kg at a rate of 25 mg/min). Seizure breakthrough requires additional benzodiazepines.

Sedation

Careful and mild sedation should be given to the agitated, hyperactive patient to prevent self-injury. A quiet patient facilitates ventilator support and diagnostic procedures. Small

TABLE 168–1. Emergency Laboratory Tests in Metabolic Coma

I. **Immediate Tests**
  A. Venous blood
    1. Glucose
    2. Electrolytes (sodium, potassium, chloride, carbon dioxide, phosphates)
    3. Urea and creatinine
    4. Osmolality
  B. Arterial blood (check color)
    1. pH
    2. Po_2
    3. Pco_2
    4. Bicarbonate
    5. Carboxyhemoglobin (if available)
  C. Cerebrospinal fluid
    1. Gram's stain
    2. Cell count
    3. Glucose
  D. Electrocardiogram

II. **Deferred Tests** (Initial Blood Sample, Processed Later)
  A. Venous blood
    1. Sedative and toxic drugs
    2. Liver function tests
    3. Coagulation studies
    4. Thyroid and adrenal function
    5. Blood cultures
    6. Viral titers
  B. Urine
    1. Sedative and toxic drugs
    2. Culture
  C. Cerebrospinal fluid
    1. Protein
    2. Culture
    3. Viral and fungal titers

doses of intravenous benzodiazepines, such as intramuscular haloperidol (1 mg as often as hourly until desired effect) or intravenous morphine (2 to 4 mg), are appropriate. In the ventilator-supported patient, the effects set in quickly, can be reversed, and are short-lasting.

Antidotes

Drug overdose is the largest single cause (30%) of coma in the emergency room. Most drug overdoses can be treated with supportive measures alone. Certain antagonists, however, specifically reverse the effects of coma-producing drugs.

Intravenous naloxone (0.4 to 2 mg) is the antidote for opiate coma. The reversal of narcotic effect, however, may precipitate acute withdrawal phenomena in an opiate addict. In suspected opiate coma, the minimum amount of naloxone should be administered to establish the diagnosis by pupillary dilation, and to reverse depressed breathing and coma. One should not attempt to reverse completely all drug effects with the first dose.

Intravenous flumazenil reverses all benzodiazepine-induced coma. It follows that coma unresponsive to 5 mg flumazenil in divided doses given over 5 minutes is not due to benzodiazepine overdose. Recurrent sedation can be prevented with 1 mg flumazenil every 20 minutes.[17]

The sedative effects of drugs with anticholinergic properties, particularly tricyclic antidepressants, can be reversed with 1 to 2 mg physostigmine given intravenously. Pretreatment with 0.5 mg atropine prevents bradycardia. Only full awakening is characteristic of an anticholinergic drug overdose, because physostigmine has nonspecific arousal properties. Physostigmine has a short duration of action (45 to 60 minutes), so its use may have to be repeated.

Body Temperature

Hyperthermia is dangerous because it increases brain metabolic demand and, at extreme levels, denatures brain proteins.[18] Elevated temperature greater than 40°C requires nonspecific cooling measures, even before the underlying etiology is determined and treated. Hyperthermia most often indicates infection but may be due to intracranial hemorrhage, anticholinergic drug intoxication, or heat exposure. A body temperature below 34°C should be slowly elevated to above 35°C to prevent cardiac dysrhythmia. Hypothermia accompanies profound sepsis, sedative-hypnotic drug overdose, near-drowning, hypoglycemia, and Wernicke's encephalopathy.

History

Once vital functions have been protected and the patient's condition is stable, clues to the cause of coma must be sought by interviewing relatives, friends, bystanders, or medical personnel who may have observed the patient before or during the decline in consciousness. The history should cover the following areas:

1. *Witnessed events*—head injury, seizure, details of a motor vehicle accident, circumstances under which the patient was found.
2. *Evolution of coma*—abrupt or gradual, headache, progressive or recurrent weakness, vertigo, nausea and vomiting.
3. *Recent medical history*—surgical procedures, infections, current medication.
4. *Past medical history*—epilepsy, head injury, drug or alcohol abuse, stroke, hypertension, diabetes, heart disease, cancer, uremia.
5. Previous psychiatric history—depression, suicide attempts, social stresses.
6. *Access to drugs*—sedatives, psychotropic drugs, narcotics, illicit drugs, drug paraphernalia, empty medicine bottles.

General Physical Examination

A systematic, detailed physical examination is helpful and necessary in the approach to the comatose patient, who is in no condition to describe prior or current medical problems. This examination is an extension of the initial evaluation and includes the following items:

1. Repeated assessment of vital signs to determine efficacy of resuscitation measures.
2. External evidence of trauma.
3. Evidence of acute or chronic medical illnesses.
4. Evidence of ingestion or self-administration of drugs (needle marks, alcohol on breath).
5. Evaluation of nuchal rigidity. Care is required if severe neck injury is possible or has not been excluded.

Neurologic Profile

The establishment of the nature of coma is critical for appropriate management. It requires the correct interpretation of neurologic signs that reflect the integrity or impairment of various functional levels of the brain. The neurologic profile helps determine whether the pattern and evolution of these signs are best explained by a supratentorial or infratentorial structural lesion, a metabolic-toxic encephalopathy, or a psychiatric cause (Tables 168–2 and 168–3).

The clinical neurologic functions that provide the most

TABLE 168–2. Neurologic Profile (A Modified Glasgow Coma Scale)

Verbal Responses	Spontaneous Eye Movement
Oriented speech	Orienting
Confused conversation	Roving conjugate
Inappropriate speech	Roving dysconjugate
Incomprehensible speech	Miscellaneous abnormal movements
No speech	None
Eye Opening	***Oculocephalic Responses***
Spontaneous	Normal (unpredictable)
Response to verbal stimuli	Full
Response to noxious stimuli	Minimal
None	None
Motor Responses	***Oculovestibular Responses***
Obeys	Normal (nystagmus)
Localizes	Tonic conjugate
Withdraws (flexion)	Minimal or dysconjugate
Abnormal flexion	None
Abnormal extension	***Deep Tendon Reflexes***
None	Normal
Pupillary Reactions	Increased
Present	Absent
Absent	

useful information in making a categorical diagnosis are outlined in Table 168-4. These indices are easily and quickly obtained. Furthermore, they have a high degree of interexaminer consistency, and when applied serially, they accurately reflect the patient's clinical course. Once the cause of coma can be assigned to one of these four categories—supratentorial mass lesion, subtentorial structural lesion, metabolic-toxic coma, psychogenic coma—specific radiographic, electrophysiologic, or chemical laboratory studies can be used to make a disease-specific diagnosis and to detect existing or potential complications.

Specific Management

Supratentorial Mass Lesions

If the cause of coma is a presumed supratentorial mass, the severity and rate of evolution of signs must be determined. A relatively stable patient next requires an emergency CT scan or magnetic resonance imaging (MRI) of the head. Carotid angiography is considerably less informative; a skull x-ray is a waste of time. The priority in deep coma or established or threatened transtentorial herniation is successfully to apply medical treatment of intracranial hypertension. Brief hyperventilation to a $Paco_2$ between 25 and 30 mm Hg is the most rapid method to lower elevated ICP; this is achieved by adjusting the ventilation rate to 10 to 16 per minute and the tidal volume to 12 to 14 mL/kg. Because the vasoconstrictive effect is transient, lasting less than an hour, an osmotic agent must be administered concurrently. Sustained hyperventilation to a $Paco_2$ of less than 30 to 35 mm Hg removes all future value of this procedure. Our view is that as mannitol is infused, the ventilator should be turned down to resume a higher steady-state $Paco_2$ of 34 to 37 mm Hg. The preferred osmotic agent is a 20% mannitol solution as an intravenous bolus of 1 g/kg. Maximum reduction in ICP occurs within 20 to 60 minutes, and the effect of a single bolus lasts about 6 hours.

TABLE 168–3. Correlation Between Levels of Brain Function and Clinical Signs

Structure	Function	Clinical Sign
Cerebral cortex	Conscious behavior	Speech (including any sounds) Purposeful movement Spontaneous To command To pain
Brain stem activating and sensory pathways (reticular activating system)	Sleep-wake cycle	Eye opening Spontaneous To command To pain
Brain stem motor pathways	Reflex limb movements	Flexor posturing (decorticate) Extensor posturing (decerebrate)
Midbrain cranial nerve (CN) III	Innervation of ciliary muscle and certain extraocular muscles	Pupillary reactivity
Pontomesencephalic medial longitudinal fasciculus	Connects pontine gaze center with CN III nucleus	Internuclear ophthalmoplegia
Upper pons		
CN V	Facial and corneal	Corneal reflex-sensory response
CN VII	Facial muscle innervation	Corneal reflex-motor response Blink Grimace
Lower pons		
CN VIII (vestibular portion) connects by brain stem pathways with CN III, IV, and VI	Reflex eye movements	Doll's eyes Caloric responses
Pontomedullary junction	Spontaneous breathing Maintained blood pressure	Breathing and blood pressure do not require mechanical or chemical support
Spinal cord	Primitive protective responses	Deep tendon reflexes Babinski reflex

TABLE 168–4. Characteristics of the Categories of Coma

I. ***Supratentorial Mass Lesion Affecting Diencephalon and Brain Stem***
- Initial focal cerebral dysfunction
- Dysfunction progresses rostral to caudal
- Signs reflect dysfunction at one level
- Signs often asymmetric

II. ***Subtentorial Structural Lesion***
- Symptoms of brain stem dysfunction or sudden-onset coma
- Brain stem signs precede or accompany coma
- Cranial nerve and oculovestibular dysfunction
- Early onset of abnormal respiratory patterns

III. ***Metabolic-Toxic Coma***
- Confusion or stupor precedes motor signs
- Motor signs usually symmetric
- Pupil responses generally preserved
- Myoclonus, asterixis, tremulousness, and generalized seizures common
- Acid-base imbalance common with compensatory ventilatory changes

IV. ***Psychogenic Coma***
- Eyelids squeezed shut
- Pupils reactive or dilated, unreactive (cycloplegics)
- Oculocephalic reflex unpredictable; nystagmus on caloric tests
- Motor tone normal or inconsistent
- No pathologic reflexes
- Awake-pattern electroencephalogram

Corticosteroids are not indicated in the emergent, empirical management of elevated ICP, because their full effects are observed only after a few hours. Furthermore, because steroids are effective only for certain lesions (e.g., edema around a brain tumor or abscess), their use can be delayed until a diagnosis has been made through head CT. Following initial ICP management, a head CT or MRI scan is required; the scan will demonstrate the nature of the supratentorial lesion and associated mass effect. Arrangements must be made to evacuate an epidural or subdural hematoma promptly. Intraparenchymal masses that acutely produce deep stupor or coma initially are best managed nonsurgically. If steroids are indicated, a dexamethasone bolus should be given (up to 100 mg IV), followed by 6 to 24 mg every 6 hours.

The patient's vital signs and neurologic condition necessitate repeated examination. The head should be kept slightly elevated. Mannitol administration may be repeated, if necessary, every 4 to 6 hours; serum electrolytes and fluid balance must be monitored.

When patients with presumed increased ICP do not demonstrate the expected clinical response to medical management or when obstructive hydrocephalus complicates a supratentorial mass lesion, we favor placement of a ventriculostomy into the lateral ventricle. The ventriculostomy allows accurate measurement of intraventricular ICP and provides a method for drainage of cerebrospinal fluid (CSF), if necessary. The placement of a ventriculostomy allows calculation of cerebral perfusion pressure (mean systemic arterial pressure minus ICP), a critical determinant of cerebral blood flow and, therefore, of oxygen and substrate delivery. Monitoring of ICP also allows adjustment of therapeutic intervention before clinical deterioration occurs in patients with diminished intracranial compliance. Drainage of CSF aims to relieve high ICP to maintain cerebral perfusion pressure (more than 80 mm Hg) and to improve intracranial compliance. The risk of ventricular infection (predominantly with *Staphylococcus epidermidis*) can be reduced by removing or changing the ventriculostomy catheter every 5 to 7 days. After increased ICP has responded to emergency management and the patient's condition has stabilized, definitive treatment of the mass lesion is required as deemed appropriate.

Infratentorial Lesions

The evolution of neurologic symptoms and signs and the results of the neurologic examination generally give sufficient information to localize the lesion to the posterior fossa; the lesions themselves may be intrinsic or extrinsic to the brain stem.

Rapid neurologic deterioration of a patient in whom an infratentorial lesion is suspected sometimes demands emergency treatment before head CT scanning is performed. Treatment of a presumed extrinsic compressive lesion of the brain stem entails measures that decrease ICP as outlined previously. In patients who are stuporous or are showing signs of progressive brain stem compression from a cerebellar hemorrhage or infarction, urgent evacuation is required. Intrinsic brain stem lesions are best treated conservatively; an incompleted stroke may benefit from heparin anticoagulation. Posterior fossa tumors are managed initially with osmotic agents and steroids; definitive treatment consists of surgery, irradiation, or both. The placement of a ventricular catheter for acute hydrocephalus must be considered cautiously and in consultation with a neurosurgeon; the procedure carries the risk of potentially fatal upward transtentorial herniation.[11]

Metabolic-Toxic Coma

The task of the physician in first contact with the patient in metabolic coma is to preserve the brain and protect it from permanent damage. Metabolic and toxicologic studies must be performed on the first blood specimens drawn (see Table 168–1).

Treatable conditions that quickly and irreversibly damage the brain are as follows:

- Hypoglycemia
- Acid-base imbalance
- Hypoxia
- Acute bacterial meningitis
- Drug overdose

Hypoglycemia

As previously noted, glucose (50 mL of a 50% solution IV) should be administered during emergency treatment, before the results of blood tests are known. Prolonged hypoglycemic coma that has considerably damaged the brain is not reversed by a glucose load; a glucose bolus may transiently worsen hyperglycemic, hyperosmolar coma. In contrast, the osmolar load of IV glucose may transiently decrease elevated ICP and lighten nonhypoglycemic coma. A glucose infusion is needed to prevent recurrent hypoglycemia.

Acid-Base Imbalance

The hyperventilating comatose patient with acute, severe metabolic acidosis and threatening cardiovascular collapse requires emergency treatment. For accurate assessment arterial blood gas analysis must be performed. An intravenous infusion of sodium hydroxide ($NaHCO_3$) (1 mEq/kg body weight) can be lifesaving; simultaneously, a search for, and specific treatment of, the cause must be conducted.

Hypoxia

Suspected, or proven, carbon monoxide poisoning requires hyperoxygenation with 100% oxygen to facilitate excretion of this toxin. Blood pressure and cardiac rhythm must be closely monitored, and abnormalities corrected.

Idiopathic or drug-induced methemoglobinemia is treated

with methylene blue; 1 to 2 mg/kg IV is given over a few minutes and repeated after 1 hour if needed.

Anemia alone does not cause coma but exacerbates other forms of hypoxia. Transfusion of packed red blood cells or whole blood is appropriate for severe anemia (hematocrit value <25%).

Cyanide poisoning causes histotoxic hypoxia of the brain. Treatment entails amylnitrite (vapor or crushed ampule inhaled every minute) and sodium nitrite (300 mg IV) followed by sodium thiosulfate (12.5 g IV).

Acute Bacterial Meningitis

A lumbar puncture must be considered for any unconscious patient with fever, signs of meningeal irritation, or both. If possible, an emergency head CT scan should be obtained prior to lumbar puncture in a comatose patient to rule out unexpected mass lesions. Increased ICP is present in all cases of bacterial meningitis, but a lumbar puncture is not contraindicated when this diagnosis is suspected.

Cerebral herniation seldom, if ever, occurs except in small children with *Haemophilus influenzae* meningitis.[19] Clinical correlates of impending herniation demand a more cautious approach to lumbar puncture; they are coma or rapidly deteriorating level of arousal; focal neurologic signs; and tonic or prolonged fits. (Papilledema is rare in acute bacterial meningitis.) Should unexpected herniation occur after lumbar puncture, treatment with hyperventilation and IV mannitol is indicated. Appropriate antibiotic treatment can usually await the results of CSF Gram's stain. If the Gram's stain result is negative but a bacterial etiology is suspected, empirical, broad-spectrum antibiotic treatment with a third-generation cephalosporin and vancomycin is appropriate.

Drug Overdose

Certain general principles apply to all patients suspected of having ingested sedative drugs.[20, 21] Most drug overdoses are treated with emergency measures (already discussed) and supportive measures (Table 168-5). Once vital signs are stable, attempts should be made to remove, neutralize, or reverse the effects of the drug.

Patients in coma from recent drug ingestion require gastric lavage after endotracheal intubation. A large, preferably double-lumen, gastric tube must be placed orally. The patient is placed in the head-down position on the left side. The procedure is performed with a 200- to 300-mL bolus of tap water or half-normal saline and is continued until the return is clear. After lavage, 1 or 2 tablespoons of activated charcoal are passed down the lavage tube.

With meticulous supportive measures, patients with uncomplicated drug-induced coma should recover without neurologic deficit. The recovery from coma due to massive doses of barbiturates or glutethimide can be hastened by hemodialysis.

General Measures for Metabolic-Toxic Coma

Constant vigilance and attention to the patient's condition, with timely and appropriate diagnostic and therapeutic evaluation, ensures the best possible outcome of metabolic coma. Effective care demands meticulous attention to the maintenance of tissue perfusion and oxygenation, the documentation and anticipation of acute neurologic events (particularly, diminished cerebral perfusion, herniation, or seizures), aggressive, rapid treatment of initial or subsequent infections, and prevention of agitation. Deep venous thrombosis can be prevented with either subcutaneous heparin (5000 units every 12 hours) or full-leg-length pneumatic compression sleeves. Enteral or parenteral feeding within 36 to 48 hours is required to satisfy nutritional needs. Corneal injury can be prevented by protecting the eyes with lubricants and taping the lids shut.

Prediction of Outcome of Coma

A complete evaluation of the comatose patient must include an estimate of prognosis. The outcome in a given comatose patient cannot be predicted with absolute certainty. Available serial data are not sufficiently specific or selective to help in establishing the prognosis in an individual patient. Guidelines on the outcome of coma have been compiled from serial examinations. Although the status of the comatose patient on admission is valuable in providing early, informed discussion with relatives of patients and medical colleagues, that moment in most instances does not provide sufficient information to withhold immediate therapy. The early establishment of a highly probable poor outcome, however, ideally should be made within 24 hours of hospital admission, in order to ration intensive care services and protect families from false hope in futile cases. A logical and sensible approach to prognostication comprises an etiologic subcategorization into (1) medical, (2) drug-induced, and (3) traumatic coma.

Medical Coma

Factors that are useful in determining the outcome of medical coma are the cause, the depth, and the duration of coma. Certain clinical signs, particularly those involving brain stem, motor, and verbal function, are the most helpful and best-validated predictors (confidence interval, 0.95).[22–25]

Overall, only 15% of patients in established medical coma for 6 hours make a good or moderate recovery; others die (61%), remain in a vegetative state (12%), or become permanently dependent on others for daily living (11%). Prognosis depends on the etiology of medical coma. Patients in coma due to a stroke, subarachnoid hemorrhage, or cardiorespiratory arrest have only about a 10% chance of achieving independent function. Thirty-five per cent of patients achieve moderate to good recovery from coma due to other metabolic reasons, including infection, organ failure, and biochemical disturbances. As noted previously, almost all patients who reach the hospital after sedative overdose or exposure to other exogenous agents will recover moderately or completely.

The depth of coma affects the individual prognosis. Patients who open their eyes in response to noxious stimuli after 6 hours of coma have a 20% chance of making a good recovery but only a 10% chance if their eyes remain closed.

The longer coma persists, the less likely are the chances for recovery; 15% of patients in a coma for 6 hours make a good or moderate recovery, but only 3% who remain unconscious at 1 week recover. Coma following head trauma has a somewhat better prognosis (see later).

The severity of signs of brain stem dysfunction on admission inversely correlates with the chance of good recovery in medical coma. Absence of pupillary responses at any time after onset of coma and, except in barbiturate or phenytoin poisoning, absence of caloric-vestibular reflexes 1 day after onset indicate a poor prognosis (<2% recovery). Except for patients in coma due to sedative drug poisoning, no patient with absence of pupillary light reflexes, corneal reflexes, or oculocephalic or caloric responses or with lack of a motor response to noxious stimulation at 3 days after onset is likely to ever regain independent function. Patients who are likely to recover will, within 1 to 3 days, speak words, open their eyes to noise, show nystagmus on caloric testing, or have spontaneous eye movements.

Postanoxic *convulsive status epilepticus* (CSE) or *myoclonic status epilepticus* (MSE) reflects a poor prognosis. Occasional patients recover consciousness but remain handicapped. Most die or become vegetative.[26, 27] Associated clinical findings, such as loss of brain stem reflexes or eye-opening at the onset of myoclonic jerks, and sinister EEG patterns, such

TABLE 168–5. Neurologic Manifestations of Common Drug Poisoning

Drug	Signs and Symptoms	Diagnostic Test	Treatment
Carbon Monoxide	Confusion; agitation; headache; convulsions; coma; respiratory failure; cardiovascular collapse	History; carboxyhemoglobin level	Remove patient from area (100% oxygen until carboxyhemoglobin levels fall to <5%); hyperbaric oxygen if central nervous system affected; treat cerebral edema with hyperventilation, diuretics, and cerebrospinal fluid drainage if necessary
Salicylate	Tinnitus; hyperpnea; confusion; convulsions; coma; hyperthermia	Blood	Supportive care; gastric lavage; charcoal; systemic alkalinization; hemodialysis for coma or seizures
Cyanide	Agitation; confusion; headache; vertigo; hypertension; hypotension; seizures; paralysis; apnea; coma	Blood	Amyl nitrate; sodium nitrate; sodium thiosulfate; 100% oxygen; hyperbaric oxygen for refractory signs; vitamin B_{12} injection
Anticonvulsants			
Phenytoin Carbamazepine Phenobarbital (see "Barbiturates") Valproic acid Primidone Ethosuximide Felbamate Clonazepam (see "Benzodiazepines")	Drowsiness; ataxia; nystagmus; tremulousness; coma; dysrhythmias with carbamazepine or phenytoin overdose	Blood; ammonia level in patients taking valproic acid	Supportive care; gastric lavage; charcoal; watch for withdrawal seizures
Sedative Hypnotics			
Benzodiazepines Barbiturates Chloral hydrate Meprobamate Ethchlorvynol (Placidyl)	Confusion; lethargy; ataxia; nystagmus; hypothermia; dysarthria; respiratory depression; coma; pupillary reactions preserved except in instances of deep barbiturate coma; possible withdrawal seizures	Blood	Supportive care; gastric lavage; flumazenil for benzodiazepine overdose; hemoperfusion for extreme barbiturate intoxication
Methaqualone	Agitation; hypertonic; hyperreflexia; ataxia; hallucinations; convulsions	Blood	Supportive care; gastric lavage; charcoal
Ethanol	Confusion; agitation; delirium; ataxia; nystagmus; dysarthria; coma	Blood; breath	Supportive care; lavage if within 1 hour of ingestion; thiamine; glucose
Opioids	Lethargy; small reactive pupils; hypothermia; hypotension; urinary retention; shallow, irregular respirations; convulsions	Urine; response to naloxone	Naloxone, 0.4 mg IV or IM; continuous naloxone infusion, if necessary; supportive care with intubation as necessary; lavage if overdose is by ingestion
Stimulants			
Amphetamine Methylphenidate Cocaine	Hypervigilance; paranoia; violent behavior; tremulousness; dilated pupils; hyperthermia; tachycardia or arrhythmia; focal neurologic signs secondary to stroke or CNS hemorrhage; seizures	Blood; urine	Supportive care; sedation with benzodiazepines; treat hypertensive crisis with sodium nitroprusside or labetalol; watch for rhabdomyolysis
Psychedelics			
LSD, mescaline, PCP	Delirium; delusions; marked agitation; hallucinations; hyperactivity; dilated pupils; hyperreflexia; nystagmus	Blood; measurement of PCP levels in gastric juice	Gastric lavage; charcoal; benzodiazepines and haloperidol for sedation

TABLE 168–5. Neurologic Manifestations of Common Drug Poisoning *Continued*

Drug	Signs and Symptoms	Diagnostic Test	Treatment
Antidepressants			
Tricyclic antidepressants	Anticholinergic effects: dry mouth; agitation; restlessness; ataxia; tachycardia or arrhythmias; hyperthermia; hysteria; convulsions; mydriasis	Blood; urine	Cardiac monitoring; gastric lavage; charcoal; mild systemic alkalinization; physostigmine for refractory arrhythmias; anticonvulsants for seizures
Monoamine oxidase inhibitors	Drowsiness; ataxia; seizures; hypertensive crisis; hypotension with severe overdose	Blood	Symptomatic care; gastric lavage; avoid narcotics
Neuroleptics	Dystonia; drowsiness; coma; convulsions; hypotension; miosis; tremor; hypothermia; neuroleptic malignant syndrome	Urine	Gastric lavage Treat extrapyramidal signs with diphenhydramine or benztropine mesylate; treat neuroleptic malignant syndrome with dantrolene or bromocriptine
Lithium	Lethargy; tremulousness; weakness; polyuria; polydipsia; ataxia; seizures; coma	Blood	Hemodialysis for delirium, seizures, or coma
Methanol, ethylene glycol	Drunkenness; hyperventilation; stupor; convulsions; coma; blindness with methanol use	Blood	Symptomatic care; gastric lavage; ethanol infusion; hemodialysis; for methanol intoxication, 4-methylpyrazole under investigation
Antihistamines	Anticholinergic effects: dry mucosa; flushed skin; hyperthermia; dilated pupils; delirium; hallucinations; seizures; coma	Blood	Supportive care; gastric lavage; control of seizures with benzodiazepines; physostigmine for life-threatening anticholinergic effects
Organophosphates	Cholinergic crisis: cramps; excessive secretions; diarrhea; bronchoconstriction; later, tremulousness; fasciculations; weakness; convulsions; hypertension; tachycardia; confusion; anxiety; coma	RBC cholinesterase level	Symptomatic care; decontamination; atropine; pralidoxime

CNS = central nervous system; LSD = lysergic acid diethylamide; PCP = phencyclidine; RBC = red blood cell.

as suppression or burst-suppression, confirm a grim neurologic outcome in this group. Autopsy studies show that cerebral and cerebellar damage can be ascribed to the initial ischemic hypoxic event; there is no evidence that status epilepticus further contributes to this damage. We initially treat patients with an intravenous loading dose of a major anticonvulsant (phenytoin, 13 to 18 mg/kg at 25 mg/min and/or phenobarbital, 20 mg/kg at 50 mg/min). MSE is generally resistant to therapy; we give intermittent doses of benzodiazepines (lorazepam, 2 to 4 mg, or clonazepam, 0.5 mg) intravenously as needed to suppress particularly severe myoclonus that interferes with ventilatory support. Anesthetic agents are rarely indicated and are unlikely to alter outcome.

The most accurate prediction of outcome for a patient in medical coma is obtained from the use of a combination of clinical signs.[22, 23] Within the first week, it is hard to justify the withdrawal of therapy from patients in medical coma unless they are already brain-dead or lack all signs of brain stem function. After that, the probability of being able to predict the quality of life increases steadily.

A multi-society task force of neurologists and neurosurgeons has obtained a large number of data concerning the *persistent vegetative state* (PVS) that provide guidelines to outcomes in patients who remain in the vegetative state 1 month following severe head trauma or coma-producing medical illness (mostly anoxic).[14] Among adults with head trauma who were in a vegetative state at 1 month (n = 434), 33% died, 15% remained in a vegetative state, and 28% suffered severe disability at 1 year. Among children vegetative for 1 month after trauma (n = 106), 9% died, 29% remained in a PVS, and 35% were severely disabled at 1 year; only 27% attained moderate to good recovery.

Results for nontraumatic (medical) coma were even worse. Among 169 adults with nontraumatic brain injury and vegetative state at 1 month, 53% died within a year, 32% remained in a vegetative state, and only 14% made a moderate to good recovery. Outcome for 45 children in similar circumstances showed 22% dead, 65% still in a vegetative state, and only 6% with a moderate to good recovery at 1 year.

Details addressing early qualities that predict good or poor late recoveries are beyond the scope of this chapter. Levy and colleagues[23] discuss specific indicators that improve one's capacity to predict outcomes during the first few weeks or months following severe nontraumatic brain injury.

In a fraction of patients, it is possible to predict within the first week who will recover, who will die in coma or enter a vegetative state, and who will survive with severe disability. Patients in anoxic coma who are in a vegetative state at 1 month never recover their full pre-anoxic physical or cognitive function.

Metabolic-Toxic Coma

Patients in coma due to *exogenous agents* (except carbon monoxide poisoning) carry an overall good prognosis, provided that circulation and respiration are protected by avoiding or correcting cardiac dysrhythmia, aspiration pneumonia, and respiratory arrest. Despite absence of brain stem reflexes (electrocerebral silence on EEG), patients with deep sedative drug intoxication have the potential for complete recovery. Therefore, in the emergent situation the patient in a coma of uncertain etiology should be supported vigorously until the precise cause of coma has been fully established.

Traumatic Coma

The outcome of traumatic coma is generally better than that of medical coma, and prognostic criteria are somewhat different,[14, 28, 29] because (1) many patients with head injury are young; (2) prolonged, post-traumatic unconsciousness of up to several months does not always preclude a satisfactory outcome; and (3) patients in traumatic coma recover more completely than patients in medical coma.

Patients in coma for longer than 6 hours after head injury have a 40% chance to recover to moderate disability or better at 6 months; the most reliable predictors of outcome at 6 months are as follows:

- Patient age (worse outcome with old age, especially after 60 years)
- Depth and duration of coma (an inverse correlation with Glasgow Coma Scale score)
- Pupil reaction and eye movements (absence at 24 hours predicts death or a vegetative state in 90%)
- Motor response in the first week of injury

An independent poor prognostic indicator is sustained, uncontrollably increased ICP (more than 20 mm Hg).

Factors in traumatic coma that appear to have little influence on outcome are the cause of head injury; the presence of skull fractures; lateralization of damage to one hemisphere; and the extent of extracranial injury.

THE ROLE OF SPECIAL INVESTIGATIONS

Neurodiagnostic Imaging

Once the patient with an altered mental status is appropriately resuscitated and stabilized, further investigation may be necessary to document the location of the lesion and to provide guidance for therapeutic intervention. CT and MRI provide an anatomic assessment, functional assessment, or both, of the central nervous system (CNS) and yield helpful information for defining the localization of lesions that produce coma.

Computed Tomography

CT scanning is currently the most expedient imaging technique and gives the most rapid information about possible structural lesions with the least risk to the patient. The value of the CT scan in demonstrating mass lesions, hemorrhage, and hydrocephalus is well established. Axial cuts (10 mm for the cerebral hemispheres, 5 mm for the posterior fossa) are sufficient initially; intravenously administered iodinated dye highlights areas of breakdown in the blood-brain barrier, such as tumor, abscess, and subacute strokes, and may be necessary to better define such lesions.

A noncontrast head CT scan is indispensable in the management of acute head injury and acute stroke. CT can delineate calvarial fractures and intracranial hematomas (epidural, subdural, intraparenchymal, intraventricular, subarachnoid), which may require acute neurosurgical intervention. CT shows tissue shifts due to intracranial intercompartmental pressure gradients but, compared with MRI, may underestimate the anatomy of herniation and its associated syndrome.[10]

Certain lesions, such as early infarction (<12 hours' duration), encephalitis, and isodense subdural hemorrhage, may be difficult to visualize. Posterior fossa pathology may be somewhat obscured by bone artifact inherent in the CT technique. Raised ICP is suggested by effacement of cortical sulci, a narrow third ventricle, and obliteration of the suprasellar or quadrigeminal cisterns but cannot be otherwise quantified.

Magnetic Resonance Imaging

MRI may be performed, depending on the clinical setting and the stability of the patient's condition. The use of MRI is limited in the urgent setting of coma evaluation because of (1) the length of time required to perform the imaging, (2) image degradation by even a slight movement of the patient, and (3) the relative inaccessibility of the patient for emergencies that may occur during the imaging process. Nevertheless, MRI provides superb visualization of the posterior fossa and its contents, which is useful when intrinsic brain stem lesions are suspected as the cause of coma.[10] MRI visualizes anatomic lesions, such as those resulting from acute stroke, encephalitis, central pontine myelinolysis, and traumatic shear injury, with greater resolution and at an earlier time than CT scanning.

The injection of the paramagnetic substance gadolinium helps delineate areas of blood-brain barrier breakdown and may augment the sensitivity of MRI. The "diffusion" technique detects changes in the hydrogen atom (read water) distribution between the intracellular and extracellular spaces and can demonstrate ischemic brain virtually immediately. Sagittal MRI views are particularly useful in the documentation of the extent of supratentorial or infratentorial herniations and may enable intervention before clinical deterioration (Fig. 168–1).[10] Newer MRI techniques allow functional imaging of the central nervous system by measurement of cerebral blood flow to a particular region. Future application of this technique may allow rapid determination of diminished cerebral blood flow, such as that occurring in stroke or vasospasm, and will probably be useful in assessing the effect of therapeutic interventions.

Electroencephalography

The EEG is a qualitative indicator of cerebral function that sometimes gives useful additional information in the evaluation of the unresponsive patient. With metabolic and toxic disorders, the EEG changes generally reflect the degree and severity of altered arousal or delirium, characterized by a decreased frequency of the background rhythm and the appearance of diffuse slow activity in the theta range (4 to 7 Hz), delta range (1 to 3 Hz), or both. Bilaterally synchronous and symmetric, medium-voltage to high-voltage, broad triphasic waves are seen in various metabolic encephalopathies, most often in hepatic coma. Rapid beta activity (>13 Hz) in a comatose patient suggests the ingestion of sedative hypnotics, such as barbiturates and benzodiazepines. Acute, focally destructive lesions show focal slow activity; when periodic lateralized epileptiform discharges appear acutely in one or both temporal lobes, herpes simplex encephalitis must be strongly considered. A nonreactive, diffuse alpha pattern in a comatose patient usually implies a poor prognosis and is most often seen after anoxic insults to the brain or acute, destructive pontine tegmental damage.[30, 31] A normally reactive EEG in an unresponsive patient suggests psychiatric disease; however, a relatively normal EEG can accompany the locked-in

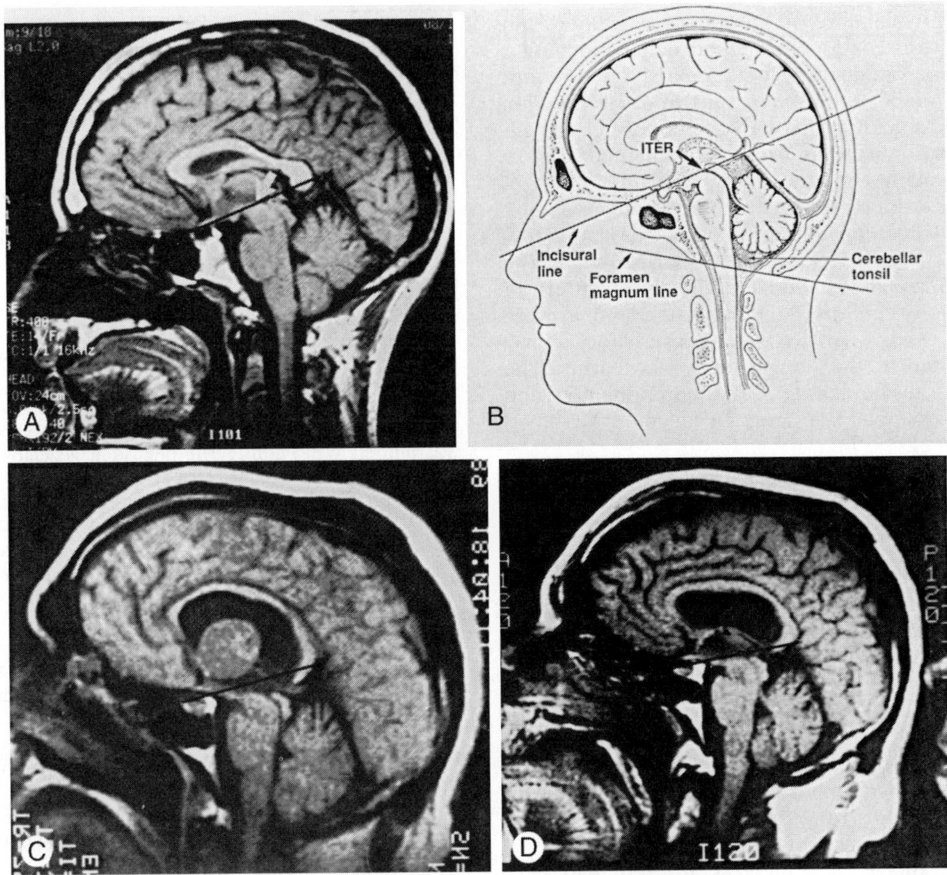

Figure 168–1. Midsagittal magnetic resonance imaging (MRI) views of a normal adult brain and of a brain with reversible downward transtentorial herniation. MRI view of a normal adult male brain (*A*) with accompanying diagram (*B*). The opening of the tentorium of the cerebellum or anterior cerebellar notch lies along a line (incisural line) defined anteriorly by the anterior tubercle of the sella turcica and posteriorly by the junction of Galen's vein, the inferior sagittal sinus, and the confluence of the straight sinus. The proximal opening of the aqueduct of Sylvius, the iter ad infundibulum (*arrow*), lies within 2 mm of the incisural line. The foramen magnum line is defined between the inferior tip of the clivus anteriorly and the bony base of the posterior lip of the foramen magnum. *C,* A 47-year-old man who experienced 1 week of headache, nausea, vomiting, and gait ataxia presented with abrupt-onset coma, palsy of cranial nerve III, hyperreflexia, and bilateral extensor plantar responses. MRI revealed a third ventricular mass, obstructive hydrocephalus, and displacement of the iter ad infundibulum inferiorly by 6.5 mm. The cerebellar tonsils were not displaced. *D,* Subsequent MRI view in the patient in *C* 2 weeks after surgical removal of a colloid cyst. The iter ad infundibulum is 1.2 mm below the incisural line. The patient had full neurologic recovery. (*A, C,* and *D,* From Reich JB, Sierra J, Camp W, et al: Magnetic resonance imaging measurements and clinical changes accompanying transtentorial and foramen magnum brain herniation. Ann Neurol 1993; 33:159–170.)

syndrome, some examples of akinetic mutism, and catatonia, all of which can be caused by structural brain lesions.

Attempts to correlate the pattern and frequency spectra of the post-resuscitative EEG with neurologic outcome have been unsatisfactory, because the EEG's predictive value is, at best, 88% accurate.[32] At present, the most useful information regarding patient prognosis is still obtained by the correct interpretation of physical signs.

Nonconvulsive generalized status epilepticus and repeated complex partial seizures may produce altered levels of awareness or arousal; the EEG is an indispensable tool in the diagnosis and management of both of these disorders. Continuous EEG monitoring optimizes management of status epilepticus, because clinical assessment is insufficiently sensitive to detect continued electrographic seizures. Furthermore, continuous EEG monitoring in the intensive care unit setting has shown an unsuspected high incidence of electrographic seizure activity in critically ill neurologic patients.[33, 34]

Jugular Venous Oximetry

Changes in jugular venous oxygen saturation measure the relationship between cerebral metabolic rate and cerebral blood flow.[35] Placement of a fiberoptic catheter into the internal jugular vein provides continuous measurements of venous oxygen saturation. Jugular venous oximetry catheters should be inserted on the side of dominant venous drainage, with the tip position high in the jugular bulb. The most common complications of catheter insertion are malposition and carotid puncture.

Normal jugular venous oxygen saturation is 50% to 75%. A value less than 50% indicates critical ischemia. A value greater than 75% indicates hyperemia. This form of monitoring offers the potential to minimize secondary insults after traumatic brain injury by providing warning of cerebral ischemia. Other applications are monitoring after other forms of brain injury and during neurosurgical procedures. When jugular venous oximetry is used with other continuous measurements, including ICP, a logical approach to the treatment of brain injury becomes possible.

Transcranial Doppler Ultrasonography

Transcranial Doppler (TCD) ultrasonography allows noninvasive measurement of blood flow velocity in basal cerebral arteries.[36] The high dynamic resolution of the technique, and its confirmed correlation with other hemodynamic modalities, encourages increasing numbers of neurointensivists to adopt it. The importance of TCD ultrasonography in early detection of vasospasm in subarachnoid hemorrhage is now clearly established; increased flow velocity can be documented prior to neurologic deterioration and thus allow early institution of therapy. Velocity also increases when there is augmentation of flow due to collateral contributions to other vascular territories, or supply to a large arteriovenous malformation. At the time of brain death, a characteristic and diagnostic pattern of flow has been demonstrated by TCD ultrasonography in large basal intracranial vessels.[37] An oscillating reverbatory movement has been noted in the flow velocity waveforms. The diagnosis is made from the finding of the reflux phenomenon during late systole following anterograde injection of blood into the vascular tree.

Evoked Potentials

Evoked potentials (EPs) are used to follow the level of functioning of the CNS in comatose patients.[38] Clinical use of brain stem auditory evoked potentials (BAEPs) and short-latency somatosensory evoked potentials (SEPs) stems from the close correlation between EP waveform and specific anatomic structures. The SEP shows special promise in the intensive care field, because it enables components generated supratentorially in the thalamus and primary sensory cortex to be identified and followed over time. Shifts of intracranial structures that lead to herniation syndromes are reflected in abnormalities of SEPs, whereas BAEPs are generated entirely at or below the lower midbrain and are less often affected.

EPs have the advantage of being less affected than EEG readings by sedative medications and septic or metabolic encephalopathies, factors that commonly confound interpretations in comatose patients. Anatomic specificity and physiologic and metabolic immutability are the basis of clinical utility of EPs. Abnormalities demonstrated by these tests, however, are etiologically nonspecific and must be carefully integrated into the clinical situation by a physician familiar with their clinical use. Studies have shown that all patients with anoxic coma and bilateral absence of SEPs had died or remained in a PVS.[39] In traumatic coma, absence of SEPs may be a less definitive prognostic indicator, because recovery of consciousness has been reported in some patients.[40] Also, caution is needed in the interpretation of SEPs to ensure that the absence is not due to technical problems. Repeat SEPs are also useful in following patients' progress. A progressive decline in amplitude appears to be associated with a poor prognosis. Furthermore, a comatose patient, especially one who has motor response of flexor posture or better, with an initial poor prognostic EEG pattern but normal SEPs, may have the potential for recovery and should be supported until the patient's condition has changed to a more prognostically definitive category.[40]

References

1. Plum F, Posner JB: The Diagnosis of Stupor and Coma. 3rd ed. Philadelphia, FA Davis, 1980.
2. Brodal A: Neurological Anatomy in Relation to Clinical Medicine. 3rd ed. Oxford, Oxford University Press, 1981.
3. Steriade M, McCarly RW: Brain Stem Control of Wakefulness and Sleep. New York, Plenum Publishing, 1990.
4. McCormick DA, Von Krosigk M: Corticothalamic activation modulates thalamic firing through glutamate "metabotropic" receptors. Proc Natl Acad Sci U S A 1992; 89:2774–2778.
5. Sejnowski TJ, McCormick DA, Steriade M: Thalamocortical oscillations in sleep and wakefulness. *In:* The Handbook of Brain Theory and Neural Networks. Arbib MA (Ed). Cambridge, Mass, The MIT Press, 1995, pp 976–980.
6. Kales A: Pharmacology of Sleep. Handbook of Experimental Pharmacology Series. Vol 116. Berlin, Springer, 1995.
7. Tinuper P: Idiopathic recurring stupor: A case with possible involvement of the gamma aminobutyric acid (GABA) ergic system. Ann Neurol 1992; 31:503–506.
8. Plum F: Coma. *In:* Encyclopedia of Neuroscience. Vol I. Adelman G (Ed). Boston, Birkhauser Boston, Inc, 1998 (in press).
9. Cuneo RA, Caronna JJ, Pitts L, et al: Upward transtentorial herniation: Seven cases and a literature review. Arch Neurol 1979; 36:618–623.
10. Reich JB, Sierra J, Camp W, et al: Magnetic resonance imaging measurements and clinical changes accompanying transtentorial and foramen magnum brain herniation. Ann Neurol 1993; 33:159–170.
11. Kase CS, Wolf PA: Cerebellar infarction: Upward transtentorial herniation after ventriculostomy. Stroke 1993; 24:1096–1098.
12. Jennett WB, Plum F: The persistent vegetative state: A syndrome in search for a name. Lancet 1972; 1:734–737.
13. Council on Scientific Affairs and Council on Ethical and Judicial Affairs: Persistent vegetative state and the decision to withdraw or withhold life support. JAMA 1990; 263:426–430.
14. Multi-Society Task Force on PVS: Medical aspects of the persistent vegetative state: Statement of a multi-society task force. N Engl J Med 1994; 330:1499–1508.
15. Cairns H: Disturbances of consciousness with lesions of the brain stem and diencephalon. Brain 1952; 75:109–146.
16. Goldberg S: The Four Minute Neurologic Exam. Miami, Medmaster, 1992.
17. Winkler E, Shlomo A, Kriger D, et al: Use of flumazenil in the diagnosis and treatment of patients with coma of unknown etiology. Crit Care Med 1993; 21:538–542.
18. Hund EF, Lehman-Horn F: Life-threatening hyperthermic syndromes. *In:* Neurocritical Care. Hacke W (Ed). Berlin, Springer-Verlag, 1994, pp 888–896.
19. Rennick G, Shann F, de Campo J: Cerebral herniation during bacterial meningitis in children. BMJ 1993; 306:953–955.
20. Howell JM, Altieri M, Jagoda AS, et al: Emergency Medicine. Philadelphia, WB Saunders, 1998, pp 1377–1538.
21. Ellenhorn MJ, Schonwald S, Ordog G, et al: Ellenhorn's Medical Toxicology: Diagnosis and Treatment of Human Poisoning. 2nd ed. Baltimore, Williams & Wilkins, 1997.
22. Levy DE, Bates D, Caronna JJ, et al: Prognosis in non-traumatic coma. Ann Intern Med 1981; 94:293–301.
23. Levy DE, Caronna JJ, Singer BH, et al: Predicting outcome from hypoxic-ischemic coma. JAMA 1985; 253:1420–1426.
24. Edgren E, Hedstrand U, Sutton-Tyrrel K, Safar P: Assessment of neurological prognosis in comatose survivors of cardiac arrest. Lancet 1994; 343:1055–1059.
25. Longstreth WT, Diehr P, Init S: Prediction of awakening after out of hospital cardiac arrest. N Engl J Med 1983; 308:1378–1382.
26. Young GB, Gilbert JJ, Zochodine DW: The significance of myoclonic status epilepticus in postanoxic coma. Neurology 1990; 40:1843–1848.
27. Wijdecks EFM, Parisi JE, Scarborough P: Prognostic value of myoclonus status in comatose survivors of cardiac arrest. Ann Neurol 1994; 35:239–243.
28. Jennett B, Teasdale G, Braakman R, et al: Prognosis of patients with severe head injury. Neurosurgery 1979; 4:283–301.
29. Marshall LF, Gautille T, Klauber MR, et al: The outcome of severe head injury. J Neurosurg 1991; 75(Suppl):S28–S36.
30. Austin EG, Walkus RJ, Longstreth WT: Etiology and prognosis of alpha coma. Neurology 1988; 38:773–777.
31. Synek VM: Prognostically important EEG coma patterns in diffuse anoxic and traumatic encephalopathies in adults. J Clin Neurophysiol 1988; 5:161–174.
32. Edgren E, Hedstrend U, Nordin M, et al: Prediction of outcome after cardiac arrest. Crit Care Med 1987; 15:820–825.
33. Young GB, Jordan KG, Doig GS: An assessment of non-convulsive seizures in the intensive care unit using continuous EEG monitoring: An investigation of variables associated with mortality. Neurology 1996; 47:83–89.
34. Lowenstein DH, Aminoff MJ: Clinical and EEG features of status epilepticus in comatose patients. Neurology 1992; 42:100–104.

35. Souter MJ, Andrews PJD: A review of jugular venous oximetry. Intensive Care World 1996; 13:32–38.
36. DeWitt LD, Wechsler LR: Transcranial Doppler. Stroke 1988; 19:915–921.
37. Ropper AH, Kehne SM, Wechsler LR: Transcranial Doppler in brain death. Neurology 1987; 37:1733–1735.
38. Chiappa KH, Hoch DB: Electrophysiologic monitoring. *In:* Neurological and Neurosurgical Intensive Care. 3rd ed. Ropper AH (Ed). New York, Raven Press, 1993, pp 147–183.
39. Chen R, Bolton CF, Young GB: Prediction of outcome in patients with anoxic coma: A clinical and electrophysiologic study. Crit Care Med 1996; 24:672–678.
40. Lindsay K, Pasaoglu A, Hirst D, et al: Somatosensory and auditory brainstem conduction after head injury: A comparison with clinical features in prediction of outcome. Neurosurgery 1990; 26:278–285.

169

Seizures in Critically Ill Patients

Thomas P. Bleck, MD, FCCM • Christopher J. Dunatov, MD

Seizures complicate the course of about 3% of adult intensive care unit (ICU) patients admitted for nonneurologic conditions. The medical and economic impact of such seizures confers importance on them out of proportion to their incidence. A seizure is often the first indication of a central nervous system (CNS) complication; thus, rapid diagnosis is mandatory. In addition, since epilepsy affects 2% of the population, patients with preexisting seizures occasionally enter the ICU for other problems. Since the initial treatment of these patients is the province of intensivists, these physicians must be familiar with seizure management as it affects critically ill patients. Patients with status epilepticus (SE) often require the care of a critical care specialist in addition to a neurologist.

Seizures have been recognized at least since Hippocrates' day, but their relatively high rate of occurrence in critically ill patients was recognized only recently. Seizures complicating critical care treatments (e.g., lidocaine use) are also a recent phenomenon. Early attempts at treatment included bromides[1] and morphine[2] as well as ice applications. Barbiturates were first employed in 1912 and phenytoin in 1937.[3] Paraldehyde was popular in the next two decades.[4] More recently, emphasis has shifted to the benzodiazepines, which were introduced in the 1960s.[5] Newer agents for treatment of seizures in critically ill patients include the phenytoin prodrug fosphenytoin and the anesthetic agent propofol.

The term status epilepticus refers to prolonged seizure episodes. SE may be the primary indication for admission to the ICU, or it may occur in any ICU patient with CNS disease. The definitions employed in studies of SE have varied substantially. Although conventional definitions of SE have used a cutoff of 30 or 60 minutes duration of sustained seizure, or discrete seizures without recovery, clinicians should recognize that most seizures terminate spontaneously within a few minutes. Seizures that persist longer than 5 to 7 minutes should probably be treated as SE.

EPIDEMIOLOGY

Limited data are available on the epidemiology of seizures in the ICU. A 10-year retrospective study of all ICU patients with seizures at the Mayo Clinic revealed that seven patients per 1000 ICU admissions had seizures.[6] Our 2-year prospective study of medical ICU patients identified 35 with seizures per 1000 admissions.[7] These two studies are not exactly comparable, as the patient populations and methods of detection differed. Seizures are probably even more frequent in pediatric ICUs. One study has reported that SE accounted for 1.6% of admissions to a pediatric ICU over a 10-year period.[8]

As many as 34% of hospital inpatients who experience a seizure die during their hospitalization.[6] Our prospective study of neurologic complications in medical ICU patients showed that having even one seizure while in the ICU for a nonneurologic reason doubled in-hospital mortality.[9] This effect on prognosis principally reflected the cause of the seizure. Table 169–1 summarizes the relative frequency of the causes of SE in adults and children. Incidence estimates for generalized convulsive SE (GCSE) in the United States vary from 50,000 cases per year[10] to 195,000 cases per year.[11] Some portion of this difference can be accounted for by different definitions; however, the latter estimate represents the only

TABLE 169–1. Causes of Status Epilepticus Presenting from the Community

Adults		Children	
History of Seizures	*No History of Seizures*	*History of Seizures*	*No History of Seizures*
Common Causes			
Subtherapeutic anticonvulsant Ethanol-related Intractable epilepsy	Ethanol-related Drug toxicity CNS infection Head trauma CNS tumor	Subtherapeutic anticonvulsant Intractable epilepsy	Febrile seizures CNS infection Head trauma
Less Common Causes			
CNS infection Metabolic aberration Drug toxicity Stroke CNS tumor Head trauma	Metabolic aberration Stroke	Anoxic brain injury Head trauma Metabolic aberration	CNS infection Intractable epilepsy Metabolic aberration

CNS = central nervous system.

TABLE 169–2. International Classification of Epileptic Seizures

I. Partial seizures (seizures beginning locally)
  A. Simple partial seizures (consciousness not impaired; SPS)
    1. With motor symptoms
    2. With somatosensory or special sensory symptoms
    3. With autonomic symptoms
    4. With psychic symptoms
  B. Complex partial seizures (with impairment of consciousness; CPS)
    1. Beginning as SPS and progressing to impairment of consciousness
      a. Without automatisms
      b. With automatisms
    2. With impairment of consciousness at onset
      a. With no other features
      b. With features of SPS
      c. With automatisms
  C. Partial seizures (simple or complex), secondarily generalized
II. Primary generalized seizures (bilaterally symmetric, without localized onset)
  A. Absence seizures
    1. True absence ("petit mal")
    2. Atypical absence
  B. Myoclonic seizures
  C. Clonic seizures
  D. Tonic seizures
  E. Tonic-clonic seizures (grand mal; GTC)
  F. Atonic seizures
III. Unclassified seizures

Adapted from Bleck TP: Status epilepticus. *In:* Textbook of Clinical Neuropharmacology. 2nd ed. Klawans HL, Goetz CG, Tanner CM (Eds). New York, Raven Press, 1992, pp 65–73.

population-based data available and may be more accurate. Mortality estimates similarly vary, from 1% to 2% in the former study to 22% in the latter. This disagreement follows from a conceptual discordance; the smaller number describes mortality, which the authors attribute directly to SE, while the larger figure estimates the overall mortality rate, even though death was frequently caused by the underlying disease rather than by SE itself. Mortality rates from SE in children admitted to a pediatric ICU have been reported to be 6% while in the ICU and 9% at 1 year.[8]

Three major factors determine outcome of SE: (1) the type of SE, (2) its cause, and (3) its duration.[12] GCSE carries the worst prognosis for neurologic recovery, and myoclonic SE after an anoxic episode indicates a very poor prognosis for survival. Complex partial SE (CPSE) can produce limbic system damage, usually manifested as a memory disturbance. Causes associated with increased mortality included anoxia, intracranial hemorrhages, tumors, infections, and trauma. The mortality associated with SE increases with the duration of the seizure: SE lasting longer than 1 hour carried a mortality of 32% as compared with 2.7% for a duration less than 1 hour.

Data are limited in regard to the functional abilities of GCSE survivors, and no data reliably permit a distinction between the effects of SE and those of its causes. One review concluded that intellectual ability declined as a consequence of SE.[13] Survivors of SE frequently seem to have memory and behavioral disorders whose extent is out of proportion to the structural damage produced by the cause of their seizures. Extensive experimental data support this observation, emphasizing strongly the benefit of rapid and effective control of SE. Case reports of severe memory deficits after prolonged CPSE have also been published.[14] Whether treatment of SE reduces the risk of subsequent epilepsy remains unclear. Experimental studies indicate that SE lowers the threshold for subsequent seizures.

CLASSIFICATION

The most frequently used classification scheme is that of the International League Against Epilepsy (Table 169–2).[15] This scheme allows classification on clinical criteria without implying cause. *Simple partial seizures* start focally in the cerebral cortex without invading other structures. The patient is aware throughout the episode and appears otherwise unchanged. Bilateral limbic dysfunction produces a *complex partial seizure;* awareness and ability to interact are diminished but may not be completely abolished. *Automatisms* (movements that a patient makes without awareness) may occur. *Secondary generalization* results from invasion by epileptic electrical activity of the other hemisphere or subcortical structures.

Primary generalized seizures arise from the cerebral cortex and diencephalon at the same time; no focal phenomena are visible, and consciousness is lost at the onset. *Absence seizures* are frequently confined to childhood, they consist of abrupt onset of a blank stare that usually lasts 5 to 15 seconds, after which the patient abruptly returns to normal. *Atypical absence seizures* occur in children with the Lennox-Gastaut syndrome. *Myoclonic seizures* start with brief synchronous jerks, without alteration of consciousness initially, followed by a generalized convulsion. They frequently occur in genetic epilepsy; in the ICU, they commonly follow anoxia or metabolic disturbances.[16] *Tonic-clonic seizures* start with tonic extension, evolve to bilaterally synchronous clonus, and conclude with a postictal phase. Clinical judgment is required to apply this system in the ICU. The nature of the partial seizures of patients whose consciousness has already been altered by drugs, hypotension, sepsis, or an intracranial lesion may be difficult to classify.

SE is classified by a similar system that has been altered to match observable clinical phenomena (Table 169–3).[17] GCSE is the most common type encountered in the ICU, and it poses the greatest risk to the patient. It may either be primarily generalized, as in drug-intoxicated patients, or secondarily generalized, as in brain abscess patients who develop GCSE. *Nonconvulsive SE* (NCSE) in the ICU after follows partially treated GCSE. Some use the term for all cases of SE that involve altered consciousness without convulsive movements;

TABLE 169–3. Clinical Classification of Status Epilepticus (SE)

I. Generalized seizures
  A. Generalized convulsive SE (GCSE)
    1. Primary generalized SE
      a. Tonic-clonic SE
      b. Myoclonic SE
      c. Clonic-tonic-clonic SE
    2. Secondarily generalized SE
      a. Partial seizure with secondary generalization
      b. Tonic SE
  B. Nonconvulsive SE (NCSE)
    1. Absence SE (petit mal status)
    2. Atypical absence SE (e.g., in the Lennox-Gastaut syndrome)
    3. Atonic SE
    4. NCSE as a sequel of partially treated GCSE
II. Partial SE
  A. Simple partial SE
    1. Typical
    2. Epilepsia partialis continua (EPC)
  B. Complex partial SE (CPSE)
III. Neonatal SE

Adapted from Lothman EW: The biochemical basis and pathophysiology of status epilepticus. Neurology 1990; 40(Suppl 2):13–23.

this blurs the distinctions among absence SE, partially treated GCSE, and CPSE, which have different causes and treatments. Epilepsia partialis continua (a special form of partial SE in which repetitive movements affect a small area of the body) sometimes lasts months or years.

PATHOGENESIS AND PATHOPHYSIOLOGY

The causes and effects of SE at the cellular, brain, and systemic levels are interrelated, but their individual analysis is useful for understanding them and their therapeutic implications. Longer-duration SE produces more profound alterations with increasing likelihood of permanence and of becoming refractory to treatment. The processes involved in a single seizure and the transition to SE have been reviewed.[18]

The pathophysiologic events of a seizure follow the opening of ion channels coupled to excitatory amino acid receptors. From the standpoint of the intensivist, three channels are particularly important because their activation may raise intracellular free calcium to toxic concentrations:

- α-Amino-3-hydroxy-5-methyl-4-isoxazole propionic acid (AMPA)
- *N*-methyl-D-aspartate (NMDA)
- Metabotropic channels

These excitatory amino acid systems are crucial for learning and memory. Many drugs that block these systems are available but are too toxic for long-term use. The deleterious consequences of SE, and the brief period for which treatment would be needed, suggest that such agents may have a role in SE. Counterregulatory ionic events are triggered by the epileptiform discharge as well, such as the activation of inhibitory interneurons, which suppress excited neurons via γ-aminobutyric acid ($GABA_A$) synapses.

The cellular effects of excessive excitatory amino acid channel activity include the following:

1. Generation of toxic concentrations of intracellular free calcium.
2. Activation of autolytic enzyme systems.
3. Production of oxygen free radicals.
4. Generation of nitric oxide, which both enhances subsequent excitation and serves as a toxin.
5. Phosphorylation of enzyme and receptor systems, making seizures more likely.
6. An increase in intracellular osmolality that produces neuronal swelling. If adenosine triphosphate (ATP) production fails, membrane ion exchange ceases and neurons swell further. These events produce the neuronal damage associated with SE.

Many other biophysical and biochemical alterations occur during and after SE. The intense neuronal activity activates immediate-early genes and produces heat shock proteins, providing indications of the deleterious effects of SE and insight into the mechanisms of neuronal protection.[19] The mechanisms by which SE damages the nervous system have been reviewed.[20] Absence SE is an exception among these conditions; it consists of rhythmically increased inhibition and produces no clinical or pathologic abnormalities.

The mechanisms that terminate seizure activity are poorly understood. The leading candidates are inhibitory mechanisms, primarily GABAergic neuronal systems. Clinical observation supports the contention that human SE frequently follows withdrawal from GABA agonists (e.g., benzodiazepines).

The electrical phenomena of SE at the whole-brain level, as seen in the scalp electroencephalogram, reflect the seizure type that initiates SE (e.g., absence SE begins with a 3-Hz wave-and-spike pattern). During SE, this rhythm slows, but the wave-and-spike characteristic remains. GCSE goes through a sequence of electrographic changes (Table 169–4).[21] The initial discharge becomes less well formed, implying that neuronal firing loses synchrony. The sustained depolarizations that characterize SE alter the extracellular milieu, most importantly by raising extracellular potassium. The excess potassium ejected during SE exceeds the buffering ability of astrocytes, and the rising extracellular potassium level contributes to the production of more seizures.

TABLE 169–4. Electroencephalographic and Clinical Correlations in Generalized Convulsive Status Epilepticus

Stage	Typical Clinical Manifestations*	Electroencephalographic Features
1	Tonic-clonic convulsions; hypertension and hyperglycemia common	Discrete seizures with interictal slowing
2	Low- or medium-amplitude clonic activity, with rare convulsions	Waxing and waning of ictal discharges
3	Slight but frequent clonic activity, often confined to the eyes, face, or hands	Continuous ictal discharges
4	Rare episodes of slight clonic activity; hypotension and hypoglycemia become manifest	Continuous ictal discharges punctuated by flat periods
5	Coma without other manifestations of seizure activity	Periodic epileptiform discharges on a flat background

Data from Treiman DM: Generalized convulsive status epilepticus in the adult. Epilepsia 1993; 34(Suppl 1):S2–S11.

*The clinical manifestations may vary considerably, depending on the underlying neuropathophysiologic process (and its anatomy), systemic diseases, and medications. In particular, stages of the electrographic progression may be sufficiently brief to be overlooked. Partially treating SE may dissociate the clinical and electrographic features.

The increased cellular activity of SE elevates demand for oxygen and glucose, and blood flow initially increases. After about 20 minutes, however, energy supplies become exhausted. This causes local catabolism to support ion pumps (in an attempt to restore the internal milieu); this is a major cause of epileptic brain damage. The brain contains systems to terminate seizure activity; GABAergic interneurons and inhibitory thalamic neurons are both important in this respect.

SE produces neuropathology even when patients are paralyzed with neuromuscular blockade, ventilated, and maintained at normal temperature and blood pressure. The hippocampus, a crucial area for memory, contains the most susceptible neurons, but other regions are also vulnerable. In addition to damaging the CNS, GCSE produces life-threatening systemic effects.[22] Excess secretion of epinephrine and cortisol causes systemic and pulmonary arterial pressures to rise dramatically at seizure onset and to produce hyperglycemia. Muscle work raises blood lactate levels. Both airway obstruction and abnormal diaphragmatic contractions impair respiration. Carbon dioxide excretion falls while its production increases markedly. Muscle work accelerates heat production; concomitantly, skin blood flow falls. This combination can raise core temperature dangerously.

The combined respiratory and metabolic acidoses frequently lower the arterial blood pH to 6.9 or lower. The acidemia may produce hyperkalemia; in addition to its deleterious effects on cardiac electrophysiology, the elevated extracellular potassium level helps to propagate seizure activity. Coupled with hypoxemia and the elevation of circulating catecholamine concentrations, these conditions rarely can produce cardiac arrest. This sequence probably accounts for some cases of epileptic sudden death; neurogenic pulmonary edema is the likely cause of many others. The severity of the acidosis may prompt consideration of bicarbonate administration. When it is attempted, however, the likelihood of pulmonary edema is inordinately high. Rapid termination of seizure activity is the most appropriate treatment; the restitution of ventilation and the metabolism of lactate quickly restore pH to normal.

After about 20 minutes, motor activity begins to diminish and ventilation usually improves; body temperature however, may continue to increase. Hyperglycemia diminishes; after 1 hour, gluconeogenesis can fail, producing hypoglycemia. Patients with GCSE often aspirate oral or gastric contents, producing chemical pneumonitis or bacterial pneumonia. Rhabdomyolysis is common and may lead to renal failure. Compression fractures, joint dislocations, and tendon avulsions are other sequelae.

CLINICAL MANIFESTATIONS

Three problems complicate seizure recognition:

1. Complex partial seizures in the setting of impaired awareness.
2. Seizures in patients with pharmacologically induced paralysis.
3. Misinterpretation of other abnormal movements as seizures.

ICU patients often have depressed consciousness in the absence of seizures, as a result of their disease, its complications (such as hepatic[23] or septic[24] encephalopathy), or drug administration. A further decline in alertness may reflect a seizure; electroencephalography is required to confirm that one has occurred.

Patients receiving neuromuscular junction-blocking agents do not manifest the usual signs of seizures. Because most such patients receive sedation with GABA agonists, the likelihood of seizures is small. One nondepolarizing agent, atracurium, has a metabolite that is potentially epileptogenic in some animals. No human electroencephalographic (EEG) studies have been performed to determine whether patients are susceptible. Autonomic signs of seizures (hypertension, tachycardia, pupillary dilatation) may also be the effects of pain or the response to inadequate sedation. Thus, patients who have a potential for seizures (e.g., those with intracranial lesions) and who manifest these signs should undergo electroencephalography. The actual incidence of this problem is unknown.

Patients with metabolic disturbances or anoxia may demonstrate abnormal movements. Some can be distinguished from seizures by observation; if doubt about their nature persists, however, electroencephalography should be performed. Psychiatric disturbances in the ICU occasionally resemble complex partial seizures. Prolonged EEG monitoring may be required if the problem is intermittent.

Manifestations of Status Epilepticus

The manifestations of SE depend on the type and, for partial SE, the cortical area of abnormality. Table 169-3 presents the types of SE encountered and focuses on those seen most frequently in the ICU.

Primary GCSE begins as tonic extension of the trunk and extremities without preceding focal activity. No aura is reported, and consciousness is lost immediately. After several seconds of tonic extension, the extremities start to vibrate; clonic (rhythmic) extension of the extremities quickly follows. This phase wanes in intensity over a few minutes. The patient may then repeat the cycle of tonus followed by clonic movements or may continue to experience intermittent bursts of clonic activity without recovery. Less common forms of GCSE are *myoclonic SE* (bursts of myoclonic jerks that increase in intensity and lead to a convulsion) and *clonic-tonic-clonic SE* (clonic activity precedes the first tonic contraction). Myoclonic SE is usually seen in patients with anoxic encephalopathy or metabolic disturbances.

Secondarily generalized SE begins with a partial seizure and progresses to a convulsive activity. The initial focal clinical activity may be overlooked. This seizure type implies a structural lesion, so care must be taken to elicit evidence of lateralized movements.

Of the several forms of generalized NCSE, the one of greatest importance to intensivists is NCSE as a sequel of inadequately treated GCSE. When a patient with GCSE is treated with anticonvulsants (often in inadequate doses), visible convulsive activity may stop, although the electrochemical seizure continues. Patients begin to awaken within 15 to 20 minutes after successful termination of SE; many regain consciousness much faster. Patients who do not start to awaken after 20 minutes should be assumed to have entered NCSE. Careful observation may disclose slight clonic activity. NCSE is an extremely dangerous problem because the destructive effects of SE continue even without obvious motor activity. NCSE demands emergent treatment guided by EEG monitoring to prevent further cerebral damage, since there are no clinical criteria to indicate whether therapy is effective.

Failure to recognize NCSE is common in patients with nonspecific neurobehavioral abnormalities such as delirium, lethargy, bizarre behavior, cataplexy, or mutism.[25] A high suspicion for this disorder should be maintained in patients with unexplained altered level of consciousness or cognition admitted to the ICU.

Partial SE in ICU patients often follows a stroke or occurs with the rapid expansion of brain masses. Clonic motor activity is most easily recognized, but the seizure takes on the characteristics of adjacent functional tissue. Therefore, somatosensory or special sensory manifestations occur, and the ICU patient may be unable to report such symptoms. *Aphasic SE* occurs when a seizure begins in a language area, and it can resemble a stroke. Epilepsia partialis continua involves repetitive movements confined to a small region of the body. It may be seen with nonketotic hyperglycemia[26] or with focal brain disease; anticonvulsant treatment is seldom useful. Complex partial SE presents with diminished awareness. The diagnosis often comes as a surprise when an electroencephalogram is obtained.

DIAGNOSTIC APPROACH

When an ICU patient has a seizure, the natural tendency is to try to stop the event. This leads to both diagnostic obscuration and iatrogenic complications. Beyond protecting the patient from harm, one can accomplish very little rapidly enough to influence the course of the seizure. Padded tongue blades and similar items should not be placed in the patient's mouth; they are more likely to obstruct the airway than to preserve it. The seizures of most patients stop before any medication can reach the brain in an effective concentration.

Observation is the most important measure to perform when a patient has a single seizure. This is the time to collect evidence of partial onset to implicate structural brain disease. The postictal examination is similarly valuable; language, motor, sensory, or reflex abnormalities after an apparently generalized seizure are evidence of a focal lesion.

Seizures in ICU patients have several potential causes that must be investigated. Drugs are a major cause of ICU seizures, especially in the setting of diminished renal or hepatic function or when the blood-brain barrier is breached. Theophylline frequently produces seizures or SE when it has been inadvisedly rapidly loaded or when concentrations of the drug are high; however, occasionally these complications arise at "therapeutic" levels. Renal failure or an altered blood-brain barrier increases the seizure likelihood of patients receiving imipenem-cilastatin, but other patients receiving this antibiotic (or GABA antagonists, such as penicillin) are also at risk. Transplant recipients, especially those receiving cyclosporine, are also at increased risk.

Drug withdrawal is another frequent offender. Although ethanol withdrawal is common, discontinuing any hypnosedative agent can prompt convulsions 1 to 3 days later. One report suggests that narcotic withdrawal may produce seizures in critically ill persons.[6]

The physical examination should obviously emphasize assessment for both global and focal abnormalities of the CNS. Evidence of cardiovascular disease or systemic infection should be sought, and the skin and fundi examined closely. Particular attention should be given to the funduscopic examination of infants presenting from the community with seizures, because retinal hemorrhages may be the only evidence of brain trauma induced by child abuse, the shaken baby syndrome.

Patients with unexplained seizures should be screened for illicit drugs. Cocaine is becoming a major cause of seizures.[27] Serum glucose and electrolyte concentrations and serum osmolality should also be measured. Nonketotic hyperglycemia can precipitate both focal and generalized seizures.[28, 29] Seizure activity may be the first presenting sign of diabetes mellitus; however, hypocalcemia rarely causes seizures beyond the neonatal period. Its identification on analysis *must not* signal the end of the diagnostic workup. Hypomagnesemia has an equally unwarranted reputation as a cause of seizures in malnourished alcoholic patients.

The need for imaging studies in these seizure patients has been an area of uncertainty. A prospective study of neurologic complications in medical ICU patients determined that 38 to 61 patients (62%) had a vascular, infectious, or neoplastic explanation for their seizures.[7] Thus, computed tomography (CT) or magnetic resonance imaging (MRI) should be performed on most ICU patients with new seizures. Patients with seizures and either hypoglycemia or nonketotic hyperglycemia might be treated for the metabolic disturbance and observed if they do not present other evidence of focal disease. With current technology, almost all patients can undergo CT. Although MRI is preferable in most situations, the magnetic field precludes the use of infusion pumps and other metal devices. Whether to administer contrast medium for CT depends on the clinical setting and on the appearance of the unenhanced CT scan.

Electroencephalography is a vital diagnostic tool for evaluating seizure patients. Partial seizures usually have EEG abnormalities that begin in the area of cortex that produces seizures. Primary generalized seizures appear to start over the entire cortex simultaneously. Postictal slowing and depressed amplitude provide clues to the focal cause of the seizures, and epileptiform activity helps to classify the type of seizure and to guide treatment. Emergent electroencephalography is necessary to exclude NCSE in patients who do not begin to awaken soon after seizures have apparently been controlled (Fig. 169–1).

Considering the causes of seizures in the ICU setting, patients who need cerebrospinal fluid (CSF) analysis usually require CT first. When CNS infection is suspected, empirical antibiotic treatment should be started while these studies are being performed.

In contrast to the patient who has one or a few seizures, the SE patient requires concomitant diagnostic and therapeutic efforts. Although 20 minutes of continuous or recurrent seizure activity usually defines SE, one should not stand by waiting for this period to pass before instituting treatment. Since most seizures in critically ill patients stop within 2 to 3 minutes, it is reasonable to start treatment after 5 minutes of continuous seizure activity or after the second or third seizure occurs without recovery between the spells.

GCSE can occasionally be confused with decerebrate posturing, but observation usually makes the distinction straightforward. Tetanus patients are awake during their spasms, and flex the arms, rather than extending them as seizure patients do.

Treatment of SE should not be delayed for electroencephalography. A variety of findings may be present on the EEG, depending on the type of SE and its duration (see Table 169–4). CPSE patients are often without such organized discharges of GCSE; instead, they have waxing and waning rhythmic activity in one or several brain regions. A diagnostic trial of intravenous benzodiazepine therapy is often necessary to confirm the diagnosis of CPSE. Patients with refractory SE or seizures during neuromuscular junction blockade require continuous EEG monitoring.

Continuous paperless EEG monitoring has become available, which allows detection of seizure activity over a long period. Subclinical seizures have been observed in patients receiving aggressive treatment for SE and even in patients treated with barbiturates to a burst-suppression EEG pattern. The clinical significance of these subclinical seizures and their effect on prognosis remain uncertain.

MANAGEMENT APPROACH

Isolated Seizures

Making the decision to administer anticonvulsants to an ICU patient who experiences one or a few seizures requires consideration of a provisional cause, estimation of the likelihood of recurrence, and recognition of the utility and limitations of anticonvulsants. For example, the occurrence of seizures during ethanol withdrawal does not indicate the need for long-term treatment, and giving phenytoin does not prevent further withdrawal convulsions. The patient may need prophylaxis against delirium tremens, but the few seizures themselves seldom require treatment. Patients with convulsions during barbiturate or benzodiazepine withdrawal, in contrast, should usually receive short-term treatment with lorazepam to prevent SE. Prolonged or frequent seizures caused by metabolic disturbances may be treated temporarily with benzodiazepines while the abnormality is being corrected. Seizures in these settings are notoriously resistant to treatment with phenytoin. In particular, treatment of partial seizures related to nonketotic hyperglycemia should be directed at correction of the hyperglycemia and hypovolemia rather than anticonvulsant therapy.[29]

The ICU patient with CNS disease who has even one seizure should usually be given chronic anticonvulsant therapy, and this approach should be reviewed before he or she is discharged. Initiating this treatment after the first *unprovoked* seizure may help to prevent subsequent epilepsy,[30] although there is considerable difference of opinion on this concept.[31] Starting therapy after the first seizure in a critically ill patient at risk for seizure recurrence may be even more important,

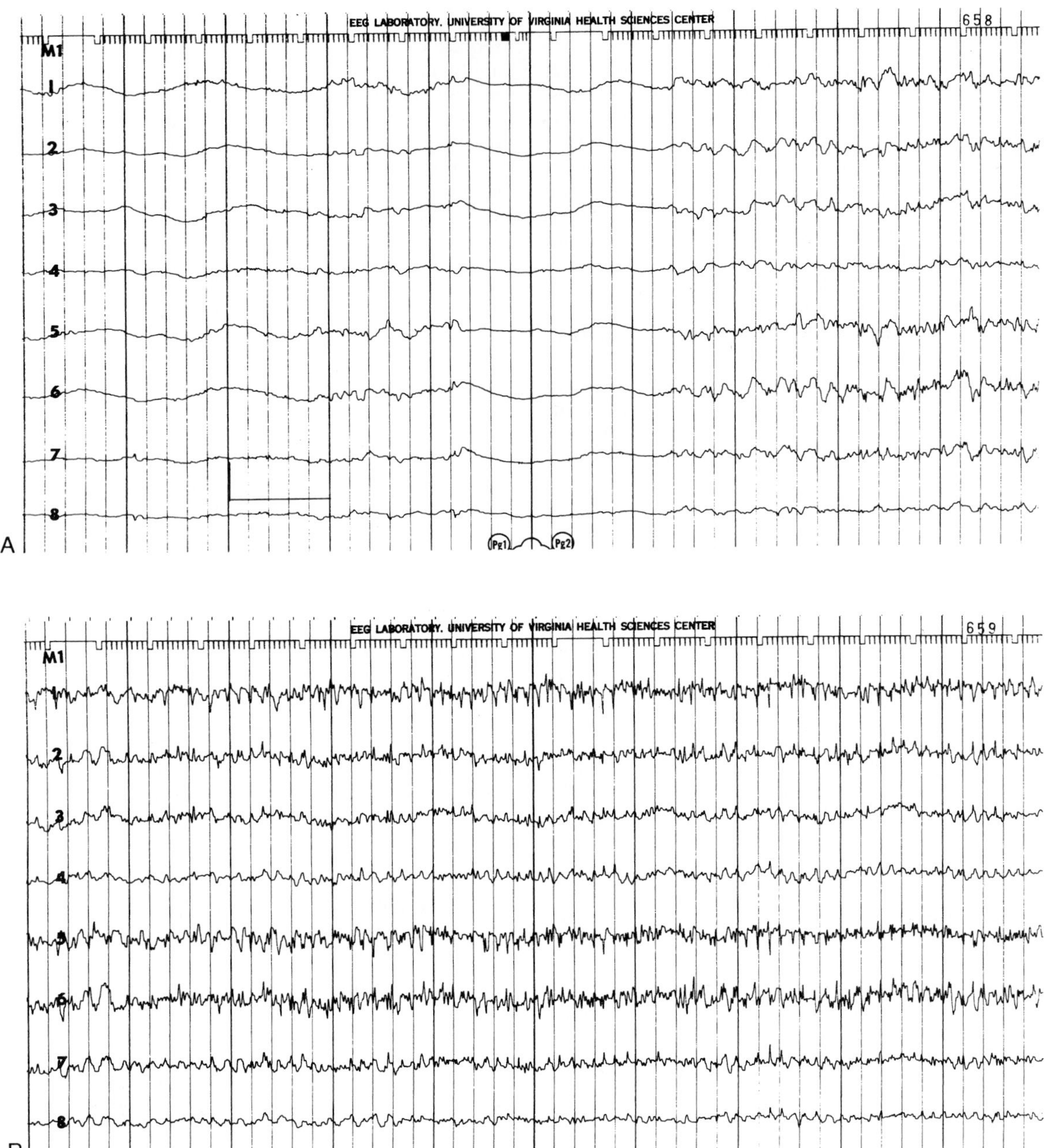

Figure 169–1. Electroencephalographic recording during status epilepticus. The first panel *(A)* illustrates onset of the seizure; subsequent panels *(B–D)* show its evolution. Montage: longitudinal bipolar; channels 1–4, left temporal, and channels 5–8, left parasagittal. Calibration: vertical, 50 μV; horizontal, 1 second.

especially if the condition would be seriously compromised by a convulsion.

In the ICU setting, phenytoin is frequently selected for its ease of administration and lack of sedative effects. Hypotension and arrhythmias may complicate intravenous administration and can usually be prevented by slowing the infusion to less than 25 mg/min. Because of the rare occurrence of third-degree atrioventricular block, an external cardiac pacemaker should be available when patients with conduction abnormalities receive intravenous phenytoin. Propylene glycol in the parenteral formulation of phenytoin is the probable cause of these effects. Additionally, the parenteral formulation of phenytoin is alkaline, and this is thought to contribute to pain, burning, and redness at the injection site.

The new phenytoin prodrug fosphenytoin is water-soluble, and its vehicle does not contain propylene glycol; adverse effects are less common with fosphenytoin than with intravenous phenytoin.[32, 33] Fosphenytoin is dosed by phenytoin equivalent units (PE); therefore, no dose adjustments are needed when patients switch from phenytoin to fosphenytoin. Fosphenytoin can be administered by intramuscular injection or by intravenous infusion at a rate of up to 150 mg PE/min. Fosphenytoin is rapidly converted to phenytoin in vivo, and free phenytoin levels after fosphenytoin administration are not markedly different from those of phenytoin.

When phenytoin *or* fosphenytoin is used, the serum phenytoin concentration should be kept in the "therapeutic" range of 10 to 20 μg/mL (corresponding to an unbound or "free"

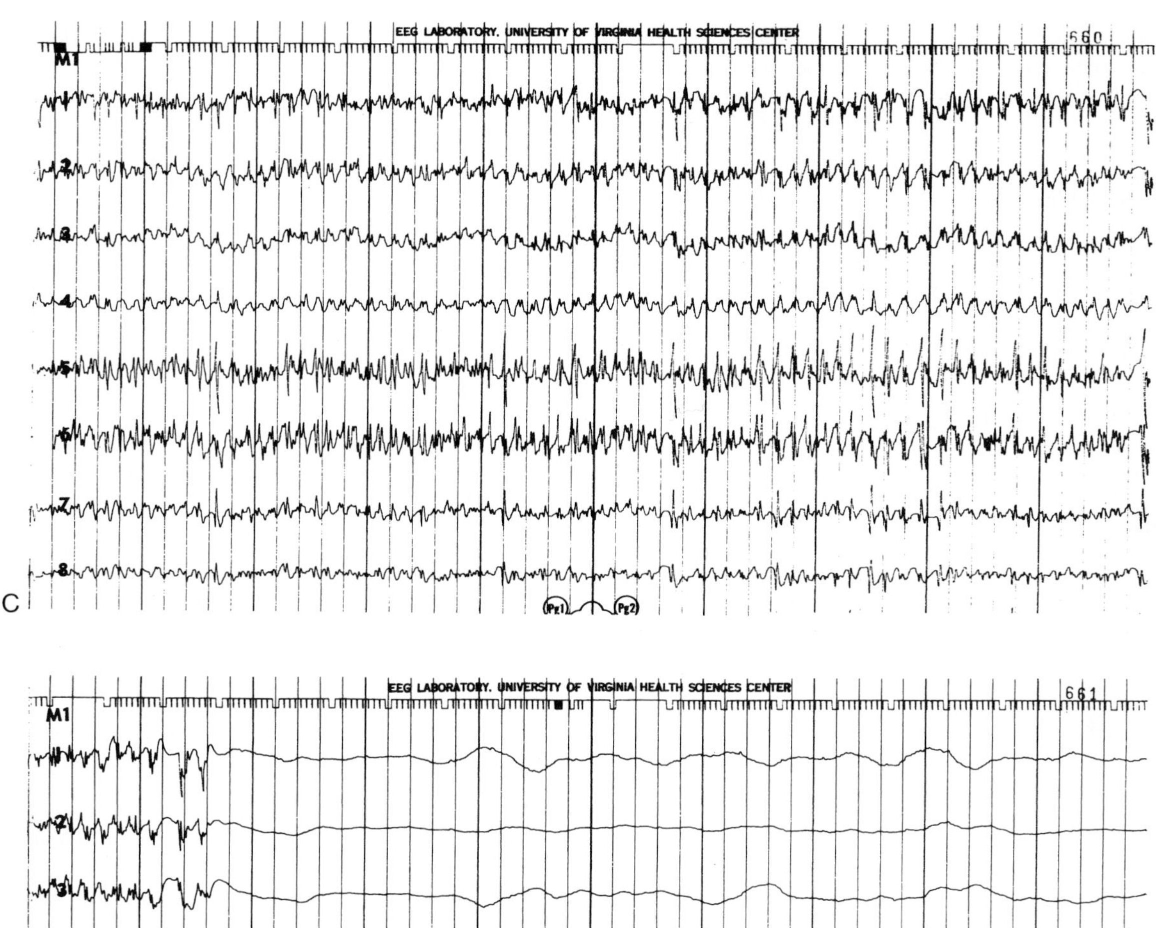

Figure 169–1 *Continued*

concentration of 1 to 2 μg/mL) unless further seizures occur, in which event the level may be increased until signs of toxicity appear. Failure to prevent seizures at a concentration of 25 μg/mL is usually an indication to add phenobarbital to the regimen. When fosphenytoin is administered, phenytoin concentrations should not be measured until the biologic conversion to phenytoin is complete: 2 hours after an intravenous infusion or 4 hours after an intramuscular injection of fosphenytoin.

Phenytoin is approximately 90% protein-bound in normal hosts. Patients with renal dysfunction have lower total phenytoin levels at a given dose because the drug is displaced from binding sites, but the unbound level is not affected. Thus, patients with renal failure and perhaps others who are receiving strongly protein-bound drugs (which compete for binding) may benefit from determination of the free phenytoin level. Because only the free fraction is metabolized, the dose is not altered by changes in renal function. The clearance half-time with normal liver function varies from about 12 to 20 hours (intravenous form) to over 24 hours (extended-release capsules), so that a new steady-state serum concentration occurs in 3 to 6 days.

Phenytoin need not be given more frequently than every 12 hours. Hepatic dysfunction mandates a decrease in the maintenance dose. Hypersensitivity is the major adverse effect of concern to intensivists. This can manifest itself solely as fever, but signs commonly include rash and eosinophilia. Adverse reactions to phenytoin and other anticonvulsants have been reviewed elsewhere.[34]

Phenobarbital remains a useful anticonvulsant for persons intolerant to phenytoin or who have persistent seizures after *adequate* phenytoin administration. The target for phenobarbital in the ICU should be a serum concentration of 20 to 40 μg/mL. Hepatic and renal dysfunction alter phenobarbital metabolism. Because its usual clearance half-time is about 96 hours, maintenance doses of this agent should be given once a day. A steady-state level takes about 3 weeks to become established. Sedation is the major adverse effect; drug allergy is rare.

Carbamazepine therapy is seldom started in the ICU because its insolubility precludes parenteral formulation. Oral loading in conscious patients may produce coma that lasts several days. This drug also causes hyponatremia in patients who take it over the long term.

Status Epilepticus

GCSE obviously constitutes a medical emergency; however, NCSE and CPSE are also emergencies but are more difficult to recognize. In each circumstance, one must act quickly to prevent additional cerebral damage. Figure 169–2 shows a management algorithm for SE, and Table 169–5 presents a sample management protocol for drug administration.[35] Patients with simple partial SE or epilepsia partialis continua are at less risk for development of widespread cerebral damage and are also less likely to respond to the aggressive approach outlined in Table 169–5. In these patients, correcting underlying problems such as nonketotic hyperosmolar hyperglycemia is crucial. Errors in terminating SE include (1) inadequate dosing of effective drugs and (2) continued use of drugs that are ineffective in the case in question.

The conventional agents used in first-line of treatment of SE are the benzodiazepines (especially lorazepam, diazepam, and midazolam), phenytoin, and phenobarbital. SE that is refractory to the traditional agents is treated with continuous infusions of the short-acting barbiturates, midazolam, or propofol. A recent multicenter clinical trial comparing lorazepam alone, phenytoin alone, diazepam followed by phenytoin, and phenobarbital alone as the initial drug treatment for GCSE has been reported.[36] In this study, the highest rate of successful treatment of "overt" GCSE was achieved with lorazepam. There was no demonstrable difference among these four drug regimens in the initial treatment of "subtle" GCSE. Lorazepam has been our agent of first choice for terminating SE for many years and remains so with support from this study.

Advantages of lorazepam over diazepam are its duration of action against SE (4 to 14 hours instead of 20 minutes) and its higher initial response rate. Europeans often use midazolam or clonazepam initially. Midazolam is useful for refractory SE.[37] Respiratory depression is the major adverse effect of the benzodiazepines, especially when they are given together with barbiturates or paraldehyde.

Phenytoin is an effective anti-SE agent; however, the constraint on the rate of intravenous administration is a concern in treatment of SE. Phenytoin has a long duration of action when an adequate dose is given (a 20-μg/kg dose produces a serum level above 20 μg/mL for 24 hours). Adding 5 μg/kg may be useful when 20 μg/kg fails to stop SE.[44] Fosphenytoin can be administered by a more rapid intravenous infusion and has fewer cardiovascular side effects than phenytoin. Free phenytoin levels reach a therapeutic range 10 to 20 minutes after infusion of fosphenytoin is started.[38, 39] Intramuscular injection of fosphenytoin in SE patients may be supported by the known pharmacokinetics of this route, but it should not be considered acceptable therapy for SE and should be reserved for those rare circumstances in which intravenous access cannot be achieved. Fosphenytoin will probably supplant phenytoin for emergency management of SE.[40]

Some advocate use of phenobarbital as a first-line drug,[41] but typically it was used as a third-line agent, after administration of a benzodiazepine and phenytoin.[42] Although this approach has been widely accepted by the neurologist community, for two reasons we rarely use phenobarbital: (1) Only a small percentage of patients who have not benefited from treatment with two anticonvulsants respond to a third conventional agent,[43] and (2), at least an additional 20 minutes is required to obtain control in the few patients who do respond. Phenobarbital remains an important drug in the man-

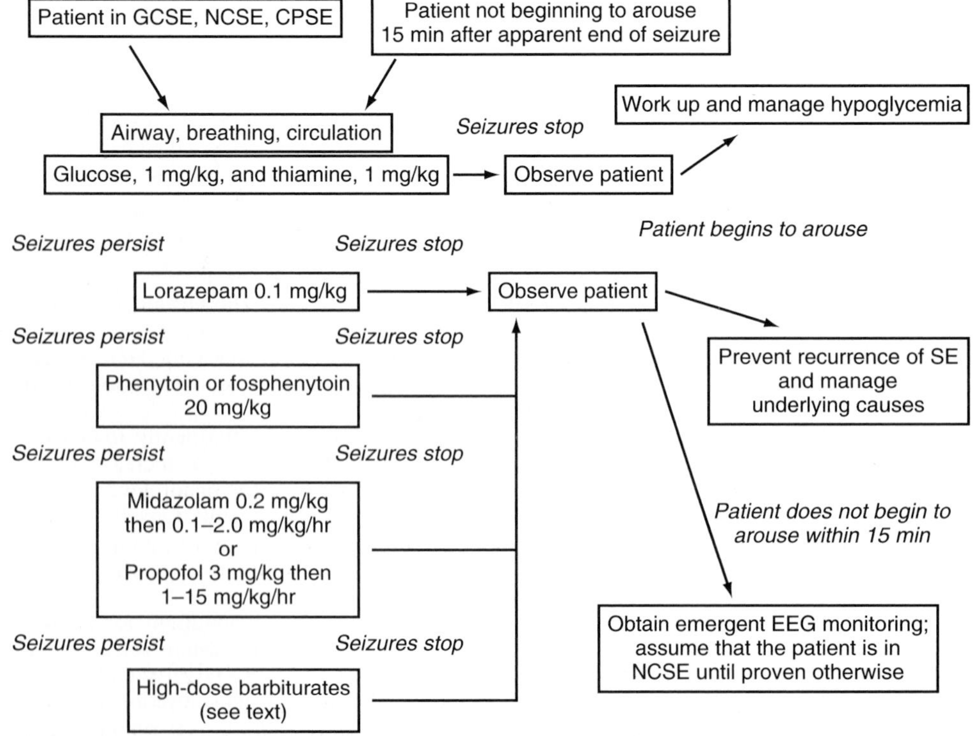

Figure 169–2. Management algorithm for status epilepticus. GCSE = generalized convulsive status epilepticus; NCSE = nonconvulsive status epilepticus; CPSE = complex partial status epilepticus; EEG = electroencephalogram.

TABLE 169–5. Suggested Protocol for Treatment of Status Epilepticus

1. Establish an airway, provide oxygen, and ensure ventilation. If neuromuscular junction blockade is required for intubation, use a short-acting agent (e.g., succinylcholine or vecuronium).
2. Determine blood pressure. If the patient is hypotensive, begin volume replacement or the use of vasoactive agents (or both) as indicated. Patients with generalized convulsive SE (GCSE) who present with hypotension usually require admission to a critical care unit. Do not treat hypertension until SE is controlled, since terminating SE usually substantially corrects it, and many of the agents used to terminate SE can produce hypotension.
3. Unless the patient is known to be normoglycemic or hyperglycemic, administer dextrose (1 mg/kg) and thiamine (1 mg/kg).
4. Terminate SE. The following sequence is recommended (see text for details). Be cognizant of the potential of these drugs to eliminate the visible convulsive movements of GCSE when leaving the patient in nonconvulsive SE. Patients who do not begin to respond to external stimuli 15 minutes after the apparent termination of GCSE should be considered at risk for nonconvulsive SE and should undergo emergent electroencephalographic (EEG) monitoring.
   a. Give lorazepam (0.1 mg/kg) at a rate of 0.04 mg/kg/min. This drug should be diluted in an equal volume of the solution being used for IV infusion, as it is quite viscous. Most adult patients who respond do so by a total administered dose of 8 mg. The latency of effect is debated, but lack of response after 5 minutes should indicate failure.
   b. If SE persists after lorazepam administration, begin fosphenytoin (20 mg/kg) at 150 mg/min (dosed by phenytoin equivalent). Many investigators believe that an additional 5-mg/kg dose of phenytoin should be administered before the next line of therapy is attempted.
   c. If SE persists, administer midazolam (0.2 mg/kg) as a bolus, followed by an infusion of 0.1 to 2.0 mg/kg/hr to achieve seizure control (as determined by EEG monitoring). Intubate the patient at this stage if this has not already been accomplished. A patient reaching this stage should be treated in a critical care unit.
   d. Should the seizure not be controlled with midazolam, administer propofol or pentobarbital. Propofol is given as a continuous infusion at a rate of 1 to 15 mg/kg/hr to achieve seizure control (as determined by EEG monitoring). A bolus dose of propofol (3.0 mg/kg) is often given but may increase the occurrence of hypotension. Pentobarbital is given as a bolus dose of 12 mg/kg at a rate of 0.2 to 0.4 mg/kg/min as tolerated, followed by an infusion of 0.25 to 2.0 mg/kg/hr, as determined by EEG monitoring (with an initial goal of burst-suppression; in some cases, an isoelectric electroencephalogram may be required to eliminate all electrical seizures). Most patients require systemic and pulmonary arterial catheterization, with fluid and vasoactive drug therapy as indicated to maintain blood pressure. For other complications of this treatment, see text.
5. Prevent recurrence of SE. The choice of drugs depends greatly on the cause of SE and the patient's medical and social situation. In general, patients not previously receiving anticonvulsants whose SE is easily controlled often respond well to long-term treatment with phenytoin or carbamazepine. In contrast, others (e.g., patients with acute encephalitis) will require two or three anticonvulsants at "toxic" levels (e.g., phenobarbital, >100 μg/mL) to be weaned from midazolam or pentobarbital and may still have occasional seizures.
6. Manage complications.
   a. Treat rhabdomyolysis with vigorous saline diuresis to prevent acute renal failure; urinary alkalinization may be a useful adjunct. If definitive treatment of GCSE takes longer than expected because of hypotension or arrhythmias, consider neuromuscular junction blockade under EEG monitoring.
   b. Hyperthermia usually remits rapidly after termination of SE. External cooling usually suffices if core temperature remains elevated. In rare instances, cool peritoneal lavage or extracorporeal blood cooling may be required. High-dose pentobarbital generally produces poikilothermia.
   c. The treatment of cerebral edema occurring secondary to SE has not been well studied. When substantial edema is present, suspect that SE and cerebral edema are both manifestations of the same underlying condition. Hyperventilation and mannitol may be valuable if edema is life-threatening. Edema due to SE is vasogenic in origin; thus, steroids may be useful as well.

agement of simple partial SE and for patients who are being weaned from high-dose midazolam or anesthetic barbiturates.

Pentobarbital and thiopental infusions are usually reserved for refractory SE.[38] Although these drugs are effective in sufficiently large doses, their side effects can limit their use and may be fatal.[44] They are important, however, when other modalities have failed (see Table 169–5). Endotracheal intubation and mechanical ventilation are mandatory when large doses of barbiturates are used, and both continuous EEG and invasive hemodynamic monitoring are strongly recommended. Severe hypotension is the most frequent side effect of pentobarbital therapy, and its occurrence is associated with increased risk of death.[45] An increased incidence of nosocomial respiratory tract infections has been reported in patients treated with pentobarbital infusion.[46] An effect on leukocyte function by the barbiturates (and other sedative agents) has been postulated. Despite these side effects, barbiturate anesthesia should not be rapidly discontinued if it is successful in terminating refractory SE; rather, continuing therapy for at least 48 hours, gradual tapering of the infusion dose, and administering phenobarbital during the drug taper are recommended.[47]

Although intravenous paraldehyde has been abandoned, it is still useful. The current formulation is licensed only for enteral use. It can be given every 3 hours through a polytef (Teflon)-coated nasogastric tube or rectally via a rubber catheter. The enteral form can be filtered for intramuscular injection; it should be delivered deep into the lateral gluteal muscles while special care is taken to avoid the sciatic nerves. This route of administration should be confined to a few doses, when rectal or oral treatment is not feasible.

Isoflurane, an inhaled anesthetic agent, controls refractory SE; however, it is difficult to deliver such a gas outside the operating suite or the recovery area. It has no known advantage over intravenous anticonvulsants, and it can raise intracranial pressure.

Propofol has been reported to be effective in the treating of refractory SE but has not been directly compared with other compounds.[48, 49] It may offer lower risk of ventilatory depression and promote more rapid awakening, as compared with other drugs, when it is discontinued. Early fears of a possible proconvulsant effect appear to be unfounded, although withdrawal convulsions may occur if the drug is abruptly terminated. A dose range of 1 to 15 mg/kg/hour has been studied,[50] although the actual upper limit is unknown. Acidosis and oxygenation difficulties have been reported in children,[51] but the drug can also be useful in this setting.[52] Careful monitoring of creatine kinase and oxygen saturation would be prudent.

Special Considerations in Children

Treatment of seizures or SE in critically ill children generally parallels that for adults. Intravenous access is often more difficult to achieve in children. Lorazepam and diazepam can both be administered by the rectal route in doses similar to those used for intravenous administration for acute treatment of seizures (usually 0.5 mg/kg per rectum for both agents). Lorazepam is probably the first-choice agent for terminating SE in children, as for adults. One group reported that children receiving diazepam for SE required intubation more often than did comparable children receiving lorazepam. Another group has reported that in the prehospital setting fewer follow-up doses were required for control of seizures with lorazepam than with diazepam.[53] Midazolam administered by continuous infusion is effective in refractory SE in children, and one group reported successful treatment of 24 children with midazolam infusion at 1 to 18 μg/kg per minute without the need for endotracheal intubation or mechanical ventilation.[54]

As with adults, rapid control of SE in children achieved with benzodiazepines should be followed by administration of a longer-acting agent, such as intravenous phenytoin (20 mg/kg), fosphenytoin (20 mg PE/kg), or phenobarbital (10 to 20 mg/kg).[55] The rate of conversion of fosphenytion to phenytoin is probably the same in children as in adults. Intramuscular injection of fosphenytoin may be particularly advantageous for preventing recurrent seizures in children without intravenous access.

References

1. Wilks S: Bromide and iodide of potassium in epilepsy. Med Times Gaz (Lond) 1861; 2:635–636.
2. Gowers WR: Epilepsy and other chronic convulsive diseases: Their causes, symptoms, and treatment. London, J and A Churchill, 1881.
3. Bleck TP, Klawans HL: Mechanisms of epilepsy and anticonvulsant action. *In:* Textbook of Clinical Neuropharmacology. Klawans HL, Goetz CG, Tanner CM (Eds). New York, Raven Press, 1992, pp 23–30.
4. Weschler IS: Intravenous injection of paraldehyde for control of convulsions. JAMA 1940; 114:2198.
5. Gastaut H, Naquet R, Poiré R, Tassinari CA: Treatment of status epilepticus with diazepam (Valium). Epilepsia 1965; 6:167–182.
6. Wijdicks EFM, Sharbrough FW: New-onset seizures in critically ill patients. Neurology 1993; 43:1042–1044.
7. Bleck TP, Smith MC, Pierre-Louis JC, Jares JJ, Murray J, Hansen CA: Neurologic complications of critical medical illnesses. Crit Care Med 1993; 21:98–103.
8. Lacroix J, Deal C, Gauthier M, et al: Admissions to a pediatric intensive care unit for status epilepticus: A 10-year experience. Crit Care Med 1994; 22:827–832.
9. Aminoff MJ, Simon RP: Status epilepticus: Causes, clinical features and consequences in 98 patients. Am J Med 1980; 69:657–666.
10. Hauser WA: Status epilepticus Epidemiologic considerations. Neurology 1990; 40(Suppl 2):9–13.
11. DeLorenzo RJ, Hauser WA, Towne AR, et al: A prospective study of status epilepticus in Richmond, Virginia. Neurology 1996; 46:1029–1035.
12. Logroscino G, Hesdorffer DC, Cascino G, Annegers JF, Hauser WA: Short-term mortality after a first episode of status epilepticus. Epilepsia 1997; 38:1344–1349.
13. Lothman EW, Bertram EH: Epileptogenic effects of status epilepticus. Epilepsia 1993; 34 (Suppl 1):S59–S70.
14. Treiman DM, Delgado-Escueta AV: Complex partial status epilepticus. Adv Neurol 1983; 34:69–81.
15. Commission on Classification and Terminology of the International League Against Epilepsy: Proposal for revised clinical and electroencephalographic classification of epileptic seizures. Epilepsia 1981; 22:489–501.
16. Bleck TP: Metabolic Encephalopathy. *In:* Emergent and Urgent Neurology. 2nd ed. Weiner WJ, Shulman LM (Eds). Philadelphia, Lippincott, 1999, pp 223–253.
17. Bleck TP: Status epilepticus. *In:* Textbook of Clinical Neuropharmacology. 2nd ed. Klawans HL, Goetz CG, Tanner CM (Eds). New York: Raven Press, 1992, pp 65–73.
18. Lothman EW: The biochemical basis and pathophysiology of status epilepticus. Neurology 1990; 40 (Suppl 2):13–23.
19. Lowenstein DH, Simon RP, Sharp FR: The pattern of 72-kDa heat shock protein-like immunoreactivity in the rat brain following fluothyl-induced status epilepticus. Brain Res 1990; 531:173–182.
20. Wasterlain CG, Fujikawa DG, Penix L, Sankar R: Pathophysiological mechanisms of brain damage from status epilepticus. Epilepsia 1993; 34 (Suppl 1):S37–S53.
21. Treiman DM: Generalized convulsive status epilepticus in the adult. Epilepsia 1993; 34 (Suppl 1):S2–S11.
22. Walton NY: Systemic effects of generalized convulsive status epilepticus. Epilepsia 1993; 34 (Suppl 1):S54–S58.
23. Ficker DM, Westmoreland BF, Sharbrough FW: Epileptiform abnormalities in hepatic encephalopathy. J Clin Neurophysiol 1997; 14:230–234.
24. Bolton CF, Young GB, Zochodne DW: The neurologic complications of sepsis. Ann Neurol 1993; 33:94–100.
25. Kaplan PW: Nonconvulsive status epilepticus in the emergency room. Epilepsia 1996; 37:643–650.
26. Singh BM, Strobos RJ: Epilepsia partialis continua associated with nonketotic hyperglycemia: Clinical and biochemical profile of 21 patients. Ann Neurol 1980; 8:155–160.
27. Rowbotham MC, Lowenstein DH: Neurologic complications of cocaine use. Annu Rev Med 1990; 41:417–422.
28. Morres CA, Dire DJ: Movement disorders as a manifestation of nonketotic hyperglycemia. J Emerg Med 1989; 7:359–364.
29. Hennis A, Corbin D, Fraser H: Focal seizures and non-ketotic hyperglycemia. J Neurol Neurosurg Psychiatry 1992; 55:195–197.
30. First Seizure Trial Group: Randomized clinical trial of the efficacy of antiepileptic drugs in reducing the risk of relapse after a first unprovoked tonic-clonic seizure. Neurology 1993; 43:478–483.
31. Musicco M, Beghi E, Solari A, Viani F: Treatment of first tonic-clonic seizure does not improve the prognosis of epilepsy. First Seizure Trial Group (FIRST Group). Neurology 1997; 49:991–998.
32. Browne TR: Fosphenytoin (Cerebyx). Clin Neuropharmacol 1997; 20:1–12.
33. Fierro LS, Savulich DH, Benezra DA: Safety of fosphenytoin sodium. Am J Health Syst Pharm 1996; 53:2707–2712.
34. Smith MC, Bleck TP: Toxicity of anticonvulsants. *In:* Textbook of Clinical Neuropharmacology. 2nd ed. Klawans HL, Goetz CG, Tanner CM (Eds). New York, Raven Press, 1992, pp 45–64.
35. Ford G, Bleck TP: Seizures in the intensive care unit. *In:* Current Therapy in Critical Care Medicine. 3rd ed. Parrillo JE (Ed). Toronto, BC Decker, 1997, pp 318–323.
36. Treiman DM, Meyers PD, Walton NY, et al: A comparison of four treatments for generalized convulsive status epilepticus: Veterans Affairs Status Epilepticus Cooperative Study Group. N Engl J Med 1998; 339:792–798.
37. Chuilli DA, Ternfrup TE, Kanter RK: The influence of diazepam or lorazepam on the frequency of endotracheal intubation in childhood status epilepticus. J Emerg Med 1991; 9:13–17.
38. Osorio I, Reed RC: Treatment of refractory generalized tonic-clonic status epilepticus with pentobarbital anesthesia after high-dose phenytoin. Epilepsia 1989; 30:464–471.
39. Leppik IE, Boucher BA, Wilder BJ, et al: Pharmacokinetics and safety of a phenytoin prodrug given IV or IM. Neurology 1990; 40:456–460.
40. Runge JW, Allen FH: Emergency treatment of status epilepticus. Neurology 1996; 46(Suppl 1):S20–S23.
41. Shaner DM, McCurdy SA, Herring MO, Gabor AJ: Treatment of status epilepticus: A prospective comparison of diazepam and phenytoin versus phenobarbital and optional phenytoin. Neurology 1988; 38:202–206.
42. Yaffe K, Lowenstein DH: Prognostic factors of pentobarbital therapy for refractory generalized status epilepticus. Neurology 1993; 43:895–900.
43. Bleck TP: Status epilepticus. Univ Rep Epilepsy 1992; 1:1–7.
44. Bleck TP: Therapy for status epilepticus. Clin Neuropharmacol 1983; 6:255–268.
45. Bleck TP: High-dose pentobarbital treatment of refractory status epilepticus: A meta-analysis of published studies. Epilepsia 1992; 33:5.
46. Sato M, Tanaka S, Suzuki K, et al: Complications associated with barbiturate therapy. Resuscitation 1989; 17:233–241.
47. Krishnamurthy KB, Drislane FW: Relapse and survival after barbi-

turate anesthetic treatment of refractory status epilepticus. Epilepsia 1996; 37:863–867.
48. Mackenzie SJ, Kapadia F, Grant IS: Propofol infusion for control of status epilepticus. Anaesthesia 1990; 45:1043–1045.
49. Kuisma M, Roine RO: Propofol in the prehospital treatment of convulsive status epilepticus. Epilepsia 1995; 36:1241–1243.
50. Stecker MM, Skaar DJ, Dulaney E, O'Meeghan R, Raps EC, Kramer TH: Treatment of refractory status epilepticus with propofol: Clinical and pharmacokinetic findings. Epilepsia 1998; 39:18–26.
51. Hanna JP, Ramundo ML: Rhabdomyolysis and hypoxia associated with prolonged propofol infusion in children. Neurology 1998; 50:301–303.
52. Harrison AM, Schunk JE, Lugo RA: Treatment of convulsive status epilepticus with propofol: Case report. Pediatr Emerg Care 1997; 13:420–422.
53. Appleton R, Sweeney A, Choonara I, et al: Lorazepam versus diazepam in the acute treatment of epileptic seizures and status epilepticus. Develop Med Child Neurol 1995; 37:682–688.
54. Rivera R, Segnini M, Baltodano A, et al: Midazolam in the treatment of status epilepticus in children. Crit Care Med 1993; 21:991–994.
55. Segeleon JE, Haun SE: Status epilepticus in children. Pediatr Ann 1996; 25:380–386.

170

Pediatric Neurosurgical Emergencies

Derek A. Bruce, MB, ChB • Dale Swift, MD
Charles Teo, MD • William J. Morris, MD

Most neurosurgical emergencies, sudden deteriorations in nervous system function that require immediate intervention, are a result of or are associated with elevated intracranial pressure (ICP). Understanding the normal physiologic mechanisms that maintain the balance between pressure and volume inside the dural sac is necessary to understand what occurs under pathologic circumstances.

INTRACRANIAL CONTENTS

The intradural space consists of the intraspinal space plus the intracranial space. The volume of this space in an adult is approximately 1700 mL, of which approximately 10% is spinal fluid, 10% blood volume, and 80% brain and spinal cord tissue. In a neonate, this volume is about 400 mL. The spinal dural sac is not always fully distended, and some increase in volume of the intradural space can be achieved at the expense of compression of the spinal epidural veins, thus permitting some distention of the spinal dural sac. In an infant with an open fontanelle and open sutures, some small increase in volume of the intradural space can be achieved by separation of the sutures and distention of the fontanelle. This increase in volume is not great and, if the rise in intracranial volume is rapid, is not adequate to prevent the occurrence of very high intracranial pressure.

Volume-Pressure Relationship

Once the dural sac is fully distended, any further increase in volume of one component of the intracranial space must be offset by a decrease in volume of one of the other components if the pressure is to remain constant. The contents of the intracranial space are brain, blood, and spinal fluid. When a formula is used to represent the intracranial volume-pressure relationships, a term is often included to represent the presence of any other intracranial mass (e.g., tumor or hematoma); as follows[1]:

$$V_{csf} + V_{blood} + V_{brain} + V_{other} = V_{constant} = V_{eq} + V_e$$

where V_{csf} is volume of cerebrospinal fluid, V_{blood} is volume of blood in cerebral vessels, V_{brain} is volume of brain tissue, V_{eq} is total volume of the intracranial space, and V_e is the elastic component of the intracranial contents. This relationship is graphically represented in Figure 170–1. When the volume of one component increases, the others decrease, and the pressure remains constant. The most effective compensations are displacement of cerebrospinal fluid (CSF) from the cranial space to the spinal space and reabsorption of CSF across the arachnoid villi. As the ICP rises, some decrease in CSF production may occur, further aiding compensation. The next major volume compensation is that of a decrease in the intracranial pial blood volume. The pial venous blood is displaced into the venous sinuses, thereby serving to maintain the ICP. Finally, the brain itself can be compressed to compensate for increases in volume. This is most easily demonstrated in the setting of acute hydrocephalus, in which the brain is compressed by the CSF, resulting in ventricular enlargement; or in the case of an acute epidural hematoma, in which the brain is compressed and distorted by the mass of the hematoma. The compressibility of the brain depends on several factors that affect the elasticity of the brain (V_e), these include the water content, the extent of myelination, and the vascular turgor from systemic arterial pressure.

As a result of these compensatory mechanisms, a certain increase in one or several of the components of the intracranial space can occur with little change in the ICP. The volume increase that can be tolerated depends on the rate of increase and the number of the components that are increasing. Once this volume is exceeded, any further increase in volume is

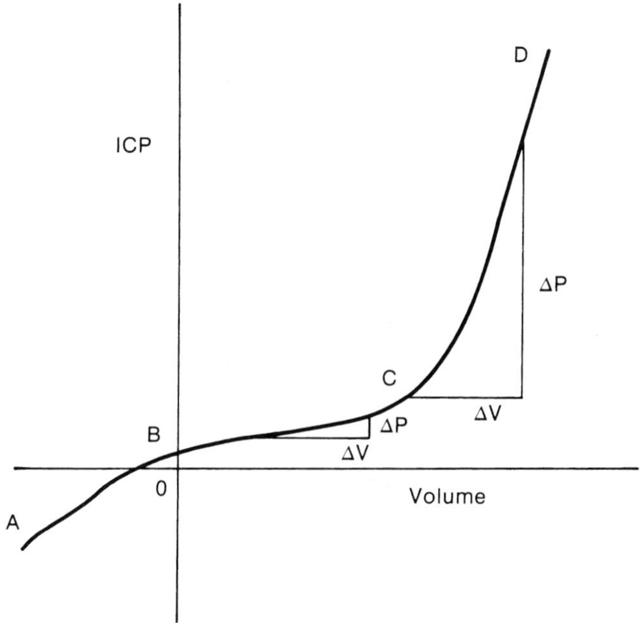

Figure 170–1. An idealized pressure-volume curve. The area on the *left* below 0, AB, represents the period during which the spinal sac is not fully distended. BC = period of volume compensation; CD = period of exhausted compensation.

tolerated less well, and some rise in pressure occurs because less volume compensation can occur; this is best demonstrated in Figure 170-1, which illustrates a biexponential curve showing a segment of little change in pressure despite an increase in volume, followed by a progressively steeper increase in pressure for each equal change in volume. This later segment, the area of limited or absent volume compensation, is increasingly dependent on the elastic properties of the intracranial contents to prevent major increases in ICP.

Anatomy of the Intracranial Space

The intradural space is divided into a series of compartments by the foramen magnum and the folds of the dura, the falx, and the tentorium. The frontal fossa is separated from the middle fossa by the lesser wing of the sphenoid bone. The right half of the supratentorial space is separated from the left by the falx cerebri, and the supratentorial space is separated from the infratentorial space by the tentorium. Finally, the intracranial space becomes the intraspinal canal at the foramen magnum. These compartments are important because rises in pressure in one compartment can result in distortion and displacement of brain into another compartment, with consequent tissue and vascular compression that can result in brain dysfunction and brain damage.

Frontal mass lesion can cause herniation across the lesser wing of the sphenoid, with resultant compression of the intracranial carotid artery and subsequent ischemia *(transalar herniation)*. Expanding lesions on one side of the supratentorial space can cause herniation of the pericallosal gyrus to the other side, under the falx cerebri, with compression of the anterior cerebral arteries and resultant ischemia *(subfalcine herniation)*. The most common cerebral herniation occurs at the tentorial hiatus, with distortion and displacement of the mesial temporal lobe or lobes, forcing the parahippocampal gyrus through the tentorial notch and producing compression of the brain stem–perforating vessels, the posterior cerebral arteries, and the perforating vessels to the thalamus *(transtentorial herniation)*. A mass in the posterior fossa can occasionally cause herniation of the cerebellar vermis upward through the tentorial notch and compression of the brain stem and posterior cerebral and thalamic perforating vessels *(upward herniation)*; this is most commonly precipitated by drainage of the lateral ventricles in the presence of a posterior fossa mass. Finally, herniation can occur at the foramen magnum, with displacement of the cerebellar tonsils through the foramen magnum and compression of the vertebral and posterior inferior cerebellar arteries and the medulla (*foramen magnum* or *cerebellar tonsilar herniation*).

It is clinically difficult to confirm the diagnosis of transalar herniation or subfalcine herniation, because they usually occur in an already comatose patient. Transtentorial herniation is recognized from a progression of symptoms that, in the awake patient, begin with increasingly severe headache, often coming in waves of pain, followed by somnolence and, eventually, loss of consciousness. The signs are of pupillary dilation, usually of the ipsilateral pupil (80%), due to compression of cranial nerve III, followed by hemiparesis of the opposite side due to compression and ischemia of the cerebral peduncle.

If the lesion is untreated, dilation of the opposite pupil occurs, with bilateral compression of cranial nerve III, bilateral hemiparesis, decerebrate posturing, bradycardia, hypertension, and, ultimately, apnea and death as a result of progressive compression of the brain stem, pons, and medulla. In children, the initial hemiparesis occurs on the side ipsilateral to the herniation 50% of the time, presumably because in the other 50%, the anatomy of the tentorial notch is such that the opposite cerebral peduncle is impacted against the tentorial edge, resulting in an ipsilateral hemiparesis. This discrepancy between the side of the enlarged pupil and the side of the hemiparesis can cause clinical confusion as to which side the mass lesion is on. This is easily resolved with a neuroimaging study.

Foramen magnum herniation may be identified from complaints of headache and neck pain. The pain may initially be relieved by extension of the neck. As herniation progresses, the medulla oblongata is compressed, with resulting hypertension, bradycardia, bradypnea, and, finally, apnea. The onset of apnea may be preceded only be severe headache or neck pain with no clinical signs.

Cerebral Blood Flow and Elevated Intracranial Pressure

As well as causing distortion and focal vascular compression, elevated ICP can affect general cerebral blood flow (CBF). The cerebral blood vessels exhibit autoregulation in response to changes in perfusion pressure. Perfusion pressure (CPP) is calculated as follows:

$$\text{CPP} + \text{MAP} - \text{MICP}$$

where MAP is mean systemic arterial pressure and MICP is mean intracranial pressure.

The cerebral vessels respond to decreases in perfusion pressure by vasodilating, decreasing resistance to flow and thus maintaining the same CBF despite either a decline in arterial pressure or an increase in ICP. The exact limits of autoregulation through the period of infancy and childhood are not known but probably range between 35 and 40 mm Hg at the lower end and greater than 100 mm Hg at the upper end. Below the limits of autoregulation, the CBF falls as the CPP is lowered. Cerebral metabolism is preserved to a CBF of about 50% of normal, after which some cerebral ischemia begins. As blood flow falls below 25% of normal, irreversible damage begins. Thus, autoregulation is a brain-protective mechanism against alterations in CPP. Trauma in children often leaves autoregulation intact, whereas ischemia seems more likely to abolish autoregulation, making the CBF more sensitive to small changes in the CPP.

Unfortunately, the status of autoregulation is not known in the clinical setting, and thus therapy is directed at maintaining normal or nearly normal ICP and MAP in hopes of preserving CBF. If the ICP is high enough or the MAP low enough, the CPP will be inadequate to maintain cerebral perfusion, and cerebral ischemia will result. The grossest manifestation of this situation is the cessation of CBF and death of the brain and thus the child.[2]

The common denominator for many neurosurgical emergencies is intracranial hypertension, with resultant cerebral herniation and focal ischemia or globally elevated ICP and diffuse cerebral ischemia. A cycle of problems occurs as the ICP rises. As noted earlier, during the early period of compensation, the addition of volume to the cranium may be tolerated. Over time, however, as compensation becomes exhausted, the addition of a similar volume may lead to a pressure wave that may rise to the level of the arterial pressure and result in cessation of CBF. As cerebral herniation progresses and the subarachnoid spaces are occluded, the transmission of pressure within the craniospinal axis is impeded. This results in a further loss of compensation and a larger increase in pressure for any given increase in volume. Frequent waves of elevated ICP may further abolish pressure autoregulation and make the brain more prone to ischemia at the same CPP. A progressive loss of compensatory ability often follows an intracranial catastrophe, and an increase in pressure that was tolerated in the first few hours after the insult may not be tolerated 24 hours later because of the gradual exhaustion of the compensatory mechanisms.

In a clinical setting, it is rare that the balance between one intracranial component and the others is preserved, because alterations in volume in all three components often occur in the same direction at the same time. After head injury, subarachnoid hemorrhage blocks the CSF pathways, interfering with pressure transmission, and increases CSF outflow resistance by clogging the arachnoid villi. CSF compensation is markedly limited. Intracranial hematomas or contusions result in greater brain volume, and the cerebral blood volume is increased as a result of hyperemia. All three components are affected at the same time, resulting in a very limited compensatory ability; therefore, increased ICP is common after severe head injury. A similar series of events—disturbance of the balance of equilibrium in several of the components of the intracranial space at the same time—occurs with many of the lesions that lead to the need for urgent neurosurgical treatment. The result of disturbed volume-pressure homeostasis is typically that of intermittent waves of ICP rather than continuously elevated pressure. The signs and symptoms can wax and wane such that the urgent need for therapy may not be recognized.

Resuscitation of a child with a neurosurgical catastrophe addresses the usual concerns about airway patency, ventilation, and circulation. The use of specific therapy to lower the ICP (e.g., mannitol or glycerol) depends on the evidence for elevated ICP and a history of rapid deterioration of level of consciousness with signs of cerebral herniation. The history is often the deciding factor, because absolute signs of intracranial hypertension are few and may not be present, depending on the rate of increase in ICP. Papilledema is a sure sign of intracranial hypertension but is often absent because of the rapidity of the onset of symptoms or because the anatomy of the subarachnoid space in the optic nerve is such that papilledema does not occur. After trauma, acute loss of consciousness is rarely the result of increased ICP, and there is no indication for routinely giving an osmotic diuretic to children in coma after head trauma.

When intracranial hypertension is suspected in a comatose child, endotracheal intubation is performed after bag-and-mask hyperventilation with 100% oxygen, followed by a nondepolarizing, short-acting muscle relaxant and sodium pentothal or a similar anesthetic. Once the airway is secured, the head is maintained in the midline position to avoid jugular vein compression, and if the blood pressure is in the normal range for age, the head is elevated 20% to 30%. If continued elevation of the ICP is an immediate concern, an ICP monitor can easily be placed after resuscitation.

Further therapy to lower the ICP is then given if necessary. In general, there is no single therapy for elevated ICP, which can have many possible causes. The selection of therapy should be based on the specific disorder causing the increased pressure; for example, ventricular drainage if there is hydrocephalus. Current recommendations to direct therapy to maintain a specific cerebral perfusion pressure[3] are misleading in children. The ideal CPP varies at different ages and is not established for any age of child. It is safer and more defined to attempt to maintain an ICP close to the normal range for the age of the child and a MAP at the high end of the normal range for age. Lowering the ICP is the appropriate direction for therapy when the primary disorder is a disturbance of the intracranial pressure-volume homeostasis. Raising the MAP is appropriate if there is systemic hypotension or suspected intracranial vasospasm. If the ICP cannot be adequately lowered, attempts to improve the CPP by manipulating the arterial pressure are reasonable even in the absence of suspected vasospasm.

The use of controlled hyperventilation is a very effective way to lower accurately elevated ICP, and despite the current concerns that too much hyperventilation can be dangerous,[4, 5] high ICP is certainly dangerous and can often result in the rapid death of the child. There are no reports proving that hyperventilation is bad for the patient, and this is a mode of therapy that is very effective and should not be discarded.[6, 7]

TRAUMA

Traumatic unconsciousness is a neurologic emergency that rarely requires immediate surgical intervention. Elevated ICP is rarely the cause of unconsciousness after trauma but is a common associated phenomenon. The initial treatment is standard resuscitation. Twenty per cent to 30% of children with a Glasgow Coma Scale score of 8 or less (coma) require surgical therapy for the following disorders:

- Epidural, subdural, and intracerebral hematomas,
- Compound depressed skull fractures,
- Penetrating trauma to the brain or spinal cord.

Traumatic injuries to the brain occur throughout childhood and adolescence, but the etiology of trauma and the physiologic response vary with age.

Birth Trauma

Intracranial hematomas are rarely encountered in the neonatal period. Epidural hematomas occur in the supratentorial and infratentorial spaces, and if they produce significant cerebral compression, such hematomas require evacuation. Before any surgery is performed in a neonate, clotting studies must be done and any abnormalities corrected.

Subdural hematomas are best treated by medical means to control the ICP before resorting to surgery. Surgery to drain subdural hematomas in neonates can be very difficult because of the very high water content of the neonate's brain. It is very difficult to prevent the brain from swelling through the dural opening with resulting increased injury to the cortex. Subdural taps can relieve some of the pressure, and every effort is made to avoid open surgery unless the situation is life-threatening.

Most intracerebral hematomas in neonates are hemorrhagic infarctions or venous hemorrhages, for which surgery is rarely indicated. The brain is 90% water, and achieving hemostasis during surgery can be very difficult. In addition, the pia mater and cerebral vessels can be easily peeled off the brain by the suction apparatus, resulting in greater damage.

Intraventricular hemorrhage is seen most commonly in the preterm infant and rarely requires acute intervention. Efforts at ventricular drainage in the first few days are rarely helpful, because the blood is clotted. The use of agents to dissolve the clots does not appear to be of value. As the clots spontaneously resolves, hydrocephalus develops in a number of the infants and requires a subgaleal reservoir or a subgaleal shunt for temporary relief until the patients are large enough for a permanent ventricular shunt. If a baby is taking enteric nutrition, the permanent shunt can be placed once the baby weighs more than 1000 g. In most cases of intracranial hemorrhage occurring around the time of birth, surgery is a last resort.

Non–Birth-Related Trauma

Compound Depressed Skull Fracture

Compound depressed skull fractures are, potentially, open wounds of the brain and require urgent surgical debridement as soon as a patient is stabilized. These fractures are the most common reason for surgery after trauma in children. The aims are as follows:

1. To debride the brain of contamination, including bone fragments.
2. To remove any associated hematomas.
3. To repair the dura in order to prevent cerebral herniation.
4. To reconstruct the skull either with the fragments present or with split cranial bone.

It is usually possible to replace the fragments and avoid a second, reconstructive operation.

Other forms of penetrating skull trauma require surgical exploration (e.g., dog bites, dart injuries). Gunshot wounds of the head and brain are increasingly common in children and usually require surgery to debride the bone fragments from the brain, remove intracranial hematomas, and repair the dura and cranium. The indications for surgery depend on whether the child is likely to survive the injury. Nothing is to be gained by operating on a child who is clearly going to die as a result of the gunshot.

Epidural Hematoma

Epidural hematomas are either venous (a result of bleeding from the diploic space of the skull after fracture) or arterial (from rupture of branches of the middle meningeal or posterior meningeal arteries). They are found in 6% to 8% of children who undergo computed tomography (CT) scanning after head injury. Epidural hematomas in children are almost equally divided into three clinical presentations; one third of the patients are never unconscious, one third are unconscious from the time of injury, and one third demonstrate a lucid period followed by unconsciousness. Early CT scanning to identify the lesion is important, because the recovery is closely correlated with the level of consciousness at the time of surgical evacuation of the clot and with the presence of other cerebral injury.

The location of the typical epidural hematoma in children younger than 8 years is rather higher in the parietal and temporal parietal area than the typical anterior temporal location seen in adults; thus, blindly placing bur holes is rarely advisable. A CT scan should be obtained whenever possible to pinpoint the exact location of the lesion and to identify other intracranial lesions. If a child with a skull fracture is showing signs of rapidly progressing herniation, and surgery must be done emergently without a CT scan, the craniotomy should be centered over the middle of any fracture. Most epidural hematomas require surgical removal by craniotomy, but small lesions (especially frontal ones) in the presence of normal consciousness are often treated conservatively.[8] These latter lesions often resolve in a week or two with no therapy.

Subdural Hematomas

Subdural hematomas are usually the result of either tearing of the bridging cortical veins from acceleration-deceleration injury or tearing of the cerebral cortical arteries from brain laceration. The incidence varies from 5% to 30% in children hospitalized for head injury. The highest frequency is in children younger than 1 year, and the cause of trauma is usually child abuse.

In infants and toddlers, the lesions are usually small, bilateral, and interhemispheric, and they rarely require surgery. In a child who has an open fontanelle and is in extremis, the fontanelle can be tapped and bloody fluid removed, immediately lowering the ICP. The major problem in the abused babies is usually the underlying brain swelling, and treatment with endotracheal intubation, ICP monitoring, and medical management of the increased ICP is the mainstay of therapy. The finding of an acute subdural hematoma and retinal hemorrhages is pathognomonic of child abuse, except when a high-speed accident has occurred and has been witnessed (e.g., automobile accident). This statement is not necessarily true for infants with chronic subdural hematomas or with dilated extracerebral spaces that predated the trauma.

In older children, subdural hematomas are usually the result of severe acceleration-deceleration injuries that result in tearing of the cerebral cortex and arterial rupture. They are usually associated with severe brain swelling and elevated ICP, and the child is usually comatose. Many of these lesions do not require surgery because the goal of treatment is to control the brain swelling and ICP. In general, if the brain distortion is considerably more than the width of the subdural hematoma and the subdural hematoma is less than 1 cm, surgery is not performed; however, the indications for surgery vary with the condition of the child and the neurosurgeon's individual criteria for surgery in this setting. Even if surgery is performed, postoperative brain swelling can be expected, and ICP monitoring and medical control of the ICP are likely to be necessary in the postoperative period.

Intracerebral Hematomas and Contusions

Most intracerebral hematomas occur following severe head trauma, often in association with diffuse axonal injury. They are encountered in 3% to 5% of postinjury CT scans in children with a Glasgow Coma Scale score below 8. Many hematomas or contusions are in the deep white mater or basal ganglia, and it is rare that surgical evacuation is necessary or advisable. Affected children are at risk for elevated ICP and may require intense medical treatment to control brain swelling and edema.[2] Large, more superficial hematomas are occasionally identified, and they may require surgical evacuation to control herniation and severely elevated ICP. Surgery, if necessary, should focus on evacuation of the hematoma, preserving as much brain tissue as possible.

Acute cerebral contusions are relatively rarely reported after head injury in children and in general do not need surgical resection, primarily because of the risk of removing brain that could recover. In follow-up studies of children with moderate or severe head injuries, a high incidence of contusions has been identified (50%), the majority in the frontal area, followed by the anterior temporal tip.[9] Although some of these lesions were visible on the original CT scans, the majority were not. These findings imply that contusions are common after head trauma in children but rarely require surgery.

Post-traumatic subarachnoid hemorrhage, brain swelling, brain edema, arterial spasm, and focal strokes do not require surgery.[10] Spasm is probably more common than has been appreciated, and the use of blood pressure elevation can be helpful for improving cerebral perfusion in this setting.[11-13] The vascular spasm that lends itself to such therapy is believed to occur after 24 to 48 hours. The earliest-measured CBF value after head trauma, however, is usually the lowest recorded,[14] and it is not clear whether some or all of this decrease is the result of acute vasospasm, metabolic depression, or a combination of both. The role of vasopressor therapy in the first few hours after trauma has not been evaluated. Some delayed traumatic lesions can require immediate surgery; they include delayed intracranial hemorrhage, after 7 to 10 days; ruptured traumatic aneurysm, with a peak incidence around 10 to 14 days; and post-traumatic hydrocephalus, which can occur anytime up to 1 year after the trauma but most commonly requires treatment in the first 3 months.

Nonaccidental Trauma

Any child under 2 years of age who presents to the emergency department (ED) with altered consciousness and the following features must be regarded as having sustained a possible nonaccidental injury.

No "good" history explaining the injury

- A history of minor trauma
- Unwitnessed trauma
- Trauma that is inappropriate for the child's age and developmental level

Infants with unexplained respiratory arrest, seizures, fevers, and somnolence are also at high risk for having sustained an abusive injury.

The early examination must include a look at the optic fundus to evaluate the presence or absence of retinal hemorrhages as well as a complete physical examination looking for any other evidence of trauma. If retinal hemorrhages are seen, a tentative diagnosis of nonaccidental injury must be considered, and the assumption made that severe brain injury may have occurred. The fundus should be examined before lumbar puncture is performed and before therapy appropriate to control or prevention of intracranial hypertension is stated. Such therapy consists of endotracheal intubation, head elevation, mild hyperventilation, moderate fluid replacement with isotonic solutions, and antiseizure medications if the child has seizures. Sudden infant death syndrome (SIDS) may also be a manifestation of child abuse, and appropriate examination of all such cases should be performed before the death is dismissed as accidental.[15]

VASCULAR LESIONS

In neonates, early, high-output cardiac failure can occur with vascular lesions in the cranium associated with high volume shunting of blood from the arterial to the venous circulations. The most common lesion is a *vein of Galen aneurysm*, which is a malformation of the vessels that supply the choroid plexus of the third ventricle. It is usually not a true arteriovenous malformation but is a direct shunting of branches of any or all of the following vessels into the vein of Galen: anterior cerebral, posterior lateral and medial choroidal, thalamic and hypothalamic perforators, posterior cerebral, anterior choroidal, and least likely the middle cerebral artery. The term *aneurysm* is misleading: The aneurysm is of the internal cerebral veins or the vein of Galen and the straight sinus, and is not arterial. This lesion rarely bleeds in the first few months of life, and the goal of therapy is to control the heart failure, which can often be accomplished by medical means. If medical therapy is unsuccessful, selective embolization of particular arterial feeders with coils or balloons may help cut down the flow and permit control of the cardiac failure.

Another option is embolization of the venous aneurysm via a transvenous route or directly through the torcula. Rarely is open operation to control the feeders successful in the first few days of life. If the heart failure can be controlled for 6 weeks or more and then recurs, direct surgery to occlude the shunting arteries can be successfully accomplished. The options for venous or arterial embolization remain open at any age and are possibly less dangerous, although the risks of hemorrhage, pulmonary embolization by the coils, and heart attack remain concerns with any mode of therapy.

Other arteriovenous shunts that occur in neonates usually affect the dura mater, with or without cerebral involvement. Early treatment focuses on control of the heart failure with embolization if necessary. Early open surgery is rarely advisable because of the high risk of excessive blood loss.

Arteriovenous Malformations

Arteriovenous malformations (AVMs) are congenital anomalies of the vascular system that can occur anywhere in the cerebrum, brain stem, cerebellum, and spinal cord. Lesions in the spinal cord are rare in children. An AVM becomes a neurosurgical emergency as a result of rupture of usually venous components of the AVM and ensuing acute hemorrhage of blood at arterial pressure into either the subarachnoid space, the cerebral substance, or the ventricular system.

AVMs are four times more likely to be the cause of intracranial hemorrhage in children than aneurysms.[16, 17] The result of AVM hemorrhage is a sudden increase in ICP, manifested clinically by the sudden onset of severe headache or sudden loss of consciousness. The signs and symptoms depend on the location of the hemorrhage and can include hemiparesis, aphasia, hemisensory loss, or hemianopsia if the hemorrhage occurs into the supratentorial brain, or focal brain stem symptoms or acute hydrocephalus if the hemorrhage is in the posterior fossa. The only manifestation may be acute loss of consciousness. The mortality from the first bleed of an AVM has been reported to be as high as 24% in children.[5]

Standard resuscitation is followed by a CT scan to confirm the diagnosis of intraventricular or intraparenchymal hemorrhage. Treatment varies according to the clinical state of the patient. With signs of progressive herniation and impending death, immediate evacuation of the hematoma may be necessary. Although obtaining an angiogram to identify the anatomy of the AVM is ideal, it is not always possible because of the rate of neurologic deterioration, especially if the deterioration cannot be reversed despite hyperventilation and osmotic diuretics. The aim of this initial surgery is evacuation of the clot to provide relief of the ICP and reverse any herniation. If an obvious nidus of AVM is encountered, it may be possible to remove it also; more often, the safer course is to stop after evacuation of the clot. Arteriography can then be performed, and a second operation performed to resect the lesion.

Acute rebleeding from an AVM is rare, and urgent surgery therefore is not necessary to prevent a rebleed. If the blood is predominantly in the ventricle, an intraventricular catheter is required to monitor the ICP and provide for CSF drainage. In the acute period, as little CSF as possible is drained to prevent the catheter's becoming clogged by blood clot. The ICP is controlled by a combination of therapy. When a patient is stable and has recovered consciousness, arteriography and definitive therapy can be undertaken. When the clot is parenchymal and the ICP and herniation can be controlled by medical means, it is advisable to postpone surgery until the clot has liquefied and the brain swelling and edema have subsided. This hiatus makes the surgery much safer and allows adequate investigation and planning of therapy. Therapy is either surgery, surgery preceded by embolization, or, for smaller deep lesions, focused radiation therapy.

In a small percentage of cases, no obvious site of hemorrhage is identified. A repeat arteriogram some months later is required to be certain that a residual lesion was not overlooked because of compression by the acute hemorrhage.

The rebleeding rate for AVMs is 2% per year. In children in whom no lesion is identified, the rebleed rate is close to zero.[18] Even in children in whom a complete resection has been achieved, there is a regrowth and rebleeding rate of approximately 5% over 10 years, and it is not clear whether a second arteriogram is required or when it should be performed.

Aneurysm

As noted earlier, intracranial hemorrhage in children is less commonly a result of rupture of an aneurysm than of an

AVM.[19] Aneurysms may be congenital or mycotic and may be found on the feeding arteries of an AVM. Aneurysms occur in the subarachnoid space, and thus, subarachnoid hemorrhage rather than intraparenchymal hemorrhage is the usual result of rupture. The signs and symptoms are typically sudden onset of unendurable headache followed by stiff neck and photophobia and, in about 50% of cases, by coma. Diagnosis is made from the history, which in a child triggers the performance of a CT scan to rule out a parenchymal clot such as would occur with an AVM. The CT scan may appear normal or may show subarachnoid hemorrhage. The definitive diagnosis is then made with lumbar puncture.

Because aneurysms tend to rebleed in 24 to 48 hours,[20–22] the next step after diagnosis of subarachnoid hemorrhage is cerebral arteriography. Magnetic resonance angiography (MRA) is not adequate to visualize a small aneurysm. Although the most common location is at the bifurcation of the carotid, many aneurysms occur distally in children, and they are often giant. Mycotic aneurysms in particular occur on the distal branches of the cerebral vessels; the rare post-traumatic aneurysm can occur on any vessel but is most commonly on the anterior cerebral artery over the corpus callosum.

The grading system for aneurysms in adults is quite adequate for children.[23] Low-grade aneurysms are usually treated by acute surgery to clip or trap the aneurysm before rebleeding, because with each rebleed, the mortality rate rises. After rebleeding, the next major complication is cerebral ischemia as a result of cerebrovascular spasm.[24] This is treated with volume expansion, calcium blockers, and induced arterial hypertension.[24, 25] Because of the need to elevate the blood pressure to treat spasm, it is currently believed that early clipping of the aneurysm makes this therapy to reverse or prevent ischemia safer. The use of free radical scavengers has been reported to markedly improve outcome in patients with subarachnoid hemorrhage.

Rarely, acute hemorrhage from the nose, mouth, or ear can occur as a result of a traumatic aneurysm of the internal carotid artery. It requires emergency arteriography and either embolization or surgical ligation, depending on the location of the lesion.

Cavernous Angiomas and Venous Angiomas

Although both cavernous and venous angiomas can manifest as the acute onset of a new neurologic deficit and headache, it is rare that they require emergency surgery. Venous angiomas rarely bleed in the supratentorial space but must be considered when the hematoma is in the posterior fossa. Brain stem compression can be sufficiently severe to require emergency treatment by clot removal. The large draining vein that is the center of the venous anomaly should not be occluded, because it is often the only venous drainage from a large area of the cerebellum, and its occlusion could result in venous infarction.

The diagnosis is usually established from a noncontrast CT scan, which shows acute hemorrhage, and a contrast-enhanced scan, which in the case of a cavernoma may demonstrate enhancement, and in the case of a venous angioma shows the large vein and its tributaries. Both these lesions are well demonstrated on magnetic resonance imaging (MRI), which shows evidence of old hemorrhage and the surrounding edema. Cerebral arteriography usually shows no lesion in the case of the cavernous malformation but demonstrates the caput of draining veins and the single large vein of the venous angioma.

Acute hydrocephalus can occur as a result of a posterior fossa hematoma and may require treatment with a ventriculostomy. The ventricle should be drained slowly, and the supratentorial pressure should be kept above 15 mm Hg to prevent upward herniation of the cerebellar vermis. There is a risk of upward herniation whenever a ventricular drain is required for relief of acute hydrocephalus secondary to a posterior fossa mass.

Anticonvulsants are necessary in patients who present with seizures. The value of prophylactic anticonvulsants is unknown, and they are used at the discretion of the attending neurosurgeon. Corticosteroids are helpful to treat the cerebral edema that is often present. It is rare that severe intracranial hypertension is present. In most cases, definitive resection of the cavernous angioma is the treatment of choice, once the hematoma and brain edema have subsided. The best treatment for venous angiomas often is to leave them alone unless repeated bleeding occurs, in which case a small AVM is often present and may be resected without damaging the venous drainage.

CONGENITAL LESIONS

Most congenital anomalies of the central nervous system are not true neurosurgical emergencies, but they are often considered by the newborn's family to be catastrophes and therefore require acute pediatric neurosurgical consultation.

Craniofacial Anomalies

The severe anomalies of the craniofacial skeleton that engender an often horrific reaction are those that involve amniotic band syndromes, facial clefts, cloverleaf skull appearance, or congenital absence of the nose or eyes. Children with severe Crouzon's disease or Apert's or Pfeiffer's syndrome also appear dramatically abnormal, and a correct initial diagnosis is often not made. Despite their appearance, few of these children require emergency neurosurgery. The acute problem is most often the airway, because choanal atresia or marked hypoplasia of the midface may interfere with ventilation.

Endotracheal intubation can be very difficult, and a tracheostomy may occasionally be required to save a child's life. The globes of the eyes occasionally are completely dislocated out of the orbit, with closure of the lids posterior to the globe; this situation results in exposure and ischemia of the globes and requires immediate treatment with lubricant and plastic wrap to keep the conjunctiva moist. Tarsorrhaphy is required to protect the conjunctiva. Early surgery with supraorbital rim advancement is rarely adequate to make a significant difference, and surgery is usually delayed until the child is 6 months or older.

Newborns with the cloverleaf skull anomaly usually have hydrocephalus and generalized suture closure, and many require a craniectomy or a shunt in the first week of life to lower the ICP and to allow unrestricted brain growth. In general, craniofacial surgery for children with severe anomalies is delayed until after 6 months of age, unless they show evidence of intracranial hypertension. It is almost impossible to adequately correct any aspect of the facial anomaly before 6 months, even in the upper orbital area. If surgery before 6 months of age is required in a child with pan-suture synostosis and raised ICP, the tendency is to expand the posterior aspect of the skull and preserve the forehead and orbits for later surgery, at 1 year of age.

Encephaloceles

Encephalocoeles occur at a rate of 1 in 10,000 live births in North America.[26] Most (70%), occur in the posterior region of the cranium and are can be either supratentorial or infratentorial. Although they often have a dramatic external appearance, most encephaloceles are not surgical emergencies. Those that are not completely skin-covered and are leaking CSF or displaying visible brain tissue require urgent closure in 24 hours if the general condition of the neonate is otherwise stable. In the interim, the exposed lesion is covered with sterile saline-soaked sponges, and broad-spectrum antibiotic therapy in begun.

CT scanning or MRI or both are required to define the anatomy of the encephalocele and the intracranial brain. Prognosis is best correlated with the size and anatomic appearance of the residual intracranial brain rather than the size of the encephalocele. The more normal the size of the head and the appearance of the brain, the more favorable the intellectual prognosis. The herniated cerebral tissue is not normal, and no effort is made to replace it within the cranial cavity; the abnormal tissue is removed, sparing the intracranial vasculature, and the dura closed.

Hydrocephalus is common but usually does not need therapy in the first few days. When the hydrocephalus is severe to insertion of a shunt and decompression of the brain before is preferable a definitive operation is performed on the encephalocele. Anterior encephaloceles that manifest on the surface are usually resected in the first few days of life by an extradural approach. Those that occur in the nose or mouth, often in association with a cleft palate, can produce acute airway obstruction and feeding problems that require tracheostomy. In such cases, it is advisable to postpone definitive surgery for as long as several months, if possible, to make the procedure safer. If there is a significant CSF leakage, a CSF-diverting shunt, either ventricular or lumbar, may be required as a temporary measure.

Aplasia Cutis Congenita

Aplasia cutis congenita is an area of the skull in which bone and skin fail to form, leaving exposed and occasionally slightly herniating dura, most commonly in the midline, associated with a suture or venous sinus. This is not an encephalocele, and because the dura is intact, it often can be treated conservatively until a child is older, at which time surgery to rotate skin over the lesion is usually necessary. Smaller lesions can be treated by immediate surgical closure of the skin.

Teratomas and Choristomas

Teratomas and choristomas are rare lesions but they can manifest at birth as emergencies because of airway obstruction or feeding problems. The most common location is in the tongue or fauces. These lesions are usually small at birth and grow rapidly in the first few days of life, yet they are rarely malignant. Tracheostomy and a feeding tube are often required during the early life-threatening phase. Those lesions that come to neurosurgical attention usually involve the intracranial space and exit from the cranium through the cranial nerve foramina, most commonly the trigeminal or superior or inferior orbital fissures, and are evident in the mouth and neck. Such lesions can usually be completely removed in a single operation in the first few months of life, with cure of the lesions.

It is unclear whether teratomas and choristomas should be categorized as congenital or neoplastic lesions, and in some cases, true tumors are found. Affected children should be treated only by craniofacial teams with the support systems to perform such surgery and, if necessary, to carry out reconstruction in infants.[27] Other congenital face and neck tumors are neurofibromas, neuroblastomas, and sarcomas.

Myelomeningocele

Failure of closure of the skin, muscle, bone, and spinal cord constitutes a myelomeningocele. Such a lesion can occur at any level of the spinal canal but is most common in the lumbar area. Myelomeningoceles often have disruption of the thin covering of arachnoid over the placode and are leaking CSF. There is no real emergency about closing such lesions, but in most pediatric neurosurgical centers, they are closed within 24 to 48 hours after birth, assuming that the neonate is otherwise stable.[28] If closure is to be delayed more than a few hours, the lesions are covered with sterile saline-soaked sponges, and broad-spectrum antibiotic therapy is begun. A sonogram of the head and kidneys is usually obtained prior to surgery to evaluate the intracranial state and to ensure that the kidneys are present.

Hydrocephalus

It is unusual for hydrocephalus in a newborn to constitute a neurosurgical emergency. Because hydrocephalus is present prenatally, the brain accommodates it, the sutures split, and the cranium significantly enlarges. Thus, there is usually time to make an accurate diagnosis of the cause of the hydrocephalus and to perform a shunt procedure electively. In the patient with signs such as apnea or bradycardia that are believed to be the result of increased ICP, the ventricle can easily be tapped through the fontanelle, and the pressure relieved until shunt can be placed electively. With the routine use of sonography in pregnant women, the diagnosis of hydrocephalus is increasingly made predelivery. Unless there are gross congenital anomalies of the brain, the prognosis cannot be made accurately. In about 30% to 50% of cases, hydrocephalus is not a surgical problem at birth, and currently, there is no evidence that intrauterine shunting is of any value.

Acute hydrocephalus due to congenital and acquired causes can manifest later in life in a child with closed skull sutures. In this case, rapid diagnosis and therapy may be required to prevent either death or serious brain damage.[29] The cranium in such a child cannot expand, and by the time a child presents for medical care, the compensatory mechanisms for volume and pressure balance are usually exhausted and waves of elevated ICP are occurring with a risk of sudden death. This situation occurs also in children who have a CSF shunt and in whom a shunt malfunction has occurred. The difficulty with diagnosis in this group of patients is the lack of definitive signs that confirm the diagnosis. The diagnosis of shunt malfunction or acute intracranial hypertension due to hydrocephalus is essentially based on the history and often confirmed only by a neuroimaging study (CT or MRI) that shows ventricular dilatation.

In a small group of children with shunts, the ventricles either do not enlarge or enlarge only minimally in the presence of a shunt dysfunction, *slit ventricle syndrome*.[30, 31] In such a child, it is important to compare the current scan with a previous scan, if possible; if comparison is not possible, one must act on the basis of the history and assume a shunt malfunction.

Because autoregulation of CBF is typically intact in a child presenting with acute hydrocephalus, the ICP waves that occur are often unassociated with any signs. The symptoms are severe, episodic headache that may be associated with vomiting or visual obscurations. The major pain may be behind the eyes or in the back of the neck as a result of tonsillar herniation. The headache may be relieved by vomiting, which triggers hyperventilation and thus a decrease in ICP that can abort the pressure wave. A child who is not having a wave of pressure at the time of the examination may appear perfectly normal, and even with a wave of high pressure, there may be nothing to identify other than the pain of the headache, which is, of course, subjective. The examination may reveal papilledema, but as mentioned earlier, the absence of papilledema does not rule out intracranial hypertension of a life-threatening degree. Decreased level of consciousness, either accompanying the headache or present continuously, may occur, as may a stiff neck due to tonsillar herniation, sixth cranial nerve palsy due to diffuse ICP, or, more rarely, a third cranial nerve palsy.

Visual acuity may be decreased as a result of chronic papilledema, or optic atrophy may be present. Vital signs changes, such as bradycardia and hypertension, may be seen but are often late manifestations that occur only at the time of brain stem decompensation and cannot be relied on as clinical indicators of increased ICP. The only way to confirm or refute the diagnosis is to obtain a CT scan and to look for evidence of ventricular enlargement. When elevated ICP is suspected, it is always preferable to avoid sedation of the child if possible or, if sedation is needed, to give the least amount possible and to realize that sedation may decrease ventilation, increase arterial partial pressure of carbon dioxide, and precipitate further pressure waves. A plan to treat these complications should be in place before sedation is given.

When hydrocephalus is present, urgent therapy is required to abort the waves of increased ICP. Therapy ranges from acute administration of corticosteroids in the patient with a tumor to ventriculostomy or an emergency shunt procedure. In patients who do not have a tumor or preexisting shunt and in whom an acute or chronic central nervous system (CNS) infectious process is not suspected, the ideal treatment is insertion of a shunt as an emergency procedure. This is the final as well as the initial therapy and avoids the risk of an infection from a temporary ventriculostomy. The critical factor is to appreciate the urgency of the situation and not to procrastinate.

In children with a preexisting shunt, a radiographic shunt survey to evaluate the intactness and position of the shunt system is necessary in addition to the scan. If there is question about a shunt block, the shunt system can be tapped, and the site of block identified as proximal or distal to the shunt reservoir. In children with the slit ventricle syndrome, in whom very little fluid is present in the ventricle and the ability to remove fluid is therefore limited, it is often better to test the proximal catheter by back-injecting contrast medium into the ventricle to establish the patency of the proximal shunt catheter. The distal end of the shunt can be checked by measuring the runoff pressure with a manometer. When the shunt is blocked proximal to the valve system such that CSF cannot be withdrawn, it is safer to revise the shunt immediately rather than to wait until the next day. If the shunt is blocked distal to the valve, adequate ventricular decompression can be attained by tapping the reservoir and removing CSF. In this setting, the shunt revision may be postponed until the next convenient opening in the operating schedule, and acetazolamide and dexamethasone may be used to slow CSF production during the waiting period. Any severe headaches need to be treated with further fluid withdrawal from the shunt, not with narcotics; if headaches continue, shunt revision is urgently required.

Pseudotumor Cerebri

A syndrome of elevated intracranial pressure in the absence of any mass lesions, pseudotumor cerebri can occur at any age of childhood. The underlying pathophysiology is believed to be a disturbance of CSF outflow resistance. In children, the only symptom may be visual, either sixth cranial nerve palsy or a decrease in visual fields or acuity or both. Headaches may be minor and are often dismissed by parents and physicians as being insignificant. In most children with this syndrome, the diagnosis is made by funduscopy, which shows papilledema or optic atrophy. Treatment is typically with repeated lumbar punctures, acetazolamide (Diamox), and steroids. In the child with significant reductions in central visual fields and visual acuity at diagnosis or with episodic losses of vision usually precipitated by a change in posture, emergency relief of the raised ICP is indicated. It is usually accomplished by the insertion of a lumboperitoneal shunt. If the visual loss is unilateral, an optic nerve decompression may relieve the pressure.

NEOPLASIA

In only a few cases are brain tumors neurosurgical catastrophes, but these must be rapidly identified and treated. Even in children's hospitals, the occasional child dies in the intensive care unit or on the ward as a result of a pressure wave associated with a brain tumor.[29] These children are usually admitted with a history of headache, nausea, and vomiting, and they suffer herniation while awaiting evaluation for a suspected gastrointestinal lesion. This unfortunate scenario occurs despite the availability of CT and MRI. Other children are admitted and a lesion is identified on scan, but the symptoms of increased ICP are ignored because of the absence of objective signs; this scenario results in clinical herniation and, occasionally, death. The problem is exactly as described in children with hydrocephalus, in whom autoregulation of CBF is intact and very high pressures can be tolerated without apparent signs. Many of the tumors that present this way are posterior fossa tumors producing hydrocephalus.

In 5% to 10% of cases of tumor, hemorrhage occurs into the tumor, producing acute deterioration that is no different from that related to other types of intracranial hemorrhage.[32] Tumors in the supratentorial compartment are easier to diagnose because of accompanying local signs (e.g., hemiparesis, visual field cut). Rarely is an emergency operation necessary, but in the presence of progressive herniation, repeated pressure waves, or unconsciousness, rapid surgical debulking of the tumor may be required. As noted previously, ventricular drainage in the presence of a large posterior fossa tumor can result in upward herniation; thus, resection of the tumor may be required at the time of insertion of the ventricular drain. In patients with less acute symptoms, corticosteroids usually bring about rapid clinical improvement, permitting surgery to be performed electively.

A final presentation of tumor that requires emergency surgery is the rapid progression of visual loss. It may be due to local compression of the optic nerves, chiasm, or tracts by tumor and can occur as a result of hemorrhage into such tumors as optic gliomas or pituitary tumors or can simply result from a tumor mass, as in craniopharyngioma or meningioma. Such rapid visual loss that is the result of local compression is an indication for emergency surgical decompression of the optic apparatus. The other setting in which rapid visual loss can occur results from papilledema. In this setting, ventricular drainage or shunting plus steroids is usually chosen over emergency tumor resection, in an effort to lower the ICP gradually and prevent the acute blindness that can occasionally occur after posterior fossa decompression. Rarely, in children, do tumors erode into adjacent structures, but epistaxis or bleeding from the ear occasionally is the first manifestation of a large skull base tumor. These lesions rarely require acute neurosurgical intervention, but if bleeding is severe or hard to control, CT or MRI may be necessary to make the diagnosis, and acute embolization or vessel ligation may be required to attain hemostasis.

INFECTIONS

The most common infectious process that requires emergency neurosurgery is a brain abscess.[33, 34] The presentation consists of either focal neurologic deficit or the signs of intracranial hypertension. The aim of therapy is dual, (1) to obtain a specimen for culture and (2) to evacuate any intracranial mass. CT usually identifies the lesion, and the therapy is usually drainage with or without leaving a catheter in situ for further drainage. It is rare for an attempt at abscess removal to be performed as the primary procedure, unless the abscess is superficially located in the brain. Even then, because of the surrounding edema, it is generally preferable simply to drain the lesion, treat with antibiotics, and monitor with scanning. Indeed, in many cases, craniotomy is never necessary, and the abscess can be treated simply with antibiotics with or without repeated needle drainage.

Subdural Empyema and Epidural Empyema

Epidural empyema usually occurs with either severe air sinus infections or osteomyelitis of the skull.[35] The mass effect is usually small, and immediate drainage is only rarely necessary. With an empyema in the frontal area, drainage of the frontal sinus often results in drainage of the epidural abscess also.

Subdural empyema is a much more catastrophic situation, with underlying pial and often cerebral inflammation, septic thrombophlebitis, and brain edema. In the past, this disorder was always treated with urgent craniotomy and aspiration of the pus.[35, 36] Currently, with earlier diagnosis made possible by CT, bur hole aspiration for culture of the fluid and immediate relief of mass effect is often all the surgery that is required, followed by antibiotics and corticosteroids.[37] In children, subdural empyemas commonly recur, often in a slightly different location, and may require repeated surgical drainage or extensive craniotomy if resolution is not achieved by medical management. Small lesions may require no surgery.

Meningitis

It is rare for meningitis to be an acute neurosurgical emergency, but acute hydrocephalus can occur with bacterial meningitis, requiring ventricular drainage. Hydrocephalus most often occurs in tuberculous meningitis but also occurs with the more common infections and presumably results from obliteration of the subarachnoid space by pus and the obstruction of the arachnoid villi by white cells. Increased outflow resistance to CSF results, along with raised ICP with or without ventricular dilation.

Viral Encephalitis

Despite antiviral agents, brain biopsy is occasionally necessary in focal encephalitis to aid in diagnosis and choice of therapy. Biopsy is more often performed in more chronic encephalitis associated with other immune disturbances, such as in an organ transplant recipient or a child with acquired immunodeficiency syndrome. High ICP occurs, especially in the hemorrhagic encephalitides (e.g., herpes simplex, Rocky Mountain spotted fever), and ICP monitoring may be required to aid in management. Rarely is there a role for acute surgical resection of inflamed tissue.

Shunt Infection

Most shunt infections do not require emergency shunt removal but do need shunt tap and appropriate antibiotics. In the child with an acute abdomen as a result of the shunt infection, emergency exteriorization of the abdominal end of the shunt may be required. When the infecting organism is *Staphylococcus,* elective removal and replacement of the shunt is usually required. With other organisms, the shunt can often be saved by appropriate antibiotic therapy.

CATASTROPHIC EPILEPSY

Epilepsy, even status epilepticus, is rarely an acute neurosurgical disease. In certain epileptic syndromes of infancy and childhood, however, the question of emergency surgery arises. In most cases, this occurs in infants who have infantile spasms that are uncontrolled with medication and in whom rapid neurologic deterioration is occurring.[38, 39] Video-electroencephalographic (EEG) monitoring, MRI, and position emission tomography (PET) or single photon emission computed tomography (SPECT) are used to identify the epilepsy as focal or unihemispheric.[40–42] The usual pathologic lesions are Sturge-Weber syndrome, hemimegalencephaly, focal cortical dysplasia, and Rasmussen's encephalitis. Occasionally, no MRI abnormality is present, yet a single hemisphere is involved and surgery is suggested. Even after hemispherectomy, no pathologic diagnosis is made in some cases.[40]

Alper's syndrome, which consist of liver failure and associated intractable epilepsy, often appears as a focal cortical involvement early in the course of the disease. Unfortunately, no evidence of liver dysfunction may be apparent at this stage so that surgery can be recommended. Surgery is at best a temporary measure; the seizures recur from a different area of the brain, and in a few months, death occurs. Chronic or subacute herpes simplex infection in infants can also manifest in similar fashion, but the findings on EEG are usually bilateral; the surgery for these lesions is usually some form of cerebral hemispherectomy.

MISCELLANEOUS CAUSES OF NERVOUS SYSTEM DYSFUNCTION

The possibility of child abuse being disguised as SIDS has already been discussed. A 1996 report has identified medium-chain acyl-CoA dehydrogenase (MCAD) deficiency as a preventable cause of SIDS in 5% to 6% of cases.[43] The emergency department (ED) physician should be aware of this entity.

Hemorrhagic shock and encephalopathy syndrome (HSE) is another cause of sudden catastrophic illness in children that is often hard to identify.[44, 45] The onset is usually acute, with fever, loss of consciousness, and seizures. Disseminated intravascular coagulopathy is often present with no obvious infectious process. The CT scan can show diffuse areas of low density throughout the brain. Outcome is usually fatal. The presumed pathology is believed to be an overactivation of the inflammatory cytokine system of unknown primary etiology. Although there is no neurosurgical therapy for HSE, the pediatric neurosurgeon may be called for consultation because of the acute alteration of consciousness of a child with the disorder.

SPINE CATASTROPHES

Most acute surgical problems of the spinal canal and cord are a result of trauma or neoplasia. The majority of spinal injuries do not require emergency neurosurgical intervention other than external stabilization with a halo device or skull tongs.[46]

Children with deteriorating neurologic findings and evidence of spinal cord compression on CT or MRI are the patients most likely to require surgical decompression and stabilization. Occasionally, an acute spinal epidural hematoma can occur that requires emergency evacuation. Surgical exploration is usually required in penetrating injuries of the spine, although this is often not the case for bullet wounds.

Spinal cord compression by tumor is usually slowly progressive, but worsening can occur suddenly. A child who is complaining of difficulty standing or walking or who has back pain plus incontinence must be taken seriously, and a careful examination and appropriate neuroimaging performed, usually MRI. It is rare for such complaints to be hysterical; however, children are still sent out of emergency departments with that presumed diagnosis, only to return within a short time with a complete spinal cord lesion. The importance or early identification of spinal cord compression is that the greater the amount of neurologic deficit present preoperatively, the less the chance for neurologic recovery. The lesions that most often produce spinal cord compression and that manifest acutely are neuroblastoma, lymphoma, bone tumors (e.g., aneurysmal bone cysts), and, least often, intrinsic spinal cord tumors. Ependymomas of the conus medullaris or filum terminale may manifest as only leg pain and back pain and can be difficult to identify. Progressive or nonresolving back pain in a child needs to be investigated. During the wait for surgery, corticosteroid therapy is begun if a neurologic deficit is present.

Vascular lesions of the spinal cord are uncommon in children, but aneurysms, cavernous angiomas, and AVMs do occur and can manifest either as acute subarachnoid hemorrhage or acute spinal cord compression. The possibility of a spinal cord lesion must be kept in mind if no intracranial site for hemorrhage is found. Spinal vascular lesions can usually be operated on electively, but with an acute intraspinal hematoma, emergency surgery may be indicated after appropriate neuroradiologic studies have defined the problem.

Acute cervical disk syndrome in children is usually the result of inflammation and acute calcification of the intervertebral disk space. Surgery is rarely required even in the presence of long tract signs, because rapid resolution of the lesion is the norm, with absorption of the prolapsed, calcified, extruded disk. In rare cases in which symptoms are progressive, are not resolving, or are producing weakness, surgery is required.

Acute lumbar or thoracic disk herniation is rare in children and adolescents. In the lumbar area, the precipitating factor is often weight lifting. The compression is usually central, and thus, radicular symptoms may be absent. Central back pain with pain on leg extension or refusal to flex the spine may be the only signs. The etiology is usually fracture of the epiphyseal plate rather than soft disk herniation.

Acute infections are rare, but epidural abcess can occur in the absence of bony or disk space infections.[47] If such an abscess is diagnosed early, antibiotic therapy is all that is required. If there is a major motor weakness or progressive symptoms of cord compression, surgery is required. Apparently, the neurologic deficits are often due to septic thrombophlebitis, and improvement following surgical decompression is variable.

Congenital lesions of the spine rarely manifest as emergencies, but they must always be considered, and an appropriate examination must be performed. Acute compression of the spinal cord can occur in children with Down's syndrome because of C1-C2 instability and acute subluxation. Such acute symptoms in a child with achondroplasia require investigation for compression of the spinal cord by a small foramen magnum and invaginating bone from the lateral and posterior margins of the foramen magnum. In achondroplasia, the whole spinal canal may be narrow, and spinal cord compression manifesting as intermittent weakness or claudication can occur. In children with craniofacial syndromes, especially Crouzon's disease, tonsillar herniation at the foramen magnum and spinal cord compression can be the cause of acute spastic quadriparesis, sleep apnea, or swallowing problems.

Acute paraplegia or loss of bladder and bowel function can occasionally develop in children with occult spinal dysraphism. It is usually precipitated by an episode of hip flexion, for example, the first pelvic examination with positioning in stirrups. The most common lesion is a lipomeningocele, which is usually visible as a fatty mass overlying the sacrum. Diastematomyelia can occasionally manifest as the acute onset or exacerbation of neurologic deficit. A hairy patch over the lumbar or thoracic sign is often present as a diagnostic clue.

POSTOPERATIVE NEUROSURGICAL EMERGENCIES

The postoperative neurosurgical catastrophes that are encountered in children depend on the location and type of surgery performed but can be divided the following categories: (1) hemorrhage, (2) edema, (3) cerebrovascular spasm or occlusion, (4) new neurologic deficits, (5) seizures, and (6) metabolic problems.

The results of postoperative hemorrhage are similar to acute intracranial hemorrhage (described earlier). After posterior fossa surgery, the most significant risk is the occurrence of acute hydrocephalus, which can manifest only as a headache until a fatal pressure wave occurs. As with other causes of hydrocephalus, the medical personnel caring for children who have undergone posterior fossa surgery must be aware of the lack of signs associated with hydrocephalus and must be ready to repeat the CT scan to identify ventricular enlargement. Treatment is usually with ventricular drainage.

Local signs of posterior fossa compression—swallowing difficulty, diplopia, cranial nerve palsies, occasional mutism, or deteriorating consciousness—may require direct evacuation of a posterior fossa clot. Intraventricular hemorrhage, like posterior fossa hemorrhage, can produce only headache and pressure waves or may result in the sudden onset of coma. Treatment is usually symptomatic, consisting of ventricular drainage and control of the ICP until the clot resolves. Intracerebral or epidural hemorrhage requires surgical evacuation if it is large enough to produce symptoms and signs.

Arterial spasm is usually associated with aneurysm or AVM surgery, and its treatment has been discussed. Brain edema usually develops over several days, and its treatment is rarely surgical. Steroids, ventilation, sedative drugs, and osmotic agents all may be required in severe cases. Seizures are uncommon in the postoperative period but, when they occur, should be vigorously treated. It is always necessary to check blood glucose, calcium, and electrolyte levels, because if one of these is the cause, anticonvulsants may not be necessary. If no metabolic derangements are found, the drug of choice is phenytoin or phosphenytoin, because neither of these agents produces any significant alteration in the level of consciousness.

Most acute metabolic problems are related to disturbances of pituitary axis function. Diabetes insipidus, the most common, occurs when the pituitary stalk is manipulated or divided, as in resection of craniopharyngioma. By combining careful fluid management and, if necessary, intravenous 1-deamino-(8-D-arginine)-vasopressin, effective control of serum sodium and osmolality can usually be achieved.

BRAIN DEATH

The diagnosis and confirmation of death as a result of irreversible brain damage are no more difficult in children than in adults.[48] Minimum anecdotal evidence suggests that in premature infants and neonates, and possibly during the first 1 month of life, the signs of brain death (absence of neurologic findings, lack of ventilation, flat EEG, absence of CBF) can occur, yet survival and recovery of the infant still be possible.[49] After that period, however, the absence of all neurologic function other than spinal reflexes for longer than 6 hours, ICP equal to the arterial pressure for longer than 1 hour, the absence of CBF, and a flat electroencephalogram all are as meaningful in a child as in an adult. Other than the ICP equal to the arterial pressure and the absence of CBF, the determinants of death depend on a known history or diagnosis of the event precipitating the death and the absolute absence of any medication or drugs that could influence the results of the examination.

There is no reason to prolong the life-support process in a dead child, and the reasons for failing to act by declaring death and removing the cardiovascular support from a dead child are almost always based on the inability of the medical attendants to accept the state of affairs. The situation is no more reversible in a child than in an adult, and by not allowing the child's family to start the grieving process once death has occurred does them a disservice. Finally, despite the apparent difficulty some physicians still have in approaching families for organ donation, studies have shown that this ability to help a living child in a situation of despair is often the one event that can help the family feel that something good has come from the tragedy of losing their own child.

References

1. Avezaat CJJ, Van Eijhdhoven JHM: Cerebrospinal Fluid Pulse Pressure and Craniospinal Dynamics: A Theoretical and Experimental Study. The Hague, A Gonabloed en zoon, 1984.
2. Bruce DA: Pathophysiology of intracranial pressure. *In:* Diseases of the Nervous System. Vol 2. Asbury AK, McKhann GM, McDonald WI (Eds). Philadelphia, WB Saunders, 1986, pp 1044–1062.
3. Rosner MJ, Rosner SD, Johnson AH: Cerebral perfusion pressure: Management protocol and clinical results. J Neurosurg 1995; 83:949–962.
4. Gopinath SP, Robertson CS, Constant CF, et al: Jugular venous desaturation and outcome after head injury. J Neurol Neurosurg Psychiatry 1994; 57:717–723.
5. Skippen P, Seear M, Poskitt K, et al: Effect of hyperventilation on regional cerebral blood flow in head injured children. Crit Care Med 1997; 25:1402–1409.
6. Cruz J: The first decade of continuous monitoring of jugular bulb oxyhemoglobin saturation: Management strategies and clinical outcome. Crit Care Med 1998; 26:344–351.
7. Chestnut R: Hyperventilation versus cerebral perfusion pressure management: Time to change the question. Crit Care Med 1998; 26:210–212.
8. Bejjani GK, Donahue DJ, Rusin J, Broemeling LD: Radiological and clinical criteria for the management of epidural hematomas in children. Pediatr Neurosurg 1996; 25:302–308.
9. Mendelsohn D, Levin HS, Bruce D, et al: Late MRI after head injury in children: Relationship to clinical features and outcome. Childs Nerv Syst 1992; 8:445–452.
10. Bruce DA: Head injuries in the pediatric population. Curr Probl Pediatr 1990; 20:67–107.
11. Zurynski YA, Dorsch NW, Pearson I: Influence and effects of increased blood flow velocity after severe head injury: A transcranial Doppler ultrasound study: I. Prediction of post-traumatic vasospam and hyperemia. J Neurol Sci 1995; 134:33–40.
12. Zurynski YA, Dorsch NW, Fearnside MR: Influence and effects of increased blood flow velocity after severe head injury: A transcranial Doppler ultrasound study: II. Effect of vasospam and hyperemia on outcome. J Neurol Sci 1995; 134:41–46.
13. Romner B, Bellner J, Kongstad P, Sjoholm H: Elevated transcranial Doppler flow velocities after severe head injury: Cerebral vasospasm or hyperemia? J Neurosurg 1996; 85:90–107.
14. Adelson PD, Clyde B, Kochanek PM, Wisniewski SR, Marion DW, Younas H: Cerebrovascular response in infants and young children following severe traumatic brain injury: A preliminary report. Pediatr Neurosurg 1997; 26:200–207.
15. Botash AS, Fuller PG, Blatt SD, Cunningham A, Weinberger HL: Child abuse, sudden infant death syndrome, and psychosocial development. Curr Opin Pediatr 1996; 8:195–200.
16. Humphreys RP: Special article: Hemorrhagic stroke in childhood. Riv Neurosci Pediatr 1986; 2:1–5.
17. Humphreys RP, Hoffman HJ, Drake JM, Rutka JT: Choices in the 1990s for the management of pediatric cerebral arteriovenous malformations. Pediatr Neurosurg 1996; 25:277–285.
18. Ondra SL, Troupp H, George ED, et al: The natural history of symptomatic arteriovenous malformations of the brain: A 24 year follow up assessment. J Neurosurg 1990; 73:387–391.
19. Meyer FB, Sundt TM, Fode NC, et al: Cerebral aneurysms in childhood and adolescence. J Neurosurg 1989; 70:420–425.
20. Hijdra A, vanGijn J, Nagelkerke NJ, et al: Prediction of delayed cerebral ischemia, rebleeding and outcome after aneurysmal subarchnoid hemorrhage. Stroke 1988; 19:1250–1256.
21. Kassell NF, Torner JC, Haley C Jr, et al: The international cooperative study of the timing of aneurysm surgery: Part I Overall management results. J Neurosurg 1990; 73:18–36.
22. Kassell NF, Torner JC, Jane JA, et al: The international cooperative study of the timing of aneurysm surgery: Part 2. Surgical results. J Neurosurg 1990; 73:37–47.
23. Drake CG: Report of World Federation of Neurological Surgeons Committee on a universal subarachnoid grading scale. J Neurosurg 1988; 68:985–990.
24. Kassell NF, Peerless SJ, Durward QJ, et al: Treatment of ischemic deficits from vasospasm with intravascular volume expansion and induced arterial hypertension. Neurosurgery 1982; 11:337–343.
25. Petruk KC, West M, Mohr G, et al: Nimodipine treatment in poor grade aneurysm patients; results of a multicenter double-blind placebo controlled trial. J Neurosurg 1988; 68:505–517.
26. David DJ, Proudman TW: Cephaloceles: Classification, pathology and management. World J Surg 1989; 13:349–357.
27. Fearon JA, Munro IR, Bruce DA, et al: Massive teratomas involving the cranial base: Treatment and outcome—a two-center report. Plast Reconstr Surg 1992; 91:223–228.
28. Charney E, Weller S, Sutton JN, et al: Management of the newborn with myelomeningocele: Time for a decision making process. Pediatrics 1985; 75:58–64.
29. Shemie S, Jay V, Rutka J, Armstrong D: Acute obstructive hydrocephalus and sudden death in children. Ann Emerg Med 1997; 29:524–528.
30. Coker SB: Cyclic vomiting and the slit ventricle syndrome. Pediatr Neurol 1987; 3:297–299.
31. Serlo W, Heikkinen E, Saukkonen AL, et al: Classification and management of the slit ventricle syndrome. Childs Nerv Syst 1985; 1:194–199.
32. Laurent JP, Bruce DA, Schut L: Hemorrhagic brain tumors in pediatric patients. Childs Brain 1981; 8:263–266.
33. Hirsch JF, Roux FX, Sainte-Rose C, et al: Brain abscess in childhood: A study of 34 cases treated by puncture and antibiotics. Childs Brain 1983; 10:251–255.
34. Neilsen H: Cerebral abscess in children. Neuropediatrics 1983; 14:76–81.
35. Smith HP, Hendrick EB: Subdural empyema and epidural abscess in children. J Neurosurg 1983; 58:392–395.
36. Hockley AD, Williams B: Surgical management of subdural empyema. Childs Brain 1983; 10:294–297.
37. de Falco R, Scarano E, Cigliano A, Russo G, Profeta L, Annicchiarico L: Surgical treatment of subdural empyema: A critical review. J Neurosurg Sci 1996; 40:53–58.
38. Wyllie E: Surgery for catastrophic localization-related epilepsy in infants. Epilepsia 1996; 37(Suppl 1):S22–S25.
39. Peacock WJ, Wehby-Grant MC, Shields WD, Shewmon DA, Chugani HT, Sankar R, Vinters HV: Hemispherectomy for intractable seizures in children: A report of 58 cases. Childs Nerv Syst 1996; 12:376–384.
40. Carmant L, Kramer U, Riviello JJ, Helmers SL, Mikati MA, Madsen

JR, Black PM, Lombroso CT, Holmes GL: EEG prior to hemispherectomy: Correlation with outcome and pathology. Electroencephalogr Clin Neurophysiol 1995; 94:265–270.
41. Zupanc ML: Neuroimaging in the evaluation of children and adolescents with intractable epilepsy: I. The role of MRI. Pediatr Neurol 1997; 17:19–26.
42. Zupanc ML: Neuroimaging in the evaluation of children and adolescents with intractable epilepsy: II. Neuroimaging and pediatric epilepsy. Pediatr Neurol 1997; 17:111–121.
43. Kemp PM, Little BB, Bost RO, Dawson DB: Whole blood levels of dodecanoic acid, a routinely detectable forensic marker for a genetic disease often misdiagnosed as sudden infant death syndrome (SIDS): MCAD deficiency. Am J Forensic Med Pathol 1996; 17:79–82.
44. Shida K, Matsuo M, Sato T, Maeda Y, Tasaki H, Miyazaki S: Extensive white matter involvement in hemorrhagic shock and encephalopathy syndrome. Acta Paediatr Jpn 1996; 38:270–273.
45. Little D, Wilkins B: Hemorrhagic shock and encephalopathy syndrome: An unusual cause of sudden death in children. Am J Forensic Med Pathol 1997; 18:79–83.
46. Dickman CA, Rekate HL, Sonntag VKH, et al: Pediatric spinal trauma: Vertebral column and spinal cord injuries in children. Pediatr Neurosci 1989; 15:237–256.
47. Tacconi L, Lohnston FG, Symon L: Spinal epidural abscess—review of 10 cases. Acta Neurochir (Wien) 1996; 138:520–523.
48. Ad Hoc Committee on Brain Death: Determination of brain death. J Pediatr 1987; 100:15–19.
49. Volpe JJ: Brain death determination in the newborn. Pediatrics 1987; 80:292–297.

171

Intracranial Hemorrhage

Howard Yonas, MD

SUBARACHNOID HEMORRHAGE

The leakage of blood into the subarachnoid space, known as subarachnoid hemorrhage (SAH), has many possible causes. Although the most common cause in all age groups is cranial trauma, this chapter focuses on spontaneous subarachnoid hemorrhage, which can be either primary or secondary. Primary SAH is due to the direct release of blood into the subarachnoid space, as most commonly occurs with aneurysm rupture. Secondary SAH is due to the leakage of blood products from an intracerebral hemorrhage either directly into the subarachnoid space or via the ventricular system.

Primary Causes

The primary causes of spontaneous SAH are (1) aneurysms and (2) arteriovenous malformations (AVMs), with a 10:1 ratio. Less common causes are (1) infectious aneurysms, (2) primary metastatic or meningeal neoplasms, (3) dural AVMs, (4) cavernous and venous angiomas, and (5) nonstructural abnormalities, such as bleeding diatheses, iatrogenic coagulopathies, and systemic infections. The incidence of primary SAH varies according to the study cited, ranging from 1.4 to 27.3 new cases per 100,000 population annually.[1, 2]

Aneurysms

Epidemiology

The incidence of unruptured aneurysms in the population ranges from 1% to 2%; therefore, they are not rare occurrences. Although smaller aneurysms that are found incidentally are rarely associated with subsequent SAH, aneurysms larger than 1 cm are associated with a significant (~4%) yearly risk of bleeding. Aneurysms of any size can, however, be responsible for an SAH; very small aneurysms are not quite as common but are just as lethal as larger ones. Women tend to have a higher rate of SAH than men, and the incidence appears to increase linearly with advancing age.[1] Of patients who present with aneurysmal SAH, 10% to 15% have multiple intracranial aneurysms.

A few risk factors for SAH have been identified. Although some aneurysms were previously described as congenital, the incidence of aneurysms occurring with clear genetic linkage is relatively rare. In some families, the incidence is more than coincidental, and studies have suggested an abnormality of collagen regulation.[3] When two first-degree relatives have known aneurysms, it would appear reasonable to screen other close relatives. Direct angiography has been the only way to screen for aneurysms in the past; both magnetic resonance imaging (MRI) and computed tomographic (CT) angiography offer the promise of being able to screen for aneurysms measuring more than a few millimeters. Other risk factors are long-term exposure to smoking and short-term exposure to alcohol and vasoactive drugs, such as cocaine. It is probable that cocaine causes not only acute hypertension but also a vasculitis that weakens intracranial arteries and predisposes hemorrhage either due to primary arterial rupture or due to aneurysm formation and secondary rupture of the aneurysm.[4, 5]

Premonitory Signs

The prognosis for patients with SAH remains poor because almost 50% of patients die within 48 hours of bleeding irrespective of therapy. The ability to identify patients at risk for a devastating hemorrhage is critical to reducing the morbidity and mortality of SAH. The phenomenon of a "warning bleed" is a common occurrence, and proper identification of the significance of this event should help improve the early diagnosis of SAH due to aneurysm rupture.

Patients with a frank SAH often give a history of having had an unusual headache for several weeks prior to the definitive event. Patients do not often seek medical attention for these symptoms, but even when they do, the pain is often ascribed to tension headache or cervical arthritis. Patients presenting with an unusual headache should be considered candidates for a CT scan. CT findings are abnormal in 90% of SAH cases on day 1. The diagnostic sensitivity falls to 72% by day 5.[6] The diagnostic capability is about 45% in patients who have a "warning leak."[7] Lumbar puncture is therefore indicated for any patient with a history consistent with SAH if CT findings are normal. The equal or increasing presence of blood in all sample tubes of cerebrospinal fluid (CSF) is often adequate for confirming the diagnosis of SAH. Although the presence of xanthochromia provides further confirmation of the diagnosis of SAH, the disorder is not often present within a few hours of bleed. A D-dimer assay is an additional, very sensitive study capable of defining the presence of older blood products and thereby helping to discriminate a traumatic SAH from a true SAH.[8]

An enlarging aneurysm may also produce neuronal compression syndromes, which must be recognized because rupture frequently follows within hours to days. Compression of the optic nerve can produce retro-orbital pain and unilateral visual loss, whereas enlargement of a posterior communicating artery aneurysm can compress the third cranial nerve. The latter event commonly causes retro-orbital discomfort, pupillary dilation, ptosis, and oculomotor deficits. This etiologic mechanism must be distinguished from a third nerve palsy due to

TABLE 171–1. World Federation of Neurological Surgery Scale for Clinical Grading After Subarachnoid Hemorrhage (SAH)

Grade	Glasgow Coma Scale Score	Presentation Following SAH
I	15	No headache or focal deficit
II	15	Headache, nuchal rigidity; no focal signs
III	13–14	Can have headache, nuchal rigidity; no focal signs
IVa	13–14	Can have headache, nuchal rigidity, or focal signs
IVb	9–12	Can have headache, nuchal rigidity, or focal signs
V	8 or less	Can have headache, nuchal rigidity, or focal signs

diabetes, which results from small vessel disease within the nerve and is less likely to cause pupillary changes.

Clinical Presentation and Diagnosis

The classic presentation for a patient with SAH is the sudden onset of the "worst headache" in the patient's life. Even if the patient has a history of headaches, the pain due to SAH is usually distinctly different. SAH due to aneurysm rupture is commonly accompanied by a period of unconsciousness, from which 50% of patients do not awaken.[9] Patients who do awaken, minutes or hours later, typically complain of a severe headache, nuchal rigidity, and photophobia. A subhyoid hemorrhage (a preretinal globular accumulation of blood) is often evident on funduscopic examination and is pathognomonic for SAH.

Grading of the severity of clinical deficits combined with knowledge about the time of onset of the bleed has proved useful in guiding subsequent clinical management. The patient may appear normal with only a headache or may be comatose, depending on the volume of blood released at hemorrhage, the presence of an intraparenchymal or intraventricular hemorrhage, and the development of hydrocephalus. A critical anatomic feature is whether the blood is localized to a single subarachnoid cistern (compartment) or whether it spreads throughout the entire subarachnoid space before extraluminal pressure equals intraluminal pressure and stops the bleeding.

A number of scales have been established for the clinical grading of patients following SAH. These scales consider the patient's mental status and neurologic deficit. A widely utilized scale was developed by the World Federation of Neurological Surgery (Table 171–1).

After the diagnosis of SAH has been made, angiography remains the standard diagnostic technique for defining the source of the bleed (Fig. 171–1). When angiography defines more than one aneurysm, treatment should be directed toward the aneurysm adjacent to the densest collection of blood. When the SAH is not focal, treatment should first be directed to the largest or most irregular aneurysm.[10] A patient with both an AVM and an aneurysm is usually assumed to have bled from the aneurysm. In the patient for whom surgical intervention is emergently necessary for evacuation of a massive, life-threatening hemorrhage, a contrast-enhanced CT scan obtained immediately after the initial CT scan can often determine whether an aneurysm or AVM is present and must be dealt with when the hematoma is evacuated.[11]

In about 10% of patients, arteriograms obtained following SAH reveal no source for the bleeding. Intense scrutiny of these patient's arteriograms is warranted, because one study has indicated that as many as 16% of such results are false-

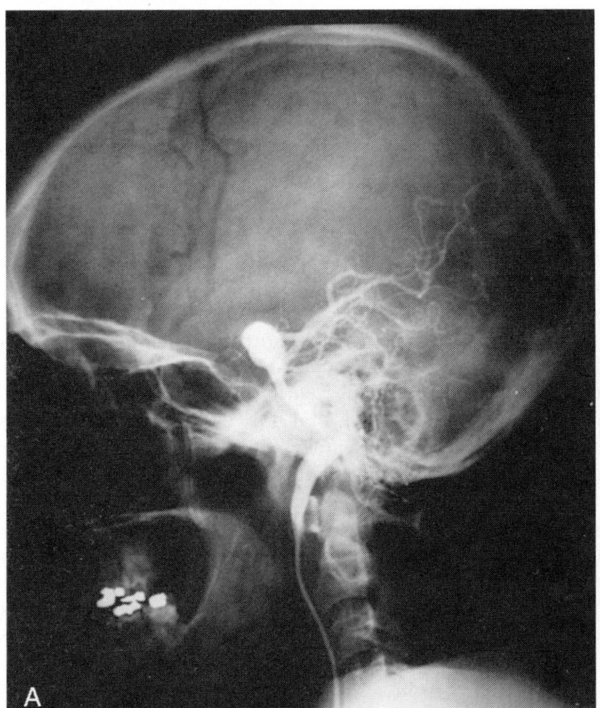

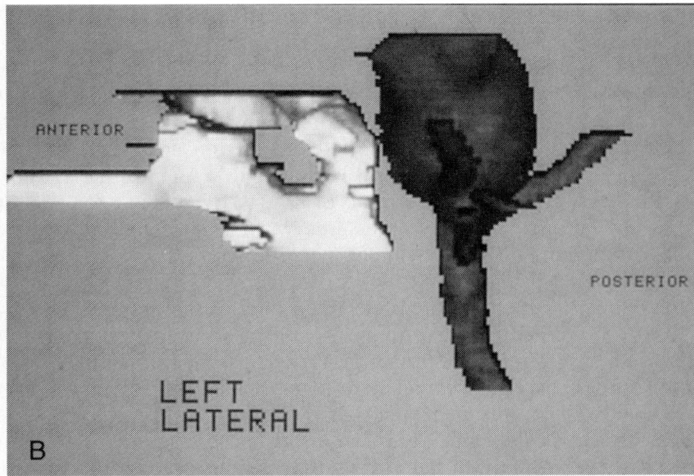

Figure 171–1. Standard angiography. Contrast medium is injected directly into the cerebral vessels through a catheter inserted into the groin. Injection of the vertebral artery resulted in demonstration of an aneurysm at the apex of the basilar artery. *B,* CT angiography involves the intravenous injection of contrast and rapid helical CT scanning. CT angiography elucidates not only the arterial anatomy in three dimensions but also the relationship to the skull base.

negative.[12] In some cases, the presence of blood in the interhemispheric or sylvian fissures may appropriately guide surgical exploration into the region about the anterior communicating or the middle cerebral arteries, respectively. Conversely, the presence of blood primarily about the perimesencephalic cisterns combined with negative angiography is highly prognostic of a good outcome; in such cases, an aneurysm is highly unlikely to be found on follow-up studies.[13]

Treatment

The treatment of SAH involves primarily (1) identifying and eliminating the causative lesion and thereby preventing rebleeding; (2) treating hydrocephalus; and (3) preventing and treating vasospasm.

The traditional management of patients with aneurysmal SAH dictated delayed surgery, at least 10 to 14 days after the SAH. Patients were managed medically in the interval, with surgery being delayed until after the peak period of vasospasm. Management consisted of bed rest, minimal stimulation, and heavy sedation. Prevention of rebleeding was attempted with the use of antifibrinolytic agents, although subsequent studies have shown that these agents significantly increased the risk of delayed ischemic injuries. In patients awaiting surgery, vasospasm was treated by intravascular volume expansion. Serial angiography or transcranial Doppler ultrasonography studies were used to document the extent of vessel narrowing, and surgery was delayed until results of these studies suggested that vasospasm had passed. Although this approach is still considered acceptable, especially for high-grade lesions, newer thinking on many of these practices is rapidly changing the standard of care.

Prevention of Rebleeding

In contrast with the earlier belief that rebleeding peaked at about day 7 after the SAH, newer data have clarified that the peak incidence of rebleeding is during the initial 24 hours after SAH, with 20% of patients experiencing rebleeding within 14 days.[14] Rebleeding occurs at a higher incidence with advancing age,[15] and patients who have a warning or mild initial bleed are just as likely to have a life-threatening event with rebleeding.

Because rebleeding occurs from an imbalance between the hemodynamic forces that are stressing the lumen of the aneurysm and the clot that has temporarily sealed the rupture point, efforts to minimize the disruptive forces are indicated. In the patient who has regained a good level of function (Hunt and Hess grades 1 and 2), blood pressure should be maintained at the lowest level consistent with a stable neurologic status. Support for the importance of early blood pressure control is provided by computer models of cerebral hemodynamics, which suggest that pressures within the aneurysm can be significantly greater than pressures within the parent vessels (Sclabassi, unpublished data). Similar studies have also shown that antihypertensive agents that function to slow the heart rate and accelerations of flow (β-blockade) can significantly reduce the peak pressures within an aneurysm dome, in comparison with a similar mean pressure generated with agents that primarily produce a peripheral vasodilation.

In an effort to decrease the incidence of rebleeding as well as allow a more vigorous treatment of vasospasm, many have supported early surgical intervention. Patients are operated on as early after arrival as is clinically reasonable. The theoretical advantage is that a greater degree of hypertension and volume expansion can begin earlier. Surgical intervention also makes possible the evacuation of blood from the subarachnoid space as well as opening of the CSF cisterns, allowing for a more rapid removal of the remaining blood products. Aggressive CSF drainage can also be maintained through the period of peak spasm in order to maximize cerebral blood flow. The theoretical disadvantage of this approach is that the surgical procedure is more difficult in a friable and swollen brain with a greater propensity for intraoperative rupture.

The International Cooperative Study on Timing of Aneurysm Surgery showed that there is essentially no difference between early surgery and delayed surgery in the hands of a large number of neurosurgeons worldwide.[16, 17] Although rebleeding was reduced in the early surgery group, the incidence of vasospastic complications was increased. Conversely, although fewer patients survived to operation in the delayed surgery group, those undergoing surgery appeared to have a better chance of a good functional outcome. The overall management and mortality were nearly identical for the two groups.

In a reanalysis of the data from the North American centers, it was reported that the rate of "good" recovery for patients with aneurysmal SAH was significantly better (70.9% versus 61.7%) in patients with planned surgery on day 0 to 3.[18] The mortality rate was higher for patients operated on between days 7 and 10 after bleeding, reinforcing the historic concept of greater surgical risk during the period of greatest vasospasm. Several groups have, however, reported that equally good results can now be obtained with immediate aneurysm surgery and aggressive antispasm therapy regardless of the time since SAH.[19-21]

Vasospasm

The incidence of symptomatic vasospasm after SAH is said by some researchers to be as high as 33% and by others to be closer to 10%.[22, 23] The incidence depends on the criteria for making the diagnosis; criteria based on clinical and indirect measures of cerebral perfusion yield the higher incidence, and criteria based on a definition of ischemia yield the lower incidence.[24] The onset of vasospasm is customarily delayed for at least 48 to 72 hours following SAH, and the risk of vasospasm continues for at least 2 weeks following hemorrhage. Patients at risk for development of vasospasm can be identified from the volume of subarachnoid clot shown on CT.[25] The Cooperative Study demonstrated that the proportion of patients with vasospasm increases with age, the highest incidence (57%) being in patients 60 to 69 years old.[15]

Vasospasm is a focal or diffuse narrowing of intracranial vessels thought to arise from the local presence of blood products, which produces decreased cerebral blood flow (CBF) and thereby may cause ischemia-induced neurologic deficits. As demonstrated by Grubb and colleagues,[26] ischemia results only after a decompensation of collateral and metabolic systems. As feeding vessels to a region of the brain become narrowed, CBF is maintained by a progressive vasodilation of the arterial bed (increased cerebral blood volume [CBV]). Continued compromise of perfusion pressure is compensated for by a greater extraction of vital nutrients (increased oxygen extraction fraction [OEF]). A neurologic deficit does not occur until nutrients essential for maintaining metabolic needs are exhausted.

Because maximal vasodilation accompanies the early loss of perfusion pressure, the critical supply of nutrients directly depends on the perfusion pressure. Thus, an early spontaneous response to vasospasm is the spontaneous elevation of blood pressure in an attempt to maintain homeostasis. If this system fails to supply enough flow, the pharmacologic elevation of blood pressure can reverse deficits. Infarction will result, depending on the depth and duration of the ischemic challenge. Thus, the timely diagnosis and treatment of ischemia due to vasospasm are essential goals of the postoperative management of aneurysms.

The basis for the current strategy of the medical management of vasospasm is calcium channel blocking agents combined with "triple-H" (hypervolemia, hemodilution, hypertension) therapy. The use of calcium channel blockers has emerged as an effective prophylaxis against ischemic complications due to vasospasm, although nimodipine has not been shown capable of causing angiographic dilation of cerebral vessels.[27] In the British trial of this agent, oral nimodipine reduced the incidence of cerebral infarction from 33% to 22% and decreased the rate of poor outcome from 33% to 20%.[28]

The standard of care following surgical clipping of an aneurysm consists of hypervolemia and hemodilution. The objective of hypervolemia is to maintain an adequate blood volume so that the patient has the fluid status needed to spontaneously maintain an optimum perfusion pressure. Directing the hematocrit value into the range of 30% to 35% attains an optimum ratio of viscosity to oxygen-carrying capacity. Volume expansion, usually with crystalloid, accomplishes both of these objectives. Although a central venous pressure (CVP) measure is usually sufficient for monitoring the adequacy of fluid loading, it is often necessary, especially in the elderly, to use a Swan-Ganz catheter to most accurately achieve the optimum blood volume without causing heart failure and pulmonary edema.

A CVP of 8 to 12 mm Hg or a pulmonary wedge pressure of 12 to 16 mm Hg is the commonly utilized goal of fluid therapy. When infusion of crystalloid does not maintain an adequate filling pressure, colloid solutions combined with an elevation of hematocrit are often sufficient. Whereas therapeutic regimens and local preferences may vary among treatment centers, it is increasingly clear that prophylactic attention to fluid balance and pressor therapy is superior to "catch-up" therapy after the onset of a delayed ischemic deficit.[19, 29]

When symptoms due to ischemia develop, hypertensive therapy is able to reverse the symptoms in many patients.[30] The introduction of hypertensive therapy must be timely, because the reversibility of an ischemic injury is related to the time and depth of the insult. In many institutions, there may be no alternative to maintaining blood pressure elevation for a few days and basing the withdrawal of medication on the careful monitoring of symptom recurrence. A preferential strategy now being used integrates objective measures of CBF to establish the diagnosis and to avoid the many complications associated with hypertensive therapy unless it is required. In one series, the diagnosis of symptomatic vasospasm based on clinical and transcranial Doppler ultrasonography information was in error 50% of the time in identifying patients who had symptoms due to territorial ischemia.[31] Because waiting until hypertensive therapy fails to progress to more definitive treatments has often resulted in the delayed treatment of areas that are already infarcted, some researchers have adopted a strategy of using hypertensive therapy only as long as needed to transport the patient to a center where interventional neuroradiology is available.[23]

The latest addition to the management of ischemia due to vasospasm is transluminal angioplasty with intra-arterial papaverine. Patients with an onset of ischemia due to vasospasm (ideally established with an objective measure of CBF) who are dependent on hypertensive therapy to ward off an irreversible ischemic injury or in whom such therapy fails are candidates for endovascular therapy[32, 33] (Fig. 171–2) (see Color Figure). Although papaverine infusion can dilate intracranial vessels, the desired effect is often transient, and treatments must be repeated every 12 to 18 hours.[34] Angioplasty, in contrast, appears to produce a long-term benefit through reversing the vasoconstriction of proximal vessels. Although the numbers are small at present, improvement of neurologic function has been reported in 69% to 80% of selected patients undergoing transluminal angioplasty.[23] This technique is currently limited by the number of centers qualified to perform it.

A significant number of patients with aneurysmal SAH are elderly. There is no question that age has a negative impact on surgical morbidity and mortality; the chance of a good outcome is 11% in patients older than 70 years, compared with 24% in all younger individuals.[35] Factors that have identified patients more likely to have a poor outcome are prolonged unconsciousness after SAH and evidence of cerebral atherosclerosis.[33, 36] It is now the policy of many institutions to offer aneurysm surgery for patients, irrespective of age, who are not moribund, especially if they are demonstrating any neurologic improvement, often with placement of an external ventricular drain following SAH.

Some studies have explored the role of surgical intervention in patients with poor neurologic status (World Federation Scale grade IV or V) at presentation. Although the traditional view is that the outcome, especially for grade V patients, is bleak,[37] the nimodipine study showed a 29% good outcome in poor-grade patients treated with nimodipine, compared with 9.0% in the control group. Bailes and associates[38] adopted an aggressive approach to grade IV and V patients, which consisted of ventriculostomy placement, early operation, and rapid institution of triple-H therapy; they report good outcome in 45% of grade IV patients and 18% of grade V patients.

Hydrocephalus

Proper management of the volume of CSF remains a vital part of the care of patients after SAH. Because CSF is produced at a constant rate of 0.34 mL/min, any obstruction of CSF dynamics can result in an increased CSF volume, which has an inverse relationship with blood volume. Blood volume in turn, has a direct effect on brain recovery immediately following the bleed as well as during the week of peak risk from vasospasm-induced ischemia.

In the initial hours after the hemorrhage, acute hydrocephalus can account for a progressive neurologic deterioration or for a persistence of the initial coma state that commonly accompanies a severe SAH. If the ventricles are significantly enlarged and the patient is not improving, a ventriculostomy can be lifesaving. Care must be taken not to lower intracranial pressure (ICP) too rapidly, and many clinicians would maintain a significant back-pressure of 30+ cm H_2O while the aneurysm remains unclipped. Rapid lowering of ICP, especially if the blood pressure remains elevated, can significantly increase the risk of rebleeding.[9] A ventriculostomy or a lumbar drain is commonly used during surgery to relax the brain and allow approach to the aneurysm with minimal retraction. Subsequent to surgery, CSF many physicians maintain drainage to minimize CSF-generated pressure that might limit brain perfusion. During the period of maximal vasospasm, attention to avoiding hydrocephalus is a key part of minimizing the incidence of ischemia due to vasospasm.

During the weeks and months following SAH, communicating hydrocephalus develops in 10% to 20% of patients. One report suggests that this rate may be increased in patients who receive early aggressive CSF drainage.[39] Follow-up CT scans obtained at subsequent clinic visits allow the monitoring of this problem, which can be effectively treated with CSF diversion (ventriculoperitoneal or lumbar peritoneal shunt).

Surgical Technique

Surgical procedures for the elimination of intracranial aneurysms involves gaining access to the feeding artery with minimal disturbance of the aneurysm. Skull base surgical concepts are integrated with microsurgical techniques to obtain needed exposure with minimal brain retraction. Usually, moderate

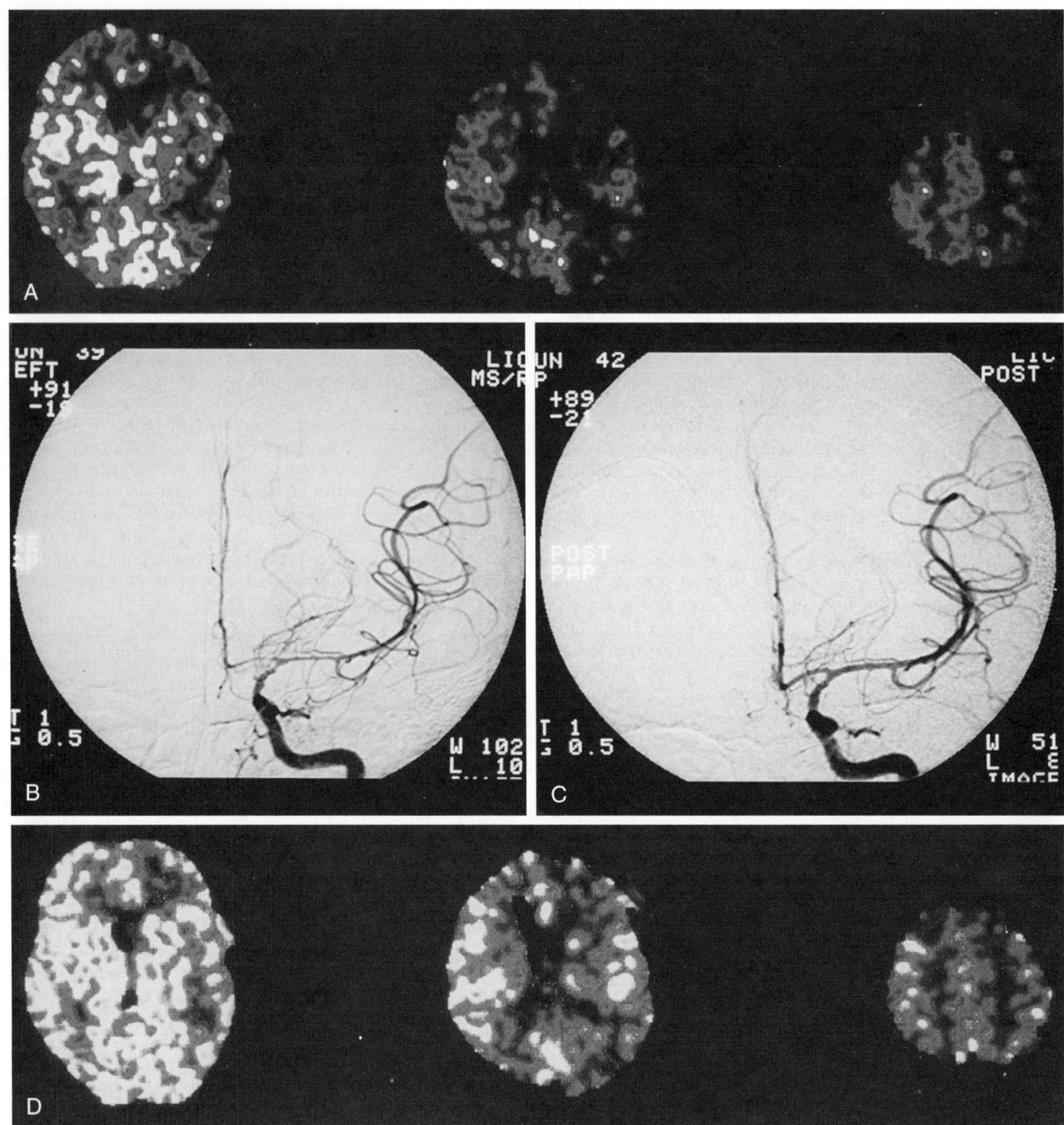

Figure 171–2. *A,* A three-level xenon/CT cerebral blood flow study obtained in a 40-year-old patient 8 days after a subarachnoid hemorrhage and 1 hour after the onset of aphasia and a new weakness of the right arm. *B,* The left internal carotid artery injection revealed severe narrowing of the anterior cerebral and middle cerebral arteries. *C,* After intra-arterial infusion of papaverine, the vascular narrowing is dramatically improved. *D,* The xenon/CT cerebral blood flow study obtained immediately after papaverine infusion revealed a dramatic improvement of perfusion within the anterior and middle cerebral territories. (*A* and *D,* See Color Figure.)

hypothermia is utilized to maximize the tolerance to brain retraction and temporary ischemia. Temporary occlusion of feeding arteries is frequently used to relax the dome and thereby permit dissection of the neck with protection of all surrounding large and small vessels. Neurophysiologic monitoring is helpful for determining whether temporary occlusion is causing ischemia. If that is the case, neuroprotection with barbiturate-induced reduction of cerebral metabolism at burst suppression level is usually sought, accompanied by an effort to minimize occlusion time. For very large, complex aneurysms that are likely to require more than 15 minutes of temporary occlusion time for dissection, profound hypothermia with cardiac arrest can prolong the safe arrest of the brain circulation to 50 minutes.

The intent of aneurysm surgery is to eliminate all elements of the aneurysm from the circulation.[40] Absence of flow within the aneurysm must be confirmed at surgery. This can be accomplished by simply puncturing the dome, which also relieves the pressure that the dome may be putting on adjacent structures. Surgical approaches that integrate skull base surgical principles have been important in making accessible aneurysms that are even more difficult to reach. Interventional neuroradiology approaches to proximal temporary occlusion have also proved helpful.

Endovascular Techniques

Endovascular approaches to treating intracranial aneurysms are evolving rapidly. Although initial reports suggested that detachable balloons could be placed within many aneurysms in order to protect patients from the risk of future rupture,[41] a subsequent series has been less successful.[42] Detachable coil systems have won favor at many centers as a treatment option for many aneurysms, especially those located at the basilar apex.[43] This is a promising technology that, as it continues to evolve, will certainly play a major role in the treatment of patients with cerebral aneurysms.

Vascular Malformations

Vascular malformations that produce SAH are parenchymal AVMs, dural AVMs, venous angiomas, and cavernous angiomas.

Parenchymal Arteriovenous Malformations

Parenchymal AVMs are congenital lesions that consist of direct shunts between abnormal arteries and veins without an intervening capillary network. No neurologic function is attributed to the malformation or to the brain tissue that is located either within or immediately around the nidus. Clinical presentation is usually due to bleeding either within the substance of the brain or into the subarachnoid space, to epilepsy, or to a "steal phenomenon" (blood taken by the malformation from surrounding normal brain).

The incidence of symptomatic AVMs in North America is 1.8 per 100,000 population.[44] SAH from AVMs is clearly much rarer than from aneurysms and appears at a younger age. In one study, 8.6% of all SAHs were due to AVMs; however, only 4% of them occurred in patients older than 60 years.[45]

The clinical presentation of an AVM is similar to that of an aneurysmal hemorrhage, except that the bleeding tends to be less violent and most often has a significant intraparenchymal component. The incidence of vasospasm and of rebleeding due to AVMs is significantly less than with aneurysms. The incidence of rebleeding in AVMs is so low that early surgical intervention is indicated only for patients with life-threatening bleeds due to severe mass effect. The majority of patients are as younger individuals with seizures or focal neurologic deficits.

The diagnosis of an AVM is definitively made with four-vessel angiography, which can be used to examine all of the feeding and draining vessels of the malformation. High-quality angiography is indicated because definition of the AVM is necessary not only for treatment planning but also for the assessment of feeding vessels, which commonly harbor aneurysms. In a patient with SAH who has both an AVM and an aneurysm, the aneurysm is more often the source of bleeding and must be attended to emergently. In contrast, treatment planning for an AVM differs because the rebleed rate is far lower, as is the incidence of vasospasm. Thus, a conservative approach to a technically difficult AVM within functionally eloquent brain regions is often acceptable.

The cumulative risk of rebleeding in a patient who has suffered a primary AVM hemorrhage is 3% to 4% per year. Unlike with aneurysms, the risk is no greater in the acute period after hemorrhage of an AVM. In young individuals with surgically accessible lesions, this risk becomes appreciable, and surgical intervention is easily justifiable. In older individuals or for AVMs that are identified as incidental findings or as part of an evaluation for epilepsy, the decision for surgical intervention has to be weighed carefully. In this setting, alternative therapies, such as radiosurgery, have won a role in the treatment of patients with AVMs.

Once an AVM that has hemorrhaged is deemed to be appropriate for surgical intervention because of its location, the complexity of its feeding and draining vessels, and the surgical experience of the operating team, surgery is often delayed several weeks.[46] At that time, the brain is usually more relaxed, and the hemorrhage has become liquid so that it can be easily separated from the fragile vessels of the AVM. The goal of surgery is complete resection; any retained AVM is consistent with a continued potential for rebleeding.

At surgery, the plan is to (1) occlude and section all feeding vessels first, (2) dissect the AVM within the glial plane about the AVM, and (3) section the draining veins. Preoperative embolization of feeding arteries that are especially difficult to reach can make AVM resection safer. Despite optimal surgical resection, postoperative deficits are common, but they most often resolve within a few days to weeks.[47]

The optimum management of nonoperative AVMs remains an open question. Although embolization has proved useful as a surgical adjunct, embolization alone has failed to become a primary treatment because it is rarely able to totally eliminate the lesion. Radiosurgery has assumed a major role in the treatment of many AVMs, especially for an inaccessible lesion or for the residual of operative cases.[48] Although radiosurgery, like surgical intervention, provides no risk reduction from recurrent hemorrhage until the AVM is totally eliminated, lesions less than 3 cm in diameter are usually eliminated totally within 2 years.

Dural Arteriovenous Malformations

Dural AVMs are developmental and occur from spontaneous thrombosis of a dural venous channel followed by capillary ingrowth, clot lysis, and the establishment of a direct arterial shunt into the previously occluded venous segment. Symptoms and signs depend on the degree of recanalization of the normal dural venous channels and the route by which the arteriovenous shunt drains. If drainage is via the normal venous system, a bruit due to the high-flow state is the normal cause of clinical presentation. If the drainage is instead to the cortical veins that normally would feed into the venous segment, cortical venous hypertension results, and interparenchymal hemorrhage may occur. On angiography an aggressive dural AVM would be shown to have leptomeningeal, galenic, and/or variceal venous dilations both within and over the cortex.[49, 50]

Patients who present with SAH or intraparenchymal hemorrhage from a dural AVM are at high risk for rebleed, and aggressive therapy is indicated. Treatment usually involves a combination of endovascular and surgical intervention designed to totally eliminate the venous segment into which arterial blood is flowing.

Cavernous Angiomas

Cavernous angiomas are readily evident on MRI as areas of hemorrhage and rehemorrhage. Bleeds of cavernous angiomas are more self-limiting than those of AVMs, perhaps because of the very small size of the arterial inputs to these relatively slow-flow lesions. The frequency of bleeding from an incidentally found cavernous angioma ranges from 0.25% to 0.7% per year.[51, 52] On the basis of these data, elective excision is recommended primarily in cases of gross hemorrhage, intractable seizures, or development of a significant mass lesion.[52]

Surgical excision of a cavernous angioma is straightforward and far less problematic than that of an AVM. Deep-seated or small lesions can be readily resected with the aid of stereotactic surgical technology.

Venous Angiomas

Venous angiomas are normal venous channels that take anomalous routes, often through the substance of the brain. Thus, incidentally found venous angiomas are not surgically removed.[53, 54] Hemorrhage can occur in association with a venous AVM; when it does, hemorrhage is believed to be due to a cavernous angioma that is adjacent to the much larger venous abnormality. If surgery is indicated for removal of hemorrhage, it is necessary to avoid occlusion of the anomalous venous channels.

Other Causes of Subarachnoid Hemorrhage

Infection

Mycotic aneurysms typically form from septic embolization of the vasa vasorum of an intracranial artery.[55] Infective endocarditis is assumed to be the source in most cases; blood culture results are often positive, and vegetations of the heart valves are commonly found on echocardiography. Mycotic aneurysms occur on secondary or tertiary vessels, in contrast to "berry" aneurysms, which occur at bifurcations of primary vessels.

It has been recommended that all patients with known endocarditis and a focal neurologic deficit should undergo selective angiography.[56] The treatment of an incidentally found small mycotic aneurysm is intravenous antibiotic therapy, which results in resolution of the vascular lesion in the majority of cases. For larger aneurysms or aneurysms that are associated with hemorrhage, surgical resection of the abnormal vascular segment is often required. In some cases, arterial occlusion can be accomplished by an endovascular route.

Systemic Causes

An association between SAH and sickle cell anemia has been reported.[57] SAH has been observed as the first sign of this disease or in association with other clinical manifestations. A careful family and patient history and appropriate coagulation studies should be performed in patients with SAH.

Primary SAH is being increasingly seen in patients with a history of drug abuse. Amphetamines are notorious offenders; they cause a vasculitis that can lead to either primary vessel rupture or aneurysm formation accompanied by rupture. The increased blood pressure that accompanies the use of these agents adds to the risk of rupture.

INTRACEREBRAL HEMORRHAGE

Spontaneous *intracerebral hemorrhage* (ICH) refers to parenchymal hematoma that is not associated with trauma. Although only 17% of all strokes are caused by ICH, this entity accounts for a disproportionate morbidity and mortality, resulting in death at a rate of 40 per 100 cases.[58-61] Presenting symptoms are variable, depending on the size and location of the ICH, and the risk of ICH increases with age, doubling with each decade.[62]

The diagnosis of ICH is straight forward, because CT is exquisitely sensitive to intraparenchymal blood. MRI, CT angiography, and conventional angiography are additional studies that can help define the source of bleeding.

The causes of ICH are many, and treatment depends on an understanding of the possible etiologies.

Differential Diagnosis

Hypertension is the most important single risk factor for ICH. A typical location of ICH and microvascular changes is seen in patients with hypertension. The basal ganglia are involved in 65% of ICHs, followed by the deep white matter in 10% to 20%, the pons in 10% to 15%, and the cerebellum in 8% to 10%.

Etiology

The mechanism for the development of ICH is debatable. Miliary aneurysms, described by Charcot and Bouchard in 1868, are found at the origins of the middle cerebral lateral striae as well as basilar paramedian branch arteries in 50% of patients with hypertension who are older than 66 years.[63-66] A more likely cause, which is more commonly found within the substance of the ICH, is destruction of the tunica media through a process described as *fibrinoid necrosis*.[62, 66-69]

Aneurysms, Arteriovenous Malformations

Aneurysms and AVMs are the causes of about 25% of ICHs. Although aneurysms more often cause SAH, 5% to 20% of aneurysm domes are buried within brain substance and manifest as either ICH or a combination of ICH and SAH. An aneurysm source for ICH must be expected when the base of the hemorrhage is in continuity with the large vessels of the circle of Willis. Although angiography is the traditional technology used for defining the vasculature, CT angiography or simply an enhanced CT scan is often adequate to guide surgical intervention, especially when the patient is deteriorating rapidly. AVMs manifest as ICH within potentially any portion of the brain.[70] The clinical course is usually less rapid than with an aneurysm and the clinical outcome is better.

Amyloidosis

Amyloidosis predominantly affects the elderly and accounts for up to 10% of ICHs.[70] Pathologic studies reveal the deposition of beta-amyloid protein in the media and adventitia of small cortical vessels, which commonly rupture, producing lobar, subcortical hemorrhages.[71] A lobar bleed in an elderly, nonhypertensive patient is strongly suggestive of the diagnosis of cerebral amyloidosis.[72] A common differential diagnosis is a *malignancy,* which also manifests as hemorrhage into the subcortical white matter. Tumors that commonly manifest in this way are glioblastoma multiforme, malignant melanoma, choriocarcinoma, renal cell carcinoma, and bronchogenic carcinoma.[73-75] Although the presence on CT scan of edema around the ICH very early after a bleed should raise the suspicion of an underlying malignancy, a small tumor can produce a large hemorrhage that can mask edema. Often, only follow-up imaging studies obtained after the ICH has resolved can answer the question of an underlying malignancy.

Coagulopathy

Coagulopathic states with or without an associated infarction account for nearly 10% of ICHs.[58] All antiplatelet, anticoagulant, and thrombolytic therapies have been implicated as causes of ICH,[76] and nearly 2% of patients receiving anticoagulation therapy experience ICH.[71] Systemic illnesses that produce a coagulopathic state, such as hepatic failure, thrombocytopenia, and the leukemias, are associated with a higher incidence of ICH.

An increasingly common cause of ICH results from the use of recombinant tissue plasminogen activator (rt-PA) in the treatment of myocardial and cerebral infarctions. A tenfold increase in ICH occurs in patients treated with IV rt-PA within 3 hours of the onset of an ischemic cerebral infarction. Patients most likely to develop ICH have been those with delayed therapy, elevated blood pressure, a severe stroke with a National Institutes of Health (NIH) Stroke Scale score of greater than 20, and evidence of mass effect on the baseline CT scan.

Infection

Infections account for a small percentage of ICHs and result from direct invasion of the arteries, either from basilar meningitis, due to emboli consisting of infected material, or from hemorrhagic encephalitis. Fungal basilar meningitis commonly causes cortical and subcortical hemorrhage, whereas a mycotic aneurysm of a usually more peripheral artery may cause both ICH and SAH. Herpes simplex virus produces an acute, necrotizing, hemorrhagic encephalitis that preferentially affects the temporal and frontal lobes.

Sinus Thrombosis and Drug Use

Two increasingly common causes of ICH are major venous sinus occlusion and the use of illicit drugs. Sinus thrombosis is associated with a variety of medical conditions, including pregnancy, systemic infection, sickle cell trait, contraceptive use, and protein C deficiency. Parasagittal ICH, especially involving both hemispheres, is a common CT finding in a patient with sagittal sinus thrombosis. The diagnosis can be confirmed with a contrast-enhanced CT scan that reveals no contrast within the sinus (delta sign).

Sympathomimetic drugs, such as cocaine, amphetamines, pseudoephedrine, and phenylpropanolamine, are frequently implicated in cases of ICH.[77, 78]

Other Causes

Spontaneous migration of a cerebral embolism is a common source of ICH. *Reperfusion* of an ischemic bed may result in the subtle leakage of blood products into the region of infarction, producing a hemorrhagic infarction or a frank hemorrhage. The former is often not associated with additional clinical deterioration, but the latter is. Fear of causing an ICH is a common reason for delaying carotid endarterectomy after an ischemic event in a patient with high-grade carotid stenosis. In the absence of postoperative hypertension, however, hemorrhage is uncommon in this setting.

Treatment

Management of ICH involves attention to all of the treatable causes of ICH, with the option of surgical intervention being reserved for the patient with the potential for a useful outcome who is deteriorating because of extreme mass effect. Initially, hypertension should be rapidly treated, with blood pressure values corrected to the prebleed level or to approximately 20% less than those at presentation.[62] Abnormalities in the coagulation profile are rapidly addressed.

Imaging studies are essential for definition of the hemorrhage, because a small bleed within critical pathways can produce profound deficits from the onset of bleed, and a large bleed within the frontal or temporal lobes can produce surprisingly little deficit. For most small bleeds, there is little evidence that surgery or any specific medical therapy should play a role, except for control of severe hypertension. With the onset of brain stem compression, care must to be directed toward reducing ICP. Intubation, moderate hyperventilation, and diuresis are appropriate. Although a ventriculostomy is critical for treating hydrocephalus in the patient with a cerebellar bleed, ventricular drainage for a patient with a supratentorial bleed can increase tentorial herniation. In this setting, a ventricular catheter can provide insight into the intracranial pressure, but only removal of the clot itself and appropriate tissues (i.e., temporal lobe with uncus) can be beneficial.

The role of surgery in the treatment of hypertensive ICH is controversial. Although a Japanese trial suggested a benefit from very early surgical intervention,[64] a larger prospective trial showed that survival following deep nuclear ICH was poor and that, in most cases, surgery did not improve outcome.[79] Another trial suggested a benefit of surgery for individuals with neurologic deficits scored between 7 and 10 on the Glasgow Coma Scale, although survivors were severely disabled. Surgery is probably most indicated for patients who present with moderate disabilities and then deteriorate owing to mass effect from extension of hemorrhage into less functionally critical areas, such as the temporal lobe. Additionally, refractory intracranial hypertension in a young patient favors surgical intervention. Factors that work against surgical treatment are severe coagulopathy, significant underlying medical disease, and age older than 75 years.

For patients with nonhypertensive ICH, definition of the cause of the bleeding is an essential first step in planning therapy. Aneurysms and AVMs may be assessed by angiography, CT angiography, or MRI. Often, more than one modality is needed to provide a full understanding of the complexity of an AVM. For most cases, it is preferable to evacuate only the hematoma and to leave the AVM for nonemergent treatment; however, this is not always possible, and if bleeding is not readily stopped, total excision of the AVM may be necessary. The treatment of some AVMs and aneurysms today is achieved through an endovascular route; especially in the patient who is a poor surgical risk, endovascular placement of coils within the aneurysm is proving to be an acceptable therapy.

When a hemorrhage is encountered within the subcortical white matter in a pattern not typical of a hypertensive ICH, a tumor must be considered as the etiology. For that reason, as the clot is removed, attention should be paid to the wall of the clot cavity for any unusual tissue that warrants biopsy. Even in the absence of clearly abnormal tissue, a biopsy is warranted in the elderly patient with a large polar bleed, because making the pathologic diagnosis of amyloid angiopathy is important for long-term management.

Because ICH is today commonly associated with the use of potent thrombolytic agents, such as recombinant tissue-plasminogen activator (rt-PA), it is important for the critical care team to be aware of the specific needs of patients with ICH from this cause. The factors that correlate with an increased risk of bleed include the dose of thrombolytic agent, the delayed time to treatment onset, and elevated blood pressure prior to treatment. In the National Institute of Neurologic Disorders (NINDS) study, two factors were associated with higher risk of symptomatic ICH:

1. A severe stroke, as measured by an NIH Stroke Scale score of greater than 20.
2. CT findings of acute hypodensity and mass effect at baseline status.[80-82]

If hemorrhage occurs with any of these treatments, the thrombolytic drug infusion is stopped and the team prepares for the administration of cryoprecipitate and platelets. If an emergent repeat CT scan defines a new ICH, 6 to 8 units of cryoprecipitate and 6 to 8 units of platelets are indicated (NINDS trial protocol). Because of the potential need for neurosurgical consultation as well as blood products, it is generally recommended that patients who receive intravenous rt-PA either should be admitted to a hospital where such consultation is available or should be transferred to such a hospital shortly after rt-PA therapy is started.

References

1. Torner JC: Epidemiology of subarachnoid hemorrhage. Semin Neurol 1984; 4:354-369.
2. Pakarinen S: Incidence, etiology and prognosis of primary subarachnoid hemorrhage: A study based on 589 cases diagnosed in a defined urban population during a defined period. Acta Neurol Scand (Suppl) 1967; 29:1-128.
3. Chyatte D, Lewis I: Gelatinase activity and the occurrence of cerebral aneurysms. Stroke 1997; 28:799-804.

4. Daras M, Tuchman AJ, Koppel BS, et al: Neurovascular complications of cocaine. Acta Neurol Scand 1994; 90:124-129.
5. Kibayashi K, Mastri AR, Hirsch CS: Cocaine induced intracerebral hemorrhage: Analysis of predisposing factors and mechanisms causing hemorrhagic strokes. Hum Pathol 1995; 26:659-663.
6. Adams HP Jr, Kassell NF, Torner JC, et al: CT and clinical correlations in recent aneurysmal subarachnoid hemorrhage: A preliminary report of the Cooperative Aneurysm Study. Neurology 1993; 33:981-988.
7. Macdonald A, Mendelow AD: Xanthochromia revisited: A re-evaluation of lumbar puncture and CT scanning in the diagnosis of subarachnoid haemorrhage. J Neurol Neurosurg Psychiatry 1988; 41:342-344.
8. Lang DT, Berberian LB, Lee S, et al: Rapid differentiation of subarachnoid hemorrhage from traumatic lumbar puncture using the D-dimer assay. Am J Clin Pathol 1990; 93:403-405.
9. Pare L, Delfino R, Leblanc R: The relationship of ventricular drainage to aneurysmal rebleeding. J Neurosurg 1992; 76:422-427.
10. Wood EH: Angiographic identification of the ruptured lesion in patients with multiple cerebral aneurysms. J Neurosurg 1964; 21:182-198.
11. LeRoux PD, Dailey AT, Newell DW, et al: Emergent aneurysm clipping without angiography in the moribund patient with intracerebral hemorrhage: The use of infusion computed tomographic scans. Neurosurgery 1993; 33:189-197.
12. Iwanage H, Wakai S, Ochiai C, et al: Ruptured cerebral aneurysms missed by initial angiographic study. Neurosurgery 1990; 27:45-51.
13. Rinkel GH, Wijdicks EFM, Vermeulen M, et al: Nonaneurysmal perimesencephalic subarachnoid hemorrhage: CT and MR patterns that differ from aneurysmal rupture. AJR Am J Roentgenol 1991; 157:1325-1326.
14. Kassell NF, Torner JC: Aneurysmal rebleeding: A preliminary report from the cooperative study. Neurosurgery 1983; 13:479-481.
15. Sahs AL, Nibbelink DW, Torner JC: Aneurysmal Subarachnoid Hemorrhage: Report of the Cooperative Study. Baltimore, Urban & Schwarzenberg, 1981.
16. Kassell NF, Torner JC, Haley EC, et al: The International Cooperative Study on the Timing of Aneurysm Surgery: Part 1. Overall management results. J Neurosurg 1990; 73:18-36.
17. Kassell NF, Torner JC, Jane JA, Haley EC, Adams HP, and participants: The International Cooperative Study on the Timing of Aneurysm Surgery: Part 2. Surgical results. J Neurosurg 1990; 73:37-47.
18. Haley EC Jr, Kassell NF, Torner JC: The International Cooperative Study on the Timing of Aneurysm Surgery. Stroke 1992; 23:205-214.
19. Solomon RA, Fink ME, Lennihan L: Prophylactic volume expansion therapy for the prevention of delayed cerebral ischemia after early aneurysm surgery. Arch Neurol 1988; 45:325-332.
20. Solomon RA, Fink ME, Lennihan L: Early aneurysm surgery and prophylactic hypervolemic hypertensive therapy for the treatment of aneurysmal subarachnoid hemorrhage. Neurosurgery. 1988; 34:699-704.
21. Symon L: Evaluation of and controversies in surgical therapies. J Stroke Cerebrovasc Dis 1992; 2:56-60.
22. Kassell NF, Sasaki T, Colohan ART, et al: Cerebral vasospasm following aneurysmal subarachnoid hemorrhage. Stroke 1985; 16:562-572.
23. Firlik AD, Kaufmann AM, Jungreis CA, et al: Effect of transluminal angioplasty on cerebral blood flow in the management of symptomatic vasospasm following aneurysmal subarachnoid hemorrhage. J Neurosurg 1997; 86:830-839.
24. Clyde BL, Field M, Rutigliano M, et al: Screening for vasospasm with CT/Xe CBF prior to angiography (Abstract). J Stroke Cerebrovasc Dis 1997; 6:440.
25. Fisher CM, Kistler JP, Davis JM: Relation of cerebral vasospasm to subarachnoid hemorrhage visualized by computed tomographic scanning. Neurosurgery 1980; 6:1-9.
26. Grubb RL Jr, Raichle ME, Eichling JO, et al: Effects of subarachnoid hemorrhage on cerebral blood volume, blood flow and oxygen utilization in humans. J Neurosurg 1997; 46:446-453.
27. Allen GS, Ahm HS, Prezioisi TJ: Cerebral arterial spasm—a controlled trial of nimodipine in patients with subarachnoid hemorrhage. N Engl J Med 1983; 308:619-624.
28. Pickard JD, Murray GD, Illingworth R, et al: Effect of oral nimodipine on cerebral infarction and outcome after subarachnoid hemorrhage: British aneurysm nimodipine trial. Brit Med J 1989; 398:636-642.
29. Origitano TC, Wascher TM, Reichman OH, et al: Sustained increased cerebral blood flow with prophylactic hypertensive hemodilution ("triple-H" therapy) after subarachnoid hemorrhage. Neurosurgery 1990; 27:729-740.
30. Kassell NF, Helm G, Simmons N, et al: Treatment of cerebral vasospasm with intraarterial papaverine. J Neurosurg 1992; 77:848-852.
31. Darby JM, Yonas H, Marks EC, et al: Acute cerebral blood flow response to dopamine-induced hypertension after subarachnoid hemorrhage. J Neurosurg 1994; 80:857-864.
32. Higashida RT, Halbach VV, Cahan LD, et al: Transluminal angioplasty for treatment of intracranial arterial vasospasm. J Neurosurg 1989; 71:648-653.
33. Nornes H, Wikeby P: Results of microsurgical management of intracranial aneurysms. J Neurosurg 1979; 41:608-614.
34. Firlik KS, Kaufman AM, Firlik AD, et al: Intraarterial papaverine for the treatment of cerebral vasospasm following aneurysmal subarchnoid hemorrhage. Surg Neurol in press.
35. Amacher AL, Drake CG: Aneurysm surgery in the seventh decade. *In:* Present Limits of Neurosurgery. Fusek I, Kinc Z, (Eds). New York, American Elsevier Publishing, 1972, pp 263-266.
36. Hugosson R: Intracranial arterial aneurysms: Considerations on the upper age limit for surgical treatment. Acta Neurochir (Wien) 1973; 28:157-164.
37. Seifert V, Trost HA, Stolke D: Management morbidity and mortality in grade IV and V patients with aneurysmal subarachnoid hemorrhage. Acta Neurochir (Wien) 1990; 103:5-10.
38. Bailes JE, Spetzler RF, Hadley MN, et al: Management, morbidity and mortality of poor-grade aneurysm patients. J Neurosurg 1990; 72:559-566.
39. Kasuya H, Shimizu T, Kagawa M: The effect of continuous drainage of cerebrospinal fluid in patients with subarachnoid hemorrhage: A retrospective analysis of 108 patients. Neurosurgery 1991; 28:56-59.
40. Fujiwara S, Fujii K, Nishio S, et al: Long term results of wrapping of intracranial ruptured aneurysms. Acta Neurochir (Wien) 1990; 103:27-29.
41. Romodanov A, Shcheglov VI: Endovascular method of excluding from the circulation saccular cerebral arterial aneurysms, leaving intact vessels patent. Acta Neurochir Suppl 1979; 28:312-315.
42. Higashida RT, Halbach VV, Barnwell SL, et al: Treatment of intracranial aneurysms with preservation of the parent vessel: Results of percutaneous balloon embolization in 84 patients. AJNR Am J Neuroradiol 1990; 11:633-640.
43. Guglielmi G, Vinuela F, Dion J, et al: Electrothrombosis of saccular aneurysms via endovascular approach: Part 2. Preliminary clinical experience. J Neurosurg 1991; 75:8-14.
44. Mohr JP: Neurological manifestations and factors related to therapeutic decisions. *In:* Intracranial Arteriovenous Malformations. Wilson CB, Stein BM (Eds). Baltimore, Williams & Wilkins, 1984, p 1.
45. Perret G, Nishioka H: Report on the Cooperative Study of Intracranial Aneurysms and Subarachnoid Hemorrhage: Section VI. Arteriovenous malformations. J Neurosurg 1966; 25:467-490.
46. Spetzler RF, Zabramski JM: Grading and staged resection of cerebral arteriovenous malformations. Clin Neurosurg 1988; 36:318-337.
47. Heros RC, Korosue K, Diebold PM: Surgical excision of cerebral arteriovenous malformations: Late results. Neurosurgery 1990; 26:570-578.
48. Ogilvy CS: Radiation therapy for arteriovenous malformations: A review. Neurosurgery 1990; 26:725-735.
49. Awad IA, Little JR, Akrawi WP, et al: Intracranial dural arteriovenous malformations: Factors predisposing to an aggressive neurological course. J Neurosurg 1990; 72:839-850.
50. Awad IA: The diagnosis and management of intracranial dural arteriovenous malformations. Contemp Neurosurg 1991; 13:1-6.
51. Curling OD, Kelly DL, Elster AD, et al: An analysis of the natural history of cavernous angiomas. J Neurosurg 1991; 75:702-708.
52. Robinson JR, Awad IA, Little JR: Natural history of the cavernous angioma. J Neurosurg 1991; 75:709-714.

53. Garner TB, Curling OD, Kelly DL, et al: The natural history of intracranial venous angiomas. J Neurosurg 1991; 75:715–722.
54. Rigamonti D, Spetzler RF, Medina M, et al: Cerebral venous malformations. J Neurosurg 1990; 73:560–564.
55. Bohmfalk GL, Story JL, Wissinger JP, et al: Bacterial intracranial aneurysm. J Neurosurg 1978; 48:369–382.
56. Salgado AV, Furlan AJ, Keys TF: Mycotic aneurysm, subarachnoid hemorrhage, and indications for cerebral arteriography in infective endocarditis. Stroke 1987; 18:1057–1060.
57. Wood DH: Cerebrovascular complications of sickle-cell disease. Curr Concepts Cerebrovasc Dis 1978; 9:73–75.
58. Cahill DW, Ducker TB: Spontaneous intracerebral hemorrhage. Clin Neurosurg 1982; 29:722–799.
59. Kurtzke JF: Epidemiology of Cerebrovascular Disease. Berlin, Springer-Verlag, 1969.
60. Mohr JP, Caplan LR, Melski JW, et al: The Harvard Cooperative Stroke Registry: A prospective registry. Neurology 1978; 28:754–762.
61. Toole JF, Patel AN: Cerebrovascular Disorders. 2nd ed. New York, McGraw-Hill, 1967.
62. Ojemann RG, Heros RC: Spontaneous brain hemorrhage. Stroke 1983; 14:468–475.
63. Fisher CM: Cerebral miliary aneurysms in hypertension. Am J Pathol 1972; 66:313–330.
64. Kaneko M, Tanaka K, Shimada T, et al: Long-term evaluation of ultra-early operation for hypertensive intracerebral hemorrhage in 100 cases. J Neurosurg 1983; 58:838–842.
65. Newton TH, Potts DG (Eds). Radiology of the Skull and Brain. St Louis, CV Mosby, 1971.
66. Okizaki H: Fundamentals of Neuropathology: Morphologic Basis of Neurologic Disorders. 2nd ed. New York, Igaku-Shoin, 1989.
67. Fisher CM: Pathological observations in hypertensive cerebral hemorrhage. J Neuropathol Exp Neurol 1971; 30:536–550.
68. Kase CS, Mohr JP: General features of intracerebral hemorrhage. *In:* Stroke: Pathophysiology, Diagnosis and Management. Barnett HJM, Stein BM, Mohr JP, Yatsu FM (Eds). New York, Churchill Livingstone, 1986, pp 497–523.
69. Rosenblum WI: Miliary aneurysms and "fibrinoid" degeneration of cerebral vessels. Hum Pathol 1977; 8:133–139.
70. Vinters HB, Gilber JJ: Amyloid angiography: Its incidence and complications in the aging brain. Stroke 1981; 12:118–120.
71. Castel JP, Kissel P: Spontaneous intracerebral and infratentorial hemorrhage. *In:* Neurological Surgery. 3rd ed. Youmans J (Ed). Philadelphia, WB Saunders, 1990, pp 1890–1917.
72. Ropper AH, Davis KR: Lobar cerebral hemorrhages: Acute clinical syndromes in 26 cases. Ann Neurol 1980; 8:141–147.
73. Acosta-Sison H: Extensive cerebral hemorrhage caused by the rupture of a cerebral blood vessel due to a chorionepithelioma embolus. Am J Obstet Gynecol 1956; 71:1119.
74. Dublin AB, Norman D: Fluid-fluid level in cystic cerebral metastatic melanoma. J Comput Assist Tomogr 1979; 3:650–652.
75. Scott M: Spontaneous intracerebral hematoma caused by cerebral neoplasms. J Neurosurg 1975; 42:338–342.
76. Aldrich MS, Sherman SA, Greenberg HS: Cerebrovascular complications of streptokinase infusion. JAMA 1985; 253:1777–1779.
77. Harrington H, Heller A, Dawson D, et al: Intracerebral hemorrhage and oral amphetamines. Arch Neurol 1983; 40:503–507.
78. Levin S: Cocaine and stroke: Current concepts of cerebrovascular disease. Stroke 1987; 22:25–29.
79. Batjer HH, Reisch JS, Plazier LJ, et al: Failure of surgery to improve outcome in hypertensive putaminal hemorrhage: A prospective randomized trial. Arch Neurol 1990; 47:1103–1106.
80. Levy DE, Brott TG, Haley EC, et al: Factors related to intracranial hematoma formation in patients receiving tissue-type plasminogen activator for acute ischemic stroke. Stroke 1994; 25:291–297.
81. National Institute of Neurologic Disorders and Stroke rt-PA Stroke Study Group: Tissue plasminogen activator for acute ischemic stroke. N Engl J Med 1995; 333:1581–1587.
82. Wolpert SM, Bruckmann H, Greenlee R, Wechsler L, Pessin MS, del Zoppo GJ, and the rt-PA Acute Study Group: Neuroradiological evaluation of patients with acute stroke treated with recombinant tissue plasminogen activator. AJNR Am J Neuroradiol 1993; 14:3–13.

172

Management of Acute Ischemic Stroke

Lawrence R. Wechsler, MD
Carol A. Barch, MN, CRNP, CNRN

Until recently, the only treatment available for stroke was prevention. Most strokes are due to ischemia, but approximately 20% are caused by intracerebral or subarachnoid hemorrhage. Stroke is the third leading cause of death and the leading cause of adult disability in the United States. More than 700,000 new strokes occur each year,[1] and the direct and indirect annual costs of stroke are estimated at more than $40 billion. Anything that reduces the disability after stroke is an important contribution to health care.

In 1995, the National Institute of Neurological Disorders and Stroke (NINDS) study of tissue plasminogen activator (t-PA) was published,[2] demonstrating for the first time in a randomized controlled trial a reduction in stroke morbidity with acute treatment. Other treatments, such as intra-arterial thrombolytics and neuroprotective agents, are currently under active investigation. At present, intravenous t-PA is beneficial if it is given within 3 hours of stroke onset. Ongoing studies may extend the therapeutic window, particularly for neuroprotective agents without the potential for hemorrhagic complications.

The rationale for acute stroke treatment is based on the concept of the ischemic penumbra. When an arterial occlusion occurs, an area of infarcted brain is surrounded by a region that has reduced blood flow, impairing function but not sufficiently severe to result in irreversible infarction. If adequate blood flow can be restored within a critical time frame, this area at risk may return to normal function. Experimental models of stroke indicated that lower levels of blood flow are tolerated for brief times, whereas slightly higher blood flow can be maintained for several hours without development of infarction. The precise relationships between blood flow levels and duration for human stroke are not known; but clearly, the sooner flow is restored, the more likely the involved tissue will be spared.

STROKE MECHANISMS

Appropriate treatment of ischemic stroke depends on identification of the mechanism of stroke. The duration of symptoms or the time course is not as important as the underlying cause of the ischemic syndrome. Ischemic strokes are generally classified as large-vessel or small-vessel thrombotic or embolic. An embolic occlusion of a major intracranial artery may require a therapeutic approach different from that for an atherosclerotic occlusion. Similarly, small-vessel thrombosis has different implications for treatment, and prognosis is better than for large-vessel thrombosis.

Unfortunately, in the first few hours after stroke, identification of stroke mechanisms may be difficult or impossible. Even distinguishing ischemic stroke from cerebral hemorrhage may be hazardous on the basis of clinical evaluation alone. Information obtained from history and rapid examination provides clues to the pathophysiologic process,[3] but definitive diagnosis usually requires additional testing, such as ultrasound and imaging examinations. Large-vessel thrombotic strokes are often preceded by transient ischemic attacks or a stepwise progression of deficits. Risk factors include hypertension, smoking, diabetes, and elevated cholesterol level. Clinical deficits typically correspond to the territory of major cerebral arteries or their border zones. In embolic strokes, the onset is usually sudden, although a stepwise progression occurs in occasional cases in the first few hours. Atrial fibrillation, rheumatic heart disease, or a recent myocardial infarction raises the probability of embolism.

Several clinical syndromes are attributable to small-vessel thrombotic or lacunar stroke. These include pure motor stroke involving face, arm, and leg; pure sensory stroke; ataxia; hemiparesis; and dysarthria-clumsy hand. Other syndromes may also be due to lacunar strokes, but the mechanism is less certain in such cases, illustrating the hazards of deciding on the stroke mechanism from clinical findings alone.

Pathophysiologic diagnosis is greatly enhanced by imaging modalities, including computed tomography (CT) and magnetic resonance imaging (MRI). These studies take time to complete, delaying administration of acute stroke therapy and potentially leading to irreversible brain injury before the diagnosis can be established. Thus, the time needed for imaging studies must be weighed against the benefit of the information obtained. Studies need to be performed rapidly with minimal delay, and the results must be used to decide on optimal treatment. It is likely that acute stroke treatment will differ according to the underlying mechanism, and therefore rapid imaging modalities should become increasingly important in acute stroke management.

PREHOSPITAL EVALUATION OF STROKE

The success of acute stroke management begins when a patient's family member or a bystander recognizes the symptoms of stroke (Table 172-1) and calls 911 immediately. When there was no acute treatment for stroke—only primary and secondary preventive measures—health care professionals did little to educate the public in recognizing stroke, identifying risk factors, or promoting stroke prevention. On average, across the United States, stroke patients arrive at the hospital 24 hours after symptom onset. A huge effort is under way to educate the public at large of the warning signs of stroke, especially those at risk and their family members (Table 172-2). The key message is how to recognize stroke, to take action, and to get to the hospital immediately.

Only recently have pre-hospital systems across the United States begun to implement an acute stroke protocol. The protocol is published in the 1997-1999 American Heart Association Advanced Cardiac Life Support (ACLS) manual.[4] An algorithm for acute stroke was developed from the experience of conducting acute stroke trials.[5-7] Like the concept of time-focused field management of myocardial infarction, acute stroke is now being approached as a medical emergency. The key elements for pre-hospital personnel are:

- Rapid identification of stroke within 6 hours
- Appropriate field assessment
- Management
- Rapid transport
- Prenotification of the incoming stroke patient to the receiving emergency department (ED)

The process begins at dispatch. Any call with complaints of "weakness, numbness, changes in speech, headache, confusion, found down or unconscious" is considered a possible stroke, and an ambulance crew is immediately sent to the scene.

TABLE 172–1. Stroke Recognition

Sudden onset of
Numbness or weakness of the face, arm, or leg
Slurred speech or difficulty with speech
Blurred vision or loss of vision in one or both eyes
Severe headache
Clumsiness or loss of balance

On arrival, the pre-hospital team should complete a quick assessment. The assessment includes following the basics of the ABC-N: airway, breathing, circulation, and neurology evaluation. Oxygen saturation should be maintained at least at 96% to provide adequate oxygenation to the brain tissue. Continuous monitoring by electrocardiography is recommended because approximately 30% of ischemic patients have arrhythmias, such as atrial fibrillation. Blood pressure should be monitored, but treatment is considered only if blood pressure is above 220/120 mm Hg. Intravenous access should be established if this does not delay transport to the ED. If intravenous fluids are being administered use only isotonic solutions, such as normal saline or lactated Ringer's. Glucose is to be avoided in intravenous fluids. Glucose may be detrimental to ischemic brain tissue and can lead to unnecessary cerebral edema. Hypoglycemia can mimic stroke symptoms, however, and serum glucose concentration should be checked. Glucose should be administered if hypoglycemia is found. Hyperglycemia needs to be treated on patient arrival in the ED.

The pre-hospital personnel should gather information about the onset of the stroke symptoms. First and foremost, it is crucial to determine the time at onset of the symptoms. This is important because the ED may not have access to individuals who were present at the onset. Time at onset is determined by when the patient was last seen without a neurologic deficit. When the deficit is present on awakening, the time at onset is considered the previous night before the patient went to bed. If thrombolytic treatment is considered, it is important to obtain a history of trauma or falling when the symptoms occurred. One checks for any signs of ecchymosis or laceration. Also, a history of seizure activity is obtained after the onset of symptoms. *Todd's paralysis,* a syndrome that follows seizure, can often be confused with stroke symptoms.

For assessment of the patient's neurologic status, the best tool to use in the field is the Pre-Hospital Stroke Scale, developed by The University of Cincinnati (Table 172-3). This quick screen allows for uniformity in assessing stroke deficits, which clarifies communication of the results to the receiving team at the hospital.

Information communicated to the receiving hospital should include age, sex, past medical history, current medications, presenting problem, onset time, neurologic status, vital signs, estimated time of arrival at the hospital, and any concerns while in transport. Field work can save precious minutes of

TABLE 172–2. Resources for Public Stroke Education

National Stroke Association (NSA) 1-800-STROKES
American Heart Association (AHA) 1-800-AHA-USA1
National Institute of Neurological Disorders and Stroke (NINDS) www.nih.gov

TABLE 172–3. The Cincinnati Pre-Hospital Stroke Scale

Facial droop: Have patient show teeth or smile.
Normal: both sides of face move equally
Abnormal: one side of the face does not move as well as the other side

Arm drift: Patient closes eyes and holds both arms out.
Normal: both arms move the same or both arms do not move at all
Abnormal: one arm does not move or one arm drifts down compared with the other

Speech: Have patient say, "you can't teach an old dog new tricks."
Normal: patient uses correct words with no slurring
Abnormal: patient slurs words, uses inappropriate words, or is unable to speak

additional work in the ED. The importance of care given by paramedics should not be underemphasized.

EMERGENT STROKE EVALUATION

General Assessment

Emergent assessment of the stroke patient begins immediately on arrival in the ED. If prenotification is obtained from the emergency medical service, a physician should meet the patient at triage in the ED and begin the evaluation. Initial concerns include assessment of respiratory function, cardiovascular stability, and level of consciousness.

An adequate airway must be established to ensure proper ventilation, particularly in obtunded or comatose patients. Aspiration, a serious concern, leads to subsequent pneumonia and is a major cause of morbidity and mortality during hospitalization.[8] Supplemental oxygen is often administered, but the benefit is uncertain when oxygenation is already adequate. However, hypoxemia should be corrected immediately and the source aggressively investigated. Arrhythmias are not uncommon in the setting of acute stroke. Bradycardia may signal underlying increased intracranial pressure or cardiac ischemia. Atrial fibrillation associated with rapid ventricular response often impairs cardiac output, requiring immediate treatment. Atrial fibrillation may also be an embolic source for stroke. Ventricular tachycardia or fibrillation rarely occurs with stroke[9] and, when present, is usually due to coexistent myocardial infarction. Hypotension should be corrected with intravenous fluids and seizures controlled with anticonvulsants. The physician's initial evaluation should be completed within 15 minutes.

Blood Pressure Management

Hypertension is a common accompaniment of both ischemic and hemorrhagic stroke.[10] In most cases of ischemic stroke, abrupt lowering of blood pressure is not advised because of the risk of causing further impairment of perfusion in the ischemic region. When a systemic or cardiac reason for reducing blood pressure is present, such as aortic dissection or acute myocardial infarction, the relative importance of the systemic and neurologic issues must be considered. Hypertensive encephalopathy is a syndrome of extreme hypertension, papilledema, altered mental status, microangiopathic hemolytic anemia, and renal insufficiency that responds to lowering of blood pressure. In the absence of papilledema or systemic features, it is unlikely that acute neurologic deficits are due to hypertensive encephalopathy, and acutely lowering blood pressure is more likely to worsen deficits than improve them.

When thrombolytic therapy is considered, reducing blood pressure within limits is necessary. Before thrombolytic therapy is administered, systolic blood pressure should be below 185 mm Hg, diastolic below 110 mm Hg.[11] Labetalol is typically administered in increasing doses every 5 to 10 minutes to control blood pressure. If β-blockers cannot be used, enalapril is a reasonable alternative. If these agents do not provide adequate control, thrombolytic therapy should probably be avoided. Although some authors recommend limiting treatment to one or two doses of labetalol before excluding the patient from thrombolytics, we generally proceed with treatment as long as the blood pressure is controlled within the time frame for treatment with thrombolytic therapy.

Triage and Laboratory Studies

The immediate concern for the ED evaluation after initial cardiovascular stabilization is confirming the diagnosis of stroke, excluding stroke mimics, and establishing whether the patient is a candidate for acute stroke intervention. It is crucial to establish the time at onset with certainty. The onset time should be considered the time the patient was found with the deficit. If the deficits were present on awakening, the onset time should be considered the previous night when the patient was last seen to be neurologically normal. This may exclude some patients who otherwise would benefit, but it avoids the risk of causing hemorrhage in those with long-established infarction. For intravenous t-PA, the window for treatment is currently 3 hours. The evaluating physician must allow time needed for CT scanning and interpretation as well as for preparing and administering t-PA. Completion of CT scanning should take no more than 25 minutes from the time of arrival, and interpretation should be completed within 45 minutes. Treatment with t-PA should be initiated within 1 hour of arrival in the ED.

The physician must consider conditions other than stroke that cause acute neurologic deficits before proceeding with acute stroke treatment. On occasion, intracranial mass lesions present with acute deficits. Migraine, seizures, and metabolic aberrations, such as hypoglycemia, may present with focal neurologic signs. A brief history obtained from the patient or family usually excludes these possibilities. Two intravenous lines should be established as soon as possible. Blood glucose level should be checked and corrected if needed. Additional blood tests obtained immediately include coagulation studies, complete blood count, and electrolyte determinations.

Stroke Team

A stroke team consists of individuals from multiple disciplines with specialized knowledge and interest in acute stroke care. The team approach brings together the necessary skills to emergently administer whatever care is best suited to the situation and divides the workload so that tasks can be performed simultaneously rather than sequentially. Ideally, a stroke team consists of a neurologist, a nurse coordinator, and a neurosurgeon. Not all hospitals will have the resources necessary to provide a complete stroke team at all times, but at least one individual should be available with the ability to acutely evaluate the neurologic status of a stroke patient, interpret the CT findings, and institute acute stroke therapy in appropriate cases. The more components of the team involved in acute stroke care, the more rapidly treatment can be initiated. The stroke team is usually responsible for confirming the onset time, evaluating the CT, establishing the diagnosis, reviewing the inclusion and exclusion criteria for thrombolytic therapy, and making the final decision to go ahead with treatment.

IMAGING OF ACUTE STROKE

Evaluation of patients with acute stroke depends heavily on imaging. Although imaging of stroke by CT and MRI is a component of standard stroke care, emergent imaging of stroke raises several new issues. Of primary importance is differentiating ischemic stroke from cerebral hemorrhage before deciding on the use of thrombolytic agents. In the future, selection of appropriate neuroprotective agents may also depend on the presence of hemorrhage. Although still investigational, it is likely that identification of an arterial occlusion and information about cerebral blood flow and perfusion will help triage acute stroke patients to a treatment regimen most likely to produce benefit while limiting the potential for complications.

At present, selection of patients for thrombolytic therapy or other acute stroke therapy is based entirely on clinical evaluation and historical time at onset. It is likely, however, that some patients within the 3-hour time window already have established infarction that will not reverse with thrombolysis and in fact may result in hemorrhage because of reperfusion of infarcted brain. In contrast, others may have salvageable brain tissue despite a greater than 3-hour interval since onset. A physiologic estimate of tissue viability would be preferable to a fixed time interval, if a study were found that reliably predicts viability of brain after stroke.[12] Both CT and MRI have the potential to provide this information.

Computed Tomography

CT has been the imaging procedure of choice for a patient with a recent stroke to exclude hemorrhage as the etiologic factor. However, CT has the potential to provide a great deal more information in an acute stroke patient. Subtle parenchymal abnormalities show evidence of early edema or infarction. Spiral CT allows CT angiography (CTA) and imaging of the intracranial and extracranial circulation. Cerebral perfusion can be examined with stable xenon CT and mapped to the arterial distribution of the major cerebral arteries. This battery of tests is performed without moving the patient from the CT scanner, which minimizes the time delay before optimal treatment is decided.

Not all patients can complete the entire battery of tests. CTA requires the administration of a contrast agent and cannot be performed in patients with allergies. There is a potential problem in patients undergoing angiography for possible intra-arterial therapy after CTA in that the dye load is increased by the combination of procedures. However, if digital angiography is used and arterial contrast is minimized, the contrast load should not be prohibitive. Xenon CT has few limitations, but excessive movement reduces the accuracy of the acquired blood flow information. Thus, blood flow data may not be reliable in agitated patients. Vomiting occasionally occurs after xenon inhalation, and care must be taken to avoid aspiration.

Early CT Changes

It was previously thought that parenchymal changes did not occur on CT imaging for at least 6 hours after ischemic stroke. However, studies indicate that early changes of ischemia not infrequently occur within a few hours of stroke onset and have been seen as early as 1 hour after stroke.[13] These changes include:

- Hyperdense middle cerebral artery
- Reduced attenuation in the basal ganglia
- Loss of gray-white differentiation, particularly in the insular region[14]
- Low density in the cortex and subcortical white matter
- Loss of sulcal markings suggesting early mass effect and edema[15] (Fig. 172-1*A* and *B*)

A hyperdense middle cerebral artery is seen in 20% to 37%,[16] indicating acute thrombus within the artery, but it rarely occurs without at least one other early CT abnormality. Hyperdensity in the basilar artery associated with thrombosis has also been reported.[17] In 100 patients studied within 14 hours of stroke onset (mean, 6.4 hours), early CT changes were found in 94%. Multiple early abnormalities correlated with size of subsequent infarct and poor outcome.[16] In the European Cooperative Acute Stroke Study (ECASS) trial of t-PA for acute stroke (see later), early CT changes correlated with larger subsequent infarct volume[18] and a greater likelihood of hemorrhagic conversion after t-PA.[19] Similarly, in the NINDS t-PA trial, patients with early CT changes treated with t-PA had a greatly increased incidence of symptomatic hemorrhage (31% versus 6%).[20] On the basis of these results, some experts recommend management without thrombolytic therapy in patients with extensive early CT changes.[21] However, whether these abnormalities represent irreversible brain infarction remains unknown. One report of a patient with hypodensity in 60% of the middle cerebral artery territory and clinical as well as CT resolution after reperfusion with intra-arterial urokinase suggest that this is not always the case.[22]

Computed Tomographic Angiography

CTA can be performed with use of spiral CT technology, adding only 15 to 20 minutes to the routine CT examination. Either the intracranial or extracranial circulation may be imaged. In a patient with acute stroke, the intracranial study may be sufficient to diagnose proximal artery occlusion. When extracranial carotid disease is suspected, both parts of the circulation can be studied. A single bolus of contrast agent, similar to that used for a contrast-enhanced CT study, is given for this examination, which limits use in patients with renal failure or contrast hypersensitivity. In the setting of acute stroke, CTA has been shown to be highly reliable for diagnosis of intracranial occlusions and correlates well with other imaging modalities[23, 24] (Fig. 172-1*C* and *D*).

Examination of the carotid bifurcation with CTA provides a three-dimensional view of carotid lesions and shows eccentric lesions or ulceration not seen on conventional angiography.[25] When CTA is used in combination with conventional CT imaging and xenon CT, the major limitation is tube heating. The studies must be sequenced properly and the area of interest on CTA selected carefully to minimize the number of slices needed to obtain the necessary anatomic information.

CTA in acute stroke patients provides important information about arterial occlusions and possibly collateral blood flow.[26] It may be useful for triage of patients with large proximal occlusions to thrombolytic therapy as well as for avoiding such treatment in those without demonstrable arterial occlusions. It is hoped that future acute stroke trials will incorporate these imaging modalities to assess the value of triage of patients on the basis of anatomic evidence of occlusion.

Xenon CT

Measurement of brain perfusion should be particularly beneficial in patients with stroke. Several methods of measuring cerebral blood flow are available, including:

- Stable xenon CT
- Single-photon emission computed tomography (SPECT)
- Positron emission tomography (PET)
- Transcranial Doppler ultrasonography

Quantitative blood flow can be obtained only with xenon CT or PET. PET has the advantage of providing corresponding

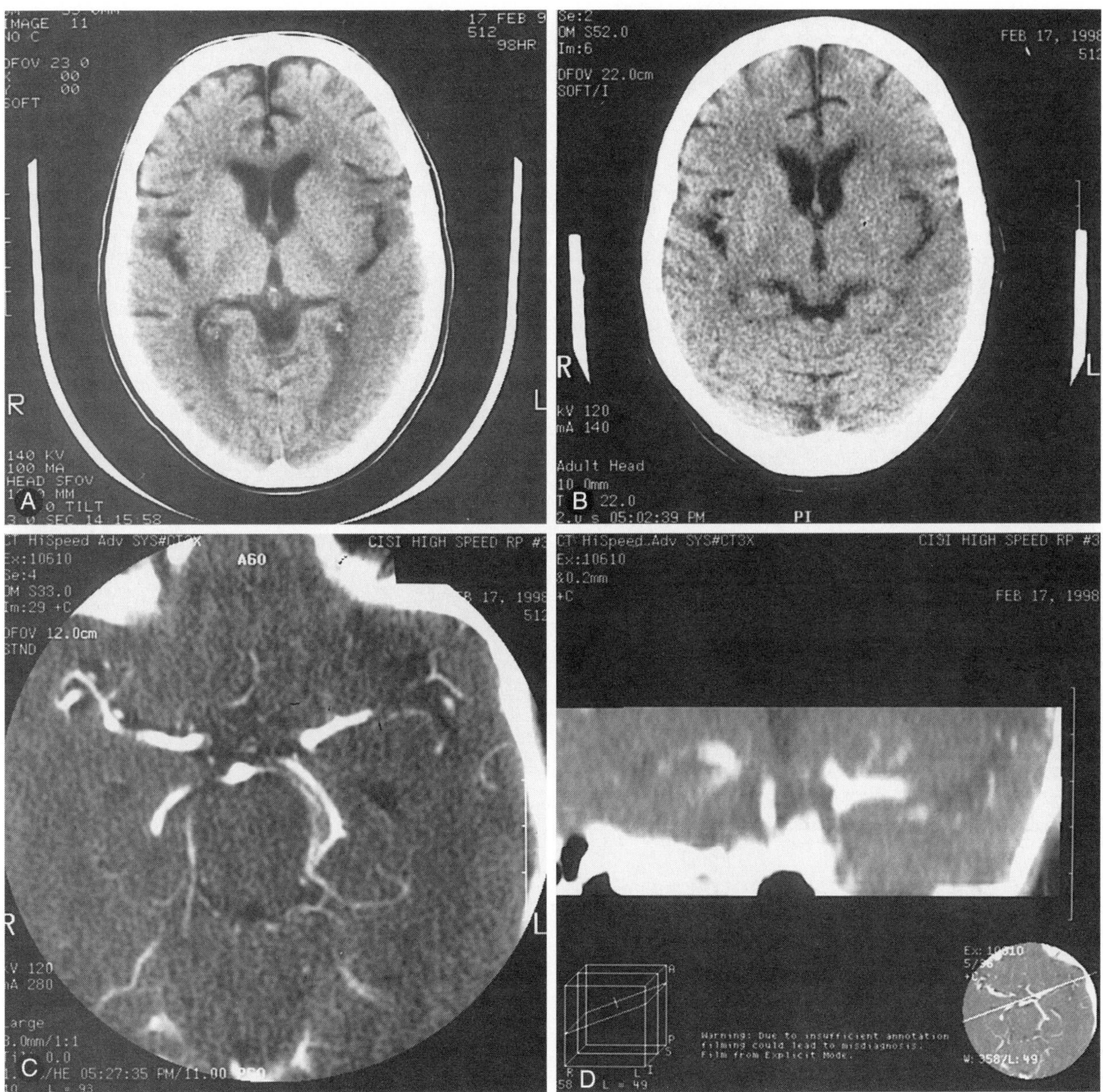

Figure 172–1. *A,* Normal CT scan of the brain 2 hours after onset of aphasia and left hemiparesis. *B,* Another CT scan 5 hours after stroke onset demonstrates early CT changes, including basal ganglia hypodensity, loss of the insular ribbon, and slight effacement of the sulci on the left. *C,* CT angiogram 5 hours after stroke onset showing complete occlusion of the left middle cerebral artery. *D,* Rapid reconstruction of the CT angiogram again demonstrates occlusion of the left middle cerebral artery.

metabolic data, but it is more difficult to perform, particularly in acutely ill patients with stroke.

Stable xenon is an inert gas inhaled as a mixture of 27% xenon and 73% oxygen. During a 4-minute inhalation, rapid scanning is performed, and pixel-by-pixel blood flow values are calculated at three brain levels. Corresponding brain CT sections allow anatomic correlation. Regions of reduced blood flow reflect arterial occlusion with inadequate collateral circulation. In acute stroke patients, xenon CT identifies ischemic regions in patients without acute changes on CT. Patients with occlusion of the proximal middle cerebral artery have significantly lower cerebral blood flow in the middle cerebral artery distribution than do those with more distal occlusion[27] (Fig. 172–2). In addition, normal cerebral blood flow in a patient with acute ischemic deficit is associated with rapid clinical improvement.[28] Xenon CT cerebral blood flow studies require about 15 minutes for completion. Reconstruction of images is accomplished within 5 minutes.

Magnetic Resonance Imaging

In many hospitals, MRI is available on an emergent basis and reliably identifies cerebral ischemia. Compared with CT, MRI is more sensitive to cerebral infarction, particularly in the brain stem and deep white matter.[29-31] Most comparisons, however, preceded the recognition of early CT changes and thus may unfairly favor MRI for diagnosis of cortical infarction. Absence of flow in major cerebral arteries suggests occlusion or slow flow in that artery. This provides important information about arterial occlusion even without angiography that may be valuable, particularly in the setting of acute stroke.

The major drawback of MRI is the difficulty in identifying

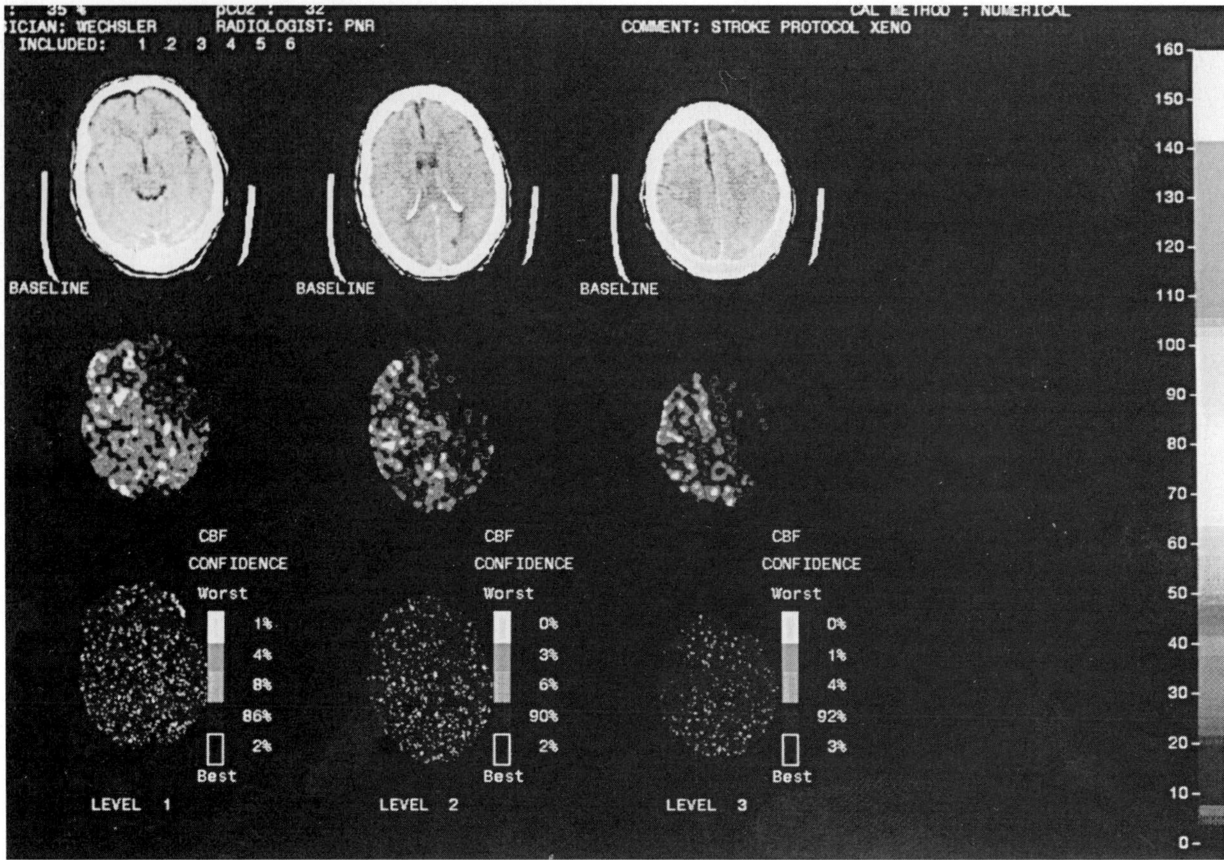

Figure 172–2. Xenon CT blood flow study of a patient with large left hemisphere stroke 3 hours after onset of symptoms. Flow is nearly absent throughout the middle cerebral artery territory on the left.

hemorrhage. MRI signal abnormalities vary, depending on the age of the hemorrhage.[32] Knowledge of the signal characteristics of hemorrhage of varying ages on specific imaging sequences is necessary for accurate diagnosis. More knowledge, experience, and skill are needed for MRI interpretation of hemorrhage than for CT evaluation. There is uncertainty about the reliability of MRI for detection of hyperacute hemorrhage and subarachnoid hemorrhage, although it is likely that experienced readers will make few mistakes.[33, 34] However, for general evaluation of acute stroke and differentiation of ischemia from hemorrhage, CT remains the test of choice.

Diffusion-Weighted Imaging and Perfusion Imaging

Diffusion-weighted imaging (DWI) shows parenchymal abnormalities earlier than do conventional T2-weighted images in patients with acute stroke.[35] Perfusion imaging is based on transit times for the contrast agent through brain parenchyma. Diffusion imaging detects the diffusion of water in the brain and shows hyperintensity in areas of reduced diffusion (Fig. 172–3). As water moves from the extracellular to the intracellular space, there is less movement of water and loss of signal, resulting in hyperintensity.[36]

DWI has potential advantages in the evaluation of acute stroke. First, early detection of lesions helps differentiate cerebral ischemia from other conditions that mimic stroke, such as seizures or toxic-metabolic states.[37] However, hyperintensity on DWI may not be entirely specific for ischemia,[38] and at least one false-negative DWI scan has been reported (although a perfusion abnormality was present).[39] Second, combining DWI with perfusion imaging may identify reversibly ischemic tissue. In some cases, the area of perfusion abnormality is larger than the DWI abnormality, indicating a region of brain that has impaired flow but has not yet become totally ischemic. This might identify patients most likely to benefit from acute stroke therapy. Expansion of DWI abnormalities between the first few hours after stroke and repeated studies many hours later also suggests the existence of tissue at risk.[40] Several studies found that the size of DWI abnormalities correlated with clinical outcome.[41] However, whether DWI abnormalities are truly irreversible is unclear. In animal models of stroke, reduction in the size of DWI abnormalities after treatment has been demonstrated,[42, 43] and similar findings have been reported in humans after treatment with neuroprotective agents.[44] Progression to infarction is a complex phenomenon that depends on many factors in addition to tissue perfusion and cerebral blood flow.[45] Whether DWI and perfusion imaging will become useful predictors of outcome or response to therapy awaits further study and randomized controlled trials.

Magnetic Resonance Angiography

Magnetic resonance angiography (MRA) provides a noninvasive method of imaging the intracranial and extracranial circulation. Several techniques are available, but most require no contrast enhancement and are based on time-of-flight techniques.[46] This method highlights flowing blood by signal suppression from all stationary tissues. The arteries composing the circle of Willis and the extracranial vertebral and carotid arteries can be examined, allowing detection of occlusions in the setting of acute stroke. Occlusions of small peripheral branch arteries may not be detected by MRA. Patients with

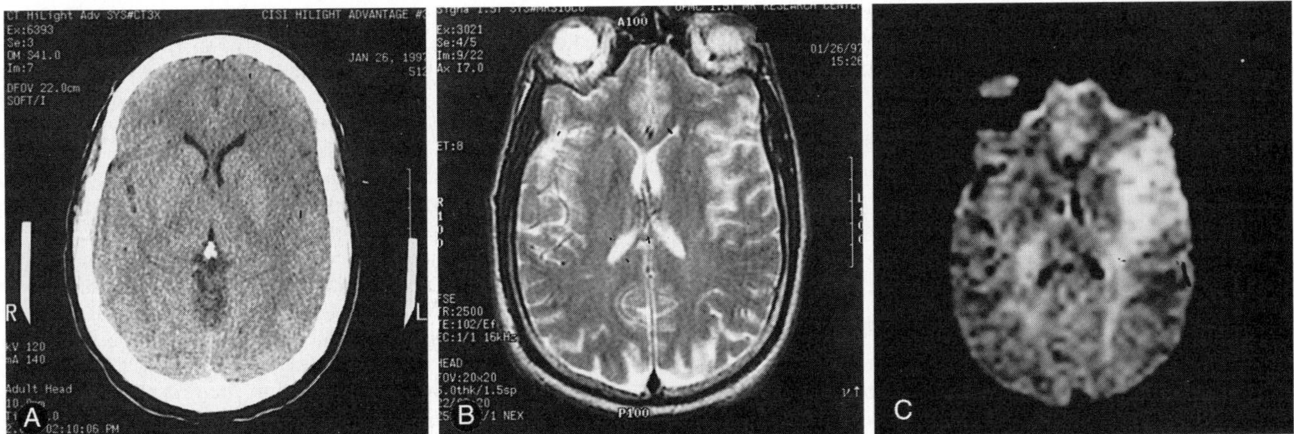

Figure 172–3. *A,* CT scan of the brain in a patient with sudden onset of expressive speech difficulty and right arm weakness 2½ hours after onset of symptoms. Early low density and sulcal effacement are present in the perisylvian region. *B,* T2-weighted magnetic resonance image of the same patient 5 hours after stroke onset. Subtle increased signal intensity is seen in the perisylvian region. *C,* Diffusion-weighted image also at 5 hours after stroke onset. A larger area of signal abnormality is present in the left hemisphere.

claustrophobia or implanted metal devices, such as pacemakers, cannot undergo MRA. Artifacts in some cases obscure proper identification of arterial pathologic processes. Signal dropout at the site of arterial stenosis may be due to the effects of turbulent flow. If an artery is tortuous, it may extend out of the imaging section and appear occluded. In addition, construction of maximal intensity projections is subject to a variety of errors.[47] Experience and careful examination of studies typically avoid these pitfalls.

In patients with stroke, MRA correlates well with angiographic evidence of stenosis or occlusion of arteries in both the intracranial[48, 49] and extracranial circulation.[50, 51] In patients undergoing MRI and particularly DWI and perfusion imaging, the addition of MRA to the armamentarium provides evidence of arterial disease and may add important diagnostic information in the consideration of treatment options.

TREATMENT OF ACUTE STROKE

Intravenous Thrombolytic Agents

Trials of intravenous thrombolytic agents in acute stroke date back to the early 1960s. At that time, several trials of streptokinase,[52] fibrinolysin,[53] and urokinase[54] were performed and demonstrated either no effect or higher mortality in patients treated with thrombolysis. These studies preceded CT scanning; thus, patients with hemorrhage were not necessarily excluded. The discouraging results inhibited further acute stroke trials until the 1980s, when several reports appeared of favorable outcomes with intra-arterial thrombolytic therapy within a few hours of stroke onset.[55, 56] This in turn led to small randomized trials and feasibility studies of intravenous thrombolytics.[57, 58] The results of two multicenter randomized controlled trials of intravenous t-PA for acute ischemic stroke have been published, with one demonstrating for the first time a beneficial effect of acute stroke treatment given within 3 hours of onset.

The NINDS acute stroke study included more than 600 patients with acute ischemic stroke within 3 hours of onset.[59] Half the patients were treated within 90 minutes. Patients were randomly assigned to receive either intravenous t-PA, 0.9 mg/kg up to a maximum of 90 mg, or intravenous placebo. Primary outcome measures were favorable outcomes at 90 days measured by the National Institutes of Health stroke scale (NIHSS) Barthel index, Glasgow outcome scale, and Rankin scale. By all four measures, significantly more patients had a favorable outcome at 90 days in the t-PA group compared with the group receiving placebo. Intracerebral hemorrhage with clinical deterioration occurred in 6.4% of t-PA-treated patients but in only 0.6% of placebo-treated patients. Despite the increase in hemorrhages, there was no significant increase in mortality or severe disability in the t-PA group compared with the placebo group. When strokes were classified according to initial impression of stroke subtype, all types of strokes had more favorable outcomes with t-PA. There were no clear factors that predicted response to t-PA,[60] but those with large strokes (NIHSS $>$ 20) and the evidence of early low density or edema on CT had a higher rate of hemorrhage after t-PA.[61]

The other major trial of intravenous t-PA for acute stroke, ECASS, was also a blinded, randomized, controlled trial including 620 patients treated within 6 hours of stroke onset.[62] This trial differed from the NINDS trial in several important ways. In addition to the longer time window for treatment, the ECASS trial used a higher t-PA dose of 1.1 mg/kg. Patients with early signs of infarction on initial CT scanning, including extensive low density, mass effect, and sulcal effacement, were intended to be excluded. However, many protocol violations occurred, particularly inclusion of patients with early CT changes. The primary analysis was based on intent to treat, but a target population was prospectively identified, including only those patients without protocol violations. The primary endpoints were improvement on the Rankin scale and Barthel index at 90 days. In the intent-to-treat group, there was no significant difference between the t-PA-treated patients and those receiving placebo on either of the primary endpoints. However, in the target population, there was a significant benefit in favor of t-PA as evidenced by improvement in the Rankin scale. Mortality was greater in t-PA-treated patients, but the difference did not reach statistical significance (17.9% versus 12.7%, $P = .08$). Intracerebral hemorrhage occurred in 19.8% of those treated with t-PA and 6.5% of patients given placebo ($P < .001$). The inclusion of patients with early CT abnormalities contributed to this increased risk.[63]

Although only one study clearly demonstrated a benefit, in June 1996 the Food and Drug Administration approved intravenous t-PA for treatment of stroke within 3 hours of onset. Since then, reports of small groups of patients suggest that similar efficacy can be obtained at community hospitals without an increase in hemorrhages as long as the NINDS protocol is used for selection of patients.[64]

Not all patients respond to intravenous t-PA. In a dose excalation trial of intravenous Duteplase (Burroughs Wellcome t-PA), angiography was performed before thrombolysis in all patients, documenting the site of arterial occlusion, and repeated 2 hours later.[65] Only 31% of arterial occlusions recanalized. Proximal occlusions in the middle cerebral artery opened less frequently than did distal branch occlusions, and only 8% of carotid occlusions recanalized. The resistance of carotid occlusion to intravenous thrombolysis has also been noted by others.[66]

Intra-arterial Thrombolytic Agents

An alternative approach to intravenous thrombolysis is direct arterial delivery of thrombolytic agents by a microcatheter embedded in the clot.[67] The advantages of the intra-arterial route include the ability to visualize the site of arterial occlusion and to titrate the amount of thrombolytic agent used on the basis of recanalization of the artery. Less lytic agent should be used, minimizing activation of systemic thrombolytic activity and, it is hoped, reducing bleeding complications (Fig. 172–4). In addition, if no clot is found, thrombolytic treatment is not needed. The major disadvantage is the additional time needed to transport the patient to angiography, prepare the groin, thread the catheter through the femoral artery, and place the catheter within the clot. In a small series of patients randomized to receive either intravenous t-PA or placebo followed by angiography and, if necessary, intra-arterial infusion of t-PA,[68] the average time to start of infusion was 1.8 hours. An average of another 1.8 hours was needed for clot lysis. In our institution, catheter placement can be performed in 45 minutes from arrival in the ED, and lysis typically occurs in 60 to 90 minutes. However, both these scenarios introduce a significant time delay that may sacrifice potentially salvageable brain tissue.

Intra-arterial thrombolysis can be accomplished with a number of agents, including t-PA, urokinase, and prourokinase. To date, most reports of intra-arterial therapy have used urokinase. Although no studies directly compare intra-arterial urokinase with t-PA, there does not appear to be a major difference in recanalization rate or hemorrhagic complications. Most reports of intra-arterial therapy include small groups of patients usually with severe strokes and variable clinical and CT follow-up. Recanalization rates vary from 50% to 100%, and outcome is typically better in those with recanalization.[69-72] Most hemorrhage rates are less than 5%, although rates as high as 28% have been reported in individual small series.[73]

Prourokinase is a precursor of urokinase that is preferentially activated at the clot surface by conversion to urokinase. This results in less activation of systemic thrombolytic activity and fewer systemic bleeding complications. Prourokinase was used in the only randomized controlled trial to date of intra-arterial thrombolysis for acute stroke.[74] Forty patients with occlusion of the M1 or M2 segment of the middle cerebral artery within 6 hours of stroke onset were treated with either intra-arterial urokinase or a saline injection in a 2:1 randomization through a catheter imbedded in the first third of the clot. Arteriography was repeated after infusion to assess recanalization. Median NIHSS was 17 in the prourokinase group and 19 in the saline control patients. Median time from stroke onset to start of infusion was 5.5 hours. Overall, partial or complete recanalization was achieved in 58% of patients with prourokinase and in 14% of those treated with saline infusion. There was a trend toward more favorable outcomes in the prourokinase patients, but this was not statistically significant (Barthel index of 9 or 10, 42% versus 36%; $P = .75$). Symptomatic hemorrhage occurred in 15.4% of those receiving prourokinase and in 7.1% of those with saline infusion. Although the frequency of symptomatic hemorrhage was greater in the patients receiving prourokinase than in patients treated with t-PA in the NINDS trial, the relative increase in hemorrhages compared with the nontreated group was considerably less (approximately two times for prourokinase and 10 times for t-PA). These preliminary results suggest that intra-arterial prourokinase may be effective and reasonably safe for treatment of proximal middle cerebral artery occlusion. The Prourokinase in Acute Cerebral Thromboembolism occlusion (PROACT) II study is now in progress randomizing a larger group of patients with M1 or M2 occlusion to a higher dose of prourokinase (9 mg versus 6 mg in PROACT I).

Occlusion of the basilar artery has been the focus of several investigations of patients treated with intra-arterial thrombolysis. In patients with basilar artery occlusion, outcome is rarely favorable and mortality is high.[75] In contrast, when the basilar

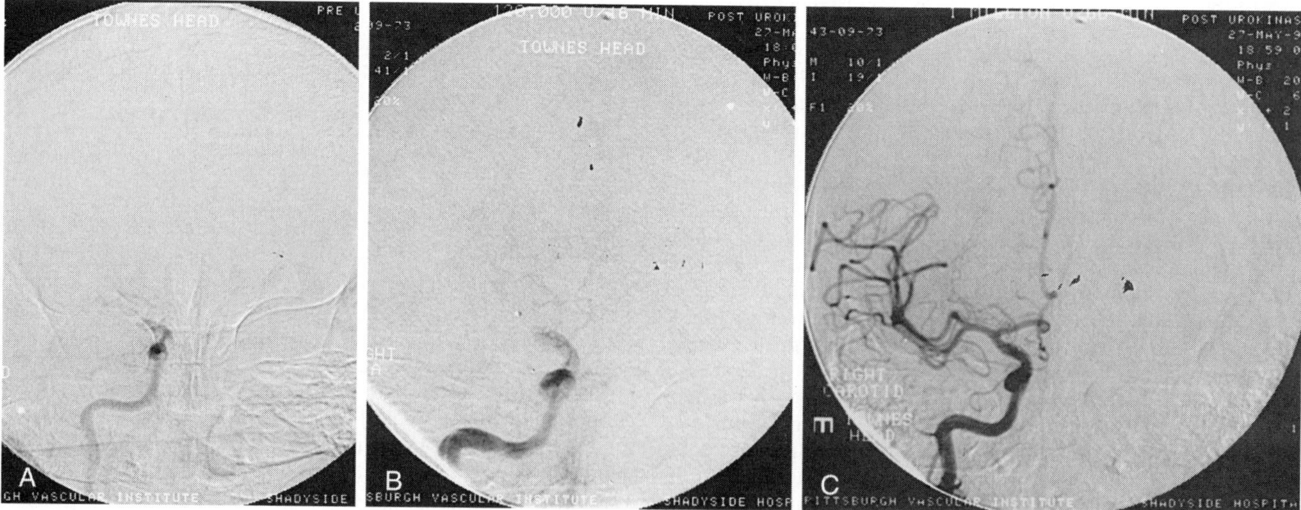

Figure 172–4. *A,* Right carotid angiogram of a patient with embolic occlusion of the right middle cerebral artery 4 hours after onset of symptoms. *B,* Angiogram of the same patient after placement of a microcatheter into the middle cerebral artery clot and infusion of 120,000 units of urokinase. There is no recanalization. *C,* Angiogram after infusion of 1 million units of urokinase directly into the clot demonstrates complete recanalization of the middle cerebral artery.

artery recanalizes with intra-arterial thrombolysis, favorable outcomes are seen in 25% to 50% of patients.[76-78] Clinical improvement has been reported in patients with basilar artery thrombosis treated with intra-arterial thrombolysis many hours beyond the usual 6-hour time window.[79] However, favorable outcome after intravenous t-PA has also been reported in patients with stroke due to vertebrobasilar artery thrombosis.[80] Only one of these cases, however, had documented basilar artery thrombosis before treatment. Other series have shown that some patients with angiographically proven basilar artery occlusion survive without interventional treatment.[81] Ultimately, only a randomized controlled trial will establish the benefit of thrombolytic therapy in this group of patients. A trial of intra-arterial urokinase for basilar artery occlusion was initiated in Australia, but thus far the trialists have been unable to enter sufficient patients to produce meaningful results.

Neuroprotective Agents

The extent of ischemic injury in the brain depends on the quantity of cerebral blood flow in the affected territory. Blood flow levels less than 10 mL/100 g/min are probably tolerated only for minutes, whereas intermediate levels of blood flow in the range of 15 to 20 mL/100 g/min may be tolerated for several hours before irreversible changes occur.[82] During ischemia, there is insufficient energy for maintenance of normal membrane pump activity. Sodium diffuses into the cell, causing depolarization of the membrane potential and impairing the ability of the neuron to generate an action potential. In addition, there is a tremendous outpouring of excitatory neurotransmitters, particularly glutamate.[83] Glutamate then activates *N*-methyl-D-aspartate (NMDA) and non-NMDA receptors, causing influx of calcium into neurons.[84] Calcium is also released from mitochondria, tremendously increasing the intracellular calcium concentration. This results in production of toxic products, including nitric oxide and free radicals, and activation of phospholipases. Membrane depolarization leads to additional calcium influx and a progression over time to cell death. The duration of this reversible ischemic state is uncertain, but animal models of focal stroke suggest that it is only a few hours.[85]

Neuroprotective therapy is designed to interfere with a cascade of cellular events that results in cell death. Blocking any of the events involved in ischemic cell death may preserve function or prolong the time window for restoration of blood flow by other means, such as thrombolysis.

Several neuroprotective agents have undergone clinical trials, and others are currently in phase II or phase III trials. NMDA receptor antagonists have been most extensively tested. Despite promising results in animal models of stroke, results of clinical trials have been disappointing. Phase II and phase III trials of NMDA antagonists were terminated or unsuccessful primarily because of undesirable side effects, such as hallucinations, confusion, and agitation.[86, 87]

Lubeluzole is a benzothiazole derivative that interferes with nitric oxide–induced glutamate toxicity, but the exact mechanism of action is uncertain.[88] A phase II trial showed a significant reduction in mortality in patients receiving lubeluzole.[89] These promising results led to a randomized controlled trial of lubeluzole versus placebo in patients treated within 6 hours of stroke onset. There was a nonsignificant trend toward reduced mortality in the patients treated with lubeluzole and a significant improvement in neurologic outcome.[90] However, a subsequent phase III trial failed to show any benefit.

Citicoline is a precursor for the synthesis of phosphatidylcholine, an important component of cell membranes. During ischemia, phosphatidylcholine is metabolized, causing release of free fatty acids and generation of oxygen free radicals. Citicoline reverses the process by increasing formation of phosphatidylcholine and reducing free fatty acids.[91] The increase in phosphatidylcholine may also protect neurons by stabilizing cell membranes and promoting recovery from ischemic injury. In a randomized controlled trial of three doses of oral citicoline given for 6 days versus placebo in patients within 24 hours of stroke onset, a significant improvement in outcome was found at 12 weeks for the 500-mg and 2000-mg doses after adjustment for differences in the NIHSS.[92] No significant improvement was found in the 1000-mg treatment group. The reason for the different results in individual dosing groups is unclear and clouds the significance of the positive findings in the low-dose and high-dose groups. In addition, there were fewer patients with severe strokes in the 500-mg treatment group, possibly confounding the favorable outcome in this group. Further phase III trials are planned and, it is hoped, will clarify the benefit of this treatment.

A number of other neuroprotective therapies have been tested in acute stroke. Nimodipine, a calcium channel blocker, has undergone several randomized controlled trials in patients treated within 24 to 48 hours of stroke onset.[93, 94] No significant benefit was demonstrated in these studies, although a meta-analysis suggested that nimodipine may be effective if it is given within 12 hours.[95] Hypervolemic hemodilution has also been subjected to randomized controlled trials in acute stroke. Treatment did not improve outcome, although maximum hemodilution was typically not achieved for 24 to 48 hours.[96, 97] Treatment with GM_1 ganglioside[98] and Enlimomab,[99] an anti-intercellular adhesion molecule, were similarly ineffective in improving outcome.

Surgical Decompression

Cerebral edema with herniation is the most frequent cause of death from stroke in the first few days.[100] Cerebral edema usually gradually increases and peaks 2 to 3 days after stroke onset. Steroids do not effectively reduce edema due to stroke, and antiedema measures, such as mannitol or hyperventilation, are of limited benefit. Control of intracranial pressure is associated with improved outcome, but whether intracranial pressure monitoring to guide therapy is helpful is uncertain.

Surgical decompression of large hemispheric infarcts causing edema and increased intracranial pressure is a logical method of treatment because the edema is usually self-limited. If herniation can be avoided, recovery may occur as in stroke without severe edema.

Several approaches to decompression have been proposed. Rengachary and colleagues[101] reported a marked reduction in mortality with hemicraniectomy in patients with severe edema after stroke. In a group of 32 patients with a large infarct of the nondominant hemisphere, mortality was reduced to 40% and long-term disability was only moderate after hemicraniectomy.[102] Kalia and Yonas[103] reported the results of "strokectomy" based on results of xenon CT cerebral blood flow studies in four patients with cerebral edema after stroke and impending herniation. Blood flow studies identify areas of nearly absent flow. This is a more reliable indicator than CT changes of irreversibly damaged brain and helps guide surgical removal, avoiding areas of intact cortex. This procedure prevents fatal herniation, but whether long-term outcome is truly improved must be determined by randomized clinical trials. Until then, surgical decompression for hemispheric infarction should be considered for younger patients with a greater potential for recovery from massive stroke, particularly in the nondominant hemisphere.

The optimal timing of decompression is uncertain. If herniation is already in progress, irreversible brain stem damage may occur, limiting the benefit of the procedure. On the other hand, early edema may not progress to herniation, and surgery could be performed unnecessarily. Xenon CT findings of extensive areas of nearly absent cerebral blood flow may help identify patients liable to suffer massive edema and herniation[104] and help select those most likely to require surgical decompression.

Cerebellar infarction is a special case that clearly requires urgent surgical intervention.[105] Compression of the brain stem and fourth ventricle leading to hydrocephalus or severe pontomedullary compromise can be reversed by rapid surgical decompression of the infarcted cerebellum. The clinical syndrome of inferior cerebellar artery occlusion including vertigo and imbalance maybe mistaken for a vestibulopathy, and CT changes may be subtle or nonexistent. Thus, it is crucial to suspect this diagnosis in patients at risk for cerebrovascular disease because surgical intervention may be lifesaving with little residual deficit.

SUMMARY

The availability of effective treatment to alter outcome within the first few hours after stroke onset necessitates dramatic changes in the evaluation of stroke. Patients with symptoms suggestive of cerebral ischemia must be treated emergently from the pre-hospital encounter to the ED. Imaging must be performed rapidly and provide useful information for the decision-making process. It is hoped that treatments in addition to t-PA will prove effective in acute stroke, increasing the time window for initiation of therapy and the benefit of such treatment. It is likely that ultimately, combinations of thrombolytic therapy, neuroprotective agents, and perhaps interventional therapy in appropriate cases will maximize the probability of limiting ischemic injury.

References

1. Broderic J, Brott T, Kothari R, Miller R, Khoury J, Pancioli A, Gebel J, Mills D, Minneci L, Shukla R: The greater Cincinnati/northern Kentucky stroke study: Preliminary first-ever and total incidence rates of stroke among blacks. Stroke 1998; 29:415-421.
2. The National Institute of Neurological Disorders and Stroke rt-PA Stroke Study Group: Tissue plasminogen activator for acute ischemic stroke. N Engl J Med 1995; 333:1581-1587.
3. Mohr JP, Sacco RL: Classification of ischemic strokes. *In:* Stroke: Pathophysiology, Diagnosis, and Management. 2nd ed. Barnett HJM, Mohr JP, Stein BM, Yatsu FM (Eds). New York, Churchill Livingstone, 1992, pp 271-283.
4. Advanced Cardiac Life Support 1997-1999: Acute stroke. Dallas, American Heart Association, 1997, pp 10-1-10-20.
5. National Institutes of Neurological Disorders and Stroke: Prehospital emergency medical care systems. *In:* Rapid Identification and Treatment of Acute Stroke. NIH publication 97-4239. Bethesda, Md, The Institute, 1997, pp 17-48.
6. Kotari R, Barson W, Brott T, et al: Frequency and accuracy of pre-hospital diagnosis of stroke. Stroke 1995; 26:937-941.
7. Rapp K, Bratina P, Barch C, et al: Code stroke: Rapid transport, triage and treatment using rt-PA therapy. J Neurosci Nurs 1997; 29:361-366.
8. Silver F, Norris JW, Lewis A, Hachinski V: Early mortality following stroke: A prospective review. Stroke 1995; 26:937-941.
9. Di Pasquale G, Pinelli G, Andreoli A, et al: Holter detection of cardiac arrhythmias in intracranial subarachnoid hemorrhage. Am J Cardiol 1987; 59:596-600.
10. Wallace JD, Levy LL: Blood pressure after stroke. JAMA 1981; 246:2177-2180.
11. Adams HP Jr, Brott TG, Furlan AJ, Gomez CR, Grotta J, Helgason CM, Kwiatkowski T, Lyden PD, Marler JR, Torner J, Feinberg W, Mayberg M, Thies W: Guidelines for thrombolytic therapy for acute stroke: A supplement to the guidelines for the management of patients with acute ischemic stroke. Stroke 1996; 27:1711-1718.
12. Baron JC, von Kummer R, del Zoppo GJ: Treatment of acute ischemic stroke: Challenging the concept of a rigid and universal time window. Stroke 1995; 26:2219-2221.
13. Tomura N, Uemura K, Inugami A, Fujita H, Higano S, Shishido F: Early CT finding in cerebral infarction: Obscuration of the lentiform nucleus. Radiology 1988; 168:463-467.
14. Truwit CL, Barkovich AJ, Gean-Marton A, Gibri N, Norman D: Loss of the insular ribbon: Another early CT sign of acute middle cerebral artery infarction. Radiology 1990; 176:801-806.
15. Moulin T, Cattin F, Crepin-Leblond T, Tatu L, Chavot D, Piotin M, Viel JF, Rumbach L, Bonneville JF: Early CT signs in acute middle cerebral artery infarction: Predictive value for subsequent infarct locations and outcome. Neurology 1996; 47:366-375.
16. Moulin T, Besson G, Crepin-Leblond T, Gramier P, Tau L, Chavot D: Hemorrhagic transformation in the MAST-E trial: Predictive factors. Cerebrovasc Dis 1996; 6:182.
17. Ehsan T, Hayat G, Malkoff M, Selhorst JB, Martin D, Manepalli A: Hyperdense basilary artery: An early computed tomography sign of thrombosis. J Neuroimaging 1994; 4:200-205.
18. Von Kummer R: Determination of the individual therapeutic time window by early computed tomography (Abstract). Cerebrovasc Dis 1996; 6:180.
19. Von Kummer R, Bozzao L, Bastianello S, Manelfe C, for the ECASS Group: Extent of ischemic brain edema and the response to plasminogen activator in acute hemispheric stroke (Abstract). Stroke 1997; 28:270.
20. The NINDS t-PA Stroke Study Group: Intracerebral hemorrhage after intravenous t-PA therapy for ischemic stroke. Stroke 1997; 28:2109-2118.
21. Adams HP, Brott TG, Furlan AJ, Gomez CR, Grotta J, Helgason HG, Kwiatkowski T, et al: Guidelines for thrombolytic therapy for acute stroke: A supplement to the guidelines for the management of patients with acute ischemic stroke. Circulation 1996; 94:1167-1174.
22. Tarr R, Taylor CL, Selman WR, Lewin JS, Landis D: Good clinical outcome in a patient with a large CT scan hypodensity treated with intra-arterial urokinase after an embolic stroke. Neurology 1996; 47:1076-1078.
23. Shrier DA, Tanaka H, Numaguchi Y, Konno S, Patel U, Shibata D: CT angiography in the evaluation of acute stroke. Am J Neuroradiol 1997; 18:1011-1020.
24. Knauth M, von Kummer R, Jansen O, Hahnel S, Dorfler A, Sartor K: Potential of CT angiography in acute ischemic stroke. Am J Neuroradiol 1997; 18:1001-1010.
25. Lev M, Ackerman RH, Chehade R, et al: The clinical utility of spiral computed tomographic angiography in the evaluation of carotid artery disease (Abstract). Stroke 1996; 27:179.
26. Wildermuth S, Knauth M, Brandt T, Winter R, Sartor K, Hacke W: Role of CT angiography in patient selection for thrombolytic therapy in acute hemispheric stroke. Stroke 1998; 29:935-938.
27. Firlik AD, Kaufmann AM, Wechsler LR, Firlik KS, Fukui MB, Yonas H: Quantitative cerebral blood flow determinations in acute ischemic stroke: Relationship to computed tomography and angiography. Stroke 1997; 28:2208-2213.
28. Firlik AD, Rubin G, Wechsler LR, Yonas H: Selection of patients for acute stroke therapy: Early detection of patients with deficits that will resolve using cerebral blood flow measurements. Neurology 1998; 50:A260.
29. Bryan RN, Levy LM, Whitlow WE, et al: Diagnosis of acute cerebral infarction: Comparison of CT and MR imaging. AJNR Am J Neuroradiol 1991; 12:611-620.
30. Kertesc A, Black SE, Nicholson L, Carr T: The sensitivity and specificity of MRI in stroke. Neurology 1987; 37:1580-1585.
31. Kinkel PR, Kinkel WR, Jacobs L: Nuclear magnetic resonance imaging in patients with stroke. Semin Neurol 1986; 6:43-52.
32. Gomori JM, Grossman RI, Goldberg HI, et al: Intracranial hematomas: Imaging by high-field MR. Radiology 1985; 157:87-93.
33. Patel MR, Edelman RR, Warach S: Detection of hyperacute primary intraparenchymal hemorrhage by magnetic resonance imaging. Stroke 1996; 27:2321-2324.
34. Chrysikopoulos H, Papanikolaou N, Pappas J, Papandreou A, Roussakis A, Vassilouthis J, Andreou J: Acute subarachnoid haem-

orrhage: Detection with magnetic resonance imaging. Br J Radiol 1996; 69:601-609.
35. Moseley ME, Kucharczyk J, Mintorovitch H, Cohen Y, Kurhanewicz J, Derugin N, Asgari H, Norman D: Diffusion-weighted MR imaging of acute stroke: Correlation with T2-weighted and magnetic susceptibility-enhanced MR imaging in cats. Am J Neuroradiol 1990; 11:423-429.
36. Mintorovitch J, Baker LL, Yang GY, Shimizu H, Weinstein PR, Moseley ME, Kucharczyk J: Diffusion-weighted hyperintensity of early cerebral ischemia: Correlation with brain water content and ATPase activity (Abstract). Proc Soc Magn Reson Med 1991; 10:329.
37. Libman RB, Wirkowski E, Alvir J, Rao TH: Conditions that mimic stroke in the emergency department. Arch Neurol 1995; 52:1119-1122.
38. Hasegawa Y, Formato JE, Latour LL, Gutierrez JA, Liu KF, Garcia JH, Sotak CH, Fisher M: Severe transient hypoglycemia causes reversible change in the apparent diffusion coefficient of water. Stroke 1996; 27:1648-1655.
39. Tong DC, Yenari MA, Albers GW, O'Brien M, Marks MP, Moseley ME: Correlation of perfusion and diffusion weighted MRI with NIH SS score in acute ischemic stroke. Neurology 1998; 50:864-870.
40. Baird AE, Benfield A, Shlaug G, et al: Enlargement of human cerebral ischemic lesion volumes measured by diffusion-weighted magnetic resonance imaging. Ann Neurol 1997; 41:581-589.
41. Lovblad KO, Baird AE, Schlaug G, et al: Ischemic lesion volumes in acute stroke by diffusion-weighted magnetic resonance imaging correlate with clinical outcome. Ann Neurol 1997; 42:164-170.
42. Muller TB, Haraldseth O, Jones RA, et al: Perfusion and diffusion-weighted MR imaging for in vivo evaluation of treatment with U74389G in a rat stroke model. Stroke 1993; 24:2074-2081.
43. Kucharczyk J, Mintorovitch J, Moseley ME, et al: Ischemic brain damage: Reduction by sodium-calcium ion channel modulator RS-87476. Radiology 1991; 179:221-227.
44. Warach S, Benfield A, Schlaug G, Siewart B, Edelman RR: Reduction of lesion volume in human stroke by citicoline detected by diffusion weighted MRI: A pilot study. Ann Neurol 1996; 40:527-528.
45. Powers WJ: Hemodynamics and metabolism in ischemic cerebrovascular disease. Neurol Clin 1992; 10:31-48.
46. Ruggieri PM, Masaryk TH, Ross JS: Magnetic resonance angiography: Cerebrovascular applications. Stroke 1992; 23:774-780.
47. Wilock DJ, Jaspan T, Worthington BS: Problems and pitfalls of 3-D TOF magnetic resonance angiography of the intracranial circulation. Clin Radiol 1995; 50:526-532.
48. Patrux B, Laissy JP, Jouini S, Kawiecki W, Coty P, Thiebot J: Magnetic resonance angiography (MRA) of the circle of Willis: A prospective comparison with conventional angiography in 54 subjects. Neuroradiology 1994; 36:193-197.
49. Korogi Y, Takahashi M, Mabuchi N, Miki H, Shiga H, Watabe T, O'Uchi T, Nakagawa T, Horikawa Y, Fugiwara S, et al: Intracranial vascular stenosis and occlusion: Diagnostic accuracy of three-dimensional, Fourier transform, time-of-flight MR angiography. Radiology 1994; 103:187-193.
50. Qureshi AI, Isa A, Cinnamon J, Fountain J, Ottenlips JR, Braimah J, Frankel MR: Magnetic resonance angiography in patients with brain infarction. J Neuroimaging 1998; 8:65-70.
51. Liberopoulos K, Kaponis A, Kokkinis K, Pagratis N, Nicolakopoulou Z, Douskou M, Stringaris K, Clonaris C, Balas P: Comparative study of magnetic resonance angiography, digital subtraction angiography, duplex ultrasound examination with surgical and histological findings of atherosclerotic carotid bifurcation disease. Int Angiol 1996; 15:131-137.
52. Meyer JS, Gilroy J, Barnhart MI, et al: Anticoagulants plus streptokinase therapy in progressive stroke. JAMA 1963; 189:373.
53. Meyer JS, Gilroy J, Barnhart MI, Johnson JF: Therapeutic thrombolysis in cerebral thromboembolism. Neurology 1963; 13:927-937.
54. Fletcher AP, Alkjaersig N, Lewis M, et al: A pilot study of urokinase therapy in cerebral infarction. Stroke 1976; 7:135-142.
55. Hacke W, Zeumer H, Ferbert A, et al: Intra-arterial thrombolytic therapy improves outcome in patients with acute vertebrobasilar occlusive disease. Stroke 1988; 19:1216-1222.
56. Del Zoppo GJ, Ferbert A, Otis S, et al: Local intra-arterial fibrinolytic therapy in acute carotid territory stroke. Stroke 1988; 19:307-313.
57. Mori E, Yoneda Y, Tabuchi M, et al: Intravenous recombinant tissue plasminogen activator in acute carotid territory stroke. Neurology 1992; 42:976-982.
58. Haley EC Jr, Brott TG, Sheppard GL, et al: Pilot randomized trial of tissue plasminogen activator in acute ischemic stroke. Stroke 1993; 24:1000-1004.
59. The National Institute of Neurological Disorders and Stroke rt-PA Stroke Study Group: Tissue plasminogen activator for acute ischemic stroke. N Engl J Med 1995; 333:1581-1587.
60. The NINDS t-PA Stroke Study Group: Generalized efficacy of t-PA for acute stroke: Subgroup analysis of the NINDS t-PA stroke trial. Stroke 1997; 28:2119-2125.
61. The NINDS t-PA Stroke Study Group: Intracerebral hemorrhage after intravenous t-PA therapy for ischemic stroke. Stroke 1997; 28:2109-2118.
62. Hacke W, Kaste M, Fieschi C, et al, for the European Cooperative Acute Stroke Study Group: Intravenous thrombolysis with recombinant tissue plasminogen activator for acute hemispheric stroke. JAMA 1995; 274:1017-1025.
63. Larrue V, von Kummer R, Hoxter G, et al: Predictors of hemorrhagic transformation in the ECASS trial (Abstract). Cerebrovasc Dis 1996; 6:181.
64. Chiu D, Drieger D, Villar-Cordova C, Kasner SE, Morgenstern LB, Bratina PL, Yatsu FM, Grotta JC: Intravenous tissue plasminogen activator for acute ischemic stroke: Feasibility, safety and efficacy in the first year of clinical practice. Stroke 1998; 29:18-22.
65. Del Zoppo GJ, Poeck K, Pessin MS, et al: Recombinant tissue plasminogen activator in acute thrombotic and embolic stroke. Ann Neurol 1992; 32:78-86.
66. Jansen O, von Kummer R, Forsting M, Hacke W, Sarto K: Thrombolytic therapy in acute occlusion of the intracranial internal carotid artery bifurcation. Stroke 1996; 27:785-786.
67. Jungreis CA, Wechsler LR, Horton JA: Intracranial thrombolysis via a catheter embedded in the clot. Stroke 1989; 20:1578-1580.
68. Emergency Management of Stroke (EMS) Investigators: Combined intra-arterial and intravenous t-PA for stroke (Abstract). Stroke 1997; 28:273.
69. Zeumer H, Freitag JJ, Grzyska V, et al: Interventional neuroradiology: Local intraarterial fibrinolysis in acute vertebrobasilar thromboembolic disease. Am J Neuroradiol 1983; 4:401-404.
70. Ezura M, Kagawa S: Selective and superselective infusion of urokinase for embolic stroke. Surg Neurol 1992; 38:353-358.
71. Higashida RT, Halback VV, Barnwell SL, Dowd CF, Hieshima GB: Thrombolytic therapy for acute stroke. J Endovasc Surg 1994; 1:4-15.
72. Satoh K, Matsubara S, Ueda S, Matsumoto K: Local thrombolytic therapy in 153 cases of acute major cerebral artery occlusion (Abstract). Cerebrovasc Dis 1996; 6:184.
73. Nakagaware J, Hyogo T, Katsumi S, Nakamura J: A superselective intra-arterial trial using rt-PA for embolic stroke. Cerebrovasc Dis 1996; 6:184.
74. Del Zoppo GJ, Higashida RT, Furlan AJ, Pessin MS, Rowley HA, Gent M, and the PROACT Investigators: PROACT: A phase II randomized trial for recombinant pro-urokinase by direct arterial delivery in acute middle cerebral artery stroke. Stroke 1998; 29:4-11.
75. Hornig CR, Buttner T, Hoffman O, Dorndorf W: Short-term prognosis of vertebrobasilar ischemic stroke. Cerebrovasc Dis 1992; 2:273-281.
76. Hacke W, Zeumer H, Ferbert A, et al: Intra-arterial thrombolytic therapy improves outcome in patients with acute vertebrobasilar occlusive disease. Stroke 1988; 19:1216-1222.
77. Zeumer N, Freitag HJ, Zanella F, et al: Local intraarterial fibrinolytic therapy in patients with stroke: Urokinase versus recombinant tissue plasminogen activator (r-TPA). Neuroradiology 1993; 35:159-162.
78. Wijdicks EFM, Nichols DA, Thielen KR, et al: Intra-arterial thrombolysis in acute basilar artery thromboembolism: The initial Mayo Clinic experience. Mayo Clin Proc 1997; 72:1005-1013.
79. Zeumer H, Freitag HJ, Grzyka U, Neunzig HP: Local intraarterial fibrinolysis in acute vertebrobasilar occlusion: Technical developments and recent results. Neuroradiology 1989; 31:336-340.

80. Grond M, Rudolf J, Schmulling S, Stenzel C, Neveling M, Heiss WD: Early intravenous thrombolysis with recombinant tissue-type plasminogen activator in vertebrobasilar stroke. Arch Neurol 1998; 55:466–469.
81. Brandt T, Pessin MS, Kwan ES, Caplan LR: Survival with basilar artery occlusion. Cerebrovasc Dis 1995; 5:182–187.
82. Astrup J, Siesjo BK, Symon L: Thresholds in cerebral ischemia: The ischemic penumbra. Stroke 1981; 12:723–725.
83. Benveniste H, Drejer J, Schousboe A, Diemer NH: Elevation of the extracellular concentrations of glutamate and aspartate in rat hippocampus during transient cerebral ischemia monitored by intracerebral microdialysis. J Neurochem 1984; 43:1369–1374.
84. Simon RP, Swan JH, Griffiths T, Meldrum BS: Blockade of *N*-methyl-D-aspartate receptors may protect against ischemic damage in the brain. Science 1984; 226:850–852.
85. Jones TH, Morawetz RB, Crowell RM, et al: Thresholds of focal cerebral ischemia in awake monkeys. J Neurosurg 1981; 12:723–725.
86. Albers GW, Atkinson RP, Kelley RE, et al: Safety, tolerability and pharmacokinetics of the *N*-methyl-D-aspartate antagonist dextrorphan in patients with acute stroke. Dextrorphan Study Group. Stroke 1995; 26:254–258.
87. Davis SM, Albers GW, Diener HC, Lees KR, Norris J: Termination of Acute Stroke Studies Involving Selfotal Treatment. ASSIST Steering Committee. Lancet 1997; 349:32.
88. De Ryck M, Keersmaekers R, Duytschaever H, Claes C, Clincke G, Janssen M, Van Reet G: Lubeluzole protects sensorimotor function and reduces infarct size in a photochemical stroke model in rats. J Pharmacol Exp Ther 1996; 279:748–758.
89. Diener HC, Hacke W, Hennerici M, et al: The effects of lubeluzole in the acute treatment of ischemic stroke: Results of a phase 2-trial (Abstract). Stroke 1995; 26:185.
90. Grotta J: Lubeluzole treatment of acute ischemic stroke. The US and Canadian Lubeluzole Ischemic Stroke Study Group. Stroke 1997; 28:2338–2346.
91. Weiss GB: Metabolism and actions of CDP-choline as an endogenous compound and administered exogenously as citicoline. Life Sci 1995; 56:637–660.
92. Clark WM, Warach SJ, Pettigrew LC, Gammans RE, Sabounjian LA, for the Citicoline Stroke Study Group: A randomized dose-response trial of citicoline in acute ischemic stroke patients. Neurology 1997; 49:671–678.
93. The American Nimodipine Study Group: Clinical trial of nimodipine in acute ischemic stroke. Stroke 1992; 23:3–8.
94. Trust Study Group: Randomized, double-blind, placebo-controlled trial of nimodipine in acute stroke. Lancet 1990; 336:1205–1209.
95. Gelmers HJ, Hennerici M: Effect of nimodipine on acute ischemic stroke: Pooled results from five randomized trials. Stroke 1990; 21:IV81–IV84.
96. Aichner FT, Fazekas F, Brainin M, Polz W, Mamoli B, Zeiler K: Hypervolemic hemodilution in acute ischemic stroke: The Multicenter Austrian Hemodilution Stroke Trial (MAHST). Stroke 1998; 29:743–749.
97. The Hemodilution in Stroke Study Group: Hypervolemic hemodilution treatment of acute stroke: Results of a randomized multicenter trial using pentastarch. Stroke 1989; 20:317–323.
98. Lenzi GL, Grigoletto F, Gent M, Roberts RS, Walker MD, Easton JD, Carolei A, Dorsey FC, Focca WA, Bruno R, et al: Early treatment of stroke with monosialoganglioside GM-1: Efficacy and safety results of the Early Stroke Trial. Stroke 1994; 25:1552–1558.
99. The Enlimomab Acute Stroke Trial Investigators, Sherman DG: The Enlimomab acute stroke trial: Final results. Neurology 1997; 48:A270.
100. Bounds JV, Wiebers DO, Whisnant JP, Okazaki H: Mechanism and timing of deaths from cerebral infarction. Stroke 1981; 12:474–477.
101. Rengachary SS, Batnitzky S, Morantz RA, Arjunan K, Jeffries B: Hemicraniectomy for acute massive cerebral infarction. Neurosurgery 1981; 8:321–328.
102. Rieke K, Krieger D, von Kummer R, Aschoff A, Hacke W: Decompressive surgery in space occupying hemispheric infarction. Crit Care Med 1995; 73:1576–1587.
103. Kalia KK, Yonas H: An aggressive approach to massive middle cerebral artery infarction. Arch Neurol 1993; 50:1293–1297.
104. Firlik AD, Yonas H, Kaufmann AM, Wechsler LR, Jungreis CA, Fukui MB, Williams RL: Relationship between cerebral blood flow and the development of swelling and life-threatening herniation in acute ischemic stroke. J Neurosurg 1998; 89:243–249.
105. Heros RC: Surgical treatment of cerebellar infarction. Stroke 1992; 23:937–938.

173

Neuromuscular Disorders in Critical Care

Vern C. Juel, MD • Thomas P. Bleck, MD, FCCM

Abnormal neuromuscular function may precipitate a patient's admission to an intensive care unit or may develop as a consequence of another critical illness and its treatment. This chapter focuses primarily on respiratory failure as a consequence of neuromuscular disease but also addresses autonomic dysfunction occurring in this setting. To facilitate understanding of the concepts involved, a brief review of the motor unit and its physiology is provided, and specific muscles critical to ventilation are identified.

THE MOTOR UNIT AND ITS PHYSIOLOGY

Central nervous system activity destined to produce motor output is conducted to the lower motor neuron, also known as the alpha motor neuron. A motor unit is composed of a motor neuron and the muscle fibers it innervates. The cell bodies of the motor neurons are located in the brain stem for the cranial musculature and in the anterior horn of the spinal cord for the other somatic muscles. At the level of the brain stem or spinal cord, the motor neurons receive various excitatory and inhibitory inputs. Motor axons project through the subarachnoid space and penetrate the dura mater as nerve roots. They may join with other motor axons and with sensory and autonomic fibers in a plexus, and then travel in peripheral nerves to the muscles they innervate. Alpha motor neurons are myelinated, a feature that accelerates nerve impulse propagation. The multiple terminal ramifications of the motor neuron synapse on individual muscle fibers.

The motor axon communicates with muscle via a specialized area termed the *neuromuscular junction*. On the presynaptic side of the neuromuscular junction, the neurotransmitter acetylcholine is synthesized, packaged in vesicles, and stored for release. Depolarization of the axon opens presynaptic voltage-gated calcium channels, which activate the molecular machinery responsible for drawing the vesicles to the presynaptic membrane. The vesicles then fuse with the membrane and release acetylcholine into the synaptic cleft. Acetylcholine molecules bind to receptors on the postsynaptic membrane and cause an influx of sodium, which in turn increases the muscle end-plate potential. When the end-plate potential exceeds the threshold level, the muscle membrane becomes depolarized. The depolarization releases calcium ions from the sarcoplasmic reticulum, and through a process known as *excitation-contraction coupling*, muscle contraction occurs. After activating the acetylcholine receptor complex, the acetylcholine molecule is degraded by cholinesterase; the choline released by this reaction is then recycled by the presynaptic neuron.

MUSCLES OF RESPIRATION

Three muscle groups may be defined on the basis of their importance for respiration, as follows[1] (Fig. 173–1):

- Upper airway muscles: palatal, pharyngeal, and lingual
- Inspiratory muscles: sternomastoid, diaphragm, scalenes, external and parasternal intercostals
- Expiratory muscles: internal intercostal muscles (except for parasternals) and abdominal muscles

The upper airway muscles receive their innervation from the lower cranial nerves. Sternomastoid innervation arrives predominantly from cranial nerve XI, with a small contribution from C-2. The phrenic nerve originates from cell bodies located between C-3 and C-5, with a maximum contribution from C-4, and innervates the diaphragm. Innervation to the scalenes arises from C-4 to C-8, whereas that of the parasternal intercostals is from T-1 to T-7. The intercostal muscles receive innervation from T-1 to T-12, and the abdominal musculature from T-7 to L-1. Reference to this innervation scheme is important in understanding the effects of spinal cord and nerve root injuries on respiration and for the differential diagnosis of disorders producing apparently diffuse weakness.

CLINICAL PRESENTATION OF NEUROMUSCULAR RESPIRATORY FAILURE

Patients experiencing respiratory dysfunction due to neuromuscular disease typically present with a combination of upper airway dysfunction and diminished tidal volume (VT). Difficulty with swallowing liquids, including respiratory secretions, is the most typical presentation of pharyngeal weakness, although some patients have an equal or greater degree of difficulty with solid food. A hoarse or nasal voice may also signal problems with the upper airway. These conditions are noted in patients who are at risk for aspiration and present difficulty with attempts at negative-pressure ventilation (cuirass[2] or iron lung), because the weakened muscles may not be able to keep the airway open as the pressure falls. *Paradoxical abdominal movement* (inward movement of the abdomen during inspiration) is an important sign of diaphragmatic weakness.[3]

Loss of VT occurs most dramatically with diaphragmatic weakness but also follows insults that affect the ability of the paraspinal intercostal muscles to keep the chest wall expanded against negative intrapleural pressure. This is most apparent in patients with lower cervical spinal cord injuries; they commonly have atelectasis despite preservation of phrenic nerve function (this problem usually diminishes over weeks as the muscles develop spasticity).

Patients with progressive generalized weakness (e.g., with the Guillain-Barré syndrome [GBS]) commonly begin to lose VT before upper airway weakness develops. In order to maintain minute ventilation (and therefore carbon dioxide excretion), a patient's respiratory rate increases. Respiratory rate is thus one of the most important clinical parameters to monitor. As the vital capacity (VC) falls from the norm of about 65 mL/kg to about 30 mL/kg, the patient's cough weakens and clearing secretions becomes difficult. A further decrease of VC to 20 to 25 mL/kg results in an impaired ability to sigh, with progressive atelectasis; hypoxemia may be present because of ventilation-perfusion mismatching and because an increasing percentage of VT is used to ventilate dead space. Before the VC reaches 15 mL/kg, the patient should be in an intensive care unit because respiratory failure is imminent, and endotracheal intubation should be considered. The precise point at which mechanical ventilation is necessary varies with the patient, the underlying condition, and especially the likelihood of a rapid response to treatment.

Regardless of the VC, however, indications for intubation are evidence of fatigue, hypoxemia despite supplemental oxygen administration, and difficulty with secretions. Although a rising arterial partial pressure of carbon dioxide (Pa_{CO_2}) usually suggests the need for intubation and mechanical ventilation, occasional patients (e.g., those with myasthenia gravis [MG]) can be managed under very close observation in an intensive care unit without such assistance or with less invasive techniques (e.g., bilevel positive airway pressure [biPAP]).

In addition to the VC, trended measurements of the maximum inspiratory pressure (PImax, more typically recorded as negative inspiratory force [NIF]) are useful indicators of ventilatory capacity. Inability to maintain a PImax greater than 20 to 25 cm H_2O usually indicates a need for mechanical ventilatory assistance. Although the maximum expiratory pressure (PEmax) is a more sensitive indicator of weakness,[4] it has

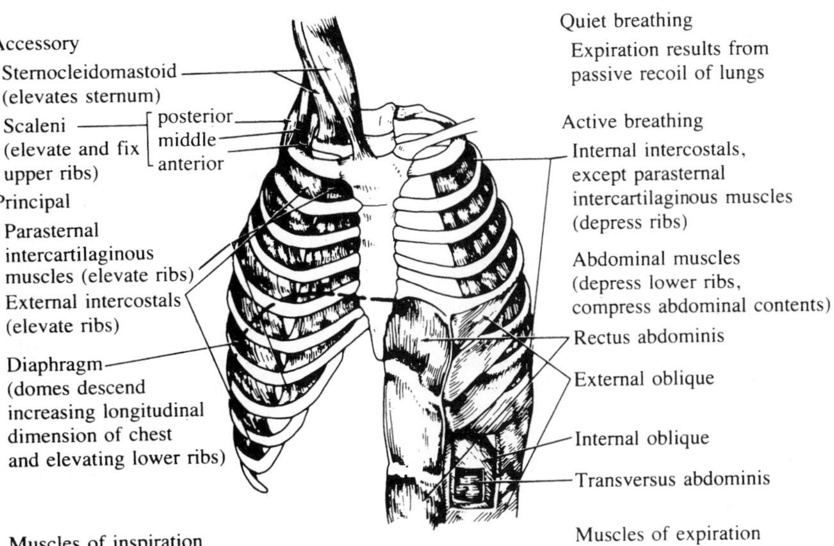

Figure 173–1. Major respiratory muscles. Inspiratory muscles are indicated on the left and expiratory muscles are indicated on the right. (From Garrity ER: Respiratory failure due to disorders of the chest wall and respiratory muscles. *In*: Respiratory Intensive Care. MacDonnell KF, Fahey PJ, Segal MS [Eds]. Boston, Little, Brown & Co, 1987, p 313. Published by Little, Brown & Company.)

not proved to be as useful as an indicator of the need for mechanical ventilation. A more detailed discussion of these variables and their use may be found elsewhere.[5, 6]

Because a patient with neuromuscular respiratory failure has intact ventilatory drive,[7] the fall in VT is initially matched by an increase in respiratory rate, keeping the $Paco_2$ normal or low until the VC becomes dangerously small. Many patients initially maintain a $Paco_2$ in the range of 35 mm Hg because of either a (1) subjective sense of dyspnea at low VT or (2) hypoxia from atelectasis and increasing dead space. When the $Paco_2$ begins to rise in this circumstance, abrupt respiratory failure may be imminent.

The modest degree of hypoxia in most of these patients worsens when the $Paco_2$ begins to rise, displacing more oxygen from the alveolar gas; however, aspiration pneumonia and pulmonary embolism are also common causes of hypoxemia in these patients. To determine the relative contributions of these conditions to a patient's hypoxemia, one can use a simplified version of the alveolar gas equation as follows (derived elsewhere).[5, 6]

$$PAO_2 = PIO_2 - (Paco_2/R)$$

PAO_2 is the alveolar partial pressure of oxygen; PIO_2 is the partial pressure of inspired oxygen (in room air, 150 mm Hg); and R is the respiratory quotient (on most diets, about 0.8). This allows one to estimate the alveolar-arterial oxygen difference ($PAO_2 - PaO_2$). Under ideal circumstances in young people breathing room air, this value is about 10 mm Hg, but it rises to about 100 mm Hg when the fraction of inspired oxygen (FIO_2) is 1.0. The alveolar gas equation allows one to factor out the contribution of hypercarbia to the decrease in arterial partial pressure of oxygen (PaO_2); it should be used to determine whether there is a cause of significant hypoxemia in addition to the displacement of oxygen by carbon dioxide.

Patients with weakness of the orbicularis oris may have artifactually low VC and NIF measurements because they cannot form a tight seal around the mouthpieces of the measuring devices. The need for nursing and respiratory therapy personnel who are experienced in the care of such patients is thus underscored. It is also important for physicians to observe these patients directly rather than relying solely on reported measurements. The physical findings associated with neuromuscular respiratory failure are reviewed elsewhere.[5, 6] Among the most important findings are rapid, shallow breathing,[8] the recruitment of accessory muscles, and paradoxical movement of the abdomen during the respiratory cycle. Fluoroscopy of the diaphragm is occasionally valuable for the diagnosis of diaphragmatic dysfunction.[9]

Autonomic dysfunction commonly accompanies some of the neuromuscular disorders requiring critical care, such as GBS, botulism, and porphyria (Table 173-1). In GBS (discussed later), dysautonomia is common and may arise synchronously with weakness or may follow the onset of the motor disorder after a week or more.

NEUROMUSCULAR DISORDERS

Many chronic neuromuscular disorders and other conditions affecting the suprasegmental innervation and control of respiratory muscles eventually compromise ventilation. This chapter, however, emphasizes the more common acute and subacute neuromuscular disorders that precipitate or prolong critical illness due to ventilatory failure and autonomic dysfunction. A more complete listing of neuromuscular diseases appears in Table 173-1; reviews of this subject[10, 11] and the references listed in Table 173-1[14-26] may be consulted for details of the more rare disorders. Some of the diseases listed (e.g., the Lambert-Eaton myasthenic syndrome) rarely cause respiratory failure in isolation but may be contributing causes in the presence of other conditions,[12] such as neuromuscular junction blockade intended only for the duration of a surgical procedure.[13]

Neuromuscular Diseases Precipitating Critical Illness

Guillain-Barré Syndrome

The Guillain-Barré syndrome, also called *acute inflammatory demyelinating polyradiculoneuropathy* (AIDP), is a predominantly motor peripheral neuropathy with a subacute onset, monophasic course, and nadir within 4 weeks. Although the precise etiology is unknown,[14-26] GBS is immune-mediated and presumably is due to antibodies directed against peripheral nerve components. Approximately 1.7 cases occur per 100,000 population per year.[27] Most patients suffer a demyelinating neuropathy, but in about 5% of cases the condition is a primary axonopathy.[28] Numerous antecedents have been implicated[29]; the more common ones are listed in Table 173-2. The association of antecedent infections suggests that certain agents may elicit immune responses involving antibodies that cross-react with peripheral nerve gangliosides. In particular, the development of ganglioside antibodies has been observed in GBS following *Campylobacter jejuni* infections, such as GM_1 antibodies in axonal forms of GBS,[30] and GQ_{1b} antibodies in the Miller Fisher variant of GBS.[31]

The initial findings in patients with GBS are subacute and progressive weakness, usually most marked in the legs, associated with sensory complaints but without objective signs of sensory dysfunction.[32] Deep tendon reflexes are often significantly reduced or absent at presentation, but this finding may take several days to develop. The cerebrospinal fluid (CSF) typically reveals an albuminocytologic dissociation, or elevated protein content without pleocytosis; this finding may not evolve until the second week of illness. The major reason to examine the CSF is to preclude other diagnoses. CSF lymphocytic pleocytosis (20 to 50 cells/mm^3) may suggest the possibility of acute human immunodeficiency virus infection.[33] Findings on electrodiagnostic studies (consisting of motor and sensory nerve conduction studies and needle electromyography), which may be normal initially, often reflect segmental nerve demyelination with multifocal conduction blocks, dispersed compound muscle action potential (CMAP) amplitudes, slowed conduction velocity, and prolongation or absence of F waves.[34] Differential diagnostic considerations for patients with suspected GBS are primarily those listed in the "Peripheral nerve" section of Table 173-1.

The components of treatment for patients with GBS are as follows:

1. Management of ventilatory failure.
2. Management of autonomic dysfunction.
3. Meticulous nursing care.
4. Psychologic support.
5. Physical and occupational therapy.
6. Prevention of deep venous thrombosis.
7. Nutritional support.
8. Early planning for rehabilitation.
9. Treatment of the immunologic lesion that produced the condition.

Patients with GBS in whom respiratory failure is developing should generally be intubated when the VC falls to about 15 mL/kg or when difficulty with secretions begins because the response to treatment is slow. If a patient has been immobile for several days before intubation and neuromuscular junction

TABLE 173–1. Neuromuscular Causes of Acute Respiratory Failure

Location	Disorder*	Associated Autonomic Dysfunction?
Spinal cord	Tetanus[14]	Frequently
Anterior horn cell	Amyotrophic lateral sclerosis[15]	No
	Poliomyelitis	No
	Rabies	Frequently
Peripheral nerve	Guillain-Barré syndrome	Frequently
	Critical illness polyneuropathy	No
	Diphtheria	No, but cardiomyopathy and arrhythmias occur
	Porphyria	Occasionally
	Ciguatoxin (ciguatera poisoning)	Sometimes
	Saxitoxin (paralytic shellfish poisoning)	No
	Tetrodotoxin (pufferfish poisoning)	No
	Thallium intoxication	No
	Arsenic intoxication[16, 17]	No
	Lead intoxication	No
	Buckthorn neuropathy	No
Neuromuscular junction	Myasthenia gravis	No
	Botulism[18]	Frequently
	Lambert-Eaton myasthenic syndrome[19]	Yes, dry mouth and postural hypotension
	Hypermagnesemia[20]	No
	Organophosphate poisoning	No
	Tick paralysis	No
	Snakebite	No
Muscle	Polymyositis/dermatomyositis	No
	Acute quadriplegic myopathy	No
	Eosinophilia-myalgia syndrome[21]	No
	Muscular dystrophies[22]	No (but cardiac rhythm disturbances common)
	Carnitine palmitoyl transferase deficiency	No
	Nemaline myopathy[23]	No
	Acid maltase deficiency[24]	No
	Mitochondrial myopathy[25]	No
	Acute hypokalemic paralysis	No
	Stonefish myotoxin poisoning	
	Rhabdomyolysis	No
	Hypophosphatemia[26]	No

*Superscript numbers refer to chapter references.

blockade is needed, a nondepolarizing agent should be used to avoid transient hyperkalemia. The oral route for intubation is again being viewed as preferable to the nasal route, because the endotracheal tube is commonly required for a week or longer, raising the risk of sinusitis with nasal intubation.

Many patients are too weak to trigger the ventilator; in such cases, the assist/control or intermittent mandatory ventilation mode is initiated. Weaning patients with GBS from mechanical ventilation must wait for adequate improvement in strength. We usually shift to pressure support ventilation for weaning, although evidence of its superiority over intermittent mandatory ventilation or synchronized intermittent mandatory ventilation modes is at present only anecdotal. Although the majority of patients require mechanical ventilation for less than 4 weeks, as many as 20% need 2 or more months of support before they can breathe without assistance. Improvement in VC to more than 15 mL/kg and in NIF to more than 25 cm H_2O suggests that a patient has improved enough to begin weaning from the ventilator. A formula using a combination of ventilatory and gas exchange variables may allow more accurate determination of a patient's ability to be weaned.[35]

Autonomic dysfunction most typically manifests as a hypersympathetic state and is often heralded by unexplained sinus tachycardia. The blood pressure may fluctuate wildly. Patients

TABLE 173–2. Major Antecedent Causes of Guillain-Barré Syndrome

Common	Uncommon	Questionable
Upper respiratory tract infections	Mycoplasma infection	Hepatitis B vaccine
Diarrheal illness due to *Campylobacter jejuni*	*Leptospira icterohaemorrhagiae* infection	Influenza vaccine
Cytomegalovirus infection	Surgery	Hyperthermia
Epstein-Barr virus infection	Salmonellosis	Epidural anesthesia
Hepatitis A infection	Rabies vaccine	
Hepatitis B infection	Tetanus toxoid	
Hepatitis C infection	Bacille Calmette-Guérin immunization	
Human immunodeficiency virus infection	Sarcoidosis	
Borrelia burgdorferi infection	Systemic lupus erythematosus	
Lymphoma		
Trauma		

may rarely experience bradycardic episodes, which may require temporary pacing. Autonomic surges during tracheal suctioning or due to a distended viscus may be very dramatic and should be minimized. Autonomic failure and pulmonary embolism are now the major causes of mortality in GBS.

Nursing care for patients with GBS is similar to that for other paralyzed and mechanically ventilated patients, but special care must be taken to remember that patients with GBS are completely lucid. In addition to explaining any procedures carefully, arranging for distractions during the daytime (e.g., television, movies, conversation, visitors) and adequate sleep at night are very important. For the most severely affected patients, sedation should be considered. In concert with physical and occupational therapists, passive exercise should be performed frequently throughout the day.

Deep venous thrombosis is a significant danger for patients with GBS. Episodic arterial desaturation is a common event, presumably owing to transient mucus plugging; submassive pulmonary emboli may therefore be overlooked. Adjusted-dose heparin (to slightly prolong the partial thromboplastin time) should be given, and sequential compression devices should be used on the legs; therapeutic anticoagulation may be considered. The risk of fatal pulmonary embolism extends through the initial period of improvement until patients are ambulatory.

Nutritional support should commence as soon as a patient is admitted, with appropriate concern for the risk of aspiration.[36] Most mechanically ventilated patients with GBS can be fed via soft, small-caliber gastric feeding tubes; autonomic dysfunction affecting the gut occasionally requires total parenteral nutrition.

Specific treatments for GBS include removal of autoantibodies with plasma exchange (PEx) or immune modulation with high-dose intravenous immune globulin (IVIg). The efficacy of plasma exchange has been demonstrated in several large clinical trials.[37–41] In the North American trial,[37] PEx and supportive care were compared in GBS patients who lost the ability to walk. Treated patients underwent four to five plasma exchanges for a total exchange volume of 200 to 250 mL/kg over 1 to 2 weeks. The time needed to improve one clinical grade (being weaned from the ventilator or being able to walk) was reduced by 50% in the PEx group in comparison with the control group. There was no significant benefit when PEx was begun later than 2 weeks following symptom onset. The optimal number of plasma exchanges has been assessed in patients with mild (unable to run), moderate (unable to stand without assistance), and severe (requiring mechanical ventilation) GBS by the French Cooperative Group.[42] On the basis of this trial, two exchanges are better than none in mild GBS; four are better than two in moderate GBS; and six are no better than four in severe GBS. Albumin is the preferred replacement solution.[39]

IVIg has been evaluated in GBS in several clinical trials. In 1992, the Dutch Guillain-Barré Study Group reported that IVIg (0.4 g/kg/day × 5 days) was equivalent or superior to PEx for GBS.[43] In this study however, the PEx-treated group exhibited outcome results similar to those of the control group in the North American GBS trial. Some smaller series at that time suggested a greater likelihood of disease progression[44] and severe relapses[45] in patients with GBS treated with IVIg. Subsequently, a prospective trial of 50 patients treated with either IVIg or PEx demonstrated no significant difference in outcome or in relapse rate.[46] The complication rate was somewhat higher in the PEx group, however. A large, international, multicenter, randomized trial compared PEx (50 mL/kg × five exchanges over 8 to 13 days), IVIg (0.4 g/kg/day × 5 days), and PEx followed by IVIg.[47] No significant outcome differences between these therapies was found with respect to functional improvement at 4 weeks or at 48 weeks. Complication rates were similar in all groups. In light of these trials, the decision whether to employ PEx or IVIg in the treatment of acute GBS may no longer hinge on therapeutic efficacy, but rather on avoiding potential side effects. Patients with congestive heart failure, renal failure, hyperviscosity, or immunoglobulin A (IgA) deficiency may be more susceptible to complications of IVIg treatment, whereas PEx may be complicated in patients with labile blood pressure, septicemia, and significant venous access problems.

Corticosteroids or immunosuppressive agents used in isolation for GBS do not improve outcome.[48] The lack of efficacy of high-dose methylprednisolone has been demonstrated in a multicenter trial.[49] In the same trial, no additional benefit was observed when high-dose methylprednisolone was added to PEx. Because of the encouraging findings in a pilot trial of combined treatment using IVIg and high-dose methylprednisolone,[50] a European trial is examining the combined treatment in a large group of patients at several centers.[51] When a specific antecedent illness (e.g., Lyme disease, *C. jejuni* enteritis) is identified, its appropriate treatment may accelerate recovery.

Myasthenia Gravis

Myasthenia gravis (MG) is a consequence of an autoimmune attack on the acetylcholine receptor complex at the postsynaptic membrane of the neuromuscular junction. This process results in clinical weakness with a fluctuating pattern that is most marked after prolonged muscle exertion. The reported prevalence is 14.2 cases per 100,000 population,[52] and up to 20% of affected patients have myasthenic crises with respiratory failure requiring mechanical ventilation.[53] MG has a predilection to affect young women and older men. Thymic abnormalities are associated with its immunopathogenesis. Thymomas are present in about 10% of patients, and thymic hyperplasia is observed in the majority of the remainder. Intensivists may encounter patients with MG because of crisis and ventilatory failure, aspiration, or complications of immunomodulating treatment, or for postoperative care following thymectomy and other surgical procedures. In a 1994 series, the most common identifiable precipitants of myasthenic crisis were bronchopulmonary infections and aspiration.[54]

MG typically involves ocular muscle weakness, which produces ptosis and diplopia, as well as bulbar muscle weakness, which results in dysphagia and dysarthria. This diagnosis should be considered in patients who have acute respiratory failure with these cranial nerve findings. In this setting, botulism (a presynaptic disorder of neuromuscular transmission) is an important differential diagnostic concern.[18] Most patients with MG and respiratory failure, however, already have an established diagnosis.[53]

In myasthenic crisis, excessive dosing with cholinesterase inhibitors may superimpose a cholinergic crisis, resulting in increased weakness that may be accompanied by abdominal cramping, diarrhea, muscle fasciculations, and thick bronchial secretions. Cholinergic crisis probably does not develop outside the context of myasthenic crisis or other serious underlying impairment of neuromuscular transmission. When there is a question of cholinergic excess contributing to respiratory insufficiency, it is most prudent to discontinue all cholinesterase inhibitors, protect the airway, and support respiration as necessary.[55] At times other than during myasthenic crisis or with the patient intubated, cholinergic excess may be assessed by blinded administration of a short-acting anticholinesterase (e.g., edrophonium [Tensilon], 10 mg) and placebo, with pre-test and post-test measurements of muscle strength (e.g., degree of ptosis, VC, or NIF). The edrophonium test should be conducted with the assistance of an experienced neurologist, because many variables affect its interpretation. A positive test result (i.e., strength improves) suggests that a higher dose of a cholinesterase inhibitor (e.g., pyridostigmine) may be useful. If a patient becomes weaker, with administration of edrophonium, the dosage of cholinesterase inhibitor should be reduced.

Patients with MG in whom ventilatory failure is developing but who are not experiencing upper airway problems may at times be managed with *permissive hypercapnea* under close observation in an intensive care unit. The criteria for intubation and mechanical ventilation are similar to those discussed earlier for GBS. If the upper airway is competent and the patient is not experiencing difficulty handling secretions, intermittent nasal biPAP may be a useful temporizing measure. The majority of patients who experience hypercapnea in myasthenic crisis require intubation, however, as do those who are becoming fatigued. Because patients beginning treatment with corticosteroids may experience a transient myasthenic exacerbation, they should be monitored for signs of deterioration during the first several days after initiation of corticosteroid treatment.

Once a patient is committed to mechanical ventilation, many experts withdraw cholinesterase inhibitors for several days. Corticosteroids or other immunomodulators are continued. Plasma exchange is often employed as an effective short-term treatment in managing myasthenic exacerbations and crises. We typically obtain five exchanges of 2 to 4 L every other day. Enteral feeding and prophylaxis for pulmonary embolism are started, and patients are allowed to rest for 2 to 4 days. The details of ventilatory support and the weaning strategy are similar to those for GBS. If a patient is not weaned within 1 week, the cholinesterase inhibitor is typically reintroduced at a lower dose. Corticosteroids (e.g., prednisone, 1 mg/kg/day) are considered for more long-term immunomodulation in patients who have not been receiving them. The details of treating these challenging patients have been reviewed.[53]

A large number of drugs are reported to worsen or unmask MG[56]; the more important of these are listed in Table 173-3. The disease also affects the response to pharmacologic neuromuscular junction blockade; patients are exceptionally sensitive to nondepolarizing agents but resistant to depolarizing agents.[57]

Thymectomy may result in long-term improvement in patients with a suspected thymoma or with a life expectancy of more than 10 years. A patient in acute respiratory failure is generally considered a poor operative risk, however, and thymectomy is usually delayed until the patient's condition has improved.[58] Post-thymectomy pain control and ventilatory function may be improved by postoperative administration of epidural morphine.[59]

TABLE 173–3. Drugs That May Increase Weakness in Myasthenia Gravis

Definite	Likely	Rare or Questionable
Neomycin	Gentamicin	Ciprofloxacin
Streptomycin	Amikacin	Atenolol
Kanamycin	Tobramycin	Phenytoin
Lincomycin	Lidocaine	
Quinidine	Lithium	
Propranolol		
Phenothiazines		
Penicillamine		
Procainamide		

Neuromuscular Diseases Secondary to Critical Illness and Its Treatment

Critical Illness Polyneuropathy

Critical illness polyneuropathy (CIP) is a widespread axonal peripheral neuropathy that develops in the context of multiple organ failure and sepsis. This entity was recognized by several investigators in 1983[60–62] and has been further characterized in large part by Bolton and colleagues.[63, 64] In a prospective series of 43 consecutive patients with sepsis and multiple organ failure, 70% demonstrated electrophysiologic evidence of a sensorimotor axonal neuropathy, and 15 patients had difficulty with weaning from mechanical ventilation as a consequence of the neuropathy.[65] CIP is possibly the most common neuromuscular cause of prolonged ventilator dependency in patients without prior known neuromuscular disease.[66] Given the limitations detailed clinical motor and sensory examinations in the setting of critical illness, the clinical features of CIP (extremity muscle weakness and wasting, distal sensory loss and paresthesias) may not be recognized. Deep tendon reflexes are generally reduced or absent. In the setting of superimposed central nervous system (CNS) insult with pyramidal tract dysfunction, however, deep tendon reflexes may be normal or increased.[67]

Electrodiagnostic studies are important in establishing a diagnosis of CIP because the clinical findings may be unobtainable or indeterminate in this setting.[67] Nerve conduction findings include normal or near-normal conduction velocity and latency values and significantly reduced CMAP and sensory nerve action potential (SNAP) amplitudes. Needle electrode examination reveals denervation changes that are most marked in distal muscles, including fibrillation potentials, positive sharp waves, and reduced recruitment of motor unit potentials.[68] With recovery over time, the spontaneous activity abates and motor unit potentials become polyphasic and enlarged. Peripheral nerve histopathology has revealed widespread, primary axonal degeneration in distal motor and sensory fibers, and skeletal muscle has exhibited fiber-type grouping.[64]

Although the clinical history is usually adequate to distinguish between CIP and GBS, the latter has developed in the context of recent surgery complicated by infection.[69] In some such instances, it may be necessary to differentiate between these two peripheral neuropathic disorders in a patient with extremity weakness and inability to wean from mechanical ventilation. Although only a few severe cases of CIP have been associated with facial weakness,[70] facial and oropharyngeal weakness are common in GBS.[69] Dysautonomia and, occasionally, external ophthalmoplegia are also observed in GBS but have virtually never been attributed to CIP.[70]

Electrophysiologic findings are also helpful in distinguishing these two disorders. Features of segmental demyelination may be observed in GBS on nerve conduction studies (e.g., reduced conduction velocity, prolonged distal and F wave latencies, conduction block, and temporal dispersion of CMAPs); these findings are not observed in CIP. Needle electromyographic findings may differ, in that relatively less spontaneous activity is observed in clinically weak muscles within the first few days in GBS.[68] Although electrophysiologic studies are quite helpful in demonstrating the classic, demyelinating form of GBS, an electrophysiologic distinction between axonal forms of GBS and CIP may not be reliable. The mean cerebrospinal fluid protein in patients with GBS is significantly higher than in patients with CIP, although there is overlap between these populations.[68] Peripheral nerve histopathology may also distinguish between these two groups, as segmental demyelination and inflammatory changes may be observed in GBS and are not seen in critical illness polyneuropathy.[64]

Although overall prognosis in CIP depends on recovery from the underlying critical illness, most patients who survive experience a functional recovery from the neuropathy within several months.[64] CIP may prolong ventilator dependence but it does not worsen long-term prognosis.[67] Proper positioning and padding are important to prevent compression neuropathies, because prognosis from superimposed compression neuropathies in the context of CIP is less favorable.[67]

The pathophysiology of CIP is currently unknown. No clear metabolic, drug, nutritional, or toxic factors have been identified,[64] although the severity of CIP has been correlated with the amount of time in the intensive care unit, the number of invasive procedures, an increased glucose level, a reduced albumin level,[65] and the severity of multiple organ failure.[71] Given the common antecedents of multiple organ failure and sepsis in which significant release of various cytokines occurs, greater microvascular permeability has been postulated to ultimately result in axonal hypoxia and degeneration as a consequence of endoneurial edema.[72]

Prolonged Effects of Neuromuscular Blocking Agents

Prolonged neuromuscular blockade may occur with nondepolarizing agents, particularly when hepatic or renal function is impaired. In one study, administration of vecuronium for 2 or more consecutive days resulted in prolonged neuromuscular blockade and paralysis lasting from 6 hours to 7 days.[73] Although vecuronium is hepatically metabolized, patients with renal failure were susceptible to prolonged effects owing to delayed excretion of the drug's active 3-desacetyl metabolite. Acidosis and elevated serum magnesium levels were also associated with prolongation of the paralytic effects of vecuronium. A peripheral nerve stimulator may be used to monitor muscle twitch responses to a train of four stimuli during the use of neuromuscular blocking agents. Drug dosage should be titrated to preserve one or two twitches to avoid overdosing. Two to three Hertz repetitive nerve stimulation studies may also be used to confirm neuromuscular blockade when it is suspected.

Acute Quadriplegic Myopathy

The syndrome currently known as acute quadriplegic myopathy[74] (AQM), or *acute myopathy of intensive care*[75] (AMIC), was originally described in 1977 in a young woman who experienced severe myopathy following treatment of status asthmaticus with high-dose corticosteroids and pancuronium.[76] Subsequent to that report, there have been numerous citations of an acute myopathy developing in critically ill patients without preexisting neuromuscular disease. AQM has occurred most commonly in the setting of severe pulmonary disorders, in which pharmacologic paralysis is used to facilitate mechanical ventilation and high-dose corticosteroids are concurrently administered. In a majority of the reported cases, paralysis was achieved with nondepolarizing neuromuscular blocking agents used for more than 2 days.[74-84] The development of acute, necrotizing myopathy with myosin loss also occurs, however, in patients receiving high-dose corticosteroids and hypnotic doses of propofol and benzodiazepines to induce paralysis.[85] This observation highlights the significance of high-dose corticosteroid exposure in the development of this syndrome and suggests that paralyzed muscles may be generally susceptible to the toxic effects of corticosteroids. The occurrence of AQM following organ transplantation may be due to the use of high-dose corticosteroids to prevent graft rejection along with perioperative exposure to neuromuscular blocking agents.[86] Although most cases of AQM have been associated with critical illness, high-dose corticosteroids, and paralytic agents, AQM has also developed after isolated corticosteroid exposure,[74, 87-90] isolated nondepolarizing neuromuscular blocking agent use,[84, 88, 91] or neither.[92] Factors that may impair neuromuscular transmission (e.g., hypermagnesemia, aminoglycoside exposure), factors that may slow the elimination of nondepolarizing neuromuscular blocking agents (e.g., hepatic or renal failure), and factors associated with critical illness (e.g., sepsis, acidosis) have also been associated with AQM, although not consistently.[77]

In typical cases, a diffuse, flaccid quadriparesis with involvement of respiratory muscles and muscle wasting evolves after several days of induced paralysis. External ophthalmoparesis has rarely been noted.[93] Sensation remains intact, but deep tendon reflexes are reduced or absent. Creatinine kinase is commonly elevated, but the elevation may not be observed if creatinine kinase is measured well after the myopathy has developed. Although the paralysis may be quite severe and may necessitate or prolong mechanical ventilation, the prognosis from the myopathy itself is good, with functional recovery over several weeks to months.[79] Electromyographic findings include reduced CMAPs with normal SNAPs and normal nerve conduction velocities. M-wave amplitude improvement accompanies clinical recovery.[84] Repetitive nerve stimulation studies may yield significant decremental responses while the residual effects of nondepolarizing neuromuscular blocking agents or their active metabolites persist.[77, 84] Needle electromyography often reveals small, low-amplitude, polyphasic motor unit potentials exhibiting early recruitment, sometimes along with positive sharp waves and fibrillation potentials.

A spectrum of muscle histologic changes may be observed, ranging from type II fiber atrophy and loss of adenosine triphosphatase (ATPase) reactivity in atrophic fibers to fiber necrosis in severe cases. The distinctive finding in most cases of AQM, however, is an extensive loss of thick filaments corresponding to myosin loss.[74, 78, 83, 87, 92] This finding may be demonstrated with immunohistochemical staining or electron microscopy. Calpain, a calcium-activated protease, may represent the primary enzyme for myosin degradation in this syndrome.[92] In an animal analog of AQM, a reversible myopathy characterized by myosin loss occurs in rat muscles reversibly denervated by nerve crush when high-dose glucocorticoids are concurrently administered.[94] The increased expression of steroid receptors in denervated and immobilized muscle[95] may render these muscles susceptible to the toxic catabolic effects of steroids.[74]

Given the growing recognition of AQM, the use of high-dose corticosteroids should be avoided when induced paralysis is required. When this regimen is medically necessary, creatinine kinase levels should be monitored every 3 days during paralysis as surveillance for developing myopathy.

References

1. Garrity ER: Respiratory failure due to disorders of the chest wall and respiratory muscles. *In*: Respiratory Intensive Care. MacDonnell KF, Fahey PI, Segal MS (Eds). Boston, Little, Brown & Co, 1987, pp 312–320.
2. Jackson M, Kinnear W, King M, et al: The effect of five years of nocturnal cuirass-assisted ventilation in chest wall disease. Eur Respir J 1993; 6:630–635.
3. Mier-Jedrzejowicz AK, Brophy C, Moxham J, et al: Assessment of diaphragm weakness. Am Rev Respir Dis 1988; 137:877–883.
4. Black LF, Hyatt RE: Maximal static respiratory pressures in generalized neuromuscular disease. Am Rev Respir Dis 1971; 103:641–650.
5. Rochester DF, Truwit JD: Respiratory muscle failure in critical illness. *In*: Textbook of Critical Care, 3rd ed. Ayres SM, Grenvik A, Holbrook PR, et al (Eds). Philadelphia, WB Saunders, 1995, pp 637–643.
6. Alex CG, Tobin MJ: Assessment of pulmonary function in critically ill patients. *In*: Textbook of Critical Care, 4th ed. Ayres SM,

Grenvik A, Holbrook PR, et al (Eds). Philadelphia, WB Saunders, 1999.
7. Borel CO, Teitelbaum JS, Hanley DF: Ventilatory failure and carbon dioxide response in ventilatory failure due to myasthenia gravis and Guillain-Barré syndrome. Crit Care Med 1993; 21:1717-1726.
8. Yang KL, Tobin MJ: A prospective study of indexes predicting the outcome of trials of weaning from mechanical ventilation. N Engl J Med 1991; 324:1445-1450.
9. Loh L, Goldman M, Newsom-Davis J: The assessment of diaphragm function. Medicine 1977; 56:165-169.
10. Bennett DA, Bleck TP: Diagnosis and treatment of neuromuscular causes of respiratory failure. Clin Neuropharmacol 1988; 11:303-347.
11. Kelly BJ, Luce JM: The diagnosis and management of neuromuscular diseases causing respiratory failure. Chest 1991; 99:1485-1494.
12. Bleck TP, Smith MC, Pierre-Louis JC, et al: Neurologic complications of critical medical illnesses. Crit Care Med 1993; 21:98-103.
13. Breucking E, Mortier W: Anesthesia in neuromuscular diseases. Acta Anaesthesiol Belg 1990; 41:127-132.
14. Bleck TP, Brauner JS: Tetanus. *In*: Infections of the Central Nervous System, 2nd ed. Scheld WM, Whitley RJ, Durack DT (Eds). New York, Raven Press, 1997, pp 629-654.
15. Kuisma MJ, Saarinen KV, Teirmoa HT: Undiagnosed amyotrophic lateral sclerosis and respiratory failure. Acta Anaesthesiol Scand 1993; 37:628-630.
16. Donofrio PD, Wilbourn AJ, Albers JW, et al: Acute arsenic intoxication presenting as Guillain-Barré like syndrome. Muscle Nerve 1987; 10:114-120.
17. Greenberg C, Davies S, McGowan T, et al: Acute respiratory failure following acute arsenic poisoning. Chest 1979; 76:596-598.
18. Bleck TP: *Clostridium botulinum*. *In*: Principles and Practice of Infectious Diseases. Mandell GM, Bennett JE, Dolin R (Eds). New York, Churchill Livingstone, 1995, pp 2178-2182.
19. Peolsi G, Perili V, Sollazzi L, et al: Lambert-Eaton myasthenic syndrome: A clinical contribution. Acta Anaesthesiol Belg 1991; 42:41-44.
20. Gambling DR, Birmingham CL, Jenkins LC: Magnesium and the anaesthetist. Can J Anaesth 1988; 35:644-654.
21. Swygert LA, Back EE, Auerbach SB, et al: Eosinophilia-myalgia syndrome: Mortality data from the U.S. national surveillance system. J Rheumatol 1993; 20:1711-1717.
22. Curran FJ, Colbert AP: Ventilator management in Duchenne muscular dystrophy and postpoliomyelitis syndrome: Twelve years' experience. Arch Phys Med Rehabil 1989; 70:180-185.
23. Sasaki M, Yoneyama H. Nonaka I: Respiratory involvement in nemaline myopathy. Pediatr Neurol 1990; 6:425-427.
24. Barohn RJ, McVey AL, DiMauro S: Adult acid maltase deficiency. Muscle Nerve 1993; 16:672-676.
25. Kim GW, Kim SM, Sunwoo IN, et al: Two cases of mitochodrial myopathy with predominantly respiratory dysfunction. Yonsei Med J 1991; 32:184-189.
26. Newman JH, Neff TA, Ziporin P: Acute respiratory failure associated with hypophosphatemia. N Engl J Med 1977; 296:1101-1103.
27. Kennedy RH, Danielson MA, Mulder DW, et al: Guillain-Barré syndrome: A 42-year epidemiologic and clinical study. Mayo Clin Proc 1978; 53:93-99.
28. Gupta SK, Taly AB, Surmh TG, et al: Acute idiopathic axonal neuropathy (AIAN): A clinical and electrophysiological observation. Acta Neurol Scand 1994; 89:220-224.
29. Ropper AH, Wijdicks EFM, Truax BT: Guillain-Barré Syndrome. Philadelphia, FA Davis, 1991.
30. Griffin JW, Li CY, Ho TW, et al: Pathology of the motor-sensory axonal Guillain-Barré syndrome. Ann Neurol 1996; 39:17-28.
31. Yuki N, Sato S, Tsuji S, et al: Frequent presence of anti-GQ_{1b} antibody in Fisher's syndrome. Neurology 1993; 43:414-417.
32. Hughes RA: The spectrum of acquired demyelinating polyradiculoneuropathy. Acta Neurol Belg 1994; 94:128-132.
33. Cornblath DR, McArthur JC, Kennedy PGE, et al: Inflammatory demyelinating peripheral neuropathies associated with human T-cell lymphotrophic virus type III infection. Ann Neurol 1987; 21:32-40.
34. Albers JW, Kelly JJ: Acquired inflammatory demyelinating polyneuropathies: Clinical and electrodiagnostic features. Muscle Nerve 1989; 12:435-451.
35. Jabour ER, Rabil DM, Truwit JD, et al: Evaluation of a new weaning index based on ventilatory endurance and the efficiency of gas exchange. Am Rev Respir Dis 1991; 144:531-537.
36. Roubenoff RA, Borel CO, Hanley DF: Hypermetabolism and hypercatabolism in Guillain-Barré syndrome. J Parenter Enteral Nutr 1992; 16:464-472.
37. Guillain-Barré Study Group: Plasmapheresis and acute Guillain-Barré syndrome. Neurology 1985; 35:1096-1104.
38. McKhann GM, Griffin JW, Cornblath DR, et al: Plasmapheresis and Guillain-Barré syndrome: Analysis of prognostic factors and the effect of plasmapheresis. Ann Neurol 1988; 23:347-353.
39. French Cooperative Group on Plasma Exchange in Guillain-Barré Syndrome: Efficacy of plasma exchange in Guillain-Barré syndrome: Role of replacement fluids. Ann Neurol 1987; 22:753-761.
40. French Cooperative Group on Plasma Exchange in Guillain-Barré Syndrome: Plasma exchange in Guillain-Barré syndrome: One-year follow-up. Ann Neurol 1992; 32:94-97.
41. Osterman PO, Lundemo G, Pirskanen R, et al: Beneficial effects of plasma exchange in acute inflammatory polyradiculoneuropathy. Lancet 1984; 2:1296-1299.
42. French Cooperative Group on Plasma Exchange in Guillain-Barré Syndrome: Appropriate number of plasma exchanges in Guillain-Barré syndrome. Ann Neurol 1997; 41:298-306.
43. van der Meche FGA, Schmitz PIM, Dutch Guillain-Barré Study Group: A randomized trial comparing intravenous immunoglobulin and plasma exchange in Guillain-Barré syndrome. N Engl J Med 1992; 326:1123-1129.
44. Castro LHM, Ropper AH: Human immune globulin infusion in Guillain-Barré syndrome: Worsening during and after treatment. Neurology 1993; 43:1034-1036.
45. Irani DN, Comblath DR, Chaudry V, et al: Relapse in Guillain-Barré syndrome after treatment with human immune globulin. Neurology 1993; 43:873-875.
46. Bril V, Ilse WK, Pearce R, et al: Pilot trial of immunoglobulin versus plasma exchange in patients with Guillain-Barré syndrome. Neurology 1996; 46:100-103.
47. Plasma Exchange/Sandoglobulin Guillain-Barré Syndrome Trial Group: Randomized trial of plasma exchange, intravenous immunoglobulin, and combined treatments in Guillain-Barré syndrome. Lancet 1997; 349:225-230.
48. Buchman AS: Inflammatory demyelinating polyneuropathies. *In*: Textbook of Clinical Neuropharmacology and Therapeutics. Klawans HL, Goetz CG, Tanner CM (Eds). New York, Raven Press, 1992, pp 497-504.
49. Guillain-Barré Syndrome Steroid Trial Group: Double-blind trial of intravenous methylprednisolone in Guillain-Barré syndrome. Lancet 1993; 341:586-590.
50. Dutch Guillain-Barré Study Group: Treatment of Guillain-Barré Syndrome with high-dose immune globulins combined with methylprednisolone: A pilot study. Ann Neurol 1994; 35:749-752.
51. van der Meche FGA, van Doorn PA: The current place of high-dose immunoglobulins in the treatment of neuromuscular disorders. Muscle Nerve 1997; 20:136-147.
52. Phillips LH, Torner JC, Anderson MS, et al: The epidemiology of myasthenia gravis in central and western Virginia. Neurology 1992; 42:1888-1893.
53. Fink ME: Treatment of the critically ill patient with myasthenia gravis. *In*: Neurological and Neurosurgical Intensive Care. Ropper AH (Ed). New York, Raven Press, 1993, pp 351-362.
54. Thomas CE, Mayer SA, Gungor Y, et al: Myasthenic crisis: Clinical features, mortality, complications, and risk factors for prolonged intubation. Neurology 1997; 48:1253-1260.
55. Sanders DB, Scoppetta C: The treatment of patients with myasthenia gravis. Neurol Clin 1994; 12:343-368.
56. Wright RB: Myasthenia. *In*: Textbook of Clinical Neuropharmacology and Therapeutics. Klawans HL, Goetz CG, Tanner CM (Eds). New York, Raven Press, 1992, pp 505-516.
57. Cullen DJ, Bigatello LM, DeMonaco HI: Anesthetic pharmacology and critical care. *In*: The Pharmacologic Approach to the Critically Ill Patient, 2nd ed. Chernow B (Ed). Baltimore, Williams & Wilkins, 1994, pp 291-308.
58. Turani E, Szathmary I, Molnar J, et al: Myasthenia gravis: Prognostic significance of clinical data in the prediction of post-thymectomy respiratory crises. Acta Chir Hung 1992-1993; 33:353-360.

59. Kirsch JR, Diringer MN, Borel CO, et al: Preoperative lumbar epidural morphine improves postoperative analgesia and ventilatory function after transsternal thymectomy in patients with myasthenia gravis. Crit Care Med 1991; 19:1474–1479.
60. Rivner MH, Kim S, Greenberg M, et al: Reversible generalized paresis following hypotension: A new neurological entity (Abstract). Neurology 1983; 33(Suppl 2):164.
61. Bolton CF, Brown JD, Sibbald WJ: The electrophysiologic investigation of respiratory paralysis in critically ill patients (Abstract). Neurology 1983; 33(Suppl 2):240.
62. Roelofs RJ, Cerra F, Bielka N, et al: Prolonged respiratory insufficiency due to acute motor neuropathy: A new syndrome (Abstract)? Neurology 1983; 33(Suppl 2):240.
63. Bolton CF, Gilbert JJ, Hahn AF, Sibbald WJ: Polyneuropathy in critically ill patients. J Neurol Neurosurg Psychiatry 1984; 47:1223–1231.
64. Zochodne DW, Bolton, CF, Wells GA, et al: Critical illness polyneuropathy: A complication of sepsis and multiple organ failure. Brain 1987; 110:819–842.
65. Witt NJ, Zochodne DW, Bolton CF, et al: Peripheral nerve function in sepsis and multiple organ failure. Chest 1991; 99:176–184.
66. Spitzer AR, Giancarlo T, Maher L, et al: Neuromuscular causes of prolonged ventilator dependency. Muscle Nerve 1992; 15:682–686.
67. Hund EF, Fogel W, Krieger D, et al: Critical illness polyneuropathy: Clinical findings and outcomes of a frequent cause of neuromuscular weaning failure. Crit Care Med 1996; 24:1328–1333.
68. Bolton CF, Laverty DA, Brown JD, et al: Critically ill polyneuropathy: Electrophysiological studies and differentiation from Guillain-Barré syndrome. J Neurol Neurosurg Psychiatry 1986; 49:563–573.
69. Arnason BGW, Soliven B: Acute inflammatory demyelinating polyradiculoneuropathy. *In*: Peripheral Neuropathy, 3rd ed. Dyck PJ, Thomas PK (Eds). Philadelphia, WB Saunders, 1993, pp. 1437–1497.
70. Leijten FS, de Weerd AW: Critical illness polyneuropathy: A review of the literature, definition and pathophysiology. Clin Neurol Neurosurg 1994; 96:10–19.
71. Leitjen FS, de Weerd AW, Poortvliet DC, et al: Critical illness polyneuropathy in multiple organ dysfunction syndrome and weaning from the ventilator. Intensive Care Med 1996; 22:856–861.
72. Bolton CF, Young GB, Zochodne DW: The neurological complications of sepsis. Ann Neurol 1993; 33:94–100.
73. Segredo V, Caldwell JE, Matthay MA, et al: Persistent paralysis in critically ill patients after long-term administration of vecuronium. N Engl J Med 1992; 327:524–528.
74. Hirano M, Ott MD, Raps EC, et al: Acute quadriplegic myopathy: A complication of treatment with steroids, nondepolarizing blocking agents, or both. Neurology 1992; 42:2082–2087.
75. Lacomis D, Giuliani MJ, Van Cott A, Kramer DJ: Acute myopathy of intensive care: Clinical, electromyographic, and pathological aspects. Ann Neurol 1996; 40:645–654.
76. MacFarlane IA, Rosenthal FD: Severe myopathy after status asthmaticus. Lancet 1977; 2:615.
77. Barohn RJ, Jackson CE, Rogers SJ, et al: Prolonged paralysis due to nondepolarizing neuromuscular blocking agents and corticosteroids. Muscle Nerve 1994; 17:647–654.
78. Danon MJ, Carpenter S: Myopathy with thick filament (myosin) loss following prolonged paralysis with vecuronium during steroid treatment. Muscle Nerve 1991; 14:1131–1139.
79. Gooch JL: Prolonged paralysis after neuromuscular blockade. Muscle Nerve 1995; 18:937–942.
80. Kaplan PW, Rocha W, Sanders DB, et al: Acute steroid-induced tetraplegia following status asthmaticus. Pediatrics 1986; 78:121–123.
81. Lacomis D, Smith TW, Chad DA: Acute myopathy and neuropathy in status asthmaticus: Case report and literature review. Muscle Nerve 1993; 16:84–90.
82. Op de Coul AAW, Lembregts PCLA, Koeman J, et al: Neuromuscular complications in patients given Pavulon (pancuronium bromide) during artificial ventilation. Clin Neurol Neurosurg 1985; 87:17–22.
83. Waclawik AJ, Sufit RL, Beinlich BR, Schutta HS: Acute myopathy with selective degeneration of myosin filaments following status asthmaticus treated with methylprednisolone and vecuronium. Neuromuscul Disord 1992; 2:19.
84. Zochodne DW, Ramsay DA, Saly V, et al: Acute necrotizing myopathy of intensive care: Electrophysiological studies. Muscle Nerve 1994; 17:285–292.
85. Hanson P, Dive A, Brucher JM, et al: Acute corticosteroid myopathy in intensive care patients. Muscle Nerve 1997; 20:1371–1380.
86. Campellone JV, Lacomis D, Kramer DJ, et al: Acute myopathy after liver transplantation. Neurology 1998; 50:46–53.
87. Al-Lozi MT, Pestronk A, Yee WC, et al: Rapidly evolving myopathy with myosin-deficient muscle fibers. Ann Neurol 1994; 35:273–279.
88. Gutmann L, Blumenthal D, Schochet SS: Acute type II myofiber atrophy in critical illness. Neurology 1996; 46:819–821.
89. Sher JH, Shafiq SA, Schutta HS: Acute myopathy with selective lysis of myosin filaments. Neurology 1979; 29:100–106.
90. Van Marle W, Woods KL: Acute hydrocortisone myopathy. Br Med J 1980; 281:271–272.
91. Gooch JL, Moore MH, Ryser DK: Prolonged paralysis after neuromuscular junction blockade: Case reports and electrodiagnostic findings. Arch Phys Med Rehabil 1993; 74:1007–1011.
92. Showalter CJ, Engel AG: Acute quadriplegic myopathy: Analysis of myosin isoforms and evidence for calpain-mediated proteolysis. Muscle Nerve 1997; 20:316–322.
93. Sitwell LD, Weinshenker BG, Monpetit V, Reid D: Complete ophthalmoplegia as a complication of acute corticosteroid- and pancuronium-associated myopathy. Neurology 1991; 41:921–922.
94. Massa R, Carpenter S, Holland P, Karpati G: Loss and renewal of thick myofilaments in glucocorticoid-treated rat soleus after denervation and reinnervation. Muscle Nerve 1992; 15:1290–1298.
95. Du Bois DC, Almon RR: A possible role for glucocorticoid in denervation atrophy. Muscle Nerve 1981; 4:370–373.

174

Brain Death—Definition, Determination, and Physiologic Effects on Donor Organs

David J. Powner, MD, FCCM • German D. DeJoya, MD
Joseph M. Darby, MD

Therapy provided for patients with severe brain injury or insult is always directed toward preservation and restoration of neuronal function. Those injuries or insults and their treatment have been reviewed (see Chapters 27, 168, 171, and 172). When this primary treatment is unsuccessful and the patient's clinical condition evolves to brain death, the critical care physician also has (1) the responsibility to offer the patient's family the opportunity to donate organs and/or tissues and (2) the obligation to unknown recipients to provide the best possible organs and tissue. This chapter addresses that part of the intensivist's continuum of care that includes not only brain death but also the complex physiologic changes that occur during the evolution of this condition.

DEFINITIONS OF DEATH

The medical diagnosis of death has changed throughout medical history.[1] Often, the methods utilized by physicians to confirm a diagnosis of death have become the medical and social criteria used to define it. Historically, death was defined by the presence of putrefaction or decapitation, failure to respond to painful stimuli, or the apparent loss of observable cardiorespiratory action, as these were the simple observations available to physicians and lay practitioners. As medical technology and instrumentation changed, supplemental criteria evolved and death was redefined as the absence of heart sounds (after invention of the stethoscope), the presence of hypothermia (following development of the thermometer), or display of an isoelectric electroencephalogram (EEG) (as electroencephalography emerged).

Thus, the medical diagnosis and definition of the absence of life have been and continue to be defined by the measuring tools of medicine. However, many of the elements integral to common definitions of life cannot be fully measured by such tools. The "personhood" of a human is such an element and cannot be measured by medicine. It has been linked to mental cognition and is assumed to be absent when coma is present. Therefore, as the medical diagnosis of coma implies the absence of cognition, it also presumes the absence of personhood. This presumed linkage allows some to define death by the absence of cognition in the unconscious state of a patient in a permanent vegetative condition.

Societal norms have, in general, accepted the equivalency of patient death and certain medical evaluative tests of brain anatomy or function despite such philosophical controversy. This acceptance has been codified in all states of the United States through enactment of the Uniform Determination of Death Act or similar legislation: "An individual who has sustained either (1) irreversible cessation of circulatory and respiratory functions, or (2) irreversible cessation of all functions of the entire brain, including the brain stem, is dead."

The statute requires documented failure of the entire brain, but it does not stipulate what these "whole brain" criteria should be. No federal or national definition or criteria exist. Most states, therefore, leave this decision to the policy of individual hospitals and medical staffs. Many criteria lists have been published[2] and uniformly include a list of physiologic conditions (e.g., shock, hypothermia) or intoxicants that must be excluded before other testing can proceed. A careful physical examination to exclude any evidence of neuronal function in the cortex and brain stem is also required. Variations among policies include the number of examinations required, time intervals between examinations, requirements for and the type of confirmatory tests, and the number and qualifications of physicians who must corroborate the clinical diagnosis of brain death. Whole brain death criteria, as required in the United States, should include some confirmatory test of cortical anatomy or function.

"Brain-stem" death[3, 4] as accepted elsewhere and most notably in the United Kingdom, equates patient death to the absence of brain stem function in a comatose patient. Other than unresponsiveness to verbal stimuli and absent cognition, no confirmatory test of cortical function is required.

At this time no legislative, judicial, or institutional organization permits death to be defined only by the permanent loss of cortical function while neuronal activity continues in the brain stem.[5]

DETERMINATION OF BRAIN DEATH

Policies that stipulate tests, examination methods, and other criteria for declaring or certifying brain death are issued by individual hospitals or institutions in the United States and by authoritative groups or agencies elsewhere in the world. Guidelines for testing have been provided by many authors.[2, 6, 7]

In general, the process for brain death certification includes:

1. Identification of historical or physical examination findings that provide a clear etiology for brain dysfunction.

TABLE 174–1. Conditions That May Confound the Clinical Diagnosis of Brain Death

- Shock/hypotension
- Hypothermia <32°C
- Drugs known to alter neurologic and/or neuromuscular function or electroencephalographic testing:
  - Anesthetics
  - Paralytics
  - Methaqualone
  - Barbiturates
  - Diazepam
  - High-dose bretylium
  - Mecloqualone
  - Amitriptyline
  - Meprobamate
  - Trichloroethylene
  - Alcohols
- Brain stem encephalitis
- Guillain-Barré syndrome[8]
- Encephalopathies associated with hepatic failure, uremia, and hyperosmolar coma
- Severe hypophosphatemia

2. Exclusion of any condition that might confound the subsequent examination of cortical or brain stem neuronal function. Table 174–1 lists those conditions that *must* be excluded so as to ensure reliable testing by physical examination or by those confirmatory tests dependent on neurologic function (see Table 174–3).

3. Performance of a complete neurologic examination. Table 174–2 highlights components, technical performance issues, and other limitations of the physical examination.

4. Performance of additional confirmatory tests, as required by local policy, if no brain function is detected during the physical examination. Table 174–3 categorizes confirmatory tests used by some institutions. Limitations of the use or interpretation of confirmatory tests also exist[6, 10]; some of these limitations are shown in Table 174–4.

TABLE 174–2. Examination Criteria of Brain Death and Methods of Examination*

1. Absence of spontaneous movement, decorticate or decerebrate posturing, seizures, shivering, response to verbal stimuli, and response to noxious stimuli administered through a cranial nerve pathway. Spinal reflexes may persist.
2. Absent pupillary reflex to direct and consensual light; pupils need not be equal or dilated. The pupillary reflex may be selectively altered by eye trauma, cataracts, high-dose dopamine, glutethimide, scopolamine, atropine, bretylium, or monoamine oxidase inhibitors.
3. Absent corneal, oculocephalic, cough, and gag reflexes. The corneal reflex may be altered as a result of facial weakness.
4. Absent oculovestibular reflex when tested with 20 to 50 mL of ice water irrigated into an external auditory canal clear of cerumen and after elevating the patient's head 30°. Labyrinthine injury or disease, anticholinergics, anticonvulsants, tricyclic antidepressants, and some sedatives may alter responses.
5. Failure of the heart rate to increase by more than 5 beats/min after 1 to 2 mg of atropine intravenously indicates absent function of the vagus nerves and nuclei.
6. Absent respiratory efforts in the presence of hypercarbia (partial pressure of carbon dioxide >50–60 mm Hg) or, in rare circumstances, carefully monitored hypoxemia (e.g., in patients with severe chronic obstructive pulmonary disease). Many protocols for apnea testing have been advocated to prevent hypoxemia during testing.[9]

*Neurologic examination should be performed only after consideration of those factors listed in Table 174–1.

TABLE 174–3. Confirmatory Tests in Whole-Brain Criteria

1. *Evaluate neuronal function**
   a. Electroencephalogram or cerebral function monitor
   b. Evoked potentials
2. *Evaluate intracranial blood flow*
   a. Contrast angiography,[10] magnetic resonance imaging,[11] computed tomography, or positron emission tomography[12]
   b. Contrast radionuclide perfusion studies using technetium, cranial radionuclide angiography, and technetium-HMPAO scintigraphy[13]
   c. Xenon-enhanced computed tomography[13]
   d. Digital subtraction angiography and venography[14]
   e. Ophthalmic artery blood flow
   f. Transcranial Doppler studies[15]
3. *Miscellaneous criteria*
   a. Mean intracranial pressure higher than mean blood pressure
   b. Sustained cerebral perfusion pressure <5 mm Hg

*Reliability is altered by factors listed in Table 174–1.

5. Repetition of testing may be required by local policy after specified intervals.

6. Final certification of the diagnosis of brain death by one or more physicians as stipulated by local policy after all indicated testing confirms no function of the entire brain. This certification is the pronouncement of death in accord with state statutes.

7. After pronouncement of death by brain death criteria, further actions may proceed, including organ procurement or withdrawal of remaining cardiopulmonary support.

Despite elaborate standards and procedures, considerable evidence shows that in some patients, residual neuronal function continues even though a patient has fulfilled whole-brain criteria. Such evidence includes:

1. Maintenance of body temperature (i.e., not all patients become poikilothermic).

2. Spontaneous neuronal membrane depolarization, detected by deeply placed electrodes, even with an isoelectric cortical EEG.[19]

3. Continuing or inducible pituitary or hypothalamic hormone production after four-vessel angiography has shown no intracranial blood flow.[20]

4. Resumption of intracranial blood flow during postmortem examination of patients whose brain death was confirmed by the prior absence of blood flow during angiography.[19]

Therefore, those who demand absolute proof that all cellular function of the entire brain is absent before brain death is confirmed acknowledge that no set of criteria is sufficiently detailed for that purpose. Most commonly, the potential that residual cellular and tissue function may exist is recognized, but confirmation not specifically sought. The criteria described earlier generally are restricted to adults and children older than 5 to 7 years of age. Specific criteria considered useful in infants and young children have been published by the Task Force for the Determination of Brain Death in Children[21] and have subsequently been evaluated[22]

TABLE 174–4. Issues Affecting Utilization and Interpretation of Some Confirmatory Tests of Brain Death

1. Xenon and technetium radionuclide blood flow studies primarily assess only supratentorial cerebral flow and poorly visualize the posterior fossa and vertebrobasilar circulation. Variant flow patterns in both tests may limit interpretation.
2. Electroencephalographic testing must be done at maximum electronic gain in accord with standards established by the American Electroencephalographic Society.[2] Technical issues and inter-rater variability may affect reliability.[16]
3. Brain stem auditory evoked potentials evaluate only the brain stem and are useful only if apnea testing fails to show spontaneous breathing.[17]
4. Transcranial Doppler testing of intracranial blood flow should be attempted only when the systolic blood pressure is greater than 100 mm Hg.[17]
5. Although cerebral oxygen extraction falls in brain death, it is not useful as a confirmatory test.[18]

PHYSIOLOGIC CONSEQUENCES OF BRAIN DEATH

Substantial evidence from animal experimentation and patient observation suggests that during the evolution of brain death, significant systemic physiologic changes occur that may damage organs considered for transplantation. Such injury may also contribute to later rejection of the transplanted organ by the recipient.[23] Tissue injury may result from thermal, hormonal, ischemic, and electrolyte changes in the milieu of extracranial organs distant from the brain. Suggested mechanisms for injury include:

1. Hypotension and systemic hypoperfusion following ischemic myocardial injury precipitated by intense spasm of coronary arterioles. This spasm is thought to be due to high plasma catecholamine levels or an accentuated discharge of the sympathetic nervous system.

2. Hypothyroidism and low glucocorticoid levels secondary to loss of pituitary function and abnormal amounts and response to insulin.

3. Hypothermia after loss of hypothalamic temperature centers.

4. Electrolyte abnormalities and hypovolemia or hypoperfusion secondary to polyuria.

5. Generalized vasoparalysis and hypotension.

Animal models have acutely induced brain death by subdural balloon catheter inflation,[24-27] expanding cerebrospinal fluid (CSF) volume,[28] or after global ischemia.[29] These experiments have usually focused on the effects of brain death on myocardial performance, seeking to explain the profound hypotension that is commonly observed in human patients who rapidly progress to brain death. Table 174–5 lists the significant findings and postulated mechanisms of injury from these important animal studies.

Similarly, observations in human patients following the evolution of brain death have confirmed changes in the donor heart:

1. Abnormal alignment of contractile elements occurs within biopsy specimens taken before heart removal in 43% of donor hearts. These abnormal findings are correlated with early and late mortality in recipients and with increased requirements for postoperative inotropic support in recipients of those hearts.[31]

2. Contraction bands (foci of compressed contraction fibrils, necrosis, and mononuclear cell infiltration) are scattered throughout the myocardium after sudden brain death,[24] after less severe brain injury,[32] in conditions associated with high catecholamine levels, following myocardial infarction, and after death from other causes.[33]

3. Primary cardiac failure after implantation leads to recipient death or emergent retransplantation in 4% to 12% of transplanted hearts.

4. Higher troponin-T levels in donors are correlated with requirements for greater ionotropic support in recipients.[34]

5. Abnormal "coupling" between β-receptors and adenyl cyclase results in decreased systolic performance in donor hearts.[35]

TABLE 174–5. Physiologic Findings after Induced Brain Death in Animals

1. A sequential cardiovascular response of initial bradycardia, increased systemic and pulmonary vascular resistances, elevated systemic and wedge pressures, and arrhythmias is followed by hypotension, decreased vascular resistances, and reduced ventricular contractility. Acute inflation of a subdural balloon produces a more severe cardiovascular response than gradual inflation but likely simulates the rapid occurrence of brain death encountered in some patients.
2. Reduced right and left ventricular compliance and/or contractility after brain death is suggested by decreased left ventricular volume in response to experimentally elevated afterload.
3. Lower myocardial blood flow and preload sensitive stroke work is present after brain death.
4. Excessive sympathetic nervous system discharge may produce regional coronary artery constriction and calcium-mediated myocardial ischemia.
5. Reduced myocardial adenosine triphosphate levels occur after brain death.[30]

Other changes in the hormonal, electrolyte, thermal, and general milieu of the heart and other organs have also been documented in both animal experiments and humans. These abnormalities, which possibly affect all organs and tissues, are listed in Table 174–6.

This complex array of physiologic changes during the evolution of and following brain death presents significant challenges to those providing care for these patients. Patient care options are similarly complex and are discussed next.

TREATMENT IMPLICATIONS

Throughout the patient's treatment, standard intensive care practices remain important; these include:

1. Invasive hemodynamic monitoring (i.e. arterial, central venous, or pulmonary artery catheterization) may be essential for adequate fluid resuscitation and titration of therapy. Radial arterial catheters are preferred in multiple organ procurement because the femoral site may be needed during some organ procurement procedures. Pulmonary artery catheters may increase the risk of endocardial injury.

2. Hypotension should first be treated by volume expansion. The choice of crystalloid, colloid, or blood products depends on coexisting electrolyte abnormalities, disorders of free water conservation, or anemia. Vasoactive drugs should be chosen carefully and used judiciously to avoid vasoconstriction and possible ischemic damage to donor organs.[42]

3. Cardiac arrest itself does not exclude organ donation, but failure to promptly reestablish oxygen delivery leads to ischemic damage. Epinephrine, isoproterenol, or transcutaneous or transvenous pacing is employed for hemodynamically significant bradyarrythmias because atropine is ineffective after loss of vagal nuclei. If cardiac function cannot be quickly reestablished, open cardiac massage, cardiopulmonary bypass or emergent organ removal should be considered.

4. Standard respiratory therapy is appropriate, including positioning the endotracheal tube to avoid injury to the area of subsequent airway anastomoses in a potential lung donor, close monitoring of fluid balance to avoid pulmonary congestion, and maintenance of minute ventilation to normalize arterial pH.

5. Diabetes insipidus does not develop in all brain-dead patients but may result in significant hypotonic polyuria, hyperosmolality, electrolyte abnormalities, hypovolemia, and hemodynamic instability. The patient's free water deficit should be corrected with hypotonic solutions. Dextrose-containing fluids should be administered carefully to prevent significant hyperglycemia, which may promote further osmotic diuresis. Exogenous vasopressin may be required to replace circulating antidiuretic hormone after brain death. Intravenous desmopressin acetate (DDAVP) is recommended. Alternatively, a continuous intravenous infusion of aqueous pitressin may be used and titrated to its lowest effective dose. Urine output should be maintained at 100 to 250 mL/hr.

6. Hypothermia is best managed through prevention, but passive and active rewarming with blankets, heated inspired gas, or warmed intravenous fluids may be required.

In addition to these accepted "standards of care" for these patients, several more controversial treatment options have been proposed. Novitsky and coworkers[43] have advocated thyroid hormone administration to the donor and recipient. Other investigators[36, 44] have confirmed low triiodothyronine and variable thyroxine levels in patients but have not shown their correlation with decreased cardiac function in the donor or recipient and do not advocate thyroid hormone administration. Fewer hemodynamic, electrocardiographic, and histologic changes were recorded in five baboons pretreated with verapamil than in 11 control animals before induced acute brain death.[45] Hearts from these animals were not transplanted

TABLE 174–6. Factors Influencing Organ and Tissue Homeostasis During the Evolution of Brain Death

1. Low serum triiodothyronine levels with low or normal thyroxine levels are present in patients with severe brain injury but do not differ from patients who have sustained brain death.[36] Low cortisol and insulin levels found in an experimental model[24] have not been confirmed in humans.[36]
2. Circulating levels of dopamine and norepinephrine vary greatly in brain-dead and similarly injured patients but do not appear to correlate with clinical myocardial dysfunction.[37]
3. The effects of overstimulation of the sympathetic nervous system have not been separable from other signs of global catecholamine excess in humans, although a period of hypertension and tachycardia in the final phases of brain death is suggestive. This period of hypertension during the evolution of brain death, of particular interest as a potential indicator of myocardial stress or injury, is commonly seen and is usually followed by marked hypotension. The etiology for these dramatic changes is thought to be a sympathetic nervous system discharge followed by a form of "neurogenic shock," a cerebrospinal "disconnection" occurring after brain death.
4. Poikilothermia (loss of hypothalamic temperature regulation) usually produces hypothermia because of lower room temperatures, cold intravenous fluids, and other factors. Temperatures as low as 27°C have been reported, although more commonly hypothermia is mild. Possible consequences include electrocardiographic changes, decreased cardiac contractility, reduced glomerular filtration, pancreatitis, and altered cellular metabolism.
5. Polyuria is common after brain death and may be due to a "physiologic diuresis" following resuscitation, osmotic agents used during intracranial pressure control, hyperglycemia, or diabetes insipidus. Polyuria from the latter three causes produces a higher free water loss than natriuresis, leading to hypernatremia. Secondary losses of potassium, magnesium, phosphorus, and calcium during high volume fluid loss in diabetes insipidus may produce changes in serum or total body concentrations of those electrolytes and resultant dysrhythmias or cellular injury. Hypovolemia after uncontrolled fluid loss may produce secondary injury to organs.
6. Although long-term support of brain-dead patients is possible and well documented,[38] occasional patients do sustain an unexpected bradycardic cardiac arrest, especially when brain death has evolved rapidly.
7. A high incidence of positive cultures has been documented from donors even without evidence of active infection. Bacteria, fungi, and viruses are transferable to the recipient.[39–41]

or otherwise evaluated beyond the 6-hour experiment. No other animal or human study has evaluated calcium channel blocker protection for the heart.

Novitzky and colleagues[46] also showed a decreased number of contraction bands in eight baboons after cardiac sympathectomy but before brain death was induced. Similarly, after receiving β-receptor blockade intravenously, one animal demonstrated less hemodynamic change and fewer contraction bands.[24] Similar protection was not observed in one animal following adrenalectomy before brain death, suggesting a greater role for regional sympathetic influences than for circulating catecholamines.[24] No human studies describe β blockade or use of calcium channel blocking agents before or during the evolution of brain death as protective treatment. The use of free radical scavengers in cardioplegic solutions to decrease reperfusion injury to the heart after organ preservation has been described.[47] However, this intervention has not been evaluated as pretreatment in the donor or as therapy for the hypothesized ischemia-reperfusion cycle after brain death.[23]

Because it is unknown when cardiac injury may occur after the donor's brain injury, the optimal time to provide any intervention is also unknown. On the basis of experimental data and clinical impression, it appears that injury to potentially transplantable organs, including the heart, may occur during the final phases of brain death evolution, before brain death can be certified. Effective prophylaxis of such injury probably must be administered well before brain death occurs.

Ethical considerations have historically separated treatment of the brain-injured *patient* from management of the organ *donor*. In cases of severe brain injury, however, the possibility and even likelihood of brain death can and should be recognized early. As in any disease process in which alternative outcomes are possible and acknowledged, accepting the possibility that the patient may become an organ donor before brain death is certified is not unethical or improper. Therapy directed toward organ support, even before brain death, in the attempt to maximize treatment of the primary injury or disease so as to restore normal brain function is, likewise, not unethical. As long as any therapy does not diminish the primary goal of restoring brain function, it may be considered as part of the primary patient care plan. Therefore, it is appropriate to prevent or treat regional or systematic catecholamine surges and other hormonal or metabolic changes that occur after severe brain injury. In so doing, the physician may prevent or minimize hemodynamic or physiologic instability that may influence recovery of the patient or injure organs that may be subsequently donated and transplanted.

ORGAN-SPECIFIC CONSIDERATIONS

As reviewed, the heart and cardiovascular system have been extensively investigated during the process of brain death development because of their pivotal role in causing hypotension. Aside from the obvious harmful consequences of hypoperfusion to all organs and the general issues already discussed, some data about the protection or enhancement of other organs have been offered:

Kidneys

1. Hydroxyethylstarch, used as a volume expanding agent in donors, appears to cause "osmotic-nephrosis-like" lesions in the renal tubules and is associated with greater dialysis requirements in the recipient.[48]

2. A retrospective comparison indicated that a mean dopamine infusion of 7.25 ± 0.88 μg/kg/min was associated with delayed graft function.[49]

3. Repeated bolus administration of DDAVP with fluid support versus fluid administration alone in a matched prospective group was associated with a higher incidence of primary dysfunction after implantation.[50]

4. In correlating donor levels of plasma renin activity, aldosterone, atrial natriuretic peptide, and vasopressin with postimplantation outcome, only low levels of vasopressin were associated with oliguria in the recipient. Rowmsky and coworkers recommend prophylactic use of vasopressin during donor management.[51]

5. Donor pretreatment with intravenous lidocaine prior to kidney procurement leads to decreased incidence of early graft dysfunction, decreased need for dialysis, fewer dialysis treatments when necessary, and earlier return of renal function compared with control groups. The mechanism for the lidocaine effect was suggested to be related to the drug's vasodilating, platelet-disaggregating, and calcium channel-blocking properties.[52]

Pancreas and Intestines

1. Pancreas graft survival was adversely affected by the duration of brain death prior to procurement, length of donor admission, and donor age above 40 years.[53]

2. Pancreas islet cell yield was higher if the donor's blood glucose level was at least 120 mg/dL and if blood pressure was maintained.[54]

3. Donor hyperglycemia appears to be a minor risk factor in pancreatic allograft survival. Use of dopamine during treatment of the donor is an independent risk factor and adversely affects the longevity of technically successful allografts.[55]

4. High levels of vasopressor (unspecified) and high serum sodium (unspecified) decreased early intestinal graft survival and increased histologic evidence of ischemic injury.[56]

Liver

1. Multivariate analysis in 14 patients of 21 variables found only high levels of alanine transaminase, ICU stay longer than 3 days, and high glucose levels (mean, 431 ± 217) at the time of donor admission were correlated with poor initial graft function.[57]

2. Glycogen repletion prior to or during liver removal through glucose loading provides suggestive benefit, as measured by bile flow and reduced "hepatocyte necrosis" after implantation.[58]

SUMMARY

The critical care physician is charged with a primary duty to promote neuronal recovery in patients with brain injury or illness. The continuum of care provided to the patient and family in some cases extends throughout worsening of the neurologic status, during the process of brain death certification, and to the time for organ or tissue removal for transplantation. The evolution of irreversible neuronal death of the entire brain, including the brainstem, is often accompanied by a series of extreme physiologic changes that affect all other organs and tissues. These changes require the continued skill of the intensivist to provide the titrated care needed to assure that the patient's or family's wishes to provide organs or tissue will be fulfilled.

References

1. Powner DJ, Ackerman BM, Grenvik A: Medical diagnosis of death in adults: Historical contributions to current controversies. Lancet 1996; 348:1219.
2. Powner DJ: The diagnosis of brain death in the adult patient. J Intensive Care Med 1987; 2:181.
3. Pallais C: Further thoughts on brainstem death. Anaesth Intensive Care 1995; 23:20.
4. Criteria for the diagnosis of brainstem death. J R Coll Physicians Lond 1995; 29:381.
5. Hoffenberg R, Lock M, Tilney N, et al: Should organs from patients

in permanent vegetative state be used for transplantation? Lancet 1997; 350:1320.
6. Practice parameters for determining brain death in adults: Report of the Quality Standards Subcommittee of the American Academy of Neurology. Neurology 1995; 45:1012.
7. Dobb GJ, Weekes JW: Clinical confirmation of brain death. Anaesth Intensive Care 1995; 23:37.
8. Hughes R, McGuire G: Neurologic disease and the determination of brain death: The importance of a diagnosis. Crit Care Med 1997; 25:1923.
9. Wijdicks EFM: Determining brain death in adults. Neurology 1995; 45:1003.
10. Paolin A, Manurali A, DiPaola F, et al: Reliability in diagnosis of brain death. Intensive Care Med 1995; 21:657.
11. Matsumura A, Meguro K, Tsuruchima H, et al: Magnetic resonance imaging of brain death. Neurol Med Chir 1996; 36:166.
12. Meyer MA: Evaluating brain death with positron emission tomography. J Neuroimaging 1996; 6:117.
13. Monsein LH: The imaging of brain death. Anaesth Intensive Care 1995; 23:44.
14. Braum M, Duerocq X, Huot JC, et al: Intravenous angiography in brain death: Report of 140 patients. Neuroradiology 1997; 39:400.
15. Dominguez-Roldan JM, Murillo-Cabezas F, Munoz-Sanchez A, et al: Changes in the Doppler waveform of intracranial arteries in patients with brain-death status. Transplant Proc 1995; 27:2391.
16. Buchner H, Schuchardt V: Reliability of electroencephalogram in the diagnosis of brain death. Eur Neurol 1990; 30:138.
17. Nau R, Prange HW, Klingel Lofer J, et al: Results of four technical investigations in fifty clinically brain dead patients. Intensive Care Med 1992; 18:82.
18. Dominguez-Roldan JM, Murillo-Cabezas F, Santamaria-Mifsut JL, et al: Cerebral oxygen extraction ratio: A useful determination for the diagnosis of brain death. Transplant Proc 1995; 27:2393.
19. Pallis C: Brainstem death: The evolution of a concept. Semin Thorac Cardiovasc Surg 1990; 2:135.
20. Arita K, Uozumi T, Oki S, et al: The function of the hypothalamo-pituitary axis in brain dead patients. Acta Neurochir (Wien) 1993; 123:64.
21. Guidelines for determination of brain death in children. Arch Neurol 1987; 44:587.
22. Mejia RE, Pollack MM: Variability in brain death determination practices in children. JAMA 1995; 274:550.
23. Halloran PF, Homik J, Goes N, et al: The "injury response": A concept linking nonspecific injury, acute rejection, and long-term transplant outcomes. Transplant Proc 1997; 29:79.
24. Novitzky D, Wicomb WN, Cooper DKC, et al: Electrocardiographic, hemodynamic and endocrine changes occurring during experimental brain death in the Chacma baboon. J Heart Transplant 1984; 4:63.
25. Shivalkar B, Vanloon J, Wieland W, et al: Variable effects of explosive or gradual increase of intracranial pressure on myocardial structure and function. Circulation 1993; 87:230.
26. Chen EP, Bittner HB, Kendall SWH, et al: Hormonal and hemodynamic changes in a validated animal model of brain death. Crit Care Med 1996; 24:1352.
27. Bittner HB, Chen EP, Kendall SWH, et al: Brain death alters cardiopulmonary hemodynamics and impairs right ventricular power reserve against an elevation of pulmonary vascular resistance. Chest 1997; 111:706.
28. Huber TS, Groh MA, Gallagher KP, et al: Myocardial contractility in a canine model of the brain-dead organ donor. Crit Care Med 1993; 21:1731.
29. Myers CH, D'Amico TA, Peterseim DS, et al: Effects of triiodothyronine and vasopressin on cardiac function and myocardial blood flow after brain death. J Heart Lung Transplant 1993; 12:68.
30. Pinelli G, Mertes PM, Carteaux JP, et al: Consequences of brain death on myocardial metabolism: Experimental study using 3IP-nuclear magnetic resonance spectroscopy. Transplant Proc 1995; 27:1650.
31. Darracott-Cankovic S, Stovin PGI, Wheeldon D, et al: Effect of donor heart damage on survival after transplantation. Eur J Cardiothoracic Surg 1989; 3:525.
32. Virmani R, Farb A, Brurke A: Contraction-band necrosis: New use for an old friend. Lancet 1996; 347:1710.
33. Adomain GE, Laks MM, Billingham ME: The incidence and significance of contraction bands in endomyocardial biopsies from normal human hearts. Am Heart J 1978; 95:348.
34. Anderson JR, Hossein-Nia M, Brown P, et al: Donor cardiac troponin-T predicts subsequent inotrope requirements following cardiac transplantation. Transplantation 1994; 58:1056.
35. White M, Wiechmann RJ, Roden RL, et al: Cardiac beta-adrenergic neuroeffector systems in acute myocardial dysfunction related to brain injury. Circulation 1995; 92:2183.
36. Powner DJ, Hendrick A, Lagler R, et al: Hormonal changes in brain dead patients. Crit Care Med 1990; 18:702.
37. Powner DJ, Hendrick A, Nyhuis A, et al: Changes in serum catecholamines in brain dead patients. J Heart Lung Transplant 1992; 111:1046.
38. Kinoshita Y, Okamoto K, Yahata K, et al: Clinical and pathological changes of the heart in brain death maintained with vasopressin and epinephrine. Pathol Res Pract 1990; 186:173.
39. Sole-Violan J, Rodriguez de Castro F, Rey A, et al: Comparison of bronchoscopic diagnostic techniques with histological findings in brain dead organ donors without suspected pneumonia. Thorax 1996; 51:929.
40. Pacholczyk MJ, Lagiewska B, Meszaros J, et al: Bacterial infections transmitted from the donor: Antibiotic prophylaxis in the donor. Transplant Proc 1996; 28:184.
41. Coll P, Montserrat I, Ballester M, et al: Epidemiologic evidence of transmission of donor-related bacterial infection through a transplanted heart. J Heart Lung Transplant 1997; 16:464.
42. Hunt SA, Baldwin J, Baumgartner W, et al: Cardiovascular management of a potential heart donor: A statement from the Transplantation Committee of the American College of Cardiology. Crit Care Med 1996; 24:1599.
43. Novitzky D: Selection and management of cardiac allograft donors. Curr Opin Cardiol 1996; 11:174.
44. Goarin JP, Cohen S, Riou B, et al: The effects of triiodothyronine on hemodynamic status and cardiac function in potential heart donors. Anesth Analg 1996; 83:41.
45. Novitzky D, Cooper DKC, Rose AG, et al: Prevention of myocardial injury by pretreatment with verapamil hydrochloride prior to experimental brain death. Am J Emerg Med 1987; 5:11.
46. Novitsky D, Wicomb WN, Cooper DKC, et al: Prevention of myocardial injury during brain death by total cardiac sympathectomy in the Chacma baboon. Ann Thorac Surg 1986; 41:520.
47. Grinyo JM: Reperfusion injury. Transplant Proc 1997; 29:59.
48. Cittanova ML, Leblanc I, Legendre C, et al: Effect of hydroxyethylstarch in brain-dead kidney donors on renal function in kidney transplant recipients. Lancet 1996; 348:1620.
49. Grekas D, Alivanis P, Derveniotis V, et al: Influence of donor data on graft function after cadaveric renal transplantation. Transplant Proc 1996; 28:2957.
50. Hirschl MM, Matzner MP, Huber WO, et al: Effect of desmopressin substitution during organ procurement on early renal allograft function. Nephrol Dial Transplant 1996; 11:173.
51. Rowinski W, Lao M, Cajzner S, et al: The influence of endocrine changes in donors and recipients on immediate outcome of kidney transplantation. Transplant Proc 1996; 28:3494.
52. Walaszewski J, Rowinski W, Pacholczyk M, et al: Multiple risk factor analysis of delayed graft function (ATN) after cadaveric transplantation: Positive effect of lidocaine donor pretreatment. Transplant Proc 1991; 23:2475.
53. Douzdjian V, Gugliuzza KG, Fish JC: Multivariate analysis of donor risk factors for pancreas allograft failure after simultaneous pancreas-kidney transplantation. Surgery 1995; 118:73.
54. Fiedor P, Goodman ER, Sung RS, et al: Factors that can affect cadaveric islet graft function include hemodynamic changes in the donor prior to organ harvest. Transplant Proc 1996; 28:169.
55. Gores PF, Viste A, Hesse UJ, et al: The influence of donor hyperglycemia and other factors on long-term pancreatic allograft survival. Transplant Proc 1990; 22:437.
56. Furukawa H, Smith C, Lee R, et al: Influence of donor criteria on early outcome after intestinal transplantation. Transplant Proc 1997; 29:690.
57. Lee YJ, Lee SG, Kwon TW, et al: Donor characteristics for liver transplantation and risk factors for early poor graft function and survival. Transplant Proc 1996; 28:1663.
58. Driscoll DF, Palombo J, Bistrian BR: Nutritional and metabolic considerations of the adult liver transplant candidate and organ donor. Curr Concepts in Clin Nutr 1995; 11:255.

175

History and Organization of Organ Transplantation

Brian A. Broznick, CPTC
Susan A. Stuart, RN, BSN, MPM, CPTC
Ake Grenvik, MD, PhD, FCCM

More than 40 years have passed since the first successful kidney transplantation occurred in Boston. Since that time, transplantation has evolved from an experimental process to an accepted and successful lifesaving therapy. The ability to replace a diseased organ with a healthy one from a living or cadaveric donor has become routine. In the United States alone, on the average, someone receives a solid-organ transplant every 30 minutes.[1] However, even though more patients are afforded a second chance at life today than 10 years ago, more patients also die awaiting their chance at transplantation. Every 2 to 3 hours of each day, another patient dies before being provided this lifesaving gift.[1] Of all patients awaiting heart transplantation worldwide, 30% die within 9 to 12 months after acceptance on a waiting list.[2] Additionally, hundreds of thousands of individuals each year receive a cornea transplant, bone graft, skin graft, or other type of human tissue that provides severely disabled individuals with the ability to lead a productive and active life. However, the need for cadaveric organs and tissues continues to exceed the numbers donated.

Although success rates in organ transplantation have reached heights of greater than 80% 1-year patient survival,[3] the successes have not come without obstacles along the way. Before 1980, advances in transplantation were painfully slow. During the latter part of the 1960s and well into the 1970s, a 1-year renal allograft survival rate of 65% was achieved but also carried a recipient mortality rate as high as 20%.[3]

New discoveries in the field of immunology with development of better immunosuppressive therapy led to greater success rates in transplantation and a decline in patient mortality. Because both graft and patient survival have greatly increased, physicians have become more willing to recommend transplantation to their patients. As a consequence, waiting lists for transplantation have more than tripled during the past 7 years.[3] Two factors that inhibit the more rapid growth of this field of medicine are:

- Not ensuring that every family is given the opportunity to donate organs or tissues when appropriate
- Families refusing to donate organs and tissues when the opportunity arises

In December 1998, more than 65,000 individuals were awaiting some type of solid-organ transplant. This figure represents a 67% increase in the number of those waiting during the past 4½ years. Because of the number of patients waiting and the lack of available organs, a formalized distribution system and organization of transplant centers and affiliated organizations had to be developed. Such arrangements need to take into account the limitations of organ preservation and transplant center resources; most important, they must keep the needs of the patient in mind. To achieve public trust and support of transplantation, a fair and equitable distribution system of available organs had to be organized.

This chapter recounts the development of the system that existed in the United States in 1992, the achievements that have been gained, and current issues of concern.

THE EARLY YEARS

Clinical trials in transplantation began in the 1940s. Achievements were made rapidly. In 1945, for example, Landsteiner, Hufnagel, and Hume[4] performed what some consider a transplantation by connecting a cadaveric kidney to a brachial artery and cephalic vein of a woman who was experiencing acute renal failure. The graft was removed 48 hours later. No significant amounts of urine were produced, but fortunately the patient's own kidneys resumed function within a few hours of the procedure.

In 1954, Murray and associates[5] performed the first successful kidney transplantation between two identical twins. The technique used by this team was adapted for similar procedures in allotransplantation of other organs. Murray was awarded the Nobel Prize in Medicine in 1990 for his pioneering transplantation research, together with Thomas and colleagues, who initiated and refined the technique for bone marrow transplantation.[6]

Through the 1960s, improved organ retrieval, surgical technique, and immunosuppression were important developments. The most common problems confronting transplantation were rejection and infection. In the late 1960s, Starzl and associates[7] began clinical trials using antilymphocyte serum to counteract rejection. During this same time period, different transfusion techniques on prospective kidney recipients and removal of the patient's spleen were carried out. Although these procedures provided some benefits, partially through donor-specific transfusions, the risk of sensitizing a patient against a transplanted graft was also identified.

THE ROLE OF HISTOCOMPATIBILITY

During the 1960s, donor-recipient compatibility in transplantation surgery became increasingly obvious. It was observed that a recipient's and donor's tissue types were critical to the outcome of a transplanted graft. The human leukocyte antigen (HLA) system was discovered by a large number of renowned researchers, and the designation HLA was agreed on at a World Health Organization meeting in New York in 1968.[8] It soon became apparent that a large recipient pool would be necessary to obtain the best HLA match between donated organs and the waiting patients. During this time, however, relatively few patients were waiting for kidney transplantation. Because renal transplantation was still considered experimental, only a few centers funded by National Institutes of Health grants were performing transplantations.

FORMATION OF A TRANSPLANTATION SYSTEM

In the late 1960s, a regional transplantation system began to take form. Successful sharing of kidneys based on HLA matching was accomplished, but few transplantation centers participated. The Medical College of Virginia, University of Virginia, Duke University, and Johns Hopkins University were initially involved. In 1968, what was probably the first long-distance transport of a donor organ took place when a kidney was sent from Richmond to Atlanta, where it was successfully transplanted. Transportation for this mission was carried out by the Virginia Air National Guard based in Richmond. During this period, preservation of kidneys consisted of simple cold-storage techniques, which permitted only brief organ preservation, making time a critical factor between procurement and transplantation.

In 1969, the Medical College of Virginia applied for and was awarded a contract from the Kidney Disease Control Agency (KDC) of the Public Health Service, with David Hume designated as the principal investigator. Other participating centers included Duke University, Georgetown University, University of North Carolina, University of Maryland, University of Virginia, Johns Hopkins University, Emory University, and Danville Memorial Hospital. This particular contract specified a feasibility study to be conducted regarding the recovery of kidneys in a remote location, preservation of these organs, and identification of HLA specificity of the donor and the best-matched recipient for the organs. At the same time, techniques for expanding the preservation time of kidneys were also being developed, using pulsatile perfusion.

A considerable number of projects were initiated simultaneously in the early phase of the KDC contract. Policies were developed for kidney sharing, studies were begun to determine the best means of kidney preservation, and thought was given to designing a computerized system for recipient matching with donated organs. The General Electric time-sharing system was ultimately selected to work with the originating centers to develop this matching system. Each original member was equipped with a terminal to connect it with the General Electric system, which became operational in late 1969 as the Southeastern Regional Organ Procurement Program (SEROPP).*

At the time the system became operational, fewer than 100 patients were awaiting transplantation. As with any new system, flaws were identified, but the new system represented the first on-line computer matching technique, operating over a fairly large geographic area. Formal criteria were developed for transplantation of donated kidneys based on the best available match. Several patients were on occasion identified with equal matches, and tie-breaking criteria were developed using patient waiting times. Thus, the patient who waited the longest was offered first opportunity for transplantation. It became apparent that funding and reimbursement were to become extremely important for the success of this system. Transplantation centers began to discuss finances with insurance companies and the federal government. Acquisition charges for the recovery, preservation, and transportation of kidneys were developed at this time.

Because SEROPP demonstrated success, it grew in importance. By showing better success rates in transplantation and the development of more refined techniques for organ preservation, the number of programs performing transplantations continued to grow, and most of these programs joined SEROPP. Some of the financial restraints were lifted in 1972, when amendments to Medicare legislation allowed for payment of cost incurred for dialysis treatment as well as kidney procurement, transportation, and transplantation.

ORGAN-SHARING SYSTEMS DEVELOP

In 1975, charter members of SEROPP decided to incorporate into a new organization known as the Southeastern Organ Procurement Foundation (SEOPF). The computer programs that were developed and remaining funds from the original KDC contract were transferred to SEOPF. During this time, other organ-sharing systems appeared in the United States and in Europe. Euro-Transplant and other programs in the United Kingdom, Germany, France, and Scandinavian countries were developed. It soon became evident that transplantation and organ sharing could not be contained within one geographic boundary but had to be expanded to include entire nations or possibly even continents. The need for this type of expansion was recognized in the United States by SEOPF, whose board of directors authorized the organization and incorporation of the United Network for Organ Sharing (UNOS).

THE GROWTH YEARS

Clinical successes in other types of organ transplantations were also achieved. However, two major obstacles continued to plague the transplantation community: graft rejection and organ shortage. During this time, many new developments took place. Improved surgical techniques and organ preservation and the development of new immunosuppressive drugs caused a tremendous growth in this field during the late 1970s and early 1980s.

In 1976, Borel[9] outlined the immunosuppressive properties of cyclosporine, which offered new hope for transplant recipients. Specifically, this drug possessed selectivity for T lymphocytes and proved far more effective than agents previously used. The initial trials with cyclosporine were conducted by Calne and colleagues.[10] Their findings, however, suggested that cyclosporine was highly toxic. Further investigative studies conducted by Starzl and coworkers[11] indicated that cyclosporine could be safely used and could be an effective immunosuppressive drug for combating organ rejection. Indeed, the development and use of cyclosporine made transplantation a useful and lifesaving form of therapy in the early 1980s.

Success rates for heart and liver transplantation achieved during this time had only been previously accomplished with renal transplantation. With this increased success rate in transplantation, more and more suitable recipients were identified. A mechanism was needed to ensure equitable sharing of all organs. It was not uncommon during the early part of the 1980s to encounter individuals bidding for lifesaving organs on television or radio or in the printed media. Livers needed for children awaiting transplantation were commonly announced in the media during this time. In addition, instances of inequitable organ distribution were being described. Although a well-organized and responsibly fair system was in place, the public demanded greater accountability and equitability in organ distribution and transplantation.

FEDERAL GOVERNMENT RESPONSE

In 1984, in response to public pressure, the U.S. Congress passed Public Law 98-507. This law became known as the National Organ Transplant Act.[12] The law called for the formation of a task force on organ procurement and transplantation, which was charged with the comprehensive examination of all aspects of human organ donation, procurement, and transplantation. The task force's role was to assess current public and private efforts to secure organs for transplantation and identify factors that diminished the number of organs available. In addition, the task force was to evaluate the problems in coordinating the procurement of transplantation organs and tissues.

This act further established procedures for certifying organ procurement organizations (OPOs). The task force would report to and work under the Secretary of Health and Human Services. Requirements for OPOs were expanded to include

*Armata T: History of the Southeastern Organ Procurement Foundation, "SEOPF." Personal communication, December 1992.

specific criteria regarding board composition, defined geographic areas for organ procurement, equitable allocation of organs recovered, and fiscal responsibilities. Additionally, the law called for the establishment of a nationwide organ procurement and transplant network (OPTN) to which all transplant centers, organ procurement organizations, and histocompatibility laboratories would have to belong. For the first time, all entities involved in transplantation would come together under one central organization. In addition, a scientific registry was established to provide accurate data on transplantation numbers, graft survival, and equity in organ sharing.

The task force published its written report in April 1986.[13] Most of the recommendations were implemented within a 2-year period. Certification of OPOs was initiated, and a 1-year contract was offered for the development and implementation of the OPTN. This contract, along with the scientific registry contract, was awarded to UNOS, based in Richmond. By the end of the first fiscal year, UNOS had implemented a nationwide organ distribution system, and the network became fully operational in October 1987.

UNITED NETWORK FOR ORGAN SHARING

UNOS now represents a formalized system for organ distribution. Besides maintaining a 24-hour, 365-day service to facilitate the placement of available organs with waiting recipients, UNOS developed membership criteria, organ recovery standards, and qualification requirements for transplantation surgeons and physicians. Histocompatibility needs and OPO requirements were also established. A board of directors was elected, comprising not only health care professionals involved in the transplantation arena but also the lay public, delegates from voluntary health organizations, and perhaps most important, patient representatives.

Independent registries for kidney, liver, heart, lung, pancreas, and bone marrow transplantation were incorporated into UNOS. Information on all organ donors and recipients became available under one unified system. This system, for the first time, allowed for the collection of comprehensive statistics that provide quality assurance and further advancement and refinement of transplantation technology.

One of the most difficult tasks that faced UNOS as a new contractor for the OPTN was establishing a fair and equitable system for distributing available organs. During the start-up time of UNOS, Starzl and associates[14] in Pittsburgh instituted a system for equitable organ allocation. This system provided "points" or "credits" to transplantation candidates based on waiting time accrued, quality of antigen match, logistic considerations, and urgency. Because this system proved fairly effective in Pittsburgh, it was adopted by UNOS. Although the system has undergone numerous changes, the primary purpose remains the same.

Under this system, each organ is matched somewhat differently. Kidneys, for example, are matched by ABO compatibility, tissue antigen matching, a negative serum–white blood cell crossmatch between donor and recipient, and waiting time. The patient with the best match, especially in relation to the donor's HLA, receives the kidney. Livers are distributed in a different manner. Because there is no effective, permanent mechanical support for patients with end-stage liver disease, histocompatibility is usually not tested before transplantation. The patients are selected based on compatibility of blood type and organ size. Waiting time and urgency of need are also factors that have important roles in the selection of recipients for liver transplantation.

Four categories exist for prioritizing patients awaiting liver transplantation. The most urgent category is status one. Patients in this category are those who are hospitalized, who are in critical condition, and whose life expectancy is less than 72 hours. All of these patients must be receiving intensive care. The next most critical category is status two, which is reserved for patients who are hospitalized but are not in an intensive care unit. These patients cannot care for themselves at home and must wait in the hospital for an available organ. Status three patients are those who are home bound but do not have the ability to work and may need some specialized care. The final category is status four, which is reserved for patients who have end-stage liver disease but are still fairly self-sufficient.

For patients awaiting heart transplantation, only two categories are recognized. *Status one* is reserved for patients in the most critical condition. These are patients who are hospitalized and need some type of supportive measure, either a mechanical support device or inotropic drug administration. *Status two* includes all patients awaiting transplantation outside the hospital. Hearts, like livers, are matched by ABO compatibility and size. Waiting time also plays an important role in heart transplantation.

For those awaiting lung transplantation, no categorization currently exists. These patients are matched solely on ABO and size compatibility. The only other factor that is taken into consideration is the length of waiting time. This is also true of patients awaiting combined heart-lung transplants.

Pancreata are distributed in a somewhat different manner from other organs but in a manner similar to that of kidneys. Because most clinicians believe that histocompatibility is important, pancreas recipients have criteria to meet that are similar to those awaiting renal transplantation. In many cases, patients receive a combined kidney-pancreas transplant.

With the exception of perfectly matched kidney and kidney-pancreas transplants, distribution of organs is carried out locally first, then regionally, and finally nationally. Organs recovered within an OPO service area are first offered to patients waiting for transplantation at centers with which the OPO has an affiliation. If for some reason the organs cannot be allocated locally, they are offered to patients within the region in which the OPO resides. Currently, 11 regions have been designated throughout the United States. Finally, if regional allocation is not feasible, organs are entered into the national pool.

ORGAN DONATION ISSUES

Although progress has been made in ensuring equitable distribution of donated organs, increasing survival rates for patients receiving a transplant, providing better immunosuppressive drugs, and improving preservation of organs, one major problem remains in ensuring everyone an opportunity for transplantation: the shortage of suitable organs for transplantation.

As part of the OPTN contract, UNOS was recently requested to develop methods for increasing organ donation. The first step taken by UNOS was to study factors that led to increased accomplishments by some OPOs. Although all areas of operation of OPOs were reviewed, very few conclusions could be drawn to distinguish why some OPOs perform better than others.[15] It was apparent, however, that a close relationship between organ procurement coordinators and donor hospitals had a positive effect on increasing donation within these hospitals. The number of years of experience and the type of background of the executive director of the OPO also seemed related to increased donation. After this study, the committee within UNOS that carried out this survey recommended that OPOs develop a way to identify their specific donor pool. Additionally, potential donor availability studies should be undertaken by every OPO, with subsequent strategies developed to maximize donation based on obtained data. The committee also believed that it was important to examine the operations of those OPOs with the highest procurement rates and disseminate its findings to all other OPOs.

UNOS has also invited most organizations involved in transplantation to develop a national campaign for increasing organ donation. This coalition has been accepted by the National Advertising Council and received nearly $30 million of free advertising between 1994 and 1996. In 1996, basketball star Michael Jordan became a spokesperson for organ donation. It is hoped that this will stimulate an increase in organ donation.

Approximately 54,000 patients were waiting for some type of solid-organ transplant in July 1997: 36,852 patients were waiting for a kidney; 8371 for a liver; 3797 for a heart; 339 for a pancreas; 1542 for combined kidney-pancreas; 227 for combined heart-lungs; 2429 for a single or double lung; and 91 for a small bowel.[16] On the average, one of these patients is dying every 4 hours. In 1996, there were 5416 organ donors, resulting in 16,801 organ donations. However, this represents an increase in donation of only 11% over 1993, while the number of potential recipients increased by 54% (Fig. 175–1). Therefore, the gap between the number of patients receiving transplants and the number of those awaiting transplantation continues to increase.[17] Intensified work needs to be carried out to gain public acceptance of donation if all patients awaiting transplantation are to be afforded an opportunity for continued life.

As mentioned before, organ donation is not keeping pace with the rapidly increasing need. Difficult problems continue to arise regarding organ allocation. One issue that needs to be further addressed in the near future is recipient selection criteria. Although the tendency has been to treat critically ill patients first because of the shortage of available organs, statistical evidence suggests that healthier patients at the time of transplantation benefit more than do critically ill patients. However, transplantation performed too early may not benefit the recipient more than conventional therapy.

A well-designed and well-executed approach needs to be planned in regard to both professional and public education. Thousands of organs are wasted needlessly every year simply because of lack of understanding, with no request for organ donation being made at the time of death. Health care professionals, including physicians such as neurologists, intensivists, traumatologists, anesthesiologists, and surgeons, must shoulder the responsibility for donor identification. They do not, however, need to assume responsibility for approaching families. Organ procurement coordinators are specifically trained and readily available to do this. Additionally, new avenues of donation must be explored. Obviously, by increasing the donor pool, more patients in need of transplantation can receive this form of treatment.

Year	Total Donors	Total Patients Waiting
1988	4084	16026
1989	4019	19095
1990	4512	21914
1991	4528	24719
1992	4521	29415
1993	4861	33352
1994	5100	37609
1995	5355	43937
1996	5416	49715

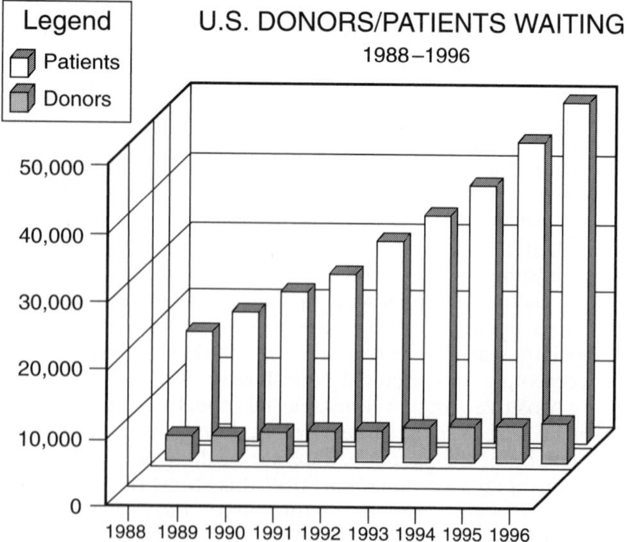

Figure 175–1. Donors and patients waiting for transplantation in the United States (1988 to 1996).

WHAT THE FUTURE MIGHT HOLD

Under the current criteria, approximately 12,000 potential organ donors with brain death exist in the United States in any given year,[18] but only about 5000 donations take place annually. One of the most important factors inhibiting an increase in the number of organ donations is that many families are never asked.[19] The second largest problem is that families approached say no.

In an attempt to ensure that every family is provided with the opportunity to donate, some states have amended their Uniform Anatomical Gift Act to mandate referrals of all inpatient hospital deaths to the regional OPO and to control who approaches families regarding donation. Pennsylvania was the first state to pass such legislation.[20] New Jersey and Tennessee passed similar legislation. At the present time, the federal government is considering this type of legislation nationally.

A possible way to provide more organs for transplantation is to look at other nontraditional types of donations. The criteria used in regard to organ donation have been greatly expanded in the past few years. Organs are increasingly being recovered from patients in their late 60s and their 70s and used for transplantation for recipients above 50 years of age. Most of these organs are kidneys, but in some cases they are also livers. Additionally, patients with a history of diabetes or hypertension are no longer ruled out for donation. Although these disease processes may affect some organ systems, they do not affect all. Many organs can be recovered from these patients and transplanted successfully.

The use of living organ donors may be expanded in the future. Although living donation was for many years limited to kidneys, the tail of the pancreas of living donors has been used, and lobes of livers or lungs have also been recovered and transplanted (e.g., from parents to their children). Even a heart can be procured from a living donor. This occurs when a patient receives a combined heart-lung transplant. If the heart of the recipient of a heart-lung block is healthy, it may be transplanted into a second recipient, so-called domino transplantation. However, this technique is seldom used because a patient with a healthy heart will only receive transplantation of the lungs.

Although difficult medicolegal problems surround donation of organs from anencephalic infants, this particular type of patient can also be used for possible donation. Many parents of anencephalic babies wish to see a donation carried out to provide some meaning to the birth of such a grossly deformed child. In some countries, such as Germany, anencephalic infants have not been considered to be alive and procurement of organs is permitted while the heart is still beating and the organs are perfused. Successful kidney transplantation from such cases has been reported.[21]

Another potential for increasing the donor pool is to return to organ recovery from non–heart-beating donors, which was commonly used in the 1960s. This is frequently done in those Asian countries where brain death is not yet recognized as death of the individual. Some Western countries (e.g., Holland) have continued to use non–heart-beating donors primarily for kidneys. In the United States, this donor category includes patients who have suffered lethal brain injuries and are not yet certified brain dead but are under evaluation for brain death when cardiac arrest occurs. If consent has been obtained, the patient is transported urgently to the operating room for immediate organ recovery. However, death must be certified on the basis of cessation of cardiopulmonary function before removal of donated organs.

Another category comprises terminally ill patients whose family decides to have life-support treatment withdrawn and wishes to donate organs. After cessation of cardiopulmonary function, the patients are declared dead and organ recovery can take place.

Non–heart-beating donors may also be patients who are admitted to the hospital in full cardiac arrest and cardiopulmonary resuscitation is either unsuccessful, contraindicated, or unwanted by the patient or his or her surrogate. If agreement has been reached in advance or if the patient's surrogate agrees to organ donation at the time, an aortic cannula can be inserted via the femoral artery for infusion of cold preservation solution for so-called in situ preservation. Similarly, an inferior vena cava cannula is inserted for drainage. The patient can then be taken to the operating room for urgent organ recovery.

Occasionally, patients who have undergone cardiac surgery cannot be weaned successfully from cardiopulmonary bypass. In some of these cases, cardiopulmonary bypass has been stopped and the patients have been certified dead, based on cardiopulmonary criteria. If consent for donation is obtained, these patients may also provide lifesaving organs for transplantation.

The foregoing are examples of possible indications for increasing the donor pool. These and other potential donor categories will no doubt continue to be discussed as the need for organs continues to outstrip the number of organs available for transplantation.

SUMMARY

Since the first successful kidney transplantation, transplantation has become a highly beneficial form of therapy, but this achievement has come at great cost. Only by ensuring equitable access to organs can this fascinating and rapidly changing medical field continue its successful growth. Trust and support are of utmost importance if this lifesaving therapy is to be offered to the many thousands of patients in need.

The federal government held public hearings to discuss changes in the allocation of livers. Although no findings have been published to date, this represents the first time that the government took interest in the allocation issue since the passage of the National Organ Transplant Act in 1984. These hearings represent the first attempt to allow the public to provide input in the allocation of this limited resource. This is a milestone and should open the door for a national organ-sharing policy.

Although the future is bright for most transplant recipients, it is not for those who die waiting for a second chance at life. As we gain more knowledge and experience in transplantation, new avenues must be explored to meet the needs of these patients. Xenografting and cell transplantation are two new areas being explored. Controversies about these procedures are numerous, but promising experiments continue to be carried out. Efforts by both involved health care professionals and the lay public need to increase significantly if transplantation is to advance further.

References

1. UNOS Update, Special Edition, Vol 8, Richmond, December 1992.
2. Markmann JF, Barker CF: Basic and clinical considerations in use of xenografts. Curr Probl Surg 1994; 31:390.
3. Smith CM, Ellison MD, Daily OT, White R: UNOS 1995 Annual Scientific Registry Report. Richmond, United Network for Organ Sharing, 1995.
4. Hume DM, Merrill JP, Miller BF, et al: Experiences with renal homotransplantation in the human: Report of nine cases. J Clin Invest 1955; 34:327.
5. Murray JE, Merrill JB, Harrison JH: Renal homotransplantation in identical twins. Surg Forum 1955; 6:432.
6. Thomas ED, Ashley CA, Lochte HL, et al: Intravenous infusion of bone marrow in patients receiving radiation and chemotherapy. N Engl J Med 1957; 257:491.
7. Starzl TE, Marchioro TL, Porter KA, et al: The use of heterologous anti-lymphoid agents in canine renal and liver homotransplantation in a human renal transplantation. Surg Gynecol Obstet 1967; 124:301.
8. Terasaki PL (Ed): History of HLA: 10 Recollections. Los Angeles, UCLA Tissue Typing Laboratory, 1990.
9. Borel J: Comparative study of in vitro and in vivo drug effects on cell-mediated cytotoxicity. Immunology 1976; 31:631.
10. Calne RY, White D, Rolles K: Prolonged survival of pig orthotopic heart grafts treated with cyclosporine A. Lancet 1978; 1:1183.
11. Starzl TE, Weil R III, Iwatsuki S, et al: The use of cyclosporin A and prednisone in cadaver transplantation. Surg Gynecol Obstet 1980; 151:17.
12. National Organ Transplant Act. Public Law 98-507, U.S. Congress, 1984.
13. Jonasson O: Organ Transplantation Issues and Recommendations: Report of the Task Force on Organ Transplantation. Department of Health and Human Services, Public Health Service, Health Resources and Services Administration, 1986.
14. Starzl TE, Shapiro R, Tepperman C: The point system for organ distribution. Transplant Proc 1989; 21:3432.
15. Alexander JW, Broznick B, Ferguson R: Organ procurement organization function. UNOS Newsletter 1992; 8:2.
16. UNOS Bull 1997; 2.
17. Association of Organ Procurement Organizations (AOPO): Voluntary Fax 1996 Survey Report. Washington, DC, AOPO, January 1997.
18. Nathan HM, Jarrell BE, Broznick BA, et al: Estimated potential organ donor pool in Pennsylvania. Nephrol News Issues 1990; 4:22.
19. Gortmaker S, Beasley C, Brigham L, Evanisko M, Franz H, Garrison N, Lucas B, Patterson R, Sobol A, Grenvik A: Organ donor potential and performance: The size and nature of the organ donor shortfall. Crit Care Med 1996; 24:432.
20. Amendments to the Pennsylvania Uniform Anatomical Gift Act. PA Act 102 of 1994, December 1994.
21. Holzgreve W, Beller FK, Uchholz B, et al: Kidney transplantation from the anencephalic donor. N Engl J Med 1987; 316:1068.

176

Alternative Organ Donor Categories

David J. Powner, MD, FCCM • Francis X. Whalen, MD
John A. Daller, MD, PhD • Ake Grenvik, MD, PhD, FCCM

Refined surgical techniques, improved immunosuppression, and advancements in critical care therapy have permitted organ transplantation to become the definitive treatment for some end-stage organ diseases, genetic defects, and malignancies. However, transplantation continues to be limited by a lack of acceptable donor organs, and, in contrast to remarkable recipient survival rates, patients frequently die while awaiting organs. The discrepancy between need and availability of donor organs is highlighted by the following data:

1. In 1996, 19,066 single or combined organ transplantation procedures were performed in the United States, an increase of 886 (4.8%) from 1995.[1] Table 176–1 summarizes the specific organs implanted during most of 1996.
2. At the close of 1996, the registration list total for donor organs was 50,130, an increase of 6,193 (14.1%) over 1995[2]; by October 31, 1997, this total had risen to 55,789.[2]
3. In 1995, 84% of all organs transplanted came from cadaveric sources and 16% came from living donors; these percentages were identical to the resources utilized in 1994, 1993, and 1992.[1]
4. Corresponding increases in actual transplantations performed and the registration lists of patients awaiting organs are shown in Table 176–2. (Some patients may register at more than one center, so that the number of registrations may be higher than actual number of patients and the same patient receiving sequential transplanted organs may be counted more than once.)
5. In 1996, more than 4000 patients in the United States died awaiting organ donation.

As transplantation emerges and expands throughout the world, the same disparity is noted.[3] The total number of organs transplanted worldwide in 1995 was approximately 50,000. However, despite an estimated potential of 50 donors per million population per year, the number of people on waiting lists is estimated at three times the number of actual transplantations. In 1995, more than 6700 patients worldwide died while awaiting an organ.

TABLE 176–1. Organ Transplantation in the United States, 1996*

Organ	No.
Kidney only	10,957
Liver only	3,934
Kidney–pancreas	849
Heart only	2,319
Lung only	849
Heart–lung	38
TOTAL (includes combinations)	19,205

Data from UNOS Update, Fall 1997, p. 36.
*Through December 11, 1996.

LEGISLATIVE POLICIES OR GUIDELINES

The widening worldwide discrepancy between the need for and availability of organ resources has occurred despite aggressive educational and legislative efforts through established organ procurement organizations (OPOs). Numerous surveys show that most private citizens have positive views about organ donation, yet the actual number of donors remains low. Legislative attempts to increase organ procurement frequency, similarly, have not been successful. Therefore, a variety of proposals have been presented and approved to increase the availability of organs. These include:

1. The Uniform Anatomic Gift Act (UAGA). Proposed in 1968 and widely enacted by state legislatures, this act allows individuals over 18 years of age to donate all or parts of their body after death.[4] Initial dramatic gains in donations after its enactment have not been sustained.
2. The evolving use of advance directives, such as donor cards, or organ donor status indicated on drivers' licenses to establish the intent of the individual to make anatomic gifts. This form of giving is also termed the "opting-in" approach.[5]
3. Required request policies, whereby hospitals are required by state law to ensure that family members are provided the opportunity to donate.
4. Routine inquiry rules, supported by the model UAGA, in which hospitals ask each patient whether he or she is an organ donor.
5. Presumed consent policies or attempted statutes, wherein all patients are assumed to be donors unless a specific declaration otherwise is made by the individual. This proposal is also known as an "opting-out" approach.[5] On the basis of the premise that most individuals are more willing to donate their own organs than those of another, it was anticipated that presumed consent policies would be accepted by most legislatures. However, such statutes have generally not been accepted within the United States.[4] Presumed consent has been effective in some parts of Europe.[6]
6. Mandated choice or required response recommendations. These would require that all persons choose whether or not to be an organ donor. Such a choice would be recorded on the driver's license and tax records and would supersede family opinion.[7, 8]
7. Authorized incentive systems[4, 9] have been proposed as:
   a. *Posthumous sale.* The donor would agree to the donation of organs or tissues after death and receive payment before death or after death as a contribution to his or her estate.
   b. *Living donor sale.* Nonvital organs (e.g., a single kidney) could be sold by individual donors at any time. Vital organs may be contracted by patients who are near death.
   c. *Combination.* A combined system to provide commercial support of donors with assured distribution to those potential recipients who cannot afford to purchase an organ.
   d. *Restrictions.* Restricted reimbursement methods wherein compensation is limited to funeral, hospitalization, or other costs related to the donor's lethal injury or illness. Indirect benefits in the form of contribution to the donor's or family's favorite charity have also been considered.
8. Organ conscription, a statutory demand by government that suitable organs must be made available for transplantation. This proposal holds that the needs of society supersede the rights of an individual to withhold such organs.[5]

TABLE 176–2. Increasing Transplantation and Waiting Lists

Year	Total Organs Transplanted	Percent Increase	Registration Lists	Percent Increase
1992-1993	16,040-17,524	9.3	29,415-33,394	13.5
1993-1994	17,524-18,180	3.7	33,394-37,684	12.8
1994-1995	18,180-19,066	4.8	37,684-43,937	16.6
1995-1996*	19,066-19,205	0.7	54,504†	

Data from UNOS Update, Fall 1997, p 36; and UNOS Bull Vol 2(2), February 1997, and November 1997.
*Through December 11, 1996.
†On August 31, 1997.

Medical, legal, and ethical concerns currently limit many of these options in the United States. Therefore, the major stimulus to motivate individuals and families to favor organ donation continues to be altruism.

ALTERNATIVE SOURCES OF DONOR ORGANS

Alternative sources of organs have been used historically and continue to be explored as a way of providing this valued resource. Organ survival and performance after implantation are profoundly affected by the duration of relative or absolute hypoperfusion while at body temperature, the so-called "warm ischemia time," to which the organ is subjected prior to explantation. Table 176–3 categorizes current alternative resources based on organ removal during continued perfusion or after cessation of circulation.

Heart-beating Donors

Living Related Donors

The first successful kidney transplantation was accomplished from a living, related donor in 1954 by Merrill and colleagues.[10] During the 1960s, a living related donor was the preferred source of organs in kidney transplantation because of the minimal risks for the donor and better results for the recipient compared with cadaveric non-heart-beating donors. As results for cadaveric organ transplantation using heart-beating, brain-dead donors improved, a trend developed in the United States away from living donors and toward brain-dead donors. Today, however, in the United States a slight resurgence of the earlier preference has occurred, as 21% of kidneys were obtained from living donors in 1990 and 27% in 1995.[1] Organ transplantation usually from living related donors has now expanded beyond renal transplantation to include one lung or a single lobe[11, 12] and parts of the pancreas,[3] intestine,[13] or liver.[14]

When living donors (specifically, related donors) are considered, the recipient's waiting period for an organ is optimized. If a potential donor is identified, only suitability testing is needed. Thereafter, the transplantation can be scheduled at the appropriate time in the progression of the recipient's disease rather than determined by the availability of an organ and the waiting list status of the recipient. Other technical advantages include minimizing procurement and preservation injury to the transplanted organs and providing sufficient time to complete ABO and human leukocyte antigen (HLA) matching. As expected, because of a short ischemia time, potentially improved tissue matching and the health status of the donor, living related donor transplantation outcomes for recipient and graft survival are generally better than when other categories of heart-beating donors are used. The ideal living related donor, of course, is an identical twin.

Extensive discussions[15, 16] have been published about the psychologic and emotional ramifications to the related donor and recipient. Of particular concern is the issue of informed consent, free of emotional coercion, for the donor. These multiple issues must be balanced against the enhanced graft and recipient benefits.

TABLE 176–3. Alternative Organ Resources

Heart-beating donors
Living related
Living unrelated
Brain-dead donors
Anencephalic patients
Non-heart-beating donors
Animal donors

Living Unrelated Donors

Bone Marrow and Blood Products

These important biologic products are usually made available from donors without significant reward to unrelated, and usually unknown, recipients and comprise a special category.[4] Bone marrow transplantation is fully discussed elsewhere in this text.

Emotionally Related Donors

Although donation rarely occurs from individuals for purely altruistic reasons[17] to unknown recipients, most living-unrelated organ donations in the United States occur between spouses or from donors who know the recipient.[18] A variation of this type of gifting is also the directed donation from a brain-dead patient to a specified recipient usually known to the donor or donor family. These combinations obviously are limited by the constraints of immunohistocompatibility and, thus, occur infrequently. Recipient and organ survival after donation from living, unrelated donors is usually better than those from other heart-beating cadaver categories because of shorter warm ischemia time and because the donor is usually healthy.[18–20]

Commercial Donation

"Compensated" donation or "rewarded gifting" is recognized in at least three forms:

1. Donor reimbursement only to offset lost wages, expenses of the procedure, etc. but no further tangible gain is received.
2. Donor reimbursement plus an additional financial or other material gain which may act as an incentive for the sale of the organs.
3. Reported instances of non-financial incentives[21] or alleged organ removal from unwilling individuals without commercial gain to the "donor" but to those who procured the organs.[22]

All forms of compensated donation are prohibited in the United States and most other countries.[4, 7, 23] Opinion has been expressed, however, that such exchanges are ethical based on the right of the individual to make such a donation and that such donations may benefit others.[23] Data from renal transplantations from such paid donors indicate increased mortality, higher surgical complications, and significant infections including acquisition of human immunodeficiency virus (HIV) infection than experienced from other categories of living donors.[17]

Brain-Dead Organ Donors

This category has been extensively reviewed in Chapter 174, and constitutes the largest current resource for all transplanted organs. Included in that chapter is a discussion of alternative definitions of brain death and similar proposals to utilize organs from patients who remain in a permanent "vegetative" condition.[4, 6, 24]

Other Heart-beating Donors

A variety of other alternative or expanded resources from heart-beating donors have been reported. These include options from both living and cadaveric donors:

1. Retransplantation of a functioning previously implanted organ from a recipient who became brain-dead from an unrelated injury has been successful.[25, 26]
2. Separating the liver from brain-dead donors into two parts allows two recipients to benefit from a single donor organ.[27, 28]
3. Implantation of both kidneys to one recipient from brain-dead donors whose older age would have precluded a single renal transplantation to a single recipient has been reported.[29]
4. Expansion of the donor pool by changing the criteria for accepting donor organs has been evolving for several years.[3] These changes include accepting organs from older donors and utilization of organs from donors with concurrent diseases or causes of death that were previously excluded.[30]
5. Completing coronary artery bypass concurrently with heart removal from donors with good ventricular function and asymptomatic coronary artery disease has been successful.[31]
6. The heart may be transplanted from living patients in the "domino" procedure, during which a heart-lung recipient donates his or her native healthy heart for transplantation into another heart recipient.[32]

Within all groups of living donors, the well-being of the donor must also be considered during and after organ removal. Donor mortality after unilateral nephrectomy is less than 0.03% and morbidity is 10% to 20%. Postoperative morbidity includes respiratory compromise, wound and urinary tract infections, and nerve injuries in the surgical field.[19] Long-term studies have noted the development of proteinuria or hypertension in only a small number of living kidney donors after nephrectomy.[19] It is important to note that donors of one paired organ are fully evaluated for normal functioning of both organs before procurement. Living donors have also contributed segments of the pancreas, liver, lung, and small intestine. These procedures technically are more complex than donor nephrectomy and may be associated with greater risk for the donor.

Anencephalic Donors

Anencephalic infants are born without a cerebrum but often with sufficient brain stem activity to sustain cardiac and respiratory function. By current definition in the United States, they are not brain-dead; however, because they do not have the capacity for cognition, the ability to experience human senses, or the capability of ever acquiring those characteristics of "personhood," philosophic questions have been raised as to whether they are truly "alive."[33]

Because death by cessation of cardiorespiratory function is inevitable in anencephalic infants, it has been proposed and legislatively enacted[34] that they be considered organ donors. Management of these infants as donors has been approached in three ways:

1. Full cardiopulmonary life support until brain death has occurred using traditional criteria.
2. Minimal support until severe hemodynamic or respiratory instability has produced brain stem death, after which cardiopulmonary support is instituted and brain death diagnosed.
3. Removal of organs while the infant is on full support and before brain stem functioning has ceased.[35]

Each option has limitations. When full cardiopulmonary support is initiated soon after birth, deterioration of the brain stem may not occur for a prolonged period, during which infection or other complications may occur that contraindicate transplantation of their organs. If cardiopulmonary function is not supported, hypotension may produce organ ischemia before brain stem death occurs, making all organs unsuitable for transplantation. Although successful renal transplantation from anencephalic donors has been reported when cardiopulmonary support has been provided and the kidneys have been removed while the brain stem function continues,[35] this method is controversial because continued function of the brain stem excludes certification of death by most criteria.

None of these options is now available in the United States.[4] Opposition to the use of anencephalic infants as donors is based on reluctance to consider these patients to be dead and on the low numbers of potential donations from this organ donor category. Because the diagnosis of anencephaly in utero can be made by ultrasonic examination, abortions are more common and the number of infants born alive with anencephaly is low and declining.[35] The option of prolonging gestation when anencephaly is recognized in utero solely for the subsequent procurement of usable organs has been uniformly decried.

Non–heart-beating Donors

Cessation of cardiorespiratory function prior to organ removal defines this category of organ donors. The period during which organ perfusion may have been inadequate prior to cardiopulmonary arrest and the time needed to cool the organ before and during explantation defines the warm ischemia time. Continued cellular metabolism during this period of inadequate or absent nutrient supply and waste removal may lead to limitations in organ function and survival in the recipient. Nevertheless, as a method to increase the availability of organs, utilization of this organ resource continues and in selected circumstances is increasing.

The major categories of non–heart-beating donors include[36]:

1. Hopelessly ill patients for whom withdrawal of life-sustaining cardiorespiratory support is planned and will be followed by organ or tissue donation. Early recipient and renal graft survival are comparable to transplantation from brain dead donors.[37, 38] Extensive discussions about this category have been published and emphasize public policy issues, protocols, and ethics as well as the medical aspects of organ and recipient morbidity and mortality.
2. Patients sustaining unanticipated cardiorespiratory arrest and unsuccessful resuscitation efforts associated with an acceptable ischemia time may be considered. Renal transplantation after various forms of unanticipated cardiac arrest has shown varying results, including no difference,[39] higher graft failure in the first month after implantation, and higher frequency of early hemodialysis due to delayed graft function.[40]

3. Trauma patients who sustain cardiac arrest during resuscitation efforts but whose injuries permit rapid in situ perfusion have been advocated as potential donors.[41]

In each of these options, successful outcomes have been dependent on a focused protocol that incorporates prospective or rapid patient identification and a coordinated multidisciplinary response to minimize warm ischemia time. Overall, these series are small but provide sufficiently positive outcomes to justify continuing debate and discussion.

Xenotransplantation

Xenografting was performed in 1905 by Princeteau with insertion of slices of rabbit kidney into a child who survived 16 days.[42] Subsequent attempted cross-species transplantation to humans has included:

1. Baboon renal implantation by Lungar in 1923.[42]
2. Lamb renal implantation by Neuhof in 1923.[42]
3. Chimpanzee kidney with early immunosuppression during the 1960s.[42]
4. Baboon heart transplantation to a neonate and survival of the recipient for 20 days[45] in 1985.
5. Baboon liver implantation in 1992 with survival of the recipient for 70 days.[46]

A variety of issues remain unresolved in the area of xenotransplantation. These include immunologic incompatibility, cross-species transmission of infection (zoonoses), surgical implantation methods, and ethical concerns about animal utilization for this purpose. No xenografting program utilizing human recipients is presently active.

SUMMARY

It is generally agreed that even with increased utilization of many of the alternative resources discussed in this chapter, neither existing nor anticipated increased needs for organs can be met. A fundamental expansion must occur in giving by individuals either directly, through advance directives, or in discussion with family members who will follow the wishes of the deceased individual. These issues are discussed elsewhere in this book and remain a most important challenge of organ procurement organizations worldwide.

Alternatively, legislation mandating some required choice or required donation, supported by the principles of societal need, may be effective. It is unlikely, however, that current ethical and political forces will enable such enactments. Therefore, expanded efforts in many areas must continue to attempt to match needs and resources. Any new or expanded resource, although making a small contribution to the number of donated organs, still makes a tremendous qualitative contribution to the life of a recipient. While organ donation from a dying patient should never become the primary motive for medical, social, or political decision making, it is a significant opportunity to create a medical, social, and political benefit.

References

1. United Network for Organ Sharing (UNOS) Update. (Richmond). Fall, 1997, p 36.
2. United Network for Organ Sharing (UNOS) Bulletin. (Richmond.). Vol 2, No. 2 and No. 11, 1997.
3. Hauptman PJ, O'Connor KJ: Procurement and allocation of solid organs for transplantation. N Engl J Med 1997; 336:422.
4. Banks GJ: Legal and ethical safeguards: Protection of society's most vulnerable participants in a commercialized organ transplant system. Am J Law Med 1995; 21:45.
5. Spital A: Ethical policy issues in altruistic living and cadaveric organ donation. Clin Transpl 1997; 11:77.
6. Roels L, DeMeester J: The relative impact of presumed-consent legislation on thoracic organ donation in the Eurotransplant area. J Transplant Coordination 1996; 6:174.
7. Chelminski PR: The procurement of vital organs: A synopsis of policy from various nations and the ethical implications of policy options. Ren Fail 1996; 18:151.
8. Spital A: Mandated choice for organ donation: Time to give it a try. Ann Intern Med 1996; 125:66.
9. Council on Ethical and Judicial Affairs–American Medical Association: Financial incentives for organ procurement. Arch Intern Med 1995; 155:581.
10. Merrill J, Murray J, Harrison J, et al: Successful homotransplantation of the human kidney between identical twins. JAMA 1956; 160:277.
11. Goldsmith MF: Mother to child: First living donor lung transplant. JAMA 1990; 264:2724.
12. Barr ML, Schenkel FA, Cohen RG, et al: Bilateral lobar transplantation utilizing living related donors. Artif Organs 1996; 20:1110.
13. Tesi R, Bech R, Lambiase L, et al: Living-related small-bowel transplantation. Transplant Proc 1997, 29:686.
14. Drews D, Sturm E, Latta A, et al: Complications following living-related and cadaveric liver transplantation in 100 children. Transplant Proc 1997; 29:421.
15. Whitington PF: Living donor liver transplantation: Ethical considerations. J Hepatol 1996; 24:625.
16. Mayer AD: The argument against live-donor liver transplantation. J Hepatol 1996; 24:628.
17. Salahudeen AK, Woods HF, Pingle A, et al: High mortality among recipients of bought living-unrelated donor kidneys. Lancet 1990; 336:725.
18. Dominguez J, Zayas E, Malave M, et al: Living emotionally related donor transplantation as an approach to donor shortage in Puerto Rico. Transplant Proc 1997; 29:187.
19. Alfani D, Pretagostini R, Rossi M, et al: Living unrelated kidney transplantation: A 12-year single center experience. Transplant Proc 1997; 29:191.
20. Terasaki PI, Cecka JM, Gjertson DW, et al: High survival rates of kidney transplants from spousal and living unrelated donors. N Engl J Med 1995; 333:333.
21. Hsieh H, Yu TJ, Yang WC, et al: The gift of life from prisoners sentenced to death: Preliminary report. Transplant Proc 1992; 24:1335.
22. Delpin EAS: Allegations of organ commerce in middle America. Transplant Proc 1996; 28:3370.
23. Marshall PA, Thomasma DC, Daar AS: Marketing human organs: The autonomy paradox. Theor Med 1996; 17:1.
24. Powner DJ, Ackerman B, Grenvik A: Medical diagnosis of death in adults: Historical considerations to current controversies. Lancet 1996; 348:1219.
25. Tantawi B, Cherqui D, Duvoux C, et al: Reuse of a liver graft five days after initial transplantation. Transplantation 1996; 62:868.
26. Moreno Gonzalez E, Gomez R, Gonzalez Pinto I, et al: Reuse of liver grafts after early death of the first recipient. World J Surg 1996; 20:309.
27. Rogiers X, Malago M, Gawad K, et al: In situ splitting of cadaveric livers: The ultimate expansion of a limited donor pool. Ann Surg 1996; 224:331.
28. Azoulay D, Astarcioglu I, Bismith H, et al: Split-liver transplantation: The Paul Brousse policy. Ann Surg 1996; 224:737.
29. Johnson LB, Kuo PC, Schweitzer EJ, et al: Double renal allografts successfully increase utilization of kidneys from older donors within a single organ procurement organization. Transplantation 1996; 62:1581.
30. Satterthwaite R, Ozgu I, Shidban H, et al: Risks of transplanting kidneys from hepatitis B surface antigen–negative, hepatitis B core antibody–positive donor. Transplantation 1997; 64:432.
31. Laks H, Gates RN, Ardetiali A, et al: Orthotopic heart transplantation and concurrent coronary bypass. J Heart Lung Transplant 1993; 12:810.
32. Smith JA, Williams JJ, Rabinov M, et al: Combined heart-lung transplantation including the "domino" donor procedure in the single lung transplant era. Transplant Proc 1992; 24:2264.
33. Cefalo RC, Ingelhardt MT: The use of fetal and ancephalic tissue for transplantation. J Med Philos 1989; 14:25.

34. Holzgreve W, Beller FK, Buchholz B, et al: Kidney transplantation from anencephalic donors. N Engl J Med 1987; 316:1069.
35. Medical Task Force on Anencephaly: The infant with anencephaly. N Engl J Med 1990; 332:669.
36. Kootstra G, Daemen JHC, Oomen APA: Categories of non-heart beating donors. Transplant Proc 1995; 27:2893.
37. Pacholczyk MJ, Lagiewska B, Szostek M, et al: Transplantation of kidneys harvested from non-heart-beating donors: Early and long-term results. Transpl Int 1996; 9(Suppl 1):S81.
38. Alonso A, Buitron JG, Gomez M, et al: Short and long term results with kidneys from non-heart-beating donors. Transplant Proc 1997; 29:1378.
39. Shiroki R, Hoshinaga K, Horiba M, et al: Favorable prognosis of kidney allografts from unconditioned cadaveric donors whose procurement was initiated after cardiac arrest. Transplant Proc 1997; 29:1388.
40. Nicholson ML, Horsburgh T, Doughman TM, et al: Comparison of the results of renal transplants from conventional and non-heart beating cadaveric donors. Transplant Proc 1997; 29:1386.
41. Wisner DH, Lo B: The feasibility of organ salvage from non-heart-beating trauma donors. Arch Surg 1996; 131:929.
42. Reemtsma K, McCracken BH, Schlegel JU, et al: Renal heterotransplantation in man. Ann Surg 1964; 160:384.
43. Bailey LL, Nehlsen-Cannarella SL, Concepcion W, Jolley WB: Baboon-to-human cardiac xenotransplantation in an neonate. JAMA 1985; 254:3321.
44. Starzl TE, Fung J, Tzakis A, et al: Baboon-to-human liver transplantation. Lancet 1993; 341:65.
45. Dorling A, Riesbeck K, Warrens A, et al: Clinical xenotransplantation of solid organs. Lancet 1997; 349:867.
46. Perico N, Remuzzi G: Xenotransplantation: Problems and prospects. Nephrol Dial Transplant 1997; 12(Suppl 1):59.

177

Multiple Organ Procurement

Ignazio Roberto Marino, MD, FACS • Howard R. Doyle, MD
Yoogoo Kang, MD • Robert L. Kormos, MD
Thomas E. Starzl, MD, PhD

Solid-organ transplantation (heart, lung, liver, kidney, pancreas, and intestine) has become a successful and widely accepted treatment for a variety of conditions. However, the shortage of cadaveric organs is hindering the larger use of this therapeutic option. In spite of the progressive evolution of public and professional understanding and acceptance of organ donation during the past 30 years, only a little more than 25% of potential brain-dead organ donors actually donate.[1-3] As of October 31, 1997, 55,789 transplant candidates were registered on the national organ waiting list compiled and managed by the United Network for Organ Sharing (UNOS), the agency that coordinates organ allocation in the United States.[4] This statistic represents a 580% increase from the 9,632 patients who were waiting in December 1986, whereas the supply of organ donors underwent only a moderate increase between 1988 and 1996 (from 4,083 to 5,417)[5-7] (Fig. 177–1).

It is estimated that every day seven potential organ recipients in the United States die before a suitable organ is found.[8] Consequently, although the need has increased dramatically, we observe with mounting concern the persistent wastage of available organs and the death of potential recipients. These are both mainly related to an unwillingness to donate or a lack of awareness regarding donation, as well as delays or failure by the medical staff to consider organ donation.[3] Other forces at work also have significantly decreased organ availability for the sicker patients, such as a policy implemented by UNOS in 1991 that substantially changed previous allocation criteria.[9] As a result of this, an even more limited number of organs are available for the most severely ill patients, and some advocate their outright exclusion from transplant candidacy in favor of the elective cases.[10, 11]

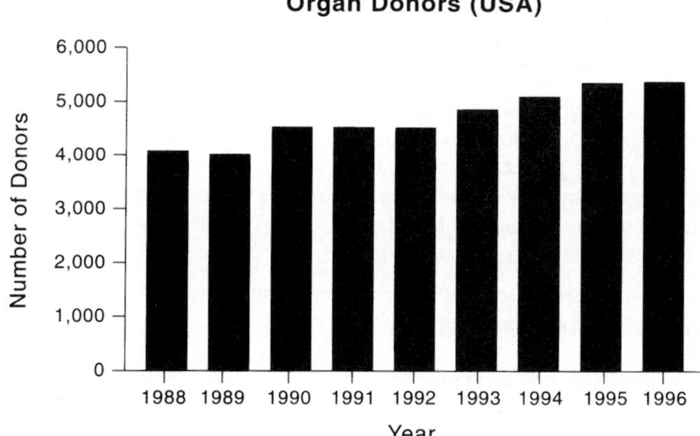

Figure 177–1. Organ donor supply in the United States from 1988 through 1996.

Many routes have been explored in an attempt to remedy this situation, including the development of artificial organs,[12] utilization of living donors even for extrarenal organs,[13-15] xenotransplantation,[16-18] and non-heart-beating donors.[19] However, a more immediate impact on organ shortage could be achieved by improving our current mechanisms for organ recovery and the management of potential donors.

ORGAN RECOVERY

Standardized criteria for the determination of brain death were defined by the Ad Hoc Committee of the Harvard Medical School[20] and have been the subject of a more recent report.[21] The concept of brain death and the management of the brain-dead donor are discussed in detail in Chapter 174.

Once a potential organ donor is identified, the multiple organ procurement process should be triggered. This starts by contacting the local organ procurement organization (OPO) as soon as the irreversibility of brain injury has been established. As of July 1, 1997, there were 54 OPOs and 280 transplant centers in the United States. These represent the largest organ procurement and transplant network in the world. Most intensive care units (ICUs) have the telephone number of the local agency available. However, the telephone number and location of area OPOs can be obtained from UNOS, which has a 24-hour telephone hot line (800-355-SHARE).

These OPOs, originally set up to organize the recovery of kidneys, now also coordinate the complex logistics of multiple organ recovery and their distribution within a predetermined geographic area. They are also responsible for the payment of all charges incurred during the process of organ donation, ensuring that donor families are not billed for any of them. Once contacted, the local OPO sends a procurement coordinator to the referring hospital. These coordinators perform a number of administrative and technical functions, covering every aspect of the donation process. On receiving a referral, they perform an evaluation and discuss organ donation with the potential donor's family, making sure the relatives have a complete and satisfactory explanation of the diagnosis of brain death and a clear understanding of the organ procurement process.

Families should be informed separately but as soon as possible after the irreversibility of the lethal brain damage has been established and should be given a clear explanation of the prognosis. This measure will give them time to accept the patient's death and allow them to deal with their grief. It is important to respect this phase, because it has been demonstrated that consent for donation increases from 18% to 60% if the family is allowed to absorb the concept of brain death first and if the issue of organ donation is brought up later.[3] Religious beliefs about human life, the dead body, and life after death are important considerations for those involved in organ donation and transplantation. No major religion specifically prohibits organ donation, although in some situations there may be restrictions. Table 177–1 summarizes some of the major religious and cultural beliefs associated with organ donation and transplantation.[22] Families may feel the need to discuss the matter with a church representative before making a decision.

If the family decides to donate, a consent for donation form is supplied by the hospital or by the procurement coordinator, and it is completed and signed by the next of kin. In addition, the coordinator ensures that all medicolegal requirements are met, from adequate documentation of brain death in the chart to securing permission from the coroner when necessary. Medical staff privileges for the recovery teams are also arranged. Hospitals differ in their policies for granting such privileges. Some hospitals do not consider the organ procurement a surgical procedure because a determination of brain death has been made. In this circumstance, temporary privileges are not required for outside surgeons.

At the same time, the procurement coordinator assumes control of three main activities:

- Donor evaluation
- Coordination of donor and recipient matching
- Donor operation and organ preservation and shipment to the recipient's hospital

The role of the coordinator in each of these is critical, because the most important issue in organ procurement, once the decision to proceed has been made, is to have someone who "directs traffic," maintaining clear lines of communication between the members of the different teams involved. A lack of communication at this point can disrupt donor care and compromise organ stability. Therefore, the needs and protocols of the individual teams should be discussed in detail before any donor surgery begins. If possible, the logistic arrangements between teams should be expedited so that no time constraints are placed on the host team. On the other hand, the host team must be tolerant because different organs often have to be flown to distant parts of the country, and some recipient surgery may be quite complex and time-consuming. To facilitate matters, the host team should make available basic information on the donor to expedite the evaluation by the visiting teams (Fig. 177–2).

DONOR EVALUATION AND MANAGEMENT

There are few absolute contraindications to organ donation, and they can be grouped into three broad categories:

1. Severe trauma.
2. Malignancy outside the central nervous system (CNS).
3. Active infections.

Trauma refers only to major injury to the organ itself and does not preclude donation of those organs not affected. Even in the case of a major trauma, however, the final decision to use or discard the organ should be made only after surgical examination of the donor and careful examination of the organ's anatomy. In the case of a liver trauma, for example, many organs can be saved if the donor team is experienced in liver surgery. Minor, and even major, parenchymal lesions can be repaired in situ, and the vascular anatomy can be precisely determined during the final preparation of the organ. Techniques of transplantation of liver segments have been

TABLE 177–1. Major Religious and Cultural Beliefs Associated with Organ Donation and Transplantation

Group	Donation	Transplantation
Amish	Reluctant if transplant outcome uncertain	Acceptable for the well-being of the candidate
Baha'i	Acceptable	Acceptable
Baptist	Individual decision	Acceptable
Buddhist	Individual decision	Buddha's teachings on the middle path (i.e., the avoidance of extremes) could be applicable to this
Christian Science	Individual decision	Individual decision
Episcopal	Encouraged	Encouraged
Evangelical Covenant	Encouraged	Encouraged
Greek Orthodox	Acceptable (although not for research)	Acceptable for the well-being of the candidate
Gypsies	Against	Against
Hinduism	Individual decision	Individual decision
Islam	Acceptable (organs of Moslem donors must be transplanted immediately, and not stored in organ banks)	Acceptable
Jehovah's Witness	Individual decision (not encouraged)	May be considered acceptable (organs should be completely drained of blood before transplantation)
Judaism	Generally encouraged	Encouraged
Latter-day Saints (Mormon Church)	Individual decision	Individual decision
Protestant denominations	Individual decision	Acceptable
Society of Friends (Quakers)	Individual decision	Individual decision
Roman Catholic	Encouraged	Acceptable
Unitarian Universalist	Acceptable	Acceptable
United Methodist	Encouraged	Acceptable

Donor Information — Donor ID# — UNOS ID#

Name ______
Age: ______ Sex: ______ Race: ______
Date of Birth: ______
Next of Kin: ______
Relationship: ______
Address: ______
______
______
Next of Kin Phone: ______

Admitting Date: ______ Referral Date: ______
Recovery Date: ______ Clamp Time: ______ AM PM
Hospital: ______
City/State: ______
Referred By: ______
Phone #: ______
Program: ______
Program 24 hr #: ______
Attending: ______
Consulting: ______
Medical Records No.: ______
Pronouncement Date: ______ Time: ______

Consent For: ______
______

Cause of Death: ______

Past Medical History: (Complete history please)

Heart Disease: (Y/N) ______
Liver Disease: (Y/N) ______
Renal Disease: (Y/N) ______
Diabetes: (Y/N) ______
Neurological: (Y/N) ______
Cancer: (Y/N) ______
Lung Disease: (Y/N) ______
Arthritis or Joint Disease: (Y/N) ______
Recent Flu-like Symptoms: (Y/N) ______
Unexplained Weight Loss: (Y/N) ______
Toxic Exposure: (Y/N) ______
Drug Use: Prescribed or Other: (Y/N) ______
Alcohol Abuse: (Y/N) ______
Smoker: (Y/N) ______
Blood Transfusion History: (x 2 yrs.) (Y/N) ______
Previous Surgery: (Y/N) ______
Immunization or Vaccinated: (x 6 mo.) (Y/N) ______
Travel outside U.S.A. since 1977: (Y/N) ______
Homosexual or Bisexual: (Y/N) ______
Received pit-hGh: (Y/N) ______
Recent Infections: (Y/N) (if yes give treatment) ______
______
G.I. Disorders: (Y/N) ______
Hematologic Disorders: (Y/N) ______
Under Physician's Care: (Y/N) ______
Physician, Phone #, Address: ______

Donor Information — Donor ID#

ABO: ______ HLA: ______ DR: ______ LE Type: ______ WT: ______ HT: ______
Chest Cir: ______ Girth: ______ RC/BRR: ______ LC/BLR: ______

Hospital History (Include E.R., V/S, Arrests, O.R. Procedures, Injuries, Infection, ect.)
______
______
______

EKG, Echo & Cardiac Consult:
______
______

Chemistries					Urinalysis				ABG'S & Lytes			
Date					Date				Date			
BUN					Color				pH			
Creat.					Appear.				PO2			
T. Bil.					pH				PCO2			
D. Bil.					Sp. Grav.				O2 Sat.			
SGOT					Glucose				FIO2			
SGPT					Protein				PEEP			
LDH					Blood				VT			
GGT					RBC				Rate			
Amylase					WBC				Na +			
CPK					Epith.				K +			
Glucose					Casts				Cl -			
Hgb/Hct.					Bact.				Ca ++			
PT												
PTT												
Plat.												
WBC												

Blood Pressure (Note B/P< 90.Time)	Urine Output (Note Anuria/Oliguria)	Med. During ADM
		Blood & Blood Products

Serology

Date	Time	Test	Pre	Post Result	Local/Import	Reported By	Reported To
		RPR/VDRL					
		HBs Ag					
		HAA					
		HIV					
		HTLV-I					
		CMV					
		HCV					

Cultures (Blood, Urine, Sputum) Date, Results
______
______

Figure 177–2. Donor data sheet used by the Western Pennsylvania Organ Procurement Organization, CORE (Center for Organ Recovery and Education). (Courtesy of Brian Broznick.)

described and successfully used, particularly in pediatric patients. These techniques may be used to rescue a liver partially damaged by trauma.

Malignancy, other than primary CNS tumors, is an absolute contraindication to organ donation.

The presence of active *infections* is an exclusionary criterion that deserves close attention. Systemic sepsis, active tuberculosis, viral encephalitis, and Guillain-Barré syndrome are contraindications to organ donation, as well as active hepatitis or the presence of the hepatitis B surface antigen. Past infection with the hepatitis B virus (HBV), as evidenced by the presence of antibodies, was not considered a contraindication to organ donation until recently. Early in 1995, a study showed the transmission of hepatitis B in eight of 13 liver recipients (negative for HBV infection before the liver transplant) transplanted with livers from hepatitis B core antibody-positive donors.[23] Our policy at the Pittsburgh Transplantation Institute is to use these donors only for hepatitis B core antibody-positive recipients.

Whether organs should be used if the donor has hepatitis C antibodies has been the subject of controversy in the past few years, as there is evidence of hepatitis C virus (HCV) transmission after transplantation.[24] However, the organ shortage is so severe that the use of HCV antibody-positive donors must be seriously considered, at least for life-saving organs such as the liver, heart, and lungs.[25] Obviously, for active disease to be ruled out, a prospective HCV antibody-positive donor absolutely requires a frozen section examination of the liver before implantation.

The human immunodeficiency virus (HIV) has greatly affected the field of transplantation. After the screening enzyme immunoassay became available in March 1985, a number of positive kidney, heart, and liver recipients were quickly reported.[26] However, the extent of the problem was clearly defined only after a large study of 1043 transplant patients was completed at the University of Pittsburgh. It was found that, overall, 1.7% were positive for HIV, with the incidence in liver transplant patients being 2.6%. Only a third of these patients were positive before the transplantation, as determined by testing stored pretransplant sera.[27] Donors who test positive for HIV antibody are now automatically rejected.

Prospective donors should also have a Venereal Disease Research Laboratory (VDRL) test as well as cytomegalovirus (CMV) titers, determined as soon as possible. The significance of a positive VDRL test is difficult to ascertain, but it is our practice to treat recipients of VDRL-positive donors with a course of benzathine penicillin. The CMV status of the donor has prognostic significance regarding the incidence and severity of subsequent CMV infections. Recipients of organs harvested from seronegative donors have a lesser chance of developing a CMV infection, regardless of their own serologic status.[28, 29] Epstein-Barr virus and varicella-zoster virus (VZV) are not part of the routine donor viral screening. The only situation in which these viruses become relevant is when the donor has active disease related to them (infectious mononucleosis or systemic VZV infection). In these cases, organ donation should not be considered.

Donors with infections under control or those affecting organs not specifically considered for donation (i.e., an abdominal organ donor suffering from pneumonia) may still be suitable. Children who die as a result of bacterial meningitis related to *Haemophilus influenzae* or *Neisseria meningitidis* can still be considered for donation if the organism and its sensitivity are known beforehand.

Prolonged organ ischemia related to severe hypotension or cardiac arrest might represent a contraindication to donation. However, it is the policy of the Pittsburgh Transplantation Institute to critically evaluate all donors, including those with cardiac arrest and prolonged cardiopulmonary resuscitation (CPR). In fact, many of these donors have been found acceptable by post-CPR physiologic and biochemical criteria, and their organs have been successfully transplanted.[19, 30]

Other patients who may not be acceptable as donors are those with a long-standing history of diabetes mellitus, hypertension, and cardiac or peripheral vascular disease. Again, however, the donor and organ viability should be assessed on a case by case basis. A patient who is not acceptable as a heart or lung donor might still be an excellent abdominal organ donor. Sometimes the suitability of individual organs can be assessed only after direct examination by the donor surgeon at the time of procurement.

The donor's age deserves special mention. The chronologic age is less important than the physiologic age in assessment. For some organs, age may not be an important limiting factor.[31–32] We have successfully used livers from donors as old as 75 years. In 1985, Popper[33] dedicated an extensive review to the aging of the liver. According to his study, the liver's great functional reserve, its regenerative capacity, and its large blood supply are the key factors in its delayed aging compared with other organs. Based on these considerations, it has long been thought that the liver is less affected than other organs by senescence.[31, 32] However, the demonstration that satisfactory livers can be obtained from donors well into the seventh decade of life or beyond was followed by a flurry of confirmatory reports, countered by descriptions of degraded results using geriatric livers.

Less has been written about the effect of the donor's sex on outcome of liver transplantation. Extensive literature, summarized by Neugarten and Silbiger,[34] shows poorer results with kidney allografts from female donors.

We have examined the effects of donor age and sex on the outcome of a consecutive series of 462 liver transplants, which included the use of 54 donors aged 60 years or older. Nine other donor variables and eight recipient variables were also analyzed, with the endpoint of the analysis being *graft failure* (defined as either patient death or retransplantation). Graft failure was significantly associated with donor age and donor sex. The effect of donor age was evident only when the donors were aged 45 years or older. Livers from female donors yielded significantly poorer results, with the 2-year graft survival of the female to male combination being 55%, female to female 64%, male to male 72%, and male to female 78%.[35]

We believe that older female donors (≥60 years) are questionable for liver procurement because in them the adverse effects of age and gender are at least additive. Because of the current organ shortage crisis, we believe that these livers should still be used, but under circumstances that are adjudicated on a case by case basis. For example, many liver transplant centers in North America and in Europe exclude from recipient candidacy patients who are HIV-positive, HBV carriers with evidence of deoxyribonucleic acid (DNA) replication, and others with risk factors that predictably degrade patient and graft survival. These patient categories would certainly be better helped by receiving geriatric female livers rather than being automatically excluded from transplantation. Table 177–2 shows the age guidelines for individual organs used in our institution. In general, it is rare to find a suitable heart or lung allograft from donors older than 60 years of age because of the increased incidence of coronary artery disease and chronic pulmonary disease.

In summary, given the enormous need for organs and the few criteria that absolutely disqualify a potential donor, the local OPO should be contacted in virtually every case. Figure 177–2 shows the data collection form used by the Center for Organ Recovery and Education, which is the organ procure-

TABLE 177–2. Age Guidelines for Organ and Tissue Donation Used at the Pittsburgh Transplantation Institute

Organ/Tissue	Age (yr)
Heart	≤60 yr*
Heart-lung	≤60 yr*
Lung	≤60 yr*
Kidney	1 month–75 yr*
Liver	≤75 yr*
Pancreas	≤65 yr*
Intestine†	
Bone	15–65 yr
Bone marrow	≤75 yr
Cornea	1–65 yr
Skin	15–65 yr
Heart valve	≤55 yr

*Donors beyond these age limits could be accepted on the basis of the individual organ function. Female donors aged 60 years or older are questionable for liver procurement because in them the adverse effects of age and gender are at least additive.

†No age limits have been set for intestinal donors. Intestines should be available from most organ donors and are always evaluated on an individual basis.

ment agency for western Pennsylvania, southern New York, and West Virginia. These data should be promptly faxed to those involved in the evaluation process.

Individual Organ Assessment: Abdominal Organs

The criteria used to determine the suitability of kidneys are very flexible. As shown in Table 177–2, a kidney donor can be between 1 month and 75 years of age. Serum creatinine and blood urea nitrogen (BUN) are used as markers of donor renal function and should be normal. Obviously, donors with chronic renal disease are not considered for kidney donation. However, patients with transient creatinine and BUN elevations related to dehydration, hypotension, or both are not excluded from kidney donation if the BUN and creatinine fall after appropriate volume correction.

Attempts at predicting liver allograft function after transplantation based on donor information have met with little success. The diverse literature devoted to the topic is testimony to our lack of a clear understanding, one that can translate into well-informed decision making during donor evaluation.[25, 35–46] As a rule, the donor should have normal or near-normal serum aspartate transaminase (AST), serum alanine transaminase (ALT), bilirubin, and prothrombin time, but we have successfully used livers from donors with AST and ALT that were 10 times greater than the upper limit of normal. The important parameter is not an isolated AST or ALT value, but the trend established since the ICU admission.[47] The bilirubin can be elevated as a result of massive blood transfusions used during the resuscitation of a shocked patient. A history of hepatitis or alcoholism is certainly a warning sign but does not preclude the use of the liver. In general, in the case of a marginal liver donor, the intraoperative assessment by the donor surgeon is the best single piece of information.

There is only one absolute exclusion criterion in the evaluation of a pancreas donor: a history of diabetes mellitus. Amylase elevations have been seen in as many as 39% of pancreas donors without any evidence of pancreatitis, and thus isolated hyperamylasemia does not contraindicate the use of the pancreas.[48] The serum glucose may be falsely elevated in donors receiving steroid therapy or as a result of decreased circulating insulin.[49]

Intestinal transplantation is emerging as a valuable modality for the treatment of patients with intestinal failure. Early in 1993, UNOS formed a subcommittee responsible for systematizing the listing of recipients, helping identify suitable donors, and establishing guidelines for the equitable allocation of intestinal grafts at both the local and national levels. Because of the time constraints, it is impossible to perform a functional assessment of the donor bowel. Relatively young age, hemodynamic stability, and donor-recipient size match are the critical parameters used in evaluating an intestinal donor.[50] At our institution, preference was initially given to infant and juvenile donors with stable hemodynamics. However, the age range has gradually expanded, providing the donor is stable and receiving minimal vasopressor support (≤10 $\mu g/kg^{-1}/min^{-1}$ of dopamine). Size matching is always given special consideration. The majority of intestinal transplant recipients have undergone extensive intestinal resections, leading to a significant reduction in the size of the abdominal cavity. Therefore, donors are chosen who weigh 15% to 40% less in body weight than the selected recipients.[50]

Individual Organ Assessment: Thoracic Organs

Aside from a negative history of cardiac disease and a normal chest x-ray film, the donor should have a normal heart physical examination and 12-lead electrocardiogram. However, a number of electrocardiographic changes may be detected in brain-dead patients, which do not preclude thoracic organ donation.[51, 52] A brain-dead patient who is able to maintain a systolic blood pressure greater than 90 mm Hg with a dopamine requirement less than 10 $\mu g/kg^{-1}/min^{-1}$ is considered a suitable candidate for heart donation.[53, 54] Cardiac isoenzymes are recommended in the case of chest trauma, to rule out myocardial contusion, and when the potential donor has suffered a cardiac arrest or prolonged hypotension. In male donors older than 35 years of age, the incidence of coronary artery disease increases, especially with risk factors such as hypercholesterolemia, a family history of heart disease, and a history of smoking. Coronary angiography may be helpful in the evaluation of high-risk and older donors, but it is not routinely required and most hospitals find the logistics of performing it prohibitive. Therefore, a decision must be made based on a cardiologic consultation, evaluating the history, electrocardiogram, and echocardiogram.

As is the case for the liver, and because of the severe shortage, it is prudent, even in high-risk donors, for the heart to be examined on the operating table following sternotomy. Visualizing and palpating the coronary arteries provides a significant amount of information with respect to the incidence of coronary artery disease. If plaques are felt along the left main coronary artery or left anterior descending artery, the heart, in most cases, is not suitable for transplantation. In extreme cases of a sick recipient, however, the transplantation team may decide to use this heart. Isolated cases of coronary artery bypass being performed at the time of transplantation have been reported. Reports exist of cases of isolated mild coronary artery disease in which the donor allograft functions well, with no increase in early mortality.

Transesophageal echocardiography has been demonstrated to be an important adjuvant in the evaluation of a potential cardiac donor. Severe cardiac hypertrophy, valvular defects, and global myocardial dysfunction or segmental wall abnormalities have been diagnosed in what appeared to be otherwise reasonable cardiac donors. At this time, limited information is available about the use of such hearts. In most cases, it is prudent to avoid the use of a heart with demonstrated wall-motion abnormalities.[55] In general, minor changes in the electrocardiogram or echocardiogram, localized infection,[56] transitory hypotension, brief cardiac arrest, and thoracic trauma do not contraindicate heart donation. The importance of donor-recipient weight mismatch greater than 20% is critical only in the face of high pulmonary vascular resistance. In carefully selected donors, survival after transplantation with a donor between 40 and 55 years of age is no different than that observed in the case of younger donors.[57] As the limits for donor selection are extended, it becomes more evident that it is safe to extend donor age up to 55 to 60 years and ischemic time longer than 4 to 5 hours.[58-60]

The presence or absence of cardiac or cardiopulmonary arrest in itself is not a contraindication to the use of a heart for transplantation. Especially in the pediatric population, it has been found that even in donors who have undergone extended CPR (up to 125 min), as long as cardiac function at the time of cardiectomy is normal, there does not appear to be an increased risk for performance of the heart or survival of the recipient after transplantation.

All of the selection criteria mentioned in the case of a heart donor also apply to heart-lung or isolated single or double lung donors. In addition, a donor is not acceptable for lung or heart-lung donation when there is a history of heavy smoking, chronic lung disease, or pulmonary aspiration. The height, weight, and chest circumference of the heart-lung donor should closely match those of the recipient. A number of physiologic parameters can be used when assessing a lung donor, including the partial pressure of arterial oxygen/fraction of inspired oxygen (PaO_2/FIO_2) ratio ($\geq$250 mm Hg) and peak airway pressure (<30 cm H_2O with 15 mL/kg of tidal volume and 5 cm H_2O of positive end-expiratory pressure [PEEP]).[61-63] Aspiration pneumonia is frequent in the brain-dead patient, and thus the character of the sputum is a critical piece of information. The role of bronchoscopy is still being debated; it is considered mandatory by some authors,[64] whereas others believe it is indicated only when there is a question of foreign-body aspiration or to obtain sputum for Gram's stain and culture.[49] Bronchoscopy, however, provides important culture information to guide appropriate antibiotic therapy after transplantation. If frank purulence is noted on bronchoscopy, the lungs are not suitable. However, one lung may be salvaged for transplantation from a set in which one appears to be more infected than the other.

COORDINATION OF DONOR AND RECIPIENT MATCHING

Once the coordinator finishes the donor evaluation, there are still many hours of intense work before completing the process. After obtaining the appropriate consent, therapeutic efforts should be geared to protect the donated organs until the actual retrieval is accomplished. Their integrity should be maintained by optimal organ perfusion, avoidance of further damage, and subsequent removal and preservation with minimal ischemic injury. Care of the donor during organ procurement, therefore, requires a continuation of the intensive care that was provided before brain death was declared, followed by a precise surgical procurement procedure. Whereas in the 1970s and early 1980s donor management mainly, if not exclusively, addressed kidney function, the patient now must always be approached as a multiple donor, and this can present a real challenge to the physician managing the case.

The physician should keep the patient hemodynamically stable with optimal organ perfusion and oxygenation. This is not easy because of the loss of many body reflexes and the dramatic changes in the hormonal milieu.[65] Several studies have shown a significant reduction of cortisol,[66] insulin,[66] and thyroid hormones.[51, 66-70] About 50% to 70% of brain-dead patients suffer from diabetes insipidus.[71, 72] A number of protocols that call for the use of hormones such as triiodothyronine, cortisol, or insulin during donor management have given conflicting results.[49, 52, 67, 69, 70, 73]

The details of donor management are provided in Chapter 174 and are not repeated here. We stress only a few points we believe are important. Adequate perfusion should always be maintained while keeping the use of vasoactive drugs to a minimum. This may require the administration of several liters of fluid to obtain adequate filling pressures. Replacement therapy with fresh frozen plasma, platelets, and cryoprecipitate may be used if a serious bleeding diathesis is present. However, even if fibrinolysis is suspected, ε-aminocaproic acid should be avoided because it can induce microvascular thrombosis in the donor organs.

During this phase, the procurement coordinator asks local transplantation programs about their needs for organs. Under the current system, local programs have first priority, and only when organs are not used locally are inquiries made at the regional and national levels. An exception to this rule is when a prospective kidney recipient who resides in another region is found to have a so-called six-antigen match. These kidneys have to be sent away, with the receiving transplantation center "paying back" at a later date. Organ allocation is a very complicated and controversial subject, and what system should be used is presently being debated.[10] As of this writing, amendments to the National Organ Transplant Act (NOTA) are being discussed in Congress, and it is not clear what changes will be implemented.

A point system for renal transplantation was developed in Pittsburgh in 1985. Credit points were given to renal transplant candidates for time waiting, quality of antigen match, degree of immunologic sensitization, medical urgency, and logistic considerations of getting the donor organ and the recipient together within the time limitations of safe organ preservation. The system began in western Pennsylvania on January 1, 1986.[9] Although initially adopted by UNOS on November 1, 1987, the point system never went into effect at the national level because of difficulties encountered in reconciling it with a myriad of local interests. A similar point system was developed for liver transplantation, having been in place in Pittsburgh since January 1987. Our experience with organ allocation based on point systems, in which organs go to those who have been waiting longer or are sicker, has been most favorable.[10, 11] Graft and patient survivals have not suffered by giving organs to sicker or older patients. At the same time, our observations provide some assurance that the concepts of equitable access and efficient use of a scarce societal resource are not mutually exclusive.

Although human leukocyte antigen (HLA) matching is not a critical issue for extrarenal organs, we routinely perform HLA typing on all extrarenal organs, a practice at variance with what most other institutions do in the United States. Although it is expensive, we consider it important because it allows us to determine the presence of microchimerism in the recipient, information that may be extremely useful in the future when deciding how to manage the immunosuppression.[74]

When the recipients for all the abdominal and thoracic organs are identified, an operating room (OR) time in the donor hospital is arranged. The procurement coordinator contacts the recipient institutions to arrange for the simultaneous arrival of all the harvesting teams. Kidneys have been procured by local teams for many years and shipped if they were not used locally. Today, a similar practice is being adopted in the United States for other organs, particularly livers.[75]

The intestinal donor should receive intravenous ampicillin and cefotaxime at the appropriate doses when first evaluated and every 6 hours after that. The last dose is given in the OR at the time of harvesting. Polyethylene glycol-electrolyte solution (GoLYTELY) is administered through the nasogastric tube to flush the intestine. The total amount ranges from 250 to 2000 mL, depending on the recipient's body size (250 mL in the infant and 2000 mL in the adult), and the administration rate is 10 to 30 mL/min. After the intestinal flushing, an antibiotic mixture that includes polymixin E (100 mg), tobramycin (80 mg), and amphotericin B (500 mg) is given through the nasogastric tube every 4 hours until procurement. In pediatric donors, the doses are halved, whereas infants receive only one fourth of the dose. Newborns receive no intestinal preparation. If preharvest flushing cannot be performed, this is done after procurement, using cold lactated Ringer's solution. Polymixin B or kanamycin can be substituted for polymyxin E, if the latter is not available at the donor hospital.

MULTIPLE DONOR OPERATION

Anesthesia

The donor operation can be time-consuming, and the role of the anesthesiologist is very important, especially if we compare the multiple organ procurement that is now usually performed with those carried out in the past, when the kidneys were often the only organs removed. A complete review of the anesthetic aspects of organ donation was recently published,[76] and we will restrict ourselves to its salient points.

The goal of medical management during organ procurement is to avoid ischemic organ damage by optimizing organ perfusion. Therefore, care of the donor is a continuation of the intensive care that was provided before brain death (see Chapter 174). The most important issue is the clear communication between the members of the procurement team because the surgical procedure and procurement protocol may differ depending on the procurement team and the specific organ. For the preoperative evaluation of the donor, the anesthesiologist should review the medical and surgical histories, including the cause of brain death, condition and supportive measures of vital organs, drug allergies, and medications. Cardiopulmonary function is assessed by means of the hemodynamic profile, requirement of inotropic support, efficiency of gas exchange, degree of ventilatory support, chest radiograph, electrocardiogram, arterial blood gas tensions, and acid-base state. Renal function is evaluated by urine output, BUN, and serum levels of creatinine and electrolytes. Hepatic function is evaluated by AST, ALT, and bilirubin, and pancreatic function is evaluated by blood glucose level and serum amylase. Hemoglobin concentration and the blood type of the donor are identified to prepare blood products. In addition, the validity of brain-death certification, consent from family members, and permission from the coroner are verified. The transition from the ICU to the OR is a crucial period, and the donor is continuously monitored, ventilated, and treated.

Intraoperative care of the donor is essentially similar to that of other critically ill patients undergoing major surgery, although management of pathophysiologic changes unique to the donor should be clearly understood. In general, equipment and medications routinely available for general anesthesia are satisfactory for the management of donors. However, a volume ventilator may be needed for donors requiring high levels of PEEP or airway pressure. The OR should be kept warm, and a warming blanket and blood warmer are necessary to prevent hypothermia. A large volume of crystalloids and colloid solutions (e.g., 5% albumin, plasma protein fraction, or hetastarch) and five units of packed red blood cells should be prepared. The electrocardiogram is monitored, preferably using lead V_5, to detect arrhythmias or myocardial ischemia, particularly in heart donors. Blood pressure is monitored by an indwelling catheter in the radial artery or brachial artery. The femoral artery cannulation is avoided because the aorta will be cross-clamped. Central venous pressure (CVP) monitoring is essential,[77] and a pulmonary arterial catheter is useful in unstable donors. Two-dimensional transesophageal echocardiography may be used to assess preload and cardiac contractility in unstable heart donors. Urine output and body temperature are monitored, and all or some of the following laboratory tests may be needed: hemoglobin and hematocrit, arterial blood gas tensions and acid-base state, serum electrolytes, ionized calcium, lactate, and blood glucose level.

General anesthetic agents are required to blunt sympathetic response that occurs during surgery.[78] This so-called mass reflex is caused by neurogenic vasoconstriction and stimulation of the adrenal medulla by the spinal reflex arc and manifests as tachycardia hypertension, perspiration, and involuntary movements. These movements, also known as the *Lazarus sign,* which includes arm and hand movements toward the body, can be disturbing to those involved in the organ recovery, and muscle relaxants should be administered ahead of time.

Isoflurane is the agent of choice because the degree of myocardial depression is less than with other inhalation agents. Halothane is avoided in liver donors because hepatotoxicity may be a concern in the presence of potential hepatic ischemia. Enflurane is avoided in kidney donors because it increases the blood level of inorganic fluoride. Short-acting narcotics, such as fentanyl (5 to 10 μg/kg), may be used in hemodynamically unstable donors. In addition, muscle relaxants (pancuronium bromide, 0.05 to 0.1 mg/kg, or vecuronium bromide, 0.05 to 0.1 mg/kg) are required to provide satisfactory abdominal muscle relaxation and to abolish involuntary movements. Other pharmacologic interventions include systemic heparinization (300 to 500 U/kg) before cannulation of the aorta, mannitol (0.25 to 0.5 g/kg), and furosemide (40 mg) to induce diuresis before division of the renal pedicle and prevent ischemia-induced acute tubular necrosis.[79–81] Alpha-adrenergic receptor blockers, such as phenoxybenzamine, may be used to promote renal vasodilation and prevent vasospasm.[82] However, these blockers are not recommended in multiple organ procurement because their effects on other organs are unknown. Prophylactic administration of antibiotics such as broad-spectrum cephalosporins is recommended by some centers,[83, 84] although its efficacy is controversial.[47, 85]

Specific goals of ventilatory care are to maintain a Pao_2 between 70 and 100 mm Hg, an oxygen saturation of arterial hemoglobin greater than 95%, and a partial pressure of arterial carbon dioxide within the range of 35 to 45 mm Hg to avoid pulmonary complications. In hypothermic donors, a mild respiratory alkalosis (pH 7.4 to 7.5) may be preferred to improve tissue perfusion.[86, 87] This goal frequently is achieved by ventilating with a tidal volume of 10 to 15 mL/kg, a respiratory rate of fewer than 20 breaths/min, FIO_2 of 30% to 40%, and a low level of PEEP (<5 cm H_2O). However, when pulmonary complications interfere with gas exchange, the tidal volume is increased up to 20 mL/kg, the respiratory rate is increased up to 20 breaths/min, and the PEEP is increased up to 10 cm H_2O. In general, an increase in FIO_2 is preferred to an excessive tidal volume and high PEEP to maintain venous return and splanchnic blood flow.

The goal of circulatory care is to preserve perfusion of all organs that are to be procured by maintaining systolic blood pressure between 100 and 120 mm Hg, with a CVP less than 10 cm H_2O and minimal vasopressor support.[51, 88, 89] Hypotension (systolic blood pressure < 80 mm Hg or mean arterial pressure < 40 mm Hg) is associated with an increased incidence of acute tubular necrosis and nonfunction of the donor kidneys[90, 91] as well as poor function of the liver.[92] However, maintaining a satisfactory blood pressure is difficult to achieve at times because of altered circulatory physiology in the brain-dead donors. Preload frequently is decreased because of blood loss, vasomotor paralysis, diuretic therapy, or diabetes insipidus. Tachycardia, bradycardia, and arrhythmias caused by massive sympathetic discharge are not unusual, and myocardial contractility frequently is impaired by myocytolysis, coronary spasm, and reduction of myocardial energy storage.[93] Afterload may be increased by excessive sympathetic tone or decreased by vasomotor paralysis.

Intravascular volume is adjusted with the guidance of the CVP (<10 cm H_2O). Fluid deficit is corrected with the infusion of a balanced electrolyte solution (e.g., lactated Ringer's solution) or a colloid solution (5% albumin or hetastarch).[94] Urine output and insensible losses are replaced by a hypotonic solution with glucose (e.g., 5% dextrose in 0.45% sodium chloride [NaCl], 1 mL/kg^{-1}/hour^{-1}). Adjustment of intravascular volume may decrease the need for vasopressors in many cases,[95] but acute volume expansion may increase myocardial oxygen consumption, congestive heart failure, arrhythmias, and the need for inotropic support because the compliance of the heart is decreased in most donors.[91] Excessive urine output (>200 to 250 mL/hour) is replaced by a hypotonic electrolyte solution with supplementation of potassium chloride (KCl, 20 mmol/L). When hypotension persists even after adequate volume replacement, vasopressors may be required. Dopamine (2 to 5 μg/kg^{-1}/min^{-1} and up to 10 μg/kg^{-1}/min^{-1}) is the first choice to improve cardiac contractility. Other inotropes include dobutamine (2 to 10 μg/kg^{-1}/min^{-1}) and isoproterenol (0.1 to 1 μg/kg^{-1}/min^{-1}), but these drugs may dilate peripheral vascular beds, decreasing blood pressure. Alpha-vasopressors (phenylephrine, norepinephrine bitartrate, or metaraminol bitartrate) are avoided because they may decrease splanchnic and coronary blood flow.[96, 97] In addition, the oxygen-carrying capacity to the peripheral tissues is improved by transfusion of packed red blood cells (1 to 3 U) to maintain the hematocrit between 25% and 30%.[98]

Severe cases of tachycardia and hypertension caused by the mass reflex may be controlled by the administration of general anesthetics, a beta antagonist, such as labetalol or esmolol, or a calcium channel blocker, such as verapamil.[66] Occasionally, an α-blocker, such as hydralazine or sodium nitroprusside, may be given to reduce afterload. Supraventricular or ventricular arrhythmias are treated with conventional antiarrhythmic drugs. Circulatory arrest, which occurs in 10% of potential donors and in 66% of referred donors,[99] is treated according to conventional circulatory resuscitative measures. If bradycardia is a concern, a direct-acting agent, such as isoproterenol or epinephrine, is used because donors are unresponsive to centrally acting chronotropic drugs, such as atropine.

Progressive hypothermia, which is seen in up to 86% of donors because of the loss of hypothalamic function.[51] results in sinus bradycardia, atrioventricular dissociation, and ventricular arrhythmias. At a temperature lower than 28°C, prolonged PR and QT intervals and wide QRS complexes are replaced by T-wave inversion, ST-segment depression, and a rise of ventricular fibrillation. Other effects of hypothermia are a leftward shift in the hemoglobin-oxygen dissociation curve, an increase in blood viscosity, a decrease in splanchnic blood flow and glomerular filtration, hyperglycemia, and metabolic and respiratory acidosis. Body temperature is kept within the normal range (>35°C) by increasing the room temperature, infusing all fluids through a blood warmer, and using a warming blanket and a heated humidifier in the inspiratory limb of the ventilation circuit.

Adequate diuresis (>0.5 mL/kg^{-1}/hour^{-1}, preferably 1 to 1.5 mL/kg^{-1}/hour^{-1}) is important because urine output is an indirect indication of preload and a prognostic indicator for renal graft and hepatic function.[100] The administration of fluid or dopamine may be effective in maintaining adequate renal perfusion and diuresis. However, a high dose of dopamine (>10 μg/kg^{-1}/min^{-1}) may lead to acute tubular necrosis and nonfunction of the renal graft.[90] For persistent oliguria, furosemide (1 to 2 mg/kg) and mannitol (0.5 g/kg) may be administered. Diabetes insipidus, caused by a nonfunctioning pituitary gland, results in polyuria, hypovolemia, and electrolyte imbalance. Excessive urine output is replaced with a hypotonic solution (0.45% NaCl with KCl, 20 mmol/L), and supplemental antidiuretic hormone is administered to maintain urine output in the range of 100 to 250 mL/hour. The synthetic analog of vasopressin, desmopressin acetate (DDAVP), is preferred (0.5 to 1 U/hour) because of its long duration of action and a low pressor/antidiuretic effect ratio.[101] However, the pressor activity in excessive doses of DDAVP may increase the risk of acute tubular necrosis[102] and reduce hepatic blood flow.[103] DDAVP increases the sensitivity to catecholamines,[103] and catecholamine doses should be reduced when DDAVP is given to the donor. Hyperglycemia is a complication of diabetes insipidus and is treated by an infusion of insulin (5 to 10 U).

Metabolic acidosis caused by inadequate tissue perfusion may be compounded by respiratory acidosis. Because of potential myocardial depression, metabolic acidosis is corrected by administration of sodium bicarbonate. When hypernatremia is a concern, tromethamine, or *tris*(hydroxymethyl) aminomethane (THAM) may be used instead of sodium bicarbonate:

$$0.3 \text{ mol THAM (mL)} = \text{body weight (kg)} \times \text{base deficit (mmol/L)}$$

Electrolyte imbalances (hypernatremia, hypokalemia, hypocalcemia, hypophosphatemia, and hypomagnesemia) caused by fluid shifts and diabetes insipidus may result in arrhythmias and myocardial dysfunction. Hypernatremia and hypokalemia are treated by administration of a hyponatremic solution (0.45% NaCl) and KCl (20 mmol/L). Ionized hypocalcemia caused by large blood transfusions is corrected by the administration of calcium chloride or calcium gluconate to preserve cardiac contractility. Hypomagnesemia is treated with magnesium sulfate (50 mg/kg), also to preserve myocardial contractility[104] Glucose metabolism is relatively well maintained, although hyperglycemia may occur as the result of a decreased level of insulin and as a complication of diabetes insipidus. Serum levels of triiodothyronine, insulin, and cortisol are low in animal models, and the administration of triiodothyronine improves hemodynamic stability by maintaining myocardial stores of energy and glycogen; however, the beneficial role of triiodothyronine is unclear in clinical settings.[52, 68]

Coagulopathy may occur in organ donors. Dilutional coagulopathy is caused by the shift of intravascular volume, consumption coagulopathy may result from the release of tissue thromboplastin from injured tissues and the ischemic organs, and fibrinolysis results from intravascular coagulation or the release of tissue plasminogen activator from the ischemic tissues. Disseminated intravascular coagulation (DIC) has been reported in 80% of donors with head injury,[105] but its clinical significance is unknown. Coagulation abnormalities are treated conservatively.

Once cardioplegia is induced, no further supportive care is necessary. After cross-clamping of the aorta (the time is recorded by the procurement coordinator) (Fig. 177-3), mechanical ventilation and monitoring are discontinued and all cannulas are removed. The organs are swiftly removed in the following sequence: heart, lungs, liver, pancreas, intestine, and kidneys. No supportive care is needed for procurement of corneas or bones because these tissues tolerate a prolonged ischemia without significant injury.

Recovery Data — Donor ID#

Surgeons

		Assisting:
Renal:	______	______
Hepatic:	______	______
Cardiac:	______	______
Heart/Lung:	______	______
Pancreas:	______	______

Coordinators/Technicians (Tissue): ______ ______

In O.R. ______ AM PM   Incision ______ AM PM   Depart O.R. (0) ______ AM PM   Depart O.R. (T) ______ AM PM

Condition During Surgery (include: Blood Pressure, Urine Output, Complications, Comments)

______

______

______

Operating Room Drugs (include dosage and time)

Methylprednisolone: ______   Mannitol: ______   Furosemide: ______

Heparin: ______   Vasodilator: ______   Blood Products ______

Antibiotics: ______   Others: ______

Nephrectomy Data

En Bloc: Y/N   In Situ: Y/N

Flush Sol'n: ______ Vol: ______

Final Flush (Sol'n Vol): ______

Storage Sol'n: ______

	R	L
Art Clamp:	______	______
Flush Start	______	______
Flush End:	______	______
Warm Ischemia Time	______	______
Clamps Off:	______	______
Cold Ischemia Time	______	______

Hepatectomy Data

Precool Start ______

Sol'n/Vol: ______

Portal Flush Start: ______

Sol'n/Vol: ______

Aortic Flush Start: ______

Sol'n/Vol: ______

Final Flush (Sol'n/Vol) ______

Clamps Off: ______

Cold Ischemia Time ______

Anatomy: ______

______

Cardiectomy Data

Infusion Start: ______

Sol'n/Vol. ______

Clamps Off: ______

Cold Ischemia Time ______

Heart Lung Data

Infusion Start (R) ______

Sol'nVol: ______

Infusion Start (L) ______

Sol'n/Vol: ______

Clamps Off: ______

Cold Ischemia Time ______

Single or Double Lung Data

Infusion Start: ______

Sol'n/Vol. ______

Clamps Off: ______

Cold Ischemia Time ______

Pancreas Data

Infusion Start: ______

Sol'n/Vol. ______

Final Flush; (Sol'n/Vol) ______

Clamps Off: ______

Cold Ischemia Time ______

Anatomy ______

Renal Anatomy

R ______ ______ ______ ______

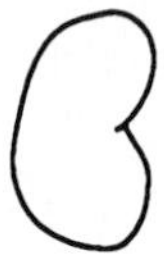

L ______ ______ ______ ______

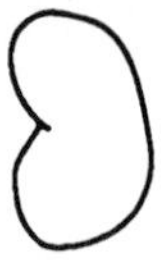

Biopsy Results: ______

______

Organs and Tissues Recovered (Check appropriate box and circle "T" for Transplant, "R" for Research)

☐ **R-KI** T/R ☐ **L-KI** T/R ☐ **LI** T/R ☐ **LU** T/R ☐ **PA** T/R ☐ **HR** T/R ☐ **HV** T/R ☐ **MV** T/R ☐ **Bones** T/R

☐ **BM** T/R ☐ **Veins** T/R ☐ **Skin** T/R ☐ **Cornea** T/R ☐ **INT** T/R ☐ **Other** T/R

Figure 177–3. Intraoperative data collection sheet used by the Western Pennsylvania Organ Procurement Organization, CORE (Center for Organ Recovery and Education). (Courtesy of Brian Broznick.)

Donor Operation

Before starting a multiple procurement, the different surgical teams must discuss the techniques and sequence they want to adopt. A detailed discussion of the surgical procedure is critical because, after aortic cross-clamping, time is of the essence. Everything should proceed as smoothly and expeditiously as possible to minimize organ damage. The basic principle of any donor operation is the core cooling of the organs to be removed. Cooling of a solid organ at the time of donor circulatory arrest was described for experimental liver transplantation nearly 40 years ago.[106] Cooling was then promptly applied to kidney preservation in clinical transplantation,[107] and it still represents the single most important aspect of any organ preservation technique. The first solution used was chilled lactated Ringer's solution, replaced in the late 1960s by the so-called Collins' solution, characterized by an electrolyte composition close to the intracellular one.[108] This solution was successfully used for about 20 years until the introduction of the University of Wisconsin solution,[109, 110] which extended the duration of organ viability. The easiest way to achieve almost immediate internal core cooling of the donor organs is by in situ infusion of the preservation solution, chilled to 4°C, at the time of the circulatory arrest. The remaining technical aspects of organ retrieval are secondary to this critical maneuver.

The surgical procedure for multiple cadaveric organ procurement has undergone a progressive evolution. In 1984, when procurement of extrarenal organs was becoming more common, the Pittsburgh group[111] published a technique that required a meticulous in vivo dissection of the donor organs and extensive manipulation of the abdominal viscera. A subsequent refinement of this technique was introduced in 1986.[112] This improved technique is used today and is basically characterized by a "no-touch en bloc removal" of the core cooled solid organs. The technical details of this operation lie outside the scope of this chapter, and we will only describe the major points.

A complete midline incision is performed from the suprasternal notch to the pubis (Fig. 177–4) (see Color Plate). As soon as the thoracic and abdominal organs are visualized, the procurement coordinator collects the first information on the appearance of the donor organs and relays it to the local OPO so that it can be made available to the recipient teams. The aorta is then exposed and encircled either immediately above or below the diaphragm (Fig. 177–5) (see Color Plate). The inferior mesenteric vein is encircled and cannulated for infusion of the cold portal perfusate. The aorta is then dissected for 2 cm at the level of the origin of the inferior mesenteric artery, which is tied and divided. The aorta is encircled at this level and prepared for cannulation. Figure 177–6 shows the donor inferior mesenteric vein and the infrarenal aorta cannulated for the cold perfusate (see Color Plate). The common bile duct is tied distally and transected close to the upper margin of the duodenum, and the gallbladder is incised and washed free of bile to prevent autolysis of the mucosa of the biliary tract.

The arterial anatomy of the liver should be carefully examined for possible anomalies. Prior knowledge of any anomaly is helpful in preventing mistakes during organ removal. At this point, the basic initial dissection is completed (Fig. 177–7) (see Color Plate) and the thoracic team prepares the chest organs for removal. The pleural spaces are opened widely after initial mediastinal dissection. Very little initial dissection is done around the inferior and superior vena cava and aorta other than to place sutures for the expected cannulation of the aorta for cardioplegia or the main pulmonary artery if the lungs are being harvested as well. The lungs are quickly examined through the pleural spaces, and little dissection is required thereafter. It should be noted that the donor's heart has continued beating spontaneously and maintained circulation of all organs.

As soon as the thoracic team completes its dissection, 300 to 500 U/kg of heparin is given intravenously, and the aorta is cannulated after ligating it distal to the inferior mesenteric artery (see Fig. 177–6). The thoracic team then occludes the superior vena cava, and the aorta is simultaneously clamped proximal to the innominate artery and just above or below the diaphragm (Fig. 177–8) (see Color Plate). The cold infusion is started, the inferior vena cava is vented, and the heart is separately perfused with cold cardioplegic solution. The heart is removed first. If the lungs are being harvested simultaneously, cold flush is started through the pulmonary artery, venting the solution through the left atrial appendage.

Once cardioplegic solution has been administered, the aorta is transected, and the rest of the lung perfusion solution is allowed to drain through the open aorta. Mediastinal dissection is then carried out, removing the lungs and heart en bloc if the block is to be used for a heart-lung transplant. The more common situation is one in which the heart is harvested by one group and the lungs are used for separate transplants. In this situation, once the cardioplegia and lung perfusion have

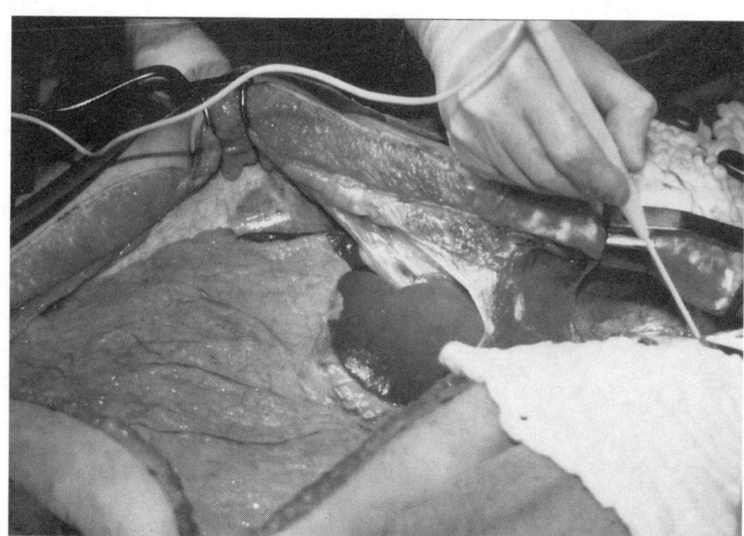

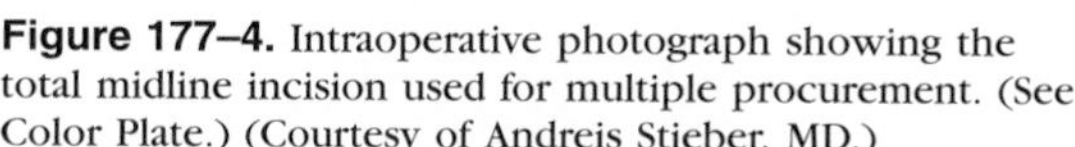

Figure 177–4. Intraoperative photograph showing the total midline incision used for multiple procurement. (See Color Plate.) (Courtesy of Andreis Stieber, MD.)

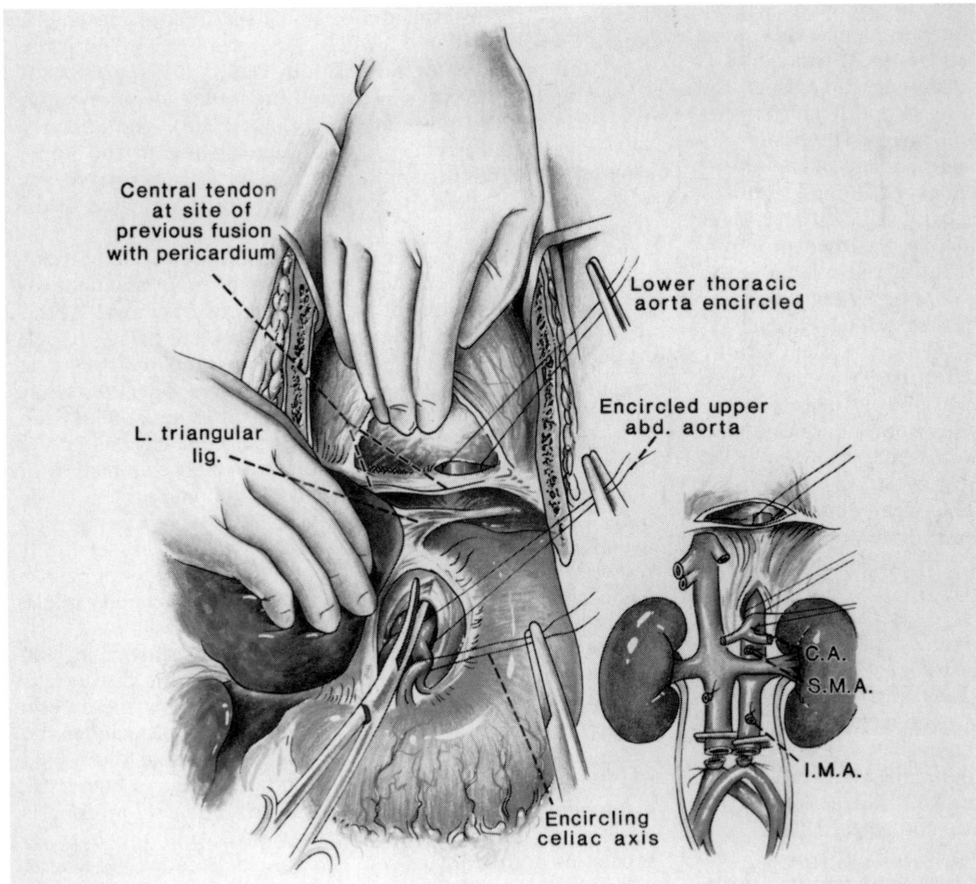

Figure 177–5. The aorta is dissected and encircled just above (or, alternatively, just below) the diaphragm. L. triangular lig. = left triangular ligament; encircled upper abd. aorta = encircled upper abdominal aorta; C.A. = celiac axis; S.M.A. = superior mesenteric artery; I.M.A. = inferior mesenteric artery. (See Color Plate.)

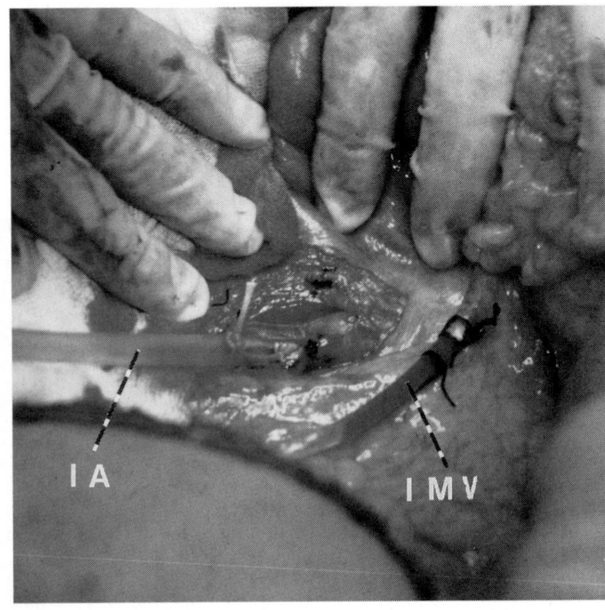

Figure 177–6. Intraoperative photograph showing cannulas for cold perfusion inserted into the dissected donor inferior mesenteric vein (IMV) and the infrarenal aorta (IA). (See Color Plate.) (Courtesy of Andreis Stieber, MD.)

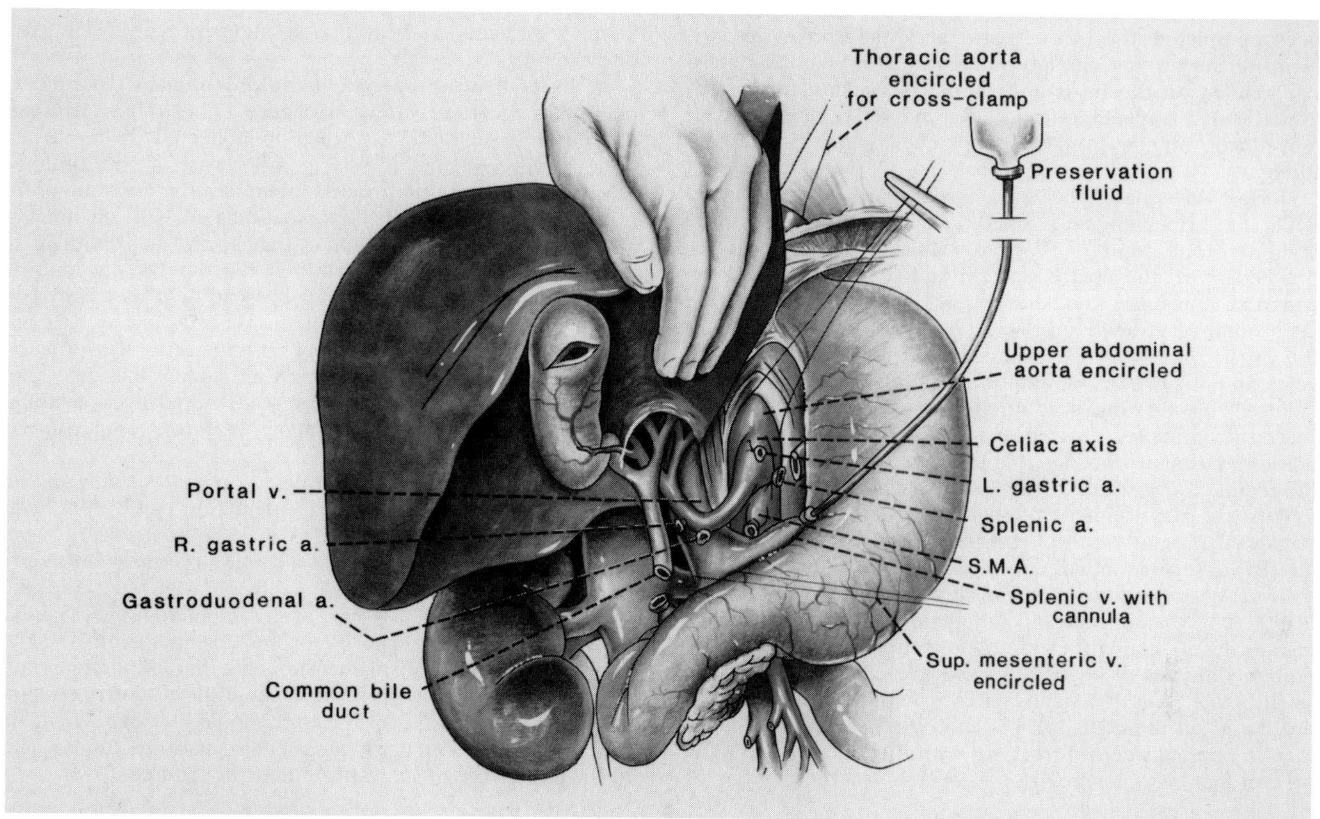

Figure 177–7. Liver hilar dissection, transection of the common bile duct, and incision of the gallbladder fundus to prevent autolysis of the mucosa of the biliary tract. In this drawing, the splenic vein is cannulated; however, the inferior mesenteric vein can be cannulated alternatively, as shown in Figure 177–6. Portal v. = portal vein; R. gastric a. = right gastric artery; Gastroduodenal a. = gastroduodenal artery; L. gastric a. = left gastric artery; Splenic a. = splenic artery; S.M.A. = superior mesenteric artery; Splenic v. with cannula = splenic vein with cannula; Sup. mesenteric v. encircled = superior mesenteric vein encircled. (See Color Plate.)

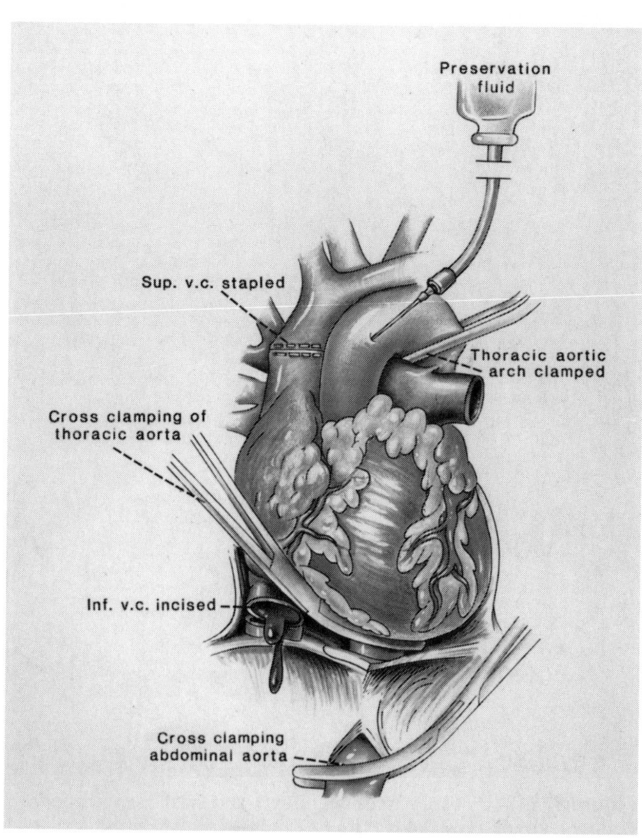

Figure 177–8. Occlusion of the superior vena cava inflow and simultaneous clamping of the aorta proximal to the innominate artery. The aorta is also simultaneously clamped just above or below the diaphragm. Cardioplegic solution infused through the ascending aorta is allowed to run only in the heart. Sup. v.c. stapled = superior vena cava stapled; Inf. v.c. incised = inferior vena cava incised. (See Color Plate.)

been completed, the heart is carefully dissected by the two teams, ensuring that enough pulmonary artery and left atrial cuff remain on the heart and the lungs, making them both available for transplantation. After the heart has been removed, the lung team can then proceed with extraction of the lungs.

During this phase, the abdominal organs are untouched while they are exsanguinated and the cold perfusion is continued. After removal of the thoracic organs, the abdominal team proceeds with the final dissection and removal of the liver, pancreas, intestine, and kidneys. The technical steps have been outlined elsewhere by us[50, 111-114] and others.[115-117] After the organ recovery, long segments of the iliac arteries and veins, inferior vena cava, and aorta[118] (and carotid arteries in children) should always be removed and stored under hypothermic conditions. This ensures the ability to deal with all possible vascular problems that might be encountered during the recipient operations.[118-123]

With the development of the intestinal and multivisceral transplant program at the University of Pittsburgh (see Chapter 184), a technique was developed for the removal of essentially the entire abdominal visceral bloc (Fig. 177-9) (see Color Plate).[50, 124] Anatomic considerations are fundamental during intestinal and multivisceral procurement because recipients require different types of intestinal transplantation (isolated small bowel, liver and small bowel, true multivisceral, and so on) based on different diseases and needs.[124] These procurement techniques do not interfere with those of other organs. In our first 35 intestinal donor operations, there were 62 kidneys, 35 livers, 18 hearts, and 3 lungs procured simultaneously.[50]

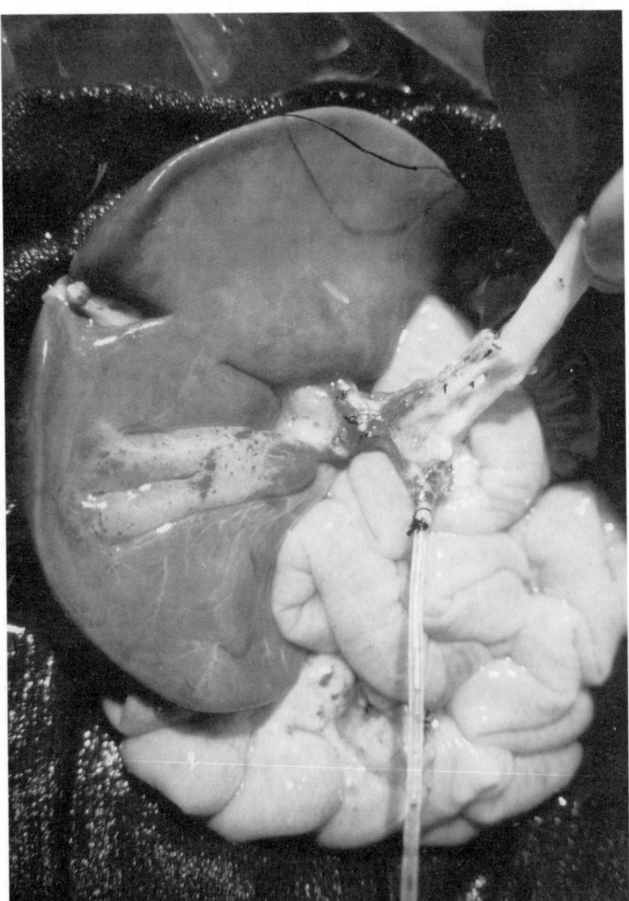

Figure 177–9. En bloc harvesting of liver and small bowel from a pediatric donor. (See Color Plate.)

At the end of the operation, the procurement coordinator completes the form shown in Figure 177-3. These data and the other basic donor information collected earlier in the donor procurement process (Fig. 177-2) are of critical importance in the selection of the recipient and the outcome of the transplantation. The risk factors associated with an unfavorable outcome, at least in some organs, may be identified by the information readily available at the time of the multiple organ procurement. This knowledge can help us stratify prospective donor-recipient combinations according to their predicted risk of failure, providing insight as to the probable outcome of individual patients and the factors that determine it. It can also be used to describe study populations, stratified according to their risk, and allow uniform comparison of outcomes.

In Pittsburgh, we have completed an analysis determining that the outcome of a liver transplantation can be predicted at the time of the surgery. This may be achieved by using information obtained as part of a routine pretransplant recipient and donor work-up, which is always available at the time of organ allocation.[125] Because of the interaction of two different biologic systems—the donor and the recipient—the outcome of an organ transplantation is a complex phenomenon. Therefore, the various aspects of multiple donor organ procurement discussed in this chapter should be carefully considered in each potential procurement scenario as fundamental to the success of the transplantation procedure.

ACKNOWLEDGMENT

The authors were aided by research grants from the Veterans Administration and Project Grant No. DK 29961 from the National Institutes of Health, Bethesda, Maryland.

References

1. Data from United Network for Organ Sharing Research Department. UNOS Update 1992; 8:20-27.
2. Evans RW, Orians CE, Ascher NL: The potential supply of organ donors. JAMA 1992; 267:239-246.
3. Garrison RN, Bentley FR, Raque GH, et al: There is an answer to the shortage of organ donors. Surg Gynecol Obstet 1991; 173:391-396.
4. UNOS Bull 1997; 2:8.
5. Evans RW: Organ procurement expeditures and the role of financial incentives. JAMA 1993; 269:3113-3118.
6. Orians CE, Evans RW, Ascher NL: Estimates of organ-specific donor availability for the United States. Transplant Proc 1993; 25:1541-1542.
7. UNOS 1997 Annual Report: Data Highlights. Washington, DC, Department of Health and Human Services, 1998, p 3.
8. Donation and Transplantation: Medical School Curriculum. Richmond, United Network for Organ Sharing, 1992.
9. Starzl TE, Shapiro R, Teperman L: The point system for organ distribution. Transplant Proc 1989; 21(Suppl 3):3432-3436.
10. Eghtesad B, Bronsther O, Starzl TE, et al: Disease gravity and urgency of need as guidelines for liver allocation. Hepatology 1994; 20:56S-62S.
11. Marino IR, Doyle HR, Rakela J, et al: Orthotopic liver transplantation: Indications and results. *In:* Textbook of Bilio-Pancreatic Diseases. Vol III. Hess W, Berci G (Eds). Padua, Italy, Piccin Publisher, 1997, pp 2107-2125.
12. Galletti PM: Bioartificial organs. J Artif Org 1992; 16:55-60.
13. Caplan A: Must I be my brother's keeper? Ethical issues in the use of living donors as sources of liver and other solid organs. Transplant Proc 1993; 25:1997-2000.
14. Kirchner SA: Living related lung transplantation: A new observation in single lung transplantation. AORN J 1991; 54:712-714.
15. Marino IR, Doyle HR: Surgical techniques and innovations in

living-related liver transplantation. *In:* New Technologies for Liver Resections. Dionigi R, Madariaga J (Eds). Basel, Karger AG, 1997, pp 132–145.
16. Starzl TE, Rao AS, Murase N, et al: Will xenotransplantation ever be feasible? J Am Coll Surg 1998; 186:383–387.
17. Starzl TE, Fung JJ, Tzakis A, et al: Baboon to human liver transplantation. Lancet 1993; 341:65–71.
18. Marino IR, Doyle HR, Nour B, Starzl TE: Baboon liver xenotransplantation in humans: Clinical experience and principles learned. *In:* Xenotransplantation: The Transplantation of Organs and Tissues Between Species. 2nd ed. Cooper DKG, Kemp E, Platt JL, White DJG (Eds). Berlin, Springer-Verlag, 1997, pp 793–811.
19. Anaise D, Rapaport FF: Use of non-heart-beating cadaver donors in clinical organ transplantation logistics, ethics and legal consideration. Transplant Proc 1993; 25:2153–2155.
20. Ad Hoc Committee of the Harvard Medical School: A definition of irreversible coma: Report of the Ad Hoc Committee of the Harvard Medical School to examine the definition of brain death. JAMA 1968; 205:337–340.
21. Guidelines for the determination of death: Report of the medical consultants on the diagnosis of death to the President's Commission for the Study of Ethical Problems in Medicine and Biomedical and Behavioral Research. JAMA 1981; 246:2184–2186.
22. Childress J: Attitudes of major western religious traditions towards uses of the human body and its parts. *In:* Justice and the Holy: Essays in Honor of Walter Harrelson. Knight DA, Paris PJ (Eds). Atlanta, Scholar Press, 1989.
23. Dickson R, Ishitani M, Caldwell S, et al: Hepatitis B core antibody positive liver donors are at high risk for transmitting hepatitis B infection to liver recipients. Twenty-first Annual Scientific Meeting of the American Society of Transplant Surgeons, Abstract book, Chicago, May 17–19, 1995, p 43.
24. Kirk AD, Heisey DM, D'Alessandro AM, et al: Clinical hepatitis after transplantation of hepatitis C virus-positive kidneys. Transplantation 1996; 62:1758–1762.
25. Pruim J, Klompmaker IDSJ, Haagsma EB, et al: Selection criteria for liver donation: A review. Transpl Int 1993; 6:226–235.
26. Prompt CA, Reis MM, Grillo FM, et al: Transmission of AIDS virus at renal transplantation. Lancet 1985; 2:672.
27. Dummer JS, Erb S, Breinig MK, et al: Infection with human immunodeficiency virus in the Pittsburgh transplant population: A study of 583 donors and 1043 recipients, 1981–1986. Transplantation 1989; 47:134–139.
28. Fox AS, Tolpin MD, Baker AL, et al: Seropositivity in liver transplant recipients as a predictor of cytomegalovirus disease. J Infect Dis 1988; 157:383–385.
29. Haagsma EB, Klompmaker IJ, Grond J: Herpes virus infection after orthotopic liver transplantation. Transplant Proc 1987; 19:4054–4056.
30. Yanaga K, Kakizoe S, Ikeda T, et al: Procurement of liver allografts from non-heart beating donors. Transplant Proc 1990; 22:275–278.
31. Teperman L, Podesta L, Mieles L, et al: The successful use of older donors for liver transplantation. JAMA 1989; 262:2837.
32. Marino IR, Doyle HR, Doria C, et al: Outcome of liver transplantation using donors 60 to 79 years of age. Transplant Proc 1995; 27:1184–1185.
33. Popper H: Aging and the liver. *In:* Progress in Liver Diseases. Vol 8. Popper H, Levy GL (Eds). New York, Grune & Stratton, 1985, pp 659–683.
34. Neugarten J, Silbiger SR: The impact of gender on renal transplantation. Transplantation 1994; 58:1145–1152.
35. Marino IR, Doyle HR, Aldrighetti L, et al: Effect of donor age and sex on the outcome of liver transplantation. Hepatology 1995; 22:1754–1762.
36. Kakizoe S, Yanaga K, Starzl TE, et al: Frozen section of liver biopsy for the evaluation of liver allografts. Transplant Proc 1990; 22:416–417.
37. Kakizoe S, Yanaga K, Starzl TE, et al: Evaluation of protocol before transplantation and after reperfusion biopsies from human orthotopic liver allografts: Considerations of preservation and early immunological injury. Hepatology 1990; 11:932–941.
38. Adam R, Azourlay D, Astarciuglu I, et al: Reliability of the MEGX test in the selection of liver grafts. Transplant Proc 1991; 23:2470–2471.
39. Bowers JL, Teramoto K, Clouse ME: 31P NMR assessment of orthotopic liver transplant viability: The effect of warm ischemia (Abstract). Presented at the Tenth Annual Meeting of the Society of Magnetic Resonance in Medicine, San Francisco, 1991.
40. Kanetsuna Y, Fujita S, Tojimbara T, et al: Usefulness of 31P-MRS as a method of evaluating the viability of preserved and transplanted rat liver. Transpl Int 1992; 5(Suppl 1):S379–S381.
41. Oellerich M, Burdelski M, Ringe B, et al: Lignocaine metabolite formation as a measure of pre-transplant liver function. Lancet 1989; 1:640–642.
42. Ozaki N, Gubernatis G, Ringe B, et al: Arterial blood ketone body ratio as an indicator for viability of donor livers. Transplant Proc 1991; 23:2487–2489.
43. Reding R, Feyaerts A, Wallemacq P, et al: Liver graft assessment in organ donors by the lidocaine monoethyglycinexylidide test is unreliable. Br J Surg 1992; 79(Suppl 1):S142.
44. Yamaoka Y, Taki Y, Gubernatis G, et al: Evaluation of the liver graft before procurement: Significance of arterial ketone body ratio in brain-dead patients. Transpl Int 1990; 3:78–81.
45. Burdelski M, Oellerich M, Raude E, et al: A novel approach to assessment of liver function in donors. Transplant Proc 1988; 20(Suppl 1):591–593.
46. Makowka L, Gordon RD, Todo S, et al: Analysis of donor criteria for the prediction of outcome in clinical liver transplantation. Transplant Proc 1987; 19:2378–2382.
47. Stock PG, Najarian JS, Ascher NL: Liver transplantation. *In:* Critical Care State of the Art. Gallagher TJ, Shoemaker WC (Eds). Fullerton, Calif, Society of Critical Care Medicine, 1988, pp 21–24.
48. Hesse UJ, Najarian JS, Sutherland DER: Amylase activity and pancreas transplants. Lancet 1985; 2:726–728.
49. Darby JM, Stein K, Grenvik A, et al: Approach to management of the heart beating brain dead organ donor. JAMA 1989; 261:2222–2228.
50. Furukawa H, Smith C, Lee R, et al: Influence of donor criteria on early outcome after intestinal transplantation. Transplant Proc 1997; 29:690.
51. Griepp RB, Stinson EB, Clark DA, et al: The cardiac donor. Surg Gynecol Obstet 1971; 133:792–798.
52. Novitzky D, Cooper DKC, Reichart B: Hemodynamic and metabolic responses to hormonal therapy in brain dead potential organ donors. Transplantation 1987; 43:852–854.
53. Copeland JG, Emery RW, Levinson MM, et al: Selection of patients for cardiac transplantation. Circulation 1987; 75:2–9.
54. Renlund DG, Bristow MR, Lee HR, et al: Medical aspects of cardiac transplantation. J Cardiothorac Anesth 1988; 2:500–512.
55. Stoddard MF, Logaker RA: The role of transesophageal echocardiography in cardiac donor screening. Am Heart J 1993; 125:1676–1681.
56. Lammermeier DE, Sweeney MS, Haupt HE, et al: Use of potentially infected donor hearts for cardiac transplantation. Ann Thorac Surg 1990; 50:222–225.
57. Luciani GB, Livi U, Faggian G, et al: Clinical results of heart transplantation in recipients over 55. J Heart Lung Transplant 1992; 11:1177–1183.
58. Pflugfelder PW, Singh NR, McKenzie FN, et al: Extending cardiac allograft ischemic time and donor age: Effect on survival and long-term cardiac function. J Cardiovasc Surg (Torino) 1991; 32:46–49.
59. Menkis AH, Novick RJ, Kostuk WJ, et al: Successful use of the "unacceptable" heart donor. J Heart Lung Transplant 1991; 10:28–32.
60. Sweeney MS, Lammermeier DE, Frazier OH, et al: Extension of donor criteria in cardiac transplantation: Surgical risk versus supply-side economics. Ann Thorac Surg 1990; 50:7–10.
61. Harjula A, Starnes VA, Oyer PE, et al: Proper donor selection for heart-lung transplantation. J Thorac Cardiovasc Surg 1987; 94:874–880.
62. Tarazi RY, Bonser RS, Jamieson SW: Heart-lung transplantation. *In:* Critical Care State of the Art. Gallagher TJ (Ed). Fullerton, Calif, Society of Critical Care Medicine, 1988, pp 55–72.
63. Todd RJ: Pulmonary transplantation. *In:* Critical Care State of the Art. Gallagher TJ (Ed). Fullerton, Calif, Society of Critical Care Medicine, 1988, pp 41–53.
64. Detterbeck FC, Mill MR, Williams W, et al: Organ donation and

the management of the multiple organ donor. Contemp Surg 1993; 42:281-285.
65. Soifer BE, Gelb AW: The multiple organ donor: Identification and management. Ann Intern Med 1989; 110:814-823.
66. Novitzky D, Wicomb WN, Cooper DKC, et al: Electrocardiographic, hemodynamic and endocrine changes occurring during experimental brain death in the Chacma baboon. J Heart Transplant 1984; 4:63-69.
67. Pennefather SH, Bullock RE: Triiodothyronine treatment in brain-dead multiorgan donors: A controlled study (Letter). Transplantation 1993; 55:1443.
68. Macoviak JA, McDougall IR, Bayer MF, et al: Significance of thyroid dysfunction in human cardiac allograft procurement. Transplantation 1987; 43:824-826.
69. Gifford RRM, Weaver AS, Burg JE, et al: Thyroid hormone levels in heart and kidney cadaver donors. J Heart Transplant 1986; 5:249-253.
70. Wahlers T, Fieguth HG, Jurmann M, et al: Does hormone depletion of organ donors impair myocardial function after cardiac transplantation? Transplant Proc 1988; 20(Suppl 1):792-794.
71. Nygaard CE, Townsend RN, Diamond DL: Organ donor management and organ outcome: A six-year review from a level I trauma center. J Trauma 1990; 30:728-732.
72. Bodenham A, Park GR: Care of the multiple organ donor. Intensive Care Med 1989; 15:340-348.
73. Novitzky D, Cooper DKC, Morrell D, et al: Change from aerobic to anaerobic metabolism after brain death, and reversal following triiodothyronine therapy. Transplantation 1988; 45:32-36.
74. Starzl TE, Demetris AJ, Trucco M, et al: Cell migration and chimerism after whole organ transplantation: The basis of graft acceptance. Hepatology 1993; 17:1127-1152.
75. Miller CM, Teodorescu V, Harrington M, et al: Regional procurement and export of hepatic allografts for transplantation. Mt Sinai J Med 1990; 57:93-96.
76. Kang YG, Kormos RL, Casavilla A: Organ procurement from donors with brain death. *In:* Trauma Anesthesia and Critical Care. Grande C (Ed). Philadelphia, WB Saunders, 1993, pp 1013-1024.
77. Luksza AR: Brain-dead kidney donor: Selection, care and administration. Br Med J 1979; 1:1316-1319.
78. Wetzel RC, Setzer N, Stiff JL, et al: Hemodynamic responses in brain dead organ donor patients. Anesth Analg 1985; 64:125-128.
79. Dahlager JL, Bilde T: The integrity of tubular cell function after preservation in Collins' solution: Canine kidneys. Transplantation 1976; 21:365-369.
80. Rijksen JFWB: Preservation of Canine Kidneys: The Effect of Various Preservation Fluids on Renal Morphology and Function (Master's thesis). The Netherlands, University of Leiden, 1972.
81. Schloerb PR, Postel J, Mortiz ED, et al: Hypothermic storage of the canine kidneys for 48 hours in a low chloride solution. Surg Gynecol Obstet 1975; 141:545-548.
82. Miller CH, Alexander JW, Smith EJ, et al: Salutary effect of phentolamine (Regitine) on renal vasoconstriction in donor kidneys: Experimental and clinical studies. Transplantation 1974; 17:201-210.
83. Abramowicz M: The choice of antimicrobial drugs. Med Lett 1982; 24:21-23.
84. Abramowicz M: Choice of cephalosporins. Med Lett 1983; 25:57-60.
85. Schuler S, Parnt R, Warnecke H, et al: Extended donor criteria for heart transplantation. J Heart Transplant 1988; 7:326-330.
86. Kroncke GM, Nichols RD, Mendenhall JT, et al: Ectothermic philosophy of acid-base balance to prevent fibrillation during hypothermia. Arch Surg 1986; 121:303-304.
87. Swain JA: Hypothermia and blood pH: A review. Arch Intern Med 1988; 148:1643-1646.
88. Flanigan WJ, Ardon LF, Brewer TE, et al: Etiology and diagnosis of early post-transplantation oliguria. Am J Surg 1976; 132:808-815.
89. Toledo-Pereyra LH, Simmons RL, Olson LC, et al: Cadaver kidney transplantation effect of hypotension and donor pretreatment with methylprednisolone and phenoxybenzamine. Minn Med 1979; 62:159-161.
90. Whelchel JD, Diethelm AG, Phillips MG, et al: The effect of high-dose dopamine in cadaver donor management on delayed graft function and graft survival following renal transplantation. Transplant Proc 1986; 18:523-527.
91. Wicomb WN, Cooper DKC, Lanza RP, et al: The effects of brain death and 24 hours storage by hypothermic perfusion on donor heart function in the pig. J Thorac Cardiovasc Surg 1986; 91:896-909.
92. Busuttil RW, Goldstein LI, Danovitch GM, et al: Liver transplantation today. Ann Intern Med 1986; 104:377-389.
93. Novitzky D, Rose AG, Cooper DKC: Injury of myocardial conduction tissue and coronary artery smooth muscle following brain death in the baboon. Transplantation 1988; 45:964-966.
94. Davidson I, Berglin E, Brynger H: Perioperative fluid regimen, blood and plasma volumes, and colloid changes in living-related donors. Transplant Proc 1984; 16:18-19.
95. Kormos RL, Donato W, Hardesty RL, et al: The influence of donor organ stability and ischemia time on subsequent cardiac recipient survival. Transplant Proc 1988; 20:980-983.
96. Slapak M: The immediate care of potential donors for cadaveric organ transplantation. Anaesthesia 1978; 33:700-709.
97. Levinson MM, Copeland JG: The organ donor: Physiology, maintenance, and procurement considerations. Contemp Anesth Pract 1987; 10:31-45.
98. Hardesty RL, Griffith BP: Multiple cadaveric organ procurement for transplantation with emphasis on the heart. Surg Clin North Am 1986; 66:451-457.
99. Emery RW, Cork RC, Levinson MM, et al: The cardiac donor: A six-year experience. Ann Thorac Surg 1986; 41:356-362.
100. Lucas BA, Vaughn WK, Spees EK, et al: Identification of donor factors predisposing to high discard rates of cadaver kidneys and increased graft loss within one year post transplantation. Transplantation 1987; 43:253-258.
101. Richardson DW, Robinson AG: Desmopressin. Ann Intern Med 1985; 103:228-239.
102. Schneider A, Toledo-Pereyra LH, Seichner WD, et al: Effect of dopamine and pitressin on kidneys procured and harvested for transplantation. Transplantation 1983; 36:110-111.
103. Cowley AW, Monos E, Guyton AS: Interaction of vasopressin and the baroreceptor reflex system in the regulation of arterial blood pressure in the dog. Circ Res 1974; 34:505-514.
104. Davis S, Olichwier KK, Chakko SC: Reversible depression of myocardial performance in hypophosphatemia. Am J Med Sci 1988; 295:183-187.
105. Kaufman HH, Hui KS, Mattson JC, et al: Clinicopathologic correlations of disseminated intravascular coagulation in patients with severe head injury. Neurosurgery 1984; 15:34-42.
106. Starzl TE, Kaupp HA Jr, Brock DR, et al: Reconstructive problems in canine liver homotransplantation with special reference to the postoperative role of hepatic venous flow. Surg Gynecol Obstet 1960; 111:733-743.
107. Starzl TE: Experience in Renal Transplantation. Philadelphia, WB Saunders, 1964.
108. Collins GM, Bravo-Shugarman M, Terasaki PI: Kidney preservation for transportation. Lancet 1969; 2:1219-1222.
109. Belzer FO, Southard JH: Principles of solid organ preservation by cold storage. Transplantation 1988; 45:673-676.
110. Todo S, Tzakis A, Starzl TE: Preservation of livers with UW or Euro Collins' solution (Letter). Transplantation 1988; 46:925-926.
111. Starzl TE, Hakala TR, Shaw BW Jr, et al: A flexible procedure for multiple cadaveric organ procurement. Surg Gynecol Obstet 1984; 158:223-230.
112. Starzl TE, Miller C, Broznick B, et al: An improved technique for multiple organ harvesting. Surg Gynecol Obstet 1987; 165:343-348.
113. Marino IR, Doyle HR, Fung JJ: Liver. *In:* The Multi-Organ Donor: Selection and Management. Higgins RSD, Sanchez JA, Lorber M, Baldwin JC (Eds). Malden, Mass, Blackwell Science, 1997, pp 241-264.
114. Yanaga K, Podesta L, Broznick B, et al: Multiple organ recovery for transplantation. *In:* Atlas of Organ Transplantation. Starzl TE, Shapiro R, Simmons RL (Eds). New York, Gower Medical Publishing, 1992, pp 3.2-3.49.
115. Schwartz ME, Podesta L, Morris M, et al: Donor management, techniques and procurement. *In:* The Handbook of Transplantation Management. Makowka L (Ed). Austin, Tex, R.G. Landes Company, 1991, pp 44-71.

116. Marsh CL, Perkins JD, Sutherland DE, et al: Combined hepatic and pancreaticoduodenal procurement for transplantation. Surg Gynecol Obstet 1989; 168:254–258.
117. Esquivel CO, Nakazato PZ, Concepcion W: Liver transplantation: Modern techniques in donor and recipient operations. *In:* Surgical Technology International. Braverman MH (Ed). San Francisco, Surgical Technology International, Thomas F. Lazslo Publisher, 1992, pp 315–321.
118. Starzl TE, Halgrimson CG, Koep LJ, et al: Vascular homografts from cadaveric organ donors. Surg Gynecol Obstet 1979; 149:76–77.
119. Todo S, Makowka L, Tzakis AG, et al: Hepatic artery in liver transplantation. Transplant Proc 1987; 19:2406–2411.
120. Tzakis A, Mazzaferro V, Pan C, et al: Renal artery reconstruction for harvesting injuries in kidney transplantation: With particular reference to the use of vascular allografts. Transpl Int 1988; 1:80–85.
121. Tzakis A, Todo S, Starzl TE: The anterior route for arterial graft conduits in liver transplantation (Letter). Transpl Int 1989; 2:121.
122. Stieber AC, Zetti G, Todo S, et al: The spectrum of portal vein thrombosis. Ann Surg 1991; 213:199–206.
123. Marino IR, Doyle HR, Starzl TE: Orthotopic liver transplantation. *In:* Textbook of Bilio-Pancreatic Diseases. Vol III. Hess W, Berci G (Eds). Padua, Italy, Piccin Publisher, 1997, pp 1779–1807.
124. Scotti-Foglieni C, Marino IR, Starzl TE, et al: Human intestinal-multivisceral transplantation. *In:* Liver Transplantation. D'Amico DF, Bassi N, Tedeschi U, et al (Eds). Milan, Masson, 1994, pp 235–254.
125. Marino IR, Morelli F, Doria C, et al: Preoperative assessment of risk in liver transplantation: A multivariable analysis in 2,376 cases of the UW era. Transplant Proc 1997; 29:454–455.

178

Principles of Immunosuppression

Ajai Khanna, MD, FRCS • Alan J. Rosenbloom, MD
Clark Andrew Bonham, MD • John J. Fung, MD, PhD

Recent advances in molecular biology and immunology have unraveled mechanisms of antigen-presenting cell (APC) and T cell interactions. This includes elucidation of molecular mechanisms involved in the activation and turning off of T cells and interleukin-2 (IL-2) gene transcription and translation. Studies leading to novel ways of inhibiting T cell activation have focused on various subunits (α, β, and γ) of the IL-2 receptor. This has led to an explosion of trials of these agents in combinations with more conventional immunosuppressive drugs.

BASIC PRINCIPLES

Optimal immunosuppression consists of drug therapy that enables graft acceptance while suppressing systemic immunity as little as possible and producing the least systemic toxicity. Immunosuppression predisposes to infection and malignancy, in addition to other side effects that are inherent risks with all the currently available immunosuppressants. Blood level monitoring and titration of immunosuppression are limited to only a few immunosuppressive agents, and in practice too much or too little immunosuppression almost invariably becomes apparent only in retrospect. Surrogate biologic assays, such as suppression of the mixed lymphocyte reaction, are either impractical or do not have proven clinical correlates.

The timing, dosing, and selection of immunosuppressive agents differ much. Current protocols use multiple drugs, each directed at a discrete site in the T cell-activation cascade.[1] Most immunosuppressive regimens are combinations of drugs, often with different modes of action and toxicity. This approach allows giving smaller doses of each drug. Transplantation immunosuppression can be (1) *pharmacologic*, consisting of drugs like corticosteroids, cytokine suppressive agents, antiproliferative agents, and cytotoxic agents or (2) *biologic*, consisting of monoclonal and polyclonal antilymphocyte antibodies and anti-cytokine receptor antibodies.[2] Newer agents are being introduced.

Tacrolimus (Tac) or cyclosporine (CyA) with steroids forms the backbone of most immunosuppressive regimens being used today. An antiproliferative agent or an antilymphocyte antibody, or both, may be added. When acute cellular rejection occurs, it is common to treat it with large doses of steroids or antilymphocyte antibodies, or both.

In general, the early postoperative period calls for the greatest degree of immunosuppression. As time goes on, many patients can maintain graft function with smaller quantities of immunosuppressive agents. Some patients can tolerate complete withdrawal of therapy without exhibiting rejection[3]; however, this is best done as a protocol-based strategy with patients under strict supervision.

OVERVIEW OF TRANSPLANT IMMUNOBIOLOGY

Lymphocytes are preprogrammed as they develop in the thymus to recognize foreign antigen. Antigen specificity is determined by an antigen-binding unit on the T cell surface, the T cell receptor (TCR). The specificity and diversity of the binding site of the TCR derive from its amino acid composition and the variations in this composition from T cell to T cell. The gene sequence that codes for the TCR rearranges during development, so each T cell ends up with a different TCR-binding specificity. Because the gene rearrangements are completely random, a huge library of binding sites capable of recognizing both *self* and *foreign* molecules is generated. Thymocytes with TCRs that bind to self molecules (and thus potentiate the development of autoimmunity) are subsequently destroyed, by mechanisms that are poorly understood.

Lymphocytes recirculate at a rate of 1% to 2% per hour, migrating through all tissues of the body. Recirculation routes are not random. Specialized cell-surface "homing" molecules on T lymphocytes mediate attachment to specific endothelial molecules in targeted tissues. Once inside tissue, antigen-presenting cells (APCs), such as macrophages, make intimate contact with the lymphocytes and present foreign antigen that has been processed in the cells by the APCs. The APCs phagocytose foreign proteins and cleave foreign protein enzymatically into small peptides of eight to 12 amino acids length. These peptides are loaded onto a class of specialized carrier molecules known as the *major histocompatibility complex* (MHC). MHC molecules carry the peptide fragments to the cell surface, where they are displayed to T cells.

The TCR is a cell-surface molecule. The TCR associates with "accessory" molecules, including CD3 and either CD4 or CD8. The TCR-CD3 complex interacts with the peptide fragment in the binding groove of the MHC molecule of the APC, and this complex is stabilized by the CD4 or CD8 molecule of the T cell. This interaction produces the signal that initiates activation of the T cell, leading to proliferation of that T cell clone, which recognizes the particular antigen fragments of foreign protein. The basis for MHC-restricted antigen recognition is the requirement for antigen presentation by APCs bearing an MHC molecule specific to the host.

Antigen-directed proliferation of T cell clones is absolutely necessary for an effective immune response. It is driven by a positive feedback loop between T cells and a soluble autocrine hormone. Cells that recognize antigen make the potent growth factor (IL-2) and simultaneously become responsive to IL-2 by expressing the IL-2 receptor. This dual synthesis allows the cells to stimulate their own "autocrine" clonal expansion.

During an ongoing immune response, proliferating T cells recruit many other cell types and immune mechanisms into action. T cells produce IL-1 through IL-6, IL-9, and IL-10 plus interferons, tumor necrosis factors α and β (TNF-α, TNF-β), granulocyte colony-stimulating factor (G-CSF), and granulocyte-monocyte colony-stimulating factor (GM-CSF).[4] These substances have at least three important functions.

First, cytokines can attract and activate other leukocytes. For example, CD4 helper T cell cytokines attract macrophages and CD8-bearing cytotoxic lymphocytes into rejecting allografts.[5] They also trigger macrophage activation and CD8 lymphocyte cell maturation. The resulting multicellular tissue infiltration has traditionally been referred to as the *delayed-type hypersensitivity* (DTH) response. CD4 helper T cell cytokines are also responsible for the activation of B cells and, thus, indirectly for the majority of antibody production.

Second, cytokines up-regulate both MHC molecules on tissues and adhesion molecules on endothelium. This enhances entry and accumulation of leukocytes in the tissue and accelerates recognition of foreign molecules.

Third, cytokines activate distant organ responses, such as the hepatic acute-phase response, bone marrow phagocyte synthesis, and the hypothalamic-pituitary axis, producing the systemic signs of inflammation.

Once the antigen is consumed or removed, the process is down-regulated. A number of sensitized memory T cells remain and contribute to a stronger secondary response on repeat challenge with the same antigen. Other mechanisms of T cell regulation that relate to expression of regulatory molecules (such as Fas ligand) may also play an important role in T cell–mediated responses.

In the case of transplanted solid organs, recipient T lymphocytes enter the graft rapidly. Conversely, donor APCs also exit the graft immediately after reperfusion. Thus, recipient lymphocytes have the potential to become sensitized to donor (foreign) antigens both inside and outside the transplanted organ.

Evidence now suggests the existence of at least two subpopulations of CD4-bearing T cells in humans. Helper T subset 1 (T_H1) cells preferentially drive cell-mediated immunity. Helper T subset 2 (T_H2) cells stimulate B cell antigen production. The two subsets produce different sets of cytokines. Some of the T_H1 cytokines down-regulate the production of T_H2 cytokines, and vice versa. Thus, the two distinct responses represented by these subsets are somewhat mutually exclusive. The predominance of one subset or the other is believed to affect the character of the immune response to a particular challenge. The mechanisms that determine the choice between T_H1 and T_H2 are under investigation.

Molecular mechanisms that elaborate IL-2 gene transcription and structure of the IL-2 receptor (IL-2R) have led to IL-2 receptor–targeted therapy. As knowledge of molecular biology has advanced, investigators have gained greater understanding of the workings of many immunosuppressants. More important, new strategies guided by this knowledge have resulted in site-directed immunosuppression. Virtually every known step of the immune process can be targeted, and many new drugs are now in various stages of development.

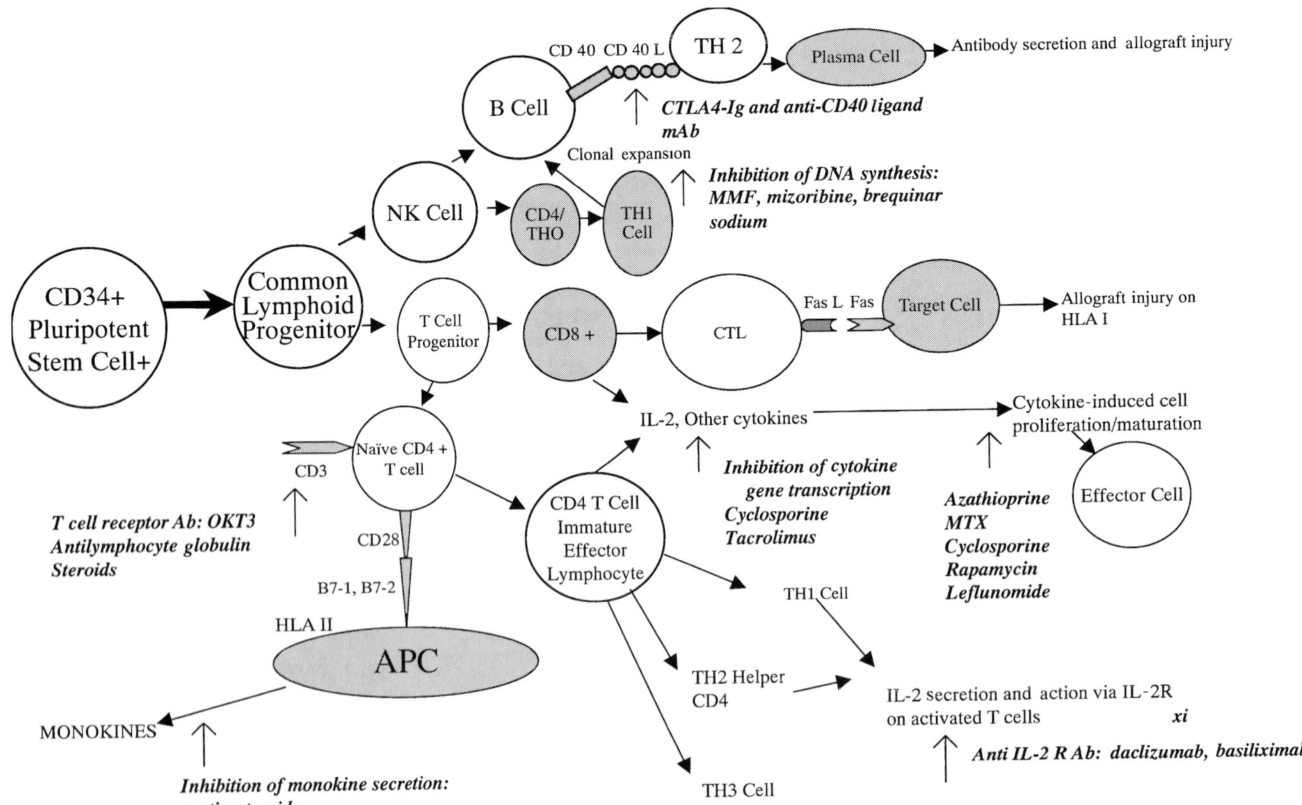

Figure 178–1. Sites of action of common immunosuppressants and immune pathways during antigen-presenting cell (APC) and T cell interaction. IL = interleukin; MTX = methotrexate; DNA = deoxyribonucleic acid; MMF = mycophenolate mofetil.

STRATEGIES IN INDUCTION OF TRANSPLANT TOLERANCE

Various therapeutic strategies are either currently in clinical use or are undergoing laboratory tests. Their putative or known mechanisms of action (Fig. 178–1) are listed next:

1. Corticosteroids cause inhibition of monokine production by APCs.
2. OKT3, OKT4, OKT8, and antilymphocyte globulin (ALG) are T cell–receptor antibodies and act by blocking accessory molecules.
3. Immunosuppressive drugs
   a. Tacrolimus (Tac) and cyclosporine: calcineurin inhibitors inhibit cytokine gene transcription.
   b. Azathioprine (AZA), methotrexate, and cyclophosphamide are antiproliferative agents.
   c. Rapamycin (RPM, Sirolimus) and leflunomide inhibit cytokine action.
   d. Mycophenolate mofetil (MMF), mizorabine, and brequinar sodium inhibit DNA synthesis.
4. Allotrap peptides to limit APC–T cell interactions bind with MHC class II complex to limit its interaction with T cells.
5. Direct treatment with T_H2 cytokines IL-10, transforming growth factor beta (TGF-β), and IL-13 to limit T_H1 response.
6. Donor-specific blood transfusion and donor bone marrow infusion promote immunomodulation and enhancement of microchimerism.
7. CD95 (Fas or Apo-1) ligand mediates immunosuppression to target activated effector T cells.
8. IL-10– and TGF-β–directed gene therapy to the graft site via retroviral vectors causes down-regulation of MHC class II receptors and activation and growth of T_H1 cells.
9. Co-stimulatory blockade
   a. Cytotoxic T lymphocyte antigen 4 (CTLA4-Ig) and anti-CD40 ligand are chimeric fusion proteins that block co-stimulation of APC and CD4 T cells.
   b. Anti-B7.1 and anti-B7.2 antibodies block signal I co-stimulation.
10. Monoclonal antibody therapy
    a. Anticytokine antibodies (anti–IL-2 and anti–TNF-α).
    b. Anticytokine receptor antibodies, including anti-TNF, anti–IL-1, and anti–IL-2 receptor (IL-2R) antibodies. Anti–IL-2R antibodies, daclizumab (Zenapax), and basiliximab (Simulect) are directed against the alpha subunit (CD25) of IL-2R, whereas AG 490 is directed against the gamma subunit of IL-2R
    c. Anti–intracellular adhesion molecule (anti-ICAM) antibody (enlimonab), T1039 (anti–T cell receptor), anti–lymphocyte function antigen (LFA) (anti-CD11a, anti-CD18) are antibodies against adhesion molecules.
11. FTY 720 is directed against adhesion molecules on the surfaces of activated lymphocytes.
12. Antisense oligonucleotides against ICAM-1, when given at the time of organ retrieval, prevent lymphocyte binding to the allograft.

SPECIFIC AGENTS

Corticosteroids

Corticosteroids are used extensively in brief but high doses for the reversal of acute rejection episodes. They are also used extensively in clinical immunosuppression protocols for both induction and maintenance phases.[6] Four principal glucocorticosteroid compounds are used in transplantation: (1) hydrocortisone, (2) prednisone, (3) prednisolone, and (4) methylprednisolone.

Because hydrocortisone has the most pronounced mineralocorticoid activity per unit of glucocorticoid activity, its routine application in transplantation has been relatively limited. The three other agents have more glucocorticoid activity in proportion to their mineralocorticoid activity.

Prednisone has oral bioavailability of about 80% and is metabolized in the liver to its active form, prednisolone. Oral prednisolone has bioavailability of 100%. The serum half-life of both prednisone and methylprednisolone is about 2 to 3 hours[7]; however, suppression of cytokine production persists for 24 hours or more.

There is no universally accepted dosing regimen. Rather, the dose is often dictated by local preference. In one study by Tornatore and coworkers, threefold variation in methylprednisolone clearance and twofold range in the volume of distribution in kidney transplant recipients during the early post-transplant period was noted.[7] This suggests that anything short of pharmacokinetic guidance for corticosteroid dosing is essentially empiric. A preoperative dose of 250 to 1000 mg may be given, followed by 20 to 200 mg/day during the first week. Acute rejection may be treated with one to three large doses—250 mg to 1 g IV methylprednisolone—or by a regimen started at 200 mg/day and tapered to baseline maintenance doses over 3 to 6 days. There is evidence that doses smaller than those traditionally used may be equally effective. In combination regimens, steroid doses can often be reduced to 10 or 20 mg/day or less and perhaps given every other day.

Corticosteroids have broad effects on many cell types. They interfere with the production of IL-1 and IL-2, blocking the early steps of T cell activation. Other immune system effects include:

1. Antagonism of inflammatory mechanisms by stabilization of leukocyte lysosomal membranes, decreased capillary permeability, and inhibition of histamine release and the kinin and complement systems.
2. Drastic reductions of lymphocyte traffic and circulating immunoglobulin levels and reductions in numbers of neutrophils and eosinophils.
3. Inhibition of leukocyte adhesion to endothelium.

Prednisone and prednisolone have much less mineralocorticoid activity than the naturally occurring glucocorticoids; however, sodium retention, edema, hypertension, potassium loss, and hypokalemic alkalosis can be associated with prolonged use of these drugs. Suppression of the hypothalamic-pituitary-adrenal axis can occur with all steroids, but it varies among patients. Acute adrenal insufficiency can develop unexpectedly when the patient is stressed, even as long as 12 months after steroids are withdrawn.

Unfortunately, the adverse effects of corticosteroids are many and cause considerable morbidity. An increased incidence of serious infections is well documented. Impaired fibroblast growth and collagen synthesis contribute to poor wound healing; thus, surgical wounds and anastomoses are at increased risk, and gastrointestinal (GI) ulcers tend to heal slowly, which places the patient at increased risk of perforation and rebleeding. Spontaneous GI tract ulceration occurs in approximately 2% of patients taking steroids. Because signs of inflammation are suppressed, the diagnosis of intra-abdominal infection and peritonitis can be significantly delayed, sometimes with disastrous consequences. Decompensation of glucose tolerance is often dramatic. Generalized protein catabolism and bone demineralization can produce a debilitated state. Atherosclerosis may be accelerated. The risks of cataract and of increased intraocular pressure (glaucoma) are increased. Central nervous system effects such as euphoria and mood swings are well known. Soft-tissue and dermal changes such as fat redistribution, skin atrophy, "moon face," and striae produce the characteristic cushingoid appearance.

Cytotoxic Drugs

Agents commonly used for immunosuppression in transplantation include antimetabolites such as azathioprine (AZA), and alkylating agents such as cyclophosphamide (CPM). AZA, a thio analog of the purine adenine, inhibits purine metabolism. Purines are required for deoxyribonucleic acid (DNA) and ribonucleic acid (RNA) synthesis. Also, AZA can be incorporated into DNA in place of natural purines. The altered DNA molecule does not function properly, allowing strand breaks in the chromosomes. Thus, not surprisingly, AZA is most toxic to proliferating cells that are making new DNA. In contrast, CPM nonspecifically damages cellular macromolecules by alkylating them, particularly DNA. Thus, CPM is toxic to both resting and dividing cells.

The precise mechanism of immunosuppression mediated by cytotoxic drugs is not known; however, the antiproliferative effects on lymphocytes are believed to inhibit generation of antigen-specific T cell clones. As one would expect, an increased risk of malignancies with the long-term use of these agents is a concern.

Azathioprine

AZA can be used in maintenance immunosuppressive regimens. It has no use in the treatment of acute rejection episodes.[8] Its oral bioavailability is about 40%. Metabolism of AZA is complex. The parent drug is inactive, but it is rapidly converted to several metabolites.[9] Thio-inosinic acid is an inhibitor of purine synthesis. The 6-thioguanine nucleotides (TGN) are known to become incorporated into DNA. TGN has a very long tissue half-life, perhaps on the order of 13 days. On this basis, once-daily dosing is logical. The inactive end metabolite is 6-thiouric acid, which is excreted by the kidneys. With congenital deficiency of the enzyme thiopurine methyltransferase (incidence one in 300 patients) or renal failure, accumulation of TGN causes increased toxicity. The drug is usually given orally. The starting dose is between 3 and 5 mg/kg once daily by mouth. For brief periods, it can be given intravenously at half the dose. Typical maintenance oral dosage after transplantation is 2 to 3 mg/kg/day. Tapering to 1 to 2 mg/kg/day is often possible as time goes on. In combination regimens, AZA can be reduced to 0.25 to 0.5 mg/kg/day.

Dose-limiting myelosuppression usually occurs 1 to 2 weeks into therapy. Pancytopenia and thrombocytopenia with megaloblastic anemia are the usual patterns. White blood cell counts below 3000 cells/mm^3 warrant discontinuation of the drug or dose reduction. As with other antiproliferative drugs, nausea, vomiting, and hair loss may occur. Hepatic injury can occur in one of two patterns: a reversible hepatitis or a rare but serious hepatic veno-occlusive disease that can cause irreversible damage. AZA therapy has also been associated with increased risk of pancreatitis, which is believed to be due to a hypersensitivity reaction. The role of AZA, however, has been questioned in both of these.[10, 11] Hypersensitivity to AZA has been reported to cause a variety of manifestations. Diagnosis of these disorders has been based largely on clinical findings.

Allopurinol inhibits xanthine oxidase, one of the enzymes involved in degradation of AZA metabolites, and can increase its toxicity. Allopurinol should be added cautiously to an immunosuppressive regimen containing AZA. When allopurinol must be used, reduction (by more than 50%) of AZA doses should be implemented.

Cyclophosphamide

CPM (Cytoxan) has been used in place of AZA, particularly when AZA-associated hepatitis is suspected. CPM is also the most widely used preparatory treatment for bone marrow recipients. It is useful in large doses to incapacitate the recipient's immune system and to prevent rejection of grafted marrow and as effective chemotherapy for neoplastic diseases that require marrow transplantation.

Oral CPM is absorbed efficiently (87% to 96%); concentrations peak in 1 hour.[12] CPM is activated on metabolism in the liver. Several metabolites are formed. The ultimately active metabolite, phosphoramide mustard, is eliminated by spontaneous hydrolysis and has an intracellular half-life of 40 to 50 minutes. Blood half-life is about 5 to 7 hours. Neither impaired renal function nor liver failure requires dose adjustment. CPM is removed by hemodialysis. CPM used in transplant regimens is administered in small doses (3 to 5 mg/kg/day), significantly smaller than the 60-mg/kg/day doses used for chemotherapy.

As with all antiproliferative agents, patients can experience nausea, vomiting, and hair loss. Hemorrhagic cystitis is a well-known side effect of CPM, but the reported incidence is very variable (0.5% to 40%). Cystitis can be limited by giving thiosulfate or, apparently just as good, by providing aggressive hydration.

Side effects are considerably more common and serious with the large-dose therapy used for bone marrow transplantation. Virtually all patients taking these large doses experience nausea, vomiting, and hair loss. As many as 15% of them experience clinically significant cardiac dysfunction. Infertility has also been associated with such doses. The side effects generally are not seen in solid organ transplant recipients, who take much smaller doses. CPM levels or effects can be increased by allopurinol or cimetidine, but not ranitidine. CPM potentiates the effects of succinylcholine.

Cytokine-Suppressive Agents

When a T lymphocyte is activated by antigen, a coordinated program of multiple gene activations is set in motion that eventuates in proliferation of the activated cell. Cyclosporine blocks the transcription of 10 genes of at least 60 that are activated. These include IL-2, IL-3, and IL-4, granulocyte-macrophage colony-stimulating factor (GM-CSF), and interferon gamma. The inhibition of the production of IL-2, which acts as a potent T cell growth factor, is likely the key effect, and it has been documented extensively. The drug is known to block activation of the IL-2 gene, ultimately preventing synthesis of IL-2. At this level, both cyclosporine and tacrolimus act alike; further, they both interfere with the binding of specific transcription factors to the promoter (control region) of the IL-2 gene, preventing RNA synthesis.

The occurrence of cyclosporine-like substances appears to be remarkably universal—and evolutionarily conserved. Specific receptors for cyclosporine are present in most cells. They have even been observed in a wide range of cell types in plants. As these drugs are studied in greater detail, it becomes clear that they have multiple effects on many processes in lymphocytes and other cells.

Cyclosporine

Before the introduction of cyclosporine (Sandimmune, Neoral), immunosuppression protocols relied heavily on steroids and cytotoxic drugs. These regimens had the disadvantage of producing broad suppression of the immune and inflammatory cascades. Cyclosporine introduced a new era of immunosuppression, being a potent, relatively T cell-specific, noncytotoxic suppressor of T cell activation.

Cyclosporine is a cyclic polypeptide of 11 amino acids and molecular weight of 1202 daltons. The drug is insoluble in water and thus must be dissolved in an organic solvent. Currently, two formulations are available: Sandimmune and Neoral. In both healthy volunteers and a variety of patient populations, absorption is substantially faster with Neoral than with Sandimmune: overall time to peak cyclosporine concentration (t_{max}) is reduced, peak concentrations (C_{max}) are higher, and area under the curve (AUC) is increased. The lipophilic nature of Sandimmune is responsible for its variable bioavailability.

Oral bioavailability is about 30%, but there is much individual variability (range, 10% to 60%). Small intestinal absorption decreases with bowel dysfunction or reduced bile flow.[14] The volume of distribution of cyclosporine is large and variable. Hepatic metabolism is the only significant elimination mechanism. Drug alteration occurs via the cytochrome P_{450} IIIA enzymes. With normal liver function the mean terminal half-life is 19 hours. At least 17 metabolites have been identified, and at least a few are immunosuppressive, although considerably less so than the parent compound. The half-life increases with hepatic failure and is changed significantly by co-administration of any of a large number of other drugs that can cause unexpected increases or decreases in serum levels, by induction or by competitive inhibition of P_{450}.[15] Many other drugs also potentiate cyclosporine's renal toxicity (Table 178–1). For all of these reasons, it is essential that levels be monitored regularly and dosage adjusted accordingly.

Monitoring cyclosporine levels is not without problems. Measuring it in blood or plasma with radioimmunoassay (RIA) and with high-pressure liquid chromatography (HPLC) give different results. No method is clearly superior; thus, there are no universally accepted standard blood levels, and target levels may vary much from center to center. Depending on the mode of testing[16] desired levels are roughly these: by RIA in serum or plasma, 150 to 250 ng/mL at the time of transplantation, tapered to 50 to 100 ng/mL after 3 to 6 months; by HPLC in whole blood, 100 to 300 ng/mL initially, tapered to 80 to 200 ng/mL.

Typically cyclosporine administration is begun 12 to 24 hours before heart or kidney transplantation and just after liver graft reperfusion. A typical dose is 4 to 5 mg/kg/day IV. This amount can be given in two doses, each over 2 to 6 hours. Alternatively, some prefer to use slow, continuous infusion over 24 hours. The changeover to oral dosing usually requires a dose three times larger (i.e., about 12 to 15 mg/kg/day). After 1 to 2 weeks, the dose can be slowly tapered as a result of equilibration within body fat stores. Many patients' dose is tapered to as little as 3 mg/kg/day by 6 months after transplantation. Liver transplant recipients who have a T tube, which diverts some bile flow, require larger oral doses because of decreased absorption. In addition, pediatric patients require 50% to 100% larger doses, weight for weight, than adults.

TABLE 178–1. Drugs That Alter Cyclosporine Concentrations

Increase	Decrease
Diltiazem	Rifampin
Nicardipine	Carbamazepine
Verapamil	Phenobarbital
Fluconazole	Phenytoin
Itraconazole	Ticlopidine
Ketoconazole	Nafcillin
Clarithromycin	Octreotide
Erythromycin	Isoniazid
Tacrolimus	
Methylprednisolone (in large doses)	
Bromocriptine	
Danazol	

Several adverse effects are seen early with the administration of cyclosporine. Significant acute nephrotoxicity and hypertension, probably resulting from vasoconstrictive effects on the afferent arterioles of the kidney, is a major problem.[17] The mechanism of this effect is under debate.[18, 19] This nephrotoxicity is transient and is reversible by reducing the dose or discontinuing the drug.[20] The incidence of nephrotoxicity varies from approximately 25% to 32%, 37%, and 38%, respectively, in kidney, heart, and liver transplant recipients.[21] Hypertension occurs frequently and within weeks of commencing therapy. The incidence of hypertension varies much in different patient populations, between 10% and 80%.[21] It is hypothesized that this is due to a vasoconstrictive effect of cyclosporine in both the renal and systemic circulations,[22] perhaps the result of antagonism of endothelium-derived relaxation factors or increased synthesis of endothelin, a vasoconstrictor. Physiologically, the hypertension is responsive to sodium restriction; therapies incorporating diuretics or calcium channel blockers have been advocated.[19] Minor neurotoxicity (tremor) is common (prevalence 10% to 55%) and sometimes abates over time without a change in therapy.

More severe symptoms, such as seizures and encephalopathy, have also been associated with cyclosporine, but often it is not clear whether the association is causal.[23] Several reports detail a rare syndrome of confusion and cortical blindness in both liver and bone marrow transplant recipients. Hypomagnesemia and hypocholesterolemia are believed to be risk factors for cyclosporine neurotoxicity.[18] Cyclosporine is diabetogenic, although analysis of this effect is confounded by the frequent intercurrent use of steroids with cyclosporine. Other metabolic effects include hypochloremic alkalosis and changes in serum potassium, magnesium, prolactin, and testosterone values. Hepatotoxicity, manifested by an increased cholestatic profile, may be quite common,[18] but a reduction in dosage often improves this effect, and it does not appear to be a major problem. Connective tissue side effects are common and can be distressing to the patient. These include hirsutism, seen over 2 to 4 weeks in 20% to 45%, gingival hyperplasia in 4% to 16%, and coarsening of facial features.[24]

Long-term administration of cyclosporine has been associated with a nonreversible nephrotoxicity. The incidence is estimated at 15% to 40%.[25] The pathologic lesion resembles nephrosclerosis.[26]

Neoral, a microemulsion formulation of cyclosporine, has superior pharmacokinetics, does not require bile excretion for bioavailability, and is better dispersed and absorbed than Sandimmune. The relative bioavailability of Neoral, as compared with that of Sandimmune, is increased between 74% and 139%.[27] The total AUC is increased by 30%.[28] The results presented at the International Neoral advisory consensus in Vancouver in November 1997 reported that the most sensitive predictor of cyclosporine outcome in patients was the AUC value to guide therapeutic monitoring of Neoral. Neoral simplifies the management of cyclosporine therapy, is easily dispersed, and has pharmacokinetic advantages over Sandimmune in both adult and pediatric transplantation.

Tacrolimus

Tacrolimus, Prograf [Fujisawa Pharmaceutical, Osaka, Japan], a new immunosuppressive agent, is a macrolide antibiotic produced by the fungus *Streptomyces tsukubaensis*. The Food and Drug Administration (FDA) approved Tac for use in liver transplantation in 1994 and for kidney transplantation in 1997. It is also used in small-bowel, pancreas, heart, and lung transplantation.

The molecular structure of Tac is not related to that of

cyclosporine, and the two drugs have different cytosolic binding sites.[29, 30] Although both inhibit T lymphocyte activation, there are functional differences in the two. Tac can be used to reverse ongoing, established rejection but cyclosporine cannot. Tac was first used for uncontrolled liver allograft rejection, which situation was considered treatment failure by conventional immunosuppression. The results of this experience revealed a marked ability to reverse ongoing rejection, even when chronic changes were observed in the allograft.[31-34] Between 50% and 70% of patients treated by conversion to Tac had both clinical and histopathologic responses. In a long-term follow-up of 113 patients with chronic rejection, 75% of patients were still alive 3 years after Tac conversion and 65% of liver allografts were still functioning.[34]

The U.S. Multicenter FK-506 Liver Study Group analyzed the prognostic factors for successful conversion from cyclosporine to Tac-based immunosuppressive therapy for refractory rejection.[35] Ninety-one patients were converted from cyclosporine to Tac for chronic rejection. In this series, the 1- and 2-year actuarial patient survival rates after conversion were 84% and 81%, respectively. The corresponding actuarial graft survivals at 1 and 2 years were 70% and 49%.

Three randomized trials have been performed (a single-center study at the University of Pittsburgh and two others in both the United States and Europe), that compared Tac with cyclosporine in primary liver transplantation.[36-38] Although the immunosuppressive regimens in each trial had unique features, all studies revealed that the clinically relevant end points, including freedom from rejection and failure of the defined treatment to prevent and control rejection, findings favored Tac over cyclosporine.

Long-term follow-up (more than 2 years) revealed a modest increase in patient and graft survival in the Tac limb,[39, 40] and the good results in the cyclosporine limb were attributed in part to the ability of Tac to control rejection in the cyclosporine group.[41] In a comparison of transplant patients' half-lives, Tac-treated patients had a calculated half-life of 25.1 years, as compared with 15.2 years for cyclosporine-treated patients.[40] The freedom from rejection remained statistically greater in the Tac-treated group over all periods studied. In addition, patients treated with Tac did not have to use steroids, and they had lower rates of hypertension, hypercholesterolemia, and hypertriglyceridemia.

The application of FK-506 rescue to kidney transplantation was an extension of the experience gained in liver transplantation.[42, 43] The main difference between the two organ systems is the predominance of arteriopathy and sclerosis of epithelial structures in kidney allografts involved with effects of chronic rejection. This was found to limit the ability of Tac to rescue grafts so damaged. In a series of 169 patients with median follow-up of 37 months, 125 patients (74%) were successfully switched (mean serum creatinine of 2.3 mg/dL) with a reduction of corticosteroid doses from 28 to 8.5 mg/day.[42]

Based on encouraging pilot studies using Tac in kidney transplantation,[44] two subsequent United States and European multicenter randomized trials compared Tac-based immunosuppression to cyclosporine-based immunosuppression.[45, 46] Although the 1-year actuarial patient and graft survival rates for the Tac and cyclosporine regimens were roughly equivalent, the rejection rate in the Tac-based regimen was statistically significantly lower than that for the cyclosporine-based regimen.

Armitage and coworkers at the University of Pittsburgh reported their experience with Tac-based immunosuppression after heart transplantation.[47, 48] Tac was used as rescue therapy for eight patients suffering from persistent, refractory cardiac rejection with cyclosporine, AZA, and steroid treatment. While receiving cyclosporine therapy, all eight patients had received one or more courses of antilymphocyte therapy that failed. In keeping with previous experiences with rescue therapy, all of these patients had demonstrated improvement in the histopathologic appearance after Tac conversion. The U.S. Multicenter Study Group reported on Tac rescue for cyclosporine intolerance or rejection on cyclosporine for 16 heart transplant patients. Six-month patient and graft survivals were 100%, and the majority of recipients (60%) had one subsequent rejection or none.[49]

Seventy-two adult patients were given Tac as primary immunosuppression after heart transplantation.[48] The 1-year patient and graft survival rates were both 92%. The freedom from rejection at 90 days was 41% and at 180 days, 34%. Renal dysfunction was frequently noted, and the mean serum creatinine level 6 months after transplantation was 2.2 mg/dL. The incidence of diastolic hypertension was 54%, but this was considered mild: treatment consisted of a single agent in all cases. The incidence of new-onset diabetes was 20% in this group of patients.

Tac therapy has also been applied to pancreas allograft recipients. Acute rejection rates for recipients of simultaneous pancreas-kidney (SPK) transplants ranged from 64% to 100% under cyclosporine.[50-52] A recent multicenter retrospective report by Gruessner[53] analyzed 154 pancreas recipients (of isolated organs, organs received after previous kidney transplants, or SPKs) who were treated with Tac for induction and rescue therapy. Patient survival for SPK recipients was 90% at 6 months. Graft survival in the same time period was 87% with Tac and 70% with cyclosporine ($P = .04$). The incidence of first reversible episodes of acute rejection in the first 6 months under Tac therapy was 35%. Although this study is somewhat limited in length of follow-up, it shows that Tac seems to be associated with a low rate of graft loss from rejection, a high rate of graft salvage, and a very low rate of insulin-dependent diabetes mellitus. In addition, it demonstrated successful use of Tac in pancreas transplantation without the need for induction therapy.

Tac is not without limitations. Toxicity profiles for Tac are similar to those of cyclosporine, perhaps because of similar mechanisms of action (i.e., calcineurin inhibition). A detailed analysis and review of the adverse effects of Tac appear elsewhere.[54, 55] Both Tac and cyclosporine have been associated with side effects, many of which are similar and some of which are peculiar to a given organ.

Clearly, both cyclosporine and Tac are highly effective immunosuppressants; the ultimate deciding factor may be the respective side effects and toxicity of the two. Precise quantitation of Tac toxicity and comparison with cyclosporine are confounded by multiple factors. Early studies with Tac used doses that were too large. The complex and variable pharmacokinetics of Tac, like those of cyclosporine, make estimating appropriate doses difficult, and blood level monitoring is very important. Many technical difficulties in obtaining and interpreting Tac levels further complicated early use of the drug. These are gradually being resolved. As the drug is being used more, and as laboratory monitoring methods improve, a clearer picture will inevitably emerge.

Absorption of an oral dose of Tac varies from 5% to 67%. GI absorption of Tac depends less on bile flow compared with cyclosporine absorption; thus, there is no need to decrease the dose when the T tube is clamped after liver transplantation.[56] The drug is metabolized by the liver, and elimination is markedly slowed with liver dysfunction. In one study of liver transplant patients,[57] the half-life ranged from 3.5 to 40.5 hours. The volume of distribution also varied much—from 5.6 to 65 L per kilogram of body weight. Tac inhibits hepatic cytochrome P_{450} reductase, which metabolizes it, potentially decreasing its own metabolism and causing an increase in blood levels. The clinical importance of this phenomenon is not known. Inhibitors of P_{450} may increase Tac blood levels by suppressing cytochrome P_{450} activity. Conversely, inducers of P_{450} may decrease Tac levels. Because Tac can cause significant toxicity, frequent determinations of blood levels are crucial, particularly for patients with hepatic dysfunction.

Tac is started intravenously with a slow, continuous infusion over 24 hours.[57] The initial dose is 0.05 mg/kg/day for liver transplants, 0.10 mg/kg/day for kidney transplants, and 0.15 mg/kg/day for pancreas and small-bowel transplants. The intravenous drug is discontinued when the patient can take Tac by mouth. The oral dose is started at 0.15 mg/kg/day in two doses.[58] Subsequent dosing is modified to maintain Tac levels between 10 and 20 ng/mL by whole blood monitoring. Tac has nephrotoxic potential, and the degree of its expression depends on other factors, such as use of other nephrotoxic drugs, pretransplant renal function, and factors associated with the development of acute tubular necrosis (ATN), such as hypotension. The mechanism is not yet clear. Increased endothelin synthesis may play a role.[59] Early studies suggest that this effect reverses with dose reduction or switching to the oral route, or both.[60] The incidence of long-term renal injury with cyclosporine is not known. Hypertension appears to be about half as common with Tac as with cyclosporine.[58]

Neurotoxicity of Tac appears comparable to that of cyclosporine; both minor and major toxic effects are seen.[61] Minor toxicity, such as tremor, insomnia, and dysesthesias, is common and, as with cyclosporine, is seen in about 20% to 30% of patients. Major toxicity, such as encephalopathy that can progress to coma, seizures, psychosis, and other neurologic deficits, is less common; estimated prevalences are 3% to 5%, depending on the organ being transplanted. Patients are particularly prone to major neurotoxicity after liver transplantation, (approximately 8%), but not after heart, lung, or kidney transplantation.

GI side effects—diarrhea, anorexia, bloating, flatulence—are similar to those seen with cyclosporine. Some investigators have regarded Tac as more diabetogenic than cyclosporine; however, a report from the University of Pittsburgh showed that 3 years after pancreas transplantation Tac was no more diabetogenic than was cyclosporine. Both drugs inhibit insulin release in a rat model. Hyperkalemia, sometimes severe enough to prompt the use of fludrocortisone acetate (Florinef), has been noted with Tac[53] and is a recognized side effect of cyclosporine. One of the major advantages of Tac appears to be the smaller corticosteroid doses.

Tac is tolerated well in pregnancy. Pregnancy in "liver-transplanted" mothers was possible with Tac medication and was associated with surprisingly low rates of hypertension, pre-eclampsia, and other maternal complications historically associated with such gestations. Preterm deliveries were common; however, fetal growth for gestational age and infant growth for postpartum age values were normal.[62]

There are many ways to measure Tac levels. The first one described used enzyme-linked immunosorbent assay with solid-phase extraction in plasma.[63] The turnaround time for Tac levels is between 24 and 48 hours. The drug is trapped in high concentration inside red blood cells in a temperature-dependent fashion. Thus, whole blood levels can be eight to 10 times higher than plasma levels, and there is much variability (3.6 to 39 ng/mL).[56] Somewhat higher, more consistent plasma levels can be obtained by equilibration of the sample at 37°C before analysis. HPLC and mass spectroscopy are being investigated, as is the use of whole blood. One study of whole blood versus plasma showed that whole blood levels were more stable than were plasma levels and more reliably elevated with nephrotoxicity.

Mycophenolate Mofetil

MMF (RS-61443, CellCept Syntex Research, Palo Alto) is an analog of mycophenolic acid and an immunosuppression agent[64] with enhanced oral bioavailability.[65] Like mycophenolic acid, MMF noncompetitively inhibits inosine monophosphate dehydrogenase (IMPDH) and guanosine monophosphate (GMP) synthetase, both key enzymes that regulate the purine nucleotide salvage pathway.[66] As compared with resting lymphocytes, activated T or B cells exhibit marked increases in IMPDH and in production of guanine nucleotides, which are essential for nucleic acid and protein synthesis, and cause accumulation of cells at the G1-S interface of the cell cycle. Thus, in vitro it has inhibitory effects on both B and T lymphocytes.[67] Mycophenolic acid (MPA) may also interfere with the expression of adhesion molecules on leukocytes.

MPA initially was used to treat refractory psoriasis.[68] This drug was tolerated relatively well, the principal side effects being leukopenia, mucositis, and GI upset. Patients reportedly had a higher than normal incidence of upper respiratory tract infections, and, over the long term, more skin cancers.

MMF has also been studied in clinical trials as primary therapy, along with cyclosporine and steroids, for kidney transplantation and for rescue therapy for refractory organ rejection.[69] Findings suggested that this drug is tolerated relatively well in doses up to 3.5 to 4.0 g/day. Several rescue studies have suggested that MMF is capable of stabilizing or reversing ongoing rejection in as many as 80% of cases when added to cyclosporine-based immunosuppression.

MMF has been approved by the FDA as an agent to prevent rejection of kidney transplants. Three multicenter, prospective, double-blind trials,[70-72] in addition to other trials,[69, 73] showed a reduction of approximately 40% in episodes of acute rejection. MMF administration in doses of 2 to 3 g/day, in combination with maintenance cyclosporine and corticosteroids as triple therapy after antithymocyte gamma globulin (ATGAM) induction therapy, has been more effective than an otherwise identical regimen that includes AZA instead of MMF in preventing acute allograft rejection in first-time cadaver kidney recipients.

MMF significantly reduced the rates of biopsy-proven rejection and other treatment failures during the first 6 months after renal transplantation and was tolerated well. MMF administered in combination with pulsed corticosteroids significantly decreases the subsequent use of antilymphocyte therapy to treat acute rejection of a first renal allograft. Although graft and patient survivals were initially similar, by 2 and 3 years the groups that received MMF were beginning to show a long-term advantage.[74]

Another trial[75] using Tac plus MMF plus steroids or Tac plus steroids after OKT3 induction regimens revealed a significantly lower incidence (10% versus 20%) of rejection in the first 6 months in the triple-therapy group. Although actuarial patient and graft survival rates at 1 year were not statistically significant, this combination in another study had significant GI tract or hematopoietic side effects that required a 30% reduction in dose.[76]

MMF has been used[73] to treat acute episodes of liver rejection that are resistant to cyclosporine, AZA, prednisolone, *and* OKT3. There was a 91% response rate, and two thirds of these patients showed resolution of rejection. MMF had no effect on chronic rejection. Other studies suggest that MMF may be useful for treating or preventing acute and chronic rejection of liver allografts.[77]

MMF has also been used as rescue therapy for acute and chronic rejection of cardiac transplants.[78] A randomized trial[79] in heart transplant recipients demonstrated a lower incidence of rejection, improved survival, and larger coronary artery luminal area in those who received MMF as compared with those who received AZA. The incidence of rejection decreased significantly ($P < .0001$) after MMF treatment. MMF trough levels (>3 μg/mL) seem to correlate directly with a markedly decreased incidence of rejection.

MMF has been used in combination with Tac in both kidney[75] and liver[76] transplantation. The mean daily dose of Tac was significantly lower in the triple-therapy group as compared with the Tac-plus-steroid group, and the actuarial patient survival rates at 1 year were 98% and 96%, respectively, in the two groups in first study. In the latter study the 2-year patient and liver graft survivals were 83% and 76% for the double-therapy and 85% and 78% for the triple-therapy group.

MMF is cleared more quickly in children than in adults. Consequently, children do better with thrice-daily dosing than with the twice-daily dosing used for adults.[80] MMF is considered to be a safe alternative to AZA as it does not cause hepatotoxicity or myelotoxicity. Side effects reported with MMF predominantly include GI disturbances—gastritis, ileus, nausea, and vomiting. No significant nephrotoxicity or hepatotoxicity has been reported.

Other Agents

Rapamycin

Rapamycin (RPM, Sirolimus) is a macrolide antibiotic that is structurally related to Tac. It binds to FKBP-12 but does not inhibit cytokine gene transcription in T cells. It blocks signals transduced to the nucleus from the IL-2 receptor and other growth factors by acting on phosphatidylinositol kinases called *targets of rapamycin* (Tor1p and Tor2p). It also inactivates p70S6 kinase, resulting in selective inhibition of the synthesis of new ribosomal proteins and prolonging cell cycle progression from G1 to G2. Thus, the mechanism of action differs significantly from that of either Tac or cyclosporine, as RPM does not block transcription of cytokine messenger RNA but, rather, inhibits the translation in RNAs. The use of rapamycin (RPM) for clinical immunosuppression is under investigation.[81-83]

The drug is clearly an extraordinarily potent immunosuppressant. It inhibits DTH and both B and T cell responses to alloantigen. In animal models, RPM prolongs survival of MHC-incompatible grafts and can arrest ongoing rejection. There is evidence that the drug may be synergistic with cyclosporine, and perhaps additive with Tac, although under some conditions RPM and Tac are antagonistic.[83]

RPM has poor bioavailability when taken by mouth. Very low plasma levels (currently below detection) are therapeutic. Drug delivery, stability, and monitoring remain problematic and must be resolved before RPM can be introduced for human use. RPM has been used in phase I, II, and III trials for maintenance and treatment of acute rejection. These studies have shown significant reduction in acute rejection when RPM is used in combination with cyclosporine.[84] A prospective, randomized, double-blind, double-dummy, multicenter clinical trial compared the safety and efficacy of RPM (2 to 5 mg/day) to those of AZA (2 to 3 mg/kg/day) added to an immunosuppressive regimen of cyclosporine and corticosteroids in recipients of primary cadaver or mismatched living donor renal allografts. Overall patient and graft survival were both 98% on the RPM regimen.[84] SDZ RAD, a new rapamycin derivative currently under phase I evaluation, is being introduced and is expected to overcome the wide interindividual pharmacokinetic variations associated with oral administration.[85]

The side effects with RPM include GI disturbances, diabetes mellitus, myocardial necrosis, and testicular atrophy. When RPM is given in combination with cyclosporine-based immunosuppression, significant elevations in serum cholesterol and triglyceride levels have also been reported.[86]

Deoxyspergualin

Deoxyspergualin (DSG), a semisynthetic analog of spergualin, acts by disrupting antigen processing and antigen presentation by APCs. It has been used successfully as first-line treatment for steroid-resistant acute rejection in three living related liver transplant recipients.[87] DSG was discovered in Japan by a drug development program investigating antitumor agents.[88-91] The drug was very active against lymphoid tumors and later was found to be immunosuppressive. The molecular basis for the action of DSG is unknown, but it appears to be different from that of all previously known immunosuppressing drugs and may block alloantigen presentation on APCs. DSG has performed well in animal models of xenograft transplantation and did better than Tac or cyclosporine. In a human trial[88] with one haplotype-matched renal transplant, the incidence of accelerated rejection was significantly decreased when DSG was combined with cyclosporine.

The drug must be given intravenously. In renal transplant patients, the half-life varied between 39 and 55 hours, about twice that reported from earlier studies in cancer patients. In a clinical trial DSG was used to reverse rejection in doses ranging from 80 to 220 mg/m²/day. The optimal dose appeared to be 180 mg/m²/day. In a small comparative study, the drug appeared similar in efficacy to OKT3 for reversing steroid-resistant rejection.[92] In other studies of DSG in combination with AZA, cyclosporine, and steroids for maintenance of immunosuppression, the dosage was 3 to 5 mg/kg/day.

Toxicity is decreased by slow infusion over 4 to 5 hours. Transplant recipients exhibited toxicity in the central nervous system (facial dysesthesias) and GI tract (anorexia, nausea), reversible bone marrow suppression (lymphocytes and thrombocytes), and reversible hypotension. Reversible bone marrow suppression appears to be the most significant side effect.

Leflunomide

After administration, leflunomide is converted to an active metabolite, butenamide. It inhibits proliferation of T and B lymphocytes and smooth muscle cells by inhibiting either T cell receptor or cytokine receptor–associated tyrosine kinase activity. It was tolerated well by patients in phase II trials for rheumatoid arthritis and holds promise as an effective immunosuppressant in clinical islet cell transplantation.[93]

Mizoribine

Mizoribine (MZB, Bredinin), an imidazole nucleotide antibiotic, undergoes phosphorylation to effect the inhibition of both inosine 5-monophosphate dehydrogenase and guanosine 5-monophosphate synthetase during purine synthesis.[94] It inhibits RNA and DNA synthesis, thus inhibiting both humoral and cellular immune responses. Limited clinical trials using mizoribine in place of AZA and with cyclosporine and steroids have shown decreasing rates of graft loss to chronic rejection after renal transplantation.[95]

MZB has been used as a maintenance agent in combination with cyclosporine and steroids, principally in renal transplant patients.[96] The drug appears to have advantages over AZA, in particular less myelotoxicity and hepatotoxicity.[97]

The drug is administered once daily in oral doses of 50 to 300 mg. With a normal GI tract, peak blood levels are achieved 2 to 3 hours after oral dosing. Absorption of MZB is delayed in the presence of GI disease. The major elimination pathway of MZB is renal. There is little hepatic metabolism, and 85% of a dose is excreted unchanged in the urine. Clearance of the drug is thus markedly affected by renal failure. In 26 kidney transplant patients with an average creatinine clearance rate of 50 mL/min (range, 22 to 93 mL/min), the half-life was 4 hours (range, 1.6 to 8.2 hours).

Brequinar

Brequinar (BQR) is an antimetabolite with broad antineoplastic activity that has been tested in humans with cancer.[98, 99] It is an inhibitor of dihydrorotate dehydrogenase, a mitochondrial enzyme that participates in the de novo synthesis pathway of pyrimidines. Dose-limiting toxicities include thrombocytopenia and severe desquamative dermatitis. The antiproliferative effects of the drug appear to be mediated by depletion of pyrimidine precursors needed for DNA and RNA synthesis. BQR was a potent immunosuppressant in a rat model[100] and appears to act synergistically, at least in vitro, with cyclosporine and RPM.[101]

BIOLOGIC AGENTS

Antilymphocyte Antibodies

Antithymocyte Globulin and Anti-CD3 Monoclonal Antibody

Antilymphocyte antibodies[102–105] such as ALG were first produced by immunizing animals against purified lymphocyte preparations, producing multispecificity polyclonal antibodies. Antibodies that cross-reacted with other cellular molecules in blood were removed by extensive absorption to blood components. Because of variability among immunized animals, substantial amounts of ALG are pooled to produce a more homogeneous preparation. Many of the limitations of antithymocyte globulin (ATG, ATGAM) preparations were related to variability in potency; leukopenia, thrombocytopenia, and anemia associated with those products were due to contaminating antibodies. Hybridoma technology later allowed the development of single-specificity monoclonal antibodies (e.g., OKT3 [Orthoclone]) directed against one particular epitope of a single cell-surface molecule). These drugs are much more uniform, standardized, and potent.[106–108]

The place of immunoglobulin therapy in immunosuppressive regimens is in a state of flux. These agents were originally shown to be effective in reversing acute rejection. For this use, OKT3 is more effective than large doses of steroids. More recently, these agents have been introduced into some maintenance regimens.

The strategy of using antilymphocyte antibodies immediately after transplantation has been referred to as *prophylactic* or *induction therapy.* This practice is based on the idea that theoretically, early incapacitation of the immune system may reduce the likelihood of subsequent rejection. Claimed benefits are delayed onset of acute rejection, fewer episodes of rejection, and no significant increase in infectious complications in these studies.[109–110] The related concept of *sequential therapy* was introduced in response to the significant renal toxicity of cyclosporine observed in liver, heart, and kidney transplant recipients. The practice is to use antibody therapy in the first 1 to 2 weeks after transplantation in lieu of cyclosporine. It is during this period that renal injury is most likely to occur, from a variety of insults. Cyclosporine therapy is begun later. Proponents cite a reduced incidence of early renal dysfunction. The impact of this strategy on long-term renal function is much less clear.

This early intensification of immunosuppression is not universally accepted. Some voice concern over the well-known associations of antilymphocyte antibody therapy and immunosuppression in general with infection and malignancy.[111, 112] Others describe no benefit, greater expense,[113] or successful use of regimens that avoid induction altogether.[114] Compromise strategies involve using prophylaxis only in high-risk patients and use of one dose of OKT3, followed by early evaluation of renal function; antibody is discontinued unless ATN is imminent.[115]

Immunoglobulin therapy is given either intravenously or intramuscularly. Equine ATG is given in the dose range of 10 to 15 mg/kg/day in a single dose. Therapy of acute rejection is usually continued for 14 days. With OKT3, the dose of 5 mg/day for 10 to 14 days is typical. Prophylactic OKT3 regimens use the same dose, usually for 7 to 10 days. Polyclonal preparations cause a high incidence of febrile reactions with the first few doses. Antihistamines, antipyretics, and sometimes steroids are given as premedication. Because the antibodies react with other blood cells, leukopenia (~14%) and thrombocytopenia (~30%) are seen. Anaphylaxis occurs in fewer than 1%. Nonetheless, a skin test is recommended beforehand. Skin rash is fairly common (10% to 30%).

OKT3 is by far the most extensively studied of the monoclonal antibodies. With the first one or two doses there is profuse intravascular release of cytokines by lymphocytes. This *first-dose effect* frequently causes fever, chills, tachycardia, GI tract disturbances, bronchospasm, and elevation or depression of blood pressure. These effects can largely be blocked by pretreatment with a 1-g IV bolus of methylprednisolone given 15 to 60 minutes before OKT3 infusion.[116]

Individuals vary in the amount of endogenous antibody they form against the mouse antibody. Intermediate and high-titer responders form a significant titer of blocking antibodies. This antibody production can be decreased by continuing other immunosuppressant therapy during administration of monoclonal antibody. Repeated treatment often succeeds when larger doses of antibody are used for subsequent courses. Those who produce the very highest antibody titers, probably about 5% to 20% of patients, fail to respond even to increased-dose therapy. Some advocate monitoring of CD3+ cell counts with flow cytometry for patients on OKT3. If CD3+ cells reach 10%, it is recommended either that the dose of OKT3 be increased (to as much as 15 mg/day) or that treatment be discontinued. Others suggest monitoring anti-OKT3 antibody titers.

Antibodies to surface molecules on lymphocytes interfere with lymphocyte function in the immune response by several possible mechanisms. Lymphocytes are known to be removed from the circulation rapidly after treatment with antilymphocyte antibodies and to be phenotypically and functionally altered. Treatment with OKT3 (anti-CD3 specific for CD3, a protein closely associated with the TCR complex) modulates the CD3-TCR complex, causing co-capping and internalization of the complex. After the initial disappearance of cells bearing the target molecule, those lymphocytes that reappear do not display the molecule on the surface, despite the fact that they are capable of producing it, unless OKT3 therapy is halted for at least 48 hours. Obviously, lymphocytes that pack the antigen receptor cannot react to antigen.

The potent suppression of T lymphocyte populations is known to be associated with increased rates of viral infection and lymphoproliferative disorders. It is not clear whether antibody therapy is any worse than other immunosuppression strategies in this regard. Some evidence suggests that problems arise because antibodies are used too long, when treatment of refractory rejection is begun too late in the course, or when the immunosuppression burden is already high.

Anti–IL-2 Receptor Monoclonal Antibodies

Anti–IL-2R and monoclonal antibodies have been used in clinical trials in Europe and the United States in combination with conventional immunosuppressive agents. Preliminary results have shown promising results in renal transplantation. T cell activation is initiated when appropriately processed and presented antigen interacts with the 90-kD polymorphic heterodimeric T cell surface receptor for the specific antigen. This is followed by the expression of IL-2 and high-affinity IL-2R by the T cell. IL-2 exerts its effects on T lymphocytes by binding to the IL-2R. The IL-2R is composed of three discrete membrane components: the alpha chain (T cell activation antigen or Tac), the beta chain, and the gamma chain. The genes that encode these receptors have been cloned and characterized.

The first murine monoclonal IgG2a (murine anti-Tac [MAT]) was found to bind to IL-2Ra based on its ability to bind to activated human T cells but not to resting T cells. Kirkman and coworkers[117] showed that treating mice with murine anti–IL-2R antibody (either M7/20 or AMT-13) prolongs cardiac allograft survival in experimental models. Kupiec-Weglinski and associates[118] reported similar results for another anti-IL-R antibody (ART18). Reed and colleagues[119] demonstrated that administration of MAT significantly prolonged the survival of renal allografts in cynomolgus monkeys.

Whereas animal studies demonstrated the efficacy of IL-2R antibodies, results of clinical trials were quite variable. Kirkman and associates[120] established that adding MAT to standard immunosuppressive treatment (with reduced cyclosporine but same doses of azathioprine and prednisone) in renal transplant patients significantly prolonged the time to first rejection (from 7.6 ± 6.3 days to 12.5 ± 6.3 days), but there were no differences in actual or actuarial graft or patient survivals between the two groups. The principal limitation of MAT is its immunogenicity, which quickly rendered this therapy ineffective.

Daclizumab

Daclizumab (Zenapax) is a unique hybrid monoclonal antibody, the variable region (binding site for the IL-2Ra) of which is retained as murine, whereas the remainder of the immunoglobulin molecule is human (IgG1). Only 10% of the hybrid molecule is of murine origin. This results in a milder immune response to the foreign protein and a longer half-life.

In a multi-institutional trial looking at the influence of IL-2 receptor blockade in renal transplantation, Vincenti and coworkers[121] showed that daclizumab prophylaxis, together with standard immunosuppressive treatment with cyclosporine, prednisone, and AZA, resulted in a significant reduction in the incidence of biopsy-documented acute rejection during the first 6 months (22%, versus 35% in the placebo group). The proportion of patients with presumptive or biopsy-confirmed acute rejection and the number of rejection episodes per patient were also lower in the daclizumab group, and the time to first rejection was longer. Daclizumab was not associated with any immediate side effects. The patient survival rates at 1 year were 98% for the daclizumab group and 96% for the placebo group. The 1-year graft survival rates in the daclizumab and placebo groups were 95% and 90%, respectively. This humanized anti-Tac (HAT), given in doses of 1 mg/kg every other week for a total of five weeks, may provide therapeutic HAT concentration levels and result in good saturation of Tac receptors for at least 12 weeks after transplantation. Its long serum half-life (20 days) and lack of immunization could make it a very useful immunosuppressive drug.[122] It was recently approved by the FDA for prophylaxis in primary kidney transplantation.

Basiliximab

Basiliximab (Simulect) is a chimeric anti-IL-2 receptor antibody with a mechanism of action similar to that of daclizumab. Unlike daclizumab, this hybrid monoclonal antibody is produced in vitro by continuous culture fermentation of a murine myeloma cell line transfected with plasmid-borne recombinant gene constructs that code for murine variable regions and human constant (C) regions. The resulting monoclonal antibody has even fewer murine amino acid sequences than daclizumab.

In clinical trials reported by Kovarik's group, basiliximab was tolerated well and produced no evidence of the cytokine-release syndrome, hypersensitivity reactions, or anti-idiotype antibody response in primary cadaver kidney recipients given steroids, AZA, and cyclosporine immunosuppression.[123] In one European trial, it was established that prophylaxis with a total of 40 mg of basiliximab reduces the incidence of acute rejection episodes significantly and produces no clinically relevant safety or tolerability hazards.[124] Nashan and coworkers reported the results of a randomized clinical trial involving basiliximab (20 mg infusions on the day of transplant and 4 days later) versus placebo for control of acute cellular rejection in renal allograft recipients. The rates of biopsy-proven acute rejection 6 months after transplantation were 51 of 171 (29.8%) in the basiliximab group and 73 of 166 (44%) in placebo group (P = .02). In addition, patients given basiliximab also had a significantly lower rate of steroid-resistant rejection (i.e., requiring OKT3). At 12 months, there were no differences in patient or graft survival. No increase in side effects was associated with basiliximab therapy.

Anti-CD4 Antibody

Selective disruption of MHC class II–CD4 interaction can prolong allograft survival and induce tolerance in animal models.[125] These antibodies have been demonstrated to reduce synovial inflammation in rheumatoid arthritis and to cause profound and long-term immunosuppression.[126] Use of anti-CD4 in conjunction with CTLA4-Ig prolongs the survival of hamster liver xenografts in rats.[127] Use of murine OKT4 in cadaver kidney transplantation has not shown promise.[128] A human anti-mouse antibody (HAMA) response of more than three times the pretreatment level was observed in 84% of patients. The rejection rate was high (37%), and several adverse events were reported. Other humanized anti-CD4 monoclonal antibodies are being evaluated for clinical trials.

Anti-CD45 Antibody

CD45 epitope plays a role in the regulation of T cell activation. The CD45RB monoclonal antibody has been shown effectively to prevent allograft rejection in animal models and in the future may have some application to humans.

Anti-CD40 Ligand or Anti-CD40 Antibody

Kirk[129] and Larsen[130] and their associates have recently shown that CD40 or CD40L-specific mAbs can reproducibly prevent and even reverse acute allograft rejection, leading to prolongation of major histocompatibility complex-mismatched renal allografts in primates without the need of chronic maintenance immunosuppression. Sun and associates[131] have shown that anti-CD40 ligand (anti-CD40L) or anti-CD40 mAb, when given with CTLA-4 immunoglobulin, forestalled evolution of chronic rejection in a mouse aortic allograft model.

Monoclonal Antibodies Against Adhesion Molecules

Leukocyte function–associated antigen 1 (LFA-1) plays an important role in adhesion of leukocytes to endothelial cells and to a variety of targets on immunocompetent cells during the effector phase of the immune response. Hourmant and colleagues found that the immunosuppressive effect of anti-LFA1 (anti-CD11a, anti-CD18) monoclonal antibody was similar to that of rabbit antithymocyte globulin as induction therapy in renal allograft recipients. Fewer patients required dialysis in the anti-LFA1 monoclonal antibody group, possibly owing to prevention of endothelial cell activation and the consequent protection of the allograft from ischemic damage.[132] Xu and colleagues[133] showed that a combination of the anti-intracellular adhesion molecule ICAM-1 monoclonal antibody and anti-LFA-1 monoclonal antibody induced tolerance to murine cardiac allografts.

Recombinant Fusion Molecules

CTLA4-Immunoglobulin

CTLA4-Ig is a chimeric fusion protein that blocks the B7-CD28/CTLA4 pathway. Azuma and associates[134] showed that it prevents development of chronic renal allograft rejection in animal models. Pearson and associates showed that CTLA4-Ig, together with donor bone marrow, induces long-term allograft survival and donor-specific unresponsiveness in the murine model.[135] Clinical trials using CTLA4-Ig together with humanized anti-CD40-L (MR1) are currently being contemplated to study the efficacy of this molecule in solid organ transplantation. Kirk and associates have shown that a combination of CTLA4-Ig with a humanized version of MR1 can prevent or reverse acute allograft rejection in primates without promoting chronic immunosuppression.[129]

OTHER NOVEL STRATEGIES AND EXPERIMENTAL AGENTS

Other strategies are being considered as potential areas for investigation for immunosuppression:

1. *T1039 (anti-T cell receptor) antibodies against T cell receptor.*
2. *FTY 720.* A sphingosine analog directed against adhesion molecules on the surface of activated lymphocytes, FTY 720 is being used in experimental models to mitigate antigen recognition and thus alter the homing pattern of T cells and encourage indirect antigen recognition.
3. *Antisense oligonucleotides against ICAM-1.* When given at the time of organ retrieval, they reduce the risk of rejection by preventing protein translation of activated genes.
4. *Peptides.* DQ65-79 is an immunomodulatory peptide that blocks cell cycle progression from G1 to S phase. Allotrap peptides are alpha-helix peptides that are a part of the human leukocyte antigen (HLA) molecule. Treatment with these results in blockade of peptide binding sites of HLA molecule, theoretically preventing antigen presentation and the immune response.
5. *Gene therapy.* Experimental studies are being conducted using retrovirus-mediated gene transfer of allogeneic MHC class I or II genes into autologous bone marrow.
6. *Chimerism.* Chimerism is necessary for the development of tolerance. Animal models have demonstrated the utility of inducing tolerance, which usually is done by introducing hematopoietic stem cells into the recipient before or at the time of transplantation. Clinical trials utilizing bone marrow augmentation at the time of solid organ transplantation have produced encouraging preliminary outcomes. Perhaps in the future the utility of nonspecific immunosuppression will be to help induce chimerism, which would obviate long-term immunosuppression (see Chapter 188, Complementary Modalities of Care).

SUMMARY

Immunosuppressive therapy for organ transplantation is rapidly undergoing changes as immune mechanisms of allograft rejection are dissected and biotechnology yields molecules that can inhibit immune responses at various points in the rejection cascade. Advances in therapeutic drug monitoring are helping clinicians to "fine tune" immunosuppressive therapy and commence early weaning. Nevertheless, the importance of immunosuppressive drug therapy based on clinical judgment cannot be overstated.

References

1. Sharma VK, Li B, Khanna AS, et al: Which way for drug-mediated immunosuppression? Curr Opin Immunol 1994; 6:784.
2. Ciancio G, Burke GW, Roth D, et al: Update in transplantation—1997. *In* Clinical Transplants 1997. Cecka, Terasaki, (Eds). Los Angeles, UCLA Tissue Typing Laboratory, 1997, p 241.
3. Mazariegos GV, Reyes J, Marino IR, et al: Weaning of immunosuppression in liver transplant recipients. Transplantation 1997; 63:243.
4. Hall BM: Cells mediating allograft rejection. Transplantation 1991; 51:1141.
5. Goust JM, Stevenson HC, Galbraith RM, et al: Immunosuppression and immunomodulation. Immunol Ser 1990; 50:481.
6. Boitard C, Bach JF: Long-term complications of conventional immunosuppressive treatment. Adv Nephrol 1989; 18:335.
7. Tornatore KM, Reed KA, Venuto RC: Methylprednisolone and cortisol metabolism during the early post-renal transplant period. Clin Transplant 1995; 9:427.
8. Schwartz R, Dameshek W: The effects of 6-mercaptopurine on homograft reactions. J Clin Invest 1960; 39:952.
9. Chan GL, Erdmann GR, Gruber SA, et al: Azathioprine metabolism: Pharmacokinetics of 6-mercaptopurine, 6-thiouric acid and 6-thioguanine nucleotides in renal transplant patients. J Clin Pharmacol 1990; 30:358.
10. Liano F, Moreno A, Matesanz R, et al: Veno-occlusive hepatic disease of the liver in renal transplantation: Is azathioprine the cause? [see Comments]. Nephron 1989; 51:509.
11. Frick TW, Fryd DS, Goodale RL, et al: Lack of association between azathioprine and acute pancreatitis in renal transplantation patients. Lancet 1991; 337:251.
12. Moore MJ: Clinical pharmacokinetics of cyclophosphamide. Clin Pharmacokinet 1991; 20:194.
13. Henderson DJ, Naya I, Bundick RV, et al: Comparison of the effects of FK-506, cyclosporin A and rapamycin on IL-2 production. Immunology 1991; 73:316.
14. Freeman DJ: Pharmacology and pharmacokinetics of cyclosporine. Clin Biochem 1991; 24:9.
15. Watkins PB: The role of cytochrome P_{450} in cyclosporine metabolism. J Am Acad Dermatol 1990; 23:1301.
16. Keown PA: Optimizing cyclosporine therapy: Dose, levels, and monitoring. Transplant Proc 1988; 20:382.
17. Remuzzi G, Bertani T: Renal vascular and thrombotic effects of cyclosporine. Am J Kidney Dis 1989; 13:261.
18. Rush DN: Cyclosporine toxicity to organs other than the kidney. Clin Biochem 1991; 24:101.
19. Keown PA, Stiller CR, Wallace AC: Effect of cyclosporine on the kidney. J Pediatr 1987; 111:1029.
20. American Hospital Formulary Service (AHFS): AHFS Drug Information 91. 33rd ed. Bethesda, American Society of Hospital Pharmacists, 1991.
21. Luke RG: Mechanism of cyclosporine-induced hypertension. Am J Hypertens 1991; 4:468.
22. Mason J: The pathophysiology of Sandimmune (cyclosporine) in man and animals. Pediatr Nephrol 1990; 4:554.
23. Scott JP, Higenbottam TW: Adverse reactions and interactions of cyclosporin. Med Toxicol Adverse Drug Exp 1988; 3:107.
24. Reznick VM, Lyons Jones K, Durham BL, et al: Changes in facial appearance during cyclosporine treatment. Lancet 1987; 1:1405.
25. Lorber MI: Cyclosporine: Lessons learned—future strategies. Clin Transplant 1991; 5:505.
26. Kopp JB, Klotman PE: Cellular and molecular mechanisms of cyclosporin nephrotoxicity. J Am Soc Nephrol 1990; 1:162.
27. Levy G, Grant D: Potential for CsA-Neoral in organ transplantation. Transplant Proc 1994; 26:2932.
28. Kovarik JM, Mueller EA, van Bree JB, et al: Cyclosporine pharma-

cokinetics and variability from a microemulsion formulation: A multicenter investigation in kidney transplant patients. Transplantation 1994; 58:658.
29. Siekierka JJ, Hung SHY, Poe M, et al: A cytosolic binding protein for the immunosuppressant FK506 has peptidyl-prolyl isomerase activity but is distinct from cyclophillin. Nature 1989; 341:755.
30. Harding MW, Galat A, Uehling DE, et al: A receptor for the immunosuppressant FK506 is *cis-trans* peptidyl-prolyl isomerase. Nature 1989; 341:758.
31. Fung JJ, Todo S, Jain A, et al: Conversion from cyclosporin to FK506 in liver allograft recipients with cyclosporine related complications. Transplant Proc 1990; 22:6.
32. Fung JJ, Todo S, Tzakis A, et al: Conversion of liver allograft recipients from cyclosporine to FK506-based immunosuppression: Benefits and pitfalls. Transplant Proc 1991; 23:14.
33. Holland R, Sorrell M, Langnas A, et al: Chronic rejection in liver transplant recipients: Does conversion to FK506 confer a survival benefit? (Abstract). Hepatology 1993; 18:74.
34. Fung JJ, Jain A, Hamad I, et al: Long term effects of FK506 following conversion from cyclosporine to FK506 for chronic rejection in liver transplant recipients (Abstract). Hepatology 1993; 18:74.
35. Sher LS, Cosenza CA, Michel J, et al: Efficacy of tacrolimus as rescue therapy for chronic rejection in orthotopic liver transplantation: A report of the U.S. Multicenter Liver Study Group. Transplantation 1997; 64:258.
36. Fung J, Eliasziw M, Todo S, et al: The Pittsburgh randomized trial of tacrolimus compared to cyclosporine for hepatic transplantation. J Am Coll Surg 1996; 183:117.
37. The European FK506 Multicenter Liver Study Group: Randomized trial comparing tacrolimus and cyclosporin in prevention of liver allograft rejection. Lancet 1994; 334:423.
38. The United States Multicenter FK506 Liver Study Group: A comparison of tacrolimus (FK506) and cyclosporine for immunosuppression in liver transplantation. N Engl J Med 1994; 331:1110.
39. Pichlmayr R, Winkler M, Neuhaus P, et al: Three year follow-up of the European multicenter tacrolimus (FK506) liver study. Transplant Proc 1997; 29:2499.
40. Wiesner R for the U.S. FK506 Study Group: Long-term comparison of tacrolimus versus cyclosporine in liver transplantation. Transplant Proc 1998; 30:1399.
41. Starzl TE, Donner A, Eliasziw M, et al: Randomised trialomania? The multicentre liver transplant trials of tacrolimus. Lancet 1995; 346:1346.
42. Jordan ML, Naraghi R, Shapiro R, et al: Tacrolimus rescue therapy for renal allograft rejection—five year experience. Transplantation 1997; 63:223.
43. Woodle ES, Thistlethwaite JR, Gordon JH, et al: A multicenter trial of FK506 (tacrolimus) therapy in refractory acute renal allograft rejection: A report of the Tacrolimus Kidney Transplantation Rescue Study Group. Transplantation 1996; 62:594.
44. Starzl TE, Fung JJ, Jordan ML, et al: Kidney transplantation under FK506. JAMA 1990; 264:63.
45. FK506 Kidney Transplant Study Group: A comparison of tacrolimus (FK506) and cyclosporine for immunosuppression after cadaveric kidney transplantation. Transplantation 1997; 63:977.
46. Mayer AD, Dmitrewski J, Squifflet JP, et al: Multicenter randomized trial comparing tacrolimus and cyclosporine in the prevention of renal allograft rejection: A report of the European tacrolimus multicenter renal study group. Transplantation 1997; 64:436.
47. Armitage JM, Kormos RL, Fung J, et al: The clinical trial of FK506 as primary and rescue immunosuppression in adult cardiac transplantation. Transplant Proc 1992; 23:3054.
48. Armitage JM, Kormos RL, Morita S, et al: Clinical trial of FK506 immunosuppression in adult cardiac transplantation. Ann Thorac Surg 1992; 54:205.
49. Mentzer RM, Jahania MS, Lasley RD: Tacrolimus as a rescue immunosuppressant after heart and lung transplantation. The U.S. Multicenter FK506 Study Group. Transplantation 1998; 65:109.
50. Corry RJ, Egidi MF, Shapiro R, et al: Tacrolimus without antilymphocyte induction therapy prevents pancreas loss from rejection in 123 consecutive patients. Transplant Proc 1998; 30:521.
51. Jordan ML, Shapiro R, Gritsch HA, et al: Long-term results of pancreas-transplantation under tacrolimus immunosuppression. Presented at the 24th Annual Scientific Meeting of the American Society of Transplant Surgeons, May 13–15, 1998. Transplantation (in press).
52. El-Ghoroury M, Hariharan S, Peddi VR, et al: Efficacy and safety of tacrolimus versus cyclosporine in kidney and pancreas transplant recipients. Transplant Proc 1997; 29:649.
53. Gruessner RWG for the Tacrolimus Pancreas Transplant Study Group: Tacrolimus in pancreas transplantation: A multicenter analysis. Clin Transplant 1997; 11:299.
54. Cillo U, Alessiani M, Fung JJ, et al: Major adverse effects of FK506 used as an immunosuppressive agent after liver transplantation. Transplant Proc 1993; 25:628.
55. Fung JJ, Alessiani M, Abu-Elmagd K, et al: Adverse effects associated with the use of FK506. Transplant Proc 1991; 23:3105.
56. Venkataramanan R, Jain A, Warty VS, et al: Pharmacokinetics of FK506 in transplant patients. Transplant Proc 1992; 23:2736.
57. Abu-Elmagd K, Fung J, Draviam R, et al: Four-hour versus 24-hour intravenous infusion of FK506 in liver transplantation. Transplant Proc 1992; 23:2767.
58. Fung JJ, Abu-Elmagd K, Todo S, et al: FK506 in clinical organ transplantation. Clin Transplant 1991; 5:517.
59. Moutabarrik A, Ishibashi M, Kameoka H, et al: FK506 mechanism of nephrotoxicity: Stimulatory effect on endothelin secretion by cultured kidney cells. Transplant Proc 1992; 23:3133.
60. McCauley J, Takaya S, Fung J, et al: The question of FK506 nephrotoxicity after liver transplantation. Transplant Proc 1991; 23:1444.
61. Eidelman BH, Abu-Elmagd K, Wilson J, et al: Neurologic complications of FK-506. Transplant Proc 1991; 23:3175.
62. Jain A, Venkataraman R, Fung JJ, et al: Pregnancy after liver transplantation under tacrolimus. Transplantation 1997; 64:559.
63. Warty VS, Venkataramanan R, Zendehrough P, et al: Practical aspects of FK506 analysis (Pittsburgh experience). Transplant Proc 1992; 23:2730.
64. Jain A, Khanna A, Molmenti E, et al: Immunosuppressive therapy: New concepts. Surg Clin North Am (in press).
65. Lee WA, Gu L, Miksztal AR, et al: Bioavailability improvement of mycophenolic acid through amino ester derivation. Pharmacol Res 1990; 7:161.
66. Franklin TJ, Cool JM: The inhibition of nucleic acid synthesis by mycophenolic acid. Biochem J 1989; 113:515.
67. Allison AC, Almquist SJ, Muller CD, et al: In vitro immunosuppressive effects of mycophenolic acid and an ester prodrug, RS-61443. Transplant Proc 1991; 23(Suppl):10.
68. Mariani R, Fleischmajer R, Schragger AH, et al: Mycophenolic acid in the treatment of psoriasis. Arch Dermatol 1977; 113:930.
69. Sollinger HW, Deierholi MH, Belzer FO, et al: RS-61443—a phase I clinical trial and pilot rescue study. Transplantation 1992; 53:428.
70. Sollinger HW for the US Renal Transplant Mycophenolate Mofetil Study Group: Mycophenolate mofetil for the prevention of acute rejection in primary cadaveric renal allograft recipients. Transplantation 1995; 60:225.
71. European Mycophenolate Mofetil Cooperative Study Group: Placebo-controlled study of mycophenolate mofetil combined with cyclosporin and corticosteroids for prevention of acute rejection. Lancet 1995; 345:1321.
72. Pescovitz MA for the Mycophenolate Mofetil Acute Renal Rejection Study Group. Mycophenolate mofetil for the treatment of a first acute renal allograft rejection. Transplantation 1998; 65:235.
73. The Mycophenolate Mofetil Renal Refractory Rejection Study Group: Rescue therapy with mycophenolate mofetil. Clin Transplant 1996; 10:131.
74. Keown PA for The Tricontinental Mycophenolate Mofetil Renal Transplantation Study Group: A blinded, randomized clinical trial of mycophenolate mofetil for the prevention of acute rejection in cadaveric renal transplantation. Transplantation 1996; 61:1029.
75. Shapiro R, Jordan ML, Scantlebury VP, et al: A prospective, randomized trial of tacrolimus/prednisone versus tacrolimus/prednisone/mycophenolate mofetil in renal transplant patients—first report. J Urol (in press).
76. Jain A, Fung JJ, Hamad I, et al: Adult primary liver transplantation: Prospective randomized trial of tacrolimus and steroid vs

tacrolimus, steroid and mycophenolate mofetil: A preliminary report. Transplantation (in press).

77. McDiarmid SV: Mycophenolate mofetil in liver transplantation. Clin Transplant 1996; 10:140.
78. Kirklin JK, Bourge RC, Nattel DC, et al: Treatment of recurrent heart rejection with mycophenolate mofetil: Initial clinical experience. J Heart Lung Transplant 1995; 13:444.
79. Kobashigawa JA: Mycophenolate mofetil in cardiac transplantation. Curr Opin Cardiol 1998; 13:117.
80. Khanna A, Venkataraman R, Molmenti E, et al: Pharmacokinetics of mycophenolic acid in pediatric small bowel transplant patients. Program and Abstracts of the 5th International Symposium on Intestinal Transplantation (Abstract No. 42). Cambridge, UK, August 1997.
81. Morris RE: Rapamycins: Antifungal, antitumor, antiproliferative and immunosuppressive macrolides. Transplant Rev 1992; 6:39.
82. Morris RE, Meiser BM, Wu J, et al: Use of rapamycin for the suppression of alloimmune reactions in vivo: Schedule dependence, tolerance induction, synergy with cyclosporine and FK 506, and effect on host-versus-graft and graft-versus-host reactions. Transplant Proc 1991; 23:521.
83. Dumont FJ, Melino MR, Staruch MJ, et al: The immunosuppressive macrolides FK-506 and rapamycin act as reciprocal antagonists in murine T cells. J Immunol 1990; 144:1418.
84. Phase III trials, Kahan BD: A phase III comparative efficacy trial of rapamune in renal allograft recipients. The Rapamune U.S. Study Group (Abstract No. 198). Program and Abstracts of the 17th World Congress of The Transplantation Society, Montreal, July 1998.
85. Schuurman HJ, Cottens S, Fuchs S, et al: SDZ, a new rapamycin derivative. Transplantation 1997; 64:32.
86. Murgia MG, Jordan S, Kahad BD: The side effect profile of sirolimus: A phase I study in quiescent cyclosporine-prednisone–treated renal transplant recipients. Kidney Int 1996; 49:209.
87. Katoh H, Ohkohchi N, Orii T, et al: Effectiveness of 15-DSG on steroid resistant acute rejection in living related transplantation. Transplant Proc 1997; 29:533.
88. Takahashi K, Ota K, Tanabe K, et al: Effect of a novel immunosuppressive agent, deoxyspergualin, on rejection in kidney transplant recipients. Transplant Proc 1990; 22:1606.
89. Ochiai T, Nakajima K, Sakamoto K, et al: Comparative studies on the immunosuppressive activity of FK506, 15-deoxyspergualin, and cyclosporine. Transplant Proc 1989; 21:829.
90. Okazaki H, Sato T, Jimbo M, et al: Prophylactic use of deoxyspergualin in living related renal transplantation. Transplant Proc 1991; 23:1094.
91. Koyama I, Amemiya H, Taguchi Y, et al: Prophylactic use of deoxyspergualin in a quadruple immunosuppressive protocol in renal transplantation. Transplant Proc 1991; 23:1096.
92. Okubo M, Tamura K, Kamata K, et al: 15-Deoxyspergualin "rescue therapy" for methylprednisolone-resistant rejection of renal transplants as compared with anti–T cell monoclonal antibody (OKT3). Transplantation 1993; 55:505.
93. Guao Z, Chong ASF, Shen J, et al: Leflunomide, a potential immunosuppressant for pancreatic islet transplantation. Transplant Proc 1997; 29:1206.
94. Turka LA, Dayton J, Sinclair G, et al: Guanine ribonucleotide depletion inhibits T cell activation: Mechanism of action of the immunosuppressive drug mizoribine. J Clin Invest 1991; 87:940.
95. Lee HA, Slapak M, Venkataraman G, et al: Mizoribine as an alternative to azathioprine in triple-therapy immunosuppressant regimens in cadaver renal transplantation. Transplant Proc 1993; 25:2699.
96. Kokado Y, Ishibashi M, Jiang H, et al: A new triple-drug induction therapy with low dose cyclosporine, mizoribine and prednisolone in renal transplantation. Transplant Proc 1989; 21:1575.
97. Mita K, Akiyama N, Nagao T, et al: Advantages of mizoribine over azathioprine in combination therapy with cyclosporine for renal transplantation. Transplant Proc 1990; 22:1679.
98. Anderson LW, Strong JM, Cysyk RL: Cellular pharmacology of DUP-785: A new anticancer agent. Cancer Communications 1989; 1:381.
99. Arteaga CL, Brown TD, Kuhn JG, et al: Phase I clinical and pharmacokinetic trial of brequinar sodium (DuP 785; NSC 368390). Cancer Res 1989; 49:4648.
100. Cramer DV, Chapman FA, Jaffee BD, et al: The effect of a new immunosuppressive drug, brequinar sodium, on heart, liver and kidney allograft rejection in the rat. Transplantation 1992; 53:303.
101. Kahan BD, Tejpal N, Gibbons-Stubbers S, et al: The synergistic interactions in vitro and in vivo of brequinar sodium with cyclosporine or rapamycin alone and in triple combination. Transplantation 1993; 55:894.
102. Woodreff MFA, Anderson NA: Effect of lymphocyte depletion by thoracic duct fistula and administration of antilymphocyte serum on the survival of skin homograft in rat. Nature 1963; 200:702.
103. Najarian J, Simmons R, Condie R, et al: Seven years experience with antilymphoblast globulin for renal transplants from cadaver donors. Ann Surg 1976; 184:352.
104. Starzl TE, Marchioro TL, Porter KA, et al: The use of heterologous antilymphoid agents in canine renal and liver homotransplantation and in human renal homotransplantation. Surg Gynecol Obstet 1967; 24:301.
105. Griepp R, Stinson E, Dong E, et al: The use of antithymocyte globulin in human heart transplantation. Circulation 1972; 45(Suppl):147.
106. Cosimi A, Burton R, Colvin R, et al: Treatment of acute allograft rejection with OKT3 monoclonal antibody. Transplantation 1981; 32:535.
107. Fung JJ, Demetris AJ, Porter KA, et al: Use of OKT3 with cyclosporin and steroids for reversal of acute kidney and liver allograft rejection. Nephron 1987; 46(Suppl):19.
108. Kreis H, Legendre C, Chatenoud L: OKT3 in organ transplantation. Transplant Rev 1991; 5:181.
109. Millis JM, McDiarmid SV, Hiatt JR, et al: Randomized prospective trial of OKT3 for early prophylaxis of rejection after liver transplantation. Transplantation 1989; 47:82.
110. Goldman M, Abramowicz D, De Pauw L, et al: Beneficial effects of prophylactic OKT3 in cadaver kidney transplantation: Comparison with cyclosporin A in a single-center prospective randomized study. Transplant Proc 1991; 23:1046.
111. Cockfield SM, Preiksaitis J, Harvey E, et al: Is sequential use of ALG and OKT3 in renal transplants associated with an increased incidence of fulminant posttransplant lymphoproliferative disorder? Transplant Proc 1991; 23:1106.
112. Taylor RM: Monoclonal and polyclonal antibodies: Clinical aspects. Immunol Lett 1991; 29:113–116.
113. Barr ML, Sanchez JA, Seche LA, et al: Anti-CD3 monoclonal antibody induction therapy: Immunological equivalency with triple-drug therapy in heart transplantation. Circulation 1990; 82:IV291.
114. Menkis AH, McKenzie FN, Thomson D, et al: Benefits of avoidance of induction immunosuppression in heart transplantation. J Heart Transplant 1989; 8:311.
115. Thistlethwaite JR Jr, Heffron TG, Stuart JK, et al: Selective OKT3 induction therapy in adult cadaveric-donor renal transplant recipients. Am J Kidney Dis 1989; 14:28.
116. Chatenoud L, Gerran C, Legendre C, et al: In vivo cell activation following OKT3 administration. Transplantation 1990; 49:697.
117. Kirkman RI, Barrett LV, Gaulton GN, et al: Administration of an anti-interleukin-2 receptor monoclonal antibody prolongs cardiac allograft survival in mice. J Exp Med 1985; 162:358.
118. Kupiec-Weglinski, Padberg, Uhteg W, et al: Selective immunosuppression with anti-interleukin-2 receptor-targeted therapy: Helper and suppressor cell activity in rat recipients of cardiac allografts. Eur J Immunol 1987; 17:313.
119. Reed MH, Shapiro ME, Strom TB, et al: Prolongation of primate renal allograft survival by anti-Tac, an anti-human IL-2 receptor monoclonal antibody. Transplantation 1989; 47:55.
120. Kirkman RL, Shapiro ME, Carpenter CB, et al: A randomized prospective trial of anti-Tac monoclonal antibody in human renal transplantation. Transplantation 1991; 51:107.
121. Vincenti F, Kirkman R, Light S, et al, for the Daclizumab Triple Therapy Study Group: Interleukin-2-receptor blockade with daclizumab to prevent acute rejection in renal transplantation. N Engl J Med 1998; 338:161.
122. Vincenti F, Lantz M, Birnbaum J, et al: A phase I trial of humanized anti-interleukin-2 receptor antibody in renal transplantation. Transplantation 1997; 63:33.
123. Kovarik J, Wolf P, Cisterine JM, et al: Disposition of basiliximab,

an interleukin-2 receptor monoclonal antibody, in recipients of mismatched cadaver renal allografts. Transplantation 1997; 64:1701.
124. Nashan B, Moore R, Amlot P, et al: Randomised trial of basiliximab versus placebo for control of acute cellular rejection in renal allograft recipients. Lancet 1997; 350:1193.
125. Arim T, Lehmann M, Wayne Flye M: Induction of donor specific transplantation tolerance to cardiac allograts following treatment with nondepleting (RIB 5/2) or depleting (OX-38) anti-CD4 mAb plus intrathymic or intravenous donor alloantigen. Transplantation 1997; 63:284.
126. Tak PP, van der Lubbe PA, Cauli A, et al: Reduction of synovial inflammation after anti-CD4 monoclonal antibody treatment in rheumatoid arthritis. Arthritis Rheum 1995; 38:1457.
127. Yin DP, Sankary HS, Chong ASF, et al: Effect of anti-CD4 monoclonal antibody combined human CTLA-4Ig on the survival of hamster liver and heart xenografts in Lewis rats. Transplantation 1997; 64:317.
128. Cooperative Clinical Trials in Transplantation Research Group: Murine OKT4 immunosuppression in cadaver donor renal allograft recipients. Transplantation 1997; 63:1087.
129. Kirk AD, Harlan DM, Armstrong NN, et al: CTLA4-Ig and anti-CD40 ligand prevent allograft rejection in primates. Proc Natl Acad Sci 1997; 94:8789.
130. Larsen CP, Elwood ET, Alexander DZ, et al: Long-term acceptance of skin and cardiac allografts after blocking CD40 and CD28 pathways. Nature 1998; 381:434.
131. Sun H, Subbotin VM, Chen C, et al: Prevention of chronic rejection in mouse aortic allografts by combined treatment with CTLA4-Ig and anti-CD40L monoclonal antibody. Transplantation 1997; 64:1838.
132. Hourmant M, Bedrossian J, Durand D, et al: A randomized multicenter trial comparing LFA-1 with rabbit antithymocyte globulin as induction treatment in first kidney transplantations. Transplantation 1996; 62:1565.
133. Xu XY, Honjo K, Devore-Carter D, et al: Immunosuppression by inhibition of cellular adhesion mediated by leukocyte function-associated antigen-1/intercellular adhesion molecule-1 in murine cardiac transplantation. Transplantation 1997; 63:876.
134. Azuma H, Chandraker A, Nadeu K, et al: Blockade of T-cell costimulation prevents development of experimental chronic renal allograft rejection. Immunology 1996; 93:1239.
135. Pearson TC, Alexander DZ, Hendrix R, et al: CTLA4-Ig plus bone marrow induces long-term allograft survival and donor-specific unresponsiveness in the murine model. Transplantation 1996; 61:997.

179

Critical Care of Kidney Transplant Recipients

Lakshmipathi Chelluri, MD, MPH • Ron Shapiro, MD
Jerry McCauley, MD

The kidney is the most commonly transplanted solid organ, and 12,000 to 13,000 renal transplant procedures are performed annually in the United States. The combination of better immunosuppression and infection prophylaxis has led to improved patient and graft survival rates. The 1- and 5-year patient survival rates in 51,442 cadaveric donor renal transplant procedures done between 1987 and 1994 were 95% and 86%, respectively. Graft survival rates in the same patient group were 81% and 58%. Patient and graft survival rates are better for living related donor procedures with 1- and 5-year survival rates of 98% and 93% for patients and 91% and 75% for grafts.[1] Kidney transplantation is a less expensive therapy than dialysis for patients with end-stage renal disease and is associated with both an improved quality of life and economic rehabilitation. It is estimated that a successful renal transplant can result in savings of $245,000 per patient compared with dialysis over a 10-year period.[2–4]

The surgical techniques and principles of perioperative management for kidney transplant recipients have been standardized, and most patients do not, in fact, need postoperative monitoring in the intensive care unit (ICU). Patients with specific medical problems or those experiencing complications during the preoperative, perioperative, or postoperative period may require management in an ICU. This chapter describes the care of straightforward patients undergoing kidney transplantation and those complications requiring management in an ICU.

PREOPERATIVE EVALUATION

Evaluation of patients for kidney transplantation is usually done on an outpatient basis.[5, 6] Potential candidates meet with the transplant surgeon, nephrologist, social worker, and transplant coordinator. A complete history and physical examination are recorded, and certain laboratory tests are performed. Important elements of the history include questions about previous transplants, complications after transplantation, blood transfusions, urologic problems, and dialysis status. Patients need not be on dialysis to undergo transplantation; patients with newly diagnosed end-stage renal disease may be evaluated and have the procedure before dialysis becomes necessary. Additional medical problems (e.g., diabetes mellitus, hypertension, cardiac or pulmonary disease, liver, pancreatic, gastrointestinal problems, neurologic or musculoskeletal disorders, infections, and malignancies) are all specifically addressed. Active infections or malignancies are absolute contraindications to transplantation. Patients at high risk for coronary artery disease and those with history of diabetes undergo noninvasive evaluation for coronary artery disease and cardiac catheterization if necessary. Patients with significant coronary artery disease may require coronary angioplasty or coronary artery bypass grafting before transplantation.[7–9] A psychosocial evaluation by a social worker is of enormous importance, particularly with regard to issues of compliance and recreational drug use.

Routine laboratory studies, in addition to the usual chemistry and hematology panels, include serologic evaluation for cytomegalovirus (CMV); hepatitis A, B, and C, and human immunodeficiency virus (HIV). Human leukocyte antigen (HLA) typing is performed, and panel-reactive antibody (PRA) levels are assessed to measure the degree of sensitization. Routine radiologic studies, in addition to a chest x-ray film, include ultrasonography of the gallbladder and native kidneys. A voiding cystourethrogram is performed only if indicated. Other tests, such as noninvasive peripheral arterial Doppler examination, pulmonary function tests, and upper and lower digestive tract endoscopy are performed when indicated.

There is no absolute lower or upper age limit for renal transplantation. Recipients have ranged in age from 8 months to 84 years. When evaluation is completed, patients are presented before the evaluation committee, and a decision is made to place the patient on the waiting list, to reject the patient, or to order further tests. Once a patient is on the waiting list, the dialysis unit sends blood on a monthly basis for crossmatching. Kidneys are allocated according to a computerized point system that takes into account quality of antigen matching, waiting time, and the panel-reactive antibody level. Patients of a suitable blood type are crossmatched when a kidney becomes available, and the patient who is highest on the list with a negative crossmatch receives the organ. The system is formally unbiased with regard to gender, age, race, and socioeconomic status.

PERIOPERATIVE MANAGEMENT

When a kidney becomes available, the selected recipient is admitted to the hospital and immediately evaluated by the surgeon, nephrologist, and anesthesiologist. In addition to an interval history and physical examination, routine tests (serum electrolyte levels, blood urea nitrogen, creatinine, electrocardiogram, chest radiograph) are obtained. Hyperkalemia and pulmonary edema on physical examination or chest radiograph, or both, are indications for preoperative dialysis. Although mild hyperkalemia (serum potassium, 5 to 5.5 mEq/L) may be treated with anion exchange enema (sodium polystyrene sulfonate [Kayexalate]), dialysis is generally preferred because anion exchange may not be effective rapidly enough, it can impose an additional sodium load, and it might precipitate or worsen pulmonary edema. Anticoagulation during dialysis is limited to prevent bleeding complications during and after surgery.

In the absence of significant cardiopulmonary dysfunction, central venous pressure (CVP) and noninvasive arterial pressure monitoring are used. Diabetic patients with autonomic neuropathy may have a higher risk of experiencing cardiovascular instability and may require additional hemodynamic monitoring.[10] Patients are maintained in a euvolemic state during surgery with guidance from CVP monitoring. The diseased kidneys are not usually removed unless they are infected or unless there is another specific indication for nephrectomy.[11]

Kidneys are generally transplanted heterotopically in the iliac fossa. The external iliac artery and vein are exposed in a retroperitoneal manner. The renal vein and artery are then anastomosed, usually end to side to the iliac vessels. Intravenous furosemide (1 mg/kg) and mannitol (1 g/kg) are given while the vascular anastomoses are being performed. Systolic arterial pressure is maintained between 120 and 140 mm Hg to ensure adequate perfusion of the transplanted kidney. After revascularization of the allograft, the transplanted ureter is implanted into the recipient's bladder. Antibiotic prophylaxis with first-generation cephalosporins, both systemic and topical, is routine.

In the immediate postoperative period, urine output is used to guide fluid replacement. Renal function is variable after transplantation; some patients have an immediate diuresis with urine volumes exceeding 1000 mL/hour, and others produce no urine at all. For patients with urine output greater than 300 mL/hour, 80% of the urine volume is replaced with normal saline, or 5% or 1% glucose with half-normal saline. (Some transplant surgeons prefer to add some sodium bicarbonate to the intravenous fluid.) For patients with urine output less than 300 mL/hour, all of the urine output is replaced with the same solution. Additional fluid is generally not indicated. Diuretics such as furosemide are given if urine output remains low and the intravascular volume is adequate. Maintenance intravenous fluid in the presence of oliguria is discouraged because it can be associated with fluid overload and development of pulmonary edema. In diabetic patients, insulin therapy is guided by frequent blood glucose monitoring. Occasionally, a continuous infusion of insulin is necessary.

General postoperative care is not particularly different from that of nontransplant patients. An oral diet is resumed after return of gastrointestinal function. Intravenous fluids can be discontinued once the patient is tolerating oral fluids well. Wound care differs only in that skin staples, if used, are left for 3 weeks instead of 1 week, to account for slower healing associated with steroid medication.

Transplant patients require a large number of medications in the initial post-transplantation period. Immunosuppressive agents (e.g., cyclosporine, tacrolimus, mycophenolate mofetil, azathioprine, prednisone) are given to prevent rejection. Antilymphocyte preparations, such as OKT3 or antithymocyte globulin (ATG), are used for induction in some centers; in other programs, they are used only for steroid resistant rejection.

Cyclosporine or tacrolimus-based immunosuppressive therapy has been associated with a 1-year patient survival between 90% and 100% and 1-year graft survival of 80% to over 90%. The variability is a function of patient selection, quality of the donor organ, skill in adjusting immunosuppression, and quality of follow-up. Cyclosporine is associated with a number of side effects; the most important of these is nephrotoxicity, although hypertension, metabolic problems, and cosmetic derangements are also seen.[12] Tacrolimus is similar in its mechanism of action and has a similar toxicity profile but somewhat better immunosuppressive efficacy.[13, 14] Mycophenolate mofetil, a mycophenolic acid derivative and a new immunosuppressive agent, has been evaluated as a substitute for azathioprine and offers better immunosuppressive efficacy.[15] Several other agents are at an earlier stage of development.

In addition to antirejection medication, patients routinely receive a number of medications to prevent opportunistic infections, such as nystatin for *Candida*, acyclovir for herpes simplex, gancyclovir for cytomegalovirus, and trimethoprim-sulfamethoxazole for *Pneumocystis carinii*. Prophylaxis for peptic ulcer is provided with histamine$_2$ (H_2) receptor blockers, antacids, sucralfate and hydrogen pump inhibitors, if necessary. Calcium, phosphorus, magnesium are supplemented as needed, and allopurinol is used to treat high uric acid levels. Over time, most of these medications can be tapered or eliminated.

INDICATIONS FOR ADMISSION TO THE INTENSIVE CARE UNIT

Most patients undergoing renal transplantation do not need to be admitted to an ICU in the immediate postoperative period. The indications for admission to an ICU can be classified into (1) those occurring during the operative and early postoperative periods and (2) those occurring in the late postoperative period (>3 months after transplantation). We evaluated admissions from the renal transplant service to the surgical ICU over a 1-year period.[16] During the year, there were 86 admissions of 71 patients and a total of 178 kidney transplants were performed. Twenty-seven (31%) admissions were in the immediate postoperative period. The indications were a history of coronary artery disease (11 patients), intraoperative cardiac ischemia (two), hyperkalemia (three), and miscellaneous causes (the rest), such as a history of heart transplantation, intraoperative cardiac arrest, pulmonary edema, failure to extubate postoperatively, altered mental status, and hypoxia. Mean Acute Physiologic and Chronic Health Evaluation (APACHE II) score was 18 ± 5, and the ICU length of stay was 5.1 ± 7.5 days. Seventeen (63%) of the 27 patients received renal replacement therapy, seven (26%) patients required mechanical ventilation, and one (3.7%) patient died in the hospital.

Forty-four (62%) patients had previously undergone renal transplantation and had 59 admissions to the ICU for various complications. These complications include infection (14), encephalopathy (11), congestive heart failure (nine), respiratory failure (four), nontransplant surgery (four), and others (17). The mean APACHE II score in this group was 19.4 ± 6, and the ICU length of stay was 7 ± 10 days. Mechanical ventilation and renal replacement therapy were needed in 34% of the patients. Nine (20.5%) patients in this group died in the hospital. Infection was the cause death in six (67%) of the patients.

Indications for Perioperative Intensive Care

Cardiac Problems

Patients with significant cardiac dysfunction (i.e., a left ventricular ejection fraction less than 30%) or significant coronary artery disease may need perioperative hemodynamic monitoring. This is usually accomplished with a Swan-Ganz catheter, inserted via a jugular vein, and a radial arterial catheter. Although the femoral artery and vein can be cannulated for such monitoring, the femoral vessels on the same side as the transplant should not be used because of the potential for compromising the vascular supply to the allograft. Maintaining adequate cardiac filling pressures and using inotropic agents can improve cardiac function and facilitate management of these patients during the perioperative period. Patients with hemodynamic instability during the transplant procedure need postoperative monitoring and assessment in the ICU for myocardial injury. Iatrogenic pulmonary edema secondary to fluid overload during the transplantation is a complication that should be avoided. Occasionally, emergency dialysis or continuous renal replacement therapy (CRRT) may be required to remove excess fluid and to improve pulmonary gas exchange.

Hypertension

Hypertension requiring parenteral therapy is occasionally necessary and can be the result of sudden inadvertent withdrawal of pretransplant antihypertensive medications or excessive fluid administration. Often, restitution of antihypertensive medications and occasional use of sublingual nifedipine (10 mg) are sufficient. Calcium channel blockers, such as verapamil and diltiazem, may increase levels of cyclosporine and tacrolimus and should be used cautiously. Intravenous nitroprusside can be used in patients with hypertension that is resistant to oral agents. Thiocyanate levels should be monitored as needed, particularly when the allograft is functioning poorly. Labetolol and esmolol are useful in controlling blood pressure but can be problematic because β-blockers can cause hyperkalemia.[17] Angiotensin-converting enzyme (ACE) inhibitors can also be used, but caution is necessary because acute tubular necrosis of the allograft is reported with use of these agents.[18]

Pulmonary Problems

Most of the patients undergoing renal transplantation are extubated immediately after the operation and do not need mechanical ventilatory support postoperatively. Patients with significant pulmonary dysfunction preoperatively or pulmonary edema perioperatively may need prolonged mechanical ventilation and respiratory therapy with bronchodilators. One report of 110 patients undergoing renal transplantation suggested that 37% of the recipients experienced pulmonary complications. Most of these were infectious complications, with 69% occurring in the first 4 months.[19] Deep venous thrombosis in the ipsilateral venous system and pulmonary embolism also have been reported, and occasionally a Greenfield vena caval filter may be needed. Greenfield filters have been used in patients after kidney transplantation without significant deterioration in kidney function.[20, 21]

Renal Failure

Early allograft dysfunction is not an uncommon problem. *Delayed* graft function, defined as need for dialysis during the first postoperative week, occurred in 23.8% of the 37,216 patients undergoing renal transplantation between 1985 and 1992 in the United States. Delayed graft function is associated with an increased incidence of acute rejection and is also associated with worse graft survival.[22] Oliguria in the early postoperative period may be related to problems with the donor prior to organ recovery, prolonged ischemia, hypovolemia or perioperative hemodynamic instability in the recipient, vascular thrombosis, and hyperacute rejection. In addition, external obstruction secondary to hematoma or obstruction of the ureter or Foley catheter can also be causes of low or no urine output postoperatively.

Renal ultrasonography and flow scans are useful in assessing blood flow in the renal vessels and kidney function. Allograft function usually improves over time (7 to 21 days) if the cause of oliguria is acute tubular necrosis. Patients with delayed graft function routinely undergo biopsy 1 week after transplantation to rule out occult acute rejection. Fluid restriction and close monitoring of electrolytes are needed in patients with oliguria or anuria.

Pulmonary edema and hyperkalemia are important complications that obviously require immediate therapy, including hemodialysis, which is also performed postoperatively for indications such as volume overload, nonresponse to diuretic therapy, and severe azotemia. Because dialysis may be associated with hypotension and exacerbation of acute tubular necrosis, routine dialysis on a thrice-weekly basis is avoided if possible. In the early postoperative period, the decision about dialysis is made on a daily basis unless the patient is oliguric or anuric. Even in the latter situation, if the patient has a potentially correctable reason for oliguria, such as cyclosporine or tacrolimus toxicity or presence of rejection, the need for dialysis is evaluated on a daily basis.

Hemodynamically stable patients can undergo dialysis to remove fluid; in hemodynamically unstable patients, bicarbonate-buffered dialysate solutions, which are associated with less hemodynamic instability than acetate-buffered solutions, can be used.[23–24] Patients who have been on peritoneal dialysis preoperatively can be put on low-volume, frequent-exchange peritoneal dialysis if peritoneal integrity has been maintained during the transplantation procedure. One complication of dialysis is hypoxemia. Therefore, patients with significant pulmonary dysfunction may need increased supplemental oxygen during hemodialysis.[25]

In critically ill patients who may not be able to tolerate dialysis, continuous renal replacement therapy techniques, such as continuous arteriovenous or venovenous hemofiltration (CAVF or CVVF) with or without dialysis, and slow continuous ultrafiltration (SCUF), with or without dialysis, are useful. These methods of renal replacement therapy are particularly useful in patients who receive large volumes of fluid because of parenteral nutrition and antibiotic therapy.[26] At the University of Pittsburgh Medical Center, continuous renal replacement therapy is performed with a double-lumen venous catheter and a roller pump to achieve the desired flow through the system.

Hyperkalemia

In the postoperative period, hyperkalemia may be caused by tissue trauma during surgery, excessive bleeding, transfusions, and, occasionally, the use of β-blockers for treatment of hypertension. Beta-blockade prevents entry of potassium into the cell and may promote hyperkalemia.[17] Although ion exchange resins can be used to decrease serum potassium levels, they have high sodium content and may worsen pulmonary edema. Colonic and small intestinal perforation has been reported with the use of Kayexalate in renal transplant recipients. Sorbitol crystals have been noted at the site of histologic necrosis in such patients. For this reason, we avoid using Kayexalate for the treatment of hyperkalemia in the early postoperative period.[27, 28] Because sorbitol may be the cause of necrosis, it is theoretically possible to use the Kayexalate with saline. Dialysis is, however, the treatment of choice in patients with hyperkalemia, particularly when hyperkalemia is associated with fluid overload.

Rejection

One of the common causes of graft dysfunction is rejection, which can occur in 50% or more of patients. Current immunosuppressive therapy at the University of Pittsburgh Medical Center includes tacrolimus and steroids as primary therapy. A trial is in progress to assess the utility of adding mycophenolate mofetil. Tacrolimus is a relatively new immunosuppressive agent and has been shown to be superior to cyclosporine in its ability to prevent rejection. Tacrolimus is more potent and somewhat more efficacious than cyclosporine. It allows the eventual elimination of steroids in 60% to 70% of patients. It is comparable to cyclosporine in terms of nephrotoxicity, neurotoxicity, and diabetogenicity, although the early incidence of diabetes may be higher. The incidence of hypertension is lower, and cholesterol levels are lower than in patients receiving cyclosporine. Both agents have significant dose-related toxicity and significant drug interactions.[29–31] Blood levels should be monitored closely to avoid such problems.

There are four types of rejection.

Hyperacute rejection is rare and should never occur with the availability of pretransplant crossmatching techniques; it is mediated by preformed antibodies. These antibodies bind to the donor organ endothelium and initiate a cascade of events that lead to graft thrombosis within minutes of transplantation. When it occurs, immediate allograft nephrectomy is required.

Accelerated rejection is similar but occurs within the first few days (rather than minutes) after transplantation. The outcome is usually, but not always, the same as with hyperacute rejection.

Acute rejection generally occurs from 1 week to several months after transplantation (although it can also occur later) and can manifest as a rise in creatinine with or without decreasing urine volume. The definitive diagnosis is made by renal biopsy. Acute rejection is managed by steroids or antilymphocyte preparations, such as OKT3 or ATG. Patients receiving OKT3 need to be monitored closely because OKT3 can cause fever, an increase in cardiac output, and a decrease in systemic vascular resistance (mediated by cytokine release, especially tumor necrosis factor [TNF]), hypotension, pulmonary edema, and, rarely, anaphylactic shock.[32–35]

Chronic rejection occurs late after transplantation; it is poorly understood and difficult to treat and leads to eventual loss of the allograft.

Technical Complications

Technical complications are unusual but need to be recognized early and may require operative intervention. Postoperative bleeding may be secondary to inadequate hemostasis or a bleeding diathesis secondary to uremia. Desmopressin acetate (DDAVP, 0.3 μg/kg), conjugated estrogens intravenously (0.6 mg/kg/day for 5 days), hemodialysis, and cryoprecipitate improve platelet function and decrease perioperative bleeding. In an uncomplicated transplantation, they are not needed.[36–39]

Vascular complications include arterial and venous thrombosis, stenosis, and disruption. Arterial stenosis may occur late after surgery and can be treated with angioplasty. The other vascular complications usually result in loss of the allograft. Ureteral complications include urinary leak from the ureter or bladder secondary to technical error or ureteral ischemia, resulting in necrosis, stenosis with obstruction, bladder outflow obstruction, ureteral stones, and urinary tract infections.

Ghasemian reported 98 urologic complications in 669 patients undergoing renal transplantation in one institution over a 6-year period, and Shoskes reported 71 complications in 1000 consecutive patients. Many of these complications require reoperation.[40–41] A lymphocele may occur because of disruption of lymphatics and can be manifested as ipsilateral leg edema with a fluid collection around the kidney detected by ultrasonographic examination. A lymphocele is usually treated by the creation of a peritoneal window to drain the lymph into the peritoneal cavity.

Indications for Late Postoperative Intensive Care

Late complications requiring intensive care are usually related to immunosuppression and its complications, most importantly the development of opportunistic infections.[42] Hypoalbuminemia is common and is an independent predictor for increased mortality after transplantation.[43]

Infectious Complications

Infection is the most common complication of immunosuppression and one of the two leading causes of death; the other is cardiac disease. Patients are at particularly high risk for various infections during the first few months after transplantation because of the large quantity of immunosuppressive agents administered during this period. Peterson reported that about one third of the patients acquired an infection within 4 years after transplantation; half of the infections were viral, and one third were bacterial.[44] Infections during the first month are usually bacterial, with fungal and opportunistic infections unusual. Other causes of infection during this period include donor-related (rare) or preexisting infection in the recipient. Viral infections, especially cytomegalus virus (CMV), are common 1 to 6 months after transplantation. Infections after 6 months again are usually bacterial. A small percentage of patients may have chronic viral infections, and another small percentage of patients who experience allograft rejection and who need increased immunosuppressive therapy may develop opportunistic infections.[45] An important principle in renal transplant patients with severe infectious complications is that the kidney is expendable; thus, immunosuppression therapy is routinely discontinued if there is any question of life-threatening infection.

Bacterial Infections

Although opportunistic infections are common in immunosuppressed patients, bacterial infections are also relatively common. Early and aggressive antibiotic therapy is crucial; at the same time, care must be taken not to overuse antibiotics because of the frequent development of resistance or antibiotic-associated diarrhea (pseudomembranous colitis). Wound infections are uncommon, and deep infections rarely occur, with appropriate antibiotic prophylaxis. Urinary tract infections are not uncommon and must be treated aggressively to prevent ascending infections; bladder catheterization should be avoided if possible.

Mycobacterial infections are unusual but can be life-threatening. Patients with a positive purified protein derivative (PPD) test result should receive prophylaxis with isoniazid and vitamin B_6 for 1 year after transplantation. Any transplant patient admitted with newly diagnosed pneumonia should be placed in respiratory isolation until three sputum samples are negative for acid-fast bacilli by smear and staining. Bronchoalveolar lavage (BAL) may be necessary to confirm a diagnosis.

Treatment of active tuberculosis includes three-drug or four-drug therapy (isoniazid, ethambutol, pyrazinamide, and rifampin) and cessation of immunosuppression.[46] *Legionella* pneumonia can be nosocomial or community-acquired.[47] Traditional treatment with high-dose erythromycin has more recently been replaced by the quinolones, ciprofloxacin, or ofloxacin. Immunosuppression is usually decreased. Erythromycin interferes with metabolism of immunosuppressive agents and increases their levels. Prophylactic trimethoprim-sulfamethoxazole therapy for *P. carinii* (see later) may also be useful for preventing *Legionella* infections.

Viral Infections

Viral infections are common after transplantation.[48–52] Four main types of viral pathogens are recognized:

- Herpesviruses (Epstein-Barr virus, CMV, varicella zoster, herpes simplex).
- Adenovirus
- Papovavirus
- Viral hepatitis

Cytomegalovirus

CMV is the most common viral infection. Its prevention is still problematic. Previous studies have reported the efficacy of high-dose acyclovir and CMV hyperimmune globulin, or both, but reliable prophylaxis, especially in seronegative recipients who receive organs from seropositive donors, has not been uniform. Some reports have suggested that administration of (high-dose) oral ganciclovir may be the most useful prophylactic technique, but there is no consensus on this issue. New modalities for the early diagnosis of asymptomatic CMV with early therapy before it progresses to symptomatic disease, such as CMV antigenemia or polymerase chain reaction (PCR), may be useful in limiting the morbidity associated with this virus.[53]

CMV can cause primary infection in a seronegative recipient of a kidney from a seropositive donor or can occur as a reactivation infection. The clinical spectrum of CMV ranges from asymptomatic infection to serious systemic disease. Early diagnosis is now made by antigenemia or PCR testing. Occasionally bronchoalveolar lavage (BAL) or upper gastrointestinal biopsy is required. If CMV infection develops despite prophylactic measures, intravenous ganciclovir, 5mg/kg twice daily, with adjustment for renal dysfunction, is given.

The prognosis of CMV pneumonia is grave if oxygenation is poor, and mechanical ventilatory support is required. In patients with severe systemic CMV disease, immunosuppression should be stopped, even if it results in loss of the allograft.[54, 55] In the preganciclovir era, death used to be seen but should be rare today because most CMV infections respond relatively well to ganciclovir therapy.

Herpes simplex infections usually present as mucocutaneous infections; low-dose acyclovir (200 mg orally twice daily) is effective prophylaxis. Active infections respond to intravenous acyclovir. Herpes zoster varicella infections (shingles) usually present as a vesicular rash along a single dermatome. Intravenous acyclovir (10 mg/kg every 8 hours with adjustment for renal dysfunction) is the treatment of choice.

Epstein-Barr virus can be associated with post-transplant lymphoproliferative disorder, which can result in serious systemic complications, multiple organ failure, or death. Immunosuppressive therapy is withdrawn, and high-dose intravenous acyclovir (500 mg/m^2 every 8 hours) or ganciclovir is administered.

Protozoal Infections

P. carinii is the most common protozoal pathogen causing pneumonia in immunosuppressed patients. Prophylactic therapy with trimethoprim-sulfamethoxazole (80/400 mg), given once or twice a day, or inhalational pentamidine (300 mg once a month) essentially eliminates the disease. Established pneumonia is treated with cessation of immunosuppression and intravenous trimethoprim-sulfamethoxazole (20 mg/kg/day with adjustment for renal dysfunction) or pentamidine (4 mg/kg/day). Patients with renal dysfunction and oliguria require close monitoring in view of the high obligatory fluid requirements associated with administration of these drugs. Patients with severe pulmonary infection require mechanical ventilatory support, and the prognosis is poor.[56, 57]

Fungal Infections

In immunosuppressed patients, saprophytic fungi can cause infections. [58–62] *Candida* is the most common fungal pathogen. Oral candidiasis is prevented by low-dose oral nystatin (5mL four times a day). *Candida* esophagitis can respond to high-dose oral nystatin (20 mL four times a day), although a short course of amphotericin B (0.25 mg/kg/day for 3 to 5 days) is often also necessary. Rarely, *Candida* infection can present as a mycotic pseudoaneurysm of the arterial suture line of the allograft. This can result in massive hemorrhage. The usual treatment of this complication consists of allograft nephrectomy and ligation of the iliac artery; arterial bypass of that vessel may also be necessary.

Systemic fungal infections resulting in pneumonia or brain abscesses are found in debilitated patients who have received a great deal of immunosuppression therapy and multiple broad-spectrum antibiotics. *Mucor, Aspergillus*, or *Cryptococcus* may be the cause of other important fungal infections and can cause severe pulmonary and cerebral complications. Systemic fungal infections are usually treated with full-dose amphotericin B. Other fungal agents, such as flucytosine and fluconazole, may be useful adjunctive agents. Patients with brain abscesses may require more aggressive treatment with drainage and placement of an Omaya reservoir for direct delivery of the drugs into the cerebrospinal fluid or actual resection of the lesion; the mortality is extremely high.

Gastrointestinal Complications

The range of gastrointestinal problems after transplantation is enormous.[63–66]

Esophagus

The most common esophageal problem, *Candida* esophagitis, has been discussed. Esophageal reflux, usually a preexisting problem, can be exacerbated by steroids and is treated with the same agents used for peptic ulcer disease.

Stomach and Duodenum

The stomach is often the site of post-transplant complications. The necessity for high-dose steroids makes peptic ulcer disease more likely. Routine prophylaxis with H_2 blockers, sucralfate, and antacids minimizes the incidence of ulcer formation. Omeprazole is effective in patients without adequate response to H_2 blockers. Patients can present with bleeding or, less commonly, perforation, but these should be uncommon with adequate prophylaxis.[67] *H. pylori* is also seen in this group of patients with symptoms and needs treatment with appropriate antibiotics.[68] CMV (see earlier) can affect both the stomach and duodenum; diagnosis and treatment are as described earlier. Diabetic patients are prone to gastroparesis; cisaparide is often effective in managing this problem. In some patients, erythromycin, 250 mg three times daily, has been useful.

Small Intestine and Colon

The large intestine is more often a source of complications than the small intestine.[69, 70] Exacerbations of preexisting disease, such as diverticulitis or even occult carcinoma, can occur and are handled according to standard surgical principles. Immunosuppression may have to be decreased or discontinued temporarily.

An important early colonic problem is pseudo-obstruction, or *Ogilvie's syndrome.* It tends to occur in patients with nonfunctioning kidneys and can lead to perforation, most commonly of the cecum. This is a devastating complication that can result in sepsis and even death. Avoidance is the goal; when it does occur, early, aggressive colonoscopy with placement of a decompression tube can be of enormous help in preventing perforation.

Perforation is treated according to the usual surgical principles. Invasive CMV disease in the colon can present as bleeding, particularly from a cecal ulcer. Post-transplant lymphoproliferative disorder can present as single or multiple masses in the colon or small intestine, or both, with or without bleeding. Both are treated as described earlier. In a report of 34 episodes of colonic perforations in 30 patients among 1401 consecutive renal transplants, the mortality rate after colonic perforation was 38%.[71]

Liver

Viral hepatitis secondary to hepatitis B or C is an important cause of morbidity and mortality after renal transplantation. Patients with quiescent preexisting disease may experience an exacerbation related to immunosuppression. New-onset disease can also occur. Progression to end-stage liver disease and the need for liver transplantation, although uncommon, can certainly occur. Treatment with interferon-alpha has been tried, with disastrous results, including a high incidence of allograft loss.

Although generally a less serious problem, gallbladder disease can be a source of significant morbidity. Gallstones noted in the pretransplant evaluation are best treated by cholecystectomy before transplantation. Post-transplant complications of preexisting cholelithiasis can include acute inflammation, pancreatitis, and even perforation. New formation of gallstones after transplantation is not uncommon, particularly under cyclosporine immunosuppression. The availability of laparoscopic cholecystectomy is an attractive option in the immunosuppressed transplant patient.

An important point should be made in patients taking original formulation of cyclosporine (Sandimmune) who require common bile duct exploration. With this cyclosporine excreted by the liver, an open T tube significantly decreases cyclosporine levels and appropriate dosage adjustment is required. The new oral formulation of cyclosporine (Neoral) may not be associated with this problem.

Pancreatitis

Pancreatitis after transplantation can be related to multiple causes. Slakey and colleagues reported an incidence of 1.3%.[72] The most important offender is steroids, although azathioprine, pentamidine, and trimethoprim-sulfamethoxazole can also cause pancreatitis in addition to hypercalcemia or biliary disease. Post-transplant pancreatitis can be a serious problem and may lead to severe morbidity and even death. Withdrawal of the offending agent and supportive care, with attention to fluid and electrolyte balance and adequate nutrition, usually lead to resolution. Immunosuppression treatment may need to be reduced or temporarily stopped as well. Somatostatin may be useful in the treatment of severe pancreatitis.[73]

Neurologic Complications

Neurologic complications are usually related to drug toxicity or infections.[74–77] Metabolic encephalopathy, hypertensive encephalopathy, cerebrovascular events, and new-onset seizures have all been reported. Infections can be caused by *Listeria, Cryptococcus, Nocardia, Aspergillus,* and *Mucor. Toxoplasma, Coccidia,* CMV, and herpes infections are also reported. Cerebral hemorrhage can occur secondary to septic emboli or intracerebral aneurysms. Early detection and aggressive management are needed to improve survival.

Seizures after transplantation may be related to inadvertent withdrawal of antiseizure medications or to drug toxicity or metabolic problems. Traditional antiseizure medications, such as phenobarbital and diphenylhydantoin, can, by virtue of accelerating the cytochrome P_{450} pathway in the liver, lead to a marked decrease in cyclosporine or tacrolimus levels and may require increased dosing, guided by close monitoring of blood levels.

SUMMARY

Most of the patients undergoing renal transplantation have a relatively unremarkable postoperative course and are usually discharged from the hospital within 4 to 10 days. This chapter has addressed both routine management and the diagnosis and treatment of complications resulting in admission to the ICU. Close collaboration among the transplant surgeon, nephrologist, and intensivist is needed to provide optimal care and improve outcome.

References

1. Cecka JM, Terasaki PI: The UNOS Scientific Renal Transplant Registry. *In:* Clinical Transplants 1995. Terasaki PI, Cecka JM (Eds). Los Angeles, UCLA Tissue Typing Laboratory, 1996, p 1.
2. Eggers P: Comparison of treatment costs between dialysis and transplantation. Semin Nephrol 1992; 12:284.
3. Simmons RG, Anderson CR, Abress LK: Quality of life and rehabilitation differences among four end-stage renal disease therapy groups. Scand J Urol Nephrol 1990; 131:7.
4. United States Renal Data System (USRDS): USRDS 1996 Annual Data Report. Bethesda, Md, National Institutes of Health, National Institute of Diabetes and Kidney Diseases, 1996; and Am J Kidney Dis 28(Suppl 2), 1996.
5. Hunt J: Pretransplant evaluation and outcome. Semin Nephrol 1992; 12:227.
6. Peddi VR, First MR: Primary care of patients with renal transplants. Med Clin North Am (Renal Disease). 1997; 81:767.
7. Braun WE, Marwick TH: Coronary artery disease in renal transplant recipients. Cleve Clin J Med 1994; 61:370.
8. Philipson JD, Carpenter BJ, Itzkoff J, et al: Evaluation of cardiovascular risk for renal transplantation in diabetic patients. Am J Med 1986; 81:630.
9. Weinrauch LA, D'elia JA, Monaco AP, et al: Preoperative evaluation for diabetic renal transplantation: Impact of clinical, laboratory, and echocardiographic parameters on patient and allograft survival. Am J Med 1992; 93:19.
10. Burgos LG, Ebert TJ, Asiddao C, et al: Increased intraoperative

cardiovascular morbidity in diabetics with autonomic neuropathy. Anesthesiology 1989; 70:591.
11. Darby CR, Cranston D, Raine AE, et al: Bilateral nephrectomy before transplantation: Indications, surgical approach, morbidity and mortality. Br J Surg 1991; 78:305.
12. Kahan BD: Cyclosporine. N Engl J Med 1989; 321:1725.
13. Starzl TE, Fung JJ, Jordan M, et al: Kidney transplantation under FK 506. JAMA 1990; 264:63.
14. Shapiro R, Jordan M, Scantlebury V, et al: FK 506 in clinical kidney transplantation. Transplant Proc 1991; 23:3065.
15. Hood KA, Zarembski DG: Mycophenolate mofetil: A unique immunosuppressive agent. Am J Health Syst Pharm 1997; 54:285.
16. Sadaghdar H, Chelluri L, Bowles SA, et al: Outcome of renal transplant recipients in the ICU. Chest 1995; 107:1402.
17. Bia MJ, Lu D, Tyler K, et al: Beta adrenergic control of extrarenal potassium disposal: A beta-2 mediated phenomenon. Nephron 1986; 43:117.
18. Garcia TMP, Cardeal da Costa JA, Costa RS, et al: Acute tubular necrosis in kidney transplant patients treated with enalapril. Ren Fail 1994; 16:419.
19. Edelstein CL, Jacobs JC, Moosa MR: Pulmonary complications in 110 consecutive renal transplant recipients. S Afr Med J 1995; 85:160.
20. Vacharajani TJ, Asari AJ, Tucker B, et al: Ipsilateral deep thrombosis in renal transplant recipients: The need for prolonged anticoagulation. Nephrol Dial Transplant 1997; 12:627.
21. Pasquale MD, Abrams JH, Najarian JS: Use of Greenfiled filters in renal transplant patients: Are they safe? [brief communication]. Transplantation 1993; 55:439.
22. Ojo AO, Wolfe RA, Held PJ, et al: Delayed graft function: Risk factors and implications for renal allograft survival. Transplantation 1997; 63:968.
23. Hampl H, Paeprer H, Unger V, et al: Hemodynamic changes during hemodialysis, sequential ultrafiltration, and hemofiltration. Kidney Int 1980; 18:S83.
24. Campese VM: Cardiovascular instability during hemodialysis. Kidney Int 1988; 33:S186.
25. Broe M, DeBacker W: Pathophysiology of hemodialysis-associated hypoxemia. Adv Nephrol 1989; 18:297.
26. Lauer A, Alvis R, Avram M: Hemodynamic consequences of continuous arteriovenous hemofiltration. Am J Kidney Dis 1988; 12:110.
27. Scott TR, Graham GM, Schweitzer EJ, et al: Colonic necrosis following sodium polystyrene sulfonate (Kayexalate) sorbitol enema in a renal transplant patient. Dis Colon Rectum 1993; 36:607.
28. Wooton FT, Rhodes DF, Lee WM, et al: Colonic necrosis with Kayexalate-sorbitol enemas after renal transplantation. Ann Intern Med 1989; 111:947.
29. Fung JJ, Alesiani M, Abu-Elmagd K, et al: Adverse effects associated with the use of FK 506. Transplant Proc 1991; 23:3105.
30. Ichihashi T, Naoe T, Yoshida H, et al: Hemolytic uremic syndrome during FK 506 therapy. Lancet 1992; 340:60.
31. Baciewicz AM, Baciewicz FA: Cyclosporine pharmacokinetic drug interactions. Am J Surg 1989; 157:264.
32. Deierhoi MH, Barber HW, Curtis JJ, et al: A comparison of OKT3 antibody and corticosteroids in the treatment of acute renal allograft rejection. Am J Kidney Dis 1988; 11:86.
33. Thistlethwaite JR, Stuart JK, Mayes JT, et al: Monitoring and complications of monoclonal therapy: Complications and monitoring of OKT3 therapy. Am J Kidney Dis 1988; 11:112.
34. Stein KL, Ladowski J, Kormos R, et al: The cardiopulmonary response to OKT3 in orthotopic cardiac transplant recipients. Chest 1989; 95:817.
35. Abramowicz D, Crusiaux A, Goldman M: Anaphylactic shock after retreatment with OKT3 monoclonal antibody. N Engl J Med 1992; 327:736.
36. Mannucci PM, Remuzzi G, Pusineri F, et al: Deamino-8-D-arginine vasopressin shortens the bleeding time in uremia. N Engl J Med 1983; 308:8.
37. Remuzzi G: Bleeding disorders in uremia: Pathophysiology and treatment. Adv Nephrol 1989; 18:171.
38. Shemin D, Elnour M, Amarantes B, et al: Oral estrogens decrease bleeding time and improve clinical bleeding in patients with renal failure. Am J Med 1990; 89:436.
39. Greger B, Bockhorn H, Reeb A, et al: Treatment of perioperative bleeding after kidney transplantation by conjugated estrogen. Transplant Proc 1987; 19:3704.
40. Ghasemian SMR, Guleria AS, Khuwand NY, et al: Diagnosis and management of the urologic complications of renal transplantation. Clin Transpl 1996; 10:218.
41. Shoskes DA, Hanbury D, Cranston D, et al: Urological complications in 1,000 consecutive renal transplant recipients. J Urol 1995; 153:18.
42. Boitard C, Bach JF: Long-term complications of conventional immunosuppressive treatment. Adv Nephrol 1989; 18:335.
43. Guijarro C, Massad ZA, Widerkehr MR, et al: Serum albumin and mortality after renal transplantation. Am J Kidney Dis 1996; 27:117.
44. Peterson PK, Ferguson R, Fryd DS, et al: Infectious diseases in hospitalized renal transplant recipients: A prospective study of a complex and evolving problem. Medicine 1982; 61:360.
45. Hibberd PL, Rubin RH: Renal transplantation and related infections. Semin Respir Infect 1993; 8:216.
46. Hall CM, Wilcox PA, Swanepoel CR, et al: Mycobacterial infection in renal transplant recipients. Chest 1994; 106:435.
47. Wilczek H, Kallings I, Nystrom B, et al: Nosocomial legionnaires' disease following renal transplantation. Transplantation 1987; 43:847.
48. Englund JA, Sullivan CJ, Jordan C, et al: Respiratory syncytial virus infection in immunocompromised adults. Ann Intern Med 1988; 109:203.
49. Sherry MK, Klainer AS, Wolff M, et al: Herpetic tracheobronchitis. Ann Intern Med 1988; 109:229.
50. Jenkins D, Wicks A: Herpes simplex esophagitis in a renal transplant patient: The need for antiviral therapy. Am J Gastroenterol 1988; 83:331.
51. Kharsa G, Degott C, Degos F, et al: Fulminant hepatitis in renal transplant recipients. Transplantation 1987; 44:221.
52. Quarto M, Germinario C, Fontana A, et al: HIV transmission through kidney transplantation from a living related donor. N Engl J Med 1989; 320:1754.
53. Cunningham R, Harris A, Frankton A, et al: Detection of cytomegalovirus using PCR in serum from renal transplant recipients. J Clin Pathol 1995; 48:575.
54. Balfour HH, Chace BA, Stapleton JT, et al: A randomized, placebo-controlled trial of oral acyclovir for the prevention of cytomegalovirus disease in recipients of renal allografts. N Engl J Med 1989; 320:1381.
55. Zaia JA: Prevention and treatment of cytomegalovirus pneumonia in transplant recipients. Clin Infect Dis 1993; 17:S392.
56. Masur H: Prevention and treatment of pneumocystis pneumonia. N Engl J Med 1992; 327:1853.
57. Fox BC, Sollinger HW, Belzer FO, et al: A prospective, randomized, double-blind study of trimethoprim-sulfamethoxazole for prophylaxis of infection in renal transplantation: Clinical efficacy, absorption of trimethoprim-sulfamethoxazole, effects on the microflora, and the cost-benefit of prophylaxis. Am J Med 1990; 89:255.
58. Nampoory MRN, Zhan ZU, Johny KV, et al: Invasive fungal infections in renal transplant recipients. J Infect 1996; 33:95.
59. Terrell CL, Hermans PE: Antifungal agents used for deep-seated mycotic infections. Mayo Clin Proc 1987; 62:1116.
60. Perfect JR, Durack DT, Gallis HA: Cryptococcemia. Medicine 1983; 62:98.
61. Martinez EJ, Cancio MR, Sinnott JT, et al: Nonfatal gastric mucormycosis in a renal transplant recipient. South Med J 1997; 90:341.
62. Morduchowicz G, Shmueli D, Shapira Z, et al: Rhinocerebral mucormycosis in renal transplant recipients: Report of three cases and review of the literature. Rev Infect Dis 1986; 8:441.
63. Tavli S, Kekec Y, Tokyay R, et al: Severe surgical complications after kidney transplantation. Transplant Proc 1992; 24:1859.
64. Santiago-Deplin EA, Morales-Otero LA, Gonzalez ZA: Gastrointestinal complications and appendicitis after kidney transplantation. Transplant Proc 1989; 21:3745.
65. Castaneda MA, Garvin PJ: General surgical procedures in renal allograft recipients. Am J Surg 1986; 152:717.
66. Komorowski RA, Cohen EB, Kauffman HM, et al: Gastrointestinal complications in renal transplant recipients. Am J Clin Pathol 1986; 86:161.
67. Sarosdy MF, Saylor R, Dittman W, et al: Upper gastrointestinal bleeding following renal transplantation. Urology 1985; 26:347.
68. Teenan RP, Burgoyne M, Brown IL, et al: *Helicobacter pylori* in renal transplant patients. Transplantation 1993; 56:100.

69. Stylianos S, Forde KA, Benvenisty AI, et al: Lower gastrointestinal hemorrhage in renal transplant recipients. Arch Surg 1988; 123:739.
70. Murphy BJ, Weinfeld A: Innocuous pneumatosis intestinalis of the right colon in renal transplant recipients: Report of three cases. Dis Colon Rectum 1987; 30:816.
71. Stelzner M, Vlahakos DV, Milford EL, et al: Colonic perforations after renal transplantation. J Am Coll Surg 1997; 184:63–69.
72. Slakey DP, Johnson CP, Cziperle DJ, et al: Management of severe pancreatitis in renal transplant patients. Ann Surg 1997; 225:217.
73. Gjorup I, Roikjaer O, Andersen B, et al: A double-blinded multicenter trial of somatostatin in the treatment of acute pancreatitis. Surg Gynecol Obstet 1992; 175:397.
74. Eiedelman B: Neurologic complications. *In:* Renal Transplantation. Shapiro R, Simmons R, Starzl T (Eds). Stamford, Conn, Appleton & Lange, 1997, p 333.
75. Gottrand F, Largilliere C, Farriaux J: Cyclosporine neurotoxicity. N Engl J Med 1991; 324:1744.
76. Eck P, Silver SM, Clark EC: Acute renal failure and coma after a high dose of oral acyclovir. N Engl J Med 1991; 325:1178.
77. Eidelman BH, Abu-Elmagd K, Wilson J, et al: Neurologic complications of FK 506. Transplant Proc 1991; 23:3175.

180

Intensive Care of Liver Transplant Recipients

David J. Kramer, MD • George V. Mazariegos, MD
John J. Fung, MD, PhD

Orthotopic liver transplantation (OLTX) has become a recognized therapeutic option for patients with end-stage liver disease (ESLD). It affords the opportunity for a disabled person to return to a full and active life. Although expensive, OLTX may well be more cost effective than the routine medical care of terminally ill liver failure patients.[1, 2] The first OLTX in humans was performed by Starzl in 1963[3]; however, significant progress was not made until the advent of more potent immunosuppressives. Still, the success of OLTX and its acceptance as a routine procedure were not acknowledged until 1981 with the introduction of cyclosporine (formerly, cyclosporin A, CyA).[4] Technical improvements in surgical approach and organ preservation, combined with increasingly sophisticated anesthetic and intensive care management, have provided 30-day survival rates of nearly 90%.

In this chapter, we outline the many developments that have occurred in this field. Major advances in defining risk categories for candidates, managing patients with cirrhosis and pulmonary hypertension, and novel immunosuppressive strategies are described. Since the third edition of this textbook, two major philosophical approaches to transplantation have evolved and crystallized. These center on how to define *best* outcome. Indeed, what constitutes the best outcome depends on whether it is the graft survival or the survival of all potential recipients that is under consideration. The graft will fare best if only the most ideal organs are donated, accepted, and implanted into the healthiest recipients. The operative risk is smallest for this group, and 1-year survival best. However, the overall benefit to the group of less sick patients is less than for the sicker candidates. In centers where extremely ill patients undergo OLTX, survival rates are initially lower than for healthier patients, although many survive and return to their families and jobs.

The benefit of the procedure is much greater, in the aggregate, for this group of patients. Furthermore, the operative risks are assumed for patients who have very little chance of surviving without OLTX. Obviously, smaller and less experienced programs focus more on the first objective and refer the sicker patients to larger, more experienced centers that have adopted the latter philosophy. Organ allocation policies may enhance or frustrate each of these approaches. The current United Network for Organ Sharing (UNOS) policy of regional allocation of organs and the absence of national organ sharing favors the more conservative approach that emphasizes graft viability. This policy is currently under review, with the U.S. Secretary of Health and Human Services proposing changes in allocation policies, including a national list.[5]

CANDIDATE SELECTION

The best candidates are those for whom the risk of surgery is far outweighed by the potential improvement in their quality of life. Furthermore, the risk of recurrence of the primary disease should be low.[6, 7] Not surprisingly, those who are at highest risk from surgery also enjoy the greatest gains when they survive. Unfortunately, high-risk patients have higher mortality rates and require significantly greater resources, particularly for intensive care and rehabilitation. Ultimately, who gets which donated organ is largely a function of institutional bias and organ availability. Indeed, programs in the nascent stages should not be expected to assume care of high-risk patients until they have demonstrated mastery of basic cases. This should not mean that the more difficult patients are not cared for, but rather that they are referred to centers with more experience.

Organ allocation, therefore, is pivotal. When donors are available or a change in technique makes available previously discarded organs, the threshold for working with high-risk patients can be lowered. When, however, organs are scarce or are not distributed according to need, patients who are at high risk often have to wait so long that transplantation is by then no longer feasible.

The University of Pittsburgh recognizes few absolute contraindications to OLTX, but certain factors have been identified that significantly increase the risk and should be recognized as relative contraindications (Table 180–1). From the surgical perspective, a history of right upper quadrant abdominal surgery, particularly biliary reconstruction, renders the procedure technically more difficult. Patients who are sicker (U.S. UNOS, Status 1),[8] particularly those with fulminant hepatic failure (FHF), fare worse. In that regard, those with higher Acute

TABLE 180–1. Contraindications to Liver Transplantation

Absolute	Relative
Extrahepatic malignancy	Cholangiocarcinoma
Extrahepatic infection	HIV infection (in the absence of AIDS)
Hepatitis B with active replication	Hepatitis B without evidence of active replication
Brain death (in patients with FHF)	Elevated intracranial pressure associated with hemodynamic instability in FHF; portal venous thrombosis; extrahepatic organ system failure not related to ESLD; pulmonary hypertension; hepatopulmonary syndrome

HIV = human immunodeficiency virus; AIDS = acquired immunodeficiency syndrome; FHF = fulminant hepatic failure; ESLD = end-stage liver disease.

Physiology and Chronic Health Evaluation (APACHE) II scores, those in an intensive care unit (ICU), and particularly those who require mechanical ventilation or hemodialysis or both, fare worst of all. Not surprisingly, in such circumstances medical therapy is even less successful.

Patients with cirrhosis and underlying hepatocellular carcinoma are candidates for OLTX when (1) the disease is limited to the liver and the lesions are small, (2) there is no evidence of major intrahepatic venous invasion, (3) the disease is unilobar, and (4) local nodal disease is absent. Extensive radiologic staging of these patients to stratify them by tumor stage is imperative so that the risk of postoperative recurrence can be estimated. Biliary tract cancers such as cholangiocarcinoma have very high rates of recurrence.[9, 10] Whether more extensive resection, including the liver, a portion of small bowel, and the pancreas, will more successfully control recurrence of these tumors is doubtful.[11, 12]

Graft recipients with chronic hepatitis B virus (HBV) infection almost always suffer recurrence of the disease in the graft.[13] The time course varies much, and some investigators have argued that the enormity of the problem, from a worldwide perspective, the speed with which viral inhibitors are being developed, and the varied post-transplant courses argue for an attempt at OLTX.[14, 15] Adjuvant therapy with hepatitis B immune globulin[15] has been reported to be of benefit, particularly when it is guided by titers. The benefit accrued is small, however, and other inhibitors (e.g., thymosin) are under active investigation.[16] Lamivudine reduces active viral replication and is being investigated for perioperative and postoperative use.[17-19] For reasons that are unclear, transplant recipients who already had hepatitis B fare worse at each postoperative stage than those with ESLD of other causes.[20]

At present, patients with evidence of active viral replication including serum HBV deoxyribonucleic acid (DNA) or who are hepatitis B E-antigen positive are not candidates for OLTX at the University of Pittsburgh Medical Center. Patients who respond to antiviral therapy and no longer exhibit active HBV replication are eligible for transplantation.

Although, given the need for additional immunosuppression, patients who are infected with the human immunodeficiency virus (HIV) at the time of OLTX might be expected to have a disastrous postoperative course, this has not been the case. Indeed, the survival rate *is* lower than that for HIV-negative OLTX patients, but only slightly so.[8, 21] Improved antiretroviral therapy with the addition of protease inhibitors[22] has changed the natural history of this infection, making more aggressive medical support appropriate. Concern is greatest for the operating surgeons, anesthesiologists, and intensivists who routinely perform invasive procedures on such patients and the operating room and intensive care nurses and other caregivers. At our center, only patients with advanced disease (i.e., acquired immunodeficiency syndrome [AIDS]-related complex or established AIDS) are denied OLTX.

Thrombosed portal veins present a formidable surgical challenge. Superior mesenteric artery (SMA) angiography is in order, with venous phase studies to demonstrate patency of the superior mesenteric vein (SMV). SMV occlusion usually precludes liver transplantation, although an innovative approach undertakes to anastomose the donor portal vein to the recipient inferior vena cava (IVC) and to place a proximal caval ligature to sustain portal flow. Mesenteric venous hypertension is not addressed directly, but portal decompression and enhanced coagulation reduce the risk of bleeding. Combined hepatic and intestinal transplantation and/or multivisceral transplantation are alternatives.[23]

FHF (i.e., liver failure with encephalopathy developing within 8 weeks in a patient who previously had no known liver disease)[24] is increasingly being managed with OLTX. With this surgical option, survival has improved from 20% to 75%.[25, 26] Such patients are critically ill at the time of transplantation. They require intensive preoperative hemodynamic and neurologic monitoring. Intracranial pressure monitoring[27-31] and cerebral blood flow determination are used routinely at our institution. The condition of some patients improves with supportive care (e.g., those with acetaminophen intoxication, *Amanita* poisoning, or hepatitis A), but most deteriorate. Progressive encephalopathy with sustained intracranial hypertension resulting in inadequate cerebral perfusion precludes successful OLTX because brain death will result.[32] Such patients are also prone to develop pancreatitis, which, when severe, makes OLTX unacceptably risky. Cardiovascular instability,[33] atrial or ventricular arrhythmia,[34] and respiratory insufficiency are common complications of FHF that make the operative risk significantly higher. Patients who require high-dose vasopressor support (e.g., more than 1 μg/kg/min epinephrine) and those with severe adult respiratory distress syndrome (ARDS), who need positive end-expiratory pressure (PEEP) of more than 10 cm H_2O or a fraction of inspired oxygen (FIO_2) greater than 70% are at unacceptable operative risk. Pancreatitis, which is common in patients with FHF, should resolve before OLTX is undertaken.

ESLD that is severe enough to make a person eligible for OLTX often progresses precipitously, so that the patient must be admitted to the ICU. Common precipitants are infection (particularly pneumonia and spontaneous bacterial peritonitis) and gastrointestinal bleeding (e.g., from esophageal or gastric varices, portal hypertensive gastropathy, gastric or duodenal ulceration). Although these events herald the impending demise of the patient and intensify the search for an organ, they also further compromise the potential recipient and may lead to multisystem organ failure (MSOF), and subsequently death.

Deciding when a patient is "too sick" to undergo OLTX is fraught with complexity. Patients with unresolved extrahepatic infection and those with high vasopressor requirements should not undergo transplantation. Although they might survive the operation, the graft is likely to fail quickly, resulting in death. Short of this disastrous scenario, we have successfully transplanted patients with MSOF who were in renal failure and required dialysis, who had respiratory failure requiring mechanical ventilation, and who had grade IV encephalopathy and profound coagulopathy. When graft function is good, MSOF resolves.

DONOR SELECTION AND OPERATION

Assessing potential donor graft function is still a very inexact exercise. Obviously, potential donors who have a malignancy or HIV or hepatitis B infection are eliminated. Other considerations include age beyond 65 years (although some such grafts have clearly functioned acceptably) and direct liver trauma. Evidence of chronic liver disease in the donor should be sought, but often it may not become evident until gross inspection of the organ or after procurement. Donor livers with biopsy-proven microvesicular steatosis are not routinely accepted. Liver function test results are not sufficiently discriminating to warrant refusing a graft. Other measures, such as lidocaine clearance,[35, 36] are not routinely available soon enough.

Brain death results in marked changes in homeostasis. Hemodynamic instability is common and may result, in part, from massive fluid loss secondary to diabetes insipidus. Correction with desmopressin, adequate hemodynamic monitoring, and intervention are essential to preserving vital organ function. Anesthetic techniques that blunt the response to surgical stimulation are also essential.

Skilled surgical dissection—rapid identification of the hepatic vessels,[37] including the hepatic arterial anomalies observed in 20% of the population, cannulation and perfusion with University of Wisconsin (UW) solution, and rapid cooling—is essential for graft preservation. Although cold ischemia of less than 16 hours' duration is preferable, up to 24 hours' ischemia is still compatible with adequate graft function.[38]

RECIPIENT OPERATION

The recipient operation has become a highly refined procedure. Improvements in anesthetic and surgical practice have made evident the importance of the other factors described previously (candidate selection and donor organ quality), in the recipient's outcome. The surgical procedure may be divided into three stages: hepatectomy, anhepatic, and postreperfusion. Each demands special consideration from anesthesiologist and surgeon.

Recipient monitoring for such cases includes pulse oximetry, electrocardiography, arterial pressure (often from two vessels), and pulmonary arterial pressure. Maintenance of large-bore central venous catheters (e.g., two No. 8.5 French introducers) and the ability to infuse whole blood at up to 2 L/min with the rapid infusion system are essential to maintaining hemodynamic stability during the occasional episode of massive blood loss.

Right ventricular function may be compromised by the presence of pulmonary hypertension, which can develop suddenly during reperfusion.[39-42] Titration of intravenous fluid and vasopressors may be more effectively guided by the right ventricular ejection fraction and end-diastolic volume. These values can be obtained through the REF1 oximetric pulmonary artery catheter (Baxter-Edwards).

Additional cardiovascular assessment is provided by frequent use of transesophageal echocardiography. This provides the anesthesiologist a dynamic on-line picture of the adequacy of resuscitation. For patients with FHF, who are prone to experience intracranial hypertension, intracranial pressure monitoring is essential. Cerebral blood flow measurements are difficult to obtain in the operating room but may be estimated from the arterial-jugular venous oxygen gradient.

Cerebral blood flow can also be assessed by transcranial Doppler ultrasound to measure the velocity of flow in the middle cerebral artery. Continuous electroencephalography (EEG) and compressed spectral array are under investigation as monitoring techniques in this setting.

Anesthesia is often induced with etomidate and maintained with a balanced technique of inhalational agents (isoflurane), muscle relaxants (vecuronium), and judicious use of narcotics (fentanyl) and benzodiazepines (midazolam).[43]

Monitoring of the recipient's coagulation capacity is complicated by profound derangements and the need for rapid correction. Depletion of coagulation factors and thrombocytopenia are common. Furthermore, excessive fibrinolysis, which may be evident early in the procedure but not clinically important, may assume a major role after significant blood loss, particularly during reperfusion. Standard measures of coagulation—prothrombin time (PT), partial thromboplastin time (PTT), platelet count—are very sensitive; however, transfusion based solely on abnormalities in these measures results in overtransfusion. Furthermore, there is often a significant delay in obtaining these measurements.

Kang and colleagues introduced the thromboelastograph for routine use during OLTX. It provides the anesthesiologist rapid assessment of the coagulation status, the presence or absence of fibrinolysis, and the effects of intervention with protamine or ε-aminocaproic acid, an inhibitor of fibrinolysis.[44-46]

The surgical procedure involves meticulous dissection, which is often hampered by severe portal hypertension and substantial bleeding from venous collaterals. Insufficient control results in significant blood loss. Identification of the hilar structures may be complicated by adhesions from previous biliary tract surgery. Recipient vessel patency and the adequacy of blood flow must be assessed before the graft is placed into the surgical field. An arterial graft for the hepatic artery may be chosen when the recipient anatomy is anomalous or of diminished caliber or when the presence of atherosclerosis makes stenosis of the celiac trunk or native hepatic artery likely. Other indications include a marked size discrepancy and inadequate donor artery length. Portal venous thrombosis may be managed with a "jump" graft from the superior mesenteric vein when the portal vein cannot be "declotted."[47] The donor and recipient caval veins are usually anastomosed end to end above and below the liver.

Another technique, "piggyback,"[48-50] may be preferred in settings of marked hemodynamic instability—using only portal bypass—or when there is a marked size discrepancy between donor and recipient. The technique requires isolating the hepatic veins of the recipient without interrupting flow in the IVC. Venovenous bypass is routinely used in our center (Fig. 180-1) to minimize hemodynamic instability, portal hypertension, and venous congestion of the intestines.[51] The biliary anastomosis is fashioned after the vascular anastomoses are completed and the graft reperfused.

Two options currently used are (1) choledochocholedochostomy and (2) creation of a midjejunal Roux-en-Y limb with a choledochojejunostomy (Fig. 180-2). The former is faster and anatomically more pleasing. Unfortunately, there is a significant rate of restenosis. Care must also be taken not to create such an anastomosis when the bile duct is involved in the primary disease process, as with primary sclerosing cholangitis.

In approximately 10% of patients, reperfusion is accompanied by nearly complete cardiovascular collapse.[52] Although the exact mechanism is undefined, marked shifts occur in electrolytes (hyperkalemia and hypocalcemia) and temperature, perhaps in reaction to the preservative solution. A hypocontractile left ventricle complicates the loss of vasomotor tone. Volume resuscitation and inotropes (epinephrine) plus replenishment of calcium guided by ionized calcium analysis is usually sufficient to recover. Fortunately, this event is usually short lived. Nevertheless, significant insults to the graft, heart, kidneys, and brain can occur that require postoperative attention.

POSTOPERATIVE MANAGEMENT

As might be surmised from the preceding discussion, the postoperative management of the OLTX recipient is governed largely by the patient's preoperative condition, the adequacy of the donor organ, and operative success of the recipient surgical and anesthesia teams. Indeed, the function of the graft is the predominant factor in the patient's recovery.

Liver Allograft Function

Early graft function is usually assessed by measurement of total bilirubin, transaminases, canalicular enzymes, and clotting factors. The schematic presented by the University of Toronto is useful for assessing graft function by these parameters (Table 180-2).[53] Parameters such as the arterial ketone body ratio (AKBR)[54] and oxygen consumption[55] correlate with graft survival. However, even in a retrospective review of our patients, Doyle and colleagues were unable to define one predictor with adequate sensitivity and specificity to render it 100% predictive of outcome for an individual patient.[56] Other

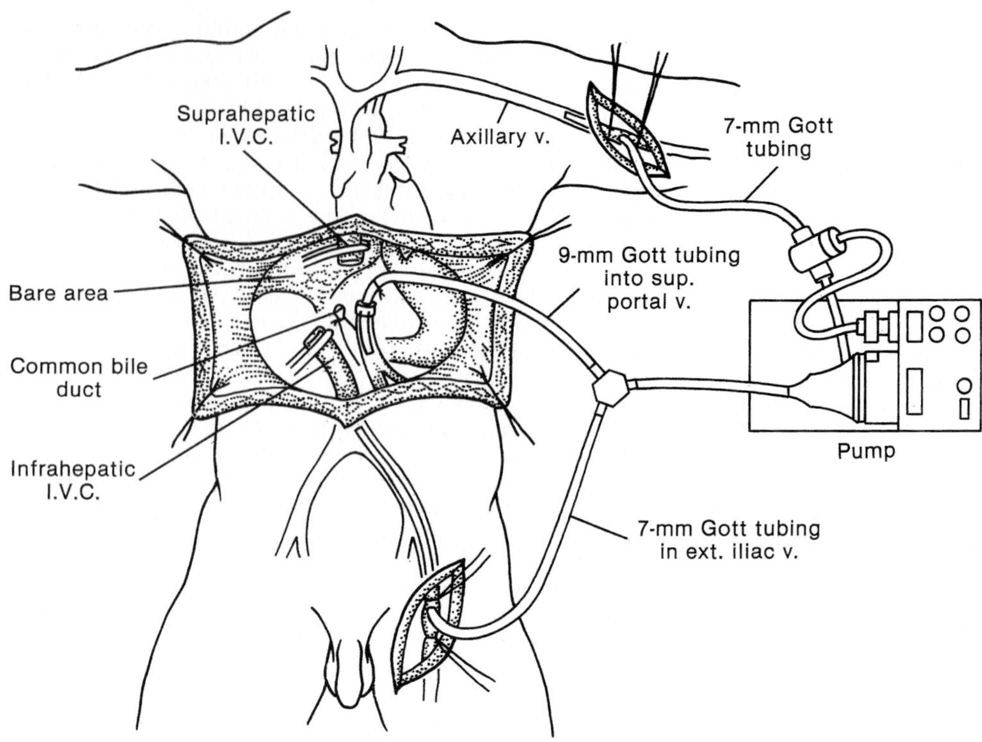

Figure 180–1. Venovenous bypass. I.V.C. = inferior vena cava; ext. iliac v. = external iliac vein. (From Starzl TE, Griffith BP, Shaw BW Jr, et al: Veno-venous bypass without systemic anticoagulation for transplantation of the human liver. Surg Gynecol Obstet 1985; 160:270, by permission of Surgery, Gynecology, & Obstetrics.)

TABLE 180–2. Classification of Graft Function After Orthotopic Liver Transplantation

Variable	Grade I	Grade II	Grade III	Grade IV
SGOT SGPT	<1000	>1000 initially <1000 at 48 hr	>2500 for 48 hr	>2500 and rising
PT	Normal	Mild prolongation	Very abnormal	Severe coagulopathy
Bile	>40 mL/day	<40 mL/day	Minimal	None

Data from Greig PD, Woolf GM, Sinclair SB, et al: Treatment of primary liver graft nonfunction with prostaglandin E_1. Transplantation 1989; 48:447–453.
SGOT = serum glutamic-oxaloacetic transaminase; SGPT = serum glutamate pyruvate transaminase; PT = prothrombin time.

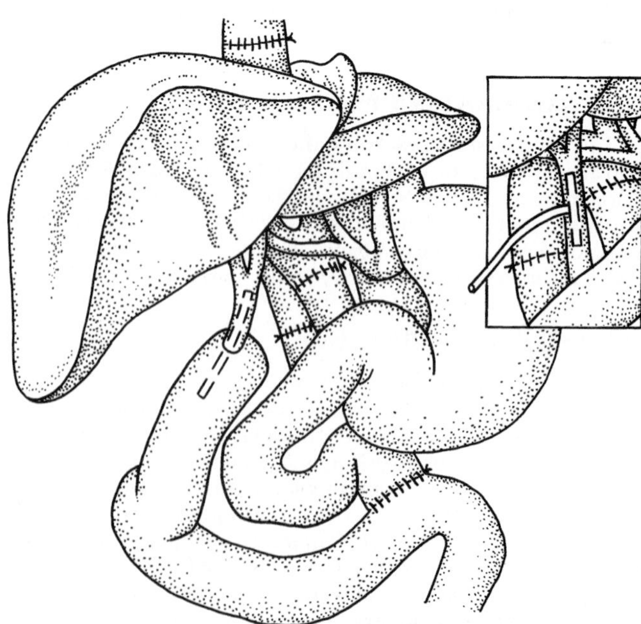

Figure 180–2. Choledochojejunostomy and choledochocholedochostomy. (From Starzl TE, Demetrius AJ, Van Thiel D: Liver transplantation. N Engl J Med 1989; 321:1014, 1092.)

techniques, such as neural network modeling, are under active investigation.[57] An alternative approach is to use a composite acuity score to predict graft and patient survival. We investigated APACHE II, a widely used acuity score for critically ill patients, in liver transplant recipients. Although the model was not developed for such patients, with recalibration predicted and observed mortality, both hospital and 1-year outcomes correlate well.[58, 59]

Typically, an elevated bilirubin level in the first few days reflects preoperative values and the consequences of the procurement. In the absence of severe harvest injury, it typically falls to normal during the first week. An injury pattern is evidenced by transaminase elevations. Aspartate aminotransferase (AST) and alanine aminotransferase (ALT) levels peak during the first 3 days and thereafter return to normal slowly. Canalicular enzymes (γ-glutamyl transpeptidase and alkaline phosphatase) typically rise to four or five times normal values and return to normal over the course of the next few weeks. Marked injury that occurs during procurement and is believed to reflect an ischemic insult results in a more extensive and more prolonged abnormality. Thus, the transaminase peak is higher, the bilirubin value remains abnormal, sometimes for weeks, and the canalicular enzymes are elevated for a long time.

Unless the liver is irreversibly damaged, synthetic function seems to normalize after the third day and the AKBR returns toward 1.0. Although the values may normalize, occasionally graft dysfunction may be evidenced only by the patient's failure to thrive. In particular, MSOF can develop or may fail to resolve. Retransplantation may then be the only option.

Knowledge of the details of procurement and implantation should color the interpretation of liver function abnormalities in the early postoperative period. Technical problems should always be sought before an immune mechanism is implicated. Even with the widespread use of percutaneous liver biopsy, histologic impressions will prove incorrect when a vascular or biliary problem is present. Furthermore, a misdiagnosed technical problem that is mistakenly treated as rejection leads to intensification of the patient's immunosuppressive regimen and places him or her at grave risk for infectious complications. Although some processes produce a typical enzyme pattern, one caveat is that these patterns are not sufficiently sensitive or specific to allow foregoing a diagnostic work-up.

The diagnostic work-up for a patient with liver function abnormalities in the perioperative period should include a Doppler ultrasound examination to determine patency of all involved vessels. Concern about the adequacy of flow should prompt angiography. Other abnormalities are often present but are not specific. Early occlusion of the hepatic artery may be addressed by immediate surgery, and the graft salvage rate is nearly 50%.[60] It presents with a precipitous deterioration in a patient's hemodynamic status, abrupt development of respiratory failure (ARDS), and severe coagulopathy, all associated with markedly elevated transaminase values. Bacteremia is common. Delayed hepatic artery thrombosis is often less dramatic in its presentation.[61] Indeed, some patients are asymptomatic. Others show destruction of the biliary duct system with multiple intrahepatic strictures, bilomas, and intrahepatic abscesses. Recurrent bacteremia, in the absence of another source, may be the only indication of hepatic artery thrombosis.

The presentation of portal venous thrombosis is usually much less dramatic. In the early postoperative period the most frequent manifestation is persistent ascites. Enteric congestion and bleeding as a consequence of portal hypertension may also occur. Later, portal vein thrombosis should be considered if variceal hemorrhage develops. Although IVC occlusion related to thrombosis in the retrohepatic vena cava does occur, it is uncommon. More common are anastomotic strictures. Stenosis at the lower anastomosis of the IVC is manifested solely by lower extremity edema and renal dysfunction. Stenosis at the upper anastomosis may present as a syndrome similar to Budd-Chiari, with marked passive congestion of the liver, ascites, lower extremity edema, and renal failure. The diagnosis may be suggested by ultrasound examination, but more often the clinical picture prompts catheterization and measurement under fluoroscopy of IVC pressures above and below the anastomoses. When the presence of strictures is confirmed, the approach is commonly surgical, but balloon dilation has been accomplished in some cases.

Competency of the biliary tract should be confirmed by cholangiography, which is simple when a T tube drains the choledochocholedochostomy but must be performed percutaneously in patients with choledochojejunostomy, for which T tubes are not used, or when elevated canalicular enzymes and persistent jaundice are unexplained. Disruption of the biliary anastomosis is rare but typically occurs near the end of the first week and may indicate thrombosis of the hepatic artery, which interrupts the blood supply to the donor part of the choledochus. It may be heralded by the sepsis syndrome and a disproportionate rise in bilirubin concentration.

Graft rejection may occur at any point after OLTX. Hyperacute rejection is noticeably rare, if it occurs at all with OLTX. Nevertheless, a humoral component of rejection may be evidenced by antibody deposition in the arterial endothelium and by persistence or recrudescence of a positive crossmatch.[62] More often, *acute cellular rejection* (ACR) develops. This is often evident after the first week but has been known to occur within the first few days—or several years—after OLTX. Thus, the usual description, "acute" is a misnomer. Although a periductal lymphocytic infiltrate associated with the development of a cellular infiltrate around the central veins is the histologic criterion for diagnosis of ACR,[63] such changes may be evident to a lesser degree even in the absence of clinical abnormalities. In a graft with stable function, rejection is typically associated with a rise in bilirubin associated with elevations in the transaminase and canalicular enzyme values. Other clinical findings include signs of the sepsis syndrome, diarrhea, suddenly increasing ascites, and laboratory findings of thrombocytopenia, hemolysis, and eosinophilia.

The term "chronic rejection," also a misnomer because it can occur at any point, refers to the development of arteriopathy and vanishing bile ducts. Its presentation is insidious, and signs of terminal liver disease may develop slowly.

Immunosuppression

The approach to rejection is divided into two phases: prophylaxis and treatment.[64] Prophylaxis is achieved by the combination of corticosteroids and cyclosporine or tacrolimus (FK-506). These agents inhibit interleukin-2 (IL-2) expression and block T cell recruitment. They offer a selective approach to immunosuppression in solid organ transplantation. Tacrolimus was incorporated into our routine clinical practice in 1989. Prospective, randomized trials comparing tacrolimus-based and cyclosporine-based regimens demonstrate that tacrolimus affords better rejection prophylaxis, is associated with fewer cases of steroid-resistant rejection and need for OKT3,[65, 66] and is less costly when total medical care in the first post-transplant year is considered.[67]

Azathioprine, used before the advent of newer immunosuppressives, is reserved for recurrent rejection episodes and for patients who are unable to tolerate necessary doses of the newer agents. Mycophenolate mofetil is hydrolized in vivo to mycophenolic acid, which inhibits inosine monophosphate dehydrogenase, resulting in selective inhibition of T and B

TABLE 180–3. Immunosuppression for Orthotopic Liver Transplant Recipients: University of Pittsburgh Regimen

Agent	Dose	Timing
Methylprednisolone	1 g	At operation
	200 mg/day taper to 20 mg/day over 6 days	Daily
PGE_1	0.6 μg/kg/hr IV infusion	5–7 days
FK-506*	0.05 mg/kg IV	Continuous infusion over 24 hr until oral intake (whole blood 10–20 ng/mL)
	0.10 mg/kg PO	Twice daily
Cyclosporine*	6 mg/kg IV	Continuous infusion over 24 hr until oral intake
	10 mg/kg PO	Twice daily
Mycophenolate	1 g	Twice daily (adjunct with FK-506 or cyclosporine ± prednisone)
Azathioprine†	2 mg/kg PO or IV	Daily (adjunct with FK-506 or cyclosporine ± prednisone)
OKT3	5–10 mg	Daily for 3–5 d for treatment of acute cellular rejection

*Either FK-506 or cyclosporine is selected.
†Used in addition to cyclosporine or FK-506.

cell proliferation.[68] Mycophenolate is more expensive than azathioprine and has significant gastrointestinal side effects (diarrhea) but less bone marrow toxicity. Preliminary data in liver transplant recipients treated with tacrolimus and prednisone versus tacrolimus, prednisone, and mycophenolate suggest that the three-drug regimen is no more toxic and may make it possible to reduce the tacrolimus dose.[69] Newer immunosuppressive agents and techniques are under development. The current regimen at the University of Pittsburgh is outlined in Table 180–3. The regimen for prophylaxis is initiated during surgery with 1 g of IV methylprednisolone followed by a rapid taper from 200 mg/day to 20 mg/day in divided doses. OKT3 is reserved for steroid-resistant ACR.[70] The approach is similar for crossmatch-positive patients, who may reject more quickly and severely,[71] but may also include prostaglandin E_1 (PGE_1, Prostin).[72] When mild, ACR is treated with a bolus of methylprednisolone and larger tacrolimus doses. If this is not adequate, we elect to use the steroid taper. OKT3 is used when rejection resistant to these measures is evident. It is used for a short course, and the tacrolimus dose is increased. Usually, chronic rejection is not amenable to intensification of therapy. One exception appears to be the improvement in graft function that occasionally attends the switch from cyclosporine to tacrolimus.[73, 74]

The major side effects of cyclosporine and tacrolimus are similar: both cause significant nephrotoxicity and neurotoxicity.[75] The insults to the kidneys incurred by the transplant procedure and the immunosuppressive regimen are evident in more than 90% of patients.[76] Ten per cent of OLTX patients require some dialysis intervention postoperatively, and a few require long-term hemodialysis. Neurotoxicity is more evident in elderly persons and is compounded by electrolyte disturbances, particularly hyponatremia and hypomagnesemia.[77] Impairments range from mild expressive aphasia to tremors, confusion, coma, and seizures. Other side effects of cyclosporine, such as hypertension and hirsutism, are less common with tacrolimus. Because tacrolimus is a more potent agent, many patients are able to have corticosteroids tapered, if not completely discontinued.[78, 79]

Abnormal liver function can attend systemic illness. For example, marked hyperbilirubinemia may occur with septic episodes, even in patients who have never received a transplant. Infections may or may not involve the liver directly; however, jaundice can occur with the development of pneumonia or may herald an abscess. Other systemic processes, such as disseminated fungal infections (*Candida* or *Aspergillus*) and herpesvirus infections (herpes simplex or herpes zoster), may result in profound derangement of liver function. A systemic process that can also affect the liver is lymphoma. A unique post-transplant lymphoproliferative disease (PTLD) has been described in these patients that can involve the liver.

HEMODYNAMIC CHANGES

The characteristic hemodynamic changes of ESLD resolve slowly after OLTX. The exact timing is not known, and the controversy likely reflects the preoperative status of some patients. Thus, these problems may resolve more slowly in patients with profoundly deranged liver function and incipient, if not established, MSOF than in recipients who are not as sick at the time of transplantation. A vasodilated hyperdynamic state is typical[80–84] and rarely normalizes completely in the immediate postoperative period. Patients who are unable to mount a hyperdynamic response fare worse, such as those who have sustained an ischemic cardiac injury or who have a restrictive cardiomyopathy, as may be seen in amyloidosis or in hemochromatosis. This observation has also been made in other postsurgical, critically ill patients; however, the magnitude of the hemodynamic changes is much greater in patients with ESLD in the post-OLTX phase.

Marked elevations in right-sided cardiac pressures compromise allograft function. Hepatic congestion results in hyperbilirubinemia. Portal vein pressure is elevated simultaneously, perhaps resulting in bacterial translocation and endotoxemia with further graft dysfunction. Depressed cardiac output causes decreased hepatic arterial and portal vein flow and allograft ischemia. Careful management of intravascular volume, with ventricular filling pressures optimized by cardiac output or stroke work index, is combined with judicious use of inotropes.

The selection of inotropic and vasopressor agents is governed by the degree of arterial vasodilatation and cardiac dysfunction. Although we favor dopamine and dobutamine, alone or in combination, it is clear that more potent agents (norepinephrine and epinephrine) may be required. In the setting of pulmonary hypertension with predominantly right-sided heart failure, more intensive monitoring of ventricular size and function with transesophageal echocardiography, including measurement of the right ventricular ejection fraction, is essential to guide titration of intravascular volume and vasoactive medication.

Marked arterial vasodilatation, which requires treatment with vasopressors, particularly when it occurs in the face of improving graft function, should prompt an evaluation for a focus of inflammation, infection, pancreatitis, and graft rejection.

In the differential diagnosis of the low cardiac output syndrome associated with high filling pressures, cardiac tamponade should be excluded at an early stage. There are surgical and medical factors that increase the potential for tamponade. These include the superior aspect of the Mercedes incision (which may violate the pericardial parietal reflection), right atrial engraftment of the inferior vena cava anastomosis, and the medical complications of depressed coagulation, thrombocytopenia, and renal failure. Cardiac tamponade usually presents with low cardiac output, elevated and equalized central venous pressure, pulmonary artery diastolic pressure and pulmonary occlusion pressure with high systemic vascular resistance, and wide arterial oxygen gradient. In patients with abnormal liver function, however, tamponade physiology may present with a deceptively normal cardiac output, calculated systemic vascular resistance, and arterial venous oxygen gradient. This paradox reflects the hyperdynamic vasodilatation present before the onset of tamponade.

Hypertension may occur in the postoperative period. It commonly reflects inadequate analgesia or sedation,[13] impaired gas exchange, and hypoglycemia, although hypotension is more common. However, hypertension may persist once these factors are addressed, and attention should then be focused on cyclosporine[85, 86] and tacrolimus. Given the vasoconstrictive properties of both medications, one likely mechanism is activation of the renin-angiotensin pathway. This complication is more common with cyclosporine than with tacrolimus (30% versus 10%) and is more resistant to antihypertensive therapy.[78, 87, 88] Antihypertensive therapy is initiated for systolic blood pressures greater than 160 mm Hg or diastolic pressure greater than 95 mm Hg and consists of calcium channel blockade with nifedipine or combined α- and β-receptor blockade with labetalol. Long-term management rests on a combination of angiotensin-converting enzyme inhibition, alpha-adrenergic blockade, and calcium channel blockade. Hypertension resistant to the first-line agents is usually managed in the ICU with stronger vasodilators, such as nitroprusside, perhaps in combination with an alpha-blocking agent.

PULMONARY CONSIDERATIONS

Pulmonary complications of ESLD are common and relate to the combination of physiologic and immune system derangements that are practically always present.[89] Thus, atelectasis, pleural effusion, reduced functional residual capacity, and limited vital capacity related to ascites are often present preoperatively. The operative procedure in the upper abdomen, placement of a "normal"-sized graft in the site of a shrunken, cirrhotic liver, and postoperative ileus may further decrease vital capacity. Inadequate pain control results in splinting and atelectasis and increases the risk of pneumonia; however, long-term pulmonary sequelae are rare, and most patients have improved pulmonary function tests when studied more than 1 year after OLTX.

Prompt evaluation of pulmonary infiltrates in these patients is mandatory. Although a primary pneumonic process should be considered, many pulmonary infiltrates do not reflect infection. Pulmonary edema—hydrostatic and nonhydrostatic—is common. Nonhydrostatic pulmonary edema, ARDS, when associated with decreased lung compliance and increased FIO_2, may result from a primary pulmonary infection but more often is associated with intra-abdominal inflammation such as peritonitis or pancreatitis. Graft failure, whether caused by rejection or primary nonfunction or a vascular catastrophe such as hepatic artery thrombosis, can also produce ARDS. When liver failure per se is identified as the cause, ARDS will resolve after successful transplantation. ARDS can also develop during treatment of rejection with OKT3.[90]

We routinely use bronchoscopic techniques to aid the clinical assessment of pulmonary infiltrates and to establish the diagnosis of pneumonia.[91] Despite the severe derangement of coagulation in these patients, bronchoalveolar lavage (BAL) may be performed without significant risk of hemorrhage. Quantitative cultures are obtained, and bacterial isolates in excess of 100,000 colony-forming units (CFU) per milliliter are considered diagnostic of pneumonia. The BAL is sensitive but lacks specificity. In certain cases when the identity of the primary offending agent must be determined, we quantitatively culture a protected brush specimen. Quantitative cultures are obtained, and isolates in excess of 1000 CFU/mL are considered positive. Complications have been rare, but we have avoided this technique in patients with severe coagulopathy. In only one third of cases of suspected pneumonia did we obtain bronchoscopic confirmation.[92] Although antibiotic administration confounds the results in some patients, in most cases negative results force evaluation for other sites of infection or inflammation.

Liver-lung interactions have been described by Matuschak and associates.[93, 94] Acute lung injury is common with advanced liver failure.[95] Patients with liver failure who develop ARDS have a very high mortality rate and are usually disqualified for liver transplantation. In a small group of patients, when we excluded the common causes of ARDS, liver transplantation was successful and lung injury resolved quickly.[96]

Two additional pulmonary complications—the hepatopulmonary syndrome and pulmonary hypertension—can also develop in patients with liver disease, specifically portosystemic shunting resulting from portal hypertension. Cyanosis has been recognized in patients with cirrhosis.[97] Several explanations have been tendered. Anatomic right-to-left shunts have been described: intrapulmonary[98, 99] and between the portal venous system and pulmonary veins via esophageal veins.[100] An increase in closing volume, resulting in air trapping, has been observed. A leftward shift of the oxyhemoglobin saturation curve has also been reported.[101] Most important, many patients have a diffusion defect. Furthermore, hypoxic pulmonary vasoconstriction is impaired. These findings correlate with anatomic studies showing dilated intrapulmonary capillaries[102] and multiple inert gas studies demonstrating significant ventilation-perfusion mismatch. Patients with the hepatopulmonary syndrome have dilated capillaries, which impair diffusion. Furthermore, increased dispersion in the ventilation-perfusion relation results in a mismatch such that many poorly ventilated units are excessively perfused.[103] This does not constitute a true right-to-left shunt, and hyperoxia will result from prolonged exposure to high FIO_2.

The most useful preoperative test is contrast echocardiography, a "bubble" study. Early appearance of contrast in the left atrium is diagnostic.[104] Such patients may successfully receive a transplant with resolution of the shunt, although they may have a prolonged postoperative ICU stay. High FIO_2 may be necessary to maintain adequate arterial saturation. Oxygen consumption must be minimized. Once graft function is restored, gas exchange improves, although complete resolution may take more than a year. If the patient does not improve, pulmonary angiography should be used to identify a single shunt large enough to be embolized.[105]

Pulmonary hypertension occurs more often in patients with cirrhosis than in controls and is called *portopulmonary hypertension*.[106] No precipitant has been identified. The histopathologic abnormalities in the lungs are typical of primary pulmonary hypertension, which is a clinical diagnosis of exclusion. Once the diagnoses of left ventricular failure, intracardiac shunting with increased cardiac output, autoimmune disease, and pulmonary embolism have been ruled out, liver-related pulmonary hypertension should be considered. It may be difficult to distinguish advanced portopulmonary hypertension from primary cardiac failure with secondary venous congestion and hepatic failure. In contrast to patients with primary pulmonary hypertension, patients with portopulmonary hypertension have little change in response to acute pharmacologic intervention directed at reducing the pulmonary arterial pressures. Therapeutic measures such as nitrates, nitroprusside, and calcium channel blockade fail to reduce pulmonary artery pressures and have been complicated by systemic hypotension. Systemic hypotension may result in right ventricular ischemia and worsening of right ventricular function. We found patients to be unresponsive to inhaled nitric oxide,[107] although others have reported benefit.[108, 109]

An alternative approach builds on the experience of continuous infusion of prostacyclin (PGI_2) for patients with primary pulmonary hypertension. Prolonged infusion with gradual upward titration[110] slowly reduces pulmonary artery pressures without causing systemic hypotension. Cardiac remodeling ensues with increased cardiac output, reduced tricuspid regurgitation, and normalization of central venous pressures. It still is not clear whether continuous prostacyclin infusion achieves sufficient normalization of the pulmonary artery pressures to enable liver transplantation, nor whether this is a reversible process, even after successful OLTX.

Although pulmonary hypertension may resolve in some patients without treatment after successful liver transplantation,[111] progressive pulmonary disease has been observed in others despite successful transplantation.[112] Patients with mild pulmonary hypertension undergo OLTX without significant complications, but the picture is bleak for those with moderate to severe pulmonary hypertension (Table 180–4). Most transplant recipients with severe pulmonary hypertension die during reperfusion or during the early recovery phase. Such patients tolerate massive fluid shifts poorly. Right ventricular overload and failure develop abruptly, particularly upon reperfusion of the graft. This rapidly compromises the graft, resulting in massive liver and bowel congestion. Low cardiac output results in graft ischemia. These patients succumb quickly in the face of acute MSOF and are not currently considered candidates for liver transplantation (Fig. 180–3).

Pulmonary hypertension that develops de novo during or soon after liver transplantation may result from embolic phenomena at the time of transplantation. Transesophageal echocardiography may be particularly useful for demonstrating large emboli. Patients both with and without an acute cause can be successfully managed with attention to sustaining right ventricular myocardial perfusion, adequate mean arterial pressure and avoidance of central venous hypertension to the extent that it may compromise graft function. Pulmonary hypertension may develop late after liver transplantation and may overlap with the portopulmonary syndrome.[113]

Liver transplant recipients often require mechanical ventilatory support preoperatively. Intubation may be necessary when the patient cannot protect the airway because of encephalopathy or massive upper gastrointestinal hemorrhage. Respiratory failure may be precipitated by volume overload and pulmonary edema, infection with high ventilatory requirements, or profound muscle weakness. These same factors govern the decision on extubation. One must balance the risk of pulmonary infection associated with an endotracheal tube and impaired clearance of secretions with the risks of aspiration and infection secondary to poor cough effort after extubation. Before extubation the patient's mental state should be clear and liver function values should be improving. The median duration of intubation after transplantation is 2 or 3 days. Early postoperative extubation is the goal, and immediate postoperative extubation is possible in persons who were least sick preoperatively and who have uncomplicated surgery.[114]

TABLE 180–4. Pulmonary Hypertension and Liver Disease

Category	Mean Pulmonary Artery Pressure (mm Hg)	Systolic Pulmonary Artery Pressure (mm Hg)
Mild	25–34	35–44
Moderate	35–44	45–59
Severe	45–75	60–100
Very severe	>75	>100

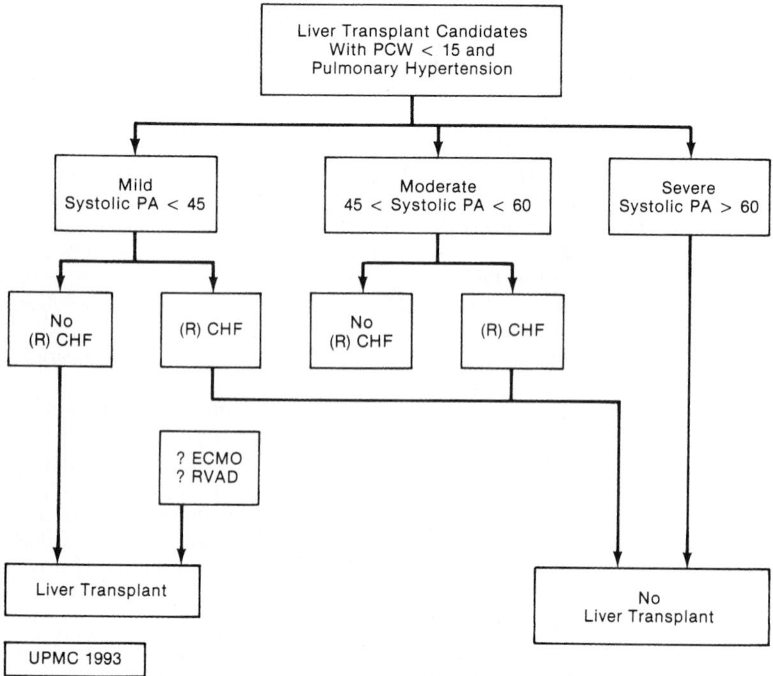

Figure 180–3. Management algorithm for patients with ESLD and pulmonary hypertension. PCW = pulmonary capillary wedge pressure; PA = pulmonary artery; CHF = congestive heart failure; ECMO = extracorporeal membrane oxygenation; RVAD = right ventricular assist device.

Prolonged need for postoperative mechanical ventilation invariably reflects an infectious complication or marginal graft function. Ventilator dependence may result from multiple insults and resolves as the primary process is treated and as the benefits of physical therapy and nutritional support are realized. In the management of hypoxemia, the benefit accrued from increased mean airway pressure obtained with PEEP or decreased expiratory time must be weighed against its variable effect on right atrial pressure, which, in addition to the effect on venous return, is reflected in the hepatic venous and portal venous pressures. In the setting of hypoxemia, in which airway pressure is reflected efficiently in venous pressure, as in patients with intrapulmonary shunt, we favor increasing FIO_2 rather than airway pressure.

RENAL CONSIDERATIONS

Renal dysfunction in patients with liver disease frequently goes unrecognized. Liver dysfunction and malnutrition make elevations in blood urea nitrogen and creatinine unimpressive despite significant derangements in glomerular filtration. In the post-transplant period, several factors conspire to impair renal function, including preoperative renal failure such as the hepatorenal syndrome, episodic hypotension resulting in tubule damage, medication such as cyclosporine, tacrolimus, and vasopressors, which cause renal arterial vasoconstriction, and amphotericin, which causes tubule damage.[115] Furthermore, liver allograft dysfunction may lead to a functional impairment of the kidneys analogous to the hepatorenal syndrome.

Dialysis support is required for approximately 10% of patients and is usually temporary. We prefer to use continuous ultrafiltration, with or without dialysis, to manage fluid balance in hemodynamically unstable patients with renal failure.

Once discharged from the ICU, such patients are managed as indicated with conventional hemodialysis. Protective measures such as perioperative dopamine, calcium channel blockade, and PGE_1 have not been efficacious in our setting when applied indiscriminately.

GASTROINTESTINAL CONSIDERATIONS

Enteral nutrition may be started early in the postoperative period for patients with a choledochocholedochostomy; it is usually deferred for 72 hours for patients with a choledochojejunostomy, because the latter also have a jejunojejunostomy (see Fig. 180-2). When parenteral nutrition is required, we use crystalline amino acids and supply one third of the nonprotein calories as fat. This minimizes glucose intolerance, which is common in the early post-OLTX period.

Upper gastrointestinal bleeding in OLTX recipients is uncommon, but prompt investigation is mandatory when it occurs. Gastritis and stress ulceration are common causes. Recurrence of esophageal and gastric varices often reflects diminished portal vein blood flow or complete thrombosis. Bleeding which is distal to the ligament of Treitz may be from the site of the jejunojejunostomy, in which case surgical control may be problematic, and we elect to optimize the coagulation status and hemodynamics before re-exploration.

Bleeding from the gastrointestinal tract weeks or months after surgery should prompt a work up for infectious causes such as cytomegalovirus (CMV) or *Clostridium difficile* enterocolitis. In addition to the considerations outlined previously, however, bleeding may be a manifestation of neoplastic gastrointestinal involvement with lymphoma (PTLD). Patients may acquire fistulas from a hepatic arterial graft or splenic artery aneurysms. Angiography may confirm the diagnosis in more stable patients but should not delay exploration because rapid operative intervention is mandatory.

Pancreatitis is a feared complication of OLTX. Although nearly 20% of patients demonstrate biochemical abnormalities (e.g., elevated amylase or lipase levels), only 5% have clinically significant pancreatitis.[116] Conservative measures are usually effective in mild cases. Management of severe pancreatitis is as controversial in this setting as in patients without OLTX. The role of somatostatin and operative débridement with continuous lavage remains to be defined.

NEUROLOGIC CONSIDERATIONS

Patients with minimal pretransplant hepatic encephalopathy who have an uncomplicated operation and receive a well-functioning graft usually exhibit rapid normalization of neurologic function after the effects of general anesthesia resolve. Changes in mental status in such patients require aggressive evaluation. Most commonly, the side effects of immunosuppressives such as cyclosporine A and tacrolimus may be identified and resolve with adjustment of medication. Focal deficits make embolic or hemorrhagic complications a concern. Intracranial infection is rare in the early postoperative period but must be ruled out in patients who present with headache and confusion.

Patients with early graft dysfunction also often have changes in mentation. Graft swelling may result in some portal congestion and portosystemic shunting. Frequently, this is difficult to demonstrate. Routine measures that result in lower ammonia levels are ineffective. Flumazenil may produce a "more awake" but still encephalopathic patient. The exact mechanism remains to be elucidated.

Medication side effects assume a much greater role in such patients. Clearance of commonly used immunosuppressives, analgesics, and sedative-hypnotics is impaired. The amnestic effects of some agents may compound the problem. We favor short-acting narcotics such as fentanyl for analgesia and short-acting benzodiazepines such as midazolam for sedation. Severe agitation often does not respond to such measures until the patient is unconscious. Haloperidol or droperidol is preferred in such settings. Careful cardiac monitoring is required during parenteral use because ventricular arrhythmias may develop, albeit rarely. An alternative approach to sedation, small doses of propofol, is rapidly gaining favor in other patient populations[117]; however, data for patients with liver failure are limited.

A small but significant incidence of seizures has been recognized in this population. Medications play a major role in the differential diagnosis because several lower the seizure threshold, including cyclosporine, tacrolimus, OKT3, and haloperidol.[118, 119] Electrolyte abnormalities, such as hyponatremia and hypomagnesemia, are common and further lower the seizure threshold. Hypoglycemia must also be considered, and treated rapidly. Although we elect to correct such abnormalities in the early postoperative period, it is unclear whether efforts at oral replenishment of magnesium are effective later in the course. Sometimes such electrolyte abnormalities are the only causative factor to be identified.

Nonconvulsive or akinetic seizures, although rare, are much more common in this ICU population than in others. It is essential that seizures, in fact status epilepticus, be part of the differential diagnosis of the comatose patient. We enjoy strong EEG support and frequently monitor such patients for long periods to define the process and to determine the effects of therapy.

Patients with FHF require special neurologic consideration. They have some elements of γ-aminobutyric acid–mediated portosystemic encephalopathy[120] of chronic liver disease but, importantly, also have intracranial hypertension and cerebral edema.[121] We elect routinely to monitor patients in grade III and grade IV coma with an epidural intracranial pressure monitor and measure cerebral blood flow with the inhalation xenon techniques during computed tomography (CT) and cerebral oxygen consumption after placing a jugular bulb catheter for oxygen content determination.[122] Continuous EEG monitoring is added once pentobarbital has been required to control intracranial hypertension. Patients are considered viable candidates for OLTX as long as EEG activity is preserved and adequate cerebral perfusion pressure can be maintained with sustained cerebral blood flow. Intraoperative monitoring includes these measures, combined with the transcranial Doppler examinations,[123] which facilitate moment-to-moment titration of anesthetics and vasopressors.

Although the initial period of graft reperfusion is the most hazardous, cerebral hyperemia and intracranial hypertension may persist for several days postoperatively. These abnormalities usually resolve with good graft function. Such intensive neurologic monitoring and careful exclusion of candidates who are at high risk for herniation have resulted in only one postoperative brain death and no apparent neurologic sequelae, even in patients transplanted in grade IV coma.

Liver transplant recipients are at risk for neuromuscular dysfunction. In a prospective study of 100 liver transplant recipients, we used electromyography and muscle biopsy to supplement the physical examination of patients who were weak. We determined a 7% incidence of clinically relevant weakness, defined as weakness that required prolonged mechanical ventilatory support. Electromyography demonstrated that this was a myopathic, rather than a neuropathic, process, and diffuse myocyte necrosis was evident in muscle biopsies taken from five patients.[124] Predisposing factors included "patient acuity" postoperatively, as judged by the APACHE II score, poor graft function at 1 week, and the requirement for dialysis and larger doses of steroids. Patients who required early retransplantation seemed to be at particular risk.

INFECTIOUS COMPLICATIONS

Rejection of the allograft is treated aggressively. Such measures are complicated by intercurrent development of infections. Heavily immunosuppressed patients die, not of rejection, but of infection. Thus, it should be appreciated that the patient with liver failure who undergoes liver transplantation is at tremendous risk for infection. In the early postoperative period, bacterial and fungal infections are common. The areas most frequently involved are the operative site and the lungs. Perioperative antimicrobial prophylaxis is currently provided as 48 hours of ampicillin plus sulbactam (Unasyn). Prophylactic regimens vary among centers. The most common microorganisms isolated in our infected patients are *Pseudomonas, Acinetobacter, Klebsiella, Enterobacter, Staphylococcus, Enterococcus,* and *Candida* species. Unfortunately, antimicrobial resistance is common, and isolates in patients who die of an infectious process are occasionally resistant to all known antimicrobials.[125]

Fungal colonization is also common. Patients whose surgical procedures are prolonged and difficult and who are heavily transfused seem to be at higher risk for fungal infection, as are patients who undergo retransplantation.[126, 127] We currently use low-dose amphotericin (10 to 20 mg/day) for 14 days, although its efficacy is unproven and fungal infections remain a significant problem. Full-dose amphotericin is appropriate for patients with *Candida* growing at multiple sites. Patients with significant *Candida* growth on quantitative culture of BAL fluid often require a full course of amphotericin.[128, 129] The outcome has improved for liver transplant recipients in whom *Aspergillus* infections develop. This previously fatal infection[130] seems to respond better to liposomal amphotericin, such as amphotericin B liposomal complex (ABLC), and we have followed prolonged intravenous therapy with a prolonged course of oral itraconazole.

Later after transplantation, infections reflect the specific effects of immunosuppressive agents on T cell function. Although bacterial and fungal infections occur, viral and opportunistic pathogens become the principal threats. Pneumonia caused by *Pneumocystis carinii* was common before prophylaxis with trimethoprim-sulfamethoxazole became routine. It occurs only in those for whom prophylactic measures have been stopped.

CMV infections are common in the transplant population[131, 132]; however, the clinical severity of infection—whether it is asymptomatic, presents with a viral syndrome, involves only one organ (e.g., lungs, gastrointestinal tract, liver), or involves multiple organs—is very variable. Patients who are seronegative before OLTX and who receive an organ from a seropositive donor are at highest risk for CMV infection. Whether patients who are seropositive before OLTX experience reactivation of latent virus or are infected by another CMV strain is a matter of some debate. In addition to the morbidity and mortality attributed directly to CMV, it should be appreciated that patients with CMV disease also have higher rates of bacterial and fungal infections. It is not clear whether it is CMV per se or the antecedent heavy immunosuppression, particularly with OKT3, which is associated with a higher incidence of CMV, that is the cause. Seroconversion may not occur until T cell immunosuppression is withdrawn.[133]

Prophylactic measures to prevent symptomatic CMV disease are under investigation. One regimen recently studied at our institution compared 2 weeks of ganciclovir followed by large doses of acyclovir with large doses of acyclovir alone.[134] At 24 weeks, CMV infection was evident in 60% and disease in 40% of those treated with acyclovir alone, but in the ganciclovir group infection decreased to 28% and disease to 12%. Surprisingly, these benefits were not realized in the highest-risk group: seronegative recipients. Additional measures such as CMV immunoglobulin administration are under investigation.[135, 136]

An alternative strategy is to monitor patients closely for evidence of CMV disease. This approach minimizes unnecessary treatment of those who will not develop CMV disease but minimizes treatment delay for those who need it. CMV antigenemia can be recognized very early by means of the pp65 antigen.[137] Serial determinations in transplant recipients with a sufficiently low threshold—10 CMV-positive cells per 200,000 white blood cells for seropositive recipients and *any* positive cells in seronegative recipients—have good sensitivity and specificity. We treat with ganciclovir until the pp65 antigen becomes negative. We use foscarnet in cases of clinical progression despite adequate ganciclovir treatment or when pancytopenia is refractory and reflects drug toxicity rather than a primary effect of the CMV.

ENDOCRINE CONSIDERATIONS

Hyperglycemia is common in the early postoperative period and reflects the combination of stress and of taking corticosteroids. Patients are routinely managed with continuous infusions of insulin, the dose being adjusted according to a sliding scale. For patients who manifest glucose intolerance conversion to six doses daily and then to twice daily therapy with regular and NPH insulin is achieved after discharge from the ICU. Although smaller doses of steroids are needed with tacrolimus than with cyclosporine, both tacrolimus and cyclosporine impair glucose tolerance. The fact that atherosclerosis is increased in transplant recipients makes tight control of the blood glucose level desirable. Unfortunately, hypoglycemia can be precipitated by liver allograft failure because gluconeogenesis is impaired. The sudden development of marked hyperglycemia or symptomatic hypoglycemia that is not iatrogenic should prompt evaluation for infection.

Adrenal insufficiency is well recognized in patients receiving steroids. An additional consideration in these patients is that the right adrenal gland is often sacrificed during transplantation. Adrenal gland infection may be caused by CMV. Adrenal hemorrhage has been observed in patients with profound coagulopathy or gram-negative sepsis. A depressed cortisol response to the corticotropin analog, cosyntropin, has been a useful test for the diagnosis of adrenal insufficiency and for the clinical decision to maintain corticosteroid supplementation.

Thyroid dysfunction, particularly hypothyroidism, is common in patients with primary biliary cirrhosis or autoimmune hepatitis. Sometimes this diagnosis is not considered preoperatively and becomes apparent in the postoperative period, being manifested as changes in mental status, depressed cardiac output, and arrhythmias, which prompt evaluation.

As with other critical illness, the euthyroid sick syndrome is commonly identified in OLTX patients when the thyroxine value is low and thyroid-stimulating hormone value is normal. When newly diagnosed and treated, an addisonian crisis can be averted with adequate corticosteroid replacement.

SUMMARY

Patients with terminal liver disease can successfully undergo transplantation. With adequate organ availability, even critically ill patients with ESLD show dramatic improvement. Intensive care of such patients is demanding but very rewarding. Future developments will focus on better candidate selection and alternative means of immunosuppression. Determining how sick someone needs to be before a lifesaving transplant should be withheld requires understanding the chance of such a patient's survival, graded for quality of life. This must be compared with transplantation for a less sick recipient who must assume the current risk of the procedure or choose the greater, but delayed, risk of waiting. The intensivist must be an active participant in this review, so that the enormous expense of intensive care is focused on those patients who can successfully undergo OLTX.

References

1. Gordon RD, Starzl TE: Changing perspectives on liver transplantation in 1988. *In:* Clinical Transplants. Terasaki PI (Ed). Los Angeles, UCLA Tissue Typing Laboratory, 1988.
2. National Institutes of Health Consensus Conference on Liver Transplantation. Bethesda, Md, 1983.
3. Starzl TE, Porter KA, Brettschneider L, et al: Clinical and pathologic observations after orthotopic transplantation of the human liver. Surg Gynecol Obstet 1969; 128:327.
4. Iwatsuki S, Starzl TE, Todo S, et al: Experience in 1000 liver transplants under cyclosporin-steroid therapy: A survival report. Transplant Proc 1988; 20(Suppl 1):498.
5. *New York Times,* February 27, 1998.
6. Van Thiel DH, Gavaler JS: Recurrent disease in patients with liver transplantation: When does it occur and how can we be sure? Hepatology 1987; 7:181.
7. Polson RJ, Portmann B, Neuberger J, et al: Evidence for disease recurrence after liver transplantation for primary biliary cirrhosis: Clinical and histologic follow-up studies. Gastroenterology 1989; 97:715.
8. United Network for Organ Sharing: A report of the Board of Directors meeting. Baltimore, November 12–13, 1997.
9. Starzl TE, Demetrius AJ, Van Thiel D: Liver transplantation (parts I and II). N Engl J Med 1989; 321:1014.
10. Koneru B, Cassavila A, Bowman J, et al: Liver transplantation for malignant tumors. Gastroenterol Clin North Am 1988; 17:177.
11. Starzl TE, Todo S, Tsakis A, et al: Abdominal organ cluster transplantation for the treatment of upper abdominal malignancies. Ann Surg 1989; 210:374.
12. Starzl TE, Towe M, Todo S, et al: Transplantation of multiple abdominal viscera. JAMA 1989; 261:449.
13. Dindzans VJ, Schade RR, Van Thiel DH: Medical problems before and after transplantation. Gastroenterol Clin North Am 1988; 17:19.
14. Todo S, Demetrius AJ, Van Thiel D, et al: Orthotopic liver transplantation for patients with hepatitis B virus (HBV) related disease. Hepatology 1991; 13:619.
15. Lauchart W, Muller R, Pichlmayer R: Long-term immunoprophylaxis of hepatitis B virus reinfection in recipients of human liver allografts. Transplant Proc 1987; 19:4051.
16. Mutchnick MG, Appelman HD, Chung HT, et al: Thymosin treatment of chronic hepatitis B: A placebo controlled pilot trial. Hepatology 1991; 14:409.
17. Grellier L, Mutimer D, Ahmed M, et al: Lamivudine prophylaxis against reinfection in liver transplantation for hepatitis B cirrhosis. Lancet 1996; 348:1212.
18. Perrillo RP: Treatment of posttransplantation hepatitis B. Liver Transplant Surg 1997; 3(5 Suppl 1):S8.
19. Nevens F, Main J, Honkoop P: Lamivudine therapy for chronic hepatitis B: A six-month randomized dose-ranging study. Gastroenterology 1997; 113:1258.
20. Terrult NA, Wright TL: Hepatitis B virus infection and liver transplantation. Gut 1997; 40:568.
21. Dummer SJ, Erb S, Breinig M, et al: Infection with human immunodeficiency virus in the Pittsburgh transplant population. Transplantation 1990; 47:134.
22. Molla A, Japour A: HIV protease inhibitors. Curr Opin Infect Dis 1997; 10:491.
23. Abu-Elmagd K, Reyes J, Todo S, et al: Clinical intestinal transplantation: New perspectives and immunologic considerations. J Am Coll Surg 1998; 186:512.
24. Trey C, Davidson CS: The management of fulminant hepatic failure. *In:* Progress in Liver Disease. Popper H, Shaffner F (Eds). New York, Grune & Stratton, 1970.
25. Bismuth H, Samuel D, Guenheim J, et al: Emergency liver transplantation for fulminant hepatitis. Ann Intern Med 1987; 107:337.
26. Kramer DJ, Aggarwald S, Martin M, et al: Fulminant hepatic failure: Management options. Transplant Proc 1991; 23:1895.
27. Hoofnagle JH, Carithers RL Jr, Shapiro C, Ascher N: Fulminant hepatic failure: Summary of a workshop. Hepatology 1995; 21:240.
28. O'Grady JG, Gimson AES, O'Brien CJ, et al: Controlled trials of charcoal hemoperfusion and prognostic factors in fulminant hepatic failure. Gastroenterology 1988; 94:1186.
29. O'Grady JG, Alexander GJM, Hayllar KM, et al: Early indicators of prognosis in fulminant hepatic failure. Gastroenterology 1989; 97:439.
30. Potter D, Peachey T, Eason J, et al: Intracranial pressure monitoring during orthotopic liver transplantation for acute liver failure. Transplant Proc 1989; 21:3528.
31. Canalese J, Gimson AES, Davis C, et al: Controlled trial of dexamethasone and mannitol for the cerebral oedema of fulminant hepatic failure. Gut 1982; 23:625.
32. Forbes A, Alexander GJ, O'Grady JG, et al: Thiopental infusion in the treatment of intracranial hypertension complicating fulminant hepatic failure. Hepatology 1989; 10:306.
33. Abelmann WH, Kowalski HJ, McNeely WF: Cardiovascular studies during acute infectious hepatitis. Gastroenterology 1954; 27:61.
34. Weston MJ, Talbot IC, Howorth PJN, et al: Frequency of arrhythmias and other cardiac abnormalities in fulminant hepatic failure. Br Heart J 1976; 38:1179.
35. Oellerich M, Raude E, Burdelski M, et al: Monoethylglycine xylidede formation kinetics: A novel approach to assessment of liver function. J Clin Chem Clin Biochem 1987; 25:845.
36. Burdelski M, Oellerich M, Lamesch P, et al: Evaluation of quantita-

tive liver function tests in liver donors. Transplant Proc 1987; 19:3838.
37. Starzl TE, Hakala TR, Shaw B, et al: A flexible procedure for multiple cadaveric organ procurement. Surg Gynecol Obstet 1984; 158:223.
38. Todo S, Nery J, Yanaga K, et al: Extended preservation of human liver grafts with UW solution. JAMA 1989; 261:711.
39. Dewolf A: Does ventricular dysfunction occur during liver transplantation? Transplant Proc 1991; 23:1922.
40. Kang Y, Freeman J, Aggarwal S, et al: Hemodynamic instability during liver transplantation. Transplant Proc 1989; 21:3489.
41. Dewolf A, Gasior T, Kang Y: Pulmonary hypertension in a patient undergoing liver transplantation. Transplant Proc 1991; 23:2000.
42. Dewolf A, Begliomin B, Gasior T, et al: Right ventricular function during liver transplantation. Anesth Analg 1993; 76:562.
43. Stoelting RK, Blitt CD, Cohen PJ, et al: Hepatic dysfunction after isoflurane anesthesia. Anesth Analg 1987; 66:147.
44. Kang YG, Martin DJ, Marquez J, et al: Intraoperative changes in blood coagulation and thromboelastographic monitoring in liver transplantation. Anesth Analg 1985; 64:888.
45. Marquez JM, Martin D: Anesthesia for liver transplantation. *In:* Hepatic Transplantation: Anesthetic and Perioperative Management. Winter PM, Kang YG (Eds). New York, Praeger, 1986.
46. Rettke SR, Chantigian RC, Janossy TA, et al: Anesthesia approach to hepatic transplantation. Mayo Clin Proc 1989; 64:224.
47. Tzakis A, Todo S, Stieber A, et al: Venous jump grafts for liver transplantation in patients with portal vein thrombosis. Transplantation 1989; 48:530.
48. Figueras J, Sabate A, Fabregat J, et al: Hemodynamics during the anhepatic phase in orthotopic liver transplantation with vena cava presentation: A comparative study. Transplant Proc 1983; 25:2588.
49. Kang Y: Hemodynamic changes during intra-abdominal organ transplantation. Transplant Proc 1993; 25:2583.
50. Stieber AC, Marsh JW Jr, Starzl TE: Preservation of the retrohepatic vena cava during recipient hepatectomy for orthotopic transplantation of the liver. Surg Gynecol Obstet 1989; 168:542.
51. Denmark W, Shaw BW, Starzl TE, et al: Veno-venous bypass without systemic anticoagulation in canine and human liver transplantation. Surg Forum 1983; 34:380.
52. Aggarwal S, Kang Y, Freeman J, et al: Post reperfusion syndrome: Cardiovascular collapse following hepatic reperfusion during liver transplantation. Transplant Proc 1987; 19:54.
53. Greig P, Woolf GM, Sinclair SB, et al: Treatment of primary liver graft nonfunction with prostaglandin E_1. Transplantation 1989; 48:447.
54. Asonuma K, Takaya S, Selby R, et al: The clinical significance of the arterial ketone body ratio as an early indicator of graft viability in human liver transplantation. Transplantation 1991; 51:164.
55. Takaya S, Nonami T, Selby R, et al: The relationship of systemic hemodynamics and oxygen consumption to early allograft failure after liver transplantation. Transplant Int 1993; 6:73.
56. Doyle HR, Marino IR, Jabbour N, et al: Early death or retransplantation in adults following orthotopic liver transplantation: Can outcome be predicted? Transplantation 1994; 57:1028.
57. Doyle HR, Dvorchik I, Mitchell S, et al: Predicting outcome after liver transplantation: A connectionist approach. Ann Surg 1994; 219:408.
58. Angus DC, Colantonio A, Kramer DJ, Byrne MC, Pinsky MR, and the Liver Transplant Intensive Care Group: Outcome prediction with the APACHE II system in liver transplantation (Abstract). Crit Care Med 1993; 21:S176.
59. Angus DC, Clermont G, Kramer DJ, Linde-Zwirble WT, Lombardero M, Pinsky MR: Short and long term outcome prediction with the APACHE II system after orthotopic liver transplantation. Crit Care Med (in press).
60. Yanaga K, Lebeau G, Marsh JW, et al: Hepatic artery reconstruction for hepatic artery thrombosis after orthotopic liver transplantation. Arch Surg 1990; 125:628.
61. Yanaga K, Makowka L, Starzl TE: Is hepatic artery thrombosis after liver transplantation really a surgical complication? Transplant Proc 1989; 21:511.
62. Manez R, Kobayashi M, Takaya S, et al: Humoral rejection associated with antidonor lymphocytotoxic antibodies following liver transplantation. Transplant Proc 1993; 25:888–890.
63. Starzl TE, Demetris AJ: Liver transplantation: A 31-Year Perspective. Chicago, Year Book, 1990.
64. Rosenbloom AJ, Kramer DJ, Stern KL, et al: Immunosuppressive therapy of transplant patients. *In:* The Pharmacologic Approach to the Critically Ill Patient. 3rd ed. Chernow B (Ed). Baltimore, Williams & Wilkins, 1994.
65. European FK506 Multicentre Liver Study Group: Randomised trial comparing tacrolimus (FK506) and cyclosporin in prevention of liver allograft rejection. Lancet 1994; 344:423.
66. The U.S. Multicenter FK506 Liver Study Group. A comparison of tacrolimus (FK506) and cyclosporine for immunosuppression in liver transplantation. N Engl J Med. 1994; 331:1110.
67. Lake JR, Gorman KJ, Esquivel CO, Wiesner RH, Klintmalm GB, Miller CM, Shaw BW, Gordon JA: The impact of immunosuppressive regimens on the cost of liver transplantation—results from the U.S. FK506 multicenter trial. Transplantation 1995; 60:1089.
68. Mycophenolate mofetil—a new immunosuppressant for organ transplantation. Med Lett 1995; 37:84.
69. Jain A, Fung JJ, Todo S, Reyes J, Kramer D, Rakela J, Starzl TE: More than 7 years actual follow up: Primary adult liver transplantation under tacrolimus (Abstract 162.). Liver Transplant Surg 1997; 3:C-71.
70. Starzl TE, Iwatsuki S, Shaw B, et al: Orthotopic liver transplantation in 1984. Transplant Proc 1985; 17:250.
71. Doyle HR, Marino IR, Morelli F, Doria C, Aldrighetti L, McMichael J, Martell J, Gayowski T, Starzl TE: Assessing risk in liver transplantation: Special reference to the significance of a positive cytotoxic crossmatch. Ann Surg 1996; 224:168.
72. Takaya S, Iwaki Y, Starzl TE: Liver transplantation in positive cytotoxic crossmatch cases using FK506, high-dose steroids, and prostaglandin E_1. Transplantation 1992; 54:927.
73. Demetrius AJ, Fung JJ, Todo S, et al: Conversion of liver allograft recipients from cyclosporin to FK 506 immunosuppressive therapy: A clinicopathologic study of 96 patients. Transplantation 1992; 53:1056.
74. McDiarmid SV, Klintmalm GB, Busuttil RW: FK506 conversion for intractable rejection of the liver allograft. Transplant Int 1993; 6:305.
75. Backman L, Nicar M, Levy M, Distant D, Eisenstein C, Renard T, Goldstein R, Husberg B, Gonwa TA, Klintmalm G: FK506 trough levels in whole blood and plasma in liver transplant recipients: Correlation with clinical events and side effects [see comments]. Transplantation 1994; 57:519.
76. McCauley J, Van Thiel D, Starzl TE, et al: Acute and chronic renal failure after liver transplantation. Nephron 1990; 55:121.
77. Thompson CB, Sullivan KM, June CH, et al: Association between cyclosporin neurotoxicity and hypomagnesaemia. Lancet 1984; 2:1116.
78. Todo S, Fung JJ, Tzakis A, et al: One hundred ten consecutive primary orthotopic liver transplants under FK 506 in adults. Transplant Proc 1991; 23:1397.
79. European FK506 Multicentre Liver Study Group: Randomized trial of FK506 and cyclosporin in prevention of liver allograft rejection. Lancet 1994; 344:423.
80. Bayley TJ, Segel N, Bishop JM: The circulatory changes in patients with cirrhosis of the liver at rest and during exercise. Clin Sci 1964; 26:227.
81. Kowalski HJ, Abelmann WH: The cardiac output at rest in Laennec's cirrhosis. J Clin Invest 1953; 32:1025.
82. Murray JF, Dawson AM, Sherlock S: Circulatory changes in chronic liver disease. Am J Med 1958; 24:358.
83. Claypool JG, Delp M, Lin TK: Hemodynamic studies in patients with Laennec's cirrhosis. Am J Med Sci 1957; 234:48.
84. Martin D: Hemodynamic monitoring during liver transplantation. *In:* Hepatic Transplantation: Anesthetic and Perioperative Management. Winter PM, Kang YG (Eds). New York, Praeger, 1986.
85. Curtis JJ, Luke RG, Jones P, et al: Hypertension in cyclosporin treated renal transplant recipients is sodium dependent. Am J Med 1988; 85:134.
86. Bennett WM, Porter GA: Cyclosporin-associated hypertension (Editorial). Am J Med 1988; 85:131.
87. Fung J, Todo S, Abu-Elmagd K, et al: Randomized trial in primary liver transplantation under immunosuppression in FK 506 or cyclosporin. Transplantation Proc 1993; 25:1130.
88. McCauley J, Fung JJ, Brown H, et al: Renal function after conver-

sion from cyclosporin to FK 506 in liver transplant patients. Transplant Proc 1991; 23:3148.
89. Krowka MJ, Cortese DA: Pulmonary aspects of chronic liver disease and liver transplantation. Mayo Clin Proc 1985; 60:407.
90. Fagon JY, Chastre J: Hospital acquired pneumonia. *In:* Pathophysiologic Foundations of Critical Care. Pinsky MR, Dhamaut JF (Eds). Baltimore, Williams & Wilkins, 1993, pp 545–570.
91. Griffin JJ, Meduri GU: New approaches in the diagnosis of nosocomial pneumonia. Med Clin North Am 1994; 78:1091.
92. Chaparala R, Kramer DJ, Miro A, et al: Comparison of clinical score, bronchoalveolar lavage and protected brush specimen for the diagnosis of bacterial pneumonia in critically ill patients with liver disease. Am Rev Respir Dis 1993; 147:A38.
93. Matuschak GM, Rinaldo JE, Pinsky MR, et al: Effect of end-stage liver failure on the incidence and resolution of the adult respiratory distress syndrome. J Crit Care 1987; 2:162.
94. Matuschak GM: Lung-liver interactions in sepsis and multiple organ failure syndrome. Clin Chest Med 1996; 17:83.
95. Bihari DJ, Gimson AE, Williams R: Cardiovascular, pulmonary and renal complications of fulminant hepatic failure. Semin Liver Dis 1986; 6(2):119.
96. Doyle HR, Marino IR, Miro A, et al: Adult respiratory distress syndrome secondary to end stage liver disease: Successful outcome following liver transplantation. Transplantation 1993; 55:292.
97. Krowka MJ, Cortese DA: Pulmonary aspects of liver disease and liver transplantation. Clin Chest Med 1987; 10:593.
98. Hales MR: Multiple small arteriovenous fistulas of the lungs. Am J Pathol 1956; 32:927.
99. Robin ED, Laman D, Horn BR, et al: Platypnea related to orthodeoxin caused by true vascular lung shunts. N Engl J Med 1976; 294:941.
100. Calabresi P, Abelmann WH: Portocaval and portopulmonary anastomosis in Laennec's cirrhosis in heart failure. J Clin Invest 1957; 36:1257.
101. Caldwell PRB, Fritts HW, Courmans A: Oxyhemoglobin dissociation curve in liver disease. J Appl Physiol 1965; 20:316.
102. Davis HH, Schwartz DJ, Letrak SS, et al: Alveolar capillary oxygen disequilibrium in hepatic cirrhosis. Chest 1978; 73:507.
103. Rodriguez-Roisin R, Roca J, August AGN, et al: Gas exchange and pulmonary vascular reactivity in patients with liver cirrhosis. Am Rev Respir Dis 1987; 135:1085.
104. Dansky HM, Schwinger ME, Cohen MV: Using contrast enhanced echocardiography to identify abnormal pulmonary arteriovenous connections in patients with hypoxemia. Chest 1992; 102:1690.
105. Poterucha JJ, Krowka MJ, Dickson ER, et al: Failure of hepatopulmonary syndrome to resolve after liver transplantation and successful treatment with embolotherapy. Hepatology 1995; 21:96.
106. Krowka MJ, McGoon MD: Portopulmonary hypertension: The next step. Chest 1997; 112:869.
107. DeWolf A, Scott V, Bjerke R, Kang Y, Kramer D, Miro A, Fung JJ, Dodson F, Gayowski T, Marino IR, Firestone L: Hemodynamic effects of inhaled nitric oxide in four patients with severe liver disease and pulmonary hypertension. Liver Transplant Surg 1997; 3:594.
108. Mandell MS: Scenario number two: Pulmonary hypertension. Liver Transplant Surg 1996; 2:320.
109. Mandell MS, Duke J: Nitric oxide reduces pulmonary hypertension during hepatic transplantation. Anesthesiology 1994; 81:1538.
110. Kuo PC, Johnson LB, Plotkin JS, et al: Continuous infusion of epoprostenol for the treatment of portopulmonary hypertension. Transplantation 1997; 63:604.
111. Scott V, DeWolf A, Kang Y, Martin M, Selby R, Fung J, Doyle H, Ziady G, Paradis I, Miro A, Kramer D: Reversibility of pulmonary hypertension after liver transplantation: A case report. Transplant Proc 1993; 25:1789.
112. Ramsay MA, Simpson BR, Nguyen AT, et al: Severe pulmonary hypertension in liver transplant candidates. Liver Transplant Surg 1997; 3:494.
113. Mandell MS, Groves BM, Duke J: Progressive plexogenic pulmonary hypertension following liver transplantation. Transplantation 1995; 59:1488.
114. Mandell MS, Lockrem J, Kelley SD: Immediate tracheal extubation after liver transplantation: Experience of two transplant centers. Anesth Analg 1997; 84:249.
115. McCauley J, Van Thiel D, Starzl TE, et al: Acute and chronic renal failure after liver transplantation. Nephron 1990; 55:121.
116. Alexander JA, Demetrius AJ, Gavaler JS, et al: Pancreatitis following liver transplantation. Transplantation 1988; 45:1062.
117. Carmichael FJ, Crawford MW, Khayyam N, et al: Effect of propofol infusion on splanchnic hemodynamics and liver oxygen consumption in the rat: A dose response study. Anesthesiology 1993; 79:1051.
118. de Groen PC, Aksamit AJ, Rakela J, et al: Central nervous system toxicity after liver transplantation. N Engl J Med 1987; 318:861.
119. Adams DH, Gunson B, Honigsberger L, et al: Neurologic complications following liver transplantation. Lancet 1987; i:949.
120. Jones EA, Basile AS, Mullen KD, et al: Flumazonil: Potential implications for hepatic encephalopathy. Pharmacotherapy 1990; 45:331.
121. Ware AJ, D'Agostiono AN, Combes B: Cerebral edema: A major complication of massive hepatic necrosis. Gastroenterology 1971; 61:877.
122. Aggarwal S, Kramer D, Yonas H, et al: Cerebral hemodynamic and metabolic changes in fulminant hepatic failure. Hepatology 1994; 19:80.
123. Aggarwal S, Witt JP, Kang Y, et al: Transcranial Doppler waveform analysis: A new approach to predict ICP in patients with fulminant hepatic failure. Hepatology 1993; 18:735.
124. Campellone JV, Lacomis D, Kramer DJ, Van Cott AC, Giuliani MJ: Acute myopathy following liver transplantation. Neurology 1998; 50:46.
125. Linden P, Pasculle AW, Kusne S, et al: Therapy and clinical outcome of vancomycin resistant *Enterococcus faecium* (VREF) in a liver transplant recipient population. Proceedings of the 32nd Interscience Conference on Antimicrobial Agents and Chemotherapy (ICAAC). (Abstract 1171). Los Angeles, October 1992, p 306.
126. Kusne S, Dummer JS, Singh N, et al: Infection after liver transplantation: An analysis of 101 consecutive cases. Medicine 1988; 67:132.
127. Kusne S, Dummer JS, Singh N, et al: Fungal infections in liver transplantation recipients. Transplantation 1985; 40:347.
128. Linden P, Kramer DJ, Mazariegos G, Marsh W, Casavilla A, Pinna A, Fung J, Kusne S: Low-dose amphotericin B (LDA) for the prophylaxis of serious *Candida* infection in high risk liver recipients. Proceedings, 36th International Conference on Antimicrobial Agents and Chemotherapy (ICAAC). (Abstract No. J47.) American Society for Microbiology, New Orleans, September 15–18, 1996, p 227.
129. Linden P, Kramer DJ, Pasculle W: The correlation of quantitative bronchoalveolar lavage fungal cultures with active or incipient invasive candidiasis (Abstract). Presented at ALA/ATS International Conference, New Orleans, May 10–15, 1996. Am J Respir Crit Care Med 1996; 153:411.
130. Torre-Cisneros J, Manez R, Kusne S, et al: The spectrum of aspergillosis in liver transplant patients: Comparison of FK 506 and cyclosporine immunosuppression. Transplant Proc 1991; 23:3040.
131. Balfour HH, Chace BA, Stapleton JT, et al: A randomized, placebo-controlled trial of oral acyclovir for the prevention of cytomegalovirus disease in recipients of renal allografts. N Engl J Med 1989; 320:1381.
132. Pomeroy C, Englund JA: Cytomegalovirus: Epidemiology and infection control. Am J Infect Control 1987; 15:107.
133. Manez R, Breinig MK, Kusne S, et al: Anomalous pattern of IgG antibody response to primary cytomegalovirus infection after solid organ transplantation. Transplantation 1995; 59:1220.
134. Martin M, Manez R, Linden P, et al: A prospective randomized trial comparing sequential ganciclovir-high dose acyclovir to high dose acyclovir for prevention of cytomegalovirus disease in adult liver transplant recipients. Transplantation 1994; 58:779.
135. Syndman DR, Werner BG, Heinze-Lacey B, et al: Use of cytomegalovirus immunoglobulin to prevent cytomegalovirus disease in renal transplant recipients. N Engl J Med 1987; 317:1049.
136. Martin M: Prophylactic cytomegalovirus management strategies. Transplant Proc 1995; 27:23.
137. Grossi P, Kusne S, Rinaldo C, St. George K, Magnone M, Rakela J, Fung J, Starzl TE: Guidance of ganciclovir therapy with pp65 antigenemia in cytomegalovirus-free recipients of livers from seropositive donors. Transplantation 1996; 61:1659.

181

Heart Transplantation

G. Daniel Martich, MD • J. David Vega, MD

December 3, 1997, marked the 30th anniversary of an event that captured the world's attention like no other medical advancement had previously. Christiaan Barnard of Cape Town, South Africa, had performed the first human heart transplant procedure. Although the patient, Louis Washkansky, died 18 days later of infectious complications, it was now a proven medical fact that a healthy human heart from one individual could be transplanted into and support the circulation of another individual. In the next 13 months, more than 100 heart transplants were performed worldwide. The results were poor by today's standards, as nearly two thirds of the patients died within 3 months of overwhelming rejection or infection. Most surgeons became disillusioned, and the procedure was largely abandoned in the 1970s, with fewer than 50 transplants performed per year worldwide. These failures only served as an impetus to Norman Shumway, at Stanford University, and Richard Lower, at the Medical College of Virginia, who persisted in their efforts to overcome the obstacles precluding long-term success with cardiac transplantation.

Today, more than 40,000 heart transplant procedures have been performed worldwide. Refinements in surgical technique, organ preservation, donor and recipient selection and management, immunosuppression, and postoperative care have led to the success of heart transplantation (Figs. 181–1 and 181–2). As a result of these advancements, heart transplantation has evolved from an experimental procedure to a viable therapeutic alternative for patients with end-stage heart disease. Current 1-year actual survival approximates 85%, according to the International Society for Heart and Lung Transplantation.[1] The majority of patients have an improved quality of life, and more than 40% of patients return to work after 2 years.[2]

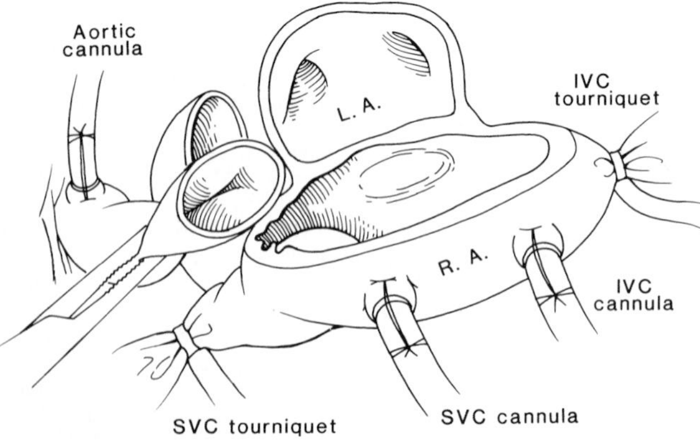

Figure 181–1. View of the chest cavity after native heart explantation in preparation for orthotopic heart transplantation. Right and left atrial cuffs remain intact in the most common surgical approach. The aorta is cross-clamped, and cardiopulmonary bypass cannulas are in place. SVC = superior vena cava; IVC = inferior vena cava; R.A. = right atrium; L.A. = left atrium. (Illustration by Jon Coulter.)

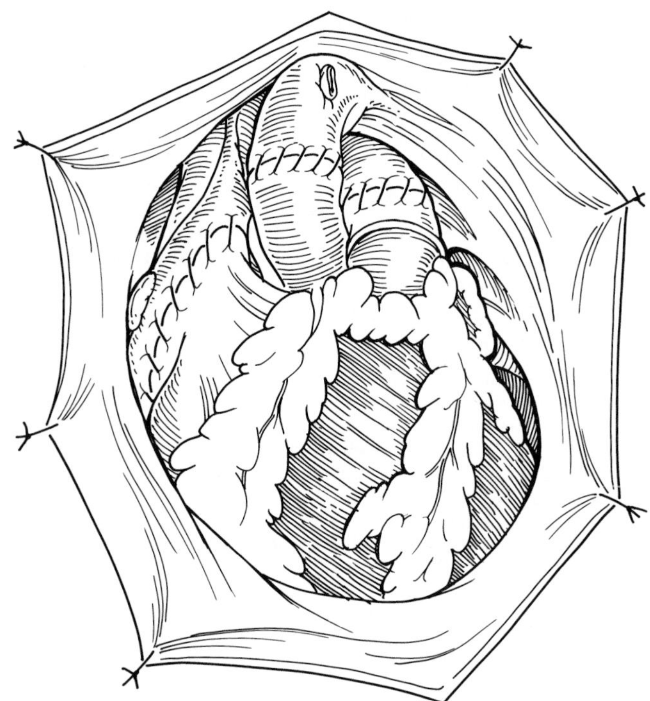

Figure 181–2. View of open pericardium with newly implanted orthotopic heart. Suture lines are easily visible along the right atrium, aorta, and main pulmonary artery. The left atrial suture line is not visible. (Illustration by Jon Coulter.)

The postoperative care of heart transplant recipients has become almost "routine" at experienced centers. This "routine" care includes optimization of hemodynamics with judicious use of fluids and inotropes, ensuring satisfactory gas exchange, correction of electrolyte abnormalities, maintenance of satisfactory urine output and renal function, prophylaxis against and surveillance for infectious complications, and adjustment of immunosuppression based on the patient's clinical status. The postoperative care of the heart transplant recipient requires attention to detail and communication among health care professionals just as the management of any other critically ill patient.

HEMODYNAMIC SUPPORT

Two important hemodynamic considerations in the immediate postoperative period influence management decisions: (1) the transplanted heart is completely denervated, and (2) the early graft function is affected by the length of the ischemic insult that just occurred. The transplanted heart may temporarily suffer from decreased diastolic compliance and diminished systolic function with impaired contractility. Because of decreased diastolic compliance, increased filling pressures are necessary to maintain satisfactory cardiac output. It is not unusual to require a pulmonary capillary wedge pressure (PCWP) of 15 to 20 mm Hg for the first 24 hours postoperatively. Diminished systolic function with impaired contractility, secondary to cold ischemia (time to procurement and implantation), cardiopulmonary bypass, and reperfusion injury, necessitates the use of inotropic support to ensure an adequate cardiac output.

Heart Rate and Arrhythmias

The initial inotrope chosen is usually dobutamine or isoproterenol. Inotropic support is usually necessary for 3 to 5 days postoperatively, depending on the donor heart function. The stroke volume of the newly transplanted heart is relatively fixed, and therefore the cardiac output is very dependent on heart rate. Both of these inotropes have the added benefit of being chronotropic agents as well. In addition, intraoperative placement of temporary atrial and ventricular pacing wires is utilized to maintain the heart rate greater than 90 beats/min. The need for temporary pacing has been reported to be as high as 27% following heart transplantation. Permanent pacemaker requirements are much lower (2% to 11%) and are almost divided equally between sinoatrial (SA) and atrioventricular (AV) node dysfunction.[3]

An additional factor that may begin to affect the inherent donor heart rate after 2 to 3 days is whether the recipient was receiving amiodarone preoperatively. Amiodarone accumulates rapidly in the transplanted myocardium of heart transplant recipients and peaks during the second postoperative week.[4] Oral beta agonists, such as Alupent and theophylline, may be necessary for several weeks to maintain an adequate heart rate after intravenous chronotropic agents are discontinued.

The occurrence of atrial or ventricular dysrhythmias after heart transplantation is uncommon. Dysrhythmias occurring early in the postoperative period are usually due to electrolyte abnormalities and may resolve with potassium or magnesium supplementation. Other possible etiologic factors include inotropic agents and the pulmonary artery catheter. Treatment options include reduction of inotropic support and removal of the pulmonary artery catheter. Cardiac rejection should be considered for dysrhythmias that occur more than 7 days after transplantation.

Treatment strategies for tachyarrhythmias and bradyarrhythmias that occur following heart transplantation need to take into consideration that the heart is completely denervated; therefore, medications that act directly on the heart and not through the sympathetic or parasympathetic systems are used. Drugs from each of the four major antiarrhythmic classifications have some direct effect on the heart. Both calcium channel blockers and β-blockers possess negative inotropic effects and must be used with caution. Adenosine is useful in treating supraventricular tachyarrhythmias, but because of increased sinus node sensitivity, the starting dose should be one-quarter to one-half normal. Atropine has no effect on atrial or atrioventricular conduction in the denervated heart and is not useful in the treatment of bradyarrhythmias. Digoxin has no effect on atrioventricular conduction when given in the early postoperative period because its mechanism of action is vagally mediated, but it may exert some effect when given chronically.

Hypotension

Acute right ventricular heart failure following cardiac transplantation is an uncommon but potentially fatal hemodynamic complication. It can occur in the operating room during weaning from cardiopulmonary bypass or postoperatively within the first 48 hours. It occurs when the right ventricle of the donor heart, which is a volume chamber, must work acutely against an excessive pulmonary vascular resistance. Early recognition and prompt treatment are mandatory. Clinical evidence includes hypotension, low cardiac output, elevated central venous pressure, and low urinary output. This condition can be confused with cardiac tamponade. Transesophageal echocardiography can rapidly distinguish between the two clinical entities.

Treatment maneuvers include reversal of acidosis, ensuring adequate oxygenation, and hyperventilation to decrease P_{CO_2}, which has the beneficial effect of pulmonary vasodilatation. Pharmacologic measures include the use of milrinone lactate, a phosphodiesterase inhibitor, which is a pulmonary vasodilator as well as an inotropic agent. Nitroglycerin, sodium nitroprusside, isoproterenol, or prostaglandin E_1 can all be selectively administered as intravenous infusions to lower the pulmonary vascular resistance. Care must be taken to avoid profound peripheral vasodilatation and subsequent hypotension. Inhaled nitric oxide has been shown to be a profound pulmonary vasodilator without systemic hemodynamic sequelae.[5] Right-sided mechanical circulatory support is indicated if these measures fail to reverse the process.

Cardiac tamponade from excessive bleeding can occur after any heart operation. Patients undergoing cardiac transplantation are at increased risk for several reasons. Many patients have been receiving warfarin preoperatively because of severe left ventricular dysfunction, many have had previous cardiac operations, and many have diminished coagulation factors due to chronic liver congestion. In addition, the donor heart often does not fill the enlarged pericardial space, thereby allowing room for blood to accumulate. The clinical characteristics of cardiac tamponade are the same as acute right ventricular failure. Diastolic equalization of pressures often is not present. Transesophageal echocardiography may be useful in establishing the diagnosis. Operative exploration should be undertaken if the diagnosis is entertained or in doubt.

IMMUNOSUPPRESSION

Most transplant centers have immunosuppressive protocols that were developed from institutional experience in treating transplant recipients. Immunosuppression can be considered in two distinct phases. The first phase consists of induction therapy, and the second phase includes maintenance therapy.

Induction therapy protocols vary from center to center. Many centers utilize a triple-drug regimen consisting of cyclosporine or tacrolimus in addition to azathioprine and corticosteroids. An equal number of centers utilize, in addition to the three-drug regimen, a short course of cytolytic therapy with antithymocyte globulin (ATG), antilymphocyte globulin (ALG), or the murine monoclonal antibody OKT3. No induction protocol has been superior to others with regard to the incidence of early rejection, infection, survival, or the development of graft vasculopathy.[6]

Most heart transplant centers utilize a triple-drug regimen for maintenance immunosuppression. In most centers in the United States, this regimen is cyclosporine-based, in combination with azathioprine and prednisone. Cyclosporine inhibits lymphokine synthesis and the generation of cytotoxic T cells. At the University of Pittsburgh Medical Center and other select centers, tacrolimus has replaced cyclosporine in the triple-drug regimen. Studies have demonstrated that patients receiving tacrolimus, which also inhibits lymphokine synthesis, have a lower incidence of hypertension and an improved quality of life.[7] There may be a higher incidence of glucose intolerance, neurotoxicity, and nephrotoxicity in patients receiving tacrolimus compared with those receiving cyclosporine. Many of the toxic effects of these drugs are dose-dependent.

Careful monitoring of blood levels is imperative. Drugs that either inhibit or induce the cytochrome P_{450} system subsequently increase or decrease the blood levels of these drugs. Because of the many potential drug interactions, one must exercise caution when adding or withdrawing medications from the transplant patient's regimen (Tables 181-1 and 181-2).

REJECTION

Acute Cellular Rejection

Acute cellular rejection (ACR) is potentially a life-threatening complication of cardiac transplantation. The diagnosis of ACR

TABLE 181–1. Drugs Known to Interact with Cyclosporine

Increase Cyclosporine Levels	Decrease Cyclosporine Levels
Amiodarone	Carbamazepine
Cimetidine	Nafcillin
Diltiazem	Octreotide
Erythromycin	Phenobarbital
Ketoconazole	Phenytoin
Metoclopramide	Rifampin
Nicardipine	Sulfamethoxazole
Tacrolimus	
Verapamil	

From Martich GD, Boujoukos AJ: Adult cardiac transplantation. J Intensive Care Med 1996; 11:79–89.

is based on both histologic and clinical criteria. ACR can be defined as any clinical event that necessitates augmentation of immunosuppression. The average rejection frequency during the first year following transplantation is 1.3 ± 0.7 episodes. The risk of rejection varies for each individual but has been higher in female recipients.[8]

The endomyocardial biopsy has become the standard method for diagnosis of cardiac rejection. In 1990, a standardized nomenclature based on histologic criteria to grade the severity of cardiac rejection was established by the International Society for Heart and Lung Transplantation (Table 181-3). This standardized grading system allows for comparison of results between institutions and also for uniform reporting in the literature. The frequency of surveillance endomyocardial biopsies varies between institutions, but they are usually performed weekly for the first month after transplantation when the risk of rejection is greatest. The frequency decreases to every 1 to 2 months for the remainder of the first year. A significant change in clinical status, such as dyspnea, pedal edema, or dysrhythmia, would prompt an earlier endomyocardial biopsy. Treatment of rejection depends on histologic grade and clinical status. Hemodynamically stable ACR is usually treated with a pulse dose of methylprednisolone (500 to 1000 mg/day) for 3 days with possible augmentation of the maintenance immunosuppression. Hemodynamically unstable ACR is usually treated with a pulse dose of methylprednisolone and lymphocytotoxic therapy, such as OKT3. Refractory ACR has been treated successfully with a variety of methods, including lymphocytotoxic therapy and total lymphoid irradiation.

Vascular Rejection

Vascular rejection (VR), also known as *antibody-mediated* or *humoral rejection,* is a potentially fatal, but fortunately rare early complication of cardiac transplantation. Biopsy findings include evidence of endothelial cell proliferation and swelling by light microscopy and vascular deposition of immunoglobulin by immunofluorescence. Whether preformed antidonor antibodies cause hyperacute rejection in heart transplant recipients is controversial, but evidence suggests that preformed antibodies can cause cardiac rejection. Previous reports have suggested that 10% of heart transplant recipients demonstrated positive crossmatches against donor cells. Few of these patients suffered from hyperacute rejection, but long-term graft survival was significantly worse than in patients with negative crossmatches.[9] Vascular rejection is a clinically more aggressive type of rejection than ACR. Overt congestive heart failure often results from graft dysfunction.

Treatment strategies are twofold: (1) circulatory support and (2) reversal of rejection. Options for circulatory support include aggressive use of inotropes, vasopressors, possible mechanical support, and consideration of retransplantation. Aggressive treatment of rejection is warranted. Strategies include pulse steroids, lymphocytotoxic therapy, cyclophosphamide, and plasmapheresis to reduce the level of circulating preformed antibodies. Despite aggressive measures, VR is associated with a much higher mortality than ACR because of the secondary injury associated with complement activation, vasoconstriction, platelet aggregation, and stimulation by polymorphonuclear leukocytes.

TABLE 181–2. Drugs Known to Interact with Tacrolimus*

Increase Tacrolimus Levels	Decrease Tacrolimus Levels
Ciprofloxacin	Carbamazepine
Clotrimazole	Phenobarbital
Cyclosporine	Phenytoin
Diltiazem	Rifampin
Erythromycin	
Fluconazole	
Ketoconazole	

From Martich GD, Boujoukos AJ: Adult cardiac transplantation. J Intensive Care Med 1996; 11:79–89.[12]

*Drug interaction studies with tacrolimus have not been conducted. These medications may affect tacrolimus levels based on clinical experience and their effects on the cytochrome P_{450} system.

TABLE 181–3. Standardized Grading System for Classifying Cellular Rejection on Endomyocardial Biopsy Specimens

Grade	New Nomenclature	Old Nomenclature
0	No rejection	No rejection
IA	Focal (perivascular or interstitial infiltrate) without necrosis	Mild rejection
IB	Diffuse but sparse infiltrate without necrosis	
II	One focus only with aggressive infiltration and/or focal myocyte damage	Focal moderate rejection
IIIA	Multifocal aggressive infiltrates and/or myocyte damage	Low to moderate rejection
IIIB	Diffuse inflammatory process with necrosis	Borderline or severe rejection
IV	Diffuse aggressive polymorphous ± infiltrate ± edema, ± hemorrhage, ± vasculitis, with necrosis	Severe acute rejection

From Billingham ME, Cary NR, Hammond ME: A working formulation for the standardization of nomenclature in the diagnosis of heart and lung rejection: Heart rejection study group. J Heart Transplant 1991; 9:587–592.[13]

INFECTION

Despite the introduction of new antibacterial and antiviral agents, infection is still a significant cause of morbidity and mortality after heart transplantation. A delicate balance exists between the immunosuppression necessary to ensure graft survival and the subsequent alterations in cell-mediated immunity that predispose the transplant recipient to infection.

Infectious complications can occur early or late following heart transplantation.

Early Complications

Early usually refers to the first month, and these complications are most often bacteria-mediated (e.g., pneumonia, catheter-related infections, wound infections, and urinary tract infections). Risk factors for early nosocomial infections include the protracted need for central venous catheters, intubation, or chest tube drainage. Organisms most often responsible for these nosocomial infections include *Staphylococcus aureus, Pseudomonas aeruginosa,* enterococci, and members of the Enterobacteriaceae family. *Candida* may also cause early infectious complications. These infections are related to the extended use of antibiotics and central venous catheters.

The choice of prophylactic antibiotics in the perioperative period varies among institutions but usually consists of a cephalosporin with or without the addition of vancomycin. Administration of prophylactic antibiotics for more than 48 hours serves only to increase the risk of resistant organisms and should be discouraged. A conscious effort should be made to remove all indwelling lines and catheters as soon as possible. Treatment with antibiotics should be based on appropriate culture and sensitivity reports.

Late Complications

Late infectious complications in the heart transplant recipient usually occur after the first month but within the first year. These infections are usually opportunistic in origin and include cytomegalovirus (CMV), *Pneumocystis carinii,* and *Legionella* species. Late fungal infections include aspergillosis, histoplasmosis, and cryptococcal infection. These types of infections are most likely to occur within the first 6 months after transplantation when maintenance immunosuppression levels are highest and during periods of augmented immunosuppression for treatment of rejection.

The prophylactic treatment of patients at risk for reactivation or primary infection with CMV remains controversial. Most centers do not routinely use prophylactic ganciclovir to prevent reactivation of CMV except during lymphocytotoxic therapy for rejection. The use of ganciclovir prophylaxis for CMV seronegative patients who receive CMV seropositive donor hearts depends on the institution. We currently wait for manifestations of CMV disease before initiating therapy. These clinical manifestations often include fever, malaise, myalgias, and gastrointestinal complaints. Bone marrow suppression in the form of leukopenia and thrombocytopenia can also occur.

Many centers routinely use prophylactic trimethoprim-sulfamethoxazole during the first year to prevent *Pneumocystis* pneumonia. Trimethoprim-sulfamethoxazole has the added benefit of being active against *Nocardia, Toxoplasma, Legionella,* and *Listeria.* Recipients who are seronegative for *Toxoplasma gondii* and receive a heart from a seropositive donor have a risk as high as 57% for development of serious *Toxoplasma* infection. Prophylaxis with a 6-week course of pyrimethamine and folinic acid is warranted in this patient population. This infection can manifest as meningoencephalitis and myocarditis and may be rapidly fatal. If disease develops, treatment consists of clindamycin or sulfadiazine with higher doses of pyrimethamine.

EXTRACARDIAC COMPLICATIONS

The rate of extracardiac complications following heart transplantation varies between 9.5% and 38%. A 30-day mortality of nearly 10% due to intra-abdominal catastrophes following heart transplantation has been reported previously. Most extracardiac complications involve the gastrointestinal tract, and between 4% and 20% may require general surgical intervention.[10] These complications include gastrointestinal bleeding, viscus perforation, diverticulitis, pancreatitis, cholecystitis, and *Clostridium difficile* pseudomembranous colitis. The high incidence of these complications is most assuredly related to the immunosuppression. Oftentimes, symptoms are discounted because of their seemingly mild nature. Unfortunately, symptoms of impending intra-abdominal emergencies are masked by immunosuppressive agents, especially steroids. A high index of suspicion is warranted. Complaints of abdominal pain or the clinical findings of abdominal tenderness or ileus requires an aggressive diagnostic approach beginning with imaging studies of the abdomen.

POST-TRANSPLANT LYMPHOPROLIFERATIVE DISORDER

Etiology

Post-transplant lymphoproliferative disorder (PTLD) is a proliferation of B lymphocytes that occurs in immunosuppressed transplant recipients. It is usually associated with infection by the Epstein-Barr virus (EBV) and is a consequence of nonspecific immunosuppression. The spectrum of lymphoproliferation ranges from mild polyclonal lymphoid hyperplasia (as in infectious mononucleosis) to frank lymphoma that is indistinguishable from non-Hodgkin's lymphoma. In normal individuals, this lymphoproliferation is controlled by multiple defense mechanisms, the most important of which is the proliferation and activity of cytotoxic T lymphocytes. This important defense mechanism of T lymphocytes is suppressed by antirejection agents, including cyclosporine and tacrolimus. Therefore, there is serious impairment of the ability to control the B-lymphocyte proliferation.

The incidence of PTLD in all solid organ transplants is approximately 2%. At the University of Pittsburgh, the incidence in heart transplant recipients is 4%. Risk factors for development of PTLD in the recipient include the use of lymphocytotoxic therapy and EBV seronegativity. The lungs, bone marrow, gastrointestinal tract, central nervous system, and lymph nodes are the most common sites of PTLD. A significant number of patients present with disseminated disease.

Treatment

PTLD may occur early (<1 year) or late (>1 year) after transplantation. Patients with *early PTLD* (peak occurrence at 3 to 4 months post transplant) have approximately a 25% mortality rate, but up to 89% respond to a reduction in immunosuppression, which is the initial treatment strategy. This reduction in immunosuppression requires an increased frequency of surveillance biopsies to monitor for rejection. *Late PTLD* rarely, if ever, responds to reduction in immunosuppression, and the associated mortality rate is greater than 70%.[11] Failure to respond to a reduction in immunosuppression necessitates a more aggressive approach with traditional radiation therapy or chemotherapy.

A new treatment strategy involves the use of lymphokine activated killer cells. In this treatment, the patient's lymphocytes are harvested from the peripheral blood by plasmapheresis. These lymphocytes are cultured in vitro with interleukin-2 (IL-2) for 2 weeks, then harvested and infused back into the patient. Preliminary reports are encouraging.

ALLOGRAFT VASCULAR DISEASE

Allograft vascular disease (AVD) is the major cause of late mortality following cardiac transplantation. AVD refers to the concentric narrowing and obstruction of the coronary arteries of the transplanted heart. It is often a diffuse disease that begins in the intramyocardial vessels and propagates proximally into the epicardial vessels. Some studies have estimated an incidence of 5% to 10% per year with 30% to 80% of patients affected within 5 years. AVD has been shown to occur in heart transplant recipients of all ages and to occur as early as 2 months after transplant. Most studies have found no statistically significant difference in the incidence of AVD based on the etiology of the pretransplant heart disease.

Etiology

The cause of AVD is unknown, but it is most likely multifactorial. Reports have implicated rejection, CMV infection, ischemia and reperfusion injury, hypertension, age, and hyperlipidemia as possible causative factors. Acute cellular rejection, vascular rejection, and even delayed hypersensitivity (type 4 cell-mediated rejection) have all been proposed as possible etiologic mechanisms.

The role of CMV in the development of AVD is controversial, but three mechanisms have been suggested: (1) direct vascular injury, (2) transformation of smooth muscle cells in the vessel wall, and (3) immunomodulation. Endothelial cell injury by ischemia and reperfusion has been demonstrated in several models, but its role in the development of AVD remains undefined. Although hypertension is a known risk factor for the development of native coronary artery disease, it has not been shown to be an independent predictor for AVD despite its high prevalence in the transplant patient population. There have been studies to support and refute recipient age as a risk factor for AVD.

Of the possible causative factors listed here, hyperlipidemia is the one generally accepted to be an independent predictor for the development of AVD. An aggressive approach to hyperlipidemia is warranted. Treatment strategies include lipid-lowering agents, adherence to a low-fat diet, and an exercise program.

Clinical Manifestations

Manifestations of AVD include congestive heart failure, arrhythmias, and sudden death. Unexplained graft dysfunction may also be the first indication of AVD. There may be new evidence of ischemia or infarction on the electrocardiogram (ECG). Angina is usually not due to denervation of the heart. Because of the subtle onset of AVD, most centers routinely screen for it with annual coronary angiography. Coronary angiography often underestimates the severity of AVD because of the diffuse, concentric nature of the disease. In some centers, intravascular ultrasound is being used to detect AVD earlier. Whether earlier detection impacts long-term outcome remains to be determined.

Treatment

Current treatment strategies include improving maintenance immunosuppression to minimize acute rejection episodes, aggressive use of lipid-lowering agents, and controlling hypertension. Diltiazem, a calcium channel blocker, appears to delay the onset of AVD, possibly via enhanced immunosuppressive effect or regulation of lipoprotein-receptor synthesis or a combination. Some patients with focal stenosis may be candidates for revascularization with percutaneous transluminal coronary angioplasty, coronary artery bypass grafting, or transmyocardial laser revascularization. Patients who have progressive AVD may be candidates for retransplantation, but the limited donor pool precludes this on a large-scale basis.

HETEROTOPIC HEART TRANSPLANTATION

Heart transplantation in the heterotopic position is a technique that is utilized primarily for patients with severe fixed pulmonary hypertension. This form of hypertension indicates a transpulmonary gradient (mean pulmonary artery pressure − PCWP) above 15 mm Hg or a pulmonary vascular resistance above 6 to 8 Wood units after aggressive vasodilator therapy. The risk of severe fixed pulmonary hypertension after orthotopic cardiac transplantation is acute right ventricular heart failure, because the unconditioned right ventricle cannot overcome the elevated pulmonary vascular resistance. Technically, this is a more challenging operation because the native heart is left in situ and the donor heart is placed in the right hemithorax. The donor heart is anastomosed to the native heart in parallel fashion with side-to-side anastomoses between the donor and native atria and with end-to-side anastomoses between donor and native pulmonary artery and aorta (Figure 181–3). In this manner, the donor left ventricle supports most of the systemic circulation and the native right ventricle supports the pulmonary circulation.

Heterotopic transplant recipients display two distinct ECGs with different heart rates and, frequently, different rhythms (Figs. 181–4 and 181–5). Careful lead placement may be able to isolate one heart rhythm over the other. In addition to increased technical difficulty, two other reasons preclude widespread application of heterotopic heart transplantation: (1) There is a problem with atelectasis of the right lower lobe because the donor heart is placed on top of it, and (2) lifelong anticoagulation is necessary because of the propensity for thrombus formation in the native left ventricle. Hemodynamic monitoring with a Swan-Ganz catheter allows for measurement of pulmonary artery pressures and mixed venous oxygen saturation, but placement of the catheter's infusion port within the common right atrium is essential for accurate cardiac output determinations by thermodilution.

The immunosuppression protocol, need for endomyocardial biopsy, and postoperative management are otherwise the same as for the standard orthotopic cardiac transplant recipient. Interestingly, the previously "fixed" pulmonary hypertension often returns to normal or near normal pressures after 3 months.[12, 13]

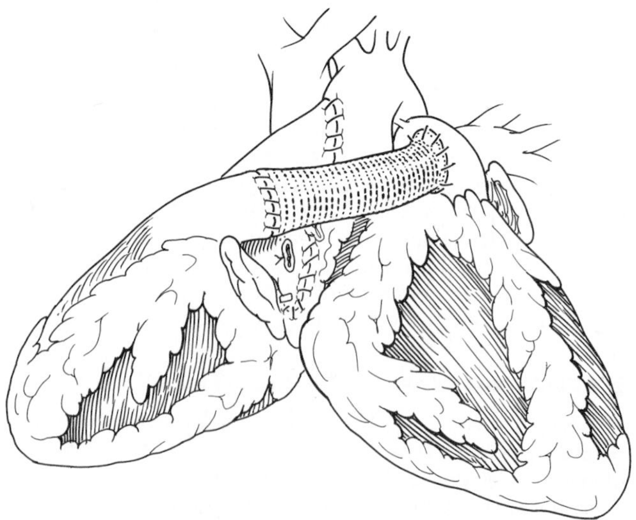

Figure 181–3. Heterotopic heart transplantation with heterotopic heart on the *left* side of the picture (in the right chest) with side-to-side anastomoses of atria and end-to-side aortic connection. Another end-to-side anastomosis is shown from the heterotopic pulmonary artery to the native main pulmonary artery with an interposition graft. The left atrial suture line is not visible. (Illustration by Jon Coulter.)

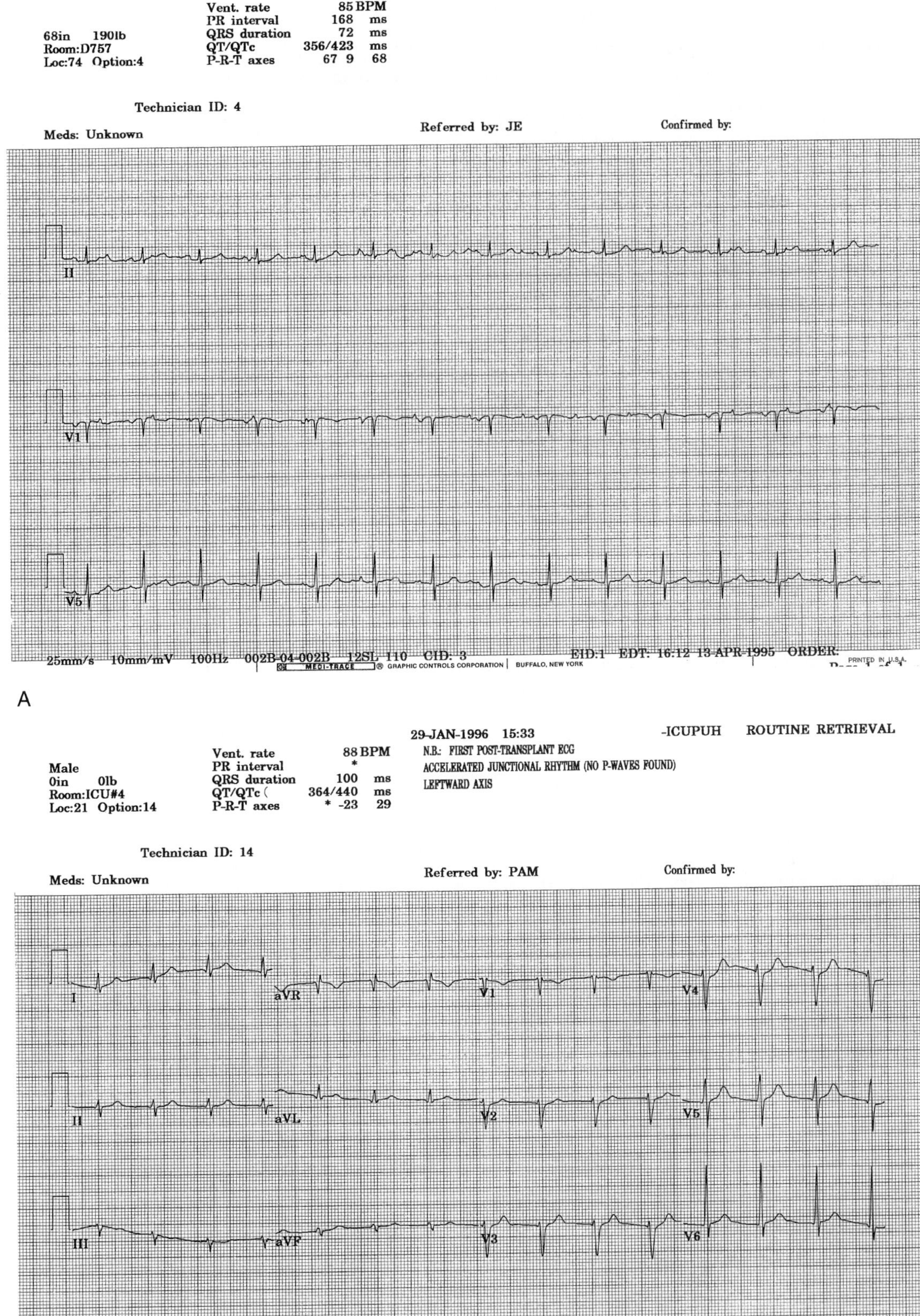

Figure 181–4. Electrocardiograms of patients after orthotopic heart transplantation may display any of the following characteristics. *A,* Three-lead rhythm strip showing two distinct P waves. One P wave is from the donor atria and is followed by the QRS complex in a sinus mechanism. The second P wave is dissociated with the QRS complex. *B,* Twelve-lead electrocardiogram with rhythm strip. Junctional rhythm devoid of P waves entirely. Any combination of the above may occur, as can atrial arrhythmias in either the donor or native atria.

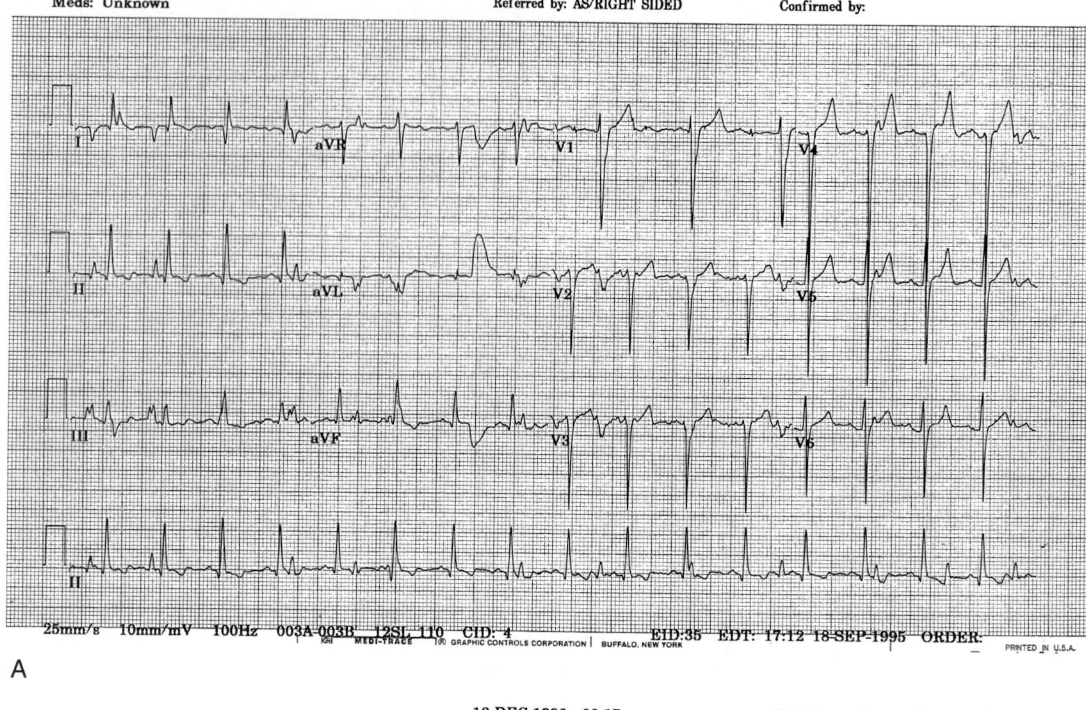

A

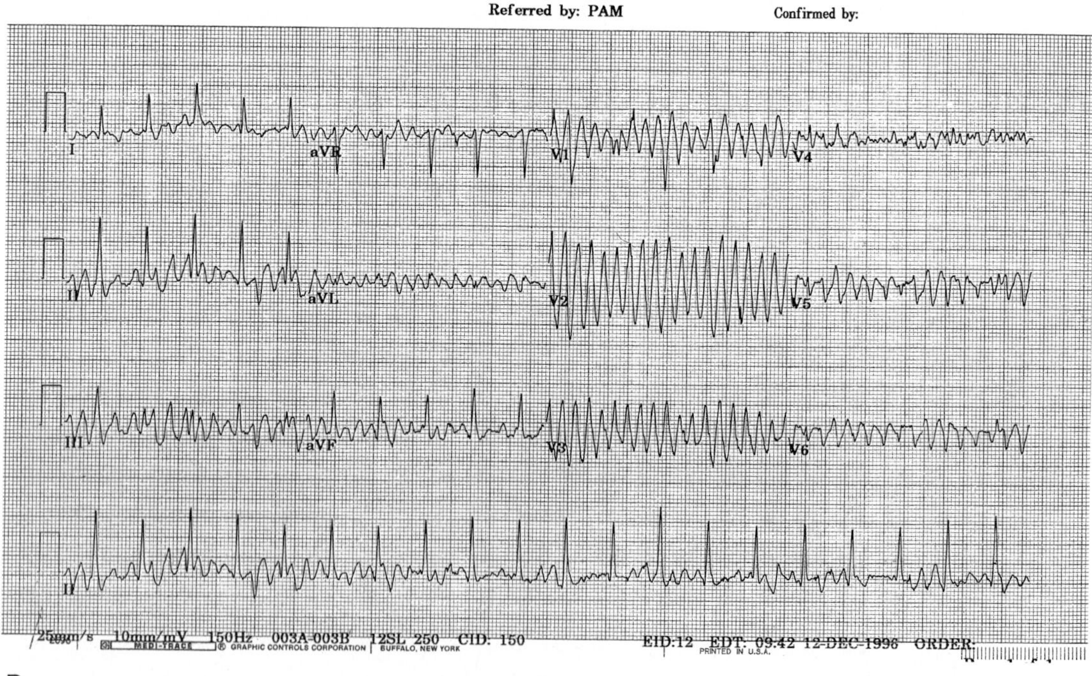

B

Figure 181–5. Electrocardiograms of patients after heterotopic heart transplant may display two distinct rhythms, making interpretation of each underlying rhythm difficult. Shown are two 12-lead electrocardiograms with rhythm strips from patients following heterotopic heart transplantation at the University of Pittsburgh Medical Center. *A,* The donor heart is in sinus rhythm, and the native heart's rhythm is atrial fibrillation. *B,* The donor heart is in sinus tachycardia, and the native heart's rhythm is ventricular fibrillation (patient was hemodynamically unchanged with these rhythms).

SUMMARY

The results of heart transplantation have markedly improved over the past 30 years. The 1-year actuarial survival now approaches 95% at many centers in the United States. In addition, the quality of life for these patients is better. Much of the success is due to the improvements in caring for these critically ill patients in the immediate postoperative period. Research continues to improve immunosuppressive agents to further reduce the incidence of acute rejection. New strategies are necessary to prevent, detect, and treat allograft vascular disease to improve long-term survival.

References

1. Keck BM, Bennett LE, Frol BS, et al: Worldwide thoracic organ transplantation: A report from the UNOS/ISHLT International Registry for Thoracic Organ Transplantation. *In* Clinical Transplants. Cecka and Teraski (eds). Los Angeles, UCLA Tissue Typing Laboratory, 1997.
2. Hosenpud JD, Bennett LE, Keck BM, et al: Registry of the International Society for Heart and Lung Transplantation: Fourteenth Official Report, 1997. J Heart Lung Transplant 1997; 16:691–712.
3. Scott CD, Omar I, McComb JM, et al: Long-term pacing in heart transplant recipients is usually unnecessary. PACE 1991; 14:1792–1796.
4. Nanas JN, Anastasiou-Nana MI, Margari ZJ, et al: Redistribution of amiodarone in heart transplant recipients treated with the drug before operation. J Heart Lung Transplant 1997; 16:387–389.
5. Auler JO Jr, Carmona MJ, Bocchi EA, et al: Low doses of inhaled nitric oxide in heart transplant recipients. J Heart Lung Transplant 1996; 15:443–450.
6. Frazier OH, Macris MP: Management of the transplant recipient. *In:* Support and Replacement of the Failing Heart. Frazier OH, Macris MP, Radovancevic B (Eds). Philadelphia, Lippincott-Raven, 1996.
7. Dew MA, Harris RC, Simmons RG, et al: Quality-of-life advantages of FK 506 vs conventional immunosuppressive drug therapy in cardiac transplantation. Transplant Proc 1991; 23:3061–3064.
8. Esmore D, Keogh A, Spratt P, et al: Heart transplantation in females. J Heart Lung Transplant 1991; 10:335–341.
9. Dunn MJ, Rose ML: Antibody mediated rejection following cardiac transplantation. *In:* Immunology of Heart and Lung Transplantation. Rose ML, Yacoub MY (Eds). London, Edward Arnold, 1993.
10. Augustine SM, Yeo CJ, Buchman TG, et al: Gastrointestinal complications in heart and heart-lung transplant patients. J Heart Lung Transplant 1991; 10:547–556.
11. Armitage JM, Kormos RL, Stuart RS, et al: Posttransplant lymphoproliferative disease in thoracic organ transplant patients: Ten years of cyclosporine-based immunosuppression. J Heart Lung Transplant 1991; 10:877–887.
12. Martich GD, Boujoukos AJ: Adult cardiac transplantation. J Intensive Care Med 1996; 11:79–89.
13. Billingham ME, Cary NR, Hammond ME: A working formulation for the standardization of nomenclature in the diagnosis of heart and lung rejection: Heart rejection study group. J Heart Transplant 1991; 9:587–592.

182

Critical Care Aspects of Lung Transplantation

David R. Nunley, MD, FCCP
Robert J. Keenan, MD, FRCSC
James H. Dauber, MD, FCCP

After the first single lung transplantation procedure in 1963, improvements in organ procurement and preservation and in surgical technique slowly advanced this therapeutic option for patients with end-stage lung disease. In the early 1980s the discovery of cyclosporine revolutionized immunosuppressive drug regimens and enhanced survival of organ allografts. In the 1990s lung transplantation increased initially, but most recently it has plateaued. Single-lung, bilateral-lung, and heart-lung procedures peaked at 1423 in 1995.[1] As more transplant centers are now skilled in caring for lung transplant recipients, donor availability is today the limiting factor for availability of the procedure. Likewise, the involvement of the critical care physician has increased as lung recipients require expert management not only in the crucial postoperative period but when critical illness develops later as a consequence of long-term immunosuppression.

PREOPERATIVE EVALUATION

Recipient Selection

The criteria for recipient selection are similar in large transplant centers.[2–4] These criteria can be organized into three areas that are crucial in determining the suitability of a person for lung transplantation:

1. The patient's general medical condition.
2. The specific pulmonary disorder.
3. Psychosocial factors.

General Medical Condition

The patient's general medical condition is assessed for factors that might affect the transplantation procedure or its long-term success. Conditions that represent contraindications to transplantation are listed in Table 182–1.

Patients with unstable medical conditions, particularly those who use mechanical ventilation, are not generally considered to be candidates because there are too few organs to permit transplantation when a proper operative evaluation cannot be performed and the risk of a poor outcome owing to underlying disease is unacceptably high. Baseline renal, hepatic, and bone marrow function are assessed because the stress of surgery and the toxicity from immunosuppression will have strong negative impact on these organ systems, failure of any one of which will jeopardize the outcome.

Renal function is assessed with serum creatinine and 24-hour creatinine clearance values. A clearance of less than 50 mL/min is grounds for exclusion at most centers.

Hepatic function is assessed by measuring serum levels of bilirubin, transaminases, and alkaline phosphatases. Although there are no strict exclusion criteria for hepatic function, a total bilirubin value greater than 3 mg/dL portends a poor outcome.[5]

Adequate reserves in the bone marrow for platelets and

TABLE 182–1. Contraindications to Lung Transplantation

Unstable clinical status (including acute respiratory failure)
Severe dysfunction of major organs
Kidney
Liver
Central nervous system
Bone marrow
Heart (left ventricular dysfunction or coronary artery disease)
Active malignancy
Uncontrollable systemic infection
Pulmonary infection with resistant organisms
Multidrug-resistant *Pseudomonas aeruginosa*
Burkholderia cepacia
Patient unable to walk more than 600 feet in 6 minutes or having no potential for rehabilitation
Ideal body weight less than 80% or greater than 120% of normal
Severe osteoporosis that does not respond to therapy
Active tobacco abuse
Drug or alcohol dependency
History of poor compliance with medical regimens
Inadequate social and financial support

granulocytes are important for homeostasis and host defense. An emerging cause of thrombocytopenia in transplant candidates is epoprostenol (Flolan) given to treat pulmonary hypertension. Platelet counts in these persons usually return to normal after dosing is stopped. Thrombocytopenia in patients on epoprostenol per se does not warrant exclusion from transplantation unless there is evidence of bone marrow hypoplasia.

Cardiac assessment is crucial to determine function of the left and right ventricles, degree of pulmonary hypertension, and presence of coronary artery disease. Nuclear imaging techniques or ultrasonography is used to measure the ejection fraction of the right and left ventricles. An ejection fraction less than 35% for the left ventricle precludes isolated lung transplantation. The lower limit of right ventricular function that precludes isolated pulmonary transplantation still has not been defined.[6, 7]

Echocardiography often provides an excellent estimate of pulmonary artery pressures, but if there is doubt about the degree of pulmonary hypertension in subjects with end-stage parenchymal lung disease, catheterization of the right side of the heart is indicated. It is obviously mandatory in persons with pulmonary vascular diseases, but it need not be repeated during the evaluation if recent results are available.

Left-sided heart catheterization with coronary angiography is performed in all patients who are considered at risk for coronary artery disease (generally men older than 40 years and women older than 50). Cardiac catheterization is also indicated for subjects with congenital heart disease who are being considered for heart-lung or isolated lung transplantation when there is any doubt about the nature of the defect.

Patients with a history of malignancy typically are not accepted for evaluation until at least 3 years after the disease has gone into remission. For breast cancer, melanoma, and colorectal cancer a longer disease-free interval is preferable, owing to the tendency toward late recurrences of these neoplasms. The only potential exception for active malignancy is bronchioloalveolar cell carcinoma. There are isolated reports of long-term survival after lung transplantation, but the tumor has also recurred in the lung allografts. More experience must be accumulated with this relatively uncommon tumor before a definitive statement can be made.

Since one of the major goals of lung transplantation is to restore recipients to a nearly normal lifestyle, candidates must have the potential to be rehabilitated in the postoperative period. An excellent measure of this potential is the ability of the candidate to walk before the transplant operation. Candidates who are not ambulatory owing to neurologic or musculoskeletal problems that cannot be corrected after the transplant generally are excluded. Those whose ambulatory status is severely impaired owing to limitation of cardiac output should not be excluded a priori. Outcome after transplantation seems to be strongly linked to the candidate's pretransplant ambulatory status. Survival is superior for those who can walk more than 600 feet just before transplantation.[8] Consequently, poor ambulatory status without the potential for substantial rehabilitation may disqualify a candidate. The correlation between ambulatory status and outcome also underscores the importance of rehabilitation in the *preoperative* period, which should be incorporated whenever feasible.

Metabolic disturbances are also assuming greater importance. Severely malnourished candidates have less favorable outcomes, for a variety of reasons. Appropriate measures for repletion applied vigorously while the candidate is waiting usually overcome this problem. Gross obesity increases the risk of any surgical procedure and interferes with achievement of normal functional status after transplantation. Reliance on corticosteroids for immunosuppression in the postoperative period only aggravates the problem of obesity.

Candidates also undergo serologic screening for herpes simplex virus, cytomegalovirus (CMV), Epstein-Barr virus (EBV), and (heart-lung candidates only) *Toxoplasma.* The results of these studies determine the type of infectious prophylactic regimen that will be used postoperatively.

Pulmonary Assessment

A wide variety of end-stage diseases may be treated successfully with lung transplantation. Pulmonary parenchymal diseases such as emphysema, cystic fibrosis, and idiopathic pulmonary fibrosis represent the majority of cases (Table 182–2). Pulmonary hypertension, either primary or secondary to congenital heart disease, is another major indication for isolated pulmonary transplantation, so long as there is no impairment of left ventricular function and the cardiac defect is correctable at the time of transplantation.

Optimal timing for transplantation during the course of a patient's illness is a challenge. The patient should not be so desperately ill that surviving the procedure is unlikely, yet all reasonable medical and surgical therapies should be exhausted before transplantation is recommended. This "transplant window" is best estimated from the natural history of the primary diseases and from close monitoring of the patient. Once cachexia, total inactivity, and multisystem organ dysfunction occur, the probability of a successful outcome diminishes dramatically. Most candidates should have a life expectancy of less than 1 to 2 years, which coincides with the average waiting period at most transplant centers. One objective measure that recently has shown some utility in predicting survival to transplant is the 6-minute walk.[9] Candidates who are unable to walk at least 400 m in 6 minutes are at higher risk of dying before transplantation than those who can exceed 400 m in 6 minutes. Walking less than 300 m is associated with even higher risk of death and warrants urgent listing if the candidate meets the usual criteria. It is always better to err on the side of referring too early rather than too late, and patients who are "too healthy" for a transplant when an organ becomes available can have their candidacy inactivated until their condition deteriorates to the point where transplantation must be undertaken soon to ensure an optimal outcome.

Previous therapy for the underlying disease can affect the transplantation procedure. Thoracotomy for lung biopsy, resection, or pleurectomy can result in extensive pleural and mediastinal adhesions, which hamper the removal of the na-

TABLE 182–2. Indications for Lung and Heart-Lung Transplantation

	Procedure					
	Single-Lung		*Double-Lung*		*Heart-Lung*	
Indication	N	%	N	%	N	%
Emphysema/COPD	1744	44.3	437	17.2	92	4.2
α_1-Antitrypsin deficiency	468	11.9	277	10.9	57	2.6
Idiopathic pulmonary fibrosis	791	20.1	175	6.9	63	2.9
Cystic fibrosis	63	1.6	859	33.8	340	15.6
Primary pulmonary hypertension	232	5.9	264	10.4	586	26.9
Congenital heart disease					650	29.8
Retransplantation	134	3.4	71	2.8	65	3.0
Other	504	12.8	460	18.1	325	14.9

Extracted from the Registry of the International Society of Heart Lung Transplantation, 14th Annual Data Report, July 1997.
COPD = chronic obstructive pulmonary disease.

tive lungs and put crucial structures such as the recurrent laryngeal, phrenic, and vagus nerves at risk. These adhesions can also result in life-threatening bleeding, particularly when cardiopulmonary bypass is necessary.

Prolonged corticosteroid therapy is common before transplantation for obstructive and restrictive lung diseases. At one time, even small doses of steroids were considered to be a contraindication to lung transplantation owing to negative effects on wound healing, particularly at the airway anastomosis. Most centers today accept patients for transplantation who are still taking moderate doses of prednisone (not more than 0.3 mg/kg/day), as the frequency and severity of dehiscence of the bronchial anastomosis have diminished significantly thanks to improved surgical techniques. These patients must be assessed carefully to determine the extent of toxicity induced by long-term steroid therapy, because they will be at higher than expected risk for similar toxicities in the post-transplantation period.

One such toxicity that is assuming much greater importance is osteoporosis.[10] Candidates who have significant osteoporosis before transplantation have a much greater risk of fracture in the postoperative period, when the effects of large doses of corticosteroids combined with other drugs, most notably cyclosporine, accelerate bone loss.[11] Such fractures drastically hinder rehabilitation and functional status. Unless there is a good response to the treatment of osteoporosis in the preoperative period, based on measurement of bone density by dual-beam adsorption spectrophotometry, transplantation candidates with advanced bone disease should be disqualified.

Chronic or recurrent administration of antibiotics also plays an important role in the treatment of several pulmonary diseases, most notably cystic fibrosis. Such patients can become colonized with bacteria that are highly resistant to antibiotics. Preoperative determination of the sensitivities of organisms isolated from candidates with septic lung disease is essential if rational antibiotic prophylaxis is to be provided during the postoperative period. In addition, multiple drug resistance is considered by most centers to be a contraindication to transplantation, since infection with these organisms after surgery is difficult to treat. Infection with the organism *Burkholderia cepacia* (formerly *Pseudomonas cepacia*) is a concern in most centers, as the organism often becomes resistant to all antibiotics after attempts to eradicate it. Although it may not be as virulent as *Pseudomonas aeruginosa,* this agent has been associated with an unacceptable rate of life-threatening infection in recipients who harbored it before transplantation.[12, 13]

Psychosocial Assessment

The transplantation process is a source of considerable stress for patients who have already contended with hardships imposed by end-stage lung disease. Psychiatric disorders are relatively common in lung transplant candidates and include mood disorders, depression, severe anxiety, and substance abuse. A careful review of these issues during the evaluation is essential.

When there is doubt about the type or severity of a psychiatric disorder, the candidate should undergo formal evaluation by a psychiatrist who is knowledgeable about lung transplantation. Candidates must also be screened carefully for ongoing tobacco or alcohol abuse and, if indicated, monitored for abstinence during the waiting period. Different stresses are encountered at different stages of the process—evaluation for listing, waiting for the transplant, the perioperative period, and out-of-hospital follow-up. Psychologic stability and strong family support are essential if the patient is to cope with the stresses at each stage of the process.

Finally, adequate financial support is becoming increasingly critical. Having sufficient resources to get through just the transplant procedure itself is no longer adequate. The cost of postoperative care is becoming increasingly important as recipients live longer and all too frequently encounter expensive complications such as chronic rejection.

Donor Selection

As with many other types of organ transplants, the availability of suitable donor lungs is a major limiting factor. It has been estimated that only 15% of potential donors' lungs are acceptable for transplantation.[14]

Ideally, potential donors must have no history of smoking or chronic lung disease. In addition, they may not have a systemic illness such as sepsis or malignancy that could affect the recipient. They must be without serologic evidence of hepatitis, syphilis, and human immunodeficiency virus (HIV). The lungs themselves must have (1) no evidence of injury or infection, as demonstrated by a clear chest radiograph; (2) good gas exchange, as determined by arterial blood gas analysis; and (3) normal pulmonary mechanics. Bronchoscopy is generally performed to ensure that the airways are free of purulent secretions, inflammation, aspirated material, and other lesions.[15]

Once the donor organs have been found to be acceptable, a recipient is matched on the basis of immunocompatibility (ABO blood type) and size. Size is assessed based on the donor's height, weight, and thoracic dimensions as determined by chest radiography. In heart-lung and double-lung transplantation, it is particularly important to avoid using lungs that are too large, because compressive atelectasis and marked hemodynamic instability could result. A single oversized lung may be transplanted to the recipient's left side, where the hemidiaphragm can descend somewhat to accommodate it.[16]

Once the donor transplant is found to be compatible, airway secretions are obtained for culture to guide perioperative antibiotic therapy. Serologic studies are performed for CMV, EBV, herpes simplex virus, and *Toxoplasma*. Because of the scarcity of organs, these studies are not used prospectively to match recipients but rather to guide the postoperative use of prophylactic measures such as ganciclovir.

OPERATIVE ISSUES

Lung Preservation

Although rapid advances in surgical technique and immunosuppression have increased the clinical success of lung and heart-lung transplantation, many issues surrounding lung preservation remain poorly understood. The earliest procedures required that the donor be brought to the transplant center so that the lungs could be removed and immediately placed into the recipient without having to be preserved.[17] Remote procurement of organs was necessary to expand the donor pool and to simplify the procedure; thus, various techniques for lung preservation had to be developed. Direct comparison of these techniques has been difficult because of the lack of consensus on an appropriate experimental model, transplantation technique, and measures of adequacy of preservation. Nevertheless, a few common principles have emerged.[18]

Hypothermic Preservation

Hypothermia is crucial to retard cellular metabolism and to depress the activity of intracellular enzymes that lead to cell death during ischemic preservation.[19] Two methods have been used to achieve pulmonary hypothermia. Core cooling of the donor can be accomplished by placing the donor on cardiopulmonary bypass.[20, 21] This technique is complex because it may require that a portable cardiopulmonary bypass unit be brought to the donor hospital. Furthermore, once hypothermic cardiac arrest occurs, pulmonary perfusion ceases, and bronchial arterial perfusion becomes unreliable. Therefore, uniform pulmonary cooling may be impossible to achieve with cardiopulmonary bypass alone. For these reasons this technique has not been widely applied.

The most common technique for achieving hypothermia involves flushing the donor lung after it has been removed with a cold preservative solution through the pulmonary artery. Generally, a vasodilator such as prostacyclin or prostaglandin E_1 is also used to ensure uniform perfusion of the organ with the hypothermic solution. The preservative flush[22] may include:

- Modified Euro-Collins
- Blood-based, low-potassium and low-dextran
- University of Wisconsin (UW) solutions

For transport to the recipient, the lungs are placed in cold saline or ice. The ideal temperature has not been established, and it has not been determined whether the lungs should be inflated or remain deflated during transport.[22] Furthermore, the benefit of supplemental oxygen for inflating donor lungs during transport has not been established.

Adjunctive Measures

Several other measures have also been considered to reduce the injury during preservation and reperfusion. The inflammatory cascades that lead to such injury have not been clearly defined. Nevertheless, a variety of anti-inflammatory agents have been used during various stages of procurement and reimplantation of the lungs.[22] For example, not only are prostaglandin E_1 and prostacyclin used in many centers for their vasodilatory properties, as outlined earlier, but these agents also have anti-inflammatory effects that may be beneficial.[23, 24] Similarly, corticosteroids have been of some benefit in animal models.[25]

Cytotoxic oxygen free radicals are widely believed to play an important role in ischemia-reperfusion injury to the lung.[24] Various measures have been contemplated as means of preventing free radical injury. For example, because leukocytes may be a source of the free radicals, leukocyte depletion using filters during procurement and reimplantation has been proposed.[26] The application of such techniques is likely to be limited, as they require that cardiopulmonary bypass be used in both donor and recipient. A much more practical approach would be to administer agents that act as free radical scavengers, such as allopurinol,[27] superoxide dismutase,[28] catalase,[29] and dimethylthiourea.[30] In addition, because iron plays a role in the generation of free radicals, chelating agents such as deferoxamine may be useful.[31] Each of these agents has been shown to be of benefit in animal models, but they have not been widely applied for transplantation in humans.

One of the major concerns in lung preservation is the inability to suitably flush the systemic (bronchial) circulation and its effect on airway healing. Recent investigations using experimental pig lung models suggest that retrograde perfusion through the left atrium results in improved flow to bronchial arterioles.[32, 33] Flow to the airway walls is increased as compared with antegrade flow, even with the addition of vasodilators such as prostacyclin. This technique has recently been adopted by many transplant programs, and on several occasions clots have been flushed from the pulmonary arterial circulation that would not have been identified with an antegrade technique.

Transplantation Options

Initially, lung transplantation was performed only in combination with heart transplantation. Although effective, it was impractical for patients with isolated lung disease, and as heart transplantation became increasingly widespread fewer heart-lung en bloc transplants were available. Single- and double-lung transplantations eliminated the need for extraneous heart transplantation and expanded the use of available donor lungs. Lobar transplantation from both cadavers and living, related donors is currently being performed on increasing numbers of pediatric and adult patients.[34] The availability of each of these choices allows the operation to be tailored to the individual needs of the recipient.

Heart-lung transplantation is currently performed for patients with complex congenital heart disease. It is also performed for patients suffering from pulmonary parenchymal or vascular disorders intercurrent with coronary artery disease or poor left ventricular function (e.g., left ventricular ejection fraction ≤35%). Double-lung transplantation must be utilized for septic pulmonary disorders (i.e., cystic fibrosis and bronchiectasis) because a single-lung allograft would be at risk for infectious complications resulting from the spread of purulent secretions from the remaining native lung. Other indications for double-lung transplantation include primary pulmonary hypertension and secondary pulmonary hypertension due to simple cardiac defects that may be corrected at the time of transplantation. In addition, double-lung transplantation may be indicated for bullous emphysema.

Single-lung transplantation has been performed in patients

with various parenchymal and vascular pulmonary diseases. It was once believed to be contraindicated in cases of emphysematous lung disease because of concerns about severe hyperinflation of the remaining native lung and ventilation-perfusion mismatch.[35] However, subsequent experience showed that such concerns had been overstated and that the procedure could be performed in patients with emphysema due to chronic obstructive pulmonary disease or α_1-antitrypsin deficiency. Although such recipients may not achieve as much improvement in lung volume as those receiving double-lung transplants, they do experience significant improvements in gas exchange and exercise tolerance.[36, 37] Given the scarcity of donor organs, single-lung transplantation for emphysema is a reasonable option.

Single-lung transplantation has recently been performed in patients with pulmonary hypertensive disorders. After transplantation, most of the blood flow is directed toward the allograft, whereas ventilation is directed toward both lungs. Nevertheless, recipients have experienced decreases in their pulmonary artery pressures, improvements in gas exchange, and recovery of right ventricular function.[38] A concern has been the increased operative risk and the lack of reserve afforded by the native lung when infection or rejection occurs in the allograft.[39] In such circumstances, ventilation-perfusion mismatch can result in severe hypoxemia. These concerns may not be warranted given recent experience. In one review of single and bilateral lung transplantation for pulmonary hypertension, it was found that single-lung recipients fared as well as their "bilateral transplant" counterparts in overall survival and functional improvement.[40]

Few guidelines exist for determining which of the native lungs to replace with a lung transplant. One approach is to perform preoperative ventilation-perfusion scanning. If ventilation and perfusion are significantly decreased in one lung, that organ is generally replaced. In emphysema patients it may be preferable to replace the right lung. The high compliance of the native lung, coupled with expiratory airflow limitation, can cause hyperinflation and compression of the newly transplanted allograft. Compression is less likely when the native lung remains in the left hemithorax because of the ability of the left hemidiaphragm to descend and thus accommodate the hyperinflated lung.

Technical Considerations

Cardiopulmonary Bypass

Cardiopulmonary bypass, although associated with risks and complications, is a necessary part of heart-lung or single-lung transplantation for pulmonary hypertension. When double-lung transplantation was initially described, implantation of both lungs en bloc also necessitated the use of bypass.[41] This procedure was later refined, and each lung is now implanted separately (Fig. 182–1).[42, 43] When a preoperative perfusion scan indicates a marked discrepancy between the right and left lungs of the recipient, the lung with the least perfusion is replaced first. As each lung is isolated, its pulmonary artery is clamped and the effects on the recipient's hemodynamic status and ability to maintain acceptable gas exchange are closely monitored. If the clamping is tolerated, cardiopulmonary bypass can successfully be avoided. A similar approach is taken with single-lung transplantation[44, 45] so that cardiopulmonary bypass is reserved for recipients who are unable to tolerate single-lung ventilation of the contralateral native lung.

Incision

Lateral thoracotomy through the fifth or sixth intercostal space is used for single-lung transplantation. For double-lung or heart-lung transplantation, a bilateral transverse thoracotomy, or "clamshell" incision, is used (Fig. 182–2). This requires transection of the sternum with division and ligature of both internal mammary arteries.

Airway Anastomoses

The integrity of the airway anastomoses has been a major concern in pulmonary transplantation. Complications such as dehiscence and stricture have necessitated several changes in surgical technique. Nutrient blood is supplied to the large airways via the bronchial circulation, which originates from the aorta and upper intercostal arteries.[46] During removal of

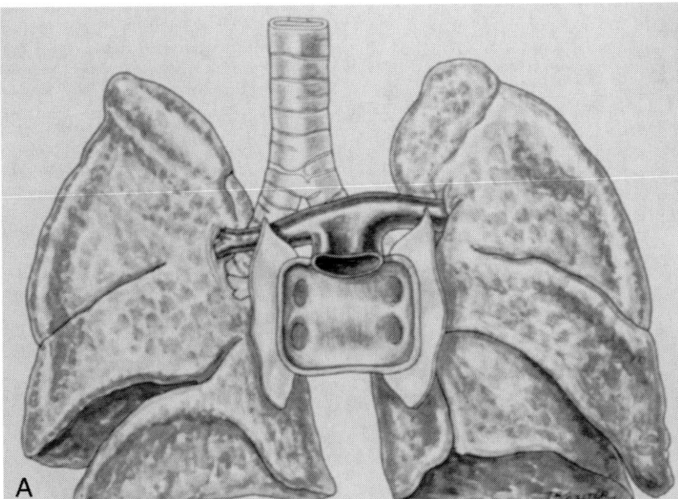

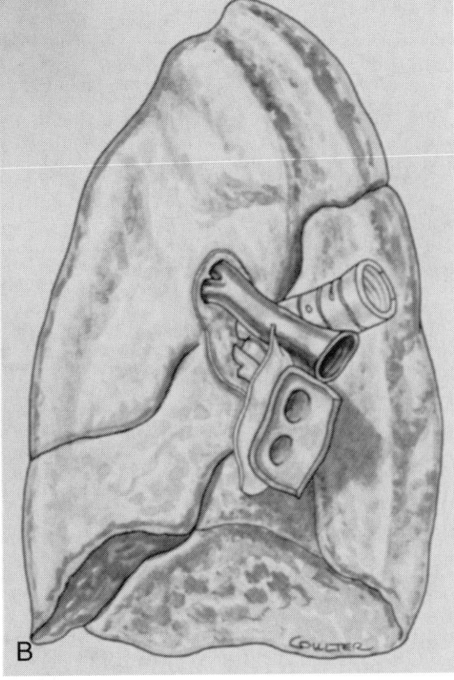

Figure 182–1. *A,* In the donor, the lungs are removed with the airway divided at the trachea, the pulmonary artery is severed proximal to its bifurcation, and the pulmonary veins are harvested as a cuff of the left atrium. *B,* Division of the mainstream bronchi, pulmonary artery, and atrial cuff yields the right and left lungs for implantation. The right lung is shown here.

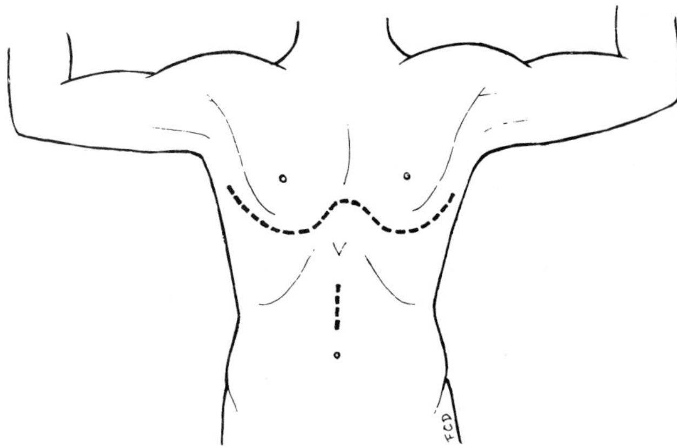

Figure 182–2. "Clam shell" incision used for double lung transplantation. The midline abdominal incision is made if the surgeon wishes to use an omentopexy. (From Egan TM, Detterbeck FC: Technique and results of double lung transplantation. Chest Surg Clin North Am 1993; 3:89–111.)

the lungs this supply is interrupted, so the airways become dependent on deoxygenated pulmonary arterial blood after transplantation. Consequently, ischemia is believed to play a major role in the development of airway complications.

Several measures can enhance the integrity and vascularity of the airway anastomoses. Dissection about the airways is minimized during removal of the native lungs to preserve the bronchial circulation as much as possible. Reconnection of the donor bronchial circulation to the recipient aorta has been performed but is technically complex and prolongs the procedure.[47] Although the tracheal anastomosis performed with heart-lung transplantation has proved to be relatively free of complications, the same anastomosis performed for double-lung transplantation has been less successful.[48] The reasons for this discrepancy are unclear, although it may relate to the loss of coronary-carinal collateral vessels that supply the lower trachea. Nevertheless, for double-lung transplantation bilateral main bronchial anastomoses are preferred.[42, 43, 49, 50]

Generally, the airways are joined by telescoping the mainstem bronchus of the donor airway into that of the recipient[51] to reinforce the juncture (Fig. 182–3). Before the development of the telescoping technique, many centers chose to wrap the anastomoses in either omentum or a pedicle of intercostal muscle or internal mammary artery.[52] This was done to provide additional reinforcement, contain any potential dehiscence, and improve revascularization.

Vascular Anastomoses

In heart-lung transplantation, the recipient aorta and a cuff of right atrium containing the vena cava recipient provide for the vascular anastomoses (Fig. 182–4). In single-lung and sequential double-lung procedures, the pulmonary artery of the side to be transplanted is joined to the pulmonary artery segment of the donor. Pulmonary veins are procured with a cuff of donor left atrium that is joined to the left atrium of the recipient (Fig. 182–5). The characteristics of the anastomoses can be assessed postoperatively with transesophageal echocardiography, radionuclide scanning, or pulmonary angiography.

Alternatives to Traditional Lung Transplantation

"Living Related" Lobar Transplantation

The success of lung transplantation for a variety of pulmonary disorders has led to a tremendous imbalance between the large number of potential recipients and a very limited supply of cadaver donors. Two recent surgical developments have proved successful in treating certain patient groups, both benefiting them and possibly increasing the supply of cadaver lungs for recipients with other lung diseases.

Pulmonary lobe transplantation was first developed as an alternative for pediatric organ recipients.[53] The technique has also been applied to adults whose major indication is cystic fibrosis. Patients with pulmonary hypertension, pulmonary fibrosis, and obliterative bronchiolitis have also undergone lobar transplantation.[54] The unique aspect of lobar transplantation is that two living donors each donate only a part of their lungs. The lower lobes have been most suitable for lobar transplantation, so one donor gives a right lower lobe and the

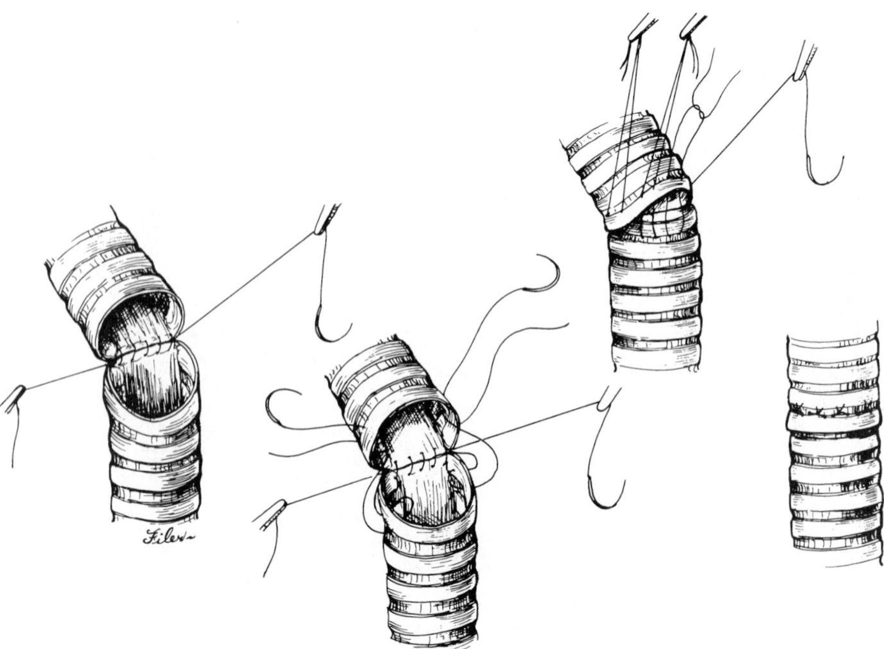

Figure 182–3. Anastomosis of the airway begins with a continuous approximation of the membranous portions and is completed with the placement of interrupted horizontal mattress sutures from the larger airway in such a way that the smaller airway is telescoped. (From Griffith BP, Magee MJ: Single lung transplantation. Chest Surg Clin North Am 1993; 3:75–88.)

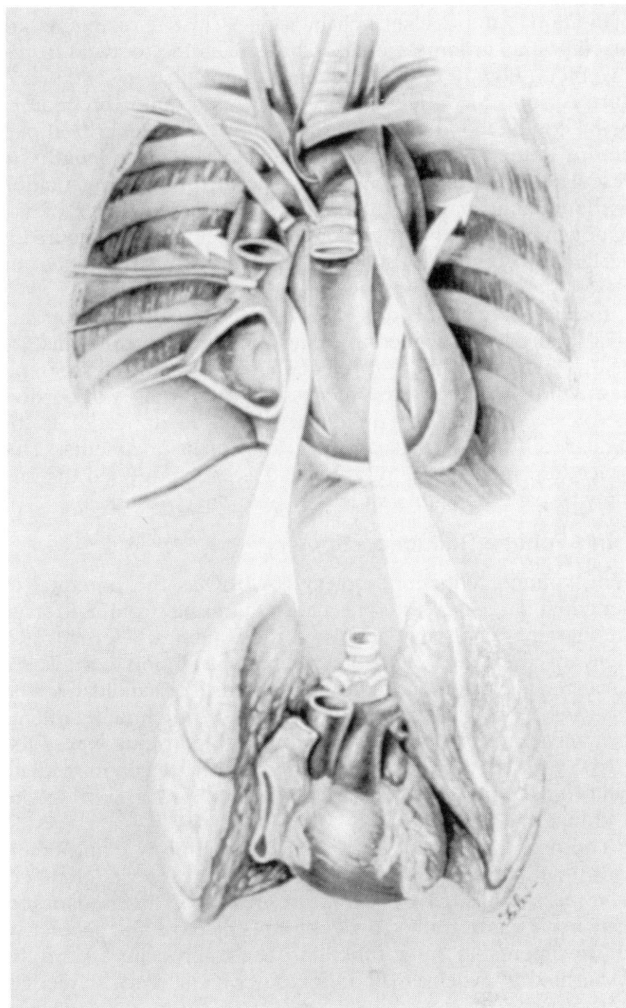

Figure 182–4. With heart-lung transplantation, the donor organs are inserted with anastomoses of the trachea, aorta, and right atrial cuff.

other the left lower lobe. For ethical and moral reasons, donors are usually relatives who share the same blood type as the recipient and have been thoroughly examined to determine that they are healthy enough to withstand donating a lobe and do so willingly. The procedure is plausible because the donors are selected to be larger than the recipient, so that their lobes will be equivalent in size to both lungs of the recipient.

For the recipient undergoing transplantation, this innovative procedure is very similar to traditional bilateral lung trans-

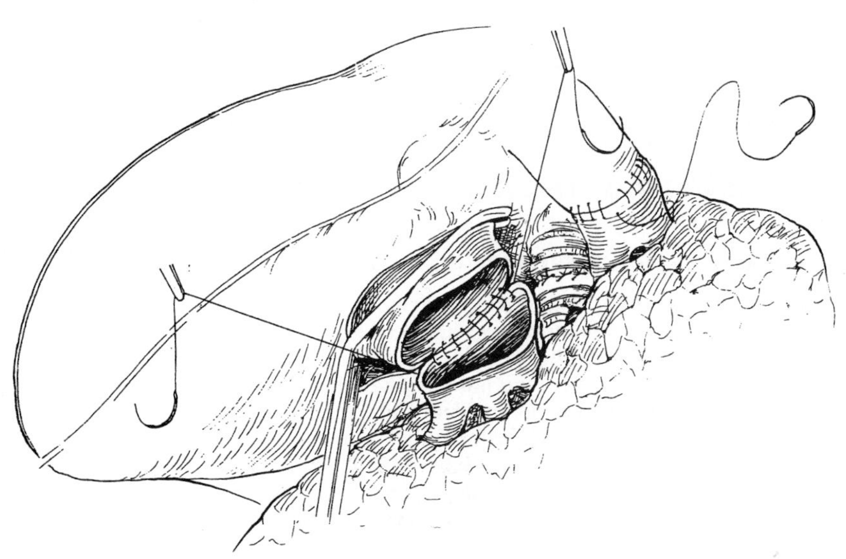

Figure 182–5. Completion of a left lung transplantation. The atrial cuff of the donor is being sewn to that of the recipient. The bronchial and pulmonary arterial anastomoses are completed. (From Griffith BP, Magee MJ: Single lung transplantation. Chest Surg Clin North Am 1993; 3:75–88.)

plantation. After a clamshell incision is made, recipients are placed on a cardiopulmonary bypass machine to avoid excessive blood flow to either lobe during implantation. The procedure is performed electively, recipient and donor procedures being conducted in adjacent operating suites. The critical part of the donor lobectomies is to obtain sufficient lengths of vascular and bronchial tissue to perform the implantation without compromising blood flow to the remainder of the donor lung. The timing of donor and recipient procedures is designed to minimize ischemia time and reduce potential injury.

Intermediate results reported recently revealed a 1-year survival rate of 68%, infection being the predominant cause of death.[55] The incidence of rejection was 0.8 episodes per patient, and all were treated successfully with pulses of corticosteroids. Postoperative pulmonary function appeared to be similar to that of cadaver lung transplant recipients. This procedure holds great promise and is being applied increasingly to patients with a variety of pulmonary diseases.

Lung Volume Reduction Surgery

Lung volume reduction surgery (LVRS) has the potential to benefit a large group of patients suffering from end-stage emphysema who have exhausted their medical alternatives.[56] Many of them are ineligible for transplantation because of advanced age or other medical conditions. For candidates who are eligible for transplantation the pool of potential recipients far exceeds the supply of donors, resulting in long waits, and possibly death. For them, LVRS offers a way to gain immediate symptomatic improvement as an alternative, or as a bridge, to eventual transplantation.

The procedure relies on resection of diffusely emphysematous tissue to reduce dyspnea and improve exercise tolerance. LVRS, accomplished by stapled resection of diseased tissue, has been demonstrated to yield both objective and subjective improvements in lung function. These procedures can be performed by video-assisted thoracoscopic surgery or median sternotomy.

Candidates should show evidence of hyperinflation on chest radiography, with well-demarcated areas of trapped air or dead space as determined by computed tomography and ventilation-perfusion scanning. These areas should be associated with both wash-in and washout abnormalities and hypoperfusion.

Stapler resection of portions of the lung is performed, the goal being to reduce the overall volume of each lung by 25% to 30%. Sites of resection are predetermined by the imaging studies; the least functional lung is chosen for resection first. The procedure produces significant improvements in airflow and lung volumes. Patients also exhibit a significant increase in oxygenation and reduced arterial carbon dioxide. Significant improvement in pulmonary mechanics is seen, and patients express significant symptomatic benefit.

MANAGEMENT IN THE INTENSIVE CARE UNIT

Respiratory Management

The basic principles of airway and ventilatory management for lung transplant recipients are no different from those for other critically ill patients. The use of supplemental oxygen and adjuncts (both invasive and noninvasive) for ensuring adequate ventilation are frequently necessary. After surgery, recipients have impaired cough reflexes owing to the disruption of afferent nerve fibers and thus have difficulty mobilizing respiratory secretions. Because many recipients have bronchorrhea and bronchoconstriction, aggressive pulmonary toilet is crucial. Frequent airway suctioning and aerosolized bronchodilators are widely utilized while the patient is still receiving mechanical ventilatory support. After extubation, recipients require early ambulation, cough and deep breathing maneuvers, and possibly continued use of aerosolized bronchodilators to help mobilize respiratory secretions and prevent atelectasis.

TABLE 182–3. Causes of Respiratory Insufficiency After Lung Transplantation

Preservation injury	Hyperinflation
Ischemia-reperfusion injury	Pneumonia
Pulmonary edema	Rejection
Pulmonary venous obstruction	Phrenic nerve dysfunction
Ventilation-perfusion mismatch	

Varying degrees of respiratory insufficiency may develop in the early postoperative period. Numerous factors can cause respiratory failure at this time, and these are outlined in Table 182–3. The development of infiltrates on the chest radiograph in the early postoperative period, combined with poor gas exchange and abnormal respiratory mechanics, was initially referred to as the *reimplantation response*.[57]

Mechanical Ventilation

In uncomplicated cases, most lung recipients can be extubated 24 to 36 hours after surgery when conventional criteria for extubation have been met and the recipient is able to protect the airway. During the period of mechanical ventilation, adequate oxygenation is ensured with supplemental oxygen and positive end-expiratory pressure while control of the arterial partial pressure of carbon dioxide ($Paco_2$) and pH is achieved by providing adequate minute ventilation at the lowest possible airway pressures. Recipients who were hypercapnic before surgery usually remain so temporarily after the transplant procedure. Function eventually normalizes over several weeks as the medullary respiratory center readjusts. Therefore, while the patient requires mechanical ventilatory support, the $Paco_2$ is adjusted accordingly to maintain adequate pH. Indeed, there is a strong correlation between duration of mechanical ventilation and length of intensive care unit (ICU) stay in single-lung recipients.[58]

Differential lung ventilation (DLV) utilizing a double-lumen endotracheal tube is a strategy employed by many transplant centers for single-lung recipients when a clear mechanical disparity exists between the native diseased lung and the allograft (e.g., in recipients with emphysema or pulmonary fibrosis). The concern with these recipients is that, with conventional mechanical ventilation and employing a single-lumen tube, the lung with the greatest compliance preferentially receives the majority of the gas flow. This may lead to hyperinflation of the more compliant lung with resulting mediastinal shift and compression of the contralateral lung. Furthermore, as the more compliant lung becomes hyperinflated, the increased airway pressure results in compression of the vascular bed with preferential redistribution of pulmonary blood flow to the collapsed lung, allowing for significant ventilation-perfusion mismatch.[59–61]

When acute lung injury (i.e., from ischemia and reperfusion) complicates the function of the allograft, this ventilation-perfusion mismatch may worsen, as most of the pulmonary blood flow is shunted toward the native lung to a greater degree than the accompanying ventilation.[62] DLV has been used successfully to treat ischemia-reperfusion injury in recipients after single-lung transplantation.[63] It has also been demonstrated that independent ventilation of the allograft via a double-lumen tracheostomy tube with spontaneous ventilation of the native lung has been used successfully for extended periods to treat ischemia-reperfusion injury.[64] At our institution, DLV is routinely employed during the first 24 hours after single-lung transplant surgery. If gas exchange remains good without signs of ischemia-reperfusion injury, the recipient is switched to conventional ventilation and efforts are made to move toward extubation.

Weaning the lung transplant recipient from mechanical ventilation may be hampered by any of the usual problems encountered in critically ill patients (e.g., infections, electrolyte imbalances, nutritional deficiencies). In addition to these, the lung transplant recipient may also be at risk for injury to the phrenic nerves secondary to the surgical procedure. In recipients with inflammatory lung disease, dense pleural adhesions may require delicate dissection during transplantation. The phrenic nerves may be damaged by traction or even inadvertently cut. Such an injury may go unnoticed in the immediate postoperative period, while the recipient is on positive-pressure ventilation, but its consequences soon become apparent when weaning is initiated. Fluoroscopy or ultrasonography of the diaphragm helps make the diagnosis.

Dysfunction of the allograft, either in the immediate postoperative period or later as a result of infection or rejection, may be so severe that, despite maximal ventilatory support, the recipient's gas exchange is inadequate. In these situations extracorporeal membrane oxygenation (ECMO) has been employed. In lung recipients who require ECMO, survival has been associated with earlier initiation of ECMO after transplantation (i.e., <7 days). Survival to hospital discharge in these recipients has been as high as 70%, and most ultimately attain normal graft function.[65] Survival also appears to be associated with treatable and reversible causes that require a shorter duration of ECMO support.[66]

Ischemia-Reperfusion Injury

Ischemia-reperfusion injury of the transplanted lung is a common problem. It occurs to some degree in all recipients and causes severe morbidity in as many as 20%. During the ischemic period decreasing endothelial adenosine triphosphate (ATP) levels inhibit activation of the xanthine oxidase pathway. Reestablishing blood flow at the time of implantation allows for oxygen, in the presence of calcium influx, to activate this pathway, resulting in the formation of uric acid along with byproducts such as superoxide anion and oxygen free radicals (hydrogen peroxide and hydroxyl anion). Toxic oxygen free radicals are also produced by the recipient's neutrophils, which become activated and adhere to the altered endothelium of the donor lung vessels. These activated neutrophils then generate superoxide anions, and the cytokines generate tumor necrosis factor-alpha and interleukin-1_{β}.[67]

The release of these metabolites is ultimately responsible for increased capillary permeability, interstitial alveolar edema, and altered vascular tone. Additionally, significant dysfunction of type II alveolar pneumocytes has been demonstrated during ischemia-reperfusion injury, which alters the composition, function, and metabolism of surfactant, resulting in further alveolar edema and hypoxemia.[68]

Clinically, ischemia-reperfusion injury of the lung presents as progressive hypoxemia, pulmonary hypertension, decreased lung compliance, and high-permeability pulmonary edema. Although usually reversible, this injury to the lung allograft is associated with increased need for mechanical ventilation, longer ICU stay, and increased morbidity and mortality.[69] Furthermore, there is some evidence to suggest that ischemia-reperfusion injury may predispose the allograft to earlier rejection.[70]

The radiographic appearance of ischemia-reperfusion injury is quite typical.[71] Generally, reticular interstitial or alveolar infiltrates develop within the first 48 hours after surgery. The infiltrates are principally in the perihilar and lower lung regions and are maximal in density by the third postoperative day. Biopsy specimens from the allograft during this period generally reveal nonspecific diffuse alveolar damage.[72] These findings begin to clear between the 4th and 7th postoperative days, and complete resolution is usually seen by day 14.

More than 90% of recipients with ischemia-reperfusion injury survive this initial lung injury. Treatment is generally supportive and often employs diuretics, positive end-expiratory pressure, and alternative modes of mechanical ventilation. Occasionally, vasodilating agents such as dobutamine, nitroglycerin, and prostaglandin E_1 may be beneficial. Inhaled nitric oxide may also be helpful by decreasing pulmonary hypertension and improving ventilation-perfusion mismatch.[73] ECMO is required by 4% to 5% of all lung transplant recipients, and survival for this group drops to approximately 70%.

Pulmonary Edema

For several reasons, the transplanted lung is particularly susceptible to development of pulmonary edema in the immediate postoperative period. First, the increases in intravascular and total body fluid volume required to maintain hemodynamic stability during the procedure result in hydrostatic forces that favor development of pulmonary edema. Any cardiac dysfunction can exacerbate this problem. Additional postoperative fluid requirements, such as transfusions for hemorrhage or blood products to correct coagulopathy, also contribute to volume overload.

Second, increases in capillary permeability related to ischemia-reperfusion injury or the use of cardiopulmonary bypass[74] further increase lung water volumes.

Third, disordered fluid clearance related to the disruption of the pulmonary lymphatic circulation may play a role in the development of pulmonary edema.

Last, it has been postulated that pulmonary edema may develop in recipients of single-lung allografts whose native lung disease results in pulmonary hypertension (either primary or secondary). After vascular reanastomosis in these recipients, the pulmonary circulation of the allograft becomes the low-pressure sink, allowing for the majority of the cardiac output to go preferentially and immediately to the new organ. This favors formation of edema fluid.[75] Recently, however, it has been suggested that the radiographic appearance of the resulting ischemia-reperfusion injury and pulmonary infiltrates may not be exacerbated by continued high volume blood flow through the allograft in recipients with primary pulmonary hypertension.[69]

For these reasons, fluid administration is minimized in the postoperative period. When necessary, vasoactive agents are added to maintain blood pressure. Diuretics are often administered when the patient is hemodynamically stable; however, care must be taken lest significant intravascular volume depletion be induced. The development of prerenal azotemia in conjunction with the use of nephrotoxic immunosuppressive and antimicrobial medications can lead to the development of acute renal failure.

The possibility of pulmonary venous obstruction must also be considered when pulmonary edema develops in the allograft.[76] This can occur as a result of kinking of the pulmonary veins or of thrombosis of a narrow venous anastomosis. When pulmonary venous obstruction is diagnosed, surgical correction is necessary. The diagnosis can be made at the bedside by measuring pulmonary venous flow from the transplanted lung with Doppler transesophageal echocardiography. Alternatively, delayed transit of contrast medium may be detected with pulmonary angiography.[77]

Ventilation-Perfusion Mismatch

In recipients of a single-lung transplant, conditions may arise that favor ventilation-perfusion mismatch, resulting in significantly abnormal gas exchange. Normally during the first few weeks after single-lung transplantation, both perfusion and ventilation slowly shift to the allograft. When the underlying native lung disease was characterized by primary or secondary pulmonary hypertension, after single-lung transplantation the majority of the cardiac output goes immediately to the allograft, allowing for a lower ventilation-perfusion ratio. Because differences in pulmonary compliance between the native lung and the allograft are usually small, ventilation initially tends to be equally split. This results in suboptimal gas exchange, but usually not to such an extent that the patient is impaired. When infiltrates develop in the allograft (e.g., secondary to ischemia-reperfusion injury, rejection, or pneumonia), serious ventilation-perfusion mismatch can result. When the allograft is compromised by such infiltrates, ventilation tends to be directed toward the native lung, whereas most of the pulmonary blood flow continues to the allograft. In recipients who have emphysema, perfusion may slowly switch back to the native lung, allowing for improved ventilation-perfusion match; however, in recipients with pulmonary hypertension, blood flow continues preferentially to the allograft, perpetuating the severe ventilation-perfusion inequalities.[69, 78] Differential lung ventilation and selective application of positive end-expiratory pressure and other techniques may be necessary to achieve adequate oxygenation and ventilation.

Hyperinflation

When single-lung transplantation is performed for lung disease complicated by obstructive impairment, the recipient is left with markedly different respiratory mechanics in each hemithorax. The allograft has either normal mechanics or, when an injury such as pulmonary edema or rejection occurs, some degree of restrictive impairment. In contrast, the native lung continues to exhibit obstructive impairment that necessitates a long expiratory time for full emptying because of expiratory airflow limitation and high compliance. Furthermore, increased compliance results in a disproportionate increase in the tidal volume directed to the native lung. This abnormal distribution of the tidal volume, coupled with the need for a prolonged expiration time, can result in serious hyperinflation.

The major potential consequence is progressive compression of the allograft. When this condition occurs and goes unrecognized, the mediastinum can be shifted so much that hemodynamic compromise results. For this reason, some transplant programs utilize differential lung ventilation in the immediate postoperative period, allowing customized tidal volumes, flow rates, and inspiratory-expiratory ratios to be delivered to each lung. Administration of bronchodilators to the native lung should continue. Finally, because positive-pressure ventilation exacerbates these problems, the patient should be extubated as soon as he or she is clinically able to tolerate spontaneous breathing.

Early Allograft Infections

Infectious complications have consistently been shown to be the major cause of morbidity and mortality after lung transplantation.[79-81] Transplant recipients are susceptible to pneumonia and bronchial infections, for several reasons.

First, the systemic immunosuppression necessary to prevent graft rejection also suppresses vital components of the host response, including T lymphocyte and granulocyte function.

Second, clearance of secretions from the allograft may be impaired by several mechanisms—dysfunctional ciliary motility and a depressed cough reflex secondary to denervation of the graft. Additionally, sloughing of respiratory tract mucosa at the site of the bronchial anastomosis can produce plugging of the bronchus that further impedes clearance of secretions.

Third, the disruption of pulmonary lymphatics alters normal migration of immune effector cells.

Fourth, colonization or infection of the donor lung can result in infection in the allograft. In one series, organisms recovered from the donor lung at the time of harvest were responsible for more than 20% of subsequent infections in the graft.[82] In single-lung transplantation, the native lung can become infected or harbor pathogens that promote infections in the allograft.[83]

Finally, the recipient's native airway (e.g., proximal trachea and sinuses) may be a source of infection to the allograft. This is especially a concern in recipients with septic lung disorders such as cystic fibrosis.[84, 85]

The development of pneumonia is quite common in the early postoperative period. Between one third and one half of these infections occur within the first 2 weeks after transplantation, most being secondary to bacterial pathogens.[86, 87] Pneumonia from CMV, fungi, or *Pneumocystis carinii* organisms is also possible, but it tends to occur later, often after the recipient has been discharged from the critical care unit. The diagnosis of pneumonia may be difficult, as recipients may have infiltrates on chest radiographs secondary to noninfectious complications such as ischemia-reperfusion injury or pulmonary edema. The use of bronchoscopy with transbronchial biopsy, bronchoalveolar lavage, and protected specimen brush catheters to obtain samples for staining, quantitative cultures, and histologic examination can help to distinguish between these entities.[88]

The consequences of early postoperative pneumonia can be quite severe. Autopsy studies have suggested that as many as 50% of the deaths in the first 30 days after transplantation may be due to pneumonia in the allograft.[89] Survivors of early pneumonia may be at increased risk for chronic allograft rejection, especially when the infections were intercurrent with episodes of acute rejection.[90] For these reasons, prophylactic antibiotics are generally given during the immediate postoperative period. Antibiotic selection is based on specimens obtained from the donor lung or from early postsurgical bronchoscopic surveillance. Recipients with septic lung disorders are generally treated with antibiotics that are effective against organisms isolated in cultures of sputum obtained before transplantation.

Bronchoscopy

Both flexible fiberoptic bronchoscopic and rigid bronchoscopic capability are often necessary in caring for lung transplant recipients. While rigid bronchoscopy most often falls within the domain of the thoracic surgeon, the critical care physician may be called on to perform frequent fiberoptic examinations. Immediately after surgery, dysfunction of the allograft may occur, accompanied by dense pulmonary infiltration on chest radiographs. To help distinguish between infection, ischemia-reperfusion injury, and rejection, fiberoptic bronchoscopy with biopsy is often necessary. Fiberoptic bronchoscopy has proved invaluable in the diagnosis of allograft infection and, when combined with transbronchial biopsy, is now the preferred procedure for diagnosing allograft rejection.[91] The sensitivity in diagnosis of acute rejection has ranged between 61% and 94%, with specificity of 90% to 100%.[92, 93] In fact, during the first 2 postoperative years, routine surveillance via fiberoptic bronchoscopy with biopsy has been beneficial in the diagnosis of allograft rejection, even in the absence of symptoms and radiographic findings.[94, 95] The technique of bronchoalveolar lavage, especially when combined with protected specimen brushing, has enhanced the ability to identify and quantify pathogens infecting the allograft.[96]

The fiberoptic bronchoscope is also utilized to maintain

good bronchial hygiene. In the first few weeks after transplantation, accumulation of secretions that the recipient is unable to clear may promote infection or atelectasis. Also, sloughing of the respiratory epithelium tends to occur at the level of the bronchial anastomosis, which may allow thick, obstructing concretions to form that could lead to complete atelectasis of the allograft. Routine fiberoptic bronchoscopy with vigorous therapeutic saline lavage and suctioning can reduce these complications. Sometimes granulation tissue forms at the bronchial anastomosis and leads to severe stenosis. When a fiberoptic laser filament is passed through the working channel of the flexible bronchoscope, this granulation tissue can be eliminated. If bronchial stenosis becomes severe, placement of an endobronchial stent may be necessary. This is usually accomplished with a rigid bronchoscope that affords controlled ventilation of the recipient during the endobronchial procedure.

Allograft Rejection

Rejection of the allograft may take one of three forms:

- Hyperacute
- Acute
- Chronic

Hyperacute Rejection

Hyperacute rejection is caused by preexisting recipient antibodies directed at antigens in the donor graft. Such antibodies usually arise in response to pregnancy, blood transfusions, or transplant procedures. These antibodies rapidly attach to the vascular endothelium of the graft, subsequently activating complement and resulting in vascular thrombosis with graft failure. Hyperacute rejection has been virtually eliminated as a complication of lung transplantation by ensuring appropriate ABO tissue matching and by screening the recipient's serum for antibodies against a standard panel of reactive antigens.

Acute Rejection

Acute rejection is mediated by helper T lymphocytes, which recognize the major histocompatibility antigens of the donor organ. Cytokines liberated in this reaction induce graft injury by activating cytotoxic T lymphocytes.[97] Extremely common in the first 3 weeks after transplantation and reported as early as postoperative day 3, acute rejection is often heralded by cough, dyspnea, a low-grade fever, a fall in oxygenation of more than 10 mm Hg, reduction of Pa_{O_2} below baseline, and a new or changing radiographic infiltrate in the allograft.[98] In one series, 60% of heart-lung recipients had histologic evidence of acute rejection during the first postoperative month, and 60% of all acute rejection episodes occurred during the first 3 months after transplantation.[99]

The chest radiograph may be helpful in diagnosing acute rejection in the first month after transplantation, but it tends to be less useful later. In a series of heart-lung recipients who had histologically confirmed acute rejection, the chest radiograph was abnormal in 74% of the episodes during the first month but was normal in 77% of acute rejection episodes that occurred later than that.[100] A radiographic picture that is compatible with acute rejection typically reveals alveolar infiltrates in the middle to lower lung zones, and sometimes pleural effusions.

Chronic Rejection

Chronic allograft rejection is characterized clinically by irreversible airflow obstruction and histologically by obliterative bronchiolitis (OB). Since OB has never been diagnosed before postoperative day 60, the critical care physician may not experience this complication during the recipient's initial ICU admission. However, the prevalence of OB is estimated to be between 20% and 40% for long-term survivors and mean time to onset between 8 and 12 months. Thus, recipients with chronic rejection may later require admission to the ICU because of respiratory failure.[101, 102]

Chronic rejection is the leading cause of late mortality in lung transplant recipients.[1] Although no therapy is fully effective for OB, stabilization or transient improvement may be seen in response to corticosteroids or antilymphocyte preparations.[103] Because OB is often complicated by infection or microbial colonization of the allograft, most authorities recommend prophylactic antimicrobial therapy during periods of intensive immunosuppression. If the recipient has a history of CMV infection, prophylaxis should cover it as well.[98]

Hemodynamic Management

The principles of hemodynamic management for transplant recipients are similar to those for other critically ill patients. The goals are to ensure adequate organ perfusion, as evidenced by adequate blood pressure, cardiac index, mixed venous oxygen saturation, and end-organ function. Vasoactive agents are added when appropriate, to maintain mean arterial pressure. Inotropic agents are needed to support cardiac output in recipients of heart-lung transplants and sometimes to support right ventricular output after transplantation when the recipient had preexisting right ventricular dysfunction. Vasodilators such as prostaglandin E_1 occasionally must be used to control elevated pulmonary artery pressure. Supraventricular arrhythmias such as atrial fibrillation that follow lung transplantation are managed with conventional therapies.

Because of alterations in pulmonary capillary permeability and therefore the propensity to develop pulmonary edema, volume administration is generally kept to a minimum after lung transplantation. Occasionally it is necessary to replace blood components, especially when the surgical procedure is complicated by postoperative bleeding. In the early days of lung transplantation, postoperative bleeding was a major cause of early morbidity and mortality.[104] Today, excessive bleeding may follow extensive lysis of pleural adhesions or systemic heparin therapy during cardiopulmonary bypass, and in patients with chronically engorged mediastinal vessels (i.e., Eisenmenger's syndrome). The ability to avoid bypass has been a major factor in reducing the incidence of hemorrhage after lung transplantation.

Management of Kidney Function

Renal function is optimized through support of the circulation, as described earlier. Because of the need to minimize lung water, recipients receive diuretics as soon as they are hemodynamically stable. When urine output is poor after surgery, use of nephrotoxic immunosuppressive agents such as cyclosporine and tacrolimus (formerly known as FK-506) is often delayed and immunosuppression is initiated with corticosteroids and antilymphocyte agents. Whereas some degree of renal insufficiency develops in most recipients sustained on these medications, some investigators have suggested that reduced cardiac output and renal perfusion before transplantation may enhance the risk of chronic cyclosporine nephropathy.[105]

Gastrointestinal and Nutritional Considerations

Like all critically ill patients, transplant recipients should receive prophylaxis against upper gastrointestinal stress ulcers. Small bowel ileus often develops in the immediate postoperative period, and it frequently delays institution of enteral feedings. Since it is known that gut transit decreases in cystic fibrosis, these recipients often experience further delays in gut motility as a result of the stress from surgery.

Gastroparesis has been reported to be a complication of heart-lung transplantation and is thought to be secondary to vagal injury.[106, 107] However, vagal injury should not occur during single or bilateral sequential lung transplantation. Despite this, gastroparesis has been reported to complicate lung transplantation in approximately a quarter of recipients, average time to onset of symptoms being 3 months. It has been suggested that the neurotoxicity of cyclosporine may contribute.[108] Resulting gastroesophageal reflux and microaspiration of food particles can be quite deleterious to the allograft, and some investigators have suggested that these may contribute to the development of OB.[109] Prokinetic agents such as metoclopramide and cisapride may help.

While no specific guidelines have been established for nutritional supplementation for lung transplant recipients, critical care physicians should recognize that many of these recipients are nutritionally depleted as a result of the chronic lung disease that made transplantation necessary. Consequently, these nutritional deficiencies and resulting respiratory muscle dysfunction may complicate weaning from mechanical ventilation.

Poor preoperative nutritional status (defined as *body mass index* below the 25th percentile*) correlates with mortality for recipients whose initial ICU stay exceeded 5 days.[110] Recipients with pancreatic insufficiency, such as those with cystic fibrosis, need to continue pancreatic enzyme supplementation once enteral feedings have begun. If a recipient with cystic fibrosis requires jejunal feeding, elemental feeding (i.e., reduced oligopeptide) formulations may obviate pancreatic enzyme supplementation. In the pediatric population with cystic fibrosis, lung recipients with a rapid and significant postoperative weight gain have improved 1-year survival. Furthermore, in this population, gastrostomy tube feedings have been more effective than oral feeding in achieving significant weight gain after transplantation.[111]

Infectious Disease Considerations

Infections are important causes of both early and late complications. Prophylactic antimicrobials are important in preventing these complications. Prophylaxis measures are summarized in Table 182–4.

Bacterial pneumonia is the most common infection in the early postoperative period. Colonization of the donor airway may produce infection in the recipient. Because donors are at risk for aspiration pneumonia and nosocomial pneumonia, prophylactic antibiotics are aimed at organisms that cause such infections (e.g., clindamycin with third-generation cephalosporin and vancomycin for *Staphylococcus aureus*). Administration of antibiotics continues until results of cultures from the donor trachea are known. When bacterial growth is demonstrated in the donor, the recipient's antibiotic regimen is modified as necessary and continued for 7 days.

For patients with cystic fibrosis, prophylactic antibiotics are chosen to cover organisms detected in cultures obtained during the pretransplantation period or directly from the trachea at the time the recipient lungs are removed. Organisms such as *B. cepacia* and some strains of *P. aeruginosa* that are resistant in vitro to multiple classes of antibiotics pose major threats. For patients with these organisms antibiotic therapy should be carefully tailored to known sensitivities and synergy between antibiotics in vitro. Appropriate drug therapy is often

*Body mass index is calculated by dividing body weight (kilograms) by the square of height (meters).

TABLE 182–4. Postoperative Infection Prophylaxis

Organism	Prophylaxis
Bacteria	
Nonseptic lung disease	Ceftazidime/clindamycin
Cystic fibrosis, bronchiectasis	Antibiotics based on sensitivities of organisms isolated preoperatively or intraoperatively
Candida species	Fluconazole or low-dose amphotericin B
Positive donor culture	
Multiple isolates from recipient	
CMV	
D^+/R^-	IV ganciclovir for 90 days
D^-/R^+	IV ganciclovir for 21 days
D^+/R^+	IV ganciclovir for 21 days
P. carinii	TMP/SMZ 3 days/wk, dapsone weekly
Herpes simplex virus	Acyclovir for 3 mo unless ganciclovir is given
Toxoplasma (heart-lung recipient)	Sulfadiazine, pyrimethamine, and folinic acid

D = donor; R = recipient; TMP/SMZ = trimethoprim-sulfamethoxazole.

continued as long as 14 days, or at least until the patient has been extubated and is doing well. Special attention must be given to treatment of sinus infections because the sinuses are a reservoir for pathogens that can produce recurrent pulmonary infection throughout the entire postoperative period.

Cultures indicating heavy growth of *Candida* in the donor have been linked to invasive candidiasis in the recipient.[112] Prophylaxis for up to 6 weeks with small doses of amphotericin B (0.3 mg/kg/day) or oral fluconazole (400 mg/day) is appropriate in this setting. *Candida* organisms from the recipient may also produce serious infection of the bronchial anastomosis and proximal donor airway. This is a more common problem in recipients who have been taking moderate doses of corticosteroids just before transplantation. Isolation of *Candida* organisms from several sites in the recipient is also an indication for prophylaxis.

Both the donor's and the recipient's serologic CMV status must be determined because these findings dictate the approach to prophylaxis against the virus. Recipients whose status is seronegative and who receive an organ from a seropositive donor are at risk for a primary infection, which before the advent of ganciclovir was an important cause of death. Recipients who are seropositive and who receive an organ from a seropositive donor are at risk for "reactivation" of latent virus or infection with a new viral strain. All of these situations require prophylaxis, which at most centers involves intravenous ganciclovir.

For recipients at risk for primary infection, there is a tendency to give ganciclovir daily for as long as 3 months, whereas in the other situations the duration is 3 weeks. Since CMV infection does not occur in the very early post-transplant period, and because of the potential nephrotoxicity of ganciclovir, prophylactic therapy is typically delayed until the fifth postoperative day for all recipients who need it. The roles of oral ganciclovir and of CMV hyperimmune globulin for prophylaxis remain to be defined. Recipients who are seronegative and who receive an organ from a seronegative donor do not require prophylaxis but should not receive blood products from which they could contract a primary infection.

Immunosuppression

Immunosuppression is typically more intense in the early postoperative period than in the late postoperative period.

Triple-drug therapy is the rule at this time. The mainstay of therapy is either cyclosporine (Sandimmune or Sandimmune Neoral) or tacrolimus (Prograf). Corticosteroids and azathioprine are the other agents used at most centers, but a recently approved drug, mycophenolate mofetil, has replaced azathioprine in some centers, with good results. Induction therapy with cytolytic antilymphocyte globulins, such as OK-3 and horse antihuman thymocyte globulin (Atgam), is used at some centers. Although this approach reduces the rate of early acute rejection and may delay the onset of chronic rejection, it is associated with higher rates of infection and lymphoma.[113]

Cyclosporine or tacrolimus is given intravenously as soon as the recipient demonstrates adequate renal function and then by the oral route as soon as liquids are tolerated. Levels of these agents in whole blood must be monitored at least daily to prevent toxicity and ensure that immunosuppression is adequate. Unfortunately there still is no clinical test to identify an optimal level of immunosuppression. Consequently, the dosing of immunosuppressive agents is determined by the severity of drug toxicity and freedom from rejection. Levels of these drugs often vary much in the early postoperative period when absorption is erratic but tend to be more predictable after the recipient assumes a more normal lifestyle. Administration of other drugs that modify the metabolism of cyclosporine and tacrolimus also alter blood levels. For this reason, the potential for drug interactions must be considered before any new agent is given. Previously, there was much more concern about the negative impact of corticosteroids on healing of airway anastomoses. Improvements in surgical techniques and appropriate selection of recipients have much reduced the rate of dehiscence in the early postoperative period. Accordingly, most centers give intravenous methylprednisolone in the perioperative period and convert to oral prednisone (0.3 mg/kg) as soon as the recipient can take liquids.

Acute rejection does not usually develop until the second postoperative week. Diagnosis should be confirmed whenever possible by transbronchial lung biopsy, but a "clinical" diagnosis can be made without biopsy if all other causes for the decline in allograft function have been reasonably excluded. Treatment of acute rejection usually involves large doses of corticosteroids, most often intravenous methylprednisolone, 500 to 1000 mg/day for 3 days. Oral prednisone may be given for less severe episodes, usually starting at 100 mg and tapering by 10 mg/day to the previous baseline dose.

The response to therapy typically is rapid, with improvement in symptoms and radiographic infiltrates within 24 hours. Assessment of the response to therapy after 10 to 21 days by transbronchial biopsy is critical because persistence of histologically significant acute rejection is common.

LATE COMPLICATIONS

Infection

Infection is a constant risk in immunosuppressed graft recipients, and vigilance for this complication is particularly crucial after intensification of immunosuppression for the treatment of rejection. Although bacterial pneumonia is the most common infectious complication in the first 30 days, thereafter other causes must be considered.

Cytomegalovirus

The prophylactic regimens described earlier have not eliminated CMV infection, but they do delay onset until the recipient is better able to tolerate the insult.[86, 114] The spectrum of CMV infection runs from asymptomatic shedding of virus to fatal pneumonitis and colitis. Shedding of virus in the allograft of a recipient who was seropositive at the time of transplantation usually does not require therapy. Detection of virus in lavage fluid or blood from high-risk recipients (R^-/D^+, R^-/D^-)* warrants treatment with intravenous ganciclovir for 2 to 3 weeks, even in the absence of symptoms, because primary infections are associated with much higher mortality and morbidity rates than are infections in "low-risk" recipients (R^+/D^+ and R^+/D^-).† Relapse is also more common in this group.

Persistent infection raises the possibility of ganciclovir resistance. Foscarnet can be used in this setting but causes much more toxicity than ganciclovir. Ganciclovir should also be given during treatment of rejection in high-risk recipients at any time in the first postoperative year. Short courses (5 to 7 days) suffice for treating rejection with corticosteroids. The duration of cytolytic therapy should be longer (10 to 14 days). When immunosuppression has been intensive owing to persistence of rejection, even low-risk recipients may develop life-threatening CMV infection.

Pneumocystis carinii

P. carinii infection has become unusual since the widespread application of prophylaxis, which for most recipients consists of oral trimethoprim-sulfamethoxazole (TMP-SMZ) taken three times a week.[115] Recipients who are intolerant to this agent usually can take dapsone 100 mg/week, with good results. The diagnosis should be suspected in recipients who after discontinuing prophylaxis demonstrate diffuse infiltrates in the transplanted lungs. Fiberoptic bronchoscopy with bronchoalveolar lavage is usually sufficient to confirm the diagnosis. Treatment with intravenous TMP-SMZ is very effective.[87]

Fungi

A variety of fungi cause infections in lung transplant recipients, but the vast majority of cases are due to *Candida* or *Aspergillus* organisms. *Candida* infections are generally limited to the early postoperative period, whereas infections with *Aspergillus* are encountered throughout the post-transplant period. The major targets of *Candida* are the bronchial anastomosis and the proximal donor airway. This type of infection occurs early after transplantation in recipients with ischemic airway injury and may take weeks to respond to therapy. Other risk factors include large doses of corticosteroids in the immediate pretransplantation period, isolation of *Candida* organisms from multiple sites in the recipient, and prolonged administration of broad-spectrum antibiotics. In a few instances, the infected airway anastomosis manifests dehiscence and, subsequently, spread of the infection to the mediastinum. Primary infection of the parenchyma of the transplanted lung is rare. Mycotic aneurysms of vascular anastomoses have also been reported,[116] but with more aggressive prophylaxis measures this complication has become exceedingly rare.

Aspergillus species and *Aspergillus fumigatus* in particular cause a variety of infections in lung recipients. In the early postoperative period, the bronchial anastomosis is the principal target. This infection tends to occur in recipients who harbored *Aspergillus* in the respiratory tract before transplantation. The infected anastomosis often is covered by a pseudomembrane, which not infrequently is black. Diagnosis is confirmed by culture of bronchial washings and endobronchial biopsy demonstrating tissue invasion by branching, septate hyphae.

Treatment includes oral itraconazole and inhaled amphotericin B. Intravenous amphotericin should be used if the infection is extensive, the airway anastomosis appears to be at risk

---

*Recipient negative/donor positive, recipient negative/donor negative.

†Recipient positive/donor positive, recipient positive/donor negative.

for dehiscence, or there is significant bleeding from the infected anastomosis. Primary infection of the lung allograft usually occurs in recipients who have been treated with multiple pulses of immunosuppression for recurrent rejection. Isolation of *Aspergillus* organisms in bronchial washings or bronchoalveolar lavage fluid is perplexing in this setting, since it is often difficult to distinguish between colonization and true invasion. Whenever *Aspergillus* is isolated from a recipient with chronic radiographic evidence of pulmonary infiltrates who is heavily immunosuppressed, treatment with intravenous amphotericin is warranted.

Another site of infection that is assuming greater importance is the native lung of single-lung allograft recipients.[117] Invasive aspergillosis is not uncommon in this poorly defended organ. New infiltrates in the native lung warrant aggressive diagnostic measures, and the demonstration of *Aspergillus* by bronchoscopy or fine-needle aspiration biopsy must not be ignored.

Finally, *Aspergillus* can cause cerebral abscesses. Typically they occur in heavily immunosuppressed recipients from whom *Aspergillus* was previously isolated. Any change in mental status or new neurologic abnormalities in this type of recipient warrant imaging of the brain.

Toxoplasma

In heart-lung transplantation, transmission of *Toxoplasma gondii* in the heart allograft and subsequent infection of the recipient is possible when the donor is seropositive and the recipient seronegative. In this setting prophylaxis with sulfadiazine and pyrimethamine, in combination with folinic acid to reduce marrow suppression, is mandatory.

Chronic Rejection

As the name implies, chronic rejection occurs later in the post-transplant period than acute rejection, but the two can occur simultaneously. Chronic rejection may emerge as early as the third postoperative month, but more typically it is delayed until the sixth month or later. By the end of the second postoperative year, the prevalence is 40% to 50% and virtually all recipients seem to be at risk for this complication.[118, 119]

The clinical hallmark is progressive dyspnea secondary to increasing airflow obstruction, which is best monitored by measuring the forced expiratory volume in one second (FEV_1). Pathologically, it is characterized by obliterative bronchiolitis, which may be demonstrated by transbronchial biopsy, but this approach is not as sensitive for chronic rejection as it is for acute cellular rejection. For this reason a clinical diagnosis of the bronchiolitis obliterans syndrome is made when a recipient exhibits a progressive decline in airflow rates that cannot be ascribed to any other cause.[120]

Pathogenesis

The pathogenesis of chronic rejection remains incompletely defined. It is widely accepted that a response to donor antigens is central to the process but that this response differs from the mechanism of acute rejection. The leading risk factors for the development of chronic rejection in all series reported to date are the frequency and severity of previous episodes of acute rejection.[118, 121-123] Recipients who experience more than three episodes of acute rejection in the first 6 to 12 months are at the highest risk for chronic rejection. Other factors that may predispose to chronic rejection are an episode of CMV pneumonia and severe ischemic injury to the allograft in the early postoperative period.[124] The process may also be promoted by actions of immunosuppressive drugs and recurrent aspiration of gastric contents, which is not uncommon after lung transplantation.

All recipients should be monitored carefully for the development of dyspnea and for a subclinical decline in allograft function. The latter is most conveniently achieved by training recipients to use a hand-held microspirometer, having them measure and record the values for the forced vital capacity (FVC) and FEV_1 several times each week, and, most important, reporting any decline in either value greater than 10% that is sustained over several days. A decline in home spirometry values should be confirmed with formal pulmonary function tests performed in a qualified laboratory.

Symptomatic recipients and those with an unexplained decline in lung function should be evaluated with bronchoscopy and transbronchial lung biopsy. Infection of the lung allograft often causes a decline in airflow rates and may mask the typical histologic finding of OB. For recipients with infection, appropriate therapy should be given and pulmonary function tests repeated in 3 to 4 weeks. If airflow rates have not increased at this time, bronchoscopy should be repeated.

Treatment

Treatment of chronic rejection is similar to that for acute rejection; namely, augmenting the level of immunosuppression. Typically, the first line of therapy is pulsed doses of corticosteroids, usually intravenous methylprednisolone. Maintenance immunosuppression is usually increased to tolerance. The majority of recipients do not show an adequate response to these measures and require additional therapy with the same cytolytic agents used to treat recurrent acute rejection.[125] This approach usually achieves only stabilization of lung function while much increasing the risk for life-threatening opportunistic infections.

Even with all measures, about 5% to 10% of recipients experience an inexorable decline in lung function ending in death from respiratory failure. The overall mortality rate is about 30% to 35%, making chronic rejection the leading cause of death in the late post-transplant period.[118] It also predisposes to many of the fatal infections during this period. For this reason, increasing efforts are required to develop more effective therapies and prevent chronic rejection entirely. Prevention and better control of acute rejection are potential strategies for avoiding chronic rejection. Regional immunosuppression via inhalation of an aerosol of cyclosporine may hold promise. In a single-center trial it was quite effective in controlling persistent acute rejection and preventing progression to chronic rejection.[126]

Airway Complications

Obstruction of airflow in the lung allograft can also result from stenosis of the proximal donor airway that arises through one of several mechanisms.[127] In the first 3 months the most common cause for bronchial stenosis is granulation tissue arising on the anastomosis. Later in the postoperative period but usually within 6 months, the main mechanism is concentric scarring, which leads to marked narrowing. Still later, functional stenosis can be due to bronchomalacia.

The loss of cartilage in the involved segment permits the airway to collapse during forced expiration and coughing. Granulation tissue responds well to laser ablation. Scarring requires dilatation followed by placement of a bronchial stent. Functional stenosis due to dynamic airway collapse also requires a stent. Recently, endovascular balloons inflated briefly for dilatation and implanted self-expanding wire stents have been used more widely to treat this form of bronchial stenosis (P. D. Orons, personal communication).

Post-transplant Lymphoproliferative Disorders

Most cases of lymphoma encountered in lung recipients are related to primary infection with EBV.[128] This type of lymphoma is thought to be due to the "immortalizing" effect of the virus on B cells and inadequate immune surveillance to control the proliferation of the transformed cells. Because most adult recipients and donors are already seropositive for EBV at the time of transplantation, primary EBV infection is unusual, but when it does occur the risk for B cell lymphoma exceeds 75%. The infection may produce symptoms consistent with infectious mononucleosis, but more often it is asymptomatic. It may be detected within the first month, but most often is not detected until the sixth postoperative week. Reactivation of a latent EBV infection with subsequent emergence of post-transplant lymphoproliferative disorder (PTLD) may be a consequence of intensive and prolonged immunosuppression, but fortunately this is relatively rare.

The use of reverse transcriptase–polymerase chain reaction to detect EBV RNA in peripheral blood is becoming more widespread, and there seems to be a correlation between the amount of RNA and the severity of PTLD.[129] Tumor deposits are found principally in the lungs, both native and allograft, intestinal tract, and lymph nodes.[130] Tumor deposits in the lung are usually asymptomatic, but perforation of a viscus is not uncommon.

The first line of treatment is to reduce the level of immunosuppression, often stopping all drugs as long as several weeks. Most cases respond to this approach, but as might be expected it carries a substantial risk for severe rejection. Chemotherapy is ineffective and is no longer employed to treat cases related to EBV infection. Although most cases respond to treatment, PTLD remains a significant cause of morbidity and mortality in lung recipients. For this reason, some centers question whether adults who are seronegative for EBV should undergo transplantation.[128]

OUTCOME

The International Society for Heart and Lung Transplantation has maintained a registry of data on patients who have received heart-lung and lung transplants since 1983. As of February 1997, information has been collected on 2186 heart-lung recipients, 2543 double-lung recipients, and 3939 single-lung recipients.[1] Survival at 1, 3, 5, and 10 years is shown in Figure 182–6. Survival rates are lower at virtually all points in time after heart-lung transplantation than after isolated lung transplantation, but at 5 years the slight difference in survival between single- and double-lung transplantation is not statistically significant. Survival after isolated lung transplantation has improved since 1988. In the period 1988 to 1992 survival after 48 months was only 42%, whereas from 1992 to 1996 it approached 60%. Those who received a single lung for emphysema had better 2-year survival (70%) than those who had idiopathic pulmonary fibrosis (56%) or primary pulmonary hypertension (58%).

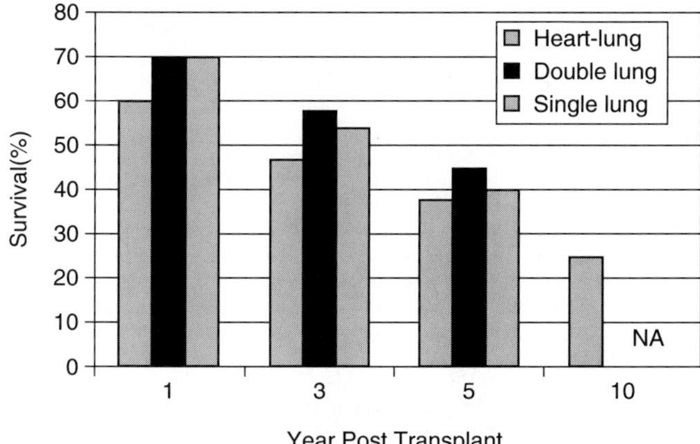

Figure 182–6. Survival following lung transplantation. (Abstracted from the Registry of the International Society of Heart Lung Transplantation, 14th Annual Data Report, July 1997.)

Infection is the leading cause of death during the first 90 days, being responsible for 29% of all deaths in this period. In contrast, rejection accounts for only 5% of deaths. After 90 days, however, rejection assumes a much more important role, being responsible for 29% of all deaths.[131] Infection continues to be an important cause of death in this time frame, too: it causes 29% of all deaths. Many deaths from infection occur in association with chronic rejection and intensive immunosuppression aimed at slowing the progress of the rejection. Clearly, this is becoming the bane of lung transplantation. Unless chronic rejection can be better controlled, outcomes of lung transplantation will continue to lag behind those of other solid organ allograft procedures.

A brief comment about retransplantation is in order, since it is often considered when a lung allograft is failing. Experience is limited, with fewer than 250 procedures having been reported. Nearly 60% of retransplants have been performed for late graft failure from chronic rejection. The remainder have been performed for early graft failure secondary to acute rejection, airway complications, and primary graft failure. During the first 4 years, survival is barely 50% of that for first-time transplant recipients. By the third year after retransplantation, 70% of recipients have developed chronic rejection and the majority have a severe degree of airway obstruction.[132] Such poor outcomes have led many centers to deny retransplantation, an approach that is consistent with optimal use of a scarce resource and reasonable cost containment. On the other hand, it is difficult not to offer a lifesaving procedure to a recipient when the transplant center already has made an initial commitment.

This issue will likely not be settled for some time because of the emotional nature of the debate. Realistically, however, retransplantation will likely become less frequent as the waiting list of candidates grows more rapidly than the donor pool.

Despite recent improvement in outcomes, at least three formidable challenges of pulmonary transplantation must be addressed. The first is one that faces the entire field of transplantation, namely, the disparity between the numbers of candidates and of donors. Clearly, for all solid organs, the former is growing much faster than the latter. Better organ preservation, and a decrease in the rate of primary graft failure, will help to alleviate the donor shortage, but increasing the pool of donors will not easily be achieved.

The second major challenge is to improve immunosuppression. Better control—and ultimately prevention—of rejection are sorely needed. New immunosuppressive drugs and antibodies directed at critical receptors on T lymphocytes that are important for activation seem to hold real promise in this area.

Accomplishing the second goal will also help to meet the third major challenge, that of controlling and preventing infection. Induction of true donor-specific tolerance would much help to reduce the impact of infection.

Unless the second and third complications can be managed successfully, there is a chance that pulmonary transplantation will not be considered a cost-effective treatment for end-stage lung disease.

ACKNOWLEDGMENT

This chapter is dedicated to the memory of Dr. Morris Bierman, whose contributions to critical care medicine and the University of Pittsburgh earned him the enduring esteem of his colleagues.

References

1. Hosenpud JD, Bennett LE, Keck BM, et al: The registry of the international society for heart and lung transplantation: Fourteenth official report—1997. J Heart Lung Transplant 1997; 16:691-712.
2. Morrison DL, Maurer JR, Grossman RF: Preoperative assessment for lung transplantation. Clin Chest Med 1990; 11:207-215.
3. Coordinating Committee: Maurer JR, Frost AE, Estenne M, et al: J Heart Lung Transplant 1998; 17:703-709.
4. Mannes GPM, de Boer WJ, van der Bij W, et al: Three hundred patients referred for lung transplantation: Experiences of the Dutch Lung Transplantation Program. Chest 1996; 109:408-413.
5. Kramer MR, Marshall SE, Tiroke A, et al: Clinical significance of hyperbilirubinemia in patients with pulmonary hypertension undergoing heart-lung transplantation. J Heart Lung Transplant 1991; 10:317-321.
6. Bando K, Armitage JM, Paradis IL, et al: Indications for and results of single, bilateral and heart-lung transplantation for pulmonary hypertension. J Thorac Cardiovasc Surg 1994; 108:1056-1065.
7. Pasque MK, Trulock EP, Cooper JD, et al: Single lung transplantation for pulmonary hypertension: Single institution experience in 34 patients. Circulation 1995; 92:2252-2258.
8. Manzetti JD, Hoffman LA, Sereika SM, et al: Exercise, education, and quality of life in lung transplant candidates. J Heart Lung Transplant 1994; 13:297-305.
9. Kadikar A, Maurer J, Kesten S: The six minute walk test: A guide to assessment for lung transplantation. J Heart Lung Transplant 1997; 16:313-319.
10. Aris RM, Neuringer IP, Weiner MA, et al: Severe osteoporosis before and after lung transplantation. Chest 1996; 109:1176-1183.
11. Epstein S, Shane E, Bilezikian JP: Organ transplantation and osteoporosis. Curr Opin Rheumatol 1995; 7:255-261.
12. Snell G, de Hoyos A, Krajden M, et al: *Pseudomonas cepacia* in lung transplant recipients with cystic fibrosis. Chest 1993; 103:446-471.
13. Noyes BE, Michaels MG, Kurland G, et al: *Pseudomonas cepacia* empyema necessitatis after lung transplantation in two patients with cystic fibrosis. Chest 1994; 105:1888-1891.
14. Harjula A, Baldwin JC, Starnes V, et al: Proper donor selection for heart-lung transplantation: The Stanford experience. J Thorac Cardiovasc Surg 1987; 94:874-880.
15. Riou B, Guesde R, Jacquens Y, et al: Fiberoptic bronchoscopy in brain-dead organ donors. Am J Respir Crit Care Med 1994; 150:558-560.
16. Miyoshi S, Schaefers HJ, Trulock EP, et al: Donor selection for single and double lung transplantation: Chest size matching and other factors influencing posttransplantation vital capacity. Chest 1990; 98:308-313.
17. Pearson FG: Lung transplantation: Samuel Jason Mixter lecture. Arch Surg 1989; 124:535.
18. Kirk AJ, Colquhoun IW, Dark JH: Lung preservation: A review of current practice and future directions. Ann Thorac Surg 1993; 56:990-1000.
19. Cooper JD, Vreim CE: NHLBI workshop summary: Biology of lung preservation for transplantation. Am Rev Respir Dis 1992; 146:803-807.
20. Baumgartner WA, Williams GM, Fraser CD, et al: Cardiopulmonary bypass with profound hypothermia: An optimal preservation method for multiorgan procurement. Transplantation 1989; 48:882-886.
21. Yacoub MH, Kaghani A, Banner N, et al: Distant organ procurement for heart and lung transplantation. Transplant Proc 1989; 21:2548-2550.
22. Novick RJ, Menkis AH, McKenzie FN: New trends in lung preservation: A collective review. J Heart Lung Transplant 1992; 11:377-392.
23. Harjula AL, Baldwin JC, Stinson ET, et al: Clinical heart-lung preservation with prostaglandin E-1. Transplant Proc 1987; 19:4101-4102.
24. Griffith BP, Zenati M: The pulmonary donor. Clin Chest Med 1990; 11:217.
25. Hooper TL, Jones MT, Thomson DS, et al: Modulation of ischemic lung injury by corticosteroids. Transplantation 1990; 50:530-532.
26. Pillai R, Bando K, Schueler S, et al: Leukocyte depletion results in excellent heart-lung function after 12 hours of storage. Ann Thorac Surg 1990; 50:211-214.
27. Bonser RS, Fragomeni LS, Harris K, et al: Acute physiologic changes after extended pulmonary preservation. J Heart Transplant 1990; 9:220-229.
28. Bando K, Tago M, Teraoka H, et al: Extended cardiopulmonary preservation for heart-lung transplantation: A comparative study of superoxide dismutase. J Heart Transplant 1989; 8:59-66.
29. Paull DE, Keagy BA, Kron EJ, et al: Reperfusion injury in the lung preserved for twenty-four hours. Ann Thorac Surg 1989; 47:187-192.
30. Detterbeck FC, Keagy BA, Paull DE, et al: Oxygen free radical scavengers decrease reperfusion injury in lung transplantation. Ann Thorac Surg 1990; 50:204-210.
31. Conte JV, Katz NM, Foegh ML, et al: Iron chelation therapy and lung transplantation: Effects of deferoxamine on lung preservation in canine single lung transplantation. J Thorac Cardiovasc Surg 1991; 101:1024-1029.
32. Baretti R, Bitu-Moreno J, Beyersdorf F, et al: Distribution of lung preservation solutions in parenchyma and airways: Influence of atelectasis and route of delivery. J Heart Lung Transplant 1995; 14:80-91.
33. Varela A, Montero CG, Cardoba M, et al: Improved distribution of pulmonary flush solution to the tracheobronchial wall in pulmonary transplantation. Eur Surg Res 1997; 29:1-4.
34. Starnes VA, Lewiston JN, Luikart H, et al: Current trends in lung transplantation: Lobar transplantation and expanded use of single lungs. J Thorac Cardiovasc Surg 1992; 104:1060-1066.
35. Stevens PM, Johnson PC, Bell RL, et al: Regional ventilation and perfusion after lung transplantation in patients with emphysema. N Engl J Med 1970; 282:245-249.
36. Low DE, Trulock EP, Kaiser LR, et al: Morbidity, mortality and early results of single versus bilateral lung transplantation for emphysema. J Thorac Cardiovasc Surg 1992; 103:1119-1126.
37. Patterson GA, Maurer JR, Williams TJ: Comparison of outcomes of double and single lung transplantation for obstructive lung disease: The Toronto Lung Transplant Group. J Thorac Cardiovasc Surg 1991; 101:623-632.
38. Pasque MK, Kaiser LR, Dressler C, et al: Single lung transplantation for pulmonary hypertension: Technical aspects and immediate hemodynamic results. J Thorac Cardiovasc Surg 1992; 103:475-481.
39. Levine SM, Jenkinson SG, Bryan CL, et al: Ventilation-perfusion inequalities during graft rejection in patients undergoing single lung transplantation for primary pulmonary hypertension. Chest 1992; 101:401-405.
40. Gammie JS, Keenan RJ, Pham SM, et al: Single- versus double-lung transplantation for pulmonary hypertension. J Thorac Cardiovasc Surg 1998; 115:397-403.
41. Patterson GA, Cooper JD, Goldman B, et al: Technique of successful clinical double-lung transplantation. Ann Thorac Surg 1988; 45:626-633.
42. Pasque MK, Cooper JD, Kaiser LR, et al: Improved technique for bilateral lung transplantation: Rationale and initial clinical experience. Ann Thorac Surg 1990; 49:785-791.
43. Bisson A, Bonnette P: A new technique for double lung transplantation: "Bilateral single lung" transplantation. J Thorac Cardiovasc Surg 1992; 6:40-46.
44. Raffin L, Michel-Cherqui M, Sperandio M, et al: Anesthesia for bilateral lung transplantation without cardiopulmonary bypass: Initial experience and review of intraoperative problems. J Cardiothorac Vasc Anesth 1992; 6:409-417.
45. Hirt SW, Haverich A, Wahlers T, et al: Predictive criteria for the need for extracorporeal circulation in single-lung transplantation. Ann Thorac Surg 1992; 54:676-680.

46. Schreinmakers HH, Weder W, Miyoshi S, et al: Direct revascularization of bronchial arteries for lung transplantation: An anatomical study. Ann Thorac Surg 1990; 49:44-54.
47. Couraud L, Baudet E, Martigne C, et al: Bronchial revascularization in double-lung transplantation: A series of eight patients: Bordeaux Lung and Heart-Lung Transplant Group. Ann Thorac Surg 1992; 53:88-94.
48. Patterson GA, Todd TR, Cooper JD, et al: Airway complications after double lung transplantation: Toronto Lung Transplant Group. J Thorac Cardiovasc Surg 1990; 99:14-21.
49. Metras D, Noirclerc M, Baillant A, et al: Double lung transplant: The role of bilateral bronchial suture. Transplant Proc 1990; 22:1477-1478.
50. Kaiser LR, Pasque MK, Trulock EP: Bilateral sequential lung transplantation: The procedure of choice for double-lung replacement. Ann Thorac Surg 1991; 52:438-446.
51. Calhoon JH, Grover FL, Gibbons WJ, et al: Single lung transplantation: Alternative indications and technique. J Thorac Cardiovasc Surg 1991; 101:816-825.
52. Turrentine MW, Kesler KA, Wright CD, et al: Effect of omental, intercostal, and internal mammary artery pedicle wraps on bronchial healing. Ann Thorac Surg 1990; 49:574-579.
53. Starnes VA, Barr ML, Cohen RG: Lobar transplantation: Indications, technique and outcomes. J Thorac Cardiovasc Surg 1994; 108:403-411.
54. Starnes VA, Barr ML, Schenkel FA, et al: Experience with living-donor lobar transplantation for indications other than cystic fibrosis. J Thorac Cardiovasc Surg 1997; 114:917-922.
55. Starnes VA, Barr ML, Cohen RG, et al: Living-donor lobar lung transplantation experience: Intermediate results. J Thorac Cardiovasc Surg 1996; 112:1284-1291.
56. Rogers RM, Sciurba FC, Keenan RJ: Lung reduction surgery in chronic obstructive lung disease. Med Clin North Am 1996; 80:623-644.
57. Reitz BA, Wallwork JL, Hunt SA, et al: Heart-lung transplantation: Successful therapy for patients with pulmonary vascular disease. N Engl J Med 1982; 306:557-564.
58. Kang HL, Martich GD, Boujoukos AJ, et al: Predicting ICU length of stay following single lung transplantation. Chest 1996; 110:1014-1017.
59. Carlon CG, Kahn R, Howland W, et al: Acute life-threatening ventilation. Perfusion inequality: An indication for independent lung ventilation. Crit Care Med 1978; 6:380-383.
60. Rivara D, Bourgain JL, Rieu P, et al: Differential ventilation in unilateral lung disease: Effects on respiratory mechanics and gas exchange. Intensive Care Med 1979; 5:189-191.
61. Stow PJ, Grant I: Asynchronous independent lung ventilation: Its use in the treatment of unilateral lung disease. Anaesthesia 1985; 40:163-166.
62. Stevens PM, Johnson PC, Bell RL, et al: Regional ventilation and perfusion after lung transplantation in patients with emphysema. N Engl J Med 1970; 282:245-249.
63. Adoumie R, Shennib H, Brown R, et al: Differential lung ventilation. J Thorac Cardiovasc Surg 1993; 105:229-233.
64. Gavazzeni V, Gaetano I, Mashceroni D, et al: Prolonged independent lung respiratory treatment after single lung transplantation in pulmonary emphysema. Chest 1993; 103:96-100.
65. Glassman LR, Keenan RJ, Fabrizio MC, et al: Extracorporeal membrane oxygenation as an adjunct treatment for primary graft failure in adult lung transplant recipients. J Thorac Cardiovasc Surg 1995; 110:723-727.
66. Whyte RI, Deeb GM, McCurry KR, et al: Extracorporeal life support after heart or lung transplantation. Ann Thorac Surg 1994; 58:754-759.
67. Lefer AM, Lefer DJ: Pharmacology of the endothelium in ischemia-reperfusion and circulatory shock. Ann Rev Pharmacol Toxicol 1993; 33:71-90.
68. Novick RJ, Gehman KE, Imtiaz SA, et al: Lung preservation: The importance of endothelial and alveolar type II cell integrity. Ann Thorac Surg 1996; 62:302-314.
69. Boujoukos AJ, Martich GD, Vega JD, et al: Reperfusion injury in single-lung transplant recipients with pulmonary hypertension and emphysema. J Heart Lung Transplant 1997; 16:439-448.
70. Shackleton CR, Ettinger SL, McLoughlin MG, et al: Effect of recovery from ischemic injury on class I and class II MHC antigen expression. Transplantation 1990; 49:641-643.
71. Anderson DC, Glazer HS, Semenkovich JW, et al: Lung transplant edema: Chest radiography after lung transplantation: The first 10 days. Radiology 1995; 195:275-281.
72. Zenati M, Yousem SA, Dowling RA, et al: Primary graft failure following pulmonary transplantation. Transplant 1990; 50:165-167.
73. Date H, Triantafillou AN, Trulock EP, et al: Inhaled nitric oxide reduces human lung allograft dysfunction. J Thorac Cardiovasc Surg 1996; 111:913-919.
74. Royston D, Minty BD, Higenbottam T, et al: The effect of surgery with cardiopulmonary bypass on alveolar-capillary barrier function in human beings. Ann Thorac Surg 1985; 40:139-143.
75. Pasque MK, Kaiser LR, Dressler C, et al: Single lung transplantation for pulmonary hypertension: Technical aspects and immediate hemodynamic results. J Thorac Cardiovasc Surg 1992; 103:475-481.
76. Haydock DA, Trulock EP, Kaiser LR, et al: Management of dysfunction in the transplanted lung: Experience with seven clinical cases: Washington University Lung Transplant Group. Ann Thorac Surg 1992; 53:635-641.
77. Malden ES, Kaiser LR, Gutierrez FR: Pulmonary vein obstruction following single lung transplantation. Chest 1992; 102:645-647.
78. Levine SM, Jenkinson SG, Bryan CL, et al: Ventilation-perfusion inequalities during graft rejection in patients undergoing single lung transplantation for primary pulmonary hypertension. Chest 1992; 101:401-405.
79. Dummer JS, Montero CG, Paradis IL, et al: Infections in heart-lung transplant recipients. Transplantation 1986; 41:725-729.
80. Dauber JH, Paradis IL, Dummer JS, et al: Infectious complications in pulmonary allograft recipients. Clin Chest Med 1990; 22:291-308.
81. Maurer JR, Tullis E, Grossman RE, et al: Infectious complications following isolated lung transplantation. Chest 1992; 101:1056-1059.
82. Low DE, Kaiser LR, Haydock DA, et al: The donor lung: Infectious and pathologic factors affecting outcome in lung transplantation. J Thorac Cardiovasc Surg 1993; 106:614-621.
83. Horvath J, Dummer S, Loyd J, et al: Infection in the transplanted and native lung after single lung transplantation. Chest 1993; 104:681-685.
84. Lewiston N, King V, Umetsu D, et al: Cystic fibrosis patients who have undergone heart-lung transplantation benefit from maxillary sinus antrostomy and repeated sinus lavage. Transplant Proc 1991; 23:1207-1208.
85. Nunley DR, Williams PA, Bauldoff GS, et al: *Pseudomonas* colonization and infection in cystic fibrosis lung transplant recipients. Chest 1998; 113:1235-1243.
86. Paradis IL, Williams P: Infection after lung transplantation. Semin Respir Infect 1993; 8:207-215.
87. Zenati M, Dowling RD, Dummer JS, et al: Influence of donor lung on development of early infections in lung transplant recipients. J Heart Transplant 1990; 9:502-509.
88. Paradis IL, Duncan SR, Dauber JH, et al: Distinguishing between infection, rejection, and the adult respiratory distress syndrome after human lung transplantation. J Heart Lung Transplant 1992; 11:S232-S236.
89. Husain AN, Siddiqui MT, Reddy VB, et al: Postmortem findings in lung transplant recipients. Mod Pathol 1996; 9:752-761.
90. Milne DS, Gascoigne AD, Ashcroft T, et al: Organizing pneumonia following pulmonary transplantation and the development of obliterative bronchiolitis. Transplantation 1994; 57:1757-1762.
91. Higenbottam T, Stewart S, Penketh A, et al: Transbronchial lung biopsy for the diagnosis of rejection in heart-lung transplant patients. Transplantation 1988; 46:532-539.
92. Trulock EP, Ettinger NA, Brunt EA, et al: The role of transbronchial lung biopsy in the treatment of lung transplant recipients: An analysis of 200 consecutive procedures. Chest 102:1049-1054.
93. Pomerance A, Madden B, Burke MM, et al: Transbronchial biopsy in heart and lung transplantation: Clinicopathological correlations. J Heart Lung Transplant 1995; 14:761-773.
94. Kesten S, Chamberlain D, Maurer J: Yield of surveillance transbronchial biopsies performed beyond two years after lung transplantation. J Heart Lung Transplant 1996; 15:384-388.
95. Gulinger RA, Paradis IL, Dauber JH, et al: The importance of

bronchoscopy with transbronchial biopsy and bronchoalveolar lavage in the management of lung transplant recipients. Am J Respir Crit Care Med 1995; 152:2037-2043.
96. Chan CC, Abi-Saleh WJ, Arroliga AC, et al: Diagnostic yield and therapeutic impact of flexible bronchoscopy in lung transplant recipients. J Heart Lung Transplant 1996; 15:196-205.
97. Bradley JA, Bolton EM: The T-cell requirements for allograft rejection. Transplant Rev 1992; 6:115-129.
98. Trulock EP: Management of lung transplant rejection. Chest 1993; 103:1566-1576.
99. Hutter JA, Despins P, Higenbottam T, et al: Heart-lung transplantation: Better use of resources. Am J Med 1988; 85:4-11.
100. Millet B, Higenbottam TW, Flower CDR, et al: The radiographic appearance of infection and acute rejection of the lung after heart-lung transplantation. Am Rev Respir Dis 1989; 140:62-67.
101. Scott JP, Higenbottam TW, Sharples L, et al: Risk factors for obliterative bronchiolitis in heart-lung transplant recipients. Transplantation 1991; 51:813-817.
102. McCarthy PM, Starnes VA, Theodore J, et al: Improved survival after heart-lung transplantation. J Thorac Cardiovasc Surg 1990; 99:54-60.
103. Paradis IL, Duncan SR, Dauber JH, et al: Effect of augmented immunosuppression on human chronic lung allograft rejection (Abstract). Am Rev Respir Dis 1992; 145:A705.
104. Griffith BP, Hardesty RL, Trento A, et al: Heart-lung transplantation: Lessons learned and future hopes. Ann Thorac Surg 1987; 43:6-16.
105. Goldstein J, Thoua Y, Wellens F, et al: Cyclosporine nephropathy after heart-lung transplantation. Proc Eur Dialysis Transplant Assoc Eur Ren Assoc 1985; 21:973-981.
106. Au J, Hawkins T, Venables C, et al: Upper gastrointestinal dysmotility in heart-lung transplant recipients. Ann Thorac Surg 1993; 55:94-97.
107. Augustine SM, Yeo CJ, Buchman TG, et al: Gastrointestinal complications in heart and heart-lung transplant patients. J Heart Lung Transplant 1991; 10:547-556.
108. Berkowitz N, Schulman LL, McGregor C, et al: Gastroparesis after lung transplantation. Potential role in postoperative respiratory complications. Chest 1995; 108:1602-1607.
109. Reid KR, McKenzie FN, Menkis AH, et al: Importance of chronic aspiration in recipients of heart-lung transplants. Lancet 1990; 336:206-208.
110. Plochl W, Pezawas L, Artemiou O, et al: Nutritional status, ICU duration and ICU mortality in lung transplant recipients. Intensive Care Med 1996; 22:1179-1185.
111. Fulton JA, Orenstein DM, Koehler AN, et al: Nutrition in the pediatric double lung transplant patient with cystic fibrosis. Nutr Clin Pract 1995; 10:67-72.
112. Zenati M, Dowling RD, Dummer JS, Griffith BP: Influence of the donor lung on development of early infections in lung transplant recipients. J Heart Transplant 1990; 9:502-509.
113. Griffith BP, Hardesty RL, Armitage JM: Acute rejection of lung allografts with various immunosuppressive protocols. Ann Thorac Surg 1992; 54:846-851.
114. Duncan SR, Grgurich WF, Iacono AT, et al: A comparison of ganciclovir and acyclovir to prevent cytomegalovirus after lung transplantation. Am J Respir Crit Care Med 1994; 150:146-152.
115. Gryzan S, Paradis IL, Zeevi A, et al: Unexpectedly high incidence of *Pneumocystis carinii* infection after lung-heart transplantation. Am Rev Respir Dis 1988; 137:1268-1274.
116. Dowling RD, Baladi N, Zenati M, et al: Disruption of the aortic anastomosis after heart-lung transplantation. Ann Thorac Surg 1990; 49:118-122.
117. Frist WH, Loyd JE, Merrill WH, et al: Single lung transplantation: A temporal look at rejection, infection, and survival. Am Surg 1994; 60:94-102.
118. Bando K, Paradis IL, Konishi H, et al: Obliterative bronchiolitis after lung and heart-lung transplantation: An analysis of risk factors and management. J Thorac Cardiovasc Surg 1995; 110:4-13.
119. Sundaresan S, Trulock EP, Mohanankumar T, et al: Prevalence and outcome of bronchiolitis obliterans syndrome after lung transplantation. Ann Thorac Surg 1995; 60:1341-1346.
120. Cooper JD, Billingham M, Egan T, et al: A working formulation for the standardization of nomenclature and for clinical staging of chronic dysfunction in lung allografts. J Heart Lung Transplant 1993; 12:713-716.
121. Scott JP, Higenbottam TW, Clelland CA, et al: Natural history of chronic rejection in heart-lung transplant recipients. J Heart Transplant 1990; 9:510-515.
122. Yousem SA, Dauber JH, Keenan R, et al: Does histologic acute rejection in lung allografts predict the development of bronchiolitis obliterans? Transplantation 1991; 52:306-309.
123. Sharples LD, Tamm M, McNeil K, et al: Development of bronchiolitis obliterans syndrome in recipients of heart-lung transplantation—early risk factors. Transplantation 1996; 61:560-566.
124. Keenan RJ, Lega ME, Dummer JS, et al: Cytomegalovirus serologic status and postoperative infection correlated with risk of developing chronic rejection after pulmonary transplantation. Transplantation 1991; 51:433-438.
125. Snell GI, Esmore DS, Williams TJ: Cytolytic therapy for the bronchiolitis obliterans syndrome complicating lung transplantation. Chest 1996; 109:874-878.
126. Iacono AT, Smaldone GC, Keenan RJ, et al: Dose-related reversal of acute lung rejection by aerosolized cyclosporine. Am J Respir Crit Care Med 1997; 155:1690-1698.
127. Ross DJ, Belman MD, Mohsesnifar Z, et al: Obstructive flow-volume loop contours after single lung transplantation. J Heart Lung Transplant 1994; 13:508-513.
128. Walker RC, Marshall WF, Strickler JG, et al: Pretransplantation assessment of the risk of lymphoproliferative disorder. Clin Infect Dis 1995; 20:1346-1353.
129. Pellenz M, Zambello R, Semenzato G, Loughran TP Jr: Detection of Epstein-Barr virus by PCR analysis in lymphoproliferative disease of granular lymphocytes. Leuk Lymphoma 1996; 23:371-374.
130. Armitage JM, Kormos RL, Stuart RS, et al: Posttransplant lymphoproliferative disease in thoracic organ transplant patients: Ten years of cyclosporine-based immunosuppression. J Heart Lung Transplant 1991; 10:877-886.
131. Trulock EP: State of the art: Lung transplantation. Am J Respir Crit Care Med 1997; 155:789-818.
132. Novick RJ, Stitt L, Schafers H-J, et al: Pulmonary retransplantation: Does the indication for operation influence postoperative lung function? J Thorac Cardiovasc Surg 1996; 112:1504-1513.

183

Pancreas Transplantation

Robert J. Corry, MD • M. Francesca Egidi, MD
Stephen D. Bowles, MD

Pancreas transplantation, as a definitive treatment modality for type I diabetes, has become more established since the last edition of this text. Refinement of surgical techniques and experience with tacrolimus, a more effective immunosuppressive agent than other drug combinations, have been responsible for the improved patient and graft survival rates of 97% and 85% (insulin-independent), respectively, at 1 year.[1]

Although precise operative technique and appropriate management of tacrolimus are required, of equal importance is the immediate postoperative management in the intensive care unit (ICU). Careful monitoring of a variety of parameters, including hemodynamics, electrolytes, blood glucose levels, fluid losses (both external and third-space), and radiologic assessment (Doppler ultrasonography, radionuclide scans) are essential.

This chapter describes the surgical aspects of pancreas transplantation and emphasizes the intensive care management of these critically ill patients during the first postoperative 4 to 5 days.

BRIEF HISTORY

The first human pancreas transplantation procedure was performed by Kelly and associates from the University of Minnesota in 1966.[2] Both the kidney and pancreas were transplanted simultaneously and functioned, but the patient subsequently died of complications of sepsis at 4½ months. Ten additional patients underwent transplantation at Minnesota, and the results were presented at the International Congress of the Transplantation Society in The Hague in 1970. Eight of the 10 patients died of sepsis or surgical complications.[3] Because it was concluded that transplantation of the whole pancreas, with a long segment of duodenum and jejunum, was responsible for the morbidity and mortality, work began in the early 1970s on a variety of techniques to transplant only the tail of the pancreas based on the splenic artery. Essentially, the pancreas was divided at its neck, the splenic artery was sutured to the recipient iliac artery, and the splenic vein was joined to the iliac vein. Exocrine drainage was established by means of a pancreatic enteric anastomosis, similar to the reconstruction following a Whipple procedure for pancreatic cancer, or by polymer injection into the divided pancreatic duct.[4] The donor spleen was removed prior to closure.

Centers for transplantation of the partial pancreas (tail) were established in a few universities in Europe, principally Lyon, Cambridge, Munich, and Stockholm, and Minnesota, Colorado, Wisconsin, Cincinnati, Iowa, and others in the United States. Although morbidity was high, a few long-term successes showed that the procedure was possible even with relatively primitive immunosuppression by today's standards.

In 1984, Starzl and colleagues, by this time at the University of Pittsburgh, published a small series of pancreatic duodenal transplants, a modification of the original Minnesota operation.[5] Only a short segment of duodenum, however, was transplanted. This procedure was adopted in the mid 1980s at Minnesota, Iowa, and Wisconsin, while the European centers continued to work at perfecting the technique of transplanting the pancreatic tail. The Iowa team, utilizing the Pittsburgh technique, presented a series of 20 combined pancreas-kidney transplants at the American College of Surgeons Annual Meeting in 1985 with good results.[6]

Further progress of a significant nature has occurred in the early 1990s as experience has been gained with the use of tacrolimus as the principal immunosuppressive agent for pancreatic transplantation. A multicenter retrospective analysis from centers using tacrolimus was presented by Gruessner at the American Society of Transplant Surgeons Annual Meeting in 1996.[7] This report illustrated that the current survival statistics have been achieved with drug combinations based on tacrolimus, which represented an improvement over prior drug therapy utilizing cyclosporine.

SELECTION OF TRANSPLANT RECIPIENTS

Generally, any patient with type I diabetes is a potential candidate. Approximately 80% of patients referred also have end-stage renal disease as well as other complications of diabetes, including vasculopathy, neuropathy, and gastroenteropathy. Most of the patients have impaired vision and have undergone numerous laser treatments to the retina. The crucial factor in the selection process is whether the potential recipient has critical coronary artery disease, which, if severe and not correctable, could render the risk greater than the potential benefit.

In addition to the routine pretransplant work-up, which includes a peripheral vascular evaluation, histocompatibility testing, gastrointestinal examination, and other tests, a thorough noninvasive cardiac work-up consisting of a dipyridamole (Persantine) or adenosine thallium stress test is performed. If results are positive, a cardiac consultant usually recommends coronary arteriography. Angioplasty, bypass, or stent placement can usually correct a critical lesion. If the coronary disease is advanced and uncorrectable, the patient is not accepted for pancreas transplantation. In most centers, 70% to 80% of patients are able to be selected for transplantation, but the acceptance rate is largely a determinant of the referral pattern. By a careful recipient selection strategy, morbidity and mortality can be significantly reduced.

DONOR SELECTION

Brain-dead victims who are physiologically stable are considered suitable pancreas donors. Donor age has been considered an important criterion by some centers. However, if the physiologic condition of an older donor in one's 60s prior to the establishment of brain death has been good, the pancreas can be utilized. On the other hand, a donor in one's 40s with obesity and arteriosclerosis might not be suitable. Generally, donors weighing below 25 kg are not ideal because of the small size of the organ and the reduced islet cell mass. Because most pancreas donors are also liver donors, a bifurcation iliac artery graft from the same donor is required to add length to the splenic and superior mesenteric arteries for subsequent transplantation and the caliber of the splenic arterial anastomosis can be quite small in pediatric donors and subject to thrombosis after implantation.

Other contraindications to donor selection include excessive and prolonged use of vasopressor agents. High-dose vasopressors constrict the small arterioles in the pancreas, which can impair blood flow through the pancreatic parenchyma after revascularization, a condition that increases the likelihood of thrombosis. Excessive obesity is a relative contraindication because the pancreas may be infiltrated with fat, which leads to thrombosis as a result of fat necrosis, edema, and pancreatitis after revascularization. Prolonged hypotension in the donor with ischemia of the organ may also lead to ischemic pancreatitis postoperatively.

Our group has advocated a rapid en bloc retrieval technique of the pancreas and liver that limits both operative and total ischemic time.[8] Separation of the liver and pancreas occurs under iced solutions.

OPERATIVE PROCEDURE

Donor Procedure

Donor operations should be attended by two teams, thoracic and abdominal. After a long midline incision is made from the xiphoid to the symphysis, the liver and pancreas are removed en bloc following aortic perfusion with chilled University of Wisconsin solution. The only required dissection in the porta hepatis is carried out principally to determine whether a replaced right hepatic artery exists. After separation of the two organs, the pancreas is packaged and sent to the recipient hospital together with an iliac artery Y-graft and a segment of common iliac vein.

The bench work on the pancreas is performed under chilled solution and consists of (1) removing excess fat, (2) shortening the duodenum to a length of 7 to 10 cm, (3) dividing the proximal duodenum just below the pylorus and the distal duodenum a few centimeters beyond the ampulla of Vater, (4) ligating the vessels at the root of the mesentery, (5) lengthening the vessels by joining the iliac vein graft to the portal vein, and (6) suturing the internal iliac artery of the Y-graft to the splenic and external iliac artery to the superior mesenteric artery. Many alternative ways to reconstruct the vessels are available, depending on the vascular anatomy of the organ.

Recipient Procedure

The recipient operation is straightforward. It consists of joining the extended artery to the iliac artery of the recipient and the extended portal vein to the iliac vein. Either a primary duodenocystostomy or duodenoenterostomy is used for drainage of the pancreatic exocrine secretions (Fig. 183–1).[9, 10]

The operation can be performed through a midline incision or an oblique incision in the right or left lower quadrant, similar to the one used for a kidney transplant. The pancreas is placed intraperitoneally and positioned appropriately to avoid kinking or twisting of the vessels.

MANAGEMENT IN THE INTENSIVE CARE UNIT

Pancreas transplant recipients require close observation in the early postoperative period. We begin patients on a continuous intravenous tacrolimus infusion aiming for target levels of 20 to 25 ng/mL. Methylprednisone is begun at 200 mg/day and tapered to 20 mg/day over the first week. Mycophenolate mofetil is also started during the first week.

Multiple antibiotic prophylactic regimens have been proposed. Most early infections are wound and intra-abdominal, and broad-spectrum antibiotic coverage against enteric flora is employed for 3 days. Pancreatic endocrine function is monitored with frequent blood glucose determinations. The blood glucose level should generally be between 80 and 150 mg/dL within a few hours after the completion of transplantation. It is best to avoid treatment of elevated blood glucose, if possible, because this obscures valuable information regarding endocrine function. In patients with bladder drainage of pancreatic exocrine secretions, urinary amylase levels are observed. A reduction in amylase levels of 25% to 50% indicates graft dysfunction.

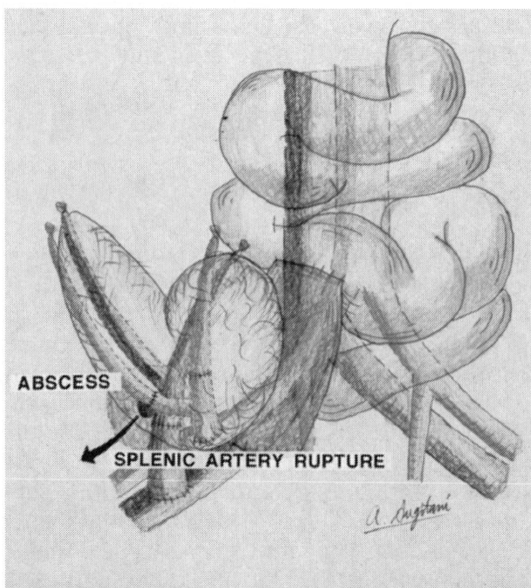

Figure 183–1. Rupture of mycotic aneurysm at splenic artery anastomosis adjacent to an abscess. Vascular and enteric anastomoses are also shown in a typical pancreas transplant in the right lower quadrant.

During the first postoperative, day a baseline radionuclide blood flow study of the pancreas is obtained, and baseline Doppler ultrasonography of the allograft vasculature may also be performed. Any sign of pancreatic dysfunction necessitates urgent repetition of these studies and early operative intervention. Serum amylase and lipase levels, while good indicators of allograft pancreatitis (which commonly occurs postoperatively) are of little value in assessing islet cell function.

Significant attention should be paid to ensuring that perfusion of the allograft is adequate. Unlike other transplanted solid organs, the pancreas is a low-flow organ, and decreased blood flow through a pancreas graft can result in thrombosis. Vasopressor therapy should be avoided unless absolutely necessary. Moderate hypertension, with systolic blood pressure up to 180 mm Hg, is usually acceptable. Because many of these patients have baseline hypertension, postoperative antihypertensive therapy must be cautiously administered. Maintaining a euvolemic state and assessing the patient's blood volume status are often complicated by significant third-space shifts owing to allograft pancreatitis and by the presence of renal insufficiency, particularly in patients receiving a simultaneous kidney that may not yet be functioning.

Dialysis, with rapid intravascular fluid removal, should be avoided. Urine output is replaced with intravenous fluids, but the patient must be closely monitored for signs of pulmonary edema secondary to mobilization of third-space fluid. Strict bed rest should be maintained for a few days to prevent kinking of vascular allografts that may result from a position shift of the pancreas.

Aspirin is routinely employed to prevent vascular thrombosis; however, if a low-flow state of the graft is perceived, additional antiplatelet therapy (e.g., low-molecular-weight dextran or full anticoagulation with intravenous heparin) may be indicated. Since bleeding from the pancreatic surface is not unusual, anticoagulation has been avoided in most cases. Drainage of pancreatic exocrine secretions in the urine can result in significant bicarbonate loss, dehydration, and electrolyte disturbances. In these patients, a Foley catheter must be left in place for at least the first week to prevent distention of the bladder and leakage from the bladder anastomosis.

Allograft pancreatitis can cause significant pain. Narcotics and benzodiazepines must be cautiously used in the presence of renal insufficiency. Despite the exclusion of patients with severe coronary artery disease, myocardial ischemia and infarction are not rare. Measures such as pain and blood pressure control must be employed, and vigilance for the diagnosis of myocardial ischemia is important, particularly if pulmonary edema occurs.

MANAGEMENT DURING THE FIRST MONTH

After the ICU stay, which generally varies from 2 to 4 days depending on the stability of the patient, care on the transplant unit consists of routine monitoring and standard postoperative management. By the 5th day, a liquid diet is usually started and advanced as appropriate. Although some patients have left the hospital as early as 6 days postoperatively, the mean length of stay is 11 days.

Close follow-up in an outpatient unit occurs for the first 10 to 14 days following discharge, during which time tacrolimus dosages based on target blood levels are adjusted. Oral tacrolimus is given twice a day to achieve whole blood through levels of 20 to 25 ng/mL during the first 2 weeks and 15 to 20 ng/mL during the second 2 weeks and is tapered slowly thereafter to achieve levels of 8 to 12 ng/mL by 2 to 3 months.[11] The recommended strategy is to give higher doses of tacrolimus in the first few weeks, with a relatively rapid taper thereafter.

Steroids are also tapered to 20 mg of prednisone by 1 week, and doses are reduced slowly thereafter. At 2 years, 68% of our patients are totally off steroids. Mycophenolate mofetil has been used as a third drug since 1996 and has reduced the rejection rate to half.[12] Rejection is monitored by fine-needle aspiration biopsy of the pancreas or core needle biopsy of the kidney.[13]

COMPLICATIONS

Complications related to pancreas transplantation are usually surgical. The standard complications that can occur in all organ transplant recipients who are immunosuppressed, such as those with opportunistic infections, are not covered here.

The earliest complication following pancreas transplantation is hemorrhage. The pancreas parasitizes its blood supply from arteries leading to other organs, namely the splenic and superior mesenteric arteries. If a ligature works its way off of one of these large end arteries early after surgery, the patient generally does not have time to return to the operating room; the incision should be opened in the ICU to clamp the vessel as a lifesaving procedure prior to a return to the operating room. In addition, several smaller vessels on the surface of the pancreas may bleed postoperatively, particularly if the patient has received anticoagulants to prevent graft thrombosis. If bleeding is slow, medical management with transfusion can be attempted; if it is persistent, however, the patient must return to the operating room so that the clot can be evacuated and the bleeding controlled. Occasionally, a large hematoma can exert pressure on the vein, causing venous thrombosis. In addition, hypotension is of concern because a low-flow state to the pancreas ensues that can also lead to thrombosis. Early return to the operating room can never be criticized even if medical management with transfusions might have worked.

Another complication within the first 48 hours is venous thrombosis of the pancreas. In this case, relatively prompt pancreatectomy is necessary to avoid subsequent sepsis and the acute respiratory distress syndrome. The pancreas is a low-flow organ, and ischemic damage to the parenchyma with edema and pancreatitis can lead to sluggish blood flow through the organ. This can cause venous pressure in the iliac venous system to exceed the pressure in the extended portal vein outflow vessel, resulting in reversal of venous flow and graft thrombosis. Additional causes of thrombosis are twisting of the vein or artery, inappropriate length of either vessel (i.e., either too short or too long), or extrinsic pressure on either the vein or artery. If the venous clot is incomplete, the organ can be salvaged on rare occasions by thrombectomy.

By the end of the first week, an anastomotic fistula can occur, from either the duodenoenterostomy or the duodenocystostomy, which is usually related to localized impairment of the blood supply to a segment of duodenum at either the anastomosis or the closed end of the duodenum. Peritonitis generally necessitates peritoneal lavage and conversion to a Roux-en-Y if the original operation has been an enteric drainage procedure. More commonly, bladder-related fistulas can be managed conservatively with closed sump drainage. Both types of fistulas require readmission to the ICU when the patient is hemodynamically unstable. Intraperitoneal wound abscesses should be drained and can be detected by computed tomography (CT). An arterial fistula from one of the many arterial anastomoses involving the pancreas is commonly related to undrained sepsis and requires urgent graft removal (see Fig. 183-1).

In about 20% of bladder-drained patients, severe dehydration and acidosis can occur secondary to large losses of bicarbonate in the urine. Acidosis does not occur in the enteric-drained pancreas recipient because bicarbonate in the pancreatic secretion is reabsorbed by the intestine. Other surgical complications can occur, including intestinal obstruction, bladder and enteric anastomotic bleeding, and other conditions not necessarily related to pancreas transplantation.

RESULTS

Most pancreatic transplantation procedures performed in the United States since 1987 have been *simultaneous pancreas-kidney* (SPK) transplants (87%). *Pancreas transplants alone* (PTA) account for 3%, while 10% are *pancreas after kidney* (PAK) transplants. In the most recent era, from 1994 to 1997, the patient survival rate was 94% at 1 year, which represents a substantial improvement compared with all previous eras. Current pancreas survival rates are 82% for SPK, 71% for PAK, and 62% for PTA.[1] Pancreas "survival" implies insulin independence with normal carbohydrate metabolism.

Today's improved survival statistics, in large part, are related to the use of tacrolimus as the primary immunosuppressant agent. In addition, the technical failure rate (nonimmunologic) has steadily decreased over time, a function of surgical teams gaining more experience and appropriate recipient and donor selection. The technical failure rate (i.e., early graft thrombosis) remains at 10% when older donors with cardiovascular disease are chosen. Not only have pancreas transplant survival rates improved since 1994, but kidney graft success rate at 1 year is 90% in the SPK group.[1]

By November 1997, close to 10,000 pancreatic transplantations had been performed worldwide and more than 7500 of them were performed in United States centers. Although there are approximately 5000 brain-dead donors per year in the United States, only about 1000 pancreatic transplantations are performed annually. There is no shortage of recipients, since 25% of patients with end-stage renal failure have diabetes. Improved strategies for increasing retrieval of pancreases from the existing donor pool, particularly from low-risk suitable donors, must be established to increase the volume of these transplantations per year. This is particularly important because pancreas transplant results match the success rates of other solid-organ transplants, rendering the procedure therapeutic rather than experimental. It is hoped that Medicare and third-party coverage will occur, but other barriers need to be overcome as well. These include the willingness of local organ procurement organizations to share a kidney with a pancreas sent to another region. The concept of local primacy for a particular organ, such as a kidney or liver, should be changed so that patients in greatest need of an organ, regardless of geographic location, are prioritized. In essence, a national list of recipients would permit utilization of all suitable organs. In addition, strategies to increase both donor awareness and the consent rate beyond the current 50% should be developed.

References

1. Gruessner AC, Sutherland DER: Pancreas transplants for United States (U.S.) and non-U.S. cases as reported to the International Pancreas Transplant Registry (IPTR) and to the United Network for Organ Sharing (UNOS). *In:* Clinical Transplants 1997. Cecka M, Terasaki PL (eds). Los Angeles, UCLA Tissue Typing Laboratory pp 45–59.
2. Kelly WD, Lillehei RC, Merkel FK, et al: Allotransplantation of the pancreas and duodenum along with the kidney in diabetic nephropathy. Surgery 1967; 61:827–837.
3. Lillehei RC, Simmons RL, Najarian JS, et al: Pancreatico-duodenal

allotransplantation: Experimental and clinical experience. Ann Surg 1970; 172:405-436.
4. Land W, Landgraf R, Illner WD, et al: Improved results in combined segmental pancreatic and renal transplantation in diabetic patients under cyclosporine therapy. Transplant Proc 1985; 17:317-324.
5. Starzl TE, Iwatsuki S, Shaw B, et al: Pancreaticoduodenal transplantation in humans. Surg Gynecol Obstet 1984; 159:265-272.
6. Corry RJ, Nghiem DD, Schulak JA, et al: Surgical treatment of diabetic nephropathy with simultaneous pancreatic duodenal and renal transplantation. Surg Gynecol Obstet 1986; 162:547-555.
7. Gruessner RWG: Tacrolimus in pancreas transplantation: A multicenter analysis, Clin Transpl 1997; 11:299-312.
8. Dodson F, Pinna A, Jabbour N, et al: Advantages of the rapid en-bloc technique for pancreas/liver recovery. Transplant Proc 1995; 27:3050.
9. Nghiem DD, Corry RJ: Technique of simultaneous renal pancreaticoduodenal transplantation with urinary drainage of pancreatic secretion. Am J Surg 1987; 153:405-406.
10. Corry RJ, Egidi MF, Shapiro R, et al: Enteric drainage revisited. Transplant Proc 1995; 27:3048-3049.
11. Corry RJ, Egidi MF, Shapiro R, et al: Tacrolimus without antilymphocyte induction therapy prevents pancreas loss from rejection in 123 consecutive patients. Transplant Proc 1998; 30:521.
12. Gritsch HA, Egidi MF, Sugitani A, et al: Comparison of azathioprine and mycophenolate mofetil in pancreas transplantation. Transplant Proc 1998; 30:526.
13. Egidi MF, Corry RJ, Sugitani A, et al: Enteric-drained pancreas transplants monitored by fine-needle aspiration biopsy. Transplant Proc 1997; 29:674-675.

Bibliography

Ames SA, Bowers VD, Corry RJ: Diagnosis of pancreas transplant rejection: Use of non-invasive tests to assess initial dysfunction in combined pancreas-kidney transplants. Transplant Proc 1989; 21:3639-3642.

Bartlett ST, Schweitzer EJ, Johnson LB, et al: Equivalent success of simultaneous pancreas kidney and solitary pancreas transplantation: A prospective trial of tacrolimus immunosuppression with percutaneous biopsy. Ann Surg 1996; 224:440-452.

Cooper MM, Wright FH, Smith JL, et al: Successful treatment of a high-output fistula with a somatostatin analogue following pancreas transplantation. Transplantation Proc 1989; 3738-3741.

Corry RJ: Pancreatic-duodenal transplantation with urinary tract drainage. *In:* Pancreatic Transplantation. Groth C (Ed). London, Grune & Stratton, 1988, pp 147-153.

Corry RJ, Zehr P: Quality of life in diabetic recipients of kidney transplants is better with the addition of the pancreas. Clin Transplant 1990; 4:238-241.

Douzdjian V, Abecassis MM, Cooper JL, et al: Incidence, management and significance of surgical complications after pancreatic transplantation. Surg Gynecol Obstet 1993; 177:451-456.

Gaber AO, El-Gebely Sdiman, Sugaltran P, et al: Early improvement in cardiac function occurs for pancreas-kidney but not diabetic kidney alone transplant recipients. Transplantation 1995; 59:1105-1112.

Georgi BA, Bowers VD, Smith JL, et al: Comparison of cholesterol levels between diabetic recipients: Pancreas-kidney and kidney transplantation. Diabetes 1989; 38 (Suppl 1):260-261.

Marsh CL, Perkins JD, Sutherland DER, et al: Combined hepatic and pancreaticoduodenal procurement for transplantation. Surg Gynecol Obstet 1989; 168:254-258.

Nghiem DD, Pitzen RH, Corry RJ: Evaluation of techniques for controlling exocrine drainage after segmental pancreatectomy in dogs: Implications for pancreatic transplantation. Arch Surg 1985; 120:1132-1137.

Nghiem DD, Gonwa TA, Corry RJ: Metabolic effects of urinary diversion of exocrine secretions in pancreas transplantation. Transplantation 1987; 43:70-73.

Nghiem DD, Schulak JA, Corry RJ: Duodenopancreatectomy for transplantation. Arch Surg 1987; 122:1201-1206.

Smith JL, Hunsicker LG, Yuh WTC, et al: Appearance of type II diabetes mellitus in type I diabetic recipients of pancreas allografts. Transplantation 1989; 47:304-311.

184

Intestinal and Multiple Organ Transplantation

Jorge Reyes, MD • Robert Selby, MD
Kareem Abu-Elmagd, MD, PhD • Satoru Todo, MD
George V. Mazariegos, MD • Javier Bueno, MD
Thomas E. Starzl, MD, PhD

The evolution of intestinal transplantation has distantly paralleled that for kidney and liver transplantation. Though the introduction of cyclosporine made other organ transplants a clinical reality, success with intestinal transplantation remained almost nonexistent due to a high incidence of graft loss from rejection, infection, and technical complications.[1]

The experimental studies on intestinal transplantation, reported by Lillehei and colleagues in 1959 as an isolated organ graft in dogs[2] and subsequently by Starzl and Kaupp with the multivisceral graft in dogs (liver, stomach, pancreaticoduodenal complex, small and large intestine),[3] supported a unidirectional paradigm of transplantation and immunology similar to that found after bone marrow transplantation.[4] These experiments predicted that graft-versus-host disease (GVHD) would be precipitated through the immunocytes in the lymphoid-rich major histocompatibility complex (MHC) disparate intestinal allografts.[5]

Numerous attempts at clinical intestinal transplantation, performed after 1964 under azathioprine and steroid and subsequently cyclosporine immunosuppression, were largely unsuccessful. In 1987, a 3-year-old girl received a multivisceral abdominal graft that contained the stomach, duodenum, pancreas, small bowel, colon, and liver; she had an extended survival of 6 months with good intestinal graft function.[6]

A modified application of this operation was the transplantation of a "cluster" of organs in 1989.[7] This allograft consisted of liver and pancreaticoduodenal complex used after upper abdominal exenteration for malignancy (Fig. 184-1). Viability of varying lengths of intestine with these clusters was proven, as was evidence of regeneration after severe rejection-induced injury. The inclusion of the liver in this type of graft was believed to protect the other organs transplanted from the same donor against rejection.[8, 9] Consequently, an even longer survival of 1 year was obtained in a recipient of a liver and small-bowel graft treated by Grant and associates.[10] Until 1990, there had been only two survivors of isolated cadaveric intestinal grafting.[11, 12]

The success of the new immunosuppressant tacrolimus (FK-506 [Prograf]) in 1989 after clinical trials with liver and kidney transplantation allowed the transplantation of human intestinal grafts (alone or a part of a multivisceral graft) almost with routine success.[13, 14] Successful intestinal transplantation then permitted the appreciation of the two-way paradigm of transplantation immunology[15]; it was postulated that two cell populations (of recipient and donor origin) reciprocally modulate immune responsiveness (host-versus-graft and graft-versus-host), including the induction of mutual nonreactivity with consequent organ allograft acceptance.[16]

INDICATIONS

Loss of intestinal function may be acute (e.g., necrotizing enterocolitis, volvulus, mesenteric thrombosis) or chronic

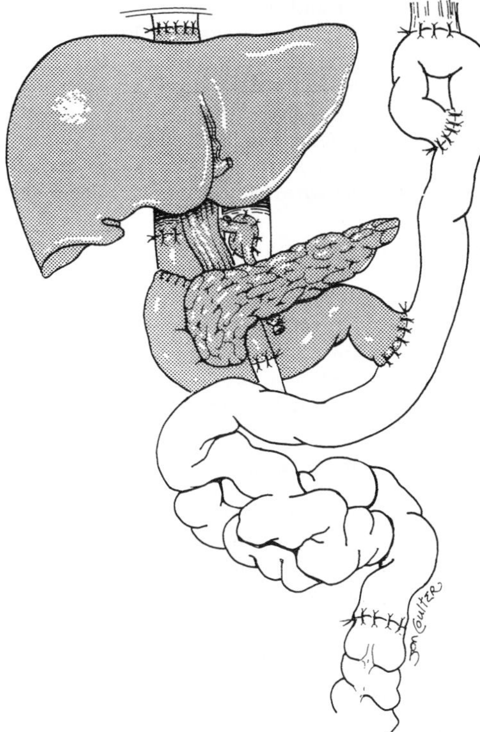

Figure 184–1. Cluster allograft (*shaded portion*), including the liver, pancreas, and duodenal segment of small intestine. (From Starzl TE, Todo S, Tzakis A, et al: Abdominal organ cluster transplantation for the treatment of upper abdominal malignancies. Ann Surg 1989; 210:374–386.)

(e.g., Crohn's disease, radiation enteritis). Disease classification can be better viewed with an arbitrary division of *surgical* (short gut) and *nonsurgical* etiologic factors. Patients with surgical causes generally suffer from loss of bowel length after resections for atresias, infarctions (e.g., volvulus, vascular catastrophes, necrotizing enterocolitis), or strictures and fistulas as with Crohn's disease. With nonsurgical causes of intestinal failure, the anatomic length and gross morphology may be normal. These causes include motility disorders (e.g., intestinal pseudo-obstruction, Hirschsprung's disease), absorptive insufficiencies (e.g., microvillus inclusion disease), polyposis syndromes, and "incarcerating" desmoid tumors.

Total parenteral nutrition (TPN) is the standard of care for patients who are unable to maintain a normal nutritional state by use of the gastrointestinal tract alone (intestinal failure).[17] Transplantation of the intestine, either alone or accompanied by other intra-abdominal organs (liver, stomach, pancreas), may be beneficial in patients who do not respond to this therapy. The stability and duration of TPN support are variable, and failure of TPN can manifest with complicating factors, such as infection, metabolic disorders, difficulty with vascular access (from extensive venous thrombosis), and liver cirrhosis with end-stage liver disease. This has resulted in an inestimable rate of morbidity and mortality.

The decision regarding allograft composition focuses on the integrity of the remaining gut and other abdominal organs, both functionally and anatomically. Guidelines used in substantiating the need for concomitant liver replacement in these intestinal transplantation candidates are:

- Biochemical dysfunction (hyperbilirubinemia, transaminase abnormalities, hypoalbuminemia, and coagulopathy)
- Pathologic processes (fibrosis or cirrhosis on liver biopsy)
- The clinical presence of portal hypertension, as manifested by hepatosplenomegaly, ascites, or esophageal varices and portal hypertensive gastroenteropathy

TABLE 184–1. Partial and Complete Intestinal Allografts

Organ Transplanted	Indication
Multivisceral (stomach, duodenum, pancreas, liver, small bowel, colon)	Pseudo-obstruction/aganglionosis syndrome with hepatic failure; diffuse splanchnic venous thrombosis and hepatic failure
Liver and small intestine	Hepatic failure after prolonged hyperalimentation for short gut syndrome
Liver, duodenum, and pancreas (organ cluster transplantation)	After upper abdominal exenteration for malignancy
Small intestine	Congenital or acquired absence or dysfunction

Patients deficient in protein S, protein C, and antithrombin III (liver-derived) may be candidates for a combined liver/small intestine allograft in the absence of clinical liver disease.[18] Recipients lacking these substances experience diffuse thromboses within the splanchnic system and undergo transplantation for mesenteric venous hypertesion rather than for intestinal failure. Patients with motility disorders or neoplasms that involve extensive lengths of the gastrointestinal tract are also candidates for replacement of this entire system (Table 184–1).

Table 184–2 lists the causes of intestinal failure in patients who have undergone transplantation at the University of Pittsburgh. Inability to continue TPN because of the development of hepatic cirrhosis or venous access limitations were the most frequent indications for transplantation.

ABDOMINAL VISCERAL PROCUREMENT

The grafts were obtained from ABO-blood type identical brain-dead donors; matching of human leukocyte antigen (HLA) was random. No attempts were made to modulate the lymphoid tissue in the intestinal allograft by either irradiation or antilymphoid antibody treatment. University of Wisconsin solution was used for graft preservation.

The safe procurement of multiple visceral organs, either en bloc or as separate components, hinges on a few fundamental precepts. Conceptually, the focus is to isolate and cool the organs, thus preserving their vascular and parenchymal anatomy and function. Multivisceral en bloc retrieval, including the stomach, duodenum, pancreas, liver, and small intestine,

TABLE 184–2. Indications for Composite and Isolated Intestinal Transplantation in 98 Patients at the University of Pittsburgh (May 1990 to August 1997)

Pediatric Patients (60)		Adult Patients (38)	
Necrotizing enterocolitis	6	Crohn's disease	8
Gastroschisis	16	Thrombotic disorder	13
Volvulus	15	Trauma	7
Pseudo-obstruction	6	Pseudo-obstruction	1
Hirschsprung's disease	4	Radiation enteritis	1
Intestinal atresia	8	Desmoid tumor	4
Microvillus inclusion disease	3	Familial polyposis	1
		Volvulus	1
Trauma	1	Gastrinoma	1
Intestinal polyposis	1	Ulcerative colitis	1

is the parent operation, and the assembled components have been likened by Starzl and colleagues to a large clump of individual grapes from the whole.[19] An appreciation of the fundamental strategy of multivisceral organ retrieval leads to an understanding of the lesser variant operations (i.e., liver, small intestine, combined liver/small intestine, and organ cluster—liver, duodenum, and pancreas—transplantation). A more complete discussion of the specifics of organ procurement is presented in Chapter 177.

RECIPIENT OPERATIONS

Most patients who need intestinal or multiorgan replacements have undergone multiple forays into the abdominal cavity for intestinal resections, lengthening procedures, and treatment of complications. This results in volume contraction of the abdominal cavity and severe adhesions. Consequently, the organs of the donor need to be smaller than those of the recipient to ensure proper abdominal closure. This allows for donor weight discrepancies of usually no greater than 20% than the recipient weight unless graft reduction can be surgically accomplished.

Previous operations may complicate the removal of the recipient's organs, especially if cirrhosis, portal hypertension, or inferior vena caval thromboses are present, all of which may be sequelae of the original disease or of prior operations. The recipient operation consists of removal of the failed organs with exposure of the vascular anatomy and, finally, allograft implantation. Following is a brief description of the salient features of the recipient operations.

Multivisceral Transplantation

After abdominal exenteration and exposure of the retroperitoneal aorta and inferior vena cava have been performed, the multivisceral graft (Fig. 184-2*A*) is connected by its vascular attachments: first the suprahepatic attachment, then infrahepatic vena caval connections (or "piggyback" to the skeletonized recipient vena cava), and finally the arterioaortic anastomosis (using an aortic interposition homograft). The recipient's portal vein and its inflow organs (gastrointestinal tract, pancreas, and liver) are removed with the enterectomy. The donor portal vein retains its continuity via the liver in the procurement of the allograft; thus, no portal vein anastomosis is required in this procedure. Patients with a normal native liver can receive a modified multivisceral procedure that excludes the allograft liver as part of the composite of organs, with portal venous return directed into the recipients portal vein (Fig. 184-2*B*).

Restoration of intestinal continuity requires an esophagogastric anastomosis and a coloenteric anastomosis with the distal ileum allograft. Initially, the patient also receives an ileostomy. Takedown of the ileostomy can be performed after several months, when oral nutrition is consistently adequate, a stable immunosuppressant regimen has been achieved, and there is no further need for frequent endoscopic surveillance.

Liver and Small Bowel

Liver and small intestine are removed in these patients, but the remainder of the foregut (stomach, duodenum, pancreas) is retained. When possible, the liver is removed with the retrohepatic vena cava preserved in situ.[20]

After the enterectomy, the composite allograft is implanted by anastomosing the suprahepatic vena cava of the donor, including the hepatic veins (so-called piggyback liver transplantation) end-to-side to the recipient's vena cava; the donor infrahepatic vena cava can then be ligated (Fig. 184-3*A*). The double arterial stem of the celiac and superior mesenteric arteries (via the Carrel patch technique) is connected to the infrarenal aorta (with an aortic conduit or iliac artery homograft), with subsequent graft reperfusion. Because the axial stem of the portal vein between the donor organs has remained intact, all that is required for the completion of portal flow is attachment of the portal vein of the remnant foregut in the recipient to the intact portal stem of the donor. This may not be possible, however, because of size discrepancy or difficult anatomic relationships between donor and recipient portal veins. In this case, a permanent portocaval shunt is performed (Fig. 184-3*B*). The intestinal anastomoses are then

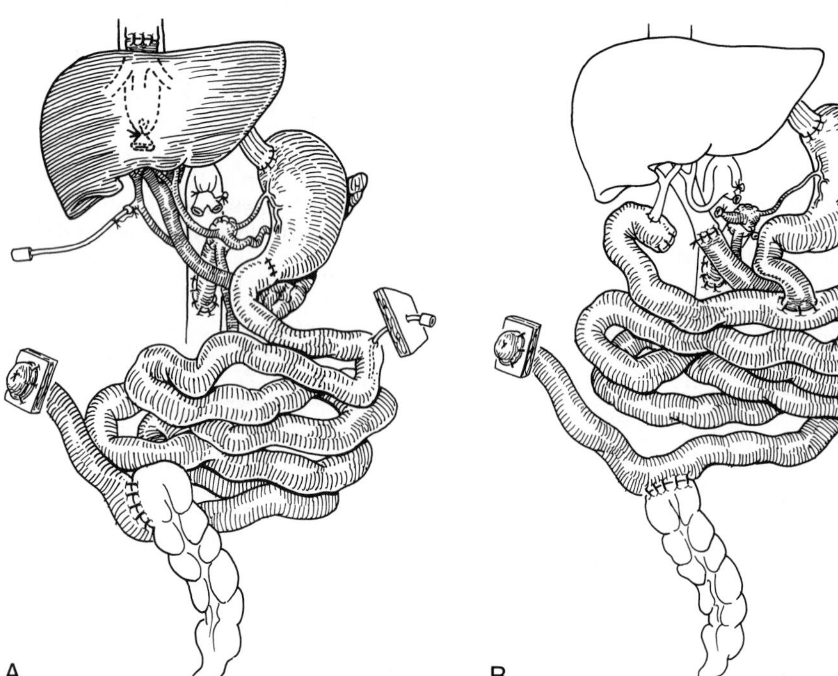

Figure 184–2. Diagrams of multivisceral donor organs: complete multivisceral (*A*) and modified multivisceral (*B*). (From Reyes J, Bueno J, Kocoshis S, et al: Current status of intestinal transplantation in children. J Pediatr Surg 1998; 33:243-254.)

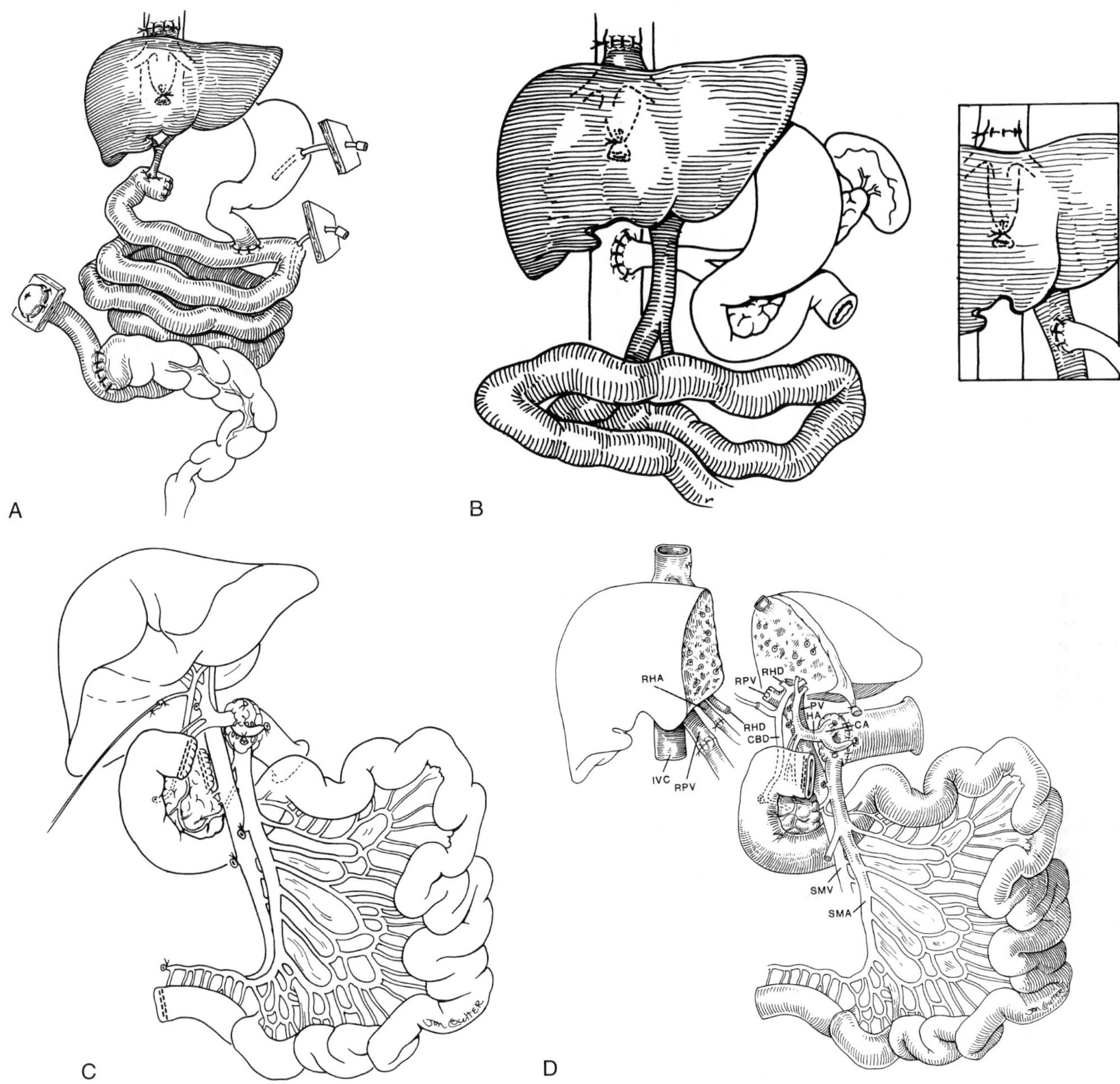

Figure 184–3. Modifications of the liver/small intestinal allograft.

A, Combined liver/small intestinal allograft.

B, Systemic porta caval shunt or recipient portal vein to donor portal vein shunt (*inset*) allows venous outflow of retained pancreas and stomach from recipient. (From Reyes J, Bueno J, Kocoshis S, et al: Current status of intestinal transplantation in children. J Pediatr Surg 1998; 33:243–254.)

C, Composite liver and intestine graft with preservation of the duodenum in continuity with the graft jejunum and hepatic biliary system. The allograft pancreas is transected to the right of the portal vein. (From Abu-Elmagd K, Reyes J, Todo S, et al: Clinical intestinal transplantation: New perspectives and immunologic considerations. J Am Coll Surg 1998; 186:512–527.)

D, In situ split liver graft that maintains the left lateral segment in continuity with the hepatic hilus and duodenum, with transection of allograft pancreas. (From Reyes J, Fishbein T, Bueno J, et al: Reduced sized orthotopic composite liver. Intestinal allograft: Rationale and *in situ* split technique in an initial experience. Transplantation 1998; 66:489–492.)

completed with a proximal jejunojejunostomy, an ileocolostomy, a temporary distal ileostomy, and a Roux-en-Y biliary anastomosis.

To avoid a biliary anastomosis (with its potential for complications), a modification of the original "cluster" allograft, as depicted in Figure 184–1, has been applied to the liver/small-bowel allografts. Here, the allograft duodenum remains in continuity with the allograft biliary system and varying lengths of allograft jejunum-ileum (Fig. 184–3*C*). In one such graft, a reduced segment of allograft liver (the left lateral segment) was successfully used after an in situ split was performed to overcome a donor-recipient size mismatch in a critically ill pediatric recipient (Fig. 184–3*D*).

Isolated Small Bowel

In cases of surgical short gut, the proximal and distal remnants of the intestine are identified; when there is functional disease

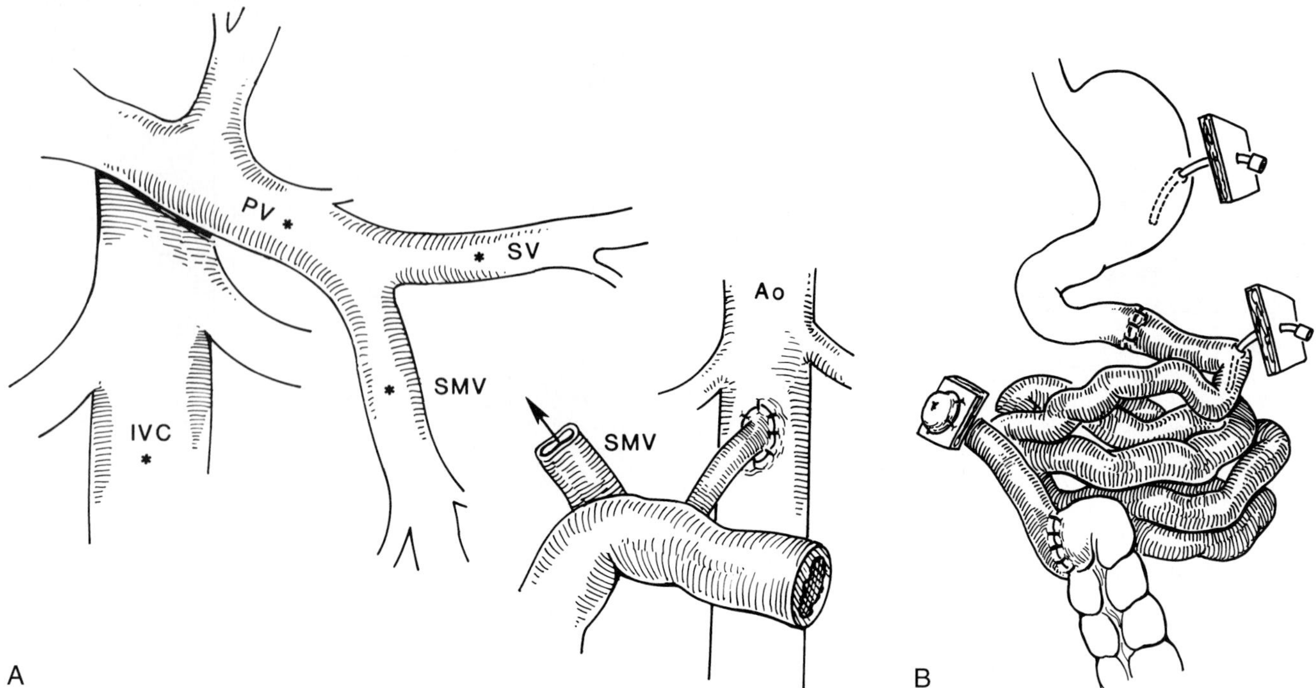

Figure 184–4. *A,* Arterialization and potential venous drainage options of the isolated small intestine allograft. *B,* Isolated small-bowel graft; the distal ileal chimney allows easy access to bowel mucosa. PV = portal vein; SV = splenic vein; SMV = superior mesenteric vein; IVC = inferior vena cava. (From Reyes J, Bueno J, Kocoshis S, et al: Current status of intestinal transplantation in children. J Pediatr Surg 1998; 33:243–254.)

or neoplasm, the recipient's diseased small intestine is removed. The superior mesenteric artery of the donor bowel is sewn to the infrarenal aorta, and the donor superior mesenteric vein to the recipient portal vein, superior mesenteric vein, splenic vein, or inferior vena cava (Fig. 184–4*A*). This may be facilitated by the use of an interposition venous graft. Reperfusion of the intestinal graft is effected after the vascular anastomoses. Intestinal continuity is completed with proximal and distal anastomoses, and access to the ileum for endoscopic examination is provided by a temporary "chimney" ileostomy (Fig. 184–4*B*).[21]

Cold ischemia refers to the time between procurement and implantation of the allograft and has ranged from 2.8 to 17 hours. *Warm ischemic time* for the allograft (sewing-in time) is about 30 minutes and is also a determinant of preservation injury to the intestine. In an attempt to reduce graft dysmotility, a segment of large intestine was included in 32 allografts. This technique was abandoned after 1994, and subsequently the enteric and celiac ganglia have been preserved for the last 16 grafts.

IMMUNOSUPPRESSION

Immunosuppression is similar in recipients of small-bowel, liver/small bowel, cluster, and multivisceral transplants. Intravenous methylprednisolone is given immediately after graft reperfusion (1 g in adults, 10 mg/kg in children). Administration of tacrolimus (0.15 mg/kg/day) is then begun by continuous intravenous infusion, with steady-state whole blood levels (microparticle enzyme immunoassay) between 15 and 25 ng/mL as targets. A steroid taper of methylprednisolone is started at a dose of 5 mg/kg/day (for children) or 200 mg/day (for adults) and reduced over a period of 5 days to 1 mg/kg/day (for children) or 20 mg/day (for adults). In some cases, azathioprine may be added to mitigate the nephrotoxicity and neurotoxicity of tacrolimus. A series of 23 patients completed a trial of cyclophosphamide (Cytoxan), which was given at a dose of 2 mg/kg/day for 4 weeks. The patients were then switched to mycophenolate mofetil (15 to 30 mg/kg/day) or azathioprine (1 to 2 mg/kg/day). As gastrointestinal motility resumes, oral tacrolimus given twice daily may be used to supplement the intravenous regimen, which is gradually tapered.

Induction therapy as well as chronic maintenance therapy involves the use of two and often three drugs. If organ tolerance with minimal rejection episodes is demonstrated, however, gradual reduction and even cessation of steroid therapy may be possible.

Prostaglandin E_1 (Prostin) is administered, 0.003 to 0.009 mg/kg/min, for the first 5 postoperative days. This is given for its beneficial effects on renal perfusion as well as its prevention of microvascular thromboses, the damage-mediating event in acute cellular rejection and procurement injury.[22] Rejection was treated with optimization of tacrolimus level, supplemental steroids, and, if necessary, OKT3.

BONE MARROW AUGMENTATION

The phenomenon of donor and recipient cell migration observed in this patient population was later confirmed to occur after transplantation of all solid organs. These "chimeric" composites form the basis of the two-way paradigm of transplantation immunology, with mutually canceling effects of donor and recipient cell populations producing eventual allograft acceptance.[15] According to this hypothesis, augmentation of leukocyte chimerism was performed with unaltered adjuvant donor bone marrow cells recovered from donor thoracolumbar vertebral bodies and infused postoperatively in a single infusion of 3 to 5 $\times$ 10^8 cells/kg body weight, as previously described.[23, 24]

Monitoring of *chimerism* (the presence of donor cells) was performed serially after transplantation using the recipient's peripheral blood by either flow cytometry or polymerase chain reaction (PCR).[25] Graft-versus-host disease (GVHD) surveillance was studied in all suspected skin and gastrointestinal lesions by routine histology, with the detection of donor cells by immunohistologic staining for donor-specific human leukocyte antigen (HLA) antigens, and in situ hybridization technique using the Y-chromosome–specific probe, as previously described.[15]

POSTOPERATIVE CARE

Recipients of multivisceral, liver/small-bowel, or cluster grafts commonly suffer from severe liver failure. Therefore, the care with respect to lungs, infection surveillance, and liver graft function is similar to that for routine liver transplant recipients. Recipients of isolated small-bowel transplants who have stable liver function have a lesser preoperative medical acuity.

Ventilatory Management

Extubation can often be accomplished within 48 hours of transplantation. Unusual circumstances, such as graft malfunction, sepsis, inability to close the abdominal wall, and severe preoperative hepatic failure, may prevent early extubation. Because the operation is quite long (8 to 18 hours) and the patients are often in a weakened nutritional state preoperatively, a careful assessment of weaning parameters is required. The inspiratory force, forced vital capacity, and spontaneous minute ventilation are most important. It is wise to observe the patients for several hours while they remain intubated on continuous positive airway pressure (CPAP) to make certain that they can tolerate the withdrawal of mechanical support and extubation.

Incisional pain, ascites, and pleural effusions may compromise ventilation and the ability to cough. Muscle wasting and malnutrition, partial or complete paralysis of the right hemidiaphragm,[26] and occasional discrepancies in donor-recipient size that produce an increased intra-abdominal volume with compression of the thoracic cavity may be factors responsible for respiratory impairment. These patients often require low doses of intravenous narcotics, repeated thoracentesis and paracentesis, and supplemental extensive respiratory therapy if they are to avoid the need for reintubation.

Many patients have required tracheostomies because of the need for prolonged ventilatory support. Rarely (two cases), severe rejection of isolated small intestine allografts with systemic venous drainage into the inferior vena cava has been heralded by respiratory insufficiency and picture of acute respiratory distress syndrome (ARDS).

Renal Function

Most intestinal transplant candidates have experienced some measure of renal injury due to multiple episodes of infection, antibiotic requirements, and liver failure. Early after transplantation, there is significant interstitial accumulation of fluid into the graft, lung, and peripheral tissues; this accumulation peaks at 48 to 72 hours. Extensive volume shifts into the transplanted bowel (related to preservation injury) and heavy ascites production (related to mesenteric lymphatic leakage) lead to intravascular volume depletion and can exacerbate the nephrotoxicity of tacrolimus and certain antibiotics. Continuous central venous pressure measurement, often for weeks following transplantation, provides important information for maximizing graft perfusion and preserving the integrity of the kidneys. Two children have undergone inclusion of an allograft kidney with their primary intestine transplant, and one long-term pediatric survivor has required sequential kidney transplantation.

Infection Control

Recipients of isolated or composite small-bowel grafts receive prophylactic, broad-spectrum intravenous antibiotics. Any history of recent nosocomial infections before transplantation should be addressed with the administration of appropriate specific antibiotics. Colonizing organisms growing from enterocutaneous fistulous tracts should be treated perioperatively.

All recipients are given a preoperative and postoperative "cocktail" of oral nonabsorbable antibiotics every 6 hours for 2 weeks; the mix includes amphotericin B, gentamicin, and polymyxin E and is intended to achieve selective bowel decontamination.[27] Surveillance stool specimens are obtained for culture weekly. When organisms grow in quantitative cultures to colonies of greater than 10^8 organisms in the presence of signs of systemic sepsis, or ongoing acute cellular rejection of the allograft, specifically directed intravenous antibiotics are added to the regimen to treat the presumed translocating organisms. This most commonly occurs during episodes of acute rejection, when the mucosal barrier of the allograft has been immunologically damaged; however, it may also be seen with enteritis associated with Epstein-Barr virus (EBV).[28]

The antiviral prophylactic strategy has evolved during this study period and presently includes a 2-week course of intravenous ganciclovir with concomitant CMV-specific hyperimmune globulin (Cytogam).[29] Lifetime oral trimethoprim-sulfamethoxazole is used as prophylaxis for *Pneumocystis carinii* pneumonia.

Nutritional Support

Full nutritional support is initially provided via standard TPN. TPN is tapered gradually as oral or enteral feedings (via gastric or jejunal tube) are advanced. Tube feedings are initiated with an isotonic dipeptide formula containing medium-chain triglycerides and glutamine. This formula is later converted to a lactose-free and gluten-free diet that contains dietary fibers to promote normalization of intestinal motility and function. Most patients do not voluntarily eat adequate amounts early after the operation, and variations to this existed among the various intestinal transplant cohorts. Most impressive has been the resistance to resumption of oral feedings in pediatric recipients.[30] Therefore, enteral supplementation is required when the intestinal tract becomes functional. Management is highly "individualized," since the simplicity of an uneventful post-transplantation course may suddenly change with any surgical or immunologic complication. These complications can be manifested with serious fluid, caloric, protein, and trace element deficits.

Assessment of Graft Status

A judgment of the anatomic and functional integrity of the graft begins in the operating room. The normal appearance of the mesentery and intestine is pink and nonedematous, with the intestine occasionally demonstrating contractions. Alterations from this appearance can be observed in the operating room and in the ileal stoma postoperatively.

Surveillance of intestinal graft rejection focuses on clinical evaluation and gross morphologic examination of the stoma and the distal ileum. Frequent routine enteroscopic surveillance has been the most reliable tool for the early diagnosis of intestinal rejection.[31] Endoscopic evaluations are performed routinely twice a week through the allograft ileostomy; upper endoscopy is performed when clinical changes are not elucidated by distal allograft evaluation. Grossly, the bowel reacts to insult in nonspecific ways with edema, cyanosis, congestion, and increased stomal output; these alterations should signal a broad differential to include preservation injury, systemic sepsis, rejection, and enteritis.

The stomal output is assessed for volume, consistency, and the presence of reducing substances, which can be seen in the event of rejection, bacterial overgrowth, or malabsorption. Typical stomal output of a clear, watery effluent within the first week of implantation is 1 to 2 L/day for adults and 40 to 60 mL/kg/day for children. If these volumes are exceeded and no significant pathology is present, paregoric, loperamide, pectin, somatostatin, or oral antibiotics may be used singly or in combination to control the diarrhea. The presence of blood in the stool is always an ominous sign and indicates rejection until proven otherwise.

Serum tests are important in assessing injury to the liver (bilirubin, aspartate aminotransferase, and alanine aminotransferase), but no such tests exist for the intestinal grafts. Serum markers for nutritional adequacy and anabolic status (transferrin, albumin, retinoic acid) are of limited value, whereas specific tests of the absorptive ability of the graft are good measures of overall function. Assessment of small-bowel function relies on absorption studies of D-xylose and tacrolimus and on the quantitation of fat in the stool. Most patients show satisfactory absorption curves for D-xylose within the first postoperative month, with absorption improving over time. Abnormal results obtained after 1 month should always prompt an aggressive search for underlying pathology, especially rejection.

The maintenance of satisfactory tacrolimus whole blood trough levels of 15 to 25 ng/mL with oral therapy alone is a good indicator of adequate absorption. In our patients, this level has occurred at a mean of 28 days after transplantation and tends to be delayed longer in recipients of multivisceral grafts.[32] The excretion of fat in the stool has been abnormal in almost all patients, but clinical steatorrhea has not been a problem.

Radiologic evaluations by standard barium gastrointestinal examination are valuable in assessing mucosal pattern and motility and are performed routinely after the first postoperative week. A normal mucosal pattern is expected. Intestinal transit time is about 2 hours. Intestinal graft rejection, when mild, can be suspected when evidence of mucosal edema exists. Severe rejection, with exfoliation of the mucosa, ablates the normal mucosal pattern and can be seen as segments of "tubulized" intestine and strictures (Fig. 184-5).

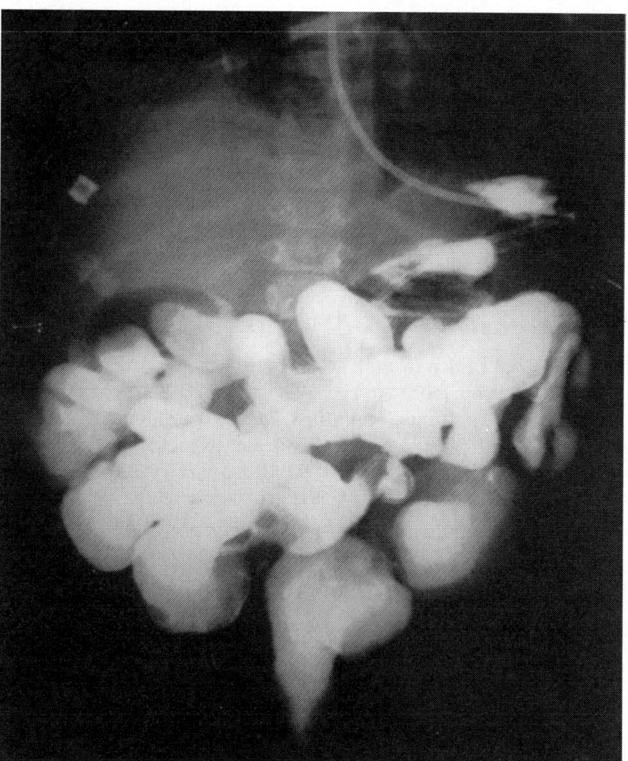

Figure 184–5. Severely damaged allograft intestine in a recipient of a liver–small bowel after multiple episodes of rejection. Diffuse tubulized gut, strictures, and significant distention of the native duodenum are seen.

COMPLICATIONS

Before the various potential complications are described, it is important to impart a general perspective on the care of these patients. Comprehensive management of intestinal recipients requires a multidisciplinary approach by surgeons, anesthesiologists, nurses, critical care physicians, pathologists, and a host of internal medicine subspecialists. Easy access to diagnostic and therapeutic modalities is paramount, including mechanical ventilation, hemodialysis, bronchoscopy, gastrointestinal endoscopy, thromboelastography, percutaneous cholangiography, ultrasonography, invasive and noninvasive contrast radiography, and sophisticated hemodynamic monitoring systems.

More important than the preceding, however, is a vigilance about patient care and attention to detail on the part of both physicians and nurses. Problems in these patients can originate from a multiplicity of sources. We can make several assumptions about these patients based on our experience:

1. Preoperative deterioration of physical performance status predisposes to various organ system failure that persists in the postoperative period even though allograft function may be acceptable.
2. Treating transplant recipients is a labor-intensive task, requiring aggressive respiratory therapy, nutritional and antibiotic support, fluid management, and nursing care, often for prolonged periods in the intensive care unit.
3. Immunotherapy doses in patients with multivisceral transplants tend to be higher than in patients with single organ transplants.
4. Most patients experience episodes of infection and rejection after transplantation, often concomitantly. Any subjective complaints or objective abnormalities should be vigorously pursued until a cause is found or until these problems resolve.

Graft Rejection

Intestinal allograft rejection can present as an array of symptoms that include fever, abdominal pain, distention, nausea, vomiting, and a sudden increase in stomal output. The stoma may become edematous, erythematous, and friable. Gastrointestinal bleeding can occur in cases of severe uncontrollable rejection in which ulcerations and sloughing of the intestinal mucosa occur. Septic shock or ARDS may develop. Bacterial or fungal translocation can occur during intestinal allograft rejection as a result of disruption of the intestinal mucosal barrier. Gut decontamination must be instituted during these episodes.[33]

Endoscopically, the transplanted intestinal mucosa loses its velvety appearance. It may become hyperemic or dusky as well as hypoperistaltic. Erythema may be focal or diffuse. The mucosa becomes friable, and diffuse ulcerations appear (Fig. 184-6) (see Color Plate).

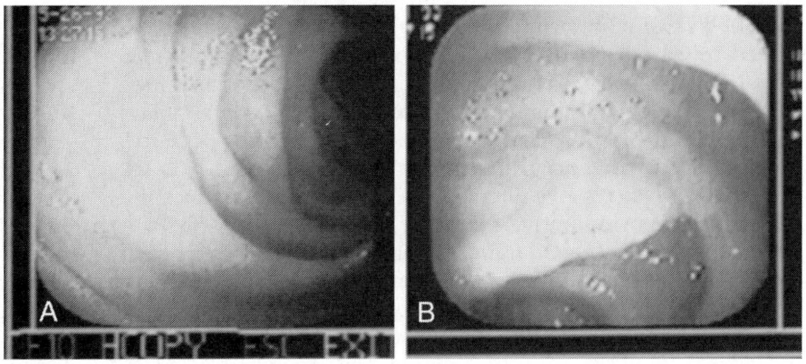

Figure 184–6. *A,* Normal endoscopic appearance of the transplanted small intestine. *B,* Moderate acute cellular rejection of an intestinal allograft demonstrating diffuse edema and focal erythema. (See Color Plate.)

Histologically, there is variable presence of lamina propria edema and villous blunting. However, the mononuclear cell infiltrates and cryptitis with apoptosis and regeneration are necessary for establishing the diagnosis of rejection. Neutrophils, eosinophils, and macrophages may be seen traversing the muscularis mucosa.[34, 35] The degree of epithelial and crypt cell damage varies. Complete mucosal sloughing and crypt destruction are seen in grafts with severe rejection. The mucosal surface is partially replaced by inflammatory pseudomembranes and granulation tissue (Fig. 184–7). This event may precipitate continuous blood loss as well as intermittent septic episodes from the damaged intestine.

Chronic rejection has been observed in patients with persistent intractable rejection episodes. Clinically progressive weight loss, chronic diarrhea, intermittent fever, and gastrointestinal bleeding dominate the presentation. Histologically, villous blunting, focal ulcerations, epithelial metaplasia, and scant cellular infiltrate are present on endoscopic mucosal biopsies. Full-thickness biopsy specimens show obliterative thickening of intestinal arterioles.

The incidence of acute intestinal allograft rejection during the first 90 days after transplantation is reported to be 92% in isolated small-bowel transplant recipients and 66% in recipients of composite graft (multivisceral, liver/small bowel), suggesting that the liver is "protective" of the intestine, as seen experimentally.[8, 36] Interestingly, the incidence of acute liver allograft rejection in recipients of composite grafts is 43%, a rate similar to that seen after isolated liver transplantation.[30]

Mild graft rejection is treated initially with intravenous methylprednisolone; moderate or severe rejection is treated with a methylprednisolone taper. Tacrolimus trough levels in whole blood should reach 15 to 25 ng/mL by either the oral or intravenous route. OKT3 is used when rejection has progressed with a steroid taper; however, it should be entertained as the initial therapeutic agent in cases of severe mucosal injury and crypt damage. The use of cyclophosphamide-mycophenolate mofetil induction therapy or bone marrow augmentation has had no beneficial effect on the frequency of rejection.[30, 36]

Postoperative Hemorrhage

Coagulopathy is more often an intraoperative problem that relates to liver dysfunction, qualitative and quantitative plate-

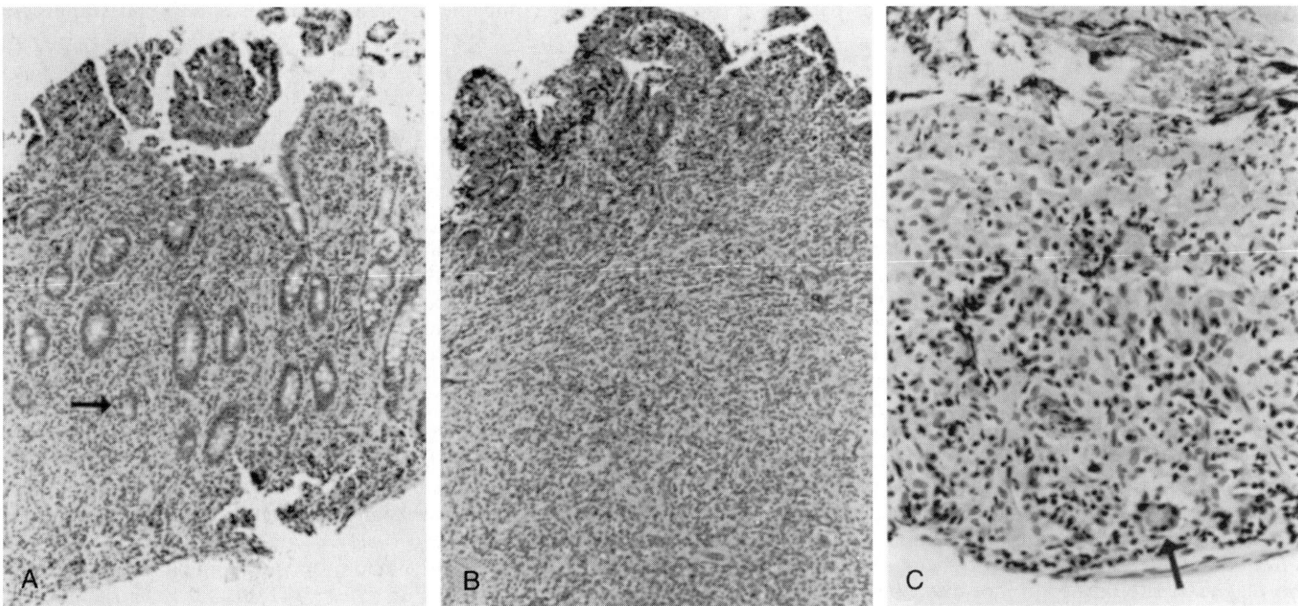

Figure 184–7. Acute cellular rejection. *A,* Endoscopic biopsy obtained 14 days after transplantation showed widening of the lamina propria with increased mononuclear cells, which were often cuffed around small vessels and infiltrating the crypt epithelium (*arrow*). (Hematoxylin and eosin, ×140.) *B,* The reaction was more intense in biopsy specimens that contained lymphoid nodules and where blastogenesis, focal ulcerations, congestion, and neutrophil plugging of capillaries were also seen (moderate acute cellular rejection). (Hematoxylin and eosin, ×140.) *C,* Uncontrolled acute rejection eventually resulted in widespread mucosal destruction; the mucosa was replaced by granulation tissue. Note the overlying inflammatory pseudomembrane (*arrow*). (Hematoxylin and eosin, ×350.)

let defects, and fibrinolysis.[37] Intraoperative bleeding is furthered by vascularized adhesions from previous surgery and portal hypertension. Temporary graft reperfusion coagulopathy mediated by plasminogen activators from the graft may occur.[38] Efforts are taken to normalize these global aspects of coagulation by the end of the operative procedure, so that in the absence of liver dysfunction, the coagulopathy is usually minor in the postoperative period.

Postoperative intra-abdominal bleeding is most often a technical problem, arising from vascular anastomoses or extensive, raw peritoneal surfaces. Certainly, coagulation should be normalized if postoperative bleeding occurs; if bleeding is proved, the origin should be presumed surgical and managed as such by early exploration.

Biliary Complications

Continuity of the biliary axis is preserved in multivisceral and cluster grafts as well as the modified liver/small-bowel graft. The standard liver/small-bowel graft requires a Roux-en-Y choledochojejunostomy. Correspondingly, these grafts can result in biliary system–related surgical complications (i.e., leaks and obstructions).

Biliary leaks usually occur within the first 2 weeks after liver/small-bowel transplantation and may herald their presence with bilious drainage from the abdominal wound or drains or merely with unexplained sepsis. The response to external bilious drainage should be immediate exploration with surgical revision of the biliary dehiscence. In the case of unexplained sepsis in any intestinal transplant recipient, all surgical anastomoses should be radiographically inspected (with percutaneous cholangiography); if leakage is suspected, the anastomoses should be openly revised. There is no place for percutaneous diversion of biliary or intestinal leakage in these patients, because both wound healing and antimicrobial immunity are impaired by multimodal immunotherapy.

Biliary obstruction generally follows an anastomotic stricture and is a delayed complication, but any clinical picture that resembles cholangitis or biliary obstruction should be investigated with cholangiography to prove patency, regardless of the timing after transplantation.

Vascular Complications

Major arterial thrombosis is a disastrous complication that leads to massive necrosis of the organs correspondingly supplied. Elevation of hepatic enzymes and pallor of the intestinal stoma are accompanied by clinical deterioration, fulminant sepsis, and hepatic coma. Isolated small-bowel grafts can be removed with the expectation of patient recovery; however, in patients with composite grafts, the event is usually fatal unless early retransplantation can be performed. Patency of the arteries can be rapidly confirmed with Doppler ultrasound examination.

Because the superior mesenteric vein/portal vein axis is preserved in the composite grafts, venous outflow thrombosis is less likely to occur in these recipients. Isolated small-bowel grafts have an anastomosis of these veins that can potentially occlude. Ascites, stomal congestion, and, ultimately, mesenteric infarction would be the end result.

Neither of these problems produces subtle clinical signs, and diagnosis should be prompt and obvious. In our series, isolated thrombosis of the hepatic artery has occurred in a pediatric recipient of a liver/small-bowel graft, with consequent hepatic gangrene. This patient required retransplantation of the liver component of the graft, even though a full liver/small-bowel graft was desirable.

Incomplete obstruction of major inflow or outflow vessels may be suspected on biopsy or based on clinical and laboratory evidence of organ dysfunction. Contrast vascular x-ray studies are confirmatory, and the correction is surgical or, in some cases, with balloon dilatation.

Gastrointestinal Complications

Gastrointestinal bleeding after intestinal transplantation is an ominous sign that requires prompt attention. Rejection or infection is probable cause and should be immediately diagnosed or ruled out on the basis of enteroscopic biopsy results. The diagnosis of rejection relies not only on histologic evidence but also on the endoscopic appearance (see Figs. 184-6 and 184-7). Bleeding from ulcerated Epstein-Barr virus– or cytomegalovirus (CMV)-induced lesions can be easily differentiated by gross endoscopic examination. Empirical therapy for rejection is not acceptable.

Leakage of either the proximal or distal gastrointestinal anastomosis can occur in any recipient, but it is more common in children than in adults. Any fresh surgical margin, including native duodenal and colonic stumps and gastrostomy sites, are vulnerable to poor wound healing and subsequent leakage. Presentation is often dramatic (florid sepsis), with confirmation by radiologic contrast imaging. Surgical revision, evacuation of peritoneal soilage, and often reexploration are required to eliminate the contamination effectively. Again, sepsis without an obvious source should prompt the performance of contrast studies to document the integrity of all gastrointestinal anastomoses; if the findings are inconclusive, diagnostic laparotomy is indicated.

Native gastric atony and pylorospasm that produce early satiety or vomiting are common and self-limiting. The evolution of motility patterns in the denervated allograft intestine is not fully understood, although it is clear that various pathologic processes may alter the individual baseline. Hypermotility of the allograft intestine occurs early after transplantation; in the absence of rejection or bacterial overgrowth, it can be controlled with agents such as paregoric, loperamide, or pectin. Sudden changes in intestinal motility, particularly when accompanied by abdominal distention and vomiting in the case of decreased motility, should initiate a search for rejection.

Infections

The frequency of infectious complications is high and is responsible for significant morbidity and mortality after intestinal transplantation. This reflects the relatively higher level of immunosuppression required to maintain the graft in these intestinal recipients. Other predisposing factors include the severity of the preoperative liver failure and the presence of intra-abdominal, pulmonary, or intravenous line–induced sepsis before transplantation. Also, technically more difficult transplantation procedures with increased operative time, transfusion requirements, and likelihood of reexploration reflect the advanced disease of these patients. Recipients of small-bowel grafts have the lowest incidence of complications because of the more elective nature of their candidacy.

Infectious pathogens include bacteria, fungi, and viruses. Infections are related (in order of frequency) to intravenous lines, the abdominal wound, deep abdominal abscesses, peritonitis, and pneumonia. Bacterial translocation in grafts damaged by rejection illustrates the need for concomitant antirejection and antimicrobial therapy and is a frequent source of infection.

Of the bacterial pathogens, staphylococci and enterococci are common, whereas gram-negative rods usually accompany polymicrobial infections. Not uncommonly, separate sources of infection occur simultaneously, or mixed infections from the same source are present. This leads to multiple antibiotic regimens and sets the stage for the development of resistant organisms. Particularly problematic has been the nascent strain of panresistant enterococci. Persistence of a physiologic hyperdynamic state in a patient being treated for proven infection should raise the suspicion of retained phlegmonous material in the abdomen or the possibility of rejection.[39]

Fungal infections become problematic after heavy treatment of rejection, massive antibiotic usage, intestinal leaks, and multiple surgical explorations. We routinely employ low-dose amphotericin B prophylaxis in patients with these complications. Established fungal infections require long-term, full-dose antibiotic therapy and reduction of immunotherapy. All recipients with persistent sepsis are potential candidates for moderation of immunosuppressant dosages if no coexistent cellular rejection is present. However, complete withdrawal of immunosuppression has been impossible in this recipient population because of a high incidence of rebound rejection, which then requires augmentation of immunotherapy.

Clinical CMV infection has occurred in 36% of intestinal graft recipients and often involves the allograft intestine. Although the incidence and distribution of disease, according to donor and recipient CMV serologic status, are similar in adults (44%) and children (31%), the clinical course has been dramatically better in children. Successful clinical management has been accomplished in 88% of episodes with ganciclovir alone or in combination with CMV-specific hyperimmunoglobulin. Immunosuppression was maintained at baseline and reduced only in the face of deteriorating clinical disease, thus indicating rebound rejection.[29] A CMV-positive donor graft transplanted into a CMV-negative recipient is a significant risk factor, but intense baseline immunosuppression with high tacrolimus levels and cumulative doses of pulse steroids is a constant feature.[40] Clinical presentation has generally been enteritis of variable severity with focal ulcerations and bleeding (Fig. 184-8) (see Color Plate). We currently avoid CMV-positive grafts only for CMV-negative candidates who are awaiting isolated intestinal grafts. However, CMV-negative candidates awaiting the larger composite grafts, because they are at risk for death from liver failure, may still receive a CMV-positive graft.[29]

Less commonly, respiratory syncytial virus, adenovirus, and parainfluenza virus have occurred in children. All viral infections are opportunistic and have as a "common denominator" the need for aggressive treatment of rejection episodes in complicated patients with high Acute Physiologic and Chronic Health Evaluation (APACHE) scores.

Post-transplantation lymphoproliferative disease (PTLD) associated with the Epstein-Barr virus has occurred in 20% of all patients, with children (27%) being at a significantly higher risk than adults (11%). Presentation varies from totally asymptomatic observations at routine endoscopy, nonspecific intestinal and systemic symptoms, bleeding, lymphadenopathy, and tumors, to fulminant disease. Risk factors other than age included the type of graft, splenectomy, and the use of OKT3. Therapy included the reduction and withdrawal of immunosuppression, antivirals (ganciclovir, acyclovir, hyperimmunoglobulin), cytokines (interferon-alfa), and chemotherapy. However the disease was lethal in 45% of our patients. Rebound rejection was a significant contributor to mortality.[30, 36, 41]

Graft-Versus-Host Disease

Skin changes consistent with graft-versus-host disease were confirmed by histopathologic criteria in five of our patients (5%), only one of whom had received adjunct bone marrow. This was confirmed by immunohistochemical studies visualizing donor cell infiltration into the lesions on two occasions. One child died with hereditary immunoglobulin (IgG and IgM) deficiency,[42] and one adult had a complex chronic GVHD in association with PTLD. All other cases have been self-limited and resolved spontaneously.

Present Status and Future

The causes of graft and patient loss are invariably multifactorial and complex. The evolution of technical and clinical management factors have improved outcome. However, the interplay between the need for high levels of immunosuppression, the high incidence of immunosuppression, the high incidence of rejection, and the opportunistic infections consequent to this remain the major stumbling blocks to further progress.

The experience accumulated over the last 8 years of this study has allowed the development of clinical and surgical strategies that has benefited a very clinically complex group of patients. Our reserved optimism is taken in light of previous experience with intestinal transplantation as well as the grim outcome of patients not receiving transplants. Nonetheless,

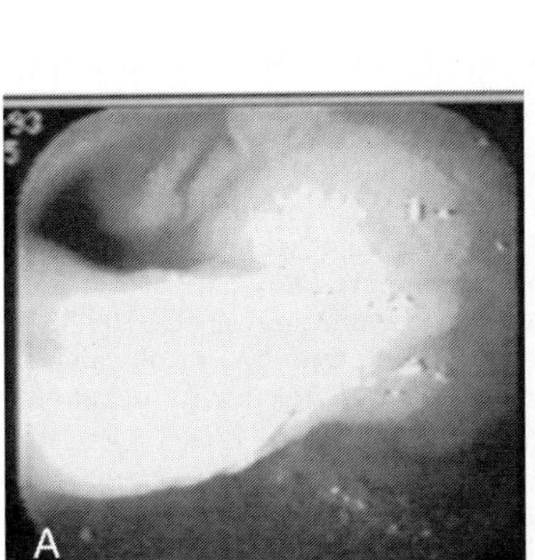

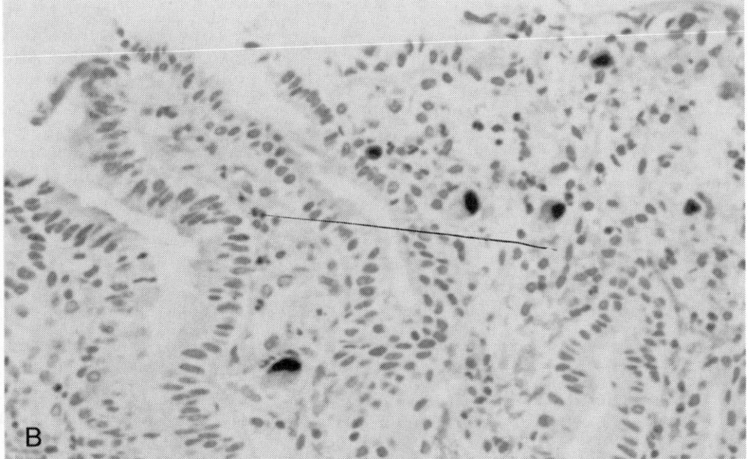

Figure 184–8. *A*, Endoscopic appearance of cytomegaloviral enteritis is characterized by hyperemic erosions. *B*, The diagnosis was confirmed histologically by the presence of characteristic inclusions, by staining for viral antigens, or both. Note the focal neutrophilic inflammation. (Immunoperoxidase for cytomegalovirus antigens, ×350.) (See Color Plate.)

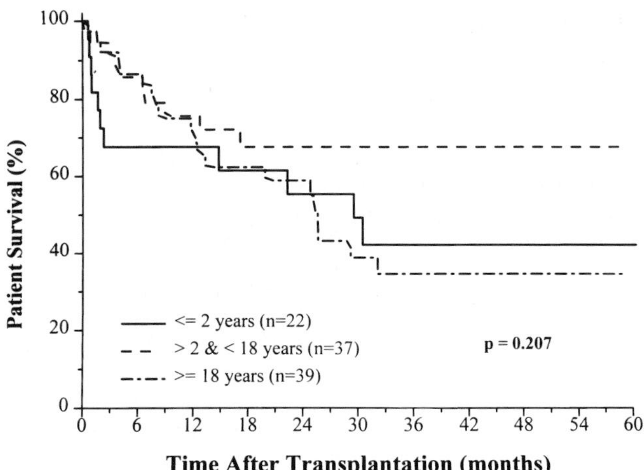

Figure 184–9. Patient survival with age distribution. (From Abu-Elmagd K, Reyes J, Todo S, et al: Clinical intestinal transplantation: New perspectives and immunologic considerations. J Am Coll Surg 1998; 186:512–527.)

the overall actuarial survival at 1 and 5 years has been 72% and 48%, respectively, with full nutritional support having been achieved in 91% of surviving patients. Improved results were achieved in the pediatric population between 2 and 18 years of age (65% at 5 years)[36] (Fig. 184–9).

The transplantation of the isolated intestinal graft has provided better patient survival at all follow-up times. However, because of a higher incidence of rejection with this type of graft, the long-term outcome of all types of grafts (isolated intestine or composite grafts) has been similar and is estimated at about 40% at 5 years[30, 36] (Fig. 184–10).

Although the augmentation of donor leukocyte chimerism with bone marrow infusion did not alter patient or graft survival, it was not responsible for any significant morbidity, thus establishing its safety as an adjunct procedure. It has provided insights into the fate of the coexisting leukocyte populations (donor or recipient); however, further immunomodulatory strategies will be necessary to advance the field of intestinal transplantation.

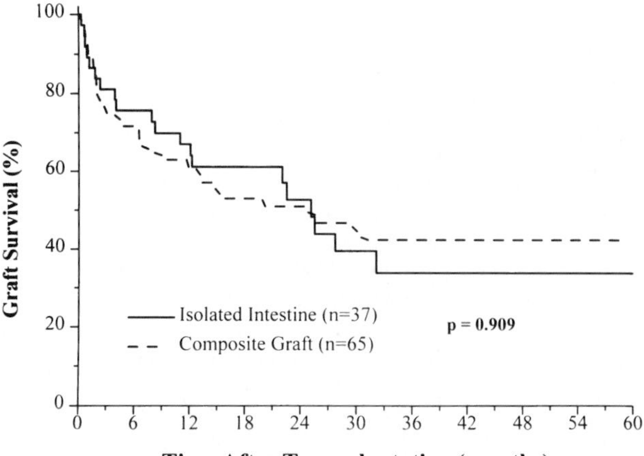

Figure 184–10. Graft survival with intestine alone, or as a composite with the liver allograft. (From Abu-Elmagd K, Reyes J, Todo S, et al: Clinical intestinal transplantation: New perspectives and immunologic considerations. J Am Coll Surg 1998; 186:512–527.)

Under the best of circumstances, the outlay of financial and time expenditures in composite and isolated small-bowel transplant recipients is impressive. For best possible results, candidates who have optimal nutritional status and who are free of active infection should be selected. Donor organs should be discarded if they are less than perfect. Even with technically perfect operations, the managing physician should expect a panoply of postoperative difficulties and should be prepared to support these patients fully for an indefinite period. Managing the balance between excessive and inadequate immunosuppression in the face of potentially virulent infections, the pursuit of rejection and sources of infection, and maintenance of comprehensive critical care support are the most challenging tasks.

References

1. Grant D: Intestinal transplantation: Current status. Transplant Proc 1989; 21:2869–2871.
2. Lillehei RC, Goott B, Miller FA: The physiologic response of the small bowel of the dog to ischemia including prolonged in vitro preservation of the bowel with successful replacement and survival. Ann Surg 1959; 150:543–560.
3. Starzl TE, Kaupp HA Jr: Mass homotransplantation of abdominal organs in dogs. Surg Forum 1960; 11:28–30.
4. Billingham RE: Reactions of grafts against their host; transplantation immunity works both ways—hosts destroy grafts and grafts may harm hosts. Science 1959; 130:947–953.
5. Monchik GJ, Russell PS: Transplantation of the small bowel in the rat: Technical and immunologic considerations. Surgery 1971; 70:693–702.
6. Starzl TE, Rowe M, Todo S, et al: Transplantation of multiple abdominal viscera. JAMA 1989; 261:1449–1457.
7. Starzl TE, Todo S, Tzakis A, et al: Abdominal organ cluster transplantation for the treatment of upper abdominal malignancies. Ann Surg 1989; 210:374–386.
8. Calne RY, Sells RA, Pena JR, et al: Introduction of immunologic tolerance by porcine liver allograft. Nature 1969; 223:472–474.
9. Kamada N, Davies HS, Wight D, et al: Liver transplantation in the rat: Biochemical and histological evidence of complete tolerance induction in nonrejector strains. Transplantation 1983; 35:304–311.
10. Grant D, Wall W, Mimeault R, et al: Successful small-bowel/liver transplantation. Lancet 1990; 335:181–184.
11. Deltz E, Schroeder P, Gebhard H, et al: Successful clinical small bowel transplantation: Report of a case. Clin Transplant 1989; 3:89.
12. Goulet OK, Revillon Y, Jan D, et al: Small-bowel transplantation in children. Transplant Proc 1990; 22:2499–2500.
13. Murase N, Demetris AJ, Mutsuzaki T, et al: Long survival in rats after multivisceral versus isolated small bowel allotransplantation under FK506. Surgery 1991; 110:87–98.
14. Todo S, Tzakis AG, Abu-Elmagd K, et al: Cadaveric small bowel and small bowel-liver transplantation in humans. Transplantation 1992; 53:369–376.
15. Starzl TE, Demetris AJ, Trucco M, et al: Cell migration and chimerism after whole-organ transplantation: The basis of graft acceptance. Hepatology 1993; 17:1127–1156.
16. Starzl TE, Demetris AJ, Murase N, et al: The lost chord: Microchimerism and allograft survival. Immunol Today 1996; 17:577–584.
17. Howard L, Ament M, Fleming RC, et al: Current use and clinical outcome of home parenteral and enteral nutrition therapies in the United States. Gastroenterology 1995; 109:355–365.
18. Casella JF, Lewis JH, Bontempo FA, et al: Successful treatment for homozygous protein C deficiency by hepatic transplantation. Lancet 1988; i:435–438.
19. Starzl TE, Todo S, Tzakis A, et al: The many faces of multivisceral transplantation. Surg Gynecol Obstet 1991; 172:335–344.
20. Tzakis A, Todo S, Starzl TE: Piggyback orthotopic liver transplantation with preservation of the inferior vena cava. Ann Surg 1989; 210:649–652.
21. Todo S, Tzakis A, Abu-Elmagd K, et al: Intestinal transplantation in composite visceral grafts or alone. Ann Surg 1992; 216:223–234.

22. Takaya S, Iwaki Y, Starzl TE: Liver transplantation in positive cytotoxic crossmatch cases using FK506, high dose steroids, and prostaglandin E_1. Transplantation 1991; 54:927-933.
23. Starzl TE, Demetris AJ, Rao As, et al: Spontaneous and iatrogenically augmented leukocyte chimerism in organ transplant recipients. Transplant Proc 1994; 26:3071-3076.
24. Rao AS, Fontes P, Zeevi A, et al: Augmentation of chimerism in whole organ recipients by simultaneous infusion of donor bone marrow cells. Transplant Proc 1995; 27:210-212.
25. Fontes P, Rao A, Demetris AJ, et al: Augmentation with bone marrow of donor leukocyte migration for kidney, liver, heart, and pancreas islet transplantation. Lancet 1994; 344:151-155.
26. Karavias D, Jabbour N, Felekouras E, et al: Right diaphragmatic paralysis following orthotopic liver transplantation. Submitted.
27. Reyes J, Abu-Elmagd K, Tzakis A, et al: Infectious complications after human small bowel transplantation. Transplant Proc 1992; 24:1249-1250.
28. Sigurdsson L, Green M, Putnam P, et al: Bacteremia frequently accompanies rejection following pediatric small bowel transplantation (Abstract). J Pediatr Gastroenterol Nutr 1995; 21:356.
29. Bueno J, Green M, Kocoshis S, et al: Cytomegalovirus infection after intestinal transplantation in children. Clin Infect Dis 1997; 25:1078-1083.
30. Reyes J, Bueno J, Kocoshis S, et al: Current status of intestinal transplantation in children. J Pediatr Surg 1998; 33:243-254.
31. Garau P, Orenstien SR, Neigut DA, et al: Role of endoscopy following small intestinal transplantation in children. Transplant Proc 1994; 26:136-137.
32. Reyes J, Tzakis AG, Todo S, et al: Nutritional management of intestinal transplant recipients. Transplant Proc 1993; 25:1200-1201.
33. Abu-Elmagd K, Tzakis A, Todo S, et al: Monitoring and treatment of intestinal allograft rejection in humans. Transplant Proc 1993; 25:1202-1203.
34. Lee RG, Nakamura K, Tsamauda ACm, et al: Pathology of human intestinal transplantation. Gastroenterology 1996; 1820-1834.
35. White FV, Reyes J, Jaffe R, et al: Pathology of intestinal transplantation in children. Am J Surg Pathol 1995; 19:687-698.
36. Abu-Elmagd K, Reyes J, Todo S, et al: Clinical intestinal transplantation: New perspectives and immunologic considerations. J Am Coll Surg 1998; 186:512-527.
37. Kang YG, Martin DJ, Marquez JM, et al: Intraoperative changes in blood coagulation and thromboelastographic monitoring in liver transplantation. Anesth Analg 1985; 64:888-896.
38. Stahl RL, Duncan A, Hooks MA, et al: A hypercoagulable state follows orthotopic liver transplantation. Hepatology 1990; 12:553.
39. Green M, Reyes J, Nour B, et al: Early infectious complications of liver-intestinal transplantation in children: Preliminary analysis. Transplant Proc 1994; 26:1420-1421.
40. Manez R, Kusne S, Green M, et al: Incidence and risk factors associated with the development of cytomegalovirus disease after intestinal transplantation. Transplantation 1995; 59:1110-1114.
41. Reyes J, Tzakis A, Bonet H, et al: Lymphoproliferative disease after intestinal transplantation under FK506 immunosuppression. Transplant Proc 1994; 26:1426-1427.
42. Reyes J, Todo S, Green M, et al: Graft-versus-host disease after liver and small bowel transplantation in a child. Clin Transpl 1997; 11:345-348.

185

Future of Transplantation (Including Xenografting)

John J. Fung, MD, PhD • Abdul S. Rao, MD, DPhil
Ernesto P. Molmenti, MD • S. Forrest Dodson, MD
Ake Grenvik, MD, PhD, FCCM • Thomas E. Starzl, MD, PhD

In Chapter 175, a detailed history of organ transplantation is provided. In order to foster the appreciation and understanding of the forces that will drive advances in transplantation into the next century, this chapter focuses on a few of the past developments in transplantation that have helped to shape current transplant practices (Fig. 185-1). The beginning of solid-organ transplantation can be traced back to the technical achievement of Alexis Carrel[1]; in 1902, he described the techniques of vascular anastomosis, thus ushering in accounts of autologous and homologous transplantation. Although a number of animal-to-human kidney transplants were reported in the ensuing three decades, a human donor organ was not used until 1933, by the Russian surgeon Voronoy.[2] This and other attempts at using human kidneys for transplantation failed owing to acute tubular necrosis and rejection. The first successful human transplant was performed on December 23, 1954, by the Boston team of Moore, Murray, Merrill, and Harrison.[3] The transplantation of an identical twin kidney from one brother to another was the immunologic advantage that distinguished the early successes in kidney transplantation from those that otherwise were doomed to fail.

Gibson and Medawar[4] ascribed an immunologic basis to the rejection of tissues between genetically nonidentical individuals. In 1960, Calne and Murray[5] used azathioprine, developed several years earlier by Burroughs-Wellcome, in attempts to gain success in unrelated kidney transplantation using immunosuppressive agents. Starzl and colleagues[6] then modified the immunosuppressive regimen by adding corticosteroids for rejection and began routinely to achieve success. This success led to growing attempts at human kidney transplantation, aggravating the shortage of organs to use for transplantation. A number of animal-to-human transplantations were attempted. The longest survivor was a 23-year-old woman who lived for 9 months after receiving kidneys from a chimpanzee.[7]

In 1968, the Ad Hoc Committee of the Harvard School of Medicine proposed the concept of "irreversible coma."[8] Further clarification of the pathophysiology of irreversible brain stem injury and subsequent somatic death followed, as did objective criteria to document irreversible brain injury. The brain death concept has eventually been accepted throughout the United States (see Chapter 174). The details of brain death evaluation and certification vary from state to state but require a clinical picture of (1) coma not due to drug overdose (e.g., alcohol) or to physical reasons (e.g., hypothermia) and (2) lack of cranial nerve reflexes. Confirmatory tests are used to document the absence of blood flow to the brain and the lack of cerebral and brain stem electric activity. The use of brain-dead donors, with optimal hemodynamic parameters, offers the possibility of better-quality organs with minimum damage from warm ischemia. It has also allowed procurement of extrarenal organs in a systematic manner.[9] Another improvement in the area of donor management was the development of preservation solutions, first Collins solution[10] and currently

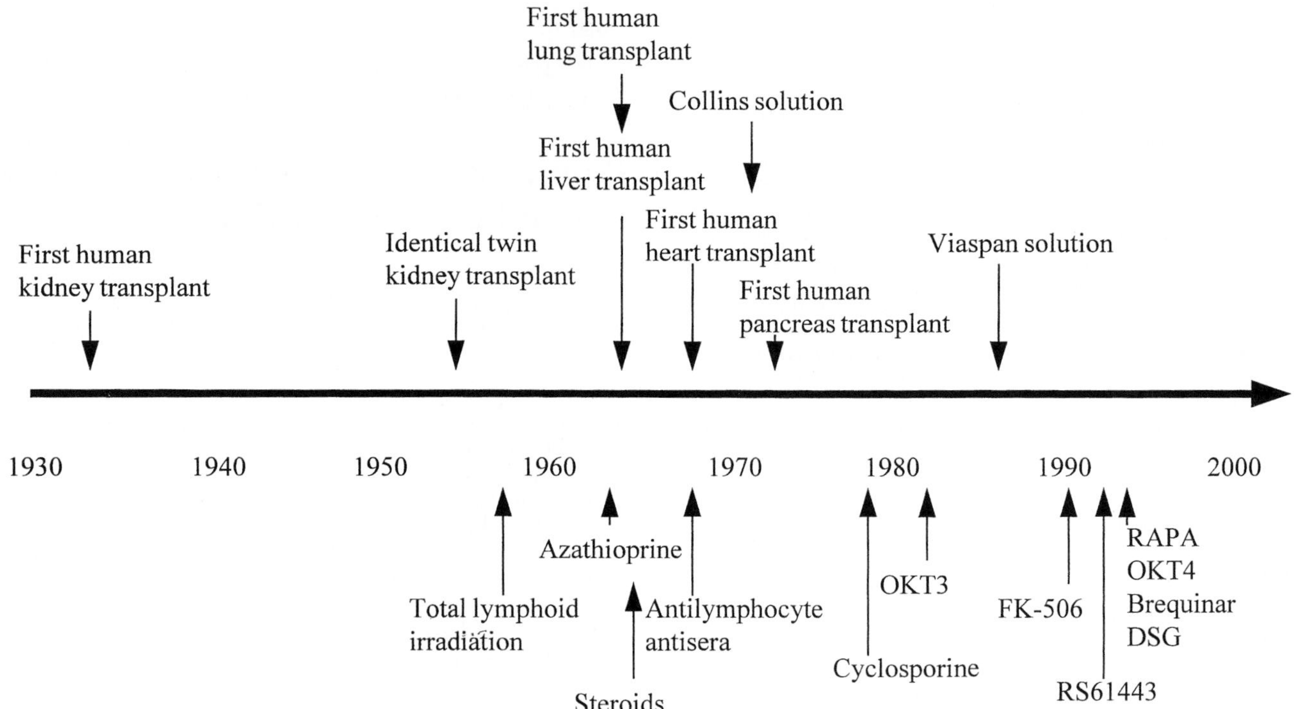

Figure 185–1. Abbreviated chronologic summary of significant milestones in transplantation.

Viaspan, developed by Belzer and Southard[11] at the University of Wisconsin (see Chapter 178).

The next advancement in the field of transplantation came with the discovery of the immunosuppressive qualities of cyclosporine, described by Borel and colleagues.[12] Clinical trials of this agent were conducted in England by Calne and colleagues[13] and shortly thereafter in the United States by Starzl and colleagues.[14] The combination of cyclosporine and steroids was soon introduced into clinical transplantation, and the impact on liver, heart, and kidney transplantation was felt almost overnight. With the introduction of cyclosporine into clinical transplantation, survival rates for patients and grafts improved dramatically (see Chapter 178).

Nevertheless, allograft rejection and the consequences of the treatment of rejection continue to constitute one of the most common causes of retransplantation or death. Clinical rejection occurs in as many as 80% of recipients of solid-organ allografts, who are maintained on a cyclosporine and steroid regimen. In addition, a number of toxicities, including nephrotoxicity, may limit the optimal use of cyclosporine. Chronic renal damage and functional impairment have been shown to occur in transplant recipients, and hypertension requiring antihypertensive therapy occurs in the majority of these patients. Alterations in clinical immunosuppression to prevent or reverse these and other side effects have included (1) reduction of cyclosporine dose and (2) the addition of azathioprine, antilymphocyte antibodies, or other agents, with concomitant reductions in the cyclosporine dose. These methodols have their inherent dangers, increasing susceptibility to both rejection and infection.

Organ transplantation is now accepted as a therapeutic modality for treatment of various end-stage organ diseases. The cost of kidney transplantation has been paid by Medicare and the End-Stage Renal Disease Program for more than 15 years. The costs of liver, heart, and heart-lung transplantations have been paid by a majority of third-party insurances for more than 10 years; Medicare has also recognized the benefits of these procedures and has developed entitlement programs covering these procedures. Pancreas, lung, and intestinal transplantations have not yet been universally subscribed to by third-party payers, but as experience accumulates and the efficacy of these procedures is proved, it is likely that these procedures will also be covered by Medicare. As experience in organ transplantation grows and the experimental procedures also become accepted, the pressure exerted on a limited donor pool continues to increase. Donors who have not previously been used are being considered, and more attention is focused on artificial support systems and the area of xenotransplantation.

This chapter attempts to put into perspective some of the areas of research and development that may affect the future of transplantation. References to other chapters detail the developments in those areas that are worth mentioning in the context of future developments in the field of organ transplantation. It is not possible here to mention all of the various fields that may affect the future of transplantation, and omission of an area of interest does not in any way suggest that such an area is not important.

UPDATE ON SUCCESSFUL SOLID-ORGAN TRANSPLANTATION

In 1984, the National Organ Transplant Act (NOTA) was passed by the Congress of the United States. This act called for formation of an organ procurement network and a scientific registry (see Chapter 175). In 1987, the United Network of Organ Sharing (UNOS) was awarded a contract by the Health Resources and Services Administration to maintain a scientific registry for organ transplantation. One of the purposes of the registry is to collect and analyze data regarding the success of organ transplantation and the factors that are important in determining success. This registry represents one of the first attempts to examine the role of donor and recipient characteristics, as well as center-specific parameters, that affect organ transplantation. The factors analyzed have included (1) age and race of the recipient, (2) risk factors in the recipient population, and (3) the medical urgency of the recipient population. These factors were then applied to national and center-specific outcomes. In 1992, the first Report of Center-Specific Graft and Patient Survival Rates was published[15]; it was followed by two additional analyses, in 1994[16] and 1997.[17] The data cited in the following pages have been abstracted from published UNOS statistics in the 1997 Annual Report for the United States experience.[18] In all organ transplant types, the registry has recorded an improvement in patient and graft survival during the period that has been analyzed. This improvement is in part related to better medical management, greater experience at the individual transplant centers, and changing recipient characteristics.

Kidney

The current 1-year patient survival rate for cadaveric kidney transplants is 94.7%, which is slightly lower, at 88%, by 3 years after transplantation; The 1- and 3-year graft survival rates are 86.6% and 72.1%, respectively. A patient whose kidney allograft fails can be put back on dialysis support, accounting for the significant differences between patient and graft survival rates.

The following factors appear to adversely affect the success of cadaveric kidney transplants:

1. Repeat transplants (~6% worse 3-year graft survival than first-time kidney transplant).
2. Blacks as recipients (~10% worse 3-year graft survival rates compared with white recipients; ~15% worse 3-year graft survival rates compared with Asian recipients).
3. Poor histocompatibility (HLA) matching (14% worse 3-year graft survival rates in the worst match compared with the best match).
4. Very young (<5 years of age) or very old (>65 years of age) recipients.

The corresponding biologic explanations for these risk factors are as follows:

1. Greater likelihood of sensitization of the recipient in repeated transplantation.
2. Worse matching characteristics in the black population than in white and Asian populations.
3. The role of histocompatibility, as determined by HLA matching, in the intensity of the rejection process.
4. Concurrent medical problems in the elderly and greater technical complications in the very young.

Living donors have been used for kidney transplantation since the earliest attempts at kidney transplantation. The overall graft and patient survival rates for recipients of living donor kidneys are better than for recipients of cadaveric kidney transplants. The 1- and 3-year patient survival rates for living donor recipients are 97.9% and 94.7%, respectively; the corresponding 1- and 3-year graft survival rates are 93.3% and 85.2%. Many of the risk factors that adversely influence graft survival in cadaveric kidney recipients also apply in living donor recipients. The biologic explanation for the better graft and patient survival rates in the living donor group compared with the cadaveric organ recipients is principally related to closer HLA matching and better-quality kidney allografts, with improved early graft function. The onset of early acute tubular necrosis after kidney transplantation, from either preservation or immunologic causes, has a deleterious effect on graft survival.

Liver

The current 1- and 3-year patient survival rates after liver transplantation are 87.0% and 77.4%, respectively; the corresponding graft survival rates are 79.1% and 66.4%. Unlike failure of kidney transplantation, failure of a liver graft results in a patient's death unless the patient undergoes retransplantation.

The risk factors associated with poorer outcomes in liver transplantation are as follows:

1. Older (>65 years of age) recipient age (3-year patient survival rate for this group is 8% less than the mean rate).
2. Repeat transplants (3-year survival rate for recipient of previous transplants was 23.5% less than for those receiving only one transplant).
3. Asian race (3-year survival rate for this group was 11.4% less than the mean rate).
4. Severity of medical illness at the time of liver transplantation (3-year survival rate of the most critically ill was 24.3% less than for those with little stigmata of chronic liver disease).
5. Primary diagnosis of malignant neoplasm (3-year survival rate for this group is 31.7% less than the mean rate).

For graft survival, the risk factors were similar, although the very young (<1 year of age) recipients had the lowest graft survival (3-year graft survival rate is approximately 9% less than the mean rate).

The corresponding biologic explanations for these risk factors are as follows:

1. Concurrent medical conditions in the elderly.
2. Greater severity of illness in those receiving more than one liver transplant.
3. Higher incidence of hepatitis B and C as well as the presence of primary liver tumors in the Asian recipients compared with other races.
4. Higher risk in sicker patients, related to other organ system involvement such as respiratory or renal failure.

In the pediatric population, a higher rate of technical complications in liver transplantation accounts for the higher graft loss in this group. For several risk factors, the effect on both patient and graft survival appears to occur in the immediate post-transplant period, without a disproportionate loss after the first 3 months.

Heart

The 1- and 3-year patient survival rates after heart transplantation are 85.1% and 76.2%, respectively; the corresponding graft survival rates are 84.5% and 74.2%. The similarity between patient and graft survival rates in heart transplantation is due to the limited retransplantations performed. For heart transplantation, the risk factors that adversely affect both patients and graft survival rates are as follows, listed in order of importance:

1. Very young age (<1 year); both patient and graft survival rates were 14% less in this age group compared with the mean.
2. Severity of medical illness at the time of heart transplantation; recipients with the most critical need for heart transplantation have a 9% worse 3-year outcome than those with minimum heart disease.
3. Women have approximately 3% to 4% worse patient and graft survival rates than men.

The corresponding biologic explanation for the first and third risk factors is the difficulty in obtaining heart grafts of appropriate size for children and for women. The second factor can be explained by the presence of concurrent medical illnesses in those who are critically in need of heart transplantation, as well as the use of biomechanical devices to maintain such patients until transplantation.

Pancreas

Pancreas transplantation has been used in the following three scenarios:

- Pancreas alone, as treatment of type I juvenile-onset diabetes mellitus, without overt renal failure
- Pancreas combined with simultaneous kidney transplantation (SPK), for diabetic patients with renal failure
- Pancreas after successful kidney transplantation (PAK)

Overall, the current 1- and 3-year graft function rates for all pancreas transplants are 79.6% and 67.4%, respectively. In the national experience, patients undergoing SPK have fared the best, with 1- and 3-year graft survival rates of 80.8% and 70.5%, compared with 63.5% and 40.2%, respectively, for pancreas alone; and 72.8% and 41.6%, respectively, for PAK. The biologic explanation for these differences lies in the difficulties in assessing pancreas rejection. In pancreas transplantation, elevation of the serum glucose is often a late sign of rejection, because only 10% of the islet mass may be present before overt diabetes mellitus reappears. Thus, reversal of rejection may not recover sufficient islet function to ensure long-term graft function. In SPK, the kidney has been used as a "window" to assess pancreas rejection. It has been assumed that treatment of kidney rejection will also treat rejection of the pancreas, which is occurring at the same time. In PAK, monitoring of pancreas rejection has been less successful; usually, the HLA types of the original kidney donor and of the pancreas donor are significantly different.

The 1- and 3-year patient survival rates for pancreas transplantation are 93.2% and 86.4%, respectively. For SPK, the corresponding survival rates are 93.2% and 86.4%, which are approximately 1.5% to 11.7% worse than for patients who receive kidney grafts alone. The higher morbidity and mortality rates associated with adding a pancreas transplant at the time of kidney transplantation are related to technical factors in pancreas grafting, such as a higher rate of infections after pancreas transplantation.

Heart-Lung

The number of heart-lung transplants has actually fallen, in part because of a shift of some candidates to just lung transplantation. The patient survival rate is almost identical to the graft survival rate, because retransplantation is rare. The 1- and 3-year survival rates are 74% and 51%, respectively. Because experience with this procedure is limited, detailed analysis of the risk factors is meaningless.

Lung

The patient survival rate after lung transplantation is also similar to the graft survival, owing to the limited experience with retransplantation. The 1- and 3-year patient survival rates are 77% and 58%, respectively; the corresponding graft survival rates are 76% and 55%, respectively. Males tend to have poorer patient and graft survival rates (approximately 4% to 5% lower 1- and 3-year survival rates than for women). The biologic explanation for this difference is not clear but may be related to differences in the indications for lung transplantation between men and women.

Controversies

One of the principal controversies about the meaning of the data cited in this discussion is the effect on national policies regarding organ allocation and possible restriction of transplant services to selected groups of recipients.[19-21] Some researchers have argued that the transplant community should restrict transplants to the patients who have the greatest likelihood of long-term survival, whereas others have viewed transplantation as a means to provide life-saving therapy to patients who have the most to gain (i.e., the most critically ill). For example, the greatest net benefit of liver transplantation is for those patients whose outcomes without transplantation are poor. The net benefit is the difference in survival between those who receive transplants and those who do not. Data derived from UNOS have already shown that this difference (i.e., net benefit) is greater for the sicker patients (on the order of 50% at 1 year) compared with the patients in whom transplantation was performed on the most elective basis (i.e., no difference in survival between those who received transplants and those who remained on the waiting list for more than 2 years).[22]

On April 2, 1998, the U.S. Department of Health and Human Services (DHHS) issued final regulations regarding organ allocation.[23] These regulations require that policies that govern organ allocation must embody the following principles:

1. Equity for patients awaiting organ transplantation as measured by waiting time.
2. Access to transplant center data for patients.
3. A "level playing field" through definition of standard listing and status criteria.
4. Reaffirmation of the role of government oversight as public advocacy.
5. Encouragement of patient participation in transplant issues.

These principles have been advanced by impartial panels. For example, in 1977, the American Medical Association Council on Ethical and Judicial Affairs[24] affirmed that, "Organs should be considered a national, rather than a local or regional, resource. Geographical priorities in the allocation of organs should be prohibited."[24] In 1984, NOTA called for the fair and equitable national allocation of organs. The 1986 recommendations by the U.S. Task Force on Organ Transplantation clearly stated the need to avoid using geography as the basis for organ distribution. Currently, these issues are being debated within the transplant community, and UNOS is leading the opposition to adoption of these regulations; the likelihood that these regulations will be implemented is still unknown. However, in a 1998 editorial published in *The Lancet,* Horton[25] wrote, "UNOS would better serve the transplant community if it abandoned its stance and began working with DHHS to draw up allocation policies that are practical and fair."

IMMUNOLOGIC ADVANCES

Several new developments in the area of immunology and immunosuppression promise to affect organ transplantation in the near future. Chapter 178 has been devoted to the discussion of immunosuppressive agents; attention is given here to two areas that will influence our immunosuppressive management of recipients of solid-organ transplants.

Chimerism

Billingham and colleagues[26, 27] first associated tolerance to skin grafting with hematopoietic mixing or chimerism in freemartin cattle and subsequently verified this finding by injecting viable allogeneic spleen cells into fetuses of the recipient strain. Ildstad and Sachs[28] demonstrated the ability to duplicate mixed allogeneic lymphodendritic chimerism and subsequent tolerance by allogeneic bone marrow transplantation. The concept of natural microchimerism, which develops after solid-organ transplantation, was first suggested by clinical observations of acquisition of delayed-type hypersensitivity in recipients after successful kidney transplantation.[29] This hypothesis was documented years later, after technologic advances allowed for detection of small numbers of donor cells (outside the grafted organ) through the use of immunostaining or polymerase chain reactions (PCRs), in which donor deoxyribonucleic acid is amplified.[30] This pattern of migration of donor-derived cells after transplantation was subsequently found in experimental animal models[31] and in other human organ transplant models, such as liver and small-bowel transplantation.

The functionality of these cells was suggested in a study by Starzl and coworkers,[30] in which an unexpected benefit of transplantation of the liver for type IV glycogen storage disease resulted in reversal of the deposition of the insoluble defective polysaccharide. In this study, donor-derived cells were detected in the heart and other tissues in two patients receiving liver transplants for type IV glycogen storage disease. Similar findings were noted in a transplant recipient with a deficiency of the lysosomal enzyme B glucocerebrosidase, which causes type 1 Gaucher's disease.

A more systematic survey of long-term survivors after liver transplantation was performed with the use of immunostaining and polymerase chain reaction.[32] Of a group of 22 surviving liver transplant recipients who had received their transplants more than 10 years before being studied, all demonstrated systemic tissue microchimerism. The immunologic privilege of the liver, its ability to induce systemic hyporesponsiveness and to protect other organs from rejection, may lie in the relative abundance of migratory cells in the liver compared with other organs, such as the kidney and heart. If this hypothesis is correct, strategies can be developed to identify the cell type and the optimal source of these cells and then to enhance their migration, in an attempt to accentuate the immunomodulating effect of the cells on the recipient immune response.

The effect of the migratory donor cells on the recipient immune response is not clear. It is likely that a number of factors determine the ultimate effect of these cells on allograft survival. First, if insufficient immunosuppression is given in the early phases after transplantation, these cells may be immunogenic and may accentuate the rejection process. Second, if the recipient is made immunoincompetent shortly before transplantation, either by cytoablation or by an imbalance in the number of immunocompetent donor cells given, a graft-versus-host disease (GVHD) process may occur, in turn further suppressing the immunocompetence of the recipient.[33] Third, if an appropriate balance of immunosuppression is given, along with a sufficient number of migratory cells or their precursor stem cells, a phase in which the donor cells can migrate and take residence in the recipient follows a phase in which peripheral anergy or coexistence may occur.[34] Put into an immunologic perspective on tolerance (ranging from chronic infection to autoimmune diseases to transplantation), the outcome of immune effector functions after antigen exposure depends on the dose, timing, route, and localization of the antigen.[35]

A number of observations have suggested these cells are of bone marrow origin. Donor-specific blood transfusions (DSTs) have been shown to enhance long-term graft survival in living donor kidney transplants since the 1970s. Cochrum and associates[36] reported that DSTs improved 1-year graft survival by 57% to 95%. Even in the cyclosporin era, Salvatierra and coworkers[37] reported a 1-year graft survival of 93% in DST-treated patients, compared with 82% in non–DST-treated patients. In addition, Reed and colleagues[38] reported a benefit of DST in reducing both rejection and the need for steroids.[38] Protocols have been developed to infuse donor bone marrow at the time of solid-organ transplantation. Several groups, including ours at the University of Pittsburgh, are currently using cadaveric bone marrow infusion, along with solid-organ transplantation from the same donor, in attempts to enhance the chimerism observed after solid-organ transplantation alone.[39–41]

University of Pittsburgh Experience

At the University of Pittsburgh, since 1992, 226 primary allograft recipients have received perioperative infusion of a single dose of 300 to 500 million unmodified donor bone marrow cells per kg of body weight. The mean recipient and donor ages are 40 years and 29 years, respectively, and follow-up periods have ranged from 3 to 2023 days.

Since April 1996, 39 organ recipients have been included in a protocol involving three daily sequential perioperative infusions of unmodified BM cells (200 million cells/kg/day) from day 0 to 2 post-transplantation. The mean recipient age in this group is 45 years, and the follow-up period has ranged from 4 to 790 days. Control subjects were those organ transplant recipients for whom bone marrow was not available ($n = 131$). Standard immunosuppression in this study consisted of tacrolimus and steroids. Mycophenolate mofetil (MMF) was used in 53 study patients and 17 control patients. In addition to serial monitoring of clinical parameters, peripheral blood from the recipients was screened for the presence of donor cell chimerism (by flow cytometry and PCR) and cellular immune responses (by mixed leukocyte reaction [MLR]). Infusion of bone marrow cells was safe in all cases, and of the 55 grafts (21%) lost in study patients, none could be attributed exclusively to bone marrow infusion. Thirty-one (24%) of the control patients experienced loss of the allograft. A slightly higher incidence (77% versus 63%) of mild to moderate acute cellular rejection (ACR) was observed in the control group.

Heart recipients demonstrated a statistically significant ($P = .006$ by Fisher's exact test) decrease in rejection episodes after BM infusion. Sixty-two per cent of study patients (as opposed to 18% of control patients) were free of rejection (grade 3A or higher) in the first 6 months after transplantation. Lung transplant recipients in the study group also showed a statistically lower incidence of obliterative bronchiolitis (3.8%) than the control group (31%).

Mild, easily reversible GVHD was observed in 1% ($n = 2$) of patients receiving single bone marrow infusions. Contrarily, fulminant GVHD was encountered in 1 of 39 recipients of multiple bone marrow infusions. This individual was a liver recipient, and in patients undergoing liver transplantation, we have reinstituted the single infusion strategy. In those patients evaluated at least 1 year after transplantation, a slightly higher incidence of steroid-free existence was noted in the bone marrow study group (53% versus 40%). This finding was associated with a higher incidence of multilineage donor cell chimerism in study patients (95% of total study group) compared with the controls (53% of total control group). In an evaluation using one-way MLR assays, donor-specific hyporeactivity was witnessed in 57% of bone marrow–augmented liver, lung, and kidney recipients compared with 44% of controls.

Ricordi and colleagues[42] are conducting a similar study at the University of Miami. They have modified the infusion protocol to include the use of one or more donor bone marrow infusions during the early post-transplantation period. This group has suggested that multiple bone infusions are associated with a lower incidence of acute rejection and higher levels of chimerism.[42] In both of these trials, the conclusive clinical endpoint will be to determine the ability to wean bone marrow–infused and control transplant recipients from immunosuppression completely and to determine the incidence of the subsequent development of chronic rejection.

Sirolimus (Rapamycin)

Sirolimus (rapamycin) is a natural fermentation product (macrolide antibiotic) with immunosuppressant properties that acts by inhibiting growth factor signal transduction.[43] Its specific mechanism of action is the blockade of T and B cell responses to stimulating cytokines, thus preventing cell cycle progression in the phase of the cell cycle G_1 and subsequent cellular proliferation.[44] Like cyclosporine, sirolimus is metabolized in the cytochrome P_{4503A} pathway and is a substrate for p-glycoprotein countertransport.[45] Animal studies have shown that when combined with standard immunosuppressive therapy, sirolimus allows for the reduction of individual drug dosages and leads to a remarkable decrease in the incidence of acute rejection.[46] Although some studies found sirolimus levels to be consistently higher when the drug was administered concomitantly with cyclosporine,[45] others found no pharmacokinetic interaction between the two agents.[47] Sirolimus prevented accelerated atherosclerosis in synergism with mycophenolic acid and reduced transplant vasculopathy.[48, 49] This drug has also been said to have a putative beneficial role in the treatment and prevention of obliterative bronchiolitis when used in combination with other immunosuppressive agents in heart-lung transplantation.[50]

Toxicities associated with sirolimus include thrombocytopenia, leukopenia, increased cholesterol levels, elevated triglyceride levels, anorexia, vomiting, diarrhea, diabetes mellitus, myocardial necrosis, and testicular atrophy.[44, 51-54] Hypertension, nephrotoxicity, and hepatotoxicity have not been reported,[52, 55] although potentiation of cyclosporine nephrotoxicity by sirolimus has been reported.[56] In vitro studies suggest that it may also have neurotoxic potentials.[57] Sirolimus is now in phase III trials for renal transplant recipients; preliminary results indicate a decrease in acute rejection when sirolimus is used in combination with cyclosporine.[58]

SDZ RAD (40-O-(2-hydroxyethyl)-rapamycin), a rapamycin analog, also acts by inhibiting growth factor–driven cell proliferation. Although it has less in vitro activity compared with sirolimus, SDZ RAD has similar immunosuppressive properties when given orally.[59, 60] Clinical trials of this agent are currently under way.

APPLICATIONS TO NEW ORGAN TRANSPLANTATION

One way to assess the impact of a new immunosuppressive agent in transplantation is the ability to successfully transplant organs that were not considered feasible for transplantation with standard immunosuppression. This was certainly the situation when cyclosporine was introduced to liver transplantation. Chapters 182 to 184 deal with the topics of lung, pancreas, and intestinal transplantation, respectively; a brief reference to the impact of tacrolimus in these organ transplants is provided here.

Intestinal Transplantation

Success with intestinal transplantation using cyclosporine immunosuppression has been sporadic.[61-63] A growing experience of small-bowel transplantation, either alone or combined with other abdominal organs, with tacrolimus immunosuppression has been accumulated at the University of Pittsburgh,[64-66] the University of Miami,[67] the University of Nebraska,[68] and the University Hospital in London, Ontario.[69] At the University of Pittsburgh, small-bowel allografts have been transplanted alone (n = 37), along with livers (n = 50), or as part of multivisceral clusters (n = 17) using tacrolimus immunosuppression. Of the 98 patients who received these 104 allografts, 48% were alive at a mean follow-up of 32 months. The actuarial 1- and 5-year patient survival rates are 72% and 48%, respectively. Graft function was satisfactory, with 91% of survivors being enterally sustained and the other 9% relying on supplemental parenteral nutrition. Rejection was common; 90% of the patients had at least one episode of rejection of the intestinal allograft. The high incidence of rejection may be altered by the addition of some of the newer immunosuppressive agents discussed in Chapter 178.

Lung Transplantation

Lung transplantation is a rapidly developing procedure that has been limited for technical, preservation, and immunologic reasons. A prospective, randomized trial of primary adult pulmonary transplantation using tacrolimus immunosuppression was conducted at the University of Pittsburgh.[70] Sixty-six patients were randomly assigned to receive tacrolimus immunosuppression, and 66 patients to receive cyclosporine immunosuppression. Although 1- and 2-year patient survival rates were not statistically significantly different for the two regimens, there was a trend toward increased survival in the tacrolimus group. In addition, obliterative bronchiolitis developed in significantly fewer patients in the tacrolimus group (22%) than in the cyclosporine group (38%).

In light of the lung allograft shortage, the utility of single lung transplantation rather than double lung transplantation for pulmonary hypertension has been established,[71] although other indications, such as cystic fibrosis, preferentially require double lung transplantation.[72] The organ shortage is reflected by a high incidence of deaths of patients on the waiting list.[73] Other approaches to increasing lung allograft availability are the development of living related donor bilateral lobar lung transplantation.[74, 75] The results reported from the University of Southern California revealed survival outcomes similar to those for transplantation from cadaveric donors, with no donor mortality and a complication rate of 10%.[74]

Islet Cell Transplantation

For treatment of type I diabetes mellitus, islet cell transplantation would be preferable to whole pancreas transplantation. The morbidity and mortality associated with transplantation of the exocrine component of whole pancreas are well known. A number of investigators have developed automated systems of enzymatic and mechanical separation that have improved previous methods of islet cell isolation.[76, 77] Application of this technique has proved to be applicable to clinical situations through infusion of purified islets into liver allografts, during combined liver-islet transplantation, and has resulted in long-term islet function in selected cases of surgically induced diabetes mellitus.[78] The early experience with islet transplantation for treatment of juvenile-onset type I diabetes mellitus was less successful, although C-peptide secretion was almost uniformly observed.[79] With improved isolation and immunosuppression, several cases of exogenous insulin freedom have been noted in patients undergoing combined kidney–islet cell transplantation.[80] The technical and immunologic factors are still being investigated.[81, 82] However, its general clinical application awaits demonstration of improvements in long-term insulin freedom.[83]

ADVANCES AND INNOVATIONS IN SUPPORT SYSTEMS

Extracorporeal Liver Assist Device

Acute liver insufficiency can present as either fulminant hepatic failure (FHF) or primary nonfunction (PNF) of liver allografts after liver transplantation. The clinical presentation is acute liver failure complicated by hepatic encephalopathy either in a previously healthy person (FHF) or after liver transplantation (PNF). Survival with either FHF or PNF is poor, particularly for patients suffering advanced encephalopathy with development of the hepatorenal syndrome, systemic lactic acidosis, and severe coagulopathy. The morbidity and mortality of FHF and PNF cannot be underestimated. The mortality rate of FHF is 60% to 95%; it is higher for FHF owing to virus or toxic exposure, and lower in patients with FHF owing to acetaminophen overdose. PNF occurs in up to 10% of patients after liver transplantation; contributing factors include donor instability and length of preservation times, although many cases of PNF have no predisposing factors. Mortality associated with PNF is approximately 40% to 50%, even after retransplantation.

Management of both PNF and FHF is challenging and is aimed at prevention and treatment of complications, including infections, brain edema, hemodynamic instability, pulmonary and renal failure, acid-base disturbances, and coagulopathy. Orthotopic liver transplantation has increasingly been used for selected patients with FHF, whereas orthotopic retransplantation is the only procedure of choice in patients with PNF.

The concept of using mechanical devices to maintain patients with PNF or FHF until transplantation is an attractive one. Nevertheless, dialysis and charcoal hemoperfusion are not of proven benefit because (1) the multiple biochemical functions are not being replaced and (2) their use has not decreased the mortality in patients with FHF.[84, 85] Three proposed systems have used a hybrid device containing metabolically active liver cells.

Laboratory models have attempted to use primary hepatocyte cultures isolated from either animal or human livers; however, the inability to grow such cells in vitro has limited the practicality of this source of cells. Rozga and coworkers[86] have used a liver support system consisting of plasma separation and perfusion through a charcoal filter and hollow-fiber cartridge with porcine hepatocytes attached to collagen-coated dextran microcarrier beads, which are then placed into the extracapillary space of a hollow-fiber cartridge. Plasma is passed through the intracapillary space, and the porcine hepatocytes are separated from the plasma by the cartridge membrane. In a case report of a patient with FHF, total hepatectomy with extracorporeal liver support was able to support the patient until orthotopic liver transplantation could successfully be completed. In this case, intracranial pressures and serum ammonia were thought to be controlled with the use of the porcine hepatocyte–extracorporeal liver assist device (ELAD) system.

Watanabe and colleagues,[87] in a phase I clinical trial, reported encouraging results with the extracorporeal bioartificial liver. Their experience involved a total of 31 patients. Of 18 patients with a diagnosis of FHF, 16 were maintained successfully until transplantation and one until recovery of native liver function. Of three patients with PNF, all were successfully maintained by the device until retransplantation. The remaining 10 patients had a diagnosis of acute exacerbation of chronic liver disease. Two of these were successfully maintained until recovery and transplantation. The other eight did not qualify for transplantation but were successfully treated with the bioartificial liver prior to their deaths. There were decreases in ammonia, bilirubin, and transaminase levels after treatment with the liver assist device. Coagulation parameters, including prothrombin time, did not improve. There was an improvement (increase) in the ratio of branched chain amino acids to aromatic amino acids.

The system described by Sielaff and colleagues[88] at the University of Minnesota is similar in concept to the porcine hepatocyte–ELAD described above but uses a three-compartment collagen gel entrapment of porcine hepatocytes in the lumens of hollow-fiber cartridges. Blood is passed through the extracapillary space, but the hepatocytes are protected from immune damage by the cartridge membrane.[89] This system is being launched for phase I human trials.

The third ELAD system is based on the use of a subclone of HepG2 (HepG2/C3), a human hepatoblastoma cell line that expresses nearly normal levels of several central metabolic pathways and has the morphology and polarity characteristic of human hepatocytes.[90] HepG2/C3 can be grown in hollow-fiber cartridges, with the intention of developing an extracorporeal liver assist device (C3-ELAD). Six human patients have been treated with C3-ELAD.[91] All of the patients had advanced encephalopathy at the start of therapy, and all were in an intensive care unit (ICU). The devices were used for between 24 hours and 6 days. Improved clinical status, such as mental status, was noted in three of the six patients. One patient recovered completely from FHF, apparently as a result of C3-ELAD. Two other patients first improved but died of non–liver-related causes, one from sepsis 3 days after discontinuation of C3-ELAD therapy, and the other of brain death following a period of hypotension not thought to be related to C3-ELAD therapy. The remaining three patients died, one during an unrelated diagnostic procedure, one owing to technical inability to continue C3-ELAD therapy, and one because of advanced metabolic derangements related to liver failure.

A larger trial of this device was performed at the King's College Hospital, where a randomized trial of C3-ELAD was compared with a control regimen. Although the patients receiving C3-ELAD therapy were noted to have a higher level of improvement in encephalopathy, survival was not different.[92] Unfortunately, the unknown risk that immunosuppressed patients may be inoculated with tumor cells in the advent of a break in the hollow fibers, along with logistic difficulties, ended this trial.

Hepatocytes obtained from livers considered unsuitable for transplantation have been isolated and determined to be viable.[93] All organs had been excluded primarily because of steatosis, although advanced donor age was a significant secondary consideration. These cells exhibited decreased length of viability in cell culture compared with hepatocytes obtained from fresh surgical specimens. However, evidence of hepatocyte-specific function was shown by their ability to metabolize diazepam and lidocaine. Intrasplenic hepatocyte transplantation has been shown to improve the survival of laboratory animals with liver failure and to lead to an improvement in associated physiologic liver-based abnormalities.[94] The exact use of isolated hepatocytes and their human application is still to be determined.

Strom and coworkers[95] have used human hepatocytes to maintain patients with FHF until liver transplantation. Five hepatocyte-treated patients were successfully maintained until liver transplantation, with improvement in cerebral perfusion and cardiac stability. In one published report, the use of allogeneic hepatocytes partially reversed a liver disease due to an inborn error of metabolim, Crigler-Najjar syndrome.[96]

Some investigators have expressed concern for risk of disease transmission from the use of animal hepatocytes, although human blood does not directly contact the animal hepatocytes. Swine herds can be maintained in specific pathogen-free facilities, and known pathogens, such as *Brucella,* can be screened out. The discovery of a pig endogenous retrovirus (PERV)[97] that can be transmitted to human cells in culture, however, has raised safety concerns.[98] Given the issues related to organ shortage and the need for support of patients with acutely failing livers, cautious exploration of bioartificial liver support devices appears warranted, in order to identify those areas that will require further study. Technologic advances and better screening tools are likely to identify donor livers that may harbor latent infections.

Bioartificial Pancreas

Unlike totally artificial pancreas devices (in which exogenous insulin is placed into a pump and delivered via a glucose sensor),[99] bioartificial pancreas devices rely on the presence of the natural glucose homeostasis mechanisms of the beta cell. Biohybrid artificial pancreatic devices have been made in which cultured cell lines derived from pancreatic islet cells were placed within three-layered encapsulating microbeads, were inserted subcutaneously, and functioned in a rat model.[100] Bioartificial constructs with transformed cells have also been suggested as an alternative, given the scarcity of islets cells.[101] Encapsulated xenografted islets were found to control carbohydrate metabolism in pregnant diabetic animals and may eliminate the higher incidence of fetal malformations observed in diabetic pregnancies.[102]

Artificial Heart Assist Devices

Owing to the success of heart transplantation, artificial heart assist devices have been used primarily to maintain patient survival until the time of transplantation. Power supplies and the complications arising from the interaction of a foreign surface with the blood remain major issues still to be resolved. Animal studies have employed electromechanical artificial hearts of reduced dimensions driven by transcutaneous energy systems that may evolve into devices of permanent implantation for humans. Several systems (Novacor, Thoratec, HeartMate) have been tested in humans, primarily as bridges to heart transplantation.[103-105] Although these devices are effective in restoring cardiac output and reversing the sequelae of cardiogenic shock, major complications have included driveline infection and thromboembolic strokes.

The U.S. Food and Drug Administration (FDA) granted approval for the use of a Ventricular Assist Device (VAD) System in patients recovering from open-heart surgery. The device, manufactured by Thoratec Laboratories of Pleasanton, Calif., has already been approved for use as a bridge prior to cardiac transplantation. This makes the VAD System the only device clinically available in the United States for the treatment of patients on a short-term or long-term basis. It remains to be determined whether these devices will be cost effective compared with heart transplantation and prolonged medical therapy.[106]

EXPANSION OF THE DONOR POOL

Non–Heart-Beating Donors

Before the acceptance of brain death, the heart function of any organ donor was required to have ceased before the organs could be procured for transplantation. In some countries where brain death legislation has not been passed, non-heart-beating donors (NHBDs) represent the principal source of organs for transplantation. Four distinct populations of NHBDs have been identified and are classified as follows by Kootstra[107]:

1. Uncontrolled cardiopulmonary arrest—dead on arrival.
2. Uncontrolled cardiopulmonary arrest—declared dead following unsuccessful cardiac resuscitation in hospital.
3. Cardiac arrest under conditions of removal from life support, without fulfillment of criteria for brain death.
4. Cardiac arrest in a brain-dead patient.

The first situation is unlikely to generate usable organs, because the warm ischemic time would be unknown. In the second scenario, reasonable expectation of organ survival would require either immediate procurement of organs or infusion of preservation solution into the individual pronounced dead in a setting where family consent may not be available. A pilot study of such a procedure has been initiated by the Regional Organ Bank of Illinois; it is based on in situ perfusion of the abdominal aorta with a double-balloon catheter.[108] The fourth situation does not require any consideration except expedient procurement of organs, because consent for organ donation has generally been obtained.

The third situation is that of using organs from a patient who does not yet fulfill brain death criteria but for whom a desire has been expressed, by either the patient or the family, for the removal of life support so that the patient may become an organ donor after the declaration of death. Such a protocol has been developed by the University of Pittsburgh Medical Center and the Center for Organ Recovery and Education, which is the organ procurement organization associated with the geographic area of Pittsburgh. This protocol was developed in response to a perception that some families wished to have the right to terminate life support and to donate organs. After lengthy review, a protocol was implemented in 1992.

The details of this protocol are worth discussing, because they may form a foundation for further developments in this field. The interest in using NHBDs is indicated by the development of protocols among organ procurement organizations (OPOs) in the United States and the potential controversies they generate.[109, 110] In 1997, in Cleveland, Ohio, the lack of clarity in one set of protocols for organ procurement generated controversy that resulted in their withdrawal by the OPO concerned.[111] In addition, the lack of uniform criteria and policies for NHBDs was the topic of the 1997 hearings conducted by the Institute of Medicine (IOM) and of its subsequent report.[112] This issue is particularly important given the growing utilization of NHBDs in the United States. According to the 1997 Annual UNOS Report, NHBDs accounted for 1% of all cadaveric donors from 1994 to 1996 (162 of 15,874).[18]

A number of principles have been suggested for a NHBD protocol to ensure that patients, health care providers, and potential recipients are safeguarded.[112] The most important recommendations are summarized here:

1. Written, locally approved NHBD protocols.
2. Public openness of NHBD protocols.
3. Case-by-case decisions on anticoagulants and vasodilators.
4. Family consent for premortem cannulation.
5. Safeguards against conflict of interest—separate times and personnel for important decisions.
6. Determination of death in controlled NHBDs as cessation of cardiopulmonary function for at least 5 minutes as indicated by electrocardiographic and arterial pressure monitoring.
7. Family options (e.g., attendance at life support withdrawal) and financial protection.

A report by Yokoyama and coworkers[113] from Japan revealed that the 1-year graft survival rates of 110 kidney allografts taken from NHBDs were similar to those reported for organs from brain-dead NHBDs. At the University of Pittsburgh, similar results have been obtained for both kidney and liver allografts taken from NHBDs.[114] Cho and associates[115] compared the early function and survival of more than 200 kidneys from NHBDs with those of more than 8700 control grafts from donors with heart beats. Graft survival rate at 1 year was 83% for the former and 86% for the latter; 48% of recipients of NHBD kidneys required dialysis within the first week after transplant, compared with 22% of the control group. Despite the delayed function, however, survival rates were high for both groups. Primary failure rate was 4% for NHBD kidneys and 1% for kidneys from donors with heart beats. Among NHBD kidneys, grafts from donors who died as a result of trauma had a statistically significant better 1-year survival than grafts from donors who had died of other causes.[115]

Xenotransplantation

To understand the trends in the development of xenotransplantation, we must realize that potential donors for cross-species transplantation into humans can be separated into two groups. Donors can be considered either discordant or concordant. A *discordant* combination is characterized by the presence of a preformed antibody in the recipient, usually at high titers, that reacts and causes hyperacute rejection of the donor organ. *Concordant* combinations are generally characterized by low or nonexistent antibodies, so that the resultant rejection process resembles that of an allograft.[116] For example, transplants from primates into humans are usually concordant, whereas cross-species transplant from a pig into a human would be discordant.

In animal studies, the organ rejection in concordant combinations usually occurs in a different time frame from that in discordant combinations. Livers and hearts from an untreated discordant combination are rejected by antibodies within minutes to hours after revascularization. These organs would be rejected days to weeks after transplantation in an untreated concordant combination. We also realize that liver grafts are less susceptible to antibody-mediated injury than kidney or heart grafts. This difference has been used in some attempts at clinical xenotransplantation, with the expectation that liver xenografts may be more likely to succeed than other types of xenografts.

If one follows this train of thought, liver xenografts may be envisioned in three different clinical settings. The first would be to use liver xenografts as a temporary support, either until the liver recovers from injury or as a "bridge" to transplantation. These organs could be perfused outside the recipient, in an ex vivo manner. Such an approach was reported in a number of early experiences in the 1960s and again by the Johns Hopkins University and Duke University groups.[117] In the second situation, heterotopic liver xenotransplantation might be envisioned as a bridging method until an appropriate human liver is found. Finally, permanent orthotopic replacement of a diseased liver with a liver xenograft can be considered as a definitive procedure that may potentially expand the donor pool.

Several general therapeutic considerations may be taken into account in xenotransplantation. The first deals directly with the selection of an appropriate donor species. If an initial high titer of cytotoxic antibodies is noted in the recipient, these antibodies must be depleted. The depletion can be achieved either specifically, by immunoabsorption, or nonspecifically, by removal of plasma immunoglobulins. Once a suitable environment is created, in which the likelihood of hyperacute rejection is reduced, one must sustain a low titer of cytotoxic xenoantibody levels in the early post-transplant period, usually by pharmacologic methods. The second consideration is to minimize the inflammatory cascades that amplify the immune system. Specifically, complement activation leads to a number of inflammatory mediators that are difficult to control. Agents that can interfere with this cascade and the subsequent inflammatory mediators must be developed. Finally, sustained suppression of cell-mediated rejection is important to minimize the long-term damage to the xenograft that may occur via lymphocyte-derived cytokines.

Other considerations regarding the success of xenotransplants depend on the compatibility of proteins between the donor and recipient species[118] as well as potential for infectious diseases.[119] These are areas of immense interest to physicians studying xenotransplantation. Although three liver xenotransplantations have failed, the longest remaining viable for 72 days, important facts about the pathology, immunology, compatibility, and physiology were obtained and will aid in future attempts.[120-122] Although the baboon-to-human xenotransplants were encouraging, the limiting factors in the pursuit of concordant xenotransplantation are "humanization of primates," limited availability, donor size incongruity, and the theoretical risk of transmitting infectious agents. These concerns have prompted a quest to seek alternative sources of animals for clinical xenotransplantation.

Pigs are available in sufficient quantities, are similar in anatomy and physiology to humans, and can be bred under conditions where they can be genetically modified. These factors have prompted the consideration of this species as a source for clinical xenotransplantation, but hyperacute rejection mediated by naturally occurring antibodies (also called "preformed xenoantibodies") presents a formidable challenge. Because of the difficulty in controlling hyperacute rejection, novel approaches are required to overcome this barrier to successful discordant xenotransplantation.

One strategy that has been utilized is the removal of preformed antibodies from the recipient's blood prior to transplantation (a process known as *plasmapheresis*). Although this approach has been utilized in ABO blood type–incompatible human-to-human transplants with some success, its application in xenotransplantation has been limited, owing to the rapidity with which the preformed xenoantibodies are produced, resulting in rapid restoration of xenoantibody levels and leading to hyperacute rejection.[122] Strategies to eliminate xenoantibody production have not been successful, and alternative approaches must therefore be taken. Preformed xenoantibodies play a vital role in mediating hyperacute rejection, but they are not the effector molecules responsible for the observed damage in discordant xenografts. Antibody binding to the xenograft results in activation of another family of proteins, complement, which is normally present in circulating blood. These proteins exist in an inactive form but are activated when antibody binds to the target cells, resulting in damage to the cell. Normally, this process is self-limited by a process of inactivation by a group of cell surface–associated proteins called *complement inhibitory proteins*. Why, then, is activated complement in the discordant xenograft not rendered inert by these complement inhibitory proteins?

Complement inhibitory proteins can interact only with complement of the same species and not with that of different species *(homologous species restriction)*; this limitation may play an important role in liver xenotransplantation, because the liver is the primary source of complement synthesis.[123] Thus, following pig-to-human xenotransplantation, activated human complement will not be inactivated by the complement inhibitory proteins found on pig cells. One unique approach to this problem entails expressing human complement inhibitory proteins on pig cells; this has been achieved by generating genetically modified pigs that carry the genes for human complement inhibitory proteins. Organs obtained from these transgenic pigs enjoy prolonged survival when transplanted across discordant barriers, suggesting that the human complement inhibitory proteins inserted genetically into the pig organ can overcome hyperacute rejection.[124-126] In these recipients, however, xenograft rejection still occurs by less understood mechanisms, including antibody-directed cell-mediated cytotoxicity. This finding suggests that additional approaches must be employed to overcome the immunologic barrier of xenotransplantation.[127]

SUMMARY

The field of transplantation has grown tremendously in the 45 years since the first successful human organ transplant. A better understanding of the immune mechanisms that cause graft damage, as well as new immunosuppressive agents, has helped put transplantation in a therapeutic realm. Unfortunately, with the success of transplantation, the scarcity of donor organs remains one of the principal limitations for broader applications. More than 7000 patients die every year while waiting for an organ; in the United States, for every individual who receives a transplant, three others are added to the waiting list. Efforts are constantly made to expand the donor pool, either by the use of donors who do not fulfill the criteria once applied to living donors or by xenotransplantation. Each of the next advances in the expansion of the donor pool is likely to generate controversy and will require careful scientific approaches to ensure the safety of the recipients. Other developments in the areas of bioartificial—totally artificial support devices and xenotransplantation—are of significant interest, because their successful development will address the organ shortage problem.

References

1. Carrel A: La technique opératoire des anastomose vasculares et la transplantation des viscères. Lyon Médicine 1902; 98:859.
2. Voronoy VV: Blocking the reticuloendothelial system in man in some forms of mercuric chloride intoxication and transplantation of the cadaver kidney as a method of treatment for the anuria resulting from the intoxication. Transplant Sci 1991; 1:71.
3. Merrill JP, Murray JE, Harrison JH, et al: Successful homotransplantation of the human kidney between identical twins. JAMA 1956; 160:277.
4. Gibson T, Medawar PB: Fate of skin homografts in man. J Anat 1942; 77:299.
5. Calne RY, Murray JE: Inhibition of the rejection of renal homografts in dogs by Burroughs Wellcome 57-222. Surg Forum 1961; 12:118.
6. Starzl TE, Marchioro TL, Waddell WR: The reversal of rejection in human renal homografts with subsequent development of homograft tolerance. Surg Gynecol Obstet 1963; 117:385.
7. Reemtsma K, McCracken BH, Schlegel JU, et al: Renal heterotransplantation in man. Ann Surg 1964; 160:384.
8. Report of the Ad Hoc Committee of the Harvard Medical School: A definition of irreversible coma. JAMA 1968; 205:537.
9. Starzl TE, Miller C, Broznick B, et al: An improved technique for multiple organ harvesting. Surg Gynecol Obstet 1987; 165:343.
10. Collins GM, Bravo-Shugarman M, Terasaki PI: Kidney preservation for transportation. Lancet 1969; 2:1219.
11. Belzer FO, Southard JH: Principles of solid organ preservation by cold storage. Transplantation 1988; 45:673.
12. Borel JF, Feurer C, Gubler HU, et al: Biological effects of cyclosporin A: A new antilymphocytic agent. Agents Actions 1976; 6:468.
13. Calne RY, Rolles K, White DJG, et al: Cyclosporin A initially as the only immunosuppressant in 34 recipients of cadaveric organs: 32 kidneys, 2 pancreata, and 2 livers. Lancet 1979; 2:1022.
14. Starzl TE, Weil R, Iwatsuki S, et al: The use of cyclosporin A and prednisone in cadaveric kidney transplantation. Surg Gynecol Obstet 1980; 151:17.
15. U.S. Department of Health and Human Services (DHHS): 1991 Report of Center-Specific Graft and Patient Survival Rates. Washington, DC, DHHS, 1991.
16. U.S. Department of Health and Human Services (DHHS): 1994 Report of Center-Specific Graft and Patient Survival Rates. Washington, DC, DHHS, 1994.
17. U.S. Department of Health and Human Services (DHHS): 1997 Report of Center-Specific Graft and Patient Survival Rates. Washington, DC, DHHS, 1997.
18. United Network for Organ Sharing (UNOS) and the U.S. Department of Health and Human Services (DHHS): 1997 Annual Report: The U.S. Scientific Registry of Transplant Recipients and the Organ Procurement and Transplantation Network. Washington, DC, DHHS, 1997.
19. Gaston RS, Ayres I, Dooley LG, et al: Racial equity in renal transplantation: The disparate impact of HLA-based allocation. JAMA 1993; 270:1352.
20. Bronsther O, Fung JJ, Tzakis A, et al: Prioritization and organ distribution for liver transplantation. JAMA 1994; 271:140.
21. Burdick JF, Klein AS, Harper AM, et al: How should livers be allocated in the United States? *In:* Clinical Transplants 1996, Cecka JM, Terasaki PI (Eds). Los Angeles, UCLA Tissue Typing Laboratory, 1997, p 321.
22. Edwards EB, Bennett LE, Daily OP, et al: The relative risk of mortality for UNOS Status 3 liver recipients: A comparison of the risk post-transplant to the risk on the waiting list (Abstract). Presented at the 16th International Congress of the Transplantation Society, Barcelona, August 25–30, 1996.
23. U.S. Department of Health and Human Services: Organ Procurement and Transplantation Network (42 CFR, § 121)—Final Rule. RIN: 0906-AA 32, Docket No: 98-HRSA-01. 63 Federal Register 16295–16338 (1998).
24. American Medical Association (AMA) Council on Ethical and Judicial Affairs: Code of Medical Ethics—Current Opinions with Annotations. Chicago, AMA, 1997, pp 31–32.
25. Horton R: Changing the U.S. transplant system (Editorial). Lancet 1998; 352:79.
26. Billingham R, Lampkin G, Medawar P, et al: Tolerance of homografts, twin diagnosis, and the freemartin condition in cattle. Heredity 1956; 6:201.
27. Billingham RE, Brent L, Medawar PB: "Actively acquired tolerance" of foreign cells. Nature 1953; 172:603.
28. Ildstad ST, Sachs DH: Reconstitution with syngeneic plus allogeneic or xenogeneic bone marrow leads to specific acceptance of allografts or xenografts. Nature 1984; 307:168.
29. Wilson WEC, Kirkpatrick CH: Immunologic aspects of renal homotransplantation. *In:* Experience in Renal Transplantation. Starzl TE (Ed). Philadelphia, WB Saunders, 1964, p 239.
30. Starzl TE, Demetris AJ, Trucco M, et al: Chimerism after liver transplantation for type IV glycogen storage disease and type I Gaucher's disease. N Engl J Med 1992; 328:745.
31. Murase N, Demetris AJ, Woo J, et al: Lymphocyte traffic and graft-versus-host disease after fully allogeneic small bowel transplantation. Transplant Proc 1991; 23:3246.
32. Starzl TE, Demetris AJ, Trucco M, et al: Systemic chimerism in human female recipients of male livers. Lancet 1992; 340:876.
33. Starzl TE, Demetris AJ, Trucco M, et al: Cell migration and chimerism after whole organ transplantation: The basis of graft acceptance. Hepatology 1993; 17:1127.
34. Nagler A, Ilan Y, Amiel A, et al: Systemic chimerism in sex-mismatched liver transplant recipients detected by fluorescence in situ hybridization. Transplantation 1994; 57:1458.
35. Starzl TE, Zinkernagel RM: The regulation of immune function by antigen migration and localization: With particular reference to infectious and transplantation tolerance. N Engl J Med, in press.
36. Cochrum KC, Salvatierra O, Belzer FO: Correlations between MLC stimulation and graft survival in living related and cadaver transplants. Ann Surg 1974; 180:617.
37. Salvatierra O, Metzer J, Vincenti F: Donor-specific blood transfu-

sions versus cyclosporine—the DST story. Transplant Proc 1987; 19:160.
38. Reed A, Pirsch JD, Armbrust MJ, et al: A comparison of donor-specific and random transfusions in living-related renal transplantation and their effect on steroid withdrawal. Transplant Proc 1991; 23:1321.
39. Rao AS, Fontes P, Zeevi A, et al: Enhancement of donor cell chimerism in whole organ allograft recipient by adjuvant bone marrow transplantation. Transplant Proc 1995; 27:3387.
40. Ricordi C, Karatzas T, Selvaggi G, et al: Multiple bone marrow infusions to enhance acceptance of allografts from the same donor. Ann N Y Acad Sci, 1995; 770:345.
41. Shapiro R, Rao AS, Fontes P, et al: Combined kidney/bone marrow transplantation—evidence of augmentation of chimerism. Transplantation 1995; 59:306.
42. Ricordi C, Karatzas T, Nery J, et al: High-dose donor bone marrow infusions to enhance allograft survival: The effect of timing. Transplantation 1997; 63:7.
43. Suthanthiran M, Strom TB: Mechanisms and management of acute renal allograft rejection. Surg Clin North Am 1998; 78:77.
44. Kelly PA, Gruber SA, Behbod F, et al: Sirolimus, a new, potent immunosuppressive agent. Pharmacotherapy 1997; 17:1148.
45. Kaplan B, Meier-Kriesche HU, Napoli KL, et al: The effects of relative timing of sirolimus and cyclosporine microemulsion formulation coadministration on the pharmacokinetics of each agent. Clin Pharmacol Ther 1998; 63:48.
46. Stepkowski SM, Tian L, Wang ME, et al: Sirolimus in transplantation. Archiv Immunol Ther Exp 1997; 45:383.
47. Ferron GM, Mishina EV, Zimmerman JJ, et al: Population pharmacokinetics of sirolimus in kidney transplant patients. Clin Pharmacol Ther 1997; 61:416.
48. Goggins WC, Risher RA, Cohen DS, et al: Effect of single-dose rapamycin-based immunosuppression on the development of cardiac allograft vasculopathy. J Heart Lung Transplant 1996; 15:790.
49. Schmid C, Heemann U, Azuma H, et al: Rapamycin inhibits transplant vasculopathy in long-surviving rat heart allografts. Transplantation 1995; 60:729.
50. Fahrni JA, Berry GJ, Morris RE, et al: Rapamycin inhibits development of obliterative airway disease in a murine heterotopic airway transplant model. Transplantation 1997; 63:533.
51. Goodyear N, Napoli KL, Murthy JN, et al: Radioreceptor assay for sirolimus in patients with decreased platelet counts. Clin Biochem 1997; 30:539.
52. Murgia MG, Jordan S, Kahan BD: The side effect profile of sirolimus: A phase I study in quiescent cyclosporine-prednisone-treated renal transplant patients. Kidney Int 1996; 49:209.
53. Brattstrom C, Sawe J, Tyden G, et al: Kinetics and dynamics of single dose of sirolimus in sixteen renal transplant recipients. Ther Drug Monit 1997; 19:397.
54. Brattstrom C, Wilczek H, Tyden G, et al: Hyperlipidemia in renal transplant recipients treated with sirolimus (rapamycin). Transplantation 1998; 65:1272.
55. Andoh TR, Burdmann EA, Fransechini N, et al: Comparison of acute rapamycin nephrotoxicity with cyclosporine and FK506. Kidney Int 1996; 50:1110.
56. Andoh TF, Lindsley J, Franceschini N, et al: Synergistic effects of cyclosporine and rapamycin in a chronic nephrotoxicity model. Transplantation 1996; 62:311.
57. Serkova N, Christians U, Flogel U, et al: Assessment of the mechanism of astrocyte swelling induced by the macrolide immunosuppressant sirolimus using multinuclear nuclear magnetic resonance spectroscopy. Chem Res Toxicol 1997; 10:1359.
58. Kahan BD for the Rapamune U.S. Study Group: A phase III comparative efficacy trial of Rapamune in renal allograft recipients (Abstract). Presented at the 17th World Congress of The Transplantation Society, Montreal, July 12–17, 1998.
59. Schuler W, Sedrani R, Cottens S, et al: SDZ RAD, a new rapamycin derivative: Pharmacological properties in vitro and in vivo. Transplantation 1997; 64:36.
60. Schuurman HJ, Cottens S, Fuchs S, et al: SDZ RAD, a new rapamycin derivative: Synergism with cyclosporine. Transplantation 1997; 64:32.
61. Deltz E, Schroeder P, Gebhardt H, et al: Successful clinical small bowel transplantation: Report of a case. Clin Transplant 1989; 3:89.
62. Grant D, Wall W, Mimeault R, et al: Successful small bowel/liver transplantation. Lancet 1990; 335:181.
63. Schroeder P, Goulet O, Lear PA: Small bowel transplantation: European experience (Letter). Lancet 1990; 336:110.
64. Todo S, Tzakis AG, Abu-Elmagd K, et al: Cadaveric small bowel and small bowel–liver transplantation in humans. Transplantation 1992; 53:369.
65. Todo S, Tzakis AG, Abu-Elmagd K, et al: Intestinal transplantation in composite visceral grafts or alone. Ann Surg 1992; 216:223.
66. Abu-Elmagd K, Reyes J, Todo S, et al: Clinical intestinal transplantation: New perspectives and immunologic considerations. J Am Coll Surg 1998; 186:512.
67. Weppler D, Khan R, Fragulidis GP, et al: Status of liver and gastrointestinal transplantation at the University of Miami. *In:* Clinical Transplants 1996. Cecka JM, Terasaki PI (Eds). Los Angeles, UCLA Tissue Typing Laboratory, 1997, pp 187–202.
68. Vanderhoof JA, Langnas AN: Short-bowel syndrome in children and adults. Gastroenterology 1997; 113:1767.
69. Asfar S, Atkison P, Ghent C, et al: Small bowel transplantation: A life-saving option for selected patients with intestinal failure. Dig Dis Sci 1996; 41:875.
70. Keenan RJ, Konishi H, Kawai A, et al: Clinical trial of tacrolimus versus cyclosporine in lung transplantation. Ann Thorac Surg 1995; 60:580.
71. Gammie JS, Keenan RJ, Pham SM, et al: Single- versus double-lung transplantation for pulmonary hypertension. J Thorac Cardiovasc Surg 1998; 115:397.
72. Mendeloff EN, Huddleston CB, Mallory GB, et al: Pediatric and adult lung transplantation for cystic fibrosis. J Thorac Cardiovasc Surg 1998; 115:404.
73. Grover FL, Fullerton DA, Zamora MR, et al: The past, present, and future of lung transplantation. Am J Surg 1997; 173:523.
74. Barr ML, Schenkel FA, Cohen RG, et al: Bilateral lobar transplantation utilizing living related donors. Artif Organs 1996; 20:1110.
75. Starnes VA, Barr ML, Cohen RG, et al: Living-donor lobar lung transplantation experience: Intermediate results. J Thorac Cardiovasc Surg 1996; 112:1284.
76. Ricordi C, Lacy PE, Finke EH, et al: An automated method for the isolation of human pancreatic islets. Diabetes 1988; 37:413.
77. Lakey JR, Warnock GL, Brierton M, et al: Development of an automated computer-controlled islet isolation system. Cell Transplant 1997; 6:47.
78. Carroll PB, Rilo HL, Alejandro R, et al: Long-term (>3-year) insulin independence in a patient with pancreatic islet cell transplantation following upper abdominal exenteration and liver replacement for fibrolamellar hepatocellular carcinoma. Transplantation 1995; 59:875.
79. Ricordi C, Tzakis AG, Carroll PB, et al: Human islet isolation and allotransplantation in 22 consecutive cases. Transplantation 1992; 53:407.
80. Secchi A, Socci C, Maffi P, et al: Islet transplantation in IDDM patients. Diabetologia 1997; 40:225.
81. Jaeger C, Brendel MD, Hering BJ, et al: Progressive islet graft failure occurs significantly earlier in autoantibody-positive than in autoantibody-negative IDDM recipients of intrahepatic islet allografts. Diabetes 1997; 46:1907.
82. Rastellini C, Shapiro R, Corry R, et al: An attempt to reverse diabetes by delayed islet cell transplantation in humans. Transplant Proc 1997; 29:2238.
83. Sutherland DE: Pancreas and islet cell transplantation: Now and then. Transplant Proc 1996; 28:2131.
84. Hughes RH, Williams R: Clinical experience with charcoal hemoperfusion and resin hemoperfusion. Semin Liver Dis 1986; 6:164.
85. O'Grady JG, Gimson AES, O'Brien CJ, et al: Controlled trials of charcoal hemoperfusion and prognostic factors in fulminant hepatic failure. Gastroenterology 1989; 94:1186.
86. Rozga J, Podesta L, LePage E, et al: Control of cerebral edema by total hepatectomy and extracorporeal liver support in fulminant hepatic failure. Lancet 1993; 342:898.
87. Watanabe FD, Mullon CJP, Hewitt WR, et al: Clinical experience with a bioartificial liver in the treatment of severe liver failure: A phase I clinical trial. Ann Surg 1997; 225:484.
88. Sielaff TD, Nyberg SL, Rollines MD, et al: Characterization of the three-compartment gel-entrapment porcine hepatocyte bioartificial liver. Cell Biol Toxicol 1997; 13:357.

89. Nyberg SL, Platt JL, Shirabe K, et al: Immunoprotection of xenocytes in a hollow fiber bioartificial liver. ASAIO J 1992; 38:M463.
90. Thrift RN, Forte TM, Cahoon BE, et al: Characterization of lipoproteins produced by the human liver cell line, HepG2, under defined conditions. J Lipid Res 1986; 27:236.
91. Sussman NL, Chong MG, Koussayer T, et al: Reversal of fulminant hepatic failure using an extracorporeal liver assist device. Hepatology 1992; 16:60.
92. Ellis AJ, Hughes RD, Wendon JA, et al: Pilot-controlled trial of the extracorporeal liver assist device in acute liver failure. Hepatology 1996; 24:1446.
93. Hewitt WR, Corno V, Eguchi S, et al: Isolation of human hepatocytes from livers rejected for whole organ transplantation. Transplant Proc 1997; 29:1945.
94. Kobayashi N, Ito M, Nakamura J, et al: Hepatocyte transplantation improves liver function and prolongs survival in rats with decompensated liver cirrhosis (Abstract). Presented at the American Society of Transplant Physicians, Chicago, May 13–15, 1998.
95. Strom SC, Fisher RA, Thompson MR, et al: Hepatocyte transplantation as a bridge to orthotopic liver transplantation in terminal liver failure. Transplantation 1997; 63:559.
96. Fox IJ, Chowdhury JR, Kaufman SS, et al: Treatment of the Crigler-Najjar syndrome type I with hepatocyte transplantation. N Engl J Med 1998; 338:1422.
97. Akiyoshi DE, Denaro M, Zhu H, et al: Identification of a full-length cDNA for an endogenous retrovirus of miniature swine. J Virol 1998; 72:4503.
98. Patience C, Takeuchi Y, Weiss RA: Infection of human cells by an endogenous retrovirus of pigs. Nature Medicine 1997; 3:282.
99. Jaremko J, Rorstad O: Advances toward the implantable artificial pancreas for treatment of diabetes. Diabetes Care 1998; 21:444.
100. Kawakami Y, Inoue K, Hayashi H, et al: Subcutaneous xenotransplantation of hybrid artificial pancreas encapsulating pancreatic B cell line (MIN6): Functional and histological study. Cell Transplant 1997; 6:541.
101. Benson JP, Papas KK, Constantinidis I, Sambanis A: Towards the development of a bioartificial pancreas: Effects of poly-L-lysine on alginate beads with BTC3 cells. Cell Transplant 1997; 6:395.
102. Hunter SK, Wang Y, Weiner CP, et al: Encapsulated beta-islet cells as a bioartificial pancreas to treat insulin-dependent diabetes during pregnancy. Am J Obstet Gynecol 1997; 177:746.
103. Koul B, Solem JO, Steen S, et al: HeartMate left ventricular assist device as bridge to heart transplantation. Ann Thorac Surg 1998; 65:1625.
104. Griffith BP, Kormos RL, Nastala CJ, et al: Results of extended bridge to transplantation: Window into the future of permanent ventricular assist devices. Ann Thorac Surg 1996; 61:396.
105. Holman WL, Bourge RC, Spruell RD, et al: Ventricular assist devices as a bridge to cardiac transplantation. A prelude to destination therapy. Ann Surg 1997; 225:695.
106. Cloy MJ, Myers TJ, Stutts LA, et al: Hospital charges for conventional therapy versus left ventricular assist system therapy in heart transplant patients. ASAIO J 1995; 41:M535.
107. Kootstra G: The asystolic, or non-heartbeating, donor. Transplantation 1997; 63:917.
108. Anaise D, Smith R, Ishimaru M, et al: An approach to organ salvage from non-heartbeating donors under existing legal and ethical requirements for transplantation. Transplant Proc 1990; 22:290.
109. Youngner SJ, Arnold RM: Ethical, psychosocial, and public policy implications of procuring organs from non-heart-beating cadaver donors. JAMA 1993; 269:2769.
110. Arnold RM, Youngner SJ (Eds): Ethical, psychosocial, and public policy implications of procuring organs from non-heart-beating cadavers. Kennedy Institute of Ethics Journal 1993; 3:103.
111. Funk J, Mazzolini J: Clinic puts controversial transplant plan on hold. *Cleveland Plain Dealer*, April 4, 1997, p 1.
112. Non-Heart-Beating Organ Transplantation: Medical and Ethical Issues in Procurement. Washington, DC, Division of Health Care Services, Institute of Medicine, National Academy Press, 1997.
113. Yokoyama I, Uchida K, Tominaga Y, et al: Ten-year experience in the use of double balloon catheter for kidney procurement from non-heart beating donors in cadaveric kidney transplant. Clin Transplant 1993; 7:258.
114. Casavilla A, Ramirez C, Shapiro R, et al: Experience with liver and kidney allografts from non-heart beating donors. Transplantation 1995; 59:197.
115. Cho YW, Terasaki PI, Cecka JM, et al: Transplantation of kidneys from donors whose hearts have stopped beating. N Engl J Med 1998; 338:221.
116. Calne RY: Organ transplantation between widely disparate species. Transplant Proc 1970; 2:550.
117. Chari RS, Collins BH, Magee JC, et al: Brief report: Treatment of hepatic failure with ex vivo pig-liver perfusion followed by liver transplantation. N Engl J Med 1994; 331:234.
118. Celli S, Valdivia LA, Fung JJ, et al: Early recipient-donor switch of the complement type after liver xenotransplantation. Immunol Invest 1997; 26:589.
119. Michaels M, Simmons R: Xenotransplant-associated zoonoses. Transplantation 1994; 57:1.
120. Starzl TE, Fung J, Tzakis A, et al: Baboon-to-human liver transplantation. Lancet 1993; 341:65.
121. Manez R, Kelly RH, Marino IR, et al: Complement activation correlates with graft damage in baboon-to-human liver xenotransplantation. Transplant Proc 1994; 26:1249.
122. Makowaka L, Cramer DV, Hoffman A, et al: The use of a pig liver xenograft for temporary support of a patient with fulminant hepatic failure. Transplantation 1995; 59:1654.
123. Valdivia LA, Fung JJ, Demetris AJ, et al: Donor species complement after liver xenotransplantation: The mechanism of protection from hyperacute rejection. Transplantation 1994; 57:918.
124. White DJ, Yannoutsos N: Production of pigs transgenic for human DAF to overcome complement-mediated hyperacute xenograft rejection in man. Res Immunol 1996; 147:88.
125. Heckl-Ostreicher B, Binder R, Kirschfink M: Functional activity of the membrane-associated complement inhibitor CD59 in a pig-to-human in vitro model for hyperacute xenograft rejection. Clin Exp Immunol 1995; 102:589.
126. Fodor W, Williams BL, Matis LA, et al: Expression of a functional human complement inhibitor in a transgenic pig as a model for the prevention of xenogeneic hyperacute organ rejection. Proc Natl Acad Sci U S A 1994; 91:11153.
127. Starzl TE, Rao AS, Murase N, et al: Will xenotransplantation ever be feasible? J Am Coll Surg 1998; 186:383.

186

Utilization and Allocation of Critical Care Resources

I. Alan Fein, MD • Sandra L. Fein, MA, RN

OVERVIEW: THE ETHICS OF UTILIZATION

Utilitarianism is the ethical theory that holds that an action is right if it achieves the greatest good for the greatest number of people. Although the concept of the "greatest good" first appeared in Richard Cumberland's 1672 tract "De Legibus Naturae," it was through Jeremy Bentham in the late 1700s that the term "utilitarianism" originated and became well known. Bentham died in 1832, and his mummified remains have been preserved in a glass case at University College, still dressed in his professorial attire and sitting in his favorite chair. On special occasions, he is trundled out to share a glass of sherry with the university dons. Although Bentham's spirit is with us, he remains trapped in his glass box.

The contemporary medical philosopher Albert Jonsen[1] has likened Bentham's situation to the current dilemmas facing those personnel confronted with the demands of medical resource allocation. Reconciling the needs of the individual with the needs of society has always been problematic, but perhaps never more so than for those now directly confronted with the realities of the utilization and allocation of health care resources. Jonsen notes that "modern health planners are not avid readers of Bentham, Mill, or Sidgewick; they are not utilitarians in theory. But they are, to some extent, utilitarians in practice; the question they ask is whether a particular technology can be shown, in some quantitative way, to effect more benefit than harm in relation to alternatives."

The glass box entrapping modern-day physicians is the conflict between what Jonsen[1] calls the "rule of rescue," or the innate desire to do something, anything, for those in dire need, and Bentham's deontologic imperatives, the inescapable demands to limit care, to not do everything in every single case, so that the greater good for the greatest number prevails. How these conflicting imperatives are reconciled is the challenge for those responsible for the utilization and allocation of critical care resources. Although this statement is true for all branches of medicine, critical care, as the most technology-intensive and most costly of specialties, is under particular scrutiny and pressure to justify its practice and utility.

Economics and Allocation

Critical care medicine came of age in a time when all health care in the United States was and is still undergoing dramatic change. The confluence of multiple forces, including an aging population, a battered economy, technologic advances, and a general awareness that the per capita cost of health care in America far exceeds that of other nations, has acutely forced a reassessment of health care delivery. Indeed, the military-industrial complex of the 1950s and 1960s has now been replaced by the medical-industrial complex as arguably the single predominant industry in the United States. Whereas the restructuring of the health care industry has been ongoing for some years now, resulting in a free-market melange of private practice, health maintenance organizations (HMOs), preferred provider organizations (PPOs), independent practice associations (IPAs), and managed care associations, the demand for change will only accelerate in the immediate future. By its very nature an expensive, technology-driven specialty, critical care will be at the center of the vortex of evolution.

The demand for reform of health care is driven by two powerful forces: The first, and perhaps more potent, is the rapidly escalating cost of health care delivery, clashing with an economy in flux; the second is an aging yet educated population whose expectations of the miracles of modern science border on the unrealistic. Health care costs in the United States exceed $1 trillion, more than 14% of the gross domestic product, and they are increasing at a rate greater than that of inflation. This situation has caused the public and legislators to take serious notice, and many echo the sentiments of the former Governor of Colorado Richard Lamm,[2] who said, "Medical care is a fiscal black hole into which a nation can pour endless wealth. We should not transfer more national assets to health care."

Serious federal attempts to reform health care and control costs began in the early 1970s. One of the major efforts was the passage of the Health Planning and Resource Development Act by Congress in 1974. This act gave states and local agencies the authority to review hospital capital expenditures through "certificates of need." Ostensibly, the goal was to reduce costs by eliminating duplication of services and by generally making institutions "think twice" before they undertake major capital purchases or engage in new construction. It has been estimated that this process has slowed the rate of increase of expenditures by 2% to 3% at best and has significantly increased bureaucracy.[3] Despite all efforts, including the introduction of the Medicare Prospective Payment System in 1983, health care expenditures continued to rise at a rate estimated at threefold to fivefold that of inflation.

By 1990, the United States was spending $2566 per capita on health care—more than twice the average for the Organization for Economic Cooperation and Development, our European counterparts. The United States outspent Canada by 45%, France by 67%, Germany by 73%, Japan by 119%, and the United Kingdom by some 164%.[4] What makes these figures remarkable is that despite these extraordinary expenditures, the United States ranked ninth in hospitalizations per capita of 11 Western industrialized nations examined; ninth in life expectancy at birth for women (11th for men); and 11th for both infant mortality and the incidence of low infant birth weight. Indeed, Sweden's infant mortality rate was 58% that of the United States.[5] In an attempt to explain these apparent discrepancies and to bring the problem into focus, one health care analyst[6] at a national public policy forum made the following suggestion:

> *The areas where the United States has excelled are principally those areas fueled by our inflated spending in health care: medical technology, high-tech therapies, and for-profit medical provider systems. Unfortunately, with an estimated 36 million people uninsured, and an equal number reportedly under-insured, the population as a whole has not received the benefits of this success. In fact, the focus by our leading health care institutions and the media on the success of unusual, high-tech, and expensive therapies serves to underscore the inequities in our current system, where many have limited access to these technologies.*

Ongoing studies continue to document the discrepancies in cost, suggesting that cultural, political, and organizational variations in the delivery of health care underlie these differences.[7]

Intense examination of the U.S. health care system is already under way, and those segments consuming disproportionately large amounts of the health care funds are being examined most closely. Because critical care accounts for more than 20% of acute care hospital charges and for about 1% of the nation's gross domestic product,[8] it is inevitable that this segment of the medical industry will come under the most careful scrutiny. A number of studies have already shown that most health care expenditures are incurred during the last few months of life, suggesting that allocation of resources is less than appropriate.[9]

Surprisingly, for a field that represents such a disproportionately large amount of this nation's resources, very little is known about the efficacy, appropriateness, allocation, or even utilization of expenditures for critical care. Indeed, in a national point-in-time survey of intensive care units (ICUs), the response rate was only 38.7%.[10] It might be speculated that this survey was biased, in that the more functional and organized units would be more likely to respond than those without well-organized leadership. Indeed, the entire issue of the relationships among organization, efficacy, and performance has yet to be clarified.

Public Policy and Allocation

As the intensity of the health care crisis has increased, discussion of "rationing" of health care services has become widespread and now permeates the literature. Although the rationing of health care services remains a politically dangerous concept, de facto rationing by practitioners and policymakers is generally conceded to be common.[11] National public policy seminars have addressed the issue, and one state, Oregon, is engaging in what has been described as "social experimentation" with the rationing of Medicaid expenditures.[12]

In the 1980s, Oregon, like many other states, found that the Medicaid budget was far from adequate and that some 450,000 Oregonians were left without health care coverage. During the 1987 legislative session, Oregon lawmakers decided that the state could no longer afford to spend its Medicaid dollars on high-cost, low-success treatment modalities, such as bone marrow transplantation, if it were to provide more poor Oregonians with health care coverage. Several months later, a young boy receiving Medicaid benefits died after he was denied a bone marrow transplantation procedure. This event elicited a widespread debate that became the focus of tremendous media attention. A variety of committees were established to study the health care issue, including numerous public forums. By 1989, the Oregon Health Plan was passed by the legislature. The approved plan languished in bureaucracy awaiting federal action. In 1993, Oregon obtained a federal waiver that allowed it to proceed with the reallocation of Medicaid funds and that would do the following:

1. Extend Medicaid eligibility to all persons with incomes below the federal poverty level.
2. Define a basic minimum health care package based on a rank-ordered listing of 709 paired medical conditions and treatments. (Treatments were ranked according to estimates of clinical effectiveness, social importance, and quality of life.)
3. Provide a liability shield for medical providers that protects them from both criminal and civil prosecution as well as from professional disciplinary action when they do not provide those services that the legislature has chosen not to fund.

The Oregon Health Plan has great implications for how critical care is provided, regardless of its ultimate success or failure. It has already significantly raised public consciousness about the problems arising from a growing demand for a supply of resources that is no longer unlimited. The term "rationing" has now become part of the medical public policy lexicon and has become the subject of much media attention. It is now common to openly discuss sensitive issues that were usually avoided just a few years ago. As the debate expands and both the general public and the medical and nursing communities become better informed, it becomes possible to develop meaningful policies and solutions to these difficult problems.

When the issue of rationing medical care for the critically ill was discussed at United States public policy development seminars held at the Brookings Institution in 1986 and in 1991, two themes became apparent[13]:

1. Can better ICU management, quality of care, efficiency, and cost containment make unnecessary a national policy that restricts costly but beneficial life-sustaining care, or will critical care units be the motivating force in the evolution of a system similar to that in Great Britain, where beneficial services are limited by overall centralized government budgeting?
2. Should physicians be the ultimate gatekeepers for society in distributing medical services, or should they remain merely the agents for the patients' own medical goals, as called for in Hippocratic tradition? Who else should participate in decisions to limit beneficial services, if at all?

Critical care is an expensive resource that must be managed effectively if we are to avoid compromising the quality of care delivered. Although there is general agreement about this matter, there is little agreement and less information about what constitutes quality care and even less about what is cost effective care. Consequently, rationing not only exists but is growing. Medical ethicists have taken up the issue of rationing and the allocation of resources, as attested by the proliferation of papers on the subject. It is the attending physician, nurse, and patient, however, who are caught between the hammer of reality and the anvil of policy; this is even more true for the nurse and physician directors of critical care units. Their primary responsibility in managing the units is to ensure the appropriateness of care, the quality of care, and, ultimately, the allocation of both care and valued scarce resources.

APPROPRIATENESS OF CARE

It has been suggested,[10, 11] and it is probably safe to assume, that if all health care rendered were appropriate, rationing would not need to be discussed. "Appropriateness" is a difficult term to define and even more difficult to measure, and attempts to do so have not been particularly encouraging.[14] A group from the RAND Corporation attempted a large-scale survey and meta-analysis of the literature to assess the "appropriateness" in health care delivery.[12] They were confronted with a lack of and low quality of information in the literature, but their findings nonetheless are interesting.

Appropriate care can generally be defined as care whose benefits exceed its cost or negative consequences. The definition and measurement of benefit and cost remain elusive yet important goals. *Benefits* usually comprise increased longevity, better quality of life, decreased pain and anxiety, and improved functional capacity. *Costs* should be separated into monetary and nonmonetary categories. Nonmonetary costs, or risks, generally are morbidity, mortality, decreased quality of life, pain, and anxiety. The RAND group suggested that the following three approaches can be used to assess appropriateness, the first two being explicit approaches:

- The *benefit-risk approach,* which excludes monetary cost

- The *benefit-cost approach,* which incorporates the cost both to the patient and society
- The *implicit approach,* which relies on the physician providing service to judge its appropriateness

This last approach is even more subjective than the first two and has the additional hazard of potentially being influenced by monetary benefits to the rating physician. The RAND group found "at least double-digit levels" of inappropriate care [in every study]. . . . In particular, perhaps as much as one fifth to one quarter of acute care services were felt to be used for equivocal or inappropriate reasons."[15] Although most of the studies they examined were not of the ICU setting, there is little to suggest that the findings there would be different.

In a key paper published in 1983, Robin[16] critically examined the workings of ICUs and specifically excluded any discussion of cost effectiveness. He questioned whether critical care resources were, in fact, properly utilized. He suggested that five subpopulations of patients are found in ICUs, as follows[16]:

1. Terminally or hopelessly ill patients for whom intensive care simply prolongs the process of dying.
2. Seriously ill patients who will benefit significantly from improvements in the quantity and quality of life furnished by the interventions provided them in the ICU.
3. Patients who will recover, whether care is provided in the critical care unit or elsewhere.
4. Patients whose lives are shortened or who are made less well specifically because of ICU-related iatrogenic complications.
5. Patients whose lives are shortened or who are made less well because of iatrogenic misadventures not necessarily attributed to their ICU admission.

Robin's concern was that despite the extraordinary expenditures and resources allocated to the care of the critically ill, there is very little information about outcomes and appropriateness of care. There was and continues to be a spectacular paucity of information regarding the utilization of our resources. As Robin concluded:

The purpose of patient management is to optimize the possibility of happy and productive lives for patients. Much of ICU management, like much of modern medicine, may function tangentially to this main purpose. Physicians do harm as well as good. It is important to recognize this, not for the purpose of mea culpa, *but so that the harm can be detected and minimized. The actual balance between good and harm has not been established in ICUs. Many patients admitted are irreversibly ill and some would benefit maximally by not being admitted to an ICU. Some patients are clearly salvaged by ICU admission; others are clearly harmed. The relative distribution of these patients is important to establish in guiding our approach to ICUs generally.*[13]

Since Robin's comments were published in 1983, awareness of the need to examine health care delivery practices for the critically ill has grown, and numerous studies and commentaries, especially in the area of medical ethics, have been made. Indeed, a veritable proliferation of papers focuses largely on those groups of patients whom Robin identified as either not benefiting or actually suffering as a result of admission to the ICU. The withdrawal and withholding of care have received attention, as has the concept of "futile care." Identifying patients for whom further care or admission to the ICU would be futile is important to ensure the appropriate utilization of a scarce resource. The difficulty arises in defining the term futile care and in identifying those patients with a high degree of certainty. Schneiderman and colleagues[17] commented that "futile care" is not necessarily a hopeless effort but, rather, interventions whose expectation of success "is either predictably or empirically so unlikely that its exact probability is often incalculable." The Ethics Committee of the Society of Critical Care Medicine (SCCM)[18] has taken a different stance, suggesting that "treatments should be defined as futile only when they will not accomplish their goal. Treatments that are extremely unlikely to be beneficial, are extremely costly, or are of uncertain benefit may be considered inappropriate and hence inadvisable, but should not be labeled futile."[18]

How mortality prediction models, such as the Acute Physiology and Chronic Health Evaluation (APACHE) and the Mortality Probability Model (MPM) tools, figure into the decision-making process remains to be seen, but they have already contributed significantly to the discussion.[19] The applicability of statistical tools that may be 95% or 99% reliable to real-world decisions raises thorny moral, ethical, and social issues. On the other hand, even when outcome probability data are available, physicians do not necessarily make use of the information, and lengths of stay in the ICU are not necessarily reduced.[20] Indeed, in spite of the advent of evidence-based medicine and the availability of both academic and commercial assessment tools, determining with any certainty what constitutes *appropriate care* remains maddeningly elusive.[21]

UTILIZATION OF CRITICAL CARE UNITS

Although more than 4000 critical care units exist in the United States[10] and these units consume about 1% of the national gross domestic product, it is remarkable that there is so little verified information available regarding the utilization of these expensive resources. It is more than likely that, apart from the types of inappropriate care previously discussed, some populations of patients admitted to critical care units could be cared for in less costly environments. This information is slowly coming to light, and it is clear that a need exists for a national, if not international, data base of information about how health care is delivered to the critically ill.

Henning and associates[22] reviewed 706 medical-surgical patients in ICUs and found that 40% of the medical patients and 30% of the surgical patients never received any ICU intervention and had been admitted strictly for monitoring purposes. These researchers characterized patients using the Acute Physiology Score and found that those with low scores received significantly fewer interventions. Henning and associates[22] also found that as many as 45% of all ICU patients were admitted because they were believed to be at risk for medical or postoperative complications, yet fewer than one third of this subgroup actually required therapeutic interventions. These researchers concluded that the organization and design of critical care units should include provisions for these "low-intervention patients," possibly in the form of intermediate or stepdown monitoring units.

Oye and Bellamy[23] also found skewed distributions of resource consumption. They observed that some 41% of patients admitted to ICUs received no acute interventions but consumed less than 10% of resources as measured using the Therapeutic Intervention Scoring System (TISS). They found that reducing the number of patients admitted for monitoring purposes would have relatively little impact on overall hospital charges and, consequently, on costs. However, the top 8% of admitted patients accounted for some 50% of all resource consumption, and their mortality rate was 70.6%. Oye and Bellamy[23] concluded that the key to better utilization was a "better understanding of the prognosis by physicians, patients, and their families . . . [to] reduce the amount of futile care. One approach to this is to regularly reassess the prognosis after patients are admitted to the unit. An additional approach is to discuss diagnosis, prognosis, and likelihood of benefit from treatment with hospitalized patients at risk for transfer to the ICU." However, surveys have shown that the majority of patients who wanted to communicate with their physician about life support had not done so.[24]

Unfortunately, it seems that transforming data, even when evidence-based, into alterations in practice patterns and improved ICU utilization is not an easily surmountable challenge. Paz and colleagues[25] attempted to alter ICU utilization by educating physicians regarding the uniformly abysmal outcomes of patients undergoing bone marrow transplants in whom acute respiratory failure develops. These patients have a survival rate of less than 4%, and their ICU length of stays are at least three times longer than those of bone marrow transplant recipients without respiratory failure. This information was presented to both oncologists and medical intensivists in multiple formats, and there was apparently general agreement regarding the relative futility of intubating and ventilating such patients when they have respiratory failure. Nonetheless, after this educational session, patients and families were rarely, if ever, counseled about the possibility of respiratory failure and the outcomes if intubation were performed. No change in ICU utilization patterns was observed following these educational efforts.[25]

Furthermore, the concept of utilization of ICUs is far more complex than utilization review managers would care to admit. What is the fate of patients denied admission to the ICU? How is "premature discharge" defined, and what are its consequences? When ICU performance is assessed, how does one account for patients who die on medical floors after discharge from the ICU? Does denial of admission to or premature discharge from the ICU result in prolonged hospital length of stay or increased complications? The existing studies suggest that standardized mortality ratios and ICU lengths of stay are simplistic tools that reveal only the tip of the iceberg and may be inadequate for the restructuring of policies and guidelines.[26, 27] Finally, outcome-oriented tools demonstrate little about the process of care. If the outcomes are poor or exemplary, there is little to indicate why.

Careful examination and documentation of current practices in critical care on a large scale are urgently needed to assess the type of care delivered and the patient populations receiving it. Indeed, as Chernow wrote in an editorial,[28] the need for information is acute. Only when this need has been satisfied can guidelines for the utilization of care be developed.

QUALITY OF CARE

Measuring and assessing the quality of care delivered are essential components of the management of critical care units. It appears that for adult medical-surgical patients, two objective measures are emerging that can be used for quality care assessment. The MPM II[29] provides information regarding the likelihood of survival at the time of admission to the ICU on the basis of 15 objective variables. The APACHE III assesses severity of illness and probability of both survival and ICU length of stay on the basis of 17 physiologic variables, age, and up to seven comorbid conditions occurring during the first day of ICU stay.[30] The Pediatric Risk of Mortality (PRISM), now in its third incarnation,[31] has been used to compare and assess pediatric ICUs. These tools and the process of outcomes prediction are discussed in detail elsewhere in this book.

Although these tools have been tested in hundreds of hospitals worldwide, they are not in widespread use. In fact, there is no consensus as to how the tools should be used. Can they be used to determine admission to or discharge from units?[32, 33] Can they be used to determine when to discontinue life support? Can they be used in selecting likely candidates for triage? Or are they simply devices for retrospective analysis of the aggregate quality of care delivered to select patient populations?

The debate continues, but few unambiguous answers are available.[34, 35] Although these tools are measures of expected mortality, it is less than clear that expected mortality is the only or best index of quality of care. To date, a universally accepted definition of a "high-performance" critical care unit has not been established. Cost and resource utilization are at least two other important reflections of performance, but they are not easily measured, if they can be measured at all. It seems imperative that a range of performance measures be developed and agreed on and that the process of unit management be evaluated as well. Some methods have already been proposed to meet these needs.[36, 37]

Zimmerman and colleagues[38] studied in detail the organizational structures of nine ICUs as part of a larger study of 42 units located throughout the United States. Using the APACHE III scoring system, they attempted to relate organizational structure with efficiency and risk-adjusted survival. They were able to characterize superior organizational practices that seemed to be more prevalent in better-performing ICUs, defining "high performance" as the attainment of superior risk-adjusted mortality ranks; that is, in high-performance units, the actual survival rates of patients exceeded the predicted survival rates. The researchers found that "superior organizational practices among these ICUs were related to a patient-centered culture, strong medical and nursing leadership, effective communication and coordination, and open, collaborative approaches to solving problems and managing conflict."[38] These units typically had the following features:

- Strong shared visions
- Empowered nursing staffs
- Ongoing educational programs
- A strong sense of collegiality among nurses, physicians, and administrative staff
- Supportive, visible leadership
- A generally defined concept of collaborative practice.

In lower-performance units, less collaboration was present, management was "top-down" and remote, and staff were more concerned about hospital rules, procedural issues, job security, hours, and pay than about patients and their well-being. This study, however, was not able to relate efficacy with efficiency or efficacy and efficiency with organizational characteristics. This could be a result of the small number of units studied or of the inadequacy of the measures of performance and organization.

If the extensive case studies performed in the non–health care business world are at all valid, strong cause-and-effect relationships exist among organization, management, and performance. Critical care units are extraordinarily complex environments with multiple constituencies and stakeholders. It will be difficult, but not impossible, to identify measurable parameters of performance, efficiency, cost, appropriateness, culture, and organization as well as perceived elements, such as patient, family, and staff satisfaction, leadership, communication, coordination, and collaboration. Management of critical care units in the era of health care reform will depend on these measures' being well defined, accepted, validated, and reliable in the near future.

ALLOCATION OF CARE

Even in the best of circumstances, when resources are used appropriately and effectively, the demand may and inevitably will occasionally exceed the supply. The responsibility to *tri-*

age (ensuring adequate care and appropriate allocation of scarce resources) falls directly on the shoulders of the unit directors. The Joint Commission on Accreditation of Healthcare Organizations[39] mandates the appointment of unit directors and that there be written, functional policies that govern action when the patient population's demands exceed operational capacity. This second issue was mandated in response to the growing realization that the allocation of resources is typically performed in an ad hoc manner, not necessarily with initial consideration of the best interests of the patient or the population as a whole. A revealing study by Marshall and colleagues[40] of the admission practices of a surgical ICU during times of overcrowding concluded that "surgical attending physicians rarely used other open in-house ICU beds when surgical ICU beds were unavailable. Political power, medical provincialism, and income maximization overrode medical suitability in the provision of critical care services."[40] It is highly unlikely that this study represents an isolated, anomalous situation.

The need to allocate resources in a reasonable manner has legal implications. Thus far, the courts have had little to say on the issue, but this situation is likely to change. A few cases have already come to light, and more are to be expected. A prime example is the case of a young female trauma victim who was admitted to an ICU in Florida in the early 1980s. The unit was overcrowded; during the night, the patient was accidentally disconnected from the ventilator and suffered irreversible brain damage. A lawsuit was brought before the court. During the trial that followed, it became apparent that inadequate staffing was largely the result of an alleged failure to perform triage. After the young woman's admission, a nearly brain-dead patient was kept in the unit rather than being transferred to a regular ward, and two new patients were admitted rather than being diverted to another institution. The court ruled that the hospital was obligated to perform triage in order to continue to provide an appropriate level of care to patients already admitted.[41] Commenting on the court's decision, Englehardt and Rie[42] wrote, "Depending on what probability of what benefits is afforded a patient already in a bed, the time of discharge can be advanced hour by hour in order to make a bed available to a newcomer who may be in slightly greater need or have a slightly greater likelihood of benefiting by admission."

The very concept of allocating scarce resources and determining "medical suitability" (i.e., who lives and who dies) invokes many medical, legal, and ethical issues that have been explored extensively in the literature. Teres[43] reviewed many of these issues from a practical perspective and offered the following suggestions:

1. An ICU medical director, designee, or supervisory nurse should be empowered as the gatekeeping officer.
2. The basis for regulating admission to, discharge from, or triage away from the special care unit should be medical suitability (from the utilitarian or egalitarian view). Conditions of limited medical suitability are as follows:
   a. High-probability estimate of hospital mortality or persistent vegetative state.
   b. Full do-not-resuscitate order (patient has not responded to aggressive medical therapy).
   c. Patient is clinically unsalvageable (no marginal benefit) due to a rapidly fatal underlying condition or Alzheimer's disease.
3. During high-level triage, when all ICU patients are receiving active therapy, these decisions should override the individual primary physician–patient relationship.
4. The guidelines should follow the "congestive heart failure" treatment analogy, as follows:
   a. Preload reduction: Hold high-risk patients in the postanesthesia care unit of emergency department, postpone surgery, or hold transfers in outlying ICUs.
   b. Improve cardiac performance: Increase efficiency and decrease workload per patient by performing fewer invasive procedures and transporting fewer patients for abdominal computed tomography scans.
   c. Afterload reduction: Keep unstable patients in the postanesthesia care unit, send sicker patients to intermediate care units, send "stable" ventilator-dependent patients to general medical-surgical units, and transfer, or resolve issues regarding patients whose condition is "hopeless."

The great difficulty for ICU directors is that triage and rationing place them in a position in which a serious potential for conflict of interest exists, especially if the director is personally caring for patients in the critical care unit. As Levinsky[44] has commented, "Physicians cannot serve two masters. . . . [They] are required to do everything they believe may benefit each patient without regard to costs or other social considerations. . . . It is society, not the individual practitioner that must make the decision to limit the availability of medical care."[44]

In an extensive discussion of utilization strategies for ICUs, Kalb and Miller[45] suggest that although this concept is firmly entrenched and "precludes physicians from rationing in their role as care givers, it does not preclude hospital-based rationing policies, nor does it preclude physician involvement in setting hospital policy." If we take this one step further, it becomes obvious not only that hospitals must have clear and unambiguous policies regarding the allocation of resources but also that the role of the critical care unit directors must also be clearly defined to maximize effectiveness and minimize the possibility of conflicts of interest.

Consequently, the Ethics Committee of the Society of Critical Care Medicine[18] has recommended that communities take a legitimate interest in allocating medical resources by limiting inadvisable treatment and that health care organizations and third-party payers should participate in this process and share accountability. Methods for doing so should be explicit, equitable, and democratic, and they should not place the poor and disenfranchised at a disadvantage. Furthermore, policies should be disclosed in the public record, reflect moral values acceptable to the community, not be based exclusively on prognostic scoring systems, articulate appellate mechanisms, and finally, be recognized by the courts.[18]

MANAGING CRITICAL CARE UNITS

The issues confronting critical care units are both legion and complex and will have serious consequences in the future if they are not vigorously confronted. As the problems of ensuring appropriate and quality care and the allocation of resources are examined, it is apparent not only that these issues have economic, medical, legal, and ethical implications but also that they are closely interrelated. None of these issues can be considered in isolation; rather, they are systematic problem areas that are closely interconnected and interdependent. For these issues to be dealt with in a timely manner, the critical care unit must be viewed as a single but not isolated system, an organization with multiple constituents and stakeholders contained in the larger framework of the hospital and its stakeholders, which in turn constitute the regional and national health care economies.

Critical care providers have long dealt solely with the disease processes of individual patients. Patients must now be regarded as part of a larger whole, and a systems approach to care provision must be entertained. The challenge to every hospital and to every director of a critical care unit is to effect change so that decision-making policies regarding the appropriateness, quality, and allocation of care can be instituted. The patient, the critical care unit, society, and the allocation of care are all inextricably interrelated. As Zimmerman and colleagues[38] concluded, critical care "will continue to be costly and the ethical issues surrounding the use of ICU resources will continue to grow. ICUs will need to become organizationally and managerially competent in order to deal with these challenges."

Implementing a management structure that can deal effectively with these issues is simple in theory but difficult in practice. A primary function of the management structure is to align and develop the internal capabilities and policies of the critical care unit with the pressures and forces generated by the multiple external environments in which the unit is embedded. Every hospital and every critical care unit have unique cultures that resist change, as do the practices of medicine and nursing themselves. Implementing changes in clinical practice is difficult enough, but when organizational structures are changed, such as moving from an open unit to a closed one, or employing a full-time intensivist or director of critical care, a significant change in thinking is required, that is, a change in the organizational culture not only of the ICU but also of the medical staff, the nurses, the ancillary staff, and the hospital administrators. A slowly growing body of evidence strongly suggests that full-time intensivist and management structures that tightly control the utilization of critical care resources not only can improve the outcomes of patients but also can control costs and resource consumption as well.[46-48]

SUMMARY

The forces of change, driven by the health care economic crisis, mandate that critical care units no longer be managed in the laissez faire mode of the past. The future requires that a comprehensive, multidisciplinary, systematic approach be taken to the management of all health care, but especially to those areas that demand the most resources. Critical care specialists must provide the leadership to ensure the optimal utilization and allocation of these vital resources.

References

1. Jonsen AR: Bentham in a box: Technology assessment Health Care allocation. Law Med Health Care 1986; 14:172–174.
2. Lamm R: The crisis in health care. *New York Times,* February 19, 1987.
3. Dranove D, Cone K: Do state rate setting regulations really lower hospital expenses? J Health Econ 1985; 4:159–165.
4. Scheiber G, Pouillier J-P: International health spending: Issues and trends. Health Aff (Millwood) 1991; 10:109.
5. Center for Health Policy Research, American Medical Association: International Health Systems: A Chartbook Perspective. Chicago, American Medical Association, 1991, pp 12–25.
6. Taylor R: Rationing healthcare in other countries. Presented at the Employee Benefit Research Institute (EBRI) Education and Research Fund Policy Forum (Rationing Health Care—Making Choices and Allocating Resources in the Health Care Delivery System: Implications for Access, Quality, and Costs), Washington, DC, December 1, 1992.
7. Angus DC, Sirio CA, Clermont G, Bion J: International comparisons of critical care outcome and resource consumption. Crit Care Clin 1997; 13:389–407.
8. Intensive care units (ICUs): Clinical outcomes, costs, and decision-making. (Health Technology Case Study 28.) Washington, DC, Congress of the United States, Office of Technology Assessment, 1984.
9. Gaumer GL, Stavins J: Medicare use in the last 90 days of life. Health Serv Res 1992; 26:725–742.
10. Groeger JS, Guntupalli KK, Strosberg M, et al: Descriptive analysis of critical care units in the United States: Patient characteristics and intensive care unit utilization. Crit Care Med 1993; 21:279–291.
11. Strauss MJ, LoGerfo JP, Yeltlatzie JA, et al: Rationing of intensive care unit services: An everyday occurrence. JAMA 1986; 225:1143–1146.
12. Strosberg MA, Weiner JM, Baker R, et al: Rationing America's Medical Care: The Oregon Plan and Beyond. Washington, DC, The Brookings Institution Press, 1992.
13. Strosberg MA, Fein IA, Carroll JD (Eds): Rationing of Medical Care for the Critically Ill. Washington, DC, The Brookings Institution Press, 1989.
14. Naylor CD: What is appropriate care? N Engl J Med 1998; 338:1918–1920.
15. Brook RH, Kamberg C, Mayer-Oakes A, et al: Appropriateness of acute medical care for the elderly: An analysis of the literature. *In:* Health Care Quality Management for the 21st Century. Couch JB (Ed). Tampa, Fla., American College of Physician Executives, 1991.
16. Robin ED: A critical look at critical care. Crit Care Med 1983; 11:144–148.
17. Schneiderman U, Jecker NS, Jonsen AR: Medical futility: Its meaning and ethical implications. Ann Intern Med 1990; 112:949–954.
18. The Ethics Committee of the Society of Critical Care Medicine: Consensus statement of the Ethics Committee of the Society of Critical Care Medicine regarding futile and other possibly inadvisable treatments. Crit Care Med 1997; 25:887–892.
19. Knaus WA, Wagner DP, Lynn J: Short-term mortality predictions for critically ill hospitalized adults: Science and ethics. Science 1991; 253:1-6.
20. The SUPPORT Principle Investigators: A controlled trial to improve care for seriously ill hospitalized patients. JAMA 1995; 274:1591–1598.
21. Shekelle PG, Kahan JP, Bernstein SJ, et al: The reproducibility of a method to identify the overuse and underuse of medical procedures. N Engl J Med 1998; 338:1888–1895.
22. Henning RJ, McClish D, Daly B, et al: Clinical characteristics and resource utilization of ICU patients: Implications for organization of intensive care. Crit Care Med 1987; 15:264–267.
23. Oye RK, Bellamy FE: Patterns of resource consumption in medical intensive care. Chest 1991; 99:685–689.
24. Frankl D, Oye RK, Bellamy PE: Attitudes of hospitalized patients toward life support: A survey of 200 medical inpatients. Am J Med 1989; 86:845–848.
25. Paz HL, Garland A, Weinar M, et al: Effect of clinical outcomes data on intensive care unit utilization by bone marrow transplant patients. Crit Care Med 1998; 26:66–70.
26. Goldhill DR, Sumner A: Outcome of intensive care patients in a group of British intensive care units. Crit Care Med 1998; 26:1337–1345.
27. Wallis CB, Davies HT, Shearer AJ: Why do patients die on general wards after discharge from intensive care units? Anaesthesia 1997; 52:9–14.
28. Chernow B: The practice of critical care: Describing who we are, evaluating what we do, and computing the cost. Crit Care Med 1993; 21:1413–1415.
29. Lemeshow S, Teres D, Klar J, et al: Mortality probability models (MPM II) based on an international cohort of intensive care patients. JAMA 1993; 270:2478–2486.
30. Knaus WA, Wagner DP, Zimmerman JE, et al: Variations in mortality and length of stay in intensive care units. Ann Intern Med 1993; 118:753–761.
31. Pollak MM, Patel KM, Ruttimann UE: PRISM III: An updated pediatric risk of mortality score. Crit Care Med 1996; 24:743–752.
32. Zimmerman JE, Wagner DP, Draper EA, et al: Improving intensive care unit discharge decisions: Supplementing physician judgement with predictions of next day risk for life support. Crit Care Med 1994; 22:1373–1384.
33. Bone RC, McElwee NE, Eubanks OH, et al: Analysis of indications for early discharge from the intensive care unit. Clinical Efficacy Assessment Project: American College of Physicians. Chest 1993; 104:1812–1817.

34. Becker RB, Zimmerman JE: ICU scoring systems allow prediction of patient outcomes and comparison of ICU performance. Crit Care Clin 1996; 12:503–514.
35. Sherk JP, Shatney CH: ICU scoring systems do not allow prediction of patient outcomes or comparison of ICU performance. Crit Care Clin 1996; 12:514–523.
36. Rapoport J, Teres D, Lemeshow S, et al: A method for assessing the clinical performance and cost-effectiveness of intensive care units: A multicenter inception cohort study. Crit Care Med 1994; 22:1385–1391.
37. Teres D, Higgins T, Loiacano L, et al: Defining a high-performance ICU system for the 21st century: A position paper. J Intensive Care Med 1998; 13:195–205.
38. Zimmerman JE, Shortell SM, Rousseau DM, et al: Improving intensive care: Observations based on organizational case studies in nine units: A prospective, multicenter study. Crit Care Med 1993; 21:1443–1451.
39. Joint Commission on Healthcare Organizations: Accreditation Manual for Hospitals: Special Care Units. Chicago, Joint Commission on Healthcare Organizations, 1992.
40. Marshall ME, Schwenzer KJ, Orsina M, et al: Influence of political power, medical provincialism, and economic incentives on the rationing of surgical intensive care beds. Crit Care Med 1992; 20:387–394.
41. Von Stettina v. Florida Medical Center, 2 Fla Supp 2d 55 (Fla 17th Cir 1982) a 436 So Rptr 3rd 1022 (1983).
42. Englehardt HT, Rie MA: Intensive care units, scarce resources, and conflicting principles of justice. JAMA 1986; 255:1159–1164.
43. Teres D: Civilian triage in the intensive care unit: The ritual of the last bed. Crit Care Med 1993; 21:598–606.
44. Levinsky NG: The doctor's master. N Engl J Med 1984; 311:1573–1575.
45. Kalb ME, Miller OH: Utilization strategies for intensive care units. JAMA 1989; 261:2389–2395.
46. Manthous CA, Amoateng-Adjepong Y, Al-Kharat T, et al: Effects of a medical intensivist on patient care in a community teaching hospital. Mayo Clin Proc 1997; 72:391–399.
47. Marini JJ: Streamlining critical care: Responsibilities and cost-effectiveness in intensive care unit organizations. Mayo Clin Proc 1997; 72:483–485.
48. Carson SS, Stocking C, Podsadecki T, et al: Effects of organizational change in the medical intensive care unit of a teaching hospital: A comparison of "open" and "closed" formats. JAMA 1996; 276:322–328.

187

Building Bedside Collaborative Practice

Maurene A. Harvey, RN, MPH, CCRN, FCCM
Tisha Fujii, DO • Richard W. Carlson, MD, PhD, FCCM

In the last half of the 20th century, the industrialized world has evolved rapidly under the pressure of social forces and scientific advances. We now operate in an increasingly sophisticated environment in which specialization and communication have dominant influences on human activity. As the division of labor increases in our society, mechanisms to integrate complex behavior into a functional whole become increasingly important. Accordingly, harmonious and efficient integration of personnel and their respective tasks in the critical care environment is an important goal to ensure optimal delivery of intensive care. In this chapter, we explore the traditional and present-day barriers to the growth of collaborative practice, national and local efforts developed to facilitate collaborative practices and their effects on clinical outcomes as well as techniques to implement similar models in day-to-day practice. Finally, we make predictions for up-grading collaboration in critical care in the future.

HISTORICAL PERSPECTIVE

Health care delivery systems have been slow to adapt to the increasingly interdependent, complex environment of personnel required to implement clinical care. The inertia displayed by these systems seems rooted in the broad trusteeship for health care that has been assumed by physicians,[1] who traditionally have directed all aspects of care in a vertical hierarchy in which communication and planning are unidirectional. This arrangement has fostered conflict among other health professionals, especially nurses, who have operated under a restricted scope of activities and who have been dependent on physicians' direction for providing various aspects of care (Fig. 187–1).

Recent changes in practice environments, however, have led to a greater identification and reliance on the knowledge, expertise, and services of other practitioners, especially professional nurses. In fact, patients are often admitted to hospitals because they need nursing care. In addition, as nurses and other caregivers involved in critical care (such as respiratory therapists) have developed distinctive identities through parallel research and professional activities, their contributions have ever more affected patient management. This evolution has necessitated the development of integrated health care practices. Moreover, as society assumes a larger role in shaping health care policy, health care providers find themselves under increasing economic and regulatory pressure to provide comprehensive, efficient, and effective care. Although the need for a smoothly run team effort is self-evident in the critical care setting, several factors can hamper the achievement of harmonious coordination of care in the intensive care unit (ICU).

We are in the midst of a revolution that is permanently altering how health care is delivered and how its quality is assessed. There is now an emphasis on primary, preventive, and holistic care, and the rise of managed care has substantially altered the roles and philosophies of many health professionals. Nurses and others have become primary care providers. Physicians in many specialties are in oversupply. Outcomes research, patient autonomy and advocacy, and a heightened awareness of ethical issues have eroded the paternalistic image of the physician, and many physicians who

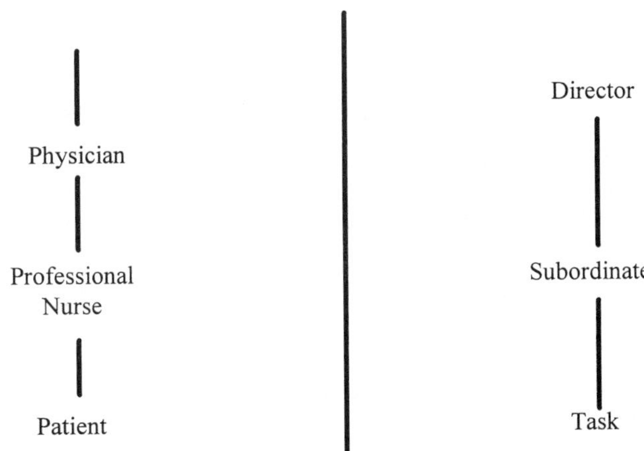

Figure 187–1. Traditional, hierarchical medical model of care.

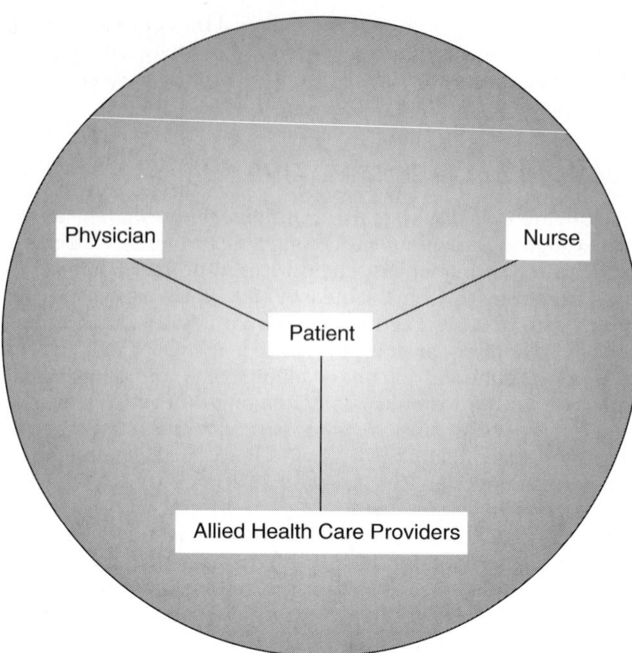

Figure 187–2. Collaborative or horizontal medical model of care.

work in managed care settings report a loss of autonomy.[2-4] The growth of large practice groups and managed care systems has also destroyed the traditional model of independent private practice. Increasing numbers of physicians are now employed, and the distinction between ambulatory practice and the services provided in hospitals continues to sharpen and shape the economics and careers of health professionals. The extent of penetration of managed care into the health care market has affected bedside decision making as caregivers struggle to observe fiscal restraint without compromising quality of care.[5, 6] This struggle is highlighted in the complex and technical environment of the modern special care unit.[7, 8]

Both nurses and physicians have come to realize that communication and a collegial relationship are essential to effective practice; however, interactions among those involved in patient care are often less than optimal, as pointed out by Prescott and coworkers.[9] Factors cited as undermining working relationships include changing economic and social status, shared practice domains, and unfamiliarity with other professions.

Traditional divisions between professional groups have attracted attention at the national level and have led to programs designed to foster bedside collaboration. As Weiss and Davis observed, "Collaboration represents the optimum of maintaining assertiveness while cooperating. Balancing these elements allows the knowledge and skills of both professions to synergistically influence the care being provided."[10] Such collaboration led to horizontal organizational models in which participants (clinicians) could be viewed as partners or colleagues in providing care (Fig. 187–2) The widespread development and use of clinical pathways have fostered positive interprofessional relationships, respect for the contributions of other team members, problem-solving skills, and collaboration.

COMPONENTS OF COLLABORATIVE PRACTICE

The body of knowledge concerning collaboration can be traced to the fields of group and institutional psychology and to industrial management. Important elements that were identified were communication, competence and accountability, trust, and administrative support.

The development of collaboration using these essential factors has a natural history, beginning with the movement away from practice in isolation toward practice in concert with other health care providers. Increasing contact favors open communication, which is essential for staff development. Increasing contact can automatically lead to greater collaboration and communication, whether they are consciously pursued or not. Communication is much more likely to be optimal, however, when it reflects a deliberate effort to identify and clarify goals and mutually overlapping roles. Through exchange of ideas and expertise, practitioners become familiar with the nature and scope of one another's practice. In this way, each practitioner is better able to assess individual competence. Once clinical expertise is demonstrated, trust can be established and negotiation of new roles for both parties in the critical care environment becomes possible.

In this regard, areas of nursing activities that are dependent, independent, and interdependent, as outlined in the American Association of Critical-Care Nurses (AACN) standards of care, must be clearly established (Table 187–1). *Dependent* nursing interventions are defined as those directed primarily by physicians through orders and medical care plans. *Independent* nursing interventions are those that are unique to nursing, such as nursing assessment and diagnosis, teaching, counseling, and manipulation of the patient's environment. Interdependent activities reflect areas of shared interest and thus include quality assurance and mutual responsibility for unit operation, organization, and administration. A close look at the ICU environment reveals increasing evidence of interdependent activities of nurses and physicians.

When dependent, independent, and interdependent areas of activity are all considered, a clearer understanding of professional obligations and responsibilities emerges. Greater emphasis on shared structure and interactions may have not only professional and ethical implications but also legal ones, as suggested by Helms and Mazur.[11] All participants must be willing to accept legal and moral responsibility for their own actions, and to some extent for, the actions of the entire patient care team.[12]

MILESTONES IN NURSE-PHYSICIAN COLLABORATION

In the late 1960s and early 1970s, the social dimension of the nurse-physician relationship was explored in many studies.[1, 6, 7]

TABLE 187–1. Classification of Nursing Functions in Relation to Physician Activities

Dependent
Is directed by physicians by means of orders and medical care plan
Independent
Performs unique nursing assessment and diagnosis
Develops care plans and outcomes
Supervises and delegates nursing functions
Interdependent
Has areas of shared responsibility (e.g., quality assurance, unit administration and operation, technology acquisition)

Adapted from Kuhn R (Ed): Outcome Standards for Nursing Care of the Critically Ill. Newport Beach, Calif, American Association of Critical-Care Nurses, 1990, pp 163–164.

TABLE 187–2. Five Prerequisites to Effective Collaboration

Communication
Competence
Accountability
Trust
Administrative support

Adapted from Devereux P: Essential elements of nurse-physician collaboration. J Nurs Admin 1981; 11:19–23.

Physicians clearly had a dominant position in the hospital environment, and both nurses' and physicians' behavior preserved this order. Stein and others popularized this hierarchical arrangement between doctors and nurses and the problems it created, calling it the "doctor-nurse game."[13–15] Stein and colleagues reviewed the topic some 24 years later and concluded that a number of factors have modified the relationship.[16] However, despite the fact that the omnipotence of omniscienct physicians has been undermined, Stein's group concluded that nurse-physician relationships remain problematic. Forte stated bluntly, "Conflict between nurses and physicians is counterproductive to patient care."[17]

In response to emerging interest in collaboration, the American Medical Association and the American Nursing Association formed the National Joint Practice Commission (NJPC) in 1972 to identify factors that would promote close working relationships.[18] The NJPC also identified five essential steps to establishing a collaborative practice environment.[19] Several practice models evolved from the NJPC; however, five essential prerequisites to effective collaboration were recognized (Table 187–2).

In 1977, under the guidance of the NJPC, a demonstration project was developed in which clinical elements incorporating these ideas were introduced simultaneously into certain hospital settings. Several years after the practice environment was restructured, participants were surveyed about their preferences in practice models. Although objective measures of performance were not obtained, general support was expressed for collaborative practice and satisfaction with patient outcome was high among those involved in the project.[20]

Following the NJPC's lead, the Society of Critical Care Medicine (SCCM) and the AACN established a task force to identify factors necessary to foster collaboration in the intensive care environment. The task force, or the Interorganization Liaison Group (ILG), has met at intervals since that time and has prepared several position papers, which were subsequently adopted by each parent organization. The first result of their activities was a joint practice statement released in 1982 (Table 187–3). The statement stressed the importance of physician and nurse autonomy in their respective fields and of accountability of all health care professionals. The statement also affirmed that nurse and physician directors of a unit should have equal authority in the organization of critical care units.[21] These societies continue to explore various practice models as part of their ongoing commitment to problem solving and collaboration. Accordingly, over the years the ILG has developed position statements on other topics of mutual concern that were subsequently affirmed by both the SCCM and the AACN.[22, 23]

Endorsement of a multidisciplinary approach to critical care also came from a consensus conference held at the National Institutes of Health (NIH) in 1983.[24] Collegial practice was supported at all levels, and the conference attendees recommended that the organizational structure of an ICU promote collaboration. In addition, the Joint Commission on Accreditation of Hospitals (JCAH) has recognized the value of integrated practice by mandating a multidisciplinary approach to the management of critical care units.[25]

COLLABORATIVE PRACTICE AND OUTCOME

Although support for joint practice activity is strong in demonstration models, objective assessment of improved patient outcome has been reported only occasionally. In a landmark study completed in 1986, Knaus and colleagues[26] evaluated the outcomes of more than 5000 patients cared for in various intensive care environments. Using the Acute Physiology and Chronic Health Evaluation (APACHE II) scoring system to stratify risks, the investigators found significant differences in institutional outcomes that were not predictable on the basis of

TABLE 187–3. Jointly Approved Society of Critical Care Medicine/American Association of Critical Care Nurses Position Statement—1982

Principles:

1. Responsibility and accountability for effective functioning of critical care unit must be vested in physician and nurse directors who are on an equal decision-making level.
2. These directors must be appropriately prepared and educated. In addition to competence in patient management, they need knowledge and experience in the following areas: management principles, resource management, and skills in interpersonal relationships (including conflict resolution).
3. The organizational structure of a critical care unit must ensure that physicians are autonomous when dealing with issues that affect medical practice.
4. The organizational structure of a critical care unit must ensure that nurses are autonomous when dealing with issues that affect nursing practice.
5. Some aspects of patient care require interdependence between physicians and nurses. These aspects must be identified and addressed jointly.
6. Every critically ill person requires medical and nursing care. The services of additional disciplines may also be required in specific situations. To provide a holistic approach, the care delivered by other health team members must be coordinated by the physician and nurse directors.
7. Unit support services must be organized to enable the directors to optimally carry out their primary responsibilities in the practice of their respective disciplines (i.e., patient care).
8. The directors are accountable for the evaluation of the quality and efficiency of care and the financial provision of that care. They must develop a unit-specific system for the evaluation of care on a timely basis.
9. The directors are responsible for creating and maintaining an environment in which individuals have opportunities to realize their potential.
10. Close collaboration between the directors is essential for successful management. This collaboration can be enhanced by daily rounds, weekly meetings, and other means that will ensure continuous, open communication.

severity of illness. An analysis of variables suggested that this unexplained outcome did not depend on technologic capability but was affected by administrative structure. The units with the highest degrees of staff involvement and positive physician-nurse interactions demonstrated the most favorable mortality rates, suggesting that the process of care affected patient outcomes.

A second project performed under the auspices of the AACN attempted to measure and relate various aspects of unit structure, process, and outcome. The demonstration unit, established in a small, nonprofit, community-based hospital, emphasized decentralized administration, expertise through critical care certification, participation in decision making, and broad guidelines for nurses' autonomy.[27] Standardized mortality ratios were derived from the APACHE II scoring system. The results revealed a strikingly favorable discrepancy with the anticipated mortality for the demonstration unit, which supported the belief that organizational characteristics can significantly affect outcome. Moreover, when patient and nursing opinions were gauged by various measurement tools, a high degree of satisfaction was demonstrated in both groups. This finding translated into less than expected turnover in nursing staff and decreased use of nurse-controlled consumable supplies.[18]

In the highly complex ICU environment some adverse events and errors are unavoidable; however, the extent to which such mishaps occur has only recently been subjected to careful scrutiny. Moreover, the effects of collaboration and communication between nurses and doctors on the frequency of such misadventures has not been rigorously examined. Nevertheless, data are emerging that indicate that better collaboration and communication will have beneficial effects on errors in the ICU. Brennan and others[28-31] have shown that errors are common in the hospital environment.[28-31] As many as 1.7 errors per patient per day may occur, and there is significant risk of serious events. The authors concluded that many of these errors could be avoided by better communication between nurses and physicians. In turn, a more collaborative atmosphere in these units should foster prompt reporting and discussion of errors. We agree and suggest that the implementation of an integrated medical record, clinical pathways and protocols, and other products of a more collaborative arrangement may help to reduce the rate and effect of errors. These effects should ultimately translate to improved outcomes.

Newer data further support the notion that increased collaboration may be associated with positive outcomes in the intensive care environment.[32-36] Baggs[37] demonstrated that transfer decisions that were agreed on jointly by nurses and physicians were associated with decreased readmission rates in the ICU and lower in-hospital mortality. We, and others, have postulated that the implementation of full-time ICU teams and a "closed unit" approach to ICU management would favorably alter the ICU environment in the direction of more efficient care and improved outcomes.[38-41]

In the most comprehensive study reported to date, Carson and colleagues[42] compared hospital mortality and mortality predicted by APACHE II scores, duration of mechanical ventilation, length of stay, charges, and other variables before and after the institution of a closed-unit setup with full-time ICU physician teams at University of Chicago facilities. They found striking improvements in all aspects of care that were measured. The authors speculate that a major factor in these results was the reorganization of physician services, but they also report greater nursing satisfaction and confidence in the full-time physician team. Accordingly, the results suggest that not only was there more efficient medical organization but that this fostered greater overall efficiency and improved function of the entire professional team.

Rosenthal and colleagues[43] studied 30 teaching and nonteaching hospitals. Mortality, length of stay, and other factors were significantly more favorable for the teaching hospitals. Overall hospital performance was also better for teaching institutions. The authors suspected that the findings might stem from differences in organization and delivery of care. We believe that they derive from parallel improvements in collaborative team efforts in teaching institutions. Physicians may be more likely today to accept a collaborative, mutually respectful relationship with professional nurses than they were even a few years ago.

NURSE RETENTION

Studies that reviewed factors affecting nursing retention have demonstrated that collaborative practice ranks high among the qualities that nurses deem important.[44, 45] When one considers that the estimated cost for recruitment and training of a nurse in a specialty care area may be more than $20,000, significant economic benefit can be realized from improving nursing retention for an institution.[46]

DIFFERENT PERSPECTIVES, DIFFERENT PERCEPTIONS

Bucknell and Thomas[47] examined nurses' perceptions of decision making in Australian ICUs. Nurses were often dissatisfied with treatment decisions, disagreements with medical staff about issues of autonomy, constraints on nursing care, and demands of new technology on knowledge bases. As many as half of the nurses frequently reported such difficulties; however, there is evidence that efforts to improve communication and collaboration and reduce barriers between physicians and nurses can enhance perceptions. Baggs and Schmitt[48] found that mutual respect, and a receptive and open attitude toward collaboration fostered better relationships and perceived improvements in patient care.

Poor communication between nurses and doctors may be related to the openness of communication, the accuracy of information communicated, and the timeliness of the interaction.[49] The ability to affect decisions is also an issue for many critical care nurses.[50]

Finally, it seems reasonable to conclude that patients and families will be better satisfied and more trusting of caregivers when care is provided in an atmosphere of co-operation. Achieving these goals remains an active area of investigation for nursing and other health care researchers.

NURSE AND PHYSICIAN ROLE MODELS AND PRACTICE

Despite empirical and objective support for collaborative practice, the pace of implementing collaborative models on a larger scale has been slow. Progress in this area has been hampered by entrenched and enduring patterns of physician dominance and nurse deference, plus a heightened sense of competition between professional groups.[9]

There are multiple causes for the perpetuation of these interprofessional conflicts and the social forces that abet them.[1, 9, 14, 15] Relationships between nurses and physicians are not static; they change in response to social and scientific advances. In particular, the past 30 years have been very turbulent for the nursing profession. The role and image of nurses held by most in society have changed dramatically during this time. In addition, dramatic changes have occurred in the professional and educational development of professional nurses. These changes have added new dimensions to the practice of nursing and have created heightened awareness of the profession's contributions to health care. These changes have come at a time when greater demands are placed on professional nurses as a result of emerging technologies, greater "patient acuity," and rising societal expectations. Nurses nevertheless continue to perceive their primary task in a positive light.[51-53] Although the issue of gender still affects how nurses and physicians interact, it appears to be abating as more men become nurses and more women physicians.

In the critical care environment, the nursing profession has responded to these challenges principally through educational initiatives and team building, which approaches have promoted a stronger sense of autonomy and clarity of purpose.[54] Formalization of the nursing process has been developed in the AACN's *Standards for Nursing Care of the Critically Ill*.[55] Under these guidelines, the profession has increasing responsibility for coordination of care and evaluation of patients' responses to the disease process and for associated interventions.

The character of nursing practice is also changing rapidly, as evidenced by the emergence of nurse practitioners, primary care nurses, and clinical nurse specialists. Accordingly, conflict related to the nurse-physician relationship is inevitable.

Physicians (unlike their nursing counterparts, who are enjoying a period of professional ascendancy) have witnessed the erosion of their traditional prerogatives on many fronts. Patient-consumers are demanding a greater voice in health care decisions. The legal profession and the insurance industry are increasingly reviewing patient management and outcomes. Cumbersome government regulations and changing reimbursement patterns are also affecting how physicians deliver care. The independence and autonomy of physicians have been eroded by the rise of managed care and health maintenance organizations (HMOs). More physicians are currently employed by organizations than practice independently. Increasingly, physicians work in groups and interact not only with their peers but also with other health care providers. In particular, hospital-based physicians, such as intensivists, are more likely than other physicians to be employed. In 1983, 24.2% of all physicians were employed; by 1996, this proportion had risen to 42.3% and the trend is expected to continue.[56]

The growth of the "hospitalist" movement is another trend that is altering the careers of many physicians and the relationships between nurses and these physicians, who now share their working environment full time.[57] We suspect that this new breed of physicians may be more likely to accept and promote a collaborative relationship with professional nurses. Many hospitalists are intensivists, so the effect on collaborative practice will be an interesting one to observe over the next few years. Many predict that the impact will, in the main, be positive.[58]

Problems may develop related to the manner in which nurses and physicians organize their time. Nurses plan their activities around the total needs of a few patients. Constant attendance at the patient's bedside allows the nurse to assess individual needs and responses. Conversely, physicians have traditionally divided their interests, which limits their contact with patients. Doctors must thus rely on nurses to summarize data and provide ongoing assessment of patients' status.

In a similar fashion, protocols and care maps are tools that foster collaboration and team building, although physicians[59] may view such devices as further eroding independent practice. Protocols may empower nurses but they require that physicians agree to one common order set for "routine" patients. The evolution of benchmarking and best practice initiatives often dictate more standardized care. The development and implementation of an integrated medical record is another example of a process that not only may improve communication but may be perceived as a threat by physicians. Nevertheless, an integrated medical record has been cited as an excellent example of a tool that should foster collaboration.[19]

Competitive interactions have, unfortunately, become a natural outgrowth of these changing professional relationships. In a descriptive study, Prescott and associates[9] found that conflict resolution in these situations is often dominated by aggressive, inflexible postures, and settlement reached only by imposed authority. Collaboration and accommodation emerged as alternative strategies that represented varying degrees of assertiveness and cooperation. Of the two, accommodation occurred more frequently than collaboration in the nurse-physician relationship, particularly in situations when patient welfare was not an issue. Unfortunately, the authors found few examples of collaboration in problem solving. In fact, collaboration occurred in only 14% of instances as perceived by physicians, whereas nurses described 7% of their interactions as collaborative.

Compromise and avoidance complete the repertoire of alternative responses to conflict resolution, although they are regarded as least desirable and are resorted to infrequently. However, disagreement and competition are not always undesirable; in fact, they often result in positive outcomes. Nevertheless, flexible postures and an emphasis on problem solving are more beneficial to all participants. In the ideal collaborative practice model, all groups receive recognition and key concerns are not compromised.

In a given unit a small number of nurse and physician champions of collaborative practice can be instrumental in establishing and role modeling such practice. These leaders can guide discussions that elaborate both the advantages of collaborating and the consequences of not collaborating. Miccolo[8] lists the following key goals of collaborative practice:

1. Providing superior care.
2. Maximizing productivity.
3. Enhancing professional development.
4. Increasing staff satisfaction.

The risks of not collaborating are inferior, inefficient, ineffective care, and decreased staff development and satisfaction.

IMPLEMENTING COLLABORATIVE PRACTICE

Organizational Structure

Collaborative practices do not arise spontaneously but grow out of commitment to a cooperative enterprise and dedication to common goals. These themes must be anchored in an organizational and managerial structure that facilitates team building.[60]

The organizational factors identified by the NJPC that contribute to collaboration include primary nursing and clear definitions of the unit's environment. That is, each unit must identify the patient population it serves best and attempt to minimize care for patients who do not "match" the facilities and expertise of the unit.

The mix of professional and technical personnel in the unit may also affect its organization and effectiveness. Opinions differ over whether units should use nursing support personnel, and how to achieve acceptable delegation of nursing tasks while ensuring responsibility and quality of care.[44, 45] The NJCP concluded that registered nurses are ideally situated to implement and evaluate all aspects of care and to serve as the pivotal knowledge brokers for other health care providers.

Others, including the Interorganization Liaison Group, and ultimately the AACN, have defined *support personnel* in the ICU and have developed a framework for their activities based on skills, knowledge base and organizational structure of unit management.[22, 23]

Defining the nature of the population served is a key consideration in the implementation of primary nursing in a critical care setting. If patient needs are accurately characterized, nursing requirements can be assessed, mechanisms can be developed to adjust to changing patient acuity, and teams can be created that have the necessary mix of skills. Controlled access through clearly articulated admission and discharge policies helps to define unit goals and preserve unit integrity.

Managerial factors can be divided into two broad categories: (1) programming and (2) feedback mechanisms. Programming involves standardization of work and skills (i.e., development of procedures and protocols), thus enabling the organization to respond to routine situations in a predictable manner. Through the development of stereotypical responses, a high level of staff coordination and cooperation can be achieved, as in modern cardiovascular ICUs.

Feedback mechanisms become important when novel situations are encountered. In the ICU environment, much patient instability and uncertainty about outcomes are likely to exist. In these instances, programmed responses cannot be relied on to cover all contingencies. Thus, the organizational structure must allow for discretionary activity, means for self-adjustment, and development. Standardization of knowledge and skills are important first steps in this process. Corrective, positive feedback through supervision and group coordination can optimize patient outcomes.[26]

Implementation

Incorporating these concepts into the day-to-day activities of special care areas continues to be a challenge. Both nursing and medical staffs must be prepared for this period of transition. In the process of developing these frameworks, the team members in each unit should discuss issues, shared values, and potential areas of conflict. Each service should develop a mission statement to define the practice model, create standards of care, outline admission and discharge criteria, and develop protocols for caring for patients with difficult problems such as severe or recurring pain or terminal illness.[61, 62] Miccolo[8] suggests developing a contract for collaboration that defines lines of communication, responsibilities, and accountabilities.

Other significant steps to improve collaboration that were endorsed by the NJPC include integration of the patient practice committees and creation of joint care review panels.[18] Implementation of an integrated medical record obviates nurse and physician progress notes. Team members may thus read the evaluations of others, and communication is enhanced and unnecessary duplication of information avoided. Many clinicians favor a problem- or system-oriented approach as a way to facilitate interprofessional communication.

The next step is independent clinical decision making, which allows the nursing staff to take full advantage of their clinical skills. Areas in which independent assessment and judgment may be employed must be clearly delineated. Nursing practice policies should be specifically tailored to the needs and requirements of a particular area and must be jointly crafted by nurse and physician administrators in keeping with legislated practice boundaries.[39] Although many ICUs currently have routine multidisciplinary rounds, some are simply designed to comply with JCAH standards or to focus on cost containment. In units with a culture that values and embraces collaboration, these rounds afford an indispensable opportunity to share and collaborate at a basic and important level.

King and colleagues[63] proposed a model for critical care that considers antecedent variables for conflict resolution: independent variables such as demographics and intervening mediators of variables related to working relationships and outcome variables that involve not only patient outcome but also cost and nurses' satisfaction and retention. The structure they propose takes into account many of the elements, prerequisites, and factors cited by the Interorganization Liaison Group, the NJPC, and others (Fig. 187–3).

A strong, ongoing commitment from hospital administration and the nursing and medicine departments is essential for the continued development of this practice model.[64, 65] Such

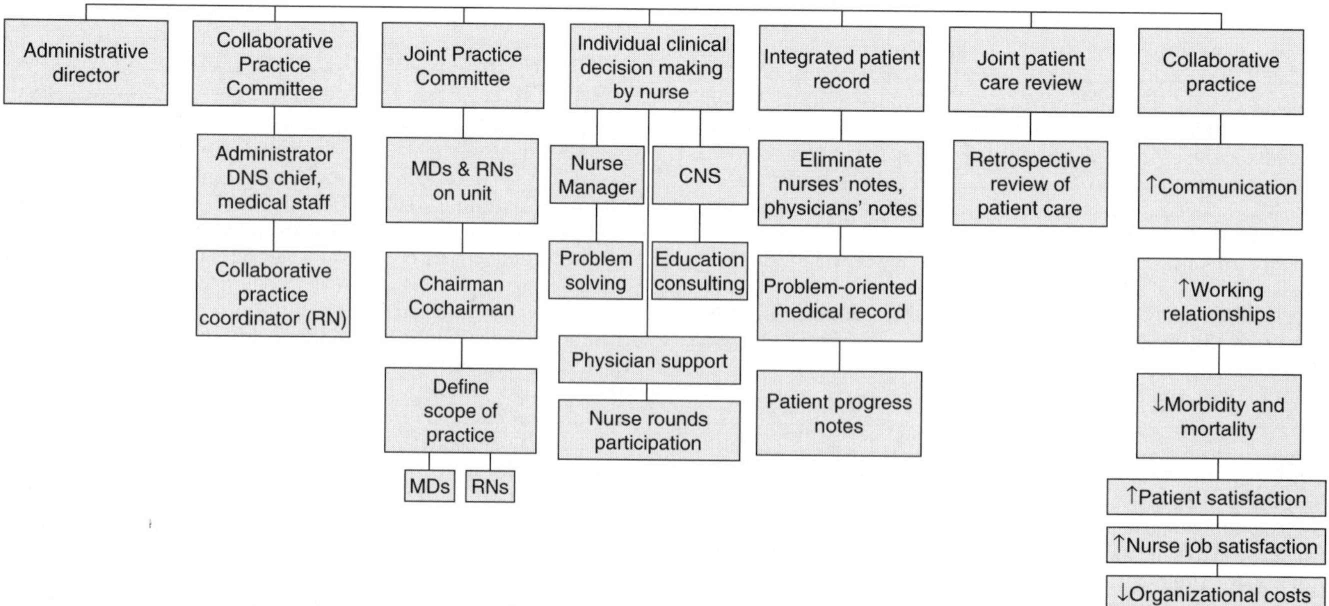

Figure 187–3. Proposed structure for establishing a collaborative practice model of care in the intensive care unit. (From King ML, Lee JL, Henneman E: A collaborative practice model for critical care. Am J Crit Care 1993; 2: 448).

commitment may take the form of seminars and workshops that define areas of competence, update skills, or stress concepts of professional practice. Support can also be demonstrated through the creation of joint practice committees charged with continuous monitoring of nurse-physician relationships and the evolution of strategies that support joint practice. These committees should have a balanced rotating membership, to decrease the likelihood that any one group will dominate the team's agenda.[66] Through ongoing self-examination, these groups develop a certain structure, definition, and direction that deflect attention from the individual members and sharpen the focus of health care delivery.

This model can also be buttressed through joint record review in which nurses and physicians jointly scrutinize care provided patients. This form of collaboration also affords an opportunity for the development of informal and formal clinical case conferences, which in turn reinforce practice guidelines, develop group competence, and promote clinical problem solving.[67] The dedicated assignment to the unit of others routinely involved in patient care, such as dietitians, pharmacists, and respiratory therapists, also contributes to the team identity.

The use of a consultant in team development provides yet another alternative to building collaboration. Having no vested interest, the consultant can take a neutral view of team functions, working relationships, and patterns of communication and can identify strengths and weaknesses of the group.[68] Activities or individuals who have negative influences on group development can be identified, and remedial action taken. Attention has recently focused on strategies that can be used to develop team orientation. Recognizing social and job-related stressors and evolving strategies to mollify their effects are measures that can avoid the consequences of the issues of unrelated events spilling over into the workplace and exaggerating interpersonal conflicts. Learning to feel tension as it develops and taking measures to reduce stress may prevent such over-reactions and the negative work-related interactions or perceptions that ensue.

Minimizing the inevitable effects of individual conflicts and personal biases is particularly difficult in intensive care, where the egos of nurses and physicians attracted to the specialty are typically quite strong. Critical care practitioners are often accustomed to independent decision making and have a strong sense of accountability. In these situations, sensitivity to each other's perspectives can be fostered by role-playing activities incorporated into unit retreats, orientation sessions for new nurses and physicians, grand rounds presentations, and continuing critical care education programs. Mechanisms should also be established to defuse unresolved conflicts without exacerbating them.[69] Third parties and ad hoc committees are useful in this regard, as long as they are professionally balanced and otherwise neutral. The object should be, not to select a winner or a loser, but to provide the best available alternative. When guided by the motto, "There are no unsolvable problems in life, only unselected alternatives," no issue appears insurmountable.

COLLABORATIVE PRACTICE IN ACTION

In response to the perceived need for greater interdisciplinary cooperation in the management of the hopelessly ill, practitioners at Wayne State University developed the Comprehensive Supportive Care Team in 1985.[70-72] The need arose when it became clear that these patients were best suited to a humane but conservative approach to management that would maximize the opportunity for family interaction and grief counseling while creating a comfort-oriented approach to management that would allow critical care resources to be marshaled more appropriately to other patients.[73, 74]

The team has achieved control in continuous operation as an example of collaborative practice that addresses a specific group of critically ill patients and has achieved a unique degree of nurse-physician partnership.

The team consists of a clinical nurse specialist and a limited number of rotating physicians who, in collaboration, provide broad support for hopelessly ill patients and their families. Specific plans are developed jointly that satisfy both nursing and medical goals. The team evaluate and revise the therapeutic plan in response to the patient's changing needs. Nursing, pastoral care, and social services staff are encouraged to participate in the decision-making process to ensure that the comfort and the psychologic and spiritual aspects of care are being provided. Close contact with the family is maintained through a designated team spokesman. The patient remains on the service until death, discharge, or a significant change in status occurs that necessitates re-evaluation.

Since its inception, the Comprehensive Supportive Care Team has provided consistent care to more than 1400 patients. Despite the nature of the population being served, acceptance and satisfaction among team and family members remains high. Moreover, by identifying the special needs of this group, costly care has been curtailed, resulting in better resource allocation in the institution.[74]

SUMMARY

The ICU is a dynamic environment that requires a coordinated effort to optimize patient outcomes. Through conscientiously applied principles of collaboration, medicine, nursing, and allied health practices can be integrated as the interests of each group are preserved. In today's health care environment, working together gives bedside practitioners a stronger voice in ensuring that patients receive the best possible care.

Concrete steps that can be taken to implement this practice model have been outlined by the NJPC, the Interorganization Liaison Group, and others. The effectiveness of these policies and techniques has been demonstrated in numerous settings and can be expected to be a common feature of future hospital environments, as providers explore ways to control costs, provide comprehensive care, promote professionalism, and ensure patient and family satisfaction.

We predict that collaborative practice will continue to evolve, become more robust, and grow in special care units. These improvements in human engineering will enhance the scientific and technical advances in critical care. Collaborative activities should increase faster, as we believe the breakpoint of inertia to collaborative practice has been passed. Critical care should thus become progressively dominated by highly efficient teams of nurses and physicians who are dedicated to maximizing the skills, knowledge, and input of all members of the team.

References

1. McGraw RW: Interdisciplinary teamwork for medical care and health services: Components in organization. Ann Intern Med 1968; 69:821.
2. Daugrid A, Spencer D: Physician reaction to the health care revolution. Arch Fam Med 1996; 5:497.
3. Donelan K, Blendon RJ, Lundberg GD, et al: The new medical marketplace: Physician's views. Health Aff 1997; 16:139.
4. O'Connor SJ, Lanning JA: The end of autonomy: Reflections on the postprofessional physician. Health Care Manage Rev 1992; 17:63.
5. English T: Personal paper: Medicine in the 1990s needs a team approach. BMJ 1997; 314:661.

6. Fagin CM: Collaboration between nurses and physicians: No longer a choice. Acad Med 1992; 67:295.
7. Cohen IL, Fitzpatrick M, Booth FV: Critical care medicine opportunities and strategies for improvement. Jt Comm J Qual Improve 1996; 22:85–103.
8. Miccolo MA, Spanier AH: Critical Care Management in the 1990's: Making collaborative practice work. Crit Care Clin 1993; 9:443.
9. Prescott P, Bowen S: Nurse/physician relationships. Ann Intern Med 1985; 103:127.
10. Weiss S, Davis P: Validity and reliability of the collaborative practice scales. Nurs Res 1985; 34:299.
11. Helms A, Mazur D: Physician collaboration dilemma. DCCN Dimens Crit Care Nurs 1992; 11:213.
12. Lumb PD: Management and the art of politics. Crit Care Clin 1993; 9:425.
13. Stein L: The doctor/nurse game. Arch Gen Psychiatry 1967; 16:699.
14. Pellegrino ED: What's wrong with the nurse-physician relationship in today's hospitals? A physician's view. Hospitals 1966; 40:70.
15. Bates B: Doctor and nurse: Changing roles and relations. N Engl J Med 1970; 283:129.
16. Stein LI, Watts DT, Howell T: The doctor-nurse game revisited. N Engl J Med 1990; 322:546.
17. Forte PS: The high cost of conflict. Nurs Econ 1997; 15:119.
18. Devereux P: Essential elements of nurse-physician collaboration. J Nurs Adm 1981; 11:19.
19. National Joint Practice Commission (NJPC): Guidelines for Establishing Joint or Collaborative Practice in Hospitals. Chicago, NJPC, 1981.
20. Devereux P: Does joint practice work? J Nurs Adm 1981; 11:39.
21. Interorganization Liaison Group: Focus on Critical Care. 1983; 10:43.
22. Wlody G: The organization of human resources in critical care units. Focus Crit Care 1983; 1:43.
23. Wlody G: Use of technical personnel in the critical care setting. Focus Crit Care 1984; 11:43.
24. Critical care medicine: Consensus conference. JAMA 1983; 250:798.
25. Joint Commission on Accreditation of Hospitals (JCAH): Accreditation Manual of Hospitals. Chicago, JCAH, 1982.
26. Knaus W, Draper E, Wagner D, et al: An evaluation of outcome from intensive care in major medical centers. Ann Intern Med 1986; 104:410.
27. Mitchell P, Armstrong S, Simpson T, et al: American Association of Critical-Care Nurses Demonstration Project: Profile of excellence in critical care nursing. Heart Lung 1989; 18:219.
28. Brennan TA, Leape LL, Laird NM, et al: Incidence of adverse events and negligence in hospitalized patients. N Engl J Med 1991; 324:370.
29. Leape LL, Brennan TA, Laird N, et al: The nature of adverse events in hospitalized patients. N Engl J Med 1991; 324:377.
30. Giraud T, Dhainaut JF, Vaxelaire JF, et al: Iatrogenic complications in adult intensive care units: A prospective two-center study. Crit Care Med 1993; 21:40.
31. Donchin Y, Gopher, D, Olin M, et al: A look into the nature and causes of human errors in the intensive care unit. Crit Care Med 1995; 23:294.
32. Spodick DH (Ed): The CCRN-CCMD partnership: Advancing the quality of patient care. Heart Lung 1993; 22:381.
33. Mallick R, Strosberg M, Lanbrinos J, Groeger JS: The intensive care unit medical director as manager: Impact on performance. Med Care 1995; 33:611.
34. Zimmerman JE, Rousseau DM, Duffy J, et al: Intensive care at two teaching hospitals: An organizational analysis. Am J Crit Care 1994; 2:129.
35. Zimmerman JE, Shortell SM, Rousseau DM, et al: Improving intensive care: Observations based on organization case studies in nine intensive care units: A prospective multicenter study. Crit Care Med 1993; 21:1443.
36. Wacksman R, Bachmeier J, Hoed RC, et al: Financial impact of a multidisciplinary critical care service (Abstract). Crit Care Med 1996; 24:A21.
37. Baggs JG: The association between interdisciplinary collaboration and patient outcomes in a medical intensive care unit. Heart Lung 1992; 21:18.
38. Reynolds HN, Haupt MT, Thill-Baharozian MC, et al: Impact of critical care physician staffing on patients with septic shock in a university hospital medical intensive care unit. JAMA 1988; 260:3446.
39. Carlson RW, Haupt MT: Organization of critical care services. Acute Care 1987; 13:2.
40. Carlson RW, Weiland DE, Srivathsan K: Does a full time 24-hour intensivist improve care and efficiency? Crit Care Clin 1996; 12:525.
41. Rainey TG: Critical care beyond the ivory tower. Crit Care Med 1993; 22:1035.
42. Carson SS, Stocking C, Podsadecki T, et al: Effects of organizational change in the medical intensive care unit of a teaching hospital. JAMA 1996; 276:322.
43. Rosenthal GE, Harper DL, Quinn LM, et al. Severity-adjusted mortality and length of stay in teaching and nonteaching hospitals. JAMA 1996; 276:322.
44. Baggs J, Ryan S: ICU nurse-physician collaboration and nursing satisfaction. Nurs Econ 1990; 8:386.
45. Everly GS, Fulcione R: Perceived dimensions of job satisfaction for staff registered nurses. Nurs Res 1976; 25:346.
46. Evans SA, Carlson RW: Nurse/physician collaboration: Solving the nursing shortage crisis. Am J Crit Care 1992; 1:25.
47. Bucknell T, Thomas S: Nurses' reflections on problems associated with decision-making in critical care settings. J Adv Nurs 1997; 25:229.
48. Baggs JG, Schmitt MH: Nurses' and resident physicians' perceptions of the process of collaboration in an MICU. Res Nurs Health 1997; 20:71.
49. Anderson FD, Maloneyu JP, Oliver DL, et al: Nurse-physician communication: Perceptions of nurses at an Army medical center. Mil Med 1996; 161:411.
50. Baggs JG, Schmitt, MH, Mushlin AI, et al: Nurse-physician collaboration and satisfaction with the associated process in three critical care units. Am J Crit Care 1997; 6:393.
51. Mohl PC, Denny NR, Mote TA, et al: Hospital unit stressors that affect nurses: Primary task vs. social factors. Psychosomatics 1992; 23:366.
52. Cronin-Stubbs D, Rooks C: The stress, social support and burnout of critical care nurses: The results of research. Heart Lung 1985; 14:31.
53. Martino JH, MacIntosh NJ: Effects of patient characteristics and technology on job satisfaction and stress of intensive care and intensive care nurses. Heart Lung 1985; 14:300.
54. Davidhizer R: Self-confidence: A requirement for collaborative practice. DCCN Dimens Crit Care Nurs 1993; 14:218.
55. Kuhn R (Ed): Outcome Standards for Nursing Care of the Critically Ill. Newport Beach, Calif, American Association of Critical-Care Nurses, 1990, pp 163–164.
56. Kletke PR, Emmons DW, Gillis KD: Current trends in physicians' practice arrangements: From owners to employees JAMA 1996; 276:555.
57. Wachter RM, Goldman L: The emerging role of 'hospitalists' in the American health care system. N Engl J Med 1996; 335:514.
58. Moore JD: The inpatient's best friend: 'Hospitalists' are physicians who care for the sick only in hospitals. Mod Healthcare 1997; 27:54.
59. Sheenan-Schreck P, Josker JS, Norris MK: The CarePlan Cord: Building collaboration in medicare and nursing orders. DCCN 1994; 13:90.
60. Fein IA: The critical care unit: In search of management. Crit Care Clin 1993; 9:401.
61. Wocial LD: Achieving collaboration in ethical decision making: Strategies for nurses in clinical practice. DCCN 1996; 15:150.
62. Ethical awareness, understanding and collaboration (Editorial). Intensive Crit Care Nurs 1993; 9:1.
63. King L, Lee JL, Henneman E: A collaborative practice model for critical care. Am J Crit Care 1993; 2:444.
64. Baggs JG: Development of an instrument to measure collaboration and satisfaction about critical care decisions. J Adv Nurs 1994; 20:176.
65. Keough V, Jenrich J, Holm K, Marshall W: A collaborative program for advanced practice in trauma/critical care nursing. Crit Care Nurse 1996; 16:120.
66. Burchell RC, Thomas D, Smith H: Some considerations for implementing collaborative practice. Am J Med 1983; 74:9.

67. Kallenbach AM, Meyer DS: Patient care conference: A coordinated, collaborative effort. Crit Care Nurse 1996; 16:77.
68. Chamberlain J: The use of a consultant in team development. J Contin Educ Nurs 1976; 7:25.
69. Caswell D, Cryer HG: Case studies: When the nurse and physician don't agree. J Cardiovasc Nurs 1995; 9:30.
70. Carlson RW, Devich L, Frank R: Development of a comprehensive supportive care team for the hopelessly ill on a university hospital service. JAMA 1988; 259:378.
71. Field BE, Devich L, Carlson RW: Impact of a comprehensive supportive care team on management of hopelessly ill patients with multiple organ failure. Chest 1989; 96:353.
72. Campbell ML, Carlson RW: Terminal weaning from mechanical ventilation: Ethical and practical considerations for management. J Crit Care 1992; 1:52.
73. Brody H, Campbell ML, Faber-Langendoen K, et al: Withdrawing intensive life-sustaining treatment. N Engl J Med 1997; 336:652.
74. Campbell ML, Frank RR: Experience with an end-of-life practice at a university hospital. Crit Care Med 1997; 25:197.

188

Complementary Modalities of Care: A Future That Is Here Now

Carole Birdsall, EdD, ANP, CCRN, FCCM
Arline Reinking-Hanf, RN, MS, CCRN, CEN, HNC

Since the mid-1960s and the birth of critical care, practitioners have struggled to incorporate strategies that humanize care and to ensure that in the highly technical or "high-tech" environment, "high-touch" care is also given. As critical care practice matured, we learned more about human responses and recognized that the loss of the fine art of touching was detrimental to the patient. It is appropriate to introduce the types of modalities that can be used at the bedside to augment traditional Western medicine. The history of critical care is replete with comments such as, "The ICU [intensive care unit] nurse must be alert to the patient's need for stress reduction" (p. 384).[1] In fact, critical care medicine has been and will remain at the forefront of new and untried treatments to foster positive patient outcomes. Therefore, the concept of complementary care is not new to critical care practitioners.

Complementary modalities are best thought of as adjunctive, synergistic, and supportive and an enhancement to what is used scientifically to manage the patient's care. Complementary modalities offer a softness that allows the bedside practitioner to help the patient deal with anxiety, pain, depression, devastation, diagnosis, or loss in a concrete personal way that is comforting to both the patient and the family. For these reasons, we offer basic information on the use of (1) massage therapy, (2) music therapy, and (3) therapeutic touch.

All three of these complementary modalities are effective, yet do not interfere with the medical plan of care. Because the modalities enhance—rather than disrupt—the plan of care, each is highly suitable for the critical care arena. Each modality is unique, and research demonstrates that patient and family acceptance is high with the use of these adjunctive modalities. Each complementary modality can contribute to establishing a relationship of trust and caring. In many instances, the effect of the complementary modality may be to help patients accept the highly technical aspect of critical care, leading to better patient outcomes.

MASSAGE THERAPY

Massage comes from the Greek word *masso,* which means "to knead" and has its roots in ancient civilization. Massage has been used as a form of therapy since the beginning of recorded time. In fact, during the height of Greek civilization, Hippocrates, the father of medicine, wrote of the therapeutic effects of massage and gave instructions for carrying it out. It has been reported that he too was a recipient of frequent massage. As modern medicine emerged, fewer and fewer people looked to the old ways for interventions to deal with health problems. In the United States, for example, seeking health care in the current era is often synonymous with getting a prescription to "fix" or eliminate symptoms. Massage therapy provides a rediscovered complementary modality of care and affords the opportunity to explore the more traditional healing therapies.

Massage is a healing art. It is a unique way of communicating without words. By touching another person, we may communicate the fact that we care, empathize, and want to support them. Massage therapy is the skillful and specific application of direct hand pressure and motion achieved by a rubbing or kneading-like action of a practitioner's hands applied to a patient's skin and underlying muscle tissue.

Therapeutic massage promotes physical and psychologic relaxation. In addition, research supports the belief that massage can improve circulation, relieve sore muscles, enhance comfort, and alleviate pain. The overall beneficial effects increase emotional stability by eliminating the negative affect seen with depression, agitation, irritability, anger, and frustration. In addition, massage therapy can be used for diversion or distraction during a painful procedure, such as insertion of an arterial line. The most important aspect of massage therapy for critical care application is that massage potentiates the therapeutic effects of other conventional treatments.

Types of Massage

One of the most common types of massage, *Swedish massage,* consists of effleurage, petrissage, friction, percussion (tapotement), and vibration. Each of these strokes can be used individually or in combination to facilitate general relaxation or to address specific problematic areas.

Effleurage consist of long, smooth, gliding-type strokes applied horizontally in relation to the tissues. The applied pressure is varied and appropriate to the patient so that it is adequate to support comfort, relief, and relaxation.

Petrissage, also known as kneading, refers to strokes that lift, roll, and squeeze the soft tissues. Just as effleurage is focused horizontally on the body, petrissage functions vertically.

Friction consists of small deep movements performed on a local area. The movement in friction is usually transverse to the fiber direction.

Percussion, also known as tapotement, is achieved by delivery of a series of brisk blows following each other in a rapid, alternating, and downward fashion.

Vibration is a fine tremulous movement, made by the hand or fingers placed firmly against a body part that causes the part to oscillate in a rhythmic manner.

Another well-known type of therapeutic massage is *acupressure,* which originated from the Taoist philosophy that began centuries ago in China. Having discovered how touch could relieve the pain from an injury, Chinese physicians and philosophers discovered that life energy, also known as *chi,* flows through the body in 12 defined paths, or *meridians.* Acupressure is based on the assumption that "not well," or disease, states result in obstructed or blocked energy flow; in healthy states, the energy flow proceeds unblocked and is well distributed throughout the meridian pathways. Fundamental to the concept of meridians in Chinese medicine is not only their function as imaginary lines linking a series of points on the skin that become sensitive in the presence of organic or functional disorders but also their function as actual energy pathways. This energy circulates throughout the body in a well-defined cycle, moving in a prescribed sequence from meridian to meridian and from organ to organ, flowing partly at the periphery and partly in the interior of the body.

The meridian system provides for a continuous flow of vital energy and nutrients to all parts of the body. In this method, the fingers are used to press key points, known as *acupoints,* on the surface of the skin located along the various meridians as a means to stimulate the body's natural self-curative abilities. When these points are pressed, they release muscular tension and promote the circulation of blood and the body's life force to aid healing. *Acupuncture* and acupressure use the same points; however, acupuncture employs needles, whereas acupressure uses the gentle but firm pressure of hands (and even feet). This is done as a means to release energy blockages as well as to maintain and enhance continuity of energy flow. Although acupressure is a form of massage, in this chapter only Swedish massage techniques are addressed.

Purpose

The overall intent of massage therapy is to achieve some degree of muscle relaxation or to stimulate the release of endogenous endorphins as a means of evoking the relaxation response. Massage is not considered replacement therapy in critical care practice; instead, it is used adjunctively in combination with conventional therapies.

Contraindications and Risk Factors

The use of massage is questionable with hemodynamically compromised patients. Research to date has indicated that massage can result in an endogenous short-term release of catecholamines, causing alterations in heart rate, blood pressure, and respiratory rate. Such physiologic changes increase the body's oxygen demands, predisposing to further hemodynamic compromise. Patients who have significant coronary artery obstruction and are awaiting cardiac surgery, as well as those with impaired volume states (pump failure), are not usually good candidates for massage therapy treatments because of the risk of fluid shifts related to peripheral vasodilation and potential alterations in cardiac output. However, one author (A.R.) provides massage therapy to coronary artery bypass graft (CABG) patients in the immediate postoperative recovery phase by use of massage to the hands and feet without any changes in hemodynamic status or noted complications. Once definitive treatment is initiated and the immediate threat of hypoperfusion is addressed, full massage therapy can be reconsidered.

Additionally, massage therapy should be used with extreme caution in patients who are at risk for thrombus formation. In such situations, very gentle, light massage strokes can be administered ever so cautiously to the back, shoulder, posterior neck areas, hands, and feet, while avoiding calf, upper leg, and arm muscles in attempts to promote relaxation. However, massage therapy treatments are definitely contraindicated in patients with thromboembolism.

When the clinician is preparing to administer massage therapy treatments to acutely ill patients, general medical history information and current physiologic and psychologic status are assessed. For critically ill patients receiving paralytic agents and/or sedation, determining the comfort level or anxiety level is problematic, but massage therapy offers a means to maximize comfort.

It is imperative that specific precautions or contraindications and risk factors be identified to guarantee patient safety. For example, massage therapy is not given to a critically ill patient writhing in pain. A list of precautions and contraindications can be identified by hospitals or caregivers when massage therapy is in use in order to avoid further patient compromise or injury. Such contraindications are for patients with an unstable cervical spine, low platelet count, or trauma associated with loss of tissue integrity. An example of a *risk factor* is in a patient prone to thromboembolic phenomena; in this instance, massage of the legs is avoided. A complete assessment identifies those body areas to avoid, such as areas of heavy bruising or tissue sloughing, wounds, including surgical incisions, hematomas, and sites where vascular lines are placed (Box 188–1).

Usually, a massage therapy referral is completed by the nurse or physician prior to administering the treatment. Explanation of massage therapy and its potential benefits is shared with patients as a means to better prepare them for the experience. During discussions with the patient, body areas to be avoided are often identified by the patient as are areas perceived as "tense" or painful. Return visits can be as often as twice a day for the duration of massage therapy; however, this schedule is based on the availability of staff who are skilled in massage. The massage therapist determines the length of treatment time. On average, a 15- to 30-minute session is appropriate for a critically ill patient; however, the therapist must carefully assess response to therapy and make appropriate decisions with each and every session. Time duration varies greatly with the patient's change in physical or emotional status and thus is individually determined.

Plan of Treatment

The therapist develops a workable plan of care. Decisions about whether to use an oil or massage lotion with or without combined aroma therapy are made when the assessment is complete. For example, if the patient is nauseated, various fragrances can trigger further distress and are avoided. On the other hand, an anxious patient can benefit from the use of lavender aroma or any of the citrus oils. Lotion provided by the hospital or brought in by the patient's family or significant other is used when doing massage for patients with allergies. Areas to focus on during massage therapy treatments are determined by the massage therapist through information obtained in communication with the patient, family, or significant other in collaboration with caregivers and review of the medical record. Body areas most appropriate for massage of

BOX 188–1
STEP-BY-STEP APPROACH TO THERAPEUTIC MASSAGE

The following is a brief step-by-step approach to the application of therapeutic massage:

1. Assess multisystem involvement, types of medications (anticoagulants, narcotics), and equipment used to maintain or monitor hemodynamic stability, and ensure that there are no risk factors, precautions, or medical contraindications.
2. Seek physician approval, and obtain written order.
3. Explain massage therapy and potential benefits to the patient.
4. Obtain the patient's consent.
5. Develop a plan of care.
6. Create the therapeutic environment.
7. Monitor patient response to therapy.

critical care patients are hand, foot, and selected back, shoulder, and neck areas. Areas to be avoided are identified, and care is taken not to accidentally disconnect or dislodge any therapeutic equipment, such as monitoring leads or lines. It is usual to target bony prominences and healthy skin surrounding areas of tissue breakdown.

Assisting the patient into positions of comfort and establishing an appropriate environment to enhance the relaxation response are additional pretreatment steps. Creating this comforting environment enhances or maximizes the effects of therapeutic massage. Consideration for room temperature, body warmth (such as an extra blanket), quiet background music, dimming lights, closing the door, and placing a "Do Not Disturb" sign (with private rooms) are preparatory steps required. If patients choose, family members may observe the relaxation with massage. This can support the family's own comfort level and enhances trust in relationship to caregivers. Practitioners coordinate the plan of the massage treatment into the general plan of care to provide a maximum opportunity for uninterrupted therapy and a period of rest upon completion of the treatment.

Assessment

Assessing the patient's response during massage therapy is vital. The degree of pressure applied, types of strokes, and treatment time are determined in accordance with individual patient needs. Monitoring of the patient's verbal, nonverbal, and somatic cues is crucial. This step includes observing for negative cues, such as facial grimacing and withdrawing, as massage is given and for positive responses, such as smiles, relaxed breathing, and sighs of relief. Throughout the massage, the therapist uses good observational skills to make appropriate modifications and to gauge effectiveness of the treatments.

At the end of the session, the patient is placed in a comfortable position with safety factors addressed, including raised side rails and a call bell and personal items within reach. The therapist encourages the relaxation response by leaving the patient in a quiet environment with the lights turned down. Appropriate chart documentation and communication to the direct care provider about the effectiveness of and response to the treatment complete the session.

Research Findings

Massage therapy has been used on multiple patient types of all ages in all types of settings with an intent to improve pain control as well as to decrease anxiety, fear, frustration, depression, and irritability. Those who have received massage therapy report improved sleep, decreased muscle tension, headache relief, better circulation, and a decrease in peripheral edema. Massage has previously been used to help patients cope more effectively with the stress of hospitalization. It has also proved beneficial for the psychologic well-being of cancer patients and generally results in increased relaxation.

In their seminal work, Bauer and Dracup[2] evaluated the effects of back massage on 25 hemodynamically stable patients after myocardial infarction. Physiologic indicators were not affected by the massage, no negative effects were seen, and 24 of the 25 patients expressed positive reactions to the intervention. Stevensen[3] completed a randomized control study of 100 patients after cardiac surgery. The groups consisted of (1) no intervention, (2) support group, (3) oil massage, and (4) aromatherapy massage. Physiologic parameters and anxiety were assessed, but no differences were noted. No differences were seen between the two massage groups, but both groups derived a positive psychologic benefit from the therapy, in that relaxation was enhanced.

Dunn and colleagues[4] completed an experimental, randomized, controlled study on 122 patients admitted to a general ICU. The three groups received massage, aromatherapy, or rest at least one time and maximally four times over 5 days. Physiologic assessment of vital signs as well as anxiety, mood, and ability to cope were evaluated. There were no effects on physiologic variables but all three therapies had a positive impact on anxiety, mood, and coping ability.

Ironson and colleagues[5] examined the effects of 1 month of daily massage therapy on immune system function in homosexual men affected with human immunodeficiency virus (HIV) (20 HIV-positive, nine HIV-negative). Daily massages were given for 1 month. A subset of 11 of the HIV-infected subjects served as their own control group (1 month with and 1 month without massages). Major immune system findings after the month of massage included a significant increase in natural killer (NK) cell number, NK cell cytotoxicity, soluble CD8, and the cytotoxic subset of CD8 cells. There were no changes in HIV disease progression markers. Major neuroendocrine findings, measured via a 24-hour urine specimen, included a significant decrease in cortisol, and nonsignificant trends toward decrease of catecholamines. There were also decreases in anxiety and increases in relaxation that correlated significantly with increases in NK cell number. Thus, there appears to be an increase in cytotoxic capacity associated with massage.

Labyak and Metzger[6] completed a meta-analysis to evaluate the efficacy of massage and its role as a nursing therapy (Table 188–1). Techniques were used to statistically integrate the

TABLE 188–1. Research Findings on Massage Therapy

Author	Subjects	Design	Measurement	Result
Bauer and Dracup (1987)	25 stable myocardial infarction patients	Semiexperimental: convenience, under patient's own control	Vital signs, muscle tension, skin conductance, temperature	No adverse effects; no physiologic changes; positive patient self-report of well-being
Stevensen (1994)	100 post-cardiac surgery patients	Randomized control: 4 groups	Physiologic variables; anxiety	No changes in physiologic variables; positive effect on patient relaxation
Dunn et al. (1995)	122 patients in intensive care unit	Experimental, randomized, 3 treatment groups	Physiologic variables; mood; anxiety	No changes in physiologic variables; positive effect on mood, anxiety, sense of well-being
Ironson et al. (1996)	29 homosexual men	2 cohorts; within subject's design	Biologic blood; urine; psychologic mood; anxiety	Decreased cortisol levels; decreased anxiety and stress

findings of nine studies in which the physiologic effects of changes in systolic blood pressure, diastolic blood pressure, heart rate, and respiratory rate of effleurage back rub were examined and to learn how the findings differed by gender and the presence of cardiovascular disease. Three-minute effleurage back massages were associated with a decline in all four values and a continued reduction during the 5-minute post-massage rest period. Subjects undergoing CABG demonstrated atypical rise in blood pressure during the back massage, and their data were excluded from this portion of the analysis. Ten-minute massages were associated with maximum reductions in heart rate and respiratory rate, followed by a subsequent rise toward pretreatment levels during the 10-minute rest period. The greatest reductions in blood pressure were noted following the 3-minute massage.

A significant gender effect could be inferred in all of the studies that compared male and female responses regardless of health status. Female subjects demonstrated a rise in blood pressure during the first 3 to 5 minutes of the massage followed by a decline in blood pressure during the 10-minute rest period. In male subjects, 5 minutes of massage was associated with a decline in blood pressure and continued reductions during the 10-minute rest period. In contrast to blood pressure, heart and respiratory rates declined immediately in both men and women and remained well below baseline values throughout the massage. Both sexes experienced a rise toward pretreatment baseline in heart and respiratory rates across the 10-minute rest period.

Implications for Critical Care Practice

In all of these studies, massage has been found to have only a positive effect on patients. Back rubs and massage have long been nursing traditions but lost favor since the 1980s with the advent of high technology care. Although critical care practitioners should continue to evaluate the effects of complementary and adjunctive therapies through well-designed studies in order to ensure quality care, the use of massage therapy should enable nurses to remain in contact with patients, enhancing "hands-on care," and to provide opportunities to develop therapeutic relationships.

MUSIC THERAPY

Music therapy is the controlled use of music as an interventional noninvasive modality to achieve a desired effect. Music influences physiologic, psychologic, and emotional responses in people. Music is an effective nonthreatening means of communication that is viewed positively in all cultures. For most people, music provides relaxation and pleasure as well as a social diversion. Music can be enjoyed alone or with others. Through familiar music, an individual can evoke positive memories of past experiences and family that can be soothing, relaxing, and therapeutic. With music therapy, the practitioner can create an environment for the patient that results in a positive response. Without moving from the bedside and by using headphones, patients can experience pleasure and comfort.

Music, as a diversion, remains an effective therapeutic tool; it also exerts its own effect on the brain. Music can alter perceptions, modulates emotions, leads to the release of endorphins, enhances relaxation, and lets the right and left sides of the brain work together.[7-9]

A critical care environment creates anxiety and fear in patients. The nature of the care provided is often painful. Pain interferes with eating, exercising, deep breathing, coughing, and sleeping, thus placing the patient at risk for potential complications and a longer stay. Pain and fear of pain lead to higher levels of anxiety that have many undesirable outcomes. Anxiety interferes with effective pain relief, sleep, appetite, and normal coping mechanisms leading to feelings of loss of control, negative emotions, and alterations in physiologic patterns. Pain theory teaches that music can be used as a diversion so that pain awareness is decreased because the mind is focused on the music. Music is both a distraction and diversion that can reduce preoccupation with actual experiences and surroundings. Music can be used to filter out unpleasant sounds in the critical care environment and can decrease isolation, anxiety, pain, pain intensity, and the need for additional medication. The overall effect of music therapy is a generalized relaxation response.

Choice of Music

Choosing a type of music that is soothing and relaxing is critical to its effectiveness. High-pitched sounds increase tension. The tempo of relaxing music for some people is between 60 and 80 beats/min and matches the heart rate; however, the patient must want to listen to the type of music offered. If the music is familiar and pleasing to the patient, it will be relaxing. Providing music that the patient does not like is not therapeutic. Because the type of music must appeal to the patient, a varied selection is needed. Some common types of music used in music therapy are country and western, instrumental, strings, classical, popular, and music specifically made to be soothing and relaxing, such as the sound of running water. Johnston and Rohaly-Davis[9] and Updike[7] present a comprehensive list of music used for therapy. In addition, depending on the age, ethnic background, and culture of the patient, it may be necessary to ask the family to bring in familiar music that is relaxing for the patient.

Financial support needed for this therapy is minimal, as the necessary equipment can easily be purchased with a small grant or help from the volunteer department of the hospital. Music therapy is planned and is scheduled during the day and at bedtime. Personal needs of the patient, such as toileting or taking appropriate pain medication, should be met before music therapy is initiated. The patient should be positioned comfortably to facilitate rest. Once the patient selects a type of music, the lights should be dimmed and both extraneous noise and needless interruptions are eliminated. Headsets are then placed on the patient, and the volume is adjusted to the patient's preference (loud volume causes pain); however, young people may enjoy loud music. Music should not be played continuously; otherwise, it can be an annoyance rather than a pleasure. Music therapy sessions vary in length from 30 to 90 minutes, depending on patient preference. With the nonalert patient, the headset should be removed periodically and the therapy reinstituted several times during the 24-hour day.

Research Findings

Barnason and colleagues[8] evaluated the effects of music therapy on 96 patients after CABG surgery (Table 188-2). Patients were randomly assigned to one of three groups: music, music videos, or rest. Physiologic measures, anxiety, and mood were measured before and after intervention on postoperative days 2 and 3. There was no significant impact on the physiologic variables but an overall relaxation response was noted. In addition, all three groups showed reduced anxiety and mood improvement.

Dubois and coworkers[10] evaluated music and comfort during bronchoscopy. In a prospective randomized trial, 21 patients received music therapy and 28 patients served as controls. Physiologic variables, comfort, cough, and the amount

TABLE 188–2. Research Findings on Music Therapy

Author	Subjects	Design	Measurement	Result
Updike (1990)	20 ICU patients; non-ventilator-dependent; awake	Pretest, post-test	Physiologic variables; rhythm; pain medication dose; emotional response	Reduced blood pressure, mean arterial pressure; improved mood; no dysrhythmias; positive overall effect
Barnason et al. (1995)	96 post-CABG patients	Quasiexperimental; random to 3 groups: music, music videos, rest	Anxiety; mood; physiologic variables	Improved mood, decreased anxiety, generalized relaxation effect in all 3 groups
Dubois et al. (1995)	49 elective bronchoscopy patients	Prospective, randomized; 2 groups: music, control	Physiologic variables; comfort; cough; dyspnea; medications	Less cough, greater comfort in music group; no difference in physiologic variables or dyspnea
Chlan (1995)	20 mechanically ventilated	Pretest, post-test; repeated measures; 2 groups: music, headphones only	Physiologic variables; mood rhythm	Decreased heart rate and respiratory rate; improved mood; no dysrhythmias

ICU = intensive care unit; CABG = coronary artery bypass graft.

of medication given were all measured. Results indicated no difference in physiologic variables. Although the medications given did not differ in the two groups, the music group rated their overall comfort significantly higher and their cough significantly lower compared with the nonmusic group.

Chlan[11] used a two-group experimental design with pretest, post-test and repeated measures with 40 mechanically ventilated patients to evaluate response to music. Twenty patients received music therapy, and 20 were in the nonmusic headphones-only group. Physiologic parameters and mood were measured. Music listening improved mood and decreased heart and respiratory rates, findings that seemed to indicate improved relaxation.

Implications for Critical Care Practice

For many people, music is an important part of life. It is often used unconsciously to block out sounds in the home or environment. Certainly, the use of music for distraction is justified in a noisy critical care unit. Music therapy offers an opportunity for the family to get involved in doing something to help their loved one by selecting music and perhaps supplying headphones. All the care provider has to do is ask. By involving the family and the patient in the selection process and allowing both some input into the frequency and duration of the music therapy, the care provider contributes to the overall long-term goals of patient- and family-centered care. The use of music therapy in critical care practice is an inexpensive and effective way to maximize the beneficial effects of pharmacotherapy and to provide patients and their families with something that is familiar to them. For these reasons, music therapy is an effective complementary modality of care.

BOX 188–2
BASIC STEPS IN THERAPEUTIC TOUCH (KRIEGER/KUNZ METHOD)

1. Centering
2. Assessment or scanning
3. Unruffling (clearing)
4. Treatment (balancing, rebalancing, and intervention)
5. Evaluation

THERAPEUTIC TOUCH

One of the most novel complementary modalities of care is Therapeutic Touch. The roots of therapeutic touch rest within Eastern medicine. In the 1960s, individuals with reputations as healers gained some public recognition for the work they were doing through the laying on of hands. During this era, Grad, a biochemist, became interested in the concept of laying on of hands and initiated research demonstrating that some type of energy was involved in the process.[12, 13] In 1972, Delores Krieger, a nurse, and Dora Kunz, a clairvoyant who has worked with physicians in paranormal diagnosis and counseling, together developed the Krieger/Kunz method[14] of Therapeutic Touch. Although other methods of therapeutic touch and healing are in use today, the Krieger/Kunz model is described here.

The Krieger/Kunz method facilitates energy interaction between practitioner and patient. The practitioner's goal is to help repattern, realign, and smooth out the patient's own energy field so that the energy field is healthy or healing in nature. Therapeutic Touch is perceived as a healing art that facilitates self-healing through a process of *resonance* rather than energy exchanging.[15, 16] No direct contact with the skin is required, although some practitioners prefer direct physical contact. It is customary for the practitioner to hold the hands 2 to 6 inches away from the patient's body.

The entire treatment takes about 15 minutes. The patient does not have to be "a believer" or even to be conscious of the treatment for the therapy to exert a positive effect. It is a skill that can be learned and refined with practice. The practitioner should be taught the correct method. Health care providers can seek additional information about learning the Krieger/Kunz method from most university-based schools of nursing in the United States and from nurse healers.*

No negative effects have been reported for either the practitioner or the patient when therapy is done properly. The outcome is usually relaxation, decreased pain, decreased anxiety and stress, and a greater sense of well-being.

Procedure

Five basic steps are used in the Krieger/Kunz method (Box 188–2). Experienced practitioners are able to use these steps simultaneously.

*Nurse Healers–Professional Associates, Inc., 1211 Locust Street, Philadelphia, PA 19107.

Centering

Initially, the care provider engages in *centering,* a meditation process used by the practitioner to focus on the task at hand. Some practitioners use deep breathing to achieve a sense of self-cleansing while centering. The practitioner develops an inner calm to quiet the body and to free the mind from extraneous thoughts. It is a form of self-relaxation that extends that concept to also being receptive to the patient. Centering is done without mental effort. If a practitioner uses Therapeutic Touch without the centering technique, the practitioner becomes tired and the results are not effective. As the practitioner centers, he or she allows the benefits of Therapeutic Touch to emerge into the conscious mind.

Scanning the Energy Field

The second step is the assessment or scanning of the patient's energy field through the use of the practitioner's hands. This sensing of the energy field is not mystical or difficult to achieve. The sensation can be likened to the effect all people feel when they gently cup their own hands and move them toward each other in a very slow clapping-like action without actually touching the skin of one hand to the other. As the hands are moved toward each other and then back out, the body of air between the hands starts to warm and starts to feel larger to the person using the clapping-like motion, even though there is nothing but air between the hands. This action provides evidence that the energy field of a person does not end at the skin.

An energy field can also be related to the sensation one experiences when someone else comes into the room even though we never heard them enter. The individual is sensing the energy field of the other person. The skilled practitioner gently cups the hands, which are usually held 2 to 6 inches away from the patient's body, then moves the hand in a symmetric, downward motion from head to feet while sensing the patient's energy field. The practitioner is seeking an area or areas in which the differences in the energy field can be felt. Although these sensations are subtle and the interpretation is subjective, skilled practitioners use knowledge of the patient's illness, intuition, and somatic cues to locate problem areas. Practitioners report sensing tingling, vibrating, and temperature changes or differences over the various areas where the energy field is altered. It is primarily those problem areas on which the practitioner focuses attention; the practitioner also validates the effects with the patient. The practitioner facilitates the flow of energy by serving as a conduit.

Clearing the Energy Field

In the next two steps, the practitioner attempts to clear, or unruffle, the energy field and give treatment. The intent is to intervene to help the patient's body balance areas of the energy field that are disrupted. In this phase, a sweeping motion of the hands is used to clear the blockage wherever it occurs. The practitioner may use imagery along with a flicking or brushing hand and finger motion to dispel the blocked field and smooth out the patient's energy field.

Balancing Energy

Energy is directed to any area in which the energy flow is sensed as being sluggish or blocked. The practitioner holds the hands over the area in an attempt to modulate and balance the energy based on the continuous flow of life energy.

Evaluating the Outcome

In the evaluation phase, the practitioner senses the improvement over the energy field through the use of the hands. Both intuition and judgment are necessary to determine when to terminate the treatment. It is usual for both the practitioner and the patient to feel a sense of relaxation, positive energy, calmness, and well-being upon completion of the session. Therapeutic Touch can be given to anyone at any time. Patients invariably choose to repeat the experience and express satisfaction with the therapy.[14, 16]

Research Findings

Therapeutic Touch has been used in multiple patient types since the early 1970s. Many research papers are published as to its effectiveness and efficacy (Table 188–3). However, there are different approaches in common use, including faith healing, laying on of hands, modified therapeutic touch, and the Krieger/Kunz method. Despite the variation, multiple research reports (some more scientific than others) lend credence to the use of this modality of care. Looking back over 30 years to the origins of varied types of therapeutic touch provides a sense that although there are many confounding variables that interfere with controlled, random trials, most research and multiple anecdotal reports indicate positive effects on patients.

Grad and colleagues[12] removed skin from 300 mice; a local healer treated half the mice, and they reported accelerated wound healing in this group. In another study, Grad had the healer hold a beaker of normal saline and treat one third of a sample of barley seeds.[13] For one third of the seeds, a non-

TABLE 188–3. Research Findings on Therapeutic Touch

Author	Subjects	Design	Measurement	Result
Gagne and Toye (1994)	31 psychiatric inpatients	Random; 2 groups: therapeutic touch with relaxation; therapeutic touch placebo	Anxiety; motor activity; patient expectations	Decreased anxiety in both groups; relaxation, reduced motor activity; no correlation to expectancy
Wirth et al. (1997)	44 healthy subjects	Experimental, double-blinded	Multisite electromyographic activity	Rise in magnetic activity with Qigong; decreased muscle energy with therapeutic touch
Olson and Sneed (1995)	40 caregiver students	Experimental; 4 groups; repeated measures	Anxiety; mood	Reduction of anxiety in high anxiety group with therapeutic touch; statistical significance not achieved
Quinn and Strelkauskas (1993)	4 bereaved patients	Pilot study	Anxiety; affect; lymphocyte levels	Modulation of lymphocyte subsets (small sample)

healer held the saline, and one third of the seeds were not treated. Seedlings that were given the saline and treated by the healer grew faster, stronger, and taller. This experiment was replicated many times in varied scenarios. It was concluded that some type of energy was involved that could penetrate the glass and influence the plants.

Wirth[17] described the effect of a modified form of therapeutic touch by evaluating the healing rates of 46 punch biopsy sites. The true intent was not revealed to the physician or technician in this study. Each subject entered an isolated room and placed the arm (site of the biopsy) into a sleeve built into a wall. The patient could not see into the other room, and the physician and technician thought the bioelectric properties of healing were being measured. In this research protocol, the practitioner only focused on the unhealed wound rather than on the entire patient, as in the Krieger/Kunz method. The control group inserted the arm into an empty room for 5 minutes, and the treated group was given the modified therapeutic touch for 5 minutes by the unseen practitioner. This procedure was continued for 16 days. The technician measured the wound size on the day of surgery, on day 8, and on day 16. On day 1, the measurement was identical for all patients. In the modified therapeutic touch group, the wound was 10 times smaller on day 8 than in the untreated group. On the last day of the study, the average size of the wound in the treated group was 0.418 mm^2; in the untreated group, the size was 5.855 mm^2, a statistically significant difference. Of the 23 subjects treated by touch, 13 were healed by day 16. No subjects in the untreated group were healed. Although this was not the Krieger/Kunz method as defined in this chapter, this work clearly identified that energy was involved in the therapeutic touch process that somehow influenced the healing rate. Wirth's later work, also using modified therapeutic touch, demonstrated that subjects experienced a modest decrease in overall muscle energy.[18]

Olson and Sneed used a four-group repeated measures experimental design on 40 healthy professional caregivers and students to test Therapeutic Touch.[19] They measured three self-report measures of anxiety (Profile of Moods State, the Speilberger State/Trait Anxiety Inventory, and a visual analog scale). Results demonstrated reduced anxiety.

Quinn[20] tested the concept of mimic therapeutic touch versus actual Therapeutic Touch to demonstrate the effectiveness of the therapy. All sessions were videotaped. Evaluators were unable to identify the mimic and real forms. In this study the mimic practitioners did not center, made no attempt to assess the patient, and did not repattern or rebalance the energy field. A self-administered pre-questionnaire and a post-questionnaire revealed a greater decrease in post-test state anxiety scores in the subjects who received Therapeutic Touch; thus, the intent of the practitioner, not the motions of the body and hands, contributed to effective therapy.

In another study Quinn and Strelkauskas,[15] summarizing the past use of Therapeutic Touch, reported that it increased hemoglobin level, induced relaxation, decreased anxiety and pain, improved wound healing, increased feelings of well-being, and altered select immunologic parameters.

Gagne and Toye[21] examined the effects of Therapeutic Touch on anxiety in psychiatric patients. The result was a reduction of anxiety, as noted with self-report.

At present, Quinn and Strelkauskas are researching the psychoimmune effects of Therapeutic Touch. Larger sample size and repeated studies are needed to more fully explicate the results of their efforts.

Implications for Critical Care Practice

Anecdotal accounts of the effect of Therapeutic Touch are often reported in the literature. For example, Mills[22] reported on a case study in which a patient with an infected right foot who had an adverse reaction to antibiotics wrote anecdotal notes while receiving Therapeutic Touch. The patient documented a feeling of warmth, decreased pain, and increased relaxation and well-being. The positive patient reaction to the therapy and the expressed satisfaction of receiving the treatment are themselves justification for concerned practitioners to explore the potential use of this complementary modality of care. All practitioners recognize the negative effects of the critical care environment on the alert patient. Anything that reduces pain, anxiety, or stress or that enhances medical care should be offered to the patient. The focus of Therapeutic Touch is based on the desire to help with healing to facilitate wholeness of the patient. Thus, this is a safe, effective bedside technique that can be used by a practitioner with minimal effort and no cost (other than time) to help achieve positive patient outcomes. The question is: How can the intensivist afford not to encourage bedside practitioners to use this therapy?

SUMMARY

For patients in an ICU, sensory overload, lack of privacy, absence of family, loss of daylight patterning, and pain and discomfort result in much stress. Practitioners dedicated to caring for these patients need to find new and creative ways to deal with this stress. Massage therapy has been used as long as recorded time and has been effective in relieving human distress. All research to date clearly identifies positive patient benefits with no ill effects on the critically ill patient.

Music is a necessary part of life for many people. For patients in the critical care environment, music therapy offers a safe, economical, and effective way to complement medical care. Music therapy requires very little to be effective and affords the family an opportunity to contribute to the patient's well-being. There is no reason to deny this therapy to most critically ill patients. The caregiver just has to get the family involved, the intensivist just has to suggest it and the therapy can be initiated. Finally, Therapeutic Touch is an effective and well-used modality that can augment the medical plan of care by facilitating relaxation.

Complementary modalities of care are being used both with and without the knowledge of physicians. These therapies expand our horizons in an attempt to use whatever else may be available to improve patient outcomes. The time is here to supplement the care provided by the medical model with the use of these effective adjunct treatments.

References

1. Meltzer LE, Abdellah FG, Kitchell JR: Concepts and Practices of Intensive Care for Nurse Specialists. Bowie, Md, Charles Press, 1969, pp 371-385.
2. Bauer WC, Dracup KA: Physiologic effects of back massage in patients with acute myocardial infarction. Focus Crit Care 1987; 14:42-46.
3. Stevensen CJ: The psychophysiological effects of aromatherapy massage following cardiac surgery. Complementary Ther Med 1994; 2:27-35.
4. Dunn C, Sleep J, Collett D: Sensing an improvement: An experimental study to evaluate the use of aromatherapy, massage and periods of rest in an intensive care unit. J Adv Nurs 1995; 21:34-40.
5. Ironson G, Field T, Scafidi F, Hashimoto M, Kumar M, Kumar A, Price A, Goncalves A, Burman I, Tetenman CY, Patarca R, Fletcher M: Massage therapy is associated with enhancement of the immune system's cytotoxic capacity. Int J Neurosci 1996; 84:205-217.
6. Labyak S, Metzger B: The effects of effleurage backrub on the physiological components of relaxation: A meta-analysis. Nurs Res 1997; 46:59-62.

7. Updike P: Music therapy results for ICU patients. Dimens Crit Care Nurs 1990; 9:39–45.
8. Barnason S, Zimmerman L, Nieveen J: The effects of music interventions on anxiety in the patient after coronary artery bypass grafting. Heart Lung 1995; 24:124–132.
9. Johnston K, Rohaly-Davis J: An introduction to music therapy: Helping the oncology patient in the ICU. Crit Care Nurs Q 1996; 18:54–60.
10. Dubois JM, Bartter T, Pratter MR: Music improves patient comfort level during outpatient bronchoscopy. Chest 1995; 108:129–130.
11. Chlan LL: Psychophysiologic responses of mechanically ventilated patients to music: A pilot study. Am J Crit Care 1995; 4:233–238.
12. Grad B, Cadoret RH, Paul GI: An unorthodox method of wound healing in mice. Int J Parapsychol 1961; 3:5–24.
13. Grad B: A telekinetic effect on plant growth. Int J Parapsychol 1963; 5:117–133.
14. Therapeutic Touch Teaching Guidelines: Krieger/Kunz Method. Allison Park, Pa, Nurse Healers–Professional Associates, Inc.
15. Quinn JF, Strelkauskas AJ: Psychoimmunologic effects of Therapeutic Touch on practitioners and recently bereaved recipients: A pilot study. Adv Nurs Sci 1993; 15:13–26.
16. Steckel CM, King RP: Nursing grand rounds. J Cardiovasc Nurs 1996; 10:50–54.
17. Wirth D: The effects of non-contact therapeutic touch on the healing rate of full thickness dermal wounds. Subtle Energies 1990; 1:1–20.
18. Wirth DP, Cram JR, Chang BA: Multisite electromyographic analysis of therapeutic touch and Qigong therapy. J Alternative Complementary Med 1997; 3:109–118.
19. Olson M, Sneed N: Anxiety and therapeutic touch. Issues Ment Health Nurs 1995; 16:97–108.
20. Quinn J: The seniors Therapeutic Touch education program. Holistic Nurs Pract 1992; 7:32–37.
21. Gagne D, Toye RC: The effects of TT and relaxation therapy in reducing anxiety. Arch Psychiatr Nurs 1994; 8:184–189.
22. Mills A: Therapeutic touch—case study: The application, documentation and outcome. Complementary Ther Med 1996; 4:127–132.

189

Preventing Complications in the Intensive Care Unit

Elizabeth A. Henneman, RN, PhD, CCRN

The prevention of complications in the critically ill patient is one of the greatest challenges for health care providers working in the intensive care unit (ICU). The high cost of complications—to patients, their families, and health care institutions—has heightened interest in the development and evaluation of methods for ameliorating such events.

Preventing all complications in critically ill patients is, perhaps, impossible. Minimizing complications, however, demands that critical care staff adopt an aggressive approach to managing what are sometimes considered the mundane aspects of patient management, such as skin care or patient positioning. Successful complication prevention requires a multidisciplinary commitment to the development and monitoring of standards of care with a preventive focus. Many of the interventions aimed at preventing complications are now being performed by unlicensed assistants (e.g., nurses aides, technicians). It is imperative that these caregivers be well-trained and closely supervised in carrying out these important responsibilities.[1]

Standards of care should reflect current research findings and should be appropriate for the population of the unit. Unit-based standards should incorporate national or international guidelines when available, such as *International Standards for Safety in the Intensive Care Unit*,[2] the Society of Critical Care Medicine's *Guidelines for Standards of Care for Patients with Acute Respiratory Failure on Mechanical Ventilatory Support*,[3] and the guidelines recommended by the Centers for Disease Control and Prevention (CDC).[4] In addition to being theoretically sound, these standards must also be feasible for the fast-paced, chaotic ICU environment. The effectiveness of the standards in achieving goals must also be evaluated continually through a unit-based program (e.g., continuous quality improvement).

Interventions aimed at preventing complications must be instituted as early as possible in the patient's admission process or before admission (e.g., in patients undergoing elective surgery), when feasible. Standardized admission order forms are useful to ensure that certain procedures are carried out routinely, especially in settings with a significant learning curve, such as teaching hospitals.

The variety and number of potential complications in critically ill patients is tremendous. This chapter reviews those that occur most often, are pertinent to the majority of critically ill patients, and in most cases are predictable—and therefore preventable. These complications include skin and mucosal breakdown, musculoskeletal injury, pulmonary complications, and ICU psychosis. No attempt has been made to cover the almost limitless list of complications that may arise in critically ill patients secondary to their illness or treatment. For example, complications associated with disease processes (e.g., arrhythmias), procedures (e.g., pneumothorax), treatments (e.g., fluid overload), and surgery (e.g., bleeding) are not covered. Stress ulcers, deep vein thromboses, and nosocomial infections, among the most common complications of ICU patients, are addressed in other chapters of this book.

SKIN AND MUCOSAL BREAKDOWN

Alterations in the integrity of the skin and mucous membranes are among the best-recognized complications in critically ill patients. They are visible and constant reminders of the consequence of clinicians' actions or inaction. The patient in the ICU is at risk for skin and mucosal problems because of the underlying illness and ICU treatment modalities. Table 189–1 lists risk factors commonly seen in critically ill patients that may lead to the development of skin and mucosal injury.

TABLE 189–1. Risk Factors for Skin and Mucosal Injury in Critically Ill Patients

Risk factor
Immobility
Decreased oxygen delivery or consumption
Impaired nutritional status
Extremes of age (<1 yr, >60 yr)
Obesity
Edema
Diabetes mellitus
Immunosuppression
Infection
Decreased level of consciousness
Impaired sensation
Hyperthermia or hypothermia
Pre-existing illness
Incontinence
Invasive therapies
Nasogastric tubes
Endotracheal or tracheostomy tubes
Rectal tubes
Vasopressor medications

Pressure Ulcers

Pressure ulcers are lesions caused by unrelieved pressure that results in damage to underlying tissue. The incidence of pressure ulcers in the critical care setting has been reported to be as high as 29%.[5] Treatment costs of up to $40,000 per patient have been reported.[6] Prevention of pressure ulcers requires multidisciplinary standards of care that recognize the potential for all critically ill patients to develop this complication. A comprehensive care plan demands early assessment, intervention, and evaluation of skin integrity. Unfortunately, because of the critical nature of the patient's condition on admission to the ICU, skin problems generally are a low priority. The patient who survives a critical illness yet dies from sepsis secondary to a pressure ulcer is a sad reminder of the irony of this situation.

Assessment of the patient's risk for pressure ulcers should be performed as early as possible in the patient's hospital stay. Elective surgery patients should be evaluated preoperatively, and preventive interventions should begin before the operation. For example, heart surgery patients, who are at risk for sacral pressure ulcers, should have special dressings or padding placed over the sacrum preoperatively in preparation for lying flat on their backs for long periods.

Tools to determine a patient's risk of developing pressure ulcers have been devised; however, their predictive value in critically ill patients has not been well-established. Modification of scoring instruments such as the Braden Scale[7] have been tested for use in critically ill patients.[8] Such tools can help to identify patients at risk for the development of pressure ulcers (see Table 189–1). ICUs should incorporate these scoring tools into their standards and protocols for maintenance of skin integrity.

Interventions to prevent skin breakdown must also be instituted early in the patient's ICU course. Unit standards should address preventive measures appropriate for various patient populations. The most effective standards are ones that delineate specific (e.g., mattress overlay) rather than vague (e.g., skin care precautions) interventions.

Because immobility is a major risk factor for the development of pressure ulcers, interventions to decrease this complication are typically aimed at maximizing patient mobility. Unfortunately, many critically ill patients must remain relatively immobile. As a result, much effort has been directed at determining ways of decreasing or relieving pressure in these immobile patients with special mattresses. Debate continues over the most effective method of pressure reduction and relief, and various mattress overlays, replacement mattresses, and specialty beds are now marketed for this purpose. Table 189–2 lists these products, their indications, and their advantages and disadvantages.

The cost-benefit ratio for the prophylactic use of these products has yet to be determined; however, the high risk of ulcers in critically ill patients has led some experts to suggest the use of universal pressure ulcer precautions, that is, special pressure-reduction beds, for all critically ill patients. The significant cost of special beds demands that an assessment of the individual patient's needs be ongoing to determine appropriate strategies for pressure reduction. For example, the use of a mattress overlay for a nominal one-time charge seems a reasonable preventive approach for all critically ill patients, but the decision to use a very expensive, low–air loss bed requires serious consideration of the cost-benefit ratio. As the patient's condition changes, the appropriateness of all pressure-reduction strategies must be examined and interventions made accordingly.

Clinical practice guidelines have been published that provide both clinicians and patients with useful information on the prevention of pressure ulcers in adults.[9] These guidelines may be useful when unit-based standards are developed for pressure ulcer prevention.

Device-Related Injury

The use of invasive therapies in critical care is plagued by numerous potential complications involving skin and mucosal injury. Indwelling devices such as endotracheal, tracheostomy, nasogastric, and rectal tubes present special problems in critically ill patients.

Endotracheal Tubes

Low-pressure cuffs on endotracheal tubes allow these tubes to be left in place longer with less concern for tracheal damage, but this practice increases the patient's risk of pressure sores in the mouth or nares. This problem is compounded when monitoring devices such as end-tidal carbon dioxide monitors are clamped onto the endotracheal tube, adding to traction and pressure. Furthermore, skin breakdown can occur on the face from the adhesive tape used to secure the tube, or lip necrosis when the lip is caught between the tube and the tape.

Management of this problem requires unit standards that call for frequent tube repositioning, support to decrease traction on the endotracheal tube, and facial skin protection. Our standard is to reposition oral endotracheal tubes (from side to side) every 24 to 48 hours. Rolled-up towels are used to prop up ventilator tubing and prevent traction on the mouth or nose from the ventilator circuitry and heavy attachments. To protect the skin, we apply Duoderm (Conva Tec, Princeton, N.J.) beneath the tape on the face of any patient who may require long-term intubation or who has friable skin (Fig. 189–1). An alternative would be to use Velcro endotracheal tube holders; however, we have not had success with this method in restless or agitated patients.

Tracheostomy Tubes

The problems of traction from the weight of ventilator tubing and other devices also occur with tracheostomy tubes. Because patients with these tubes are often more mobile than

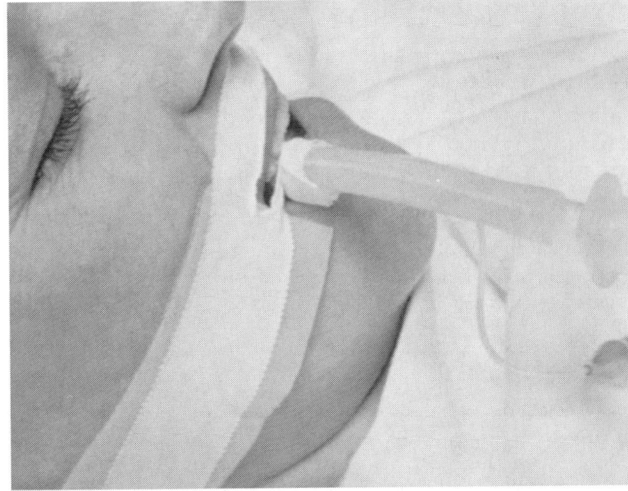

Figure 189–1. Use of a protective barrier under adhesive tape decreases the incidence of skin breakdown in high-risk patients (e.g., patients undergoing long-term intubation or those with friable skin).

TABLE 189–2. Pressure Reduction and Relief Devices

Device	Indications	Advantages	Disadvantages	Comments
Mattress Overlay	Patients at low to moderate risk who are expected to be on bed rest >24 hr. May be used as a prophylactic strategy on all ICU beds.			
Foam (3–4 inches thick and of appropriate density)*		Comfortable. One-time charge or low cost. No daily maintenance. Less user error than with plastic overlays. Less friction and shear than with standard hospital bed.	Potentially flammable. Difficult to reposition patient. Difficult to fit sheets on thick mattresses. Added height makes getting patient out of bed difficult. Require incontinence devices to prevent permanent soiling.	
Plastic		One-time charge or low cost. Potentially more effective than foam with heavy patients. Easy to clean.	Ensuring proper inflation level is cumbersome and subjective. Increased perspiration. Patient discomfort. Leaks if punctured.	
Water overlay		One-time charge or low cost. Conforms to body contours.	Set-up cumbersome. Set-up time required. Leaks if punctured. May reduce effectiveness of CPR.	
Alternating-Pressure Mattress		Provides alternating pressure. Easy to clean. User friendly.	Plastic increases perspiration. Motor requires an electric source.	
Replacement Mattress		No maintenance by nursing staff.	Initial cost.	Used in place of hospital mattress. Designed for multiple patient use.
Low–Air Loss Bed	Patients who are immobile and cannot be turned at regular intervals or who are at high risk in other areas.	Surface fabrics are low-friction materials. Built-in scales available on most models.	High daily cost. Reduce patient mobility (patient "sinks" in bed). Difficult to transfer in and out of bed. Difficult to transfer patient in bed (heavy). Difficult to perform CPR.	Consists of multiple rows of air-filled cushions that can be programmed for each patient to provide maximum pressure relief. Tissue interface pressures are maintained below the recommended 25 mm Hg.
Air-Fluidized Bed	Immobility associated with wounds (e.g., stage IV pressure ulcers, burns, or grafts).	Pressure relief.	Potential dehydration from high air flow. Spontaneous patient movement restricted. Difficult to secure Fowler's position (uses foam wedges, which slip). Difficult patient transfer in and out of bed. Bed extremely heavy. Cleaning process cumbersome (beads blown into air).	A fluid-like environment is created by passing air under silicone-coated beads, which are covered by a semipermeable sheet.

TABLE 189–2. Pressure Reduction and Relief Devices *Continued*

Device	Indications	Advantages	Disadvantages	Comments
Pulsating Bed		Pressure relief plus potential for improved venous return.	Same as for Low-Air Loss Bed.	
Kinetic Therapy				
Oscillating bed: low-air loss	Severe hemodynamic instability or pulmonary conditions that would benefit from frequent turning.	May be effective in management of pulmonary process.	High cost. Conscious patients may not tolerate constant motion or turning.	Air cushions are alternately inflated and deflated to allow for gentle patient turning, or the bed frame rotates.

*Two-inch foam eggcrate mattresses do not reduce pressure and are intended for patient comfort only.
CPR = cardiopulmonary resuscitation; ICU = intensive care unit.

those with ventilator tubes, extra care must be taken during transfers and repositioning to ensure that the tubes are positioned properly. Tracheostomy tubes pose the additional problem of skin breakdown secondary to secretions that ooze from the tracheostomy incision or from twill ties applied too tightly. The combination of the two (i.e., wet, tight tracheostomy ties) can seriously macerate the skin. Products are now available that use wide, soft material with Velcro fasteners, which we have found to be quite effective in securing tracheostomy tubes.

Feeding Tubes

Most skin breakdown problems resulting from feeding tubes can be avoided with proper positioning and taping. In efforts to adequately secure them, tubes are often flexed upward, out of the patient's face. This maneuver can produce upward traction on the patient's nares and eventual skin breakdown at the nostrils (Figs. 189–2 and 189–3). Although usually not life-threatening, this complication causes an avoidable disfiguration and is an unfortunate reminder of the patient's stay in the ICU.

Proper positioning and protective skin barriers, such as those previously recommended for endotracheal tubes, are useful in decreasing the skin breakdown associated with these tubes. A variety of methods of securing feeding tubes are used in the ICU. Researchers have suggested that adhesive tape ("pink tape") is more effective than others for securing tubes.[10]

Rectal Tubes

Rectal tubes are used for critically ill patients with unremitting diarrhea. Although the goal of these tubes is to increase patient comfort and decrease skin breakdown, other consequences must be considered. The high pressure of the cuff used to prevent dislodgment of the tube can cause breakdown of the rectal mucosa and damage to the sphincter. Appropriate use of these tubes demands that a strict schedule of balloon deflation be adhered to (e.g., a half hour every 4 hours). Alternatives to rectal tubes, such as rectal bags, should be used whenever possible. An aggressive approach to the assessment and management of diarrhea is the most important step in limiting use of such devices.

Wound Drainage or Fistulas

Exudates from draining wounds or enterocutaneous fistulas can be extremely irritating to surrounding skin. Gastrointestinal contents (e.g., bile) pose serious threats to skin integrity. Prevention of skin breakdown requires that the surrounding skin be meticulously cleared of exudate. This goal is accomplished with frequent dressing changes and protective skin barriers such as transparent or hydro-occlusive dressings.

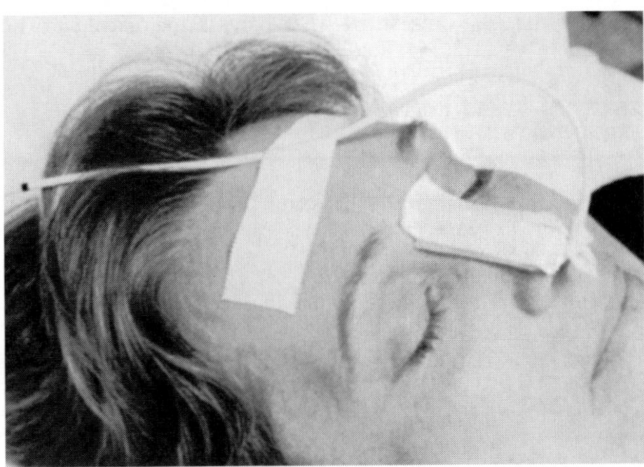

Figure 189–2. Incorrect positioning of a nasogastric tube. Upward flexion of the tube places pressure on patient's nares.

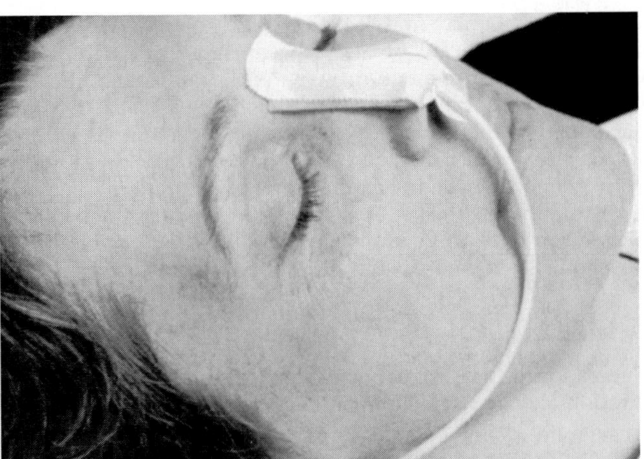

Figure 189–3. Correct nasogastric tube positioning. A protective barrier is also used under the adhesive tape.

Gravity drainage bags are often useful for channeling large amounts of drainage away from the skin.

MUSCULOSKELETAL COMPLICATIONS

Muscle weakness was once believed to result solely from prolonged immobility and catabolism associated with critical illness. Research now suggests that critically ill patients may suffer from a phenomenon called *critical illness polyneuropathy* (CIP), which exacerbates muscle weakness in this group of patients at risk. This syndrome of acute reversible neuropathy has been reported in as many as 70% of patients with sepsis and multiple organ system failure.[11] Recognition of the syndrome underscores the importance of efforts aimed at maintaining muscle function in critically ill persons.

Neuromuscular junction–blocking agents are considered an important adjunct in the treatment of severe respiratory failure or increased intracranial pressure. These drugs have been associated with muscle weakness and prolonged paralysis.[12] As a result, even closer attention should be paid to aggressive preventive management of muscle atrophy when these drugs are used.

Prevention of musculoskeletal complications requires frequent repositioning of the limbs and passive range-of-motion exercises. Maintaining proper body alignment and performing passive range-of-motion exercises are typically the responsibility of the critical care nurse, who integrates these interventions into other aspects of the patient's care (e.g., bathing).

A variety of commercially available devices or high-top sneakers can be used to help to prevent foot drop. Their use requires that the staff pay careful attention to the proper fit and positioning of the foot inside the device or sneaker. In particular, the staff must check the integrity of the skin of the foot. Patients with pedal edema or poor circulation are at increased risk for skin breakdown.

Involvement of the physical therapist is vital to ensuring a comprehensive patient care plan. In addition to evaluating the appropriateness and effectiveness of the exercise program, the physical therapist can evaluate the patient's progress and can make recommendations that address the patient's ongoing needs.

Family members who have expressed an interest in participating in the patient's care should be instructed on performing bedside exercises. Posting exercise instructions (i.e., "how-to" diagrams) and schedules can help motivate staff, patients, and families to follow these regimens.

PULMONARY COMPLICATIONS

The critically ill patient is at high risk for pulmonary complications secondary to the disease process, surgery, or debilitation or to use of equipment that supports the patient through the illness (e.g., ventilators, endotracheal tubes). Guidelines developed by the Society of Critical Care Medicine for patients with acute respiratory failure[2] may help to decrease the number of pulmonary complications by standardizing the management of this high-risk population. The following section reviews some complications common in ICUs: atelectasis, nosocomial pneumonia, and unplanned extubation.

Atelectasis

The patient who is immobile or unable to breathe deeply may develop atelectasis, a common complication in the postoperative period, especially after abdominal or thoracic surgery. The mainstay of prophylaxis for atelectasis is to encourage the patient to breathe deeply on a regular basis. Although this recommendation seems straightforward, this goal is difficult to achieve for a very ill patient, whose consciousness may be altered, whose mobility is limited, and who is in pain.

For an awake patient, deep breathing is usually sufficient for preventing atelectasis. Maintaining a sustained maximal inspiration has been found to be the optimal means of preventing postoperative pulmonary complications.[13, 14] Devices such as incentive spirometers may help to motivate the patient but are of little value unless they are accompanied by specific instructions, monitoring, and support from the nurse or respiratory therapist.

The patient with a decreased level of consciousness requires alternative forms of therapy to prevent atelectasis, including frequent repositioning, intermittent positive-pressure breathing, and chest physiotherapy. Turning the patient from side to side, either manually or via kinetic therapy, helps to prevent atelectasis in the dependent lung. Routine use of intermittent positive-pressure ventilation in a lucid, co-operative postoperative patient is inappropriate; incentive spirometry is as effective and less costly. Intermittent positive-pressure ventilation is, however, indicated when the patient is unable spontaneously to perform deep-breathing maneuvers.

Routine use of chest physiotherapy (postural drainage, vibration, percussion) for the prevention of atelectasis has not been supported by research; however, atelectasis secondary to mucous plugs has been shown to be reversed with the use of chest physiotherapy.[15] Routine use of chest physiotherapy in all postoperative and ICU patients should be replaced by thoughtful consideration of each patient's needs. In many instances, deep breathing and increased mobility adequately prevent atelectasis.

Pain is often a major obstacle to patient compliance with deep-breathing maneuvers. Effective pain management and using pillows to splint incisions may enhance patient cooperation. Patient-controlled anesthesia devices allow patients to relieve their pain during deep-breathing exercises.

Nosocomial Pneumonia

The ICU is the hospital setting where most nosocomial pneumonias develop. The occurrence of a nosocomial infection has been demonstrated to increase the risk of death in critically ill patients.[16] Risk factors related to both the ICU patient and the environment are noted in Table 189–3. Traditionally, strategies for preventing pneumonia were aimed at optimizing the patient's potential to fight infection and at managing the environment to prevent the introduction of organisms and cross-contamination. Despite these efforts, the incidence of nosocomial infection remains high, especially in patients receiving mechanical ventilation.[17, 18] New research suggests that colonization of the gastrointestinal tract plays a major role in the

TABLE 189–3. Risk Factors for Nosocomial Infections in Critically Ill Patients

Immobility
Impaired nutritional status
Extremes of age (<1 yr, >60 yr)
Diabetes mellitus
Immunosuppression
Decreased level of consciousness
Decreased cardiac output
Use of invasive therapies
Nasogastric tubes
Endotracheal or tracheostomy tubes
Rectal tubes
Vascular access devices
Use of mechanical ventilation
Proximity of patients

development of pneumonia, and efforts have been directed at developing ways to decrease the occurrence of this phenomenon.

Patients who are intubated and receiving mechanical ventilation are especially vulnerable to pneumonia because they lack normal protective mechanisms such as a cough reflex and functional cilia. Endotracheal and nasogastric tubes also inhibit normal mechanisms such as chewing and swallowing that prevent colonization of the oral cavity. Patients with depressed levels of consciousness from sedation or neurologic injury are at risk for aspiration of colonizing organisms.

Because patients in the ICU are also at risk for gastric stress ulcers and bleeding, they often receive prophylactic histamine blockers or antacids. Antacids have been demonstrated to increase the risk of pneumonia in patients receiving mechanical ventilation, presumably by increasing the pH above 4, a level inadequate for inhibition of bacterial growth.[17]

Other researchers have suggested that aspiration of contaminated nasopharyngeal secretions may not be the major cause of nosocomial pneumonia. Recent findings indicate that ischemic mucosal injury and the associated translocation of enteric bacteria may play a more critical role.[19] Clearly, more research is needed into the pathogenic mechanisms active in the development of nosocomial pneumonia before optimal strategies can be created for preventing it.

Interventions aimed at maximizing patient defenses have included meticulous oral care and methods of preventing stasis of secretions, which serve as a reservoir for growth of organisms. Routine interventions include turning, coughing, deep breathing, chest physiotherapy, and, more recently, the use of kinetic beds. Although these techniques may be theoretically sound, their effectiveness in preventing pneumonia is not consistently supported in the literature.

The most recent technologic advance in the prevention of pneumonia has been the development of kinetic, or "self-rotating," beds of various designs. Enthusiasm for these beds is based on the notion that, if frequent turning is good for the patient, then constant turning is better. Several such beds allow repositioning of patients who otherwise could not be turned (e.g., those with unstable spine injuries). Some beds alternately inflate and deflate cushions in the mattress to gently reposition the patient; in others, the entire bed frame moves. The newest models incorporate pressure-relief features as well as kinetic therapy. Few data exist to support the efficacy of these beds in achieving such outcomes as decreased incidence of pressure ulcers, of length of hospital stay, or of mortality rates.[20]

Managing the environment to prevent nosocomial infection requires appropriate standards for infection control. The CDC offers guidelines for the development of such standards.[21] Significant progress can be made toward preventing pneumonia if regimens designed to prevent cross-contamination are in place and are strictly enforced. Of these, proper hand washing is most important for prevention of nosocomial infections.

Recently, attention has been directed at eradicating organisms in the gastrointestinal tract to prevent nosocomial pneumonia, a technique called *selective decontamination of the digestive tract*. This intervention is based on the theory that respiratory infections appear to be related to colonization of the upper gastrointestinal tract and subsequent spillover of gastrointestinal contents into the respiratory tract. Research supports the effectiveness of selective decontamination of the digestive tract in decreasing colonization and infection rates in various patient populations[22, 23]; however, data demonstrating a relationship between selective decontamination of the gastrointestinal tract and patient outcomes remain controversial.[24, 25] Nonetheless, interest in the use of selective decontamination of the digestive tract is high, and the approach is worthy of further investigation to determine which patient groups might benefit from it.

Aspiration pneumonia is a significant concern in ICU patients. Routine procedures, such as checking placement of nasogastric tubes before feedings and positioning patients properly, can be effective in decreasing the incidence of aspiration pneumonia.

Although aspiration of gastric contents is used routinely to ensure correct nasogastric tube placement or measure nasogastric aspirate, it is not always a reliable way of making these determinations.[26] In patients with small-bore feeding tubes the technique is fraught with problems, because the tubing collapses down onto itself when aspiration is attempted. A chest radiograph should always be obtained to verify placement of small-bore tubes before the first tube feeding.

Clinicians often assume (erroneously) that an inflated cuff on the endotracheal tube prevents aspiration of gastric contents into the lungs. As a result, patients may be laid supine, which increases the risk of aspiration. Research suggests that placing the patient at a 45° angle can be effective in reducing aspiration of gastric contents.[27]

Unplanned Extubation

Regardless of how well an endotracheal tube is secured, partial or complete unplanned extubation can occur.[28, 29] Partial extubation typically occurs when an agitated and restless patient mouths the tube, slowly moving it up and out of position. Partial extubation can also occur in a patient whose cough is strong or during repositioning of the tube. Unplanned extubation (i.e., when the tube comes out entirely) generally occurs in agitated or confused patients.

The basic requisite for the prevention of either type of extubation is avoidance of situations that produce anxiety and confusion. Every attempt must be made to inform the patient of the purpose of the endotracheal tube, if possible before it is inserted. Procedures such as suctioning should be explained before they are performed so that patients know what to expect. Judicious use of sedatives, in addition to explanations, is frequently warranted; however, indiscriminate application of restraints (either physical or chemical) to all intubated patients is ill-advised. A variety of methods exist for securing endotracheal tubes. Studies to date have not demonstrated any one method to be superior.[30, 31]

The proper position for the endotracheal tube at the teeth or gums should be noted and documented to ensure that partial extubations do not occur. Patients with a strong cough may benefit from more frequent suctioning or, if secretions are not the cause of the cough, from the addition of intratracheal lidocaine (Xylocaine). Endotracheal tube repositioning should always be performed with two staff members present, one to secure the tube and the other to apply the tape.

INTENSIVE CARE UNIT PSYCHOSIS

The psychologic complications of ICU care are perhaps the least understood, but potentially the most devastating, of all complications. *ICU psychosis* is the term traditionally used to describe the delirium that occurs between the 3rd and 7th days in the ICU.[32] It has been described as a fluctuating state of consciousness characterized by features such as fatigue, confusion, distraction, anxiety, and hallucinations. Some investigators have suggested that the development of ICU psychosis is related to three factors: the patient, drugs, and the ICU environment. The fact that the psychosis typically resolves within 2 days after ICU discharge suggests that modifying the

TABLE 189–4. Contributing Factors to Intensive Care Unit Psychosis and Preventive Measures

Problem: Unfamiliar Environment or Personnel

Solution

1. Orient patient and family to ICU as soon as possible after admission (preoperatively for elective surgery patients).
2. Use patient-family information booklets or videos as needed (e.g., American Association of Critical-Care Nurses booklet, *It's Critical That You Know**).
3. Minimize the number of personnel that come into contact with the patient.
4. Adopt models of care that maximize consistency of staff and promote continuity of care (e.g., primary nursing).

Problem: Lack of Patient or Family Control over Environment

Solution

1. Provide patient and family with ongoing information regarding diagnosis, treatment plan, and prognosis. Use simple, straightforward communication style. Avoid medical jargon.
2. Allow patient and family decision making regarding care plan and daily activities (e.g., number of visitors, bathing times, aggressiveness of care).

Problem: Isolation

Solution

1. Institute unrestricted visiting practices: modify based on patient and family needs.
2. Encourage family participation in routine activities (e.g., mouth care, foot massage).
3. Encourage family to bring in "comfort" items from home (e.g., pillow, drawings, photographs).
4. Ensure that patient has a means of communicating needs to staff (e.g., call bell, communication board).
5. If patient requires isolation precautions, provide patient and family with explanation as to need and purpose of such measures. Avoid unnecessary isolation procedures.

Problem: Noise

Solution

1. Limit staff conversation at the bedside to patient and family discussions and necessary patient care discussion.
2. Adjust audible bedside alarms to appropriate level. Set alarm limits to reasonable levels.

Problem: Altered Sleep Patterns

Solution

1. Cluster activities and interventions to allow for periods of uninterrupted sleep.
2. Obtain vital signs and perform interventions only as necessary.
3. Maximize the use of natural lighting. Dim lights at night.
4. Plan activities to allow sleep at night (e.g., wean during day if fatigue is an issue).
5. Administer sleep medications as needed.

*American Association of Critical-Care Nurses: It's Critical That You Know: A Resource for Families of Critically Ill Patients. Newport Beach, Calif, American Association of Critical Care Nurses, 1987.

ICU environment and the routines may significantly affect the patient's psychological outcome.[32]

Table 189–4 lists some of the common causes of ICU psychosis and suggests ways of preventing or minimizing this complication. In general, the patient and family must be included in the patient's day-to-day care, and, most important, they must be given clear, consistent information about the patient's progress and treatment plan. This often requires that ICU staff repeat the same information (e.g., time and place when orienting the patient) several times a day or during a shift. Even more effort is required when patients are intubated and cannot communicate easily. In some instances, a pencil and paper is all that is needed, so that the patient can write down questions and concerns. When the patient cannot write, more creative ways of facilitating communication must be used, such as eye blinks and communication boards. Speaking valves (e.g., Passy-Muir valves) should be used whenever possible to enable the patient to communicate verbally. These valves can be used in tracheostomy patients both on and off the ventilator.[33-35]

The patient should be given as much control as possible over his or her environment and schedule. All too frequently, the "patient's" schedule (e.g., preparing laboratory blood work, bathing, eating, weaning) is based on the convenience of the staff rather than the patient's needs.

Pain and discomfort can exacerbate ICU psychosis. The high incidence of pain in critically ill persons is well-established.[36] Unfortunately, pain is frequently viewed as an inevitable consequence of being critically ill. A common sentiment expressed in critical care units is that a little pain is a small price to pay for wellness. Inadequately managed, however, pain not only contributes to delirium but also has a deleterious effect on the patient's physiologic state.

Effective management of pain in a critically ill patient presents challenges, but they are not insurmountable. Communication difficulties and unstable cardiopulmonary function are but two of the many obstacles to optimal pain management in critically ill persons. Table 189–5 suggests strategies for providing appropriate pain management in the ICU. Patients who are unable to communicate their pain because of factors such as sedation, neurologic injury, or the use of a paralytic agent, are at a disadvantage in the ICU because they cannot express their complaints or give feedback on the effectiveness of their pain medications. Research suggests that many patients with diagnoses not typically associated with pain (e.g., congestive heart failure, chronic obstructive pulmonary disease, cirrhosis) reported having moderate to severe pain that was often treated inadequately.[36]

TABLE 189–5. Pain Management in Critically Ill Patients: Problems and Solutions

Problem: Inability to Assess Pain in Noncommunicative Patient

Solution

1. Be alert to routine circumstances, procedures, and interventions that may cause pain (e.g., immobility, turning, weighing, blood drawing, suctioning).
2. Assess for signs and symptoms of acute pain (e.g., increased heart rate, blood pressure, and respiratory rate; cool clammy skin; crying, moaning, grimacing). Be aware that over time adaptation occurs, and these signs may no longer be present.

Problem: Pain Medication Withheld Because of Concerns of Hypotension and/or Respiratory Depression

Solution

1. Be aware that severe pain may contribute to hypotension.
2. Monitor blood pressure frequently during narcotic administration (especially in patients with cardiac disease, hypovolemia, and pre-existing hypotension).
3. Slowly administer small, incremental intravenous doses of narcotics.
4. Monitor respiratory rate frequently during narcotic administration. Use apnea monitors as needed.

Although many tools have been developed for rating pain, they are typically too cumbersome to use or are not applicable to many ICU patients. Clinicians in the ICU must rely on indirect physiologic indices of pain, such as increased heart rate or blood pressure. Unfortunately, many mechanisms other than pain can lead to alterations in these variables, and they are valid indices only during the period of very acute illness.

SUMMARY

Preventing complications in the ICU requires the concerted efforts of a highly skilled, multidisciplinary group. Unit-based standards of care and a preventive approach are important for ensuring early assessment and intervention for all patients. Ongoing evaluation of these standards, through quality-improvement monitoring, is necessary to ensure that desired patient outcomes are achieved.

References

1. Turner SO: Competency-based skill building curriculum for *unlicensed* assistive personnel. Aliso Viejo, Calif, American Association of Critical-Care Nurses, 1996.
2. The International Task Force on Safety in the Intensive Care Unit: International standards for safety in the intensive care unit. Crit Care Med 1993; 21:453–456.
3. Task Force on Guidelines, Society of Critical Care Medicine: Guidelines for Standards of Care for Patients with Acute Respiratory Failure on Mechanical Ventilatory Support. Anaheim, Calif, Society of Critical Care Medicine, 1990.
4. Pearson ML: Guideline for prevention of intravascular-device related infections. Infect Control Hosp Epidemiol 1996; 17:438–472.
5. Clarke M, Kadhom HM: The nursing prevention of pressure sores in hospital and community patients. J Adv Nurs 1988; 13:365–373.
6. Inman KJ, Sibbald WJ, Rutledge FS, Clark BJ: Clinical utility and cost-effectiveness of an air suspension bed in the prevention of pressure ulcers. JAMA 1993; 269:1139–1143.
7. Bergstrom N, Braden BJ, Laguzza A, Holman V: The Braden Scale for predicting pressure sore risk. Nurs Res 1987; 36:205–210.
8. Jirick MK, Ryan P, Caravalho MA, Bukvich J: Pressure ulcer risk factors in an ICU population. Am J of Crit Care 1995; 4:361–367.
9. Pressure Ulcers in Adults: Prediction and Prevention: Clinical Practice Guideline No. 3. Publication No. 92-0047. Rockville, Md, U.S. Department of Health and Human Services: Agency for Health Care Policy and Research, 1992.
10. Burns SM, Martin M, Robbins V, Friday T, Coffindaffer M, Burns SC, Burns JE: Comparison of nasogastric tube securing methods and tube types in medical intensive care patients. Am J Crit Care 1995; 4:198–203.
11. Witt NJ, Zochodne DW, Bolton CF, Grand'Maison F, Wells G, Young B, Sibbald WJ: Peripheral nerve function in sepsis and multiple organ failure. Chest 1991; 99:176–184.
12. Gooch JL, Suchyta MR, Balbierz JM, et al: Prolonged paralysis after treatment with neuromuscular junction blocking agents. Crit Care Med 1991; 19:1125–1131.
13. Breslin E: Prevention and treatment of pulmonary complications in patients after surgery of the upper abdomen. Heart Lung 1981; 10:511–519.
14. Risser N: Preoperative and postoperative care to prevent pulmonary complication. Heart Lung 1980; 9:57–67.
15. Sutton P, Pavia D, Bateman J, et al: Chest physiotherapy: A review. Eur J Respir Dis 1982; 62:188–210.
16. Bueno-Cavanillas A, Delgado-Rodriguez M, Lopez-Luque A, et al: Influence of nosocomical infection on mortality rate in an intensive care unit. Crit Care Med 1994; 22:55–60.
17. Du Moulin GC, Paterson DG, Hedley-Whyte J, et al: Aspiration of gastric bacteria in antacid-treated patients: A frequent cause of postoperative colonization of the airway. Lancet 1982; i:242–245.
18. Jimenez P, Torres A, Rodriguez-Roisin R, et al: Incidence and etiology of pneumonia acquired during mechanical ventilation. Crit Care Med 1989; 17:882–885.
19. Fiddian-Green RG, Baker S: Nosocomial pneumonia in the critically ill: Product of aspiration or translocation. Crit Care Med 1992; 19:763–769.
20. Choi SC, Nelson LD: Kinetic therapy in critically ill patients: Combined results based on meta-analysis. J Crit Care 1992; 7:57–62.
21. Guidelines for prevention of nosocomial pneumonia. Centers for Disease Control and Prevention. MMWR Morb Mortal Wkly Rep 1997; 46:1–79.
22. Rodriguez-Roldan JM, Altuna-Cuesta A, Lopez A, et al: Prevention of nosocomial lung infection in ventilated patients: Use of an antimicrobial pharyngeal nonabsorbable paste. Crit Care Med 1990; 18:1239–1242.
23. Hartenauer U, Thulig B, Diemer W, et al: Effect of selective flora suppression on colonization, infection, and mortality in critically ill patients: A one-year, prospective consecutive study. Crit Care Med 1991; 19:463–473.
24. Hammond JM, Potgieter PD, Saunders GL: Selective decontamination of the digestive tract in multiple trauma patients—Is there a role? Results of a prospective, double-blind, randomized trial. Crit Care Med 1994; 22:33–39.
25. Tetteroo GWM, Wagenvoort JHI, Mulder PGH, et al: Decreased mortality rate and length of hospital stay in surgical intensive care unit patients with successful selective decontamination of the gut. Crit Care Med 1994; 21:1692–1698.
26. Dobranowski J, Fitzgerald JM, Baxter F, Woods D: Incorrect positioning of nasogastric feeding tubes and the development of pneumothorax. Can Assoc Radiol J 1992; 43:35–39.
27. Torres A, Serra-Batlles J, Ros E, et al: Pulmonary aspiration of gastric contents in patients receiving mechanical ventilation: The effect of body position. J Am Coll Physicians 1992; 116:540–543.
28. Vassal R, Anh NGD, Gabillet JM, Guidet B, Staikowsky F, Offenstadt B: Prospective evaluation of self extubations in a medical intensive care unit. Intensive Care Med 1993; 19:340–342.
29. Christie JM, Dethlefsen M, Cane RD: Unplanned extubations in the intensive care unit. J Clin Anesth 1996; 8:289–293.
30. Kaplow R, Bookbinder M: A comparison of four endotracheal tube holders. Heart Lung 1994; 23:59–66.
31. Levy H, Griego L: A comparative study of oral endotracheal tube-securing methods. Chest 1993; 104:1537–1540.
32. Ballard KS: Identification of environmental stressors for patients in a surgical intensive care unit. Issues Mental Health Nurs 1981; 3:89–108.
33. Manzano JL, Lubillo S, Henriquez D, Martin JC, Perez MC, Wilson DJ: Verbal communication of ventilator dependent patients. Dimens Crit Care Nurs 1991; 10:115–122.
34. Connolly MA: Communicating with ventilator-dependent patients. Dimens Crit Care Nurs 1991; 10:115–122.
35. Williams ML: An algorithum for selecting a communication technique with intubated patients. Dimens Crit Care Nurs 1992; 11:222–229.
36. Desbiens NA, Wu AW, Bergner M, et al: The six month pain experience of critically and seriously ill hospitalized adult patients. Clin Res 1992; 40:555A.
37. American Association of Critical-Care Nurses (AACCN): It's Critical That You Know: A Resource for Families of Critically Ill Patients. Newport Beach, Calif, AACCN, 1987.

190

Barriers to Effective Patient Care

Virginia R. Carlson, MSN, MBA, RN, FCCM
Ingrid Mroz, MS, RN, CCRN, ARNP

THE CHALLENGE

Critical care units are designed to support and promote healing in acutely ill populations; however, they may also contain barriers to maximizing the healing process. Critical care units vary greatly by population (age or physical systems), by type of institution (academic or community), by site (urban or rural), by financial structure (profit or nonprofit), or by physician management (intensivist or private physician). The monitoring of factors that contribute to or inhibit healing has been ongoing. This chapter is intended to heighten the reader's awareness of potential barriers in his or her own practice environment and to offer suggestions for corrective strategies.

Critical care units have been data-driven since their inception. Continuous monitoring of physiologic parameters and patient observation have been the hallmarks of the critical care unit. During the 1980s, measuring success was primarily carried out with a focus on mortality and morbidity. Knaus and colleagues began using the same data to determine physiologic predictors of successful outcomes. The 1990s, however, have taken on a different emphasis. The measurement of success is determined by the evaluation of patient outcomes and determination of quality and satisfaction with services provided.[1] Investigators have looked at circumstances that affect patient care beyond the classic symptom/system/physiologic parameters by examining conditions that support or enhance the processes of healing. The atmosphere of each critical care unit is as unique as the combination of the factors that make it special, including all the individuals involved: patients, family, visitors, and health care providers.

The future challenge is to minimize barriers to optimal patient-centered care resulting in cost-effective quality outcomes. Payers, professional organizations, and health care institutions and agencies are evaluating the delivery of care and the customer's satisfaction level against quantifiable benefit.[2]

EXPERIENTIAL INFLUENCES

External and Environmental Factors

Design Concepts

Critical care units have been recognized as stress-invoking environments since their beginning because of their focus on the prevention of, or intervention in, life-threatening events. In critical care, we support patients through physiologic crises, providing life-saving techniques when appropriate. The very nature of our high technology care is an alien environment for our patients, families, and staff. In these stimulus-rich environments are physiologically unstable patients with diminished resources and intense physiologic and psychologic needs. Despite our ability to address and reverse life-threatening events, our environment may place additional demands on these patients with diminished resources.[3] The essence of healing remains within the patient's own ability to muster internal resources to gain "health." We are merely supporting them through this period of life. Critical care unit design should strive to provide physical and psychologic comfort for patients, families, and staff members.[4]

Since the early 1990s, professional organizations have acknowledged the need to create more humane and caring environments. Suggestions to improve our environments with the purpose of enhancing healing for patients, families, and caregivers were made at a consensus conference sponsored by the Society of Critical Care Medicine (SCCM),[5] for example[4, 5]:

1. Incorporate and enhance warmth and comfort in planning unit design.
2. Provide natural light and outside views.
3. Include mirrors reflecting the view when the bed faces away from the window.
4. Supply quiet, relaxing colors, adequate space, and auditory and visual flexibility for privacy.
5. Encourage the patient to display cherished personal items and pictures prior to hospitalization to diminish dehumanizing the individual.

The opportunity to build a new unit is an expensive undertaking, and those who are planning to do so have several resources to help create an environment that is conducive to healing. The American Association of Critical Care Nurses (AACN) and the SCCM have developed joint statements in supporting health system changes and unit design that are excellent resources.[6, 7] Additionally, site visits should be made to units that have been opened within 5 years prior to planning. On average, a unit opens 1 to 5 years after initial conceptualization. Visiting units opened prior to this time period might not provide the necessary "state of the art" perspective. State health departments and local architectural firms can provide guidelines to help design a unit that complies with fire and safety codes. Including interior design personnel in the planning may help create a technologically advanced unit with an esthetically comfortable environment. Designing comfortable space with pleasing surroundings while simultaneously permitting employment of technologic advances can be accomplished and will decrease environmental stress for patients, families, and health care providers.[4]

Common Environment

One category of stressors is purely environmental and related to the physical construction of the space. Although practitioners can identify environmental barriers, such as open wards, poor acoustic designs and mixed-age populations, they may feel the challenge of improving the healing environment is overwhelming. However, many environmental changes can be quite simple, especially if we view the environment not only from the standpoint of clinical efficiency but also from the standpoint of patients and families. Many units use fluorescent lighting, which is associated with business or commercial environments. A simple solution would be to increase the number of incandescent lights that can be controlled by patients and families; this would increase comfort and familiarity for the critically ill adult.[4] In open wards, where noise control is impossible to maintain, allowing patients the use of earplugs or earphones with music of their choice may alter their exposure to sensory overload and allow prolonged periods of rest.

Noise

Despite frequent and ongoing studies, two complaints are repeatedly and consistently reported by patients: noise and sleep disturbances. Patients and families, unlike the unit staff, do not have the ability to walk away from noxious stimuli. They tolerate inappropriate conversations, loud sounds, frequent alarms, whooshing ventilator cycles, television programs they would never choose, and so on. Signals from patient call systems, alarms from monitoring equipment, and telephones add to the sensory overload in critical care units. The International Noise Council recommends that noise levels should not exceed 45 decibels (dB) in the daytime, 40 dB in the evening, and 20 dB during the night.[3] Noise measured in one ICU was 62 to 72 dB, with noisy equipment and conversations being the main contributors.[8, 9] Suggestions to abate noise include floor coverings that absorb sound; walls and ceilings constructed of materials with high sound absorption capabilities; alarms modulated to a level sufficient to alert staff members, yet rendered less noxious; ceiling soffets and baffles to help reduce echoed sounds; and private cubicles with doorways offset to reduce sound transmission. Counters, partitions, and glass doors are also effective in reducing noise levels.[8, 10] Lower volume on telephone bells and the elimination of overhead paging systems effectively lower sound and noise stimuli in the ICU. The patient's sense of powerlessness can be only partly overcome by increased sensitivity of staff to the issues of noise as an environmental stressor.

Some investigators have examined the effects of altering the sensory stimulation of sound by using music.[11-14] They have found that music may provide a recreational and social diversion from the monotony and isolation of hospitalization.[13] It alters the experiences of sound and, if chosen correctly, can be associated with a decrease in physiologic parameters such as heart and respiratory rates.[11]

Overstimulation

The other common complaint expressed by patients following a stay in the critical care unit is the inability to rest and sleep.[9] The "action-oriented subculture," in addition to peer pressure, conflicting priorities, and external influences, often places promotion of sleep low on a list of priorities in care planning.[15] Sleep deprivation experienced by the ICU patient can lead to the development of impaired cognition; manifestations can range from apathy to delirium, which may lead to an increased patient morbidity.[8] Studies within a respiratory unit identified bursts of sounds disrupting sleep and poor management of sleep-wake cycles as contributors to poor weaning.[16] Chronobiologic studies of normal biologic rhythms have demonstrated normally lower urine output during customary sleep time and decreased responsiveness to pharmacologic agents during sleep due to lowered metabolism. Using chronobiologic principles can raise the provider's awareness related to parameters that we observe on a continuum and may enhance the appropriateness of interventions.[3]

Developing a well-formulated plan for sleep is as important as many of the other interventions we provide, as perceived by patients.[17] Discussions by staff with family members about the patient's sleep history and habits, including length of time and frequency of naps provides valuable information. Here are some steps to include:

1. Ensure that the documentation tools (flowsheets and critical paths) include sleep periods, plans, and strategies.
2. Schedule periods of rest and sleep.
3. Provide social interventions and visiting during normal waking cycles, and avoid the same stimulus during sleep cycles.
4. Collaborate with other departments, staff, and services to prevent sleep period interruptions.

Dimming lights at night simulates darkness but also encourages staff to decrease noise. Providing patients with assurance that the clinician is continuously watching them and encouraging or giving them permission to sleep are also effective.[15] Whether sleep directly promotes healing or not is controversial; however, sleeplessness has been demonstrated to impair cognitive functioning in healthy persons under laboratory testing conditions.[10]

Patterns of stimuli in the critical care environment differ greatly from patterns of a patient's customary prehospitalization environment. There is little we can do to change the functional schedules demanded by rapidly changing physiology and the constant vigilant monitoring that occurs in a 24-hour care unit. However, increasing our awareness of chronobiologic principles often enhances the delivery of patient care. Two aspects of patient-environment interactions are especially pertinent:

1. The aspect of "environmental docility"— the mutual acting and being acted upon. For example, the patient exhibits physiologic changes that are acted upon by the health care providers, which results in a response by the patient. The patient has little or no control over the interactions and cannot leave the environment voluntarily.
2. *Entrainment,* which occurs when the patient's biologic rhythms become synchronized with new time patterns. This aspect has not been studied adequately in critical care, but in normal subjects the process of entrainment creates impaired function similar to "jet lag."[3, 10] This process can have a considerable impact on a patient's healing abilities in the critical care unit, if it is found to be a similar experience for patients. Entrainment does not usually occur in less than 5 days, but for patients with prolonged stays, it may become an important factor.[3]

PATIENT EXPERIENCES

Pain and Anxiety

Patients are subjected to the critical care environment in order to avert life-threatening events. Many patients are not prepared for the experiences they encounter. Despite the health care professional's best efforts to provide quality, patient-centered care, some of the challenges patients experience (e.g., pain, procedural distress, anxiety, confusion) become barriers to effective care. Inadequate pain management has been identified as a major problem and has gained increased attention from researchers, clinicians, and policymakers.

Many researchers evaluating the ICU experience have found that pain and anxiety are frequently reported and recalled.[19-21] These findings should alert health care providers to our inability to adequately address these often harmful and potentially serious experiences. Heney reported that the patient's fear of pain is second only to fear of death.[22]

A patient's experience of pain is related to the acute illness, injury, diagnostic procedures, and treatments.[20] In one study, preoperative information about personal sensory experiences, such as pain and oral hygiene, is important in decreasing concerns related to an elective critical care experience.[18] Pain has been identified as a primary source of stress and concern for ICU patients.[18, 19]

Pain is an unpleasant sensory and motor experience that arises from actual or potential tissue damage.[23] It is a subjective human response with quantifiable features, including intensity, quality, time course, impact, and personal meaning.[24] Pain and anxiety can further tax a person's resources to recover. Physiologic responses to pain can have a negative impact on patients by creating a "stress hormone response." This response may include an increased metabolic rate, impaired immune function, and a triggered "fight or flight" response of the sympathetic nervous system. The physiologic and psychologic risks of untreated pain may be greatest in patients with other illnesses as they undergo major procedures.[25]

Pain can be exaggerated by the stressors inherent in the critical care environment as well as by the patient's inability to describe symptoms as a result of altered airway or cognition.[21, 26] The patient's experience of pain may be compounded by the nature of the treatments.

The Agency for Health Care Policy and Research[25] guidelines state that patients have the right to treatment that includes the prevention and adequate relief of pain. The management of pain, procedural distress, and anxiety can present formidable challenges to the most experienced critical care practitioner. However, a structured, planned, collaborative approach by the interdisciplinary care team can minimize these stressful and potentially harmful experiences. The management plan should be individualized for each patient. Establishing open communications with the patient in a cooperative caring manner is crucial to obtaining honest subjective reporting of the extent of painful symptoms. Proactive planning for the treatment of symptoms is more effective than reacting to the experience of pain.[25] Clearly defined goals of analgesia and sedation should be planned and communicated with all members of the team. Educating and preparing the patient for procedures and potential sensory experiences increase the patient's coping ability and decrease psychologic distress.[25]

Thousands of patients undergo diagnostic and therapeutic procedures each day outside of operating rooms in emergency departments, clinics, hospital inpatient units, and critical care units that may or may not result in pain, distress, or anxiety. A structured approach should take into consideration the type of procedure, anticipated range of responses (intensity and duration of pain and anxiety), and individual factors (age, physical condition). For painful procedures, the plan should incorporate both pharmacologic and nonpharmacologic approaches that will result in preventing or reducing pain and anxiety. Although research regarding practices related to procedural pain in critical care units is scant, it is believed that medications may be underprescribed and underadministered.[27]

Sometimes pain cannot be prevented or treated prophylactically. But with the prevalence of reports of poorly managed pain, it is imperative that the clinician be prepared to treat it appropriately and quickly when it occurs. A careful history of the patient's previous experience and use of prescriptions or over-the-counter preparations to treat pain (i.e., headaches, backaches, arthritis) can help the practitioner understand underlying influences. Previous experiences of the patient are influential, as are the clinician's own attitudes toward and knowledge of pain.[24] General principles of effective pain management include assessment, treatment, and determination of effectiveness.

Management of Pain and Anxiety

The first of these principles is *careful and planned assessment of pain or anxiety and its relief.* The most common reason for unrelieved pain is the failure of staff to routinely assess pain and pain relief.[25] A routine assessment procedure should include a measurement scale that is simple, easy to use, and validated. The most reliable indicator of pain is the patient's self-report.[25] The measurement of self-reported pain intensity and distress may be accomplished with assessment tools that are easy to use and realistic, such as numerical rating, visual analog scale, or adjective rating scale. The report of family members, particularly if they have been the care provider before hospitalization, can be meaningful. Careful observation of the patient's behaviors is particularly important in patients who cannot verbally communicate. The clinician should observe facial expressions of grimacing, wrinkling of the forehead, vocalizations of sighing and moaning, verbalizations (praying or counting), and body actions of rubbing, rocking, and thrashing. One must consider the possibility that the aforementioned may be signs of coping responses to pain and anxiety. The monitoring of physiologic parameters may demonstrate alterations during the experience of pain, such as elevations of heart rate and blood pressure. Often nurses rely more on the changes in vital signs and nonverbal body language than on the actual patient report of pain.[28] However, pain is purely a subjective experience based on what the patient says it is, existing whenever the person says it does.[28]

Anxiety is much more difficult to assess because no practical assessment tool has been developed. The nurse must rely on objective observations of signs and symptoms.[29] The signs and symptoms demonstrated are:

1. Changes in cognitive ability, such as disruption in perceiving, thinking, and conceptualizing.
2. Physiologic indicators (sympathetic nervous system stimulation).
3. Behaviors such as anger, avoidance, and joking.

Anxiety can be on a continuum from mild to severe panic. This range in experience can be evidenced by mild (heightened awareness), moderate (increased heart and respiratory rate and frequent body position changes), severe (sense of impending doom, hyperventilation and profound tachycardia), or panic (extreme discomfort, fear of dying, dyspnea, chest pain).[29]

The second major management principle is *determination of treatment options* and *implementation of the treatment plan*. The patient history and family information is particularly helpful in deciding the choice of treatments to be initiated. If possible, one should treat anticipated pain or anxiety prophylactically. Particularly in the treatment of pain, prevention is more effective than treating pain once it is established. Pain is more difficult to suppress.[25] If pharmacologic interventions are selected, sufficient lead time must be allowed for a full therapeutic effect.

The type of pharmacologic agent selected is determined, in part, by the goal of therapy.

1. *Analgesics* are used to *diminish* the perception of pain and include nonsteroidal anti-inflammatory drugs, narcotics, and opioids.
2. *Anesthetics* are used to *abolish* the perception of pain (general and local).
3. *Anxiolytics* can be sedatives that blunt the response to situations but do not alleviate pain.
4. *Hypnotics* and *sedative-hypnotics* such as benzodiazepines and propofol, induce sleep or drowsiness.

The route of administration should not be painful. Underreporting of pain by patients has been a result of their aversion to injections.

Nonpharmacologic methods employed with pharmacologic agents may supplement the effects of relief. Physical methods include transcutaneous electrical nerve stimulation (TENS), application of cold or heat, massage, immobilization, acupuncture, or acupressure. Cognitive methods may also be employed to enhance the agents used to treat pain, such as music therapy,[13] relaxation, and guided imagery. Hypnosis and biofeedback are behavioral approaches that may be available depending on the setting.

The third major pain management principle is *assessment of the patient's perception of the effectiveness of the intervention*. Documentation of success or changes in therapy must be communicated clearly. The design and success of a pain-anxiety treatment plan may take many trials. If professionals do not communicate the ongoing attempts and failures, a successful outcome of relief may never be achieved.

Barriers to the effective treatment of pain and anxiety have been encountered.[24, 25] These barriers include:

1. The nurse's or physician's disbelief that a problem exists.
2. Lack of knowledge about current pain management practices.
3. Personal beliefs and attitudes about pain and its treatment.
4. Concern regarding legal liability and addiction.
5. Communication and knowledge deficits regarding adequate assessment and interventions.

Effective management of pain and anxiety requires a partnership between patients, nurses, physicians, and other members of the health care team committed to quality care of critically ill patients.

Aging

The elderly, once considered a special population within critical care, now make up more than 50% of patients in most adult critical care units.[30] Promoting the functional status of older people in the acute care setting is important for several reasons[31]:

1. Older people fear the prospect of dependency.
2. Care for dependent people is often more costly because it is labor-intensive.
3. People with functional impairments need more individualized social service and nursing interventions to promote their remaining capabilities.

In a study of 60 functionally independent individuals, 75 years of age or older, who were admitted to the hospital from their home for acute illness, 75% were no longer independent on discharge.[32] Improving the quality of critical care should focus efforts and energy on promoting the functional ability of the older population.

The normal aging process is associated with changes that increase susceptibility to various stresses. The elderly are vulnerable and stand at the threshold of functional disability, at risk of being propelled over that threshold when stressed.[32] The physiologic changes seen with normal aging include a decrease in muscle strength and aerobic capacity, vasomotor instability, decreased bone density, decreased ventilation, decreased sensory continence, altered thirst and nutrition, fragile skin and a tendency for urinary incontinence.[32] Older people present a growing challenge in the critical care setting, not only because of compelling demographics but also because of the sophistication of knowledge required to provide specialized, comprehensive care. The complex interaction of many dynamic systems requires care based on diverse and sound knowledge.[33] Acute illness can affect the normal aging process and, in view of comorbidities, can present a formidable challenge to the critical care practitioners. Once critically ill, older patients experience an increased incidence of complications, a longer hospital stay, and higher mortality and morbidity rates.[30, 33] Comorbidities affecting the normal aging process make this population more complex than others. Two conditions that complicate all clinical situations are (1) skin ulcerations and breakdown and (2) delirium or acute confusion.

Critical care is a life-sustaining environment, particularly in patients experiencing cardiopulmonary system failures. The integumentary system is not a focus during the treatment of the elderly in ICUs, as is demonstrated by the prevalence of pressure ulcerations (30% to 82%) in these patients.[34] As a result of normal physiologic changes, skin fragility becomes further compromised by urinary incontinence. Diminished circulation and limited mobility further contribute to the potential for skin breakdown and decreased effectiveness of skin as a barrier to infection. The primary cause of ulceration is pressure, but shearing forces, friction, inadequate nutrition, and moisture are also contributing factors.[33] Specialty beds have been used to prevent or treat skin ulceration, particularly in high-risk populations. Specialty beds themselves do not prevent pressure ulcerations.[34] Adequate skin care and frequent repositioning of the patient remain the best preventive measures for averting skin breakdown.

Psychologic and Emotional Responses

Critical care patients who exhibit confusion, agitation, and combativeness are common and difficult to manage. The environment of critical care is foreign and threatening to patients. Altered sensory exposure and exhaustion prevail, challenging the most resilient patient. The elderly have fewer resources than younger individuals to cope with and resist the bombardment of environmental stimuli. Initial reactions to hospitalization by the elderly can range from fear of the ICU as a precursor to death[31] to relief at having ventilatory support provided for the air-hungry patient with chronic obstructive pulmonary disease.[35]

The statistics related to the development of acute confusion or delirium in the elderly are impressive. Almost half of the elder population in the ICU will have symptoms of delirium, and 70% of those symptoms are not identified or treated appropriately.[36] Because the risk of these conditions is high, evaluation of potential causative factors from the time of admission assessment is necessary. The history of the elderly patient's underlying cognitive ability and psychologic status is key in determining the possible category and reversibility of altered cognition demonstrated during critical illness.

It is important to differentiate between chronic dementia, underlying depression, and acute confusion[37]:

1. *Delirium* is an acute confusional state characterized by an abrupt onset that can develop over hours, a fluctuating mental status, and an inability to maintain attention.[36]
2. *Dementia* usually occurs gradually, and memory problems worsen over time. Patients with the chronic confusion of dementia are alert and able to maintain attention until later in the course of the disease.
3. In *acute confusion*, the primary hallmark is inattention.

Although acute confusion was once viewed as a transient disorder, evidence now suggests that symptoms may persist long after discharge, affecting rehabilitation, cognition, and independent functioning.[38]

Delirium may be multifactorial in origin, multifaceted in presentation, and embedded in a complex host of acute and chronic conditions and their treatments.[36] Any condition that can affect brain function can cause delirium. Factors that can contribute to the development of confusion can be organic, psychologic, or environmental:

1. The *organic factors* may be (a) primary cerebral disease, such as meningitis or stroke, (b) systemic diseases, such as congestive heart failure, pneumonia, hypoglycemia and thyroid disease, (c) exogenous toxic substances, such as in medication intoxication, and (d) withdrawal from sedative-hypnotic agents or alcohol.
2. *Psychologic factors* may be emotional stress in dealing with pain, anxiety, grief, and depression.
3. *Environmental factors* can be sleep deprivation, sensory deprivation and overload, immobility, social isolation, and unfamiliarity with the critical care environment.[38]

The presentation of delirium may be highly variable, ranging from quiet disorientation to a severely agitated state. The *hyperactive* or *hyperalert* state attracts the most attention of staff because of the patient's increased motor activity and restlessness. The *hypoactive* or *hypoalert* state, exhibited by slow speech, lethargy, and decreased psychomotor activity, may not alert the health care providers to the altered mental state and may account for the high incidence of misdiagnosis. Some patients exhibit symptoms of both states.[38]

Management of Altered Cognition

If symptoms of altered cognition are not part of the patient's prehospital condition, preventive measures and early detection within the critical care environment are crucial. Nurses are in the best position to discern subtle changes in patient status and can play a key role in the early detection and treatment of delirium.[36, 37] Providing measures that increase patient comfort within the environment, such as direct eye contact, therapeutic touch, and a calm approach, communicates to the patient that he or she is in the hands of a competent and caring practitioner. Respect for the person's need for modesty and warmth requires little effort, yet supports the patient's self-esteem.[35] Early recognition that the patient is experiencing acute confusion and initiating a physician consultation to determine the cause may contribute to early diagnosis and treatment.[39]

Management of acute confusion or delirium is based on two major approaches:

- Eliminating any underlying causes
- Providing support through comfort, safety, and prevention of complications

A comprehensive review of the history and physical examination are important. It is particularly important to include an extensive review of all medications. Eliminating or safely reducing the number of drugs or doses may be the first step in successfully treating delirium. Involving a clinical pharmacist in the evaluation and selection of pharmacologic treatment is a valuable step in a multidisciplinary approach to problem solving in this circumstance. In view of the many compounding and often conflicting factors that exist for the elderly requiring critical care, a multidisciplinary approach often results in the best treatment plan.

Treatment may be as simple as promoting sleep and establishing sleep-wake cycles or providing patients with their own sensory aids, such as eyeglasses and hearing devices. Controlling extremes of sensory input or deprivation can be helpful. The family may be pivotal in helping the patient stay focused on reality by their presence and through provision of familiar objects that may be comforting for the patient. Orientation to time, date, and place, in addition to clocks, calendars, and windows, is important in helping the patient connect with reality. Communication should be slowly paced, simple, and face-to-face. Giving orienting information, such as introductions including the date and time unobtrusively, helps the patient to connect to reality. Repeated interrogations about day, time, and place can be threatening to the confused patient and may increase agitation.[36]

The acute care environment, the acute illness experience, and the stresses of hospitalization seem to induce or exacerbate confused mental status in the elderly. The primary recipients of restraint application are older patients who interfere with medical treatments or devices, who demonstrate disruptive behaviors, or who are perceived to be at risk for falls.[40] There is growing evidence that restraint use as a therapy not only is outmoded but also is potentially so harmful that the benefits rarely outweigh the risks. Previous publications report incidents of strangulation, skin irritation and breakdown, incontinence, impaired circulation, nerve damage, constipation, aspiration pneumonia, and increased agitation.[40]

Arguments in favor of restraint use often point to the risk of litigation if patients should harm themselves; however, a review of the patient's record may prove that alternatives were not attempted before application of physical restraints. This can lead to further litigation for violation of the patient's rights. Inadequate staffing levels have also been the stimulus for the use of physical restraints. If units are using the appropriate documentation now mandated by external agencies, the application of restraints may actually increase the nurse's workload. Alternatives to the application of physical restraints should always be attempted first, and that should include family support.[40]

FAMILY EXPERIENCES

Patients are members of a family long before they become participants in the environment of critical care. As a member of a family, the patient carries out a role and receives support from the family. When patients are admitted to critical care, they continue to need the nurturing, care, and support of their family system. Encouraging families to visit and participate in care can assist patients in maintaining their cognitive integrity and contact with reality. Despite research spanning two decades that supports including and embracing the family as part of the healing environment, many critical care staff members see the family as obstructive to the care process. The impending and dramatic changes in health care delivery will provide the opportunity to develop family-focused health care.[41] By the year 2000, hospitals without family-focused programs of care will be as "respectable" as today's hospitals without good medical records.[42] A quality approach to care sees illness, and the discrete event of critical illness, as part of the patient's entire life span, thereby supporting the concept of family inclusion in the plan of care.

Development of Family-Focused Care

Families of critically ill patients have discrete needs for support because of the uncertainty, anxiety, and stress of having a critically ill family member. The crisis event often occurs without warning, giving families little time to employ coping strategies. Ineffective coping, potentiated by the fear of the loss of a loved one, may engender behaviors perceived as barriers to effective care.

During the initial treatment of an acutely unstable patient, the critical care staff is focused almost solely on saving the individual's life. The team members become so intent on that goal that they may be unable to expand their view to include the family. Yet, simple methods of encouraging the family's support can be used, such as having a partner or significant other speak to the patient during the acute phase of illness, which may be a pivotal experience for the patient.

Quality care is focused on the perception of the hospital experience by patients and families. Family-focused care is designed through identification of family roles and responsibilities, as defined by the patient and significant others, and the individualized interactions among family members to meet the needs of the critically ill patient within the context of family.[43] Directing efforts to promoting family-centered care may provide an institution with an advantage over competing institutions.

Molter's landmark and descriptive work[44] has been the basis for identifying family needs. The development of the Critical

Care Family Needs Inventory (CCFNI) described five dimensions of a family's need:

- Support
- Comfort
- Information
- Proximity
- Reassurance

Subsequent studies have substantiated Molter's findings and have further refined them into three major categories.[45-51] Leske's analysis[46] of cumulative data suggests families have three primary needs:

- Assurance
- Proximity
- Information

Previous studies not only identified needs of families but also reported their experiences within a timeline of a critical illness. The first 24 hours presents the family with a sudden crisis, initiating feelings of fear, worry, anger, exhaustion, and despair.[52] These emotions can create a need for close proximity, which can be perceived as hovering by the staff. This hovering is caused by a sense of confusion, stress, and uncertainty while the family waits to see the patient in the ICU.[53] The stress experienced by families peaks at the time of ICU admission and reaches a plateau at day 6, followed by a progressive drop until day 28.[54] At the outset of the critical care experience, families are in profound crisis that can be addressed only by a planned multidisciplinary intervention program.

Interventional Strategies

Interventions should be focused on the promotion of coping[52] and should address major family needs. As the number of unmet needs increases, so may emotional distress.[48] The assessment of the patient on admission should include a family evaluation. The family assessment provides information and data for the development of a family-focused plan of care. Baseline data on family constellation and roles, family perceptions and coping mechanisms, economic and social resources, and health maintenance activities can provide fruitful information for use during the critical illness and the patient's entire hospital stay.[54] This question-and-answer process provides family inclusion in the care plan and can be perceived as assuring.[50]

Assurance is defined as the quality of inspiring confidence, security, and freedom from doubt.[46] The family wants to know that their loved one is receiving the highest quality of care.[51] Relatives need caring attitudes to be shared by staff and concerns voiced by them to be acknowledged as important.[55] Incorporating chaplain and social worker services in the support of families is often a source of reassurance; this sense of inclusion can help them become familiar with the environment and with the critical care routines.

Proximity is another major need of families. The need of the family to be near the patient has been repeatedly reported and is a need that is frequently unmet.[47, 51] Visual reassurance of the patient's status and care are paramount to a family's sense of security. This need for reassurance can be met only through flexible visitation.[53] Open visitation has been positively associated with decreasing anxiety.[49] The family's fear of leaving the ICU is based on their perception that they may be needed for information, communication, decision making, or patient comfort.[55] Having unlimited visitation, attractive and comfortable waiting rooms, areas for privacy and reflection, and adequate space for family meetings is important in providing the family with a sense of being welcomed and supported.

Information is also rated high in family needs assessments.[44, 45, 47] Health care providers can minimize stress associated with the hospitalization of relatives by anticipating family needs for information and resources,[53] which have been reported to increase satisfaction.[56] Printed brochures about the hospital, available services, and critical care structures and routines are a valuable tool in supplying families with concrete, consistent information.[57] Regularly scheduled meetings between the family and critical care staff can provide ongoing support but also provide for timely and consensus-driven decision making.[58] Families need to know how the patient is being treated, exactly what is being done, specific facts about the patient's progress, and why procedures are being performed.[59] At the bedside, families consider it important for staff to give directions about what family members can do for the patient.[60] Directing them to talk to and touch the patient is necessary in an environment with multiple invasive therapies. Allowing the family to assist in the delivery of personal care can be among the most supportive activities in meeting their needs to feel important in promoting healing. Encouraging family members to talk to the patient regarding home activities can be important in avoiding the patient's sense of alienation from the preadmission life.

Families can present considerable barriers for the staff in the attempt to provide quality patient care. Relatives who become angry, vociferous, bitter, or resentful toward the staff can take up undue amounts of time and energy, diverting resources away from patient care. The critical care staff is a powerful force in developing family inclusion in care and in preempting perceived family barriers. Inconsistencies in family treatment (visitation, care provision, information) can be problematic for families and may have a negative impact on family trust and cooperation.[61] Most health care providers agree that humanistic, family-oriented care requires that families be given as much access as possible to critically ill patients. Family visitation is not a privilege granted by hospitals. It is a necessary adjunct to a therapeutic regimen.[62] If critical care practitioners truly believe in a health care system driven by the needs of patients and their families, changes need to be made in philosophy of care, policies, and physical structure of our critical care units to support this vision.

STAFF EXPERIENCES

Many health care environments provide challenge and stimulation, creating a sense of accomplishment for employees. Critical care units provide all of these in abundance, but the environment and patients create special challenges and often obstacles for health care providers. The life-and-death decisions and actions require constant vigilance and timely interventions to assist patients through adverse events. Besides providing demanding specialized care to critically ill patients, a number of stress-invoking factors exist in the ICU milieu for the health care provider.[63-70]

Physicians

Physicians identified some stressors such as the following:

1. The demoralizing situation of patient's not getting better despite the practitioner's best efforts.
2. Unrealistic expectations of families.
3. Lack of beds and need to make triage decisions.
4. Conflict resolution.
5. Poor support services.
6. Ethical dilemmas.
7. Issues of death and dying.

Physicians found the most taxing issues in the critical care setting were not patient-related at all, however, but were administrative hassles. In order, they were (1) conflict resolution, (2) bed-finding, and (3) lack of support services.[66]

Nurses

A study of critical care nurses, however, found that patient care issues were rated very high and related to a perception of lack of control. Nurses reported that the major contributors to stress were (1) the unnecessary prolongation of life, (2) sudden emergency changes in patient status, and (3) the trajectory of illness rather than death itself.[68]

In multiple studies of nurse satisfaction management and organizational issues rated moderately high in importance, this coincides with physician reports of administrative stressors. In particular, nurses reported insufficient and malfunctioning equipment, noise, and communications difficulties with nursing leadership.[68] Additionally, work content and work environment variables appear to have a stronger relationship with satisfaction than either the economic or individual difference variables.

Administrators

Administrators and nurse managers have more control over work content variables (through job redesign) or work environment variables (through appropriate leadership and human resource management practices) than over external labor market factors or internal, individual factors.[71] Successful managers focus improvement efforts on system failures that increase frustration and challenge the care team. It is important to continuously evaluate sources of tension and ways to enhance individual input at the unit level and to implement changes where possible.[70] In turn, a more satisfied and less stressed team will improve the quality of care delivery to patients and families. Future studies need to be conducted to identify the factors that contribute to quality. It indeed may be found that our greatest assets are the people who are involved in the delivery of our care product rather than in the length of stay and cost per patient-day statistics that are currently in focus.

SUMMARY

Despite the challenges confronted by all participants in the critical-care environment, barriers to effective patient care can be minimized. Sensitivity of health care providers to barriers that may exist in their individual environments can be addressed through a planned and focused approach. Each team needs to identify their prevalent barriers and create improvement projects to address them. However, major themes have emerged in averting barriers to effective care:

1. A comprehensive and multidisciplinary patient admission assessment.

2. A cohesive team approach to patient care (including the family).

3. Presence of a resilient, sensitive, critical care team.

As we move into the 21st century, we need to demonstrate cost-effective, patient-centered care. Acknowledging and preventing barriers will be instrumental in achieving this goal.

References

1. Eagleton BB, Goldman L: The quality connection: Satisfaction of patients and their families. Crit Care Nurs 1997; 17:76-80, 100.
2. Cohen IL, Fitzpatrick M, Booth FV: Critical care medicine: Opportunities and strategies for improvement. J Comm J Qual Improv 1996; 22:85-103.
3. Felver L: Patient-environment interactions in critical care. Crit Care Nurs Clin North Am 1995; 7:327-335.
4. Gregory MM: On humanizing the critical care environment. Crit Care Nurs Q 1993; 16:1-6.
5. Harvey MA, Ninos NP, Adler DC, et al: Results of the Consensus Conference on Fostering More Humane Critical Care: Creating a healing environment. AACN Clin Issues Crit Care Nurs 1993; 4:484-549.
6. American College of Critical Care Medicine, Society of Critical Care Medicine: Guidelines for intensive care unit design. Crit Care Med 1995; 23:582-588.
7. Society of Critical Care Medicine and American Association of Critical Care Nursing: Joint Position Statement: Essential provisions for critical care in health system reform. Crit Care Med 1994; 22:2017-2019.
8. Krachman SL, D'Alonzo GE, Criner GJ: Sleep in the intensive care unit. Chest 1995; 107:1713-1720.
9. Aaron JN, Carlisle CC, Carskadon MA, et al: Environmental noise as a cause of sleep disruption in an intermediate respiratory care unit. Sleep 1996; 19:707-710.
10. Topf M, Bookman M, Arand D: Effects of critical care unit noise on the subjective quality of sleep. J Adv Nurs 1996; 24:545-551.
11. Chlan LL: Psychophysiologic responses of mechanically ventilated patients to music: A pilot study. Am J Crit Care 1995; 4:233-238.
12. Barnason S, Zimmerman L, Nieveen J: The effects of music intervention on anxiety in the patient after coronary bypass grafting. Heart Lung 1995; 24:124-132.
13. Johnston K, Rohaly-Davis J: An introduction to music therapy: Helping the oncology patient in the ICU. Crit Care Nurs Q 1996; 18:54-60.
14. Zimmerman L, Nieveen J, Barnason S, Schnaderer M: The effects of music interventions on postoperative pain and sleep in CABG patients. Scholarly Inquiry Nurs Pract 1996; 10:153-170.
15. Evans JC, French DG: Sleep and healing in intensive care settings. Dimens Crit Care Nurs 1995; 14:189-193.
16. Meyer TJ, et al: Adverse environmental conditions in the respiratory and medical ICU settings. Chest 1994; 105:1211-1216.
17. Parker KP: Promoting sleep and rest in critically ill patients. Crit Care Nurs Clin North Am 1995; 7:337-349.
18. Watts S, Brooks A: Patients' perceptions of the preoperative information they need about events they may experience in the intensive care unit. J Adv Nurs 1997; 26:85-92.
19. Turner JS, Briggs SJ, Springhorn HE, et al: Patients' recollection of ICU experience. Crit Care Med 1990; 18:966-968.
20. Porter L: Procedural distress in critical care settings. Crit Care Nurs Clin North Am 1995; 7:307-314.
21. Puntillo K: Pain in the Critically Ill: Assessment and Management. Gaithersburg, Md, Aspen Publishers, 1991, pp 3-7.
22. Heney LL: Music therapy—a nursing intervention for the control of pain and anxiety in the ICU: A review of the research literature. Dimens Crit Care Nurs 1995; 14:295-303.
23. International Association for the Study of Pain: Pain terms: A list of definitions and notes on usage. Pain 1979; 6:249.
24. Gujol MC: A survey of pain assessment and management practices among critical care nurses. Am J Crit Care 1994; 3:123-128.
25. Agency for Health Care Policy and Research (AHCPR): Acute Pain Management Guidelines Panel: Acute pain management: Operative or medical procedures and trauma. Clinical Practice Guidelines 1994. Rockville, Md, U.S. Department of Health and Human Services.
26. Puntillo K: Dimensions of procedural pain and its analgesic management in critically ill surgical patients. Am J Crit Care 1994; 3(2):116-122.
27. Dracup K, Bryan-Brown C: Pain in the ICU: Fact or fiction? Am J Crit Care 1995; 4:337-339.
28. McCaffrey M, Beebe A: Pain: Clinical Manual for Nursing Practice. St. Louis, CV Mosby, 1989.
29. Clark S, Fontaine DK, Simpson T: Recognition, assessment, and treatment of anxiety in the critical care setting. Crit Care Nurse Suppl 1994: 2-6.
30. Walker MK: The physiology of normal aging: Implications for nursing management of critically compromised adults. *In*: Critical

Care Nursing of the Elderly. Fulmer TT, Walker MK (Eds). New York, Springer-Verlag, 1992, p 32.
31. Girard NH: Gerontological nursing in acute care settings. *In*: Gerontological Nursing: Concepts and Practice. 2nd ed. Matteson MA, McConnell ES, Linton AD (Eds). Philadelphia, WB Saunders, 1997, p 855.
32. Creditor MC: Hazards of hospitalization of the elderly. Ann Intern Med 1993; 118:219–223.
33. Rauen CA, Britt TL: Elderly patients. *In*: Critical Care Nursing. 2nd ed. Clochesy JM, Breu C, Cardin S, et al. (Eds). Philadelphia, WB Saunders, 1996, pp 1493–1509.
34. Shannon ML, Lehman CA: Protecting the skin of the elderly patient in the intensive care unit. Crit Care Nurs Clin North Am 1996; 8:17–28.
35. Stanley M, Burggraf: Nurses' role with the elderly in acute care setting. *In*: Gerontological Nursing. Stanley M, Beare PG (Eds). Philadelphia, FA Davis, 1995, p 80.
36. St. Pierre J: Delirium in hospitalized elderly patients: Off track. Crit Care Clin North Am 1996; 8:53–60.
37. Foreman MD, Kleinpell K: Medical intensive care. *In*: Critical Care Nursing of the Elderly. Fullmer TT, Walker MK (Eds). New York, Springer-Verlag, 1992, p 105.
38. Kelley FJ: Planning care for acutely confused critically ill older persons. Crit Care Nurs Q 1996; 19:41–46.
39. Stockton P, Burke MM: Cognition and mood. *In*: Wholistic Care of the Older Adult. Burke MM, Walsh MB (Eds). St. Louis, Mosby-Year Book, 1997, p 478.
40. Wilson EB: Physical restraints of elderly patients in critical care. Crit Care Nurs Clin North Am 1996; 8:61–69.
41. Chesla CA, Stannard D: Breakdown in the nursing care of families in the ICU. Am J Crit Care 1997; 6:64–71.
42. Sigmond RM: Hospital planning should provide for a family role in care. Hospitals 1981; 55:63–113.
43. Titler MG, Bombei C, Schuatte DL: Developing family-focused care. Crit Care Nurs Clin North Am 1995; 7:375–386.
44. Molter N: Needs of relatives of critically ill patients: A descriptive study. Heart Lung 1979; 8:332–339.
45. Leske JS: Internal psychometric properties of the critical care family needs inventory. Heart Lung 1991; 20:236–244.
46. Leske JS: Overview of family needs after critical illness: From assessment to intervention. AACN Clin Issues 1991; 2:220–226.
47. Kleinpell RM: Needs of families of critically ill patients: A literature review. Crit Care Nurs 1991; 11:34–40.
48. Foss KR, Tenholder MF: Expectations and needs of persons with family members in an intensive care unit as opposed to a general ward. South Med J 1993; 86:380–384.
49. Freismuth CA: Meeting the needs of families of critically ill patients: A comparison of visiting policies in the intensive care setting. Heart Lung 1986; 15:309–310.
50. Simpson T: Needs and concerns of families of critically ill adults. Focus Crit Care 1989; 16:388–397.
51. Hickey M: What are the needs of critically ill patients? A review of the literature since 1976. Heart Lung 1990; 19:401–415.
52. Kleiber C, Halm M, Titler M, et al: Emotional responses of family members during a critical care hospitalization. Am J Crit Care 1994; 3:70–76.
53. Jamerson PA, Scheibmeir M, Bott MJ, et al: The experience of families with a relative in the intensive care unit. Heart Lung 1996; 25:467–474.
54. Halm MA, Titler MG, Johnson SK, et al: Behavioral responses of family members during critical illness. Clin Nurs Res 1993; 2:414–437.
55. Olson D: Paging the family: Using technology to enhance communication. Crit Care Nurs 1997; 17:39–41.
56. Hennemann EA, McKenzie JB, Dewa CS: An evaluation of interventions for meeting the informational needs of families. Am J Crit Care 1992; 1:85–93.
57. Medland JJ, Ferrans CE: Effectiveness of a structured communication program for family members of patients in an ICU. Am J Crit Care 1998; 7:24–29.
58. Dracup KA, Breu CS: Using research findings to meet the needs of grieving spouses. Nurs Res 1978; 4:212–216.
59. Leske JS: Needs of family members after critical illness: Prescriptions for interventions after critical illness: Crit Care Nurs Clin North Am 1992; 4:587–596.
60. Clarke SP: Increasing the quality of family visits to the ICU. Dimens Crit Care Nurs 1994; 14:200–212.
61. Kirchhoff KT, Pugh E, Calame RM, et al: Nurses' beliefs and attitudes toward visiting in adult critical care settings. Am J Crit Care 1993; 2:238–245.
62. Cleveland AM: ICU visitation policies. Nurs Manage 1994; 25:80–84.
63. Blegen MA: Nurses' job satisfaction: A meta-analysis of related variables. Nurs Res 1993; 42:36–41.
64. Collins MA: The relation of work stress, hardiness, and burnout among full-time hospital staff nurses. J Nurs Staff Dev 1996; 12:81–85.
65. Erlen JA: Critical care nurses, ethical decision-making and stress. J Adv Nurs 1997; 26:953–961.
66. Guntupalli KK, Fromm RE: Burnout in the internist-intensivist. Intensive Care Med 1996; 22:625–630.
67. Hibbert M: Stressors experienced by nurses while caring for organ donors and their families. Heart Lung 1995; 24:399–407.
68. Sawatsky JV: Stress in critical care nurses: Actual and perceived. Heart Lung 1996; 25:409–417.
69. Stechmiller JK, Yarandi HN: Predictors of burnout in critical care nurses. Heart Lung 1993; 22:534–540.
70. van Servellen G, Leake B: Burn-out in hospital nurses: A comparison of acquired immunodeficiency syndrome, oncology, general medical, and intensive care unit nurse samples. J Prof Nurs 1993; 9:169–177.
71. Irvine DM, Evans MG: Job satisfaction and turnover among nurses: Integrating research findings across studies. Nurs Res 1995; 44:246–251.

191

Impact of Health Care and Technology Trends on Critical Care Practice

Ginger Schafer Wlody, RN, MS, EdD, FCCM

The next 20 years will continue to be critical times for health care and the specialty practice of caring for critically ill patients. Global shifts in power, immigration, the changing economic and political climates, and soaring health care costs will continue to affect delivery of critical care.

In this chapter we discuss current and future trends that affect the practice of critical care and set forth multidisciplinary strategies to help critical care practitioners maximize resources. These strategies are designed to address the changing health care environment by assuming a proactive stance. First, global trends and United States trends will be addressed, then health care costs and factors that affect those costs. Subsequently, technology and its benefits and liabilities will be addressed. Guidelines for technology assessment will be presented, and, finally, the role of the critical care manager in creating a safe, healing environment will be discussed. Four major strategies for maximizing resources in the current and future critical care environment will be presented.

GLOBAL TRENDS

In discussing health care and the future it is important to note global trends that affect health care—and, consequently, critical care practice. Worldwide societal and economic changes are occurring at an accelerating rate. A "mosaic society" has emerged, in which "minorities" are the majority, jobs are information based rather than industrial, high-technology skills are required, the population is aging, women outnumber men, and illiteracy is growing. The globe continues to shrink as communication technology advances. That which affects one country soon affects another. The impact of the European Common Market continues to change the way business is done across European borders. The recent downturn in the Asian stock markets affected markets worldwide.

Economic and communications changes subsequently affect health care. The economic rise of the Pacific Rim countries is startling, and Naisbett and Aburdene[1] point to it as a powerful global presence. Scientific advances in one country are quickly adopted in other countries across the globe. Diseases, too, spread rapidly. The travels of the human immunodeficiency virus (HIV) were traced from Africa to all nations of the world. We all face problems related to acquired immunodeficiency syndrome (AIDS), an issue of awesome impact for the world population. In the year 2001 it is projected that there will be 6 million persons with AIDS.[2] In the future, advances in medical and nursing care and in the associated technology will continue to have global, rather than local, implications.

HEALTH CARE TRENDS IN THE UNITED STATES

Although global changes affect the practice of critical care, this chapter focuses on practice in the United States. Current health care trends in the United States can be divided into six areas: trends related to the financial climate; changes in health care services; technologic advances; changes in health care management; the emerging concept of an "ethical environment"; and burgeoning legal concerns. Triage, resource allocation, and rationing currently take various forms.

Technologic and scientific advances in health care have propelled complex financial issues to the forefront. As we have increased our ability to diagnose and treat illness, and to sustain life indefinitely, we have encountered increasing financial and ethical dilemmas. The current state of technology reveals that advances have occurred in every aspect of medical and health care. As we have become more proficient in prolonging life, replacing body parts, predicting genetic defects, treating the fetus in utero, and using embryonic tissue to combat specific illnesses, we learned that each new technology engenders a multitude of conflicts, dilemmas, and legal and financial questions. Ethical issues continue to play an increasingly important role in health care. Another important trend that will affect delivery of critical care services more directly in the future is the growing aging population. Rowe and coworkers assert, "Estimates of the number of older Americans who will need specialized care by the year 2000 and the number of physicians who will be trained to provide that care foretell a serious disparity."[3] It is estimated that the number of people older than 85 years, now 2.1 million, will double by the end of the 20th century. The health care needs of this aging population differ substantially from those of younger persons.[4]

OVERALL HEALTH CARE TRENDS

Overall health care trends include downsizing in American hospitals, increased patient "acuity," increased complexity of home care, increased use of primary care, increased use of ambulatory services, and delivery of services to more underprivileged people. For example, ambulatory surgery centers, which opened in the early 1970s, have dramatically increased in numbers since that time. Procedures such as cholecystectomy are frequently performed on an outpatient basis. Reimbursement policies have changed the way health care is delivered because reimbursement for ambulatory procedures has increased while reimbursement for in-hospital procedures has decreased.[5] The proportion of hospital beds devoted to care of the critically ill has continued to increase as the acuity of hospitalized patients increases. More health care services are delivered to chronically ill persons in their homes. The increased numbers of HIV-infected patients have caused changes in hospital services for these patients, which may or may not include increased critical care services and greater demand for hospice care as more patients wish to die at home. Thanks to new drugs, many AIDS patients are living longer and requiring less time in the ICU. Improvements in techniques and continued progress in organ transplantation have been tremendous during the last decade, and these patients will continue to require critical care services. Noninvasive technologic devices will increase, thereby decreasing costs and risks related to invasive procedures.

Other advances in technology, as in genetic engineering to create new drugs and solve other health care problems, will continue. Such advances then require changes in educational needs and patient care delivery systems. A paradigm shift in the methods of patient care management and payment systems is occurring as managed care (use of health maintenance organizations [HMOs] and preferred provider organizations [PPOs]) becomes more the rule. Most analysts in the health care field today have deemed this shift necessary. Technologic advances are also resulting in escalating computerization of systems and in trends toward use of bedside computers for all data gathering and analysis. Use of quality and performance measurement techniques has increased and will continue to escalate as data systems provide information needed to monitor quality of care.

Current Health Care Trends

Naisbett and Aburdene[1] said, "We're poised on the threshold of a great era of biotechnology" (p. 241). Three major directions in biotechnology today affect critical care:

- Genetic manipulation of crops and farm animals
- Identification and manipulation of inherited characteristics
- Genetic engineering to conquer diseases for which there are now no cures

According to the U.S. Commerce Department, spiraling health care costs led to health spending of $661.3 billion in 1990 in the United States.[6] Problems related to widespread lack of insurance, an aging population, and waves of low-income immigrants forced restructuring of the United States health care system. During the past few years, the health care delivery system has changed dramatically. A large percentage of care in the United States is now delivered through a variety of managed care and preferred provider plans. Rosner[7] wrote in 1997: "The need for health care reform in the United States is obvious. The costs of medical care continue to escalate despite utilization review, quality assurance, and the diagnostic group prospective payment system for hospital care." Many see the growth of enrollment in managed care organizations as a cost-containment strategy, in and of itself. Other concerns Rosner expressed are related to the large numbers of Americans who are uninsured or underinsured and to inequities in physician reimbursement and health services utilization. This leads to disparities in the cost of health care in different areas and to restrictions on a patient's choice of physician.[7] Indemnification insurance plans offer free choice of physicians. They manage care by monitoring claims and denying or reducing payment for claims deemed unjustifiable.[8] Alternative

TABLE 191–1. Alternative Systems for Provision of Health Care

1. Single-payer model of a national health care system (e.g., Canadian system)
2. "Play or pay" approach—employers are obligated to provide basic health care benefits for their employees/dependents or to finance a public program for the uninsured.
3. Expansion of Medicare to all Americans
4. Oregon-type initiative to ration very expensive medical services that benefit only a few patients in order to provide basic health care services for all citizens

Data from Rosner F: The ethics of managed care. Mt Sinai J Med 1997; 64:8–19.[7]

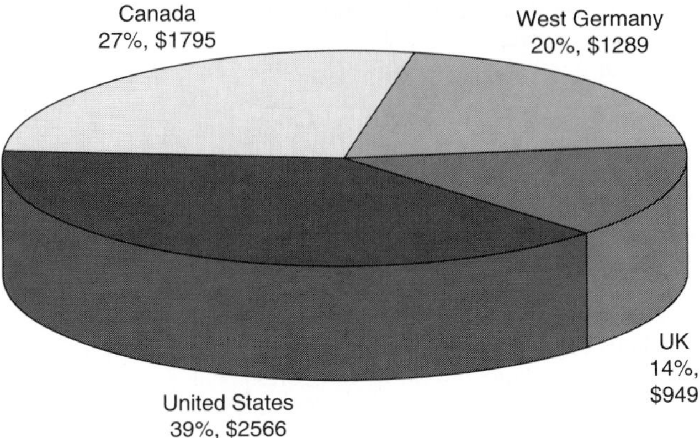

Figure 191–1. Comparison of United States health care spending per person with other countries in U.S. dollars (1990).

systems for the provision of health care outlined by Rosner (1997)[7] are listed in Table 191–1.

Advanced medical equipment and technology is viewed as a strategic asset for attracting both physicians and patients to a hospital or health care institution. Health care institutions demonstrate their belief in the importance of technology by their rising technologic investment. Health care providers spent $8.25 billion on capital equipment in 1988, as compared with $8.21 billion in 1987.[9] In fact, the culprit most often cited for the increases in health care costs is technology.[10] In 1993 in the United States, 60% to 70% of medical professionals practiced in specialties and 30% to 40% in general practice. These ratios have drastically shifted in the direction of general practice and physicians' being employed by others.[11] Postoperative infections and septic complications continue to be major contributors to poorer clinical outcomes for patients after operations. This occurs despite improvements in techniques for the management of surgical infection and development of more powerful antibiotics.[12]

Critical Care Trends

Critical care services have been extended to care for patients at home. Patients are discharged connected to ventilators and other high-technology equipment. Macready and Evans[13] wrote this:

New technologies evolve in response to the demands of the marketplace. In their quest to economize, clinicians today are trying to provide patient care more efficiently and, whenever possible, in the least expensive setting, be that an ICU, a hospital general care unit, a skilled nursing facility, or an outpatient clinic. Even a patient's home is becoming the site for many types of care or monitoring that were once provided only by hospitals. This has created a demand for portable, versatile medical devices that can travel easily from the ICU all the way to the homecare setting.

Fewer invasive procedures will be performed on critically ill patients, but more assistive devices (e.g., pulmonary or cardiac) will be used. There have been increases in telemetry and intermediate care (stepdown units) to cope with the increasing number of high-acuity patients.[13] More and more critical care physicians have to choose to work for hospitals or large practice groups because of the changes in health care reimbursement.

FINANCIAL CLIMATE AND TRENDS

Since 1968, there has been a rapid increase in hospital care expenditures that can be attributed to inflation in prices of medical goods and services and medical care of high intensity being provided to a larger population. In 1988 health care expenditures ran close to 12% of the gross national product[14] and in 1991 it was as high as 14%.[15] Many view technology as the main cause of these increases.

Until recently, health care costs continued to escalate and no end was in sight. They comprised 14% of the gross national product in 1993, and it was predicted they would soar toward 20% if drastic action was not taken. When compared with other countries the United States spends more on health care (Fig. 191–1).[15] Oregon was the first state to attempt to completely restructure health care at the state level. At a meeting in Sacramento in 1991, John Kitzhaber, M.D., president of the Oregon state senate, told the California Health Forum that the United States health system is "fundamentally flawed and failing." He noted, "Thirty-five million Americans are without health insurance in a system that spends 1.5 billion daily."[15]

Problems that affect financial trends in our health care system today include lack of universal access to care, cost shifting (disguised as cost containment), and increasing reliance on technology with limited assessment of its value and little motivation in Congress to change the technology assessment system. Oregon implemented a state health care system that provided a basic level of benefits to all citizens based on effectiveness of care rather than ability to pay. The Oregon plan, the first of its kind in the country, based its public policy on several assumptions (Table 191–2) and has been fairly successful.[15]

The Health Care Services Commission in Oregon established the priority list of services, which was then approved by the governor. Dr. Kitzhaber stated, "Hospitals don't drive the costs of health care up, physicians do, by sending patients there."[15]

TABLE 191–2. Assumptions in the Oregon Health Care Proposal

1. Health care allocations made as part of the overall budgetary allocation process
2. Clear accountability
3. Universal access for all citizens
4. Society to finance a certain level of care for those who cannot themselves afford it
5. A clearly defined process to determine the basic level of care
6. Health care to be publicly debated
7. Creation of incentives to use effective medical procedures
8. Funding explicit and economically sustainable

*Data from Treatment for the American Health Care System: Universal access? Calif Hosp 1991; 18:25.

Long-term evaluation will provide data about the success of this bold venture.

Changes in Health Care Costs and Services

Current reimbursement policies have changed the way health care is delivered. Reimbursement for outpatient ambulatory services has increased; that for inpatient services has declined. This reimbursement mechanism has forced hospitals to convert many procedures from inpatient to outpatient services.[5] Hospitals are being closed or drastically downsized. Problems of recruitment and retention of professional nurses changed the way care is delivered to patients. Increased complexity in the health care system led to new initiatives and programs such as case management. Such programs provided more opportunities for nurses in roles such as "acute care nurse practitioner" and various other areas of advanced practice.

The American Association of Critical-Care Nurses (AACN) projects that 400,000 nurses will be required to meet the demands in the 21st century.[16] There is already greater delegation of non-nursing activities to non-licensed staff such as patient technicians. Critical care education will place more emphasis on management and training for both physician and nurse managers. Use of advanced-practice nurses as acute care- and family nurse practitioners will continue to increase as payors try to reduce the costs of health care services.

CHANGING BELIEFS ABOUT HEALTH CARE

Although technologic advances have occurred very rapidly during the past 25 years, societal and cultural belief systems have not kept pace. During this time, societal changes have occurred in attitudes toward access to care, beliefs about the infallibility of the physician, attitudes toward death and dying, informed consent, and handicapped persons. Universal access to care was a major issue in the early 1960s, when Medicare was created because the Great Society believed that everyone was entitled to equal access to care. President Lyndon Johnson took advantage of the Democratic gains in the 1964 congressional elections to push through landmark health care legislation. Medicare was established to provide care for aged and disabled citizens, and Medicaid to guarantee some medical care for indigent ones.[17] In the late 1960s the phrase *health care industry* began to be heard, and national health expenditures reached $46.3 billion in 1966 and $75 billion in 1970.[17] President Jimmy Carter's attempt to impose price controls on hospitals in 1979 was narrowly defeated in Congress. In the Reagan administration attention shifted to the economic incentives for efficiency.

Today, our society has returned to the concept of limited access to care and to patients' personal responsibility to provide for their own care. The phrase *equal access to care* has been replaced by *equitable access to care*.[18] On October 1, 1983, the Medicare program began phasing in a new plan to pay hospitals on the basis of diagnosis-related groups of illnesses. In this model, Medicare paid hospitals a set fee for each diagnostic category. The incentive was monies left over when care was provided more efficiently or at less expense. The idea was to slow the growth of expenditures for hospital care, which are the bulk of Medicare costs.[19] A study by Russell and Manning found that prospective payment has substantially reduced Medicare's hospital costs.[19] Purchasing new technology must be more carefully considered because hospitals can no longer as easily bill patients for such purchases. The current environment is one of competition among health care institutions and providers for patients' business, rather than of cooperation and collaboration.

The issues discussed so far are ones of macroallocation that deal with patients in the aggregate. Microallocation issues affect individual patients and their health care providers. Scarce or decreasing resources have the effect of forcing those in health care to make difficult choices in a strained fiscal environment.

The Ethical Environment

Three major struggles are seen as being primary between individuals, caregivers, and society. The three broad major ethical issues that will continue to plague us in critical care into the 21st century are related to the struggle between (1) individual autonomy and beneficence, (2) individual autonomy and utilitarianism, and (3) struggles related to individual rights in general. Currently there are disparities in level of health care services, and, as resources become more scarce and there is increased control of physicians by payors, individual choice is becoming more limited.

We are currently in an era of strong patients' rights: patients are still frequently able to choose what level and type of care they want or can afford. In the future our choices will be limited further toward the end of more universal health care services. These tensions relate to the increasing number of patients who will require care (e.g., more older persons and persons with AIDS) and the scarcity of resources. These problems affect critical care nurses, physicians, other providers, and health care organizations.

Patient autonomy must be preserved as much as possible, and the physician's ability to practice must be sustained to the extent necessary. The use of informed consent has been greatly expanded. The Patient Self-Determination Act, which required that patients be given information on advance directives, should result in an increase in patients' wishes being followed when they are unable to make their own decisions. Surrogates will be more readily identified, thus shortening delays in decisions altering care and the withdrawal of care. A recent study funded by the Robert Wood Johnson Foundation, however, noted that care at the end of life is less than optimal, particularly in the ICU.[20]

The struggle will continue—between patients and families on one hand and the health care team on the other. Ultimately, patients' autonomy will be limited by their respective health care plans. Other ethical struggles that are impacting critical care include the controversial topics of physician-assisted suicide and euthanasia. Supporters of these options have become increasingly vocal, and an assisted suicide referendum was defeated only narrowly in California in 1992. On June 26th, 1997 the U.S. Supreme Court ruled that no constitutionally protected right to physician-assisted suicide exists, but this does not prohibit individual states from legalizing physician-assisted suicide. This has implications for the ICU and for better end-of-life care, including pain management; comprehensive, compassionate physical care; and at times, the foregoing of life-sustaining therapy.

The third major ethical struggle has to do with maximizing limited resources. As the costs of health care delivery and services have increased, it has become impossible to ensure that all health care needs of all citizens are met. Scarcity of resources will necessitate use of decision-making strategies that, although localized, will need to be coordinated, perhaps on the regional or national level. Decisions made at the local level are best and support the public demand for local control. Kassirer[21] believes that the government already has a substantial role in medical practice and expresses concern that medical care decisions not be made by politicians. He believes the role of government is to protect its citizens by ensuring health care for vulnerable persons, access to emergency services, effective grievance procedures in health plans, and availability of information about contracting physicians.

TECHNOLOGIC ADVANCES IN CRITICAL CARE

Definitions

Technology is the popular word used to describe the apparatus and the procedures that are based on modern science, in contrast with the supposedly simpler and more humane healing arts. Diagnostic technology, in contrast to therapeutic technology, involves the use of expensive "scientific" machines, radioisotopes, electronics, and the like, to make diagnoses. Therapeutic technology is viewed (in the popular context) as complex surgical procedures such as organ transplantation and insertion of devices such as pacemakers, and special procedures such as dialysis therapy.[10] Medical technology assessment means (at a minimum) a systematic evaluation of safety and efficacy, but it can also include evaluations of economic, social, and ethical factors.[22]

Technologic Problems

Technologic advances have moved beyond society's ability to cope with the financial and ethical dilemmas they have induced. Technology is not inherently evil,[1] but how we use it is key. Anderson and Steinberg[23] describe the technologic arsenal already in place in hospitals and relate it to the eagerness with which physicians have incorporated new procedures into their practice and to the frequency with which such procedures have become part of patient-physician encounters. Technologic advances, although they are awesome and help many patients, also require tremendous investments of highly skilled personnel and costly equipment to support them. Ramifications of the technologic imperative in health care today will be discussed, as will problems related to developing, introducing, assessing, and utilizing new technologies. Additionally, current and proposed models of technology assessment will be explored.

A growing trend in critical care is the expansion of the field of organ transplantation, which has moved rapidly from an experimental therapy to the standard of care for some cases of end-stage kidney, heart, lung, and liver disease. As the benefits of transplantation have become increasingly apparent and the medical barriers have fallen, the demand for transplantation has far outstripped the supply of organs.[24] As transplantation options expand, the need for critical care nurses in transplantation increases. Critical care nurses are involved in preparing patients and families for transplantation and for postoperative care and the necessary psychological and social adjustments. Awareness has increased, and the number of organ transplants has been phenomenal during the past decade and will increase exponentially in the future.

Organ donations are increasing, but there is currently a chronic shortage in the United States. More than 22,000 men, women, and children are waiting for organs. Of those, 5000 will die before an organ becomes available.[25] Randall[26] estimated in 1991 that as many as 30% of the more than 3000 patients then awaiting heart or liver transplantation would die before an organ donor could be found. Every year about 15,000 people die under circumstances that would allow their organs to be transplanted, yet fewer than 4000 donations occur.

THE TECHNOLOGIC IMPERATIVE

Ronald Bayer, Ph.D., associate for policy studies at the Hastings Institute, noted, "As technology becomes available there is an ineluctable dynamic that makes it intolerable to have the technology and not use it."[18] He went on to say that, once one subset of the population has access to a technology, society finds it intolerable to watch people who need it die. This was demonstrated recently by the case of a young child whose insurance would not pay for an experimental procedure to treat her fatal condition. The family sued the insurance company and appeared on television to garner support for their cause. There is a similar compulsion in hospitals to utilize high-tech interventions. Administrators blame "a pervasive American infatuation" with technology but continue to purchase new items as soon as they become available. Although the managed care environment has taken the public emphasis away from high-technology invasive care, such care continues to be a priority.

Koenig[27] discusses the technologic imperative, observing that many believe that the mere existence of a dramatic new medical device constitutes mandate for its use. She studied the social processes that contribute to the operation of a technologic imperative in medical practice and identified a social "routinization" of a technical medical procedure and the creation of social rituals related to the technology. These social rituals supported continued use of a technology and its acceptance as "normal." Koenig found that the "new" standard of care became a moral and a technical obligation. Siegal,[28] in a piercing article, reviewed the development of coronary care units (CCUs) as a paradigm for the uncritical acceptance of technology in medical services. In studies comparing CCUs with other settings for treating acute myocardial infarctions intensive care was not shown to offer a consistent benefit over more conservative treatment. The author related the proliferation of CCUs to corporate involvement in medical research: corporations that build monitoring devices "lobbied" for the development of CCUs.

Problems Related to Inadequate Technology Assessment

This immediate and enthusiastic acceptance of new technology—the technologic imperative— creates a host of problems related to inadequate assessment, increased cost, lack of expertise, technology diffusion, and inadequate planning. Profits from the use of new technologies are very high, and many large hospitals race to be the first to have the latest in the technologic armamentarium, sometimes before adequately assessing a device or technique. The *Los Angeles Times*,[30] in a front-page story, described the 1984 purchase by Humana Inc. of six lithotripters ($1.6 million each) soon after they were approved by the federal government. Lithotripters are machines that pulverize kidney stones with shock waves. The technique works, but only relatively few patients have kidney stones. Soon, lithotripter owners began looking for other uses for their machines and focused on gallstones. Every year a million Americans have a gallbladder attack because of stones. Studies from clinical trials now show that lithotripsy works for only 10% to 25% of gallstone patients. Thus, the majority required surgery. The treatments also caused disturbing side effects such as hematuria and hypertension. This example points out the fact that expensive new technology is adopted with few guidelines and little agreement on application. A model for technology assessment in critical care should include such factors as technologic capability, range of possible uses, therapeutic impact, diagnostic and therapeutic accuracy, impact on the health care provider, and patient outcome.

New technologies usually do not decrease costs at all; rather, physicians add the new technology to their armamentarium and utilize several methods of diagnosis instead of one. For example, the computed tomography (CT) scanner or the magnetic resonance imager may be much more accurate than conventional x-ray studies at detecting blood clots in the brain, but, more often than not, physicians use all three. Costs then quickly get out of hand.[30] A third concern related to the rate of introduction of new technology is the need for standards for training those who use it. These authors say that frequently a new technology becomes available and is introduced to the medical community so rapidly that those who acquire the new device, administer the new drug, or perform the new procedure are not competent to use it effectively.

The diffusion of a new technology into practice is a fourth problem that has been described.[31] Because technology assessment involves examining techniques before they are released *and* their subsequent diffusion into practice, follow-up studies must be done. Anderson and Lomas[30] analyzed coronary artery bypass graft (CABG) surgery in the province of Ontario, Canada. They found that the annual number of procedures increased 52% over a 7-year period from 1979 through 1985. Interestingly, large increases in CABG rates among persons older than 65 years accounted for more than half of the increase in procedures, yet increased rates of surgery in this population were unlikely to be related to increased prevalence of coronary artery disease. The authors felt that the increase was related to a change in the clinical attitude toward the use of CABG.

A fifth problem of rapid adoption of new health care technology is inadequate planning. The reimbursement system has fostered the use of technology related to patient procedures rather than on new technology to cut the cost of caring for patients in the hospital. In the past, capital purchases focused on technologic devices for which patients could be charged directly. For example, hospital information systems are lagging far behind available technology.[31] Bedside data systems would provide safer, more efficient care by nursing and other personnel, but when interviewed a hospital leader stated, "I see nobody really willing to go into investment to put in bedside computers, which would certainly cut down on the problem of charting and improve the quality of care."[31] Costly, rapidly emerging technologies that are seen as "must haves" preclude planning for and purchasing "everyday" equipment. Thus, available funds go for the new technologies.

Current and Proposed Approaches to Technology Assessment

Technology assessment is frustrating to hospital executives, who know that they must examine new technologies for their clinical use, cost effectiveness, and "fit" within hospital marketing strategies. The largest medical centers used formal technology assessment procedures, but small rural institutions simply do not have the resources for technology assessment. Frequently, hospitals rely on their physicians for information on emerging technologies, but this, too, is becoming problematic as the pace of change accelerates. Some multihospital or large hospital systems have directors of technology assessment. Others utilize committees of physicians and administrators, supplemented by a staff of researchers,[32] and in very small hospitals it is the chief executive officer who makes decisions on technology acquisition.

A number of approaches to technology assessment have been recommended. Patricia Harris, Secretary of the Department of Health and Human Services in 1980, announced that new health technologies should be subjected to cost-benefit analyses before Health and Human Services would agree to fund their wide distribution.[33] Dorsey recommends that some expectation of minimal benefit, in terms of longevity, improved functional capacity, or socially useful productivity, justifies application of a very expensive technology.[33] Disler[34] suggests developing a system of technology distribution that would focus on the benefit that a particular technology would confer on a given group, on the basis of certain health standards. Re[35] believes that it does not appear possible to wait for all technologies to be thoroughly tested in studies of cost and efficacy before they are introduced into clinical use. He feels that, somehow, a "golden mean" must be found, a new approach that would reduce excessive use while "fostering innovation and providing for a pluralistic evaluation of technology . . . seeking care that has been demonstrated to be effective on the basis of cost-efficacy analysis."

Groups that are involved in technology assessment or have information to guide others include the U.S. Office of Technology Assessment, the Advanced Treatment and Bionics Institute (a private organization), the American Hospital Association's Division of Clinical Services and Technology, the Institute of Medicine's Council on Health Care Technology, and the Johns Hopkins Program for Medical Technology and Practice Assessment. These programs are costly, particularly for smaller institutions, because of the expertise and paperwork required.

Guyatt[36] proposed guidelines for assessment of technology (Table 191-3). The criteria developed would lead to the conclusion that a diagnostic technology is ready for dissemination. These six criteria can be considered as a hierarchy of incrementally rigorous evaluation. Models such as that presented by Guyatt[36] should be developed and utilized to prevent unnecessary further escalation of health care costs.

The Future

As costs escalate, more and more issues related to therapy technology will have to be addressed. According to Perry,[31]

TABLE 191–3. Guidelines for Technology Assessment

Criterion	Definition
Technologic capability	The ability of the technology to perform to specifications in a laboratory setting has been demonstrated.
Range of possible uses	The technology promises to provide important diagnostic information in a number of clinical situations.
Diagnostic accuracy	The technology provides information that allows the health worker to make a more accurate assessment of the presence and severity of disease.
Impact on the health care provider	The technology results in health care workers' being more confident of their diagnoses and thus decreases anxiety and increases comfort for the health care provider.
Therapeutic impact	The therapeutic decisions made by the health care provider are altered as a result of application of the technology.
Patient outcome	Application of the technology results in benefit to the patient.

Data from Guyatt G: Guidelines for the general and economic evaluation of health care technologies. Social Sci Med 1986; 22:393–408.

hospitals that have high Medicare and Medicaid populations will not be able to afford more "technology." Transplantation costs will continue to escalate as the demand for replacement of defective body parts increases. In 1985 more than 1 million people received artificial body parts.[37] Today the annual number is much increased, and it will continue to grow. Questions such as these may be raised in an attempt to determine how much health care technology Americans want:

1. How much health care technology are we willing to pay for?
2. Will our pervasive American infatuation with high technology come at the expense of elderly, disabled, and mentally ill persons who need less "glamorous" care?
3. Can we accept cost containment in health care?
4. Can we, and will we, establish an equitable process for rationing?
5. Will use of increasingly complex technology continue to drive our health care system and overshadow health care efficacy and patient needs?
6. Will mechanisms of technology assessment that are "fair" be developed in our capitalistic, profit-oriented society?
7. Will health care institutions utilize mechanisms and models of technology assessment? Will managed care directly or indirectly decrease use of technology in critical care?

Society will continue to struggle with these issues. Consumers will identify their priorities and communicate them to government and health care leaders, physicians, nurses, and insurers.

MANAGEMENT ENVIRONMENT FOR THE FUTURE

Management in critical care is affected by hospital, medical center, and university governing bodies (for those in affiliated teaching centers). Recently, management trends include "flattening" of the organization, greater worker involvement, quality improvement and effectiveness, and increasing attention to selecting effective, well-prepared managers. There is greater commitment on the part of leadership to increased effectiveness and a focus on meeting customers' needs. These concepts were promoted by Deming in the United States and then became popular in Japan during the 1980s. Today the concepts of total quality improvement (TQI) and total quality management (TQM) are being espoused by health care leaders and those who set the standards in hospitals, the Joint Commission for the Accreditation of Hospitals (JCAH). Other management trends include utilization of concepts related to TQM or TQI, a movement from "quality assurance" to quality "assessment and improvement," "performance measurement," and the use of interdisciplinary health care teams for solving problems that prevent effective delivery of patient care. Rosabeth Moss Kantor, former editor of the *Harvard Business Review*,[38] recommends a newer model for managing businesses in the future. She recommends fewer levels of bureaucracy, so there is more contact between "top" and "bottom," more focus on teamwork across areas, more interest in external alliances, more sharing of resources with other organizations, and more stimulation of creativity. To create the ICU of the future, it will be necessary to create a clinical practice environment that promotes excellence in patient care and intertwines components of the healing environment, the professional practice environment, the financial environment, and the interactive or communication environments.

Clinical practice is the essence of patient care. To manage it, factors that promote a patient-centered environment must be present. Today, critical care managers are operating in a highly technical and competitive health care market, and they need to be both effective and efficient. It is important to help critical care managers to create an environment that, although highly technical, is nevertheless compassionate and humanistic. The nurse manager must have the concepts, tools, and strategies to create a clinical practice environment in which excellence in patient care is not only highly valued but also actually provided. It is the patient-centered, "customer-oriented" healing environment created by the nurse manager that empowers staff to deliver excellent patient care, that is based on recognized standards, shared processes, and measurable outcomes.

Knowledge, methods, and systems for assisting critical care managers must be in place so that they can meet the challenges of managing nursing care for a group of critically ill patients. It is helpful to utilize the nursing role framework of CARE components (*c*linical, *a*dministrative, *r*esearch, and *e*ducational nursing roles). The components of a healing environment, from the practical new methods related to TQI to the philosophy of TQM, are important to consider. If management strategies are implemented, resource use will be maximized and patient care enhanced.

SUMMARY

Major changes in health care are occurring and will continue into the 21st century. As health care costs continue to soar, more than 30% of people in the United States remain uninsured. Global trends have been addressed, and multidisciplinary strategies for critical care nurses at the hospital or unit level have been put forth. As we move into the 21st century, nurses have unique opportunities to create environments where patients' needs can be met. In the current health care environment, where managers are challenged daily by economic, administrative, and ethical issues, it is essential to create and sustain excellence in management of critically ill patients. It is the patient-centered, "customer-oriented," healing environment created by nurse managers that empowers staff to deliver excellence in patient care, excellence based on recognized standards, shared processes, and measurable outcomes.

Strategies for maximizing resources at the hospital and the unit level include nurse-physician collaboration, creation of a healing environment, development of a professional practice environment, survival of the economic environment, and creation of an interactive environment. Specific activities to support these strategies have been discussed. Future health care changes aimed at cost containment include streamlining care services, regionalization of care,[39] decreasing the overall number of hospital beds, increasing the number of critical care and intermediate care (step-down) units, and increased use of appropriate technology at the bedside.

References

1. Naisbett J, Aburdene P: Megatrends 2000: Ten Directions for the 1990's. New York; William Morrow, 1990.
2. Chulay M: Critical care nursing in the 21st century. Presented at Cleveland Clinic Symposium, Cleveland, April 5, 1993.
3. Rowe JW, Grossman E, Bond E: Academic geriatrics for the year 2000: An IOM report. N Engl J Med 1992; 316:1425–1428.
4. Schneider EL, Williams TF: Geriatrics and gerontology: Imperatives in education and training. Ann Intern Med 1986; 104:432–435.
5. Ferguson A: Critical care nurses magnified in crystal ball of health care. Nat Employment Rev 1991; 36:91.
6. Rehm A: Legislative Update (Organizational letter). Newport Beach, Calif, American Association of Critical-Care Nurses, 1990.
7. Rosner F: The ethics of managed care. Mt Sinai J Med 1997; 64:8–19.

8. Relman AS: Controlling costs by "managed competition"—would it work? N Engl J Med 1993; 328:133–135.
9. Wagner S: Promoting high tech equipment. Mod Health Care November 19, 1989, pp 39–50.
10. Mc Gregor M: Technology and the allocation of resources. N Engl J Med 1989; 320:118–120.
11. Don't expect health care reform any time soon. *USA Today*, 11A, April 6, 1993.
12. Senkal M, Mumme A, Eickhoff U, Geier B, Spath G, Wulfert D, Joosten U, Frei A, Kemen M: Early postoperative enteral immunonutrition: Clinical outcome and cost-comparison analysis in surgical patients. Crit Care Med 1997; 25:1489–1496.
13. Macready N, Evans A: Flexible monitoring: Mobilizing critical care. Am J Crit Care 1997; 6(Suppl):3–15.
14. Reagan M: Health care rationing: What does it mean? N Engl J Med 1988; 319:149–51.
15. Health cost keep skyrocketing. *USA Today*, 11A, April 6, 1993.
16. American Association of Critical-Care Nurses (AACN): Summary Analysis of Critical Care Nurse Supply and Requirements. Newport Beach, Calif, AACN, 1988.
17. Millenson M: Health care in America. Mod Health Care September 9, 1988, pp 58–74.
18. Richards G: Technology, costs and rationing issues. Hospitals 1984; 80–86.
19. Russell L, Manning CL: The effects of prospective payment on medicine expenditures. N Engl J Med 1989; 320:439–444.
20. The support principal investigators: A controlled trial to improve care for seriously ill hospitalized patients. JAMA 1995; 274:1591–1598.
21. Kassirer JP: Practicing medicine without a license: The new intrusions by congress. N Engl J Med 1997; 336:1747.
22. Rose M, Liebenluft RF: Antitrust implications of medical technology assessment. N Engl J Med 1989; 314:1490–1493.
23. Anderson G, Steinberg E: To buy or not to buy? Technology acquisition under prospective payment. N Engl J Med 1984; 311:182–185.
24. Margreiter R: What can be done about the insufficient supply of grafts? Transplant Proc 1987; 19:79–87.
25. Evans SA: Organ donors needed. *Tallahassee Opinion*, May 1991, p 4.
26. Randall T: Too few human organs for transplantation, too many in need . . . and the gap widens. JAMA 1991; 265:1223–1227.
27. Koenig B: The technological imperative in medical practice: The social creation of a routine treatment. *In*: Biomedicine Examined. Locke M, Gordon D (Eds). Boston, Kluwer, 1988.
28. Siegal DM: The high cost of medical technology: Getting at the heart of the matter. Med Care 1987; 25:979–987.
29. Chen R: Technology costs. *Los Angeles Times*, February 28, 1990, p 1.
30. Anderson G, Lomas J: Monitoring the diffusion of a technology: Coronary artery bypass surgery in Ontario. Am J Pub Health 1988; 78:251–254.
31. Perry L: Challenges of '89. Mod Health Care January 6, 1989, pp 28–36.
32. Evans RW: Health care technology and the inevitability of resource allocation and rationing decisions. JAMA 1983; 249:2047–2052.
33. Dorsey: The other health care revolution. Arch Pathol Med 1986; 110:264–268.
34. Disler DG: Rationing scarce resources. N Engl J Med 1989; 320:1629–1630.
35. Re R: Technology and the allocation of resources (Letter to the Editor). N Engl J Med 1989; 32:1629.
36. Guyatt G: Guidelines for the general and economic evaluation of health care technologies. Social Sci Med 1986; 22:393–408.
37. *Glamour*. New York, Conde Nast, 1985, p 456.
38. Flower J: How to be a business athlete: A conversation with Rosabeth Moss Kanter. Healthcare Forum J 1990; January/February, pp 39–42.
39. Treatment for the American health care system: Universal access? Calif Hosp 1991; 18:25.

192

Critical Care Applications of Large Data Bases

Howard Belzberg, MD, FCCM, FCCP, FACP
Danila Oder, BA • Jacquard Guenon, MS

OVERVIEW

Although large data bases allow for rapid access to large volumes of data, to convert raw data to information, large numbers of data points must be correlated into a descriptive pattern that can be interpreted by the user. Data bases must be constructed so that the raw data can be reliably extracted into a format that supports analysis of events in a meaningful, objective, and reproducible manner. Data bases must be responsive to a variety of users, without demanding unrealistic amounts of effort on those responsible for data entry. Standard protocols that are now in various stages of development will make data bases easier to use and more reliable. Data base management tools, such as the Internet and the National Library of Medicine, will become more integrated into the practice of critical care medicine at all levels, including administration, clinical care, and research.

This chapter describes of the capabilities and difficulties associated with large data bases. The major areas of use of large data bases in the hospital setting are administration, bibliography, patient care, research, and education. Each of these areas has different requirements and is supported by different types of data bases. In this chapter, we review (1) the advantages and disadvantages of linear, relational, and object-oriented data bases; (2) issues relating to methods of data entry; (3) the accuracy and reliability of data; and (4) the challenges involving integration of various sources of data and the interfacing of devices.

Advanced information management systems are necessary in order to apply the increased capacity of the diagnostic and therapeutic tools available in the modern intensive care unit (ICU). The large volumes of data acquired from physiologic monitoring and laboratory analysis must be presented in a format that can be applied to clinical decision making. Data from a variety of sources must be integrated in order to make advances in the understanding of the underlying causes of physiologic decompensation. Such processes as adult respiratory distress syndrome (ARDS), hyperdynamic septic shock, and the systemic inflammatory response syndrome (SIRS)[1–3] have been identified, largely as a result of analyses dependent on large data bases. Recent advances in the identification of markers of diseases as varied as ARDS, vertigo, and diabetes[4, 5] are based on extensive and sophisticated use of data bases. Advanced applications include looking at patterns of physiology in acute disease, comorbid variables in chronic disease, and genetic markers in hereditary disease.[6–9]

The ability to manipulate large volumes of data is the critical component of advancing the understanding of complex systems in many health care arenas, including hospital management, information management, and clinical research. Advanced data base management must be specifically geared to the unique problems and environment of each of these areas.[10, 11] Because this diversity is necessary, integrating these requirements and capabilities is one of the major challenges of system design. System integration is the major emphasis of much of the current research and development activity in the computer sciences. A variety of groups, including the Institute of Medicine, the Institute of Electrical and Electronics Engineers (IEEE), and the American Society for the Testing of Materials (ASTM) have established working committees to establish standards that will allow computer systems to communicate.

In order to identify the interrelations between seemingly diverse events, data must be available for processing in a fashion that allows for analysis from a variety of perspectives. For example, a patient with a positive blood culture who needs surgery is of interest to several individuals.[12] The manager wants to be able to predict operating room utilization from early indicators (positive blood culture), the clinician wants to be forewarned of the potential need for surgical intervention based on a positive marker (positive blood culture), and the researcher wants to understand the relation of an administered drug (prophylactic antibiotics) to a positive blood culture and subsequent need for surgery. To provide the most significant impact, each of these users will receive the input to allow for the conversion of data to information that will be useful to the various users.[13]

The use of clinical data bases is the essential step in comparing patients and in decision making regarding the multiple events that make up a complex disease process.[14] Large data bases greatly facilitate comparison of patients with similar patterns[15] and acuity of illness. Of current interest are efforts using data base analysis to make these comparisons in real time,[16, 17] which would improve the ability to predict outcome during the hospital course rather than inform retrospectively.

The most powerful application of the large data base is subjecting massive amounts of data to advanced analytic methods, such as trajectory analysis, neural networking, and artificial intelligence.[18]

In this chapter, we discuss the following:

- Categories of data available
- Acquisition of data
- Available methods for storage and access
- System applications
- Future applications of information management

In particular, we highlight the design features being developed that will improve the health care user's ability to employ these powerful tools.

TYPES OF DATA BASES

Patient Information

The Hospital Information System (HIS) is the basis of many hospital computer systems. The HIS is usually a large commercial package that operates on large, mainframe-type computers. They are commonly designed with functional blocks to support various activities throughout the hospital. These functional blocks consist of various specialized capabilities such as accounting, billing, materials management, and admission/discharge/transfer (ADT). These systems routinely include a demographic profile of the patient that consists of relatively static information that is updated only intermittently, usually in a batch fashion rather than in real time. This type of system is well suited to supporting the business functions of the hospital, but it routinely lacks the detail or emphasis on clinical data to support research into the mechanisms and process of individual patient diseases. The design of these large systems is based on the intermittent acquisition of integral data points rather than the continuous streams of data that are characteristic of physiologic systems monitoring. Nevertheless, these data bases are widely used and serve vital demographic functions. In particular, the HIS is the most common method for electronic reporting of basic diagnostic data to centralized data bases and is essential for financial and demographic purposes.

These large hospital-based data bases are central to the identification of incidence and prevalence of general information on diagnoses and demographics. The data are often collected into regional or statewide registries (e.g., in Maryland, North Carolina, and Pennsylvania). The strength of these systems lies in their large numbers of data points and long periods of collection. Unfortunately, these data bases lack fine definition of physiologic data. Typically, only discharge diagnosis and complications noted on discharge summaries are captured.

The nomenclature systems most frequently utilized to collect and report these discharge data points are the International Classification of Disease (ICD) and Current Procedural Terminology (CPT) codes. Although these potentially robust systems have a tree structure that theoretically allows for very specific and detailed descriptions,[19] in practice the accuracy of the data is usually limited to a relatively gross level of resolution. In particular, the accuracy of the hospital course is limited to the specified complications, with inadequate information on the physiologic course of the disease. In addition, these data bases usually depend on the *discharge summary* of the patient. The discharge summary is a retrospective abstraction, colored by the perception of the individual and variability in the criteria used for a diagnosis. The discharge summary must be used with serious skepticism, and, for statistical purposes, only the most objective data are reliable. Items such as demographics, length of stay, basic discharge diagnosis, and admission diagnosis are routinely used in epidemiologic research, and the large numbers of patients allow these data to be considered as reliable reflections of the large trends. Unfortunately, interval diagnoses, such as infection and pulmonary embolism, are rarely available.

Abstracted and episodic data are the basis of much current data base design activity. Efforts are concentrated in two areas:

- Improved accuracy and definition of the description of diagnosis
- Standardization of markers of physiologic status

In both areas, there are multiple attempts to create scoring systems that will allow for comparison of patients.[14, 20, 21] These systems range from grading of traumatic injuries to various organs to overall physiologic measures, to combinations of physiologic and anatomic weighted systems.[22, 23] These systems are discussed later.

Bibliographic Support

Although the use of large data bases for bibliographic support is primarily a concern of library science, the interface with clinical applications is important. Integration of bibliographic data with clinical information systems allows for improved teaching and decision making. In addition, automated bibliographic data are available through several sources to identify potential interactions and new indications or potential complications.

The volume of published literature pertaining to patient care is overwhelming.[24] The National Library of Medicine has taken a leading role in electronically cataloguing the medical literature. In the time span of electronic cataloguing, a significant increase in the number of periodicals and articles has occurred. Current applications of sophisticated data base utilization are directed at improving the utility of the massive amounts of data archived.[25] One of the major design challenges is facilitating the use of a huge data base, such as the National Library of Medicine's MEDLINE, by a large number of individuals with varying levels of expertise. A number of public, proprietary, and research projects are now available or in development to address the central issue of searching and making available the contents of a large data base. The design challenges are to provide a "search engine" that responds to queries with all appropriate data and a minimum of irrelevant data and allows the queries to be formulated by people with limited expertise.

The use of advanced "front ends" and search tools is critical in the management of any complex large data base. In the setting of the bibliographic data base, these efforts involve the use of a "metathesaurus" [26-30] based on attempts to create a unified lexicon known as the Unified Medical Language System (UMLS),[31] linked to attempts to provide automation of searching through a semantic network and an information services map. Tools such as Grateful Med[32] and others help to ease and organize access and use of bibliographic data bases.

Among medical bibliographic databases, MEDLINE and the other National Library of Medicine data bases are preeminent, but other bibliographic data bases may also fulfill specific needs, including full-text, medical specialty programs and systems design for certain problem sets.[33-36] Various tools to ease access are available or will be, such as Loansome Doc[37, 38] and voice recognition software to reduce the need for keyboard entry.[39] An increasing number of publications are available electronically, allowing for more efficient integration of current literature resources into electronic data bases for analysis and distribution.

The accessibility of the bibliographic data bases is rapidly advancing. A variety of proprietary services offer access to large bibliographic data bases, such as MEDLINE. A number of proprietary bibliographic services use either the MEDLINE data base or other sets of bibliographic references. These services, such as OVID,[40] may offer full text as well as selected content. Many journals are rapidly becoming available in electronic versions and are therefore accessible for searching by data bases; these include *New England Journal of Medicine, CHEST, Annals of Internal Medicine, the Lancet, British Medical Journal*, and *Journal of the American Medical Association*.[41]

Of significant interest is the implication of the bibliographic data bases in the development of "evidence-based medicine." This approach to resolving clinical problems and establishing treatment standards depends on extensive review and analysis of published studies. Searching a variety of bibliographic data bases is usually the first step in determining the available literature that will be considered for further analysis.[42]

Basic Science

Large data bases have become a major tool of the basic sciences. Because they solve specific problems, basic science applications are significantly different from the more general applications used by clinicians. Basic science data bases commonly allow for more complex and specific data acquisition and analytic functions. These design features improve the efficiency of data base use. However, the automation of data acquisition by advanced laboratory equipment and the extensive backlog of data have increased the need for central processing unit (CPU) capacity and storage. The demand for this power is increasingly being met by (1) distributed processing, including the use of the Internet, and (2) the use of supercomputers.[43, 44]

For extremely complex problems, the Internet allows segmentation of large processes on a variety of computers throughout the world in a distributed fashion. Internet technology is well suited to performing multiple analysis on segments of large data sets. For example, several applications are available for using the Internet in describing gene pairs as parts of various genome projects.[45, 46]

DATA ACQUISITION: PROBLEMS AND PRACTICE

Accuracy and Reproducibility of Data

The most basic rule of computer systems is "garbage in, garbage out." The decisions of clinicians, researchers, and administrators depend on accurate data. In large data bases, the validity of entered data may be compromised in several ways, transcription error being the most common. If a data base is large enough, an occasional erroneous data point will be outweighed by large numbers of correct data points. These errors proportionally reduce the confidence that can be placed in any conclusions reached, and they continually threaten the data's credibility, which must be reevaluated in each situation for which it is used.

The reliability of large data bases can be compromised by variations in accuracy and reproducibility of entered data. The level of accuracy limits the types of conclusions that may be drawn from the data base. For example, if time on a ventilator is recorded in days only, the clinician cannot assess the impact of interventions that induce changes over a time span of minutes. This lack of accuracy may lead to conclusions implying relationships that may not exist; further, the accuracy or level of detail may not reflect significant changes.

It is essential that data be reproducible as well as accurate and finely detailed. The value of clinical observations depends on accurate description and recording. Unfortunately, many clinical observations are highly subjective, severely limiting the comparability of observations between patients and across time.

These problems have led to the evolution of a large group of "scoring systems" that attempt to provide objective markers to describe complex and often subtle findings.[15] One of the most commonly used systems is the Glasgow Coma Scale. It attempts to quantify the neurologic examination by expressing three sets of reproducible observations (eye opening, verbalization, and motor activity) as a numeric value. Many of these scoring systems have in turn spawned large data bases, initially for validation and subsequently for analysis. Among these are the Acute Physiology and Chronic Health Evaluation (APACHE) I, II, and III[21]; the Mortality Prediction Model (MPM)[47]; and the Multiple Trauma Outcome Study (MTOS).[48] Validation of these tools depends on showing that different observers will independently arrive at the same value, indicating that the tool has a high level of "reproducibility." ("Reproducibility" also applies to different techniques for measurement arriving at the same value, with a given technique achieving the same value on a variety of occasions.)

A number of documentation tools have been developed to reduce the subjectivity and improve the reproducibility of clinical observations. Descriptive anatomic systems for grading injuries, pathologic lesions, and radiologic findings are widely available.[49] Other clinical tools are directed at defining the course of physiologic progression of disease, including APACHE, for example.

Several outcome scores attempt to predict both severity and probability of survival.[50] The usefulness of these scoring systems depends on the ability to reproducibly identify similar conditions in different patients. Although we do not individually review all the available scoring systems here, it is crucial to recognize that within the context of applying large data bases to these scoring systems, reducing the conclusions to an individual patient is neither statistically valid nor clinically reliable. Attempts to apply the findings of large models to individual cases have often been invalid.[49]

Analysis of large sets of data is often unreliable because of a lack of reproducibility. The reproducibility in data acquisition is a major entry point for error and bias in large data bases. In particular, retrospective abstraction of medical records is often an inaccurate reflection of the patient's course, since the reproducibility of the abstraction is low.[10, 51] Accurate description of the course and outcome of different groups of pathologies depends on variable perceptions of the importance of a variety of factors or different emphasis on these factors. Any subjective components of a data set are subject to both the clinical experience and the projection of the observer.[52]

Several principles are central to the acquisition and analysis of the large number of components in any physiologic system. First, data acquired concurrently are the most likely to be reliable. That is, data entered immediately at the time of collection from physiologic monitors are less subject to errors of subjectivity or recall. The ideal of all data entry should be capture and recording simultaneous with the occurrence of the event.

Direct acquisition of data is a feature of many modern information systems. Integrated systems that directly enter a variety of data into electronic format have been made possible by advances in interfaces and data base design. One of the early examples of integration is the HELP system developed at Latter Day Saints Hospital in Salt Lake City.[53] Subsequent advances in computer technology and networking have supported integration of various data sources (e.g., bedside, laboratory, pharmacy, HIS). This integration varies among institutions and systems and is the source of much of the effort being invested in system design and development by individual institutions, national organizations, and proprietary vendors.[54]

Accuracy is also crucial; it involves the level of detail, which must be individualized for types of data and goal of analysis. For example, data for studies of overall demographics of automobile accidents may have adequate accuracy based on number of long-bone, lower-extremity fractures, whereas studies involving the same group of patients but targeted at orthopedic stabilization techniques must have much more defined descriptors of the type and extent of fracture.

Integration of Data Sources

Integrating complex systems of communication and validation requires a variety of devices. This is difficult in the medical environment owing to the diversity of data sources and the variety of formats that must be consolidated. For example, both analog signals, such as the electrocardiogram (ECG), and digital signals such as ventilator data, yield continuous measurements. In critically ill patients, as many as eight to 10 continuous waveforms may be monitored, including ECG, arterial blood pressure, central venous pressure, pulmonary artery pressure, intracranial pressure, respiratory motion, exhaled gases, pulse oximetry, and transcutaneous oxygenation.[55]

Large volumes of intermittent data (usually in a digital format) are also available for most critically ill patients as a feature of ICU devices and the clinical information system. Intermittent data may be divided into two categories:

- Data generated at the bedside (e.g., respirator data)
- Data generated at a distant site (e.g., laboratory data)

Some form of integration among the various bedside devices is necessary to ensure that temporal relationships and physiologic phenomena are accurately related. In many systems today, it is possible to combine the data from the bedside monitoring system with some of the data from separate or independent bedside devices. Data generated at a distant site may be entered into the data base by a system of interfaces developed either locally or through a proprietary system.

Much effort has been devoted to developing systems and standards to integrate the various devices at the bedside in order to allow for rapid and simple interchange of data. For many years, the IEEE has been attempting to establish a standard using a system of cards for the devices (the Device Controller Card [DCC]), which would then integrate with a centralized card (the *bedside controller card* [BCC]), which would provide a common interface standard. This approach has not been practically implemented, and its future is doubtful.

As mentioned, much additional information is generated at sites distant from the bedside, such as the laboratory, pharmacy, radiology department, and HIS. The most likely solution to the challenge of integrating these systems is a standardized communication protocol, such as Health Language 7 (HL7), combined with advanced networking solutions, such as Internet and Transport Control Protocol/Internet Protocol (TCP/IP) protocols, and hardware-driven networks.[55–57]

Full utilization of the capacities of large data base technology will depend on continued improvements in the accuracy, reliability, reproducibility, and interfacing of data from a variety of sources throughout the hospital and the health care system.

DATA BASE STRUCTURE AND DESIGN

As in other areas of hospital computer applications, the use and design of large data bases should be driven by the demands and capacities of the users. Each data base is distinguished by how the data points are stored and interrelated. The way in which data are grouped determines how they can be accessed. In some data bases, data are stored in groups or files that favor discrete, integer-type data. Other systems treat data as packets of information, and still others use an "object-oriented" system that treats each piece of data as a specifically defined entity.

The data base structure determines how data may be analyzed. Data stored linearly are rapidly accessible and efficiently organized for viewing a particular record but are extremely difficult to compare with other records. Many electronic medical record storage systems in use, such as those designed predominantly for vital sign storage or nursing functions, share this failing.

The primary alternative method of data storage is generically known as a "relational" data base, which enables linking of similar data points from a variety of records. Relational data bases are far more useful than linear data bases for most research activities that involve comparing groups of patients. However, relational data bases require data be entered in rigid formats and are limited to comparing data that fit the predetermined formats. New searching tools allow for the analysis of data from relational data bases by formulating standard "queries" using advanced systems generally known as "Structured Query Language" (SQL).[58]

Advances in relational data bases also allow combination of data from different sources into a single data base. This combination may occur within the data base or via a "data bridge." The data bridge provides a pathway using both hardware and software for transferring data to the main relational data base from a second linear, relational, or object-oriented data base.

Object-oriented data bases have much potential for future

utilization. These data bases are dependent on designing systems that allow each data point to be treated as either a unique entity or part of a unique grouping. Object-oriented data bases depend on development of new software tools and new hardware capabilities. Currently, some systems utilize object-oriented processing as one component of their data base. Manipulation of object-oriented data is still difficult because of the nonstandard nature of the data and because of the lack of software tools to support analysis.

STRUCTURAL CONSIDERATIONS FOR LARGE DATA BASES

Supportive "general knowledge" data bases (e.g., bibliographic search engines, drug references) are fairly well developed. They are not considered further here, except to the extent that they need to be integrated at a process-to-process level into the decision making surrounding patient care. This integration will probably occur via the World Wide Web or a similar high-speed interconnect protocol that allows the maintenance of a central, up-to-date reference data base.

There are two general uses for data base technology in a clinical setting.

1. An individual patient data base for direct patient care. A data base of all of a patient's current (and perhaps prior) clinical information is required. This data base is focused on a single patient's information. The data base itself is complex, utilizing multimedia technology (x-ray studies, heart sounds, video clips, tracings for replay, text for notes), flat file arrangements (for voluminous monitored values that are date-stamped and time-stamped), hierarchical information (e.g., one hospital stay of multiple days), relational information (a laboratory value code pointing to the flat file of laboratory values) and object-oriented structures and design. The great diversity in size and structure of patient data demands an object-oriented approach, such as demographic information versus binary large objects (BLOBs), such as images or video.
2. A research and statistical setting. Patients are considered together in a cohort and are used to discern patterns of illness, intervention, and outcome, which can be used for traditional reporting (outcome studies) as well as for more sophisticated artificial intelligence rule derivation.

Some consider a third general use. For example, the individual patient data (illness, intervention, and outcome) may be compared to some external reference (e.g., standards of care) and a resulting score may then be used to update the individual patient data. This use falls in both categories, depending on the user's point of view. For the caregiver, this use falls in the category of individual patient data; for the researcher evaluating the standard of care, this use falls in the statistical category.

Individual Patient Data

The clinician looks for changes in trends in patient information. This is the major design feature for the data base management technology supporting direct patient care. Voluminous data can be managed and displayed. When data are reduced and summarized (the right information at the right time in the right format, in front of the right person), they become information.

Data become information when a decision needs to be made. This decision-making process is what drives the "right information in the right format" criteria. The same data might be displayed in vastly different forms according to the type of decision that needs to be made (see, for example, Tufte's excellent works, *Envisioning Information* and *The Visual Display of Quantitative Information)*. The preservation of confidentiality is a major element of the conversion of patient records to electronic format. This problem is both a technologic[59] and a policy issue.[60] The technologic problems are being addressed by evolving encryption processes, limiting access to systems by electronic protection (e.g., passwords) and mechanical barriers (isolation of systems from outside access).[60] The policy issues involve the statutory regulation of access to medical records to third-party payers and government agencies[61] and the availability of encryption technology.[62]

Statistical Data

The major problem with viewing aggregated patient data is the necessary speed required to process large volumes of data in a "very short" space of time. Very short refers to the time needed to make a therapeutic decision and still change the patient outcome.

Multidimensional analysis is a data base technique used to reduce this time demand at the bedside. It preprocesses the data along anticipated analysis dimensions so that the final analysis has to reduce an already preprocessed matrix along the needed dimensions.

Statistical data bases are also fundamental to the artificial intelligence effort (e.g., rule derivation and training of neural nets). The rules, or heuristics, of artificial intelligence are derived from past experience. The data collected must adhere to certain standards to enable comparability. When this rule derivation process itself becomes automated and demonstrably reliable, there will be a tendency to use more closed loop applications.

Bandwidth and Time

An underlying assumption of this data base technology in the clinical setting is the existence of large amounts of secure network bandwidth for the movement and retrieval of information in support of the clinical decision-making process. Given such bandwidth, patient data can be stored anywhere on the network. However, the practical reality (system failures) dictates that as much information as possible be stored on a bedside or ward device that has an almost 100% uptime.

Another underlying assumption in clinical data management is the strict data-stamping and time-stamping of all information regarding events, measurements, and interventions. This is the most crucial dimension in clinical information, and its importance cannot be overemphasized. This time importance scales all the way to the epidemiologic use of clinical data. For example, with complete online medical data, the Centers for Disease Control and Prevention (CDC) can track the spread of symptoms in a population in almost real time.

The data base technology needed to support clinical applications on all fronts (e.g., closed loop applications) is not yet mature enough for complete adoption, but developments in hardware, software, and networking are converging in the right directions.

The requirements of hospital management are largely served by the conventional data bases that are well suited for financial and inventory functions. These capacities translate well from business applications. Although these data bases have a significant capacity for relational analysis, their weakness is the difficulty applying them to continuous variables and linking them to close time frames.

SUMMARY

Large data bases are powerful tools that can serve many needs in the health care setting, and are critical supports for administration, clinical care, education, and research. To meet the needs of these areas and to maximize the benefit of large data bases, each component of the hospital and all other interested parties must cooperate and support interfacing with other systems without compromising the essential functions of each component.

In the future, these data bases should become more efficient and will be used for advanced analysis of physiologic and pathologic states driven by faster processors. Novel approaches to logical processing (artificial intelligence, neural networks, fuzzy logic) will enhance data base power and flexibility. Whatever the advances, the most basic rules of data management—accuracy, reliability, reproducibility, and ease of use—will drive our ability to maximize the potential benefits of these powerful tools.

GLOSSARY

APACHE (Acute Physiology and Chronic Health Evaluation): a system for scoring physiologic parameters of acute injury, intended to reduce subjectivity in diagnosis.

BCC/DCC (bedside controller card/device controller card): Components of the Medical Information Bus of the IEEE, they would process output (DCC) from bedside devices and accept (BCC) input from all devices at the bedside and process them into a format that can be entered into a central data base.

BLOB (binary large object): a large amount of binary data that is treated as a whole, such as a graphic image.

Closed loop application: A process that receives data, makes decisions, and implements actions without input from the outside.

CPT (current procedure terminology): The most common method of coding performed procedures and diagnosis; used for epidemiologic information and retrospective research.

Front-end: A simple access tool superimposed on a more complex tool to ease entry and use.

Fuzzy logic: A system of decision making that allows for imperfect matches, overlapping definitions of data, and training of neural networks.

Grateful Med: A user-friendly microcomputer software package for searching National Library of Medicine data bases.

HIS (Hospital Information System): An information system that supports data management throughout the hospital including logistic support, patient care, accounting, and so on.

HL7 (Health Language 7): A protocol for formatting, transmitting, and receiving data in a health care environment.

ICD (International Classification of Disease): A lexicon of diseases classified in hierarchical groupings, updated by the World Health Organization. Version 9 is standard, and version 10 is being finalized.

IEEE (Institute of Electrical and Electronics Engineers): The largest professional society for these fields of endeavor.

Linear data base: A data base in which the patient record is a unit. Patient records can be accessed and stratified by a few keywords, such as name, date of admission, and diagnosis, but clinical and research use is very limited.

Loansome Doc: A feature of Grateful Med allowing microcomputer users to order full-text articles form National Library of Medicine data bases, including MEDLINE.

MEDLINE: The data base compiled by the National Library of Medicine containing abstracts from most peer-reviewed medical journals since 1966. It can be searched by keyword over the Internet.

Metathesaurus: A thesaurus based on the Unified Medical Language System (UMLS).

MPM (Mortality Prediction Model): Statistical models of hospital mortality for ICU patients on the basis of clinical variables.

Network bandwidth: The capacity of an electronic network to transmit data rapidly.

Neural networks: Self-training and self-regulating electronic systems based on "fuzzy" logic; useful for finding relationships and identifying patterns in data.

Object-oriented data base: A data base that stores each element of a patient record separately, allowing for complete flexibility in retrieving and displaying data.

Real time: Data output occurring concurrently with an event.

Relational data base: A data base in which clinical information about various patients can be accessed and compiled. The patient record is a conglomeration of fields that are separately accessible.

SAPS (Simplified Acute Physiology Score): A scoring system that uses 14 physiologic and demographic variables for classifying patients.

Search engine: A program that allows a user to search a data base. The user can perform only those types of searches allowed by the search engine.

SQL (Structured Query Language): A software system that allows users to extract data from data bases using commands based on English rather than writing in computer language. SQL is much easier than older languages, but much training is required.

TCP/IP (Transport Control Protocol/Internet Protocol): A family of related protocols designed to transfer information across a network and provide information about a network; the language and communication standard for the Internet.

UMLS (Unified Medical Language System): A unified lexicon for searching medical data bases, developed by the National Library of Medicine.

Uptime: Time in which a computer system is fully operational.

References

1. Siegel JH, Stoklosa JC, Borg U, et al: Quantification of asymmetric lung pathophysiologies as a guide to the use of simultaneous independent lung ventilation in post-traumatic and septic adult respiratory distress syndrome. Ann Surg 1985; 202:425.
2. Bone RC, Fisher CJ Jr, Clemmer TP, et al: Sepsis syndrome: A valid clinical entity. Crit Care Med 1989; 17:389.
3. Barriere SL, Lowry SF: An overview of mortality risk prediction in sepsis. Crit Care Med 1995; 23:376.
4. Adams MD, Kerlavage AR, Fleischmann RD, et al: Initial assessment of human gene diversity and expression patterns based upon 83 million nucleotides of cDNA sequence. Nature 1995; 377(6547 Suppl):3.
5. Moszer I, Glaser P, Danchin A: SubtiList: A relational database for the *Bacillus subtilis* genome. Part 2. Microbiology 1995; 141:261.
6. Kaye JJ: Radiographic assessment of rheumatoid arthritis. Rheum Dis Clin North Am 1995; 21:395.
7. Newcombe J, Cuzner ML: Organization and research applications of the U.K. Multiple Sclerosis Society Tissue Bank. J Neural Transm Suppl 1993; 39:155.
8. Kiejna A: Applications of computer database in prospective studies on the mortality of patients with diagnosis of schizophrenia. Psychiatria Polska 1993; 27:85.
9. Kentala E, Pyykko I, Auramo Y, et al: Database for vertigo. Otolaryngol Head Neck Surg 1995; 112:383.
10. DeGaetano A, Castegneto M, Mingtone G, et al: PC-based differential model fitting as a support for clinical research. Int J Clin Monit Comput 1994; 11:35.
11. DeGaetano A, Coleman WP, Pizzi R, et al: Hydra: A C-language environment for real-time DOS multitasking at the bedside. Int J Clin Monit Comput 1993; 10:147.
12. Coleman WP, Siegel JH, Giovannini I, et al: Computational logic: A method for formal analysis of the ICU knowledge base. Int J Clin Monitor Comput 1993; 10:67.
13. Bishop CW, Ewing PD: Transferring knowledge from one system

to another. Proceedings of the Annual Symposium on Computer Applications in Medical Care, 1994, p 967.
14. Watts CM, Knaus WA: The case for using objective scoring systems to predict intensive care unit outcome. Crit Care Clin 1994; 10:73.
15. Castella X, Artigas A, Bion J, et al: A comparison of severity of illness scoring systems for intensive care unit patients: Results of a multicenter, multinational study. The European/North American Severity Study Group. Crit Care Med 1995; 23:1327.
16. Becker RB, Zimmerman JE, Knaus WA, et al: The use of APACHE III to evaluate ICU length of stay, resource use, and mortality after coronary artery by-pass surgery. J Cardiovasc Surg 1995; 36:1.
17. Le Gall JR, Loirat P, Alperovitch A: The simplified acute physiology score (SAPS). Problems in critical care: Prognostic scoring systems in the ICU. 1989; 3:578.
18. Buchman TG, Kubos KL, Seidler AJ, et al: A comparison of statistical and connectionist models for the prediction of chronicity in a surgical intensive care unit. Crit Care Med 1994; 22:750.
19. Kingma J, TenVergert E, Werkman HA, et al: A Turbo Pascal program to convert ICD-9CM coded injury diagnoses into injury severity scores: ICDTOAIS. Percept Mot Skills 1994; 78(3 Pt 1):915.
20. Tuchschmidt JA, Mecher CE: Predictors of outcome from critical illness: Shock and cardiopulmonary resuscitation. Crit Care Clin 1994; 10:179.
21. Rutledge R, Fakhry S, Rutherford E, et al: Comparison of APACHE II, Trauma Score and Injury Severity Score as predictors of outcome in critically injured trauma patients. Am J Surg 1993; 166:244.
22. Bowes CL, Wilson AJ: Information management systems for intensive care. Comput Methods Programs Biomed 1994; 44:1.
23. Kingma J, TenVergert E, Klasen HJ: SHOWICD: A computer program to display ICD-9CM coded injury diagnoses and their corresponding injury severity scores for a particular patient. Percept Mot Skills 1994; 78(3 Pt 1):39.
24. Humphreys BL, McCutcheon DE: Growth patterns in the National Library of Medicine's serials collection and in Index Medicus journals, 1966–1985. Bull Med Libr Assoc 1994; 82:18.
25. Hersh W, Hickam D: Information retrieval in medicine: The SAPHIRE experience. Medinfo 1995; 8(Pt 2):1433.
26. Nelson SJ, Cole WG, Tuttle MS, et al: Recognizing new medical knowledge computationally. Proceedings of the Annual Symposium on Computer Applications in Medical Care 1993, p 409.
27. Radow DP, Blake M, Howard E, et al: Using the Metathesaurus for bibliographic retrieval: A pre-implementation study. Proceedings of the Annual Symposium on Computer Applications in Medical Care, 1994, p 980.
28. Kingsland LC III, Harbourt AM, Syed EJ, et al: Coach: Applying UMLS knowledge sources in an expert searcher environment. Bull Med Libr Assoc 1993:81:178.
29. Harbourt AM, Syed EJ, Hole WT, et al: The ranking algorithm of the Coach browser for the UMLS metathesaurus. Proceedings of the Annual Symposium on Computer Applications in Medical Care, 1993, p 720.
30. Schuyler PL, Hole WT, Tuttle MS, et al: The UMLS metathesaurus: Representing different views of biomedical concepts. Bull Med Libr Assoc 1993; 81:217.
31. McCray AT, Aronson AR, Browne AC, et al: UMLS knowledge for biomedical language processing. Bull Med Libr Assoc 1993; 81:184.
32. Jachna JS, Powsner SM, Miller PL: Augmenting Grateful Med with the UMLS metathesaurus: An initial evaluation. Bull Med Libr Assoc 1993; 81:20.
33. Miller PL, Frawley SJ, Wright L, et al: Lessons learned from a pilot implementation of the UMLS information sources map. J Am Med Inform Assoc 1995; 2:102.
34. Hersh WR, Hickam DH, Haynes RB, et al: A performance and failure analysis of SAPHIRE with a MEDLINE test collection. J Am Med Inform Assoc 1994; 1:51.
35. Guidi JN: Matching references with MEDLINE via TCP/IP. Proceedings of the Annual Symposium on Computer Applications in Medical Care, 1993, p 606.
36. Jean FC, Engelmann U, Sauquet D, et al: The HELIOS Medical Connection Services. Comput Methods Programs Biomed 1994; 45(Suppl):S117.
37. Wood EH: MEDLINE: The options for health professionals. J Am Med Inform Assoc 1994; 1:372.
38. Lovas I: A look at Loansome Doc service. Bull Med Libr Assoc 1994; 82:176.
39. Sherertz DD, Tuttle MS, Olson NE, et al: Accessing oncology information at the point of care: Experience using speech, pen, and 3-D interfaces with a knowledge server. Medinfo 1995; 8(Pt 1):792.
40. Schoonbaert D: SPIRS, WinSPIRS, and OVID: A comparison of three MEDLINE-on-CD-ROM interfaces. Bull Med Libr Assoc 1997; 85:57.
41. Marik PE: Keeping up-to-date in the electronic age. Crit Care Med 1998; 6:307.
42. Haynes RB, Sackett DL, Gray JA, et al: Transferring evidence from research into practice: 2. Getting the evidence straight. ACP J Club 1997; 126:A14.
43. Butler B: Nucleic acid sequence analysis software packages. Curr Opin Biotechnol 1994; 5:19.
44. Nakai K, Tokimori T, Ogiwara A, et al: Gnome—an Internet-based sequence analysis tool. Comput Applications Biosci 1994; 10:547.
45. Singh GB, Nelson JE, Maclinden TP, et al: ISWAC: Proposed system for the integrated assembly of chromosomes. DNA Seq 1994; 5:67.
46. Tachinardi U, Furuie SS, Bertozzo N, et al: Hypermedia patient data retrieval and presentation through WWW. Proceedings: The Annual Symposium on Computer Applications in Medical Care, 1995, p 551.
47. Teres D, Lemeshow S, Harris D, et al: Mortality prediction models (MPM) for ICU patients. Problems in critical care: Prognostic scoring systems in the ICU. 1989; 3:585.
48. Garber BG, Hebert PC, Wells G, et al: Validation of trauma and injury severity score in blunt trauma patients by using a Canadian trauma registry. J Trauma 1996; 40:733.
49. Walder AD, Yeoman PM, Turnbull A: The abbreviated injury scale as a predictor of outcome of severe head injury. Intensive Care Med 1995; 21:606.
50. Rothwell PM, Lawler PG. Prediction of outcome in intensive care patients using endocrine parameters. Crit Care Med 1995; 23:78.
51. Kooijman CJ, Klaassen-Leil CC. Extraction, preparation, and presentation of patient classification data for the benefit of management overviews. Medinfo 1995; 8(Pt 2):1382.
52. Martin-Baranera M, Planas I, Palau J, et al: IMASIS computer-based medical record project: Dealing with the human factor. Medinfo 1995; 8(Pt 1):333.
53. Gibson R, Haug P: Linking the Computerized Severity Index (CSI) to coded patient findings in the HELP system patient database. Proceedings of The Annual Symposium on Computer Applications in Medical Care, 1993, p 673.
54. van Mulligen EM, Cornet R, Timmers T: Problems with integrating legacy systems. Proceedings of the Annual Symposium on Computer Applications in Medical Care, 1995, p 747.
55. Lindberg DA: Global information infrastructure. Intl J Biomed Comput 1994; 34:13.
56. LaCroix EM, Backus JE, Lyon BJ: Service providers and users discover the Internet. Bull Med Libr Assoc 1994; 82:412.
57. Miller PL, Nadkarni PM, Kidd KK, et al: Internet-based support for bioscience research: A collaborative genome center for human chromosome 12. J Am Med Inform Assoc 1995; 2:351.
58. Hooymans MP, Liefkes H, Schipper JA, et al: Retrieval from a large, integrated HIS database through formal descriptions and SQL. Medinfo 1995; 8(Pt 1):478.
59. Masys DR, Baker DB: Patient-Centered Access to Secure Systems Online (PCASSO): A secure approach to clinical data access via the World Wide Web. Proceedings/AMIA Annual Fall Symposium, 1997, p 340.
60. Marwick C: Increasing use of computerized recordkeeping leads to legislative proposals for medical privacy. JAMA 1996; 276:270.
61. Woodward B: The computer-based patient record and confidentiality. N Engl J Med 1995; 333:1419.
62. Stehle W: Reliable cryptology as a means for confidentiality and safety in medical communication and documentation (transl). Zentralbl Gynakol 1998; 120:350.

193

Appraising and Using Evidence in Critical Care

John A. Kellum, MD • Nagarajan Ramakrishnan, MBBS
Derek C. Angus, MB, ChB, MPH

The practice of medicine is changing constantly, and the pace of change is ever-increasing. Among the many forces for change, the rapid increase in information is perhaps the most important. Although the majority of medical practitioners do not engage in research themselves, they are consumers of research information and must therefore understand how research is conducted to apply this information to their patients. Fellowship programs in critical care, as in various other fields of medicine, emphasize education in this area to varying degrees. The traditional approach has been to require fellows to actively participate in a research project, either clinical or basic science. However, there has also been a growing interest in developing methods to evaluate the existing literature and standards by which to compare individual studies.

In recent years, this approach has been popularized under the banner of "evidence-based medicine" (EBM),[1] although this is arguably not a new concept.[2-4] Application of the principles of epidemiology and biostatistics to improve the care of a given patient is the foundation of clinical epidemiology.[4] This field can claim Sydenham, Osler, and even Hippocrates as its early heroes. However, the birth of modern decision analysis occurred in the early 1980s when a number of clinicians and researchers sought to apply the basic science of clinical epidemiology to better understand how to care for individual patients. Like other basic sciences, such as pathology, clinical epidemiology has certain techniques that, once learned, can be applied across many fields of clinical science. Instead of the frozen section and the hematoxylin and eosin stain, clinical epidemiology uses the odds ratio and posterior probability.

However, even armed with the skills to appraise a given article, we are still left with the challenge of dealing with the sheer volume of medical literature. There are now more than 20,000 medical journals containing more than 2 million articles annually.[1] Even in one's own field, the most avid reader can barely scan every study published, let alone render a critical appraisal. Accordingly, physicians must rely on summaries of the literature presented through a variety of approaches. These approaches have traditionally included didactic tools such as local grand rounds and journal clubs, society conferences, newsletters, review articles, and textbooks. However, such approaches cannot guarantee systemized, unbiased reviews of entire topics, nor can they guarantee effective delivery of information to key decision makers in a timely manner. Thus, new approaches, including computerized systematic and statistically based literature scans, Internet-based continued medical education endeavors, and hospital computer-based decision support systems, are increasingly being promoted as the tools that will lead to more rational and contemporary medical education, research, and patient care.

In this chapter, we review the methodology, applications, and limitations of the current techniques used for appraising, combining, and summarizing evidence. We also consider the use of these techniques in the practice of critical care medicine and discuss some of the unique aspects of its application to this field.

GATHERING, APPRAISING, AND SUMMARIZING EVIDENCE

Individual Study Design and Assessment

Randomized Clinical Trials

Randomized clinical trials (RCTs), also referred to as experimental or interventional studies, are the cornerstones of medical evidence. Physicians place considerable faith in the results of RCTs.[5, 6] This faith is placed with good reason because randomization remains perhaps the best solution to avoid misinterpreting the effect of a therapy in the presence of confounding variables.[7] When participants are allocated to groups at random, factors other than the variable of interest (e.g., a new sepsis agent) that are likely to affect the outcome of interest are usually distributed equally to both groups. For example, with randomization, the number of patients with underlying comorbidity, which of course may adversely affect outcome, should be similar in each study arm, presuming sample size is appropriate. A special advantage of randomization is that this equal distribution will occur for all variables (excluding the intervention) whether these variables are identified by the researcher or not, and thus it maximizes the ability to determine the effect of the studied intervention.

However, RCTs are expensive, difficult, and sometimes unethical to conduct with the consequence that less than 20% of clinical practice is based on the results of RCTs.[8] Moreover, many important questions, such as determining the optimal timing of a new therapy or determining the effects of health care practices, cannot practically be studied by RCTs.

The field of critical care medicine has particularly unique problems with regard to the use of RCTs. During the past 20 years, multiple RCTs of new therapies in sepsis and the acute respiratory distress syndrome (ARDS) have failed to demonstrate benefit despite advances in both the development of new therapies and trial design.[9-11] Some have argued that this is because there is not yet enough understanding of the underlying mechanisms of sepsis and organ dysfunction and that consequently more basic research is required.[10-14] Whereas this is no doubt true, others have also emphasized the need to further examine and improve the design of RCTs in critical care.[10, 11, 13] In particular, attention has been focused on which patients should be selected, whether the process of care should be standardized, and whether the choice of endpoints is correct.

Added to these problems, there is now increasing attention on the impact a new therapy will have on health care practice and spending. The size of an effect measured under the rigorous conditions of a tightly controlled trial (efficacy) is often criticized as too optimistic of an estimate of the likely effect in the real world (effectiveness). Reasons for effectiveness falling short of efficacy include differences in the selection of patients, timing and dosing of therapy, and use of concomitant therapies, all of which represent the realities of the world in which we live. Furthermore, as rising health care costs bring increasing pressure to bear on the consideration of the costs and benefits of new therapies, the value of new therapies is measured differently. A therapy would previously have been deemed valuable purely on the basis of its effect, whereas value is now seen more as a trade-off of the costs incurred per effect gained.[15]

Observational Studies

Thus, an RCT is neither always possible nor always applicable. The principal alternative approach to the RCT involves observation rather than experimentation. Prior experience has biased us to favor RCTs, but partly in response to the increasing need to answer questions unanswerable by an RCT, the design and execution of observational outcome studies have become much more sophisticated. In critiquing such studies, it is necessary to consider carefully the different elements most susceptible to bias.

First, the data source must be considered. Observational outcome studies are often performed on large data sets wherein the data were collected for purposes other than research. This can lead to error because of either lack of pertinent information or a bias in the information recorded.[16] It is important to appreciate that the data should be considered separately from the trial design, that lack of accuracy of certain data may or may not be important depending on their pertinence to the question asked. Second, one must consider how the investigators attempt to control for confounding. The measured effect size of a variable on outcome (e.g., the effect of the pulmonary artery catheter on mortality) can be confounded by the distribution of other known or unknown variables.

There are several techniques that attempt to account for known variables, including matching, stratification, and regression modeling. All have advantages and disadvantages, and it is incumbent on the investigators to defend the rationale for their choice and present evidence supporting how well their technique performed.[17] Even if the investigators have devised a reliable and valid technique to adjust for known confounders, they still have the problem of controlling for unknown variables. Although there are methods that attempt to measure the extent to which an unmeasured variable may be present in an observational outcome study (e.g., by inserting imaginary variables), there is no well-accepted test for this. The reader must therefore ask, Is there anything unaccounted for in this study that I believe could explain the magnitude and direction of effect otherwise attributable to the intervention?

It may appear that the alternative to randomization is burdensome. However, observational outcome studies are powerful tools for addressing many questions that RCTs cannot address, including measuring the effect of harmful substances (e.g., tobacco smoke and other carcinogens), organizational structures (e.g., payer status, open versus closed intensive care unit [ICU]), and geography (e.g., rural versus urban access to health care). Investigators have recently reproduced many of the large cardiology intervention trials in the Duke Cardiovascular Registry using observational outcome techniques, exploring the effectiveness of therapies previously tested only under tightly controlled (efficacy) conditions. Investigators have also explored the effects of different therapies that are already accepted, but used variably, in clinical practice.[18] Randomization would be an ethical problem in such situations.

Thus, as questions not addressable by RCTs become more important, it becomes necessary to embrace the challenge to adopt and understand observational outcome studies as part of the methodologic toolset. Finally, it may even be necessary to deal with situations in which a well-conducted RCT and a well-conducted observational outcome study on the same intervention yield opposite results and to conclude that both studies are correct. In other words, the RCT demonstrated that a therapy had a significant effect under ideal conditions, but the observational outcome study demonstrated that the effect was lost in the real world. Either study alone would tell only part of the story. The combined information would allow policymakers and clinicians to examine practice patterns and devise strategies to ensure that the therapy was used properly in the real world to realize the potential seen in the experimental setting.

Critical Appraisal Methods

Determining which studies provide information useful in the care of patients is largely a question of deciding whether a study is valid and, if it is, whether its results can be applied to the patients in question. One format for appraising individual studies is the critically appraised topic (CAT) format that has been popularized as part of evidence-based medicine. The purpose of the CAT format is to evaluate a given study or set of studies with use of a standardized approach. Studies that address etiology, diagnosis, prognosis, therapy, and cost effectiveness all have a separate CAT format.[4] An example is shown in Table 193-1 for studies that address therapy.

The CAT format for these studies asks several questions intended to address the issues of validity and clinical utility. Studies that fail to achieve these measures are not generally useful, although studies do not necessarily have to fulfill every criterion, depending on the nature of the topic. For example, a study that examines the effect of walking once a day for the prevention of stroke would not be expected to include a detailed examination of side effects or cost effectiveness. However, a study comparing streptokinase with placebo for treatment of stroke would be expected to do so because of the excessive risks and costs associated with such therapy. For example, blinding may not always be possible, and the effects of the investigators being unblinded can be minimized by separating them from the clinicians making the treatment decisions or by establishing standard treatment protocols that are applied to both the study and control groups. Alternatively, a study would be "fatally flawed" if it failed in terms of randomization or was not analyzed as "intention to treat" (see Appendix A). A number of other useful tools are available for assessing study design and for quantifying effect size and cost effectiveness. In general, these are the tools of epidemiology and biostatistics and, as such, are beyond the scope of this chapter, but a basic primer and glossary of terms are included as Appendix A.

Another popular method of appraising evidence is to set a hierarchy for studies on the basis of their design and size. Perhaps the most widely used scheme is the one detailed in Table 193-2. Under this classification, it is assumed that the results of a level I study overrule any lower level study. However, the quality of individual studies must also be considered (see Table 193-1). At present, rules for integrating study quality and study level have not been established. Presumably, a perfect level III study would not necessarily be dismissed by

TABLE 193–1. Critical Appraisal of the Literature

Are the results of the study valid?
- Were the patients correctly randomized?
- Were all the patients accounted for?
- Was follow-up complete?
- Were patients analyzed according to how they were randomized (i.e., intention to treat)?
- Were all people involved in the study blinded?
- Were the groups similar at the start?
- Were the groups treated equally apart from the experimental intervention?

Are the results clinically useful?
- How large was the treatment effect?
- How precise was the estimate of the treatment effect?
- Are the patients similar to the "norm"?
- Were all clinically important outcomes considered?
- Was a cost-benefit analysis performed?

Adapted from Sackett DL, Haynes RB, Guyatt GH, Tugwell P: Clinical Epidemiology: A Basic Science for Clinical Medicine. 2nd ed. Boston, Little, Brown & Co, 1991.

TABLE 193–2. Levels of Evidence

Level I	Randomized trials with low false-positive (α) and low false-negative (β) error (i.e., high power)
Level II	Randomized trials with high α error or low power
Level III	Nonrandomized concurrent cohort studies
Level IV	Nonrandomized historic cohort studies
Level V	Case series

Adapted from Cook DJ, Guyatt GH, Laupacis A, Sackett DL: Rules of evidence and clinical recommendations on the use of antithrombotic agents. Antithrombotic Therapy Consensus Conference. Chest 1992; 102:305–311S.

a questionable level I trial. Furthermore, the hierarchy in Table 193–2 would seem to imply that even a small (and thus underpowered) level II study would be preferable, and indeed superior, to all level III and level IV studies. Strictly adhering to this strategy would suggest that a single small RCT with the spurious result that cigarette smoking was associated with improved health would invalidate the entire "observational" literature on smoking. Thus, although this grading system may offer an attractive rubric by which to rate, or rank, different studies, a thorough understanding of the issue being addressed will still be required.

Multiple Study Assessment

Narrative Literature Reviews

Clinicians often correctly point out that there are studies both for and against many of the treatments they prescribe. A familiar refrain of the busy clinician goes something like this: "I can show you six articles, three for and three against. However, in my experience this therapy almost always helps. . . ." Such statements attempt to invalidate the entire body of research in a given area simply because the studies show conflicting results. The conclusion is that there is no "proof" of anything and therefore the clinician's experience is the only guide to decision making. This may be appropriate in many cases, particularly when rare diseases are present or when combinations of conditions exist, but it is more often the case that when several articles exist, the literature can guide much more than personal experience. Still, clinicians must either appraise and integrate the results of various studies themselves or rely on the various systems available for this purpose.

The most common system is the familiar "review" article or collection of reviews. This textbook is an example of the latter. These articles or chapters combine the information from several primary articles, sometimes a few hundred, in a way that is digestible by the average reader. Reviews may be focused on recent advances, or they may provide a complete tutorial on a given subject. In either case, in the traditional method known as the *narrative review,* the methodology is the same: an author, presumably someone knowledgeable of the subject matter, reviews the existing literature in some way, formulates an opinion, and disseminates this opinion along with references to support each argument. This approach is also used in the discussion section of most original articles in which the authors attempt to discuss their findings in the context of the existing literature.

Narrative reviews have several limitations, the most important being that evidence used to support the author's positions is not collected, evaluated, and compared in an organized and reproducible manner. There is no way to ensure that the information is complete or that it is judged in an unbiased manner. Journal articles are often peer-reviewed, which provides some limited oversight for completeness and lack of bias, but this is far from perfect. Furthermore, review articles and textbook chapters are not generally subject to vigorous review and therefore may be the least reliable sources of information, particularly current information. For example, by 1988, 15 studies had been reported on the use of prophylactic lidocaine in acute myocardial infarction. Although no single study was definitive, pooled data from the nearly 9000 patients showed that the practice was useless at best. Nonetheless, by 1990, there were still more recommendations for its use than against it appearing in textbooks and review articles.[2] The advantage of the narrative review is that it provides a detailed qualitative discussion, usually by an expert with years of experience (Table 193–3).

Systematic Reviews

In contrast to a narrative review, a *systematic literature review* involves a more systematic search, assembly, and appraisal of existing literature and combines the results of multiple studies. In this type of review, studies are identified, included, and excluded according to explicit criteria. The reasons for these criteria are also made explicit. For example, a systematic review typically uses an electronic data base (e.g., MEDLINE) and may also include other sources, such as bibliographies, personal files, and the like. The search terms and key words are provided, and thus some degree of reproducibility is established. Set criteria are used for inclusion and exclusion of individual studies. Although these criteria may be subjective, they are clearly stated and thus open to scrutiny. For example, studies that use physiologic endpoints (e.g., renal blood flow, urine output) may be excluded from a review that focuses on the effects of a given therapy on patient outcomes (e.g., need for dialysis).[19]

Finally, individual studies are usually graded according to some predetermined scheme, such as the one presented in Table 193–2. The disadvantage of the systematic as opposed to the narrative review is that whereas the former is more objective, the latter contains more qualitative assessment. However, narrative reviews may use objective search strategies, and systematic reviews may contain a discussion of studies that did not fit the precise inclusion criteria. One can argue, therefore, that the best reviews should incorporate elements from both approaches such that they are objective in their analysis and subjective in their discussion.

Meta-analyses

In contrast to the systematic review, which combines study results, the *meta-analysis* combines actual data from several

TABLE 193–3. Literature Review Methods

	Narrative Review	Systematic Review	Meta-analysis
Indentification of studies	Unspecified Subjective	Specified Objective	Specified Objective
Inclusion and exclusion criteria	Unspecified Subjective	Specified Objective	Specified, restrictive Objective
Analysis	Subjective	Objective	Statistical
Interpretation	Expert opinion	Limited	Limited
Value	Qualitative		Quantitative

Many published reviews have both narrative and systematic elements.

small but high-quality studies. This approach places greater emphasis than the systematic review on statistical methods.[20] The term meta-analysis has been used in several ways.[21-23]

Components

Briefly, the basic components of meta-analysis are: (1) A pre hoc decision regarding study selection and ranking of quality combined with (2) a pre hoc choice of formal statistical techniques to combine and analyze reported data with a goal to (3) garner statistically significant inferences through the combination of "like" studies previously unable to conclude with significance because of inadequate sample size. Summarizing available information in these instances may provide valuable information by merely increasing the number of subjects studied and thereby increasing the power.

Results

The results of a meta-analysis may help authors decide if it is worth conducting further trials to address a particular question. A striking example is shown in Figure 193–1. However, sometimes the results of meta-analyses have been significantly different from subsequent large RCTs.[24-26] It is likely that this is, in part, a reflection of the bias in selection of source articles for meta-analyses. Another cause appears to be whether primary or secondary endpoints are used. Overall, large RCTs disagree with meta-analysis 10% to 23% of the time.[25]

This discrepancy is only one of several issues that have been raised regarding the utility of meta-analyses (Table 193–4). Concerns are often raised as to whether a meta-analysis is purely an objective and mechanical exercise and whether some allowance should be made for the quality of each trial included in the meta-analysis. Obviously, the validity of a meta-analysis is a reflection of the validity and quality of the studies included, and hence study selection is an important step in performing meta-analysis. Identifying studies for meta-analysis, with specific efforts at minimizing biases and random errors, remains a challenge.

In addition, the popular search techniques to identify studies are inherently limited by the fact that unpublished studies

TABLE 193–4. Issues with Performing a Meta-analysis

Identification of Studies
Appropriate search techniques
Inclusion of unpublished trials (i.e., avoiding publication bias)
Inclusion of trials published in journals not included in "popular" data bases
Quality of Studies Included
Evaluate appropriateness of randomization techniques, statistical methods, and endpoints
Improper to attribute quality of study to the journal where published
Meta-analytical Techniques
Asking a relevant question
Choosing right endpoints
Choosing the right statistical techniques

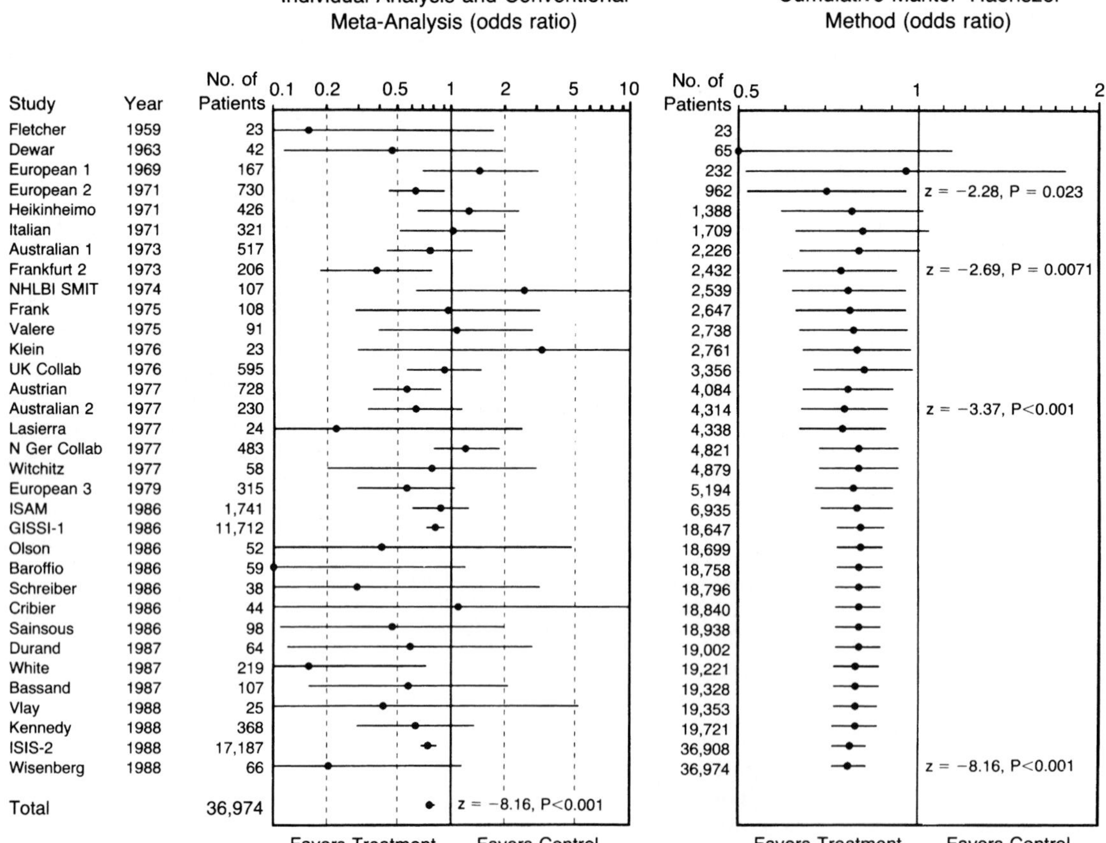

Figure 193–1. Conventional and cumulative meta-analyses of 33 trials of intravenous streptokinase for acute myocardial infarction. The odds ratios and 95% confidence intervals for an effect of treatment on mortality are shown on a logarithmic scale. (From Lau J, Antman EM, Jimenez-Silva J, et al: Cumulative meta-analysis of therapeutic trials for myocardial infarction. N Engl J Med 1992; 2327:248–254.)

are unaccounted for in any review (publication bias). This has led authors to propose maintenance of study registries in which all RCTs are registered irrespective of their publication status.[27] This would help to include smaller studies and those studies published in journals that are not listed in cumulative *Index Medicus,* MEDLINE, and other popular data bases. This could also aid performance of cumulative meta-analyses, when a new meta-analysis is performed by repeated pooling of studies every time a new trial is added to a series of trials in the registry.[28] However, the statistical implications of this approach have not been fully explored. A problem analogous to an α error may occur if no further studies are added once significance is achieved.

Improving the Quality of Meta-analyses

Its proponents argue that meta-analysis is a valuable technique in exploring well-studied yet unresolved questions because it can be conducted quickly, easily, and at low cost. The alternative, it is argued, is usually a large, expensive, and time-consuming RCT—which may yield no more new information than the meta-analysis. However, the inherent limitations already outlined have led authors to look at ways to increase the rigor of meta-analysis, even though this might involve considerable increase in time, expense, and logistic burden.[25, 29] In particular, the Cochrane work group proposes that meta-analysis use individual patient data as the yardstick against which all systematic reviews should be measured.[30, 31] Although it was proposed many years ago, the feasibility of this approach remains to be tested[32] because this could be so cumbersome as to offset many of the advantages of meta-analysis.

APPLYING EVIDENCE

Medical Education

It is easy to see that systematic reviews are valuable resources to practicing clinicians who cannot possibly review and grade every individual study. However, the value of each review is limited by its applicability to the individual patients the clinician cares for. Therefore, the most useful reviews consider the clinical circumstances in which the information can be used. For example, there are studies available to guide the choice of antibiotic therapy in hospital-acquired pneumonia. These studies can be reviewed in a systematic way, and evidence-based conclusions can be reached[33]; however, antibiotic sensitivity patterns vary by hospital. Therapy that is based on evidence of efficacy in one population may not be applicable to another. Here, the more knowledgeable the authors are of the specific clinical issues involved, the more applicable will be the review.[33] Nonetheless, systematic reviews are more likely than narrative reviews to contain an objective appraisal of the literature. The individual clinician still needs to determine how this information should be integrated into the care of his or her patients.

A potentially useful application of evidence-based medicine is in the familiar journal clubs common in training programs and among some individual group practices. The appraisal of a paper on a given topic can be greatly enhanced and objectified by using techniques of evidence-based medicine. Furthermore, these critiques can be disseminated to colleagues or even published. Such applications are well established in some fields and are growing rapidly in critical care (see Appendix B).

Bedside Decision Making

In addition to its application as a resource for staying up to date on the medical literature, evidence-based medicine can be used for bedside decision making. Here the assumption is that the individual patient's problems can be addressed by existing literature and that application of this literature can augment clinical judgment.[34] The emphasis on the word "augment" is important, as is the distinction from the word "replace." As in the previous example, clinical knowledge and experience are required to understand how to apply the results of studies to individual patients.

The tool used for this application is the CAT format described before. The appraisal exercise itself requires significant understanding of the disease process and its effects on the individual patient. Even judging the validity of a study requires this understanding. To answer questions such as whether the groups were treated equally apart from the experimental intervention requires detailed knowledge of which co-interventions are essentially equal and which are likely to have an impact on the disease process or the outcome of interest. Serious mistakes can be made if the results of quality studies are applied to the wrong patients or clinical scenarios.

Guidelines and Protocols

Perhaps a natural extension of evidence-based medicine is the desire to standardize care when evidence can be found that certain treatments or diagnostic procedures are superior in effect or cost effectiveness. When such therapeutic or diagnostic strategies exist, they should be widely applied and a convenient way to ensure this is to develop a protocol or a guideline. Although this application of evidence appraisal has produced useful information to guide therapy[35] or further research,[36] it has also generated considerable controversy.[37-39] The disagreement is not specifically over the recommendation of practices on the basis of sound evidence but, instead, about the perception that when evidence is lacking, these practices should be avoided. Thus, clinicians are weary of being told that they and their patients cannot pursue diagnostic and therapeutic choices because there is no evidence that these practices work. In this regard, it is important to note a basic principle: Not finding an effect is not the same as finding no effect. That is, the lack of evidence that something works is not evidence that it does not work. This issue is particularly relevant to critical illness in which, by definition, patients are seriously ill and often do not respond to therapy. Should treatment that is possibly effective be withheld from patients with otherwise lethal conditions on grounds that it is unproved?

For new therapies, there are already evidence-based standards in place for evaluation and approval.[40] However, numerous therapies are in use in the ICU today without proven efficacy, and many others for which there may be proof in one population of patients are being prescribed in another. Unfortunately, there may be significant barriers to obtaining evidence for these practices. For example, funding agencies and corporations may be unwilling to study therapies that are no longer patented. Furthermore, placebo-controlled studies are often impossible to conduct because clinicians find it unethical to withhold "standard" therapies. Efforts to use "lack of evidence" to justify withholding these therapies should be tempered by these and the following considerations:

1. Are alternatives available that are proven to be effective?
2. Is there evidence that the treatment or procedure is potentially harmful?
3. What is the natural history of the disease without treatment?
4. In the case of prophylaxis, what is the risk for development of disease?
5. What is the cost of treatment as well as of not treating?

Clinicians routinely grapple with these issues even for therapies proven effective. The risk-benefit ratio for any therapy is patient specific, and the clinician must judge the probability for benefit or harm to each individual patient. Evidence-based guidelines can be useful in helping clinicians and patients make these decisions, but they cannot take the place of clinical judgment. Obviously, treatments that are proven to be useless or even harmful should be avoided unless compelling evidence exists for their use in a specific patient. However, restrictions on existing therapy on the grounds that this therapy is unproven will need to be developed with great caution.

Research Methodology

The final application for evidence appraisal techniques is in research. Discussion sections in original articles are now frequently using an evidence-based approach to explain the state of the field and what new information the current study provides. This application of evidence can be useful because it places the article in the context of the existing literature and identifies areas of research that are lacking. Yet, if the discussion ends here, there will be no conjecture or speculation. These traditional aspects of the discussion section can spark new research to which the existing evidence never pointed. We agree with those who have argued that a traditional narrative is still valuable.[26]

Barriers to Applying Evidence

Not unlike the experience with combining other fields of science, clinical medicine is not easily or happily married with epidemiology and biostatistics. Most clinicians lack sufficient experience with these basic sciences to use them efficiently. Furthermore, a basic problem in medical training is that physicians are educated as independent thinkers.

A complementary problem exists when epidemiologists, biostatisticians, or medical economists try to interpret the medical literature. Studies may be valid from a statistical and design standpoint but still fatally flawed from a medical perspective. This may occur when inappropriate outcome measures are used. For example, the rate of resolution of infection might be an appropriate outcome for studies comparing two types of antibiotics in patients in widely different conditions. However, mortality rates would not be appropriate for comparison. Similarly, subtle nuances in the field may be important in understanding what studies can and cannot be combined. For example, some studies on the use of enteral antibiotics for selective decontamination of the gastrointestinal tract have cultured the stool to ensure that virulent organisms were, in fact, suppressed, whereas others have not.[41] Pooling the data from all these studies might lead to serious errors in interpretation. Another example would be the evaluation of outcomes in patients with bacteremia without consideration of the source, such as line infections versus pneumonia. Finally, even well-performed studies from both the medical and statistical viewpoints can still be misinterpreted.

ASSESSING AND USING EVIDENCE IN THE INTENSIVE CARE UNIT

Evidence assessment has been penetrating all fields of medicine and allied specialties for some time. Much as one can accept the rationale in applying the literature to bedside care, intensivists in particular are disturbed by its impracticality because we are often amidst emergent medical situations requiring immediate care and decision making. The issue is complicated by the fact that most illnesses dealt with in ICUs are not single diseases but, rather, heterogeneous combinations of conditions and comorbidities. We have a tendency to consider conditions such as systemic inflammatory response syndrome (SIRS), multiorgan dysfunction syndrome (MODS), and ARDS as diseases when in fact they are syndromes and poorly defined at that. Whether we want to better define the optimal level of intensive care or simply understand whether a new therapy is superior to conventional therapy, we need to have a reliable and valid way to identify and classify ICU patients.

Yet, for all of our efforts in this area, we are as plagued by contradiction and vagueness today as we were 20 years ago. Studies of sepsis and SIRS from around the world continue to show unacceptable differences in the incidence, outcome, and interrelationships of SIRS, sepsis, severe sepsis, and septic shock.[42–45] These differences are almost certainly due to problems with definitions. ARDS is similarly plagued by a lack of consensus on definition,[46, 47] and the very number of alternative organ failure and dysfunction scores[48–51] further highlights this problem. It is unknown whether the results from studies examining the effects of treatment for one disease can be applied to patients with combinations of diseases or conditions. Although the ability to study certain therapies and programs in large RCTs can at least ensure that groups of patients are likely to be comparable and more homogeneous, extrapolation of results to the real world where heterogeneity of patients is the rule can be misleading. Furthermore, the study of anything outside an RCT will likely be fraught with hazard until we can better attribute definitions to our patients that are more closely related to their underlying mechanisms of disease.

Not only do we have problems defining who our patients are; we are also faced with a problem of understanding their outcomes.[52, 53] It is well known, and indeed generally well accepted, that the patients enrolled in sepsis or ARDS RCTs vary widely in both their demographic characteristics and underlying diseases. The reason this variance has been tolerated is the underlying premise that the sepsis or organ failure, and not the underlying disease, is the principal threat to short-term outcome. However, each patient brings a constellation of features that contribute to his or her short-term risk of death, including age, primary diagnosis, comorbid illnesses, presence of concomitant complications, and infectious agents. Because many of these features pose a risk that cannot be diminished by a new therapy targeted at reversing the sepsis or respiratory failure, the ability of a new anti-sepsis strategy to decrease mortality may be less than might have been anticipated during the design of the study. Figure 193–2 illustrates this point.

In other fields, one can employ a Bayesian consideration of prior evidence in determining effect size and the needed sample size in an RCT.[54] But this is exceedingly difficult in the ICU because there have been no successful trials for therapy in sepsis or multiple organ failure on which to base such predictions. Estimates of plausible effect and, therefore, sample size are exceedingly arbitrary under these conditions. Animal studies may provide little help because most animal studies are conducted on animals that are well before the induction of sepsis or acute organ injury.[55] Indeed, in the few studies conducted on animals in which chronic illness was induced before the induction of sepsis or acute organ dysfunction, mortality was much higher and much less open to manipulation by otherwise promising therapies.[55, 56]

In other words, with the advances in the delivery of critical care during the last 30 years, we may now be approaching the point where only a small proportion of the risk of death can be modified by therapies provided in the ICU. Consequently, against a background "noise" of highly varying mortality rates (due to heterogeneity of patients with different underlying diseases), we must search for a small effect "signal." However, the size of this signal-to-noise problem is difficult to estimate, other than to say that we probably have to conduct very large studies.

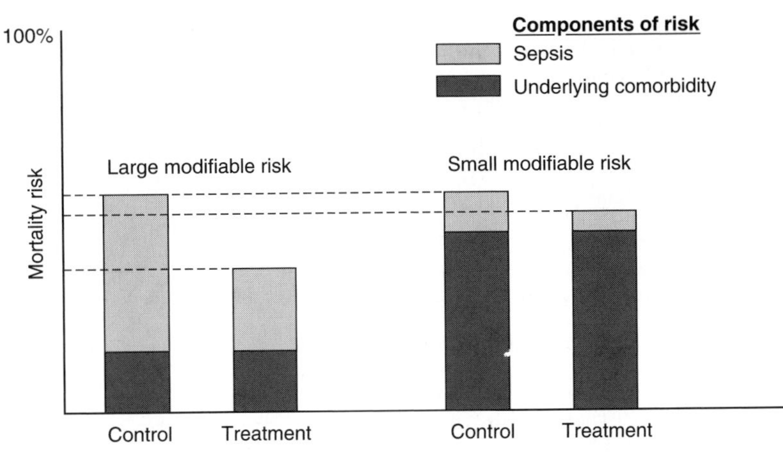

Figure 193–2. Attributable risk: alternative scenarios for a sepsis study with a therapy that has a strong effect on the sepsis process. The implications for sample size in randomized clinical trials are profound. The typical randomized clinical trial in sepsis and adult respiratory distress syndrome has been conducted on fewer randomized clinical trials than 1500 patients and often on only several hundred patients. Typically, these studies are designed with the assumption that septic patients have a hospital mortality of around 40% and that the therapy under consideration will reduce that mortality by 25%, an absolute change of 10%, to 30%. When constructed to have 80% power, this would require 750 patients; at 90% power, 1200 patients are required. In the GUSTO (Global Utilization of Streptokinase and Tissue Plasminogen Activator for Occluded Coronary Arteries) study, on the other hand, detecting a 12.5% relative difference (1% absolute difference) at 90% power required 40,000 patients. If the same *relative* change is applied to a sepsis trial (i.e., to drop mortality from 40% to 35%), 3000 patients will be required at 80% power and 3700 at 90% power. A sepsis study designed to detect a similar *absolute* change (i.e., a 1% drop from 40% to 39%) would require 76,000 patients at 80% power and 100,000 patients at 90%! (Adapted from Angus DC: Discource on method: Measuring the value of new therapies in intensive care. *In:* Yearbook of Intensive Care and Emergency Medicine. Vincent JL [Ed]. Heidelberg, Springer-Verlag, 1998; pp 263–279.)

PERSPECTIVES ON THE FUTURE

There can be little doubt that the recent social upheaval in medicine has fueled interest in evidence-based medicine. Throughout the past three decades, hospitals have steadily increased charges to patients to maintain revenues. Accordingly, the 1990s have seen a new strategy—the reduction of services. However, the emphasis in the future, and already a growing force, will be on increasing efficiency.[57, 58] This goal will require the sophisticated tools available through clinical epidemiology and health services research. In this way, evidence-based initiatives can be seen as the outgrowth of the quality improvement initiatives of this decade.[59]

However, the medical literature is for clinicians and not for hospital administrators.[1, 60] Physicians caring for patients remain the target audience for most reviews and editorials written today, and clinicians continue to be in control of the majority of clinical practice. Unfortunately, this traditional arrangement is being eroded not only by the demands of hospitals, governments, and third-party payers but also by the sheer amount of information now available to all parties including the patients. The dissemination and evaluation of this information has become an increasingly difficult undertaking. Clinicians are being asked to justify their practice as never before.

A frequent misunderstanding about reviewing evidence is the notion that the methodology is fixed. Indeed, the current methodology of evidence-based medicine has serious limitations that are perhaps most obvious in its application in the ICU. Evidence appraisal must evolve to solve these problems, and the techniques will need to be further refined and improved. However, these same problems exist across the entire spectrum of clinical research in the ICU today. Unless a better way is found to identify the correct patients, much larger trials than are currently performed will be needed.

Unfortunately, many logistic problems exist with this approach. In addition, economic pressures demand that we determine not only efficacy but also effectiveness and cost. Solutions to the first problem limit our ability to solve the second. Approaches to measure effectiveness require even larger trials and may therefore force us to include observational outcome studies and simulation models in our current methodology toolset. Although well established in other fields, these methods have played little role in ICU research to date. By further refining our techniques for evaluating and applying evidence, we may be able to realize a goal of Sir William Osler "to blend the art of medicine with the science of probability."

SUMMARY

Clinicians are required to effectively interpret the evidence in their fields. It is much easier to teach a physician how to use the tools of clinical epidemiology and biostatistics than it is to teach a nonphysician medicine. With clinician leadership, efforts to improve the practice of medicine can succeed, not just from a financial standpoint. However, the techniques for evaluating and applying evidence are not panaceas. They are, like the medical literature itself, only tools for clinicians to use to best care for their patients. Experience and consensus are equally important and will still have a role in modern decision analysis. Evidence is no more or less important than these, although it is by definition more objective.

Is evidence-based medicine a tool of clinicians or a leash held by hospital administrators, insurance companies, and government bureaucracies? It is likely to be both, but in the hands of the clinician, it can be much more powerful and accurate.

References

1. Evidence Based Medicine Working Group: Evidence based medicine: A new approach to teaching the practice of medicine. JAMA 1992; 268:2420–2425.
2. Mulrow C: Rationale for systematic reviews. *In:* Systematic Reviews. Chalmers I, Altman DG (Eds). London, BMJ Publishing, 1995, pp 1–8.
3. Rangachari PK: Evidence-based medicine: Old French wine with a new Canadian label? J R Soc Med 1997; 90:280–284.
4. Sackett DL, Haynes RB, Guyatt GH, Tugwell P: Clinical Epidemiology: A Basic Science for Clinical Medicine. 2nd ed. Boston, Little, Brown & Co, 1991.
5. Ware JH, Antman EM: Equivalence trials. N Engl J Med 1997; 337:1159–1161.
6. Lamas GA, Pfeffer MA, Hamm P, Wertheimer J, Rouleau JL, Braunwald E: Do the results of randomized clinical trials of cardiovascular drugs influence medical practice? The SAVE Investigators. N Engl J Med 1992; 327:241–247.
7. Lavori PW, Louis TA, Bailar JCI, Polansky M: Designs for experiments—parallel comparisons of treatments. *In:* Medical Uses of Statistics. Bailar JI, Mosteller F (Eds). Waltham, Mass, NEJM Books, 1986, pp 41–66.
8. Committee for Evaluating Medical Technologies in Clinical Use, Division of Health Sciences Policy, Division of Health Promotion and Disease Prevention, Institute of Medicine: Assessing Medical Technologies. Washington, DC, National Academy Press, 1985.

9. Brun-Buisson C: The HA-1A saga: The scientific and ethical dilemma of innovative and costly therapies. Intensive Care Med 1994; 20:314-316.
10. Sibbald WJ, Vincent J: Roundtable conference on clinical trials for the treatment of sepsis. Chest 1995; 107:522-527.
11. Dellinger RP: From the bench to the bedside: The future of sepsis research. Executive Summary of an American College of Chest Physicians, National Institute of Allergy and Infectious Disease, and National Heart, Lung, and Blood Institute Workshop. Chest 1997; 111:744-753.
12. Bone RC: Why sepsis trials fail. JAMA 1996; 276:565-566.
13. Opal SM: Lessons learned from clinical trials of sepsis. J Endotoxin Res 1995; 2:221-226.
14. Eidelman LA, Sprung CL: Why have new effective therapies for sepsis not been developed? Crit Care Med 1994; 22:1330-1334.
15. Russell LB, Gold MR, Siegel JE, Daniels N, Weinstein MC: The role of cost-effectiveness analysis in health and medicine. Panel on Cost-Effectiveness in Health and Medicine. JAMA 1996; 276:1172-1177.
16. Iezzoni LI, Foley SM, Daley J, Hughes JS, Fisher ES, Heeren T: Comorbidities, complications, and coding bias. Does the number of diagnosis codes matter in predicting in-hospital mortality? JAMA 1992; 267:2197-2203.
17. Angus DC, Pinsky MR: Risk prediction—judging the judges. Intensive Care Med 1997; 23:363-365.
18. McClellan M, McNeil BJ, Newhouse JP: Does more intensive treatment of acute myocardial infarction in the elderly reduce mortality? Analysis using instrumental variables. JAMA 1994; 272:859-866.
19. Kellum JA: The use of diuretics and dopamine in acute renal failure: A systematic review of the evidence. Crit Care 1997; 1:53-59.
20. Cook DJ, Sackett DL, Spitzer WO: Methodologic guidelines for systematic reviews of randomized control trials in health care from the Potsdam Consultation on Meta-analysis. J Clin Epidemiol 1995; 48:167-171.
21. Rosenfel RM: How to systematically review the medical literature. Otolaryngol Head Neck Surg 1996; 15:53-63.
22. Parmar MKB, Stewart LA, Altman DG: Meta-analyses of randomised trials: When the whole is more than just the sum of the parts. Br J Cancer 1996; 74:496-501.
23. D'Agostino RB, Weintraub M: Meta-analysis: A method of synthesizing research. Clin Pharmacol Ther 1995; 58:605-616.
24. LeLorier J, Gregoire G, Benhaddad A, Lapierre J, Derderian F: Discrepancies between meta-analyses and subsequent large randomized, controlled trials. N Engl J Med 1997; 337:536-542.
25. Ioannidis JPA, Cappelleri JC, Lau J: Issues in comparisons between meta-analyses and large trials. JAMA 1998; 279:1089-1093.
26. Bailar JC: The promise and problems of meta-analysis. N Engl J Med 1997; 337:559-560.
27. Pignon JP, Arriagada R: Meta-analysis of randomized clinical trials: How to improve their quality. Lung Cancer 1994; 10:S135-S141.
28. Lau J, Schmid CH, Chalmers TC: Cumulative meta-analysis of clinical trials builds evidence for exemplary medical care. J Clin Epidemiol 1995; 48:45-57.
29. Powe NR, Turner JA, Maklan CW, Ersek M: Alternative methods for formal literature review and meta-analysis in AHCPR Patient Outcomes Research Teams. Med Care 1994; 32:JS22-JS37.
30. Chalmers I: The Cochrane collaboration: Preparing, maintaining and disseminating systematic reviews of the effects of health care. Ann N Y Acad Sci 1993; 203:156-165.
31. Stewart LA, Clarke MJ: Practical methodology of meta-analyses (overviews) using updated individual patient data. Stat Med 1995; 14:2057-2079.
32. Ramakrishnan N, Angus DC, Clermont G, Linde-Zwirble WT, Fine MJ, Pinsky MR: Tracing original data for meta-analyses: Is it possible? Am J Respir Crit Care Med 1998; 157:A300.
33. Campbell GD, Niederman MS, Broughton WA, et al: Hospital-acquired pneumonia in adults: Diagnosis, assessment of severity, initial antimicrobial therapy, and preventative strategies: A consensus statement. Am J Respir Crit Care Med 1996; 153:1711-1725.
34. Cook DJ, Hebert PC, Heyland DK, et al: How to use an article on therapy or prevention: Pneumonia prevention using subglottic secretion drainage. Crit Care Med 1997; 25:1502-1513.
35. Cook DJ, Guyatt GH, Laupacis A, Sackett DL: Rules of evidence and clinical recommendations on the use of antithrombotic agents. Antithrombotic Therapy Consensus Conference. Chest 1992; 102:305-311S.
36. Sibbald WJ, Vincent JL: Roundtable Conference on clinical trials for the treatment of sepsis. Crit Care Med 1995; 23:394-399.
37. Cassiere HA, Groth M, Niederman MS: Evidence-based medicine: The wolf in sheep's clothing. *In:* Yearbook of Intensive Care and Emergency Medicine. Vincent JL (Ed). Heidelberg, Springer-Verlag, 1998, pp 744-749.
38. Charlton BG: Restoring the balance: Evidence-based medicine put in its place. J Eval Clin Pract 1997; 3:87-98.
39. Sullivan FM: Evidence in consultations: Interpreted and individualized. Lancet 1996; 348:941-943.
40. Eddy DM: Investigational treatments: How strict should we be? JAMA 1997; 278:179-185.
41. Stoutenbeek CP, van Saene HKF: Selective decontamination of the digestive tract. *In:* The Splanchnic Circulation: No Longer a Silent Partner. Pinsky MR, Dhainaut JF, Artigas A (Eds). Berlin, Springer-Verlag, 1995; pp 165-174.
42. Brun-Buisson C, Doyon F, Carlet J, et al: Incidence, risk factors, and outcome of severe sepsis and septic shock in adults: A multicenter prospective study in intensive care units. JAMA 1995; 274:968-974.
43. Rangel-Fruausto MS, Pittet D, Costigan M, Hwang T, Davis CS, Wenzel RP: The natural history of the systemic inflammatory response syndrome (SIRS): A prospective study. JAMA 1995; 273:117-123.
44. Salvo I, de Cian W, Musicco M, et al: The Italian SEPSIS study: Preliminary results on the incidence and evolution of SIRS, sepsis, severe sepsis and septic shock. Intensive Care Med 1995; 21:S244-S249.
45. Sands KE, Bates DW, Lanken PN, et al: Epidemiology of sepsis syndrome in 8 academic medical centers. JAMA 1997; 278:234-240.
46. Rubenfeld GD, Doyle RL, Matthay MA: Evaluation of definitions of ARDS. Am J Respir Crit Care Med 1995; 151:1270-1271.
47. Kollef MH, Schuster DP: The acute respiratory distress syndrome. N Engl J Med 1995; 332:27-37.
48. Knaus WA, Wagner DP, Draper EA, et al: The APACHE III prognostic system: Risk prediction of hospital mortality for critically ill hospitalized adults. Chest 1991; 100:1619-1636.
49. Le Gall JR, Klar J, Lemeshow S, Saulnier F, Alberti C, Artigas A, Teres D: The logistic organ dysfunction system: A new way to assess organ dysfunction in the intensive care unit. JAMA 1996; 276:802-810.
50. Marshall JC, Cook DJ, Christou NV, Bernard GR, Sprung CL, Sibbald WJ: Multiple organ dysfunction score: A reliable descriptor of a complex clinical outcome. Crit Care Med 1995; 23:1638-1652.
51. Knaus WA, Draper EA, Wagner DP, Zimmerman JE: Prognosis in acute organ system failure. Ann Surg 1985; 202:685-693.
52. Metcalfe MA, Sloggett A, McPherson K: Mortality among appropriately referred patients refused admission to intensive-care units. Lancet 1997; 350:7-11.
53. Angus DC: Discource on method: Measuring the value of new therapies in intensive care. *In:* Yearbook of Intensive Care and Emergency Medicine. Vincent JL (Ed). Heidelberg, Springer-Verlag, 1998; pp 263-279.
54. Hornberger J, Wrone E: When to base clinical policies on observational versus randomized trial data. Ann Intern Med 1997; 127:697-703.
55. Piper RD, Cook DJ, Bone RC, Sibbald WJ: Introducing *critical appraisal* to studies of animal models investigating novel therapies in sepsis. Crit Care Med 1996; 24:2059-2070.
56. Galanos C, Freudenberg MA: Mechanisms of endotoxin shock and endotoxin hypersensitivity. Immunobiology 1993; 187:346-356.
57. Berwick DM: Continuous improvement as an ideal in health care. N Engl J Med 1989; 320:53-56.
58. Ellwood PM: Shattuck Lecture—outcomes management. N Engl J Med 1988; 318:1549—1556.
59. Blumenthal D: Quality of health care. Part 4: The origins of the quality-of-care. N Engl J Med 1996; 335:1146-1149.
60. Cook DJ, Sibbald WJ, Vincent J-L, Cerra FB: Evidence based critical care medicine: What is it and what can it do for us? Crit Care Med 1996; 24:334-337.

Appendix A for Chapter 193

DEFINITIONS AND EQUATIONS

Study Design: The research methodology used. There are basically four categories. From weakest to strongest, these are:

1. Case series.
2. Case-control study.
3. Cohort study.
4. Randomized clinical trial.

Two-by-Two Table:

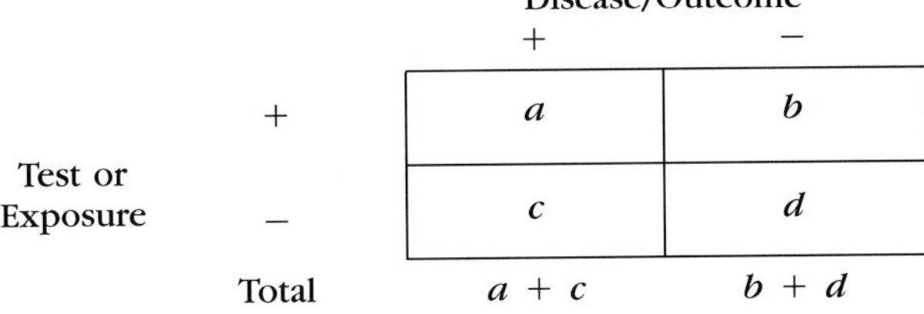

		Disease/Outcome +	Disease/Outcome −
Test or Exposure	+	*a*	*b*
	−	*c*	*d*
	Total	*a* + *c*	*b* + *d*

For Diagnostic Tests

Sensitivity: Probability that the test will be (+) when the disease is present. $a/a+c$

Specificity: Probability that the test will be (−) when the disease is absent. $d/b+d$

Positive Predictive Value: Probability that the disease is present given a (+) test. $a/a+b$

Negative Predictive Value: Probability that the disease is absent given a (−) test. $d/c+d$

For Association (with Exposure or Therapy)

Relative Risk (RR): Estimates the magnitude of an association between exposure and disease (or in the case of therapy, the negative association between treatment and morbid outcome). The relative risk indicates the likelihood of development of disease in the exposed group relative to those who were not exposed (also called risk ratio).

$$\text{RR} = \frac{\text{incidence in exposed group}}{\text{incidence in unexposed group}} = \frac{a/(a+b)}{c/(c+d)}$$

Relative Risk Reduction (RRR): Expressed as a percentage reduction in events in treated versus untreated groups.

$$\text{RRR} = (1 - [a/(a+b)]/[c/(c+d)]) \times 100\%$$

Odds Ratio (OR): For case-control studies, RR cannot be used because participants are selected on the basis of disease, not exposure. The RR can be estimated by the OR, however.

$$\text{OR} = \frac{a/c}{b/d} = \frac{ad}{bc}$$

Attributable Risk (AR): A measure of association that provides information about the absolute effect of the exposure or the excess risk of disease in those exposed compared with those unexposed.

$$\text{AR} = (\text{incidence in exposed group}) - (\text{incidence in unexposed group}) = [a/(a+b)] - [c/(c+d)]$$

Absolute Risk Reduction (ARR): A measure of the treatment effect. Note the *order* is reversed compared with AR.

$$\text{ARR} = [c/(c+d)] - [a/(a+b)]$$

Number Needed to Treat (NNT): The inverse of the ARR: 1/ARR.

$$\text{NNT} = \frac{1}{[c/(c+d)] - [a/(a+b)]}$$

Biostatistics

Type I Error (alpha): A difference between study and control groups is found when in reality there is none. Standard = 5%.

Type II Error (beta): No difference between study and control groups is found when in reality there is a difference. Standard = 20%.

Types of Data

Nominal: Numbers are arbitrary.

Ordinal: Numbers denote rank order only.

Interval: Numbers denote units of equal magnitude and rank order.

Parametric: Interval data in a *normal* distribution.

Standard Deviation (SD): Measure of the scatter of data in a *normally* distributed sample; 95.44% of the data will fall within 2 SD of the mean. SD = square root of the variance.

Standard Error of the Mean (SE): SE = $SD/\sqrt{n}$. Used to calculate confidence intervals, but not a measure of scatter. Should *not* be used in place of SD.

Confidence Interval (CI): The estimated range of values likely to include the true value for the entire population. The standard is 95%.

Power Calculation ($1 - \beta$): Statistical power is the ability of an experiment to find a significant difference between groups when in fact one exists. *Note:* As α increases, so does power. As n is increased, β decreases and power increases, that is, the chance of either a type I or type II error is reduced.

Intention-to-treat Analysis: All data are analyzed according to what group the subject was assigned to regardless of what treatment the subject actually received: "analyzed as randomized."

Appendix B for Chapter 193

The following is a partial list of some of the best Web sites and other sources of information available on evaluating and using evidence in medicine.

EVIDENCE USE AND APPRAISAL RESOURCES ON THE INTERNET

Centre for EBM, Oxford	http://cebm.jr2.ox.ac.uk/
The Health Information Research Unit, McMaster University	http://hiru.mcmaster.ca/
The Unit for Evidence-Based Practice and Policy, London	http://www.ucl.ac.uk/primcare-popsci/uebpp/uebpp.htm
Cochrane Collaboration	http://www.cochrane.de/
The SCHARR Guide to Evidence-Based Medicine on the Internet	http://panizzi.shef.ac.uk/auracle/links.html
Oregon Health Sciences University	http://www.ohsu.edu/bicc-informatics/ebm/
Bandolier, Oxford	http://www.jr2.ox.ac.uk/Bandolier/index.html
Emory University Health Sciences Center Library	http://www.gen.emory.edu/MEDWEB/

JOURNALS CLUBS ON THE INTERNET

Critical Care

MCCTP, Pittsburgh	http://www.anes.upmc.edu/mcctp
SORAHSN, Ontario	http://ahsn.lhsc.on.ca/cat/index.html
PedsCCM EB Journal Club	http://PedsCCM.wustl.edu/EBJournal__club.html

Other

Wayne State University Journal Club	http://www.phypc.med.wayne.edu/jfp/jcindex.htm
Journal Club on the Web	http://www.webcom.com/mjljweb/jrnlclb/index.html
Health Reviews for Primary Care Providers	http://www.auhs.edu/library/resource/reviews/revw__ind.htm
Journal of Family Practice—POEMs	http://jfp.msu.edu/jclub/jclub.htm

ON-LINE JOURNALS

Critical Care Forum	http://biomednet.com/forum/cc/
Evidence-Based Medicine	http://www.bmjpg.com/data/ebm.htm
ACP Journal Club	http://www.acponline.org/journals/acpjc/jcmenu.htm

OTHER USEFUL RESOURCES

Journal Series

1. Journal of the American Medical Association
   Oxman AD, et al: 1993; 270:2093–2095
   Guyatt GH, et al: 1993; 270:2598–2601
   Guyatt GH, et al: 1994; 271:59–63
   Jaeschke R, et al: 1994; 271:703–707
   Levine MS, et al: 1994; 271:1615–1619
   Laupacis A, et al: 1994; 272:234–237
   Oxman AD, et al: 1994; 272:1367–1371
   Richardson WS, et al: 1995; 273:1292–1295
   Richardson WS, et al: 1995; 273:1610–1613
   Hayward R, et al: 1995; 274:570–574
   Wilson MC, et al: 1995; 274:1630–1632
   Guyatt GH, et al: 1995; 274:1800–1804
   Naylor CD, et al: 1996; 275:554–558
   Naylor CD, et al: 1996; 275:1435–1439
2. Canadian Medical Association Journal
   Oxman AD, et al: 1994; 150:1249–1254
   Oxman AD, et al: 1994; 150:1417–1423
   Oxman AD, et al: 1994; 150:1575–1579
   Oxman AD, et al: 1994; 150:1793–1796
   Oxman AD, et al: 1994; 150:1971–1973
3. Critical Care Medicine
   Cook DJ, et al: 1996; 24:334–337
   Cook DJ, et al: 1996; 24:1757–1768

Textbooks

1. Panzer RJ, Black ER, Griner PF (Eds). Diagnostic Strategies for Common Medical Problems. Philadelphia, American College of Physicians Press, 1991.
2. Sackett DL, Haynes RB, Guyatt GH, Tugwell P: Clinical Epidemiology: A Basic Science for Clinical Medicine. 2nd ed. Boston, Little, Brown & Co, 1991.
3. Fletcher RH, Fletcher SW, Wagner EH: Clinical Epidemiology: The Essentials. 3rd ed. Baltimore, William & Wilkins, 1996.
4. Sackett DL, Richardson WS, Rosenberg W, Haynes RB: Evidence-Based Medicine: How to Practice and Teach EBM. London, Churchill Livingstone, 1996.

Computer Software

1. Scientific American Medicine on CD (SAM-CD). 800-545-0554
2. Best Evidence on CD-ROM. Available through the American College of Physicians. http://www.acponline.org
3. Cochrane Library. BMJ Publishing Group. 800-523-1546, +44-0-171-383-6245

194

Severity of Illness Indices and Outcome Prediction: Development and Evaluation

Thomas L. Higgins, MD, FACP, FCCM

And he will manage the cure best who has foreseen what is to happen from the present state of matters. . . .[1]

Predicting outcome is a time-honored duty of physicians, dating back at least to the time of Hippocrates. The need for a scientific approach to outcome prediction, however, is more recent. In addition to the natural desire of a patient or family members to know the prognosis, there is an increasing need for measuring medical care outcomes and for adjusting these outcomes to the presenting condition of the patient. In today's highly competitive health care environment, such information may be publicly disseminated or used to award contracts for care. The Health Care Financing Administration (HCFA) released annual reports comparing hospital mortality rates with predicted rates until concerns about inadequate adjustment for severity of illness[2, 3] stopped the process. Local and regional initiatives to assess the quality of care are becoming increasingly common.[4] Many of these "report cards" specifically address the performance of intensive care units (ICUs) using existing ICU risk stratification systems, so it is essential that the clinician understand these systems and how they are properly applied. A focus on report cards, however, may detract from other potential uses for risk stratification, including more precise risk-benefit decisions, prognostication, efficient assessment of new therapy and technology, and modifications to the management plan based on severity of illness.

Prognostication based on clinical judgment may be affected by memory of recent events, inaccurate estimation of the relative contributions of factors, false beliefs, and human limitations such as fatigue.[5] An outcome prediction model, on the other hand, always produces the same estimate from a given data set and correctly values relevant data. In an environment where clinical judgment may be questioned owing to financial or legal issues, an objective prediction of outcome becomes especially important. This chapter addresses the methods by which models are developed and the application of commonly used models in clinical practice.

Early efforts at adjusting clinical outcomes for the presenting condition of the patient, such as the American Society of Anesthesiologists (ASA) Physical Status Classification,[6] the Glasgow Coma Scale,[7] and the Killip Classification for myocardial infarction,[8] were limited to specific situations. Outcome may also be predicted by serial albumin measurements, endocrine profiles, hemodynamics, and gastric pH in subsets of ICU patients. An organized approach to comparing outcomes should stratify results by the patient's initial condition, be relevant to a heterogeneous population, and rely only on data routinely collected for clinical purposes. Unlike those in other areas of medicine, where risk stratification is nonexistent or is based only on administrative data, the ICU physician can choose from a number of robust, mature models developed on clinical data and subjected to rigorous statistical evaluation. These models are valid for a wide range of ICU diagnoses and can provide a probability of survival even for patients with multisystem disease.

OUTCOMES OF INTEREST

Mortality is a commonly chosen outcome, since it is easily defined and readily available. It is insufficient as the sole outcome measure, however, since it does not reflect important issues such as return to work, quality of life, or even costs, because early death may result in a lower cost than prolonged hospitalization. The use of complication rates to judge quality of care has not been well evaluated, and there may be poor correlation between hospital rankings based on death and those based on complications.[9] Morbidities such as myocardial infarction, prolonged ventilation, stroke and other central nervous system complications, renal failure, and serious infection are also difficult to collect, and administrative records may not reflect all relevant events.[10] There is also little standardization of the definition of morbidity. Outcomes must be clinically relevant, unambiguous, reliably collected, and independent of therapeutic decisions. Well-defined endpoints are preferred (e.g., elevations in laboratory values, days on mechanical ventilation, number of ICU days). Other endpoints may be germane: ICU or hospital length of stay, resource use, return to work, quality of life, and 1- to 5-year survival. Patient satisfaction is an outcome highly valued by purchasers of health care but is subjective[11] and costly to evaluate. The European Consensus Conference in Critical Care has recommended augmenting mortality data with generic health status and quality-of-life measures.[12]

DATA BASES AND DEFINITIONS

The quality of a risk stratification system depends on the quality of the data base from which it was developed. Outcome analysis can be either retrospective, relying on existing medical records and administrative data bases, or prospective, using data collected concurrently with patient care. Retrospective studies using existing data are quicker and less expensive to conduct but may be compromised by missing data, imprecise definitions, and changes in medical practice over the time period considered.

Data derived from discharge summaries or insurance claims data may not adequately capture the presence of comorbid disease[13] or may be discordant with data collected clinically.[14] Because some discharge reports limit the number of reportable events, diagnoses may be missed, and this coding bias is most apparent in severely ill patients.[10] Coding errors and use of computer programs to optimize Diagnostic-Related Group (DRG) reimbursement can also reduce the validity of claims-derived data. Recent work, however, suggests that augmentation of administrative data with laboratory values can produce quality models.[15]

Ideally, outcome analysis should utilize strict, accurate diagnostic criteria and account for severity of illness at hospital admission, since subsequent treatment can skew results.[16] Clear, unambiguous definitions are essential for consistent data collection between institutions and over time in one institution.

The outcome study should also report on any quality checks that were performed to ensure accuracy of the data base. A variety of appropriate methods exist, such as reabstraction of a sample of charts by personnel blinded to the initial results, or electronic comparison with an independent data base. In many institutions, mortality statistics are collected for multiple purposes, and administrative data bases may be readily available to cross-check against clinical data bases. Kappa analysis, a method of examining the rate of discrepancies between measurements (values) of the same variable in different data bases (i.e., original and reabstracted), quantifies agreement, where zero (0) represents no agreement (or random) results and 1.0 is perfect agreement.[17]

MODEL DEVELOPMENT

Once data integrity is ensured, a number of approaches for adjusting outcome by presenting condition are possible. Some early ICU models were distillations of practical clinical wisdom that assigned arbitrary point values for clinical findings thought to increase risk. This theoretical approach can be augmented using statistical techniques to allocate point values to the variables considered. The empirical approach is to use a large data base and to subject the data to a series of statistical manipulations (Table 194–1). The initial step is to determine the endpoint (typically death, a morbidity, or resource consumption) that defines outcome. Factors thought to predict outcome *(independent variables)* are then evaluated against the specific outcome *(dependent variable)*, using univariate tests (*chi*-square, Fisher's exact, Student's *t*-test) to establish the magnitude and significance of any relationship.

The independent variables should reflect patient condition independent of therapeutic decisions. *Measured variables*, such as cardiac index and hematocrit, are preferred over *process variables*, such as use of inotropes and transfusion given, because the criteria for intervention may vary by provider or hospital. Variables that are part of the outcome should not be used to predict that outcome (e.g., use of cardiac enzyme values to predict myocardial infarction when enzymes are part of the diagnostic criteria). Current models rely on *measured physiologic variables*, such as heart rate, blood pressure, neurologic status, and common *laboratory values*, such as creatinine and white blood cell count. In addition, terms are generally included to reflect age, physiologic reserve, and general health status.

Items chosen for inclusion in a scoring system should be readily available and clinically relevant to clinicians involved in the care of these patients, and variables that have neither clinical nor statistical bearing on outcome should not be included. This may necessitate use of more than one scoring system when a patient population (certain surgical, pediatric, burn, trauma, and cardiac patients) demonstrates markedly different characteristics from the general ICU population. For example, left ventricular ejection fraction and reoperative status are important predictors of outcome in the cardiac surgical population but are not routinely measured or are irrelevant to other population groups.[18] If the independent variable is dichotomous *(yes - no, male - female)*, a two-by-two table can be constructed to examine the odds ratio, or the influence of the independent variable on the outcome (Table 194–2). If multiple variables are being considered, the level of significance is generally set smaller than $P = .05$, often using a Bonferroni correction[19] to determine a more appropriate P value.

When the independent variable under consideration is a continuous variable (e.g., age) a Student's *t*-test is one appropriate choice for statistical comparison. Care must be taken with continuous variables when the *relationship* of the variable *to outcome* is not linear. Figure 194–1 demonstrates the relationship of serum bicarbonate values at ICU admission to mortality outcome for cardiac surgery patients when the data points have been averaged with adjacent values to produce

TABLE 194–1. Developing a Severity of Illness Model

1. Precisely define outcome or outcomes of interest.
2. Identify and define candidate predictor variables.
3. Collect data and ensure their accuracy (reabstraction, kappa analysis).
4. Examine continuous variables, and transform or dichotomize as necessary.
5. Univariate analysis (*chi*-square, Fisher's exact, Student *t*-test).
6. Multivariate analysis (multiple logistic regression, neural nets, Bayesian, others).
7. Examine for and adjust for interactions.
8. Develop score or equation that relates independent variables to outcome.
9. Test calibration of model (goodness of fit).
10. Test discrimination of model (receiver operating characteristic C statistic, sensitivity, and specificity).
11. Validate model with independent data, split sample, or jacknife techniques.
12. External validation in new setting.
13. Peer-reviewed publication.

TABLE 194–2. Two-by-Two Contingency Table

Predictor Variable: History of CHF	Outcome Variable: Multisystem Organ Failure	
	Yes	***No***
Yes	121	846
No	166	2697

Data from Higgins TL, Estanfanous FG, Loop FD, et al: ICU admission score for predicting morbidity and mortality risk after coronary bypass grafting. Ann Thorac Surg 1997; 64:1050–1058.

A two-by-two contingency table examining the relationship of multisystem organ failure after open heart surgery (outcome) to a history of congestive heart failure (CHF) (predictor) in 3830 patients. The odds ratio is defined by cross-multiplication $(121 \times 2697) \div (846 \times 166)$. The odds ratio of 2.3 indicates that patients with CHF are 2.3 times as likely to develop postoperative organ system failure as those without prior CHF. This univariate relationship can then be tested by *chi*-square for statistical significance.

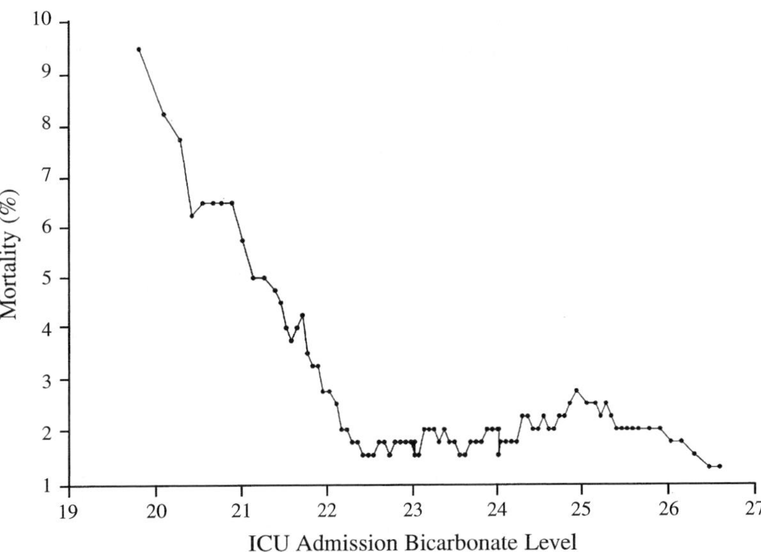

Figure 194–1. A locally weighted smoothing scatterplot (LOWESS) analysis of the relationship between intensive care unit admission bicarbonate level (*x*-axis) and mortality (*y*-axis). Individual patient data are grouped and averaged with surrounding data to produce a smooth plot. In this instance, the mortality rate appears to be stable with admission bicarbonate levels of 22 and above but rises rapidly with lower values. Admission bicarbonate levels below 21 mmol/L were given prognostic weight in the model that used these data. (From Higgins TL, Estafanous FG, Loop FD, et al: ICU admission score for predicting morbidity and mortality risk after coronary artery bypass grafting. Ann Thorac Surg 1997; 64:1050-1058.)

a locally weighted smoothing scatterplot (LOWESS) graph.[20] Serum bicarbonate values above 22 mEq/L at ICU admission imply a relatively constant risk. Below this value, the risk of death rises sharply. Analysis of this LOWESS[21] graph suggests two ways of dealing with the impact of serum bicarbonate on mortality: (1) making bicarbonate on admission a dichotomous variable (i.e., ≥22 mEqL or ≤21 mEqL) and (2) transforming the data via a logarithmic equation to make the relationship more linear. Cubic splines analysis, another statistical smoothing technique, may also be used to assign weight to physiologic variables.

Univariate analyses assess the predictive weight of variables without regard to possible correlations or interactions between variables. Linear discriminant and logistic regression techniques[22] can evaluate and correct for overlapping influences on outcome. For example, a history of congestive failure and a depressed left ventricular ejection fraction are both known predictors of poor outcome in candidates for cardiac surgery.[23] As might be expected, there is considerable overlap between the population with congestive heart failure and patients with low ejection fraction. The multivariate analysis in this specific instance eliminates congestive heart failure as a predictor and retains only ejection fraction in the final equation.

Because linear discriminant techniques require certain assumptions about data, logistic techniques are used more often. Subjecting the data to multiple logistic regression produces an equation with a constant, a beta coefficient and standard error, and an odds ratio that calculates each term's effect on outcome. Table 194-3 displays the results of the logistic regression used in the Mortality Probability Model (MPM) II ICU admission model. There are 15 variable terms and a

TABLE 194–3. Variables in the Admission Mortality Probability Model (MPM_0*) with Estimated Coefficients, Standard Errors, Adjusted Odds Ratios, and 95% Confidence Intervals for the Adjusted Odds Ratios

Variable	β (SE)	Estimate Adjusted Odds Ratio (95% Confidence Interval)
Constant	−5.46836	†
Physiology (coma or deep stupor)	1.48592 (0.079)	4.4 (3.8-5.2)
Heart rate ≥150 beats/min	0.45603 (0.145)	1.6 (1.2-2.1)
Systolic blood pressure ≤90 mmHg	1.06127 (0.079)	2.9 (2.5-3.4)
Chronic diagnoses		
Chronic renal insufficiency	0.91906 (0.105)	2.5 (2.0-3.1)
Cirrhosis	1.13681 (0.126)	3.1 (2.4-4.0)
Metastatic neoplasm	1.19979 (0.098)	3.3 (2.7-4.0)
Acute diagnoses		
Acute renal failure	1.48210 (0.089)	4.4 (3.7-5.2)
Cardiac dysrhythmia	0.28095 (0.068)	1.3 (1.2-1.5)
Cerebrovascular incident	0.21338 (0.089)	1.2 (1.0-1.5)
Gastrointestinal bleeding	0.39653 (0.094)	1.5 (1.2-1.8)
Intracranial mass effect	0.86533 (0.088)	2.4 (2.0-2.8)
Other		
Age (10-year odds ratio)	0.03057 (0.002)	1.4 (1.3-1.4)
Cardiopulmonary resuscitation prior to admission	0.56995 (0.112)	1.4 (1.3-1.4)
Mechanical ventilation	0.79105 (0.056)	2.2 (2.0-2.5)
Nonelective surgery	1.19098 (0.074)	3.3 (2.8-3.8)

From Lemeshow S, Teres D, Klar J, et al: Mortality Probability Model (MPM II) based on an international cohort of intensive care unit patients. JAMA 1993; 270:2478. Copyright 1993, American Medical Association.

*MPM_0 indicates system admission model.

†Not applicable.

constant term, each with a beta value, that plug into an equation that calculates probability of mortality. The odds ratios reflect the increased risk of mortality when a factor is present. Generally accepted practice is to limit the number of terms in the logistic regression model to 10% of the number of patients with the outcome of interest, in order to avoid "overfitting" the model to the developmental data set. In a population of 5000 patients with a mortality rate of 3%, there will be 150 deaths. One tenth of 150, or 15, is the maximum number of terms that could usefully be included in a logistic regression model for this sample size. It is important to identify interactions between variables that might be additive, subtractive (canceling), or synergistic and that would require additional terms in the final model.

The type of disease is an important determinant of outcome, but there are two philosophies on how disease status should be addressed by a severity adjustment model.

One approach is to define principal diagnostic categories and add a weighted term to the logistic regression equation for each illness. This approach acknowledges the different impacts of physiologic derangements, depending on diagnosis. For example, patients with diabetic ketoacidosis have markedly altered physiology but low expectation of death; a patient with a leaking abdominal aneurysm may show little physiologic abnormality and yet be at high risk for death or morbidity. Too many diagnostic categories, however, may produce too few patients in each category to allow statistical analysis in the typical ICU.

The other approach is to ignore disease status and assume that factors such as age, general health status, and altered physiologic function suffice to explain outcome in large groups of patients. This method avoids the requirement to pick one diagnosis in patients with multiple problems and the need for lengthy lists of coefficients but could result in a model that depends more on having an "average" case mix. Regardless of the general approach, age and comorbidities (metastatic or hematopoietic cancer, immunosuppression, cirrhosis) are included in the popular ICU models to account for the patient's physiologic reserve, or ability to recover from acute illness.

VALIDATION AND TESTING MODEL PERFORMANCE

After the multivariate logistic model has been developed, it should be tested, ideally on an independent data set. Other methods, including jackknife or bootstrap validation,[24] randomly and repeatedly remove subjects from the population, recalculate the model, and can assess the coefficients and predictive validity of multiple models when a validation data set is not available. A split sample technique, which divides the available data into developmental and test (validation) subsets, is often used. This type of validation should be considered internal because testing is done at the same hospitals using the same data collection techniques.

Two criteria are important in assessing model performance. The first is *calibration*, or how well the model tracks outcomes across its relevant range. A model may be very good at predicting good outcomes in healthy patients and poor outcomes in very sick patients, yet be unable to distinguish outcome for patients in the middle range. The Hosmer-Lemeshow goodness-of-fit test[25] assesses calibration by stratifying the data into categories (usually deciles) of risk. The number of patients with an observed outcome is compared to the number of predicted outcomes at each risk level (Table 194–4). If the observed and expected outcomes are very close at each level across the range of the model, the sum of *chi*-squares is low, indicating good calibration. The P value for the Hosmer-Lemeshow goodness-of-fit test *increases* with better calibration and should be insignificant (i.e., $P > .05$).

The second measure of model performance is *discrimination*, or how well the model predicts the correct outcome. A classification table (Table 194–5) displays four possible outcomes that define sensitivity and specificity of a model with a binary (died/survived) prediction and outcome. Sensitivity (true-positive rate) and specificity (the true-negative rate, or 1 minus the false-positive rate) are measures of discrimination, but they depend on what percentage or decision point is chosen to distinguish between outcomes when a model produces a continuous range of possibilities. We can recalculate the classification table for a range of outcomes by choosing various decision points—for example, 10%, 25%, 50%, 75%, and 95% mortality risk. At each decision point, the true-positive rate (proportion of deaths correctly predicted) and the false-negative rate (proportion of survivors incorrectly predicted to die) and the overall correct classification rate can be presented.

The C statistic, or area under a receiver operating characteristic (ROC) curve, is a convenient way of summarizing sensitivity and specificity at various decision points.[26, 27] A graph of the true-positive proportion (sensitivity) against the false-positive proportion (1 minus specificity) across the range of

TABLE 194–4. Hosmer-Lemeshow Goodness-of-Fit Testing in the Mortality Probability Model (MPM-II) on Admission to the Intensive Care Unit*

Probability of Dying	Survived, No. (n = 9978)		Died, No. (n = 2632)	
	Observed	*Expected*	*Observed*	*Expected*
.000–.031	1196	1185.3	16	26.7
>.031–.045	1259	1259.2	49	48.8
>.045–.064	1180	1177.9	66	68.1
>.064–.086	1182	1180.2	93	94.8
>.086–.117	1140	1134.6	121	126.4
>.117–.162	1080	1087.9	182	174.1
>.162–.224	1011	1017.9	249	242.1
>.224–.338	916	918.1	348	345.9
>.338–.572	691	702.7	568	556.3
>.572–.999	323	314.3	940	948.7

From Lemeshow S, Teres D, Klar J, et al: Mortality Probability Model (MPM II) based on an international cohort of intensive care unit patients. JAMA 1993; 270:2478. Copyright 1993, American Medical Association.

*Goodness of fit = 6.21 (eight degrees of freedom); $P = .623$

†The low goodness-of-fit value and the nonsignificant P value indicate good calibration across 10 deciles of risk.

TABLE 194–5. Classification Table for Determining Sensitivity, Specificity, and Accuracy

Predicted Outcome	Actual Outcome: Died	Actual Outcome: Survived
Died	a	c
Survived	b	d

True-positive ratio = a/(a+b) (sensitivity)
False-positive ratio = c/(c+d)
True-negative ratio = d/(c+d) (specificity)
False-negative ratio = b/(a+b)
Accuracy (total correct prediction) = (a+d)/a+b+c+d

the model produces the ROC (Fig. 194-2). A model with equal probability of producing the correct or incorrect result (e.g., flipping a coin) produces a straight line at a 45° angle that encompasses half (0.5) of the area under the curve. Models with better discrimination incorporate larger areas under the curve, to a theoretical maximum of 1.0. Most ICU models have ROC areas of 0.8 to 0.9 in the development set, although the ROC area usually decreases when models are applied prospectively to new data sets. The ROC is valid only if the model has been first shown to calibrate well.

A model may discriminate and calibrate well on its development data set yet fail when applied to a new population. Discrepancies in performance can relate to differences in surveillance strategies and definitions[28] and can occur when a population is skewed because an unusual number of patients have certain risk factors, as they might in a specialized ICU.[29] Models can also deteriorate over time owing to changes in medical practice. These explanations should be considered before one concludes that quality of care in the original and in later applications of a model was different.

SCORING SYSTEMS

Logistic regression is a statistically sound way to express the relationship between independent and dependent variables

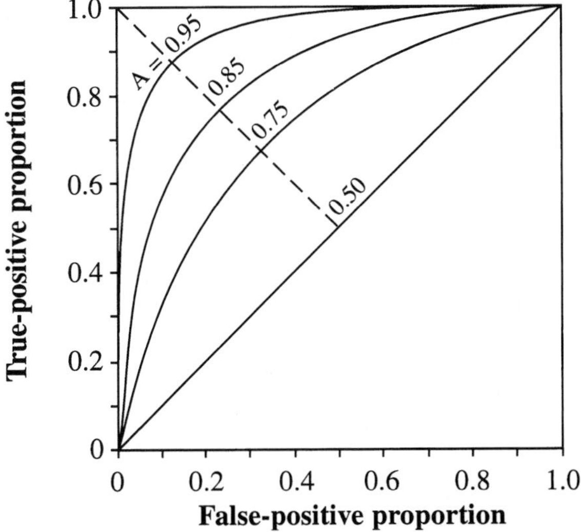

Figure 194–2. Relative operating characteristic (ROC) curves. A coin toss gives an ROC of 0.5. In models that discriminate outcome, an increasing area under the curve, also called the C-statistic, is enclosed. (Adapted from Swets JA: Measuring the accuracy of diagnostic systems. Science 1988; 240:1285–1294.)

but requires a computer or programmable calculator for application. It is possible to use either the beta coefficients or the odds ratios from the logistic regression results to assign integer values based on relative importance of independent variables to create a score that will be useful at the bedside. The validity of a simplified score can be confirmed when the clinical score is subjected to the same discrimination and calibration tests as the multiple logistic regression model.[20]

STANDARDIZED MORTALITY RATIOS

Application of a severity of illness index involves comparison of observed outcomes with those predicted by the model. The *standardized mortality ratio* (SMR) is defined as observed mortality divided by expected mortality. It is generally expressed as a mean value plus or minus 95% confidence intervals, which depend on the number of patients in the sample. SMR values of 1.0 (± the confidence interval) indicate that the mortality rate, adjusted for presenting illness, is at the expected level. SMR values significantly lower than 1.0 indicate better than expected performance. Small differences in scores, such as those that could be caused by consistent errors in scoring elements or timing of data collection, may cause important changes in the SMR.[30]

SCORING SYSTEMS BASED ON RESOURCE UTILIZATION

One approach to ranking severity of illness is to assess resource utilization, on the assumption that more severely ill patients will need more nursing time, more invasive monitoring, and more therapeutic interventions. The Therapeutic Intervention Scoring System (TISS)[31] quantifies the number of interventions to estimate severity of illness. The original TISS scored 57 therapeutic interventions with point values of 1 to 4, and patients at highest risk had scores of more than 40 points. Variations on TISS include the *intermediate* TISS, designed for stepdown areas,[32] and a *simplified* TISS-28, which reduces the number of variables.[33] Medicus, a proprietary product, is based on the same premise as TISS, and it is commonly used to assess nursing workload and nursing staffing patterns. Because interventions can be driven by local custom, TISS scores generally are not used for prognosis or quality assessment. Physiologic predictors of outcome can be correlated with observed TISS scores to produce estimates of resource utilization in ICU patients. Estimates of staffing requirements based on TISS vary with the type of ICU.[34]

MODELS BASED ON PHYSIOLOGIC DERANGEMENT

Three widely utilized general-purpose ICU outcome systems are based on physiology:

- The Acute Physiology and Chronic Health Evaluation (APACHE-I, APACHE-II,[35] APACHE-III[36])
- The Mortality Probability Model (MPM-I,[37] MPM-II,[38] including MPM_0, and MPM_{24})
- The Simplified Acute Physiology Score (SAPS-I,[39] SAPS-II[40])

These models are all based on the premise that more critically ill patients have values that deviate more from physiologic normal for a variety of common parameters such as heart rate, blood pressure, and neurologic status, and laboratory values and that they also have altered physiologic reserve with advanced age and chronic illness.

Acute Physiology and Chronic Health Evaluation

APACHE II Model

APACHE II was developed from studies of 5815 medical and surgical ICU admissions at 13 hospitals. APACHE II score severity was based on 12 routine physiologic measurements plus the patient's age and previous health status (Fig. 194–3). Scoring is based on the most abnormal measurements during the first 24 hours in the ICU. The maximum score is 71 points, although more than 80% of patients have scores of 29 or less.[35] APACHE II represents a reduction in variables and an improvement in performance over the original APACHE based on multivariate regression analysis. Figure 194–3 shows the correlation between physiologic abnormalities and the acute physiology score and contains the information needed to generate an APACHE II score. The relationship between APACHE II scores and hospital mortality differs for surgical and nonsurgical patients (Fig. 194–4), since the prognostic impact of altered physiology is less severe in postoperative patients.

APACHE II was developed on a data base of medical and surgical patients that excluded coronary artery bypass grafting, coronary care, burn, and pediatric patients. Knaus and coworkers note, "It is crucial to combine the APACHE II score with a precise description of disease," and provide coefficients to adjust the APACHE II score for 29 nonoperative and 16 postoperative diagnostic categories.[35] They also caution that disease-specific mortality predictions should be derived from at least 50 patients in each diagnostic category. These appropriate precautions have not always been observed in application of APACHE II.

Another common misunderstanding is the use of APACHE II, calibrated on unselected ICU admissions, to a patient sample selected by other criteria, such as need for mechanical ventilation.[36] APACHE II does not control for pre-ICU management, which can restore a patient's altered physiology and lead to a lower score, thus underestimating a patient's true risk. Subsequent investigators have demonstrated that the admission source predicts hospital death independent of the APACHE II score.[16] In a study of 235 medical patients scored with APACHE II, the actual mortality was the same as predicted mortality only for patients admitted directly from the emergency room. The actual mortality rate was higher than predicted for transfers from hospital floors, stepdown units, and other hospitals. Multivariate logistic regression analysis confirmed the independent association between admission source and outcome (odds ratio, between 3 and 5). The authors note that failure to consider the source of admission may lead to erroneous conclusions about the quality of medical care.[16]

APACHE III Model

APACHE III, published in 1991,[36] addresses the limitations of APACHE II, specifically the impact of treatment location before ICU admission, and it expands the number of separate disease categories from 45 to 78. APACHE III was developed on a representative national data base of 17,440 patients at 40 hospitals, including 14 tertiary facilities that volunteered for the study and 26 randomly chosen hospitals. As in the previous version, pediatric, burn, and coronary artery bypass patients are excluded, and scoring is based on the "worst" value obtained during the initial 24 hours of intensive care. The weighting of variables was estimated by multivariate logistic regression and, as compared with APACHE II, defines narrower ranges of physiologic "normal" and increases the weighting to extreme deviations (Fig. 194–5). Interactions between variables were considered, five new ones (blood urea nitrogen, urine output, serum albumin, bilirubin, and glucose) were added, and serum potassium and bicarbonate were dropped from the score. Information was also collected on 34 chronic health conditions, seven of which (acquired immunodeficiency syndrome, hepatic failure, lymphoma, solid tumor with metastasis, leukemia or multiple myeloma, immunocompromise, cirrhosis) were significant in predicting outcome.

APACHE III scoring ranges from zero to 299, and a 5-point increase represents a significant increase in risk of hospital death. In addition to the APACHE III *score*, which provides an initial risk estimate, there is an APACHE III *predictive equation* that uses the APACHE III score and proprietary reference data on disease category and treatment location before ICU admission to provide individual risk estimates for ICU patients. This risk estimate is within 3% of observed outcome for 95% of ICU admissions. Overall correct classification at a 50% estimate for mortality risk is 88.2%, with an ROC area of 0.90, significantly better than APACHE II.[36] Sequential APACHE III scoring can update the daily risk estimate, although most of the variation in observed death rates is accounted for by the initial APACHE III score.

APACHE III equations assign different weights for measurements past the initial 24-hour period. The single most important factor in daily risk of hospital death is the updated APACHE III score, but the change in the APACHE III score, the admission diagnosis, the age and chronic health status of the patient, and previous treatment are also important. A predicted risk of death in excess of 90% on any of the first 7 days is associated with a 90% mortality rate.

Detailed instructions for calculating an APACHE III *score* (Table 194–6; see Fig. 194–5) are readily available.[36] The re-

TABLE 194–6. Components of the APACHE III Score

	Points
***Acute Physiology Score** (0–252 points)*	
Mean blood pressure	0–23
Respiratory rate adjusted for mechanical ventilation	0–18
Temperature	0–20
Pulse	0–17
Neurologic status	0–48
24-hour urine output	0–15
Hematocrit	0–3
White blood count	0–19
Arterial pH adjusted for P_{CO_2}	0–12
Arterial P_{O_2} or A_{ADO_2}, if ventilated	0–15
Serum sodium	0–4
Serum albumin	0–11
Serum glucose	0–9
Serum creatinine	0–10
Blood urea nitrogen	0–12
Serum bilirubin	0–16
***Age, yr** (0–24 points)*	
≤44	0
45–59	5
60–64	11
65–69	13
70–74	16
75–84	17
≥85	24
Chronic Health Condition (0–24 points)*	
Acquired immunodeficiency syndrome	23
Hepatic failure	16
Lymphoma	13
Metastatic cancer	11
Leukemia/multiple myeloma	10
Immunosuppression	10
Cirrhosis	4

Adapted from Knaus WA, Wagner DP, Draper EA, et al: The APACHE III Prognostic System. Risk prediction of hospital mortality for critically ill hospitalized adults. Crit Care Med 1985; 13:519.

*Excluded for elective surgery patients.

THE APACHE II SEVERITY OF DISEASE CLASSIFICATION SYSTEM

PHYSIOLOGIC VARIABLE	HIGH ABNORMAL RANGE					LOW ABNORMAL RANGE			
	+4	+3	+2	+1	0	+1	+2	+3	+4
TEMPERATURE — rectal (°C)	≥41°	39°-40.9°		38.5°-38.9°	36°-38.4°	34°-35.9°	32°-33.9°	30°-31.9°	≤29.9°
MEAN ARTERIAL PRESSURE — mm Hg	≥160	130-159	110-129		70-109		50-69		≤49
HEART RATE (ventricular response)	≥180	140-179	110-139		70-109		55-69	40-54	≤39
RESPIRATORY RATE — (non-ventilated or ventilated)	≥50	35-49		25-34	12-24	10-11	6-9		≤5
OXYGENATION: A-aDO$_2$ or PaO$_2$ (mm Hg) a. FiO$_2$ ≥0.5 record A-aDO$_2$	≥500	350-499	200-349		<200				
b. FiO$_2$ <0.5 record only PaO$_2$					PO$_2$ >70	PO$_2$ 61-70		PO$_2$ 55-60	PO$_2$ <55
ARTERIAL pH	≥7.7	7.6-7.69		7.5-7.59	7.33-7.49		7.25-7.32	7.15-7.24	<7.15
SERUM SODIUM (mMol/L)	≥180	160-179	155-159	150-154	130-149		120-129	111-119	≤110
SERUM POTASSIUM (mMol/L)	≥7	6-6.9		5.5-5.9	3.5-5.4	3-3.4	2.5-2.9		<2.5
SERUM CREATININE (mg/100 ml) (Double point score for **acute** renal failure)	≥3.5	2-3.4	1.5-1.9		0.6-1.4		<0.6		
HEMATOCRIT (%)	≥60		50-59.9	46-49.9	30-45.9		20-29.9		<20
WHITE BLOOD COUNT (total/mm3) (in 1,000s)	≥40		20-39.9	15-19.9	3-14.9		1-2.9		<1
GLASGOW COMA SCORE (GCS): Score = 15 minus actual GCS									
[A] Total ACUTE PHYSIOLOGY SCORE (APS): Sum of the 12 individual variable points									
Serum HCO$_3$ (venous-mMol/L) [Not preferred, use if no ABGs]	≥52	41-51.9		32-40.9	22-31.9		18-21.9	15-17.9	<15

[B] AGE POINTS:
Assign points to age as follows:

AGE(yrs)	Points
≤44	0
45-54	2
55-64	3
65-74	5
≥75	6

[C] CHRONIC HEALTH POINTS

If the patient has a history of severe organ system insufficiency or is immuno-compromised assign points as follows:

a. for nonoperative or emergency postoperative patients — 5 points

or

b. for elective postoperative patients — 2 points

DEFINITIONS

Organ Insufficiency or immuno-compromised state must have been evident **prior** to this hospital admission and conform to the following criteria:

LIVER: Biopsy proven cirrhosis and documented portal hypertension; episodes of past upper GI bleeding attributed to portal hypertension; or prior episodes of hepatic failure/encephalopathy/coma

CARDIOVASCULAR: New York Heart Association Class IV.

RESPIRATORY: Chronic restrictive, obstructive, or vascular disease resulting in severe exercise restriction, i.e., unable to climb stairs or perform household duties; or documented chronic hypoxia, hypercapnia, secondary polycythemia, severe pulmonary hypertension (>40mmHg), or respirator dependency

RENAL: Receiving chronic dialysis

IMMUNO-COMPROMISED: The patient has received therapy that suppresses resistance to infection, e.g., immuno-suppression, chemotherapy, radiation, long term or recent high dose steroids, or has a disease that is sufficiently advanced to suppress resistance to infection, e.g., leukemia, lymphoma, AIDS

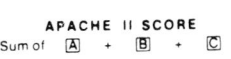

APACHE II SCORE

Sum of [A] + [B] + [C]

[A] APS points

[B] Age points

[C] Chronic Health points

Total APACHE II

Figure 194–3. The APACHE II Classification System. Normal physiologic values do not receive points; high or low abnormal values receive increasing points according to the above chart, which defines the Acute Physiology Score. Adding points for Age and Chronic Health status produces the APACHE II score, which can then be related to outcome (see Fig. 194–4). (From Knaus WA, Draper EA, Wagner DP, Zimmerman JE: APACHE II: A severity of disease classification system. Crit Care Med 1985; 13:818–829.)

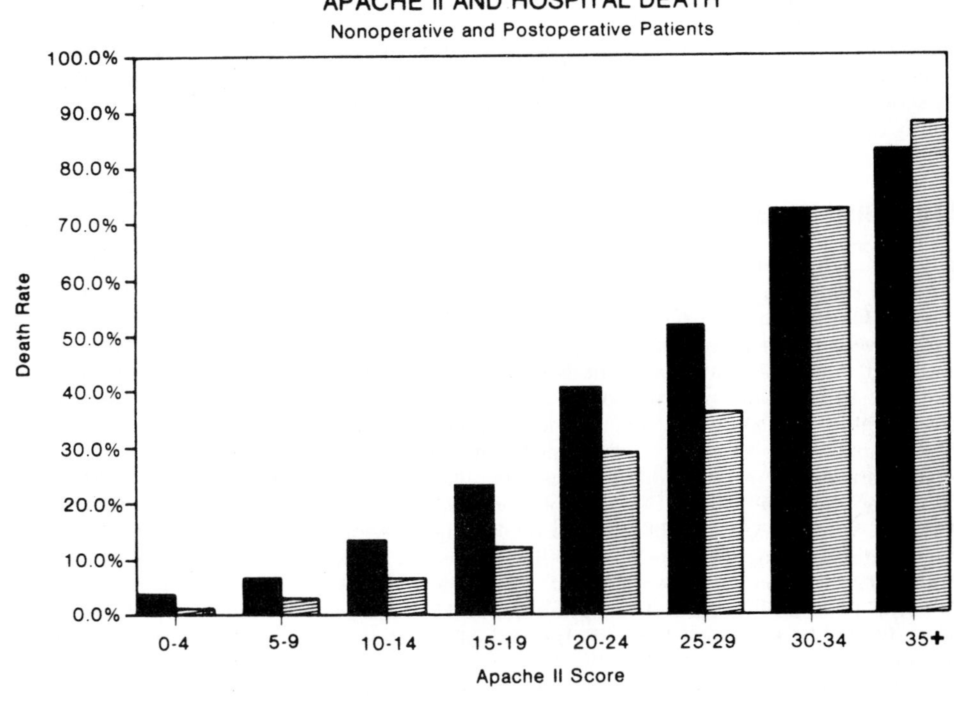

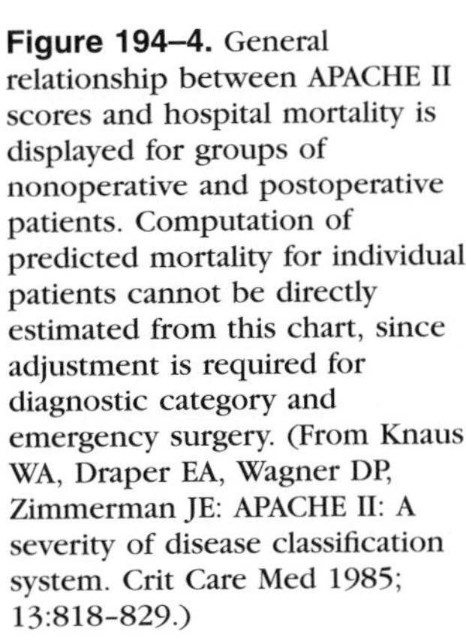

Figure 194–4. General relationship between APACHE II scores and hospital mortality is displayed for groups of nonoperative and postoperative patients. Computation of predicted mortality for individual patients cannot be directly estimated from this chart, since adjustment is required for diagnostic category and emergency surgery. (From Knaus WA, Draper EA, Wagner DP, Zimmerman JE: APACHE II: A severity of disease classification system. Crit Care Med 1985; 13:818–829.)

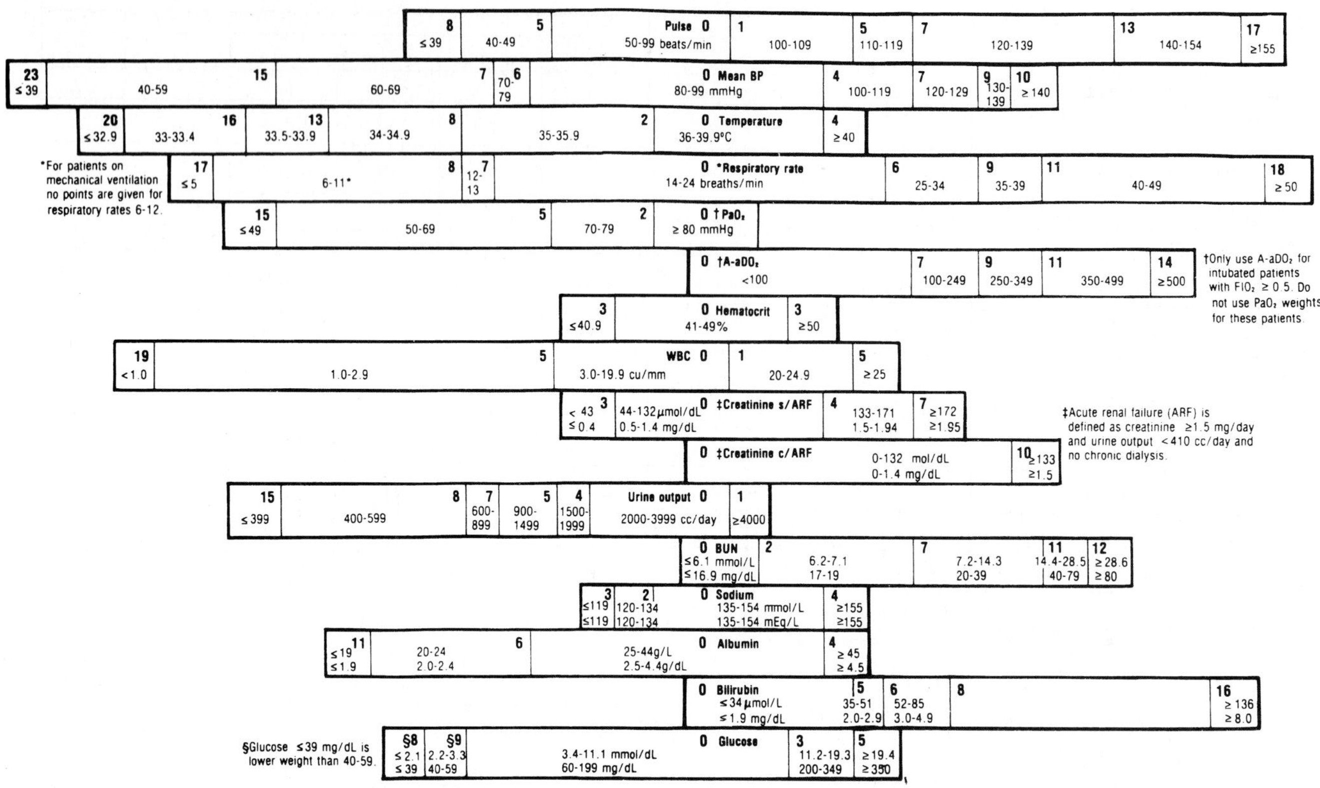

Figure 194–5. The APACHE III Classification System. Variables, point values, and scoring ranges have changed from APACHE II. The APACHE III score generated from this table can be related to hospital risk of death with additional weighting for diagnostic category. (From Knaus WA, Wagner DP, Draper EA, et al: The APACHE III Prognostic System: Risk prediction of hospital mortality for critically ill hospitalized adults. Chest 1991; 100:1619–1636.)

gression coefficients and detailed definitions for calculating predicted risk of hospital mortality are proprietary and require subscription to a software-based clinical information system. The TISS and nursing benchmarks that are tied to the APACHE III score represent observed practice rather than an independently determined ideal.

Mortality Probability Models

The original MPM was developed from 755 patients at a single hospital, using multiple logistic regression to assign weights to variables predicting hospital mortality.[37] The MPM II models were developed on an international sample of 12,610 patients and then validated on a subsequent sample of 6514.[38] MPM, like APACHE, excludes pediatric, burn, and coronary and cardiac surgical patients and estimates hospital mortality risk based partly on physiologic derangement, but considers a smaller number of variables. MPM II uses data obtained at ICU admission (MPM_0) and at the end of the first 24 hours (MPM_{24}), whereas APACHE II or III is scored using the worst data obtained during the first 24 hours. The admission model (Table 194–3) contains 15 variables; the 24-hour model (MPM_{24}, Table 194–7), uses five of the 15 MPM_0 variables plus eight additional ones. Age and chronic health status are included in both MPM_0 and MPM_{24}.

While APACHE generates a score and then, with additional information, converts that score into a probability estimate of survival, MPM directly calculates a probability of survival from the available data. Both versions of MPM assigned weights to variables by statistical techniques. The MPM_{24} recognizes that patients who remain in the ICU 24 hours or longer differ from those who die or are well enough to be discharged. This line of reasoning has been further extended to create 48- and 72-hour models.[41] Additional variables in MPM_{24}, MPM_{48}, and MPM_{72}, but not MPM_0 are prothrombin time, urine output, creatinine, arterial oxygenation, continuing coma or deep stupor, confirmed infection, mechanical ventilation, or intravenous vasoactive drug therapy.

In an evaluation of 3023 patients from Massachusetts and New York, the probability of death was found to increase at 48 and 72 hours even when the MPM variables and coefficients were unchanged, reflecting the clinical impression that the mortality risk is increasing in patients whose clinical profile remains unchanged over time.[41] MPM_{48} and MPM_{72} adjust for this observation by changing the β_0 (the constant term) in the MPM_{24} equation.

The most important difference between MPM and other systems is that the MPM_0, with the exception of information related to cardiopulmonary resuscitation, produces a probability estimate that is available at ICU presentation and is independent of ICU treatment. MPM does not require specifying a diagnosis, which can be an advantage in "complex" ICU patients, but it may also make it more sensitive to changes in the case mix. MPM II calibrates well and has ROC areas of 0.837 for the admission model and 0.844 for the MPM_{24}.

Simplified Acute Physiology Score

The simplified acute physiology score (SAPS I), which uses a subset of the original APACHE variables, was developed from a population of 679 consecutive patients admitted to eight multidisciplinary ICUs in France. Like the APACHE system, SAPS uses the worst values collected during the first 24 hours after ICU admission.

SAPS II was developed from experience with 13,152 patients at 137 adult medical or surgical ICUs in Europe and North America. Like MPM and APACHE, SAPS excludes burn patients, patients younger than 18 years, coronary care patients, and cardiac surgery patients. The outcome measure for SAPS II is vital status at hospital discharge. Seventeen variables are used in the model: 12 physiologic variables, age, type of admission, and the presence of acquired immunodeficiency syndrome, metastatic cancer, or hematologic malignancy (Table 194–8). The area under the ROC curve is 0.88 in the developmental sample and 0.86 in the validation sample. The model calibrates well by goodness-of-fit testing. Like MPM, the SAPS II can be scored without specifying a primary diagnosis and can be fully implemented from published information.

SPECIALIZED MODELS

APACHE, MPM, and SAPS, while useful for general medical-surgical ICUs, exclude patients younger than 18, burn patients, and coronary care and cardiac surgical patients. Murphy-Filkins and colleagues[29] have demonstrated that severity of illness models may become invalid when the percentage of patients with abnormal findings exceeds a critical limit, as might be seen in specialized intensive care units. Of the patients in the MPM II data base, 20% were aged 75 or older. If this percentage of elderly patients is arbitrarily changed to 42%, the model would no longer predict accurately. Similar changes are seen when the proportion of patients with cardiac arrhythmias, cerebrovascular disease, intracranial mass effects, coma, cardiopulmonary resuscitation before ICU admission, emergency admission, or gastrointestinal bleeding rises above the critical values. Thus, severity of illness scoring system should be used with caution when units become highly specialized. The European Consensus Conference recommends that severity indices be validated and customized, if needed, when applied to a new setting such as a particular country or type of ICU.[12]

To address this problem, specific models have been developed for pediatric,[42] trauma,[43, 44] and cardiac surgical populations.[20] The cardiac surgical population differs from the general ICU population because admission physiology data can be misleading in a population routinely subjected to hypothermia, hemodilution, and deliberate control of hemodynamics by the operating room team. Crucial factors for predicting outcome in cardiac surgery include ventricular function, coronary anatomy and heart valve pathology, reoperation status, and the degree of extracardiac vascular disease.[18]

Four cardiac surgical models based on preoperative data have been prospectively compared on an independent data set and found to be accurate; however, each has shortcomings, with marked discrepancies in individual patient prediction.[45] The ROC C statistics of the original models on their development samples range from 0.72 to 0.86, but in prospective evaluation this range drops to 0.70 to 0.74. The preoperative models are useful for evaluating the entire hospital course of a population of patients undergoing cardiac surgery, but they do not specifically address the quality of ICU care. Operating room events can neutralize or amplify preoperative risk, depending on such events as opening the chest in a "reoperative" patient, hemodynamic management in an emergency patient, and the degree of myocardial protection. Analysis of 5000 patients undergoing coronary artery bypass grafting identifies eight risk factors available at ICU admission that predict hospital mortality, and another five that also predict morbidity.[20] Similar to MPM_0, this model relies on admission data, not the worst values over 24 hours. The 13 mortality or morbidity variables, identified by logistic regression, were simplified into a clinical score (Fig. 194–6, Table 194–9) that applies equally well to patients undergoing coronary artery bypass grafting alone, or combined with a valve or carotid

TABLE 194–7. Variables in the 24-Hour Mortality Probability Model (MPM_{24})* with Their Estimated Coefficients, Standard Errors, Adjusted Odds Ratios, and 95% Confidence Intervals for the Adjusted Odds Ratios

Variable	β (SE)	Estimate Adjusted Odds Ratio (95% Confidence Interval)
Constant	−5.64592	†
Variables ascertained at admission		
Age, 10-yr odds ratio	0.03268 (0.002)	1.4 (1.3–1.4)
Cirrhosis	1.08745 (0.135)	3.0 (2.3–3.9)
Intracranial mass effect	0.91314 (0.095)	2.5 (2.1–3.0)
Metastatic neoplasm	1.16109 (0.112)	3.2 (2.6–4.0)
Medical or unscheduled surgery admission	0.83404 (0.080)	2.3 (2.0–2.7)
24-hr assessments		
Coma or deep stupor at 24 hr	1.68790 (0.082)	5.4 (4.6–6.4)
Creatinine >176.8 μmol (2.0 mg/dL)	0.72283 (0.078)	2.1 (1.8–2.4)
Confirmed infection	0.49742 (0.070)	1.6 (1.4–1.9)
Mechanical ventilation	0.80845 (0.067)	2.2 (2.0–2.6)
Partial pressure of oxygen (Po_2) <7.98 kilopascal (60 mmHg)	0.46677 (0.077)	1.6 (1.4–1.9)
Prothrombin time >3 sec above standard	0.82286 (0.088)	2.3 (1.9–2.7)
Urine output <150 mL in 8 hr	0.82286 (0.088)	2.3 (1.9–2.7)
Vasoactive drugs ≥1 hr intravenously	0.71626 (0.065)	2.0 (1.8–2.3)

From Lemeshow S, Teres D, Klar J et al: Mortality Probability Model (MPM II) based on an international cohort of intensive care unit patients. JAMA 1993; 270:2478. Copyright 1993, American Medical Association.

*MPM_{24}, system 24-hr model.

†Not applicable.

TABLE 194–8. Variables and Definitions for Simplified Acute Physiology Score (SAPS II)

Variable	Definition	Points
Age	Age (in years) at last birthday	0–18
Heart rate	Use the worst value in 24 hours, either low or high heart rate: if it varied from cardiac arrest (11 points) to extreme tachycardia (7 points), assign 11 points.	0–11
Systolic blood pressure	Use the same method as for heart rate: e.g., if it varied from 60 mm Hg to 205 mm Hg, assign 13 points	0–13
Body temperature	Use the highest temperature	0–3
Pao_2/FIO_2 ratio	If the patient is ventilated or on continuous positive airway pressure, use the lowest value of the ratio	0–11
Urinary output	If the patient is in the intensive care unit for less than 24 hours, make the calculation for 24 hours: e.g., 1 L in 8 hours = 3 L in 24 hours	0–11
Serum urea or serum urea nitrogen level	Use the highest value in mmol/L for serum urea, in mg/dL for serum urea nitrogen	0–10
WBC count	Use the worst (high or low) WBC count	0–12
Serum potassium level	Use the worst (high or low) value in mmol/L	0–3
Serum sodium level	Use the worst (high or low) value in mmol/L	0–5
Serum bicarbonate level	Use the lowest value in mEq/L	0–6
Bilirubin level	Use the highest value in μmol/L or mg/dL	0–9
Glasgow Coma Scale	If the patient is sedated, record the estimated Glasgow Coma Scale score before sedation.	0–26
Type of admission	Unscheduled surgical,* scheduled surgical,† or medical‡	8, 0, or 6
AIDS	Yes, if HIV-positive with clinical complications such as *Pneumocystis carinii* pneumonia, Kaposi's sarcoma, lymphoma, tuberculosis, or *Toxoplasma* infection	17
Hematologic malignancy	Yes, if lymphoma, acute leukemia, or multiple myeloma	10
Metastatic cancer	Yes, if proven metastasis by surgery, computed tomography, or any other method	9

From Le Gall J-R, Lemeshow S, Saulnier F: A new Simplified Acute Physiology Score (SAPS II) based on a European/North American multicenter study. JAMA 1993; 270;2957–2963. Copyright 1993, American Medical Association.

*Patients added to operating room schedule within 24 hours of the operation.

†Patients whose surgery was scheduled at least 24 hours in advance.

‡Patients having surgery within 1 week of admission to the intensive care unit.

FIO_2 = fraction of inspired oxygen; WBC = white blood cell; AIDS = acquired immunodeficiency syndrome; HIV = human immunodeficiency virus.

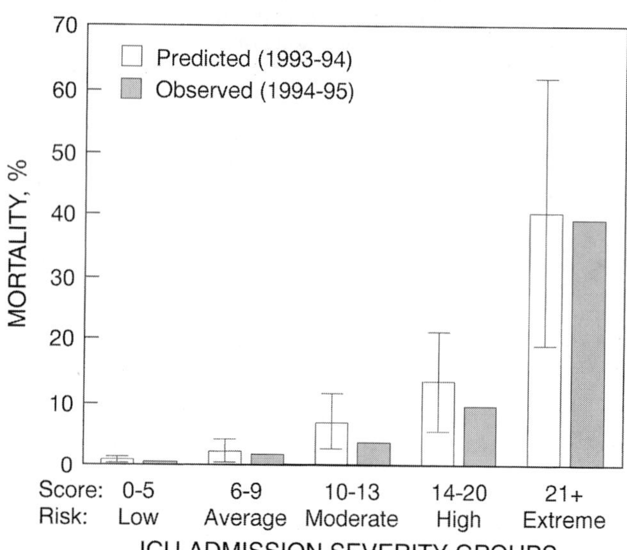

Figure 194–6. Mortality following cardiac surgery by intensive care unit (ICU) admission risk group. Risk is estimated by summing the individual elements from Table 194–9. Results are displayed for the development set (1993 to 1994) and prospective validation (1994 to 1995). Note the width of the 95% confidence intervals in the highest risk groups; only 136 patients (5.6% of the data set) had scores of 14 or above. (From Higgins TL, Estanfanous FG, Loop FD, et al: ICU admission score for predicting morbidity and mortality risk after coronary artery bypass grafting. Ann Thorac Surg 1997; 64:1050–1058.)

TABLE 194–9. Intensive Care Unit (ICU) Risk Stratification Score for Cardiac Surgery

Variable	Value
Preoperative Factors	
Small body size (BSA <1.72 m²)	1
Prior heart operation	
One	1
Two or more	2
History of operation or angioplasty for peripheral vascular disease	3
Age ≥70 yr	3
Preoperative creatinine ≥1.9 mg/dL	4
Preoperative albumin <3.5 mg/dL	5
Intraoperative Factors	
CPB time ≥160 minutes	3
Use of IABP after CPB	7
ICU admission physiology	
A − a O_2 gradient ≥250 mmHg	2
Heart rate ≥100 beats/min	3
Cardiac index <2.1 $L\text{-}min^{-1}\text{-}m^{-2}$	3
CVP ≥17 mmHg	4
Arterial bicarbonate <21 mmol/L	4

From Higgins TL, Estafanous FG, Loop FD, et al: ICU admission score for predicting morbidity and mortality risk after coronary artery bypass grafting. Ann Thorac Surg 1997; 64:1050–1058.

A − a, alveolar-arterial; BSA, body surface area; CPB = cardiopulmonary bypass; CVP = central venous pressure; IABP = intra-aortic balloon pump.

procedure. The C statistic was 0.86 for the mortality model and 0.82 for predicting morbidity, with good calibration by Hosmer-Lemeshow goodness-of-fit testing.

A modified APACHE III has also been used successfully for cardiac surgery in a prospective multicenter study of 2435 patients.[46] Independent predictors of hospital mortality included the APACHE score, age, emergency or reoperation status, the number of bypass grafts, and the gender of the patient. This model, which has an ROC area of 0.85, can be used to evaluate ICU length of stay and resource use as well as mortality risk.

COMPARISONS OF MODELS

Surprisingly little has been published that compares the current versions of the three general prognostic systems, and comparisons of older versions[47, 48] may no longer be relevant. From their review of published articles, Lemeshow and Le Gall[49] concluded that the newer models (APACHE III, MPM II, SAPS II) were based on rigorous research and reported performance sufficient to justify use in assessing prognosis, comparing ICU performance, and in stratifying patients for clinical trials. Castella and colleagues compared APACHE II and III, SAPS I and II, and MPM I and II in a multicenter, multinational study of 14,745 patients in 137 ICUs (Table 194–10).[50] None of the older models calibrated well, but the revised systems were consistently superior to their earlier ones, as judged by both ROC area and goodness of fit. The newer systems all posted adequate discrimination where this could be assessed. This study evaluated patients from the same data base used for the development of SAPS II and MPM II. Even though comparisons were made using a subset of 4685 patients not part of the development samples, the data collection techniques and definitions would have been identical, a situation unlikely to be replicated by others.

Moreno and Morais recently compared the performance of SAPS II and of APACHE II in an independent data base of 1094 patients in 19 Portuguese ICUs.[51] Discrimination by ROC testing was better for SAPS II, but neither model calibrated well by Hosmer-Lemeshow goodness-of-fit testing. In a comparison of APACHE systems in 1144 British ICU patients, APACHE II had better calibration but APACHE III had better discrimination.[52] Hospital mortality was higher than predicted with either model, agreement being closest in "respiratory" patients and the least in trauma patients. The authors note that differences in trauma care infrastructure between the United States and the United Kingdom might account for some of this discrepancy. APACHE II had superior risk estimates for surgical patients.

Finally, APACHE II has been compared to clinical assessment by nurses and house staff working in the ICU.[53] Sensitivity, specificity, correct prediction, and area under the ROC curve were compared, and no significant differences were noted between ROC areas for APACHE II and nurses, fellows, residents, or interns.

The current APACHE, SAPs, and MPM scores are highly specific (better than 90% ability to predict survival) but relatively insensitive in predicting death. Such information should not be used as a rationale for relying on clinical judgment and forgoing formal scoring. The existing severity indices, despite their flaws, do provide useful, objective information for comparing groups of patients for quality improvement, purchasing decisions, research, and ICU management. Further, although use for individual outcome prediction is more constrained, the severity indices can be used to guide individual prognosis

TABLE 194–10. Comparison of Severity Models on a Common Data Set

	Discrimination (ROC Area)	Calibration	Sample Size
		GOF (H Statistic)	
APACHE II*	0.853	<.0001	12899
APACHE III	0.848	Not available	12899
MPM_0I	0.766	<.0001	4605
MPM_0II	0.805	.0143	4605
$MPM_{24}I$	0.815	<.0001	4101
$MPM_{24}II$†	0.833	.0247	4101
SAPS I	0.784	Not applicable	4605
SAPS II*	0.847	.1019	4605

Adapted from Castella X, Artigas A, Bion J, et al: A comparison of severity of illness scoring systems for intensive care unit patients. Crit Care Med 1995; 23:1327.

*Discrimination and calibration assessed on probability estimate, not score.

†Lower P value implies poor fit. For example, the newer MPM_{24} at $P = 0.0247$ calibrates than the original MPM_{24} at $P < .0001$. All P values approach significance owing to the size of the data base.

SAPS = Simplified Acute Physiology Score; MPM = Mortality Probability Model; ROC = receiver operating characteristic; APACHE = Acute Physiologic and Chronic Health Evaluation; GOF = goodness of fit.

and triage decisions, bearing in mind that patient autonomy and medical ethics may force a different conclusion than the severity of illness model might suggest.

USES OF SEVERITY ADJUSTMENT

Prediction of Individual Outcome

The difficulty in using scoring systems for individuals arises from attempts to apply a probability estimate, which may range from 0 *to* 1, to an individual whose result will be 0 *or* 1. No model is accurate enough to predict that a given patient will certainly either survive or die, so the use of scoring systems alone to direct therapy is not recommended. An article suggesting that APACHE II could be used to limit provision of total parenteral nutrition (TPN)[54] was widely criticized by physicians who pointed out exceptions to the rules and the danger of self-fulfilling prophecies.[55] The adjustments needed to avoid false predictions of death reduce the sensitivity of APACHE II so as to render it useless.[56] It is unlikely that any score calculated within 24 hours of ICU admission would ever perfectly predict outcome, since the patient's individual response to therapy clearly plays a role. In patients with perforated gastrointestinal viscus, the development of overt multiple organ failure was a better predictor of death than the APACHE III score.[57]

Sequential prognostic estimates, an approach explored by both APACHE[58] and MPM,[41] holds promise, but neither sequential model has been validated prospectively, and this use raises the possibility of creating a negative feedback loop where a declining risk of survival could precipitate withdrawal or limitation of care. Objective predictions of the need for next-day life support can inform triage and discharge decisions,[59] but further study of this approach is still needed.[60]

Point estimates of survival should always be presented with confidence intervals, which may be very wide under the circumstances. The European Consensus recommends against the use of existing scoring systems for making predictions in individual patients.[12]

Clinical Research

Existing data bases and severity adjustment make possible hypothesis-generating observations and conclusions about therapeutic choices in situations where randomized, prospective evaluations might not be permitted or funded. For prospective studies, severity scoring indices can be used to "risk stratify" the population before randomization, thus reducing the number of patients and the cost of clinical trials.[61] Representative examples of this approach include risk stratification for comparison of different antibiotic regimens[62] and anticytokine therapies.[63] Acute physiologic abnormalities are the most important prognostic factors influencing outcome in patients who meet criteria for sepsis syndrome.[64] Correlations have been noted between the MPM_0 II sepsis score[65] and interleukin 6 plasma levels, and between APACHE III scores and plasma levels of tumor necrosis factor-sR, interleukin-6, and C-reactive protein.[66] Nonsurvivors have significantly higher MPM II or APACHE III scores at any time during sepsis.

Quality Improvement

Quality improvement, like research, requires a severity adjustment method to control for differences in the presenting characteristics of patients when one is assessing outcome. A study of 13 tertiary care centers found that outcome, after adjustment using APACHE II, may have correlated with the degree of co-ordination in the ICU.[67] Resource utilization,[46] cost variations,[68] and reimbursement strategies[69] can also be analyzed using a severity adjustment approach; these are covered in more detail in Chapter 195.

Outcomes Reporting

Rankings of hospital quality range from the annual report on "America's Best Hospitals" published by *U.S. News and World Report*,[70] to government-mandated medical outcomes data.[71] Critical care outcomes are beginning to attract national attention,[72] and a number of local initiatives utilize ICU severity adjustment to produce reports available to the general public.[69, 73] Cleveland Health Quality Choice,[73] a regional program for health market reform, uses APACHE III to report hospital mortality and length of stay for ICU patients at individual hospitals. Interestingly, in the reporting period covering March 1993 to 1994, 14 of the 29 hospitals were reported to have ICU mortality lower than predicted, reflecting an aggregate trend toward lower hospital mortality.[73] Whether this represents true improvement or better attention to scoring risk factors is open to question. Public reporting of outcome data may have unexpected consequences such as increased referral of seriously ill patients to tertiary care centers.[74, 75]

Managed care organizations and group practices are keenly interested in outcomes. Data specific to ICU practice may not be widely collected yet, but 15% of health plans and 50% of large group practices and hospitals collect and distribute medical outcomes data.[76] Unfortunately, some methods lack statistical sophistication, and simplistic methods may lead to faulty conclusions.[77] Obtaining good information is expensive,[78] and cost constraints may dictate less than optimal data collection approaches, such as reliance on claims data.[10, 13, 14] Increasing automation of medical records will eventually make use of clinical data for outcome assessment routine and cost effective.

PITFALLS APPLICATION

Like any tool, severity of illness indices can become a dangerous weapon when misapplied. The use (and abuse) of data bases for profiling ICUs or individual physicians is growing, despite flaws in administrative data bases and problems identified with application of statistical models.[2, 3, 9, 10, 13, 14, 27, 28, 30, 47, 75, 79] Assuming use of a properly developed model, the potential pitfalls in application fall into four major categories: data collection and entry errors, misapplication of the model (especially related to case mix), use of mortality as the sole criterion of outcome, and failure to account for sample size and chance variability when reporting results (Table 194-11). Determination of the diagnosis is prone to bias.[80] Models that assess performance using a patient's condition at 24 hours are not truly independent of treatment. When the characteristics of patients are markedly different from those of a general population, the resulting case mix bias alters model performance.[29] Less obvious is the fact that all models start the clock with ICU admission, a clinical decision that itself may be arbitrary and influenced by local conditions such as ICU bed availability. Also, ICUs do not function in isolation in the process of care, and the recent trend toward aggressive use of stepdown facilities and off-site chronic ventilation and rehabilitation units raises the question of whether hospital mortality is valid when patients may be transferred alive, but still technology-dependent, to other facilities.

The issue of lead time bias (pre-ICU stabilization) was mentioned earlier; assessment is further complicated for patients with multiple admissions to intensive care. Which ICU stay should be counted in the patient who has ICU observation after an uneventful vascular procedure and then experiences

TABLE 194–11. Potential Pitfalls in the Application and Reporting of Severity-Adjusted Outcome

Data Collection and Entry

Inclusion of ineligible patients
Missing variables and data management errors
Substitution of available for properly timed data
Transcription and data entry errors
Wrong diagnosis selected
Administrative data may not reflect clinical condition
Deliberate "gaming" of the system

Models

Case mix differences (critical threshold exceeded)
Application to subsets of development population
Changes in weighting over time
Small clinical changes can translate into large risk increments when continuous data are categorized.
Lead-time bias

Outcomes

Insufficient range of outcomes reported
Use of proxy outcomes that inadequately reflect true status
Patient lost to follow-up
Chance variability masquerading as true difference
Relationships of scores to resource utilization and costs reflect observed practice, not ideal.

Reporting

Confidence intervals not reported
Inadequate sample size used
Physician of record misidentified
Computational errors
Misapplication of group data to individuals
Misinterpretation of statistical as clinical significance

complications that require ICU readmission on the fifth postoperative day? It is increasingly necessary to evaluate the performance of an ICU *system*, which includes pre-ICU, ICU, and post-ICU care.[81] Rules for starting times and end points of evaluation remain to be defined.

SUMMARY

APACHE II and III, MPM II, and SAPS II are highly developed, prospectively validated tools useful for comparison of ICU performance in the care of groups of patients. Specialized models are available for burn, trauma, sepsis, coronary, cardiac surgery, and pediatric patients. When used as intended, these models allow stratification of patients for quality improvement, research, utilization management, and dissemination of outcome results. Important implementation considerations include careful data collection, appropriate matching of the model and the population under study, and use of proper sample sizes and confidence intervals in reporting results.

None of the models are, or are ever likely to become, 100% accurate when applied to individual patients; however, this limitation is true of almost any test used in medicine, and it need not preclude the use of prognostic estimates for clinical decision support. Work now under way on sequential probability estimates and customized models may increase the acceptance of objective measurements in defining potentially ineffective care. Physicians must be alert to the limitations of severity adjustment models in performance-based assessment, because case mix differences, inadequate sample sizes, or systematic errors in data collection can generate erroneous conclusions about the quality of care.

References

1. Struss MB: Familiar Medical Quotations. Boston, Little, Brown & Co, 1968, p 460.
2. Green J, Wintfeld N, Sharkey P, Passman LJ: The importance of severity of illness in assessing hospital mortality. JAMA 1990; 263:241–246.
3. Jencks SF, Daley J, Draper D, et al: Interpreting hospital mortality data: The role of clinical risk adjustment. JAMA 1988; 260:3611–3616.
4. Higgins TL: Assessing ICU quality of care in 1997: A North American perspective. Clin Intensive Care 1997; 8:76–80.
5. Dawes RM, Faust D, Meehl PE: Clinical versus actuarial judgment. Science 1989; 243:1668–1674.
6. Owens WD, Felts JA, Spitznagel EL: ASA Physical Status Classifications: A study of consistency of ratings. Anesthesiology 1978; 49:239–243.
7. Bastos PG, Sun X, Wagner DP, et al: Glasgow Coma Scale score in the evaluation of outcome in the intensive care unit: Findings from the Acute Physiology and Chronic Health Evaluation III study. Crit Care Med 1993; 21:1459–1465.
8. Killip T, Kimball JT: Treatment of myocardial infarction in a coronary care unit. Am J Cardiol 1967; 20:457–460.
9. Silber JH, Rosenbaum PR, Schwartz JS, et al: Evaluation of the complication rate as a measure of quality of care in coronary artery bypass graft surgery. JAMA 1995; 274:317–323.
10. Iezzoni LI, Foley SM, Daley J, et al: Comorbidities, complications, and coding bias: Does the number of diagnosis codes matter in predicting in-hospital mortality? JAMA 1992; 267:2197–2203.
11. Gill TM, Feinstein AR: A critical appraisal of the quality of quality-of-life measurements. JAMA 1994; 272:619–626.
12. Second European Consensus Conference in Intensive Care Medicine: Predicting outcome in intensive care unit patients. Clin Intensive Care 1994; 11:148–151.
13. Greenfield S, Aronow HU, Elashoff RM, Watanabe D: Flaws in mortality data: The hazards of ignoring comorbid disease. JAMA 1988; 260:2253–2255.
14. Jollis JG, Ancukiewicz M, DeLong ER, et al: Discordance of databases designed for claims payment versus clinical information systems. Ann Intern Med 1993; 119:844–850.
15. Pine M, Norusis M, Jones B, Rosenthal GE: Predictions of hospital mortality rates: A comparison of data sources. Ann Intern Med 1997; 126:347–354.
16. Escarce JJ, Kelley MA: Admission source to the medical intensive care unit predicts hospital death independent of APACHE II score. JAMA 1990; 264:2389–2394.
17. Cohen J: A coefficient of agreement for nominal scales. Educ Psychol Measure 1960; 20:37–46.
18. Higgins TL: Cardiac surgery "report card" modelling. Curr Opin Crit Care 1997; 3:169–174.
19. Meinert CL: Clinical Trials. Design, Conduct and Analysis. New York, Oxford University Press, 1986, pp 213–214.
20. Higgins TL, Estafanous FG, Loop FD, et al: ICU admission score for predicting morbidity and mortality risk after coronary artery bypass grafting. Ann Thorac Surg 1997; 64:1050–1058.
21. Cleveland WS: Robust locally weighted regression and smoothing scatterplots. J Am Stat Assoc 1979; 74:829–836.
22. Kiefe C: Statistical methods used by ICU prognostic indices. Prob Crit Care 1989; 3:514–527.
23. Higgins TL, Estafanous FG, Loop FD, et al: Stratification of morbidity and mortality outcome by preoperative risk factors in coronary artery bypass patients: A clinical severity score. JAMA 1992; 267:2344–2348.
24. Efron B, Tibshirani RJ: An Introduction to the Bootstrap. New York, Chapman and Hall, 1993, pp 141–152.
25. Lemeshow S, Hosmer DW: A review of goodness of fit statistics for use in the development of logistic regression models. Am J Epidemiol 1982; 115:92–106.
26. Swets JA: Measuring the accuracy of diagnostic systems. Science 1988; 240:1285–1294.
27. Hanley JA, McNeil BJ: The meaning and use of the area under a receiver-operating characteristic. Radiology 1982; 143:29–32.
28. Charlson ME, Ales KL, Simon R, MacKenzie R: Why predictive indexes perform less well in validation studies: Is it magic or methods? Arch Intern Med 1987; 147:2155–2161.

29. Murphy-Filkins RL, Teres D, Lemeshow S, Hosmer DW: Effect of changing patient mix on the performance of an intensive care unit severity-of-illness model: How to distinguish a general from a specialty intensive care unit. Crit Care Med 1996; 24:1968–1973.
30. Goldhill DR, Withington PS: Mortality predicted by APACHE II: The effect of changes in physiological values and post-ICU hospital mortality. Anaesthesia 1996; 51:719–723.
31. Cullen DJ, Civetta JM, Briggs BA, Ferrara LC: Therapeutic intervention scoring system: A method for quantitative comparison of patient care. Crit Care Med 1974; 2:57–60.
32. Cullen DJ, Nemeskal AR, Zaslavsky AM: Intermediate TISS: A new Therapeutic Intervention Scoring System for non-ICU patients. Crit Care Med 1994; 22:1406–1411.
33. Miranda DR, de Rijk A, Schaufeli W: Simplified Therapeutic Intervention Scoring System: The TISS-28 items—results from a multicenter study. Crit Care Med 1996; 24:64–73.
34. Dick W, Pehl S, Tzanova I, et al: Physician and nursing (personnel) requirements for ICUs: Therapeutic Intervention Scoring System (TISS) versus time requirements for patient care—a comparative study in an interdisciplinary surgical intensive care unit. Clin Intensive Care 1992; 3:116–121.
35. Knaus WA, Draper EA, Wagner DP, Zimmerman JE: APACHE II: A severity of disease classification system. Crit Care Med 1985; 13:818–829.
36. Knaus WA, Wagner DP, Draper EA, et al: The APACHE III Prognostic System: Risk prediction of hospital mortality for critically ill hospitalized adults. Chest 1991; 100:1619–1636.
37. Lemeshow S, Teres D, Pastides H, et al: A method for predicting survival and mortality of ICU patients using objectively derived weights. Crit Care Med 1985; 13:519–525.
38. Lemeshow S, Teres D, Klar J, et al: Mortality Probability Model (MPM II) based on an international cohort of intensive care unit patients. JAMA 1993; 270:2478–2486.
39. Le Gall, J-R, Loirat P, Alperovitch A, et al: A simplified acute physiology score for ICU patients. Crit Care Med 1984; 12:975–977.
40. Le Gall J-R, Lemeshow S, Saulnier F: A new Simplified Acute Physiology Score (SAPS II) based on a European/North American multicenter study. JAMA 1993; 270:2957–2963.
41. Lemeshow S, Klar J, Teres D, et al: Mortality probability models for patients in the intensive care unit for 48 or 72 hours: A prospective, multicenter study. Crit Care Med 1994; 22:1351–1358.
42. Pollack MM, Ruttimann UE, Getson PR: Pediatric risk of mortality (PRISM) score. Crit Care Med 1988; 16:1110–1116.
43. Baker SP, O'Neil B, Haddon W, Long WB: The Injury Severity Score: A method for describing patients with multiple injuries and evaluating emergency care. J Trauma 1974; 14:187–196.
44. Champion HR, Sacco WJ, Copes WS, Gann DS, Gennarelli TA, Flanagan ME: A revision of the trauma score. J Trauma 1992; 33:417–423.
45. Orr RK, Maini BS, Sottile FD, et al: A comparison of four severity-adjusted models to predict mortality after coronary artery bypass graft surgery. Arch Surg 1995; 130:301.
46. Becker RB, Zimmerman JE, Knaus WA, et al: The use of APACHE III to evaluate ICU length of stay, resource use, and mortality after coronary artery by-pass surgery. J Cardiovasc Surg 1995; 36:1–11.
47. Rowan KM, Kerr JH, Major E, et al: Intensive Care Society's Acute Physiology and Chronic Health Evaluation (APACHE II) study in Britain and Ireland: A prospective, multicenter, cohort study comparing two methods for predicting outcome for adult intensive care patients. Crit Care Med 1994; 22:1392–1401.
48. Schafer J-H, Maurer A, Jochimsen F, et al: Outcome prediction models on admission in a medical intensive care unit: Do they predict individual outcome? Crit Care Med 1990; 18:1111–1117.
49. Lemeshow S, Le Gall J-R: Modeling the severity of illness of ICU patients: A systems update. JAMA 1994; 272:1049–1055.
50. Castella X, Artigas A, Bion J, et al: A comparison of severity of illness scoring systems for intensive care unit patients: Results of a multicenter, multinational study. Crit Care Med 1995; 23:1327–1335.
51. Moreno R, Morais P: Outcome prediction in intensive care: Results of a prospective, multicentre, Portuguese study. Intensive Care Med 1997; 23:177–186.
52. Beck DH, Taylor BL, Millar B, Smith GB: Prediction of outcome from intensive care: A prospective cohort study comparing Acute Physiology and Chronic Health Evaluation II and III prognostic systems in a United Kingdom intensive care unit. Crit Care Med 1997; 25:9–15.
53. Kruse JA, Thill-Baharozian MC, Carlson RW: Comparison of clinical assessment with APACHE II for predicting mortality risk in patients admitted to a medical intensive care unit. JAMA 1988; 260:1739–1742.
54. Chang RWS, Jacobs S, Lee B: Use of APACHE II severity of disease classification to identify intensive care unit patients who would not benefit from total parenteral nutrition. Lancet 1986; 1:1483–1487.
55. Bion J: Prediction by APACHE score (Letter to the Editor). Lancet 1986; p 286.
56. Rogers J, Fuller HD: Use of daily Acute Physiology and Chronic Health Evaluation (APACHE) II scores to predict individual patient survival rate. Crit Care Med 1994; 22:1402–1405.
57. Barie PS, Hydo LJ, Fischer E: Development of multiple organ dysfunction syndrome in critically ill patients with perforated viscus. Arch Surg 1996; 131:37–43.
58. Wagner DP, Knaus WA, Harrell FE, et al: Daily prognostic estimates for critically ill adults in intensive care units: Results from a prospective, multicenter, inception cohort analysis. Crit Care Med 1994; 22:1359–1372.
59. Zimmerman JE, Wagner DP, Draper EA, Knaus WA: Improving intensive care unit discharge decisions: Supplementing physician judgment with predictions of next day risk for life support. Crit Care Med 1994; 22:1373–1384.
60. Bone RC, McElwee NE, Eubanks DH, Gluck EH: Analysis of indications for early discharge from the intensive care unit: Clinical efficacy assessment project. American College of Physicians. Chest 1993; 104:1812–1817.
61. Knaus WA, Wagner DP: Multiple systems organ failure: Epidemiology and prognosis. Crit Care Clin 1989; 5:221–232.
62. Solomkin JS, Dellinger EP, Christou NV, Busuttil RW: Results of a multicenter trial comparing imipenem/cilastatin to tobramycin/clindamycin for intra-abdominal infections. Ann Surg 1990; 212:581–591.
63. Knaus WA, Harrell FE, Fisher CJ, et al: The clinical evaluation of new drugs for sepsis: A prospective study design based on survival analysis. JAMA 1993; 270:1233–1241.
64. Knaus WA, Harrell FE, LaBrecque JF, et al: Use of predicted risk of mortality to evaluate the efficacy of anticytokine therapy in sepsis. Crit Care Med 1996; 24:46–56.
65. Le Gall J-R, Lemeshow S, Leleu G, et al: Customized probability models for early severe sepsis in adult intensive care patients. JAMA 1995; 273:644–650.
66. Presterl E, Staudinger T, Pettermann M, et al: Cytokine profile and correlation to the APACHE III and MPM II scores in patients with sepsis. Am J Respir Crit Care Med 1997; 156:825–832.
67. Knaus WA, Draper EA, Wagner DP, Zimmerman JE: An evaluation of outcome from intensive care in major medical center. Ann Intern Med 1986; 104:410–418.
68. Thomas JW, Ashcraft MLF: Measuring severity of illness: Six severity systems and their ability to explain cost variations. Inquiry 1991; 28:39–55.
69. Lockrem JD, Sirio CA: The use of intensive care unit severity scoring systems in reimbursement strategies. Crit Care Clin 1994; 10:145–156.
70. Rosenthal GE, Chren MM, Lasek RJ, Landefeld CS: The annual guide to "American's Best Hospitals": Evidence of influence among health care leaders. J Gen Intern 1996; 11:366–369.
71. Chassin MR, Hannan EL, DeBuono BA: Benefits and hazards of reporting medical outcomes publicly. N Engl J Med 1996; 334:394–398.
72. The SUPPORT Principal Investigators: A controlled trial to improve care for seriously ill hospitalized patients: The study to understand prognosis and preferences for outcomes and risks of treatment (SUPPORT). JAMA 1996; 274:1591–1598.
73. Summary Report: A Summary of Information from the Cleveland-Area Hospital Quality Outcome Measures and Patient Satisfaction Report. Quality Information Management Corporation. December 7, 1994; pp 1–36.
74. Clough JD, Kay R, Gombeski WR, et al: Mortality of patients transferred to a tertiary care hospital. Cleve Clin J Med 1993; 60:449–454.

75. Omoigui NA, Miller DP, Brown KJ, et al: Outmigration for coronary bypass surgery in an era of public dissemination of clinical outcomes. Circulation 1996; 93:27–33.
76. Doyle E: New breed of report cards turns up the heat on doctors. ACP Observer 1995; 15:1–12.
77. Localio AR, Hamory BH, Sharp TJ, et al: Comparing hospital mortality in adult patients with pneumonia: A case study of statistical methods in a managed care program. Ann Intern Med 1995; 122:125–132.
78. Iezzoni LI: How much are we willing to pay for information about quality of care? Ann Intern Med 1997; 126:391–393.
79. Kassirer JP: The use and abuse of practice profiles (Editorial). N Engl J Med 1994; 330:634–635.
80. Cowen JS, Kelley MA: Errors and bias in using predictive scoring systems. Crit Care Clin 1994; 10:53–72.
81. Teres D, Higgins T, Steingrub J, et al: Defining a high-performance ICU system for the 21st century: A position paper. J Intensive Care Med 1998; 13:195–205.

195

Benchmarking and Clinical Reengineering in the Intensive Care Unit

Jack E. Zimmerman, MD, FCCM • Michael G. Seneff, MD

Benchmarking, a process by which performance is compared to a standard, is an important part of any organization's integrated quality improvement plan. Hospital-based physicians have become increasingly interested in benchmarking techniques because of shrinking revenues, an oversupply of inpatient beds, and the need to reduce costs and at the same time improve the quality of care. One response to these constraints has been to indiscriminately downsize and cut costs evenly throughout the hospital. Unfortunately, this approach often leads to inefficient resource use, unhappy patients and staff, and financial disappointments. Another approach has been to use *operational reengineering,*[1, 2] a technique used by manufacturing and service corporations, to streamline operations in order to improve quality and decrease costs. *Reengineering* is defined as a fundamental rethinking and radical redesign of processes to achieve dramatic improvement in performance; when it is adapted to the health care delivery process, the term *clinical reengineering* is used.[3]

Reengineering is a multistage process involving identification, mobilization, assessment, redesign, implementation, and measurement (Fig. 195–1). When an opportunity to improve a clinical process is identified, reengineering begins with mobilization of a multidisciplinary team of staff members who are involved in the process to be improved. The assessment phase is the benchmarking process in which current care and outcomes are compared to existing practices, particularly those that have been identified as "best practices." The team next redesigns the existing process, often adopting some or all of the practices associated with superior performance, implements the changes, and then sets up a measurement process to continuously assess quality improvement. Each reengineering effort has unique features, but the general principles of the process are shown in Table 195–1.[2]

The intensive care unit (ICU) is a logical setting for clinical reengineering. Substantial cost reduction is possible, because critical care accounts for 10% to 15% of all inpatient beds; utilizes 25% of hospital resources; and accounts for 20% of all United States health care dollars.[4] In addition, the critical care team is often a tightly focused multidisciplinary group who are able to work together in solving problems. Potential ICU performance benchmarks that might be targets for reengineering are (1) the rate of complications, (2) mortality, (3) length of stay, (4) duration of mechanical ventilation, and (5) the use of ancillary resources such as radiologic or laboratory tests. Although mortality is important to patients and physicians as a marker of quality of care, it has a limited role in reengineering, for the following reasons[5, 6]:

1. Most ICUs have observed hospital mortality rates that are at or below the expected rate.
2. Survival after critical illness is influenced by care given on the regular floors as well as by ICU care processes.
3. Focusing on mortality alone provides little opportunity to improve efficiency and care processes.

In this chapter, therefore, we focus on nonmortality benchmarks.

There are three major barriers to improving ICU efficiency and resource use with benchmarking and clinical reengineering. First, information about optimal protocols and processes is often lacking. Identifying best practices may not be possible if a care process is unique to an individual ICU or if the team is developing novel care pathways. Second, information systems and data collection are commonly inadequate or incomplete. For example, determining whether an ICU's intravenous catheter-related infection rate is excessive can be difficult, because so many factors influence infection rate.

Third, to avoid "comparing apples with oranges," benchmarks must be adjusted for differences in case-mix, as defined by diagnosis, severity of illness, and other important outcome determinants. Possible approaches to case-mix adjustment are as follows:

1. A single ICU's performance can be compared over time. Provided that there is no major difference in case-mix, changes over time will be worthy of investigation. An example of this type of comparison includes assessment of the impact of the addition of an intensivist to an ICU's medical staff.[7–9]
2. An ICU's performance can be compared to that of units that have "similar" characteristics. Comparing the process of ICU care after cardiac surgery, for example, is possible because the patients, hospitals, and ICUs are often similar.
3. A scoring system can be used to compare an ICU's observed outcomes to a case-mix–adjusted standard. Scoring systems use statistical techniques to predict outcomes that are adjusted to reflect differences in diagnosis, severity of illness, and other important outcome determinants. The patient data on which these case-mix–adjusted outcome predictions are based provides the standard or benchmark, which is then compared with observed outcome.[3] Examples of scoring sys-

TABLE 195–1. Clinical Reengineering Principles

1. Use a multidisciplinary approach.
2. Reduce unnecessary administrative tasks.
3. Eliminate redundancies, non-value-added steps, unnecessary quality assurance, and approval layers.
4. Simplify points of contact and minimize movement of patients.
5. Establish accountability for all elements of the process.
6. Modernize information management systems and automate wherever possible.

Adapted with permission from Greeson D, Lowenhaupt M: A benchmark strategy. The Physician Executive, October 1996, p 10.

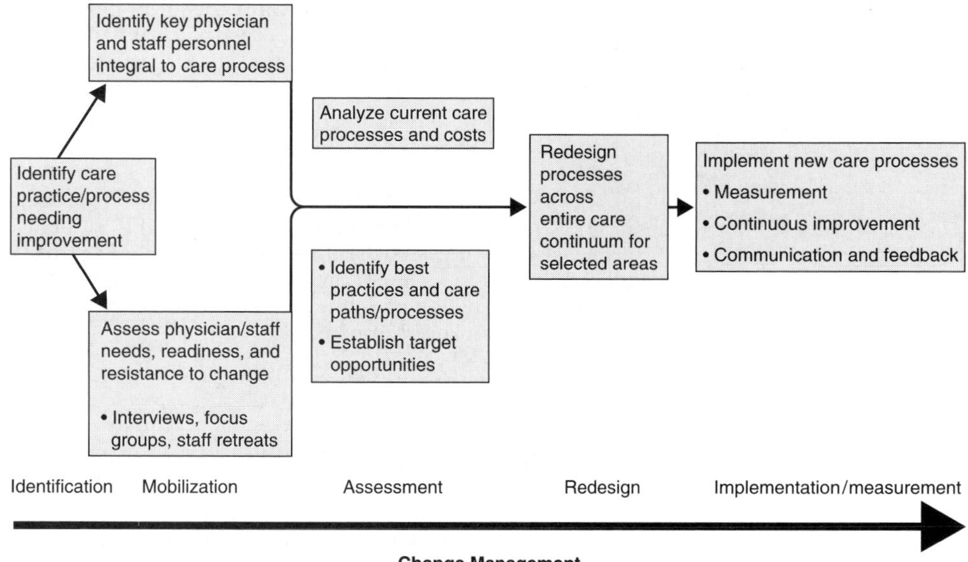

Figure 195–1. Phases of clinical reengineering. (Adapted from Greeson D, Lowenhaupt M: A benchmark strategy. The Physician Executive October 1996, p 10.)

tems that have been used in this manner are the Acute Physiology and Chronic Health Evaluation (APACHE) system and the Mortality Prediction Model (MPM).[10-13]

We emphasize that strict reliance on benchmarking to identify best practices can restrict a quality improvement team's thinking to the framework of what is already being done at other institutions. By aspiring only to be as good as the best, the team in effect sets a limit on its own ambitions, and benchmarking becomes a tool for catching up, not for jumping ahead. In our opinion, benchmarking is a useful tool for documenting how well an ICU can perform a particular service, and for initiating dialogue on how to achieve maximal performance. Reengineering, however, should focus on using any and all methods to improve, without regard to whether the process was already in existence at another institution or is radically new and unique.

In this chapter, we use the "fast-tracking" protocols that were developed for patients undergoing coronary artery bypass surgery as a model of successful benchmarking and clinical reengineering. We then summarize how benchmarks for ICU effectiveness and efficiency are being used to evaluate organizational and administrative structure and to improve the efficiency and quality of care in individual ICUs. Finally, we review how the latest benchmarks and process changes are being used to improve the use of specific ICU services.

BENCHMARKING AND REENGINEERING AFTER CORONARY ARTERY BYPASS SURGERY

The benchmarking and clinical reengineering techniques used for patients undergoing coronary artery bypass graft (CABG) surgery provide an excellent prototype for both the potential and the pitfalls of these methods. CABG surgery, because of high cost, large number of procedures, and varied outcomes, was an early target for assessment of risk-adjusted morbidity and mortality. During the past decade, multiple models were developed to compare observed and predicted mortality[14-18] and to evaluate postoperative complications[19-21] after CABG surgery. The benchmarks established by these risk-adjusted outcome predictions have each demonstrated institutional variations that are independent of case-mix. Benchmarking data have been publicly released in New York[22] and Pennsylvania[23] to help guide patients and referring physicians in selecting where they should seek care. The public release of risk-adjusted CABG mortality data, also known as "scorecards" or "report cards," has been highly controversial and engendered considerable criticism regarding methodology and ability to adjust for case-mix.[23-25]

Although many of these criticisms are valid, risk-adjusted mortality following CABG surgery did decrease after release of the data. This improvement in outcome has been attributed to (1) the public release of risk-adjusted mortality data,[22] (2) a shift of patients away from low-volume surgeons with high risk-adjusted mortality,[26] and (3) data feedback, training in continuous quality improvement, and focused observations by surgeons at other medical centers.[27] In a later report, however, similar decreases in CABG surgery mortality were identified in Massachusetts, a state with no program for quality improvement or public outcome reporting.[28] It is therefore possible that decreases in risk-adjusted mortality after CABG surgery are related to secular trends (i.e., widespread improvements over time) rather than to public reporting or quality improvement programs.

The publication of observed and predicted mortality data has been accompanied by a less controversial but equally important application of benchmarking. Faced with decreasing reimbursement for one of their economically most important services, hospitals have sought to improve their efficiency and reduce the cost of CABG surgery. Their major focus in accomplishing this goal was to shorten ICU and hospital length of stays. To do this, cardiac surgeons and anesthesiologists reengineered perioperative care using a combination of previously described clinical processes that were associated with a reduced hospital stay.[29-31] The reduced length of stay for these patients became a performance benchmark, and the reengineered clinical process was called "fast tracking" because it reduced the time patients remained intubated and shortened ICU and hospital length of stay. Many patients having elective CABG surgery are now extubated early (1 to 6 hours), stay in the ICU for 12 to 24 hours, and leave the hospital after 4 to 5 days. A prospective, randomized, controlled trial showed that fast tracking has reduced total costs per patient by 25%, predominantly through decreases in nursing and ICU costs.[32] Since their introduction, these protocols have been refined, their lack of impact on hospital morbidity and mortality in comparison with conventional care has been documented,[33, 34] and their impact on cost and resource use has been quantitated.[29, 32, 35]

Widespread adoption of fast-tracking protocols has been possible because the patients who receive this type of postoperative care are similar and their surgery is performed in hospitals and ICUs with similar characteristics. Although fast tracking was an economically motivated change in practice, the availability of case-mix-adjusted morbidity and mortality benchmarks made it possible to demonstrate that improved efficiency and reduced cost could be achieved with either no change or an improvement in patient outcomes.

The results of fast tracking after CABG surgery compare favorably with those of the widely criticized 1-day discharge after vaginal delivery, a practice that was implemented with little attention to impact on patient outcome.[36, 37] Despite doubts about the credibility of publicly released CABG mortality data, a consensus about these outcome measures has emerged, which can be summarized as follows[24, 38]:

- It is now widely accepted that outcomes should be measured.
- Patient care is a process that can be reengineered to improve results.
- Performance benchmarks are helpful in improving and achieving high-value health care.

We believe that the mortality and length of stay benchmarks and fast-tracking protocols used for CABG surgery represent a model for how benchmarking and clinical reengineering can be used to improve the effectiveness and efficiency of care for other ICU patient groups.

IMPROVING ICU PERFORMANCE: BENCHMARKING ACTIVITIES FOR THE INDIVIDUAL ICU

Previous experience with benchmarking and reengineering activities provides valuable lessons about how an individual ICU can improve its performance. These experiences suggest that efficiency can be improved by (1) changing management and administrative structure, (2) improving patient selection, (3) decreasing length of stay, and (4) optimizing resource use and the care of patients within specific diagnostic groups. Here, we discuss each of these topics separately and review how benchmarking and clinical reengineering techniques can be used to improve an ICU's structure and efficiency.

Management and Administrative Structure

The management and administrative structure of an ICU is the way in which an ICU is governed, its hierarchy, the characteristics of its staff, their tools, and how patient care decisions are made. Studies have demonstrated that certain ICU managerial and administrative structures are associated with better quality and more efficient care.[10, 39–42] The presence of a full-time medical director empowered to make triage decisions,[7, 9, 10] an on-site dedicated critical care team providing 24-hour coverage,[8] and conversion of an ICU management policy from an "open" to "closed"[42, 43] are examples of changes in structure that have improved efficiency. In our opinion, a first step in quality improvement for many ICUs should be to modify the administration and organization to reflect a more effective model (as discussed later), because units without these structural characteristics may be limited in their ability to adapt clinical reengineering techniques.

An excellent example of the importance of ICU management and administrative structure in performance was provided by a survey conducted in the University Health System Consortium (UHC). A benchmarking survey was conducted at 84 adult ICUs in 51 UHC hospitals across the United States in May and June 1996.[44, 45] The survey used the APACHE III prognostic scoring system to determine case-mix-adjusted ICU and hospital mortality, length of stay, and frequency of admissions of low-risk patients only for monitoring.[46, 47] The goals of the UHC project were to (1) support organizational improvement, (2) identify best practices, (3) develop systems to change clinical practice, and (4) maximize the value of patient care.

The best-performing ICUs in this survey had lower than expected risk-adjusted mortality rates, an average ICU length of stay less than expected with an average or lower readmission rate, and a lower than average frequency of low-risk monitoring admissions. ICUs with the best performance (top 10%) were asked to complete a questionnaire in order to identify their best practices. Although the UHC survey was limited because it involved only 125 to 200 admissions per unit, it yielded potentially useful information. The best-performing ICUs believed that their effectiveness and efficiency were associated with several structural characteristics:

- A critical care team empowered to make triage decisions
- A "closed" versus "open" ICU
- Access to an intermediate care or stepdown unit

These conclusions are supported by numerous other studies.[7–10, 42, 43, 48–52]

Improving Patient Selection for Intensive Care

Admitting only those patients who are most likely to benefit from ICU care could improve efficiency, reduce cost, and have little impact on mortality. Because such a strategy is perceived as "rationing" (not providing all the care expected to be beneficial to all patients), U.S. clinicians have avoided these methods.[53–55] ICU clinicians in the United States have instead focused on the ethical allocation of ICU resources.[56, 57] Although rationing does occur, it usually happens in individual cases and is not based on systematic guidelines.[58–60] In this discussion, we review some of the approaches for selecting patients for ICU admission that have been recommended to improve resource allocation. The methods for improving patient selection can be grouped into four general categories: (1) the use of outcome studies, (2) the use of prognostic scoring systems, (3) the use of futility guidelines, and (4) the development of alternatives to intensive care.

Outcome Studies

The first approach to improving selection for ICU care has been to avoid admitting patients who have been identified in outcome studies as being "unlikely" to benefit from intensive care.[61–63] Table 195-2 lists these patient groups and the published studies[64–89] indicating that such groups are likely to have a poor outcome from ICU care. Unfortunately, data are unavailable for most ICU patients, and the majority of the published data is not sufficient to accurately predict nonsurvival before ICU admission. As a result, patients with a poor prognosis usually receive a trial of ICU therapy. ICU admission is generally precluded only for patients who refuse therapy, are in a chronic vegetative state, or are brain-dead and not candidates for organ donation.[57, 63]

Prognostic Scoring Systems

A second approach to improving ICU resource allocation has been the proposed use of prognostic scoring systems to identify patients who have a low probability of survival.[63, 90] Be-

TABLE 195–2. Patient Groups That Are Unlikely to Benefit from Intensive Care

Patient Group	Chapter References	Limitations*
Respiratory failure after bone marrow transplant	64-66	Knowledge of poor prognosis has not influenced care[67]
Prolonged multiple organ system failure	68-70	Prognosis must reflect outcome from current therapy
Nontraumatic coma	71-74	Must exclude drugs or metabolic coma; highly publicized exceptions[75, 76]
Cardiac arrest	77-80	Poor communication about end-of-life decisions[81, 82]
Chronic liver disease	83-85	Prognosis can vary with new therapies[85]
Metastatic or hematologic malignancy and respiratory failure	66, 86-88	Different perceptions about prognosis[89]

*Superscript numbers indicate chapter references.

cause these systems were developed using data from patients who actually received ICU care, they cannot be used to determine whether a patient should be admitted to an ICU. In addition, the estimates provided by these systems were neither designed nor intended for individual prognostication.[11, 12] Severity systems, which use daily changes in physiology over time as a measure of response to therapy, may, however, assist physicians in deciding whether treatment should be escalated, maintained, or withdrawn after an individual patient has received a trial of therapy.[91-95] Nevertheless, these prognostic estimates cannot determine whether a patient should be admitted or whether a patient will live or die. In addition, there is little evidence that accurate prognostic data influence decision-making[82] or that the use of such data would affect the use of ICU resources.[82, 96]

Futility Guidelines

A third method for improving ICU resource allocation has been the proposed development of a rigorous definition of "medical futility." The Ethics Committee of the Society of Critical Care Medicine[97] defined futile treatment as treatment that has no beneficial physiologic effect. When defined in this fashion, futile treatment is rare and constitutes a small fraction of ICU care.

Schneiderman and colleagues[98-100] proposed a less restrictive definition. They regarded therapy as futile if it had been useless in the last 100 cases or had merely preserved permanent unconsciousness or continued ICU dependence. This proposal has been criticized because of a lack of consensus regarding definition, its value-laden content, prognostic uncertainty, and the potential for conflict with patient autonomy and religious beliefs.[101-103] To avoid some of these problems and to forge a consensus among medical professionals and the public, community guidelines for the use of intensive care are being developed in Denver, Colorado,[104] and a multi-institutional futility policy has actually been implemented in the greater Houston area.[105]

We object to the futility concept, for four reasons. First, prognostication is too imprecise. For example, among patients in the APACHE III and SUPPORT data bases, the median predicted chance of survival for 2 months was *14% to 17% on the day before actual death.*[106] Second, patient autonomy is a core value in our society, and most patients and physicians have not communicated about preferences for end-of-life care.[92, 107] Third, educational programs that emphasize an extremely poor prognosis (e.g., mechanical ventilation for bone marrow transplant recipients) do not alter practice even when physicians agree that likely outcome is dismal.[67] Fourth, although physicians are not ethically required to provide futile care, the legal status of physician refusal of requested care has not been fully established.[108, 109]

Alternatives to Intensive Care

A fourth approach to improving ICU resource allocation has been the development of intermediate or stepdown care units to provide graded care options that meet patient care needs.[110-112] The reported advantages of admission to an intermediate care unit include an improvement in ICU utilization,[52, 112-114] a reduction in ICU readmissions,[115] and a decrease in mortality on hospital wards.[113] The impact of intermediate care units on costs, however, is uncertain.[116]

Admitting patients to intermediate care units avoids the problems associated with formal ICU rationing policies but also requires an ability to identify candidates for early discharge from the ICU or patients who can safely be managed in an intermediate care unit rather than an ICU. Decisions about admission for intensive versus intermediate care and about ICU discharge are currently based on physician judgment alone. Reviews of the indications for ICU admission and discharge,[63, 90] however, have emphasized the need for objective methods to identify candidates for early ICU discharge or admission to an intermediate care unit. The methods of identifying these patients use diagnosis, age, severity of illness, and other patient characteristics to assess a low risk for mortality as well as a low (<10%) risk for receiving active life-supporting therapy.[47, 117] These studies have concentrated on the 20% to 77% of adult patients who are admitted to ICUs for monitoring rather than active life-supporting treatment.[47, 118-122] We emphasize that these risk predictions were designed to retrospectively identify groups of patients admitted for monitoring who were at a low risk for mortality and active treatment rather than to make ICU admission decisions for individual patients.

In the previously described UHC benchmarking survey of adult ICUs, an average of 19% of medical patients (range, 7% to 37%), 30% of surgical patients (range, 5% to 52%), and 29% of medical-surgical patients (range, 14% to 46%) admitted to ICUs for monitoring only were at a low (<10%) risk of receiving active life-supporting treatment.[44, 45] These data, obtained in May and June 1996, confirm that a substantial proportion of patients admitted to ICUs are at low risk and require monitor only, and that there are large variations in the frequency of admission for these patients among hospitals. Regression analysis of these data showed that two factors were associated with a lower proportion of low-risk monitoring admissions[45]:

- An intensivist who provided the majority of patient care
- A higher ICU occupancy rate (i.e., a lack of excess ICU capacity)

Table 195-3 summarizes the strategies that have been suggested by top-performing UHC ICUs for reducing low-risk monitoring admissions. Other reports suggest that a reduction

TABLE 195–3. Suggested Strategies for Reducing Frequency or Length of Stay in the Intensive Care Unit (ICU) for Low-Risk Monitoring Admissions

1. *Develop alternatives to ICU care.*
   a. Intermediate care unit (3–4:1 nurse-patient ratio)
   b. Acute care floor (9 nursing hours/patient/day)
   c. Flexible staffing in ICU, stepdown unit, and floor
2. *Restructure the ICU.*
   a. Number of low-risk monitor admissions is fewer in closed units.
   b. Full-time intensivists are associated with fewer low-risk monitoring admissions.
   c. Decrease excess ICU capacity; ICUs with high occupancy have fewer low-risk monitor admissions
3. *Improve patient selection for intensive care.*
   a. Develop detailed ICU admission and discharge criteria.
   b. Have critical care team screen all ICU admissions.
   c. Empower ICU medical director to enforce admission and discharge criteria.

in the proportion of low-risk monitoring patients results in better use of ICU resources and a modest reduction in cost.[47, 111, 118] Analysis of the services received by low-risk monitoring patients can also assist in planning and assessing the services provided in intermediate care units.[121, 122]

Decreasing ICU Length of Stay

To meet the challenges posed by decreases in reimbursement, hospitals have attempted to improve patient throughput.[123, 124] To do this, they have reduced hospital length of stay by streamlining admission and discharge practices and by standardizing care processes with care maps and guidelines.[125–127] In an analysis of more than 20,000 ICU admissions at 147 ICUs in 82 U.S. hospitals, both case-mix adjusted and unadjusted mean duration of hospital stay was 3.4 days shorter during 1993 to 1996 compared with a 1988 to 1990 benchmark.[128] For the same patients, however, case-mix–adjusted mean ICU length of stay during 1993 to 1996 did not differ significantly from the 1988–1990 benchmark.[129] Although not different in aggregate, ICU stays were significantly shorter for patients admitted for acute myocardial infarction, unstable angina, and rhythm disturbances; and longer for patients with pneumonia, subarachnoid hemorrhage, stroke, and diabetic ketoacidosis.

What can ICU clinicians do to reduce ICU length of stay? At present, we believe the example provided by CABG surgery represents the best prototype for achieving a safe reduction in ICU stay. Like cardiac surgeons, we now have reliable and valid tools to assess risk-adjusted mortality for multidiagnostic patient groups in adult,[46, 130] pediatric,[131] and neonatal[132] ICUs. We also have case-mix–adjusted measures of ICU length of stay for adult[46, 129] and pediatric[133] ICU patients. We understand that intensive care is expensive care and we can begin to reengineer care using methods similar to those used by cardiac surgeons.

Fast tracking is no longer a process unique to CABG surgery; there are now similar protocols for reducing ICU length of stay following liver transplantation,[134] carotid endarterectomy,[135, 136] and nonaortic arterial surgery.[137, 138] In addition, multi-institutional benchmarking data can now be used to (1) identify ICUs with a significantly shorter case-mix–adjusted ICU length of stay and (2) assess the practices that might account for these findings. Table 195–4 lists the strategies for reducing ICU stay suggested by the best-performing ICUs (top 10%) in the UHC survey.[44] Multidisciplinary teams seeking to reduce their ICU's length of stay can use these suggestions in their clinical reengineering efforts.

Improving Resource Use in the ICU

Virtually any disease treatment pathway or practice involving the use of ICU resources can be clinically reengineered. A major barrier to reengineering, however, is the lack of benchmarks that are case-mix adjusted. Sicker patients necessarily utilize more laboratory, radiologic, and therapeutic resources, and make comparisons invalid if the benchmark is not based on data from similar patients. One way to avoid this problem is to compare overall utilization within a single ICU prior to and then after a particular intervention. For example, the number of laboratory requests at one institution was decreased after redesign of the request form.[139] As long as admitting and referral patterns were unchanged, the conclusion that request form redesign was responsible for the decrease in laboratory utilization is probably valid.

Later efforts have emphasized the adaptation of clinical reengineering techniques to development of comprehensive protocols and practice guidelines that govern appropriate disease-specific test ordering and insertion of arterial catheters.[140–142] Roberts and colleagues[142] used a management data base to track the use of 123 laboratory investigations during a 7-month period, and targeted nine frequently ordered tests for reduction. Specific guidelines for ordering these tests were developed by a multidisciplinary committee and then were applied for all patients admitted to the ICU for a 1-year intervention and 2-year follow-up period. There was a significant reduction for all nine of the targeted tests as well as in 13 of the 114 nontargeted tests, with an estimated annual cost savings of more than $150,000 Canadian. Because the authors were unable to identify any significant change in the study population before and after intervention (comparing age, sex, APACHE II score, and admitting diagnosis), it is likely that the reduction in laboratory tests was actually due to a change in physician ordering behavior rather than differences in case-mix.[142]

In our ICU, we have initiated a multistage clinical reengineering project designed to improve laboratory utilization. We use an equation that predicts laboratory utilization on ICU day 2 on the basis of severity of disease and other patient characteristics from ICU day 1. The predicted number of blood samples drawn on ICU day 2 is used as a case-mix–adjusted benchmark for laboratory utilization that is based on a sample of more than 17,000 admissions from 42 ICUs in the United States.[143] Stage 1 of the project involved an initial assessment of current risk-adjusted blood-sampling practices.

TABLE 195–4. Suggested Strategies for Reducing Length of Stay in the Intensive Care Unit (ICU)

1. *Reengineer the patient transfer process.*
   a. Make "night before" ICU discharge decisions.
   b. Empower the ICU director to make decisions.
   c. Develop a multidisciplinary team to identify and solve systematic problems.
2. *Identify alternatives to ICU care.*
   a. Provide access to intermediate or acute care units.
   b. Develop special units for chronic critical illness.
   c. Implement "sitter" programs for confused, agitated, or potentially suicidal patients.
3. *Develop physician incentives.*
   a. Prolonged ICU stay is costly for hospitals but generates revenue for physicians; indirect rewards (e.g., office space, secretarial support) can be funded using savings from reductions in ICU stay.

Our multidisciplinary critical care staff then developed and instituted comprehensive, literature-based protocols governing insertion and removal of arterial catheters, use of insulin infusions and anticoagulation nomograms, ordering of routine laboratory tests, and measurements of antibiotic drug levels. These protocols were collated into a handbook that is given to all house officers at the start of their ICU rotations. We are now measuring the impact of these protocols on laboratory utilization, with the intent of continuously monitoring and altering the protocols as necessary. We will also continue to monitor risk-adjusted hospital mortality to assess the impact of a reduction in laboratory utilization on these outcomes.[143]

Other ICU activities in which benchmarking and clinical reengineering have been applied to improve performance include ventilator weaning,[144-146] catheter-related infection,[147] and antibiotic utilization.[148-152]

Ventilator Weaning

A decrease in duration of ventilation through introduction of weaning protocols has been documented in several studies. These studies have included trials of respiratory therapist–determined spontaneous breathing (using continuous positive airway pressure or T pieces)[144, 145] and the use of a bedside work-of-breathing monitor.[146] For example, Kollef and associates[145] conducted a randomized, controlled trial in patients requiring mechanical ventilation to compare the existing method of physician-directed weaning to a new protocol involving nurses and respiratory therapists. The ICU medical directors developed the new protocol, and nursing and respiratory staff participated in a 1-month training period prior to its implementation. Outcomes for the group receiving protocol-directed weaning (179 patients), including duration of ventilation and complications, were compared with those for the group receiving traditional physician-directed weaning (178 patients). Mortality was 22.3% and median duration of weaning was 35 hours in the protocol group, versus 23.6% and 44 hours, respectively, in the traditional care group. Total hospital cost savings for the patient group who had protocol-directed weaning was $42,960 compared with the patient group that had physician-directed weaning.[145] This study is a good example of an effective reengineering process that used existing staff and unit resources to achieve a significant cost savings and an improvement in patient care.

Catheter-Related Infections

Catheter-related infection (CRI) is a common nosocomial complication that adds significantly to a patient's overall cost of care and length of hospital stay. The rate of infection is affected by many variables, including the route of catheter insertion, method of disinfection, type of catheter, dressing, operator experience, and use of sterile technique.[153] Studies have shown that CRIs can be decreased by improving sterile technique (triple barriers),[154] using chlorhexadine gluconate for site preparation,[155] or using antibiotic-impregnated catheters.[156]

In our experience, many institutions do not have uniform catheter insertion or management protocols, and this lack represents one clear opportunity to affect patient care favorably and reduce expenditures. Many studies have proved that the incidence of CRI decreases dramatically after the introduction of relatively simple guidelines, protocols, and educational programs.[157] For example, Civetta and associates,[147] using continuous quality improvement management techniques, developed new catheter insertion and maintenance protocols to be used with antibiotic-coated or antiseptic-coated catheters. They were able to demonstrate a reduction in CRIs and significant cost savings in their critical care practice.[147]

Utilization of Antibiotics

A final example of performance improvement using benchmarking and clinical reengineering is their use in improving antibiotic utilization.[148-152] Pestotnik and coworkers[152] developed a comprehensive antibiotic management program that used computer-assisted decision support programs and clinician-derived consensus guidelines. Prescribing guidelines were developed for prophylactic, empiric, and therapeutic uses of antibiotics. Over a 7-year period, antibiotic use improved, antibiotic-associated costs decreased, the emergence of antimicrobial resistance patterns stabilized, and there was improvement or no change in outcomes and antibiotic complications.[152] The same researchers have reported similar success using a computer-assisted program for antibiotic use in a 12-bed surgical intensive care unit.

Rifenburg and associates[150] used benchmarking techniques to analyze the strategies hospitals use to control antibiotic expenditures. They demonstrated that a policy of formulary restriction is ineffective in significantly reducing antibiotic costs and may even aggravate resistance problems. Schentag and colleagues[149, 151] developed a protocol that allows clinicians to choose the empirical antibiotic of their choice on day 1, as long as the antibiotic is changed on day 3 to a more selective agent (or oral form) on the basis of culture results.[149, 151] All antibiotic dosing and changes are based on nomograms and clinical recommendations provided by an antibiotic consultation service. Implementation of this strategy saved the group's hospital more than $1 million yearly in antibiotic costs alone, with stabilized to improved resistance patterns.[149] Given the emergence of dangerous organisms, such as vancomycin-resistant enterococci and vancomycin-methicillin–resistant staphylococci, all hospitals need to employ strategies that improve antibiotic utilization.

CLINICAL CARE PATHWAYS

Clinical care pathways are an adaptation of the critical path method of project planning that was originally developed for use in industry in the mid-1950s.[158] Care pathways use a multidisciplinary perspective to develop methods for improving the quality and cost effectiveness of care delivery. Although care pathways may be limited to the establishment of protocols for existing care, their optimal development requires the application of clinical reengineering and benchmarking techniques. The use of care pathways, also known as "care maps," "critical paths," and "case management," was introduced to the hospital setting in the early 1990s and is most often applied to patients within specific diagnostic groups. Examples of diagnosis-specific care pathways that have been successful in standardizing patient care while decreasing length of stay and hospital costs are those used after CABG surgery, total hip or knee replacement, subarachnoid hemorrhage, chronic obstructive pulmonary disease, and prolonged mechanical ventilation.[158-160] As discussed previously, fast tracking utilized in CABG surgery is essentially a care pathway that has now been adapted to other procedures, such as carotid endarterectomy and nonaortic vascular surgery.

SUMMARY

Clinical reengineering techniques are increasingly being used in critical care medicine to improve quality and efficiency and control costs of care as well as to help hospitals remain competitive in the modern health care environment. Benchmarking is an important tool and part of an integrated reengineering program, but participants in the process must be careful to not be limited by striving only to be better. The intensive care unit is an ideal area in which to apply reengineering efforts because of the high cost of critical care and the presence (optimally) of a highly committed and focused multidisciplinary health care team. Fast tracking after CABG surgery is an excellent example of a successful benchmarking and reengineering program. Similar techniques can be applied to many facets of intensive care, and we have provided examples of how they have been used to improve patient selection, decrease length of stay, optimize resource utilization, and streamline the care for specific diagnoses. Critical care physicians and nurse managers need to be familiar with reengineering and benchmarking techniques so that they can lead the efforts within their own institutions to improve the efficacy and efficiency of patient care.

FINANCIAL DISCLOSURE

Dr. Zimmerman is a founder and equity shareholder of, and receives research support from, APACHE Medical Systems (AMS) Inc., a for-profit Delaware-based corporation. AMS markets a software-based clinical information system for critical care units and holds the commercial copyright on the APACHE III data base and several of the predictive equations discussed in this chapter. Dr. Seneff is an equity shareholder of AMS and also receives financial support from AMS in the form of research grants.

References

1. Hammer M, Champy J: Reengineering the Corporation. New York, Harper Collins, 1993.
2. Greeson D, Lowenhaupt M: A benchmark strategy. The Physician Executive; October 1996, p 10.
3. Dobb GJ: "Benchmarking" in intensive care. Intensive Care World 1996; 13:88.
4. Coalition for Critical Care Excellence: ICU Cost Reduction: Practical Suggestions and Future Considerations. Society of Critical Care Medicine, 1994, pp 1–49.
5. Jiang HJ, Fielselmann JF, Hendryx MS, et al: Assessing the impact of patient characteristics and process performance on rural intensive care unit hospital mortality rates. Crit Care Med 1997; 25:773.
6. Josephson MA, Agger WA, Bennett CL, et al: Performance measurement in pneumonia care: Beyond report cards. Mayo Clin Proc 1998; 73:5.
7. Mallick R, Strosberg M, Lambrinos J, et al: The intensive care unit director as manager: Impact on performance. Med Care 1995; 33:611.
8. Carlson RW, Weiland DE, Srivathsan K: Does a full-time, 24-hour intensivist improve care and efficiency? Crit Care Clin 1996; 12:525.
9. Manthous CA, Amoateng-Adjepong Y, Al-Kharrat T, et al: Effects of a medical intensivist on patient care in a community teaching hospital. Mayo Clin Proc 1997; 72:391.
10. Zimmerman JE, Shortell SM, Rousseau DM, et al: Improving intensive care: Observations based on organizational case studies in nine intensive care units: A prospective, multicenter study. Crit Care Med 1993; 21:1443.
11. Knaus WA, Wagner DP, Draper EA, et al: The APACHE III prognostic system: Risk prediction of hospital mortality for critically ill hospitalized adults. Chest 1991; 100:1619.
12. Lemeshow S, Teres D, Klar J, et al: Mortality probability models (MPM II) based on an international cohort of intensive care unit patients. JAMA 1993; 270:2478.
13. Rapoport J, Teres D, Lemeshow S, et al: A method for assessing the clinical performance and cost-effectiveness of intensive care units: A multicenter inception cohort study. Crit Care Med 1994; 22:1285.
14. Hannan EL, Kilburn H, O'Donell JF, et al: Adult open heart surgery in New York State: An analysis of risk factors and hospital mortality rates. JAMA 1990; 264:2768.
15. O'Connor GT, Plume SK, Olmstead EM, et al: A regional prospective study of in-hospital mortality associated with coronary artery bypass grafting. JAMA 1991; 266:803.
16. Higgins TL, Estafanous FG, Loop FD, et al: Stratification of morbidity and mortality outcome by preoperative risk factors in coronary artery bypass patients: A clinical severity score. JAMA 1992; 267:2344.
17. Becker RB, Zimmerman JE, Knaus WA, et al: The use of APACHE III to evaluate ICU length of stay, resource use, and mortality after coronary artery bypass surgery. J Cardiovasc Surg 1995; 36:1.
18. Clark RE: The STS cardiac surgery national database: An update. Ann Thorac Surg 1995; 59:1376.
19. Geraci JM, Rosen AK, Ash AS, et al: Predicting the occurrence of adverse events after coronary artery bypass surgery. Ann Intern Med 1993; 118:18.
20. Silber JH, Rosenbaum PR, Schwartz S, et al: Evaluation of the complication rate as a measure of quality of care in coronary artery bypass graft surgery. JAMA 1995; 274:317.
21. Shaughnessy TE, Mickler TA: Does acute physiologic and chronic health evaluation (APACHE II) scoring predict need for prolonged support after coronary revascularization? Anesth Analg 1995; 81:24.
22. Hannan EL, Kilburn H, Racz M, et al: Improving the outcomes of coronary artery bypass surgery in New York State. JAMA 1994; 271:761.
23. Schneider EC, Epstein AM: Influence of cardiac surgery performance reports on referral practices and access to care. N Engl J Med 1996; 335:251.
24. Topol EJ, Califf RM: Scorecard cardiovascular medicine: Its impact and future directions. Ann Intern Med 1994; 120:65.
25. Green J, Wintfeld N: Report cards on cardiac surgeons: Assessing New York State's approach. N Engl J Med 1995; 332:1229.
26. Hannan EL, Siu AL, Kumar D, et al: The decline in coronary artery bypass graft surgery mortality in New York State: The role of surgeon volume. JAMA 1995; 273:209.
27. O'Connor GT, Pume SK, Olmstead EM, et al: A regional intervention to improve the hospital mortality associated with coronary artery bypass surgery. JAMA 1996; 275:841.
28. Ghali WA, Ash AS, Hall RE, et al: Statewide quality improvement initiatives and mortality after cardiac surgery. JAMA 1997; 277:379.
29. Krohn BG, Kay JH, Mendez MA, et al: Rapid sustained recovery after cardiac operations. J Thorac Cardiovasc Surg 1990; 100:194.
30. Cotton P: Fast-track improves CABG outcomes. JAMA 1993; 270:2023.
31. Anderson RP, Guyton SW, Paull DL, et al: Selection of patients for same-day coronary bypass operations. J Thorac Cardiovasc Surg 1993; 105:444.
32. Cheng DCH, Karske J, Peniston C, et al: Early tracheal extubation after coronary artery bypass graft surgery reduces costs and improves resource use: A prospective, randomized, controlled trial. Anesthesiology 1996; 85:1300.
33. Engelman RM: Mechanisms to reduce hospital stays. Ann Thorac Surg 1996; 61(Suppl):S26.
34. Reyes A, Vega G, Blancas R, et al: Early vs conventional extubation after cardiac surgery with cardiopulmonary bypass. Chest 1997; 112:193.
35. Cheng DCH: Early extubation after cardiac surgery decreases intensive care unit stay and cost. J Cardiothorac Vasc Anesth 1995; 9:460.
36. Annas GJ: Women and children first. N Engl J Med 1995; 333:1647.
37. Braveman P, Kessel W, Egerter S, et al: Early discharge and evidence-based practice: Good science and good judgment. JAMA 1997; 278:334.
38. Jencks SF: Can large-scale interventions improve care (Editorial)? JAMA 1997; 277:419.
39. Knaus WA, Draper EA, Wagner DP, et al: An evaluation of outcome from intensive care in major medical centers. Ann Intern Med 1986; 104:410.
40. Shortell SM, Zimmerman JE, Rousseau DM, et al: The perfor-

mance of intensive care units: Does good management make a difference? Med Care 1994; 32:508.

41. Bastos PG, Knaus WA, Zimmerman JE, et al: The importance of technology for achieving superior outcomes from intensive care. Intensive Care Med 1996; 22:664.
42. Carson SS, Stocking C, Podsadecki T, et al: Effects of organizational change in the medical intensive care unit of a teaching hospital: A comparison of "open" and "closed" formats. JAMA 1996; 276:322.
43. Multz AS, Samson I: A "closed" ICU is more efficient compared to an "open" ICU (Abstract). Crit Care Med 1997; 25:A106.
44. Sirio CA, Coleman MB: Results of the University Health System Consortium adult ICU benchmarking survey. *In* Proceedings of the Fifth Annual APACHE User Group, San Diego, April 18–20, 1997.
45. Sirio CA, Coleman MB, McGrath B, et al: The impact of intensivists and ICU occupancy on rates of low risk-monitor-only admissions to the ICU (Abstract). Chest 1997; 112(Suppl):16S.
46. Knaus WA, Wagner DP, Zimmerman JE, et al: Variations in mortality and length of stay in intensive care units. Ann Intern Med 1993; 118:753.
47. Zimmerman JE, Wagner DP, Knaus WA, et al: The use of risk predictions to identify candidates for intermediate care units: Implications for intensive care utilization and cost. Chest 1995; 108:490.
48. Rafkin H, Powner M, Hoyt J: Twenty four hour coverage decreases length of stay in the intensive care unit (ICU) without compromising survival. Crit Care Med 1997; 25:A106.
49. Pollock MM, Katz RW, Ruttimann UE, et al: Improving the outcome and efficiency of intensive care: The impact of an intensivist. Crit Care Med 1988; 16:11.
50. Rapoport J, Teres D, Lemeshow S, et al: A comparison of resource utilization in Alberta and western Massachusetts. Crit Care Med 1995; 23:1336.
51. Brown JJ, Sullivan G: Effect on ICU mortality of a full-time critical care specialist. Chest 1989; 96:127.
52. Byrick RJ, Mazer D, Caskennette FM: Closure of an intermediate care unit: Impact on critical care utilization. Chest 1993; 104:876.
53. Osborne M, Patterson J: Ethical allocation of ICU resources: A view from the U.S.A. Intensive Care Med 1996; 22:1009.
54. Kalb PE, Miller DH: Utilization strategies for intensive care units. JAMA 1989; 261:2389.
55. Snider GL: Allocation of intensive care: The physician's role. Am J Respir Crit Care Med 1994; 150:575.
56. Lanken PM, Terry PB, Osborne ML: Ethics of allocating intensive care unit resources. New Horiz 1997; 5:38.
57. Society of Critical Care Medicine Ethics Committee: Consensus statement on the triage of critically ill patients. JAMA 1994; 271:1200.
58. Singer DE, Carr PL, Mulley AG, et al: Rationing intensive care: Physician responses to a resource shortage. N Engl J Med 1983; 309:1155.
59. Strauss MJ, LoGerfo JP, Yeltlatzie JA, et al: Rationing of intensive care unit services: An everyday occurrence. JAMA 1986; 225:1143.
60. Marshall MF, Schwenzer KJ, Orsina M, et al: Influence of political power, medical provincialism, and economic incentives on the rationing of surgical intensive care unit beds. Crit Care Med 1992; 20:387.
61. Streat S, Judson JA: Cost containment: New Zealand. New Horiz 1994; 2:392.
62. Teres D: Civilian triage in the intensive care unit: The ritual of the last bed. Crit Care Med 1993; 21:598.
63. Bone RC, McElwee NE, Eubanks DH, et al: Analysis of indications for intensive care unit admission: Clinical Efficacy Project, American College of Physicians. Chest 1993; 104:1806.
64. Crawford SW, Petersen FB: Long-term survival from respiratory failure after marrow transplantation for malignancy. Am J Respir Crit Care Med 1992; 145:510.
65. Paz HL, Crilley P, Weinar M, et al: Outcomes of patients requiring medical ICU admission following bone marrow transplantation. Chest 1993; 104:527.
66. Rubenfeld GD, Crawford SW: Withdrawing life support from mechanically ventilated recipients of bone marrow transplantation: A case for evidence-based guidelines. Ann Intern Med 1996; 125:625.
67. Paz HL, Garland A, Weinar M, et al: Effect of clinical outcomes data on intensive care unit utilization by bone marrow transplant patients. Crit Care Med 1998; 26:66.
68. Knaus WA, Draper EA, Wagner DP, et al: Prognosis in acute organ-system failure. Ann Surg 1985; 202:685.
69. Zimmerman JE, Knaus WA, Wagner DP, et al: A comparison of risks and outcomes for patients with organ system failure: 1982–1990. Crit Care Med 1996; 24:1633.
70. Villar J, Manzanno JJ, Blazquez MA, et al: Multiple system organ failure in acute respiratory failure. J Crit Care 1991; 6:75.
71. Levy DE, Bates D, Caronna JJ, et al: Prognosis in nontraumatic coma. Ann Intern Med 1981; 94:293.
72. Hamel MB, Goldman L, Teno J, et al: Identification of comatose patients at high risk for death or severe disability. JAMA 1995; 273:1842.
73. Edgren E, Hedstrand U, Kelsey S, et al: Assessment of neurological prognosis in comatose survivors of cardiac arrest. Lancet 1994; 343:1055.
74. Tuhrim S, Horowitz DR, Sacher M, et al: Validation and comparison of models predicting survival following intracerebral hemorrhage. Crit Care Med 1995; 23:950.
75. The Multi-Society Task Force on PVS: Medical aspects of the persistent vegetative state. N Engl J Med 1994; 330:1572.
76. Childs NL, Mercer WN: Late improvement in consciousness after post-traumatic vegetative state. N Engl J Med 1996; 334:24.
77. Bedell SE, Delbanco TL, Cook EF, et al: Survival after cardiopulmonary resuscitation in the hospital. N Engl J Med 1983; 309:569.
78. Levy DE, Caronna JJ, Singer BH: Predicting outcome from hypoxic-ischemic coma. JAMA 1985; 253:1420.
79. Gray WA, Capone RJ, Most AS: Unsuccessful emergency medical resuscitation—are continued efforts in the emergency department justified? N Engl J Med 1991; 325:1393.
80. Murphy DJ, Finucane TE: New do-not-resuscitate policies. Arch Intern Med 1993; 153:1641.
81. Murphy DJ, Burrows D, Santilli S, et al: The influence of the probability of survival on patients' preferences regarding cardiopulmonary resuscitation. N Engl J Med 1994; 330:545.
82. Phillips RS, Wenger NS, Teno J, et al: Choices of seriously ill patients about cardiopulmonary resuscitation: Correlates and outcomes. Am J Med 1996; 100:128.
83. Goldfarb G, Novel O, Poynard T, et al: Efficacy of respiratory assistance in cirrhotic patients with liver failure. Intensive Care Med 1983; 16:671.
84. Shellman RG, Fulkerson WJ, DeLong E, et al: Prognosis of patients with cirrhosis and chronic liver disease admitted to the medical intensive care unit. Crit Care Med 1988; 16:671.
85. Zimmerman JE, Wagner DP, Seneff MG, et al: Intensive care unit admissions with cirrhosis: Risk stratifying patient groups and predicting individual survival. Hepatology 1996; 23:1393.
86. Schuster DP, Marion JM: Precedents for meaningful recovery during treatment in a medical intensive care unit: Outcome in patients with hematologic malignancy. Am J Med 1983; 75:402.
87. Peters SG, Medows JA, Gracey DR: Outcome of respiratory failure in hematologic malignancy. Chest 1988; 94:99.
88. Schapira DV, Studnicki J, Bradham DD, et al: Intensive care, survival, and expense of treating critically ill cancer patients. JAMA 1993; 269:783.
89. Poses RM, Bekes C, Copare FJ, et al: The answer to "what are my chances, doctor?" depends on whom is asked: Prognostic disagreement and inaccuracy for critically ill patients. Crit Care Med 1989; 17:827.
90. Bone RC, McElwee NE, Eubanks DH, et al: Analysis of indications for early discharge from the intensive care unit: Clinical Efficacy Project, American College of Physicians. Chest 1993; 104:1812.
91. Wu AW, Damiano AM, Lynn J, et al: Predicting future functional status for seriously ill hospitalized adults: The SUPPORT prognostic model. Ann Intern Med 1995; 122:342.
92. The SUPPORT principal investigators: A controlled trial to improve care for seriously ill hospitalized patients. JAMA 1995; 274:1591.
93. Wagner DP, Knaus WA, Harrell FE, et al: Daily prognostic estimates for critically ill adults in intensive care units: Results from

a prospective, multicenter, inception cohort analysis. Crit Care Med 1994; 22:1359.
94. Esserman L, Belkora J, Lenert L: Potentially ineffective care: A new outcome to assess the limits of critical care. JAMA 1995; 274:1544.
95. Cher DJ, Lenert LA: Method of medicare reimbursement and the rate of potentially ineffective care of critically ill patients. JAMA 1997; 278:1001.
96. Teno JM, Murphy D, Lynn J, et al: Prognosis-based futility guidelines: Does anyone win? J Am Geriatr Soc 1994; 42:1202.
97. The Ethics Committee of the Society of Critical Care Medicine: Consensus statement of the Society of Critical Care Medicine's Ethics Committee regarding futile and other possible inadvisable treatments. Crit Care Med 1997; 25:887.
98. Schneiderman LJ, Jecker NS, Jonsen AR: Medical futility: Its meaning and ethical implications. Ann Intern Med 1990; 112:949.
99. Schneiderman LJ, Jecker NS: Futility in practice. Arch Intern Med 1993; 153:437.
100. Schneiderman LJ, Jecker NS, Jonsen AR: Medical futility: Response to critiques. Ann Intern Med 1996; 125:669.
101. Truog RD, Brett AS: The problem with futility. N Engl J Med 1992; 327:1560.
102. Loewy EH, Carlson RA: Futility and its wider implications: A concept in need of further examination. Arch Intern Med 1993; 153:429.
103. Curtis JR, Park DR, Krone MR, et al: Use of the medical futility rationale in do-not-attempt-resuscitation orders. JAMA 1995; 273:124.
104. Murphy DJ, Barbour E: GUIDe (Guidelines for the Use of Intensive Care in Denver): A community effort to define futile and inappropriate care. New Horiz 1994; 2:326.
105. Halevy A, Brody BA: A multiinstitutional collaborative policy on medical futility. JAMA 1996; 276:571.
106. Lynn J, Harrell F, Cohn F, et al: Prognoses of seriously ill hospitalized patients on the days before death: Implications for patient care and public policy. New Horiz 1997; 5:56.
107. Hofmann JC, Wenger NS, Davis RB, et al: Patient preferences for communication with physicians about end-of-life decisions. Ann Intern Med 1997; 127:1.
108. Luce JM: Physicians do not have a responsibility to provide futile or unreasonable care if the patient or family insists. Crit Care Med 1995; 23:760.
109. Civetta JM: Futile care or caregiver frustration? A practical approach. Crit Care Med 1996; 24:346.
110. Popovich J: Intermediate care units: Graded care options. Chest 1991; 99:4.
111. Elpern EH, Silver MR, Rosen RL, et al: The noninvasive respiratory care unit: Patterns of use and financial implications. Chest 1991; 99:205.
112. Mazer CD, Byrick RJ, Sibbald WJ, et al: Postoperative utilization of critical care services by cardiac surgery: A multicenter study in the Canadian healthcare system. Crit Care Med 1993; 21:851.
113. Franklin CM, Rackow EC, Mamdani B, et al: Decreases in mortality on a large urban medical service by facilitating access to critical care: An alternative to rationing. Arch Intern Med 1988; 148:1403.
114. Byrick RJ, Power JD, Ycas JO, et al: Impact of an intermediate care area on utilization after cardiac surgery. Crit Care Med 1986; 14:869.
115. Durbin CG, Kopel RF: A case-control study of patients readmitted to the intensive care unit. Crit Care Med 1993; 21:1547.
116. Keenan SP, Massel D, Inman KJ, et al: A systematic review of cost-effectiveness of noncardiac transitional care units. Chest 1998; 113:172.
117. Zimmerman JE, Wagner DP, Draper EA, et al: Improving intensive care unit discharge decisions: Supplementing physician judgment with predictions of next day risk for life support. Crit Care Med 1994; 22:1373.
118. Wagner DP, Knaus WA, Draper EA: Identification of low-risk monitor admissions to medical-surgical ICUs. Chest 1987; 92:423.
119. Groeger JS, Guntupalli KK, Strosberg M, et al: Descriptive analysis of critical care units in the United States: Patient characteristics and intensive care unit utilization. Crit Care Med 1993; 21:279.
120. Oye RK, Bellamy PE: Patterns of resource consumption in medical intensive care. Chest 1991; 99:685.
121. Zimmerman JE, Wagner DP, Sun X, et al: Planning patient services for intermediate care units: Insights based on care for intensive care unit low-risk monitor admissions. Crit Care Med 1996; 24:1626.
122. Zimmerman JE, Junker CD, Becker RB, et al: Neurological intensive care unit admissions: Identifying candidates for intermediate care and the services they receive. Neurosurgery 1998; 42:91.
123. Schwartz WB, Mendelson DN: Hospital cost containment in the 1980s: Hard lessons learned and prospects for the 1990s. N Engl J Med 1991; 324:1037.
124. Parisi VM, Meyer BA: To stay or not to stay? That is the question. N Engl J Med 1995; 333:1635.
125. Hay JA, Lyubashevsky E, Elashoff J, et al: Upper gastrointestinal hemorrhage clinical guideline—determining the optimal hospital length of stay. Am J Med 1996; 100:313.
126. Hay JA, Maldonado L, Weingarten SR, et al: Prospective evaluation of a clinical guideline recommending hospital length of stay for upper gastrointestinal tract hemorrhage. JAMA 1997; 278:2151.
127. Weingarten SR, Riedinger MS, Conner L, et al: Practice guidelines and reminders to reduce duration of hospital stay for patients with chest pain: An interventional trial. Ann Intern Med 1994; 120:257.
128. Zimmerman JE, Rosenberg AL, Wagner DP, et al: Changes in hospital length of stay for ICU admissions 1988–1990 vs. 1993–1996 (Abstract). Crit Care Med 1997; 25 (Suppl):A107.
129. Rosenberg AL, Zimmerman JE, Seneff MG, et al: Differences in hospital mortality and resource use for ICU admissions over a five year period (Abstract). Crit Care Med 1997; 25 (Suppl):A107.
130. Zimmerman JE, Wagner DP, Draper EA, et al: Evaluation of acute physiology and chronic health evaluation (APACHE) III predictions of hospital mortality in an independent database. Crit Care Med 1998; 26:1317.
131. Pollack MM, Patel KM, Ruttimann UE: PRISM III: An updated pediatric risk of mortality score. Crit Care Med 1996; 24:743.
132. Hobar JD: The Vermont-Oxford Neonatal Network: Integrating research and clinical practice to improve the quality of medical care. Semin Perinatol 1995; 19:124.
133. Ruttimann UE, Pollack MM: Variability in duration of stay in pediatric intensive care units: A multiinstitutional study. J Pediatr 1996; 128:35.
134. Mandell MS, Lockrem J, Kelley SD: Immediate tracheal extubation after liver transplantation: Experience of two transplant centers. Anesth Analg 1997; 84:249.
135. Kraiss LW, Kilberg L, Critch S, et al: Short-stay carotid endarterectomy is safe and cost-effective. Am J Surg 1995; 169:512.
136. Morasch MD, Hodgett D, Burke K, et al: Selective use of the intensive care unit following carotid endarterectomy. Ann Vasc Surg 1995; 9:229.
137. Katz SG, Kohl RD: Selective use of the intensive care unit after nonaortic arterial surgery. J Vasc Surg 1996; 24:235.
138. Chandra M, Wagner WH, Shabot M: ICU care after infrainguinal arterial surgery: An analysis of indications and outcomes. Am Surg 1995; 61:904.
139. Wong ET, McCarron MM, Shaw ST: Ordering of laboratory tests in a teaching hospital. Can it be improved? JAMA 1983; 249:3076.
140. Kelly JT: Role of clinical practice guidelines and clinical profiling in facilitating optimal laboratory use. Clin Chem 1995; 41:1234.
141. Pilon CS, Leathley M, London R, et al: Practice guideline for arterial blood gas measurement in the intensive care unit decreases numbers and increases appropriateness of tests. Crit Care Med 1997; 25:1308.
142. Roberts DE, Bell DD, Ostryzniuk T, et al: Eliminating needless testing in intensive care—an information based team management approach. Crit Care Med 1993; 21:1452.
143. Zimmerman JE, Seneff MG, Sun X, et al: Evaluating laboratory usage in the intensive care unit: Patient and institutional characteristics that influence frequency of blood sampling. Crit Care Med 1997; 25:737.
144. Ely EW, Baker AM, Dunagan DP, et al: Effect on the duration of mechanical ventilation of identifying patients capable of breathing spontaneously. N Engl J Med 1996; 335:1864.

145. Kollef MH, Shapiro SD, Silver P, et al: A randomized, controlled trial of protocol-directed versus physician-directed weaning from mechanical ventilation. Crit Care Med 1997; 25:567.
146. Kirton OC, DeHaven B, Hudson-Civetta J, et al: Re-engineering ventilatory support to decrease days and improve resource utilization. Ann Surg 1996; 224:396.
147. Civetta JM, Hudson-Civetta J, Ball S: Decreasing catheter-related infection and hospital costs by continuous quality improvement. Crit Care Med 1996; 24:1660.
148. Evans RS, Pestotnik SL, Classen DC, et al: A computer-assisted management program for antibiotics and other antiinfective agents. N Engl J Med 1998; 338:232.
149. Schentag JJ: Optimizing antibiotic use in the critical care unit. Pathol Crit Care 1997; 2:1.
150. Rifenburg RP, Paladino JA, Hanson SC, et al: Benchmark analysis of strategies hospitals use to control antimicrobial expenditures. Am J Health Syst Pharm 1996; 53:2054.
151. Schentag JJ, Ballow CH, Fritz AL, et al: Changes in antimicrobial agent usage resulting from interactions among clinical pharmacy, the infectious disease division, and the microbiology laboratory. Diagn Microbiol Infect Dis 1996; 16:255.
152. Pestotnik SL, Classen DC, Evan RS, et al: Implementing antibiotic practice guidelines through computer-assisted decision support: Clinical and financial outcomes. Ann Intern Med 1996; 124:884.
153. Pearson ML: Hospital Infection Control Practices Advisory Committee: Guideline for prevention of intravascular-device-related infections. Infect Control Hosp Epidemiol 1996; 17:438.
154. Raad II, Hohn DC, Gilbreath J, et al: Prevention of central venous catheter-related infections by using maximal sterile barrier precautions during insertion. Infect Control Hosp Epidemiol 1994; 15:231.
155. Mimoz O, Pieroni L, Lawrence C, et al: Prospective, randomized trial of two antiseptic solutions for prevention of central venous or arterial catheter colonization and infection in intensive care unit patients. Crit Care Med 1996; 24:1818.
156. Kamal GD, Pfaller MA, Rempe LE, et al: Reduced intravascular catheter infection by antibiotic bonding: A prospective, randomized, controlled trial. JAMA 1996; 265:2364.
157. Parras F, Ena J, Bouza E, et al: Impact of an educational program for the prevention of colonization of intravascular catheters. Infect Control Hosp Epidemiol 1994; 15:239.
158. Hofmann P: Critical path method: An important tool for coordinating clinical care. J Qual Imp 1993; 19:235.
159. Thompson K: Building a critical path for ventilator dependency. Am J Nurs 1991; 7:28.
160. Kong GK, Belman MJ, Weingarten S: Reducing length of stay for patients hospitalized with exacerbation of COPD by using a practice guideline. Chest 1997; 111:89.

196

Evaluating Pediatric Critical Care

Anne L. Naclerio, MD • Murray M. Pollack, MD

OVERVIEW

There have been many changes in the care of critically ill children over the past two decades. Since the early 1980s, remarkable growth has occurred in the number of pediatric intensive care units (PICUs) and in the diversity of their organization, structure, and the types of patients that they care for. Concurrently the number of pediatric critical care fellowship training programs and of intensivists has grown. Since 1987, the American Board of Pediatrics has recognized Pediatric Critical Care as a specialty field, and a certification examination was instituted to help further define and control the expertise required to practice in the field. The 1990s brought new forces into the medical arena. While health care costs consumed increasing proportions of the gross domestic product, the population's health status lagged behind that of other countries with lesser health care expenditures. The desire to control medical costs became national in scope and has shaped the recent evolution of all areas of medicine, including critical care. Except for the cases of the most severely ill, cost-saving efforts have shifted care to outpatient settings, reducing the demand for inpatient beds.

Increased awareness of "efficiency" and of "quality" of care have accompanied the efforts to control medical costs. "Benchmarks" and national "standards" are being used increasingly for comparisons and goals for hospitals to use, both internally and externally. This chapter reviews the current trends in pediatric intensive care and discusses ways to evaluate pediatric ICU performance that enable internal comparisons to other time intervals, and external comparisons to other institutions, to be made.

THE NATIONAL PERSPECTIVE

The 1980s saw rapid growth in the number of pediatric ICUs and pediatric ICU beds in the United States. There was an increase from 211 pediatric ICUs with 1600 beds in 1980 to 335 pediatric ICUs with 2900 beds in 1990 (59% and 76%, respectively). During the same period, the numbers of pediatric inpatient facilities and pediatric hospital beds declined by 16% and 24%, respectively (Figs. 196–1, 196–2). These trends have continued but at a slower rate over the last 5 years. As of 1995, 342 hospitals reported having pediatric ICUs with 3190 beds, only 2.1% and 2.0% increases since 1990. The number of pediatric inpatient resources has continued to decline; as of 1994, the number of pediatric inpatient units decreased by 9%, to 2174 facilities. Overall, the proportion of inpatient care devoted to pediatric intensive care has risen sharply, from 3.1% in 1980 to 7.9% in 1994, an increase of more than 150%. The effect of this expansion on quality and efficiency of care is not known.

Most recently, there appears to be an increase in the number of small ICUs in community hospitals, as these hospitals attempt to preserve or increase the number of pediatric inpatients by providing a larger range of services. This allows them to refer fewer patients to the other centers and to compete with other local hospitals that do not offer a full range of services. A complete range of services may also make hospitals more competitive for pediatric managed care contracts.

An analysis by Groeger and coworkers of ICUs across the country showed that pediatric ICUs are still regional referral centers but that occupancy rates for pediatric ICUs were less than 80%.[1] The occupancy rate for pediatric ICUs was lower than that for adult or neonatal ICUs, suggesting that overexpansion had occurred. In 1989, Pollack and colleagues surveyed 235 pediatric ICUs to determine the amount of diversity that existed in the structure and organization of units.[2] They found substantial diversity with potentially important ramifications for issues such as quality and efficiency. Most (40%) pediatric ICUs were small, having a capacity of four to six beds, whereas only 6% had more than 18 beds. The organization within pediatric ICUs also varied. For instance, only 79.6% of pediatric ICUs had full-time medical directors, 73.2% had a pediatric intensivist available to the unit and only 48.5% had 24-hour-a-day physician coverage. The percentage of units with full-time medical directors, pediatric intensivists, and 24-hour-a-day dedicated physician coverage increased as the size of the unit increased. Moreover, the larger centers were more likely to have a medical school affiliation with a responsibility for training students.

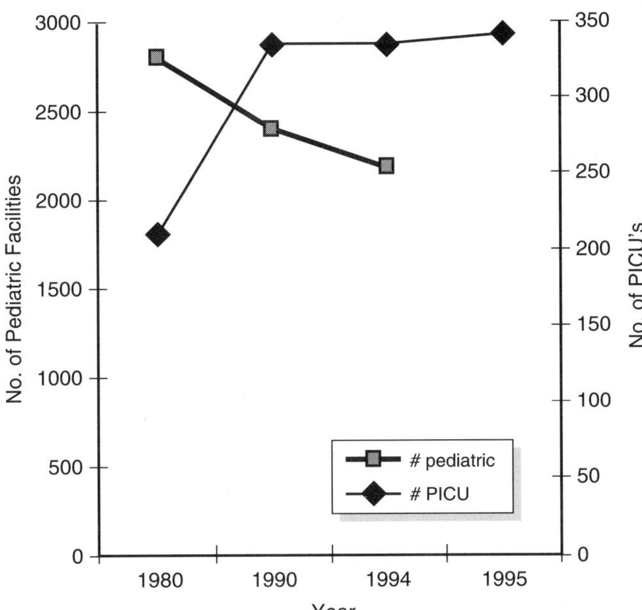

Figure 196–1. Pediatric facilities: changes over time for pediatric intensive care units (PICUs). (Data from the American Hospital Association.)

Concomitant with the growth in the number of pediatric ICUs, there has been significant growth in intensive care training programs nationally. From 1980, the number of pediatric critical care training programs has grown from 14 to 63. Since the first certification examination was given in 1987, the American Board of Pediatrics has certified 869 physicians. At the most recent examination in 1998, of the 250 physicians who registered, 155 passed the exam. If the current rate continues, the number of board-certified pediatric intensivists will double by the year 2010.

Will the trend toward increasing pediatric intensivist numbers slow? Today there are competing forces. There are pressures on hospitals to eliminate or at least limit graduate medical education (GME). The federal government recently enacted financial incentives to limit training, managed care companies are refusing to contribute toward the funding of GME, and there is increasing awareness of the need for attending physicians to be at the bedside to bill for critical care time and procedures. On the other hand, the standard of care in larger ICUs is becoming 24-hour in-house physician coverage, many smaller hospitals are opening new units that will require staffing, and physician burnout, which has been well documented in pediatric ICUs previously,[3] may increase as the current pressures cause inceases in night-time coverage and decreases in the number of fellows being trained.

The diversity of units has many implications for pediatric intensive care. Organizational and structural aspects of pediatric ICUs have been associated with quality. Children cared for in pediatric ICUs, as opposed to adult ICUs, have a significantly lower mortality rate,[4] especially the most seriously ill children, for whom increased physician, nursing, and unit competency are most likely to make a significant difference.

Specific care factors have been associated with improved pediatric ICU outcomes. The presence of a pediatric intensivist has been associated with improved outcomes as compared with pediatric ICUs without pediatric intensivists.[5] Pediatric ICUs where care is delivered by residents were associated with worse outcomes than units without residents, and units associated with fellowship programs also had better outcomes than those without fellowship programs.[6] The increasing use of alternative labor sources to improve efficiency and cost-effectiveness of ICUs is also being evaluated. The use of a ventilatory management team, composed of an ICU physician, a Registered Nurse (RN), and a respiratory therapist, was found to decrease the number of days of mechanical ventilation, ICU length of stay, number of arterial blood gas determinations, and number of indwelling arterial catheters resulting in significant cost savings and improved ICU efficiency.[7] Because hospitals are a labor-intensive industry, increasing productivity has largely involved improving labor productivity.

The use of "extenders" was popularized in the 1980s, when the nursing supply became tight. Several economic studies have evaluated hospitals' production functions and have shown that all-RN nursing staffs had the worst productivity performance and that the use of nurse extenders reduced wasted labor and enhanced productivity, especially in areas with tight nursing markets.[8] Studies to assess their effect on outcomes are still lacking. Other factors, such as the volume of pediatric ICU patients cared for, have not been associated with outcome differences.

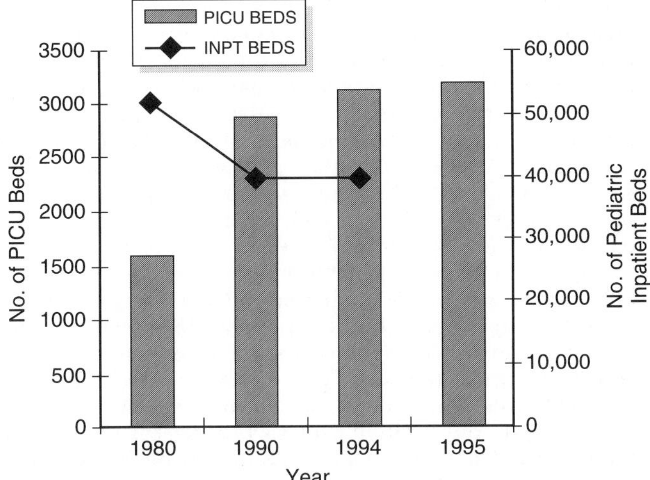

Figure 196–2. Pediatric beds: changes over time for beds in the pediatric intensive care unit (PICU). (Data from the American Hospital Association.)

THE LOCAL PERSPECTIVE

The evaluation of individual pediatric ICUs is undertaken to assess both effectiveness and efficiency. Unit effectiveness includes traditional quality assessment, and unit efficiency assesses care delivery—cost effectiveness *and* unit efficiency. Efficiency has become more important as the efforts to reduce costs have become more rigorous. Both quality and efficiency can be used to benchmark pediatric ICUs. *Benchmarking* is a process by which comparisons are made, either to "self" (internal benchmarking) or to others (external benchmarking). Data used for benchmarking should be adjusted appropriately for severity of illness and other case mix factors. Institutions are sometimes uncomfortable with benchmarking, fearing that public knowledge could affect referral patterns.

Confidential evaluations enable sites to understand how they perform in comparison with other sites and take steps to do better if necessary. The "best practice philosophy" proposes that institutions strive to achieve the results of the institutions with the best results. This is the basic philosophy behind the ORYX initiative by the Joint Commission on the Accreditation of Healthcare Organizations (JCAHO). This program mandates severity and case mix–adjusted data appropriate and meaningful for organizational benchmarking to be collected. Over time, ORYX will require increasing number of variables involving an increasing proportion of patients.

MEASURING QUALITY

Quality of pediatric ICU care can be assessed in many ways. Although this chapter focuses on standardized mortality ratios, other methods are common. Commonly used outcomes include accidental extubation, medication errors, adverse event reports, and nosocomial infections. Each should be adjusted to ensure that future comparisons would be meaningful. For example, accidental extubations should be standardized for the number of mechanical ventilation days, and medication errors should be standardized for the total number of medication administrations. Nosocomial infection rates should be standardized for a variety of case and therapeutic factors, including severity of illness, use of invasive lines and antimicrobial therapy, nutritional support, and other medications.[9]

In pediatric ICU medicine the outcome measure most often used to assess quality is survival or death. Pediatric ICUs vary much in their crude mortality rate, by a factor of at least 800%. This difference is mainly secondary to differences in the severity of illness of patient populations; however, some of the differences are due to real quality differences. Therefore, methods must adjust these crude mortality rates for the severity of illness and other case mix factors in the underlying population. Physiology-based scoring systems enable adjustment for severity of illness. Along with case mix variables such as selected diagnoses, they accurately predict mortality for pediatric ICU populations. These predicted outcomes are compared to actual outcomes to attain outcome ratios termed *standardized mortality ratios* (SMRs)

Severity of illness assessment stems from the idea that increasing organ system failures coincide with increasing mortality rates. In pediatric ICUs the mortality rates for one, two, three, and four or more organ system failures are approximately 1%, 10%, 50%, and 75%, respectively.[10] Modern measures of severity of illness assessment evolved from the observation that the degree of physiologic derangement coincides with the probability of dying. Individual physiologic variables, when combined using multivariate statistical techniques, can accurately assess mortality risk. The main pediatric mortality risk assessment is the Pediatric Risk of Mortality (PRISM) score, and the most current version of this score is the PRISM III score. PRISM III was developed and validated from a database of more than 11,000 patients from 32 pediatric ICUs. This score has 17 physiologic variables subdivided into 26 ranges and applies to the first 12 hours of stay (PRISM III-12) and the first 24 hours of stay (PRISM III-24), allowing both early and accurate prediction of mortality risk.[11]

When an institution decides to assess their SMR for quantitative quality assurance, the process is as follows. First, a consecutive patient sample must be acquired. The power to detect differences between observed and expected outcomes will be related to the size of the sample, and especially to the number of least common outcomes (deaths). The expected numbers of survivors and deaths are calculated by summing the individual patients' mortality risks. The SMR is the observed number of deaths divided by the expected number of deaths.

Multiple methods have been recommended for comparisons between the observed numbers of ICU survivors and deaths and expected numbers of ICU survivors and deaths. First, the total number of observed outcomes is compared to the number of expected outcomes. Statistical tests such as the Z-score proposed by Flora are used for this comparison.[12] A second method is the goodness-of-fit test, which evaluates both the distribution of outcomes and the total numbers of outcomes.[13] This follows the simple observation that a larger proportion of the sicker patients would be expected to die than of the healthier patients. When the patients are divided into mortality risk groups based on the estimated mortality risk, both the total number of outcomes and the distribution of outcomes can be evaluated with a goodness-of-fit test based on the chi-square statistic. Other methods are based on receiver-operating-characteristic (ROC) curve analysis. Institutions where the discrimination of the predictor is better, on the basis of ROC analysis, are "better" than those with lower-ROC curve analyses.

If the observed number and distribution of outcomes are similar to the predicted number and distribution of outcomes, then the institution's performance is equivalent to the performance of institutions in the multi-institutional studies upon which the predictor was initially validated. If the performance of the institution is different from what was expected, an explanation must be sought. As with any test, physicians using this quality assurance method need to understand (1) its strengths and limitations, (2) when false-positive and false-negative results can occur, (3) confounding variables, and (4) peculiarities of the method. If the goodness-of-fit method is used, a specific mortality risk interval can be targeted for detailed chart reviews.

When "too few" deaths occur, it could indicate that the care delivered in the ICU was better than that delivered in the institutions validating the scores. However, other explanations must be sought. The investigation of deaths detected by the mortality predictors may or may not indicate that medical misadventures have occurred. There are legitimate explanations for "extra" ICU deaths. For example, when the ICU population is skewed for toward diagnostic groups that have not been tested extensively, the scores may not be applicable. Subjective chart reviews may determine that the deaths were not unexpected. For example, a logical explanation for underestimation of deaths in low–severity of illness strata might be that many physiologically stable patients with terminal conditions were admitted.

MEASURING EFFICIENCY AND STANDARDIZED LENGTH-OF-STAY RATIOS

Unlike other industries, medicine has not prided itself on efficiency of output. Until recently, quality has been the most important measure. Health care costs in the United States grew at a rate that outpaced inflation and was almost double the rate of growth in all other sectors of the economy over the same period. Medical expenditures have gone from 9.2% of the Gross National Product (GNP) in 1980 to 14% of the GNP in 1994, and they continue to rise.[14] ICU costs have consistently increased faster than costs in other inpatient care areas. Although ICU beds account for fewer than 10% of inpatient beds, they account for 22% of hospital costs, which equates to about 1% of the GNP.[15, 16]

Historically, the system of health care reimbursements in the United States provided little incentive for patients or providers to limit spending. As cost containment efforts have become more visible, there has been a large increase in managed care organizations and, with them, a change in focus to managed costs. The general tenet behind the managed care philosophy is the institution of an economic structure and philosophy that stimulates cost-conscious behavior among both providers and enrollees.[17] Changes in the way hospitals are reimbursed for care by insurers is a catalyst for hospitals to move toward greater fiscal accountability. For example, although 15 years ago it was unheard of, today it is commonplace for managed health plans to request information pertinent to the efficient utilization of ICUs before contracting with hospitals.

Evaluation of efficiency in the ICU has thus become as important as evaluation of quality measures. There are reasons to believe that there are too many PICU beds and that they are being utilized inefficiently. Groeger's study of all types of ICUs nationally found that utilization was lowest in pediatric ICUs.[18] The low mortality rates for many pediatric ICUs implies that many patients who are relatively healthy are admitted. In general, when the mortality rates of pediatric ICUs differ much (e.g., by more than 100%), the inefficiency of bed utilization changes in the opposite direction. When there are too many ICUs and ICU beds, the severity of admitted patients' conditions declines. In Marshall's study of surgical ICUs, number of beds and severity of illness were inversely proportional.[19]

Two main strategies for assessing appropriateness of pediatric ICU resource use have developed. First, efficiency may be computed based on daily use of ICU-unique therapies.[20] *Unique therapies* are those ideally suited to delivery in an ICU, such as mechanical ventilation and vasoactive infusions. Monitoring modalities, however, are not included in this group, as philosophies on their use differ greatly. "Low-risk monitor patients" are those who do not receive an active ICU intervention during their pediatric ICU stay. While the initial efforts at measuring efficiency required rather substantial data collections, the approach has been simplified and the result is reliable comparisons of efficiency among pediatric ICUs. The following equation is currently used to measure efficiency:

$$\text{efficiency} = \frac{\text{total patient days of care using either mechanical ventilation or vasoactive agent infusions}}{\text{total patient days of care}}$$

A study of eight similar pediatric ICUs found efficiency rates to vary from 55% to 90%. Low-risk monitor patients ranged from 18% to 58% and consumed 5% to 35% of the days of care, whereas patients who could have been discharged sooner accounted for another 12% to 29% of patients and consumed 5% to 17% of the days of care.[21] The variation in utilization in dissimilar units may be expected to be even greater. This diversity in efficiency continues today.[21]

The second assessment method, severity-adjusted length of stay (LOS), can be used to compute standardized length-of-stay ratios (SLOSR). Observed LOS is compared to the expected LOS after adjustment for severity and case mix factors. The prediction model for severity and case mix–adjusted LOS was developed using PRISM to adjust for severity of illness; today PRISM III is used. In the initial studies, SLOSR varied from 0.83 to 1.25, with more than 20% of pediatric ICUs displaying significantly ($P < .05$) longer stays than predicted and more than 20% displaying significantly shorter stays than predicted.[22] Factors associated with shorter stays were presence of an intensivist, presence of residents, and co-ordination of care. Increased LOS was associated with increased PICU-hospital bed ratios. There is excellent agreement between direct measurement of efficiency and SLOSRs. The severity-adjusted LOS method, however, is less time consuming, because the information is collected only on the first day of care. Using this method, data collected in the first 24 hours can be used to accurately reflect both ICU efficiency (SLOSR) and quality (SMR).

Pediatric ICUs function within a hospital environment. Influences on that environment may have effects on the performance of the ICU, especially its efficiency. For example, during times of high hospital census, ICUs may be unable to discharge patients as quickly as they might wish and may, therefore, experience reduced efficiency. Severity-adjusted LOS is an important measure of ICU resource utilization, but it is not the only one. For example, laboratory, radiology, and pharmacy use are also important, as ICUs depend much more on ancillary services than other hospital areas do.[23]

LOS outliers are patients whose stay is greater than the 95 percentile for LOS. Nationally, this is longer than 12 days. These patients represent important resource consumption. Long-stay patients have been found to have significantly higher mortality rates (both PICU and hospital), and although they are less than 10% of the PICU population, they consume 50% of the resources.[24] In a more recent study, patients who died were found to have stayed almost twice as long and used more than twice as many diagnostic tests per day, and their costs for tests were twice as much as for the survivors.[25]

Utilization of resources is amenable to change. In one study, the availability of daily severity-of-illness assessments to physicians resulted in significant reduction in resource utilization.[26] In another study, the availability of daily patient-related charges to providers resulted in a change in practice patterns that produced a decrease in patient charges and improved cost containment in the pediatric ICU studied.[27] For these reasons, emphasis is currently being placed on the use of critical pathways and new technologies in the hope that they will have similar effects. Managed care organizations in the United States have promised to provide equal or better care at lower cost by increasing efficiency. However, studies to date of almost 90,000 ICU admissions have shown that severity-adjusted LOS has not been shortened under managed care.[28]

SUMMARY

When comparing ICU performance, adjustments for severity of illness and other case-mix variables are important. The rigorous, multi-institutional validation of PRISM III is the backbone of its use in outcome-based, quantitative quality assurance. These same validation methods are available to individual hospitals and regions with commonly available computer technology and appropriate software. Such methods are not designed to replace other quality assurance tasks, such as evaluations of nosocomial infections, and unplanned extubations; however, they are designed to provide objective, outcome-based measures of quality—and more recently efficiency—because they overcome the difficulties in using crude mortality rates and unadjusted LOS. They are becoming more important for benchmarking and continuous quality improvement.

Our economy is moving toward limiting overutilization of expensive resources and inefficient delivery of care. The measures described in this chapter can serve as national benchmarks for pediatric ICUs and their practitioners.

References

1. Groeger JS, Guntupalli KK, Strosberg M, et al: Descriptive analysis of critical care units in the United States: Patient characteristics and intensive care unit utilization. Crit Care Med 1993; 21:279–299.
2. Pollack MM, Cuerdon TC, Getson PR: Pediatric intensive care units: Results of a national survey. Crit Care Med 1993; 21:607–612.
3. Fields AI, Cuerdon TS, Brasseux CD, et al: Physician burnout in pediatric critical care medicine. Crit Care Med 1995; 23:1425–1429.
4. Pollack MM, Alexander SR, Clarke N, et al: Improved outcomes from tertiary center pediatric intensive care: A statewide comparison of tertiary and non-tertiary care facilities. Crit Care Med 1991; 19:150–159.

5. Pollack MM, Cuerdon TC, Patel KM, et al: Impact of quality of care factors on pediatric ICU mortality. JAMA 1994; 227:941-946.
6. Ibid.
7. Cohen IL, Bari N, Strosberg MA, et al: Reduction of duration and cost of mechanical ventilation in an intensive care unit by use of a ventilatory management team. Crit Care Med 1991; 19:1278-1284.
8. Estaugh S: Hospital nursing technical efficiency: Nurse extenders and enhance productivity. Hosp Health Services Admin 1990; 35:561-573.
9. Singh-naz N, Sprague BM, Patel KM, Pollack MM: Risk factors for nosocomial infection in critically ill children: A prospective cohort study. Crit Care Med 1996; 24:875-878.
10. Wilkinson JD, Pollack MM, Ruttiman UE, et al: Outcome of pediatric patients with multiple organ system failure. Crit Care Med 1986; 14:271-274.
11. Pollack MM, Patel KM, Ruttiman UE: PRISM III: An updated pediatric risk of mortality score. Crit Care Med 1996; 29:743-752.
12. Flora JD: A method for comparing survival of burn patients to a standard survival curve. J Trauma 1978; 18:701-705.
13. Lameshow S, Hosmer DW: A review of goodness-of-fit statistics for use in the development of logistic regression models. Am J Epidemiol 1982; 115:92-102.
14. Chalfin DB: Cost containment issues in the United States: Critical care medicine in managed competition and a managed care environment. New Horiz 1994; 2:275-282.
15. Halpern NA: Federal and nationwide intensive care units and healthcare costs: 1986-1992. Crit Care Med 1994; 22:2001-2007.
16. Pollack MM, Getson PR: Pediatric critical care cost containment: Combined actuarial and clinical program. Crit Care Med 1991; 19:12-20.
17. Chalfin DB: Cost containment issues in the United States: Critical care medicine in managed competition and a managed care environment. New Horiz 1994; 2:275-282.
18. Groeger JS, Guntupalli KK, Strosberg M, et al: Descriptive analysis of critical care units in the United States: Patient characteristics and intensive care unit utilization. Crit Care Med 1993; 21:279-299.
19. Marshall MF, Schwenzer KJ, Orsina M, et al: Influence of political power, medical provincialism, and economic incentives on the rationing of surgical intensive care unit beds. Crit Care Med 1992; 20:387-394.
20. Pollack MM, Getson PR, Ruttimann UE, et al: Efficiency of intensive care: A comparative analysis of eight pediatric intensive care units. JAMA 1987; 258:1481-1486.
21. Pollack MM: Pediatric intensive care unit evaluations database. 1998, unpublished data.
22. Ruttimann UE, MM Pollack: Variability in duration of stay in pediatric intensive care units: A multi-institutional study. J Pediatr 1996; 128:35-44.
23. Winkel P, Statland BE: Assessing cost savings when unnecessary utilization of laboratory tests can be abolished. Am J Clin Pathol 1984; 82:418-423.
24. Pollack MM, Wilkinson JD, Glass NL: Long-stay pediatric intensive care unit patients: Outcome and resource utilization. Pediatrics 1987; 80:855-860.
25. Klem SA, Pollack MM, Getson PR: Cost, resource utilization, and severity of illness in intensive care. J Pedaitr 1990; 116:231-237.
26. Pollack MM, Getson PR: Pediatric critical care cost containment: Combined actuarial and clinical program. Crit Care Med 1991; 19:12-20.
27. Sachdeva RC, Jefferson LS, Coss-Bu J, et al: Effects of availability of patient-related charges on practice pattern and cost containment in the pediatric intensive care unit. Crit Care Med 1996; 24:501-506.
28. Angus DC, Linde-Zwirble WT, Sirio CA, et al: The effect of managed care on ICU length of stay: Implications for Medicare. JAMA 1996; 276:1075-1082.

197

Legal Issues in the Delivery of Critical Care Medicine

Karen N. Swisher, MS, JD

BACKGROUND

With the advent of advanced and complex medical technology, and an ever increasing concern over patients' rights to make informed medical decisions, it is not surprising to see a concomitant increase in litigation over medical care decisions. These are not, however, the traditional medical malpractice cases with which most American courts are relatively familiar. Rather, these cases involve complex ethical, legal, and medical issues concerning a patient's "right to die" and right to demand or reject appropriate medical care. Since the mid to late 1970s, thousands of cases throughout the United States have been labeled in the popular literature as "right to die cases." These cases are decided according to state statutory and judicial law and culminate in a variety of legal opinions with little consensus among the courts.

Judicial cases in this area have become so numerous and contradictory that the federal government enacted the Patient Self-Determination Act (PSDA) of 1991.[1] The intent was to reduce the number of patient and medical provider controversies being resolved in the courts. This Act represents significant legislation. It requires all hospitals, skilled nursing facilities, home health agencies, hospice programs, and health maintenance organizations (HMOs) receiving Medicaid or Medicare funding to give written information to all incoming patients regarding their right to create a "living will" or a medical power of attorney under applicable state laws.[2] According to the PSDA, a medical facility need not actually assist patients in making these advance directives, but each medical facility must have a written policy informing its patients of the assistance they can receive in adopting or rejecting these advance directives. Because these advance directives are created by state law, the PSDA has a secondary purpose: that of encouraging state legislatures to reassess and revise their statutes based on newer empirical, ethical, and legal trends in medical decision making.

Despite good intentions and widespread publicity, the PSDA has done little to reduce the amount of litigation regarding "end of life" medical decisions. The reasons are varied and complex. Fewer than 15 per cent of the population have living wills, and those who do seldom have the documents available during emergencies. Most living wills are written in vague, statutorily prescribed language, giving little guidance on patient values when the patient becomes incompetent. Research indicates that families and health care providers often ignore living wills, and treatment decisions are based primarily on physician values rather than patient values. Few state statutes allow for pediatric advance directives. Most state statutes limit the freedom of incompetent patients to have life-sustaining treatment withdrawn if they are pregnant. There remains inconsistency in many states over what medical treatments can be withheld or withdrawn. Finally, confusion remains when one state must honor the living will document created in another state.

When courts are asked to resolve these conflicts, they typically hear cases dealing with five general areas of concern, namely:

1. Medical treatments and modalities that can be withheld, withdrawn, or provided.
2. Who can make medical decisions on behalf of incompetent patients.
3. Legal tests used to determine how a surrogate decision maker will make a medical decision for an incompetent patient.
4. The type of evidence necessary to determine medical choices made on behalf of an incompetent patient.
5. Interests of the state that may overrule patient choice.

Each of these interrelated categories is discussed next.

DECISION MAKING BY COMPETENT ADULTS

Competent adult patients have the legal right to consent to or refuse medical treatment and to be free of medical intervention, even at the risk of death. This principle has been upheld by the U.S. Supreme Court in two cases determining the constitutionality of physician-assisted suicide. Although the Court ruled that individual states may limit or ban physician-assisted suicide, such states cannot limit a patient's right to consent to or refuse medical treatments, even life-sustaining treatments:

> *... at common law, even the touching of one person by another without consent and without legal justification was a battery ... informed consent is generally required for medical treatment (and) ... the common-law doctrine of informed consent is viewed as generally encompassing the right of a competent individual to refuse medical treatment.... Therefore, for our purposes we assumed that the United States Constitution would grant a competent person a constitutionally protected right to refuse life saving hydration and nutrition ... we acknowledged that competent, dying persons have the right to direct the removal of life-sustaining medical treatment and thus hasten death.*[3]

For patient consent to be legally valid, however, patients must receive relevant information regarding the proposed treatment on which to base their decision. At a minimum, this information must address:

1. Risks and benefits of treatment.
2. Alternatives to treatment.
3. Consequences of forgoing such treatment.

When patients are given this information, courts will uphold patients' rights to consent to or refuse medical treatment. The respect for patient autonomy as part of informed consent has also been codified and adopted by the American Medical Association (AMA). The AMA states: "The social commitment of the physician is to sustain life and relieve suffering. Where the performance of one duty conflicts with the other, the preferences of the patient should prevail."[4]

Every good physician knows that informed consent is a process of communication, not just a legal form for the patient to sign. The problem with informed consent, however, rests in knowing how much information must be disclosed to a particular patient. The timing of such information is also critical in order to avoid adding stress to patients whose conditions are otherwise already compromised by illness. A case in California demonstrates the difficulty in determining what type of information is relevant.

CASE HISTORY

Miklos Arato was a successful 42-year-old electrical contractor when his internist confirmed the diagnosis of a failing kidney and pancreas. A follow-up examination revealed a malignancy, and the patient was referred to a group of oncologists. During his initial visit to the oncologists, Mr. Arato filled out a multipage questionnaire. Among the 150 questions asked was whether he wished to be told the truth about his condition. He stated that he *did* want to know the truth. The oncologists recommended a course of treatment including chemotherapy and radiation therapy. Mr. Arato and his wife agreed to the course of treatment. The patient, however, was *not* given any information regarding statistical data for his life expectancy. The treatment was not successful, and Mr. Arato died shortly thereafter. His estate brought suit, alleging that Mr. Arato's physicians had failed to disclose important information to him, including his statistical probability of survival. Had the patient known the futility of this experimental procedure, it was alleged, he would not have consented to this experimental medical treatment but would have spent his remaining time with his family and gotten his financial affairs in order.

The California Supreme Court declined to require that such specific information be disclosed in the medical context as a matter of law:

the contexts and clinical settings in which physician and patient interact and exchange information material to therapeutic decisions are so multifarious, the informational needs and degree of dependency of individual patients so various, and the professional relationship itself such an intimate and irreducibly judgment-laden, that we believe it is unwise to require as a matter of law that a particular species of information be disclosed.[5]

This case demonstrates the complexities of informing patients of their medical choices when patients are under the physical and mental stress of a life-threatening condition.[6]

Physicians are still confused over what types of treatments patients can refuse. Classifying treatments as either being "active" or "passive," choosing to withhold or withdraw treatment, and choosing "ordinary" or "extraordinary" treatment are becoming anachronisms in the law just as they have become anachronisms in ethical discussions. Generally, any treatment offered in a health care setting can be withheld or withdrawn at the patient's request, including hydration and nutrition. Whereas most states recognize the patient's right to refuse medical treatment, some states still limit the patient's choice of treatment.

Finally, most courts agree that the patient can consent to or refuse medical treatment regardless of the patient's medical condition. Some physicians believe that patients can refuse medical treatment only if they are considered "terminally ill." Patients can refuse medical treatment for a variety of reasons, based on religious values, fear of pain, or cost. Although it is good medical practice to inquire why patients may refuse treatment (since many of these reasons can be remedied), courts and physicians still adhere to the general rule respecting patient autonomy.[7] Thus, in the case of *Bartling v. Superior Court,*[8] a California appellate court held that a competent adult person with a serious illness, probably incurable but not classified as terminal, had the legal right, over the objections of his physicians and the hospital, to have life-support equipment disconnected, even though withdrawal of such medical devices would hasten his death.

MEDICAL DECISION MAKING ON BEHALF OF INCOMPETENT ADULTS

The right to refuse medical treatment is not abated when patients lose their capacity to make decisions. An incompetent patient may express this intent through a prior living will document, a durable power of attorney, or the surrogate decision making of a relative.[9]

When patients lose their capacity to make medical decisions, or for those patients who never had the capacity for medical choice, the law must address three significant issues that determine the form and the outcome of proxy decision making for incompetent patients:[10]

1. Selection of the surrogate or proxy decision maker.
2. The substantive principles that must guide that decision maker.
3. The process to be followed when the proxy decision maker is appointed and when the decision is made.

For some patients (e.g., those under anesthesia or in a persistent vegetative state), determining lack of capacity for making medical decisions is elementary. For most patients, the capacity to make medical decisions is questioned only when they disagree with their physician's recommendation or differ significantly with their physician's values.[11]

It is important for physicians to note that the law distinguishes patients who are incompetent from those who lack the capacity for medical decisions. Some patients may be incompetent by a court of law, yet still have capacity to refuse indicated medical treatment. Capacity for medical decisions is based on the patient's ability to understand the elements of informed consent. Patients do not lose their right to informed consent even when adjudicated incompetent. According to an article written by Roth and associates,[12] five tests for competency have been proposed:

1. Evidencing of a choice.
2. "Reasonable outcome" of choice.
3. Choice based on "rational" reasons.
4. Ability to understand.
5. Actual understanding.

The *evidencing of a choice* test for competency is set at a very low level and is the most respectful test for the autonomy of patient decision making. Under this test, the competent patient is one who evidences a preference for, or against, treatment. The test focuses not on the quality of the patient's decision but on the presence or absence of a decision. This test of competency encompasses, at a minimum, the unconscious patient. In psychiatry, it encompasses the mute patient who cannot or will not verbally express an opinion.

The *reasonable outcome* of choice test involves an evaluation of a patient's capacity to reach the reasonable, right, or responsible decision. The emphasis is on the outcome rather than the decision itself or how it was reached. Thus, the patient who does not make a decision that a reasonable person under similar circumstances would make is viewed as incompetent.

The choice based on a *rational reasons* test is is based on whether the reasons for the patient's decision are "rational" (i.e., whether the patient's decision is a product of mental illness). As in the reasonable outcome test, if the patient decides in favor of appropriate medical treatment, the issue of the patient's competency seldom arises because of the medical profession's bias toward consent to treatment and its countervailing bias against refusal of treatment. In this test, the quality of a patient's thinking is the salient feature.

The *ability to understand* test, which consists of ascertaining the ability of the patient to understand the risks, benefits, and alternatives to treatment (including refusal of treatment), is most consistent with the law of informed consent. Decision making need not be rational in either process or outcome, and unwise choices are permitted. Nevertheless, the patient, at a minimum, must manifest evidence of a sufficient ability to understand the information about medical treatment, even if the patient weighs this information differently from his or her attending physician.

The fifth test is the *actual understanding* test. Under this test, the physician has an obligation to educate the patient and to ascertain whether the patient has understood the risks and benefits of medical treatment or nontreatment. This test arguably requires a fairly high level of competency and sophisticated understanding by the patient that may be difficult to achieve.

The 1980 President's Commission on Making Health Care Decisions perceived the elements of patient capacity in this manner:

In the view of the Commission, any determination of the capacity to decide on a course of treatment must relate to the individual abilities of a patient, the requirements of the task at hand, and the consequences likely to flow from the decision. Decision-making capacity requires, to greater or lesser degree: (1) possession of a set of values and goals; (2) the ability to communicate and to understand information; and (3) the ability to reason and to deliberate about one's choices.[13]

Although patient competency to make an informed medical decision thus appears to be an extremely complex and difficult issue to determine, it actually is not that complicated for a number of reasons. First, many states have enacted statutory definitions that cover patient competency and capacity. These statutory definitions are generally broadly drafted to provide interpretive room for the person making the ultimate decision regarding patient capacity, and that person frequently is the attending physician who is involved in providing his or her patient with the elements of informed consent. In Virginia, for example, "incapable of making an informed decision" means:

inability of an adult patient, because of mental illness, mental retardation, or any other mental or physical disorder, which precludes communication or impairs judgment and which has been diagnosed and certified in writing by his attending physician and a second physician or licensed clinical psychologist after personal examination of such patient, to make an informed decision about providing, withholding or withdrawing a specific medical treatment or course of treatment because he is unable to understand the nature, extent or probable consequences of the proposed medical decision, or to make a rational evaluation of the risks and benefits of alternatives to that decision.[14]

Physicians also apply their own common sense test in determining patient capacity for informed consent. If the physician recommends an indicated medical treatment and the patient agrees, capacity is presumed to exist. If the physician recommends a medical treatment and the patient disagrees, the physician might question the patient's reasons and the patient's capacity for making this contrary choice.

Choosing a Surrogate

Once a determination is made that the patient does not have the capacity to make medical decisions, the courts must apply additional legal tests to determine who will make such medical decisions in lieu of, and on behalf of, the incompetent patient. There are three ways by which surrogates are selected:

1. Power of attorney.
2. Relatives.
3. Guardian ad litem.

First, patients may designate in advance who their surrogate should be by having a durable power of attorney document for health care. This legal document is often incorporated within a living will, whereby a capable patient determines in writing who will make medical decisions on his or her behalf and determines the scope and parameters of those decisions.[15]

Because most patients do not have advance directives, many state statutes allow for immediate family members to make such decisions. Families are a logical choice for medical decisions because family members most often know of, and reflect, a patient's values and preferences.

Finally, proxy persons may be appointed by the court using a guardian ad litem. This person is not technically a guardian, and this similarity in title has confused judges as well as those who have been appointed to serve in these two distinct roles. A guardian ad litem is a lawyer who acts as legal counsel during the course of the litigation on behalf of the subject of such litigation. A guardian may have responsibilities beyond the litigation, both in time and scope. Guardianships are used as a last resort when patients have no families or when family members express serious differences in treatment options for the patient.

Once the surrogate decision maker is identified, the second inquiry is to determine how that surrogate will make decisions. Usually, the proxy person makes a decision based on what the patient would have wanted, had the patient been competent to make such a decision independently. This legal standard for surrogate decision making is called the *substituted judgment test.* For example, in the highly regarded and influential case of *In re Conroy,*[16] the New Jersey Supreme Court held that life-sustaining medical treatment could be withheld or withdrawn from an incompetent patient when the particular patient would clearly have refused the treatment under the circumstances involved. The seminal question in the Conroy case is not what a reasonable or average person would have chosen to do under the circumstances but what the particular patient would have chosen if able.

The patient's intent can be ascertained in various ways. First, under a *limited-objective test,* life-sustaining treatment may be withheld or withdrawn from a patient when trustworthy evidence exists that the patient would have refused the treatment and when the decision maker is satisfied that the burdens of the patient's continued life, with the treatment, clearly outweigh the benefits of life to the patient. This limited-objective standard thus permits the termination of treatment for patients who had not unequivocally expressed their desires before becoming incompetent, when it is clear that the treatment in question would merely prolong suffering. This test also requires trustworthy evidence that patient would have wanted the medical treatment terminated.

In the absence of such trustworthy evidence or in the absence of any evidence that the patient would have declined the treatment, lifesaving medical treatment may still be withheld or withdrawn from a formerly competent person if a *pure-objective test* is satisfied. Under this test, the net burdens of such treatment should outweigh any benefits that the patient might receive from continued life. Further, the pain and suffering of continued treatment should be so severe that administering life-sustaining treatment would be inhumane.

The *Conroy* court expressly declined to authorize surrogate decision making based on assessments of the patient's personal worth, or social utility, or on the value of that life to others. Under the *Conroy* test, the primary focus should be the patient's desires and experiences of pain and enjoyment, not the type of treatment involved.

Should incompetent patients in persistent vegetative states also be bound by the *Conroy* test? In two subsequent decisions,[17, 18] the New Jersey Supreme Court stated that, by definition, patients in persistent vegetative states do not experience the benefits and burdens that the *Conroy* balancing tests were intended to appraise and, therefore, these *Conroy* tests should not be applied. Moreover, if close and caring family members are willing to make this medical decision on behalf of the incompetent patient, a guardian need not be appointed.

Thus, a surrogate decision maker attempts to establish, with as much accuracy as possible, the decision the patient would make if he or she were competent to do so. Employing this theory, the surrogate decision maker first tries to determine whether or not the patient had expressed any explicit intent regarding the type of medical treatment preferred before becoming incompetent. If no clear intent exists, the patient's personal value system must guide the surrogate decision maker.

In the *Brophy* case, for example,[19] the Massachusetts Supreme Court held that food and hydration could be withheld from a comatose adult patient based on a substituted-judgment, surrogate decision-making test that included the following factors:

1. The patient's expressed preferences.
2. His religious convictions and their relation to a refusal of medical treatment.
3. The impact on the family.
4. The probability of adverse side effects.
5. The intrusiveness of the procedure, such as the need to use a feeding tube.

Although Brophy had never specifically discussed whether the gastrostomy feeding tube should be withdrawn if he were to be in a persistent vegetative state after surgery, the surrogate decision maker inferred that if Brophy were presently competent, he would choose to forgo artificial nutrition and hydration by means of a gastrostomy tube.

Traditionally, physicians and the courts look to the patient's family as appropriate surrogate decision makers. The family is usually the most knowledgeable about the patient and desires to do what is best for the patient. The President's Commission suggests five reasons for this deference to family members as surrogate decision makers[21]:

1. The family is generally the most concerned about the good of the patient.
2. The family is usually most knowledgeable about the patient's goals, preferences, and values.
3. The family deserves recognition as an important social unit that ought to be treated, within limits, as a responsible decision maker in matters that intimately affect its members.
4. Especially in a society in which many other traditional forms of community have eroded, participation in a family is often an important dimension of personal fulfillment.
5. Because a protected sphere of privacy and autonomy is required for the flourishing of this interpersonal union, institutions and the state should be reluctant to intrude, particularly regarding matters that are personal, and on which a wide range of opinion in society exists.[20]

Consulting with family members also neutralizes the possibility of subsequent medical malpractice claims, and this element also accounts for its current popularity.

Families have traditionally, legally, and morally made a vast number of important decisions concerning other family members in many related areas of family law.[22] It is unfortunate, therefore, that the good intentions of the family were almost totally disregarded by the court in the *Cruzan* case, which held that individual states could establish tough evidentiary hurdles for surrogate decision makers to cross when deciding on behalf of an incompetent patient.[23] It would have been more logical, more humane, and more in keeping with prior family law precedent for the court to have established a "rebuttable presumption" that family members are making the best choice for the patient, as is true in most states. Therefore, from a legal standard, it is generally presumed that the family is acting in the best interests of the patient and the burden to prove otherwise shifts to the person protesting the family's decision.

Problems may still arise when family members disagree as to what would constitute appropriate medical treatment for the incompetent patient. Problems also arise when family members may not be acting in the best interests of the patient or when a patient has never had the capacity to make medical decisions. Many state statutes provide for a hierarchy of family members authorized to make medical care decisions. These statutes typically require the majority of family members in the same hierarchy to agree on a treatment choice. Unfortunately, when family members cannot agree, the case often goes to court, leaving everyone dissatisfied in the end.

Some patients never have had capacity for medical choice. Examples include infants and small children, patients born with severe mental illnesses, or mentally retarded patients. For such patients, many courts are increasingly using a *best interests* test, as enunciated in the *Saikewicz* case.[24] The "best interests" of an incompetent person are not necessarily served by imposing on such persons aggressive medical treatments that most competent people would refuse.

It does not advance the interest of the state or the patient to treat the incompetent patient as a person of lesser status or dignity than others. . . . If a competent person, faced with death, may choose to decline treatment which not only will not cure the person, but which may substantially increase suffering in exchange for a possible yet brief prolongation of life, then it cannot be said that it is always in the "best interests" of the incompetent patient to require submission to such treatment.

One major problem with the best interests test is that many courts apparently have a difficult time conceding to the reality of an impending death in the same manner that many Americans evidence a general denial of death. Thus, when court-appointed guardians are used to determine the best interests of the incompetent patient, they often choose to continue aggressive medical care despite poor outcomes or despite additional suffering by the patient. The debatable logic behind this questionable approach is that any prolongation of life is a better "interest" than is death and any act that can be performed to prolong life, despite the medical futility and suffering of the patient, is defined as being in the best interest of the patient. The assumption that all people under these circumstances would choose aggressive medical treatments, regardless of the quality of life they may hope to achieve, has come under increased scrutiny.

Like any other test, the best interests test should use a flexible approach. It should be based on the facts surrounding each patient, the "totality of the circumstances," and not a small measure of basic common sense and human compassion. It is an approach best left to the family of an incompetent patient, as his or her surrogate decision maker, and to the patient's attending physician.[25] As a concurring and dissenting judge in the Maryland appellate case of *Mack v Mack*[26] aptly observed:

The best interests test mandates that the decision to terminate life support be made relying on objective criteria rather than the family members' opinions as to what the patient would have chosen if the patient could choose. Perhaps the best interests test has applicability (1) where there is no available surrogate decision maker who is familiar with the patient; and (2) as a safeguard against bad faith or improper decisions by family members to terminate life support. Where a family's motives are suspect, a court could refuse to effectuate the family's decision to terminate life support if the court finds that decision is contrary to the patient's best interests.

The best interests test may also be helpful where there are conflicting opinions by family members regarding appropriate medical treatment. Measuring contrasting opinions against the objective criteria of the best interests test may aid the courts in resolving such conflict.

The Burden of Proof

The final issue to be resolved by the courts in determining treatment options for incompetent patients relates to the amount of evidence needed, the weight of such evidence in determining the "best interests" of the patient, and what the patient would have wanted (substituted judgment). Courts have concluded that whoever requests life-sustaining treatment to be discontinued in the case of an incompetent patient must present clear and convincing evidence regarding the patient's wishes. This was the very issue that the U.S. Supreme Court upheld in the *Cruzan* case—that state statutes can require a very rigid burden of proof, even for family members who all acknowledged acting in the best interests of the patient.

In defining its clear and convincing standard, a New York court announced that this standard requires proof

"sufficient to persuade the trier of fact that the patient held a firm and settled commitment to the termination of life supports" under the circumstances like those presented. As a threshold matter, the trier of fact must be convinced, as far as is humanly possible, that the strength of the individual's beliefs and the durability of the individual's commitment to those beliefs makes a recent change of heart unlikely.[27]

Utilizing this standard is another manifestation of the presumption that life should be maintained under virtually all circumstances.

What evidence do courts require to determine patients' wishes? First, courts are receptive to written documents, including a living will, a durable power of attorney, or another written statement of patient choice. Unfortunately, for the few patients who do have living wills, these documents often do not clearly state specific treatment choices.[28] Oral statements made to family and friends are more common evidence, but courts typically discount many oral statements. Sometimes family members present their own values as a reflection of the patient's values simply because the patient is a member of the family. Studies indicate that even close family members are not always accurate in predicting patient values and preferences.[29] With these obstacles in mind, courts are disinclined to discontinue life support treatment under the clear and convincing standard.

JUDICIAL LIMITATIONS ON A PATIENT'S MEDICAL CHOICE

The legal right to consent to or refuse any medical treatment is based on state constitutions and state common law, and it is not absolute. The right to individual autonomy may be narrowed, limited, and defined by independent interests of the state to protect its citizens. These interests include:

- Preserving life
- Preventing suicide
- Protecting innocent third persons, such as children
- Preserving the integrity of the medical profession
- Encouraging the charitable and humane care of afflicted persons

In balancing the individual's right to privacy and right to choose one's own destiny against the state's responsibility to protect its citizens, courts must consider not only the strength of the state's interests but also the means by which the state has chosen to further those interests through regulation. The varied nature of the judicial attempts to define such state interests is a reflection of diversified values in a pluralistic American society.

State's Interest in Preservation of Life

The state's interest in preserving life is considered a significant state interest. Translating this obligation of a government to protect its citizens, however, to a governmental obligation to protect patients near death is another matter. It may be seen as embracing two separate but related concerns: (1) an interest in preserving the life of the particular patient and (2) an interest in preserving the sanctity of all life.

One of the first cases in which a court had to weight the state's interest in the preservation of life against a patient's right to choose was the case of Karen Quinlan, a 22-year-old woman who was confirmed to be in a persistent vegetative state. The court held that

. . . the claimed interests of the state in this case are essentially the preservation and sanctity of human life. . . . Ultimately there comes a point at which the individual's rights overcome the state interest, it is for that reason that we believe Karen's choice if she were competent to make it, would be vindicated by law.[30]

The difficulty in defining this obligation is nowhere more apparent than in the *Cruzan* case. The Supreme Court upheld the state's right to protect all life regardless of the quality of life that the patient may suffer. As one Justice stated in his dissent:

The only state interest asserted here is a general interest in the preservation of life. But the state has no legitimate general interest in someone's life, completely abstracted from the interest of the person living that life, that could outweigh the person's choice to avoid medical treatment. The state's general interest in life must accede to Nancy Cruzan's particularized and intense interest in self-determination in her choice of medical treatment. There is simply nothing legitimately within the state's purview to be gained by superseding her decision.[31]

State's Interest in Prevention of Suicide

The state's responsibility to protect its citizens from suicide, and from the influence of suicide, has been hotly debated in recent U.S. Supreme Court cases on the legalization of physician-assisted suicide for terminally ill patients. In the older "right to die" cases, courts had struggled to distinguish between the affirmative act of taking one's life and the act of discontinuing artificial life support to let nature take its course. The case of *McKay v Bergstedt* illustrates this point.

CASE HISTORY

The patient, 31-year-old Kenneth Bergstedt, was a respirator-dependent quadriplegic. For 10 years, his parents had cared for him at home. After the death of his mother, and faced with the imminent death of his father from cancer, Kenneth petitioned his local court for an order permitting the removal of his respirator by a medical professional who could also administer a sedative to relieve his pain. He sought an order of legal immunity for any person assisting him and a court decree that his actions would not constitute suicide. Kenneth's father reluctantly approved of his son's actions. The state of Nevada contested this action as promoting "state-sponsored suicide."

The Supreme Court of Nevada held (posthumously) that Kenneth had a right to refuse treatment, even if the refusal would result in his death. The court used three factors to distinguish the action desired by Kenneth from suicide: patient attitude; physical condition; and prognosis. The Nevada court concluded that Kenneth did not wish to commit suicide but simply wished to live only as long as his condition would permit without artificial support. Refusing medical intervention merely allows the disease or the effects of an injury to take a natural course; death, therefore, would be the result of the underlying disease or injury, not the result of self-inflicted injury.[32]

As the Kevorkian cases have demonstrated, courts continue to grapple with the issue of patients wishing to end their pain, as opposed to wishing to end their lives. The more recent cases focus on the state's compelling interest in preventing persons from committing suicide because of depression or coercion by third parties. The U.S. Supreme Court stated:

patients whose physical pain is inadequately treated will be more likely to request assisted suicide. Encouraging the development and ensuring the availability of adequate pain treatment is of utmost importance; palliative care, however, cannot alleviate all pain and suffering. As death becomes more imminent, pain and suffering become progressively more difficult to treat. An individual adequately informed of the care alternatives thus might make a rational choice for assisted suicide. For such an individual, the state's interest in preventing potential abuse and mistake is only minimally implicated.[33]

State's Interest in Protecting Innocent Third Parties

The state's interest in protecting innocent third parties is intended to protect the most vulnerable of its citizens: children, mentally and physically incapacitated persons, the poor, and the elderly. The state's interest goes beyond protecting the vulnerable from coercion; it extends to protecting disabled and terminally ill people from prejudice, negative and inaccurate stereotypes, and societal indifference. Those patients in severe pain are most vulnerable to requests for assistance in dying. The U.S. Supreme Court stated:

The state claims interests in protecting patients from mistakenly and involuntarily deciding to end their lives, and in guarding against both voluntary and involuntary euthanasia. Leaving aside any difficulties in coming to a clear concept of imminent death, mistaken decisions may result from inadequate palliative care or a terminal prognosis that turns out to be in error; coercion and abuse may stem from the large medical bills that family members cannot bear or unreimbursed hospitals decline to shoulder.[34]

Courts have always taken a strong interest in the protection of children. Therefore, when parents refuse to consent for medical treatment deemed necessary to save the life of a child, courts often overrule the parents' desires, whether they are based on religious convictions or other reasons. Courts may also invoke this state interest when parents cannot agree on a treatment decision for a terminally ill child. The case of *In re Jane Doe, A Minor* involved a 13-year-old terminally ill child in a nearly complete unconsciousness state. One parent consented to a *do-not-resuscitate* order, but the other parent refused to consent. Because the parents could not agree on the care to be provided, the hospital requested a hearing. An independent guardian ad litem was appointed to represent the child's interests.

The court found that if either parent decided to continue medical support, that decision must be respected. The integrity of the family was the issue that the court wished to protect, stating:

A court ruling authorizing termination against the wishes of one parent at the behest of another parent could be very detrimental to family harmony and create a serious precedent allowing courts to interfere in such major familial decision, all in violation of public policy.[35]

Protecting the Integrity of the Medical Profession

Historically, state courts and legislatures have deferred to the medical profession's own internal management. State regulatory boards, composed mostly of physicians, determine the appropriate practice of medicine in each state, and the courts require other physicians to testify in medical malpractice cases regarding the appropriate standard of medical care. For example, a 1977 Massachusetts Supreme Court decision involving withdrawal of care from an incompetent mentally retarded patient stated:

The state interest requiring discussion is that of the maintenance of the ethical integrity of the medical profession as well as allowing hospitals the full opportunity to care for people under their control. The force and impact of this interest is lessened by the prevailing medical ethical standards. Prevailing medical ethical practice does not, without exception, demand that all efforts toward life prolongation be made in all circumstances. Rather, the prevailing ethical practice seems to be to recognize that the dying are more often in need of comfort than treatment.

The U.S. Supreme Court, in the two physician-assisted suicide cases, has reexamined the meaning of protecting the integrity of the medical profession and states:

The fear is that a rule permitting physicians to assist in suicide is inconsistent with the perception that (the physicians) serve their patients solely as healers. But for some patients, it would be a physician's refusal to dispense medication to ease their suffering and make their death tolerable and dignified that would be inconsistent with the healing role.[36]

PHYSICIAN-ASSISTED SUICIDE IN THE UNITED STATES

In June 1997, the U.S. Supreme Court rendered two unanimous decisions concerning physician-assisted suicide. It is important to understand the legal reasoning behind these decisions, since they will surely have great impact on the delivery of critical care medicine in the future. The only issue presented by the two U.S. Supreme Court cases was whether the federal Constitution required or compelled the states to legalize physician-assisted suicide (at least for competent, terminally ill patients who requested it), not whether the states were permitted to do so. In the first case, the Supreme Court was asked to decide whether mentally competent, terminally ill patients have a constitutionally protected right to receive suicide assistance from their physicians. Washington State law made it a crime for anyone to assist in a suicide. The Court ruled there is no federally protected *right to die* under the federal Constitution and that any laws legalizing physician-assisted suicide should come from state legislatures.

In rendering this seminal decision, the Justices stated that constitutional rights must be clearly articulated and clearly defined. An examination of the nation's history, legal traditions, and legal practices demonstrates that Anglo-American law has punished, or otherwise disapproved of, assisting suicide for more than 700 years and that rendering such assistance is still a crime in almost every state. The Court encouraged continued debate on the morality and legality of physician-assisted suicide and still left the door open for individual states to amend their laws reflective of this debate.

In examining the role of the state in protecting its citizens from abuse, the Justices noted that many people who request assistance in dying do so because they suffer from depression or uncontrolled pain. However, living will statutes and medical ethical canons encourage physicians to treat depression and provide sufficient pain medication to their patients. The Court noted the AMA's formal statement that "physician-assisted suicide is fundamentally incompatible with the physician's role as health provider." At the same time, the AMA also endorses the practice of terminal sedation ("the administration of sufficient dosages of pain killing medication to terminally ill patients to protect them from excruciating pain even when it is clear that the time of death will be advanced)." The purpose of terminal sedation, the Court acknowledged, is to ease suffering of the patient, not to advance the death of the patient. The Court was persuaded that most states allow and encourage physicians to alleviate anxiety and discomfort when withdrawing artificial life support by administering medication that may hasten death even more quickly. State laws generally permit physicians to administer medication to patients in terminal conditions when the primary intent is to alleviate pain and when the patient chooses to receive it with the understanding that the medication is so powerful as to hasten death.

The Justices were concerned about the "slippery slope" effect of legalizing physician-assisted suicide for competent patients. Concern was expressed that physicians might not be the best judge in distinguishing patients in true need from those severely influenced because of stress, financial problems, or family conflict. There is a subjective line between assistance in suicide and euthanasia. Justice Souter stated:

[T]his difficulty could become the greater by combining with another fact within the realm of plausibility, that physicians simply would not be assiduous to preserve the line. They have compassion, and those who would be willing to assist in suicide at all might be the most susceptible to the wishes of a patient, whether the patient was technically quite responsible or not. Physicians, and their hospitals, have their own financial incentives, too, in this new age of managed care. The case for the slippery slope is fairly made out here, not because the recognition of one due process right would leave a court with no principled basis to avoid the recognition of another. It is, rather, because there is a plausible case that the right claimed would not be readily containable by reference to facts about the mind that are matters of difficult judgment, or by gatekeepers who are subject to temptation, noble or not.

Thus, the U.S. Supreme Court clearly is *not* willing to infer additional fundamental rights or liberty interests regarding assistance in dying. It restates, however, the general rule that patients have a right to consent to or refuse medical treatment, even life-sustaining treatment. The Court also recognized that states have a responsibility to protect their citizens against abuse and to defer to the clearly articulated standards of medical care developed by the medical profession.

In the second case, respondents argued that New York's statute, making assisted suicide a crime, denied certain patients "equal protection" under the law. Under New York's living will laws, terminally ill patients may refuse life-sustaining medical treatment, thereby hastening death. Other terminally ill patients, not connected to respirators or feeding tubes, cannot hasten death without physician assistance. They argued that such contradictions in law are unfair and deny equal treatment of all terminally ill patients. Again, the Supreme Court disagreed. The federal Constitution's Equal Protection Clause provides that states must treat like cases alike but may treat unlike cases accordingly. Neither the assisted-suicide ban nor the law permitting patients to refuse medical modalities treats anyone differently or draws any distinctions between persons. Competent patients, regardless of physical condition, are entitled to refuse unwanted lifesaving medical treatment, and no one is permitted to assist a suicide.

The Justices discussed at length the distinction between letting a patient die (e.g., by removal of a feeding tube or ventilator), and assisting a patient in death by administering a bolus of drug. Again, the Court looked to the medical profession and found such a distinction recognized. The AMA, for example, has emphasized the "fundamental difference between refusing life-sustaining treatment and demanding a life-ending treatment."

Although the outcome is the same for both patient categories, the intent of the physician is different: "When a doctor provides aggressive palliative care, in some cases, painkilling drugs may hasten a patient's death, but the physician's purpose and intent is, or may be, only to ease the patient's pain. A doctor who assists a suicide, however, must necessarily and indubitably, intend primarily that the patient be made dead." The law has long used the person's intent or purpose to distinguish between two acts that may have the same outcome. Although this distinction may be difficult to recognize, it is one that the majority of states have defined.

The U.S. Supreme Court clearly determined that regulation surrounding physician-assisted suicide is within the sole jurisdiction of state legislatures and state courts and left open the possibility of legalized physician-assisted suicide by some states in the future. As of this writing, only Oregon has legalized physician-assisted suicide but other states may soon follow. The justices were deferential to those ethical cannons memorialized by the AMA and clinical research published on this subject. The justices believed that individual states do provide for appropriate pain management statutes for their patients, and they encouraged physicians to aggressively treat pain. However, some Justices acknowledged that for some patients pain medications cannot alleviate suffering. In these cases, assistance in dying may indeed be the only option. These patients may have to resort to the courts again for guidance, "where the legal circumstances different were state law to prevent the provision of palliative care, including the administration of drugs as needed to avoid pain at the end of life—then the law's impact upon serious and otherwise unavoidable physical pain would be more directly at issue."

Some commentators have maintained that the U.S. Supreme Court seemed to endorse a limited right to die for people in great pain. Patients undergoing severe pain and suffering may have a constitutionally recognizable interest in obtaining relief from distress, even if that relief may hasten their death. Some may imply that the Fourteenth Amendment Due Process Clause may not allow a state to prevent patients from receiving the palliative care they need to avoid pain at the end of life. But a right to gain access to pain relief and management is a different right, and a narrower one, than the right to assistance in suicide.

RISK MANAGEMENT GUIDELINES

With the recent litigation involving conflicts in medical management regarding patient choice, physicians may find little comfort in the way courts render these decisions using an adversarial system of litigation or in the subjective way that legal standards are applied to such cases. In addition, litigation is costly for all parties and is a sure way to erode the trust established between patient and physician. Litigation leaves bitter and permanent scars on the living who may survive the experience. For these reasons, physicians should take a proactive stance in avoiding conflict with patients and their families that can be resolved only in a legal system.

Physicians can do much to help patients, their families, and themselves reach consensus on an appropriate treatment plan. For some, this is called good risk management; for others it is called good practice of medicine.

1. *Inquire early whether or not a patient has a living will or durable medical power of attorney.* The PSDA requires that hospitals, on patient admission, present these options, but it is much better for the physician to present these options before hospitalization. There remains much confusion sur-

rounding living wills and their limited effectiveness. The better option is to encourage patients to have a durable medical power of attorney and to express their values, including religious preferences, with the family and the physician.

2. *Take a "values" history from patients; better yet, give a values statement to your patients.* Many values-history forms have been developed to help physicians understand their patients better. Most address issues relating to a patient's quality of life, religious values, financial concerns, family relationships, and philosophy on medicine and mortality.[37] Patients are often more concerned about quality-of-life issues surrounding any treatment than selection of the treatment modality itself (which they would prefer to leave to the expertise of the physician). Knowing this, however, some experts suggest that it is better for patients to know the values and treatment philosophy of the physician than vice versa. Patients naturally feel more comfortable working with physicians who possess values similar to their own.

3. *Emphasize treatment goals, rather than treatment modalities, to patients.* When physicians find there is little medically they can do to improve the condition of terminally ill patients, they sometimes choose to intervene with suggestions on treatment options intended only to prolong the dying process. Families have unknown or unrealistic expectations regarding these treatment modalities, and everyone loses perspective on the final outcome. If treatment goals are discussed, for example, stabilizing patients so that they can go home to die or managing severe pain during the dying process, modalities become important only if they fulfill those goals. A discussion concerning goals helps patients, families, and physicians focus on the truth of the patient's diagnosis and prognosis.

4. *Recognize that informed consent should focus on treatment options and their relationship to quality-of-life issues.* Informed consent is meaningful only if patients know their options, particularly those concerning conservative treatment and pain management. Patients can choose treatments based on their own subjective criteria for how these treatment options will affect their quality of life.

5. *If a conflict between a patient and you persists, get help from others.* Most conflicts are, and should be, resolved within the health care environment. If a conflict persists, most hospitals have ethics consult services to help mediate conflicts. In addition, do not forget that pastoral services, social services, and other physicians as consultants can help diffuse an impasse between a physician and a patient.

6. *Know your state laws on living wills and informed consent.* Physicians should know their state health laws and should understand how they work. Risk managers, hospital attorneys, or even insurance carriers can assist in walking through the nuances of state statutes on medical care.

7. *Manage pain assertively and aggressively.* Studies clearly indicate that patients are being undermedicated or inappropriately managed for pain during the last few days of life. Many hospitals now have pain management centers, and many physicians specialize in pain management. Get a second opinion, and treat pain aggressively.

8. *Obtain a psychiatric consultation and treat patients for depression.* In addition to pain management, depression is a large issue. Hospices and other facilities working with terminally ill or severely ill patients know that depression is common in patients and their caregivers. Treatment with medications as well as with social services should be part of any treatment plan for such patients.

9. *Understand the difference between pain and suffering, and treat accordingly.* Terminally ill patients sometimes feel little physical pain, but they suffer greatly. They suffer because of fear over the costs of medical care and because their caregivers and family members are under much stress. If they are older and alienated from mainstream society because they are dying, these patients suffer because their friends are deceased and their support groups are gone. Hospices and social workers can provide services to complement physical pain management. Religious support systems are also helpful. Often physical pain becomes controllable when emotional distress is alleviated.

10. *Understand your own values relating to the goals of medicine and your role in the care-versus-cure debate.* Studies indicate that contemporary physicians do not have sufficient training in palliative care, and they are not taught how to care for patients when a cure is no longer an option. Many medical schools are alleviating this deficiency, and many offer continuing medical education in the art of caring for patients with an added focus on communication and compassion.

11. *Tell patients the truth about their diagnosis and prognosis.* Even though patients seem to want to know the truth about their condition, few patients are willing or able to bring up the subject. Physicians have a responsibility to give patients an opportunity to discuss their diagnosis, prognosis, and treatment plan. Again, the art of communication can only enhance the doctor-patient relationship.

12. *Accept your own mortality and understand the role you play and how you affect the patient's views on mortality.* For some physicians, a denial of a patient's impending death is a denial of their own death. Worse yet, it is sometimes perceived as a confirmation of the physician's limited ability to cure all patients at all times. Many hospitals are experimenting with physician "bereavement" support groups, which help physicians cope with the death of their patients.

13. *Listen to patients.* Some physicians do not listen to their patients, making assumptions regarding their patients' preferences when in reality they do not know them. Physicians should ask patients questions and should listen for responses, both direct and subtle. Sometimes all patients really need or want is for someone to simply listen to them express themselves.

As the population ages, as medical technology continues to expand, as health care systems consolidate and compete for "covered lives," and as health care reform progresses, the potential for conflicts to arise in determining treatment options for patients will continue to increase. Health care rationing by governmental and private insurers will undoubtedly constitute the next horizon of judicial involvement in this brave new medicolegal world. However, one thing that will never change is the ethical responsibility the physician has to advocate for the best medical interest of the patient.

References

1. Omnibus Budget Reconciliation Act of 1990, Pub L No. 101-508, 42 USCA §1395.
2. 42 USCA §1395cc (a) (1) (1) (A).
3. Washington, et al, Petitioners v Harold Glucksberg et al, 65 LW 4660 at 4675 (June 26, 1996).
4. AMA Op. 2.20 (June 1994). Also see Decisions Near the End of Life, JAMA 1992; 267:2229.
5. Arato v Avedon, 858P.2d 598 (Cal. 1993) at 606.
6. Schaeffer M, Drantz D, Wichman A, Masur, H, Reed E: The impact of disease severity on the informed consent process in clinical research. Am J Med 1996; 100:261.
7. Brock DW, Wartman SA: When competent patients make irrational choices. N Eng J Med 1990; 322:1595.
8. Bartling v. Superior Court, 163 Cal App3d 186, 209 Cal Rptr 220 (1984).
9. Childress JF: Refusal of lifesaving treatment by adults. J Fam L 1984; 23:191.
10. Steven M. Richard, Note: Someone make up my mind: The troubling right to die issues presented by incompetent patients with

no prior expression of a treatment preference. Notre Dame Law Rev 1989; 64:394, 396-397.
11. Kevin R. Wolff, Note: Determining patient competency in treatment refusal cases. Ga L Rev 1990; 24:733,750.
12. Roth LG, Meisel A, Lidz CW: Tests of competence to consent to treatment. Am J Psychiatry 1977; 134:279.
13. President's Commission for the Study of Ethical Problems in Medicine and Biomedical and Behavioral Research: Making Health Care Decisions. Washington, DC, U.S. Government Printing Office, 1982, p 57.
14. §54.1-2982 of the Virginia Health Care Decisions Act (1996).
15. Schmitt MN, Hatfield SA: The durable power of attorney: Applications and limitations. Mil Law Rev 1991; 132:203, 204.
16. In re Conroy, 98 NJ 321, 486 A2d 1209 (1985).
17. In re Jobes, 108 NJ 394, 529 A2d 434 (1987).
18. In re Peter, 108 NJ 365, 529 A2d 419 (1987).
19. Brophy v New England Sinai Hospital, Inc, 398 Mass 417, 497 NE2d 626 (1986).
20. President's Commission: Deciding to Forgo Life-Sustaining Treatment. Washington, DC, U.S. Government Printing Office, 1983, p 127.
21. Furrow BR, Johnson SH, Jost TS, et al: Bioethics: Health Care Law and Ethics. St. Paul, West Publishers, 1991, p 280.
22. Gregory JD, Swisher PN, Scheible SL: Understanding Family Law. New York, Matthew Bender, 1995, pp 161-183.
23. Cruzan v Director, Missouri Department of Health, 110 S Ct 2841, 497 U.S. 260 (1990).
24. Superintendent of Belchertown State School v Saikewicz, 373 Mass 728, 370 NE2d 417 (1977).
25. Suhl J, Simmons P, Reedy T, et al: Myth of substituted judgment: Surrogate decision making regarding life support is unreliable. Arch Intern Med 1994; 154:90.
26. Mack v Mack 329 Md 188, 618 A2d 744 (Md Ct App 1993).
27. In re Westchester County Med Ctr, 534 N.Y.S.2d 886, 531 N.E.2d 607, 613 (NY 1988).
28. Sugarman J, Weinberger M, Samsa G: Factors associated with veterans' decisions about living wills. Arch Intern Med 1992; 152:343.
29. Uhlmann RF, Pearlman RA, Cain KC: Physicians and spouses' predictions of elderly patients' resuscitation preferences. Gerontology 1988; 431:M115, M116.
30. In re Quinlan, 70 NJ 10,355 A2d 266 (1976).
31. Cruzan, Id. At 313-14, 110 S. Ct. at 2869-70.
32. McKay v Bergstedt, 801 P2d 617 (Nov 1990).
33. Dennis C. Vacco, Attorney General of New York v Timothy Quill, MD 65 LW 4695 at 4703) (NY 1997).
34. Washington v Glucksberg, supra at 4692.
35. In re Jane Doe, A Minor Civil Action No. D-93064, Super Ct of Fulton County, Georgia (Order, October 17, 1991).
36. Washington v Glucksberg, supra at 4693.
37. Lambert P, et al: The values history: An innovation in surrogate medical decision making. Law Med Health Care 1990; 18:202.

198

Medical Futility

Stuart J. Youngner, MD

Since the 1980s, our society has established the primacy of informed consent to medical treatment. Implied in the doctrine of *informed consent* is the patient's right not only to choose between alternative treatments but also to decide to have no treatment at all. Of course, decisions to refuse treatment are most weighty when the medical interventions being refused are lifesaving or life-prolonging. After struggling with this issue for almost 20 years, we have reached a broad consensus that competent adult patients may refuse any and all life-sustaining interventions—from dialysis and mechanical ventilation to the technical provision of fluids and nutrition. If physicians disagree with a patient's treatment refusals and have explained their reasons to no avail, they have but two morally acceptable alternatives: either to transfer care to another physician or to follow the patient's wishes.

However, what is the *physician's* role when he or she determines that additional or continued life-sustaining measures are futile? Physicians are concerned that too often they are forced into giving futile end-of-life interventions, such as cardiopulmonary resuscitation (CPR). Must such measures be offered to patients and their families? Must they be given when patients or families ask for or demand them? Can physicians simply say no? These questions, under the general rubric of *medical futility*, have been hotly debated in the medical literature during the 1990s.

Increasingly, physicians, hospitals, professional organizations,[1,2,3] and even some state legislatures[4] have endorsed or adopted policies that recognize that limits exist as to a physician's obligation at the end of a patient's life, regardless of the wishes of the patient or family. Many think that the pendulum has swung too far in the direction of consumerism and away from professional responsibility. They believe that physicians should shoulder more of the weight, relieving families of unnecessary guilt and protecting patients from "high-technology placebos."[5] Interest in medical futility has been greatly enhanced by growing concerns about efficiency and resource allocation in the health care system.

Nonetheless, many questions about futility remain unanswered. For instance, little agreement exists about the definition of futility:

- If a right to treatment does exist, how should we understand that right?
- Once physicians have determined that a given intervention is futile, how should they proceed?
- Should physicians inform the patient that the intervention will not be given, or should they wait for the patient to bring it up?
- Could do-not-resuscitate orders be written not only without patient or family permission but without informing them as well?
- What is the difference between futility and rationing?
- Why would patients or families demand interventions that competent and compassionate health professionals have told them will do no good and may well cause considerable harm?
- How can we better communicate with patients and families to avoid confrontations about futility?

The rest of this chapter attempts to answer some of these difficult questions.

HISTORICAL CONTEXT

The discussion of treatment limitation in the United States has largely taken place in the context of patient autonomy and the right to refuse treatment. Famous court cases, from Karen Quinlan in the 1970s to Nancy Cruzan in the 1990s, have centered on patients or families who sought to limit life-sustaining treatment in opposition to physicians who insisted that it be continued. These court cases and dozens of others have established the right of patients or appropriate surrogates to refuse life-sustaining treatment. Patients' rights were elevated almost to the level of a movement. During this period, malpractice litigation (and with it, the physician's legal paranoia) grew dramatically.

At the same time, critical care physicians were learning

from experience that patients at the end stage of chronic illness or those with multisystem organ failure rarely benefited from aggressive interventions such as CPR. And although the famous cases involved patients and families who refused treatment when physicians wanted it to continue, more often patients, and families in particular, demanded aggressive interventions when physicians had decided that sufficient treatment had been administered. Because of legal fears and a mistaken notion of patients' rights, we have established an unfortunate tradition of asking the question, "Do you want us to do everything?" and then following this direction when the answer comes back, "Yes."

POSITIVE VERSUS NEGATIVE RIGHTS AND THE INTEGRITY OF THE MEDICAL PROFESSION

It is a fallacy that because patients have a moral right to refuse life-sustaining treatment they have an unqualified right to demand it. The rights defined in the treatment refusal court cases were *negative* rights—the right that no treatment be given to the patient. *Positive* rights, conversely, "in the physician-patient context—the right that something *be* done—endorse the patient's right to select a particular intervention and implies a coexisting obligation of the physician to make that intervention available."[6] Claims to negative rights are generally considered to be more powerful than those to positive rights, and they can be traced to different areas of moral theory and the law.

The right to refuse treatment is found in the constitutional rights of privacy and liberty or in the common law right against battery. The negative right to refuse treatment has been firmly established and rooted in our constitutional and common law heritage. Positive rights to have treatment may exist; but if they do, they must be understood and justified separately from the right to refuse treatment. In fact, in a nation that is currently debating the appropriate level of access to beneficial health care, it seems a cruel irony that we feel obliged to give nonbeneficial care to persons in critical care environments simply because they demand that we do so.

The doctrine of informed consent specifies that patients have a right to an informed choice or a refusal of treatments offered to them within the standard of medical care; it does not say that they have a right to ask for any and all treatments in a physician's armamentarium. This observation is confirmed in everyday medical practice. A surgeon who has determined that a patient would not benefit from surgery does not feel obligated to ask: "Do you want me to do it anyway?" Nor must an internist prescribe antibiotics for a viral upper respiratory infection or give vitamin B_{12} injections because the patient wants them. As Brett and McCullough[6] wrote, the patient's ability to exercise positive rights to treatment is limited by the physician's clinical judgment:

> *Because the physician is a necessary element in the dyad, his or her moral and medical values obviously are not extraneous factors in clinical decision making. The foundation of the clinical encounter is a specified body of knowledge and expertise about what is beneficial for patients. When a patient seeks to exercise a positive right to an intervention, a necessary condition is that there is either an established or theoretical medical basis for this patient's request.*[6]

Society has entrusted physicians with the responsibility for making clinical judgments. Physicians are held accountable for those judgments, and they are also given some authority to make them. In fact, these judgments form the basis of the medical profession. Physicians are more than technicians who follow the orders of patients, and medicine has goals that the physician must promote—above all, to benefit patients and do them no harm. Furthermore, by offering desperately ill persons and their families futile treatments, we hardly promote the ideal of patient autonomy. The act of offering a futile intervention sends a mixed message that may actually undermine patient autonomy.[7] After all, why would a physician offer a treatment if it was not going to be successful?

DEFINING FUTILITY

Although the word *futility* has a categorical ring, it is difficult to define precisely. Some elements of the definition are clear, however. Futility must always be discussed in relation to an identified goal. Intervention A is futile if it is not successful in achieving goal B. Intervention A may not be futile in relation to goal C. Thus, the futility of an intervention is difficult to determine without identification of the goal.

Numerous possible goals may be identified for any given intervention.[8] For example, we can understand an intervention purely in *physiologic* terms. By this standard, we would judge the administration of intravenous bicarbonate futile if it failed to correct an electrolyte disturbance. Other potential goals include postponing the moment of death, extending life for a specific period of time, and achieving an acceptable quality of life. We might also define futility by the *probability* of a given intervention's achieving a goal. Below a certain probability, an intervention would be considered futile.

Thus, communicating using the word "futility," without first identifying goals, can be confusing and misleading. Moreover, the farther we get away from physiologic futility (e.g., by defining it in terms of length or quality of life) and a zero probability of achieving a worthwhile goal, the more we begin to introduce value judgments about the worthiness of the goals we can achieve or the requisite probability that distinguishes an unacceptably low chance from a chance worth taking. But if value judgments inevitably come into play, whose values should be determinant: those of the patient and family or those of the physician?

Some authors have argued that physicians have a right and, indeed, an obligation to act on value judgments both about the probability of achieving certain goals and about whether the goals themselves are worthy. Tomlinson and Brody[9] claim that "physicians must be able to restrict the alternatives made available to patients and must be able to employ value judgments in doing so." Schneiderman and colleagues[10] distinguish between the effects of an intervention and its benefits: "We believe that the goal of medical treatment is not merely to cause an effect on some portion of the patient's anatomy, physiology, or chemistry, but to benefit the patient as a whole." They argue that futility should be defined within the context of evolving standards of care and that the goal of medicine is to achieve a benefit above a certain minimum *qualitative* or *quantitative* threshold.[10] They have proposed specific standards for determining futility in both of these dimensions.

They define as *qualitatively futile* "any treatment that merely preserves permanent unconsciousness or that fails to end total dependence on intensive medical care"[10] and consider both of these results to be of no benefit to the patient. *Quantitative futility* is "any effort to achieve a result that is possible but that reasoning or experience suggests is highly improbable and that cannot be systematically produced."[10] More specifically, they propose: "When physicians conclude (either through personal experience, experiences shared with colleagues, or consideration of reported empirical data) that in the last 100 cases a medical treatment has been useless, they should regard that treatment as futile."[10]

They justify this position by noting that although observing no successes in the last 100 trials does not mean that the treatment never works, such an observation would serve as a point estimate of the probability of success, and using statistical methods, a range of values that include the true success rate can be estimated with a specified probability. Thus, if no successes have occurred in 100 consecutive cases, the clinician can be 95% confident that no more than three successes would occur in each of 100 comparable trials.[10]

Schneiderman and colleagues thus acknowledged that their proposals would be controversial and invited "examination and challenge" to them, a response that was quickly forthcoming. Truog and coworkers[11] challenged the Schneiderman statistical approach. They pointed to the literature that documented problems with physicians' estimates of prognosis. Asking physicians to remember their last 100 similar cases is probably unrealistic, but even if empirical studies identify 100 consecutive patients who did not respond to a given treatment, the authors asked, "How similar must the patients be?" In assessing the efficacy of mechanical ventilation to treat pneumonia, for example, is it sufficient simply to recall the 100 most recent patients who received artificial ventilation for pneumonia, or must this group be stratified according to age, etiologic organism, or coexisting illness?[11]

Callahan[12] raised a more general concern.[12] He likened futility to other issues that have both factual and value elements, (e.g., abortion and the definition of death), noting that "no social 'ought' can be drawn from a scientific 'is.'" Lantos and his colleagues[13] made a similar point: "Because futility determinations . . . combine technical considerations, patient values, and clinical judgments, the framework for these determinations should be one of shared decision-making."

Others have criticized Schneiderman and colleagues' notion of qualitative futility. Veatch and Spicer,[14] for example, argued that when a medical intervention will prolong life and physicians think continued life is not beneficial, the "situation must be resolved with a bias in favor of life." Addressing Schneiderman and colleagues' assignment of permanent unconsciousness to the realm of futility, they replied,

Life-prolonging care is fundamental, precisely because we can imagine ourselves in the minority desiring this care, and we would go to great lengths to assure that if we were in the minority, we would have some opportunity to gain access. . . . Even those not usually identified with pro-life positions would recognize how offensive it must be to a patient who believes in the ultimate value of biological life to be prohibited access to life-prolonging care by one's clinician.[14]

Schneiderman and colleagues' other example of nonbeneficial (hence, qualitatively futile) treatment is keeping someone alive who is totally dependent on intensive care. Sometimes, however, prolonging life does allow time for good-byes and settling of unfinished business. It is difficult to understand how these goals are not beneficial or how critical care physicians could turn off a ventilator or stop vasopressor administration for a patient who wanted to be kept alive for these purposes.

Clearly, although widespread sympathy with the notion of medical futility exists, little agreement exists about how to define it.

UNITED STATES COURT CASES

Few cases of futility have been tested in the courts.[15] The first to capture national attention was the case of Helga Wanglie.

Helga Wanglie

A woman in her nineties, Mrs. Wanglie was ventilator-dependent and in a persistent vegetative state.[16] After several months, her physicians at Hennepin County Hospital recommended that mechanical ventilation be discontinued and that she be allowed to die.[17] Her husband objected and reported that she would have wanted to live as long as possible under the current circumstances. The hospital went to court to have an independent conservator appointed. The patient's husband objected, and the court appointed him as conservator.[18]

Because the patient died shortly after this ruling, the right of the physicians to override the husband's wishes was never directly addressed by the court. Some persons hailed the outcome of the Wanglie case as a victory for the rights of families.[19] Others, sympathetic to the notion of futility, nonetheless thought a tactical error had been committed because this first major case hinged on such a subjective notion of futility, that is, a judgment that the patient's quality of life was unacceptable.

Baby K

Baby K[20] was born in 1992 with anencephaly, and, contrary to usual custom, her mother (who had refused abortion when a diagnosis of anencephaly had been made in utero) insisted that Baby K be kept alive by all means possible. The diagnosis and prognosis were not in dispute. The physicians and hospital took the case to federal court where it was first heard by the U.S. District court and then the U.S. Court of Appeals. Both courts upheld the mother's right to demand treatment.[20]

Catherine Gilgunn

The third case was decided by a jury in a civil suit.[21] Catherine Gilgunn was a 71-year-old woman at the end stage of several chronic illnesses, including diabetes, heart disease, Parkinson's disease and a stroke. When she lapsed into a coma, her physicians at Massachusetts General Hospital suggested that a do-not-resuscitate order be written. A representative of the hospital's ethics committee, called in by Mrs. Gilgunn's physician, wrote a note in the chart supporting unilateral action by the physicians. The ethics committee's representative did not attempt to mediate the dispute. In fact, he did not speak with the patient's family. Against the expressed wishes of the patient's family and the patient's previously stated wishes that she wanted everything done, Mrs. Gilgunn died after her physicians wrote unilateral orders for both do-not-resuscitate and discontinuation of mechanical ventilation.

Discussion

Although many, if not most, persons would not insist on aggressive treatment in situations such as those illustrated in these three court cases, a small minority of our citizens would. In the Baby K and Wanglie cases, the families specifically cited religious beliefs to support their positions. In the case of Baby K, the lower court specifically cited religious freedom as a factor in its decision.[22] And while many advocates of unilateral futility decisions by physicians hail the Gilgunn decision as a victory, critics point out that a jury decision in one case in one state hardly establishes a legal standard. Moreover, as Capron argues, the jury's verdict can be explained by the judge's narrow charge to the jury that treatment is futile if it does not provide cure.[23] Capron is also critical of the hospital's failure to provide even minimal mechanisms for resolving the dispute. The Massachusetts General Hospital ethics committee did not follow standards now suggested for ethics consultation.[24]

Johnson and colleagues conclude, in their review of the subject, that case law does not "reveal, a core area of consensus on the issue of medical futility. Treatment decisions, conflict resolution, and policy drafting must take place in the context of a lack of consensus."[15]

DANGERS OF APPLYING FUTILITY

Several other concerns have been raised about physicians' using futility as a rationale for unilaterally limiting treatment. First, because determinations of futility are value-laden, until standards (such as those of Schneiderman and colleagues) are set for the profession as a whole, definitions of futility will likely vary from physician to physician. If all physicians unilaterally acted on their judgments about futility, similar cases would be treated differently,[25] opening the way for accusations of abuse and prejudice.

Second, some argue that condoning unilateral decision making by physicians would set back shared decision making between patient, family, and physician, returning us to an earlier era of unbridled paternalism, which our society has found unsatisfactory.[11, 13, 14] Even strong proponents of futility (like Schneiderman and colleagues[10] and Tomlinson and Brody[9]) agree that physicians should not *act* unilaterally until a much broader public discussion of the issues has occurred. Such a public discussion could be stimulated by several methods, including:

1. Formulation of institutional policies on futility after wide discussion within the hospital and the community of persons it serves.
2. Publishing and disseminating standards or guidelines by professional groups.
3. Taking of selected cases to court.
4. Educating health professionals and the general public about these issues.

Third, concern exists that *rationing* and *futility* are becoming confused.[8, 11, 26] This issue is important because both futility and rationing have different meanings, moral implications, and methods of resolution. Jecker and Schneiderman[26] as well as Morreim[27] described the common economic, historical, and demographic factors that have brought both concepts into the foreground, including:

1. A dramatic and continuing increase in health care costs and a concomitant call for measures to stop it.
2. The development of high-technology medicine and increased options for aggressive intervention.
3. An aging society that requires more and more medical care.
4. A general recognition of the limits of individual autonomy as the needs of the greater society become more pressing (e.g., allocation of scarce medical resources).

The differences between futility and rationing are important. A futile treatment is one that offers no benefit to the patient. *Rationing* implies denial of beneficial treatment to some persons because the treatment is not available in sufficient quantities to treat these persons. Limiting futile treatments may in fact help conserve resources and may make our health care system more efficient, but futile treatments could and should be limited, even in times of resource abundance.[26] "Circumstances of rationing always presuppose scarcity," Jecker notes, and "ethical rationing must meet standards articulated in theories of distributive justice."[26] Conversely, *futility* implies a cause-and-effect relationship between a medical intervention and its intended outcome in a specific patient. The distribution of scarce resources (rationing) is a matter for society, not individual physicians, to decide. Physicians owe their allegiance to their patients, who trust them to look after their interests, not the interests of others.[28] Rationing is an extremely sensitive topic; in our pluralistic society, little agreement exists about who should be excluded from treatment when insufficient quantities of the treatment exist. As Jecker and Schneiderman wisely caution, futility can become a "subterfuge for allocation decisions."[26]

MOTIVES FOR DEMANDING FUTILE TREATMENT

Most troubling, perhaps, is that instead of learning to understand the reasons why patients and their families demand futile interventions, physicians may use medical futility as a shortcut to decision making. Too often, the discussion of futility in the medical literature concerns cases in which extreme positions have already been taken—patients or their families demanding interventions that physicians have determined are useless.[29] However, these cases do not adequately portray the historical, social, and personal context in which these situations arise that motivate people to demand futile treatment. Better understanding of these motives will not resolve the futility debate, but it can prevent a confrontation about medical futility from occurring in many cases. Understanding what motivates people to ask for or demand futile therapy offers physicians an opportunity to provide optimal care for dying patients and their families and to promote shared decision making.

Failure to Set Timely Treatment Goals

In their discussions with patients, families, and each other, physicians too often focus on specific treatments rather than on the goals they may or may not achieve.[7, 8, 29]

CASE HISTORY

Mrs. Smith
Mrs. Smith, a 95-year-old woman with severe dementia and a diagnosis of metastatic adenocarcinoma, was admitted to the hospital from a nursing home because of sepsis, renal failure, congestive heart failure, and gastrointestinal bleeding. Meeting the family for the first time, a house officer tells them the serious nature of patient's condition and then asks the question, "Do you want us to do everything?"

Mr. Jones
Mr. Jones, an otherwise healthy 70-year-old man, was admitted to a cardiac monitoring unit with chest pain. The house officer approached his wife with the question, "If your husband's heart stops, do you want us to try to start it again?" "Of course I want you to try," she replied. Later, she told her family physician about the incident. "What did that young man think? That I wanted my husband to die?"

The questions posed by the house officers in these two cases are meaningless or even misleading until the potential goals of treatment have been clarified and set. As we have seen, whatever one's definition of futility, it must be defined in relationship to a specific goal. Interventions such as the use of ventilators, vasopressors, or CPR are not ends in themselves but are means to ends that have been chosen through shared decision making.

Of course, patients and their families most often seek the goal of saving and restoring life. Sometimes, the highest priority is to help them realize that this goal is not achievable. Physicians often have difficulty with this task and postpone it until the last days or hours before the patient dies. Some physicians feel a sense of failure when they cannot save their patients' lives, whereas for others the illusion of control brings a sense of power or narcissistic gratification. In both cases, to admit that the patient is going to die is to admit failure.

Discussing death and dying is also emotionally difficult and time-consuming, and many physicians avoid it. Effectively talking about these issues requires great interpersonal skills, self-awareness, and timing. It is little wonder, then, that families and patients demand treatment when they have understood neither the reality of the patient's overall condition nor the various goals individual treatments may or may not serve.

Worthwhile goals might include keeping the patient comfortable while allowing death to occur as quickly as possible, restoring the patient to a previous satisfactory quality of life, keeping the patient alive long enough to say good-bye to loved ones, and achieving a reduced, but still satisfactory, quality of life. Undesirable goals might include keeping the patient alive for a short while but with great pain, suffering, and indignity; restoring the patient to a quality of life that was, and remains, unacceptable to the patient; and achieving a reduced quality of life (e.g., bedridden, incontinent, dependent on others) that is unacceptable to the patient. Individual treatments may achieve some of these goals and not others. Of the goals that are achievable, some may be desired by the patient, others not.

Discussions with patients and their families are most effective if they identify goals first and the treatments that may or may not achieve them second.

Ignorance

Sometimes people demand futile treatment when they simply do not understand the facts. When Mr. Jones' wife was outraged by the house officer's implication that she might not have wanted to "start up" her husband's heart if it stopped, she had little notion of what this process might involve or what the likely outcome would be if her husband were to receive full CPR.

In the report of a study of multiply impaired, elderly nursing home residents, Murphy[30] found that do-not-resuscitate orders were written in the charts of only 10%. He changed the way the issue was approached by encouraging discussion and avoiding misleading language such as, "Would you want us to do everything to save your life if your heart stopped beating?" When he spoke candidly to patients and families about their medical conditions, poor prognoses, and the unpleasant realities of dying in an intensive care unit, they uniformly (23 of 24 patients and all but one relative) rejected the use of CPR.[30] By acting proactively, Murphy empowered his patients and avoided a later confrontation over medical futility.

Confusion

People sometimes demand futile treatment because they are confused, often because they have been given inconsistent and contradictory information from health professionals.[29] Several causes exist for such confusion.

First, no evidence exists that practicing physicians agree on a single definition of futility. A patient will inevitably be confused after speaking with clinicians who have different thresholds for determining either qualitative or quantitative futility; such differences exist between different services (e.g., the experimental oncology ward and the intensive care unit).[31] Oncologists have initiated treatments with patient and family consent and are less willing to call off aggressive interventions when the patient's condition deteriorates than are their critical care colleagues, who have not invested as much in the initial treatment and see more failures of cancer therapy than successes.

Second, the phenomenon of multiple consultants breeds confusion. Patients in critical care units in large tertiary medical centers may have many consultants, each of whom watches the progress of one problem. A steady stream of consultant teams passes by the patient's bedside, examining one part of the patient, one part of the chart, and one part of the laboratory results. Comments to the family, similarly, reflect a narrow focus—"the patient is no longer bleeding," "there is no sign of infection," "the heart is beating stronger today"—failing to convey an overall picture of the patient's deterioration. Such inadequate communication only exacerbates the patient and family's preoccupation with treatments or laboratory values as if they were ends in themselves while the overall treatment plan is ignored.

Finally, confusion is exacerbated by the fragmentation of care that results from monthly rotations of house officers and attending physicians and from shift changes for nurses. These characteristics of the health care system make it likely that patients and families will hear different facts, different interpretations of similar facts, and different prognoses. Physicians should not unfairly give futility as a justification when patients and families have been confused by multiple messages.

Mistrust

Patients may not accept physicians' pronouncements of futility because they do not trust the physicians.[27] Some people are mistrusting by nature; others may have heard previous predictions of doom that did not materialize.

More important, perhaps, is how socioeconomic and cultural factors influence perceptions and attitudes. African Americans, for example, have many reasons to mistrust both the medical profession and the institutions where they receive their care. The Tuskegee medical experiments and the fact that most hospital wards, until recently, were segregated provide historical reasons for mistrust. Unfortunately, subtler forms of racial and economic discrimination persist. Few nurses and physicians are African American, and many poor and minority patients have inadequate access to health care unless they are critically ill.[32–34]

Some data demonstrate that minority status and lower socioeconomic status are associated with preferences for more aggressive care.[35, 36] By understanding the motives that lead to requests for futile treatment, physicians can take steps to prevent a confrontation near the end of a patient's life. By helping patients and families set treatment goals, physicians can avoid meaningless debates about the utility of specific interventions. By giving full disclosure about the invasiveness and poor outcomes (in most situations) of CPR, they can reduce unreasonable demands for this procedure. By providing continuity and consistency of care, they can minimize the confusion that too often results in unrealistic demands for treatment. Mistrust, however, is a more difficult problem that cannot be overcome until we have more minority health professionals and a more equitable health care system.

FUTURE TRENDS

There seems to be growing opinion that a clear definition of futility is an elusive goal about which our society is unlikely to reach consensus.[15, 37, 38] One suggested alternative is that instead of setting a rigid definition of futility on which health professionals could act unilaterally, entire communities develop a common policy that emphasizes a fair process for resolving disputes.[37, 39]

It is hoped that physicians will use what we have learned from the futility debate to communicate more effectively with patients and their families, thereby avoiding unproductive and painful confrontation. Perhaps, as more institutions and professional societies develop medical futility policies, our society will recognize the difference between the negative right to refuse treatment and the positive right to demand it, letting physicians exercise professional judgment in order to determine when end-of-life interventions offer little or no benefit.

Undoubtedly, the courts will hear more futility cases, and they are unlikely to give physicians the formal power to make unilateral futility judgments in any but the most narrow physiologic meanings of futility. At the same time, increasing pressure to conserve medical resources will make overt rationing an inevitability. (We covertly ration now—by ability to pay.) In fact, two community policies about futility openly acknowledge a rationing component, a development made more palatable because the policies grew out of a discussion that included, at least to some degree, the general public.[37, 39]

However, in a society where great inequity, racial division, and a pluralism of religious and cultural values exist, the confusion between futility and rationing will frequently manifest itself. Clinical studies will identify more situations in which outcomes are poor, and statistical models will better predict hopeless situations,[40] but most dying patients will continue to fall into ambiguous categories. Physicians may have less, rather than more, time to optimally plan with their patients, who, because of the nature of our health care system, will often be strangers to them.[41]

References

1. American Thoracic Society: Withholding and withdrawing life-sustaining therapy. Ann Intern Med 1991; 115:478–486.
2. Task Force on Ethics, Society of Critical Care Medicine: Consensus report on ethics of forgoing life-sustaining treatments in the critically ill. Crit Care Med 1990; 18:1435–1439.
3. Council on Ethical and Judicial Affairs, American Medical Association: Guidelines for the appropriate use of do-not-resuscitate orders. JAMA 1991; 265:1868–1871.
4. The Virginia Health Care Decisions Act of 1992. Virginia Code 8. {Section}54.1-2990.
5. Blackhall LJ: Must we always use CPR? N Engl J Med 1987; 317:1281–1285.
6. Brett AS, McCullough LB: When patients request specific interventions: Defining the limits of the physician's obligation. N Engl J Med 1986; 315:1347–1351.
7. Tomlinson T, Brody H: Ethics and communication in do-not-resuscitate order. N Engl J Med 1988; 318:43–46.
8. Youngner SJ: Who defines futility? JAMA 1988; 260:2094–2095.
9. Tomlinson T, Brody H: Futility and the ethics of resuscitation. JAMA 1990; 264:1276–1280.
10. Schneiderman LJ, Jecker NS, Jonsen AR: Medical futility: Its meaning and ethical implications. Ann Intern Med 1990; 112:949–954.
11. Truog RD, Brett AS, Frader J: The problem of futility. N Engl J Med 1992; 326:1560–1564.
12. Callahan D: Medical futility, medical necessity: The-problem-without-a-name. Hastings Cent Rep 1991; 21:30–35.
13. Lantos JD, Singer PA, Walker RM, et al: The illusion of futility in clinical practice. Am J Med 1989; 87:81–84.
14. Veatch RM, Spicer CM: Medically futile care: The role of the physician in setting limits. Am J Law Med 1992; 18:15–36.
15. Johnson SH, Gibbons VP, Goldner JA, et al: Legal and institutional policy responses to medical futility. J Health and Hosp Law 1997; 30:21–36.
16. *In re Wanglie* No. PX-91-283, 4th JD, Hennepin County, Minn, July 1991.
17. Miles SH: Informed demand for "non-beneficial" medical treatment. N Engl J Med 1991; 325:512–515.
18. Brennan TA: Physicians and futile care: Using ethics committees to slow the momentum. Law Med Health Care 1992; 20:336–339.
19. Angell M: The case of Helga Wanglie: A new kind of "right to die" case. N Engl J Med 1991; 325:511–512.
20. Annas GJ: Asking the courts to set the standard of care: The case of Baby K. N Engl J Med 1994; 330:1542–1545.
21. Gilgunn v. Massachusetts General Hospital. Super. Ct. Civ. Action No. 92-4820, Suffolk Co. Mass., verdict, 21 April 1995.
22. Post S: Baby K: Medical futility and the free exercise of religion. J Law Med Ethics 1995; 23:5–11.
23. Capron AM: Abandoning a waning life. Hast Cent Rep 1995; 25:24–26.
24. Report of the SHHV-SBC Task Force on Standards for Bioethics Consultation (in press).
25. McCrary SV, Swanson JW, Youngner SJ, et al: Physicians' qualitative assessment of medical futility. J Clin Ethics 1994; 5:100–105.
26. Jecker NS, Schneiderman LJ: Futility and rationing. Am J Med 1992; 92:189–196.
27. Morreim EH: Profoundly diminished life: The casualties of coercion. Hastings Cent Rep 1994; 24:33–42.
28. Angell M: Cost containment and the physician. JAMA 1985; 254:1203–1207.
29. Youngner SJ: Applying futility: Saying no is not enough. J Am Geriatr Soc 1994; 42:887–889.
30. Murphy DJ: Do-not-resuscitate orders: Time for reappraisal in long-term-care institutions. JAMA 1988; 260:2098–2101.
31. Youngner SJ, Allen M, Montenegro H, et al: Resolving problems at the intensive care unit/oncology unit interface. Perspect Biol Med 1988; 31:299–308.
32. Wenneker MB, Weissman JS, Epstein AM: The association of payer with utilization of cardiac procedures in Massachusetts. JAMA 1990; 264:1255–1260.
33. Buckle JM, Horn SD, Oates VM, et al: Severity of illness and resource use differences among white and black hospitalized elderly. Arch Intern Med 1992; 152:1596–1603.
34. Braverman PA, Egerter A, Bennett R, et al: Differences in hospital resource allocation among sick newborns according to insurance coverage. JAMA 1991; 266:3300–3308.
35. Danis M, Patrick DL, Southerland LI, et al: Patients' and families' preferences for medical intensive care. JAMA 1988; 260:797–802.
36. Garrett JM, Harris RP, Norburn JK, et al: Life-sustaining treatment during terminal illness: Who wants it? J Gen Intern Med 1993; 8:361–368.
37. Halevy A, Brody B. Multi-institutional collaborative policy on medical futility. JAMA 1996; 267:571–574.
38. Tomlinson T, Czlonka D: Futility and hospital policy. Hast Cent Rep 1995; 25:28–35.
39. Murphy DJ, Finncane TE: New do-not-resuscitate policies: a first step in cost control. Arch Intern Med 1993; 153:1641–1648.
40. Rubenfeld GD, Crawford SW: Withdrawing life support from mechanically ventilated recipients of bone marrow transplants: a case for evidence-based guidelines. Ann Intern Med 1996; 8:625–633.
41. Youngner SJ: Medical futility and the social contract (who are the real doctors on Howard Brody's island?). Seton Hall Law Rev 1995; 25:1015–1026.

199

Forgoing Life-Sustaining Therapy in Intensive Care

Michael A. DeVita, MD • Ake Grenvik, MD, PhD, FCCM

As technology keeps advancing, it is more common for patients to die in institutions. In 1939, 37% of all deaths in the United States occurred in hospitals; in 1989, as many as 85% did. Approximately 70% to 90% of these deaths have followed a decision to either withhold or withdraw some form of therapy.[1, 2] Because limitations to the level of care occur so frequently, it is important for the intensive care practitioner to understand the rationale for such a conclusion, to assist patients and surrogates in their decision making, and to carry out therapeutic options in a way that preserves patient dignity and prevents suffering. This chapter reviews the rationale for forgoing life-sustaining therapy and provides practical comments about making such decisions.

WITHHOLDING LIFE SUPPORT: A BRIEF HISTORY

The origins of withholding support are found in ancient times. In *The Art*, Hippocrates stated that the role of medicine was "to do away with the sufferings of the sick, to lessen the violence of their diseases, and to refuse to treat those who are overmastered by their diseases, realizing that in such cases, medicine is powerless." Thus, the physician must try to cure those who may be cured, decrease morbidity of diseases when possible, and if unable to do so, he or she should ensure comfort for a patient. Finally, when a disease has "won" and a patient is destined to die, the physician is obligated to recognize this and to ease the dying process. This characterization remains peculiarly pertinent to intensive care more than two millennia since the time of Hippocrates.

During the long history of medicine and until very recently, the physician has been accorded the responsibility of dictating therapy to be considered and then choosing the course for a patient to follow. The patient, in turn, was obligated to follow "doctor's orders."

While physicians have always attempted to forestall death, it was not until the 1950s that physicians could significantly alter the course of a disease process. In fact, it is now possible to prevent death without influencing the likelihood of recovery for some individuals. That is, with the advent of techniques that support failing organs for an indefinite period of time, physicians can now provide breathing, the pumping of blood, the excretion of wastes, and nutrition for their patients. A new category of patient has been created as a result of medical advancement: the "nearly dead," one who is alive only because he or she is receiving life support in the intensive care unit (ICU).

When ICUs were first created, they were filled not with old patients but, rather, young patients who were more likely to benefit from the interventions provided in those sites, such as mechanical ventilation.[3] As the benefits became more apparent, older and sicker patients were also treated in these ICUs. In the early 1960s, cardiopulmonary resuscitation and dialysis made a major impact on public and medical expectations and results. With these new interventions, death could be forestalled for long periods (e.g., in a patient with the previously fatal condition of renal failure) and lethal processes could be reversed. The decisions in the United States to provide dialysis for all patients with renal failure and to widely train people in cardiopulmonary resuscitation have created an expectation that all individuals have a right to all possible therapy.

With the advance of technologic capability, virtually all organs were able to be supported nearly indefinitely. Cancers could be treated more aggressively, failing organs replaced with artificial or transplanted new ones, and infections cured with better antibiotics. However, some "survivors" could not recover and return to society. The new dilemma of how to deal with the incurable, life-supported ICU patient was recognized.

For example, patients who had sustained a lethal brain injury and, in fact, had irreversibly absent brain function could be kept "alive" on ventilators.[4, 5] Breathing was provided by a ventilator, and even the heart could be supported by a pacemaker. In this situation, physicians realized that lack of cardiac function should not be an absolute criterion included in the definition of death. Several conventions of physicians and ethicists[6, 7] and legislative actions[8] forwarded the concept of *brain death* (see Chapter 174). This currently well-accepted term equates irreversible cessation of all brain function with death of the individual. The original purpose of such a concept and legislation was to allow physicians to ethically and legally terminate support and to enable these patients to donate viable organs for procurement and transplantation after death has been established.

The late 1960s thus brought the willingness to terminate "life support" using an ethical justification that relied on a patient already being declared dead. In the 1970s, other individuals on life-sustaining support who were not dead but clearly could and would not benefit from continued treatment became the focus of a national medical and ethical debate. One such patient was Karen Ann Quinlan,[9] a young woman with severe anoxic encephalopathy following a drug overdose and cardiac arrest, which responded to cardiopulmonary resuscitation. Her parents wished to have her life support terminated, stating that she would never have wanted such support in her current condition and would never have agreed to it. The resultant New Jersey Supreme Court ruling indicated that patients have the right to refuse even life-supporting therapy based on their autonomy and the right to decide what should be allowed to happen to their bodies; essentially, this is grounded in the legal and ethical basis of *informed consent*. It is also important to realize that physicians have no obligation to treat diseases when there is no hope of recovery.

In 1991, the U.S. Congress passed and implemented the Patient Self-Determination Act, which further supports the right of patients to refuse therapy and recommends the use of advance directives to make their wishes known. The U.S. Supreme Court, in *Cruzan v. Missouri Department of Health*,[10] has affirmed the constitutional right of patients to refuse unwanted therapy, although states may regulate the criteria used to determine patient preferences. Thus, at present, removal of life support for patients who are not expected to benefit from this therapy is widely accepted.

THE DISTINCTION BETWEEN WITHHOLDING AND WITHDRAWING SUPPORT

The discussion of terminating life-sustaining therapy in hopelessly ill patients has been an emotional one from its onset. Many health care professionals have been uncomfortable with removal of such support from these patients, believing that by doing so they become active agents of death. Some prefer to withhold support rather than to withdraw it. Withholding support is defined as never providing the patient with the therapy in question. For example, a patient in irreversible renal failure would require dialysis for continued life. Physicians who prefer to withhold support would never initiate dialysis for patients unlikely to benefit. They believe that in this scenario the renal failure causes the patient to die.

Withdrawing support refers to discontinuing already instituted therapy. Proponents may feel more comfortable withdrawing support than withholding it because the therapy has already been shown not to benefit the patient. Those favoring this approach believe that withdrawing the therapy results in the capability of the underlying disease to overwhelm the patient.

Forgoing therapy refers both to the withdrawing and the withholding of therapy. Because both the withdrawing and the withholding of therapy result in unimpeded progression of the disease, and because the justification for withdrawing support is almost always satisfactory for withholding support as well, the two actions can be considered ethically equivalent. However, many families and clinicians, despite understanding this equivalence, may feel more uncomfortable terminating support because of the temporal relationship between the removal of support and the patient's death, which usually occurs as a consequence. The involved physicians and nurses should be aware of the potential for this emotional response and should try to help families and coworkers deal with their feelings.

Interventions *intended* to hasten death directly constitute *active euthanasia*, which is illegal in most countries, including the United States (with the exception of capital punishment). By contrast, *forgoing therapy* is considered passive because the disease, not the intervention, causes death. An example of active euthanasia is the delivery of a lethal intravenous dose of potassium chloride, which directly causes cardiac arrest.

Assisted suicide is defined as helping a person to take his or her own life but not directly performing the action that causes death. An example would be placement of an intravenous catheter, supplying the lethal medication, and instructing the patient in how to use it to commit suicide. Although assisted suicide is not equivalent to euthanasia per se, the two terms are often considered together because of the intention and active induction of death as their goals. In the United States, the practice is prohibited by law in most states; in recent years, however, these statutes have been challenged in some areas. In particular, the state of Oregon has legalized physician-assisted suicide. Recently, the status of this legislation was being challenged at both the state and federal level. The federal Department of Justice and the Food and Drug Administration (FDA) are considering possible actions in this area.

WITHDRAWING AND WITHHOLDING MECHANICAL VENTILATORY ASSISTANCE

Withdrawing and withholding respiratory support require special attention because of the emotional nature and the significant distress that forgoing support can cause for the patient, family, and professional staff. Therefore, removal of ventilatory assistance is discussed separately from the withdrawal of other types of life support.

The primary goal of removing ventilatory assistance is the withdrawal of unwanted therapy while maintaining a patient's comfort. The responsible physician and nurse are not trying to cause death, although that is the usual and expected consequence of withdrawing support. When ventilatory assistance is withdrawn or withheld, patients are likely to suffer respiratory distress unless the physician anticipates this occurrence and acts to prevent and treat it.

Sedation in the form of narcotics administration (to suppress feelings of dyspnea and, perhaps, to provide euphoria) and the use of anxiolytics (to suppress anxiety) are almost always necessary. In dosing these medications, it is important to remember the therapeutic goals. It is crucial that comfort be maintained, even if providing the needed medication also hastens death. This has been referred to as the "double effect." For example, a hypotensive patient who has respiratory discomfort should still receive narcotics, even though this causes both further hypotension and diminished respiratory drive and, as a result, death may occur sooner. The physician's *primary* intent—to relieve suffering by decreasing respiratory drive—is crucial to legitimize giving medications that may also hasten death as a secondary unintended, albeit expected, effect.

Withholding ventilatory assistance from patients with severe lung disease can also be difficult. Sooner or later, such patients experience respiratory distress if they are not prepared adequately. If insufficient medication to prevent distress is not available, a crisis may emerge. Physicians, patients, or families may panic, reverse their opinion, and demand endotracheal intubation and mechanical ventilation as a way of relieving the distress. Anger, hostility, and a sense of physician incompetence or abandonment may ensue. For patients refusing intubation and mechanical ventilation, sufficient quantities of sedatives and or opiates (rather than intubation) must be delivered beforehand to prevent distress, since it is difficult or impossible to reverse severe respiratory distress quickly without intubation.

DeVita and Friedman[11] have reported the use of face mask continuous positive airway pressure (CPAP) instead of intubation and ventilation as a method of providing sufficient ventilatory assistance to relieve distress and enable the physician and nurse to give appropriate medication. CPAP can provide some comfort and creates time needed for discussion (if the patient has not already made a decision) or for sufficient medication to be delivered and to ensure comfort. Once a decision is made and comfort is ensured, the physician can discontinue CPAP. Sometimes large doses of opiates or sedatives may be needed.

Most physicians choose to give morphine or diazepam, or both, to relieve anxiety and to prevent dyspnea before they initiate therapy withdrawal.[12] As withdrawal of mechanical ventilation progresses, more sedation is usually required. Physicians and nursing staff must carefully monitor the patient for signs of problems and must alleviate any distress immediately. It is important to recognize that hypoxia and hypercarbia are potent forces of distress. In addition, many patients in the ICU have developed some tolerance to opioids and sedatives; therefore, surprisingly large doses of these medications may be required.[13] Campbell and Carlson[14] describe morphine drip dosages up to 70 mg/hr, and some patients may ultimately need hundreds of milligrams of morphine if adequate control is to be achieved.[15] Experienced physicians are able to titrate the sedation to prevent rather than relieve discomfort, a laudable practice. As long as the patient remains comfortable, weaning from ventilatory support may proceed, but the rate of progression is dependent on patient tolerance.

Sample orders for sedation and comfort during terminal weaning are presented in Table 199–1. These orders are directed at *preventing* distress through the continuous delivery of medication. An alternative approach directed at *alleviating* distress would use less (or no) continuous sedative infusion and require administration of sedatives as needed in response to any perceived distress. Both approaches to adequate provision of sedatives and or narcotics for prevention and allevia-

TABLE 199–1. Sample Orders for Withdrawal of Mechanical Ventilatory Assistance

1. Patient to receive comfort measures only.
2. Morphine, 5 mg, and diazepam 5 mg intravenously immediately.
3. Begin continuous morphine intravenous infusion at 5 mg/hr.
4. Change ventilator mode to intermittent mandatory ventilation.
5. Decrease ventilator rate by four breaths every 5 minutes.
6. When ventilator rate is decreased to zero, discontinue ventilator and extubate the patient.
7. If patient's respiratory rate is greater than 20 breaths per minute, give morphine, 5 mg intravenously every 5 minutes, until respiratory rate is less than or equal to 20, and increase morphine infusion by 5 mg/hr.
8. Do not withhold medications for treatment of low blood pressure.

*The doses of medication are not recommendations but are used for illustrative purposes only.

tion are directed toward maintaining patient comfort during terminal weaning from the ventilator.

Weaning from mechanical ventilation followed by extubation is preferred by physicians (53%) over either weaning alone (33%) or extubation without first weaning from the ventilator (13%)[12]. The decision whether to extubate the patient must be considered jointly by the medical team, the patient, and the family. The endotracheal tube may have symbolic value for the patient, family, or physician that may dictate whether the tube should remain in place or be removed. If it is removed, the clinician must prevent acute airway obstruction, which will cause suffocation and distress. An oral or nasal airway or positioning the patient to avoid airway obstruction is usually sufficient for this purpose. Reintubation is rarely, if ever, necessary but should be discussed in advance, because in our experience most patients and families prefer heavier sedation to reintubation.

The physician should remain at the bedside to titrate the medications.[12] Careful documentation of dosage and of the rationale for the medication is warranted. Some nurses who are experienced in the withdrawal of life support are able to enact terminal weaning orders as long as an experienced physician is readily available to oversee and assist this activity.

The goal of ventilator withdrawal is to remove the unwanted or nonbeneficial therapy while guaranteeing patient comfort and dignity. In the United States, it is unlawful to intend to cause or to directly cause patient death, although death is the expected outcome of removing ventilatory support. In some instances, physicians have stopped withdrawing mechanical ventilation because of poor patient tolerance. The involved physician or nurse was usually reluctant to provide the large doses of narcotics and sedatives required for comfort because of fear of "killing" the patient. Thus, physicians in this situation have been unable to withdraw unwanted therapy.

Some caregivers consider patient sedation and hastening death as therapeutic objectives. Wilson[16] reported that 36% of physicians ordered and 39% of nurses delivered sedation with the intention of hastening of death. Such intention to hasten or cause death remains illegal and is outside the accepted practice standards of nurses and physicians in most, but not all, countries.

When physicians, nurses, and respiratory therapists at the University of Pittsburgh Medical Center wean a patient from a ventilator, they usually employ intermittent mandatory ventilation. Assist-control ventilation is not used because attempts to breathe trigger a full machine breath. In this mode, decreased ventilatory support can result only from eradication of all respiratory effort or suppression of the patient's ability to trigger the ventilator. In contrast, pressure support, inspired oxygen concentration, and end-expiratory pressure can all be reduced gradually or rapidly.

WITHDRAWING NONVENTILATORY LIFE SUPPORT

In addition to mechanical ventilation, other forms of life-sustaining support can be forgone. Physicians discontinue left ventricular assist devices,[17] implanted cardioverter-defibrillators,[18] vasopressor and inotropic support, dialysis, antibiotics, nutrition, and oxygen.[19] Intravenous medical therapy with antibiotics, blood products, and antiarrhythmic agents is usually discontinued abruptly and painlessly. Although there is no great controversy or difficulty in forgoing most of these forms of therapy, removal of other therapies may be more emotional because of some special symbolism or significance. Discontinuation of artificial hydration and nutrition have been particularly difficult to rationalize for some,[20, 21] but the majority of physicians,[22-26] court opinions,[10, 27] and the public[28] ethically and legally equate all forms of medical therapy. That is, all therapy (with the exception of comfort measures) can be considered to sustain life. For example, mechanical ventilation and assisted circulation, on the one hand, and artificial feeding and fluid administration, on the other, are therapies that sustain life. It can be argued that the primary ethical difference between these therapies is the immediacy of the effects of their deprivation on a patient. Removal of mechanical ventilation *feels* different from discontinuing antibiotics because the patient is likely to die quickly after the former therapy is stopped. Both therapies, when stopped, however, allow the disease process to advance unchecked.

Just as discontinuation of mechanical ventilation requires sufficient ethical justification, so does the withdrawal of other mechanical, hemodynamic, or homeostatic support. Once the decision to withdraw life-sustaining therapy is made, the patient's comfort must be maintained as a primary goal. However, most nonventilatory therapies do not have the same potential to cause distress as does withdrawal of ventilatory support. Discontinuation of antibiotics and blood products, for example, is not associated with pain or discomfort. For therapies that may cause distress when removed, the physician must consider this possibility and treat or preferably prevent its occurrence. For example, hunger may be caused by the discontinuation of feedings, or patients who understand that treatment is being discontinued may experience anxiety. Physicians should treat or prevent these feelings with anxiolytics, sedatives, or opiates, all of which are able to suppress such sensations. We recommend administering anxiolytics and narcotics to those patients who *possibly* may experience such sensations.

Other examples of support whose withdrawal does not typically cause distress are (1) cardiac bypass (because the patient is typically anesthetized), (2) dialysis, and (3) cardiac pacing. Examples of therapies whose discontinuation sometimes may be associated with discomfort are nutrition (hunger), hydration (thirst), use of pressor and inotropic agents, artificial heart devices, and dialysis in patients with volume overload (dyspnea from pulmonary vascular congestion).

As is the case in withdrawal of mechanical ventilation, forgoing other therapies always requires careful discussion with the patient's family and, if possible, with the patient. Early communication, before any decisions are made, builds trust and is effective in educating the involved persons about legal, medical, ethical, religious, and prognostic considerations. The discussions enable the physician and patient and family to create a rational framework for agreeing on therapy that involves all of these considerations.

Families have demonstrated the ability to rationalize various combinations of therapy that are acceptable to them. For example, the prognosis for two patients was poor for recovery from pneumonia and persistent vegetative conditions. Both patients were intubated and mechanically ventilated. Careful discussion with one patient's family revealed the patient's desire not to be kept alive by machines if there was no hope of recovery, but the patient approved of all other therapies, such as the administration of antibiotics and prophylaxis for bedsores. The second family reported that their loved one would not desire further therapy but did not want the ventilator disconnected because the patient believed that this was placing "God's work into man's hands." The physicians discontinued the former patient's ventilator therapy only and the latter patient's medical and diagnostic therapy but not mechanical ventilation. In both cases, the families believed that the correct decision had been made, and the physicians were comfortable that nonbeneficial or unwanted therapy had been appropriately withdrawn.

ATTITUDES TOWARDS FORGOING LIFE-SUSTAINING THERAPY

Solomon and coworkers[29] reported that physicians commonly provide care to patients not expected to benefit. In this study, physicians also reported a reluctance to remove such patients from life support even if the patients or their families had expressed a desire to forgo such support. This dichotomy of understanding that continued therapy may not be in a patient's best interest but still not stopping that therapy points out the ethical and social tension and ambiguous reasoning that physicians may exhibit.

Vincent[30] surveyed European ICU physicians about similar issues. Thirty-one per cent of responding physicians indicated that they discuss Do Not Resuscitate (DNR) status with the patients, whereas 57% instead stated that they discuss this issue only with the families. DNR orders were frequently given but were usually oral and not written. Eighty-three per cent of the responding physicians included withholding of support as part of their practice, 63% withdrew initiated therapy if no longer indicated or wanted, and 36% stated that they practice euthanasia. In the example of an irreversibly ill and comatose patient whose family wants "everything done," more than 100 of the 242 respondents stated they would withhold support, and more than 30 would withdraw therapy anyway. While this practice may be acceptable in some countries with socialized medicine, it is not recommended in the United States, where the patient's wishes are paramount.

Miller[31] has supported the physician's role in the dying process and, further, calls for recognition of the obligation the physician has to the dying. When appropriate, the physician must actively choose not to try to prevent death and, in fact, must help facilitate it if the autonomy or dignity of the individual is threatened. Osler demonstrated this when caring for his patients and at the time of his own death. Hinohara[32] cites Osler's approval of the use of medications under certain circumstances when a patient is terminally ill. Osler, as his own death approached, turned from the use of medications for his chronic bronchitis to the use of opium, which made him comfortable. He recognized the importance of dying as a process, which must be psychologically and, if necessary, medically supported to eliminate suffering—whether it be spiritual, physical, or mental.

It is possible that the nursing staff may be working with an understanding and goal of therapy different (although rational) from those of the physician. For this reason, it is important to include the nursing staff in family discussions and the decision-making process. At the very least, the physician must discuss the plan with the nursing staff once a decision is made. Without such communication, the ordered and intended therapy may not be the same as the delivered therapy. Nurses may give less or more medication than required based on their own interpretation, which may be differ from the intent of the physician or patient. Nurses spend more time at patients' bedsides and with families than physicians do, and frequently nurses possess insights to patient and family attitudes and preferences that will provide important information to end-of-life discussions.

Patient preferences for ICU management clearly support the desire to survive if that outcome is likely. It is equally clear that if the outcome is expected to be poor, most patients disagree with the continuation of life support. However, fully 25% of the patients in one study preferred life support even in the face of either a permanent vegetative state or terminal illness.[33]

Although many physicians and nurses may be concerned about the ethics and legality of forgoing life-sustaining therapy, the clinician in virtually all cases does not need a judge to permit such activity. In 1990, Mishkin[34] reported that no physician had ever been found liable for terminating treatment at the request of a competent adult. This is because all interventions require consent, which reflects the voluntary nature of the patient's participation. This effectively precludes the physician from liability. Still, physicians may fear litigation. In this situation, Mishkin argues that the courts and judges are not adequately trained to handle and lack the experience to confront such biomedical-ethical situations. It is the responsibility of hospitals to design policies regarding the management of such problems.

On the other hand, by *not* complying with a request to terminate treatment, the physician does become vulnerable to a new type of legal action: the "right-to-die" suit. In fact, in such a situation, physicians have been found liable for pain and suffering caused by unwanted care.[34]

Several groups have attempted to facilitate removal of life support from hopelessly ill patients. Some have focused on creating a comprehensive supportive care team[35] that provides an alternative to the ICU or ward environment by concentrating on the physical and psychosocial needs of the dying patient. Kwack and Grenvik have created a plan modeled after a practice observed in Korea.[36] This plan allows patients (or families) to decide whether to have life support withdrawn at home, with family members present, thereby lessening the intrusion of technology into an intensely personal and emotional event. Others have created so-called "futility" policies, which support the duty of the physicians, nurses, and other health professionals to treat patients only when a reasonable hope of benefit is expected. Comfort and hygienic measures should always be provided. These policies permit physicians to withdraw futile (nonbeneficial) therapy even if the patients themselves or their families request continued treatment.[37-40] Although the decision to terminate life support is usually made jointly by the physician, patient, and family (or surrogates), some reports describe involvement of third parties, whose goal is to prevent withdrawal of therapy.[41-43]

EUTHANASIA AND ASSISTED SUICIDE

The rationale for forgoing therapy has been framed in terms of enhancing patient autonomy or avoiding futile therapy while allowing death to occur with dignity and quality at the end of the patient's life. Supporters have argued that euthanasia fosters the same principles.

Euthanasia (Greek, "good death") has received greatest acceptance by society when it is considered for patients who have terminal illness and are unresponsive to therapeutic interventions that are acceptable (to the patient). These patients commonly suffer from pain or unremitting psychologic anguish. Miller[31] has stated that "the physicians, [patients,] and surrogates must be ready and willing to decide not to intervene in the dying process, indeed to hasten it when they see the autonomy and dignity of patients threatened." However, hastening death remains an illegal action in the United States as well as in most other countries. Unfortunately, current laws depend on the physician's intentions as well as specific actions. Cameron writes that "the difference between euthanasia and letting the patient die by omitting life-sustaining treatment is a moral quibble."[44] That is, the actions are different while the intentions may be quite similar.

Colloquially, euthanasia is an active intervention intended to hasten the death of an individual. Groups such as Choice in Dying have been formed to support social acceptance and foster legislation permitting euthanasia. They have been active in promoting the same goals for forgoing support as well.

Euthanasia and assisted suicide have received considerable media attention. Jack Kevorkian, a retired pathologist, has become renowned because he has helped several patients to commit suicide. His actions have caught the attention of lay people, legislators, and ethicists throughout the United States and the world. States such as Michigan have passed statutes making assisting suicide a felony offense. The U.S. Supreme Court has ruled that there is no *constitutional* right to physician assisted suicide.[45, 46] However, it has declined to review the case challenging the constitutionality of the Oregon referendum legalizing physician assisted suicide.[47] Therefore, the constitutionality of state laws permitting physician assisted suicide is still untested, and it appears that states may set the standard. The Oregon statute has now been implemented despite a variety of procedural and regulatory obstacles. The U.S. Drug Enforcement Administration is considering criminal charges for violating federal narcotics laws for physicians engaging in physician assisted suicide. The U.S. Justice Department is reviewing the statute as well. Pharmacists may be at risk for dispensing medications prescribed for assisting suicide, and physicians' and pharmacists' associations have not endorsed the practice.

In his book *Final Exit*, Derek Humphrey[48] argues that "when cure is no longer possible and the patient seeks relief through euthanasia, the help of physicians is most appropriate." In contrast, a trustee of the American Medical Association was quoted as saying that the assistance of suicide or euthanasia by physicians would destroy the therapeutic relationship of trust necessary for patients and physicians. Others contend that making these options widely available would raise the likelihood that individuals would inappropriately commit suicide or even permit murder.[49] Humphrey's book is explicit with regard to step-by-step methods, dosages, and pitfalls in suicide and euthanasia. As a testament to the public interest in this matter, in 1992 the book made the *New York Times* bestseller list.

In the Netherlands, physicians have helped thousands of patients commit suicide and have also participated in euthanasia of patients. Although not legal, the practice currently is not prosecuted. The Dutch Parliament has implemented a law that protects physicians from legal sanction if they participate in assisted suicide or euthanasia, provided that accepted guidelines are followed.[50] Thus, engaging in this practice does not result in prosecution.

The Dutch have created a set of practice guidelines that seek to ensure that only "appropriate" patients are considered for euthanasia. The request must be made voluntarily by the patient, who must be well informed about the procedure and alternatives; he or she must be suffering unbearably, without hope of recovery. Furthermore, the patient's decision must remain unchanged over time. The hope is to prevent depressed or impulsive individuals from acting on a poorly grounded decision. The physician must consult with at least one colleague experienced in these matters, and adequate written documentation must demonstrate that the noted requirements have been met.

Yet, not all Dutch physicians are pleased with the Parliament's decision; 11% state that they would refuse to participate,[50] and one physician has said, "Today, the Netherlands abolished the Hippocratic oath."[51] Many assert that requests for euthanasia and assisted suicide are manifestations that care for patients at the end of life is inadequate. Concern about improving end-of-life care has led to increasing inquiry into patient needs and preferences and has resulted in the burgeoning field of "palliative care." Improved attention to a patient's psychosocial needs and palliation of symptoms may decrease the perception that suicide and euthanasia are ever necessary. Critical care clinicians should expect and support initiatives to enhance care for dying patients.

HOSPITAL POLICY FORMATION

In the United States, legislation requiring hospitals to adopt policies regarding advance directives has given further impetus to the trend toward the development of policies concerning withdrawal of support. Since 1975, the University of Pittsburgh Medical Center (UPMC) has had a policy that provides guidelines for the withdrawal of support.[52] In 1986 and 1997, those guidelines were revised (see the Appendix of this chapter). There are several major changes from past versions.

First, a specific mechanism for a decision-making process now exists for individuals who are unable to speak for themselves, whose wishes are unknown, and for whom there are no surrogates. Before the policy revision, such cases were decided by the courts or by the clinicians based on a loose "best interest of the patient" premise, or they were left undecided. The new policy requires existing hospital and community resources, especially the clinicians and the ethics committee, which represent both patient and clinician perspectives and viewpoints, to make a decision without involving the judicial system. To date, the mechanism has been effective and has provided an effective forum for all viewpoints to be considered.

The second major change involves level of care. The new policy has three levels: (1) all appropriate measures, (2) limited measures, and (3) comfort measures only. This policy recognizes the fact that patients and their families place different values on various therapies. For instance, patients may decide on various components of resuscitation (e.g., endotracheal intubation but not chest compressions) because of their likelihood of, or lack of, success and because of the values that these therapies may have for them. The policy allows patients and physicians to specify which therapies are to be provided and which are to be forgone.

Increasingly, families and physicians seem to be unable to reach an agreement regarding further provision of care.[38, 53, 54] When the patient or family wants care but the physician believes that the therapy is not indicated, a stalemate of sorts may ensue. The UPMC policy, which is based on patient autonomy and cooperation, may sometimes be ill suited to deal with this problem. A stalemate may still occur, even though a policy may explicitly state that patients and surrogates may not compel physicians to provide therapy that the physician judges to be nonbeneficial (as stated in the UPMC policy [see Appendix]).

Therefore, some institutions have policies[38] or committees[53] that serve as a mechanism to withdraw care without family consent or over family refusal. Usually, a third-party review is required by another physician and by an ethicist, and some sort of formal discussion of the problem is necessary. Stell[54] cites the need to inform the surrogates of such a decision before its implementation, allowing the surrogates the opportunity to appeal or to transfer care to another physician or institution. The formalization of the process and the assurance that it seems to provide physicians appear to have resulted in lifting the burden of decision making from families unable to reach these decisions on their own. The policy has resulted in increasing communication and diminishing conflict between surrogates and caregivers.[54] However, to date, no higher court decisions in the United States have supported or refuted the applicability of such intrainstitutional policies.

A final change regards invasive interventions in patients who refuse resuscitation or intubation. The policy states that surgery for patients who refuse to be resuscitated is ethical and legal even if the patient remains a no-resuscitation candidate. Conversely, it also supports temporarily rescinding the no-resuscitation order during the perioperative interval in appropriate circumstances. The UPMC policy continues the resuscitate order until the physician resumes the prior orders or after a specific time interval, whichever comes first. In all cases, discussion between the surgeon, anesthesiologist, and patient or surrogate is necessary.

Compliance with the Patient Self-Determination Act (PSDA) has been a problem for institutions. The PSDA requires that hospitals educate patients about the advance directive, permit patients to create one, and obtain copies of existing advance directive documents. Now the Joint Commission for the Accreditation of Healthcare Organizations (JCAHO) requires that three attempts to obtain an existing advance directive are documented. If one is obtained, the physician is required to document the discussion held with the patient or the patient's family (or surrogate) and to define the resulting medical and nursing care plan. Appropriate orders must follow.

SUMMARY

Forgoing therapy in the ICU is a common practice in the United States and is accepted in most countries. However, the legality, practice, and societal acceptance of this option vary widely among and within countries. Because physicians are now empowered with newer and increasingly more effective therapies to prevent death, more hopelessly ill patients die only following an active decision not to provide some or all life-sustaining therapy. Already, most hospitalized patients die following a decision to forgo some therapy. The physician must be aware of the rationale for forgoing support and must effectively prevent pain and distress as much as possible as the end of life approaches. Physicians must be just as prepared to approach the making of such decisions as they are in approaching other medical dilemmas.

Many resources available to caregivers can facilitate the decision-making process. Advance directives provide a framework for collaborative decision making. Ethics consultants may be helpful. Nurses and social workers can provide insight into patient and family attitudes, perceptions, and preferences. Effective ICU patient management includes creating appropriate policies and utilizing a team approach to deal with decisions of an ethical nature. The team may include nurses, physicians, social workers, clergy, patient representatives, family members, and, of course whenever possible, the patients themselves.

References

1. Faber-Langendoen K, Bartels D: Process of forgoing life-sustaining treatment in a university hospital: An empirical study. Crit Care Med 1992; 20:570.
2. Prendergast TJ, Luce JM: Increasing incidence of withholding and withdrawal of life support from the critically ill. Am J Respir Crit Care Med 1997; 155:15.
3. Rapin M: The ethics of intensive care (Editorial). Intensive Care Med 1987; 13:300.
4. Lofstedt S, von Reis G: Intracranial lesions with abolished passage of x-ray contrast through the internal carotid arteries. Opuscula Med 1956; 8:199.
5. Mollaret P, Goulon M: Le coma dépassé. Rev Neurol (Paris) 1959; 101:3.
6. Wolstenholme G, O'Connor M (Eds): 1966 Ciba Foundation Symposium: Ethics in Medical Progress with Special Reference to Transplantation. Boston, Little, Brown & Co, 1966.
7. Beecher H: A definition of irreversible coma: Special communication. Report of the Ad Hoc Committee of the Harvard Medical School to Examine the Definition of Brain Death. JAMA 1968; 205:337.
8. Wasmuth CE, Stewart BH: Medical and legal aspects of human organ transplantation. Cleveland-Marshall Law Review 1965; 14:464.
9. *In re Quinlan*, 355 A 2d647 (NJ 1976).
10. *Cruzan v Director, Missouri Department of Health*, 110 S Ct 284 (1990).
11. DeVita M, Friedman Y, Petrella V: Mask continuous positive airway pressure in AIDS. Crit Care Clin 1993; 9:137.
12. Faber-Langendoen K: The clinical management of dying patients receiving mechanical ventilation: A survey of physician practice. Chest 1994; 106:880.
13. Carlson JP: Managing pain and suffering in the dying patient. Minn Med 1990; 73:35.
14. Campbell ML, Carlson RW: Terminal weaning from mechanical ventilation: Ethical and practical considerations for patient management. Am J Crit Care 1992; 1:52.
15. DeVita M, Grenvik A: Personal communication, June 1, 1993.
16. Wilson WC, Smedira NG, Fink C, et al: Ordering and administering of sedatives and analgesics during the withholding and withdrawal of life support from critically ill patients. JAMA 1992; 267:949.
17. Powell TP, Oz MC: Discontinuing the LVAD: Ethical considerations. Ann Thorac Surg 1997; 63:1223.
18. Quill TE, Barold SS, Sussman BL: Discontinuing an implantable cardioverter defibrillator as a life sustaining treatment. Am J Cardiol 1994; 74:205.
19. Wood GG, Martin E: Withholding and withdrawing life sustaining therapy in a Canadian intensive care unit. Can J Anaesth 1995; 42:186.
20. Ramsey P: The indignity of "death with dignity." *In*: Death Inside Out: The Hastings Center Report. Steinfels P, Veatch RM (Eds). New York, Harper & Row, 1974, pp 81–96.
21. Rosner F: Withholding therapy and anti-cruelty policies (Letter). Ann Intern Med 1986; 105:468.
22. Steinbrook R, Lo B: Artificial feeding: Solid ground, not a slippery slope. N Engl J Med 1988; 318:286.
23. Council on Ethical and Judicial Affairs of the American Medical Association: Guidelines for the appropriate use of do-not-resuscitate orders. JAMA 1991; 265:1868.
24. Orentlicher D: The right to die after Cruzan. JAMA 1990; 264:2444.
25. Lo B, Dornbrand L: The case of Claire Conroy: Will administrative review safeguard incompetent patients? Ann Intern Med 1986; 104:869.
26. O'Rourke K: The AMA statement on tube feeding: An ethical analysis. America 1986; 155:321.
27. *In re Conroy*, 98 NJ 321, 486 A 2d 1209 (1985).
28. Pinkney D: N.Y. law allows home-bound patients to refuse resuscitation. *American Medical News*, August 12, 1991, p 3.
29. Solomon MZ, O'Donnell LO, Jennings B: Decisions near the end of life: Professional views on life-sustaining treatments. Am J Public Health 1993; 83:14.
30. Vincent JL: European attitudes towards ethical problems in intensive care medicine: Results of an ethical questionnaire. Intensive Care Med 1990; 16:256.
31. Miller PJ: Death with dignity and the right to die: Sometimes doctors have a duty to hasten death. J Med Ethics 1987; 13:81.
32. Hinohara S: Sir William Osler's philosophy on death. Ann Intern Med 1993; 118:638.
33. Elpern EH, Patterson PA, Gloskey D, et al: Patients' preferences for intensive care. Crit Care Med 1992; 20:43.
34. Mishkin DB: You don't need a judge to terminate treatment. J Intensive Care Med 1990; 5:201.
35. Field BE, Devich LE, Carlson RW: Impact of a comprehensive supportive care team on management of hopelessly ill patients with multiple organ failure. Chest 1989; 96:353.
36. Kwack IY, Grenvik A: Personal communication, September 3, 1989.
37. Paris JJ, Crone RK, Reardon F: Physician refusal of requested treatment. N Engl J Med 1990; 322:1012.
38. Stell LK: Stopping treatment on grounds of futility: A role for institutional policy. St. Louis University Public Law Review 1992; 11:481.
39. Hansen-Flaschen JH: When life support is futile (Editorial). Chest 1991; 100:1191.
40. Marsh FH, Staver A: Futile cardiopulmonary resuscitation and physician authority for unilateral do-not-resuscitate orders. J Crit Care 1991; 6:221.

41. McCormick RA: "Moral considerations" ill considered. America 1992; 166:210.
42. Swanson H: Murder and the right to die. *Newsweek* 1989; 113:33.
43. Burnell GM: My mother wants to die: A lawyer won't let her. Med Econ 1988; 65:57.
44. Cameron DCS: The Truth About Cancer. Englewood Cliffs, NJ, Prentice-Hall, 1956, p 116.
45. *Washington v. Glucksberg*, 117 S. Ct. 2258(1997).
46. *Vacco v. Quill*, 117 S.Ct. 2293(1997).
47. *Lee v. Harcleroad*, 66 U.S.L.W. 3278(1997).
48. Humphrey D: Final Exit. Secaucus, NJ, Hemlock Society, 1991.
49. Henry WA III: Do-it-yourself death lessons. *Time* 1991; 138:55.
50. Simons M: Dutch parliament approves law permitting euthanasia. *New York Times*, February 10, 1993, p A5.
51. Steinfels P: Help for the helping hands in death. *New York Times*, February 14, 1993, Section 4, p 1.
52. Meisel A, Grenvik A, Pinkus RL, et al: Hospital guidelines for deciding about life-sustaining treatment: Dealing with health "limbo." Crit Care Med 1986; 14:239.
53. Brennan TA: Do-not-resuscitate orders for the incompetent patient in the absence of family consent. Law Med Health Care 1986; 14:13.
54. Stell LK: Personal communication, May 4, 1993.

Appendix:

Summary of University of Pittsburgh Medical Center Guidelines on Forgoing Life-Sustaining Treatment (1992 Revision of Previously Published Guidelines)

PURPOSE

The purpose of this summary is to provide access to information contained in the University of Pittsburgh Medical Center Guidelines on Forgoing Life-Sustaining Treatment. It is not to be used as a substitute for those guidelines, which should be referred to when specific medical-ethical dilemmas occur.

INTRODUCTION

No ethically relevant distinction exists between failing to institute new treatment and discontinuing treatment that has already been initiated. Therefore, the term "forgo" is used to include stopping treatment already begun as well as not starting a new treatment. These guidelines are applicable to all kinds of life-sustaining treatment and are not limited to decisions to forgo cardiopulmonary resuscitation.

STATEMENT OF GENERAL PRINCIPLES

General Principles Governing Decision Making

As a general rule, all adult patients who do not lack decision-making capacity may decline any treatment or procedure. Patients who lack decision-making capacity have the same ethical and legal rights as do patients who possess such capacity, but health care decisions must be made on their behalf by a surrogate decision maker. Provision is made for a process to make decisions for patients who do not have surrogates. This process includes ethics committee review. It is the ethical and legal right of an individual physician to decline to participate in the limitation or withdrawal of therapy, if he or she considers this action inappropriate. However, no physician may abandon his or her patient until care by another physician has been secured. Further, a patient or his or her surrogate may not compel the physician to provide any treatment which in the physician's professional judgment is unlikely to provide the patient with significant benefit; i.e., the treatment is not medically indicated. Procedures for assessing decision-making capacity, for selecting a surrogate decision maker, and for Ethics Committee consultation are outlined in this section.

ADVANCE DIRECTIVES

The definition of, weight to be given to, and procedures for handling advance directives (living wills) are outlined in this section.

Documentation of Decisions and Entry of Orders

When it has been determined that a particular life-sustaining procedure is to be forgone, the resulting order must be written into the patient's medical record and an appropriate progress note written, including information on diagnosis, prognosis, patient's or surrogate's wishes, the recommendations of the treating team, and a description of the patient's decision-making ability. It is the physician's responsibility to communicate this information to other members of the health care team.

Detailed orders are usually required. Three categories of care are outlined.

All Appropriate Therapy: These patients are treated vigorously, using indicated diagnostic and therapeutic interventions.

Limited Therapy: This category includes patients for whom the decision has been made to forgo some therapy. Therapy already initiated will be limited by specific written order only. Patients, their families or surrogates, and their physicians will accord different values, risks, benefits, and burdens imposed by various therapies and diagnostics. Thus, it is reasonable to allow involved parties to choose the appropriate interventions for that particular group of individuals. For example, patients with similar problems and prognoses may choose with their doctors to have in one case mechanical ventilation, but not hemodynamic support, and in another, the reverse. It is important for the physician to document such decisions and their rationale in the patient medical record.

Comfort Measures Only: These patients will receive only nursing, hygienic care, and medications appropriate to maintain comfort as ordered. Therapy (e.g., administration of narcotics) which is necessary for comfort may be utilized even if it contributes to cardiorespiratory depression. Therapies already initiated will be reviewed by the physician and discontinued if not related to comfort or hygiene.

Selection of a Surrogate Decision Maker

When there is no appropriate person to serve as a surrogate and the patient has not previously designated a surrogate and/or executed an advance directive, it is recommended that the

Ethics Consultation Service and Legal Services be consulted. When it is decided not to request judicial appointment of a surrogate, forgoing life-sustaining treatment is ethically acceptable if each of the following conditions is satisfied:

a. Reasonable efforts have been made to identify an appropriate person (e.g., a family member or a friend) to serve as a surrogate, and those attempts have been unsuccessful.

b. There is a consensus among physicians involved with the case that there is no significant chance of meaningful recovery and life-sustaining treatment is of no expected benefit to the patient.

c. Conditions (a) and (b) are clearly documented in the patient's chart (progress notes).

d. There is a consensus at a meeting of the Medical Ethics Committee that: (i) reasonable efforts have been made to identify an appropriate person to serve as a surrogate, (ii) considering the patient's condition and prognosis, a reasonable person would conclude that life-sustaining treatment is of no expected benefit and therefore, not want it, and (iii) reasonable efforts have been made to determine whether pertinent members of the health care team object to the forgoing of life-sustaining treatment for this patient, and insufficient reasons have been offered to conclude that forgoing treatment is ethically unacceptable. For the purposes of this meeting, a quorum shall consist of: the Chair of the Medical Ethics Committee or his or her designee, a representative from the Ethics Consultation Service, a nurse, a representative from Legal Services, a representative from Clinical Social Work, a lay representative, and an additional physician not involved with the case. Representation from Patient Relations and Pastoral Care is recommended.

Temporary Reversal of Do Not Resuscitate Orders

Some patients who have chosen not to receive life-sustaining procedures may nevertheless be candidates for invasive procedures intended to promote comfort and quality of life. Such procedures may involve use of anesthesia that requires temporary use of endotracheal intubation, ventilator support, or intravenous medication. Before such procedures are performed, it is appropriate to consider temporarily rescinding orders to forgo resuscitation during the perioperative period. It is not necessary to rescind a code status in order for a procedure to occur. However, a patient may not compel a physician to perform a procedure when the patient has do not resuscitate orders. The patient may be transferred to another physician who is willing to perform the procedure under those conditions.

The prior code status is resumed following a physician order to do so, or 24 hours after the procedure if the physician has not done so.

200

The Ethics of Resource Allocation in the Intensive Care Unit

Stephen M. Ayres, MD • Karen N. Swisher, MS, JD

Many physicians, particularly intensivists, are intuitively compelled to ration scarce resources on a daily basis. The demand for well-staffed and well-equipped intensive care unit (ICU) beds frequently exceeds the local supply, and physicians must provide ICU care for some, knowing that they may in the process deny care to others who might benefit from that care. Using only their professional knowledge and a sense of equity, intensivists regularly decide whether to admit one more patient to a crowded ICU, transfer a patient to a less well-staffed unit in favor of one who shows greater promise of benefiting from ICU treatment, or transfer a patient who now shows little chance of benefit from ICU treatment.[1] Although ethicists, attorneys, and others worry about the legal and ethical bases for rationing care, intensivists practice rationing of ICU resources regularly. Because these patients are seriously ill, the reason for rationing is almost always based on the scarcity of resources rather than on the insurance status of the patients.

Strauss and coworkers,[2] in a 1986 study entitled "Rationing of Intensive Care Unit Services: An Every Day Occurrence," analyzed admission decision making in an 18-bed general ICU in a hospital associated with a medical school. Admission decisions were made by two specified physicians, the senior surgical resident and senior medical resident assigned to the unit. A statistically significant inverse correlation existed between bed availability and the age and severity of illness among those admitted to the unit. Patients admitted when beds were scarce were significantly sicker than those admitted when beds were plentiful! No significant differences were observed in the percentage of patients intubated, the ICU death rate, and the total length of stay in the hospital after ICU discharge. Discharges from the unit were 3.4 times more likely when no empty beds were available compared with when five empty beds were available. In economic terms, admission to the ICU was elastic in relation to bed availability.

Medical directors of special care units and other physicians are increasingly asked to make administrative decisions, such as determining the appropriateness of the admission of one patient over another to an ICU bed. Continuing pressures from regulators, administrators, and third-party payers will intensify the need for physicians as well as other clinical professionals to make decisions about the cost effectiveness of diagnostic and treatment procedures.[3]

Many hospitals have decentralized their administrative and management functions, creating more opportunities for clinician-managers. Hospitals are placing greater responsibility upon clinicians in a number of ways: (1) through reorganization, so that allocation decisions are delegated to front-line health professionals; (2) in the creation of programs to provide cost information to physicians and other health professional decision makers; and (3) by changing physician behavior through utilization management programs that attempt to improve their efficiency and effectiveness.[4] Physicians assigned to these new roles are frequently poorly prepared for the ethical consequences of such resource allocation decisions. They are traditionally trained to be advocates for individual patients, and their frame of reference emphasizes patient and professional autonomy. Frequently, their insistence on individual patient needs comes into conflict with the financial needs of the institution.

Hiller[5] has provided a useful description of the physicians' dilemma by classifying the levels of their ethical conflicts. *Microlevel conflicts* are those that involve individual or professional values, *mesolevel conflicts* are those that involve institutional values, and *macrolevel conflicts* are those that involve community or cultural values. Physicians asked to make mesolevel or macrolevel decisions often feel that such considerations inevitably compromise the traditional doctor-patient relationship. Physicians perceive conflict between their role as clinicians and their role as advocates for the hospital. On a personal level, physician conflicts may include (1) expectations by hospital administration of actions that are incongruent with the orientations and values of the individual physician; (2) time overloading, if various role expectations exceed the available times and resources; and (3) role ambiguity, if information regarding the scope of responsibilities or the expectations of others are uncertain.[6]

Administrators and clinicians must realize the potential role conflict experienced by those clinicians who now must make allocation choices. They can never hope to achieve a sound policy that purports to enhance quality of patient care in a time of resource limitation. Manager-physicians must broaden their ethical perspective and training to include the implications of their actions. Clinical ethical training has only a limited role to play here.

In 1984, Hiller[5] noted that no comprehensive framework existed in the literature for the study of ethics in health care administration. Hospital administrators themselves are frequently poorly trained in business ethics and can offer little guidance to clinicians embarking upon a new career.

The demand for increased rationality in the matching of available resources to patients' needs requires increased communication, understanding, and integration of clinical and business ethics among all health care professionals.

ALLOCATION, RATIONING, AND THE BUSINESS OF HEALTH CARE

Health care services have never been considered a basic American right. Instead, health care is considered to be a commodity that is, just like any other commodity, allocated and rationed through the marketplace. Services are available to those who can afford health care; those who cannot afford it frequently go without. The long-delayed move to health care reform has been fueled in large part by the belief held by many Americans that it is unfair and unjust to link access to health care to socioeconomic status.

Important distinctions between allocation and rationing can be made. *Allocation* decisions determine to what extent a society devotes its resources to a particular service. Funding levels for Medicare and Medicaid in the United States or those for national health systems in other countries are examples of "macrolevel" allocation policies. Conversely, *rationing* is usually a "microlevel" issue because decisions are made as to who receives resources for a particular purpose. Through rationing, a society decides who gets a particular heart transplant and who can go on dialysis. Obviously, allocation decisions affect rationing decisions; the almost universal availability of hemodialysis through Medicare reduces the need for rationing decisions.

Federal and state allocation decisions, in turn, have a major impact on the strategic planning of hospitals and other health care organizations. The more resources allocated for a given clinical problem, the more profitable it is to provide such services. Hospitals attempt to increase their market share of reimbursed services by vigorously promoting their programs in transplantation or cardiac surgery but not for poorly reimbursed services such as treatments for multiple injury.

The implicitly accepted idea that the intensivist serves as the agent of rationing suggests that some agreed-on definition of the word "rationing" itself exists. The definition espoused by the Catholic Health Association is "the withholding of potentially beneficial health care services because practices and policies establish limits on the resources available for health care."[7] A contrasting definition is "not all care expected to be beneficial is provided to all patients." The Catholic Health Association definition clearly indicates that it is the issue of "potential benefit" that determines whether the limitation of certain services is actually rationing. The patients discharged earlier from the ICU studied by Strauss and coworkers[2] apparently did not experience rationing because there was no evidence of unfavorable outcome after they were transferred. Although ethicists may set rules for rationing, by this definition, only physicians can define the potential benefit of an intervention and know, therefore, whether rationing has actually occurred.

Henry J. Aaron, the Brookings Institution scholar who wrote *The Painful Prescription: Rationing Hospital Care* with William Schwartz in 1984, has an even more limiting definition of rationing. He believes that rationing can be said to exist only when the limited activity is known to be beneficial and is not available to individuals even if they could pay for it.[8]

A major emotional distinction exists between statistical and identifiable lives when rationing is under consideration. Governments and insurers make decisions whether to pay for a specific procedure on the basis of population statistics and the number of lives that might be spared or lost as a result of these decisions. In contrast, when a particular child who requires organ transplantation dies while the family is trying to raise funds for the procedure, the child becomes a very identifiable individual. Furrow and coworkers have pointed out that,

> *It is a commonplace that society will expend almost limitless resources to save the identifiable life, but is willing to sacrifice statistical lives at a much lower cost. The more overtly and explicitly a government is responsible, the more difficulty the government will face in saying no, in refusing to provide the resource necessary to save a life or to relieve suffering. This distinction is related to the preceding one, in that allocation decisions usually affect statistical lives—rationing, identifiable lives.*[9]

Health care reform is shifting rationing and allocation decisions from the marketplace to the political arena. Such a shift has great impact on the legal system. Once government makes eligibility for a specific procedure conditional, litigation inevitably increases as individuals are given the right to appeal conditional decisions. Health care reform will almost certainly create much more litigation in the health care industry than has been seen under the present system, in which most legal action is related to the allegation of medical malpractice.

THE IMPACT OF THE LEGAL SYSTEM ON ALLOCATION AND RATIONING

Physicians and hospitals are gravely concerned about the rising frequency and severity of medical malpractice claims. Physicians are held to a standard of care for all patients. How well the courts will consider and incorporate the realities of rationing and allocation into these decisions is not clear. Physicians rightly fear that the limitation of ICU beds at any given moment will not be fully understood by the courts when a particular physician is forced to deny a particular patient access to one of these beds.

This issue was tested in the Maryland courts in 1993, when a 3-year-old child with a long history of complex seizure disorders that were often life-threatening required urgent admission to a hospital. The protocol for the emergency medical service used by the family required that the child be transported to the nearest hospital, where he would be stabilized and then transferred to Johns Hopkins Hospital for further treatment. The physicians at Johns Hopkins Hospital, in cooperation with the child's parents, developed a new protocol that would allow the child to be transported directly to the hospital, even though the child was not stable. The physician treating the child wrote a letter in 1991 describing the procedure and stating that

it would be better to transport the child directly to the Hopkins Pediatric Emergency Room with advance warning by radio to the emergency room and pediatric neurology. There are always risks in transporting a seizing child, but I feel that they are in this case justified. These risks have been explained to the parents who understand and support this decision. . . .

In 1992, the child began to have seizures and was taken by ambulance to the designated helicopter for transportation. During transport, the ambulance called Johns Hopkins Hospital to inform physicians there of the child's impending arrival. The call was transferred directly to the staff of the pediatric ICU which replied that they could not admit the child because the unit was on "fly-by" status (i.e., new patients were not to be accepted because of staff and facilities shortages). Following hospital policy, the resident stated that the child should be taken to the nearest hospital or to Children's Hospital in Washington, D.C., only 6 minutes farther away. The father of the child refused and insisted that the child go to Johns Hopkins Hospital.

The Johns Hopkins physicians then conferred briefly about the possibility of creating a place for the child. They agreed that the director of the pediatric ICU, who alone had the authority to suspend the fly-by status, should be called at her home. That physician reaffirmed that the child should be taken to Children's Hospital. Again the father demanded that the child be brought to Johns Hopkins. The unit director then stated, "Tell them to come on, I guess; I don't know what else to do; there's refusal to go to Children's Hospital." Immediately thereafter, that physician spoke to the charge nurse and determined which of the 11 children in the unit could be moved out of the unit with the least risk. One child was transferred out of the pediatric ICU, and the convulsing child was moved in. He was stabilized but suffered permanent brain damage in the course of his seizures.

The parents sued the hospital, alleging that the 5- to 10-minute delay occasioned by the initial refusal to accept the child caused the damage. The court ruled on behalf of the hospital, stating that "a hospital is under no duty to accept a person with an emergency condition where there are no facilities available to treat the person properly. A hospital cannot be placed in the position where the admission of an additional patient will jeopardize the care of its existing patients." The hospital won its case, in large part owing to a well-established hospital policy regarding fly-by status and to an elaboration of the responsibility of the pediatric ICU director in making exceptions to the policy.[10]

In another legal case, H. Tristam Engelhardt, an ethicist, and Michael Rie, a physician,[1] discussed the ethical and legal consequences of inadvertent and perhaps inept rationing of scarce resources to a patient already in an ICU bed. They describe a $13 million court award to the survivors of Susan Von Stetina, a previously healthy 27-year-old woman who was accidently disconnected from a respirator. She had been injured in an automobile accident and suffered a fracture of the right femur and complete transsection of the pancreas. Respiratory distress syndrome developed on the fourth day after trauma; the patient was intubated, placed on a mechanical ventilator, and pharmacologically paralyzed to permit control of ventilation. She was successfully resuscitated after ventilation was restored but never regained consciousness because of chronic anoxic brain injury; however, she made a complete recovery from her traumatic injuries.

The court, in reaching its verdict, was influenced by evidence that only three nurses were available for the care of seven patients, even though the patient required the full attention of one nurse. Evidence presented at the trial indicated that one patient in the unit almost met the criteria for brain death and died 36 hours later. Two patients were to be electively discharged the next morning. In addition, three other hospitals in the community probably were better staffed at the moment and could have provided care for the patient. However, neither a medical director nor an administrative policy for dealing with census/staff relationships was available to address triage or transfer issues. If the facts in this case were those presented at trial, it certainly appeared that a breakdown occurred in the implicit or explicit rationing of scarce resources on the basis of expected benefit to be realized by ICU treatment.

These two cases, the outcome of one for and that of the other against the hospital, demonstrate the need for published policies that provide prescribed rules for making allocation and rationing decisions. Physicians can be required only to provide the standard of care that is appropriate under the circumstances, and sometimes understaffing, fly-by status, or the need to triage patients for limited ICU beds requires physicians to refuse to admit patients to their unit. The development of criteria for admission is important but controversial. Most physicians would agree that the likelihood of potential benefit should guide such decision making, but issues of patient desire, sex, income, age, preexisting illness, and social worth frequently make it almost impossible for them to develop universally acceptable criteria.

THEORIES OF JUSTICE

Although physicians make clinical decisions based on the ethical concepts of patient autonomy, nonmaleficence, beneficence, and confidentiality, management decisions regarding allocation and rationing are heavily premised on theories of distributive justice. This principle states that benefits and burdens should be distributed equitably, that resources should be allocated fairly, and that one should act in such a manner that no one person or group bears a disproportionate share of benefits or burdens. Physicians frequently wonder whether it is morally right to prioritize patient admissions based on some criterion such as potential benefit. Ethicists Arras and Rhoden[11] point out that such judgments frequently lead to a win-lose framework and ignore the moral impact of the decision on each patient involved:

. . . Relativism, if taken seriously, has the odd implication that all moral reflection and deliberation are in fact quite irrelevant. Take the all-too-frequent medical dilemma concerning whether it would be wrong to terminate the life of a patient who is slowly and painfully dying. Ethical relativism would not have us search for a solution based upon consideration of mercy nor would it ask us what we would do if we were in the patient's place. Rather, it would seem that ethical relativism would have us consult a sociologist, for our dilemma could only be resolved by discovering the prevailing societal attitudes. In turn, this points to another difficulty with ethical relativism, namely, that often there is no prevailing attitude. . . . But we don't take this split as an indication that there is no right or wrong in these matters; rather we take it as an indication

that, for the moment at least, we don't know what is right and what is wrong in these cases.[11]

Many formulations of rationing draw heavily on the concept of justice put forth by John Rawls in his many writings and in his comprehensive work, *A Theory of Justice*.[12] Rawls begins by discussing "justice as fairness" and suggests that "society is well-ordered when it is not only designed to advance the good of its members but when it is also regulated by a public conception of justice." He states that most people agree with the need for a general code of justice but frequently disagree over what principles should determine the assignment of "basic rights and duties" and "the proper distribution of the benefits and burdens of social cooperation." Since part of the disagreement over the distribution of societal goods is based on each individual's position in society, Rawls suggests that such decisions be made behind a "veil of ignorance," when one does not know whether he will become rich or poor, healthy or ill. This concept must be:

. . . understood as a purely hypothetical situation characterized so as to lead to a certain conception of justice. Among the essential features of this situation is that no one knows his place in society, his class position, or social status, nor does anyone know his fortune in the distribution of natural assets and abilities, his intelligence, strength, and the like. . . . The principles of justice are chosen behind a veil of ignorance. This insures that no one is advantaged or disadvantaged in the choice of principles by the outcome of natural chance or the contingency of social circumstances. Since all are similarly situated and no one is able to design principles to favor his particular condition, the principles of justice are the result of a fair agreement or bargain (p 12).[12]

Rawls then suggests that these principles of justice be embodied in a social contract between the body politic and the social institution or country. He rejects classic utilitarianism, which suggests that "society is rightly ordered and therefore just, when its major institutions are arranged so as to achieve the greatest net balance of satisfaction summed over all the individuals belonging to it." This suggests that some members of a group are forced to make sacrifices for others in order to maximize the success of the whole. Whereas this may be a useful concept in times of national struggle, it does not fit Rawls' idea of justice as fairness. He summarizes his views in two principles of justice:

1. Each person is to have an equal right to the most extensive basic liberty compatible with a similar liberty for others.
2. Social and economic inequalities are to be arranged so that they are both (a) reasonably expected to be to everyone's advantage and (b) attached to positions and offices open to all (p 60).[12]

Rawls repeatedly rejects the utilitarian views that disadvantages in power or income of one group may be tolerated if they are outweighed by the advantages of another. Instead, he insists that "social and economic inequalities, for example inequalities of wealth and authority, are just only if they result in compensating benefits for everyone, and in particular for the least advantaged members of society," (p 14).[12] Rawls' interpretation of justice as fairness is based on "Kant's notion of autonomy" and his "idea that moral principles are the objects of rational choice." It is little wonder, therefore, that Kantian ethical theories have achieved predominance in the field of bioethics.

APPLIED JUSTICE IN HEALTH CARE POLICY

Norman Daniels in his provocatively entitled book, *Just Health Care*,[13] suggests that Rawls' approach to justice as fairness may be applied to health care by claiming that such care, like education, is necessary to ensure equality of opportunity. One of us (SMA)[14] has argued that health care should be distributed on the basis of need and that its use be limited "to those who could benefit from it." In this view, either underutilization or overutilization is wrong. Daniels accepts this "functional" approach to the distribution of health care, but points out that the existence of significant "need" itself is not morally sufficient because it does not explain why the need for health care is different from any other human preference or need.

Daniels points out that each individual's genetic make-up provides him or her with a "normal opportunity range." It is considered "morally acceptable that there are winners and losers, even in races where the prize is a share of important social goods, provided the race is *fair* to all participants." Disease and disability reduce the range of available opportunities, and measures that reverse or moderate these disadvantages can be morally justified because they help provide a more "level playing field." However, society cannot provide every health care service that an individual might like; thus, agreement on what are *essential* health care services is necessary. He summarizes his view of the opportunity principle:

I urge the fair equality of opportunity principle as an appropriate principle to govern macro decisions about the design of our health care system. Such a principle defines, from the perspective of justice, what the moral function of the health care system must be—to help guarantee fair equality of opportunity.[13]

THE PRESIDENT'S COMMISSION FOR THE STUDY OF ETHICAL PROBLEMS

As the United States and other countries embark on the road of major health care reform, a full national debate on access to such care and related issues is necessary. The federal government has regularly advanced such debates over a wide range of issues in health care by establishing national interdisciplinary commissions to marshal the facts and arguments that relate to each issue and often to make recommendations for governmental action. The ethical problems of unequal access to health care have concerned most of the nations of this world.

A 1932 report of the national Committee on the Costs of Medical Care pointed out that "many persons do not receive service which is adequate either in quantity or quality, and the costs of service are inequably distributed. The result is a tremendous amount of preventable physical pain and mental anguish, needless deaths, economic inefficiency, and social waste."[15]

A half century later, in 1974, the President's Commission for the Study of Ethical Problems in Medicine and Biomedical and Behavioral Research was created; the Commission completed its work in 1978.[16] In addition to making recommendations, the Commission concluded that equity in health care can be realized only by providing an adequate level of care for all Americans. It is not surprising for readers to see an analogy between the President's Commission's requirement for adequate levels of care for all Americans as an example of John Rawls' interpretation of a social contract:

Understanding equitable access to health care to mean that everyone should be able to secure an adequate level of care has several strengths. Because an adequate level of care may be less than "all beneficial care" and because it does not require that all needs be satisfied, it acknowledges the need for setting priorities within health care and signals a clear recognition that society's resources are limited and that there are other goods besides health care. Thus, interpreting equity as access to adequate care does not generate an open-ended obligation. One of the chief dangers of interpretations of equity that require virtually unlimited resources is that they encourage the view that equitable access is an impossible ideal.

Defining equity as an adequate level of care for all avoids an impossible commitment of resources without falling into the opposite error of abandoning the enterprise of seeking to ensure that health care is in fact available for everyone.[16]

The Commission's letter to the President and to the leaders of Congress stated that "In examining the special nature of health care, we discern in our country's traditional commitment to fairness an ethical obligation on the part of society to ensure that all Americans have access to an adequate level of health care without the imposition of excessive burdens."

Thus, the President's Commission appears to support rationing (the withholding of potentially beneficial care) for certain individuals on the grounds that certain kinds of beneficial care do not need to be provided for everyone because they exceed the definition of what is adequate. There is a clear suggestion in the report that the kind of care that may be ethically denied is care that is too expensive and therefore cannot be provided from public resources for economic reasons.

The final paper in the appendix to the President's report is a fascinating discussion, entitled "Health Care and the 'Deserving Poor'" by George Sher.[17] Because intensivists frequently care for injured drunken drivers and gunshot wound victims who are involved in criminal activity, Sher's discussion is quite relevant. He begins by recalling that "the idea that some poor persons deserve to be helped while others do not has long been influential in this country" and that "the blameworthy poor—the paupers were relegated to poorhouses," whereas the "blind, the deaf-mute and other blameless classes of the poor were helped in much less humiliating ways." The fact that some people are believed to be poor because of their own actions and that others become ill because of drinking, smoking, reckless driving, inappropriate sexual activity, or other risky behavior makes it attractive to create a class of "undeserving poor" or "undeserving ill" who might be excluded from governmentally funded health care services. Although people should expect their "desserts," he doubts whether American society is ready to withhold care from those who have squandered their ability to obtain health insurance because it seems "inhumane, and indeed indecent, to let someone suffer or die for lack of easily available care." Even the undeserving poor should have access to the "adequate" care proposed by the President's Commission.

Although many of these recommendations will surely be considered by the Clinton administration, the President's Commission of 1974 is not without its limitations. Daniel Callahan[18] criticized the Commission as limiting itself to a description of the rights and privileges of individuals exercising their individual autonomy but failed entirely to provide procedures or mechanisms for how such autonomous choices should be made. He states:

We have gone through an important era that has established many new rights and privileges in the face of the power and potency of biomedicine. We have been told that we are autonomous and can make free choices—that autonomy is a key ingredient in the thread of consensus that runs through the reports of the President's Commission. In the next stage, we must begin work on the content of that freedom. For it is here that consensus will most desperately be needed; otherwise, the newly gained freedoms will turn out to be either empty or dangerous.[18]

State governments, perhaps, have made more significant progress toward consensus on bioethical issues, particularly those dealing with allocation of medical resources, than has the federal government. A year after the President's Commission completed its report, the state of New York developed its own Task Force on Law and Life. This task force has released several comprehensive reports. Although other states have followed New York's lead in developing interdisciplinary commissions, Oregon is perhaps best known for its attempt to actually implement rationing of care to its poorest citizens.

In the early 1990s, the state of Oregon decided to limit Medicaid costs by rank-ordering 709 diagnosis-treatment pairs out of the more than 10,000 diagnoses. The pairs were ranked by estimates of net benefit, but the cutoff was arbitrarily placed at the 587th pair based on the state's budgeted amount for Medicaid expenditures. No consideration was given to the intensity or appropriateness of care for each individual. This is what some—but not all—would consider rationing. State employees and other insured people could receive whatever their physicians believed to be necessary, whereas Medicaid recipients were limited to whatever the state could afford. Oregon leaders soon realized the important difference between statistical lives and individuals' lives as public outcry subjected the state government to what some might call "symbolic blackmail."

The impetus for formal health care rationing arose from the shifting of funding from organ transplantation to comprehensive prenatal care. In 1987, one child—Coby Howard—was turned into a "national martyr" when attempts to collect donations for a needed bone marrow transplant failed and he died. In 1990, a chastened Oregon restored Medicaid funding for organ transplants. The Oregon plan to ration health care for the poor but not the affluent ran into considerable opposition on both political and moral grounds. It uses an arbitrary ranking system to redistribute health care resources among the poor. Current Medicaid recipients receive less care, the uninsured poor receive more care, and the insured continue to receive their same level of benefits. The Bush Administration declined to support the Oregon plan on the basis of noncompliance with the Americans with Disabilities Act of 1990. Interestingly, it was the requirement for a treatment to return an individual to "asymptomatic" life that caused the greatest concern. An asymptomatic existence suggested a quality of life test, and the Clinton Administration insisted on its removal before it granted the necessary waiver.

Fox and Leichter, writing in the summer of 1993, concluded:

Three lessons emerge from the Oregon experience. The first is that citizen participation is a politically and legally flawed strategy to gain widespread acceptance for innovative reform. The second is that specificity (the infamous "List") can become a political albatross. No state has emulated the list or seems likely to do so soon. . . . The final lesson of Oregon is ironic. Oregon lawmakers backed into defining a minimum basic package of services. In so doing, they showed that it is possible to design and implement a plan that puts a floor of coverage under everyone in the state.[19]

In 1993, a federal court maintained that Medicaid had to fund all children in need of transplants, thus adding unanticipated millions into state Medicaid budgets. It is anticipated that litigation for patient rights of access to federal programs will only increase during health care reform.

In an article entitled "Why a Two-Tier System of Health Care Delivery is Morally Unavoidable," Engelhardt probably spoke for many others when he congratulated the authors of the Oregon plan and suggested that it

. . . provides a heuristic (philosophic jargon for "method") for resolving the public policy challenge. The creation of a basic adequate package through communal funds can be regarded as a prudent act of self-insurance, as a limited act of solidarity with others, or as a limited act of altruism. These and probably other reasons and goals will motivate citizens to create a basic package whose secular authority will be derived from a communal decision. The existence of a private luxury tier, supported through private insurance and direct out-of-pocket payments, represents a recognition of the limits of communal authority to define the proper ways in which justice and fairness ought to be achieved; the right of

individuals to deploy their private resources and energies as they wish, once they have discharged their limited civic duties; and the diversity of human values with regard to health, disease, health care, and the avoidance of risks.[20]

THEORIES OF JUSTICE AND THE PRACTICE OF CRITICAL CARE MEDICINE

Theories of justice are most useful in making health care policy decisions but have limitations when clinician managers are faced with the decision as to whether to admit the individual with a myocardial infarction and unstable blood pressure or the gunshot victim to the last monitored bed in the ICU. These physicians are making distributive decisions, and such decisions are almost always based on the chances of clinical benefit to the patient. If survival rates appear to be similar, physicians usually start considering the patients' preexisting health status, their age, and the likelihood of full restoration of health.

In recent years, attempts have been made to measure health status in order to better understand the allocation of resources. Conceptions of good health vary from person to person, and Kaplan and Bush[21] at the University of California at San Diego have attempted to quantify levels of health or well-being. Their general health policy model includes mortality and quality of life and may be expressed as a continuum, using arbitrary values. The quality of life measure may then be modified by the likelihood of serious illness and its successful treatment and multiplied by the estimated years of remaining life to arrive at an estimate of "quality-adjusted life-years." Engelhardt and Rie,[1] in discussing the Von Stetina case, suggested using the potential benefit of a treatment (P), the quality of life expected (Q), and the remaining length of life (L) divided by the cost (C) to develop an "ICU treatment entitlement index (ICU-EI)":

$$\text{ICU} - \text{EI} = \frac{\text{PQL}}{\text{C}}$$

Preparing for the inevitable criticism over the use of such a mathematical analysis, Engelhardt and Rie concluded:

The point remains that some calculation of an index for treatment is better than no such calculation. Only through such an index, however informally drawn, will one be able to provide a basis for creating a society-endorsed and implementable policy regarding the use of scarce resources in general, and ICU resources in particular.[1]

Consistent with their belief that a two-tier system is morally unavoidable, they also argue that the ICU-EI could be specified for government-guaranteed health policy contracts and that the affluent could be permitted to purchase a lower level of permissible ICU-EI.

JUSTICE AND COST

The concept of "health," to use the jargon of the economist, is clearly elastic. The Rand Health Insurance Study estimated that 80% of the general population has no dysfunction but that 88% of the population will report symptoms at any time. Because the presence of symptoms leads to physician intervention, it is essential to distinguish between the "ill" and the "worried well." The total cost to the nation of all health care is dependent on how much care is given to those without serious illness as well as to the 20% of Americans who are ill. It could, for example, cost the nation far more to treat headaches with aspirin than to perform heart, kidney, lung, and bone marrow transplantations on relatively few patients. Thus, total cost is "elastic" to the perception of medical need and the cost of medical intervention, but the usual market expectation of demand driving down cost almost never occurs. The perverse incentives of fee-for-service practice, which have rewarded physicians for satisfying the desires of patients for increasing amounts of "magic," high-technology care, have prevented them from doing what is "right." Little has been written, in a market-organized economy, to emphasize how much the competition to perform expensive and, presumably, useful techniques has raised the cost of health care. If it is morally necessary to calculate the numerator of Engelhardt and Rie's equation[1] (PQL), is it not also morally necessary to define appropriate cost?

Analysis of the prevalence of coronary artery bypass surgery demonstrates how the proliferation of technology-rich tertiary care has increased the cost of medical care while probably decreasing its quality. In 1986, 702 hospitals performed bypass surgery; only one third of them performed more than 100 procedures. Both mortality rates and medical costs were substantially lower in those hospitals that performed more than 100 procedures. By 1993, 827 hospitals in the United States were performing bypass surgery. Los Angeles County alone had 37 "open heart centers," as they became called, but many of these only performed a few operations. A survey of American hospitals revealed almost nine cardiac surgical units for every trauma unit, presumably because the payment system favors care for heart disease over trauma care.

In the mid-1980s, Luft and associates[22] and Showstack and colleagues[23] discovered that the results of some operations depended on how often a surgeon actually performed surgery. The Luft study found substantially higher death rates for hospitals that performed fewer than 200 bypass operations compared with those that performed more. Whereas practice seems to make perfect, results also appeared to differ among surgeons. A careful study conducted by the Northern New England Cardiovascular Disease Study Group[24] showed that even when the severity of a patient's condition was taken into consideration, the mortality rates for individual surgeons ranged from about 2% to greater than 9%!

TOWARD AN ETHIC FOR RESOURCE ALLOCATION

The frustrations experienced by intensivists charged with the allocation of a fixed number of ICU beds are similar to those of many other clinician-managers. Lemieux-Charles and colleagues[25] attempted to deal with these issues through a series of focus groups held at the University of Toronto. Twenty-eight clinician-managers were asked to discuss what they perceived to be the ethical issues affecting their daily practice. These issues were then classified by Hiller's taxonomy.[5] Microlevel issues dealt with the conflicts between their moral obligation to provide high-quality care and the interest of the institution in cost containment. They pointed to conflicts between physician payment incentives and institutional objectives, and to their own interpersonal conflicts regarding the various roles they were asked to assume. Macrolevel issues included determining priorities for care, conflicts between standards of individual health professions, conflict between clinicians and clinician-managers, relationship of unit activities to the hospital's mission, and the equitable allocation of resources throughout the hospital. They identified the needs of the community versus the needs of the hospital as their major macrolevel issue.

The Lemieux-Charles observations[25] have important implications for health care organizations and their professionals. The authors suggest the following:

(1) Organizational approaches that aim to control expenditures

and improve quality of care will be more successful if both roles and their obligations are treated as separate but related problems; (2) Ethical considerations should be acknowledged early in the development of any process of institutional change and considered regularly as part of a hospital's strategic planning, implementation, and evaluation of such changes; (3) Role expectations and the obligations they create should be the subject of both informal and formal hospital discussions within the institution; (4) Mechanisms for orientation and education should be developed at all hospitals to address conflicts experienced by individuals as well as those in working groups or treatment teams.

It is important for institutional interdisciplinary committees to create written policies regarding major rationing and allocation choices. Such policies should specify not only who makes such decisions but also the criteria on which these decisions are based. These policies should become part of the medical standard of care, thereby decreasing liability for physicians and hospitals that follow such policies. The role of hospital ethics committees should be extended from its traditional emphasis on individual patient care decisions to one that analyzes the way that institutions respond to the complex moral issues that they regularly encounter. The stakes in allocation ethics are high, and, to the most practical extent possible, such policies should be published and debated within the population served by the hospital. Objective information is critical to resource allocation and to decision making on the part of both health professionals and their patients. Only when accurate assessments of the outcomes of treatment on the duration and quality of subsequent life are available will it be possible to allow society to adopt the morally appealing principle of providing potentially beneficial care to all who require it.

The relationships among access to care, cost of such care, and appropriate levels of care for any given population should be freely debated by the public. Cost issues cannot be ignored, of course, and common sense would always dictate a less expensive approach if the same outcome could be achieved. Reducing cost and increasing the precision of medical decision making will permit society to adopt the morally appealing principle of providing potentially beneficial care to all who require it. Institutional ethics committees need to address the ethical dilemmas that they face as part of their business planning, as well as clinical ethical dilemmas. Finally, academic institutions training hospital administrators and clinicians must include training in allocation ethics into their curricula. The substantial benefits anticipated in the "brave new world" of health care reform will only be realized if structural change is accompanied by broad interdisciplinary training of the individuals who are expected to perform expanded roles that extend far beyond the traditional health professional–patient relationship.

References

1. Engelhardt HT, Rie MA: Intensive care units, scarce resources, and conflicting principles of justice. JAMA 1986; 255:1159–1164.
2. Strauss MJ, LoGerfo JP, Yeltazie JA, et al: Rationing of intensive care unit services: An every day occurrence. JAMA 1986; 255:1143–1146.
3. Begun JW, Lippincott RC: Strategic Adaptation in the Health Professions: Meeting the Challenges of Change. San Francisco, Jossey-Bass, 1993.
4. Leatt P, Vayda E, Williams JI: Medical Staff Organization in Canadian Hospitals. Unpublished research report prepared for the Social Sciences and Humanities Council of Canada, Toronto, 1987.
5. Hiller MD: Ethics and health care administration: Issues in education and practice. J Health Admin Educ 1984; 2:148–192.
6. Ruelas E, Leatt P: The roles of physician-executives in hospitals: A framework for management education. J Health Admin Educ 1985; 3:151–169.
7. With Justice For All? The Ethics of Healthcare Rationing. St. Louis, Catholic Health Association of the United States, 1991.
8. Aaron HJ: The Oregon experiment. *In:* Rationing America's Medical Care: The Oregon Plan and Beyond. Strosberg MA, Wiener JM, Baker R, et al (Eds). Washington, DC, Brookings Institution, 1992, p 107.
9. Furrow BR, Johnson SH, Jost TS, et al: Bioethics: Health Care Law & Ethics. St. Paul, West, 1991.
10. *Davis v Johns Hopkins Hospital*, 622 A2d 128 (Md 1993).
11. Arras J, Rhoden N: Ethical Issues in Modern Medicine. 3rd ed. Mountain View, Calif, Mayfield, 1989, pp 6–28.
12. Rawls J: A Theory of Justice. Cambridge, Belknap Press, 1971, pp 3–60.
13. Daniels N: Just Health Care. Cambridge, Mass, Cambridge University Press, 1985, pp 37–41.
14. Ayres S: Rationality, not rationing in health care. *In:* Rationing America's Medical Care: The Oregon Plan and Beyond. Strosberg MA, Wiener JM, Baker R, et al (Eds). Washington, DC, Brookings Institution, 1992, p 136.
15. Committee on the Costs of Medical Care: Medical Care for the American People. Washington, DC, Department of Health, Education, and Welfare, 1932, publication No. 28. New York, Arno Press, 1972 (reprinted).
16. President's Commission for the Study of Ethical Problems in Medicine and Biomedical and Behavioral Research: Securing Access to Health Care. Vol 1. Washington, DC, U.S. Government Printing Office, publication No. 83-600501, 1983, p 20.
17. Sher G: Health care and the "deserving poor." *In:* Securing Access to Health Care. Vol 2. President's Commission for the Study of Ethical Problems in Medicine and Biomedical and Behavioral Research. Washington, DC, U.S. Government Printing Office, publication No. 82-600637, 1983, pp 293–301.
18. Callahan D: Morality and contemporary culture: The President's Commission and beyond. Cardozo Leg Rev 1984; 6:347.
19. Fox DM, Leichter HM: The ups and downs of Oregon's rationing plan. Health Aff (Millwood) 1993; 12:66–70.
20. Engelhardt R: Why a two-tier system of health care delivery is morally unavoidable. *In:* Rationing America's Medical Care: The Oregon Plan and Beyond. Strosberg MA, Wiener JM, Baker R, et al (Eds). Washington, DC, Brookings Institution, 1992, p 197.
21. Kaplan RM, Bush JW: Health-related quality of life measurement for evaluation research and policy analysis. Health Psychol 1982; 1:61–80.
22. Luft HS, Bunker J, Enthoven A: Should operations be regionalized? The empirical relationship between surgical volume and mortality. N Engl J Med 1979; 301:1364.
23. Showstack JA, Rosenfeld DW, Garnick DW, et al: Association of volume with outcomes of coronary artery bypass graft survival: Scheduled versus non-scheduled operations. JAMA 1987; 257:785.
24. O'Connor GT, Plume SK, Olmstead EM, et al: A regional prospective study of in-hospital mortality associated with coronary artery by-pass grafting. JAMA 1991; 266:803–809.
25. Lemieux-Charles L, Meslin EM, Aird C, et al: Ethical issues faced by clinician/managers in resource-allocation decisions. Hosp Health Serv Admin 1993; 38:267.

201

Legal and Risk Management Issues Surrounding Managed Care

Karen N. Swisher, MS, JD • Peter N. Swisher, MA, JD

THE RISE OF MANAGED CARE IN THE UNITED STATES

Many readers may recall the joke about three nurses going to Heaven that was circulated on the Internet and was widely heard on National Public Radio. Three nurses go to Heaven and wait at the Pearly Gates for St. Peter to admit them. The first nurse tells St. Peter that she worked her whole life in a public hospital helping the poor and the sick. "You are a good nurse and may enter Heaven" St. Peter tells her. The second nurse states she has worked her whole career in a hospice comforting the dying and their families. "You are a good nurse and may enter Heaven," St. Peter tells her. The third nurse states she has devoted her career to utilization review functions for a health maintenance organization (HMO). St. Peter reviews her paper work and tells her, "I can approve you for a 5-day stay."

(We might add that the nurse attempted to appeal this decision, but her risk retention benefits contract with St. Peter stated that his decision was final and was not appealable under state, federal, or heavenly law.)

Physicians currently practicing medicine and students of medicine and health administration may believe that managed care, as applied to medicine, is a recent phenomenon in the otherwise long history of American medicine, but such is not the case. Paul Starr, in his classic work, *The Social Transformation of American Medicine,* describes the onset of "prepaid health care practice" models developed almost 100 years ago for the benefit of various mining, lumber, and railroad industries. Despite organized medicine's initial opposition to such "insurance" for health care, the trend of prepaid insurance continued to progress in the 1930s and 1940s. Probably the most recognized name in managed care, Kaiser-Permanente, was founded during this time. After World War II, employers interested in attracting and maintaining good workers with augmented salaries and benefits sought various forms of prepaid health insurance as a way of offering "fringe" benefits to their employees. At that time, most people in the United States did not have any sort of health insurance, and for a nominal fee each month it seemed like a good investment. Although premiums for these health insurance plans were slightly higher than for other forms of insurance, coverage was comprehensive and there were few medical exclusions, limits, or copayments. By the 1960s, prepaid health care insurance enjoyed a small but stable niche in the health care marketplace.

The 1960s saw a significant change in the financing of health care as the federal government became a major payer in establishing Medicare and Medicaid. The vast majority of health care was paid for under the traditional fee-for-service plans in which physicians and hospitals were reimbursed prospectively for whatever they charged their patients. Medical technology and medical services expanded, and for a variety of reasons the cost of health care began to skyrocket. Dr. Paul Ellwood coined the term health maintenance organizations* in the 1970s, as the Nixon administration looked for solutions to the health care crisis in America. In 1973, Congress passed the Health Maintenance Organization Act. This legislation provided financing and other support for the development of HMOs. Among other things, the HMO Act required companies with more than 25 employees that offered health insurance to provide at least one qualifying HMO as an alternative to conventional health insurance if such an HMO was located in the area. (Incidentally, health insurance benefits have never been a legal requirement for employers.)

President Nixon's hope of expanding the HMO market in a few years was never realized during his tenure as President.[1] Indeed, rather than controlling costs, the HMO Act established a relatively regulated and more costly form of health coverage. By 1980, approximately 15 million persons were enrolled in HMOs, a figure that had not changed appreciably for more than a decade.[2]

The development of this modern managed care revolution in the 1980s and early 1990s was the result of a number of factors. Costs for providing health care and health care insurance continued to climb, so that by 1996 health care accounted for almost 14% of the gross national product. The purchasing power of many employers greatly expanded during this time, and employers saw these health care benefits not only as fringe benefits but also as a significant component in the cost of doing business. There also emerged a general public concern about the quality of health care in the United States, coinciding with a public reaction against perceptions of high medical fees and profits of both hospitals and physicians.

Finally, during this time the legal system created a favorable environment for the expansion of managed care. First, a federal law, entitled the Employee Retirement Income Security Act (ERISA), allowed employers to bypass the commercial health insurance system in favor of self-funded models. Under ERISA, employers could create their own health benefit plans and condition physicians' access to employees and patients according to the physician's willingness to accept greatly discounted rates and extensive administrative oversight. Second, federal antitrust and fraud laws encouraged sectors of the health care industry, providers, and payers to integrate vertically to form integrated delivery systems (IDSs). As Congress began to prohibit economic incentives among independent medical groups, the movement toward the formation of large companies selling discounted health services to unregulated corporate purchasers dominated the health care area.[3]

Today more than 65 million Americans are members of HMOs. Roughly 90 million other Americans are enrolled in similar MCOs, such as preferred provider organizations (PPOs).[4] In addition, more than 80% of the practicing physicians are either employed by or have entered into at least one contractual arrangement with a managed care plan.[5] With this kind of market penetration, profits for managed care companies soared, and the 1990s showed a significant change in the HMO environment. This was a time of rapid growth of for-profit HMOs, increased consolidations of HMOs, rapid growth in network and individual physician practice association (IPA) models, declining community rating methods, altered payment arrangements with physicians, increased patient cost sharing,

---

*In this chapter, the terms HMO and MCO (maintenance care organization) are used generically to describe any form of managed care organization. While there are many such models of managed care, all are defined as any health coverage arrangement in which, for a preset fee, a company sells a defined package of benefits to a purchaser, with services furnished to enrolled members through a network of participating providers who operate under written contractual or employment agreements and whose selection and authority to furnish covered benefits is controlled by the managed care company.

declining hospital use, and increased use of clinical guidelines.[6]

As with all types of revolutions, the HMO revolution was immediately followed by a popular backlash against HMOs. This was exemplified by hundreds, then thousands, of lawsuits under a variety of legal theories, and a proliferation of state and federal legislation attempting to "right the wrongs" against Americans insured by a managed care system. Some perceived a system that encouraged profits over care and that created an onerous bureaucracy intruding on the traditional physician-patient relationship. One cannot pick up a newspaper, read a popular news magazine such as *Time* or *Newsweek,* or watch television shows such as "60 Minutes," "Dateline," "ER," or "Chicago Hope," for example, without featured stories about a helpless patient posed against a heartless HMO.

Physicians who practice in HMOs with their patients insured by HMOs are also alarmed by the amount of litigation in this arena. They are concerned about the quality of care their patients may or may not receive and about the sometimes oppressive utilization review and scrutiny employed. They are concerned about being excluded from a network that insures a significant number of their patients. They are concerned about "gag orders" on what they can or cannot tell their patients about treatment options. Finally, physicians worry about how they are being compensated for their medical services, not only with medical incomes being ratcheted down but also with the possible effect of creative risk-sharing mechanisms on how they practice medicine.

This chapter briefly reviews legal liability issues facing physicians practicing within a managed care environment. By understanding and analyzing these legal issues, physicians can develop risk management techniques for avoiding legal liability and, at the same time, advocate better quality care for their patients.

THE ERISA VACUUM: WHY MANY PATIENTS ARE NOT PROTECTED BY ADEQUATE REGULATORY LAWS

Because managed care involves both medical care practice and insurance regulation, each state, through its state insurance department and state insurance code, is empowered to regulate aspects of an HMO managed care entity that pertains to the "business of insurance"[7] under applicable state insurance law.[8] Although state insurance regulation of managed care entities has been uneven from state to state, a growing number of states in recent years have increasingly become more active in the regulation of managed care arrangements by providing regulatory oversight of managed care plans operating in each state, specifically relating to financial, performance, and quality-related activities.[9]

However, a serious problem involves the regulation of managed care entities when such managed care plans are self-insured risk retention arrangements. For example, many employers have self-insured their employees for health insurance coverage and other employee benefits. Although traditional health insurers are heavily regulated by state insurance laws, ERISA contains a serious loophole.[10] Under federal preemption principles, ERISA supersedes "any and all State laws insofar as they relate to any employee benefit plan"[11] for self-insured entities. Consequently, ERISA imposes virtually no regulations or requirements for managed care self-insured, risk retention plans to provide for adequate standardized health care benefits or procedures. This lack of federal or state regulation for self-insured, risk retention managed care plans has created a critical regulatory vacuum.[12]

Moreover, for a state law to avoid federal preemption under ERISA, even involving commercially insured managed care health insurance plans, the state must "regulate insurance" within the meaning of ERISA. States do have an important legitimate interest in regulating managed care delivery, including the selection and credentialing of physicians, quality of care measures, consumer protection, financial solvency requirements, and many other related issues. But the crucial question remains: "[A]t what point state law ceases being the "regulation of insurance" and begins to encroach on preempted [ERISA] areas."[13] Until Congress provides more guidance by enacting much needed legislative reform to ERISA or until the courts provide adequate judicial remedies, this unfortunate ERISA vacuum will continue to plague health care managers, health care providers, and their patients.[14]

LIABILITY ISSUES AND PATIENTS WHO ARE DENIED MEDICAL CARE

There is nothing more disheartening to both patient and physician as when medical treatment coverage and payment, recommended by the physician, is denied by a health insurance company. Likewise, nothing is more disheartening to a health insurance company as the unwanted, and often unwarranted, media publicity when such actions become public. Many cases have come under media scrutiny when "Jane Doe," with her two children and a loving, supportive husband, is denied health insurance funding for an autologous bone marrow transplant and she dies shortly thereafter while her family frantically tries to raise the money privately. Or little "Jimmy," whose parents publish emotional pleas for contributions to a fund for a third liver transplantation because the health insurance carrier has refused to fund a third organ transplant procedure. Although it seems that both the public and the insurance companies are exposed to this kind of publicity all too often, it is worth noting that these types of cases—many of which go into litigation—are a relatively new phenomenon in the health care industry.

Under the standard indemnity-type health insurance plans, insurers rarely interfered with a physician's medical recommendation or patient's demand for medical treatment. The few denials that the insurer made were based on the specific contractual language in the insurance policy between patient and insurer that clearly stated which treatments were excluded from coverage and which were not. Treatment for certain medical conditions, such as acquired immunodeficiency syndrome (AIDS) or infertility, for example, was clearly excluded in the health insurance contract. When lawsuits did arise, courts used general principles of insurance contract law, and the courts generally upheld these exclusions unless they were contrary to federal or state antidiscrimination laws.

In the early 1980s, as managed care began to take hold of the health insurance industry, dramatic changes began to take place:

1. Costs of medical services skyrocketed.
2. A number of expensive and hazardous treatments for severe illnesses were developed.
3. Medical researchers began to question the validity of many of these treatments.
4. Physicians themselves began publicly to question the efficacy of many heroic treatments for seriously ill patients.

All this culminated in health insurance policy changes incorporating general language for denying treatment that was now labeled "educational," "experimental," or not "medically necessary."[15]

Accordingly, the number of lawsuits coming before various state and federal courts has also proliferated. While each case is based on individual factual issues, legal analysis of these cases basically involves three major legal issues:

1. Courts are often asked to define the substantive meaning of the terms "medical necessity" and "experimental medical treatment."[16]

2. Courts look behind the insurance contract to determine the process by which the insurance company defines these terms, and what—in some states—the "reasonable expectations" of the insured to coverage might entail *vis-à-vis* the written contract.[17]

3. Courts must look at how health insurance companies review their own denials of payment under these contractual terms and the burden of proof that the patient must demonstrate when a claim is denied.[18]

In general, courts look at these cases as a contract dispute between the parties.[19] Because health insurance contracts are usually negotiated between employer and insurance company, with the patient-beneficiary having little or no say in what is covered or excluded in the health benefit contract, courts often hold such health insurance contracts to be "contracts of adhesion," with any ambiguities in the health insurance contract being construed against the contract drafter (i.e., the health insurance company).[20] Courts also realize the significant imbalance of power and knowledge between health insurance companies and their patient-policyholder, and their holdings often have been sympathetic in favor of the patient-policyholder by finding the insurance company has fiduciary responsibility to its policyholders.[21] Despite what may appear to be a favorable ground for many patient-policyholders to sue in court, many patients who would otherwise have a valid legal cause of action against their health insurance company do not sue. Some policyholders simply do not question the ruling of the insurance company's denial of coverage. If they do sue, these individuals must often pay thousands of dollars in legal expenses; if they do win, they usually receive only what they are otherwise entitled to by way of benefits.[22] Contract law generally does *not* provide for punitive, exemplary, or pain and suffering damages, absent an insurer's "bad faith" or the insurer's egregious and willful conduct[23]; legal expenses may not be covered; and the benefits granted to the patient-policyholder after long litigation often are too little and too late.

THE DEVIL MADE ME DO IT: UTILIZATION REVIEW LIABILITY

Although MCOs come in a variety of models, all have a primary goal of reducing health care costs and maximizing the value of health care to both patient and payer. The most common strategy to control such costs is the aggressive use of utilization review and management. Utilization review, designed to evaluate medical necessity and those medical procedures covered or excluded under the terms of the contract, can occur before, during, or after medical services are rendered. The MCO may perform these functions in-house, or it may contract with a third party to oversee the utilization review process. These functions can be quite elaborate and may require physicians and patients to jump many hurdles to prove that appropriate medical care should be provided under the terms of the contract.[24] Indeed, more than a few physicians have been exasperated and intimidated with this sometimes "inhumane" bureaucratic process.[25]

During the past decade, there have been a string of cases holding MCOs directly liable for faulty review systems.[26] MCOs have a direct responsibility to make decisions in accordance with appropriate medical standards of care, not based solely on cost containment parameters, to have systems of review in place, and to educate physicians as to these review procedures. Reviewers' decisions cannot arbitrarily ignore or unreasonably disregard the treating physician's treatment concerns and plans.

On the other hand, physicians treating patients in MCOs have additional legal and ethical responsibilities to advocate for their patients and to avail themselves of the utilization review process, including appealing decision denials if physicians believe that such denials are contrary to the best interest of their patients. Although a number of physicians sued by their patients have attempted to defend their own negligence by stating that "the HMO made me do it," most courts are not sympathetic to this defense. In one case, for example, a group of psychiatrists who had agreed to participate in a pilot program with prospective and concurrent utilization review objected to the incentives created by the program. The physicians argued that the MCO provided "powerful economic incentives for a physician to disregard his best judgment at the behest of one not licensed to render medicine . . ."[27]

It is clear that these cases hold that the legal responsibility for appropriate patient care, including discharge from a hospital, rests with the treating physician. As a California court held in 1986,

> *The patient who requires treatment, and who is harmed when care which should have been provided is not provided, should recover for injuries suffered from all those responsible for the deprivation of such care, including, when appropriate, health care payors. The physician who complies without protest with the limitations imposed by a third-party payor, when his medical judgment dictates otherwise, cannot avoid his ultimate responsibility for his patient's care. He cannot point to the health care payor as the liability scapegoat when the consequences of his own determinative medical decisions go sour.*[28]

"GAG CLAUSES": WHAT PATIENTS DON'T KNOW CAN HARM THEM

Few who saw him on the Phil Donahue television show in 1995 will forget Dr. David Himmelstein's discussion of his relationship with U.S. Healthcare. At approximately the same time, Dr. Himmelstein presented a slide show to the National Managed Health Care Congress to demonstrate what the so-called gag clause in his contract with U.S. Healthcare was preventing him from doing for his patients. U.S. Healthcare was not happy with this unwelcome publicity, and on December 1, 1995, three days after the Phil Donahue show aired, U.S. Healthcare terminated Dr. Himmelstein's contract with them without cause. This public issue created an explosion of controversy over whether a managed care organization's use of gag clauses is unethical or even illegal.[29]

Gag clauses are controversial contract provisions which restrict physicians from disclosing certain information to their patients or the public. While the language varies, typical gag clauses prevent health care providers from revealing how they are paid by the MCO or from recommending treatment options that are not covered by the MCO even if the physician deems it to be the best treatment. Dr. Himmelstein's contractual agreement with U.S. Healthcare, for example, stated: "Physician shall agree not to take any action or make any communication which undermines the confidence of enrollees, potential enrollees, their employers, their unions, or the public in U.S. Healthcare or the quality of U.S. Healthcare coverage."[30]

MCOs defend the use of gag clauses by arguing that they protect propriety information regarding how they financially contract with their plan providers. Yet some physicians state that gag clauses prevent them from performing their ethical and legal responsibility of providing informed consent to the patient by preventing them from discussing all alternatives and medical choices, including those that might not be covered by the MCO. To date, at least 16 states have passed laws that attempt to ban such clauses.* (A proposed federal Patient Bill of Rights Act is pending in Congress, and may be enacted in the near future). Although these state statutes are laudable, they still do not protect most Americans who are receiving health insurance under self-insured, risk retention plans that are preempted under federal ERISA law. More than 50% of all Americans are so covered.

Physicians who violate gag clauses risk (1) termination, (2) refusal by the MCO to renew their contracts, to refer patients, and to compensate the provider for covered patients and (3) other retaliatory actions.[31] As the result of widespread negative publicity, several MCOs have dropped gag clause provisions from their contracts with physicians. However, a number of other MCOs have retained and strengthened their gag clauses. The gag clause controversy and litigation continue.

EASY COME, EASY GO: PROVIDER SELECTION AND DESELECTION

Although hospitals have long had the direct legal responsibility to properly credential physicians for privileges, more recently this duty has extended to MCOs as well.[32] The fact that courts now hold MCOs liable for negligent selection of panel members and for negligent supervision of panel members should come as no surprise to anyone. As patient choice in selecting a physician is limited by the MCO's panel of physicians, and as the patient explicitly relies on the MCO rather than the physician for comprehensive medical care, liability transfers to the MCO even though these physicians are not employed by the MCO.[33]

Contemporary credentialing of physicians in MCOs is every bit as elaborate as the process in hospitals. Accrediting bodies, such as the National Committee for Quality Assurance (NCQA) and the Accreditation Association for Ambulatory Health Care, define and set standards for credentialing. The NCQA requires that MCOs have written policies and procedures for credentialing, recredentialing, recertification, or reappointment of physicians.[34] Physicians remained "qualified" to participate in MCOs, but many physicians were finding themselves denied contractual privileges. Consequently, a number of states have enacted "any willing provider" statutes to protect such physicians. For example, the Louisiana "any willing provider" statute mandates that: "no licensed provider . . . who agrees to the terms and conditions of the preferred provider contract shall be denied the right to become a preferred provider."[35] In Virginia, the statute states in part:

> *Any such insurer shall establish terms and conditions that shall be met by a hospital, physician or type of provider . . . These terms and conditions shall not discriminate unreasonably against or among such health care providers. No hospital, physician or type of provider . . . willing to meet the terms and conditions offered to it or him shall be excluded.*[36]

As with many other state regulatory statutes designed to give protection to patients and providers participating in managed care, however, "any willing provider" statutes may be preempted by ERISA, and thus would not apply to the majority of Americans participating in ERISA self-insured, risk retention plans.

A larger concern for many physicians is not their initial participation in MCO plans but being "deselected" for a variety of reasons or for no reason at all. One of the more controversial grounds for selecting or deselecting physicians from participating in MCO plans is the practice of "economic credentialing."[37] The debate continues as to the definition of economic credentialing because many factors may legitimately relate to both the cost and quality of delivering health care. Despite this continuing debate, however, most hospitals surveyed state that they intend to continue considering relevant economic data in defining staff privileges. Similarly, MCOs remain very conscious of economic data when selecting and deselecting physicians on their panels.

The relationship between the physician and the MCO is usually contractual in nature. These contracts typically contain termination provisions with or without cause and with a relatively short time frame for written notice of termination. In *Harper v. Healthsource,* for example, Dr. Harper, a physician, had such a written notice of termination and was terminated without cause. After exhausting his internal appeals with Healthsource, he appealed his case to the New Hampshire courts. He asserted that the contractual termination without cause provision in his MCO contract was void as against state public policy, and the New Hampshire Supreme Court agreed with Dr. Harper's contention.[38]

In addition to judicial intervention, some states, including California, have enacted statutes giving physicians some protection from arbitrary deselection. California requires a provision for fair hearing rights and maintenance of grievance systems, and appeal procedures for disputes between MCOs and enrollees. Additional California legislation requires MCOs to disclose their termination or deselection contractual policies with their health care provider enrollees.[39] While other states are expected to follow California's lead in giving protection to both patients and health care providers in MCOs, the ultimate effectiveness of these statutes will almost certainly come under judicial scrutiny, especially in light of federal preemption issues involving ERISA mandated rights and remedies.

RISK MANAGEMENT TECHNIQUES FOR REDUCING LIABILITY

MCOs as well as physicians are very interested in reducing the possibility of a malpractice suit against them. There are many things that physicians can do to reduce the possibility of a lawsuit. Physicians often feel at a great disadvantage when contracting with MCOs; they sometimes believe that they must sign any contract put before them or risk losing their patient population without such contracts. Physicians often sign several such contracts without fully understanding the ramifications of these contracts until a dispute arises.

The first thing a physician should do is to read and *understand* the contract before signing. These are usually "boilerplate" or standardized contracts, and physicians may feel there is little they can do to change the terms. This is far from the truth. "Knowledge is power," and we offer the following suggested techniques to help physicians realize that by understanding (1) the contracting process, and (2) the terms and provisions generally utilized in managed care contracts, and (3) their own medical practice costs and patterns, physicians can enter into rewarding and long-term contracts for the benefit of their patients and themselves. Here's how:

- Prepare for the negotiating process. Several references are helpful in preparing for a negotiating strategy with an MCO (e.g., *A Practical Guide to Negotiation*[40] and *Managed Care Handbook*[41]).
- Determine how you are insured for medical malpractice. If you are an employee, you will probably have insurance through your company. If the MCO tightly manages your practice patterns, even if you are an independent pro-

*California, Colorado, Delaware, Georgia, Indiana, Maine, Maryland, Massachusetts, New Hampshire, New York, Pennsylvania, Rhode Island, Tennessee, Vermont, Virginia, and Washington.

vider, you may be able to negotiate malpractice insurance provisions.

- Determine how you are being paid. Can you live with these limits? Risk-based financing and physician incentives are the "bread and butter" of managed care contracts. Physicians need to know their own costs in running their medical practice before they sign for such incentives. A good consulting company can help you understand your own costs of doing business.
- How are financial outliers handled? Is there insurance for them?
- Determine the treatment philosophy of the MCO. Do you agree with it? What are the definitions of "medical necessity" and "experimental" or "educational" procedures? What right of appeal do you and your patients have when denials are made?
- What practice standards are utilized? Do they conform to the community standard of medical practice?
- Is there a clearly documented process for utilization review? Can you follow it?
- Are there any restrictions on your duty of informed consent, including alternatives to treatment not covered by the policy? Can you live with them?
- Does the MCO provide educational services for its panel members?
- Do physicians have input in the allocation of services? What is the MCO's policy with regard to specialist referrals?
- Are patients educated regarding the benefits of their plan?
- What are the specific structural characteristics of the MCO (i.e., profit status, chain-affiliation, or model type)? Are these acceptable to you?
- What is the claims history of the HMO? What is the financial rating and security of the MCO? Is it solvent?
- What is the history of the MCO with the applicable state insurance regulatory agency? Are documented complaints or other legal issues involved?
- Is the MCO publicly traded? If so, does the available information (i.e., annual reports, 10-K filings) reflect a well run organization?
- How does the MCO assess quality? Is the organization accredited by the NCQA?
- How is patient and physician satisfaction measured? What do the most recent data show with regard to these satisfaction levels?
- What is the network composition (i.e., primary care and specialist ratios, number of inpatient facilities, alternative health providers)? What are the credentialing requirements? Do you have medical staff privileges at the facilities included in the network? What rights do you have if you are deselected from the provider network?
- What types of references do other physicians and health care providers give the MCO?

This list is not intended to be exhaustive. Several other practical guide references can aid the reader in determining the best risk management techniques.[42] Finally, the Internet is a wonderful source of information and references, for example:

American Association of Health Plans (*http://www.aahp.org*)
Consumer Coalition for Quality Health Care (*http://www.consumers.org*)
Families USA (*http://www.familiesusa.org*)
Integrated Healthcare Association (*http://www.iha.org*)
National Committee for Quality Assurance (*http://www.ncqa.org*)
National Organization of Physicians Who Care (*http://www.hmopage.org*)
Patient Access to Specialty Care Coalition (*http://www.home.patientaccess.com/pac*)
President's Advisory Commission on Consumer Protection and Quality in the Health Care Industry (*http://www.hcqualitycommission.gov*)

References

1. Miller RH, Luft HS: Managed care plan performance since 1980: A literature analysis. JAMA 1994; 272:1512.
2. General Accounting Office, Employers Turn to Managed Care to Control Costs, p 3, cited in Rosenblatt RE, Law SA, Rosenbaum S: Law and the American Health Care System. Westbury, NY, Foundation Press, 1997, p 549.
3. Frankford DM: Creating and dividing the fruits of collective economic activity: Referrals among health care providers. Columbus L Rev 1989; 89:1861.
4. Noah B: The managed care dilemma: Can theories of tort liability adapt to the realities of cost containment? Mercer L Rev 1997; 48:1219, 1220.
5. Segal D: Doctors who dodge a managed care stampede. *Washington Post,* May 20, 1996, p 5 (Health Section).
6. Gabel J: Ten ways HMOs have changed during the 1990s. Health Aff 1997; 16:134.
7. This would include the regulation of the managed care entity, including the financial requirements for operation, solvency requirements, rules covering the relationship between an insurer and an insured, rules related to the spreading of risk over covered persons, and so forth. See Rosenblatt RE, et al, supra note 1 at 630-636.
8. The federal McCarran-Ferguson Act, 15 U.S.C. Sec. 1101 et seq. generally authorizes state regulation of insurance law unless such laws are preempted by federal law.
9. Horvath J: Emerging Challenges in State Regulation of Managed Care. Portland, Me, National Academy of State Health Policy, 1996, p 7.
10. 29 U.S.C. Sec. 1001 et seq.
11. 29 U.S.C. Sec. 1003(a).
12. Widiss A, Gostin J: What's wrong with the ERISA vacuum? The case against unrestricted freedom for employers to terminate employee health care plans and to decide what coverage is to be provided when risk retention plans are established for health care. Drake L Rev 1992; 41:635.

    A 1996 study conducted for the Henry J. Kaiser Family Foundation reported a trend that more employers are reducing their reliance on self-insured health plans in favor of commercially insured managed care plans due in part to self-insured managed care solvency and liability issues. Nevertheless, more than half of American employees are presently enrolled in fully or partially self-insured health plans. Derek Liston and Martha Priddy Patterson, Analysis of the Number of Workers Covered by Self-Insured Health Plans Under ERISA (Henry J. Kaiser Family Foundation Study, Menlo Park, Calif. 1996) at 3-6.
13. See Rosenblatt et al. *supra* note 1 at 635–636.
14. Bilimoria NM: Beware HMOs: The future of HMO medical malpractice liability is uncertain. DePaul J Health Care Law 1997; 1:711.
15. Hall MA, Anderson GF: Health insurers' assessment of medical necessity. U Penn L Rev 1992; 140:1637.
16. See Adams v. Blue Cross/Blue Shield of Maryland, 757 F. Supp. 661 (D. Ct. Md. 1991); and Holder v. Prudential Insurance Co. of America, 951 F.2d 89 (5th Cir. 1992).
17. See Abraham K: Judge-made law and judge-made insurance: Honoring the reasonable expectations of the insured. Va L Rev 1981; 67:1151. But see also Swisher P: Judicial interpretations of insurance contract disputes: Toward a realistic middle ground approach. Ohio St LJ 1996; 57:543. See generally Windt AD: Insurance Claims and Disputes. 3d ed. Colorado Springs, Shepards-McGraw Hill, 1995.
18. Fischer E, Swisher P: Principles of Insurance Law. 2nd ed. Sec 5.08 New York, Matthew Bender, 1994.
19. See authority cited in note 17, supra.
20. See generally Allan Windt, Insurance Claims and Disputes. 3d ed. Vol. 1, Sec. 6.03, 1995.

21. Rosenblatt et al., supra note 1 at 213.
22. This is especially true with ERISA-related lawsuits. See, e.g., Pilot Life Insurance Co. v. Dedeaux, 481 U.S. 41 (1987) (holding that ERISA's civil enforcement remedies were intended to be exclusive, and cannot be supplemented or supplanted by varying state laws); and McManus v. Traveler's Health Network of Texas, 742 F. Supp. 377 (W.D. Texas 1990) (similar holding).
23. Shernoff W, Gage S, Levine H: Insurance Bad Faith Litigation, 1985.
24. Schlessler CE: Liability implications of utilization review as a cost containment mechanism. J Contemp Health Law Policy 1992; 8:379.
25. Milstein A, et al: *In:* Pursuit of Value: American Utilization Management at the Fifteen-Year Mark in Making Managed Healthcare Work: A Practical Guide to Strategies and Solutions. Boland P (Ed). Gaithersburg, Md, Aspen Publishers, 1993.
26. Hughes v. Blue Cross of Northern California, 215 Cal. App. 3d 832, 263 Cal. Rptr. 850 (1989); see also Blum JD: An analysis of legal liability in health care utilization and care management. Houston L Rev 1989; 26:191.
27. Varol v. Blue Cross and Blue Shield, 708 F. Supp. 826 (E.D. Mich. 1989).
28. Wickline v. State, 192 Cal. App.3d 1630 at 1645 (Cal. 1986).
29. Myron JL: Comment: HMOs' use of gag clauses: An unethical threat to America's health. Dickinson L Rev 1997; 101:729.
30. Woolhandler S, Himmelstein D: Extreme risk: The new corporate proposition for physicians. N Engl J Med 1995; 333:1706.
31. Martin JA, Bjerknes LK: The legal and ethical implication of gag clauses in physician contracts. Am J Law Med 1977; 22:433.
32. Harrell v. Total Health Care, Inc. No. WD 39809, slip op (Mo. Ct. App. 1989), affirmed 781 S.W.2d 58 (Mo. 1989).
33. McClellan v. HMO of Pennsylvania, 604 A.2d 1053 (Pa. Super. Ct. 1992).
34. National Committee for Quality Assurance, Standards for Accreditation 46, 1995.
35. CIGNA Healthplan of Louisiana, Inc., v. State of La. Ex rel. Ieyoub, 82 F. 3d 642 (5th Cir. 1996).
36. Virginia Code Ann. Section 38.2-3407, as cited in Stuart Circle Hospital v. Aetna Health Management, 995 F.2d 500 (4th Cir. 1993).
37. Blum JD: Economic credentialing: A new twist in hospital appraisal process. J Legal Med 1991; 12:427.
38. Harper v. Healthsource, 674 A.2d 962 (N.H. 1996).
39. Kadzielski M: Symposium: Provider deselection and decapitation in a changing healthcare environment. St Louis L J 1997; 41:891.
40. Guernsey TF: A Practical Guide to Negotiation. South Bend, Ind, National Institute for Trial Advocacy, 1966. e-mail: NITA.1@nd.edu.
41. American Academy of Hospital Attorneys, Managed Care Committee: Managed Care Handbook. Chicago, American Hospital Association, 1993.
42. Dasco ST, Dasco CC: Managed Care Answer Book. 2nd ed. New York, Panel Publishers, 1997.

202

Caring for a Child in an Adult Intensive Care Unit

Ann E. Thompson, MD

Historically, many children have received treatment in adult intensive care units (ICUs). Initially, this was due to the lack of pediatric intensive care units (PICUs) and appropriately trained personnel; more recently, the practice has continued because of an inability to transfer a child to a PICU or because of a lack of conviction that such a transfer was necessary. In addition, today's concern about the cost of care has created additional pressure to admit children to adult ICUs to avoid transfer or to maintain a high census in local facilities. This chapter reviews current issues related to this matter.

The clear priority, about which there can be little controversy, is to provide optimal care for critically ill children. Wherever such care is being provided, those involved intend to deliver highest quality care. However, it is becoming increasingly clear that outcome for children receiving treatment in ICUs, other than tertiary-care PICUs, is inferior to results for patients matched for severity of illness and treated in tertiary PICUs.

Such observations should not be surprising given the evidence in many fields, within and outside of medicine, showing that "practice makes perfect." There is a growing literature that shows that hospitals or units that care for many patients with a given disorder have better results overall than those caring for fewer patients, even when relatively "simple" disorders or procedures are concerned.[1-4] Potential advantages of regionalized care include (1) better-trained, more experienced, and more highly skilled personnel; (2) more depth in 24-hour staffing; (3) greater opportunity for recognition of the characteristics of best practice and standardization of care; and (4) enhanced clinical research into improving outcome.[5] In addition, there can be greater depth in pediatric subspecialty consultants, virtually all of whom are clustered in major pediatric centers.

Fortunately, relatively fewer children (than adults) require intensive care. Those who do can be concentrated in a limited number of highly regionalized centers with adequate volume to allow development and maintenance of the expertise needed for optimal outcome. Several studies have suggested a need for approximately one PICU bed per 27,000 to 32,000 children, or 20 beds per million children per day.[6-7] A corollary is that relatively few centers are needed to provide care for these infants and children. Admitting children to adult ICUs and developing multiple small PICUs has great potential to weaken the competence of every center.

A common reason to transfer patients to another center is the perceived need for technology or a specialist not available at the referring hospital. Unfortunately, the need for a pediatric intensivist is frequently unrecognized. However, an early study showed that introduction of a pediatric intensivist to a tertiary pediatric facility led to increased efficiency in the PICU and a lower severity-of-illness-adjusted mortality rate.[8]

Several studies have demonstrated the value of highly structured PICU services. A statewide comparison of outcome in children with respiratory failure and head trauma receiving care in other centers, in contrast to those cared for in a tertiary PICU, showed an *increase* in mortality ranging from 2.4-fold to eightfold in moderate-risk to high-risk patients in the nontertiary, non-PICUs.[9] Patients who died in the nontertiary units were older and frequently had suffered trauma, providing evidence against the common practice of keeping older children in adult units. Several studies provide additional evidence for improved outcome in children with blunt trauma treated in pediatric trauma centers compared with those cared for in adult trauma units.[10-11] A dedicated PICU is a necessary component of these centers, and only a fraction of the patients require surgical intervention. Only the group composed of adolescents with penetrating injuries had as good an outcome in adult centers as in pediatric trauma centers. The authors suggest that management of similar injuries in children is frequently different from that in adults.

A study of children treated from 1994 to 1995 in Victoria, Australia, and Trent, England, showed a similar rate of admission to ICUs, but a longer length of stay and an increased mortality rate in Trent after adjustment for severity of illness.[12]

Striking differences between the two regions include highly centralized care in Victoria (two PICUs) and highly fragmented care in Trent (13 ICUs, three designated as PICUs). As would be predicted, many fewer children were admitted to each of the English ICUs. Other striking differences between the two regions included the absence in Trent of pediatric intensivists even in the PICUs, specifically trained nursing personnel, and house staff dedicated to the units. The differences noted were great enough that the excess deaths were sufficient to impact overall child mortality.

One would hope that early triage using an available severity of illness scoring system would indicate which patients require transfer to a tertiary PICU. Unfortunately, the study by Pearson and coworkers[12] showed that the greatest excess mortality occurred in *low-risk* and *medium-risk* patients. In a nationwide study of pediatric intensive care in the Netherlands, there was an increased risk of mortality in *medium-risk* to *high-risk* patients treated in nontertiary hospitals.[13] It is reasonable to conclude, then, that all critically ill infants and children should be transferred to high-volume tertiary PICUs.

Concern regarding the risks of transporting a critically ill child is sometimes cited as a reason not to transfer a child to a PICU. However, the state of the art of transporting such patients is such that even desperately ill infants and children can be safely transferred.[14] During the period from 1982 to 1997, a pediatric transport team that has transported nearly 15,000 infants and children, many of whom were being moved from an emergency department or another PICU in very unstable condition to a major tertiary/quarternary PICU, and at particularly high risk, had fewer than 10 deaths during transport during this entire period.[15] Where such transport systems are absent, the relative risk of skilled transport versus continuing to care for a child in a suboptimal setting strongly encourages their development.

The Pediatric Section of the Society of Critical Care Medicine and the American Academy of Pediatrics Critical Care Section and Committee on Hospital Care have defined levels of ICU care for children.[16] These guidelines indicate that pediatric intensive care is primarily provided at a single level but recognizes that there may be value in a second level in areas of low population density to permit stabilization prior to transfer or to avoid long-distance transfer for children with less complex disorders or lesser acuity. In general, these guidelines were not intended as a statement of the ideal but, rather, as recommendations for what is "current, necessary, and attainable." They do not have the force of regulation or law, but they do represent the opinion of these two organizations and their members and offer the best approximation of a standard of care currently available.

Personnel requirements include 24-hour availability of a pediatric intensivist and multiple medical and surgical pediatric subspecialists, dedicated nursing leadership with pediatric critical care training, staff nurses, respiratory therapists, and other professionals with pediatric training and experience. Specialized diagnostic services are also necessary, including laboratory, radiologic, cardiology and neurologic studies.

There is now strong evidence that a centralized system, staffed by full-time physician and nurse specialists in pediatric critical care, can deliver higher-quality care with greater efficiency than appears possible with decentralized, fragmented care. Providers sometimes raise the concern that transfer of critically ill children away from their homes and family support systems is itself detrimental and likely to be resisted. Experience, however, clearly shows that parents will go to great lengths to obtain the best treatment for their children. If made aware of the likely benefit of transfer to a tertiary PICU, few would accept any other alternative.

The adult ICU that cares for children is advised to adhere to the American Academy of Pediatrics/Society of Critical Care Medicine recommendations. High-quality care and organizational or equipment requirements may prove to be too costly to maintain. Fortunately, the availability of transport systems can allow for the smooth and safe transfer of critically ill infants and children to centers best equipped to address their needs. In the current environment, state-of-the-art pediatric intensive care is best delivered in tertiary pediatric centers.

References

1. Flood AB, Scott WR, Ewy W: Does practice make perfect? I. The relation between hospital volume and outcomes and other hospital characteristics. Med Care 1984; 22:98–114.
2. Hughes R, Hunt SS, Luft HS: Effects of surgeon volume and hospital volume on quality of care in hospitals. Med Care 1987; 25:489–503.
3. Showstack J, Rosenfeld K, Garnick D, et al: Association of volume with outcome of coronary artery bypass graft surgery. JAMA 1987; 257:785–789.
4. Hannan E, O'Donnell J, Kilburn H: Investigation of the relationship between volume and mortality for surgical procedures performed in New York State hospitals. JAMA 1989; 262:503–510.
5. Thompson DR, Clemmer TP, Applefeld JJ, et al: Regionalization of critical care medicine: Task Force report of the American College of Critical Care Medicine. Crit Care Med 1994; 22:1306–1313.
6. Milne E, Whitty P: Calculation of the need for paediatric intensive care beds. Arch Dis Child 1995; 73:505–507.
7. Yeh TS: Regionalization of pediatric critical care. Crit Care Clin 1992; 8:23–35.
8. Pollack MM, Katz RW, Getson PR, et al: Improving the outcome and efficiency of intensive care: The impact of an intensivist. Crit Care Med 1988; 16:11–17.
9. Pollack MM, Alexander SR, Clarke N, et al: Improved outcomes from tertiary center pediatric intensive care: A state-wide comparison of tertiary and non-tertiary care facilities. Crit Care Med 1991; 19:150–59.
10. Hall JR, Reyes HM, Meller JL, et al: The outcome for children with blunt trauma is best at a pediatric trauma center. J Pediatr Surg 1996; 31:72–77.
11. Haller JA, Shorter N, Miller D, et al: Organization and function of a regional pediatric trauma center: Does a system of management improve outcome. J Trauma 1983; 23:691–696.
12. Pearson G, Shann F, Barry P, et al: Should paediatric intensive care be centralized? Trent versus Victoria. Lancet 1997; 349:1213–1217.
13. Gemke RJBJ, Bonsel GJ: The Pediatric Intensive Care Assessment of Outcome (PICASSO) Study Group: Comparative assessment of pediatric intensive care: A national multicenter study. Crit Care Med 1995; 23:238–245.
14. Britto J, Nadel S, Maconochie I, et al: Morbidity and severity of illness during interhospital transfer: Impact of a specialized paediatric retrieval team. BMJ 1995; 311:836–839.
15. Orr RA, Singleton C: Personal communication, 1998.
16. Committee on Hospital Care and Pediatric Section of the Society of Critical Care Medicine: Guidelines and Levels of Care for Pediatric Intensive Care Units. Pediatrics 1993; 92:166–175.

INDEX

Page numbers in *italics* refer to illustrations; page numbers followed by b refer to boxed material, and those followed by t to tables.

ISBN 0-7216-7246-9